FUNDAMENTAL IMMUNOLOGY

FOURTH EDITION

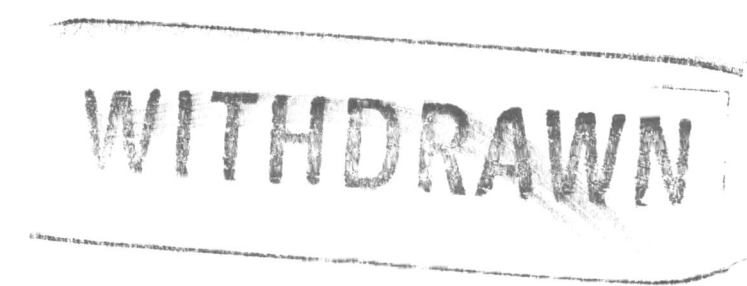

FUNDAMENTAL IMMUNOLOGY

FOURTH EDITION

Editor

WILLIAM E. PAUL, M.D.

Laboratory of Immunology
National Institute of Allergy and Infectious Diseases
National Institutes of Health
Bethesda, Maryland

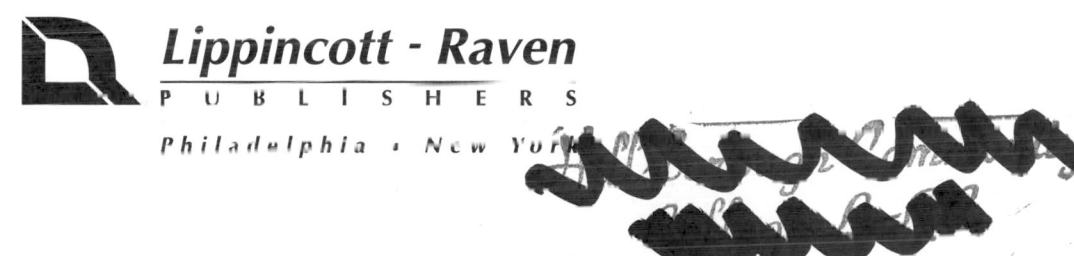

Lippincott - Raven
PUBLISHERS
Philadelphia • New York

Acquisitions Editor: Ruth W. Weinberg
Developmental Editor: Ellen DiFrancesco
Manufacturing Manager: Kevin Watt
Supervising Editor: Liane Carita
Production Service: Colophon
Compositor: Lippincott–Raven Desktop Division
Printer: Courier-Westford

Printed in the United States of America

9 8 7 6 5 4 3 2 1

Library of Congress Cataloging-in-Publication Data
Fundamental immunology / editor, William E. Paul. — 4th ed.
　　　　p.　　cm.
　　Includes bibliographical references and index
　　ISBN 0-7817-1412-5
　　1. Immunology.　I. Paul, William E.
　　[DNLM: 1. Immunity.　QW 540 F981 1998]
　QR181.F84　　1998
　616.07′9—dc21
　DNLM/DLC
　for Library of Congress　　　　　　　　　　　　　98-3611
　　　　　　　　　　　　　　　　　　　　　　　　CIP

Care has been taken to confirm the accuracy of the information presented and to
describe generally accepted practices. However, the authors, editors, and publisher are
not responsible for errors or omissions or for any consequences from application of the
information in this book and make no warranty, express or implied, with respect to the
contents of the publication.
　The authors, editors, and publisher have exerted every effort to ensure that drug
selection and dosage set forth in this text are in accordance with current
recommendations and practice at the time of publication. However, in view of ongoing
research, changes in government regulations, and the constant flow of information
relating to drug therapy and drug reactions, the reader is urged to check the package
insert for each drug for any change in indications and dosage and for added warnings
and precautions. This is particularly important when the recommended agent is a new or
infrequently employed drug.
　Some drugs and medical devices presented in this publication have Food and Drug
Administration (FDA) clearance for limited use in restricted research settings. It is the
responsibility of the health care provider to ascertain the FDA status of each drug or
device planned for use in their clinical practice.

To Baruj Benacerraf—
in gratitude and friendship

Contents

Regulation of the Immune Response

Effector Mechanisms of Immunity

Mechanistic Basis of Immunology

Contributors

Rafi Ahmed, Ph.D., *Director, Emory Vaccine Center, Emory University School of Medicine, Rollins Research Building, 1510 Clifton Road, Atlanta, GA 30322*

Michael A. Apicella, M.D., *Professor and Head, Department of Microbiology, The University of Iowa, 51 Newton Road, Iowa City, IA 52242*

Hugh Auchincloss, Jr., M.D. *Associate Professor, Department of Surgery, Harvard Medical School and Massachusetts General Hospital, 55 Fruit Street, Boston, MA 02114-2696*

Christophe Benoist, M.D., Ph.D., *Director of Research, Department of Immunology, Institut de Génétique et de Biologie Moléculaire et Cellulaire, 1 rue Laurent Fries, 67400 Illkirch, C.U. de Strasbourg, France*

Claudia Berek, Ph.D., *Deutsches Rheuma ForschungsZentrum, Monbijoustrasse 2, D-10117 Berlin, Germany*

Ira J. Berkower, M.D., Ph.D., *Chief, Laboratory of Immunoregulation, Office of Vaccines, Center for Biologics Evaluation and Research, Food and Drug Administration, NIH Campus, Bethesda, MD 20892*

Jay A. Berzofsky, M.D., Ph.D., *Chief, Molecular Immunogenetics and Vaccine Research Section, Metabolism Branch, National Cancer Institute, National Institutes of Health, 10 Center Drive, Bethesda, MD 20892-1578*

Christine A. Biron, Ph.D., *Esther Elizabeth Brintzenhoff Professor of Medical Science, Department of Microbiology and Immunology, Division of Biology and Medicine, Brown University, Providence, RI 02912*

Jeffrey A. Bluestone, Ph.D., *Charles B. Huggins Professor, Ben May Institute for Cancer Research, University of Chicago, 5841 S. Maryland, Chicago, IL 60637*

David E. Briles, Ph.D., *Professor, Department of Microbiology, University of Alabama at Birmingham, 658 BBRB, UAB Station, Birmingham, AL 35294-2170*

Eric J. Brown, M.D., *Department of Internal Medicine, Division of Infectious Diseases, 660 S. Euclid Avenue, Washington University School of Medicine, St. Louis, MO 63110*

Rebecca H. Buckley, M.D., *J. Buren Sidbury Professor of Pediatrics, Departments of Pediatrics and Immunology, Duke University School of Medicine, 363 Jones Building, Durham, NC 27710-0001*

J. Donald Capra, M.D., *President and Scientific Director, Oklahoma Medical Research Foundation, Oklahoma City, OK 73104*

Yueh-Hsiu Chien, Ph.D., *Department of Microbiology and Immunology, Stanford University School of Medicine, Stanford, CA 94305-5428*

Stephen P. Cobbold, Ph.D., *Sir William Dunn School of Pathology, University of Oxford, South Parks Road, Oxford OX1 3RE, United Kingdom*

Oren Cohen, M.D., *Laboratory of Immunoregulation, National Institute of Allergy and Infectious Diseases, National Institutes of Health, 10 Center Drive, Bethesda, MD 20892-1876*

Philip L. Cohen, M.D., *Departments of Medicine and Microbiology/Immunology, University of North Carolina, 3330 Thurston Building, Chapel Hill, NC 27599-7280*

xi

Mark M. Davis, Ph.D., *Professor, Department of Microbiology and Immunology, Stanford University School of Medicine, Howard Hughes Medical Institute, Beckman Center, Stanford, CA 94305-5428*

Anthony L. DeFranco, M.D., Ph.D., *Professor of Microbiology and Immunology, University of California, San Francisco, 3rd and Parnassus Avenues, San Francisco, CA 94143-0552*

Manfred P. Dierich, M.D., *Institut für Hygiene, University of Innsbruck, Fritz-Pregl-Str. 3, Innsbruck, A-6020, Austria*

Louis Du Pasquier, Ph.D., *Basel Institute for Immunology, Grenzacherstrasse 487, CH-4005 Basel, Switzerland*

Suzanne L. Epstein, Ph.D., *Chief, Molecular Immunology Laboratory, Division of Cellular and Gene Therapies, Center for Biologics Evaluation and Research, Food and Drug Administration, 1401 Rockville Pike, Rockville, MD 20852-1448*

Anna Erdei, Ph.D., *Department of Immunology, Eötvös Lorand University, Jávorka S. 14, Göd, H-2131, Hungary*

Anthony S. Fauci, M.D., *Director, National Institute of Allergy and Infectious Diseases, National Institutes of Health, 31 Center Drive, Bethesda, MD 20892-2520*

Fred D. Finkelman, M.D., *Division of Immunology, University of Cincinnati Medical Center, P.O. Box 670563, Cincinnati, OH 45267-0563*

Martin F. Flajnik, Ph.D., *Department of Microbiology and Immunology, University of Maryland, Baltimore MD 21201-1559*

J. Kimble Frazer, M.D., *Department of Molecular Immunogenetics, Oklahoma Medical Research Foundation, Oklahoma City, OK 73104*

Stephen J. Galli, M.D., *Director, Division of Experimental Pathology, Department of Pathology, Beth Israel Deaconess Medical Center, 330 Brookline Avenue, Boston, MA 02215-5491*

John I. Gallin, M.D., *Director, Warren G. Magnusen Clinical Center; Associate Director for Clinical Research, National Institutes of Health; Chief, Laboratory of Host Defenses, National Institute of Allergy and Infectious Diseases, National Institutes of Health, 10 Center Drive, Bethesda, MD 20892-1504*

Ronald N. Germain, M.D., Ph.D., *Laboratory of Immunology, National Institute of Allergy and Infectious Diseases, National Institutes of Health, 10 Center Drive, Bethesda, MD 20892-1892*

Lisa K. Gilliland, Ph.D., *Sir William Dunn School of Pathology, University of Oxford, South Parks Road, Oxford OX1 3RE, United Kingdom*

Siamon Gordon, M.B., Ch.B., Ph.D., *Professor, Sir William Dunn School of Pathology, University of Oxford, South Parks Road, Oxford OX1 3RE, United Kingdom*

Geoffrey Hale, Ph.D., *Sir William Dunn School of Pathology, University of Oxford, South Parks Road, Oxford OX1 3RE, United Kingdom*

Pierre A. Henkart, M.D., *Experimental Immunology Branch, National Cancer Institute, National Institutes of Health, Bethesda, MD 20892-1360*

Samuel L. Jones, D.V.M., Ph.D., *Department of Molecular Microbiology, Division of Infectious Diseases, Washington University School of Medicine, 660 S. Euclid Avenue, St. Louis, MO 63110*

Stefan H.E. Kaufmann, Ph.D., *Professor and Chair, Department of Immunology, Max-Planck-Institute for Infection Biology, Monbijoustrasse 2, D-10117 Berlin, Germany*

Roli Khattri, Ph.D., *Ben May Institute for Cancer Research, University of Chicago, 11219 NE 53rd Street, Kirkland, WA 98033*

Hiroshi Kiyono, D.D.S., Ph.D., *Department of Mucosal Immunology, Research Institute for Microbial Diseases, Osaka University, 3-1 Yamadaoka, Suita, Osaka 565, Japan*

Teresa Krakauer, Ph.D., *Department of Immunology and Molecular Biology, USAMRIID, Fort Detrick, Frederick, MD 21702-1201*

Chris S. Lantz, Ph.D., *Department of Pathology, Harvard Medical School and Beth Israel Deaconess Medical Center, 330 Brookline Avenue, Boston, MA 02215-5419*

Warren J. Leonard, M.D., *Chief, Laboratory of Molecular Immunology, National Heart, Lung, and Blood Institute, National Institutes of Health, 10 Center Drive, Bethesda, MD 20892-1674*

Frederik P. Lindberg, M.D., Ph.D., *Department of Internal Medicine, Division of Infectious Diseases, Washington University School of Medicine, 660 S. Euclid Avenue, St. Louis, MO 63110*

David H. Margulies, M.D., Ph.D., *Molecular Biology Section, Laboratory of Immunology, National Institute of Allergy and Infectious Diseases, National Institutes of Health, 10 Center Drive, Bethesda, MD 20892-1892*

Diane Mathis, M.D., Ph.D., *Universite de Strasbourg, BP 163, Institut de Génétique et de Biologie Moléculaire et Cellulaire, 67400 Illkirch, C.U. de Strasbourg, France*

Edward E. Max, M.D., Ph.D., *Laboratory of Cell and Viral Regulation, Center for Biologics Evaluation and Research, Food and Drug Administration, 8800 Rockville Pike, Bethesda, MD 20892-0001*

Jerry R. McGhee, Ph.D., *Director, Department of Microbiology, The University of Alabama at Birmingham, Bevill Biomedical Research Building, 845 19th Street South, Birmingham, AL 35294-2170*

Fritz Melchers, Ph.D., *Director, Basel Institute for Immunology, Grenzacherstrasse 487, CH-4005 Basel, Switzerland*

Richard A. Miller, M.D., Ph.D., *Department of Pathology, University of Michigan, 1500 East Medical Center Drive, Ann Arbor, MI 48109-0946*

Timothy M. Mosmann, Ph.D., *Professor, Department of Medical Microbiology and Immunology, Heritage Medical Research Center, University of Alberta, Edmonton, Alberta T66 2H7, Canada*

Moon H. Nahm, M.D., *Departments of Pediatrics, Pathology, and Internal Medicine, University of Rochester, 601 Elmwood Avenue, Rochester, NY 14642-8777*

G.J.V. Nossal, M.D., Ph.D., *Professor Emeritus, Department of Pathology, The University of Melbourne, Royal Parade, Parkville, Victoria 3052, Australia*

Joost J. Oppenheim, M.D., *Chief, Laboratory of Molecular Immunoregulation, National Cancer Institute, FDRDC, Frederick, MD 21702-1201*

William E. Paul, M.D., *Chief, Laboratory of Immunology, National Institute of Allergy and Infectious Diseases, National Institutes of Health, 10 Center Drive, Bethesda, MD 20892-1892.*

Edward J. Pearce, M.D., Ph.D., *Department of Microbiology and Immunology, Cornell University College of Veterinary Medicine, Ithaca, NY 14853*

Louis J. Picker, M.D., *Associate Professor of Pathology, Department of Pathology, University of Texas Southwestern Medical Center, 5323 Harry Hines Boulevard, Dallas, TX 75235-9072*

Wolfgang M. Prodinger, M.D., *Institut für Hygiene, University of Innsbruck, Fritz-Pregl-Str. 3, Innsbruck, A-6020, Austria*

Antonius Rollnk, Ph.D., *Basel Institute for Immunology, Grenzacherstrasse 487, CH-4005 Basel, Switzerland*

Helene F. Rosenberg, M.D., Ph.D., *Investigator, Laboratory of Host Defenses, National Institute of Allergy and Infectious Diseases, National Institutes of Health, 10 Center Drive, Bethesda, MD 20892-1888*

David H. Sachs, M.D., *Department of Surgery, Transplantation Biology Research Center, Harvard Medical School and Massachusetts General Hospital, 13th Street, Boston, MA 02129*

Hans Schreiber, M.D., Ph.D., *Department of Pathology, The University of Chicago, 5841 S. Maryland Avenue, Chicago, IL 60637-1463*

Ronald H. Schwartz, M.D., Ph.D., *Chief, Laboratory of Cellular and Molecular Immunology, National Institute of Allergy and Infectious Diseases, National Institutes of Health, 9000 Rockville Pike, Bethesda, MD 20892-0420*

Phillip A. Scott, Ph.D., *Department of Pathobiology, School of Veterinary Medicine, University of Pennsylvania, 3800 Spruce Street, Philadelphia, PA 19104*

Robert A. Seder, M.D., *Acting Chief, Clinical Immunology Section, Laboratory of Clinical Investigation, National Institute of Allergy and Infectious Diseases, National Institutes of Health, 10 Center Drive, Bethesda, MD 20892-1880*

Alan Sher, Ph.D., *Immunobiology Section, Laboratory of Parasitic Diseases, National Institute of Allergy and Infectious Diseases, National Institutes of Health, 9000 Rockville Pike, Bethesda, MD 20892-1360*

Ethan M. Shevach, M.D., *Laboratory of Immunology, National Institute of Allergy and Infectious Diseases, National Institutes of Health, 10 Center Drive, Bethesda, MD 20892-1892*

Mark H. Siegelman, M.D., Ph.D., *Assistant Professor, Department of Pathology, University of Texas Southwestern Medical Center, 5323 Harry Hines Boulevard, Dallas, TX 75235-9072*

Arthur M. Silverstein, Ph.D., *Professor Emeritus, Institute of the History of Medicine, Johns Hopkins University School of Medicine, 1900 East Monument Street, Baltimore, MD 21205*

Clifford M. Snapper, M.D., *Department of Pathology, Uniformed Services University of the Health Sciences, 4301 Jones Bridge Road, Bethesda, MD 20814*

Ralph M. Steinman, M.D., *Laboratory of Cellular Physiology and Immunology, Rockefeller University, 1230 York Avenue, New York, NY 10021-6399*

Megan Sykes, M.D., *Department of Surgery, Transplantation Biology Research Center, Harvard Medical School and Massachusetts General Hospital, 13th Street, Boston, MA 02129*

Craig B. Thompson, M.D., *Howard Hughes Medical Institute, Department of Medicine, University of Chicago, 924 E. 57th Street, Chicago, IL 60637-5420*

Gijs A. van Seventer, Ph.D., *Department of Pathology, University of Chicago, 5841 South Maryland Avenue, Chicago, IL 60637*

Jan Vilcek, M.D., Ph.D., *Professor of Microbiology, New York University Medical Center, 550 First Avenue, New York, NY 10016*

Herman Waldmann, M.D., *Head of Department, Sir William Dunn School of Pathology, University of Oxford, South Parks Road, Oxford OX1 3RE, United Kingdom*

Arthur Weiss, M.D., Ph.D., *Department of Medicine, Howard Hughes Medical Institute, University of California, San Francisco, 3rd and Parnassus Avenues, San Francisco, CA 94143-0795*

Drew Weissman, M.D., Ph.D., *Division of Infectious Diseases, University of Pennsylvania Medical Center, 536 Johnson Pavilion, Philadelphia, PA 19104*

Reinhard Würzner, M.D., Ph.D., *Institut für Hygiene, University of Innsbruck, Fritz-Pregl-Str. 3, Innsbruck, A-6020, Austria*

Wayne M. Yokoyama, M.D., *Professor, Howard Hughes Medical Institute, Department of Rheumatology, Washington University School of Medicine, 600 S. Euclid Avenue, St. Louis, MO 63110*

Acknowledgments

The preparation of the *Fourth Edition* of *Fundamental Immunology* required the efforts of many individuals. I particularly wish to thank each of the authors; their contributions, prepared in the midst of extremely busy schedules, are responsible for the value of this book. Ruth Weinberg and Ellen DiFrancesco of Lippincott–Raven not only saw that the process of receiving, editing, and assembling the chapters went as smoothly as possibly, they provided valuable advice at key junctures in the preparation of this edition. I wish to gratefully acknowledge the efforts of the editorial and production staffs at Lippincott–Raven.

Preface

When I first undertook the editing of *Fundamental Immunology*, culminating in the *First Edition,* which appeared in 1984 and was 809 pages in length, I thought there was a good possibility that immunological science was completing a phase of explosive growth that would be followed by a period of consolidation, the main features of which would be the expansion and broadening of the concepts that had already been enunciated. Simple reference to the length of each succeeding edition indicates that the idea was wrong. The fourth edition of *Fundamental Immunology* is 1616 pages in length. This increase in size reflects the continued explosive growth of immunological science. The fields of immunoregulation, cytokine biology, antigen-processing, and T-cell recognition, among others, have yielded entirely new insights into the means through which the immune system functions. Equally impressive has been the growing recognition of the role immune mechanisms play in prevention and pathogenesis of disease. In 1984, it was certainly clear that the immune system had great relevance to the initiation and propagation of a wide range of diseases, but its true impact was more hinted at than understood. Even today, we are far from a complete understanding of the impact of the immune and inflammatory systems on many diseases. Perhaps most telling, in 1984 AIDS had only recently been recognized, and HIV was only being discovered. The great and growing impact of HIV infection tragically emphasizes how important the immune system is in the battle against the pathogenic microbes with which we share our environment.

As with previous editions of *Fundamental Immunology,* this *Fourth Edition* is not simply an updating of the previous edition. It is an entirely new book that responds to the new and changed situation that exists in the study of the immune system. This may be appreciated in the organizational structure of this edition, which is quite different from that of the *Third Edition*, which was based on introducing the cellular elements of the immune system, and then progressing to the key molecular components that control cellular functions. This was largely based on the reality that we had a deeper understanding of the cells than of many of the key molecules. In the last four years, our understanding of the structure and function of the molecular components of immunity has expanded greatly. It now seems more appropriate to discuss the key molecules, particularly the receptors of the T and B cells and the major histocompatibility complex molecules, before attempting to integrate this knowledge into a discussion of cellular function. Accordingly, the order of sections in the *Fourth Edition* is different than in the third edition. This edition begins as previous editions with the section *Introduction,* in which Chapter 1, "The Immune System: An Introduction", reviews the major issues of contemporary immunology so that the reader with limited background in immunology can profitably read the succeeding chapters. An insightful chapter on the history of immunology is also included in this section. The next section, *Immunoglobulins and B Lymphocytes,* progresses from the chemistry, interactions, and molecular biology of immunoglobulins to a discussion of the biology of B-cell development and of B-cell activation, differentiation, and function. This is followed by a section on *T Lymphocytes* which fully incorporates major histocompatibility complex molecules and antigen-processing as central to the T-cell recognition process rather than treating them as a stand-alone topic, as they were in prior editions. This section also presents discussions of T-cell receptors and T-cell development, function, and activation with particular emphasis of the role of accessory or costimulatory molecules. The book then considers the immune system on a broader scale in the section *Organization of the Immune System*. This section also presents discussions of other major cellular elements of the immune system including dendritic cells, macrophages, and NK cells and considers the fascinating subject of the evolution of the immune system.

With the basic elements of the immune system in place, the book goes on to deal with the very large topic of *Regulation of the Immune Response,* which considers the issues of immunogenicity and tolerance, discusses the key molecular determinants of immune regulation, the cytokines, and then emphasizes to individual subjects that play a central role in understanding how the immune system is regulated, including apoptosis, immunoglobulin class switching, affinity maturation, control of T-cell phenotype, mucosal immunity, and the immunology of aging. From there, the book moves to a consideration of the key *Effector Mechanisms of Immunity,* including the complement system, phagocytosis, cytotoxicity, and inflammation. The *Fourth Edition* concludes with a long section on the *Mechanistic Basis of Clinical Immunology*. This section is not a detailed discussion of clinical immunology, which would be beyond the scope of even this very large book. Rather, it presents those mechanisms that have been elucidated by the study of basic immunology that make important contributions to our understanding of the role of the immune system in disease prevention and pathogenesis. It contains chapters on systemic and organ specific autoimmunity, allergy, transplantation, and tumor immunology. These are followed by chapters on various aspects of the immunity to infectious agents, including immunoparasitology, immunity to viruses, immunity to intracellular bacteria, immunity to extracellular bacteria, and vaccines, with a final comprehensive chapter on HIV infection. The section closes with chapters on primary immuno-deficiency and on the use of immune mechanisms therapeutically.

The contributors to *Fundamental Immunology, Fourth Edition,* are all leaders in their respective fields of immunology. They write their chapters from this vantage point, paying particular attention to the very rapid pace at which their subjects are progressing. They grapple with issues of great importance but on which a scientific consensus may not yet have been reached. Inevitably, this leads to circumstances in which different authors may express different points of view on the same subject. My position in editing this edition is that as long as the basis for the conclusion is well laid out, the presentation of differing views is useful. As I have stated in the prefaces to previous editions, I leave it to the reader to judge such differences of opinion and to follow the developments in the field to determine the resolution of these issues. I welcome comments by readers regarding *Fundamental Immunology, Fourth Edition*. Such input will be of great value in improving the book as it enters subsequent editions.

William E. Paul
Bethesda, MD

Discovery consists of seeing what everybody has seen and thinking what nobody has thought.

Albert Szent-Gyorgyi

. . . the clonal selection hypothesis . . . assumes that. . . there exist clones of mesenchymal cells, each carrying immunologically reactive sites . . . complementary . . . to one (or possibly a small number of) potential antigenic determinants.

Sir Macfarlane Burnet,
The Clonal Selection Theory of Acquired Immunity

In the fields of observation, chance favors only the mind that is prepared.

Louis Pasteur,
Address at the University of Lille

In all things of nature there is something of the marvelous.

Aristotle,
Parts of Animals

FUNDAMENTAL IMMUNOLOGY

FOURTH EDITION

Fundamental Immunology, Fourth Edition,
edited by William E. Paul
Published by Lippincott–Raven Publishers, Philadelphia 1999.

CHAPTER 1

The Immune System: An Introduction

William E. Paul

Introduction
Key Characteristics of the Immune Response
Cells of the Immune System and their Specific Receptors and Products
B-Lymphocytes and Antibody
T-Lymphocytes
Cytokines
The Major Histocompatibility Complex and Antigen Presentation
Effector Mechanisms of Immunity
Conclusion

INTRODUCTION

The immune system is a remarkable defense mechanism, found in its most advanced form in higher vertebrates. It provides the means to make rapid, highly specific, and often very protective responses against the myriad potentially pathogenic microorganisms that inhabit the world in which we live. Indeed, the tragic example of severe immunodeficiencies, as seen in both genetically determined diseases and in acquired immunodeficiency syndrome (AIDS), graphically illustrates the central role the immune response plays in protection against microbial infection. There is growing reason to believe that the immune system also has an important role in the rejection of tumors, but most immunologists would agree that the evolutionary pressure that has principally shaped the immune system is the challenge of the microbial world.

Fundamental Immunology has as its goal the authoritative presentation of the basic elements of the immune system; of the means through which the mechanisms of immunity act in a wide range of clinical conditions, including recovery from infectious diseases, rejection of tumors, transplantation of tissue and organs, autoimmune and other immunopathologic conditions, and allergy; and how the mechanisms of immunity can be martialled by vaccination to provide protection against microbial pathogens.

The purpose of the opening chapter is to provide readers with a general introduction to our current understanding of the immune system. It will thus be of particular importance for those with a limited background in immunology, providing them with the preparation needed for subsequent chapters of the book. Indeed, rather than providing extensive references in this chapter, each of the subject headings will indicate the chapters that deal in detail with the topic under discussion. Those chapters will not only provide an extended treatment of the topic but will also furnish the reader with a comprehensive reference list.

KEY CHARACTERISTICS OF THE IMMUNE RESPONSE

Primary Responses

Immune responses are initiated by the encounter of an individual with a foreign antigenic substance, generally an infectious microorganism. The infected person rapidly responds with the production of antibody molecules specific for the antigenic determinants of the immunogen and with the expansion and differentiation of antigen-specific regulatory and effector T-lymphocytes. The lat-

W. E. Paul: Laboratory of Immunology, National Institute of Allergy and Infectious Diseases, National Institutes of Health, Bethesda, MD 20892.

ter include both cells that produce cytokines and killer T cells, capable of lysing infected cells. Generally, the initial immune response is sufficient to control and eradicate the microbe. Indeed, the most effective function of the immune system is to mount a response that eliminates the infectious agent from the body.

Secondary Responses and Immunologic Memory

As a consequence of the initial response, the immunized individual develops a state of immunologic memory. If the same (or a closely related) microorganism is encountered again, a secondary response is made. This generally consists of an antibody response that is more rapid, greater in magnitude, and composed of antibodies that bind to the antigen with greater affinity and are more effective in clearing the microbe from the body. A similar enhanced and often more effective T-cell response ensues. One effect is that an initial infection with a microorganism initiates a state of immunity in which the individual is protected against a second infection. In the majority of situations, the protection is provided by high-affinity antibody molecules that rapidly clear the reintroduced microbe. This is the basis of vaccination; the great power of vaccines is illustrated by the elimination of small pox from the world and by the complete control of polio in the Western Hemisphere (see Chapter 42).

The Immune Response Is Highly Specific and the Antigenic Universe Is Vast

The immune response is highly specific. Primary immunization with a given microorganism evokes antibodies and T cells that are specific for the antigenic determinants found on that microorganism but that usually fail to recognize (or recognize only poorly) antigenic determinants expressed by unrelated microbes. Indeed, the range of antigenic specificities that can be discriminated by the immune system is enormous.

The Immune System Is Tolerant of Self Antigens

One of the most striking and important features of the immune system is its ability to discriminate between antigenic determinants expressed on foreign substances, such as pathogenic microbes, and antigenic determinants expressed by the tissues of the host. The capacity of the system to ignore host antigens is an active process involving the elimination or inactivation of cells that could recognize self antigens through a process designated immunologic tolerance.

Immune Responses Against Self Antigens Can Result in Autoimmune Diseases

Failures in establishing immunologic tolerance or unusual presentations of self antigens can give rise to tissue-damaging immune responses directed against antigenic determinants on host molecules. These often result in autoimmune diseases. It is now recognized that a range of extremely important diseases are autoimmune or have major autoimmune components, including systemic lupus erythematosus, rheumatoid arthritis, insulin-dependent diabetes mellitus, multiple sclerosis, myasthenia gravis, and regional enteritis. Efforts to treat these diseases by modulating the autoimmune response are a major theme of contemporary medicine.

AIDS Is an Example of a Disease Caused by a Virus That the Immune System Generally Fails to Eliminate

Immune responses against infectious agents do not always lead to elimination of the pathogen. In some instances, a chronic infection ensues in which the immune system adopts a variety of strategies to limit damage caused by the organism or by the immune response. One of the most notable infectious diseases in which the immune response generally fails to eliminate the organism is acquired immune deficiency syndrome (AIDS), caused by the human immunodeficiency virus (HIV).

Major Principles of Immunity

The major principles of the immune response are listed as follows:

Highly specific recognition of foreign antigens coupled with potent mechanisms for elimination of microbes bearing such antigens
A vast universe of distinct antigenic specificities
The capacity of the system to display immunologic memory
The tolerance of self-antigens

The remainder of this introductory chapter will describe briefly the molecular and cellular basis of the system and how these central characteristics of the immune response may be explained.

CELLS OF THE IMMUNE SYSTEM AND THEIR SPECIFIC RECEPTORS AND PRODUCTS

The immune system consists of a wide range of distinct cell types, each with important roles. The lymphocytes occupy central stage because they are the cells that determine the specificity of immunity. It is their response that orchestrates the effector limbs of the immune system. Cells that interact with lymphocytes play critical parts both in the presentation of antigen and in the mediation of immunologic functions. These cells include the monocyte/macrophages, dendritic cells, and the closely related Langerhans' cells, as well as natural killer (NK) cells, mast cells, basophils, and other members of the myeloid lineage of cells. In addition, a series of specialized epithelial and stromal cells provide the anatomic environment in which immunity occurs, often by secreting critical factors that regulate growth and/or gene activation in cells of the immune system. Such cells also play direct roles in the induction and effector phases of the response.

The cells of the immune system are found in peripheral organized tissues, such as the spleen, lymph nodes, Peyer's patches of the intestine, and tonsils. It is within these tissues that immune responses occur. Lymphocytes are also found in the central lymphoid organs, the thymus, and bone marrow, where they undergo the developmental steps that equip them to mediate the myriad responses of the mature immune system. A substantial portion of the lymphocytes and macrophages comprise a recirculating pool of cells found in the blood and lymph, providing the means to deliver immunocompetent cells to sites where they are needed and to allow immunity that is generated locally to become generalized.

Individual lymphocytes are specialized in that they are committed to respond to a limited set of structurally related antigens. This commitment, which exists before the first contact of the immune system with a given antigen, is expressed by the presence on the lymphocyte's surface membrane of receptors specific for determinants (epitopes) on the antigen. Each lymphocyte possesses a population of receptors, all of which have identical combining sites. One set, or clone, of lymphocytes differs from another clone in the structure of the combining region of its receptors and thus differs in the epitopes, expressed on immunogenic substances, that it can recognize. The ability of an organism to respond to virtually any nonself antigen is achieved by the existence of a very large number of different clones of lymphocytes, each bearing receptors specific for a distinct epitope. As a consequence, lymphocytes are an enormously heterogeneous group of cells. Based on reasonable assumptions as to the range of diversity that can be created in the genes encoding antigen-specific receptors, it seems virtually certain that the number of distinct combining sites on lymphocyte receptors of an adult human can be measured in the millions.

Lymphocytes differ from each other not only in the specificity of their receptors but also in their functions. Two broad classes of lymphocytes are recognized: the B-lymphocytes, which are precursors of antibody-secreting cells, and the T (thymus-derived) lymphocytes. T-lymphocytes express important regulatory functions, such as the ability to help or, in some cases, inhibit the development of specific types of immune responses, including the production of antibody by B cells and the increase in the microbicidal activity of macrophages. Other T-lymphocytes are involved in direct effector functions, such as the lysis of virus-infected cells or certain neoplastic cells.

B-LYMPHOCYTES AND ANTIBODY (Chapters 3–7)

B-Lymphocyte Development (Chapter 6)

B-lymphocytes derive from hematopoietic stem cells by a complex set of differentiation events that are only partially understood

(Fig. 1). A detailed picture has been obtained of the molecular mechanisms through which committed early members of the B lineage develop into mature B-lymphocytes. These events occur in the fetal liver and, in adult life, principally in the bone marrow. Interaction with specialized stromal cells and their products, including cytokines such as interleukin (IL)-7, are critical to the normal regulation of this process.

The key events in B-cell development occur in cells designated pro-B cells and pre-B cells. They center about the assembly of the genetic elements, encoding the cell surface receptor of B cells, which are immunoglobulin (Ig) molecules specialized for expression on the cell surface. Igs are heterodimeric molecules consisting of heavy (H) and light (L) chains, both of which have regions (variable [V] regions) that contribute to the binding of antigen and that are highly variable from one Ig molecule to another (Fig. 2). In addition, H and L chains contain regions that are nonvariable or constant.

The genetic elements encoding the variable portions of Ig H and L chains are not contiguous in germline DNA or in the DNA of nonlymphoid cells (Fig. 3). In pro- and pre-B cells, these genetic elements are translocated to construct an expressible V-region gene. This process involves a choice among a large set of potentially usable variable (V), diversity (D), and joining (J) elements in a combinatorial manner. Such combinatorial translocation, together with a related set of events that add diversity in the course of the joining process, results in the generation of a very large number of distinct H and L chains. The pairing of H and L chains in a quasi-random manner further expands the number of distinct Ig molecules that can be formed.

The H-chain variable region is initially expressed in association with the product of a constant (C)-region gene element designated

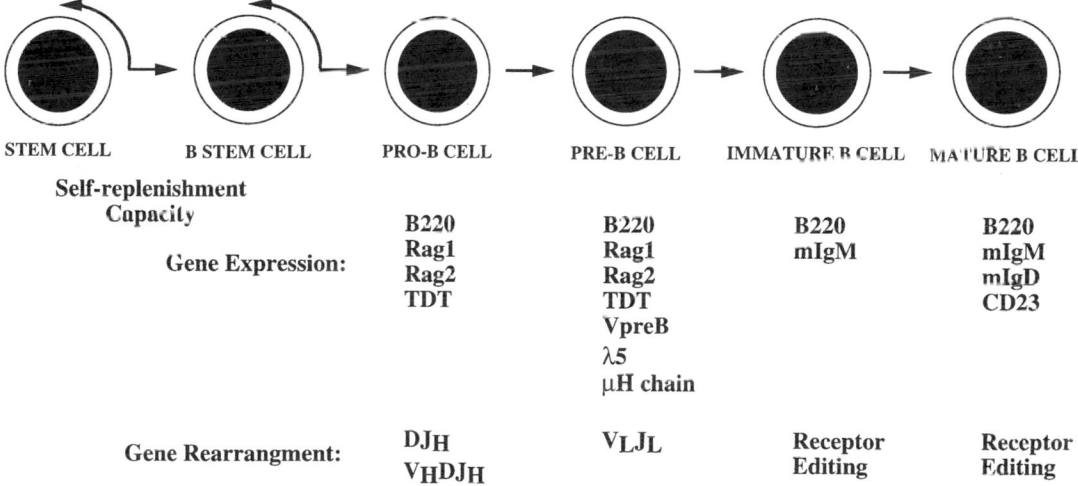

	STEM CELL	B STEM CELL	PRO-B CELL	PRE-B CELL	IMMATURE B CELL	MATURE B CELL
Self-replenishment Capacity						
Gene Expression:			B220 Rag1 Rag2 TDT	B220 Rag1 Rag2 TDT VpreB λ5 μH chain	B220 mIgM	B220 mIgM mIgD CD23
Gene Rearrangment:			DJH VHDJH	VLJL	Receptor Editing	Receptor Editing

FIG. 1. Pathway of B-cell development. B cells develop from hematopoietic stem cells. These cells and the proposed B stem cell (i.e., a self-replenishing cell with a differentiation capacity largely limited to the B lineage) give rise to the more identifiable members of the lineage. Both the stem cell and the B stem cell are capable of self-renewal. The first clearly identifiable member of the B lineage is the pro-B cell. This cell has begun the process of Ig gene rearrangement, largely limited to H-chain genes. It expresses genes encoding the B-cell form of CD45 (B220), the recombinase activating genes Rag-1 and Rag-2, and terminyl deoxynucleotidyl transferase (TDT), the enzyme responsible for N-region addition. The successful completion of VHDJH rearrangement and expression of μ H chains signals the end of the H-chain gene rearrangement and the onset of L-chain gene rearrangement. It marks the boundary between pro-B cell and pre-B cell states. Pre-B cells continue to express CD45 and Rag 1 and Rag-2 but extinguish expression of TDT. They express genes that encode surrogate light chains (VpreB and λ5) that can be expressed on the cell surface with μ H chains. Once L-chain rearrangement has yielded an expressible L chain that can pair with the expressed μ H chain, the cell may be considered to be an immature B cell bearing cell surface IgM. With the further expression of the δ H chain (and thus of membrane IgD) and of a set of other markers, of which CD23 is one, the cell may be regarded as having entered a state of maturity.

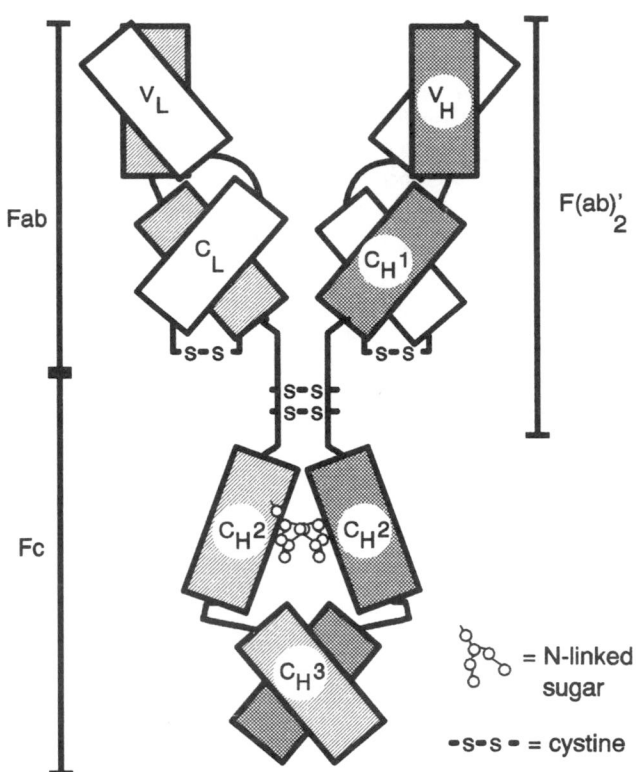

FIG. 2. Schematic structure of an Ig molecule. A schematic representation of an Ig molecule indicating the means through which the V regions and the CH1 and CL regions of H and L chains pair with one another and how the the CH2 and CH3 regions of the H chains pair. (This figure also appears in Chapter 3.)

Cellular Expression   ## Protein Products

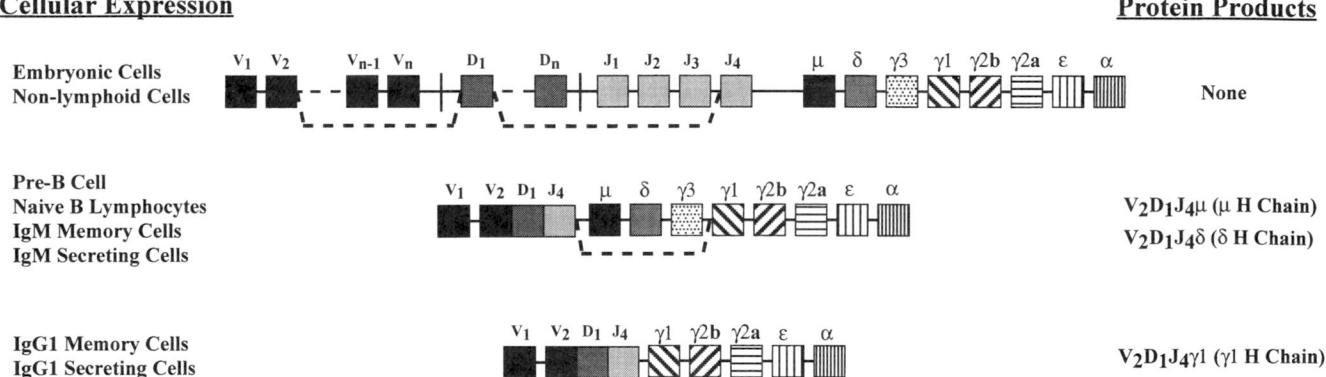

FIG. 3. Organization and translocation of mouse IgH genes. Ig H chains are encoded by four distinct genetic elements: Igh-V (V), Igh-D (D), Igh-J (J), and Igh-C genes. The V, D, and J genes together specify the variable region of the H chain. The Igh-C gene specifies the C region. The same V region can be found in association with each of the C regions (e.g., μ, δ, γ3, γ1, γ2b, γ2a, ε, and α). In the germline genome, the V, D, and J genes are far apart and there are multiple forms of each of these genes. In the course of lymphocyte development, a VDJ gene complex is formed by translocation of individual V and D genes so that they lie next to one of the J genes, with the excision of intervening genes. This VDJ complex is initially expressed with μ and δ C genes but may subsequently be translocated so that it lies near one of the other C genes (e.g., γ1) and in that case leads to the expression of a VDJ γ1 chain.

μ. Together these elements encode the μ IgH chain, which is used in Igs of the IgM class.

The successful completion of the process of Ig gene rearrangement and the expression of the resultant IgM on the cell surface marks the transition between the pre-B– and B–cell states (Fig. 1). The newly differentiated B cell initially expresses surface Ig solely of the IgM class. The cell completes its maturation process by expressing on its surface a second class of Ig (IgD) composed of the same variable (VDJ) region but of a different constant region; this second Ig H chain is designated δ, and the Ig to which it contributes is designated IgD.

The differentiation process is regulated at several steps by a system of checks that determines whether prior steps have been successfully completed. These checks depend on the expression on the surface of the cell of appropriately constructed Ig or Ig-like molecules. For, example, in the period after an Igμ chain has been successfully assembled but before a light chain has been assembled, the μ chain is expressed on the cell surface in associ-

Cognate T Cell- B Cell Help

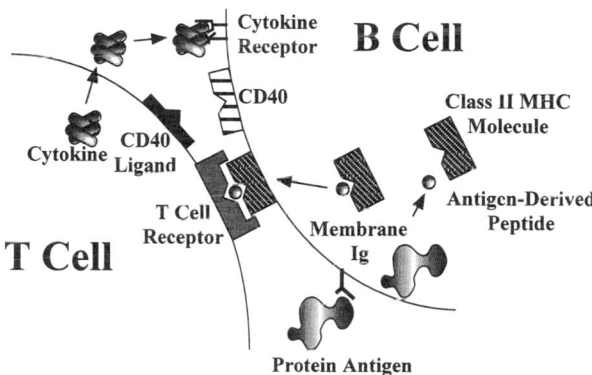

Cross-linkage-dependent B Cell Activation

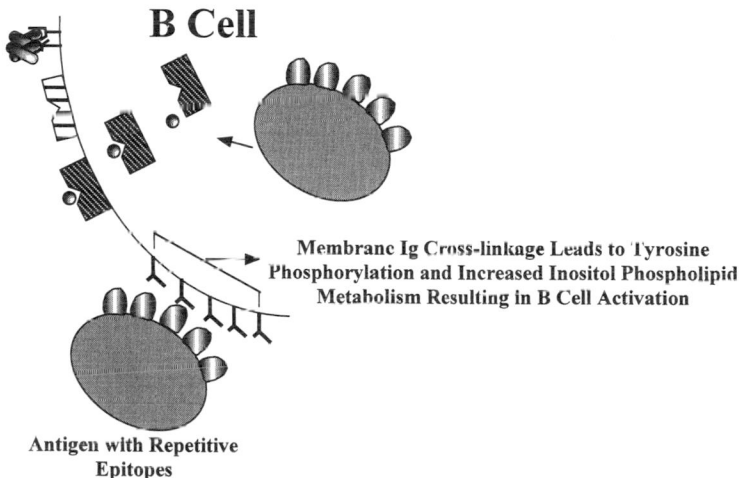

FIG. 4. Two forms of B-cell activation. **A:** Cognate T-cell/B-cell help. Resting B cells can bind antigens that bear epitopes complementary to their cell surface Ig. Even if the antigen cannot cross-link the receptor, because it does not possess more than one copy of the recognized epitope, it will be endocytosed and enter late endosomes and lysosomes, where it will be degraded to peptides. Some of the peptides will be loaded into class II MHC molecules and brought to the cell surface, where they can be recognized by CD4+ T cells that bear receptors specific for the B cell's peptide/class II protein complex. This interaction in turn allows the activation ligand on the T cell (CD40 ligand) to bind to its receptor on the B cell (CD40) and signal B-cell activation. In addition, the T cells secrete several cytokines that regulate the growth and differentiation of the stimulated B cell by binding to cytokine receptors on the B cell. **B:** Cross-linkage–dependent B-cell activation. When B cells encounter antigens that bear multiple copies of an epitope that can bind to their surface Ig, the resultant cross-linkage stimulates biochemical signals within the cell, including tyrosine phosphorylation and increased inositol phospholipid metabolism. These responses, together with the action of cytokines, cause B-cell activation, growth, and differentiation. The B cell continues to express class II MHC molecules loaded with peptide. The latter may derive from the antigen or from other sources but does not appear to play a direct role in this activation process. Similarly, it does not appear that the CD40 is directly involved in cross-linkage – dependent activation. As noted in the text, in many instances, B cell activation events may use both pathways of activation.

ation with a surrogate light chain. Cells that fail to express this μ/surrogate L-chain complex do not move forward to future differentiation states or do so very inefficiently. It is generally believed that the expression of this cell surface molecule implies the existence of a ligand and that the binding of this ligand determines that the cell may move to the next step of the differentiation process.

B-Lymphocyte Activation (Chapter 7)

A mature B cell can be activated by an encounter with an antigen that expresses epitopes that are recognized by its cell surface Ig (Fig. 4). The activation process may be a direct one, dependent on cross-linkage of membrane Ig molecules by the antigen (cross-linkage–dependent B-cell activation), or an indirect one, occurring most efficiently in the context of an intimate interaction with a helper T cell, in a process often referred to as cognate help.

Because each B cell bears membrane Ig molecules with identical variable regions, cross-linkage of the cell surface receptors requires that the antigen express more than one copy of an epitope complementary to the binding site of the receptor. Although many simple protein antigens do not express repeating antigenic determinants, such a requirement is fulfilled by polysaccharides and other antigens with repetitive epitopes. Among these antigens are the capsular polysaccharides of many medically important microorganisms such as pneumococci, streptococci, and meningococci. Similar expression of multiple identical epitopes on a single immunogenic particle is a property of many viruses because they express multiple copies of envelope proteins on their surface. Cross-linkage–dependent B-cell activation is a major protective immune response mounted against these microbes. The binding of complement components (see Chapter 29) to antigen or antigen/antibody complexes can increase the magnitude of the cross-linkage–dependent B-cell activation due to the action of a receptor for complement, which, together with other molecules, increases the magnitude of a B-cell response to limiting amounts of antigen.

Cognate help allows B cells to mount responses against antigens that cannot cross-link receptors and, at the same time, provides the costimulatory signals that rescue B cells from inactivation when they are stimulated by weak cross-linkage events. Cognate help is dependent on the binding of antigen by the B cell's membrane Ig, the endocytosis of the antigen, and its fragmentation into peptides within the endosomal/lysosomal compartment of the cell. Some of the resultant peptides are loaded into a groove in a specialized set of cell surface proteins, the class II major histocompatibility complex (MHC) molecules. The resultant class II/peptide complexes are expressed on the cell surface. As will be discussed below, these complexes are the ligands for the antigen-specific receptors of a set of T cells designated CD4+ T cells. CD4+ T cells with receptors specific for the class II/peptide complex expressed on the B-cell surface recognize and interact with that B cell. That interaction results in the activation of the B cell through the agency of cell surface molecules expressed by the T cells (e.g., the CD40 ligand [CD40L]) and cytokines produced by the T cell (Fig. 4). The role of the B-cell receptor for antigen is to create the T-cell ligand on the surface of antigen-specific B cells; activation of the B cell derives largely from the action of the T cell. However, in many physiologic situations, receptor cross-linkage stimuli and cognate help synergize to yield more vigorous B-cell responses.

B-Lymphocyte Differentiation (Chapters 6, 7, 24, and 25)

B-cell activation prepares the cell to divide and to differentiate either into antibody-secreting cells or into memory cells, so that there are more cells specific for the antigen used for immunization and these cells have new properties. The production of antibody under these circumstances accounts for primary antibody responses. The memory cells give rise to antibody production upon rechallenge of the individual. The hallmark of the antibody response to rechallenge (a secondary response) is that it is of greater magnitude, occurs more promptly, is composed of antibodies with higher affinity for the antigen, and is dominated by Igs expressing gamma, alpha, or epsilon C regions (Cγ, Cα or Cε) rather than by IgM, which is the dominant Ig of the primary response.

Division and differentiation of cells into antibody-secreting cells is largely controlled by the interaction of the activated B cells with T cells expressing CD40L and by their stimulation by T cell–derived cytokines, including IL-4, IL-5, and IL-6 or IL-2.

The differentiation of activated B cells into memory cells occurs in a specialized microenvironmental structure in the spleen and lymph node, the germinal center. The process through which increases in antibody affinity occur also takes place within the germinal center. The latter process, designated affinity maturation, is dependent on somatic hypermutation with antigen-mediated selection of cells, whose receptors have heightened avidity for the antigen.

The process through which a single H-chain V region can become expressed with genes encoding C regions other than μ and δ is referred to as Ig class switching. It is dependent on a gene translocation event through which the C-region genes between the genetic elements encoding the V region and the newly expressed C gene are excised, resulting in the switched C gene being located in the position that the Cμ gene formerly occupied (Fig. 3). The excised genes are often found in the form of large circular DNA.

B1 or CD5+ B-Lymphocytes (Chapter 6)

A second population of B cells has been described that differs from the dominant (or conventional) B-cell population in several important respects. These cells were initially recognized because some express a cell-surface protein, CD5, not generally found on other B cells but expressed by virtually all T cells. In the adult mouse, B1 B cells are found in relatively high frequency in the peritoneal cavity but are present at very low frequency in the spleen and lymph node. B1 B cells are quite numerous in fetal and perinatal life.

Evidence has been obtained that suggests that B1 B cells may emerge from a separate set of stem cells found in the fetal liver but absent from (or present only at low frequency in) the adult bone marrow. This suggests that B1 B cells cannot be replenished during adult life. Rather, it appears that B1 B cells are self-renewing, in contrast to conventional B cells in which division and memory are antigen driven.

The unique functional attributes of conventional and B1 B cells are still matters of intense study, but B1 B cells have a relatively high propensity to recognize autoantigens, and they may be responsible for the production of a large fraction of the IgM found in the serum of normal mice.

B-Lymphocyte Tolerance (Chapter 20)

One of the central problems facing the immune system is that of being able to mount a highly effective immune response to the anti-

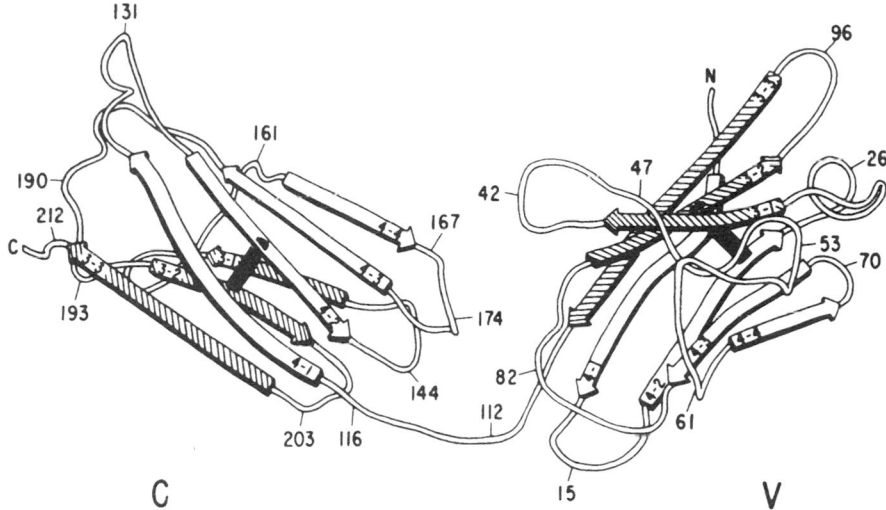

FIG. 5. Schematic drawing of the V and C domains of a light chain. The β strands participating in the antiparallel β-pleated sheets of each domain are represented as arrows. The β strands of the three-stranded sheets are shaded, whereas those in the four-stranded sheets are white. The β strands are numbered according to the scheme of Edmundson. The intradomain disulfide bonds are represented as black bars. Selected amino acids are numbered, with position 1 as the N terminus. (Reprinted with permission from Edmundson AB, Ely KR, Abola EE, Schiffer M, Panagiotopoulous N. Rotational allomerism and divergent evolution of domains in immunoglobulin light chains. *Biochemistry* 1975;14:3953–3961.)

gens of foreign, potentially pathogenic, agents while ignoring antigens associated with the host's own tissues. The mechanisms ensuring this failure to respond to self-antigens are now recognized to be complex and to involve a series of strategies. Chief among them appears to be elimination of cells capable of self-reactivity or the inactivation of such cells. The encounter of immature, naive B cells with antigens with repetitive epitopes capable of cross-linkage of membrane Ig can lead to elimination of the B cells, particularly if no T-cell help is provided at the time of the encounter. This elimination of potentially self-reactive cells is often referred to as clonal elimination. However, there are many self-antigens that are not encountered by the developing B-cell population or that do not have the capacity to cross-link B-cell receptors to a sufficient degree to elicit the clonal elimination process. Such cells, even when mature, may nonetheless be inactivated through a process that involves cross-linkage of receptors without the receipt of critical costimulatory signals. These inactivated cells may be retained in the body but are unresponsive to antigen and are referred to as anergic. When removed from the presence of the anergy-inducing stimulus, such cells regain responsiveness.

Immunoglobulins (Chapters 3–5)

Structure (Chapter 3)

The antigen-specific membrane receptors and secreted products of B cells are Ig molecules. Ig molecules are members of a large family of proteins designated the immunoglobulin supergene family. Members of the Ig supergene family have sequence homology, a common gene organization, and, where studied, similarities in three-dimensional structure. The latter is characterized by a structural element referred to as the Ig fold, generally consisting of a set of seven β-pleated sheets organized into two apposing layers (Fig. 5). Many of the cell surface proteins that participate in immuno-

logic recognition processes, including the T-cell receptor (TCR), the CD3 complex, and molecules associated with the B-cell receptor (Igα and Igβ), are members of the Ig supergene family.

The Igs themselves are constructed of a unit that consists of two H chains and two L chains (Fig. 2). The H and L chains are composed of a series of domains, each consisting of approximately 110 amino acids.

The L chains, of which there are two types (κ and λ), consist of two domains. The carboxy-terminal domain is essentially identical among L chains of a given type and is referred to as the constant (C) region. As already discussed, the amino-terminal domain varies from L chain to L chain and contributes to the binding site of antibody. Because of its variability, it is referred to as the variable (V) region. The variability of this region is largely concentrated in three segments, designated the hypervariable or complementarity-determining regions (CDRs). The CDRs contain the amino acids that are the L chain's contribution to the lining of the antibody's combining site. The three CDRs are interspersed among four regions of much lower degree of variability, designated framework regions (FRs).

The H chains of Ig molecules are of several classes (μ, δ, γ [of which there are several subclasses], α, and ε). An assembled Ig molecule, consisting of one or more units of two identical H and L chains, derives its name from the H chain that it possesses. Thus, there are IgM, IgD, IgG, IgA, and IgE antibodies. The H chains each consist of a single amino-terminal V region and three or four C regions. In many H chains, a hinge region separates the first and second C regions and conveys flexibility to the molecule, allowing the two combining sites of a single unit to move in relation to one another so as to promote the binding of a single antibody molecule to an antigen that has more than one copy of the same epitope. Such divalent binding to a single antigenic structure results in a great gain in energy of interaction. The H-chain V region, like that of the L chain, contains three CDRs lining the combining site of the antibody and four FRs.

The C region of each H-chain class conveys unique functional attributes to the antibodies that possess it. Among the distinct biologic functions of each class of antibody are the following:

1. IgM antibodies are potent activators of the complement system (Chapter 29).
2. IgA antibodies are secreted into a variety of bodily fluids and are principally responsible for immunity at mucosal surfaces (Chapter 27).
3. IgE antibodies are bound by specific receptors (FcεRI) on basophils and mast cells. When cross-linked by antigen, these IgE/ FcεRI complexes cause the cells to release a set of mediators responsible for allergic inflammatory responses (Chapter 35).
4. IgD antibodies act virtually exclusively as membrane receptors for antigen.
5. IgG antibodies, made up of four subclasses in both humans and mice, mediate a wide range of functions including transplacental passage and opsonization of antigens through binding of antigen/antibody complexes to specialized Fc receptors on macrophages and other cell types.

IgD, IgG, and IgE antibodies consist of a single unit of two H and L chains. IgM antibodies are constructed of five or six such units, although they consist of a single unit when they act as membrane receptors. IgA antibodies may consist of one or more units. The antibodies that are made up of more than a single unit generally contain an additional polypeptide chain, the J chain, which plays an important role in the multiunit structure.

Each of the distinct Igs can exist as secreted antibodies and as membrane molecules. Antibodies and cell surface receptors of the same class made by a specific cell have identical structures except for differences in their carboxy-terminal regions. Membrane Ig possesses a hydrophobic region, spanning the membrane, and a short intracytoplasmic tail, both of which are lacking in the secretory form.

Immunoglobulin Genetics (Chapter 5)

The genetic makeup of the Ig H-chain gene has already been alluded to. The IgH chain gene of a mature lymphocyte is derived from a set of genetic elements that are separated from one another in the germline. The V region is composed of three types of genetic elements: V_H, D, and J_H. More than 100 V_H elements exist; there are more than 10 D elements and a small number of J_H elements (four in the mouse). An H-chain $V_H DJ_H$ gene is created by the translocation of one of the D elements on a given chromosome to one of the J_H elements on that chromosome, generally with the excision of the intervening DNA. This is followed by a second translocation event in which one of the V_H elements is brought into apposition with the assembled DJ_H element to create the $V_H DJ_H$ (V region) gene (Fig. 3). Although it is likely that the choice of the V_H, D, and J_H elements that are assembled is not entirely random, the combinatorial process allows the creation of a very large number of distinct H-chain V-region genes. Additional diversity is created by the junctional imprecision of the joining events and by the deletion of nucleotides and addition of new, untemplated nucleotides between D and J_H and between V_H and D, forming N regions in these areas. This further increases the diversity of distinct IgH chains that can be generated from the relatively modest amount of genetic information present in the germline.

The assembly of L-chain genes follows generally similar rules. However, L chains are assembled from V_L and J_L elements only. Although there is junctional diversity, no N regions exist for L chains. Additional diversity is provided by the existence of two classes of L chains, κ and λ.

An Ig molecule is assembled by the pairing of IgH-chain polypeptide with an IgL-chain polypeptide. Although this process is almost certainly not completely random, it allows the formation of an exceedingly large number of distinct Ig molecules, the majority of which will have individual specificities.

The rearrangement events that result in the assembly of expressible IgH and IgL chains occur in the course of B-cell development in pro-B cells and pre-B cells, respectively (Fig. 1). This process is regulated by the Ig products of the rearrangement events. The formation of a μ chain signals the termination of rearrangement of H-chain gene elements and the onset of rearrangement of L-chain gene elements, with κ rearrangements generally preceding λ rearrangements. One important consequence of this is that only a single expressible μ chain will be produced in a given cell, since the first expressible μ chain shuts off the possibility of producing an expressible μ chain on the alternative chromosome. Comparable mechanisms exist to ensure that only one L-chain gene is produced, leading to the phenomenon known as allelic exclusion. Thus, the product of only one of the two alternative allelic regions at both the H- and L-chain loci are expressed. The closely related phenomenon of L-chain isotype exclusion ensures the production of either κ or λ chains in an individual cell, but not both. An obvious but critical consequence of allelic exclusion is that an individual B cell makes antibodies, all of which have identical H- and L-chain V regions, a central prediction of the clonal selection theory of the immune response.

Class Switching (Chapter 24)

An individual B cell can continue to express the same IgH-chain V region but, as it matures, can switch the IgH-chain C region it uses (Fig. 3). Thus, a cell that expresses receptors of the IgM and IgD classes may differentiate into a cell that expresses IgG, IgA, or IgE receptors and then into a cell-secreting antibody of the same class as is expressed on the cell surface. This process allows the production of antibodies capable of mediating distinct biologic functions but that retain the same antigen-combining specificity. When linked with the process of affinity maturation of antibodies, Ig class switching provides antibodies of extremely high efficacy in preventing reinfection with microbial pathogens or in rapidly eliminating such pathogens. These two associated phenomena account for the high degree of effectiveness of antibodies produced in secondary immune responses.

The process of switching is known to involve a recombination event between specialized switch (S) regions, containing repetitive sequences, that are located upstream of each C region (with the exception of the δ C region). Thus, the S region upstream of the μ C_H region gene (Sμ) recombines with an S region upstream of a downstream isotype, such as Sγ1, to create a chimeric Sμ/Sγ1 region resulting in the deletion of the intervening DNA (Fig. 6). The genes encoding the C regions of the various γ chains (in the human γ1, γ2, γ3, and γ4; in the mouse γ1, γ2a, γ2b, and γ3), of the α chain, and of the ε chain are located 3′ from the Cμ and Cδ genes.

The induction of the switching process is dependent on the action of a specialized set of B-cell stimulants. Of these, the most widely studied are bacterial lipopolysaccharide (LPS) and CD40L, expressed on the surface of activated T cells. The targeting of the C

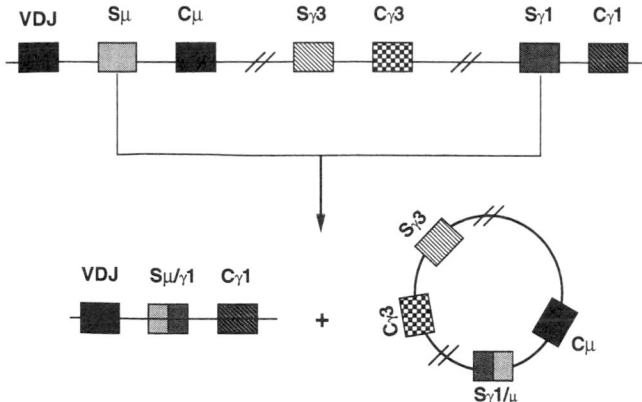

FIG. 6. Ig class switching. The process through which a given VDJ gene in a stimulated B cell may switch its C-region gene from μ to another, such as γ1, is illustrated. A recombination event occurs in which DNA between a cleavage point in Sμ and one in Sγ1 forms a circular episome. This results in Cγ1 being located immediately downstream of the chimeric Sμ/γ1 region, in a position such that transcription initiating upstream of VDJ results in the formation of VDJCγ1 mRNA and γ1 H-chain protein.

region that will be expressed as a result of switching is largely determined by cytokines. Thus, IL-4 determines that switch events in the human and mouse will be to the ε C region and to the γ4 (human) or γ1 (mouse) C regions. In the mouse, interferon-gamma (IFN-γ) determines switching to γ2a and transforming growth factor-beta (TGF-β) determines switching to α. A major goal is to understand the physiologic determination of the specificity of the switching process. Because cytokines are often the key controllers of which Ig classes will represent the switched isotype, this logically translates into asking what regulates the relative amounts of particular cytokines that are produced by different modes of immunization.

Affinity Maturation and Somatic Hypermutation (Chapters 14 and 25)

The process of generation of diversity embodied in the construction of the H- and L-chain V-region genes and of the pairing of H and L chains creates a large number of distinct antibody molecules, each expressed in an individual B cell. This primary repertoire is sufficiently large so that most epitopes on foreign antigens will encounter B cells with complementary receptors. Thus, if adequate T-cell help can be generated, antibody responses can be made to a wide array of foreign substances. Nonetheless, the antibody that is initially produced usually has a relatively low affinity for the antigen. This is partially compensated for by the fact that IgM, the antibody initially made, is a pentamer and thus, through multivalent binding, high avidities can be achieved even if individual combining sites have only modest affinity (see Chapter 4). In the course of T cell–dependent B-cell stimulation, particularly within the germinal center, a process of somatic hypermutation is initiated that leads to a large number of mutational events, largely confined to the H-chain and L-chain V-region genes and their immediately surrounding introns.

During the process of somatic hypermutation, mutational rates of 1 per 1,000 base pairs (bp) per generation may be achieved. This implies that, with each cell division, close to one mutation will occur in either the H- or L-chain V region of an individual cell. This cre-

ates an enormous increase in antibody diversity. Although most of these mutations will either not affect the affinity with which the antibody binds its ligand or will lower that affinity, some will increase it. Thus, some B cells emerge that can bind antigen more avidly than the initial population of responding cells. Because there is an active process of apoptosis in the germinal center from which B cells can be rescued by the binding of antigen to their membrane receptors, cells with the most avid receptors should have an advantage over other antigen-specific B cells and should come to dominate the population of responding cells. Thus, upon rechallenge, the affinity of antibody produced will be greater than that in the initial response. As time after immunization elapses, the affinity of antibody produced will increase. This process leads to the presence in immunized individuals of high-affinity antibodies that are much more effective, on a weight basis, in protecting against microbial agents and other antigen-bearing pathogens than was the antibody initially produced. Together with antibody class switching, affinity maturation results in the increased effectiveness of antibody in preventing reinfection with agents with which the individual has had a prior encounter.

T-LYMPHOCYTES (Chapters 10–12)

T-lymphocytes constitute the second major class of lymphocytes. They derive from precursors in hematopoietic tissue, undergo differentiation in the thymus (hence the name thymus-derived [T] lymphocytes), and are then seeded to the peripheral lymphoid tissue and to the recirculating pool of lymphocytes (see Chapter 14). T cells may be subdivided into two distinct classes based on the cell surface receptors they express. The majority of T cells express TCRs consisting of α and β chains. A small group of T cells express receptors made up of γ and δ chains. Among the α/β T cells are two important sublineages: those that express the coreceptor molecule CD4 (CD4+ T cells) and those that express CD8 (CD8+ T cells). These cells differ fundamentally in how they recognize antigen but also tend to mediate different types of regulatory and effector functions.

CD4+ T cells are the major regulatory cells of the immune system. Their regulatory function depends both on cell surface molecules such as CD40L, induced upon these cells when they are activated, and on the wide array of cytokines they secrete when activated. CD4+ T cells tend to differentiate, as a consequence of priming, into cells that principally secrete the cytokines IL-4, IL-5, IL-6, and IL-10 (T$_{H2}$ cells) or into cells that mainly produce IL-2, IFN γ, and lymphotoxin (T$_{H1}$ cells). T$_{H2}$ cells are very effective in helping B cells develop into antibody-producing cells, whereas T$_{H1}$ cells are effective inducers of cellular immune responses, involving enhancement in microbicidal activity of monocytes and macrophages and consequent increased efficiency in lysing microorganisms in intracellular vesicular compartments.

T cells also mediate important effector functions. Some of these are determined by the patterns of cytokines they secrete. These powerful molecules can be directly toxic to target cells and can mobilize potent inflammatory mechanisms. In addition, T cells, particularly CD8+ T cells, can develop into cytotoxic T-lymphocytes (CTLs) capable of efficiently lysing target cells that express antigens recognized by the CTLs.

T-Lymphocyte Antigen Recognition (Chapters 8–10)

T cells differ from B cells in their mechanism of antigen recognition. Immunoglobulin, the B-cell's receptor, binds to individual antigenic epitopes on soluble molecules or on particulate surfaces.

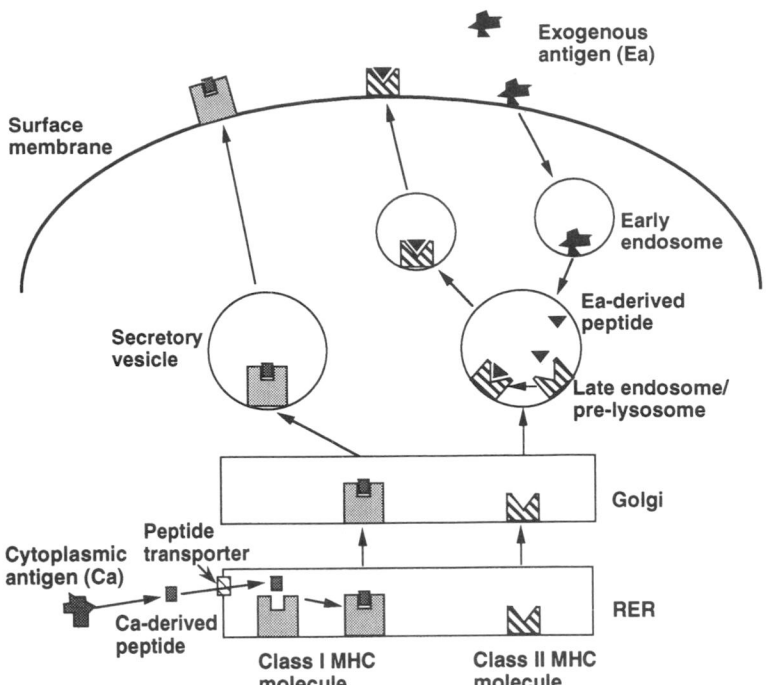

FIG. 7. Pathways of antigen processing. Exogenous antigen (Ea) enters the cell via endocytosis and is transported from early endosomes into late endosomes or prelysosomes, where it is fragmented and where peptide resulting from it (Ea-derived peptide) is loaded into class II MHC molecules. The latter have been transported from the rough endoplasmic reticulum (RER) through the Golgi apparatus to the peptide-containing vesicles. Class II MHC molecule/Ea-derived peptide complexes are then transported to the cell surface, where they may be recognized by TCR expressed on CD4+ T cells. Cytoplasmic antigens (Ca) are degraded in the cytoplasm and then enter the RER through a peptide transporter. In the RER, Ca-derived peptides are loaded into class I MHC molecules that move through the Golgi apparatus into secretory vesicles and are then expressed on the cell surface, where they may be recognized by CD8+ T cells. (Reprinted with permission from Paul WE. In: Gallin JI, Goldstein I, Snyderman R, eds. *Inflammation*. New York: Raven, 1992:776.)

B-cell receptors see epitopes expressed on the surface of native molecules. Antibody and B-cell receptors evolved to bind to and to protect against microorganisms in extracellular fluids.

By contrast, T cells invariably recognize antigens on the surface of other cells and mediate their functions by interacting with and altering the behavior of these antigen-presenting cells (APCs). Indeed, the TCR does not recognize antigenic determinants on intact, undenatured molecules. Rather, it recognizes a complex consisting of a peptide, derived by proteolysis of the antigen, bound into a specialized groove of a class II or class I MHC protein. Indeed, what differentiates a CD4+ T cell from a CD8+ T cell is that the CD4+ T cells only recognize peptide/class II complexes, whereas the CD8+ T cells recognize peptide/class I complexes.

The TCR's ligand (i.e., the peptide/MHC protein complex) is created within the APC. In general, class II MHC molecules bind peptides derived from proteins that have been taken up by the APC through an endocytic process (Fig. 7). These endocytosed proteins are fragmented by proteolytic enzymes within the endosome/lysosomal compartment, and the resulting peptides are loaded into class II MHC that traffic through this compartment. These peptide-loaded class II molecules are then expressed on the surface of the cell, where they are available to be bound by CD4+ T cells with TCRs capable of recognizing the expressed cell surface complex. Thus, CD4+ T cells are specialized to largely react with antigens derived from extracellular sources.

In contrast, class I MHC molecules are mainly loaded with peptides derived from internally synthesized proteins, such as viral proteins. These peptides are produced from cytosolic proteins by proteolysis by the proteasome and are translocated into the rough endoplasmic reticulum. Such peptides, generally nine amino acids in length, are bound into the class I MHC molecules and are brought to the cell surface, where they can be recognized by CD8+ T cells expressing appropriate receptors. This property gives the T-cell system, particularly CD8+ T cells, the ability to detect cells expressing proteins that are different from, or produced in much larger amounts

than, those of cells of the remainder of the organism (e.g., viral antigens [whether internal, envelope, or cell surface] or mutant antigens [such as active oncogene products]), even if these proteins, in their intact form, are neither expressed on the cell surface nor secreted.

T-Lymphocyte Receptors (Chapters 10 and 12)

The TCR is a disulfide-linked heterodimer (Fig. 8). The constituent chains (α and β, or γ and δ) are Ig supergene family members. The TCR is associated with a set of transmembrane proteins, collectively designated the CD3 complex, that play a critical role in

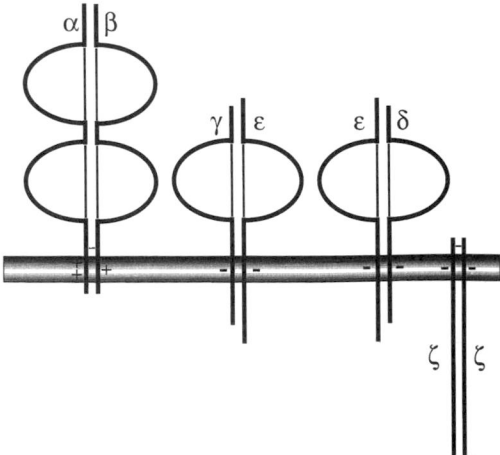

FIG. 8. The T-cell antigen receptor. Illustrated schematically is the antigen-binding subunit composed of an α/β heterodimer, and the associated invariant CD3 γ, δ, and ε chains, as well as the ζ chains. Acidic (−) and basic (+) residues located within the plasma membrane are indicated.

signal transduction. The CD3 complex consists of the γ (note that the CD3 γ and δ chains and the TCR γ and δ chains are distinct polypeptides that, unfortunately, have similar designations), δ, and ε chains and is associated with a homodimer of two ζ chains or a heterodimer of ζ and η chains. CD3 γ, δ, and ε consist of extracellular domains that are Ig supergene family members. The cytosolic domains of CD3 γ, δ, and ε and of ζ and η contain a signaling motif—the immunoreceptor tyrosine-based activation motif (ITAM) (D/ExxYxxLxxxxxxxYxxL/I)—that is found in a variety of chains associated with immune recognition receptors. This motif appears to be very important in the signal transduction process.

The TCR chains are organized much like Ig chains. Their N-terminal portions are variable and their C-terminal portions are constant. Furthermore, similar recombinational mechanisms are used to assemble the V-region genes of the TCR chains. Thus, the V region of the TCR β chain is encoded by a gene made of three distinct genetic elements (Vβ, D, and Jβ) that are separated in the germline. Although the relative numbers of Vβ, D, and Jβ genes differ from that for Ig, the strategies for creation of a very large number of distinct genes by combinatorial assembly are the same. Both junctional diversity and N-region addition further diversify the genes, and their encoded products. One major difference is that TCR β has fewer V genes than IgH but much more diversity centered on the D/J region, which encodes the equivalent of the third CDR of Igs. The α chain follows similar principles, except that it does not use a D gene.

The genes for TCR γ and δ chains are assembled in a similar manner except that they have many fewer V genes from which to choose. Indeed, γ/δ T cells in certain environments, such as the skin and specific mucosal surfaces, are exceptionally homogeneous. It has been suggested that the TCRs encoded by these essentially invariant γ and δ chains may be specific for some antigen that signals microbial invasion and that activation of γ/δ T cells through this mechanism constitutes an initial response that aids the development of the more sophisticated response of α/β T cells.

T Lymphocyte Activation (Chapter 12)

T-cell activation is dependent on the interaction of the TCR/CD3 complex with its cognate ligand, a peptide bound in the groove of a class I or class II MHC molecule. Through the use of chimeric cell surface molecules that possess cytosolic domains largely limited to the signaling motif alluded to above, it is clear that cross-linkage of molecules containing such domains can generate some of the signals that result from TCR engagement. Nonetheless, the molecular events set in motion by receptor engagement are complex ones. Among the earliest steps appears to be the activation of tyrosine kinases leading to the tyrosine phosphorylation of a set of substrates that control several signaling pathways. Current evidence suggests that early events in this process involve the src family tyrosine kinases p56^{lck}, associated with the cytosolic domains of the CD4 and CD8 coreceptors, p59^{fyn} associated with CD3, and ZAP-70, a Syk family tyrosine kinase, that binds to the phosphorylated ITAM of the ζ chain, as well as the action of the protein tyrosine phosphatase CD45, found on the surface of all T cells.

A series of important substrates are tyrosine phosphorylated as a result of the action of the kinases associated with the TCR complex. These include a set of adapter proteins that link the TCR to the ras pathway; phospholipase Cγ1, the tyrosine phosphorylation of which increases its catalytic activity and engages the inositol phospholipid metabolic pathway, leading to elevation of intracellular free calcium

concentration and activation of protein kinase C; and a series of other important enzymes that control cellular growth and differentiation.

In general, normal T cells and cloned T-cell lines that are stimulated only by TCR cross-linkage fail to give complete responses. Indeed, TCR engagement by itself may often lead to a response in which the key T cell–derived growth factor, IL-2, is not produced and in which the cells enter a state of anergy such that they are unresponsive or poorly responsive to a subsequent competent stimulus (see Chapter 20). Full responsiveness of a T cell requires, in addition to receptor engagement, an accessory cell–delivered costimulatory activity. The engagement of CD28 on the T cell by CD80 and/or CD86 on the APC appears to provide a potent costimulatory activity. Inhibitors of this interaction markedly diminish antigen-specific T-cell activation in vivo and in vitro, indicating that the CD80/86–CD28 interaction is physiologically very important in T-cell activation (see Chapter 13).

The interaction of CD80/86 with CD28 increases cytokine production by the responding T cells. For the production of IL-2, this increase appears to be mediated both by enhancing the transcription of the IL-2 gene and by stabilizing IL-2 messenger RNA (mRNA). These dual consequences of the CD80/86–CD28 interaction cause a striking increase in the production of IL-2 by antigen-stimulated T cells.

CD80/86 has a second receptor on the T cell, CTLA-4, that is expressed later in the course of T-cell activation. The bulk of evidence indicates that the engagement of CTLA-4 by CD80/86 leads to a set of biochemical signals that terminate the T-cell response.

T-Lymphocyte Development (Chapter 11 and 20)

Upon entry into the thymus, T-cell precursors do not express TCR chains, the CD3 complex, or the CD4 or CD8 molecules (Fig. 9). Because these cells lack both CD4 and CD8, they are often referred to as double-negative (DN) cells. Thymocytes develop from this DN pool into cells that are both CD4$^+$ and CD8$^+$ (double-positive cells) and express low levels of TCR and CD3 on their surface. In turn, double-positive cells further differentiate into relatively mature thymocytes that express either CD4 or CD8 (single-positive cells) and high levels of the TCR/CD3 complex.

The expression of the TCR depends on complex rearrangement processes that generate TCR α and β (or γ and δ) chains. Once expressed, these cells undergo two important selection processes. One, termed "negative selection," is the deletion of cells that express receptors that bind with high affinity to complexes of self-peptides with self-MHC molecules. This is a major mechanism through which the T-cell compartment develops immunologic unresponsiveness to self antigens. In addition, a second major selection process is positive selection, in which T cells with receptors capable of recognizing self-MHC molecules are selected, thus forming the basis of the T-cell repertoire for foreign peptides associated with self-MHC molecules. It appears that T cells that are not positively selected are eliminated in the thymic cortex by apoptosis. Similarly, T cells that are negatively selected as a result of high-affinity binding to self-peptide/self-MHC complexes are also deleted through apoptotic death. These two selection processes result in the development of a population of T cells that are biased toward the recognition of foreign peptides in association with self-MHC molecules from which those cells that are potentially autoreactive (capable of high-affinity binding of self-peptide/self-MHC complexes) have been purged.

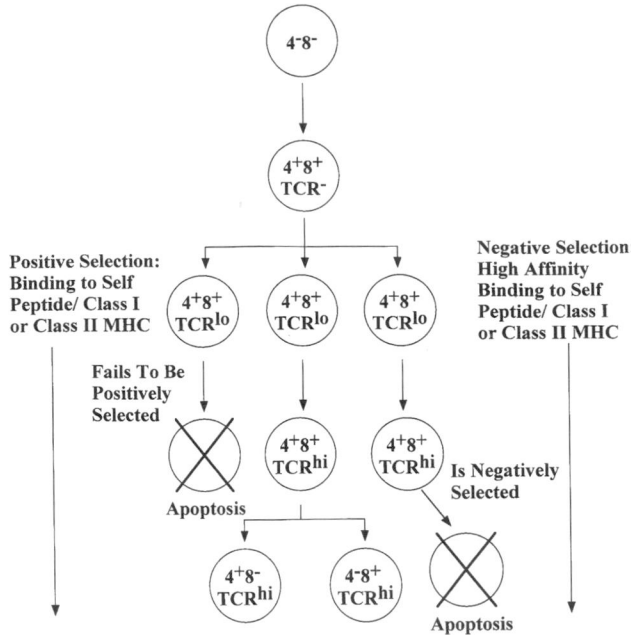

FIG. 9. Development of α/β T cells in the thymus. Double-negative T cells (4⁻8⁻) acquire CD4 and CD8 (4⁺8⁺) and then express α/β TCRs, initially at low levels. Thereafter, the degree of expression of TCRs increases and the cells differentiate into CD4 or CD8 cells and are then exported to the periphery. Once the T cells have expressed receptors, in order to survive they must recognize peptide/MHC class I or class II molecules with an affinity above some given threshhold. If they fail to do so, the cells undergo apoptosis. These cells have failed to be positively selected. Positive selection is also associated with the differentiation of 4⁺8⁺ into CD4 or CD8 cells. Positive selection by recognition of peptide/class I MHC molecules leads to the development of CD8 cells, whereas positive selection by peptide/class II MHC molecules leads to the development of CD4 cells. During this process, if a T cell recognizes a peptide/MHC complex with high affinity, it is also eliminated via apoptosis (it is negatively selected). The precise timing of positive and negative selection events is still not established.

One important event in the development of T cells is their differentiation from double-positive cells into CD4⁺ or CD8⁺ single-positive cells. This process appears to be due to the selection of double-positive thymocytes by accessory cells in the thymus through interaction with class II or class I MHC molecules. Indeed, CD4 binds to monomorphic sites on class II molecules, whereas CD8 binds to comparable sites on class I molecules. The capacity of the TCR and CD4 (or of the TCR and CD8) to bind to a class II MHC (or a class I MHC) molecule on an accessory cell leads to the differentiation of double-positive thymocytes into CD4⁺ (or CD8⁺) single-positive T cells.

Less is understood about the differentiation of thymocytes that express TCRs composed of γ/δ chains. These cells fail to express either CD4 or CD8. However, γ/δ cells are relatively numerous early in fetal life; this, together with their limited degree of heterogeneity, suggests that they may comprise a relatively primitive T-cell compartment.

T-Lymphocyte Functions (Chapters 11, 14, 21, 26, and 31)

T cells mediate a wide range of immunologic functions. These include the capacity to help B cells develop into antibody-produc-

ing cells, the capacity to increase the microbicidal action of monocyte/macrophages, the inhibition of certain types of immune responses, direct killing of target cells, and mobilization of the inflammatory response. In general, these effects depend on their expression of specific cell-surface molecules and the secretion of cytokines.

Helper T Cells (Chapters 11 and 26)

Helper T cells are cells that stimulate B cells to make antibody responses to proteins and other T cell–dependent antigens. T cell–dependent antigens are immunogens in which individual epitopes appear only once or only a limited number of times so that they are unable to cross-link the membrane Ig of B cells or do so inefficiently. B cells bind the antigen through their membrane Ig, and the complex undergoes endocytosis. Within the endosomal and lysosomal compartments, the antigen is fragmented into peptides by proteolytic enzymes and one or more of the generated peptides are loaded into class II MHC molecules, which traffic through this vesicular compartment. The resulting complex of class II MHC molecule and bound peptide is exported to the B-cell surface membrane. T cells with receptors specific for the peptide/class II molecular complex recognize that complex on the B-cell surface.

B-cell activation depends not only on the binding of the T cell through its TCR but also on the interaction T-cell CD40L with CD40 on the B cell. T cells do not constitutively express CD40L; rather, it is induced as a result of an interaction with an APC that expresses both a cognate antigen recognized by the TCR of the T cell and CD80 or CD86. CD80/86 is generally expressed by activated but not resting B cells so that the helper interaction involving an activated B cell and a T cell could lead to efficient antibody production. In many cases, however, the initial induction of CD40L on T cells is dependent on their recognition of antigen on the surface of APCs that constitutively express CD80/86, such as dendritic cells. Such activated helper T cells can then efficiently interact with and help B cells. Cross-linkage of membrane Ig on the B cell, even if inefficient, may synergize with the CD40L/CD40 interaction to yield vigorous B-cell activation.

The subsequent events in the B-cell response program, including proliferation, Ig secretion, and class switching either depend on or are enhanced by the actions of T cell–derived cytokines. Thus, B-cell proliferation and Ig secretion are enhanced by the actions of IL-4 and IL-5, as well as IL-2. Ig class switching is dependent both on the initiation of competence for switching, which can be induced by the CD40L/CD40 interaction, and on the targeting of particular C regions for switching, which is determined, in many instances, by cytokines. The best studied example of this is the role of IL-4 in determining switching to IgG1 and IgE in the mouse and to IgG4 and IgE in the human. Indeed, the central role of IL-4 in the production of IgE is demonstrated by the fact that mice that lack the IL-4 gene or the gene for the IL-4 receptor α chain, as a result of homologous recombination-mediated gene knockouts, have a marked defect in IgE production.

Although CD4⁺ T cells with the phenotype of T_{H2} cells (i.e., IL-4, IL-5, IL-6, and IL-10 producers) are efficient helper cells, T_{H1} cells also have the capacity to act as helpers. Because T_{H1} cells produce IFN-γ, which acts as a switch factor for IgG2a in the mouse, T_{H1}-mediated help often is dominated by the production of IgG2a antibodies.

Induction of Cellular Immunity (Chapters 15, 21, 22, and 26)

T cells also may act to enhance the capacity of monocytes and macrophages to destroy intracellular microorganisms. In particular, IFN-γ enhances several mechanisms through which mononuclear phagocytes destroy intracellular bacteria and parasites, including the generation of nitric oxide and induction of tumor necrosis factor (TNF) production. T_{H1}-type cells are particularly effective in enhancing microbicidal action because they produce IFN-γ. By contrast, two of the major cytokines produced by T_{H2} cells, IL-4 and IL-10, block these activities. Thus, T_{H2} cells often oppose the action of T_{H1} cells in inducing cellular immunity and in certain infections with microorganisms that are intracellular pathogens of macrophages, a T_{H2}-dominated response may be associated with failure to control the infection.

Suppressor T Cells

There has been a long-standing interest in the capacity of T cells to diminish as well as to help immune responses. Cells that mediate such effects are often referred to as suppressor T cells. There is little doubt that the potent regulatory activities of T cells leads to inhibition of certain types of responses. However, much of the phenomena that were formerly believed to be controlled by the action of specialized suppressor cells may reflect the fact that sets of T cells with distinct cytokine-producing phenotypes oppose one another's actions. As already discussed, this is particularly true of T_{H1} and T_{H2} CD4+ T cells. Thus, IFN-γ blocks many of the effects of IL-4, including the induction of class switching and secretion of antibodies. IL-4 and IL-10 also act as inhibitors of IFN-γ production and function. Thus, the action of a set of T cells in the immune response may be to deviate it in a particular direction. If the T-cell or B-cell function that is measured is diminished as a result of such deviation, one might conclude that the response had been suppressed when it had only been redirected.

In other situations, T cells capable of producing the cytokine TGF-β, which has broad antiinflammatory and immunosuppressive actions, can certainly act as specific suppressor T cells.

Cytotoxic T Cells (Chapter 31)

One of the most striking actions of T cells is the lysis of cells expressing specific antigens. Most cells with such cytotoxic activity are CD8+ T cells that recognize peptides derived from proteins produced within the target cell, bound to class I MHC molecules expressed on the surface of the target cell. However, CD4+ T cells can express CTL activity, although in such cases the antigen recognized is a peptide associated with a class II MHC molecule; often such peptides derive from exogenous antigens.

The molecular mechanisms of lysis have been considerably clarified recently. Two major mechanisms are now recognized. One involves the production by the CTL of perforin, a molecule that can insert into the membrane of target cells and promote the lysis of that cell. Perforin-mediated lysis is enhanced by a series of enzymes produced by activated CTLs, referred to as granzymes. Many active CTLs also express large amounts of fas ligand on their surface. The interaction of fas ligand on the surface of the CTL with fas on the surface of the target cell initiates apoptosis in the target cell, leading to the death of these cells

CTL-mediated lysis appears to be a major mechanism for the destruction of virally infected cells. If activated during the period in which the virus is in its eclipse phase, CTLs may be capable of eliminating virus and curing the host with relatively limited cell destruction. On the other hand, vigorous CTL activity after a virus has been widely disseminated may lead to substantial tissue injury because of the large number of infected cells and thus the large number of cells that could be killed by the action of the CTLs. Thus, in many infections, the disease is caused by the destruction of tissue by CTLs rather than by the virus itself. One example is hepatitis B, in which much of the liver damage represents the attack of HBV-specific CTLs on infected liver cells.

It is usually observed that CTLs that have been induced as a result of a viral infection or intentional immunization must be reactivated in vitro through the recognition of antigen on the target cell. This is particularly true if some interval has elapsed between the time of infection or immunization and the time of test. This has led to some question being raised as to the importance of CTL immunity in protection against reinfection and how important CTL generation is in the long-term immunity induced by protective vaccines.

CYTOKINES (Chapters 21, 22, and 26)

Many of the functions of cells of the immune system are mediated through the production of a set of small proteins referred to as cytokines. These proteins can now be divided into several families. They include the type I cytokines that encompass many of the interleukins (i.e., IL-2, IL-3, IL-4, IL-5, IL-6, IL-7, IL-9, IL-11, IL-12, IL-13, and IL-15), as well as several hematopoietic growth factors; the type II cytokines, including the interferons and IL-10; the TNF-related molecules, including TNF and lymphotoxin; Ig superfamily members, including IL-1; and the chemokines, a growing family of molecules playing critical roles in a wide variety of immune and inflammatory functions.

Many of the cytokines are T-cell products; their production represents one of the means through which the wide variety of functions of T cells are effected. Most cytokines are not constitutive products of the T cell. Rather, they are produced in response to T-cell activation, usually resulting from presentation of antigen to T cells by APCs in concert with the action of a costimulatory molecule, such as the interaction of CD80/86 with CD28. Although cytokines are produced in small quantities, they are very potent, binding to their receptors with equilibrium constants of approximately 10^{10} M^{-1}. In some instances, cytokines are directionally secreted into the limited space between the T cells and the APCs, so that they act in a paracrine manner and have limited action at a distance from the cell that produced them. This appears to be particularly true of many of the type I cytokines. However, other cytokines act by diffusion through extracellular fluids and blood to target cells that are distant from the producers. Among these are cytokines that have proinflammatory effects, such as IL-1, IL-6, and TNF.

THE MAJOR HISTOCOMPATIBILITY COMPLEX AND ANTIGEN PRESENTATION (Chapters 8 and 9)

The MHC has already been introduced in this chapter in the discussion of T-cell recognition of antigen-derived peptides bound to specialized grooves in class I and class II MHC proteins. Indeed, the class I and class II MHC molecules are essential to the process

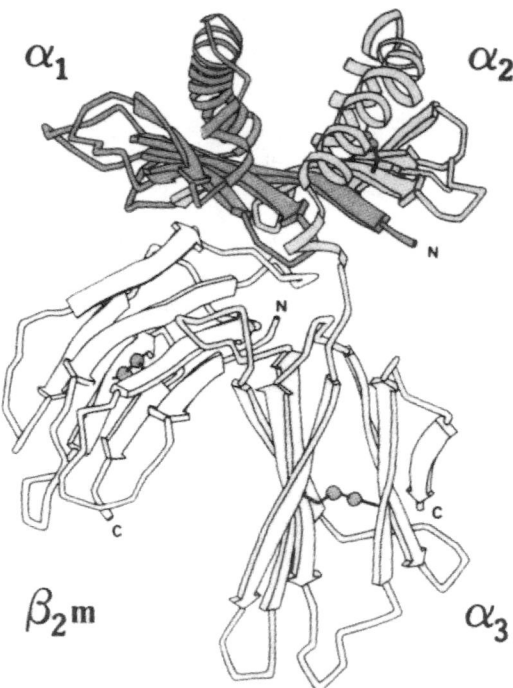

FIG. 10. Model of class I HLA-A2 molecule. A schematic representation of the structure of the HLA-A2 class I MHC molecule. The polymorphic $\alpha 1$ and $\alpha 2$ domains are at the top; they form a groove into which antigen-derived peptides fit to form the peptide/MHC class I complex that is recognized by TCRs of CD8[+] T cells. (Reprinted with permission from Bjorkman PJ et al. *Nature* 1987;329:506–512.)

of T-cell recognition and response. Nonetheless, they were first recognized not for this reason but because of the dominant role that MHC class I and class II proteins play in transplantation immunity (see Chapter 36). Because of their high degree of polymorphism and the wide array of peptides associated with class I and class II molecules, MHC proteins are the principal targets of immune responses that result in the rejection of organ and tissue allografts.

When the genetic basis of transplantation rejection between mice of distinct inbred strains was sought, it was recognized that although multiple genetic regions contributed to the rejection process, one region played a dominant role. Differences at this region alone would cause prompt graft rejection, whereas any other individual difference usually resulted in a slow rejection of foreign tissue. For this reason, the genetic region responsible for prompt graft rejection was termed the major histocompatibility complex.

In the human, the MHC is found on chromosome 6 and in the mouse on chromosome 17. In all higher vertebrates that have been thoroughly studied, a comparable MHC exists. The defining features of the MHC are the transplantation antigens that it encodes. These are the class I and class II MHC molecules. However, the MHC also includes other genes, particularly genes for certain complement components, often designated class III MHC molecules. In addition, genes for the cytokines TNF-α and lymphotoxin (also designated TNF-β) are found in the MHC.

Class I MHC Molecules (Chapter 8)

Class I MHC molecules are membrane glycoproteins expressed on the great majority of cells. They consist of an α chain of approx-

imately 45,000 daltons in noncovalent association with $\beta 2$-microglobulin, a 12,000-dalton molecule (Fig. 10). The gene for the α chain is encoded in the MHC, whereas that for $\beta 2$-microglobulin is not. Both the α chain and $\beta 2$-microglobulin are Ig supergene family members. The α chain is highly polymorphic, with the polymorphisms found mainly in the regions that constitute the binding sites for antigen-derived peptides and that are contact sites for the TCR.

The class I α chain consists of three extracellular regions or domains, each of similar length, designated $\alpha 1$, $\alpha 2$, and $\alpha 3$. In addition, α chains have a membrane-spanning domain and a short carboxy-terminal cytoplasmic tail. The solution of the crystal structure of several class I molecules indicates that the $\alpha 1$ and $\alpha 2$ domains form a site for the binding of peptides derived from antigens. This site is defined by a floor consisting of β sheets and bounded by α-helical walls. As noted above, the polymorphisms of the class I molecule are mainly in these areas.

In the human, three loci encoding classical class I molecules have been defined: these are designated HLA-A, HLA-B, and HLA-C. All display high degrees of polymorphism. A similar situation exists in the mouse. In addition, there are a series of genes, defined principally in the mouse, that encode class I–like molecules (class Ib molecules). Recently, some of these also have been shown to have antigen-presenting activity for formylated peptides, suggesting that they may be specialized to present certain prokaryotic antigens. In addition, the class Ib molecule CD1 has been shown to have antigen-presenting function for mycobacterial lipids, providing a mechanism through which T cells specific for such molecules can be generated. In the mouse, CD1 has been shown to be recognized by a novel class of T cells (NK T cells) that produce large amounts of cytokines upon immediate stimulation.

Class II MHC Molecules (Chapters 8)

Class II MHC molecules are heterodimeric membrane glycoproteins. Their constituent chains are designated α and β; both chains are immunoglobulin supergene family members, and both are encoded within the MHC. Each chain consists of two extracellular domains ($\alpha 1$ and $\alpha 2$; $\beta 1$ and $\beta 2$, respectively), a hydrophobic domain, and a short cytoplasmic segment. The overall conformation of class II MHC molecules appears to be quite similar to that of class I molecules. However, the solution of the three-dimensional structure of class II molecules indicates certain distinctive features that explain differences in the length of peptides that the two types of MHC molecules can bind: class I molecules generally bind peptides with a mean length of nine amino acids, whereas class II molecules can bind substantially larger peptides. The peptide-binding site of the class II molecules is contributed to by the $\alpha 1$ and $\beta 1$ domains; it is within these domains that the majority of the polymorphic residues of class II molecules are found.

In the mouse, class II MHC molecules are encoded by genes within the I region of the MHC. These molecules are often referred to as I region–associated antigens. Two sets of class II molecules exist, designated I-A and I-E, respectively. The α and β chains of the I-A molecules (Aα and Aβ) pair with one another, as do the α and β chains of I-E (Eα and Eβ). In general, cross-pairing between I-A and I-E chains does not occur, although exceptions have been described in vitro. In heterozygous mice, α and β chains encoded on alternative chromosomes (i.e., Aα^b and Aβ^k) may cross-pair so that heterozygous mice can express both parental and hybrid class II molecules. However, the degree of cross-pairing is allele specific, and thus not all hybrid pairs are formed with equal efficiency.

In the human, there are three major sets of class II molecules, encoded in the DR, DQ, and DP regions of the HLA complex. Pairing occurs between the β chain(s) encoded in a given region and the α chain encoded in that region.

Class II molecules have a more restricted tissue distribution than do class I molecules. Class II molecules are found on B cells, macrophages, epidermal Langerhans' cells, dendritic cells, thymic epithelial cells, and, in the human, activated T cells. Levels of class II molecule expression are regulated in many cell types by interferons and in B cells by IL-4. Indeed, interferons can cause expression of class II molecules on many cell types that normally lack these cell surface molecules. Interferons also can cause striking upregulation in the expression of class I MHC molecules. Thus, immunologically mediated inflammation may result in aberrant expression of class II MHC molecules and heightened expression of class I molecules. Such altered expression of MHC molecules can allow cells that do not normally function as APCs for CD4+ T cells to do so and enhances the sensitivity of such cells to CD8+ T cells. This could have important consequences for immunopathologic responses and for autoimmunity.

Antigen Presentation (Chapter 9)

As already discussed, the function of class I and class II MHC molecules is to bind and present antigen-derived peptides to T cells whose receptors can recognize the peptide/MHC complex that is generated. There are two major types of antigen-processing events, specialized to deal with distinct classes of pathogens that the T cell system must confront (Fig. 7).

Extracellular bacteria, viruses that have not yet integrated into cells, and extracellular proteins enter APCs by endocytosis or phagocytosis. The antigen is fragmented in endosomes or lysosomes, and peptides derived from the antigen are loaded into class II MHC molecules as these proteins traverse the vesicular compartments in which the peptides are found. The loading of peptide into a class II MHC molecule is important in stabilizing the structure of that molecule. The acidic pH of the compartments in which loading occurs appears to facilitate the loading process. However, once the peptide-loaded class II molecules reaches neutral pH, such as at the cell surface, the peptide/MHC complex is very stable. Peptide dissociation from such class II molecules is very slow, with a half-time measured in hours. The peptide/class II complex is recognized by T cells of the CD4 class with complementary receptors. As already pointed out, the specialization of CD4+ T cells to recognize peptide/class II complexes is due to the affinity of the CD4 molecule for monomorphic determinants on class II molecules. Obviously, this form of antigen processing can only apply to cells that express class II MHC molecules. Indeed, APCs for CD4+ T cells principally include cells that normally express class II MHC molecules, including B cells, macrophages, and dendritic cells.

T cells also can recognize proteins that are produced within the cell that presents the antigen. The major pathogens recognized by this means are viruses and other obligate intracellular (non–endosomal/lysosomal) microbes that have infected cells. In addition, proteins that are unique to tumors, such as mutant oncogenes, also can be recognized by T cells. Endogenously produced proteins are fragmented in the cytosol by the proteases in the proteasome. The resultant peptides are transported into the rough endoplasmic reticulum, through the action of a specialized transport system. These peptides are then available for loading into class I molecules. In contrast to the loading of class II molecules, which is facilitated by the acid pH of

the loading environment, the loading of class I molecules is controlled by interaction of the class I α chain with β2-microglobulin. Thus, the bond between peptide and class I molecule is generally weak in the absence of β2-microglobulin, and the binding of β2-microglobulin strikingly stabilizes the complex. (It also should be pointed out that the binding of β2-microglobulin to the α chain is markedly enhanced by the presence of peptide in the α chain groove.) The peptide-loaded class I molecule is then brought to the cell surface. In contrast to peptide-loaded class II molecules that are recognized by CD4+ T cells, peptide-loaded class I molecules are recognized by CD8+ T cells. This form of antigen processing and presentation can be performed by virtually all cells because, with a few exceptions, class I MHC molecules are universally expressed.

Although the specialization of class I molecules to bind and present endogenously produced peptides and of class II molecules to bind and present peptides derived from exogenous antigens is generally correct, there are exceptions, many of which have physiologic importance.

T-Lymphocyte Recognition of Peptide/MHC Complexes Results in MHC-Restricted Recognition (Chapters 9, 10, 20 and 36)

Before the biochemical nature of the interaction between antigen-derived peptides and MHC molecules was recognized, it was observed that T-cell responses displayed MHC-restricted antigen recognition. Thus, if individual animals were primed to a given antigen, their T cells would be able to recognize and respond to that antigen only if a source of APCs were present that shared MHC molecules with the individual that had been immunized. The antigen would not be recognized when presented by APCs of an allogeneic MHC type. This can now be explained by the fact that the TCR recognizes peptide bound to an MHC molecule. MHC molecules display high degrees of polymorphism, and this polymorphism is concentrated in the regions of the class I and class II molecules that interact with the peptide and that can bind to the TCR. Differences in structure of the MHC molecules derived from different individuals (or different inbred strains of mice) profoundly affect the recognition process. Two obvious explanations exist to account for this. First, the structure of the grooves in different MHC molecules may determine that a different range of peptides are bound or, even if the same peptide is bound, may change the conformation of the surface presented to the TCR. Second, polymorphic sites on the walls of the α-helices that are exposed to the TCR can either enhance or diminish binding of the whole complex, depending on their structure. Thus, priming an individual with a given antigen on APCs that are syngeneic to the individual will elicit a response by T cells specific for a given peptide (derived from the antigen) with a given conformation and adapted to the exposed polymorphic residues of the MHC molecule. When the same antigen is used with APCs of different MHC type, it is unlikely that the same peptide/MHC surface can be formed, and thus the primed T cells are not likely to bind and respond to such stimulation.

Indeed, this process also occurs within the thymus in the generation of the T cell repertoire, as already discussed. T cells developing within the thymus undergo a positive selection event in which those T cells capable of recognizing MHC molecules displayed within the thymus are selected (and the remainder undergo programmed cell death). This leads to the skewing of the populations of T cells that emerge from the thymus so that they are specialized to respond to peptides on self MHC molecules. One of the unsolved enigmas of positive selection within the thymus is how the vast array of T cells with receptors capable of reacting with a very large set of foreign peptides associated with self MHC molecules are chosen by self MHC molecules that can only display self peptides. It is believed that a high degree of cross-reactivity may exist so that T cells selected to bind a given class I (or class II) molecule plus self peptide A can also bind a set of other peptides bound to the same MHC molecule.

Our modern understanding of T-cell recognition also aids in explaining the phenomenon of immune response (Ir) gene control of specific responses. In many situations, the capacity to recognize simple antigens can be found in only some members of a species. In most such cases, the genes that determine the capacity to make these responses have been mapped to the MHC. We would now explain Ir gene control of immune responses based on the capacity of different class II MHC molecules (or class I MHC molecules) to bind different sets of peptides. Thus, for simple molecules, it is likely that peptides can be generated that are only capable of binding to some of the polymorphic MHC molecules of the species. Only individuals that possess those allelic forms of the MHC will be able to respond to those antigens. It is also possible that mice of the nonresponder MHC type may bind peptide to their MHC molecules but that no TCRs are found in the T-cell population capable of recognizing that particular peptide/MHC molecule complex. In either case, one would observe that some individuals are nonresponders because of the failure to generate a peptide/MHC molecule complex that can be recognized by the T-cell system.

This mechanism also may explain the linkage of MHC type with susceptibility to various diseases. Many diseases show a greater incidence in individuals of a given MHC type. These include reactive arthritides, gluten-sensitive enteropathy, insulin-dependent diabetes mellitus, and rheumatoid arthritis (see Chapter 34). One explanation is that the MHC type that is associated with increased incidence may convey altered responsiveness to antigens of agents that cause or exacerbate the disease. Indeed, it appears that many of these diseases may be due to enhanced or inappropriate immune responses.

EFFECTOR MECHANISMS OF IMMUNITY

The ultimate purpose of the immune system is to mount responses that protect the individual against infections with pathogenic microorganisms or, where it is not possible to eliminate such infections, to control their spread and virulence. In addition, the immune system may play an important role in the control of the development and spread of some malignant tumors. The responses that actually cause the destruction of the agents that initiate these pathogenic states (e.g., bacteria, viruses, parasites, tumor cells) are collectively the effector mechanisms of the immune system. Several have already been alluded to. Among these is the cytotoxic action of CTLs, which leads to the destruction of cells harboring viruses and, in some circumstances, expressing tumor antigens. In some cases, antibody can be directly protective by neutralizing determinants essential to a critical step through which the pathogen establishes or spreads an infectious process. However, in most cases, the immune system mobilizes powerful nonspecific mechanisms to actually mediate its effector function.

Effector Cells of the Immune Response (Other than T and B Lymphocytes) (Chapters 15, 17, 29, 30, 31, and 32)

Among the cells that mediate important functions in the immune system are cells of the monocyte/macrophage lineage, NK cells, mast cells, basophils, and granulocytes. It is beyond the scope of this introductory chapter to present an extended discussion of each of these important cell types. However, a brief mention of some of their actions will help in understanding their critical functions in the immune response.

Monocytes and Macrophages (Chapter 15)

Cells of the monocyte/macrophage lineage play a central role in immunity. As already discussed, they are important APCs. This appears to be particularly true for the presentation of antigens derived from bacteria and other microbial agents that have established infections within macrophages. Indeed, one of the key goals of cellular immunity is to aid the macrophages in eliminating organisms that have established such intracellular infections. In general, nonactivated macrophages are inefficient in destroying intracellular microbes. However, the production of IFN-γ and other mediators by T cells can enhance the capacity of macrophages to eliminate such microorganisms. Several mechanisms exist for this purpose, including the development of reactive forms of oxygen, the development of nitric oxide, and the induction of a series of proteolytic enzymes, as well as the induction of cytokine production.

Natural Killer Cells (Chapter 17)

Natural killer cells play an important role in the immune system. Indeed, in mice that lack mature T and B cells due to the *scid* mutation, the NK system appears to be highly active and to provide these animals a substantial measure of protection against infection. NK cells appear to be closely related to T cells. They lack conventional TCR (or Ig) but express two classes of receptors. They have a set of positive receptors that allow them to recognize features associated with virally infected cells or tumor cells. They also express receptors for MHC molecules that shut off their lytic activity. Thus, tumor cells or virally infected cells that attempt to escape the surveillance of cytotoxic T cells by downregulating or shutting off expression of MHC molecules then become targets for efficient killing by NK cells because the cytotoxic activity of the latter cells is no longer shut off by the recognition of particular alleles of MHC class I molecules.

In addition, NK express a receptor for the Fc portion of IgG (FcγRIII). Antibody-coated cells can be recognized by NK cells, and such cells can then be lysed. This process is referred to as antibody-dependent cellular cytotoxicity (ADCC).

NK cells are efficient producers of IFN-γ. A variety of stimuli, including recognition of virally infected cells and tumor cells, cross-linkage of FcγRIII, and stimulation by the macrophage-derived cytokines TNF and IL-12, cause striking induction of IFN-γ production by NK cells.

Mast Cells and Basophils (Chapter 35)

Mast cells and basophils play important roles in the induction of allergic inflammatory responses. They express cell surface receptors for the Fc portions of IgE (FcεRI) and for certain classes of IgG (FcγR). This enables them to bind antibody to their surfaces, and when antigen capable of reacting with that antibody is introduced, the resultant cross-linkage of FcεRI and/or FcγR results in the prompt release of a series of potent mediators such as histamine, serotonin, and a variety of enzymes that play critical roles in initiating allergic and anaphylactic-type responses. In addition, such stimulation also causes these cells to produce a set of cytokines, including IL-3, IL-4, IL-5, IL-6, granulocyte-macrophage colony-stimulating factor (GM-CSF), and TNF, that have important late consequences in allergic inflammatory responses.

Granulocytes (Chapter 32)

Granulocytes have critical roles to play in a wide range of inflammatory situations. Rather than attempting a cryptic discussion of these potent cells, it may be sufficient to say that in their absence it is exceedingly difficult to clear infections with extracellular bacteria and that the immune response plays an important role in orchestrating the growth, differentiation, and mobilization of these crucial cells.

The Complement System (Chapter 29)

The complement system is a complex system of proteolytic enzymes, regulatory and inflammatory proteins and peptides, cell surface receptors, and proteins capable of causing the lysis of cells. The system can be thought of as consisting of three arrays of proteins. Two of these sets of proteins, when engaged, lead to the activation of the third component of complement (C3) (Fig. 11). The activation of C3 releases proteins that are critical for opsonization (preparation for phagocytosis) of bacteria and other particles and

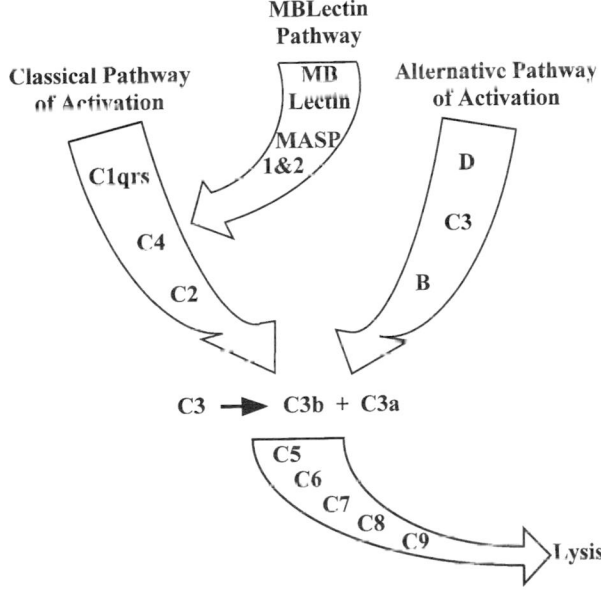

FIG. 11. The complement system. The classical pathway of complement activation, usually initiated by the aggregation of C1 by binding to antigen/antibody complexes, results in the formation of an enzyme, a C3 convertase, that cleaves C3 into two fragments, C3b and C3a. The classical pathway also can be initiated by the aggregation of MBLectin as a result of binding sugars expressed in the capsules of many pathogenic microbes. The components of the MBLectin pathway appear to mimic the function of C1qrs. The alternative pathway of complement activation provides a potent means of activating complement without requiring antibody recognition of antigen. It results in the formation of a distinct C3 convertase. The fragments formed by cleaving C3 have important biologic activities. In addition, C3b, together with elements of the classical pathway (C4b, C2a) or the alternative pathway (Bb, properdin), forms enzymes (C5 convertases) that cleave C5, the initial member of the terminal family of proteins. Cleavage of C5 leads to the formation of the membrane attack complex that can result in osmotic lysis of cells.

engages the third set of proteins that insert into biologic membranes and produce cell death through osmotic lysis. In addition, fragments generated from some of the complement components (e.g., C3a and C5a) have potent inflammatory activities.

The Classical Pathway of Complement Activation

The two activation systems for C3 are referred to as the classical pathway and the alternative pathway. The classical pathway is initiated by the formation of complexes of antigen with IgM or IgG antibody. This leads to the binding of the first component of complement, C1, and its activation, creating the C1 esterase that can cleave the next two components of the complement system, C4 and C2.

C4 is a trimeric molecule, consisting of α, β, and γ chains. C1 esterase cleaves the α chain, releasing C4b, which binds to surfaces in the immediate vicinity of the antigen/antibody/C1 esterase complex. A single C1 esterase molecule will cause the deposition of multiple C4b molecules.

C2 is a single polypeptide chain that binds to C4b and is then proteolytically cleaved by C1 esterase, releasing C2b. The resulting complex of the residual portion of C2 (C2a) with C4b (C4b2a) is a serine protease whose substrate is C3. Cleavage of C3 by C4b2a (also referred to as the classical pathway C3 convertase) results in the release of C3a and C3b. The amplification nature of this system is implicit in the capacity of a single antigen/antibody complex and its associated C1 esterase to produce a large number of C3 convertases (i.e., C4b2a complexes) and thus to cleave a large number of C3 molecules.

The components of the classical pathway can be activated by a distinct, non–antibody-dependent mechanism. The mannose-binding lectin (MBLectin) is activated by binding to (and being cross-linked by) repetitive sugar residues such as N-acetylglucosamine or mannose. The activation of MBLectin recruits the MBL-associated serine proteases MASP-1 and MASP-2, which are homologues of two of the constituent chains of C1 (C1r and C1s). This results in the activation of C4 and C2 and the formation of the classical pathway C3 convertase. Because the capsules of several pathogenic microbes can be bound by MBLectin, this provides an antibody-independent pathway through which the complement system can be activated by foreign microorganisms.

The Alternative Pathway of Complement Activation

Although discovered more recently, the alternative pathway appears to be the evolutionarily more ancient system of complement activation. Indeed, it can be regarded as providing individuals with a primitive type of nonspecific immune system. The alternative pathway can be activated by a variety of agents such as insoluble yeast cell wall preparations and bacterial lipopolysaccharide. Antigen/antibody complexes also can activate the alternative pathway. The C3 convertase of the alternative pathway consists of a complex of C3b (itself a product of cleavage of C3) bound to the b fragment of the molecule factor B. C3bBb is produced by the action of the hydrolytic enzyme, factor D, that cleaves factor B; this cleavage only occurs when factor B has been bound by C3b.

Apart from the importance of the alternative pathway in activating the complement system in response to nonspecific stimulants, it also can act to amplify the activity of the classical pathway because the C3 convertase of the classical system (C4b2a) provides a source of C3b that can strikingly enhance formation of the alternative pathway convertase (C3bBb) in the presence of factor D.

The Terminal Components of the Complement System

C3b, formed from C3 by the action of the C3 convertases, possesses an internal thioester bond that can be cleaved to form a free sulfhydryl group. The latter can form a covalent bond with a variety of surface structures. C3b is recognized by receptors on various types of cells, including macrophages and B cells. The binding of C3b to antibody-coated bacteria is often an essential step for the phagocytosis of these microbes by macrophages.

C3b is also essential to the engagement of the terminal components of the complement system (C5 through C9) to form the membrane attack complex that causes cellular lysis. This process is initiated by the cleavage of C5, a 200,000-dalton two-chain molecule. The C5 convertases that catalyze this reaction are C4b2a3b (the classical pathway C5 convertase) or a complex of C3bBb with a protein designated properdin (the alternative pathway C5 convertase). Cleaved C5, C5b, forms a complex with C6 and then with C7, C8, and C9. This C5b/C9 complex behaves as an integral membrane protein that is responsible for the formation of complement-induced lesions in cell membranes. Such lesions have a donutlike appearance, with C9 molecules forming the ring of the donut.

In addition to the role of the complement system in osponization and in cell lysis, several of the fragments of complement components formed during activation are potent mediators of inflammation. C3a, the 9,000-dalton fragment released by the action of the C3 convertases, binds to receptors on mast cells and basophils, resulting in the release of histamine and other mediators of anaphylaxis. C3a is thus termed an anaphylotoxin, as is C5a, the 11,000-dalton fragment released as a result of the action of the C5 convertases. C5a is also a chemoattractant for neutrophils and monocytes.

Finally, it is important to note that the process of activation of the complement cascade is highly regulated. Several regulatory proteins (e.g., C1 esterase inhibitor, decay accelerator factor, membrane cofactor protein) exist that function to prevent uncontrolled complement activation. Abnormalities in these regulatory proteins are often associated with clinical disorders such as hereditary angioedema and paroxysmal nocturnal hemoglobinuria.

CONCLUSION

This introductory chapter should provide the reader with an appreciation of the overall organization of the immune system and of the properties of its key cellular and molecular components. It should be obvious that the immune system is highly complex, that it is capable of a wide range of effector functions, and that its activities are subject to potent, but only partially understood, regulatory processes. As the most versatile and powerful defense of higher organisms, the immune system may provide the key to the development of effective means to treat and prevent a broad range of diseases. Indeed, the last section of this book deals explicitly with immunologic mechanisms in disease. The introductory material provided here should be of considerable help to the uninitiated reader in understanding the immunologic mechanisms brought into play in a wide range of clinical conditions in which immune processes play a major role in pathogenesis.

Fundamental Immunology, Fourth Edition,
edited by William E. Paul
Lippincott–Raven Publishers, Philadelphia © 1999.

CHAPTER 2

The History of Immunology

Arthur M. Silverstein

Early Theories of Acquired Immunity
  Expulsion Theories · Depletion Theories
The Origins and Research Program of Early Immunology
  Preventive Immunization · Cellular Immunity · Serotherapy · Cytotoxic Antibodies and Autoimmunity · Serology and Immunodiagnosis · Allergy and Immunopathology · Immunohematology · Ehrlich's Side-Chain Theory · The Cellular Versus Humoral Controversy · Transplantation and Immunogenetics
Immunology in Transition, 1912–1950s
  The Fate of the Early Immunological Research Program · The Rise to Dominance of Immunochemistry · Theory Follows Mindset: Instruction Theories · The Scope and Influence of the Immunochemical Research Program
The Immunobiological Revolution
  Selection Theories of Antibody Formation · The Immunological Synthesis
Nobel Prize Highlights in Immunology
  1901, von Behring · 1905, Koch · 1908, Metchnikoff and Ehrlich · 1913, Richet · 1919, Bordet · 1930, Landsteiner · 1951, Theiler · 1957, Bovet · 1960, Burnet and Medawar · 1972, Porter and Edelman · 1977, Yalow · 1980, Benacerraf, Dausset, and Snell · 1984, Milstein, Köhler, and Jerne   1987, Tonegawa · 1996, Doherty and Zinkernagel
Bibliography

EARLY THEORIES OF ACQUIRED IMMUNITY

It is clear that humankind must have known the ravages of epidemic disease from the very start of its social organization. Thus, the Babylonian Epic of Gilgamesh from about 2000 B.C. records visitations of disease and pestilence, and severe epidemics are recorded in the annals of the early dynasties of Egypt. In most early societies, however, and even today among more primitive peoples, both humans and nature were thought to function under the magical influences of spirits and demons, or under the mystical influences of the gods. It was only natural, then, that disease came to be considered a punishment for some infraction of a tribal taboo or some sin against the gods. Both the Babylonians and the ancient Egyptians included in their pantheons a god of disease, and throughout the Old Testament, God is continually smiting those who trespass against Him, often employing pestilential disease as a punishment. Thus, God brought down a pestilence not only on His own chosen people as punishment of David's sin of numbering the people (II Samuel 24), but also on their various enemies, including the Egyptians (Exodus 9:9), the Philistines (I Samuel 5:6), and King Sennacherib's Assyrians (Isaiah 37:36). Even in ancient Greece the sun god, Phoebus Apollo, was supposed to have caused the plague of Thebes because it had been tainted by the misdeeds

of Oedipus Rex. Apollo was supposed also to have rained plague arrows on the Greek army before Troy because their leader Agamemnon had abducted the daughter of Apollo's priest.

Although the nature of these various epidemics and their relationship to one another were unknown, the keen observer could not fail to notice that those who had once survived a disease might often be spared further involvement on its return. This phenomenon was described well by the historian Thucydides in his account of the plague of Athens of 430 B.C., when he wrote, "Yet it was with those who had recovered from the disease that the sick and the dying found most compassion. These knew what it was from experience, and had now no fear for themselves; for the same man was never attacked twice—never at least fatally." Although this "plague" was most probably not due to *Pasteurella pestis*, the plague of Justinian some thousand years later was more likely to have been bubonic plague, and of this the historian Procopius said, "At a later time it [the plague] came back; then those who dwelt round about this land, whom formerly it had afflicted most sorely, it did not touch at all." In time, this resistance to reinfection came to be known by the term *immunity*, from the Latin *immunitas*, which in ancient Rome originally described the exemption of an individual from service or duty to the state.

The view of disease as originating from a vengeful deity contains within it an implicit theory of immunity. If disease be considered a punishment for sin, then being spared during a raging epidemic (i.e., *natural immunity*) would automatically be viewed as

A. M. Silverstein: Institute of the History of Medicine, Johns Hopkins University School of Medicine, Baltimore, Maryland 21205.

the inevitable result of having led a pious life. But a significant change occurred in early Christian times. Now not only did God punish the sins of humans with disease, but He might also employ disease to cleanse humans of their sins. If, then, disease was viewed as an expiation and purgative, then the recovery from a deadly plague would imply not only that the sins had been minor, but also that once cleansed of these sins the individual would not deserve further punishment when the plague returned (*acquired immunity*). Given the fervent religiosity of the times, such a concept of immunity may have been so ingrained as not to require explicit statement.

It was only during the last millennium that explicit theories of acquired immunity were advanced, most of them highly imaginative and each of them eminently consistent with the then-prevailing notion of disease pathogenesis. Because smallpox was one of the earliest diseases to be identified clinically, and because the lifelong immunity that it conferred could hardly escape notice, it is not surprising that most early theories of immunity would be couched in terms of this disease.

Expulsion Theories

The first clear clinical description of smallpox was given by the tenth century Islamic physician Rhazes. Not only did Rhazes differentiate smallpox from measles and other exanthematous diseases for the first time, but he also stated clearly that recovery from smallpox infection provides lasting immunity. To explain this phenomenon, he advanced the first explicit theory of acquired immunity that we have been able to find in the literature. Like all of his contemporaries, Rhazes followed the Hippocratic tradition, which held that disease was due to quantitative imbalances among the four humors (blood, phlegm, yellow bile, and black bile), to changes in their temperature and consistency, or even to their fermentation. Smallpox was believed to affect the blood, and Rhazes claimed that the disease was due to a fermentation of this humor, which helped to dispel the "excess moisture" that he thought was present in the blood of the young. He proposed that the pustules that formed on the skin during this disease and broke to release fluid were the mechanism whereby the body expelled the excess moisture contained in the blood. He compared the maturation of an individual to the fermentation of wine from grape juice (must) and even suggested that smallpox disease itself might assist in this normal process! Thus he wrote:

> I say then that every man, from the time of his birth till he arrives at old age, is continually tending to dryness; and for this reason the blood of children and infants is much moister than the blood of young men, and still more so than that of old men. . . . Now the smallpox arises when the blood putrefies and ferments, so that superfluous vapors are thrown out of it and it is changed from the blood of infants, which is like must, into the blood of young men, which is like wine perfectly ripened; as to the blood of old men, it may be compared to wine which has now lost its strength and is beginning to grow vapid and sour; and the smallpox itself may be compared to the fermentation and the hissing noise which takes place in must at that time. And this is the reason why children, especially males, rarely escape being seized with this disease, because it is impossible to prevent the blood's changing from this state into its second state, just as it is impossible to prevent must . . . from changing.

This curious theory appeared to explain well all that was known about smallpox: (a) Substantially everyone is affected, especially during youth (since then the blood is most moist); (b) the disease is seldom seen in adults and almost never in old age (because by then the normal aging process would have sufficiently dried the blood, so that it no longer could support the infection); and (c) a single infection would lead to lasting immunity, and recurrence of the disease would be impossible (since the initial attack would have expelled all of the "excess moisture" that the theory required as a prerequisite for the disease process). It is interesting that Rhazes presented the smallpox of the tenth century as an almost benign childhood disease, and even as a salutory phenomenon that appeared to aid the normal development from infancy to adulthood.

During the eleventh century, Avicenna hinted at another interesting theory of acquired immunity, which was expanded on some 500 years later by the Italian physician Girolamo Fracastoro in his 1546 book *On Contagion*. Fracastoro claimed that all disease was caused by small seeds or germs (*seminaria*) which might spread from person to person, each of which possesses a specific affinity for a given plant or animal, and for a given organ or humor. He claimed that the germ of smallpox has an affinity for and caused the fermentation only of that trace of menstrual blood contaminant that he supposed tainted all mammalian young *in utero*. When a (young) person was infected, the menstrual contaminant would ferment, rise to the surface beneath the skin in the form of pustules, and be expelled when the pustules broke. He wrote,

> This ebulition is a kind of purification of the blood . . . infection contracted by the child from the menstrual blood of the mother's womb is localized by means of this sort of ebulition and its putrefaction, and the blood is thus purified by a sort of crisis provided by nature. That is why almost all of us suffer from this malady, . . . and this fever is of itself seldom fatal [*sic*!], but is rather a purgation . . . the malady usually does not recur because the infection has already been secreted in the previous attack.

Thus Fracastoro's theory appeared also to explain satisfactorily all that was then known about smallpox. In this instance, acquired immunity would result from the expulsion during the first illness of the menstrual blood contaminant that he thought we all are born with, and without which the disease could not recur. But Fracastoro felt that his theory also implied a simultaneously acquired immunity to other exanthematous diseases, such as measles, and this was criticized by Heironymus Mercurialis, who made perhaps the earliest statement about immunologic specificity. Mercurialis pointed out that Fracastoro's theory could not be correct because, among other objections, measles and smallpox could not *both* be based on a menstrual blood contaminant, since infection with one should have cleansed the blood of the contaminant and conferred immunity to the other disease also; such "cross-immunity" was, Mercurialis noted, contrary to fact.

Several other variants of the menstrual blood expulsion theory should be noted, each proposing an analogous pathogenesis of smallpox and a comparable basis for acquired immunity. Thus, in place of menstrual blood contaminant, it has variously been proposed that amniotic fluid or umbilical blood is the culprit. In each instance, the disease was felt to involve the putrefaction of the contaminating substance, its expulsion via the pustules, and lifelong immunity due to the absence of further substrate upon which a new infection might act.

Depletion Theories

The introduction of variolation as a prophylactic measure (the inoculation of live virus from a diseased smallpox victim) led to renewed interest in the nature and in the mechanism of acquired immunity early in the eighteenth century. The inoculation of crusts derived from the pustules of "favorable" cases of smallpox had apparently been practiced widely in the folk medicine of many cultures in Asia and Africa and even in the rural areas of Western Europe. The practice may have originated among the Chinese, who advised the blowing of the infected matter into the nose of the recipient through a silver tube, the left nostril being used for males and the right one for females. Elsewhere, it was more customary to make a small incision in the skin and therein to insert the infected crust, or to run into the skin a thread that had been dipped in infected pustular fluid.

Although the practice of inoculation was inveighed against on both religious and medical grounds, it did attain a degree of acceptance, especially in England, thanks to the example set by the Prince and Princess of Wales in 1722 in permitting their children to be inoculated. Inoculation proved especially popular during periods of epidemic smallpox, when the mortality rate often reached 15% to 20% of those infected and the rate of disfigurement was even higher. In contrast, inoculation protected well against reinfection, most frequently involved no facial scarring, and was accompanied by at most a 2% to 3% death rate. The famous Voltaire observed the practice during his travels in England and waxed enthusiastic about its efficacy in his *Lettres Philosophiques,* crediting (probably erroneously) Lady Mary Wortley Montagu with its introduction into England. Voltaire speculated that inoculation might have originated with the Circassians to protect the beauty of their daughters, whom they could not sell pock-marked into the harems of the Ottoman Empire.

Thus it was that when the practice of inoculation was given currency in the pages of the Philosophical Transactions of the Royal Society, and especially after the prestigious demonstrations that attended the inoculation of the royal family, many were tempted to try the new procedure, and a few were led to speculate on its meaning. As early as 1721, the New England divine Cotton Mather convinced his friend Dr. Zabdiel Boylston to undertake the practice during an epidemic in Boston. Mather subsequently advanced a theory of acquired immunity in the following florid prose:

> Whereas, the *Miasms* of the *Small-Pox* being admitted in the Way of *Inoculation,* their Approaches are made only by the *Outerworks* of the Citadel, and at a Considerable Distance from the Center of it. The Enemy [smallpox], tis true, getts in so far as to make Some Spoil, yea, so much as to satisfy him, and leaves no *Prey* in the Body of the Patient, for him ever afterwards to seize upon . . . tho' not without a *Surrender* of those Humours in the Blood, which the Invader makes a Seizure on, they oblige him *to march out the same way he came in,* and are sure of never being troubled with him any more.

Mather thus suggests that some unidentified substrate is depleted during either natural infection or following inoculation, its absence thenceforth inhibiting the development of the disease a second time.

It was in this context of three-quarters of a century of smallpox inoculation that Edward Jenner published in 1798 his epoch-making report on a safer and even more efficacious vaccine against smallpox, derived from cowpox pustules. The rapidity with which Jennerian vaccination (Latin *vaccus,* cow) swept the world is truly impressive; only a few years later, when Jenner interceded with the French enemy on behalf of an English prisoner, Napoleon remarked that he could refuse nothing to this great benefactor of humankind. Unfortunately, Jenner appears never to have specu-

lated on why his vaccine caused immunity, perhaps influenced by the earlier advice of his eminent teacher John Hunter: "Why think? Why not try the experiment?"

One of the more fanciful concepts of disease pathogenesis, and thus of disease immunity, that arose during the seventeenth and eighteenth centuries was that of the "innate seed." Humans (and animals) were held to be born with the seeds (*ovula*) for every different disease to which they were subject, each of which could be fertilized specifically by the appropriate contagious agent to produce the given disease. As Thomas Fuller so elegantly summarized the theory:

> Because these Ovula are of distinct Kinds, . . . therefore the Pestilence can never breed the Small Pox, nor the Small Pox the Measles. . . . The Ovula always lie quiet and unprolific, till impregnated, and therefore these Distempers seldom come without Infection, which is as it were the Male, and the active Cause. The Ovula of each particular Fever, are all, and every individual one of them, usually impregnated at once. . . . And when these have been impregnated, and delivered of their morbid Foetus, there is an End of them; . . . Upon this Account no Man can possibly . . . be infected with any of the respective Distempers any more than once.

Thus Fuller not only recognized specific etiology, but also offered a plausible explanation of acquired immunity that is at once specific and also long-lasting.

This view that immunity was based on the depletion of some substance necessary to support the disease process was repeated often during the eighteenth century. Thus, one finds statements in the literature such as the following by M. Maty in 1755: "I lately tried this experiment [inoculation] upon myself, . . . and it had no effect upon my blood, as it had been sufficiently *defecated* 15 years before." Again, a contemporary commentator, Angelo Gatti, compared susceptibility to smallpox with a body which a single spark might set afire, but which thenceforth has become "incombustible" although surrounded by flames, and thus immune to further infection.

The 1870s saw increasing acceptance of the germ theory of disease and, thanks to the efforts of Louis Pasteur, Robert Koch, and others, the identification of the specific agents of many diseases and the elucidation of their modes of action. The newer concepts of disease pathogenesis, and especially Pasteur's demonstration in 1880 that acquired immunity could be induced against fowl cholera with an attenuated strain of organisms, overthrew all earlier concepts of the mechanism of immunity. Stimulated by his observations on immunity, and knowing something of the kinetics of bacterial growth in culture, the ever-imaginative Pasteur advanced his own explanation for acquired immunity, which held sway briefly. Pasteur recognized that bacterial growth *in vitro* rapidly terminates following its initial log phase multiplication and attributed this to the depletion of critical trace substances for which each bacterial species was thought to have specific requirements. At a time when the only known vaccines consisted of live attenuated organisms, Pasteur suggested that infection of the host either naturally or by immunization would rapidly deplete the body of those unique nutrients required for the continued growth of the infectious agent. Absent these necessary substances in the previously depleted host, it would be impossible to establish a second infection with the same agent, and acquired immunity would persist in the host so long as the substances were not renewed. The subsequent demonstrations by Theobald Smith that dead organisms would suffice for the vaccine, and by Emil von Behring and Shibasaburo Kitasato that even the supernatants from the culture growth of diphtheria or tetanus organisms would confer immunity, quickly demonstrated the inadequacy of Pasteur's depletion theory.

THE ORIGINS AND RESEARCH PROGRAM OF EARLY IMMUNOLOGY

Preventive Immunization

The science of immunology was born in the laboratory of Louis Pasteur in the context of Pasteur's dedicated commitment to the germ theory of disease. Pasteur's earlier work on the agents responsible for certain diseases in the French silkworm and wine industries had convinced him that each disease is the reproducible result of an infection by a specific microorganism. Moreover, he held that not only does spontaneous generation not exist, but that these pathogenic agents are constant and specific in their ability to cause a given disease and cannot undergo transformation to yield some other disease picture. Then, in collaboration with Emile Roux, Pasteur discovered variations in the pathogenicity of different strains of a given organism, such that one strain might produce a much less severe disease than another. Pasteur and Roux devised techniques for the attenuation of cultures of virulent bacteria, working most notably with the organism responsible for the disease chicken cholera. By one of those happy instances of serendipity in science, it was discovered that chickens that had recovered from a mild attack of chicken cholera induced by an attenuated strain were thenceforth protected from challenge with more lethal strains.

This report in 1880 was the first generalization on Edward Jenner's use of cowpox vaccine to protect against smallpox, and it opened up an entirely new research program of prophylactic immunization. Pasteur was quick to seize upon these possibilities, as his subsequent work on anthrax, rabies, and other diseases amply testifies. Over the next quarter-century, as the specific pathogens of different diseases were reported with increasing frequency in the journals, scientists throughout the world endeavored to develop appropriate preventive vaccines, using Pasteurian approaches.

Cellular Immunity

The second significant step in the expansion of the immunological research program of the nineteenth century came in 1884 with Ilya Metchnikoff's cellular theory of immunity. Based upon purely Darwinian evolutionary principles, Metchnikoff suggested that the primitive intracellular digestive functions of lower animal forms had persisted in the capacity of the mobile phagocytes of metazoa and higher forms to ingest and digest foreign substances. Metchnikoff proposed that the phagocytic cell is the primary element in *natural* immunity (the first line of defense against infection) and is critical also for *acquired* immunity (the heightened protection conferred by preventive immunization or prior infection).

Metchnikoff's theory had several far-reaching consequences for biology and medicine. First, it introduced the notion that *inter*specific conflict might contribute as importantly to evolution as the classical Darwinian notion of *intra*specific competition. Here, the struggle for survival was between the infected host and the offending pathogen, with the phagocyte entering the lists as champion of the former.

Another notable contribution of the phagocytic theory was to the field of general pathology. At the time, most believed that inflam-

mation was a damaging component of the disease process itself; Metchnikoff, on the other hand, suggested that the inflammatory response was in fact an evolutionary mechanism designed to protect the organism. Whereas Metchnikoff's idea of the protective role of inflammation eventually triumphed, his cellular theory of immunity stimulated much opposition from those who claimed that humoral (blood-borne) factors were by far the more important. The debate between these two camps over the next two to three decades was fierce, as will be outlined below.

Serotherapy

A notable advance was achieved in 1888, when Emile Roux and Alexandre Yersin demonstrated that a soluble toxin could be isolated from the supernatants of cultures of the diphtheria organism. This toxin alone produced all of the symptoms of typical diphtheria in experimental animals, and it became evident that at least in some situations it was not the organism per se, but an exotoxin elaborated by it that caused the disease. It did not take long for von Behring and his colleague Kitasato to exploit this observation, with their reports in 1890 that animals immunized with diphtheria and tetanus toxins produced something in their blood that could neutralize or destroy the toxin, thus preventing disease. Antitoxic sera from experimental animals were quickly tested in infected children and were shown to produce remarkable and rapid cures, especially when administered during the early stages of the disease. The substance that acted against the toxin was called an *antitoxin,* and soon the more general and noncommittal term *antibody* was used to describe this new class of substances. The material responsible for generating these antibodies came to be known as the *antigen*.

von Behring's demonstration of antitoxic therapy took the medical world by storm, and the generality of the approach appeared to receive support from Paul Ehrlich's finding that neutralizing antitoxins could be formed by the immunization of animals with the plant toxins ricin and abrin. Here was a remarkable new addition to the medical armamentarium, and it offered great therapeutic promise in combating a variety of infectious diseases. The new so-called serotherapy stimulated an explosion of laboratory and clinical experimentation and of high expectation, in recognition of which von Behring received the first Nobel Prize in 1901.

Cytotoxic Antibodies and Autoimmunity

The fourth significant area that occupied early immunologists stemmed from the demonstration by Jules Bordet in 1899 that antibodies specific for erythrocytes could cause their destruction (hemolysis) in conjunction with the nonspecifically acting serum factor complement. Here was a clear explanation of one of the important mechanisms of protective immunity—the direct destruction of bacterial pathogens through the cooperation of these two immunologic factors. But other far-reaching implications were seen in Bordet's observation. For the first time, the cells and tissues of the immunized host itself were seen possibly to be at risk by an "aberrant" immune response against self components. With little delay, scientists in almost every active laboratory began to immunize experimental animals with suspensions or extracts of almost every tissue or organ in the body, in an attempt to find cytotoxic antibodies that might be responsible for one or another local disease. Soon the journals were filled with reports of such experiments, and indeed much of the 1900 issue of *Annales de l'Institut Pasteur* was devoted to this question. While it was quickly discovered that *xeno*antibodies and *iso*antibodies were often formed, and might be cytotoxic against the target tissue or organ, *auto*antibodies were, with few exceptions, rarely produced. This led Paul Ehrlich to formulate his famous dictum of *horror autotoxicus,* which held that, for reasons unknown, an individual is unable to mount a destructive immune response against self-constituents. Nevertheless, for years thereafter, the possibility was seriously entertained that such cytotoxic antibodies might play an important role in the pathogenesis of a number of diseases, both as pure autoimmune phenomena and as secondary contributors to the lesions seen in such diseases as syphilis and sympathetic ophthalmia. Indeed, Donath and Landsteiner reported in 1904 on the first observation of a true autoimmune disease—paroxysmal cold hemoglobinuria.

Serology and Immunodiagnosis

The discovery in 1896 of the phenomenon of bacterial agglutination was quickly recognized to provide a powerful tool for the bacteriologist. Not only could bacteria be identified and differentiated with the use of appropriate antisera, but the serum of patients could be tested for their ability to agglutinate a given organism, thus testing for prior exposure to that organism and for the degree of immunity against infection that the individual might possess. The discovery of the precipitin reaction extended this approach even further, now to include the assay of antigens and antibodies in systems involving bacterial products, or even nonbacterial agents. This technique was nowhere more elegantly applied than by G. H. F. Nuttall, who showed by the reactions and cross-reactions of antisera prepared against animal and plant proteins that immunology might be usefully applied to the study of taxonomic relationships, and even for forensic purposes.

When Bordet showed that immune hemolysis might be mediated by antierythrocyte antibodies and complement, and that the components of the reaction could be titrated precisely, he opened the door to a new approach to the diagnosis of disease. Now the blood of patients could be examined for the presence of even those antibodies that do not agglutinate or precipitate their respective antigens, but do fix complement. Thus, not only could prior exposure to a pathogen be assessed, but the course of a disease might even be followed serologically. This approach was brilliantly exploited by August von Wassermann and his colleagues in the development of a serodiagnostic complement fixation test for syphilis, and soon thereafter many other adaptations of complement fixation were proposed for the qualitative and quantitative analysis of both antibodies and antigens.

Allergy and Immunopathology

A seminal discovery in the history of immunology was made in 1902 by physiologists Paul Portier and Charles Richet. Until that time, the immune response had been viewed as a purely benign set of mechanisms whose only function was to protect the organism against exogenous pathogens; the work of those searching for cytotoxic antibodies had done little to alter this view. It had been found only a few years earlier that an immune response could be stimulated by other than bacterial antigens and toxins. Now came Portier and Richet to demonstrate that even bland substances could, when injected into presensitized individuals, cause severe systemic shocklike symptoms and even death. They termed this phenomenon *ana*phylaxis, in an attempt to distinguish it from the usual *pro*phylactic results expected of the immune system. Shortly thereafter, Maurice Arthus demonstrated that bland antigens could cause local necrotizing lesions when they react with specific antibody in the skin of test animals, the so-called Arthus phenomenon. Then, in 1906 Clemens von Pirquet and Bela Schick demonstrated that the pathogenesis of so-called serum sickness depends upon an antibody response by the host to the injection of large quantities of foreign protein antigens, such as accompanied the administration of horse antidiphtheria toxin according to von Behring's serotherapeutic doctrine. It could not be argued that these were only artificial laboratory phenomena; soon thereafter it was demonstrated that two of the significant curses of humankind—hayfever and asthma—also belong to this same group of specific antibody-mediated diseases.

It is interesting to consider the ambivalence with which early immunology viewed the many manifestations of allergy or hypersensitivity. Here was a system, presumably evolved for defensive functions, that somehow "went astray" to produce a variety of pathological conditions. This teleologic view of immunity was so deeply ingrained that for over half a century the mechanisms of allergy were treated as quite separate from those of immunity. Only with an increased understanding of the immunologic contributions to the pathogenesis of such diseases as tuberculosis and leprosy, and the development of experimental models of such diseases as Masugi nephritis, experimental allergic encephalomyelitis, and lymphocytic choriomeningitis, was immunopathology incorporated into the broader context of immunologic phenomena.

Immunohematology

The initial demonstration in the late 1890s that antibodies directed against erythrocytes might mediate their agglutination and hemolysis early focused attention on these cells as antigens, and many studies were undertaken to immunize animals with erythrocytes, both within and across species lines. It was soon found that many animal sera contained "natural" isoantibodies capable of agglutinating the erythrocytes of certain other members of the same species. In a series of studies starting in 1901, and for which he gained the Nobel Prize, Karl Landsteiner showed that humans could be divided into several groups, depending on the presence in their sera of agglutinins specific for the erythrocytes of other humans. These groupings were quite distinct and served as the basis for the ABO system of blood types, later shown to be genetically determined by three allelic genes. The theoretical importance of this observation on genetically determined antigenic polymorphism was soon overshadowed by its clinical implications, since it permitted the beginning of a rational approach to blood typing and modern blood transfusion techniques. Landsteiner followed up this observation in the 1920s by discovering, with Philip Levine, the M, N, and P blood groups, and in 1940 he and Alexander Wiener discovered the rhesus factor, important in both blood transfusions and as the principal contributor to the transplacental disease of the newborn, erythroblastosis fetalis. Since that time, many other minor erythrocyte antigens have been identified, and immunohematology has contributed significantly to theoretical immunology, to forensic medicine, and to anthropologic studies of racial relationships and mass migrations.

Ehrlich's Side-Chain Theory

The term *antibody* (*antikörper*) was originally a noncommittal one, employed to designate whatever it was in immune serum that had the capacity to neutralize toxins and pathogenic bacteria. With the demonstration of the ability to transfer immunity passively by means of serum, it quickly became apparent that antibody must be a discrete substance somehow formed within the immune host, and thus the mechanism of its formation became a valid topic for speculation and study. At the outset, the plausible explanation was advanced that antigen itself carried the information for antibody specificity by somehow being incorporated into the antibody molecule in such a manner that it would thenceforth react specifically with other similar molecules of antigen. Such a theory could not long survive the early quantitative studies that showed that much more antibody was formed than could be accounted for by the quantity of antigen injected, and that antibody formation would continue, once started, without further administration of antigen. It remained for Paul Ehrlich to propose a comprehensive theory of antibody formation in 1897, which he first appended to his epoch-making study on the measurement of diphtheria toxin and antitoxin, and which was later elaborated in great detail by Ehrlich and his students.

Ehrlich believed that antibodies are macromolecules whose specificity for antigen and even complement depends upon the presence of certain sterochemical configurations, whose complementarity with analogous structures on the antigen permits specific interaction. He suggested that these antibodies are naturally occurring products of the body that function as specific receptors on the surface membrane of the cell, there to fulfill normal physiologic functions similar to those served by hypothetical food receptors in digestion (or by drug receptors, in his later theories of chemotherapy). Ehrlich postulated that these antibody receptors would be selected for specifically by an appropriate antigen, leading to their loss from the surface and thereby stimulating a compensatory overproduction of receptors that would appear in the blood as circulating antibody. Ehrlich's imaginative theory held great sway for many years and, especially in Germany, influenced conceptual thought in many different fields of medicine. Few were troubled at the time by any hint that the potential size of the immunologic repertoire of antigens and antibodies presented any problem, since the only antibodies known in the mid-1890s were thought to be antitoxins directed against a rather limited number of human and animal pathogens. But two changes occurred in immunology over the succeeding decades to cast doubt on Ehrlich's theory. The first of these was the flood of studies that showed that antibodies could be produced against a wide variety of even benign, naturally occurring animal and plant substances, including many to which the host would normally never be exposed. Then, in the second decade of the twentieth century came the observation of F. Obermeyer and E. P. Pick, greatly extended by Karl Landsteiner, that showed that antibodies could be formed against almost any artificial chemical capable of being coupled as a hapten onto a protein carrier. Thus, it began to appear unreasonable that an individual could make specific antibodies spontaneously against so great a number of foreign and even artificial structures.

The Cellular Versus Humoral Controversy

Historians of science recognize that very often the eras that mark the most significant advances in a field are those characterized by disputes between two opposing schools, in which each is stimulated to devise experiments designed to uphold its own position and to challenge the opposing view. Such conflicts arose during the early days of immunology, involving the nature of the antigen–antibody interaction and the mode of action of complement, and these provided notable stimuli for the rapid advance of immunologic knowledge. But perhaps no dispute lasted so long and had such important consequences for the future development of immunology as did that between the proponents of a cellular theory of immunity and those who argued that all immunity was based on the action of humoral elements. This immunologic dispute was, however, not an isolated event; it was rather part of a larger conceptual revolution in medicine in the nineteenth century that concerned the very basis of normal and abnormal physiologic processes. For more than 2,000 years, medicine had been under the domination of the Greek humoralist view that disease was based on quantitative or qualitative imbalances in the essential bodily humors. Only in the nineteenth century was the importance of the cells that comprise the various tissues appreciated, and Virchow's cellular pathology (which held that disease is based on abnormal cellular function) was scarcely 30 years old when immunologists chose sides in their own modification of this larger conflict.

It was the zoologist Ilya Metchnikoff who first suggested clearly in 1884 that leukocytes might play an important role in the body's defense against infectious diseases, by virtue of their phagocytic capabilities. Metchnikoff based his thesis on observations that even marine invertebrates possess macrophages capable of ingesting and destroying foreign substances or invading bacteria, or at least of walling them off by the formation of giant cells and granulomatous reactions. Metchnikoff suggested that the vertebrate phagocytic cells perform a similar protective function and in fact are the most important contributors to both natural and acquired immunity. This work impressed Pasteur, who invited Metchnikoff to join him at the newly constructed Pasteur Institute in Paris, where Metchnikoff and a succession of distinguished students spent the next decades working productively and imaginatively to verify and extend the cellular (phagocytic) theory of immunity.

Metchnikoff's cellular theory quickly excited opposition. In the first place, it was advanced at a time when most pathologists considered the inflammatory reaction, and the microphages and macrophages that accompanied it, to be deleterious rather than protective responses. It was even thought at the time that although phagocytic cells might indeed ingest infectious organisms, the result was not the destruction of these agents but rather their transport throughout the body to cause dissemination of the disease. Then, in 1888 Nuttall observed that the serum of normal animals contains substances that are naturally toxic for certain microorganisms and that these antibacterial properties are much enhanced in the immunized host. Then Koch's student Richard Pfeiffer described the phenomenon that bears his name, in which circulating antibody (even that passively transferred to a normal recipient) would cause the specific lysis of cholera vibrios injected into the peritoneal cavity of immune guinea pigs. Two different humoral substances were found to cooperate in bacterial lysis: (a) heat-stable serum antibody and (b) the thermolabile factor called complement, or alexin (Greek *aleksein*, to defend).

But perhaps the most telling blow to the cellular theory of immunity came with the description by von Behring and Kitasato in 1890 of immunity to diphtheria and tetanus, clearly mediated by circulating antibody rather than by phagocytic cells. As time went on, circulating antibodies were found for most of the new pathogenic organisms that were rapidly being discovered, and Paul Ehrlich not only showed in the diphtheria antitoxin system how these antibodies might be measured, but also published pictures of them that made readers feel that they understood what an antibody was and how it acted. Finally, when Metchnikoff's own student Bordet described the lysis of erythrocytes by humoral antibody and complement, most investigators were tempted to agree with Koch that the humoralists had carried the day.

Metchnikoff and his students were by no means silent in the face of these strong attacks against the phagocytic theory. In paper after paper, these workers showed that there is often no relationship between the bactericidal powers of the blood and host resistance to infection against a given organism. Rather, species resistance can often be directly correlated with the ability of its phagocytes to ingest the pathogen, as in the case of anthrax, and ingenious experiments were devised to show that microorganisms enclosed within little sacks of filter paper that protected them from phagocytes would remain virulent, although bathed in antibody-containing tissue fluids. Metchnikoff also showed that the creation of a macrophage-rich peritoneal exudate, with the attendant activation of these macrophages, would protect the host against intraperitoneal injection of otherwise lethal doses of different bacterial pathogens, an early forerunner of the modern practice of nonspecific immunotherapy. But the tide had obviously turned against the phagocytic theory during the 1890s, and Metchnikoff's last-ditch attempt to reestablish the importance of phagocytosis with the publication in 1901 of his famous book, *Immunity in the Infectious Diseases,* came too late. The book was widely admired for its scholarship, but made few converts among the unbelievers.

If we analyze the immunologic literature of the first decade of the twentieth century, it becomes apparent that by their choice of subjects, most investigators had voted for the humoral theory of immunity and against the cellular theory. Except for Metchnikoff and his immediate adherents, most chose to study antibodies, which were more easily measured and worked with, and few devoted themselves to the more difficultly manipulable cells. Even so, two attempts were made during this period to mediate the cellular–humoral dispute. In 1908, the Swedish Academy conferred the Nobel Prize in Medicine jointly to Metchnikoff, the champion of cellularism, and to Ehrlich, the then-leading exponent of humoralist doctrines. In England somewhat earlier, Sir Almroth Wright and S. R. Douglas attempted to rationalize the differences between these two schools by their extensive work on the process of opsonization (Greek *opsonein,* to render palatable). These investigators claimed that both humoral and cellular factors were equally important and interdependent, in that humoral antibody appears to interact specifically with its target microorganism to render it more susceptible to phagocytosis by macrophages.

Wright's espousal of this doctrine became so popular in England that his friend Bernard Shaw used it as the subject of his play *The Doctor's Dilemma.* In his *Preface on Doctors,* Shaw summarized Wright's approach in an otherwise scathing castigation of the medical profession:

> Sir Almroth Wright, following up one of Metchnikoff's most suggestive biological romances, discovered that the white corpuscles or phagocytes, which attack and devour disease germs for us, do their work only when we butter the disease germs appetizingly for them with a natural sauce which Sir Almroth named opsonin.

But partly because his techniques were so difficult to perform and their results difficult to reproduce, Wright's opsonic indices and

therapeutic approaches soon fell out of favor, and his efforts to revivify the cellular theory of immunity had little long-lasting effect.

The fact that the humoral theory of immunity carried the day over the cellular theory around the turn of the century had long-term implications for future developments in the young discipline of immunology. It is generally the case in science that the most imaginative and productive investigators tend to choose their problems based on what they (or their teachers) feel is most significant in their field, and during the early decades of the twentieth century it was clear to most workers that antibody held the key to an understanding of immunity. In the humoralist context of the times, many approachable problems in cellular immunology were thus neglected as being "uninteresting."

Transplantation and Immunogenetics

Transplantation research occupies a curious place in the history of immunology. Pursued since the turn of the century, it produced throughout its course valuable information of great potential significance to immunology. However, those who worked in the area were not immunologists but surgeons, oncologists, biologists, and geneticists with little connection to contemporary immunology, and thus the significance of their results generally went unrecognized by mainstream immunology for over 50 years.

Surgeons have dreamed of replacing missing or defective tissues and organs since the Middle Ages, and the miracle of the transplantation of a leg by Saints Cosmas and Damian was often celebrated by Renaissance painters. But through the centuries, all attempts failed, save for the occasional success with corneal grafts. Then, at the end of the nineteenth century, it was shown that tumors could be passaged in experimental animals. But these grafts usually failed—the recipients were held to be "immune"—and tumor biologists saw in this phenomenon an approach to the solution of the problem of human cancer. If they could unravel the secrets of tumor graft rejection, then perhaps humans could be induced to reject their own tumors as well. Thus, at the turn of the century, a massive effort began to study the rejection of tumor grafts. These studies generally employed normal tissues such as skin as a control, to establish that it was the host and not some peculiarity of cancer tissues that accounted for rejection.

In not much more than a decade, the general rules of graft rejection had been worked out and were summarized in 1912 in a remarkable book, *Heteroplastic and Homoplastic Transplantation,* by Georg Schöne: (a) Transplantation into a foreign species (heteroplastic = xenogeneic) invariably fails; (b) grafts to unrelated members of the same species (homoplastic = allogeneic) usually fail; (c) autografts almost invariably succeed; (d) in an allogeneic recipient, there is a primary take and delayed rejection of a first graft; (e) rejection of a second graft from the same donor is accelerated, as is that in a recipient preimmunized with other donor material; (f) the closer the "blood relationship" between donor and recipient, the more likely is successful transplantation; and (g) these rules apply to normal as well as tumor tissues. There is no question that Schöne viewed rejection as an active response on the part of the host's immune system; indeed, he coined the term *transplantation immunity.*

These early findings were reconfirmed and extended in a 1916 review, *Tumor Immunity,* by E. E. Tyzzer, who pointed out that studies with inbred mice showed the genetic nature of donor–recipient incompatibility, and that this was not inherited as "a single Mendelizing factor." Moreover, morphologic data showed that the inflammatory infiltrate was predominantly lymphocytic, and not merely *exudative,* but *proliferative* as well. James Murphy, who worked initially with Peyton Rous, wrote a monograph in 1926–*The Lymphocyte in Resistance to Tissue Grafting, Malignant Disease, and Tuberculous Infection.* Murphy showed that immune rejection did not function in embryos; that while a tumor might grow in a "privileged site" like the brain, cotransplantation of lymphoid tissue would induce rejection even there; and that X-irradiation would inhibit the rejection process.

It was a similar interest in the tumor problem that stimulated Clarence C. Little to found the Jackson Laboratories in Bar Harbor, Maine, devoted to genetic studies of tumor transplantation. Here, in the 1930s and 1940s, George Snell "invented" the congenic mouse and helped to define the major histocompatibility complex (MHC), based originally on the demonstration by Peter Gorer that graft rejection in mice was accompanied by the production of antibodies specific for an (erythrocyte) antigen, which he labeled antigen-II. But while much was learned about the immunology of tissue graft rejection in all of these studies, it appeared increasingly to have little to offer toward a solution of the problem of human tumors. It is interesting that all of this immunologic activity on the part of the surgeons, tumor biologists, and geneticists went substantially unnoticed by the immunologists of the day. In this era of chemically oriented activity in immunology (see below), investigators were little interested in the more biological aspects of autoimmunity and transplantation, but worked primarily on antibody and antigen chemistry, on the specificity of serologic reactions, and on quantitative immunochemistry.

Of the three groups that had worked on the problem of transplantation, the surgeons left the field first, due to the apparent impracticability of tissue and organ grafting in the human. Similarly, the tumor biologists found no way to apply the knowledge derived from animal experiments to humans, and they too moved on to other aspects of the cancer problem. The shift in interest of the geneticists was more subtle. At the outset, they had viewed the inbred mouse as the perfect tool to study human tumor susceptibility and, ultimately, therapeutic approaches. But if the early work to identify the histocompatibility loci in mice was aimed at understanding the immune response to tumor grafts, it quickly lost its oncologic and even immunologic motivations and became a study in pure genetics. They now devoted themselves to establishing the size and polymorphism of the MHC and the rules of segregation. Only later, when their practical applicability to tissue typing and histocompatibility matching was established, would the investigations return to the realm of transplantation biology.

IMMUNOLOGY IN TRANSITION, 1912–1950s

The Fate of the Early Immunological Research Program

We have seen that during the period 1880 to about 1910, the young and highly productive field of immunology had organized itself predominantly in terms of a number of major areas of interest. By the beginning of the First World War, while most of its practitioners might not yet have called themselves "immunologists," institutionalization of the discipline had begun in earnest. An institute devoted to its aims had been established for Paul Ehrlich in Frankfurt, and departments and services dedicated to the discipline

had been formed within many of the leading research institutions around the world. Sections devoted to one or another component of the immunologic program were to be found at International Congresses of Medicine or Hygiene, and an "invisible college" existed, involving informal exchange among its practitioners. While the pages of the *Annales de l'Institut Pasteur* had long been devoted to immunological reports, the discipline was more formally recognized by the founding in 1908 of the *Zeitschrift für Immunitätsforschung* and of the *American Journal of Immunology* in 1916. The commonality of interest of this subgroup of scientists and practitioners was recognized, at least in America, by the founding of the American Association of Immunologists in 1913.

Let us now look at developments within each of the components that composed the early immunological research program. Preventive immunization had seen its great victories in the case of chicken cholera, anthrax, rabies, plague, and several other important diseases. But increasingly, pathogenic organisms were being described for which it was proving impossible to prepare efficacious vaccines. These included not only such important agents as the tubercle and leprous bacilli, the cholera vibrio, and the spirochete of syphilis, but also the important group of disease-producing gram-positive organisms, to say nothing of a number of newly described diseases due to viruses and parasites that so ravaged humans and animals. Thus, by 1910 the great early promise of pasteurian immunization was no longer being fulfilled; new successes would thenceforth be few and far between and achieved only with great difficulty. Work in this area very rapidly left the "classical" immunology laboratory and was taken over by bacteriologists, virologists, and parasitologists interested more in organisms than in immunologic mechanisms.

The study of cellular immunology and of Metchnikoff's phagocytic theory, as we have seen, went into decline early in the century at the hands of proponents of humoralist theories. Cells were much more difficult to work with than were humoral antibodies, and no such antibody techniques as agglutination, the antigen–antibody precipitin reaction, immune hemolysis, and the ability to transfer antibody passively from one animal to another existed in the field of cell studies. Indeed, the cell was still considered something of a mystery, whereas Ehrlich's pictures of antibodies and their specific combining sites could almost convince one that the antibody was a "real" entity whose structure and properties were readily understood.

The techniques of serotherapy for the prevention or cure of disease suffered a fate similar to that of preventive immunization. After the remarkable demonstration of the efficacy of horse antidiphtheria and antitetanus sera in the treatment of these diseases, no significant further victories were recorded in this area. While laboratories throughout the world continued to produce these two antisera (the Pasteur Institute helped support itself with its stable of immunized horses), interest in this approach waned, since there were so few other significant diseases that were caused by exotoxins and thus amenable to this approach. When, much later, passive transfer of antibody would be employed, it would be by hematologists using human gamma-globulin to prevent erythroblastosis fetalis or by pediatricians employing convalescent sera to deal with poliomyelitis.

As for the interest in cytotoxic antibodies and autoimmunity, this proved to be ephemeral. Despite all attempts to implicate antitissue and antiorgan antibodies in the pathogenesis of disease, with the exception of antierythrocyte antibodies responsible for hemolytic anemias, no convincing demonstrations were forthcoming, and immunologists even forgot about Donath and Landsteiner's demonstration of the pathogenesis of paroxysmal cold hemoglobinuria as the possible tip of an autoimmune disease iceberg. By 1912, the study of immune cytotoxic phenomena had left the immunology laboratory to be pursued only within essentially unrelated clinical specialty areas such as ophthalmology, with its interest in sympathic ophthalmia and autoimmune disease of the lens.

Developments within the area of serodiagnosis represent a more typical example of disciplinary differentiation for the sociologist of science. These techniques had developed within the very heart of an immunologic enterprise interested in immunity in the infectious diseases, which therefore not only demanded an understanding of disease pathogenesis, but also required the ability to diagnose these diseases. Syphilis remained the mainstay of serodiagnostic laboratories, and work to perfect the technique and extend it to other diseases continued throughout the period under discussion. But very quickly, the technique became quite routine and applied, and immunologists interested in basic mechanisms soon lost interest in the area. Work in this field was taken over by classical bacteriologists, and in fact those who devoted themselves to this and other aspects of serodiagnosis soon began to call themselves "serologists" and worked principally in diagnostic laboratories rather than in those devoted to basic immunologic research.

Soon after their discovery, anaphylaxis and its related diseases had also become an intimate concern of immunologic experimentalists. They were interested in the nature of the antibodies responsible for these phenomena and in the basic mechanisms involved in the diseases that resulted from their action. But after a short and essentially unsuccessful struggle with the paradox of a system presumably evolved to protect now being demonstrated to *cause* disease, the immunologists soon deserted the field to others. In the main, those upon whom these interests devolved were clinicians interested in hayfever and asthma. Clinical allergy was established as a medical subspeciality, and it was primarily in the laboratories of allergists that further progress was realized in sorting out the mechanisms involved and in developing skin tests and therapeutic approaches to the treatment of human allergies. In addition to these, however, the study of anaphylactic and related phenomena was of great interest to physiologists such as Sir Henry Dale, who was interested in the physiologic mechanisms involved in such diseases, and also to a large group of experimental pathologists, who were interested in the comparative study of the lesions that accompanied these diseases.

The Rise to Dominance of Immunochemistry

Thus, the immunologic research program waned in all of its interest areas, so far as the basic scientist was concerned, and several of these areas devolved upon others. Now we shall see how the general field itself experienced a devolution into the hands of a new *Denkkollektiv*. The seeds of the future interest in the chemistry of antigens and antibodies can be traced back to the fertile imagination of Paul Ehrlich. Ehrlich's side-chain theory of antibody formation pictured antigen, antibody, and complement as true chemical molecules, and their combining sites as stereochemically complementary structures that would account for the specificity of their interactions. At the time, however, little was known of the structure and precise composition of protein molecules, and appropriate techniques were unavailable to translate Ehrlich's theory into laboratory experiments.

It is common in most textbooks to ascribe the paternity of the field of immunochemistry to the famous physical chemist Svante Arrhenius, because he coined the term *immunochemistry* in a series of lectures with that title in 1904. Like many another physical scientist, Arrhenius was attracted by the mysteries and the confusion that existed in biology and felt that he could bring some order to the chaos by the introduction of the rigorous laws of chemistry and physics. Through his Danish colleague Madsen, Arrhenius became interested in the problem of diphtheria toxin-antitoxin titration and proposed that these interactions are reversible, like the interactions that he had described for weak acids and weak bases that had contributed so much to his earlier fame. But it would probably be erroneous to attribute the fatherhood of the field to Arrhenius, because his contributions were purely theoretical, could not be adequately tested at the time, and had little immediate influence on subsequent events.

Perhaps the true turning point came in 1906, with the demonstration by Obermeyer and Pick that protein antigens could be modified chemically to alter their immunological specificity. For example, when nitrated proteins were employed to immunize animals, the specificity of the resulting antibodies appeared to be directed no longer at the original protein, but at the added nitro groups. In an encyclopedic review of this area in 1912, Pick showed that a number of different synthetic groupings (called *haptens*) might be joined to a carrier protein to serve as antigenic determinants. Here was a powerful new tool, with which the small molecules produced in the organic chemistry laboratory could be used to dissect intimately the nature of immunologic specificity and the character of the combining site on antibody. No one exploited this approach more assiduously or to better effect than polymath Karl Landsteiner, who in 1917 published two papers that illustrated the power of this approach and that helped to define both his own work during the next 37 years and much of the domain of immunochemistry as well. Now the biological basis of antibody formation and the biological effects of antigen–antibody interactions took a back seat to interest in the chemical nature of antigens and antibodies.

Another approach to the chemistry of antigens and antibodies was opened up in the 1920s by organic chemist Michael Heidelberger. Working initially in the context of a bacteriological laboratory, Heidelberger was able to show that, contrary to the classical view that antibodies could only be formed against protein antigens, the capsular polysaccharides of the pneumococcus could also stimulate a specific antibody response. This led Heidelberger to study the chemical differences among the polysaccharide antigens of different strains of pneumococcus, in pursuit of which he developed over many years an impressive set of quantitative techniques that helped establish immunology as a more exact science.

Theory Follows Mindset: Instruction Theories

We saw above that during the early biomedical era of immunology, the first theory of immunity advanced by Ilya Metchnikoff, trained in zoology, followed strict Darwinian evolutionary principles, and the first theory of antibody formation proposed by Paul Ehrlich, trained in medicine, was similarly based. But the chemically oriented investigators who dominated immunology after the First World War had little interest in the biological basis of immunity. They were, however, interested in antibodies and their formation, and new theories of antibody formation were not slow to appear. These new theories no longer focused on the *function* of antibodies, but on their chemical *structure,* and more specifically on the question of how such a large group of specific molecules able to interact with an ever-growing universe of potential antigens could possibly be produced within the vertebrate host. This was the rock upon which Ehrlich's side-chain theory had foundered: the improbability that evolution could have accounted for the spontaneous production of so many different antibodies, the greater portion of which were directed against bland and even artificial antigens of no obvious evolutionary selective force.

It is not surprising, therefore, that the new chemical theories of antibody formation were quite Lamarckian in nature; in contrast to the molecules of the biologist, those of the chemist generally have no evolutionary history. The first of the new theories to be advanced was that of biochemist Felix Haurowitz, in 1930. In this, it was proposed that only the antigen itself contains all of the information necessary for antibody formation and imposes a complementary structure on a nascent protein by acting as a template for the synthesis of a unique sequence of amino acids. This was the first so-called instruction theory of antibody formation. Here was a ready explanation not only for the tremendous diversity of different antibodies, but also for how so fine a specificity could be imparted to the antibody molecule. This instructive theory of antibody formation was further refined in 1940 by chemical physicist Linus Pauling, who proposed that the antigen serves as a template upon which the nascent amino acid chain coils to form a protein molecule.

But these chemical theories did not explain, to the satisfaction of the biologist, how antibody production might persist in the apparent absence of antigen, nor did they attempt to explain why a second exposure to the same antigen should result in an enhanced booster response. Moreover, these theories provided no explanation for newer data that showed that repeated immunization might produce changes in the *quality* of the antibody, in some instances sharpening specificity and in other instances considerably broadening the potential for serologic cross-reactions. It was the biological shortcomings of the direct template theories that disturbed virologist Macfarlane Burnet and caused him to advance an instructionist alternative in 1941. With the growing recognition of the importance of enzymes in synthesis as well as in digestion, Burnet suggested that the function of antigen might be to stimulate an adaptive modification of those enzymes necessary for globulin synthesis, such that a unique protein molecule with the required specificity would result. This adaptive enzyme theory had the advantage of explaining not only the large repertoire in terms of initial instruction by antigen, but also the persistence of antibody formation and the booster antibody response, by allowing replication of the adaptive enzymes within an expanding population of proliferating daughter cells, all capable of antibody formation. This latter point is especially noteworthy, since Burnet was perhaps the first to stress the important role of continuing cellular function and of cell replication in antibody production.

With an increasing understanding of the probable genetic role of nucleic acids, Burnet and Frank Fenner advanced a modification of this theory in 1949, still impelled by essentially biological considerations. They now suggested that antigen might impress the information for its specific determinant directly on the (?RNA) genome, against which indirect template a specific antibody might be formed. Not only would this new genocopy persist within the cell, but it would also be reproduced from mother to daughter cells during proliferation, thus explaining persisting antibody formation

and a heightened booster response. It is interesting that so ingrained in the collective immunological psyche of the times were these chemical ideas that even biologist Burnet, in his first two theories of antibody formation, felt obliged to employ Lamarckian instructive approaches.

The Scope and Influence of the Immunochemical Research Program

The application of synthetic haptens to the study of antibody specificity led to progress in clarifying the size and structure of antigen and antibody combining sites and in defining the thermodynamic parameters of their interaction. These studies were facilitated by the development of quantitative techniques for the measurement of these reactions and by the identification of antibody as a gamma-globulin protein, paving the way for the development of chemical purification methods.

The scope of the field of immunology from the 1920s to the early 1960s is perhaps best epitomized by five of the leading books of the period: Well's *The Chemical Aspects of Immunity* in 1924; Marrack's *The Chemistry of Antigens and Antibodies* in 1934; Landsteiner's *The Specificity of Serological Reactions* in 1937; Boyd's *Fundamentals of Immunology* in 1943; and Kabat and Mayer's *Quantitative Immunochemistry* in 1949. These were the reference books from which a generation of young immunologists learned their trade, and little attention was paid in any of them to the biological or medical aspects of the field. If a Max Theiler developed a new vaccine in the mid-1930s against yellow fever, this was of interest only to virologists and students of infectious diseases. If a Hans Zinsser or an Arnold Rich studied allergic reactions to bacteria, or if a Louis Dienes or a Simon and Rackemann developed models of delayed hypersensitivity lesions to simple proteins in the 1920s and 1930s, this was interest only to bacteriologists and experimental pathologists. Finally, if a Thomas Rivers developed an experimental model of allergic encephalomyelitis as early as 1933, this seemed to excite no one at the time. These and other similar excursions into areas of biomedical interest lay out of the mainstream of contemporary immunology, were usually published in "outside" journals, and made little impression upon the governing *Denkkollektiv*. Only a later generation of immunologists more attuned to biological questions would identify these contributions as landmarks in immunological progress.

This is not to suggest that all work along the classical lines described above ceased during the immunochemical era. It has been pointed out that, ". . . research areas which have become well established take a long time to die out altogether. There is always some work that can be done." Thus, as described above, the clinical allergists gave new life to the study of anaphylactic phenomena by redefining the field along new lines; continued progress was made in the preparation of better toxoids and better modes of immunization; serologists continued to improve and expand the application of serodiagnostic procedures; and from time to time, an effective vaccine would be developed against one or another disease of humans or animals.

THE IMMUNOBIOLOGICAL REVOLUTION

The research program that governed the normative science of the immunochemical era between the 1920s and 1950s produced interesting results. It had gone far to define the chemical nature of both antigens and antibodies and the precision of their specific interactions. Increasingly, however, biologists working on the fringes of immunology made observations whose explanation was not to be found in the received wisdom of instructionist theories of antibody formation. How, they asked, could antibody formation persist in the apparent absence of antigen? Why should a second exposure to antigen result in an enhanced booster response that is much more productive than is the primary response to antigenic stimulus? How can repeated exposure to antigen change the very quality of the antibody, in many instances sharpening its specificity by increasing its affinity for the antigenic determinant employed? Finally, how is it possible that immunity to some viral diseases appears to be unrelated to the presence of circulating antiviral antibodies? These and other biologically based questions began seriously to challenge the immunochemical paradigm, most notably through the pen of Macfarlane Burnet in his two books entitled *The Production of Antibodies* (1941 and 1949). Burnet complained repeatedly that the chemical theories, while quite elegant, failed to explain the more functional biological aspects of the immune response.

By the 1950s, the stage seemed to be set for a large-scale confrontation such as described by Thomas Kuhn in his book *The Structure of Scientific Revolutions*. On the one hand was the immunochemical tradition, guided by theories that could no longer satisfactorily explain all of the phenomena of the field, and employing approaches that yielded results of increasingly parochial interest and of decreasing marginal value. Challenging this classical tradition was a growing group of biomedical scientists seeking answers to a set of new and important questions that traditional immunochemical theory and practice were ill prepared to answer.

In the 1940s, Peter Medawar "rediscovered" the laws of transplantation, demonstrating that the rejection of tissue transplants was a purely immunologic phenomenon, but one unrelated to humoral antibody. In 1945, Ray Owen described the paradoxical situation of dizygotic twin calves that were incapable of responding to one another's antigens. The explanation of this phenomenon lay in the ontogeny of the immune response in the vertebrate fetus, leading Burnet and Fenner to postulate the existence of a cell-based immunological tolerance, a hypothesis that Peter Medawar (still at the time a zoologist) and colleagues confirmed experimentally, and for which Burnet and Medawar shared the Nobel Prize in 1960. Yet another observation, for which no ready explanation was available in classical theory, involved the description in the early 1950s of a group of immunological deficiency diseases in humans, the explanation of which would go to the very heart of the biological basis of the immune response. Finally, after a hiatus of some 40 years or more, interest in autoimmune diseases was reawakened by new demonstrations of autoimmune hemolytic anemias, experimental and human autoimmune thyroiditis, and allergic encephalomyelitis.

While these new phenomena provided a sufficient basis to question the old values, such questions could only be answered by the development of new methods, and these were rapidly forthcoming. The techniques of immunofluorescent staining and of hemolytic plaque assay permitted the tissue localization and quantitative enumeration of antibody-forming cells. The technique of passive cell transfer and especially that of cell culture permitted for the first time the analysis of cell–cell interactions and immunocyte dynamics. Here was a true revolution in the offing, awaiting only the appearance of a theoretical leader to lead the charge against the old regime and its outmoded paradigm. That theoretician was Macfarlane Burnet.

Selection Theories of Antibody Formation

Burnet and Fenner's indirect template theory of 1949 had pointed up another crucial biological fact that had to be dealt with by any theory of antibody formation—the recently described phenomenon of acquired immunologic tolerance. It now became important to explain theoretically not only how antibody formation could be stimulated, but also the mechanisms whereby it might be aborted.

The first of the purely biological selection theories of antibody formation was outlined by Niels Jerne in 1955, in what he called a "natural selection" theory. Jerne proposed, as had Paul Ehrlich before him, that the host could indeed synthesize small quantities of each of the antibody specificities in the entire repertoire, which would appear spontaneously in the blood as "natural antibodies." The function of these natural antibodies would be to interact selectively with their appropriate antigen and thereby transport that antigen into cells somewhere in the body where the antibody would signal the reproduction of molecules identical to itself; that is, it would initiate the formation of large amounts of specific antibody. The booster antibody response was thus readily explained by the presence, after initial immunization, of an increased number of antibody "carriers," whose presence would also favor the selection by antigen of those antibodies with the higher affinity, thus also explaining changes in the quality of antibody following repeated immunization. The phenomenon of immunologic tolerance was also neatly dealt with for the first time by postulating that any natural antibodies formed against self-antigens would at the outset immediately be absorbed by the tissues of the body, and thenceforth would be unavailable to mediate autoantibody formation.

Although Jerne's natural selection theory converted few believers in instruction theories, its historical importance lies in the stimulus that it provided to biologically oriented theoreticians. This stimulus did not lie dormant very long, for within a few years Burnet gave birth to the clonal selection theory of antibody formation. Central to this concept was the postulate that antibodies are natural products that appear on the cell surface as receptors, with which antigen reacts selectively. The interaction of antigen with the surface receptors then signals a clonal proliferation of a population of cells phenotypically restricted for the given antibody specificity, some daughter cells of the clone differentiating into antibody-forming cells and others remaining as immunologic memory cells able to participate in later booster responses. Finally, the theory suggested that immunologic tolerance was due to a "clonal abortion," mediated specifically by self-antigens or by those introduced from without at a critical period in the embryonic maturation of the clonal precursors. Burnet's theory received important support and elaboration from David Talmage and Joshua Lederberg. It was Talmage alone who addressed the questions of antibody specificity and repertoire size, pointing out that a limited number of different antibody specificities (later clonotypes) might distinguish a far greater number of antigenic determinants. Lederberg, on the other hand, considered the genetic implications of clonal selection and suggested that antibody diversity might depend upon a high rate of somatic mutation of the "immunoglobulin gene."

Within a very few years, it became clear that the clonal selection theory of antibody formation had attained wide acceptance, thanks in part to the application of newer techniques for the study of cells, and thanks also to developments in the new genetics. Once the DNA control of antibody structure was accepted, and the amino acid sequences of the immunoglobulin chains elucidated, the clonal selection theory generated its own repertoire controversy. This involved a lengthy debate by those who maintained that the entire specificity repertoire is encoded in the germ line and by others who argued that immunologic diversity is generated by the somatic mutation or recombination of a highly restricted number of germ-line genes. The resolution of this repertoire problem is one of the triumphs of twentieth century molecular biology. It involves the variable combination of a number of minigene segments, assisted by mutations, to form the large universe of antibody light and heavy chains.

The Immunological Synthesis

We have defined three distinct eras in the 110-year history of the discipline of immunology. The first, extending from 1880 to about the First World War, centered around the new bacteriology and infectious diseases and had a distinctly medical orientation. Several of the components of the original research program in immunology failed to maintain their original momentum or to fulfill their initial high promise, and went into decline. These included the development of new vaccines, serotherapeutic approaches, the study of cellular immunity, and the study of diseases that might be mediated by cytotoxic antibodies. Two other subprograms followed a somewhat different course; the study of anaphylaxis and related diseases passed primarily into the hands of clinical allergists, while the development and adaptation of serodiagnostic techniques passed into the hands of the new discipline of serology.

As interest in the components of the old program was falling away, there developed a new area of interest in immunology. Leadership in the field devolved upon a new group of individuals with a predominantly chemical orientation to the study of antigens and antibodies, who pursued a research program and developed a theoretical base that reflected this orientation well. A science does not change its precepts and approaches spontaneously; it is moved to the new position by those who explore fertile new areas. But while the earlier immunological program had interacted extensively with many different fields of biology and medicine, the immunochemical era was characterized by a relative introversion, interacting little with other biomedical disciplines. We can date this second era from about the First World War until the late 1950s and early 1960s.

There then occurred an abrupt transition in the field of immunology, which may well be called a scientific revolution. Since the old theories and old techniques could not satisfactorily explain newer observations, the biologists took over command of the discipline from the chemists. Chemical approaches and chemically oriented theories rapidly lost ground to the new biomedical paradigm, which, guided by the clonal selection theory, now asked a markedly different set of questions involving the biological basis and biomedical implications of the immune response.

Eventually, there occurred a synthesis of the two positions. The chemists (who had approached the system by working back from the final molecular product, the antibody) and the biologists (who had worked forward from the initial cellular interactions) found that their different questions and diverse techniques were really aimed at two aspects of the *same* system. They reached a common ground in the chemistry and molecular biology of T- and B-cell receptors and of lymphokines; together they have clarified the major questions about antibody formation and structure, the dynamics and chemistry of cell–cell interactions, and the mechanisms of regulation of the immune response.

Immunology once again touches many other disciplines. It has offered classical evolutionary theory the elegant model of an extremely complicated mechanism that is even able to anticipate the appearance of new pathogens, rather than merely slowly adapting its response to their presence. Indeed, this peculiarity of evolution occurred not just once, but twice—once for the immunoglobulin B-cell receptor and again somewhat differently for the T-cell receptor. It has offered to geneticists the unique example of an immunoglobulin gene superfamily whose components exercise a broad range of interrelated activities extending even beyond the immune response, and whose mechanism for the generation of immunologic diversity has shown how a gene product can be assembled by the variable splicing of many different DNA segments. In its study of lymphokines and cytokines, modern immunology has offered to the physiologist a variety of examples of how cells may communicate with and influence one another. Finally, the new immunology has assisted many medical subspecialties in defining the pathogenesis of some of their most important diseases, and it has pointed the way as well to the development of preventive measures or therapeutic modalities to combat these diseases, as the following chapters will demonstrate.

NOBEL PRIZE HIGHLIGHTS IN IMMUNOLOGY

1901, von Behring

The first Nobel Prize in Medicine was awarded to Emil von Behring (1854–1917). von Behring studied under Robert Koch at Koch's Institute in Berlin. Following Löffler's isolation of the diphtheria bacillus in 1883 and the identification of diphtheria exotoxin by Roux and Yersin in 1888, von Behring, with his colleagues Kitasato and Wernicke, showed in 1890 to 1892 that diphtheria and tetanus immunity were due to the formation of circulating antitoxins. He showed that passive administration of antitoxin serum to diseased patients might effect a cure, thus opening the way for serum immunotherapy in a number of diseases. His citation read, "For his work on serum therapy, especially its application against diphtheria, by which he has opened a new road in the domain of medical science and thereby placed in the hands of the physician a victorious weapon against illness and death."

1905, Koch

The prize was awarded to Robert Koch (1843–1910), "for his investigations and discoveries in regard to tuberculosis." Koch had been a small-town physician in Germany when his private investigations on the life cycle of the anthrax bacillus and the etiology of anthrax excited the medical profession in 1876. He was given first a laboratory and then an institute in Berlin, and it was there, with the help of a distinguished series of students, that he made bacteriology a true science, by his development of stringent bacterial isolation and culture techniques and by his emphasis on the famous Koch postulates for proof of etiology. Koch devoted himself to the study of a number of different diseases, but it was his identification of the tubercle bacillus and of tuberculin, and his continuing devotion to the study of tuberculosis, that earned him the Nobel Prize. Both the immunodiagnostic tuberculin reaction and the "Koch phenomenon," involving the excessive dermal reaction to tubercle bacilli in the skin of sensitized animals, played major roles in the later elucidation of the mechanisms of cellular immunity.

1908, Metchnikoff and Ehrlich

The prize this year was shared by Elie Metchnikoff (1845–1916) and Paul Ehrlich (1854–1915), "in recognition for their work on immunity." Metchnikoff was born in the Russian Ukraine and studied zoology with an emphasis on comparative embryology. In 1884, working in a marine biology laboratory in Italy, he made the initial observations on the phagocytic cells of starfish larvae that provided the basis for his cellular (phagocytic) theory of immunity. When Metchnikoff left Russia for political reasons, Pasteur offered him a position at his new institute in Paris, where Metchnikoff devoted the rest of his life to an impressive series of investigations in support of his phagocytic theory, and to its vigorous defense from the many attacks of those who favored the view that immunity was based upon humoral (i.e., antibody–complement) mechanisms.

Paul Ehrlich was born in Germany, studied medicine, and early became interested in the staining reactions of cells in tissues, devising some of the most useful stains for the tubercle bacillus and for blood leukocytes. In 1891, he became an assistant to Koch at the Institute for Infectious Diseases, where he commenced his immunologic studies. Following early work on the antibody response to the plant toxins abrin and ricin, Ehrlich made his most notable early contribution to immunology in 1897, with publication of his paper describing the first practical method for standardization of diphtheria toxin and antitoxin preparations. This same publication contained also the outline of his famous side-chain theory of antibody formation, which greatly influenced immunologic theories for several decades. With Julius Morgenroth, he published an important series of papers on the mechanism of immune hemolysis. Shortly after the turn of the century, Ehrlich gave up most of his activities in immunology to pursue his interests in the chemical treatment of disease, making important discoveries in the treatment of trypanosomiasis and syphilis (Salvarsan—the "magic bullet") and helping to found scientific pharmacology.

1913, Richet

The prize was awarded to Charles Richet (1850–1935), "for his work on anaphylaxis." Richet was a Parisian who studied medicine and became especially interested in physiology. These interests led him, while cruising on the yacht of the Prince of Monaco, to study the physiologic effects on mammals of marine invertebrate poisons. With his colleague Paul Portier, he discovered the phenomenon of anaphylaxis, dependent not upon the toxic properties of the substance injected, but only upon its function as an antigen in the previously sensitized animal. In so doing, he opened up a new and, at the time, surprising vista in medicine, by showing that the "protective" mechanisms of immunity might function also to cause disease. The later demonstration of the relationship between experimental anaphylaxis and other more familiar human allergies made this observation clinically as well as theoretically important to immunology.

1919, Bordet

The prize was awarded to Jules Bordet (1870–1961), "for his studies in regard to immunity." Bordet was a Belgian physician who, at the age of 24, went to study with Metchnikoff at the Pasteur Institute in Paris. He made important early contributions to an understanding of the mechanism of complement-mediated bacteriolysis, and in 1899 he discovered the phenomenon of specific hemolysis. Shortly thereafter, in collaboration with his assistant and brother-in-law Octave Gengou, Bordet described the phenomenon of complement fixation and its diagnostic possibilities. This soon developed into a powerful tool in the diagnosis of infectious diseases, most notably in the hands of August von Wasserman and his colleagues in their complement-fixation test for syphilis. Bordet made many other important contributions to immunology, and he is known also for his famous debates with Ehrlich on the nature of antigen–antibody–complement interactions.

1930, Landsteiner

The prize was awarded to Karl Landsteiner (1868–1943), "for his discovery of the human blood groups." Landsteiner was a Viennese physician who developed a keen interest in structural organic chemistry before embarking on a career in immunology. From the very outset, Landsteiner seemed always to choose important areas in which to work, or to make important those subjects to which he turned his attention. In early studies of antierythrocyte antibodies, he described in 1901 the set of human isoagglutinins that now comprise the ABO system of blood groups. In 1926, Landsteiner and Philip Levine discovered the MNP system, and with Albert Wiener in 1940 the Rh system of blood groups. He was the first to demonstrate that poliomyelitis could be produced in nonhuman primates, and he was one of the first to make the same observation for syphilis. During the First World War, he became interested in the antibody response to chemically defined haptens, and over the next quarter-century, primarily at the Rockefeller Institute in New York, he contributed impressively to an understanding of the chemical basis for antigen–antibody interactions, as summarized in his famous book *The Specificity of Serologic Reactions*. While acknowledging the importance of his discovery of blood groups, Landsteiner is said to have felt that his 1930 Nobel Prize should rather have been awarded for his work on antibody–hapten interactions.

1951, Theiler

The prize was awarded to Max Theiler (1899–1972), "for his development of vaccines against yellow fever." Theiler was a South African who studied medicine in Britain and then moved to the United States in 1922, first to the School of Tropical Medicine at Harvard and then to the Rockefeller Institute in New York. It was he who showed that yellow fever was caused by a filterable virus, and his description of the mouse protection test (in which serum antibody mixed with the virus protects a mouse from the lethal effects of intracerebral inoculation) provided a very important tool for epidemiology and other studies of yellow fever. In the late 1930s he succeeded in developing attenuated strains of yellow fever virus by serial passage *in vitro* in mouse and chick embryo tissue cultures. By these means, strains were developed that retained their immunogenicity, but were devoid of pathogenicity, the basis of the currently effective yellow fever vaccines.

1957, Bovet

The prize was awarded to Daniel Bovet (1907–), Swiss physiologist and pharmacologist, "for his development of antihistamines in the treatment of allergy." The discovery of the Schultz-Dale phenomenon, in which a strip of sensitized uterine tissue could be caused to contract under the action of antigen, provided a useful *in vitro* model for allergic reactions and for the clarification of the physiologic mechanisms involved. This led to the finding that histamine was the most significant agent released in anaphylaxis, along with serotonin and other active substances. Bovet must have been exposed to immunology and allergy while working under Emile Roux at the Pasteur Institute in Paris, and he published extensively on the response of the autonomic nervous system to various chemicals. It was this that led him to a study of agents that might counter the effects of histamine, and from this emerged the drugs that were to prove so useful in the treatment of asthma and hayfever. Even had he not become famous for his work on antihistamines, his South American adventures with curare and its mode of action and his development of curare-like relaxants, tranquilizing drugs, and anesthetics would have given him a secure place in the annals of medicine.

1960, Burnet and Medawar

The prize was awarded to F. Macfarlane Burnet (1899–1985) and Peter B. Medawar (1915–1987), "for the discovery of acquired immunological tolerance." The Second World War stimulated basic research in a number of sciences, among them the search to improve the survivability of skin and other tissue grafts on burn and wound victims, and to explain their rejection. Medawar, who had trained in zoology and pathology at Oxford, was interested in tissue repair and thus in problems of tissue transplantation. His initial work established conclusively that the rejection of foreign skin grafts followed all of the rules of immunologic specificity, and this was in fact based upon the same mechanisms responsible for protection against bacterial and viral infections. The follow-up work that he and a series of distinguished students (most notably Rupert Billingham and Leslie Brent) undertook firmly established transplantation immunobiology as an important subdiscipline, yielding many later dividends in the field of clinical organ transplantation. Then, in 1945 to 1947, Ray Owen reported the curious observation that dizygotic cattle twins that had shared the same circulatory system *in utero* had become blood-cell chimeras, unable to respond immunologically to one another's antigens. This observation was seized upon by the Australian physician-virologist Macfarlane Burnet, not only a productive investigator, but also a wide-ranging theoretician. Burnet had published in 1941 a stimulating book, *The Production of Antibodies,* and was now preparing a revision of this book with his colleague Frank Fenner. The new book (1949) not only proposed a novel indirect template theory of antibody formation, but also provided a theoretical explanation for Owen's findings. Burnet and Fenner suggested that immunologic responses arise fairly late in embryonic life and involve a cataloguing by a system of "self-markers" of those antigens then present, to which the host thenceforth would be tolerant and unable to respond immunologically. Any antigens not so catalogued would be "nonself" and could later stimulate an active immune response. The suggestion was made that any antigen introduced during this critical period would be adopted as self, would induce tolerance, and thus would be unable later to activate the immunologic apparatus. These concepts were further developed by Burnet in his clonal selection theory of antibody formation. Burnet and Fenner's suggestion on tolerance was put to the test by Medawar and his colleagues, and in 1953 they provided ample confirmation of the Burnet-Fenner hypothesis using inbred strains of mice, a phenomenon to which Medawar gave the name *acquired immunological tolerance.*

1972, Porter and Edelman

This prize was awarded to Rodney R. Porter (1917–1985) of Oxford University and Gerald M. Edelman (1929–) of the Rockefeller University, "for their work on the chemical structure of antibodies." The demonstration by A. Tiselius and E. A. Kabat that antibodies were high-molecular-weight gamma-globulins made it clear that it would be extremely difficult to define chemically the basis for either their primary immunologic specificity or for their secondary biological functions. Porter undertook to cleave the antibody molecule with enzymes in an attempt to obtain smaller, active fragments, and he succeeded in 1958 in accounting for the entire molecule in terms of papain cleavage into two identical Fab fragments and a third Fc fragment, the former containing the antibody-binding sites and the latter responsible for the secondary biological activity of antibodies. Edelman then showed that homogeneous myeloma globulin could be reductively cleaved into its component polypeptide chains, comprising both light (L) and heavy (H) chains. He also showed that the L chains of different guinea pig antibodies had different electrophoretic mobility patterns, and further that the Bence Jones protein of multiple myeloma was similar to the L chains of antibody. Porter and his colleagues next demonstrated that the immunoglobulin molecule was composed of two L and two H chains, leading to the now-accepted model for IgG. The isolation of immunoglobulin chains and fragments now permitted an approach to their primary amino acid sequencing, and this was hotly pursued in the laboratories of Porter, Edelman, and many other investigators. From this work emerged an understanding of the existence of both variable and constant regions on the L and H chains and the ability to compare primary sequences among different antibody specificities, different isotypes, and even different species. Finally, in 1969 Edelman and his co-workers succeeded in working out the primary sequence of an entire immunoglobulin molecule, helping to define not only the location of the active site, but also the location of the "domains" responsible for the secondary biological activities of antibodies.

1977, Yalow

This prize was awarded to Rosalyn Yalow (1921–), "for the development of radio immunoassays of peptide hormones" (shared with Roger Guillemin and Andrew Schally, "for their discoveries concerning the peptide hormone production of the brain"). Beginning in the early 1950s, Yalow and her long-term collaborator Solomon Berson investigated the causes of insulin resistance in diabetes. They discovered that diabetics treated with insulin formed antibodies specific for this insulin, but their initial attempt to publish this important observation was rejected in the belief that so small a molecule was incapable of being immunogenic. Berson (who died in 1972) and Yalow then showed that the addition of increasing amounts of unlabeled insulin to an immune complex of antiinsulin and its radiolabeled antigen resulted in a measurable displacement of the labeled insulin. This discovery formed the basis of the first radioimmunoassay of a hormone, capable of estimating nanogram or even picogram quantities. Since then, this assay system has been applied to other hormones and biologically active substances and has become a valuable tool for much basic and clinical research. It was this technique that contributed importantly to the isolation and characterization of hypothalamic hormones by Guillemin and Schally.

1980, Benacerraf, Dausset, and Snell

This prize was awarded to Baruj Benacerraf (1920–), Jean Dausset (1916–), and George Snell (1903–), "for their work on genetically determined structures of the cell surface that regulate immunologic reactions." The demonstration that the ability of mice to reject tumors was genetically determined stimulated geneticist Snell to search for methods to study the genes responsible for this phenomenon. This led Snell in the mid-1940s "to invent the idea of congenic mice," animals that are bred to be genetically identical except at a single locus or genetic region. In collaboration with Peter Gorer, Snell identified a locus important for allograft rejection, designated H (histocompatibility)-2, subsequently shown to be a complex of many closely linked genes, with many different alleles occurring at each locus. The work of many investigators has since contributed to a better understanding of the composition and many of the functions of this complicated stretch of DNA, now called the major histocompatibility complex (MHC). In the 1950s, Jean Dausset of France found isoantibodies against leukocyte antigens in the blood of transfusion recipients, helping to demonstrate the analogy between the H-2 complex of the mouse and the human leukocyte antigen (HLA) system in humans and providing a powerful tool to define individual HLA antigens. In 1965, Dausset and his co-workers described a system of some ten human antigens encoded for in the histocompatibility complex, containing "subloci," each of which specified a limited number of antigenic alleles. It was this approach that finally opened the way for the definition and genetic location of those major and minor antigens responsible for histoincompatibility. But the importance of the genes in the HLA and H-2 complexes had thus far been restricted to the somewhat unphysiologic practices of tissue and blood transplantation. It remained for Benacerraf, McDevitt, and others to demonstrate that many of the genes located within the major histocompatibility complex may also control active immune responses to various antigenic stimuli. Utilizing simple antigens, such as synthetic polypeptides, Benacerraf found that the ability of an animal to respond immunologically to a given antigen was controlled by specific genes—called Ir (for immune response) genes—subsequently shown by others to reside within the I region of the MHC. Since then, work in Benacerraf's and many other laboratories has shown the importance of I-region genes in controlling the intercommunication among immunocytes responsible for the regulation of the immune response, and the importance of some MHC genes in predisposing for certain chronic diseases.

1984, Milstein, Köhler, and Jerne

The prize this year was shared by Cesar Milstein (1927–) and Georges F. Kohler (1946–1995), for development of the technique of monoclonal antibody formation, and Niels K. Jerne (1912–1994), for his theoretical contributions that have shaped our concept of the immune system. Henry Kunkel and co-workers showed in 1955 that myeloma tumors produced monoclonal antibodies, and Michael Potter showed in 1962 that such plasma-cell

tumors could be induced in mice, while others were able to adapt such tumors to grow indefinitely in culture. In 1974, Köhler started a postdoctoral fellowship in Milstein's laboratory in Cambridge, and the two undertook to immortalize antibody-forming cells by fusing them with myelomas, in order to study the genetic basis of antibody diversity. It was hoped that the tumor cell would endow the otherwise short-lived antibody-forming cell with the capacity for long-term survival in the resulting hybrid (called a *hybridoma*). The key to success in this venture was the development of a selective technique to recover only fused cells, employing a mutant myeloma cell line deficient in the enzyme hypoxanthine phosphoribosyltransferase. Without this enzyme, the cells would die in a medium containing hypoxanthine, aminopterine, and thymidine (HAT), but the hybrid cells would survive and could be selected, since the normal antibody-forming cell component of the hybrid would contribute the enzyme required. Isolation of a hybridoma clone would thus yield large quantities of monoclonal antibodies specific for a single antigenic determinant. The availability of such pure reagents has provided one of the most powerful tools of the current revolution in molecular biology, and has opened up new avenues of investigation in many basic and clinical sciences.

Niels Jerne's contributions to immunology are almost too numerous to record, and his influence on the field is impossible to exaggerate. While still a student, Jerne made important observations on the avidity of antibodies and on the changing quality of antibodies in response to successive booster immunizations. In 1963, Jerne and Albert Nordin described the hemolytic plaque assay method for enumerating antibody-forming cells, a technique that would receive broad application in studies of the cellular events underlying the antibody response. But it was Jerne's theoretical contributions that helped to bring immunology and immunologists to their current important position in the biomedical sciences. In 1955, Jerne was the first modern scientist to challenge the then-current instructive theories of antibody formation, by proposing a selective theory in which antigen functions to *select* specifically from a *preexisting* repertoire of antibody-forming capabilities. While the particulars of Jerne's hypothesis might require correction, his theory served as the critical stimulus to Macfarlane Burnet's clonal selection theory of antibody formation. In 1971, Jerne made another conceptual leap to explain the development of the repertoire of T-cell specificities. He postulated that the principal driving force that stimulates lymphocytes to divide and mutate at a high rate in the thymus is the individual's MHC antigens. Once again, a Jerne conceptual leap served as an important stimulus to experimental and conceptual progress in the field. The third, and perhaps the most profound, of Jerne's theories was his idiotype network theory of 1974. Jacques Oudin, Henry Kunkel, and Philip Gell had previously shown that the antibody combining site possesses unique antigenic determinants (idiotypes). Jerne's proposal was that the balanced production of a cascading network of idiotypes and antiidiotypes might constitute one of the principal regulatory mechanisms governing the immune response. This theory, eminently testable, has profound implications for the physiology of the immune system, and for its regulation of such pathological states as autoimmunity.

1987, Tonegawa

This prize was awarded to Susumu Tonegawa (1939–), for his work on the molecular biology of immunoglobulin genes, demonstrating how antibody diversity is generated. It had always been difficult to believe that all of the genes required to generate the remarkable diversity of antibodies could be present in the germ line; thus, most investigators favored a somatic mutation theory acting upon only a very limited number of germ-line genes. In 1965, Dreyer and Bennett proposed that less DNA might be required, if multiple variable (V)-region genes could combine with a single constant (C)-region gene for a given isotype (the two gene–one polypeptide theory). This speculation was confirmed in 1976 by Tonegawa and Hozumi, by showing that C-region and V-region genes were separate in embryonic DNA. Tonegawa, Gilbert, and Maxam then showed that combination of these two genes in differentiated cells still involves their separation by a noncoding DNA sequence (an "intron"). It was further found by Tonegawa, and also by Philip Leder and his colleagues, that the V-region polypeptide chain contains more amino acids than is encoded in the V-region DNA of the L chain, suggesting that yet another DNA segment might be needed to encode the complete V-region. Tonegawa and his colleagues soon located the missing DNA segment, which was designated J (for *joining*). Thus, the combination of a single C-region segment with one of several J segments and one of many V-region segments would suffice to generate a wide range of different L chains. In studying the assembly of the genes for the H chains of antibody, it was found by both Tonegawa and Leroy Hood that now three separate DNA segments must be joined to complete the sequence for the H-chain V-region. In addition to the V and J segments, a third group of DNA segments, termed D (for *diversity*), was involved. In addition to the ability to choose among multiple V, D, and J elements, additional variability is introduced into the H chain by permitting splicing in the middle of a triplet codon, resulting in a translation shift. The demonstration by Hood and others that mutations in these gene segments could also occur appeared finally to complete the picture of how the immense repertoire of antibody specificities is generated. Tonegawa's work, and that of others, has had important implications in other areas, including the structure and formation of T-cell receptors and the DNA rearrangements that might be responsible for lymphomas and leukemias.

1996, Doherty and Zinkernagel

The prize was awarded to Peter Doherty (1940–) and Rolf Zinkernagel (1944–) for their demonstration of the MHC restriction of cytotoxic T-cell recognition of viral antigens on infected cells. The 1950s were years of great ferment in immunology. On the one hand, Burnet's notion of immunological tolerance focused attention on the "immunological self," a term that would eventually take on more than just metaphorical implications. On the other hand, the differences between the familiar functions of antibody and the role of cells in delayed-type hypersensitivity and in destroying the cells bearing allogeneic transplantation antigens would lead to the separation of B- and T-cell lineages and functions. Indeed, it was Mitchison in 1954 who speculated that cellular recognition of skin-sensitizing antigens occurred only when these were present on the surface membranes of autochthonous cells, thus mimicking foreign transplantation antigens. It was the suggestion by Lewis Thomas that these cellular mechanisms had evolved to control tumor formation (immunological surveillance) that led Sherwood Lawrence to extend the idea to include protection from all intracellular parasites. In an imaginative conceptual leap, Lawrence went on to propose that immunological recognition

might involve the parasitic (viral) antigen only in association with a self-antigen, the so-called *self plus X* hypothesis. The scene now moves forward to the early 1970s when prospective surgeon Zinkernagel stopped in Canberra on his *Wanderjahr* and was, for lack of adequate space, assigned to share the same laboratory with prospective veterinarian Doherty. The project upon which they collaborated was then a highly popular one; it involved the study of the mechanism of damage caused by virus-immune cytotoxic cells in lymphocytic choriomeningitis virus (LCMV) disease of mice. It had recently been reported that many aspects of the immune response to certain antigens was controlled by *Ir-genes*, known to be a part of the MHC, and, more specifically, that susceptibility to LCMV disease might be related to the particular MHC of the infected mouse. Doherty and Zinkernagel chose for their experiments an *in vitro* system that measures the ability of virus-immune effector cells to destroy virus-infected target cells. When the two cell types originated in the same strain of mice, death of the infected cells was efficient. When, however, the virus-specific cytotoxic cells and the virus-infected target cells came from mice of different MHC haplotypes, destruction of the targets generally failed to take place. The investigators were then able to conclude that the effector cell must recognize two signals on a virus-infected cell, one derived from the virus and the other from the MHC molecule normally present on the cell. The past two decades have amply confirmed the Doherty-Zinkernagel observation. It has been found that the T-cell receptor is so constructed that it is able to bind tightly to a polypeptide breakdown product of the virus, which lies in a special cleft characteristic of the surface of the MHC molecule. Thus, T-cell recognition is truly "in the context of self."

BIBLIOGRAPHY

Primary Sources

Arrhenius S. *Immunochemistry.* New York: Macmillan, 1970.
Bordet J. *Studies on immunity.* Gay, F, translator. New York: John Wiley and Sons, 1909.
Bordet J. *Traité de l'immunité dans les maladies infectieuses.* Paris: Masson, 1920.
Burnet FM. *The Production of Antibodies.* 1st ed. Melbourne: Macmillan: 1941.
Burnet FM. *The clonal selection theory of acquired immunity.* Cambridge: The University Press, 1959.
Burnet FM, Fenner F. *The production of antibodies.* 2nd ed. Melbourne: Macmillan, 1949.
Ehrlich P. The Croonian lecture: on immunity. *Proc Soc Lond Biol* 1900;66:424.
Ehrlich P. *Collected studies in immunity.* New York: John Wiley and Sons, 1905.
Ehrlich P. *Collected papers of Paul Ehrlich.* vol 2. New York: Pergamon Press, 1957.
Landsteiner K. *The specificity of serological reactions.* Boston: Harvard University Press, 1945.
Marrack JR. *The chemistry of antigens and antibodies.* London: H. M. Stationery Office, 1934.
Metchnikoff E. *Lectures on the comparative pathology of inflammation.* London: Kegan, Paul, Trench, Trübner, 1893.
Metchnikoff E. *Immunity in the infectious diseases.* New York: Macmillan, 1905.
Murphy JB. *The lymphocyte in relation to tissue grafting, malignant disease, and tuberculous infection.* New York: Rockefeller Inst. Monograph #21, 1926.
Nuttall GHF. *Blood immunity and blood relationships.* Cambridge: The University Press, 1904.
von Pirquet C, Schick B. *Serum sickness.* Baltimore: Williams & Wilkins 1951.

Secondary Sources

Bibel DJ. *Milestones in immunology.* New York: Springer-Verlag, 1988.
Brent L. *A history of transplantation immunology.* San Diego: Academic Press, 1997.
Bulloch W. *The history of bacteriology.* London: Oxford University Press, 1938.
Castiglioni A. *A history of medicine.* New York: Knopf, 1947.
Foster WD. *A history of medical bacteriology and immunology.* London: Heinemann, 1970.

Marks GM, Beatty WK. *Epidemics.* New York: Scribner, 1976.

Marquardt M. *Paul Ehrlich.* New York: Schuman, 1957.

Mazumdar PMH. Immunity in 1890. *J Hist Med Allied Sci* 1972;27:312.

Mazumdar PMH. The antigen-antibody reaction and the physics and chemistry of life. *Bull Hist Med* 1974;48:1.

Mazumdar PMH. *Species and specificity.* Cambridge: The University Press, 1995.

Metchnikoff O. *Life of Elie Metchnikoff.* Boston: Houghton Mifflin, 1921.

Miller G. *The adoption of inoculation for smallpox in England and France.* Philadelphia University of Pennsylvania Press, 1957.

Moulin A-M. *Le dernier langage de la médicine: histoire de l'immunologie de Pasteur au SIDA.* Paris: Presse Universitaire, 1991.

Parascandola J, Jasensky R. Origins of the receptor theory of drug action. *Bull Hist Med* 1974;48:199.

Parrish HJ. *A history of immunization.* Edinburgh: Livingstone, 1965.

Rubin LP. Styles in scientific explanation: Paul Ehrlich and Svante Arrhenius on immunochemistry. *J Hist Med* 1980;35:397.

Silverstein AM. *A history of immunology.* New York: Academic Press, 1989.

Silverstein AM. The dynamics of conceptual change in twentieth century immunology. *Cell Immunol* 1991;132:515.

Speiser P, Smekal FG. *Karl Landsteiner.* Vienna: Brüder Hollinek, 1975.

Tauber AI, Chernyak L. *Metchnikoff and the origins of immunology.* New York: Oxford University Press, 1991.

Topley WWC, Wilson GS. *The principles of bacteriology and immunity,* 2d ed. Baltimore: Wood, 1936.

Vallery-Radot R. *Life of Pasteur.* London: Constable, 1906.

Woodruff MFA. *The transplantation of tissues and organs.* Springfield, IL: Charles C. Thomas Publisher, 1960.

Zinsser H. *Infection and resistance.* New York: Macmillan, 1914.

Fundamental Immunology, Fourth Edition,
edited by William E. Paul, Philadelphia
Lippincott–Raven Publishers, Philadelphia © 1999.

CHAPTER 3

Immunoglobulins: Structure and Function

J. Kimble Frazer and J. Donald Capra

INTRODUCTION

Immunoglobulin is the crux of the humoral immune response. As a cell surface receptor on B lymphocytes, immunoglobulin is responsible for instigating cellular processes as diverse as activation, differentiation, and even programmed cell death. As secreted antibody in plasma and other bodily fluids, immunoglobulin is able to bind foreign antigen, thereby either neutralizing it directly or initiating steps necessary to arm and recruit effector systems such as complement or antibody-dependent cell cytolysis by monocytic phagocytes. The ability of immunoglobulin to perform such a wide array of duties can be attributed to evolution's clever usage of a structural paradigm the immunoglobulin domain—and its duplication, diversification, and elaboration upon that design to endow it with an assortment of functional qualities.

Despite the variety of purposes served by immunoglobulin molecules, one feature remains common to virtually all considerations of immunoglobulin structure and function: immunoglobulins have an amazing capacity to interact with other molecules. In one sense, immunoglobulins must be able to effectively bind a finite set of invariant partners, such as Fc receptors, signal-transducing molecules, and components of the complement cascade. In another sense, immunoglobulins, collectively, must meet the challenge of

being able to recognize an essentially infinite array of antigenic determinants. More remarkable, perhaps, is the fact that immunoglobulin is frequently called upon to fulfill both of these binding responsibilities simultaneously, and in such a way as to mediate significant biological effects. As such, immunoglobulin molecules may be viewed as a marriage between the constraints engendered by biological continuity and the quest for diversity superimposed upon this evolutionary framework.

The lengths to which evolution has gone in order to bestow immunoglobulin with these conflicting capabilities has been the subject of intense scientific scrutiny, and has yielded innumerable fascinating insights into immunology, genetics, protein chemistry, and the discipline of biology as a whole. In trying to understand how antibody is able to recognize such a multitude of different specificities, science has benefited from the discovery of both VDJ recombination (see Chapter 5) and somatic hypermutation (see Chapter 25). In an attempt to reconcile the incongruity entailed by the observation of highly divergent N-terminal regions coupled to constant C-terminal domains, research has gained not only the once-heretical "two genes, one polypeptide" hypothesis (1), but also the concept of isotype switching (see Chapter 24). Thus, studies into immunoglobulin diversity have proven to be extremely profitable scientific endeavors. In addition, while diversity has been a hallmark of the study of immunoglobulin since it was first recognized to be a salient feature, several aspects that derive from immunoglobulins' underlying uniformity have been used to glean understanding into protein structure–function relationships in general.

Immunoglobulins were the first molecules described from the ancestral immunoglobulin superfamily (IgSF) (2–4). As an ever-

　J.K. Frazer: Graduate Program in Molecular Microbiology and Medical Scientist Training Program, University of Texas Southwestern Medical School, Dallas, TX 75235-9110.
　J.D. Capra: President and Scientific Director, Oklahoma Medical Research Foundation, Oklahoma City, OK 73104.

expanding gene family, members of the IgSF have been shown to be vital to issues of cell–cell interaction and molecular recognition in a variety of cell types and across several taxonomic boundaries. Many molecules central to the functioning of the immune system, including the antigen-specific chains of the T-cell receptor (TCR) (see Chapter 10) and the class I and II major histocompatibility complex (MHC) antigens (see Chapter 8), are counted among this group. Common to all members of the superfamily is the presence of one or more immunoglobulin-like domains. Three-dimensional structural analyses of proteins containing these regions have demonstrated that the conserved amino acid sequences that make up an immunoglobulin homology domain comprise a recurring structural motif that can fold into a compact globular subunit. These subunits, in turn, are capable of integrating into complex macromolecules (5,6). As a result, different immunoglobulin molecular structures are similar not only to each other, but also to a multitude of other important proteins.

Because such a concerted scientific effort has been made to understand the way in which immunoglobulin functions, a large volume of sequence information—at both the nucleotide and amino acid levels—is available in both the literature and public databases. Indeed, immunoglobulins have likely been sequenced more frequently than any other class of gene or protein. Similarly, immunoglobulins have been well represented in structural studies, crystallographic and otherwise, to an unprecedented degree. This mass of work has allowed a number of conclusions regarding structure–function relationships of immunoglobulins to be made. Specifically, the aim of this chapter is not to compile an exhaustive catalogue of all extant work on the topic of immunoglobulin sequences, but rather to present the essential features of immunoglobulin structure and their relation to immunologic function as is currently understood. Further, because immunoglobulin proteins have been so evolutionarily valuable, they can be found, in one form or another, throughout vertebrate species. Many of these molecules are only now being characterized, and surely many more are yet to be identified. As a consequence of this diversity, however, it is impossible to relate all of the details of immunoglobulin structure and function in their entirety. Instead, unless otherwise noted, the examples of human and murine immunoglobulins will be used as models to convey the general conclusions garnered from scientific insight and experimentation into this important and fascinating class of proteins. The organization of this discussion will begin, following an introduction to basic immunoglobulin features, with a consideration of the primary structure of antibody molecules and proceed through the secondary, tertiary, quaternary, and higher order immunoglobulin structural topics that derive from its sequence. Once this foundation has been laid, the functional attributes of immunoglobulin will be considered, with an eye to correlating an antibody's capacities—to the extent which it is possible—with that of its structure. A section on the IgSF follows, which will briefly address its evolution and also specifically detail particular IgSF members critical to immune responses that are not explicitly covered elsewhere in this volume.

GENERAL IMMUNOGLOBULIN STRUCTURE, NOMENCLATURE, AND HISTORY

Structural Considerations

Figure 1 presents a diagrammatic representation of an antibody molecule. The typical immunoglobulin monomer is comprised of

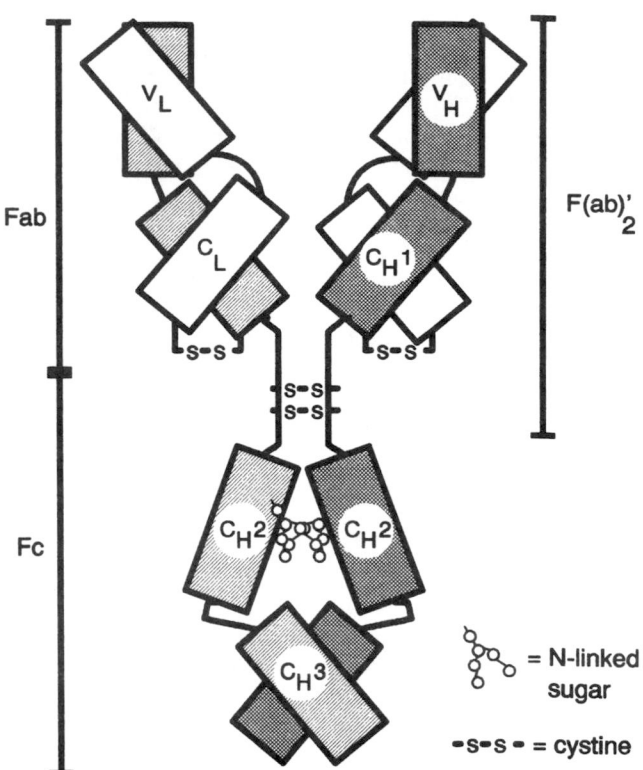

FIG. 1. Schematic representation of a prototypic immunoglobulin monomer. Each box symbolizes a complete immunoglobulin domain from either the heavy (*shaded boxes*) or light (*unshaded*) chain. Labeling of domains follows standard nomenclature, as outlined in the text. Interchain disulfide bonds are denoted by *black bars*. Note that these bonds are present between both heavy and light chain pairs and between the two heavy chains. Conserved N-linked carbohydrate occurs on all C_H2 domains as shown, although some immunoglobulins are also glycosylated at additional sites elsewhere in the molecule. Also of note is the fact that all of the domains associate to form dimeric modules (V_H/V_L, C_H1/C_L, and C_H3/C_H3), except C_H2 domains. The Fab, Fc, and F(ab)'₂ proteolytic fragments are demarcated by *bars* to either side of the diagram. (From ref. 6a, with permission.)

four polypeptide chains complexed together via hydrophobic interactions and stabilized by disulfide bonds. Due to allelic exclusion (see Chapters 5 and 6) B lymphocytes usually express only one functionally rearranged heavy chain gene and only one light chain polypeptide as well. Consequently, complete immunoglobulin proteins are composed of two identical heavy chain polypeptides of approximately 55 kD and two identical light chains of 25 kD. Each heavy and light chain pair is joined by one or more interchain disulfide bonds, and also relies upon noncovalent interactions to properly orient the two chains relative to each other. One such "half-antibody" contains a single antigen binding site (i.e., it is monovalent). The complete four polypeptide chain monomer is formed by similar hydrophobic bonding between the two heavy chains, and it also utilizes one or more disulfide bonds to stabilize the complex. Thus, a complete immunoglobulin molecule is bivalent with two identical sites for potential binding of antigen. As such, an immunoglobulin may be thought of as a "dimer of a heterodimer," although these half-molecules do not occur naturally.

Each individual polypeptide chain consists of two to five domains of approximately 110 amino acids (7), each capable of folding independently. These domains form compact, protease-resistant structures which serve as the fundamental unit of immunoglobulin structure. The interactions that allow for the formation of the aforementioned immunoglobulin monomer almost exclusively occur in pair-wise fashion between domains of two different polypeptide chains (see Fig. 1), such that the functional modules of an antibody are in fact dimerized domains. In addition, as each domain of an antibody molecule is encoded by a separate exon, immunoglobulin domains also serve as the essential element of antibody genetics. In this light, it is easy to recognize how evolution has used the prototypical immunoglobulin domain as a substrate for experimentation, and as a result different domains have attained distinct structural and functional attributes. Moreover, the presence of one or more "immunoglobulin homology domains" also proves to be the distinguishing characteristic for inclusion in the immunoglobulin gene superfamily. Thus, the duplication and adaptation of the Ig homology domain has occurred not only within the context of formal "immunoglobulin genes," but also in the greater scope of the IgSF, which far predates the emergence of antibody. In either case, the archetypal immunoglobulin domain has clearly proven to be a powerful evolutionary tool, as will be detailed below and in greater detail throughout this chapter.

The hallmark of all Ig domains is the presence of a structural motif termed the *immunoglobulin fold*. This characteristic feature is actually a specialized "β-barrel" typically comprised of seven polypeptide strands, which form antiparallel β-pleated sheets in the folded domain. This configuration is depicted in Fig. 2, which was deduced from x-ray diffraction studies of an immunoglobulin light chain (8). Each Ig domain is composed of two β-pleated sheets, one containing four β strands, the other consisting of at least three β strands (represented by arrows in Fig. 2). Loops of variable length connect the different strands, allowing the β sheets to form. The two β-pleated layers are oriented in a sandwich, enclosing a hydrophobic interior. Further stability is provided by a disulfide bond near the domain's core, which covalently links the two sheet layers. The cysteines that contribute this bond are conserved in all immunoglobulins, and in almost all proteins that possess Ig-like domains. Two residues, a tryptophan in strand 3-1 and an aromatic residue that precedes the second half-cystine, are also maintained consistently and serve to protect the disulfide bond in the three-dimensional structure. Other conserved features include hydropho-

bic core residues, which stabilize the inside of the sandwich, and glycine and proline loop residues, which provide the flexibility necessary for the formation of these interconnecting sequences (9–12).

Since the hydrophobic core residues are predominantly responsible for promoting the folding of the β sheets, and thus the entire immunoglobulin fold, the sequences of the loop residues are free to vary considerably. This, in turn, grants loop residues the freedom to serve as substrates for selection, at the level of selection of a particular antibody in an immune response and at the level of natural selection in phylogeny. In this way, the prototypical immunoglobulin homology domain serves as a potent cofactor for the evolution of both organismal immunity and that of the species in general.

Immunoglobulin Nomenclature

Light chains contain two such immunoglobulin domains, whereas a heavy chain is made up of either four or five domains, depending on the type of heavy chain (isotype) used by the antibody in question. Different immunoglobulin domains possess different structural and functional characteristics, and their naming, in part, reflects these differences. The amino-terminal domain of each chain, whether of the heavy or light type, is termed a *variable* (V) region due to the discovery of extensive sequence divergence between different antibody proteins in this part of the molecule. These are designated V_H and V_L for heavy and light chains, respectively. V regions have been demonstrated to be responsible for the antigenic specificity of the immunoglobulin.

Carboxy-terminal domains, on the other hand, display considerably less sequence variation within a given isotype and are referred to as *constant* (C) regions. Heavy chain C regions are numbered C_H1, C_H2, and so on, beginning with the most V region-proximal domain. The constant region domains of the heavy chain have been shown to be responsible for many aspects of antibody function, including interaction with Fc receptors, complement fixation, transplacental transfer, the ability to multimerize, and the capacity to be secreted on mucosal surfaces. Because different heavy chain isotypes have different C region domains (i.e., the C_H3 domains of different isotypes are distinct), these capabilities vary with the class of the particular antibody. Five major classes of heavy chain C regions exist: alpha (α), gamma (γ), delta (δ), epsilon (ε), and mu (μ). As a direct consequence of the correlation between the

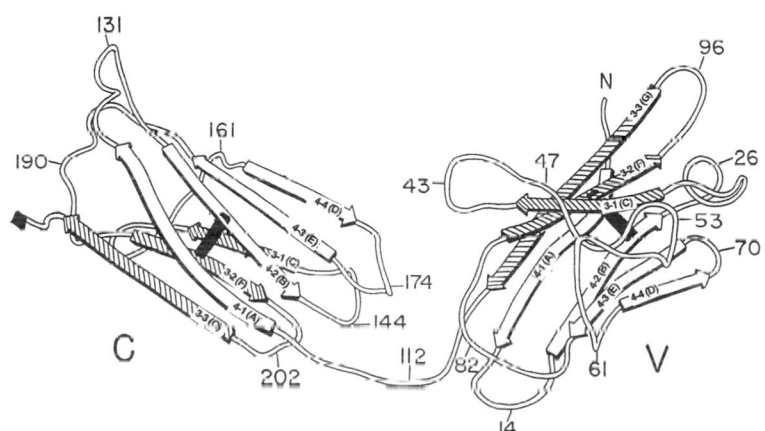

FIG. 2. Ribbon drawing of the V and C domains of a light chain. β strands are depicted as *arrows*, with those of the four-stranded face *unshaded* and those of the three-stranded face *shaded*. Strands are numbered according to Edmundson and lettered (*in parentheses*) according to Hood. Intrachain disulfide bonds are represented as *black bars*. Selected amino acids are numbered, with position 1 being the N-terminus. Residues 26, 53, and 96 correspond to amino acids in CDRs 1, 2, and 3, respectively. The dimerization surfaces of each domain (four-strand side of the C domain, three-strand side of the V domain) face upwards. (Adapted from ref 8, with permission.)

heavy chain class of an antibody and its resultant effector functions, immunoglobulins are named according to their heavy chain, using an English-letter terminology (IgA, IgG, IgD, IgE, IgM), which corresponds to their Greek letter isotypes. Specific domains of C regions are often designated according to the class of heavy chain from whence they originate as well (i.e., the C_H3 domain of a μ antibody is signified by $C_\mu3$). Owing to the propensity of immunoglobulin domains to evolve independent of one another, oftentimes a particular domain of a specific isotype may be responsible for one or more functional characteristics of the entire antibody, making this naming system particularly relevant. On the other hand, the constant regions of light chains, possessing only one C domain, are usually simply denoted by C_L. The two light chain classes, kappa (κ) and lambda (λ), may be indicated by the use of C_κ or C_λ designations. No distinct functional attributes have as yet been ascribed to either the κ or λ light chain isotypes.

Finally, immunoglobulins also have hinge regions located C-terminal to the C_H1 domains of their heavy chains. In the case of heavy chains of the μ and ε isotypes, the hinge is so elongated that it is actually an extra immunoglobulin domain, explaining the presence of a fifth C domain in these molecules. Other heavy chain classes use shorter stretches of protein, which are thought nonetheless to have evolved from the $C_{\mu/\varepsilon}2$ domain. Consistent with the independent evolution of the other domains of immunoglobulin genes, hinge regions are generally encoded by individual exons as well. As the name implies, the hinge permits a generous degree of flexibility between the antigen-binding and effector-interacting components of the molecule. Thus, the hinge domain facilitates linking of the two disparate elements of immunoglobulin function: the ability to interact with an endless array of structural determinants on antigenic surfaces (mediated by V regions) and the capacity to interact with a limited number of effector-activating molecules (mediated by C regions). In addition, disulfide bridges between the two heavy chains typically occur within the boundaries of the hinge region, allowing the complete tetrameric complex to form.

Hence, in many cases, the discrete elements of immunoglobulin structure defined both genetically and structurally as immunoglobulin domains are also responsible for specific functional qualities. Moreover, in addition to the one-domain-per-exon correlation that exists for immunoglobulins, in both heavy and light chains the V region domain and the domains of the different C regions are in fact distinct genes (13). This type of genetic arrangement allows the ability to recognize a specific antigen to be united with the effector functions that are most appropriate for that particular immune response at that particular time. In this regard, then, it is clear that antibodies truly embody the linkage of structure to that of function.

An Historical Perspective

Long before x-ray diffraction of crystals had yielded the keys to dissecting the structure of immunoglobulin, other seminal studies had been performed that, in retrospect, agree completely with the conclusions drawn from crystallization analysis. Many of these experiments focused on the basic protein chemistry of pooled IgG, using the techniques of proteolysis, reduction, and denaturation. First, it was revealed that papain digestion of IgG would render two types of protein fragments: Fab, a monovalent antigen binding fragment, and Fc, an easily crystallizable fragment (14). Soon after, it was recognized that pepsin treatment of IgG produced an antigen-binding fragment designated $F(ab)'_2$ which had bivalent activity (15). Furthermore, if this fragment was treated with reducing agents, two univalent Fab' fragments could be obtained. These different fragments are schematically represented in Fig. 1. Reduction and dissociation of IgG also demonstrated that identical heavy and light chains were complexed via disulfide bonds (16). This and other work eventually allowed investigators to decipher a working model for immunoglobulin structure consisting of four polypeptide subunits—two identical heavy chains and two identical light chains—stabilized by multiple interchain disulfide bonds (17,18), which we now know to be correct.

Early studies of a different type also proved successful in revealing information about antibodies; these experiments focused upon utilizing the immune system itself as a means to decode aspects of immunoglobulin structure (reviewed in refs. 19–21). As large glycoproteins, antibodies themselves are potent immunogens capable of eliciting vigorous humoral immune responses. Investigators used immunoglobulin preparations (initially either heterogeneous total serum immunoglobulin or homogeneous myeloma or plasmacytoma proteins, and later monoclonal antibodies from hybridomas) as antigens to generate antibody responses by injecting them into animals of differing species or different animals of the same species. The antibodies produced by these immunization protocols proved useful in resolving several key elements of immunoglobulin structure, and many of the antigenic determinants recognized by these antisera have subsequently been shown to correlate exactly with known structural features of immunoglobulins.

A three-tiered serological classification scheme for immunoglobulin was devised using these antisera (after adsorption) as reagents to categorize antibody molecules into distinct groups. The first tier of organization is that of the *isotype*. Isotypes define C region determinants and, as such, distinguish heavy and light chain constant regions from one another. Initially, five heavy chain classes were recognized and given the Greek letter designations mentioned in the previous section. The presence of these five isotypes in virtually all mammals for which immunoglobulin profiles have been determined indicates that the divergence of C region genes occurred at an early stage of mammalian evolution. Similarly, light chain constant regions were also divided into discrete κ and λ classes. Soon after, refinements made clear that two of the human heavy chain classes, α and γ, in fact contained several related members that could be further divided into subclasses. Human IgA is separated into $\alpha1$ and $\alpha2$ subclasses, and human IgG is separated into four γ subclasses: $\gamma1$, $\gamma2$, $\gamma3$, and $\gamma4$. Murine IgG is also composed of four γ subclasses ($\gamma1$, $\gamma2a$, $\gamma2b$, and $\gamma3$), although their structural and functional characteristics—and their abbreviated designations—do not agree with their human counterparts, thus indicating this diversification occurred after these species' evolutionary divergence. Each different isotype (whether class or subclass) is represented by a separate C region gene in the haploid genome, and all isotypes are present in the sera of all normal individuals of a given species.

Allotypes, on the other hand, refer to determinants found on the antibodies of some, but not all, members of a species. These determinants are encoded by one allele of a particular C region gene (either heavy or light chain) and are inherited in typical Mendelian fashion as autosomal dominant traits. Compilations of human allotypes are summarized in ref. 22 and are covered more extensively in ref. 23. Whereas isotypes and allotypes are localized to the C regions of immunoglobulins, *idiotypes* are antigenic determinants found on the V regions of antibodies, and they frequently correlate with binding specificity. Generally, idiotypes are present only in an individual member of a given species, and these antigenic epitopes reflect the uniqueness of each individual immunoglobulin molecule. An idiotypic determinant defined by a monoclonal antibody is called an *idiotope*. Idiotypes are not always restricted to the individual, however. Occasionally, when two individuals are challenged with the same antigen, they will produce antibodies that share the same idiotypic determinant(s). In such cases, the idiotype is called a *cross-reactive*, or *public*, *idiotype* (24). Cross-reactive idiotypes represent the usage of the same V gene segment by different individuals. Thus, idiotypes may be best thought of as being restricted not to the individual organism, but to the individual immunoglobulin molecule.

Obviously, a tremendous amount of effort, using a variety of scientific approaches, has been focused upon attempts to understand immunoglobulin structure. It is remarkable, though, that the vast majority of this early work, whether utilizing protein chemistry to resolve basic structural characteristics or manipulating the humoral immune response to generate reagents to classify immunoglobulin proteins relative to one another, has in fact identified, and in many cases answered, many of the crucial questions of immunoglobulin structure correctly. As shall be discussed in the following sections, many of the crucial structural features of the antibody—from primary sequence to quaternary associations—were first inferred from these initial landmark studies.

IMMUNOGLOBULIN STRUCTURE

Primary Structure—Two Genes, One Polypeptide

The assertion that each immunoglobulin chain derived from two distinct genetic entities was a novel and provocative hypothesis at the time it was proposed (1), and it has proven to be correct. Owing to this genetic independence, the structures of the V and C regions of immunoglobulin will be treated separately here as well, although they obviously share numerous commonalties.

Among the most remarkable discrepancies between V and C regions are the differences in their genetic organization. While the different heavy and light chain C regions are encoded by fewer than 20 genes, V region genes (V_H, V_κ, and V_λ) number in the hundreds. Further distinguishing the V region loci is the fact that genes for complete V_H or V_L domains are not present in the genome originally, but are "recombined" at the genetic level according to the processes of somatic diversification described in Chapter 5. This recombination of V, D, and J elements to form functional heavy chain genes (or V and J in the case of light chains) imposes another degree of diversity upon the V regions. Due to these complexities, sequence variability is in fact the hallmark of variable region domains. In addition to the differences between V and C domains in their genetic design and construction, V region sequences also have uniquely identifiable characteristics. One of the most easily recognizable features is the fact that V regions are approximately 16 residues longer than the prototypic 110 amino acid immunoglobulin domain. These extra residues allow V regions to form a distinctive immunoglobulin fold structure using two additional β strands, which distinguishes V domains from C domains and also has implications for V region function. Also, the processes of V(D)J recombination can further alter the germline–encoded length of V regions, subtly affecting V domain structure and function as well.

V regions form the amino-terminal domains of heavy and light chains, and their primary responsibility is the binding of antigen.

The promotion of the capacity to recognize antigenic determinants has been the driving force behind the evolution of V genes, both at the structural level of individual genes and for the evolution of the different V loci. When sequence data first became available from antibody proteins (see Fig. 3), it was apparent that great variation existed between V regions relative to that found between C regions. A means was developed to quantitate this variation whereby variability was defined as the number of different amino acids observed at a given position divided by the frequency of the most common amino acid at that position (25). Using this equation, an invariant residue would have a variability equal to one, whereas the theoretical upper limit for a position occupied by each of the 20 amino acids in a random fashion would be 400. This can be illustrated graphically by plotting the variability scores of a particular protein against its residue number, as is demonstrated in Fig. 4. Variability plots of this type established not only that V regions were characterized by diversity in their sequences, but that this variation was principally clustered in three regions, which were deemed *hypervariable regions* (HVRs). It was hypothesized that these highly variable segments of heavy and light chains would coordinate in such a way as to form the antigen-combining site

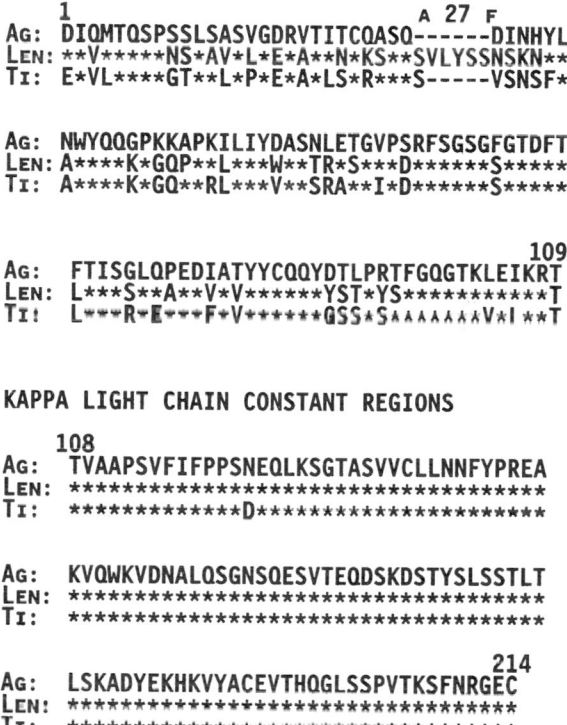

FIG. 3. Amino acid sequences of human antibody light chains. *Dashes* denote gaps introduced to optimally align sequences; *asterisks* represent identity relative to the top sequence. These are among the first immunoglobulin sequences ever obtained, demonstrating the dramatic differences in variation between V and C regions. The appearance of clusters of conserved residues within the different V domains also illustrates the necessity of a system to accurately quantify variations between several sequences (see Fig. 4). (Developed from the sequence compendium of Kabat et al. in ref. 24a.)

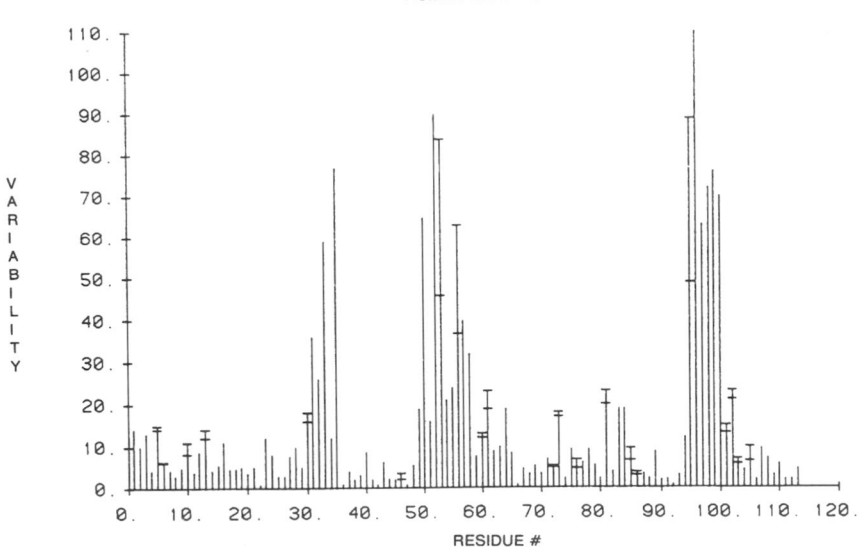

FIG. 4. Variability plot of human heavy chains. The hypervariable regions are apparent as the three obvious peaks in the graph. (From ref. 24a, with permission).

(reviewed in ref. 26); thus they were termed *complementarity-determining regions* (CDRs) as well.

Variability analysis also determined that other stretches of V region sequence were reasonably well conserved from protein to protein; these were presumed to perform basic structural functions necessary for proper folding of all V domains. Accordingly, they were dubbed *framework regions* (FRs) because they provide the platform that supports the CDRs. Structural analyses have confirmed that the FRs largely coincide with the β strands of the immunoglobulin fold, while CDRs, on the other hand, chiefly correspond to the loops that join β strands on the C region-distal end of the V domain. A linear representation of this association is shown in Fig. 5; note that CDRs 1, 2, and 3 join β strands B and C, C and D, and F and G, respectively. Significant sequence motifs are also apparent in this comparison of six V region proteins: a W/F-G-X-G motif in FR4 that is common to all V domains (27), the V_H-specific G-L-E-W-hydrophobic stretch in FR2 (28), and the V_L-specific sequence P-hydrophilic-hydrophobic-L-hydrophobic in the analogous FR2 location (28). These motifs are vital for proper dimerization of domains and will be discussed further in the section on quaternary immunoglobulin structure. Another important distinction between heavy and light chain V region sequences is also apparent in Fig. 5: relative to V_L domains, V_H regions generally utilize longer FR1 and CDR2 segments and shorter CDR1 and FR2 stretches. While the vast number of V genes precludes the ability to definitively assign boundaries for FRs and CDRs that are constant among all immunoglobulin V regions, Table 1 summarizes the traditional positions that delineate these areas for both heavy and light chains.

The presence of hundreds of different germline V region genes obviously contributes greatly to the sequence diversity of different variable domains. However, the somatic process of V(D)J recombination (see Chapter 5) further accentuates V region variability, specifically targeting the CDR3 of the protein (29). In this system, approximately 100 unique V genes (V_H, V_κ, or V_λ loci) encode the N-terminal FR1-CDR1-FR2-CDR2-FR3-5′CDR3 portions of V regions, while four to six "joining" (J) minigenes code for the carboxy-terminal 3′CDR3-FR4 segments. Heavy chains also incorporate one of about 30 short "diversity" (D) gene segments between V and J genes to generate complete V region domains. The relationship between rearranged V(D)J gene segments and the FR/CDR organization of the V region is schematically represented in Fig. 6. The combinatorial assortment of gene segments to form complete heavy and light chains, followed by the combinatorial assortment of heavy and light chains with each other to form antigen-binding V_H/V_L dimers, results in a practically limitless number of V domain structures. Moreover, during the recombination process itself, the activity of exonucleases and untemplated N-segment additions (29), templated P-nucleotide incorporation (30), and D-D fusion events (31) can boost the diversity of CDR3 even further. Finally, superimposed on these aspects of "combinatorial" and "junctional" diversity-generating mechanisms, somatic hypermutation (32,33; see Chapter 25) serves to introduce still more variation by altering residues throughout the V region.

Despite—and perhaps as a result of—the seemingly endless number of possible V region sequences, sophisticated schema have emerged for their classification. These groupings are based upon homology-based hierarchies that directly reflect the evolution of the antibody gene loci. Members of a group are more similar to each other than to all other sequences from other groups and share linked amino acid substitution patterns, which serve as "identifiers" for the various classifications. The most evolutionary distant grouping is, of course, that of the V regions themselves, followed by the V_H, V_κ, and V_λ distinctions, which represent the separate V gene loci. In humans, the heavy chain locus is found on chromosome 14, and the κ and λ loci are found on chromosomes 2 and 22, respectively (34–36). In the mouse, these genes are located on chromosomes 12, 6, and 16 (37–39). Other stratifications for V region organization also mirror the evolution of the antibody gene loci. The use of "clans" to categorize V genes has demonstrated the

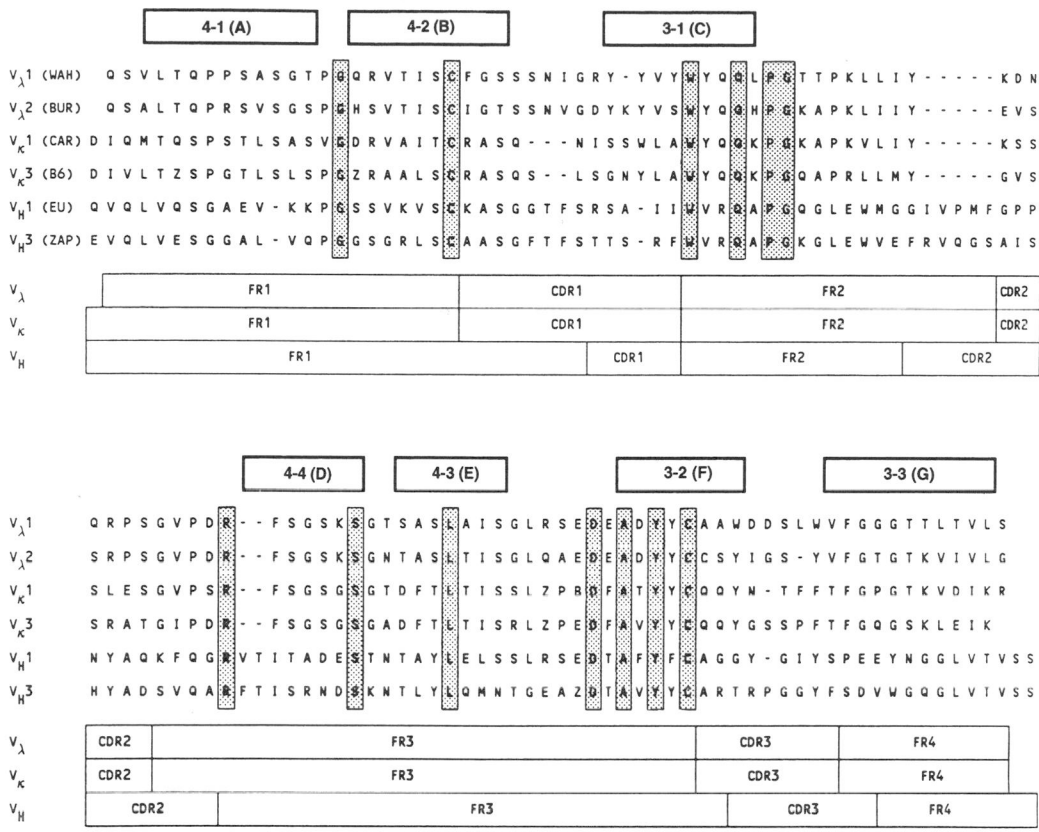

FIG. 5. Sequence alignment of six human V regions. Boxes above sequences represent β strands of the domains. Strands are numbered according to Edmundson and lettered (*in parentheses*) according to Hood. Gaps introduced to maximize homology are represented by *dashes*. Amino acids conserved among all six proteins are *boxed* and *shaded*. Boxes beneath the sequences depict the statistical boundaries of V region subdomains (see Table 1). Note differences in the lengths of the FR1, CDR1, FR2, and CDR2 segments between the four light chains and two heavy chains.

TABLE 1. *Boundaries delineating the statistical and structural subdomains of variable regions*

Subdomain region	Ig Chain	Residue positions	Boundaries of structural loop
FR1	Heavy	1–30	
	Light	1–23	
CDR1	Heavy	31–35*	H1: 26–32
	Light	24–34*	L1: 26–33
FR2	Heavy	36–49	
	Light	35–49	
CDR2	Heavy	50–65*	H2: 53–55
	Light	50–56	L2: 50–52
FR3	Heavy	66–94*	
	Light	57–88	
CDR3	Heavy	95–102*	H3: 96–101
	Light	89–97*	L3: 91–96
FR4	Heavy	103–113	
	Light	98 107*	

FR1–4 (framework regions), CDR1-3 (complementarity-determining regions), H1-3 (heavy chain variable loops), and L1-3 (light chain variable loops) are numbered according to Kabat et al (1) using an alignment giving priority to conserved residues. Asterisks indicate regions which may have length variations depending upon germline V gene usage and/or junctional diversity. Data for the table were compiled from Kabat et al. (24a) and Chothia and Lesk (28a).

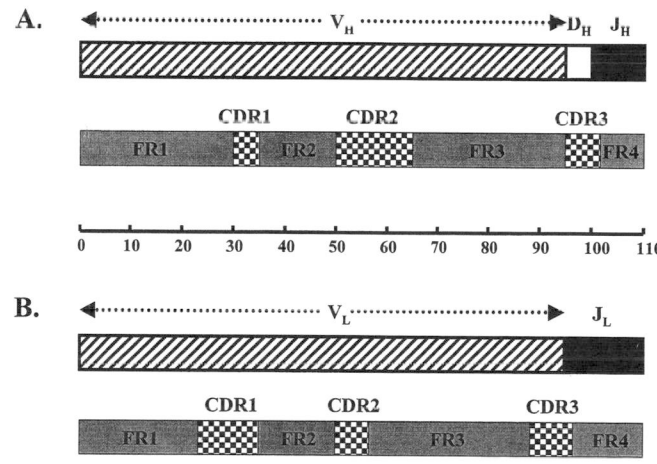

FIG. 6. Comparison of the gene structures and protein subdomains of rearranged V regions. (**A**) Heavy chain V domain. (**B**) Light chain V domain. The V_H and V_L gene segments are represented as *hatched boxes*, the D_H gene segment as a *white box*, and the J_H and J_L gene segments as *black boxes*. Framework regions (FRs) are displayed as *shaded boxes* and complementarity-determining regions (CDRs) are pictured as *checkered boxes*. An approximate amino acid scale separates the two diagrams.

development of V loci across several vertebrate species (see Fig. 7) for both heavy and light chains (40–44). Three V_H clans have been recognized using nucleotide sequence homology comparisons across the FR1 6–24 codon interval. While this stretch of FR1 sequence is conserved within a clan, a similar span (the 67–85 codon interval of FR3) can also be used to discriminate between V_H genes that belong to the same clan but differ in regard to the next level of classification, that of the family.

Classically, families are the groupings that have been used most frequently to identify and categorize V region genes relative to one another (reviewed in refs. 45–47). Members of a V region family share about 80% identity at the DNA level. Historically, when genomic Southern blotting was used to work out approximate family sizes, this degree of homology allowed for sufficient cross-hybridization to occur under low-stringency conditions, accounting for the utility of the family designation. At the protein level, this translates to levels of about 75% identity between gene products from the same family and less than 70% homology for proteins belonging to different families. Using these criteria, human V_H genes may be segregated into seven families, V_κ into four major families, and V_λ into ten families. The murine system (which contains larger absolute numbers of V genes) is more complicated, as evidenced by the fact that 14 V_H and 20 V_κ families have been recognized. Example sequences from several human V_κ and V_H gene families are aligned in Fig. 8. Note the presence of numerous "shared substitutions" within pairs of sequences belonging to the same family that are not present in the other sequences. These serve as distinctive "signature residues," which facilitate rapid identification of a particular sequence's "family of origin." The sequences in Fig. 8 also demonstrate another important characteristic of V gene families: Different families frequently possess different CDR lengths. Thus, independent of amino acid sequence, V

region families intrinsically possess differing binding-site structures, thereby affecting their functional capabilities.

Shared substitutions have also been used to further refine families into subfamilies. Subfamilies, as are all classification schema to some extent, are particularly arbitrary divisions, largely because the parameters used to define subfamilies are not standardized. Generally, the features that describe a particular subfamily are esoteric and depend upon the specific characteristic(s) being studied. Finally, at the most descriptive level of classification, the work of Rabbitts, Winter, Honjo, and many others (46–50) has resulted in the identification, mapping, and—to some extent—sequencing of presumably most, if not all, human V region genes. Within a family, single V gene segments may be compared against a consensus sequence representing that family (Fig. 9). When such a comparison is performed, it becomes clear that individual V genes' divergence is focused primarily in their CDR1 and CDR2 segments (42). Thus, on the basis of primary sequence structural information, even closely related V genes may be predicted to adopt similar framework cores but differ in terms of their CDR1 and CDR2 loops such that a plethora of potential antigenic specificities are encoded genomically. In fact, even at the level of the individual V gene variability persists in this system. As one might expect with "variable" genes, allelic variation and polymorphism of the antibody loci exists as well—such that it is probably safe to conclude that all of the possible incarnations of immunoglobulin V genes will never truly be identified and categorized. Suffice to say, then, that the variable gene loci, clans, families, subfamilies, and even individual V genes themselves all derive from gene duplication events; only the period in evolutionary time at which the duplication occurred truly separates one gene or group of genes from any another.

While V regions provide the surfaces that interact with "foreign" antigenic determinants, constant regions perform the function of

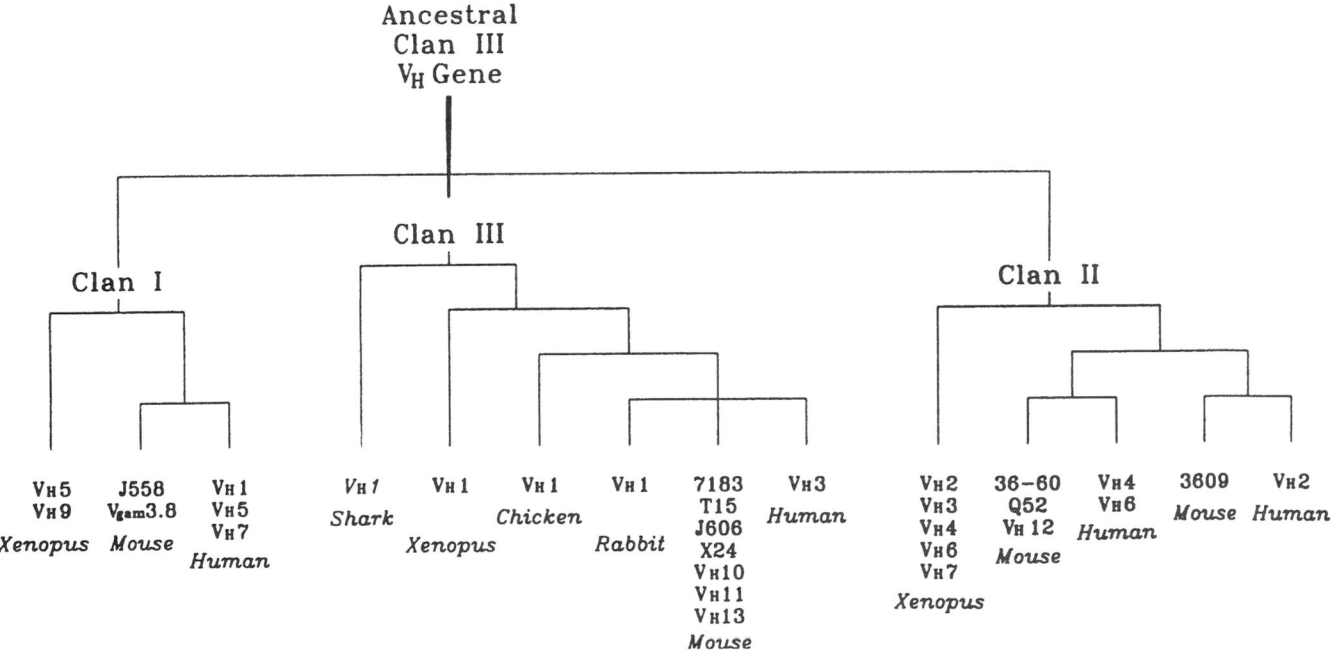

FIG. 7. Clan groupings segregate V_H genes across vertebrate species into distinct clusters of sequences. Note that several different V_H families in a given species can be present within a single clan, reflecting their underlying structural similarity. The lines depicting evolutionary relatedness are not drawn to scale. (From ref. 42, with permission).

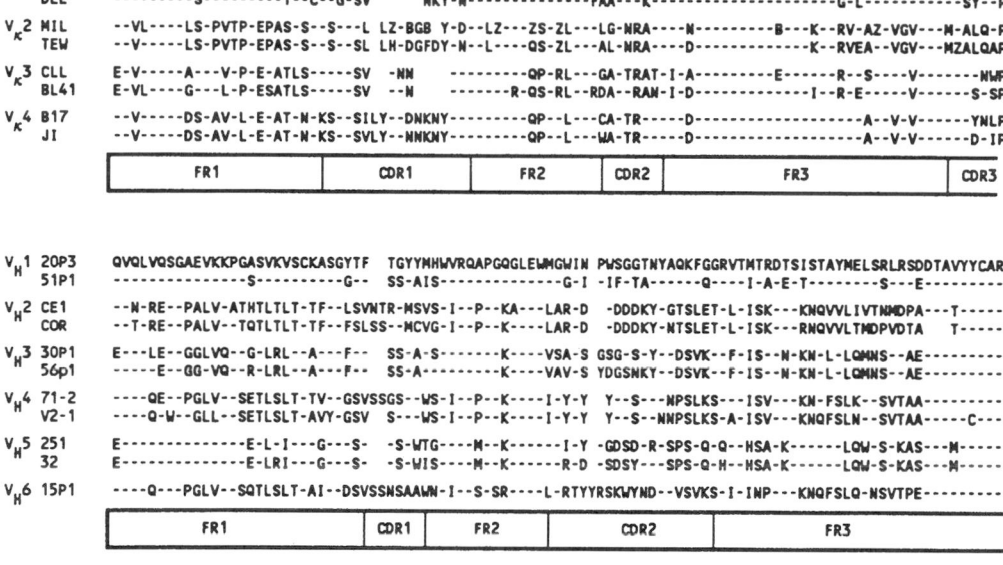

FIG. 8. Representative sequences from several human V_κ and V_H families. Gaps introduced to optimally align the sequences are indicated by *blank spaces*. Identity between residues in the top sequence and those below it is signified by *dashes*. Canonical boundaries for FRs and CDRs are schematized beneath both the light chain and heavy chain sequence groupings. Note the presence of many "shared substitutions" (amino acids common to two sequences belonging to the same family, but absent in sequences from other families).

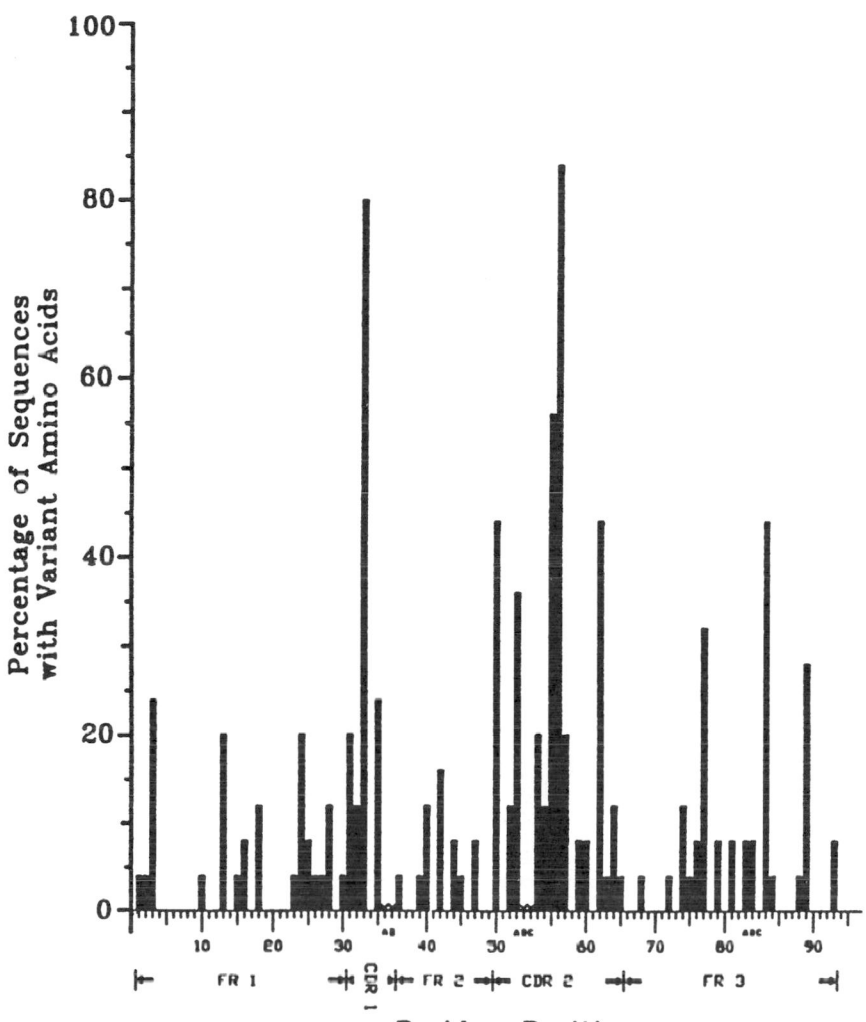

FIG. 9. Sequence variation within a V region family. Twenty-five unique germline sequences from the murine V_H 7183 family were used to generate a consensus sequence for the family. Divergence from the consensus 7183 sequence is represented as the percentage of sequences having a variant amino acid (an amino acid different from the consensus residue) at a particular position. Like the variability plot of heavy chains from multiple families (see Fig. 4), highly divergent positions within the same family also tend to localize to the CDRs. (From ref. 42, with permission.)

binding to the "self" molecules that mediate physiologic and immunologic effector pathways. Light chains have one constant region domain (either C_κ or C_λ) C-terminal to the V_L. The C_L pairs with the first constant region domain of the heavy chain (C_H1) using hydrophobic and disulfide interactions to stabilize heavy and light chain coupling. C_L is not known to specifically bind any other biological moities; therefore, no known effector properties are attributable to light chain C regions. By contrast, all known quaternary associations, biologic characteristics, and physiologic functions of immunoglobulins are governed by heavy chain C regions. Depending upon antibody isotype, heavy chain C regions consist of either three or four C_H domains. The first domain (C_H1) mediates association with C_L as detailed above and is part of the Fab fragment, while the following two (or three) C-terminal domains participate in interchain binding between heavy chain molecules and collectively comprise the Fc. Connection between C_H1 domains of μ and ε antibodies and their respective Fc is accomplished by specialized C_H domains ($C_\mu2$ or $C_\varepsilon2$) that allow for flexibility of the Fabs, yet maintain features of other Ig constant domains. Antibodies of the γ, α, and δ classes, however, utilize a shorter flexible hinge segment for this purpose, which will be specifically detailed elsewhere.

While initial studies indicated that C region sequences were reasonably highly conserved—at least relative to V regions (refer to Fig. 3)—their designation as "constant" is actually somewhat of a misnomer. For instance, studies comparing V and C regions from primitive species have suggested that the lengths of the loops connecting the β strands of constant regions actually vary more than do those of variable regions (51). Furthermore, between different isotypes of the same species, C_H regions share only about 30% sequence identity overall (Fig. 10). C region domains differ in

regard to their interclass homologies such that different domains show various levels of sequence conservation. C_H1 domains are the most similar between isotypes; this may derive from the fact that all share the common function of pairing with immunoglobulin light chains. Similarly, the carboxy-terminal domains of μ, α, and γ ($C_\mu4$, $C_\alpha3$, and $C_\gamma3$) are substantially more related than the average for their Fc as a whole. As x-ray studies have indicated close contact exists between the C-terminal domains of the Fc, this sequence conservation may result from similar constraints as for the C_H1/C_L situation. Moreover, in the case of the μ and α chains, the relatively higher homology likely reflects the common role of the last domain in multimer formation. Also note that the $C_\mu4$ and $C_\alpha3$ domains each possess an 18-amino acid "tailpiece" at their C-termini. The penultimate cysteine residue in each sequence contributes to an intersubunit disulfide bond, allowing IgM and IgA polymerization (52). Much like the V region paradigm, a hierarchy of shared substitutions can be used to distinguish sequences of different domains, classes, and subclasses. In all comparisons between isotypes, however, it is apparent that the majority of conserved residues are localized to the β strands. As was the situation with the V region FRs, these strands are responsible for the proper folding of the domain. In addition, the two cysteines that form the intrachain disulfide bond, and the tryptophan which protects it from solvent reduction, are preserved among all C_H sequences as well.

In analogous fashion to V region evolution, the five heavy chain isotypes likely arose by duplication and diversification of a common gene precursor. This probably occurred in an ancestral organism that preceded mammalian speciation, because examples of all five classes appear in all mammals. Actually, interspecies sequence comparisons of a given isotype demonstrate their similarity far exceeds that of the different isotypes within a species (compare

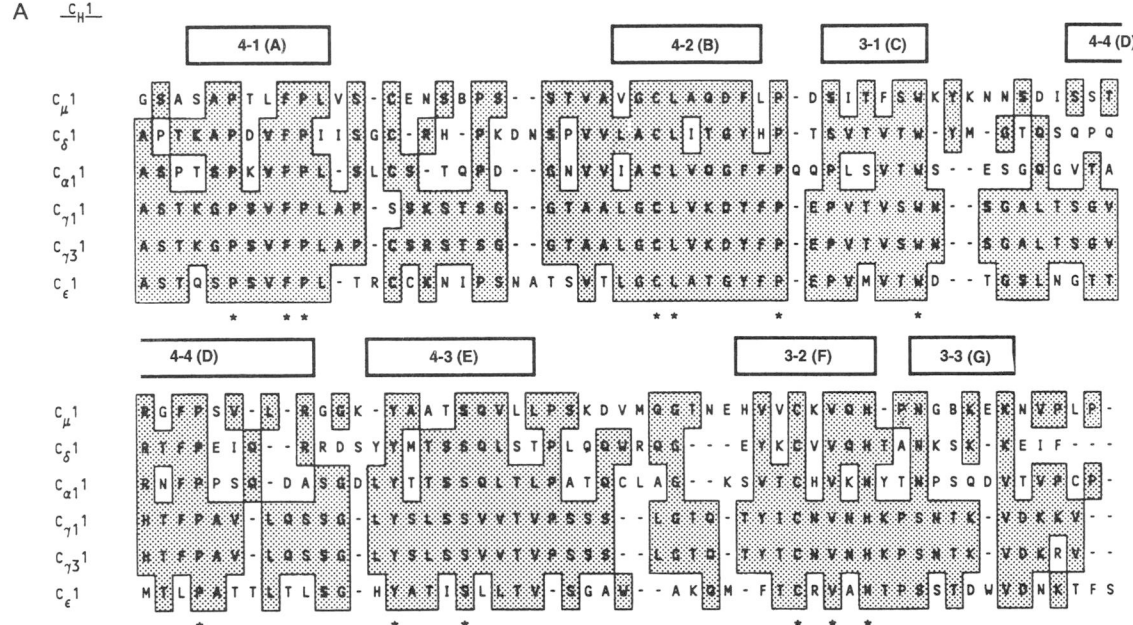

FIG. 10. Comparison of the amino acid sequences of the (A) C_H1 and (B) Fc regions of all human isotypes (excluding the γ2, γ4, and α2 subclasses). *Boxed* and *shaded* amino acids represent residues shared by two or more isotypes. *Asterisks* mark amino acids conserved among all six sequences. *Dashes* indicate gaps introduced to maximize homology between sequences. β strands are numbered according to Edmundson and lettered (*in parentheses*) according to Hood in *white boxes* above the alignments.

Figs. 10A and 11). Subclasses represent more recent gene duplication events. Accordingly, distinct subclass profiles exist in various mammalian species. For instance, while humans have two α loci and hence two IgA subclasses (53), murine species have only one α gene, and rabbits have 13 (54)! Due to their later evolutionary divergence, heavy chain subclasses display greater sequence similarity—on the order of 60% to 90%—as evidenced by the γ1 and γ3 alignments depicted in Fig. 10. Despite the high levels of concordance between C regions of related subclasses, even slight differences can have profound functional repercussions. As an example, among the four human IgG subclasses (whose sequences are over 95% identical to one another), IgG1 and IgG3 bind to macrophages and other phagocytes with ease, while IgG2 and IgG4 bind very poorly. This binding is mediated by an Fcγ receptor that has been extensively characterized (detailed later within this chapter). Similar subtle sequence differences are also involved in functional properties affecting immunoglobulin catabolism, placental transfer, and reactivity with staphylococcal protein A (SPA). It is this selective pressure for the ability to perform in a variety of functional capacities that has both maintained the five major C_H classes throughout mammalian species and also driven the evolution of subclasses to their points of divergence in these same

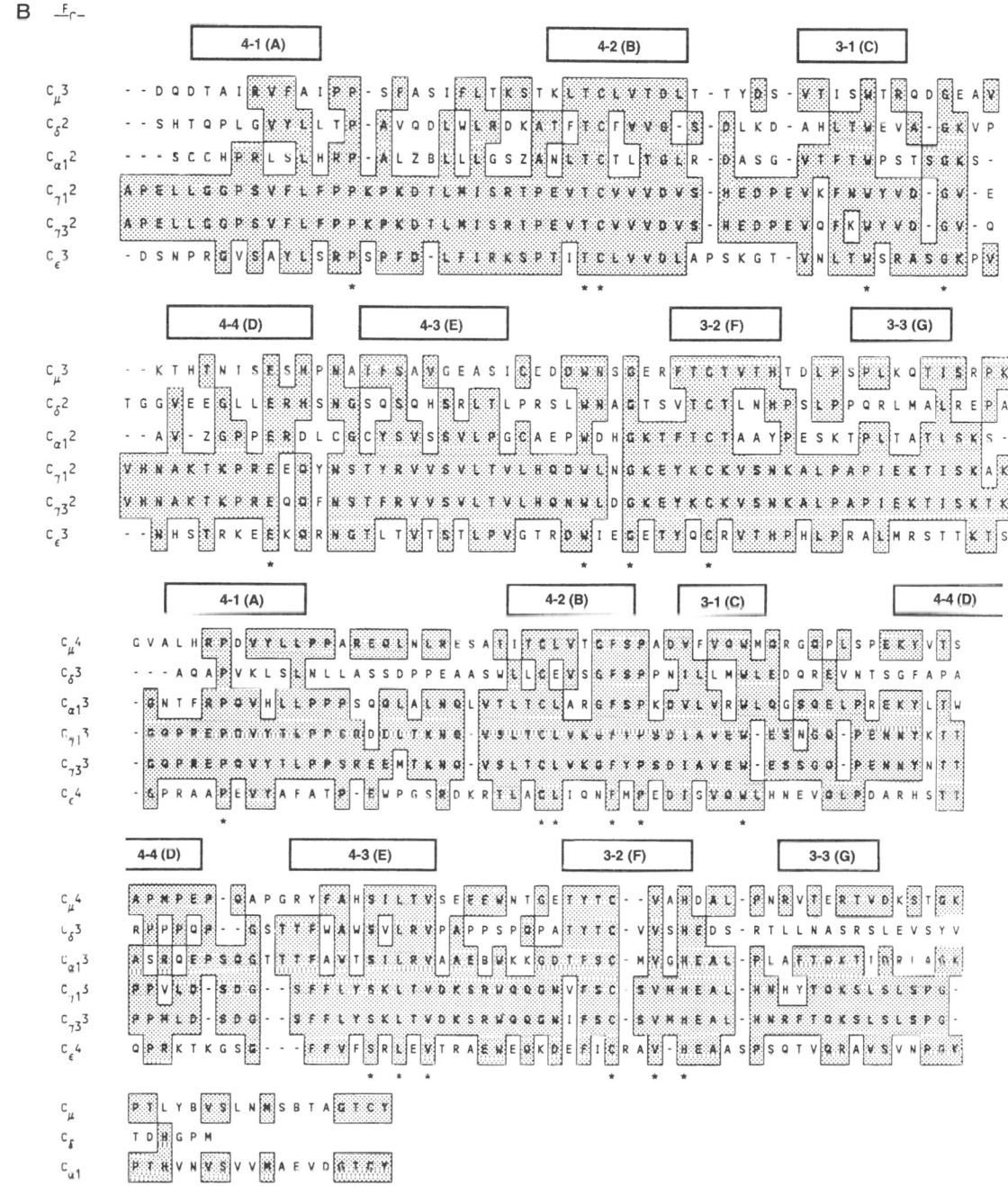

FIG. 10. *Continued*

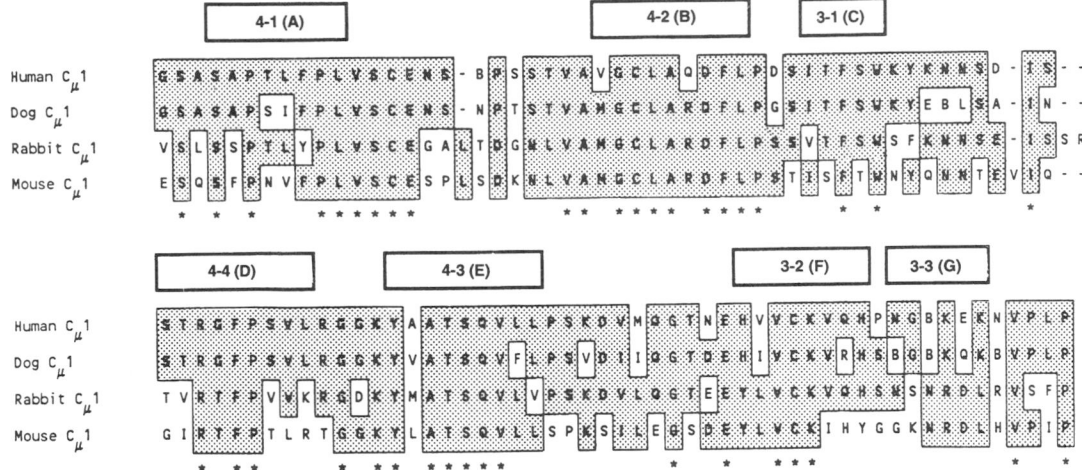

FIG. 11. Protein sequence alignments of the $C_\mu 1$ domains from four mammalian species. Labels are as for Fig. 10. Note the paucity of gapping required and also the high number of absolutely conserved residues (*) across species relative to the alignments of the different human $C_H 1$ isotypes in Fig. 10A.

species. Collectively, these evolutionary changes have bestowed upon the different isotypes the ability to respond to antigenic challenge in a variety of immunologically productive ways.

Despite the absence of evidence to suggest that light chain C regions participate in biologically significant interactions (other than coupling with heavy chains), multiple forms of C_L have also been identified. First, the light chain isotypes C_κ and C_λ—while functionally indistinguishable—exist as separate genetic loci with their own complement of possible V and J gene segment partners. This is in contrast to the situation with the heavy chain locus, in which any rearranged VDJ can potentially become associated with any C_H isotype via the process of class switching (see Chapter 24). While the use of κ versus λ isotypes seems to be inconsequential as to the antibody's efficacy, differences in their utilization are nonetheless present. In human immunoglobulins the $\kappa:\lambda$ ratio is approximately 70:30, while in murine systems about 95% of antibody is of the κ class (20). The reasons for these imbalances are yet to be definitively explained, but are probably related to the number of V_κ and V_λ genes available for use in the respective genomes of these organisms. As was the case for heavy chain C regions, light chain isotypes are well conserved across species (Fig. 12). In addition, within a species, κ and λ classes are more similar to each other (about 38%) than were the different C_H isotypes (compare Figs. 10 and 12). Note also the presence of a terminal (C_κ) or penultimate (C_λ) cysteine residue in these sequences. This half-cystine is responsible for the light chain's contribution to the H–L interchain disulfide bond. A second point of variation within C_L regions concerns C_λ subclasses. While only a single C_κ gene is present in human and mouse, five or four λ-chain subclasses exist in human or murine genomes, respectively. A final deviation from "constancy" involves the C_κ domain. While only one κ constant region gene is found in the locus, three human κ allotypes have been identified. These alleles differ in regard to their residues at the surface-exposed positions 153 and 191, such that these allotypic markers are able to serve as antigenic determinants (55).

As mentioned previously, hinges—either as distinct domains in the cases of the μ and ϵ chains or as shorter specialized segments for α, γ, and δ antibodies—connect the Fab and Fc portions of the immunoglobulin molecule. However, the lack of extensive hinge structure in nonmammalian heavy chain sequences indicates that the evolution of this function largely occurred after mammalian radiation (51). Consequently, discussion here is restricted to mammalian hinges as typified by human sequences.

Hinge regions not only connect Fab to Fc, but also contain the disulfide bonds that covalently link the two heavy chains (discussed further in the section on quaternary structure) in the Fc portion of the antibody molecule. They display great variability between isotypes and are generally encoded by unique exons. For example, the hinges of human IgG1, IgG2, and IgG4 are each produced from a single short exon encoding a peptide of between 12 and 15 amino acids. Alternatively, the IgG3 hinge derives from four distinct exons, resulting in a hinge region that spans approximately four times as many residues as the other γ isotypes (56). Owing to similarities between the different hinge sequences and the extra C_μ and C_ϵ domain sequences, it is thought that hinges evolved from the $C_{\mu/\epsilon}2$ domain; unfortunately the hinge sequences are too short and the homologies too weak to trace hinge lineage with certainty. It is clear from sequence comparisons, however, that the $C_\gamma 3$ hinge evolved from the $C_\gamma 1$ hinge by multiple duplication (further substantiated by the aforementioned $C_\gamma 1$ and $C_\gamma 3$ hinge exon arrangements). Figure 13 aligns the extra domains of C_μ and C_ϵ, in addition to the hinges of several other human isotypes.

In addition to the variable, constant, and hinge regions of antibodies, other primary sequence features must also be considered. For instance, both heavy and light chains of immunoglobulin are synthesized with a leader peptide (almost entirely encoded by a separate exon upstream of the V region) of 16 to 26 amino acids in length. During translation, this leader (more generally referred to as a signal peptide) directs the mRNA/ribosome/polypeptide complex to the rough endoplasmic reticulum (RER) where translation is completed. During the synthesis and extrusion of the nascent polypeptide through the RER membrane, the signal peptide is then removed by specific proteolytic cleavage.

Finally, for a comprehensive discussion of primary immunoglobulin structure, mention must be made of sequences present exclusively in the case of surface immunoglobulin expression. Heavy

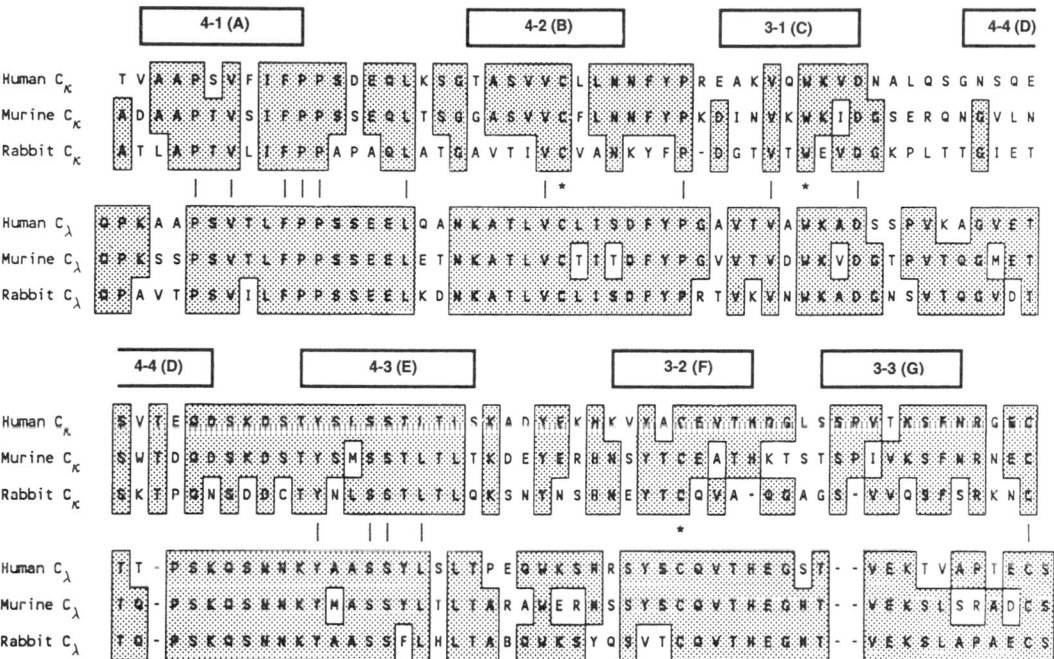

FIG. 12. Comparison of the C_κ and C_λ domains from three mammalian species. Labeling is as for Figs. 10 and 11, except *vertical lines* now represent amino acids shared among all six sequences and *asterisks* specifically denote the invariant tryptophan and cysteines at the core of the domain (also shared by all sequences). As in Fig. 11, little gapping is needed and high homology persists across species.

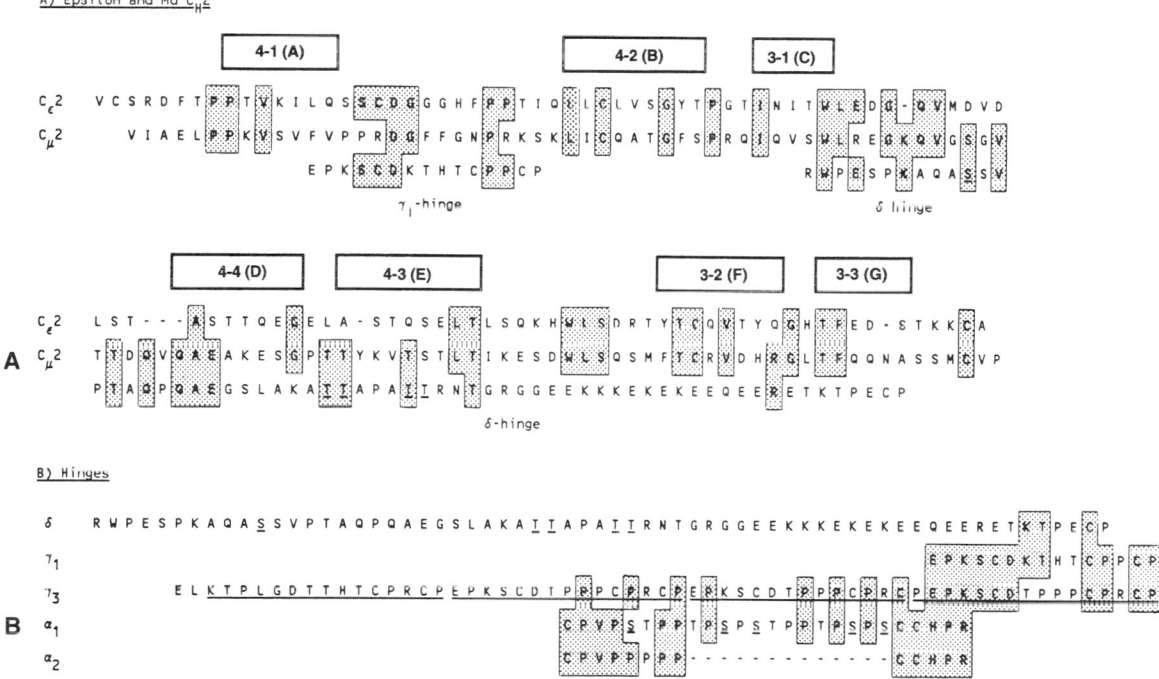

FIG. 13. Alignment of the amino acid sequences of (**A**) the human $C_\mu 2$ and $C_\epsilon 2$ domains and the $\gamma 1$ and δ hinges and (**B**) several human immunoglobulin hinge regions. Labeling is as for Figs. 10–12. In (**A**), the $C_{\mu/\epsilon}2$ domains are compared with the hinges of two different isotypes to display their potential, although limited, evolutionary relationship. Part (**D**) demonstrates several features of hinge regions. Note the high proline, cysteine, and serine/threonine content of the hinges, which consists of the bulk of the homologies between isotypes. This interclass homology is reasonably low, whereas intersubclass homologies (compare $\gamma 1$ to $\gamma 3$ and $\alpha 1$ to $\alpha 2$) are considerably higher. Note the fourfold duplication of the $\gamma 1$ hinge in $\gamma 3$ (the repeating unit is *underlined*). Also note the deletion within the $\alpha 2$ hinge relative to $\alpha 1$. O-linked glycosylation sites in the δ and $\alpha 1$ hinges are also *underlined*.

chains of all isotypes can exist either as secreted antibody or as membrane-bound immunoglobulin (mIg), which serves as the central component of the antigen-specific B cell receptor (BCR). The choice between mIg and secreted immunoglobulin is manifest at the level of alternative mRNA splicing at the 3′ end of the message. Differential processing in favor of the surface immunoglobulin form results in the replacement of the hydrophilic carboxy-terminal residues of secreted antibody with a stretch of hydrophobic amino acids (which anchors the immunoglobulin in the cell membrane) and a short cytoplasmic tail (57,58). Expression of these sequences not only tethers the immunoglobulin to the cell surface, but also governs the ability of mIg to interact with other constituents of the BCR necessary for signal propagation and eventual activation by antigen (see Chapter 7). As such, the regulation of this splicing event and its ultimate protein products is tightly controlled through the stages of B lymphocyte differentiation so as to ensure the proper production of membrane immunoglobulin versus secreted antibody at the appropriate developmental stage of the B cell (see Chapters 5 and 6).

Secondary Structure—The Immunoglobulin Fold

With the exceptions of the hinge and cytoplasmic tail, the properties of the immunoglobulin fold as a protein motif dominate all aspects of immunoglobulin structure, from primary to quaternary. In regard to secondary structure, this refers to the different patterns of β-pleated sheet formation assumed by the V and C regions. As explained earlier, all immunoglobulin folds are composed of two layers of antiparallel β sheet arranged in a sandwich (or β-barrel) that encloses a hydrophobic interior. Early on, it was recognized that each immunoglobulin domain contains seven polypeptide β strands, four of which comprise one β-pleated sheet, the other sheet consisting of the remaining three strands. Accordingly, a nomenclature was developed that reflected within which β sheet (four-stranded or three-stranded) a particular strand was located, using numbering (3-1, 3-2, 3-3 and 4-1, 4-2, 4-3, 4-4). Subsequent stud-

ies revealed that superimposed upon this secondary structural organization shared by all immunoglobulin folds was a discrepancy between V and C region immunoglobulin folds; some of the "extra" amino acid residues found in variable regions actually participated in β sheet formation, giving rise to two additional β strands. Consequently, the immunoglobulin folds of V domains actually form a barrel using five-stranded (analogous to the C region three-strand sheet) and four-stranded β-pleated sheet layers. A second naming system using letter designations (A, B, C, C′, C″, D, E, F, and G) for the different strands of immunoglobulin fold β-pleated sheets makes allowance for these extra β strands. Figure 14 displays "unfolded" immunoglobulin folds of each type so as to schematically represent the secondary structure of both V and C immunoglobulin domains. Note that while the letter nomenclature proceeds in accordance with the primary structure of the protein (A, B, C, D, etc.), the numbering system of β strands is nonlinear with respect to the primary sequence (4-1, 4-2, 3-1, 4-4, 4-3, 3-2, 3-3). Rather, this naming system is designed so as to coincide with the three-dimensional orientation of the strands in the context of the fully folded immunoglobulin domain (refer back to Fig. 2), which will be discussed in greater detail below.

Tertiary Structure—The Immunoglobulin Domain

Logically, if the β sheets of the immunoglobulin fold are the dominant secondary structural protein motif of the antibody, then the fully-folded tertiary structural correlate of this paradigm is that of the immunoglobulin domain. As has been explained, Ig domains are founded upon the premise of two layers of β-pleated sheet, sandwiched around a core of hydrophobic side chains, to form a compact globular structure. Of course, upon this general structural framework, Ig domains vary considerably. Still, certain features common to all Ig domains of actual immunoglobulin molecules (as opposed to Ig domains of other IgSF members) are invariant. Central to the Ig domain, both literally and figuratively, is the presence of the two cysteines that form the intradomain disulfide bond and

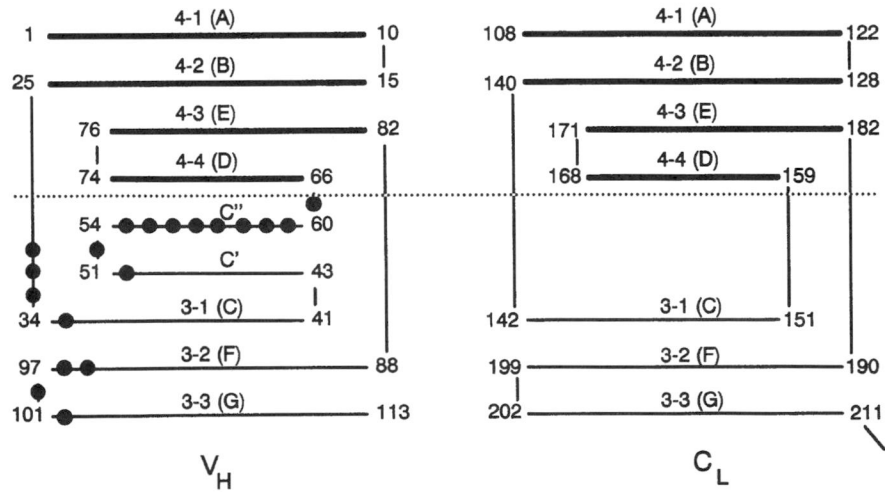

FIG. 14. Schematic diagram of the secondary structure of "unfolded" immunoglobulin domains. β strands are represented by *horizontal lines,* loops connecting β strands are depicted as *vertical lines. Bold horizontal lines* are in the four-stranded face of the domain, *light horizontal lines* are in the three- (five-) stranded β sheet. *Dotted regions* denote CDRs. Strands are numbered according to Edmundson and lettered (*in parenthesis*) according to Hood. In three dimensions, immunoglobulin domains are folded with the *light horizontal strands* under the *bold horizontal strands* using the dotted line as an axis.

the tryptophan which protects this bond from hydrolysis. All domains of immunoglobulin—variable region or constant, heavy chain or light–conserve these three key residues, and they occupy homologous positions in the different domains of the fully-folded protein.

Beyond these key core residues, however, different Ig domains are still able to maintain similar tertiary structures in the face of dramatic differences in their primary sequences. This chiefly derives from the fact that the identity of a particular residue at a particular position is not nearly so important to proper Ig domain folding as is the character of the particular residue at that position. In other words, as long as amino acids with side chains compatible with β-pleated sheet formation are present in the proper locations and those necessary to terminate β strands are similarly in the correct places, their actual identity appears not to be crucial.

There are, of course, other residues essential to proper folding and functioning of Ig domains, but these are specific to particular domains and not common to all Ig domains within immunoglobulin. For example, the FR4 motif W/F-G-X-G is widely conserved, but only among V regions, where it serves to create a "β bulge" necessary for proper V_H/V_L dimerization. Similarly, the V_H-specific (G-L-E-W-hydrophobic) and V_L-specific (P-hydrophilic-hydrophobic-L-hydrophobic) FR2 sequence motifs—and their accompanying β bulges—are also conserved tertiary structures among their respective subsets of Ig domains. Finally, as was discussed in secondary structure, V and C domains also differ in terms of their basic arrangement of the immunoglobulin fold such that V domains are composed of a four-strand (A, B, E, and D) and a five-strand (C", C', C, F, and G) layer, whereas C domains consist of four-stranded (A, B, E, and D) and three-stranded (C, F, and G) β sheets. Clearly, this distinguishes variable and constant domains at the tertiary structural level as well.

Once again, as with primary and secondary structural considerations, examination of tertiary structure can be facilitated by distinguishing between V and C domains. In the case of variable regions, whether from heavy or light chains, obviously no single protein structure will ever fully suffice in describing the entire group. This is because each domain, V_H or V_L, is in effect a new structure, and unless solved crystallographically, can only be postulated. Nonetheless, two broad generalities as pertains to V region tertiary structure are evident. First, the similarity between two different V domain structures tends to closely parallel their relatedness at the genetic level; that is, one can reasonably predict that two different V_H structures will be more similar to each other than to a V_L structure, two V_H domains belonging to the same clan will be more similar than to one from a different clan, and so on. Colorplates 1 and 2, which compare molecular models of FR1 regions from antibodies belonging to the same and different clans, are particularly compelling in this regard. While undoubtedly exceptions exist where two proteins are genetically similar but diverge at a few key residues with important structural consequences, in most instances this rule is valid for extrapolating the tertiary structures of unsolved V domains. In this context, it is perhaps also important to note that the FR1 region utilized to assign clan identity is solvent exposed and distal to the antigen-binding site, while the FR3 region which correlates best with family designation is immediately adjacent to the binding site, and capable of affecting its conformation and even interacting with antigen directly (42). In light of several reports linking over-representation of certain families in the repertoires reactive against particular antigenic specificities, the tertiary

structural predictions available by this means perhaps take on added significance.

The second pervasive trend which is apparent upon scrutiny of V region tertiary structures is the tendency of the antigen-binding site to represent a "nested gradient of antibody diversity" (42). Recall, investigations into the very first antibody proteins identified nonconserved "hypervariable" regions and reasonably well-conserved "framework" regions, which were in turn postulated to correspond to the antigen-binding and structural foundations, respectively, of the molecule. These hypotheses proved correct, as the FRs were demonstrated to coincide with the β strands, and the CDRs were shown to derive from the variable loops that interconnect the strands. Moreover, current understanding of antibody structure makes it possible to recognize that, as a general rule, the most variable residues of an immunoglobulin V region localize immediately proximal to the antigen-binding site, whereas those that are most conserved tend to be distant to that site. Colorplate 3 provides one such example of this concept. Thus, the three-dimensional context in which amino acids interact to create a platform for ligand-binding (paratope) diverges dramatically from antibody to antibody.

There are several factors that influence the tertiary structure of the paratope itself, and their composite effect can be complex. First, sequence variation of two types in the loops can profoundly alter antigenic specificity and affinity. CDRs vary considerably in length, both as a function of V gene usage (affecting primarily CDRs 1 and 2) and as a consequence of junctional diversity (affecting only CDR3). Second, CDRs obviously differ significantly in terms of their sequence composition, due once again to gene usage and junctional diversity, and in addition to somatic hypermutation. In this way, diversity-generating mechanisms target amino acid variability to the CDR loops where they are most apt to change both the physical shape and chemical nature of the combining site. Also, because FR residues near CDR boundaries frequently interact with antigen directly (59), alterations in these positions affect structural variety as well. Even glycosylation of CDR asparagine residues has been implicated in changing loop conformation and antigen binding (60,61). Conformational variability can also play a critical role in diversifying the paratope surface, as CDR loops have been shown to interact extensively with adjacent FR amino acids and with each other (62,63). These studies, and failed attempts to engineer antibodies by simply swapping CDRs onto different FR backbones without appreciably affecting affinity for antigen, have further demonstrated that while V regions can be conveniently dissected into FRs and CDRs at the primary structural level, in actuality these elements cooperate to facilitate antigen-binding rather than acting as discrete elements.

While the limitless capacity of the immune system to generate new variable region domains makes impossible the absolute elucidation of all potential V region structures, the relatively smaller number of constant regions has allowed reasonable progress to be made in terms of assigning definitive tertiary structures to the C region domains. To date, x-ray diffraction analysis has resulted in a high resolution structure for only the Fc fragment of IgG1 (11). An α-carbon backbone of this structure is shown in Fig. 15A. Additionally, one whole immunoglobulin (an unusual IgG1 molecule with a hinge deletion) has been crystallized (64). Other Fc isotypes, based on the Fcγl paradigm, can be modeled (see Fig. 15B) using sequence homology with IgG and energy minimization calculations (65). Otherwise, almost all three dimensional studies have utilized Fab fragments or Fv fragments, often produced in

A

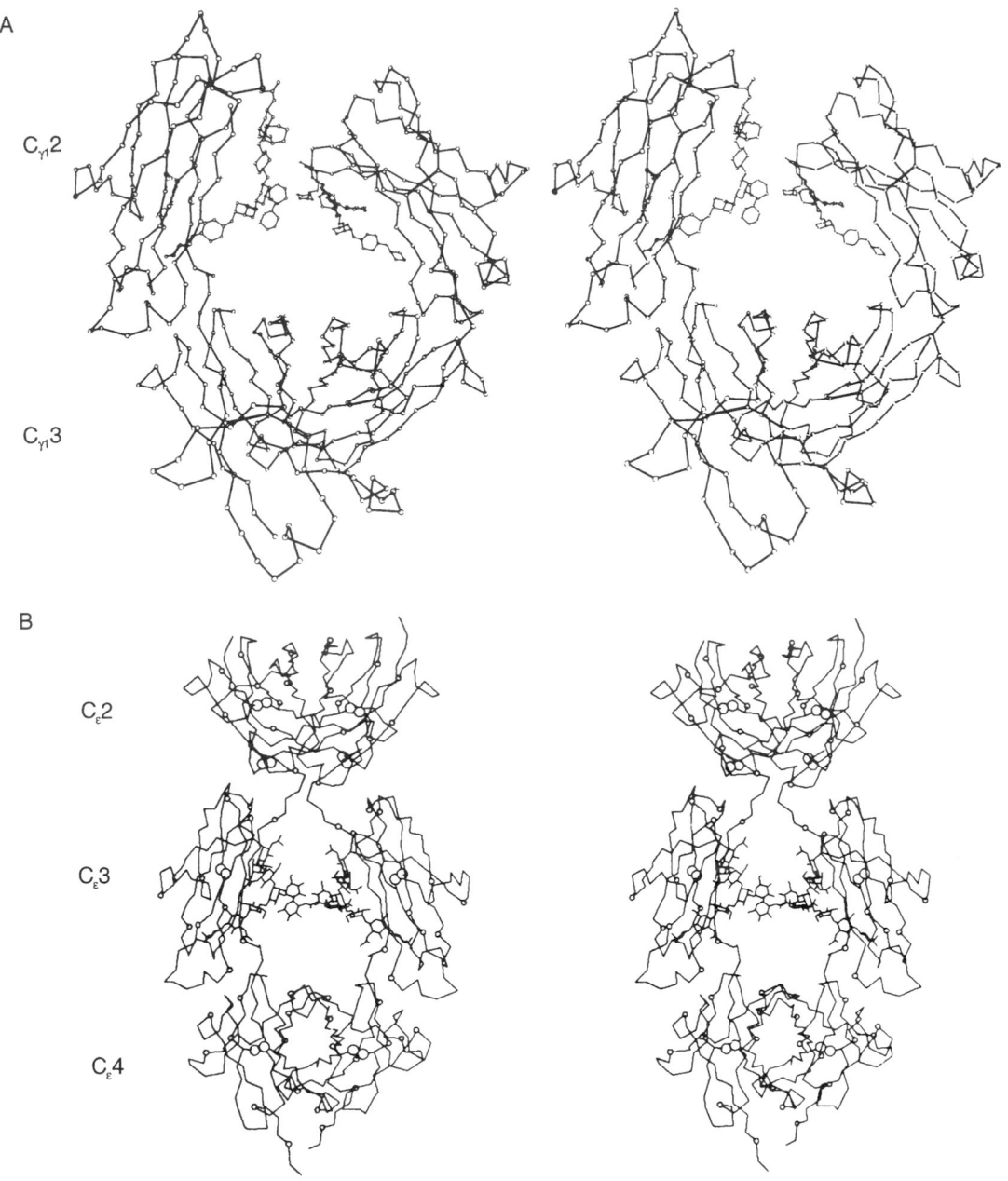

$C_{\gamma}2$

$C_{\gamma}3$

B

$C_{\varepsilon}2$

$C_{\varepsilon}3$

$C_{\varepsilon}4$

FIG. 15. Stereoviews of the α-carbon backbones of (**A**) Fcγ1 and (**B**) Fcε. In both cases, the C-terminal domains dimerize, but the penultimate domains ($C_{\gamma}2$ or $C_{\varepsilon}3$) contact their counterparts only via their carbohydrate moieties. The Fcε structure is a prediction modeled on the IgG1 crystal. As IgG has no $C_{\varepsilon}2$ domain equivalent, the $C_{\varepsilon}2$ structure is less reliable conjecture than is the rest of the molecule. (From refs. 12 and 65, with permission.)

bacteria. Of note, the IgG Fc crystal has also been solved as a co-crystal with staphylococcal protein A (SPA) (12). Importantly, this structure reveals the binding of SPA between both the $C_{\gamma}2$ and $C_{\gamma}3$ domains. This is contrary to the notion originally promulgated that single domains would perform IgG functions. Another example of sharing of function between domains is the Fcα receptor binding site on human IgA, which also involves both $C_{\alpha}2$ and $C_{\alpha}3$ (66). Surprising results such as these demonstrate the need for continuing investigation—by both crystallographic and other means—into the structural intricacies of all of the immunoglobulin isotypes. In

any case, in the intervening time, the general properties of Fc topology, though proven only for IgG, are reasonably generalized to the other isotypes, since the residues involved in the various contacts are largely conserved.

As for the V region domains, constant region domain structure is governed by general principles that tend to hold true in most examples of C region domains thus far studied. The overriding consideration in this regard, as for the V domains, concerns the relative concentration of variability outside the β strands. C regions conserve a much higher percentage of residues from domain to

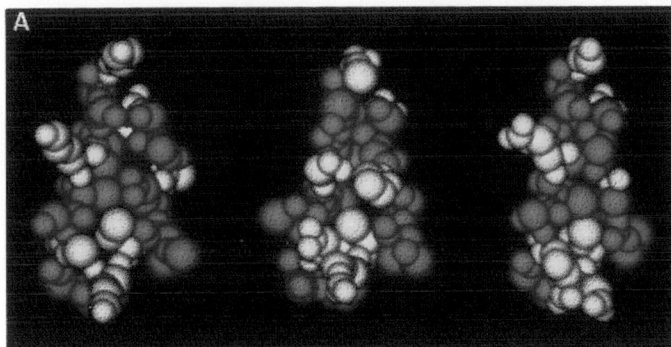
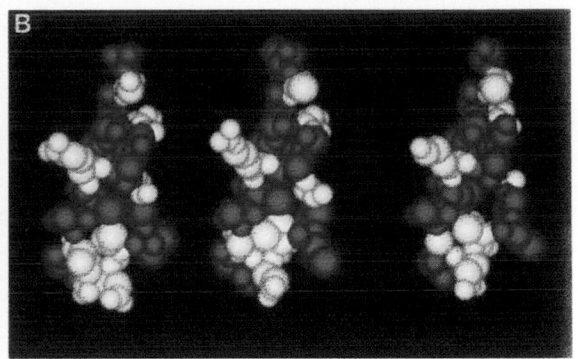

COLORPLATE 1. Three-dimensional models of immunoglobulin FR1 regions. Space-filling representations of amino acids 6–24 are displayed with orientation such that the CDRs would be above, and the C_H1 domain below, the models. Amino acid residues 6, 9, 12, 13, 16, 19, and 23 are colored *yellow* for reference. In (**A**), antibodies deriving from each of the three clans—clan I HyHEL-5 (*left*), clan II NEW (*middle*), and clan III KOL (*right*)—are presented. Clearly these structures differ in their structural characteristics. In (**B**), three clan III antibodies—human V_H3 family KOL (*left*), murine V_HT15 family MCPC603 (*middle*), and murine V_HX24 family J539 (right)—are compared. Note the similarity of these three FR1 loops relative to those in part (**A**). (From ref. 41, with permission.)

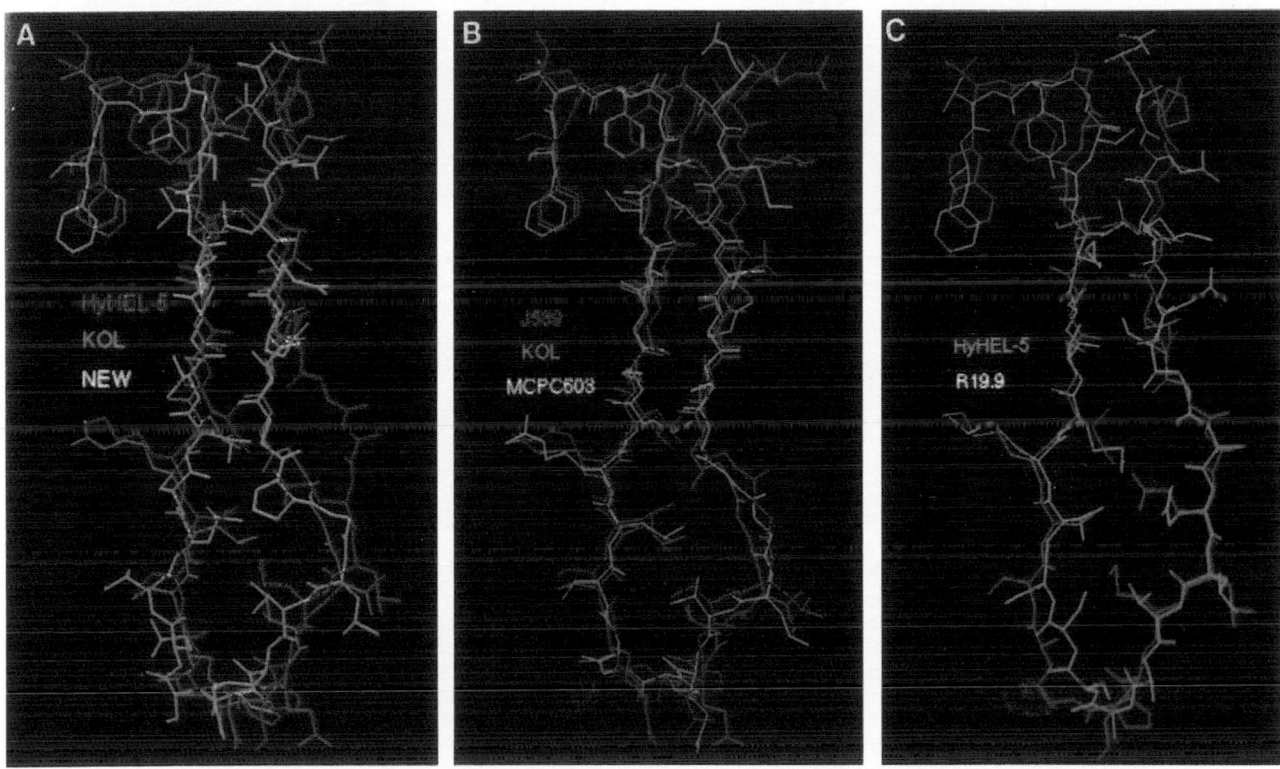

COLORPLATE 2. Superposition of FR1 regions from antibodies of (**A**) different, and (**B,C**) the same, clans. Stick diagrams of amino acid residues and their respective side chains are overlayed to facilitate comparisons. In (**A**), clan I HyHEL-5 and clan II NEW are superimposed on clan III KOL. These molecules can be seen to vary significantly. In (**B**), clan III antibodies MCPC603, J539, and KOL are modeled. Note that the agreement between structures even extends to side-chain sizes and orientations. In (**C**), clan I R19.9 antibody is superimposed on clan I HyHEL 5 with similar results. (From ref. 41, with permission.)

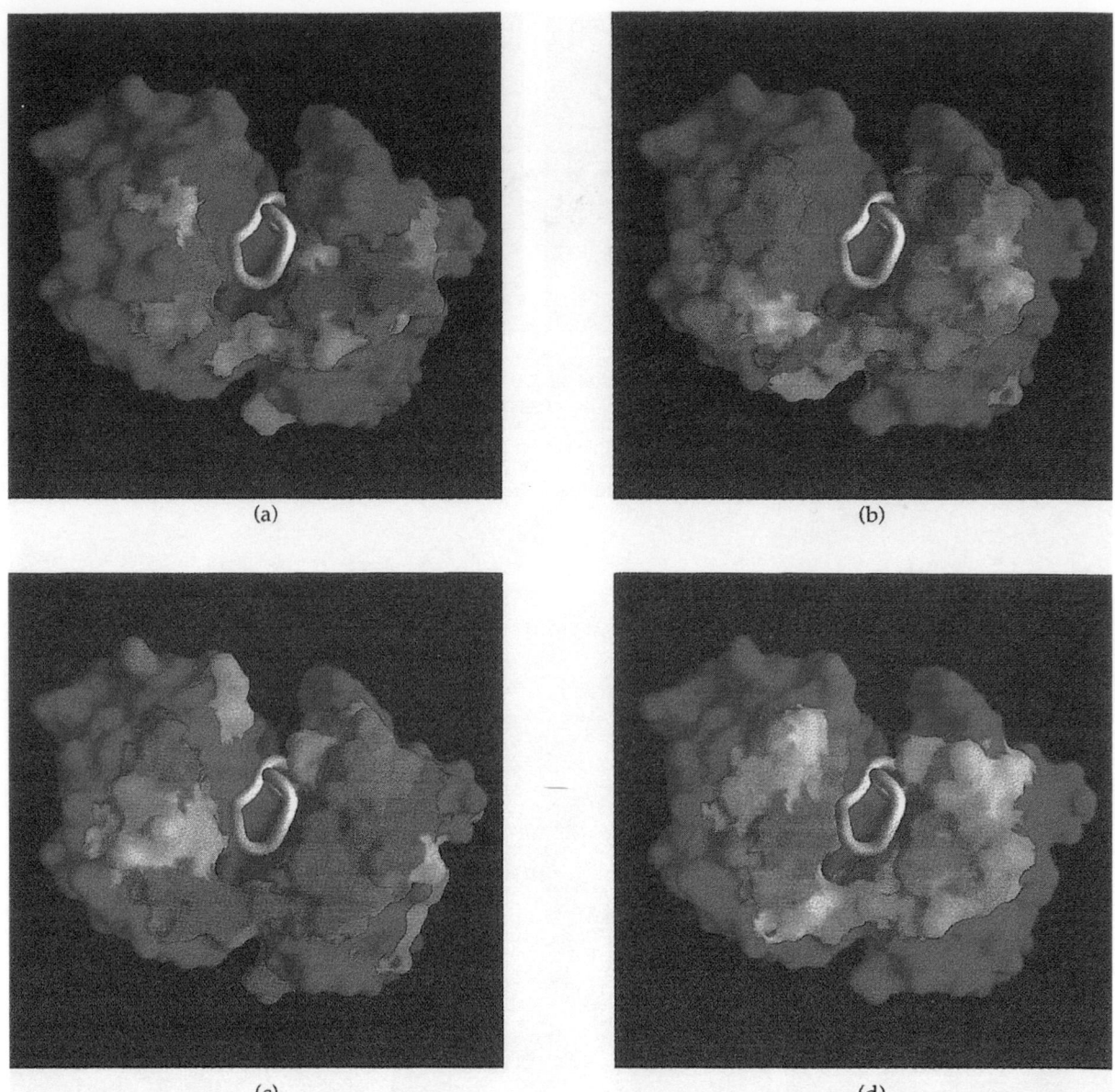

COLORPLATE 3. The antigen-combining site is the product of a nested gradient of diversity. Antibody sequence variation is mapped on the template of the surface of the antibody POT using a scale of *blue* (highly conserved) to *red* (highly divergent). The V_κ domain is to the left of each model, and the V_H domain is on the right. The most highly variable CDR3 loop of the V_H is depicted as a *gray ribbon* in the center of the diagrams; the highly variable V_κ CDR3 is not shown in these representations. In (**A**), germ-line diversity is displayed. In (**B**), diversity introduced by somatic hypermutation is presented. In (**C**), the sum of these two diversities is depicted. Note that in all cases, variation is predominantly restricted to the antigen-binding site, and diversity is highest in close proximity to the V_H CDR3. In (**D**), residues that have been demonstrated to make direct side-chain contacts with antigen in 21 separate crystals are plotted on the same *blue* (zero contacts) to *red* (up to 16 contacts) scale. Thus, the presence of diversity and the tendency to contact antigen are intimately related. (From ref. 58a, with permission.)

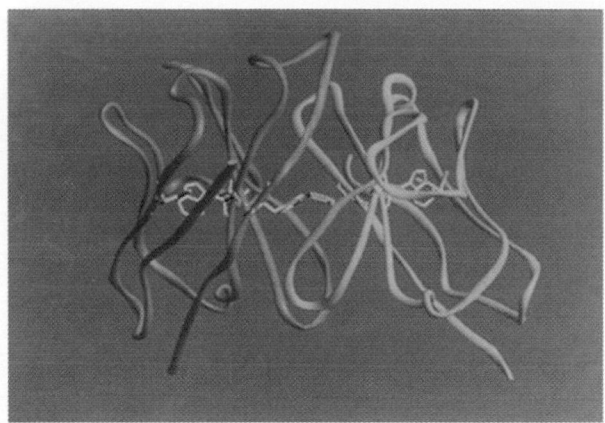

COLORPLATE 4. Ribbon diagram of the α-carbon backbone of an immunoglobulin Fv fragment. The heavy chain is shown in *blue,* and the light chain is represnted in *violet.* The invariant cysteines, tryptophans, and aromatic residues at the core of the V$_H$ and V$_L$ domains are shown in *yellow.* Orientation of the Fv is such that the antigen-binding site is at the *top,* and the C$_H$I/C$_L$ domains would lie at the *bottom,* of the plate. (From ref. 42, with permission.)

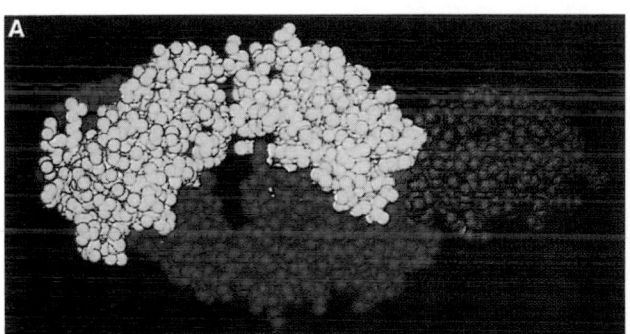

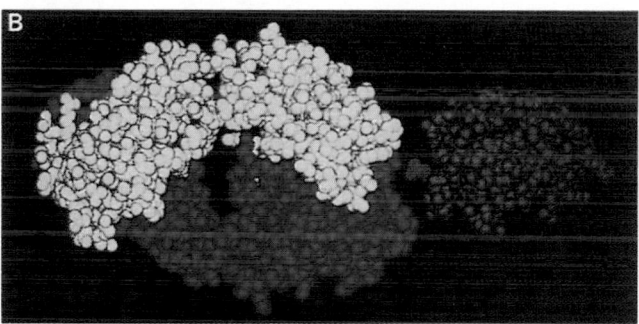

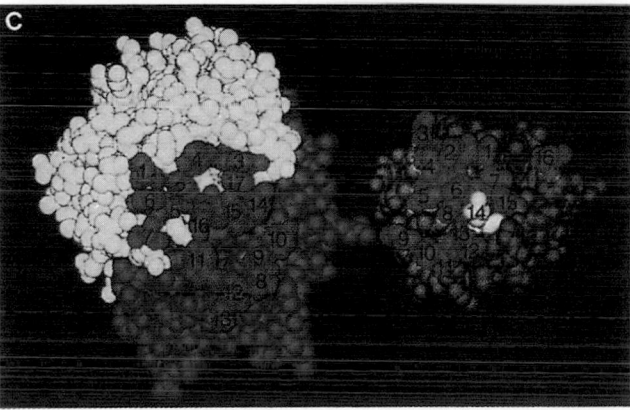

COLORPLATE 5. Model of the lysozyme–antilysozyme antibody (Fab D1.3) complex. The lysozyme molecule is depicted in *green,* and its glutamine-121 residue in *red.* The D1.3 heavy chain is shown in *blue,* and the light chain in *yellow.* In (**A**), the complex is seen as it was in the crystal—as a blunt, end-to-end interface of the two molecules. In (**B**), the two proteins have been separated to demonstrate their structural complementarity. In (**C**), the molecules have been rotated toward the viewer to allow visualization of important contact amino acids (now portrayed in *red,* Gln-121 in *violet*). (From ref. 109a, with permission.)

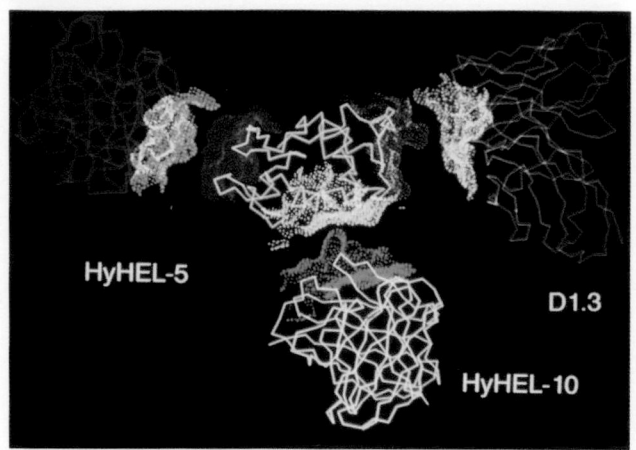

COLORPLATE 6. Model of lysozyme and three antilysozyme complexes. The Fab D1.3 (see Colorplate 5) is included for reference along with two additional antibodies: HyHEL-5 (*left*) and HyHEL-10 (*below*) Molecules are shown as α-carbon backbones except for colored van der Waals surfaces involved in binding. (From ref. 110 with permission.)

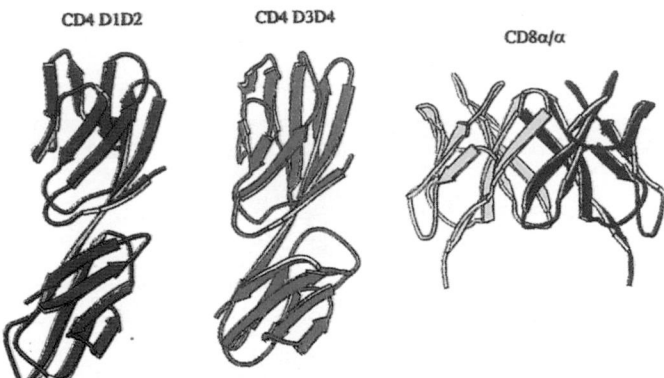

COLORPLATE 7. Ribbon diagrams of CD4 D1D2 (*red*), CD4 D3D4 (*green*), and a CD8α/α homodimer (one subunit *yellow*, the other *blue*). Note the continuous β strand that links domains D1 to D2 and D3 to D4 in CD4. This causes the D1D2 and D3D4 segments to be rigid structurally. (From ref. 207, with permission.)

domain—across immunoglobulin class and even across species—than do individual V regions (refer back to Figs. 10–12), but even so, stretches of relatively lower identity can be localized to distinct parts of the protein. Even though C domains are not formally delineated into framework and hypervariable regions, the tenets used to classify the subdomains of V regions are still applicable when discussing C regions. In Fig. 10A, for example, which compares different human C_H1 domains, note the areas of not only lower conservation but also where gapping is necessary to preserve alignment. Without exception, these regions are most prevalent between strands, especially the loops connecting strands 4-1 and 4-2 (A and B), 4-2 and 3-1 (B and C), 3-1 and 4-4 (C and D), 4-4 and 4-3 (D and E), and 4-3 and 3-2 (E and F). Conversely, the areas of highest conservation are found within the β strands (especially 4-1, 4-2, 3-1, 4-3, and 3-2), where, in addition to the residues needed for the intradomain disulfide linkage present in all Ig domains, the amino acids necessary for main-chain folding, stabilization, and dimerization of the domain reside.

Therefore, as was the case for V regions, the least conserved segments of antibody C domains coincide with the loops that interconnect the different β strands in the fully-folded protein. In the case of C region domains, this refers to divergent loops found at each end of the Ig domain, unlike V regions, where the CDRs are clustered at one end of the domain. Not surprisingly, these loops are also where the preponderance of functional interactions have been localized in binding studies. For instance, the binding site on IgG for the FcγRI receptor is located near the hinge region in just such a loop of the $C_\gamma2$ domain. Likewise, the previously mentioned binding of SPA with IgG Fc involves similar loops in both the $C_\gamma2$ and $C_\gamma3$ regions (12). In another example, although no crystal structure is available for IgA, by modeling the IgA sequence on the IgG Fc three-dimensional structure, an exposed loop in the $C_\alpha3$ domain is predicted to be the binding site for the polymeric immunoglobulin receptor.

Thus, the areas of greatest divergence between different C domains are also those implicated in mediating the different biological effects that distinguish one class or subclass of antibody from another. It is fair to speculate that, like the pressures driving the evolution of diversity-generating mechanisms in V regions, similar forces have used the template of the C region Ig domain to select for a variety of distinct binding capabilities and functional attributes, and have utilized a similar region of the domain for these purposes. In a manner analogous to that seen for variable region tertiary structure, those parts of the C region domain that are most malleable structurally are the very same selected evolutionarily for the acquiescence of new biological characteristics.

Quaternary Structure—The Immunoglobulin Monomer

Although, as stated previously, immunoglobulin domains are each capable of folding independently into stable tertiary globular structures, neither individual Ig domains alone nor entire heavy or light chains are ever encountered under normal physiological circumstances. Rather, the simplest form of this protein that occurs naturally is that of the immunoglobulin monomer schematically depicted in Fig. 1. The complete "monomeric" antibody molecule is actually a four-chain dimer of a heterodimer covalently linked by multiple interchain disulfide bonds. In almost all cases, the heavy and light chains are joined by a single cystine to form a "half-

monomer" with one complete antigen-binding site, and one or more disulfide bonds in the hinge regions (or hinge domains) link the two heavy chains to form the bivalent tetramer.

Figure 16 represents in two dimensions a member of each of the five classes of human immunoglobulin. Notice that the primary differences between these structures are the presence of the extra C domain in the IgM and IgE isotypes and the number and placement of disulfide linkages and carbohydrate derivatives among the different molecules. Like the intrachain disulfide bond considered in tertiary structure, the interchain cystine attaching heavy and light chains is highly conserved. The cysteines participating in this bond are located at the N-terminal end of C_H1 and the C-terminal end of C_L. IgG1 is an exception where the cysteine donated by the heavy chain is found at the carboxyl end of C_H1 (55). Another exception to the typical bonding pattern is found in the A2m(1) allotype of IgA2. Distinctively, this particular isotype utilizes H–H and L–L disulfide pairing to stabilize the four chains instead of the usual H–L linkage (67). The interchain cystines joining the heavy chains are more variable in both number and position between different isotypes. Generally, H–H bonds are formed between the hinge regions or, in the cases of IgM and IgE, analogous positions in $C_\mu2$ or $C_\epsilon2$ domains, respectively. In addition, both IgM and IgA have two additional half-cystines that have dual roles, depending upon whether the antibody is incorporated into a polymeric form of immunoglobulin. An extra cysteine near the C-terminus is involved in a disulfide bond occurring during J chain–mediated polymerization; another half-cystine in the $C_\mu3$ or $C_\alpha2$ domain forms an inter-subunit cystine in the case of IgM or IgA multimers. The disulfide bonds formed by these cysteines in the monomeric forms of IgM and IgA are either interchain (μ and α) or intrachain (α only).

Once interchain disulfide bonds have cemented the four chains into a complete immunoglobulin monomer, the quaternary structure of these molecules can once again be best understood using a domain-by-domain analysis to examine the entire protein. Recall that at this structural level, individual domains interact in such a way that an antibody actually consists of a series of dimeric modules (reviewed in ref. 27). These dimerized domains define the smallest structural and functional units of native immunoglobulin as demonstrated by proteolysis and x-ray diffraction studies. Accordingly, these modules will be reviewed in this context, beginning with the most amino-terminal domain pair, the Fv fragment—or V_H/V_L dimer.

The Fv (see Colorplate 4) is the variable part of the Fab fragment, and as such, constitutes the minimal antigen-binding unit of an antibody. Likely due to this specific functional necessity, V domains dimerize in a manner unlike the strategy employed by all other immunoglobulin domains. In β-pleated sheets, consecutive amino acid side chains protrude on alternating sides at right angles to the plane of the sheet. In most proteins, one side of the sheet packs against another part of the protein (i.e., it is hydrophobic) and the other face of the sheet is exposed to solvent (hydrophilic), leading to a sequence of alternating hydrophobic–hydrophilic residues. In immunoglobulin domains that dimerize, however, this alternating pattern is broken by one of the domain's two β sheets. The sheet that makes up the dimerizing face must interact with both the other β sheet in its own domain and the dimerization face of the adjacent domain. Thus, hydrophilic residues are replaced by hydrophobic side chains that support the dimerization event. While the feature of breaking the alternating hydrophilicity pattern is common to both types of Ig domains that form dimers, V domains interact in a fashion not only specific to V_H and V_L, but also—at

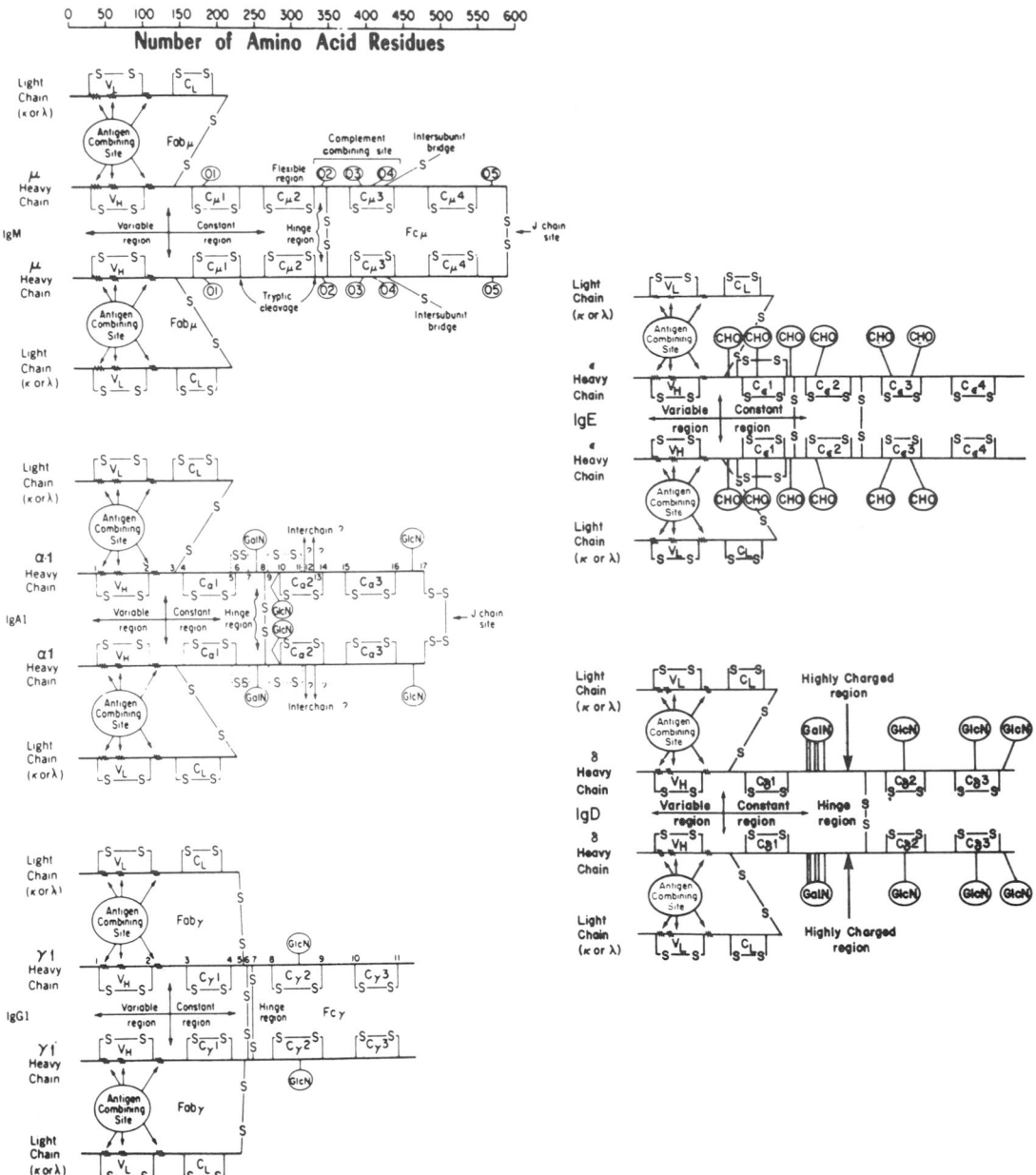

FIG. 16. Schematic representation of the five human immunoglobulin classes. Positions of disulfide bonds and glycosylation are shown for each antibody. (From ref. 66a, with permission.)

the time it was first recognized—unique among all known protein structures (28). Unlike C domains, V domains utilize the five-stranded β-pleated sheet (recall these are unique to V domains) as a dimerization surface (68). The actual V_H/V_L interface consists of the four strands C'-C-F-G on each V domain.

This singular dimerization tactic has profound structural repercussions. In the section detailing tertiary structure, three different β bulges were cited: one common to all V regions found in strand G, one specific to V_H domains located in strand C', and a third unique to V_L also in strand C'. Note that all of these bulges occur in strands at the edges of their respective β sheets. Normally, β sheets pack such that residues in the middle strands form most of the contacts between layers. On account of these conserved β bulges, however, V domain edge residue side chains protrude into the dimer's interior, preventing a close association of V_H and V_L. The loose packing of the Fv has the effect of creating a hydrophilic groove into which small molecules can fit. This groove, which is primarily lined by residues of the HVRs, and the remaining CDR loops at the end of the V regions form a potential antigen-binding site whose surface area is approximately 2000 to 3000 Å^2 (69).

Many of the residues consistently responsible for V_H/V_L interdomain contacts have been localized. About half of the hydrophobic core contacts are formed between FR2 of one chain and FR4 of the other. The majority of remaining interactions involve CDR3 of one chain and the FR2 and/or CDR3 of the complementary domain. Overall 12 to 21 V_L and 16 to 22 V_H residues participate in interchain stabilization (69). Given the extensive contribution of HVRs to these interactions (28), one might expect that the affinity of H–L pairing might also be variable. Nonetheless, a number of studies using heavy and light chains from different individuals, or even different species, have demonstrated the capacity of heterologous H–L pairs to form stable associations. This implies that the conservation of the basic structural features of V_H and V_L domains has persisted throughout evolution, or at the very least not diverged to the point where the C_H1 and C_L elements are unable to anchor productive interactions between these disparate entities.

Between the Fv and Fb (C_H1/C_L dimer) fragments, a short polypeptide stretch exists that is vital to both the Fv's ability to bind antigen productively and to the ability of C_H1/C_L domains—and all constant domains C-terminal to them—to dimerize properly. This region, comprising the carboxy-terminal amino acids of the V region contiguous with the N-terminal residues of the C region, connects Fv to Fb in the complete Fab fragment and is known as the *elbow peptide*. Collectively, the two elbows of an immunoglobulin Fab are also referred to as the *switch peptide*. Several Fab crystal structures have demonstrated the switch to be a flexible segment permitting considerable bending between the V and C domains (70). This is thought to be important in allowing Fabs to bind epitopes of varying spatial arrangement. An equally important feature of the individual elbow peptides is the fact that they make possible a remarkable 180-degree rotation in the quaternary structure of antibody domains that is essential for the correct orientation of all C domains in order for dimer formation between them (8).

These 180-degree rotations occur at the elbows between V_H-C_H1 and V_L-C_L, and are necessary to properly position the C regions. The most N-terminal C domains, C_H1 and C_L, are then able to combine to form the Fb fragment. C_H1 and C_L are prototypes for the C type Ig domain. Like all C domains, they lack the C' and C" strands present in the V domain five-stranded sheet. Like V domains, they also break the alternating hydrophilicity pattern in one of their two β sheets, but in the case of these domains, this occurs on the four-stranded face of the immunoglobulin fold (A-B-E-D) instead. As a result—and due to the permissive rotations at the elbows—C_H1 and C_L utilize the opposite (relative to V_H and V_L) sides of their domains to dimerize (68). The less-polar residues at the core of these dimeric C modules are conserved in both C_H1 and C_L across species (8–10,12), and in this case (unlike V domains), they tend to reside primarily in the middle strands (B and E), where they mediate a much "tighter" association. Consequently, the Fb is often perceived as a compact anchor for the V domains, forming a stable platform upon which antigen binding can occur. Fb, together with the hinge, also serves as a spacer between the Ag combining site and the bulky Fc region.

Between the Fab and Fc regions, immunoglobulin hinges (or extra domains) are critical determinants of overall antibody structural and functional properties. Structurally, hinges are extended segments of dimeric peptide held together by one or more disulfide bonds and dominated by prolines, serines, and threonines. This amino acid composition gives hinges flexibility and gives the Fab arms of an antibody flexional (71) and torsional (72) mobility. Hinge flexibility allows the Fabs to conform to the arrangement of epitopes in order to bind bivalently—presumably giving an antibody greater avidity and versatility. The degree of flexing permitted correlates strongly with hinge length between the end of C_H1

and the first interheavy disulfide bridge (the "upper hinge") (71,73); thus IgG3 is more flexible than IgG1. Hinge length and flexibility also reduce the steric barrier that Fabs may present to the access of C_H2 by other molecules. For example, while normal human IgG1 activates complement effectively, the hinge-deleted variant IgG1 paraprotein *Mcg* is unable to fix complement because the Fabs rest too close to the C1q-binding site on C_H2 to allow interaction.

The hinge, being an extended peptide, is the most proteolytically labile part of an immunoglobulin; recall that the early studies that resulted in the understanding of Fab and Fc relied on proteolytic digestion of the hinge. For instance, the δ isotype, with its long, charged hinge, is very susceptible to proteolysis, which may explain its short serum half-life (74). This issue is of critical importance to IgA, which serves its primary function at mucosal surfaces where proteases from bacterial and host sources are prevalent. For example, the α1 hinge contains five carbohydrate attachment sites within a stretch of only 17 amino acids (75), rendering IgA1 resistant to cleavage by intestinal proteolytic enzymes. However, several strains of bacteria secrete proteases that specifically target the α1 hinge. Presumably as an evolutionary consequence, the hinge of IgA2 has undergone a 13-amino acid deletion, restoring its resistance to this second form of proteolytic challenge (53,76,77). Similarly, structural features unique to hinges of each of the different isotypes may have evolved so as to confer their respective immunoglobulins with specific functional characteristics.

C-terminal to the hinge, the Fc region resides. In the cases of IgG, IgA, and IgD, the Fc is a dimer of two C_H2–C_H3; in IgM and IgE it consists of paired C_H2–C_H3–C_H4 domains. Structurally, $C_{\mu/\epsilon}3$ is equivalent to $C_\gamma2$, and $C_{\mu/\epsilon}4$ is homologous to $C_\gamma3$. As has been described above, the vast majority of sites that define the function and physiology of a particular isotype map to the Fc region. The first striking quaternary structural feature of the Fc is that $C_\gamma2$ (and its structural homologues) fail to dimerize. Analysis of these regions demonstrates that C_H2 domains possess a hybrid structure intermediate between V and C domains. Whereas V domains are five-strand/four-strand sandwiches (dimerizing on the five-strand face) and C domains are three strand/four strand sandwiches (dimerizing on the four-strand face), $C_\gamma2$ is a four-strand/four-strand sandwich. Moreover, substitutions present in outward-pointing side chains on both sides of the domain prevent dimerization along either face (11). Another mixed feature observed is that the β strands of $C_\gamma2$ are of lengths longer than those of V domains, yet shorter than those of either $C_\gamma1$ or $C_\gamma3$ domains. Finally, all C_H2 domains are derivitized by an N-linked oligosaccharide near the middle of the domain (refer back to Fig. 1), except $C_\alpha2$, where it is found nearer to the carboxy-terminal end of the domain. Hydrogen bonding between these sugars serves as the only contact between C_H2 domains. Moving C-terminally, another important distinction concerning C_H2 is that longitudinal contact with the C_H3 domain (about 340 Å² surface area/domain) prevents little interdomain bending (12), unlike the flexible elbows between Fv/Fb and the hinge separating Fab and Fc.

The final domains of the Fc, $C_\gamma3$ and its structural equivalents, pair in the manner described for C_H1 and C_L. Studies using limited proteolysis, reduction, and denaturation originally designated this fragment, a dimer of C_H3 domains, as pFc'. C_H3 domains, like the Fb, dimerize with tight association between them (1100 Å²/domain), using the four-stranded faces of each domain (11). Also like C_H1 and C_L, all C_H3-domain isotypes show conservation of core residues involved in this pairwise domain interaction.

Structurally, the only feature that makes a marked distinction between the different C_H3 domain homologues is the presence of the 18-amino acid "tail-piece" that exists at the carboxy-termini of the $C_\alpha3$ and $C_\mu4$ domains. This sequence is important to polymerization and will be discussed further in the section on higher-order immunoglobulin structure. Taken together, the Fc can thus be thought of as an approximation of the Fab, having two pseudo-V regions (the C_H2s) at its amino-terminus, and a module of C-terminal constant regions (the C_H3s) dimerized in the mode characteristic of classic C-type domains.

Although similar in many ways at the protein level, one of the properties that most notably differentiates the quaternary structures of the five classes of Fc is their pattern of glycosylation—with significant functional ramifications. For instance, while the oligosaccharide moiety of the IgG molecule accounts for only 2% to 3% of its mass, it has been shown to be essential for optimal activation of effector mechanisms leading to the clearance and destruction of pathogens (78–80). As introduced above, all human antibody molecules of the IgG class have N-linked oligosaccharide attached at the amide side chain of Asn 297 on the β-4 bend (between β strands D and E) of the inner face of the C_H2 domain of the Fc region (81). This oligosaccharide moiety is of the complex biantennary type, having a hexasaccharide "core" structure (GlcNAc2Man3GlcNAc) and variable outer arm "noncore" sugar residues, such as fucose, bisecting N-acetylglucosamine, galactose, and sialic acid (see Fig. 17). In all, a total of 36 structurally unique oligosaccharide chains may be attached at each Asn 297 residue. It is likely, but not certain, that the precise fidelity of this glycosylation is important.

The site for this C_H2 carbohydrate is a conserved feature for all mammalian IgGs, and glycosylation occurs at a homologous position in human IgM, IgD, and IgE molecules. As stated above, IgA is also glycosylated within its $C_\alpha2$ domain, but at a site further C-terminal. Human IgM, IgA, IgE, and IgD molecules also bear additional N-linked oligosaccharide moieties attached to the C domains of their heavy chains. Furthermore, IgA1 and IgD proteins also possess multiple O-linked sugars in their extended hinge regions, attached to the hydroxyl groups of serine and threonine residues. Glycosylation, in one form or another, is in fact characteristic of all heavy chain C regions and remains one of the most active areas of research in immunoglobulin structural biology.

The structural and functional consequences of Fc oligosaccharides have begun to be assessed experimentally by comparison of

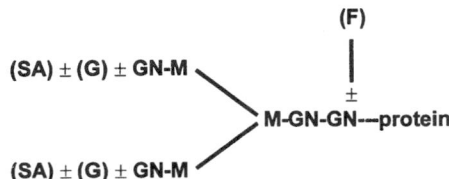

FIG. 17. Schematic representation of N-linked sugars attached to all C_H2 domains. The core carbohydrate moiety of the complex form of oligandosaccharides is represented by the sugar residues in *open type*. The possible outer-arm residues are *in parenthesis*. All possible combinations are observed. SA, sialic acid; G, galactose; GN, N-acetylglucosamine; M, mannose; F, fucose. Attachment of oliosaccharide occurs on the amide side chain of the Asn-X-Ser/Thr sequon (X ≠ Pro). The Ser/Thr residue forms hydrogen bond(s) with the amide group in order to activate it for attachment to the primary *N*-acetylglucosamine residue of the dolichol intermediate (catalyzed by oligosaccharyltransferase). (From ref. 81a, with permission.)

glycosylated and aglycosylated forms of IgG. The latter is ordinarily generated by growing IgG-producing *E. coli* in the presence of tunicamycin (a glycosylation inhibitor) or by protein engineering of the carbohydrate acceptor sequence. One characteristic apparently affected by the sugar moieties found on antibodies is the duration of these proteins' existence *in vivo*. Studies of the blood clearance of glycosylated and aglycosylated mouse/human chimeric IgG1 molecules in mice reveal accelerated clearance for the aglycosylated form despite similar half-lives. Additionally, galactosylated and agalactosylated IgG have been investigated to determine the role of outer-arm sugars in complement (C1q)-mediated lysis. The agalactosylated form, produced following exposure to β-galactosidase, has an observed two fold lower activity than the galactosylated form (82). Related studies have substantiated these conclusions (83).

The vital importance of correct glycosylation was further provided by a study using a human/mouse chimeric IgG1 molecule produced in yeast cells, and anticipated to have high mannose-type oligosaccharide attached at Asn 297. The yeast IgG1 product was unable to activate C1q to trigger human complement-mediated lysis of targets, while the same chimeric IgG1 construct expressed in rodent cells (and therefore glycosylated normally) was effective in that regard. A direct role for oligosaccharide in activating the complement cascade is apparent with mannan-binding protein, a lectin that can function as a surrogate C1 component. The specificity of mannan-binding protein is for mannose and N-acetylglucosamine residues, and it has been shown that it can access and bind to terminal N-acetylglucosamine residues exposed on agalactosyl IgG (84).

Studies utilizing the three types of human Fcγ receptors (FcγRI, FcγRII, and FcγRIII) have also attested to the significance of oligosaccharide modifications on antibodies. The IgG subclass specificity of the FcγR suggests that recognition is correlated with the presence or absence of carbohydrate derivatives. This conclusion is supported by the demonstration that aglycosylated human chimeric IgG3 has a reduced interaction with all three Fcγ receptors. Moreover, at the level of function, while haptenated RBCs sensitized with this same aglycosylated IgG3 antibody could still trigger superoxide production by U937 cells, higher levels of sensitization were required compared to normally glycosylated IgG3. The aglycosylated IgG3 also was not recognized by human FcγRII expressed on K562 and Daudi cells, had reduced rosette formation (mediated through FcγRII expressed on human NK cells), and essentially abolished antibody-dependent cellular cytotoxicity (85,86). Clearly these conclusions illustrate that proper Fc glycosylation is—at least in some cases—necessary for normal structural recognition and biologic function of immunoglobulins.

Glycosylation is potentially important outside of the Fc region as well. It has been estimated that up to 30% of polyclonal IgG molecules are also derivitized by oligosaccharide within the Fab region. Since there are no known sites for sugar attachment in $C_\gamma1$ or C_L, this is most likely in the V regions. Of interest in this regard, an analysis of the DNA sequences of 83 functional human germline V_H gene segments revealed five that encoded potential glycosylation sites. Some, but not all, of these are known to be glycolyslated. In one study of protein and cDNA V_H and V_L sequences, about 25% had potential glycosylation sequences, some of which had arisen as a result of somatic mutation and antigenic selection (87). In most circumstances of V region glycosylation studied thus far, the oligosaccharide moiety does not contribute directly to ligand binding, but can exert a subtle influence on protein tertiary and quaternary structure that is essential for full activity of the antibody. Thus, oligosaccharides occur in many places on immunoglobulin molecules and can affect antibody characteristics as disparate as antigen-binding and the assortment of different Fc-associated functions.

Higher-Order Immunoglobulin Structure—Polymeric Immunoglobulin

One of the most fascinating structural attributes of immunoglobulin is the ability of two classes of heavy chain, IgM and IgA, to form higher order multimeric complexes. IgM and IgA antibodies do not always form polymers, however; monomeric α and μ isotypes exist in forms analogous to those for the γ, δ, and ε isotypes, as well. In addition, polymeric immunoglobulin (pIg) can typically come in a variety of manifestations. The most common forms of these molecules are dimeric (IgA) and pentameric (IgM), although other polymers have also been described. Electron micrographs of murine pentameric and hexameric IgM and human dimeric and trimeric IgA molecules are presented in Fig. 18. Multimerization obviously increases the number of potential antigen-binding sites

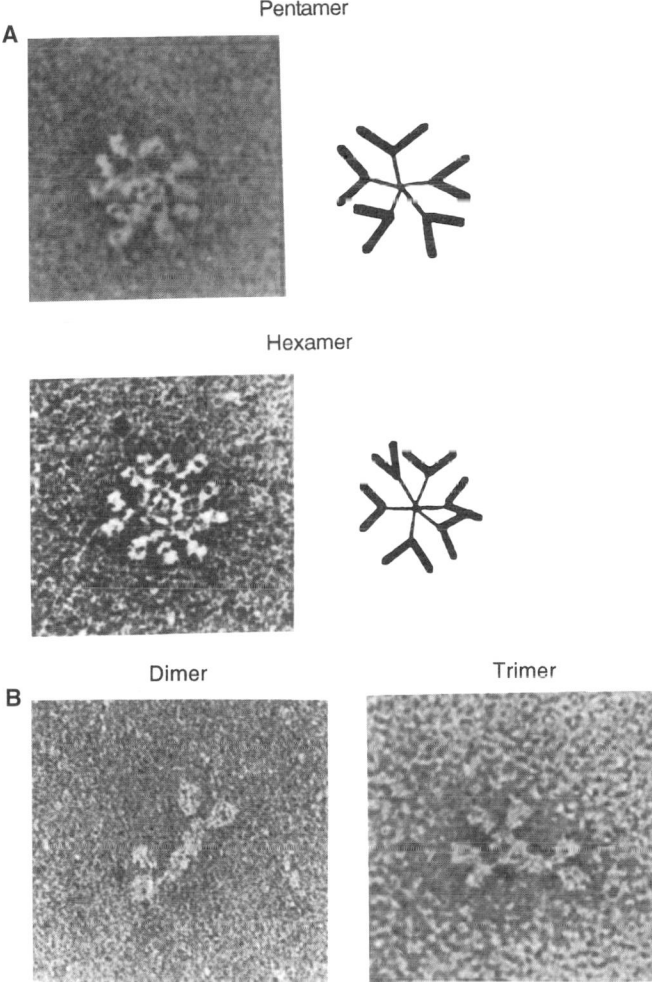

FIG. 18. Electron micrographs of immunoglobulin multimers. In (**A**), a murine IgM pentamer and interpretive diagram (*top*) and a murine IgM hexamer and diagram (*bottom*) are displayed. In (**B**), a human IgA dimer (*top*) and trimer (*bottom*) are presented. All magnifications are ×600,000. (From ref. 87a, with permission, and courtesy of K. H. Roux.)

available on the antibody, and this increase in valence translates into enhanced avidity for polymeric, low-affinity epitopes. This is particularly beneficial for antibodies of the μ and α classes, which serve as the first line of defense at mucosal surfaces where encounter with this type of pathogenic target (i.e., cell-wall polysaccharides) is most frequent. Moreover, IgM, which is the antibody characteristic of primary humoral responses when affinity maturation has not yet occurred, is reliant upon this increased avidity to mediate its functional responsibilities. In addition to raising the apparent affinity for antigen binding, polymeric IgM's juxtaposition of several Fc regions in close proximity also likely plays a role in its efficacy in fixing complement components of the classical pathway. Mechanistically, assembly and secretion of pIg involves the covalent linkage of concatomers of prototypic immunoglobulin monomers, and two accessory proteins termed *J (joining) chain* and *secretory component* (SC) play key roles in these processes.

J chain is a 137-amino acid polypeptide synthesized by pIg-producing plasma cells. J chain covalently interacts with one or more cysteines of immunoglobulin monomers undergoing multimerization (88). It is a proteolytically labile molecule with a high content of negatively charged amino acids and has eight cysteine residues involved in both intra- and interchain disulfide bonds (89). The high level of conservation between J chains of human (90), murine (91), rabbit (92), and even amphibian (93) origin implies that there is a powerful selective pressure to maintain J chain structure. A report identifying J chains in invertebrates which have no known correlate to antibody proteins (94) also indicates that the J chain probably performs some basic protein function that predates its eventual development of the ability to interact with immunoglobulin. In any event, structural studies imply that despite the fact that J chain lacks any significant sequence homology with immunoglobulin, it likely folds into a β-barrel structure similar to that of an immunoglobulin fold (95). Besides the intrachain cystines which stabilize the J chain itself, additional cysteine residues form disulfide bridges to the tailpiece of one or more immunoglobulin monomers during multimer assembly (89). Although the actual details of polymerization have not as yet been elucidated, it is known that the 18-amino acid $C_{\mu/\alpha}$ tailpiece and its penultimate cysteine residue are necessary for the process (52,96).

The stoichiometry of multimer assembly is such that one J chain is present per polymer (whether dimer, trimer, pentamer, etc.). While not always a part of pIgM molecules, J chain is probably absolutely necessary for formation of polymeric IgA, as it is always present in the complex. J chain synthesis is known to be highly regulated (97), and it is thought to be linked to the B cell's activation state as well (98). High levels of J chain expression have been shown to result in production of normal J chain–associated pentameric IgM, while low J chain synthesis results in secretion of hexameric IgM lacking the protein. Intriguingly, this hexameric IgM is actually 20-fold more potent at promoting lysis by complement than is the usual pentamer (99).

The second accessory molecule associated with the secretion of multimeric antibodies actually derives from another protein belonging to the IgSF—the pIg receptor (pIgR)—and is not even made by cells of the B lineage. Secretory component (also called *secretory piece*) was initially discovered as a polypeptide found tightly complexed to the Fc of secreted forms of IgA and IgM (100); subsequently, it was recognized that SC is actually a portion of the larger transmembrane pIgR protein (101). The entire cDNA sequence of the pIgR reveals a protein consisting of seven domains: the first five are extracellular and structurally similar to immunoglobulin V regions, the sixth contains a transmembrane segment and is partially homologous to immunoglobulin V domains, and the seventh contains an unrelated C-terminal intracellular domain (102). The first five domains of the pIgR are in fact the secretory piece originally co-isolated as part of the secreted immunoglobulin complex.

The pIgR is synthesized in epithelial cells of the respiratory, gastrointestinal, and genitourinary tracts and is expressed on their basolateral aspect, where it binds to pIgA and pIgM in a high-affinity interaction. It is known that the N-terminal domain of the pIgR confers binding specificity, and it is thought that both J chain and Fc $C_\alpha3/C_\mu4$ determinants are recognized by the receptor. Interestingly, although the precise molecular locations of pIg/SC interaction have not been identified, there is evidence that, at least structurally, the site is well conserved. Studies have shown, for instance, that human SC binds not only human pIgA and pIgM (103,104), but also several other mammalian species' IgM and IgA (105), and even chicken IgA (106). This cross-reactivity, however, may be mediated by the J chain rather than the Fc regions.

Regardless, following the initial interaction between domain 1 of the pIgR and the C-terminal domain/J chain of the pIg, secondary contact occurs between pIgR domains 3, 4, and 5 with the antibody, consumated by formation of a disulfide linkage between the SC and $C_\alpha2/C_\mu3$. This covalent bond is between Cys 467 in domain 5 of the pIgR and Cys 311 located in the $C_\alpha2$ domain of one IgA subunit's heavy chain (an IgA dimer would have four $C_\alpha2$ domains overall) (107). After a stable interaction has been established, endocytosis of the complex occurs via clathrin-coated pits. Next, following cleavage between domains 5 and 6 of the pIgR, the poly-Ig /SC (now formally termed *secretory immunoglobulin*) is exocytosed at the apex of the cell, releasing the secretory immunoglobulin onto the mucosal surface (108). Current thinking holds that SC's most important function, outside the realm of its role as the pIg-binding portion of the pIgR, is to help protect secretory immunoglobulin in harsh mucosal environments.

Structurally then, polymeric antibodies represent the pinnacle of complexity in terms of immunoglobulin's expansion upon the Ig homology domain concept. From the fundamentals of a simple 110-amino acid domain with a few conserved core residues and a basic structural topology, an intricate molecule such as pentameric IgM (containing 70 different Ig domains of both V and C types, not to mention Ig domains contributed by SC!) is constructed. A molecule capable of recognizing as many as ten (although steric constraints usually dictate less) identical specific antigenic determinants, and also able to mediate several different important biologic functions—all of which will be detailed in the following section.

IMMUNOGLOBULIN FUNCTION

Throughout this chapter thus far, many of the differing functional capacities of antibodies have already been alluded to, as pertains to the identification of the specific structural determinants responsible for particular interactions. Still, the plethora of biologic activities performed by immunoglobulin is best treated as a separate section, in which the many and varied aspects of immunoglobulin function can be detailed and integrated in a physiologic context. Collectively, secreted antibodies are able to activate both the classical and alternative complement cascades (see Chapter 29), transcytose across epithelial cell layers to provide a

barrier to pathogens at mucosal surfaces (see Chapter 27), travel transplacentally to confer maternal humoral immunity to the fetus and neonate, induce phagocytosis by macrophages and granulocytes via the process of opsonization (see Chapters 30 and 41), foster antibody-dependent cellular cytotoxicity by lymphocytes and NK cells (see Chapters 17 and 31), encourage antiparasite immune responses by eosinophils (see Chapter 38), and promote degranulation by mast cells and basophils (see Chapters 32 and 35)—not to mention antibody's ability to bind and inactivate foreign antigenic entities directly (see Chapter 39)!

Even this imposing list of attributes neglects to mention the myriad effects mediated by surface immunoglobulin that include, but are not limited to, the induction(s) of activation (see Chapter 7), differentiation (see Chapter 6), anergy (see Chapter 20), and even apoptosis (see Chapter 23) of B lymphocytes, which are detailed elsewhere in this volume. Surface Ig on memory B cells also has the ability to act as a high-affinity receptor for the recognition, internalization, degradation, and eventual presentation of specific antigens to T cells (see Chapter 9). This allows memory B cells to act as *antigen-specific* antigen-presenting cells (APC), which makes them uniquely efficient among this class of cells. Moreover, emerging fields of study, such as the growing body of literature concerning intracellular antibodies, indicate that new functional capacities for immunoglobulin are likely yet to be discovered.

As for the preceding sections on immunoglobulin structure, the biologic capabilities of immunoglobulin are best treated by dissecting the molecule into the portions responsible for each of its different functional characteristics. While there are some exceptions, in general, specific functions of antibodies can be ascribed to individual domains of the molecule. In the case of variable regions, this requires consideration of the two V domains (V_H and V_L) whose primary function is the binding of antigen. Additionally, it has also been appreciated that certain "superantigens" bind to the V domains as well. In the case of constant regions, because no effector properties have been linked to C_L domains, this entails discussion of each of the heavy chain isotypes (IgM, IgD, IgG, IgA, and IgE), whose functional differences must be a direct result of their structural heterogeneity.

Variable Region Functions

The two V regions (either V_H/V_λ or V_H/V_κ) together form the variable domains of an antibody molecule and provide the specificity for targeting the effector arms of immune response. In general, both V regions are needed to provide specificity and high affinity. There are many examples of individual variable regions binding antigen, but clearly, when the two chains act in concert, the exquisite specificity and affinity of interaction between antibody and foreign antigen is dramatically enhanced.

The concept of hypervariable regions and complementarity-determining regions is pertinent here. In general, most of the contacts between the V domains and antigen take place between amino acid residues in the CDRs and the major epitopes on the antigen (109). However, more recent studies have documented considerable contact between so-called framework residues and antigen. This is most dramatically seen in the lysozyme–antibody crystal (see Colorplate 6) where many residues (especially in the heavy chain FR3 region) are in direct contact with the antigen (110). The generalization that the CDRs provide *all* of the contact residues grew out of the early work involving hapten/anti-hapten systems. When only small organic haptens are the "antigen," then the CDRs can easily provide a "pocket" in which antigen engages antibody (recall that the peculiar dimerization strategy employed by V domains has the propensity to generate such pockets). Closer inspection of the lysozyme Ag-Ab complex—in particular, lysozyme residue Gln 121—is instructive in this regard. Gln 121 protrudes into the cleft between V_H and V_L much like haptens fit into the groove described above. However, other non-groove residues still appear to provide the bulk of the interacting surface for this antibody. In fact, other antibodies that are also reactive with lysozyme (see Colorplate 6) have further borne out this face-to-face binding concept (59). It is fair to say, then, that generally when large molecules such as proteins complex with antibody, the interaction is one of two protein "faces" coming together. In that instance, the notion of a pocket is less appropriate, and as such, non-CDR residues (especially in FR1 and FR3) are also frequently involved.

As with all molecular associations, antigen–antibody interactions occur only if the binding reaction releases enough free energy to be thermodynamically favored. The affinity of interaction is exponentially related to changes in free energy (see Chapter 4). Free energy changes are the sum of changes in both entropy and enthalpy, with increases in entropy and decreases in enthalpy favoring binding. Few association reactions are able to fulfill both of these requirements, however. Instead, a favorable change in one component compensates for a less unfavorable change in the other. When antibodies bind their ligands, the freedom of one molecule to move relative to the other is lost (an unfavorable decrease in entropy). Stabilization of most conformational motions of both the epitope and the backbone and side chains of the paratope surface lowers entropy even further. Thus, to encourage binding to antigen, antibodies must attempt to limit decreases in entropy and offset these losses by potentiating decreases in enthalpy. At the amino acid level, this leads to a selection for Tyr, Trp, Ser, and Asn in combining sites (111,112), because these residues have lower conformational freedom, and hence less entropy to lose upon binding. Additionally, the side chains of these residues foster the varied chemical interactions that drive changes in enthalpy necessary to promote binding energetically.

Specifically, the antigen–antibody interaction involves a variety of forces, including electrostatic (the attraction between opposite charges), hydrogen bonds (hydrogen shared between electronegative atoms), van der Waals forces (the fluctuations in electron clouds around molecules oppositely polarize neighboring atoms), and hydrophobic forces (hydrophobic groups interact unfavorably with water and tend to pack together to exclude water molecules) (113). Of course, salt bridges and other forms of interaction also come into play in some specific immunoglobulin–ligand complexes as well. It is also important to appreciate that rarely do covalent bonds occur between antigen and antibody. Thus, antigen–antibody complexes are readily dissociated by solvents that break the above bonds, such as high salt, organic solvents, urea, and so on.

Thermodynamic considerations for ligand binding are favored by large interacting surfaces of both antibody and antigen, which are packed as closely as possible. Large interaction areas exclude more bound water, somewhat opposing losses in protein entropies with gains in solvent entropy. Surprisingly then, some antigen–antibody complexes actually retain water molecules in their interfaces. However, rather than interfering with binding, these frequently contribute to the interaction by hydrogen bonding to both surfaces (114). More important than entropic changes, the overriding impetus for large contact areas of antibody and antigen is their

ability to bring about large decreases in enthalpy. This effect is mediated by allowing many chemical interactions of all kinds to occur simultaneously between the epitope and paratope.

A model for interaction outside the realm of typical antibody–antigen binding has recently come into vogue, that of the "superantigen." Superantigens were first appreciated in the context of T cell activation. Certain molecules (particularly bacterial products) were found to interact with many different T cell receptors (TCRs) having a variety of specificities (115). Thus, superantigens were originally defined as intact proteins that stimulated large numbers of T cells by binding the V region of a specific family of V_β chains (the heavy chain of the TCR) outside its normal binding groove. Typical T cell superantigens simultaneously stimulate 5% to 25% of the T lymphocyte population, compared with 0.01% stimulation of T cells by a conventional antigen.

More recently, this concept has been extended to B cells (116,117). SPA is a prototype of a B cell superantigen. Although SPA was known to bind to certain immunoglobulin C regions—it has long been used as a mitogen for human B cells—it has been shown that SPA also binds to certain human V_H3-encoded antibodies (118,119). It also binds to the Fab region of murine immunoglobulins, particularly those of the J606 and S107 V_H gene families (which belong to the same clan as human V_H3). SPA binds independently of D, J_H, and light chain utilization, although some light chains influence the extent of binding. Since the interaction is independent of the specificity of the antibody, and since SPA in general does not block antigen binding, it is considered a B cell superantigen. SPA is even able to deliver activation signals to stimulate the differentiation of those B cells containing V_H3-encoded receptors, and SPA also stimulates antibody production. More recent work (120) has documented that SPA simultaneously interacts with FR1, CDR2, and FR3 on the V_H region (Fig. 19).

Other superantigens have also been described that are able to bind immunoglobulin in regions apart from the traditional antigen-

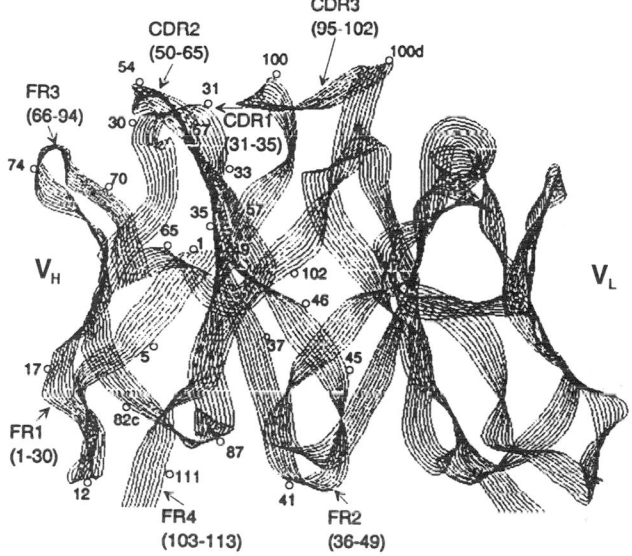

FIG. 19. Ribbon drawing of the Fv fragment of the V_H3 antibody KOL. The FR1, CDR2, and FR3 subdomains of the heavy chain (*left*) are juxtaposed in a manner forming a solvent-exposed face which allows SPA binding. (From ref. 120, with permission.)

combining site (based on their broad specificities). These include the HIV envelope protein gp120 (121), which like SPA binds V_H3-encoded antibodies, and the TCR-associated molecule CD4 (122). Like the circumstance with antigen binding, superantigens generally require both V_H and V_L domains (even though the particular identity of the light chain is unimportant). Individual heavy chains do not bind the B cell superantigens that have been described to date, indicating that light chains must influence their conformations appreciably. Finally, the report of a crystal structure (an IgM rheumatoid factor Fab complexed to its autoantigen, an IgG Fc) showing residues at the edge of the conventional binding site mediating interaction indicates that still more novel paradigms for antibody–antigen binding possibly exist as well (123).

Constant Region Functions

Because mammalian species each utilize the same major classes of antibody (although their organization of subclasses differs), it is reasonable to presume that each isotype subserves some vital biologic function(s). Along these same lines, it should be remarked that even in "lower" species, where only one type or one copy of heavy chain gene is present, the protein product resulting from this element is typically heterogeneous. In other words, although fish, amphibians, and reptiles all possess fewer immunoglobulin isotypes than do mammals at the genomic level, greater than one C region protein is produced per gene. For example, sharks make both monomeric and polymeric IgM; in skate, turtle, and duck there are truncated and full-length versions of the immunoglobulin polypeptide; *Xenopus* immunoglobulin comes in both glycosylated and aglycosylated forms (51). Clearly, evolution has recurrently employed the strategy of adopting more than one type of antibody

to perform the multitude of biologic responsibilities that are required by species for effective immunologic functioning.

In a broad sense, Fc-mediated effector functions can be classified into three general categories: (a) activation of complement, (b) interaction with effector cells, and (c) transport and compartmentalization of immunoglobulins. In addition, different isotypes have different stabilities *in vivo*, such that this is an important variable as well. In the following sections, the five classes of human immunoglobulins are each discussed separately with respect to function. Table 2 presents a summary of key properties for each class of human antibody, and Fig. 20 compares the circulating serum levels for each of the five major isotypes.

IgM

IgM is the most versatile antibody and almost certainly the first type of immunoglobulin to have developed evolutionarily. Heavy chains of the μ class are the first type expressed during B cell development, and IgM is the isotype produced in primary immune responses. IgM, in the form of surface immunoglobulin, is also an important receptor on immature B lymphocytes and on mature, naive B lymphocytes. Total serum Ig consists of 5% to 10% IgM, and second to IgA it is the major isotype of mucosal immunity. Originally named due to their description as _m_acroglobulins, IgM molecules are thought to serve similar functions in all mammalian species. In fact, IgM-like (polymeric, having five domain heavy chains with large carbohydrate content, and present as a cell surface receptor on most B cells) antibodies have even been identified in most non-mammalian vertebrates other than the jawless fish (51). Unquestionably, the polymeric structure of IgM has been conserved in evolution, probably due to its higher avidity for antigen compared with that of the monomer.

TABLE 2. *Physical, chemical, and biological properties of human heavy chain immunoglobulin classes*

Property	IgM	IgD	IgG	IgA	IgE
Molecular form	Pentamer, hexamer	Monomer	Monomer	Monomer, dimer	Monomer
Number of C region domains	4	3	3	3	4
Tailpiece	+	−	−	+	−
Accessory chains	J chain, SC	None	None	J chain, SC	None
Subclasses	None	None	G1,G2,G3,G4	A1,A2	None
Molecular weight	950 kD, 1150 kD	175 kD	150 kD	160 kD, 400 kD	190 kD
Carbohydrate content (%)	10	9	3	7	13
Percentage of total serum Ig	5–10%	0.3%	75–85%	7–15%	0.02%
Average adult free serum level (mg/ml)	0.7–1.7	0.04	9.5–12.5	1.5–2.6	0.0003
Synthesis rate (mg/kg/d)	7	0.4	33	65	0.016
Serum half-life (d)	5	3	23	6	2.5
Antibody valence	10, 12	2	2	2, 4	2
Bacterial lysis	+	?	+	+++	?
Placental transfer	−	−	+	−	−
Mast cell/basophil binding	−	−	−	−	+
Macrophage binding	−	−	+	+	−
Classical complement activation	++	−	+	−	−
Alternate complement activation	−	+	+	A1+,A2−	−
Other biological properties	Primary Ab responses; Secretory immunoglobulin	Unknown; Useful as a B cell marker	Hallmark of secondary immune responses	Main secretory immunoglobulin	Allergic and anti-parasite responses

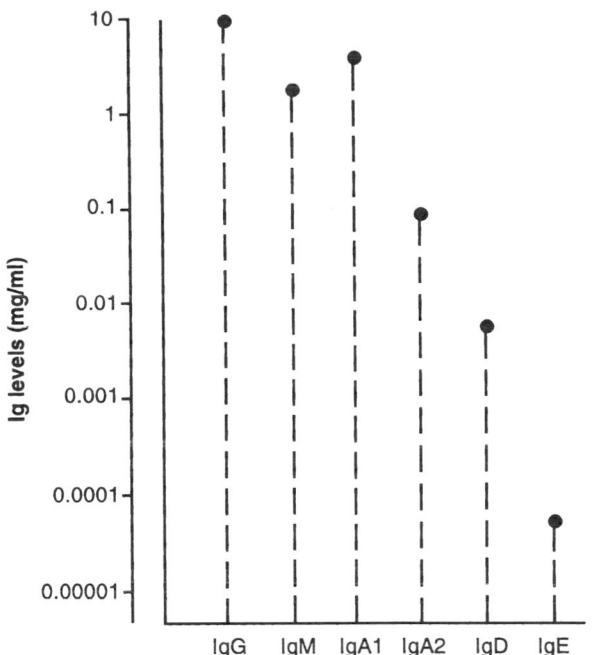

FIG. 20. Circulating levels of different human immunoglobulin isotypes. Note the log scale of the graph and that both human IgA isotypes are represented. (From ref. 123a, with permission.).

The two most common forms of IgM are the membrane-bound monomeric form and the secreted pentamer. The cell-surface version of IgM serves as the antigen-specific receptor for B cell activation, although the activation signal is actually transmitted by the transmembrane accessory molecules Igα and Igβ (124). It is unclear whether the $C_\mu 4$ domains of surface IgM participate in the interaction with the α/β heterodimer, but it is more likely that the important associations lie in the transmembrane and cytoplasmic regions of IgM that are specific to the cell-surface form (125). The surface form of IgM is also important in the development of the B cell. During pre-B stages, μ heavy chains are associated (via a disulfide linkage in $C_\mu 1$) with the "surrogate" light chains V_{preB} (analogous to a V_L domain) and λ5 (a C_λ analogue) (126,127). This complex, once again through accessory molecules, is able to transduce signals thought to be necessary for allelic exclusion of the other heavy chain locus and for subsequent light chain rearrangement (detailed in Chapter 5). Eventually, of course, the IgM heavy chains become associated with either λ or κ light chains.

Polymeric IgM also has its own catalogue of functional attributes. IgM antibodies are the first to be secreted from plasma cells upon challenge by antigen; since IgM is not secreted in large quantities from memory B cells, elevated IgM is indicative of recent antigenic exposure. As stated earlier, IgM antibodies generally have low affinity, as they have not gone through the processes of somatic hypermutation and affinity selection. Nonetheless, the high avidity of pIgM renders it capable of efficiently binding antigen. Similarly, a single polymeric IgM molecule is able to effectively initiate classical complement fixation, even though the affinity of C1q for Cμ is very low. The C1q-binding site of IgM has been localized to the $C_\mu 3$ domain (128) and appears to be dependent upon carbohydrate found there for potent binding (129). While $C_\mu 3$ domains (and their structural homologues) are not well conserved evolutionarily, the ability

to mix IgM and complement from different species and retain activity indicates that the complement recognition sites on vertebrate immunoglobulins may be similar. In fact, even *Xenopus* IgM has been demonstrated to fix mammalian complement components (130)! IgM has also been shown to interact with C3b via its $C_\mu 1$ domain, thereby allowing antibody–antigen complexes containing IgM to indirectly mediate phagocytosis. By this mechanism, C3b, once fixed, can promote uptake via complement receptors found on macrophages.

The high avidity of IgM for both antigen and complement is crucial in the context of its role as a front-line defense mechanism. IgM not only is the humoral agent of primary immune responses, but also—like IgA—is transported by the pIgR across epithelia such that it serves a role as a secretory immunoglobulin at mucosal surfaces. Since secretory immunoglobulins are present in breast milk as well, IgM also participates significantly in protecting the newborn from intestinal pathogens until such time as the neonatal immune system is fully functioning. A role for IgM in mucosal immunity must have developed early in evolution, as it is the sole immunoglobulin in some animals.

IgD

IgD is present in serum in very low amounts (less than 0.5% of total serum Ig). Although synthesis of IgD is also very low (at least an order of magnitude lower than that of IgM, IgG, and IgA), IgD's pronounced susceptibility to proteolytic degradation is probably also responsible for its scarcity in plasma and other bodily fluids. The unusually long hinge region linking Fab to Fc in IgD is thought to be largely accountable for its short half-life. IgD is secreted neither during an immune response, nor following mitogenic stimulation of IgD+ B cells, although in the form of immune complexes it is known to be able to activate the alternative complement cascade. IgD's low levels make this complement fixation unlikely to be important in the *in vivo* context. In fact, no specific functions unique to IgD have been definitively assigned to the δ Fc region in either its membrane-bound or soluble forms. That notwithstanding, the fact that the IgD class is maintained in all mammals, has a high level of conservation across species (131), and the existence of an Fcδ receptor, all suggest that it may have some distinct purpose. Still, two independently derived strains of IgD knockout mice have failed to ascribe to it a convincing immunologic role. In one strain, in which a premature stop codon was introduced into the $C_\delta 3$ domain, a subtle reduction in the total number of peripheral B cells was noted (132). In the other, which carried an insertion in its $C_\delta 1$ exon and a frameshift in $C_\delta 3$, delayed affinity maturation during T cell-dependent antigen responses was demonstrated (133).

Although not known to have any unique function, IgD, together with IgM, is a major surface component on many B cells. Because the C region genes for μ and δ are both transcribed in the same primary RNA message, differential splicing to produce either IgM or IgD is required. This particular genomic organization facilitates their coexpression, which is not possible for any other isotypes (reviewed in Chapter 5). Mature, naive B cells migrate from the bone marrow as IgM+/IgD+ cells (134) and make up about 90% of peripheral B cells in both the murine and human systems (see Chapter 6). Similarly, B cells in the primary follicles of secondary lymphoid organs coexpress IgM and IgD, but as they mature to memory cells, IgD expression is typically lost (135,136). Curiously, studies of IgM+/IgD+ splenic B cells reflect that IgD surface expression is actually tenfold higher than IgM levels (137). This is particularly puzzling, given that δ message levels are lower than are μ mRNAs, and IgD (at least in the serum) is known to be so proteolytically labile. Perhaps helping to explain this high level of IgD expression is that fact that IgD does not need to complex with other proteins for transport to the cell surface, distinguishing it from all other immunoglobulin classes (138). It is possible that IgD's high levels of surface expression and intrinsic flexibility (139) afford it a role in the early response to antigen (123a,140).

In addition to their coexpression, IgM and IgD have a number of commonalties in terms of their function as B cell antigen receptors. Like IgM, IgD is non-covalently associated with Igα/Igβ heterodimers, which serve as the signaling component of their BCR (138). Not surprisingly then, ligation of either IgM or IgD by antigen can independently mediate activation, deletion, or anergy of B cells (141), and likewise, the signals propagated by IgM or IgD BCR seem to be the same, albeit with different kinetics (see Chapter 7). Specifically, signals transmitted through surface IgD have been reported to cause induction of APC function (142); upregulation of coreceptors B7-1 and B7-2 (143); class switching to IgM, IgG1, IgG2, IgG3, and IgA (144); and increased secretion of IgE (145). The biologic significance of many of these findings remains unclear. In fact, reports (146,147) describing a new class of germinal center IgD+ B cells (having evidence of up to 80 different somatic mutations within their V regions!) demonstrate just how little is still understood about the cells expressing—and the protein—IgD.

IgG

IgG is the predominant immunoglobulin in blood, lymph, peritoneal fluid, and cerebrospinal fluid. Collectively, it makes up more than 75% of serum immunoglobulin and is synthesized at a high rate (over 30 mg/kg/d, second only to IgA). The presence of high-affinity IgG is the hallmark of secondary humoral immune responses. Electrophoretically, IgG proteins migrate to the γ range of serum globulins, hence IgG's earlier designation as gammaglobulin. Actually, IgG is composed of four subclasses of antibody, whose salient features are summarized in Table 3. The selection of IgG subclass by a particular immune response does not appear to be random: in murine systems, anti-carbohydrate specificities tend to be IgG3, anti-protein IgG1, and anti-viral IgG2a (148,149). In man, reactivities against polysaccharide immunogens are skewed toward IgG1 and IgG2, while anti-protein and anti-viral γ antibodies are biased in the direction of IgG1, IgG3, and IgG4 (150). As

an offshoot of these phenomena, clinical syndromes in which specific IgG subclasses are absent are known to present themselves as characteristic immunodeficiencies (see Chapter 43).

Perhaps the most studied feature of the IgG isotypes is their ability to activate the classical complement pathway. Although all four are capable of initiating the classical cascade, they do so to varying degrees (G3>G1>G2>G4) (150,151). Understanding the means by which the different IgG subclasses interact with specific components of complement has been difficult, complicated by many confounding reports. Results indicating that C1q is unable to bind either IgG2 or IgG4 antibodies (152) were perplexing, given that both are able to activate the classical cascade. Similarly, despite Fcγ3's higher affinity for C1q (152), IgG1 is more effective at potentiating complement-mediated cytolysis. When the site for C1q-binding was mapped to the C-terminal portion of the $C_\gamma 2$ domain near the hinge region (153,154), investigators surmised that differences in the IgG subclasses' abilities to activate complement were likely attributable to steric freedom, or lack thereof, conferred by the particular hinge of the antibody (155,156). For this reason, the longer hinge of the γ3 C region was thought to account for IgG3's higher affinity for C1q, relative to that of IgG1. Still, hinge-deletion (157) and hinge-swapping (158) experiments have yielded data that contradict the notion of the hinge being a key determinant for complement activation. Be that as it may, recall that proper glycosylation within the $C_\gamma 2$ domain is accepted as an obligatory element for fixation of complement as well.

The explanation for the difference in efficacy of lysis by complement between IgG1 and IgG3 (paradoxical, given their affinities for C1q) is even more convoluted. It may reflect that other differences between the IgG1 and IgG3 C1q sites are present that affect complement activation. Alternatively, it may derive from differences in a second, separate site in the $C_\gamma 1$ domains of these molecules which, like IgM, binds activated C3b and protects it from inhibition. This second site also likely explains the capacity of IgG2 and IgG4 to activate the classical pathway, despite an inability to bind C1q. Finally, note that IgG4 is able to efficiently recruit and activate the alternative complement cascade, distinguishing it from the other three subclasses.

Another means by which IgG antibodies communicate with the effector arms of the immune system is via the Fcγ receptors (FcγRs). A number of different IgG FcR exist (covered specifically in the section on the IgSF), each of which have their own profile and affinities for binding of the different IgG subclasses, expression patterns on different cell types, and different biologic responsibilities (159). Among the immunologic cell types implicated as

TABLE 3. *Properties of Human IgG subclasses*

Property	IgG1	IgG2	IgG3	IgG4
Disulfide linkages	2	4	5–15	2
Molecular weight	146 kD	146 kD	165 kD	146 kD
Percentage of total serum immunoglobulin	34–87%	5–56%	0.5–12%	7–12%
Average adult free serum level (mg/ml)	5.9 ± 2.6	3 ± 2.5	0.6 ± 0.55	0.9 ± 0.25
Macrophage binding by FcγR	+	−	+	+
Placental transfer	+	++	+	++
ADCC	+++	+	+++	+
Classical complement activation	+++	++	++++	+
Alternative complement activation	+	+	+	+++

Adapted from Simard and Mak (140).

important binders of IgG are macrophages, polymononuclear cells, and lymphocytes (including B cells). Interactions with these receptors cause many functional effects, including phagocytosis (160) and antibody-dependent cell-mediated cytotoxicity (161), both of which ultimately lead to the destruction of the bound antigen. Specifically, the hierarchy for ADCC by mononuclear cells is IgG1, IgG3 > IgG2, IgG4 (152,162). Signals transmitted via FcγR also modulate lymphocyte function by means of up-regulation or down-regulation of antigen presentation, cytokine release, cytokine receptor expression and/or sensitivity, and even immunoglobulin secretion. Even soluble FcγR are known to bind IgG, although the significance of this finding is unclear (163). Finally, IgG FcR also permit transplacental movement of maternal antibodies during gestation (164). This provides the developing fetus with a source of high-affinity serum immunoglobulin that is able to interact with complement to mediate biologic effects at a time at which it has no other form of specific humoral immunity. It should not be overlooked that IgG molecules are the most stable isotype in serum (with a half-life of over 3 weeks), further maximizing their utility in this endeavor—even into the post-natal period.

Binding of the four IgG subclasses by the different FcγR varies in terms of the specific contact residues involved for each respective ligand–receptor pair. Generally, although the IgG binding sites for the FcR are thought to largely overlap, the precise elements responsible for interaction likely have subtle differences. By consensus, research into these issues has suggested that the sites are bipartite, consisting of a site on the C-terminal portion of the hinge and also reliant upon residues found in the portion of the $C_\gamma 2$ domain already implicated in C1q-binding (86,165). Because the four IgG isotypes differ considerably in these regions, this would fit nicely with their noted differential binding of the varied FcγR.

IgA

IgA is the major immunoglobulin in external secretions such as saliva, mucus, sweat, gastric fluid, and tears. Moreover, it is also the major immunoglobulin of colostrum and breast milk, where it provides the neonate with a readily available source of intestinal protection against pathogens (167). The secretory forms of IgA are exclusively polymeric, including J chain and SC in the manner described previously. In addition, IgA—present predominantly in its monomeric form—is also an important component of serum Ig, where it makes up 10% to 15% of the total. The synthetic rate of IgA is roughly double that of IgG, such that total daily IgA production outpaces that of all other immunoglobulins combined. The majority of IgA synthesized is in the secretory form, with the largest fraction of IgA plasma cells residing in the subepithelial mucosa of the small intestine. Because secretory IgA coats all external surfaces except skin, it is rightly considered a first line of defense against organisms that would invade via mucosal routes. IgA's role in mucosal immunity (see Chapter 27) is phenotypically evident in persons with the most common genetic defect of the humoral immune system, IgA deficiency (see Chapter 43). Individuals with this condition are susceptible to invasion across mucosal barriers and typically present clinically with recurrent infections of this type.

Serum and secreted IgA originate from separate pools of B lymphocytes: plasma cells in specialized sites of the respiratory, urogenital, gastrointestinal, and mammary tissues produce the IgA found in secretions, while the IgA in serum emanates from plasma cells in the bone marrow, lymph nodes, and spleen. Despite this compartmentalization of production, antigenic exposure occurring at either mucosal or systemic sites will prime the development of both secretory and serum IgA responses simultaneously (168).

In humans, the two IgA subclasses, IgA1 and IgA2, show an interesting division of expression which affects their resultant biologic utilities. IgA1 exists primarily as a monomeric molecule, and accordingly is the main IgA isotype in plasma (refer to Fig. 20). In bone marrow, about 90% of IgA-secreting plasma cells make IgA1 (169). IgA2, on the other hand, is usually found as a polymer. Recall that the main structural difference between these two isotypes is localized to the hinge. Whereas the IgA1 subclass has a higher concentration of carbohydrate in its hinge region (protecting it from most forms of proteolytic degradation), the IgA2 isotype has deleted much of that hinge region—presumably as an evolutionary response to bacterial IgA1-specific proteases (170). Thus, it is consistent that the broadly protease-resistant form (IgA1) should predominate in serum to maximize its lifespan, while the targeted protease-resistant subclass (IgA2) should prevail where bacterial exposure is more common.

IgA does not efficiently induce inflammatory responses. Rather, it is believed to protect primarily by exclusion, binding and cross-linking pathogens to prevent their uptake across epithelia and facilitating their expulsion in mucus excretions (123a,140). It is noteworthy that inflammatory responses localized to mucosa would likely be detrimental to barrier function, as tissue damage could compromise the integrity of epithelial surfaces. While IgA does have the ability to fix complement via the alternate cascade, this ability is restricted to IgA1. IgA can also opsonize antigens for phagocytosis; this is accomplished via a specific Fcα receptor (FcαR) found on macrophages, monocytes, and neutrophils. This provides a mechanism for IgA immune complexes that accumulate at mucosal surfaces to be engulfed and processed. The FcαR is known to bind secretory IgA with higher affinity than serum IgA, but strangely, the site on IgA that is recognized seems to be unrelated to the J chain or SC which distinguish the secretory and serum forms (66). Rather, in a manner unique from all other IgSF FcR, which see a hinge-proximal site in the $C_H 2$ (or equivalent) domain, the FcαR sees a site bridging the domain boundary between $C_\alpha 2$ and $C_\alpha 3$, reminiscent of SPA binding (66). Finally, IgA has also been shown to induce eosinophil degranulation via the FcαR, implicating it in antiparasite immunity. Given that many parasites gain access to host tissues by crossing mucosal barriers, this is a logical biologic activity for IgA as well.

IgE

IgE is present in serum in the lowest concentration of all the immunoglobulins. Its rate of synthesis is between 25- and 2,000-fold less than each of the other isotypes, it has the shortest serum half-life, is unable to activate either the classical or alternative complement cascades, and lacks the ability to opsonize antigens. Nonetheless, IgE's biological effects more than compensate for these shortcomings, due to the profound efficiency of its behavior. The principle function of IgE is to arm basophils and mast cells with specific antigen receptors. These cells in turn act as potent dispensers of inflammatory reactions (see Chapter 32).

Plasma cells that produce IgE are chiefly found in the lung and skin. Upon its release from these B cells, circulating IgE is quickly bound by a high-affinity Fcε receptor (FcεRI, K_D 10^{-10} M) found on these granulocytes, allowing the IgE molecules to stably remain on the cells for weeks or months. Once primed with many such antigen-specific receptors (recognize that cells bearing FcεRI can have IgE molecules of many different reactivities on their surfaces, unlike the case for antigen-specific B cells), multivalent antigen can then cross-link the bound IgE, indirectly cross-linking the FcεRI molecules as well. Ultimately, this causes mast cells and basophils to release granules containing inflammation-mediating substances and chemoattractants for a variety of cell types. The granule contents of mast cells and basophils are powerful, able to induce rapid responses—including mucous secretion, coughing and sneezing, vomiting, diarrhea, and inflammation. While this type of response can be vital in the clearance of parasites (see Chapter 38), it has the unfortunate consequences of also causing allergy (see Chapter 35) and anaphylaxis in predisposed individuals. In such atopic individuals, it has been seen that increased amounts of IgE are synthesized and found on the surfaces of mast cells and basophils, likely explaining their predilection for these inappropriate responses.

Other cells types also express the high-affinity FcεRI, including Langerhan's cells (171,172) and eosinophils (173), but the rationale for its presence there is yet to be definitively elucidated. In addition, the CD23 surface antigen has also been shown to be a low-affinity IgE receptor (designated FcεRII). Among other cell types, CD23 is known to be expressed on monocytes and some follicular B cells. In fact, monocytes can even be induced to secrete a soluble form of FcεRII (174), but once again the significance of this finding is unclear. Considering the low levels of circulating IgE, the relatively low affinity of the receptor, and the fact that CD23 is known to interact with CD11/CD18, there is doubt as to whether IgE is even an important ligand for this receptor *in vivo*.

Like the pIgR and several of the FcγRs, the FcεRI molecule is also a member of the IgSF (detailed further in the following section). Interaction between IgE and its high-affinity receptor was the first well-characterized Ig-FcR ligand–receptor pair of this type. Originally, studies using synthetic peptides as specific inhibitors of IgE–FcεRI binding identified a 76-amino acid polypeptide spanning $C_\varepsilon2$–$C_\varepsilon3$ as the FcR recognition site on IgE (175). Subsequently, this localization was refined further to a site in $C_\varepsilon3$ analogous to the FcγR site on $C_\gamma2$. Unlike the binding situation for IgG that was also dependent upon residues in the hinge regions (see above discussion), the extra $C_\varepsilon2$ hinge domain of IgE is not believed to play a significant role in the interaction (176).

THE IMMUNOGLOBULIN SUPERFAMILY

Evolution of the Immunoglobulin Superfamily

Soon after the sequencing and structural analyses of antibodies revealed the protein motif of the immunoglobulin domain (7,177), it became apparent that evolution had incorporated Ig homology domains in a variety of other important molecules as well. The sequencing of MHC genes, TCRs, and the pIgR, among others, demonstrated the use of both V region- and C region-type domains by a number of cell-surface proteins of the immune system. Contemporaneously, a number of cell adhesion molecules (CAMs) involved with neurite outgrowth in developing axons were also found to contain Ig-like domains (reviewed in ref. 178). It was quickly recognized that a large family of genes that contained putative immunoglobulin folds existed (2,3,179), whose members were globally implicated in issues of molecular recognition and/or cel-

lular adhesion. Comprised of several multigene families in their own right (V_H, V_L, TCRα, TCRβ, TCRγ, TCRδ, MHC I, MHC II, Sialoadhesin, CAM, etc.), the term *immunoglobulin superfamily* was adopted to refer to this diverse group of genes, which each contained one or more Ig homology domains.

Currently the IgSF encompasses well over 100 genes, and extends across several phylogenetic boundaries (reviewed comprehensively in ref. 4). Disparate species in which IgSF members have been identified include chicken, zebrafish, tunicates, grasshoppers, squid, *C. elegans,* sponges, and *S. cerevisiae.* In addition, reports identifying proteins containing structures reminiscent of immunoglobulin homology domains from prokaryotic organisms (180,181) raise the possibility that this archetypal structure antedates even eukaryote evolution. The discovery of new molecules with novel functional attributes (for this class of proteins) also continues to expand the role of IgSF members. For instance, while the preponderance of immunoglobulin homology domain-containing proteins that have been identified are either cell surface or secreted proteins involved in recognition and adhesion events, a newer class of intracellular muscle proteins (titin, telokin, etc.) belonging to the IgSF demonstrate that the immunoglobulin fold structure is adaptable to an assortment of functional capacities.

The evolution of the IgSF has been the subject of considerable scientific speculation and potentially has implications for both the development of the vertebrate immune system and the process of organogenesis in general. Based upon the overwhelming number of IgSF members that possess adhesive qualities, it has been proposed that the first IgSF molecules were simply single Ig domain extracellular proteins that served as primordial "cellular glues" (2,3). Substantiating this argument is the noted stability of the compact β-barrel structure of the immunoglobulin fold, which would foster its utility in harsh extracellular environments. Further bolstering this hypothesis is the fact that numerous IgSF proteins participate in both homotypic and heterotypic interactions with other IgSF molecules, demonstrating their potential to act as adhesion molecules.

Some evidence suggests that IgSF proteins have promoted clustering of cells since the earliest stages of eukaryotic development. For example, the yeast *S. cerevisiae* uses the IgSF glycoprotein α-agglutinin to mediate cell–cell contact during mating (182). IgSF forebears may have also allowed the first examples of rudimentary organogenesis in phylogeny. The slime mold *Dictyostelium,* which bridges the gap between unicellular and multicellular eukaryotes, uses a protein possessing a region with striking similarity to an immunoglobulin domain for the purpose of forming aggregations called "fruiting bodies" when conditions are nutrient-scarce (183,184).

Finally, it has also been put forth that ancestral IgSF glycoproteins may have mediated the first evolutionary examples of allorecognition in colonial invertebrates (185). In defense of this proposition, it is noteworthy that two examples of metazoan receptor tyrosine kinases with purported recognition functions have been shown to possess extracellular Ig-like domains, one from the cnidarian *Hydra vulgaris* and the other from the marine sponge *Geodia cydonium.* From these data, then, it is possible to make tentative, yet tenable, conjecture that the complex cellular and molecular interactions of the vertebrate immune system (mediated in no small part by members of the IgSF) may in fact be an outgrowth of this primitive allorecognition. In this light, the notable analogy between vertebrate graft acceptance/rejection reactions and colonial invertebrate fusion/rejection phenomena perhaps takes on new significance (see Chapter 18).

Regardless of its derivation, the immunoglobulin domain has obviously proven to be a pliable evolutionary substrate, amenable to mutation and diversification for a number of important reasons. First, as was noted for the actual domains of immunoglobulins, the primary structure of these units can vary dramatically without appreciably altering their tertiary structure (186,187). This is particularly evident in the interconnecting loops that join the β strands, allowing them to diverge rapidly to perform a multitude of distinct functions. Second, most Ig domains are encoded by discrete exons, facilitating their duplication by relatively simple genetic events. This one-domain-per-exon rule is also conducive to alternative splicing phenomena, encouraging differential expression of IgSF molecules as well. This is further accommodated by a splicing convention followed by most IgSF exons: The 3′ end of one exon is always the first position of a codon, while the 5′ end of the next tandem unit begins with the second position of a codon. Thus, immunoglobulin homology domains of IgSF proteins may be easily duplicated in tandem (the *C. elegans* muscle protein twitchin contains 26 Ig-like domains) and shuffled to create new genes with the capacity to diversify both somatically and evolutionarily. Finally, the propensity of Ig domains to form homotypic and/or heterotypic dimers (also demonstrated by immunoglobulin proper) forms the basis for proteins which serve as receptor and ligand molecules. These combinatorial associations enhance their diversification potentials still further.

Despite the inherent complexity in a gene superfamily containing such vast disparities in its members' functional qualities, it was recognized early on that IgSF proteins could be subdivided into distinct "sets" on the basis of sequence and structural analyses (2). These groupings are based upon the arrangement of the β strands of the immunoglobulin fold and are schematized in Fig. 21. Note that while V-set domains are composed of a four-strand sheet and a five-strand sheet (as detailed earlier), C-set domains have four-strand and three-strand layers; these are discriminated on the basis of placement of the D strand in the sheet of strands A, B, and E (the C1 set) or with the layer formed by strands G, F, and C (the C2 set). However, studies with the IgSF muscle protein telokin have revealed a new "I set," which has domain features that are intermediary between the V and C1 sets (188). Moreover, many IgSF adhesion molecules and cell-surface receptors likely belong to this I set, rather than to the sets to which they were previously ascribed. In any case, the IgSF remains a fascinating collection of proteins with structural similarities but a wide array of functional abilities. While immunoglobulin remains the definitive example of this class of molecules, a number of IgSF proteins are also of particular significance to humoral immune responses, and their structural and functional characteristics are briefly summarized in the following sections.

Fc Receptor Molecules

FcR allow antibodies to interact with cells of both the specific and non-specific immune systems. In so doing, FcR connect humoral immune responses to cellular immune responses, and more globally, acquired immunity to that of innate immunity. These contacts play two vital roles in the biology of immune functioning. First, FcR allow antibodies to act as "flags" signaling the need for certain cellular effector events, such as phagocytosis and ADCC. Second, the different FcR facilitate antibody acting as a mediator of overall immune regulation. The signals they transmit can induce changes in cytokine secretion, expression of cell-surface receptors, and extensive differentiation programs (189).

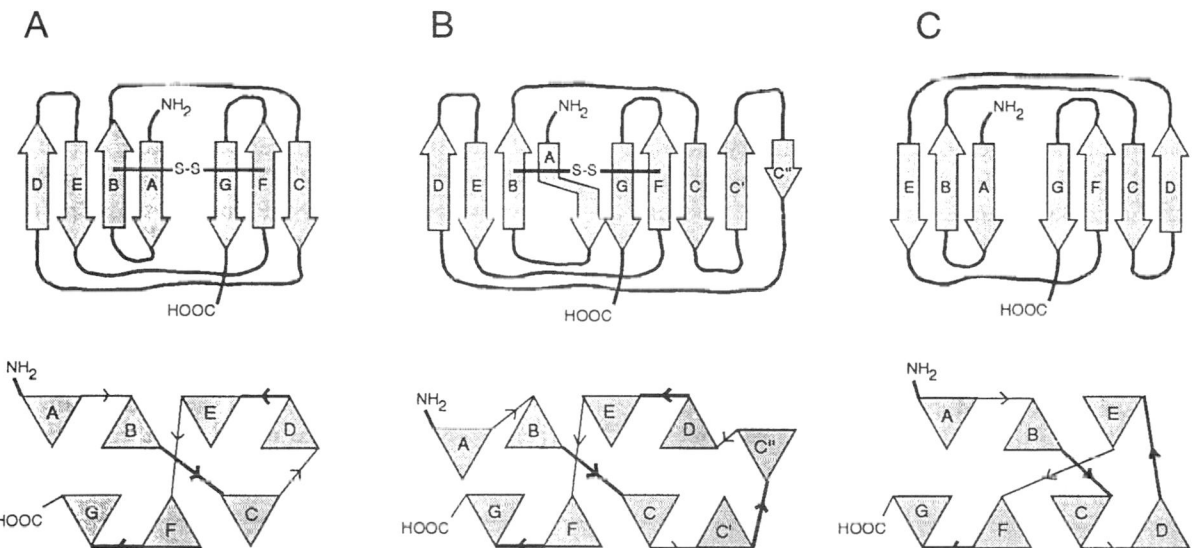

FIG. 21. Topology of different immunoglobulin domain types. Diagrams of the (**A**) C1 set, (**B**) V set, and (**C**) C2 set are presented. In the upper part of the figure, β strands are depicted as *broad arrows* and their intervening loops by *thin lines.* Note that the V-type domains have five- and four-stranded faces, while C1- and C2-type domains have four- and three-strand faces. The C region-like structures are discriminated on the basis of placement of their D strand. In the lower part of the figure, an end-on view of the different β-barrels is shown. *Triangles (with their apex at the top)* symbolize β strands running out of the plane of the paper; *triangles (whose apex points down)* are β strands traveling into the paper. *Bold lines* represent connecting loops at the top of the immunoglobulin fold; *thin lines* indicate connections at the bottom of the domain. (From ref. 4, with permission.)

Three large classes of molecules can bind Fc regions: glycosyl-transferases, which recognize oligosaccharide derivatives on antibodies, lectin-like molecules, and receptors belonging to the IgSF. Of the "true" FcR that recognize antibody protein determinants rather than carbohydrate, all FcR thus far identified belong to the IgSF, other than the low-affinity IgE receptor (CD23/FcεRII). These molecules include FcγR I, II, and III (CD64, CD32, and CD16), FcεRI, FcαR (CD89), and the pIgR, which has already been discussed. All cells of lymphoid origin express FcRs, although the profiles and isotype specificities between lineages can vary greatly (reviewed in refs. 190 and 191). While receptors for all classes of immunoglobulin have been described as biological activities, human FcμR and FcδR have not yet been cloned. Thus far, the FcγR proteins and FcεRI are the most well characterized examples of these molecules.

FcγR Molecules

Receptors for the Fc portion of IgG are of three types (reviewed in ref. 192). FcγRI (CD64) is a high-affinity receptor and the only one able to bind monomeric IgG. It possesses three extracellular Ig-like domains. FcγRII (CD32) and FcγRIII (CD16) are both low-affinity receptors that bind IgG-containing immune complexes. They each have only two extracellular Ig homology domains. Schematic diagrams of the FcγRI, FcγRII, FcγRIII complexes, along with the FcεRI and FcαR complexes, are presented in Fig. 22.

FcγRI is a 70-kD glycoprotein that is constitutively expressed at low levels on monocytes and macrophages. IFN-γ upregulates its levels on these cells, and also can induce its expression by neutrophils. FcγRI's affinity for IgG is highest for the IgG1 and IgG3 subclasses ($K_D = 10^{-8}$ M), tenfold lower for IgG4, and will not bind IgG2. Functionally, the primary effect of cross-linking FcγRI molecules appears to be the potentiation of both ADCC and phagocytosis. As IFN-γ enhances both of these activities by the cell types known to express FcγRI, this would fit well with their being important roles for the receptor.

Like surface immunoglobulin, FcγRI requires accessory proteins in order to transmit signals. This is, in fact, a common feature of most FcRs (except for FcγRII) and an interesting parallel between the IgSF antigen receptors (BCR and TCR) and the IgSF "indirect"

antigen receptors (the FcR), which use antibody to bridge the span between FcR and antigen (193). In the specific case of FcγRI, the actual signaling molecule is a 12γ-kD transmembrane protein designated the "γ-subunit" or, more generally, FcRγ. This nomenclature can be particularly confusing, as the "γ" of FcRγ refers not to the fact that it is part of the of FcγR complex (the receptor for γ-class immunoglobulin), but rather to γ as an individual subunit of a multi-molecule complex. In any case, for the FcγRI *complex,* the α subunit is the actual IgSF protein FcγRI, and the γ subunit is FcRγ, which forms a disulfide-linked homodimer. Complicating terminology further, FcRγ is also a subunit of other FcR complexes, including that of the FcγRIIIA and those of the non-FcγR, FcεRI and FcαR. Intriguingly, FcRγ is a close homologue of the TCR-associated protein CD3ζ. In fact, CD3ζ cannot only heterodimerize with FcRγ, but also has been shown to be capable of functionally substituting for FcRγ as the signal-transducing subunit of the FcγRIIIA receptor complex (194).

The situation for FcγRII (CD32) is even more complex. FcγRII is the product of three distinct but homologous genes: FcγRIIA, FcγRIIB, and FcγRIIC. This is further complicated by the fact that at least two of the FcγRII genes are alternatively spliced to generate multiple isoforms (195). The FcγRIIA gene gives rise to two transcripts: FcγRIIa1, which has a transmembrane domain, and FcγRIIa2, which lacks it. The FcγRIIB gene has three isoforms—FcγRIIb1, FcγRIIb2, and FcγRIIb3—generated by differential splicing and alternative polyadenylation processing. Collectively, the FcγRII variants are the most ubiquitously expressed FcγRs, being present on monocytes, macrophages, neutrophils, B lymphocytes, megakaryocytes, and platelets. Specifically, megakaryocytes express FcγRIIA (both isoforms), B lymphocytes express FcγRIIB (b1 and b2 transcripts) and FcγRIIC, and cells of myelomonocyte derivation produce at least one or more isoforms from all three genes (195).

Functionally, due to their expression on many cell types, FcγRII signals cause diverse effects. When cell surface FcγRII engage IgG immune complexes (all subclasses, with varying affinities), they potentiate several biologic changes, most immunoregulatory in nature. Generally, these signals down modulate IgG-, IgA-, and IgE-mediated activations of a number of cell types, including monocytes and macrophages, granulocytes, mast cells, and Langerhans and other dendritic cells. They also induce platelet aggregation at the site of immune complexes and effect B cell feedback inhibition by down-

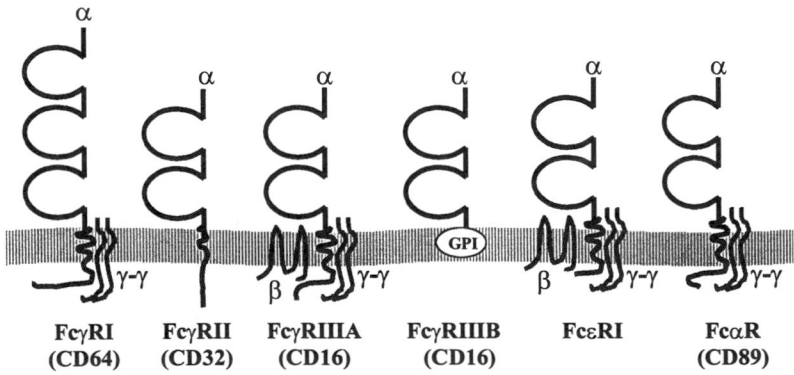

FIG. 22. Schematic diagram of human immunoglobulin Fc receptors belonging to the IgSF. Each Ig domain is depicted as a *rounded bulge.* The α chains are the components of the receptor complex that determine binding specificity. β and γ chains are responsible for association and signal propagation by the receptor(s).

regulating both proliferation and antibody production. Specifically, FcγRIIB are known to suppress BCR-mediated activation signals when the two are coaggregated (196). The signal for this inhibition is brought about in a manner unique among all IgSF FcR. As single-chain receptors without accessory proteins, FcγRII are able to transduce their own signals. They do so by way of an immunoreceptor tyrosine-based inhibition motif (ITIM) present in the cytoplasmic region of the protein (197).

Specific binding of IgG by FcγRII was initially mapped to the C-terminal portion of the second extracellular Ig-like domain of the receptor (198). This primary site, comprising residues Asn 154–Ser 161, has since been revised to also include domain 2 stretches Ser 109–Val 116 and Phe 129–Thr 135, along with domain 1 contacts (199). In sum, a three-dimensional model of the entire FcγRII extracellular region predicts that loops of both Ig-like domains that co-localize to the domain interface are responsible for the recognition of IgG.

The final IgG FcR is the FcγRIII (CD16). FcγRIII has two extracellular Ig-like domains and is encoded by two separate genes whose expression varies by cell type. On monocytes, macrophages, and NK cells, it is a transmembrane glycoprotein called FcγRIIIA. The FcγRIIIA receptor protein has three accessory proteins with which it is complexed. The first is a 30-kD "β-subunit" having four transmembrane regions, which is also a component of the FcεRI complex. The other protein(s) associated with FcγRIIIA is a homodimer of FcRγ subunits, which, as explained earlier, is also part of the receptor complexes of FcγRI, FcεRI, and FcαR (200). The other FcγRIII gene encodes a glycophosphoinositol-linked protein termed FcγRIIIB that is expressed on neutrophils. Individuals deficient in this gene suffer from a condition called paroxysmal nocturnal hemoglobinuria, characterized by increased susceptibility to infection and delayed clearance of immune complexes (201). FcγRIII's binding preference is for IgG1 and IgG3, both of which it binds with low affinity only in the form of immune complexes. Biologic activities fostered by FcγRIII include ADCC, phagocytosis, and transport of internalized Ab-Ag complexes to the antigen-presentation pathway.

FcεRI and FcαR Molecules

The high-affinity IgE receptor (FcεRI) was the first and best characterized of the FcR (202). FcεRI is a transmembrane protein having two extracellular Ig homology domains and, like previous examples, associates with accessory proteins for signal-transmission purposes. It is expressed on mast cells, basophils, eosinophils, Langerhans cells, and on the monocytes of atopic individuals (203). The proteins associated with FcεRI are the same as for FcγRIIIA: one β subunit and a homodimer of FcRγ proteins. Gene targeting experiments to verify the roles these proteins play in the FcεRI complex have yielded reassuring results: homozygous deletion of the IgSF chain of the receptor created animals that were predictably resistant to anaphylaxis (204); disruption of FcRγ caused the same phenotype, plus defects in ADCC and phagocytosis consistent with the γ-subunit's participation in other receptor complexes (205,206).

The Fcε-binding site on FcεRI has been localized to three regions of the second extracellular Ig domain (198). It is important to remember that serum IgE binds to the receptor in a high-affinity interaction not dependent on antigen (unlike all other antibody isotypes, which must first bind antigen in order to be recognized by

their respective FcR). This allows polyvalent immunogens to bind effector cells directly, without the need for conformational change of the immunoglobulin and/or immune complex formation. This contributes to the rapidity of the response exhibited by cells expressing FcεRI. The specific biologic effects of cross-linking the receptor were discussed previously in the section on IgE function.

The final FcR of the IgSF to be covered is that for IgA. The FcαR (CD89) is the most recently identified and least characterized of the different Ig receptor classes. It possesses two extracellular Ig domains and is expressed by monocytes, macrophages, neutrophils, and eosinophils. Several isoforms have been identified: a cell surface FcαRa form, which has intracellular and transmembrane domains, an FcαRb form lacking these domains that is both secreted and associated with the cell surface (by an unknown mechanism), and even an isoform lacking the membrane-proximal Ig-like domain. Structurally, the FcαR has homology with the FcγR molecules. Like FcγRI, FcγRIII, and FcεRI, the IgA receptor complex includes the FcRγ homodimer as a signaling component. The particulars of the receptor binding site on the FcαR are not yet determined. The site it recognizes on IgA and the effects mediated by FcαR-binding were detailed in the section on IgA function.

Coreceptor CD4 and CD8 Molecules

Antigen-recognition functions in the body are not limited to immunoglobulin but are also performed by receptors on T cells (TCR), which bind antigenic peptides. In a defining event of immune responses, these antigenic fragments are "presented" to T cells within the context of molecules of the MHC. Recognition of MHC/antigen by TCR is the fundamental biologic interaction responsible for initiation, perpetuation, and mediation of cellular immunity. As pertains to antibody, binding of MHC/peptide complexes by TCR is also vital for recruitment of T cell help needed in many humoral immune responses. While the details and effects of these vital interactions are well beyond the scope of this chapter (see Chapters 8–13), many IgSF proteins play key roles in assuring its productive functional outcome. Of these, the TCR "coreceptors" CD4 and CD8 are crucial components worthy of mention here.

CD4 and CD8 were among the first non-immunoglobulin IgSF members for which structural information became available (reviewed in ref. 207). These molecules are each expressed on the surface of T cells, where they participate in TCR/MHC interactions (schematized in Fig. 23) by engaging non-polymorphic regions of the MHC in low-affinity interactions (208,209). T cells break down into two major functional subclasses—helper T cells and cytotoxic T cells—characterized by different responses to antigen. Both T cell types utilize the same group of TCR genetic elements to compose their specific antigen-receptors, however. Ordinarily, although there are notable exceptions, T cell effector functions correlate with the type of MHC protein with which they interact. MHC I molecules specify cytotoxic T cell responses and are found on most cell types of the body. MHC II molecules, on the other hand, dictate helper T cell functioning and are more restricted in their expression, typically found only on "professional" antigen-presenting cells. CD8 molecules bind to class I MHC proteins, while CD4 molecules mediate interaction with class II; thus, these two proteins play an important role in determining what type of response a particular T cell is likely to mediate.

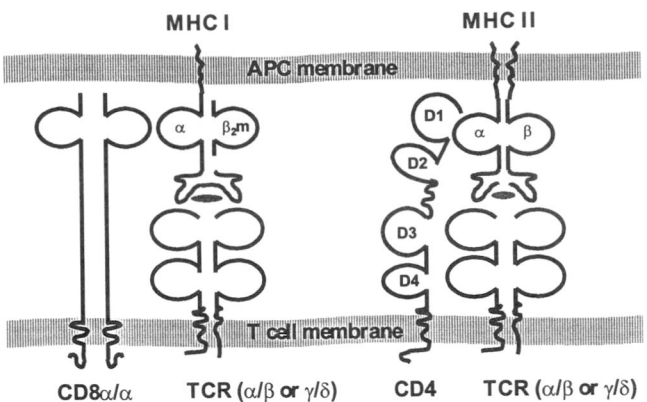

FIG. 23. Schematic diagram of the CD8 and CD4 coreceptor molecules. The figure shows both TCR/MHC coreceptor complexes on the same membrane, although T cells express either CD8 or CD4 for the majority of their lifetime. *Bulges* represent Ig domains, and *gray ovals* signify peptide presented by MHC molecules. Only the CD8α/α homodimer is schematized here, although the CD8α/β heterodimer presumably binds MHC I in similar fashion. The models demonstrate the simplest stoichiometry for association; other possible modes of interaction are discussed in the text.

Both CD8 and CD4 are glycoproteins and, in their most common incarnations, possess transmembrane segments and short cytoplasmic tails (210). The intracytoplasmic regions of both molecules interact with the src-like tyrosine kinase p56[lck] (211), which presumably serves to allow signal-transduction necessary for proper thymic selection (212) and activation (213) of T cells. Reinforcing this idea is the fact that co-ligation of CD4 or CD8 with TCR greatly enhances stimulation of T cells relative to that of cross-linking TCR alone (see Chapters 12 and 13). In addition, CD8 and CD4 also increase the avidity of interaction between TCR and MHC, by virtue of their action as adhesion molecules between the two cell membranes. Collectively, these behaviors have been estimated to boost antigen recognition over 100-fold from that of basal levels (TCR engagement by MHC/Ag only). However, despite these similarities in their biologic effects, structurally CD8 and CD4 have many important differences. While many details are still unresolved, a number of crystals involving these two proteins have been solved by x-ray diffraction, permitting a thorough examination of their salient characteristics.

CD8

CD8 exists as a disulfide-linked dimer in one of two forms. A homodimer of two CD8α subunits was the first human isoform identified (214). Subsequently, a CD8α/β heterodimer was described as well (215,216). Both proteins are 34-kD and have homologous (although only 17% identical) N-terminal Ig-like domains, extended hinge regions of 50 (α) and 30 (β) amino acid residues, single transmembrane stretches, and short cytoplasmic tails. While the CD8β chain lacks residues necessary for interaction with p56[lck], the heterodimer is still capable of interacting with it via the α subunit. Nevertheless, several lines of evidence indicate that a specific role for the heterodimer may exist, apart from that of the homodimer. Differences in functional effects (217), thymic selection (218), avidity for MHC (219), and p56[lck] activity (220) have all been attributed to the CD8β chain. In addition, there are differences in expression of the different isoforms: thymocytes and peripheral T cells are CD8α/β+, TCR γ/δ+ intraepithelial lymphocytes (IEL) are primarily CD8α/α+, and TCR α/β+ IEL express either of the two molecules. Finally, investigations into CD8β have divulged that there are actually two genes encoding this protein (221) (i.e., the locus has been recently duplicated), which—along with alternative splicing phenomena—results in as many as seven unique CD8β isoforms being expressed (222). Four of these transcripts lack the transmembrane region of the message, raising the possibility that some forms of CD8β may be secreted. In sum, the story of this protein subunit, and of the CD8 heterodimer that derives from it, is still an active area of research that is yet to be clarified.

The enumeration of the CD8α/α homodimer, thanks in large part to two crystal structures, is somewhat further along. The primary advance in this regard was the solving of the amino-terminal domains of human CD8α/α (223). This study revealed that these 113-amino acid segments formed V-type Ig domains consisting of four- and five-strand layers (see Fig. 24). In agreement with its V region-type topology, CD8α domains were shown to dimerize with one another via their five-strand faces, as do immunoglobulin V domains (see Colorplate 7). Two significant structural disparities between CD8α and immunoglobulin V regions were also recognized. First, the C'-C" loop (corresponding to CDR2) is extended in the α subunit (note the right side of Fig. 24D). Second, while the usual intradomain disulfide bridge between β strands B and F was identified, an unpaired cysteine in strand C is also conserved. In rodent CD8α this residue has been shown to form the intradomain cystine together with the Cys of strand B (224). The α subunit hinge region is extensively glycosylated (via O-linkages), and this is thought to promote its adopting an extended structure (223,225–227). This is particularly important because an elongated conformation of the hinge would be necessary to allow the N-terminal Ig domain to interact with the MHC I molecule appropriately (refer back to Fig. 23).

The other important structural features of CD8 concern its interaction with class I MHC molecules. Initial experiments into these questions indicated that the CDR-like loops of CD8α were involved with recognizing a negatively-charged region on the α3 domain of MHC I (228). The aforementioned crystal structure supported this conclusion by demonstrating that these same loops were the only region on CD8 where positive charge was localized. Mutational studies performed after the crystal was solved also implicated residues in the A and B strands of the CD8α protein as contact points with the α2 domain of MHC I (229). As each CD8 homodimer has two α chains, and as the A and B strands of each chain are not on the dimerizing face of the subunit, this implied that CD8's interaction with MHC I could be bivalent (i.e., one CD8α/α and two MHC class I proteins). The publication of a crystal structure of the complex containing CD8α/α and MHC I plus peptide has seemingly resolved these issues (230). The homodimer was shown to have contacts with not only the α3 domain, but also the α2 domain, and even with the β2-microglobulin subunit of MHC class I. Strikingly, the negatively-charged region of the α3 MHC I protein fits between the CDR-like loops of the two CD8α subunits in the fashion of classical antibody–antigen interactions! However, because both CD8 subunits are needed for the binding of one such loop, it would appear that the stoichiometry of the CD8/MHC I interaction is in fact 1:1. Because the clustering of receptor complexes is likely an important feature for the generation of intracellular signals, this is a crucial piece of information, as shall be seen for CD4.

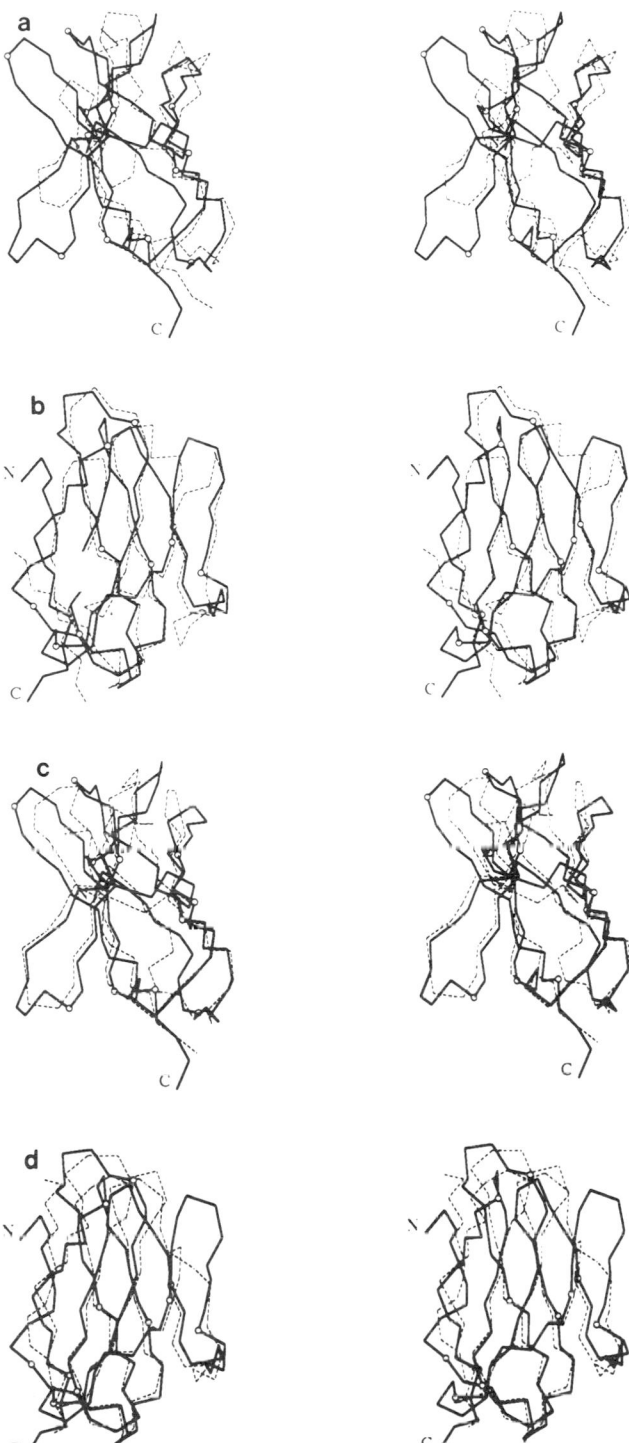

FIG. 24. Stereoviews of the α-carbon backbones of CD8α, CD4 domain 1, and the V_L of the antibody REI. In (**a,b**) the Ig domain of CD8α (*solid lines*) is superimposed on domain 1 of CD4 (*dashed lines*). In (**c,d**) V_L (now in *dashed lines*) is overlaid by CD8α. Parts (**a**) and (**c**) are side views (parallel to the dimerization surface); (**b**) and (**d**) are perpendicular to the β-sheet faces. In all cases, the CDR loops are at the top of the figure. Comparing parts (**a**) to (**c**) illustrates the truncation of the F–G (*top left*) and C–C′ (*bottom left*) loops of CD4 D1 relative to CD8α and V_L. Comparison of the N-termini [left edge of (**b**) and (**d**)] shows the shortening of CD4 D1's A strand as well. The CDR2-like C′–C″ loop [upper right of (**b**) and (**d**)] demonstrates that this segment is elongated in both CD8α and CD4 D1 relative to V_L. (From ref. 207, with permission.)

CD4

CD4 has four extracellular Ig homology domains (D1–D4) and is thought to exist as a 55-kD monomer on the cell surface (231). Scientifically, CD4 became the center of intense scrutiny when it was demonstrated to be the molecule utilized by HIV for attachment to T cells. Like immunoglobulin, proteolytic analyses established that CD4 generated stable fragments upon cleavage. These, in turn, were the initial substrates for crystallographic study. The amino-terminal (and T cell membrane-distal) D1D2 segments were the first regions of CD4 structurally determined, as they had been shown to contain the HIV-binding site. These studies (232,233) described an N-terminal V-type Ig domain (D1) and a smaller, unusual Ig-like domain (D2), each with features unique among previously reported IgSF structures.

D1 is a four- and five-strand domain (see Colorplate 7) that maintains the normal core intradomain disulfide bond and its associated residues. However, by comparison with immunoglobulin V regions, it became apparent that part of the A strand was missing (see Fig. 24). Similarly, the two loops connecting β strands C to C′ and F to G were both shortened in length. Since amino acids in these positions of immunoglobulin (and CD8) participate in dimerization events, this was taken to be reflective of the fact that CD4 was not known to dimerize. Like CD8, the CDR2-homologous C′-C″ loop of CD4 D1 is also extended relative to immunoglobulin (compare the right edges of Figs. 24B and 24D). In fact, a Phe residue found on this lengthened segment has been shown to be crucial for binding of HIV gp120 to CD4. Another interesting characteristic of these crystals concerns the D1 to D2 domain connection. Note in Colorplate 7 that the G strand of D1 is contiguous with D2's A strand (contrast with the elbow peptides connecting V and C domains). As a result, D1 and D2 have a large amount of longitudinal contact and, accordingly, little flexibility to move relative to one another.

The D2 domain is even more peculiar. D2 is smaller than most Ig domains, and it consists of only seven β strands, like Ig C-set domains (see Colorplate 7). Unlike the canonical C-type domain, D2 has switched the placement of one of its strands from one face to the other (i.e., it belongs to the C2 set; refer back to Fig. 21). Remarkably, D2 also fails to conserve the core residues necessary for the typical intradomain cystine. Curiously, its intradomain disulfide linkage is between cysteines found in the same β-stranded sheet (i.e., its disulfide bond is *intra*sheet instead of the usual *inter*sheet). Despite this idiosyncratic arrangement, D2 forms an Ig fold consistent with other Ig domains—a powerful testimony to the principle of tertiary structural conservation in the face of primary structural variation, embodied by the IgSF.

The remaining two Ig domains of CD4—D3 and D4—have also been crystallized (albeit the rat CD4 homologue) and their structures elucidated by x-ray diffraction (234,235). Remarkably, the D3D4 fragment adopts a conformation resembling that of the D1D2 portion of the molecule (see Colorplate 7), embracing prior hypotheses that CD4 arose by way of duplication of a two-domain precursor (236). D3 is a larger V-type domain homologous to D1, and D4 is a smaller module reminiscent of D2. Once again, the D3 G strand is contiguous with the A strand of D4, closely approximating the two domains and limiting the flexibility between them. However, D3 does have characteristics which distinguish it from the D1 domain. First, D3 fails to conserve the intradomain disulfide bond, resulting in a "relaxed" domain, which is packed less tightly. Second, unlike D1, the C to C′ and F to G loops of D3 are not shortened relative to immunoglobulin V regions. Still, these loops are unlikely to mediate dimerization of D3 domains (as they did in the Fv fragment of immunoglobulin), on account of an N-linked glycosylation site on the F strand of D3's inner face that would interfere with such interactions. Recently, a recombinant soluble form of human CD4 has also been solved crystallographically (237). While consistent with previous conclusions, this report makes the added contribution of definitively establishing the D1D2 to D3D4 junction as a hinge-like region of the protein. Thus, the rod-like two domain portions of CD4 (D1D2 and D3D4) are able to bend at a point of flexion akin to the scenario for Fab–Fc bending at the antibody hinge.

Studies have also examined the means by which CD4 binds to MHC II proteins (refer back to Fig. 23). CD4 contacts the α2 and β2 domains of class II molecules using a variety of residues in the D1 and D2 domains. Most evidence points to a large surface of CD4, involving both lateral faces of D1 and the F–G loop of the D2 domain, being implicated in MHC II binding (238–240). Once more the question of the stoichiometry of interaction between coreceptor and MHC is of interest. As both sides of the D1 domain appear to contact the class II molecule, the prospect of a bivalent complex (one CD4 protein with two MHC II molecules) is once again at issue. Given that crystal studies of class II proteins have demonstrated a dimeric association between MHC II molecules, this seems a plausible mode of complex formation. Contrarily, the crystal of soluble human D1–D4 (237) has revealed a homodimeric association between D4 domains of CD4. This implies that—as had been proposed by others (241)—opposite faces of a CD4 dimer may interact with two separate class II molecules. Regardless of the specifics of their dimeric interactions, it is reasonable to conclude that multiple surfaces of CD4 are responsible for binding, and that the majority of these amino acids reside in the D1 domain.

CONCLUSION

Although these discussions only scratch the surface of structure–function relationships within the immunoglobulin superfamily of proteins, it is hoped that this chapter has served to introduce the reader to the inherent utility—and exquisite beauty—of the immunoglobulin domain as both an evolutionary tool and molecular motif. While antibody proteins have been structurally characterized and functionally probed to an unparalleled degree by the concerted and persistent efforts of the scientific community, the continued emergence of unexpected findings indicates that a great wealth of knowledge is yet to be tapped in their inquiry. Moreover, the TCR and MHC IgSF proteins occupy an even greater role in terms of immune system functioning, and their investigations have been fruitful fields for study, as well. Other molecules, like CD4 and CD8, while not the focus of attention for the prolonged duration that has been the case for immunoglobulin, have nonetheless seen seminal findings in the pursuit of their understanding, and have served to broaden our comprehension of the IgSF's variety and capacity. Still others, like the antigen-receptor signaling proteins Igα, Igβ, and CD3 subunits, or the co-stimulatory molecules B7-1 (CD80), B7-2 (CD86), CTLA-4, and CD28 have only recently been described in detail and will no doubt be centers of concentration in the immediate future. Given the unequivocal fact that new and exciting IgSF members are yet to be discovered, when one considers the pervasiveness of this class of proteins in

immunology—and in biology as a whole—it is perhaps accurate to surmise that the study of the immunoglobulin superfamily is still only in its infancy.

REFERENCES

1. Dreyer WJ, Bennett JC. The molecular basis of antibody formation: a paradox. *Proc Natl Acad Sci USA* 1965;54:864–869.
2. Williams AF, Barclay AN. The immunoglobulin superfamily—domains for cell surface recognition. *Annu Rev Immunol* 1988;6:381–405.
3. Hunkapiller T, Hood L. Diversity of the immunoglobulin superfamily. *Adv Immunol* 1989;44:1–63.
4. Brummendorf T, Rathjen FG. Cell adhesion molecules 1: immunoglobulin superfamily. *Protein Profile* 1995;2:963–1108.
5. Hilschmann N, Craig LC. Amino acid sequence studies with Bence-Jones proteins. *Proc Natl Acad Sci USA* 1965;53:1403–1409.
6. Silverton EW, Navia MA, Davis DR. Three-dimensional structure of an intact human immunoglobulin. *Proc Natl Acad Sci USA* 1977;74:5140–5144.
6a. Carayannopoulous L, Capra JD. Immunoglobulins: structure and function. In: Paul WE, ed. *Fundamental Immunology,* 3rd ed. New York: Raven Press Ltd., 1993.
7. Hill RL, Delaney R, Fellows RE, Lebovitz HE. The evolutionary origins of the immunoglobulins. *Proc Natl Acad Sci USA* 1966;56:1762–1769.
8. Edmundson AB, Ely KR, Abola EE, Schiffer M, Panagiotopoulos N. Rotational allomerism and divergent evolution of domains in Ig light chains. *Biochemistry* 1975;14:3953–3961.
9. Davies DR, Padlan EA, Segal DM. Immunoglobulin structures at high resolution. *Annu Rev Biochem* 1975;44:639–667.
10. Amzel LM, Poljak RJ. Three dimensional structure of immunoglobulins. *Annu Rev Biochem* 1979;48:961–997.
11. Deisenhofer J, Colman PM, Epp O, Huber R. Crystallographic structural studies of a human Fc fragment. *Hoppe-Zeylers Z Physiol Chem* 1976;357:1421–1434.
12. Deisenhofer J. Crystallographic refinement and atomic models of a human Fc fragment and its complex with fragment B of protein A from *Staphylococcus aureus* at 2.9 and 2.8 Å resolution. *Biochemistry* 1981;20:2361–2370.
13. Federation of American Society for Experimental Biology Symposium, "Two Genes, One Polypeptide Chain." *Fed Proc* 1972;31:176–209.
14. Porter RR. Separation and isolation of fractions of rabbit γ-globulin containing the antibody and antigenic combining sites. *Nature* 1958;182:670–671.
15. Nisonoff A, Wissler FC, Lipman LN. Properties of the major component of a peptic digest of rabbit antibody. *Science* 1960;132:1770–1771.
16. Palmer JL, Nisonoff A. Dissociation of rabbit γ-globulin into half-molecules after reduction of one labile disulfide bond. *Biochemistry* 1964;3:863–869.
17. Fleischman JB, Porter RR, Press E. The arrangement of the peptide chains in γ-globulin. *Biochem J* 1963;88:220–228.
18. Nisonoff A, Thorbecke GJ. Immunochemistry. *Annu Rev Biochem* 1964;33:355–402.
19. Natvig JB, Kunkel HG. Human Igs: classes, subclasses, genetic variants, and idiotypes. *Adv Immunol* 1973;16:1–59.
20. Nisonoff A, Hopper JE, Spring SB. *The antibody molecule.* New York: Academic Press, 1975.
21. Kindt TJ, Capra JD. *The antibody enigma.* New York: Plenum Press, 1984.
22. Hasemann CA, Capra JD. Immunoglobulins: structure and function. In: Paul WE, ed. *Fundamental immunology,* 2nd ed. New York: Raven Press, 1989.
23. Weir DM, ed. *Handbook of experimental immunology,* vol. 3, *Genetics & molecular immunology.* London: Blackwell Scientific Press, 1986.
24. Williams RC Jr, Kunkel HG, Capra JD. Antigenic specificities related to the cold agglutinin activity of gamma M globulins. *Science* 1968;161:379–381.
24a. Kabat EA, Wu TT, Perry HM, Gottesman KS, Foeller C. *Sequences of proteins of immunological interest.* Washington, DC: US Department of Health and Human Services, 1991.
25. Wu TT, Kabat EA. An analysis of the sequences of the variable regions of Bence-Jones proteins and myeloma light chains and their implications for antibody complementarity. *J Exp Med* 1970;132:211–250.
26. Capra JD, Kehoe JM. Hypervariable regions, idiotypy, and the antibody-combining site. *Adv Immunol* 1975;20:1–40.
27. Colman PM. Structure of antibody-antigen complexes: implications for immune recognition. *Adv Immunol* 1988;43:99–132.
28. Chothia C, Novotny J, Bruccoleri R, Karplus M. Domain association in immunoglobulin molecules. *J Mol Biol* 1985;186:651–663.
28a. Chothia C, Lesk AM. Canonical structures for the hypervariable regions of immunoglobulins. *J Mol Biol* 1987;196:901–917.
29. Tonegawa S. Somatic generation of antibody diversity. *Nature* 1983;302:575–581.
30. Meier JT, Lewis SM. P nucleotides in V(D)J recombination: a fine-structure analysis. *Mol Cell Biol* 1993;13(2):1078–1092.
31. Meek KD, Hasemann CA, Capra JD. Novel rearrangements at the immunoglobulin D locus. *J Exp Med* 1989;170:39–57.
32. McKean D, Huppi K, Bell M, Staudt L, Gerhard W, Weigert M. Generation of antibody diversity in the immune response of BALB/c mice to influenza virus hemagglutinin. *Proc Natl Acad Sci USA* 1984;81:3180–3184.

33. Neuberger MS, Milstein C. Somatic hypermutation. *Curr Opin Immunol.* 1995; 7:248–254.
34. Croce CM, Shander M, Martinis J, et al. Chromosomal location of the genes for human immunoglobulin heavy chains. *Proc Natl Acad Sci USA* 1979;76: 3416–3419.
35. Malcolm S, Barton P, Murphy C, Ferguson-Smith MA, Bentley DL, Rabbitts TH. Localization of human immunoglobulin kappa light chain variable region genes to the short arm of chromosome 2 by *in situ* hybridization. *Proc Natl Acad Sci USA* 1982;79(16):4957–4961.
36. Erickson J, Martinis J, Croce CM. Assignment of the genes for human λ immunoglobulin chains to chromosome 22. *Nature* 1981;294:173–175.
37. D'Eustachio P, Pravtcheva D, Marcu K, Ruddle FH. Chromosomal location of the structural gene cluster encoding murine immunoglobulin heavy chains. *J Exp Med* 1980;151(6):1545–1550.
38. Swan D, D'Eustachio P, Leinwand L, Seidman J, Keithley D, Ruddle FH. Chromosomal assignment of the mouse κ light chain genes. *Proc Natl Acad Sci USA* 1979;76(6):2735–2739.
39. D'Eustachio P, Bothwell AL, Takaro TK, Baltimore D, Ruddle FH. Chromosomal location of structural genes encoding murine Ig λ light chains. *J Exp Med* 1981;153(4):793–800.
40. Schroeder HW Jr, Hillson JL, Perlmutter RM. Structure and evolution of mammalian V_H families. *Int Immunol* 1990;2:41–50.
41. Kirkham PM, Mortari F, Newton JA, Schroeder HW Jr. Immunoglobulin V_H clan and family identity predicts variable domain structure and may influence antigen binding. *EMBO J* 1992;11:603–609.
42. Kirkham PM, Schroeder HW Jr. Antibody structure and the evolution of immunoglobulin V gene segments. *Semin Immunol* 1994;6:347–360.
43. Kirkham PM, Elgavish RA, Schroeder HW Jr. Structure and evolution of mammalian $V_κ$ families. *J Immunol* 1993;150:151a.
44. Kroemer G, Helmberg A, Bernot A, Auffray C, Kofler R. Evolutionary relationship between human and mouse immunoglobulin κ light chain variable region genes. *Immunogenetics* 1991;33:42–49.
45. Pascual V, Capra JD. Human immunoglobulin heavy-chain variable region genes: organization, polymorphism, and expression. *Adv Immunol* 1991;49: 1–74.
46. Zachau HG. The immunoglobulin κ locus—or—what has been learned from looking closely at one-tenth of a percent of the human genome. *Gene* 1993;135: 167–173.
47. Frippiat JP, Williams SC, Tomlinson IM, et al. Organization of the human immunoglobulin λ light-chain locus on chromosome 22q11.2. *Hum Mol Genet* 1995;4(6):983–991.
48. Cook GP, Tomlinson IM, Walter G, et al. A map of the human immunoglobulin V_H locus completed by analysis of the telomeric region of chromosome 14q. *Nat Genet* 1994;7(2):162–168.
49. Matsuda F, Shin EK, Nagaoka H, et al. Structure and physical map of 64 variable segments in the 3' 0.8 megabase region of the human immunoglobulin heavy chain locus. *Nat Genet* 1993;3:88–94.
50. Matsuda F, Honjo T. Organization of the human immunoglobulin heavy chain locus. *Adv Immunol* 1996;62:1–29.
51. Hsu E. The variation in immunoglobulin heavy chain C regions in evolution. *Semin Immunol* 1994;6:383–391.
52. Davis AC, Roux KH, Pursey J, Shulman MJ. Intermolecular disulfide bonding in IgM: effects of replacing cysteine residues in the μ heavy chain. *EMBO J* 1989;8:2519–2526.
53. Mestecky J, Russell MW. IgA subclasses. *Monogr Allergy* 1986;19:277–301.
54. Burnett RC, Hanly WC, Zhai SK, Knight KL. The IgA heavy chain gene family in rabbit: cloning and sequence analysis of 13 Cα genes. *EMBO J* 1989;8: 4041–4047.
55. Poljak RJ. X-ray diffraction studies of immunoglobulins. *Adv Immunol* 1975;21: 1–33.
56. Huck S, Fort P, Crawford DH, Lefranc MP, Lefranc G. Sequence of a human IgG3 heavy chain C region gene: comparison with the other human Cγ genes. *Nucleic Acids Res* 1986;14:1779–1789.
57. Kocher HP, Bijlenga RK, Jaton JC. Biosynthesis and structure of membrane and secretory immunoglobulins. *Mol Cell Biochem* 1982;47:11–22.
58. Rogers J, Choi E, Souza L, et al. Gene segments encoding transmembrane carboxyl termini of Ig γ chains. *Cell* 1981:19–27.
58a. Tomlinson IM, Walter G, Jones PT, Dear PH, Sonnhammer ELL, Winter G. The imprint of somatic hypermutation on the repertoire of human germline V genes. *J Mol Biol* 1996;256:813–817.
59. Davies DR, Padlan EA, Sheriff S. Antigen-antibody complexes. *Annu Rev Biochem* 1990;59:439–473.
60. Wright A, Tao MH, Kabat EA, Morrison SL. Antibody variable region glycosylation: position effects on antigen binding and carbohydrate structure. *EMBO J* 1991;10:2717–2723.
61. Middaugh CR, Litman GW. Atypical glycosylation of an IgG monoclonal cryo-Ig. *J Biol Chem* 1987;262:3671–3673.
62. Chothia C, Lesk AM, Tramontano A, et al. Conformations of immunoglobulin hypervariable regions. *Nature* 1989;342:877–883.
63. Strong RK, Campbell R, Rose DR, Petsko GA, Sharon J, Margolies MN. Three-dimensional structure of murine anti-p-azophenylarsonate Fab 36–71. *Biochemistry* 1991;30:3739–3748.
64. Guddat LW, Herron JN, Edmundson AB. Three-dimensional structure of a

human immunoglobulin with a hinge deletion. *Proc Natl Acad Sci USA* 1993;90:4271–4275.
65. Padlan EA, Davies DR. A model of the Fc of IgE. *Mol Immunol* 1986;10: 1063–1075.
66. Carayannopoulos L, Hexham JM, Capra JD. Localization of the binding site for the monocyte IgA-Fc receptor (CD89) to the domain boundary between $C_α2$ and $C_α3$ in human IgA1. *J Exp Med* 1996;183:1579–1586.
66a. Putnam FW. *The plasma proteins: structure, function, and genetic control*, vol 3, 2nd ed. New York: Academic Press, 1977.
67. Grey HM, Abel CA, Yount WJ, Kunkel HG. A subclass of human γA-globulins (γ-A2) which lacks the disulfide bonds linking heavy and light chains. *J Exp Med* 1968;128:1223–1236.
68. Saul FA, Amzel LM, Poljak RJ. Preliminary refinement and structural analysis of the Fab fragment from human immunoglobulin New at 2.0 A resolution. *J Biol Chem* 1978;253:585–597.
69. Padlan EA. Anatomy of the antibody molecule. *Mol Immunol* 1994;31: 169–217.
70. Davies DR, Sheriff S, Padlan E. Comparative study of two Fab-lysozyme crystal structures. *Cold Spring Harb Symp Quant Biol* 1989;54:233–238.
71. Schumaker VN, Phillips ML, Hansen DC. Dynamic aspects of antibody structure. *Mol Immunol* 1991;28:1347–1360.
72. Wade RH, Taveau JC, Lamy JN. Concerning the axial flexibility of the Fab regions of IgG. *J Mol Biol* 1989;206:349–356.
73. Dangl JL, Wensel TG, Morrison SL, Streyer L, Herzenberg LA, Oi VT. Segmental flexibility and complement fixation of genetically engineered chimeric human, rabbit and mouse Abs. *EMBO J* 1988;7:1989–1994.
74. Spiegelberg HL. The structure and biology of human IgD. *Immunol Rev* 1977; 37:3–23.
75. Putnam FW, Liu YS, Low TL. Primary structure of a human IgA1 immunoglobulin. *J Biol Chem* 1979;254:2865–2874.
76. Plaut AG, Wistar R Jr, Capra JD. Differential susceptibility of human IgA immunoglobulins to streptococcal IgA protease. *J Clin Invest* 1974;54: 1295–1300.
77. Plaut AG, Gilbert JV, Artenstein MS, Capra JD. *Neisseria gonorrhoeae* and *Neisseria meningitidis*: extracellular enzyme cleaves human IgA. *Science* 1975;190: 1103–1105.
78. Dwek R. Glycobiology—towards understanding the function of sugars. *Biochem Soc Trans* 1995;23:1–25.
79. Jenkins M, Curling E. Glycosylation of recombinant proteins: problems and prospects. *Enzyme Microb Technol* 1995;16:354–361.
80. Schaffner G, Haase M, Geiss S. Criteria for investigation of the product equivalence of monoclonal antibodies for therapeutic and *in vivo* diagnostic use in case of change in manufacturing process. *Biologicals* 1995;23:253–259.
81. Beale D, Feinstein A. Structure and function of the C regions of immunoglobulins. *Q Rev Biophys* 1976;9:135–180.
81a. Jefferis R, Lund J. Glycosylation of antibody molecules: structural and functional significance. *Chem Immunol* 1997;65:111–128.
82. Tsuchiya N, Endo T, Matsuta K, et al. Effects of galactose depletion from oligosaccharide chains on immunological activities of human IgG. *J Rheumatol* 1989;16:285–290.
83. Tao MH, Morrison SL. Studies of aglycosylated chimeric mouse-human IgG. *J Immunol* 1989;143:2595–2601.
84. Wright A, Morrison SL. Effect of altered C_H2-associated carbohydrate structure on the functional properties and *in vivo* fate of human IgG1. *J Exp Med* 1994; 180:1087–1096.
85. Lund J, Winter G, Jones PT, et al. Human FcγRI and FcγRII interact with distinct but overlapping binding sites on the human IgG. *J Immunol* 1991;147: 2657–2662.
86. Canfield SM, Morrison SL. The binding affinity of human IgG for its high affinity Fc receptor is determined by multiple amino acids in the C_H2 domain and is modulated by the hinge region. *J Exp Med* 1991;173:1483–1491.
87. Jefferis R, Lund J, Goodall M. Recognition sites on human IgG for Fcγ receptors: the role of glycosylation. *Immunol Lett* 1995;44:111–117.
87a. Davis AC, Roux KH, Shulman MJ. On the structure of polymeric IgM. *Eur J Immunol* 1988;18:1001–1008.
88. Mole JE, Bhown AS, Bennett JC. Primary structure of human J chain: alignment of peptides from chemical and enzymatic hydrolyses. *Biochemistry* 1977;16: 3507–3513.
89. Koshland ME. The coming of age of the immunoglobulin J chain. *Annu Rev Immunol* 1985;3:425–453.
90. Max EE, Korsmeyer SJ. Human J chain gene. *J Exp Med* 1985;161:832–849.
91. Cann GM, Zaritsky A, Koshland ME. Primary structure of the immunoglobulin J chain from the mouse. *Proc Natl Acad Sci USA* 1982;79:6656–6660.
92. Hughes GJ, Frutiger S, Paquet N, Jaton JC. The amino acid sequence of rabbit J chain in secretory IgA. *Biochem J* 1990;271:641–647.
93. Mikoryak CA, Margolies MN, Steiner LA. J chain in *Rana catesbeiana* high molecular weight Ig. *J Immunol* 1988;140:4279–4285.
94. Takahashi T, Iwase T, Takenouchi N, et al. The joining (J) chain is present in invertebrates that do not express immunoglobulins. *Proc Natl Acad Sci USA* 1996;93:1886–1891.
95. Zikan J, Novotny J, Trapane TL, et al. Secondary structure of the immunoglobulin J chain. *Proc Natl Acad Sci USA* 1985;82:5905–5909.
96. Davis AC, Collins C, Yoshimura MI, D'Agostaro G, Shulman MJ. Mutations of

the mouse μ chain which prevent polymer assembly. *J Immunol* 1989;143:
1352–1357.

97. Mather EL, Alt FW, Bothwell A, Baltimore D, Koshland ME. Expression of J chain RNA in cell lines representing different stages of B lymphocyte differentiation. *Cell* 1981;23:369–378.

98. Randall TD, Parkhouse RM, Corley RB. J chain synthesis and secretion of hexameric IgM is differentially regulated by LPS and IL5. *Proc Natl Acad Sci USA* 1992;89:962–966.

99. Randall TD, King LB, Corley RB. The biological effects of IgM hexamer formation. *Eur J Immunol* 1990;20:1971–1979.

100. Underdown B. Transcytosis by the receptor for polymeric immunoglobulin. In: Metzger H, ed. *Fc receptors and the action of antibodies.* Washington, DC: American Society for Microbiology, 1990.

101. Mostov KE, Blobel G. A transmembrane precursor of secretory component. *J Biol Chem* 1982;257:11816–11821.

102. Mostov KE, Friedlander M, Blobel G. The receptor for transepithelial transport of IgA and IgM contains multiple immunoglobulin-like domains. *Nature* 1984;308:37–43.

103. Brandtzaeg P. Human secretory IgM. *Immunology* 1975;29:559–570.

104. Weicker J, Underdown BJ. A study of the association of human secretory component with IgA and IgM proteins. *J Immunol* 1975;114:1337–1344.

105. Mach J-P. *In vitro* combination of human and bovine free secretory component with IgA of various species. *Nature* 1970;228:1278–1282.

106. Bienenstock J, Perey DY, Gauldie J, Underdown BJ. Chicken γA: physiochemical and immunochemical characteristics. *J Immunol* 1973;110:524–533.

107. Fallgreen-Gebauer E, Bebauer W, Bastian A, et al. The covalent linkage of secretory component to IgA. *Biol Chem Hoppe Seyler* 1993;374:1023–1028.

108. Bakos MA, Kurosky A, Goldblum RM. Characterization of a critical binding site for human polymeric immunoglobulin on secretory component. *J Immunol* 1991;147:3419–3426.

109. Hasemann C, Capra JD. Mutational analysis of arsonate binding by a CRIA+ antibody. *J Biol Chem* 1991;266:7626–7632.

110. Amit AG, Mariuzza RA, Phillips SEV, Poljak RJ. Three-dimensional structure of an antigen-antibody complex at 2.8 Å resolution. *Science* 1986;233:747–753.

110a.Davies DR, Sheriff S, Padlan EA, Silverton EW, Cohen GH, Smith-Gill SJ. Three-dimensional structures of two Fab complexes with lysozyme. In: Smith-Gill SJ, Sercarz EE, eds. *The immune response to structurally define proteins: the lysozyme model.* Schenectady, NY: Adenine Press, 1989.

111. Padlan EA. On the nature of antibody combining sites: unusual structural features that may confer on these sites an enhanced capacity for binding ligands. *Proteins* 1990;7:112–124.

112. Mian IS, Bradwell AR, Olson AJ. Structure, function and properties of antibody binding sites. *J Mol Biol* 1991;217:133–151.

113. Mariuzza RA, Poljak RJ, Schwarz FP. The energetics of antigen-antibody binding. *Res Immunol* 1994;145:70–72.

114. Braden BC, Poljak RJ. Structural features of the reactions between antibodies and protein antigens. *FASEB J* 1995;9:9–16.

115. Herman A, Kappler JW, Marrack P, Pullen AM. Superantigens: mechanism of T-cell stimulation and role in immune responses. *Annu Rev Immunol* 1991;9:745–772.

116. Pascual V, Capra JD. B-cell superantigens? *Curr Biol* 1991;1:315.

117. Silverman GJ. Superantigens and spectrum of unconventional B-cell antigens. *The Immunologist* 1994;2:51–57.

118. Biguzzi S. Fcγ-like determinants on immunoglobulin variable regions: identification by staphylococcal protein A. *Scand J Immunol* 1982;15:605–618.

119. Sasso EH, Silverman GJ, Mannik M. Human IgM molecules that bind staphylococcal protein A contain V_HIII H chains. *J Immunol* 1989;142:2778–2783.

120. Potter KN, Li Y, Capra JD. Staphylococcal protein A simultaneously interacts with FR1, CDR2, and FR3 on human V_H3-encoded Igs. *J Immunol* 1996;157:2982–2988.

121. Berberian L, Goodglick L, Kipps TJ, Braun J. Immunoglobulin V_H3 gene products: natural ligands for HIV gp120. *Science* 1991;261:1588–1591.

122. Lenert P, Kroon D, Spiegelberg H, Golub ES, Zanetti M. Human CD4 binds immunoglobulins. *Science* 1990;248:1639–1643.

123. Corper AL, Sohi MK, Bonagura VR, et al. Structure of human IgM rheumatoid factor Fab bound to its autoantigen IgG Fc reveals a novel topology of antibody-antigen interaction. *Nat Struct Biol* 1997;4:374–381.

123a.Simard J, Mak TW. Immunoglobulins and the B cell receptor. In: *Genetic basis of immune responses* (in press).

124. Hombach J, Lottspeich F, Reth M. Identification of the genes encoding the IgM-α and Ig-β components of the IgM antigen receptor complex by amino-terminal sequencing. *Eur J Immunol* 1990;20:2795–2799.

125. Williams GT, Venkitaraman AR, Gilmore DJ, Neuberger MS. The sequence of the μ transmembrane segment determines the tissue specificity of the transport of IgM to the cell surface. *J Exp Med* 1990;171:947–952.

126. Karasuyama H, Kudo A, Melchers F. The proteins encoded by the VpreB and λ5 pre-B cell-specific genes can associate with each other and with μ heavy chain. *J Exp Med* 1990;172:969–972.

127. Tsubata T, Reth M. The products of pre-B cell-specific genes (λ5 and VpreB) and the immunoglobulin μ chain form a complex that is transported onto the cell surface. *J Exp Med* 1990;172:973–976.

128. Arya S, Chen F, Spycher S, Isenman DE, Shulman MJ, Painter RH. Mapping of amino acid residues in the C_μ3 domain of mouse IgM important in macromole-

cular assembly and complement-dependent cytolysis. *J Immunol* 1994;152:1206–1212.

129. Wright JF, Shulman MJ, Isenman DE, Painter RH. C1 binding by mouse IgM. *J Biol Chem* 1990;265:10506–10513.

130. Du Pasquier L, Wabl MR. Antibody diversity in amphibians: inheritance of isoelectric focusing antibody patterns in isogenic frogs. *Eur J Immunol* 1978;8:428–433.

131. Lin LC, Putnam FW. Primary structure of the Fc region of human IgD: implications of evolutionary origin and biologic function. *Proc Natl Acad Sci USA* 1981;78:504–508.

132. Nitschke L, Kosco MH, Kohler G, Lamers MC. IgD-deficient mice can mount normal immune responses to thymus-independent and -dependent antigens. *Proc Natl Acad Sci USA* 1993;90:1887–1891.

133. Roes J, Rajewsky K. Immunoglobulin D (IgD)-deficient mice reveal an auxiliary receptor function for IgD in antigen-mediated recruitment of B cells. *J Exp Med* 1993;177:45–55.

134. Forster I, Vieira P, Rajewsky K. Flow cytometric analysis of cell proliferation dynamics in the B cell compartment of the mouse. *Int Immunol* 1989;1(4):321–331.

135. Black SJ, van der Loo W, Loken MR, Herzenberg LA. Expression of IgD by murine lymphocytes. Loss of surface IgD indicates maturation of memory B cells. *J Exp Med* 1978;147:984–996.

136. McHeyzer-Williams MG, Nossal GJ, Lalor PA. Molecular characterization of single memory B cells. *Nature* 1991;350:502–505.

137. Havran WL, DiGiusto DL, Cambier JC. mIgM:mIgD ratios on B cells: mean mIgD expression exceeds mIgM by 10-fold on most splenic B cells. *J Immunol* 1984;132:1712–1716.

138. Venkitaraman AR, Williams GT, Dariavach P, Neuberger MS. The B-cell antigen receptor of the five immunoglobulin classes. *Nature* 1991;352:777–781.

139. Nezlin R. Internal movements in immunoglobulin molecules. *Adv Immunol* 1990;48:1–40.

140. Simard J, Mak TW. Immunoglobulins and the B cell receptor. In: *Genetic basis of immune responses* (in press).

141. Brink R, Goodnow CC, Crosbie J, et al. IgM and IgD antigen receptors are both capable of mediating B lymphocyte activation, deletion, or anergy after interaction with specific antigen. *J Exp Med* 1992;176:991–1005.

142. Morris SC, Lees A, Finkelman FD. *In vivo* activation of naïve T cells by antigen-presenting B cells. *J Immunol* 1994;152:3777–3785.

143. Brink R, Goodnow CC, Basten A. IgD expression on B cells is more efficient than IgM but both receptors are functionally equivalent in up-regulating CD80/CD86 co-stimulatory molecules. *Eur J Immunol* 1995;25:1980–1984.

144. Swenson CD, Van Vollenhoven RF, Xue B, Siskind GW, Thorbecke GJ, Coico RF. Physiology of IgD. *Eur J Immunol* 1988;18:13–20.

145. Finkelman FD, Snapper CM, Mountz JD, Katona IM. Polyclonal activation of the murine immune system by a goat antibody to mouse IgD. *J Immunol* 1987;138:2826–2830.

146. Liu Y-J, de Bouteiller O, Arpin C, et al. Normal human IgD+/IgM+ germinal center B cells can express up to 80 mutations in the variable region of their IgD transcripts. *Immunity* 1996;4:603–613.

147. Billian G, Bella C, Mondiere P, Defrance T. Identification of a tonsil IgD+ B cell subset with phenotypical and functional characteristics of germinal center B cells. *Eur J Immunol* 1996;26:1712–1719.

148. Perlemutter RG, Hansburg D, Briles DE, Nicolotti RA, Davis JM. Subclass restriction of murine anti-carbohydrate antibodies. *J Immunol* 1978;121:566–571.

149. Coutelier J-P, van der Logt JTM, Heessen FWA, Warnier G, Van Snick J. IgG2a restriction of murine antibodies elicited by viral infections. *J Exp Med* 1987;165:64–69.

150. Papadea C, Check IJ. Human IgG and IgG subclasses: biochemical, genetic, and clinical aspects. *Crit Rev Clin Lab Sci* 1989;27:27–58.

151. Brekke OH, Michaelsen TE, Sandlie I. The structural requirements for complement activation by IgG: does it hinge on the hinge? *Immunol Today* 1995;16:85–90.

152. Bruggemann M, Williams GT, Bindon CI, et al. Comparison of the effector functions of human immunoglobulins using a matched set of chimeric antibodies. *J Exp Med* 1987;166:1351–1361.

153. Duncan AR, Winter G. The binding site for C1q on IgG. *Nature.* 1988;332:738–740.

154. Tao M-H, Canfield SM, Morrison SL. The differential ability of human IgG1 and IgG4 to activate complement is determined by the COOH-terminal sequence of the C_H2 domain. *J Exp Med* 1991;173:1025–1028.

155. Tan LK, Shopes RJ, Oi VT, Morrison SL. Influence of the hinge region on complement activation, C1q binding, and segmental flexibility in chimeric human immunoglobulins. *Proc Natl Acad Sci USA* 1990;87:162–166.

156. Sandlie I, Michaelsen TE. Engineering monoclonal antibodies to determine the structural requirements for complement activation and complement mediated lysis. *Mol Immunol* 1991;28:1361–1368.

157. Brekke OH, Michaelsen TE, Sandin R, Sandlie I. Activation of complement by an IgG molecule without a genetic hinge. *Nature* 1993;363:628–630.

158. Norderhaug L, Brekke OH, Bremnes B, et al. Chimeric mouse-human IgG3 antibodies with an IgG4-like hinge region induce complement-mediated lysis more efficiently than IgG3 with normal hinge. *Eur J Immunol* 1991;21:2379–2384.

159. Kimberly RP, Salmon JE, Edberg JC. Receptors for IgG. *Arthritis Rheum* 1995;38:306–314.

160. Indik ZK, Park JG, Hunter S, Schreiber AD. Structure/function relationships of Fcγ receptors in phagocytosis. *Semin Immunol* 1995;7:45–54.

161. Unkeless JC. Function and heterogeneity of human Fc receptors for IgG. *J Clin Invest* 1989;83:355–361.

162. Michaelsen TE, Aase A, Norderhaug L, Sandlie I. Antibody dependent cell-mediated cytotoxicity induced by chimeric mouse-human IgG subclasses and IgG3 antibodies with altered hinge region. *Mol Immunol* 1992;29:319–326.

163. Galon J, Bouchard C, Fridman WH, Sautes C. Ligands and biological activities of soluble Fcγ receptors. *Immunol Lett* 1995;44:175–181.

164. Saji F, Koyama M, Matsuzaki N. Current topic: human placental Fc receptors. *Placenta* 1994;15:453–466.

165. Sarmay G, Lund J, Rozsnyay Z, Gergely J, Jefferis R. Mapping and comparison of the interaction sites on the Fc region of IgG responsible for triggering ADCC through different types of human Fcγ receptor. *Mol Immunol* 1992;29:633–639.

166. Canfield SM, Morrison SL. The binding affinity of human IgG for its high affinity Fc receptor is determined by multiple amino acids in the C$_H$2 domain and is modulated by the hinge region. *J Exp Med* 1991;173:1483–1491.

167. Tomasi TB, Grey HM. Structure and function of IgA. *Prog Allergy* 1972;16:81–213.

168. Lehner T, Bergmeier LA, Tao L, et al. Targeted lymph node immunization with simian immunodeficiency virus p27 antigen to elicit genital, rectal, and urinary immune responses in nonhuman primates. *J Immunol* 1994;153:1858–1868.

169. Mestecky J, McGhee JR. Immunoglobulin A (IgA): molecular and cellular interactions involved in IgA biosynthesis and immune response. *Adv Immunol* 1987;40:153–245.

170. Qiu JZ, Brackee GP, Plaut AG, Sneller MC, Strober W. Analysis of the specificity of bacterial IgA proteases by a comparative study of ape serum IgAs as substrates. *Infect Immun* 1996;64:933–937.

171. Wang B, Rieger A, Kilgus O, et al. Human epidermal Langerhans cells from normal human skin bind monomeric IgE via FcεRI. *J Exp Med* 1992;175:1353–1365.

172. Bieber T, de la Salle H, Wollenberg A, et al. Human epidermal Langerhans cells express the high affinity receptor for IgE (FcεRI). *J Exp Med* 1992;175:1285–1290.

173. Gounni AS, Lamkhioued B, Ochiai K, et al. High-affinity IgE receptor on eosinophils is involved in defense against parasites. *Nature* 1994;367:183–186.

174. Hashimoto S, Koh K, Tomita Y, et al. TNF-α regulates IL-4-induced FcεRII/CD23 gene expression and soluble FcεRII release by human monocytes. *Int Immunol* 1995;7:705–713.

175. Helm B, Marsh P, Vercelli D, Padlan E, Gould H, Geha R. The mast cell binding site on human immunoglobulin E. *Nature* 1988;331:180–183.

176. Nissim A, Eshhar Z. The human mast cell receptor binding site maps to the third constant domain of IgE. *Mol Immunol* 1992;29:1065–1072.

177. Edelman GM, Cunningham BA, Gall WE, Gottlieb PD, Rutishauser U, Waxdal MJ. The covalent structure of an entire γG immunoglobulin molecule. *Proc Natl Acad Sci USA* 1969;63:78–85.

178. Brummendorf T, Rathjen FG. Structure/function relationships of axon-associated adhesion receptors of the immunoglobulin superfamily. *Curr Opin Neurobiol* 1996;6:584–593.

179. Edelman GM. CAMs and Igs: cell adhesion and the evolutionary origins of immunity. *Immunol Rev* 1987;100:11–45.

180. Hultgren SJ, Jacob-Dubuisson F, Jones CH, Branden CI. PapD and superfamily of periplasmic immunoglobulin-like pilus chaperones. *Adv Protein Chem* 1993;44:99–123.

181. Bateman A, Eddy SR, Chothia C. Members of the immunoglobulin superfamily in bacteria. *Protein Sci* 1996;5:1939–1941.

182. Wojciechowicz D, Lu CF, Kurjan J, Lipke PN. Cell surface anchorage and ligand-binding domains of the *Saccharomyces cerevisiae* cell adhesion protein alpha-agglutinin, a member of the IgSF. *Mol Cell Biol* 1993;13:2554–2563.

183. Ohno S. The origin of Igs and T-cell receptors is likely to be the cell death sensor of macrophages. *Res Immunol* 1996;147:247–252.

184. Noegel A, Gerisch G, Stadler J, Westfal M. Complete sequence and transcript regulation of a cell adhesion protein from aggregating *Dictyostelium* cells. *Embo J* 1986;5:1473–1476.

185. Mokady O. Occam's Razor, invertebrate allorecognition and immunoglobulin superfamily evolution. *Res Immunol* 1996;147:241–246.

186. Lesk AM, Chothia C. Evolution of proteins formed by β-sheets. *J Mol Biol* 1982;160:325–342.

187. Chothia C, Lesk AM. The relation between the divergence of sequence and structure in proteins. *EMBO J* 1986;5:823–826.

188. Harpaz Y, Chothia C. Many of the IgSF domains in cell adhesion molecules and surface receptors belong to a new structural set which is close to that containing variable domains. *J Mol Biol* 1994;238:528–539.

189. Kolsch E, Oberbarnscheidt J, Bruner K, Heuer J. The Fc receptor: its role in the transmission of differentiation signals. *Immunol Rev* 1980;49:61–78.

190. Fridman WM. Fc receptors and immunoglobulin binding factors. *FASEB J* 1991;5:2684–2690.

191. Unkeless JC, Scigliano E, Freedman VH. Structure and function of human and murine receptors for IgG. *Annu Rev Immunol* 1988;6:251–281.

192. Sandor M, Lynch R. The biology and pathology of Fc receptors. *J Clin Immunol* 1993;13:237–246.

193. Keegan AD, Paul WE. Multichain immune recognition receptors: similarities in structure and signaling pathways. *Immunol Today* 1992;13:63–68.

194. Lanier L, Yu G, Phillips J. Analysis of FcγRIII (CD16) membrane expression and association with CD3ζ and FcεRI-γ by site directed mutation. *J Immunol* 1991;146:1571–1576.

195. Cassel DL, Keller MA, Surrey S, et al. Differential expression of FcγRIIA, FcγRIIB and FcγRIIC in hematopoietic cells: analysis of transcripts. *Mol Immunol* 1993;30:451–460.

196. Heyman B. The immune complex: possible ways of regulating the antibody response. *Immunol Today* 1990;11:310–313.

197. Vivier E, Daeron M. Immunoreceptor tyrosine-based inhibition motifs. *Immunol Today* 1997;18:286–291.

198. Hogarth PM, Hulett MD, Ierino FL, Tate B, Powell MS, Brinkworth RL. Identification of the immunoglobulin binding regions of FcγRII and FcεRI. *Immunol Rev* 1992;125:21–35.

199. Hulett MD, Witort E, Brinkworth RI, McKenzie IF, Hogarth PM. Multiple regions of human FcγRII (CD32) contribute to the binding of IgG. *J Biol Chem* 1995;270:21188–21194.

200. Letourneur O, Kennedy IC, Brini AT, Ortaldo JR, O'Shea JJ, Kinet JP. Characterization of the family of dimers associated with Fc receptors (FcεRI and FcγRIII). *J Immunol* 1991;147:2652–2656.

201. Selvaraj P, Rosse WF, Silber R, Springer TA. The major Fc receptor in blood has a phosphatidylinositol anchor and is deficient in paroxysmal nocturnal haemoglobinuria. *Nature* 1988;333:565–567.

202. Metzger H. The receptor with high affinity for IgE. *Immunol Rev* 1992;125:38–48.

203. Maurer D, Fiebiger E, Reininger B, et al. Expression of functional high affinity IgE receptors (FcεRI) on monocytes of atopic individuals. *J Exp Med* 1994;179:745–750.

204. Dombrowicz D, Flamand V, Brigman K, et al. Abolition of anaphylaxis by targeted disruption of the high affinity IgE receptor alpha chain gene. *Cell* 1993;75:969–976.

205. Takai T, Li M, Sylvestre D, et al. FcR γ chain deletion results in pleiotropic effector cell defects. *Cell* 1994;76:519–529.

206. Clynes R, Ravetch J. Cytotoxic antibodies trigger inflammation through Fc receptors. *Immunity* 1995;3:21–26.

207. Leahy DJ. A structural view of CD4 and CD8. *FASEB J* 1995;9:17–25.

208. Rosenstein Y, Ratnofshy S, Burakoff SJ, Herrmann SH. Direct evidence for binding of CD8 to HLA class I antigens. *J Exp Med* 1989;169:149–160.

209. Weber S, Karjalainen K. Mouse CD4 binds MHC class II with extremely low affinity. *Int Immunol* 1993;5:695–698.

210. Littman DR. The structure of the CD4 and CD8 genes. *Annu Rev Immunol* 1987;5:561–584.

211. Veillette A, Bookman MA, Horak EM, Bolen JB. The CD4 and CD8 T cell surface antigens are associated with the internal membrane tyrosine-protein kinase p56^{lck}. *Cell* 1988;55:301–308.

212. Wallace VA, Penninger J, Mak TW. CD4, CD8 and tyrosine kinases in thymic selection. *Curr Opin Immunol* 1983;5:235–240.

213. Janeway CA. The T cell receptor as a multicomponent signaling machine: CD4/CD8 coreceptors, and CD45 in T cell activation. *Annu Rev Immunol* 1992;10:645–674.

214. Littman DR, Thomas Y, Maddon PJ, Chess L, Axel R. The isolation and sequence of the gene encoding T8: a molecule defining functional classes of T lymphocytes. *Cell* 1985;40:237–246.

215. Norment AM, Littman DR. A second subunit of CD8 is expressed in human T cells. *EMBO J* 1988;7:3433–3439.

216. Shiue L, Gorman SD, Parnes JR. A second chain of human CD8 is expressed on peripheral blood lymphocytes. *J Exp Med* 1988;168:1993–2005.

217. Wheeler CJ, von Hoegen P, Parnes JR. An immunological role for the CD8β-chain. *Nature* 1992;357:247–249.

218. Nakayama K, Nakayama K, Negishi I, et al. Requirement for CD8β chain in positive selection of CD8-lineage T cells. *Science* 1994;263:1131–1133.

219. Renard V, Romero P, Vivier E, Malissen B, Luescher IF. CD8β increases CD8 coreceptor function and participation in TCR-ligand binding. *J Exp Med* 1996;184:2439–2444.

220. Irie HY, Ravichandran KS, Burakoff SJ. CD8β chain influences CD8α chain-associated Lck kinase activity. *J Exp Med* 1995;181:1267–1273.

221. Nakayama K, Kawachi Y, Tokito S, et al. Recent duplication of the two human CD8 β-chain genes. *J Immunol* 1992;148:1919–1927.

222. DiSanto JP, Smith D, de Bruin D, Lacy E, Flomenberg N. Transcriptional diversity at the duplicated human CD8β loci. *Eur J Immunol* 1993;23:320–326.

223. Leahy DJ, Axel R, Hendrickson WA. Crystal structure of a soluble form of the human T cell coreceptor CD8 at 2.6 Å resolution. *Cell* 1992;68:1145–1162.

224. Kirszbaum L, Sharpe JA, Goss N, Lahnstein J, Walker ID. The α-chain of murine CD8 lacks an invariant Ig-like disulfide bond but contains a unique intrachain loop instead. *J Immunol* 1989;142:3931–3936.

225. Classon BJ, Brown MH, Garnett D, et al. The hinge region of the CD8α chain: structure, antigenicity, and utility in expression of IgSF domains. *Int Immunol* 1992;4:215–225.

226. Pascale MC, Erra MC, Malagolini N, Serafini-Cessi F, Leone A, Bonatti S. Post translational processing of an O-glycosylated protein, the human CD8 glycopro

tein, during the intracellular transport to the plasma membrane. *J Biol Chem* 1992;267:25196–25201.

227. Boursier JP, Alcover A, Herve F, Laisney I, Acuto O. Evidence for an extended structure of the T-cell co-receptor CD8α as deduced from the hydrodynamic properties of soluble forms of the extracellular region. *J Biol Chem* 1993;268:2013–2020.

228. Sanders SK, Fox RO, Kavathas P. Mutations in CD8 that affect interactions with HLA class I and monoclonal anti-CD8 antibodies. *J Exp Med* 1991;174:371–379.

229. Giblin PA, Leahy DJ, Mennone J, Kavathas PB. The role of charge and multiple faces of the CD8 α/α homodimer in binding to MHC class I molecules: support for a bivalent model. *Proc Natl Acad Sci USA* 1994;91:1716–1720.

230. Gao GF, Tormo J, Gerth UC, et al. Crystal structure of the complex between human CD8α/α and HLA-A2. *Nature* 1997;387:630–634.

231. Maddon PJ, Littman DR, Godfrey M, Maddon DE, Chess L, Axel R. The isolation and nucleotide sequence of a cDNA encoding the T-cell surface protein T4: a new member of the IgSF. *Cell* 1985;42:93–104.

232. Wang JH, Yau YW, Garrett TP, et al. Atomic structure of a fragment of human CD4 containing two immunoglobulin-like domains. *Nature* 1990;348:411–418.

233. Ryu SE, Kwong PD, Truneh A, et al. Crystal structure of an HIV-binding recombinant fragment of human CD4. *Nature* 1990;348:419–426.

234. Brady RL, Dodson EJ, Dodson GG, et al. Crystal structure of domains 3 and 4 of rat CD4: relation to the NH2-terminal domains. *Science* 1993;260:979–983.

235. Lange G, Lewis SJ, Murshudov GN, et al. Crystal structure of an extracellular fragment of the rat CD4 receptor containing domains 3 and 4. *Structure* 1994;2: 469–481.

236. Williams AF, Davis SJ, He Q, Barclay AN. Structural diversity in domains of the immunoglobulin superfamily. *Cold Spring Harb Symp Quant Biol* 1989;54: 637–647.

237. Wu H, Kwong PD, Hendrickson WA. Dimeric association and segmental variability in the structure of human CD4. *Nature* 1997;387:527–530.

238. Fleury S, Lamarre D, Meloche S, et al. Mutational analysis of the interaction between CD4 and class II MHC: class II antigens contact CD4 on a surface opposite the gp120-binding site. *Cell* 1991;66:1037–1049.

239. Moebius U, Pallai P, Harrison SC, Reinherz EL. Delineation of an extended surface contact area on human CD4 involved in class II major histocompatibility complex binding. *Proc Natl Acad Sci USA* 1993;90:8259–8263.

240. Huang B, Yachou A, Fleury S, Hendrickson WA, Sekaly RP. Analysis of the contact sites on the CD4 molecule with class II MHC molecule: co-ligand versus co-receptor function. *J Immunol* 1997;158:216–225.

241. Langedijk JP, Puijk WC, van Hoorn WP, Meloen RH. Location of CD4 dimerization site explains critical role of CDR3-like region in HIV-1 infection and T-cell activation and implies a model for complex of coreceptor-MHC. *J Biol Chem* 1993;268:16875–16878.

Fundamental Immunology, Fourth Edition,
edited by William E. Paul
Published by Lippincott–Raven Publishers, Philadelphia 1999.

CHAPTER 4

Antigen–Antibody Interactions and Monoclonal Antibodies

Jay A. Berzofsky, Ira J. Berkower, and Suzanne L. Epstein

The basic principles of antigen–antibody interaction are those of any bimolecular reaction. Moreover, the binding of antigen by antibody can, in general, be described by the same theories and studied by the same experimental approaches as the binding of a hormone by its receptor, of a substrate by enzyme, or of oxygen by hemoglobin. There are several major differences, however, between antigen–antibody interactions and these other situations. First, unlike most enzymes and many hormone-binding systems, antibodies do not irreversibly alter the antigen they bind. Thus the reactions are, at least in principle, always reversible. Second, antibodies can be raised, by design of the investigator, with specificity for almost any substance known. In each case, one can find antibodies with affinities as high as and specificities as great as those of enzymes for their substrates and receptors for their hormones. The

interaction of antibody with antigen can thus be taken as a prototype for interactions of macromolecules with ligands in general. In addition, these same features of reversibility and availability of a wide variety of specificities have made antibodies invaluable reagents for identifying, quantitating, and even purifying a growing number of substances of biologic and medical importance.

One other feature of antibodies that in the past proved to be a difficulty in studying and using them, compared to, say, enzymes, is their enormous heterogeneity. Even "purified" antibodies from an immune antiserum, all specific for the same substance and sharing the same overall immunoglobulin structure (see Chapter 9), will be a heterogeneous mixture of molecules of different subclass, different affinity, and different fine specificity and ability to discriminate among cross-reacting antigens. The advent of hybridoma monoclonal antibodies (1–3) has made available a source of homogeneous antibodies to almost anything to which antisera can be raised. Nevertheless, heterogeneous antisera are still in widespread use and even have advantages for certain purposes, such as precipitation reactions. Therefore, it is critical to keep in mind throughout this chapter, and indeed much of the volume, that the principles derived for the interaction of one antibody with one antigen must be modified and extended to cover the case of heterogeneous components in the reaction.

J. A. Berzofsky: Molecular Immunogenetics and Vaccine Research Section, Metabolism Branch, National Cancer Institute, National Institutes of Health, Bethesda, Maryland 20892.
I.J. Berkower: Laboratory of Immunoregulation, Office of Vaccines, Center for Biologics Evaluation and Research, Food and Drug Administration, Bethesda, Maryland 20892.
S. L. Epstein: Molecular Immunology Laboratory, Division of Cellular and Gene Therapies, Center for Biologics Evaluation and Research, Food and Drug Administration, Bethesda, Maryland 20892.

In this chapter we examine the theoretical principles necessary for analyzing, in a quantitative manner, the interaction of antibody with antigen, and the experimental techniques that have been developed to study these interactions as well as to make use of antibodies as quantitative reagents. In addition, we explore the effects of antigen binding on the antibody molecule itself. Furthermore, we discuss the derivation, use, and properties of monoclonal antibodies.

THERMODYNAMICS AND KINETICS

The Thermodynamics of Affinity

The basic thermodynamic principles of antigen–antibody interactions, as indicated above, are the same as those for any reversible bimolecular binding reaction. We review these as they apply to this particular immunologic reaction.

Chemical Equilibrium in Solution

For this purpose, let S = antibody-binding sites, L = ligand (antigen) sites, and SL = the complex of the two. Then for the reaction

$$S + L \rightleftharpoons SL \qquad [1]$$

the mass action law states

$$K_A = \frac{[SL]}{[S][L]} \qquad [2]$$

where K_A is the association constant (or affinity) and square brackets indicate molar concentration of the reactants enclosed. The import of this equation is that, for any given set of conditions, such as temperature, pH, and salt concentration, the ratio of the concentration of the complex to the product of the concentrations of the reactants at equilibrium is always constant. Thus, changing the concentration of either antibody or ligand will invariably change the concentration of the complex, provided neither reactant is limiting (i.e., neither has already been saturated) and provided sufficient time is allowed to reach a new state of equilibrium. Moreover, since the concentrations of antibody and ligand appear in this equation in a completely symmetrical fashion, doubling either the antibody concentration or the antigen concentration results in a doubling of the concentration of the antigen–antibody complex, provided the other reactant is in sufficient excess. This proviso, an echo of the one just above, is inherent in the fact that [S] and [L] refer to the concentrations of free S and free L, respectively, in solution, not the total concentration, which would include that of the complex. Thus, if L is not in great excess, doubling [S] results in a decrease in [L] as some of it is consumed in the complex, so the net result is less than a doubling of [SL]. Similarly, halving the volume results in a doubling of the total concentration of both antibody and ligand. If the fraction of both reactants tied up in the complex is negligibly small (as might be the case for low-affinity binding), the concentration of the complex quadruples. However, in most practical cases, the concentration of complex is a significant fraction of the total concentration of antigen or antibody or both, so the net result is an increase in the concentration of complex, but by a factor of less than 4. The other important, perhaps obvious, but often forgotten, principle to be gleaned from this example is that since it is concentration, not amount, of each reactant that enters into

the mass action law (Eq. 2), putting the same amount of antigen and antibody in a smaller volume will increase the amount of complex formed, and diluting them in a larger volume will greatly decrease the amount of complex formed. Moreover, these changes go approximately as the square of the volume, so volumes are critical in the design of an experiment.

The effect of increasing free ligand concentration [L], at constant total antibody concentration, on the concentration of complex, [SL], is illustrated in Fig. 1. The mass action law (Eq. 2) can be rewritten

$$[SL] = K_A[S][L] = K_A([S]_t - [SL])[L] \qquad [3]$$

or

$$[SL] = \frac{K_A[S]_t[L]}{1 + K_A[L]} \qquad [3']$$

where $[S]_t$ is total antibody site concentration; that is, [S] – [SL]. Initially, when the complex [SL] is a negligible fraction of the total antibody $[S]_t$, the concentration of complex increases nearly linearly with increasing ligand. However, as a larger fraction of antibody is consumed, the slope tapers off and the concentration of complex, [SL], asymptotically approaches a plateau value of $[S]_t$ as all the antibody becomes saturated. Thus the concentration of antibody-binding sites can be determined from such a saturation binding curve (see Fig. 1), taking the concentration of (radioactively or otherwise labeled) ligand bound at saturation as a measure of the concentration of antibody sites.[1] This measurement is sometimes referred to as antigen-binding capacity.

The total concentration of ligand at which the antibody begins to saturate is a function not only of the antibody concentration, but also of the association constant, K_A, also called the affinity. This constant has units of M^{-1} or liters per mole, if all the concentrations in Eq. 2 are molar. Thus, the product $K_A[L]$ is unitless. It is the value of this product relative to 1 that determines how saturated the antibody is, as can be seen from Eq. 3'. For example, an antibody with an affinity of 10^7 M^{-1} will not be saturated if the ligand concentration is 10^{-8} M (product $K_A[L] = 0.1$) even if the total amount of ligand is in great excess over the total amount of antibody. From Eq. 3' the fraction of antibody occupied would be only 0.1/1.1, or about 9%, in this example. These aspects of affinity and the methods for measuring affinity are analyzed in greater detail in the next section.

Free Energy

With regard to thermodynamics, the affinity, K_A, is also the central quantity, because it is directly related to the free energy, ΔF, of the reaction by the equations

$$\Delta F^\circ = -RT \ln K_A \qquad [4]$$

$$K_A = e^{-\Delta F^\circ/RT} \qquad [4']$$

where R is the so-called gas constant (1.98717 cal/°K · mol), T is the absolute temperature (in degrees Kelvin), ln is the natural logarithm, and e is the base of the natural logarithms. The minus sign is introduced because of the convention that a negative change in free

---

[1] This point is strictly true only for univalent ligands, but most multivalent ligands behave as effectively univalent at large antigen excess, where this plateau is measured.

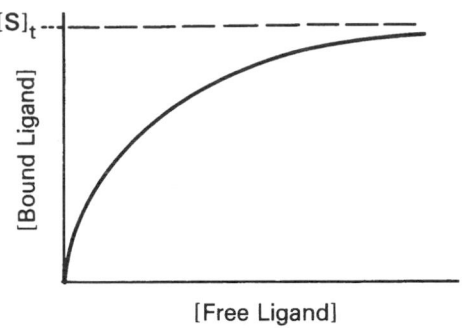

FIG. 1. Schematic plot of bound ligand concentration as a function of free ligand concentration at a constant total concentration of antibody combining sites, $[S]_t$. The curve asymptotically approaches a plateau at which [bound ligand] equals $[S]_t$.

energy corresponds to positive binding. $\Delta F°$ is the standard free-energy change defined as the ΔF for 1 mol antigen – 1 mol antibody sites combining to form 1 mol of complex, at unit concentration.

It is also instructive to note an apparent discrepancy in Eqs. 4 and 4′. As defined in Eq. 2, K_A has dimensions of M^{-1} (i.e., liters/mol), whereas in Eq. 4′, it is dimensionless. The reason is that for Eq. 4′ to hold strictly, K_A must be expressed in terms of mole fractions rather than concentrations. The mole fraction of a solute is the ratio of moles of that solute to the total number of moles of all components in the solution. Since water (55 M) is by far the predominant component of most aqueous solutions, for practical purposes, one can convert K_A into a unitless ratio of mole fractions by dividing all concentrations in Eq. 2 by 55 M. This transformation makes Eq. 4′ strictly correct, but it introduces an additional term, $-RT \ln 55$ (corresponding to the entropy of dilution), into Eq. 4. This constant term cancels out when one is subtracting ΔF values, but not when one discusses ratios of ΔF values.

An important rule of thumb can be extracted from these equations. Since $\ln 10 = 2.303$, a tenfold increase in affinity of binding corresponds to a free-energy change ΔF of only 1.42 kcal per mol at 37°C (310.15°K). (The corresponding values for 25° and 4°C are 1.36 and 1.27 kcal per mol, respectively.) This is less than one-third the energy of a single hydrogen bond (about 4.5 kcal per mol). Looked at another way, a very high affinity of 10^{10} M^{-1} corresponds to a ΔF of only 14.2 kcal/mol, approximately the bonding energy of three hydrogen bonds. (Of course, since hydrogen bonds with water are broken during the formation of hydrogen bonds between antigen and antibody, the net energy per hydrogen bond is closer to 1 kcal/mol.) It is apparent from this example that of the many interactions (hydrophobic and ionic as well as hydrogen bonding) that occur between the contact residues in an antibody-combining site and the contacting residues of an antigen (such as a protein), almost as many are repulsive as attractive. It is this small difference of a few kilocalories between much larger numbers corresponding to the total of attractive and the total of repulsive interactions that leads to net "high-affinity" binding. If ΔF were any larger, binding reactions would be of such high affinity as to be essentially irreversible. Viewed in this way, it is not surprising that a small modification of the antigen can result in an enormous change in affinity. A single hydrogen bond can change the affinity many-fold, and similar arguments apply to hydrophobic interactions and other forms of bonding. This concept is important when we discuss specificity and antigen structure later.

Effects of Temperature, pH, and Salt Concentration

It was mentioned earlier that K_A is constant for any given set of conditions, such as temperature, pH, and salt concentration. However, it varies with each of these conditions. We have already seen that the conversion of free energy to affinity depends on temperature. However, the free energy itself is also a function of temperature

$$\Delta F° = \Delta H° - T \Delta S° \qquad [5]$$

where ΔH is change in enthalpy (the heat of the reaction)[2] and ΔS is the entropy (a term related to the change in disorder produced by the reaction),[2] and T is the absolute temperature (in degrees Kelvin).

It can be shown that the association constant K_A will thus vary with temperature as follows:

$$\frac{d \ln K_A}{dT} = \frac{\Delta H°}{RT^2} \qquad [6]$$

or equivalently,

$$\frac{d \ln K_A}{d(1/T)} = \frac{-\Delta H°}{R} \qquad [6′]$$

The derivation of these equations is beyond the scope of this book (see ref. 4). However, the practical implications are as follows. First, one can determine the standard enthalpy change $\Delta H°$ of the reaction from the slope of a plot of $\ln K_A$ versus $1/T$. Second, for an interaction that is primarily exothermic (i.e., driven by a large negative ΔH, such as the formation of hydrogen bonds and polar bonds), the affinity decreases with increasing temperature. Thus many antigen–antibody interactions have a higher affinity at 4°C than at 25° or 37°C, so maximum binding for a given set of concentrations can be achieved in the cold. In contrast, apolar or hydrophobic interactions are driven largely by the entropy term, $T \Delta S$, and $\Delta H°$ is near zero. In this case, there is little effect of temperature on the affinity.

As for the effects of pH and salt concentration (or ionic strength) on the affinity, these vary depending on the nature of the interacting groups. Most antigen–antibody reactions are studied near neutral pH and at physiologic salt concentrations (0.15 M NaCl). If the interaction is dominated by ionic interactions, high salt concentration lowers the affinity.

Kinetics of Antigen–Antibody Reactions

A fundamental connection between the thermodynamics and kinetics of antigen–antibody binding is expressed by the relationship

$$K_A = \frac{k_1}{k_{-1}} \qquad [7]$$

where k_1 and k_{-1} are the rate constants for the forward (association) and backward (dissociation) reactions.

The forward reaction is determined largely by diffusion rates (theoretical upper limit 10^9 L/mol · sec) and by the probability that a collision will result in binding, that is, largely the probability that both the antigen and the antibody will be oriented in the right way to produce a good fit, as well as the activation energy for binding.

---

[2]For a more complete description of these concepts, see a physical chemistry text such as Moore (4).

The diffusive rate constant can be shown (5) to be approximated by the Smoluchowski equation

$$k_{dl} = 4\pi a D(6 \times 10^{20}) \qquad [7a]$$

where a is the sum of the radii in centimeters of the two reactants and D is the sum of the diffusion constants in square centimeters per second for the individual reactants, and the constant 6×10^{20} is necessary to convert the units to $M^{-1} \cdot sec^{-1}$. For example, if $a = 10^{-6}$ cm and $D = 10^{-7}$ cm^2/sec, then $k_{dl} \sim 7.5 \times 10^8$ $M^{-1} \cdot sec^{-1}$. Association rates will generally be slower for large protein antigens than for small haptens. This observation may be due to the smaller value of D, to the orientational effects in the collision, and to other nondiffusional aspects of protein–protein interactions. Therefore association rates for protein antigens are more frequently on the order of 10^5 to 10^6 $M^{-1} \cdot sec^{-1}$ (see below). However, this observation can also be partly understood from diffusion-limited rates alone. If the radii of hypothetically spherical reactants are r_1 and r_2, then in Eq. 7a, $a = r_1 + r_2$, whereas D is proportional to $1/r_1 + 1/r_2$. The diffusive rate constant is therefore proportional to

$$(r_1 + r_2)\left(\frac{1}{r_1} + \frac{1}{r_2}\right) = \frac{(r_1 + r_2)^2}{r_1 r_2} \qquad [7b]$$

From this result it can be seen that if $r_1 = r_2 = r$, then r cancels out and the whole term in Eq. 7b is simply equal to 4. Thus, for the interaction between two molecules of equal size, the diffusive rate constant is the same regardless of whether those molecules are large or small (6). However, if one molecule is large and the other small, the rate is greater than if both molecules are large. This difference occurs because reducing the radius r_1 while keeping r_2 constant (and larger than r_1) has a greater effect on increasing the diffusion constant term D, proportional to $(1/r_1 + 1/r_2)$, in which the smaller radius produces the larger term, than it has on the term a, which is still dominated by the larger radius r_2. For example, if $r_2 = r$, as above, but $r_1 = 0.1r$, then the numerator in Eq. 7b is only reduced from $4r^2$ to $1.21r^2$, whereas the denominator is reduced from $1r^2$ to $0.1r^2$. Thus the ratio is increased from 4 to 12.1. Viewed another way, the greater diffusive mobility of the small hapten outweighs its diminished target area relative to a large protein antigen, since the larger target area of the antibody is available to both.

The dissociation rate (or "off rate") k_{-1} is determined by the strength of the bonds (as it affects the activation energy barriers for dissociation) and the thermal energy kT (where k is Boltzmann's constant), which provides the energy to surmount this barrier. The activation energy for dissociation is the difference in energy between the starting state and the transition state of highest energy to which the system must be raised before dissociation can occur.

As pointed out by Eisen (7), if one compares a series of related antigens, of similar size and other physical properties, for binding to an antibody, the association rates are all very similar. The differences in affinity largely correspond to the differences in dissociation rates.

A good example is that of antibodies to the protein antigen staphylococcal nuclease (8). Antibodies to native nuclease were fractionated on affinity columns of peptide fragments to isolate a fraction specific for residues 99 through 126. The antibodies had an affinity of 8.3×10^8 M^{-1} for the native antigen and an association rate constant, k_{on}, of 4.1×10^5 $M^{-1} \cdot sec^{-1}$. This k_{on} was several orders of magnitude lower than had been observed for small haptens (9), as discussed above. A value of k_{off} of 4.9×10^{-4} sec^{-1} was calculated using these results in Eq. 7. This is a first-order rate constant from which one can calculate a half-time for dissociation (based on $t_{1/2} = \ln 2/k_{off}$) of 23 minutes. These rates are probably typical for high-affinity ($K_A \simeq 10^9$ M^{-1}) antibodies to small protein antigens such as nuclease (MW $\simeq 17,000$). The dissociation rate is important to know in designing experiments to measure binding, since if the act of measurement perturbs the equilibrium, the time one has to make the measurement (e.g., to separate bound and free) is determined by this half-time for dissociation. For instance, a 2-minute procedure that involves dilution of the antigen–antibody mixture can be completed before significant dissociation has occurred if the dissociation half-time is 23 minutes. However, if the on rate is the same, but the affinity tenfold lower, still a respectable 8×10^7 M^{-1}, then the complex could be 50% dissociated in the time required to complete the procedure. This caution is very relevant when we discuss methods of measuring binding and affinity.

Since knowledge of the dissociation rate can be so important in the design of experiments, a word should be said about techniques to measure it. Perhaps the most widely applicable one is the use of radiolabeled antigen. After equilibrium is reached and the equilibrium concentration of bound radioactivity determined, a large excess of unlabeled antigen is added. Since any radioactive antigen molecule that dissociates is quickly replaced by an unlabeled one, the probability of a radioactive molecule associating again is very small. Therefore one can measure the decrease in radioactivity bound to antibody with time to determine the dissociation rate.[3]

AFFINITY

It is apparent from the foregoing discussion that a lot of information about an antigen–antibody reaction is packed into a single value, its affinity. In this section we examine affinity more closely, including methods for measuring affinity and the heterogeneity thereof, the effects of multivalency of antibody and/or of antigen, and the special effects seen when the antigen–antibody interaction occurs on a solid surface (two-phase systems).

Interaction in Solution with Monovalent Ligand

The simplest case is that of the interaction of antibody with monovalent ligand. We may include in this category both antihapten antibodies reacting with truly monovalent haptens, and antimacromolecule antibodies, which have been fractionated to obtain a population that reacts only with a single, nonrepeating site on the antigen.[4] In the latter case, the antigen behaves as if monovalent in its interaction with the particular antibody population under study. The proviso that the site recognized (antigenic determinant) be nonrepeating (i.e., occur only once per antigen molecule), of course, is critical.

If the combining sites on the antibody are independent (i.e., display no positive or negative cooperativity for antigen binding), then for many purposes one can treat these combining sites, reacting with monovalent ligands, as if they were separate molecules. Thus many, but not all, of the properties we discuss can be analyzed in terms of the concentration of antibody-combining sites, independent of the number of such sites per antibody molecule (two for IgG and IgA, ten for IgM).

---

[3]This method assumes that all binding sites are independent, as is generally true for antibodies and monovalent ligands. If there were either negative or positive cooperativity in binding, then the change in receptor occupancy that occurs when a large excess of unlabeled antigen is added would probably perturb the dissociation rate of radiolabeled antigen molecules already bound to other sites.

[4]Such fractionated antibodies may contain mixtures of antibodies to overlapping sites within a domain on the antigen, but as long as no two antibody molecules (or combining sites) can bind to the same antigen molecule simultaneously, the antigen still behaves as effectively monovalent.

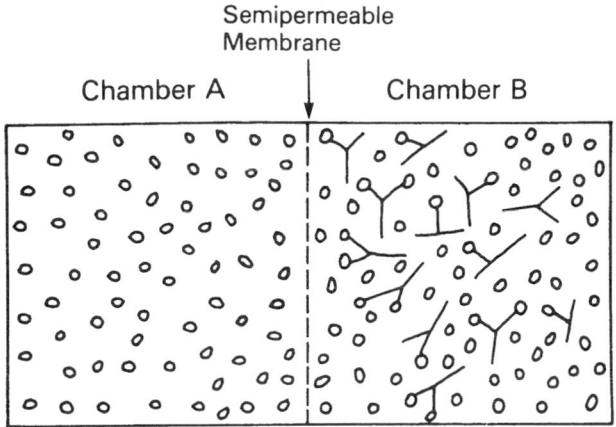

Semipermeable
Membrane

Chamber A   Chamber B

FIG. 2. Equilibrium dialysis. Two chambers are separated by a semipermeable membrane that is freely permeable to ligand but not at all to antibody. Antibody is placed in one chamber (*B*), and ligand is placed in one or both chambers. Regardless of how the ligand is distributed initially, after sufficient time to reach equilibrium, it will be distributed as follows. The concentration of free ligand will be identical in both chambers, but chamber B will have additional ligand bound to antibody. The concentration of bound ligand is thus the difference between the ligand concentration in the two chambers, whereas the free concentration is the concentration in chamber A. Since these concentrations must obey the mass action law, Eq. 2, they can be used to determine the affinity K_A, from Eq. 3 or 3′, by any of several graphical procedures, such as Scatchard analysis (described in the text).

To determine the affinity of an antibody, one generally determines the equilibrium concentrations of bound and free ligand, at increasing total ligand concentrations, but at constant antibody concentration. Alternatively, one can vary the antibody concentration, but then the analysis is slightly more complicated. Perhaps the theoretically most elegant experimental method to determine these quantities is equilibrium dialysis (10,11), depicted and explained in Fig. 2, in which ligand (antigen) is allowed to equilibrate between two chambers, only one of which contains antibody, separated by a semipermeable membrane impermeable to antibody. The important feature of this method, as opposed to most others, is that the concentrations of ligand in each chamber can be determined without perturbing the equilibrium. The disadvantage of this method is that it is applicable only to antigens small enough to permeate freely a membrane that will exclude antibody. Another technical disadvantage is that bound antigen, determined as the difference between bound plus free antigen in one chamber and free antigen in the other, is not measured independently of free antigen.

Another category of method uses radiolabeled ligand in equilibrium with antibody and then physically separates free antigen bound to antibody and quantitates each separately. The methods used to separate bound and free antigen are discussed in the section on radioimmunoassay. These methods generally allow independent measurement of bound and free antigen but may perturb the equilibrium.

Scatchard Analysis

Once data are obtained, there are a number of methods of computing the affinity, of which we shall discuss two. Perhaps the most widely used is that described by Scatchard (12) (Fig. 3, ref.13). The mass action equilibrium law is plotted in the form of Eq. 3

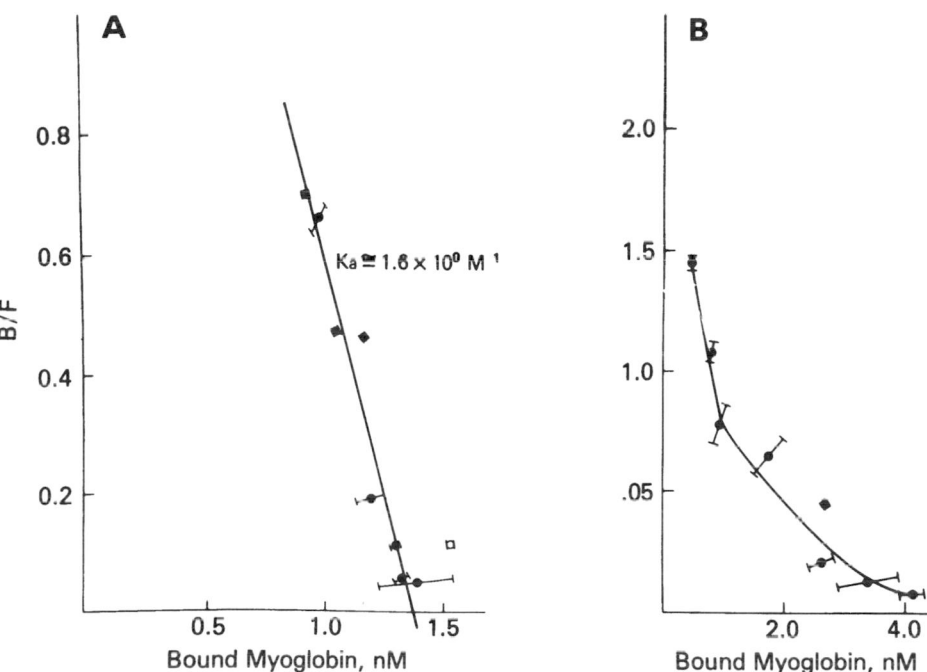

FIG. 3. Scatchard analysis of the binding of [²H]-sperm whale myoglobin by a monoclonal antibody to myoglobin (**A**) and by the serum antibodies from the same mouse whose spleen cells were fused to prepare the hybridoma (**B**). The monoclonal antibody (clone HAL 13–201E11, clone 5) produces a linear Scatchard plot, whose slope, $-1.6 \times 10^9\ M^{-1}$, equals $-K_A$, and whose intercept on the abscissa gives the concentration of antibody-binding sites. In contrast, the serum antibodies produce a curved (concave-up) Scatchard plot, indicative of heterogeneity of affinity. (From ref.13, with permission.)

$$[SL] = K_A([S]_t - [SL])[L] \qquad [3]$$

and B is substituted for [SL] and F for [L], referring to bound and free ligand, respectively. Then the Scatchard equation is

$$\frac{B}{F} = K_A([S]_t - B) \qquad [8]$$

Note that a very critical implicit assumption was made in this seemingly very simple conversion. The [SL] within the parentheses in Eq. 3 was intended to be the concentration of bound antibody sites, so that $([S]_t - [SL]) = $ free [S]. However, in Eq. 8, we have substituted B, the concentration of bound ligand. If the ligand behaves as monovalent, then this substitution is legitimate, since every bound ligand molecule corresponds to an occupied antibody site. However, if the ligand is multivalent and can bind more than one antibody site, then Eq. 8 is valid only in ligand excess where the frequency of ligands with more than one antibody bound is very low. In this section we are discussing only monovalent ligands, but this proviso must be kept in mind when the Scatchard analysis is applied in other circumstances.

From Eq. 8, we see that a plot of B/F versus B should yield a straight line (for a single affinity), with a slope of $-K_A$ and an intercept on the abscissa corresponding to antibody-binding site concentration (see Fig. 3). This is the so-called Scatchard plot. An alternative version that is normalized for antibody concentration is especially useful if the data were obtained at different values of total antibody concentration, $[A]_t$, instead of constant $[A]_t$. For this version, however, one requires an independent measure of total antibody concentration, other than the intercept of the plot. Then one divides Eq. 8 by the total concentration of antibody molecules (making no assumptions about the number of sites per molecule) to obtain

$$\frac{r}{c} = K_A(n - r) \qquad [9]$$

where r is defined as the number of occupied sites per antibody molecule, n is defined as the total number of sites per antibody molecule, and c is free ligand concentration; that is, $c = F$. Thus

$$r = \frac{B}{[\text{total antibody}]} = \frac{B}{[A]_t}$$

$$n = \frac{[\text{total sites}]}{[\text{total antibody}]} = \frac{[S]_t}{[A]_t}$$

where $[A]_t = $ total molar antibody concentration. In this form of the Scatchard plot, r/c versus r; the slope is still $-K_A$ and the intercept on the r axis is n. Thus one can determine the number of sites per molecule. Of course, if one determines $[S]_t$ from the intercept of Eq. 8, one can also calculate the number of sites per molecule by dividing $[S]_t$ by any independent measure of antibody concentration. Thus the only advantage of normalizing all the data points first to plot the r/c form arises when the data were obtained at varying antibody concentrations. If the antibody concentration is unknown but held constant, then the B/F form is more convenient and actually provides one measure of antibody (site) concentration. Since today we know the value of n for each class of antibody (two for IgG and serum IgA, ten for IgM), the concentration of sites and that of antibody are easily converted in many cases.

Heterogeneity of Affinity

The next level of complexity arises when one is dealing with a mixture of antibodies of varying affinity for the ligand. This is the rule, rather than the exception, when one deals with antibodies from immune serum, even if they are fractionated to be monospecific (i.e., all specific for the same site on the antigen). Contrast, for example, the linear Scatchard plot for a homogeneous monoclonal antibody to myoglobin (see Fig. 3A) with the curved Scatchard plot for the serum antibodies from the same mouse used to prepare the hybridoma monoclonal antibody (see Fig. 3B). This concave-up Scatchard plot is typical for heterogeneous antibodies. In a system such as hormone receptor–hormone interaction, in which negative cooperativity can occur between receptor sites (i.e., occupation of one site lowers the affinity of its neighbor), a concave-up Scatchard plot can be produced by negative cooperativity in the absence of any intrinsic heterogeneity in affinity. However, in the case of antibodies, where no such allosteric effect has been demonstrated, a concave-up Scatchard plot indicates heterogeneity of affinity.

Ideally, one would like to imagine that the tangents all along the curve correspond (in slope) to the affinities of the many subpopulations of antibodies. Mathematically, this is not strictly correct, but it is true that the steeper part of the curve corresponds to the higher affinity antibodies and the shallower part of the curve to the lower affinity antibodies. Graphical methods have been developed to analyze more quantitatively the components of such curves (14,15), and a very general and versatile computer program (LIGAND) has been developed by Munson and Rodbard (16) that can fit such curves using any number of subpopulations of different affinity. For purposes of this chapter, we discuss only the case of two affinities and then examine the types of average affinities that have been proposed when one is dealing with much greater heterogeneity. We also examine mathematical estimates of the degree of heterogeneity (analogous to a variance).

When an antibody population consists of only two subpopulations of different affinities, K_1 and K_2, then we can add the component Equation 3′ to obtain

$$r = r_1 + r_2 = \frac{n_1 K_1 c}{1 + K_1 c} + \frac{n_2 K_2 c}{1 + K_2 c} \qquad [10]$$

so that

$$\frac{r}{c} = \frac{n_1 K_1}{1 + K_1 c} + \frac{n_2 K_2}{1 + K_2 c} \qquad [10']$$

where the subscripts correspond to the two populations. Then the graph of r/c versus r can be shown to be a hyperbola whose asymptotes are, in fact, the linear Scatchard plots of the two components (Fig. 4). This situation has been analyzed graphically by Bright (17). Taking the limits as $c \to 0$ and as $c \to \infty$, it can easily be shown that the intercept on the abscissa is just $n_1 + n_2$ (or, in the form B/F versus B, the intercept is the total concentration of binding sites $[S]_t$), and the intercept on the ordinate is $n_1 K_1 + n_2 K_2$. Thus one can still obtain the total value of n or $[S]_t$ from the intercept on the abscissa. The problem is in obtaining the two affinities, K_1 and K_2, and the concentrations of the individual antibody subpopulations (corresponding to n_1 and n_2). If K_1 is greater than K_2, one can approximate the affinities from the slopes of the tangents at the two intercepts (see Fig. 4), but these will not, in general, be exactly parallel to the two asymptotes, which give the true affinities, so some error is always introduced, depending on the relative values of n_1 and n_2 and K_1 and K_2. A graphical method for solving for these exactly has been worked out by Bright (17) and computer methods by Munson and Rodbard (16).

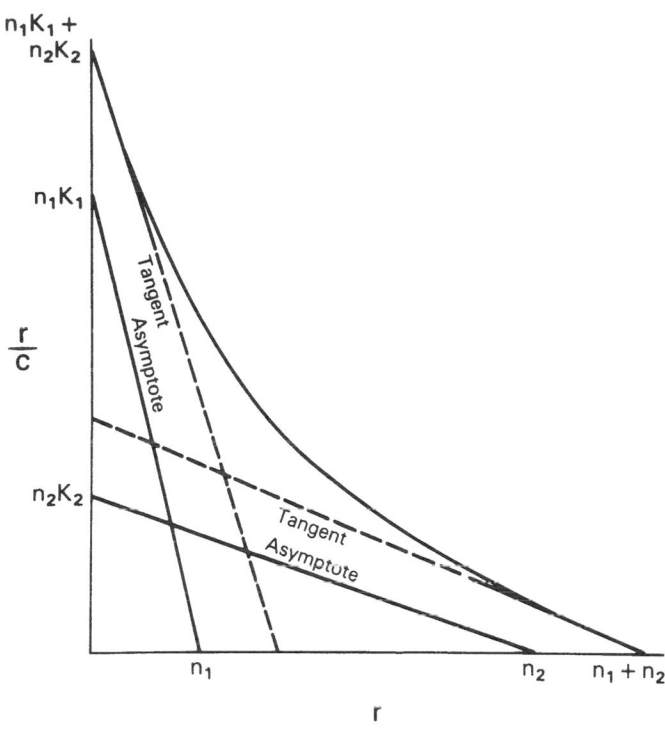

FIG. 4. Analysis of a curved Scatchard plot produced by a mixture of two antibodies with different affinities. The antibodies have affinities K_1 and K_2 and have n_1 and n_2 binding sites per molecule, respectively. r is the concentration of bound antigen divided by the total antibody concentration (i.e., bound sites per molecule), and c is the free antigen concentration. The curve is a hyperbola that can be decomposed into its two asymptotes, which correspond to the linear Scatchard plots of the two components in the antibody mixture. The tangents to the curve at its intercepts only approximate these asymptotes, so that the slopes of the tangents estimate but do not accurately correspond to the affinities of the two antibodies. However, the intercept on the r axis corresponds to $n_1 + n_2$. Note that in this case, n_1 and n_2 must be defined in terms of the total antibody concentration, not that of each component.

Average Affinities

In practice, of course, one rarely knows that one is dealing with exactly two subpopulations, and most antisera are significantly more heterogeneous than that. Therefore, the preceding case is more illustrative of principles than of practical value. When faced with a curved Scatchard plot, one usually asks what the average affinity is, and perhaps some measure of the variance of the affinities, without being able to define exactly how many different affinity populations exist.

Suppose one has m populations each with site concentration $[S_i]$ and affinity K_i, so that at free ligand concentration $[L]$, the fraction of each antibody that has ligand bound will be given by an equation of the form of Eq. 3':

$$B_i = \frac{K_i[S_i]_t[L]}{1 + K_i[L]} \qquad [11]$$

Then the bound concentrations sum to give

$$B = \sum B_i = \sum_{i=1}^{m} \frac{K_i[S_i]_t[L]}{1 + K_i[L]} \qquad [11']$$

Substituting F for [L] and dividing through by this quantity, one obtains

$$\frac{B}{F} = \sum_{i=1}^{m} \frac{K_i[S_i]_t}{1 + K_iF} \qquad [12]$$

or equivalently,

$$\frac{r}{c} = \sum_{i=1}^{m} \frac{K_i n_i}{1 + K_i c} \qquad [12']$$

These can be seen to be generalizations of Eq. 10 and 10'. Taking the limits as $F \to 0$ and $F \to \infty$, one again sees that the

$$\text{intercept on ordinate} = \sum_{i=1}^{m} K_i[S_i]_t \qquad [13]$$

and the

$$\text{intercept on abscissa} = \sum_{i=1}^{m} [S_i]_t = [S]_t \qquad [14]$$

Therefore one can still obtain the total antibody site concentration from the intercept on the abscissa (Fig. 5) (18).

Two types of average affinity can be obtained graphically from the Scatchard plot (18). Perhaps the more widely used, K_0, is actually more accurately a median affinity rather than a mean affinity. It is defined as the slope of the tangent at the point on the curve where half the sites are bound; that is, where $B = [S]_t/2$ (see Fig. 5). A second type of average affinity, which we call K_{av}, is a weighted mean of the affinities, each affinity weighted by its proportional representation in the antibody population. Thus we take the ratio

$$K_{av} = \sum_{i=1}^{m} \frac{K_i[S_i]_t}{[S]_t} \qquad [15]$$

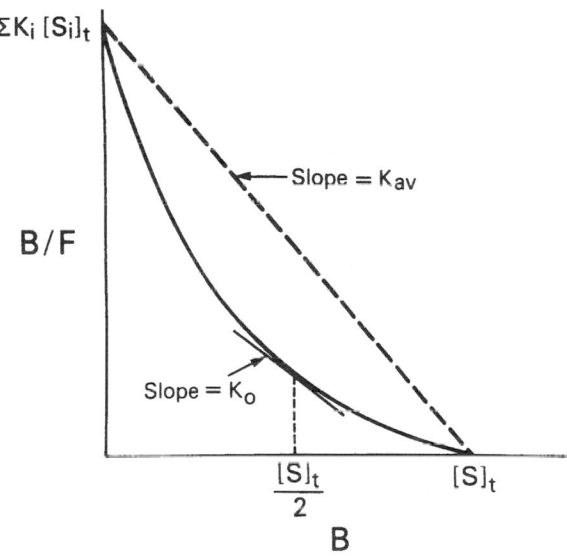

FIG. 5. Types of average affinities for a heterogeneous population of antibodies, as defined on a Scatchard plot. K_0 is the slope of the tangent to the curve at a point where $B = [S]_t/2$, that is, where half the antibody sites are bound. Thus, K_0 corresponds to a median affinity. K_{av} is the slope of the chord between the intercepts and corresponds to a weighted average of the affinities, weighted by the concentrations of the antibodies with each affinity. (Adapted from ref. 18.)

From Eqs. 13 and 14, it is apparent that K_{av} is simply the ratio of the two intercepts on the B/F and B axes, that is, the slope of the chord (see Fig. 5). This type of weighted mean affinity, K_{av}, is therefore actually easier to obtain graphically in some cases than is K_0, and we shall see that it is useful in other types of plots as well.

Indices of Heterogeneity: The Sips Plot

For a heterogeneous antiserum, one would also like to have some idea of the extent of heterogeneity of affinity. For instance, if the affinities were distributed according to a normal (Gaussian) distribution, one would like to know the variance (19,20). More complex analyses have been developed that do not require as many assumptions about the shape of the distribution (21–23), but the first and most widely used index of heterogeneity arbitrarily assumes that the affinities fit a distribution, first described by Sips (24), that is similar in shape to a normal distribution. This was applied to the case of antibody heterogeneity by Nisonoff and Pressman (25) and is summarized by Karush and Karush (26). One fits the data to the assumed binding function

$$r = \frac{n(K_0 c)^a}{1 + (K_0 c)^a} \qquad [16]$$

which is analogous to Eqs. 3′ and 11 (the Langmuir adsorption isotherm) except for the exponent a, which is the index of heterogeneity. This index, a, is allowed to range from 0 to 1. For $a = 1$, Eq. 16 is equivalent to Eq. 3, and there is no heterogeneity. As a decreases toward 0, the heterogeneity increases. To obtain a value for a graphically, one plots the algebraic rearrangement of Eq. 16:

$$\log\left(\frac{r}{n-r}\right) = a \log c + a \log K_0 \qquad [17]$$

so that the slope of $\log[r/(n-r)]$ versus $\log c$ is the heterogeneity index a.

C. DeLisi (*personal communication*) has derived the variance (second moment) of the Sips distribution in terms of the free energy $RT \ln K_0$, about the mean of free energy. The result (normalized to RT) gives the dispersion or width of the distribution as a function of a:

$$\frac{\sigma^2_{Sips}}{R^2 T^2} = \frac{\pi^2(1 - a^2)}{3a^2} \qquad [18]$$

This is useful for determining a quantity, σ_{Sips}, which can be thought of as analogous to a standard deviation, if one keeps in mind that this is not a true Gaussian distribution. In addition, as noted above, the use of the Sips distribution requires the assumption that the affinities (really the free energies) are continuously distributed symmetrically about a mean, approximating a Gaussian distribution. This assumption frequently is not valid.

The Plot of B/F Versus F or T

Another graphical method that is useful for estimating affinities is the plot of bound/free versus free or total ligand concentration, denoted F and T, respectively (18) (Fig. 6). To simplify the discussion, let us define the bound/free ratio, B/F, as R, and define R_0 as the intercept, or limit, as free ligand $F \to 0$. First, for the case of a homogeneous antibody, from Eq. 3′,

$$R = \frac{B}{F} = \frac{K[S]_t}{1 + KF} \qquad [19]$$

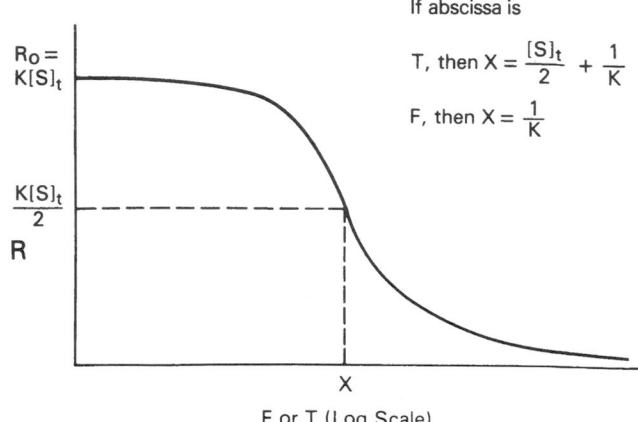

FIG. 6. Schematic plot of R, the bound/free ratio, as a function of free (F) or total (T) antigen concentration. The curves have a similar sigmoidal shape, but the midpoint (where $R = R_0/2$) of the plot of R versus T has a term dependent on antibody-site concentration ($[S]_t$), whereas the midpoint of the plot of R versus F is exactly $1/K$, independent of antibody concentration. (Adapted from ref. 18.)

and

$$R_0 = \lim_{F \to 0} \frac{B}{F} = K[S]_t \qquad [20]$$

Let us define the midpoint of the plot (see Fig. 6) as the point at which R decreases to half its initial value, R_0, that is, at which $R = K[S]_t/2$. For the case of homogeneous antibody (i.e., a single affinity), simple algebraic manipulation (18), substituting $K[S]_t/2$ (i.e., $R_0/2$) for B/F in Eq. 8, will show that at this midpoint[5]

$$F = \frac{1}{K} \qquad [21]$$

and

$$B = [S]_t/2 \qquad [22]$$

so that the total concentration, T, is

$$T = B + F = \frac{[S]_t}{2} + \frac{1}{K} \qquad [23]$$

Thus, if one plots B/F versus F, the midpoint directly yields $1/K$. However, it is frequently more convenient experimentally to plot B/F versus T. In this case, the midpoint is no longer simply the reciprocal of the affinity. As seen from Eq. 23, the assumption that the midpoint is $1/K$ will result in an error equal to half the antibody-binding site concentration. Thus in plots of B/F versus T, the midpoint will be a good estimate of the affinity only if $[S]_t/2$ is much less than $1/K$, that is, if the antibody concentration is low compared to the dissociation constant. In fact, if the affinity is so high that $1/K$ is much less than $[S]_t/2$, then one will merely be measuring the antibody concentration, not the affinity at all (18) (see Fig. 6).

---

[5]It is important to note that R_0 must be the limit of B/F as F truly approaches zero. In an RIA in which the concentration of tracer is significant compared to $1/K$, reducing the unlabeled ligand concentration all the way to zero will still not yield the true limit R_0. The tracer concentration must also be negligible. If not, R_0 will be estimated falsely low, and the affinity will also be underestimated.

In the case of a heterogeneous antiserum, we have already seen that

$$R_0 = \sum_i K_i [S_i]_t \qquad [13]$$

Therefore, at the midpoint, when $B/F = R_0/2$, it is easy to see that

$$K_{av} = \left(\frac{B}{F}\right)\left(\frac{2}{[S]_t}\right) = \frac{R_0}{[S]_t} \qquad [24]$$

Thus one can still obtain the average affinity, as defined above (18).

Regardless of average affinities, the effect of affinity heterogeneity is to broaden the curve or to make the slope shallower. This can be seen by visualizing the curve of B/F versus F as a step function. Each antibody subpopulation of a given affinity, K_i, will be titrated to 50% of its microscopic B/F at a free ligand concentration $F = 1/K_i$. The high-affinity antibodies will be titrated at low F, but the low-affinity antibodies will require much higher F to be titrated. The resulting step function is analogous to the successive transitions corresponding to different pK values in a pH titration.

Intrinsic Affinity

The affinity, K_A, that we have been discussing so far is what has been termed the *intrinsic affinity*, that is, the affinity of each antibody-combining site treated in isolation. We have been able to do this, regardless of the valence of the antibodies, by using the concentration of combining sites, [S], in our equations rather than the concentration of antibody molecules, [A], which may have more than one site. Even without any cooperativity between combining sites, there is a statistical effect that makes the actual affinity different from the intrinsic affinity if the antibody is multivalent and one uses whole antibody concentration rather than site concentration. The way this difference arises can best be seen by examining the case of a bivalent antibody, such as IgG. We assume that the two sites are equivalent and neither is affected by events at the other. The ligand, as in this whole section, is monovalent. Then there are two binding steps

$$A + L \underset{}{\overset{K_1}{\rightleftharpoons}} AL, \qquad AL + L \underset{}{\overset{K_2}{\rightleftharpoons}} AL_2 \qquad [25]$$

and the corresponding actual affinities are

$$K_1 = \frac{[AL]}{[A][L]}, \qquad K_2 = \frac{[AL_2]}{[AL][L]} \qquad [26]$$

If the intrinsic affinity of both equivalent sites is K, then K_1 will actually be twice K, because the concentration of available sites [S] will be twice the antibody concentration when the first ligand is about to bind, in step 1. However, once one site is bound, the reverse (dissociation) reaction of step 1 can occur from only one site, namely, that which is occupied. Conversely, for the second step, the forward reaction has only one remaining available site; however, in the reverse reaction, $AL_2 \rightarrow AL + L$, either site can dissociate to go back to the AL state. The second site bound need not be the first to dissociate, and since the sites are identical, one cannot tell the difference. Thus, for step 2, the apparent concentration of sites for the reverse reaction is twice that available for the forward reaction, so the affinity K_2 for the second step will be only half the intrinsic affinity, K.

It is easy to see how this statistical effect can be extrapolated to an antibody with n sites (27):

$$K_1 = nK \quad \text{and} \quad K_n = \frac{1}{n}K \qquad [27]$$

For the steps in between, two derivations are available (7,27), which yield

$$K_i = \frac{n - i + 1}{i} K \qquad [28]$$

The actual affinity, rather than the intrinsic affinity, becomes important with monovalent ligands when one is interested in the effective affinity (based on a molar antibody concentration) under conditions where [L] is so low that only one site can bind antigen. Then for IgG or IgM (with two or ten sites per molecule, respectively), the apparent affinity will be theoretically two or ten times the intrinsic affinity. For most purposes, it is easier to use site concentrations and intrinsic affinities. The analyses given above, such as B/F versus F or the Scatchard plot, whether B/F versus B or r/c versus r, will all yield intrinsic affinities. It is the intrinsic affinity that tells us something about the nature of the antibody–ligand interaction.

Once one enters the realm of multivalent ligands, the actual affinity or effective affinity involving multipoint binding between multivalent antibody molecule and multivalent ligand molecule can be much greater than the intrinsic affinity for binding at each site. This case is the subject of the next section.

Interaction with Multivalent Ligands

So far, we have discussed only situations in which the ligand is monovalent, or effectively monovalent with respect to the particular antibody under study. However, in many situations the ligand molecule has multiple repeating identical determinants, each of which can bind independently to the several identical combining sites on a divalent or multivalent antibody.[6] Although the intrinsic affinity for the interaction of any single antibody-combining site with any single antigenic determinant may be the same as that discussed in the preceding section, the apparent or effective affinity may be much higher, due to the ability of a single antibody molecule to bind more than one identical determinant of a multivalent antigen molecule. Karush (28) has termed this phenomenon *monogamous bivalency*. Such monogamous binding can occur between two molecules in solution, or between a molecule in solution and one on a solid surface, such as a cell membrane or microtiter plate. We first discuss the situation in solution and then discuss the additional considerations that apply when one of the reactants is bound to a solid surface.

Monogamous Bivalency

Suppose a divalent antibody molecule reacts with antigen that has two identical determinants. This situation has been treated in detail by Crothers and Metzger (29) and by Karush (28). Let us call the two antibody sites S and S', and the antigenic determinants D and D', with the understanding that, in actuality, we cannot distinguish S from S' or D from D'. The interaction can be broken up into two steps, a bimolecular reaction

$$\begin{array}{ccc} S & D & S - D \\ | + | & \overset{K_1}{\rightleftharpoons} & | \quad | \\ S' & D' & S' \quad D' \end{array} \qquad [29]$$

---

[6]If only the antigen is multivalent, and the antibody monovalent, such as a Fab fragment, the situation can be analyzed using the same statistical considerations discussed above.

followed by an intramolecular reaction

$$
\begin{array}{ccc}
\mathrm{S} - \mathrm{D} & & \mathrm{S} - \mathrm{D} \\
| \quad\quad | & \overset{K_2}{\rightleftarrows} & | \quad\quad | \\
\mathrm{S}' \quad \mathrm{D}' & & \mathrm{S}' - \mathrm{D}'
\end{array} \qquad [30]
$$

The association constant for the first step, K_1, is related to the intrinsic affinity, K, simply by a statistical factor of 4 due to the degeneracy (equivalence) between S and S' and between D and D'. This is a typical second-order reaction between antigen and antibody. However, the second step (Eq. 30) is a first-order reaction, since it is effectively an interconversion between two states of a single molecular complex, the reactants S' and D' being linked chemically (albeit noncovalently) through the S—D bond formed in the first step. Thus, the first-order equilibrium constant, K_2, is not a function of the concentrations of S—S and D—D in solution, as K_1 would be. Rather, the forward reaction depends on the geometry of the complex and the flexibility of the arms; in other words, the probability that S' and D' will encounter each other and be in the right orientation to react if they do come in contact depends on the distances and freedom of motion along the chain S'—S—D—D' rather than on the density of molecules in solution (i.e., concentration).

The reverse reaction for step 2, on the other hand, will have a rate constant similar to that for the simple monovalent S—D → S + D reaction, since the dissociation reaction depends on the strength of the S'—D' (or S—D) bond and is not influenced by the other S—D interaction unless there is strain introduced by the angles required for simultaneous bonds between S and D and S' and D'. Note that K_2 will inherently have a statistical factor of 1/2 compared to the intrinsic K_2' for the analogous reaction if the S'—S—D—D' link were all covalent, since in the forward reaction of Eq. 30, only one pair can react, whereas in the reverse reaction, either S'—D' or S—D could dissociate to produce the equivalent result.

We would like to know the apparent or observed affinity for the overall reaction

$$
\begin{array}{ccc}
\mathrm{S} \quad \mathrm{D} & & \mathrm{S} - \mathrm{D} \\
| \; + \; | & \overset{K_{obs}}{\rightleftarrows} & | \quad\quad | \\
\mathrm{S} \quad \mathrm{D} & & \mathrm{S} - \mathrm{D}
\end{array} \qquad [31]
$$

Since the free energies, ΔF_1 and ΔF_2, for the two steps are additive, the observed affinity will be the product of K_1 and K_2

$$
K_{obs} = K_1 K_2 \qquad [32]
$$

where we have defined K_1 and K_2 to include the statistical degeneracy factors.[7] The equilibrium constants K_1 and K_2 are each the ratios of forward and reverse rate constants, as in Eq. 7. Of these four rate constants, all are directly related to the corresponding terms for the intrinsic affinity between S and D, except for the intramolecular forward reaction of step 2, as noted above. Thus, the difficulty in predicting K_{obs} is largely a problem of analyzing the geometric (steric) aspects of K_2, assuming one already knows the intrinsic affinity, K. Crothers and Metzger (29) have analyzed this problem for particular situations. Qualitatively, we can say that whether K_2 will be larger or smaller than K will depend on factors such as the enforced proximity of S' and D' in step 2 and the distance between D and D' compared to the possible distances accessible between S and S', which in turn depends on the length of the

antibody arms and the flexibility of the hinge between them (see Chapter 3). Thus, since K_1 can be approximated by K, except for statistical factors, the apparent affinity for this "monogamous bivalent" binding interaction, K_{obs}, may range from significantly less than to significantly greater than K_2. If K_2 is of the same order of magnitude as K, then K_{obs} will be of the order of K_2, which can be huge (e.g., if K is approximately equal to 10^9 M^{-1}, K_{obs} could be approximately equal to 10^{18} M^{-1}). The half-time for dissociation would be thousands of years. It is easy to see how such monogamous bivalent interactions can appear to be irreversible, even though in practice the observed affinity is rarely more than a few orders of magnitude larger than the K for a single site, possibly due to structural constraints (30).

If apparent affinities this high can be reached by monogamous bivalency, even greater ones should be possible for the multipoint binding of an IgM molecule to a multivalent ligand. Although IgM is decavalent for small monovalent ligands, steric restrictions often make it behave as if pentavalent for binding to large multivalent ligands. However, even five-point binding can lead to enormously tight interactions. Therefore, even though the intrinsic affinity of IgM molecules tends to be lower than that of IgG molecules for the same antigen (28), the apparent affinity of IgM can be quite high.

Two-phase Systems

The same enhanced affinity seen for multipoint binding applies to two-phase systems. Examples include the reaction of multivalent antibodies with antigen attached to a cell surface or an artificial surface (such as Sepharose or the plastic walls of a microtiter plate); the reaction of a multivalent ligand with antibodies on the surface of a B cell, a Sepharose bead, or a plastic plate; and the reaction of either component with an antigen–antibody precipitate. For the reasons outlined above, "monogamous" binding can make the apparent affinity of a multivalent antibody or antigen for multiple sites on a solid surface be quite large, to the point of effective irreversibility.

However, another effect also increases the effective affinity in a two-phase system. This effect applies even for monovalent antibodies (Fab fragments) or monovalent ligands. The effect arises from the enormously high effective local concentration of binding sites at the surface, compared to the concentration if the same number of sites were distributed in bulk solution (31). Looked at another way, the effect is due to the violation, at the liquid–solid interface, of the basic assumption in the association constants, K_A, discussed above, that the reactants are all distributed randomly in the solution. (To some extent, the latter is involved in the enhanced affinity of multivalency as well.) This situation has been analyzed by DeLisi (32) and DeLisi and Wiegel (33), who break the reaction down into two steps: (a) the diffusive process necessary to bring the antigen and antibody into the right proximity and orientation to react and (b) the reactive process itself. The complex between antigen and antibody, when positioned but not yet reacted, is called the *encounter complex*. The reaction can then be written

$$
\mathrm{S} + \mathrm{D} \underset{k_-}{\overset{k_+}{\rightleftharpoons}} \mathrm{S}\cdots\mathrm{D} \underset{k_{-1}}{\overset{k_1}{\rightleftharpoons}} \mathrm{SD} \qquad [33]
$$

where S is antibody site, D is antigenic determinant, k_+ and k_- are the forward and reverse diffusive rate constants, and k_1 and k_{-1} are the forward and reverse reactive rate constants once the encounter complex is formed. If the encounter complex is in a steady state, the overall rate constants will be given by

---

[7]In some treatments, in which these statistical factors are not included in K_1 and K_2, the equivalent equation may be given as $K_{obs} = 2K_1K_2$.

$$k_f = \frac{k_1 k_+}{k_1 + k_-} \qquad [34]$$

$$k_r = \frac{k_{-1} k_-}{k_1 + k_-} \qquad [35]$$

where subscripts *f* and *r* stand for *forward* and *reverse,* respectively (32). The association constant, according to Eq. 7, is the ratio of these two, or

$$K_A = \frac{k_1 k_+}{k_{-1} k_-} \qquad [36]$$

The relative magnitudes of k_1 and k_- determine the probable fate of the encounter complex. Is it more likely to react to form SD or to break up as the reactants diffuse apart?

Now suppose that k_- is slow compared to k_1. Then the SD bound complex and the encounter complex, S···D, may interconvert many times before the encounter complex breaks up and one of the reactants diffuses off into bulk solution. If the surface has multiple antigenic sites, D, then even a monovalent antibody (Fab) may be much more likely, when SD dissociates to S···D, to rereact with the same or nearby sites than to diffuse away into bulk solution, again depending on the relative magnitudes of these rate constants. This greater probability to rereact with the surface rather than diffuse away is the essence of the effect we are describing. A more extensive mathematical treatment of reactions with cells is given in DeLisi (32) and DeLisi and Wiegel (33).

A somewhat different, and very useful, analysis of the same or a very similar effect was given by Silhavy et al. (34). These authors studied the case of a ligand diffusing out of a dialysis bag containing a protein for which the ligand had a significant affinity. Once the ligand concentration became low enough that there was an excess of free protein sites, then the rate of exit of ligand from the dialysis bag was no longer simply its diffusion rate; nor was it simply the rate of dissociation of protein–ligand complex. These authors showed that under these conditions the exit of ligand followed quasi–first-order kinetics, but with a half-life longer than the half-life in the absence of protein by a factor of $(1 + [P]K_A)$

$$t_+ = t_-(1 + [P]K_A) \qquad [37]$$

where [P] is the protein site concentration, K_A is the affinity, and t_+ and t_- are the half-lives in the presence and absence of protein in the bag.

In this case, the protein was in solution, so the authors could use the actual protein concentration and the actual intrinsic affinity, K_A. In the case of protein on a two-dimensional surface, it is harder to know what to use as the effective concentration. However, the high local concentration of protein compartmentalized in the dialysis bag can be seen to be analogous to the high local concentration attached to the solid surface. The underlying mechanism of the two effects is essentially the same and so are the implications. For instance, in the case of dialysis, a modest 10 μM concentration of antibody sites with an affinity of 10^8 M^{-1} can reduce the rate of exit of a ligand 1,000–fold. A dialysis that would otherwise take 3 hours would take 4 months! It is easy to see how this "retention effect" can make even modest affinities appear infinite (i.e., the reactions appear irreversible). This retention effect applies not only to immunologic systems, but also to other interactions at a cell surface or between cell compartments where the local concentration of a protein may be high. In particular, these principles of two-phase systems should also govern the interaction between antigen-specific receptors on the surface of T cells and antigen–major histocompatibility complex (MHC) molecule complexes on the surface of antigen-presenting cells, B cells, or target cells.

One final point is useful to note. Since these retention effects depend on a localized abundance of unoccupied sites, addition of a large excess of unlabeled ligand to saturate these sites will diminish or abolish the retention effect and greatly accelerate the dissociation or exit of labeled ligand. This effect of unlabeled ligand can be used as a test for the retention effect, although one must be aware that in certain cases the same result can be an indication of negative cooperativity among receptor sites.

RADIOIMMUNOASSAY AND RELATED METHODS

Since it was first suggested in 1960 by Yalow and Berson (35), radioimmunoassay (RIA) has rapidly become one of the most widespread, widely applicable, and most sensitive techniques for assessing the concentration of a whole host of biologic molecules. Most of the basic principles necessary to understand and apply RIA techniques have already been covered in the earlier sections of this chapter. In this section, we examine the concepts and methodologic approaches used in RIA. For a detailed methods book, we refer the reader to Chard (36), Rodbard (37), and Yalow (38).

The central concept of RIA is that the binding of an infinitesimal concentration of highly radioactive tracer antigen to low concentrations of a high-affinity specific antibody is very sensitive to competition by unlabeled antigen and is also very specific for that antigen. Thus concentrations of antigen in unknown samples can be determined by their ability to compete with tracer for binding to antibody. The method can be used to measure very low concentrations of a molecule, even in the presence of the many impurities in biologic fluids. To do this, one must prepare the appropriate high-affinity antibody and radiolabeled antigen, develop a method to distinguish bound from free labeled antigen, determine the optimal concentrations of antibody and tracer-labeled antigen to maximize sensitivity, and generate a standard curve, using known concentrations of competing unlabeled antigen, from which to read off the concentrations in unknown samples. One must also choose the best method for graphically (or numerically) representing the data. Although we do not discuss the methods for preparing antibodies or labeled antigens, we do review the other steps and pitfalls in this procedure.

Separation of Bound and Free Antigen

Whatever parameter one uses to assess the amount of competition by the unlabeled antigen in the unknown sample to be tested, it will always be a function of bound, or bound and free, radiolabeled antigen. Therefore, one of the most critical technical requirements is the ability to distinguish clearly between antibody-bound radioactive tracer and free radioactive tracer. This distinction usually requires physical separation of bound and free tracer ligand, and independent counting of radioactivity in the two fractions. If the bound fraction is contaminated by free ligand, or vice versa, enormous errors can result, depending on the part of the binding curve on which the data fall.

Solution Methods

Solution RIA methods have the advantage that binding can be related to the intrinsic affinity of the antibody. However, bound and free antigen must be separated by a method that does not perturb the equilibrium. Three basic types of approaches have been used: precipitate the antibody with bound antigen, leaving free antigen in solution; precipitate the free antigen, leaving antibody and bound antigen in solution; or separate free from antibody-bound antigen molecules in solution on the basis of size by gel filtration. This last method is too cumbersome to use for large numbers of samples and is too slow, in general, to be sure the equilibrium is not perturbed in the process. Therefore, gel filtration columns are not widely used for RIA.

Methods that precipitate antibody are perhaps the most widely used. If the antigen is sufficiently smaller (MW < 30,000) than the antibody that it will remain in solution at concentrations of either ammonium sulfate (39) or polyethylene glycol, MW 6,000 (10% W:W) (40), which will precipitate essentially all the antibody, then these two reagents are frequently the most useful. For instance, precipitation with polyethylene glycol and centrifugation can be accomplished in a total of less than 2 minutes, allowing separation of bound and free antigen before any significant dissociation has occurred due to the dilutional effect of adding the polyethylene glycol (41). (Note that if whole serum is not used, nonspecific carrier gamma-globulin must be added to produce a macroscopic pellet.) However, if the antigen is much larger than about 30,000 to 40,000 MW or is not globular in shape, then concentrations of polyethylene glycol that completely precipitate the antibody may also precipitate more than 10% of the free antigen and thus will produce unacceptably high background control values in the absence of specific antibody. If the antibody is primarily of a subclass of IgG that binds to staphylococcal protein A or protein G, one can take advantage of the high affinity of protein A or G for IgG by using either protein A (or G)–Sepharose or formalin-killed staphylococcal organisms (Cowan I strain) to precipitate the antibody. Centrifuging the beads or the staphylococci carrying the antibody and bound antigen leaves free antigen in solution (42). Finally, one can precipitate the antibody using a specific second antibody, an antiimmunoglobulin raised in another species. This method has the widest applicability but is also the most cumbersome. As will be discussed below, maximal precipitation occurs not at antibody excess, but at the "point of equivalence" in the middle of the titration curve where antigen (in this case, the first antibody) and the (second) antibody are approximately equal in concentration. Thus, one must add carrier immunoglobulin to keep the immunoglobulin concentration constant and determine the point of equivalence by titrating with the second antibody (antiimmunoglobulin). Even worse, the precipitin reaction is slow, since lattice formation and the formation of aggregates large enough to precipitate are much slower than the antigen–antibody reaction itself. Thus, the incubation with second antibody usually requires 24 to 48 hours or even longer, allowing reequilibration of the antigen–antibody interaction after dilution by the second antibody. Some of these problems can be reduced by enhancing precipitation with low concentrations of polyethylene glycol.

The other type of separation method is adsorption of free antigen to an agent that leaves antigen bound to antibody in solution. The most widely used reagents for this purpose are activated charcoal (carbon) and talc. Since binding of antigen by these agents depends on size and hydrophobicity, they are applicable only to certain antigens. Although these methods are inexpensive and rapid, they require careful adjustment and monitoring of pH, ionic strength, and temperature to obtain reproducible results and to avoid adsorption of the antigen–antibody complex. Furthermore,

since these agents have a high affinity for antigen, they can compete with a low-affinity antibody and alter the equilibrium. Also, since charcoal quenches beta scintillation counting, it can be used only with gamma-emitting isotopes such as [125]I.

Solid-phase Methods

Solid-phase RIA methods have the advantages of ease of processing large numbers of samples and potentially increased affinity (compared to the intrinsic affinity of the antibody) due to the effects at the solid–liquid interface noted above. However, they have the concomitant disadvantage that one is not measuring the true intrinsic affinity because of these same effects. The method itself is fairly simple. One binds the antibody in advance to a solid surface such as a Sepharose bead or the walls of a test tube or microtiter plate well. The latter is usually accomplished by simply incubating antibody in the plastic wells, since most proteins bind nonspecifically to plastic (polyvinyl chloride more than polystyrene), and then coating unoccupied sites with an irrelevant protein (e.g., bovine serum albumin) by the same procedure. To avoid competition from other serum proteins, one must use purified antibody in this coating step. The concentration of antibody coating the plastic can be varied by varying the antibody concentration with which the wells are incubated, or by changing the type of plastic. Once the wells (or Sepharose beads) are coated, one can incubate them with labeled tracer antigen with or without unlabeled competitor, wash, and count directly the radioactivity bound to the plastic wells or to the Sepharose. The microtiter plate method is particularly useful for processing large numbers of samples. However, since the concentration, or even the amount, of antibody coating the surface is unknown, and since the affinity is not the intrinsic affinity, one cannot use these methods for studying the chemistry of the antigen–antibody reaction itself. Also, one usually measures only bound antigen in these methods, and so rarely measures the free concentration independently. Nevertheless, if one's only purpose is to measure the concentration of unknown competitor by empiric comparison with a standard curve, the plate-binding method can be ideal. A detailed analysis of the optimum parameters in this method is given by Zollinger et al. (41).

A variation that does allow determination of affinity, based on the enzyme-linked immunosorbant assay (ELISA) described below, but equally applicable to RIA, was described by Friguet et al. (43). This uses antigen-coated microtiter wells and free antibody, but measures competition by free antigen to prevent the antibody in solution from binding to the antibody on the plate (see Fig. 9B). Thus, the antibody bound to the plastic is antibody that was free in the solution equilibrium. The affinity measured is that between the antibody and antigen in solution, not that on the plastic, so it is not directly influenced by the multivalency of the surface. However, as pointed out by Stevens (44), the determination of affinity is strictly accurate only for monovalent Fab fragments, because a bivalent antibody with only one arm bound to the plastic and one bound by antigen in solution will still be counted as free. Therefore, there will be an underestimate of the ligand occupancy of the antibody combining sites, and thus an underestimate of affinity. Stevens also points out a method to correct for this error based on binomial analysis. Subsequently, Seligman (45) showed that the nature and density of the antigen on the solid surface can also influence the estimate of affinity.

Optimization of Antibody and Tracer Concentrations for Sensitivity

The primary limitations on the sensitivity of the assay are the antibody affinity and concentration, the tracer concentration, and the precision (reproducibility) of the data. In general, the higher the affinity of the antibody, the more sensitive the assay can be made. Once one prepares the highest affinity antibody available, this parameter limits the extent to which the other parameters can be manipulated. For instance, since the unlabeled antigen in the unknown sample is going to compete against labeled tracer antigen, the lower the tracer concentration, the lower the concentration of the unknown, which can be measured, up to a point. That point is determined by the affinity, K_A, as can be seen from the theoretical considerations above (36). The steepest part of the titration curve will occur in the range of concentrations around $1/K_A$. Concentrations of ligand much below $1/K_A$ will leave most of the antibody sites unoccupied, so that competition will be less effective. Thus, there is no value in reducing the tracer concentration more than a fewfold lower than $1/K_A$. Therefore, although it is in general useful to increase the specific radioactivity of the tracer and reduce its concentration, it is important to be aware of this limit of $1/K_A$. Increasing the specific activity more than necessary for optimum sensitivity can result in denaturation of antigen, and decreasing the number of counts per minute in the assay too far would necessitate inconveniently long counting times.

Similarly, lowering the antibody concentration will also increase sensitivity, up to a point. This limit also depends on $1/K_A$ and on the background "nonspecific binding". Clearly, decreasing the antibody concentration to the point that binding of tracer in the absence of unlabeled antigen is too close to background will result in loss of sensitivity due to loss of precision. In general, the fraction of tracer bound in the absence of competitor should be kept greater than 0.2, and in general closer to 0.5 (see ref. 46).

A convenient procedure to follow to optimize tracer and antibody concentrations is first to choose the lowest tracer concentration that results in convenient counting times and counting precision for bound values of only one-half to one-tenth the total tracer. Then, keeping this tracer concentration constant, one dilutes out the antibody until the bound/free antigen ratio is close to 1.0 (bound/total = 0.5) in the absence of competitor. This antibody concentration in conjunction with this tracer concentration will generally give near-optimal sensitivities, within the limits noted above. It is important to be aware that changing the tracer concentration will require readjusting the antibody concentration to optimize sensitivity.

Analysis of Data: Graphic and Numeric Representation

We have already examined the Scatchard plot (bound/free versus bound) and the plot of bound/free versus free or total antigen concentration as methods of determining affinity. The latter lends itself particularly to the type of competition curves that constitute a RIA. In fact, the independent variable must always be antigen concentration, since that is the known quantity one varies to generate the standard curve. Let us use B, F, and T to represent the concentrations of bound, free, and total antigen, respectively. We have seen above that the plot of B/F versus F is more useful for determining the affinity, K_A, than the plot of B/F versus T. However, in RIA, the quantity one wants to determine is T, and, correspondingly, the known independent variable in generating the

standard curve is T. Another difference between the situation in RIA and that discussed earlier is that, in RIA, one has both labeled and unlabeled antigen. The dependent variable, such as B/F, is the ratio of bound tracer over free tracer, since only radioactive antigen is counted. B/F for the unlabeled antigen will be the same at equilibrium, assuming that labeled and unlabeled antigen bind the antibody equivalently, that is, with the same K_A. This assumption is not always valid and requires experimental testing. Even if it is not the case, one may still be able to read concentrations of an unknown off a standard curve, but any more detailed analysis becomes complex.

The sigmoidal shape of B/F versus F or T, when F or T (the "dose") is plotted on a log scale, has been seen in Fig. 6. The shape for B/T versus F or T would be similar. Note that since B + F = T,

$$\frac{B}{F} = \frac{B}{T-B} = \frac{B/T}{(1-B/T)} \qquad [38]$$

and

$$\frac{B}{T} = \frac{B/F}{1+B/F} \qquad [39]$$

These transformations can be useful. If one plots B/F or B/T versus F or T on a linear scale, then the shape is approximately hyperbolic, as in Fig. 7. The plot of B/F versus T (log scale) was one of the first methods used to plot RIA data and is still among the most useful. The most sensitive part of the curve is the part with the steepest slope.

It has been shown by probability analysis that if the antigen has multiple determinants, each capable of binding antibody molecules simultaneously and independently of one another, then the more such determinants capable of being recognized by the antibodies in use, the steeper will be the slope (47). This effect of multideterminant binding on steepness arises because, in RIA, an antigen molecule is scored as bound whether it has one antibody molecule attached or several. It is scored as free only if no antibody molecules are attached. Thus, the probability that an antigen molecule is scored as free is the product of the probabilities that each of its determinants is free. The effect can lead to quite steep slopes and has been confirmed experimentally (47).

A transform that allows linearization of the data in most cases is the logit transform (48,49). To use this, one first expresses the data as B/B_0, where B_0 is the concentration of bound tracer in the

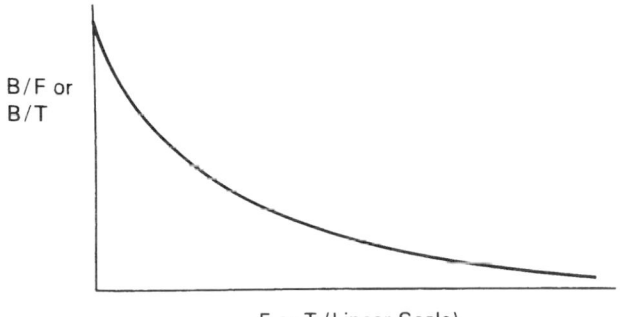

FIG. 7. Schematic plot of B/F or B/T (the bound over free or total antigen concentration) as a function of free (F) or total (T) antigen concentration, when plotted on a linear scale. Contrast with similar plot on a log scale in Fig. 6.

absence of competitor. One then takes the logit transform of this ratio, defined as

$$\text{logit}\,(Y) = \ln\left(\frac{Y}{1-Y}\right) \qquad [40]$$

where ln means the natural log (log to the base e). The plot of logit (B/B_0) versus ln T is usually a straight line (Fig. 8).The slope is usually -1 for the simplest case of a monoclonal antibody binding a monovalent antigen. The linearity of this plot obviously makes it very useful for graphical interpolation, which one would like to do to read antigen concentration off a standard curve. One additional advantage is that linearity facilitates tests of parallelism. If the unknown under study is identical to the antigen used to generate the standard curve, then a dilution curve of the unknown should be parallel to the standard curve in this logit–log coordinate system. (Of course, parallelism does not guarantee that they are identical.) If not, the assay is not valid.

These and other methods of analyzing the data are discussed further by Feldman and Rodbard (50) and Rodbard (37), including statistical treatment of data. While a number of computer programs have become available for rapid analysis of RIA data without using manual plots of standard curves, they are all based on these and similar methods, and their accurate interpretation depends on an understanding of these concepts.

Corrections for B, F, and T

Before we leave this section on analysis of RIA data, we must point out a few controls and corrections to the data without which the results may be fallacious.

First, in any method that precipitates antibody and bound antigen (or uses a solid-phase antibody), there may always be a fraction of antigen that precipitates or binds nonspecifically in the absence of specific antibody. Thus one must always run controls with normal serum (or the equivalent, depending on the form of the antibody) to determine this nonspecific or background binding. The nonspecific binding usually increases linearly with antigen dose and should constitute the same fraction of unlabeled as of labeled antigen; that is, it does not saturate. This control value should be subtracted from B but does not affect F, if F is measured independently. If F is determined as the difference of T and B (for labeled tracer), then F will be affected, since T must also be corrected by the amount of nonspecific binding. In other words, the

total antigen that is meaningful in the assay is the sum of that which is specifically bound and that which is free. Any antigen that is nonspecifically bound should be deleted from any term in which it appears.

A second correction, which may be less obvious, is that for immunologically inactive radiolabel. In many situations, the radiolabeled tracer is contaminated by either free radioisotope, isotope coupled to an antigenically inactive impurity in the antigen preparation, or isotope coupled to denatured antigen (which may have become denatured in the process of radiolabeling). The fraction of radioactive material that is immunologically reactive with the antibodies in the assay can be determined by using a constant, low concentration of labeled antigen and adding increasing concentrations of antibody. If there is no contamination with inactive material, all the radioactivity should be able to be bound by sufficient antibody. If the fraction of tracer bound reaches a plateau at less than 100% bound, then only this fraction is active in the assay. The importance of correcting for the inactive fraction can be seen from the following example. Suppose that the tracer is only 80% active and 20% inactive, and suppose that the true B/F at a certain point is 3; that is, by Eq. 39, B/T = 0.75. These values will apply only to the active 80% of the tracer. The remaining 20%, which can never be bound, will mistakenly be included in the free tracer, doubling the amount that is measured as free. Thus the measured B/F will be only 1.5 (i.e., 0.6/0.4) instead of the true value of 3 (i.e., 0.6/0.2). This factor of 2 will make a serious difference in the calculation of affinity, for instance, from a Scatchard plot. Also, it will result in a plateau in the Scatchard plot at high values of B/F, since with 20% of the tracer obligatorily free, B/F can never exceed 4 (i.e., 0.8/0.2). To correct for this potentially serious problem, the inactive fraction of tracer must always be determined for each batch of tracer and subtracted from both F and T. When B and F are measured independently and tracer T (not total ligand including unlabeled competitor) is determined as B + F, then a convenient way to make this correction without assumptions about input T is to calculate B/T = B/(B + F), correct this ratio by dividing by the fraction of tracer that is immunologically active (0.8 in the above example), and then convert to B/F by Eq. 38.

Nonequilibrium Radioimmunoassay

So far, we have assumed that tracer and unlabeled competitor are added simultaneously and sufficient incubation time is allowed to achieve equilibrium. To measure the affinity, of course, equilibrium must be assured. However, suppose one's sole purpose is to measure the concentration of competitor by RIA. Then one can actually increase the sensitivity of the assay by adding the competitor first, allowing it to react with the antibody, and then intentionally adding the tracer for too short a time to reach a new equilibrium. One is essentially giving the competitor a competitive advantage. It can be shown that the slope of the dose-response curve, B/T versus total antigen added, is increased in the low-dose range—a mathematical measure of increased sensitivity. A detailed mathematical analysis of this procedure may be found in Rodbard et al. (51). Note, however, that use of such nonequilibrium conditions requires very careful control of time and temperature.

Enzyme-linked Immunosorbent Assay

An alternative solid-phase readout system for the detection of antigen–antibody reactions is the ELISA assay (52). In principle,

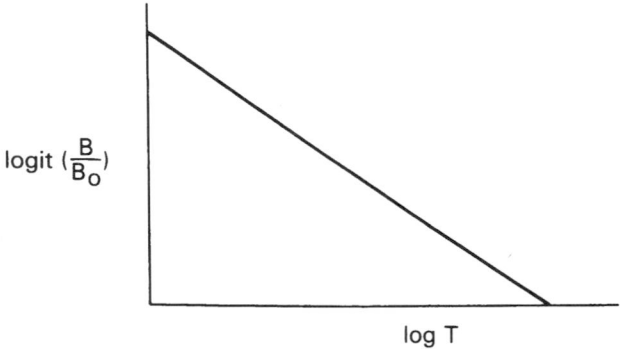

FIG. 8. Schematic logit–log plot used to linearize RIA data. B and T are bound tracer and total antigen concentration, respectively, and B_0 is the value of B when no unlabeled antigen is added to tracer. The logit function is defined by Eq. 40, logit $(Y) = \ln[Y/(1-Y)]$.

the only difference from RIAs is that antibodies or antigen are covalently coupled to an enzyme instead of a radioisotope, so that bound enzyme activity is measured instead of bound counts per minute. In practice, the safety and convenience of nonradioactive materials and the commercial availability of plate readers that can measure the absorbance of 96 wells in a few seconds account for ELISA's popularity. Since both ELISA and RIA are governed by the same thermodynamic constraints, and the enzyme can be detected in the same range of molarity as commonly used radioisotopes, the sensitivity and specificity are comparable. We consider four basic strategies for using ELISA assays to detect specific antibody, antigen, or cross-reacting antibodies.

As shown in Fig. 9A, the indirect antibody method is the simplest way to detect and measure specific antibody in an unknown antiserum. Antigen is noncovalently attached to each well of a plastic microtiter dish. For this purpose, it is fortunate that most proteins bind nonspecifically to plastic. Excess free antigen is washed off, and the wells are incubated with an albumin solution to block the remaining nonspecific protein-binding sites. The test antiserum is then added, and any specific antibody binds to the solid-phase antigen. Washing removes unbound antibodies. Enzyme-labeled antiimmunoglobulin is added. This binds to specific antibody already bound to antigen on the solid phase, bringing along covalently attached enzyme. Unbound antiglobulin–enzyme conjugate is washed off; then substrate is added. The action of bound enzyme on substrate produces a colored product, which is detected as increased absorbance in a spectrophotometer.

Although this method is quick and very sensitive, it is often difficult to quantitate. Within a defined range, the increase in optical density is proportional to the amount of specific antibody added in the first step. However, the amount of antibody bound is not measured directly. Instead, the antibody concentration of the sample is estimated by comparing it with a standard curve for a known amount of antibody. It is also difficult to determine affinity by this method, since the solid-phase antigen tends to increase the apparent affinity. The sensitivity of this assay for detecting minute amounts of antibody is quite good, especially when affinity-purified antiglobulins are used as the enzyme-linked reagent. A single preparation of enzyme-linked antiglobulin can be used to detect antibodies to many different antigens. Alternatively, class-specific antiglobulins can be used to detect how much of a specific antibody response is due to each immunoglobulin class. Obviously, reproducibility of the assay depends on uniform antigen coating of each well (which can vary), and the specificity depends on using purified antigen to coat the wells.

Figure 9B shows the competition technique for detecting antigen. Soluble antigen is mixed with limiting amounts of specific antibody in the first step. Then the mixture is added to antigen-coated wells and treated as described in Fig. 9A. Any antigen–antibody complexes formed in the first step will reduce the amount of antibody bound to the plate and hence will reduce the absorbance measured in the final step. This method permits the estimate of affinity for free antigen, which is related to the half-inhibitory concentration of antigen. Mathematical analysis of affinity by this approach was

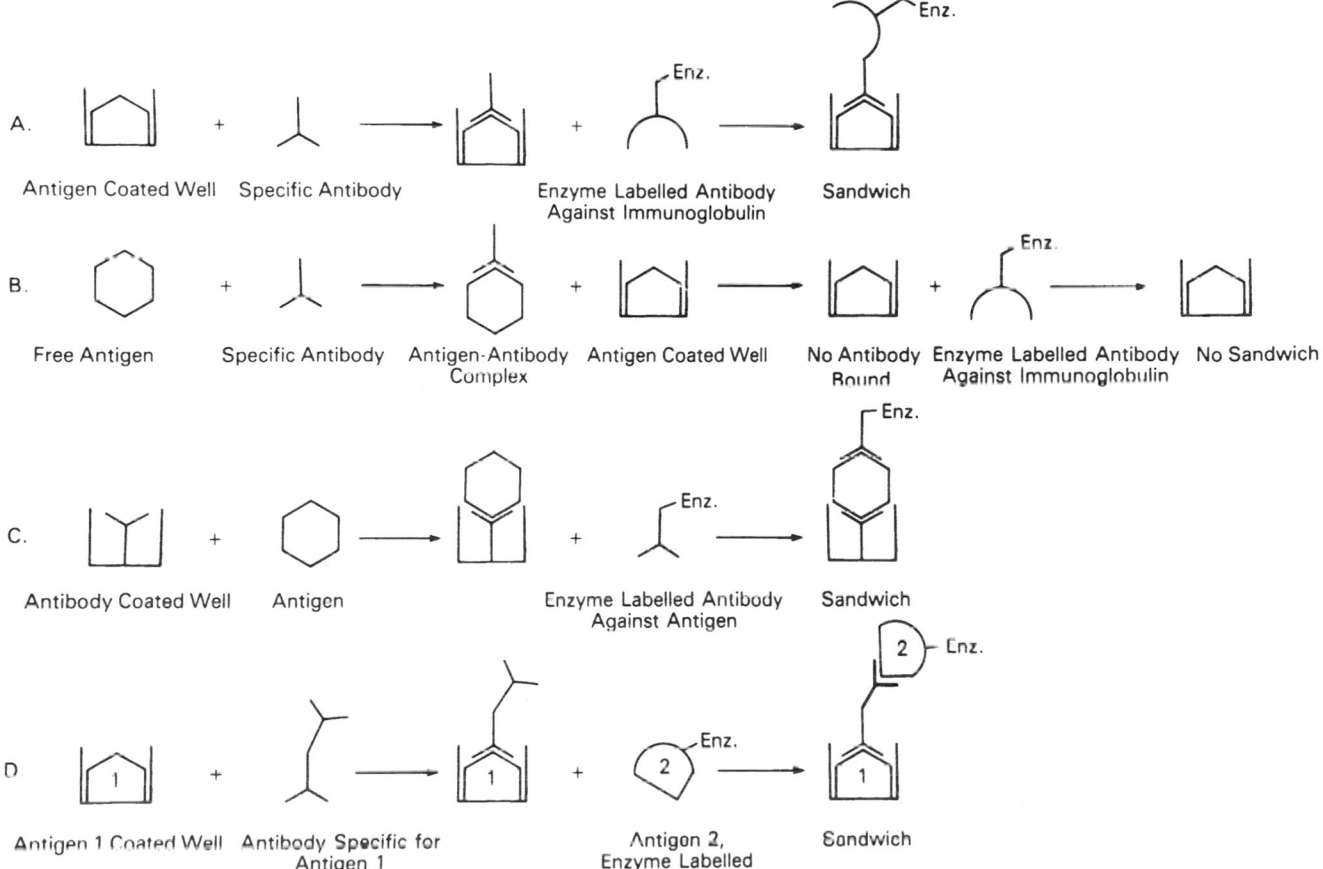

FIG. 9. Four strategies for the detection of specific antibody–antigen reactions using the ELISA technique. **A:** Direct binding. **B:** Hapten inhibition. **C:** Antigen sandwich. **D:** Antibody sandwich.

A. Antigen Coated Well — Specific Antibody — Enzyme Labelled Antibody Against Immunoglobulin — Sandwich

B. Free Antigen — Specific Antibody — Antigen-Antibody Complex — Antigen Coated Well — No Antibody Bound — Enzyme Labelled Antibody Against Immunoglobulin — No Sandwich

C. Antibody Coated Well — Antigen — Enzyme Labelled Antibody Against Antigen — Sandwich

D. Antigen 1 Coated Well — Antibody Specific for Antigen 1 — Antigen 2, Enzyme Labelled — Sandwich

described by Friguet et al. (43) with modification by Stevens (44), as discussed in the preceding section on RIA solid-phase methods. In addition, some estimate of cross-reactivity between the antigen in solution and that on the plate can be obtained.

Figure 9C shows the sandwich technique for detecting antigen. Specific antibody is used to coat the microtiter wells. Antigen is then bound to the solid-phase antibody. Finally, a second antibody, linked to enzyme, is added. This binds to the solid-phase antigen–antibody complex, carrying enzyme along with it. Excess second antibody is washed off and substrate is added. The absorbance produced is a function of the antigen concentration of the test solution, which can be determined from a standard curve. Specificity of the assay depends on the specificity of the antibodies used to coat the plate and detect antigen. Sensitivity depends on affinities as well as the amount of the first antibody bound to the well, which can be increased by using affinity-purified antibodies in the coating step. The binding of both antibodies of the sandwich depends on divalency of the antigen, or else the two antibodies must be specific for different antigenic determinants on the same antigen molecule. If the antibodies are two different monoclonal antibodies that both bind to the same monomeric antigen, this technique can be used to ascertain whether the two antibodies can bind simultaneously to the same molecule or whether they compete for the same site or sites close enough to cause steric hindrance (53).

Figure 9D shows the sandwich technique for detecting antibody cross-reactivity. The wells are coated with antigen 1, followed by the adsorption of specific antibody for antigen 1. Excess antibody is washed off, and enzyme-labeled antigen 2 is added. If bound antibody cross-reacts with both antigen 1 and antigen 2, then enzyme-labeled antigen 2 will adsorb onto the solid phase. This will be measured as increased absorbance of the enzyme-catalyzed reaction. This method has been used to assay the cross-reactivity of antiidiotype antisera for two preparations of idiotype, or for detection of anti-antiidiotype (see Chapter 3). Other arrangements of antibody and antigen are also possible. Extra layers of detecting reagents can amplify sensitivity but also tend to raise the background and introduce variability.

An example of the first method described above is the detection of human antibodies to influenza virus (54) (Fig. 10). Alternate columns were coated with influenza virus or bovine albumin. Serum was added at 1/10 dilution to the top two wells of each box and serially diluted in fourfold steps from top to bottom. The last colored well indicates the titer, whereas the absence of color in the albumin-coated wells indicates the specificity. A second use of this method is for screening culture supernatants in the production of hybridoma antibodies. The sensitivity and speed of the ELISA method make it possible to screen large numbers of wells for the production of specific antibody. Clones selected by this method tend to have high antigen affinities, perhaps due to dissociation of low-affinity antibodies during the wash steps.

An important caution when using native protein antigens to coat solid-phase surfaces (see Fig. 9A) is that binding to a surface can alter the conformation of the protein. For instance, using conformation-specific monoclonal antibodies to myoglobin, Darst et al. (55) found that binding of myoglobin to a surface altered the apparent affinity of some antibodies more than others. This problem may be avoided by using the methods of Fig. 9B and C.

ELIspot Assay

The normal ELISA assay can be modified to measure antibody production at the single-cell level. In this method, tissue culture

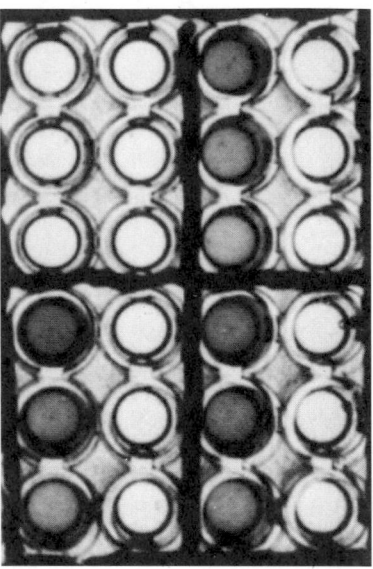

FIG. 10. Typical ELISA plate, using the direct binding method. Wells in alternate columns were coated with influenza virus or bovine serum albumin. Samples to be tested for antiinfluenza antibodies were added to the top wells of each box and serially diluted in fourfold steps from top to bottom. Enzyme-labeled goat antihuman immunoglobulin was used as detecting reagent. (Photograph courtesy of Dr. R. Yarchoan and Dr. D. L. Nelson.)

plates are coated with antigen, and various cell populations are cultured on the plate for 4 hours. During that time, B cells settle to the bottom and secrete antibodies, which bind antigen nearby and produce an analogue of the cell's footprint. The cells are then washed off, and a second antibody, such as enzyme-labeled goat antihuman IgG, is added. Finally, unbound antibody is washed off, and enzyme substrate is added in soft agar. Over the next 10 minutes, localized zones of enzyme activity convert the substrate to a dark spot of insoluble dye, where the B cell originally secreted its antibody.

Using this method, it is possible to detect as few as ten to 20 antibody-producing B cells in the presence of 10^6 spleen cells, and typical results for immunized mice range from 200 to 500 (56,57). Clearly, to work at all, this assay must be capable of detecting the amount of antibody secreted by a single immune B cell and specific enough to disregard nonspecific antibodies produced by the vast majority of nonimmune B cells. Sensitivity depends on the affinity and amount of antibodies secreted and may be optimized by titering the amount of antigen on the plate.

This type of assay is useful in analyzing the cellular requirements for antibody production *in vitro,* since the number of responding B cells is measured directly. It can also be used to detect antibodies made in the presence of excess antigen. For example, in acute infections (58) and in autoimmunity (59), when antigen may be in excess over antibody, this assay makes it possible to measure antibody-producing B cells, even though free antibody may not be detectable in circulation. It can also be used to measure local production of self-reactive antibodies in a specific tissue, such as synovium. By using two detecting antibodies, each specific for a different immunoglobulin class and coupled to a different enzyme, and two substrates producing different colored dyes, cells secreting IgA and IgG simultaneously can be detected (60). ELIspot has been used to show that bacterial DNA containing CpG sequences is a polyclonal B-cell mitogen (61).

ELIspot can also detect secreted antigens, as opposed to antibodies, by coating the plate with a capture antibody and detecting antigen with an enzyme-coupled second antibody (as in a sandwich ELISA; see Fig. 9C). For example, using plates coated with monoclonal antibody to interleukin-4 (IL-4), T cells secreting IL-4 could be detected (62). In this way, T-helper 2 cells can be measured, even though a specific antibody for a marker on these cells is currently not available.

SPECIFICITY AND CROSS-REACTIVITY

The specificity of an antibody or antiserum is defined by its ability to discriminate between the antigen against which it was made (called the *homologous antigen,* or *immunogen*) and any other antigen one might test. In practice, one cannot test the whole universe of antigens, but only selected antigens. In this sense, specificity can only be defined experimentally within that set of antigens one chooses to compare. Karush (28) has defined a related term, *selectivity,* as the ability of an antibody to discriminate, in an all-or-none fashion, between two related ligands. Thus, selectivity depends not only on the relative affinity of the antibody for the two ligands, but also on the experimental lower limit for detection of reactivity. For instance, an anticarbohydrate antibody with an affinity of 10^5 M^{-1} for the immunogen may appear to be highly selective, since reaction with a related carbohydrate with a 100-fold lower affinity, 10^3 M^{-1}, may be undetectable. On the other hand, an antibody with an affinity of 10^9 M^{-1} for the homologous ligand may appear to be less selective because any reaction with a related ligand with a 100-fold lower affinity would still be quite easily detectable.

Conversely, *cross-reactivity* is defined as the ability to react with related ligands other than the immunogen. More usually, this is examined from the point of view of the ligand. Thus, one might say that antigen Y cross-reacts with antigen X because it binds to anti-X antibodies. Note that in this sense, it is the two antigens that are cross-reactive, not the antibody. However, the cross-reactivity of two antigens, X and Y, can be defined only with respect to a particular antibody or antiserum. For instance, a different group of anti-X antibodies may not react at all with Y, so that with respect to these antibodies, Y would not be cross-reactive with X. One can also use the term in a different sense, saying that some anti-X antibodies cross-react with antigen Y.

In most cases, cross-reactive ligands have lower affinity than the immunogen for a particular antibody. However, exceptions can occur, in which a cross-reactive antigen binds with a higher affinity than the homologous antigen itself. This phenomenon is called *heteroclicity,* and the antigen that has a higher affinity for the antibody than does the immunogen is said to be heteroclitic. Antibodies that manifest this behavior are also described as heteroclitic antibodies. A good example is the case of antibodies raised in C57BL/10 mice against the hapten nitrophenyl acetyl (NP). These antibodies have been shown by Mäkelä and Karjalainen (63) to bind with higher affinity to the cross-reactive hapten, nitro-iodophenyl acetyl (NIP), than to the immunogen itself. Another example is the case of retro-inverso or retro-D peptides (64–68). By reversing the chirality from L to D amino acids, and simultaneously reversing the sequence of amino acids, one can produce a peptide that is resistant to proteolysis and has its side chains approximately in the same position as the original L amino acid peptide, with the exception of some amino acids with secondary chiral centers such as Thr and Ile. However, the backbone NH and CO moieties are reversed. Antibodies that interact with only the side chains might not distinguish these peptides, whereas antibodies that interact with the main chain as well as side chains might distinguish them, and have potentially higher or lower affinity. In a study of monoclonal antibodies to a hexapeptide from histone H3, some bound the retro-D form with higher affinity than the native sequence and some did not (66,67). The former are an example of heteroclicity. In addition to greater binding affinity, the retro-D peptides may have even greater activity *in vivo* because of their resistance to proteolysis (64–68) (and in measuring affinity differences, one must be sure that stability of the peptide in the assay is not contributing to the apparent affinity). This stability makes them more useful as drugs as well (64,65,69).

In many practical situations, cross-reactivity is detected by methods such as precipitin, especially precipitation in agar (the Ouchterlony test), or hemagglutination (see below for descriptions of both of these) or similar methods, which have in common the fact that they do not distinguish well between differences in affinity and differences in concentration. This practical aspect, coupled with the heterogeneity of immune antisera, has led to ambiguities in the usage of the terms *cross-reactivity* and *specificity*. With the advent of RIA techniques, this ambiguity in the terminology, as well as in the interpretation of data, has become apparent.

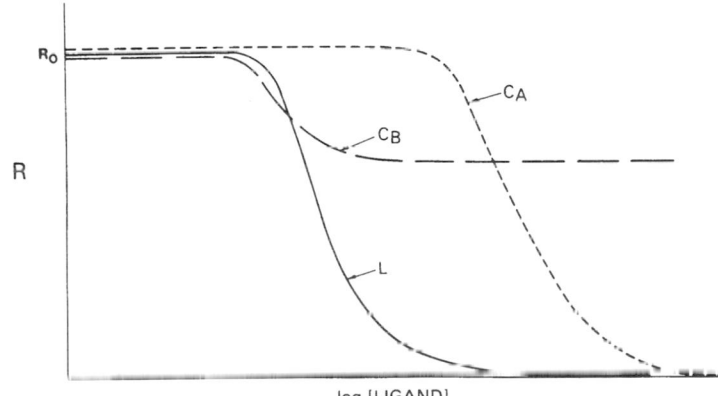

log [LIGAND]

FIG. 11. Schematic RIA binding curves for homologous ligand L and cross-reacting ligands. Cross-reacting ligand CA manifests type 1 or true cross-reactivity demonstrated by complete inhibition of tracer ligand binding, and a lower affinity. Ligand CB displays type 2 cross-reactivity or determinant sharing, as recognized from the plateau at less than 100% inhibition, but not necessarily a lower affinity. The ordinate R is the ratio of bound/free radiolabeled tracer ligand, and R_0 is the limit of R as the concentration of all ligands, including tracer, approaches zero. (From ref. 70, with permission.)

For these reasons, Berzofsky and Schechter (70) have defined two forms of cross-reactivity and, correspondingly, two forms of specificity. These two forms of cross-reactivity are illustrated by the two prototype competition RIA curves in Fig. 11. In reality, most antisera display both phenomena simultaneously.

Type 1 cross-reactivity, or *true cross-reactivity,* is defined as the ability of two ligands to react with the same site on the same antibody molecule, possibly with different affinities. For example, the related haptens dinitrophenyl (DNP) and trinitrophenyl (TNP) may react with different affinity for antibodies raised to DNP hapten. In protein antigens, such differences could occur with small changes in primary sequence (e.g., the conservative substitution of threonine for serine) or with changes in conformation, such as the cleavage of the protein into fragments (Fig. 12) (70–74). If a peptide fragment contained all the contact residues in an antigenic determinant (i.e., those that contact the antibody-combining site), it might cross-react with the native determinant for antibodies against the native form, but with lower affinity because the peptide would not retain the native conformation (see Chapter 19). This type of affinity difference is illustrated by competitor CA in Fig. 11, in which complete displacement of tracer can be achieved at high enough concentrations of CA, but higher concentrations of CA than of the homologous ligand, L, are required to produce any given degree of inhibition.

An issue separate from affinity differences is whether the cross-reactive ligand reacts with all or only a subpopulation of the antibodies in a heterogeneous serum. This second type of cross-reactivity, which we call *type 2 cross-reactivity,* or *shared reactivity,* therefore can occur only when the antibody population is heterogeneous, as in most conventional antisera. In this case, the affinity of the cross-reactive ligand may be greater than, less than, or equal to that of the homologous ligand for those antibodies with which it interacts. Therefore, the competition curve is not necessarily displaced to the right, but the inhibition will reach a plateau at less than complete inhibition, as illustrated by competitor CB in Fig. 11. As an example, let us consider the case of a protein with determinants X and Y, and an antiserum against this protein containing both anti-X and anti-Y antibodies. Then a mutant protein in which determinant Y was so altered as to be unrecognizable by anti-Y, but determinant X was intact, would manifest type 2 cross-reactivity. It would compete with the wild-type protein only for anti-X antibodies (possibly even with equal affinity), but not for anti-Y antibodies.

Occasionally, even monoclonal antibodies may appear to display type 2 cross-reactivity in situations in which secondary reactions are involved in the measurement of the antigen–antibody reaction. For example, Sharon et al. (75) and Cisar et al. (76) observed plateau values at less than 100% binding of a homogeneous myeloma or hybridoma antibody reactive with dextrans. In this case, the assay used was quantitative precipitin, in which differential solubility of different complexes could account for such a plateau. If one could directly observe the antigen–antibody interaction in solution, without the need for any secondary reaction that might be incomplete, the reaction of a homogeneous antibody with its homogeneous antigen theoretically could not reach a plateau at less than 100% reaction or inhibition. Therefore, the existence of secondary competing reactions should be considered when such plateaus are observed.

Of course, both types of cross-reactivity could occur simultaneously. A classic example would be the peptide fragment discussed in the preceding case of type I cross-reactivity. Suppose the frag-

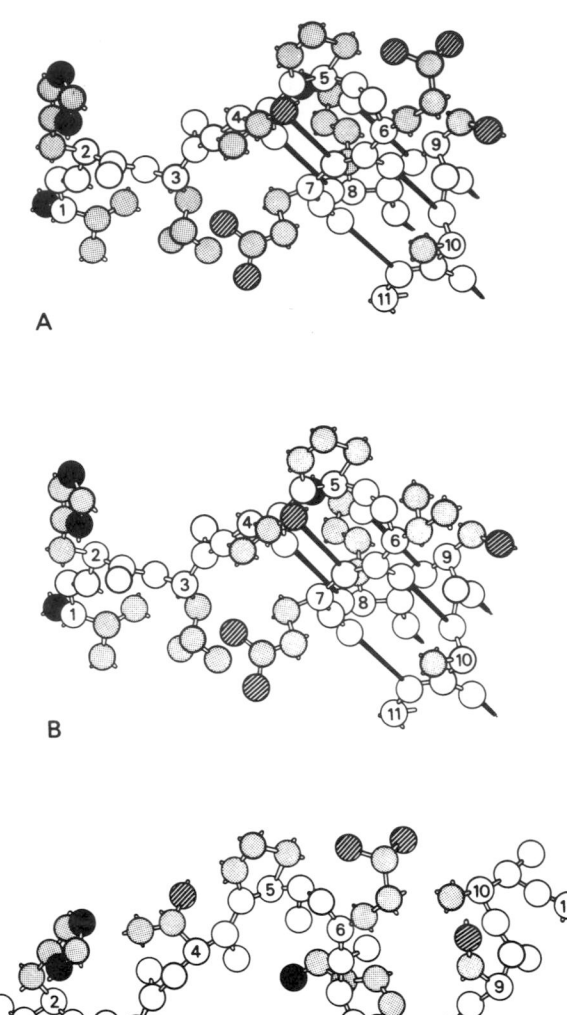

FIG. 12. An artist's drawing of the amino terminal region of the β chain of hemoglobin. **A:** The first 11 residues of the βᴬ chain. **B:** The comparable regions of the βˢ chain. The substitution of valine for the normal glutamic acid at position 6 makes a distinct antigenic determinant to which a subpopulation of antibodies may be isolated (71,72). **C:** A schematic diagram of the sequence in (A) unfolded as occurs when the protein is denatured. This region may be cleaved from the protein, or the peptide synthesized (73), resulting in changed antigenic reactivity. An antiserum prepared to hemoglobin (or the β chain thereof) might exhibit cross-reactivity with the structures shown in (**B**) and (**C**), but the molecular mechanisms would be different. Polypeptide backbone atoms are in *white* in the side chains, oxygen atoms are *hatched,* nitrogen atoms are *black,* and carbon atoms are *lightly stippled.* (Adapted from refs. 70,74.)

ment contained the residues of determinant X, albeit not in the native conformation, but did not contain the residues of a second determinant, Y, which was also expressed on the native protein. If the antiserum to the native protein consisted of anti-X and anti-Y, the peptide would compete only for anti-X antibodies (type 2 cross-reactivity) but would have a lower affinity than the native protein, even for these antibodies. Thus the competition curve would be shifted to the right and would plateau before reaching complete inhibition.[8]

In the case of a homogeneous (e.g., monoclonal) antibody in which only type 1 or true cross-reactivity can occur, one can quantitate the differences in affinity for different cross-reactive ligands by a method analogous to the B/F versus F method described previously. Suppose that ligands X and Y cross-react with homologous ligand L for a monoclonal antibody. If one plots the bound/free (B/F = R) ratio for radiolabeled tracer ligand L as a function of the log of the concentration of competitors X and Y, one obtains two parallel competition curves (Fig. 13) (70), under the appropriate conditions (below). The first condition is that the concentration of free tracer be less than $1/K_L$, the affinity for tracer. In this case, it can be shown (70) that

$$K_X \simeq \frac{1}{[X]_{free}} \qquad [41]$$

at the midpoint where $R = R_0/2$, where K_X is the affinity for X. This is analogous to Eq. 21 for the case in which unlabeled homologous ligand is the competitor. Also, in analogy with Eq. 23, it can be shown that if the total concentration of competitor, $[X]_t$, is used

instead of the free concentration, $[X]_{free}$, an error term will arise, giving

$$[X]_t \text{ (at } R = R_0/2) = \frac{1}{K_X} + \frac{[S]_t}{2} \qquad [42]$$

Thus, with competitor on a linear scale, the difference in midpoint for competitors X and Y will correspond to the difference $1/K_X - 1/K_Y$, regardless of whether free or total competitor is plotted, but the ratio of midpoint concentrations will equal K_X/K_Y only if the free concentrations are used. This last point is important if one plots the log of competitor concentration, as is usually done, since the horizontal displacement between the two curves on a log scale corresponds to the ratio $[X]/[Y]$, not the difference (70).

If a second condition also holds, namely, that the concentration of bound tracer is small compared to the antibody site concentration $[S]_t$, then the slopes (on a linear scale) of the curves at their respective midpoints (where $R = R_0/2$) will be proportional to the affinity for that competitor, K_X or K_Y (70). (Both conditions can be met by keeping tracer L small relative to both K_L and $[S]_t$.) When $[X]_{free}$ and $[Y]_{free}$ are plotted on a log scale, the slopes will appear to be equal (i.e., the curves will appear parallel), since a parallel line shifted m-fold to the right on a log scale will actually be $1/m$ as steep, at any point, in terms of the antilog as abscissa.

When the antibodies are heterogeneous in affinity, the curves will be broadened and in general will not be parallel. When heterogeneity of specificity is present, and type 2 cross-reactivity occurs, it should be pointed out that the fractional inhibition achieved at the plateau in a B/F versus free competitor plot will not be proportional to the fraction of antibodies reacting with that competitor but will be proportional to a weighted fraction, where the antibody concentrations are weighted by their affinity for the tracer (70).

---

[8]An ambiguous case could occur experimentally in which the distinction between the two types of cross-reactivity would be blurred. For example, in the case of antibodies that all react with determinant X but have a very wide range of affinities for X, some such antibodies may have such a low affinity for cross-reactive determinant X' that they would appear not to bind X' at all. Then a competition curve using X' might appear to reach a plateau at incomplete inhibition even though all the antibodies were specific for X, and the only difference between X and X' was affinity.

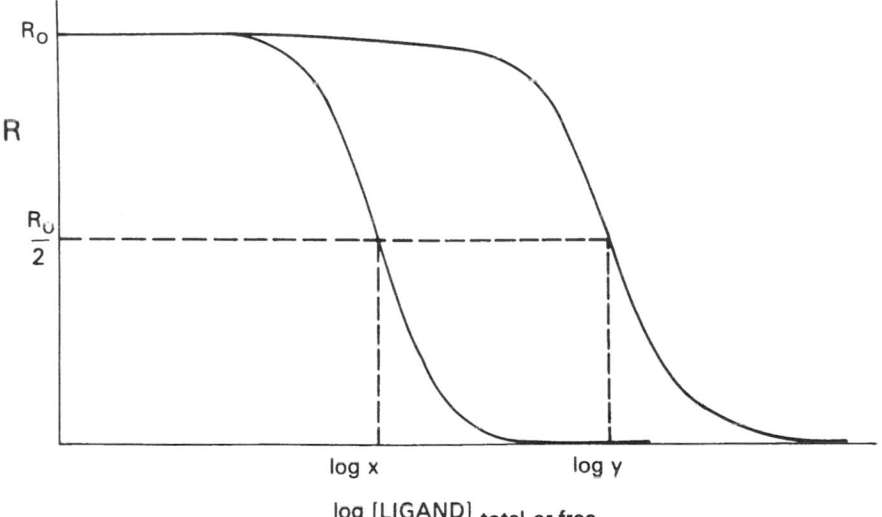

FIG. 13. Schematic RIA binding curves showing the effect of affinity on the midpoint and the slope at the midpoint, and the value of using free [ligand] rather than total [ligand]. Ordinate R is the ratio of bound/free radiolabeled tracer ligand, and R_0 is the limit of R as all ligand concentrations approach zero. If x and y are the concentrations of ligands X and Y that reduce R to exactly $R_0/2$, then if the abscissa is total ligand concentration, $x = 1/K_X + [S]_t/2$ and $y = 1/K_Y + [S]_t/2$, where $[S]_t$ is the concentration of antibody-binding sites and K_X and K_Y are the affinities of the antibody for the respective ligands. However, if the abscissa is free ligand concentration, $x = 1/K_X$ and $y = 1/K_Y$ so that the ratio x/y (or the difference log x – log y on a log plot) corresponds to the ratio of affinities K_Y/K_X. Note that the slopes at the midpoints are the same on a log scale, but that for Y would be only K_Y/K_X that for X on a linear scale. (From ref. 70, with permission.)

These two types of cross-reactivity lead naturally to two definitions of *specificity* (70). The overall specificity of a heterogeneous antiserum is a composite of both of these facets of specificity. Type 1 specificity is based on the relative affinities of the antibody for the homologous ligand and any cross-reactive ligands. If the affinity is much higher for the homologous ligand than for any cross-reactive ligand tested, then the antibody is said to be highly specific for the homologous ligand; that is, it discriminates very well between this ligand and the others. If the affinity for cross-reactive ligands is below the threshold for detection in an experimental situation, then type 1 specificity gives rise to selectivity as was discussed above (cf. ref. 28). The specificity can even be quantitated in terms of the ratio of affinities for the homologous ligand and a cross-reactive ligand (cf. ref. 77). It is this type 1 specificity that most immunochemists would call *true specificity,* just as we have called type 1 cross-reactivity *true cross-reactivity.*

The common use of the term *cross-reactivity* to include type 2 or partial reactivity leads to a second definition of *specificity,* which applies only to heterogeneous populations of antibodies such as antisera. We call this *type 2 specificity.* If all the antibodies in the mixture react with the immunogen, but only a small proportion react with any single cross-reactive antigen, then the antiserum would be said to be relatively specific for the immunogen. Note that it does not matter whether the affinity of a subpopulation that reacts with a cross-reactive antigen is high or low (type 1 cross-reactivity). As long as that subpopulation is a small fraction of the antibodies, the mixture is specific. Thus, type 2 specificity depends on the relative concentrations of antibodies in the heterogeneous antiserum, not just on their affinities. Also note that one can use these relative concentrations of antibody subpopulations to compare the specificity of a single antiserum for two cross-reactive ligands. However, it would not be meaningful to compare the specificity of two different antisera for the same ligand by comparing the fraction of antibodies in each serum that reacted with that ligand. Although type 2 specificity may appear to some a less classic concept of specificity than type 1, it is type 2 specificity that one primarily measures in such assays as the Ouchterlony double immunodiffusion test, and it carries equal weight with type 1 specificity in such assays as hemagglutination (discussed below). Type 2 specificity also leads naturally to the concept of multispecificity.

Multispecificity

The theory of multispecificity, introduced and analyzed by Talmadge (78) and Inman (79,80) and discussed on a structural level by Richards et al. (81), suggests a mechanism by which the great diversity and specificity of antisera can be explained without the need for a correspondingly large repertoire of antibody structures (or structural genes). The idea is that each antibody may actually bind, with high affinity, a wide variety of quite diverse antigens. When one immunizes with immunogen A, one selects for many distinct antibodies, which have in common only that they all react with A. In fact, each antibody may react with other compounds, but if fewer than 1% of the antibodies bind B, and fewer than 1% bind C, and so on, then by type 2 specificity, the whole antiserum will appear to be highly specific for A. Note that the subpopulation that binds B may react with an affinity for B as high as or higher than that for A, so that the population would not be type 1–specific for A. This same population would presumably be selected if one immunized with B, as well as with perhaps hundreds of other immunogens with which these antibodies react. The net result

would be that the diversity of highly (type 2) specific antisera an organism could generate would be much greater than the diversity of B-cell clones (or antibody structures) that it would require. However, this concept of multispecificity remains an interesting hypothesis without experimental validation (see ref. 70 and references therein).

OTHER METHODS

We mention only a few of the other methods for measuring antigen–antibody interactions. Other useful techniques include quenching of the tryptophan fluorescence of the antibody by certain antigens on binding (82) (a sensitive method useful for such experiments as fast kinetic studies), antibody-dependent cellular cytotoxicity, immunofluorescence including flow cytometry, immunohistochemistry, and inhibition by antibody of plaque formation by antigen-conjugated bacteriophage (83) (a method as sensitive as RIA, since inhibition of even a few phage virions can be detected).

Quantitative Precipitin

Among the earliest known properties of antibodies were their ability to neutralize pathogenic bacteria and their ability to form precipitates with bacterial culture supernatants. Both activities of the antiserum were highly specific for the bacterial strain against which the antiserum was made. The precipitates contained antibody protein and bacterial products. The supernatants contained decreased amounts of antibody protein and, under the right conditions, had lost the ability to neutralize bacteria. However, quantitation of the antibody precipitated was difficult, since the precipitate contained antigen protein as well as antibody protein. Heidelberger and Kendall (84,85) solved this problem when they found that purified pneumococcal cell-wall polysaccharide could precipitate with antipneumococcal antibodies. In this case, the amount of protein nitrogen measured in the precipitate was entirely due to antibody nitrogen. Plotting the amount of antibody protein precipitated from a constant volume of antiserum by increasing amounts of carbohydrate antigen gives the curve shown in Fig. 14.

As shown in Fig. 14A, the amount of antibody precipitated rises initially, reaches a plateau, and then falls off. The point of maximum precipitation was found to coincide with the point of complete depletion of neutralizing antibodies and is called the *equivalence point.* The amount of antibody protein in the precipitate at equivalence is considered to equal the total amount of specific antibody in that volume of antiserum. The rising part of the curve is called the *antibody excess zone* (antigen limiting), and the part of the curve beyond the equivalence point is called the *antigen excess zone.*

Careful analysis of supernatants and precipitates was carried out for each zone of antibody or antigen excess, as shown in Fig. 14B. When antigen was limiting, the precipitate contained high ratios of antibody to antigen. The supernatant in this zone contained free antibody with no detectable antigen. As more antigen was added, the amount of antibody in the precipitate rose, but the ratio of antibody to antigen fell. At equivalence, no free antibody or antigen could be detected in the supernatant. As more antigen was added, the precipitate contained less antibody, but the ratio of antibody to antigen remained constant. The supernatant now contained antigen–antibody complexes, since the complexes at antigen excess were small enough to be soluble. No unreacted antibody was detected.

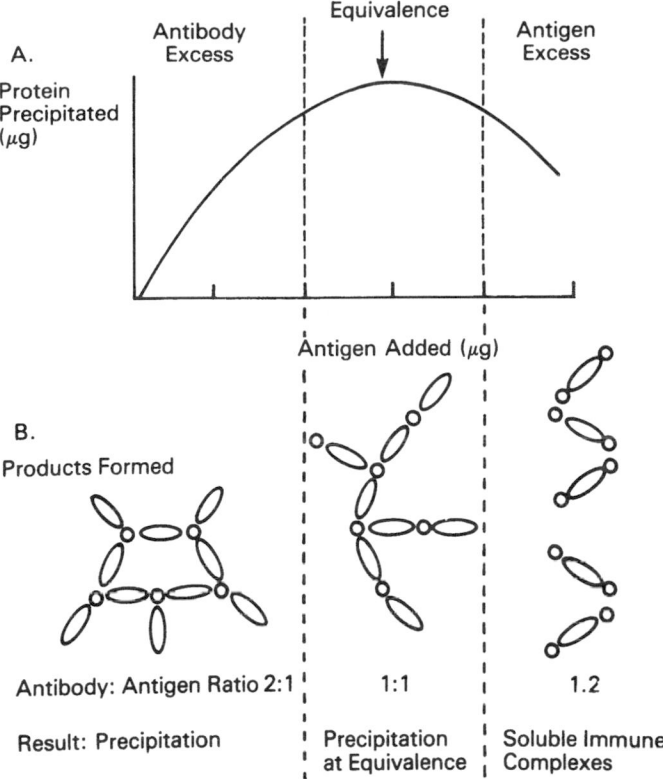

A.

Protein
Precipitated
(μg)

Antibody Excess   Equivalence   Antigen Excess

Antigen Added (μg)

B.

Products Formed

Antibody: Antigen Ratio 2:1   1:1   1.2

Result: Precipitation | Precipitation at Equivalence | Soluble Immune Complexes

FIG. 14. Quantitative immunoprecipitation. To a fixed amount of specific antibody are added increasing amounts of nonprotein antigen. The figure shows the amount of antibody protein (**A**) and the ratio of antibody to antigen (**B**) found in the precipitate. At antigen excess, soluble immune complexes are found in the supernatant, and the precipitate is decreased.

The lattice theory (84,85) is a model of the precipitation reaction that explains these observations. It assumes that antibodies are multivalent and antigens are bi- or polyvalent. Thus, long chains can form, consisting of antibody linked to antigen linked to antibody, and so on. The larger the size of the aggregate, the less soluble the product, until a precipitate is formed. In the antibody excess zone, branch points can form wherever three antibodies bind to a single antigen, giving a large and insoluble product. For example, at the antibody to antigen ratio 3:1, every antigen molecule can bind three antibody molecules in a three-dimensional lattice structure. However, when equimolar amounts of antibody and antigen are mixed (the equivalence zone), the likelihood of more than two antibodies binding each antigen molecule decreases. Thus, the number of branch points decreases, and the product consists of longer chains of alternating antibody and antigen molecules with fewer branches. As the antigen concentration reaches excess, the precipitate approaches linear chains with molar ratio 1:1. Also, at even higher antigen ratios, more antigen molecules will have zero or one antibody bound. One antibody bound is equivalent to a chain termination, so shorter chain lengths are found, until the product is small enough to remain soluble. Such soluble antigen–antibody "immune complexes" are detectable in the antigen excess zone, where no free antibody is found.

In addition to explaining the observed precipitation phenomena on a statistical basis, the lattice theory made the important predic-

tion that antibodies are bivalent or multivalent. The subsequent structural characterization of antibodies (see Chapter 3) revealed their molecular weight and valency. Antibodies are indeed bivalent, except for IgM, which is functionally pentavalent and forms precipitates even more efficiently.

Antigens can be polyvalent either by having multiple copies of the same determinant or by having many different determinants, each of which reacts with a different antibody subpopulation in a heterogeneous antiserum. A good example of the former case, which illustrates the use of precipitation, or lack thereof, to define antigenic determinants, is described in Chapter 19. The predominant antigenic determinants of polysaccharides are often the nonreducing end of the chain. Branched-chain polysaccharides have more than one end and are polyvalent. Nonbranched chains such as dextran (polymer of glucose) are monovalent for end-specific antidextran antibodies and do not precipitate them (86). However, a second group of antidextran antibodies is specific for internal glucose moieties. Since each dextran polymer consists of many of these internal units, it is polyvalent for internal $\alpha(1 \rightarrow 6)$-linked glucose-specific antibodies. Thus unbranched dextran polymer can be used to distinguish between end-specific and internal-specific antibodies, as it will precipitate with the latter antibodies but not the former (86,87). Monomeric protein antigens, such as myoglobin (see Chapter 19) or lysozyme, are examples of the second case since they behave as if they were polyvalent for heterogeneous antisera but monovalent for monoclonal antibodies. This results from the fact that each antigen molecule has multiple antigenic determinants but only one copy of each determinant. Thus, using a polyspecific antiserum with antibodies directed against each of several determinants, the antigen can bind more than one antibody and form a lattice. However, when using antibodies directed against a single determinant (such as a monoclonal antibody), no precipitate will form. In this case, antigen–antibody reactions must then be measured by some other form of binding assay, such as the RIA and ELISA methods described previously.

Immunodiffusion

One of the most useful applications of immunoprecipitation is in combination with a diffusion system (88). Diffusion could be observed by gently adding a drop of protein solution to a dish of water, without disturbing the liquid. The rate of migration of protein into the liquid is proportional to the concentration gradient times the diffusion coefficient of the protein according to Fick's law,

$$\frac{dQ}{dt} = -DA \frac{dc}{dx} \qquad [43]$$

where Q is the amount of substance that diffuses across an area A per unit time t, D is the diffusion coefficient, which depends on the size of the molecule, and dc/dx is the concentration gradient. Since antibody molecules are so large, their diffusion coefficients are quite low, and diffusion often takes 1 day or more to cover the 5 to 20 mm required in most systems. In order to stabilize the liquid phase for such long periods, a gel matrix is added to provide support without hindering protein migration. In practice, 0.3% to 1.5% agar or agarose is found to permit migration of proteins up to the size of antibodies while preventing mechanical and thermal currents. By carefully adjusting the concentration of antibody and antigen, these systems can provide a simple analysis of the number of antigenic components and the concentration of a given component. By adjusting the geometry of the reactants entering the gel, immunodiffusion can provide useful information concerning antigenic identity or difference, or partial cross-reaction, as well as the purity of antigens and the specificity of antibodies. Four commonly used arrangements of antigen and antibody are discussed next.

Single Diffusion in One Dimension

In this method, antibody is incorporated into the gel, which is formed in the lumen of a glass tube. A solution containing antigen a is layered onto the gel, and the antigen begins to diffuse into the gel matrix (Fig. 15A). Over time, the antigen a concentration reaches equivalence with the anti-a antibody in the gel, and a precipitin band forms at t_1. As more antigen diffuses, antigen excess is achieved at this position, so the precipitate at t_1 dissolves and the boundary of

equivalence moves to t_2. By integrating Fick's law, we find that the distance moved is proportional to the square root of time. If two species of antigen a and b are diffusing, and the antiserum contains antibodies to both, two independent bands will form. These will move at independent rates, depending on antigen concentration in the sample, diffusion coefficient (size), and antibody concentration in the agar. However, since the bands move with time, it becomes difficult to use this method for quantitative measurements.

Single Diffusion in Two Dimensions

In this method (89–92), antibody is incorporated in the gel as before, but the geometry of diffusion is now two dimensional (see Fig. 15B). A solution containing antigen a is placed into a small

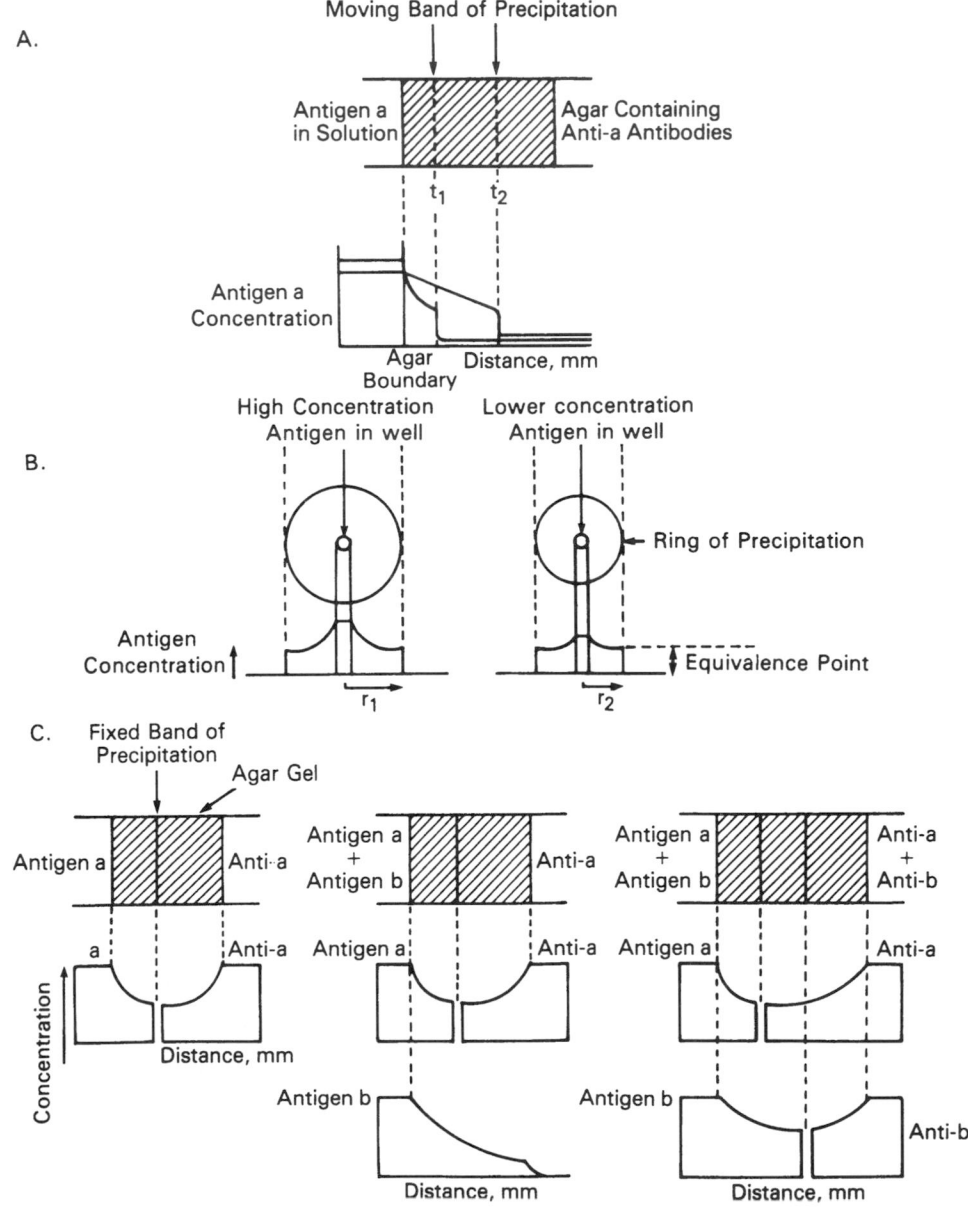

FIG. 15. Immunodiffusion. **A:** One component in one dimension. **B:** One component in two dimensions. **C:** Two components in one dimension. The vertical dimension in the lower part of each section is concentration of the diffusing component.

hole cut into a gel formed in a petri dish. Several dilutions of antigen are placed in successive wells. Over time, antigen diffuses out of each well, and a gradient forms. At a given radius of diffusion, antigen concentration will be equivalent to the antibody in the gel, and a precipitin ring will form. The higher the initial antigen concentration, the farther the antigen will diffuse before precipitating and the wider the area of the ring will be. The area of the ring is directly proportional to the initial antigen concentration. This method provides a convenient quantitative assay that is widely used to measure immunoglobulin classes, by placing test serum in the well and antiserum to each class of human immunoglobulin in the agar. Sensitivity can be increased by lowering the concentration of antiserum in the gel, giving wider rings, since the antigen must reach a lower concentration to be at equivalence. However, the antiserum cannot be diluted too far, or no precipitate will form.

Double Diffusion in One Dimension

Pure agarose is allowed to gel in the lumen of a glass tube. At one end is applied a solution containing antigen a, whereas anti-a antibody is applied to the opposite end of the gel. For the first several hours, both reactants diffuse toward each other through the gel (see Fig. 15C). Eventually, antigen molecules encounter antibody molecules; at some point in the gel, antigen diffusion and antibody diffusion will provide sufficient concentrations of both reactants for immunoprecipitation to occur. This is shown in the left panel as

a single precipitin band. Its location is the result of several factors, including the concentration of antigen and antibody, as well as the diffusion coefficient of each. The line of precipitation becomes a barrier for the further diffusion of the reactants, so the precipitin band is stable. As shown in the middle panel, the diffusion of an immunologically unrelated antigen b is unaffected by the precipitation of a-anti-a. As shown in the right panel, antigen b will form an independent precipitin line if anti-b antibody is present in the antiserum. Thus, the presence or absence of an antigenic species or its antibody is reflected in the presence or absence of a line of precipitation. The number of lines indicates the number of antigen–antibody systems reacting in the gel. The ability of immunodiffusion to separate different antigen–antibody systems gives a convenient estimate of antigen purity or antibody specificity.

Double Diffusion in Two Dimensions (Ouchterlony Method)

In this method (88), pure agarose is gelled in a glass petri dish, and three or more wells are cut in the pattern shown in Fig. 16. Antigen a or b is placed in the upper wells, whereas antiserum containing anti-a or anti-b is placed in the lower well. As in the previous system, each antigen–antibody reaction system will form its own precipitin line between the wells. As shown in Fig. 16A, this should extend an equal length on both sides of the wells. When different antigens are present in different wells (see Fig. 16C), the pre-

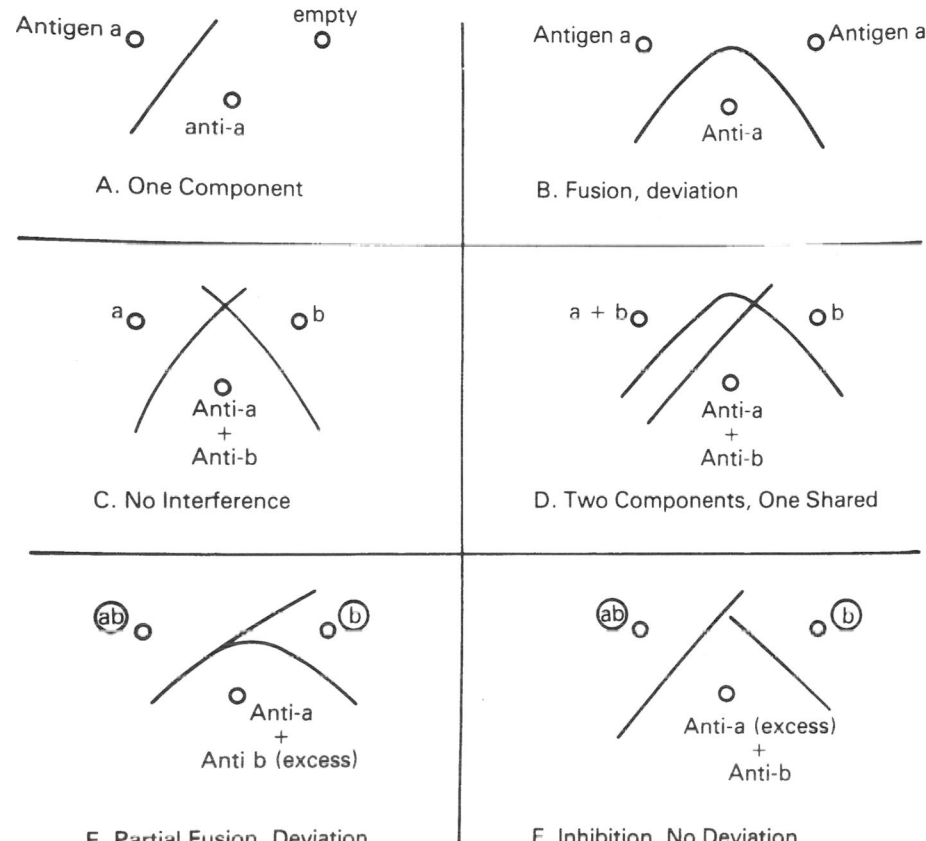

FIG. 16 (A–F). Immunodiffusion of two components in two dimensions. Cross-reactions produce inhibition (*shortened bands*) or deviation (*curved bands*). Lines of identity are shown in (**B**) and (**D**), and partial identity in (**E**) (88).

cipitating systems do not interact immunochemically, so the precipitin lines cross. However, when the same antigen is present in both wells (see Fig. 16B), each line of precipitation becomes a barrier for the antigen and antibody involved, preventing them from diffusing past the precipitin line. This shortens the precipitin line on that side of the well. In addition, antigen diffusion from the neighboring wells shifts the zone of antigen excess, causing the equivalence line to deviate downward and meet between the two wells. Complete fusion of precipitin lines with no spurs (contrast Figs. 16B and 16E) is called a *line of identity*, indicating that the antigen in each well reacts with all the antibody capable of reacting with antigen in the other well.

The great analytical power of this method is shown in Fig. 16D. When a mixed antigen sample is placed in one well, and pure antigen *b* is placed in the other well, antiserum to *a* plus *b* gives the pattern shown. Two precipitin lines form with the left well and one precipitin line with the right well. The line of complete fusion allows us to identify the second band as antigen *b;* the first band is antigen *a*. From their relative distance of migration, we can conclude that antigen *a* is in excess over antigen *b*, assuming their diffusion coefficients are comparable and both antibodies are present in equal amounts. Finally, since the precipitin line of antigen *a*-anti-*a* is not shortened at all, there is no contamination of the right sample with antigen *a*, and the two antigens do not cross-react.

Subtle interpretation of these gels may reveal additional details about partial cross-reactivity of antigens or antibodies, as shown in Figs. 16E and 16F. One antigen with two determinants *a* and *b* is placed in the left well, and antigen *b* is in the right well. Antibodies to both antigens are in the lower well. If anti-*a* antibody is in excess, the pattern in Fig. 16F is obtained. The reaction of anti-*a* with (*ab*) particles causes the precipitin line on the left. But this line also becomes a barrier to diffusion of anti-*b* antibodies, thereby shortening the precipitin line formed with the right well. But the precipitin line with *b*-anti-*b* on the right does not inhibit the migration of anti-*a* antibodies, so there is no shortening of the line to the left. Thus, a spur is formed. If anti-*b* antibody is in excess, the pattern in Fig. 16E is obtained. Both (*ab*) and *b* antigens are precipitated by the same antibody, so partial fusion and deviation occur. But a spur of anti-*a* reacting with (*ab*) is also observed. When mixed antibodies are used with partially cross-reacting antigens, the antibody component forming the leading edge of precipitation determines which pattern will occur.

It is worth reemphasizing at this point that the type of cross-reactivity detected by this Ouchterlony double immunodiffusion in agar is what we have defined previously as type 2 cross-reactivity. The method is not really suitable for measuring affinity differences required for quantitating type 1 cross-reactivity. Also, note that sensitivity can be increased by use of radioactive antigen and detection of the precipitate by autoradiography.

Immunoelectrophoresis

Some antigen–antibody systems are too complex for double immunodiffusion analysis, either because there are too many bands or because the bands are too close together. Immunoelectrophoresis combines electrophoresis in one direction (Fig. 17) with immunodiffusion in the perpendicular direction. In the first step, electrophoresis separates the test antigens according to charge, thus separating the origin of diffusion of different antigens. This is equivalent to having each antigen start in a different well, as shown in the right-hand panel. A horizontal trough is then cut into the agar and filled with antiserum to all the components. Immunodiffusion occurs between the separated antigens and the linear source of antibody. The results for a mixture of three antigens approximate those shown for three antigens in separate wells (88). Fusion, deviation, and inhibition between precipitin lines can be analyzed as described above. The resolution of each band is somewhat decreased, due to widening of the origin of diffusion during electrophoresis. However, the immunodiffusion of unseparated human serum proteins, for example, is greatly facilitated by prior electrophoresis. Starting from a single well, only the heavier bands would be visible. However, prior electrophoresis makes it possible for each electrophoretic species to make its own precipitin line. As shown in Fig. 17B, monospecific antiserum can be placed in a parallel horizontal trough, so that each band of precipitation can be identified. Immunoelectrophoresis is commonly used to diagnose myeloma proteins in human serum. The unknown serum is placed in wells and electrophoresed, followed by immunodiffusion against antihuman serum, antihuman κ, or antihuman λ antiserum. A widening in the arc of IgG precipitation with antihuman serum suggests the presence of an abnormal species. At this same electrophoretic mobility, a precipitin line with anti-κ, but not anti-λ reactivity, or vice versa, strongly suggests the diagnosis of myeloma or monoclonal gammopathy, since these proteins are known to arise from a single clone which synthesizes only one or the other light chain. All normal electrophoretic species of human immunoglobulins contain both light-chain isotypes, although κ exceeds λ by the ratio of 2:1. As shown in Fig. 17C (patient), the abnormal arc with γ mobility reacts with anti-IgG and anti-κ but not anti-λ antiserum. Thus, it is identified as an IgG-κ monoclonal protein. If the abnormal serum component of another patient reacted with anti-IgG and anti-λ, but not anti-κ, it would indicate an IgG-λ myeloma protein.

Rocket Electrophoresis

As in the method of immunodiffusion in two dimensions described above, an agarose layer containing specific antibodies is preformed on a glass slide, and antigen is placed into a small well cut in the agarose. An electric field is applied, and the charged antigen migrates into the gel, while antibody molecules, which are near their isoelectric point, remain essentially fixed in the gel. Unlike the diffusion methods described above, the electric field provides the driving force for antigen migration, rather than the gradient of antigen concentration. Since the entire sample moves out of the starting well, lower concentrations of antigen can be used. As the antigen migrates through the gel, it interacts with the local concentration of specific antibody. Initially, the antigen is in great excess, so that soluble immune complexes (Ag$_2$–Ab or Ag–Ab) are formed, and the migration of bound antigen is retarded, while excess free antigen migrates faster. As free antigen enters a zone where antibody is in equivalence, an immunoprecipitate forms. It is an empirically observed fact that the boundary of antigen–antibody precipitation forms a rocket-shaped zone pointing in the direction of the electric field, and the height of the rocket is directly proportional to the initial antigen concentration (93). This occurs because most of the antigen movement is in the direction of the electric field, and diffusion is minimal.

The great advantage of rocket electrophoresis is that it provides quantitative results and is more sensitive than single diffusion in two dimensions. Since rocket height is linearly proportional to anti-

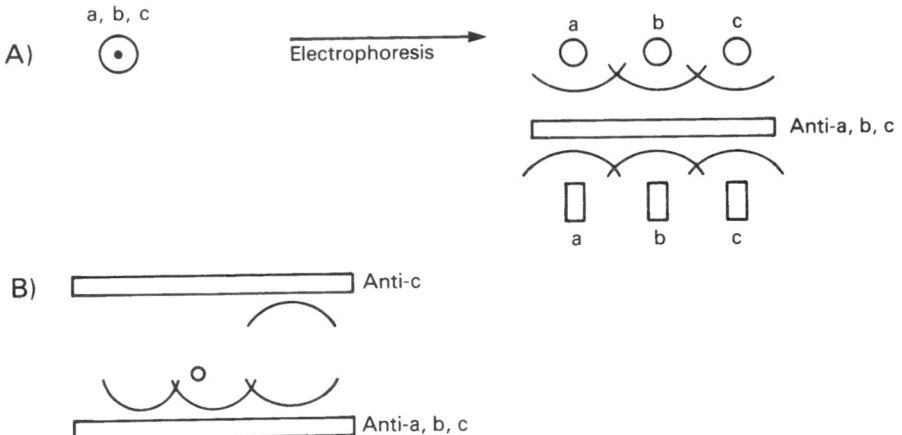

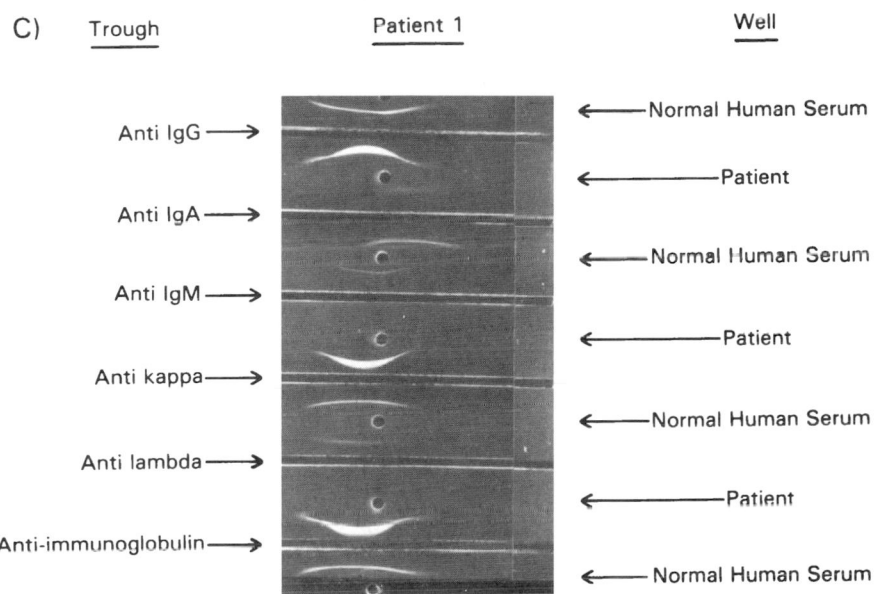

FIG. 17. Immunoelectrophoresis. A sample containing three components, *a, b,* and *c,* is electrophoresed in an agarose gel, separating the antigens in the horizontal dimension. Then a horizontal trough is cut into the gel and antiserum is added. Immunodiffusion between the separated antigens and the trough is equivalent to having three wells, each with a different antigen (**A**) (88). In (**B**), a second trough containing monospecific anti-*c* antibodies is used to identify antigen *c.* In (**C**), this technique is used to identify a myeloma protein in human serum. Sera from the patient or normal individual were placed in the circular wells and electrophoresed. Antisera were then placed in the rectangular troughs and immunodiffusion proceeded perpendicular to the direction of electrophoresis. The abnormally strong reaction with anti-IgG and anti-κ, but no reaction with anti-λ antibodies, indicates a monoclonal protein (IgG,κ), since polyclonal immunoglobulin should react with both anti–light-chain antisera. Failure to form a band with anti-IgM and a reduced band with anti-IgA show typical reduction of normal immunoglobulins in this disease. (Photographs courtesy of Theresa Wilson, NIH Clinical Chemistry Section.)

gen concentration, unknown samples can be assayed for antigen by comparison with a series of known standards over the same concentration range. For any antigen concentration, the actual rocket height, and therefore the sensitivity, can be increased by decreasing the fixed antibody concentration in the gel and thus allowing the antigen to migrate further before reaching the equivalence point. The practical limit for detection of most antigens is 1 to 10 ng.

Hemagglutination and Hemagglutination Inhibition

Hemagglutination

A highly sensitive technique yielding semiquantitative values for the interaction of antibody with antigen involves the agglutination by antibodies of red blood cells coated with the antigen (94). Because the antigen is not endogenous to the red blood cell surface, the reaction is called *passive hemagglutination*. Untreated red

blood cells are negatively charged and electrostatic forces oppose agglutination. Following treatment with tannic acid (0.02 mg/mL for 10 min at 37°C), however, they clump readily.

Untreated red blood cells are easily coated with polysaccharide antigens, which they adsorb readily. After tanning, the uptake of some protein antigens is good, giving a sensitive reagent, whereas for others it tends to be quite variable; this has been the limiting factor in the usefulness of this method for certain antigens. Apparently, slightly aggregated or partially denatured protein antigens are adsorbed preferentially (94). Antigen purity is also very important for the adsorption step, since impurities may compete for protein-binding sites. After tanning and adsorption, the red blood cells are stored in 1% serum solution to prevent spontaneous aggregation. If tanning does not work, chromic chloride treatment facilitates adsorption of some protein antigens, apparently by neutralizing negative charge on the cell surface. Finally, covalent attachment of antigens to the cell surface has been achieved through bivalent cross-linking reagents such as bis diazobenzidine or glutaraldehyde, or through carbodiimide intermediates.

The test for specific antibodies is done by serially diluting the antiserum in the U-shaped wells of a microtiter plate (Fig. 18). To this is added 0.1 mL of 1% solution of antigen-coated red cells. After mixing, the red cells are allowed to settle for 2 hours. In the presence of specific antibodies, agglutinated cells settle into an even carpet covering the round bottom of the well. Unagglutinated red cells slide down the sides and form a button at the very bottom of the well. The titer of a sample is the highest dilution at which definite agglutination occurs. Agglutinated cells form a fragile network that can even be resuspended after settling, and they would give the same endpoint on resettling. With hyperimmune antisera, inhibition of agglutination is observed at high doses of antibody, termed a *prozone effect*. Two interpretations have been given to this prozone. One is that it is similar to the prozone in quantitative precipitin: namely, at large antibody excess, each cell is coated with different antibody molecules, so cross-linking by the same antibody molecule becomes improbable. The second interpretation is the existence of some species of inefficient antibodies that occupy antigen sites without causing aggregation of cells (7). These inefficient or "blocking" antibodies are usually present in low titers, and agglutination occurs at higher dilutions. To assure antigen specificity, the antiserum should be absorbed against uncoated red cells prior to the assay, and an uncoated red cell control should be included with each assay.

The advantage of this test is that it is far more sensitive than immunoprecipitation, since molecular events are transformed into the agglutination of an entire red blood cell. Antigen specificity is the same as for immunoprecipitation. If, for example, nucleated red cells are coated with one antigen and nonnucleated red cells with another, hemagglutination of the mixture with antiserum specific for both antigens results in two types of aggregates, each containing only one type of red blood cell. A problem with the assay is variation in antigen coating, which has marked effects on the sensitivity to agglutination. In addition, IgM is up to 750 times more efficient than IgG at causing agglutination, which may affect interpretation of data based on titration. Lastly, the titer may vary by a factor of 2 simply due to subjective estimates of the endpoint.

Hemagglutination Inhibition

Once the titer of an antiserum is determined, its interaction with antigen-coated red blood cells can be used as a sensitive assay for antigen. To constant amounts of antibody (diluted to a concentration twofold higher than the limiting concentration producing agglutination) are added varying amounts of free antigen. Agglutination will be inhibited when half or more of the antibody sites are occupied by free antigen. In a similar fashion, the agglutination of antigen-coated red cells by antibody can be inhibited by prior incubation of antibody with antiidiotype antiserum. This provides a sensitive assay for the detection and quantitation of antiidiotype antibodies that react with the variable region of antibodies and sterically block antigen binding.

Immunoblot (Western Blot)

A most useful technique in the analysis of proteins is polyacrylamide gel electrophoresis (PAGE), in which charged proteins migrate through a gel in response to an electric field. When ionic detergents such as sodium dodecyl sulfate are used, the distance traveled is inversely proportional to the logarithm of molecular weight. The protein components of complex structures, such as ribosomes or viruses, appear as distinct bands, each at its characteristic molecular weight. These bands could be identified using specific antibodies. However, it is difficult for antibodies to diffuse into most polyacrylamide gels, so it is necessary to transfer the protein bands out of the gel and onto a nitrocellulose membrane support where they are readily accessible to antibodies. The locations of the antigens on the membrane are a faithful reproduction of the locations in the gel, and now it is easy to detect antibody binding to the specific bands that correspond to protein antigens (95).

One particularly important use of the immunoblot is the interaction of viral components with specific antibodies. The viral anti-

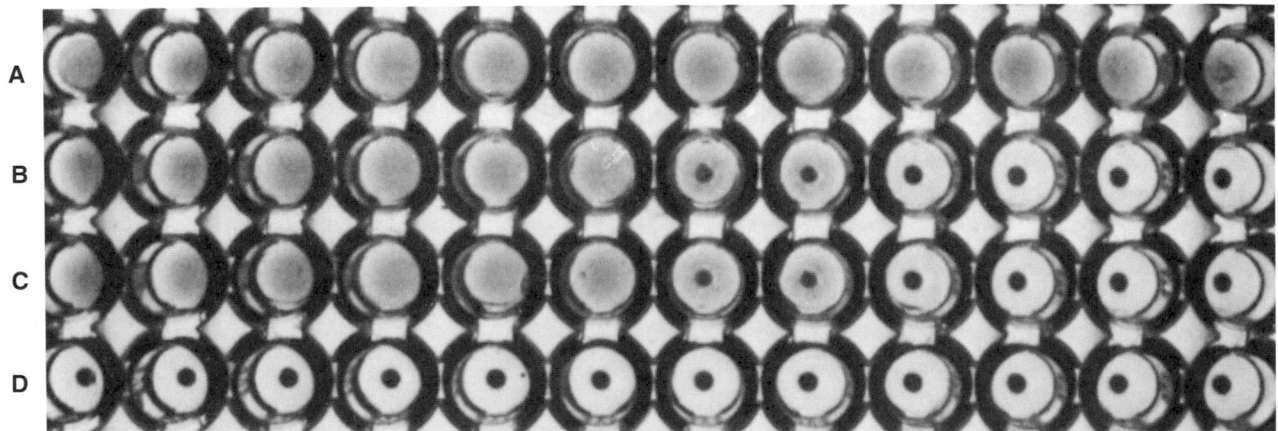

FIG. 18 (A–D). Hemagglutination of antigen-coated red blood cells with specific antibody. Antiserum is added to the wells at the far left of the plate and serially diluted from left to right. Antigen-coated red blood cells are added to each well and allowed to settle. Antibody binding prevents the red cells from settling into a tight pellet. The titer is the highest dilution still giving a carpet of red blood cells and is 212 for row B and 27 for rows C and D. Row E is a preimmune control. Row B shows a slight prozone effect in the first well. (Photograph courtesy of Dr. D. L. Nelson and Dr. R. Yarchoan.)

A

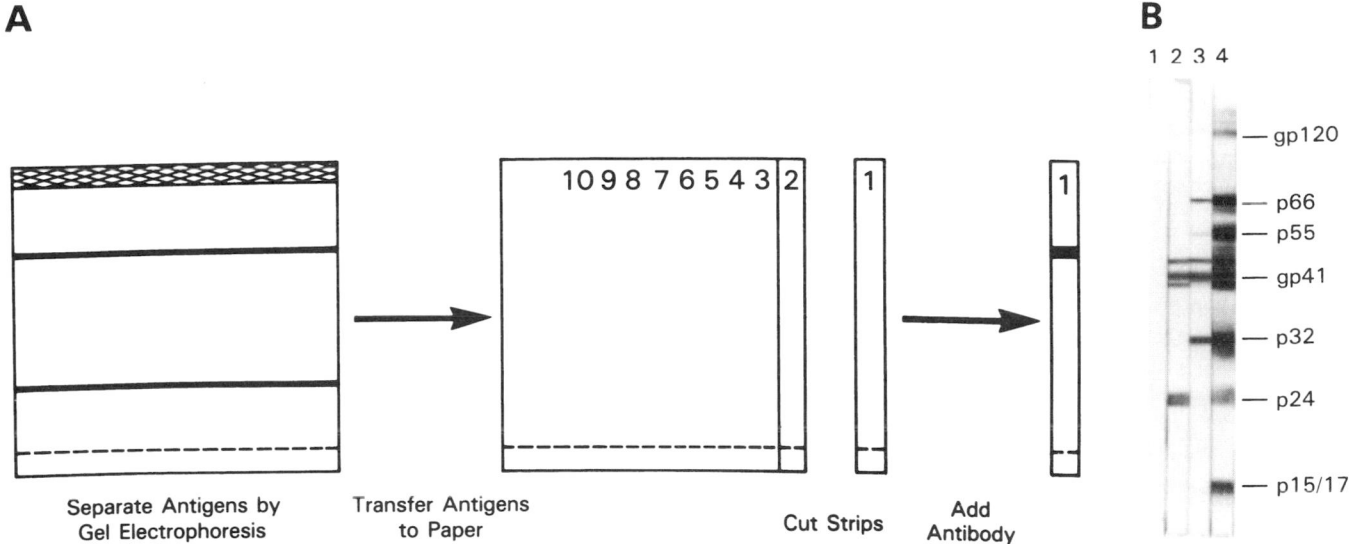

B

1 2 3 4

— gp120
— p66
— p55
— gp41
— p32
— p24
— p15/17

Separate Antigens by
Gel Electrophoresis

Transfer Antigens
to Paper

Cut Strips

Add
Antibody

FIG. 19. A: Western blot technique. The antigen preparation is run through a polyacrylamide gel, which separates its components into different bands. These bands are then transferred to paper by electrophoresis in the horizontal dimension. The paper is cut into strips. Each strip is incubated with test antibodies, followed by further incubation with enzyme-labeled second antibodies. If the test antibodies bind to the component antigens, they will produce discrete dark bands at the corresponding positions on the strip. **B:** Clinical specimens from AIDS patients tested on strips bearing HIV-1 viral antigens, showing antibodies to viral gag (p15/17, p24, and p55 precursor), pol (p66 and possibly p32), and env (gp41 and gp120) proteins. Lane 1 is the negative control, and lanes 2 to 4 are sera from three different patients.

gens are separated by PAGE, followed by lateral transfer of all bands to a nitrocellulose membrane by electrophoresis. The membrane-bound antigens are then exposed to the antibodies, which bind to the bands corresponding to each antigen. Then a second antibody, which is either enzyme conjugated or radiolabeled, is used to detect the antigen–antibody band. The enzyme causes a localized color reaction that reveals the location of the antigen band, or the radiolabel is detected by exposing the nitrocellulose to photographic film. Crude viral antigen preparations can be used, since only those bands that correspond to viral antigens to which antibodies are present will show up, and this accounts for the specificity of the assay.

Typical results are shown in Fig. 19. Human immunodeficiency virus type 1 (HIV-1) was cultured in susceptible H9 cells, and the virus concentrated from the cell supernatant by sedimentation. The viral proteins were separated by PAGE and detected by immunoblot, using the serum of infected patients. Each antigen band recognized by the antiserum has been identified as a viral component or precursor protein. Using monospecific antisera, it can be shown that the gp160 precursor is processed to the gp120 and gp41 envelope proteins, while a p66 precursor is processed to the p51 mature form of reverse transcriptase. p24 and p17 are the core antigens of the virus (96). The practical uses of such a test include diagnosing infection, screening blood units to reduce the risk of HIV transmission, and testing the immunogenicity and protective efficacy of a new vaccine.

MONOCLONAL ANTIBODIES

Homogeneous immunoglobulins have long played important roles in immunologic research. Starting in the 1960s, human and animal myeloma proteins were studied as representative immunoglobulins and recognized for the advantages they had in studies of proteins as diverse as antibodies. Potter and colleagues characterized numerous mouse myeloma tumors and identified the antigenic specificities of some of them (97). These could then be used for studies of immunoglobulin structure, function, and genetics. It was not yet possible, however, to induce monoclonal immunoglobulins of desired specificity.

This goal was achieved by the introduction of hybridoma technology by Köhler and Milstein (1,98) and by Margulies and colleagues (99) in the 1970s. Since that time, monoclonal antibodies have come to play an enormous role in biologic research and applications. They offer as advantages the relative ease of the production and purification of large quantities of antibody, the uniformity of antibody batches, and the ready availability of immunoglobulin messenger RNA (mRNA) and DNA from the hybrid cell lines.

Derivation of Hybridomas

This section presents an overview of the techniques of hybridoma derivation and a discussion of some of the issues involved. It will not attempt to provide a detailed, step-by-step protocol for laboratory use. For that purpose, the reader is referred to monographs and reviews on the subject (3,100–103), including a detailed laboratory protocol with many hints and mention of problems to avoid (104).

Hybridomas producing monoclonal antibodies are generated by the somatic cell fusion of two cell types: antibody-producing cells from an immunized animal, which by themselves die in tissue culture in a relatively short time, and myeloma cells, which contribute their immortality in tissue culture to the hybrid cell. The myeloma cells are variants carrying drug selection markers, so that only those myeloma cells that have fused with spleen cells providing the missing enzyme will survive under selective conditions. Successful hybridoma production is influenced by the characteristics of each of the cell populations, the fusion conditions, and the subsequent selection and screening of the hybrids. A diagrammatic version of the overall process of hybridoma derivation is presented in Fig. 20.

Immunization of Donor Animals

Immunization protocols for fusion purposes have been developed empirically. A wide variety of standard routes and schedules of immunization can be used, the main distinguishing feature being the use of a final intravenous boost with antigen 2 to 4 days before fusion. The importance and required timing of the intravenous boost are thought to be related to the type of cell that preferentially fuses: Peak hybridoma production was found to precede the peak plaque-forming cell and the peak of serum antibody but corresponded to the peak of proliferation (105). Some investigators feel that animals should not be given the final boost and fused when they are at peak antibody titers, but rather should be rested until antibody levels decline, and then boosted for fusion (101).

Myeloma Cell Lines Used as Fusion Partners

One technical advance necessary for successful production of hybridomas was the development of drug-sensitive variants of

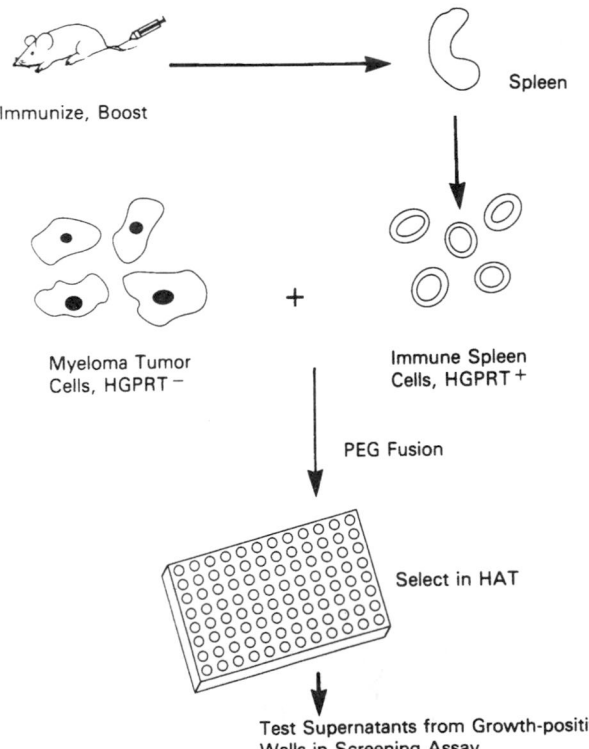

FIG. 20. Production of hybridomas. Steps in the derivation of hybridomas can be outlined as shown. Spleen cells from immunized donors are fused with myeloma cells bearing a selection marker (see Fig. 21). The fused cells are then cultured in selective medium until visible colonies grow, and their supernatants are then screened for antibody production.

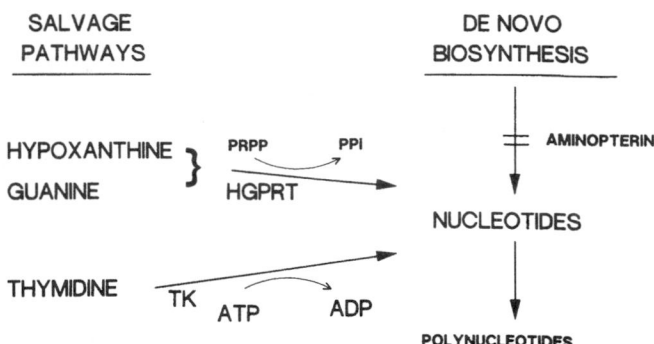

FIG. 21. Pathways of nucleotide biosynthesis showing enzymatic steps that are altered in mutant cells used as fusion partners. Mutant cells lacking HGPRT or TK cannot use the corresponding salvage pathway for nucleotide biosynthesis. Such mutants cannot survive in medium containing aminopterin to poison the de novo synthesis pathway. However, individual mutant cells that have fused with spleen cells and thus do contain the HGPRT or TK enzyme can survive in appropriate selective medium by using the salvage pathway. HGPRT, hypoxanthine guanine phosphoribosyl transferase; TK, thymidine kinase.

myeloma cell lines. A commonly used selective marker is sensitivity to medium containing hypoxanthine, aminopterin, and thymidine (HAT). The biochemical pathways involved are shown schematically in Fig. 21. Aminopterin poisons the de novo synthesis of purines. Spleen cells expressing the enzyme HGPRT necessary for the salvage pathway to recycle purines are able to survive in HAT medium, but die after a short time unless immortalized by fusion with the myeloma cell. The myeloma cells, mutagenized and selected to be HGPRT-negative, are killed by the HAT-containing medium unless they have fused and therefore contain the enzymes of the spleen cell. Thus, for several days after a fusion, there is extensive cell death; subsequently, the culture should contain only cells resulting from spleen–myeloma fusion. Other drug markers are occasionally used, for example, ouabain resistance.

Initial work used myeloma cells, which retained the capacity to secrete their own immunoglobulin products (1). Later, such fusion partners were replaced by myeloma variants that express only one endogenous chain (98) or that fail to express immunoglobulin (106,107), so that the fused cell secretes primarily or exclusively antibody of the desired specificity. This confers a large advantage since, assuming random association, a cell making two heavy chains and two light chains would make immunoglobulin of which only one-sixteenth was of the desired type.

Periodically, the myeloma cells should be cycled through selective medium such as 8-azaguanine, to assure that they have not reverted to a drug-resistant phenotype, although this would be unnecessary for cell lines in which the mutation responsible for drug sensitivity is a deletion. Incorporation of 8-azaguanine into DNA is dependent on the salvage pathway, so it selectively kills HGPRT-positive cells.

Fusion Methods

Several different agents have been used to cause cell–cell fusion. Early somatic cell fusion work used Sendai virus (1). That approach has been replaced for routine fusions by use of polyethylene glycol (PEG). Both of these methods cause random fusions; many of the donor cells fusing will not be B cells in the right state to allow antibody production by the hybrid cell, and of those producing antibody, many will not make antibody of the desired specificity.

Fusion efficiency is influenced by reagents in poorly understood ways. PEG or fetal bovine serum or other sera used in the medium must be tested in actual fusions and batches screened to select those able to support the fusion step. Ability of reagents to support cell growth is not an adequate test. Mycoplasma contamination of cell lines can also interfere, and monitoring for mycoplasma should be carried out.

Of growth-positive wells, the proportion secreting antibody of the desired specificity is quite variable. The original descriptions of fusions producing anti-SRBC antibodies reported 10% specific antibody among viable hybrids (1), but many antigens give far lower yields than that. The poor yield of desired hybridomas from random fusion methods led some investigators to attempt selective fusion of those cells expressing receptors specific for a particular antigen. Selective fusion methods involve attaching antigen to the myeloma cell, directly or indirectly, for example via an avidin–biotin bridge. Immune spleen cells are then mixed with the antigen-coated myeloma cells and cell aggregates are allowed to form. The aggregates are fused by addition of PEG (108) or by application of a strong electric field (109).

Screening Methods

Methods for testing supernatants for desired antibodies can include the same range of methods used for studying such antibodies. Fusions have been successfully screened using RIA, ELISA, or other binding assays; visual immunofluorescence or flow cytometry; cytotoxicity assays; and assays for activation or blocking of biologic effects such as cell-mediated lympholysis (CML), receptor activation, and lymphokine activity. Fusions can also be screened by hybridization to detect mRNA for immunoglobulin of certain types in the cells, rather than antibody in the supernatant (110).

The major issue in choosing a screening assay is that the assay not be subject to fluctuation, which would lead to many false-positive identifications and a large investment of effort in maintaining and cloning hybrid cells of no interest. Thus, clear-cut discrimination between positives and negatives is often more important than exquisite sensitivity. Most supernatants contain at least several milligrams per milliliter of antibody, which is enough to detect by numerous methods.

A good screening assay should be convenient to use with hundreds of samples and should give results quickly, so that cells of greatest interest are still healthy when identified. If a parameter of interest is more difficult or time consuming to measure, it is often practical to use another assay for primary screening and then evaluate likely candidates in the more demanding assay. For example, a simple binding assay can be used for primary screening, and the positives then tested by immune precipitation to determine which bind to a particular component. Multiple-pass screening is useful in many other situations in which two or more antibody characteristics are important in the choice of clones to keep.

A screening assay difficult to perform on very large numbers of samples can also be applied by testing supernatants pooled from groups of hybrids, provided the assay sensitivity would allow detection of one positive supernatant diluted in a pool of negative ones. Components of positive pools are then screened individually.

Postfusion Processing of Hybridomas

After identification of positive cultures, hybridomas must be cloned to assure production of only one antibody, and cells must be frozen for future use. Since a great deal of labor and material are consumed by processing of candidate hybridomas, an efficient strategy must be used.

It is often best to retest all hybrids before cloning any of them. Only those hybrids producing specific antibody again at the second screening are then cloned. Cloning can be performed by limiting dilution or by colony selection from soft agar. In either case, it is best to clone promptly, before possible nonproducing cells in the same well, including variants of the positive cell, can overgrow the antibody producers. Newly derived hybridomas are often unstable in their antibody production, perhaps because somatic cell hybrids are aneuploid and throw off chromosomes. The uncloned lines are maintained until active clones have been well established. Clones producing desired antibody must then be expanded, supernatant collected for antibody preparation, cells frozen, and frozen cells thawed for verification of viability and antibody secretion.

Hybridomas Derived from Species Other than Mice

Laboratory mice are the most common species immunized for hybridoma production, but for a variety of reasons, other animal species often have advantages. If an antigen of interest is nonpolymorphic in the mouse, the mouse component might be immunogenic in other species, while mice would be tolerant to it. In the case of hybridomas for clinical use, mouse antibodies have the drawback of inducing antimouse immunoglobulin immune responses with possible deleterious effects, so derivation of human hybridomas is important.

Several approaches have been taken to the derivation of hybridomas in species other than mouse. First, interspecies hybridization can be performed using mouse myeloma fusion partners. The resulting hybrids are often unstable and throw off chromosomes, but clones can sometimes be selected that produce antibody in a stable fashion. Examples of this would be rat–mouse fusion to produce antibody to the mouse Fc receptor (111), and hamster–mouse fusion to produce antibody to mouse CD3 (112). Rabbit–mouse hybridomas have also been described (113).

A second approach is the use of fusion partner cells from the desired species. Myeloma variants carrying drug selection markers are available in a number of species. A rat myeloma line adapted for this purpose, IR983F, was described by Bazin (114). This approach avoids some of the instability in interspecies hybrids and allows ascites production in homologous hosts.

Production of human hybridomas is of special importance, because their use in therapies would avoid the problem of human immune responses to immunoglobulin derived from other animal species. Due to its clinical importance, this subject will be discussed in detail in the section on applications.

Use of Gene Libraries to Derive Monoclonal Antibodies

Monoclonal antibodies produced by hybridoma technology are derived from B cells of immunized animals. An alternative technology uses gene libraries and expression systems instead. This approach has the advantages of avoiding labor-intensive immunizations of animals and the screening of antibody-containing supernatants. Another advantage of the approach is circumventing tolerance. One can derive mAbs to antigens expressed in the responding animal species, including highly conserved antigens for which there may be no available responder that does not express the antigen.

The first version of such an approach involved preparation of V_H and V_κ libraries and expression of the libraries in bacteria. In some cases, a V_H domain alone binds antigen with reasonable affinity, and so the expressed products of the gene library could be screened directly (115). Further development of the system led to use of V_H and V_L libraries made separately, and then preparation of a combinatorial library by cleaving, mixing, and religating the libraries at a restriction site (116,117). A linker can be used so that V_H and V_L can both be expressed on one covalent polypeptide; the flexibility of the linker allows association of the V_H and V_L in a normal three-dimensional configuration and thus formation of an antigen-binding site (117).

Another technical innovation involves expression of V_H and V_κ genes on the surface of bacteriophage as fusion proteins with a phage protein, to permit rapid screening of large numbers of sequences (117–119). Adsorption of antibody-bearing phage on antigen-coated surfaces allows positive selection of phage containing DNA encoding the desired Fv.

The phage technique has been applied to combinatorial variable-region gene (V-region) libraries (118,119). In one study, rearranged V_H and V_κ genes from immunized mice were used and the resulting V_H–linker–V_κ products were screened for antigen binding. By using either V_H or V_κ genes that gave activity, new sets, termed *hierarchic libraries,* were developed by pairing the known active gene segment with all elements of the library for the other chain from immunized mice. New active combinations were found by this approach (118).

Human antibody gene sequences can be recovered by polymerase chain reaction (PCR) from peripheral blood cells (120), bone marrow (121), or human cells reimmunized in SCID-hu mice (122). The phage display technique can then be used to select antigen-binding clones and derive human reagents of desired specificity, such as antibody to hepatitis surface antigen (120) or HIV envelope (121).

One limitation in the phage library technique initially was low affinity of the mAbs derived. Since they were generated by a random process and not subject to further somatic mutation, they did not achieve the exquisite fit of antibodies produced *in vivo*. Several approaches have now been used to improve affinities. Hypermutation and selection has now been achieved *in vitro* by a strategy using a bacterial mutator strain (123). The mutD5 strain of *E. coli* has an error-prone DNA polymerase III, leading to a high mutation rate, up to 10^5-fold enhanced over wild-type.

If a phage encoding antibody V regions infects such bacteria, the antibody sequence may be mutated. A single bacterium will harbor both wild-type and mutant phage, leading to mixed-sequence protein displayed on each phage. Thus, before stringent selection for high-affinity mutants, the phage must be grown in nonmutator bacteria, so that each bacterium contains only one antibody sequence and antibody expressed on a phage matches its sequence. Multiple rounds of mutation followed by growth in nonmutator bacteria and then selection for high-affinity binding led to an overall 100-fold increase in affinity (123). Improved affinity has also been achieved by use of site-directed mutagene-

sis to alter residues in hypervariable regions affecting dissociation rates (124).

Since arbitrary combinatorial possibilities of V_H and V_L can occur in the various libraries discussed, the antibodies generated do not reflect the combinations actually selected and expressed in immune responses (116). It has been suggested (118) that one could recover a "natural library" by recovering V-region genes from individual cells by PCR. However, recovering genes from a large enough number of representative cells does not seem a reasonable or efficient approach to repertoire studies. Thus, the combinatorial library technology does not replace hybridoma technology for many immunologic studies, including studies of the immune repertoire and patterns of its expression in immune responses. What combinatorial gene libraries do provide is a powerful way to derive antibody reagents of desired specificity, including some that would not occur naturally and so could not be derived by other means.

Applications of Monoclonal Antibodies

Laboratory Uses

Since monoclonal antibodies can be made easily and reproducibly in large quantities, they allow many experiments that were not previously possible or practical. They have the advantages that undesirable cross-reactions can be avoided and that very high titers can be achieved easily. However, it must be kept in mind that even monoclonal antibodies can still display unexpected type 1 cross-reactivity (see the following section on specificity and cross-reactivity). Thus, monoclonal antibodies are used in a wide variety of procedures, not only in immunology, but also in other biologic and physical sciences. This section gives only a sampling of such applications.

Affinity chromatography based on monoclonal antibodies can be used as a step in purification of molecular species that are difficult to purify chemically. Even a one-step purification can achieve enrichment adequate for some purposes. Purification on monoclonal antibody columns has been applied successfully for MHC antigens (125,126).

The approach also has advantages for purification of receptors with ligands in limited supply, making affinity chromatography on ligand impractical. This is the case for some hormones, neurotransmitters, and lymphokines.

Homogeneous antibody can be crystallized and can also be crystallized with antigen to permit the study of the structure of antibody and of antigen–antibody complexes by x-ray diffraction. Myeloma proteins were originally used for such studies, but this limited the range of antigens studied to those for which myelomas had been identified. Hybridoma proteins have permitted the extension of this approach to other antigens of interest, such as proteins like lysozyme (127,128) and influenza neuraminidase (129) (reviewed in ref. 130).

Homogeneous antibodies are very valuable in the study of antibody diversity. The ability to analyze multiple components of an antibody response has added greatly to our understanding of how antibody responses mature. Examples include sequence analysis of variable regions expressed in responses to antigens such as phosphorylcholine (131), arsonate (110,132), influenza hemagglutinin (133), and oxazolone (134). Such analyses have revealed much about the roles of somatic mutation, changes in affinity, and changes in clonal dominance in antibody responses.

Catalytic Antibodies

Another area of interest is the use of antibody molecules to catalyze chemical reactions (135). In this role, antibodies serve as an alternative to enzymes, an alternative that can be customized and manipulated more easily in some cases. Enzymes can be custom designed, too, by site-directed mutagenesis of genes for natural enzymes and selection of ones with altered properties. However, the enormous diversity of the immune repertoire provides a huge pool of possible structures not requiring individual laboratory synthesis.

The concept of antibodies as catalysts had been proposed a long time ago by D. W. Woolley (cited in ref. 135). Attempts had been made to raise antibodies with enzymatic properties. Reduced Schiff's base compounds were used in one study as stable analogues of reaction intermediates, and were used to raise polyclonal antibodies. The antibodies bound appropriate substrates and the chemical reaction could proceed at the binding site, but it was not accelerated relative to the spontaneous rate in solution (136). Use of homogeneous antibodies permitted identification of some with significant catalytic effects; MOPC167 accelerates the hydrolysis of nitrophenyl-phosphorylcholine by 770-fold (137). Polyclonal antibodies have also been reported to possess detectable enzymatic activity; cleavage of DNA by autoimmune sera was found to reside in the purified immunoglobulin fraction, and in fact in $F(ab)_2$ but not Fc (138).

With the advent of hybridoma technology, purposeful selection of antibodies with potent enzymatic function became possible. In the past few years, antibodies have been characterized that catalyze numerous chemical reactions, with rates nearing 10^8-fold above the spontaneous rate (reviewed in ref. 135). One common strategy for elicitation of such antibodies is immunization with transition-state analogues (139), although there are other strategies (140). Antibodies function as catalysts in a stereospecific manner (141), a valuable property.

Why would binding of an antibody to a compound catalyze covalent bond changes? The possibilities are similar to those for enzymes. In order to accelerate a reaction, an antibody has to lower the activation energy barrier to the reaction, which means lowering the energy of the transition state by stabilizing it. This can be achieved because of the contribution of the binding energy to the overall energy of the transition state. For this reason, an antibody that recognizes the transition state is favorable, and immunizations with analogues of the transition state have advantages.

Antibodies can serve as what has been termed an *entropy trap* (135); binding to the antibody "freezes out" the rotational and translational degrees of freedom of the substrate and thus makes a chemical reaction far more favorable energetically. Interactions with chemical groups on the antibody can neutralize charges or bury hydrophobic groups, thereby stabilizing a constrained transition state. Mechanisms of antibody-mediated catalysis vary, as do enzymatic reactions. Interactions between antibody and substrate can be electrostatic (140) or covalent (142). A variety of mechanisms of antibody catalysis have been reported, including β elimination (140) and ping-pong bi-bi (reaction of one substrate with antibody to form an intermediate with release of one reaction product, followed by reaction of a second substrate with the intermediate and release of a second product) (142).

Discovery of such catalytic antibodies opens practical opportunities: Antibodies can be customized for an application by appropriate selection and can be produced relatively cheaply and purified easily. Catalytic antibodies can be developed to perform chemical reactions for which no enzyme is available; for example, antibodies to a conformationally locked cyclohexane ring with an ethano bridge catalyzed a Diels-Alder reaction (143). They can shield intermediates from solvent, for example, allowing reactions that do not occur in aqueous solution (144). They can form peptide bonds (145), suggesting a new approach to polypeptide synthesis. Thus, catalytic antibodies will likely have many practical applications.

Bispecific Antibodies

Antibodies produced naturally by a single B cell have only one binding-site specificity. The availability of monoclonal antibodies made possible the generation in quantity of artificial antibodies as cross-linking reagents, by linking binding sites of two specificities. A variety of techniques have been used to prepare such hybrid or bispecific antibodies, and a variety of sites targeted in functional assays. Cumbersome cross-linking chemistry may also be replaced in the future by genetic engineering (146).

One of the most powerful uses of such hybrid antibodies is in redirecting cytolytic cells to targets of a defined specificity. In one early demonstration of this use (147), a monoclonal antibody specific for the Fcγ receptor and one specific for the hapten DNP were chemical cross-linked. In the presence of this hybrid antibody, FcγR-bearing cells were able to lyse haptenated target cells specifically. The FcγR played a critical role; antibody to MHC class I antigens on the cell could not be substituted.

Antibody to the T-cell receptor complex has been used extensively to redirect T-cell lysis to desired targets. For example, anti-CD3 was cross-linked to antitumor antibodies and mixed with effector cells. These "targeted T cells" were able to inhibit the growth of human tumor cells *in vivo* in nude mice (148).

Bispecific antibodies have also been used in a clever way to alter the tropism of a viral gene therapy vector (149). Interaction of α_v integrins with the viral penton base-coat protein is important for adenovirus entry into cells, but initial attachment is mediated by a different interaction, that of viral fiber-coat protein with an unidentified cellular receptor. An adenovirus vector was engineered to express a marker peptide in its penton base-coat protein. Bispecific antibodies were produced cross-linking one antibody specific for α_v integrins to another antibody to the marker peptide. When targeted by the antibody complex, this adenovirus could now efficiently infect cells that express α_v integrins but lack sufficient fiber receptors. This technique has the potential to target viral vectors to specific tissues or cell types, a potential major improvement in gene therapy.

Clinical Applications

The possible clinical uses of monoclonal antibodies are many. *In vitro*, they are widely used in RIA and ELISA measurements of substances in biologic fluids, from hormones to toxins. They are also extremely valuable in flow cytometric assays of cell populations using antibodies specific for differentiation antigens expressed on cell surfaces. Monoclonal antibodies plus complement or toxin-conjugated monoclonal antibodies have also been used to remove T cells from bone marrow prior to transplantation (150).

In vivo, monoclonal antibodies are already in use or in trials for a variety of purposes (reviewed in refs. 151,152). Monoclonal antibody OKT3 directed to a marker on human T-lymphocytes is used as a treatment for rejection reactions in kidney transplant patients (153). Other monoclonal antibodies, for example ^{111}In-labeled CYT-103, referred to as Oncoscint (154), are used as diagnostic tumor-imaging reagents. Monoclonal antibodies are being tested for a variety of therapeutic uses. Cancer therapies use either unconjugated monoclonal antibody (151,155) or toxin-conjugated (156) or radiolabeled monoclonal antibody (155,157). Other therapies studied include anti-LPS for treatment of sepsis, anti-IL-6 receptor for treatment of multiple myeloma, and anti-IgE for treatment of allergy (surveyed in ref. 152).

In the specialized case of B-cell lymphoma, monoclonal antiidiotypes against the idiotype expressed by the patient's tumor have been tested as a "magic bullet" therapy (158). Active immunization of the patient with idiotype has the advantage that escape mutants (159) are less likely to emerge because multiple idiotopes are recognized. Another approach under study is immunization using not idiotype as protein, but plasmid DNA encoding patient idiotype (160). This approach would have additional advantages, such as ease of preparing customized reagents for each patient.

Production of Human or Humanized Monoclonal Antibodies

Many of the side effects of monoclonal antibodies in clinical use are due to the foreign immunoglobulin constant regions. Recognition of foreign epitopes can lead to sensitization and so preclude subsequent use in the same individual of different monoclonal antibodies. Thus, monoclonal antibodies with some or all structure derived from human immunoglobulins have advantages.

Several approaches have been taken employing fusion of human cells with animal myelomas or with human tumor cells of various kinds (161,162), and use of Epstein-Barr virus to immortalize antibody-producing cells (163). Production of populations of sensitized human cells to be fused presents another special problem, since the donors cannot be immunized at will. In one example, *in vitro* stimulation of lymphocytes with antigen followed by fusion with mouse myeloma cells has been used to generate a series of antibodies to varicella zoster (164).

Another approach to production of monoclonal antibodies with human characteristics involves application of genetic engineering. When mouse monoclonal antibodies are used clinically, many of the complications are due to reactions to mouse immunoglobulin as a foreign protein, and thus there could be an advantage to minimizing the part of the antibody structure recognized as foreign by humans. Human constant regions can be combined with mouse V regions (165,166) or even just mouse hypervariable segments (167) by molecular genetic techniques. Antigen-binding specificity is retained in some cases, and the "humanized" chimeric molecules may have many of the advantages of human hybridomas.

Production of fully human mAbs in transgenic mice has now been achieved by multiple laboratories. The strategy has involved insertion of constructs containing clusters of human immunoglobulin V, D, J, and C genes into the mouse germ line to generate one transgenic line, and targeted disruption of the mouse heavy-chain and κ-chain loci to generate another transgenic line. From these two lines, mice are then bred that express only human antibodies.

To show feasibility of this approach, cosmids carrying parts of the human heavy-chain locus were used to make transgenic mice (168). The mice could rearrange human genes, and extensive junctional diversity was generated, demonstrating that mouse enzymatic machinery could operate on the human loci. Plasmids were used by another group to generate transgenic lines with either heavy- or light-chain human gene clusters in the mouse genome. Again, gene rearrangement and generation of diversity were seen (169), though the observed repertoire was not normal in V-gene usage and N-segment length.

More recently, the next step has been taken to produce mice carrying human genes for both heavy and light chains to generate a functional human repertoire. Several groups using different technologies constructed heavy-chain miniloci containing functional V segments representing several major V-region families, D and J segments, constant and switch regions, and enhancers. The κ-chain constructs contained multiple functional Vκ segments, the J segments, Cκ, and enhancers. One group [Lonberg et al. (170)] assembled the gene segments into plasmids. They inserted μ and γ1 C_H genes, permitting studies of class switching. Another group [Green et al. (171)] used yeast artificial chromosomes (YACs) to bring in human immunoglobulin loci. The heavy-chain locus included μ and δ constant regions.

Mice carrying the human loci but retaining intact mouse immunoglobulin loci expressed human immunoglobulin at low levels. Mice were then bred that were homozygous both for the transgene loci and for disruption of the mouse heavy-chain and κ light-chain loci; note that the mouse λ locus was left intact. They expressed far more human immunoglobulin than did the mice with intact mouse immunoglobulin loci. The human immunoglobulin genes could rearrange in the mouse genome, and expression of human immunoglobulin resulted. If these mice were immunized with a fragment of tetanus toxin, resulting antibodies included some that were fully human (171).

In the Lonberg study (170), serum contained human μ, γ1, and κ as well as mouse λ and γ. Immunization of such mice with with various antigens led to class switching, somatic mutation, and production of human antibodies of affinities of almost 10^8.

Studies in these mice demonstrate cross-species compatibility of the components involved in antibody gene rearrangement and diversification. The mice also provide a responder able to provide fully human antibodies to clinically important antigens, and have the advantage that they are not tolerant to human antigens, such as the human IgE and human CD4 used by Lonberg et al. (170).

Specificity and Cross-reactivity

Specificity of Monoclonal Antibodies

Since all of the molecules in a sample of monoclonal antibody have the same V-region structure, barring variants arising after cloning, they all have the same specificity. This uniformity has the advantage that batches of monoclonal antibody do not vary in specificity as polyclonal sera often do. The most obvious fact about cross-reactions of monoclonal antibodies is that they are characteristic of all molecules and cannot be removed by absorption without removing all activity. An exception would be an apparent cross-reaction due to a subset of denatured antibody molecules, which could be removed on the basis of that binding. The homogeneity of monoclonal antibodies allows refinement of specificity analysis that was not possible with polyclonal sera. A few examples follow.

First, one can use monoclonal antibodies to distinguish closely related ligands in cases where most antibodies in a polyclonal serum would cross-react, and so absorption of a serum would not leave sufficient activity to define additional specificities. This ability is useful in designing clinical assays for related hormones, for example. Such fine discrimination also allows the definition of new specificities on complex antigens. When large numbers of monoclonal antibodies specific for class I and class II MHC antigens were analyzed, some defined specificities that could not be defined with existing polyclonal antisera (172–174).

On the other hand, monoclonal antibodies are also a powerful tool for demonstrating similarities rather than distinctions between two antigens. In some cases, only a minor portion of an antibody response detects a cross-reaction, and so it is not detected by polyclonal reagents. For example, determinants shared by the I-A and I-E class II MHC antigens in the mouse were demonstrated using monoclonal antibodies (174), while they had been suspected but were difficult to demonstrate using polyclonal sera.

Another type of fine specificity analysis possible only with monoclonal antibodies is the discrimination of spatial sites (epitope clusters) by competitive binding. In some cases, such epitope clusters correspond to specificities that are readily distinguished by other means. However, in other cases, the epitope clusters may not be distinguishable by any serologic or genetic means. An example is the splitting of the classical specificity Ia.7 into three epitope clusters by competitive binding with monoclonal antibodies (174). The epitopes cannot be distinguished genetically, since all three are expressed on cells of all Ia.7-positive mouse strains. Thus, polyclonal sera cannot be absorbed to reveal the different specificities. Only with the use of monoclonal antibodies were the epitopes resolved from each other.

The importance of this type of analysis is shown by another example, the definition of epitope clusters on CD4, a surface molecule on a subset of human T cells that also functions as the receptor for HIV. Monoclonal antibodies to CD4 can be divided into several groups based on competitive inhibition (175). The cluster containing the site recognized by OKT4A is closely related to virus infection, since antibodies to this site block syncytium formation. The cluster recognized by OKT4, however, is not related to infection since antibodies to it do not block syncytium formation (175), and cells expressing variant forms of the CD4 molecule lacking the OKT4 epitope can still be infected by HIV (176). This information about the sites on the molecule is important in understanding the molecular interactions of virus with its receptor and may be useful in designing vaccine candidates.

Cross-reactions of Monoclonal Antibodies

Monoclonal antibodies display many type 1 cross-reactions, emphasizing that antibody cross-reactions represent real similarities among the antigens, not just an effect of heterogeneity of serum antibodies. Even antigens that differ for most of their structure can share one determinant, and a monoclonal antibody recognizing this site would then give a 100% cross-reaction. An example is the reactivity of autoantibodies in lupus with both DNA and cardiolipin (177).

It should be emphasized that sharing a "determinant" does not mean that the antigens contain identical chemical structures, but rather that they bear a chemical resemblance that may not be well understood, for example, a distribution of surface charges. Antibodies to the whole range of antigens can react with immunoglobulins in idiotype antiidiotype reactions, showing a cross-reactivity of these antibodies with proteins (the antiidiotypes) and with carbohydrates, nucleic acids, lipids, or haptens.

Polyclonal Versus Monoclonal Antibodies

When monoclonal antibodies first became available, some people expected that they would be exquisitely specific and would be superior to polyclonal sera for essentially all purposes. Further thought about the issues discussed above, however, suggests that this is not always the case and depends on the intended use of the antibodies. Not only do monoclonal antibodies cross-react, but when they do, the cross-reaction is not minor and cannot be removed by absorption. A large panel of monoclonal antibodies may be needed before one is identified with the precise range of reactivity desired for a study.

In polyclonal sera, on the other hand, each different antibody has a distinct range of reactivity, and the only common feature would be detectable reactivity with the antigen used for immunization or testing. Thus the serum as a whole may show only a low-titered cross-reaction with any particular other antigen, and that cross-reaction can be removed by absorption, leaving substantial activity against the immunizing antigen. For the purposes of an experiment, a polyclonal serum may be "more specific" than any one of its clonal parts and may be more useful. This concept is the basis of the theory of "multispecificity" (see above).

Polyclonal sera also have advantages in certain technical situations, such as immunoprecipitation in which multivalency is important. Many antigens are univalent with respect to monoclonal antibody binding but display multiple distinct sites that can be recognized by different components of polyclonal sera. Thus a greater degree of cross-linking can be achieved.

The ultimate serologic reagent in many cases may well be a mixture of monoclonal antibodies that have been chosen according to their cross-reactions. The mixture would be better defined and more reproducible than a polyclonal antiserum and would have the same advantage of overlapping specificities.

CONCLUSION

Antibodies, whether monoclonal or polyclonal, provide a unique type of reagent that can be made with high specificity for almost any desired organic or biochemical structure, often with extremely high affinity. These can be naturally divalent (e.g., in the case of IgG) or multivalent (e.g., in the case of IgM) or can be made as monovalent molecules, such as Fab or recombinant Fv fragments. They serve not only as a major arm of host defense, playing a major role in the protective efficacy of most existing antiviral and all antibacterial vaccines, but also as very versatile tools for research and clinical use. RIAs and ELISA have revolutionized the detection of minute quantities of biologic molecules, such as hormones and cytokines, and thus have become indispensable for clinical diagnosis and monitoring of patients, as well as for basic and applied research. Current solid-phase versions of these take advantage not only of the intrinsic affinity and specificity of the antibodies, but also of the implicit multivalency and local high concentration on a solid surface. Cross-reactivity of antibodies often provides the first clue to relationships between molecules that might not otherwise have been compared. Conversely, methods that use antigens to detect the presence of antibodies in serum have become widespread in testing for exposure to a variety of pathogens, such as HIV. Antibodies also provide specific reagents that are invaluable in the rapid purification of many other molecules by affinity chromatography. They have also become indispensable reagents for other branches of biology, for example, in histocompatibility typing and phenotyping of cells using a myriad of cell-surface markers that were themselves discovered with monoclonal antibodies, and for separating these cells by fluorescence-activated cell sorting, panning, or chromatographic techniques. Thus, antibodies are among the most versatile and widely used types of reagents, and their use is constantly growing. Understanding the fundamental concepts in antigen–antibody interactions has become essential not only to an understanding of immunology, but also to the effective use of these valuable molecules in many other fields.

ACKNOWLEDGMENTS

We thank Drs. Charles DeLisi, Elvin A. Kabat, and Henry Metzger for their detailed critique of the manuscript as well as many helpful discussions, and Dr. Fred Karush for valuable suggestions.

REFERENCES

1. Köhler G, Milstein C. Continuous cultures of fused cells secreting antibody of predefined specificity. *Nature* 1975;256:495–497.
2. Melchers F, Potter M, Warner NC. *Lymphocyte hybridomas.* Berlin: Springer-Verlag, 1978.
3. Kennett RH, McKearn TJ, Bechtol KB. *Monoclonal antibodies. Hybridomas: A new dimension in biological analyses.* New York and London: Plenum Press, 1980.
4. Moore WJ. *Physical chemistry,* 3rd ed. Englewood Cliffs, NJ: Prentice-Hall, 1962.
5. DeLisi C. The biophysics of ligand-receptor interactions. *Q Rev Biophys* 1980;13:201–230.
6. Fersht A. *Enzyme structure and mechanisms.* New York: Freeman, 1977.
7. Eisen HN. *Immunology,* 2nd ed. Baltimore: Harper & Row, 1980.
8. Sachs DH, Schecter AN, Eastlake A, Anfinsen CB. Inactivation of staphylococcal nuclease by the binding of antibodies to a distinct antigenic determinant. *Biochemistry* 1972;11:4268–4273.
9. Hammes GG. Relaxation spectrometry of biological systems. *Adv Protein Chem* 1968;23:1–57.
10. Eisen HN, Karush F. The interaction of purified antibody with homologous hapten. Antibody valence and binding constant. *J Am Chem Soc* 1949;71:363–364.
11. Pinckard RN. Equilibrium dialysis and preparation of hapten conjugates. In: Weir DM, ed. *Handbook of experimental immunology.* Oxford: Blackwells, 1978:17.1–17.23.
12. Scatchard G. The attractions of proteins for small molecules and ions. *Ann NY Acad Sci* 1949;51:660–672.
13. Berzofsky JA, Hicks G, Fedorko J, Minna J. Properties of monoclonal antibodies specific for determinants of a protein antigen, myoglobin. *J Biol Chem* 1980;255:11188–11191.
14. Rodbard D, Munson PJ, Thakur AK. Quantitative characterization of hormone receptors. *Cancer* 1980;46:2907–2918.
15. Thakur AK, Jaffe ML, Rodbard D. Graphical analysis of ligand-binding systems: evaluation by Monte Carlo studies. *Anal Biochem* 1980;107:279–295.
16. Munson PJ, Rodbard D. LIGAND: a versatile computerized approach for characterization of ligand-binding systems. *Anal Biochem* 1980;107:220–239.
17. Bright DS. *On interpreting spectrophotometric measurements of two quinoline-DNA complexes.* Doctoral dissertation, Colorado State University, Fort Collins, CO 1974.
18. Berzofsky JA. The assessment of antibody affinity from radioimmunoassay. *Clin Chem* 1978;24:419–421.
19. Pauling L, Pressman D, Grossberg AL. Serological properties of simple substances. VII. A quantitative theory of the inhibition by haptens of the precipitation of heterogeneous antisera with antigens, and comparison with experimental results for polyhaptenic simple substances and for azoproteins. *J Am Chem Soc* 1944;66:784–792.
20. Karush F. The interaction of purified antibody with optically isomeric haptens. *J Am Chem Soc* 1956;78:5519–5526.
21. Thakur AK, DeLisi C. Theory of ligand binding to heterogeneous receptor populations: characterization of the free-energy distribution function. *Biopolymers* 1978;17:1075–1089.
22. DeLisi C. Characterization of receptor affinity heterogeneity by Scatchard plots. *Biopolymers* 1978;17:1385–1386.
23. Thakur AK, Munson PJ, Hunston DL, Rodbard D. Characterization of ligand-binding systems by continuous affinity distributions of arbitrary shape. *Anal Biochem* 1980;103:240–254.
24. Sips R. On the structure of a catalyst surface. *J Chem Phys* 1948;16:490–495.
25. Nisonoff A, Pressman D. Heterogeneity and average combining site constants of antibodies from individual rabbits. *J Immunol* 1958;80:417–428.
26. Karush F, Karush SS. Equilibrium dialysis. 3. Calculations. In: Williams CA, Chase MW, eds. *Methods in immunology and immunochemistry.* New York: Academic Press, 1971:389–393.
27. Klotz IM. Protein interactions. In: Neurath H, Bailey K, eds. *The proteins.* New York: Academic Press, 1953:727–806.
28. Karush F. The affinity of antibody: range, variability, and the role of multivalence. In: Litman GW, Good RA, eds. *Comprehensive immunology.* New York: Plenum Publishing, 1978:85–116.
29. Crothers DM, Metzger H. The influence of polyvalency on the binding properties of antibodies. *Immunochemistry* 1972;9:341–357.
30. Hornick CL, Karush F. Antibody affinity—III. The role of multivalence. *Immunochemistry* 1972;9:325–340.
31. DeLisi C, Metzger H. Some physical chemical aspects of receptor-ligand interactions. *Immunol Commun* 1976;5:417–436.
32. DeLisi C. The effect of cell size and receptor density on ligand-receptor reaction rate constants. *Mol Immunol* 1981;18:507–511.
33. DeLisi C, Wiegel FW. Effect of nonspecific forces and finite receptor number on rate constants of ligand-cell bound-receptor interactions. *Proc Natl Acad Sci USA* 1981;78:5569–5572.
34. Silhavy TJ, Szmelcman S, Boos W, Schwartz M. On the significance of the retention of ligand by protein. *Proc Natl Acad Sci USA* 1975;72:2120–2124.
35. Yalow RS, Berson SA. Immunoassay of endogenous plasma insulin in man. *J Clin Invest* 1960;39:1157–1175.
36. Chard T. *An introduction to radioimmunoassay and related techniques.* Amsterdam: North-Holland, 1978.
37. Rodbard D. Mathematics and statistics of ligand assays: an illustrated guide. In: Langan J, Clapp JJ, eds. *Ligand assay: analysis of international developments on isotopic and nonisotopic immunoassay.* New York: Masson, 1981:45–101.
38. Yalow R. Radioimmunoassay. *Rev Biophys Bioeng* 1980;9:327–345.
39. Farr RS. A quantitative immunochemical measure of the primary interaction between I*BSA and antibody. *J Infect Dis* 1958;103:239–262.
40. Desbuquois B, Aurbach GD. Use of polyethylene glycol to separate free and antibody-bound peptide hormones in radioimmunoassays. *J Clin Endocrinol Metab* 1971;33:732–738.
41. Zollinger WD, Dalrymple JM, Artenstein MS. Analysis of parameters affecting the solid phase radioimmunoassay quantitation of antibody to meningococcal antigens. *J Immunol* 1976;117:1788–1798.
42. Kessler SW. Rapid isolation of antigens from cells with a staphylococcal protein-A-antibody adsorbent: parameters of the interaction of antibody-antigen complexes with protein A. *J Immunol* 1975;115:1617–1624.
43. Friguet B, Chaffotte AF, Djavadi-Ohaniance L, Goldberg ME. Measurements of the true affinity constant in solution of antigen-antibody complexes by enzyme-linked immunosorbent assay. *J Immunol Methods* 1985;77:305–319.
44. Stevens FJ. Modification of an ELISA-based procedure for affinity determination: correction necessary for use with bivalent antibody. *Mol Immunol* 1987;24:1055–1060.
45. Seligman SJ. Influence of solid-phase antigen in competition enzyme-linked immunosorbent assays (ELISAs) on calculated antigen-antibody dissociation constants. *J Immunol Methods* 1994;168:101–110.
46. Ekins RP. Basic principles and theory. *Br Med Bull* 1974;30:3–11.
47. Berzofsky JA, Curd JG, Schechter AN. Probability analysis of the interaction of antibodies with multideterminant antigens in radioimmunoassay: application to the amino terminus of the beta chain of hemoglobin S. *Biochemistry* 1976;15:2113–2121.
48. von Krogh M. Colloidal chemistry and immunology. *J Infect Dis* 1916;19:452–477.
49. Rodbard D, Lewald JE. Computer analysis of radioligand assay and radioimmunoassay data. *Acta Endocrinol* 1970;64:79–103.
50. Feldman H, Rodbard D. Mathematical theory of radioimmunoassay. In: Odell WD, Daughaday WH, eds. *Principles of competitive protein-binding assays.* Philadelphia: Lippincott, 1971:158–203.
51. Rodbard D, Ruder JH, Vaitukaitis J, Jacobs HS. Mathematical analysis of kinetics of radioligand assays: improved sensitivity obtained by delayed addition of labeled ligand. *J Clin Endocrinol Metab* 1971;33:343–355.
52. Voller A, Bidwell D, Bartlett A. Enzyme-linked immunosorbent assay. In: Rose NR, Friedman H, eds. *Manual of clinical immunology,* 2nd ed. Washington, DC: American Society of Microbiology, 1980:359–371.
53. Kohno Y, Berkower I, Minna J, Berzofsky JA. Idiotypes of anti-myoglobin antibodies: shared idiotypes among monoclonal antibodies to distinct determinants of sperm whale myoglobin. *J Immunol* 1982;128:1742–1748.
54. Yarchoan R, Murphy BR, Strober W, Schneider HS, Nelson DS. Specific anti-influenza virus antibody production in vitro by human peripheral blood mononuclear cells. *J Immunol* 1981;127:2588–2594.
55. Darst SA, Robertson CR, Berzofsky JA. Adsorption of the protein antigen myoglobin affects the binding of conformation-specific monoclonal antibodies. *Biophys J* 1988;53:533–539.
56. Sedgwick JD, and Holt PG. A solid phase immunoenzymatic technique for the enumeration of specific antibody-secreting cells. *J Immunol Methods* 1983;57:301–309.
57. Czerkinsky CC, Nilsson LA. A solid-phase enzyme-linked immunospot

(ELISPOT) assay for enumeration of specific antibody-secreting cells. *J Immunol Methods* 1983;65:109–121.

58. Bocher WO, Herzog-Hauff S. Regulation of the neutralizing anti-hepatitis B surface (HBs) antibody response in vitro in HBs vaccine recipients and patients with acute or chronic hepatitis virus (HBV) infection. *Clin Exp Immunol* 1996;105:52–58.

59. Ronnelid J, Huang YH. Short-term kinetics of the humoral anti-C1q response in SLE using the ELIspot method: fast decline in production in resonse to steroids. *Scand J Immunol* 1994;40:243–250.

60. Czerkinsky C, Moldoveanu Z. A novel two colour ELISPOT assay I. Simultaneous detection of distinct types of antibody-secreting cells. *J Immunol Methods* 1988;115:31–37.

61. Krieg AM, Yi AK. CpG motifs in bacterial DNA trigger direct B cell activation. *Nature* 1995;374:546

62. Ronnelid J, and Klareskog L. A comparison between ELISPOT methods for the detection of cytokine producing cells: greater sensitivity and specificity using ELISA plates as compared to nitrocellulose membranes. *J Immunol Methods* 1997;200:17–26.

63. Mäkelä O, Karjalainen K. Inherited immunoglobulin idiotypes of the mouse. *Immunol Rev* 1977;34:119–138.

64. Jameson BA, McDonnell JM, Marini JC, Korngold R. A rationally designed CD4 analogue inhibits experimental allergic encephalomyelitis. *Nature* 1994; 368:744–746.

65. Brady L, Dodson G. Reflections on a peptide. *Nature* 1994;368:692–693.

66. Guichard G, Benkirane N, Zeder-Lutz G, Van Regenmortel MHV, Briand J-P, Muller S. Antigenic mimicry of natural L-peptides with retro-inverso-peptidomimetics. *Proc Natl Acad Sci USA* 1994;91:9765–9769.

67. Benkirance N, Guichard G, Van Regenmortel MHV, Briand J-P, Muller S. Cross-reactivity of antibodies to retro-inverso peptidomimetics with the parent protein histone H3 and chromatin core particle. *J Biol Chem* 1995;270: 11921–11926.

68. Briand J-P, Guichard G, Dumortier H, Muller S. Retro-inverso peptidomimetics as new immunological probes. *J Biol Chem* 1995;270:20686–20691.

69. Häyry P, Myllärniemi M, Aavik E, et al. Stabile D-peptide analog of insulin-like growth factor-1 inhibits smooth muscle cell proliferation after carotid ballooning injury in the rat. *FASEB J* 1995;9:1336–1344.

70. Berzofsky JA, Schechter AN. The concepts of cross-reactivity and specificity in immunology. *Mol Immunol* 1981;18:751–763.

71. Young NS, Curd JG, Eastlake A, Furie B, Schechter AN. Isolation of antibodies specific to sickle hemoglobin by affinity chromatography using a synthetic peptide. *Proc Natl Acad Sci USA* 1975;72:4759–4763.

72. Young NS, Eastlake A, Schecter AN. The amino terminal region of the sickle hemoglobin beta chain. II. Characterization of monospecific antibodies. *J Biol Chem* 1976;251:6431–6435.

73. Curd JG, Young N, Schecter AN. Antibodies to an amino terminal fragment of beta globin. II. Specificity and isolation of antibodies for the sickle mutation. *J Biol Chem* 1976;251:1290–1295.

74. Dean J, Schecter AN. Sickle-cell anemia: molecular and cellular bases of therapeutic approaches. *N Engl J Med* 1978;299:752–763.

75. Sharon J, Kabat EA, Morrison SL. Immunochemical characterization of binding sites of hybridoma antibodies specific for alpha(1 6) linked dextran. *Mol Immunol* 1982;19:375–388.

76. Cisar J, Kabat EA, Liao J, Potter M. Immunochemical studies on mouse myeloma proteins reactive with dextrans or with fructosans and on human antil-evans. *J Exp Med* 1974;139:159–179.

77. Johnston MFM, Eisen HN. Cross-reactions between 2,4-dinitrophenyl and nemadione (vitamin K3) and the general problem of antibody specificity. *J Immunol* 1976;117;1189–1196.

78. Talmadge D. Immunological specificity. *Science* 1959;129:1643–1648.

79. Inman JK. Multispecificity of the antibody combining region and antibody diversity. In: Sercarz EE, Williamson AR, Fox CF, eds. *The immune system: genes, receptors, signals.* New York: Academic Press, 1974:37–52.

80. Inman JK. The antibody combining region: speculations on the hypothesis of general multispecificity. In: Bell GI, Perelson AS, Pimbley GH Jr, eds. *Theoretical immunology.* New York: Marcel Dekker Inc, 1978:243–278.

81. Richards FF, Konigsberg WH, Rosenstein RW, Varga JM. On the specificity of antibodies. *Science* 1975;187:130–137.

82. Parker CW. Spectrofluorometric methods. In: Weir DM, ed. *Handbook of experimental immunology,* 3rd ed. Oxford: Blackwell, 1978:18.1–18.25.

83. Haimovich J, Hurwitz E, Novik N, Sela M. Preparation of protein-bacteriophage conjugates and their use in detection of antiprotein antibodies. *Biochim Biophys Acta* 1970;207:115–124.

84. Heidelberger M, Kendall FE. The precipitin reaction between type III pneumococcus polysaccharide and homologous antibody. *J Exp Med* 1935;61: 563–591.

85. Heidelberger M, Kendall FE. A quantitative theory of the precipitin reaction. II. A study of an azoprotein-antibody system. *J Exp Med* 1935;62:467–483.

86. Kabat EA. *Structural concepts in immunology and immunochemistry,* 2nd ed. New York: Holt, Rinehart & Winston, 1976.

87. Cisar J, Kabat EA, Dorner MM, Liao J. Binding properties of immunoglobulin containing sites specific for terminal or nonterminal antigenic determinants in dextran. *J Exp Med* 1975;142:435–459.

88. Ouchterlony O, Nilsson LA. Immunodiffusion and immunoelectrophoresis. In:

Weir DM, ed. *Handbook of experimental immunology,* 3rd ed. Oxford: Blackwell, 1978:19.1–19.44.

89. Feinberg JG. Identification, discrimination and quantification in Ouchterlony gel plates. *Int Arch Allergy* 1957;11:;129–152.

90. Tomasi TBJ, Zigelbaum S. The selective occurrence of gamma1A globulins in certain body body fluids. *J Clin Invest* 1963;42:1552–1560.

91. Fahey JL, McKelvey EM. Quantitative determination of serum immunoglobulins in antibody-agar plates. *J Immunol* 1965;94:84–90.

92. Mancini G, Carbonara AO, Heremans JF. Immunochemical quantitation of antigens by single radial immunodiffusion. *Immunochemistry* 1965;2:235–254.

93. Laurell CB, McKay EJ. Electroimmunoassay. *Methods Enzymol* 1981;73:339–369.

94. Herbert WJ. Passive haemagglutination with special reference to the tanned cell technique. In: Weir DM, ed. *Handbook of experimental immunology.* Oxford: Blackwell, 1978:20.1–20.20.

95. Towbin H, Staehelin T, Gordon J. Electrophoretic transfer of proteins from polyacrylamide gels to nitrocellulose sheets: Procedure and some applications. *Proc Natl Acad Sci USA* 1979;76:4350–4354.

96. Schupbach J, Popovic M, Gilden RV, Gonda MA, Sarngadharan MG, Gallo RC. Serological analysis of a subgroup of human T-lymphotropic retroviruses (HTLV-III) associated with AIDS. *Science* 1984;224:503–505.

97. Potter M. Immunoglobulin-producing tumors and myeloma proteins of mice. *Physiol Rev* 1972;52:631–719.

98. Köhler G, Milstein C. Derivation of specific antibody-producing tissue culture and tumor lines by cell fusion. *Eur J Immunol* 1976;6:511–519.

99. Margulies DH, Kuehl WM, Scharff MD. Somatic cell hybridization of mouse myeloma cells. *Cell* 1976;8:405–415.

100. de St.Groth SF, Scheidegger D. Production of monoclonal antibodies: strategy and tactics. *J Immunol Methods* 1980;35:1–21.

101. French D, Fischberg E, Buhl S, Scharff MD. The production of more useful monoclonal antibodies. I. Modifications of the basic technology. *Immunol Today* 1986;7:344–346.

102. Langone JJ, Van Vunakis H. *Methods in enzymology,* vol 121. *Immunochemical techniques. Part I. Hybridoma technology and monoclonal antibodies.* Orlando: Academic Press, 1986.

103. Hämmerling GJ, Hämmerling U, Kearney JF. *Monoclonal antibodies and T-cell hybridomas. Perspectives and technical advances.* Amsterdam: Elsevier/North-Holland Biomedical Press, 1981.

104. Yokoyama WM. Production of monoclonal antibodies. In: Coligan JE, Kruisbeek AM, Margulies DH, Shevach EM, Strober W, eds. *Current protocols in immunology.* New York: John Wiley and Sons, 1995.2.5.1–2.5.17.

105. Paslay J, Roozen K. The effect of B cell stimulation on hybridoma formation. In: Hämmerling GJ, Hämmerling U, Kearney JF, eds. *Monoclonal antibodies and T-cell hybridomas, perspectives and technical advances.* Amsterdam: Elsevier/North-Holland Biomedical Press, 1981:551–559.

106. Shulman M, Wilde CD, Köhler G. A better cell line for making hybridomas secreting specific antibodies. *Nature* 1978;276:269–270.

107. Kearney JF, Radbruch A, Liesegang B, Rajewsky K. A new mouse myeloma cell line that has lost immunoglobulin expression but permits the construction of antibody-secreting hybrid cell lines. *J Immunol* 1979;123:1548–1550.

108. Gefter ML, Margulies DH, Scharff MD. A simple method for polyethylene glycol-promoted hybridization of mouse myeloma cells. *Somatic Cell Genet* 1977; 3:231–236.

109. Lo MMS, Tsong TY, Conrad MK, Strittmatter SM, Hester LD, Snyder SH. Monoclonal antibody production by receptor-mediated electrically induced cell fusion. *Nature* 1984;310:792–794.

110. Manser T, Huang S, Gefter ML. Influence of clonal selection on the expression of immunoglobulin variable region genes. *Science* 1984;226:1283–1288.

111. Unkeless JC. Characterization of monoclonal antibody directed against mouse macrophage and lymphocyte Fc receptors. *J Exp Med* 1979;150:580–596.

112. Leo O, Foo M, Sachs DH, Samelson LE, Bluestone JA. Identification of a monoclonal antibody specific for a murine T3 polypeptide. *Proc Natl Acad Sci USA* 1987;84:1374–1378.

113. Yarmush ML, Gates FT III, Weisfogel DR, Kindt TJ. Identification and characterization of rabbit-mouse hybridomas secreting specific rabbit immunoglobulin chains. *Proc Natl Acad Sci USA* 1980;77:2899–2903.

114. Bazin H. Production of rat monoclonal antibodies with the Lou rat non-secreting IR983F myeloma cell line. *Prot Biol Fluids* 1981;29:615–618.

115. Ward ES, Güssow D, Griffiths AD, Jones PT, Winter G. Binding activities of a repertoire of single immunoglobulin variable domains secreted from *Escherichia coli. Nature* 1989;341:544–546.

116. Huse WD, Sastry L, Iverson SA, et al. Generation of a large combinatorial library of the immunoglobulin repertoire in phage lambda. *Science* 1989;246: 1275–1281.

117. Clackson T, Hoogenboom HR, Griffiths AD, Winter G. Making antibody fragments using phage display libraries. *Nature* 1991;352:624–628.

118. McCafferty J, Griffiths AD, Winter G, Chiswell DJ. Phage antibodies: filamentous phage displaying antibody variable domains. *Nature* 1990;348:552–554.

119. Kang AS, Barbas CF, Janda KD, Benkovic SJ, Lerner RA. Linkage of recognition and replication functions by assembling combinatorial antibody Fab libraries along phage surfaces. *Proc Natl Acad Sci USA* 1991;88:4363–4366.

120. Zebedee SL, Barbas CFI, Hom Y L, et al. Human combinatorial antibody libraries to hepatitis B surface antigen. *Proc Natl Acad Sci USA* 1992;89: 3175–3179.

121. Burton DR, Barbas CFI, Persson MAA, Koenig S, Chanock RM, Lerner RA. A large array of human monoclonal antibodies to type 1 human immunodeficiency virus from combinatorial libraries of asymptomatic seropositive individuals. *Proc Natl Acad Sci USA* 1991;88:10134–10137.

122. Duchosal MA, Eming SA, Fischer P, et al. Immunization of hu-PBL-SCID mice and the rescue of human monoclonal Fab fragments through combinatorial libraries. *Nature* 1992;355:258–262.

123. Low NM, Holliger P, Winter G. Mimicking somatic hypermutation: affinity maturation of antibodies displayed on bacteriophage using a bacterial mutator strain. *J Mol Biol* 1996;260:359–368.

124. Thompson J, Pope T, Tung J-S, et al. Affinity maturation of a high-affinity human monoclonal antibody against the third hypervariable loop of human immunodeficiency virus: use of phage display to improve affinity and broaden strain reactivity. *J Mol Biol* 1996;256:77–88.

125. Mescher MF, Stallcup KC, Sullivan CP, Turkewitz AP, Herrmann SH. Purification of murine MHC antigens by monoclonal antibody affinity chromatography. *Methods Enzymol* 1983;92:86–109.

126. Parham P. Monoclonal antibodies against HLA products and their use in immunoaffinity purification. *Methods Enzymol* 1983;92:110–138.

127. Amit AG, Mariuzza RA, Phillips SEV, Poljak RJ. Three-dimensional structure of an antigen-antibody complex at 2.8 A° resolution. *Science* 1986;233:747–753.

128. Sheriff S, Silverton EW, Padlan EA, et al. Three-dimensional structure of an antigen-antibody complex. *Proc Natl Acad Sci USA* 1987;84:8075–8079.

129. Colman PM, Laver WG, Varghese JN, et al. Three-dimensional structure of a complex of antibody with influenza virus neuraminidase. *Nature* 1987;326:358–363.

130. Davies DR, Padlan EA, Sheriff S. Antigen-antibody complexes. *Annu Rev Biochem* 1990;59:439–473.

131. Gearhart P, Johnson N, Douglas R, Hood L. IgG antibodies to phosphorylcholine exhibit more diversity than their IgM counterparts. *Nature* 1981;291:29–34.

132. Lamoyi E, Estess P, Capra JD, Nisonoff A. Heterogeneity of an intrastrain cross-reactive idiotype associated with anti-p-azophenylarsonate antibodies of A/J mice. *J Immunol* 1980;124:2834–2840.

133. Clarke SH, Huppi K, Ruezinsky D, Staudt L, Gerhard W, Weigert M. Inter- and intraclonal diversity in the antibody response to influenza hemagglutinin. *J Exp Med* 1985;161:687–704.

134. Berek C, Griffiths G, Milstein C. Molecular events during maturation of the immune response to oxazolone. *Nature* 1985;316:412–418.

135. Lerner RA, Benkovic SJ, Schultz PG. At the crossroads of chemistry and immunology: catalytic antibodies. *Science* 1991;252:659–667.

136. Raso V, Stollar BD. The antibody-enzyme analogy. Comparison of enzymes and antibodies specific for phosphopyridoxyltyrosine. *Biochemistry* 1975;14:591–599.

137. Pollack SJ, Jacobs JW, Schultz PG. Selective chemical catalysis by an antibody. *Science* 1986;234:1570–1573.

138. Shuster AM, Gololobov GV, Kvashuk OA, Bogomolova AE, Smirnov IV, Gabibov AG. DNA hydrolyzing autoantibodies. *Science* 1992;256:665–667.

139. Tramontano A, Janda KD, Lerner RA. Catalytic antibodies. *Science* 1986;234:1566–1570.

140. Shokat KM, Leumann CJ, Sugasawara R, Schultz PG. A new strategy for the generation of catalytic antibodies. *Nature* 1989;338:269–271.

141. Pollack SJ, Hsiun P, Schultz PG. Stereospecific hydrolysis of alkyl esters by antibodies. *J Am Chem Soc* 1989;111:5961–5962.

142. Wirsching P, Ashley JA, Benkovic SJ, Janda KD, Lerner RA. An unexpectedly efficient catalytic antibody operating by ping-pong and induced fit mechanisms. *Science* 1991;252:680–685.

143. Braisted A, Schultz PG. An antibody-catalyzed bimolecular Diels-Alder reaction. *J Am Chem Soc* 1990;112:7430–7431.

144. Shabat D, Itzhaky H, Reymond J-L, Keinan E. Antibody catalysis of a reaction otherwise strongly disfavoured in water. *Nature* 1995;374:143–146.

145. Hirschmann R, Smith AB III, Taylor CM, et al. Peptide synthesis catalyzed by an antibody containing a binding site for variable amino acids. *Science* 1994;265:234–237.

146. Holliger P, Winter G. Engineering bispecific antibodies. *Curr Opin Biotechnol* 1993;4:446–449.

147. Karpovsky B, Titus JA, Stephany DA, Segal DM. Production of target-specific effector cells using hetero-cross-linked aggregates containing anti-target cell and anti-Fc γ receptor antibodies. *J Exp Med* 1984;160:1686–1701.

148. Titus JA, Garrido MA, Hecht TT, Winkler DF, Wunderlich JR, Segal DM. Human T cells targeted with anti-T3 cross-linked to antitumor antibody prevent tumor growth in nude mice. *J Immunol* 1987;138:4018–4022.

149. Wickham TJ, Segal DM, Roelvink PW, et al. Targeted adenovirus gene transfer to endothelial and smooth muscle cells by using bispecific antibodies. *J Virol* 1996;70:6831–6838.

150. Vallera DA, Ash RC, Zanjani ED, et al. Anti-T-cell reagents for human bone marrow transplantation: ricin linked to three monoclonal antibodies. *Science* 1983;222:512–515.

151. Waldmann TA. Monoclonal antibodies in diagnosis and therapy. *Science* 1991;252:1657–1662.

152. Berkower I. The promise and pitfalls of monoclonal antibody therapeutics. *Curr Opin Biotechnol* 1996;7:622–628.

153. Ortho Multicenter Transplant Study Group. A randomized clinical trial of OKT3 monoclonal antibody for acute rejection of cadaveric renal transplants. *N Engl J Med* 1988;313:337–342.

154. Collier BD, Abdel-Nabi H, Doerr RJ, et al. Immunoscintigraphy performed with In-111-labeled CYT-103 in the management of colorectal cancer: comparison with CT. *Radiology* 1992;185:179–186.

155. Sears HF, Herlyn D, Steplewski Z, Koprowski H. Effects of monoclonal antibody immunotherapy on patients with gastrointestinal adenocarcinoma. *J Biol Response Mod* 1984;3:138–150.

156. Frankel AE, Houston LL, Issell BF. Prospects for immunotoxin therapy in cancer. *Annu Rev Med* 1986;37:125–142.

157. Carrasquillo JA, Krohn JA, Beaumier P, et al. Diagnosis and therapy for solid tumors with radiolabeled antibodies and immune fragments. *Cancer Treat Rep* 1984;68:317–328.

158. Miller RA, Maloney DG, Warnke R, Levy R. Treatment of B-cell lymphoma with monoclonal anti-idiotype antibody. *N Engl J Med* 1982;306:517–522.

159. Meeker T, Lowder J, Cleary ML, et al. Emergence of idiotype variants during treatment of B-cell lymphoma with anti-idiotype antibodies. *N Engl J Med* 1985;312:1658–1665.

160. Hakim I, Levy S, Levy R. A nine-amino acid peptide from IL-1b augments antitumor immune responses induced by protein and DNA vaccines. *J Immunol* 1996;157:5503–5511.

161. Cole RJ, Morrisey DM, Houghton AN, Beattie Jr, Oettgen HF, Old LJ. Generation of human monoclonal antibodies reactive with cellular antigens. *Proc Natl Acad Sci USA* 1983;80:2026–2030.

162. Olsson L, Kaplan HS. Human-human monoclonal antibody-producing hybridomas: technical aspects. *Methods Enzymol* 1983;92:3–16.

163. Seigneurin JM, Desgranges C, Seigneurin D, et al. Herpes simplex virus glycoprotein D: human monoclonal antibody produced by bone marrow cell line. *Science* 1983;221:173–175.

164. Sugano T, Matsumoto Y, Miyamoto C, Masuho Y. Hybridomas producing human monoclonal antibodies against varicella-zoster virus. *Eur J Immunol* 1987;17:359–364.

165. Morrison SL. Transfectomas provide novel chimeric antibodies. *Science* 1985;229:1202–1207.

166. Morrison SL, Johnson MJ, Herzenberg LA, Oi VT. Chimeric human antibody molecules: mouse antigen-binding domains with human constant region domains. *Proc Natl Acad Sci USA* 1984;81:6851–6855.

167. Jones PT, Dear PH, Foote J, Neuberger MS, Winter G. Replacing the complementarity-determining regions in a human antibody with those from a mouse. *Nature* 1986;321:522–525.

168. Brüggemann M, Spicer C, Buluwela L, et al. Human antibody production in transgenic mice: expression from 100 kb of the human IgH locus. *Eur J Immunol* 1991;21:1323–1326.

169. Taylor LD, Carmack CE, Schramm SR, et al. A transgenic mouse that expresses a diversity of human sequence heavy and light chain immunoglobulins. *Nucleic Acids Res* 1992;20:6287–6295.

170. Lonberg N, Taylor LD, Harding FA, et al. Antigen-specific human antibodies from mice comprising four distinct genetic modifications. *Nature* 1994;368:856–859.

171. Green LL, Hardy MC, Maynard-Currie CE, et al. Antigen-specific human monoclonal antibodies from mice engineered with human Ig heavy and light chain YACs. *Nat Genet* 1994;7:13–21.

172. Klein J, Huang H-JS, Lemke H, Hämmerling GJ, Hämmerling U. Serological analysis of H-2 and Ia molecules with monoclonal antibodies. *Immunogenetics* 1979;8:419–432.

173. Ozato K, Mayer N, Sachs DH. Hybridoma cell lines secreting monoclonal antibodies to mouse H-2 and Ia antigens. *J Immunol* 1980;124:533–540.

174. Pierres M, Devaux C, Dosseto M, Marchetto S. Clonal analysis of B- and T-cell responses to Ia antigens. I. Topology of epitope regions on I-A^k and I-E^k molecules analyzed with 35 monoclonal alloantibodies. *Immunogenetics* 1981;14:481–495.

175. Sattentau QJ, Dalgleish AG, Weiss RA, Beverley PCL. Epitopes of the CD4 antigen and HIV infection. *Science* 1986;234:1120–1123.

176. Hoxie JA, Flaherty LE, Haggarty BS, Rackowski JL. Infection of T4 lymphocytes by HTLV-III does not require expression of the OKT4 epitope. *J Immunol* 1986;136:361–363.

177. Koike T, Tomioka H, Kumagai A. Antibodies cross-reactive with DNA and cardiolipin in patients with systemic lupus erythematosus. *Clin Exp Immunol* 1982;50:298–302.

Fundamental Immunology, Fourth Edition,
edited by William E. Paul
Published by Lippincott–Raven Publishers, Philadelphia 1999.

CHAPTER 5

Immunoglobulins: Molecular Genetics

Edward E. Max

The study of the molecular biology of immunoglobulin (Ig) genes represents one of the first triumphs of recombinant DNA technology. Before the advent of gene cloning, Ig genes could be studied only indirectly by inferences from amino acid sequences. Many perplexing questions were resolved when it became possible to examine directly the genes themselves. Recently the cloned genes have moved beyond the pure research laboratory to be used as tools for various applied engineering projects. This chapter summarizes some of these exciting advances in both the basic and applied arenas.

The unique mystery of antibody genes lies in the diversity of proteins they encode. This diversity exists at several levels.

Most striking is the diversity of antigen-combining sites of these molecules. The classic studies of Landsteiner suggested that the repertoire of binding specificities of antibodies is essentially unlimited. The diversity of binding specificities is explained by the diversity of amino acid sequences found in the N-terminal domain of both light (L) and heavy (H) chains—the variable (V) region—each containing three regions of especially high variability (hypervariable regions) which correspond to the loops of the protein that contact antigen, or complementarity determining regions (CDRs), as discussed in Chapter 3. Yet on the C-terminal end, the single domain of the L chain and the three (or four depending on isotype) domains

of H chains were found to be invariant within each class of L or H chains; these segments are designated constant (C) regions. Many models were proposed to explain the unprecedented diversity found in Ig V regions. One extreme model suggested that the immense diversity of V regions was directly encoded in the germline genome, presumably a result of gene duplication and mutation acting over evolutionary time. At the other extreme, the somatic mutation model supposed that very few V-region sequences were encoded in the genome and that a special somatic mutation mechanism operated on these sequences to increase diversity within the life span of the organism. Regardless of whether sequence diversification occurred in phylogeny (germline diversity) or ontogeny (somatic mutation), another question remained: How did the C regions of Ig genes escape such changes? In 1965, Dreyer and Bennett (1) proposed that for each class of Ig genes there might be only a single C-region gene, which was encoded in the germline separately from the multiple V-region genes; in the development of an antibody-producing cell, one of the V-region sequences would become associated with the C-region sequence, leading to a complete (V + C) gene, which the cell could then express. Thus, mechanisms that increase diversity in the isolated V-region genes might leave the single C region gene at its distant locus untouched. This model, with its proposal of gene rearrangement occurring independently in each lymphocyte, was revolutionary in that it violated the then-accepted notion that DNA is the same in all cells of the organism. Clearly, a definitive assessment of Dreyer and Bennett's proposal

E. E. Max: Laboratory of Cell and Viral Regulation, Center for Biologics Evaluation and Research, Food and Drug Administration, Bethesda, Maryland 20892.

and an evaluation of the relative significance of somatic and germline interpretations of V-region diversity required a direct analysis of the genes in question. Two additional mysteries: given the fact that each B lymphocyte should contain two copies of each gene locus (i.e., from the maternally and paternally derived chromosomes), why does the cell express only a single L chain and H chain, as if the locus on the nonexpressed chromosome were somehow silenced—the phenomenon known as "allelic exclusion"? And how can one explain the fact that affinity of serum antibodies for antigen increases over a period of weeks after antigen exposure—the phenomenon of "affinity maturation"?

Apart from the diversity of V regions in both L and H chains, H chains exhibit a different sort of diversity that also demands a molecular biologic explanation: all developing B cells synthesize IgM initially and can switch H-chain isotype from μ to γ, ε, or α only later in their maturation. As the expressed C-region "switches," the cell continues to express the same L- and H-chain V regions, so that antigen specificity remains unchanged. Thus, in addition to understanding how, in different cells, a single C region can become associated with multiple different V regions (V-C recombination), we need to consider the molecular mechanism by which, during lymphocyte development, a single V region may become associated sequentially with several C regions (H-chain switch).

A final level of diversity exhibited by Ig H chains is represented by the alternative forms of Ig found embedded in the membrane of B cells versus those in blood and secretions. Membrane Igs have C-terminal extensions containing hydrophobic amino acids that associate with membrane lipids, whereas secreted Igs lack this C-terminal piece but are otherwise identical to the membrane counterparts. Analysis of Ig genes has shown how these two forms are encoded in the genome.

This chapter will begin with a brief discussion of V gene assembly in H- and L-chain genes. We then describe the H-chain locus—including molecular explanations for the membrane forms of Ig and isotype switching—followed by descriptions of κ and λ gene loci; however, a detailed discussion of each germline V-gene locus is deferred until later in the chapter. Next we consider in detail the DNA recombination events underlying V-gene assembly and the regulation of this process to maintain allelic exclusion. The chapter continues with a discussion of the mechanisms contributing to V-region diversity: the germline V repertoire, junctional diversity, and somatic mutation. A discussion of the regulation of Ig gene expression follows. The chapter ends with several topics in the "applied science" of Ig genes.

The investigations described in this chapter have been chosen from the literature to facilitate a clear exposition of the important issues rather than to provide a comprehensive compendium of data and references on Ig genes. In these descriptions, most of the discussion focuses on murine and human Ig genes. Murine genes were studied first because of the availability of pristane-induced murine myelomas of BALB/c mice, which served as convenient monoclonal sources of Ig protein for early structural studies. The same myelomas then provided messenger RNA (mRNA) and DNA for molecular biology analysis, which was greatly facilitated by the fact that these myelomas derived from the same genetic background—the inbred BALB/c strain. Later, study of the homologous human loci showed many fundamental similarities between the Ig genes of these two species, whereas some other mammalian orders show surprisingly significant differences.

Isotype switching and somatic mutation of Ig genes are covered in more detail in separate chapters of this text (Chapters 23 and 24).

OVERVIEW OF IMMUNOGLOBULIN V-GENE ASSEMBLY

In the late 1970s, experiments on L-chain genes established that the Dreyer-Bennett hypothesis was fundamentally correct: each lymphocyte expresses only a single Ig molecule encoded by one VL and one VH gene, each having been "activated" by a recombination event that brings the V gene near its respective C-region gene. This conclusion was supported by comparisons of Ig genes from B-lymphoid cells, particularly murine myelomas, and the corresponding gene loci from "germline" DNA. (Although true germline DNA can experimentally be obtained only from sperm, any nonlymphoid DNA is assumed to be representative of germline DNA because the rearrangements of Ig genes occur only in lymphoid cells. When DNA from sperm versus other nonlymphoid tissues has been compared by Southern blots, the results have been identical. Therefore, despite the risk of some imprecision, nonlymphoid DNA samples are conventionally referred to as germline whether the DNA is from sperm, whole embryo, liver, placenta, or other nonlymphoid sources.)

Evidence from Southern Blots and Gene Cloning

Initially the myeloma and germline DNA samples were compared by Southern blotting using hybridization probes derived from myeloma complementary DNA (cDNA). As schematically shown in Fig. 1 for an analysis of κ L-chain genes, a Cκ probe detects only a single band in germline DNA, consistent with a single Cκ gene. A probe representing an expressed Vκ gene detects several bands, as though hybridizing to a family of related sequences. Moreover, although not shown in Fig. 1, probes representing different expressed Vκ genes are found to hybridize to a different set of bands, representing a different family of related Vκ genes. These observations support the hypothesis of multiple V genes, single C gene. The novel recombination postulate of the Dreyer-Bennett hypothesis is supported by the differences observed when these probes are hybridized to myeloma DNA instead of germline DNA. As shown in Fig. 1, the recombination bringing a V gene close to a C gene can cause an alteration in size of the Cκ-hybridizing restriction fragment. The new rearranged band may be larger, smaller, or fortuitously the same size as the germline band, depending on the location of the restriction sites flanking the V and C genes. One of the V-region bands may similarly be expected to be rearranged in the myeloma so as to lie on a different-sized fragment, the same fragment that hybridizes to the Cκ probe. Results like these for κ and λ genes strongly supported the Dreyer-Bennett hypothesis and forcefully challenged the concept that every cell in the body has identical genes (2,3). In panels of myelomas analyzed for Cκ recombination by Southern blotting, many showed evidence of DNA rearrangement on both allelic chromosomes. This result argued against the possibility that allelic exclusion might be explained by a mechanism that allowed recombination on only one chromosome, and it raised questions about the nature of the "second" gene rearrangement in these cells, as discussed later in this chapter.

A more complete understanding of recombination of Ig genes developed from sequence analysis of cloned myeloma versus germline DNA. The general structures of the germline V genes are similar for the three Ig loci: H chain, κ, and λ. Each V gene begins with a sequence encoding a signal peptide of about 22 amino acids. (Signal peptides are found at the N-terminus of most proteins destined for secretion or expression on the cell membranes; after rout-

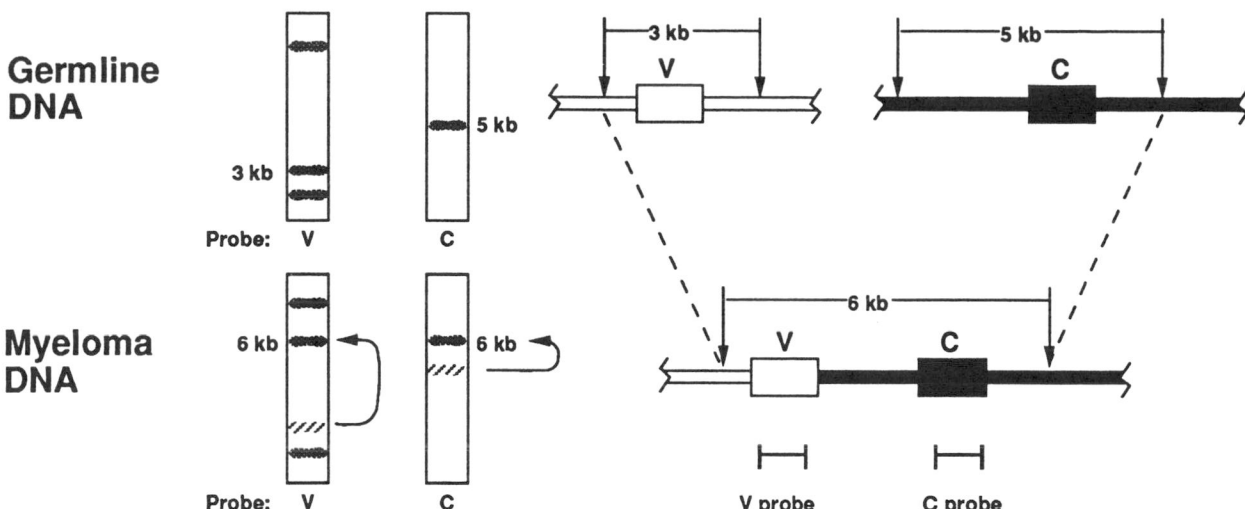

FIG. 1. Southern blot demonstration of rearrangement of Ig V and C region genes. *Eco*RI sites in this hypothetical example are indicated by arrows. In germline DNA (*upper drawings*) V and C are an unknown distance apart and are found by Southern blotting (*left*) to lie on *Eco*RI fragments of 3 and 5 kb, respectively. The V region probe hybridizes to a family of related genes (shown by bands above and below the 3-kb band). In myeloma DNA (*lower panel*), V and C genes have been brought into close proximity and, in this example, are no longer separated by *Eco*RI sites; both genes are found on the same *Eco*RI fragment of 6 kb, which is thus identified by either probe. The germline-sized fragments (hatched bands in the Southern blots) may or may not be preserved in the myeloma, depending on whether the nonexpressed homologous chromosome has remained in its germline (unrearranged) state. In many myelomas both chromosomes are present and both are rearranged.

ing the protein to the endoplasmic reticulum, the peptide is generally removed by specific peptidases.) Within codon 4 (numbering backward from the beginning of the mature protein sequence), the coding sequence is interrupted by an intron, usually 0.1 to 0.3 kb long. What was unanticipated was the discovery that each V-region gene as it exists in the germline is incomplete, and that recombination is necessary to assemble a complete V gene (4). For example, most murine κ chains have V regions 108 amino acids in length, but murine germline Vκ genes encode only about 95 of these. The remaining 13 amino acids are encoded by segments known as J (joining) regions that lie upstream of the C-region gene (5,6). An assembled Vκ gene thus results from recombination that joins one of many germline Vκ genes to one of five Jκ gene segments (Fig. 2A). A similar recombination event is necessary to assemble a complete Vλ-chain sequence from germline Vλ and Jλ genes (7). For H chains, recombination assembles a V region from three types of germline elements; between the residues encoded by germline VH and JH elements there are interposed variable numbers of amino acids—commonly from zero to eight residues—encoded by a D (diversity) region. The assembly of a complete H-chain V region occurs in two separate steps (Fig. 2B): initially one of several germline DH regions joins with one of the JH regions; then a germline VH region is added to complete the assembled VDJ H-chain gene.

How Recombination Contributes to Diversity

The V-assembly recombination contributes in two significant ways to the diversity of antigen-binding specificities. First, because there are multiple germline V regions and multiple D and J regions, the number of possible combinations of Vλ, Jλ, VH, DH, and JH is the multiplication product of the numbers of each of these five classes of germline sequence elements. This repertoire is vastly larger than could be achieved by devoting the same total lengths of

DNA sequence to preassembled V regions. A second factor that increases diversity was recognized by comparing nucleotide sequences of various myeloma genes to their germline precursors. For example, as shown in Fig. 3A, a comparison between the Vκ gene expressed in the murine myeloma MOPC41 and the corresponding germline Vκ and Jκ genes shows that the myeloma gene matches the germline precursor through the second nucleotide of codon 95; the VJ recombination junction clearly occurs at this point because sequence beyond this position in the myeloma gene clearly derives from Jκ1. Similar analyses of other myelomas show that the recombination junctions can occur at several different positions within codon 95 or 96. As shown in Fig. 3B, this flexibility of the position of the recombination junction increases the diversity of the affected codons. H-chain V regions exhibit this flexibility at both VD and DJ junctions. In addition, many H-chain VDJ junctions (and a smaller percentage of L-chain VJ junctions) show insertions of a few extra nucleotides not present in the germline precursors; the mechanism of these insertions will be discussed later in this chapter. Significantly, the three-dimensional structure of Igs established from x-ray crystallography shows that the Vλ-JL junction and the VH-DH-JH junction both form CDR3 loops that can contact antigen; thus this junctional diversity is physiologically relevant for diversifying antigen binding. The important role of D junctional amino acids for antigen binding has been verified by mutational analysis (8). In addition, many H-chain VDJ junctions (and a smaller percentage of L-chain VJ junctions) reveal insertions of a few extra nucleotides not present in the germline precursors; the mechanism of these insertions—known as N regions—will be discussed later in this chapter.

When the flexibility of the position of recombination was initially discovered, it was hard to understand how the germline elements could be joined with such variability and yet maintain the correct triplet reading frame between V and J. (An out-of-frame recombi-

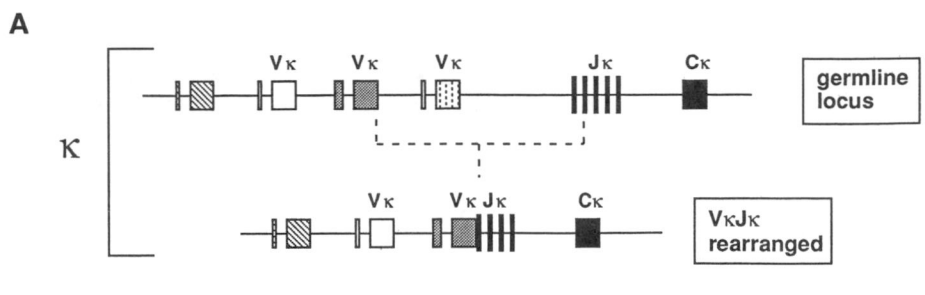

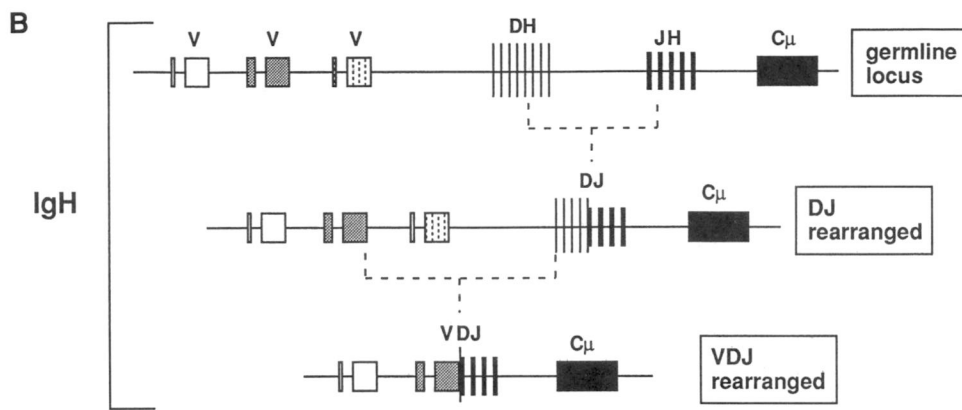

FIG. 2. V assembly recombination. **A:** In the κ locus a single recombination event joins a germline Vκ region with one of the Jκ segments. **B:** In the IgH locus an initial recombination joins a D segment to a JH segment. A second recombination completes the V assembly by joining a VH to DJH.

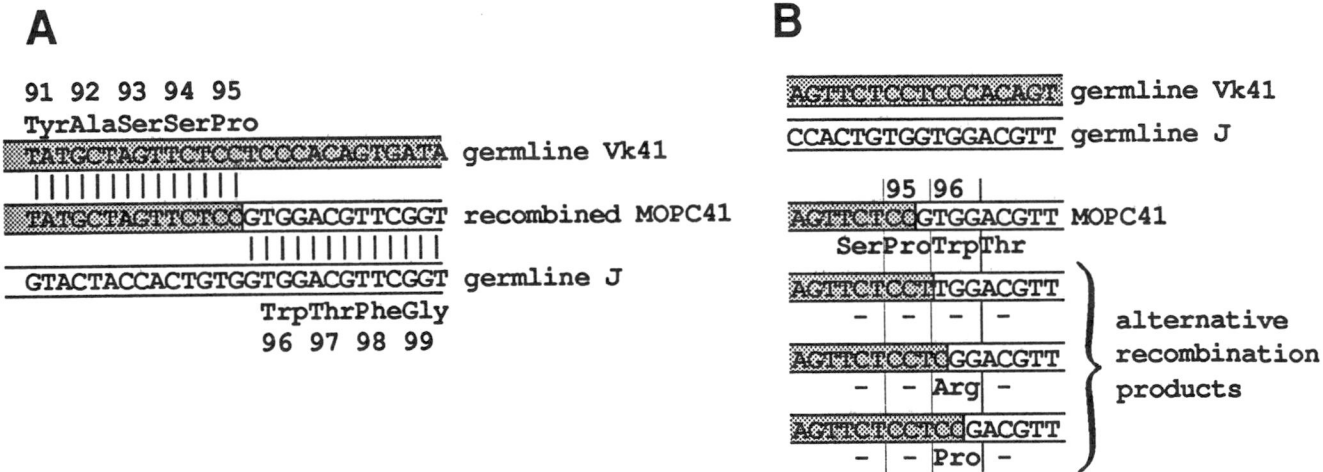

FIG. 3. Vκ-Jκ recombination at single base resolution. **A:** The sequence of the recombined MOPC41 κ gene around the VJ junction is shown at center, with the sequences of the two germline precursors (Vκ41 and Jκ1) shown above and below. The germline origins of the recombined gene are indicated by the vertical lines and the shading of the V-derived sequence. **B:** The consequences of joining the same germline sequences (from **A**) at four different positions are shown. Of the four alternative recombination products illustrated, the top one is that actually found in MOPC41. The second example has a single nucleotide difference but no change in encoded amino acid sequence. The third and fourth alternatives yield Arg or Pro at position 96; both of these amino acids have been found at this position in sequenced mouse κ chains.

nation would cause the entire C region to be read in a nonsense reading frame, so the gene would be nonfunctional.) It soon became clear, however, that if one looks beyond the subset of assembled V regions that are expressed in myeloma antibodies—a subset selected for expression of a functional L and H chain—one can find many assembled V genes with out-of-frame recombination junctions (9). Indeed, in unselected VJ recombinations the frequency of in-frame junctions is about 1/3, as predicted for a recombination mechanism insensitive to reading frame. In myelomas with rearrangements on both allelic copies of an Ig gene locus, the unexpressed recombination is generally out-of-frame or "non-productive." For H-chain VDJ recombination, one could theoretically retain the correct reading frame between V and J while allowing the interposed D-region segments to be used in all three reading frames. In murine H chains, however, only a single D-region reading frame is generally found, and several mechanisms prevent expression of antibodies with D regions in the other two reading frames (10). In human antibodies this intense selection against variant reading frames is not found (11), allowing for additional sequence diversity. The generation of V-region diversity in the three Ig gene loci (IgH, κ, and λ) is considered in more detail in a later section.

Recombination Signal Elements

Analysis of DNA sequences flanking the germline V-, D-, and J-region sequences showed two conserved sequence elements that apparently play a role in the recombination event signaling the position where the DNA should rearrange. The first signal element is a 7-mer CACTGTG that occurs as a consensus sequence 5' to the Jκ coding sequences, with its (reverse) complement CACAGTG appearing 3' to the Vκ coding sequences. The second element is a 9-mer GGTTTTTGT that appears about 23 nucleotides 5' to the Jκ 7-mer, its complement ACAAAAACC appearing about 12 nucleotides 3' to the Vκ 7-mer (5,6). The likelihood that these recombination signal sequences (RSS) are significant in the recombination is reinforced by their appearance at similar positions in L- and H-chain Ig genes throughout phylogeny as well as in T-cell receptor (TCR) genes (see Chapter 10), which undergo similar V assembly recombinations; furthermore, there are no other well-conserved sequences flanking these genes. In all of these systems the length of the spacer between the 7-mer and 9-mer appears significant. Recombination apparently occurs only between one coding sequence with a 12-bp spacer and another coding sequence with a 23-bp spacer, a requirement referred to as the 12/23 rule. The benefit of this requirement may be that futile recombinations, such as between two Vκ or two Jκ gene segments, are prevented. Although a computerized alignment of several hundred spacer sequences has detected some preferred nucleotides at specific positions (12), mutations of spacer sequences in plasmid recombination substrates have little effect on recombination frequency. The length of the spacers flanking H- and L-chain V, D, and J elements are shown in Fig. 4.

Although the complementarity of the Vκ and Jκ copies of the 7-mer and 9-mer signal elements initially led to the hypothesis that these elements might participate in the formation of a stem-and-loop intermediate in the recombination reaction, current evidence strongly favors an alternative role for the RSS: as recognition sequences for DNA-binding proteins mediating the recombination. This evidence is presented later in a detailed discussion of V(D)J recombination.

Because of the conservation of the RSS elements among κ, λ, IgH genes, and TCR genes, the enzymatic recombinase machinery that assembles complete V genes from germline precursors is believed to be the same in all these systems. This notion is reinforced by much other evidence, including the observations that germline TCR V-gene segments can be correctly rearranged when introduced into pre-B cells and that hybrid Ig-TCR rearrangement can occur (although only in abnormal cells, as discussed in a later section).

THE THREE IMMUNOGLOBULIN GENE LOCI

This section presents an overview of the three Ig loci: H chain, κ, and λ. The V regions of these loci are described in a later section on germline diversity (except that the tiny murine Vλ repertoire is discussed in the present section).

Heavy-Chain Genes

In the development of a B-lymphocyte, the cell initially produces IgM with a binding specificity determined by the productively rearranged VH and VL regions. Subsequently, each B cell and its

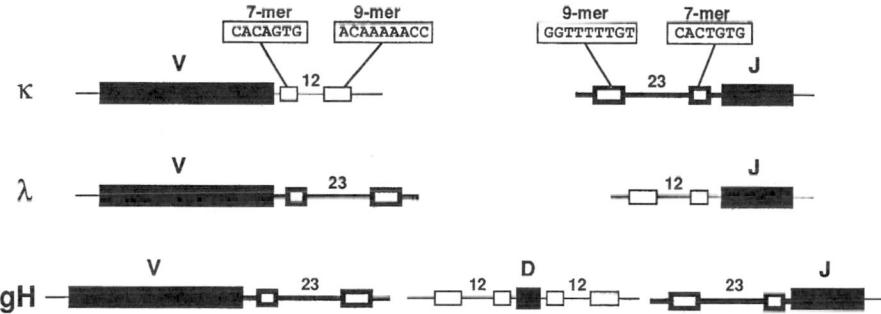

FIG. 4. Conserved elements flank germline V, D, and J region genes. Conserved 7-mer and 9-mer RSS lie adjacent to V, D, and J coding sequences and are important for targeting V(D)J recombination. The 7-mer and 9-mer elements are separated by spacer regions of about 12 bp (illustrated by thin lines in the figure) or 23 bp (thick lines). Depending on the locus, V regions may be flanked by 12- or 23-bp RSS, and similarly for J regions. But one of each type of element must be present for recombination to occur, a requirement that prevents futile recombination events (e.g., J to J).

progeny cells synthesize antibodies with the same L- and H-chain V regions; but they may later switch the isotype of the H chain. Early evidence for this developmental scheme includes (among other observations) (a) the isotype shift seen during the course of an immune response (13); (b) the ability of B-cell clones—myelomas (14,15) and splenic foci (16)—to express IgM plus another isotype, with identical VH regions; and (c) in vivo ablation studies suggesting that IgM-producing cells are the precursors of IgG producers (17). The molecular mechanism by which one part of a protein can change while another part remains unchanged has generated considerable interest.

Several groups (18–20) have demonstrated that active rearranged α, γ2b, and γ1 genes isolated from myelomas expressing the respective H chains contain—between their V and C regions—DNA sequences derived from the DNA upstream of the germline Cμ gene, including one or more JH sequences. These observations led to the model (Fig. 5) that the VH region rearranges initially to a position 5′ to the μ gene (leading to IgM production), and that when a cell expresses a new isotype the Cμ-region gene is replaced by the CH region encoding the new isotype. This isotype switch appears to result from a deletion of the CH genes between the assembled VDJ and the CH gene expressed after the switch. Early support for this deletion model came from analysis of the content of specific CH genes in myelomas that had undergone different switch recombinations. Solution hybridization kinetics or Southern blotting with cDNA-derived CH probes confirmed that switching was associated with loss of CH sequences from the cell. From the specific C regions lost in myelomas expressing different isotypes, it was possible to predict a linear order of the different CH genes on the chromosome (21,22).

A more detailed picture of the H-chain locus emerged as many laboratories reported the isolation of genomic clones for CH genes. In general, these clones were obtained in the early 1980s by screening genomic DNA libraries with cDNA probes derived from myeloma mRNA. From the wealth of data generated, we can consider only a few interesting conclusions because of space limitations.

One striking characteristic of CH genes is that the 100 to 110 amino acid domains—identified by internal homologies of amino acid sequences and by three-dimensional structural analysis (x-ray crystallography)—are encoded as intact exons, separated from other domain segments by introns of 0.1 to 0.3 kb (23–25). Thus, for example, the mouse γ2b protein has three major domains (CH1, CH2, and CH3), with a small hinge domain between CH1 and CH2. The gene structure (23,26,27) may be summarized as follows:

CH1 —intron—**hinge**—intron—**CH2**—intron—**CH3**
(292)　　(314)　(64)　(106)　(328)　(119)　(322)

where the numbers in parentheses represent the number of nucleotides in each segment. As an interesting contrast, the hinge region of the α gene is encoded contiguously with the CH2 domain

with no intervening intron (25), whereas the unusually long human γ3 hinge is encoded by three or four hinge exons (28). Analyses of genomic CH genes have led to speculations that the evolutionary history of H-chain genes may have included mutations that created or destroyed RNA splice sites and thereby converted portions of intron sequence into exon and vice versa. For example, the sequence of the intron 5′ to the hinge of the mouse γ2b gene shows a surprising degree of similarity with the sequence of CH1; this observation led to the speculation (23) that the hinge exon may have originated from a full Ig domain that became foreshortened either by the destruction of the RNA splice site at the 5′ end of the domain or the creation of a new splice site within the domain.

About 7 kb upstream from the murine Cμ gene lies a cluster of four JH segments (six JH segments in humans) that participate in VDJ recombination. Further upstream lie 13 D segments (about 27 in humans) and beyond them the VH regions. V and D regions are described later in this chapter in the section on V-region diversity.

Membrane Versus Secreted Immunoglobulin

Studies of IgH gene and cDNA structure have provided an explanation for the alternative membrane and secreted forms of the H chain. As noted earlier, the membrane-bound forms of Ig H chains are slightly larger than the secreted forms owing to an additional C-terminal hydrophobic segment that anchors the protein in membrane lipids (29). In the case of the μ chain, these two forms are products of two different mRNAs of 2.7 and 2.4 kb, which can be separated by gel electrophoresis. By comparing the DNA sequence of a genomic μ clone and μ cDNA clones corresponding to these two RNA species, several laboratories (30–33) have demonstrated that the two RNA species represent transcripts of the identical gene that have been spliced differently at their 3′ or C-terminal ends (Fig. 6). The nucleotide sequence encoding the 20 C-terminal residues of the secretory (μs) form is derived from DNA contiguous with the CH4 domain of the μ gene, whereas in the membrane mRNA (μm) the sequence after CH4 derives from two exons about 2 kb 3′ further downstream. These membrane exons encode 41 residues, including a stretch of 26 uncharged residues that span the membrane to fix the Ig to the cell surface. The same general gene structure has been found for the other CH genes (34–37), suggesting that the differential splicing mechanism probably accounts for the two forms of Ig of all isotypes.

Early B cells make substantial quantities of both μm and μs, whereas maturation to the plasma cell stage is associated with strong predominance of μs production, consistent with the function of such cells in generating the pool of circulating Ig. The balance between the two RNA splice forms of μ has been interpreted as a competition between CH4-M1 splicing and the cleavage/polyadenylation at the upstream μs poly(A) addition site. The factors influencing this balance have been studied by transfecting either early or late B cells

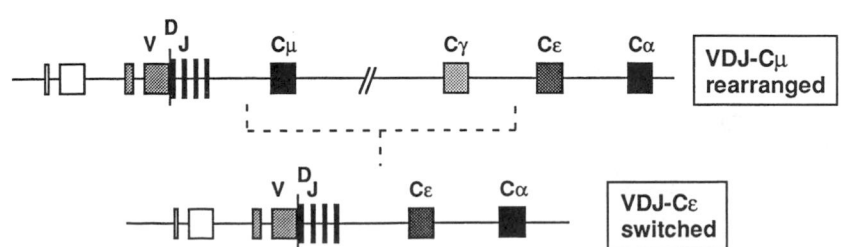

FIG. 5. Deletional isotype switch recombination. The expression of downstream H-chain genes is accomplished by a recombination event that replaces the Cμ gene with the appropriate H-chain C gene (Cε as depicted here), deleting the DNA between the recombination breakpoints.

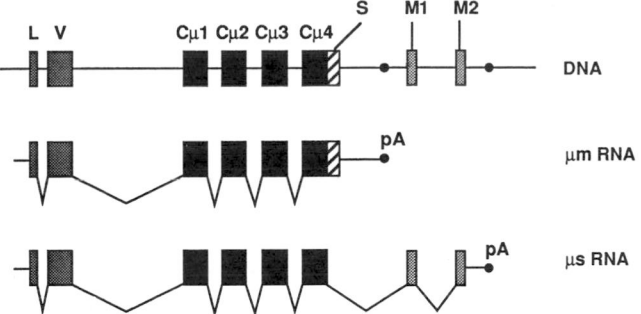

FIG. 6. Two RNAs generated from the μ gene by alternative processing. The top line illustrates the exons of the μ gene (*black rectangles*) in an expressed, rearranged μ gene. A primary transcript including all the exons present in the DNA can be processed as shown to yield either μs RNA (containing a C-terminal secreted [S] sequence) or μm RNA (containing the two membrane [M] exons).

with μ gene sequences or constructs in which the splice sites or cleavage/polyadenylation sites have been mutated, placed different distances apart, or rearranged in different order on the transfected gene construct. In some experiments constructs have been injected into frog oocytes with or without B-cell nuclei. Conflicting interpretations have emerged as to whether the critical factor influencing the μm/μs ratio is differential splicing (38) or poly(A) site choice (39,40). It does appear that the length of the intron between CH4 and M1 has an influence (41,42), that a stem-loop RNA structure at the 3' end of the CH4-M 1 intron may play a role (43), and that the mechanisms regulating this ratio may be different for different isotypes (44). Additional investigations will be necessary to explain exactly how cell maturation leads to an appropriate alteration in the ratio of the membrane and secreted forms of Ig.

Membrane Ig serves as the antigen-specific component of the B-cell receptor (BCR), which is critical for initiating the signal for lymphocyte activation on contact with antigen, as described in Chapter 7. The segments of membrane Igs (of all isotypes) that penetrate into the cytoplasm are too short to encode functional signal transduction domains. Instead, transduction is mediated by an associated protein dimer composed of the BCR components Igα and Igβ. This dimer also has important signaling roles during B-cell development before the mature BCR is assembled, as discussed later in this chapter.

Organization of CH Gene Loci

As genomic clones for the C-region genes of the H-chain loci of humans and mice were obtained, efforts were made to "link" them, i.e., to clone continuous stretches of DNA including the CH genes as well as all the DNA lying between them in the genome. The general strategy of this work was to use cDNA clones to obtain the CH genes and to use "gene walking" techniques to fill in the noncoding DNA between the genes. The murine locus was completely linked in 1982 with a report (45) of clones covering the entire region of the mouse genome—all eight CH genes—spanning about 200 kb of DNA on chromosome 12. These clones define the general structure of the region as shown in Fig. 7, where the numbers indicate the distance in kilobases between the genes. All the CH genes are oriented in the same 5' to 3' direction. Recent sequence analysis has shown several γ pseudogenes within the clustered γ genes (46).

The human CH genes also have been cloned and localized to chromosome 14q32 (47), but not completely linked as of this writing. One significant difference between the human and murine IgH loci is that a large duplication exists in the human at the 3' end of the H-chain gene locus, with two copies of a γ-γ-ε-α unit (48,49) (Fig. 7). One of the duplicated ε sequences is a pseudogene in which the CH1 and CH2 domains have been deleted (49,51). In addition, the human genome contains a third closely homologous ε-related sequence: a "processed" pseudogene found on chromosome 9 (50,51). (Pseudogenes of this type appear to have been reverse-transcribed from a processed RNA intermediate and then to have been inserted in the genome at locations unrelated to the original locus of the transcribed source gene.) A γ-related pseudogene lacking a switch region is also present in the human IgH locus between the two γ-γ-ε-α duplications (52). The map presented in Fig. 7 is based on partial contiguous overlaps and pulsed field gel

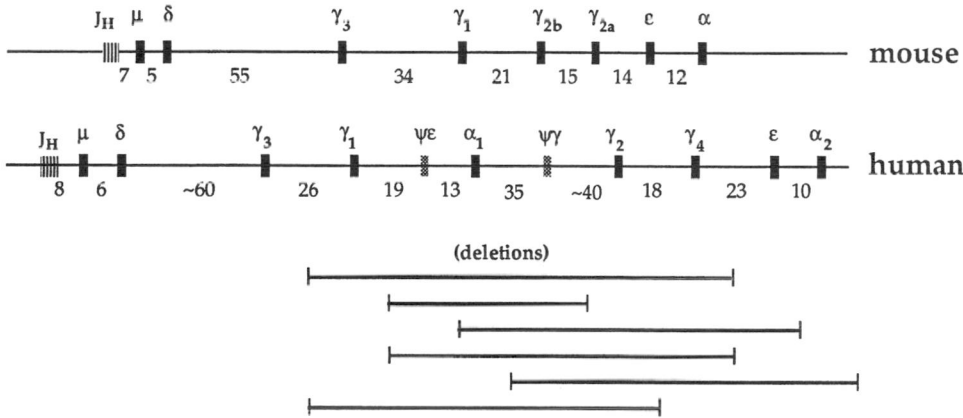

FIG. 7. H-chain constant region loci of mice and humans. The murine locus has been cloned in its entirety (45); the constant region genes are diagrammed with the approximate intergene distance indicated below (in kb). The human locus shows a large duplication at the downstream end. Although not all of the diagrammed segments have been physically linked by contiguous clones, the indicated order is supported by the deletions observed in various individuals as well as mapping by PFGE (53,54).

electrophoresis (PFGE) (53,54). PFGE allows electrophoretic separation of very large fragments—up to several megabases in length—that cannot be separated by conventional electrophoresis; fragments of this length are useful in mapping over long distances and can be generated by restriction enzymes that have unusually rare recognition sequences. The map of the human IgH locus in Fig. 7 is consistent with the known deletions in the H-chain locus (55), as diagrammed in the same figure.

The IgH locus also has been examined in several other species besides mice and humans, and several notable differences have been observed. Rabbits, for example, have 13 Cα sequences and only a single Cγ gene (56); this unusual expansion of genes contributing to mucosal immunity may be related to the peculiar habit of coprophagy in these animals. In contrast to the multiplicity of rabbit Cα genes, pigs have only one Cα gene and eight Cγ genes (57). Camels are unusual in having H chains that function in the absence of L chains (58). H-chain Ig genes (VH or CH) have been cloned from a number of other species, including rats [which are highly homologous with mice (59)], cows (56), chickens (60–63), horses (64), sharks (65), bony fish (66,67), crocodiles (68), frogs (69) and axolotls (70).

Heavy-Chain Switch

Switch Regions

The availability of genomic IgH clones allowed detailed sequence analysis of the deletional switch recombination. The active switched genes from several myelomas were compared with the corresponding germline CH genes and with the germline μ gene, with particular attention to the sequences surrounding the switch recombination site. In each case the recombination events were found to have occurred within or near regions of remarkably internally repetitive DNA sequences 5' to the CH coding sequences; these have become known as switch (S) sequences (71–74).

The S region of the mouse μ gene, Sμ, is located about 1 to 2 kb 5' to the Cμ coding sequence and is composed of numerous tandem repeats of sequences of the form (GAGCT)$_n$(GGGGT), where n is usually 2 to 5 but can be as high as 17 (74). These repeats apparently promote deletions within the Sμ region by homologous recombination events that can occur during the laboratory construction and isolation of clones containing the Sμ region. Because of such deletions, most cloned germline μ genes are found on EcoRI fragments shorter than the 12.5-kb fragment identified in genomic blots of BALB/c DNA. Deletions of the same region have been demonstrated to occur in vivo by comparison of the μ locus in different mouse strains by Southern blotting (75) and may occur especially frequently during the activity of switch recombination in normal B cells (76).

Similar internally repetitive S regions spanning 1 to 10 kb have been found 5' to all the other CH genes except Cδ. All of the S regions include occurrences of pentamers similar to GAGCT and GGGGT that are the basic repeated elements of the Sμ gene (77); in the other S regions these pentamers are not precisely tandemly repeated as in Sμ, but instead are embedded in larger repeat units. The 10-kb Sγ1 region has an additional higher order structure: two direct repeat sequences flank each of two clusters of 49-bp tandem repeats (78). S regions of human H-chain genes have been found very similar to their mouse homologs (79–81). Indeed, sequence similarity between human and mouse clones 5' to the CH genes has been found to be confined to the S regions, an observation that supports the biologic significance of these regions.

A switch recombination between, for example, μ and ε genes produces a composite Sμ-Sε sequence (Fig. 8). By examination of the germline Sμ and Sε sequences in comparison with the myeloma- or hybridoma-derived Sμ-Sε composite S region, it has been possible to localize the exact recombination sites between Sμ and Sε that occurred in different cells; similar analyses have been performed with cells producing other isotypes. These studies have indicated that there is no specific site, either in Sμ or in any other

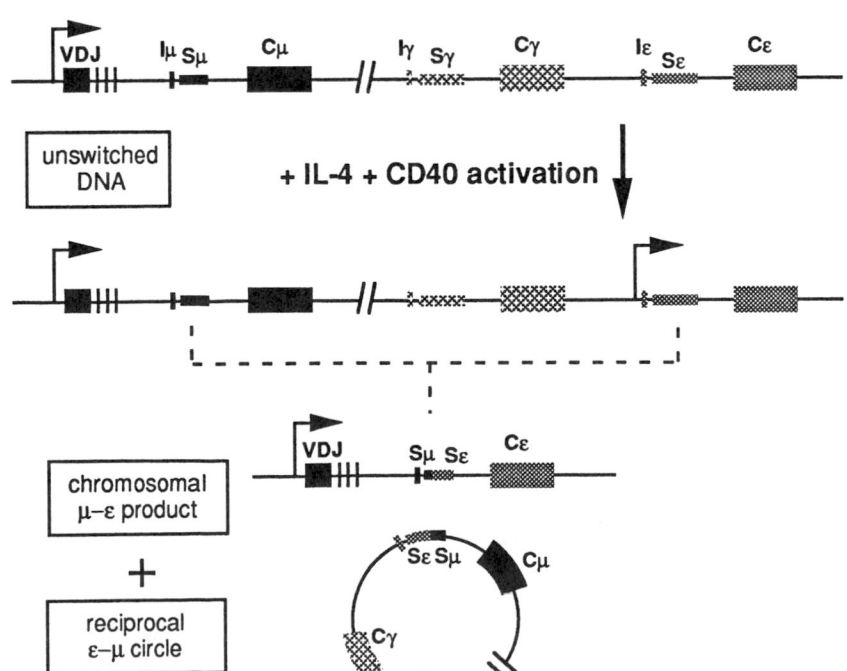

FIG. 8. Switch regions and composite switch junctions. The recombination breakpoints in isotype switch recombination fall within repetitive S regions. Stimuli that activate switch recombination (IL-4 and CD40 activation in the example shown) generally promote transcription across the target S region, initiating just upstream at the I exon. Recombination between Sμ and Sε produces two composite switch junctions: an Sμ-Sε junction retained in chromosomal DNA, and a reciprocal Sε-Sμ junction found in fractions of circular DNA. PCR amplification across either composite junction can be used to study switch recombination.

S region, where the recombination always occurs. Thus, unlike the enzymatic machinery of VJ recombination, the switch machinery can join sequences in a broad target region; this makes sense because VDJ recombination occurs within coding sequences, whereas switch recombination is less constrained because it occurs in introns. Many composite switch junction sequences show evidence of mutations at the recombination breakpoint when compared with the corresponding germline switch sequences; these mutations have been interpreted as reflecting an error-prone DNA synthesis step that may be a component of the switch recombination mechanism (82).

DNA excised by switch recombination has been detected by cloning from fractions of circular DNA isolated from cells actively undergoing isotype switch recombination (83–85). Thus, at least some of the excised DNA segments ligate their ends to form switch circles; these contain composite switch junctions that are reciprocal to the composite switch junction retained on chromosomal DNA (Fig. 8). For the example of cells switching from μ to ε, composite Sμ-Sε junctions are found on chromosomal DNA, whereas Sε-Sμ junctions can be found representing the reciprocal junctions from switch circles. Because switch circles are not linked to centromeres and may not contain origins of replication, they are not efficiently replicated. Therefore, they are not found in cells that have divided multiple times after switching, e.g., in myelomas or hybridomas.

Methods of Assaying Switching

In stable myelomas or hybridomas expressing switched isotypes, evidence of switch recombination can be obtained by gene cloning or Southern blotting. However, for studies of the regulation and mechanism of switch recombination, assays are needed that can detect switch recombination in a minority population of cells switching in culture. Some laboratories assess switching by simply measuring Ig protein of the switched isotype appearing in the culture supernatant. Alternatively, reverse-transcriptase polymerase chain reaction (RT-PCR) can be used to detect mRNA corresponding to the mature VDJ-C RNA transcripts of the switched isotype. However, because the culture conditions favoring isotype switching also may influence transcription or protein synthesis rates independently of switch recombination, RNA or protein assays may not faithfully reflect the DNA recombination events. Furthermore, switched RNA or protein cannot be assumed to reflect DNA recombination if one is exploring one of several models for nonrecombinational mechanisms for isotype switching. Therefore, two different PCR strategies have been developed to assess switch recombination at the DNA level. In one strategy, PCR primers are designed to amplify across the composite S region of interest (86). A related strategy is to amplify the reciprocal switch junctions found on circular DNA (87,88); these junctions can be used to "count" recombination events independent of proliferation if one assumes that each circle is produced as a by product of a single switch recombination event and, failing to replicate as the cells divide, is randomly partitioned to daughter cells at successive divisions after the recombination event. Because the efficiency of amplification varies for different composite switch junctions— smaller templates are amplified more efficiently, and the largest may not amplify at all—the PCR strategy described above cannot easily be adapted to assay switch recombination quantitatively. For this reason a second strategy known as digestion-circularization PCR (DC-PCR) was developed (89). In this approach DNA from switching cells is digested with a restriction enzyme, and restric-

tion fragments—including the ones bearing a composite Sμ-Sε junction—are ligated to form circles. Primers designed to amplify across the restriction site generated by ligation of the Sμ-Sε fragment ends will yield a consistent product whose size depends only on the distance between primers and the restriction site. From unswitched DNA no product is amplified because the two primers can never both hybridize to the same DNA circle. Therefore, with appropriate calibration (90), the amount of DC-PCR product formed can be used as a semiquantitative measure of the amount of composite switch junctions in a DNA sample. These methods have been used in many of the experiments described below.

Regulation of Isotype Switching

Isotype switching occurs physiologically in animals about 1 week after immunization with T-dependent antigens, at about the same time that somatic mutation of Ig genes begins. Somatic mutation (discussed later in this chapter) clearly occurs in germinal centers of lymphoid organs—a location that facilitates T- and B-cell interaction—and there is some evidence that germinal centers are a major site for isotype switching as well. As demonstrated by in vitro switching experiments, T cells promote switching by secretion of cytokines (especially interleukin [IL]-4 and transforming growth factor-β [TGF-β]) as well as by cell-to-cell contact. A major component of the cell contact signal is mediated by an interaction between the B-cell surface marker CD40 and its ligand (designated CD40L or glycoprotein [gp]39), expressed on activated T cells. The dependence of switching on this interaction is highlighted by the genetic disease known as the X-linked hyper-IgM syndrome, which was found (independently by several laboratories) to be caused by a defect in the gene encoding CD40L/gp39 (91). Patients with this syndrome have elevated concentrations of IgM in their serum and almost no Igs of other isotypes. In addition, their antibodies fail to show affinity maturation or evidence of B-cell memory responses. Mouse strains with engineered defects in CD40 or CD40L show a similar phenotype, although they respond with normal isotype switching to T-independent antigens (92); little is known about this T-independent switching pathway. The discovery of the importance of the of CD40–CD40L interaction has facilitated in vitro switching experiments in which T cells can be replaced with antibodies to CD40 or with cells engineered to express surface CD40L. One role of the CD40 stimulus is to induce B-cell proliferation. Indeed, other proliferative stimuli (e.g., lipopolysaccharide [LPS] or IgM or IgD cross-linking) can support cytokine-induced isotype switching in vitro in the absence of T cells and CD40 activation; and switching may be related to the cell cycle (93). However, CD40 has additional effects, including upregulation of IL-4 responsiveness and IL-4 receptor number (94); the signaling pathways initiated by CD40 are under active investigation (95).

Different isotypes are known to predominate in different immune responses depending on the antigen, route of antigen administration and several other parameters. As discussed more fully in Chapter 23, these different parameters act in part by influencing the cytokine milieu of the B cells. IL-4, for example, promotes the expression of IgE (and IgG1 in mice), whereas TGF β promotes switching to IgA. These lymphokines are believed to act by making the C region of the target isotype accessible to switch recombinase machinery that may be non–isotype- specific. The accessibility is associated with expression of an RNA transcript that initiates upstream of a target S region and extends through the target C region (Fig. 8). This type of RNA is designated a germline transcript because it is transcribed while the

IgH locus is in germline (i.e., unswitched) configuration; alternatively, these transcripts are called sterile (i.e., lacking a V region). After in vitro treatment of B cells with IL-4, for example, but before any switch recombination to Cε, sterile transcripts are detected with a structure that includes Cε preceded by a short exon known as Iε. The Iε sequence derives from DNA upstream of Sε, a location that would be deleted during the formation of the Sμ-Sε composite S region; in the germline transcripts the Iε region is spliced to Cε by removal of an intron containing the Sε region. Similar transcripts have been found for every isotype examined in both human and mouse systems, including μ. In each case many of the same experimental conditions (including cytokines) that favor the accumulation of sterile transcripts from a particular isotype also favor switch recombination involving the corresponding S region. In some cases the signals transduced by the cytokine receptor have been elucidated. For example, IL-4 stimulates transcription by activating the transcription factor STAT6, which attaches to one of several nuclear protein binding motifs in the promoter region upstream of Iε and Igλγ, as discussed later in this chapter. Apart from I-region promoters, sterile transcription and isotype switching are also regulated by an enhancer lying downstream of the murine Cα gene, as deduced from switching defects in mice in which this enhancer was replaced by a neomycin resistance gene in all B cells (96); defects were observed in switching to IgE and several IgG isotypes, but not to IgG1.

Studies of mouse strains in which the I region from various isotypes have been targeted by homologous recombination suggest that sterile transcription is necessary but not sufficient for recombination (97–99). The low extent of sequence conservation of the I exons and the lack of consistent open reading frames suggest that these transcripts do not encode a functional protein. What then is their role? One hypothesis is that the critical chromosomal alteration that renders an isotype locus accessible to the switch recombinase machinery is achieved by the process of transcribing through the locus, and that the transcripts themselves serve no function. A second hypothesis is that the transcripts participate in the recombination event in some way, perhaps by formation of an RNA:DNA triple helix (100). In support of this idea, cell-free transcription of S regions was found to lead to a stable association of the transcript RNA with the template DNA (101); significantly, this association occurred only with RNA transcribed from S region DNA and only when the RNA was transcribed in the physiologic orientation. Neither of these two hypotheses concerning the role of sterile transcription account well for a feature conserved in all the transcripts: the RNA splice that removes the Sx region from the mature IxCx transcript. It is noteworthy that sterile transcripts from the germline components of V(D)J assembly recombination are also synthesized just before that recombination event, and transcription is also observed from rearranging yeast DNA sequences. These observations suggest that the transcription of DNA immediately before recombination may be a general feature of recombination events common to many biologic systems. On the other hand, it is likely that cytokines regulate other aspects of the switching mechanism besides sterile transcription because several examples have been reported of cytokines up- or downregulating switch recombination without a parallel effect on sterile transcripts (102).

Mechanism of Switch Recombination

The mechanism of isotype switch recombination has been probed with a variety of strategies, so far with limited results. One approach to delineating the sequences required for switch rearrangement has been to construct plasmid substrates containing switch sequences that might undergo switch recombination when transfected into B-lineage cells either stably (103) or in transient systems (104). For example, the construct of Daniels and Lieber (105) contained the polyoma origin and T-antigen gene (to allow replication in murine cells) and fragments of Sμ and Sγ3 segments, with viral promoters upstream of each and a *supF* transfer RNA (tRNA) gene between them; expression of the *supF* tRNA gene in appropriately engineered bacteria led to blue colonies on culture plates. Plasmids undergoing Sμ-Sγ3 recombination in eukaryotic cell lines could be recovered and identified by the production of white colonies in bacteria. Although various nonlymphoid cell lines produced white colonies within the first 20 hours of transfection (perhaps resulting from DNA repair enzymes acting on nicked plasmids), continued increases in the percentage of white colonies beyond 20 hours appeared to be B cell specific. Deletion of the promoters had only minor effects on the recombination frequency, but white colonies were dramatically decreased when the promoters were arranged so that the S regions were transcribed in the nonphysiological direction. When the S regions were replaced with irrelevant DNA, the direction of transcription had no effect on recombination. The dependence of recombination frequency on transcriptional orientation of switch sequences parallels findings described above in which the RNA–DNA complex involving S regions was strand dependent.

Another strategy for elucidating the switch recombinase mechanism is to identify intermediates in the reaction, an approach that has been strikingly successful in studying VDJ recombination, as discussed later in this chapter. A single study exploring this approach has used ligation-mediated PCR (a technique described later in connection with VDJ recombination) to detect blunt, double-stranded cuts in the murine γ3 region in B cells switching in culture (106); these cuts may be generated by the switch recombinase machinery.

Possible Switch Recombinase Components

In an effort to identify components of the recombinase machinery, several laboratories have investigated proteins that bind in a sequence-specific manner to S-region sequences in vitro. Several examples are described below, although it should be emphasized that none of the components discussed in this section has been demonstrated to participate in switch recombination. LR1 is a protein found in nuclear extracts from murine splenic B-lymphocytes after induction with LPS; it binds to Sγ1, Sγ3, and Sα, as well as to the H-chain enhancer (107). The protein has been purified (108), and one component has been identified as the nucleolar protein nucleolin (109). Sμbp-2 is a ubiquitous protein, also upregulated by LPS in murine splenic B cells, which binds to a segment from the tandem repeats in Sμ. A murine cDNA clone was found to exhibit sequence similarity to genes encoding helicases; such an activity could be critical for switch recombination (110). NF-Sμ is another protein that binds to Sμ tandem repeats and is induced in splenic B cells by LPS; its binding specificity is slightly different from the other proteins already described (111). Two proteins that bind within Sγ regions to subsequences associated with a high frequency of recombination junctions have been designated SNIP and SNAP and apparently correspond (respectively) to the transcription factors NF-κB/p50 and E47, which are discussed later in this chapter (112,113). A role for NF-κB in switching is supported by experiments in B cells from a mouse strain in which the p50 gene has been disrupted by homologous recombination. In these p50 knockout mice, isotype switching to IgE and IgG3 secretion was markedly reduced; however, reduced expression of the corresponding germline transcripts could indicate that the p50 was required for promoting "accessibility" rather than for the actual recombination event (114). In these experiments switching to IgG1 expression was almost unaffected by the absence of p50, and α was the only isotype whose expression was markedly reduced in the face of normal germline transcription. A possible role for E47 in switching is supported by experiments in which expression of Id1, an antagonist of the E2A transcription factors of which E47 is a member, was found to partially inhibit spontaneous and induced switching to IgA in the murine cell line CH12.LX2 (115).

Apart from studying proteins that bind to S-region DNA, another approach to identify switch recombinase components has been to search for an enzyme activity expected to participate in the recombination. A lymphoid-specific endonuclease activity that preferentially cleaves G-rich segments of S regions has been partially purified and proposed as a possible participant in switch recombination (116).

The possibility that switch recombination depends on some of the same components that are known to participate in V(D)J recombination has been tested for several proteins (whose role in V(D)J recombination is discussed later in this chapter). Both SCID mice, which are natural mutants of DNA-dependent protein kinase (DNA-PK), and mice with homozygous knockouts of their recombinaton activating gene-2 (RAG-2) genes are impaired in developing mature B lymphocytes because of their inability to assemble V genes efficiently. However, when early B-lineage cells from these mice were allowed to proliferate *in vitro* and were then treated with IL-4 and anti-CD40, switch recombination occurred in the RAG-2 knockout cells but not in the SCID cells (116a). Thus, DNA-PK appears necessary for switch recombination but RAG-2 does not. DNA-PK binds DNA as part of a complex that also contains the protein Ku80 (also discussed later in this chapter). Recently, Ku80 was also implicated in switch recombination in experiments in which Ku80 knockout mice were crossed with mice in which recombined VκJκ and VDJ genes were "knocked in" to the respective loci by homologous recombination. Whereas "knock-in" mice with intact Ku80 genes expressed IgM encoded by the engineered Vk and VH genes and also switched to downstream isotypes, the corresponding Ku80-deficient mice made IgM but did not switch isotypes, suggesting that Ku80 is also required for switch recombination (116b).

A recent achievement that holds promise for identifying recombinase proteins is the development of a cell-free nuclear extract system that can accomplish recombination between S-region sequences in vitro (117,118). This system depends on a powerful assay in which tritium-labeled plasmid molecules containing Sγ are incubated with digoxigenin-labeled plasmid containing Sμ. Recombination between the plasmids is detected as tritium immunoprecipitable by antidigoxigenin, and the recombinant DNA structure can be verified by PCR amplification across the composite switch junctions. Optimal recombination was found to require adenosine triphosphate (ATP), both Sμ and Sγ, and nuclear extract from LPS-blasted B cells. Partial fractionation of nuclear extracts identified an active complex designated SWAP (switch activation proteins) composed of at least four proteins: nucleophosmin (which has a RecA-like DNA D-loop forming activity), poly(ADP)ribose polymerase (PARP, a nuclear protein implicated in DNA repair), nucleolin (described above as a component of the Sμ-binding protein LR1), and a novel 70 kD protein designated SWAP-70, not homologous to any known protein family (118). SWAP-70 is strongly expressed only in B cells that have been activated for switch recombination,

and binds with high affinity to the other components of the complex. The SWAP complex is a strong candidate for a switch recombinase component, but as of this writing, the definitive evidence from a knockout experiment is not yet available.

Nonstandard Switch Recombination

Thus far we have considered switch recombination to involve a simple deletion of the DNA between two S regions; although this is the most common scenario, three additional situations should be considered for completeness.

Sequential Switching. Several switch recombination events can occur sequentially on a given chromosome. One well-studied example involves sequential switching to γ1 followed by ε in mouse B-lymphocytes. The same cytokine, IL-4, promotes switching to both isotypes. After an initial switch recombination generating a composite Sμ-Sγ1 junction (leading to IgG1 expression), this composite S region can undergo a secondary switch recombination with Sε, which lies downstream. In IgE-expressing cells, evidence of the initial recombination to γ1 can be demonstrated by the presence of a composite Sμ-Sγ1-Sε junction (119), or by the detection of the reciprocal switch circle product Sε-Sγ1. To assess the quantitative importance of this pathway in IgE generation, resting B cells stimulated with IL-4 plus LPS were treated with an anti-IgG1 antibody to eliminate cells expressing this isotype from the culture; IgE secretion was inhibited about 70%, suggesting that most mouse B cells expressing IgE have undergone an intermediate stage in which they expressed IgG1 (120). However, in mutant mice with a block in γ1 switching due to a targeted deletion in the γ1 locus, the frequency of switching to ε is normal, suggesting that the sequential switching results from the simultaneous accessibility of both Sγ1 and Sε, rather than an obligatory sequential switch program (121). Sequential switching to IgE expression via IgG also occurs in human B cells (81,122), but the quantitative significance of this pathway is not known.

Inversional Recombination. Some switch recombinations apparently lead to inversion rather than deletion of the DNA between the two S regions involved (123,124). A chromosome with an inversional switch recombination would be incapable of encoding a functional H chain because the C region downstream of the VDJ region would be in inverted orientation, but the chromosome could be "rescued" by a second switch recombination to a downstream constant region. In human B-cell leukemias—which are under no selection for Ig production—inversional switch recombination has reported to occur at a frequency of about 15% (125).

Trans-Switching. Although most switch recombinations involve a single chromosome, transchromosomal switching between allelic chromosomes has been detected in rabbits at a frequency of about 5% (126). The detection of trans-switching in rabbits was facilitated by the availability of allotypic markers of C and V regions in this species; the frequency of trans-switching in other species is not known.

Switched Isotypes Without Switch Recombination

Several laboratories have reported detection of B cells expressing Ig of more than one isotype. Such double-producing cells may reflect a normal transient intermediate stage when a switched isotype may be expressed (after normal switch recombination) along with IgM that is retained in the cells because of the long half-life of the protein or its mRNA. However, some laboratories have reported a stable double-producer phenotype in cell lines without apparent switch recombination in the expressed IgH locus. For the case of μ-δ double producers, the explanation is apparently that δ transcripts can be produced by RNA splicing from a long primary transcript that includes μ and δ (127). More difficult to explain are the cell lines expressing μ along with an isotype whose C region is so distant from Cμ that an analogous long transcript would be on the order of 100 kb or more; such transcripts are longer than have been observed with current laboratory methods, although precedents for genes whose exons are spread over similar distances are known. One interesting proposal being considered to explain expression of downstream isotypes without switch recombination is that separate short transcripts of VDJ and a downstream CH gene (i.e., a sterile transcript) could be joined by a trans-splicing mechanism similar to that documented for trypanosomes and certain viruses (128,129). A nonphysiologic mechanism has been described that could account for some cases of double isotype production as a consequence of chromosomal duplication (130). Stable double-producing cell lines continue to be studied (131–133); at present we cannot be certain whether cells stably expressing this phenotype represent important physiologic counterparts of normal B cell subsets. A semiquantitative assessment of switch recombination in a population of murine B-cell switching in vitro to IgG1 indicated that DNA rearrangement can account for the IgG1 expression observed (90), suggesting that most expression of switched isotype Ig is associated with switch recombination, and that alternative nonrecombinational models for switching do not seem to be required on quantitative grounds.

Kappa Light-Chain Genes

In comparison with the H-chain genes, the κ locus is relatively simple. A single Cκ gene with a single exon and no reported alternative splice products is found in both mice and humans. Upstream of the murine Cκ gene lie five Jκ gene segments, spaced about 0.3 kb apart (5,6). Of these Jκ segments, the third encodes an amino acid sequence never observed in κ chains and is believed to be nonfunctional owing to a defect in the splice donor site that would join the corresponding RNA sequence to Cκ. The human locus is similar, with five Jκ regions upstream of Cκ; however, no homolog of the defective murine Jκ3 is present in the human Jκ cluster, whereas an additional Jκ sequence lies downstream of the sequence homologous to murine Jκ5 (134,135). Upstream of the Jκ segments in both species lie the Vκ genes, which will be described later in this chapter.

Apart from Vκ-Jκ rearrangement, an additional recombination event occurs in this locus, a recombination unique to κ genes and apparently mediated by the same 7-mer/9-mer signal elements involved in V(D)J recombination. This event, which involves deletion of the Cκ gene segment, was initially suggested by the observation that Southern blots of DNA from λ-expressing human lymphoid cells generally show no detectable Cκ sequence (136). Apparently in most B cells the Cκ genes are deleted from both chromosomes before λ gene rearrangement begins. When the boundaries of the deleted segment of DNA were examined in several human and mouse cell lines, a common sequence element was found at the downstream boundary; this element was designated RS (recombining sequence) in the mouse studies (137) and κde (kappa-deleting element) in the human studies (138). The human κde in germline DNA is located 24 kb downstream from the Cκ gene and is flanked by a 7-mer/9-mer RSS similar to that found flanking the Jκ regions (i.e., with a 23-bp spacer) (139). The similar murine RS is about 25 kb downstream from murine Cκ (140). The κde element can apparently recombine either with a Vκ gene

segment (leading to a deletion of the entire Jκ-Cκ locus) or with an isolated 7-mer element that is located in the Jκ-Cκ intron (leading to deletion of Cκ but retention of the Jκ locus). The 7-mer in the Jκ-Cκ intron is 30 bp 5' from a poorly conserved 9-mer-like sequence, a spacing that seems to violate the usual 12/23 rule. The significance of this unusual spacer is not understood, but possibly the 7-mer in these recombinations is active without a functional 9-mer, as seems to be the case for secondary VH recombinations (discussed in a later section).

A comparison between the mouse RS and human κde sequences (138,139) shows that the recombination signals are highly conserved and that downstream of these elements a region of about 500 bp is partially conserved (about 50% sequence identity). The latter region includes open reading frames of 127 (mouse) or 102 (human) codons. It is not known whether these reading frames are ever expressed as protein as a consequence of the RS/κde recombination events, but the fact that the recombination may occur with either a Vκ region or intron sequence suggests that the sequences joined by the event may be less important than the sequences deleted. RS/κde elements are consistently found to be rearranged in cells in which Cκ is deleted and λ rearrangements are found; this has led to the speculation that the RS/κde recombination event may mediate the developmental switch from κ to λ gene rearrangement, perhaps by deleting a gene for a negative regulator of λ gene rearrangement. However, current evidence argues against this view.

Lambda Light-Chain Genes

Murine λ Locus

In laboratory mouse strains, λ chains represent only about 5% of L chains, and this diminished abundance is associated with remarkably meager diversity. In contrast to the κ system with its multiple V-region families, amino acid sequence analysis of monoclonal λ chains detected only two sequences that appeared to represent germline Vλ regions. Furthermore, in contrast to the single mouse Cκ region, three nonallelic mouse isotypes are known from secreted λ chains; these are designated λ1, λ2, and λ3, in decreasing order of abundance.

The first λ gene to be cloned was a germline Vλ2 gene obtained by Tonegawa's laboratory in 1977 (141) (this was the first Ig gene cloned). The sequence of this Vλ gene (7) showed structural features that are similar to those of other germline Vλ genes, as well as Vκ and VH genes, which were discovered later. The Vλ2 coding sequence begins with a 19-amino-acid signal peptide that is interrupted within codon 4 by an intron (which was one of the first introns demonstrated). After the remaining signal peptide codons, the DNA sequence matches closely that expected based on amino acid sequence determined chemically from a λ2 myeloma L chain. However, the sequence of this germline Vλ2 gene ends abruptly 13 codons short of the expected end of the Vλ2 region, an observation that led to the first recognition of a separately encoded J region.

Cloning and long range mapping studies by pulsed field gel electrophoresis (142,143) have led to a substantial understanding of the mouse λ locus (Fig. 9). There are four Cλ genes, each with its own Jλ-region gene located about 1.3 kb 5' from the C. The J-Cλ3 and J-Cλ1 genes are arranged in one cluster about 3 kb apart with the Vλ1 gene lying about 19 kb upstream. A second Cλ cluster lying about 130 kb upstream from the Cλ3-1 locus contains J-Cλ2 and an unexpressed gene J-Cλ4. These are flanked by two upstream Vλ genes, Vλ2 and the rarely used Vx, which has an in-frame termination codon at its 3' end (144). The gene order (V2-Vx-JC2-JC4-V1-

JC3-JC1) explains the common expression of Vλ2 (or Vx) in association with Cλ2 and Vλ1 with Cλ1 or Cλ3. The Vλ2 has been found in rare association with the 190-kb distant Cλ1 locus, but the backward recombination of Vλ1 with Cλ2 has not been observed. The similarities between the four J-C genes suggest that the two clusters arose by a duplication of an ancestral V-J-Cλx-J-Cλy unit that in turn was the result of a prior J-Cλ duplication event. The ancestry of the Vx gene is uncertain because this gene is rather dissimilar to the other Vλ genes; indeed, it resembles Vκ as much as Vλ. Anti-Vλx antisera detect expression of this Vλ in all laboratory mice tested, but it may have a particular restricted function.

The sequences of genes in the λ locus have been examined for clues that might explain the relative abundance of their expressed products—λ1 > λ2 λ3 > > > (λ4) (145). The sequence of Cλ4 includes several amino acid substitutions but no termination codons that would necessarily render it nonfunctional; however, at the 3′ end of Jλ4, a mutation has destroyed the "GT . . ." found at almost all known donor splice sites, so that an RNA transcript of this gene would not be properly processed (reminiscent of the mouse Jκ3). The Jλ gene segments are all flanked on their 5′ sides by sequences similar to the 9-mer and 7-mer signal elements observed in the VH and Vκ system. The 12/23 rule discussed in relation to spacing between the signal elements in the κ locus also applies to λ, but in the λ locus the RSS elements are spaced about 23 bp apart for V regions and about 12 bp apart for J regions (the opposite of the arrangement in κ genes), as shown in Fig. 4. The decreased abundance of λ2 and λ3 relative to λ1 may be related to discrepancies between their 9-mer homology elements and the consensus 9-mer element.

Analyses of λ genes in wild mice by Southern blotting have indicated more complex and varied loci than that seen in typical laboratory strains (146). These complex λ loci may result from gene duplication events beyond those evident in laboratory strains, although the observation that at least one wild Vλ gene missing from BALB/c is similar to a human Vλ (146) suggests that some of the difference between wild and laboratory strains must be due to gene loss in that latter.

Human λ Locus

Lambda L chains are much more abundant in humans than in mice (about 40% of human L chains versus about 5% in mice). Furthermore, four isotypic forms of human λ chains have been characterized, known by their original serologic designation as Kern−Oz−, Kern−Oz+, Kern+Oz−, and Mcg; several other variants have been described, perhaps representing allelic polymorphisms.

Seven human Jλ-Cλ segments are clustered within an approximately 33-kb region of DNA that has been entirely sequenced (147–149). As shown in Fig. 9, genes for the four major expressed human λ isotypes have been localized within the major cluster and correspond to JCλ1, JCλ2, JCλ3, and JCλ7. The remaining three homologous J-C segments are apparently pseudogenes, with either in-frame stop codons or frame-shifting deletions. However, JCλ6 may be functional in some individuals (150), and the common allele—which has a 4-bp insertion leading to a deletion of the C-terminal third of the Cλ region—can nevertheless undergo Vλ-Jλ recombination, encoding a truncated protein that can associate with H chains (151). A variety of polymorphic variants of the human λ locus have been detected, apparently the result of gene duplication; as shown in Fig. 9, one to three extra λ segments have been detected on Southern blots of human DNA (152).

Three Cλ-related sequences have been discovered near the major Jλ-Cλ cluster. One of these, designated λ14.1, represents the human homolog of the murine surrogate L chain λ5. Finally, an additional weakly hybridizing DNA segment outside the linked cluster has been characterized as a processed pseudogene (153). V genes of the human λ system have been completely characterized, as discussed in a later section.

λ-Related Surrogate Light Chains

Immunoglobulin μ H chains can be detected on the surface of pre-B cells that do not make L chains. However, in mature B cells,

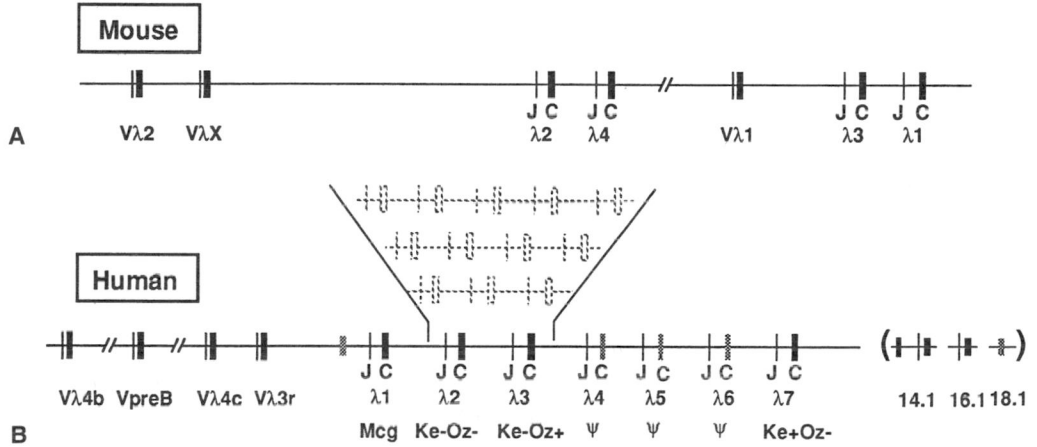

FIG. 9. Germline λ genes. The maps in this figure are schematic, i.e., not to scale. **A:** The murine λ gene system includes four JC complexes and three V genes, which have been characterized in two unlinked contig (sets of overlapping clones) as shown. **B:** The human λ locus has been characterized by complete sequence analysis. The human VpreB surrogate L-chain gene is located within the Vλ cluster. The Cλ locus includes a segment of seven JC complexes plus three additional unlinked sequences. The hatched JC complexes diagrammed above the seven linked λ sequences represent polymorphic variants with additional duplications of the JC unit as deduced from Southern blots. The 14.1 sequence—the human λ5 surrogate L chain homolog—lies downstream from the JC cluster but its location relative to the other I-like sequences is not known. Exon 1 of the 14.1 gene is homologous to a exon upstream from Jλ1 (*gray rectangle*).

Ig H chains cannot reach the cell surface if L-chain synthesis is interrupted. What allows the expression of surface H chain in pre-B cells in the absence of L chain?

The first clues to this question were uncovered in a search for genes whose expression is specific to the pre-B stage of lymphocyte development. Melchers and colleagues identified one such gene that demonstrated striking sequence similarity to the J and C regions of the λ locus; they named it λ5 because four murine Cλ genes were already known (154,155). The genomic λ5 gene includes three exons (Fig. 10): exon 1, which appears to encode a signal peptide; exon 2, whose 3′ end is homologous to Jλ; and exon3, homologous to Cλ. When flanking regions of the genomic λ5 clone were tested as probes against pre-B cell mRNA, another transcribed segment was found about 4.7 kb 5′ from λ5 (156). (Fig. 10.) Sequence analysis of the latter region showed similarities to both Vλ and Vκ; for this reason (and because of its expression in pre-B cells) it is called VpreB1. A second, nearly identical sequence in the mouse genome is named VpreB2 (157) and appears to be functional (158); a less similar VpreB3 also has been described (159). Neither λ5 nor VpreB genes show evidence of gene rearrangement in B or pre-B cells. Both genes have typical consensus splice sites and initiation and termination codons and have no apparent defects that would prevent their expression as proteins. That they are expressed and serve an important role is suggested by the conservation of homologs in every mammalian species examined.

Evidence strongly supports the notion that these genes encode surrogate L chains (SLCs) that associate with μ H chains to permit surface μ expression before the availability of L chains. Thus, when a μ H-chain gene was transfected into an Ig-negative myeloma line, no surface μ expression was observed unless λ5 and VpreB genes were also transfected (160). The surface μ chains were found to be covalently linked to the 22-kDa product of the λ5 gene, whereas the 16-kDa VpreB product was noncovalently associated. A similar complex is observed in pre-B cell lines and in normal bone marrow pre-B cells (161). The V-like VpreB gene product [also known as ι (162)] apparently associates with the Cλ-like λ5 product (also known as ω) to form an L chain-like heterodimer that can fulfill some functions of a true L chain.

One likely role for a μ-SLC complex is suggested by the observation that most Vκ-Jκ recombination occurs only in cells expressing a functional μ H chain (as discussed more fully in the section on regulation of V(D)J recombination); apparently μ-SLC expression on the cell surface can trigger the onset of Vκ-Jκ rearrangement. Evidence for this view comes from experiments in which a pre-B line that normally does not rearrange its κ locus was transfected with a construct encoding the membrane form of μ H chain (163); when the transfected μ gene was expressed in a complex containing VpreB and λ5, Vκ rearrangement was induced. In contrast, surface expression of a deleted μ gene (μΔm)—which lacked VH and CH1 and which did not associate with SLC—was ineffective in inducing Vκ rearrangement unless the μΔm protein was crosslinked by an anti-μ antibody. These results suggest that the SLC may facilitate cross-linking of surface μ chains in pre-B cells, a necessary step before the B cell can proceed to Vκ rearrangement, L-chain synthesis and mature Ig production. Further support for such a critical role is discussed later in this chapter.

Human homologs of both λ5 and VpreB have been cloned. Three λ5-like sequences are located downstream from the Cλ cluster on chromosome 22 (164), but only one (designated 14.1) appears to be functional, possessing the three-exon structure of λ5 (165–167). Interestingly, a sequence upstream of Jλ1 is homologous to exon 1 of 14.1/λ5, suggesting that 14.1 and Jλ-Cλ1 may have had a common ancestral gene that could be expressed in either of two ways: (a) by rearranging its J-like exon 2 with a V-region gene, like modern λ genes; or (b) without rearrangement, using exon 1, with the encoded protein assembling with a noncovalently linked VpreB-like subunit. The human VpreB homolog lies within the Vλ cluster (168), in contrast to murine VpreB, which lies close upstream of λ5.

V GENE ASSEMBLY RECOMBINATION

The mechanism by which germline variable-region constituents (VL and JL, or VH, D, and JH) assemble in the DNA to form a complete active V gene has been pursued ever since Ig gene recombination was first discovered. In this section we address (a) the topology of the recombinations from a "macro" viewpoint, (b) the components of the recombinase machinery (a "micro" view), and (c) the regulation of that machinery in B-cell development.

Topology of V Assembly Recombination

Deletion Versus Inversion

The earliest model for Vκ-Jκ rearrangement assumed that V segments and J segments were all oriented in the same direction of transcription and that the DNA between the recombining V and J segments was simply excised and lost from the cell (Fig.11A). However, Southern blotting of a panel of myelomas and normal κ-bearing lymphocytes showed that some cells had retained the DNA just upstream from Jκ1, a region that should have been absent from all chromosomes that underwent deletional recombination (169). Although several complex models were proposed to explain such results, the presently accepted explanation is simple: some Vκ genes are oriented in the opposite direction from the Jκ-Cκ region. This topology would allow the VJ recombination to occur by an inversion of the DNA between the recombining V and J segments (Fig. 11B), leaving the DNA upstream from Jκ1 retained on the chromosome. The same recombinase machinery can presumably rearrange the germline elements by either inversion or deletion—depending on the relative orientations of the sequences—because

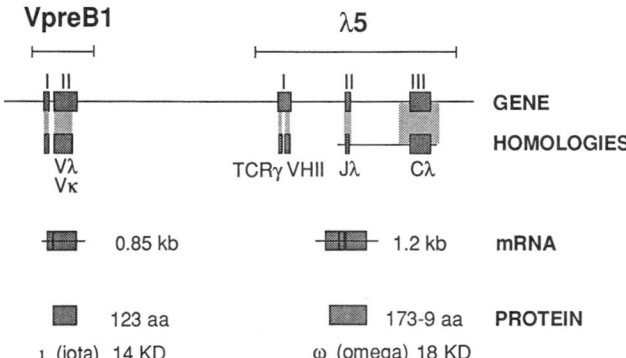

FIG. 10. λ-related genes that encode a surrogate L chain. The top line of the diagram portrays the exons of the VpreB1 gene and the λ5 gene of the mouse, which have been physically linked as shown. The second line shows sequence similarity relationships with other known Ig or TCR sequences. The expressed mRNAs and proteins that have been detected from these two genes are shown below.

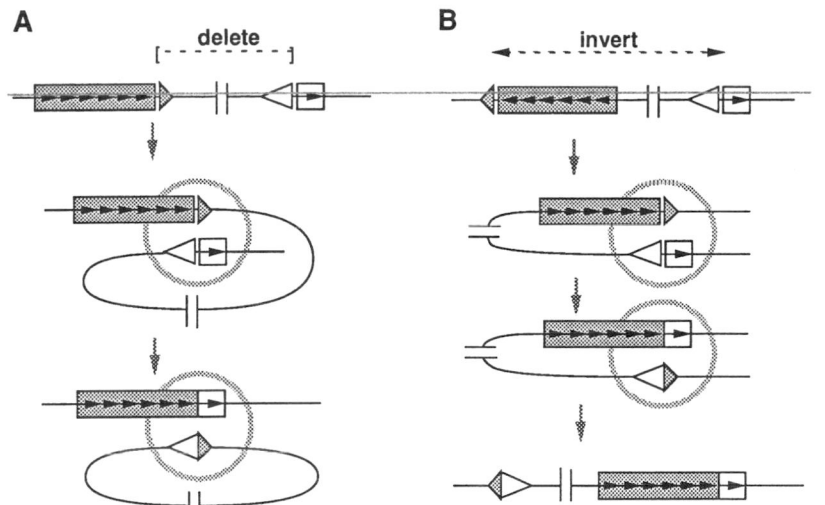

FIG. 11. The same micro mechanism of recombination can join Vκ and Jκ by deletion or inversion, depending on the relative orientation of the two precursors in germline DNA. **A:** When the V coding sequence (*shaded rectangle*) and the J coding sequence (*white rectangle*) are oriented in the same 5'→3' direction in germline DNA (*internal arrowheads*), the recombination yields a VJ coding joint plus a DNA circle containing the signal joint (*apposed triangles*). **B:** If V is oriented in the opposite direction in germline DNA, then an identical recombination reaction at the micro level (*inside shaded circle*) leaves the signal joint linked to the recombined VJ coding joint.

this enzymatic machinery "sees" only the DNA in the immediate vicinity of the recombination site (circled in Fig. 11) and is insensitive to the topology of the DNA strands far from this site. One implication of this model (Fig. 11B) is that cells that have undergone an inversional Vκ-Jκ recombination should retain on the chromosome a recombination joint with two sets of signal sequences—the RSS from downstream of the Vκ and the RSS from upstream of the Jκ segment joined together. Indeed such signal joints (also known as flank products and reciprocal joints) have been detected in several cell lines (170–172). In contrast to the flexibility observed in the position of the recombination breakpoint in the VJ segment (the coding joint), the sequences of signal joints usually show the J-derived 7-mer joined directly to the V-derived 7-mer, without even a single intervening nucleotide between them. Surprisingly, the signal joints retained on the expressed chromosome have almost always been derived from Jκ1. As additional evidence that inversion can occur in Vκ-Jκ recombinations, several laboratories (173,174) have reported that engineered gene constructs carrying Vκ and Jκ recombination signals in opposite orientation can undergo recombination by inversion when transfected into a B-lymphoid cell line.

The idea that some germline Vκ genes are oriented opposite to the Jκ-Cκ locus has been directly verified for the most J-proximal human Vκ gene segments and for one of the two large duplications in the human Vκ locus, as discussed in a later section. For the mouse Vκ locus, less is known about V orientation; but the observation of signal joints that are retained on the chromosome in murine cells can most easily be explained by inverted murine Vκ genes (175). On the other hand, in the H chain or lambda loci there is no evidence for inverted V genes or retained signal joints, so these loci probably recombine only by deletion.

When the recombination occurs by deletion, the model of Fig. 11A suggests that a signal joint is formed on a circular DNA molecule; such a DNA circle would not be attached to the main chromosome and, lacking an origin of replication and a centromere, would be expected to be lost from the progeny of the cell in which the recombination took place. Nevertheless, by isolating circular DNA from cells that are undergoing Vκ-Jκ rearrangement, it has been possible to detect the predicted molecules bearing signal joints (176), supporting the model.

Secondary Recombinations

A final issue for consideration of V assembly topology at the macro-level concerns secondary V gene recombinations. As discussed in an earlier section, the flexibility of VJ or VDJ joining causes nonproductive out-of-frame recombination with high frequency. A B-lymphocyte that rearranged its κ genes nonproductively on both parental chromosomes might be thought to have no further avenue for making a functional L chain; but the availability of upstream V genes and downstream J segments could allow additional recombinations to occur, as shown in Fig. 12A. More complex events are possible as a consequence of the inverted orientation of some Vκ genes. The occurrence of such secondary recombinations has in fact been reported for κ genes (172) and would be implied by the recovery of chromosomal signal joints that are not reciprocal to coding joints in the same cells. The preponderance of Jκ1-derived nonreciprocal flank products observed in myelomas may result from initial nonproductive recombinations between this J segment and inverted V genes, followed by successive recombinations involving more downstream J segments; by the time a productive rearrangement occurs, many myelomas will carry signal joint relics of earlier recombinations involving Jκ1 (177). In addition to lymphocytes with nonproductive VκJκ junctions on both chromosomes, cells that have assembled a productive VκJκ joint may undergo secondary recombination if the resulting VH-VL pair recognizes an autoantigen; this type of secondary recombination, known as receptor editing, is considered in more detail later in this chapter.

For H-chain genes the possibility of secondary recombination might seem to be ruled out by the fact that a VDJ rearrangement must eliminate all the 12-bp spaced signal elements from the VH locus because these elements are deleted on both sides of the D region that is retained in the recombined VDJ unit, and from all the germline D segments eliminated by the VD and DJ recombination events (Fig. 12B). Secondary DJ rearrangements should be possible before VHD recombination removes unrearranged upstream DH segments (Fig. 12B) and indeed this has been shown to occur (178). Of greater functional interest has been the demonstration (179) that upstream germline VH genes can recombine with an established VDJ unit, displacing the originally assembled V gene. This type of

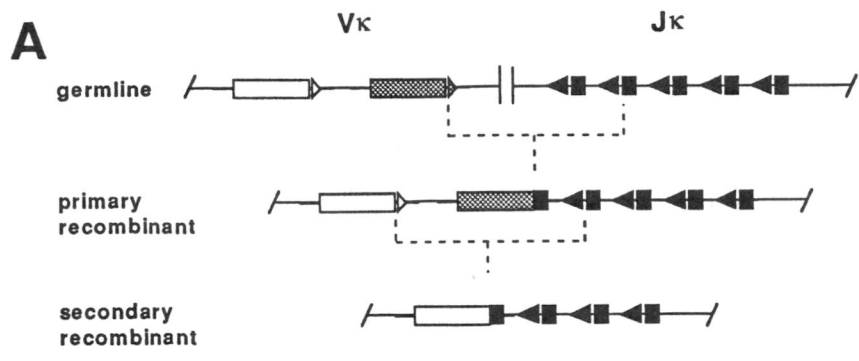

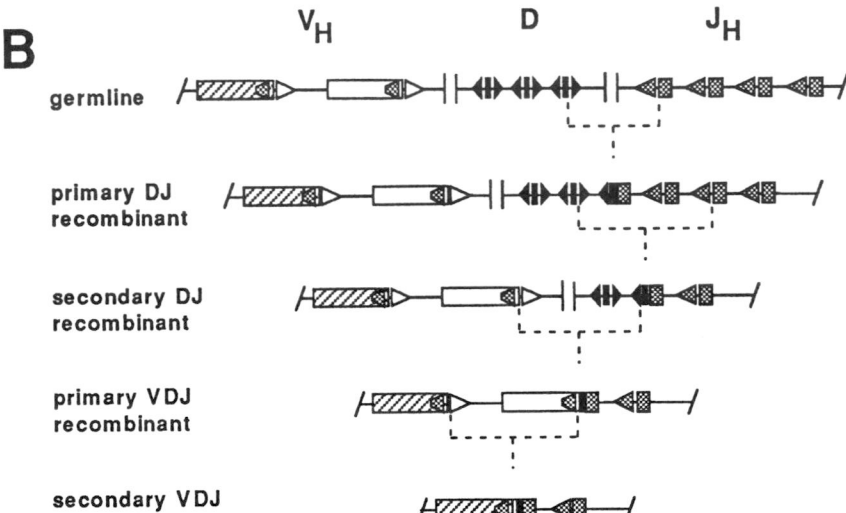

FIG. 12. Secondary recombinations. A: In the κ L-chain system, a primary recombination can be followed by recombination between an upstream V and a downstream J. B: Analogous secondary recombinations can occur in the H-chain system between upstream D and downstream J segments. After VDJ recombination eliminates all short spacer signal elements from the chromosome, secondary recombination can still occur between VH (long spacer signal) and an internal heptamer within the VH coding sequence of the VDJ unit.

recombination is apparently mediated by a sequence that closely matches the consensus signal 7-mer and that appears near the 3' end of the coding region in about 70% of VH genes (Fig. 12B) (179,180). The internal 7-mer is not found in most L-chain genes. After VH replacement, the few nucleotides remaining from the originally assembled VH could potentially contribute to diversity; such nucleotides would be difficult to distinguish from N-region nucleotides. Secondary recombination thus represents an escape mechanism for cells with nonproductive rearrangements on both H-chain chromosomes, or, as alluded to above, for cells whose antibody encodes an autoantigen (181); it is not known, however, how frequently such escapes occur in these circumstances, as opposed to the alternative path of cell death. The fact that the isolated 7-mer is apparently able to function in VH replacement recombinations without an associated 9-mer again suggests that the 7-mer is the more critical recombination signal, although it has been suggested that an additional consensus sequence upstream of the internal 7-mer (181) may contribute to VH replacement recombination.

A Micro View of the Mechanism of V Assembly Recombinase Machinery

As mentioned earlier, the same recombinase machinery is believed to mediate V gene assembly recombinations of all four types in the Ig gene systems (κ, λ, and VH-D and D-JH) as well as similar events in the four TCR gene loci. This belief is based on the observation that all these systems share the same 7-mer/9-mer RSS and follow the same 12/23 spacer rule of recombination. Furthermore, gene constructs designed to test in vitro recombination of TCR gene segments were found to be accurately recombined when transfected into B cells. The severe combined immunodeficient (SCID) mouse strain was found to have a deficiency in recombination of both Ig and TCR genes, suggesting that both systems could be affected by a single gene defect (182). Finally, the two recombination activating genes, RAG-1 and RAG-2, have been found to be key mediators of both Ig and TCR gene recombination. The assumption that the same recombinase machinery operates on these two gene families has allowed investigators to pool knowledge concerning the mechanism of the recombination gained from studies of both systems. On the other hand the assumption of a common recombinase raises the question of how B cells preferentially rearrange Ig genes (and T cells TCR genes) when both gene systems are available to be rearranged by the common recombinase in both cell lineages; this issue will be addressed later in this section. The mechanism of V gene assembly has been investigated by several different strategies: sequence analysis of normal substrates and products (germline and recombined DNA), the use of plasmid substrate constructs capable of recombination after transfection into lymphoid cells (in order to assess the effects of alterations in the substrate sequences), the study of presumed intermediates in the enzymatic reaction, purification of proteins that bind to RSS motifs or that perform enzymatic functions hypothesized to occur during the recombination, studies of mutations that affect the efficiency or fidelity of VDJ recombination, and, ultimately, cell-free in vitro studies using cell extracts or putative components of the recombination machinery.

Recombination Model

A model for the detailed mechanism of the recombination event must account for the observed features of the recombination products—the coding and signal joints—and of their germline precursors. The features in the germline precursors that appear necessary and sufficient for recombination are the 7-mer and 9-mer RSS with appropriate spacing (12 and 23 bp); model substrates containing these elements are competent to undergo recombination even in the absence of normal V, D, or J coding regions, although the efficiency of recombination can be influenced by features of the sequences replacing the coding regions. As for the products, the features of the signal joints are relatively simple: the 7-mers are joined "back-to-back," with only rare additions or deletions. The features of the coding joints are more complex, due to the flexibility of junctions as discussed earlier:

1. A variable number of bases are deleted from the ends of the coding regions (in comparison with the "complete" sequence in the germline precursor).
2. Nongermline nucleotides (N regions) unrelated to the germline precursor sequences are added in some coding joints; these are generally rich in G and C nucleotides.
3. Less frequently, extra bases are added that can be interpreted as P nucleotides; these are nucleotides that are joined to the end of an undeleted coding sequence and that form a palindrome (P) with that sequence end (183,184). P nucleotides are generally only 1 or 2 bp, but they can be longer, especially in mice with the SCID defect (185).

The recombination model first proposed by Alt and Baltimore (186) accommodates many of these observations and, with some recent modifications, can serve as a framework for consideration of the recombination mechanism (Fig. 13). The recombination is thought to begin with binding of components of the enzymatic recombinase machinery to the 7-mer–9-mer RSS adjacent to the two segments to be recombined. Both DNA segments are then cleaved at the border of the two 7-mers (a reaction now known to be catalyzed by the RAG genes). The two 7-mer ends are joined together without modification, but the ends that will form the coding joint (which are now known to exist transiently in the form of a "hairpin" loop) are digested to varying extents by an exonuclease activity. Variable numbers of nucleotides may be added to the 3′ ends through the action of terminal deoxynucleotide transferase (TdT). Then the 5′ ends are filled in by a DNA polymerase and the resulting flush ends are ligated together, completing the recombination event.

In Vitro Experiments to Investigate Substrates and Products

Investigations of the recombination mechanism have been advanced by the development of methods for following these events in vitro. Some experiments have exploited the ability of the Abelson murine leukemia virus (AMuLV) to selectively transform

pre-B cells without abolishing the active V gene assembly characteristic of this stage of lymphoid development. Several AMuLV lines have been cloned and then repeatedly subcloned in order to follow the progression of recombination events (187–189). Particularly valuable information has been gained by transfecting AMuLV lines, as well as other lymphoid and nonlymphoid cells, with artificial gene constructs capable of undergoing V(D)J recombination. Several such constructs have been designed with selectable markers whose expression depends on a recombination event. For example, Lewis et al. (190) used a retroviral construct in which a drug-resistance gene was placed between Jκ and Vκ sequences such that the gene could be expressed only after inversional VJ recombination. In another strategy, Lieber et al. (191) transfected various cell lines with a plasmid containing an ampicillin resistance gene (Amp^r) plus a chloramphenicol resistance gene (Cam^r) whose expression was blocked by a stop codon flanked by two V(D)J recombination signal sequences. In B cells, recombination between the two signal sequences deletes the stop codon, allowing expression of the Cam^r gene. When extrachromosomal circles are recovered from the cells and transfected into bacteria, the extent of recombination can be determined by the ratio of transformed Amp^r bacteria that are Cam^r. Depending on the orientation of the signal sequences in the starting construct, the recombination products represent coding or signal joints. These joints can be recovered efficiently from the Cam^r colonies for analysis; the sequences of these joints have all the characteristics of natural recombination products. One interesting outcome from such experiments was the discovery that pre-B and pre-T cells from SCID mice were capable of recombination to form signal joints but were markedly defective in their ability to join coding ends to form coding joints (192).

Indeed, from recombined engineered substrates, certain nonstandard joints also have been recovered, which, although not contributing to physiologic V gene assembly, may reflect features of the recombination mechanism (193). These nonstandard joints can be understood by appreciating that there are three topologies in which DNA that has been cut twice—generating four ends—can be rejoined. If the four ends are coding(V), signal(V), signal(J), and coding(J), the three possibilities can be defined by considering the three different ends that may join to the coding(V) end (assuming that the remaining two ends must join to each other). The possibilities are as follows:

1. coding(V)–coding(J) plus signal(V)–signal(J). This is the standard reaction product in which the coding(V)–coding(J) product encodes the assembled VJ gene and the signal(V)–signal(J) represents the signal joint.
2. coding(V)–signal(V) plus signal(J)–coding(J). These products (open and shut joints) look like the starting DNAs but can be distinguished from them if nucleotides have been added or deleted at the junctions so that they no longer hybridize to oligonucleotide probes specific for the coding/signal junction.
3. coding(V)–signal(J) plus signal(V)–coding(J). These are hybrid joints, in which the signal ends have switched places.

The fact that all these recombinations can occur readily in the transfected construct DNA—which contains little Ig gene sequence beyond the DNA immediately flanking the V and J—suggests that neither a specific chromosomal location nor extensive flanking sequences are necessary for the recombination.

The critical characteristics of the signal sequences have been explored using transfected constructs carrying various mutations (194,195). These experiments have verified the importance of the 7-

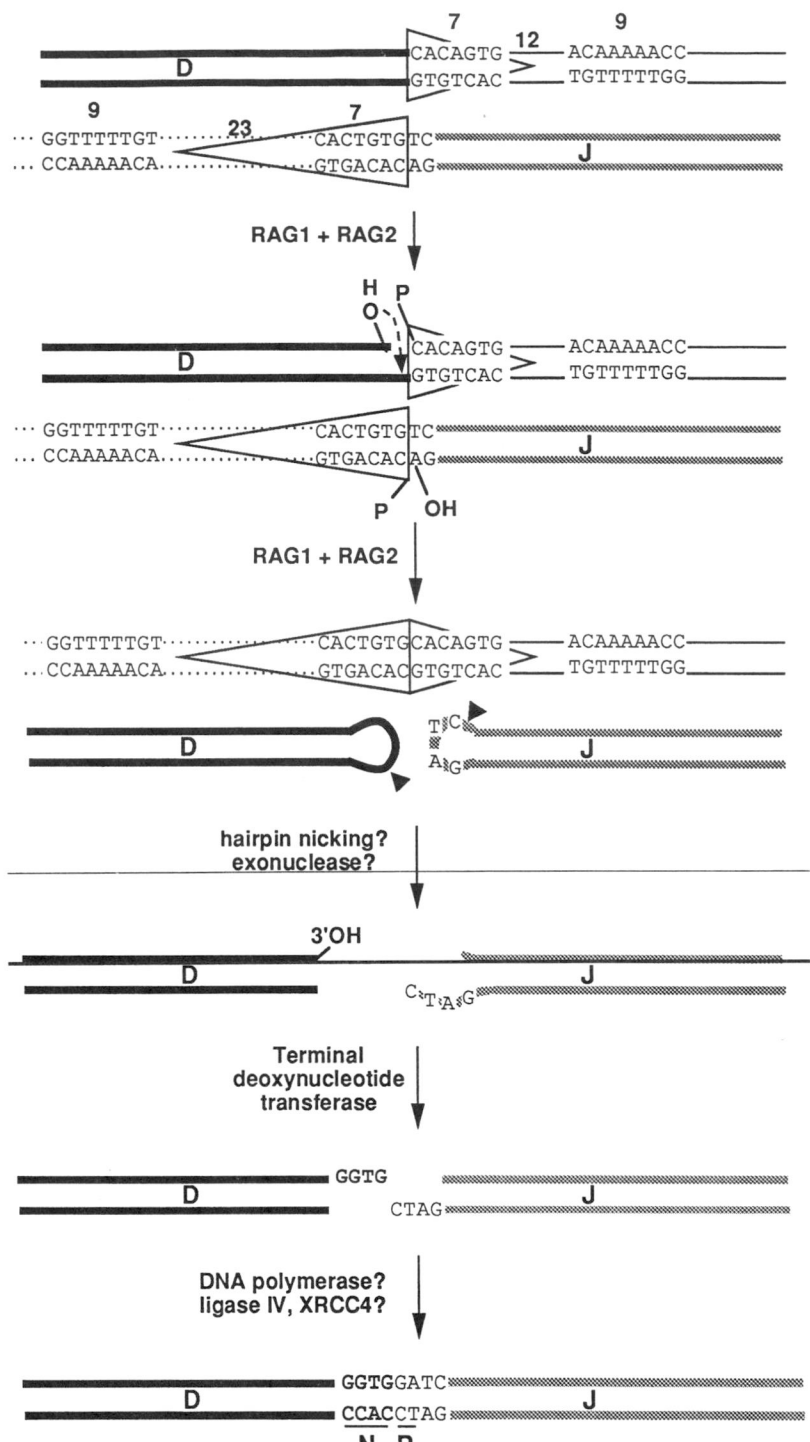

FIG. 13. Model for V assembly recombinations. All V assembly recombination reactions (in Ig and TCR genes) may proceed by a common mechanism, illustrated here by D-J recombination. The RSS 7-mers are depicted in triangles, which is the conventionally used RSS graphic. Hairpin loops are created on coding ends dependent on the action of RAG1 and RAG2.

This reaction also generates two signal ends, which are ligated together. In the example shown here, after the opening of the hairpin loops on the coding ends, the D coding sequence is nibbled by exonuclease, whereas the J coding sequence is spared and instead shows P nucleotide generation due to asymmetric hairpin cleavage. N-region addition is pictured in this example as occurring only on the D-region end, but in reality, exonuclease digestion and N nucleotide addition can occur on either (or both) coding ends. The steps in the proposed mechanism are discussed in the text.

mer/9-mer sequences and have shown that the spacer sequences are not critical as long as the spacer length (12 or 23 bp) is maintained. The 7-mer appears especially important, with the 3 bp closest to the coding sequence being most critical for signaling recombination. Recombination activity could be detected in a variety of pro-B and pre-B cells as well as pre-T lines, but was virtually absent in mature B and T cells and in cells of nonlymphoid lineages (191).

P Regions and Hairpin Intermediates

To study intermediates in V(D)J recombination, Roth et al. (196,197) designed a Southern blot strategy to detect double-strand breaks in the TCR δ locus between D and J, and applied this strategy to DNA from newborn murine thymus cells, which actively rearrange the TCR δ locus. Compared with DNA from adult liver, additional bands were found in the newborn thymus DNA, representing DNA fragments extending from a D-derived 7-mer on one end to a J-derived 7-mer on the other end. In order to characterize the sequence of the signal ends in detail, several laboratories have used ligation-mediated PCR (LM-PCR). This technique involves ligating the blunt genomic signal ends with a double-stranded oligonucleotide, followed by amplification extending from a primer sequence near the genomic signal end to the added oligonucleotide sequence; amplified products can then be cloned and their sequence determined. LM-PCR analyses of both TCR and Ig genes have defined the signal ends as blunt-ended cuts, usually exactly at the 7-mer border, leaving 5' phosphate and 3' hydroxyl groups (198,199).

In their original Southern blot assays, Roth et al. detected the signal ends from these cuts at levels representing about 2% of the thymus DNA; but the coding ends could not be visualized at all, perhaps because of rapid processing of these ends into coding joints. Based on the known defect of SCID lymphocytes in forming coding joints, Roth et al. (196) reasoned that SCID thymocytes might accumulate the cut coding ends that could not be visualized in normal thymocytes. Indeed, coding ends were detected in the SCID thymocyte DNA and, moreover, were found to have several properties suggestive of a hairpin-like structure. First, the coding ends in SCID thymocyte DNA were resistant to exonuclease treatment. Furthermore, restriction fragments bearing these in vivo–generated ends on one side were found to move on a denaturing electrophoresis gel as if they were twice as long as predicted from the size of the double-stranded fragment before denaturation. Finally, LM-PCR experiments failed to detect the coding ends unless they were pretreated with a single strand–specific endonuclease, consistent with the impossibility of ligation to a hairpin unless it was first opened. The sequences of LM-PCR products obtained after endonuclease treatment suggested that the hairpins contained the entire sequence of the coding element, without loss or gain of a single nucleotide (200).

One interpretation of these hairpin ends in the SCID DNA is that they represent normal V(D)J recombination intermediates that—in wild-type cells—are opened at variable positions within the hairpin loop by an endonuclease activity that is dependent on the normal allele of the SCID gene. P nucleotides could then result from opening the loop at an asymmetric position (Fig. 13); this model would explain the absence of P nucleotides from coding ends that have been "nibbled" after opening of the hairpin. The unusually long P nucleotide segments observed in the rare coding joints assembled in SCID mice might then be interpreted as resulting from resolution of hairpins by nonspecific nicking enzymes that, unlike the exonuclease activity dependent on the normal allele of the SCID gene, do not focus on the hairpin loops

but nick in variable positions in the double-stranded hairpin "stem" (196).

In support of the notion that the hairpin coding ends are intermediates in normal VJ recombination, Ramsden and Gellert (201), using LM-PCR, were able to detect such ends in a normal (non-SCID) B-lymphoid line engineered to sustain a high level of κ gene recombination. In this line, broken Jκ1 signal ends were detectable in amounts corresponding to 30% to 40% of the κ loci present. Coding ends were observed at 10- to 100-fold lower abundance, with both hairpin and open ends. The observed kinetics were consistent with simultaneous production of signal ends and hairpin coding ends, with rapid processing of hairpins to open coding ends and then to coding joints, but slower ligation of signal ends. This model is further supported by the observation that linear DNA molecules with hairpins at both ends can, after transfection into B-cell lines, be recovered as recircularized molecules, with the frequent creation of P insertions (202). Interestingly, SCID B cells perform about as well as normal B cells in this assay, suggesting that the protein missing in SCID cells is not the hairpin nicking enzyme itself, but rather an activity that makes natural endogenous hairpin coding ends available to the enzyme; these endogenous ends may require such an activity because of their association with recombinase or other chromosomal proteins, whereas transfected hairpins free of attached proteins may be accessible independent of the protein missing in SCID. The molecular basis of the SCID defect is considered in more detail below.

In Vitro Cell-Free VDJ Recombinase Activities

In attempts to discover components of the VDJ recombination machinery, several groups have studied endonuclease activities from lymphoid sources that cleave DNA selectively near the 7-mer element (203–205); but these experiments have not led to any breakthroughs, and it presently seems unlikely that any of these activities represent components of the recombinase.

RAG Genes

A rather unlikely experiment has led to a major breakthrough: the identification of two genes whose products are apparently critical for V(D)J recombination in B- and T-lineages. Schatz and Baltimore (206) stably transfected fibroblasts with a construct containing a selectable marker whose expression was dependent on VDJ recombination; as expected, no measurable recombination occurred in this nonlymphoid cell. However, when either human or murine genomic DNA was transfected into these fibroblasts, a small fraction of recipient cells stably expressed recombinase activity, activating the selectable marker. This suggested that a single transfected genomic DNA fragment was able to confer recombinase activity in a fibroblast. After successive rounds of transfection and selection for recombinase activity, the critical genomic fragment was identified. This fragment turned out to contain two genes, designated RAG-1 and RAG-2. These genes are not homologous to each other, and neither is strikingly similar to any other known genes, although a weak relationship between RAG-1 and a topoisomerase has been suggested. Both genes are required for activity; therefore, these genes would not have been discovered by this transfection technique if they had been situated too far apart in the genome for both to be transferred on a single DNA fragment. The genes are notable for having no introns in most species (certain fish are exceptions) and for their close association and opposite transcriptional orientation in all species examined. The close proximity of these two genes related by function but not by sequence has led to the speculation that they might have arisen from a more primitive viral or fungal recombination system (207), as discussed later in this chapter.

A crucial role for the RAG genes in V assembly recombination is supported by the conservation of these genes in a variety of Ig-producing vertebrate species, from humans to sharks (208), whereas RAG homologs have not been identified in any species that does not demonstrate Ig V gene assembly recombination. RAG-1 and RAG-2 are expressed together in pre-B and pre-T cells, specifically at the stages expressing V(D)J recombinase activity. Moreover, mouse strains in which either gene has been eliminated by homologous recombination (gene knockouts) have no mature B or T cells as the apparent result of abrogation of V(D)J recombination (209,210). Recently a subset of human patients with a SCID syndrome and no B-lymphocytes were found to have mutations in RAG genes (211).

Attempts to demonstrate activities of the RAG proteins on recombination substrates in vitro were hampered by poor solubility of the proteins, but functional analyses of mutated RAG genes—using RAG expression vectors cotransfected with recombination substrate plasmids into fibroblasts—showed that surprisingly large segments of both proteins can be deleted without eliminating recombinase activity (212); and some of the deleted proteins were soluble and could be handled relatively easily as fusion proteins. This work allowed the demonstration that in a cell-free in vitro system the two RAG proteins together can perform cleavage of substrate DNAs as well as hairpin formation on the coding end (213). The reaction occurs in two steps: first a nick occurs on one strand adjacent to the heptamer—the top strand as drawn in Fig. 13—then the 3' hydroxyl created at the nick causes transesterification by nucleophilic attack on the phosphodiester bond adjacent to the 7-mer on the bottom strand (Fig. 13), yielding a hairpin on the coding end and a new 3' hydroxyl on the 3' end of the bottom 7-mer strand (214). This transesterification mechanism is consistent with the observation that the formation of the new phosphodiester bond in the hairpin occurs in the absence of external energy source such as ATP, apparently using the energy inherent in the phosphodiester bond broken in the nucleophilic attack. The stereochemistry observed in the reaction suggests that no phosphodiester linkage to protein occurs as an intermediate, such as occurs in bacteriophage lambda integration; instead the direct transesterification mechanism resembles the μ transposition and retroviral integration, which can both produce hairpins under certain experimental conditions (214).

The actions of the RAG proteins were found to be dependent on divalent ions in the medium (215,216). In Mn^{2+} the RAG proteins catalyzed cleavage of substrates with a single RSS; but in Mg^{2+} cleavage required two RSSs and occurred most efficiently if the substrate conformed to the 12/23 rule regarding the spacing between 7-mer and 9-mer elements; thus, this rule may be a result of RAG protein specificity, although other proteins also seem to contribute to 12/23 specificity, perhaps by promoting an optimal molecular architecture (217). In Ca^{2+} the RAG proteins and a radiolabeled DNA substrate containing an RSS formed a stable complex that was apparent in an electrophoretic mobility shift assay (EMSA) and was stable to competition with unlabeled substrate, but the substrate was not nicked or cleaved. However, when Mg^{2+} was added to the stable complex, substrate cleavage occurred. (Interestingly, in the presence of Ca^{2+} human immunodeficiency virus (HIV) integrase and μ transposase also form similar stable complexes in which substrate DNA is bound but no cleavage

occurs.) The Ca^{2+}-mediated binding of RAG proteins to substrate DNA was decreased 10-fold by the elimination of the 9-mer from the RSS, so the RAG proteins must recognize both components of the RSS. In contrast, mutations in the 7-mer that altered the nucleotides closest to the coding region (residues known to be critical for supporting cleavage) had minimal effect on binding. This is consistent with other evidence (218,219), suggesting that these nucleotides, and the adjacent nucleotides in the coding region, may contribute to a local alteration in DNA helix structure that is important for the cleavage reactions. Recently, in vitro experiments have been reported in which RAG proteins supplemented with extracts from several cell lines were able to generate signal joints (220) and coding joints (221,222). In one system, RAG-1 and RAG-2 could be detected in a stable complex containing two signal ends, an HMG (high-mobility group) protein, and perhaps other proteins as well (223). These in vitro VDJ recombination experiments should allow the elucidation of other components required for the reaction, as well as its mechanism.

The double-strand DNA breaks catalyzed by the RAG proteins could be potentially deleterious if they occurred during DNA synthesis or mitosis, but this problem appears to be prevented by tight posttranscriptional regulation of RAG-2 protein levels across the cell cycle. Although the RAG-1 protein and mRNA transcripts of both RAG genes vary little across the cell cycle, a phosphorylation-dependent degradation signal mediates destruction of the RAG-2 protein (224,225), thereby preventing double-strand DNA breaks in the H-chain JH locus from occurring during M, G2, and S (199). The phosphorylation site, a threonine at amino acid 490, falls into a region of the sequence that is highly conserved across species and contains a consensus sequence characteristic of targets of cyclin-dependent kinases. This regulatory region is dispensable for enzymatic activity. In RAG-2 knockout mice carrying a transgenic RAG-2 gene with an alanine replacing the phosphorylatable threonine, RAG-2 protein and double-stranded DNA breaks were found throughout the cell cycle, demonstrating the importance of the RAG-2 degradation signal in cell cycle control of VDJ recombination (226).

Although all the binding and enzymatic activities of the RAG proteins discussed so far have required the presence of both RAG-1 and RAG-2, recent reports have suggested that RAG-1 may bind weakly to the RSS 9-mer in the absence of RAG-2 and that this binding may be mediated by a segment of RAG-1 that bears sequence similarity to the DNA binding domain of bacterial invertases (227,228). Two circumstances have been described in which only one of the two RAG genes is expressed. RAG-1 was reported to be expressed without RAG-2 at low levels in the developing central nervous system (229) (although the RAG-1–deficient mice show no obvious central nervous system defects). Conversely, RAG-2 is expressed without RAG-1 in the chicken bursa of Fabricius (230), which contains B-lineage cells at a developmental stage when their genes have already undergone V(D)J rearrangement and are in the process of being diversified by gene conversion (as discussed later in this chapter). The significance of this finding is unclear at present because RAG-2 is apparently not essential for the gene conversion itself (231).

Apart from the obvious importance of the RAG proteins in mediating the initial steps of VDJ recombination, knowledge of these proteins and their genes has allowed two major technical advances that have opened the way to many additional experiments. One such advance is the availability of the RAG-1 and RAG-2 knockout mice. These mice have no functional B cells or T cells, and are not "leaky" like SCID mice, which develop some functional B and T cells, especially as the animals age. The RAG knockouts can be used to study the importance of the innate immune system (i.e., responses that occur in the absence of antigen-specific lymphocytes) in particular immune responses. The knockouts can be used as recipients for various lymphocyte subsets to explore the roles of different cell types. They can be used to study the signals for B cell development by introducing transgenes with specific functionally recombined Ig genes and characterizing the phenotypes of lymphocytes that develop. Finally, they can be used in RAG complementation experiments designed to assess the phenotype (in lymphocytes) of various other gene knockouts (232). In RAG complementation, embryonic stem (ES) cells in which the gene of interest has been knocked out by homologous recombination are injected into homozygous RAG knockout blastocysts (RAG-/-); this procedure yields chimeric mice in which all B and T cells derive from the engineered ES cells, which are the only source of intact RAG genes to support lymphocyte development. Such animals can be made more easily than a knockout mouse line and can be used to study the effect of gene deletion in lymphocytes independent of effects the deletion may have in other cells. In particular, for cases where the gene knockout causes embryonic lethality due to effects on nonlymphoid cells, RAG complementation allows the selective knockout in lymphocytes to be studied.

The second major technical fallout from the RAG genes is the method for investigating VDJ recombination in nonlymphoid cell lines with well-characterized mutations in genes governing DNA repair; when such lines are transfected with RAG genes, the effects of these gene mutations on VDJ recombination can be assessed.

Components of Later Steps in VDJ Recombination

Clearly the RAG genes are critical for the first steps in VDJ recombination (recognition of RSS, cleavage, and hairpin formation), but additional components are required to complete the reaction; and at least some of these components may function not only in VDJ recombination but also in ubiquitous DNA repair pathways. The first clear example of such a component to be recognized was the murine SCID mutation described above. This mutation was originally identified in a mouse strain that was immunodeficient as a result of a marked impairment in VDJ recombination of both Ig and TCR genes; SCID lymphocytes can perform the RAG-mediated reactions of cleavage and hairpin formation, and can form signal joints, but are markedly defective in coding joint formation. Subsequently it was found that the SCID mutation also blocks the enzymatic mechanism responsible for repair of double-strand DNA breaks—such as those caused by ionizing radiation—in both lymphoid and nonlymphoid cells. This suggested that after RAG-mediated DNA cleavage, lymphocytes may complete the joining reactions using enzymes that function ubiquitously in DNA repair. To test this hypothesis, Taccioli et al. screened panels of Chinese hamster ovary (CHO) cell lines carrying well-characterized defects in DNA repair to see if these lines were impaired in performing VDJ recombination after transfection with the RAG genes (233). Such cells had previously been classified into x-ray cross complementation (XRCC) groups by investigating the outcome when two mutant cell lines are combined to make a somatic hybrid. If such a hybrid shows no DNA repair defect, this implies that the two original cell lines carry different mutations such that the hybrid ends up with a normal copy of each gene (the mutant cell lines cross-complemented one another). Conversely, by definition, cells in the same cross-complementation group are unable to complement each other. Of eight XRCC groups of ionizing radiation-sensitive rodent cell lines, three were known to

be defective in repair of double-strand breaks in DNA (XRCC groups 4, 5, and 7), and all three of these groups were found to be impaired in VDJ recombination after RAG transfection.

The genes mutated in XRCC 5 and XRCC 7 turned out to encode two components of a three-polypeptide complex known as the Ku complex. Originally characterized as the autoantigen recognized by a patient antiserum, Ku is composed of an approximately 70-kDa protein (Ku70) and an approximately 86-kDa protein (Ku86, often called Ku80) which, when heterodimerized, can bind to DNA (234). Then the DNA-Ku heterodimer complex can recruit the third component: an approximately 450-kDa protein with a protein kinase activity that is dependent on binding to DNA (234,234a). Some evidence suggests that DNA-PK can bind DNA even in the absence of Ku (234b). The conservation of Ku genes in drosophila and yeast suggest that the complex evolved long before VDJ rearrangement. Extensive evidence indicates that the gene defective in XRCC 5 encodes Ku80 (235,236), whereas the gene defective in XRCC 7 (which corresponds to the gene mutated in murine SCID) encodes the 450-kDa DNA-PK (237). Although the murine SCID mutation impairs primarily coding joints, this difference is probably a result of residual DNA-PK protein in the SCID cells because a more complete equine DNA-PK mutation impairs both coding and signal joints (238). Ku80 mutant cell lines are also defective in both signal and coding joint formation, as are mice with a knockout of the Ku80 gene (200). Ku70 mutants have not been detected in panels of existing XRCC mutants, but recent evidence indicates that cells with homozygous disruption of Ku70 are also defective in VDJ recombination induced by RAG gene transfection (239).

The Ku complex had previously been studied as an activity with an unusual DNA binding specificity: rather than recognizing particular nucleotide sequences in DNA, it recognizes particular topologic features of DNA, including double-stranded DNA ends (such as might be generated by double-strand breaks caused by x-rays or by recombinases). Once bound to an end, it can translocate down the length of the DNA (240). The Ku heterodimer also has been reported to have an ATP-dependent helicase (DNA-unwinding) activity (241). Several models can be envisioned for the role of this complex in VDJ recombination: the complex may bind to the hairpin coding ends and regulate hairpin opening and DNA degradation by exonucleases; it may participate in destabilizing the DNA double-helix through helicase action; and it may influence recombination by phosphorylating other proteins via the protein kinase activity of DNA-PK. Additional investigation will be necessary to clarify which (if any) of these roles is important for VDJ recombination.

The gene mutated in XRCC group 4 also has been cloned (242). It encodes a ubiquitously expressed protein of about 38 kDa predicted size that is not homologous to any known protein. The protein has recently been found to bind to and activate DNA ligase IV, suggesting that this enzyme is probably important for ligating signal and coding joints in VDJ recombination (243,244). In addition, the XRCC4 protein product interacts with DNA-PK and is phosphorylated by this kinase (244a).

Other Proteins that May Participate in V(D)J Recombination

The RAG proteins, the Ku-DNA-PK complex, and the XRCC 4 protein have all been shown to play a role in VDJ recombination because mutations that compromise these proteins impair the recombination. Various other entities have been proposed as participants in VDJ recombination; some of these are described below, although it is not clear that any of them participate in VDJ recombination.

Several laboratories have sought components of the recombinase machinery by searching for proteins that (a) are present in nuclear extracts from cells early in the B-lineage in which VDJ recombination is occurring and (b) bind in vitro to the 7-mer or 9-mer signal sequences in a sequence-specific manner. Although this would seem a reasonable approach, it is clear that binding to RSS sequences does not necessarily imply a physiologic role in the recombinase reaction. The RAG proteins, which clearly bind to RSS sequences, seem both necessary and sufficient to initiate VDJ recombination, so it is possible that no further RSS-specific components are necessary for the recombinase. An instructive cautionary example is provided by the case of the RSS-binding protein for Jκ (RBP-Jκ). This protein was purified from a murine pre-B cell line on the basis of sequence-specific binding in vitro to a Jκ 7-mer, was found in lymphoid cell lines but not in nonlymphoid lines, and bears sequence homology to bacterial integrases, which reinforced its possible role in a DNA recombination; but more recent studies suggest a function for RBP-Jκ that is unrelated to VDJ recombination (245).

With such caveats in mind, several other candidate participants in VDJ recombination can be mentioned. One protein capable of binding to a probe containing the 7-mer signal element was detected by EMSA in several pre-B cell lines, but not in myeloma, mature T-cell, monocyte, or fibroblast cell lines, consistent with a role for the protein in recombination-competent cells (246). Another RSS-binding protein has been identified by a technique known as Southwestern analysis: a protein extract is subjected to SDS-polyacrylamide gel electrophoresis, blotting onto nitrocellulose, and probing with a radioactive oligonucleotide including the RSS. By this method a 115-kDa protein was detected in extracts of immature B- and T-cell lines, but not in a myeloma line; the binding of this protein seemed markedly reduced when mutations were introduced into either the 7-mer or the 9-mer in the probe (247). Another protein, designated T160, was obtained as a cDNA clone from a protein expression library that was screened with an RSS probe having a 12-bp spacer (248). The T160 gene product, expressed as a fusion protein, was able to bind to the original screening probe but not to a probe with a mutated 7-mer or to a probe with a 23-bp spacer. Another protein has been identified as binding to the 9-mer RSS element but not to several mutated versions of the 9-mer (249). Designated NBP (nonamer binding protein), this 63-kDa protein was purified approximately 20,000-fold from calf thymus. A possibly related protein designated VDJP was identified from a lymphoid cDNA expression library by screening with a Jκ RSS probe (250). The resulting full-length cDNA represents a lymphoid-specific alternative splice form of the ubiquitous replication factor C (RF-C) mRNA; both sequences contain a region homologous to bacterial ligases. In vitro–expressed VDJP protein catalyzes a DNA joining reaction dependent on an RSS sequence in the DNA fragments that are joined (251). However, the substrates and products of this joining reaction differ in many critical respects from Ig genes, so the relevance of this protein to VDJ recombination is uncertain. A protein designated recognition component (Rc) is encoded by a cDNA that was isolated from a cDNA expression library from mouse thymocyte RNA using a radiolabeled RSS as a probe (252). The in vitro–expressed protein binds DNA as multimers, suggesting a possible role in bringing together elements to be joined by VDJ recombinase machinery (253). A 30-kDa protein recognizing both 7-mer and 9-mer of the RSS was detected in immature thymocytes enriched for pre-T cells undergoing VDJ rearrangement (254). A possibly related cDNA clone with homology to DNA helicases, designated lymphoid-specific helicase (lsh), was cloned from fetal thymus (255).

Exonuclease

Many recombined V regions are found to be missing variable numbers of nucleotides at the recombination junctions compared with the coding sequences present in their respective germline V, D, or J precursors. This observation has been proposed to result from exonuclease-induced nibbling of the cut DNA ends during the time between cleavage near the 7-mer RSS and rejoining of the cut DNA ends. Although the responsible exonuclease has been sought (256), and several exonucleases are known to exist in mammalian cells, the specific enzyme that nibbles the ends of V, D, and J segments has not been definitively identified.

N Regions and TdT

Terminal deoxynucleotide transferase, the proposed source of N-region additions, is an enzyme found in thymus and bone marrow, and also is a distinguishing characteristic of lymphoid versus myeloid leukemias. It catalyzes the addition of nucleotides onto the 3′ end of DNA strands. Although no template specificity determines the nucleotides added, the enzyme adds dG residues preferentially. This fact is consistent with a role for this enzyme in the origin of N regions found at the V-D and D-J junctions because these N nucleotides tend to be G-rich at the 3′ ends of both the upstream coding strand and the downstream noncoding strand. Both N-region addition and TdT are characteristically absent from fetal lymphocytes (257). N-region addition is common in H-chain genes but rare in murine L-chain genes, although perhaps less rare in humans (258).

The proposal that N regions result from the action of TdT has received considerable support. Lymphocytes with engineered defects in their TdT genes produced rearranged Ig V regions with almost no N additions (259,260). Conversely, when TdT expression was engineered in cells undergoing κ or λ L-chain rearrangement, the normally low level of N-region insertion in these recombinations was dramatically increased (261–263). This result suggests that the low frequency of N-region sequences in normal κ or λ recombinations is not due to the inability of these coding sequences to accept N-region nucleotides. Instead, the preferential occurrence of N regions in H-chain versus L-chain genes (in mice, at least) reflects TdT levels that are higher in early B-lineage cells undergoing H-chain rearrangement than in the later stage of L-chain recombination; indeed, mice with an engineered mutation that allows premature Vκ-Jκ joining in pro-B cells show an increased frequency of N-region nucleotides in their recombined Vκ genes (264). In normal mice the expression of a μ H chain may downregulate TdT expression (265), contributing to the reduced level during the stage of L-chain recombination.

N regions are also observed in TCR genes, in which they may be particularly significant as a source of sequence diversity in view of the lower germline V diversity and absence of somatic mutation in the TCR gene systems. Although N regions clearly enhance the diversity of Ig and TCR V regions, mice lacking TdT show no significant deficiencies in immune responses (266). The normal phenotype of such mice (apart from the absence of N regions) and the lymphoid-specific expression of TdT in normal mice both support the view that the only function of this enzyme is to diversify V-region genes. In TdT mutant mice, as well as in normal fetal lymphocytes low in TdT activity, absence of N-region addition is associated with an increase in the frequency of recombination junctions in which short stretches of nucleotides could have derived from either germline element because of an overlap of identical sequences at the coding ends. These junctions suggest a recombination intermediate in which the complementary single-stranded regions from the two coding ends hybridize to each other, much as "sticky ends" generated by restriction endonucleases can facilitate ligation of DNA fragments. Such homology-mediated recombination may restrict the diversity of neonatal antibodies. The resulting antibodies possibly are enriched in specificities for commonly encountered pathogens, or have broadened specificity, as has been reported for TCRs lacking N regions (267).

Regulation of V(D)J Recombination

The recombination events that occur among Ig genes must be among the most important events that mark the development of a B-cell clone. Regions of the genome are irrevocably deleted, and commitments are made as to which L-chain isotype and which VL-VH pair will be expressed in subsequent progeny cells. It would be expected that such significant events would be well regulated. Indeed, the observation that each B-cell line generally expresses only one L-chain isotype (isotype exclusion) and uses only one of the two homologous chromosomal loci for H- and L-chain genes (allelic exclusion) implies some form of regulation. Isotype and allelic exclusion ensure that each lymphocyte expresses a single

H_2L_2 combination and thus a single antigen-binding specificity, a crucial feature of the clonal selection model of the immune response. Furthermore, if the same recombinase machinery mediates the V-gene assembly reactions of all the Ig and TCR gene systems, then some mechanism must regulate which gene systems are susceptible to recombination in B-cell versus T-cell development. Current evidence suggests that VDJ recombination is controlled at two levels: regulation of the RAG protein levels and regulation of accessibility of the recombinase machinery to the germline substrates of rearrangement. Because RAG expression and locus accessibility are in turn regulated depending on the stage of B-cell development, a brief scheme of this development is presented below as background; a detailed account is provided in Chapter 6.

B-Lymphocyte Development

Figure 14 illustrates a scheme of B-lymphoid development as elucidated by the following:

1. Analysis of lymphoid malignancies or virally immortalized cells representing different stages of arrested development
2. Purification of subpopulations of normal cells from lymphoid organs by fluorescence-activated cell sorting (FACS), followed by analyses of different subsets

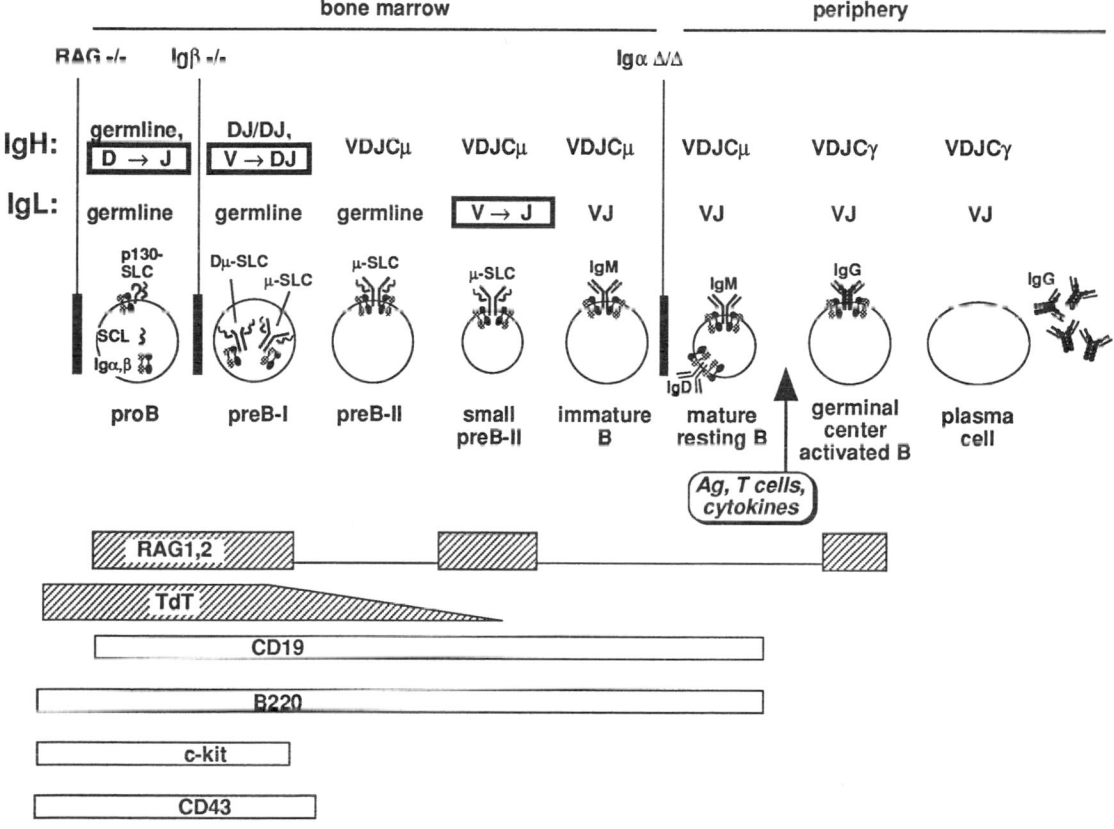

FIG. 14. Ig gene recombination in B-cell development. A simplified scheme of B-cell development is presented as a background for discussion of Ig gene recombination. The stages occurring in the bone marrow versus in the periphery (e.g., lymph nodes, spleen) are shown, along with the status of IgH and IgL genes at each stage. A graphic image depicts the Ig related proteins displayed on the surface at each stage; at the bottom, the stage-dependent expression of RAG genes and TdT—both important in V(D)J recombination—is schematically depicted, as is the expression of several other marker proteins.

3. Phenotypic analysis of mutant mice with defects in various genes critical for progression from one developmental stage to the next

4. Culture of B-cell precursors in vitro using systems that allow developmental progression.

This figure attempts a consensus of schemes from two principal laboratories (268,269). Some known differences between human and mouse B-cell development and surface markers (270) are not reflected in this simplified summary figure.

B- and T-lymphocytes differentiate from pluripotent hematopoietic stem cells in the fetal liver and bone marrow. The primordial lymphoid progenitor has the potential to differentiate into B- or T-lymphocytes or natural killer (NK) cells. Among the earliest markers that indicate B-lineage specificity are the non-Ig components of the pre-B cell receptor (pre-BCR): $Ig\alpha$, $Ig\beta$ and $\lambda 5$ (271). CD19, which functions as a coreceptor in signal transduction, first appears in large proliferating pro-B cells, which also express several other distinguishing surface markers, including c-kit (receptor for the stem cell [growth] factor [SCF]), B220 (a B-lineage form of the phosphatase CD45), TdT, and CD43 (a sialoglycoprotein known as leukosialin). In the absence of H-chain protein, the SLC is displayed on the surface membrane in association with a complex of glycoproteins, represented by a hook shape in Fig. 14, which has sometimes been called a surrogate H chain (272). The next stage, the pre-B cell, is marked by expression of the RAG genes and H-chain rearrangement, as well as loss of c-kit and then CD43 expression. Initially DJ rearrangements occur on both chromosomal loci, producing the preB-I cell; then germline V regions join to complete a VDJ gene (preB-II). The resulting μ protein appears on the B-cell surface along with the SLCs in a pre-BCR or μ-SLC complex that also includes $Ig\alpha$ and $Ig\beta$. The resulting large pre-B cells proliferate, with RAG gene expression downregulated. Then the cells become smaller, stop dividing, turn up RAG gene expression once more, undergo L-chain rearrangement, and express surface IgM (immature B cells). When they eventually also express surface IgD they become mature B cells and migrate into the periphery, ready to be triggered by antigen exposure.

Recombinational Accessibility and Transcription

What maintains the locus specificity of VDJ rearrangement—i.e., why is Ig gene recombination confined to B cells, with H-chain rearrangement before L-chain rearrangement, and why is TCR gene recombination exclusive to T cells? One possible clue is the observation that susceptibility to recombination seems to be correlated with transcriptional activity of germline gene elements. For example, Reth and Alt (273) reported that AMuLV-transformed pre-B cell lines—representing a developmental stage capable of rearranging VH to DJH—synthesize an RNA transcript that includes DJ and Cμ sequence (termed Dμ RNA). Furthermore, many germline VH genes are transcribed at the pre-B cell stage, just at the time when these genes are targets for recombination (274); these transcripts—designated sterile transcripts because they do not encode a functional Ig chain—are not seen in more mature B cells in which H-chain recombination has been terminated (275). Similar sterile transcripts have been reported for other germline Ig gene elements during the period when they are actively rearranging. Susceptibility of a segment of DNA to both transcription and recombination might be a reflection of a common chromosomal state (accessibility) required for both reactions, or transcription itself might be a prerequisite for recombination, perhaps by partially unwinding the DNA. Interestingly, a similar correlation between transcription and recombination has

been reported for the isotype switch of H-chain genes, discussed above, and recombination of yeast mating-type genes.

To further explore the relationship of transcription to recombination, several groups have deleted enhancer regions known to stimulate transcription of the murine κ or H-chain locus and found that recombination of the corresponding locus was substantially reduced. In the κ locus, one enhancer (iEκ) is located in the intron between Jκ and Cκ, and a second enhancer (3'Eκ) is located about 9 kb downstream from Cκ. When homologous recombination in ES cells was used to replace Eκ by a neomycin resistance gene (neo^r), homozygous mutant mice were found to have no κ gene rearrangements (276). It should be noted that another report suggests that replacement by neo^r may impair κ gene recombination more effectively than simple deletion (277). Compared with effects of Eκ elimination, deletion of the 3'Eκ caused a more modest reduction in κ gene rearrangement (278). Similar conclusions on the importance of gene enhancers in supporting recombination have been obtained with transgenic miniloci capable of V(D)J recombination (279) and with similar constructs stably integrated into cell lines competent for V(D)J recombination (280). However, the relationship between transcription and recombination is not simple. One report suggests that in transgenic constructs the 3'κ enhancer actually downregulates recombination (264). And in mouse strains transgenic for another κ minilocus, linkage to a rabbit iEκ substantially increased recombination even though this enhancer is inactive in upregulating transcription in mouse cells (281). Finally, two elements known as KI and KII, which are located just upstream from Jκ1 and have no known enhancer function, appear to be important for Vκ-Jκ recombination because such recombination was substantially inhibited in B cells containing disruptions in these elements, at least under certain conditions (282). Clearly, further investigation will be necessary to clarify how gene recombination is controlled by transcription and chromosomal changes. The further question of how these parameters are themselves regulated is addressed below (with respect to feedback regulation by Ig proteins) and in more detail later in this chapter.

Allelic Exclusion Models

Two general models have been proposed to explain allelic exclusion and isotype exclusion. The stochastic model interprets the observed high frequency of defective rearranged genes as a consequence of the rarity of functional rearrangements; allelic exclusion would follow from the low probability of the coincident occurrence of two rare events in the same cell (283). In this model, the low frequency of λ-producing cells in the mouse would be a stochastic consequence of the smaller repertoire of λ V regions available to rearrange. An alternative to the stochastic model, which might be called the regulated model, was first proposed by Alt and colleagues (284) and has received considerable experimental support. According to this model, the functional rearrangement of an L (or H)-chain gene in a particular B cell would inhibit further L (or H)-chain gene rearrangement in the same cell. If the inhibition occurred promptly after the first functional rearrangement, then two functional Igs could never be produced in the same cell. An initial nonproductive rearrangement would have no inhibitory effect, so recombination could continue until a functional product resulted or until the cell used up all its germline precursors.

Model for Regulated Recombination

As a framework for discussing this model in more detail, Fig. 15 illustrates four hypothetical regulatory influences that could be components of an allelic exclusion control mechanism. As shown in the upper left corner of the figure, the first Ig gene rearrangements that occur in a B-lineage cells join D to JH segments. The resulting DJ junctions are commonly seen on both chromosomes in early B-lineage cells from fetal liver or bone marrow that have been transformed by AMuLV, as well as in pro-B cells isolated from normal bone marrow by flow cytometry (285). Analyses of cells at this early stage consistently show κ and λ genes in germline configuration. The next recombination step is V→DJ. The expected frequency of VDJ joints maintaining the proper triplet reading frame from V to J is about one third, so most VDJ junctions will be nonfunctional. In addition, some rearranged H-chain genes may be nonfunctional despite in-frame VDJ junctions (286) owing to defects in the germline VH sequence. According to the model, if the initial VDJ junction is nonfunctional for any reason, then in the absence of a viable μ protein, H-chain gene recombination can continue on the other chromosome. If the VDJ recombination on the second chromosome is also nonfunctional, then the cell may have reached a dead end, leading to death by apoptosis (gray shape in Fig. 15). The apoptotic fate of such nonproductive cells has been supported by the observation that mice transgenic for the apoptosis suppression gene *bcl-x_L* harbor an expanded population of bone marrow pro-B cells with almost all nonproductive VDJ joints (9). Although secondary rearrangement may rescue some cells with two nonfunctional recombinations, it is not clear how frequently such secondary events occur.

In contrast, if the first V→DJ recombination in a pro-B cell produces a functional VDJ gene, then its expression will lead to the synthesis of μ H chain. This H chain is expressed in the surface of pre-B cells as a pre-BCR in association with the SLCs VpreB and λ5 (as discussed above) and the same Igα-Igβ heterodimer that, in mature B cells, transmits into the cell the activation signal initiated by antigen-induced cross-linking of surface IgM (see Chapter 7). This pre-BCR complex has two regulatory effects: it blocks further H-chain recombination (① in Fig. 15) and it activates κ gene rearrangement (② in Fig. 15). The μ-induced block to further H-

chain rearrangement was initially hypothesized based on the static analysis of myelomas (i.e., as an explanation for observed allelic exclusion), but more recently it has been directly supported by experimental manipulation of Ig genes. When a functionally rearranged μ transgene was inserted into the genome of a mouse strain, it was found to markedly suppress the rearrangement of endogenous H-chain genes in B-lymphocytes (287), suggesting that the protein product of the μ transgene, expressed in pre-B cells, could shut off V(D)J recombination of germline elements in the endogenous IgH locus. A transgene encoding the membrane form of μ (μ_m) was competent to suppress endogenous VDJ recombination, but one encoding only the secreted form (μ_s) was not (288–290), demonstrating that a membrane form of μ protein is required to mediate allelic exclusion. This implication is supported by the observation that allelic exclusion is lost in mouse strains that—due to gene targeting—cannot express the μ membrane exon (291) or functional λ5 protein (292) that is necessary for surface Ig expression; in these animals, individual B cells may carry two productive V(D)J junctions because any μ protein resulting from an initial recombination on one allele cannot assemble on the membrane as a pre-BCR to shut off V→DJ rearrangement of the other allele. The signal for suppressing VDJ recombination appears to be mediated by the Igα-Igβ heterodimer; a μ_m transgene in which critical residues mediating association of μ H chain with this heterodimer were mutated did not suppress endogenous VDJ recombination, but when this transgene was engineered to express the cytoplasmic domain of Igα or Igβ, the resulting chimeric transgenes were able to shut off endogenous VDJ recombination (293,294). The normal pre-BCR–induced shut-off may be mediated in part by downregulation of RAG gene expression (295). This view would be consistent with the levels of RAG gene expression detected in murine bone marrow cells sorted by flow cytometry into populations representing different stages in B-lymphocyte development: RAG-1 and RAG-2 mRNAs were detectable in pro-B and early pre-B cells (corresponding to cells undergoing D→J and V→DJ recombination), but undetectable in the large prolifer-

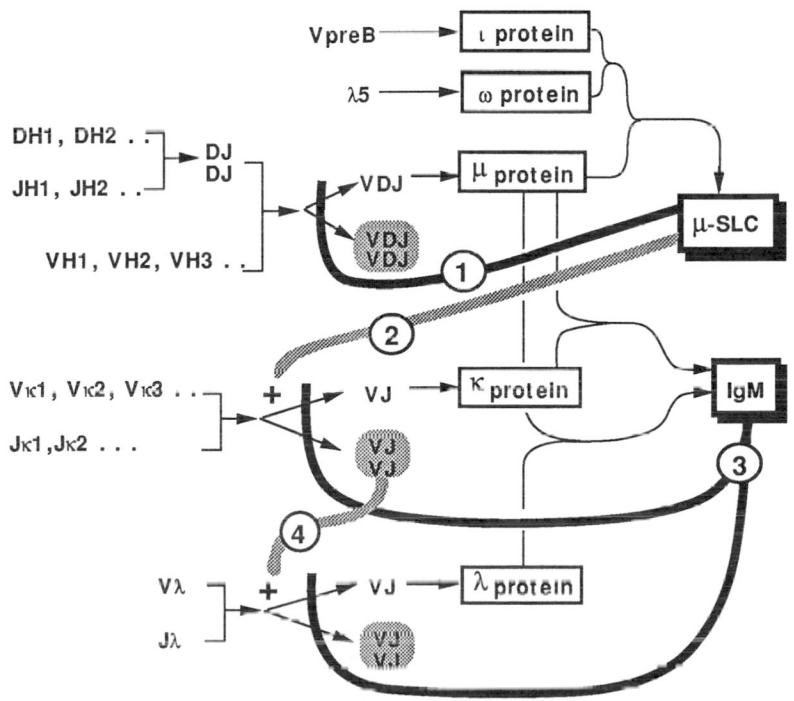

FIG. 15. Regulation of V assembly recombination. Allelic and isotypic exclusion can be explained by the four regulatory effects diagrammed here. Negative regulatory effects (*thick black lines*) prevent a second H- or L-chain recombination event from occurring after an earlier event leads to a functional protein product. Positive regulatory effects (*thick gray lines terminating in* +) switch on κ recombination only after a functional μ protein is produced, and switch on λ recombination only after nonproductive κ recombination has occurred on both chromosomes (*shaded oval area*). The latter effect has not been demonstrated unequivocally; alternatively, a functional μ protein may activate recombination in both κ and λ loci.

ating preB-II cells expressing μ-SLC. RAG gene expression then becomes detectable again in the small preB-II cells undergoing L-chain V→J recombination. In addition to effects on RAG activity, the pre-BCR may also downregulate further VDJ recombination by reducing accessibility of the H-chain locus, as indicated by reduced sterile VH gene transcription (296) and by reduced ability of RAG proteins to produce broken signal ends in nuclei incubated in vitro, as determined by LMPCR (297). Diminished accessibility of the IgH locus would prevent further V→DJ recombination during the subsequent stage when RAG proteins are upregulated to activate L-chain VJ recombination.

Interestingly, the signals mediated by the pre-BCR (μ-SLC) and the mature BCR (IgM) are critical not only for regulating VDJ recombination but also as checkpoints controlling other features of B-lymphocyte differentiation. Thus, in bone marrows of RAG knockout (298) or JH knockout mice (299), B-lymphopoiesis appears to be blocked at the earliest pro-B stage: (a) large cells stain positive for B220, CD43, and c-kit, and (b) cells with surface markers typical of mature B cells are absent from the periphery. When a recombined VDJ-Cμ H-chain transgene was introduced into a RAG-1-/- or RAG-2-/- background (300,301), the resulting μ protein allowed the progression of B-lineage cells to the stage of small preB-II cells, where L-chain recombination would normally occur. These cells could not undergo VL→JL recombination in the absence of RAG proteins but did show upregulation of sterile κ transcription, an apparent reflection of regulatory effect ② in Fig. 15. If, in addition to the μ gene, a complete recombined L-chain transgene was also added to the genome of the RAG knockout mice, then B cell development appeared to be restored, with normal numbers of B cells in the periphery, expressing mature B-cell surface markers and secreting antibody encoded by the transgenes. (An L-chain transgene alone was ineffective in "rescuing" B-cell differentiation.) The developmental block in RAG knockouts is similar to that seen in λ5 knockouts, which lack the SLC component of the pre-BCR. These mice are also arrested in pre-B cell maturation because of the absence of pre-BCR signaling. A similar immunodeficiency syndrome has recently been reported in humans with homozygous defects in the human homolog of λ5 (301a). Interestingly, the λ5 knockout mice could be rescued from their developmental arrest by a recombined κ transgene that was expressed in pre-B cells, indicating that a κ chain can substitute for the SLC in mediating maturation signals (302); indeed, even without the κ transgene, some maturation occurs in the λ5 knockout mice, a presumed result of small amounts of Vκ-Jκ recombination occurring before VDJH recombination and thus providing a κ chain that allows surface IgM expression and signaling. The permissive effect of the pre-BCR on developmental progression appears to be mediated by the Igα-Igβ heterodimer, based on results with the mutant or chimeric μ transgenes linked to Igα or Igβ cytoplasmic domains, as described above (293,294).

The hypothesis that μ protein can activate κ-chain recombination (effect ② in Fig. 15) was originally derived from static comparisons of various B-lymphoid cell lines: cells in which only μ genes are rearranged and expressed are common (pre-B cell lines), but κ-expressing cells without H-chain gene rearrangement and expression are rare, as though H-chain expression were a prerequisite for κ expression. This view has been supported by observation of AMuLV-transformed lines (187) and normal B-cell precursors cultured in vitro: these lines always rearrange H-chain genes before κ genes. In a more direct demonstration that μ protein could stimulate κ rearrangement, an AMuLV-transformed cell that could not express endogenous H chain (because of defective VDJ rearrange-

ments on both of its H-chain loci) was found to retain the κ locus stably in germline configuration until a functional μ gene was introduced; this μ gene activated κ gene rearrangement and expression (189,303). Only a gene encoding μm was effective in activating κ rearrangement and not a μs gene, again suggesting a requirement of surface pre-BCR expression for this signaling. A similar conclusion was deduced from the rescue of RAG knockout animals by a recombined VDJ-Cμ transgene, which caused upregulation of sterile κ transcription in preB-II cells, as described above. Also, a human μ transgene was found to upregulate both κ gene (sterile) transcription and Vκ-Jκ rearrangement in B-lymphoid precursors in fetal liver (296). To directly assay for accessibility of Ig loci to RAG proteins, Constantinescu et al. (297) incubated RAG-/- nuclei from different B-cell developmental stages with RAG proteins in vitro and detected broken signal ends by LMPCR; using this method, they found that introduction of a VDJ-Cμ transgene into the RAG-/- background caused a 30-fold increase in the frequency of breaks at Jκ1 observed in pre-B cell nuclei incubated with RAG proteins. Interestingly, a δ transgene is also apparently able to both inhibit endogenous VDJ rearrangement and activate κ rearrangement (304), so these effects must be mediated by properties common to δ and μ H chains. Crosslinking of the pre-BCR complex is apparently required for activation of κ recombination (163), suggesting that a ligand that occurs physiologically in the environment of the pre-B cell may bind to the pre-BCR to signal activation of gene rearrangement in the κ locus and suppression in the H-chain locus; however, no candidate ligand has been identified.

Despite all the evidence cited above, it is clear that some sterile κ gene transcription Vκ-Jκ recombination can occur in the absence of a μm-containing pre-BCR (291,305–307). This may be a consequence of some "leakiness" of the controls on L-chain recombination in early B-lymphopoiesis or may reflect a separate developmental lineage in which Vκ-Jκ recombination is activated earlier; but the low frequency of this premature Vκ-Jκ recombination would keep the possibility of L-chain double-producers violating allelic exclusion below 1% (299).

When κ recombination begins, the possibilities for functional and nonfunctional VJ rearrangements resemble those discussed above for the H chain. According to the regulatory model, if a cell initially rearranges its κ locus on one chromosome nonproductively, then it can proceed to rearrange the locus on the homologous chromosome. As soon as functional κ gene rearrangement leads to expression of a functional κ chain that can associate with μ to form a surface-expressed IgM molecule (i.e., a mature BCR), then further κ rearrangement will be suppressed (effect ③ in Fig. 15). This regulatory influence would explain the observation of allelic exclusion in κ-expressing myelomas, and it has been supported by the finding that a functional rearranged VJ-Cκ transgene can suppress rearrangement of endogenous κ genes (308). Furthermore, in murine B-lymphoma lines expressing RAG proteins, cross-linking of surface IgM with an anti-μ antibody was found to rapidly suppress RAG gene expression (309). A ligand might deliver a corresponding signal in physiologic circumstances, but this is not clear, especially because under some conditions cross-linking the BCR of pre-B cells (as might occur on binding of a self-antigen) can actually upregulate RAG gene expression to activate "receptor editing." A BCR-mediated signal seems to be required for small preB-II cells to advance to the immature B phenotype and move into the periphery because, as mentioned above, RAG knockout animals rescued with only a μ transgene were not able to advance beyond the pre-B stage, whereas a combination of μ and κ transgenes allowed normal B-cell proliferation, surface marker expression, and migration to the periphery. Igα is also apparently critical for mediating some differentiation signals of the BCR because mice with an engineered deletion in the cytoplasmic signaling domain of Igα had only 1% of the normal numbers of circulating B cells (310).

Regulatory effect ④ in Fig. 15 is rather speculative because little is known about regulation of λ gene rearrangement. The idea that λ recombination is somehow triggered by nonfunctional κ rearrangements on both chromosomes derives from the observations that most B cells show isotypic exclusion (i.e., express either κ or λ but not both) and that κ rearrangement seems to occur before λ. Thus, in studies of normal and malignant human B-lymphoid cells (136,311), in κ-expressing cells, λ genes were found to be in germline configuration, whereas in λ-expressing cells, κ genes were either rearranged (rarely) or deleted (most commonly). The κ deletions reflect the RS recombination event discussed earlier in this chapter. These results suggest that λ genes remain unrearranged until κ genes rearrange nonproductively or are deleted. The mechanism of this apparent regulation of the λ genes by the κ locus is unknown. It has been suggested that somewhere in the 24 kb between Cκ and the RS site lies a sequence that suppresses λ rearrangement but is deleted in the κ RS recombination event to alleviate this suppression. However, in contrast to this hypothesis are the observations that mice with a targeted deletion of either Cκ or the intronic κ enhancer have almost normal numbers of B cells, essentially all of which express λ despite having no loss of DNA between $C_κ$ and Rs (276,306,312).

It is assumed that membrane expression of a μ-λ IgM would shut off all further L-chain gene recombination by a similar mechanism to that in the κ locus (as illustrated by effect ③ in Fig. 15), a supposition supported by suppression of κ gene expression in λ transgenic mice (313). However, this suppression is somewhat leaky, especially in older mice (314–317), and even in normal splenocytes a small population of cells expresses both isotypes (318). These observations have led to the speculation that certain B-lymphocytes are not programmed for strict isotype exclusion. It is also possible that in some cells expressing both κ and λ, one of the isotype L chains has such a greater affinity for the expressed H-chain protein (on the basis of VH-VL compatibility) that the other isotype does not functionally contribute to surface Ig and is thus allelically excluded at the protein level. Some evidence in opposition to the strictly ordered (κ before λ) rearrangement model for L chains has been put forward (285,319), suggesting that VJ recombination is activated concurrently in both the κ and λ loci. In this model the preponderance of κ-expressing lymphocytes (in mice at least) would result from a stochastic process in which κ rearrangements are favored by the larger Vκ repertoire and other features of the κ locus, such as more active recombination signal sequences (320). Alternatively, the preponderance of κ expression may be explained by a model in which κ and λ rearrangement occurs independently, but κ recombination initiates earlier in B-cell development (321). In either of the latter two models of L-chain rearrangement, a surface IgM molecule ($H_2κ_2$ or $H_2λ_2$) would signal feedback suppression of L-chain recombination, so that both allelic exclusion and isotype exclusion would be explained by the same mechanism (and the regulatory effect ④ of Fig. 15 would not exist).

RAG Protein Production after Mature BCR Expression

Although the RAG genes are apparently downregulated through a signal mediated by the appearance of IgM on an immature B cell, there is evidence that RAG gene expression occurs in at least two later stages of B-cell development: during receptor editing of autoreactive B cells in the bone marrow and during B-cell maturation in germinal centers.

An early observation suggesting the possibility of receptor editing by secondary rearrangement of κ L-chain genes came from an analysis of circular DNAs representing the deleted segment in VJ recombination (322). It was observed that, in addition to containing the expected signal joints, many of these circles contained VJ junctions; these could have formed in an initial inversional recombination, which was then followed by a secondary deletional rearrangement that produced the observed circular DNA. Significantly, about a third of the VJ junctions analyzed showed no apparent defect, indicating that they could have produced a functional antibody that was altered by secondary recombination. Since this study, several laboratories have directly observed secondary κ rearrangements in B-cell tumors and AMuLV-transformed pre-B lines (188,323). H-chain V-gene replacement also can occur, mediated by a 7-mer embedded in the 3′ end of many VH coding regions, as described in an earlier section. As in the case of κ genes, such replacement can occur even after a productive VDJ recombination (180,324). A potential reason for replacing productively rearranged L or H chains would be to abort production of an antibody that was autoreactive. Thus, receptor editing might complement two other mechanisms for preventing autoantibodies: anergization and cell deletion by apoptosis.

Several studies have supported this interpretation using mice carrying transgenes expressing autoreactive antibodies (325,326). In one study, the JH locus was targeted for replacement by homologous recombination with the 3H9 recombined VDJ gene; this gene encodes an H chain that in combination with most (but not all) κ L chains can bind to DNA, a self antigen (181). In such mice, most B cells have replaced the 3H9 gene by an upstream VH gene, with junctions showing typical N regions and exonuclease nibbling. When inserted as a normal transgene, 3H9 also stimulates L-chain editing, as evidenced by increased frequency of Jκ5 usage and reduced diversity of Vκ genes expressed by the B cells displaying the 3H9 H chain (325). These results are consistent with the interpretation that primary rearrangements, yielding Vκ proteins capable of supporting DNA binding, were edited by secondary rearrangements involving downstream Jκs and Vκ regions incompatible with DNA binding. Receptor editing appears to occur in the immature B-cell population in the bone marrow (327,328) and is associated with increased RAG gene expression. Indeed, BCR cross-linking of a human B-cell line was found to upregulate RAG gene expression (329). As previously discussed, BCR cross-linking also has been reported to terminate RAG gene expression of surface IgM+ immature B cells to mediate allelic exclusion (309). How a cell can discriminate between a BCR-mediated signal that downregulates RAG expression to mediate allelic exclusion and a BCR-mediated signal that upregulates RAG expression to initiate receptor editing is currently not understood; but differences in receptor affinity, the precise stage of development, or costimulatory signals might be involved. Interestingly, a failure of receptor editing may contribute to the autoantibodies mediating systemic lupus erythematosis (330).

A second instance of late RAG expression occurs in germinal center (GC) B cells (331,332). RAG-1 and RAG-2 mRNA transcripts were detected by RT-PCR in FACS-purified GC cells from immunized mice, the RAG proteins were detected in GC cells by immunofluorescence, and evidence of ongoing V(D)J recombination was found in GC cells (332a,332b). RAG expression also was observed constitutively in Peyer's patch GCs (which are maintained by food antigens in the absence of intentional immunization) and in splenic B cells cultured with IL-4 plus LPS (conditions known to induce at least one other process typical of GC cells, i.e., isotype switching). GC cells appear to recapitulate expression of several surface markers characteristic of early B-lineage cells, including heat stable antigen (CD24) and λ5; so it appears that the RAG gene expression may be just one aspect of a GC-induced reversion to a primitive phenotype. What function might RAG proteins have in the GC? The primary processes that affect Ig expression in the GC are somatic mutation and isotype switching, but it is unlikely that RAG proteins are expressed in GC to function in either of these processes because both can occur in B cells of RAG-/- mice (116a,331). One possibility is that RAG-dependent receptor editing may be turned on to replace V regions that have become autoreactive as a result of GC-induced somatic mutations; further experiments will be necessary to evaluate this interpretation.

GENERATION OF DIVERSITY

One of the most interesting questions about Igs is the source of the immense variation observed in antibody-binding specificities. As discussed at the beginning of this chapter, early speculative debates about this question centered on the relative contributions of germline repertoire and somatic mutation in creating diversity. One source of diversity that was unanticipated before the recombinant DNA revolution already has been discussed in this chapter in some detail: somatic recombinational diversity. We will now focus on the germline repertoire and then consider the contribution of somatic mutation.

Germline Diversity

A comprehensive evaluation of the germline repertoire of V-gene segments requires an examination of the sequences of all germline V regions, a daunting task. However, modern molecular biology techniques—including cloning vectors allowing long genomic inserts and large-scale sequencing with fluorescent dyes and automated sample preparation—have helped realize this goal for the human κ, λ, and H-chain loci; and considerable progress has been made with the murine κ and H-chain loci. (The tiny V repertoire of the murine λ loci has already been discussed in the section on λ genes.)

Two Worldwide Web resources are devoted to providing convenient updated access to Ig germline gene sequences. The IMGT (international ImMunoGeneTics) data base (http://imgt.cnusc.fr:8104/home.html), coordinated by Marie-Paule Lefranc, includes a data base for Ig and TCR sequences, as well as a separate one for major histocompatibility complex (MHC) sequences (333). In the Ig/TCR database, all species for which data are available are included; sequences are annotated in standard formats, and map information is provided graphically. V Base Gold (http://www.mrc-cpe.cam.ac.uk/imt-doc/public/INTRO.html) is an online catalog of human V gene segments and alleles coordinated by Ian M. Tomlinson.

Germline Diversity of the Murine IgH Locus

Attempts to analyze the mouse VH repertoire began before the gene cloning era with the study of VH amino acid sequences from mouse myelomas. Initial attempts to classify the observed VHs into related groups were based on limited amino acid sequence analysis, primarily of N-termini of myeloma proteins. The current scheme classifies two V gene sequences into the same group or family if they show more than about 80% nucleotide sequence identity, and into different families if their sequences are less than

70% identical. (Empirically, few VH comparisons yield identities between 70% and 80%.) These criteria for sequence similarity correspond well with the degree of similarity that allows hybridization between a V probe and members of the same family under conditions of moderate stringency. The initial classifications based on this scheme identified seven VH families (334,335). Since that time, continuing analysis of new sequences has identified eight additional families (336–338). The families now known contribute to the bulk of the immune response: when 2,000 cDNA clones hybridizing to both Cμ and JH probes were analyzed, all had V regions from the 15 families, based on hybridization or sequence analysis, except for about 2% of the clones representing truncated or aberrant cDNA synthesis (338). The families have been further classified into three groups, or clans, based on sequence conservation in the framework I region (FR1; codons 6–24) and FR3 (codons 67–85) (339–341). (Framework amino acids are the non-CDR parts of the Ig V region that hold the CDR loops in position to contact antigens.) The clans are conserved between humans, mice, and frogs, suggesting that several fundamental steps in germline VH diversification preceded the amphibian-reptile divergence (342).

The classification of VH genes into families leads to two approachable questions: (a) How many genes in each family are available to contribute to Ig diversity? (b) How are the families arranged on the chromosome? One straightforward approach to the question of gene number is to count the number of bands visible on Southern blots. However, this method can yield only a rough estimate of gene number because of several complications in the interpretation. The number of bands may underestimate the number of VH regions for two main reasons: (a) a given DNA fragment may contain more than one V-related sequence; and (b) some observed bands may actually represent several comigrating hybridizing DNA fragments, each containing different VH genes. On the other hand, the number of bands could theoretically exceed the number of different VH genes for two reasons. First, some hybridizing sequences may not contribute effectively to sequence diversity. In particular, some nonallelic gene pairs may be so similar that the second copy provides no gain in amino acid sequence diversity. Other V sequences are nonfunctional because they have become separated from the C-region locus, even lying on a different chromosome. Still other germline clones isolated on the basis of hybridization to a V probe have turned out to contain multiple defects that would preclude their expression as functional V regions even if they underwent rearrangement (i.e., they are pseudogenes); conceivably these pseudogenes could contribute to diversity at the somatic level through gene conversion, a mechanism known to operate in chickens and rabbits as discussed later. Second, some bands could be counted twice because of hybridization to probes of two different families. This could occur if a specific DNA fragment carried germline V sequences from two different families or if hybridization occurred across group boundaries owing to a clustering of residues identical to the probe sequence.

With these caveats, Table 1, modified from a compilation by Kofler et al. (343), is presented to give an idea of the widely varying complexity of the different VH groups. Several groups have only a few members. For example the VH S107 family yields four Southern blot bands, and extensive cloning with a probe for this family has in fact detected only four germline members (of which one is apparently a pseudogene). At the other extreme, the VH J558 family shows much greater Southern blot complexity and may contain as many as 1,000 members in the BALB/c mouse. This estimate (344) was based on quantitative kinetics of hybridization using an excess of single-stranded J558 probe, whereas the lower estimate of 60 genes is based on counting Southern blot bands. If the larger estimate is accurate, then many of the bands observed on Southern blots with the VH-J558 probe must contain multiple comigrating DNA fragments; these would probably represent recent duplications in the VH locus and would be expected to encode minimally diverged VH sequences. Other strains of mice besides BALB/c seem to have smaller J558 families (345), consistent with the notion of a recent expansion of J558 VH genes in BALB/c.

The question of how the germline VH genes are arrayed on the chromosome has been approached by several different techniques. One straightforward method has been to screen phage libraries of germline DNA with VH probes and to examine clones containing more than one VH region. Application of this method to the mouse VH locus has yielded three important generalizations: adjacent VH genes are usually members of the same family; they are oriented in the same 5'-3' direction; and they are spaced about 7 to 15 kb apart (346–348). The first finding suggests that members of a given VH family are clustered together on the chromosome. Such clustering represents a simplifying principle that allows the mapping of murine VH genes to be conceptually divided into establishing the order of the family clusters on the chromosome and then establishing the order of VH genes within each cluster.

One approach to ordering the VH families has been to examine (by Southern blotting) the VH bands that are deleted in various myelomas or hybridomas. Deductions about the order of VH families can be made if the nonexpressed chromosome is deleted so that all the VH fragments observed on a Southern blot can be considered to derive from the same (i.e., the expressed) chromosome and to lie upstream from the rearranged VH gene (349–351). A powerful variant of the deletion method has used a panel of Abelson virus–transformed B-cell lines constructed from F1 animals heterozygous for allotype at the IgH locus. In most of these cell lines it was possible to distinguish deletions on the two parental chromosomes and establish an independent VH gene order for each (338,352).

Another mapping approach is brute force chromosome walking by the generation of large overlapping clones using cosmid libraries; this approach is being pursued by a number of laboratories, but is made difficult by the occurrence of recent duplications leaving nearly identical DNA segments that cannot easily be distinguished or ordered on a map. This problem should hopefully be resolved by the use of yeast artificial chromosome (YAC) clones, which can accommodate 1- to 2-Mb segments of genomic DNA. YACs have been useful in long-range mapping of the human V loci. Pulsed field gel electrophoresis also has been used to separate large fragments of genomic DNA for mapping by Southern blotting.

Studies using these techniques have been in general agreement about the order of certain murine VH families, but a complete map consistent with all data from the various mapping methods is not currently available. It is clear from several laboratories that some interdigitation between families occurs (351,353), and this could contribute to difficulties in interpretation. A representative map of 15 murine VH families is shown in Fig. 16, based on the work of Brodeur and colleagues (352,354).

Among VH maps based on different techniques, the best agreement is on the families closest to $C\mu$. The map order of these families is: S107—Q52—7183—D—J—$C\mu$, with some overlap between these three families as shown in the Fig. 16. This order is of special interest because the most proximal family cluster (designated 7183), and in particular its most proximal member (designated VH81X), is the V region that is significantly over-represented in the VDJ rearrangements occurring in fetal liver pre-B cells (355). This observation was earlier taken as evidence favoring a tracking model of V gene rearrangement [i.e., a recombinase would engage DNA near the J regions and slide 5' to find V regions to recombine (356)]; but alternative interpretations have been proposed based on more recent data (339,340,357,358).

Mouse Germline DH and JH Regions

D regions were initially hypothesized based on the highly diverse amino acid sequences in myeloma proteins between the V

TABLE 1. *VH region families of mice and humans*

	Mouse				Human	
Family number	Family name	Complexity[a]	Clan[b]	Group[c]	Family number	Complexity[d]
VH2	Q52	15				
VH3	36–60	5–8	II	I	VH2	4
VH8	3609	7–10			VH4	9
VH12	CH27	1			VH6	1
VH1	J558	6–1000				
VH9	VGAM3-8	5–7	I	II	VH1	14
VH14	SM7	3–4			VH7	5
VH15	VH15	2			VH7	5
VH4	X-24	2				
VH5	7183	12				
VH6	J606	10–12	III	III	VH3	46
VH7	S107	3				
VH11	CP3	1–6				
VH13	3609N	1				

This table is based on a compilation of murine VH regions by Kofler et al. (343), and a review of human VH regions by Pascual and Capra (822) and a paper by Mainville et al. (000). Original references for the data can be found in those sources.

[a]Complexity, an estimate of the number of VH sequences in each family.
[b]Clans of VH sequences as defined by Schroeder et al. (340)
[c]Groups, based on the classification by Tutter and Riblet (339).
[d]Complexity, based on the prototypic haplotype provided by Cook and †omlinson (381).

and J regions, as briefly discussed earlier in this chapter. Because both VH and JH were known to be flanked by signal elements of the long space type (23 bp), it was predicted that a germline D region would be flanked on both sides by short signal element spaces so that both V-D and D-J recombination would conform to the 12/23 spacer rule (359).

Finding a germline D gene with a probe corresponding to D-region sequence from one of the cloned recombined genes was technically difficult because the DNA segment encoding the few amino acids of the D region would be too short to give a usable hybridization signal. To obtain more effective probes, DNA fragments have been isolated from DJH intermediates that have not yet recombined with a VH gene, and thus retain the 5′ flanking sequences from the germline D providing a longer probe (360). A DJH intermediate cloned from the myeloma QUPC52 identified its germline D precursor—designated DQ52—0.7 kb 5′ to JH1. Its structure was very similar to expectation: a 10-nucleotide coding sequence flanked on both sides by RSS elements with a 12-bp spacing. A similar clone derived from a rearranged DJH in a T-cell line (SP2) was used as a second probe to clone nine related D regions clustered within a 60-kb region, all having 17-nucleotide coding segments and short spacing of the signal elements (361,362). A third D probe called FL16, derived similarly, identified the FL16 family, which is composed of only two germline D genes but is well represented in the rearranged IgH-chain genes that have been sequenced. Finally, a last D region, D_{ST4}, was identified through the recognition of a recurring nucleotide sequence observed between V and J in recombined VDJ regions that was not accounted for by the previously known D sequences (363). The 13 murine D regions span about 80 kb upstream from the four JH segments that in turn lie upstream from Cµ.

Apart from the additional combinatorial diversity contributed by the repertoire of germline D elements, the flexibility of the recombination site applies on both ends of the D region. Furthermore, an out-of-frame recombination at the VD junction may be compensated by the frame of the DJ junction so that a particular D element could theoretically be read in all three frames in different VDJ recombinants. As mentioned previously, this extra source of diver-

sity is used by human H chains (11), but the murine system has evolved mechanisms that strongly favor the reading frame known as RF1 (10). DJ rearrangement in RF3 is counterselected owing to frequent internal stop codons. When DJ recombination has occurred in RF2, the resulting transcripts can encode a DJ-Cµ protein (designated the Dµ protein), which can be expressed on the surface of a pre-B cell in association with the products of the VpreB and λ5 genes (364–366). Murine cells expressing Dµ protein cannot progress to normal Ig production, perhaps because the Dµ protein triggers the shut-off of VDJ recombination before V assembly is complete; therefore, expressed H-chain V regions rarely include a DJ junction in RF2 (10). This curious model is supported by the observations that RF2 suppression is not observed in λ5 knockout mice (which fail to express Dµ protein on the cell surface) (367) and that analysis of recombination in single cells by PCR failed to detect cells containing both a DJ junction in RF2 as well as a productive VDJ junction (368). In humans this mechanism is not operative because ATG initiation codons are not generally present 5′ from D regions to encode a Dµ protein. Some rearranged VDJ sequences seem to be interpretable as V-D-D-J products, even in cases where D-D recombination would seem to violate the 12/23 rule (369).

Murine Germline Vκ Locus

Although murine L-chain genes were among the first Ig genes studied by molecular biology techniques, the organization of the mouse germline Vκ locus has been less thoroughly characterized than the human. On the basis of N-terminal amino acid sequence data, Potter and colleagues classified mouse Vκ sequences into 24 groups (370). Current classification based on the nucleotide sequence criteria described above recognizes about 20 families (371). However, different classification schemes have yielded different estimates, perhaps because the Vκ genes show degrees of relatedness that are not discrete steps, but rather continuous gradations (372), as would be expected if gene duplications could occur on a time continuum and rates of sequence diversification could also vary. As described above for VH genes, some Vκ families are

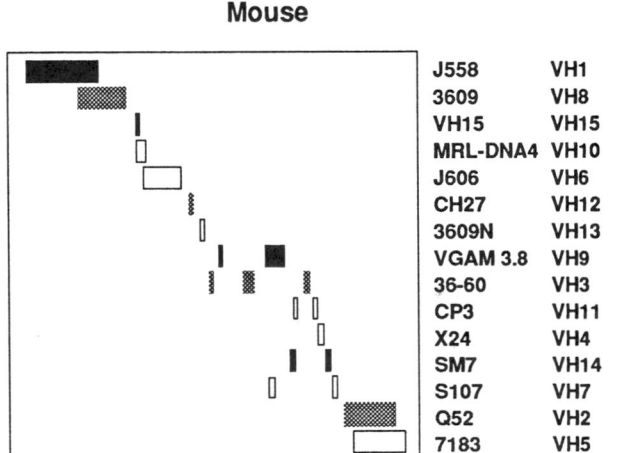
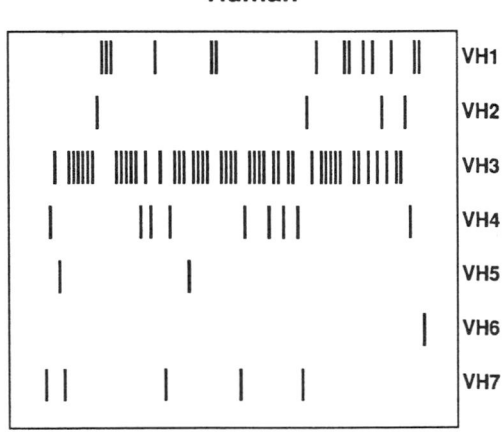

J558	VH1
3609	VH8
VH15	VH15
MRL-DNA4	VH10
J606	VH6
CH27	VH12
3609N	VH13
VGAM 3.8	VH9
36-60	VH3
CP3	VH11
X24	VH4
SM7	VH14
S107	VH7
Q52	VH2
7183	VH5

FIG. 16. Maps of the murine and human VH loci. The 15 known murine VH gene families are shown in their approximate map positions. Each rectangle represents a cluster of VH genes of the indicated family; the clan identification (340) of the VH families is indicated by the color of the rectangle: black for clan I, gray for clan II, and white for clan III. Although some interdigitation is shown by overlapping families (e.g., the Q52 and 7183 families), the families are largely clustered. In contrast, all human VH genes (*vertical lines*) of a prototypic haplotype are shown in the right panel, based on the formulation by Cook and Tomlinson (381); extensive interdigitation of families is apparent.

shared by humans and mice, suggesting that the family divisions preceded primate–rodent species divergence (373,374). The murine locus, including about 140 Vκ sequences (genes and pseudogenes), has been cloned on a series of overlapping bacterial artificial chromosome (BAC) and YAC clones, and spans about 3.5 Mb upstream from the Cκ gene on chromosome 6 (375–377). In addition, a few Vκ sequences have been localized to other chromosomes (chromosome 16 and 19), where they could not contribute to diversity and are thus considered "orphons." In the functional Vκ locus on chromosome 6, many related Vκ sequences are found to lie clustered together, although some interspersion of families also exists. As of this writing, the total number of genes (versus pseudogenes) has not been completely determined by sequence analysis.

Human Germline VH Locus

Amino acid sequences of human myeloma VH-region proteins were originally classified by Kabat into three groups. These have been found to correlate well with three families defined by sorting together VH probes that produce similar Southern blot patterns. Four additional human VH families have been found more recently using molecular genetics approaches. Several of the human VH families show sequence similarities to particular mouse VH families (378), and all can be classified within the three large clans of murine VH genes common to the mouse, human, and Xenopus; as noted above, these observations suggest that significant germline VH diversification antedated the amphibian–reptile species divergence.

Early phage and cosmid clones of human VH genes demonstrated that the human VH families are extensively interdigitated, in contrast to the family clusters characteristic of the murine locus. This interdigitated structure was confirmed by gene mapping studies involving analysis of VH deletion in B-cell lines and of PFGE-based mapping data (354,379); ultimately the complete delineation of the human VH region has been achieved through analysis of overlapping YAC clones covering the entire locus (380–382). The VH locus spans 1.1 Mb at the telomeric end of chromosome 14 and includes 95 VH sequences; of these, 51 are functional and most of the remainder appear to be pseudogenes (although the exact numbers are somewhat variable depending on the haplotype, and a few V sequences have not yet been fully characterized). Each VH region is identified by a two-digit number: the first number corresponds to the VH family and the second indicates the sequential number of the VH on the standard map (starting from the JH proximal end), with the letter P appended for pseudogenes. A particular VH locus is judged to be functional if it has no obvious defects in coding sequence and has been detected in a rearranged VDJ gene, indicating intact recombination signals. Additional polymorphic V regions are designated (using a decimal point) with reference to the JH-proximal standard VH; e.g. a polymorphic V region from the VH7 family lying between 4-4 and 2-5 is identified as 7-4.1. The entire VH locus thus extends from V 6-1, which is located about 77 kb 5′ from JH1 (383), through V 7-81, which appears to be located within a few kb of the telomeric repeat sequences marking the end of the q arm of chromosome 14. Twenty-four additional germline VH sequences have been mapped to chromosomes 15 and 16 and represent nonfunctional orphons that were apparently duplicated from the functional locus on chromosome 14 (384,385); these sequences contributed to earlier overestimates of the length of the functional human VH locus. All the VH regions whose transcriptional orientations have been determined share the same orientation characteristic of the JH regions, consistent with recombination by

deletion rather than inversion. Several regions in the locus show evidence of ancient duplications: segments in which a pattern of hybridization to different probes from nearby DNA regions is repeated elsewhere in the locus. Thus, the complete locus map may offer clues to its evolution, as well as defining the repertoire of germline VH diversity available to the immune system.

Human JH and DH Regions

Upstream of the human Cμ gene lies a set of JH-region genes, including six apparently functional JH regions (386). Interspersed among the active human JH genes are three J pseudogenes that encode amino acid sequences never found in human H chains and that lack the RNA splice signal found at the 3′ end of all active JH genes. All of the JH genes and pseudogenes demonstrate 23-bp RSS spacing (as in the mouse).

Complete sequence analysis of a 92-kb region spanning the human D regions (11) has confirmed the general structure of the locus previously deduced from partial sequence analysis and Southern blotting. One germline D gene is located in a position roughly homologous to that of the mouse DQ52, that is, 5′ to the human JH1. This human D gene, initially designated DHQ52, bears striking homology to its murine counterpart but is the only human D segment showing such human/mouse homology. All of the other human D regions fall into six families and lie in a cluster of duplicated domains about 22 kb upstream from JH1. There are 27 D regions; 24 of these are accounted for by four tandem approximate duplications of a 9.5-kb segment containing a representative of the six D families. In addition to these 24 D regions, three more D regions result from (a) an additional partial duplication of 2.8 kb, including one D; (b) an internal duplication creating one D; and (c) DHQ52, which is in a family of its own, distinct from the six duplicated families. The D regions have been renamed following a scheme similar to that used for the VH genes: a first number identifies the family, and a second identifies the sequential position in the locus. The locus starts with the 5′-most D region, D1-1, and ends with D7-27 (DHQ52). Three D regions are apparently nonfunctional as a result of mutations in RSS 7-mers, and there are two pairs of D regions with identical coding sequences (including one of the D segments with a 7-mer mutation); so there are 23 distinct D regions that can contribute to human Ig diversity. A comprehensive computer analysis of a data base of published human VH sequences showed that all of these sequences appear in the data base, many in all three reading frames. In general, one reading frame encodes primarily hydrophilic residues, one encodes hydrophobic residues, and one includes frequent stop codons. (Some D regions that contain stop codons can be used if these codons are removed by nuclease trimming before VDJ assembly is complete.)

In addition to these D regions, all flanked by signal elements with the typical 12-bp spacing, one putative family, designated DIR (D with irregular spacing), has been described, having RSS elements that could be taken with either 12- or 23-bp spacing; theoretically, DIR regions could contribute extra diversity in the form of V-D-DIR-J or V-DIR-D-J rearrangements without violating the 12/23 rule (387). However, the systematic evaluation of the data base of 893 published VH regions failed to detect expression of DIR regions (11) confirming the failure to detect such rearrangements using a sensitive PCR assay (388). Also absent from this VH data base were inverted D regions and the previously hypothesized D-D rearrangements (which would violate the 12/23 rule), although evidence that both of these can occur at low frequency has been obtained using highly sensitive PCR techniques (388,389).

Furthermore, DIR rearrangements, both direct and inverted, were found in mice transgenic for a human IgH minilocus (389a). Additional human D segments originally thought to lie upstream from the main cluster apparently lie on the duplicated orphon cluster on chromosome 15 and are thus nonfunctional (385,390).

Human Germline Vκ Locus

The human Vκ locus is located on the short arm of chromosome 2 (2p11-2). Most of its genes fall into four known V gene families: VκI, VκII, VκIII, and VκIV. Five cloned Vκ sequences have been described that would fall into three additional families (VκV through VκVII), but these sequences have apparently not contributed to known proteins and thus are probably pseudogenes. Zachau and colleagues have performed an extensive investigation of the human locus by cloning, PFGE, and sequence analysis (391,392). They have identified 76 Vκ sequences in the human Vκ locus, lying in two 0.4-Mb contigs separated by a spacer of about 0.8 Mb that is apparently devoid of Vκ sequences. The Jκ distal (upstream) segment, including 36 Vκ sequences, appears to be the result of a large duplication. Within each duplicated segment, all V regions have the same 5'-3' orientation. Remarkably, the segment distal to the Jκ-Cκ region lies in inverted orientation with respect to the proximal segment and Jκ-Cκ. Most of the duplicated Vκ sequences could be assigned to the proximal or distal segment by preparative separation of the two loci using PFGE, followed by Southern blots exploiting the rare differences in the restriction maps of the duplicated segments. Alternatively, assignments could be deduced from Southern blot bands absent from the DNA of rare individuals lacking the distal duplication. In all B-lymphoid cell lines examined, those with rearrangements involving the distal inverted Vκ segments contained retained signal joints and failed to show deletions of downstream Vκ and 5' J-flanking DNA, consistent with Vκ-Jκ recombination by inversion. Except for two insertion/deletion differences leading to one unpaired proximal Vκ and one unpaired distal Vκ, the Vκ sequences of the proximal and distal parts of the locus match their homologs with 95% to 99% sequence identity. This high degree of similarity suggests a recent origin for the duplication, which is supported by the fact that the duplication is not found in chimpanzees or gorillas (393), which are thought to have diverged from the human lineage only 6 to 8 million years ago. Between the proximal duplication and the Jκ regions lie an additional six unpaired Vκ sequences, of which the two nearest Jκ lie in inverted orientation. The most J-proximal Vκ sequence, the single gene of the VκIV family, is only 23 kb upstream from Jκ1. Members of the VκI, VκII, and VκIII family have been found to be extensively interspersed. Of the 76 Vκ sequences in the locus, 33 are without apparent defect, although some in the duplicated segments are so similar to their duplicated counterpart that they do not contribute significantly to diversity of the locus, and some may not be expressed, for unknown reasons. In an examination of 70 cDNAs from a human spleen library plus 170 cDNAs from the literature, only 21 of the Vκ genes plus five from duplicated identical genes were found to be expressed, for an expressed cDNA repertoire of 27 Vκ genes (394). Of the remaining Vκ sequences in the germline Vκ locus, 25 are unequivocal pseudogenes, demonstrating several crippling defects; in addition, 16 sequences have one or two minor defects and might be functional in some haplotypes.

Apart from the Vκ sequences in the cluster near the Jκ-Cκ locus, Zachau and colleagues have identified at least 25 orphons. One orphon cluster is located in the long arm of chromosome 2; perhaps it was separated from the major locus—on the short arm of this chromosome—by a pericentric inversion [which must have occurred rather recently in evolution because it is absent from chimpanzees and gorillas (395)]. Other orphons are located on chromosomes 1 and 22; and at least one probably nonfunctional Vκ lies about 1.5 Mb downstream from Cκ (396).

Human Germline Vλ Locus

For many years the human Vλ system was the least characterized of the V loci of human and mouse, but the relative obscurity of this locus has been dramatically reversed by recent intensive cloning, sequencing, and mapping of Vλ regions (168,397) and ultimately by the complete sequence analysis of 1,025,415 bp covering the entire locus (149). The locus contains about 36 potentially functional Vλ genes (in 10 families), 33 pseudogenes, and 34 relics, containing Vλ-like sequences severely disrupted by insertions or deletions. (As noted for other loci, exact numbers may differ depending on the haplotype and method of analysis.) Of the potentially functional genes, only about 30 have been documented to be expressed by comparison with cDNA sequences. Within the clustered Vλ sequences lies the human VpreB gene, as well as several genes and pseudogenes unrelated to the λ system. All the Vλ sequences are in the same transcriptional orientation as the J-C cluster. Analysis of the 1-Mb sequence shows several segments of internal duplications, some including Vλ regions. The largest and most frequently expressed Vλ gene families lie relatively close to the J-C cluster, mostly within the proximal 400 kb. Interestingly, these families are most similar in sequence to the Vλ genes of species that express predominantly this isotype of L chain, including chicken, horse, and sheep, whereas the Vλ genes of the BALB/c mouse are most similar to the least frequently expressed human families.

Combinatorial Diversity Estimates

Before the era of recombinant DNA technology, the source of antibody diversity was so mysterious that it was whimsically referred to as the problem of generation of diversity (GOD). Knowledge of antibody genes gained over the past 20 years has elucidated the diversity inherent in the germline V repertoire plus the diversity contributed by recombinational mechanisms (combinatorial multiplication, flexibility of recombination site, N and P nucleotides), as already discussed. Together these diversity elements provide an immense potential repertoire, one so large that to some investigators it seemed unnecessary to postulate that diversity was further increased by somatic mutation. As an exercise in estimating the contribution of germline and recombinational diversity in the human, consider the number of different antibodies that could be formed assuming 39 functional VH genes, 27 Vκ genes, and 30 Vλ genes. For κ sequences, we can multiply 27 (Vκ genes) × 5 (Jκ regions) × 2 (a conservative multiplier reflecting variability around residue 96 resulting from flexible recombination), yielding the product 270. For λ sequences, we can multiply 30 (Vλ genes) × 4 (Jλ regions) × 2 (flexibility multiplier), yielding the product 480. Thus, the total VL possibilities are 270 + 480 = 750. For VH sequences we have 39 functional germline genes × 23 (DH segments) × 4 (JH) × 4 (flexibility multiplier on both sides of the D segment) × 3 (possible reading frames of the D region) = 43,056. Assuming random association of L and H chains to form a complete L_2H_2 antibody molecule, the number of different combinations is 750 × 43,056 = 32 million. This estimate has neglected additional sources of diversity that are substantial but difficult to quantitate: the insertion of N and P nucleotides. However, even neglecting these factors the exercise demonstrates how nature has greatly enlarged the potential sequence diversity available from a limited number of total nucleotides by allowing flexible recombination between different sequence elements.

Although it is clear that the above mechanisms imply a vast repertoire, it is worth considering some qualifications that tend to reduce the actual combinatorial diversity, especially early in ontogeny. It seems unlikely, for example, that every possible combination of L and H chains yields a functional antibody molecule because in vitro L and H reassociation experiments show that certain hybrid molecules (formed from L and H chains derived from different antibodies) are relatively unstable. Similarly, association of V and J (or V, D, and J) is conceivably not completely random. Evidence of striking bias in the selection of VH genes in fetal pre-B hybridomas has been mentioned. In mice these hybridomas are biased toward the use of genes from the VH7183 and VQ52 families. In addition, fetal and newborn VDJ junctions show a paucity of N nucleotides and a tendency to form VDJ junctions across short stretches of sequence identity between the recombining sequences (homology-mediated recombination, discussed earlier in this chapter). Both of these effects reduce diversity at the recombination junctions, perhaps reflecting a mechanism that ensures the production of certain antibodies advantageous for young individuals. The neonatal bias toward usage of VH7183 and VQ52 families is not observed in adult B cells, but this bias raises the possibility that other less striking recombination biases may exist in adults, reducing the actual diversity below that calculated on simplistic assumptions. It has been reported, for instance, that mouse Jκ rearrangements use Jκ1 and Jκ2 preferentially (398,399), whereas human B cells use JH4 preferentially (400) so that the combinatorial contribution of the available J regions to diversity is probably less than it would be if all were used equally frequently.

Somatic Mutation

Some early arguments suggesting the existence of somatic mutation in antibody genes were based on claims that estimates of combinatorial diversity (as computed along the lines of the above exercise) were, although vast, still too small to account for the observed number of different antibodies. The latter number might be estimated from the percentage of B cells binding a particular antigen and the number of different antibodies—within that binding specificity—that could be distinguished by isoelectric focusing, idiotype characteristics, or analysis of the fine specificity of antigen binding. Such arguments based on global evaluations of diversity were superseded by studies of systems with restricted diversity, in which germline and expressed repertoire can be more reliably compared; these studies generated convincing evidence for somatic mutation. The brief account below summarizes some of the major features of somatic mutation; this topic is discussed in detail in Chapter 24.

Early Evidence for Somatic Mutation

Analyses of amino acid sequences of murine λ1 chains from myeloma antibodies provided the first strong support for somatic mutation, even before the era of recombinant DNA analysis. Thus, when the amino acid sequences of λ1 chains produced by 21 independently derived myelomas were analyzed (401,402), 12 were found to be identical, representing a prototype Vλ1 sequence. The remaining variants were each unique, generally differing from the prototype sequence by single amino acid substitutions that could be

accounted for by single base changes. Significantly, all but one of the amino acid substitutions were unique to a single variant sequence. The investigators concluded that the prototype sequence corresponded to a single germline gene, whereas the variants arose by somatic mutation of this gene. This interpretation seemed consistent with the observation that each variant sequence occurred only once, whereas several occurrences of the same sequence might have been expected if there were several germline Vλ1 genes. Now that gene cloning has confirmed that there is only a single Vλ1 gene, the identification of the variants as products of somatic mutation has been verified.

Subsequent studies led to similar conclusions for mouse Vκ or VH systems involving small V families whose germline members could be readily cloned. An example of such a system is the relatively restricted murine antibody response to phosphorylcholine (PC). Sequence analysis of a panel of PC-binding hybridomas and myelomas expressing a similar VH sequence showed that all IgM antibodies shared a single prototype sequence (403). In contrast, some IgA and most IgG VH regions showed scattered amino acid substitutions with respect to the prototype sequence. All of the sequence variants were unique to single cell lines. By analogy to the Vλ system discussed above, these comparisons suggested that the prototype sequences reflected a germline gene, whereas the variants were products of diverse somatic mutations. A search of the four germline VH-region genes homologous to the prototype expressed VH gene showed only one gene that could have served as a precursor for the PC-binding VH regions; and this one matched the prototype sequence exactly (404). The fact that the variant VH sequences were seen only in IgA and IgG, not in IgM, is consistent with the fact that IgM is characteristically produced early in the immune response, whereas somatic mutation occurs later in the response overlapping the stage of isotype switching; other studies have shown that somatic mutation can be seen in IgM at a low frequency.

Role of Hypermutation in Immune Responses

To understand the role of somatic mutation in the antibody response, several groups have studied the extent of somatic mutation at different times after the immunization of mice. Studies of the responses to p-azophenylarsonate (Ars), phosphorylcholine, influenza hemagglutinin, oxazalone, and several other antigens have all indicated that the initial response after primary immunization is contributed by antibodies showing no somatic mutation. About 1 week after immunization, mutated sequences begin to be observed, increasing during the next week or so. Booster immunizations yield sequences showing additional mutations.

Many hybridomas made late in the immune response produce mutated antibodies with a higher antigen affinity than the unmutated (sometimes loosely called germline) antibodies made early after immunization. The shift to higher affinity is a phenomenon long recognized at the level of (polyclonal) antisera and has been termed "affinity maturation." This phenomenon can now be explained as the result of an evolutionary mechanism selecting antibodies of progressively higher affinity from the pool of randomly mutated V sequences. According to this model, at the time of initial antigen exposure an animal has a set of B lymphocytes expressing germline (unmutated) versions of Ig sequences resulting from gene rearrangements that occurred before immunization. Because of the diversity of available VH, D, JH, VL, and JL sequences as well as the impressive recombinational potential described earlier, some B cells will express Ig molecules capable of binding the antigen with modest affinity. These cells are stimulated (by antigen binding) to proliferate and to secrete antibody. Activated B cells located in lymphoid follicles also bind antigen and receive T-cell help; at some point in the response the somatic hypermutation machinery is activated in these cells, generating random mutations in the Ig genes of stimulated cells in the GCs. Many of these mutations can be expected to reduce the resulting antibody's affinity for antigen; indeed, such mutated antibodies with markedly reduced affinity have been demonstrated (405), as have mutated antibodies that have acquired autoantibody specificity (406). As antigen clearance reduces antigen concentrations seen by the lymphocytes, only the cells displaying high affinity antibody will be effectively stimulated by antigen; cells displaying lower affinity antibodies or antibodies with affinity for self antigens may be subjected to programmed cell death (apoptosis) (407–409). The preferential proliferation of the high-affinity cells and their maturation to secreting plasma cells will be reflected in an increase in the average affinity of the antibodies in the serum. These high-affinity cells will be left as the predominant population to be represented as memory cells when antigen exposure ceases; they thus can induce the rapid, high-affinity response on secondary antigen exposure. In this model the driving force for affinity maturation—analogous to natural selection in the evolution of species—is selection for high antibody affinity in the face of low antigen concentration. The importance of this selective force is suggested by the observation that repeated injection of antigen can inhibit affinity maturation, as though by abolishing the selective pressure for high affinity (410).

Cellular Context of Somatic Mutation

Somatic mutations occur primarily in B cells of the GCs of lymphoid tissues (411,412), particularly in a subpopulation of B cells known as centroblasts. These cells proliferate in the "dark zone" of the GC and bear characteristic surface markers, including IgD, CD38, and the receptor for peanut agglutinin (413,414). Each GC appears to be populated by a small number of antigen-specific founder B cells (412) and an unusual Thy-1–negative T-cell population, also antigen specific (415). The GC environment promotes contact between the B cell and follicular dendritic cells (FDCs) which store, process, and present antigen, and T-lymphocytes, which activate somatic mutation in part via CD40–CD40L interaction (416). Proliferating GC centroblasts give rise to centrocytes, which are programmed for apoptosis unless they are rescued by FDC-presented antigen and T-cell activation via CD40 engagement (409,417). It is at this stage where positive selection for high-affinity antibodies occurs via apoptosis of cells expressing low-affinity antibodies, yet paradoxically apoptosis is also promoted by soluble antigen, perhaps functioning to select against autoantibodies (408,418,419). As mentioned earlier, receptor editing may be another fate for autoantibody-producing cells in GCs. The features of antigen signaling that select for survival versus apoptosis or editing are not fully understood. Susceptibility of GC cell populations to apoptosis is correlated with their expression of Fas, Bax, p53, and c-*myc*, all of which promote apoptosis, as well as down-regulation of the apoptosis suppressor Bcl-2. B cells of mice with engineered up-regulation of Bcl-2 expression can escape selection against autoreactivity (419a).

Germinal center B cells may undergo several successive cycles of mutation followed by selection. Such a scheme is suggested by the sequence analysis of mutated Ig genes PCR-amplified from single cells microdissected from a histologic section of a GC (420); resulting sequences can be organized into genealogical[91] trees con-

sistent with several stages of somatic mutation. Additional evidence for successive mutations has been reported in purified memory B cells (421). A computer simulation has affirmed the high efficiency of alternating periods of somatic mutation and mutation-free selection as a strategy for generating high-affinity antibodies (422). Despite the evidence that somatic mutation occurs normally in GCs, mice lacking histologically detectable GCs as a result of lymphotoxin-α-deficiency are capable of affinity maturation and somatic hypermutation (422a).

Distribution and Targeting of Mutations

To explore the mechanism of somatic hypermutation, several groups have examined the distribution of mutations around Ig genes by comparing the sequences of somatically mutated rearranged genes to their germline precursors. Mutations occur not only in sequence derived from the germline V coding sequence, but also in the J region and nearby flanking intron sequence derived from upstream of the C-region gene. The somatic mutations seem to cluster in the V(D)J region, extending upstream no further than the RNA initiation site (with few exceptions) and tapering off downstream to define a target domain of about 1.5 kb. Therefore, for VDJ units involving the 3' JH4 segment, mutations extend farther downstream than for units involving JH1 (423,424). The focal nature of the mutations suggests a specific Ig hypermutation mechanism that recognizes some feature of the DNA in or near the VDJ sequence as a target for mutations.

Exactly what feature of the V(D)J locus targets the hypermutation machinery is not understood. Unrearranged Vκ, VH, and DJ regions are generally not mutated, suggesting that the functional target probably includes elements contributed by both V and J (425–427); however, unrearranged Vλ regions can be mutated (428). This difference may be related to the fact that unrearranged Vλ genes are transcribed in B cells (429), whereas unrearranged Vκ genes are not (275). Therefore, the element that is contributed by V(D)J recombination in support of Vκ and VH hypermutation may be the proximity of the V-region promoters to enhancers lying near the C region, which can increase transcription. The specific chromosomal location of Ig genes does not seem to be necessary for hypermutation because transgenic mice carrying a rearranged expressible Ig gene—presumably inserted randomly in the genome—show somatic mutations in copies of the transgene cloned from hybridomas (430).

The appearance of hypermutation in transgenes has allowed further experimentation on the sequence requirements for mutation through studies of the effects of altered transgene structure on the mutation rate. The importance of transcription in targeting hypermutation is reinforced by studies of transgenic constructs engineered with or without either of the two transcriptional enhancers associated with the κ locus: the "intronic" enhancer lying between the Jκ segments and Cκ, and the downstream enhancer lying 3' from Cκ. Rearranged κ transgenes that included the downstream κ enhancer and other downstream elements were more highly transcribed and better somatic mutation targets than similar constructs lacking these regions (431,432,432a,432b), whereas removal of the intronic enhancer essentially abolished hypermutation (432). Furthermore, a VκJκ-Cκ transgene in which a duplicate copy of the Vκ promoter was engineered upstream from the Cκ region was found to incur mutations over 1.5-kb domains downstream from both promoters; the extra promoter created a new mutation domain extending into the Cκ region (433). However, the promotion of hypermutation does not seem to be specific to Ig promoters because replacement of the Vκ promoter with the β-globin promoter did not abolish hypermutation (432); non-Ig enhancers also can promote hypermutation (434). Furthermore, the Vκ coding sequence can be replaced by a human β-globin gene or prokaryotic *neo* or *gpt* gene without affecting the hypermutation rate downstream from the promoter (435). In contrast, a similar transgenic construct in which the Vκ gene was replaced by the CD72 gene was not targeted for hypermutation despite high levels of transcription (436), and even a highly expressed Vλ-Cλ transgene was not mutated (437). To summarize, it appears that transcription is necessary but not sufficient for targeting hypermutation, and additional requirements have not been defined as of this writing. Currently available data leave open the possibility that targeting of V genes for somatic mutation is not very specific and that some non-Ig genes that are transcribed in GC B cells also may be subject to mutation (438). Somatic mutations observed in the *bcl6* gene may represent an example of this phenomenon (438a).

Because mutations are not confined to hypervariable (CDR) regions and sometimes even occur in introns, it is apparent that the hypermutation mechanism does not distinguish coding from noncoding regions, let alone hypervariable regions from framework. The apparent clustering of mutations in the CDRs of sequenced Igs may be partly a result of selection for cells expressing primarily CDR mutations, either because framework alterations interfere with the basic folding of the protein or because CDR mutations can lead to higher affinity for antigen and thus stronger activation to clonal expansion, as discussed above. However, in Ig genes that are not selected for function (e.g., nonproductively rearranged VDJ alleles or passenger transgenes engineered with stop codons to prevent expression as a protein), mutational hot spots as well as cold spots have been recognized, apparently due to local DNA features that may promote or suppress somatic mutation within the domain of DNA targeted for hypermutation. It is possible that evolution has selected for sequences that create mutational hot spots in CDR regions to enhance the potential for diversity generation in the parts of the protein critical for antigen contact (439,440).

Molecular Mechanism of Hypermutation

The molecular mechanism of the mutations remains obscure. The observed mutations have shown little about what may have caused them. All four nucleotides have been targets for mutation, and all have been products. Both transitions (purine–purine and pyrimidine–pyrimidine interchanges) and transversions (purine–pyrimidine interchanges) have been observed, with apparent preferential targeting of G-C base pairs (441). Small insertions and deletions rarely occur. Significantly, in an unselected passenger Vκ transgene, A and G nucleotides were mutated more frequently on the coding strand than on the noncoding strand (442); this strand polarity—also observed in human VH regions (443)—suggests that the mutation mechanism may be affected by a process that can distinguish between the strands, such as transcription through the V region.

One report has argued that somatic mutations in an expressed mouse VH gene occurred by gene conversion, i.e., the clustered changes were templated by a nearby related VH region whose sequence agrees with all the observed mutations in the expressed gene (444). Apparent gene conversion also was observed in a mouse strain carrying a transgenic gene construct designed to optimize the possibility of conversion events (445). Clearly gene conversion seems to play a major role in somatic diversification of

chicken and rabbit V genes (446,447) and probably pig V genes as well (448), and it may play a role in the evolutionary diversification of the germline repertoire (449,450); but no further evidence supporting a role for gene conversion in somatic diversification of murine or human Ig genes has been reported, even in cases where such conversion events might be easily detected (451). Indeed, gene conversion could not explain many examples of somatic mutation—e.g., in Vλ1 genes and in the J regions and associated introns—because no closely related but different sequences are present in germline DNA that could donate the mutated nucleotides found in these regions of rearranged genes. This argument also applies to the prokaryotic transgenes targeted for hypermutation in the experiments described above.

The observation that the sequences near somatically mutated nucleotides in Ig genes include direct repeats and palindromic sequences has led to the suggestion that these may play a role in somatic mutation (452). It also has been proposed that mutations may be generated by an error-prone polymerase during repair of nicks or gaps in the DNA (453). Because patients or mice with several defects in DNA repair seem competent for Ig somatic hypermutation, the affected genes are apparently dispensable for this process (454,454a).

A recent model envisions the mutations as a consequence of transcription-coupled repair (433). In one version of this model, a mutator protein specific to GC B cells might load onto the transcriptional complex at the promoter and cause pausing of the complex at various positions; this pausing would induce gratuitous transcription-coupled repair that would occasionally produce errors. Multiple rounds of transcription in each cell could offer repeated opportunities for mutation by this mechanism. In each round of transcription, the mutator protein would fall off the transcription complex as a stochastic event during progression of the complex downstream, thus accounting for the irregular decline in the mutation frequency at increasing distances from the promoter. Such a model would be consistent with the strong correlation between the transcription initiation site and the 5' boundary of mutations (454b,454c).

The product of the mismatch repair gene *Pms2* (homologous to *mutL* in *E. coli*) has been implicated in somatic mutation by a recent experiment: a *Pms2* knockout allele was bred into a mouse strain—the quasimonoclonal or QM mouse—engineered with rearranged VκJκ and VDJ genes knocked-in to the respective germline loci by homologous recombination (454d). Although the *Pms2* mutation causes a general increase in mutation rate in most tissues (454e), the immunoglobulin genes in B cells showed significantly fewer somatic mutations than were seen in the QM mouse with normal *Pms2* (454d), suggesting that *Pms2* activity contributes to Ig gene hypermutation. Mismatch repair machinery could hypothetically participate in Ig gene hypermutation by switching its usual preference for correcting the newly synthesized strand, instead preserving any mutations in this strand by "correcting" the opposite strand.

An important, but as yet unclarified, role for IgD in somatic mutation is suggested by the observation that mice with a homozygous targeted disruption of their Cδ gene were impaired, although not completely deficient, in affinity maturation (455). Conversely, an IgM⁻IgD⁺ subset of GC B cells from human tonsils were found to accumulate extremely high numbers of somatic mutations (456).

Investigations of somatic mutation should be facilitated by recently described systems for observing the process in vitro in primary B cells (454f,457) or cell lines (441,458) and by the development of rapid methods for detecting somatic mutation (459).

Immunoglobulin Gene Evolution: Varying Roles for V Gene Assembly

Evolution of the Immunoglobulin Superfamily and V Assembly Recombination

The three families of Ig genes (κ, λ, and H chains) and the closely related four families of TCR genes (α, β, γ, and δ) clearly provide a powerful and flexible molecular defense mechanism that is valuable for survival in the face of the diverse pathogenic microorganisms that abound in our environment. How did such a complex and elegant system evolve? One obvious approach to elucidating Ig gene evolution is to infer genetic history from comparisons of the Ig gene systems in different modern species. The more ancient history of these genes may be approached by examining homologous non-Ig genes. The ever-growing number of non-Ig genes that demonstrate sequence similarity, and therefore presumed homology, to the Ig genes has become known as the Ig superfamily (460,461). This family name reflects the fact that the Ig genes were the first members to be sequenced and does not imply a functional relationship of the superfamily to Igs or to the immune system. The hallmark of the Ig superfamily is the Ig domain: approximately 100 amino acids, generally encoded in a single exon, and including an internal disulfide loop spanning roughly 60 to 70 amino acids. Despite some rather tenuous primary sequence similarities, the Ig domains are all assumed to share approximately the same three-dimensional structure found in Igs, comprising seven roughly parallel strands forming two layers of β-pleated sheets. This assumption has been confirmed for several members of the superfamily, including β2-microglobulin, CD4, TCR-α and -β chains, and the α3 domain of MHC class I.

Almost all of the Ig superfamily members are surface proteins that function by contacting other surface proteins in cell–cell interactions. Because Ig superfamily members mediating such interactions are found in even the most primitive metazoan organisms—e.g., cell adhesion molecules in slime molds (462)—the Ig domain is likely to be truly ancient, significantly predating the function of superfamily members in defense against microbial invasion. On the other hand, several invertebrate superfamily members have been described that do play a role in microbial defense, e.g., the molluscan defense molecule (463) and insect hemolin (464), which may even share with Ig genes some features of gene regulation by Rel family transcription factors (465). Such examples suggest that some members of the superfamily may have functioned in a primitive immune system in a common ancestor of molluscs, insects, and vertebrates.

Although the Ig domains of most currently known superfamily members are encoded in single exons, several examples (e.g., CD4, N-CAM, and the Xenopus CTX protein) are encoded in two separate exons (466,467). It is uncertain whether this structure reflects an origin of the Ig domain from association of two primordial half-domains by exon shuffling (with later loss of the intron in most current superfamily genes) or the introduction of an intron into a preexisting single-exon Ig domain. Several of the distantly related superfamily members appear to be more C-like or V-like, suggesting that they arose after the divergence between the primordial C domain and V domain. However, this sequence of events is not definitively established, and examples of both C- and V-like genes are known that show the divided half-domain structure.

Do the separated V-region elements (V, D, and J) found in modern Ig (and TCR) genes reflect an association of originally unrelated sequences or fragmentation of elements that were contiguous in an ancestral gene? Suggestive observations bearing on this question have come from an analysis of the CD8 gene. A genealogic relationship between the CD8 antigen and κ Ig is suggested not only by sequence similarity but also by the linkage of their genes on chromosome 6 of mice and chromosome 2 of humans. The CD8 gene has been found to include a segment of J-like sequence contiguous with the V-like sequence (468), suggesting that V and J sequences may have been contiguous in a primordial ancestor gene. The presently observed separation of V and J may then have resulted from insertion of DNA between them by a transposition-like event (Fig. 17), as originally proposed by Sakano et al. (6). A second similar insertion may have separated D sequence from the germline V, as shown in the Fig. 17, although an alternative hypothesis involving a single insertion event also has been proposed (469). In order for the V, (D), and J regions to be reassembled after they were rendered noncontiguous by the transposition event, one would need to assume the prior or simultaneous development of a mechanism—presumably based on the RAG proteins—for V(D)J recombination. Because there is no evidence for RAG-like genes in primitive species without V(D)J recombination, simultaneous acquisition of the RAG genes and the insertion separating germline V, (D), and J elements appears reasonable, lending favor to the speculation that the RAG genes may have been carried on a transposonlike element—flanked by 7-mer and 9-mer RSS repeats on both ends—that inserted into a primitive V region. Such a transposon might have derived by lateral transfer from a prokaryotic element. Presumably the sequence inserted roughly 400 million years ago into the genome of a primitive cartilaginous fish because RAG genes (208), as well as V(D)J recombination of Ig and TCR genes, are found in modern sharks and all higher vertebrates examined (470–472); but none of these parameters are found in the slightly more primitive lamprey and hagfish. Interestingly, the shark RAG-1 gene shows sequence similarity to the INT (integrase) gene of phage λ (as well as to the yeast DNA repair proteins RAD 16 and 18 and the human breast cancer susceptibility gene BRCA1), whereas RAG-2 shows sequence similarity to the bacterial integration host factor gene. The similarities to modern prokaryotic genes with a recombination-related function strengthens the hypothesis of a prokaryotic source for the RAG genes. Moreover, as noted earlier, the mechanism of RAG-catalyzed DNA rearrangement—with a hairpin intermediate—bears some similarity to prokaryotic DNA recombination mechanisms.

V(D)J recombination may have provided primordial Ig superfamily genes with their first potential for somatic diversification, i.e., variable junctions resulting from the flexibility of the recombination position. Presumably, as soon as diversity became functionally important for recognition of specific foreign antigens, mechanisms for clonal activation would have been developed and allelic exclusion would have become important to focus the specificity of the response. Conceivably these features arose before the divergence between Ig and TCR genes.

Diverse Evolutionary Mechanisms for Diversity

Ig genes of the shark, chicken, and rabbit provide interesting contrasts to the more familiar evolutionary paths taken by mice and humans. The shark H-chain locus consists of multiple duplicates of ~10-kb units containing separated V, D, J, and CH elements (65,473). The V, D, and J elements are associated with recombination signal elements similar to their mammalian homologs. Sequence comparisons between duplicated units demonstrate differences not only between the germline V genes but between the

CH genes as well. If VDJ recombination occurs only within one of these repeat units, as has been presumed, then diversity would derive from junctional flexibility but not from combinatorial multiplication; sharks also would lack the level of diversity afforded by the isotype switch because a particular V region would always be associated with a specific CH region. This limited system allows the shark to mount specific antibody responses, but these responses show remarkably little variation between individuals, although somatic mutation does occur. Presumably, the mechanism for clonal selection is operative in sharks.

Diversity generation in chickens follows a still different scheme. The λ system has been particularly well studied (474,475) and in the germline consists of a Vλ1 gene 1.7 kb upstream from a typical Jλ-Cλ unit. All the expressed λ protein apparently derives from VJ recombination involving this Vλ1 gene. Upstream of Vλ1 lie 25 Vλ pseudogenes. These pseudogenes cannot themselves encode viable V regions and do not rearrange with the Jλ segment. However, they contribute to diversity by donating stretches of their sequence to the rearranged Vλ1 by a somatic gene conversion process; expressed Vλ sequences show multiple patches of sequence that differ from Vλ1

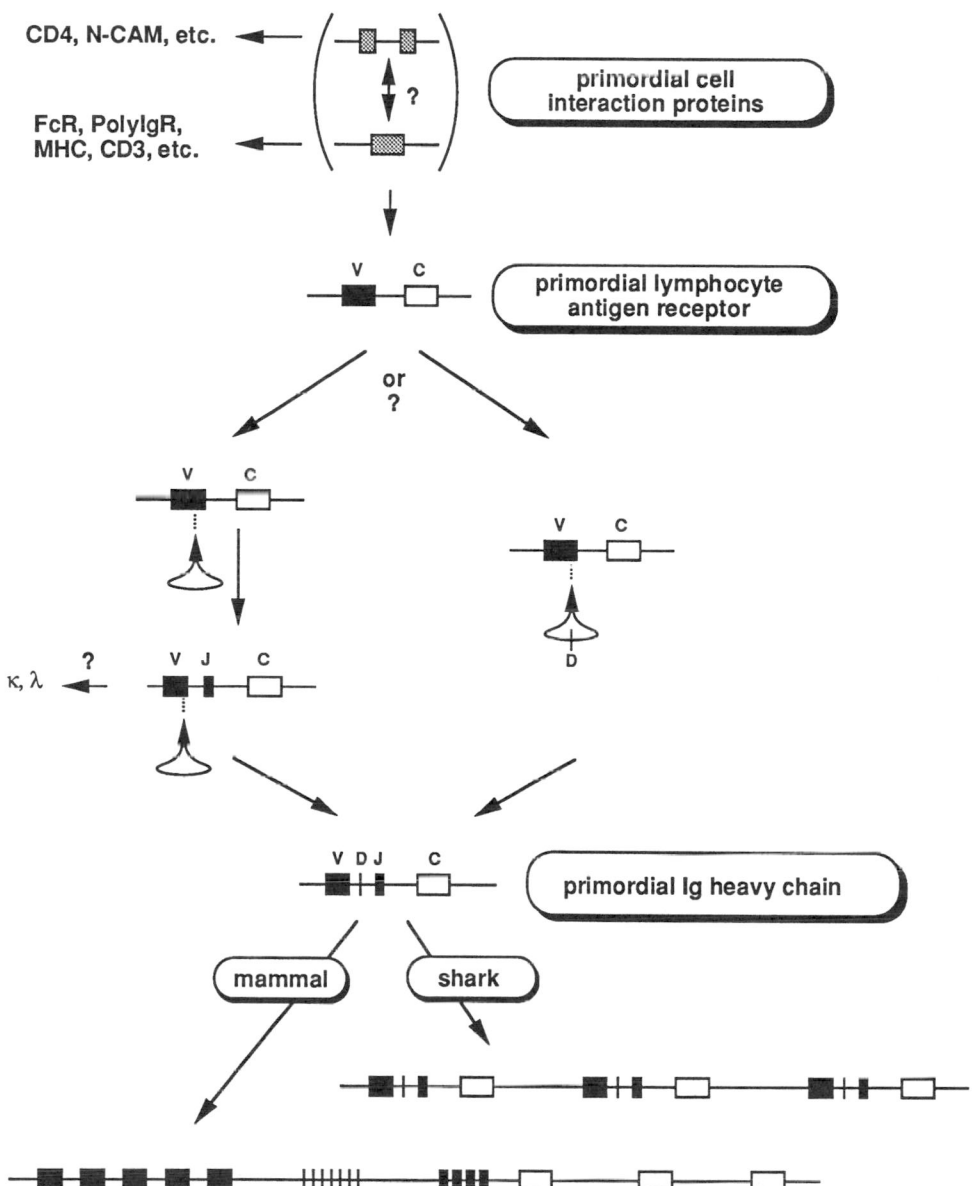

FIG. 17. Evolution of Ig genes. The Ig superfamily presumably evolved from a primordial cell interaction domain by multiple rounds of duplication followed by individual mutation and specialization by different duplicated copies. Because both Ig and TCR systems share specialized V and C domains and V assembly recombination, these features probably evolved before divergence of these two antigen receptor systems. The evolution of the split V region (requiring assembly of V, D, and J to form a functional domain) could have resulted from a single event inserting a D sequence and flanking DNA between V and J of a primordial V domain (pathway on right) or by two separate insertion events (pathway on left). The primordial H-chain gene evolved by different pathways of duplication in shark and mammalian lineages. Sharks show duplication of the entire VDJC unit, whereas in mammals separate duplication of each of these elements occurred.

but precisely match specific pseudogene sequences. Thus, in contrast to the somatic hypermutation observed in mice and humans, individual expressed chicken λ genes show no evidence of random point mutations, and no sequence alterations are found in the intron sequences flanking the rearranged VJ unit. Although combinatorial joining diversity is completely absent in this system, the chicken is capable of a highly heterogeneous λ response as a result of multiple rounds of gene conversion events operating in different regions of the V segment. A similar gene conversion mechanism is important in generating diversity in the chicken H-chain system.

Rabbit Igs might have been expected to follow the schema demonstrated for the homologous loci from the two most intensively studied mammals (mice and humans), but the facts are more interesting. A particularly puzzling feature of rabbit Ig relates to expression of VH allotypes. From 70% to 90% of rabbit antibodies display one of three serologically defined allotypes known as a1, a2, or a3. Rabbits that express one predominant allotype pass this characteristic to their progeny as though a single gene with three alleles were being transmitted as a Mendelian codominant trait; however, Southern blots of rabbit genomic DNA showed several hundred VH-hybridizing bands. How could the simple inheritance of allotype expression be explained given the large number of VH genes? The answer, as demonstrated primarily by Knight and colleagues, is that rearrangements of the most D-proximal VH region, designated VH1, account for most of the H chains expressed in rabbits, and this VH gene encodes the specific amino acids that define the VHa allotype (476). The other VH-region segments contribute to diversity primarily by gene conversion events that alter the VH1 sequence (447); somatic point mutations apparently occur as well (476a). These upstream VH regions may occasionally rearrange productively, perhaps accounting for the 10% to 30% of VHa allotype-negative antibodies in normal rabbits. The potential for such recombination is suggested by a strain of rabbits (Alicia) in which the VH1 gene was deleted; this strain nevertheless makes normal amounts of antibody, most of which is VHa allotype negative. Gene conversion also contributes to diversity in bovine Igs (477).

Undoubtedly, examination of the Ig genes of other organisms will provide additional details of the evolution of these remarkable loci and a better understanding of the differing strategies for the generation of diversity. Such studies also should help to elucidate the evolutionary relationship between Ig genes, the homologous TCR genes, and other Ig superfamily members not involved in immune defense.

REGULATION OF IMMUNOGLOBULIN GENE EXPRESSION

General Principles of Gene Regulation

The mechanisms that regulate the expression of Ig genes have been under intense investigation in recent years as part of a wide effort to understand development and differentiation in molecular terms. Immunoglobulins are synthesized only by B-lymphocytes; even within this lineage these proteins are made in differing amounts at different developmental stages. Although rates of protein synthesis can be regulated at the levels of mRNA transcription, processing, transport, stability, and translation, most attention has focused on transcription because this seems to be the limiting step in most systems that have been examined [although changes in mRNA stability can clearly play an important role (478)]. The gene loci encoding lymphocyte antigen receptors (Ig and TCR) are unique in that the complete genes do not exist in the earliest stages of lymphocyte maturation; only the germline precursors are present. Thus, the regulation of Ig gene expression must be integrated with the progress of Ig gene rearrangements. These processes are further intertwined because as discussed elsewhere in this chapter, transcription is apparently required for Ig gene rearrangement, both for V(D)J assembly and isotype switch recombination. Thus, the transcriptional regulation of nonrearranged loci also merits analysis.

Cis Regulation

Gene transcription can be regulated by cis influences—dependent on the DNA sequence of genetic elements attached to a gene—and trans influences, dependent on the environment of the gene. For most genes, regulatory studies have initially focused on the cis elements that regulate gene expression. Some insights have been gained by examining how gene expression is affected by spontaneous mutations or deletions of regulatory sequences in cells or animals. However, most advances have been made by inserting putative regulatory elements into DNA constructs containing a reporter gene—one whose expression can be conveniently assayed—and then transfecting the constructs back into eukaryotic cells; the function of the putative regulatory elements is then tested by assaying for reporter gene expression. In some experiments the assays are performed only 2 to 3 days after transfection, an interval so short that most of the DNA remains in an unstable episomal form; these are known as transient transfections. In contrast, other experiments are designed to produce stable transfectants in which the engineered DNA construct becomes inserted into the cell chromosomes. As an alternative to transfection of cells, similar constructs can be introduced into the mouse genome, thereby creating strains of transgenic mice. The expression of the introduced transgene can then be assessed in a variety of tissues in the animal to examine whether the candidate regulatory element can program the same pattern of tissue-specific expression as that observed for the gene from which the element was derived.

Through such transfection and transgene experiments three major classes of eukaryotic cis regulatory elements have been defined. A promoter is a DNA segment that is located near the transcriptional initiation site and that promotes the initiation of RNA transcription in a specific direction, i.e., toward the coding sequence of the gene. An enhancer is a DNA segment that can stimulate transcription when positioned at variable distances from the transcription initiation site and in either orientation. A silencer downregulates transcription, operating (like an enhancer) in both orientations and over variable distances via mechanisms not thoroughly understood. All three kinds of elements are generally active in only certain cell types and thus participate in regulating the tissue-specific expression of the associated gene. Two other types of cis elements have been characterized in eukaryotic chromosomes and should be noted. Matrix attachment regions (MARs) attach DNA to the chromosomal scaffold proteins and may promote local unpairing of the DNA strands (479,480). Locus control regions (LCRs), first discovered in the β-globin locus (481), are complex regulatory regions that are composed of smaller elements that individually have enhancer function. LCRs affect chromatin structure and gene activity over longer distances than enhancers are thought to act. Operationally they are defined by their ability—when tested in transgenic constructs—to program associated reporter genes for expression independent of the position of integration into chromosomal DNA; in contrast, constructs without LCRs generally are expressed at widely different levels in different transgenic mouse strains depending on integration site.

Figure 18 provides an overview of the currently known regulatory sequences of the Ig loci in the mouse (similar regions have been reported for most of the homologous human loci). Promoters are present in the flanking DNA just upstream of each V gene in all three loci: κ, λ, and H chain. In plasmacytomas only the promoter of the rearranged V region is active, whereas similar promoters of unrearranged upstream Vκ or VH regions are inactive. This observation provoked a search for an additional regulatory sequence downstream from the J that might activate the promoter of the adjacent rearranged V region. The J-C regions of the κ and H-chain loci were screened for regulatory regions, and enhancers were found in J-C introns of both loci. (The J-C introns of λ loci apparently lack enhancers.) Near the intronic enhancers of the κ and IgH loci, silencer regions have been reported that may inhibit the activity of the associated enhancers in non-B cells. After the discovery of intron enhancers, two observations led to expectations of additional enhancers 3′ from the C-region genes. First, several myelomas were found to have undergone spontaneous deletions that eliminated the J-C intronic enhancer of the expressed H-chain gene, but the myelomas nonetheless continued to express this gene at normal levels; these observations were consistent with the presence of an additional enhancer in the DNA that had not been deleted. Second, enhancers were discovered downstream from C-region genes in the related family of TCR genes. Subsequent investigation uncovered enhancers 3′ from κ and λ C-region genes, as well as an enhancer 3′ from the Cα gene, the most downstream constant gene in the H-chain locus.

These enhancers, silencers, and the V-region promoters may be sufficient to explain the transcription of complete, assembled Ig genes; but additional germline or sterile transcripts are transcribed from Ig C-region genes that are being activated for V assembly or isotype switch rearrangements. These transcripts are also controlled by promoters (Fig. 18), which in some cases have been found to be critical for regulation of the associated DNA rearrangement.

Promoters, enhancers, and silencers are composed of clusters of several short sequence motifs, each of which can be recognized by a specific nuclear protein (or proteins). Some of these motifs are present in more than one enhancer or may even be shared between enhancers and promoters. In the discussion below, several of the important murine regulatory regions and their functional motifs are described, along with nuclear protein families known to regulate Ig gene expression by binding to these motifs. Each murine regulatory region has been found to have an apparent homolog in humans, often with many of the same nuclear binding motifs conserved. The presence of multiple motifs in a given enhancer complicates the analysis of the role of any one motif. Engineered mutations in a particular motif often have very little effect on the activity of the complete enhancer, and sometimes an artificial construct containing a single functional motif often shows no enhancer activity on its own. Two strategies have been used to demonstrate the function of such motifs. In a construct with an enhancer fragment in which all but a few motifs have been deleted, the contribution of each remaining element is often detectable through the effects of mutations. Alternatively, an artificial enhancer containing several multimerized copies of a single motif may have enhancer activity when a single copy does not. The proteins that bind to enhancer motifs mediate the regulatory function by promoting (or inhibiting, in the case of silencers) the assembly of transcriptional machinery at the promoter. The proposed interactions between proteins binding enhancer and promoter imply that the intervening DNA forms a large loop. Many regulatory proteins are present in the nuclei of only certain tissues or cell types, a fact that can in principle explain the cell type specificity of the transcription

of particular genes. External stimuli that up- or downregulate Ig gene expression (e.g., cytokines or antigen binding) typically work by altering the amounts or activity of certain DNA-binding proteins.

Types of Trans Effects

Alteration in the nuclear content of DNA binding proteins that interact with cis regulatory elements represents a well-studied mechanism for trans regulation of gene expression, but other approaches to investigating trans regulation should also be mentioned. One correlate of gene activation that formally falls in the class of trans effects is the altered chromatin environment of DNA in expressed genes that is often detectable by nuclease sensitivity experiments. In these experiments isolated nuclei are treated with varying concentrations of DNase I (or a variety of other nucleases, including restriction endonucleases) and the DNA is then purified, digested with a restriction enzyme, and analyzed by Southern blotting using a hybridization probe for the genes under study. In general, when the nuclei are derived from cells expressing a particular gene, that gene is more sensitive to DNase I than unexpressed genes in the same cells; i.e., a Southern blot band carrying the expressed gene can be abolished by treatment with low concentrations of DNase that leave unexpressed genes (or their Southern blot bands) relatively unaffected. In addition, appropriate Southern blot strategies show that certain segments of DNA in expressed genes may be hypersensitive to DNase I; these segments tend to coincide with regulatory regions of genes where sequence-specific binding by regulatory proteins blocks access of these DNA regions to nucleosomes, rendering them accessible to nucleases.

Another chromatin correlate of gene activation is the extent of DNA methylation. Most cytosine residues within CpG dinucleotides are methylated in mammalian DNA, but genes that are actively expressed in a particular cell generally appear relatively undermethylated in that cell type (482). The extent of CpG methylation can conveniently be estimated for that subset of CpG dinucleotides that fall within the sequence CCGG, which is the recognition site for two restriction endonucleases: Msp I cuts at this site regardless of the methylation status of the internal cytosines, whereas Hpa II cuts only the completely demethylated site. Southern blot strategies that exploit this difference have been used to compare methylation in active and inactive genes. Both μ and κ C-region genes have been shown to be sensitive to DNase I and undermethylated in pre-B cells, B cells, and plasma cells but DNase resistant in nonlymphoid cells (483–487). Cells that are undergoing isotype switching show undermethylation of the C-region genes that are the targets of switch recombination (483,488); such undermethylation correlates with synthesis of germline transcripts from these CH genes. Of V-region genes in B cells, only the rearranged and transcribed V gene generally shows the undermethylation and DNase sensitivity characteristic of active genes (484,489). In the IgH locus, DNase I hypersensitivity sites have been found overlapping the intronic (486) and downstream enhancers (490,491). In the κ gene, hypersensitivity sites occur at the promoter and enhancer as well as at a site 5′ from the enhancer (492,493).

Methods of Studying Trans-Acting Proteins Binding to cis Regulatory Motifs

Recent studies have investigated trans-acting proteins identified by their interaction with known cis-acting promoters or enhancers. In vitro binding of nuclear proteins to specific regulatory sequence elements can be detected by several techniques, some of which can be

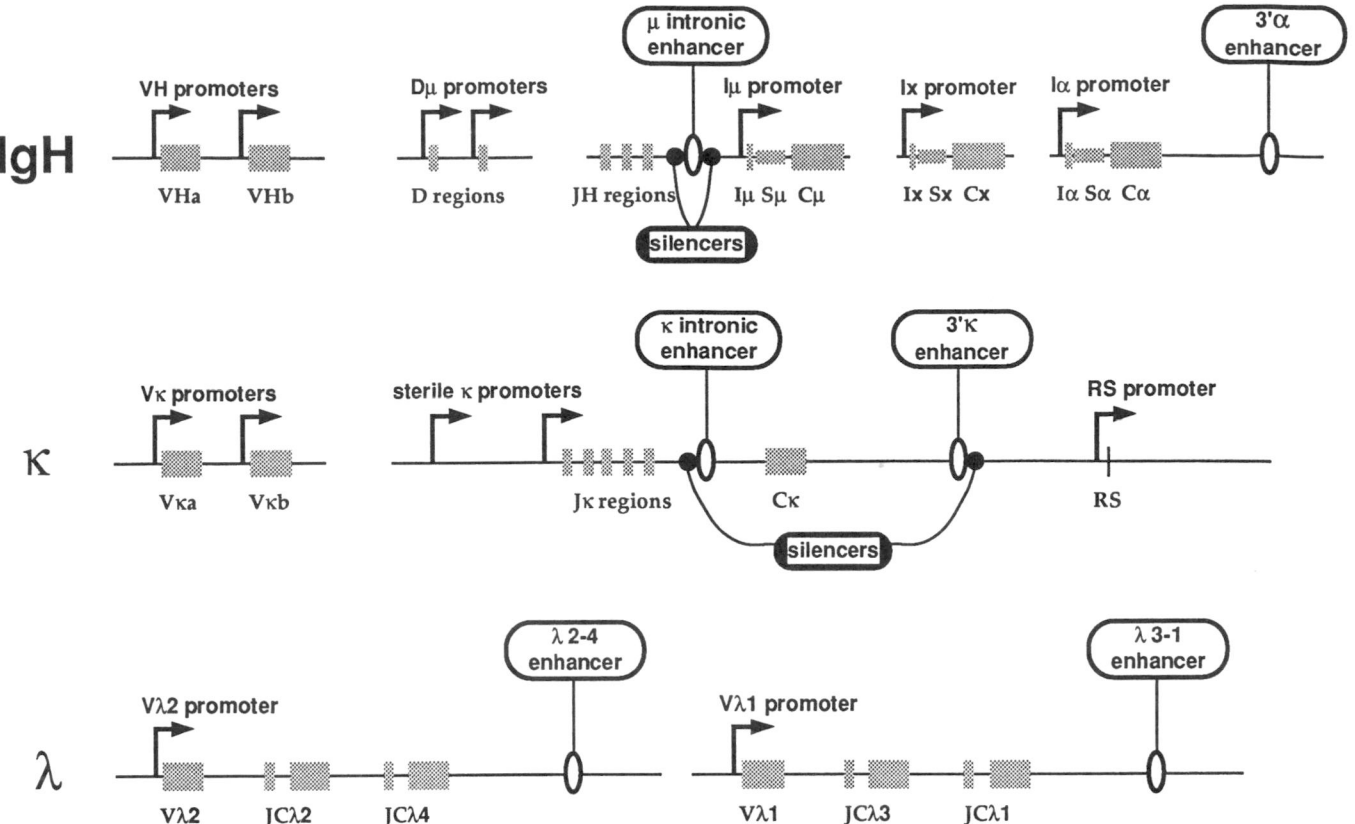

FIG. 18. Enhancers and promoters of the murine Ig loci. Schematic maps (not to scale) of the three murine Ig loci are shown: IgH (*top*), κ (*middle*), and λ (*bottom*). The six known Ig enhancers are shown as vertical ellipses, the four silencer regions by black circles, and the various promoters by arrows indicating the direction of transcription. The enhancer reported upstream from murine DQ52 (572) is not shown in the graphic image.

used to assess sequence-specific binding even in crude protein mixtures. The simplest technique is the EMSA. In this assay a short (typically 30–300 bp) radioactively labeled double-stranded DNA fragment is allowed to interact with a mixture of proteins extracted from cell nuclei by a salt solution; when the DNA is then electrophoresed in an acrylamide gel, binding of protein(s) to the DNA can be detected by the retarded mobility of the protein–DNA complexes in the gel in comparison with the mobility of the free DNA probe. Sequence specificity of the retarded band must be demonstrated by showing (a) that its intensity can be diminished by adding to the incubation mixture an unlabeled competitor oligonucleotide identical to the probe sequence, but (b) that a similar amount of oligonucleotide of unrelated sequence is without effect. Retarded complexes can be identified as containing an already characterized protein if an antibody to that protein specifically eliminates or supershifts (i.e., further retards the electrophoretic mobility) of the band. Another powerful technique, DNA footprinting, allows the visualization of the specific DNA sequence covered by a bound protein. In this technique a protein preparation is allowed to bind to a fragment of DNA that has been radioactively labeled on one end of one strand. The DNA-protein mixture is then treated with DNase under conditions so mild that on average each strand will be nicked by the enzyme only once; then the DNA is purified from the incubated proteins and electrophoresed on a denaturing acrylamide gel (along with size markers) in order to detect the positions of DNase-induced nicks in the radiolabeled strand. A nuclear protein that can bind tightly to the radioactive DNA fragment during the initial DNase incubation step

protects the region of the DNA that it contacts from nuclease attack, and so the position of the bound protein can be inferred from a region of the fragment that is relatively free of nicks (the footprint).

Once a protein has been detected that binds to a critical regulatory element in the DNA, detailed study of the protein requires molecular cloning of its gene. Two main strategies have been used for such cloning. In one approach the protein is first purified by classic fractionation procedures. EMSA or DNase footprinting assays can be used to follow the binding protein through fractionation steps. Typically, the purification includes an affinity column in which the DNA sequence representing the binding target is fixed to the column bed; the specifically interacting protein binds this DNA sequence with high affinity, separating it from contaminating material. When the protein is pure, amino acid sequences are obtained from tryptic fragments; these sequences are used to design DNA probes that can be used to isolate clones from a cDNA library. An alternative cloning strategy (494) bypasses the protein purification procedure. From a cell expressing the binding protein, a cDNA library is constructed using the vector λgt11, a bacteriophage engineered to allow transcription and translation of insert cDNA sequences in infected bacteria. A library of viral plaques imprinted onto membrane filters is screened by soaking the filters in a solution containing the target DNA binding sequence as a radioactively labeled fragment. A plaque that expresses a cDNA encoding the binding protein is able to bind the probe and thus creates a radioactive spot on an autoradiograph of the filters. Clones identified by their position on the filters are then isolated for study.

The fact that a purified nuclear protein binds in a sequence-specific manner to a regulatory DNA sequence does not prove that this protein mediates the regulatory function of the DNA sequence. However, a functional role for an enhancer-binding protein can be inferred if transfection of a clone encoding the protein induces transcription of a cotransfected reporter gene linked to the enhancer/promoter motif that is bound by the cloned protein. Such experiments have verified the function of several Ig promoter- and enhancer-binding proteins, which can therefore be considered transcription factors. Some of these occur only in B-lymphocytes and thus can account in part for the B-cell specificity of Ig gene expression. Others are more widespread. Many of these regulators of Ig genes are homologous to mammalian oncogenes as well as to genes of drosophila and yeast, suggesting ancient evolutionary origins and fundamental importance of these proteins in the regulation of cellular metabolism.

Several of these proteins will be discussed below in connection with the cis regulatory elements with which they interact. Most of this discussion is based on analysis of murine Ig genes, which have been examined most extensively.

Cis-Acting Elements in V-Region Promoters

The Octamer Motif

The transcription of assembled Ig genes initiates upstream from the V gene sequences. The promoters that regulate this initiation are, by virtue of their upstream positions, present in each germline V-region gene even before V assembly recombination. Like many eukaryotic genes, most V gene promoters contain a TATA site about 25 bp 5′ from the initiation site; TATA sites serve as binding sites for the transcription factor TFIID and related proteins and thereby play a role in specifying the exact position where RNA transcription initiates. The only other conserved feature of all classes of Ig V promoters (i.e., κ, λ, and H chain) is an octamer ATTTGCAT that is found associated with Vκ and Vλ genes, whereas the inverted complement ATGCAAAT is found 5′ from VH genes (495,496). (The same sequence is sometimes identified as a decamer TNATTTGCAT or the complementary ATGCAAATNA.) Vκ promoters generally include only the octamer plus the TATA box, whereas VH and Vλ promoters can include both of these motifs as well as other characteristic regulatory elements. The conservation of the octamer element in Ig V promoters suggested that it might play an important role in Ig gene function; indeed, when constructs containing this motif were analyzed by transfection, it became clear that the octamer is critical in conferring B-cell specificity to the promoter. Deletions or mutations in the octamer cause dramatically reduced B cell–specific promoter activity when tested either in Ig gene constructs or in heterologous genes transfected into B cells (497–501). The octamer also has been shown to be required for optimal in vitro transcription by B-cell nuclear extracts, whereas it had no effect on transcription by HeLa extracts (502). Octamers appear in the promoters of several B cell–specific genes other than Ig, including B29 (Igβ) (503), CD21 (504), and CD20 (505). A multimerized octamer can act as a B cell–specific enhancer (506).

A puzzling feature of transcriptional regulation by the octamer is that this sequence is also a functional component of promoters of several other genes whose transcription is not B cell specific. These include the herpes thymidine kinase gene, histone H2B genes, and U1 and U2 small nuclear RNA genes. To understand the puzzling relationship between octamers in Ig and non-Ig promoters, several laboratories have undertaken analyses of the trans-acting nuclear proteins that bind to these elements. Two such proteins—designated

Oct-1 and Oct-2—have been extensively characterized, initially by EMSA experiments and subsequently by gene cloning (507–510). These two proteins show differing tissue distributions. Most cells make Oct-1 (also known as OTF-1 and NFA-1), but only B cells and a few other cell types (notably, activated T cells) make Oct-2 (OTF-2, NFA-2). Several additional octamer-binding proteins specific to other tissues (e.g., in neural cells or embryonic stem cells) have been reported. The Oct proteins share a similar 160–amino acid DNA binding domain, which explains their virtually identical binding specificity. Amino acid sequences similar to this DNA binding domain have been found in several other nuclear proteins that bind to motifs resembling the octamer. This binding domain thus defines a family of nuclear factors, which has been designated the POU family (pronounced "pow"), named for the three factors in which this conserved domain was first noted: Pit-1, Oct-1/2, and the nematode gene unc86. The domain includes a 75-to 80-residue POU-specific domain (POU$_S$), a short flexible linker, and a 60–amino acid segment (POU$_H$) homologous to the homeobox domain. (Homeoboxes were first recognized in genes regulating drosophila development, but more recently have been noted in genes throughout the animal kingdom and even in plants.) The POU$_S$ domain contacts the ATGC part of the ATGCAAAT sequence, whereas the POU$_H$ domain contacts the AAAT segment (511).

The Oct proteins have been demonstrated to be transcription factors by experiments in which the corresponding genes were cotransfected into fibroblasts or HeLa cells along with reporter gene constructs driven by octamer-containing promoters. Critical activation regions, necessary for the Oct proteins to stimulate transcription, have been deduced from the effects of deletions and mutations placed in different regions of Oct proteins (512) and the effects of swapping (through genetic engineering) various domains between Oct-1, Oct-2, and other POU proteins (513–515). On the N-terminal side of the POU domain, Oct-1 and Oct-2 both contain a glutamine-rich activation region, but on the C-terminal side Oct-2 contains a feature missing from Oct-1: an activation region rich in serines, threonines, and prolines. Apparently the C-terminal differences are functionally important because swapping the N-terminal domains between Oct-1 and Oct-2 has little effect, whereas replacing the C-terminal domain of Oct-1 by that of Oct-2 confers a distinctive property of Oct-2: the ability to activate transcription from multiple octamer motifs functioning as either a promoter or an enhancer (506).

The B-cell specificity of Oct-2 suggested that this factor might be important for activity of the octamer motif in V promoters, and some evidence supports this inference. However, targeted disruption of the Oct-2 genes in a B-cell line (516) produced little effect on the expression of either endogenous Ig genes or a transfected gene driven by an octamer-containing promoter. Furthermore, although homozygous Oct-2 knockout mice (517) die without obvious pathology within a few hours of birth, they contain roughly normal numbers of B cells, which respond to activation by a T-cell clone with near normal cell proliferation and Ig secretion (518). These results suggest that Oct-2 is unnecessary for the V-region promoter activity required either for early B-cell development or for T cell–activated Ig secretion, possibly because of the redundant role of Oct-1 for these processes. On the other hand, cultured B cells from the homozygous Oct-2 knockout animals showed marked defects in LPS plus cytokine–activated Ig secretion and in anti-IgM–induced proliferation, suggesting a role for Oct-2 dependent proteins in these signaling pathways.

The B-cell specificity of Oct proteins is complicated by their interactions with additional proteins. One such protein—designated octamer coactivator from B cells (OCA-B)—was originally detected in affinity-purified preparations of either Oct-1 or Oct-2 as a factor necessary for optimal in vitro transcription from a Vκ promoter (519). The purified protein has now been cloned by several laboratories, which use several different names for it: OCA-B (520), OBF-1 (521), and Bob-1 (522). Binding of OCA-B to the octamer/Oct–protein complex apparently stimulates transcription through a transcriptional activation domain of OCA-B (523). The OCA-B protein binds to the POU domain of either Oct-1 or Oct-2, but also may contact the DNA at the fifth base of the ATGCAAAT sequence; oligonucleotides with alterations at that position bind the Oct proteins normally but cannot form a complex with OCA-B, nor can a reporter construct mutated at that position show OCA-B–induced stimulation of transcription (523,524). An important role of this protein for in vivo regulation of Ig production is suggested by the effects of OCA-B disruption by gene targeting (525,526). OCA-B knockout mice seem healthy and are fertile but show defects in B-cell maturation and Ig production. The number of mature B cells in the spleen is reduced, and the response to immunization is dramatically impaired, with reduced proliferation and a severe decrease in IgG, IgA, and IgE, apparently due to decreased Ig gene transcription in B cells that have undergone isotype switch recombination. GCs are not formed in these mice. Some of these effects are apparently mediated by decreased Ig gene transcription, whereas others may result from interference with OCA-B–dependent expression of other genes. Purified OCA-B seems to bind preferentially to Oct-1 rather than Oct-2 (527); a second coactivator has been postulated to mediate Oct-2–dependent transactivation (528).

What is the critical feature of octamer motifs in Ig promoters that confers B-cell specificity when the same motif in an H2B promoter is active ubiquitously? Although the answer is still not known, one possibility is that apart from the TATA box, octamers in Ig promoters are not associated with other important promoter motifs that might allow ubiquitous expression in ubiquitously expressed genes. Consistent with this view is the observation that the insertion of a CCAAT promoter motif to an otherwise lymphoid-specific promoter renders the promoter active in nonlymphoid cells (529). It is also possible that—as in the case of several other coactivators for Oct-1, including VP16 (530,531) and PTF (532)—sequences outside the octamer play a role in discriminating between Ig and other promoters. OCA-B may mediate some of this discrimination because OCA-B, when added to a HeLa-derived in vitro transcription system or when coexpressed in HeLa cells, could coactivate a construct driven by a Vκ promoter much more effectively than a similar construct with an H2B promoter, even though both promoter sequences supported complex formation with OCA-B (520,521). Candidate motifs that might contribute to B-cell specificity of Vκ promoters include sequences downstream from the transcription start site (532a).

In addition to its role in V promoters, the octamer also appears in the H-chain enhancer, where it can contribute to the B cell specificity of constructs transfected into various cell lines (533), although it did not appear critical for enhancer function in transgenic mice (534). This octamer may activate the enhancer under certain conditions of cell stimulation (535) and clearly plays an important role when this region functions as a promoter driving sterile transcripts of the Cμ gene (536). Additional DNA segments that are similar, but not identical, to the octamer have been found in several other regulatory regions of Ig genes, e.g., upstream of the mouse κ intron enhancer (537). However, the functional importance of most of these octamerlike motifs has not been demonstrated. The mechanism of regulation by the Oct proteins is likely

to be considerably more complex than outlined here because of the existence of several isoforms resulting from alternative RNA splicing (538–540), several phosphorylation states critical to protein function (513,541), and the ability of both OCA-B and the Oct proteins to interact with other regulatory factors ((520,542,543).

Other Elements of Ig V Promoters

Although unusual Vκ promoters that lack efficient octamer motifs have been reported to attain promoter activity through an alternative pyrimidine-rich element designated κY (544), and a motif binding early B-cell factor may contribute to some Vκ promoters (545), Vκ promoters are typically composed only of the octamer plus TATA box. In contrast, Vλ and VH promoters routinely contain additional functional elements besides the octamer and TATA box, some of which are briefly described below. In VH promoters a heptamer CTCATGA generally lying 2 to 22 bp 5′ from the octamer was found to be well conserved and required for optimum promoter activity (546). Surprisingly, although this sequence bears little resemblance to the conserved octamer ATGCAAAT, it appears to bind in vitro to both Oct-1 and Oct-2 (547–551). The heptamer binds these proteins with lower intrinsic affinity but shows cooperative interaction with occupancy of an adjacent octamer site. Cooperativity also can be demonstrated at a functional level by in vitro transcription experiments (551). Another element showing some sequence conservation in VH promoters and a role in optimal promoter function is a polypyrimidine tract located between 0 and 46 bp upstream from the heptamer (546). A motif that includes a polypyrimidine tract (GGAACCTCCCCC) has been identified as a component required for optimal function of the MOPC141 VH promoter (552). This motif, which was designated the N element, was found to bind a novel transcription factor of ubiquitous distribution. The relationship between the N element and the pyrimidine-rich κY motif is not known at present. A motif (TTANGTAA) conserved in many VH regions binds to C/EBP factors, originally identified as binding to the E motif in the μ enhancer. This motif is required for optimal transcription of VH promoter–driven transfected constructs in vivo, and the purified binding protein stimulates transcription from such promoters in vitro (553). One final VH element deserves mention. In an investigation of the mechanism by which treatment with the lymphokine IL-5 plus antigen upregulates Ig H-chain mRNA, Webb et al. (554) detected an A/T-rich element between 125 and 250 bp 5′ from the VHS107 start site that could mediate increased transcription by these agents. In an EMSA experiment this element produced a band that was upregulated in extracts obtained from cells treated with IL-5 plus antigen. In its A/T richness, the element resembles MARs, and a cloned protein corresponding to this binding activity—designated B-cell regulator of IgH transcription (Bright) (555)—partitions partly with the insoluble chromatin matrix. The significance of the Bright binding site for VH function is uncertain because most VH regions lack similar sequences within the 5′ flanking region as far as has been sequenced; furthermore, a transgenic construct driven by a related VH promoter deleted for Bright binding was still expressed in a lymphocyte-specific manner (556). Additional response elements may be discovered as the mechanisms of Ig transcriptional response to other manipulations (including other lymphokines) are investigated. To speculate further, the several VH promoter elements that are absent from VL promoters may facilitate the early transcription of germline VH genes, allowing VDJ recombination to occur at a time when VL genes are transcriptionally inactive;

however, much additional evidence would be necessary to support such a hypothesis. It is also possible that variations in the content or spacing of different elements in different VH promoters may differentially regulate V gene transcription, thereby influencing the frequency with which specific V regions are rearranged and utilized in the Ig repertoire (557–559).

Vλ promoters have received less study than Vκ or VH. When the two major murine Vλ genes were studied, the Vλ2 promoter was found to contain octamer and TATA plus an additional functional element located upstream from the octamer and not precisely conserved in Vλ1. This element, CACGTGAC, is identical to that recognized by the protein USF (upstream stimulatory factor) (560). USF is a ubiquitous transcription factor originally isolated based on its role in regulating the major late promoter of adenovirus, but since then found to regulate a wide variety of cellular genes. It belongs to the family of helix-loop-helix (HLH) transcription factors that is described in more detail below. When Vλ2 promoter activity was studied in an in vitro system with a B-cell nuclear extract, transcription was found to be reduced by passage of the extract through an anti-USF antibody column but could be restored by the addition of purified USF (561). Thus, it appears that the murine Vλ2 promoter includes a functional USF motif. Little is currently known about the functional components of human Vλ promoters or of other murine Vλ promoters except that most of them contain octamer-like sequences and TATA boxes.

Promoters of Sterile Transcripts

Ig RNA transcripts that are sterile (i.e., do not encode a complete Ig protein) are produced before V(D)J and isotype switch rearrangements, as discussed earlier in this chapter. The sterile transcription, by altering the accessibility of the DNA, may constitute part of the regulation of the corresponding gene rearrangements. Sterile transcripts including unrearranged V regions (274,562,563), Cκ (305,564,565), or Cμ (566,567) regions were initially detected, and more recently sterile transcripts of most of the downstream CH genes of the murine and human loci have been characterized. Salient features of the regulation of these transcripts are briefly outlined below.

Sterile V-Region Transcripts

The promoter of a particular V region is assumed to be identical whether sterile or mature—i.e., V(D)JC—transcripts are produced. Therefore, the earlier discussion of V-region promoters probably applies to sterile transcripts. It remains to be determined, however, what mechanisms allow the promiscuous transcription of sterile V transcripts during the developmental stage when V(D)J rearrangements are occurring, but later shut off the promoters of all but the rearranged V regions (274,275).

Sterile Cμ Transcripts

Two types of sterile μ transcripts have been described. In the first type, transcription can initiate at heterogeneous positions near the 5′ end of the JH-Cμ intronic enhancer (Eμ). When the resulting RNA transcripts are spliced to the Cμ1 exon, an Iμ exon (intron-derived) remains attached to the RNA encoding Cμ. The promoter of Iμ-Cμ transcripts has been found to be coincident with the Eμ enhancer; however, as mentioned above, the octamer motif plays a much more prominent role for this region as a promoter than it does as an enhancer (536). This promoter lacks a TATA box in both murine (536) and human (568) loci. Because the TATA box is generally

responsible for establishing a precise transcription start site, its absence from the Iμ promoter probably accounts for the heterogeneity of the 5′ ends of these transcripts. The Iμ exon is remarkable for containing multiple stop codons in all three reading frames. This feature has been hypothesized (567) to protect against the possibility that the Iμ-Cμ transcript might be translated into a protein that could prematurely provide the signal to terminate V(D)J recombination, a signal that is normally generated by a complete H-chain protein (see the discussion on allelic exclusion earlier in this chapter). After switch recombination has produced a composite switch junction (e.g., Sμ-Sγ), the Iμ promoter is retained and remains active, leading to hybrid transcripts such as Iμ-Cγ (569).

The second type of sterile Cμ transcript is derived from loci that have undergone DJ rearrangement (273); these transcripts have the structure DJ-Cμ after splicing out the JH-Cμ intron. These transcripts initiate from promoters that lie upstream of the germline DH elements (570) but have not been fully characterized. For the most JH-proximal murine D region, DQ52, an upstream promoter and enhancer have been reported (571,572). In mice, the subset of DJ-Cμ transcripts in reading frame 2 (RF2) encodes the Dμ protein that suppresses RF2 in expressed H-chain V regions, as described earlier.

Sterile Cκ Transcripts

Two types of sterile Cκ transcripts also have been described: an 8.4-kb primary transcript (564,573) that initiates about 3.5 kb upstream from Jκ1 (and is processed to a 1.1-kb RNA) and a 4.7-kb primary transcript that initiates just upstream from Jκ1 (and is processed to 0.8 kb) (573). Both of these transcripts are found in pre-B cells and are upregulated by exposure to LPS. The 5′ flanking sequences of both initiation sites contain octamer-like sequences (7/8 match to consensus) which are capable of sequence-specific binding to nuclear proteins, binding that can be competed by cold consensus octamer oligonucleotides (573). Close to the initiation site near Jκ1 there are also two binding sites for an additional protein designated KLP, which is B cell specific (574). Further experiments will be necessary to completely delineate the functional elements of these promoters and to understand how they might respond to the presence of a μ protein in the pre-B cell to activate κ transcription and subsequent κ rearrangement. A sterile JCκ transcript has been reported to encode a "V-less" κ protein analogous to the Dμ protein, which might associate with μ H chain on the surface of pre-B cells as an alternative to the VpreB-λ5 SLC complex (575). The function that such a protein might have is unclear; certainly the striking phenotype of λ5 knockout mice indicates that a JCκ protein is not redundant with the SLC.

One final transcript from the κ locus should be mentioned for completeness. To test the generality of the principle that gene rearrangements are associated with transcription of the recombination targets, the RS element involved in deletion of the Cκ gene (discussed earlier in this chapter) was examined for transcriptional activity. A transcript derived from this region was found in some pre-B cells (576). The regulation of expression of this transcript remains to be explored.

Sterile I-CH Transcripts

The regulation of sterile transcripts of downstream CH regions is being actively investigated because this regulation may be important for understanding the mechanism by which numerous factors influence the selection of specific isotypes expressed in particular immune responses (as described earlier, and discussed more fully in Chapter 23). In this view the promoter for the sterile transcript of a given isotype may be expected to contain a unique combination of motifs mediating the action of antigen, various cytokines, and other T-cell influences that are known to regulate switching to that isotype. The regulation of the IgE response has been studied intensively because of its clinical implications for allergy, and it may represent an illustrative example.

The switching of B cells from the production of μ H chains to ε is highly dependent on the cytokine IL-4, as demonstrated by the abolition of IgE synthesis in IL-4 knockout mice (577). In experiments in vitro, switching of splenic B cells to ε production requires IL-4 in the presence of an additional signal that can be supplied by several mitogenic treatments, including LPS, anti-CD40, T-cell membranes, etc. In vitro production of ε H-chain protein is preceded by synthesis of sterile Iε-Cε RNA transcripts—also known as germline ε (Gε) transcripts—which initiate at multiple start sites, apparently owing to the absence of a TATA site in the promoter (578). Significantly, the Iε promoter can confer IL-4 inducibility to reporter gene constructs. The minimum sequence with this capacity contains binding sites for two known nuclear proteins (579). One of these is STAT6, a member of the family of signal transducers and activators of transcription, which transduce signals from many cytokine receptors to mediate transcriptional regulation. STAT6 is activated by engagement of the IL-4 receptor and is required for the IL-4 effect on Iε transcription and switching to Cε, as shown by experiments in cells lacking STAT6 and in STAT6 knockout mice (580–582). The other component required in the minimal IL-4 responsive element of the Iε promoter is a binding site for the CAAT/enhancer binding protein (C/EBP) family of transcription factors. This family includes C/EBPα, expressed constitutively in liver cells, and NF-IL6 (C/EBPβ), which mediates the action of LPS and inflammatory cytokines such as IL-1, tumor necrosis factor-α (TNF-α), and IL-6. Another member of this family is the widely expressed C/EBPγ (also known as Ig/EBP), which lacks a transcriptional activator domain but can act as a transdominant negative inhibitor of other C/EBP family members by heterodimerizing with them (583). Changing ratios of different members of this family in B-cell development contribute to regulated expression of VH promoters, and the intronic enhancers of the κ and IgH loci (584).

In addition to the STAT6 and C/EBP binding sites, two nearby motifs closer to the Iε initiation sites contribute to optimal IL-4 inducibility of the promoter and also mediate the synergistic response of the promoter to CD40 engagement (585); these sites bind to the complex family of proteins known as NF-κB, which is described below in connection with the intronic κ enhancer. Elimination of both NF-κB sites from the promoter inhibits IL-4 inducibility, consistent with the absence of Iε sterile transcripts and switching to Cε expression in mice with targeted deletion of the NF-κB component p50 (586).

An additional level of IL-4 control of the promoter apparently results from an A/T-rich sequence overlapping with some of the Iε transcriptional initiation sites. This sequence confers repression of the promoter, apparently due to binding of the chromosomal protein HMG-I(Y) (587). IL-4 induces phosphorylation of this protein, perhaps thereby decreasing binding affinity and relieving the transcriptional repression (588). An additional component of the murine Iε promoter that contributes to basal activity but not to IL-4 inducibility is a binding site for the B cell–specific activator protein (BSAP) (585,589), a transcription factor described in more detail below. In the human Iε promoter, a BSAP

site apparently enhances both IL-4- and CD40-mediated promoter activity (589a). Apart from the promoter, sterile Iε transcription and isotype switching are also regulated by an enhancer lying downstream from the murine Cα gene, as deduced from abnormalities in mice in which this enhancer was replaced by a neomycin resistance gene in all B cells (96): defects were observed in switching to IgE and several IgG isotypes (but not to IgG1), with corresponding decreases in sterile transcripts of the affected isotypes.

Investigations of the regulation of sterile transcripts of other CH genes suggest promoters of similar complexity. In general, these promoters include motifs that act as response elements for signals known to promote switching to the respective isotypes; additional discussion can be found in Chapter 23.

Cis Elements of Ig Gene Enhancers

As pointed out above, enhancers are regulatory elements that stimulate transcription of nearby genes but, in contrast to promoters, can affect transcriptional initiation thousands of base pairs away and in either orientation. Enhancers have been found upstream and downstream from genes and, as is the case in the Ig genes, in introns. Although their position and orientation independence led to a variety of speculative models to explain how these sequences act to stimulate transcription, the prevailing view at present is that, like promoters, enhancers bind to nuclear proteins that facilitate assembly of a transcription initiation complex. As mentioned already, even enhancers that are positioned thousands of base pairs away from the initiation site in terms of linear distance on the DNA sequence can come close to the promoter simply by forming a large loop of DNA that doubles back on itself. Such loops have been observed by electron microscopy in several model systems.

The discussion that follows focuses on murine enhancers, which have been studied in most detail. The human homologs are briefly described at the end of this section.

Heavy-Chain Intronic Enhancer

E-Boxes and Their Binding Proteins

The enhancer located in the JH-Cμ intron was one of the first cellular (nonviral) enhancers recognized, and it continues to be a target of intense study because of its remarkable complexity (as indicated in Fig. 19A). In both the human and murine loci this enhancer, often designated Eμ, lies about 0.5 kb 3' from the most downstream JH region and appears to be spread over about 0.3 kb. This segment is 5' from the μ S region and is thus routinely retained on the expressed gene after isotype switch recombination. A major effort has been made to analyze the mechanism of action of this enhancer by analyzing the component functional motifs and their binding proteins that mediate enhancer activity.

In early work aimed at identifying the positions within the murine Eμ that might serve as binding sites for nuclear proteins, Church, Ephrussi, and colleagues (590,591) used an in vivo version of the footprinting method described above, examining the accessibility of the enhancer region to the methylating agent dimethylsulfate (DMS) in B cells versus nonlymphoid cells. These experiments located four clusters of nucleotides demonstrating B cell–specific alterations in DMS reactivity. These clusters defined a consensus octamer CAGGTGGC that appears not only at these four positions in the μ intronic enhancer (designated μE1, μE2, μE3, and μE4) but also at a fifth position not apparent on the footprint (μE5) as well as at three positions within the mouse κ enhancer (κE1, κE2, and κE3). These motifs have become known as E boxes or E motifs.

The functional significance of E motifs in the μ enhancer has been tested by transfection of DNA constructs containing the enhancer with one or more of these motifs altered by deletion or by clustered mutations. Most of the E motifs were found to be functionally redundant in that constructs containing mutations in single E motifs or even in several pairs of E motifs still retained substantial enhancer activity (533,592), but a construct with mutations in μE1, μE3, and μE4 showed loss of 98% of the normal enhancer activity. EMSA experiments established that nuclear proteins can bind specifically to the E motifs in vitro. Despite the sequence similarity of these motifs to one another, they do not all bind to the same proteins. Furthermore, although these E motifs were first noted as sites of in vivo alterations in DMS reactivity that were B cell specific, the proteins binding to these motifs were detected by EMSA experiments in nuclear extracts from a surprising variety of nonlymphoid sources.

The identification and characterization of E motif binding proteins showed a complex regulatory mechanism involving evolutionarily ancient components. A central role is played by products of the E2A gene, including two forms—known as E12 and E47—resulting from alternative RNA splicing (593). These proteins, and products of the related E2-2 and HEB genes, bind to the μE2, μE4, and μE5 motifs, as well as the similar κE2 motif from the κ intronic enhancer. All of these proteins are members of the HLH family of transcription factors. This family, now including over 200 proteins from species as diverse as drosophila, yeast, and plants, all share a common consensus binding motif—CANNTG—and the HLH domain: two 13–amino acid α-helices separated by an intervening loop. This structure mediates homo- or heterodimer formation between members of this family. Such dimerization is necessary (but not sufficient) for DNA binding; and the binding specificity and affinity for particular E boxes depends on both members of the dimer pairs. As an example, proteins derived from the E2A gene associate with MyoD (or related muscle factors) to form heterodimers that bind with high affinity to E box–like motifs in promoters of muscle-specific genes (594–596). Apparently E2A-encoded proteins, which are expressed virtually ubiquitously, may participate in tissue-specific gene regulation by binding with HLH partners with narrower tissue distribution. However, the B cell–specific E2A factor (known as BCF-1) is a homodimer of E47 subunits, which for unknown reasons seems to form uniquely in B cells despite the wide tissue distribution of E47 (597,598). Besides the HLH dimerization structure, most HLH proteins (including the E2A products) contain an additional element that is necessary for DNA binding: a segment of basic amino acids adjacent to the HLH on its N-terminal side, hence the designation bHLH for the subclass of proteins that have this basic region. In fact, HLH proteins that lack this segment—e.g., the Id group of HLH proteins (599,600))—apparently serve as physiologic inhibitors of E-motif function by dimerizing with HLH proteins and preventing their DNA binding. An additional component of some HLH proteins is a leucine zipper; this is an α-helical structure with several leucines at seven-residue intervals such that they all project from the same side of the helix. HLH proteins that include leucine zippers (bHLH-zip proteins) can dimerize to each other via hydrophobic interactions between the leucines, but they cannot dimerize to HLH

proteins lacking the zipper component (like Id, to which they are thus resistant). The bHLH-zip proteins include the Myc proteins (and their heterodimer partner Max) as well as three proteins present in B-cell nuclei that can bind to μE3 and κE3: USF, TFE3, and TFEB.

With this background on the HLH proteins, several features of their regulatory role in B cells may be considered. The critical importance of E2A proteins for B-cell development is highlighted by the phenotype of mice in which this protein was disrupted by homologous recombination (601,602) Homozygous mutant mice develop to term, but most die within a few days of birth. Strikingly, the mice fail to generate any B-lymphocytes, although the T-cell compartment is grossly normal as are other tissues like muscle in which participation of E2A proteins as heterodimers has been documented. Perhaps products of the related E2-2 gene are able to compensate for lack of E2A in muscle but not in the B-lineage. When transgenes expressing E-12 or E47 transcripts were added to the E2A knockout mice, a synergistic action of these two transcripts in B-cell development was apparent (603). Although impairment of Ig E box–dependent enhancer function may contribute to the E2A knockout phenotype—which includes marked inhibition of Iμ transcription and DJH recombination in fetal liver—this is difficult to establish because of the dramatic reduction in other transcripts important for B-cell development, including RAG-1, mb-1, CD19, and λ5. Transcription of the latter two genes is known to be regulated by the transcription factor BSAP, and expression of the gene for BSAP was also significantly reduced. Thus, impaired interactions between E2A proteins and E-box motifs in Eμ may not contribute significantly to the knockout phenotype. Other evidence for a role of E2A products in regulating Ig genes comes from experiments in which an E47 expression vector was transfected into a T-lymphocyte line (604); this caused a dramatic upregulation of Iμ transcription and DJH rearrangement (although some indirect effects may play a role in this system because expression of Oct-2 and both RAG genes was observed to be increased). E47 overexpression also caused Iμ transcription in a transfected fibroblast line (605). Regulation of E47 may be modulated by phosphorylation in non-B cells, which may reduce the ability of this protein to bind to DNA in the B cell–specific homodimer form (606).

E2-2 and HEB are similar to E2A in structure and in that they are expressed in many different cell types, but their roles in Ig expression have been less well studied. Early in B-lineage development E2-2 is more highly expressed than E2A and probably contributes more to E-box binding (607). Homozygous knockouts for E2-2 or HEB (608) showed unexplained perinatal lethality similar to that observed in E2A knockouts, but only a modest decrease in proB cell numbers; so these genes are clearly are less important for B-cell development than is E2A.

The complexity of the function of E boxes in the μ enhancer is illustrated by investigations on the function of a small fragment of the enhancer containing only μE5, μE2, and μE3 (609,610). A tetramer of this fragment is sufficient to induce enhancer activity in constructs transfected into a B cell. In this enhancer fragment, μE3 mediates a significant part of the enhancer function, and the protein that best mediates this effect is the μE3 binding protein TFE3 (611). Indeed, B cells lacking TFE3 show reduced activation of Ig secretion (612). In contrast to the activity of the tetramerized μE5-μE2-μE3 fragment in B cells, this construct showed no activity in fibroblasts; but a similar tetramer lacking μE5 was active in both B cells and fibroblasts, suggesting that μE5 confers inhibition

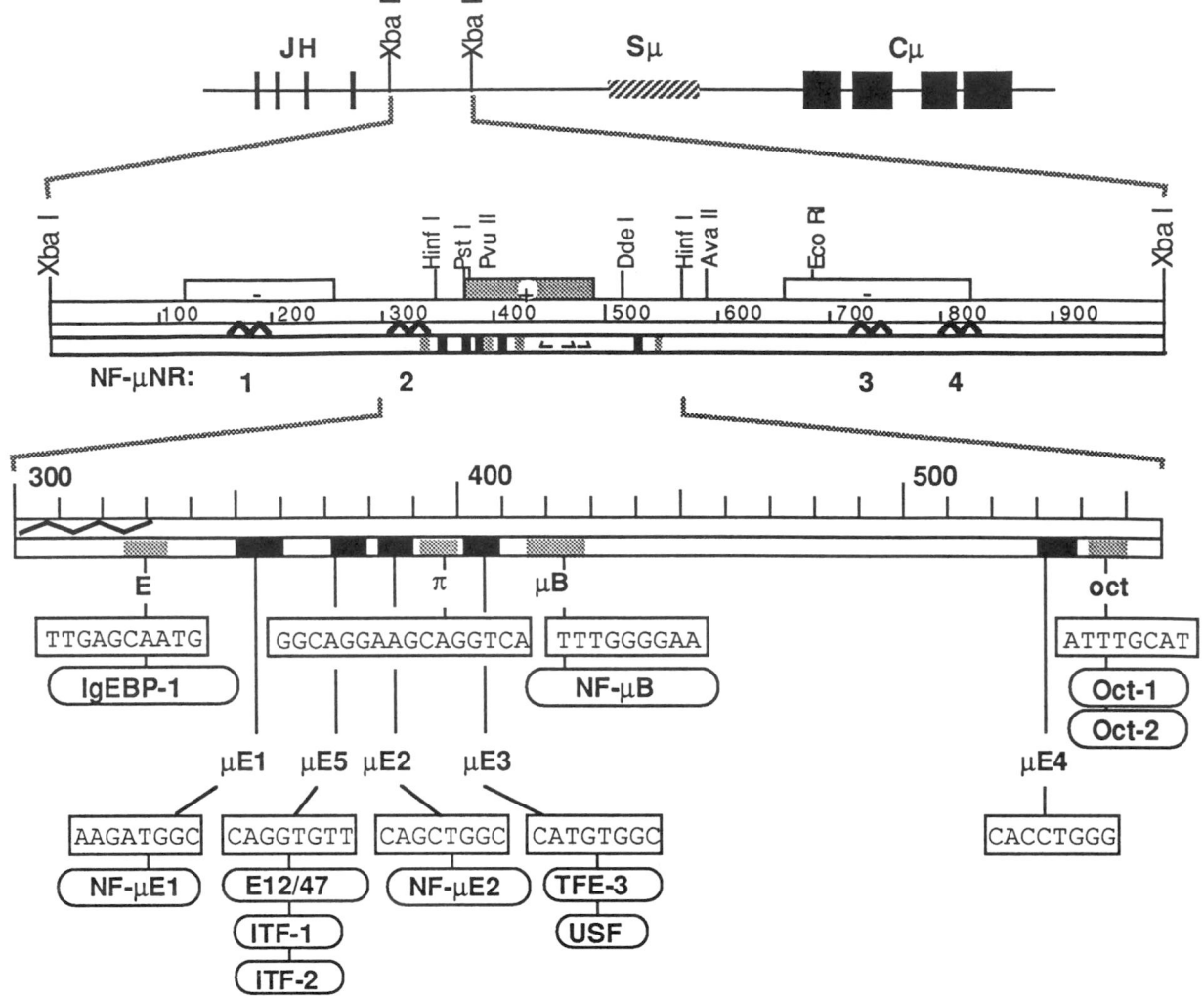

FIG. 19. Four murine Ig gene enhancers. **A:** The H-chain enhancer is located between two *Xba* I sites in the JH-Cμ intron. In the expanded diagram the scale is numbered from the 5' *Xba* I site; additional restriction sites used by various investigators are shown. The large rectangles above the numbered scale indicate locations of positive or negative regulatory regions identified by Imler et al. (631). The E motifs (*black rectangles*) and other motifs (*shaded rectangle*) are indicated, as are the four binding sites reported for the negative regulatory protein NF-μNR (*sawtooth lines*). The expanded scale at the bottom shows the central motifs with their names, DNA sequence (*rectangles*) and associated binding proteins, where known (*cartouches*).

in non-B cells. This inhibition is apparently mediated by the binding of a non-HLH protein designated ZEB to the μE5 site, allowing inhibition of TFE3. Inhibition by ZEB can be partially reversed by overexpression of the E47-like protein ITF-1, which binds to μE5 and displaces ZEB. Competition between E2A products and ZEB may similarly contribute to the B-cell specificity of the Eμ during B-cell development.

Another mechanism by which Eμ activity mediated by HLH proteins may be regulated is through the Id proteins Id1, Id2, Id3, and Id4. As mentioned above, the Id proteins are dominant negative regulators of bHLH proteins because they can heterodimerize to these transcription factors and prevent them from binding to their cognate motifs in DNA (613). Id1 and Id2 are expressed in pro-B cells at a time when E2A proteins are expressed but are not detectably bound to E boxes. Later these Id proteins are downreg-

ulated, apparently allowing bHLH activation of their target regulatory regions (599,600). The model that Id expression can suppress bHLH activation is supported by the phenotype of mice with an Id1 transgene that was designed for late B-cell expression using an mb-1 promoter and the Eμ enhancer (614); these mice showed a marked impairment in B-cell development very similar to the E2A knockout mice described earlier.

A clinically important aspect of the E2A proteins is the capacity of their genes to participate in oncogenic transformation as a consequence of translocations that fuse parts of these genes with foreign genetic material from a different chromosome. The human chromosomal locus of the E2A gene on 19p13 is the site of at least two classes of translocation events in acute lymphocytic leukemia—t(1;19)(q23;p13) and t(17;19)(q22;p13)—that produce oncogenic E2A fusion genes (615,616).

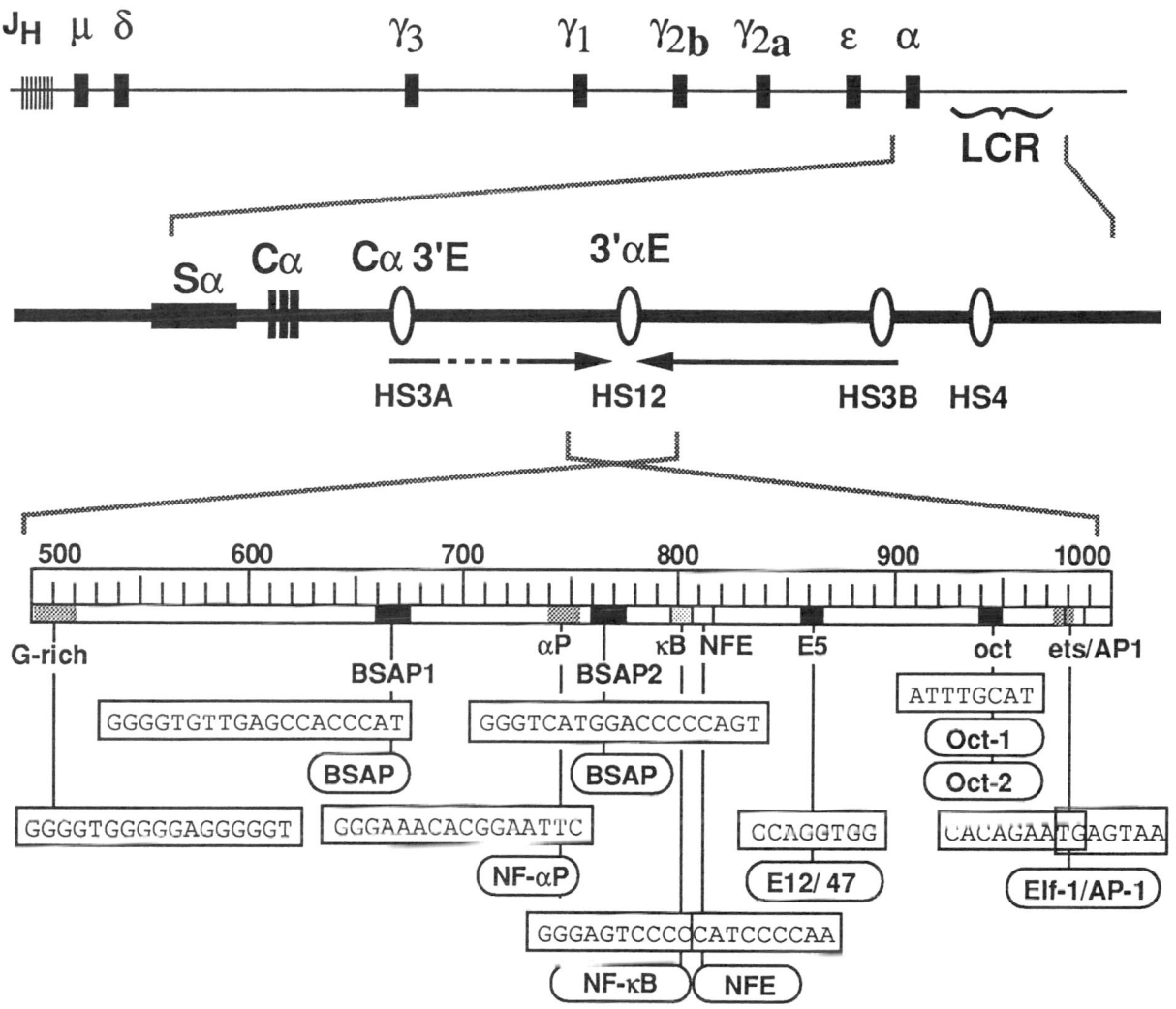

B

FIG. 19. *Continued.* B: Regulatory regions 3′ from murine Cα. The top line shows the location of an LCR downstream from Cα; this is expanded on the next line to display the reported LCR components: HS3A (Ca3′E), HS12 (3′αE), HS3B, and HS4. The arrows show the palindromic structure that surrounds HS12, the major enhancer in the locus. The component's motifs within the HS12 enhancer are shown at the bottom, using the sequence numbering from Dariavach et al. (648). This is the numbering scheme used by most investigators, but it should be noted that this sequence is in the 3′ to 5′ orientation; therefore, the orientation of the third line in the graphic is opposite from that above, and all the boxed sequences are from the antisense strand.

ETS Family Members and Their Role in Eμ

Members of another large family of transcription factors participate in Eμ regulation: the ETS proteins, which bind as monomers to the sites in Eμ known as μA (also called π) and μB (617) (Fig. 19A), as well as to similar sites in the other Ig enhancers. ETS family members share a conserved 85–amino acid DNA binding domain that recognizes DNA motifs generally containing a core GGAA sequence. Mutations at the μA site in transfected reporter constructs suggest that its integrity is crucial for Eμ activity in pre-B cells but not later in B-cell development (618). Several widely expressed ETS proteins, including Ets-1, Ets-2, Erp, and NERF, can bind to μA, although some evidence favors a physiologic role for Elf-1 at this site (619). In contrast, the μB site binds primarily to PU.1, which is expressed only in B cells and macrophages (620).

PU.1 appears to be critical for regulation of all three Ig loci and several non-Ig genes, including the mb-1 and J-chain genes. The importance of this protein for lymphoid development has been documented by PU.1 knockout mice; these mice die before birth, showing profound defects in lymphoid and myeloid lineages, although not in erythroid or megakaryocyte cells (621). Although neither μA, μB, nor the intervening μE3 show substantial enhancer activity by themselves when multimerized, the fragment containing these three adjacent motifs does show enhancer activity in B cells (617), and the spacing between the μA and μB elements is critical for activity (622). These findings as well as systematic studies of the in vivo and in vitro interactions between the proteins binding μA, μE3, and μB elements suggest that activity of this minimal enhancer depends on complex mutual interactions between these proteins and the Eμ DNA (623,624). This minimal enhancer shows

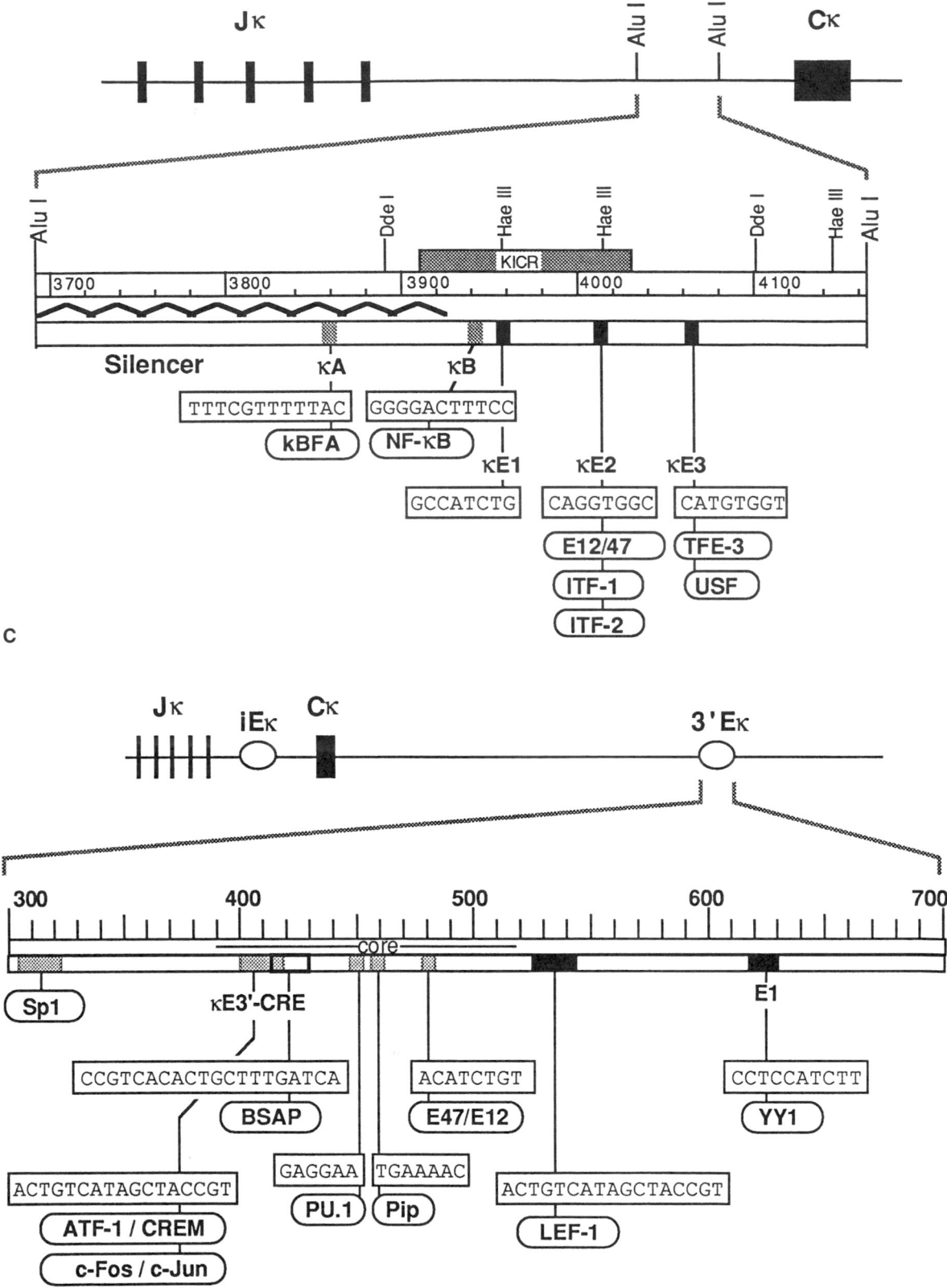

FIG. 19. *Continued.* **C:** The intronic κ enhancer. The murine κ enhancer is located between two *Alu* I sites in the Jκ-Cκ intron. In the expanded diagram the scale is numbered according to a published sequence of this region (824). The E motifs (*black rectangles*) and the κA and κB motifs (*shaded rectangles*) are shown. The shaded rectangle above the scale shows the position of the KICR (671), an island of sequence conservation observed by comparisons between the human, mouse, and rabbit Jκ-Cκ introns. **D:** The 3' κ enhancer. The motifs and corresponding binding proteins are shown, with the numbering scheme based on Muller et al. (140).

activity in macrophages as well as B cells, but inhibitory influences from flanking E boxes inactivate the enhancer in macrophages, fine tuning the cell type specificity of the enhancer. Similarly complex interactions have been reported between the μE2, μA and μE3 motifs and their binding proteins (624a).

Other Motifs in Eμ

A site in the μ enhancer known as E (unrelated to E boxes) also has been shown to be necessary for optimal enhancer activity (624b,624c). This site binds to members of the C/EBP family (discussed above), which in B cells is represented by Ig/EBP (C/EBPγ) and NF-IL6, with the latter increasing as B-cell development progresses (584). IL-6 is known to upregulate Ig secretion in B-cell lines (625), and the E site is a likely (although not yet documented) participant in this regulation through activation of NF-IL6.

Despite the initial designation of μE1 as an E box, it lacks key criterion now implied by this term, namely the canonical CANNTG motif that seems necessary for HLH protein binding. Instead, the μE1 site is apparently bound by a protein known as YY1 (626) (YinYang1), so called because it can mediate either positive or negative effects on gene expression, depending on circumstances. This protein also binds to a similar site in the 3' κ enhancer and participates in the regulation of a wide variety of genes in many tissues. YY1 has four zinc fingers (which are zinc-chelating domains found on a subset of DNA binding proteins) and both positive and negative regulatory domains (627,628). The function of this protein in Eμ has not been fully elucidated; mutations of the site decreased enhancer activity in plasmacytoma cells (533) but had no effect in other conditions (629).

Matrix Attachment Regions Flanking Eμ

Several factors apparently contribute to the B-cell specificity of the μ enhancer. As discussed above, two motifs in the enhancer bind to B cell–specific nuclear factors (μB and the octamer), and one motif (μE5) can inhibit function of μ enhancer fragment constructs in fibroblasts. However, several reports have suggested that an additional measure of B-cell specificity is conferred by sequences flanking the enhancer that suppress the activity of the central motifs in nonlymphoid cells (630–632). These suppressive sequences overlap with A/T-rich sequences that flank the core enhancer and have the properties of MARs (633). As discussed earlier, MARs are believed to represent the sites where DNA is tethered to the insoluble protein scaffold of the nuclear matrix, and they have been found near several enhancers (including the κ intron enhancer) and associated with one VH gene. A nuclear protein designated NF-μNR (nuclear factor-μ negative regulator), detected in several cell lines not expressing Ig, has been shown to bind to four A/T-rich μNR elements that lie with one pair in each of the MARs flanking the central enhancer region (Fig. 19A). In transient transfection assays, deletion of these μNR elements from enhancer constructs had little effect on transcription in B cells, which do not express NF-μNR; but in macrophages and T cells, which do express NF-μNR and cannot support activity of the intact enhancer, deletion of the μNR elements activated the enhancer, apparently releasing it from inhibition mediated by NF-μNR (634). This suggested that binding of the MARs to the matrix might be necessary for optimal enhancer function and that NF-μNR might inhibit this interaction in non-B cells. In support of this model, a matrix protein designated MAR-BP1 that might mediate this interaction has been purified from urea-sol-

ubilized matrix and has been shown capable of binding to the Eμ-associated MARs; in accordance with the model, this interaction was inhibited by purified NF-μNR (635).

Although the MARs flanking Eμ have been found to contribute little to enhancer activity in constructs transfected into B cells, they are apparently important for Eμ-driven transcription in transgenic constructs (636). When flanked by its MARs, the Eμ demonstrates a defining property of an LCR: it confers position-independent transcription on transgenic constructs integrated at various positions in the genome. Other MARs have been reported to demonstrate this property (637), but the exact relationship between MARs and LCRs is not yet understood. One possibility is that MARs may act by relieving superhelical strain because they correlate with sequences capable of becoming unpaired and nucleating unwinding (479).

There is good evidence that enhancers can stimulate transcription by approximating their binding proteins to promoter-binding proteins, looping out the intervening DNA and forming a three-dimensional transcription factor complex that facilitates formation of a transcription initiation complex. To assess whether enhancers can mediate changes in chromatin structure apart from this promoter enhancer interaction mechanism, B-cell nuclei from mouse strains harboring a variety of transgenic Eμ constructs without linked eukaryotic promoters were tested for access to DNase and prokaryotic T3 or T7 polymerases (638,639); the constructs contained promoters for the same polymerases, and some contained an MAR from the Eμ flanking region. A minimal Eμ enhancer was found to mediate local factor accessibility, but a MAR was required to extend the accessibility to a promoter 1 kb away from Eμ, implying that MARs can collaborate with an enhancer to generate a domain of chromatin accessibility even without specific interactions between enhancer- and promoter-bound proteins.

Additional insights on MAR function have been gained by studying several other proteins—besides NF-μNR—that can bind to MARs, including SATB1 (640), nucleolin (641) and Bright, as mentioned above (555). But considerable additional work will be required for a comprehensive understanding of how these elements function.

The 3' α Enhancer and LCR

Discovery of the Enhancer Complex

A complex regulatory locus has been reported to lie downstream from the murine Ig H-chain Cα gene. The existence of a regulatory region in this location was originally inferred when it was found that plasmacytomas that had undergone spontaneous deletions of Eμ nevertheless remained capable of high-level Ig secretion (642–645). Conversely, a myeloma subclone that retained the intronic enhancer but lost a segment of DNA downstream from the murine Cα gene was found to have markedly reduced H-chain gene expression (646). A systematic search in the homologous region of the rat H-chain locus showed an enhancer (647), and a homologous mouse enhancer designated 3'αE was found soon thereafter (648,649) positioned about 16 kb downstream from Cα. The mouse and rat 3'αE segments lie in opposite orientations and are flanked by inverted repeats (648). In addition to the 3'αE, Matthias and Baltimore also reported a weak enhancer in mouse lying only 4 kb downstream from Cα (650).

More recently, Madisen and Groudine (490) analyzed B cell–specific DNase I hypersensitivity downstream from Cα and detected four hypersensitive sites: HS1 and HS2 overlap the previously described 3'αE, whereas HS3 and HS4 lie further downstream and identify two new regions with somewhat weaker enhancer activity in transient transfection assays. The HS3 sequence is almost identical to that of the enhancer described by Matthias and Baltimore but in inverted orientation. This reflects the fact that the sequence surrounding the HS12-3'αE is present in the mouse in a long inverted repeat (651,652) (Fig. 19B). When constructs containing HS3, HS12, and HS4 linked to a reporter gene were transfected into a B-cell line, subsequently isolated stable transfectants were found to express the reporter gene in a position-independent manner. This suggested that the three enhancer sequences (HS12, HS3, and HS4) acted together as an LCR.

Component Motifs of the Enhancer Complex

Analyses of the regulatory regions downstream from murine Cα have identified several motifs that bind specific transcription factors to mediate different aspects of regulation of enhancer function. The 3'αE has been found to activate transcription strongly in plasmacytomas, but only weakly in earlier B-lymphoid cells. Part of this developmental change is attributable to a motif known as E5, which matches the E-box consensus binding site—CANNTG—characteristic for members of the bHLH family of transcription factors. The contribution of the E5 site to enhancer activity is inhibited in early stages of development by the dominant negative nuclear regulator Id3, which is expressed in early B-lineage cells but downregulated in plasma cells (653). At least four other motifs in the 3'αE have been reported to contribute to enhancer activity in plasmacytomas but not in early B cells. One site known as αP binds to a member of the ETS family of transcription factors designated NF-αP (654). Another is the octamer motif (ATGCAAAT) common to Ig V-region promoters and several Ig enhancers (655). A third is a κB-like site that binds to members of the NF-κB/Rel family of transcription factors described below (653). The fourth is a G-rich sequence whose function has been demonstrated by mutational analysis but for which binding proteins have not been identified (656). Activity of all four of these sites appears to be regulated by the product of the Pax-5 gene known as BSAP, mentioned earlier. This protein, which binds to two motifs in the 3'αE, is present in early B-lineage cells, in which it suppresses enhancer activity; but its loss in plasmacytomas relieves the suppression. In most contexts BSAP is a transcriptional activator, but in the 3'αE it inhibits the enhancer activity in at least two different ways. First, it prevents the binding of the transcriptional activator NF-αP to the αP site; second, it causes the octamer, G-rich, and κB-like motifs to exert an active repressive influence on transcription (654,656). Optimal activity of the κB site in the 3'αE may require interactions between NF-κB and proteins binding to an adjacent motif designated NFE (657).

Apart from the motifs mediating upregulation of the 3'αE during maturation to plasma cells, a response element in the enhancer for activation induced by BCR cross-linking has been traced to partially overlapping sites for the ETS family member Elf-1 and for members of the AP-1 transcription factor family (658). The same DNA sites represent a response element for CD40, though perhaps mediated by slightly different members of AP-1/ETS families (659). Two other motifs in the enhancer have been proposed to contribute to its regulation, but are less well documented: the μE1 and the μB motifs, which were first noted in the rat 3'αE and which are partially conserved in mice. The HS3 and HS4 enhancer regions of mice have been studied in less detail, but the HS4 enhancer apparently contains functional Oct-1 and BSAP binding sites (660,661).

A role for the 3'αE in isotype switching was suggested by experiments in which this region was replaced by a neomycin resistance gene (neo^r) through homologous recombination in ES cells that were then used to reconstitute the B-cell population in RAG-2 knockout mice. The resulting B cells showed normal V(D)J recombination but marked deficiencies in switching to IgG2a, IgG2b, IgG3, and IgE in vitro, whereas expression of IgM and IgG1 was normal (96). This observation suggests that the enhancer exerts isotype-specific effects on switch recombination, possibly by affecting the extent of germline transcription of the different isotypes before switch recombination. One caveat follows from the observation that, in neo^r replacement experiments to test the role of the κ enhancers, the neomycin resistance gene apparently affected κ expression beyond simple deletion of the enhancer (277,278); a similar effect of the neo^r gene may contribute to the phenotype observed in the 3'αE replacement mice.

Roles of the Two IgH Enhancers in B-Cell Development

From the experiments analyzing the Eμ and 3'αE, it would appear that Eμ functions primarily in early in B-cell development, with the 3'αE functioning later. Thus, B cells with targeted neo^r replacement of the Eμ enhancer (in chimeric RAG complementation mice) showed cis inhibition of germline transcription and VDJ recombination (662,663), whereas the similar 3'αE replacement just discussed showed normal VDJ recombination. The latter construct affected isotype switching, characteristic of late B-cell maturation. Moreover, as discussed above, spontaneous deletions of Eμ in plasmacytomas did not significantly affect Ig secretion, whereas spontaneous (646) or targeted (664) deletions removing the 3'αE depressed Ig secretion (in the latter study Eμ was also missing). Transfected and transgenic constructs driven by the 3'αE indicate that activity of this enhancer is specific to late, activated B cells (665–667), perhaps due in part to suppression by BSAP and Id3 early in the B-lineage (as discussed above) as well as to stimulation through motifs in the enhancer that are specifically responsive to antigen binding, T-cell stimuli, or mitogens such as LPS.

The κ Intron Enhancer and NF-κB

By transfecting deleted κ genes and constructs containing segments from the murine Jκ-Cκ intron linked to reporter genes, several groups demonstrated an enhancer lying about 0.7 kb 5' from the Cκ-region gene (668,669). This location corresponds to a B-cell specific DNase I hypersensitivity site (492,493,670) and also to a segment of the intron noted to have a remarkably high degree of sequence conservation between mice, humans, and rabbits (671). The intronic κ enhancer, sometimes designated iEκ, has been dissected by fine deletions, mutations, and protein binding studies (Fig. 17C). As mentioned above, three E boxes were recognized in this enhancer, and they seem to bind to the same proteins targeted to the corresponding Eμ motifs: κE1 binds to YY1, κE2 binds to the E2A proteins, and κE3 binds to TFE3 and related proteins. E-box mutations that reduce enhancer function abolish protein binding at this motif (533).

NF-κB

An additional motif of major importance in iEκ is the κB motif GGGACTTTCC. This motif was originally discovered as a binding site for a nuclear protein, detectable in EMSA experiments, in extracts from B cells—hence its designation NF-κB (nuclear factor-κB) (672). The presence of this protein in the same cells capable of supporting κ enhancer function provided a clue that NF-κB might be important for mediating enhancer activity. A further correlation was provided by the pre-B line 70Z/3, which has a rearranged but functionally silent κ gene. Treatment of 70Z/3 cells with LPS causes an activation of κ transcription associated with the appearance of NF-κB activity in 70Z/3 nuclear extracts (673). Mutations in the κB motif strongly reduce κ enhancer activity (533), suggesting a critical role in enhancer function. Indeed, this motif in isolation from the E-box motifs has been shown to possess enhancer activity, especially in constructs containing tandem copies of the motif (674). The enhancer activity of these constructs was much greater when transfected into a B-lymphocyte than into a fibroblast, consistent with the importance of this motif for the B-cell specificity of κ gene expression. An important physiologic role for NF-κB in mediating B-cell activation triggered by antigen recognition is suggested by the ability of surface IgM cross-linking to upregulate NF-κB activity (675). Since the discovery of the κB motif in iEκ, similar motifs have been recognized as critical functional elements regulating numerous genes outside the Ig loci. These include the genes encoding MHC class I and class II proteins and β2-microglobulin, urokinase, IL-2 and IL-2 receptor α chain, IL-6, granulocyte-macrophage colony-stimulating factor, β-interferon, inducible nitric oxide synthetase, and TNF-α and -β; the motif is also found (in tandem repeated copies) in the long terminal repeat of HIV. Many of these genes are expressed outside the B-lymphoid lineage; and indeed NF-κB was found to be inducible in T cells and HeLa by phorbol esters (673) and in other cell types by a variety of agents, including LPS, phorbol esters, TNF-α, and IL-1. Thus, rather than being B cell specific, NF-κB proteins act in many cell types, often regulated by agents associated with inflammation and often regulating inflammation-related responses. In B cells the protein regulates not only iEκ, but also the 3′αE and sites in the promoters of I regions of several H-chain isotypes, as discussed above. The complexity of NF-κB and its clinical relevance to various immune processes have inspired considerable investigation, and a large body of literature has resulted on the molecular basis of NF-κB action.

In general, the induction of NF-κB activity is not blocked by protein synthesis inhibitors, suggesting that activation must be due to modification of a preexisting protein molecule. Indeed, most cells that lack NF-κB activity in their nuclei have an inactive cytoplasmic form that is unable to bind to κB sites but can be activated when cytoplasmic extracts are treated in vitro with sodium deoxycholate (DOC) (676). DOC was found to work by abolishing the binding of an inhibitory subunit designated IκB to NF-κB (677). The active form of NF-κB initially studied is a complex of two distinct subunits of molecular weights of 50 and 65 kDa, known as p50 and p65, respectively. Thus, the initial experiments suggested a model of the inactive cytoplasmic NF-κB as a complex of p50, p65, and IκB; physiologic activators of NF-κB would abolish IκB activity, releasing the p50-p65 heterodimer to move to the nucleus, bind to κB sites, and activate transcription.

The cloning of genes encoding proteins of the NF-κB has provided a more complex and interesting picture (678). The p50 subunit and a closely related p52 protein are encoded as precursor proteins known as NF-κB1 (p105/p50) and NF-κB2 (p100/p52). The N-terminal half of both proteins share a domain of about 300 amino acids that is responsible for DNA binding. This domain is

shared by an ancient family of evolutionarily conserved proteins with functionally homologous members in drosophila. The family and the domain are designated Rel, after the v-rel oncogene from the avian reticuloendotheliosis virus, an early recognized family member (679). The C-terminal halves of both NF-κB1 and NF-κB2 contain seven repeats of a 33-residue sequence known as the ankyrin repeat; these repeats are found in diverse proteins from bacteria to mammals and often mediate protein–protein interactions. The precursor forms of NF-κB1 and NF-κB2 are inactive and restricted to the cytoplasm because a nuclear localization sequence (NLS) is occluded by the C-terminal domain; the protein is activated by proteolytic cleavage of this domain, which uncovers the NLS of p50 (or p52). The other members of the Rel family currently known contain the Rel homology domain without an inhibitory domain; they instead contain transcriptional activation domains. These proteins include RelA (which encodes p65), c-rel (the cellular homolog of the v-rel oncogene), RelB, and the two drosophila proteins Dorsal and Dif. Interacting through their Rel domains, various members of the Rel family can form heterodimers or homodimers, some showing slight differences in preferred DNA binding motif. Different members function predominantly at different stages of B-cell development; in pre-B cells (and in non-B cells) p50 and p65 are seen, with p50 and c-Rel in mature B cells and LPS-treated pre-B cells, and p52 and RelB in plasmacytoma cells (657,680–682). Despite the apparent importance of the p50 subunit in B-cell development, p50 knockout mice have grossly normal κ Ig expression with a normal ratio of κ to λ L chains, possibly because of compensation by other Rel family members. However, these mice show impairments in activated Ig production (586) and in expression of certain switched isotypes, including IgG1, IgA, and IgE (114), as mentioned earlier.

Cloning of IκB genes (683–685) showed another family of proteins, all of which share the ankyrin repeats characteristic of the C-terminal half of NF-κB1 and NF-κB2 precursor proteins. This family includes IκBα, IκBβ, bcl3, and the drosophila protein cactus. Bcl3 is unusual in that when it binds to p50 or p52 homodimers it promotes nuclear localization (686) and stimulates transcription through an activation domain (687,688); this protein is not directly involved in NF-κB function in the Igκ enhancer. IκBα or IκBβ can bind to Rel family dimers, retaining them in inactive form in the cytoplasm. Many of the same stimuli that cause proteolytic removal of the ankyrin repeat-containing C-terminal half of the Rel precursor proteins also activate Rel dimer–IκB complexes through a similar mechanism. A critical step is phosphorylation of the IκB (689), apparently by an IκB-specific kinase (690,691, 691a). The phosphorylated protein is a target for addition of the small protein ubiquitin, a modification that flags proteins for destruction by proteasomes (692). IκBα and IκBβ show somewhat different preferences for specific Rel dimers, different tissue distribution, and an interesting difference in regulation. The IκBα promoter contains multiple κB sites, which are activated when IκB destruction releases NF-κB, allowing this protein to migrate to the nucleus and stimulate IκBα resynthesis, which causes inhibition of NF-κB. Thus, in cells where IκBα predominates, NF-κB activation is short lived (693). In contrast, IκBβ is not regulated in this way, so in cells where it predominates, NF-κB activation may be more prolonged (685). The importance of NF-κB for κ expression was supported by transfection of AMuLV pre-B cell lines with an engineered form of IκB capable of suppressing both RelA and c-Rel; this dual block markedly inhibited germline κ transcription and rearrangement (694).

A MAR and Silencer Elements Upstream from iEκ

Upstream from iEκ lies an A/T-rich region that has been identified as a MAR (695). Kappa gene constructs inserted into the mouse genome as transgenes or stably integrated into B cells demonstrated that this MAR contributes to transcription of the associated gene (696,697) and to associated demethylation (698). [The demethylation also appears to be regulated by NF-κB (699).] Within the MAR an AP1 binding site has been reported (700). This site appears to be required for optimal enhancer activity when transfected into LPS-treated pre-B cells and mature B cells and shows LPS-inducible binding in EMSA experiments. In transfections into HeLa and T cells, a 232-bp fragment 5′ from the κB sequence inhibited expression of a linked gene, whereas this fragment did not affect expression in B cells (701). Thus, this fragment may contain a gene silencer that is active in non-B cells and contributes to the B-cell specificity of the enhancer. A shorter element designated κNE (negative element) lying just upstream from κB, and conserved at this position in humans and rabbits, has been reported to inhibit enhancer activity (702); this inhibition was reversed in a B cell–specific manner by another element a few base pairs upstream.

The 3′ κ Enhancer

Components of the Enhancer

As in the H-chain system, the search for a second enhancer downstream from the Cκ gene was inspired by a cell line whose expression of its endogenous κ gene seemed difficult to explain in terms of the known intronic enhancer. Thus, the myeloma S107 was found unable to support transcription of transfected constructs driven by the κ intronic enhancer because this line lacks NF-κB activity, yet it is able to transcribe its endogenous κ genes (703). A search 3′ from the Cκ gene showed a second enhancer about 9 kb downstream from Cκ (704). This enhancer is about sevenfold stronger than the κ intronic enhancer and in transfection experiments is B cell specific. Inclusion of the 3′ enhancer in transgenic constructs leads to more than 20-fold higher transgene expression than observed with constructs lacking this sequence (705). Like the iEκ, the 3′Eκ can be activated in pre-B cells by LPS. The functional elements of the murine enhancer have been dissected, demonstrating a complex set of motifs mostly clustered in a 132-bp core enhancer (Fig. 19D). One important motif identified by deletion and multimerization constructs contains the sequence CATCTGTT, which conforms to the CANNTG consensus for HLH binding motifs; indeed, this motif appears to bind to such a protein because the activity of multimerized versions of this motif, as well as the activity of the entire enhancer, can be inhibited by the HLH protein Id described above (706). The second principal motif binds PU.1, a member of the ETS domain family of transcription factors described earlier in this section. The binding of PU.1 to the enhancer recruits a second B cell–specific protein—designated PU.1 interaction protein or Pip (formerly NF-EM5)—which binds to an adjacent DNA segment whose integrity is necessary for full enhancer function (707,708). Pip is homologous to members of the interferon regulatory factor (IRF) family of transcription factors, and its binding to PU.1 is also important in the murine λ enhancers described below. The Pip-PU.1 interaction requires phosphorylation on a particular serine residue of PU.1, suggesting the possibility that the degree of phosphorylation might contribute to physiologic regulation of enhancer activity.

Upstream from these two motifs lies a sequence that was found by mutation analysis to be necessary for maximal enhancer activity and which was found, by λgt11 library screening, to bind to the transcription factors ATF-1 (activating transcription factor) and CREM (cyclic AMP response element modulator) (709). Both of these proteins can bind to PU.1 in vitro. The ability of CREM to function in the enhancer is supported by the observation that dibutyryl cAMP can increase the 3′Eκ enhancer activity. The DNA binding motif for these factors also corresponds to an AP-1 site, and the components of AP-1, c-Fos, and c-Jun were also found to activate the enhancer through this motif (710). Indeed these two AP-1 subunits can participate in a higher order complex with PU.1 and Pip that is detectable biochemically by EMSA and functionally by synergistic activation of the enhancer by these proteins when expressed in fibroblasts, in which the enhancer is normally silent. A site detected by in vivo footprinting that is occupied in pre-B and B cells, but not in plasma cells, was shown in EMSA experiments to bind a protein with characteristics of BSAP (711). At about 90 bp upstream of the core enhancer is an additional site that binds the transcription factor Sp1 and that is required for maximal enhancer activity in some constructs (712).

Just downstream from the murine 3′ κ enhancer is a negative regulatory region that seems to suppress the activity of this enhancer in pre-B cells (626). One component of this region appears to be a binding site for the zinc-finger protein YY1 or NF-E1 discussed earlier in the context of this protein's function in Eμ. An additional component may be a binding site for lymphocyte enhancer factor-1 (LEF-1), an HMG-related protein that binds in the minor groove of DNA and causes DNA bending; this protein is also a known component of TCR-α enhancer regulation. Binding activity at the presumptive LEF-1 site was depressed by treatment with LPS, suggesting the possibility that this effect may explain how the 3′Eκ enhancer activity might be upregulated by LPS in the absence of a site for NF-κB (713).

Roles of the Two κ Enhancers in B-Cell Development

The intronic κ enhancer seems critical for supporting Vκ-Jκ recombination because targeted disruption of the enhancer by neo^r replacement severely impairs or abolishes such recombination (277,714). Based on transfection experiments suggest that this enhancer is moderately active in pre-B cells but can be upregulated with activating agents such as LPS and phorbol esters, which exert their effects through NF-κB activation. Although the enhancer is active in plasmacytoma cells, its integrity does not seem critical for κ gene expression at this stage, when the 3′Eκ is more active; however, some transfection experiments suggest that the two enhancers may function synergistically in mature B and plasma cell stages (715,716). Even at the pre-B stage the 3′Eκ is active and can support lineage-specific expression of a transgenic κ gene lacking iEκ (717). Both enhancers seemed necessary to support somatic mutation in κ transgenes (432), although some of this effect may be mediated by effects on transcription. In mice with targeted disruption of 3′Eκ, decreased numbers of κ-expressing B cells were observed, as though this enhancer contributes to Vκ-Jκ recombination (278), although in transgenic animals harboring constructs capable of Vκ-Jκ joining, the 3′Eκ seemed primarily to suppress recombination. In the absence of this enhancer, recombination occurred in T cells or prematurely in pro-B cells (264). In vivo footprinting studies have shown that changes in activity of the two enhancers during B-lineage development are accompanied by changes in occupancy of specific motifs by nuclear binding proteins (711,718).

λ Enhancers

For many years the λ locus frustrated investigators searching for an enhancer in the Jλ-Cλ intron, but with the recognition of enhancers downstream from C genes, attention turned to these regions and λ enhancers were identified (719). Highly homologous B cell–specific enhancers are located 15.5 kb downstream from murine Cλ4 (the $E_{λ2-4}$ enhancer) and 35 kb downstream from Cλ1 (the $E_{λ3-1}$ enhancer). Four functional motifs were identified in each enhancer (720). Two, λA and λB, are critical for enhancer function in that mutations in either abolish activity, although neither of them are active when present in multimerized form in constructs. The λB motif binds to PU.1 and Pip (721,722), which also bind together in the 3′Eκ, as discussed above. The λA and λB elements are flanked by E box–like motifs, which may bind to HLH proteins active in other Ig enhancers.

Human Ig Enhancers

The above account of regulatory regions in the three Ig loci has focused on the mouse genes because these regions were discovered before homologous regions of other species, and they have been most thoroughly studied. Sequence analysis of homologous human regions have shown a high degree of conservation, especially in the core enhancers containing functional transcription factor binding motifs; and other enhancer properties—including DNase hypersensitivity, in vitro protein binding, and functional enhancer activity—also have been documented for human Ig enhancers. Some differences in enhancer number have resulted from gene duplications specific to mice or humans. Thus, in contrast to the two murine λ enhancers, the human λ locus includes a single enhancer downstream from Cλ7 (723–725). Conversely, the duplication of the two γ-γ-ε-α segments of the human IgH locus has led to duplicated enhancer complexes downstream from the human Cα genes (491,726). Analyses also have been conducted on the human iEκ (493,671,727–729), the human 3′Eκ (140,730), and the human Eμ (486,731–734).

Generalizations Concerning Ig Transcriptional Regulation

Each gene segment within the three Ig loci is regulated by nearby DNA regions outside the coding exons. The regulatory regions are composed of several motifs that control transcription by binding to specific nuclear factors that can stimulate or inhibit transcriptional initiation. Some of the motifs are shared between different enhancers or promoters and some are unique to one region. The presence (or activity) of the nuclear factors in different cell types often correlates with the expression of the associated gene segment. The research to date seems to have identified many components of a complex regulatory machinery, but there are many gaps in our understanding. We know little about what regulates the nuclear factors—how the known components change in response to cell maturation and to external signals such as antigens, cytokines and T cells—nor do we understand how the actions of these nuclear factors are integrated with other chromosomal changes such as histone acetylation, DNA methylation, matrix attachment, and nucleosome repositioning.

APPLIED SCIENCE OF IMMUNOGLOBULIN GENES

Up to this point, this chapter has considered how our current knowledge of Ig genes can explain the antibody response. In the present section we briefly address several examples of other areas to which this knowledge has been applied with interesting results.

Ig Genes in Lymphoid Malignancies

Many malignant tumors have been shown to derive from single transformed cells that have undergone clonal expansion with failure of normal cellular controls. Lymphoid malignancies of the B-lineage provide a classic demonstration of clonality because they derive from cells with unique genetic material (rearranged Ig genes) distinct from the bulk DNA of the same organism. Similarly, analyses of TCR genes have been valuable in establishing clonality of T-cell malignancies. Examination of both gene systems is useful in establishing the lineage of neoplasms that lack characteristic phenotypic markers and in detecting clonal rearrangements as a marker for malignancy; a huge clinical literature has accumulated (735–738).

The first general strategy to analyze clonality has been to isolate genomic DNA from neoplastic and normal tissue from the same patient and to examine it for Ig or TCR gene rearrangements using Southern blotting. A nonclonal population of B-lymphocytes contains a mixture of rearrangements so numerous that, after restriction enzyme digestion and Southern analysis, the rearranged fragments bearing the JH sequence are spread thinly throughout the length of the gel, so no specific rearranged band is detectable. In contrast, clonal expansions of a specific rearrangment as in a lymphoid malignancy will produce a distinct rearranged band, detectable even when the malignant cells are present as a minority in the cell population. Admixture experiments have demonstrated that rearranged bands can be detected when malignant clonal cells represent as little as 1% of the population, although 5% is a more typical detection limit. The Southern blotting technique can be used on peripheral lymphocytes as well as on biopsy specimens of solid tumors. More recently the power of the PCR to amplify miniscule amounts of DNA has made it possible to assess clonal rearrangements from samples as small as histologic tissue sections or to detect rare leukemic cells in a 10^5 excess of normal cells; such assessments are critical for clinically important judgments (739). Ig gene rearrangements have been demonstrated in acute lymphoblastic leukemia (ALL), chronic lymphocytic leukemia (CLL), multiple myeloma, B-cell follicular and diffuse lymphoma, hairy cell leukemia, B-cell prolymphocytic leukemia, Hodgkin's Disease, Burkitt's lymphoma, and in the blast crisis of chronic myelogenous leukemia (738).

DNA analysis has been particularly revealing in the case of ALL cells, which before the advent of DNA analysis were generally (80%) of uncertain lineage, lacking both B-and T-phenotypic markers. The majority of these null ALL samples analyzed contain rearrangements of H-chain Ig genes, and about 40% also have rearranged L-chain genes, although no surface Ig is detectable. The cells thus typically resemble the pre-B stage of lymphoid development. During the course of the disease some ALL cells show clonal evolution of additional Ig gene rearrangements, thus further matching the pre-B phenotype. When DNA from serial peripheral blood samples of pre-B ALL patients are examined by Southern blotting, the clonal rearranged band can be used as a marker of leukemic remission and relapse (740,741). Ig gene rearrangements also have been sought in T-cell ALL; rearrangement of the Ig H-chain gene occurs rarely in these malignancies, and L-chain rearrangement is not observed. Conversely, TCR gene rearrangement occurs in roughly half of pre-B cell ALL, especially at the TCR-γ locus (740). These examples of lineage infidelity may reflect a developmental stage before definitive commitment to B- or T-differentiation when both gene systems may be susceptible to the recombinase machinery.

Chromosomal Translocations Involving Ig Gene Loci

In contrast to the rearrangements in tumors discussed so far, which represent physiologic recombination events that occurred in premalignant progenitor cells, an entirely different kind of Ig gene rearrangement has been found in several lymphoid neoplasms: rearrangements that appear to have played a role in the malignant transformation itself. All except the two most recently discovered cases involve genes normally expressed in the B-cell lineage.

c-myc *Translocations in Burkitt's Lymphoma*

The first example to be elucidated—and one that still represents a prototype—was in Burkitt's lymphoma, where a consistent pattern of chromosomal translocation has been observed involving a reciprocal exchange between chromosome 8 and either chromosome 14, chromosome 2, or chromosome 22. The latter three chromosomes contain the three human Ig gene loci (H chain, κ, and λ) (47,742), and the Ig genes were mapped by in situ hybridization to the same bands involved in the chromosome 8 translocations. The translocation breakpoints have been cloned and sequenced, providing a detailed picture of these nonphysiologic recombination products (Fig. 20).

The sequence consistently donated from chromosome 8 has been found to be the c-*myc* oncogene, the mammalian cellular homolog of the oncogene first identified in avian leukosis virus (743). Translocation of c-*myc* into the IgH locus is also observed in the 12;15 translocations commonly seen in murine plasmacytomas. The CH regions most frequently involved are α (in the mouse) and μ (in human cells), generally the alleles on the nonexpressed chromosome. These translocations leave the IgH and c-*myc* genes joined head to head (in opposite orientations). As shown in Fig. 20, the first exon of the c-*myc* gene is commonly absent from the IgH-associated translocation product, but because this is a noncoding exon, such genes can still encode a functional protein. The site of the translocation can vary over a wide distance for both the c-*myc* and IgH genes, which may be separated by more than 100 kb in some 14q+ chromosomes. Generally the translocations in Burkitt's lines fall into two categories roughly paralleling the two clinical forms of the disease: the endemic African type and the sporadic type (744). The endemic Burkitt lines seem to represent an early B lymphoid stage as they make primarily membrane Ig; these lines demonstrate Ig locus breakpoints near V and J regions and c-myc breakpoints far 5' of exon 1. However, recent reports that endemic lines show evidence of somatic mutation (744a,744b), combined with the realization that VDJ recombination may be reactivated in the GC (as discussed earlier), have suggested that endemic lines may represent later stages in B-cell development than investigators initially thought. The less frequent translocations involving κ and λ bring these genes downstream from c-myc and oriented in the same 5'-3' direction, as shown in Fig. 20. Analysis of these translocations has incidentally provided an assignment of the 5'-3' orientation of the normal Ig gene loci with respect to the centromeres on their respective chromosomes.

Several observations suggest that the translocation event bringing the c-*myc* gene adjacent to the Ig gene locus participates in the malignant transformation of the progenitor lymphocyte. In normal cells the Myc protein plays a complex role in regulating cell cycle progression, probably through transcriptional activation of genes associated with cell division. The Myc protein has a structure typical for the bHLH-zip family of HLH transcription factors discussed earlier in this chapter. In association with a heterodimer partner named Max, Myc binds in vitro to a typical E-box motif CACGTG (745) and regulates several genes that might be relevant to its role in regulating proliferation (746,747). In Burkitt's lines transcription is generally maintained at relatively high steady-state levels, which could contribute to the malignant proliferation of these cells. Among somatic cell hybrids constructed between a Burkitt's lymphoma and mouse myeloma, human c-*myc* transcripts were found in hybrid cells containing the 14q+ chromosome but not in those with the normal chromosome 8; this finding suggests that translocation of the c-*myc* gene into the Ig locus was responsible for activating its transcription in cis (748). This activation could be mediated by proximity to the intronic μ enhancer in some Burkitt's lymphomas. In others, in which this intronic enhancer is absent from the translocated c-*myc* locus, c-*myc* activation might be mediated by the 3'αE and associated regulatory regions, which have been shown to be competent to stimulate transcription from the c-*myc* promoter (490). The potential long-distance regulation implied by the LCR properties of these regions may explain the dysregulation of c-*myc* expression in some Burkitt's lines even where the c-*myc* gene is relatively distant from the IgH locus. The observation of T-cell leukemias with c-*myc* translocations into the TCR-α chain locus (749) support the generality of deregulated c-*myc* expression in oncogenesis.

Other Oncogenic Translocations Involving the Immunoglobulin Loci

In addition to the translocations of the c-*myc* gene on chromosome 8, other translocations involving the IgH locus have been reported in lymphoid malignancies, and translocation breakpoints have been cloned in the hope of identifying new protooncogenes that—by analogy with c-*myc*–might be activated by the translocation. An 11;14 translocation seen in some CLLs and centrocytic B-cell lymphomas was found to join the nonexpressed IgH locus to a region of chromosome 11 that has been termed *bcl*-1 (B-cell leukemia/lymphoma-1) (750). Although attempts to detect a deregulated transcription unit in this region were initially unsuccessful, an oncogene candidate has emerged that was first discovered as a partner in a different chromosomal rearrangement, one involving the parathyroid gene (751). This oncogene, known as PRAD-1 (parathyroid adenomatosis-1) encodes cyclin D1—a regulator of cell division—and maps to the same band (11q13) involved in the translocations with the IgH locus. Cyclin D1/PRAD-1/Bcl-1 transcripts are elevated in several CLL lines with *bcl*-1 translocations (in contrast to other CLLs lacking this translocation) and in approximately 90% of mantle-cell lymphomas (752).

Another translocation involving chromosome 14 occurs in the majority of cases of follicular lymphoma and involves chromo-

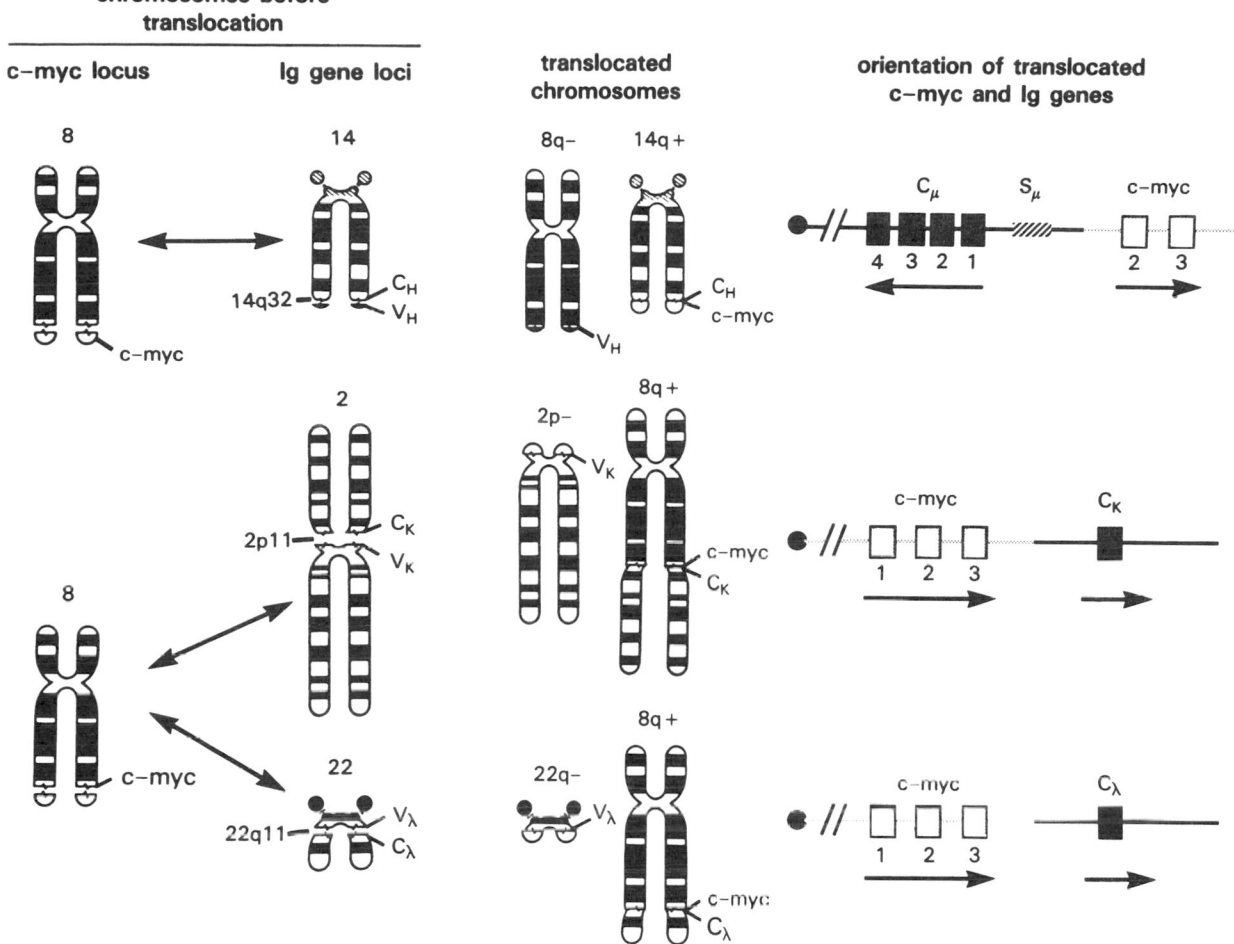

FIG. 20. Translocations between Ig genes and the c-*myc* locus observed in lymphoid malignancies. The c-*myc* gene on chromosome 8 (*left*) is associated with translocations resulting from chromosomal breaks either above (*top*) or below (*bottom*) the gene itself. In the former case, translocation to the IgH locus at 14q32 leads to a 14q+ chromosome bearing c-*myc* sequence and IgH sequence in opposite orientations (*upper right*). In the latter case translocations with the Igκ locus at 2p11 or the Igl locus at 22q11 lead to junctions in which the *myc* and Ig genes are in the same orientation.

some 18 band q21. Analysis of cloned fragments containing the translocation breakpoint led to the identification of a new oncogene designated *bcl*-2 (753). The 14;18 translocation creates a *bcl*-2–Ig fusion gene whose mRNA transcripts are elevated as a result of both transcriptional deregulation and altered RNA processing. The *bcl*-2 gene is unusual among protooncogenes in that its normal role appears not to be the promotion of cell proliferation but rather the inhibition of programmed cell death or apoptosis (754). It was the first identified member of a family of proteins that form heterodimers that stimulate or inhibit apoptosis (755). The Bcl-2 protein is expressed in tissues where some cell populations undergo apoptosis but selected subsets are spared (756). In particular, the protein can be detected in the apical light zone of GCs, where it is believed that somatic mutation of Ig genes is ongoing and only the subset of B cells displaying surface Ig with high binding affinity for antigen can survive. Bcl-2 protein is also expressed in surviving T cells in the thymic medulla. Transgenic mice with a *bcl*-2–Ig minigene developed a lymphoproliferative syndrome due to the extended life span of their lym-

phoid lineage; eventually most mice progressed to a lymphoma (757), supporting an important role of the *bcl*-2–Ig translocation in malignant transformation.

A translocation involving the IgH locus and chromosome 19 band q13.1 is a recurring but uncommon abnormality in CLL (758,759). The cloned translocation breakpoint showed a gene, designated *bcl*-3 (760), that encodes a protein containing seven of the ankyrin repeats characteristic of IκB-like proteins, and which was discussed earlier in this chapter. The recombination is often head to head near Sα in the IgH locus and leads to a marked elevation of intact Bcl-3 transcripts in CLL lines with the 14;19 translocation, as compared with lines without this abnormality. The identity of the genes regulated by Bcl-3 is not known, although presumably these genes are normally regulated by Rel family dimers.

Bcl-6 was first identified by cloning the breakpoint at the most common translocation observed in B-cell non-Hodgkin's lymphoma, that involving the IgH locus and 3q27 (761). Intact bcl-6 transcripts are increased by the translocation. The 95-kDa DNA-binding Bcl-6 protein has six zinc finger domains and is able to mediate strong transcriptional repression, largely as a result of its N-terminal POZ domain (762). Bcl-6 transcription is downregulated on B-cell activation, but the protein is detected at relatively high levels in GCs (763). Bcl-6 knockout mice fail to form GCs and do not show affinity maturation, but have diffuse inflammation with an increase in IgE-bearing lymphocytes (764,765).

The bcl-7A gene at 12q24.1 (766) and bcl-8 gene at 15q11-13 (767) were cloned from breakpoints in IgH translocations in lymphomas. The Bcl-7A sequence appears homologous to the actin-binding protein caldesmon, and the bcl-8 gene is expressed in testis and prostate; but little more is known about the function of these genes at present.

Many of the translocations described above can be detected by PCR as clonally unique amplification products, which can be used as markers for minimal residual disease (768).

Hybrid Recombinations

Another class of aberrant chromosomal rearrangements involving the IgH locus includes the chromosome 14 inversions observed in some T-cell lymphomas (769,770). These remarkable rearrangements occur between the IgH locus at 14q23 and the TCR-α locus at 14q11 and clearly appear to have been mediated by the V assembly recombinase. In one well-studied example, an Ig VH segment is joined to a TCR Jα segment on the telomeric end of the chromosome, whereas in the centromeric region a signal joint is found; because this joint is not reciprocal to the VH-Jα coding joint on the same chromosome, at least two recombination steps must have occurred. In these chromosomal inversions no oncogene sequence seems to be involved, so their relationship to the malignancy is uncertain. By PCR, similar hybrid antigen receptor recombinations can be detected at low levels in normal individuals; these recombinations are present in higher than normal frequencies in patients with ataxia telangectasia and in agricultural workers exposed to chemicals, a population with increased risk for lymphoid malignancy (771).

Abnormal Ig Gene Loci in Disease

Several immune deficiency diseases are associated with selective or global decrease in serum Ig levels. Although it might have been expected that elucidation of the Ig gene loci would clarify the molecular basis for these diseases, very few examples of genetic defects in Ig genes have been reported. Indeed, examination of restriction fragment length polymorphisms (RFLPs) detected with probes in the IgH locus have indicated that at least two genetic defects associated with Ig H chains (familial selective IgA deficiency and the hyper-IgM syndrome) are not linked to the IgH genes. Many Ig deficiencies are undoubtedly caused by cellular abnormalities in the complex mechanisms of B-cell development, T-cell interaction, lymphokine response, antigen triggering, and so forth.

In one of the rare examples of an Ig deficiency due to Ig gene mutation, defects in the Cκ genes have been described in a patient with selective deficiency of κ synthesis (772). Different point mutations in each of the Cκ alleles of a patient were observed, leading to amino acid replacements that could have disturbed the intradomain disulfide bonds critical to Ig structure.

In the H-chain locus six large deletions have been described in humans (Fig. 7), the largest involving the loss of the γ1, ψε1, α1, γ2, and γ4 genes (55); despite the complete absence of the corresponding H chains in the serum, individuals with homozygous deletions generally show no clinical evidence of immunodeficiency. However, homozygous defects in the μ gene can result in agammaglobulinemia (772a).

The contribution that specific polymorphic V genes might make to autoimmune disease has been explored by several investigators. Although human V gene sequences are remarkably well conserved between individuals, it is known that human V loci display large insertion/deletion polymorphisms in the population (381,382, 773–777). Extrapolating from this fact, it might be supposed that the presence of specific unusual germline V genes could increase the risk for certain autoimmune responses, much as certain MHC haplotypes are associated with increased risk for such diseases. However, the genes expressed in autoimmune antibodies have not proved to be rare in the population; and although some disease associations with V haplotypes have been reported (778,779), genetic variation in V genes does not appear to be a major risk factor. Specific immune defects due to the absence of specific V regions are also possible. In Navajos a defective copy of the VκA2 gene—which encodes the predominant Vκ chain in antibodies against *Haemophilus influenzae*—has been suggested as possibly contributing to the high susceptibility in this population to infections with this bacterium (780).

Genetic Engineering of Ig Genes

Using the considerable knowledge of Ig genes that has been gained from modern molecular cloning techniques, a number of investigators have been exploiting these genes as bioengineering tools for various basic research and applied science goals. Although a detailed treatment of these studies is beyond the scope of this chapter, we will briefly consider a few of the more interesting ideas.

One basic research goal is the exploration of structure–function relationships of Ig molecules by engineered modifications of Ig structure. The IgM molecule has been studied in this way initially by exploiting natural mutant hybridoma lines making abnormal antibodies. The abnormal μ genes were cloned and sequenced, and observed mutations that were candidates for causing the phenotypic abnormality were either reverted or reintroduced into normal genes by site-directed mutagenesis to verify their effects. Using this approach, a 39-bp deletion near the C-terminal end of the molecule was found to prevent pentamer formation (781) and replacement at codon 436 in the CH3 domain was found to depress complement-activated cytolysis (782). Sequences responsible for differential complement activation by human γ isotypes were identified by exchanging various residues from one isotype to another and following the resulting effects on complement activation (783). In an analysis of the mouse γ2b H chain, systematic alteration of amino acids on the surface of the CH2 domain by in vitro mutagenesis led to the identification of three residues critical for the binding of the complement factor Clq (784). A structure–function analysis of the ε H chain was undertaken by testing ε chain fragments—generated by bacterial expression of engineered segments of the ε gene sequence—for their biologic activity. A 76–amino acid fragment spanning the CH2-CH3 boundary was found to bind to mast cells in vitro and to inhibit the action of IgE *in vivo* (Prausnitz-Kustner reaction) (785). For V-region structure–function analysis, site-directed mutagenesis of V regions has been used to study the determinants of antibody affinity and specificity (786). These studies suggest that biotechnology can provide powerful methods for analyzing important features of Ig protein structure.

When structure–function relationships are sufficiently understood, the next logical engineering challenge is to improve on nature, designing Ig molecules with specific desired properties by modifying appropriate segments of Ig genes. One goal has been to combine the advantages of human and murine monoclonal antibodies to make medically useful products. Murine hybridomas grow quickly, produce large amounts of antibody and are quite stable relative to human hybridomas, which are generally poor in all three respects. Yet for many applications—like the use of antitumor antibodies in human patients—the more easily generated mouse monoclonals would be unsatisfactory because of their immunogenicity and their relative inefficiency in generating C region–dependent effector functions (such as complement fixation and antibody-dependent cellular cytotoxicity). A solution that has been tested by several laboratories is to construct chimeric genes linking a human C-region gene to a murine V region cloned from a mouse hybridoma generated against the antigen of interest; these constructs are then transfected into nonsecreting variants of mouse hybridomas yielding transfectomas that secrete humanized antibodies with murine V regions and human C regions (787–789). To reduce immunogenicity arising from the murine V-region sequences, the CDRs from a murine antibody of desired specificity can be grafted onto human V-region framework sequences (790,791). A completely different approach to obtain human antibodies using murine hybridoma technology involves engineering mice to express human antibodies (792). This ambitious goal was achieved starting with mice whose endogenous Ig κ and IgH gene loci were disrupted by homologous recombination. ES cells from these mice were then fused with yeast spheroplasts containing YAC constructs of human DNA. The resulting "xenomice" bear 66 VH regions, about 80% of the human VH repertoire, and the complete DH, JH, μ, δ, and γ2 C-region genes, including intronic and 3′α enhancers. The transferred κ locus contains most of the proximal part of the Vκ locus (32 Vκ genes), Jκs, and Cκ as well as both the intronic and 3′ enhancers and the kde. The human genes support grossly normal development of murine B cells, most of which secrete exclusively human Ig; about 15% of B cells express human H chain with mouse λ chain. The human gene loci support antigen specific antibody responses to immunization, demonstrating isotype switching and somatic mutation. Xenomice can be used to generate hybridomas that secrete human Ig but that provide all the advantages associated with their murine origin.

As further variations on Ig structure, bioengineers have designed antigen-binding molecules that do not require combining separate proteins containing the L-chain and H-chain V regions. One approach is to exploit camel Igs, which lack L chains but still can bind antigens efficiently (793). A more widely studied strategy involves single-chain Fv proteins (794,795); these can be obtained from gene constructs encoding hybridoma-derived Vκ and VH domains connected by a flexible synthetic linker of about 15 amino acids that allows these two domains to associate via the same protein–protein interactions that hold them together in a normal antibody. The two domains thus form a composite antigen-binding structure that often retains the specificity and affinity of its parent monoclonal antibody.

The paradigm has facilitated another engineering advance: a scheme for generating monoclonal antibodies without hybridoma fusions. Libraries of amplified Vκ and VH regions are cloned together into the same filamentous phage vector, which is designed to express both V regions as an Fv fusion protein on the outer surface of the phage. Such phage display libraries can then be selected for antigen binding by passage over an antigen-containing affinity column (796) or by successive precipitations with antigen (797). Phage clones selected for antigen binding contain the Vκ and VH genes encoding an effective antigen-binding domain. In several libraries of 10^6 clones, antigen-binding phage could be found only if the V-region sequences were derived from B cells that were obtained after immunization, but for considerably larger libraries, prior immunization is not necessary. Once an antigen-binding clone is obtained, it can be subjected to random mutagenesis and further rounds of selection to obtain higher affinity antigen binding (798). Mutagenesis can be achieved by chemical mutagens, by error prone PCR, by shuffling Vκ and VH chains between constructs, by passage through a mutator strain of bacteria or by a strategy of codon-based mutagenesis (799). A dramatically effective mutagenesis strategy with great promise for exploring the sequence space of antibody structures allows shuffling of mutations at different positions within a protein sequence to assemble various combinations of mutations before selection (800). Once a combination of high-affinity Vκ and VH have been selected, the individual Vκ and VH regions can be subcloned and inserted back into appropriate expression vectors to generate Ig molecules (801,802). It is debatable whether antibody sequences obtained by the phage display library strategy are typical of natural antibodies, but it is clear that the technology has general utility for producing high-affinity monoclonal antibodies of various specificities without hybridomas.

Bioengineering technologies have been used to alter the natural sequences of both C and V regions to obtain proteins with particular properties. Tinkering with C-region sequences can improve function of engineered antibodies. For example, in the CH3 domain of a γ1 monoclonal, replacement of a serine residue by cysteine led to dimerization and a dramatic improvement in function of an antileukemia antibody (803). One particularly interesting use of V-region engineering is the design of antibodies with catalytic activity. Enzymes are thought to catalyze reactions in part by reducing the activation energy—that is, stabilizing activated transition-state intermediates by strong binding interactions. Several groups have shown that, by a similar mechanism, antibodies directed against a molecule resembling the transition state of a chemical reaction can catalyze that reaction (804,805). Catalysis also can be achieved by Fv proteins (806). Site-directed mutations of V-region sequences can be used to analyze and enhance the catalytic activity (807). Indeed, if the antibody catalysis can be engineered to replace an in vivo loss mutation of an essential enzyme, random mutations of the antibody gene can be selected in vivo for improved activity (808).

In another avenue of Ig engineering, antibody domains have been added to unrelated peptide sequences in order to confer some desired Ig function to a different protein. Most commonly the V region is used to direct the unrelated polypeptide to a specific target. For example, in an attempt to improve the potency and specificity of tissue plasminogen activator (t-PA, an enzyme useful in dissolving clots in heart attack victims) an antifibrin antibody was linked to t-PA sequence to focus the plasminogen activation on fibrin clots (809). Other similar engineering projects have linked staphylococcal nuclease and Escherichia coli DNA polymerase functions to Ig molecules. A major area of applied research explores Ig-toxin hybrids, which offer the potential of delivering potent toxins to specific targets, especially cancer cells (810). A related strategy is to link a V region of one specificity to an Ig of a second specificity, creating bispecific antibodies or diabodies. Bispecific antibodies have a wide range of uses, including targeting T cells (via anti-CD3) to cells bearing a particular antigen that can be recognized by an antibody rather than by a TCR (811); they also can be used in immunoassays (812). Bispecific antibodies can be generated by transfecting the two L-chain and two H-chain genes into a single producer cell, or by fusing cells producing two antibodies; in either case the desired bispecific protein must then be purified from the resultant mixture of components. Alternatively, bispecific antibodies can be genetically engineered as two Fv proteins joined by a linker chain of amino acids (813).

Although the above examples represent uses of Ig V regions, Ig C regions also have been exploited, often fused to unrelated proteins that have their own targeting properties; such fusion proteins are known as immunoadhesins. In such constructs the Ig constant domains can confer multivalency, increased stability, and effector functions (e.g., binding to Fc receptors) that can be useful for certain applications (814). For example, the receptor for most human rhinoviruses is ICAM-1, and a soluble form of this protein might act as a decoy receptor to block infection. An ICAM-1 molecule fused to Ig H-chain domains was a much more efficient inhibitor of infection than ICAM-1 alone (815).

Antibody gene constructs have been expressed in a variety of production systems, including B-lymphoid lines (transfectomas), other mammalian lines (e.g., COS cells), and bacteria. More recent experiments have involved expression in insect cells (816) and in plants (817), where they could theoretically be ingested in an unpurified state to confer passive mucosal immunotherapy. Ig gene constructs also have been designed so that the antibody is not secreted, but instead binds (as an "intrabody") to intracellular targets (818).

The strategies described above have used the coding sequences of Ig genes, but regulatory sequences also have been used in bioengineering projects, primarily to obtain B cell–specific expression of foreign gene constructs introduced nonspecifically into multiple cell types. Transgenes, for example, are present in every cell type, but transgenic constructs linking the μ enhancer to the c-myc gene have induced malignancies specific to the B-cell lineage, in which this enhancer is active (819,820). By similar logic, a retroviral construct containing an intracellular toxin (like diphtheria toxin) programmed for B cell–specific expression might be used to treat B-cell malignancies (821).

CONCLUSION

Recombinant DNA technology has revolutionized the study of the antibody response. Initial investigations used powerful cloning and sequencing methods to define the structure of the Ig genes as they exist in the germline and in actively secreting B-lymphocytes. More recent studies have probed the mechanisms of the processes unique to these genes, i.e., rearrangements and somatic mutation. These more difficult questions will represent a challenge for a long time to come, although the recent experiments yielding VDJ and switch recombination reactions in cell-free extracts can be expected to yield valuable clues to the mechanisms of these processes. Meanwhile the knowledge already gained about Ig genes is being applied to many clinical and scientific endeavors that hold promise for exciting advances in the near future.

REFERENCES

1. Dreyer WJ, Bennett JC. The molecular basis of antibody formation. *Proc Natl Acad Sci USA* 1965;54:864–869.
2. Brack C, Hirama M, Lenhard SR, Tonegawa S. A complete immunoglobulin gene is created by somatic recombination. *Cell* 1978;15:1–14.
3. Rabbitts TH. Evidence for splicing of interrupted immunoglobulin variable and constant region sequences in nuclear RNA. *Nature* 1978;275:291–296.
4. Seidman JG, Max EE, Leder P. A kappa-immunoglobulin gene is formed by site-specific recombination without further somatic mutation. *Nature* 1979;280:370–375.
5. Max EE, Seidman JG, Leder P. Sequences of five potential recombination sites encoded close to an immunoglobulin kappa constant region gene. *Proc Natl Acad Sci USA* 1979;76:3450–3454.
6. Sakano H, Huppi K, Heinrich G, Tonegawa S. Sequences at the somatic recombination sites of immunoglobulin light-chain genes. *Nature* 1979;280:288–294.
7. Tonegawa S, Maxam AM, Tizard R, Bernard O, Gilbert W. Sequence of a mouse germ-line gene for a variable region of an immunoglobulin light chain. *Proc Natl Acad Sci USA* 1978;75:1485–1489.
8. Parhami SB, Margolies MN. Contribution of heavy chain junctional amino acid diversity to antibody affinity among p-azophenylarsonate-specific antibodies. *J Immunol* 1996;157:2066–2072.
9. Fang W, Mueller DL, Pennell CA, et al. Frequent aberrant immunoglobulin gene rearrangements in pro-B cells revealed by a bcl-xL transgene. *Immunity* 1996;4:291–299.
10. Gu H, Kitamura D, Rajewsky K. B cell development regulated by gene rearrangement: Arrest of maturation by membrane-bound D mu protein and selection of DH element reading frames. *Cell* 1991;65:47–54.
11. Corbett S, Tomlinson I, Sonnhammer E, Buck D, Winter G. Sequence of the human immunoglobulin diversity (D) segment locus: A systematic analysis provides no evidence for the use of DIR segments, inverted D segments, "minor" D segments or D-D recombination. *J Mol Biol* 1997;271:587–597.
12. Ramsden DA, Baetz K, Wu GE. Conservation of sequence in recombination signal sequence spacers. *Nucleic Acids Res* 1994;22:1785–1796.
13. Nossal BJ, Szenberg A, Ada GL, Austin CM. Single cell studies on 19S antibody production. *J Exp Med* 1964;119:485–501.
14. Wang AC, Wang IYF, McCormick MN, Fudenberg HH. The identity of light chains of monoclonal IgG and monoclonal IgM in one patient. *Immunochemistry* 1969;6:451–459.
15. Nisonoff A, Fudenberg HH, Wilson SK, Hopper JE, Wang AC. Individual antigenic specificiy in immunoglobulins: Relationship to biosynthesis. *Fed Proc* 1972;31:206–209.
16. Gearhart PJ, Sigal NH, Klinman NR. Production of antibodies of identical idiotype but diverse immunoglobulin classes by cells derived from a single stimulated B cell. *Proc Natl Acad Sci USA* 1975;72:1707–1711.
17. Kincade PW, Lawton AR, Bockman DE, Cooper MD. Suppression of immunoglobulin G synthesis as a result of antibody mediated suppression of immunoglobulin M synthesis in chickens. *Proc Natl Acad Sci USA* 1970;67:1918–1925.
18. Davis MM, Calame K, Early PW, et al. An immunoglobulin heavy-chain gene is formed by at least two recombinational events. *Nature* 1980;283:733–739.
19. Kataoka T, Kawakami T, Takahashi N, Honjo T. Rearrangement of immunoglobulin gamma 1-chain gene and mechanism for heavy-chain class switch. *Proc Natl Acad Sci USA* 1980;77:919–923.
20. Maki R, Traunecker A, Sakano H, Roeder W, Tonegawa S. Exon shuffling generates an immunoglobulin heavy chain gene. *Proc Natl Acad Sci USA* 1980;77:2138–2142.
21. Honjo T, Kataoka T. Organization of immunoglobulin heavy chain genes and allelic deletion model. *Proc Natl Acad Sci USA* 1978;75:2140–2144.
22. Cory S, Adams JM. Deletions are associated with somatic rearrangement of immunoglobulin heavy chain genes. *Cell* 1980;19:37–51.
23. Tucker PW, Marcu KB, Newell N, Richards J, Blattner FR. Sequence of the cloned gene for the constant region of murine gamma 2b immunoglobulin heavy chain. *Science* 1979;206:1303–1306.
24. Calame K, Rogers J, Early P, et al. Mouse Cmu heavy chain immunoglobulin gene segment contains three intervening sequences separating domains. *Nature* 1980;284:452–455.
25. Tucker PW, Slightom JL, Blattner FR. Mouse IgA heavy chain gene sequence: Implications for evolution of immunoglobulin hinge axons. *Proc Natl Acad Sci USA* 1981;78:7684–7688.
26. Tucker PW, Marcu KB, Slightom JL, Blattner FR. Structure of the constant and 3′ untranslated regions of the murine gamma 2b heavy chain messenger RNA. *Science* 1979;206:1299–1303.
27. Yamawaki KY, Kataoka T, Takahashi N, Obata M, Honjo T. Complete nucleotide sequence of immunoglobulin gamma2b chain gene cloned from newborn mouse DNA. *Nature* 1980;283:786–789.
28. Dard P, Huck S, Frippiat JP, et al. The IGHG3 gene shows a structural polymorphism characterized by different hinge lengths: Sequence of a new 2-exon hinge gene. *Hum Genet* 1997;99:138–141.
29. Yassalli P, Tedghi R, Lisowska-Bernstein B, Tartakoff A, Jaton JC. Evidence for hydrophobic region within heavy chains of mouse B lymphocyte membrane-bound IgM. *Proc Natl Acad Sci USA* 1979;76:5515–5519.
30. Alt FW, Bothwell AL, Knapp M, et al. Synthesis of secreted and membrane-bound immunoglobulin mu heavy chains is directed by mRNAs that differ at their 3′ ends. *Cell* 1980;20:293–301.
31. Early P, Rogers J, Davis M, et al. Two mRNAs can be produced from a single immunoglobulin mu gene by alternative RNA processing pathways. *Cell* 1980;20:313–319.
32. Kemp DJ, Harris AW, Adams JM. Transcripts of the immunoglobulin C mu gene vary in structure and splicing during lymphoid development. *Proc Natl Acad Sci USA* 1980;77:7400–7404.

33. Rogers J, Early P, Carter C, et al. Two mRNAs with different 3' ends encode membrane-bound and secreted forms of immunoglobulin mu chain. *Cell* 1980; 20:303–312.

34. Rogers J, Choi E, Souza L, et al. Gene segments encoding transmembrane carboxyl termini of immunoglobulin gamma chains. *Cell* 1981;26:19–27.

35. Tyler BM, Cowman AF, Gerondakis SD, Adams JM, Bernard O. mRNA for surface immunoglobulin gamma chains encodes a highly conserved transmembrane sequence and a 28-residue intracellular domain. *Proc Natl Acad Sci USA* 1982; 79:2008–2012.

36. Yamawaki KY, Nakai S, Miyata T, Honjo T. Nucleotide sequences of gene segments encoding membrane domains of immunoglobulin gamma chains. *Proc Natl Acad Sci USA* 1982;79:2623–2627.

37. Zhang K, Saxon A, Max EE. Two unusual forms of human immunoglobulin E encoded by alternative RNA splicing of epsilon heavy chain membrane exons. *J Exp Med* 1992;176:233–243.

38. Tsurushita N, Ho L, Korn LJ. Nuclear factors in B lymphoma enhance splicing of mouse membrane-bound mu mRNA in Xenopus oocytes. *Science* 1988;239: 494–497.

39. Galli G, Guise J, Tucker PW, Nevins JR. Poly(A) site choice rather than splice site choice governs the regulated production of IgM heavy-chain RNAs. *Proc Natl Acad Sci USA* 1988;85:2439–2443.

40. Peterson ML, Gimmi ER, Perry RP. The developmentally regulated shift from membrane to secreted mu mRNA production is accompanied by an increase in cleavage-polyadenylation efficiency but no measurable change in splicing efficiency. *Mol Cell Biol* 1991;11:2324–2327.

41. Peterson ML, Perry RP. Regulated production of mu m and mu s mRNA requires linkage of the poly(A) addition sites and is dependent on the length of the mu s-mu m intron. *Proc Natl Acad Sci USA* 1986,83.8883–8887.

42. Tsurushita N, Korn LJ. Effects of intron length on differential processing of mouse mu heavy-chain mRNA. *Mol Cell Biol* 1987;7:2602–2605.

43. Watakabe A, Inoue K, Sakamoto H, Shimura Y. A secondary structure at the 3' splice site affects the in vitro splicing reaction of mouse immunoglobulin mu chain pre-mRNAs. *Nucleic Acids Res* 1989;17:8159–8169.

44. Lassman CR, Milcarek C. Regulated expression of the mouse gamma 2b Ig H chain gene is influenced by polyA site order and strength. *J Immunol* 1992;148: 2578 2585.

45. Shimizu A, Takahashi N, Yaoita Y, Honjo T. Organization of the constant-region gene family of the mouse immunoglobulin heavy chain. *Cell* 1982;28:499–506.

46. Akahori Y, Kurosawa Y. Nucleotide sequences of all the gamma gene loci of murine immunoglobulin heavy chains. *Genomics* 1997;41:100–104

47. Kirsch IR, Morton CC, Nakahara K, Leder P. Human immunoglobulin heavy chain genes map to a region of translocations in malignant B lymphocytes. *Science* 1982;216:301–303.

48. Flanagan JG, Rabbitts TH. Arrangement of human immunoglobulin heavy chain constant region genes implies evolutionary duplication of a segment containing gamma, epsilon and alpha genes. *Nature* 1982;300:709 713.

49. Max EE, Battey J, Ney R, Kirsch IR, Leder P. Duplication and deletion in the human immunoglobulin epsilon genes. *Cell* 1982;29:691–699.

50. Battey J, Max EE, McBride WO, Swan D, Leder P. A processed human immunoglobulin epsilon gene has moved to chromosome 9. *Proc Natl Acad Sci USA* 1982;79:5956–5960.

51. Hisajima H, Nishida Y, Nakai S, Takahashi N, Ueda S, Honjo T. Structure of the human immunoglobulin C epsilon 2 gene, a truncated pseudogene: Implications for its evolutionary origin. *Proc Natl Acad Sci USA* 1983;80.2995–2999.

52. Bensmana M, Huck S, Lefranc G, Lefranc MP. The human immunoglobulin pseudo-gamma IGHGP gene shows no major structural defect. *Nucleic Acids Res* 1988;16:3108.

53. Bottaro A, DeMarchi M, Migone N, Carbonara AO. Pulsed-field gel analysis of human immunoglobulin heavy-chain constant region gene deletions reveals the extent of unmapped regions within the locus. *Genomics* 1989;4:505–508.

54. Hofker MH, Walter MA, Cox DW. Complete physical map of the human immunoglobulin heavy chain constant region gene complex. *Proc Natl Acad Sci USA* 1989;86:5567–5571.

55. Lefranc MP, Hammarstrom L, Smith CI, Lefranc G. Gene deletions in the human immunoglobulin heavy chain constant region locus: Molecular and immunological analysis. *Immunodefic Rev* 1991;2:265–281.

56. Knight KL, Becker RS. Isolation of genes encoding bovine IgM, IgG, IgA and IgE chains. *Vet Immunol Immunopathol* 1987;17:17–24.

57. Butler JE, Brown WR. The immunoglobulins and immunoglobulin genes of swine. *Vet Immunol Immunopathol* 1994;43:5–12.

58. Hamers-Casterman C, Atarhouch T, Muyldermans S, et al. Naturally occurring antibodies devoid of light chains. *Nature* 1993;363:446–448.

59. Bruggemann M, Free J, Diamond A, Howard J, Cobbold S, Waldmann H. Immunoglobulin heavy chain locus of the rat: Striking homology to mouse antibody genes. *Proc Natl Acad Sci USA* 1986;83:6075–6079.

60. Dahan A, Reynaud CA, Weill JC. Nucleotide sequence of the constant region of a chicken mu heavy chain immunoglobulin mRNA. *Nucleic Acids Res* 1983;11: 5381–5389.

61. Weill JC, Reynaud CA, Lassila O, Pink JR. Rearrangement of chicken immunoglobulin genes is not an ongoing process in the embryonic bursa of Fabricius. *Proc Natl Acad Sci USA* 1986;83:3336 3340.

62. Parvari R, Avivi A, Lentner F, et al. Chicken immunoglobulin gamma heavy chains: Limited VH gene repertoire, combinatorial diversification by D gene segments and evolution of the heavy chain locus. *EMBO J* 1988;7:739–744.

63. Reynaud CA, Dahan A, Anquez V, Weill JC. Somatic hyperconversion diversi-

fies the single Vh gene of the chicken with a high incidence in the D region. *Cell* 1989;59:171–183.

64. Schrenzel MD, King DP, McKnight ML, Ferrick DA. Characterization of horse (*Equus caballus*) immunoglobulin mu chain-encoding genes. *Immunogenetics* 1997;45:386–393.

65. Kokubu F, Hinds K, Litman R, Shamblott MJ, Litman GW. Extensive families of constant region genes in a phylogenetically primitive vertebrate indicate an additional level of immunoglobulin complexity. *Proc Natl Acad Sci USA* 1987;84: 5868–5872.

66. Amemiya CT, Litman GW. Complete nucleotide sequence of an immunoglobulin heavy-chain gene and analysis of immunoglobulin gene organization in a primitive teleost species. *Proc Natl Acad Sci USA* 1990;87:811–815.

67. Wilson MR, Marcuz A, van GF, et al. The immunoglobulin M heavy chain constant region gene of the channel catfish, *Ictalurus punctatus*: an unusual mRNA splice pattern produces the membrane form of the molecule. *Nucleic Acids Res* 1990;18:5227–5233.

68. Litman GW, Murphy K, Berger L, Litman R, Hinds K, Erickson BW. Complete nucleotide sequences of three VH genes in Caiman, a phylogenetically ancient reptile: Evolutionary diversification in coding segments and variation in the structure and organization of recombination elements. *Proc Natl Acad Sci USA* 1985;82:844–848.

69. Yamawaki KY, Honjo T. Nucleotide sequences of variable region segments of the immunoglobulin heavy chain of *Xenopus laevis*. *Nucleic Acids Res* 1987;15:5888.

70. Charlemagne J. Noninbred axolotls use the same unique heavy chain and a limited number of light chains for their anti-2,4-dinitrophenyl antibody responses. *Eur J Immunol* 1987;17:421–424.

71. Davis MM, Kim SK, Hood LE. DNA sequences mediating class switching in alpha immunoglobulins. *Science* 1980;209:1360–1365.

72. Dunnick W, Rabbitts TH, Milstein C. An immunoglobulin deletion mutant with implications for the heavy-chain switch and RNA splicing. *Nature* 1980;286: 669–675.

73. Kataoka T, Miyata T, Honjo T. Repetitive sequences in class-switch recombination regions of immunoglobulin heavy chain genes. *Cell* 1981;23:357–368.

74. Nikaido T, Nakai S, Honjo T. Switch region of immunoglobulin Cmu gene is composed of simple tandem repetitive sequences. *Nature* 1981;281:845–848.

75. Marcu KB, Banerji J, Penncavage NA, Lang R, Arnheim N. 5' flanking region of immunoglobulin heavy chain constant region genes displays length heterogeneity in germlines of inbred mouse strains. *Cell* 1980;22:187–196.

76. Winter E, Krawinkel U, Radbruch A. Directed Ig class switch recombination in activated murine B cells. *EMBO J* 1987;6:1663–1671.

77. Nikaido T, Yamawaki KY, Honjo T. Nucleotide sequences of switch regions of immunoglobulin C epsilon and C gamma genes and their comparison. *J Biol Chem* 1982;257:7322–7329.

78. Mowatt MR, Dunnick WA. DNA sequence of the murine gamma 1 switch segment reveals novel structural elements. *J Immunol* 1986;136:2674–2683.

79. Ravetch JV, Kirsch IR, Leder P. Evolutionary approach to the question of immunoglobulin heavy chain switching: Evidence from cloned human and mouse genes. *Proc Natl Acad Sci USA* 1980;77:6734–6738.

80. Rabbitts TH, Forster A, Milstein CP. Human immunoglobulin heavy chain genes: Evolutionary comparisons of C mu, C delta and C gamma genes and associated switch sequences. *Nucleic Acids Res* 1981;9:4509–4524.

81. Mills FC, Mitchell MP, Harindranath N, Max EE. Human Ig S gamma regions and their participation in sequential switching to IgE. *J Immunol* 1995;155: 3021–3036.

82. Dunnick W, Hertz GZ, Scappino L, Gritzmacher C. DNA sequences at immunoglobulin switch region recombination sites. *Nucleic Acids Res* 1993;21: 365–372.

83. Iwasato T, Shimizu A, Honjo T, Yamagishi H. Circular DNA is excised by immunoglobulin class switch recombination. *Cell* 1990;62:143–149.

84. Matsuoka M, Yoshida K, Maeda T, Usuda S, Sakano H. Switch circular DNA formed in cytokine-treated mouse splenocytes: Evidence for intramolecular DNA deletion in immunoglobulin class switching. *Cell* 1990;62:135–142.

85. von-Schwedler U, Jack HM, Wabl M. Circular DNA is a product of the immunoglobulin class switch rearrangement. *Nature* 1990;345:452–456.

86. Mills FC, Thyphronitis G, Finkelman FD, Max EE. Ig mu-epsilon isotype switch in IL-4-treated human B lymphoblastoid cells. Evidence for a sequential switch. *J Immunol* 1992;149:1075–1085.

87. Zhang K, Mills FC, Saxon A. Switch circles from IL-4-directed epsilon class switching from human B lymphocytes. Evidence for direct, sequential, and multiple step sequential switch from mu to epsilon Ig heavy chain gene. *J Immunol* 1994;152:3427–3435.

88. Malisan F, Briere F, Bridon JM, et al. Interleukin-10 induces immunoglobulin G isotype switch recombination in human CD40-activated naive B lymphocytes. *J Exp Med* 1996;183:937–947.

89. Chu CC, Paul WE, Max EE. Quantitation of immunoglobulin mu-gamma 1 heavy chain switch region recombination by a digestion-circularization polymerase chain reaction method. *Proc Natl Acad Sci USA* 1992;89:6978–6982.

90. Chu CC, Max EE, Paul WE. DNA rearrangement can account for in vitro switching to IgG1. *J Exp Med* 1993;178:1381 1390.

91. Allen RC, Armitage RJ, Conley ME, et al. CD40 ligand gene defects responsible for X linked hyper-IgM syndrome. *Science* 1993;259:990–993.

92. Xu J, Foy TM, Laman JD, et al. Mice deficient for the CD40 ligand. *Immunity* 1994;1:423–431.

93. Hodgkin PD, Lee JH, Lyons AB. B cell differentiation and isotype switching is related to division cycle number. *J Exp Med* 1996;184:277–281.

94. Siepmann K, Wohlleben G, Gray D. CD40-mediated regulation of interleukin-4 signaling pathways in B lymphocytes. *Eur J Immunol* 1996;26:1544–1552.

95. Cheng G, Cleary AM, Ye ZS, Hong DI, Lederman S, Baltimore D. Involvement of CRAF1, a relative of TRAF, in CD40 signaling. *Science* 1995;267: 1494–1498.

96. Cogne M, Lansford R, Bottaro A, et al. A class switch control region at the 3' end of the immunoglobulin heavy chain locus. *Cell* 1994;77:737–747.

97. Jung S, Rajewsky K, Radbruch A. Shutdown of class switch recombination by deletion of a switch region control element. *Science* 1993;259:984–987.

98. Bottaro A, Lansford R, Xu L, Zhang J, Rothman P, Alt FW. S region transcription per se promotes basal IgE class switch recombination but additional factors regulate the efficiency of the process. *EMBO J* 1994;13:665–674.

99. Lorenz M, Jung S, Radbruch A. Switch transcripts in immunoglobulin class switching. *Science* 1995;267:1825–1828.

100. Reaban ME, Griffin JA. Induction of RNA-stabilized DNA conformers by transcription of an immunoglobulin switch region. *Nature* 1990;348:342–344.

101. Daniels GA, Lieber MR. RNA:DNA complex formation upon transcription of immunoglobulin switch regions: implications for the mechanism and regulation of class switch recombination. *Nucleic Acids Res* 1995;23:5006–5011.

102. Snapper CM, Marcu KB, Zelazowski P. The immunoglobulin class switch: beyond "accessibility." *Immunity* 1997;6:217–223.

103. Ott DE, Alt FW, Marcu KB. Immunoglobulin heavy chain switch region recombination within a retroviral vector in murine pre-B cells. *EMBO J* 1987;6:577–584.

104. Leung H, Maizels N. Regulation and targeting of recombination in extrachromosomal substrates carrying immunoglobulin switch region sequences. *Mol Cell Biol* 1994;14:1450–1458.

105. Daniels GA, Lieber MR. Strand specificity in the transcriptional targeting of recombination at immunoglobulin switch sequences. *Proc Natl Acad Sci USA* 1995;92:5625–5629.

106. Du J, Zhu Y, Shanmugam A, Kenter AL. Analysis of immunoglobulin S gamma3 recombination breakpoints by PCR: Implications for the mechanism of isotype switching. *Nucleic Acids Res* 1997;25:3066–3074.

107. Williams M, Maizels N. LR1, a lipopolysaccharide-responsive factor with binding sites in the immunoglobulin switch regions and heavy-chain enhancer. *Genes Dev* 1991;5:2353–2361.

108. Williams M, Hanakahi LA, Maizels N. Purification and properties of LR1, an inducible DNA binding protein from mammalian B lymphocytes. *J Biol Chem* 1993;268:13731–13737.

109. Hanakahi LA, Dempsey LA, Li MJ, Maizels N. Nucleolin is one component of the B cell-specific transcription factor and switch region binding protein, LR1. *Proc Natl Acad Sci USA* 1997;94:3605–3610.

110. Mizuta TR, Fukita Y, Miyoshi T, Shimizu A, Honjo T. Isolation of cDNA encoding a binding protein specific to 5'-phosphorylated single-stranded DNA with G-rich sequences. *Nucleic Acids Res* 1993;21:1761–1766.

111. Wuerffel RA, Nathan AT, Kenter AL. Detection of an immunoglobulin switch region-specific DNA-binding protein in mitogen-stimulated mouse splenic B cells. *Mol Cell Biol* 1990;10:1714–1718.

112. Kenter AL, Wuerffel R, Sen R, Jamieson CE, Merkulov GV. Switch recombination breakpoints occur at nonrandom positions in the S gamma tandem repeat. *J Immunol* 1993;151:4718–4731.

113. Ma L, Hu B, Kenter AL. Ig S-gamma-specific DNA binding protein SNAP is related to the helix-loop-helix transcription factor E47. *Int Immunol* 1997;9: 1021–1029.

114. Snapper CM, Zelazowski P, Rosas FR, et al. B cells from p50/NF-kappa B knockout mice have selective defects in proliferation, differentiation, germ-line CH transcription, and Ig class switching. *J Immunol* 1996;156:183–191.

115. Goldfarb AN, Flores JP, Lewandowska K. Involvement of the E2A basic helix-loop-helix protein in immunoglobulin heavy chain class switching. *Mol Immunol* 1996;33:947–956.

116. Lyon CJ, Aguilera RJ. Purification and characterization of the immunoglobulin switch sequence-specific endonuclease (Endo-SR) from bovine spleen. *Mol Immunol* 1997;34:209–219.

116a. Rolink A, Melchers F, Andersson J. The SCID but not the RAG-2 gene product is required for S mu-S epsilon heavy chain class switching. *Immunity* 1996;5: 319–330.

116b. Casellas R, Nussenzweig A, Wuerffel R, et al. Ku80 is required for immunoglobulin isotype switching. *EMBO J* 1998;17:2404–2411.

117. Jessberger R, Wabl M, Borggrefe T. Biochemical studies of class switch recombination. *Curr Top Microbiol Immunol* 1996;217:191–202.

118. Borggrefe T, Wabl M, Akhmedov AT, Jessberger R. A B-Cell specific DNA recombination complex. *J Biol Chem* 1998;in press.

119. Siebenkotten G, Esser C, Wabl M, Radbruch A. The murine IgG1/IgE class switch program. *Eur J Immunol* 1992;22:1827–1834.

120. Mandler R, Finkelman FD, Levine AD, Snapper CM. IL-4 induction of IgE class switching by lipopolysaccharide-activated murine B cells occurs predominantly through sequential switching. *J Immunol* 1993;150:407–418.

121. Jung S, Siebenkotten G, Radbruch A. Frequency of immunoglobulin E class switching is autonomously determined and independent of prior switching to other classes. *J Exp Med* 1994;179:2023–2026.

122. Baskin B, Islam KB, Evengard B, Emtestam L, Smith CI. Direct and sequential switching from mu to epsilon in patients with Schistosoma mansoni infection and atopic dermatitis. *Eur J Immunol* 1997;27:130–135.

123. Greenberg R, Lang RB, Diamond MS, Marcu KB. A switch region inversion contributes to the aberrant rearrangement of a mu immunoglobulin heavy chain gene in MPC-11 cells. *Nucleic Acids Res* 1982;10:7751–7761.

124. Jack HM, McDowell M, Steinberg CM, Wabl M. Looping out and deletion mechanism for the immunoglobulin heavy-chain class switch. *Proc Natl Acad Sci USA* 1988;85:1581–1585.

125. Laffan M, Luzzatto L. Anomalous rearrangements of the immunoglobulin heavy chain genes in human leukemias support the loop-out mechanism of class switch. *J Clin Invest* 1992;90:2299–2303.

126. Knight KL, Kingzette M, Crane MA, Zhai SK. Transchromosomally derived Ig heavy chains. *J Immunol* 1995;155:684–691.

127. Maki R, Roeder W, Traunecker A, et al. The role of DNA rearrangement and alternative RNA processing in the expression of immunoglobulin delta genes. *Cell* 1981;24:353–365.

128. Shimizu A, Nussenzweig MC, Han H, Sanchez M, Honjo T. Trans-splicing as a possible molecular mechanism for the multiple isotype expression of the immunoglobulin gene. *J Exp Med* 1991;173:1385–1393.

129. Shimizu A, Honjo T. Synthesis and regulation of trans-mRNA encoding the immunoglobulin epsilon heavy chain. *FASEB J* 1993;7:149–154.

130. Mizuta TR, Suzuki N, Shimizu A, Honjo T. Duplicated variable region genes account for double isotype expression in a human leukemic B-cell line that gives rise to single isotype-expressing cells. *J Biol Chem* 1991;266:12514–12521.

131. Chen YW, Word C, Dev V, Uhr JW, Vitetta ES, Tucker PW. Double isotype production by a neoplastic B cell line. II. Allelically excluded production of mu and gamma 1 heavy chains without CH gene rearrangement. *J Exp Med* 1986;164: 562–579.

132. Akahori Y, Kurosawa Y, Kamachi Y, Torii S, Matsuoka H. Presence of immunoglobulin (Ig) M and IgG double isotype-bearing cells and defect of switch recombination in hyper IgM immunodeficiency. *J Clin Invest* 1990;85: 1722–1727.

133. Kunimoto DY, Sneller MC, Claflin L, Mushinski JF, Strober W. Molecular analysis of double isotype expression in IgA switching. *J Immunol* 1993;150: 1338–1347.

134. Hieter PA, Max EE, Seidman JG, Maizel JJ, Leder P. Cloned human and mouse kappa immunoglobulin constant and J region genes conserve homology in functional segments. *Cell* 1980;22:197–207.

135. Hieter PA, Maizel JJ, Leder P. Evolution of human immunoglobulin kappa J region genes. *J Biol Chem* 1982;257:1516–1522.

136. Hieter PA, Korsmeyer SJ, Waldmann TA, Leder P. Human immunoglobulin kappa light-chain genes are deleted or rearranged in lambda-producing B cells. *Nature* 1981;290:368–372.

137. Durdik J, Moore MW, Selsing E. Novel kappa light-chain gene rearrangements in mouse lambda light chain-producing B lymphocytes. *Nature* 1984;307: 749–752.

138. Siminovitch KA, Bakhshi A, Goldman P, Korsmeyer SJ. A uniform deleting element mediates the loss of kappa genes in human B cells. *Nature* 1985;316: 260–262.

139. Klobeck HG, Zachau HG. The human CK gene segment and the kappa deleting element are closely linked. *Nucleic Acids Res* 1986;14:4591–4603.

140. Muller B, Stappert H, Reth M. A physical map and analysis of the murine C kappa-RS region show the presence of a conserved element. *Eur J Immunol* 1990;20:1409–1411.

141. Tonegawa S, Brack C, Hozumi N, Schuller R. Cloning of an immunoglobulin variable region gene from mouse embryo. *Proc Natl Acad Sci USA* 1977;74: 3518–3522.

142. Miller J, Ogden S, McMullen M, Andres H, Storb U. The order and orientation of mouse lambda-genes explain lambda-rearrangement patterns. *J Immunol* 1988;141:2497–2502.

143. Storb U, Haasch D, Arp B, Sanchez P, Cazenave PA, Miller J. Physical linkage of mouse lambda genes by pulsed-field gel electrophoresis suggests that the rearrangement process favors proximate target sequences. *Mol Cell Biol* 1989;9: 711–718.

144. Sanchez P, Marche PN, Rueff JD, Cazenave PA. Mouse V lambda x gene sequence generates no junctional diversity and is conserved in mammalian species. *J Immunol* 1990;144:2816–2820.

145. Miller J, Selsing E, Storb U. Structural alterations in J regions of mouse immunoglobulin lambda genes are associated with differential gene expression. *Nature* 1982;295:428–430.

146. Scott CL, Mushinski JF, Huppi K, Weigert M, Potter M. Amplification of immunoglobulin lambda constant genes in populations of wild mice. *Nature* 1982;300:757–760.

147. Hieter PA, Hollis GF, Korsmeyer SJ, Waldmann TA, Leder P. Clustered arrangement of immunoglobulin lambda constant region genes in man. *Nature* 1981; 294:536–540.

148. Vasicek TJ, Leder P. Structure and expression of the human immunoglobulin lambda genes. *J Exp Med* 1990;172:609–620.

149. Kawasaki K, Minoshima S, Nakato E, et al. One-megabase sequence analysis of the human immunoglobulin lambda gene locus. *Genome Res* 1997;7:250–261.

150. Dariavach P, Lefranc G, Lefranc MP. Human immunoglobulin C lambda 6 gene encodes the Kern+Oz-lambda chain and C lambda 4 and C lambda 5 are pseudogenes. *Proc Natl Acad Sci USA* 1987;84:9074–9078.

151. Stiernholm NB, Verkoczy LK, Berinstein NL. Rearrangement and expression of the human psi C lambda 6 gene segment results in a surface Ig receptor with a truncated light chain constant region. *J Immunol* 1995;154:4583–4591.

152. Taub RA, Hollis GF, Hieter PA, Korsmeyer S, Waldmann TA, Leder P. Variable amplification of immunoglobulin lambda light-chain genes in human populations. *Nature* 1983;304:172–174.

153. Hollis GF, Hieter PA, McBride OW, Swan D, Leder P. Processed genes: A dis-

persed human immunoglobulin gene bearing evidence of RNA-type processing. *Nature* 1982;296:321–325.

154. Sakaguchi N, Melchers F. Lambda 5, a new light-chain-related locus selectively expressed in pre-B lymphocytes. *Nature* 1986;324:579–582.

155. Kudo A, Sakaguchi N, Melchers F. Organization of the murine Ig-related lambda 5 gene transcribed selectively in pre-B lymphocytes. *EMBO J* 1987;6:103–107.

156. Kudo A, Melchers F. A second gene, VpreB in the lambda 5 locus of the mouse, which appears to be selectively expressed in pre-B lymphocytes. *EMBO J* 1987;6:2267–2272.

157. Sakaguchi N, Berger CN, Melchers F. Isolation of a cDNA copy of an RNA species expressed in murine pre-B cells. *EMBO J* 1986;5:2139–2147.

158. Dul JL, Argon Y, Winkler T, ten Boekel E, Melchers F, Martensson IL. The murine VpreB1 and VpreB2 genes both encode a protein of the surrogate light chain and are co-expressed during B cell development. *Eur J Immunol* 1996;26:906–913.

159. Hagiwara S, Tsunetsugu YY, Kimoto H, Takemori T. Expression of Vpre-B3 (8HS-20) molecules by alternative RNA processing. *Int Immunol* 1996;8:1237–1244.

160. Tsubata T, Reth M. The products of pre-B cell-specific genes (lambda 5 and VpreB) and the immunoglobulin mu chain form a complex that is transported onto the cell. *J Exp Med* 1990;172:973–976.

161. Cherayil BJ, Pillai S. The omega/lambda 5 surrogate immunoglobulin light chain is expressed on the surface of transitional B lymphocytes in murine bone marrow. *J Exp Med* 1991;173:111–116.

162. Pillai S, Baltimore D. The omega and iota surrogate immunoglobulin light chains. *Curr Top Microbiol Immunol* 1988;137:136–139.

163. Tsubata T, Tsubata R, Reth M. Crosslinking of the cell surface immunoglobulin (mu-surrogate light chains complex) on pre-B cells induces activation of V gene rearrangements at the immunoglobulin kappa locus. *Int Immunol* 1992;4:637–641.

164. Bauer TJ, McDermid HE, Budarf ML, Van KM, Blomberg BB. Physical location of the human immunoglobulin lambda-like genes, 14.1, 16.1, and 16.2. *Immunogenetics* 1993;38:387–399.

165. Bossy D, Milili M, Zucman J, Thomas G, Fougereau M, Schiff C. Organization and expression of the lambda-like genes that contribute to the mu-psi light chain complex in human pre-B cells. *Int Immunol* 1991;3:1081–1090.

166. Evans RJ, Hollis GF. Genomic structure of the human Ig lambda 1 gene suggests that it may be expressed as an Ig lambda 14.1-like protein or as a canonical B cell Ig lambda light chain: Implications for Ig lambda gene evolution. *J Exp Med* 1991;173:305–311.

167. Schiff C, Milili M, Bossy D, Fougereau M. Organization and expression of the pseudo-light chain genes in human B-cell ontogeny. *Int Rev Immunol* 1992;8:135–145.

168. Frippiat JP, Williams SC, Tomlinson IM, et al. Organization of the human immunoglobulin lambda light-chain locus on chromosome 22q11.2. *Hum Mol Genet* 1995;4:983–991.

169. Van Ness BG, Coleclough C, Perry RP, Weigert M. DNA between variable and joining gene segments of immunoglobulin kappa light chain is frequently retained in cells that rearrange the kappa locus. *Proc Natl Acad Sci USA* 1982;79:262–266.

170. Hochtl J, Müller CR, Zachau HG. Recombined flanks of the variable and joining segments of immunoglobulin genes. *Proc Natl Acad Sci USA* 1982;79:1383–1387.

171. Hochtl J, Zachau HG. A novel type of aberrant recombination in immunoglobulin genes and its implications for V-J joining mechanism. *Nature* 1983;302:260–263.

172. Feddersen RM, Van NB. Double recombination of a single immunoglobulin kappa-chain allele: Implications for the mechanism of rearrangement. *Proc Natl Acad Sci USA* 1985;82:4793–4797.

173. Lewis S, Gifford A, Baltimore D. Joining of V kappa to J kappa gene segments in a retroviral vector introduced into lymphoid cells. *Nature* 1984;308:425–428.

174. Hesse JE, Lieber MR, Gellert M, Mizuuchi K. Extrachromosomal DNA substrates in pre-B cells undergo inversion or deletion at immunoglobulin V-(D)-J joining signals. *Cell* 1987;49:775–783.

175. Shapiro MA, Weigert M. How immunoglobulin V kappa genes rearrange. *J Immunol* 1987;139:3834–3839.

176. Shimizu T, Iwasato T, Yamagishi H. Deletions of immunoglobulin C kappa region characterized by the circular excision products in mouse splenocytes. *J Exp Med* 1991;173:1065–1072.

177. Selsing E, Voss J, Storb U. Immunoglobulin gene "remnant" DNA—implications for antibody gene recombination. *Nucleic Acids Res* 1984;12:4229–4246.

178. Maeda T, Sugiyama H, Tani Y, et al. Start of mu-chain production by the further two-step rearrangements of immunoglobulin heavy chain genes on one chromosome from a DJH/DJH configuration in an Abelson virus-transformed cell line: Evidence of secondary DJH complex formation. *J Immunol* 1987;138:2305–2310.

179. Reth M, Gehrmann P, Petrac F, Wiese P. A novel VH to VHDJH joining mechanism in heavy-chain-negative (null) pre-B cells results in heavy-chain production. *Nature* 1986;322:840–842.

180. Covey LR, Ferrier P, Alt FW. VH to VHDJH rearrangement is mediated by the internal VH heptamer. *Int Immunol* 1990;2:579–583.

181. Chen C, Nagy Z, Prak EL, Weigert M. Immunoglobulin heavy chain gene replacement: A mechanism of receptor editing. *Immunity* 1995;3:747–755.

182. Schuler W, Weiler IJ, Schuler A, et al. Rearrangement of antigen receptor genes is defective in mice with severe combined immune deficiency. *Cell* 1986;46:963–972.

183. Lafaille JJ, DeCloux A, Bonneville M, Takagaki Y, Tonegawa S. Junctional sequences of T cell receptor gamma delta genes: implications for gamma delta T cell lineages and for a novel intermediate of V-(D)-J joining. *Cell* 1989;59:859–870.

184. McCormack WT, Tjoelker LW, Carlson LM, et al. Chicken IgL gene rearrangement involves deletion of a circular episome and addition of single nonrandom nucleotides to both coding segments. *Cell* 1989;56:785–791.

185. Schuler W, Ruetsch NR, Amsler M, Bosma MJ. Coding joint formation of endogenous T cell receptor genes in lymphoid cells from scid mice: Unusual P-nucleotide additions in VJ-coding joints. *Eur J Immunol* 1991;21:589–596.

186. Alt FW, Baltimore D. Joining of immunoglobulin heavy chain gene segments: Implications from a chromosome with evidence of three D-JH fusions. *Proc Natl Acad Sci USA* 1982;79:4118–4122.

187. Alt F, Rosenberg N, Lewis S, Thomas E, Baltimore D. Organization and reorganization of immunoglobulin genes in A-MULV-transformed cells: Rearrangement of heavy but not light chain genes. *Cell* 1981;27:391–390.

188. Lewis S, Rosenberg N, Alt F, Baltimore D. Continuing kappa-gene rearrangement in a cell line transformed by Abelson murine leukemia virus. *Cell* 1982;30:807–816.

189. Reth MG, Ammirati P, Jackson S, Alt FW. Regulated progression of a cultured pre-B-cell line to the B-cell stage. *Nature* 1985;317:353–355.

190. Lewis S, Gifford A, Baltimore D. DNA elements are asymmetrically joined during the site-specific recombination of kappa immunoglobulin genes. *Science* 1985;228:677–685.

191. Lieber MR, Hesse JE, Mizuuchi K, Gellert M. Developmental stage specificity of the lymphoid V(D)J recombination activity. *Genes Dev* 1987;1:751–761.

192. Lieber MR, Hesse JE, Lewis S, et al. The defect in murine severe combined immune deficiency: Joining of signal sequences but not coding segments in V(D)J recombination. *Cell* 1988;55:7–16.

193. Lewis SM, Hesse JE, Mizuuchi K, Gellert M. Novel strand exchanges in V(D)J recombination. *Cell* 1988;55:1099–1107.

194. Akira S, Okazaki K, Sakano H. Two pairs of recombination signals are sufficient to cause immunoglobulin V-(D)-J joining. *Science* 1987;238:1134–1138.

195. Hesse JE, Lieber MR, Mizuuchi K, Gellert M. V(D)J recombination: a functional definition of the joining signals. *Genes Dev* 1989;3:1053–1061.

196. Roth DB, Menetski JP, Nakajima PB, Bosma MJ, Gellert M. V(D)J recombination: Broken DNA molecules with covalently sealed (hairpin) coding ends in scid mouse thymocytes. *Cell* 1992;70:983–991.

197. Roth DB, Nakajima PB, Menetski JP, Bosma MJ, Gellert M. V(D)J recombination in mouse thymocytes: Double-strand breaks near T cell receptor delta rearrangement signals. *Cell* 1992;69:41–53.

198. Roth DB, Zhu C, Gellert M. Characterization of broken DNA molecules associated with V(D)J recombination. *Proc Natl Acad Sci USA* 1993;90:10788–10792.

199. Schlissel M, Constantinescu A, Morrow T, Baxter M, Peng A. Double-strand signal sequence breaks in V(D)J recombination are blunt, 5′-phosphorylated, RAG-dependent, and cell cycle regulated. *Genes Dev* 1993;7:2320–2332.

200. Zhu C, Roth DB. Characterization of coding ends in thymocytes of scid mice: Implications for the mechanism of V(D)J recombination. *Immunity* 1995;2:101–112.

201. Ramsden DA, Gellert M. Formation and resolution of double-strand break intermediates in V(D)J rearrangement. *Genes Dev* 1995;9:2409–2420.

202. Lewis SM. P nucleotide insertions and the resolution of hairpin DNA structures in mammalian cells. *Proc Natl Acad Sci USA* 1994;91:1332–1336.

203. Desiderio S, Baltimore D. Double-stranded cleavage by cell extracts near recombinational signal sequences of immunoglobulin genes. *Nature* 1984;308:860–862.

204. Kataoka T, Kondo S, Nishi M, Kodaira M, Honjo T. Isolation and characterization of endonuclease J: A sequence-specific endonuclease cleaving immunoglobulin genes. *Nucleic Acids Res* 1984;12:5995–6010.

205. Hope TJ, Aguilera RJ, Minie ME, Sakano H. Endonucleolytic activity that cleaves immunoglobulin recombination sequences. *Science* 1986;231:1141–1145.

206. Schatz DG, Baltimore D. Stable expression of immunoglobulin gene V(D)J recombinase activity by gene transfer into 3T3 fibroblasts. *Cell* 1988;53:107–115.

207. Oettinger MA, Schatz DG, Gorka C, Baltimore D. RAG-1 and RAG-2, adjacent genes that synergistically activate V(D)J recombination. *Science* 1990;248:1517–1523.

208. Bernstein RM, Schluter SF, Bernstein H, Marchalonis JJ. Primordial emergence of the recombination activating gene 1 (RAG1): Sequence of the complete shark gene indicates homology to microbial integrases. *Proc Natl Acad Sci USA* 1996;93:9454–9459.

209. Mombaerts P, Iacomini J, Johnson RS, et al. RAG-1-deficient mice have no mature B and T lymphocytes. *Cell* 1992;68:869–877.

210. Shinkai Y, Rathbun G, Lam KP, et al. RAG-2-deficient mice lack mature lymphocytes owing to inability to initiate V(D)J rearrangement. *Cell* 1992;68:855–867.

211. Schwarz K, Gauss GH, Ludwig L, et al. RAG mutations in human B cell-negative SCID. *Science* 1996;274:97–99.

212. Sadofsky MJ, Hesse JE, McBlane JF, Gellert M. Expression and V(D)J recombination activity of mutated RAG-1 proteins. *Nucleic Acids Res* 1993;21:5644–5650.

213. McBlane JF, van GD, Ramsden DA, et al. Cleavage at a V(D)J recombination signal requires only RAG1 and RAG2 proteins and occurs in two steps. *Cell* 1995;83:387–395.

214. van Gent DC, Mizuuchi K, Gellert M. Similarities between initiation of V(D)J recombination and retroviral integration. *Science* 1996;271:1592–1594.

215. van Gent DC, Ramsden DA, Gellert M. The RAG1 and RAG2 proteins establish the 12/23 rule in V(D)J recombination. *Cell* 1996;85:107–113.

216. Hiom K, Gellert M. A stable RAG1-RAG2-DNA complex that is active in V(D)J cleavage. *Cell* 1997;88:65–72.

217. Sawchuk DJ, Weis GF, Malik S, et al. V(D)J recombination: Modulation of RAG1 and RAG2 cleavage activity on 12/23 substrates by whole cell extract and DNA-bending proteins. *J Exp Med* 1997;185:2025–2032.

218. Cuomo CA, Mundy CL, Oettinger MA. DNA sequence and structure requirements for cleavage of V(D)J recombination signal sequences. *Mol Cell Biol* 1996;16:5683–5690.

219. Ramsden DA, McBlane JF, van Gent DC, Gellert M. Distinct DNA sequence and structure requirements for the two steps of V(D)J recombination signal cleavage. *EMBO J* 1996;15:3197–3206.

220. Cortes P, Weis GF, Misulovin Z, et al. In vitro V(D)J recombination: Signal joint formation. *Proc Natl Acad Sci USA* 1996;93:14008–14013.

221. Leu TMJ, Eastman QM, Schatz DG. Coding joint formation in a cell-free V(D)J recombination system. *Immunity* 1997;7:303–314.

222. Ramsden DA, Paull TT, Gellert M. Cell-free V(D)J recombination. *Nature* 1997;388:488–491.

223. Agrawal A, Schatz DG. RAG1 and RAG2 form a stable postcleavage synaptic complex with DNA containing signal ends in V(D)J recombination. *Cell* 1997; 89:43–53.

224. Lin WC, Desiderio S. Regulation of V(D)J recombination activator protein RAG-2 by phosphorylation. *Science* 1993;260:953–959.

225. Lin WC, Desiderio S. Cell cycle regulation of V(D)J recombination-activating protein RAG-2. *Proc Natl Acad Sci USA* 1994;91:2733–2737.

226. Li Z, Dordai DI, Lee J, Desiderio S. A conserved degradation signal regulates RAG-2 accumulation during cell division and links V(D)J recombination to the cell cycle. *Immunity* 1996;5:575–589.

227. Difilippantonio MJ, McMahan CJ, Eastman QM, Spanopoulou E, Schatz DG. RAG1 mediates signal sequence recognition and recruitment of RAG2 in V(D)J recombination. *Cell* 1996;87:253–262.

228. Spanopoulou E, Zaitseva F, Wang FH, Santagata S, Baltimore D, Panayotou G. The homeodomain region of Rag-1 reveals the parallel mechanisms of bacterial and V(D)J recombination. *Cell* 1996;87:263–276.

229. Chun JJ, Schatz DG, Oettinger MA, Jaenisch R, Baltimore D. The recombination activating gene-1 (RAG-1) transcript is present in the murine central nervous system. *Cell* 1991;64:189–200.

230. Carlson LM, Oettinger MA, Schatz DG, et al. Selective expression of RAG-2 in chicken B cells undergoing immunoglobulin gene conversion. *Cell* 1991;64: 201–208.

231. Takeda S, Masteller EL, Thompson CB, Buerstedde JM. RAG-2 expression is not essential for chicken immunoglobulin gene conversion. *Proc Natl Acad Sci USA* 1992;89:4023–4027.

232. Chen J, Lansford R, Stewart V, Young F, Alt FW. RAG-2-deficient blastocyst complementation: An assay of gene function in lymphocyte development. *Proc Natl Acad Sci USA* 1993;90:4528–4532.

233. Taccioli GE, Rathbun G, Oltz E, Stamato T, Jeggo PA, Alt FW. Impairment of V(D)J recombination in double-strand break repair mutants. *Science* 1993;260: 207–210.

234. Troelstra C, Jaspers NGJ. Ku starts at the end. *Curr Biol* 1994;4:1149–1151.

234a. Wu X, Lieber MR. Protein-protein and protein-DNA interaction regions within the DNA end-binding protein Ku70-Ku86. *Mol Cell Biol* 1996;16:5186–5193.

234b. Yaneva M, Kowalewski T, Lieber MR. Interaction of DNA-dependent protein kinase with DNA and with Ku: Biochemical and atomic-force microscopy studies. *EMBO J* 1997;16:5098–5112.

235. Taccioli GE, Gottlieb TM, Blunt T, et al. Ku80: Product of the XRCC5 gene and its role in DNA repair and V(D)J recombination. *Science* 1994;265:1442–1445.

236. Errami A, Smider V, Rathmell WK, et al. Ku86 defines the genetic defect and restores X-ray resistance and V(D)J recombination to complementation group 5 hamster cell mutants. *Mol Cell Biol* 1996;16:1519–1526.

237. Blunt T, Finnie NJ, Taccioli GE, et al. Defective DNA-dependent protein kinase activity is linked to V(D)J recombination and DNA repair defects associated with the murine scid mutation. *Cell* 1995;80:813–823.

238. Shin EK, Perryman LE, Meek K. A kinase-negative mutation of DNA-PK(CS) in equine SCID results in defective coding and signal joint formation. *J Immunol* 1997;158:3565–3569.

239. Gu Y, Jin S, Gao Y, Weaver DT, Alt FW. Ku70-deficient embryonic stem cells have increased ionizing radiosensitivity, defective DNA end-binding activity, and inability to support V(D)J recombination. *Proc Natl Acad Sci USA* 1997;94:8076–8081.

240. de Vries E, van DW, Bergsma WG, et al. HeLa nuclear protein recognizing DNA termini and translocating on DNA forming a regular DNA-multimeric protein complex. *J Mol Biol* 1989;208:65–78.

241. Tuteja N, Tuteja R, Ochem A, et al. Human DNA helicase II: A novel DNA unwinding enzyme identified as the Ku autoantigen. *EMBO J* 1994;13: 4991–5001.

242. Li Z, Otevrel T, Gao Y, et al. The XRCC4 gene encodes a novel protein involved in DNA double-strand break repair and V(D)J recombination. *Cell* 1995;83: 1079–1089.

243. Critchlow SE, Bowater RP, Jackson SP. Mammalian DNA double-strand break repair protein XRCC4 interacts with DNA ligase IV. *Curr Biol* 1997;7:588–598.

244. Grawunder U, Wilm M, Wu XK, P., Wilson TE, Mann M, Lieber MR. Activity of DNA ligase IV stimulate by complex formation with XRCC4 in mammalian cells. *Nature* 1997;388:492.

244a. Leber R, Wise TW, Mizuta R, Meek K. The XRCC4 gene product is a target for and interacts with the DNA-dependent protein kinase. *J Biol Chem* 1998;273: 1794–1801.

245. Hsieh JJ, Henkel T, Salmon P, Robey E, Peterson MG, Hayward SD. Truncated mammalian Notch1 activates CBF1/RBPJk-repressed genes by a mechanism resembling that of Epstein-Barr virus EBNA2. *Mol Cell Biol* 1996;16:952–959.

246. Aguilera RJ, Akira S, Okazaki K, Sakano H. A pre-B cell nuclear protein that specifically interacts with the immunoglobulin V-J recombination sequences. *Cell* 1987;51:909–917.

247. Miyake S, Sugiyama H, Tani Y, Fukuda T, Kishimoto S. Identification of a recombinational signal sequence-specific DNA-binding protein(s) of Mr 115,000 in the nuclear extracts from immature lymphoid cell lines. *J Immunogenet* 1990;17:67–75.

248. Shirakata M, Huppi K, Usuda S, Okazaki K, Yoshida K, Sakano H. HMG1-related DNA-binding protein isolated with V-(D)-J recombination signal probes. *Mol Cell Biol* 1991;11:4528–4536.

249. Li M, Morzycka WE, Desiderio SV. NBP, a protein that specifically binds an enhancer of immunoglobulin gene rearrangement: Purification and characterization. *Genes Dev* 1989;3:1801–1813.

250. Halligan BD, Teng M, Guilliams TG, Nauert JB, Halligan NL. Cloning of the murine cDNA encoding VDJP, a protein homologous to the large subunit of replication factor C and bacterial DNA ligases. *Gene* 1995;161:217–222.

251. Guilliams TG, Teng M, Halligan BD. Site directed DNA joining. *Biochimie* 1997;79:13–22.

252. Wu LC, Mak CH, Dear N, Boehm T, Foroni L, Rabbitts TH. Molecular cloning of a zinc finger protein which binds to the heptamer of the signal sequence for V(D)J recombination. *Nucleic Acids Res* 1993;21:5067–5073.

253. Mak CH, Strandtmann J, Wu LC. The V(D)J recombination signal sequence and kappa B binding protein Rc binds DNA as dimers and forms multimeric structures with its DNA ligands. *Nucleic Acids Res* 1994;22:383–390.

254. Muegge K, West M, Durum SK. Recombination sequence-binding protein in thymocytes undergoing T-cell receptor gene rearrangement. *Proc Natl Acad Sci USA* 1993;90:4151–4155.

255. Jarvis CD, Geiman T, Vila SM, et al. A novel putative helicase produced in early murine lymphocytes. *Gene* 1996;169:203–207.

256. Kenter AL, Tredup J. High expression of a 3′–5′ exonuclease activity is specific to B lymphocytes. *Mol Cell Biol* 1991;11:4398–4404.

257. Feeney AJ. Lack of N regions in fetal and neonatal mouse immunoglobulin V-D-J junctional sequences. *J Exp Med* 1990;172:1377–1390.

258. Victor KD, Capra JD. An apparently common mechanism of generating antibody diversity: Length variation of the VL-JL junction. *Mol Immunol* 1994;31:39–46.

259. Gilfillan S, Dierich A, Lemeur M, Benoist C, Mathis D. Mice lacking TdT: Mature animals with an immature lymphocyte repertoire. *Science* 1993;261: 1175–1178.

260. Komori T, Okada A, Stewart V, Alt FW. Lack of N regions in antigen receptor variable region genes of TdT- deficient lymphocytes. *Science* 1993;261:1171–1175.

261. Landau NR, Schatz DG, Rosa M, Baltimore D. Increased frequency of N-region insertion in a murine pre-B-cell line infected with a terminal deoxynucleotidyl transferase retroviral expression vector. *Mol Cell Biol* 1987;7:3237–3243.

262. Kallenbach S, Doyen N, Fanton dAM, Rougeon F. Three lymphoid-specific factors account for all junctional diversity characteristic of somatic assembly of T-cell receptor and immunoglobulin genes. *Proc Natl Acad Sci USA* 1992; 89:2799–2803.

263. Bentolila LA, Wu GE, Nourrit F, Fanton dAM, Rougeon F, Doyen N. Constitutive expression of terminal deoxynucleotidyl transferase in transgenic mice is sufficient for N diversity to occur at any Ig locus throughout B cell differentiation. *J Immunol* 1997;158:715–723.

264. Hiramatsu R, Akagi K, Matsuoka M, et al. The 3′ enhancer region determines the B/T specificity and pro-B/pre-B specificity of immunoglobulin V kappa-J kappa joining. *Cell* 1995;83:1113–1123.

265. Wasserman R, Li YS, Hardy RR. Down-regulation of terminal deoxynucleotidyl transferase by Ig heavy chain in B lineage cells. *J Immunol* 1997;158:1133–1138.

266. Gilfillan S, Bachmann M, Trembleau S, et al. Efficient immune responses in mice lacking N-region diversity. *Eur J Immunol* 1995;25:3115–3122.

267. Gavin MA, Bevan MJ. Increased peptide promiscuity provides a rationale for the lack of N regions in the neonatal T cell repertoire. *Immunity* 1995;3:793–800.

268. Rolink A, Melchers F. B lymphopoiesis in the mouse. *Adv Immunol* 1993;53: 123–156.

269. Hardy RR, Hayakawa K. B-lineage differentiation stages resolved by multiparameter flow cytometry. *Ann N Y Acad Sci* 1995;764:19–24.

270. Melchers F, Rolink A, Grawunder U, et al. Positive and negative selection events during B lymphopoiesis. *Curr Opin Immunol* 1995;7:214–227.

271. Li YS, Wasserman R, Hayakawa K, Hardy RR. Identification of the earliest B lineage stage in mouse bone marrow. *Immunity* 1996;5:527–535.

272. Karasuyama H, Rolink A, Melchers F. A complex of glycoproteins is associated with VpreB/lambda 5 surrogate light chain on the surface of mu heavy chain-negative early precursor B cell lines. *J Exp Med* 1993;178:469–478.

273. Reth MG, Alt FW. Novel immunoglobulin heavy chains are produced from DJH gene segment rearrangements in lymphoid cells. *Nature* 1984;312:418–423.

274. Yancopoulos GD, Alt FW. Developmentally controlled and tissue-specific expression of unrearranged VH gene segments. *Cell* 1985;40:271–281.

275. Mather EL, Perry RP. Transcriptional regulation of immunoglobulin V genes. *Nucleic Acids Res* 1981;9:6855–6867.

276. Takeda S, Zou YR, Bluethmann H, Kitamura D, Muller U, Rajewsky K. Deletion

of the immunoglobulin kappa chain intron enhancer abolishes kappa chain gene rearrangement in cis but not lambda chain gene rearrangement in trans. *EMBO J* 1993;12:2329–2336.

277. Xu Y, Davidson L, Alt FW, Baltimore D. Deletion of the Ig kappa light chain intronic enhancer/matrix attachment region impairs but does not abolish V kappa J kappa rearrangement. *Immunity* 1996;4:377–385.

278. Gorman JR, van der Stoep N, Monroe R, et al. The Ig(kappa) enhancer influences the ratio of Ig(kappa) versus Ig(lambda) B lymphocytes. *Immunity* 1996;5:241–252.

279. Lauster R, Reynaud CA, Martensson IL, et al. Promoter, enhancer and silencer elements regulate rearrangement of an immunoglobulin transgene. *EMBO J* 1993;12:4615–4623.

280. Oltz EM, Alt FW, Lin WC, et al. A V(D)J recombinase-inducible B-cell line: Role of transcriptional enhancer elements in directing V(D)J recombination. *Mol Cell Biol* 1993;13:6223–6230.

281. Kallenbach S, Babinet C, Pournin S, Cavelier P, Goodhardt M, Rougeon F. The intronic immunoglobulin kappa gene enhancer acts independently on rearrangement and on transcription. *Eur J Immunol* 1993;23:1917–1921.

282. Ferradini L, Gu H, De SA, Rajewsky K, Reynaud CA, Weill JC. Rearrangement-enhancing element upstream of the mouse immunoglobulin kappa chain J cluster. *Science* 1996;271:1416–1420.

283. Coleclough C, Perry RP, Karjalainen K, Weigert M. Aberrant rearrangements contribute significantly to the allelic exclusion of immunoglobulin gene expression. *Nature* 1981;290:372–378.

284. Alt FW, Enea V, Bothwell AL, Baltimore D. Activity of multiple light chain genes in murine myeloma cells producing a single, functional light chain. *Cell* 1980;21:1–12.

285. ten Boekel E, Melchers F, Rolink A. The status of Ig loci rearrangements in single cells from different stages of B cell development. *Int Immunol* 1995;7:1013–1019.

286. Nottenburg C, St. John T, Weissman IL. Unusual immunoglobulin DNA sequences from the nonexpressed chromosome of mouse normal B lymphocytes: Implications for allelic exclusion and the DNA rearrangement process. *J Immunol* 1987;139:1718–1726.

287. Weaver D, Costantini F, Imanishi KT, Baltimore D. A transgenic immunoglobulin mu gene prevents rearrangement of endogenous genes. *Cell* 1985;42:117–127.

288. Storb U, Pinkert C, Arp B, et al. Transgenic mice with mu and kappa genes encoding antiphosphorylcholine antibodies. *J Exp Med* 1986;164:627–641.

289. Nussenzweig MC, Shaw AC, Sinn E, et al. Allelic exclusion in transgenic mice that express the membrane form of immunoglobulin mu. *Science* 1987;236:816–819.

290. Picarella D, Serunian LA, Rosenberg N. Allelic exclusion of membrane but not secreted immunoglobulin in a mature B cell line. *Eur J Immunol* 1991;21:55–62.

291. Kitamura D, Rajewsky K. Targeted disruption of mu chain membrane exon causes loss of heavy-chain allelic exclusion. *Nature* 1992;356:154–156.

292. Loffert D, Ehlich A, Muller W, Rajewsky K. Surrogate light chain expression is required to establish immunoglobulin heavy chain allelic exclusion during early B cell development. *Immunity* 1996;4:133–144.

293. Papavasiliou F, Jankovic M, Suh H, Nussenzweig MC. The cytoplasmic domains of immunoglobulin (Ig) alpha and Ig beta can independently induce the precursor B cell transition and allelic exclusion. *J Exp Med* 1995;182:1389–1394.

294. Papavasiliou F, Misulovin Z, Suh H, Nussenzweig MC. The role of Ig beta in precursor B cell transition and allelic exclusion. *Science* 1995;268:408–411.

295. Grawunder U, Leu TM, Schatz DG, et al. Down-regulation of RAG1 and RAG2 gene expression in preB cells after functional immunoglobulin heavy chain rearrangement. *Immunity* 1995;3:601–608.

296. Schlissel MS, Morrow T. Ig heavy chain protein controls B cell development by regulating germ-line transcription and retargeting V(D)J recombination. *J Immunol* 1994;153:1645–1657.

297. Constantinescu A, Schlissel MS. Changes in locus-specific V(D)J recombinase activity induced by immunoglobulin gene products during B cell development. *J Exp Med* 1997;185:609–620.

298. Shinkai Y, Rathbun G, Lam KP, et al. RAG-2-deficient mice lack mature lymphocytes owing to inability to initiate V(D)J rearrangement. *Cell* 1992;68:855–867.

299. Ehlich A, Schaal S, Gu H, Kitamura D, Muller W, Rajewsky K. Immunoglobulin heavy and light chain genes rearrange independently at early stages of B cell development. *Cell* 1993;72:695–704.

300. Spanopoulou E, Roman CA, Corcoran LM, et al. Functional immunoglobulin transgenes guide ordered B-cell differentiation in Rag-1-deficient mice. *Genes Dev* 1994;8:1030–1042.

301. Young F, Ardman B, Shinkai Y, et al. Influence of immunoglobulin heavy- and light-chain expression on B-cell differentiation. *Genes Dev* 1994;8:1043–1057.

301a. Minegishi Y, Coustan SE, Wang YH, Cooper MD, Campana D, Conley ME. Mutations in the human lambda5/14.1 gene result in B cell deficiency and agammaglobulinemia. *J Exp Med* 1998;187:71–77.

302. Pelanda R, Schaal S, Torres RM, Rajewsky K. A prematurely expressed Ig(kappa) transgene, but not V(kappa)J(kappa) gene segment targeted into the Ig(kappa) locus, can rescue B cell development in lambda5-deficient mice. *Immunity* 1996;5:229–239.

303. Reth M, Petrac E, Wiese P, Lobel L, Alt FW. Activation of V kappa gene rearrangement in pre-B cells follows the expression of membrane-bound immunoglobulin heavy chains. *EMBO J* 1987;6:3299–3305.

304. Iglesias A, Lamers M, Kohler G. Expression of immunoglobulin delta chain causes allelic exclusion in transgenic mice. *Nature* 1987;330:482–484.

305. Schlissel MS, Baltimore D. Activation of immunoglobulin kappa gene rearrangement correlates with induction of germline kappa gene transcription. *Cell* 1989;58:1001–1007.

306. Chen J, Trounstine M, Alt FW, et al. Immunoglobulin gene rearrangement in B cell deficient mice generated by targeted deletion of the JH locus. *Int Immunol* 1993;5:647–656.

307. Grawunder U, Rolink A, Melchers F. Induction of sterile transcription from the kappa L chain gene locus in V(D)J recombinase-deficient progenitor B cells. *Int Immunol* 1995;7:1915–1925.

308. Ritchie KA, Brinster RL, Storb U. Allelic exclusion and control of endogenous immunoglobulin gene rearrangement in kappa transgenic mice. *Nature* 1984;312:517–520.

309. Ma A, Fisher P, Dildrop R, et al. Surface IgM mediated regulation of RAG gene expression in E mu-N-myc B cell lines. *EMBO J* 1992;11:2727–2734.

310. Torres RM, Flaswinkel H, Reth M, Rajewsky K. Aberrant B cell development and immune response in mice with a compromised BCR complex. *Science* 1996;272:1804–1808.

311. Korsmeyer SJ, Hieter PA, Ravetch JV, Poplack DG, Waldmann TA, Leder P. Developmental hierarchy of immunoglobulin gene rearrangements in human leukemic pre-B-cells. *Proc Natl Acad Sci USA* 1981;78:7096–7100.

312. Zou YR, Takeda S, Rajewsky K. Gene targeting in the Ig kappa locus: efficient generation of lambda chain-expressing B cells, independent of gene rearrangements in Ig kappa. *EMBO J* 1993;12:811–820.

313. Doglio L, Kim JY, Bozek G, Storb U. Expression of lambda and kappa genes can occur in all B cells and is initiated around the same pre-B-cell developmental stage. *Dev Immunol* 1994;4:13–26.

314. Hagman J, Lo D, Doglio LT, et al. Inhibition of immunoglobulin gene rearrangement by the expression of a lambda 2 transgene. *J Exp Med* 1989;169:1911–1929.

315. Neuberger MS, Caskey HM, Pettersson S, Williams GT, Surani MA. Isotype exclusion and transgene down-regulation in immunoglobulin-lambda transgenic mice. *Nature* 1989;338:350–352.

316. Rudin CM, Hackett JJ, Storb U. Precursors of both conventional and Ly-1 B cells can escape feedback inhibition of Ig gene rearrangement. *J Immunol* 1991;146:3205–3210.

317. Hengstschlager M, Maizels N. Isotype exclusion in lambda 1 transgenic mice depends on transgene copy number and diminishes with down-regulation of transgene transcripts. *Eur J Immunol* 1995;25:187–191.

318. Gollahon KA, Hagman J, Brinster RL, Storb U. Ig lambda-producing B cells do not show feedback inhibition of gene rearrangement. *J Immunol* 1988;141:2771–2780.

319. Berg J, McDowell M, Jack HM, Wabl M. Immunoglobulin lambda gene rearrangement can precede kappa gene rearrangement. *Dev Immunol* 1990;1:53–57.

320. Ramsden DA, Wu GE. Mouse kappa light-chain recombination signal sequences mediate recombination more frequently than do those of lambda light chain. *Proc Natl Acad Sci USA* 1991;88:10721–10725.

321. Arakawa H, Takeda S. Early expression of Ig mu chain from a transgene significantly reduces the duration of the pro-B stage but does not affect the small pre-B stage. *Int Immunol* 1996;8:1319–1328.

322. Harada K, Yamagishi H. Lack of feedback inhibition of V kappa gene rearrangement by productively rearranged alleles. *J Exp Med* 1991;173:409–415.

323. Levy S, Campbell MJ, Levy R. Functional immunoglobulin light chain genes are replaced by ongoing rearrangements of germline V kappa genes to downstream J kappa segment in a murine B cell line. *J Exp Med* 1989;170:1–13.

324. Kleinfield R, Hardy RR, Tarlinton D, Dangl J, Herzenberg LA, Weigert M. Recombination between an expressed immunoglobulin heavy-chain gene and a germline variable gene segment in a Ly 1+ B-cell lymphoma. *Nature* 1986;322:843–846.

325. Radic MZ, Erikson J, Litwin S, Weigert M. B lymphocytes may escape tolerance by revising their antigen receptors. *J Exp Med* 1993;177:1165–1173.

326. Tiegs SL, Russell DM, Nemazee D. Receptor editing in self-reactive bone marrow B cells. *J Exp Med* 1993;177:1009–1020.

327. Chen C, Nagy Z, Radic MZ, et al. The site and stage of anti-DNA B-cell deletion. *Nature* 1995;373:252–255.

328. Hertz M, Nemazee D. BCR ligation induces receptor editing in IgM+IgD1- bone marrow B cells in vitro. *Immunity* 1997;6:429–436.

329. Verkoczy LK, Stiernholm BJ, Berinstein NL. Up-regulation of recombination activating gene expression by signal transduction through the surface Ig receptor. *J Immunol* 1995;154:5136–5143.

330. Suzuki N, Harada T, Mihara S, Sakane T. Characterization of a germline Vk gene encoding cationic anti-DNA antibody and role of receptor editing for development of the autoantibody in patients with systemic lupus erythematosus. *J Clin Invest* 1996;98:1843–1850.

331. Han S, Zheng B, Schatz DG, Spanopoulou E, Kelsoe G. Neoteny in lymphocytes: Rag1 and Rag2 expression in germinal center B cells. *Science* 1996;274:2094–2097.

332. Hikida M, Mori M, Takai T, Tomochika K, Hamatani K, Ohmori H. Reexpression of RAG-1 and RAG-2 genes in activated mature mouse B cells. *Science* 1996;274:2092–2094.

332a. Han S, Dillon SR, Zheng B, Shimoda M, Schlissel MS, Kelsoe G. V(D)J recombinase activity in a subset of germinal center B lymphocytes. *Science* 1997;278:301–305.

332b.Papavasiliou F, Casellas R, Suh H, et al. V(D)J recombination in mature B cells: a mechanism for altering antibody responses. Science 1997;278:298-301.

333. Giudicelli V, Chaume D, Bodmer J, et al. IMGT, the international ImMuno-GeneTics database. Nucleic Acids Res 1997;25:206-211.

334. Brodeur PH, Riblet R. The immunoglobulin heavy chain variable region (Igh-V) locus in the mouse. I. One hundred Igh-V genes comprise seven families of homologous genes. Eur J Immunol 1984;14:922–930.

335. Dildrop R. A new classification of mouse VH sequences. Immunol Today 1984;5:85–88.

336. Meek K, Rathbun G, Reininger L, et al. Organization of the murine immuno-globulin VH complex: Placement of two new VH families (VH10 and VH11) and analysis of VH family clustering and interdigitation. Mol Immunol 1990;27:1073–1081.

337. Tutter A, Brodeur P, Shlomchik M, Riblet R. Structure, map position, and evolution of two newly diverged mouse Ig VH gene families. J Immunol 1991;147:3215–3223.

338. Mainville CA, Sheehan KM, Klaman LD, Giorgetti CA, Press JL, Brodeur PH. Deletional mapping of fifteen mouse VH gene families reveals a common organization for three Igh haplotypes. J Immunol 1996;156:1038–1046.

339. Tutter A, Riblet R. Conservation of an immunoglobulin variable-region gene family indicates a specific, noncoding function. Proc Natl Acad Sci USA 1989;86:7460–7464.

340. Schroeder HWJ, Hillson JL, Perlmutter RM. Structure and evolution of mammalian VH families. Int Immunol 1990;2:41–50.

341. Kirkham PM, Mortari F, Newton JA, Schroeder HWJ. Immunoglobulin VH clan and family identity predicts variable domain structure and may influence antigen binding. EMBO J 1992;11:603–609.

342. Nei M, Gu X, Sitnikova T. Evolution by the birth-and-death process in multigene families of the vertebrate immune system. Proc Natl Acad Sci USA 1997;94:7799–7806.

343. Kofler R, Geley S, Kofler H, Helmberg A. Mouse variable-region gene families: Complexity, polymorphism and use in non-autoimmune responses. Immunol Rev 1992;128:5–21.

344. Livant D, Blatt C, Hood L. One heavy chain variable region gene segment subfamily in the BALB/c mouse contains 500–1000 or more members. Cell 1986;47:461–470.

345. Blankenstein T, Bonhomme F, Krawinkel U. Evolution of pseudogenes in the immunoglobulin VH-gene family of the mouse. Immunogenetics 1987;26:237–248.

346. Kemp DJ, Cory S, Adams JM. Cloned pairs of variable region genes for immunoglobulin heavy chains isolated from a clone library of the entire mouse genome. Proc Natl Acad Sci USA 1979;76:4627–4631.

347. Bothwell AL, Paskind M, Reth M, Imanishi KT, Rajewsky K, Baltimore D. Heavy chain variable region contribution to the NPb family of antibodies: Somatic mutation evident in a gamma 2a variable region. Cell 1981;24:625–637.

348. Givol D, Zakut R, Effron K, Rechavi G, Ram D, Cohen JB. Diversity of germ-line immunoglobulin VH genes. Nature 1981;292:426–430.

349. Kemp DJ, Tyler B, Bernard O, et al. Organization of genes and spacers within the mouse immunoglobulin VH locus. J Mol Appl Genet 1981;1:245–261.

350. Rechavi G, Bienz B, Ram D, et al. Organization and evolution of immunoglobulin VH gene subgroups. Proc Natl Acad Sci USA 1982;79:4405–4409.

351. Rathbun GA, Capra JD, Tucker PW. Organization of the murine immunoglobulin VH complex in the inbred strains. EMBO J 1987;6:2931–2937.

352. Brodeur PH, Osman GE, Mackle JJ, Lalor TM. The organization of the mouse Igh-V locus. Dispersion, interspersion, and the evolution of VH gene family clusters. J Exp Med 1988;168:2261–2278.

353. Blankenstein T, Krawinkel U. Immunoglobulin VH region genes of the mouse are organized in overlapping clusters. Eur J Immunol 1987;17:1351–1357.

354. Walter MA, Dosch HM, Cox DW. A deletion map of the human immunoglobulin heavy chain variable region. J Exp Med 1991;174:335–349.

355. Perlmutter RM, Kearney JF, Chang SP, Hood LE. Developmentally controlled expression of immunoglobulin VH genes. Science 1985;227:1597–1601.

356. Malynn BA, Berman JE, Yancopoulos GD, Bona CA, Alt FW. Expression of the immunoglobulin heavy-chain variable gene repertoire. Curr Top Microbiol Immunol 1987;135:75–94.

357. Feeney AJ. Predominance of VH-D-JH junctions occurring at sites of short sequence homology results in limited junctional diversity in neonatal antibodies. J Immunol 1992;149:222–229.

358. Gauss GH, Lieber MR. The basis for the mechanistic bias for deletional over inversional V(D)J recombination. Genes Dev 1992;6:1553–1561.

359. Early P, Huang H, Davis M, Calame K, Hood L. An immunoglobulin heavy chain variable region gene is generated from three segments of DNA: VH, D and JH. Cell 1980;19:981–992.

360. Sakano H, Kurosawa Y, Weigert M, Tonegawa S. Identification and nucleotide sequence of a diversity DNA segment (D) of immunoglobulin heavy-chain genes. Nature 1981;290:562–565.

361. Kurosawa Y, von BH, Haas W, Sakano H, Trauneker A, Tonegawa S. Identification of D segments of immunoglobulin heavy-chain genes and their rearrangement in T lymphocytes. Nature 1981;290:565–570.

362. Kurosawa Y, Tonegawa S. Organization, structure, and assembly of immunoglobulin heavy chain diversity DNA segments. J Exp Med 1982;155:201–218.

363. Feeney AJ, Riblet R. DST4: A new, and probably the last, functional DH gene in the BALB/c mouse. Immunogenetics 1993;37:217–221.

364. Tsubata T, Tsubata R, Reth M. Cell surface expression of the short immunoglobulin mu chain (D mu protein) in murine pre-B cells is differently regulated from that of the intact mu chain. Eur J Immunol 1991;21:1359–1363.

365. Haasner D, Rolink A, Melchers F. Influence of surrogate L chain on DHJH-reading frame 2 suppression in mouse precursor B cells. Int Immunol 1994;6:21–30.

366. Horne MC, Roth PE, DeFranco AL. Assembly of the truncated immunoglobulin heavy chain D mu into antigen receptor-like complexes in pre-B cells but not in B cells. Immunity 1996;4:145–158.

367. Ehlich A, Martin V, Muller W, Rajewsky K. Analysis of the B-cell progenitor compartment at the level of single cells. Curr Biol 1994;4:573–583.

368. Tarlinton D, Strasser A, McLean M, Basten A. DH element reading frame selection is influenced by an Ig heavy chain transgene, but not by bcl-2. J Immunol 1995;154:3341–3350.

369. Meek KD, Hasemann CA, Capra JD. Novel rearrangements at the immunoglobulin D locus. Inversions and fusions add to IgH somatic diversity. J Exp Med 1989;170:39–57.

370. Potter M, Newell JB, Rudikoff S, Haber E. Classification of mouse VK groups based on the partial amino acid sequence to the first invariant tryptophan: Impact of 14 new sequences from IgG myeloma proteins. Mol Immunol 1982;19:1619–1630.

371. Kofler R, Helmberg A. A new Igk-V gene family in the mouse. Immunogenetics 1991;34:139–140.

372. Kofler R, Duchosal MA, Dixon FJ. Complexity, polymorphism, and connectivity of mouse Vk gene families. Immunogenetics 1989;29:65–74.

373. Strohal R, Helmberg A, Kroemer G, Kofler R. Mouse Vk gene classification by nucleic acid sequence similarity. Immunogenetics 1989;30:475–493.

374. Kroemer G, Helmberg A, Bernot A, Auffray C, Kofler R. Evolutionary relationship between human and mouse immunoglobulin kappa light chain variable region genes. Immunogenetics 1991;33:42–49.

375. George JB, Li S, Garrard WT. Yeast artificial chromosome contigs reveal that distal variable-region genes reside at least 3 megabases from the joining regions in the murine immunoglobulin kappa locus. Proc Natl Acad Sci USA 1995;92:12421–12425.

376. Kirschbaum T, Jaenichen R, Zachau HG. The mouse immunoglobulin kappa locus contains about 140 variable gene segments. Eur J Immunol 1996;26:1613–1620.

377. Schupp IW, Schlake T, Kirschbaum T, Zachau HG, Boehm T. A yeast artificial chromosome contig spanning the mouse immunoglobulin kappa light chain locus. Immunogenetics 1997;45:180–187.

378. Lee KH, Matsuda F, Kinashi T, Kodaira M, Honjo T. A novel family of variable region genes of the human immunoglobulin heavy chain. J Mol Biol 1987;195:761–768.

379. Walter MA, Surti U, Hofker MH, Cox DW. The physical organization of the human immunoglobulin heavy chain gene complex. EMBO J 1990;9:3303–3313.

380. Cook GP, Tomlinson IM, Walter G, et al. A map of the human immunoglobulin VH locus completed by analysis of the telomeric region of chromosome 14q. Nature Genet 1994;7:162–168.

381. Cook GP, Tomlinson IM. The human immunoglobulin VH repertoire. Immunol Today 1995;16:237–242.

382. Matsuda F, Honjo T. Organization of the human immunoglobulin heavy-chain locus. Adv Immunol 1996;62:1–29.

383. Schroeder HJ, Walter MA, Hofker MH, et al. Physical linkage of a human immunoglobulin heavy chain variable region gene segment to diversity and joining region elements. Proc Natl Acad Sci USA 1988;85:8196–8200.

384. Nagaoka H, Ozawa K, Matsuda F, et al. Recent translocation of variable and diversity segments of the human immunoglobulin heavy chain from chromosome 14 to chromosomes 15 and 16. Genomics 1994;22:189–197.

385. Tomlinson IM, Cook GP, Carter NP, et al. Human immunoglobulin VH and D segments on chromosomes 15q11.2 and 16p11.2. Hum Mol Genet 1994;3:853–860.

386. Ravetch JV, Siebenlist U, Korsmeyer SJ, Waldmann T, Leder P. Structure of the human immunoglobulin mu locus; characterization of embryonic and rearranged J and D genes. Cell 1981;27:583–591.

387. Ichihara Y, Matsuoka H, Kurosawa Y. Organization of human immunoglobulin heavy chain diversity gene loci. EMBO J 1988;7:4141–4150.

388. Moore BB, Meek K. Recombination potential of the human DIR elements. J Immunol 1995;154:2175–2187.

389. Tuaillon N, Miller AB, Tucker PW, Capra JD. Analysis of direct and inverted DJH rearrangements in a human Ig heavy chain transgenic minilocus. J Immunol 1995;154:6453–6465.

389a.Tuaillon N, Capra JD. Use of D gene segments with irregular spacers in terminal deoxynucleotidyltransferase (TdT)+/+ and TdT-/- mice carrying a human Ig heavy chain transgenic minilocus. Proc Natl Acad Sci U S A 1998;95:1703-1708.

390. Nagaoka H, Ozawa K, Matsuda F, et al. Recent translocation of variable and diversity segments of the human immunoglobulin heavy chain from chromosome 14 to chromosomes 15 and 16. Genomics 1994;22:189–197.

391. Schable KF, Zachau HG. The variable genes of the human immunoglobulin kappa locus. Biol Chem Hoppe Seyler 1993;374:1001–1022.

392. Schable K, Thiebe R, Flugel A, Meindl A, Zachau HG. The human immunoglobulin kappa locus: Pseudogenes, unique and repetitive sequences. Biol Chem Hoppe Seyler 1994;375:189–199.

393. Ermert K, Mitlohner H, Schempp W, Zachau HG. The immunoglobulin kappa locus of primates. *Genomics* 1995;25:623–629.

394. Klein R, Zachau HG. Comparison of human germ-line kappa gene sequences to sequence data from the literature. *Eur J Immunol* 1993;23:3263–3271.

395. Arnold N, Wienberg J, Ermert K, Zachau HG. Comparative mapping of DNA probes derived from the V kappa immunoglobulin gene regions on human and great ape chromosomes by fluorescence in situ hybridization. *Genomics* 1995; 26:147–150.

396. Huber C, Thiebe R, Zachau HG. A potentially functional V kappa gene at a distance of 1.5 Mb from the immunoglobulin kappa locus. *Genomics* 1994;22: 213–215.

397. Williams SC, Frippiat JP, Tomlinson IM, Ignatovich O, Lefranc MP, Winter G. Sequence and evolution of the human germline V lambda repertoire. *J Mol Biol* 1996;264:220–232.

398. Wood DL, Coleclough C. Different joining region J elements of the murine kappa immunoglobulin light chain locus are used at markedly different frequencies. *Proc Natl Acad Sci USA* 1984;81:4756–4760.

399. Nishi M, Kataoka T, Honjo T. Preferential rearrangement of the immunoglobulin kappa chain joining region J kappa 1 and J kappa 2 segments in mouse spleen DNA. *Proc Natl Acad Sci USA* 1985;82:6399–6403.

400. Yamada M, Wasserman R, Reichard BA, Shane S, Caton AJ, Rovera G. Preferential utilization of specific immunoglobulin heavy chain diversity and joining segments in adult human peripheral blood B lymphocytes. *J Exp Med* 1991;173: 395–407.

401. Cohn M, Blomberg B, Geckler W, Raschke W, Riblet R, Weigert M. First order considerations in analyzing the generator of diversity. In: EE Sercarz, AR Williamson, CF Fox, eds. *The immune system: Genes, receptors, signals.* New York: Academic Press, 1974;89.

402. Weigert M, Riblet R. Genetic control of antibody variable regions. *Cold Spring Harb Symp Quant Biol* 1977;2:837–846.

403. Gearhart PJ, Johnson ND, Douglas R, Hood L. IgG antibodies to phosphorylcholine exhibit more diversity than their IgM counterparts. *Nature* 1981;291: 29–34.

404. Crews S, Griffin J, Huang H, Calame K, Hood L. A single VH gene segment encodes the immune response to phosphorylcholine: Somatic mutation is correlated with the class of the antibody. *Cell* 1981;25:59–66.

405. Manser T, Parhami SB, Margolies MN, Gefter ML. Somatically mutated forms of a major anti-p-azophenylarsonate antibody variable region with drastically reduced affinity for p-azophenylarsonate. By-products of an antigen-driven immune response? *J Exp Med* 1987;166:1456–1463.

406. Ray SK, Putterman C, Diamond B. Pathogenic autoantibodies are routinely generated during the response to foreign antigen: A paradigm for autoimmune disease. *Proc Natl Acad Sci USA* 1996;93:2019–2024.

407. Liu YJ, Joshua DE, Williams GT, Smith CA, Gordon J, MacLennan IC. Mechanism of antigen-driven selection in germinal centres. *Nature* 1989;342:929–931.

408. Shokat KM, Goodnow CC. Antigen-induced B-cell death and elimination during germinal-centre immune responses. *Nature* 1995;375:334–338.

409. Choe J, Kim HS, Zhang X, Armitage RJ, Choi YS. Cellular and molecular factors that regulate the differentiation and apoptosis of germinal center B cells. Anti-Ig down-regulates Fas expression of CD40 ligand-stimulated germinal center B cells and inhibits Fas-mediated apoptosis. *J Immunol* 1996;157:1006–1016.

410. Eisen HN, Siskind GW. Variations in affinities of antibodies during the immune response. *Biochemistry* 1964;3:996–1008.

411. Jacob J, Kelsoe G, Rajewsky K, Weiss U. Intraclonal generation of antibody mutants in germinal centres. *Nature* 1991;354:389–392.

412. Jacob J, Kelsoe G. In situ studies of the primary immune response to (4-hydroxy-3-nitrophenyl)acetyl. II. A common clonal origin for periarteriolar lymphoid sheath-associated foci and germinal centers. *J Exp Med* 1992;176:679–687.

413. Pascual V, Liu YJ, Magalski A, de Boutellier O, Banchereau J, Capra JD. Analysis of somatic mutation in five B cell subsets of human tonsil. *J Exp Med* 1994; 180:329–339.

414. Lebecque S, de Boutellier O, Arpin C, Banchereau J, Liu YJ. Germinal center founder cells display propensity for apoptosis before onset of somatic mutation. *J Exp Med* 1997;185:563–571.

415. Zheng B, Han S, Kelsoe G. T helper cells in murine germinal centers are antigen-specific emigrants that downregulate Thy-1. *J Exp Med* 1996;184:1083–1091.

416. Razanajaona D, van Kooten C, Lebecque S, et al. Somatic mutations in human Ig variable genes correlate with a partially functional CD40-ligand in the X-linked hyper-IgM syndrome. *J Immunol* 1996;157:1492–1498.

417. Casamayor PM, Khan M, MacLennan IC. A subset of CD4+ memory T cells contains preformed CD40 ligand that is rapidly but transiently expressed on their surface after activation through the T cell receptor complex. *J Exp Med* 1995;181:1293–1301.

418. Han S, Zheng B, Dal PJ, Kelsoe G. In situ studies of the primary immune response to (4-hydroxy-3-nitrophenyl)acetyl. IV. Affinity-dependent, antigen-driven B cell apoptosis in germinal centers as a mechanism for maintaining self-tolerance. *J Exp Med* 1995;182:1635–1644.

419. Pulendran B, Kannourakis G, Nouri S, Smith KG, Nossal GJ. Soluble antigen can cause enhanced apoptosis of germinal-centre B cells. *Nature* 1995;375: 331–334.

419a.Hande S, Notidis E, Manser T. Bcl-2 obstructs negative selection of autoreactive, hypermutated antibody V regions during memory B cell development. *Immunity* 1998;8:189–198.

420. Kuppers R, Zhao M, Hansmann ML, Rajewsky K. Tracing B cell development in human germinal centres by molecular analysis of single cells picked from histological sections. *EMBO J* 1993;12:4955–4967.

421. Decker DJ, Linton PJ, Zaharevitz S, Biery M, Gingeras TR, Klinman NR. Defining subsets of naive and memory B cells based on the ability of their progeny to somatically mutate in vitro. *Immunity* 1995;2:195–203.

422. Kepler TB, Perelson AS. Cyclic re-entry of germinal center B cells and the efficiency of affinity maturation. *Immunol Today* 1993;14:412–415.

422a.Matsumoto M, Lo SF, Carruthers CJ, et al. Affinity maturation without germinal centres in lymphotoxin-alpha-deficient mice. *Nature* 1996;382:462–466.

423. Kim S, David M, Sinn E, Patten P, Hood L. Antibody diversity: Somatic hypermutation of rearranged VH genes. *Cell* 1981;27:573–581.

424. Lebecque SG, Gearhart PJ. Boundaries of somatic mutation in rearranged immunoglobulin genes: 5′ boundary is near the promoter, and 3′ boundary is approximately 1 kb from V(D)J gene. *J Exp Med* 1990;172:1717–1727.

425. Gorski J, Rollini P, Mach B. Somatic mutations of immunoglobulin variable genes are restricted to the rearranged V gene. *Science* 1983;220:1179–1181.

426. Sablitzky F, Weisbaum D, Rajewsky K. Sequence analysis of non-expressed immunoglobulin heavy chain loci in clonally related, somatically mutated hybridoma cells. *EMBO J* 1985;4:3435–3437.

427. Giusti AM, Manser T. Hypermutation is observed only in antibody H chain V region transgenes that have recombined with endogenous immunoglobulin H DNA: Implications for the location of cis-acting elements required for somatic mutation. *J Exp Med* 1993;177:797–809.

428. Weiss S, Wu GE. Somatic point mutations in unrearranged immunoglobulin gene segments encoding the variable region of lambda light chains. *EMBO J* 1987;6:927–932.

429. Picard D, Schaffner W. Unrearranged immunoglobulin lambda variable region is transcribed in kappa-producing myelomas. *EMBO J* 1984;3:3031–3035.

430. O'Brien RL, Brinster RL, Storb U. Somatic hypermutation of an immunoglobulin transgene in kappa transgenic mice. *Nature* 1987;326:405–409.

431. Sharpe MJ, Milstein C, Jarvis JM, Neuberger MS. Somatic hypermutation of immunoglobulin kappa may depend on sequences 3′ of C kappa and occurs on passenger transgenes. *EMBO J* 1991;10:2139–2145.

432. Betz AG, Milstein C, Gonzalez FA, Pannell R, Larson T, Neuberger MS. Elements regulating somatic hypermutation of an immunoglobulin kappa gene: critical role for the intron enhancer/matrix attachment region. *Cell* 1994;77: 239–248.

432a.Goyenechea B, Klix N, Yelamos J, et al. Cells strongly expressing Ig(kappa) transgenes show clonal recruitment of hypermutation: a role for both MAR and the enhancers. *EMBO J* 1997;16:3987–3994.

432b.Klix N, Jolly CJ, Davies SL, Bruggemann M, Williams GT, Neuberger MS. Multiple sequences from downstream of the J kappa cluster can combine to recruit somatic hypermutation to a heterologous, upstream mutation domain. *Eur J Immunol* 1998;28:317–326.

433. Peters A, Storb U. Somatic hypermutation of immunoglobulin genes is linked to transcription initiation. *Immunity* 1996;4:57–65.

434. Bachl J, Wabl M. Enhancers of hypermutation. *Immunogenetics* 1996;45:59–64.

435. Yelamos J, Klix N, Goyenechea B, et al. Targeting of non-Ig sequences in place of the V segment by somatic hypermutation. *Nature* 1995;376:225–229.

436. Tumas-Brundage K, Vora KA, Giusti AM, Manser T. Characterization of the cis-acting elements required for somatic hypermutation of murine antibody V genes using conventional transgenic and transgene homologous recombination approaches. *Semin Immunol* 1996;8:141–150.

437. Hengstschlager M, Williams M, Maizels N. A lambda 1 transgene under the control of a heavy chain promoter and enhancer does not undergo somatic hypermutation. *Eur J Immunol* 1994;24:1649–1656.

438. Storb U. The molecular basis of somatic hypermutation of immunoglobulin genes. *Curr Opin Immunol* 1996;8:206–214.

438a.Migliazza A, Martinotti S, Chen W, et al. Frequent somatic hypermutation of the 5′ noncoding region of the BCL6 gene in B-cell lymphoma. *Proc Natl Acad Sci USA* 1995;92:12520–12524.

439. Goyenechea B, Milstein C. Modifying the sequence of an immunoglobulin V-gene alters the resulting pattern of hypermutation. *Proc Natl Acad Sci USA* 1996; 93:13979–13984.

440. Dorner T, Brezinschek HP, Brezinschek RI, Foster SJ, Domiati SR, Lipsky PE. Analysis of the frequency and pattern of somatic mutations within nonproductively rearranged human variable heavy chain genes. *J Immunol* 1997;158: 2779–2789.

441. Bachl J, Wabl M. An immunoglobulin mutator that targets G.C base pairs. *Proc Natl Acad Sci USA* 1996;93:851–855.

442. Betz AG, Rada C, Pannell R, Milstein C, Neuberger MS. Passenger transgenes reveal intrinsic specificity of the antibody hypermutation mechanism: Clustering, polarity, and specific hot spots. *Proc Natl Acad Sci USA* 1993;90: 2385–2388.

443. Insel RA, Varade WS. Bias in somatic hypermutation of human VH genes. *Int Immunol* 1994;6:1437–1443.

444. Dildrop R, Bruggemann M, Radbruch A, Rajewsky K, Beyreuther K. Immunoglobulin V region variants in hybridoma cells. II. Recombination between V genes. *EMBO J* 1982;1:635–640.

445. Xu B, Selsing E. Analysis of sequence transfers resembling gene conversion in a mouse antibody transgene. *Science* 1994;265:1590–1593.

446. Reynaud CA, Anquez V, Dahan A, Weill JC. A single rearrangement event gen-

erates most of the chicken immunoglobulin light chain diversity. *Cell* 1985;40: 283–291.

447. Becker RS, Knight KL. Somatic diversification of immunoglobulin heavy chain VDJ genes: evidence for somatic gene conversion in rabbits. *Cell* 1990;63: 987–997.

448. Sun J, Butler JE. Molecular characterization of VDJ transcripts from a newborn piglet. *Immunology* 1996;88:331–339.

449. Bentley DL, Rabbitts TH. Evolution of immunoglobulin V genes: evidence indicating that recently duplicated human V kappa sequences have diverged by gene conversion. *Cell* 1983;32:181–189.

450. Cohen JB, Givol D. Allelic immunoglobulin VH genes in two mouse strains: Possible germline gene recombination. *EMBO J* 1983;2:2013–2018.

451. Rogerson BJ. Somatic hypermutation of VHS107 genes is not associated with gene conversion among family members. *Int Immunol* 1995;7:1225–1235.

452. Golding GB, Gearhart PJ, Glickman BW. Patterns of somatic mutations in immunoglobulin variable genes. *Genetics* 1987;115:169–176.

453. Seidman MM, Bredberg A, Seetharam S, Kraemer KH. Multiple point mutations in a shuttle vector propagated in human cells: Evidence for an error-prone DNA polymerase activity. *Proc Natl Acad Sci USA* 1987;84:4944–4948.

454. Kim N, Kage K, Matsuda F, Lefranc MP, Storb U. B lymphocytes of xeroderma pigmentosum or Cockayne syndrome patients with inherited defects in nucleotide excision repair are fully capable of somatic hypermutation of immunoglobulin genes. *J Exp Med* 1997;186:413–419.

454a. Shen HM, Cheo DL, Friedberg E, Storb U. The inactivation of the XP-C gene does not affect somatic hypermutation or class switch recombination of immunoglobulin genes. *Mol Immunol* 1997;34:527–533.

454b. Rada C, Yelamos J, Dean W, Milstein C. The 5' hypermutation boundary of kappa chains is independent of local and neighboring sequences and related to the distance from the initiation of transcription. *Eur J Immunol* 1997;27:3115–3120.

454c. Tumas-Brundage K, Manser T. The transcriptional promoter regulates hypermutation of the antibody heavy chain locus. *J Exp Med* 1997;185:239–250.

454d. Cascalho M, Wong J, Steinberg C, Wabl M. Mismatch repair co-opted by hypermutation. *Science* 1998;279:1207–1210.

454e. Narayanan L, Fritzell MA, Baker SM, Liskay RM, Glazer PM. Elevated levels of mutation in multiple tissues of mice deficient in the DNA mismatch repair gene Pms2. *Proc Natl Acad Sci USA* 1997;94:3122–3127.

454f. Razanajaona D, Denepoux S, Blanchard D, et al. In vitro triggering of somatic mutation in human naive B cells. *J Immunol* 1997;159:3347–3353.

455. Roes J, Rajewsky K. Immunoglobulin D (IgD)-deficient mice reveal an auxiliary receptor function for IgD in antigen-mediated recruitment of B cells. *J Exp Med* 1993;177:45–55.

456. Liu YJ, de Boutellier O, Arpin C, et al. Normal human IgD⁺IgM⁻ germinal center B cells can express up to 80 mutations in the variable region of their IgD transcripts. *Immunity* 1996;4:603–613.

457. Kallberg E, Jainandunsing S, Gray D, Leanderson T. Somatic mutation of immunoglobulin V genes in vitro. *Science* 1996;271:1285–1289.

458. Denepoux S, Razanajaona D, Blanchard D, et al. Induction of somatic mutation in a human B cell line in vitro. *Immunity* 1997;6:35–46.

459. Jolly CJ, Klix N, Neuberger MS. Rapid methods for the analysis of immunoglobulin gene hypermutation: Application to transgenic and gene targeted mice. *Nucleic Acids Res* 1997;25:1913–1919.

460. Williams AF. A year in the life of the immunoglobulin superfamily. *Immunol Today* 1987;8:298–303.

461. Hunkapiller T, Hood L. Diversity of the immunoglobulin gene superfamily. *Adv Immunol* 1989;44:1–63.

462. Matsunaga T, Mori N. The origin of the immune system. The possibility that immunoglobulin superfamily molecules and cell adhesion molecules of chicken and slime mould are all related. *Scand J Immunol* 1987;25:485–495.

463. Hoek RM, Smit AB, Frings H, et al. A new Ig-superfamily member, molluscan defence molecule (MDM) from *Lymnaea stagnalis,* is down-regulated during parasitosis. *Eur J Immunol* 1996;26:939–944.

464. Sun SC, Lindstrom I, Boman HG, Faye I, Schmidt O. Hemolin: An insect-immune protein belonging to the immunoglobulin superfamily. *Science* 1990; 250:1729–1732.

465. Lindstrom-Dinnetz I, Sun SC, Faye I. Structure and expression of Hemolin, an insect member of the immunoglobulin gene superfamily. *Eur J Biochem* 1995; 230:920–925.

466. Parnes JR, Hunkapiller T. L3T4 and the immunoglobulin gene superfamily: New relationships between the immune system and the nervous system. *Immunol Rev* 1987;100:109–127.

467. Chretien I, Robert J, Marcuz A, Garcia SJ, Courtet M, Du PL. CTX, a novel molecule specifically expressed on the surface of cortical thymocytes in Xenopus. *Eur J Immunol* 1996;26:780–791.

468. Johnson P, Williams AF. Striking similarities between antigen receptor J pieces and sequence in the second chain of the murine CD8 antigen. *Nature* 1986;323:74–76.

469. Siu G, Kronenberg M, Strauss E, Haars R, Mak TW, Hood L. The structure, rearrangement and expression of D beta gene segments of the murine T-cell antigen receptor. *Nature* 1984;311:344–350.

470. Rast JP, Litman GW. T-cell receptor gene homologs are present in the most primitive jawed vertebrates. *Proc Natl Acad Sci USA* 1994;91:9248–9252.

471. Hawke NA, Rast JP, Litman GW. Extensive diversity of transcribed TCR-beta in phylogenetically primitive vertebrate. *J Immunol* 1996;156:2458–2464.

472. Rast JP, Anderson MK, Strong SJ, Luer C, Litman RT, Litman GW. Alpha, beta, gamma, and delta T cell antigen receptor genes arose early in vertebrate phylogeny. *Immunity* 1997;6:1–11.

473. Hinds KR, Litman GW. Major reorganization of immunoglobulin VH segmental elements during vertebrate evolution. *Nature* 1986;320:546–549.

474. Reynaud CA, Anquez V, Grimal H, Weill JC. A hyperconversion mechanism generates the chicken light chain preimmune repertoire. *Cell* 1987;48:379–388.

475. Thompson CB, Neiman PE. Somatic diversification of the chicken immunoglobulin light chain gene is limited to the rearranged variable gene segment. *Cell* 1987;48:369–378.

476. Knight KL, Becker RS. Molecular basis of the allelic inheritance of rabbit immunoglobulin VH allotypes: Implications for the generation of antibody diversity. *Cell* 1990;60:963–970.

476a. Lanning DK, Knight KL. Somatic hypermutation: mutations 3' of rabbit VDJ H-chain genes. *J Immunol* 1997;159:4403-4407.

477. Parng CL, Hansal S, Goldsby RA, Osborne BA. Gene conversion contributes to Ig light chain diversity in cattle. *J Immunol* 1996;157:5478–5486.

478. Jack HM, Wabl M. Immunoglobulin mRNA stability varies during B lymphocyte differentiation. *EMBO J* 1988;7:1041–1046.

479. Bode J, Kohwi Y, Dickinson L, et al. Biological significance of unwinding capability of nuclear matrix-associating DNAs. *Science* 1992;255:195–197.

480. Freeman LA, Garrard WT. DNA supercoiling in chromatin structure and gene expression. *Crit Rev Eukaryot Gene Expr* 1992;2:165–209.

481. Baron MH. Developmental regulation of the vertebrate globin multigene family. *Gene Expr* 1996;6:129–137.

482. Razin A, Riggs AD. DNA metylation and gene function. *Science* 1980;210: 604–610.

483. Rogers J, Wall R. Immunoglobulin heavy chain genes: Demethylation accompanies class switching. *Proc Natl Acad Sci USA* 1981;78:7497–7501.

484. Storb U, Wilson R, Selsing E, Walfield A. Rearranged and germline immunoglobulin kappa genes: Different states of DNase I sensitivity of constant kappa genes in immunocompetent and nonimmune cells. *Biochemistry* 1981;20:990–996.

485. Mather EL, Perry RP. Methylation status and DNase I sensitivity of immunoglobulin genes: Changes associated with rearrangement. *Proc Natl Acad Sci USA* 1983;80:4689–4693.

486. Mills FC, Fisher LM, Kuroda R, Ford AM, Gould HJ. DNase I hypersensitive sites in the chromatin of human mu immunoglobulin heavy-chain genes. *Nature* 1983;306:809–812.

487. Blackman MA, Koshland ME. Specific 5' and 3' regions of the mu chain gene are undermethylated at distinct stages of B-cell differentiation. *Proc Natl Acad Sci USA* 1985;82:3809–3813.

488. Stavnezer-Nordgren J, Sirlin S. Specificity of immunoglobulin heavy chain switch correlates with activity of germline heavy chain genes prior to switching. *EMBO J* 1986;5:95–102.

489. Pfeiffer W, Zachau HG. Accessibility of expressed and non-expressed genes to a restriction nuclease. *Nucleic Acids Res* 1980;8:4621–4638.

490. Madisen L, Groudine M. Identification of a locus control region in the immunoglobulin heavy-chain locus that deregulates c-myc expression in plasmacytoma and Burkitt's lymphoma cells. *Genes Dev* 1994;8:2212–2226.

491. Mills FC, Harindranath N, Mitchell M, Max EE. Enhancer complexes located downstream of both human immunoglobulin C-alpha genes. *J Exp Med* 1997; 186:845–858.

492. Weischet WO, Glotov BO, Schnell H, Zachau HG. Differences in the nuclease sensitivity between the two alleles of the immunoglobulin kappa light chain genes in mouse liver and myeloma nuclei. *Nucleic Acids Res* 1982;10: 3627–3645.

493. Gimble JM, Max EE. Human immunoglobulin kappa gene enhancer: Chromatin structure analysis at high resolution. *Mol Cell Biol* 1987;7:15–25.

494. Singh H, LeBowitz JH, Baldwin AJ, Sharp PA. Molecular cloning of an enhancer binding protein: Isolation by screening of an expression library with a recognition site DNA. *Cell* 1988;52:415–423.

495. Falkner FG, Zachau HG. Correct transcription of an immunoglobulin kappa gene requires an upstream fragment containing conserved sequence elements. *Nature* 1984;310:71–74.

496. Parslow TG, Blair DL, Murphy WJ, Granner DK. Structure of the 5' ends of immunoglobulin genes: A novel conserved sequence. *Proc Natl Acad Sci USA* 1984;91:2650–2654.

497. Bergman Y, Rice D, Grosschedl R, Baltimore D. Two regulatory elements for immunoglobulin kappa light chain gene expression. *Proc Natl Acad Sci USA* 1984;81:7041–7045.

498. Grosschedl R, Baltimore D. Cell-type specificity of immunoglobulin gene expression is regulated by at least three DNA sequence elements. *Cell* 1985;41: 885–897.

499. Picard D, Schaffner W. Cell-type preference of immunoglobulin kappa and lambda gene promoters. *EMBO J* 1985;4:2831–2838.

500. Ballard DW, Bothwell A. Mutational analysis of the immunoglobulin heavy chain promoter region. *Proc Natl Acad Sci USA* 1986;83:9626–9630.

501. Wirth T, Staudt L, Baltimore D. An octamer oligonucleotide upstream of a TATA motif is sufficient for lymphoid-specific promoter activity. *Nature* 1987;329: 174–178.

502. Mizushima-Sugano J, Roeder RG. Cell-type-specific transcription of an immunoglobulin kappa light chain gene in vitro. *Proc Natl Acad Sci USA* 1986;83: 8511–8515.

503. Hermanson GG, Briskin M, Sigman D, Wall R. Immunoglobulin enhancer and

promoter motifs 5′ of the B29 B-cell- specific gene. *Proc Natl Acad Sci USA* 1989;86:7341–7345.

504. Christensen SM, Martin BK, Tan SS, Weis JH. Identification of sites for distinct DNA binding proteins including Oct-1 and Oct-2 in the Cr2 gene. *J Immunol* 1992;148:3610–3617.

505. Thevenin C, Lucas BP, Kozlow EJ, Kehrl JH. Cell type- and stage-specific expression of the CD20/B1 antigen correlates with the activity of a diverged octamer DNA motif present in its promoter. *J Biol Chem* 1993;268:5949–5956.

506. Annweiler A, Muller IM, Wirth T. Oct2 transactivation from a remote enhancer position requires a B-cell-restricted activity. *Mol Cell Biol* 1992;12:3107–3116.

507. Clerc RG, Corcoran LM, LeBowitz JH, Baltimore D, Sharp PA. The B-cell-specific Oct-2 protein contains POU box- and homeo box-type domains. *Genes Dev* 1988;2:1570–1581.

508. Ko HS, Fast P, McBride W, Staudt LM. A human protein specific for the immunoglobulin octamer DNA motif contains a functional homeobox domain. *Cell* 1988;55:135–144.

509. Staudt LM, Clerc RG, Singh H, LeBowitz JH, Sharp PA, Baltimore D. Cloning of a lymphoid-specific cDNA encoding a protein binding the regulatory octamer DNA motif. *Science* 1988;241:577–580.

510. Sturm RA, Das G, Herr W. The ubiquitous octamer-binding protein Oct-1 contains a POU domain with a homeo box subdomain. *Genes Dev* 1988;2:1582–1599.

511. Klemm JD, Rould MA, Aurora R, Herr W, Pabo CO. Crystal structure of the Oct-1 POU domain bound to an octamer site: DNA recognition with tethered DNA-binding modules. *Cell* 1994;77:21–32.

512. Gerster T, Balmaceda CG, Roeder RG. The cell type-specific octamer transcription factor OTF-2 has two domains required for the activation of transcription. *EMBO J* 1990;9:1635–1643.

513. Tanaka M, Herr W. Differential transcriptional activation by Oct-1 and Oct-2: Interdependent activation domains induce Oct-2 phosphorylation. *Cell* 1990;60:375–386.

514. Yang J, Muller IM, Seipel K, et al. Both Oct-1 and Oct-2A contain domains which can activate the ubiquitously expressed U2 snRNA genes. *EMBO J* 1991;10:2291–2296.

515. Tanaka M, Lai JS, Herr W. Promoter-selective activation domains in Oct-1 and Oct-2 direct differential activation of an snRNA and mRNA promoter. *Cell* 1992;68:755–767.

516. Feldhaus AL, Klug CA, Arvin KL, Singh H. Targeted disruption of the Oct-2 locus in a B cell provides genetic evidence for two distinct cell type-specific pathways of octamer element-mediated gene activation. *EMBO J* 1993;12:2763–2772.

517. Corcoran LM, Karvelas M, Nossal GJ, Ye ZS, Jacks T, Baltimore D. Oct-2, although not required for early B-cell development, is critical for later B-cell maturation and for postnatal survival. *Genes Dev* 1993;7:570–582.

518. Corcoran LM, Karvelas M. Oct-2 is required early in T cell-independent B cell activation for G1 progression and for proliferation. *Immunity* 1994;1:635–645.

519. Pierani A, Heguy A, Fujii H, Roeder RG. Activation of octamer-containing promoters by either octamer-binding transcription factor 1 (OTF-1) or OTF-2 and requirement of an additional B-cell-specific component for optimal transcription of immunoglobulin promoters. *Mol Cell Biol* 1990;10:6204–6215.

520. Luo Y, Roeder RG. Cloning, functional characterization, and mechanism of action of the B-cell-specific transcriptional coactivator OCA-B. *Mol Cell Biol* 1995;15:4115–4124.

521. Strubin M, Newell JW, Matthias P. OBF-1, a novel B cell-specific coactivator that stimulates immunoglobulin promoter activity through association with octamer-binding proteins. *Cell* 1995;80:497–506.

522. Gstaiger M, Knoepfel L, Georgiev O, Schaffner W, Hovens CM. A B-cell coactivator of octamer-binding transcription factors. *Nature* 1995;373:360–362.

523. Gstaiger M, Georgiev O, van Lit, et al. The B cell coactivator Bob1 shows DNA sequence-dependent complex formation with Oct-1/Oct-2 factors, leading to differential promoter activation. *EMBO J* 1996;15:2781–2790.

524. Cepek KL, Chasman DI, Sharp PA. Sequence-specific DNA binding of the B-cell specific coactivator OCA-B. *Genes Dev* 1996;10:2079–2088.

525. Kim U, Qin XF, Gong S, et al. The B-cell-specific transcription coactivator OCA-B/OBF-1/Bob-1 is essential for normal production of immunoglobulin isotypes. *Nature* 1996;383:542–547.

526. Schubart DB, Rolink A, Kosco VM, Botteri F, Matthias P. B-cell-specific coactivator OBF-1/OCA-B/Bob1 required for immune response and germinal centre formation. *Nature* 1996;383:538–542.

527. Luo Y, Fujii H, Gerster T, Roeder RG. A novel B cell-derived coactivator potentiates the activation of immunoglobulin promoters by octamer-binding transcription factors. *Cell* 1992;71:231–241.

528. Pfisterer P, Annweiler A, Ullmer C, Corcoran LM, Wirth T. Differential transactivation potential of Oct1 and Oct2 is determined by additional B cell-specific activities. *EMBO J* 1994;13:1655–1663.

529. Cook GP, Neuberger MS. Lymphoid-specific transcriptional activation by components of the IgH enhancer: Studies on the E2/E3 and octanucleotide elements. *Nucleic Acids Res* 1990;18:3565–3571.

530. Stern S, Tanaka M, Herr W. The Oct-1 homoeodomain directs formation of a multiprotein-DNA complex with the HSV transactivator VP16. *Nature* 1989;341:624–630.

531. Kristie TM, Sharp PA. Interactions of the Oct-1 POU subdomains with specific DNA sequences and with the HSV alpha-trans-activator protein. *Genes Dev* 1990;4:2383–2396.

532. Murphy S, Yoon JB, Gerster T, Roeder RG. Oct-1 and Oct-2 potentiate functional interactions of a transcription factor with the proximal sequence element of small nuclear RNA genes. *Mol Cell Biol* 1992;12:3247–3261.

532a.Pelletier MR, Hatada EN, Scholz G, Scheidereit C. Efficient transcription of an immunoglobulin kappa promoter requires specific sequence elements overlapping with and downstream of the transcriptional start site. *Nucl Acids Res* 1997;25:3995–4003.

533. Lenardo M, Pierce JW, Baltimore D. Protein-binding sites in Ig gene enhancers determine transcriptional activity and inducibility. *Science* 1987;236:1573–1577.

534. Jenuwein T, Grosschedl R. Complex pattern of immunoglobulin mu gene expression in normal and transgenic mice: Nonoverlapping regulatory sequences govern distinct tissue specificities. *Genes Dev* 1991;5:932–943.

535. Yuan D, Dang T, Hawley J, Jenuwein T, Grosschedl R. Role of the OCTA site in regulation of IgH chain gene transcription during B cell activation. *Int Immunol* 1995;7:1163–1172.

536. Su LK, Kadesch T. The immunoglobulin heavy-chain enhancer functions as the promoter for I mu sterile transcription. *Mol Cell Biol* 1990;10:2619–2624.

537. Currie RA, Roeder RG. Identification of an octamer-binding site in the mouse kappa light-chain immunoglobulin enhancer. *Mol Cell Biol* 1989;9:4239–4247.

538. Kemler I, Schaffner W. Octamer transcription factors and the cell type-specificity of immunoglobulin gene activation. *FASEB J* 1990;4:1444–1449.

539. Wirth T, Priess A, Annweiler A, Zwilling S, Oeler B. Multiple Oct2 isoforms are generated by alternative splicing. *Nucleic Acids Res* 1991;19:43–51.

540. Stoykova AS, Sterrer S, Erselius JR, Hatzopoulos AK, Gruss P. Mini-Oct and Oct-2c: Two novel, functionally diverse murine Oct-2 gene products are differentially expressed in the CNS. *Neuron* 1992;8:541–558.

541. Segil N, Roberts SB, Heintz N. Mitotic phosphorylation of the Oct-1 homeodomain and regulation of Oct-1 DNA binding activity. *Science* 1991;254:1814–1816.

542. Zwilling S, Konig H, Wirth T. High mobility group protein 2 functionally interacts with the POU domains of octamer transcription factors. *EMBO J* 1995;14:1198–1208.

543. Fontes JD, Jabrane FN, Toth CR, Peterlin BM. Binding and cooperative interactions between two B cell-specific transcriptional coactivators. *J Exp Med* 1996;183:2517–2521.

544. Atchison ML, Delmas V, Perry RP. A novel upstream element compensates for an ineffectual octamer motif in an immunoglobulin V kappa promoter. *EMBO J* 1990;9:3109–3117.

545. Sigvardsson M, Akerblad P, Leanderson T. Early B cell factor interacts with a subset of kappa promoters. *J Immunol* 1996;156:3788–3796.

546. Eaton S, Calame K. Multiple DNA sequence elements are necessary for the function of an immunoglobulin heavy chain promoter. *Proc Natl Acad Sci USA* 1987;84:7634–7638.

547. Landolfi NF, Yin XM, Capra JD, Tucker PW. A conserved heptamer upstream of the IgH promoter region octamer can be the site of a coordinate protein-DNA interaction. *Nucleic Acids Res* 1988;16:5503–5514.

548. Kemler I, Schreiber E, Muller MM, Matthias P, Schaffner W. Octamer transcription factors bind to two different sequence motifs of the immunoglobulin heavy chain promoter. *EMBO J* 1989;8:2001–2008.

549. LeBowitz JH, Clerc RG, Brenowitz M, Sharp PA. The Oct-2 protein binds cooperatively to adjacent octamer sites. *Genes Dev* 1989;3:1625–1638.

550. Poellinger L, Roeder RG. Octamer transcription factors 1 and 2 each bind to two different functional elements in the immunoglobulin heavy-chain promoter. *Mol Cell Biol* 1989;9:747–756.

551. Poellinger L, Yoza BK, Roeder RG. Functional cooperativity between protein molecules bound at two distinct sequence elements of the immunoglobulin heavy-chain promoter. *Nature* 1989;337:573–576.

552. Yoza BK, Roeder RG. Identification of a novel factor that interacts with an immunoglobulin heavy-chain promoter and stimulates transcription in conjunction with the lymphoid cell-specific factor OTF2. *Mol Cell Biol* 1990;10:2145–2153.

553. Cooper C, Johnson D, Roman C, Avitahl N, Tucker P, Calame K. The C/EBP family of transcriptional activators is functionally important for Ig VH promoter activity in vivo and in vitro. *J Immunol* 1992;149:3225–3231.

554. Webb CF, Das C, Eaton S, Calame K, Tucker PW. Novel protein-DNA interactions associated with increased immunoglobulin transcription in response to antigen plus interleukin-5. *Mol Cell Biol* 1991;11:5197–5205.

555. Herrscher RF, Kaplan MH, Lelsz DL, Das C, Scheuermann R, Tucker PW. The immunoglobulin heavy-chain matrix-associating regions are bound by Bright: A B cell-specific trans-activator that describes a new DNA-binding protein family. *Genes Dev* 1995;9:3067–3082.

556. Avitahl N, Calame K. A 125 bp region of the Ig VH1 promoter is sufficient to confer lymphocyte-specific expression in transgenic mice. *Int Immunol* 1996;8:1359–1366.

557. Buchanan KL, Hodgetts SI, Byrnes J, Webb CF. Differential transcription efficiency of two Ig VH promoters in vitro. *J Immunol* 1995;155:4270–4277.

558. Stiernholm NB, Berinstein NL. A mutated promoter of a human Ig V lambda gene segment is associated with reduced germ-line transcription and a low frequency of rearrangement. *J Immunol* 1995;154:1748–1761.

559. Buchanan KL, Smith EA, Dou S, Corcoran LM, Webb CF. Family-specific differences in transcription efficiency of Ig heavy chain promoters. *J Immunol* 1997;159:1247–1254.

560. Sawadogo M, Roeder RG. Interaction of a gene-specific transcription factor with

the adenovirus major late promoter upstream of the TATA box region. *Cell* 1985;43:165–175.

561. Chang LA, Smith T, Pognonec P, Roeder RG, Murialdo H. Identification of USF as the ubiquitous murine factor that binds to and stimulates transcription from the immunoglobulin lambda 2-chain promoter. *Nucleic Acids Res* 1992;20:287–293.

562. Blackwell TK, Moore MW, Yancopoulos GD, et al. Recombination between immunoglobulin variable region gene segments is enhanced by transcription. *Nature* 1986;324:585–589.

563. Berman JE, Humphries CG, Barth J, Alt FW, Tucker PW. Structure and expression of human germline VH transcripts. *J Exp Med* 1991;173:1529–1535.

564. Perry RP, Kelley DE, Coleclough C, et al. Transcription of mouse kappa chain genes: Implications for allelic exclusion. *Proc Natl Acad Sci USA* 1980;77:1937–1941.

565. Martin D, Huang RQ, LeBien T, Van Ness B. Induced rearrangement of kappa genes in the BLIN-1 human pre-B cell line correlates with germline J-C kappa and V kappa transcription. *J Exp Med* 1991;173:639–645.

566. Nelson KJ, Haimovich J, Perry RP. Characterization of productive and sterile transcripts from the immunoglobulin heavy-chain locus: Processing of micron and muS mRNA. *Mol Cell Biol* 1983;3:1317–1332.

567. Lennon GG, Perry RP. C mu-containing transcripts initiate heterogeneously within the IgH enhancer region and contain a novel 5'-nontranslatable exon. *Nature* 1985;318:475–478.

568. Neale GA, Kitchingman GR. mRNA transcripts initiating within the human immunoglobulin mu heavy chain enhancer region contain a non-translatable exon and are extremely heterogeneous at the 5' end. *Nucleic Acids Res* 1991;19:2427–2433.

569. Li SC, Rothman PB, Zhang J, Chan C, Hirsh D, Alt FW. Expression of I mu-C gamma hybrid germline transcripts subsequent to immunoglobulin heavy chain class switching. *Int Immunol* 1994;6:491–497.

570. Alessandrini A, Desiderio SV. Coordination of immunoglobulin DJH transcription and D-to-JH rearrangement by promoter-enhancer approximation. *Mol Cell Biol* 1991;11:2096–2107.

571. Kottmann AH, Brack C, Eibel H, Kohler G. A survey of protein-DNA interaction sites within the murine immunoglobulin heavy chain locus reveals a particularly complex pattern around the DQ52 element. *Eur J Immunol* 1992;22:2113–2120.

572. Kottmann AH, Zevnik B, Welte M, Nielsen PJ, Kohler G. A second promoter and enhancer element within the immunoglobulin heavy chain locus. *Eur J Immunol* 1994;24:817–821.

573. Martin DJ, Van Ness B. Initiation and processing of two kappa immunoglobulin germ line transcripts in mouse B cells. *Mol Cell Biol* 1990;10:1950–1958.

574. Weaver D, Baltimore D. B lymphocyte-specific protein binding near an immunoglobulin kappa-chain gene J segment. *Proc Natl Acad Sci USA* 1987;84:1516–1520.

575. Frances V, Pandrau GD, Guret C, et al. A surrogate 15 kDa JC kappa protein is expressed in combination with mu heavy chain by human B cell precursors. *EMBO J* 1994;13:5937–5943.

576. Daitch LE, Moore MW, Persiani DM, Durdik JM, Selsing E. Transcription and recombination of the murine RS element. *J Immunol* 1992;149:832–840.

577. Kuhn R, Rajewsky K, Muller W. Generation and analysis of interleukin-4 deficient mice. *Science* 1991;254:707–710.

578. Rothman P, Chen YY, Lutzker S, et al. Structure and expression of germ line immunoglobulin heavy-chain epsilon transcripts: Interleukin-4 plus lipopolysaccharide-directed switching to C epsilon. *Mol Cell Biol* 1990;10:1672–1679.

579. Delphin S, Stavnezer J. Characterization of an interleukin 4 (IL-4) responsive region in the immunoglobulin heavy chain germline epsilon promoter: Regulation by NF-IL-4, a C/EBP family member and NF-kappa B/p50. *J Exp Med* 1995;181:181–192.

580. Mikita T, Campbell D, Wu P, Williamson K, Schindler U. Requirements for interleukin-4-induced gene expression and functional characterization of Stat6. *Mol Cell Biol* 1996;16:5811–5820.

581. Shimoda K, van DJ, Sangster MY, et al. Lack of IL-4-induced Th2 response and IgE class switching in mice with disrupted Stat6 gene. *Nature* 1996;380:630–633.

582. Takeda K, Tanaka T, Shi W, et al. Essential role of Stat6 in IL-4 signalling. *Nature* 1996;380:627–630.

583. Cooper C, Henderson A, Artandi S, Avitahl N, Calame K. Ig/EBP (C/EBP gamma) is a transdominant negative inhibitor of C/EBP family transcriptional activators. *Nucleic Acids Res* 1995;23:4371–4377.

584. Cooper CL, Berrier AL, Roman C, Calame KL. Limited expression of C/EBP family proteins during B lymphocyte development. Negative regulator Ig/EBP predominates early and activator NF-IL-6 is induced later. *J Immunol* 1994;153:5049–5058.

585. Iciek LA, Delphin SA, Stavnezer J. CD40 cross-linking induces Ig epsilon germline transcripts in B cells via activation of NF-kappa B: Synergy with IL-4 induction. *J Immunol* 1997;158:4769–4779.

586. Sha WC, Liou HC, Tuomanen EI, Baltimore D. Targeted disruption of the p50 subunit of NF-kappa B leads to multifocal defects in immune responses. *Cell* 1995;80:321–330.

587. Kim J, Reeves R, Rothman P, Boothby M. The non-histone chromosomal protein HMG-I(Y) contributes to repression of the immunoglobulin heavy chain germline epsilon RNA promoter. *Eur J Immunol* 1995;25:798–808.

588. Wang DZ, Ray P, Boothby M. Interleukin 4-inducible phosphorylation of HMG-I(Y) is inhibited by rapamycin. *J Biol Chem* 1995;270:22924–22932.

589. Liao F, Birshtein BK, Busslinger M, Rothman P. The transcription factor BSAP (NF-HB) is essential for immunoglobulin germ-line epsilon transcription. *J Immunol* 1994;152:2904–2911.

589a.Thienes CP, De ML, Monticelli S, Busslinger M, Gould HJ, Vercelli D. The transcription factor B cell-specific activator protein (BSAP) enhances both IL-4- and CD40-mediated activation of the human epsilon germline promoter. *J Immunol* 1997;158:5874–5882.

590. Church GM, Ephrussi A, Gilbert W, Tonegawa S. Cell-type-specific contacts to immunoglobulin enhancers in nuclei. *Nature* 1985;313:798–801.

591. Ephrussi A, Church GM, Tonegawa S, Gilbert W. B lineage–specific interactions of an immunoglobulin enhancer with cellular factors in vivo. *Science* 1985;227:134–140.

592. Kadesch T, Zervos P, Ruezinsky D. Functional analysis of the murine IgH enhancer: Evidence for negative control of cell-type specificity. *Nucleic Acids Res* 1986;14:8209–8221.

593. Murre C, McCaw PS, Baltimore D. A new DNA binding and dimerization motif in immunoglobulin enhancer binding, daughterless, MyoD, and myc proteins. *Cell* 1989;56:777–783.

594. Murre C, McCaw PS, Vaessin H, et al. Interactions between heterologous helix-loop-helix proteins generate complexes that bind specifically to a common DNA sequence. *Cell* 1989;58:537–544.

595. Lassar AB, Davis RL, Wright WE, et al. Functional activity of myogenic HLH proteins requires hetero-oligomerization with E12/E47-like proteins in vivo. *Cell* 1991;66:305–315.

596. Lin H, Yutzey KE, Konieczny SF. Muscle-specific expression of the troponin I gene requires interactions between helix-loop-helix muscle regulatory factors and ubiquitous transcription factors. *Mol Cell Biol* 1991;11:267–280.

597. Voliva CF, Aronheim A, Walker MD, Peterlin BM. B-cell factor 1 is required for optimal expression of the DRA promoter in B cells. *Mol Cell Biol* 1992;12:2383–2390.

598. Shen CP, Kadesch T. B-cell-specific DNA binding by an E47 homodimer. *Mol Cell Biol* 1995;15:4518–4524.

599. Sun XH, Copeland NG, Jenkins NA, Baltimore D. Id proteins Id1 and Id2 selectively inhibit DNA binding by one class of helix-loop-helix proteins. *Mol Cell Biol* 1991;11:5603–5611.

600. Wilson RB, Kiledjian M, Shen CP, et al. Repression of immunoglobulin enhancers by the helix-loop-helix protein Id: Implications for B-lymphoid-cell development. *Mol Cell Biol* 1991;11:6185–6191.

601. Bain G, Maandag EC, Izon DJ, et al. E2A proteins are required for proper B cell development and initiation of immunoglobulin gene rearrangements. *Cell* 1994;79:885–892.

602. Zhuang Y, Soriano P, Weintraub H. The helix-loop-helix gene E2A is required for B cell formation. *Cell* 1994;79:875–884.

603. Bain G, Robanus ME, te RH, et al. Both E12 and E47 allow commitment to the B cell lineage. *Immunity* 1997;6:145–154.

604. Schlissel M, Voronova A, Baltimore D. Helix-loop-helix transcription factor E47 activates germ-line immunoglobulin heavy-chain gene transcription and rearrangement in a pre-T-cell line. *Genes Dev* 1991;5:1367–1376.

605. Choi JK, Shen CP, Radomska HS, Eckhardt LA, Kadesch T. E47 activates the Ig-heavy chain and TdT loci in non-B cells. *EMBO J* 1996;15:5014–5021.

606. Sloan SR, Shen CP, McCarrick WR, Kadesch T. Phosphorylation of E47 as a potential determinant of B-cell-specific activity. *Mol Cell Biol* 1996;16:6900–6908.

607. Bain G, Gruenwald S, Murre C. E2A and E2-2 are subunits of B-cell-specific E2-box DNA-binding proteins. *Mol Cell Biol* 1993;13:3522–3529.

608. Zhuang Y, Cheng P, Weintraub H. B-lymphocyte development is regulated by the combined dosage of three basic helix-loop-helix genes, E2A, E2-2, and HEB. *Mol Cell Biol* 1996;16:2898–2905.

609. Ruezinsky D, Beckmann H, Kadesch T. Modulation of the IgH enhancer's cell type specificity through a genetic switch. *Genes Dev* 1991;5:29–37.

610. Genetta T, Ruezinsky D, Kadesch T. Displacement of an E-box-binding repressor by basic helix-loop-helix proteins: Implications for B-cell specificity of the immunoglobulin heavy-chain enhancer. *Mol Cell Biol* 1994;14:6153–6163.

611. Carter RS, Ordentlich P, Kadesch T. Selective utilization of basic helix-loop-helix-leucine zipper proteins at the immunoglobulin heavy-chain enhancer. *Mol Cell Biol* 1997;17:18–23.

612. Merrell K, Wells S, Henderson A, et al. The absence of the transcription activator TFE3 impairs activation of B cells in vivo. *Mol Cell Biol* 1997;17:3335–3344.

613. Benezra R, Davis RL, Lockshon D, Turner DL, Weintraub H. The protein Id: A negative regulator of helix-loop-helix DNA binding proteins. *Cell* 1990;61:49–59.

614. Sun XH. Constitutive expression of the Id1 gene impairs mouse B cell development. *Cell* 1994;79:893–900.

615. Mellentin JD, Murre C, Donlon TA, et al. The gene for enhancer binding proteins E12/E47 lies at the t(1;19) breakpoint in acute leukemias. *Science* 1989;246:379–382.

616. Inaba T, Roberts WM, Shapiro LH, et al. Fusion of the leucine zipper gene HLF to the E2A gene in human acute B-lineage leukemia. *Science* 1992;257:531–534.

617. Nelsen B, Tian G, Erman B, et al. Regulation of lymphoid-specific immunoglobulin mu heavy chain gene enhancer by ETS-domain factors. *Science* 1993;261:82–86.

618. Libermann TA, Baltimore D. Pi, a pre-B-cell-specific enhancer element in the immunoglobulin heavy-chain enhancer. *Mol Cell Biol* 1993;13:5957–5969.

619. Akbarali Y, Oettgen P, Boltax J, Libermann TA. ELF-1 interacts with and transactivates the IgH enhancer pi site. *J Biol Chem* 1996;271:26007–26012.

620. Klemsz MJ, McKercher SR, Celada A, Van BC, Maki RA. The macrophage and B cell-specific transcription factor PU.1 is related to the ets oncogene. *Cell* 1990;61:113–124.

621. Scott EW, Simon MC, Anastasi J, Singh H. Requirement of transcription factor PU.1 in the development of multiple hematopoietic lineages. *Science* 1994;265:1573–1577.

622. Nikolajczyk BS, Nelsen B, Sen R. Precise alignment of sites required for mu enhancer activation in B cells. *Mol Cell Biol* 1996;16:4544–4554.

623. Nikolajczyk BS, Cortes M, Feinman R, Sen R. Combinatorial determinants of tissue-specific transcription in B cells and macrophages. *Mol Cell Biol* 1997;17:3527–3535.

624. Rao E, Dang W, Tian G, Sen R. A three-protein-DNA complex on a B cell-specific domain of the immunoglobulin mu heavy chain gene enhancer. *J Biol Chem* 1997;272:6722–6732.

624a. Dang W, Sun XH, Sen R. ETS-mediated cooperation between basic helix-loop-helix motifs of the immunoglobulin mu heavy-chain gene enhancer. *Mol Cell Biol* 1998;18:1477-1488.

624b. Peterson CL, Eaton S, Calame K. Purified mu EBP-E binds to immunoglobulin enhancers and promoters. *Mol Cell Biol* 1988;8:4972-4980.

624c. Tsao BP, Wang XF, Peterson CL, Calame K. In vivo functional analysis of in vitro protein binding sites in the immunoglobulin heavy chain enhancer. *Nucleic Acids Res* 1988;16:3239-3253.

625. Raynal MC, Liu ZY, Hirano T, Mayer L, Kishimoto T, Chen KS. Interleukin 6 induces secretion of IgG1 by coordinated transcriptional activation and differential mRNA accumulation. *Proc Natl Acad Sci USA* 1989;86:8024–8028.

626. Park K, Atchison ML. Isolation of a candidate repressor/activator, NF-E1 (YY-1, delta), that binds to the immunoglobulin kappa 3′ enhancer and the immunoglobulin heavy-chain mu E1 site. *Proc Natl Acad Sci USA* 1991;88:9804–9808.

627. Shi Y, Seto E, Chang LS, Shenk T. Transcriptional repression by YY1, a human GLI-Kruppel-related protein, and relief of repression by adenovirus E1A protein. *Cell* 1991;67:377–388.

628. Bushmeyer S, Park K, Atchison ML. Characterization of functional domains within the multifunctional transcription factor, YY1. *J Biol Chem* 1995;270:30213–30220.

629. Kiledjian M, Su LK, Kadesch T. Identification and characterization of two functional domains within the murine heavy-chain enhancer. *Mol Cell Biol* 1988;8:145–152.

630. Wasylyk C, Wasylyk B. The immunoglobulin heavy-chain B-lymphocyte enhancer efficiently stimulates transcription in non-lymphoid cells. *EMBO J* 1986;5:553–560.

631. Imler JL, Lemaire C, Wasylyk C, Wasylyk B. Negative regulation contributes to tissue specificity of the immunoglobulin heavy-chain enhancer. *Mol Cell Biol* 1987;7:2558–2567.

632. Weinberger J, Jat PS, Sharp PA. Localization of a repressive sequence contributing to B-cell specificity in the immunoglobulin heavy-chain enhancer. *Mol Cell Biol* 1988;8.988–992.

633. Cockerill PN, Yuen MH, Garrard WT. The enhancer of the immunoglobulin heavy chain locus is flanked by presumptive chromosomal loop anchorage elements. *J Biol Chem* 1987;262:5394–5397.

634. Scheuermann RH, Chen U. A developmental-specific factor binds to suppressor sites flanking the immunoglobulin heavy-chain enhancer. *Genes Dev* 1989;3:1255–1266.

635. Zong RT, Scheuermann RH. Mutually exclusive interaction of a novel matrix attachment region binding protein and the NF-muNR enhancer repressor. Implications for regulation of immunoglobulin heavy chain expression. *J Biol Chem* 1995;270:24010–24018.

636. Forrester WC, van Genderen C, Jenuwein T, Grosschedl R. Dependence of enhancer-mediated transcription of the immunoglobulin mu gene on nuclear matrix attachment regions. *Science* 1994;265:1221–1225.

637. McKnight RA, Shamay A, Sankaran L, Wall RJ, Hennighausen L. Matrix-attachment regions can impart position-independent regulation of a tissue-specific gene in transgenic mice. *Proc Natl Acad Sci USA* 1992;89:6943–6947.

638. Jenuwein T, Forrester WC, Qiu RG, Grosschedl R. The immunoglobulin mu enhancer core establishes local factor access in nuclear chromatin independent of transcriptional stimulation. *Genes Dev* 1993;7:2016–2032.

639. Jenuwein T, Forrester WC, Fernandez HL, Laible G, Dull M, Grosschedl R. Extension of chromatin accessibility by nuclear matrix attachment regions. *Nature* 1997;385:269–272.

640. Dickinson LA, Joh T, Kohwi Y, Kohwi ST. A tissue-specific MAR/SAR DNA-binding protein with unusual binding site recognition. *Cell* 1992;70:631–645.

641. Dickinson LA, Kohwi ST. Nucleolin is a matrix attachment region DNA-binding protein that specifically recognizes a region with high base-unpairing potential. *Mol Cell Biol* 1995;15:456–465.

642. Klein S, Sablitzky F, Radbruch A. Deletion of the IgH enhancer does not reduce immunoglobulin heavy chain production of a hybridoma IgD class switch variant. *EMBO J* 1984;3:2473–2476.

643. Wabl MR, Burrows PD. Expression of immunoglobulin heavy chain at a high level in the absence of a proposed immunoglobulin enhancer element in cis. *Proc Natl Acad Sci USA* 1984;81:2452–2455.

644. Aguilera RJ, Hope TJ, Sakano H. Characterization of immunoglobulin enhancer deletions in murine plasmacytomas. *EMBO J* 1985;4:3689–3693.

644a. Klein U, Klein G, Ehlin HD, Rajewsky K, Kuppers R. Burkitt's lymphoma is a malignancy of mature B cells expressing somatically mutated V region genes. *Mol Med* 1995;1:495-505.

644b. Tamaru J, Hummel M, Marafioti T, et al. Burkitt's lymphomas express VH genes with a moderate number of antigen-selected somatic mutations. *Am J Pathol* 1995;147:1398-1407.

645. Eckhardt LA, Birshtein BK. Independent immunoglobulin class-switch events occurring in a single myeloma cell line. *Mol Cell Biol* 1985;5:856–868.

646. Gregor PD, Morrison SL. Myeloma mutant with a novel 3′ flanking region: Loss of normal sequence and insertion of repetitive elements leads to decreased transcription but normal processing of the alpha heavy-chain gene products. *Mol Cell Biol* 1986;6:1903–1916.

647. Pettersson S, Cook GP, Bruggemann M, Williams GT, Neuberger MS. A second B cell-specific enhancer 3′ of the immunoglobulin heavy-chain locus. *Nature* 1990;344:165–168.

648. Dariavach P, Williams GT, Campbell K, Pettersson S, Neuberger MS. The mouse IgH 3′-enhancer. *Eur J Immunol* 1991;21:1499–1504.

649. Lieberson R, Giannini SL, Birshtein BK, Eckhardt LA. An enhancer at the 3′ end of the mouse immunoglobulin heavy chain locus. *Nucleic Acids Res* 1991;19:933–937.

650. Matthias P, Baltimore D. The immunoglobulin heavy chain locus contains another B-cell-specific 3′ enhancer close to the alpha constant region. *Mol Cell Biol* 1993;13:1547–1553.

651. Chauveau C, Cogne M. Palindromic structure of the IgH 3′ locus control region. *Nat Genet* 1996;14:15–16.

652. Saleque S, Singh M, Little RD, Giannini SL, Michaelson JS, Birshtein BK. Dyad symmetry within the mouse 3′ IgH regulatory region includes two virtually identical enhancers (C alpha3′E and hs3). *J Immunol* 1997;158:4780–4787.

653. Meyer KB, Skogberg M, Margenfeld C, Ireland J, Pettersson S. Repression of the immunoglobulin heavy chain 3′ enhancer by helix-loop-helix protein Id3 via a functionally important F47/E12 binding site: Implications for developmental control of enhancer function. *Eur J Immunol* 1995;25:1770–1777.

654. Neurath MF, Max EE, Strober W. Pax5 (BSAP) regulates the murine immunoglobulin 3′ alpha enhancer by suppressing binding of NF-alpha P, a protein that controls heavy chain transcription. *Proc Natl Acad Sci USA* 1995;92:5336–5340.

655. Ernst P, Smale ST. Combinatorial regulation of transcription II: the immunoglobulin mu heavy chain gene. *Immunity* 1995;2:427–438.

656. Singh M, Birshtein BK. Concerted repression of an immunoglobulin heavy-chain enhancer, 3′ alpha E(hs1,2). *Proc Natl Acad Sci USA* 1996;93:4392–4397.

657. Linderson Y, Cross D, Neurath MF, Pettersson S. NFE, a new transcriptional activator that facilitates p50 and c-Rel-dependent IgH 3′ enhancer activity. *Eur J Immunol* 1997;27:460 475.

658. Grant PA, Thompson CB, Pettersson S. IgM receptor-mediated transactivation of the IgH 3′ enhancer couples a novel Elf-1-AP-1 protein complex to the developmental control of enhancer function. *EMBO J* 1995;14:4501 4513.

659. Grant PA, Andersson T, Neurath MF, et al. A T cell controlled molecular pathway regulating the IgH locus: CD40-mediated activation of the IgH 3′ enhancer. *EMBO J* 1996;15:6691–6700.

660. Michaelson JS, Giannini SL, Birshtein BK. Identification of 3′ alpha-hs4, a novel Ig heavy chain enhancer element regulated at multiple stages of B cell differentiation. *Nucleic Acids Res* 1995;23:975–981.

661. Michaelson JS, Singh M, Snapper CM, Sha WC, Baltimore D, Birshtein BK. Regulation of 3′ IgH enhancers by a common set of factors, including kappa B-binding proteins. *J Immunol* 1996;156:2828 2839.

662. Chen J, Young F, Bottaro A, Stewart V, Smith RK, Alt FW. Mutations of the intronic IgH enhancer and its flanking sequences differentially affect accessibility of the JH locus. *EMBO J* 1993;12:4635–4645.

663. Serwe M, Sablitzky F. V(D)J recombination in B cells is impaired but not blocked by targeted deletion of the immunoglobulin heavy chain intron enhancer. *EMBO J* 1993;12:2321–2327.

664. Lieberson R, Ong J, Shi X, Eckhardt LA. Immunoglobulin gene transcription ceases upon deletion of a distant enhancer. *EMBO J* 1995;14:6229–6238.

665. Singh M, Birshtein BK. NF-HB (BSAP) is a repressor of the murine immunoglobulin heavy-chain 3′ alpha enhancer at early stages of B-cell differentiation. *Mol Cell Biol* 1993;13:3611–3622.

666. Arulampalam V, Grant PA, Samuelsson A, Lendahl U, Pettersson S. Lipopolysaccharide-dependent transactivation of the temporally regulated immunoglobulin heavy chain 3′enhancer. *Eur J Immunol* 1994;24:1671–1677.

667. Arulampalam V, Furebring C, Samuelsson A, et al. Elevated expression levels of an Ig transgene in mice links the IgH 3′ enhancer to the regulation of IgH expression. *Int Immunol* 1996;8:1149–1157.

668. Picard D, Schaffner W. A lymphocyte-specific enhancer in the mouse immunoglobulin kappa gene. *Nature* 1984;307:80–82.

669. Queen C, Stafford J. Fine mapping of an immunoglobulin gene activator. *Mol Cell Biol* 1984;4:1042–1049.

670. Chung SY, Folsom V, Wooley J. DNase I-hypersensitive sites in the chromatin of immunoglobulin kappa light chain genes. *Proc Natl Acad Sci USA* 1983;80:2427–2431.

671. Emorine L, Kuehl M, Weir L, Leder P, Max EE. A conserved sequence in the immunoglobulin J kappa-C kappa intron: Possible enhancer element. *Nature* 1983;304:447–449

672. Sen R, Baltimore D. Multiple nuclear factors interact with the immunoglobulin enhancer sequences. *Cell* 1986;46:705–716.

673. Sen R, Baltimore D. Inducibility of kappa immunoglobulin enhancer-binding protein Nf-kappa B by a posttranslational mechanism. *Cell* 1986;47:921–928.

674. Pierce JW, Lenardo M, Baltimore D. Oligonucleotide that binds nuclear factor

NF-kappa B acts as a lymphoid-specific and inducible enhancer element. *Proc Natl Acad Sci USA* 1988;85:1482–1486.

675. Rooney JW, Dubois PM, Sibley CH. Cross-linking of surface IgM activates NF-kappa B in B lymphocyte. *Eur J Immunol* 1991;21:2993–2998.

676. Baeuerle PA, Baltimore D. Activation of DNA-binding activity in an apparently cytoplasmic precursor of the NF-kappa B transcription factor. *Cell* 1988;53: 211–217.

677. Baeuerle PA, Baltimore D. I kappa B: A specific inhibitor of the NF-kappa B transcription factor. *Science* 1988;242:540–546.

678. Baldwin AS. The NF-kB and IkB proteins: New discoveries and insights. *Annu Rev Immunol* 1996;14:649–681.

679. Stephens RM, Rice NR, Hiebsch RR, Bose HJ, Gilden RV. Nucleotide sequence of v-rel: The oncogene of reticuloendotheliosis virus. *Proc Natl Acad Sci USA* 1983;80:6229–6233.

680. Lernbecher T, Muller U, Wirth T. Distinct NF-kappa B/Rel transcription factors are responsible for tissue-specific and inducible gene activation. *Nature* 1993;365:767–770.

681. Liou HC, Sha WC, Scott ML, Baltimore D. Sequential induction of NF-kappa B/Rel family proteins during B-cell terminal differentiation. *Mol Cell Biol* 1994;14:5349–5359.

682. Miyamoto S, Schmitt MJ, Verma IM. Qualitative changes in the subunit composition of kappa B-binding complexes during murine B-cell differentiation. *Proc Natl Acad Sci USA* 1994;91:5056–5060.

683. Davis N, Ghosh S, Simmons DL, et al. Rel-associated pp40: An inhibitor of the rel family of transcription factors. *Science* 1991;253:1268–1271.

684. Haskill S, Beg AA, Tompkins SM, et al. Characterization of an immediate-early gene induced in adherent monocytes that encodes I kappa B-like activity. *Cell* 1991;65:1281–1289.

685. Thompson JE, Phillips RJ, Erdjument BH, Tempst P, Ghosh S. I kappa B-beta regulates the persistent response in a biphasic activation of NF-kappa B. *Cell* 1995;80:573–582.

686. Zhang Q, Didonato JA, Karin M, McKeithan TW. BCL3 encodes a nuclear protein which can alter the subcellular location of NF-kappa B proteins. *Mol Cell Biol* 1994;14:3915–3926.

687. Bours V, Franzoso G, Azarenko V, et al. The oncoprotein Bcl-3 directly transactivates through kappa B motifs via association with DNA-binding p50B homodimers. *Cell* 1993;72:729–739.

688. Fujita T, Nolan GP, Liou HC, Scott ML, Baltimore D. The candidate proto-oncogene bcl-3 encodes a transcriptional coactivator that activates through NF-kappa B p50 homodimers. *Genes Dev* 1993;7:1354–1363.

689. Naumann M, Scheidereit C. Activation of NF-kappa B in vivo is regulated by multiple phosphorylations. *EMBO J* 1994;13:4597–4607.

690. Chen JC, Parent L, Maniatis T. Site-specific phosphorylation of I-kappa B-alpha by a novel ubiquitination-dependent protein kinase activity. *Cell* 1996;84: 853–862.

691. DiDonato JA, Hayakawa M, Rothwarf DM, Zandi E, Karin M. A cytokine-responsive I-kappaB kinase that activates the transcription factor NF-kappaB. *Nature* 1997;388:548–554.

691a. Regnier CH, Song HY, Gao X, Goeddel DV, Cao Z, Rothe M. Identification and characterization of an I-kappa-B kinase. *Cell* 1997;90:373-383.

692. Chen Z, Hagler J, Palombella VJ, et al. Signal-induced site-specific phosphorylation targets I kappa B alpha to the ubiquitin-proteasome pathway. *Genes Dev* 1995;9:1586–1597.

693. Arenzana SF, Thompson J, Rodriguez MS, Bachelerie F, Thomas D, Hay RT. Inducible nuclear expression of newly synthesized I kappa B alpha negatively regulates DNA-binding and transcriptional activities of NF-kappa B. *Mol Cell Biol* 1995;15:2689–2696.

694. Scherer DC, Brockman JA, Bendall HH, Zhang GM, Ballard DW, Oltz EM. Corepression of RelA and c-rel inhibits immunoglobulin kappa gene transcription and rearrangement in precursor B lymphocytes. *Immunity* 1996;5:563–574.

695. Cockerill PN, Garrard WT. Chromosomal loop anchorage of the kappa immunoglobulin gene occurs next to the enhancer in a region containing topoisomerase II sites. *Cell* 1986;44:273–282.

696. Blasquez VC, Xu M, Moses SC, Garrard WT. Immunoglobulin kappa gene expression after stable integration. I. Role of the intronic MAR and enhancer in plasmacytoma cells. *J Biol Chem* 1989;264:21183–21189.

697. Xu M, Hammer RE, Blasquez VC, Jones SL, Garrard WT. Immunoglobulin kappa gene expression after stable integration. II. Role of the intronic MAR and enhancer in transgenic mice. *J Biol Chem* 1989;264:21190–21195.

698. Lichtenstein M, Keini G, Cedar H, Bergman Y. B cell-specific demethylation: A novel role for the intronic kappa chain enhancer sequence. *Cell* 1994;76: 913–923.

699. Kirillov A, Kistler B, Mostoslavsky R, Cedar H, Wirth T, Bergman Y. A role for nuclear NF-kappaB in B-cell-specific demethylation of the Igkappa locus. *Nat Genet* 1996;13:435–441.

700. Schanke JT, Marcuzzi A, Podzorski RP, Van NB. An AP1 binding site upstream of the kappa immunoglobulin intron enhancer binds inducible factors and contributes to expression. *Nucleic Acids Res* 1994;22:5425–5432.

701. Pierce JW, Gifford AM, Baltimore D. Silencing of the expression of the immunoglobulin kappa gene in non-B cells. *Mol Cell Biol* 1991;11:1431–1437.

702. Saksela K, Baltimore D. Negative regulation of immunoglobulin kappa light-chain gene transcription by a short sequence homologous to the murine B1 repetitive element. *Mol Cell Biol* 1993;13:3698–3705.

703. Atchison ML, Perry RP. The role of the kappa enhancer and its binding factor

704. Meyer KB, Neuberger MS. The immunoglobulin kappa locus contains a second, stronger B-cell-specific enhancer which is located downstream of the constant region. *EMBO J* 1989;8:1959–1964.

705. Meyer KB, Sharpe MJ, Surani MA, Neuberger MS. The importance of the 3'-enhancer region in immunoglobulin kappa gene expression. *Nucleic Acids Res* 1990;18:5609–5615.

706. Pongubala JM, Atchison ML. Functional characterization of the developmentally controlled immunoglobulin kappa 3' enhancer: Regulation by Id, a repressor of helix-loop-helix transcription factors. *Mol Cell Biol* 1991;11:1040–1047.

707. Pongubala JM, Nagulapalli S, Klemsz MJ, et al. PU.1 recruits a second nuclear factor to a site important for immunoglobulin kappa 3' enhancer activity. *Mol Cell Biol* 1992;12:368–378.

708. Brass AL, Kehrli E, Eisenbeis CF, Storb U, Singh H. Pip, a lymphoid-restricted IRF, contains a regulatory domain that is important for autoinhibition and ternary complex formation with the Ets factor PU.1. *Genes Dev* 1996;10: 2335–2347.

709. Pongubala JM, Atchison ML. Activating transcription factor 1 and cyclic AMP response element modulator can modulate the activity of the immunoglobulin kappa 3' enhancer. *J Biol Chem* 1995;270:10304–10313.

710. Pongubala JM, Atchison ML. PU.1 can participate in an active enhancer complex without its transcriptional activation domain. *Proc Natl Acad Sci USA* 1997;94: 127–132.

711. Roque MC, Smith PA, Blasquez VC. A developmentally modulated chromatin structure at the mouse immunoglobulin kappa 3' enhancer. *Mol Cell Biol* 1996;16:3138–3155.

712. Costa MW, Atchison ML. Identification of an Spl-like element within the immunoglobulin kappa 3' enhancer necessary for maximal enhancer activity. *Biochemistry* 1996;35:8662–8669.

713. Meyer KB, Ireland J. Activation of the immunoglobulin kappa 3' enhancer in pre-B cells correlates with the suppression of a nuclear factor binding to a sequence flanking the active core. *Nucleic Acids Res* 1994;22:1576–1582.

714. Takeda S, Zou YR, Bluethmann H, Kitamura D, Muller U, Rajewsky K. Deletion of the immunoglobulin kappa chain gene rearrangement in cis but not lambda chain gene rearrangement in trans. *EMBO J* 1993;12:2329–2336.

715. Fulton R, Van Ness B. Kappa immunoglobulin promoters and enhancers display developmentally controlled interactions. *Nucleic Acids Res* 1993;21:4941–4947.

716. Fulton R, van NB. Selective synergy of immunoglobulin enhancer elements in B-cell development: A characteristic of kappa light chain enhancers, but not heavy chain enhancers. *Nucleic Acids Res* 1994;22:4216–4223.

717. Meyer KB, Teh YM, Neuberger MS. The Ig kappa 3'-enhancer triggers gene expression in early B lymphocytes but its activity is enhanced on B cell activation. *Int Immunol* 1996;8:1561–1568.

718. Shaffer AL, Peng A, Schlissel MS. In vivo occupancy of the kappa light chain enhancers in primary pro- and pre-B cells: A model for kappa locus activation. *Immunity* 1997;6:131–141.

719. Hagman J, Rudin CM, Haasch D, Chaplin D, Storb U. A novel enhancer in the immunoglobulin lambda locus is duplicated and functionally independent of NF kappa B. *Genes Dev* 1990;4:978–992.

720. Rudin CM, Storb U. Two conserved essential motifs of the murine immunoglobulin lambda enhancers bind B-cell-specific factors. *Mol Cell Biol* 1992;12: 309–320.

721. Eisenbeis CF, Singh H, Storb U. PU.1 is a component of a multiprotein complex which binds an essential site in the murine immunoglobulin lambda 2-4 enhancer. *Mol Cell Biol* 1993;13:6452–6461.

722. Eisenbeis CF, Singh H, Storb U. Pip, a novel IRF family member, is a lymphoid-specific, PU.1-dependent transcriptional activator. *Genes Dev* 1995;9: 1377–1387.

723. Blomberg BB, Rudin CM, Storb U. Identification and localization of an enhancer for the human lambda L chain Ig gene complex. *J Immunol* 1991;147: 2354–2358.

724. Asenbauer H, Klobeck HG. Tissue-specific deoxyribonuclease I-hypersensitive sites in the vicinity of the immunoglobulin C lambda cluster of man. *Eur J Immunol* 1996;26:142–150.

725. Glozak MA, Blomberg BB. The human lambda immunoglobulin enhancer is controlled by both positive elements and developmentally regulated negative elements. *Mol Immunol* 1996;33:427–438.

726. Chen C, Birshtein BK. Virtually identical enhancers containing a segment of homology to murine 3'IgH-E(hs1,2) lie downstream of human Ig C alpha 1 and C alpha 2 genes. *J Immunol* 1997;159:1310–1318.

727. Pospelov VA, Klobeck HG, Zachau HG. Correlation between DNase I hypersensitive sites and putative regulatory sequences in human immunoglobulin genes of the kappa light chain type. *Nucleic Acids Res* 1984;12:7007–7021.

728. Potter H, Weir L, Leder P. Enhancer-dependent expression of human kappa immunoglobulin genes introduced into mouse pre-B lymphocytes by electroporation. *Proc Natl Acad Sci USA* 1984;81:7161–7165.

729. Gimble JM, Levens D, Max EE. B-cell nuclear proteins binding in vitro to the human immunoglobulin kappa enhancer: Localization by exonuclease protection. *Mol Cell Biol* 1987;7:1815–1822.

730. Judde JG, Max EE. Characterization of the human immunoglobulin kappa gene 3' enhancer: Functional importance of three motifs that demonstrate B-cell-specific in vivo footprints. *Mol Cell Biol* 1992;12:5206–5216.

731. Rabbitts TH, Forster A, Baer R, Hamlyn PH. Transcription enhancer identified near the human C mu immunoglobulin heavy chain gene is unavailable to the translocated c-myc gene in a Burkitt lymphoma. *Nature* 1983;306:806–809.

732. Hayday AC, Gillies SD, Saito H, et al. Activation of a translocated human c-myc gene by an enhancer in the immunoglobulin heavy-chain locus. *Nature* 1984; 307:334–340.

733. Okamura K, Ishiguro H, Ichihara Y, Kurosawa Y. Comparison of nucleotide sequences from upstream of the DQ52 gene to the S mu region of immunoglobulin heavy-chain gene loci between Suncus murinus, mouse and human. *Mol Immunol* 1993;30:461–467.

734. Enjoji M. Human HE2 (microB) and microA motifs show the same function as whole IgH intronic enhancer in transgenic mice. *Mol Cell Biochem* 1994;137: 33–37.

735. Waldmann TA. The arrangement of immunoglobulin and T cell receptor genes in human lymphoproliferative disorders. *Adv Immunol* 1987;40:247–321.

736. Korsmeyer SJ. B-lymphoid neoplasms: immunoglobulin genes as molecular determinants of clonality, lineage, differentiation, and translocation. *Adv Intern Med* 1988;33:1–15.

737. Felix CA, Poplack DG. Characterization of acute lymphoblastic leukemia of childhood by immunoglobulin and T-cell receptor gene patterns. *Leukemia* 1991; 5:1015–1025.

738. Veronese ML, Schichman SA, Croce CM. Molecular diagnosis of lymphoma. *Curr Opin Oncol* 1996;8:346–352.

739. Roberts WM, Estrov Z, Kitchingman GR, Zipf TF. The clinical significance of residual disease in childhood acute lymphoblastic leukemia as detected by polymerase chain reaction amplification by antigen-receptor gene sequences. *Leuk Lymphoma* 1996;20:181–197.

740. Felix CA, Wright JJ, Poplack DG, et al. T cell receptor alpha-, beta-, and gamma genes in T cell and pre-B cell acute lymphoblastic leukemia. *J Clin Invest* 1987;80:545–556.

741. Wright JJ, Poplack DG, Bakhshi A, et al. Gene rearrangements as markers of clonal variation and minimal residual disease in acute lymphoblastic leukemia. *J Clin Oncol* 1987;5:735–741.

742. Croce CM, Shander M, Martinis J, et al. Chromosomal location of the genes for human immunoglobulin heavy chains. *Proc Natl Acad Sci USA* 1979;76: 3416–3419.

743. Taub R, Kelly K, Battey J, et al. A novel alteration in the structure of an activated c-myc gene in a variant t(2;8) Burkitt lymphoma. *Cell* 1984;37:511–520.

744. Showe LC, Croce CM. The role of chromosomal translocations in B- and T-cell neoplasia. *Ann Rev Immunol* 1987;5:253–277.

745. Kato GJ, Lee WM, Chen LL, Dang CV. Max: Functional domains and interaction with c-Myc. *Genes Dev* 1992;6:81–92.

746. Galaktionov K, Chen X, Beach D. Cdc25 cell-cycle phosphatase as a target of c-myc. *Nature* 1996;382:511–517.

747. Schuldiner O, Eden A, Ben YT, Yanuka O, Simchen G, Benvenisty N. ECA39, a conserved gene regulated by c-Myc in mice, is involved in G1/S cell cycle regulation in yeast. *Proc Natl Acad Sci USA* 1996;93:7143–7148.

748. Nishikura K, ar-Rushdi A, Erikson J, Watt R, Rovera G, Croce CM. Differential expression of the normal and of the translocated human c-myc oncogenes in B cells. *Proc Natl Acad Sci USA* 1983;80:4822–4826.

749. Shima EA, Le BM, McKeithan TW, et al. Gene encoding the alpha chain of the T-cell receptor is moved immediately downstream of c-myc in a chromosomal 8;14 translocation in a cell line from a human T-cell leukemia. *Proc Natl Acad Sci USA* 1986;83:3439–3443.

750. Tsujimoto Y, Yunis J, Onorato SL, Erikson J, Nowell PC, Croce CM. Molecular cloning of the chromosomal breakpoint of B-cell lymphomas and leukemias with the t(11;14) chromosome translocation. *Science* 1984;224: 1403–1406.

751. Rosenberg CL, Wong E, Petty EM, et al. PRAD1, a candidate BCL1 oncogene: Mapping and expression in centrocytic lymphoma. *Proc Natl Acad Sci USA* 1991;88:9638–9642.

752. de Boer C, van Krieken J, Schuuring E, Kluin PM. Bcl-1/cyclin D1 in malignant lymphoma. *Ann Oncol* 1997;2:109–117.

753. Tsujimoto Y, Finger LR, Yunis J, Nowell PC, Croce CM. Cloning of the chromosome breakpoint of neoplastic B cells with the t(14;18) chromosome translocation. *Science* 1984;226:1097–1099.

754. Hockenbery D, Nuñez G, Milliman C, Schreiber RD, Korsmeyer SJ. Bcl-2 is an inner mitochondrial membrane protein that blocks programmed cell death. *Nature* 1990;348:334–336.

755. Reed JC. Regulation of apoptosis by bcl-2 family proteins and its role in cancer and chemoresistance. *Curr Opin Oncol* 1995;7:541–546.

756. Hockenbery DM, Zutter M, Hickey W, Nahm M, Korsmeyer SJ. BCL2 protein is topographically restricted in tissues characterized by apoptotic cell death. *Proc Natl Acad Sci USA* 1991;88:6961–6965.

757. McDonnell TJ, Deane N, Platt FM, et al. bcl-2-immunoglobulin transgenic mice demonstrate extended B cell survival and follicular lymphoproliferation. *Cell* 1989;57:79–88.

758. McKeithan TW, Rowley JD, Shows TB, Diaz MO. Cloning of the chromosome translocation breakpoint junction of the t(14;19) in chronic lymphocytic leukemia. *Proc Natl Acad Sci USA* 1987;84:9257–9260.

759. Michaux L, Dierlamm J, Wlodarska I, et al. t(14;19)/BCL3 rearrangements in lymphoproliferative disorders: A review of 23 cases. *Cancer Genet Cytogenet* 1997;94:36–43.

760. Ohno H, Takimoto G, McKeithan TW. The candidate proto-oncogene bcl-3 is related to genes implicated in cell lineage determination and cell cycle control. *Cell* 1990;60:991–997.

761. Baron BW, Nucifora G, McCabe N, Espinosa Rd, Le BM, McKeithan TW. Identification of the gene associated with the recurring chromosomal translocations t(3;14)(q27;q32) and t(3;22)(q27;q11) in B-cell lymphomas. *Proc Natl Acad Sci USA* 1993;90:5262–5266.

762. Seyfert VL, Allman D, He Y, Staudt LM. Transcriptional repression by the proto-oncogene BCL-6. *Oncogene* 1996;12:2331–2342.

763. Allman D, Jain A, Dent A, et al. BCL-6 expression during B-cell activation. *Blood* 1996;87:5257–5268.

764. Dent AL, Shaffer AL, Yu X, Allman D, Staudt LM. Control of inflammation, cytokine expression, and germinal center formation by BCL-6. *Science* 1997; 276:589–592.

765. Ye BH, Cattoretti G, Shen Q, et al. The BCL-6 proto-oncogene controls germinal-centre formation and Th2- type inflammation. *Nat Genet* 1997;16:161–170.

766. Zani VJ, Asou N, Jadayel D, et al. Molecular cloning of complex chromosomal translocation t(8;14;12)(q24.1;q32.3;q24.1) in a Burkitt lymphoma cell line defines a new gene (BCL7A) with homology to caldesmon. *Blood* 1996;87: 3124–3134.

767. Dyomin VG, Rao PH, Dalla-Favera R, Chaganti R. BCL8, a novel gene involved in translocations affecting band 15q11-13 in diffuse large-cell lymphoma. *Proc Natl Acad Sci USA* 1997;94:5728–5732.

768. Akasaka T, Muramatsu M, Ohno H, et al. Application of long-distance polymerase chain reaction to detection of junctional sequences created by chromosomal translocation in mature B-cell neoplasms. *Blood* 1996;88:985–994.

769. Denny CT, Yoshikai Y, Mak TW, Smith SD, Hollis GF, Kirsch IR. A chromosome 14 inversion in a T-cell lymphoma is caused by site-specific recombination between immunoglobulin and T-cell receptor loci. *Nature* 1986;320: 549–551.

770. Baer R, Forster A, Rabbitts TH. The mechanism of chromosome 14 inversion in a human T cell lymphoma. *Cell* 1987;50:97–105.

771. Lipkowitz S, Garry VF, Kirsch IR. Interlocus V-J recombination measures genomic instability in agriculture workers at risk for lymphoid malignancies. *Proc Natl Acad Sci USA* 1992;89:5301–5305.

772. Stavnezer-Nordgren J, Kekish O, Zegers BJ. Molecular defects in a human immunoglobulin kappa chain deficiency. *Science* 1985;230:458–461.

772a.Yel L, Minegishi Y, Coustan SE, et al. Mutations in the mu heavy-chain gene in patients with agammaglobulinemia. *N Engl J Med* 1996;335:1486–1493.

773. Humphries CG, Shen A, Kuziel WA, Capra JD, Blattner FR, Tucker PW. A new human immunoglobulin VH family preferentially rearranged in immature B-cell tumours. *Nature* 1988;331:446–449.

774. Chen PP, Siminovitch KA, Olsen NJ, Erger RA, Carson DA. A highly informative probe for two polymorphic Vh gene regions that contain one or more autoantibody-associated Vh genes. *J Clin Invest* 1989;84:706–710.

775. Sanz I, Kelly P, Williams C, Scholl S, Tucker P, Capra JD. The smaller human VH gene families display remarkably little polymorphism. *EMBO J* 1989;8: 3741–3748.

776. Shin EK, Matsuda F, Nagaoka H, et al. Physical map of the 3′ region of the human immunoglobulin heavy chain locus: Clustering of autoantibody-related variable segments in one haplotype. *EMBO J* 1991;10:3641–3645.

777. Walter MA, Gibson WT, Ebers GC, Cox DW. Susceptibility to multiple sclerosis is associated with the proximal immunoglobulin heavy chain variable region. *J Clin Invest* 1991;87:1266–1273.

778. Moxley G. DNA polymorphism of immunoglobulin kappa confers risk of rheumatoid arthritis. *Arthritis Rheum* 1989;32:634–637.

779. Meindl A, Klobeck HG, Ohnheiser R, Zachau HG. The V kappa gene repertoire in the human germ line. *Eur J Immunol* 1990;20:1855–1863.

780. Feeney AJ, Atkinson MJ, Cowan MJ, Escuro G, Lugo G. A defective Vkappa A2 allele in Navajos which may play a role in increased susceptibility to haemophilus influenzae type b disease. *J Clin Invest* 1996;97:2277–2282.

781. Baker MD, Wu GE, Toone WM, Murialdo H, Davis AC, Shulman MJ. A region of the immunoglobulin-mu heavy chain necessary for forming pentameric IgM. *J Immunol* 1986;137:1724–1728.

782. Shulman MJ, Collins C, Pennell N, Hozumi N. Complement activation by IgM: Evidence for the importance of the third constant domain of the mu heavy chain. *Eur J Immunol* 1987;17:549–554.

783. Tao MH, Canfield SM, Morrison SL. The differential ability of human IgG1 and IgG4 to activate complement is determined by the COOH terminal sequence of the CH2 domain. *J Exp Med* 1991;173:1025–1028.

784. Duncan AR, Winter G. The binding site for C1q on IgG. *Nature* 1988;332: 738–740.

785. Helm B, Marsh P, Vercelli D, Padlan E, Gould H, Geha R. The mast cell binding site on human immunoglobulin E. *Nature* 1988;331:180–183.

786. Roberts S, Cheetham JC, Rees AR. Generation of an antibody with enhanced affinity and specificity for its antigen by protein engineering. *Nature* 1987;328: 731–734.

787. Boulianne GL, Hozumi N, Shulman MJ. Production of functional chimaeric mouse/human antibody. *Nature* 1984;312:643–646.

788. Morrison SL. Transfectomas provide novel chimeric antibodies. *Science* 1985; 229:1202–1207.

789. Liu AY, Robinson RR, Murray EJ, Ledbetter JA, Hellstrom I, Hellstrom KE. Production of a mouse-human chimeric monoclonal antibody to CD20 with potent Fc-dependent biologic activity. *J Immunol* 1987;139:3521–3526.

790. Jones PT, Dear PH, Foote J, Neuberger MS, Winter G. Replacing the comple-

mentarity-determining regions in a human antibody with those from a mouse. *Nature* 1986;321:522–525.

791. Co MS, Avdalovic NM, Caron PC, Avdalovic MV, Scheinberg DA, Queen C. Chimeric and humanized antibodies with specificity for the CD33 antigen. *J Immunol* 1992;148:1149–1154.

792. Mendez MJ, Green LL, Corvalan JR, et al. Functional transplant of megabase human immunoglobulin loci recapitulates human antibody response in mice. *Nat Genet* 1997;15:146–156.

793. Desmyter A, Transue TR, Ghahroudi MA, et al. Crystal structure of a camel single-domain VH antibody fragment in complex with lysozyme. *Nat Struct Biol* 1996;3:803–811.

794. Bird RE, Hardman KD, Jacobson JW, et al. Single-chain antigen-binding proteins. *Science* 1988;242:423–426.

795. Huston JS, Levinson D, Mudgett HM, et al. Protein engineering of antibody binding sites: Recovery of specific activity in an anti-digoxin single-chain Fv analogue produced in *Escherichia coli*. *Proc Natl Acad Sci USA* 1988;85:5879–5883.

796. Clackson T, Hoogenboom HR, Griffiths AD, Winter G. Making antibody fragments using phage display libraries. *Nature* 1991;352:624–628.

797. Kang AS, Barbas CF, Janda KD, Benkovic SJ, Lerner RA. Linkage of recognition and replication functions by assembling combinatorial antibody Fab libraries along phage surfaces. *Proc Natl Acad Sci USA* 1991;88:4363–4366.

798. Huse WD, Stinchcombe TJ, Glaser SM, et al. Application of a filamentous phage pVIII fusion protein system suitable for efficient production, screening and mutagenesis of F(ab) antibody fragments. *J Immunol* 1992;149:3914–3920.

799. Yelton DE, Rosok MJ, Cruz G, et al. Affinity maturation of the BR96 anti-carcinoma antibody by codon-based mutagenesis. *J Immunol* 1995;155:1994–2004.

800. Crameri A, Cwirla S, Stemmer WP. Construction and evolution of antibody-phage libraries by DNA shuffling. *Nat Med* 1996;2:100–102.

801. Orlandi R, Gussow DH, Jones PT, Winter G. Cloning immunoglobulin variable domains for expression by the polymerase chain reaction. *Proc Natl Acad Sci USA* 1989;86:3833–3837.

802. Persic L, Roberts A, Wilton J, Cattaneo A, Bradbury A, Hoogenboom HR. An integrated vector system for the eukaryotic expression of antibodies or their fragments after selection from phage display libraries. *Gene* 1997;187:9–18.

803. Caron PC, Laird W, Co MS, Avdalovic NM, Queen C, Scheinberg DA. Engineered humanized dimeric forms of IgG are more effective antibodies. *J Exp Med* 1992;176:1191–1195.

804. Pollack SJ, Jacobs JW, Schultz PG. Selective chemical catalysis by an antibody. *Science* 1986;234:1570–1573.

805. Tramontano A, Janda KD, Lerner RA. Catalytic antibodies. *Science* 1986;234:1566–1570.

806. Gibbs RA, Posner BA, Filpula DR, et al. Construction and characterization of a single-chain catalytic antibody. *Proc Natl Acad Sci USA* 1991;88:4001–4004.

807. Jackson DY, Prudent JR, Baldwin EP, Schultz PG. A mutagenesis study of a catalytic antibody. *Proc Natl Acad Sci USA* 1991;88:58–62.

808. Tang Y, Hicks JB, Hilvert D. In vivo catalysis of a metabolically essential reaction by an antibody. *Proc Natl Acad Sci USA* 1991;88:8784–8786.

809. Schnee JM, Runge MS, Matsueda GR, et al. Construction and expression of a recombinant antibody-targeted plasminogen activator. *Proc Natl Acad Sci USA* 1987;84:6904–6908.

810. Thrush GR, Lark LR, Clinchy BC, Vitetta ES. Immunotoxins: An update. *Annu Rev Immunol* 1996;14:49–71.

811. Staerz UD, Bevan MJ. Hybrid hybridoma producing a bispecific monoclonal antibody that can focus effector T-cell activity. *Proc Natl Acad Sci USA* 1986;83:1453–1457.

812. Suresh MR, Cuello AC, Milstein C. Advantages of bispecific hybridomas in one-step immunocytochemistry and immunoassays. *Proc Natl Acad Sci USA* 1986;83:7989–7993.

813. Mallender WD, Voss EJ. Construction, expression, and activity of a bivalent bispecific single-chain antibody. *J Biol Chem* 1994;269:199–206.

814. Staunton DE, Ockenhouse CF, Springer TA. Soluble intercellular adhesion molecule 1-immunoglobulin G1 immunoadhesin mediates phagocytosis of malaria-infected erythrocytes. *J Exp Med* 1992;176:1471–1476.

815. Martin S, Casasnovas JM, Staunton DE, Springer TA. Efficient neutralization and disruption of rhinovirus by chimeric ICAM-1/immunoglobulin molecules. *J Virol* 1993;67:3561–3568.

816. Hasemann CA, Capra JD. High-level production of a functional immunoglobulin heterodimer in a baculovirus expression system. *Proc Natl Acad Sci USA* 1990;87:3942–3946.

817. Ma JK, Hiatt A, Hein M, et al. Generation and assembly of secretory antibodies in plants. *Science* 1995;268:716–719.

818. Mhashilkar AM, Bagley J, Chen SY, Szilvay AM, Helland DG, Marasco WA. Inhibition of HIV-1 Tat-mediated LTR transactivation and HIV-1 infection by anti-Tat single chain intrabodies. *EMBO J* 1995;14:1542–1551.

819. Knight KL, Spieker PH, Kazdin DS, Oi VT. Transgenic rabbits with lymphocytic leukemia induced by the c-myc oncogene fused with the immunoglobulin heavy chain enhancer. *Proc Natl Acad Sci USA* 1988;85:3130–3134.

820. Schmidt EV, Pattengale PK, Weir L, Leder P. Transgenic mice bearing the human c-myc gene activated by an immunoglobulin enhancer: A pre-B-cell lymphoma model. *Proc Natl Acad Sci USA* 1988;85:6047–6051.

821. Maxwell IH, Glode LM, Maxwell F. Expression of the diphtheria toxin A-chain coding sequence under the control of promoters and enhancers from immunoglobulin genes as a means of directing toxicity to B-lymphoid cells. *Cancer Res* 1991;51:4299–4304.

822. Pascual V, Capra JD. Human immunoglobulin heavy-chain variable region genes: Organization, polymorphism, and expression. *Adv Immunol* 1991;49:1–74.

823. Miwa H, Nosaka T, Kita K, et al. Immunogenotypes of lymphoid malignancies: The rearrangement of T cell receptor beta chain gene can occur before the gamma chain gene rearrangement. *Jpn J Cancer Res* 1988;79:484–490.

824. Max EE, Maizel JJ, Leder P. The nucleotide sequence of a 5.5-kilobase DNA segment containing the mouse kappa immunoglobulin J and C region genes. *J Biol Chem* 1981;256:5116–5120.

Fundamental Immunology, Fourth Edition,
edited by William E. Paul
Lippincott–Raven Publishers, Philadelphia © 1999.

CHAPTER 6

B-Lymphocyte Development and Biology

Fritz Melchers and Antonius Rolink

Diverse repertoires of antibodies, synonymously called immunoglobulins (Ig), are produced by B lymphocytes. B denotes their origin from bone marrow in mouse, humans, and other mammals, and from the bursa of Fabricius in birds. Ig molecules are made up of heavy (H) and light (L) chains, both of which have at their amino-terminal ends an Ig domain, which, in its structure, is variable (V) from one Ig to another. With these V regions, Ig molecules bind antigens. The specificity for antigen binding is made up of three complementarity-determining regions (CDRs). A majority of all B-lymphocytes displays a single combination of H and L chains with a unique set of CDRs, out of an endless number of possible combinations in the total repertoire of Ig molecules (see Chapters 3 and 4).

The diversity of antigen-binding V regions of Ig molecules is generated on the DNA level by successive rearrangements of gene segments, by insertion of P- and N-region sequences at the joints, and, potentially, by replacements of V segments within a rearranged V_H or V_L gene by other V segments (see Chapter 5). The majority of all B lymphocytes manages to rearrange only one of the two H- and L-chain alleles productively, and, hence, allelically excludes the expression of two IgH- and L-chain alleles. Consequently, the total available repertoire of antigen-recognizing Ig molecules is limited by the total number of Ig-producing B cells in the immune system.

Ig molecules can be expressed on the surface of B lymphocytes, in short called *B cells,* where they act as receptors to bind antigen-so-called B-cell receptors (BCRs). Exposure to antigen of a mature B cell can initiate the proliferation and maturation of clones, and can result in the formation of so-called plasma cells that secrete Ig molecules into the bloodstream. During the proliferation and maturation of B cells, the structure of the Ig molecules can be altered by (a) changes at the DNA level through somatic V-gene hypermutation, (b) conversion of the V_H and V_L gene regions, and (c) somatic recombination of the constant (C) regions of the H-chain genes in a process called *class switching* (see Chapters 7, 24, and 25).

As defense against an invader, the Ig molecules in the bloodstream are the antigen-specific, essential components of a humoral response of the immune system. Immunodeficiencies that affect the production of B cells and antibodies demonstrate the importance of humoral immunity (see Chapter 43). Without B cells and antibody production, humans are only protected against bacterial and other infectious diseases if they are given injections of Ig from donors, which hopefully responds against the same invaders (see Chapters 38, 39, 40, and 41). By binding to antigen, Ig molecules can fix and activate complement (see Chapter 29). At the surface of an antigen expressing invader (e.g., a bacterium), the Ig–complement complex

F. Melchers and A. Rolink: Basel Institute for Immunology, CH-4005 Basel, Switzerland.

can induce the formation of pores in the cell membrane which lyse the invading cell. Ig molecules in the form of immune complexes can also bind to F_c receptors on monocytes, macrophages, eosinophils, basophils, mast cells, and natural killer (NK) cells. Binding of immune complexes activates these cells of the innate immune system, with the result that they fight the invader by the powers of phagocytosis, cytolysis, and inflammation.

B cells develop at specific sites, called *primary lymphoid organs.* They develop from pluripotent hematopoietic stem cells (HSC), from which all the different blood-cell lineages develop. B-cell development can be subdivided into different phases. First, cells become committed to the B lineage of differentiation; thereafter, they rearrange the gene segments of the Ig H- and L-chain gene loci to produce immunoglobulins, which are deposited on B cells. The emerging repertoire of Ig-expressing B cells is then screened against specificities for autoantigens present in the primary lymphoid organs, a process called *negative selection,* leading to central tolerance. A small part of all remaining surface Ig (sIg)-expressing B cells is then allowed to emigrate from the primary into the secondary peripheral lymphoid organs (positive selection). The repertoires of sIg$^+$ B cells are once more screened against autoantigens not present in the primary lymphoid organ, but now present in the periphery (negative selection, leading to peripheral tolerance) (see Chapter 20). Only a small proportion of the immature B cells is selected into the pool of long-lived, recirculating B cells (positive selection).

During negative selection, sIg-expressing B cells reacting to autoantigens results in the death (apoptosis; see Chapters 20 and 23) or the induction of an anergic state in these B cells. Mature B cells, on the other hand, have changed their reactivity to antigen to enter proliferation, maturation to Ig-secreting cells, and generation of memory B cells. For many of the steps of this cellular development from HSCs to plasma cells and memory cells, cooperation with other cells in the environment, first with stromal cells in the primary lymphoid organs and last with helper T cells, macrophages, dendritic cells, and follicular dendritic cells in the germinal center of secondary lymphoid organs, is mandatory.

This chapter is concerned with the development of B lymphocytes from HSCs through commitment, BCR expression, cellular expansion, migration, and negative and positive selection, to the stage of a mature, antigen-reactive B cell, ready to enter T cell-dependent or T cell-independent antigenic stimulation. This development is extensively studied in mice. We therefore describe foremost the development of B cells in the mouse.

B-lymphocyte development in humans is very similar to that in mice. However, the description of B-cell development in other mammals and in birds illuminates strategies of generating and maintaining B-cell repertoires that appear to differ from those in mice and humans.

B-CELL DEVELOPMENT IN THE MOUSE

Embryonic Development and Adult Regeneration of Pluripotent Hematopoietic Stem Cells

At days 6 to 7 of mouse embryogenesis, the three germ layers—endoderm, ectoderm, and mesoderm—are formed (Fig. 1). Mesoderm is generated by the migration of epiblastic cells (ectoderm) through the primitive streak underlying the primitive endoderm, thus generating the intermediate layer of cells called *mesoderm.* After lateral expansion, mesoderm expands first in the posterior, then in the anterior direction. Intraembryonic mesoderm then

develops, among others, progenitors of endothelial cardiac cells, muscle cells, and hematopoietic cells (1). The putative common precursors of endothelial and hematopoietic cells are called hemangioblasts (2). It is the intraembryonic splanchnopleura at day 7 to 7.5 from which the aorta–gonad–mesonephros (AGM) region develops at day 10, at which HSC formation is initiated and expanded (3) (see Fig. 1). It is thought that these HSCs might rapidly colonize the yolk sac, where the first erythromyeloid cell generation is initiated. Lymphocytes, however, do not appear to be generated from yolk sac (4). HSCs from the AGM area can be put into tissue culture, where, after a first step lasting several days, the resulting cells can be cultured in a second step under conditions that favor either T-, B-, or myeloid-cell development (5). Such experiments show that the HSCs from the splanchnopleura at day 7 to 7.5 (i.e., before establishment of embryonic circulation) can give rise to erythroid, myeloid, as well as T and B lymphoid cells.

Pluripotent HSCs have been defined in a variety of experimental systems by their genotype, which distinguishes them and all their descendents from the host in which they grow up (6–14). The existence of pluripotent HSCs can also be deduced from experiments in which HSCs were marked by a specific chromosomal translocation or by a retroviral insertion (15,16). They show that a single HSC, characterized by a unique translocation or integration event, can populate all blood-cell lineages, including T and B lineages. However, they also show that the population of cell lineages is not stable and will change in different compartments at different times from marked to unmarked cells (17,18). This suggests that different HSCs are active in repopulating the lineages at different times during life. Often, not all lineages carry the marked chromosomes. This indicates different turnover rates in the different hematopoietic compartments and/or suggests that progenitor cells with renewal capacities exist that are not pluripotent but are already committed to a more or less diverse part of all hematopoietic lineages.

Embryonic stem cells (ES cells) can be used to study the commitment of primitive ectoderm to mesoderm and its subsequent development of HSCs *in vitro.* ES cells can be grown in tissue culture (19–21). ES cell lines can develop into embryoid bodies in which blood islands form. Further *in vitro* cultures of disintegrated embryoid bodies can develop erythroid, myeloid, and lymphoid cells (22–24).

ES cells can also be genetically altered *in vitro* by heterologous or homologous integration of a gene at any site in the chromosomes (25) or at the homologous site of the endogenous copy of the gene (26). These genetically altered ES cells can be injected into mouse blastocysts and the mixed blastocysts implanted into a foster mother (27,28). The offspring is chimeric. Whenever germ cells are generated from the injected ES cells, the chimeric mouse can be the founder of a new, transgenic mouse strain, carrying the integrated ES-derived mutation (29).

Injection of ES cells into blastocysts can also be used to study the effects of embryonally or neonatally lethal mutations in the lymphocytic pathway of differentiation. In this so-called blastocyst complementation assay, blastocysts of recombinase-activating gene 1 or 2–deficient (RAG-1$^{-/-}$ or RAG-2$^{-/-}$) mice are injected with ES cells carrying such lethal mutations, introduced by homologous recombination. Since the RAG mutations abolish T- and B-lymphocyte development at a point just after lineage commitment, any more mature lymphocytes developing in these mice must derive from the mutated ES cells (30). Therefore, any mutation affecting B- (and T-) lymphocyte development after the block introduced by the RAG$^{-/-}$ mutations becomes detectable.

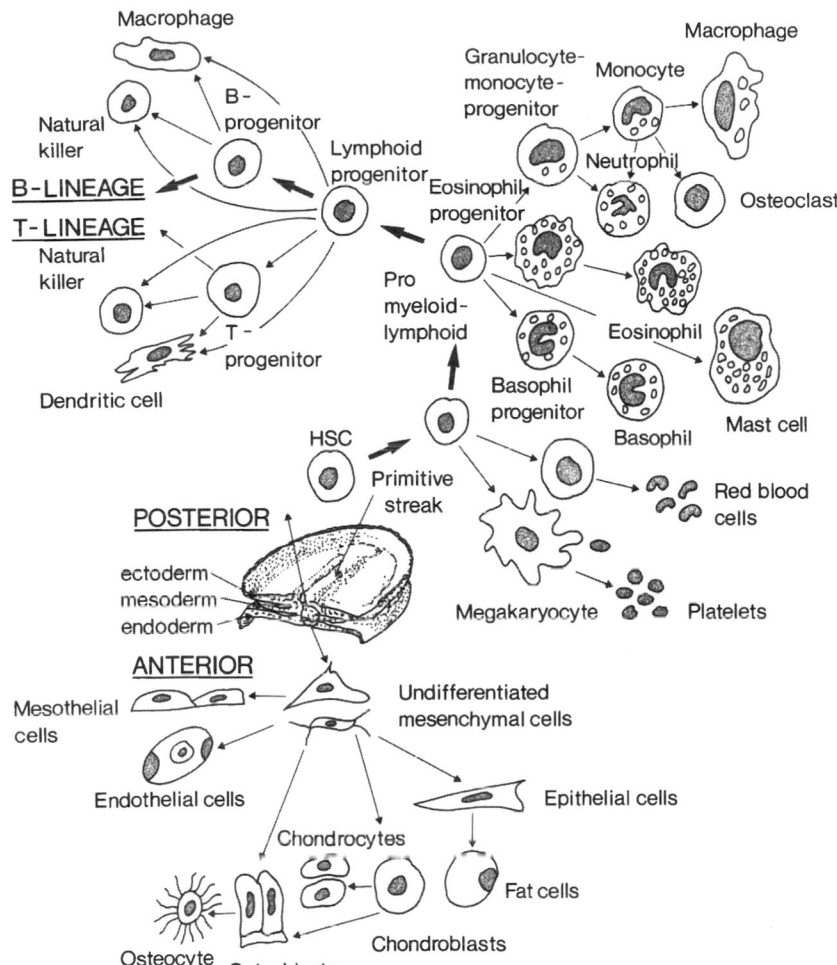

FIG. 1. B-lineage cell development from intraembryonic mesoderm through HSC and early erythroid–myeloid–lymphoid progenitor stages.

Hierarchies of Early Hematopoiesis

HSCs are defined as cells with self-renewing capacity, also after transplantation, which are capable of generating all erythro-, myelo-, and lymphocytic cell lineages. The stringent test for transplantability of HSC as HSC is a second transplantation from the primary transplant (31–36). The state of an HSC appears to be unstable when it is removed from its natural environment during these primary and secondary adoptive transfers, so that adoptive transfers from transplanted hosts are often much less successful (37). In principle, however, one HSC should retain the capacity and only one HSC should be sufficient to repopulate all hematopoietic lineages in a host for long periods of time.

HSCs have been characterized in mouse and human. In general, they do not express the markers that are specific for the different lineages of blood cells (e.g., CD19 for the B lineage, or Mac-1 for the macrophage lineage), hence they are lin$^-$ (i.e., lineage marker–negative). In the mouse, they are Sca-1$^+$ (38), c-kit^{low}, major histocompatibility complex (MHC) class I^{high}, CD71$^-$ (39), and VLA-4$^+$ (see ref. 4).

HSCs have not yet been grown in tissue culture. Hence, it is not known how often an HSC can divide and maintain its stem-cell state of differentiation. HSCs can be mobilized *in vivo* so that they appear in the bloodstream, ready to be collected for transplantation.

Stem-cell factor (SCF) (40,41), granulocyte colony-forming factor (G-CSF) (40), interleukin-8 (IL-8) (42,43), and antibodies specific for α4 integrin (44,45) are among the mobilizing reagents. Requirements for HSC mobilization can vary during fetal and adult hematopoiesis (46). It is highly likely that these mobilization strategies also activate the emergence of progenitors that are not fully pluripotent, but already committed to (a) certain lineage(s) of blood cells. Hence, SCF and IL-7 are likely to mobilize lymphoid and B lineage–committed progenitors (47,48).

HSCs can be induced to differentiate in colonies *in vitro* into the different blood-cell lineages (49). The combination of SCF and IL-6 or IL-11 or G-CSF has been found in a two-step culture system to offer optimal conditions for the generation of B-lineage cells (50). The signal-transducing gp130 subunit of the IL-6 receptor and c-kit synergize *in vitro* in the expansion of HSCs (51). The flt-3 ligand promotes their survival (52).

Decisions for Hematopoietic Stem-Cell Formation

The patterns of expression of a series of transcription factors in early hematopoietic cells and their subsequent inactivation by homologous recombination with a defective copy have been instrumental in ordering the early hierarchies of developmental pathways in hematopoiesis. Blastocyst complementation assays (30) have revealed that Rbtn-1 (53), TAL-1 (54), and GATA-2 (55–57) defective mice appear to have a general deficiency for all hematopoietic cell lineages so far known (Figs. 2 and 3). The target genes for these transcription factors involved in those early steps of hematopoiesis still need to be found. Also, the blastocyst complementation assay does not distinguish between mutations that completely abrogate development and mutations that only slow down development, since in the host RAG$^{-/-}$ mice, erythromyelocytic development is normal and lymphocytic development also remains normal to the stage of T and B lineage–committed precursors (see below). Hence, developing mutant hematopoietic progenitors must compete with, and might often be outgrown by, the endogenous, normal progenitors of the RAG$^{-/-}$ hosts.

Migrations of Hematopoietic Stem Cells to Competent Sites of Hematopoietic Differentiation

HSCs are expected to migrate during embryonic development from sites where they are generated (i.e., in the splanchnopleura and in the AGM area) to sites where primitive hematopoiesis with the generation of red cells producing fetal hemoglobin occurs (i.e., to yolk sac) and later to sites where definitive erythropoiesis of red cells producing adult hemoglobin develops (58,59). GATA-1 is essential for establishing primitive as well as definitive erythropoiesis (60,61). AML-1, CBF-β, and EKLF mutant mice all allow primitive erythropoiesis but are defective in definitive erythropoiesis (62–64) (see Fig. 2).

One day after the first HSCs have been formed, embryonic blood circulation is established at day 8 of gestation. The number of HSCs increases until day 10 in the AGM area, to decline thereafter (Fig. 4). From day 9 onward, progenitors of B-lineage cells have been detected in embryonic blood (5,65,66). They are most frequent at day 12, and then disappear. It appears reasonable to expect that HSCs migrate via the embryonic circulation to the embryonic sites (fetal liver, thymus, omentum, bone marrow), where they find the appropriate environment to be induced to a specialized program of erythroid, myeloid, or lymphoid differentiation. This migration is impaired in β$_1$-integrin$^{-/-}$ mice (67).

Flk-1$^{-/-}$ mice are defective in endothelial cell development and in vasculogenesis. Furthermore, in ES cell blastocyst complementation assay, it becomes evident that the Flk-1$^{-/-}$ cells also do not contribute to primitive erythropoiesis or definite erythropoiesis and lymphopoiesis. The progenitors cannot reach their sites of hematopoietic differentiation (a) because the blood vessels do not form and (b) because the Flk$^{-/-}$ progenitors are unable to migrate. Flk-1 therefore appears to be involved in the migration of cells from the primitive mesoderm (see Fig. 1) to the yolk sac as well as to the intraembryonic sites of early hematopoiesis (68).

Decisions between Myeloid–Lymphoid and Megakaryocyte–Platelet Differentiation

In the next step of hematopoietic differentiation, cells appear to have the option to become megakaryocytes and platelets or to retain the potential to become either myeloid or lymphoid cells (see Figs. 2 and 3). This is exemplified in PU-1 mutant mice. PU-1 is a transcription factor of the ets-domains protein family encoded by the Spi-1 protooncogene, which is specifically expressed in hematopoietic cells (69–72). Target genes for regulation of expression by PU-1 include the μH-chain gene (73), the L-chain gene (74,75), the mb-1 gene encoding Igα (75,76), and the J-chain gene (77). The mutation of the Spi-1 gene involving the deletion of the exon

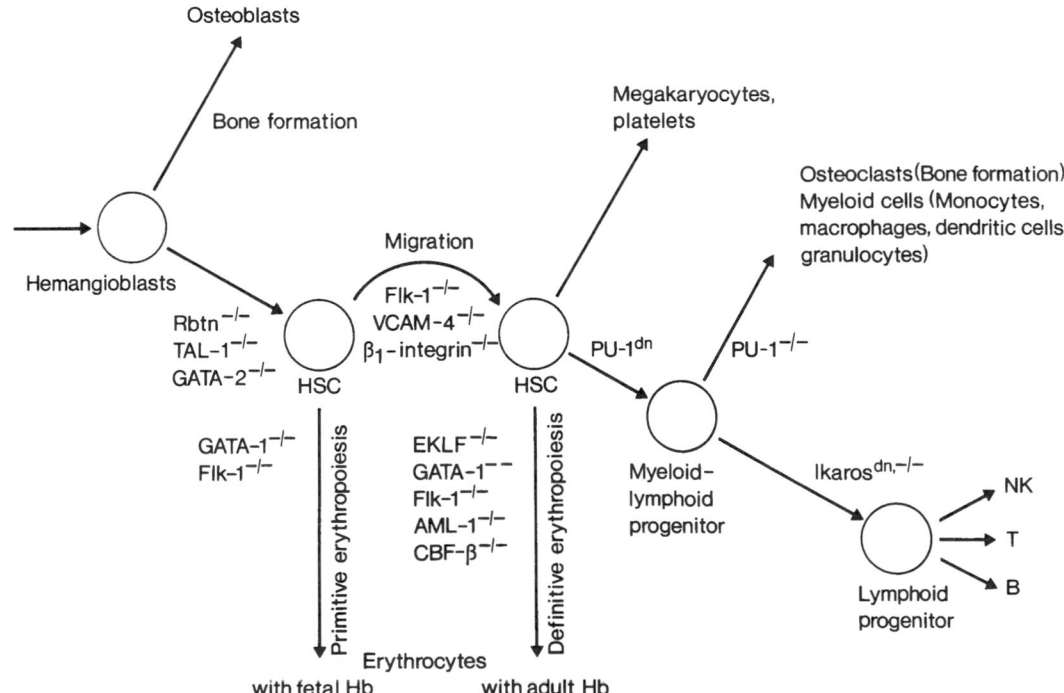

FIG. 2. Genes controlling early hematopoiesis. dn, dominant negative; –/–, homozygous defective. For details, see the text.

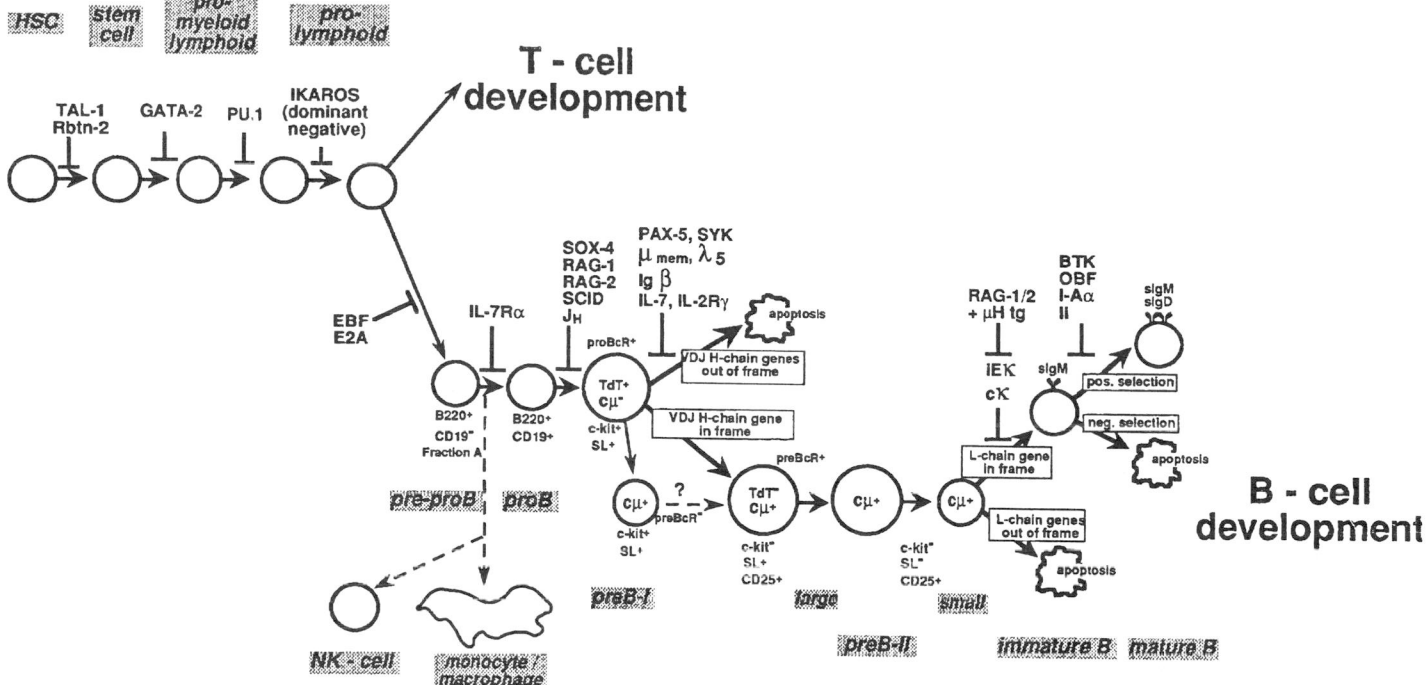

FIG. 3. Genes controlling B-lymphocyte lineage development in the mouse. For details, see the text. Large cells are predominantly in cell cycle; small cells are resting. Steps at which maturation is arrested in gene knockout mice are indicated (e.g., TAL-1 and Rbtn-2 knockouts prevent HSC maturation to stem cell).

encoding the ets-DNA binding domain might exert its effects in a dominant-negative fashion by possibly replacing the normal form of the PU-1 protein in complexes with other transcription factors. These mutant PU-1 mice develop erythrocytes, megakaryocytes, and platelets normally, but they have a severe deficiency in the development of myeloid cells, NK cells, T cells, and B cells (72,78). The block in lineage differentiation appears to be complete for the B lineage, while the mutant mice generate small numbers of neutrophils and some T-lineage cells, with age.

PU-1⁻/⁻ mutant mice, in which the expression of the Spi-1 gene has been deleted altogether, show a phenotype that is different from that of the mouse in which only the DNA binding domain has been deleted (69,79). In this null mutant mouse, the formation of macrophages and osteoclasts is inhibited (see Figs. 2 and 3). The latter defect leads to osteopetrosis. This defect can be rescued by transplantation of wild-type bone marrow cells, showing that it is cell-autonomous and that osteoclasts (and hence parts of bone formation) (see previous discussion of decisions for HSC formation) are likely to originate from a common hematopoietic progenitor (80–82). Final proof for this common progenitor, however, must await the transplantation of a single multipotent progenitor that can repair both defects.

Decisions for Lymphoid Differentiation

The decisions to enter the T- and B-lymphoid lineages of development appear controlled by the Ikaros gene (see Figs. 2 and 3). Lymphoid cell development is abrogated by a mutation of the Ikaros gene in which the high-affinity DNA-binding domain has been deleted (83). The Ikaros gene encodes a family of zinc finger DNA-binding proteins that are products of alternate splicing. Four

of the five alternate forms of proteins contain a low-avidity DNA-binding site at their amino-terminal and a high-affinity DNA-binding site at their carboxy-terminal end (84). The mutation, in which the high-affinity DNA-binding domain has been deleted, acts in a dominant-negative fashion, replacing the wild-type form in complexes with other transcription factors. Targets for the Ikaros transcription factor(s) include (a) essential components of the gene rearrangement machinery (i.e., the RAG and TdT genes), (b) the IgH- and L-chain genes, (c) the mb-1 gene encoding Igα, as well as (d) members of the CD3 complex (i.e., essential elements of the antigen-sensitive receptor complexes, TCR and BCR, and their precursor forms). This suggests that, in fact, the Ikaros dominant-negative form of mutation may be effective in generating the observed deficient phenotype by interfering with the expression of the rearrangement machinery and with early forms of TCR and BCR complex expression. In these mice, the development of erythrocytes, megakaryocytes, platelets, and myeloid cells is normal, but NK cells and T- and B-cell lineages are severely deficient. Again, the block in B-lineage development appears to be complete, since even the earliest committed B-lineage precursors are absent. The block in T-lineage development is less complete because, with age, small numbers of early T-lineage cells can be found.

The Ikaros⁻/⁻ null mutation, in which the expression of the whole gene has been abrogated, differs in phenotype. Mice homozygous for this mutation are defective in fetal T- and B-lineage development, as well as in adult B-cell development. They also lack large parts of NK cells, subsets of γ/δ TCR T cells and thymic dendritic cells. However, postnatally, CD4⁺ T cells appear to expand with age (85). It is therefore not unreasonable to expect that many of these hematopoietic deficiency inducing transcription factor gene mutations can be complemented, though at low efficiency, by another

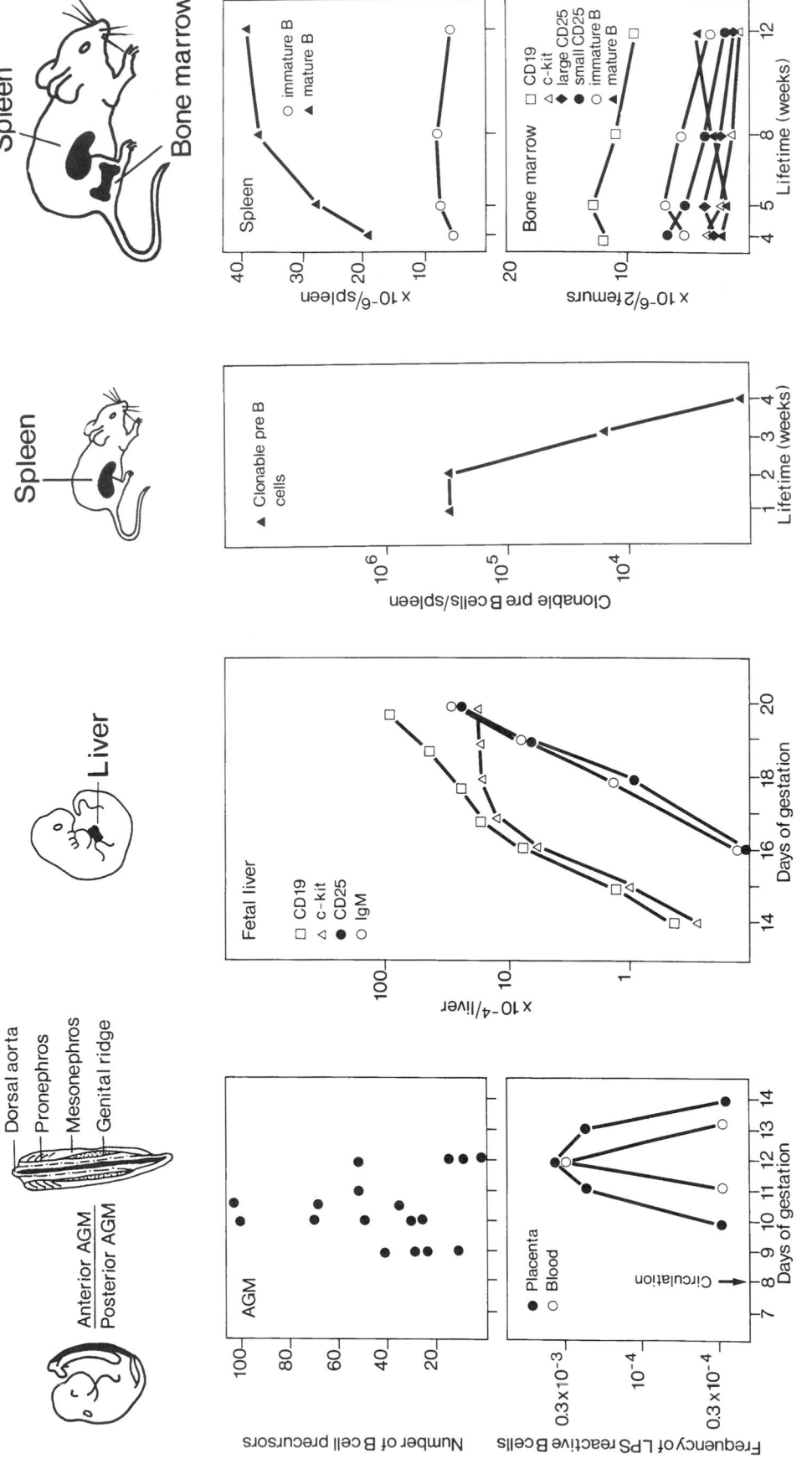

FIG. 4. Waves of B-lymphocyte development before and after birth of the mouse. The earliest site of pluripotent HSC generation with the capacity to develop into B lymphocytes develops from the splanchnopleura in the AGM region. The schematic drawing indicates the tissue constituting this region: pronephros, mesonephros, genital ridge, and dorsal aorta. The anterior portion of the AGM develops B lymphocytes. (Taken from ref. 550.) Embryonic blood and the embryonic part of the placenta vascularized by the embryonic blood are the next sites before fetal liver and omentum become B-lymphopoietic sites. Spleen contains B-lineage precursors around birth, and bone marrow becomes the site of continuous B-cell generation, which decreases with age.

gene encoding (a) transcription factor(s) with similar function(s). It is also quite possible that the selective pressures to develop the different lineage, possibly even by environmental (antigenic) influences, are different for myeloid, NK, T, and B cells. Altogether the Ikaros mutant phenotypes suggest that a lymphoid progenitor cell exists that is the common ancestor of T- and B-lineage cells (15,16,86).

Commitment to the B-Lineage Pathway

The commitment of hematopoietic progenitors to the B-lymphoid lineage of development is thought to progress, like commitment to other hematopoietic lineages, through a cascade of irreversible differentiation steps. Concomitant with commitment is thought to be a progressive loss of the capacity to differentiate into other lineages. How commitment is finally achieved is unclear at the moment. Clear signs of commitment to the lymphoid lineages are the activation and expression of the genes encoding the rearrangement machinery (i.e., of the RAG-1 and RAG-2 and in the adult of the TdT gene). The activation of the genes encoding the antigen-specific receptor complexes on precursors and on immature and mature lymphocytes (i.e., for the B lineages, the genes encoding the μH chain and the surrogate L chain of the pre-BCR), as well as the genes encoding Igα and Igβ as receptor-anchoring and signal-transducing molecules, are similarly clear signs for commitment to B-lineage versus T-lineage differentiation (Table 1).

Commitment through the Action of Transcription Factors

Just as targeted mutagenesis of specific genes has helped to identify earlier stages of hematopoiesis (see Fig. 2), so has the same experimental approach helped to characterize genes with important bottle-neck functions in the commitment and later progression of B-lymphoid lineage cells in their pathway of differentiation (see Fig. 3). Again, genes encoding transcription factors have, so far, clarified some of the earlier steps of this pathway. They are E2A, EBF, Sox-4, and PAX-5 (see Fig. 3). Their effects on B lymphopoiesis have been reviewed by Rolink et al. (87) and Opstelten (88).

By alternative splicing, the mouse E2A gene can generate two proteins of the basic helix–loop–helix (bHLH) family: E12 and E47 (89,90). The bHLH proteins form homo- or heterodimers via the HLH region and then bind to DNA via the basic region. Many of the bHLH proteins, including E12 and E47, are expressed ubiquitously. In B lymphocytes, binding sites for these E proteins have been detected in the IgH- and IgL-chain gene enhancers (89,90).

Despite its broad expression pattern in hematopoietic cells, targeted disruption of the E2A gene affects only B-cell development (89,90). Almost no B220+ cells and no $D_H J_H$ or $V_κ J_κ$ rearrangements are detectable in these mice. Moreover, transcripts of Iμ, RAG-1, mb1, CD19, λ5, and Pax-5 are absent, or at least dramatically reduced. Based on this specific and very early block in

TABLE 1. *Expression of B-lymphocyte–lineage-related markers at different stages of development*

	Pre/Pro B[a]	Pro B	Pre B-I	Large pre B-II[b] A	Large pre B-II[b] B	Small pre B-II	Immature	Mature
Markers								
B220 (CD45R)	■	■	■	■	■	■	■	■
CD19	□	■	■	■	■	■	■	■
CD25 (IL2 receptor α chain)	□	□	□	■	■	■	■/□	□
Pre B and B receptors								
Igα, Igβ	■	■	■	■	■	■	■	■
gp130		■	■					
Surrogate L chain	■	■	■	■	□	□	□	□
I cμ RNA	■	■	■	■	■	■	■	■
$D_H J_H$ DNA	■	■	■	■	■	■	■	■
$V_H D_H J_H$ DNA	□	□	(■)/□	■	■	■	■	■
I cκ RNA	□	□	□	□	■	■	■	■
$V_κ D_κ$ DNA	□	□	□	□	□	■	■	■
Surface IgM	□	□	□	□	□	□	■	■
Surface IgD	□	□	□	□	□	□	□	■
Rearrangement machinery								
RAG-1	□	□	■	□	(■)/□	■	■	□
RAG-2	□	□	■	□	(■)/□	■	■	□
TdT	□	□	■	□	□	□	□	□
Cytokine receptors								
Flk-2		■	□	□	□	□	□	□
c-kit	■	■	■	□	□	□	□	□
IL7-R	■	■	■	■	■/□	□	□	□
IFN-τR			■					
CD40	□	□	□	□	□	■/□	■	■
Intracellular signaling								
myc		■	■	■	□	□	□	■/□

Filled squares, expressed; open squares, not expressed.
[a]Pre/pro B cells are about 1% of the B220+, CD19−, cells in the bone marrow and do not express CD4, NK1.1, and MHC class II.
[b]Large pre B-II cells can be subdivided into an A fraction, which expresses the pre BCR, and a B fraction, which has lost this expression.

B-cell development, it is likely that the E2A gene plays a key role in B-lineage commitment. The finding that overexpression of E47 in a pre-T-cell line can stimulate transcription and rearrangement of the IgH-chain locus (91) supports this idea. The most convincing evidence for an important role of the E2A gene products in B-lineage commitment comes from the finding that transfection and expression of E47 in fibroblasts activates the expression of TdT and of the IgH-chain locus (92). By contrast, genes encoding PU-1 or other early-acting transcription factors do not activate these B lineage-related or -specific loci.

Early B-cell factor (EBF) was identified as a tissue-specific transcriptional activator. Within the hematopoietic lineages, its expression is restricted to the pro- and pre-B-cell stages (76,93). EBF$^{-/-}$ mice have a similar, if not identical, block in very early B-cell development, as do E2A$^{-/-}$ mice (94). Thus, only low numbers of B220$^+$ cells with IgH- and IgL-chain genes in germline configuration and without detectable levels of RAG-1, RAG-2, Hmb-1, B29, VpreB, and λ5 transcripts are found in EBF$^{-/-}$ mice. Like E2A, EBF could also play a key role in B-lineage commitment. A potential target gene for EBF is Hmb-1, which encodes Igα (76,93). However, whether the phenotype of EBF$^{-/-}$ mice is due to the lack of Hmb-1 expression is questionable, since B29$^{-/-}$ mice show a block in B-cell development significantly later than EBF$^{-/-}$ mice (B29 encodes Igβ which is the functional partner of Igα encoded by mb-1) (95).

Sox-4 encodes a protein containing an amino-terminal high-mobility group (HMG) box (which exhibits sequence specificity in DNA binding) and a serine-rich carboxy-terminus. Sox-4 can transactivate transcription through an AACAAAG motif, for which the non–DNA-binding serine-rich carboxy-terminus is indispensable (96).

During murine embryogenesis, Sox-4 is expressed at several sites, while in adult mice, expression is restricted to immature B and T cells (96). Sox-4$^{-/-}$ mice die *in utero* at day 14 of gestation due to circulatory failure (97). *In vitro* analyses using a stromal cell/IL-7 culture system revealed a strongly reduced number of cells capable of giving rise to B cells in fetal liver of Sox-4$^{-/-}$ mice at day 13 of gestation. Moreover, the growth rate of these cells was strongly reduced. Transplantation of Sox-4$^{-/-}$ fetal liver cells into irradiated normal recipients showed that erythropoiesis, myelopoiesis, and T lymphopoiesis is unaffected, while B-lymphopoiesis is blocked at a very early stage (probably when D$_H$J$_H$ rearrangements take place). Thus, Sox-4 plays an important role in B-cell development, although the *in vitro* experiments indicate that Sox-4 is not absolutely required. The potential target genes for Sox-4 in B cells are unknown.

The Pax gene family of transcription factors plays an important role in several different developmental processes. Up to eight different PAX genes are described that all share a conserved region of 128 amino acids, termed the *paired domain*, which displays the DNA-binding activity (98–100). PAX-5, a member of this family, is expressed in the midbrain–hindbrain junction, along the spinal cord in mid-gestation embryos, in adult testis, and as the only member of the family during all stages of B-cell development except plasma cells (101,102). Potential binding sites for the PAX-5 gene, which encodes the protein BSAP, are found in the promotor regions of CD19 (103), the B lymphoid-specific tyrosine kinase BLK (104), λ5 and VpreB (105), and in the 3′ IgH enhancer (106). Additional BSAP binding sites are found in several Ig switch regions (107–110). B-cell development in bone marrow of PAX-5$^{-/-}$ mice is arrested at the pre-B-I cell stage

(111) (see discussion in the section on the order of precursor cells in development). On the other hand, no progenitor or precursor B cells are detectable in the fetal liver of Pax-5$^{-/-}$ embryos. The reason(s) for this obvious difference between bone marrow and fetal liver is unknown.

In conclusion, the transcription factors E2A, EBF, SOX-4, and PAX-5 target at least some of the early genes expressed in B-lineage cells, which could commit the cells by their action. However, it remains to be worked out how control of these early genes creates the bottle-necks of development that are observed when these genes are mutated.

Waves of B-Cell Development at Different Sites

B lymphocytes are generated during embryonic development and after birth at different sites in the mouse (112–117) (see Fig. 4). The first B-lineage precursors can be found in the embryonic blood and in the organs supplied by embryonic blood, such as the embryonic part of the placenta, soon after circulation is established at day 8 of gestation (5,65,116). After days 11 and 12 of gestation, the first progenitors and then precursors of the B lineage can be detected in the omentum (118) and in fetal liver (119,120). It is thought that the HSCs generated in the AGM region of the embryo seed into these sites because they have been attracted by them. They migrate to these sites, where they are induced to a B-lineage pathway of differentiation. It is not known at the present time which decisions are made during the development from HSC to a B-lineage progenitor before the cells enter these embryonic organs, and which decisions are induced by the environment of these organs.

In fetal liver most of the B-lineage cells develop in one synchronous wave so that at day 16, the first sIgM$^+$ cells become detectable. On day 18 (i.e., around birth), the number of sIgM$^+$ mitogen-reactive B cells reach a maximum, to decline in numbers thereafter (see Fig. 4) (120–124). The kinetics of cellular development, with cell cycling times between 12 and 18 hours, make it likely that B lymphopoiesis is initiated once, and that all B-lineage cells expand by proliferation *in situ* (47). These kinetics cannot, however, rule out that a small number of cells initiate differentiation at a later time. Precursors can also be found in the spleen until 4 weeks after birth (120) (see Fig. 4). B-cell development in bone marrow begins around birth. A defective lef-1 gene leaves the embryonic waves of B-cell development intact, but abolishes development in the adult mouse (72,125). This is one of the many signs that embryonic and adult B-cell development are different.

Early waves of B-cell development in omentum and fetal liver generate H-chain repertoires in which the joints between V, D, and J segments do not contain N-nucleotide insertions because the enzyme terminal deoxynucleotidyl transferase (TdT) is not expressed in these B-lineage cells (126–130).

Within the first 4 weeks after birth, the bone marrow becomes the major site of B-cell development, increasing its number of B-lineage cells to the sizes described in Fig. 4. Thereafter, the number of B-lineage cells, especially those of the early progenitors and precursors, begins to decrease again with age. The bone marrow becomes increasingly filled with fat, reducing the spaces for hematopoiesis and B lymphopoiesis. However, HSCs and B-lineage precursors are not lost completely: bone marrow of old mice continues to be a sufficient source for successful reconstitution of the blood-cell lineages, including B-lineage cells in the bone marrow and the periphery of lethally irradiated, reconstituted hosts (120).

The Environment of B-Lymphopoiesis

The Ultrastructure of Bone Marrow and Its Generation

Bone marrow is the cellular content of the bone cavities. Bone develops from mesenchyme. At the sites of bone formation in the embryo, mesenchymal cells form a dense aggregation by proliferation in the shape of the future bone (Fig. 5). Chondroblasts secrete substances that form collagenous fibers as intercellular matrices within which chondrocytes develop. The chondrocytes become hypertrophic and begin to secrete a different matrix with different types of collagen and more fibronectin. This new matrix is thought to attract blood vessels that bring in osteoblasts. Cartilage is formed. Calcium salts are deposited in the intracellular matrix, leading to calcification of the cartilage. Some of the invading cells destroy the remaining cartilaginous matrix that has not been calcified. This leaves the calcified matrices with empty spaces inbetween to be filled by capillaries and mesenchymal cells, which differentiate into chondrocytes, osteoblasts, and osteocytes. Osteoblasts form a matrix on the calcified intracellular matrix. Osteoclasts, on the other side, which are hematopoietic in origin and differentiate from monocytes under the influence of IL-11 (80–82), destroy the central areas of the matrices in bone. The space created in the center of the bone is then filled with hematopoietic cells and with stromal cells of fibroblastic morphology, at least some of which are preadipocytes. In this marrow of the bone, hematopoiesis and lymphopoiesis are then initiated and continue to occur throughout life. This marrow is red, since erythropoiesis is part of hematopoiesis. Bones with white marrow are usually not hematopoietic, but contain only adipocytic cells producing fat. Aging hematopoietic bone marrow increases its fat-producing activity, while decreasing hematopoietic activity.

In red bone marrow the remaining matrix forms a network of trabeculae (Fig. 6). The internal bone's surface is covered by the endosteum, a single layer of osteoblasts and osteoclasts. It remains to be seen whether stromal cells with specific interactive capacities for pluripotent and early myeoloid–lymphoid progenitor stem cells are included in this endosteum.

The main blood supply, and in later life the site of immigration of mature lymphocytes, is secured by the nutrient artery, entering the marrow at about midshaft, traveling out to the two ends. The

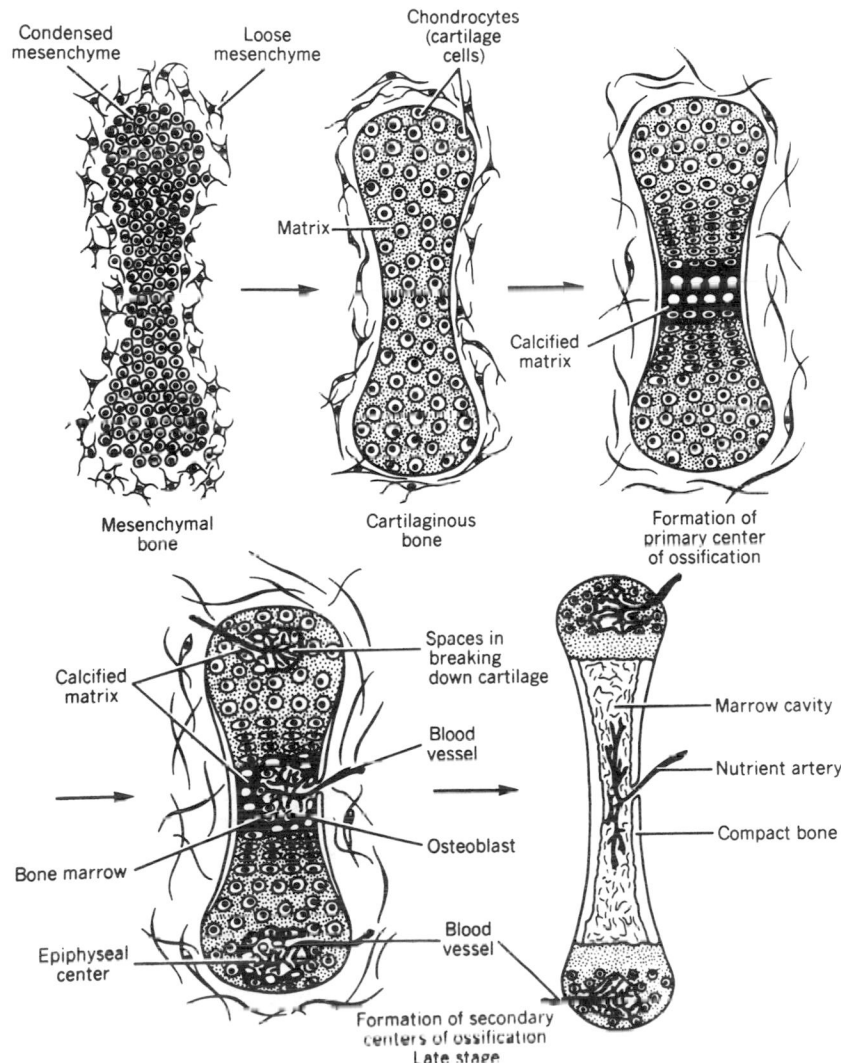

FIG. 5. Stages in the development of a long bone from undifferentiated mesenchyme. (Taken from ref. 551, as adapted from Snell HS. *Clinical embryology for medical students.* Boston: Little, Brown, 1975.)

arteries end in capillaries, which are connected with a network of venous sinuses. These sinuses collect into radial veins, which empty into the central vein that runs parallel to the central artery. The venous sinuses are special in lymphoid organs, allowing the transit of lymphocytes and other leukocytes in the marrow from the site of their production into the blood, hence from the primary organ into the peripheral secondary organs, notably into spleen (see Fig. 6).

The space between the trabeculae and the blood vessel is occupied by reticular cells and hematopoietic cells. The reticular cells form a framework of interconnected cells that is thought to provide a stroma for interactions with the hematopoietic cells. The different B-lymphocyte lineage cell populations, described later in detail, fill their compartments in marrow to defined sizes (Fig. 7).

Dynamic Equilibrium of B-Lineage Precursor Pools

The generation of B-lineage cells at different specialized sites suggests that a specialized environment of cells for B-lineage progenitors and precursors exists in these organs that supports this development (see Fig. 6). The environmental stromal cells in the B cell-generating organs are not yet well defined. *In vitro* prolifera-

tion of normal mouse precursor B cells requires contact with stromal cells, which can be preadipocytic fibroblasts (see later discussion). When these preadipocytes mature to fat-producing cells, their capacity to support precursor B-cell growth is lost. This suggests that the development of fat-producing cells and of fat not only reduces space for B lymphopoiesis, but also inactivates the B cell differentiation supportive compartments. *In vitro* growth of B-lineage precursors on stromal cells also shows that the contact with this B lymphopoiesis–competent environment actually retains these precursors in their state of development. Loss of contact with the environmental cells induces the development of more differentiated cells of the B lineage (see later discussion). It follows that the size of a given precursor B-cell compartment is dependent on the number of stromal cells and the interstitial spaces between them, in which a defined, limited number of precursor B cells can remain in contact with these stromal cells.

Support for this view also comes from measurements of the sizes of progenitor and precursor B-cell compartments in the bone marrow of mutant mice, which have B-cell development arrested at defined stages of their development (see Fig.7). In these mice, in which later stages of precursor and immature B cells are missing in the bone marrow, the numbers of earlier progenitors and precursors

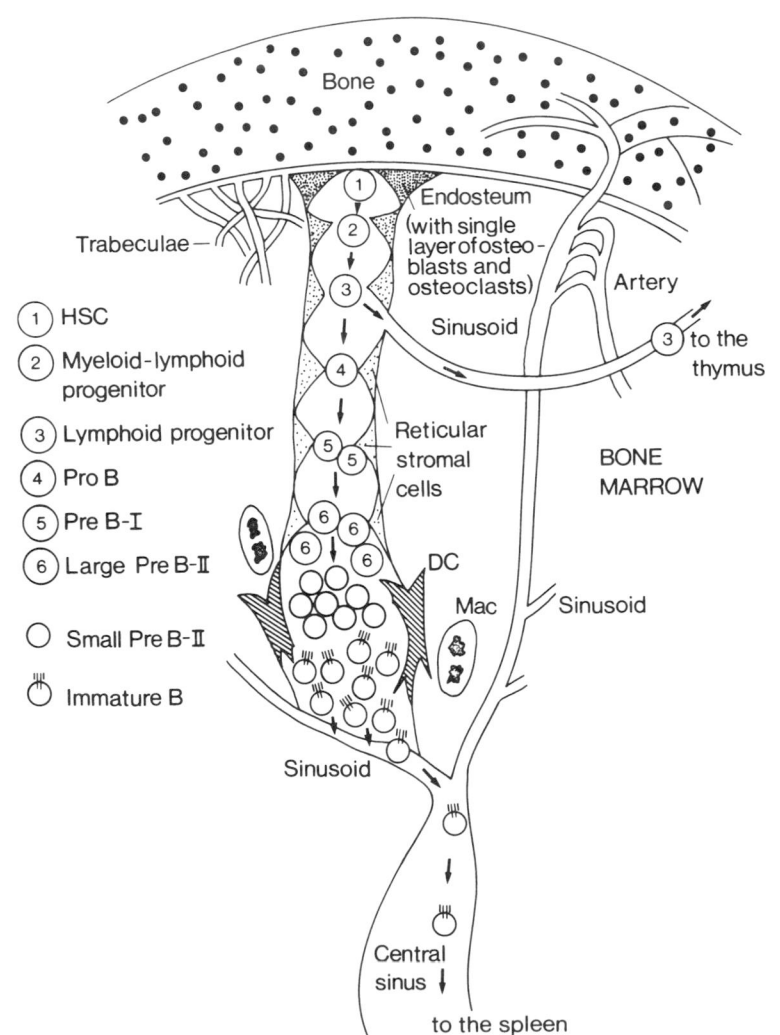

FIG. 6. Schematic drawing of the development of B-lymphocyte lineage cells in the bone marrow in interaction with different types of stromal cells **(left side)**. The earliest stages of B-lineage cells are located near the endosteum. A prolymphoid progenitor is pictured to have the choice to migrate to the thymus and enter T-lymphoid differentiation, or continue down the road of B-lymphoid differentiation. At later stages, dendritic cells (*DC*) may interact with sIg+ immature B cells in selections of repertoires, while macrophages may phagocytose apoptotic cells of the B lineage. Immature sIgM+ B cells leave the marrow via sinusoids, which enter into the central sinus, which transports the cells via venous blood to the heart, where the lymphocytes enter the main artery leading to the spleen (see also Fig. 12).

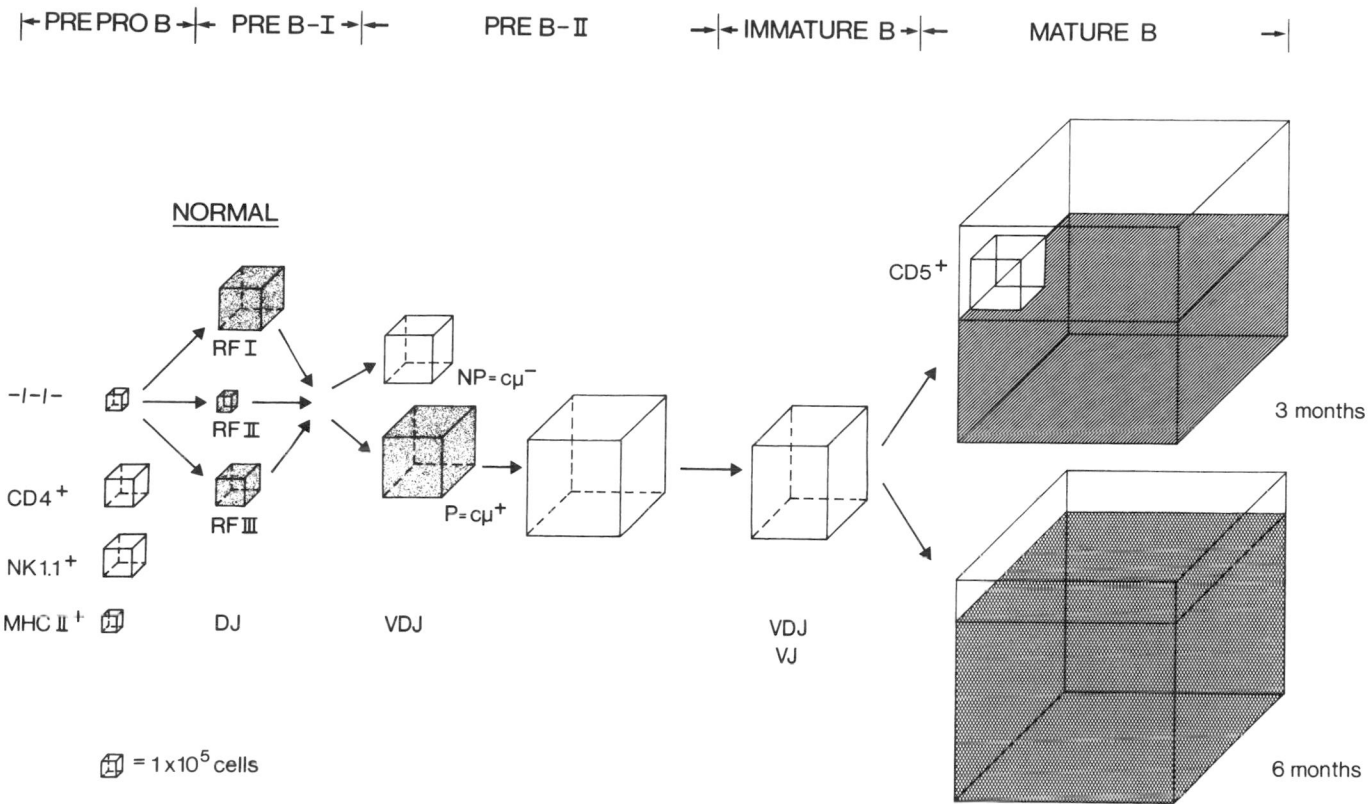

FIG. 7. Sizes of B-lymphocyte lineage compartments in bone marrow and in the periphery. *Shaded boxes* indicate cycling cells; *open boxes,* resting cells; and *dark boxes,* long-lived cells.

either remain the same or are only slightly elevated. Hence, they do not expand into the empty spaces of the bone marrow.

When a progenitor or precursor cell divides in these filled compartments, one daughter cell can be expected to remain in contact with the stroma; that is, it will remain in its state of differentiation. The other daughter cell, however, loses this contact, is pushed out of the compartment, migrates, and begins further differentiation. Hence, precursor growth might be expected to be linear, not exponential, as long as all stages of differentiation are kept within confined compartments. Precursor differentiation is induced by loss of a ligand rather than by the exposure to a new one. This will become evident from *in vitro* proliferation and differentiation studies with progenitor and precursor B cells (described in the section on the order of precursor B cells in development).

Almost nothing is known of the development, state of differentiation, regulation of activities, stability, and specificity of the stromal cells to cooperate with given differentiative states in the development of HSCs to B cells. It might well be that different types of stromal cells are specialized to interact with different types of precursors (see Fig. 6). This specialization should be manifest in a spatial order within the B cell-generating organ, which should form an assembly line for B-lineage cells. It should also be characterized by special molecular contacts between stromal cells and B-lineage cells, and by special chemokines and lymphokines produced by one type of cell and received by the other type. It is known that the most immature progenitors, including HSCs, are found preferentially accumulated in the subendosteal regions of the bone marrow (131) (see Fig. 6). However, for later

stages of hematopoiesis and B-lymphopoiesis, such a spatial order is not visible in either fetal liver or bone marrow (132,133). A three-dimensional picture of the distribution of B-lineage cells at different stages of their differentiation has not yet been constructed for either of these organs, a picture that might well reveal ordered cell assembly lines.

The sizes of the different precursor B-cell compartments, their proliferative capacities, and the rates at which programmed cell death occurs in these compartments have been measured (131,134–139). Daily production of cells in the bone marrow (140) and outflow of sIgM+ cells into the periphery (141) have been measured. With some refinements in these measurements, this should eventually allow the construction of a dynamic model of B-lymphocyte generation, turnover, and outflow in bone marrow. It will allow an estimation of the contribution of asymmetric and symmetric divisions (i.e., of linear and exponential generation of cells) in the proliferating precursor compartments to maintain the steady state of cells in the bone marrow and the continuous outflow and maturation of sIgM+ B cells.

Perturbations of the Environment

The injection of a variety of exogenous agents into a mouse can increase B-lymphocyte production in the bone marrow (134,135,142–145). The nature of these agents varies considerably, from sheep erythrocytes to mineral oil. A prolonged increase in the proliferation of early progenitors (pro- and pre-B-I cells; see later discussion) and a concomitant loss of later precursors (pre-

B-II cells) and immature B cells are observed. Chronic activation by mineral oil may be one of the factors contributing to tumor development in B-lineage cells (146–148). In these proliferating precursors, the Ig gene rearrangement machinery (TdT, RAG-1, and -2) is activated, increasing the chances for chromosomal translocations of an oncogene such as myc into the IgH- and L-chain loci (149).

B lymphopoiesis is selectively suppressed in the bone marrow of pregnant mice. Early progenitors (i.e., pro-B and pre-B cells and some pre-B-I cells; see later discussion) appear less affected than later stages (i.e., pre-B-II and immature B cells) (150). After delivery, B lymphopoiesis returns to normal pool sizes in the marrow. The sex hormones estrone, estriol, and β-estradiol all mediate this suppression (150,151). Progesterone by itself has no effect but sensitizes the action of estrogens. Genetically hypogonadal female mice that have a secondary deficiency in gonadal steroidogenesis have hyperactive B lymphopoiesis in bone marrow. This hyperactivity can be reduced by the administration of estrogen (152). Hence, sex hormones may influence the levels of B lymphopoiesis under normal conditions (153).

B1 and Conventional B Cells

Two B-cell lineages, B1 and conventional B cells, emerge from this development (154,155) (see Fig. 7). They are thought to be selected (i.e., separated from a common precursor) after sIgM has first been expressed during development (156–158). B1 cells are generated as the only lineage in omentum (118), and as the earlier of two lineages in fetal liver (B1a) and bone marrow (B1b) (154,159).

Hence, they predominate in the B-cell repertoire early in life. B1 cells preferentially populate the pleural cavities, the peritoneum, and the marginal zone of the spleen. At least some of them express CD21, but not CD23 (160). Part of the B1 cells (B1a cells) can be distinguished from conventional B cells by the selective expression of CD5 (154,161). B1-cell populations are highly and disproportionally represented in autoantibody-producing B-cell populations (162–166) and in B-cell neoplasms (118,167). Ig receptors recognizing bacterial antigens such as phosphorylcholine are frequently expressed on them (158,163, 168–171). B1 cells have the capacity of self-replenishment from the pool of sIgM$^+$ B cells at later times in life, when their generation has ceased. They express a selected V_H repertoire on H chains that might be a reflection of a selection by specific antigens (166,172–175). They are capable of cooperating with helper T cells, but their reactivity to T cell-independent antigens and to polyclonal activators differs strikingly from that of conventional B cells (164,176). In vitro, the polyclonal activator LPS strongly activates them; in vivo, it depletes them (177). On the other hand, B1 cells in the peritoneal cavity, expressing a transgenic autoreactive sIg with specificity for red blood cells, are activated by LPS to autoantibody production and secretion, which leads to autoimmune hemolytic anemia (178). Apparently these autoantibody-producing B cells are not deleted in the bone marrow and are not anergized by the presence of autoantigen in the periphery (see later discussion on immature B cells). The signal transducer and activator STAT-3 is constitutively activated in B1 cells but only inducibly expressed in conventional B cells (179). B1 cells, but not conventional B cells, require IL-12 for their development (180). The generation of B1 cells is impaired in CD19$^{-/-}$ mice (181).

The other lineage of B cells (conventional B cells) regenerates its central and peripheral compartments from sIg-negative precursors, and does so throughout life. It constitutes the major B-cell compartment in the adult, is found predominantly in the follicular regions of spleen and lymph nodes, expresses CD23 (but only low levels of CD21) (160,182), and is responsive to T cell-independent and T cell–dependent antigens and to mitogens in the normal way, as described in Chapter 7. Their repertoire is screened by negative selection against high-avidity autoantibodies in the central and peripheral lymphoid organs (see Chapter 20), and hence is mainly directed against foreign antigens, though autoantibodies with unknown avidity to autoantigens can be detected in them (183).

The Order of Precursor B Cells in Development

B-cell development from early progenitors to mature, sIg$^+$ B cells is characterized by changes in

1. their status of IgH- and L-chain gene loci rearrangements
2. the expression of intracellular and surface-bound markers, some with functions in this development
3. cell cycle status
4. in vitro growth progenitors and responsiveness to cytokines, chemokines, mitogens, and antigens
5. transplantability into suitably deficient hosts and capacity to populate these hosts
6. life expectancy in vivo

Figure 3 summarizes the different stages of B-cell development; Table 1 provides the markers that characterize B cells; Fig. 8 describes the methods to detect and separate them; and Fig. 7 gives their sizes in the marrow and in the periphery.

The studies of Osmond (131), Hardy et al. (184), Tsubata and Nishikawa (185), Rajewsky (186) and their colleagues, as well as our own (187–193) have all contributed to the characterization of the different stages of B-cell development. In this chapter, we use the nomenclature for precursor B-cell subpopulations introduced by us. The nomenclature used by other laboratories is cross-referenced in Table 2. Single-cell polymerase chain reaction (PCR) analyses of the status of rearrangements of the two H-chain, κL- and λL-chain alleles of the Ig loci have allowed us to order these B-lineage progenitors and precursors in their pathway of differentiation (194,195). The cellular analyses of a series of naturally occurring or experimentally induced mutant mouse strains, leading to changes in this B-cell developmental pathway, have supported this order (see Fig. 3). The effects of some of these mutations in B-lineage development are described in the following sections.

Early embryonic development in omentum and fetal liver can be distinguished from neonatal and adult development in bone marrow by the differential surface expression of MHC class II molecules (absent on precursors in fetal liver, and present on those in bone marrow) (196,197) and of a myosin-like light chain (present in bone marrow, and absent in fetal liver) (198). Furthermore, precursor B cells in fetal liver do not express the enzyme TdT (130), while those in bone marrow do. TdT expression in mouse bone marrow is only on during H-chain gene rearrangement, and it is shut off when L-chain genes are rearranged. Consequently, H chains of B cells made in bone marrow usually carry N regions inserted at the V to D and D to J joints, while those B cells made in fetal liver do not contain them, nor do κ or λL chains of the mouse that are made in either fetal liver or bone marrow.

TABLE 2. *Nomenclatures for B-lineage cells used by different laboratories*

Rolink and Melchers	Pro-B	Pre B-I			Large pre-B-II	Small B-II	Immature B	Mature B
Osmond	Early pro-B	Intermediate pro-B			Late pre B/large pre-B-II	Small pre-B	Immature B	Mature B
Nishikawa	B-Pro I PA6 only	B-Pro II PA6-IL7			CFU-IL-7 only			
Hardy	—	A	B	C	C'	D	Immature B	Mature B
		Pre/pro-B	Pro-B	Pro-B		pre-B		

Precursor and Progenitor B Cells

The earliest types of B-cell progenitors in the scheme of Hardy et al. (184) are found within fraction A (Fig. 8A). The B-lineage cells in this fraction are characterized by the expression of B220 and CD43 and by the absence of HSA and BP-1 (see Table 1). They constitute around 3% of total nucleated cells in bone marrow (see Fig. 7). B-lineage cells belonging to fraction A do not express CD19, while all other stages of B-cell development do (189). The vast majority of cells in fraction A do not belong to the B-cell lineage (Fig. 8B). About 30% of them are precursors of NK cells. They express NK cell markers and, more importantly, lyse NK cell targets upon stimulation with IL-2 (189). Another 30% to 40% coexpress CD4 in levels comparable to those found on T cells. However, these cells do not appear to be T-lineage cells since they do not express components of the TCR, are found in similar numbers in RAG-1– and RAG-2–deficient animals, and do not yield T cells upon transplantation into rearrangement-deficient hosts. Another 25% express MHC class II molecules on the surface. Both the CD4+ and the MHC class II+ cells of fraction A do not proliferate on stromal cells in the presence of IL-7, as do pro-B and pre-B-I cells (see discussion in the following section). Moreover, transfer of cells of either subpopulation into RAG$^{-/-}$ mice did not lead to the development of detectable numbers of B cells or any other cell type of the hematopoietic lineage in the rearrangement-deficient hosts. Thus, the origin, function, and eventual fate of these cells is presently unclear.

On the other hand, stromal cell/IL-7 reactive progenitor B cells can be detected in the remaining 30% of fraction A cells (i.e., in the B220+, CD43+, CD19–, NK1.1–, CD4– subpopulation). Upon expansion of these cells on stromal cells in the presence of IL-7, they gain the phenotype of a pre-B-I cell by changing to B220+, CD19+, CD43+, c-kit+ cells. Moreover, transfer of these cells into RAG-2$^{-/-}$ mice develops a small but significant mature B-cell compartment in the hosts. In a transgenic mouse that expresses the human IL-2 receptor α chain (CD25, TAC) under the control of the λ5 promotor (199), the pro-B and pre-B cells in fraction A express human CD25. Hence, these cells, as well as their normal counterparts in nontransgenic animals, probably also express λ5.

In summary, only a very small part of fraction A has B-cell progenitor activity. The question whether these are already committed to the B-cell lineage, or whether they still have potential for other cell lineages is still open. A more recent analysis of these early progenitor populations has shown that these B progenitors express AA4.1, Igα and Igβ, surrogate L chain, EBF, and E2A (200,201). It is this small population of pro-B and pre-B cells with B-cell progenitor activity that is absent in E2A$^{-/-}$ and EBF$^{-/-}$ mice, making E2A and EBF prime candidates for determining B-lineage commitment.

The IL-7Rα$^{-/-}$ mouse also has a major but not absolute block at this early state of B-cell development (202). Since the IL-7Rα chain is a subunit of the receptor for IL-7, as well as the thymic stromal cell-derived lymphopoietin (TSLP) (202,203), whose activities parallel those of IL-7, it is very likely that IL-7 or TSLP is required at this stage for further B-cell development at normal rates and in normal ways. Possible explanations as to why the block in B-cell development is not absolute are discussed below.

Progenitor B and Precursor B-I Cells

Successive rearrangements of first the H chain, then the L-chain gene loci of the Ig genes are hallmarks of B-cell development. However, it is not clear whether the first D_H to J_H rearrangement already irreversibly commits cells to the B lineage. Virus-transformed early cells with B-lineage and macrophage-lineage markers can give rise to precursor B-cell lines as well as macrophage lines, both of which carry $D_H J_H$-rearranged IgH-chain loci (204,205). They appear to be similar to bi-potential colony-forming cells found in fetal liver that give rise to normal precursor B cells and macrophages in the same colony (206,207).

Pre-B-I cells have long-term proliferative capacities *in vitro* on stromal cells in the presence of IL-7, have undergone $D_H J_H$ (see discussion later in this section), retain their L-chain gene loci in germline configuration, and express B220, c-kit, CD43, RAG-1 and RAG-2, the surrogate L chain and, TdT (the latter only in bone marrow, not in fetal liver). The majority of these pre-B-I cells appear to be the same as Hardy's pre–pro B-cell fractions A to C (184), Osmond's intermediate pro-B cells (185), and Nishikawa's PA-6/IL-7 pro-B cells (185) (see Fig. 8).

A block in the development of B cells is seen at the stage of pro-B cells in RAG-1$^{-/-}$, RAG-2$^{-/-}$, and severe combined immunodeficiency (SCID) mice, and at the similar but $D_H J_H$-rearranged pre-B-I cell stage in λ5$^{-/-}$ (208), μH-tm$^{-/-}$ (209), Igβ$^{-/-}$ (95), IL-2Rγ$^{-/-}$ (210), IL-7$^{-/-}$ (211), Syk$^{-/-}$ (212,213), and PAX-5$^{-/-}$ (101,102,111) mice. The block observed in μtm$^{-/-}$, Igβ$^{-/-}$, and PAX/5$^{-/-}$ mice is almost absolute, while in λ5$^{-/-}$, IL-2Rg$^{-/-}$, Syk$^{-/-}$, and IL-7$^{-/-}$ mice, later stages, including mature B cells, are found in the bone marrow and in peripheral lymphoid organs, although in lower numbers. The functional significance of these mutations is discussed below, and the functions of the pre-BCR will be considered.

Pre-B-I cells show limited proliferation potential in IL-7-containing medium in the absence of stromal cells, usually for no longer than a week. They might, under these culture conditions, be the same cells as Nishikawa's IL-7, only pro-B cells (see Table 2). Once grown *in vivo*, pre-B-I cells no longer proliferate in the presence of IL-7 alone, but remain in their state of differentiation as $D_H J_H$-rearranged, clonable pre-B-I cells (195,214–216). The pool of pre-B-I cells in the bone marrow of a young normal mouse contains between 2 and 5×10^6 cells (see Fig. 7).

Pro-B cells are phenotypically indistinguishable from pre-B-I cells. Surface and intracellular marker expression and growth properties are the same. However, their Ig loci are in germline configuration. Hence, in a RAG$^{-/-}$ mouse, the pro-B-cell compartment takes the place of the pre-B-I compartment in normal mice (see Fig. 7).

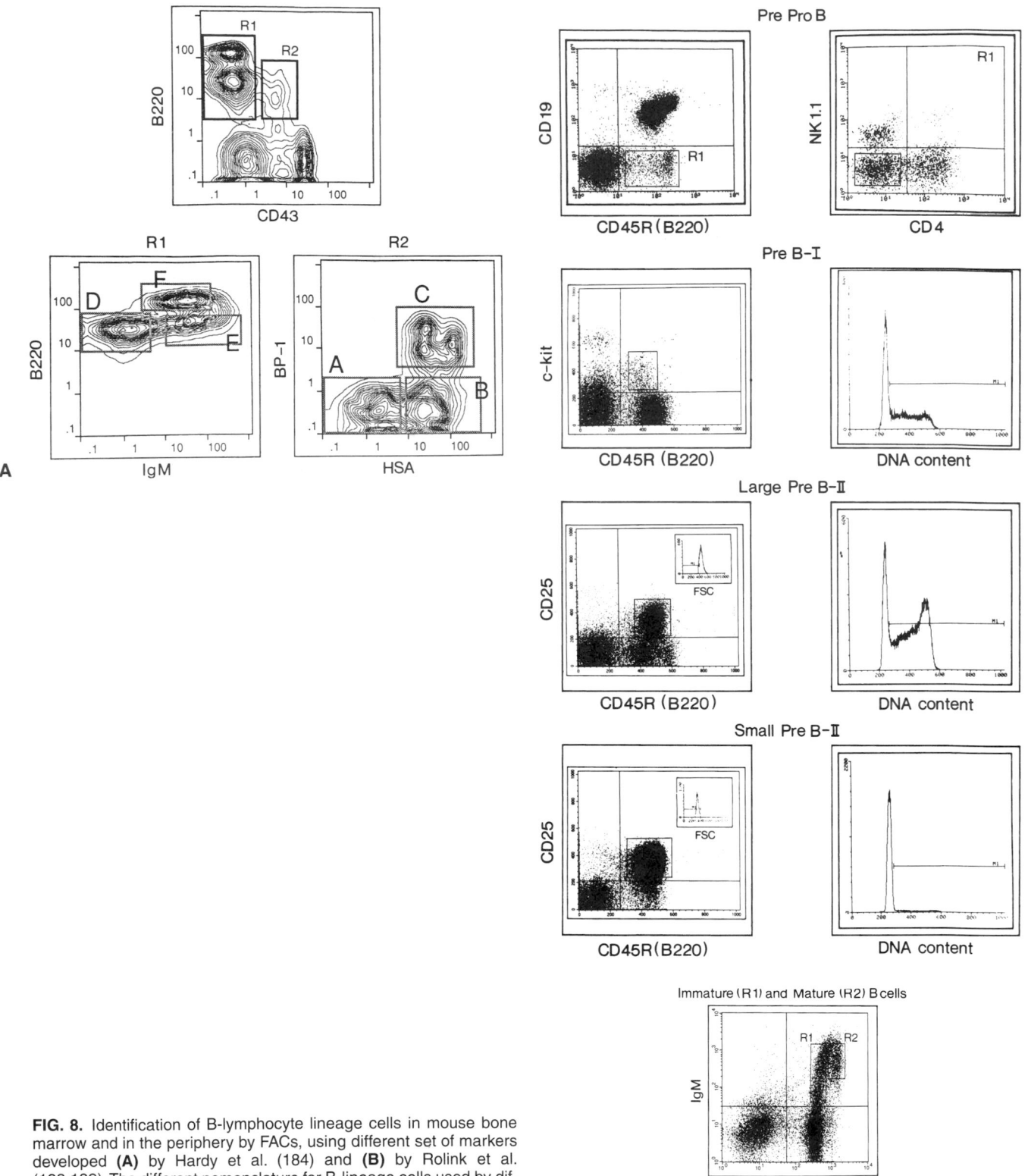

FIG. 8. Identification of B-lymphocyte lineage cells in mouse bone marrow and in the periphery by FACs, using different set of markers developed **(A)** by Hardy et al. (184) and **(B)** by Rolink et al. (188,189). The different nomenclature for B-lineage cells used by different laboratories is cross-referenced in Table 2.

Studies of the growth, differentiation, and survival properties of pre-B-I cells in tissue culture allow insights into the possible molecular and kinetic modes of B-cell development *in vivo*, as outlined in the preceding section (191,217,218).

Proliferation of Progenitor B and Precursor B-I Cells In Vitro

Pro-B and pre-B-I cells of normal and most mutant mice have the capacity to proliferate for weeks and months and to be clonable *ex vivo* and *in vitro* with near 100% plating efficiency, stimulated either by IL-7 or IL-3 (214,216) (Fig. 9). In fact, the same pro-B and pre-B-I cells expanded *in vitro* respond to both IL-7 and IL-3, as these two cytokines can be used back and forth in culture (216).

Pro-B and pre-B-I cells require contact with stromal cells to proliferate in long-term cultures and to remain in their state of differentiation. Both types of cells receive signals. Stromal cells are induced to secrete cytokines, such as IL-7, SCF, or insulin-like growth factor (IGF-1), and many express, or change the form of, adhesion molecules and ligands for receptors on pre-B cells (219–221). Adhesion molecules involved in these contacts are CD44 and hyaluronate, very late activation antigen 4, and fibronectin (222–225). Pro-B and pre-B-I cells receive signals through cytokine receptors and cell adhesion molecules to proliferate, but not to differentiate further. Cytokine receptors involved in these signaling reactions are the IL-7 receptor, the IL-3 receptor, the tyrosine kinase c-kit, which is the receptor for SCF produced by stromal cells, and the IGF-1 receptor. Their roles in the regulation of proliferation and differentiation, in concert with the other receptors and adhesion molecules, remain to be clarified. Expression of c-kit and CD43 on the cell surface is a sign that mouse pro-B and pre-B-I cells have the capacity to proliferate. In contact with stromal cells, they retain this state as an actively cycling cell population and do not express μH chains as pre-BCRs on the surface.

Antibodies specific for c-kit inhibit pro-B and pre-B-I cell proliferation *in vitro* (226) as well as hematopoiesis of many lineages *in vivo*. Curiously, the same mAb (ACK-2) that inhibits *in vitro* B lymphopoiesis actually enhances *in vivo* B lymphopoiesis (227). Since the c-kit-specific antibodies also suppress myelopoiesis, the bone marrow compartments are emptied of myeloid cells by this treatment. The increase in the number of pre-B cells in bone marrow after c-kit treatment *in vivo* may well result from an expansion of the pre-B cells into areas normally occupied by myeloid cells. This would then be different from the situation in mutant mice, which are defective in the transit from pre-B-I to pre-B-II cells, and in which the pre-B-I cell compartment is normal or only marginally expanded in size (see discussion in next section and Figs. 3 and 7). This indicates that in normal, untreated mice, the precursor compartments are confined to certain areas and thereby limited in size.

The *in vivo* outgrowth of pre-B cells under c-kit antibody treatment might indicate that not all pre-B cells use c-kit as a growth-regulating tyrosine kinase (228). This suggests that the c-kit nonresponsive subpopulation might take over and might even expand under c-kit antibody treatment.

Proliferation of pro–pre-B-I cells on stromal cells in the presence of IL-7 can also be inhibited by interferon-γ (IFN-γ) (229). Normal pro–pre-B cells die by apoptosis as a consequence of exposure to IFN-γ *in vivo*. Since Eμ-bcl-2 transgenic mice, which have B-lineage cells with very prolonged life spans *in vitro* and *in vivo* (230), have normal numbers of normally proliferating pro-B and pre-B cells (231), the effect of IFN-γ can also be studied with cells from these mice. While the proliferation of pro-B and pre-B-I cells from Eμ-bcl-2 transgenic mice is inhibited by IFN-γ, as in normal cells, these cells do not die by apoptosis. It becomes apparent that IFN-γ does not induce differentiation to more mature B-lineage cells. Both normal and Eμ-bcl-2 transgenic (tg) pre-B cells exposed to IFN-γ in the presence of stromal cells and IL-7 fail to differentiate; that is, they do not express surface immunoglobulin, they retain expression of VpreB and λ5, and they do not express the α chain of the IL-2 receptor. They retain the capacity to proliferate on stromal cells in the presence of IL-7 once IFN-γ is removed.

At least some of the pro-B and pre-B-I cell proliferative supporting stromal cells are preadipocytic fibroblasts that can differentiate to fat cells (228). When they do so, they lose the capacity to support pro-B–pre-B-I proliferation. If this happens *in vivo*, B-lymphopoietic activity is reduced.

Transplantation of B Lineage–committed Precursor Cells: Repair of B-Lineage Immunodeficiencies and Analysis of B Lineage–expressed Gene Defects in Autoimmune Disease

Pre-B-I cells isolated *ex vivo* or grown *in vitro* are useful for two practical purposes. For one, they can repopulate some of the central and peripheral compartments of B-lineage cells when transplanted into suitably immunodeficient mice (e.g., SCID or RAG−/−). Upon transplantation, the hosts develop B-cell compartments in the periphery that are responsive to T cell-independent

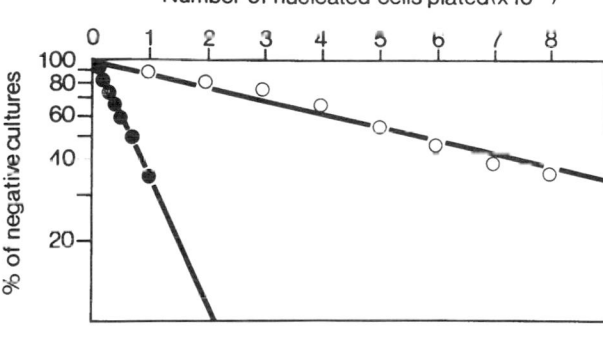

Number of nucleated cells plated(x 10⁻²)

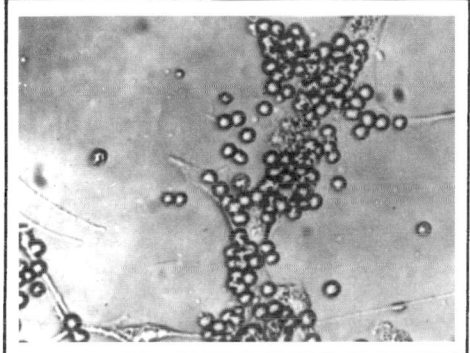

FIG. 9. Frequency of pre-B cells clonable on stromal cells in the presence of IL-7 or IL-3 in cell suspensions of fetal liver at day 18 of gestation (-●-) and in bone marrow at 15 weeks (-○-). Lower part shows a clone of pre-B cells growing on stromal cells and IL-7.

but not T cell-dependent antigens. No mature T cells develop. After 3 to 4 weeks, IgM levels reach normal levels and IgA reaches half-normal levels, but all IgG subclasses stay 20- to 50-fold lower than those of normal mice. The repopulation of the B-cell compartments is long-lasting (i.e., stable for over a year) (214,232). Cotransfer of CD4$^+$ T cells also establishes normal levels of IgG subclasses, and the peripheral B cells are now also reactive to T cell-dependent antigens. The potency of pre-B-I cells from fetal liver and bone marrow to repopulate stably, and for a long time, some of the B-lineage compartments is different. Fetal liver-derived precursors yield long-term reconstitution, but bone marrow-derived ones yield only transient repopulation of peripheral B-cell compartments (233).

The same pattern of reconstitution of the peripheral immune system can be seen when mature T and B cells are transplanted (234). The transplantation of pre-B-I cells offers the added advantage that a new repertoire of peripheral B cells can be generated from D$_H$J$_H$-rearranged precursors. Apparently, this repertoire is filtered against autoreactivities, as autoantibodies against double-stranded (ds) DNA are absent in the pre-B-I cell–transplanted mice. If the same transplantations can ever be developed for human B-lineage precursors (see later in the section on human B-cell development), then they may offer the possibility of reconstituting bone marrow transplantation patients with reactive, tolerized B-cell compartments, which often are absent in these patients with current transplantation protocols.

Pre-B-I cell transplantation into immunodeficient hosts also allows the phenotypic analysis *in vivo* of genetic defects leading to immunodeficiency and autoimmune diseases, which are expressed in B-lineage cells (235–237). One example is the (NZB × NZW)F$_1$ pre-B-I cell transplantation, which reveals the hyperreactivity of B cells and the hypergammaglobulinemia in IgM and IgG$_{2a}$ levels of the lupus erythematosus-prone mice in the transplanted SCID or RAG$^{-/-}$ hosts. Again, no T cells develop, indicating that these lupus-associated deregulations are expressed selectively in B cells. The IgG$_{2a}$ serum antibodies contain anti-ds DNA antibodies. Further dissection of the genetic contributions to these lupus-associated phenotypes can be seen when NZB pre-B-I cells lead to IgM, but not to IgG$_{2a}$ hypergammaglobulinemia, while NZW pre-B-I cells elicit IgG$_{2a}$, but not IgM hypergammaglobulinemia. Double-stranded DNA-specific antibodies are found in the NZW, but not in the NZB pre-B-I cell-transplanted hosts.

On the other hand, transplantation of pre-B-I cells of immunodeficient mice (suitable examples are given in Fig. 3) allows them to retain their immunodeficiency in the B-cell compartments upon adoptive transfer, a finding that allows defects inherently expressed in B-lineage cells to be distinguished from those that are generated by a defective interaction with T cells or with other cooperating cells of the environment. Again, these pre-B-I cell transplantations are potentially useful in the analysis, since they could offer a possible cure by transplantations of defects expressed in human B-lineage cells.

D$_H$J$_H$ Rearrangements

In the mouse genome, the D$_H$J$_H$ segments of the H-chain loci contain promoter elements at their 5′ ends that allow transcription in pre-B-I cells of a D$_H$J$_H$-rearranged H-chain gene locus (238–243). When D$_H$ is rearranged to J$_H$ in reading frame II, the corresponding messenger RNA (mRNA) potentially encodes a D$_H$J$_H$Cμ protein (244). Such a D$_H$J$_H$Cμ protein has, however, only

been found in one Abelson virus-transformed cell line, but not yet in normal pre-B cells in which D$_H$J$_H$ rearrangements have taken place (245). It therefore remains a speculation that normal cells deposit this protein on the surface membrane of pre-B cells, bound by disulfide bonds to the λ5 protein of the surrogate L chain. Human pre-B cells do not express the D$_H$J$_H$Cμ protein, suggesting that it is a peculiar and perhaps unique product of mouse B-lineage cells.

At the transition of pro-B to pre-B-I cells, D$_H$ to J$_H$ rearrangement can occur in all three reading frames (241,246–248). Reading frame I (nomenclature of ref. 239) is preferred over reading frames II and III. Several reasons can be quoted for this unequal representation of reading frames in the V$_H$ repertoire of precursor and mature B cells. First, short stretches of sequence homologies in D and J segments may mediate the alignment of the recombining DNA strands. This mechanism can select for reading frame I as long as no N regions are introduced (i.e., in fetal liver before the birth of a mouse). The preference for reading frame I and the absence of reading frame II are also visible in preexisting D$_H$J$_H$ joints found in the circular DNA, which arise as products during D$_H$ to J$_H$ rearrangements in pre-B cells (242). Ratios for reading frame I–reading frame II–reading frame III of 70:15:15 have been measured with recombination substrates (249). These ratios are close to those seen in the earliest pre-B-I cells developing without N-region insertions in fetal liver (250).

Second, in reading frame III, many D$_H$ segments contain one or more stop codons, disfavoring this reading frame (247,248).

Third, proliferation of pre-B-I cells *in vivo* in fetal liver, or *in vitro* on stromal cells, in the presence of IL-7 leads to loss of cells with reading frame II (250). This suggests that the D$_H$J$_H$Cμ protein inhibits the capacity of a pre-B cell to be clonable, just as much as a μH chain does when pre-B-I cells differentiate to pre-B-II cells (see discussion elsewhere in this section). Cells containing the other two reading frames outgrow those with reading frame II. This suppression of reading frame II is not observed in μH-tm$^{-/-}$ and in λ5$^{-/-}$ mice and their pre-B-I cells, arguing that the earlier form of a pre-BCR (i.e., the association of surrogate L chain with D$_H$J$_H$Cμ protein in its membrane-bound form) mediates reading frame II suppression.

Fourth, the pre-B receptor, in its D$_H$J$_H$Cμ-surrogate L-chain form, could signal allelic exclusion (i.e., inhibit the V$_H$ to D$_H$J$_H$ rearrangement of the second allele in a pre-B-I cell) (194). This would effectively remove them from the pool of cells that either can or do express μH chains.

Precursor B-II Cells

The next developmental stage in the B-lineage is characterized by cytoplasmic μH chain expression, which defines the pre-B-II cell stage. These typical pre-B cells have lost the expression of c-kit and TdT, and the majority also do not express CD43 (188). On the other hand, these cells have gained the expression of μH chains as well as CD25 (188).

The pre-B-II compartment can be subdivided into three different developmental stages: two that are large and cycling and one that is small and resting. Pre-B-II cells have lost the capacity to be clonable on stromal cells in the presence of IL-7 or IL-3. The first stage contains large, cycling cells that express on their surface the pre-BCR consisting of the SL chain in association with the μH chain (214,216,251). These cells do not express RAG-1 and RAG-2 and still have their IgL-chain loci in germline configuration.

The Progenitor and Precursor B-Cell Receptors

Structure

Two proteins encoded by the pre-B cell–specific genes VpreB and λ5 (252,253) can associate with each other to form an L-chain-like structure, the so-called surrogate light chain (Fig. 10) (254). The surrogate L chain can be found in association with a molecular complex of glycoproteins on the surface of μH chain-negative pro-B cells (255,256). This complex is referred to as the pro-BCR.

In the pre-BCR, the surrogate L chain is associated with μH chains (257–260) (see Fig. 10). The pre-BCR has a structure similar to the BCR, which is composed of μH chain and L chains because the accessory molecules (Igα and Igβ) that function as signal transducers are found associated with both receptors (95, 260–266) (see Fig. 10).

The genes encoding the VpreB and the λ5 proteins are found on the same chromosomes as the λ L-chain genes in both mouse (chromosome 16) and human (chromosome 22) (267,268) (see Fig. 10). In the mouse, there are two functional VpreB genes with very high sequence homology (253). The $VpreB_1$ and λ5 genes are located within 10 kb of each other, with an unknown distance from $VpreB_2$ and from the λ L-chain locus. VpreB genes show weak sequence homologies to V_H and V_L segments at the NH_2-terminal with the region equivalent to the third CDR, while the λ5 gene shows strong sequence homologies to λL-chain sequences in the J and C region-equivalent parts. The amino-terminal region of λ5 shows weak similarities to V regions in which the β-pleated sheets C, D, and E are missing, while the carboxy-terminal region of VpreB has, so far, no sequence similarity with any known gene.

In contrast to the V and J genes of the L-chain loci, the VpreB and λ5 genes do not undergo rearrangement with each other during B-cell development. The typical rearrangement signal sequences that are present immediately 3′ of the V_L-chain genes, as well as immediately 5′ of the J_L-chain genes, are missing in the VpreB and λ5 genes.

Another VpreB-like molecule has been found to be expressed in pre-B cells (earlier called 8HS20) (269), and is called $VpreB_3$ (270). In contrast to $VpreB_1$ and $VpreB_2$ genes, the $VpreB_3$ gene contains an intron separating the V-like domain into two exons. The location of this gene within the genome of the mouse has not been determined.

In human, there is only one VpreB gene within a cluster of Vλ genes (271) with 80% overall sequence identity to the mouse $VpreB_{1/2}$ genes (272). Multiple λ5-like genes have been found in humans (240,273–275). A cluster of three genes—14.1, 16.1, and Fλ1—do not rearrange during B-cell development. Another gene, the Igλ1 gene, which can rearrange during B-cell development, is also organized in a typical three-exon structure very similar to that of the λ5 and 14.1 genes (276). The 14.1 gene is transcribed and translated into a λ5-like protein. None of the other λ5-like genes has been found to be translated into protein. It is intriguing to speculate that the Igλ1 gene represents a descendent of a primordial λ5-like gene in which the rearrangement signal sequences have been integrated. It remains unclear, however, how the surrogate L-chain genes evolved relative to the λ L-chain loci as well as to the V region clusters used in rearrangements of the IgH- and κL-chain genes.

The 5′ λ5 region contains two separable elements: a 3′ part with general promotor activity and a 5′ part containing an enhancer that confers the specificity of expression. It also acts on heterologous promoters (277–280). Apparently the enhancer acts as an expression-suppressing element in later B-cell stages and in other cells. The transcription factor EBF binds to a DNA motif in the λ5 enhancer. When a 722bp-long region 5′ of the λ5 gene was coupled to the human CD25 gene, encoding the α chain of the IL-2 receptor, and a transgenic mouse was made, the reporter gene was expressed in parallel to the endogenous λ5 gene (199). This lineage fidelity of expression of a reporter gene offers the advantage to identify and study rare early B-cell progenitors in the mouse (see discussion in the previous section).

The VpreB and λ5 genes have, so far, always been found coexpressed in the same cells. In transformed cell lines of mouse and human, the expression ranges from earliest pre-B cells to $sIgM^+$ immature B cells (281), while in normal B-lineage cells, expression is more restricted, beginning with $B220^+$ $CD19^-$ precursors, continuing in pre-B-I cells and in large, pre-B receptor-expressing pre-B-II cells. Expression is terminated thereafter so that small pre-B-II cells and immature $sIgM^+$ cells no longer express surrogate L chain (254). The VpreB and λ5 genes have never been found to be expressed in any other lineage of cells, except in those of the early B lineage.

Although some reports have questioned the comparable expression patterns of surrogate L chain in mouse and human (273,282), sufficient experimental evidence now appears to conclude that the expression patterns of surrogate L chain in mouse and human show striking similarities. In both species, early pro-B and pre-B-I cells express surrogate L chain with a complex of glycoproteins as the so called pro-B receptor (283,284), and large pre-B-II cells express surrogate L chain with μH chains on the surface as the pre-B receptor (273,282,285). Normal immature $sIgM^+$ B cells of both species have not been seen to express surrogate L chain. The strikingly similar development in the bone marrow of mice and humans is described later in the section on human B-cell development.

Functions

The function of the molecular complex of the surrogate L chain in association with the gp130 molecule is unclear. Early B-lineage development prior to expression of the μH chain appears to be normal in $λ5^{-/-}$ mice (see Fig. 3), and pre-B-I cells from those mice show normal in vitro growth on stromal cells in the presence of IL-7, as well as normal modes and kinetics of differentiation.

However, one has to keep in mind that VpreB is expressed in the λ5-deficient mouse. It is possible that an early receptor complex consisting of VpreB in association with gp130, and possibly with other proteins, functions normally in the absence of the λ5 protein. This hypothesis will become testable when all three genes on chromosome 16 of the mouse (i.e., $VpreB_1$, $VpreB_2$, and λ5) have been deleted on the same chromosome. It will be interesting to see whether in such triple-defective mice B-cell development up to the pre-B-I cell stage is still normal. Likewise, the identification of the gene encoding for gp130 protein and the targeted disruption of this gene should shed light on the role of the early receptor complex in B-cell development.

When a D_HJ_H-rearranged pre-B-I cell rearranges V_H to the D_HJ_H-rearranged alleles, this rearrangement can be either in or out of frame. It has been estimated that only 10% to 15% of all pre-B-I cells end up with at least one productive μH-chain gene locus. In $λ5^{-/-}$ mice, this is the percentage of cytoplasmically μH

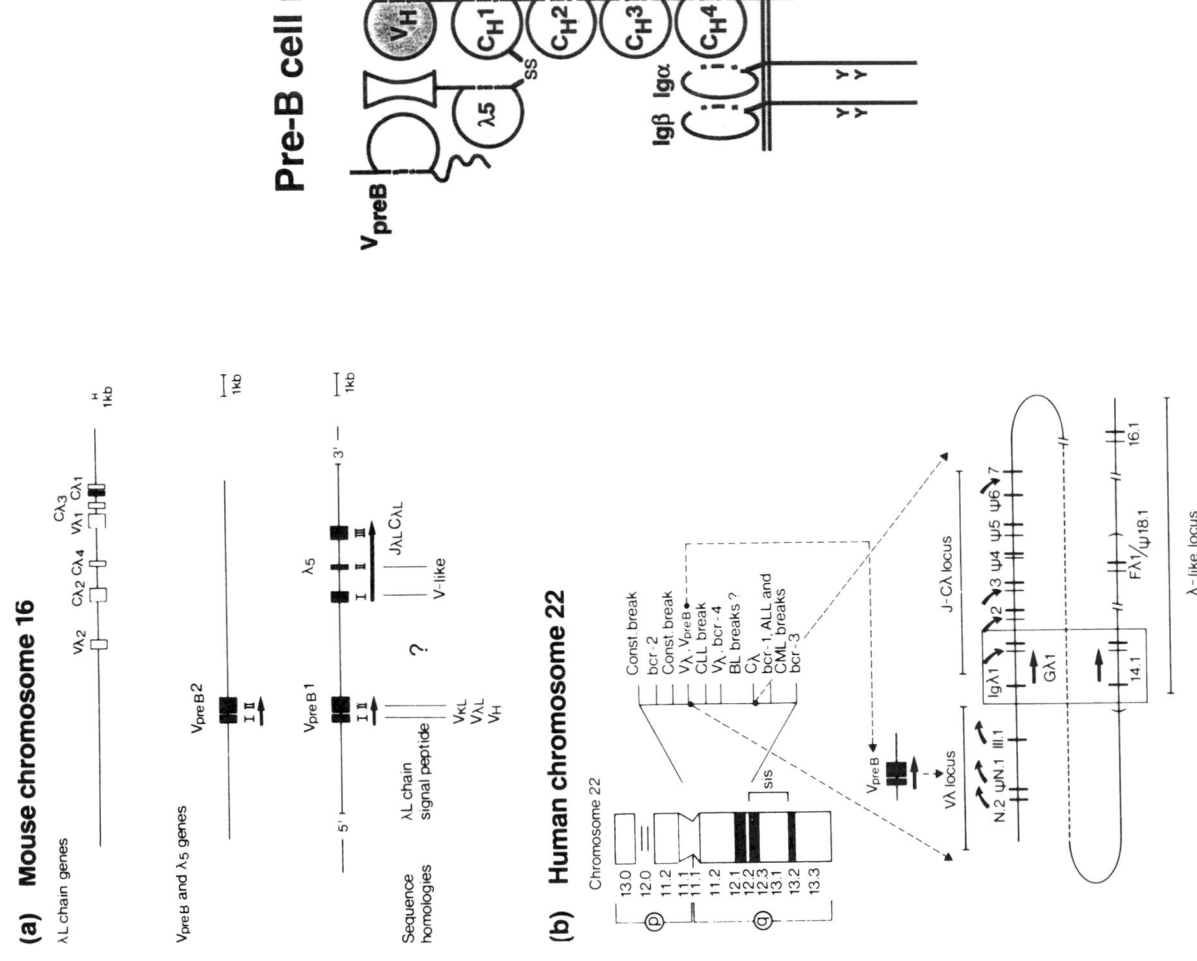

(a) Mouse chromosome 16

λL chain genes

VλB and λ5 genes

Sequence homologies

λL chain signal peptide

(b) Human chromosome 22

chain-expressing pre-B cells that can be found among the B220[+] B-lineage cells (188).

Whenever V_H to $D_H J_H$ rearrangement occurs in-frame, a μH chain can be produced that potentially can pair with surrogate L chain to form a pre-BCR. A large pre-B-II cell is generated by this productive rearrangement. It is exactly at this stage of B-cell development that two important reactions in B-lineage cells are initiated, and both appear to involve the pre-BCR. One leads to proliferative burst of all pre-B cells that express a pre-B receptor on the surface (188). The other turns off V_H to $D_H J_H$ rearrangements at the second H-chain allele, a process leading to allelic exclusion of two productively $V_H D_H J_H$-rearranged H-chain alleles (i.e., preventing two H chains being expressed by the same B-lineage cell) (286). The large, pre-B receptor-expressing pre-B-II cells are the most likely sites for these actions: They are in cell cycle and their $V_H D_H J_H$-rearrangement machinery has been turned off (287). The L-chain gene loci are not yet transcriptionally active, and the H-chain locus, which has not been $V_H D_H J_H$-rearranged, might be rendered inaccessible for further rearrangements in ways that need to be clarified.

Large pre-B-II cells and all subsequent stages of B-cell development are greatly enriched for productively $V_H D_H J_H$-rearranged H-chain loci (184,188,208). Moreover, the absolute number of cytoplasmically μH chain–expressing cells in normal mice is 10 to 15 times higher than in $\lambda 5^{-/-}$ mice (188,288). Thus, the expression of the pre-BCR ensures proliferative expansion and, in fact, constitutes a positive selection for pre-B cells with a productive $V_H D_H J_H$ rearrangement.

From the calculations described above, it seems that cells with nonproductive $V_H D_H J_H$ alleles initially form a larger pool of cells than those with a productive μH-chain rearrangement. Single-cell analyses of the rearrangement status of the H-chain alleles by Ehlich and colleagues (194) have shown that cells with two non-functionally $V_H D_H J_H$-rearranged alleles accumulate in fraction C (see Fig. 8A) of Hardy et al. (184), which contains cells expressing the surface markers CD43, HSA, and BP-1.

The death repressor gene bcl-x, which is a member of the bcl-2 family and which blocks diverse apoptotic pathways in lymphocytes, plays a crucial role at this developmental stage (289,290). Thus, bcl-x$^{-/-}$ mice have largely reduced $c\mu H^+$ pre-B-II compartments (289), while bcl-x transgenic mice have largely expanded populations of aberrantly rearranged pre-B cells (290). These findings might suggest that a signal via the pre-B receptor is inducing bcl-x expression, thereby giving productively $V_H D_H J_H$-rearranged pre-B cells a longer lifespan.

Early V_H Repertoires and Their Changes during Development

The diversity of 14 families of V_H, 13 functional D, and 4 J_H segments, which randomly rearrange with each other, and the added diversity introduced by N-region insertions into the V_H to D and D to J_H joints, provide for an immense "potential" repertoire of different μH chains in pre-BCRs (239,291–294). However, the V_H, D, or J_H segments represented in pre-B cells, and later in mature sIgM[+]/sIgD[+] repertoires, do not proportionally correlate with their representation in germline (240,247,295–298). V_H genes belonging to the $V_H 7183$ and $V_H Q52$ families are overrepresented early in development (i.e., in fetal liver B cells) (299–304). In particular, the most D-proximal functional V_H gene segment, $V_H 81X$, which is a member of the $V_H 7183$ family, predominates in repertoires early in ontogeny (300–305). In contrast, peripheral mature B-cell populations in adult mice express a V_H repertoire in which the frequency of each V_H family used correlates with its germline complexity (301,306–309). $V_H 81X$ representation declines in $V_H D_H J_H$ rearrangements during B-cell development in bone marrow of adult mice (305). Indeed, $V_H 81X$-expressing B cells are rarely found in the spleen (296,301,310). Moreover, virtually all $V_H D_H J_H$ rearrangements utilizing $V_H 81X$ genes in the splenic sIg^+ B-cell repertoire are nonproductive, while 25% to 30% of $V_H 81X$ rearrangements in sIg^- pre-B cells in the bone marrow are productive (295,296,311). This is in contrast to rearrangements using other V_H genes, which are largely productive (248,310,311).

Preferential representation of the $V_H 7183$ and $V_H Q52$ families early in B-cell development might be the result of preferential usage of these segments on the genomic level during the rearrangement process (300,302–304,307). In agreement with this notion, it has been implicated that the recombination signal sequences of $V_H 7183$ mediate recombination more frequently than do those of $V_H J558$ (312). Suppression of the representation of certain V_H segments later during B-cell generation could then be the result of the action of the pre-BCR. In fact, mutant mice defective in pre-BCR expression, such as the $\lambda 5^{-/-}$ mice, do not display the change of V_H representation in adult bone marrow. Also, pre-B cells expressing an H chain, which is incapable of pairing with the surrogate L chain (313,314), would be excluded from the repertoire.

This, in fact, can be seen at early stages of $V_H D_H J_H$-rearranged precursor B cells in bone marrow of normal mice. In a fraction of c-kit$^+$ cytoplasmic μH-chain$^+$ B cells, a V_H repertoire is expressed that is biased toward the D-proximal V_H families, $V_H 7183$ and $V_H Q52$, on the productive and the nonproductive allele (314). Only

---

FIG. 10. The organization of the VpreB and $\lambda 5$ genes on mouse chromosome 16 and human chromosome 22, and a speculative structure of the pre-BCR, relative to the BCR. The organization of the cluster of λL-chain genes of the mouse (**a**) is adapted from Carson and Wu (552), and that of the human (**b**) from Combriato and Klobeck (553). The λL-like pre-B cell–specific loci VpreB$_2$ and VpreB$_1$ and $\lambda 5$ in the mouse (**a**) and Gλ_1/Igλ\14.1, Fλ/ψ18.1 and 16.1 of human (**b**) are on the same chromosomes, at unknown distances from the λL-chain loci. The human VpreB gene is within a cluster of V_λ segments, further defined by breakpoints of chromosomal translocations found in lymphomas and leukemias. Pre-B cell–specific expression is indicated by the symbol →, and the capacity to rearrange Vλ_L to Jλ_L to form a productive (V$_L$J$_L$) λL-chain gene is indicated by the symbol ↗↘. Nucleotide sequence homologies of the mouse VpreB$_1$ $\lambda 5$ locus are indicated on the bottom of the mouse gene map. The V-like homology is detectable not by nucleotides, but by amino acid similarities. The question mark indicates that no sequence homology is detectable with any sequence published so far. In the protein structure of the pre-BCR, VpreB is drawn as if it would be an Ig V region with an unknown carboxy-terminus protruding from the region analogous to the CDR3 of a V region. $\lambda 5$ is drawn with a C region analogous to the C_L region and with a V region-like amino terminal, in which four (A, B, F, and G) of the seven β strands of an Ig domain appear to be present (254). The pre-B cell and BCRs are both anchored in the surface membrane by Igα and Igβ.

half of the μH chains expressed in these cells can form a pre-BCR. The subsequent c-kit⁻ cytoplasmic μH chain⁺, partially pre-BCR⁺, cycling pre-B-II cells show a suppression of the representation of the D-proximal V_H-gene families on the productive, but not on the nonproductive alleles. Over 95% of the μH chains expressed in these cells can form a pre-BCR. In λ5-deficient mice, the pool of cytoplasmic μH-chain⁺ precursor B cells expresses a V_H-gene repertoire biased to the D-proximal V_H families (314). Half of the μH chains can associate with the surrogate L chain. In splenic mature B cells of λ5-deficient mice, however, the representation of the D-proximal V_H-gene families is suppressed on the productive, but not on the nonproductive alleles (314). The pre-BCR appears to mediate the V_H repertoire change in normal bone marrow B-lineage cells, while the BCR does so in λ5-deficient mice. This indicates that positive selection of pre-B and B cells appears to be mediated by the capacity of H chains expressed by them to form a pre-BCR and a BCR, respectively.

Mutants with Defective Precursor B-Cell Receptors and Other Mutations That Affect the Transition from Precursor B-I to Large Precursor B-II Cells

The importance of the large pre-B-II stage of development, and particularly the expression of the pre-B receptor that ensures normal B-cell development, is best exemplified in mutants that are unable to produce this receptor. Thus, mice with a deletion in the transmembrane portion of their μH-chain μH-tm⁻/⁻ and mice with a deletion in the λ5 part of the surrogate L chain-encoding genes have no large cycling pre-B-II cells and reduced numbers of small pre-B cells (188,209,288). A similar phenotype was found in mice with a deletion in the Igβ gene (95), indicating that the association between the pre-BCR and Igβ and probably also Igα is required for the transition from pre-B-I to pre-B-II cells.

In μH-tm⁺/⁻ heterozygous mice, the capacity of the wild-type allele to insert intact μH chain into the membrane enables normal proliferative expansion and development of the pre-B-II compartment and, subsequently, the development of normal numbers of mature B cells at normal rates (208). In many B cells, however, the mutated allele is not subjected to allelic exclusion (i.e., it, also, is productively rearranged). If the membrane-bound form of μH chains is involved in signaling inhibition of further V_H to D_HJ_H rearrangements, then one might expect that in all μH-tm⁺/⁻ heterozygous B cells with two productively $V_HD_HJ_H$-rearranged IgH loci, the μH-tm⁻ allele should have rearranged first.

The tyrosine kinase Syk⁻/⁻ mouse displays a block at the pre-B-I to pre-B-II stage of B-cell development, indicating a key role for Syk in pre-BCR signaling (212,213). At this point, it is worthwhile to note that the homologous kinase ZAP-70, which is crucial in pre-TCR signaling, can replace the function of Syk in B-cell development, indicating a similar type of signal transduction in T and B cells at this stage of development (315).

PAX-5⁻/⁻ mice have a block at the same transitional stage of B-cell development in bone marrow. The number of pre-B-I cells with both IgH-chain alleles in a D_H-J_H-rearranged configuration is relatively normal in Pax-5⁻/⁻ bone marrow. However, V_H-D_HJ_H rearrangements are dramatically, if not absolutely, blocked in these mice (101,102,111). How the absence of a functional Pax-5 gene product leads to this selective block in B-cell development is unclear. Genes that might cause such a defect, like RAG-1 or -2, λ5, or VpreB, are expressed at normal levels in pre-B-I cells from

Pax-5⁻/⁻ mice (102,111). At this point, the only gene known to be affected by the absence of a functional Pax-5 gene is CD19. CD19 transcripts as well as CD19 protein are undetectable in Pax-5⁻/⁻ mice (101,102,111). However, the lack of CD19 expression cannot explain the Pax-5 phenotype, because CD19⁻/⁻ mice have relatively normal B-cell development (181,316).

The Roles of Transgenic μH Chains in Precursor B-Cell Receptors

Early expression of a number of different transgenic μH chains under the control of the Eμ enhancer leads to inhibition of V_H to D_HJ_H rearrangements of the two endogenous H-chain alleles (317). The transgenic μH chains do so regardless of whether they are inserted by homologous recombination at the proper site (i.e., by being "knocked into" the H-chain gene locus) (318) or whether they are inserted at other places in the genome by heterologous recombination. The membrane-bound form of the μH chain is required for this form of allelic exclusion, as the secreted form of a transgenic μH chain does not inhibit endogenous V_H to D_HJ_H rearrangements, and normal B-cell development (319,320). When expressed under Eμ-control, transgenic δH chains can also mediate the same inhibitory effect on $V_HD_HJ_H$ rearrangements (321). Precursor-cell development, as judged by the phenotypes and the number of pre-B-II immature and mature B cells, appears to remain normal, though the Ig repertoires of these cells are altered.

Transgenic γ2bH chains under Eμ control, however, have a differential effect on B-cell development at the pre-B-II stage (322–324). Several γ2bH-chain transgenic mouse strains show strong inhibition of endogenous V_H to D_HJ_H rearrangements, but do not allow normal cell development to mature sIg⁺ B cells. The sIg⁺ B cells, which develop at much reduced rates, all express endogenous μH chains in addition to transgenic γ2bH chains, indicating that inhibition of endogenous V_H to D_HJ_H rearrangements is partial. Crosses between γ2bH-chain and μH-chain transgenic mice develop normal numbers of pre-B and B cells, suggesting that these transgenic γ2bH chains are not toxic. These results suggest that signals for the inhibition of $V_HD_HJ_H$ rearrangements of the other (in transgenic mice of both endogenous) allele(s) and signals for proliferative expansion and further development to pre-B-II cells may be different. As μH chains and δH chains have very similar, short intracytoplasmic tails, whereas γ2bH chains have different, long ones, the structural basis for this difference in the γ2bH-transgenic situation might be sought in differential signaling properties of these intracytoplasmic tails.

The effect of transgenic μH chains on the proliferative expansion and development of the pre-B-II compartment is most clearly visible against a SCID background of SCID mice (325–329) or RAG-T⁻/⁻ (330) or RAG-2⁻/⁻ (188,331). In these mice, the introduction of four different transgenic μH chains (one of which is even a human μH chain) resulted in an apparently complete development of normal numbers of pre-B-II cells [measured either by the appearance of normal numbers of cells in Hardy's fraction D, or by the appearance of normal numbers of CD25 (TAC)⁺ pre-B-II cells]. Rolink et al. (188) also found normal numbers of large cycling and small resting cells in this pre-B-cell compartment, indicating that the transgenic μH chain induced normal proliferative expansion of cells at the transition of pre-B-I to pre-B-II cells. These results make it less likely that a specific autoreactivity for defined ligands in the bone marrow microenvironment of a special set of V_H regions expressed at the transition from pre-B-I to pre-B-II cells is involved either in the signaling for inhibition of the V_H to $D_H J_H$ rearrangements, or in the proliferative expansion of pre-B cells into the pre-B-II compartments. The fact that a conventional L-chain expressed as a transgene early in development can overcome the defect in B-cell development in the $\lambda 5^{-/-}$ mice (332–334) further supports the idea that the pre-BCR does not need to interact with a ligand in order to function.

All transgenic forms of H chains need the association with surrogate L chain into a pre-BCR to signal proliferative expansion and the development of small pre-B-II cells. A notable exception to this rule is a truncated form of a μH chain in which a $D_H J_H$-rearranged segment is joined to the 3′ end of the $C\mu_{H2}$ domain, followed by the rest of the μH chain (i.e., $C\mu_{H3}$, $C\mu_{H4}$ transmembrane and intracytoplasmic portions) (260). This truncated μH chain cannot associate with surrogate L chain, but is deposited on the cell surface of peripheral B cells (335). In the presence of $\lambda 5$, as well as in its absence, this truncated μH chain allows B-lineage cells to differentiate to pre-B-II–like cells. In contrast to a normal transgenic μH chain on a RAG-deficient background, it even allows the appearance of surface μH chain–expressing B cells in the periphery. How it does so needs to be investigated.

Allelic Exclusion at the H-Chain Gene Locus

The pre-BCR also appears to be involved in allelic exclusion, because in both the μH-tm$^{-/-}$ and the $\lambda 5^{-/-}$ mice, absence of allelic exclusion has been reported (208,286). However, in the case of the $\lambda 5^{-/-}$ mice, all double producers so far found are of a special phenotype. They produce one μH chain that can and a second that cannot pair with surrogate L chain (314,336). Furthermore, such pairing–nonpairing double producers are also found in normal mice at the same frequencies, indicating that, in fact, the $\lambda 5^{-/-}$ defect does not abolish allelic exclusion of two pairing μH chains. Since VpreB can associate with μH chain even in the absence of $\lambda 5$ protein (337), this leaves open the possibility that a VpreB/μH-chain dimer form of the pre-BCR surfaces to signal the pre-B-II cell to terminate V_H to $D_H J_H$ rearrangements at the second allele.

Initiation of L-Chain Gene Transcription and Rearrangements

In all likelihood, the pre-B-cell stage following the pre-BCR positive cells is the large cycling pre-B-II that has lost the expression of the SL chain (188,216,251). Unlike the pre-BCR–positive cells, these cells express RAG-1 and RAG-2 at the RNA level, but not yet at the protein level (287). Moreover, sterile transcripts from the κL-chain gene locus become detectable, although the L-chain gene loci in these cells are still in germline configuration (195,287).

When the large, cycling pre-B-II cells become resting and small, RAG-1 and RAG-2 expression is turned on at both the RNA and the protein level, and stays on in at least some sIg$^+$ immature B cells (287). A large proportion of the cells are found to have been rearranged at the L-chain gene loci (195). Already at this stage, the κ- and λL-chain loci are rearranged in the characteristic 10:1 ratio (195), although small pre-B-II cells do not express Ig on their surface.

Four possible explanations can be given concerning why $V_L J_L$-rearranged small pre-B-II cells do not express L-chain protein in association with μH chains as IgM molecules on the surface. First,

rearrangements could all be out of frame. Second, the L chains produced from productively rearranged alleles might not be able to pair with μH chains. Third, productive rearrangements might just have happened, but protein synthesis has not yet generated sufficient quantities of L-chain protein to be detectable on the surface. Fourth, sIgM might be downregulated as a consequence of interaction with autoantigens (see, below, the "editing" reaction of immature B cells).

Mutations that specifically affect the formation of the large, cycling pre-BCR–negative or the subsequent small resting pre-B-II compartments have not been found. It is important to realize that the large and small pre-B-II cell compartments are formed with normal cell cycle status, CD25 marker expression, and in near-normal numbers, even in mice that either cannot rearrange the κL-chain gene locus (338,339) or cannot rearrange any L-chain gene loci but express a transgenic μH chain (i.e., on a RAG$^{-/-}$ or SCID background) (see above). This shows that the pre-BCR potentiates pre-B-II cell development by proliferative expansion and that the accumulation of these cellular compartments in bone marrow occurs independently of any L-chain gene rearrangements.

The finding that the IL-7$^{-/-}$ mice have a block in B-cell development at the transition from pre-B-I to pre-B-II strongly suggests that IL-7 is the cytokine that is involved in the proliferative expansion of pre-BCR–positive pre-B-II cells (211). This idea is consistent with the finding that IL-7 transgenic mice have a largely expanded pre-B-II compartment (48).

Immature B Cells

Formation

Small pre-B-II cells with a productive κL- or λL-chain rearrangement can become sIgM$^+$ immature B cells. In the mouse, the ratio of κL to λL chain-expressing B cells is approximately 10:1 (246). In normal mice, the ratio of small pre-B-II cells to immature sIgM$^+$ B cells is approximately 1 (131,188). However, in mice that cannot undergo κL-chain rearrangement due to a targeted deletion of the intron enhancer (338) or that cannot make a κL-chain protein due the deletion of the $C\kappa$ region (339), this ratio is approximately 4, with a decrease in immature B cells. Thus, the inability to produce a κL-chain protein greatly affects the transition from small pre-B-II cells to immature sIgM$^+$ B cells. Poor efficiency of λL chains to pair with μH chains and low efficiency of λL-chain gene rearrangements, are two mutually nonexclusive possibilities that might explain this finding.

Negative Selection: The Arrest of Differentiation of Immature B Cells

Exposure of immature B cells to antigen results in the downregulation of expression of sIgM and B220 (CD45R) (Fig.11). This has been demonstrated *in vitro* as well as *in vivo* with immature B cells from transgenic mice expressing a hen egg lysozyme (HEL)-specific, highly somatically mutated IgM (340). *In vitro* exposure of anti-HEL transgenic immature B cells to thymocytes expressing a surface membrane–bound form of HEL (mHEL) results in the downregulation of sIgM and B220 expression on the transgenic, immature B cells. *In vivo*, the presence of mHEL in the bone marrow generates sIgM^{low} B220^{low} immature B cells and arrests the further differentiation of the mHEL-reactive transgenic B cells. In

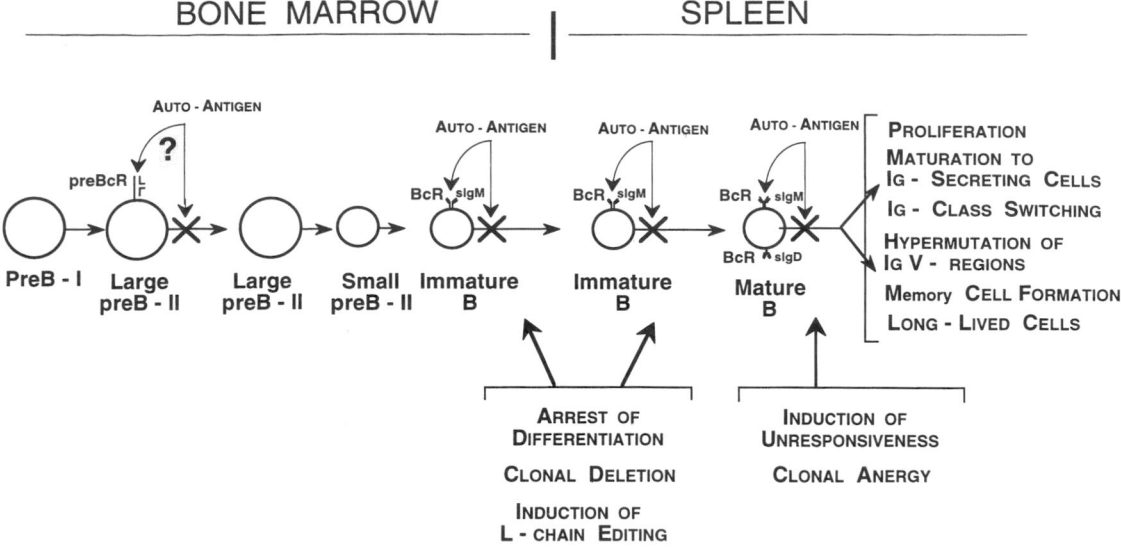

BONE MARROW | **SPLEEN**

FIG. 11. Actions of autoantigens during B-cell development in the primary (bone marrow) and secondary (spleen) lymphoid organs. The question mark denotes the speculation that the pre-BCR might recognize autoantigens, leading to arrest and deletion of large pre-B-II cells. Three target cells—immature B cells in bone marrow and in spleen and mature B cells in spleen—are subject to negative selection by autoantigens.

another transgenic mouse model, these cells have been called *transitional B cells* (341). *In vitro,* the arrested transgenic immature B cells are kept at the sIgM^{low} B220^{low} state in the presence of the antigen (e.g., when mHEL-expressing thymocytes are present). However, they will differentiate into sIgM$^+$ sIgD$^+$, mature, mitogen-, and antigen-reactive B cells expressing L-selectin, complement receptors 1 and 2, and CD22 and CD23 markers in the absence of mHEL. This also occurs *in vivo* in anti-HEL transgenic animals not expressing mHEL.

Arrest of differentiation can be seen most clearly when endogenous L-chain rearrangements are not possible (i.e., when the transgenic H- and L-chain genes are bred onto a homozygous SCID RAG-1$^{-/-}$ or RAG-2$^{-/-}$ background) (325,330,331,342,343). In three of these transgenics (325,330,343), an autoantigen can only be suspected, and its expression is uncontrollable. In a fourth case, however, the specificity of the transgenic sIgM is known (330). Transgenic sIgM$^+$, MHC class I-specific immature B cells are arrested at the IgM^{low} B220^{low} stage of differentiation in bone marrow of H2^b mice (i.e., when the specific autoantigen is present), whereas sIgM$^+$ immature and sIgM$^+$ mature B cells develop in normal numbers and with unimpaired reactivities when the autoantigen is absent, for example, in H2^d mice.

Arrest of differentiation is not seen in the 186.2 VH-µC/λ$_1$L anti-NP transgenic mice on a RAG-2 background (331). The emerging B cells are normal, mature, antigen-reactive cells. This implies either that the transgenic receptor does not recognize an (unknown) autoantigen in primary lymphoid organs, or that the signaling in immature, but not in mature B cells is impaired. So far, the analyses of these transgenic mice on normal (i.e., L-chain rearranging) genetic backgrounds have not discovered any abnormalities in their B-cell repertoires that might indicate such a defect.

An interesting situation is generated in mice with a transgenic Ig specific for mouse erythrocytes. Apparently, the CD5$^+$ B-cell lineage represented in the peritoneum (176) escapes differentiation arrest, whereas the very small number of conventional B cells

remaining in other lymphoid organs appears anergized (344). Oral administration of lipopolysaccharide activates CD5$^+$ B cells in the peritoneum and lamina propria, resulting in autoantibody secretion and thus, autoimmune symptoms of anemia (178). It could be that red cells are presented as autoantigens in a different way to that of the other autoantigens employed with transgenic mice, with the result that conventional, but not CD5$^+$ B cells are arrested, censored, and edited. Alternatively, because CD5$^+$ B cells are, at least in part, generated from fetal liver early in ontogeny (345) but most conventional CD5$^+$ B cells arise from the bone marrow throughout life, arrest of differentiation and/or censoring and editing might either not happen in this lineage, or follow different rules. Autoreactive, often activated B cells, which are found in this CD5$^+$ compartment, could be expected from such a lack of tolerance induction.

It appears that antigens, cross-reactive with autoantigens, might be able to interfere with the arrest of differentiation of immature B cells. Injection of the T-independent antigen TNP-Ficoll into the anti-TNP mAb (and cross-reactive with dsDNA)-transgenic Sp6 mouse on a rearrangement-deficient genetic background relieves the inhibition of differentiation and leads to the development of plasma cells secreting the transgenic IgM in large quantities. This points to a way by which central tolerance may be broken, or never established (343). If the foreign antigen, in this case the hapten TNP, is cross-reactive with autoantigens, in this case ds DNA, the autoantigen-specific B cells may be diverted from an arrest to further progression in differentiation to the mature B-cell stage.

A number of pathogenic bacteria are suspected to be capable of inducing an autoimmune disease (reviewed in ref. 346) because of a mimicry of bacterial antigen with an autoantigen. Many bacterial structures are known to act as T cell-independent antigens (347). They may be competitors for the interactions between an autoantigen and its immature sIg$^+$ B cells whenever they are cross-reactive with the autoantigen and whenever they manage to be present in the primary lymphoid organ (i.e., in the bone marrow).

Immunoglobulin Receptor Editing

Immature B cells cannot yet respond to antigenic or mitogenic stimulation by proliferation and maturation into Ig-secreting cells (231,348–352). They still express the RAG-1 and RAG-2 proteins and can undergo secondary L-chain rearrangements (231,287, 353–355). Secondary L-chain rearrangements are visible in a decrease of the κL/λL-chain ratio, in the changes of κL chain-expressing cells to λL chain-expressing cells, and in the changes from κL chain or λL chain expressing to sIg L-chain cells.

It even appears that at least some of the continued expression of the rearrangement machinery and the secondary L-chain rearrangements may, in fact, be induced by autoantigens present in the central lymphoid organ (e.g., in the bone marrow) (353,356, 357). The reaction of immature sIg⁺ B cells with autoantigens appears to provide a scenario in which interactions of the ligand (autoantigen) with sIg on the immature B cells do not terminate the immature state, but induce further rearrangements, as measured by increased levels of λL- over κL-chain gene rearrangements and subsequent expression, and by L-chain repertoire changes induced by the autoreactive transgenic Ig molecule. This is of potential advantage, because it gives an autoreactive B cell a chance to lose its specificity for autoantigen by changing the V region or the V and C regions of the L chain.

Whenever the peripheral, edited B-cell repertoire has been analyzed in Ig-transgenic mice on a normal (i.e., rearrangement-effective) genetic background, transgenic and endogenous L chains were often found to be coexpressed in the same cell (358). For different strains of Ig-transgenic mice, the percentage of B cells coexpressing two L chains differed. It can be expected that the immature B cells (and their descendants) that coexpressed transgenic and endogenous L chain, in fact, generated lymphoid sIgM molecules that must have given the cell a different capacity to react to autoantigen. How this interferes with editing and arrest of differentiation needs to be clarified.

Life Expectancy of B-Lineage Cells in Bone Marrow

Pro-B, pre-B-I, pre-B-II, and immature sIg⁺ cells are all produced at high rates and turn over rapidly. Their half-lives in bone marrow are estimated to be between 2 and 4 days. Only a fraction (2 to 3 million) of the immature sIgM⁺ cells is selected into the mature B-cell pool each day (141,359–363). This indicates that the majority of all cells produced in the bone marrow dies in situ, irrespective of whether they have managed to become sIgM⁺ immature B cells. It is not clear at present whether cell death occurs by apoptosis or by phagocytosis (141). Thus, while immature B cells are able to evade recognition of autoantigens by altering the antigen-binding regions of their sIgM molecules, their ability to do so remains limited because of their short lifespan, which, without successful editing away from autoreactivity, results in their death. Very little, if anything, is known of the cooperating cell adhesion molecules, cytokines, cooperating autoantigen-presenting cells, and signal transduction pathways controlling the behavior of immature B cells (349,350). Phosphorylation–dephosphorylation reactions induced by the occupancy of sIg on immature and mature B cells have been found to differ in ways that suggest that this difference is already initiated at the transmembrane level at the sIg-mediated signal transduction pathway (364–368). However, it appears that recognition of autoantigen by an immature B cell does not accelerate death to shorten even more the already short lifespan (369).

Transit of Immature B Cells from Bone Marrow to Spleen and Maturation of Immature to Mature B Cells in the Periphery

The transition from immature to mature B cells is characterized by a series of changes in marker expression (see Fig. 3 and Table 1), lifestyle, and reactivities of the B cells. Mature B cells express the L-selectin lymph node homing receptor, the complement receptors CR1 and CR2 (CD35 and CD21), CD22, CD23, and CD40 (340). They can be stimulated by T cell-dependent and T cell-independent antigens to proliferate and mature into Ig-secreting cells (see Chapter 7). Some of them become long-lived, with half-lives of 6 weeks and longer.

For a pool of 2 to 4×10^7 immature B cells in bone marrow, 2×10^7 cells are newly generated each day (131). Hence, the same number of cells will exit this pool by either apoptosis or by transit to spleen (359). Immature B cells enter the spleen via the central artery and localize in the extrafollicular and follicular areas (Fig. 12) (363,370). At these sites in the spleen, B cells are still immature and can be distinguished from their mature counterparts by their half-life (days versus weeks), their lower B220 and sIgD, and the higher HSA and sIgM expression levels (184,361).

Only 5% to 10% of the newly generated immature B cells get selected into the pool of long-lived mature B cells (141,234, 360–363). Why and how only such a small proportion of immature B cells is selected is largely unknown. By comparison to T-cell development, it is remarkable that a very similar number of CD4⁺ and CD8⁺ T cells is selected in the thymus from a very similarly sized pool of CD4⁺ CD8⁺ double-positive immature thymocytes. Hence, while it is generally accepted that positive selection of T cells into the mature pools of single-positive cells is mediated by the interaction of TCRs with MHC molecules in the thymus, positively selecting self-antigens shaping the Ig repertoire of mature B cells are unknown, although the specificity of the IgM expressed on B cells has been invoked to play a role (247,371–373). A radically different view has been voiced to explain the generation of mature lymphocytes by the argument that all blood-cell lineages are generated, and that their mature pools are maintained by homeostatic mechanisms that do not use the specificity (and signaling) of the antigen-specific receptors as molecular modes of cellular selection.

Transit of immature B cells from bone marrow to spleen is the first of two steps of a way to the mature stage of a B cell (see Fig. 3). The OBF⁻/⁻ mutant mouse (374,375) and the double-mutant CBA/N × CD40⁻/⁻ (376,377) show a major deficiency in this transition. Furthermore, mice expressing only a truncated form of Igα (mb-1) (378) have a defect in the transit, suggesting that signaling via surface Ig could be required. Moreover, A/WySnJ mice show impaired B-cell transit due to one recessive gene, called Bcmd (379,380). The identity of this gene has not yet been determined. In CD45⁻/⁻ mice, a three- to fourfold increased number of immature B cells has been observed in spleen (381). The CD45 phosphatase could be involved in an increased rate of selection from the bone marrow either by an increased survival of immature B cells in spleen, or by a decreased rate of differentiation of immature to mature cells.

Maturation of immature B cells to mature B cells in spleen, the second step in the generation of a mature B cell, is impaired in btk-deficient CBA/N mice (382,383) in B6 MHC class II I-Aα⁻/⁻ mice (384) and in invariant-chain (ii)-deficient mice (385). These genetic analyses indicate that the generation of mature from imma-

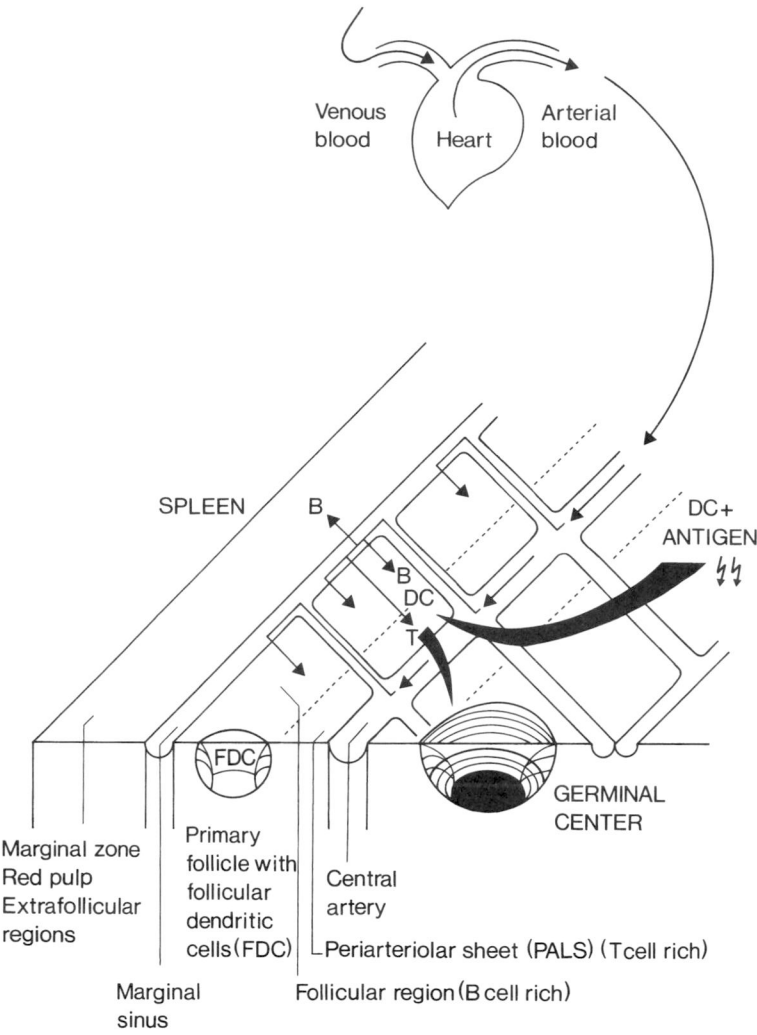

FIG. 12. Entry of B lymphocytes into the spleen. The schematic drawing shows B lymphocytes that have exited the bone marrow via the sinuses, have entered the venous blood, and have been pumped by the heart through the central artery into the spleen, entering the follicular and extrafollicular regions via the marginal sinus. T lymphocytes coming from the thymus via the same route into the spleen localize close to the main artery and form the periarteriolar lymphocyte sheet (*PALS*), while the B cells are more distant from the artery. Primary follicles within the follicular regions contain a network of follicular dendritic cells (*FDC*), which act as depositories for native antigen. When antigen enters in native form into the follicular regions, it binds to B cells via surface Ig, and to FDC as immune complexes via complement receptors. Antigen also enters in processed form as peptide–MHC class II complexes on dendritic cells (*DC*) and stimulates helper T cells in or at the boundaries of the PALS. At the boundaries of the T cell–rich PALS with the B cell–rich follicular regions, stimulation of antigen-specific B cells by helper T cells is initiated. The stimulated B cells are thought to then enter the FDC–antigen complex containing follicles, to expand by proliferation, somatic hypermutation, class-switching, and maturation to Ig-secreting cells, transforming the follicle into a germinal center.

ture cells is a multistep process that occurs at different sites within the immune system. It does not give any definitive clues as to which molecular mechanisms act on which cells, nor does it define whether the B1 or conventional B cells produced during either fetal or adult life in fetal liver or bone marrow are affected.

Differentiation of B-Lineage Cells with and without Immunoglobulin *In Vitro*

When contact with stromal cells is abolished, pro-B and pre-B-I cells differentiate *in vitro* within 2 to 3 days to sIg$^+$ immature B cells and sIg$^-$ B-lineage cells. The sIg$^-$ B-lineage cells probably arise by nonproductive V$_H$ to D$_H$J$_H$ rearrangements. Pre-B cells rearrange V$_H$ to D$_H$J$_H$ and V$_L$ to J$_L$, the latter in an initial κ/λ frequency of 10:1 (226,386), and thus become either sIg$^+$ or sIg$^-$ B cells that are no longer capable of proliferation on stromal cells in the presence of IL-7. It appears that the lack of a signal induces a pro-B or pre-B-I cell without contact to stroma to complete all H- and L-chain gene rearrangements and differentiate to sIg$^+$ and sIg$^-$ immature B cells. The differentiated cells gain the expression of CD25 and lose the expression of c-kit, CD43, and the IL-7 receptor immediately, whereas expression of surrogate L chain and

RAG-1 and RAG-2 is lost later. In fact, while expression is lost in the *in vivo* differentiation of pre-B-I to pre-B-II cells, there is a burst of upregulated expression of RAG-1 and RAG-2 when pre-B-I cells differentiate *in vitro* (231).

The analyses of the V$_H$ repertoire expressed in hybridomas derived from LPS-activated immature sIg$^+$ B cells differentiated *in vitro* from fetal liver pre-B-I cells have indicated that the 3'-located V$_H$ families V$_H$7183 and V$_H$Q52 are preferentially used during this *in vitro* differentiation (387). Hence, the *in vitro* differentiating pre-B cells express V$_H$ repertoires that are characteristic of early repertoires in fetal liver (see earlier discussion in the section on progenitor and precursor BCRs).

The sIg$^-$ pre-B cells that arise in differentiating cultures are, in fact, V$_H$D$_H$J$_H$- and V$_L$J$_L$-rearranged but out of frame, hence nonproductive either in H or L or in both Ig loci. This differentiation *in vitro* occurs in the absence of cell division. More than 95% of the still viable, differentiated cells lose their capacity to proliferate on stromal cells in the presence of rIL-7 (i.e., are no longer clonable within 2-3 days). This indicates that the vast majority of cells differentiate under these conditions.

Cells differentiating not only from normal pre-B-I cells, but also from SCID, RAG$^{-/-}$, λ5$^{-/-}$, and other mutant mice undergo programmed cell death *in vitro* and lose the capacity to proliferate on stromal cells in the presence of IL-7 (191,214). Even bcl-2 transgenic pre-B-I cells lose their clonability, although they do not die by apoptosis (231,388). That suggests that the capacity of a pro-B or pre-B-I cell to differentiate is connected neither with productive (or even attempted) Ig rearrangements, nor with the capacity of precursor B cells to enter apoptosis. While the nonproductively rearranged (i.e., sIg⁻) cells die *in vivo* in the bcl-2 transgenic mice, they remain alive in bcl-xL-transgenic mice (290). Hence, bcl-xL appears to be involved in the control of pre-B-II cell death *in vivo*. It remains to be seen which mechanism of cell death (apoptosis, phagocytosis, or other) operates *in vivo*.

In vitro differentiation of pro-B and pre-B-I cells by the removal of IL-7 occurs without cell division and results in the activation of transcription of the L-chain gene loci, regardless of whether the IgH locus has been productively, nonproductively, or not at all rearranged, and regardless of whether the L-chain gene loci can be rearranged (388). Furthermore, when CD40-specific mAb and IL-4 are added to the differentiating cells, again regardless of whether they can rearrange Ig genes and/or express Ig chains, transcription of the εH locus is induced (389). In RAG-2⁻/⁻ but not in SCID B lineage cells, Sμ–Sε switching is induced in a large part of the cells as frequently as in differentiating cells from normal mice. This indicates that Sμ–Sε switching induced by anti-CD40 and IL-4 requires the SCID gene-encoded DNA-dependent protein kinase, but not the RAG-2 protein. Equally important for an understanding of the mechanisms influencing and controlling B-cell development from the early pro-B and pre-B-I cells to Sμ–Sε-switched, mature B cells is the realization that this lineage differentiation does require the cooperative action of B-lineage cells with stromal cells and T cells, mediated by cytokines and cell–cell contacts. It does not require the expression of the antigen-specific BCR Ig (390).

HUMAN B-CELL DEVELOPMENT

Cellular Stages

B-cell development in human bone marrow is very similar to that in mouse, although the expression of various cell surface markers that characterizes the various stages is partly different (282,285,391,392). A summary is given in Fig. 13. Cells at the earliest stage of B-cell development in human bone marrow, corresponding to the mouse pro/pre-B-I compartment, are CD19⁺, CD10⁺, and CD34⁺. They express TdT and RAG intracellularly, but not yet μH chains. On the surface, these cells also express the SL chain. However, proteins with which the SL chain is associated at this stage of differentiation are not identified. Like their murine counterparts, these cells are actively in cell cycle. However, unlike with mouse cells, it has not yet been possible to grow these human cells *in vitro* on stromal cells and IL-7, or together with any other cytokine. It is also worthwhile to note that IL-7 seems to be far less important in human than in mouse B-cell development. This is based on the finding that patients with an inactive IL-2Rγ chain (which is part of the IL-7 receptor) appear to have normal B-cell development (393,394), while IL-2Rγ⁻/⁻ mice have a major block in B-cell development during the transition from pre-B-I to pre-B-II cells (210).

The second precursor cells in line in the human are equivalent to mouse pre-BCR⁺ pre-B-II cells. In the human, they are CD19⁺, CD10⁺, CD34⁻, TdT⁻, RAG-1, pre-BCR⁺ large, cycling cells. They have productively V$_H$D$_H$J$_H$-rearranged IgH-chain loci, while their

L-chain gene loci are still in germline configuration. A mutation, comparable to the λ5⁻/⁻, μH-tm⁻/⁻, IL-7Rα⁻/⁻, or Syk⁻/⁻ mutations in mice, has not yet been identified as a human B-cell immunodeficiency (see also the following description of the btk-encoded XLA phenotype). Hence, it has not been formally proven but can be assumed that the pre-BCR plays a role in human B-cell development that is similar to the one it plays in mice, namely selection proliferative expansion and allelic exclusion of V$_H$D$_H$J$_H$ in-frame rearranged pre-B cells. This assumption is based on the fact that the vast majority of pre-B cells also in human bone marrow expresses μH-chains in the cytoplasm.

The next B-lineage cell is CD19⁺, CD10⁺, CD34⁻, TdT⁻, RAG-1^low, cytoplasmic μH chain⁺, pre-BCR⁻ pre-B-II cells. However, some minor differences between mouse and human are also apparent at this stage of differentiation. Thus, a small but significant number of the large pre-BCR human pre-B-II have undergone L-chain rearrangements. Moreover, low levels of VpreB mRNA, but not proteins, are still detectable in these cells.

When the large and cycling pre-BCR human pre-B-II cells go out of the cell cycle, they upregulate RAG expression and lose the expression of VpreB. Single-cell PCR analysis has revealed that the majority of them have then rearranged their IgL-chain loci. Thus, these cells are comparable to small resting pre-B-II cells in mouse.

Collectively, these results indicate that the different stages of B-cell development in human bone marrow are very similar to those found in the mouse. The relative sizes of the different pre-B-cell compartments in young mice and young humans are also comparable. The identification of patients with impaired B-cell development at a certain stage of differentiation might help to elucidate more similarities or find differences in the involvement of transcription factors, cell surface receptors, and signaling molecules in B-cell development in mouse and human.

Embryonic and Adult Development of B Cells

As in mouse, B-cell development in humans is separable into two major phases: an early embryonic phase and a postnatal, continuous production during adulthood. While the numbers of progenitors and precursors decline with age, B cells are, nevertheless, generated throughout life (285,395). Bone marrow appears to be the major site for this adult development, which can give rise to both B1 and conventional B cells.

Pre-B cells of the various states described above can be found in fetal liver by week 8 of gestation; immature sIgM⁺ B cells are detectable at week 9, and sIgM⁺/sIgD⁺ mature B cells are detectable at week 12. Soon thereafter, IgH-chain class-switched B cells and Ig-secreting plasma cells can be detected in the embryo. Fetal lung and omentum have also been indicated as embryonic B cell-generating organs (118), though at lower efficiency. This indicates that an antigen-reactive B-cell compartment is formed well before birth (396), a fact also recognizable with prematurely delivered children (397). Active transport of Ig from the mother through the placenta commences at weeks 20 to 21 of gestation (398), so that at birth most of the serum Ig of a child is derived from the mother. It is catabolized after birth, with a half-life of 1 month, and begins to be replaced by the newborn's own Ig, so that at 3 to 6 months after birth, the lowest Ig levels are reached; normal levels of IgM are attained at 1 year, IgG at 6 years, and IgA around puberty. Responses to tetanus toxoid are detectable before 6 months, to diphtheria toxin at 6 months, and to bacterial polysaccharides not before 2 years (399–401).

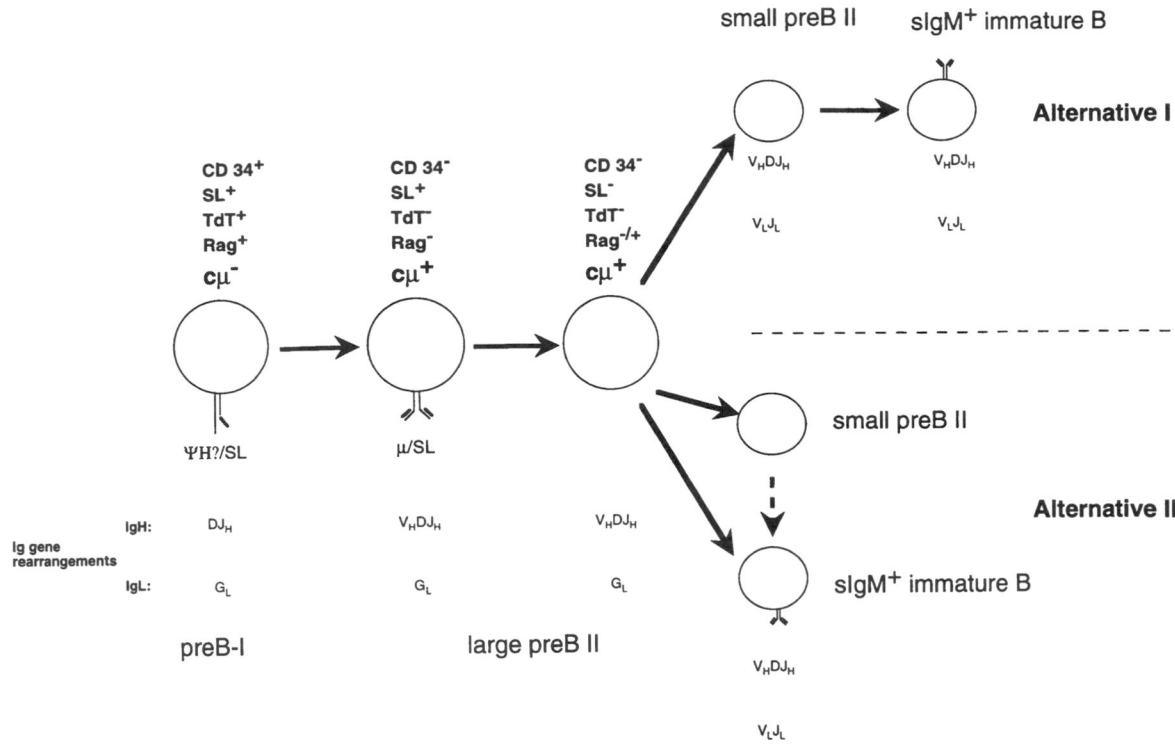

FIG. 13. Human B-cell development. Scheme of human B-cell differentiation in bone marrow. Two alternative pathways of immature B-cell generation are shown. The *dotted arrow* between small pre-B-II and sIgM⁺ immature B cells in alternative II indicates that the RAG-expressing pre-B-II cells continue to rearrange κL- and λL-chain loci. G, germline configuration. (From ref. 285, with permission.)

	Pro/pre B-I	Large pre B-II Type 1	Large pre B-II Type 2	Small pre B-II	Immature B	Mature B
CD34	+	-	-	-	-	-
CD19	+	+	+	+	+	+
CD10	+	+	+	+	+	-
SL chain	+ (association unknown)	+ (μH)	-	-	-	-
CD40	-	-	-	+	+	+
TdT	+	-	-	-	-	-
μH chain protein	-	+	+	+	+	+
RAG-1 RNA	+	nd	nd	+	+	-

Not all of the approximately 100 V_H-gene segments are expressed during development in proportion to their representation in the germline. Some are overrepresented, and others are underrepresented. Therefore, it is well possible that mechanisms of positive and negative V_H selection on the level of rearrangements, expression of the genes, and usage as protein similar to that detectable in mouse B-lineage cells (see earlier discussion) are operative in humans.

Immunodeficiency Diseases

Human SCID is defined as a group of genetically and phenotypically heterogeneous diseases (402,403), with which affected children die (without bone marrow transplantation) of severe, persistent infections (404,405). Some SCID patients have peripheral B cells; others do not.

RAG-1 and RAG-2 Mutations

RAG-1 and RAG-2 mutants, identified as RAG mutants (404,405), were first described by Hitzig et al. (406) as Swiss-type agammaglobulinemia, with severe defects in T and B cells and no serum Ig levels. The RAG-1 and RAG-2 genes, cloned on the basis of their activity to rearrange recombination substrates in fibroblasts (407–409), are highly conserved genes found in mice, humans, chickens, rabbits, and *Xenopus,* and probably also in sharks, goldfish, paddlefish, and axolotls (408,410–414). In the mouse, the two genes face each other with their 3′ ends on chromosome 2p, and the human genes, on chromosome 11p 13. They are coexpressed only in cells that are known or suspected to mediate V(D)J recombination (408,409,415–417). Their expression on protein levels is regulated with the cell cycle (418–420) and during T- and B-lymphocyte development in thymus and bone marrow (287,421).

Their function in the mechanisms of V(D)J recombination has been clarified (422–424). Targeted inactivation of the RAG-1 or RAG-2 gene in mice leads to blocks in T- and B-cell differentiation at early stages, in the B lineage at the transition from pro/pre-B-I cells to large pre-B-II cells (see Fig. 3) (425,426). No T or B cells develop.

Screening of the human RAG-1–RAG-2 locus by single-stranded conformation polymorphism analysis (427) identified three polymorphisms in the RAG-1 gene and one in the RAG-2 gene (404,428). RAG-gene mutations with loss of functions in B cell-negative SCID patients were also found (405). Of all SCID patients, 15% are B-SCID, and of those, 50% are RAG mutants. The defective genes for the other half of the B-SCID patients have not been identified. Hence, the mouse SCID mutation on chromosome 16 encoding a DNA protein kinase (429–432) has not yet been found as a defect in humans. The B-SCID patients who are not RAG mutants may include such mutations and others, such as Ikaros, EBF, E2A, and PAX-5 mutants identified in the mouse (see previous discussion).

X-linked Agammaglobulinemia–btk Mutations

Bruton first described a male child with hypogammaglobulinemia and early onset of bacterial infections (433). In X-linked agammaglobulinemia (XLA) patients, the levels of serum Ig are severely decreased but not absent. The patients have mature T cells but are severely impaired in T cell-dependent B-cell responses (434) and lack germinal centers. Development of human B cells appears to be impaired at *two* points (see Fig. 13). The first is at the transition from pro/pre-B-I to large pre-B-II cells. In XLA patients, pro/pre-B-I cells (TdT$^+$ cytoplasmic μH chain$^-$) are increased in numbers, while large pre-B-II cells (TdT$^-$ cytoplasmic μH chain$^+$) are decreased in numbers as well as proliferate activity (333,435,436). The second defect appears to lie at the transition from immature to mature B cells from bone marrow into the periphery. A much reduced number of sIgM$^+$ B cells in the periphery indicates that they have an immature phenotype and apparently do not respond to antigenic stimulation (434,437). The latter defect is comparable to the effect of the XID mutation in mouse B-cell development (382,383). The defects in human are intrinsic to the B-lineage cells and are not due to an impaired environment (434), although the heterogeneity of genetic backgrounds of human patients is not distinguishable from environmental effects, which may differ in different patients.

The gene on the X-chromosome at q22 was identified as the btk gene encoding a cytosolic tyrosine kinase (438,439). It encodes a 659-amino acid-long protein belonging to the family of Srk-related tyrosine kinase, with a pleckstin homology domain (from the amino to the carboxy-terminal end), a tec-homology domain, a src-homology region (SH) 3, an SH2 domain, and an SH1 (kinase) domain (440). Mutations are found in all domains that yield an XLA phenotype. The severity of the immunodeficiency, however, varies in different patients with different mutations. Furthermore, the same amino acid exchange in the pleckstin homology domain in mouse and human yields a severe phenotype in human and a much lighter one (XID) in mouse (382,383,441,442). The latter may be explainable if the mouse mutations affect only the second step in B-cell development, while the human mutations may affect

both. Different mutations in humans may affect the two affected steps differently, or they may be more or less severe on different genetic backgrounds and/or in different environments. Other SCID defects of humans affect B-lineage development indirectly or at later, mature stages (reviewed by 392,434).

B-CELL DEVELOPMENT IN RABBITS

Structure of the IgH- and L-Chain Gene Loci

The IgH locus of rabbit contains multiple V_H (approximately 200), D_H (more than ten), and J_H (five) segments (443–445), and a Cμ region, a Cδ region, a Cε region, and 13 Cα regions (see Chapters 3, 5, and 18). Each of the 13 Cα genes can be expressed as an IgA subclass (446–449). This multitude of IgA subclasses points to the importance of the gut-associated lymphoid tissues (GALTs) in the development and functioning of the rabbit's immune system, although the functions of the subclasses are presently not known.

Ninety percent to 95% of all rabbit Ig molecules contain κL chains and 5% to 10% λL chains. Two Cκ genes, each associated with a separate cluster of Jκ segments and most likely with a separate Vκ cluster, and a small, not precisely determined number of V_λ, J_λ and C_λ genes encode these L chains (450–455).

Preferential Usage of the 3′-located V_H1 Segment in Early B-Cell Repertoires

Approximately one half of the V_H segments are potentially functional sequences (443,456–465), but their promotors are not yet known. Several allotypes have been defined on rabbit Ig H chains (466). The a-allotypes were found to be present on IgM and IgG molecules (467), and later also on IgA molecules (468). This clearly violated the then prevailing dogma that one gene encodes one polypeptide chain. The discovery of V and C regions of Ig molecules (469) and of somatic rearrangements of gene segments encoding V and C regions of Ig molecules (470–472) made it likely that a-allotypes could be encoded by V-region segments. In fact, it is the V_H1 gene segment that encodes the a1, a2, and a3 allotypes of the rabbit; that is, it exists in three allelic forms in rabbits (473,474).

Most B cells use only this 3′ V_H segment, V_H1, in the $V_HD_HJ_H$-rearranged productive H-chain allele (475). A mutant strain, Alicia (476), has a 10-kb deletion in the IgH locus that includes the a2-allotype-bearing V_H-I-segment. Consequently, the Alicia rabbit cannot make V_H1-a2-containing Ig molecules, but has normal levels of serum Ig and B cells with other V regions (460,477), indicating that other V_H regions are functional and can be used to build up a B-cell repertoire whenever V_H-I cannot be expressed (478,479). In an (Alicia × normal) F$_1$ rabbit, the vast majority of all B cells and Ig molecules express the allotype encoded by the V_H-I gene of the wild-type allele. Hence, the preferential rearrangement of the 3′ V_H1 gene on the normal allele leads to the dominance of those B cells expressing the wild-type allele (and excluding the expression of the mutated allele) over those that express the defective Alicia allele at an apparently much lower efficiency (and excluding the expression of the wild-type allele) (476). These a-allotype-negative V_H regions make up 10% to 20% of the repertoire of the rabbit (474). They increase their representation in rabbits that have been suppressed for a-allotype expression by the injection of an allotype-specific antibody (464,480).

The preferential usage of V_H1 genes in V(D)J recombination on the IgH-chain locus in the rabbit is already observed in sIgM-cytoplasmic µH-chain$^+$ pre-B cells (445). This makes it likely that V$_H$1 is not positively selected as part of an antigen-specific Ig molecule on B cells, but predominates because of preferential rearrangement on the DNA level. Most rabbit B-lineage precursor cells V(D)J-rearrange only one allele, while the other allele either remains in germline configuration, or is only D$_H$J$_H$-rearranged (481). This is in marked contrast to the mouse, in which half of all B cells have the second allele V(D)J rearranged, while the other half is D$_H$J$_H$-rearranged (195). Hence, allelic exclusion at the H-chain locus in the rabbit is secured mainly by limited V(D)J recombination. The same preferential rearrangement and usage of V$_H$1(D)J-rearranged B cells can be seen in the rabbit's fetal repertoire (482).

Ontogeny of B-Lineage Cells

Pre-B cells appear in embryonic development of the rabbit at days 17 to 21 of gestation in fetal liver, and at day 25 in bone marrow (483,484). Pre-B cells can also be detected in the omentum (118). The peak of pre-B-cell development in fetal liver is seen shortly after birth. B-lineage cells have essentially disappeared from liver after day 10 of postnatal life.

In bone marrow, pre-B cells are highest 1 day after birth. Thereafter, they rapidly decrease (484–486). In adult rabbits, approximately 1% of all cells are pre-B cells. Despite their presence, it is suspected that they do not contribute to the maintenance and renewal of the peripheral mature B-cell compartments (461,462,487). Several observations support this view of limited B-lymphopoiesis from progenitors and precursors of the B lineage. First, all rabbit B cells express CD5, a marker that in mouse and human characterizes the B1a lineage, which is generated once early in life, but not during adulthood, and is renewed from sIgM$^+$ B cells (162,175,488; see also previous discussion). Second, neonatal suppression of B cells by allotype-specific antibody treatment has a long-term effect on CD5$^+$ cells in mice and on all B cells in rabbits, suggesting that the treatment abolishes the CD5$^+$ compartments of B1 cells (480,489). Third, V(D)J joints appear more diversified as rabbits age (487). The diversification of V(D)J-rearranged sequences of H-chain loci is expected to result from somatic gene conversion and point mutations of V(D)J-rearranged loci in sIg$^+$ B cells. Fourth, the expression of the rearrangement machinery (i.e., the RAG-1 and RAG-2 genes) is seen early but not late in life (412).

Somatic Diversification of Immunoglobulin Variable-gene Regions during Adult Life

The Ig repertoire of rabbit B cells at birth is so restricted, due to the preferential usage of the 3′-located V$_H$1 gene, that the newborn rabbit appears nonresponsive to many antigens. Responses to antigens improve with age. In parallel, the diversity of V(D)J-rearranged sequences increases. From birth until 4 or 5 weeks of age, most V(D)J sequences are still nondiversified (487). Codon insertions, codon deletions, and clustered nucleotide sequence changes indicate that gene conversion of the primary V$_H$1 D$_H$J$_H$-rearranged locus with upstream V$_H$-gene segments creates much of this somatic diversification. From 1 month of age onward, a far more diverse repertoire appears that can, at least in part, also be the consequence of somatic point mutations in V(D)J-rearranged (perhaps already gene-converted) H-chain gene loci (461,490). In germ-free rabbits, only limited diversification is observed (491,492), and these germ-free rabbits, as neonatal normal ones, are unresponsive to antigens (493).

The Gut-associated Lymphoid Tissues as Sites for Immunoglobulin Repertoire Diversification

B-lymphocytes can be found in two major areas of the GALTs: in the lamina propria and in follicles. Surgical removal of the appendix, the saccutus rotundus, and the Peyer's patches of the GALTs from newborn rabbits immunocompromised them, so that circulating B cells and serum Ig were lower, and responses to some, but not all, antigens could not be elicited (494). GALTs could be intrinsically active in promoting diversification of the Ig repertoire by somatic changes of the V regions. Alternatively, external influences (e.g., by foreign antigens) could drive this repertoire expansion. Rabbits in which the Peyer's patch-type lymphoepithelial tissue was neonatally extirpated (495) and germ-free rabbits were shown to lack antigen responsiveness. In germ-free rabbits, V(D)J diversification was also severely reduced, suggesting that antigenic stimulation is at least in large part responsible for Ig diversification and responsiveness.

B-CELL DEVELOPMENT IN FETAL LAMB AND SHEEP

The ontogeny of B-lineage cells in sheep is markedly different from that in other mammals. Lambs are born around day 150 of gestation. *In utero,* they are not exposed to the mother's serum Ig molecules because the placenta is impermeable to them (see articles in ref. 496). Hematopoiesis begins extraembryonically within the yolk sac at around day 16 of gestation, generating erythroid cells 3 to 5 days before implantation. Hematopoiesis leading to erythrocyte, megakaryocyte, and myeloid cell development, but to no detectable lymphoid cell development, is next seen in fetal liver at days 21 to 23. Fetal liver, in fact, never becomes a lymphopoietic organ. The thymus begins to develop lymphocytes at days 38 to 40. The first B lymphocytes become detectable at days 45 to 50 in spleen (497,498). They expand to occupy 20% of the spleen by day 77. Only 5% of all sIgM$^+$ cells express CD5 at day 81. The characteristic organization of a splenic white pulp with follicles was seen at day 90. A single injection of IgM-specific antibody at day 63 severely depleted sheep of B cells, not only in the spleen, but also in other organs, such as Peyer's patches (499). When these anti-IgM-treated lambs were analyzed a week before birth, they were found to contain normal numbers of T cells in their proper sites, but they had only small numbers of scattered B cells and without the normal follicular accumulation. These experiments suggested that the sIgM$^+$ B cells present at day 63 (e.g., in spleen) are progenitors of later waves of B-cell development (e.g., in Peyer's patches).

From day 100 onward, the majority of B cells appears to be made in Peyer's patches (500). Bone marrow, on the other hand, is only a minor site of lymphopoiesis after day 70 and does not assume a major B cell-generating role until late in life, when the B-cell generation in Peyer's patches has ceased (i.e., after weeks 8 to 12 of postnatal life, when the patches begin to involute, and beyond 18 months, when the patches have almost disappeared). B lymphopoiesis is seen as extensive cell proliferation in the approximately 100,000 follicles of the ileal Peyer's patches before, as well as after, birth. Surgical removal of most of the Peyer's patches from fetal lamb, and from newborn sheep during the first week after birth, leads to severe deficiency of B lymphocytes (501). These observations have been taken as evidence that Peyer's patches are primary sites of B-cell generation, in the sense that foreign antigens of the microbial flora do not stimulate this development, although the fetal lamb is responsive to foreign antigens before birth (502–504).

An analysis of the V-region sequences expressed in ileal Peyer's patch-derived B cells before and after birth showed that somatic hypermutation starts before birth (i.e., in the sterile environment of the fetus) and continues in the antigenic environment of food and bacterial antigens after birth (505). When fragments of the ileum were surgically isolated from the gut during fetal life, when fetal lamb was thymectomized, or when sheep were kept in germ-free conditions, the number of age-dependent somatic mutations in IgVl regions was essentially unaltered, and it increased with age (506). Replacement mutations altering V-region protein structure appeared favored. Hence, while there is evidence that Peyer's patches of sheep are not indifferent to external antigens, (507) the question remains whether pre-B cells generate B cells in Peyer's patches, and how sIgM$^+$ B cells in the patches are driven to proliferate, hypermutate, and be selected in the apparent absence of external foreign antigens.

B-CELL DEVELOPMENT IN CHICKEN

In birds, the bursa of Fabricius is the most important organ of B-cell generation (Fig. 14). Bursectomy in the embryo leads to severe agammaglobulinemia (9,112,508–511). In fact, lymphocytes have been named B-type also because they are *b*ursa-derived in birds.

Embryonic Development

Not only are birds unique examples for lymphocyte development, quite distinct from mouse and human, they also offer several experimental advantages for studying the development and functioning of their immune system (see articles in refs. 512, 513). The embryo is accessible to *in situ* experimentation during organogenesis, allowing a delineation of its different rudiments. In fact, development in chicken and quail is so similar that parts of their early embryos can be surgically exchanged between them, which leads to the development of chimeric birds. Cells of chicken and quail origin can be distinguished by nuclear features and by other markers (514–516). There are a large number of inbred strains of chicken with genetic allelism in gene loci with functions in the immune system.

Hematopoietic cells with the capacity to commit themselves to the B-lineage pathway of differentiation are identifiable in the birds before, during, and after the time the bursa functions as a B cell-generating organ. Consequently, prebursal, bursal, and postbursal stem cells are defined not only by their localization, but also by their capacity to restore the B-cell compartments of a depleted host upon adoptive cell transfer (517) (see Fig. 14).

Prebursal stem cells probably arrive first from mesenchymal cells in hematopoietic islands near the aorta at day 3 of incubation (518). Prebursal stem cells themselves become detectable in 7-day embryonic mesenchyme (519,520). The rudiment of the embryonic bursa is colonized between days 8 and 15 (515,521,522). The bursa develops to 10^4 follicles, each of which is colonized from between two and ten prebursal stem cells (523,524). The prebursal stem cells are probably sIg$^-$ (525). By contrast, bursal stem cells are sIg$^+$ (523,526–528). Injection of an Ig allotype-specific antibody at this bursal time of development leads to suppression of B-cell development in the bursal follicles, suggesting that the precursors that populate the bursa are already sIg$^+$. A single follicle, when finally filled, contains as many as 2 to 5 × 10^5 cells.

At day 18, the bursal B cells emigrate to the periphery, where they form the postbursal stem-cell compartments. Three weeks after hatching (which occurs at day 18), bursectomy no longer leads to agammaglobulinemia. By 6 months, the bursa has almost completely disappeared. During the colonization of the periphery, sIgM$^+$ B cells appear in bone marrow and spleen, but in these organs these cells will not be induced to the same differentiation as in the bursa. However, when postbursal sIgM$^+$ cells are adoptively transferred into recipients with a competent bursa, they are induced to the differentiation events described below. It is likely that prebursal and postbursal stem cells are committed to a different degree to B-lineage development.

Organization and Rearrangements of IgH- and L-chain Genes

Both H- and L-chain gene loci in chicken have a unique organization and pattern of rearrangements. The L-chain locus, structurally similar to λL chain, consists of one functional Vλ, one Jλ, and one Cλ segment, which rearranges to form a V$_λ$J$_λ$-rearranged master L-chain gene. Upstream of the Vλ gene segment, within 40 kb, are 25 pseudo V-gene segments, arranged in pairs with opposite orientation on the chromosome (529,530).

In the H-chain locus, one functional V$_H$1-gene segment rearranges with 16 D segments and one functional J segment to form a master H chain. Upstream of the V$_H$1-gene segment, within 60 to 80 kb, lie an estimated 80 to 100 pseudo V$_H$-gene segments, again ordered in pairs of segments in the opposite direction on the chromosome (531,532). At their 3' end, they have no recombination signals, but they do contain D-like sequences and, in some cases, even J-like sequences. Hence, they have the potential for encoding CDR3 regions of V$_H$ domains.

D elements encode eight, nine, or ten amino acids. When rearranged in three possible reading frames (rf), in rf I, they encode hydrophilic and aromatic amino acids; in rf II, they encode hydrophobic amino acids; and in rf III, stop codons abolish expression as protein (532,533). These translations in three rf resemble those of the mouse D$_{fl16}$ and D$_{sp2}$ families. Of the chicken D, the Dx is poorly expressed and counter-selected during B-cell proliferation in the bursa (532). D–D joints are seen in chicken IgH genes.

Only one allele of the IgH locus is V$_H$D$_H$J$_H$-rearranged in chicken B cells from a population of precursors that have in majority both H-chain alleles D$_H$J$_H$-rearranged. Again, only one allele of the Ig L locus is V$_H$J$_H$-rearranged (532,534). One master H chain with restricted diversity in the D-encoded CDR3 and one master L chain with very little diversity in CDR3 can form B cells with Ig molecules with two defined sets of CDR1 and CDR2 regions (i.e., an Ig molecule with restricted diversity). It has been speculated that these sets of CDR1/CDR2 may have a common binding specificity for an unknown self-antigen in the bursal epithelium, which might induce the original sIgM$^+$ B cells to proliferation and to the diversification reactions described below (531,534–536).

Immunoglobulin Diversification by Gene Conversion

The finding of the master and pseudo H- and L-chain genes in chicken and the observed heterogeneity of Ig molecules in the chicken's adult immune system made it likely that a mechanism of gene conversion had to operate to generate diversity, analogous to recombination models for generation of variability in V genes proposed by Hilschmann and Craig (469), Smithies (537), and Edelmann and Gally (538).

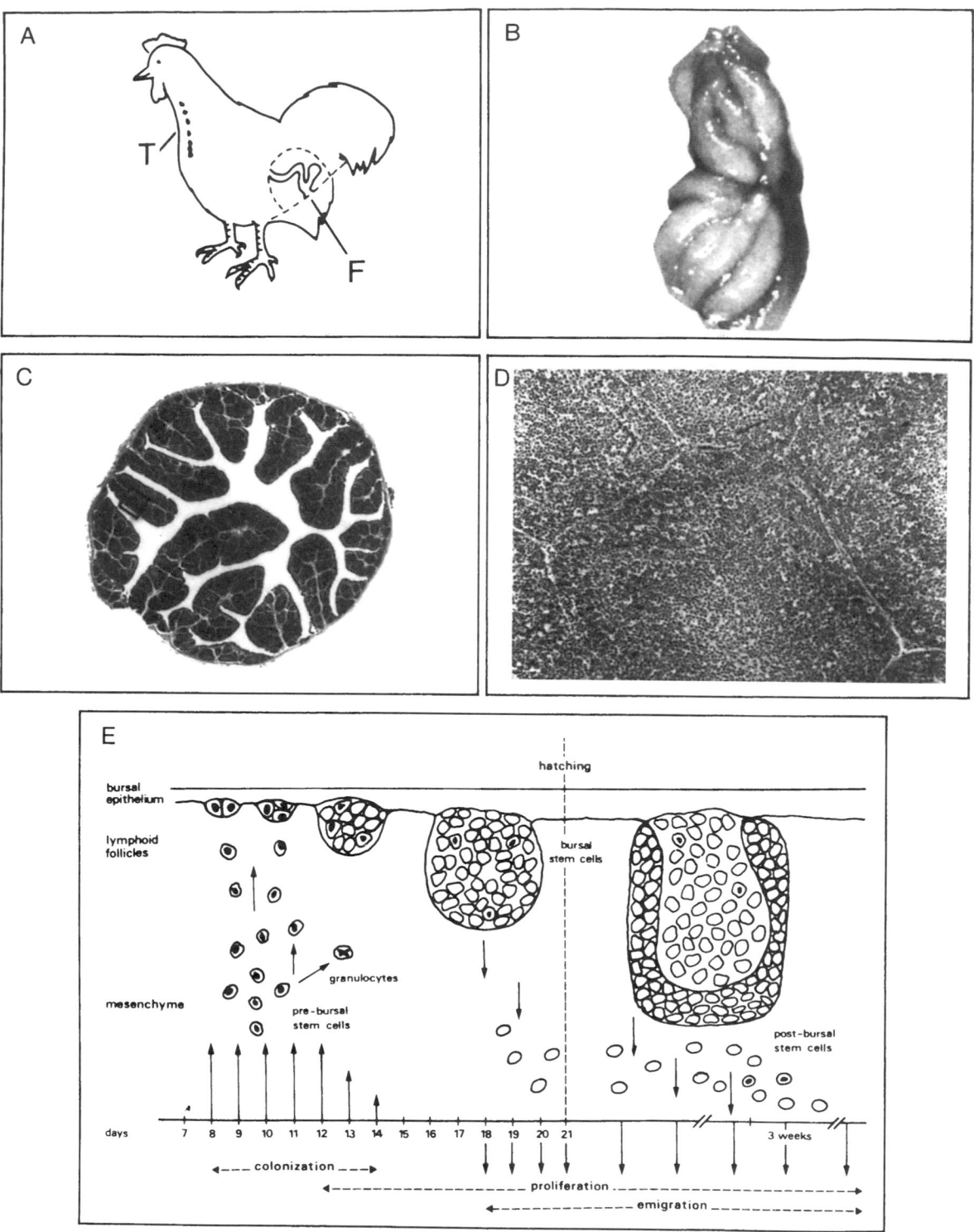

FIG. 14. (A) The locations of thymus (T) and bursa of Fabricius. **B:** The bursa of Fabricius. **C:** A cross section of the bursa of Fabricius at low-level magnification (×10). **D:** A bursal follicle (×250). **E:** A schematic drawing of the prebursal, bursal, and postbursal development of B lymphocytes in the bursa of Fabricius (taken from ref. 554).

V-region sequence analyses of Ig expressed in B cells during bursal development confirmed this proposition (530,539). Conversion events in V genes increase in time, from one to three at birth to four to six at 3 weeks after birth. From these analyses it has been estimated that one gene conversion event occurs for every 10 to 20 B-cell divisions. Using a transformed bursal-derived B-cell line, it has been found that gene conversion is independent of RAG-2 expression (540). The lengths of the converted sequences can vary from 10 to 100; in some cases there are even more nucleotides (530). In the nonconverted master gene set expressed in the early bursal B cells, D in rf I is selected. Since the D-like elements in the pseudo V_H genes are also in rf I, conversions of D regions usually do not alter significantly the V-region sequence in those areas. Different pseudo V_H and V_k genes with higher homologies to the master genes are favored. At the borders of the conversion events, nontemplated mutations can be observed. Furthermore, somatic point mutation also may occur (541). It should be remembered that all of the somatic mutation processes after V(D)J rearrangements of the two master genes occur only on one allele, which avoids the problems of allelic inclusion of a second specificity in a single B cell.

Gene Rearrangements and Gene Conversions in Prebursal, Bursal, and Postbursal Development

PCR analyses of the configurations of the H- and L-chain gene loci during chicken B-cell development have shown that D_H to J_H rearrangements begin to be performed at days 5 to 6 of incubation (i.e., at the time when hematopoietic progenitors are seen to migrate to the yolk sac). If these rearrangements are induced by the cell migration, it could be either the environment of the yolk sac or the departure from the environment of the intraembryonic, periaortic sites. When prebursal stem cells seed the various lymphoid organs, they continue with D_H to J_H rearrangements. One to 2 days later, the first cells with $V_H D_H J_H$-rearranged H-chain loci are detectable circulating in embryonic blood. These B-lineage cells appear not to be in cell cycle (532,542). The number of $D_H J_H$-rearranged progenitor B cells have been estimated to be 1,000 to 2,000 at day 8 in yolk sac (thereafter disappearing), 1 to 2.5×10^5 at day 10 in blood, increasing to 2.5 to 5×10^5 at day 13, then decreasing to 10^3 at day 17. In spleen, 2 to 5×10^3 are found at day 10, increasing to 5×10^5 at day 13, and decreasing to 2 to 4×10^4 at day 17. In bone marrow, ten to 20 can be detected at day 10, 10^5 at day 13, and 2×10^3 to 10^4 at day 17.

The only organ in which the number increases at day 17 is the bursa, with 10^2 at day 10, 10^3 at day 13, and 10^6 at day 17 (543). Whether spleen and bone marrow are functionally important intermediate stages of B-cell development or dead-end sites remains to be seen (528,543–545). $V_H D_H J_H$-rearranged H-chain loci and $V_H J_H$-rearranged L-chain loci can be found between days 10 and 13 in B cells express sIgM (i.e., at the time of original colonization of the bursa). It is, therefore, likely that at least some V(D)J rearrangements occur outside the bursa before colonization (546). No temporal difference has been seen between $V_H D_H J_H$ rearrangements on H-chain loci and $V_H J_H$ rearrangements on L-chain loci. Originally, no N regions are inserted and rf I is favored over the others. Rf representation does not change during bursal development of B cells, suggesting that any rf selection succeeding the original DNA sequence–mediated preferences should occur on the $V_H D_H J_H$-rearranged level (i.e., on H chain expressed on B cells) (532).

B cells with productively $V_H D_H J_H$- and $V_H J_H$-rearranged loci (i.e., sIgM$^+$ B cells) are selected over nonproductively rearranged sIg$^-$ cells to enter a phase of extensive proliferation. From an average of two to ten cells seeding a follicle, 1 to 2×10^5 cells are generated in an average of 15 to 16 divisions. If an original Ig recognizes a self antigen in the epithelial environment of the bursa, and if that recognition signals proliferation (see above), any cell converting its recognition specificity away from this self-recognition would stop proliferating, and at the same time gain a new, unexpected specificity. One can expect that in chicken, at birth, 10^4 follicles would produce 1 to 2×10^9 cells per day, of which at least 10^8 have converted V genes (i.e., mutated sIgM). The bursa of Fabricius thus appears to be a mutant-breeding lymphoid organ. Well before any of the structures of Ig genes were known (547), Jerne proposed such a mutant breeding organ to explain the generation of antibody diversity.

B cells in the chicken appear to be generated in one wave in the bursa, reaching a peak at birth. After birth, in postbursal B-cell development, rearrangements no longer appear detectable (533). Furthermore, since the bursa involutes, the major site for the generation of diversity by gene conversion disappears. It remains to be investigated in greater detail whether chickens can generate further diversity later in life at other sites in the somatic mutations, or whether they have to survive with the B cells (and their self-renewing capacity) that they made early in life.

RULES OF B LYMPHOPOIESIS AND THEIR VARIATIONS

It is evident that B lymphopoiesis uses different strategies in different species to generate diverse repertoires of Ig-producing cells. However, striking similarities are also apparent.

All species so far studied generate lymphocytes from pluripotent hematopoietic stem cells. After commitment to the B-lineage pathway in a competent, specific environment, the cells first use V(D)J recombination to generate sIg$^+$ cells from precursors. All species appear to use the products of the RAG-1, RAG-2, and TdT genes in this process.

In humans and mice, these V(D)J rearrangements are ordered: D_H to J_H before V_H to $V_H D_H$ and before V_H to J_H. Hence, the rearrangement machinery must be turned on, then off, then on again, and then off. By forming pre-BCRs, surrogate L chain is essential in this ordering of the rearrangement steps.

In other species, such as the chicken, all loci appear to be rearranged at once, not separable in identifiable steps in different cellular stages. Whether V(D)J recombination is ever again used after a mature B cell has been made is a possibility that needs further study (548,549).

V(D)J recombination and B lymphopoiesis begins during embryonic development in all species. It generates a first repertoire of sIgM$^+$ B cells. In rabbits and chickens, that repertoire of B cells appears to be the only one that remains for use in the system throughout life. While the replenishing of B cells in the system of these species should occur from sIg$^+$ "stem" cells in adult life, regeneration of B cells in humans and mice appears to be done from sIg$^-$ precursors, though at decreasing efficiency with increasing age. On the other hand, humans and mice also have sIg$^+$ "stem" cells from which they can regenerate at least the B1 compartments of their system, again with increasing age at decreasing rates. To which extent the repertoires of B1 and conventional B cells are screened against autoantigens, and how this screening is effected, is not clear.

V_H-segment usage in V(D)J rearrangements and V_H-region representation in early B lymphopoiesis are nonrandom, biased toward a selected set of V_H segments and expressed V_H domains on Ig molecules. In fact, chicken has only one functional V_H segment in its germline gene repertoire. It is striking how conserved these preferentially used V_H segments have remained during evolution.

The same V_H domains, which are favored early in development, are often disfavored later. Such repertoire changes can occur by replacing old cells with newly made ones. On the other hand, in a V(D)J-rearranged locus, one V can be replaced on the DNA level by another. These methods to change repertoires are used in humans and mice. Chickens and rabbits, however, change the V-region sequences in sIg+ "stem cells" by gene conversions. In sheep, hypermutation by point mutations before antigenic stimulation is yet another molecular mechanism to vary the early V-encoded repertoires.

A competent environment of a special lymphoid organ appears to be essential for repertoire development and repertoire changes. It is evident that all species use proliferative expansion from a small number of precursor sIg− or sIg+ cells to a much larger pool of more diverse sIg+ cells to build up their B-cell repertoires. Hence, the environment appears to provide inductive stimuli for B-lineage commitment, V(D)J recombination, V replacement, V conversion and/or V hypermutation, and cellular proliferation. Much needs to be learned of this inductive environment. Candidate molecules involved in these inductive stimuli include those possibly binding to pre-BCR and BCR, cytokine receptors, and cell–cell interaction molecules. Mutations in the V regions of sIg might change the interactive capacities of pre-BCR+ or BCR+ B cells and thereby alter their fate in the repertoire-generating organs.

We assume, but only know it for mouse in more detail, that emerging B-cell repertoires are subjected to negative selection by arrest of differentiation and anergy, and possibly even to positive selection. Even in mouse it is not clear how negative and positive selection shape the B1 and conventional B-cell repertoires, which are evidently different. In other species, mechanisms of negative and positive selection of B-cell repertoires still need to be investigated and defined.

The continuous developmental changes in the composition and reactivity of the B-lineage compartments of the immune system, and their unpredictable exposure to foreign antigens, make it clear that no immune system is ever the same in the course of the life of an organism. Therefore, the description of B-lymphopoiesis in any species must be related to the age of the individual in which it is analyzed.

The similarities in developmental stages of mouse and human B-lineage precursors and their pool sizes, the use of surrogate L chain in the order of this development, and the existence of a B1 and a conventional B-cell lineage in the mature B-cell pool all point to the remarkable possibility that studies on the molecular and cellular mechanisms of B lymphopoiesis in mice are applicable to humans. This is obviously important for experimental approaches in diagnosis and the eventual care of immunodeficiencies and autoimmune diseases expressed in B-lineage cells.

Even more striking are the similarities of B-cell development in bone marrow and T-cell development in thymus of mice (see Fig. 15). Thymus and bone marrow contain very similar numbers of cells. Prothymocytes (comparable with pro-B cells) and CD4−

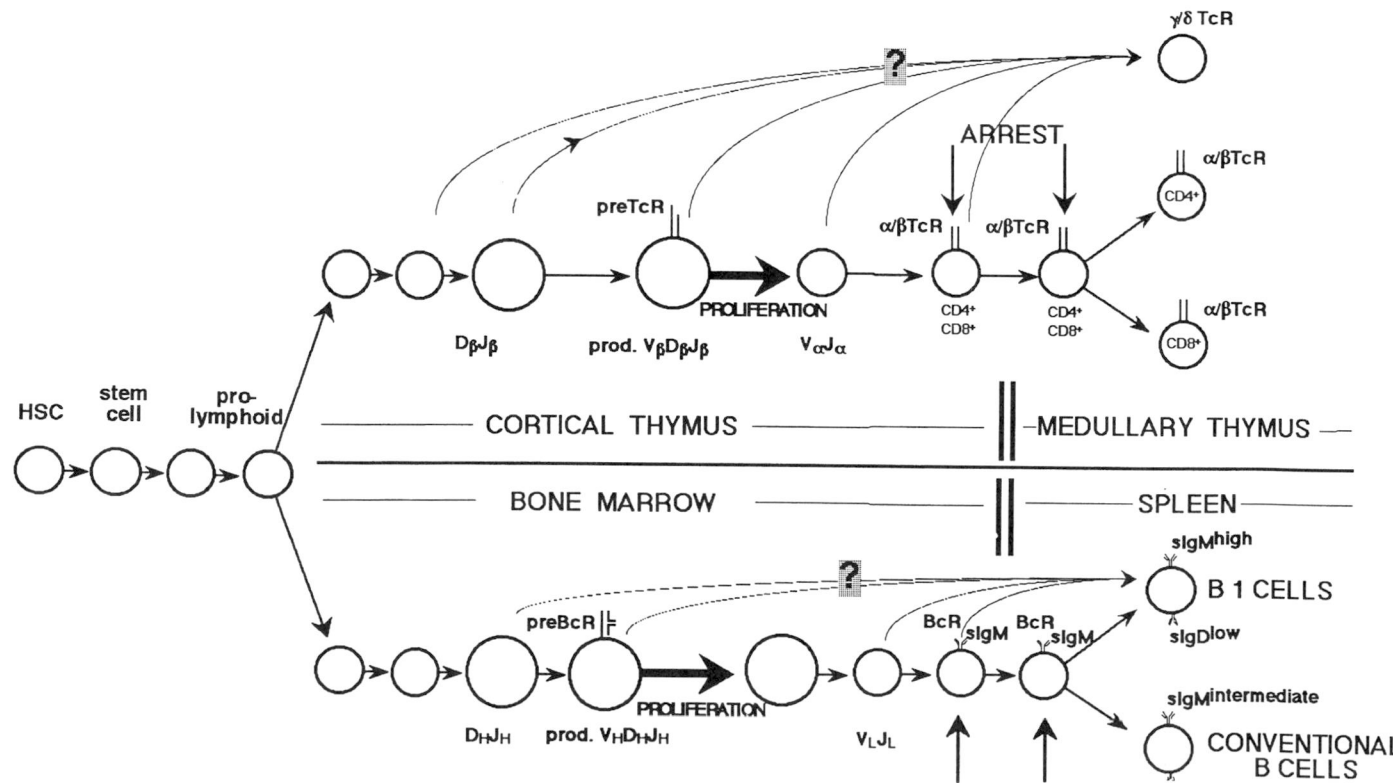

FIG. 15. Similarities between T-cell development in thymus and B-cell development in bone marrow and spleen. See text for details.

CD8⁻ thymocytes (comparable with pre-B-I cells) compose approximately 3% of all thymocytes, are actively cycling, express c-kit, and proliferate *in vitro* in response to IL-7 and SCF. The thymus of irradiated hosts can be reconstituted by c-kit⁺ precursors upon intrathymic transfer. In the first phase of proliferative expansion and establishment of thymocyte compartments before the birth of a mouse, TdT is not expressed in thymocytes. TdT begins to be expressed 3 to 5 days after birth, shortly before N-region insertions can be found in TCR gene joints.

Rearrangements of TCRβ-gene loci precede those of the α-gene loci. For monitoring V_H to $D_H J_H$ rearrangements, B- and T-lineage cells have developed a surrogate chain [surrogate L, surrogate (or pre-T) α], which they express as prelymphocyte receptors together with TCR β chains (pre-TCR) or μH chains (pre-BCR). These surrogate chains are expressed in a narrow window of lymphocyte development. In both lineages, they control proliferative expansion and, in all likelihood, also allelic exclusion. It is a fascinating question how the immune system evolved two structurally similar but distinct surrogate chains for use in the developmental pathways of two lymphocyte lineages at very similar points and for very similar purposes.

The similarities in B- and T-cell development continue to be apparent in negative selection of autoreactive cells which, are particularly impressive in rearrangement-deficient mice that express transgenic TCRβ, μH chain, or α/β TCR, or IgM molecules with specificities for autoantigens expressed in the primary lymphoid organs or in the periphery. This leads to arrest of differentiation or to anergy. In both B- and T-lineage immature, antigen receptor-expressing cells, the rearrangement machinery continues to be expressed, allowing secondary rearrangements in the L chain, and TCRα-chain gene loci, and hence, receptor editing. T-cell differentiation to the CD4/CD8 double-positive, and maybe even to the CD4⁺ or CD8⁺ single-positive, stage of differentiation can occur in the absence of V(D)J rearrangement (i.e., in RAG-deficient cells, just as it can to the mature, sμ–sε-switched state of B-lineage cells.

From a pool of approximately 5×10^7 immature, antigen receptor-expressing cells in thymus and bone marrow, a very similar number (i.e., 2 to 3×10^6 cells) are selected each day in both lineages to enter the pool of mature antigen-reactive lymphocytes in the periphery. While the rules for this positive selection (i.e., adaptation of the repertoire to MHC class I- and class II-restricted recognition) are well understood for T-lineage cell development, such rules are unknown for B-lineage development.

REFERENCES

1. Zon LI. Developmental biology of hematopoiesis. *Blood* 1995;86:2876–2891.
2. Eichmann A, Corbel C, Nataf V, Vaigot P, Breant C, Le Douarin NM. Ligand-dependent development of the endothelial and hemopoietic lineages from embryonic mesodermal cells expressing vascular endothelial growth factor receptor 2. *Proc Natl Acad Sci USA* 1997;94:5141–5146.
3. Müller AM, Medvinsky A, Strouboulis J, Grosveld F, Dzierzak E. Development of hematopoietic stem cell activity in the mouse embryo. *Immunity* 1994;1:291–301.
4. Morrison SJ, Wright DE, Cheshier SH, Weissman IL. Hematopoietic stem cells: challenges to expectations. *Curr Opin Immunol* 1997;9:216–221.
5. Cumano A, Dieterlen Lievre F, Godin I. Lymphoid potential, probed before circulation in mouse, is restricted to caudal intraembryonic splanchnopleura. *Cell* 1996;86:907–916.
6. Siminovitch L, McCulloch E, Till E. The distribution of colony-forming cells among spleen colonies. *J Cell Comp Physiol* 1963;62:327–336.
7. Wu A, Till J, Siminovitch L, McCulloch E. A cytological study of the capacity for differentiation of normal hemopoietic colony-forming cells. *J Cell Physiol* 1967;69:177–184.
8. Wu A, Till J, Siminovitch L, McCulloch E. Cytological evidence for a relationship between normal hematopoietic colony-forming cells and cells of the lymphoid system. *J Exp Med* 1968;127:455–467.
9. Cooper MD, Van Alten PJ, Good RA. Development and function of the immunoglobulin producing system. I. Effect of bursectomy at different stages of development on germinal centers, plasma cells, immunoglobulins, and antibody production. *Int Arch Allergy* 1969;35:242–252.
10. Spangrude GJ, Heimfeld S, Weissman IL. Purification and characterization of mouse hematopoietic stem cells. *Science* 1988;241:58–62.
11. Jordan CT, Lemischka IR. Clonal and systemic analysis of long-term hematopoiesis in the mouse. *Genes Dev* 1990;4:220–232.
12. Smith LG, Weissmann IL, Heimfeld S. Clonal analysis of hematopoietic stem-cell differentiation *in vivo*. *Proc Natl Acad Sci USA* 1991;88:2788–2792.
13. Moore MAS, Metcalf D. Ontogeny of the haemopoietic system: yolk sac origin of *in vivo* and *in vitro* colony forming cells in the developing mouse embryo. *Br J Haematol* 1970;18:279–296.
14. Dieterlen-Lièvre F. On the origin of haemopoietic stem cells in the avian embryo: an experimental approach. *J Embryol Exp Morphol* 1975;33:607–619.
15. Keller G, Paige C, Gilboa E, Wagner EF. Expression of a foreign gene in myeloid and lymphoid cells derived from multipotent haematopoietic precursors. *Nature* 1985;318:149–154.
16. Fulop GM, Phillips RA. Use of *scid* mice to identify and quantitate lymphoid-restricted stem cells in long-term bone marrow cultures. *Blood* 1989;74:1537–1544.
17. Keller G, Snodgrass R. Life span multipotential hematopoietic stem cells in vivo. *J Exp Med* 1990;171:1407–1418.
18. Snodgrass R, Keller G. Clonal fluctuation within the haematopoietic system of mice reconstituted with retrovirus-infected stem cells. *EMBO J* 1987;6:3955–3960.
19. Evans MJ, Kaufmann MH. Establishment in culture of pluripotent cells from mouse embryos. *Nature* 1981;292:154–156.
20. Magnuson T, Epstein CJ, Silver LM, Martin GR. Pluripotent embryonic stem cell lines can be derived from tw5/tw5 blastocysts. *Nature* 1982;298:750–753.
21. Martin G. Isolation of a pluripotent cell line from early mouse embryos cultured in medium conditioned by terratocarcinoma stem cells. *Proc Natl Acad Sci USA* 1981;78:7634–7638.
22. Potocnik AJ, Nielsen PJ, Eichmann K. *In vitro* generation of lymphoid precursors from embryonic stem cells. *EMBO J* 1994;13:5274–5283.
23. Potocnik AJ, Köhler H, Eichmann K. Hemato-lymphoid in vivo reconstitution potential of subpopulations derived from in vitro differentiated embryonic stem cells. *Proc Natl Acad Sci USA* 1997;94.10295–10300.
24. Potocnik AJ, Nerz G, Köhler H, Eichmann K. Reconstitution of B cell subset in RAG deficient mice by transplantation of in vitro differentiated embryonic stem cells. *Immunol Lett* 1997;57:131–137.
25. Gossler A, Doetschman T, Korn R, Serfling E, Kemler R. Transgenesis by means of blastocyst-derived embryonic stem cell lines. *Proc Natl Acad Sci USA* 1986;83:9065–9069.
26. Thomas KR, Capecchi MR. Site-directed mutagenesis by gene targeting in mouse embryo-derived stem cells. *Cell* 1987;51:503–512.
27. Stewart TA, Mintz B. Successive generations of mice produced from an established culture line of euploid teratocarcinoma cells. *J Embryol Exp Morphol* 1981;70:99–112.
28. Rossant J, McBurney MW. The developmental potential of a euploid male teratocarcinoma cell line after blastocyst injection. *J Embryol Exp Morphol* 1992;70:99–112.
29. Torres RM, Kühn R. *Laboratory protocols for conditional gene targeting.* Oxford: Oxford University Press, 1997.
30. Chen J. Analysis of gene function in lymphocytes by RAG-2-deficient blastocyst complementation. *Adv Immunol* 1996;62:31–59.
31. Lemischka IR, Raulet D, Mulligan RC. Developmental potential and dynamic behavior of hematopoietic stem cells. *Cell* 1986;45:917–927.
32. Harrison DE, Lerner C, Hoppe PC, Carlson GA, Alling D. Large numbers of primitive stem cells are active simultaneously in aggregated embryo chimeric mice. *Blood* 1987;69:773–777.
33. Harrison DE, Astle CM, Lerner C. Number and continuous proliferative pattern of transplanted primitive immunohematopoietic stem cells. *Proc Natl Acad Sci USA* 1988;85:822–826.
34. Pietrzyk ME, Priestley GV, Wolf NS. Normal cycling patterns of hematopoietic stem cell subpopulations: an assay using long-term *in vivo* BrdU infusion. *Blood* 1985;66:1460–1462.
35. Morrison SJ, Hemmati HD. The purification and characterization of fetal liver hematopoietic stem cells. *Proc Natl Acad Sci USA* 1995;92:10302–10306.
36. Li CL, Johnson GR. Murine hematopoietic stem and progenitor cells. I. Enrichment and biologic characterization. *Blood* 1995;85:1472–1479.
37. Spangrude GJ, Brooks DM, Tumas DB. Long-term repopulation of irradiated mice with limiting numbers of purified hematopoietic stem cells: in vivo expansion of stem cell phenotype but not function. *Blood* 1995;85:1006–1016.
38. Morrison SJ, Weissmann IL. The long-term repopulating subset of hematopoietic stem cells is deterministic and isolatable by phenotype. *Immunity* 1994;1:661–673.
39. Doi H, Inaba M, Yamamoto Y, et al. Pluripotent hemopoietic stem cells are c-kit^slow. *Immunology* 1997;94:2513–2517.
40. Bodine DM, Seidel NE, Zsebo KM, Orlic D. *In vivo* administration of stem cell factor to mice increases the absolute number of pluripotent stem cells. *Blood* 1993;82:445–455.
41. Fleming WH, Alpern EJ, Uchida N, Ikuta K, Weissman IL. Steel factor influences the distribution and activity of murine hematopoietic stem cells *in vivo*. *Proc Natl Acad Sci USA* 1993;90:3760–3764.

42. Laterveer L, Lindley IJD, Heemskerk DPM, Camps JAJ, Pauwels EKJ, Willemze R, Fibbe WE. Rapid mobilization of hematopoietic progenitor cells in rhesus monkeys by a single intravenous injection of interleukin-8. *Blood* 1997;87: 781–788.

43. Laterveer L, LI J, Hamilton MS, Willemze R, Fibbe WE. Interleukin-8 induces rapid mobilization of hematopoietic stem cells with radioprotective capacity and long-term myelolymphoid repopulating ability. *Blood* 1995;85:2269–2275.

44. Papayannopoulou T, Nakamoto B. Peripheralization of hemopoietic progenitors in primates treated with anti-VLA integrin. *Proc Natl Acad Sci USA* 1993;90: 9374–9378.

45. Papayannopoulou T, Craddock C, Nakamoto B, Priestley GV, Wolf NS. The VLA4/VCAM-1 adhesion pathway defines contrasting mechanisms of lodgement of transplanted murine hemopoietic progenitors between bone marrow and spleen. *Proc Natl Acad Sci USA* 1995;92:9647–9751.

46. Arroyo A, Yang JT, Rayburn H, Hynes RO. Differential requirements for alpha-4 integrins during fetal and adult hematopoiesis. *Cell* 1996;85:997–1008.

47. Ceredig R, ten Boekel E, Rolink A, Melchers F, Andersson J. Fetal liver organ cultures allow the proliferative expansion of pre-B receptor-expressing pre-B II cells and the differentiation of immature and mature B cells in vitro. *Intl Immunol* 1998;10:49–59.

48. Mertsching E, Grawunder U, Meyer V, Rolink T, Ceredig R. Phenotypic and functional analysis of B lymphopoiesis in interleukin-7-transgenic mice: expansion of pro/pre-B cell number and persistence of B lymphocyte development in lymph nodes and spleen. *Eur J Immunol* 1996;26:28–33.

49. Tsuji K, Lyman SD, Sudo T, Clark SC, Ogawa M. Enhancement of murine hematopoiesis by synergistic interactions between steel factor (ligand for *c-kit*), interleukin-11, and other early acting factors in culture. *Blood* 1992;11:2855–2860.

50. Hirayama F, Shih JP, Awgulewitsch A, Warr GW, Clark SC, Ogawa M. Clonal proliferation of murine lymphohemopoietic progenitors in culture. *Proc Natl Acad Sci USA* 1992;89:5907–5911.

51. Sui X, Tsuji K, Tanaka R, et al. gp130 and c-Kit signalings synergize for *ex vivo* expansion of human primitive hemopoietic progenitor cells. *Proc Natl Acad Sci USA* 1994;92:2859–2863.

52. Veiby OP, Jacobsen FW, Cui L, Lyman SD, Jacobsen SEW. The *flt3* ligand promotes the survival of primitive hemopoietic progenitor cells with myeloid as well as B lymphoid potential. *Am Assoc Immunol* 1996;157:2953–2960.

53. Warren AJ, Colledge WH, Carlton MB, Evans MJ, Smith AJ, Rabbitts TH. The oncogenic cysteine-rich LIM domain protein rbtn2 is essential for erythroid development. *Cell* 1994;78:45–57.

54. Porcher C, Swat W, Rockwell K, Fujiwara Y, Alt FW, Orkin SH. The T cell leukemia oncoprotein SCL/tal-1 is essential for development of all hematopoietic lineages. *Cell* 1996;86:47–57.

55. Orkin SH. GATA-binding transcription factors in hematopoietic cells. *Blood* 1992;80:575–581.

56. Weiss MJ, Orkin SH. GATA transcription factors: key regulators of hematopoiesis. *Exp Hematol* 1995;23:99–107.

57. Tsai FY, Keller G, Kuo FC, et l. An early haematopoietic defect in mice lacking the transcription factor GATA-2. *Nature* 1994;371:221–226.

58. Tavassoli M. Embryonic and fetal hematopoiesis: an overview. *Blood Cells* 1991;1:269–281.

59. Kennedy M, Firpo M, Choi K, et al. A common precursor for primitive erythropoiesis and definitive haematopoiesis. *Nature* 1997;386:488–493.

60. Fujiwara Y, Browne CP, Cunniff, Goff SC, Orkin SH. Arrested development of embryonic red cell precursors in mouse embryos lacking transcription factor GATA-1. *Proc Natl Acad Sci USA* 1996;93:12355–12358.

61. Onodara K, Takahashi S, Nishimura S, et al. GATA-1 transcription is controlled by distinct regulatory mechanisms during primitive and definitive erythropoiesis. *Proc Natl Acad Sci USA* 1997;94:4487–4492.

62. Okuda T, Van Deursen J, Hiebert SW, Grosveld G, Downing JR. AML1, the target of multiple chromosomal translocations in human leukemia, is essential for normal fetal liver hematopoiesis. *Cell* 1996;84:321–330.

63. Sasaki K, Yagi R, Bronson RT, et al. Absence of fetal liver hematopoiesis in mice deficient in transcriptional coactivator core binding factor β. *Proc Natl Acad Sci USA* 1996;93:12359–12363.

64. Nuez B, Michalovich D, Bygrave A, Ploemacher R, Grosveld F. Defective haematopoiesis in fetal liver resulting from inactivation of the EKLF gene. *Nature* 1995;375:316–318.

65. Melchers F, Abramczuk J. Murine embryonic blood between day 10 and 13 of gestation as a source of immature precursor B cells. *Eur J Immunol* 1980;10:763–767.

66. Delassus S, Cumano A. Circulation of hematopoietic progenitors in the mouse embryo. *Immunity* 1996;4:97–106.

67. Hirsch E, Iglesias A, Potocnik AJ, Hartmann U, Fassler R. Impaired migration but not differentiation of haematopoietic stem cells in the absence of beta-1 integrins. *Nature* 1996;380:171–175.

68. Shalaby F, Ho J, Stanford WL, et al. A requirement for Flk1 in primitive and definitive hematopoiesis and vasculogenesis. *Cell* 1997;89:981–990.

69. Klemsz M, McKercher S, Celada A, Van Beveren C, Maki R. The macrophage and B cell-specific transcription factor PU.1 is related to the ets oncogene. *Cell* 1990;61:113–124.

70. Hromas R, Orazi A, Neiman R, et al. Hematopoietic lineage- and stage-restricted expression of the ETS oncogene family member PU.1. *Blood* 1993;182: 2998–3004.

71. Goebl M. The PU.1 transcription factor is the product of the putative oncogene Spi-1. *Cell* 1990;61:1165–1166.

72. Singh H. Gene targeting reveals a hierarchy of transcription factors regulating specification of lymphoid cell fates. *Curr Opin Immunol* 1996;8:160–165.

73. Nelsen B, Tian G, Erman B, et al. Regulation of lymphoid-specific immunoglobulin μ heavy chain gene enhancer by ETS-domain proteins. *Science* 1993;261: 82–86.

74. Eisenbeis C, Singh H, Storb U. PU.1 is a component of a multi-protein complex which binds an essential site in the murine immunoglobulin λ2–4 enhancer. *Mol Cell Biol* 1993;13:6452–6461.

75. Hagman J, Grosschedl R. An inhibitory carboxyl-terminal domain in Ets-1 and Ets-2 mediates differential binding of ETS family factors to promoter sequences of the mb-1 gene. *Proc Natl Acad Sci USA* 1992;89:8889–8893.

76. Feldhaus AL, Mbangkollo D, Arvin KL, Klug CA, Singh H. BLyF, a novel cell-type-and stage-specific regulator of the B-lymphocyte gene mb-1. *Mol Cell Biol* 1992;12:1126–1133.

77. Shin M, Koshland M. Ets-related protein PU.1 regulates expression of the immunoglobulin J-chain gene through a novel Ets-binding element. *Genes Dev* 1993;7:2006–2015.

78. McKercher S, Torbett BE, Anderson KL, et al. Targeted disruption of the PU.1 gene results in multiple hematopoietic abnormalities. *EMBO J* 1996;15: 5647–5658.

79. Tondravi MM, McKercher SR, Anderson K, et al. Osteopetrosis in mice lacking haematopoietic transcription factor PU.1. *Nature* 1997;386:81–84.

80. Hayase Y, Muguruma Y, Lee MY. Osteoclast development from hematopoietic stem cells: apparent divergence of the osteoclast lineage prior to macrophage commitment. *Exp Hematol* 1997;25:19–25.

81. Hayashi S, Miyamoto A, Yamane T, et al. Osteoclast precursors in bone marrow and peritoneal cavity. *J Cell Physiol* 1997;170:241–247.

82. Girasole G, Passeri G, Jilka RL, Manolagas SC. Interleukin-11: a new cytokine critical for osteoclast development. *J Clin Invest* 1994;93:1516–1524.

83. Georgopoulos K, Bigby M, Wang JH, et al. The Ikaros gene is required for the development of all lymphoid lineages. *Cell* 1994;79:143–156.

84. Molnar A, Georgopoulos K. The *Ikaros* gene encodes a family of functionally diverse zinc finger DNA binding proteins. *Mol Cell Biol* 1994;14:8292–8303.

85. Wang J-H, Nichogiannopoulou A, Wu L, et al. Selective defects in the development of the fetal and adult lymphoid system in mice with an ikaros null mutation. *Immunity* 1996;5:537–549.

86. Müller-Sieburg CE, Whitlock CA, Weissman IL. Isolation of two early B lymphocyte progenitors from mouse marrow: a committed pre-pre-B cell and a clonogenic Thy-1lo hematopoietic stem cell. *Cell* 1986;44:653–662.

87. Rolink A, Andersson J, Ghia P, et al. Molecular mechanisms guiding B cell development. In: Ochs H, Smith E, Puck J, eds. *Primary immunodeficieny diseases: a molecular and genetic approach.* 1998 (*in press*).

88. Opstelten D. B lymphocyte development and transcription regulation *in vivo. Adv Immunol* 1996;63:197–268.

89. Bain G, Maandag EC, Izon DJ, et al. E2A proteins are required for proper B cell development and initiation of immunoglobulin gene rearrangements. *Cell* 1994;79:885–892.

90. Zhuang Y, Soriano P, Weintraub H. The helix-loop-helix gene E2A is required for B cell formation. *Cell* 1994;79:875–884.

91. Schlissel M, Voronova A, Baltimore D. Helix-loop-helix transcription factor E47 activates germ-line immunoglobulin heavy-chain gene transcription and rearrangement in a pre-T-cell line. *Genes Dev* 1991;5:1367–1376.

92. Choi JK, Shen CP, Radomska HS, Eckhardt LA, Kadesch T. E47 activates the Ig-heavy chain and TdT loci in non-B cells. *EMBO J* 1996;15:5014–5021.

93. Hagman J, Travis A, Grosschedl R. A novel lineage-specific nuclear factor regulates mb-1 gene transcription at the early stages of B cell differentiation. *EMBO J* 1991;10:3409–3417.

94. Lin H, Grosschedl R. Failure of B-cell differentiation in mice lacking the transcription factor EBF. *Nature* 1995a;376:263–267.

95. Gong S, Nussenzweig MC. Regulation of an early developmental checkpoint in the B cell pathway by Igβ. *Science* 1996;272:411–414.

96. van de Wetering M, Oosterwegel M, van Norren K, Clevers H. Sox-4, an Sry-like HMG box protein, is a transcriptional activator in lymphocytes. *EMBO J* 1993;12:3847–3854.

97. Schilham MW, Oosterwegel MA, Moerer P, et al. Defects in cardiac outflow tract formation and pro-B-lymphocyte expansion in mice lacking Sox-4. *Nature* 1996;380:711–714.

98. Walther C, Guenet JL, Simon D, et al. Pax: a murine multigene family of paired box-containing genes. *Genomics* 1991;11:424–434.

99. Stoykova A, Gruss P. Roles of Pax-genes in developing and adult brain as suggested by expression patterns. *J Neurosci* 1994;14:1395–1412.

100. Strachan T, Read AP. PAX genes. *Curr Opin Genet Dev* 1994;4:427–438.

101. Urbanek P, Wang ZQ, Fetka I, Wagner EF, Busslinger M. Complete block of early B cell differentiation and altered patterning of the posterior midbrain in mice lacking Pax5/BSAP. *Cell* 1994;79:901–912.

102. Busslinger M, Urbanek P. The role of BSAP (Pax-5) in B-cell development. *Curr Opin Genet Dev* 1995;5:595–601.

103. Kozmik Z, Wang S, Dorfler P, Adams B, Busslinger M. The promoter of the CD19 gene is a target for the B-cell-specific transcription factor BSAP. *Mol Cell Biol* 1992;12:2662–2672.

104. Zwollo P, Desiderio S. Specific recognition of the blk promoter by the B-lymphoid transcription factor B-cell-specific activator protein. *J Biol Chem* 1994; 269:15310–15317.

105. Okabe T, Watanabe T, Kudo A. A pre-B- and B cell-specific DNA-binding pro-

tein, EBB-1, which binds to the promoter of the V$_{preB1}$ gene. *Eur J Immunol* 1992;22:37–43.

106. Neurath MF, Strober W, Wakatsuki Y. The murine Ig 3′ alpha enhancer is a target site with repressor function for the B cell lineage-specific transcription factor BSAP (NF-HB, S alpha-BP). *J Immunol* 1994;153:730–742.

107. Waters SH, Saikh KU, Stavnezer J. A B-cell-specific nuclear protein that binds to DNA sites 5′ to immunoglobulin S$_\alpha$ tandem repeats is regulated during differentiation. *Mol Cell Biol* 1989;9:5594–5601.

108. Rothman P, Li SC, Gorham B, Glimcher L, Alt F, Boothby M. Identification of a conserved lipopolysaccharide-plus-interleukin-4-responsive element located at the promoter of germ line epsilon transcripts. *Mol Cell Biol* 1991;11:5551–5561.

109. Liao F, Giannini SL, Birshtein BK. A nuclear DNA-binding protein expressed during early stages of B cell differentiation interacts with diverse segments within and 3′ of the Ig H chain gene cluster. *J Immunol* 1992;148:2909–2917.

110. Xu L, Kim MG, Marcu KB. Properties of B cell stage specific and ubiquitous nuclear factors binding to immunoglobulin heavy chain gene switch regions. *Int Immunol* 1992;4:875–887.

111. Nutt SL, Urbanek P, Rolink A, Busslinger M. Essential functions of Pax5 (BSAP) in pro-B cell development: difference between fetal and adult B lymphopoiesis and reduced V-to-DJ recombination at the IgH locus. *Genes Dev* 1997;11:476–491.

112. Cooper MD, Peterson RDA, Good RA. Delineation of the thymic and bursal lymphoid systems in the chicken. *Nature* 1965;205:143–146.

113. Kincade PW. Formation of B lymphocytes in fetal and adult life. *Adv Immunol* 1981;31:177–245.

114. Owen JJT, Raff MC, Cooper MD. Studies on the generation of B lymphocytes in the mouse embryo. *Eur J Immunol* 1975;5:468–473.

115. Melchers F. Three waves of B lymphocyte development during embryonic development in the mouse. In: le Douarin N, ed. *Cell lineage, stem cells and cell determination. INSERM Symposium 10,* vol 10. Amsterdam: Elsevier Science, 1979a:281–289.

116. Melchers F. Murine embryonic B lymphocyte development in the placenta. *Nature* 1979b;277:219–221.

117. Marcos MA, Gutierrez JC, Huetz F, Martinez C, Dieterlen-Lievre F. Waves of B-lymphopoiesis in the establishment of the mouse B-cell compartment. *Scand J Immunol* 1991;34:129–135.

118. Solvason N, Kearney JF. The human fetal omentum: a site of B cell generation. *J Exp Med* 1992;175:397–404.

119. Owen JJT, Cooper MD, Raff MC. *In vitro* generation of B lymphocytes in mouse fetal liver, a mammalian "bursa equivalent". *Nature* 1974;249:361–363.

120. Rolink A, Haasner D, Nishikawa SI, Melchers F. Changes in frequencies of clonable preB cells during life in different lymphoid organs of mice. *Blood* 1993c;81:2290–2300.

121. Strasser A, Rolink T, Melchers F. One synchronous wave of B cell development in mouse fetal liver changes at day 16 of gestation from dependence to independence of a stromal cell environment. *J Exp Med* 1989;170:1973–1986.

122. Melchers F. B lymphocyte development in fetal liver. I. Development of reactivities to B cell mitogens *in vivo* and *in vitro*. *Eur J Immunol* 1977a;7:476–481.

123. Rosenberg YJ, Cunningham AJ. Ontogeny of the antibody-forming cells in mice. I. Kinetics of appearance of mature B cells. *Eur J Immunol* 1976a;5:444–447.

124. Rosenberg YJ, Cunningham AJ. Ontogeny of the antibody-forming cells in mice. II. Maturation of B cells during fetal development. *J Immunol* 1976b;117:1618–1621.

125. Clevers HC, Grosschedl R. Transcriptional control of lymphoid development: lessons from gene targeting. *Immunol Today* 1996;17:336–343.

126. Holmberg D, Anderson A, Carlsson L, Forsgren S. Establishment and functional implications of B cell connectivity. *Immunol Rev* 1989;110:889–903.

127. Gu H, Förster I, Rajewsky K. Sequence homologies, N sequence insertion and J$_H$ gene utilization in V$_H$DJ$_H$ joining: implications for the joining mechanism and the ontogenetic timing of Ly1 B cell and B-CLL progenitor generation. *EMBO J* 1990;9:2133–2140.

128. Meek K. Analysis of junctional diversity during B lymphocyte development. *Science* 1990;250:820–823.

129. Feeney A. Lack of N regions in fetal and neonatal mouse immunoglobulin V-D-J junctional sequences. *J Exp Med* 1990;172:1377–1390.

130. Gregoire KE, Goldschneider I, Barton RW, Bollum FJ. Ontogeny of terminal deoxynucleotidyl transferase-positive cells in lymphohemopoietic tissues of rat and mouse. *J Immunol* 1979;123:1347–1352.

131. Osmond DG. Proliferation kinetics and the lifespan of B cells in central and peripheral lymphoid organs. *Curr Opin Immunol* 1991;3:179–185.

132. Hermans MH, Hartsuiker H, Opstelten D. An *in situ* study of B-lymphocytopoiesis in rat bone marrow. Topographical arrangement of terminal deoxynucleotidyl transferase-positive cells and pre-B cells. *J Immunol* 1989;142:67–73.

133. Jacobsen K, Osmond DG. Microenvironmental organisation and stromal cell associations of B lymphocyte precursor cells in mouse bone marrow. *Eur J Immunol* 1990;20:2395–2404.

134. Fulop GM, Osmond DG. Regulation of bone marrow lymphocyte production. III. Increased production of B and non-B lymphocytes after administering systemic antigens. *Cell Immunol* 1983a;75:80–90.

135. Fulop GM, Osmond DG. Regulation of bone marrow lymphocyte production. IV. Cells mediating the stimulation of marrow lymphocyte production by sheep red blood cells: studies in anti-IgM-suppressed mice, athymic mice, and silica-treated mice. *Cell Immunol* 1983b;75:91–102.

136. Fulop G, Gordon J, Osmond DG. Regulation of lymphocyte production in the bone marrow. I. Turnover of small lymphocytes in mice depleted of B lymphocytes by treatment with anti-IgM antibodies. *J Immunol* 1983c;130:644–648.

137. Opstelten D, Osmond DG. Pre-B cells in mouse bone marrow: immunofluorescence stathmokinetic studies of the proliferation of cytoplasmic μ-chain-bearing cells in normal mice. *J Immunol* 1983;131:2635–2640.

138. Opstelten D, Osmond DG. Regulation of pre-B cell proliferation in bone marrow: immunofluorescence stathmokinetic studies of cytoplasmic μ-chain-bearing cells in anti-IgM-treated mice, hematologically deficient mutant mice and mice given sheep red blood cells. *Eur J Immunol* 1985;15:599–605.

139. Lu L, Osmond DG. Apoptosis during B lymphopoiesis in mouse bone marrow. *J Immunol* 1997;158:5136–5145.

140. Dejbakhsh-Jones S, Okazaki H, Strober S. Similar rates of production of T and B lymphocytes in the bone marrow. *J Exp Med* 1995;181:2201–2211.

141. Osmond DG. The turnover of B lymphocyte populations. *Immunol Today* 1993;14:34–37.

142. Fulop GM, Pietrangeli CE, Osmond DG. Regulation of bone marrow lymphocyte production: IV. Altered kinetic steady state of lymphocyte production after chronic changes in exogenous stimuli. *Exp Hematol* 1986;14:27–34.

143. Pietrangeli CE, Osmond DG. Regulation of B-lymphocyte production in the bone marrow: role of macrophages and the spleen in mediating responses to exogenous agents. *Cell Immunol* 1985;94:147–158.

144. Osmond DG, Fulop GM, Opstelten D, Pietrangeli C. *In vivo* regulation of B lymphocyte production in the bone marrow: effects and mechanism of action of exogenous stimuli on pre-B cell proliferation and lymphocyte turnover. *Adv Exp Med Biol* 1985;186:35–46.

145. Rico-Vargas SA, Potter M, Osmond DG. Perturbation of B cell genesis in the bone marrow of pristane-treated mice. Implications for plasmacytoma induction. *J Immunol* 1995;154:2082–2091.

146. Potter M. Genetics of susceptiblity to plasmacytoma development in BALB/c mice. *Cancer Surv* 1984;3:247–264.

147. Cancro M, Potter M. The requirement of an adherent cell substratum for the growth of developing plasmacytoma cells in vivo. *J Exp Med* 1976;144:1554–1567.

148. Potter M, Wax JS. Peritoneal plasmacytomagenesis in mice: comparison of different pristane dose regimens. *J Natl Cancer Inst* 1983;71:391–395.

149. Potter M, Melchers F. C-Myc in B-cell neoplasia. *Curr Top Microbiol Immunol* 1997;224:1–291.

150. Medina KL, Smithson G, Kincade PW. Suppression of B lymphopoiesis during normal pregnancy. *J Exp Med* 1993;178:1507–1515.

151. Medina KL, Kincade PW. Pregnancy-related steroids are potential negative regulators of B lymphopoiesis. *Proc Natl Acad Sci USA* 1994;91:5382–5386.

152. Smithson G, Beamer WG, Shultz KL, Christianson SW, Shultz LD, Kincade PW. Increased B lymphopoiesis in genetically sex steroid-deficient hypogonadal (hpg) mice. *J Exp Med* 1994;180:717–720.

153. Kincade PW, Medina KL, Smithson G. Sex hormones as negative regulators of lymphopoiesis. *Immunol Rev* 1994;137:119–134.

154. Kantor AB, Stall AM, Adams S, Herzenberg LA, Herzenberg LA. Differential development of progenitor activity for three B-cell lineages. *Proc Natl Acad Sci USA* 1992;89:3320–3324.

155. Kantor AB, Stall AM, Adams S, Watanabe K, Herzenberg LA. *De novo* development and self-replenishment of B cells. *Int Immunol* 1995;7:55.

156. Solvason N, Lehuen A, Kearney JF. An embryonic source of Ly1 but not conventional B cells. *Int Immunol* 1991;3:543–550.

157. Hardy RR, Hayakawa K. A developmental switch in B lymphopoiesis. *Proc Natl Acad Sci USA* 1991b;88:11550–11554.

158. Arnold LW, Pennell CA, McCray SK, Clarke SH. Development of B-1 cells: segregation of phosphatidyl choline-specific B cells to the B-1 population occurs after immunoglobulin gene expression. *J Exp Med* 1994;179:1585–1595.

159. Stall AM, Adams S, Herzenberg LA, Kantor AB. Characteristics and development of the murine B-1b (Ly 1 B sister) cell population. *Ann NY Acad Sci* 1992;651:33–43.

160. Waldschmidt TJ, Kroese FGM, Tygrett LT, Lynch C, Lynch RG. The expression of B cell surface receptors. III. The murine low affinitiy IgE FcεR is not expressed on Ly1 or "Ly1-like" B cells. *Int Immunol* 1991;3:305–315.

161. Hayakawa KRR, Hardy LA, Herzenberg LA, Herzenberg LA. Progenitors for Ly1 B cells are distinct from progenitors for other B cells. *J Exp Med* 1985;161:1554–1568.

162. Hayakawa K, Hardy RR, Honda M, Herzenberg LA, Steinberg AD, Herzenberg LA. Ly-1 B cells: functionally distinct lymphocytes that secrete IgM autoantibodies. *Proc Natl Acad Sci USA* 1984;81:2494–2498.

163. Mercolino TJ, Arnold LW, Haughton G. Phosphatidyl choline is recognized by a series of Ly1 murine B cell lymphomas specific for erythrocyte membranes. *J Exp Med* 1986;163:155–165.

164. Nisitani S, Murakami M, Honjo T. Anti red blood cell immunoglobulin transgenic mice. An experimental model of autoimmune hemolytic anemia. *Ann NY Acad Sci* 1997;815:246–252.

165. Hayakawa K, Carmack CE, Hyman R, Hardy RR. Natural autoantibodies to thymocytes: origin, VH genes, fine specificities, and the role of Thy-1 glycoprotein. *J Exp Med* 1990;172:869–878.

166. Hardy RR, Carmack CE, Shinton SA, Riblet RJ, Hayakawa K. A single V$_H$ gene is utilized predominantly in anti-BrMRBC hybridomas derived from purified Ly-1 B cells. Definition of the V$_H$11 family. *J Immunol* 1989;142:3643–3651.

167. Stall AM, Farinas MC, Tarlinton DM, et al. Ly-1 B-cell clones similar to human

chronic lymphocytic leukemias routinely develop in older normal mice and young autoimmune (New Zealand Black-related) animals. *Proc Natl Acad Sci USA* 1988;85:7312–7316.

168. Mercolino TJ, Arnold LW, Hawkins LA, Haughton G. Normal mouse peritoneum contains a large population of Ly-1⁺ (CD5) B cells that recognize phosphatidyl choline. Relationship to cells that secrete hemolytic-antibody specific for autologous erythrocytes. *J Exp Med* 1988;168:687–698.

169. Masmoudi H, Mota-Santos S, Huetz F, Coutinho A, Casenave PA. All T15 Id-positive antibodies (but not the majority of V$_H$T15⁺ antibodies) are produced by peritoneal CD5⁺ B lymphocytes. *Int Immunol* 1990;2:515–520.

170. Arnold LW, Haughton G. Autoantibodies to phosphatidylcholine. The murine antibromelain RBC response. *Ann NY Acad Sci* 1992;651:354–359.

171. Arnold LW, Spencer DH, Clarke SH, Haughton G. Mechanisms that limit the diversity of antibody: three sequentially acting mechanisms that favor the spontaneous production of germline encoded anti-phosphatidyl choline. *Int Immunol* 1993;5:1365–1373.

172. Hardy RR. Variable gene usage, physiology and development of Ly1⁺ (CD5⁺) B cells. *Curr Opin Immunol* 1992b;4:181–185.

173. Pennell CA, Mercolino TJ, Grdina TA, Arnold LW, Haughton G, Clarke SH. Biased immunoglobulin variable region gene expression by Ly-1 B cells due to clonal selection. *Eur J Immunol* 1989;19:1289–1295.

174. Tarlinton D, Stall AM, Herzenberg LA. Repetitive usage of immunoglobulin VH and D gene segments in CD5⁺ Ly-1 B clones of (NZB × NZW)F1 mice. *EMBO J* 1988;7:3705–3710.

175. Förster I, Rajewsky K. Expansion and functional activity of Ly-1⁺ B cells upon transfer of peritoneal cells into allotype-congenic, newborn mice. *Eur J Immunol* 1987;17:521–528.

176. Hardy RR, Hayakawa K. CD5 B cells, a fetal B cell lineage. *Adv Immunol* 1994a;55:297–339.

177. Paeng N, Kido N, Kato Y, et al. Marked reduction of mouse peritoneal CD5⁺ B cells by intraperitoneal administration of lipopolysaccharide. *Infect Immun* 1997;65:122–126.

178. Murakami M, Tsubata T, Shinkura R, et al. Oral administration of lipopolysaccharides activates B-1 cells in the peritoneal cavity and lamina propria of the gut and induces autoimmune symptoms in an autoantibody transgenic mouse. *J Exp Med* 1994;180:111–121.

179. Karras JG, Wang Z, Huo L, Howard G, Frank DA, Rothstein TL. Signal transducer and activator of transcription-3 (STAT3) is constitutively activated in normal, self-renewing B-1 cells but only inducibly expressed in conventional B lymphocytes. *J Exp Med* 1997;185:1035–1042.

180. Jones BM. Effect of 12 neutralizing anti-cytokine antibodies on in vitro activation of B-cells. Interleukin-12 is required by B1a but not B2 cells. *Scand J Immunol* 1996;43:64–72.

181. Rickert RC, Rajewsky K, Roes J. Impairment of T-cell-dependent B-cell responses and B-1 cell development in CD19-deficient mice. *Nature* 1995;376:352–355.

182. Oliver AM, Martin F, Gartland GL, Carter RH, Kearney JF. Marginal zone B cells exhibit unique activation, proliferative and immunoglobulin secretory responses. *Eur J Immunol* 1997;27:2366–2374.

183. Rolink AG, Radaszkiewicz T, Melchers F. The autoantigen-binding B cell repertoires of normal and of chronically graft-versus-host-diseased mice. *J Exp Med* 1987;165:1675–1687.

184. Hardy RR, Carmack CE, Shinton SA, Kemp JD, Hayakawa K. Resolution and characterization of proB and pre-pro B cell stages in normal mouse bone marrow. *J Exp Med* 1991a;173:1213–1225.

185. Tsubata T, Nishikawa S. Molecular and cellular aspects of early B-cell development. *Curr Opin Immunol* 1991a;3:186–192.

186. Rajewsky K. Early and late B-cell development in the mouse. *Curr Opin Immunol* 1992;4:171–176.

187. Rolink A, Melchers F. Molecular and cellular origins of B lymphocyte diversity. *Cell* 1991b;66:1081–1094.

188. Rolink A, Grawunder U, Winkler TH, Karasuyama H, Melchers F. IL-2 receptor a chain (CD25, TAC) expression defines a crucial stage in preB cell development. *Int Immunol* 1994;6:1257–1264.

189. Rolink A, Ten Boekel E, Melchers F, Fearon DT, Krop I, Andersson J. A subpopulation of B220⁺ cells in murine bone marrow does not express CD19 and contains NK cell-progenitors. *J Exp Med* 1996a;183:187–194.

190. Rolink A, Karasuyama H, Haasner D, et al. Two pathways of B lymphocyte development in mouse bone marrow and the roles of surrogate L chain in this development. *Immunol Rev* 1994a;137:185–201.

191. Rolink A, Ghia P, Grawunder U, et al. In vitro analyses of mechanisms of B-cell development. *Semin Immunol* 1995;7:155–167.

192. Rolink A, Melchers F. Generation and regeneration of cells of the B-lymphocyte lineage. *Curr Opin Immunol* 1993a;5:207–217.

193. Melchers F, Rolink A, Grawunder U, et al. Positive and negative selection events during B lymphopoiesis. *Curr Opin Immunol* 1995;7:214–227.

194. Ehlich A, Matin V, Müller W, Rajewsky K. Analysis of the B-cell progenitor compartment at the level of single cells. *Curr Biol* 1994;4:573–583.

195. ten Boekel E, Melchers F, Rolink A. The status of Ig loci rearrangements in single cells from different stages of B cell development. *Int Immunol* 1995;7:1013–1019.

196. Hayakawa K, Tarlinton D, Hardy RR. Absence of MHC class II expression distinguishes fetal from adult B lymphopoiesis in mice. *J Immunol* 1994;152:4801.

197. Lam KP, Stall AM. Major histocompatibility complex class II expression distinguishes two distinct B cell developmental pathways during ontogeny. *J Exp Med* 1994;180:507–516.

198. Oltz EM, Yancopoulos GD, Morrow MA, et al. A novel regulatory myosin light chain gene distinguishes pre-B cell subsets and is IL-7 inducible. *EMBO J* 1992;11:2759–2767.

199. Mårtensson I-L, Melchers F, Winkler TH. A transgenic marker for mouse B lymphoid precursors. *J Exp Med* 1997a;185:653–661.

200. Li YS, Wasserman R, Hayakawa K, Hardy RR. Identification of the earliest B lineage stage in mouse bone marrow. *Immunity* 1996;5:527–535.

201. Winkler TH, Melchers F. Structure and function of the pro- and pre-B cell receptors on B-lymphoid lineage precursor cells. In: Monroe J, Rothenberg E, eds. *Molecular biology of B and T cell development.* Clifton, NJ: Humana Press, 1997 (*in press*).

202. Peschon JJ, Morrissey PJ, Grabstein KH, et al. Early lymphocyte expansion is severely impaired in interleukin 7 receptor-deficient mice. *J Exp Med* 1994;180:1955–1960.

203. Ray RJ, Furlonger C, Williams DE, Paige CJ. Characterization of thymic stromal-derived lymphopoietin (TSLP) in murine B cell development *in vitro. Eur J Immunol* 1996;26:10–16.

204. Davidson WF, Fredrickson TN, Rudikoff EK, Coffman RL, Hartley JW, Morse HC III. A unique series of lymphomas related to the Ly-1⁺ lineage of B lymphocyte differentiation. *J Immunol* 1984;133:744–753.

205. Davidson WF, Pierce JH, Rudikoff S, Morse HC III. Relationships between B cell and myeloid differentiation. Studies with a B lymphocyte progenitor line, HAFTL-1. *J Exp Med* 1988;168:389–407.

206. Cumano A, Paige CJ. Enrichment and characterization of uncommitted B-cell precursors from fetal liver at day 12 of gestation. *EMBO J* 1992a;11:593–601.

207. Cumano A, Paige CJ, Iscove NN, Brady G. Bipotential precursors of B cells and macrophages in murine fetal liver. *Nature* 1992b;356:612–615.

208. Kitamura D, Rajewsky K. Targeted disruption of mu chain membrane exon causes loss of heavy-chain allelic exclusion. *Nature* 1992a;356:154–156.

209. Kitamura D, Roes J, Kühn R, Rajewsky K. A B cell-deficient mouse by targeted disruption of the membrane exon of the immunoglobulin μ chain gene. *Nature* 1991;350:423–426.

210. DiSanto JP, Muller W, Guy-Grand D, Fischer A, Rajewsky K. Lymphoid development in mice with a targeted deletion of the interleukin 2 receptor gamma chain. *Proc Natl Acad Sci USA* 1995;92:377–381.

211. von-Freeden-Jeffry U, Vieira P, Lucian LA, McNeil T, Burdach SE, Murray R. Lymphopenia in interleukin (IL)-7 gene-deleted mice identifies IL-7 as a nonredundant cytokine. *J Exp Med* 1995;181:1519–1526.

212. Cheng AM, Rowley B, Pao W, Hayday A, Bolen JB, Pawson T. Syk tyrosine kinase required for mouse viability and B-cell development. *Nature* 1995;378:303–306.

213. Turner M, Mee PJ, Costello PS, et al. Perinatal lethality and blocked B-cell development in mice lacking the tyrosine kinase Syk. *Nature* 1995;378:298–302.

214. Rolink A, Kudo A, Karasuyama H, Kikuchi Y, Melchers F. Long-term proliferating early pre B cell lines and clones with the potential to develop to surface-Ig positive mitogen-reactive B cells *in vitro* and *in vivo. EMBO J* 1991d;10:327–336.

215. Winkler TH, Melchers F, Rolink AG. Interleukin-3 and interleukin-7 are alternative growth factors for the same B-cell precursors in the mouse. *Blood* 1994;85:2045–2051.

216. Winkler TH, Rolink AG, Melchers F, Karasuyama H. Precursor B cells of mouse bone marrow express two different complexes with the surrogate light chain on the surface. *Eur J Immunol* 1995;25:446–450.

217. Denis KA, Witte ON. Long-term lymphoid cultures in the study of B-cell differentiation. In: Honjo T, Alt FW, Rabbits TH, eds. *Immunoglob Genes,* London: Academic Press Ltd., 1989;45–59.

218. Suda T, Ohara A, Suda S, et al. Early B cell differentiation from hematopoietic stem cells in the presence of stromal cells and interleukin-7 (IL-7). *Exp Haemtol Today* 1990;45–52.

219. Landreth KS, Narayanan R, Dorshkind K. Insulin-like growth factor-I regulates pro-B cell differentiation. *Blood* 1992;80:1207–1212.

220. Toksoz D, Zsebo KM, Smith KA, et al. Support of human hematopoiesis in long-term bone marrow cultures by murine stromal cells selectively expressing the membrane-bound and secreted forms of the human homolog of the steel gene product, stem cell factor. *Proc Natl Acad Sci USA* 1992;89:7350–7354.

221. Jacobsen K, Miyake K, Kincade PW, Osmond DG. Highly restricted expression of a stromal cell determinant in mouse bone marrow *in vitro. J Exp Med* 1992;176:927–935.

222. Bernardi P, Patel VP, Lodish HF. Lymphoid precursor cells adhere to two different sites on fibronectin. *J Cell Biol* 1987;105:489–495.

223. Miyake K, Medina KL, Hayashi S, Ono S, Hamaoka T, Kincade PW. Monoclonal antibodies to Pgp-1/CD44 block lympho-hemopoiesis in long-term bone marrow cultures. *J Exp Med* 1990a;171:477–488.

224. Miyake K, Underhill CB, Lesley J, Kincade PW. Hyaluronate can function as a cell adhesion molecule and CD44 participates in hyaluronate recognition. *J Exp Med* 1990b;172:69–75.

225. Miyake K, Weissman IL, Greenberger JS, Kincade PW. Evidence for a role of the integrin VLA-4 in lympho-hemopoiesis. *J Exp Med* 1991;173:599–607.

226. Rolink A, Streb M, Melchers F. The κ/λ ratio in surface immunoglobulin molecules on B lymphocytes differentiating from D$_H$J$_H$-rearranged murine pre-B cell clones *in vitro. Eur J Immunol* 1991c;21:2895–2898.

227. Ogawa M, Matzusaki Y, Nishikawa S, et al. Expression and function of c-kit in hemopoietic progenitor cells. *J Exp Med* 1991;174:63–70.

228. Kodama H, Nose M, Yamaguchi Y, et al. *In vitro* proliferation of primitive hemopoietic stem cells supported by stromal cells: evidence for the presence of a mechanism(s) other than that involving c-kit receptor and its ligand. *J Exp Med* 1992;176:351–361.

229. Grawunder U, Melchers F, Rolink A. Interferon-γ arrests proliferation and causes apoptosis in stromal cell/interleukin-7-dependent normal murine pre-B cell lines and clones *in vitro*, but does not induce differentiation to surface immunoglobulin-positive B cells. *Eur J Immunol* 1993a;23:544–551.

230. Strasser A, Wittingham S, Vaux DL, et al. Enforced BCL2 expression in B-lymphoid cells prolongs antibody responses and elicits autoimmune disease. *Proc Natl Acad Sci USA* 1991;88:8661–8665.

231. Rolink A, Grawunder U, Haasner D, Strasser A, Melchers F. Immature surface Ig⁺ B cells can continue to rearrange κ and λ L chain gene loci. *J Exp Med* 1993b;178:1263–1270.

232. Rolink AG, Reiniger L, Oka Y, Kalberer CP, Winkler TH, Melchers F. Repopulation of SCID mice with long-term *in vitro* proliferating pre-B-cell lines from normal and autoimmune disease-prone mice. *Res Immunol* 1994b;145:353–356.

233. Hardy RR, Shinton SA, Hayakawa K. Repopulation of SCID mice with fetal-derived B-lineage cells. *Curr Top Microbiol Immunol* 1992a;182:73–80.

234. Sprent J, Schaefer M, Hurd M, Surh CD, Ron Y. Mature murine B and T cells transferred to SCID mice can survive indefinitely and many maintain a virgin phenotype. *J Exp Med* 1991;174:717–728.

235. Reininger L, Radaszkiewicz T, Kosco M, Melchers F, Rolink AG. Development of autoimmune disease in SCID mice populated with long-term *in vitro* proliferating (NZB × NZW)F1 pre-B cells. *J Exp Med* 1992;176:1343–1353.

236. Reininger L, Winkler TH, Kalberer CP, Jourdan M, Melchers F, Rolink AG. Intrinsic B cell defects in NZB and NZW mice contribute to systemic lupus erythematosus in (NZB × NZW)F1 mice. *J Exp Med* 1996;184:853–861.

237. Oka Y, Rolink AG, Suematsu S, Kishimoto T, Melchers F. An interleukin-6 transgene expressed in B lymphocyte lineage cells overcomes the T cell-dependent establishment of normal levels of switched immunoglobulin isotypes. *Eur J Immunol* 1995;25:1332–1337.

238. Kurosawa Y, Tonegawa S. Organization, structure and assembly of immunoglobulin heavy chain diversity DNA segments. *J Exp Med* 1982;155:201–218.

239. Ichihara Y, Hayashida H, Miyazawa S, Kurosawa Y. Only D_{FL16}, D_{SP2} and D_{Q52} gene families exist in mouse immunoglobulin heavy chain diversity gene loci, of which D_{FL16} and D_{SP2} originate from the same primordial D_H gene. *Eur J Immunol* 1989;19:1849–1854.

240. Chang Y, Paige CJ, Wu GE. Enumeration and characterization of DJH structures in mouse fetal liver. *EMBO J* 1992;11:1891–1899.

241. Kaartinen M, Mäkelä O. Reading of D genes in variable frames as a source of antibody diversity. *Immunol Today* 1985;6:324–330.

242. Shimizu T, Yamagishi H. Biased reading frames of preexisting DH-JH coding joints and preferential nucleotide insertions at VH-DJH signal joints of excision products of immunoglobulin heavy chain gene rearrangements. *EMBO J* 1992;11:4869–4879.

243. Kottman AH, Brack C, Eibel H, Köhler G. A survey of protein-DNA interaction sites within the murine immunoglobulin heavy chain locus reveals a particularly complex pattern around the DQ_{52} element. *Eur J Immunol* 1992;22:2113–2120.

244. Reth MG, Alt FW. Novel immunoglobulin heavy chains are produced from DJH gene segment rearrangements in lymphoid cells. *Nature* 1984;312:418–423.

245. Tsubata T, Tsubata R, Reth M. Cell surface expression of the short immunoglobulin μ chain (D_μ protein) in murine pre-B cells is differently regulated from that of the intact μ chain. *Eur J Immunol* 1991b;21:1359–1363.

246. Cohn M, Langman RE. The protecton: the unit of humoral immunity selected by evolution. *Immunol Rev* 1990;115:7–147.

247. Gu H, Tarlinton D, Muller W, Rajewsky K, Forster I. Most peripheral B cells in mice are ligand selected. *J Exp Med* 1991a;173:1357–1371.

248. Gu H, Kitamura D, Rajewsky K. B cell development regulated by gene rearrangement: arrest of maturation by membrane-bound D_μ protein and selection of D_H element reading frames. *Cell* 1991b;65:47–55.

249. Gerstein RM, Lieber MR. Extent to which homology can constrain junctional diversity in V(D)J recombination. *Nature* 1993;363:625–627.

250. Haasner D, Rolink A, Melchers F. Influence of surrogate L chain on D_HJ_H-reading frame 2 suppression in mouse precursor B cells. *Int Immunol* 1994;6:21–30.

251. Karasuyama H, Rolink A, Shinkai Y, Young F, Alt FW, Melchers F. The expression of V_{preB}/λ_5 surrogate light chain in early bone marrow precursor B cells of normal and B-cell deficient mutant mice. *Cell* 1994;77:133–143.

252. Sakaguchi N, Melchers F. λ_5, a new light-chain-related locus selectively expressed in preB lymphocytes. *Nature* 1986;324:579–582.

253. Kudo A, Melchers F. A second gene, V_{preB} in the λ_5 locus of the mouse, which appears to be selectively expressed in preB lymphocytes. *EMBO J* 1987a;6:2267–2272.

254. Melchers F, Karasuyama H, Haasner D, et al. The surrogate light chain in B-cell development. *Immunol Today* 1993;14:60–68.

255. Karasuyama H, Melchers F, Rolink A. A complex of glycoproteins is associated with V_{preB}/λ_5 surrogate light chain on the surface of μ heavy chain-negative early precursor B cell lines. *J Exp Med* 1993;178:469–478.

256. Shinjo F, Hardy RR, Jongstra J. Monoclonal anti-λ_5 antibody FS1 identifies a 130 kDa protein associated with λ_5 and V_{preB} on the surface of early pre-B cell lines. *Int Immunol* 1994;6:393–399.

257. Kerr WG, Cooper MD, Feng L, Burrows PD, Hendershot LM. μ heavy chains can associate with a pseudo-light chain complex (XL) in human pre-B cell lines. *Int Immunol* 1989;1:355–361.

258. Karasuyama H, Kudo A, Melchers F. The proteins encoded by the V_{preB} and λ_5 preB cell specific genes can associate with each other and with μ heavy chain. *J Exp Med* 1990;172:969–972.

259. Pillai S, Baltimore D. Formation of disulphide-linked $\mu_2\omega_2$ tetramers in pre-B cells by the 18K ω-immunoglobulin light chain. *Nature* 1987;329:172–174.

260. Tsubata T, Reth M. The products of preB cell specific genes (λ_5 and V_{preB}) and the immunoglobulin μ chain form a complex that is transported onto the cell surface. *J Exp Med* 1990;172:973–976.

261. Misener V, Downey GP, Jongstra J. The immunoglobulin light chain related protein λ_5 is expressed on the surface of mouse pre-B cell lines and can function as a signal transducing molecule. *Int Immunol* 1991;3:1129–1136.

262. Brouns GS, de-Vries E, van-Noesel CJ, Mason DY, van-Lier RA, Borst J. The structure of the μ/pseudo light chain complex on human pre-B cells is consistent with a function in signal transduction. *Eur J Immunol* 1993;23:1088–1097.

263. Hombach J, Tsubata T, Leclercq L, Stappert H, Reth M. Molecular components of the B-cell antigen receptor complex of the IgM class. *Nature* 1990;343:760–762.

264. Nagata K, Nakamura T, Kitamura F, et al. The Igα/Igβ heterodimer on μ-negative proB cells is competent for transducing signals to induce early B cell differentiation. *Immunity* 1997;7:559–570.

265. Nomura J, Matsuo T, Kubota L, Kimoto M, Sakaguchi N. Signal transmission through the B cell-specific MB-1 molecule at the pre-B cell stage. *Int Immunol* 1991;3:117–126.

266. Kuwahara K, Kawai T, Mitsuyoshi S, et al. Cross-linking of B cell antigen receptor related structure of pre-B cell lines induces tyrosine phosphorylation of p85 and p110 subunits and activation of phosphatidylinositol 3-kinase. *Int Immunol* 1996;8:1273–1285.

267. Kudo A, Pravtcheva D, Sakaguchi N, Ruddle FH, Melchers F. Localization of the murine λ_5 gene on chromsome 16. *Genomics* 1987b;1:277–279.

268. Mattei MG, Fumoux F, Roeckel N, Fougereau M, Schiff C. The human pre-B-specific λ-like cluster is located in the 22q11.2–22q12.3 region, distal to the IgCλ locus. *Genomics* 1991;9:544–546.

269. Shirasawa T, Ohnishi K, Hagiwara S, et al. A novel gene product associated with μ chains in immature B cells. *EMBO J* 1993;12:1827–1834.

270. Ohnishi K, Takemori T. Molecular components and assembly of mu.surrogate light chain complexes in pre-B cell lines. *J Biol Chem* 1994;269:28347–28353.

271. Bauer SR, Huebner K, Budarf M, et al. The human V_{preB} gene is located on chromosome 22 near a cluster of $V_{\lambda1}$ gene segments. *Immunogenetics* 1988a;28:328–333.

272. Bauer SR, Kudo A, Melchers F. Structure and pre-B lymphocyte restricted expression of the V_{preB} in humans and conservation of its structure in other mammalian species. *EMBO J* 1988b;7:111–116.

273. Guelpa Fonlupt V, Tonnelle C, Blaise D, Fougereau M, Fumoux F. Discrete early pro-B and pre-B stages in normal human bone marrow as defined by surface pseudo-light chain expression. *Eur J Immunol* 1994;24:257–264.

274. Hollis GF, Evans RJ, Stafford-Hollis JM, Korsmeyer SJ, McKearn JP. Immunoglobulin λ light-chain-related genes 14.1 and 16.1 are expressed in pre-B cells and may encode the human immunoglobulin ω light-chain protein. *Proc Natl Acad Sci USA* 1989;86:5552–5556.

275. Schiff C, Bensmana M, Guglielmi P, Milili M, Lefranc MP, Fougereau M. The immunoglobulin lambda-like gene cluster (14.1, 16.1 and F λ 1) contains gene(s) selectively expressed in pre-B cells and is the human counterpart of the mouse λ_5 gene. *Int Immunol* 1990;2:201–207.

276. Evans RJ, Hollis GF. Genomic structure of the human Ig lambda 1 gene suggests that it may be expressed as an Ig lambda 14.1-like protein or as a canonical B cell Ig lambda light chain: implications for Ig lambda gene evolution. *J Exp Med* 1991;173:305–311.

277. Donohoe ME, Blomberg BB. The 14.1 surrogate light chain promoter has lineage- and stage-restricted activity. *J Immunol* 1997;158:1681–1691.

278. Mårtensson IL, Melchers F. Pre-B cell-specific lambda 5 gene expression due to suppression in non pre-B cells. *Int Immunol* 1994;6:863–872.

279. Mårtensson A, Mårtensson IL. Early B cell factor binds to a site critical for lambda5 core enhancer activity. *Eur J Immunol* 1997b;27:315–320.

280. Yang J, Glozak MA, Blomberg BB. Identification and localization of a developmental stage-specific promoter activity from the murine lambda 5 gene. *J Immunol* 1995;155:2498–2514.

281. Kudo A, Thalmann P, Sakaguchi N, et al. The expression of the mouse V_{preB}/λ_5 locus in transformed cell lines and tumors of the B lineage differentiation pathway. *Int Immunol* 1992;4:831–840.

282. Lassoued K, Nunez CA, Billips L, et al. Expression of surrogate light chain receptors is restricted to a late stage in pre-B cell differentiation. *Cell* 1993;73:73–86.

283. Meffre E, Fougereau M, Argenson JN, Aubaniac JM, Schiff C. Cell surface expression of surrogate light chain (psi L) in the absence of mu on human pro-B cell lines and normal pro-B cells. *Eur J Immunol* 1996;26:2172–2180.

284. Sanz E, de la Hera A. A novel anti-V_{preB} antibody identifies immunoglobulin-surrogate receptors on the surface of human pre-B cells. *J Exp Med* 1996;183:2693–2698.

285. Ghia P, ten Boekel E, Sanz E, de la Hera A, Rolink AG, Melchers F. Ordering of

human bone marrow B-lineage precursors by an analysis of V$_{preB}$ expression and of the status of immunoglobulin loci in single cells. *J Exp Med* 1996;184: 2217–2219.

286. Loffert D, Ehlich A, Muller W, Rajewsky K. Surrogate light chain expression is required to establish immunoglobulin heavy chain allelic exclusion during early B cell development. *Immunity* 1996;4:133–144.

287. Grawunder U, Leu TMJ, Schatz DG, et al. Down-regulation of *RAG1* and *RAG2* gene expression in preB cells after functional immunoglobulin heavy chain rearrangement. *Immunity* 1995;3:601–608.

288. Kitamura D, Kudo A, Schaal S, Müller W, Melchers F, Rajewsky K. A critical role of λ₅ in B cell development. *Cell* 1992b;69:823–831.

289. Motoyama N, Wang F, Roth KA, et al. Massive cell death of immature hematopoietic cells and neurons in Bcl-x-deficient mice. *Science* 1995;267:1506–1510.

290. Fang W, Mueller DL, Pennell CA, et al. Frequent aberrant immunoglobulin gene rearrangements in pro-B cells revealed by a$_{bcd-xl}$ transgene. *Immunity* 1996;4: 291–299.

291. Brodeur PH, Riblet R. The immunoglobulin heavy chain variable region (Igh-V) locus in the mouse. I. One hundred Igh-V genes comprise seven families of homologous genes. *Eur J Immunol* 1984;14:922–930.

292. Feeney AJ, Riblet R. D$_{ST4}$: a new, and probably the last, functional D$_H$ gene in the BALB/c mouse. *Immunogenetics* 1993;37:217–221.

293. Kofler R, Geley S, Kofler H, Helmberg A. Mouse variable-region gene families: complexity, polymorphism and use in non-autoimmune responses. *Immunol Rev* 1992;128:5–21.

294. Winter E, Radbruch A, Krawinkel U. Members of novel V$_H$ gene families are found in VDJ regions of polyclonally activated B-lymphocytes. *EMBO J* 1985;4:2861–2867.

295. Carlsson L, Övermo C, Holmberg D. Developmentally controlled selection of antibody genes: characterization of individual V$_H$7183 genes and evidence for stage-specific somatic diversification. *Eur J Immunol* 1992;22:71–78.

296. Huetz F, Carlsson L, Tornberg UC, Holmberg D. V-region directed selection in differentiating B lymphocytes. *EMBO J* 1993;12:1819–1826.

297. Reth M, Gehrmann P, Petrac E, Wiese P. A novel V$_H$ to V$_H$DJ$_H$ joining mechanism in heavy-chain-negative (null) preB cells results in heavy-chain production. *Nature* 1986;322:840–842.

298. Teale JM, Medina CA. Comparative expression of adult and fetal V gene repertoires. *Int Rev Immunol* 1992;8:95–111.

299. Wu GE, Paige CJ. V$_H$ gene family utilization in colonies derived from B and pre-B cells detected by the RNA colony blot assay. *EMBO J* 1986;5:3475–3481.

300. Yancopoulos GD, Desiderio SV, Paskind M, Kearney JF, Baltimore D, Alt FW. Preferential utilization of the most J$_H$-proximal V$_H$ gene segments in pre-B-cell lines. *Nature* 1984;311:727–733.

301. Yancopoulos GD, Malynn BA, Alt FW. Developmentally regulated and strain-specific expression of murine V$_H$ gene families. *J Exp Med* 1988;168:417–435.

302. Perlmutter RM, Kearney JF, Chang SP, Hood LE. Developmentally controlled expression of immunoglobulin V$_H$ genes. *Science* 1985;227:1597–1601.

303. Alt FW, Blackwell TK, Yancopoulos GD. Development of the primary antibody repertoire. *Science* 1987;238:1079–1087.

304. Malynn BA, Yancopoulos GD, Barth JE, Bona CA, Alt FW. Biased expression of J$_H$-proximal V$_H$ genes occurs in the newly generated repertoire of neonatal and adult mice. *J Exp Med* 1990;171:843–859.

305. Marshall AJ, Wu GE, Paige GJ. Frequency of V$_H$81x usage during B cell development: initial decline in usage is independent of Ig heavy chain cell surface expression. *J Immunol* 1996;156:2077–2084.

306. Dildrop R, Krawinkel U, Winter E, Rajewsky K. V$_H$-gene expression in murine lipopolysaccharide blasts distributes over the nine known V$_H$-gene groups and may be random. *Eur J Immunol* 1985;15:1154–1156.

307. Jeong HD, Teale JM. Comparison of the fetal and adult functional B cell repertoires by analysis of V$_H$ gene family expression. *J Exp Med* 1988;168:589–603.

308. Schulze DH, Kelsoe G. Genotypic analysis of B cell colonies by in situ hybridization. Stoichiometric expression of three VH families in adult C57BL/6 and BALB/c mice. *J Exp Med* 1987;166:163–172.

309. Sheehan KM, Brodeur PH. Molecular cloning of the primary IgH repertoire: a quantitative analysis of VH gene usage in adult mice. *EMBO J* 1989;8: 2313–2320.

310. Decker DJ, Kline GH, Hayden TA, Zaharevitz SN, Klinman NR. Heavy chain V gene-specific elimination of B cells during the pre-B cell to B cell transition. *J Immunol* 1995;154:4924–4935.

311. Decker DJ, Boyle NE, Klinman NR. Predominance of nonproductive rearrangements of V$_H$81X gene segments evidences a dependence of B cell clonal maturation on the structure of nascent H chains. *J Immunol* 1991;147:1406–1411.

312. Connor AM, Fanning LJ, Celler JW, Hicks LK, Ramsden DA, Wu GE. Mouse V$_H$7183 recombination signal sequences mediate recombination more frequently than those of V$_H$J558. *J Immunol* 1995;155:5268–5272.

313. Keyna U, Beck-Engeser GB, Jongstra J, Applequist SE, Jack HM. Surrogate light chain-dependent selection of Ig heavy chain V regions. *J Immunol* 1995;155: 5536–5542.

314. ten Boekel E, Melchers F, Rolink AG. Changes in the V(H) gene repertoire of developing precursor B lymphocytes in mouse bone marrow mediated by the pre-B cell receptor. *Immunity* 1997;7:357–368.

315. Kong GH, Bu JY, Kurosaki T, Shaw AS, Chan AC. Reconstitution of Syk function by the ZAP-70 protein tyrosine kinase. *Immunity* 1995;2:485–492.

316. Engel P, Zhou LJ, Ord DC, Sato S, Koller B, Tedder TF. Abnormal B lymphocyte development, activation, and differentiation in mice that lack or overexpress the CD19 signal transduction molecule. *Immunity* 1995;3:39–50.

317. Storb U, Engler P, Manz J, et al. Expression of immunoglobulin genes in transgenic mice and transfected cells. *Ann NY Acad Sci* 1988;546:51–56.

318. Taki S, Meiering M, Rajewsky K. Targeted insertion of a variable region gene into the immunoglobulin heavy chain locus [see comments]. *Science* 1993;262: 1268–1271.

319. Manz J, Dennis K, Witte O, Brinster R, Storb U. Feedback inhibition of immunoglobulin gene rearrangement by membrane μ, but not by secreted μ heavy chains. *J Exp Med* 1988;168:1363–1381.

320. Nussenzweig MC, Shaw AC, Sinn E, Campos-Torres J, Leder P. Allelic exclusion in transgenic mice carrying mutant human IgM genes. *J Exp Med* 1988;167: 1969–1974.

321. Iglesias A, Lamers M, Kohler G. Expression of immunoglobulin delta chain causes allelic exclusion in transgenic mice. *Nature* 1987;330:482–484.

322. Reth M, Petrac E, Wiese P, Lobel L, Alt FW. Activation of V κ gene rearrangement in pre-B cells follows the expression of membrane-bound immunoglobulin heavy chains. *EMBO J* 1987;6:3299–3305.

323. Kurtz BS, Witte PL, Storb U. Gamma 2b provides only some of the signals normally given via mu in B cell development. *Int Immunol* 1997;9:415–426.

324. Kenny JJ, Stall AM, Fisher RT, et al. Ig γ 2b transgenes promote B cell development but alternate developmental pathways appear to function in different transgenic lines. *J Immunol* 1995;154:5694–5705.

325. Reichman-Fried M, Hardy RR, Bosma MJ. Development of B-lineage cells in the bone marrow of scid/scid mice following the introduction of functionally rearranged immunoglobulin transgenes. *Proc Natl Acad Sci USA* 1990;87: 2730–2734.

326. Kotloff DB, Bosma MJ, Ruetsch NR. Scid mouse Pre-B cells with intracellular mu chains: analysis of recombinase activity and IgH gene rearrangements. *Int Immunol* 1993a;5:383–391.

327. Kotloff DB, Bosma MJ, Ruetsch NR. V(D)J recombination in peritoneal B cells of leaky scid mice. *J Exp Med* 1993b;178:1981–1994.

328. Chang Y, Bosma MJ. Effect of different Ig transgenes on B cell differentiation in scid mice. *Int Immunol* 1997;9:373–380.

329. Chang Y, Bosma GC, Bosma MJ. Development of B cells in scid mice with immunoglobulin transgenes: implications for the control of V(D)J recombination. *Immunity* 1995;2:607–616.

330. Spanopoulou E, Roman CAJ, Corcoran LM, et al. Functional immunoglobulin transgenes guide ordered B-cell differentiation in RAG-1-deficient mice. *Genes Dev* 1994;8:1030–1042.

331. Young F, Ardman B, Shinkai Y, et al. Influence of immunoglobulin heavy- and light-chain expression on B-cell differentiation. *Genes Dev* 1994;8:1043–1057.

332. Papavasiliou F, Jankovic M, Nussenzweig MC. Surrogate or conventional light chains are required for membrane immunoglobulin mu to activate the precursor B cell transition. *J Exp Med* 1996;184:2025–2030.

333. Pearl ER, Vogler LB, Okos AJ, Crist WM, Lawton AR III, Cooper MD. B lymphocyte precursors in human bone marrow: an analysis of normal individuals and patients with antibody-deficiency states. *J Immunol* 1978;120:1169–1175.

334. Rolink A, Haasner D, Melchers F, Andersson J. The surrogate light chain in mouse B cell development. *Int Rev Immunol* 1996c;13:341–356.

335. Shaffer AL, Schlissel MS. A truncated heavy chain protein relieves the requirement for surrogate light chains in early B cell development. *J Immunol* 1997;159:1265–1275.

336. ten Boekel E, Melchers F, Rolink AG. Precursor B cells showing H chain allelic inclusion display allelic exclusion at the level of pre-B cell receptor surface expression. *Immunity* 1998;8:199–207.

337. Hirabayashi Y, Lecerf JM, Dong Z, Stollar BD. Kinetic analysis of the interactions of recombinant human VpreB and Ig V domains. *J Immunol* 1995;155: 1218–1228.

338. Takeda S, Zou YR, Bluethmann H, Kitamura D, Muller U, Rajewsky K. Deletion of the immunoglobulin kappa chain intron enhancer abolishes kappa chain gene rearrangements in cis but not lambda chain rearrangements in trans. *EMBO J* 1993;12:2329–2336.

339. Chen J, Trounstine M, Kurahara C, et al. B cell development in mice that lack one or both immunoglobulin κ light chain genes. *EMBO J* 1993c;12:821–830.

340. Hartley SB, Cooke MP, Fulcher PA, et al. Elimination of self-reactive B lymphocytes proceed in two stages: arrested development and cell death. *Cell* 1993; 72:325–335.

341. Carsetti R, Kohler G, Lamers MC. Transitional B cells are the target of negative selection in the B cell compartment. *J Exp Med* 1995;181:2129–2140.

342. Roth PE, Doglio L, Manz JT, Kim JY, Lo D, Storb U. Immunoglobulin gamma 2b transgenes inhibit heavy chain gene rearrangement, but cannot promote B cell development. *J Exp Med* 1993;178:2007–2021.

343. Andersson J, Melchers F, Rolink A. Stimulation by T cell independent antigens can relieve the arrest of differentiation of immature auto-reactive B cells in the bone marrow. *Scand J Immunol* 1995;42:21–33.

344. Okamoto M, Murakami M, Shimizu A, et al. A transgenic model of autoimmune hemolytic anemia. *J Exp Med* 1992;175:71–79.

345. Hardy RR, Carmack CE, Li YS, Hayakawa K. Distinctive developmental origins and specificities of murine CD5⁺ B cells. *Immunol Rev* 1994b;137:91–118.

346. Oldstone MB. Molecular mimicry as a mechanism for the cause and a probe uncovering etiologic agent(s) of autoimmune disease. *Curr Top Microbiol Immunol* 1989;145:127–135.

347. Coutinho A, Moller G. B cell mitogenic properties of thymus-independent antigens. *Nat New Biol* 1973;245:12–14.

348. Lang J, Jackson M, Teyton L, Brunmark A, Kane K, Nemazee D. B cells are exquisitely sensitive to central tolerance and receptor editing induced by ultralow affinity, membrane-bound antigen. *J Exp Med* 1996;184:1685–1697.

349. Scott DW, Livnat D, Pennell CA, Keng P. Lymphoma models for B cell activation and tolerance. III. Cell cycle dependence for negative signalling of WEHI-231 B lymphoma cells by anti-μ. *J Exp Med* 1986;164:156–164.

350. Scott DW, Donjerkovic D, Maddox B, Ezhevsky S, Grdina T. Role of c-myc and p27 in anti-IgM induced B-lymphoma apoptosis. *Curr Top Microbiol Immunol* 1997;224:103–112.

351. Benhamou LE, Cazenave PA, Sarthou P. Anti-immunoglobulins induce death by apoptosis in WEHI-231 B lymphoma cells. *Eur J Immunol* 1990;20:1405–1407.

352. Hasbold J, Klaus GG. Anti-immunoglobulin antibodies induce apoptosis in immature B cell lymphomas. *Eur J Immunol* 1990;20:1685–1690.

353. Gay D, Saunders T, Camper S, Weigert M. Receptor editing: an approach by autoreactive B cells to escape self tolerance. *J Exp Med* 1993;177:999–1008.

354. Tiegs SL, Russell DM, Nemazee D. Receptor editing in self-reactive bone marrow B cells. *J Exp Med* 1993;177:1009–1020.

355. Ghia P, Gratwohl A, Signer E, Winkler TH, Melchers F, Rolink AG. Immature B cells from human and mouse bone marrow can change their surface light chain expression. *Eur J Immunol* 1995;25:3108–3114.

356. Radic MZ, Zouali M. Receptor editing, immune diversification, and self-tolerance. *Immunity* 1996;5:505–511.

357. Chen C, Prak EL, Weigert M. Editing disease-associated autoantibodies. *Immunity* 1997;6:97–105.

358. Rusconi S, Köhler G. Transmission and expression of a specific pair of rearranged immunoglobulin μ and κ genes in a transgenic mouse line. *Nature* 1985;314:330–338.

359. Allman DM, Ferguson SE, Lentz VM, Cancro MP. Peripheral B cell maturation. II. Heat-stable antigen(hi) splenic B cells are an immature developmental intermediate in the production of long-lived marrow-derived B cells. *J Immunol* 1993;151:4431–4444.

360. Thomas-Vaslin V, Freitas AA. Lymphocyte population kinetics during the development of the immune system. B cell persistence and life-span can be determined by the host environment. *Int Immunol* 1989;1:237–246.

361. Förster I, Rajewsky K. The bulk of the peripheral B-cell pool in mice is stable and not rapidly renewed from the bone marrow. *Proc Natl Acad Sci USA* 1990;87:4781–4784.

362. Rajewsky K. B-cell lifespans in the mouse—why to debate what? *Immunol Today* 1993;14:40–41.

363. MacLennan I, Chan E. The dynamic relationship between B-cell populations in adults [see comments]. *Immunol Today* 1993;14:29–34.

364. Igarashi H, Kuwahara K, Nomura J, et al. B cell Ag receptor mediates different types of signals in the protein kinase activity between immature B cell and mature B cell. *J Immunol* 1994;153:2381–2393.

365. Monroe JG. Tolerance sensitivity of immature-stage B cells: can developmentally regulated B cell antigen receptor (BCR) signal transduction play a role? *J Immunol* 1996;156:2657–2660.

366. Sanchez M, Misulovin Z, Burkhardt AL, et al. Signal transduction by immunoglobulin is mediated through Igα and Igβ. *J Exp Med* 1993;178:1049–1055.

367. Teh YM, Neuberger MS. The immunoglobulin (Ig)α and Igβ cytoplasmic domains are independently sufficient to signal B cell maturation and activation in transgenic mice. *J Exp Med* 1997;185:1753–1758.

368. Reth M, Hombach J, Wienands J, et al. The B-cell antigen receptor complex. *Immunol Today* 1991;12:196–201.

369. Melamed D, Nemazee D. Self-antigen does not accelerate immature B cell apoptosis, but stimulates receptor editing as a consequence of developmental arrest. *Proc Natl Acad Sci USA* 1997;94:9267–9272.

370. Chan EYT, MacLennan ICM. Only a small proportion of splenic B cells in adults are short-lived virgin cells. *Eur J Immunol* 1993;23:357–363.

371. Clarke SH, McCray SK. V_H CDR3-dependent positive selection of murine V_H12-expressing B cells in the neonate. *Eur J Immunol* 1993;23:3327–3334.

372. Ye J, McCray SK, Clarke SH. The majority of murine V_H12-expressing B cells are excluded from the peripheral repertoire in adults. *Eur J Immunol* 1995;25:2511–2521.

373. Ye J, McCray SK, Clarke SH. The transition of pre-BI to pre-BII cells is dependent on the VH structure of the mu/surrogate L chain receptor. *EMBO J* 1996;15:1524–1533.

374. Schubart DB, Rolink A, Kosco-Vilbois M, Botteri F, Matthias P. B-cell-specific coactivator OBF-1/OCA-B/Bob1 required for immune response and germinal centre formation. *Nature* 1996;383:538–542.

375. Schubart DB, Rolink A, Matthias P. 1998 (*in preparation*).

376. Oka Y, Rolink AG, Andersson J, et al. Profound reduction of mature B cell numbers, reactivities and serum immunoglobulin levels in mice which simultaneously carry the XID and CD40-deficiency genes. *Int Immunol* 1996;8:1675–1685.

377. Khan WN, Nilsson A, Mizoguchi E, et al. Impaired B cell maturation in mice lacking Bruton's tyrosine kinase (Btk) and CD40. *Int Immunol* 1997;9:395–405.

378. Torres RM, Flaswinkel H, Reth M, Rajewsky K. Aberrant B cell development and immune response in mice with a compromised BCR complex [see comments]. *Science* 1996;272:1804–1808.

379. Miller DJ, Hayes CE. Phenotypic and genetic characterization of a unique B lymphocyte deficiency in strain A/WySnJ mice. *Eur J Immunol* 1991;21:1123–1130.

380. Lentz VM, Cancro MP, Nashold FE, Hayes CE. Bcmd governs recruitment of new B cells into the stable peripheral B cell pool in the A/WySnJ mouse. *J Immunol* 1996;157:598–606.

381. Benatar T, Carsetti R, Furlonger C, Kamalia N, Mak T, Paige CJ. Immunoglobulin-mediated signal transduction in B cells from CD45-deficient mice. *J Exp Med* 1996;183:329–334.

382. Scher I. CBA/N immune defective mice: evidence for the failure of a B cell subpopulation to be expressed. *Immunol Rev* 1982a;64:117–136.

383. Scher I. The CBA/N mouse strain: an experimental model illustrating the influence of the X-chromosome on immunity. *Adv Immunol* 1982b;33:1–71.

384. Rolink A, Brocker T, Andersson J, Melchers F. MHC class II dependent, helper T cell independent generation of mature B cells. 1998 (*submitted*).

385. Shachar I, Flavell RA. Requirement for invariant chain in B cell maturation and function. *Science* 1996;274:106–108.

386. Ramsden DA, Wu GE. Mouse κ light-chain recombination signal sequences mediate recombination more frequently than do those of λ light chain. *Proc Natl Acad Sci USA* 1991;88:10721–10725.

387. Streb M. *B cell development in the mouse.* Ph.D. thesis, University of Basel, Switzerland, 1992.

388. Grawunder U, Haasner D, Melchers F, Rolink A. Rearrangement and expression of κ light chain genes can occur without μ heavy chain expression during differentiation of pre-B cells. *Int Immunol* 1993b;5:1609–1618.

389. Snapper CM, Mond JJ. Towards a comprehensive view of immunoglobulin class switching. *Immunol Today* 1993;14:15–17.

390. Rolink AG, Melchers F, Andersson J. The SCID but not the *RAG 2* gene product is required for Sμ-Sε-heavy chain class switching. *Immunity* 1996b;5:319–330.

391. Banchereau J, Rousset F. Human B lymphocytes: phenotype, proliferation, and differentiation. *Adv Immunol* 1992;52:125–262.

392. Burrows PD, Schroeder HW, Cooper MD. B-cell differentiation in humans. In Honjo T, Alt FW, eds. *Immunoglob Genes,* 2nd Ed. London: Academic Press Ltd., 1995, 3–31.

393. Gougeon ML, Drean G, Le Deist F, et al. Human severe combined immunodeficiency disease: phenotypic and functional characteristics of peripheral B lymphocytes. *J Immunol* 1990;145:2873–2879.

394. Noguchi M, Yi H, Rosenblatt HM, et al. Interleukin-2 receptor gamma chain mutation results in X-linked severe combined immunodeficiency in humans. *Cell* 1993;73:147–157.

395. Nuñez C, Nishimoto N, Gartland GL, et al. B cells are generated throughout life in humans. *J Immunol* 1996;156:866–872.

396. Silverstein AM. *Ontogeny of the immune response: a perspective.* New York: Raven Press, 1977.

397. Uhr JW, Dancis J, Franklin EC, Finkelstein MS, Lewis EW. The antibody response to bacteriophage in newborn premature infants. *J Clin Invest* 1962;41:1508–1513.

398. Kohler PF, Farr RS. Elevation of cord over maternal IgG immunoglobulin: evidence for an active placental IgG transport. *Nature* 1966;210:1070–1071.

399. Stein KE. Thymus-independent and thymus-dependent repsonses to polysaccharide antigens. *J Infect Dis* 1992;165:S49–S52.

400. Cooke JV, Holowach J, Atkins JE, Powers JR. Antibody formation in early infancy against diphtheria and tetanus toxoids. *J Pediatr* 1948;33:141–146.

401. Paton JC, Toogood IR, Cockington RA, Hansman D. Antibody response to pneumococcal vaccine in children aged 5 to 15 years. *Am J Dis Child* 1986;140:135–138.

402. Rosen FS, Wedgwood RJ, Eibl MC, et al. Primary immunodeficiency diseases. Report of a WHO scientific group. *Immunodefic Rev* 1992;3:195–236.

403. Fischer A. Severe combined immunodeficiencies. *Immunodefic Rev* 1992;3:83–100.

404. Schwarz K, Bartram CR. V(D)J recombination pathology. *Adv Immunol* 1996a;61:285–326.

405. Schwarz K, Gauss GH, Ludwig L, et al. RAG mutations in human B cell-negative SCID. *Science* 1996b;274:97–99.

406. Hitzig WH, Biro Z, Bosch H, Huser HJ. Agammaglobulinämie und Alymphocytose mit Schwund des lymphatischen Gewebes. *Helv Paediat Acta* 1958;13:551–585.

407. Schatz DG, Baltimore D. Stable expression of immunoglobulin gene V(D)J recombinase activity by gene transfer into 3T3 fibroblasts. *Cell* 1988;53:107–115.

408. Schatz DG, Oettinger MA, Baltimore D. The V(D)J recombination activating gene, RAG-1. *Cell* 1989;59:1035–1048.

409. Oettinger MA, Schatz DG, Gorka C, Baltimore D. RAG-1 and RAG-2, adjacent genes that synergistically activate V(D)J recombination. *Science* 1990;248:1517–1523.

410. Bernstein RM, Schluter SF, Lake DF, Marchalonis IJ. Evolutionary conservation and molecular cloning of the recombinase activating gene 1. *Biochemistry* 1994;205:687–692.

411. Carlson LM, Oettinger MA, Schatz DG, et al. Selective expression of RAG-2 in chicken B cells undergoing immunoglobulin gene conversion. *Cell* 1991;64:201–208.

412. Fuschiotti P, Fitts MG, Pospisil R, Weinstein PD, Mage RG. RAG1 and RAG2 in developing rabbit appendix subpopulations. *J Immunol* 1997;1997:55–64.

413. Greenhalgh P, Olesen CE, Steiner LA. Characterization and expression of

recombination activating genes (RAG-1 and RAG-2) in Xenopus laevis. *J Immunol* 1993;151:3100–3110.

414. Ichihara Y, Hirai M, Kurosawa Y. Sequence and chromosome assignment to 11p13-p12 of human RAG genes. *Immunol Lett* 1992;33:277–284.

415. Boehm T, Gonzales-Sarmiento R, Kennedey M, Rabbits TH. A simple technique for generating probes for RNA in situ hybridization: an adjunct to genome mapping exemplified by the RAG-1/RAG-2 gene cluster. *Proc Natl Acad Sci USA* 1991;88:3927–3931.

416. Guy-Grand D, Vanden Broecke C, Briottet C, Malassis-Seris M, Selz F, Vassalli P. Different expression of the recombination activity gene RAG-1 in various populations of thymocytes, peripheral T cells and gut thymus-independent intraepithelial lymphocytes suggests two pathways of T cell receptor rearrangement. *Eur J Immunol* 1992;22:505–510.

417. Turka LA, Schatz DG, Oettinger MA, et al. Thymocyte expression of RAG-1 and RAG-2: termination by T cell receptor cross-linking. *Science* 1991;253:778–781.

418. Lin W-C, Desiderio S. Regulation of V(D)J recombination activator protein RAG-2 by phosphorylation. *Science* 1993;260:953–959.

419. Lin W-C, Desiderio S. V(D)J recombination and the cell cycle. *Immunol Today* 1995b;16:279–289.

420. Schlissel M, Constantinescu A, Morrow T, Baxter M, Peng A. Double-strand signal sequence breaks in V(D)J recombination are blunt, 5′-phosphorylated, RAG-dependent, and cell cycle regulated. *Genes Dev* 1993;7:2520–2532.

421. Hoffman ES, Passoni L, Crompton T, et al. Productive T-cell receptor β-chain gene rearrangement: coincident regulation of cell cycle and clonality during development in vivo. *Genes Dev* 1996;10:948–962.

422. McBlane JF, van Gent DC, Ramsden DA, et al. Cleavage at a V(D)J recombination signal requires only RAG1 and RAG2 proteins and occurs in two steps. *Cell* 1995;83:387–395.

423. Eastman QM, Leu TM, Schatz DG. Initiation of V(D)J recombination *in vitro* obeying the 12/23 rule. *Nature* 1996;380:85–88.

424. van Gent DC, Ramsden DA, Gellert M. The RAG1 and RAG2 proteins establish the 12/23 rule in V(D)J recombination. *Cell* 1996;85:107–113.

425. Mombaerts P, Iacomini J, Johnson RS, Herrup K, Tonegawa S, Papaioannou VE. RAG-1-deficient mice have no mature B and T lymphocytes. *Cell* 1992;68:869–877.

426. Shinkai Y, Rathbun G, Lam KP, et al. RAG-2-deficient mice lack mature lymphocytes owing to inability to initiate V(D)J rearrangement. *Cell* 1992;68:855–867.

427. Orita M, Suzuki Y, Sekiya T, Hayashi K. Rapid and sensitive detection of point mutations and DNA polymorphisms using the polymerase chain reaction. *Genomics* 1989;5:874–879.

428. Nomdedeu JF, Lasa A, Seminago R, Baiget M, Soler J. Polymorphism in the RAG-1 gene identified by SSCP. *Leukemia* 1995;9:229–230.

429. Bosma GC, Custer RP, Bosma MJ. A severe combined immunodeficiency mutation in the mouse. *Nature* 1983;301:527–530.

430. Blunt T, Finnie NJ, Taccioli GE, et al. Defective DNA-dependent protein kinase activity is linked to V(D)J recombination and DNA repair defects associated with the murine *scid* mutation. *Cell* 1995;80:813–823.

431. Kirchgessner CU, Patil CK, Evans JW, et al. DNA-dependent kinase (p350) as a candidate gene for the murine SCID defect. *Science* 1995;267:1178–1183.

432. Peterson SR, Kurimasa A, Oshimara M, Dynan WS, Bradbury EM, Chen DJ. Loss of the catalytic subunit of the DNA-dependent protein kinase in DNA double-strand-break-repair mutant mammalian cells. *Proc Natl Acad Sci USA* 1995;92:3171–3174.

433. Bruton OC. Agammaglobulinemia. *Pediatrics* 1952;9:722–727.

434. Conley ME, Parolini O, Rohrer J, Campana D. X-linked agammaglobulinemia: new approaches to old questions based on the identification of the defective gene. *Immunol Rev* 1994;138:5–21.

435. Campana D, Farrant J, Inamdar N, Webster ADB, Janossy G. Phenotypic features and proliferative activity of B cell progenitors in X-linked agammaglobulinemia and selective immunoglobulin. *J Immunol* 1990;145:1675–1680.

436. Milili M, Le-Deist F, de-Saint-Basile G, Fischer A, Fougereau M, Schiff C. Bone marrow cells in X-linked agammaglobulinemia express pre-B-specific genes (λ-like and V$_{pre-B}$) and present immunoglobulin V-D-J gene usage strongly biased to a fetal-like repertoire. *J Clin Invest* 1993;91:1616–1629.

437. Conley ME. B cells in patients with X-linked aggammaglobulinemia. *J Immunol* 1985;134:3070–3074.

438. Tsukada S, Saffran DC, Rawlings DJ, et al. Deficient expression of a B cell cytoplasmic tyrosine kinase in human X-linked agammaglobulinemia. *Cell* 1993;72:279–290.

439. Vetrie D, Vorechovsky I, Sideras P, et al. The gene involved in X-linked agammaglobulinaemia is a member of the *src* family of protein-tyrosine kinases. *Nature* 1993;361:226–233.

440. Sideras P, Smith CIE. Molecular and cellular aspects of X-linked agammaglobulinemia. *Adv Immunol* 1995;59:135–223.

441. Khan WN, Alt FW, Gerstein RM, et al. Defective B cell development and function in Btk-deficient mice. *Immunity* 1995;3:283–299.

442. Kerner JD, Appleby MW, Mohr RN, et al. Impaired expansion of mouse B cell progenitors lacking Btk. *Immunity* 1995;3:301–312.

443. Currier SJ, Gallarda JL, Knight KL. Partial molecular genetic map of the rabbit V$_H$ chromosomal region. *J Immunol* 1988;140:1651–1659.

444. Becker RS, Zhai SK, Currier SJ, Knight KL. Ig VH, DH and JH germ-line gene segments linked by overlapping cosmid clones of rabbit DNA. *J Immunol* 1989;142:1351–1355.

445. Friedman ML, Tunyaplin C, Zhai SK, Knight KL. Neonatal V$_H$, D and J$_H$ gene usage in rabbit B-lineage cells. *J Immunol* 1994;152:632–641.

446. Schneidermann RD, Hanly WC, Knight KL. Expression of 12 rabbit IgA Cα genes as chimeric rabbit-mouse IgA antibodies. *Proc Natl Acad Sci USA* 1989;86:7561–7565.

447. Schneidermann RD, Lint TF, Knight KL. Activation of the alternative pathway of complement by twelve different rabbit-mouse chimeric transfectoma IgA isotypes. *J Immunol* 1990;145:233–237.

448. Spieker-Polet H, Yam PC, Knight KL. Differential expression of 13 IgA-heavy chain genes in rabbit lymphoid tissues. *J Immunol* 1993;150:5457–5465.

449. Burnett RC, Hanly WC, Zhai SK, Knight KL. The IgA heavy-chain gene family in rabbit: cloning and sequence analysis of 13 Cα genes. *EMBO J* 1989;8:4041–4047.

450. Benammar A, Cazenave PA. A second rabbit κ isotype. *J Exp Med* 1982;156:585–595.

451. Emorine L, Max EE. Structural analysis of a rabbit immunoglobulin κ2 J-C locus reveals multiple deletions. *Nucleic Acids Res* 1983;11:8877–8890.

452. Heidmann O, Rougeon F. Multiplicity of constant κ light chain genes in the rabbit genome: a b4b4 homozygous rabbit contains a κ-*bas* gene. *EMBO* J 1983;2:437–441.

453. Hole NJK, Young-Cooper GO, Mage RG. Mapping of the duplicated rabbit immunoglobulin κ light chain locus. *Eur J Immunol* 1991;21:403–409.

454. Duvoisin RM, Heidmann O, Jaton JC. Characterization of four constant region genes of rabbit immunoglobulin-λ chains. *J Immunol* 1986;136:4297–4302.

455. Hayzer DJ, Duvoisin RM, Jaton JC. cDNA clones encoding rabbit immunoglobulin λ chains. *Biochem J* 1987;245:691–697.

456. Bernstein KE, Alexander CB, Mage RG. Germline V$_H$ genes in an a3 rabbit not typical of any one V$_{HA}$ allotype. *J Immunol* 1985;134:3480–3488.

457. Gallarda JL, Gelason KS, Knight KL. Organization of rabbit immunoglobulin genes. I. Structure and multiplicity of germ-line VH genes. *J Immunol* 1985;135:4222–4228.

458. McCormack WT, Laster SM, Marzluff WF, Roux KH. Dynamic gene interactions in the evolution of rabbit V$_H$ genes: a four codon duplication and block homologies provide evidence for intergenic exchange. *Nucleic Acids Res* 1985;13:7041–7054.

459. Fitts MG, Metzger DW. Identification of rabbit genomic Ig-VH pseudogenes that could serve as donor sequences for latent allotype expression. *J Immunol* 1990;145:2713–2717.

460. Knight KL, Becker RS. Molecular basis of the allelic inheritance of rabbit immunoglobulin V$_H$ allotypes: implications for the generation of antibody diversity. *Cell* 1990;60:963–970.

461. Knight KL, Crane MA. Generating the antibody repertoire in rabbit. *Adv Immunol* 1994;56:179–218.

462. Knight KL, Winstead CR. Generation of antibody diversity in rabbits. *Curr Opin Immunol* 1997;9:228–232.

463. Roux KH, Dhanarajan P, Gotschalk V, McCormack WT, Renshaw RW. Latent a1 VH germline genes in an a²a² rabbit: evidence for gene conversion at both the germline and somatic levels. *J Immunol* 1991;146:2027–2036.

464. Short JA, Sethupathi P, Zhai SK, Knight KL. VDJ genes in V$_H$a2 allotype-suppressed rabbits: limited germline V$_H$ gene usage and accumulation of somatic mutations in D regions. *J Immunol* 1991;147:4014–4018.

465. Raman C, Spieker-Polet H, Yam PC, Knight KL. Preferential V$_H$ gene usage in rabbit immunoglobulin-secreting heterohybridomas. *J Immunol* 1994;152:3935–3945.

466. Oudin J. L'Allocypie de ceertains antigens proteindiques du serum. *CR Acad Sci* 1956;242:2606–2608.

467. Todd CW. Allotypy in rabbit 19S protein. *Biochem Biophys Res Commun* 1963;11:170–175.

468. Feinstein A. Character and allotypy of an immune globulin in rabbit colostrum. *Nature* 1963;199:1197–1199.

469. Hilschmann N, Craig LC. Amino acid sequence studies with Bence-Jones proteins. *Proc Natl Acad Sci USA* 1965;53:1403–1409.

470. Maki R, Kearney J, Paige C, Tonegawa S. Immunoglobulin gene rearrangement in immature B cells. *Science* 1980;209:1366–1369.

471. Tonegawa S, Hozumi N, Matthyssens G, Schuller R. Somatic changes in the content and context of immunoglobulin genes. *Cold Spring Harb Symp Quant Biol* 1977;41:Pt 2:877–889.

472. Tonegawa S. Somatic generation of antibody diversity. *Nature* 1983;302:575–581.

473. Dray S, Young GO, Gerald L. Immunochemical identification and genetics of rabbit γ-globulin allotypes. *J Immunol* 1963a;91:403–410.

474. Dray S, Young GO, Nisonoff A. Distribution of allotypic specificities among rabbit γ-globulin molecules genetically defined at two loci. *Nature* 1963b;199:52–54.

475. Becker RS, Knight KL. Somatic diversification of immunoglobulin heavy chain VDJ genes: evidence for somatic gene conversion in rabbits. *Cell* 1990;63:987–997.

476. Kelus AS, Weiss S. Mutation affecting the expression of immunoglobulin variable regions in the rabbit. *Proc Natl Acad Sci USA* 1986;83:4883–4886.

477. Allegrucci M, Newman BA, Young-Cooper GO, et al. Altered phenotypic expression of immunoglobulin heavy-chain variable-region (VH) genes in

Alicia rabbits probably reflects a small deletion in the VH genes closest to the joining region. *Proc Natl Acad Sci USA* 1990;87:5444–5448.

478. DiPietro LA, Short JA, Zhai SK, Kelus AS, Meier D, Knight KL. Limited number of immunoglobulin V_H regions expressed in the mutant rabbit "Alicia". *Eur J Immunol* 1990a;20:1401–1404.

479. Chen HT, Alexander CB, Young-Cooper GO, Mage RG. V_H gene expression and regulation in the mutant alicia rabbit: rescue of V_Ha2 allotype expression. *J Immunol* 1993a;150:2783–2793.

480. Mage R, Dray S. Persistent altered phenotypic expression of allelic γG-immunoglobulin allotypes in heterozygous rabbits exposed to isoantibodies in fetal and neonatal life. *J Immunol* 1965;95:525–535.

481. Tunyaplin C, Knight KL. IgH gene rearrangements on the unexpressed allele in rabbit B cells. *J Immunol* 1997;158:4805–4811.

482. Tunyaplin C, Knight KL. Fetal VDJ gene repertoire in rabbit: evidence for preferential rearrangement of V_H1. *Eur J Immunol* 1995;25:2583–2587.

483. Hayward AR, Simons MA, Lawton AR, Mage RG, Cooper MD. Pre-B and B cells in rabbits. Ontogeny and allelic exclusion of κ light chain genes. *J Exp Med* 1978;148:1367–1377.

484. McElroy PJ, Willcox N, Catty D. Early precursors of B lymphocytes. I. Rabbit/mouse species differences in the physical properties and surface phenotype of pre-B cells, and in the maturation sequence of early B cells. *Eur J Immunol* 1981;11:76–85.

485. Gathings WE, Mage RG, Cooper MD, Lawton AR, Young-Cooper G. Immunofluorescence studies on the expression of VH a allotypes by pre-B and B cells of homozygous and heterozygous rabbits. *Eur J Immunol* 1981;11:200–206.

486. Gathings WE, Mage RG, Cooper MD, Young-Cooper GO. A subpopulation of small pre-B cells in rabbit bone marrow express κ light chains and exhibit allelic exclusion b locus allotypes. *Eur J Immunol* 1982;12:76–81.

487. Crane MA, Kingzette M, Knight KL. Evidence for limited B-lymphopoiesis in adult rabbits. *J Exp Med* 1996;183:2119–2127.

488. Hayakawa K, Hardy RR, Stall AM, Herzenberg LA, Herzenberg LA. Immunoglobulin-bearing B cells reconstitute and maintain the murine Ly-1 B cell lineage. *Eur J Immunol* 1986;16:1313–1316.

489. Harrison MR, Mage R. Allotype suppression in the rabbit. I. The ontogeny of cells bearing immunoglobulin of paternal allotype and the fate of these cells after treatment with antiallotype antisera. *J Exp Med* 1973;138:764–774.

490. DiPietro LA, Knight KL. Restricted utilization of germ-line V_H genes and diversity of D regions in rabbit splenic Ig mRNA. *J Immunol* 1990b;144:1969–1973.

491. Stepankova R, Kovaru F. Development of lymphatic tissues in germfree and conventionally reared rabbits. In: Malek P, Bartos V, Weissleder H, Witc MII, eds. *Proc 6th Int Cong Lymphology*, Stuttgart: Georg Thieme; Prague: Avieenum, Czech Medical Press, 1978;290–292.

492. Stepankova R, Kovaru F. Immunoglobulin-producing cells in lymphatic tissues of germfree and conventional rabbits as detected by an immunofluorescence method. *Folia Microbiol (Praha)* 1985;30:291–294.

493. Tlaskalova-Hogenova H, Stepankova R. Development of antibody formation in germfree and conventionally reared rabbits: the role of intestinal lymphoid tissue in antibody formation to *E. coli* antigens. *Folia Biol* 1980;26:81–93.

494. Cooper MD, Perey DY, Gabrielsen AE, Sutherland DER, McKneally MF, Good RA. Production of an antibody deficiency syndrome in rabbits by neonatal removal of organized intestinal lymphoid tissues. *Int Arch Allergy* 1968;33:65–88.

495. Perey DY, Cooper MD, Good RA. The mammalian homologue of the avian bursa of Fabricius. *Surgery* 1968;64:614–621.

496. Morris B, Miyashka M. *Immunology of the sheep*. Basel: Editiones Roche, 1985.

497. Maddox JF, Mackay CR, Brandon MR. Ontogeny of ovine lymphocytes. II. An immunohistochemical study on the development of T lymphocytes in the sheep fetal spleen. *Immunology* 1987;62:107–112.

498. Press CMCL, Hein WR, Landsverk T. Ontogeny of leucocyte populations in the spleen of fetal lambs with emphasis on the early prominence of B cells. *Immunology* 1993;88:28–34.

499. Press CMCL, Reynolds JD, McClure SJ, Simpson-Morgans MW, Landsverk T. Fetal lambs are depleted of IgM$^+$ cells following a single injection of an anti-IgM antibody early in gestation. *Immunology* 1996;88:28–34.

500. Reynolds JD, Morris B. The evolution and involution of Peyer's patches in fetal and postnatal sheep. *Eur J Immunol* 1983;13:627–635.

501. Gerber HA, Morris B, Trevella W. The role of gut-associated lymphoid tissues in the generation of immunoglobulin-bearing lymphocytes in sheep. *Aust J Exp Biol Med Sci* 1986;64:201–213.

502. Miyasaka M, McCullagh P. The response of the foetal lamb to maternal lymphocytes. *J Reprod Immunol* 1982;4:217–230.

503. Silverstein AM, Prendergast RA, Kraner KL. Foetal response to antigenic stimulus. IV. Rejection of skin homografts by the foetal lamb. *J Exp Med* 1964;119:955–964.

504. Schinckel PG, Ferguson KA. Skin transplantation in the foetal lamb. *Aust J Exp Biol Med Sci* 1953;6:533–545.

505. Reynaud CA, MacKay CR, Muller RG, Weill JC. Somatic generation of diversity in a mammalian primary lymphoid organ: the sheep ileal Peyer's patches. *Cell* 1991a;64:995–1005.

506. Reynaud CA, Garcia C, Hein WR, Weill JC. Hypermutation generating the sheep immunoglobulin repertoire is an antigen-independent process. *Cell* 1995;80:115–125.

507. Renstroem HM, Press CHMCL, Trevella W, Landsverk TH. Response of leuco-

508. Glick G, Chang TS, Jaap RG. The bursa of Fabricius and antibody production. *Poult Sci* 1956;35:224–225.

509. Mueller AP, Wolfe HR, Meyer J. Precipitin production in chickens. XXI. Antibody production in bursectomized chickens and in chickens injected with 19-notestosterone on the fifth day of incubation. *J Immunol* 1959;83:507–510.

510. Cooper MD, Peterson RAA, South MA, Good RA. The functions of the thymus system and the bursa system in the chicken. *J Exp Med* 1966;123:75–102.

511. Warner NL, Uhr W, Thorbecke GJ, Ovary Z. Immunoglobulins, antibodies and the bursa of Fabricius: induction of aggammaglobulinemia and the loss of all antibody-forming capacity by hormonal buresectomy. *J Immunol* 1969;103:1317–1330.

512. Toivanen A, Toivanen P. Avian immunology basis and practice. I. Florida: Boca Raton, CRC Press, 1987a.

513. Toivanen A, Toivanen P. Avian immunology basis and practice. II. Florida: Boca Raton, CRC Press, 1987b.

514. Le Douarin N. Particularités du noyau interphasique chey la Caille japonaise (Coturnix coturnix japonica). Utilisation de ces particariés comme "marquage biologique" dans les recherches sur les interactions tissulaires et les migrations cellulaires u cours de l'ontogenese. *Bull Biol Fr Belge* 1969;103:453–468.

515. Le Douarin NM, Houssaint E, Jotereau FV, Belo M. Origin of hemopoietic stem cells in embryonic bursa of Fabricius and bone marrow studied through interspecific chimeras. *Proc Natl Acad Sci USA* 1975;72:2701–2705.

516. Le Douarin N, Maclaren A. *Chimeras in developmental biology*. Orlando: Academic Press, 1984.

517. Toivanen P, Naukkarinen A, Vainio O. Bursal and post-bursal stem cells in the chicken: functional characteristics. *Eur J Immunol* 1987;3:585–595.

518. Dieterlen-Lièvre F, Martin C. Diffuse intraembryonic hemopoiesis in normal and chimeric avian development. *Dev Biol* 1981;88:180–191.

519. Lassila O, Eskola J, Toivanen P, Martin C, Diterlen-Lièvre F. The origin of lymphoid stem cells studied in chick yolk sac-embryo chimeras. *Nature* 1978;727:353–354.

520. Lassila O, Martin C, Dieterlen-Lievre F, Gilmour DG, Eskola J, Toivanen P. Migration of prebursal stem cells from the early chicken embryo to the yolk sac. *Scand J Immunol* 1982;16:265–268.

521. Houssaint E, Belo M, Le Douarin NM. Investigations on cell lineage and tissue interactions in the developing bursa of Fabricius through interspecific chimeras. *Dev Biol* 1976;53:250–264.

522. Moore MA, Owen JJT. Chromosome marker studies in the irradiated chick embryo. *Nature* 1967;215:1081–1082.

523. Pink JRL, Ratcliffe MJH, Vainio O. Immunoglobulin-bearing stem cells for clones of B (bursa-derived) lymphocytes. *Eur J Immunol* 1985;15:617–620.

524. Pink JRL. Counting components of the chicken's B cell system. *Immunol Rev* 1986;91:113–128.

525. Szenberg A. Ontogenesis of the immune system in birds. In: Marchalonis JJ, ed. *Comparative immunology*. Oxford: Blackwell Science, 1976:419.

526. Pink JRL, Lassila O. B-cell commitment and diversification in the bursa of Fabricius. *Curr Top Microbiol Immunol* 1987;135:57–64.

527. Ratcliffe MJ, Ivanyi J. Allotype suppression in the chicken. IV. Deletion of B cells and lack of suppressor cells during chronic suppression. *Eur J Immunol* 1981;11:306–310.

528. Ratcliffe MJH, Lassila O, Pink JRL, Vainio O. Avian B cell precursors: surface immunoglobulin expression is an early, possibly bursa-independent event. *Eur J Immunol* 1986;16:129–133.

529. Reynaud CA, Anquez V, Dahan A. A single rearrangement event generates most of the chicken Ig light chain diversity. *Cell* 1985;40:283–290.

530. Reynaud CA, Anquez V, Grimal H, Weill JC. A hyperconversion mechanism generates the chicken light chain preimmune repertoire. *Cell* 1987;48:379–388.

531. Reynaud CA, Dahan A, Anquez V, Weill JC. Somatic hyperconversion diversifies the single V_h gene of the chicken with a high incidence in the D region. *Cell* 1989;59:171–183.

532. Reynaud CA, Anquez V, Weill JC. The chicken D locus and its contribution to the immunoglobulin heavy chain repertoire. *Eur J Immunol* 1991b;21:2661–2670.

533. McCormack WT, Tjoelker LW, Carlson LM, et al. Chicken Ig$_L$ gene rearrangement involves deletion of a circular episome and addition of single nonrandom nucleotides to both coding segments. *Cell* 1989a;56:785–791.

534. McCormack WT, Tjoelker LW, Barth CF, et al. Selection for B cells with productive IgL gene rearrangements occurs in the bursa of Fabricius during chicken embryonic development. *Genes Dev* 1989b;3:838–847.

535. Melchers F. *Introduction to the Annual Report of the Basel Institute for Immunology*. Basel: Basel Institute for Immunology, 1988.

536. Langman RE, Cohn M. A theory of the ontogeny of the chicken humoral immune system: the consequences of diversification by gene hyperconversion and immune system. The consequences of diversification by gene hyperconversion and its extension to rabbit. *Res Immunol* 1993;144:422–446.

537. Smithies O. *The genetic basis of antibody variability*. Cold Spring Harbor Symp Quant Biol 1967;32:161–166.

538. Edelman GM, Gally JA. Somatic recombination of duplicated genes: an hypothesis on the origin of antibody diversity. *Proc Natl Acad Sci USA* 1967;57:353–358.

539. Thompson CB, Neiman P. Somatic diversification of the chicken immunoglobu-

lin light chain gene is limited to the rearranged variable gene segment. *Cell* 1987;48:369–378.

540. Takeda S, Masteller EL, Thompson CB, Buerstedde JM. RAG-2 expression is not essential for chicken immunoglobulin gene conversion. *Proc Natl Acad Sci USA* 1992;89:4023–4027.

541. Parvari R, Ziv E, Lantner F, Heller DK, Schechter I. Somatic diversification of chicken immunoglobulin light chains by point mutations. *Proc Natl Acad Sci USA* 1990;87:3072–3076.

542. Reynaud CA, Imhof BA, Anquez V, Weill JC. Emergence of committed B lymphoid progenitors in the developing chicken embryo. *EMBO J* 1992;12: 4349–4358.

543. Reynaud CA, Bertocci B, Dahan A, Weill JC. Formation of the chicken B-cell repertoire: ontogenesis, regulation of Ig gene rearrangement, and diversification by gene conversion. *Adv Immunol* 1994;57:353–375.

544. Houssaint E, Lassila O, Vainio O. Bu-I antigen expression as a marker for B cell precursors in chicken embryos. *Eur J Immunol* 1989;19:239–243.

545. Houssaint E, Mansikka A, Vainio O. Early separation of B and T lymphocyte precursors in chick embryo. *J Exp Med* 1991;174:397–406.

546. Mansikka A, Sandberg M, Lissila O, Toivanen P. Rearrangement of immuno-globulin light chain genes in the chicken occurs prior to colonization of the embryonic bursa of Fabricius. *Proc Natl Acad Sci USA* 1990;87:9416–9420.

547. Jerne NK. The somatic generation of immune recognition. *Eur J Immunol* 1971; 1:1–9.

548. Papavasiliou F, Casellas R, Suh H, et al. V(D)J recombination in mature B cells: a mechanism for altering antibody responses. *Science* 1997;278:298–301.

549. Han S, Dillon SR, Zheng B, Shimoda M, Schlissel MS, Kelsoe G. V(D)J recom-binase activity in a subset of germinal center B lymphocytes. *Science* 1997;278: 301–305.

550. Medvinsky A, Dzierzak E. Definitive hematopoiesis is autonomously initiated by the AGM region. *Cell* 1996;86:897–906.

551. Klein J. *Immunology—the science of self–nonself discrimination.* New York: John Wiley and Sons, 1982:89.

552. Carson S, Wu GE. A linkage map of the mouse immunoglobulin lambda light chain locus. *Immunogenetics* 1989;29:173–179.

553. Combriato G, Klobeck HG. V lambda and J lambda–C lambda gene segments of the human immunoglobulin lambda light chain locus are separated by 1513–1522.

554. Weill JC. Mechanisms of B cell neoplasia. Basel: Editiones Roche, 1989:16.

Fundamental Immunology, Fourth Edition,
edited by William E. Paul
Lippincott–Raven Publishers, Philadelphia © 1999.

CHAPTER 7

B-Lymphocyte Activation

Anthony L. DeFranco

OVERVIEW OF B-CELL ACTIVATION

After their generation in the bone marrow and exit to the periphery, B cells go through a brief immature phase during which they are very sensitive to inactivation by antigen contact. This is one mechanism for inducing immunologic tolerance in the B cell compartment. After a short period in the periphery, less than 1 week, the newly generated B cells acquire a mature long-lived recirculating phenotype and are competent to make antibody responses, provided they receive the necessary signals from antigen and from other cell types. Antigen contact with the specific B cell triggers the transmembrane signaling function of the B-cell antigen receptor (BCR). This, in turn, induces early events in B-cell activation, including increased expression of class II major histocompatibility complex (MHC) molecules, exit from the resting state (G_0) into G_1 phase of the cell cycle, and, in the case of a strong antigenic stimulus, proliferation. BCR molecules are also rapidly internalized after antigen binding, leading to antigen uptake and degradation in endosomes or lysosomes. In the case of protein antigens, antigen-derived peptides bind in the groove of class II MHC molecules, after which this complex comes to the cell surface, where it serves as a stimulus for specific helper T cells. Antigen recognition by the helper T cell induces it to form a tight and long-lasting interaction with the B cell and to synthesize B-cell growth and differentiation factors. These cytokines

can be secreted directly into the narrow space between the interacting lymphocytes. In addition, the activated helper T cell expresses cell surface molecules, the most important of which is CD40 ligand (CD40L), that interact with receptors on the B cell, providing important activation signals. B cells activated in this way may either proliferate and terminally differentiate to antibody-secreting cells (also called plasma cells) in the T-cell zone of the lymphoid organ, or after initial activation may migrate to the follicular area and initiate the formation of a germinal center. It is in the germinal center that B cells activate somatic hypermutation of their immunoglobulin genes and then undergo a stringent selection for high-affinity binding to antigen, resulting in the production of memory B cells and plasma cells secreting antibody of high affinity.

Although antibody responses to protein antigens usually require B-cell collaboration with helper T cells, some antibody responses can occur independently of T-cell help. These T cell independent (TI) antigens are categorized as either type 1 or type 2 based on their properties. TI-2 antigens have highly repetitious structures, with polysaccharides being the prime examples. These antigens may be especially able to trigger vigorous or prolonged signaling by the BCR. In contrast, TI-1 antigens usually contain as part of their structures components that are very potent polyclonal activators of B cells. In immune responses to these antigens, the BCR may function primarily as a focusing component that concentrates the polyclonal activator on the surface of those B cells that specifically bind a linked epitope. For both types of T cell-independent antigens, cytokines appear to be required for the B cell to make an

A. L. DeFranco: Department of Microbiology and Immunology, University of California, San Francisco, California 94143.

antibody response, although the source may be a nonlymphoid cell type, such as the macrophage. In both cases, a particular feature of the antigen relieves or reduces the requirement for soluble and cell-bound stimuli coming from helper T cells.

REGULATION OF B-CELL ACTIVATION BY ANTIGEN

The BCR plays a central role in the generation, maturation, survival, and activation of B cells. A great deal has been learned about the structure and signaling mechanism of the BCR, although the latter is quite complicated. The use of genetic and pseudogenetic approaches in recent years has begun to elucidate how the BCR controls B-cell fate, but clearly there is a tremendous amount still to be learned.

B-Cell Antigen Receptor Structure

Newly generated B cells initially express membrane immunoglobulin M (mIgM) and soon thereafter express mIgM plus mIgD. Class switch recombination occurring during an immune response leads to the appearance of memory B cells that express other classes of mIg, e.g., IgG, IgA, or IgE. The cytoplasmic domains of mIgs are short, ranging from only three amino acid residues in the case of mIgM and mIgD (lysine-valine-lysine-COOH in each case) to 28 residues for the mIgG subclasses (1). The longer cytoplasmic domains of IgG and IgE appear to enhance the efficiency of memory B-cell responses (2,3). The mIg transmembrane segments are about 25 amino acids long and lack the potentially charged residues seen in each T cell receptor subunit. The potential for interaction with other polypeptides is present in mIg transmembrane regions, however, as they contain many hydroxyl-containing amino acids (10 of 25 residues in the case of murine mIgM). Although the transmembrane regions of the different mIg heavy chains differ considerably in sequence, amino acids lying on one side of the expected α-helix are highly conserved (1). This conserved surface of mIg transmembrane domains is likely to play a role in interactions with other components of the antigen receptor complex.

B-cell antigen receptors exist as a complex between mIg and at least two other transmembrane polypeptides, called Ig-α and Ig-β (Fig. 1). All isotypes of mIg can form a complex with Ig-α and Ig-β (4). The existence of this complex was unrecognized for many years because it is only stable in very mild detergents such as digitonin and 3-[(3-cholamidopropyl)-dimethylammonio]-1-propanesulfonate (CHAPS). More commonly used nonionic detergents such as nonidet (NP-40) and Triton X-100 quantitatively dissociate mIg from Ig-α and Ig-β. Expression in nonlymphoid Cos cells of a construct encoding the membrane form of μ heavy chain (μ$_m$) along with one encoding a light chain leads to mIgM expression in the endoplasmic reticulum (ER) but not in the plasma membrane (5). Introduction of expression vectors for Ig-α and Ig-β (the *mb-1* and *B29* gene products, respectively) along with heavy and light chain, leads to cell surface expression of the four polypeptide complex. It is believed that cell surface expression of mIgM in B cells also requires assembly into a complex with Ig-α/Ig-β. Some other isotypes of mIg, such as mIgD, are able to get to the cell surface in the absence of the accessory proteins, but nonetheless seem to be present in B cells primarily as a complex with Ig-α and Ig-β.

In the mouse, the Ig-α and Ig-β polypeptides combine to form a disulfide-linked heterodimer consisting of 34- and 40-kDa poly-

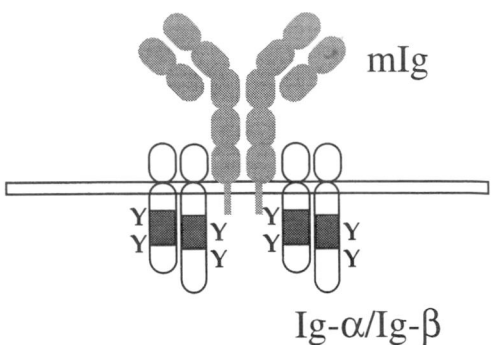

FIG. 1. B-cell antigen receptor structure. The BCR contains membrane Ig, containing two heavy chains and disulfide-linked heterodimers of the Ig-α and Ig-β accessory proteins. The latter components are required for transit of mIgM to the cell surface. ITAM sequences, represented by boxes in the cytoplasmic domains of Ig-α and Ig-β are responsible for signal transduction function. The number of Ig-α/Ig-β heterodimers associated with one mIg molecule is unknown (two are shown). Note that the sizes of the cytoplasmic domains are exaggerated relative to the sizes of the extracellular domains.

peptides, respectively (1). A minority of Ig-β molecules exist as slightly smaller polypeptides, referred to as Ig-γ. In human B cells, the relative sizes of Ig-α and Ig-β are reversed, probably due to heavier glycosylation of Ig-α. The Ig-α and Ig-β polypeptides have marked structural similarity to the three CD3 polypeptides (γ, δ, and ε). Each has a single external Ig-like domain followed by a transmembrane region and a C-terminal cytoplasmic domain of 61 (Ig-α) or 48 (Ig-β) amino acid residues. These cytoplasmic tails are large enough to mediate interactions with signaling components, and they each contain a sequence (YxxL/Ix$_7$YxxL/I; single letter code, x = any amino acid) with homology to sequences in the cytoplasmic domains of subunits of the T-cell receptor complex and most Fc receptors. This sequence is called the immunoreceptor tyrosine-based activation motif (ITAM) (1,6), and the ITAMs play a pivotal role in BCR signaling, as described below.

The *mb-1* and *B29* genes were originally isolated because they are expressed in B cells but not in T cells. They are expressed in a B-cell–specific manner from the pre-B precursor stage to the plasma cell stage, where *B29* is expressed but *mb-1* is not. In many plasmacytoma cells, mIg is not expressed on the surface, and this is due to the absence of Ig-α.

A related pre-BCR complex is formed in pre-B cells and is required for efficient development of B cells. This complex contains the μ heavy chain and Ig-α/Ig-β heterodimers just like the BCR, but the light chain is replaced by the λ5 and V$_{preB}$ surrogate light chains. In the absence of this receptor complex, as occurs in various mice with targeted mutations disrupting these components (7), B-cell development is stalled at this stage and no or very few B cells develop. The most likely hypothesis is that pre-BCR signaling allows pre-B cells to mature to the next stage of development, during which the Ig κ and λ loci rearrange. It is not known how pre-BCR signaling is triggered.

Initiation of Signaling by the BCR

The signal transduction function of the BCR is triggered by cross-linking of receptor molecules by oligomeric or multimeric

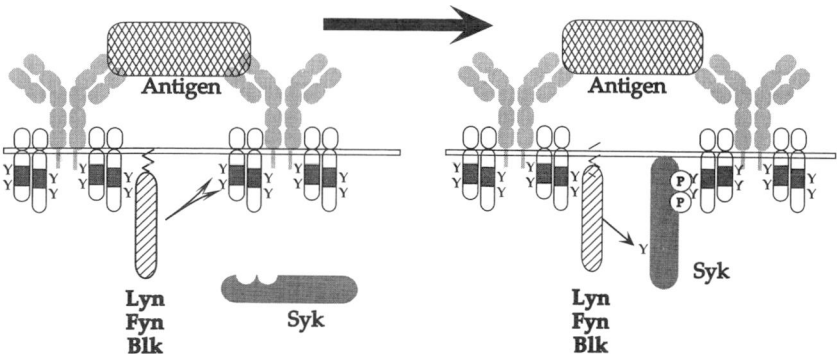

FIG. 2. Activation of tyrosine kinases by receptor oligomerization. Antigen induces oligomerization of BCRs, leading to phosphorylation of ITAM tyrosines by Src family tyrosine kinases, which may be prebound to the BCR or may simply be nearby in the plasma membrane. This provides a binding site to recruit Syk to the receptor, whereupon it becomes activated by phosphorylation of tyrosines in its kinase domain. This is shown as being performed by Src family members, but Syk can also phosphorylate other Syk molecules in trans. Src family tyrosine kinases also can bind to phosphorylated ITAMs and become activated.

antigens. Experimentally, this event is usually induced artificially with anti-Ig antibodies because this makes it possible to trigger signaling in all B cells simultaneously. Nonetheless, it should be kept in mind that real antigens may have important differences in their abilities to trigger signaling by the BCR. Such differences could result from the physical properties of the antigen, such as valency, flexibility, etc., from abilities to interact with other molecules present on the surface of the B cell (see below), or from the affinity of interaction with mIg.

The initial event observed after antigen receptor cross-linking is increased tyrosine phosphorylation of a handful of proteins, which then either directly alters their activity or leads to assembly of multi-protein signaling complexes (8,9). This phosphorylation is most readily visualized by immunoblotting with antiphosphotyrosine antibodies and can be observed as early as 5 seconds after the addition of anti-Ig to B cells. This increased phosphorylation is primarily due to activation of two types of intracellular protein tyrosine kinases: Syk and several members of the Src family, with subsequent activation of a third type of tyrosine kinase, Btk.

A widely accepted model for how BCR cross-linking activates Syk and Src family tyrosine kinases is depicted in Fig. 2. The initial event after receptor engagement and clustering is phosphorylation of the two ITAM tyrosines of Ig-α and Ig-β (9). The doubly phosphorylated ITAMs are recognized with high affinity (10) by the tandem Src-homology 2 (SH2) domains of Syk (Fig. 3), leading to the recruitment of Syk to the clustered BCR complex. The structure of the related T-cell tyrosine kinase ZAP-70 binding to a doubly phosphorylated T-cell receptor (TCR) ITAM peptide has been determined by x-ray crystallography (11) and presumably is quite similar to the equivalent region of Syk. The C-terminal SH2 of ZAP-70 binds to the first pYxxL/I (pY = phosphotyrosine) of the ITAM, whereas the second pYxxL/I sequence binds to the N-terminal SH2, with some contribution from the other SH2. The latter is an atypical arrangement because most SH2 domains are self-contained functional units. The spacing between the two tyrosines is known to be important for ITAM signaling function (12), and it can be seen from the structure that the intervening peptide is extended and that a shorter spacing would not allow binding to both SH2 domains. Src-family kinases also can bind to the phosphorylated ITAMs, although more weakly than Syk because they only have a single SH2 domain (13).

This aspect of BCR signaling illustrates a common feature of signaling by receptors that activate tyrosine kinases: phosphorylation of the receptor itself or of other proteins promotes the formation of multiprotein signaling complexes. Many signaling components

have recognizable domains of protein structure that are responsible for mediating the induced protein–protein interactions. For example, SH2 domains of signaling proteins bind to tyrosine phosphorylated regions of proteins in a manner that is dependent on both phosphorylation and the neighboring sequence context (14). As described above, the Syk SH2 domains each bind preferentially to the pYxxL or pYxxI sequences of ITAMs. Other domains of note are the Src-homology 3 (SH3) domain, which binds to proline-rich sequences and the pleckstrin-homology (PH) domain, some examples of which bind to phosphoinositides, and a subgroup of which, also called phosphotyrosine-binding (PTB) domains, bind to distinctive phosphotyrosine-containing sequences (15).

Once bound to a phosphorylated ITAM, Syk becomes phosphorylated on two adjacent tyrosines within the kinase domain (Y518 and Y519) upregulating its activity, probably by at least 10-fold. The binding of Syk to a doubly phosphorylated ITAM appears to cause a conformational change that favors this activating phosphorylation (16–18). The kinase responsible for these activating phosphorylations is not entirely known. A variety of experiments indicate that these phosphorylations can be provided either by Src family kinases or by other molecules of Syk in a transphosphory-

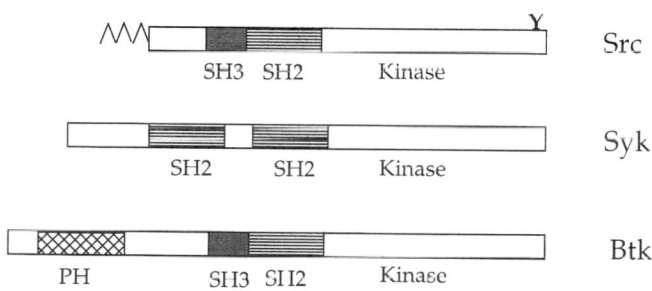

FIG. 3. Structural domains of protein tyrosine kinases involved in BCR signaling. Members of the Src family of intracellular tyrosine kinases have a kinase domain containing a positive regulatory tyrosine phosphorylation site, two other homology domains, called SH2 and SH3 (SH for Src homology), which mediate protein protein interactions, a C-terminal negative regulatory tyrosine phosphorylation site, and a unique N-terminal region containing a myristylation site, which is involved in membrane localization. In contrast, Syk and ZAP-70 have a kinase domain and two SH2 domains, but lack the SH3 domain, the myristylation site and the regulatory C-terminal tyrosine seen in Src family members. Btk has PH (pleckstrin homology), SH2 and SH3 domains, in addition to a C-terminal kinase domain.

lation reaction (19–23). This is a significant regulatory difference between Syk and its close relative in T cells, ZAP-70, because the latter absolutely requires an Src family member for its activation. Thus, BCR activation is less dependent on Src-family tyrosine kinases than is TCR signaling. This regulatory difference may be important for allowing B cells greater flexibility in responding to antigens of diverse physical forms, while restricting T cells to responding only to peptide-MHC complexes.

Although there is clearly a synergy in the interplay between Syk and Src-family tyrosine kinases, Syk appears to be the more important. For example, some residual signaling remains in a DT40 chicken B cell derivative in which the *lyn* gene, which appears to be the only Src family gene expressed in these cells, has been ablated by homologous recombination. In contrast, ablation of the *syk* gene leads to a profound defect in BCR signaling in these cells (24) and a block in development of mouse B cells (25,26). The latter effect is likely due to a Syk requirement for the signaling role of the pre-BCR in B-cell development in the bone marrow. Whereas DT40 chicken B cells appear to express only the Lyn member of the Src-family, mammalian B cells express at least three members of this family: p53/56^{lyn}, p59^{fyn}, and p55^{blk}. In addition, mature B cells express some p58^{fgr} and also a low level of p56^{lck} (27). Of these, Lyn is the predominant form, typically comprising roughly two thirds of the total Src family kinase protein and activity. Although mice in which the *blk, fyn,* or *fgr* genes have been knocked out have B cells that are relatively normal with regard to BCR signaling (28,29), *lyn*$^{-/-}$ mice have B cells that have a variety of defects (30–32). These B cells have a decreased overall content of Src family members because there is no compensatory change in the levels or activities of Fyn or Blk. Upon cross-linking of the BCR from Lyn-deficient B cells, there is a delayed tyrosine phosphorylation of Ig-α and of Syk compared with what is seen in normal B cells, although peak levels of phosphorylation are affected only to a minor degree (32). Correspondingly, some downstream signaling events (tyrosine phosphorylation of Shc, overall induced tyrosine phosphoproteins, etc.) are also delayed or decreased somewhat, but in contrast, activation of mitogen activated protein (MAP) kinase is elevated. These results, with the exception of the last one, are readily explained by the model shown in Fig. 2. As total Src family kinase levels are decreased by about threefold, slower phosphorylation of Ig-α and Syk presumably reflects a redundant role of Lyn and other Src family member(s) in performing the phosphorylations that are critical for initiating the BCR-signaling cascade. In addition, Lyn plays a role in downstream events that negatively regulate BCR signaling, as described below.

Exactly how BCR engagement leads to the initial phosphorylations of the BCR ITAMs is not well established. The simplest model is that Src-family tyrosine kinases are preassociated with the BCR such that cross-linking allows the kinase associated with one BCR complex to phosphorylate ITAMs of another complex. Each of the Src-family protein kinases has been shown to be associated with the antigen receptor complex (27), although in rather low amounts. These kinases may bind to Ig-α cytoplasmic domains either via a weak interaction between the unique N-terminal region of these kinases (Fig. 3) and a sequence found between the two tyrosines of the Ig-α ITAM, or to Ig-α or Ig-β via a stronger interaction between the SH2 domain of the kinase and an ITAM that has either tyrosine phosphorylated (33,34). The latter mode of binding requires a low level of constitutive phosphorylation, which presumably occurs as a continual balance between cellular tyrosine kinases (primarily Src family members, which are held in the mem-

brane by N-terminally attached fatty acids) and cellular tyrosine phosphatases such as CD45. In either case, the key aspect of receptor clustering is that a low amount of kinases are now held near a number of ITAMs so that the ITAMs become efficiently phosphorylated and bind Syk, as well as more Src family kinases. This increases the amount of the tyrosine kinases in the clustered receptor signaling complex, resulting in more ITAM phosphorylation in a positive feedback loop that can overwhelm phosphatase action.

A key feature of the BCR signaling mechanism is the activation of tyrosine kinases. As mentioned above, Syk bound to the cross-linked receptor complex becomes activated by phosphorylation of Y518 and Y519 in its kinase domain. Src family members bound to ITAMs also become activated, apparently by virtue of the SH2 interaction with the phosphorylated BCR cytoplasmic domains (35). Src family kinases are also negatively regulated by phosphorylation of a tyrosine near the C-terminus by the tyrosine kinase Csk. This negative regulation is relieved by removal of the phosphate by CD45 (36). Indeed, considerable circumstantial evidence indicates that CD45 is an important positive regulator of antigen receptor signaling in B cells and T cells, presumably via dephosphorylation of Src family kinases (36). Full signaling of the BCR requires activity of both Syk and Src family tyrosine kinases, although some signaling is seen in the absence of Src family members or under conditions where they are greatly inhibited, for example in the absence of CD45. As mentioned above, this may reflect the ability of Syk to be phosphorylated and activated by other Syk molecules.

Another tyrosine kinase that participates in BCR signaling is Btk (37,38). Btk is an intracellular tyrosine kinase with a distinctive structure (Fig. 3) that is defective in X-linked agammaglobulinemia, a human immunodeficiency syndrome in which there is greatly impaired B-cell development and very poor production of antibodies. A mutation in the gene for Btk is also responsible for the murine XID mouse, in which B cells are produced in substantial numbers but are functionally impaired. In particular, these B cells are unable to make antibodies to TI-2 antigens. These phenotypes suggest an important role for Btk in signaling by the pre-BCR in B-cell development and by the BCR in B-cell activation to TI-2 antigens. Indeed, BCR cross-linking leads to tyrosine phosphorylation and activation of Btk and Btk plays an important role in BCR-induced phosphoinositide hydrolysis (38,39).

Signaling Events Triggered by the BCR

The tyrosine kinases activated by BCR clustering act to trigger a complex panel of early signaling events, some of which are depicted in Fig. 4. Particularly important signaling pathways mediating BCR engagement include hydrolysis of phosphatidylinositol 4,5-bisphosphate (PIP$_2$), activation of Ras, activation of phosphatidylinositol 3-kinase (PI 3-kinase), and activation of Vav and HS-1. These signaling reactions are considered in turn.

Phosphoinositide Hydrolysis

Cross-linking of the BCR with anti-Ig antibodies leads to rapid hydrolysis of PIP$_2$ by phospholipase Cγ (Fig. 5) (8). Although in most cell types PLCγ1 predominates, in B cells PLCγ2 is the main isoform. Phosphorylation of key tyrosine residues of PLCγ1 increases its intrinsic activity considerably. Regulation of PLCγ2 is likely to be similar in this regard. In addition, in order to be fully

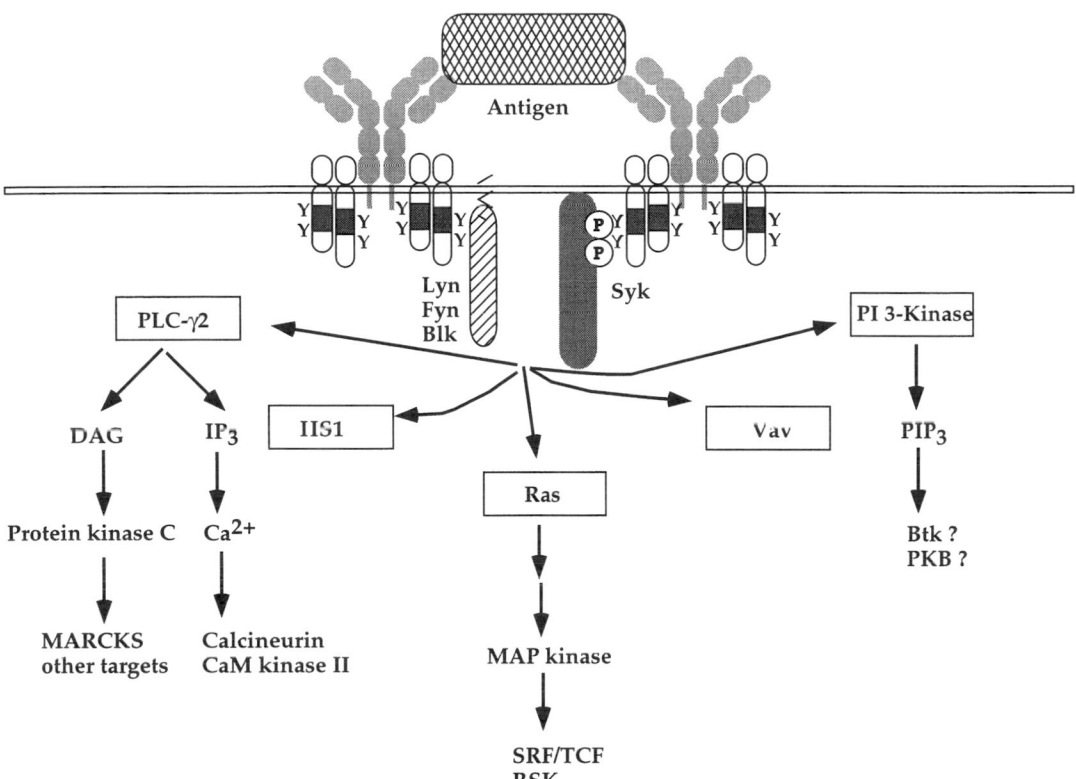

FIG. 4. Signaling pathways activated by the BCR. The major signaling pathways activated by the BCR are shown. Activation of PLCγ2 leads to PIP₂ hydrolysis, generating the second messengers diacylglycerol (DAG), which activates protein kinase C, and inositol trisphosphate (IP₃), which causes a release of Ca²⁺ from internal stores into the cytoplasm. Activation of the Ras pathway leads to activation of the Erk1/Erk2 MAP kinases. Activation of PI 3-kinase leads to generation of PIP₃, which may serve as a ligand for various signaling proteins containing PH domains, such as the tyrosine protein kinase Btk and the serine/threonine protein kinase protein kinase B (PKB, also called c-Akt). Less is known about the signaling events downstream from HS1 and Vav, but mice deficient in these signaling components have poor responses to BCR stimulation.

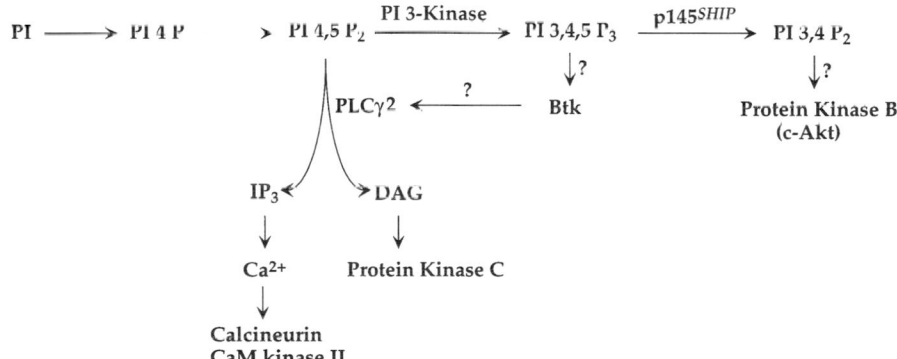

FIG. 5. Signaling pathways involving inositol-containing phospholipids. PI is phosphorylated on the 4 and 5 positions of the inositol ring to create PI 4,5P₂. This is the substrate for PLCγ2, which cleaves it to generate DAG and IP₃. The former activates most isoforms of protein kinase C, whereas the latter causes release of calcium from intracellular stores into the cytoplasm, resulting in the activation of calmodulin-dependent enzymes. PI 4,5P₂ is also the major substrate for PI 3-kinase, which phosphorylates it on the 3 position to generate PIP₃. PIP₃ is likely to be an important second messenger, perhaps by binding to PH domains of signaling components such as Btk. The SH2-containing inositol phosphatase SHIP removes the 5 phosphate from PIP₃ to generate PI 3,4P₂, which is the ligand for the PH domain of protein kinase B (c-Akt).

effective, PLCγ must be translocated from the cytosol to the plasma membrane where its substrate is located. For some receptors, this translocation is mediated by binding of PLCγ to the tyrosine phosphorylated receptor; how this is achieved in B cells is not known.

The second messengers resulting from PIP$_2$ hydrolysis are diacylglycerol and inositol 1,4,5-trisphosphate (IP$_3$). Diacylglycerol is a lipophilic compound that remains in the plasma membrane and activates most protein kinase C (PKC) isozymes, which are also activated by the tumor-promoting phorbol esters (e.g., phorbol myristate acetate [PMA]). One target of PKC in B cells is MAR-CKS (40), a protein that regulates the actin cytoskeleton (41). Other substrates of PKC in B cells are not well established, but mice with the gene for PKCβ inactivated have decreased antibody responses (42). Strikingly, the phenotype of PKCβ-deficient mice is quite similar to the phenotype of xid mice, which are defective in the tyrosine kinase Btk (38). Moreover, a direct interaction between PKCβ and Btk has been observed in mast cells (43), so it would appear that these two signaling components act in concert to promote B-cell activation. The transcription factor CREB (cyclic adenosine monophosphate [cAMP] response element binding protein) is activated upon stimulation of PKC with phorbol esters in B cells (44,45), suggesting that it is a direct or indirect target of PKC. At least one other isoform of PKC, PKCμ is also activated in BCR-stimulated B cells (46). In contrast to PKCβ, PKCμ may be a negative regulator because it can phosphorylate Syk in vitro and inhibit its ability to phosphorylate PLCγ1. Interestingly, PKCμ also has been found bound to the BCR, so it is appropriately located to perform such a negative feedback regulation.

The other second messenger released by PIP$_2$ hydrolysis is IP$_3$. This is a water-soluble second messenger that diffuses to the endoplasmic reticulum, where it interacts with receptors that cause the release of calcium ions from this intracellular compartment. This release is responsible for the initial dramatic elevation of intracellular free calcium. Intracellular free calcium, as measured by calcium-sensitive fluorescent dyes such as indo-1, fura-2, or fluo-3, rises from a resting value of about 100 nmol/L to a peak of 1 μmol/L or higher (47). Once the calcium of the intracellular stores is fully released, this causes an opening of plasma membrane calcium channels (48) via a poorly understood mechanism that is referred to as capacitative calcium entry (49). These plasma membrane channels are responsible for the sustained elevation of calcium, which either is terminated by receptor desensitization (50) or is maintained over a substantial period of time, for example in anergic B cells (51).

The elevated intracellular calcium binds to calmodulin and promotes the activation of both serine/threonine protein kinases (primarily calmodulin-dependent protein kinase II) (52) and serine/threonine-specific protein phosphatases (primarily calcineurin) (53). Again, targets of these downstream signaling enzymes are not well understood, but calcineurin appears to be the phosphatase that directly dephosphorylates the NFAT family of transcription factors (54). Although initially described as a transcription factor that is important for cytokine gene expression in TCR-stimulated T cells, NFAT is clearly present in other cell types and can be activated by BCR stimulation in B cells (55). Another transcription factor, Ets-1, becomes phosphorylated in response to BCR stimulation in a calcium-dependent manner (56). Calcium elevation also appears to participate in the activation of a number of other transcription factors, including NF-κB and ATF-2 (57).

Ras Pathway

A second major signaling pathway triggered in response to BCR engagement is the Ras pathway. Ras is an important regulator of cell growth and differentiation in many cell types (58). The activity of Ras and related superfamily members is determined by the nature of a bound guanine nucleotide. When guanosine diphosphate (GDP) is bound, Ras is inactive, whereas when guanosine triphosphate (GTP) is bound, Ras is active and promotes downstream signaling events such as activation of the classical MAP kinases Erk1and Erk2 (Fig. 6). Typically, receptors induce the translocation of regulators called nucleotide exchange factors (e.g., mSOS1 and mSOS2) from the cytoplasm to the plasma membrane, where Ras is located. The exchange factors then promote the release of GDP from Ras, making it free to bind GTP. Ras has a rather slow intrinsic GTPase activity that hydrolyzes the bound GTP to yield GDP and phosphate. Release of the phosphate molecule then converts Ras from the active to the inactive form. This step is regulated by a second class of molecules, called GTPase activating proteins (GAPs), the two principal forms of which are called RasGAP and neurofibromin (58).

BCR cross-linking leads to a rapid increase in the amount of GTP-bound Ras (59,60), and a redistribution of Ras, such that it accumulates underneath the cross-linked BCR molecules (61). The mechanism by which the BCR activates Ras is not yet established, but a favored hypothesis is that it involves the adapter protein Shc. BCR stimulation leads to rapid tyrosine phosphorylation of Shc, an adapter protein that can bind to another adapter protein, Grb-2, which in turn binds to the nucleotide exchange factors mSOS1 and mSOS2 (Fig. 6). Thus, BCR stimulation induces the formation of a multi-protein complex including Shc, Grb2, and mSOS1/2 (62–65). This complex appears to be membrane associated (62), but how this association occurs is unclear, because none of these proteins is a membrane protein. One hypothesis is that Shc in turn binds to a currently unidentified membrane protein. Phorbol diesters, which activate most isoforms of PKC, can activate Ras in hematopoietic lineage cells, including B cells, so it is possible that a portion of the Ras activation in BCR-stimulated B cells occurs via PIP$_2$ hydrolysis and PKC activation. It is not known how PKC promotes Ras activation.

Finally, although it is currently thought that the primary mechanism of activating Ras is by stimulating the action of nucleotide exchange factors, inhibition of the GAPs also may contribute to Ras activation. Alternatively, translocation of rasGAP to the plasma membrane may be a feedback inhibitory event limiting activation of Ras. BCR stimulation promotes tyrosine phosphorylation of RasGAP and its association with two other proteins, p62^{dok} and p190 (66). The p190 protein is itself a GAP for the Rac/Rho family of Ras superfamily GTPases (67), which in turn regulate the actin-based cytoskeleton. The p62^{dok} protein appears to be an adapter protein of some sort (68,69), perhaps serving to localize rasGAP near activated Ras and thereby providing a counterbalancing inhibition of Ras. Interestingly, p62^{dok} also binds to Csk, the tyrosine kinase that negatively regulates Src family kinases. The formation of the p62^{dok}–Csk complex is stimulated somewhat by BCR cross-linking and to a greater degree by coengagement of the BCR and FcγRIIb (70). Thus, p62^{dok} may be an inhibitor of signaling that brings rasGAP and Csk to the region of the cell where signaling is occurring and thereby increases the negative regulatory function of these proteins.

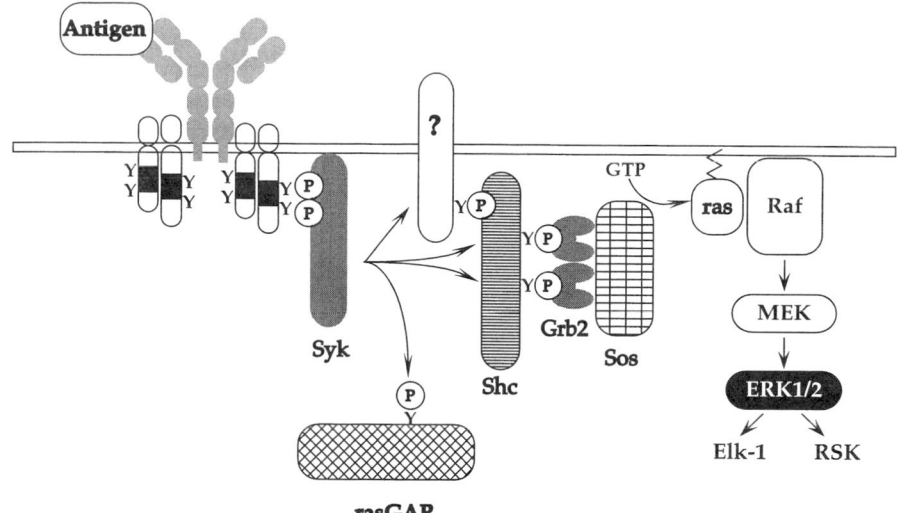

FIG. 6. The Ras signaling pathway. Ras exists in two states, an inactive state bound to GDP and an active state bound to GTP. Nucleotide exchange factors such as SOS1 and SOS2 induce the release of GDP from the Ras/GDP complex, allowing GTP to bind and Ras to become activated. It is thought that the BCR activates Ras primarily by Syk phosphorylating the adapter protein Shc, which allows Grb2 and SOS to bind to it via the SH2 domain of Grb2. Grb2 has two SH3 domains that bind to proline-rich regions of SOS. Shc is apparently held at the membrane, but how this occurs is unknown. Translocation of SOS to the membrane allows it to act on Ras. Active Ras binds to Raf, which now becomes activated by phosphorylation. Raf phosphorylates and activates MEK, which in turn phosphorylates and activates Erk1 and Erk2 MAP kinases. Downstream targets of the MAP kinases include transcription factors such as Elk-1 and the serine/threonine protein kinase RSK. BCR signaling also leads to phosphorylation of the GTPase-activating protein, RasGAP, which inactivates Ras.

Activated Ras has multiple downstream effector pathways, the best understood of which is a cascade of protein kinases from Raf to MAP kinase (71). The activation of Raf involves its binding to activated Ras followed by phosphorylation of Raf by an unidentified protein kinase (72), after which Raf phosphorylates and activates MEK1 and MEK2, which then activate the Erk1 and Erk2 MAP kinases (Fig. 6). These MAP kinases are clearly activated in B cells stimulated through the BCR (73–75). The main targets of the MAP kinases include another serine/threonine protein kinase, p90rsk, and a number of transcription factors, including the Ets family members that cooperate with serum response factor (SRF) to activate transcription at serum response elements (SREs) (76). Indeed, one of the genes rapidly induced by BCR signaling is the *egr-1* gene, which has multiple SREs, and these SREs and Ras mediate its transcriptional induction (77,78).

Phosphatidylinositol 3-Kinase Pathway

A third signaling pathway activated by the engaged BCRs is the phosphatidylinositol 3-kinase (PI 3-kinase) pathway. This enzyme adds a phosphate group to the 3 position of the inositol ring of phosphoinositides (Fig. 5). BCR stimulation leads to rapid tyrosine phosphorylation of PI 3-kinase (79,80) and accumulation of two PI 3-kinase products, PI 3,4-P_2 and PI 3,4,5-P_3 (81). PIP$_3$ increases more rapidly than does PI 3,4-P_2, suggesting that the primary substrate for PI 3-kinase *in vivo* may be PI 4,5-P_2 in preference to PI 4-P. Particularly interesting in this regard is the fact that another target of BCR-induced tyrosine phosphorylation is the inositol 5 phosphatase SHIP (SH2-containing inositol phosphatase) (82,83),

which converts PIP$_3$ to PI 3,4-P_2 (84–86), suggesting that the main route for production of PI 3,4-P_2 may be via the combined action of PI 3-kinase and SHIP (Fig. 5).

The phosphoinositides produced by PI 3-kinase and SHIP appear to be second messengers. In particular, these molecules are ligands for pleckstrin homology (PH) domains of a number of signaling components, which may show a preference for one or another phosphorylated phosphoinositide. For example, the PH domain of the tyrosine kinase Btk (Fig. 3) binds preferentially to PIP$_3$ (87), whereas the PH domain of a serine/threonine protein kinase called PKB or c-Akt binds preferentially to PI 3,4-P_2 (88,89). In the latter case, this binding event enhances the activity of PKB. A favored hypothesis is that the binding of PH domains to phosphoinositides provides a mechanism for recruiting PH-domain containing molecules to the plasma membrane. Interestingly, selection for mutations that confer upon Btk the ability to transform fibroblasts led to the isolation of a mutation in Btk's PH domain that enhances membrane association of Btk (90). This result suggests that biologically active Btk is found at the plasma membrane, perhaps as a result of its PH domain binding to PIP$_3$.

Additional Signaling Reactions Activated by the BCR

Signaling by receptors that activate tyrosine phosphorylation is characterized by the engagement of multiple downstream signaling pathways, and BCR signaling is no exception. Three additional signaling components that become tyrosine phosphorylated in response to BCR engagement and have received considerable attention are Vav (91), Cbl (92–94), and HS1 (95).

Vav is a protooncogene product expressed primarily in lymphocytes and other blood cell types. Although one group has reported evidence indicating that Vav regulates Ras, others have presented evidence against a general role of Vav in Ras regulation (96). Interesting in this regard is the fact that a region of Vav has significant homology to a domain in Dbl and other proteins, called the Dbl-homology domain. This domain in Dbl and in a number of other proteins has nucleotide exchange factor activity not for Ras (whose nucleotide exchange factors have sequences related to one another but not to Dbl), but for the Ras-related Rac family of small molecular weight GTP-binding proteins. It may be that this domain in Vav has weak exchange factor activity for Ras, but stronger activity for other proteins, such as members of the Rac family. Indeed, Vav has recently been reported to have exchange factor activity for these proteins (97,98). It may be that Vav has other functionally important activities as well, as it has a number of protein–protein interaction domains, including an SH2 domain and an SH3 domain, and thus may in part function to aid in the assembly of multiprotein signaling complexes. In agreement with this possibility, Vav has functionally important interactions with both ZAP-70 and another signaling component called SLP-76 during T-cell activation (99,100).

The Rac, CDC42, and Rho proteins constitute one of the major subfamilies of the Ras superfamily of small molecular weight GTP-binding proteins (101). Recent experiments have established roles for these proteins in controlling organization of actin-based microfilaments (102). For example, introduction of botulinis toxin into cells leads to ADP ribosylation and inactivation of Rho proteins along with loss of stress fibers, a major microfilament structure. Conversely, introduction of a mutated activated version of Rho induces formation of stress fibers in serum-starved cells, which otherwise have few such structures. Similarly, mutated activated Rac-1 and mutated dominant negative Rac-1 have opposing effects on the cortical microfilaments thought to be involved in filapodium extention. In addition, Rac 1 and CDC42 can directly interact with and activate protein kinases of the PAK65 family. Further downstream of these reactions is activation of the c-Jun N-terminal kinase (JNK) (103), which is activated in response to BCR engagement, or more strongly in response to CD40 engagement (104,105).

Another prominent target of BCR-induced tyrosine phosphorylation is Cbl, which is also a protooncogene. Cbl interacts with a number of other signaling components, but its function is not yet established. Loss of function mutations in the *Caenorhabditis elegans* homolog of *cbl, sli-1,* were isolated as genetic suppressors for vulval induction of partial loss of function mutations of *C. elegans ras* (106). One possible interpretation of the finding that loss of Cbl compensates for low Ras function is that Cbl is a negative regulator of Ras. In agreement with this idea, Cbl has been found to form a complex with the adapter protein Crk and with C3G (107,108). C3G is a guanine nucleotide exchange factor for the GTP-binding protein Rap1A, which may function as an inhibitor of Ras by competing with active Ras for effectors of Ras, and thereby preventing their activation (109).

Finally, BCR cross-linking also induces strong tyrosine phosphorylation of HS1, which is expressed primarily in cells of hematopoietic lineages. As discussed below, genetic experiments demonstrate a significant role for HS1 in B-cell responses to antigen. Recently, it has been found that BCR-induced tyrosine phosphorylation of HS1 induces it to translocate to the nucleus (110), suggesting that it may be a transcription factor activated by BCR

signaling. In addition, a protein that interacts with HS1, named HAX-1, has been isolated (111). HAX-1 is primarily localized to mitochrondria, which could reflect a role in regulating apoptosis, for example by interacting with the Bcl-2/BAX proteins, which are also present in that location.

Selection of Signaling Targets by the BCR

An important issue of current BCR signaling research is to understand the mechanism by which signaling targets are efficiently engaged upon BCR cross-linking. Studies of the tyrosine kinase growth factor receptors have established two related mechanisms for efficient engagement of signaling targets: either SH2-domain containing targets are attracted to the engaged receptor by directly binding via their SH2 domains to particular autophosphorylation sites on the receptor, or they bind to adapter proteins that use this mechanism (15,112). By analogy, antigen receptors could also efficiently attract relevant signaling components by these means. This possibility is limited, perhaps by the fact that almost all of the receptor tyrosines are present in ITAM sequences, which would be expected to bind only to one type of SH2 domain (14), those that bind to YxxL/I type sequences. Some of the targets of BCR-induced tyrosine phosphorylation fit into this category, for example the adapter protein Shc. Other targets, such as PI 3-kinase, Vav, and PLCγ2, would be expected not to bind well to phosphorylated ITAM sequences. Interesting in this regard is the observation that expression of the BCR and Syk in the nonlymphoid cell line AtT20 reconstituted Shc phosphorylation and MAP kinase activation but not PIP₂ hydrolysis or calcium elevation (113). This result suggests that BCR engagement of Shc and activation of the Ras/MAP kinase pathway does not require any additional lymphoid-specific signaling components, whereas activation of PLCγ2 does. Genetic ablation of Btk greatly decreases PIP₂ hydrolysis in DT-40 chicken B cells (39), suggesting that Btk may be a required lymphoid-specific component. Introduction of Btk into the AtT20 cells expressing the BCR and Syk did not reconstitute PIP₂ hydrolysis (J. Richards, P. Roth and A.L. DeFranco, unpublished results), however, so additional lymphoid-specific components also may be required.

Two additional mechanisms have been postulated to be important for BCR downstream signaling reactions: interactions of targets with the intracellular tyrosine kinases activated by the BCR (e.g., Syk, Btk, and the Src family members), and interaction of target SH2 domains with membrane proteins that associate with the BCR and become phosphorylated in response to BCR stimulation (8) (Fig. 7). It is entirely possible that these two mechanisms occur simultaneously, and that a large signaling complex is formed between the associated membrane protein, tyrosine kinases, and signaling targets. In this regard, it is important to recognize that most SH2-based interactions are of moderate affinity with relatively fast dissociation rates. A consequence of such a binding mechanism is that a target may bind and quickly leave the site of binding. In some cases, such interactions may last long enough for the target protein to become phosphorylated. In other cases, multiple interactions (an SH2 domain-phosphotyrosine peptide interaction plus a second interaction, either based on an SH2 or some other mechanism that is of low or moderate affinity by itself) may be necessary to form a signaling complex that is sufficiently stable to be functional (e.g., if the signaling component must be held at the membrane).

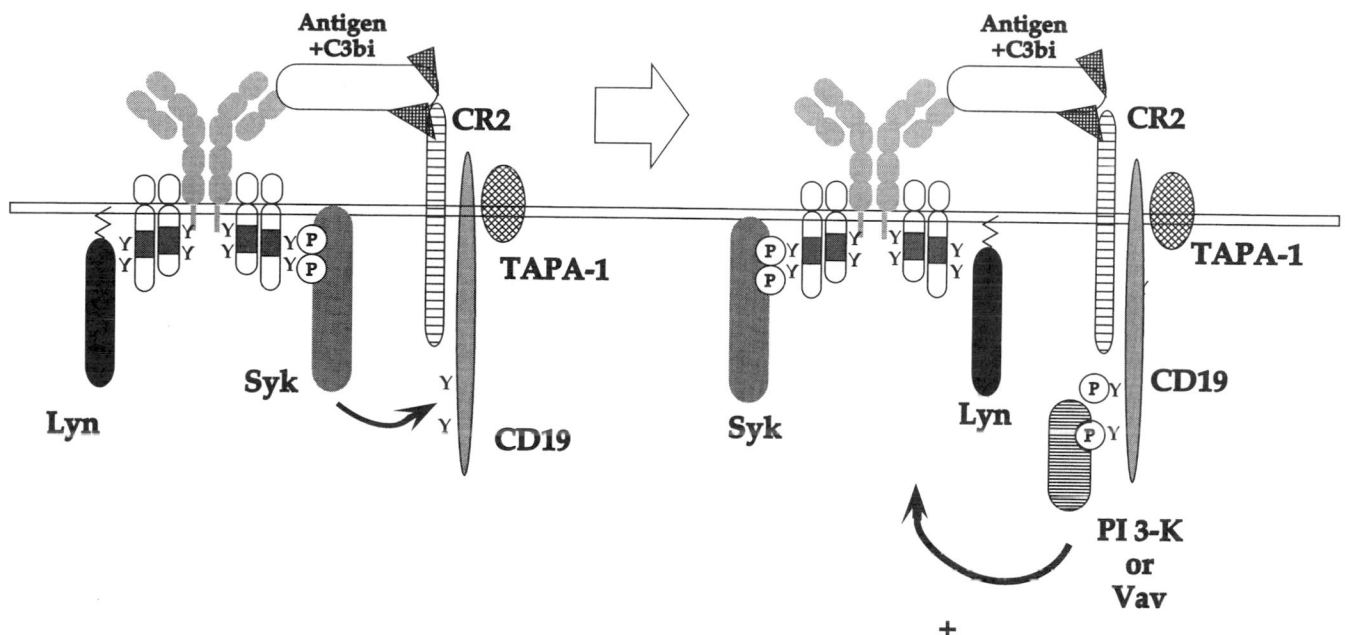

FIG. 7. Synergistic activation of B cells by antigen-complement conjugates. Antigens with fragments of C3 deposited on them can bind to both the BCR and to the CR2/CD19/TAPA-1 complex and bring them together. This promotes efficient phosphorylation of the cytoplasmic tyrosines of CD19, which then serve as binding sites for the signaling components PI 3-kinase and Vav, which enhance the response of B cells to antigenic stimulation. Syk is shown phosphorylating the cytoplasmic domain of CD19, but it is not known whether this is primarily a function of Syk or of the Src family tyrosine kinases.

Considerable circumstantial evidence exists for both of these mechanisms because many of the targets of signaling are found to associate with Syk or Lyn, as well as with BCR-associated membrane proteins such as CD19 and CD22 (114–116). For example, PLCγ2 interacts directly with Syk (117,118), whereas PI 3-kinase interacts with Lyn and Fyn (79). The relative importance of these interactions remain to be determined.

Recognition of Complex Antigens by the BCR and Coreceptors

Oligomeric antigen cross-linking the BCR triggers the signaling function of the BCR ITAMs by the mechanism described above. One advantage of the complex architecture of the BCR signaling unit, with its use of separate polypeptides for antigen recognition, tyrosine kinase activity, and tyrosine kinase localization may be that there is a considerable steric flexibility for triggering signaling. Tyrosine kinase growth factor receptors probably require dimerization in a relatively precise way to trigger their signaling function, but that is readily achieved as the ligand induces a reproducible geometry of dimerization. For the BCR, however, different antigens will induce sterically distinct oligimerization configurations depending on the shape of the antigen. Thus, in order for the B cell to respond appropriately to many different physical entities, it is important that receptor oligimerization trigger signaling with little dependence upon the particular geometry of receptor clustering.

A second and perhaps more important advantage of the antigen receptor signaling setup is that the B cell can use other cell surface receptors (coreceptors) in conjunction with the BCR to detect dec-

oration of an antigen by other elements of the immune system. This in turn can modulate BCR signaling and alter the cellular response. This principle is clearly seen in T cells with the role of the coreceptors CD4 and CD8. These coreceptors bind directly to MHC molecules. When the TCR engages a peptide/MHC complex, the coreceptor can also bind to that ligand creating a four-way complex of TCR, coreceptor, MHC molecule, and bound peptide. The consequence of this is that the cytoplasmic domains of CD4 or CD8, both of which bind Lck in relatively high stoichiometry, are brought next to the cytoplasmic domains of the TCR polypeptides. This allows for highly efficient phosphorylation of ITAMs and ITAM-bound ZAP-70 by Lck (119). In contrast, when the TCR binds to an inappropriate ligand, there is no MHC molecule to engage the coreceptor and signaling is much weaker. Thus, the CD4 and CD8 coreceptors help the T cell know whether its TCR has engaged an appropriate ligand or an inappropriate one, and to respond accordingly.

It is now clear that BCR signaling is influenced by at least two coreceptors, the complement receptor CR2 promoting B-cell activation and the Fc receptor FcγRIIb inhibiting it. The B cell's response to antigen is enhanced by decoration of the antigen by the complement system. In this case, the antigen has been identified as foreign either through the action of the alternative pathway of complement or by reaction of the antigen with preexisting low-affinity polyreactive IgM (120) and the classical pathway. A striking example of the powerful function of this coreceptor comes from experiments in which mice were immunized with either lysozyme or with lysozyme-C3d fusion proteins. The latter can induce a strong antibody response in the absence of adjuvant with at least 1,000-fold less protein than lysozyme alone (121). Alternatively, the B cell's response to antigen is dampened by an abundance of antigen-specific IgG antibodies, indicating that a further antibody response is not necessary. This mechanism limits an immune response because mice in which the gene encoding FcγRIIb has been inactivated exhibit elevated antibody responses, particularly late after immunization (122).

The CR2 Coreceptor

B cells express two receptors for C3b or its breakdown products iC3b or C3dg: complement receptors 1 and 2 (CR1 and CR2). Of these complement receptors, CR2, which is expressed primarily on B cells and follicular dendritic cells, is the one that participates in B-cell activation. CR2 is present in the membrane in two different complexes: a complex with CR1 and a complex with CD19 and TAPA-1 (CD81) (123) (Fig. 7). CD19 is also preassociated with the BCR, although in relatively low stoichiometry. Thus, antigen-induced clustering of the BCR would cocluster a small amount of CD19. However, the amount of CD19 present would be greatly increased by an antigen decorated with C3d fragments. Artificial co–cross-linking of CR2 or CD19 with the BCR leads to synergistic PIP$_2$ hydrolysis and enhanced B-cell proliferation compared with cross-linking of the BCR alone, demonstrating a significant positive role of the CR2/CD19/TAPA-1 complex as a B-cell coreceptor (124,125). CD19 is thought to be primarily responsible for this effect because a larger synergy is seen when using antibodies directed at CD19 than with antibodies directed at CR2 or TAPA-1.

Similarly, the phenotypes of mice genetically deficient for CR2 or CD19 support the conclusion that CR2 and CD19 play very important roles in promoting B-cell activation. Mice lacking CR2 exhibit markedly decreased T cell–dependent antibody responses, and this is primarily due to the loss of CR2 from B cells (126–128). CD19-deficient mice likewise have 10 to 100 times lower antibody responses to T cell–dependent antigens than littermate control mice (129,130). The response of these mice to TI-2 antigens is normal or elevated. Previous work in which complement was depleted or complement receptor function was blocked had suggested that CR2 played a role in T cell–dependent antibody responses primarily at low antigen concentrations, but the experiments described to date with both CD19-deficient and CR2-deficient mice have shown a similar decrease in antibody response at both low and high antigen doses of immunization. The extent of the defect in antibody response may be greater in the CD19-deficient mice, but this point needs to be tested by direct side-by-side comparisons of the antibody responses of these mice. If the defects are similar, this would support the argument that the main role of CD19 in the antibody response is via its participation in the CR2 complex. On the other hand, if the CD19 defect is actually greater, as appears to be the case, this would support the argument that CD19 has two roles: one requiring the CR2 complex and another independent of it. Because a modest amount of CD19 binds directly to the BCR, it is attractive to think that this pool of CD19 molecules also provides an additional positive role in B-cell activation occurring independently of the complement receptor. However, it should be noted that TI-2 antibody responses are normal in the absence of CD19 and that the in vitro proliferative responses to BCR stimulation are either normal or decreased by only about 50%, depending on the study (129,130). Thus, CD19 is not an essential component of BCR signal transduction or of BCR participation in B-cell activation.

The mechanism by which CR2 enhances B-cell responses to BCR cross-linking in vitro and to antigens in vivo is unknown.

Most studies have focused on the cytoplasmic domain of CD19 as most likely to provide the positive stimulus to BCR signaling. The cytoplasmic domain of CD19 has nine tyrosines, and BCR cross-linking leads to dramatic phosphorylation of those tyrosines. Two of these sites are recognized by the SH2 domains of PI 3-kinase (114), whereas another site is recognized by the SH2 domain of Vav (115). Thus, a leading hypothesis is that CD19 participation in BCR signaling, either at low levels constitutively or at higher levels when CR2 is coclustered with the BCR, causes selective recruitment of two signaling components—Vav and PI 3-kinase—which in some way promotes B-cell activation over negative responses. Indeed, one result of coclustering of CR2 with the BCR is to inhibit BCR-induced apoptosis (131). CD19 also associates to some degree with Lyn and Fyn (132,133), and so its participation may also enhance initial signaling events such as ITAM phosphorylation. CD19 is clearly not required for initiating tyrosine kinase action, however, because CD19-deficient B cells have relatively normal BCR-induced tyrosine phosphorylation (130).

In addition to the role of CR2 in promoting activation of B cells through the BCR, separate engagement of CR2 with a multivalent ligand can act as a growth stimulus for already activated B cells (134). In humans, CR2 also serves as the receptor for Epstein-Barr virus (135,136), which causes continual proliferation of B-lymphocytes, leading to the disease infectious mononucleosis, which, in the absence of sufficient CD8 T-cell immunity, can lead to Burkitt's lymphoma.

The FcγRIIb Coreceptor

A second coreceptor for B cells is the Fc receptor for IgG on B cells (FcγRIIb). This receptor is co-ligated with the BCR when the predominant form of antigen is an immune complex that is free in solution. This is inhibitory for BCR-induced B-cell proliferation in vitro (137) and promotes apoptosis of B cells (138). It should be noted that if an immune complex first comes in contact with a follicular dendritic cell (FDC), then the antigen can be held by the FDC via its FcγRs and presented in a positive fashion to the B cell, for example to aid in selection for higher affinity mutant B cells, as discussed in a later section.

The mechanism by which FcγRIIb inhibits B-cell activation has been studied extensively in vitro by using rabbit anti-IgM antibodies, which efficiently coligate the IgM form of the BCR with FcγRIIb. For example, addition of intact rabbit anti-IgM antibody results in much less PIP$_2$ breakdown than does addition of the F(ab')$_2$ version of the same antibody (139). The elevation of intracellular free calcium is also attenuated, due primarily to an inhibition of calcium influx (140,141).

The inhibition of BCR calcium signaling is dependent on the cytoplasmic domain of FcγRIIb, with one tyrosine and its surrounding amino acids being critical to this function (141). This region is referred to as the immunoreceptor tyrosine-based inhibitory motif (ITIM). The ITIM tyrosine becomes phosphorylated only when the FcR is coligated to the BCR (Fig. 8). This tyrosine-phosphorylated region of the FcR serves as a binding site for three SH2-containing phosphatases: the closely related tyrosine phosphatases SHP-1 and SHP-2 and the inositol 5-phosphatase SHIP (83,142–144). The relative contributions of these signaling inhibitors is controversial at the time of this writing (145). B cells from mice defective in SHP-1 (moth-eaten viable mice) appear to have lost at least some of the FcR inhibition (142), but some of it

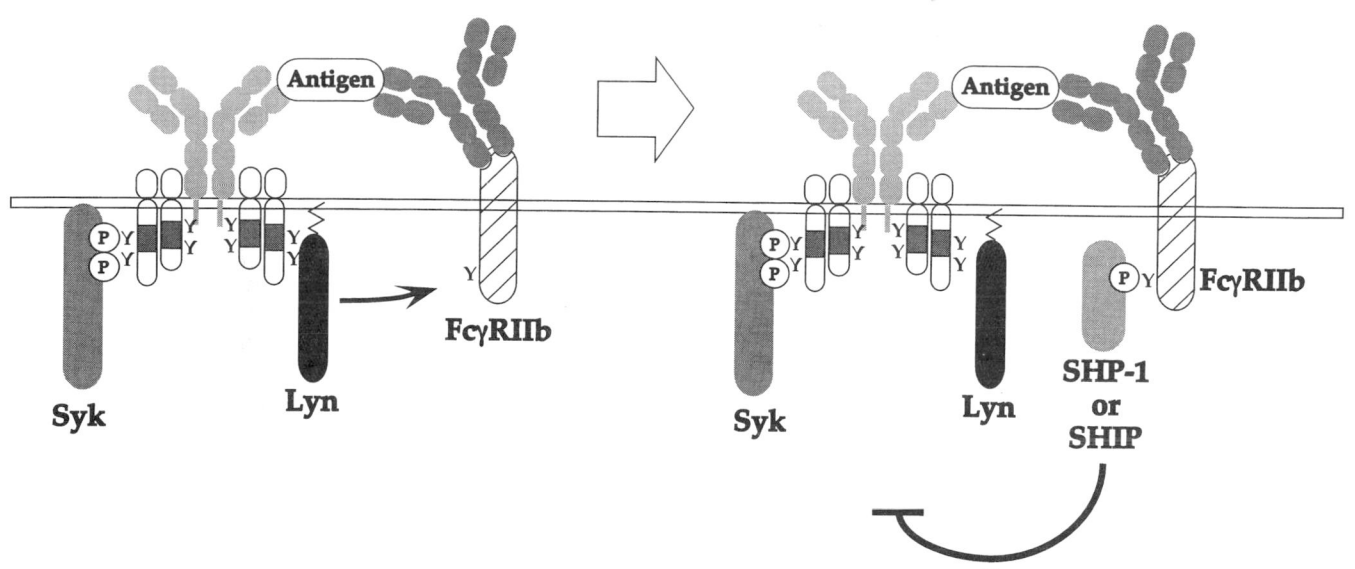

FIG. 8. Inhibition of B-cell activation by FcR engagement. When antigen is prebound to soluble IgG, then FcγRIIb1 is brought together with the BCR. This leads to phosphorylation of the ITIM tyrosine in the cytoplasmic domain of the FcR. Lyn is primarily responsible for this phosphorylation. This site now recruits the SH2-containing inositol phosphatase SHIP and the SH2-containing tyrosine phosphatase SHP-1 via their SH2 domains. Both of these components have the potential to inhibit BCR signaling reactions, although SHIP appears to be more important in this context.

is retained (146). Mast cells, which exhibit an analogous inhibition of FcεRI function by coengagement with FcγRIIb, were found to exhibit considerable inhibition even if derived from moth-eaten mice (143). This led the authors to conclude that SHIP was providing the negative regulatory function seen. Targeted deletion of the genes for SHP-1 or SHIP in the chicken DT-40 B-cell line showed a critical role for SHIP but not SHP-1 in this system (144). Conversely, when a chimeric protein was made between the extracellular domain of the FcR and the intracellular domain of an inhibitory receptor from natural killer cells that binds SHP-1 and not SHIP, it was found that inhibition was dependent on SHP-1 expression but not upon SHIP expression (144). Thus, it appears that SHIP is the major inhibitor used by FcγRIIb, but SHP-1 also can inhibit signaling by antigen receptors (Fig. 8) and does so in conjunction with the killer inhibitory receptors. It remains possible that SHP-1 contributes to FcγRIIb function in murine B cells as well.

How SHIP and/or SHP-1 inhibit BCR signaling function is not yet fully understood. Coengagement of the BCR and FcγRIIb leads to phosphorylation of the key tyrosine in the cytoplasmic domain of the FcR, and activation of Lyn or Syk is still seen at normal levels, indicating that there is not a total shutdown of BCR signaling (147,148). Tyrosine phosphorylation of CD19 is inhibited, suggesting that this may be an important target of SHP-1 (148). As described above, one of the functions of CD19 is to recruit PI 3-kinase on BCR cross-linking. Wortmannin, a reasonably specific PI 3-kinase inhibitor, also partially inhibited the BCR-induced calcium elevation, suggesting that inhibition of CD19 phosphorylation could account for the FcR inhibition of calcium influx. It should be noted that SHIP can degrade the product of PI 3-kinase, PIP3 (Fig. 5), so prevention of PI 3-kinase activation and degradation of its product could both contribute to the same end: prevention of PIP3 elevation and its consequent second messenger function.

Because Btk was found to be necessary for BCR-induced PIP2 hydrolysis in the chicken DT-40 B-cell line, a unifying model for FcγRIIb inhibition would be that CD19 recruits PI 3-kinase, resulting in production of PIP3, which may help recruit Btk to the plasma membrane where it can collaborate with Syk and Src family tyrosine kinases to activate PLCγ2. SHIP could act as an inhibitor by converting PIP3 to PI 3,4-P2, which is not a ligand for the Btk PH domain. How the phosphorylation of CD19 is prevented is unknown, but this could be the role of SHP-1. This model accounts for the ability of either SHP-1 or SHIP to inhibit BCR signaling, by postulating that they act in different ways to prevent elevation of the same second messenger, PIP3 (Fig. 5). CD19-deficient B cells still exhibit an elevation of calcium in response to BCR cross-linking (130,148), but this appears to be less than that seen in wild-type B cells and it is not inhibited by FcγRIIb coengagement (148). The residual calcium elevation seen in CD19-deficient B cells may reflect the presence of a second mechanism to activate PI 3-kinase or a second mechanism to activate PIP2 hydrolysis, which in either case is quantitatively less important than the mechanism blocked by the FcR.

Coengagement of FcγRIIb with the BCR also leads to much less Ras activation than seen in response to BCR engagement alone (149). This inhibition is accompanied by a decrease in Shc-Grb2 interaction and a large increase in association between Shc and SHIP. This interaction involves, at least in part, binding of the PTB domain of Shc to a tyrosine-phosphorylated site on SHIP. The simplest hypothesis to bring together these observations is that recruitment of SHIP to the tyrosine phosphorylated inhibitory motif of FcγRIIb brings SHIP near BCR-associated tyrosine kinases and thereby leads to its efficient phosphorylation on sites that mediate binding of Shc. Thus, SHIP appears to also be involved in the FcγRIIb inhibition of BCR-induced Ras activation, probably by preventing the formation of the Shc-Grb2-mSOS complex that is thought to be responsible for activation of Ras in response to BCR ligation (Fig. 6). Hydrolysis of PIP$_2$ and Ras activation of MAP kinase appear to both participate in BCR-induced proliferation, as discussed below, so the ability of FcγRIIb to inhibit these signaling events likely explains the inhibition of proliferation. FcγRIIb induction of apoptosis may reflect the actions of one or more additional signaling events that are not inhibited by this receptor. Recently it was found that a measles virus coat protein also binds to human FcγRII, and this interaction also suppresses B-cell activation (150).

Other Possible B-Cell Coreceptors

The signal transduction function of the BCR can be regulated by at least three other receptors on the B-cell surface: CD22, CD45, and CD5. These may be additional coreceptors for B cells, although at this point the extracellular interactions that might modulate the effects of these molecules on BCR signaling are unknown.

CD22 is an immunoglobulin superfamily member that recognizes terminal, α2,6-linked sialic acid (in human) or N-glycolyl neuraminic acid (in mouse) residues on glycoproteins or glycolipids (151,152). A subset of CD22 molecules is preassociated with the BCR, and cross-linking the BCR leads to phosphorylation of some of CD22's six cytoplasmic domain tyrosine residues (151). This in turn leads to the recruitment of SHP-1 via its SH2 domains to CD22 (151,152). Because SHP-1 is a negative regulator of BCR signaling (36), this observation suggests that CD22 is also a negative regulator of BCR signaling. Interestingly, CD22 is similar in both its structure and its ability to bind to SHP-1 to a new class of widely expressed molecules that bind both to the closely related tyrosine phosphatase SHP-2 and to tyrosine kinase growth factor receptors, and negatively regulate the latter (153). CD22 may not function completely as a negative regulator, however, because it also binds positive signaling components such as Syk, Lyn, PI 3-kinase, and PLCγl (116,154). Indeed, the phenotype of CD22 knockout mice indicates that CD22 is not purely a positive or a negative regulator (155–158). The BCR-induced calcium elevation is enhanced in CD22-deficient B cells, indicating a negative role for CD22 in this signaling reaction. BCR-induced B-cell proliferation in vitro is generally decreased in the absence of CD22, however, and T cell–independent antibody responses were also decreased. The most straightforward interpretation of these results is that they reflect multiple roles for CD22 in regulating B-cell activation, some positive and some negative. Alternatively, it has been suggested that chronic BCR stimulation due to lack of CD22 inhibition leads to an anergic phenotype of the CD22-deficient B cells, which subsequently leads to poor responsiveness to BCR stimulation (152). As mentioned above, however, calcium elevation in response to BCR stimulation is increased in the CD22-deficient B cells, in contrast to anergic B cells, where this response is decreased (51,159).

The phosphorylation of CD22 is almost completely absent in Lyn-deficient B cells, indicating that CD22 is phosphorylated by Lyn (32). Interestingly, the other negative regulator of BCR signaling, FcγRIIb1, is also primarily phosphorylated by Lyn. The deficiency in phosphorylation of FcγRIIb1 and CD22 may account for the hyperreactive phenotype of B cells from Lyn-deficient mice.

The transmembrane tyrosine phosphatase CD45 is a positive regulator of antigen receptor signaling in both B cells and T cells (36). This is thought to be due to the ability of CD45 to dephosphorylate Src family tyrosine kinases at the COOH-terminal negative regulatory tyrosine (Fig. 3). In agreement with this view, mice deficient in CD45 exhibit deficient responses to antigen, both in vitro and in vivo (160–163). Although a variety of ligands for CD45 have been identified, it is presently unclear how CD45 action on Src family tyrosine kinases or other possible targets is controlled.

Only a small subpopulation of B cells, termed the "B-1a population" (164), expresses CD5, and this is at a reduced level compared with its expression on T cells. CD5 appears to be a negative regulator of TCR signaling (165). Interestingly, CD5 appears to participate in the BCR-induced apoptosis of B-1a cells because treatment of peritoneal B cells from CD5-deficient mice does not induce apoptosis but rather leads to proliferation (166). Moreover, sequestration of CD5 molecules on normal B-1a B cells by anti-CD5 antibodies also prevents apoptosis and stimulates proliferation (166).

STIMULATION OF EARLY EVENTS OF B-CELL ACTIVATION BY THE BCR

Regulation of B-Cell Survival

Each day a large number of newly generated B cells are exported from the bone marrow into the periphery, and in each T cell–dependent humoral immune response many memory B cells are generated from expansion of very few virgin B cells. These sources of B cells must be balanced by death of B cells because the total number of B cells is held at a nearly constant level. Among the newly generated B cells, about 80% will die within 1 week, whereas the remaining 20% will enter the long-lived pool of recirculating virgin B cells (167) (Fig. 9). This is what occurs in the presence of an established peripheral B-cell population, whereas in its absence, all of these cells become long lived. These observations indicate that entry into the long-lived pool of B cells involves some sort of competition, perhaps for a limited resource such as access to primary follicles of lymphoid organs (168).

One major parameter determining which B cells survive and which B cells die is that survival appears to depend on a low level of signaling from the BCR. One piece of evidence for this idea comes from studies with B cells expressing Ig heavy- and light-chain transgenes encoding an antilysozyme Ig. These B cells normally enter a long-lived pool in the absence of lysozyme and enter a tolerized anergic state in the presence of the high-affinity ligand lysozyme. Introduction of this trangene into mice with a loss of function mutation of CD45, however, resulted in poor B-cell survival unless lysozyme was introduced, in which case long-lived B cells of a normal phenotype were obtained (169). Because the loss of CD45 is known to decrease BCR signaling (CD45 dephosphorylates a negative regulatory phosphotyrosine of Src family tyrosine kinases), these observations have been interpreted to indicate that BCR signaling resulting from interaction with self components that serve as low-affinity ligands is required for maturation of B cells and entry into a long-lived state, and this signal is absent in the CD45-mutant B cells due to decreased signaling capacity. Addition of lysozyme restores this low level signal in the CD45-mutant situation and thereby restores survival, whereas in B cells with normal CD45, lysozyme induces greater signaling and this induces anergy instead of survival. In addition, induced deletion of the IgH locus in mature B cells leads to their rapid death by apop-

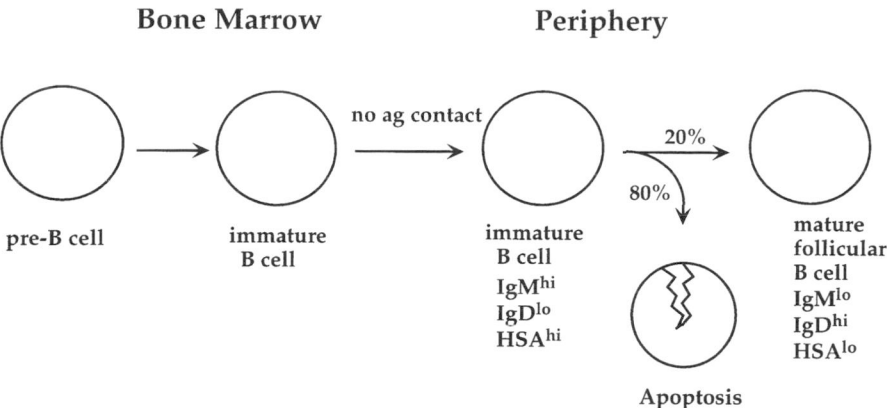

FIG. 9. Maturation of B cells. B cells are generated after successful Ig gene rearrangements in the bone marrow. Antigen contact with new immature B cells in the bone marrow causes maturational arrest and retention in the bone marrow while receptor editing occurs. In the absence of antigen contact in the bone marrow, the immature B cell exits to the periphery, where its fate is apparently dependent on appropriate BCR engagement. Most immature B cells fail to enter the long-lived mature follicular B-cell population and die by apoptosis within 1 week of export from the bone marrow, but approximately 20% mature and survive.

tosis, indicating that most peripheral B cells require some sort of signal from the BCR continuously or periodically to survive in the periphery, even after entry into the long-lived pool (170). Finally, memory B cells also appear to require their inducing antigen to survive.

Survival of nonactivated B cells is closely correlated with expression of the anti-apoptotic protein Bcl-2 (171). Immature B cells recently exported from the bone marrow express little or no Bcl-2 and are short-lived unless selected into the long-lived peripheral B-cell pool. Mature B cells express significant levels of Bcl-2, with the exception that germinal center B cells turn off Bcl-2 expression. These cells are subject to stringent selection for BCR affinity for antigen in the germinal centers with many of them dying by apoptosis. In addition, plasma cells generally do not express Bcl-2 and most of them die within a few days of terminal differentiation, the exception being plasma cells in the bone marrow or gut, which live for several weeks. Hematopoiesis is fairly normal in Bcl-2 knockout mice, but there is a catastrophic loss of peripheral lymphocytes after birth, indicating that Bcl-2 expression is required for survival of peripheral B cells and peripheral T cells (172,173). Conversely, enforced expression of Bcl-2 as a transgene driven by the IgH enhancer leads to increased levels of peripheral B cells, long-lived plasma cells that secrete antibody for a long period of time, and memory B cells that survive after adoptive transfer in the absence of antigen (171). Activation stimuli often lead to downregulation of Bcl-2 and upregulation of the closely related antiapoptotic protein Bcl-X_L (174). Although, the expression of other Bcl-2 antiapoptotic and proapoptotic family members need to be studied in more detail for a complete picture to emerge, Bcl-2 expression is clearly of critical importance for survival of resting B cells.

BCR-Induced Proliferation In Vitro

Anti-IgM or anti-IgD treatment of resting splenic B cells leads to entry into the G_1 phase of the cell cycle, as indicated by size enlargement and increased RNA synthesis. These activated B cells undergo at least one round of replication if stimulated with a high concentration of polyclonal or high-affinity monoclonal anti-Ig (175,176). Although there is some induction of the antiapoptotic protein Bcl-X_L, viability of B cells in culture is enhanced slightly or not at all (177). This may reflect a balance between the increasing levels of Bcl-X_L and the decreasing levels of Bcl-2. In the absence of additional stimuli, the proliferation induced by anti-Ig is short-lived; most cells complete one division, but many do not continue cycling. A number of different cytokines can promote proliferation of B cells stimulated in vitro via the BCR, particularly in the case of human B cells (178). For murine B cells, the best costimulant is interleukin 4 (IL-4).

IL-4 strongly promotes the viability of murine B cells in vitro. How it does so is unknown because it does not induce elevated expression of Bcl-X_L (177). IL-4 does enhance the response to the BCR, such that lower doses of anti-Ig reagents are now sufficient to induce strong proliferation for at least two to three divisions (179,180).

IL-4 promotes the early activation of B cells but is not a growth factor in the traditional sense. Pretreatment of resting B cells with IL-4 shortens the length of time required for BCR stimulation to induce entry of B cells into S phase of the cell cycle. In contrast, B cells pretreated with anti-Ig will not proliferate if subsequently incubated with IL-4 alone. Thus, IL-4 should not be considered to be a growth factor for B cells, its original name of B-cell growth factor I was a misnomer. Recent examination of expression of the proteins that control the cell cycle supports this view. BCR stimulation of resting B cells leads to rapidly induced expression of cyclins D2 and D3 and the cyclin-dependent protein kinases that interact with these cyclins, cdk4 and cdk6 (181–183). IL-4 also can induce expression of cyclins D2 and D3, but this is transient and of lower magnitude than with anti-Ig (181). IL-4 does not markedly enhance the elevation of these proteins seen in response to anti-Ig alone. Anti-Ig stimulation also leads to a considerable decrease in the expression of the cdk inhibitor p27^{Kip1}. Interestingly, this decrease is transient and goes back up at later times, when proliferation is ending. Mice deficient in p27^{Kip1} due to targeted gene knockout show lymphoid hyperplasia, indicating that this is an important regulator (184,185).

The cyclin D/cdk4 or -6 complexes induced by BCR cross-linking are important for progression through the G1 phase of the cell cycle (Fig. 10). The expression of cyclin E and cdk2 are also induced in anti-Ig–stimulated B cells; this complex is thought to be important for inducing entry into the S phase. Further progression through the cell cycle is promoted by cyclin A/cdk2 and by cyclin B/cdc2, the expression of which are also induced and correlate with proliferation (181).

How BCR signaling events promote these key viability and cell cycle regulatory events are at this point poorly understood. The tyrphostin tyrosine kinase inhibitors block B-cell activation by mIg, suggesting that tyrosine phosphorylation of proteins, the central mechanism of BCR signaling, is important for this response (186).

The best studied signaling reactions involved in BCR-induced B-cell activation are those involving PIP$_2$ hydrolysis. B-cell progression from the G$_0$ to the G$_1$ phase of the cell cycle and proliferation can be stimulated by the combination of a phorbol ester, which activates PKC, and a calcium ionophore, which elevates intracellular free Ca^{2+}, but not by either type of agent alone. In some experiments, such stimulation primarily induces purified resting B cells to enter G$_1$ phase of the cell cycle but not to proliferate (187). Addition of IL-4 results in vigorous proliferation, as is seen with a low dose of anti-Ig and IL-4 (188). Other investigators have observed vigorous proliferation with just the pharmacologic activators, perhaps mimicking the response obtained with a higher dose of anti-IgM (189). Induction of cyclin D2 and cdk4 required stimulation with both phorbol esters and calcium ionophores, as was seen for B-cell proliferation (183). Correspondingly, PKC inhibitors block B-cell activation at an early stage (187). B cells from mice with the β isoform of PKC ablated by gene targeting have considerably decreased BCR-induced proliferation (42). Thus, PKC β plays a significant role in this response. Moreover, cyclosporine A and FK-506 prevent anti-Ig–induced proliferation (190), arguing for an important role of calcium signaling via calcineurin as well.

Similarly, Bcl-X$_L$ induction in response to anti-Ig is blocked by reduction of extracellular calcium or inhibition of calcium signaling through calcineurin by cyclosporine A (177). Elevation of intracellular calcium with ionophores is not sufficient to induce

expression of Bcl-X$_L$, but the combination of phorbol esters and a calcium ionophore is sufficient. Thus, calcium/calcineurin signaling events must combine with signaling events stimulated by phorbol esters (PKC activation, Ras activation) to induce Bcl-X$_L$ expression and promote B-cell viability.

The Ras signaling pathway is activated by anti-Ig and also by phorbol esters and is thought to be important for promoting proliferation in many cell types. Indeed, inhibition of the Ras/MAP kinase pathway with the inhibitor PD098059, which inhibits the activation of the intermediary enzyme MEK-1 (Fig. 6), inhibits anti-Ig–induced proliferation (J. Richards and A.L. DeFranco, manuscript submitted). Conversely, in B cells from Lyn-deficient mice, most BCR-signaling reactions appear to be somewhat slower or decreased, but MAP kinase activation is enhanced (32). These B cells exhibit enhanced proliferation, suggesting that the Erk1 and Erk2 MAP kinases may be limiting for proliferation in splenic B cells. Taken together, these results suggest that the Ras/MAP kinase pathway is quite important for BCR-induced B-cell proliferation.

Anti-Ig–induced proliferation is decreased severalfold in B cells from mice lacking the signaling components Vav or HS1, suggesting that these components also participate in B-cell proliferation in response to BCR cross-linking (191–193). Interestingly, proliferation induced by lipopolysaccharide (LPS) or by CD40L was normal in both cases, so the roles of these signaling components are restricted to BCR stimulation.

Regulation of Gene Expression by the BCR

The regulation of B-cell survival and proliferation in response to antigen contact is probably largely dependent on changes in transcription of genes such as those encoding Bcl-X$_L$ and cyclin D2. In addition, BCR engagement triggers a number of changes in gene expression that are important for promoting interaction of B cells with helper T cells, such as increased expression of class II MHC molecules, B7-2, and adhesion molecules such as ICAM-1 (CD54), CD44, CD18 (LFA-1 β chain), and LFA-3 (194). A moderate amount is now known about how the BCR directs changes in gene expression, although our understanding is still fragmentary.

As in other cell types stimulated by other receptors, BCR-induced changes in gene expression are a composite of the effects

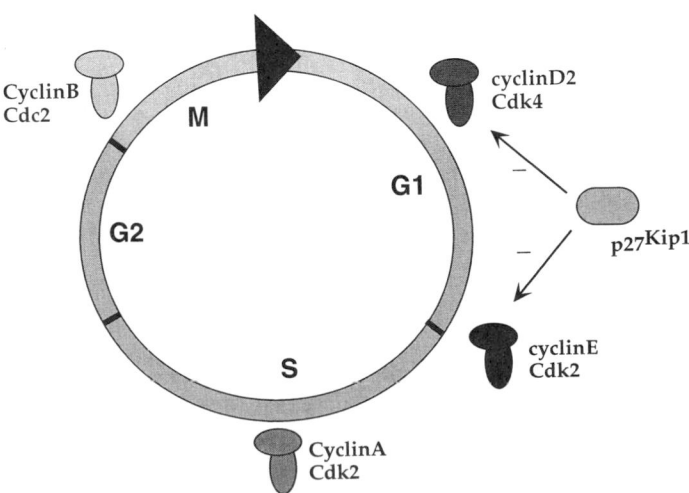

FIG. 10. Regulation of the B-cell cycle. BCR stimulation of resting mature B cells induces synthesis of proteins that regulate the cell cycle. Different pairs of cyclins and cyclin-dependent protein kinases regulate different parts of the cell cycle, as has been demonstrated in other mammalian cell types. BCR stimulation initially induces expression of cyclin D2 and Cdk4 and to a lesser extent cyclin D3 and Cdk6, which promote progress through the G1 phase. BCR stimulation also leads to a disappearance of the Cdk inhibitor p27^{Kip1}. At later times, the other cyclins and cyclin-dependent kinases appear.

of signaling reactions on constitutively expressed transcription factors, which participate in the transcription of the early response genes and secondary transcriptional events mediated by those early response genes that are transcription factors (Fig. 11). Indeed, most of the currently appreciated early response genes are transcription factors, so it is likely that many of the important downstream genes important for B-cell survival, proliferation, or interaction with helper T cells are dependent on transcription induced by the early response genes. Among the preexisting transcription factors that are directly regulated by signaling events are NF-AT, NF-κB, SRF/TCF, and CREB; these will be discussed in turn.

NF-AT, the nuclear factor of activated T cells, was initially described as a transcription factor that plays a key role in regulating transcription of IL-2. The originally defined NF-AT site in the IL-2 promoter turns out to be a composite site that binds an AP-1 transcription factor complex and the factor that is now referred to as NF-AT, which in unstimulated cells is expressed in an inactive, phosphorylated form in the cytoplasm. Antigen receptor stimulation of T cells or B cells leads to a rapid dephosphorylation of NF-AT, probably as a direct action of the Ca²⁺/calmodulin-activated serine/threonine protein phosphatase calcineurin, and this dephosphorylation permits transit to the nucleus and binding of DNA (54). NF-AT activation depends solely on elevation of cytoplasmic free calcium, and its continued activation requires continued elevation of calcium. Transcriptional activation of the IL-2 promoter NF-AT site also requires occupation of the AP-1 part of the site and AP-1 expression and function depends on other signaling events, so transcription from NF-AT sites typically requires multiple signaling events to happen concurrently.

This is an important general concept that applies to the regulation of many biological responses by receptors: receptors induce multiple signaling events, and these events often work in concert to exert changes in the cell. The cell may require two different receptors to be engaged if the response in question depends on signaling events, only a subset of which are provided by either receptor alone. Alternatively, a single receptor may provide all of the needed signaling events, but individual signaling events may be modulated by other receptors of the cell and this may have a major effect on particular responsive elements.

Four different isoforms of NF-AT have been found to date, referred to as NF-AT1 (NF-ATp), NF-AT2 (NF-ATc), NF-AT3, and NF-AT4. Lymphocytes express three of these, all but NF-AT3. NF-

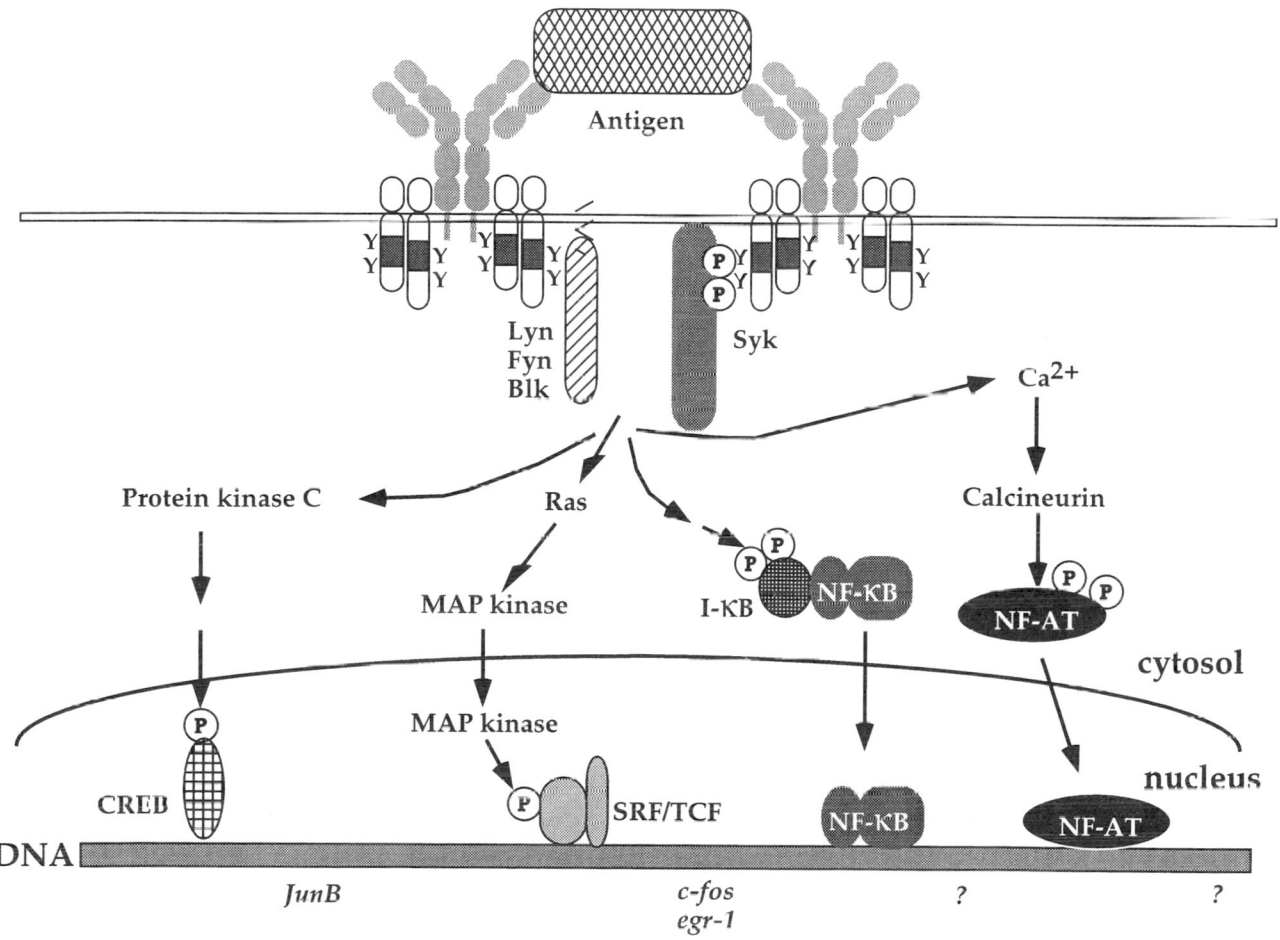

FIG. 11. Activation of transcription factors by BCR signaling. Regulation of transcription by the BCR occurs in two waves. First there is activation of preexisting transcription factors, including NF-AT, NF-κB, SRF/TCF, and CREB, as shown. These transcription factors activate transcription of a series of genes within the first hour or so of stimulation. These early response genes are mostly transcription factors as well, such as *junB, c-fos,* and *egr-1.* These induced transcription factors in turn trigger the expression of additional genes important for B-cell activation.

AT4 seems to have somewhat different DNA binding specificity compared with NF-AT1 and NF-AT2. In T cells, NF-AT is important for the induced transcription of most cytokines, as well as CD40L and FasL (54). In B cells, BCR stimulation leads to elevation of intracellular free calcium and consequent activation of NF-AT (55), but the genes regulated by NF-AT are presently unknown. The immunosuppressants cyclosporine A and FK-506 act by inhibiting the action of calcineurin, and NF-AT is a major (but not the only) target of these agents. As these immunosuppressants block BCR-induced proliferation of B cells (190), it is thought that NF-AT plays an important part in regulating one or more genes that are critical for B-cell proliferation.

BCR stimulation also leads to activation of the transcription factor NF-κB (195,196). NF-κB was originally discovered by its ability to bind to a site in the intronic enhancer of the Ig κ locus, the κB site, but was subsequently found to play a key role in many immunologic and stress responses (197). Many transformed B-cell lines express high levels of NF-κB binding activity, and it was originally postulated that this transcription factor was constitutively expressed in this lineage to promote light-chain gene expression. However, resting splenic B cells were found to have a low level of active NF-κB and to have a considerable pool of inactive NF-κB, like other cell types. Moreover, BCR stimulation activates this pool of NF-κB. In the unstimulated state, NF-κB is present in the cytoplasm as dimers, most typically as heterodimers of a p50 subunit and either a c-Rel or a RelA (p65) subunit. These dimers bind to an inhibitory subunit called I-κB. I-κB binds to the c-Rel or RelA subunit of NF-κB and both holds the complex in the cytoplasm and inhibits its DNA binding activity. Cell stimulation leads to activation of an I-κB protein kinase (198) that phosphorylates I-κB on two neighboring serine residues, which then triggers a proteosome-mediated degradation of the inhibitor. This frees NF-κB for transit to the nucleus, binding to DNA and activation of transcription by the transactivating function provided by the c-Rel/RelA subunit of the complex (Fig. 11).

The different isoforms of NF-κB appear to have distinct functions, because B cells from mice deficient in c-Rel have almost totally lost the ability to proliferate in response to BCR cross-linking (199). In these B cells, the p50/RelA form of NF-κB still is activated by BCR cross-linking, apparently in greater amounts than in wild-type cells. B cells lacking RelA show a lesser defect but still have a several-fold decreased proliferative response to BCR engagement (200). The most straightforward interpretation of these results is that p50/c-Rel and p50/RelA complexes have at least partially distinct functions, perhaps by promoting the activation of distinct genes required for full proliferation. Surprisingly, B cells lacking p50 show only a modest decrease in proliferation and do exhibit BCR-induced NF-κB DNA binding activity, which appears to be due to dimers composed of c-Rel and RelA (as homo- or heterodimers). Because these subunits contain the transactivating regions of NF-κB, their function in the absence of p50 is not entirely surprising.

BCR stimulation also activates the transcription factor CREB, which was initially discovered for its role in mediating transcriptional events induced by the second messenger cAMP. CREB is constitutively expressed and present bound to its cognate sites in the DNA, called cAMP response elements (CREs). In many cell types, elevation of cAMP activates protein kinase A, which in turn phosphorylates serine 133 of CREB, allowing it to interact with the transcriptional coactivator protein CBP (201). CREB is not solely regulated by cAMP, however, because in some circum-stances it is subject to activation by elevated cytoplasmic free Ca^{2+}. For reasons that are not known, in B cells, CREB appears to be unresponsive to elevations in cAMP, but it is activated in response to BCR stimulation. This activation also involves phosphorylation of serine 133, which appears to be dependent on PKC (44). A CRE site is found in the promoter region of the *junB* gene, which is an early response gene in BCR-stimulated B cells. Dominant negative forms of CREB block the induction of reporter genes based on the *junB* promoter, so it appears likely that CREB participates in the activation of this early response gene (202).

Downstream from the Ras/MAP kinase pathway in B cells and other cell types is the activation of transcription at serum response elements (SREs). SRE sites bind two transcription factors: serum response factor (SRF), which is constitutively bound to the SRE, and a second factor whose binding is dependent on SRF, called ternary complex factor (TCF). Two forms of TCF have been described, Elk-1 and SAP-1a, both of which are members of the Ets family of transcription factors. Both Elk-1 and SAP-1a are targets of phosphorylation by the Erk1/Erk2 MAP kinases, and phosphorylation is required for transcriptional activity (76). In addition, SRF is positively regulated by phosphorylation, probably by RSK, a serine/threonine protein kinase that is directly activated by Erk1/Erk2. Thus, SRE elements are activated by the Ras/MAP kinase pathway.

SRE elements are found in the BCR-activated early response genes *egr*-1 and *c-fos,* which are themselves transcription factors. The *egr*-1 gene has six SRE-like elements in its promoter region and they are required for BCR-induced transcription (78). Moreover, inhibition of the Ras pathway with dominant negative mutant forms of Ras block induction of Egr-1, as expected from the fact that MAP kinase appears to be the critical activator of the transcription factors that bind to the SRE. Egr-1 in turn has been shown to be important for the BCR-induced inductions of the genes encoding the cell–cell adhesion molecules ICAM-1 and CD44 (203,204), providing an example of a cascade of gene inductions in response to BCR engagement.

Another cascade of gene inductions is likely to stem from induced expression of members of the Fos/Jun family of transcription factors. Resting B cells do not express members of these families, but JunB, JunD, c-Fos, FosB, and Fra-1 are all early response genes induced in response to BCR cross-linking. In all cases, family members must dimerize via regions of protein structure called the leucine zipper to be active and bind to DNA sites referred to as TREs (TPA/PMA response elements). Jun-related members of the family can homodimerize, dimerize with other Jun members, or heterodimerize with Fos family members, whereas the latter can only heterodimerize with Jun family members. Within 2 hours of BCR stimulation, there is the appearance of dimers including JunB, JunD, c-Fos, and FosB. A further increase in the levels of these dimers is detected about 8 hours after stimulation (205). These different dimers are known to have distinct properties in participating with other transcription factors in the regulation of gene expression (206).

One interesting feature of the Fos/Jun family of transcription factors is that the regulation of expression of individual family members appears to be distinct. As described above, junB has a CRE site in its promoter and appears to be regulated by CREB activated by PKC. In contrast, c-fos appears to be primarily regulated by an SRE and the Ras/MAP kinase pathway. Therefore, the exact nature of Fos/Jun dimers will be determined by the relative strengths of a number of different signaling reactions activated by the BCR. Thus, one can imagine that regulation of these different signaling events—for example, by coreceptor participation or by expression levels of phosphatases inactivating Erk1 and Erk2—may greatly affect the response of the B cell.

Another important transcription factor that is a BCR-induced early response gene is *c-myc*. The *c-myc* gene product forms a noncovalent heterodimer with a constitutively expressed protein called Max. This complex is a transcriptional activator playing a role in inducing cell proliferation (207).

BCR stimulation also induces transcription of class II MHC genes. The enhanced expression of class II MHC is important for B-cell activation because it provides newly synthesized MHC molecules, which are routed to the endosomal compartments where they meet internalized and processed antigen. These newly synthesized MHC class II molecules bind antigen-derived peptides and then go to the cell surface, where they specify interaction with antigen-recognizing helper T cells (208). The expression of class II MHC genes is induced by either phorbol esters or by calcium ionophores, suggesting that both sides of the phosphoinositide signaling pathway play a role in this gene activation (187). Calcium elevation appears to be necessary in the context of BCR stimulation (209). Continual low-level BCR signaling appears to be responsible for at least part of the basal level of expression of MHC class I and class II molecules (170).

Antigen receptor stimulation also leads to changes in expression of receptors for cytokines and adhesion molecules. For example, anti-Ig treatment of resting B cells induces increased expression of IL-4 receptors (210). Anti-Ig also induces expression of low levels of IL-2 receptor α chain in B cells. Addition of supernatants of activated T cells to anti-Ig–stimulated B cells leads to induction of high-affinity IL-2 receptors and ability to proliferate in response to IL-2 (211). Antigen receptor stimulation also increases expression of B7-2, which is a ligand for CD28 on helper T cells and provides an important costimulatory signal to the T cell as part of antigen presentation (212). In summary, anti-Ig treatment leads to a variety of changes in B cells that are likely to influence their responsiveness to cytokines and their ability to participate in interactions with helper T cells.

DISTINCT TYPES OF ANTIBODY RESPONSES

Antibody responses to real antigens are heterogeneous with respect to mechanism. At least four different classes of antigens can readily be distinguished. For example, responses to some antigens require the presence of mature T cells and are therefore classified as T cell dependent (TD), whereas responses to other antigens do not and are classified as T cell independent (TI). This does not reflect the antigenic specificity of the B cells, but rather other properties of the antigen, such as its physical structure and its ability to interact with other receptors on the B cell. For example, TNP-dextran (TNP, trinitrophenyl, a typical hapten) induces a strong anti-TNP antibody response in nude mice, which lack mature T cells, whereas TNP-SRBCs (sheep red blood cells) induce only a weak response and TNP-protein antigens fail to induce any response at all. The latter two antigens are both T cell–dependent antigens but differ in what aspects of T-cell help are required for antibody responses, at least in vitro, as is discussed in detail below. The T cell–independent antigens are often subdivided into two categories: TI-1 and TI-2.

ANTIBODY RESPONSES TO T CELL–INDEPENDENT ANTIGENS

The initial IgM response to many infectious agents is probably largely based on T cell–independent antibody responses. As discussed below, many bacterial cell wall components fall into both TI-1 and TI-2 categories of antigens. Moreover, initial antibody responses to hepatitis B virus, vesticular stomatitis virus, and polyoma virus particles have been shown to be T cell independent (213–215).

It should be noted that the evidence for T cell–independent antibody responses is overwhelmingly derived from studies with mice. Evidence for parallel mechanisms of antibody production in humans is disappointingly scant (216). Nonetheless, a number of observations with vaccines and immunodeficiencies make it likely that T cell–independent antibody responses are important for humoral immunity in humans as in mice. For example, one characteristic of TI-2 responses in the mouse is that they are slow to appear following birth (217). Mice of approximately 3 to 6 weeks of age are quite competent at mounting a TD antibody response but fail to make TI-2 responses. A similar phenomenon appears to occur in humans. The initial vaccine to *Haemophilus influenzae* type b was a capsular polysaccharide preparation, which would clearly be a TI-2 antigen in the mouse. This vaccine induced a strong antibody response, but only in children over 2 years of age. Conjugation of this polysaccharide to an immunogenic carrier protein made the vaccine efficacious in much younger children, 2 months and older, which are an important group susceptible to *H. influenzae* infection (218). The most likely interpretation of these observations is that the protein component provides epitopes for helper T cells and thereby makes a TD response possible, whereas the original vaccine requires a TI-2 response that is not functional in young children.

Originally, the subdivision of T cell–independent antigens into TI-1 and TI-2 subgroupings was based on their ability or inability, respectively, to elicit an antibody response in another type of immunodeficient mouse, the *xid* (X-linked immunodeficiency) mouse. These mice are now known to exhibit a loss-of-function missense mutation in the gene encoding the intracellular tyrosine kinase Btk, which participates in BCR signal transduction. These mice make relatively normal responses to many T cell–dependent antigens and to some of the TI antigens, but they are severely deficient in their ability to make antibodies in response to immunization with most polysaccharide antigens. It should be noted, however, that there are circumstances in which antibody responses can be seen in *xid* mice to antigens that are by other criteria TI-2 antigens, so at this point there is no absolute empirical criterion to separate TI-1 from TI-2 antigens. Nonetheless, the categorization of TI antigens into these two groups is quite useful and almost certainly reflects important mechanistic differences in antibody responses to these two types of antigens.

TI-1 Antigens

T cell-independent type 1 antigens have the unusual and dramatic property of being polyclonal B-cell activators. Polyclonal B-cell activators, as the name implies, are directly mitogenic for murine B cells, irrespective of antigen specificity, and induce them to differentiate to antibody-secreting cells (Fig. 12). Many of these compounds are components of bacterial cell walls (LPS, peptido-

Typical Antigen

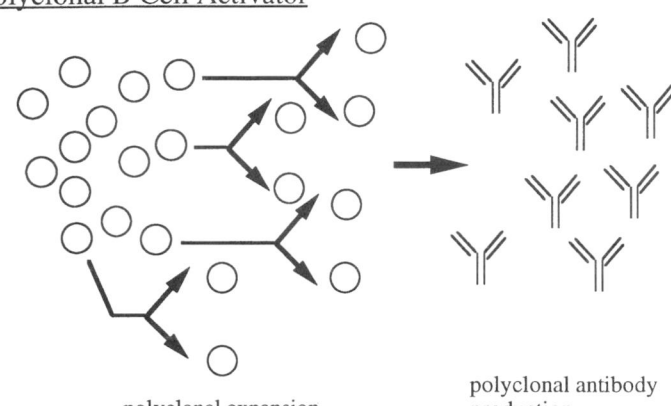

clonal expansion

specific antibody
production

Polyclonal B Cell Activator

polyclonal expansion

polyclonal antibody
production

FIG. 12. Mode of action of polyclonal B-cell activators. In an antibody response to a typical antigen, the rare antigen-specific B cells are activated to proliferate and make antibodies. In contrast, polyclonal B-cell activators such as bacterial LPS activate a sizeable fraction of B cells (as high as one in three) to proliferate and differentiate into antibody-secreting cells. At low concentrations of the activator, B cells that bind to the activator via mIg may be favored so that the antibody produced in such circumstances can be largely specific.

glycan, lipoprotein, porin, etc.), and it is likely that the ability of multicellular organisms to recognize and respond to them represents an evolved part of the immune response to bacteria (219,220). Indeed, host defense responses to LPS are present in invertebrate organisms such as *Drosophila melanogaster* and *Limulus polyphemus* as well as in vertebrates (221,222). The best studied of these compounds is LPS, a major constituent of the outer leaflet of the outer membrane of Gram-negative bacteria. At doses of LPS below those that induce polyclonal B-cell proliferation and antibody production, haptenated LPS (TNP-LPS, etc.) can induce specific antihapten antibody production. One interpretation of this phenomenon is that hapten-specific B cells bind the haptenated antigen and in so doing concentrate the LPS, providing the necessary local concentration to bind to B-cell low-affinity LPS receptors, which then drive B-cell activation. Additionally, it is possible that BCR signaling synergizes with the signal from the polyclonal B-cell activator.

The identity of LPS receptors on B cells is enigmatic, although some progress has been made in understanding how macrophages recognize LPS. Macrophages respond to LPS by the production of the cytokines IL-1, IL-6, tumor necrosis factor (TNF-α), and interferon-α; by the secretion of the chemokines IL-8 and macrophage inflammatory proteins 1 and 2; and by the release of eicosanoid mediators such as prostaglandins (223,224). One or more of these macrophage-derived mediators likely contribute to antibody responses to LPS and other TI-1 antigens (225). The macrophage responds to much lower concentrations of LPS than does the B cell, with a strong response occurring at about 1 ng/ml LPS, compared

with 10 μg/ml required by the B cell for a polyclonal B-cell response. This difference in sensitivity is due to the cell surface expression by macrophages of CD14, which can bind monomers of LPS transferred to it by the serum protein LPS-binding protein (226). CD14 is a glycosyl-phosphatidylinositol-linked protein, and as such has no transmembrane or cytoplasmic domains. It should not be able to send signals to the cell interior on its own. Moreover, macrophages lacking CD14 can still respond to LPS but require much higher concentrations (226). This has led to the hypothesis that macrophages and B cells both express low-affinity LPS receptors, which may be the same. When LPS is used at high concentrations, it can bind directly to this low-affinity receptor and stimulate most B cells to proliferate and differentiate into antibody-secreting cells: this is the polyclonal B-cell activator phenomenon. Low concentrations of LPS, in contrast, can only stimulate macrophages or B cells if another receptor—CD14 in the case of the macrophage and mIg of a specificity that can bind to an epitope on the LPS molecule in the case of B cells—is present (Fig. 13). This second receptor has a high-affinity interaction with LPS, which allows the low-affinity signaling receptor to bind and induce biologic responses: production of cytokines and other mediators in the case of the macrophage, and proliferation and differentiation in the case of the antigen-specific B cell. In this scenario, the binding of hapten to the BCR also may trigger BCR signaling reactions, which would also promote B-cell activation. Although this is an attractive model, little is known about the molecular details of how LPS activates B cells. Curiously, although LPS is a strong activator of human as well as murine macrophages, it activates only murine B

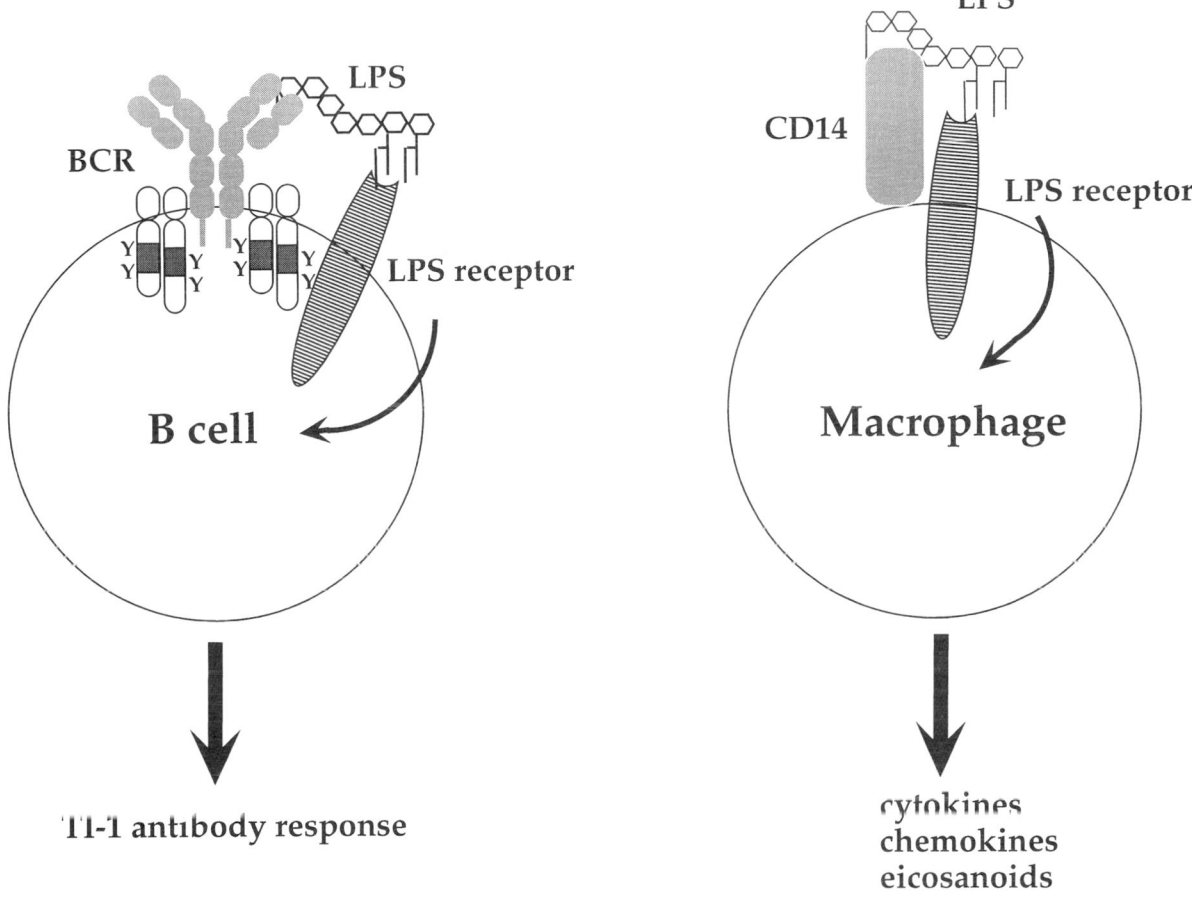

FIG. 13. Cooperation of receptors in TI-1 antibody responses. The macrophage responds to low concentrations of LPS by using CD14 to bind to LPS with high affinity. CD14 is believed not to be a signaling receptor because all of its protein is outside the cell and it is only attached to the membrane by covalently linked lipid. A putative LPS receptor binds LPS with low affinity, but can promote the response to low concentrations of LPS if the LPS is held on the membrane efficiently by CD14, increasing its effective concentration. By analogy, membrane Ig specific for epitopes on the LPS may allow for efficient antibody production in a TI-1 antibody response by binding LPS with high affinity and allowing the low-affinity LPS receptor to bind LPS more efficiently and activate the B cell.

cells. Other bacterial cell wall components are polyclonal B-cell activators in mice and humans. For example, cell walls of *Staphlococcus aureus* Cowan I strain, a Gram-positive bacterium, are potent polyclonal activators of human B cells. This response requires protein A on the surface of the *S. aureus* particles, but also requires other cell wall components (216).

TI-2 Antigens

T cell-independent type 2 antigens are typically repeating polymers such as polysaccharide antigens and lack the intrinsic polyclonal B cell–activating properties characteristic of TI-1 antigens. Bacterial cell walls contain both polyclonal B cell–activating molecules and repetitious capsular polysaccharides and hence are composites of TI-1 and TI-2 antigens. Viral particles also have antigenic epitopes displayed in a highly repetitious manner, probably explaining their ability to elicit TI IgM responses early in an immune response (227).

The physical characteristics of TI-2 antigens are important for their ability to stimulate antibody responses. For example, antibody responses to a haptenated polyacrylamide antigen require a minimum of 12 to 16 properly spaced haptens per molecule in order to induce a strong in vivo TI antibody response (228). These results were interpreted as indicating that an immunon of one antigen molecule and an oligomeric cluster of bound BCR molecules was formed on the surface of the B cell and that this complex was required to induce an efficient TI-2 antibody response. If the polymer has too few epitopes, then it induces tolerance, even during an ongoing response to a haptenated protein (T cell-dependent) antigen (229).

Highly haptenated proteins may contain a similar number of epitopes to TI-2 antigens, but still be T cell–dependent antigens, indicating that the physical form of the antigen is an important feature of the TI-2 antigen. The flexible nature of polysaccharide backbones may allow the antigen-bound BCR molecules to cluster into a structure that is very efficient at generating intracellular signaling reactions. In the case of membrane-bound virus particles, the ability of viral membrane proteins to move in the viral membrane may likewise promote the formation of efficient BCR signaling clusters.

To simulate a TI-2 antigen and thereby study the mechanism by which it activates the B cell, anti-IgM and anti-IgD have been conjugated to dextran molecules. These reagents are dramatically more potent (about 10,000 times) than soluble anti-Ig at inducing B cell proliferation and BCR signaling events such as phosphoinositide breakdown and calcium elevation (230). The requirements for induction of antibody production by anti-Ig-dextran–stimulated B cells are similar to those for TI-2 antigen–stimulated B cells in vitro, supporting the idea that this is a useful model for TI-2 antigens (217,219). Mitogenic concentrations of soluble anti-Ig antibodies rapidly cap all surface BCRs. Subsequent signaling and B-cell activation depends on the presence of high-affinity anti-Ig that can rapidly bind and induce signaling of small numbers of BCR complexes as they become expressed at the surface (175,176). In contrast, anti-Ig-dextran conjugates are fully mitogenic at doses that bind to only a minority of BCR molecules and do not downmodulate BCR expression. Therefore, the anti-Ig-dextran/BCR complexes appear to signal efficiently for a prolonged period and are internalized slowly. Thus, a key feature of TI-2 antigens may be their ability to induce the formation of persistent, efficient BCR signaling complexes (immunons) at the cell surface. The ability of TI-2 antigens to activate B cells independently of T cells, therefore, appears to reflect their superior ability to induce BCR signaling reactions (Fig. 14). Many TI-2 antigens can fix complement (either via the alternative pathway or by binding low-affinity natural antibody), and so may also bring the CR2/CD19/CD81 complex together with the BCR on the cell surface. As described above, this complex can enhance B-cell activation. However, it should be noted that mice deficient in CD19 expression have elevated TI-2 responses, not depressed ones (231), indicating that the TI-2 response is not dependent on CD19.

Stimulation of highly purified resting B cells with TI-2 antigens or dextran anti-Ig conjugates in vitro does not induce antibody production, suggesting that these responses have additional require-

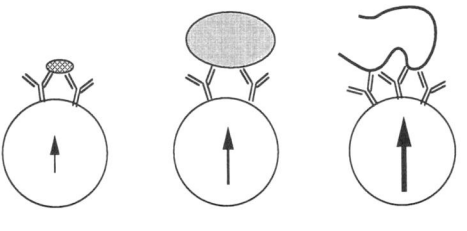

| Antigen: | soluble protein | cell-bound | polysaccharide |
| Signaling: | moderate | strong | very strong |

FIG. 14. Importance of antigen structure for BCR signaling. An attractive hypothesis to explain the different requirements for making antibody responses is that some antigens are much better than others at triggering signaling by the BCR. In particular, this hypothesis holds that soluble protein antigens can only induce moderate signaling, whereas cell-bound antigens, either by virtue of their polyvalent nature or due to participation of cell–cell adhesion molecules, can induce strong signaling. The flexible and repeating nature of polysaccharide antigens may make them especially good at triggering antigen receptor signaling, as suggested by experiments with anti-Ig molecules linked to dextran. These antigens typically demonstrate the least requirement for additional signals from helper T cells or macrophages.

ments. Addition of cytokines can support a strong antibody response (217,219). Especially important in promoting this response are IL-2, IFN-γ, IL-3, and granulocyte-macrophage colony-stimulating factor (GM-CSF), although none of these is required. IL-5 also can promote in vitro antibody responses to TI-2 antigens. Interesting in this regard is the observation that anti-Ig dextran induces expression of IL-5 receptors on B cells (232). In these in vitro responses, IFN-γ also promotes switching to IgG3, the predominant IgG subclass seen in mouse TI-2 responses, suggesting that it participates in vivo in most circumstances. The source of these cytokines in vivo is not well established, although the NK cell is one attractive possibility, especially in viral responses (219). In normal animals, T cells responding to other antigens nearby also could be the source of these cytokines.

In vitro antibody responses to TI-2 antigens or to anti-Ig-dextran conjugates are also strongly stimulated by low concentrations of a number of polyclonal B-cell activators, including LPS, porins, lipoprotein, and bacterial DNA (219). In this situation, the polyclonal B-cell activators are active at submitogenic concentrations, and this response requires the strong BCR cross-linking seen with anti-Ig-dextran because soluble anti-IgM will not substitute.

Bacterial DNA is apparently distinguished from endogenous mammalian DNA by the frequency of sequences containing unmethylated CpG dinucleotides (233). Methylation of cytosine in CpG sequences is an important gene regulatory device in vertebrate organisms. Because unmethylated CpG sequences are primarily found in the upstream regions of expressed genes, their frequency in mammalian DNA is low. Thus, the presence of large amounts of unmethylated CpG sequences is a hallmark of infection, and by stimulating TI-2 responses, it, as well as various bacterial cell wall structures, can promote the initial immune response to nearby TI-2 antigens. Thus, bacterial cell walls, which contain both repetitious polysaccharides and polyclonal B-cell activators, can stimulate B-cell activation in an extremely potent fashion by the combination of TI-2 stimulation of strong signaling via the BCR of antigen-specific B cells and the induction of terminal differentiation by the polyclonal B-cell activator components.

B Cells Responsible for TI-2 Responses

The spleen has been found to be important for the ability of mice, rats, and humans to make antibody responses to polysaccharide antigens (217,234), and this may reflect an especially important role of marginal zone B cells in making these responses. Marginal zone B cells are located at the margin between the white pulp and the red pulp in the spleen, in contrast to most B cells, which are in the follicles. The marginal zone includes a distinctive type of macrophage that can readily bind polysaccharide antigens, and marginal zone B cells, which are CD23⁻, IgMʰⁱIgDˡᵒ largely nonrecirculating cells. On the basis of repopulation after irradiation, it has been argued that marginal zone B cells represent a distinct subset of B cells, which are uniquely capable of mounting TI-2 responses (234,235). This hypothesis lacks direct support, however, because in vitro antibody responses to anti-Ig-dextran conjugates and cytokines can be efficiently mounted by cells of follicular phenotype as well as by cells of marginal zone phenotype (236). Moreover, it is striking that the phenotype and number of marginal zone B cells are very similar to the recently generated B cells that have emigrated from the bone marrow (167). Marginal zone B cells are probably a mixture of these recent emigrants and longer-lived distinctive marginal zone B cells, which are relatively sessile and include some memory cells (234,235).

B-1 B Cells: A Distinctive B-Cell Subset

Most peripheral B cells belong to the long-lived recirculating follicular B-cell population, but there are probably several other subsets of B cells as well. As is described below, newly generated B cells are functionally distinct in that they are highly susceptible to tolerance induction. In addition, these cells will all die within about 1 week of their generation unless they are selected into the long-lived follicular pool (167). Less well understood is the subset of B cells that occupy the marginal zones in the spleen, as described in the preceding section. Finally, there is a numerically small subpopulation of B cells referred to as the B-1 subset. These cells express high levels of IgM, low levels of IgD, and Mac1 (CD11b/CD18) and fail to express CD23. Some of these cells express low levels of CD5, whereas others do not; the former are referred to as B-1a cells and the latter as B-1b cells (237). B-1 cells are primarily generated during fetal life and the neonatal period and are characterized by restricted IgH gene rearrangements (164). These rearrangements primarily use a few V_H genes—those located near the D_H genes—and often they do not contain N region additions (238). Thus, their repertoire is much more limited than that of the conventional B cells. Moreover, B1 B cells are primarily located in the peritoneal and pleural cavities. None are present in lymph nodes, although a small number are found in the spleen, making up 2% to 3% of splenic B cells. Curiously, splenic B-1 cells do not express Mac-1, although their phenotype is otherwise similar to peritoneal B-1 cells (239). A substantial number of splenic B-1 cells are IgM-secreting plasma cells, and often their antibody dominates serum IgM. In addition, a substantial fraction of the IgA-producing plasma cells of the gut are probably derived from B-1 cells (240). The function of the B-1 cells remains mysterious, although the most attractive idea is that they produce antibodies that are useful for protection against ubiquitous bacteria and thus provide an immune defense early in life, before the normal adaptive immune response is fully functional. In support of this view, adoptive transfer of peritoneal B-1 cells into SCID mice reconstitutes IgA production against many gut bacteria (240).

A unique property of B-1 cells is that they have the potential to proliferate and expand almost indefinitely in vivo. With regard to B-cell activation, they are capable of making TD antibody responses but do not participate in germinal center reactions (239,241).

On the basis of their special properties, it has been argued that B-1 cells represent a separate lineage of B cells, and this view has considerable experimental support. For example, adoptive transfer of precursors from fetal liver or omentum readily reconstitutes the B-1 population, whereas precursors from adult bone marrow reconstitute conventional B cells but not B-1 cells (164,239). Thus, it appears that B-cell precursors early in life are committed to a B-1 lineage, both with regard to Ig repertoire and with regard to phenotypic properties, whereas later in life B-cell precursors are committed to make the more diverse follicular B cells.

Although certain B-cell precursors are committed to the B-1 lineage, antigen-based stimuli appear to be important for newly generated B-1 cells to become long lived, as is the case for conventional B cells (239). This possibility was initially suggested by in vitro experiments in which stimulation of splenic B cells with anti-

Ig antibodies and IL-6 was found to induce the acquisition of a B-1–like phenotype (242). Moreover, various Ig transgenic mice exhibit either many B-1 cells or almost none, a result that is most consistent with a BCR signaling requirement for production or survival of B-1 cells. For example, the antilysozyme Ig transgenic mice have almost no B-1 cells, but when this transgene was introduced into the moth-eaten viable background many B-1 cells were present (243). Moth-eaten viable is a partial loss of function mutation of the tyrosine phosphatase SHP-1. SHP-1 inhibits BCR signaling, so BCR signaling is enhanced in these mutant mice. The simplest interpretation is that some endogenous ligand interacting with the antilysozyme BCR is sufficient for entry of conventional B cells into the long-lived follicular pool but is insufficient for entry of B-1 committed precursors into the long-lived B-1 pool, but when the signaling is enhanced, then it is over the threshold and positive selection into the B-1 pool can occur. Thus, it appears that there are different signaling thresholds for positive selection of conventional and B-1 cells. This hypothesis is consistent with the fact that B-1 cells are preferentially lost in various mice in which genes encoding signaling components, including Btk, Vav, and CD19, are removed by targeted gene ablation (38). All of these components are likely to participate in BCR signaling, but conventional B cells can develop in their absence, perhaps because a lower level of signaling is required by those cells. There also may be different thresholds for negative selection as well, which could explain the frequent low-affinity self-reactivity seen in the B-1 population (239).

ANTIBODY RESPONSES TO T CELL–DEPENDENT ANTIGENS

Overview of TD Responses

Antibody responses to most protein antigens are dependent on helper T cells. For example, most such responses are not seen after immunization of athymic "nude" mice, which have very few T cells. Naive, long-lived B cells circulate through the blood and lymph nodes until they contact specific antigen, which typically would happen in the T cell area in the spleen or lymph node. Antigen is brought to this location from peripheral sites by macrophages and/or dendritic cells. Antigen contact causes B cells to stop migrating and remain in the T cell zone (244,245). Specific B cells internalize antigen via the BCR complex, process it to peptides that can combine with MHC class II molecules, and then display the resulting peptide/MHC class II complexes on the cell surface. Naive antigen-specific helper T cells are also activated in this location, probably by antigen-presenting interdigitating dendritic cells. These activated helper T cells search for and find B cells presenting the antigen. Antigen recognition by the T cell leads to formation of stable conjugates with the antigen-presenting B cell, followed by delivery of soluble and membrane-bound helper signals, as described in detail below. These signals induce B cells to proliferate and terminally differentiate into antibody-secreting cells. This response initially occurs in the T cell zone and is responsible for the first burst of IgM produced in a primary antibody response. Instead of terminally differentiating in situ, some B cells stimulated in this way migrate into the follicular region and initiate the germinal center reaction. This pathway requires the induced expression of CD40 ligand by the T cell and receipt of this signal by CD40 on the B cell. The related molecules OX40 (on the T cell) and OX40 ligand (on the B cell) may promote the nongerminal center pathway (246). The germinal center pathway involves rapid proliferation and rapid somatic mutation of the B cell's immunoglobulin genes. After somatic mutation, germinal center B cells undergo stringent selection, with only those cells expressing higher affinity mIg molecules surviving. Class switching to other Ig heavy-chain isotypes is also prominent in germinal center B cells. Finally, germinal center B cells either terminally differentiate to plasma cells or become quiescent memory cells. Most antibody-secreting plasma cells live for only a few days before undergoing programmed cell death, although plasma cells generated in the germinal center can migrate to the gut or the bone marrow, where they can live and secrete antibodies for more than 20 days.

B-Cell Presentation of Antigen to Helper T Cells

Most TD antibody responses require direct interaction between antigen-specific B cells and helper T cells. This interaction begins with the helper T cell encountering the appropriate complex of antigen-derived peptide and MHC class II molecule displayed on the surface of a B cell. If the BCR on the B cell can bind the antigen in question, then the antigen is taken up by receptor-mediated endocytosis, and the activation of antigen-specific helper T cells occurs very efficiently. If the antigen does not bind to the BCR, it is taken up inefficiently by fluid phase pinocytosis. In the latter case, 10^3- to 10^4-fold greater antigen concentrations are required to activate the T cell (247). Thus, the BCR plays a powerful role in mediating antigen uptake and thereby promoting interaction of antigen-specific B cells with helper T cells that recognize linked antigenic determinants (Fig. 15).

Antigen uptake by the BCR appears to be a consequence of continual BCR cycling between the cell surface and internal membrane compartments called endosomes. In a study with an antigen-specific EBV-transformed B-cell line, nearly one half of the BCR complexes were found in endosomes at any given time (248). When monovalent antigen (tetanus toxin) was added to these cells, the antigen was internalized with a half-time of 8.5 minutes. This internalization occurred with ligands of varying sizes. Interestingly, when free BCR complexes were internalized, very few of them were degraded before returning to the cell surface. In contrast, when tetanus toxin-bound BCR molecules were internalized, some of them returned to the surface, but some of them were degraded. Proteolysis of both antigen and mIg were evident. The

mechanism by which ligand-bound BCR is preferentially degraded is not known.

Although it is attractive to think that antigen receptor signaling promotes internalization and/or targeting of mIg-antigen complexes for proteolytic processing, current evidence argues against such roles. Although cross-linking of the BCR is usually required for signal transduction, it is not required for antigen internalization or for efficient antigen presentation (248,249). Moreover, mutations of the transmembrane region of the μ chain have yielded mIgM molecules that appear to signal normally, but are deficient in presentation of specific antigen (250). These molecules internalize the antigen but do not take it to the appropriate subcellular compartment where peptide loading of MHC class II molecules is most efficient (251).

Antigen presentation by the BCR requires Ig-α/Ig-β binding to mIg, and this function is contained in the cytoplasmic domains of Ig-α and Ig-β (252,253). This function is apparently distinct from the ITAMs, however, because mutation of tyrosines in Ig-β do not abrogate the antigen-presentation function of chimeric molecules containing the Ig-β cytoplasmic domain (252). Interestingly, chimeric molecules with the cytoplasmic domains of Ig-α or of Ig-β induce trafficking of bound antigen to different intracellular compartments, indicating distinctive functions of these cytoplasmic domains (253). Ig-α chimeras take the bound antigen into a compartment rich in newly synthesized MHC class II molecules, presumably the compartment where most peptide loading occurs (see Chapter 9). In contrast, Ig-β chimeras take the bound antigen preferentially to transferrin receptor-containing endosomes. How these two distinct targeting signals work together in the intact BCR remains to be determined. Moreover, in the case of mIgG, the cyoplasmic tail of the γ heavy chain also has a targeting signal for antigen presentation (254), so BCRs of IgG+ memory B cells have three targeting signals for antigen presentation.

Although BCR signaling may not contribute to antigen uptake, it does promote helper T cell–B cell interaction in other ways. Anti-Ig activated B cells are considerably better at presenting antigen to CD4+ T cells on a per cell basis than are resting B cells (255). In part, this may reflect induction of B7-2, which provides costimulatory signals to T cells via CD28 (256). Moreover, stimulation of resting B cells with either anti-IgM or with the phosphoinositide second messenger mimicking agents PMA, which activates PKC, and ionomycin, a calcium ionophore, leads to a rapid increase in clustering of B cells to cloned helper T cells (257). This clustering probably involves the LFA-1 and ICAM-1 adhesion molecule pair because phorbol esters rapidly increase the homotypic cell interac-

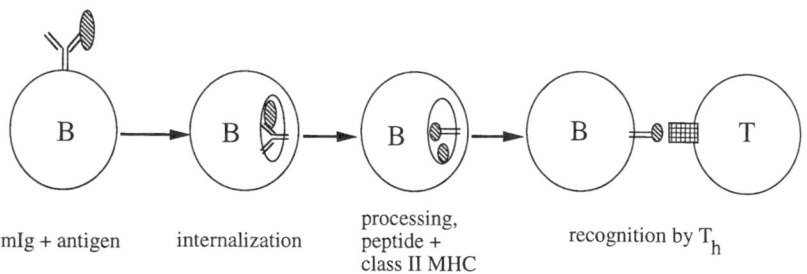

mIg + antigen   internalization   processing, peptide + class II MHC   recognition by T_h

FIG. 15. Antigen presentation by B cells. B cells that bind a particular antigen via the BCR can efficiently internalize this antigen. The internalized protein antigen is then processed by proteolysis in either late endosomes or lysosomes. Appropriate antigen-derived peptides can combine with class II MHC molecules, which are routed to late endosomes before trafficking to the cell surface. Once formed, the peptide/MHC complex can come to the cell surface, where it serves as a recognition structure for antigen-specific helper T cells.

tions of B-cell lines via these molecules. Treatment of B cells with anti-Ig also enhanced LFA-1/ICAM-1–based cell–cell adhesion (258). Presumably, BCR signaling regulates the affinity of these adhesion molecules, although the molecular mechanism has not been defined. As mentioned above, BCR signaling reactions increase the expression of class II MHC genes, and this is also likely to enhance antigen presentation by the B cell, especially because newly synthesized class II MHC molecules are primarily responsible for binding peptides in endosomes (208). To summarize, the BCR plays two roles in antigen presentation: it efficiently internalizes antigen, directing it to relevant internal compartments, and it stimulates signal transduction events that enhance adhesion and expression of class II MHC and B7-2 (Fig. 16). These and possibly other events promote the general ability of the antigen-recognizing B cell to present that antigen to specific helper T cells.

Model T Cell–Dependent Antibody Responses

Three types of model antibody responses have been used primarily to assess the nature of the signals from helper T cells that promote B cell activation. One well-studied model of antibody response uses soluble anti-Ig antibodies as a surrogate for antigen. Low concentrations of anti-Ig induce resting B cells to exit the resting G_0 state and to enter the G_1 phase of the cell cycle. Higher concentrations of high-affinity anti-Ig can induce substantial proliferation of B cells, but no antibody production. Addition of the supernatants of activated T cells to anti-Ig–stimulated B cells enhances proliferation and induces vigorous antibody production (259,260). Biochemical purification identified IL-4 as an important cytokine responsible for enhancing proliferation of anti-Ig–stimulated B cells (261). IL-2 also can have activity in this assay and, with human but not mouse B cells, IFN-γ also can enhance proliferation to anti-Ig.

The available evidence indicates that the role of IL-4 in B-cell proliferation is not as a growth factor analogous to the role of IL-2

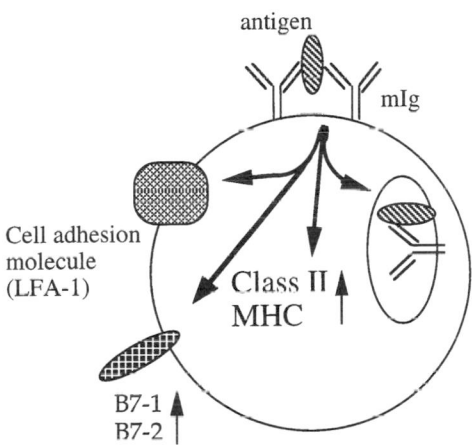

FIG. 16. Multiple roles for the BCR in antigen presentation to helper T cells. In addition to antigen uptake, as depicted in Fig. 15, antigen binding to the BCR also triggers signal transduction reactions. These reactions induce class II MHC gene expression, which provides more class II MHC molecules to the late endosomes where they can bind antigen-derived peptides. In addition, BCR signaling modulates the affinity of cell–cell adhesion molecules on the B-cell surface and induces the expression of B7-2, and thereby promotes effective interaction with helper T cells.

in promoting T-cell proliferation, but rather as an agent that enhances the response to BCR stimulation and also promotes the viability of the B cells. For example, anti-Ig must be present continuously to stimulate proliferation, whereas the effect of IL-4 requires an early presence more than a late presence (179,180). This is very different from the situation in T cells, where TCR stimulation induces IL-2 production and IL-2 receptor expression, which then drive T-cell proliferation in the absence of further TCR stimulation.

IgM production in response to anti-Ig treatment of resting B cells requires IL-4, IL-5, and a third, late-acting cytokine, which can be either IL-2 or IL-6 (Fig. 17) (262). In this response, IL-4 clearly plays a role in promoting proliferation, and IL-2 and IL-6 promote differentiation, because the latter agents can be added for the last 18 hours of culture and be fully effective. Recently, IL-6 has been shown to induce expression of the cell cycle inhibitor protein $p18^{INK4c}$, which binds to and inhibits cyclinD/cdk4 or -6 complexes, suggesting that this is how it induces growth arrest as a prelude to terminal differentiation (263). Induction of terminal differentiation presumably involves other genetic events as well. In the case of IL-2, a key molecular event controlling differentiation is the induction of the transcriptional regulator Blimp-1. This molecule is upregulated in differentiating B cells, and it induces terminal differentiation upon transfection into B cells (264,265).

The role of IL-5 in these antibody responses is less clear. It does not enhance proliferation of B cells stimulated with anti-Ig and IL-4, although it does promote proliferation of some B-cell lines and B-1 cells (266,267). One of IL-5's effects is to induce receptors for IL-2 (268). For example, resting B cells are induced to express the β and α chains of the IL-2 receptor in response to IL-4 and IL-5, respectively (269). In the BCL₁ leukemic B-cell line, IL-5 and IL-2 will cooperate to induce this cell to secrete antibody. In this system, IL-5 induces IL-2 receptors, and IL-2 is apparently responsible for activating expression of some of the genes characteristic of the differentiated secretory cell, such as the gene-encoding J chain (270). It seems likely that IL-5 also promotes differentiation on its own because in some circumstances IL-4 and IL-5 are sufficient to promote strong antibody production, for example, when anti-Ig is removed from the culture before terminal differentiation (271).

One important issue regarding these findings is which antigens behave like anti-Ig in activating B cells. In one study, hapten-specific B cells were isolated and stimulated in vitro with various haptenated antigens and IL-4. A haptenated TI-2 antigen could induce B-cell proliferation, whereas a haptenated protein antigen could not (272), suggesting that many protein antigens do not stimulate sufficient BCR signaling to support a vigorous antibody response in the presence of IL-4 + IL-5 + IL-2 or IL-6. In contrast, very potent engagement of the BCR, as is seen with anti-Ig-dextran conjugates does promote antibody responses in the presence of various cytokines, as described above. Nonetheless, soluble proteins are capable of eliciting significant BCR signaling, as evidenced by increased protein tyrosine phosphorylation, phosphoinositide breakdown, calcium elevation, and c-myc induction in antigen-specific B cells (159,273–275).

A second highly studied model system uses haptenated SRBCs as the antigen. This antigen was the first to be successfully used to generate an antibody response in vitro, and it was found that this response requires T cells, which could be replaced by supernatants of activated helper T cells (276). These supernatants were fractionated and tested for activity in this assay. It was found that the combination of IL-2 and IFN-γ was able to substitute for the helper T cell-derived supernatants (277). Interestingly, human B cells stim-

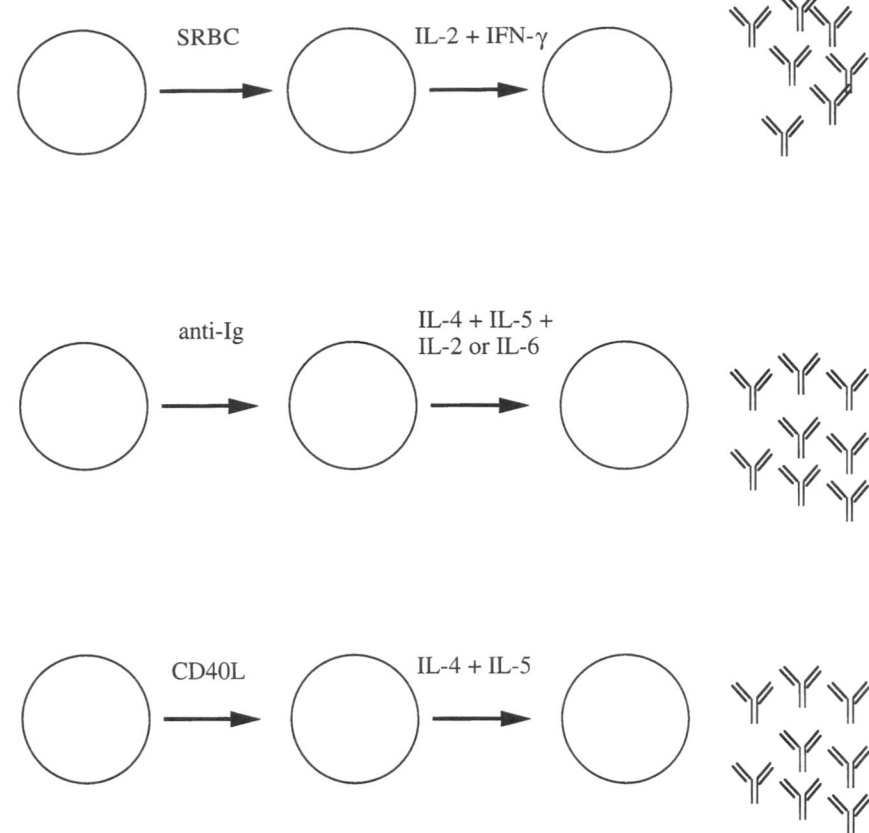

FIG. 17. Model T cell–dependent antibody responses. As described in the text, three highly studied models for TD antibody responses involve the anti-SRBC response, the polyclonal antibody response to soluble anti-Ig antibodies, and the response to CD40L. In all three models, cytokines promote proliferation and induce terminal differentiation.

ulated with *Staphylococcus aureus* Cowan I stain (SAC; the Gram-positive bacterium that expresses immunoglobulin-binding protein A on its surface) produce polyclonal antibody upon addition of IL-2 and IFN-γ (278), indicating that these two cytokines can contribute to antibody responses to several distinct types of antigens. Similarly, anti-Ig-dextran–stimulated B cells also produce antibody upon addition of IL-2 and IFN-γ, but soluble anti-Ig–stimulated B cells do not, indicating that strong BCR signaling is required for this response (219).

Although IL-2 often plays important roles in promoting antibody responses, the impact of IFN-γ is more complex. In many contexts, IFN-γ suppresses antibody responses, whereas in some cases, such as the situations listed above, IFN-γ stimulates antibody production. In particular, IFN-γ often antagonizes effects of IL-4 on B cells (279).

One surprising feature of these two model systems is that the SRBC system requires IL-2 and IFN-γ, which are products of one subset of helper T cells (T_{H1} cells), whereas the anti-Ig system requires IL-4, IL-5, and IL-6, which are produced by the other major subset of helper T cells, T_{H2} cells, and not by T_{H1} cells. The anti-Ig system also exhibits antibody production when IL-2 is substituted for IL-6, and a third subset of helper T cells, called T_{H0} cells, produces IL-2, IL-4, and IL-5, along with other cytokines. Thus, the first model system may represent B-cell activation proceeding with a T_{H2} or T_{H0} helper cell, whereas the second model system may represent a route of B-cell activation involving a T_{H1} helper cell.

In contrast to what is seen with the two model TD antibody responses described above, the antibody response to soluble protein antigens requires contact with helper T cells (280). Thus, SRBC and anti-Ig provide a signal required for B-cell activation that soluble proteins cannot provide. The most likely explanation is that the difference is a quantitative one rather than a qualitative one, i.e., that anti-Ig and SRBCs are relatively strong inducers of BCR signaling reactions, whereas soluble protein antigens are weaker inducers of these signaling reactions (Fig. 14).

In a variety of model systems, activated T_H cells can activate B cells that present antigen to them (280). Often B-cell activation is markedly improved if BCR signaling is also triggered. For example, in studies of lysozyme-specific Ig transgenic B cells, T_H specific for an alloantigen could provide help for antibody production, but this was greatly enhanced by addition of lysozyme (159). In these experiments the signal provided by the T_H cannot be provided by soluble cytokines from T cells but can be supplied by isolated plasma membranes of activated T cells, and hence is due to a cell-bound molecule.

Monoclonal antibodies that would block the T_H cell-bound signal were obtained after immunization with membranes from activated T_H cells. At about the same time, the ligand for CD40 was cloned and was found to be recognized by these antibodies (281). Moreover, a soluble CD40-Ig chimeric protein was found to block the ability of activated T_H cell plasma membranes to induce B cells to enter the G1 phase of the cell cycle. A related chimera also blocked the induction of B-cell proliferation by live T_H cells (282).

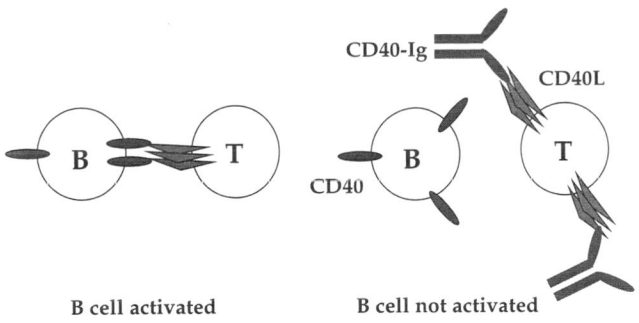

FIG. 18. Inhibition of B-cell activation by soluble CD40-Ig. B cells are stimulated by activated helper T cells in a CD40L-dependent manner. In a variety of systems where B-cell activation is dependent on contact with helper T cells (*left*), addition of a fusion protein between the extracellular domain of CD40 and the Fc portion of IgG (CD40-Ig), blocks this activation (*right*) because the fusion protein competes for binding to CD40L and thereby prevents delivery of activation signals to the B cell via its CD40.

cells can express it as well (283). TCR stimulation induces the synthesis and expression of CD40L within 1 to 2 hours, with peak levels obtained in 4 to 8 hours. B cells presenting antigen to helper T cells can form cell–cell contacts lasting for at least this long (279), and therefore would be expected to receive the CD40L signal through their CD40 molecules, which are constitutively expressed.

Stimulation of purified resting B cells with oligomeric, cross-linked, or immobilized forms of CD40L induce proliferation, and this proliferation is enhanced by a number of cytokines, especially IL-4. CD40L stimulation alone does not induce terminal differentiation to the plasma cell state, but addition of cytokines leads to vigorous antibody production, with IL-4 plus IL-5 generally being the best combination (Fig. 17) (284). The ability to respond to IL-4 and IL-5 in the absence of IL-2 or IL-6 is also seen in response to anti-Ig if the anti-Ig is removed late in the response; otherwise, IL-2 or IL-6 is required (271). As with anti-Ig stimulation, IL-2 + IFN-γ will not induce a strong antibody response in CD40L-stimulated B cells (285).

It is striking that some of the effects of CD40L on resting B cells closely parallel the effects of soluble anti-IgM stimulation of the BCR. Thus, in part, this T_H-contact-dependent signal can provide a signal in place of a moderate BCR signal. This aspect of CD40L action is likely to be important for antibody responses to soluble protein antigens that only induce fairly weak BCR signaling. Equally important, however, are the ways in which the CD40L signal and the BCR signal are distinct. For example, CD40L induces expression of Fas by B cells and sensitivity to killing by Fas ligand (FasL). BCR signaling does not induce Fas, and in fact protects B cells from killing by FasL if CD40L has already induced Fas (Fig. 19) (286). This interplay has been shown to be important for pre-

The most straightforward interpretation of these results is that the chimera binds to a ligand for CD40 on the T cells and this binding prevents the ligand from interacting with CD40 on the B cells and in this way blocks the activation (Fig. 18).

Subsequent experiments have substantiated the conclusion that the major signal resulting from activated T_H cell contact with B cells involves CD40L (also called glycoprotein [gp]39 and CD154) on the helper T cell interacting with CD40 on the B cell. CD40L is expressed primarily by activated CD4+ T cells, although certain other

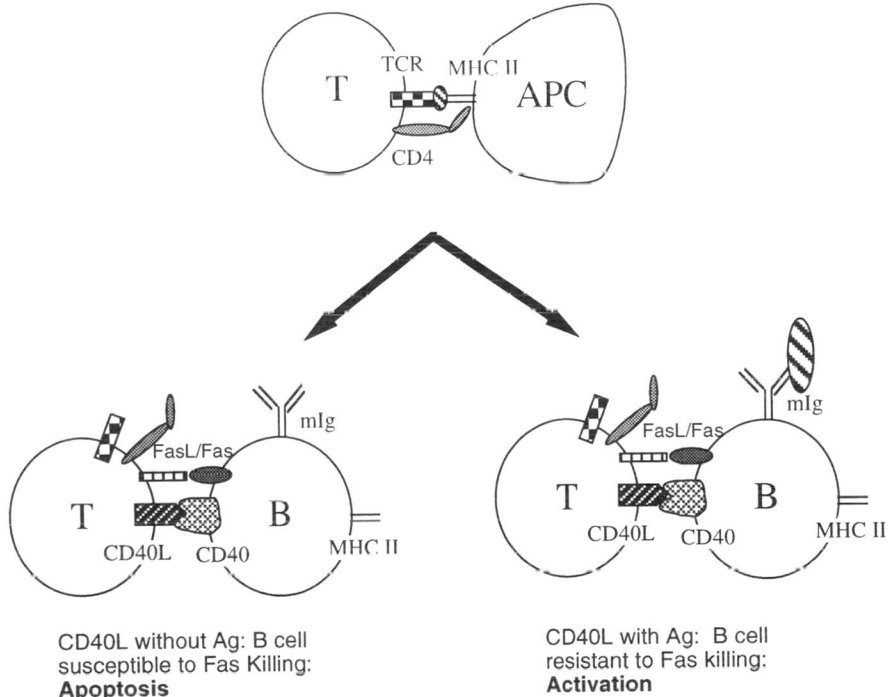

FIG. 19. Fas sensitivity of B cells stimulated via CD40. Activation of a helper T cell (*top*) causes it to rapidly induce expression of CD40L and more slowly induce expression of FasL. Contact between the activated helper T cell and a B-cell presenting antigen in the absence of BCR signaling (*lower left*) results in transient activation of the B cell via CD40 and cytokine stimulation, but at the same time the B cell upregulates expression of Fas and becomes sensitive to killing induced by FasL. The result is apoptosis, not activation, and this is the fate of anergic B cells that present antigen to helper T cells. Contact between the activated helper T cell and a B-cell presenting antigen that is also receiving signaling via its BCR (*lower right*) results in activation because the BCR signaling makes the B cell resistant to killing by FasL.

venting antibody responses by anergic B cells, as described below. Similarly, CD40L signaling is required for initiating a germinal center reaction, but BCR signaling is not sufficient for this response, and germinal center reactions are largely lacking in TI responses in the absence of T cells.

Blockage of CD40L–CD40 interactions, as achieved by administering a blocking antibody, by gene ablation in mice, or as seen in humans with naturally occurring mutations of CD40L, all result in greatly diminished TD antibody responses (284). The gene for CD40L is on the X chromosome, and humans with defective CD40L molecules suffer from a disease called X-linked hyper-IgM syndrome. These patients have very low titers of IgG, IgA, and IgE but have elevated titers of IgM. The latter are probably due to TI responses to the numerous and excessive infections experienced by these people. Mice lacking either CD40 or CD40L exhibit similar phenotypes, although IgM levels are typically not elevated. These mice make essentially no IgG, IgA, or IgE responses to TD stimuli and make markedly decreased IgM responses to TD stimuli as well, with the exception of antigens emulsified in complete Freund's adjuvant, which has polyclonal B-cell activators included among its components. Interestingly, the in vivo IgM response to SRBCs was also greatly decreased (about 20-fold), indicating that in vivo, the antibody response to SRBC mostly requires CD40L and hence contact with antigen-specific helper T cells (287). Antibody responses to polysaccharide antigens and to haptenated LPS are normal, demonstrating that TI antigens do not require stimulation through CD40.

The observations that helper T cells can provide help to B cells that are not displaying the peptide/MHC class II complex recognized by those T cells is paradoxical: How can antigen-specificity of the antibody response be maintained if helper T cells can activate any B cell? As mentioned above, in the absence of a signal from the BCR, CD40L not only stimulates the B cell but also makes it sensitive to killing by FasL. In addition, it is likely that during a real immune response in vivo, the helper T cell preferentially interacts with B cells that do display the appropriate recognition units by specifically taking up the antigen and presenting it. In part, this may result from the fact that helper T cells initially (before expression of CD40L) form strong and persistent cell conjugates only with antigen-presenting B cells (288,289).

The interactions between a B cell and a helper T cell in this initial period result in the formation of stable cell–cell conjugates only if the B cell expresses the appropriate MHC/antigenic peptide complex (288,289). The TCR, CD4, and LFA-1 molecules of the T cell concentrate in the region of cell–cell contact. These molecules may be held in this location either by their corresponding ligands on the B cell or by components of the T-cell cytoskeleton. Interestingly, the cytoskeletal protein talin also concentrates in this region of the T cell, and the microtubule organizing center points toward the contact region (289). Microtubules are thought to mediate movement of intracellular organelles. Interestingly, lymphokine secretion has been found to be directed toward the region of T-cell contact with the antigen-presenting cell (290).

A large number of molecules on the surfaces of B cells and helper T cells appear to participate in the cell–cell interaction (291). Of course, the TCR and CD4 interact with the class II MHC molecule on the B cell. In addition, the adhesion molecules LFA-1 and ICAM-1 are present on both B cells and T cells, potentially giving a bidirectional interaction, although it should be remembered that the adhesiveness of these molecules is regulated by receptor signaling events (258,292). Additional interacting mole-

cule pairs identified to date include the B7-2 molecule on activated but not resting B cells and CD28 on T cells, as well as CD40L on the T cells and CD40 on the B cell (Fig. 20).

These interacting molecule pairs are involved in crucial information transfer. The B7-2 interaction with CD28 is critical to activation of the helper T cell. If the helper T cell recognizes antigen/MHC II complexes with the TCR and does not recognize B7 with CD28, it enters an anergic state rather than being activated (212). Similarly, the importance of the CD40L interaction with CD40 on the B cell has been described above.

In addition to its role in antigen presentation to the T cell, the class II MHC molecule on the B cell also may receive an activation signal from the helper T cell. For example, antibodies to class II MHC molecules can provide a strong proliferative signal to B cells that have previously been activated with anti-Ig or anti-Ig + IL-4 (293,294). Anti–class II MHC antibodies induce cAMP elevation in resting B cells (295). In agreement with the idea that stimulation via class II MHC molecules may occur during helper T cell–B cell interactions, addition of fixed activated helper T cells to resting B cells induces a rapid elevation of cAMP (296). Interestingly, in B cells pretreated with anti-Ig, anti–class II antibodies induce phosphoinositide breakdown and a pattern of protein tyrosine phosphorylation that is indistinguishable from the pattern induced by anti-IgM (297). Because cAMP elevation is often inhibitory for B-cell activation, signaling via class II MHC molecules may reflect another mechanism to decrease activation of B cells that have not recognized antigen, and at the same, increase activation of B cells that have contacted antigen.

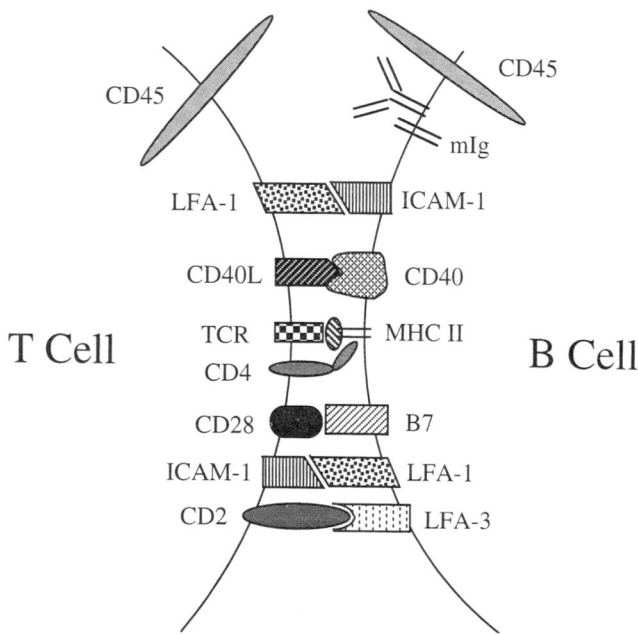

FIG. 20. Cell surface molecules involved in B cell–helper T cell interactions. A wide variety of cell surface molecules on B cells have the ability to interact with cell surface molecules on helper T cells. These include antigen-presenting and antigen recognition structures (MHC class II and the TCR + CD4), molecules involved in activating helper T cells (B7-2 and CD28), molecules involved in activating B cells (CD40 and CD40L), and cell–cell adhesion molecules. CD45 molecules are postulated to have interactions with molecules on other cells (such as CD22 on the B cell) or laterally with other cell surface molecules on the same cell.

CD40 Structure and Signaling Function

CD40 and CD40L belong to a larger family of receptor/ligand pairs, which include TNF receptors and TNF, Fas and Fas ligand, and CD30 and CD30 ligand, (298). The three-dimensional structures of two of the ligands of this family (TNF-α and lymphotoxin) were determined and found to be trimers. The homology of CD40L to these molecules makes it almost certain that CD40L also exists naturally as a trimeric ligand. Ligands of this family induce receptor oligomerization and in this way are thought to activate the signaling function of the corresponding receptors. A subset of these receptors, including TNF receptor II and CD40, appear to signal primarily by binding to members of a family of adapter molecules referred to as TNF receptor-associated factors (TRAFs). Six TRAFs have been identified to date. Receptor oligomerization induces binding of TRAF heterodimers or homodimers. In the case of CD40, TRAF2 and TRAF3 bind to engaged receptors at a site in the cytoplasmic domain corresponding to amino acids 246 to 269 (299). TRAF2 appears to be critical for activation of the transcription factor NF-κB, whereas TRAF3 is important for the isotype switch inducing properties of CD40 (198,300). In addition, a second region of the cytoplasmic domain closer to the N-terminus (amino acids 230–245) is a distinct binding site for TRAF6, which can also activate NF-κB (301).

How TRAFs activate downstream signaling events is not well understood, although rapid progress is being made in this area. As described above, activation of NF-κB involves phosphorylation of two serines in I-κB, which target it for ubiquitin-mediated destruction. This releases p50/p65 and related heterodimers to go to the nucleus, bind DNA, and activate transcription. Recently two subunits of an I-κB kinase have been identified (198), and an upstream protein kinase involved in the activation of I-κB kinase, NIK, also has been identified. Interestingly, NIK can bind to TRAFs, suggesting a direct link between TRAF binding to receptors and activation of NIK and I-κB kinase, although the details of this activation process are not yet known (Fig. 21).

CD40 signaling also may involve activation of intracellular protein tyrosine kinases, such as Lyn and Btk, although how it does so is unclear (284). The CD40 cytoplasmic domain lacks ITAMs, and it is not obviously phosphorylated on tyrosine after stimulation. Interestingly, *xid* B cells, which have a loss-of-function mutation in the gene encoding Btk, have a reduced in vitro response to CD40L (302), which would be consistent with a role of Btk in CD40 signaling. This effect could be indirect, however, and it should be noted that the TD antibody responses of *xid* mice are only partially compromised, certainly less so than are the responses of B cells lacking CD40, so it is not clear that Btk participates directly in CD40 signaling. CD40 stimulation is also a strong activator of two types of MAP kinases, the c-Jun N-terminal kinases, JNK-1 and JNK-2, and the p38 MAP kinases, and to a lesser extent the Erk1/Erk2 MAP kinases (104,303). In this respect it is complementary to BCR signaling, which activates Erk1/Erk2 more strongly and JNK and p38 MAP kinases weakly (105), although CD19 participation can increase the latter responses (304).

Regulation of Immunoglobulin Isotype Expression

In addition to their roles in B cell activation, cytokines released by helper T cells also influence immunoglobulin class switch recombination by B cells (305). In the mouse, IL-4 promotes switching of B cells to IgG1 and to IgE. The effects of blocking

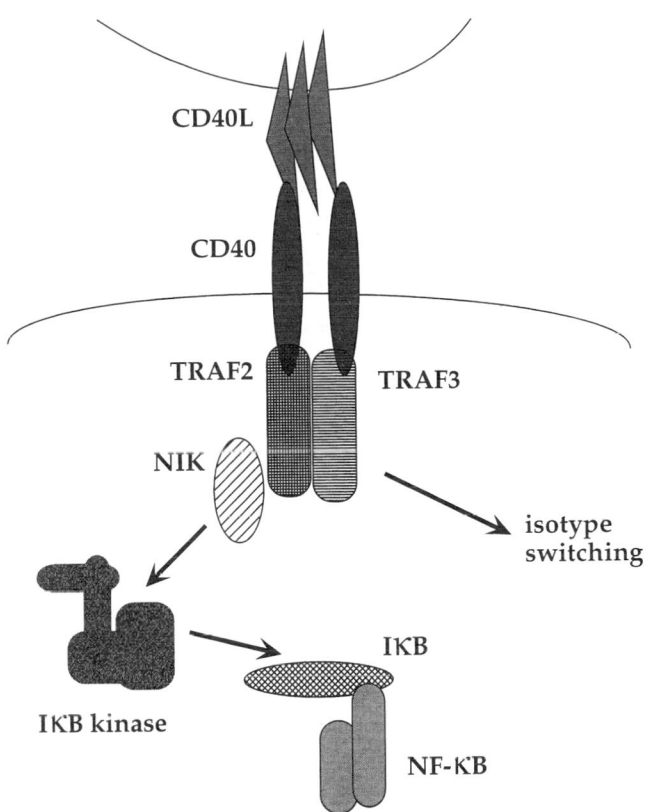

FIG. 21. CD40 signaling pathway. Oligomerization of CD40 (lower cell) by CD40L on the helper T cell (upper cell) leads to assembly of an oligomeric complex of TRAF family members associating with the cytoplasmic domains of the clustered CD40 molecules. Shown is a heterodimer of TRAF2 and TRAF3. TRAF3 promotes isotype switch recombination by an unknown mechanism, whereas TRAF2 (as well as TRAF6, which binds to a distinct site in the cytoplasmic tail of CD40, not shown) binds to a serine/threonine protein kinase called NIK, which phosphorylates and activates a large multicomponent complex called I-κB kinase. The I-κB kinase then phosphorylates I-κB on two neighboring serine residues, which provides the signal for ubiquitin- and proteasome-mediated degradation of I-κB. This releases the heterodimeric NF-κB complex to go to the nucleus where it can bind to target sites in the DNA and activate transcription.

antibodies to IL-4 both in vivo and in vitro strongly suggests that IL-4 is required for class switching to IgE, but that class switching to IgG1 can occur without IL-4. Studies with mice genetically lacking IL-4 have come to similar conclusions (306). IL-4 seems to be primarily responsible for regulation of Ig isotype expression by T$_{H2}$ cells, although IL-5 promotes IgA responses in some circumstances. This effect of IL-5 apparently reflects an effect on B cells that have already switched to IgA, and TGF-β is the major cytokine that promotes class switching to IgA. T$_{H1}$ cells promote production of other Ig isotypes. In particular, IFN-γ promotes class switching to IgG2a, and interferes with the class switching regulatory effects of IL-4. This topic is considered further in Chapter 24.

B-Cell Production of Cytokines

The major effector function of B cells obviously is the production of antibodies, but B cells also participate in cell–cell interactions with other components of the immune system such as helper

T cells and follicular dendritic cells. Thus, it is not entirely surprising that B cells produce some cytokines when stimulated. Activated B cells produce significant quantities of IL-1, TNF-α, lymphotoxin-α, and GM-CSF, and probably other cytokines as well (307). These agents may act on neighboring cells, or they may act on B cells in an autocrine fashion. Indeed, memory B cells produce nerve growth factor (NGF), and this appears to promote their survival (308). Germinal center B cells produce G-CSF, and this may act on them in an autocrine fashion as well.

In Vivo Requirements for TD Responses

Initial efforts to understand the cytokine requirement for TD antibody responses were based on in vitro experiments, using either cloned T_H cell lines or in vitro stimulated CD4$^+$ T cells. Normal T cells stimulated by antigen acquire the ability to secrete large amounts of cytokines upon restimulation several days later. Incubation of these stimulated T cells in the presence of different cytokines can lead them to acquire a T_{H1}-like, a T_{H2}-like, or a T_{H0}-like phenotype (309,310). These effector T cells are able to provide help to B cells, as described above for helper T-cell clones. The cytokine requirements for antibody production were examined by using blocking antibodies against either the cytokines or their receptors (311–313). The antibody response to T_{H0}-like and T_{H1}-like effector T cells was inhibited considerably by blocking IL-2 and to a lesser extent by blocking IL-6. The T_{H1} cells did not make any detectable IL-5, and antibodies to this cytokine had no effect here, whereas they did inhibit the response to the T_{H0} cells by about 50%. The T_{H1}-like cells did make low amounts of IL-4 and, interestingly, antibodies to IL-4 decreased the response here by about two thirds. Surprisingly, anti–IL-4 did not inhibit the antibody response seen in the presence of T_{H2}-like cells, whereas anti–IL-5 had a strong inhibitory effect. These experiments reinforce the notion that there is some redundancy in the cytokines involved in B-cell activation and, moreover, that cytokine requirements are complex and vary according to the circumstances.

Blocking antibodies and more recently gene knockouts have been used to try and dissect the in vivo requirements for antibody responses. So far the results have been surprising, although they agree to some extent with the in vitro experiments described in the previous paragraph. As described above, TD responses in vivo are almost all dependent on CD40/CD40L interactions. This reflects a positive role of CD40 signaling for B-cell activation, and it may also reflect the effects of the CD40/CD40L interaction on activation of helper T cells. For example, CD40 signaling can induce expression of B7-2 costimulatory molecules that then lead to greater cytokine production by helper T cells (284). In addition, CD40L engagement also sends direct activating signals to helper T cells (314). Although there is some evidence that other members of this family, including TNF receptors and CD30, can participate in B-cell activation, CD40 clearly provides a unique and important element of T cell–dependent antibody responses.

Efforts to understand the in vivo roles of cytokines in B-cell activation have been somewhat less successful to date. The clearest answers have emerged with regard to the roles of IL-4 and IFN-γ in regulation of isotype switching, as described above. Despite evidence for important roles for IL-2 and IL-4 in various in vitro antibody responses, genetic ablation of these genes does not materially affect the amount of antibody produced in systemic TD antibody responses (315). A defect was found in the IL-4–deficient mice in

an antibody response to a mucosal immunization (316). Interpretation of observations with the IL-4 knockout must take into account the fact that in the absence of IL-4, helper T cells all end up with T_{H1} type phenotypes. Clearly, T_{H1} cells are good helper T cells for antibody response, provided they do not produce high levels of IFN-γ, which can inhibit antibody responses. Which cytokines are critical for antibody responses driven by T_{H1} cells is unclear, particularly because IL-2 + IFN-γ is not an effective combination for CD40L-stimulated B cells (285). Moreover, antibodies to IFN-γ or the knockout of IFN or the IFN-γ receptor have minimal effects on the overall level of antibody responses (317).

Given the ability of both T_{H1} and T_{H2} cells to serve as good helper T cells, it may be important to create mutant mice in which both pathways are disrupted in order to inhibit TD antibody responses. One such effort has been made; an IL-2, IL-4 double knockout mouse strain was created and this mouse was also found to have normal antibody responses (315). Presumably, this means that T_{H1} cells produce cytokines other than IL-2 that are sufficient in concert with CD40L to drive in vivo antibody responses. Interpretations of these results are also complicated by the existence of two cytokines with very similar properties to IL-2 and IL-4, i.e., IL-15 and IL-13, respectively. Both of these cytokines share use of cytokine receptor polypeptides with IL-2 and IL-4 (IL-2R β chain and IL-4R α chain, respectively), so the use of cytokine receptor knockouts for experiments such as these might be informative.

Clearer evidence for the importance of cytokines in antibody responses has come from the IL-6 and IL-5 knockouts. TD IgG antibody responses to viral and protein challenge are decreased by five- to tenfold in IL-6–deficient mice, indicating that this factor is important for terminal differentiation of B cells in vivo as well as in vitro (316). Interestingly, the TI IgM response to VSV infection was normal in these mice. Also interesting are the results with IL-5 knockout mice. T cells in these mice should exhibit fairly normal differentiation into T_{H1} and T_{H2} effectors, but the T_{H2} effectors will lack IL-5 and hence one would expect that certain in vivo antibody responses should be affected. A similar argument would apply to IL-5R α chain mutant mice. Initial studies with the latter mice demonstrated a two- to threefold decrease in serum levels of IgM and IgG3, suggesting a partial defect in TI-2 responses (318). Indeed, in vitro antibody responses to TNP-Ficoll showed an approximately fivefold decrease without addition of cytokines and a 20-fold defect in the presence of added IL-5. In vitro proliferation of B cells to LPS or anti-IgM plus IL-4 were both normal, as expected. Clearly, studies of in vivo antibody responses in these mice, particularly in circumstances where the antibody response is dominated by IgG1 and IgE isotypes reflective of a T_{H2} response, will be quite informative. Knockouts of cytokines or their receptors are starting to provide important information about the in vivo importance of various cytokines in TD and TI antibody responses, but further studies are clearly necessary to develop a more comprehensive picture.

B-Cell Memory and the Germinal Center Reaction

When B cells contact their corresponding antigen, they stop their recirculation in the T-cell zone of the nearest secondary lymphoid organism (244,245). Activated helper T cells can recognize antigenic peptide/MHC complexes presented by the antigen-specific B cells and promote their activation. Some B cells are activated in situ, proliferate to form foci, and then differentiate to the antibody-secreting cell state. Other activated B cells migrate to the nearby follicular region, where they initiate the formation of germinal centers (Fig. 22). Germinal centers are a prominent site of B-cell proliferation upon challenge with a TD antigen and are associated with affinity maturation and production of memory B cells.

Migration of activated B cells from the T cell zone to the follicular region is currently thought to be under the influence of a chemokine that binds to a 7-transmembrane receptor called BLR1 (319), possibly the newly discovered chemokine B lymphocyte chemoattractant (BLC) (319a), and also requires that the T_H cells that stimulate the B cells receive a signal through their CD40L molecule (314). Germinal centers can be founded by one or a few, possibly up to 10, antigen-specific B cells (320). Here the activated B cells proliferate extremely rapidly, with a doubling time of 6 to 7 hours, and expand to about 10^4 cells in just a few days (320,321). At this stage, somatic hypermutation of the Ig genes of the centroblasts begins, and continued proliferation is matched by exit of cells from cell cycle and movement of these cells, now called centrocytes, into the adjacent area, called the light zone. The region of centroblast proliferation is called the dark zone, reflecting its histologic appearance in most species, although not in mice. The light zone is densely packed with processes of the follicular dentritic cells (FDC), and the centrocytes are in close contact with these processes. The FDC is a specialized cell type distinct from the interdigitating dendritic cell of the T-cell zone. A striking feature of FDCs is their ability to hold antigen on their surface in an unprocessed form for very long periods of time (more than 1 year). They are thought to do this via $Fc\gamma Rs$ and CR2. Antigen held by FDCs is almost certainly critical for the selective events that occur in the germinal center to select for B cells capable of producing high-affinity antibodies.

The process of affinity maturation, in which the average affinity of antibodies produced increases during the immune response, involves first random mutation of the immunoglobulin genes and then selection for B cells with mutations that improve antibody affinity. Somatic hypermutation is largely if not completely restricted to the germinal center (322,323) and targets the V regions of Ig genes. It generates nearly random mutations at a rate of 1 mutation per 10^2 to 10^3 base pairs per generation (324). This process generates many variants of the initial antibodies, which are generally of a low or moderate affinity. Because the higher affinity of antibodies seen late in antibody responses is often the result of changes introduced by somatic hypermutation, the germinal center reaction is thought to be central to improving the affinity of antibodies during the immune response.

The process of somatic mutation puts random mutations clustered in the V regions of the Ig genes (324). Most such mutations are likely to be deleterious, with only rare mutations increasing the affinity of Ig for the antigen. Nonetheless, the average antibody affinity increases during a secondary response. Thus, there must be a powerful mechanism to select those cells with favorable mutations and to select against those with harmful mutations. This selection appears to occur at the centrocyte stage. Centroblasts express very little membrane Ig, but centrocytes express the now mutated Ig molecules in their BCRs. Moreover, centrocytes are highly susceptible to apoptotic cell death. The light zone of the germinal center has many macrophages with tingible bodies, which are the remnants of apoptotic cells engulfed by those macrophages. Isolated centrocytes cultured in vitro die rapidly unless stimulated with anti-Ig antibodies, which prevent apoptosis for a short time, or with anti-CD40 or CD40L, which provide more prolonged protection (Fig. 23) (321,325). Thus, centrocytes appear to be destined to die unless rescued by signals that involve BCR signaling and BCR uptake of antigen and presentation of antigen to helper T cells. Those centrocytes with Ig mutations that compromise antigen binding are at a disadvantage and preferentially die by apoptosis. Apparently, the antigen that must be bound is the antigen presented by the FDCs because injection of soluble antigen at the height of a germinal center reaction leads to rapid apoptosis of many of the germinal center B cells (326–328). Thus, contact between the FDC and the centrocyte is an important element in the survival of centrocytes. B cells also must present antigen to the small number of

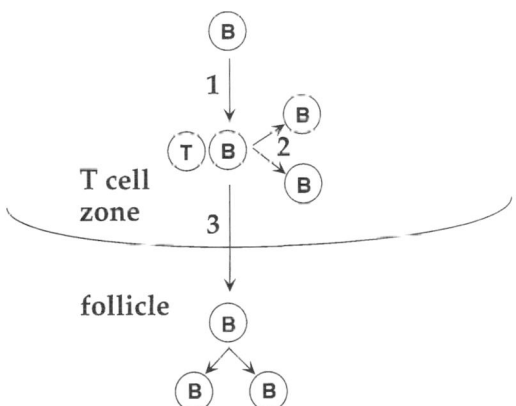

FIG. 22. Distinct T cell–dependent activation pathways for B cells. The B cell that contacts antigen travels to the T cell zone of a lymphoid organ (1) and then stops its migration there, where the MHC class II/peptide complexes on its surface are sampled by helper T cells. In the absence of interaction with specific helper T cells, the cell may die in this location, but upon interaction with an antigen-recognizing helper T cell, the B cell becomes activated and can either proliferate and differentiate in situ (2) or it can migrate to the follicular region (3) and initiate a germinal center reaction. The latter response requires CD40L/CD40 interaction, in part due to its effects on the helper T cell, whereas activation in the T cell zone, which is responsible for the initial IgM of a T cell–dependent primary response, appears to require interaction between OX40 ligand on the B cell and OX40 on the helper T cell.

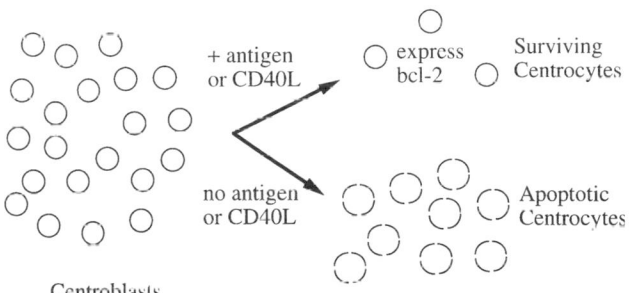

FIG. 23. Antigen-dependent survival of germinal center B cells. In the germinal center, B cells divide rapidly (centroblasts) and undergo extensive somatic mutation of their Ig genes. The postproliferative centrocytes with mutated mIg that bind antigen weakly undergo apoptosis, whereas cells with mIg that can bind antigen well are believed to receive signals from either BCR signaling or from CD40. These signals induce expression of the bcl-2 gene product and lead to cell survival. Affinity maturation can still occur in the presence of a bcl-2 transgene, suggesting that the survival signals must promote survival in other ways as well.

antigen-specific CD4$^+$ T cells present in germinal centers (321). This antigen presentation leads to expression of CD40L by the T$_H$ cells, which provides an important survival signal to the B cells. The molecular mechanisms regulating survival of the centrocyte are not yet clear. Although centrocytes have downregulated expression of the antiapoptotic protein Bcl-2 (see below), affinity maturation can occur in the face of sustained Bcl-2 production driven by the immunoglobulin heavy-chain enhancer, as well as in the absence of Fas (329,330).

The cells that give rise to germinal centers upon adoptive transfer into SCID mice express low levels of the heat stable antigen (HSA or CD24, recognized by the monoclonal antibody J11D), whereas B cells with higher levels of this marker give rise to primary IgM antibody responses but not to germinal centers (331). It is currently controversial whether this reflects the existence of a separate subset of B cells that gives rise to the germinal center response and does not give rise to the initial IgM response or whether this reflects a distribution of tendencies of cells in a single subset, e.g., the mature recirculating follicular B cells and their immature precursors.

The centrocytes that survive in the light zone due to their ability to bind antigen with sufficient affinity must ultimately decide to become either antibody-secreting cells or memory B cells. The former migrate to either the bone marrow or the gut, where they are quite long-lived (3 to 6 weeks), perhaps due to survival-promoting influences in these microenvironments (332). In vitro culture of centrocytes with helper T cells isolated from germinal centers leads to rapid acquisition of a memory B-cell surface phenotype (CD44$^+$CD23$^-$CD77$^-$) (325). The adoption of a memory B cell fate requires continued delivery of the CD40L signal to B cells, whereas terminal differentiation may require that this signal terminate at the correct point (333). One of the B-cell growth factors identified from human T cells, called high molecular weight BCGF (IL-14), stimulates proliferation and inhibits differentiation of B cells, suggesting that it also may participate in the decision between memory and terminal differentiation (334).

Once memory B cells are generated during a primary response, they can persist in a nonproliferative state for an extended period of time (335). This survival requires the continued presence of antigen, either from continued microorganism replication at a low level or from retention of antigen on the surface of FDCs. For example, adoptive transfer of purified B cells into a new host leads to rapid loss of ability to mount a secondary antibody response. This is interpreted as loss of the antigen-specific memory B cells resulting from their separation from persistent antigen during the transfer. Interestingly, when this experiment was performed with B cells from mice containing a transgenic *bcl-2* gene expressed constitutively in their B cells, memory B cells did not require antigen presence for survival (336). This observation suggests that memory B cells are also programmed to undergo apoptosis and that contact between mIg and antigen induces *bcl-2* expression and promotes their survival. IgG$^+$ or IgA$^+$ memory B cells produce nerve growth factor (NGF), and neutralization of this factor with specific antibodies caused rapid apoptotic death of the memory B cells as well as disappearance of Bcl-2 (308). The same antibody had no effect on IgM$^+$IgD$^+$ B cells, which are primarily virgin B cells, indicating that NGF is an autocrine survival factor for memory B cells but not for virgin B cells. One attractive hypothesis is that antigen contact leads to NGF production, which then promotes survival. Alternatively, NGF production might be controlled in some other way, for example by contact with FDCs

in follicles of secondary lymphoid organs, in which case it would represent a mechanism for restricting the overall number of memory B cells in the body.

Interestingly, *bcl-2* transgenic mice also exhibit greatly prolonged antibody secretion after immunization. This observation suggests that the normal fate of antibody-secreting cells is to die rather than to return to the resting B-cell pool. In the *bcl-2* transgenic mice, the expression of the transgene presumably prevents this cell death. Because the antibody-secreting cells expressing the *bcl-2* transgene do not undergo programmed cell death, they continue to secrete antibodies, with the eventual consequence of autoimmunity (337).

B-CELL ACTIVATION VERSUS INACTIVATION

In addition to the necessity of making antibody responses against foreign invaders, the immune system must avoid making antibody responses against self components. A number of distinct mechanisms act at the level of the B cell to limit the production of autoantibodies. First, there is an initial checkpoint in the maturation of B cells in the bone marrow. Immediately after rearrangement of Ig light chain genes, the newly generated immature B cell expresses its BCR, and if this BCR contacts antigen, it leads to maturational arrest, reexpression of *rag*-1 and *rag*-2, and resumption of rearrangement at the light-chain loci. This process has the potential to delete the initial successfully rearranged light-chain gene and create a new rearranged light chain gene, which may now contribute to a BCR that is not self-reactive. For this reason this regulatory event has been called receptor editing (338). It is presumed that immature B cells which have lost self-reactivity can now mature and leave the bone marrow.

A B cell that does not react strongly to a self-antigen in the bone marrow can mature further and leave the bone marrow. This immature B cell then circulates but is a short-lived cell that is very sensitive to antigen-induced apoptosis (339–341). Tolerance induction at this stage of development would occur for B cells recognizing antigens expressed in the periphery but not in the bone marrow. Strong BCR stimulation leads to death, also referred to as clonal deletion, whereas a weak BCR signal leads to a refractory state, clonal anergy (342,343). Both clonal deletion and clonal anergy are observed in Ig transgenic mice expressing an anti-self mIg on almost all of their B cells. In the limited number of cases examined to date, soluble protein antigens induce clonal anergy, whereas membrane-bound protein antigens induce clonal deletion (344). Deletion or anergy also can be induced by antigen contact with mature B cells in the absence of T-cell help. As described above, antigen contact causes the B cell to stop its migration in the T-cell zone of secondary lymphoid organs. In the absence of T-cell help, these arrested cells die more rapidly than recirculating B cells, probably due to lack of a survival signal provided in the follicular microenvironment (168).

Although deletion obviously removes the possibility that the B cell will produce antibodies, anergic B cells can be activated if antigen appears in a form that results in greater BCR signaling than the anergizing self antigen. For example, soluble hen egg lysozyme (HEL) induces anergy in B cells expressing a high-affinity antilysozyme BCR, and these anergized B cells cannot be activated by alloreactive helper T cells (reactive to the MHC of the B cell) in the presence of HEL, whereas naive antilysozyme B cells can be activated in this way (159). Addition of a membrane-bound form of

HEL in addition to the alloreactive helper T cells resulted in activation of the anergized B cells. This differential response may reflect the fact that chronic contact of the BCR with soluble antigen leads to chronic low-level signaling as well as decreased BCR signaling capability (51,159). This is manifest in induction of B7-2: HEL addition to naive antigen-specific B cells leads to induction of sufficient B7 costimulatory molecules to support activation of the T_H cells, whereas HEL stimulation of anergic B cells does not (345). A deficiency of BCR signaling is also manifest in FasL-mediated apoptosis of the B cell. CD40L stimulation of B cells induces expression of Fas and makes the B cell susceptible to killing induced by FasL. BCR stimulation of these B cells makes them resistant to Fas killing (286). HEL-specific anergic B cells fail to gain this resistance upon addition of soluble HEL. The physiologic importance of this defect in anergic B cells was revealed by examining the response in animals carrying mutations in the genes for Fas or for CD40L. In mice lacking just Fas, rather than being eliminated, the anergic B cells were activated and secreted antibody. In the absence of CD40L, elimination of anergic B cells did not occur, but activation did not occur either (346,347).

Thus, as with T cells, tolerance of self-reactive B cells occurs in both a central tolerance mode, in the case of B cells occurring in the bone marrow, and in a peripheral tolerance mode (Fig. 24). Peripheral tolerance of B cells results from contact with antigen in a way that does not promote full activation, either because the B cell is still immature and hence less responsive to B-cell activation pathways or because the B cell contacts a TD antigen in the absence of T-cell help. If the antigen contact is a weak one, the B cell becomes anergic and can only respond to antigen in a stronger form. A cross-reactive antigen present as part of a virus particle or bacterial cell surface structure would presumably succeed in stimulating antibody production from these anergic B cells. The antibody produced would likely be effective against the pathogen, but might also have self-reactivity. A hallmark of human autoimmune diseases is the chronic production of autoantibodies, so a short burst of autoantibody production in conjunction with an immune response would not necessarily create severe pathology. Autoimmune disease may require a further deregulation of the response such that it becomes greatly prolonged.

SUMMARY

Antibody production is regulated in multiple, complex ways. This complexity reflects the fact that the B cells must be able to make antibody responses to a wide range of antigens. The physical properties of these antigens can have profound effects on the B cell, both through their quantitative ability to induce BCR signal transduction events and as these properties may be important determinants of additional signals provided to the B cell, such as T cell help, bound fragments of C3b, and polyclonal activators. Successful antibody responses require second signals in addition to signals delivered via BCR. This requirement is important so that the B cell makes antibodies against foreign components but not against self components, which would lead to autoimmune destruction.

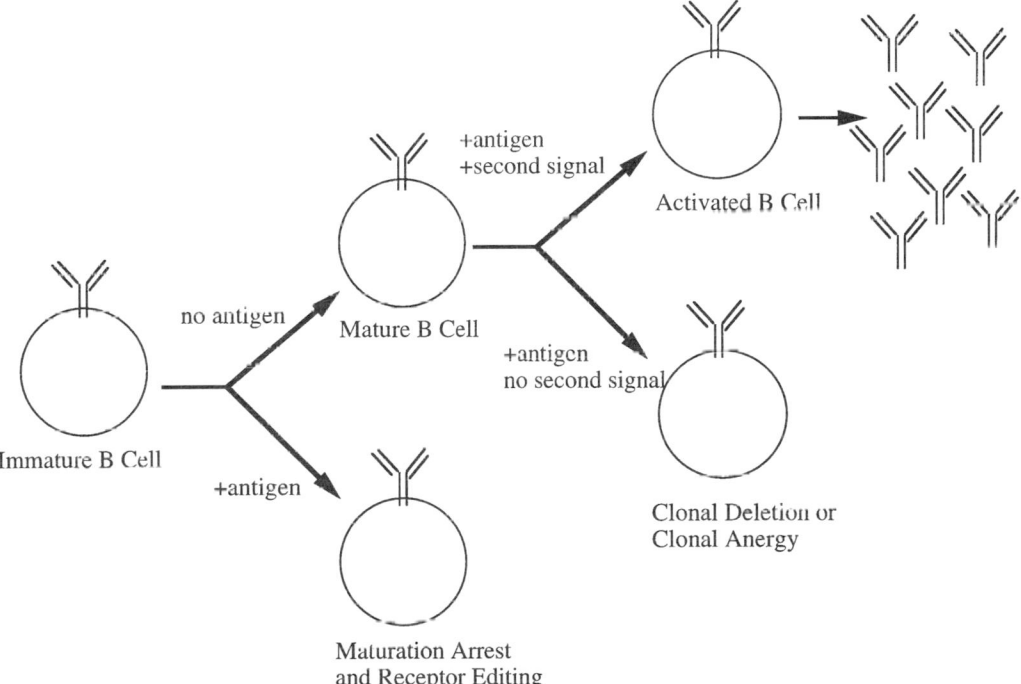

FIG. 24. Activation versus inactivation of B cells. B cells can become inactivated by antigen contact at multiple stages. If the immature B cell contacts antigen in the bone marrow, this leads to maturational arrest and receptor editing to try and change the specificity of the BCR. Once the immature B cell exits the bone marrow, it remains immature for a short period (not shown) and is highly susceptible to tolerance induction. B cells that mature and enter the long-lived pool can either become activated or inactivated by contact with antigen, depending on the availability of additional cues, or second signals, which may vary depending on the type of antigen contacted. Cells that receive appropriate second signals make antibody responses, whereas cells that contact antigen in the absence of second signals are inactivated (anergy) or are induced to commit suicide.

REFERENCES

1. Reth M. Antigen receptors on B lymphocytes. *Ann Rev Immunol* 1992;10: 97–121.
2. Kaisho T, Schwenk F, Rajewsky K. The roles of γ1 heavy chain membrane expression and cytoplasmic tail in IgG1 responses. *Science* 1997;276:412–415.
3. Achatz G, Nitschke L, Lamers MC. Effect of transmembrane and cytoplasmic domains of IgE on the IgE response. *Science* 1997;276:409–411.
4. Venkitaraman AR, Williams GT, Dariavach P, Neuberger MS. The B cell antigen receptor of the five immunoglobulin classes. *Nature* 1991;352:777–781.
5. Williams GT, Venkitaraman AR, Gilmore DJ, Neuberger MS. The sequence of the mu transmembrane segment determines the tissue specificity of the transport of immunoglobulin M to the cell surface. *J Exp Med* 1990;171:947–952.
6. Ravetch JV. Fc receptors: Rubor redux. *Cell* 1994;78:553–560.
7. Roth PE, DeFranco AL. Lymphocyte development: Intrinsic checkpoints for maturation. *Curr Biol* 1995;5:349–352.
8. DeFranco AL. The complexity of signaling pathways activated by the BCR. *Curr Opin Immunol* 1997;9:296–308.
9. DeFranco AL. Transmembrane signaling by antigen receptors of B and T lymphocytes. *Curr Opin Cell Biol* 1995;7:163–175.
10. Chen T, Repetto B, Chizzonite R, et al. Interaction of phosphorylated FceRIγ immunoglobulin receptor tyrosine activation motif-based peptides with dual and single SH2 domains of p72^{syk}. Assessment of binding parameters and real time binding kinetics. *J Biol Chem* 1996;271:25308–25315.
11. Hatada MH, Lu X, Laird ER, et al. Molecular basis for interaction of the protein tyrosine kinase ZAP-70 with the T-cell receptor. *Nature* 1995;377:32–38.
12. Sefton BM, Taddie JA. Role of tyrosine kinases in lymphocyte activation. *Curr Opin Immunol* 1994;6:372–379.
13. Law DA, Chan VWF, Datta SK, DeFranco AL. B-cell antigen receptor motifs have redundant signalling capabilities and bind the tyrosine kinases PTK72, Lyn and Fyn. *Curr Biol* 1993;3:645–657.
14. Songyang Z, Cantley L. Recognition and specificity in protein tyrosine kinase-mediated signalling. *Trends Biochem Sci* 1995;20:470–475.
15. Pawson T. Protein modules and signalling networks. *Nature* 1995;373:573–580.
16. Rowley RB, Burkhardt AL, Chao HG, Matsueda GR, Bolen JB. Syk protein-tyrosine kinase is regulated by tyrosine-phosphorylated Ig alpha/Ig beta immunoreceptor tyrosine activation motif binding and autophosphorylation. *J Biol Chem* 1995;270:11590–11594.
17. Shiue L, Zoller MJ, Brugge JS. Syk is activated by phosphotyrosine-containing peptides representing the tyrosine-based activation motifs of the high affinity receptor for IgE. *J Biol Chem* 1995;270:10498–10502.
18. Kimura T, Sakamoto H, Appella E, Siraganian RP. Conformational changes induced in the protein tyrosine kinase p72^{syk} by tyrosine phosphorylation or by binding of phosphorylated immunoreceptor tyrosine-based activation motif peptides. *Mol Cell Biol* 1996;16:1471–1478.
19. Kurosaki T. Molecular mechanisms in B cell antigen receptor signaling. *Curr Opin Immunol* 1997;9:309–318.
20. Kolanus W, Romeo C, Seed B. T cell activation by clustered tyrosine kinases. *Cell* 1993;74:171–183.
21. Chu DH, Spits H, Peyron JF, Rowley RB, Bolen JB, Weiss A. The Syk protein tyrosine kinase can function independently of CD45 or Lck in T cell antigen receptor signaling. *EMBO J* 1996;15:6251–6261.
22. Zoller KE, MacNeil IA, Brugge JS. Protein tyrosine kinases Syk and ZAP-70 display distinct requirements for Src family kinases in immune response receptor signal transduction. *J Immunol* 1997;158:1650–1659.
23. El-Hillal O, Kurosaki T, Yamamura H, Kinet JP, Scharenberg AM. syk kinase activation by a src kinase-initiated activation loop phosphorylation chain reaction. *Proc Natl Acad Sci USA* 1997;94:1919–1924.
24. Takata M, Sabe H, Hata A, et al. Tyrosine kinases Lyn and Syk regulate B cell receptor-coupled Ca^{2+} mobilization through distinct pathways. *EMBO J* 1994;13:1341–1349.
25. Turner M, Mee PJ, Costello PS, et al. Perinatal lethality and a block in the development of B cells in mice lacking the tyrosine kinase p72syk. *Nature* 1995;378: 298–302.
26. Cheng AM, Rowley B, Pao W, Hayday A, Bolen JB, Pawson T. Syk tyrosine kinase required for mouse viability and B-cell development. *Nature* 1995;378: 303–306.
27. Bolen JB. Protein tyrosine kinases in the initiation of antigen receptor signaling. *Curr Opin Immunol* 1995;7:306–311.
28. Sillman AL, Monroe JG. Surface IgM-stimulated proliferation, inositol phospholipid hydrolysis, Ca^{2+} flux, and tyrosine phosphorylation are not altered in B cells from p59^{fyn-1}-mice. *J Leukoc Biol* 1994;56:812–816.
29. Lowell CA, Soriano P. Knockouts of Src-family kinases: Stiff bones, wimpy T cells, and bad memories. *Genes Dev* 1996;10:1845–1857.
30. Hibbs ML, Tarlinton DM, Armes J, et al. Multiple defects in the immune system of Lyn-deficient mice culminating in autoimmune disease. *Cell* 1995;83: 301–311.
31. Nishizumi H, Taniuchi I, Yamanashi Y, et al. Impaired proliferation of peripheral B cells and indication of autoimmune disease in lyn-deficient mice. *Immunity* 1995;3:549–560.
32. Chan VWF, Meng F, Soriano P, DeFranco AL, Lowell CA. Characterization of the B lymphocyte populations in Lyn-deficient mice and the role of Lyn in signal initiation and downregulation. *Immunity* 1997;7:69–81.
33. Clark MR, Johnson SA, Cambier JC. Analysis of Ig-alpha-tyrosine kinase interaction reveals two levels of binding specificity and tyrosine phosphorylated Ig-alpha stimulation of Fyn activity. *EMBO J* 1994;13:1911–1919.
34. Pleiman CM, Abrams C, Gauen LT, et al. Distinct p53/56^{lyn} and p59^{fyn} domains associate with nonphosphorylated and phosphorylated Ig-alpha. *Proc Natl Acad Sci USA* 1994;91:4268–4272.
35. Johnson SA, Pleiman CM, Pao L, Schneringer J, Hippen K, Cambier JC. Phosphorylated immunoreceptor signaling motifs (ITAMs) exhibit unique abilities to bind and activate Lyn and Syk tyrosine kinases. *J Immunol* 1995;155: 4596–4603.
36. Neel BG. Role of phosphatases in lymphocyte activation. *Curr Opin Immunol* 1997;9:405–420.
37. Rawlings DJ, Witte ON. The Btk subfamily of cytoplasmic tyrosine kinases: Structure, regulation and function. *Semin Immunol* 1995;7:237–246.
38. Tarakhovsky A. Xid and Xid-like immunodeficiencies from a signaling point of view. *Curr Opin Immunol* 1997;9:319–323.
39. Takata M, Kurosaki T. A role for Bruton's tyrosine kinase in B cell antigen receptor-mediated activation of phospholipase C-gamma 2. *J Exp Med* 1996;184: 31–40.
40. Hornbeck P, Nakabayashi H, Fowlkes B, Paul W, Kligman D. A major myristylated substrate of protein kinase C and protein kinase C itself are differentially regulated during murine B- and T-lymphocyte development and activation. *Mol Cell Biol* 1989;9:3727–3735.
41. Aderem A. The MARCKS brothers: A family of protein kinase C substrates. *Cell* 1992;71:713–716.
42. Leitges M, Schmedt C, Guinamard R, et al. Immunodeficiency in protein kinase C beta-deficient mice. *Science* 1996;273:788–791.
43. Yao L, Kawakami Y, Kawakami T. The pleckstrin homology domain of Bruton tyrosine kinase interacts with protein kinase C. *Proc Natl Acad Sci USA* 1994; 91:9175–9179.
44. Xie H, Rothstein TL. Protein kinase C mediates activation of nuclear cAMP response element-binding protein (CREB) in B lymphocytes stimulated through surface Ig. *J Immunol* 1995;154:1717–1723.
45. Xie H, Wang Z, Rothstein T. Signaling pathways for antigen receptor-mediated induction of transcription factor CREB in B lymphocytes. *Cell Immunol* 1996; 169:264–270.
46. Sidorenko SP, Law C-L, Klaus SJ, et al. Protein kinase C μ (PKCμ) associates with the B cell antigen receptor complex and regulates lymphocyte signaling. *Immunity* 1996;5:353–363.
47. Cambier JC, Ransom JT. Molecular mechanisms of transmembrane signaling in B lymphocytes. *Ann Rev Immunol* 1987;5:175–199.
48. Gelfand EW, MacDougall SL, Cheung RK, Grinstein S. Independent regulation of Ca^{2+} entry and release from internal stores in activated B cells. *J Exp Med* 1989;170:315–320.
49. Penner R, Fasolato C, Hoth M. Calcium influx and its control by calcium release. *Curr Opin Neurobiol* 1993;3:368–374.
50. Cambier J, Chen Z-Z, Pasternak J, Ransom J, Sandoval V, Pickles H. Ligand-induced desensitization of B-cell membrane immunoglobulin-mediated Ca^{2+} mobilization and protein kinase C translocation. *Proc Natl Acad Sci USA* 1988; 85:6493–6497.
51. Healy JI, Dolmetsch RE, Timmerman LA, et al. Different nuclear signals are activated by the B cell receptor during positive versus negative signaling. *Immunity* 1997;6:419–428.
52. Valentine MA, Czernik AJ, Rachie N, et al. Anti-immunoglobulin M activates nuclear calcium/calmodulin-dependent protein kinase II in human B lymphocytes. *J Exp Med* 1995;182:1943–1949.
53. Schreiber SL, Crabtree GR. The mechanism of action of cyclosporin A and FK506. *Immunol Today* 1992;13:136–142.
54. Rao A, Luo C, Hogan PG. Transcription factors of the NFAT family: Regulation and function. *Ann Rev Immunol* 1997;15:707–747.
55. Venkataraman L, Francis DA, Wang Z, Liu J, Rothstein TL, Sen R. Cyclosporin-A sensitive induction of NF-AT in murine B cells. *Immunity* 1994;1:189–196.
56. Fisher CL, Ghysdael J, Cambier JC. Ligation of membrane Ig leads to calcium-mediated phosphorylation of the proto-oncogene product Ets-1. *J Immunol* 1991;146:1743–1749.
57. Dolmetsch RE, Lewis RS, Goodnow CC, Healy JI. Differential activation of transcription factors induced by Ca^{2+} response amplitude and duration. *Nature* 1997;386:855–858.
58. McCormick F. Activators and effectors of ras p21 proteins. *Curr Opin Genet Dev* 1994;4:71–76.
59. Lazarus AH, Kawauchi K, Rapoport MJ, Delovitch TL. Antigen-induced B lymphocyte activation involves the p21^{ras} and RasGAP signaling pathway. *J Exp Med* 1993;178:1765–1769.
60. Harwood AE, Cambier JC. B cell antigen receptor cross-linking triggers rapid protein kinase C independent activation of p21^{ras}. *J Immunol* 1993;151: 4513–4522.
61. Graziadei L, Riabowol K, Bar-Sagi D. Co-capping of ras proteins with surface immunoglobulins in B lymphocytes. *Nature* 1990;347:396–400.
62. Saxton TM, van Oostveen I, Bowtell D, Aebersold R, Gold MR. B cell antigen receptor cross-linking induces phosphorylation of the p21^{ras} oncoprotein activators SHC and mSOS1 as well as assembly of complexes containing SHC, GRB-2, mSOS1 and a 145-kDa tyrosine-phosphorylated protein. *J Immunol* 1994;153: 623–636.

63. Lankester AC, van Schijndel GM, Rood PM, Verhoeven AJ, van Lier RA. B cell antigen receptor cross-linking induces tyrosine phosphorylation and membrane translocation of a multimeric Shc complex that is augmented by CD19 co-ligation. *Eur J Immunol* 1994;24:2818–2825.

64. Smit L, deVries-Smits AMM, Bos JL, Borst J. B cell antigen receptor stimulation induces formation of a Shc-Grb2 complex containing multiple tyrosine-phosphorylated proteins. *J Biol Chem* 1994;269:20209–20212.

65. Harmer SL, DeFranco AL. Shc contains two Grb2 binding sites needed for efficient formation of complexes with SOS in B lymphocytes. *Mol Cell Biol* 1997;17:4087–4095.

66. Gold MR, Crowley MT, Martin GA, McCormick F, DeFranco AL. Targets of B lymphocyte antigen receptor signal transduction include the p21ras GTPase-activating protein (GAP) and two GAP-associated proteins. *J Immunol* 1993;150:377–386.

67. Settleman J, Albright CF, Foster LC, Weinberg RA. Association between GTPase activators for Rho and Ras families. *Nature* 1992;359:153–154.

68. Yamanashi Y, Baltimore D. Identification of the Abl- and rasGAP-associated 62 kDa protein as a docking protein Dok. *Cell* 1997;88:205–211.

69. Carpino N, Wisniewski D, Strife A, et al. p62dok: A constitutively tyrosine-phosphorylated, GAP-associated protein in chronic myelogenous leukemia progenitor cells. *Cell* 1997;88.197–204.

70. Vuica M, Desiderio S, Schneck JP. Differential effects of B cell receptor and B cell receptor-FcgammaRIIB1 engagement on docking of Csk to GTPase-activating protein (GAP)-associated p62. *J Exp Med* 1997;186:259–267.

71. Marshall CJ. Ras effectors. *Curr Opin Cell Biol* 1996;8:197–204.

72. Morrison DK, Cutler RE. The complexity of Raf-1 regulation. *Curr Opin Cell Biol* 1997;9:174–179.

73. Casillas A, Hanekom C, Williams K, Katz R, Nel AE. Stimulation of B-cells via the membrane immunoglobulin receptor or with phorbol myristate 13-acetate induces tyrosine phosphorylation and activation of a 42-kDa microtubule-associated protein-2 kinase. *J Biol Chem* 1991;266:19088–19094.

74. Gold MR, Sanghera JS, Stewart J, Pelech SL. Selective activation of p42 MAP kinase in murine B lymphoma cell lines by membrane immunoglobulin crosslinking. Evidence for protein kinase C-independent and -dependent mechanisms of activation. *Biochem J* 1992;286:269–276.

75. Tordai A, Franklin RA, Patel H, Gardner AM, Johnson GL, Gelfand EW. Cross-linking of surface IgM stimulates the Ras/Raf-1/MEK/MAPK cascade in human B lymphocytes. *J Biol Chem* 1994;269.7538–7543.

76. Treisman R. Regulation of transcription by MAP kinase cascades. *Curr Opin Cell Biol* 1996;8.205–215.

77. McMahon SB, Monroe JG. A ternary complex factor-dependent mechanism mediates induction of egr-1 through selective serum response elements following antigen receptor crosslinking in B lymphocytes. *Mol Cell Biol* 1995;15:1086–1093.

78. McMahon SB, Monroe JG. Activation of the p21ras pathway couples antigen receptor stimulation to induction of the primary response gene egr-1 in B lymphocytes. *J Exp Med* 1995;181:417–422.

79. Yamanashi Y, Fukui Y, Wongsasant B, et al. Activation of Src-like protein-tyrosine kinase Lyn and its association with phosphatidylinositol 3-kinase upon B-cell antigen receptor-mediated signaling. *Proc Natl Acad Sci USA* 1992;89:1118–1122.

80. Gold MR, Chan VWF, Turck CW, DeFranco AL. Membrane Ig cross-linking regulates phosphatidylinositol 3-kinase in B lymphocytes. *J Immunol* 1992;148:2012–2022.

81. Gold MR, Aebersold R. Both phosphatidylinositol 3-kinase and phosphatidylinositol 4-kinase products are increased by antigen receptor signaling in B cells. *J Immunol* 1994;152:42–50.

82. Crowley MT, Harmer SL, DeFranco AL. Activation-induced association of a 145-kDa tyrosine-phosphorylated protein with Shc and Syk in B lymphocytes and macrophages. *J Biol Chem* 1996;271:1145–1152.

83. Chacko GW, Tridandapani S, Damen JE, Liu L, Krystal G, Coggeshall KM. Negative signaling in B lymphocytes induces tyrosine phosphorylation of the 145-kDa inositol polyphosphate 5-phosphatase, SHIP. *J Immunol* 1996;157:2234–2238.

84. Damen JE, Liu L, Rosten P, Humphries RK, Jefferson AB, Majerus PW, Krystal G. The 145-kDa protein induced to associate with Shc by multiple cytokines is an inositol tetraphosphate and phosphatidylinositol 3,4,5-triphosphate 5-phosphatase. *Proc Natl Acad Sci USA* 1996;93:1689–1693.

85. Lioubin MN, Algate PA, Tsai S, Carlberg K, Aebersold A, Rohrschneider LR. p150ship, a signal transduction molecule with inositol polyphosphate-5-phosphatase activity. *Genes Dev* 1996;10:1084–1095.

86. Kavanaugh WM, Pot DA, Chin SM, et al. Multiple forms of an inositol polyphosphate 5-phosphatase form signaling complexes with Shc and Grb2. *Curr Biol* 1996;6:438–445.

87. Salim K, Bottomley MJ, Querfurth E, et al. Distinct specificity in the recognition of phosphoinositides by the pleckstrin homology domains of dynamin and Bruton's tyrosine kinase. *EMBO J* 1996;15:6241–6250.

88. Franke TF, Kaplan DR, Cantley LC, Toker A. Direct regulation of the Akt proto-oncogene product by phosphatidylinositol-3,4 bisphosphate. *Science* 1997;275:665–668.

89. Klippel A, Kavanaugh WM, Pot D, Williams LT. A specific product of phosphatidylinositol 3-kinase directly activates the protein kinase Akt through its pleckstrin homology domain. *Mol Cell Biol* 1997;17:338–344.

90. Li T, Tsukada S, Satterthwaite A, et al. Activation of Bruton's tyrosine kinase (BTK) by a point mutation in its pleckstrin homology (PH) domain. *Immunity* 1995;2:451–460.

91. Bustelo XR, Barbacid M. Tyrosine phosphorylation of the vav proto-oncogene product in activated B cells. *Science* 1992;256:1196–1199.

92. Cory GO, Lovering RC, Hinshelwood S, MacCarthy-Morrogh L, Levinsky RJ, Kinnon C. The protein product of the c-cbl protooncogene is phosphorylated after B cell receptor stimulation and binds the SH3 domain of Bruton's tyrosine kinase. *J Exp Med* 1995;182:611–615.

93. Hartley D, Meisner H, Corvera S. Specific association of the beta isoform of the p85 subunit of phosphatidylinositol-3 kinase with the proto-oncogene c-cbl. *J Biol Chem* 1995;270:18260–18263.

94. Kim TJ, Kim YT, Pillai S. Association of activated phosphatidylinositol 3-kinase with p120cbl in antigen receptor-ligated B cells. *J Biol Chem* 1995;270:27504–27509.

95. Yamanashi Y, Okada M, Semba T, et al. Identification of HS1 protein as a major substrate of protein-tyrosine kinase(s) upon B-cell antigen receptor-mediated signaling. *Proc Natl Acad Sci USA* 1993;90:3631–3635.

96. Bonnefoy-Berard N, Munshi A, Yron I, et al. Vav: Function and regulation in hematopoietic cell signaling. *Stem Cells* 1996;14:250–268.

97. Olson MF, Pasteris NG, Gorski JL, Hall A. Faciogenital dysplasia protein (FGD1) and Vav, two related proteins required for normal embryonic development, are upstream regulators of Rho GTPases. *Curr Biol* 1996;6:1628–1633.

98. Crespo P, Schuebel KE, Ostrom AA, Gutkind JS, Bustelo XR. Phosphotyrosine-dependent activation of Rac-1 GDP/GTP exchange by the vav proto-oncogene product. *Nature* 1997;385:169–172.

99. Wu J, Motto DG, Koretzky GA, Weiss A. Vav and SLP-76 interact and functionally cooperate in IL-2 gene activation. *Immunity* 1996;4:593–602.

100. Wu J, Zhao Q, Kurosaki T, Weiss A. The Vav binding site (Y315) in ZAP-70 is critical for antigen receptor-mediated signal transduction. *J Exp Med* 1997;185:1877–1882.

101. Bourne HR, Sanders DA, McCormick F. The GTPase superfamily: Conserved structure and molecular mechanism. *Nature* 1991;349:117–127.

102. Tapon N, Hall A. Rho, Rac and Cdc42 GTPases regulate the organization of the actin cytoskeleton. *Curr Opin Cell Biol* 1997;9:86–92.

103. Kyriakis JM, Avruch J. Sounding the alarm: Protein kinase cascades activated by stress and inflammation. *J Biol Chem* 1996;271:24313–24316.

104. Berberich I, Shu G, Siebelt F, Woodgett JR, Kyriakis JM, Clark EA. Cross-linking CD40 on B cells preferentially induces stress-activated protein kinases rather than mitogen-activated protein kinases. *EMBO J* 1996;15:92–101.

105. Sutherland CL, Heath AW, Pelech SL, Young PR, Gold MR. Differential activation of the ERK, JNK, and p38 mitogen-activated protein kinases by CD40 and the B cell antigen receptor. *J Immunol* 1996;157:3381–3390.

106. Yoon CH, Lee J, Jongeward GD, Sternberg PW. Similarity of sli-1, a regulator of vulval development in *C. elegans*, to the mammalian proto-oncogene c-cbl. *Science* 1995;269:1102–1105.

107. Smit L, van der Horst G, Borst J. Sos, Vav, and C3G participate in B cell receptor-induced signaling pathways and differentially associate with Shc-Grb2, Crk, and Crk-L adaptors. *J Biol Chem* 1996;271:8564–8569.

108. Ingham RJ, Krebs DL, Barbazuk SM, et al. B cell antigen receptor signaling induces the formation of complexes containing the Crk adapter proteins. *J Biol Chem* 1996;271:32306–32214.

109. McCormick F, Wittinghofer A. Interactions between Ras proteins and their effectors. *Curr Opin Biotechnol* 1996;7:449–456.

110. Yamanashi Y, Fukuda T, Nishizumi H, et al. Role of tyrosine phosphorylation of HS1 in B cell antigen receptor-mediated apoptosis. *J Exp Med* 1997;185:1387–1392.

111. Suzuki Y, Demoliere C, Kitamura D, Takeshita H, Deuschle U, Watanabe T. HAX-1, a novel intracellular protein, localized on mitochondria, directly associates with HS1, a substrate of Src family tyrosine kinases. *J Immunol* 1997;158:2736–2744.

112. Fantl WJ, Johnson DF, Williams LT. Signalling by receptor tyrosine kinases. *Ann Rev Biochem* 1993;62:453–481.

113. Richards JD, Gold MR, Hourihane SL, DeFranco AL, Matsuuchi L. Reconstitution of B cell antigen receptor-induced signaling events in a nonlymphoid cell line by expressing the Syk protein-tyrosine kinase. *J Biol Chem* 1996;271:6458–6466.

114. Tuveson DA, Carter RH, Soltoff SP, Fearon DT. CD19 of B cells as a surrogate kinase insert region to bind phosphatidylinositol 3-kinase. *Science* 1993;260:986–989.

115. Weng W-K, Jarvis L, LeBien TW. Signaling through CD19 activates Vav/mitogen-activated protein kinase pathway and induces formation of a CD19/Vav/phosphatidylinositol 3-kinase complex in human B cell precursors. *J Biol Chem* 1994;269:32514–32521.

116. Law CL, Sidorenko SP, Chandran KA, et al. CD22 associates with protein tyrosine phosphatase 1C, Syk, and phospholipase C-gamma(1) upon B cell activation. *J Exp Med* 1996;183:547–560.

117. Sillman AL, Monroe JG. Association of p72syk with the src-homology-2 (SH2) domains of PLC-γl in B lymphocytes. *J Biol Chem* 1995;270:11806–11811.

118. Law CL, Chandran KA, Sidorenko SP, Clark EA. Phospholipase C-gamma1 interacts with conserved phosphotyrosyl residues in the linker region of Syk and is a substrate for Syk. *Mol Cell Biol* 1996;16:1305–1315.

119. Weiss A, Littman DR. Signal transduction by lymphocyte antigen receptors. *Cell* 1994;76:263–274.

120. Chen X, Kearney JF. Generation and function of natural self-reactive B lymphocytes. *Semin Immunol* 1996;8:19–27.

121. Dempsey PW, Allison MED, Akkaraju S, Goodnow CC, Fearon DT. C3d of complement as a molecular adjuvant: Bridging innate and acquired immunity. *Science* 1996;271:348–350.

122. Takai T, Ono M, Hikida M, Ohmori H, Ravetch JV. Augmented humoral and anaphylactic responses in FcγRII-deficient mice. *Nature* 1996;379:346–349.

123. Matsumoto AK, Kopicky-Burd J, Carter RH, Tuveson DA, Tedder TF, Fearon DT. Intersection of the complement and immune systems: A signal transduction complex of the B lymphocyte-containing complement receptor type 2 and CD19. *J Exp Med* 1991;173:55–64.

124. Carter RH, Spycher MO, Ng YC, Hoffman H, Fearon DT. Synergistic interaction between complement receptor type 2 and membrane IgM on B lymphocytes. *J Immunol* 1988;141:457–463.

125. Carter RH, Fearon DT. CD19: Lowering the threshold for antigen receptor stimulation of B lymphocytes. *Science* 1992;256:105–107.

126. Ahearn JM, Fischer MB, Croix D, et al. Disruption of the Cr2 locus results in a reduction in B-1a cells and in an impaired B cell response to T-dependent antigen. *Immunity* 1996;4:251–262.

127. Molina H, Holers VM, Li B, et al. Markedly impaired humoral immune response in mice deficient in complement receptors 1 and 2. *Proc Natl Acad Sci USA* 1996;93:3357–3361.

128. Croix D, Ahearn JM, Rosengard AM, et al. Antibody response to a T-dependent antigen requires B cell expression of complement receptors. *J Exp Med* 1996;183:1857–1864.

129. Engel P, Zhou LJ, Ord DC, Sato S, Koller B, Tedder TF. Abnormal B lymphocyte development, activation, and differentiation in mice that lack or overexpress the CD19 signal transduction molecule. *Immunity* 1995;3:39–50.

130. Rickert RC, Rajewsky K, Roes J. Impairment of T-cell-dependent B-cell responses and B-1 cell development in CD19-deficient mice. *Nature* 1995;376:352–355.

131. Kozono Y, Duke RC, Schleicher MS, Holers VM. Co-ligation of mouse complement receptors 1 and 2 with surface IgM rescues splenic B cells and WEHI-231 cells from anti-surface IgM-induced apoptosis. *Eur J Immunol* 1995;25:1013–1017.

132. van Noesel CJM, Lankester AC, van Schijndel GMW, van Lier RAW. The CR2/CD19 complex on human B cells contains the src-family kinase Lyn. *Int Immunol* 1993;5:699–705.

133. Uckun FM, Burkhardt AL, Jarvis L, et al. Signal transduction through the CD19 receptor during discrete developmental stages of human B-cell ontogeny. *J Biol Chem* 1993;268:21172–21184.

134. Erdei A, Melchers F, Schulz T, Dierich M. The action of human C3 in soluble and cross-linked form with resting and activated murine B lymphocytes. *Eur J Immunol* 1985;15:184–188.

135. Fingeroth JD, Weis JJ, Tedder TF, Strominger JL, Biro PA, Fearon DT. Epstein-Barr virus receptor of human B-lymphocytes is the C3d receptor CR2. *Proc Natl Acad Sci USA* 1984;81:4510–4514.

136. Nemerow GR, Wolfert R, McNaughton ME, Cooper NR. Identification and characterization of the Epstein-Barr virus receptor on human B lymphocytes and its relationship to the C3d complement receptor (CR2). *J Virol* 1985;55:347–351.

137. Phillips NE, Parker DC. Fc-dependent inhibition of mouse B cell activation by whole anti-μ antibodies. *J Immunol* 1983;130:602–606.

138. Ashman RF, Peckham D, Stunz LL. Fc receptor off-signal in the B cell involves apoptosis. *J Immunol* 1996;157:5–11.

139. Bijsterbosch MK, Klaus GGB. Crosslinking of surface immunoglobulin and Fc receptors on B lymphocytes inhibits stimulation of inositol phospholipid breakdown via the antigen receptor. *J Exp Med* 1985;162:1825–1836.

140. Choquet D, Partiseti M, Amigorena S, Bonnerot C, Fridman WH, Korn H. Crosslinking of IgG receptors inhibits membrane immunoglobulin-stimulated calcium influx in B lymphocytes. *J Cell Biol* 1993;121:355–363.

141. Muta T, Kurosaki T, Misulovin Z, Sanchez M, Nussenzweig MC, Ravetch JV. A 13-amino acid motif in the cytoplasmic domain of FcγRIIB modulates B-cell receptor signaling. *Nature* 1994;368:70–73.

142. D'Ambrosio D, Hippen KH, Minskoff SA, et al. Recruitment and activation of PTP1C in negative regulation of antigen receptor signaling by FcγRIIB1. *Science* 1995;268:293–297.

143. Ono M, Bolland S, Tempst P, Ravetch JV. Role of the inositol phosphatase SHIP in negative regulation of the immune system by the receptor Fc(gamma)RIIB. *Nature* 1996;383:263–266.

144. Ono M, Okada H, Bolland S, Yanagi S, Kurosaki T, Ravetch JV. Deletion of SHIP or SHP-1 reveals two distinct pathways for inhibitory signaling. *Cell* 1997;90:293–301.

145. Scharenberg AM, Kinet JP. The emerging field of receptor-mediated inhibitory signaling: SHP or SHIP? *Cell* 1996;87:961–964.

146. Nadler MJS, Chen B, Anderson JS, Wortis HH, Neel BG. Protein-tyrosine phosphatase SHP-1 is dispensable for FcgammaRIIB-mediated inhibition of B cell antigen receptor activation. *J Biol Chem* 1997;272:20038–20043.

147. Sarkar S, Schlottmann K, Cooney D, Coggeshall KM. Negative signaling via FcgammaRIIB1 in B cells blocks phospholipase Cgamma2 tyrosine phosphorylation but not Syk or Lyn activation. *J Biol Chem* 1996;271:20182–20186.

148. Hippen KL, Buhl AM, D'Ambrosio D, Nakamura K, Persin C, Cambier JC. FcγRIIB1 inhibition of BCR-mediated phosphoinositide hydrolysis and Ca²⁺

149. Tridandapani S, Chacko GW, Van Brocklyn JR, Coggeshall KM. Negative signaling in B cells causes reduced Ras activity by reducing Shc-Grb2 interactions. *J Immunol* 1997;158:1125–1132.

150. Ravanel K, Castelle C, Defrance T, et al. Measles virus nucleocapsid protein binds to FcγRII and inhibits human B cell antibody production. *J Exp Med* 1997;186:269–278.

151. Tedder TF, Tuscano J, Sato S, Kehrl JH. CD22, a B lymphocyte-specific adhesion molecule that regulates antigen receptor signaling. *Ann Rev Immunol* 1997;15:481–504.

152. O'Rourke L, Tooze R, Fearon DT. Co-receptors of B lymphocytes. *Curr Opin Immunol* 1997;9:324–329.

153. Kharitonenkov A, Chen Z, Sures I, Wang H, Schilling J, Ullrich A. A family of proteins that inhibit signalling through tyrosine kinase receptors. *Nature* 1997;386:181–186.

154. Tuscano JM, Engel P, Tedder TF, Agarwal A, Kehrl JH. Involvement of p72syk kinase, p53/56lyn kinase and phosphatidylinositol 3-kinase in signal transduction via human B lymphocyte antigen CD22. *Eur J Immunol* 1996;26:1246–1252.

155. O'Keefe TL, Williams GT, Davies SL, Neuberger MS. Hyperresponsive B cells in CD22-deficient mice. *Science* 1996;274:798–801.

156. Otipoby KL, Andersson KB, Draves KE, et al. CD22 regulates thymus-independent responses and the lifespan of B cells. *Nature* 1996;384:634–637.

157. Sato S, Miller AS, Inaoki M, et al. CD22 is both a positive and negative regulator of B lymphocyte antigen receptor signal transduction: Altered signaling in CD22-deficient mice. *Immunity* 1996;5:551–562.

158. Nitschke L, Carsetti R, Ocker B, Kohler G, Lamers MC. CD22 is a negative regulator of B-cell receptor signalling. *Curr Biol* 1997;7:133–143.

159. Cooke MP, Heath AW, Shokat KM, et al. Immunoglobulin signal transduction guides the specificity of B cell-T cell interactions and is blocked in tolerant self-reactive B cells. *J Exp Med* 1994;179:425–438.

160. Justement LB, Campbell KS, Chien NC, Cambier JC. Regulation of B cell antigen receptor signal transduction and phosphorylation by CD45. *Science* 1991;252:1839–1842.

161. Kishihara K, Penninger J, Wallace VA, et al. Normal B lymphocyte development but impaired T cell maturation in CD45-exon6 protein tyrosine phosphatase-deficient mice. *Cell* 1993;74:143–156.

162. Benatar T, Carsetti R, Furlonger C, Kamalia N, Mak T, Paige CJ. Immunoglobulin-mediated signal transduction in B cells from CD45-deficient mice. *J Exp Med* 1996;183:329–334.

163. Byth KF, Conroy LA, Howlett S, et al. CD45-null transgenic mice reveal a positive regulatory role for CD45 in early thymocyte development, in the selection of CD4⁺CD8⁺ thymocytes, and in B cell maturation. *J Exp Med* 1996;183:1707–1718.

164. Kantor AB, Herzenberg LA. Origins of murine B cell lineages. *Annu Rev Immunol* 1993;11:501–538.

165. Tarakhovsky A, Kanner SB, Hombach J, et al. A role for CD5 in TCR-mediated signal transduction and thymocyte selection. *Science* 1995;269:535–537.

166. Bikah G, Carey J, Ciallella JR, Tarakhovsky A, Bondada S. CD5-mediated negative regulation of antigen receptor-induced growth signals in B-1 B cells. *Science* 1996;274:1906–1909.

167. Allman DM, Ferguson SE, Lentz VM, Cancro MP. Peripheral B cell maturation. II. Heat-stable antigen(hi) splenic B cells are an immune developmental intermediate in the production of long-lived marrow-derived B cells. *J Immunol* 1993;151:4431–4444.

168. Cyster JG, Goodnow CC. Antigen-induced exclusion from follicles and anergy are separate and complementary processes that influence peripheral B cell fate. *Immunity* 1995;3:691–701.

169. Cyster JG, Healy JI, Goodnow CC. Regulation of B lymphocyte negative and positive selection by tyrosine phosphatase CD45. *Nature* 1996;381:325–328.

170. Lam K-P, Kuhn R, Rajewsky K. In vivo ablation of surface immunoglobulin on mature B cells by inducible gene targeting results in rapid cell death. *Cell* 1997;90:1073–1083.

171. Cory S. Regulation of lymphocyte survival by the Bcl-2 gene family. *Ann Rev Immunol* 1995;13:513–543.

172. Veis DJ, Sorenson CM, Shutter JR, Korsmeyer SJ. Bcl-2-deficient mice demonstrate fulminant lymphoid apoptosis, polycystic kidneys, and hypopigmented hair. *Cell* 1993;75:229–240.

173. Nakayama K, Nakayama K, Negishi I, et al. Disappearance of the lymphoid system in Bcl-2 homozygous mutant chimeric mice. *Science* 1993;261:1584–1588.

174. Boise LH, Thompson CB. Hierarchical control of lymphocyte survival. *Science* 1996;274:67–68.

175. Goroff DK, Stall A, Mond JJ, Finkelman FD. In vitro and in vivo B lymphocyte-activating properties of monoclonal anti-delta antibodies. I. Determinants of B lymphocyte-activating properties. *J Immunol* 1986;136:2382–2392.

176. Mongini PKA, Blessinger CA, Dalton JP. Affinity requirements for induction of sequential phases of human B cell activation by membrane IgM-cross-linking ligands. *J Immunol* 1991;146:1791–1800.

177. Anderson JS, Teutsch M, Dong Z, Wortis HH. An essential role for Bruton's tyrosine kinase in the regulation of B-cell apoptosis. *Proc Natl Acad Sci USA* 1996;93:10966–10971.

mobilization is integrated by CD19 dephosphorylation. *J Immunol* 1997;130:602–606.

178. Callard RE. Cytokine regulation of B-cell growth and differentiation. *Br Med Bull* 1989;45:371–388.

179. Rabin EM, Ohara J, Paul WE. B-cell stimulatory factor 1 activates resting B cells. *Proc Natl Acad Sci USA* 1985;82:2935–2939.

180. Oliver K, Noelle RJ, Uhr JW, Krammer PH, Vitetta ES. B-cell growth factor (B-cell growth factor I or B-cell stimulating factor, provisional I) is a differentiation factor for resting B cells and may not induce cell growth. *Proc Natl Acad Sci USA* 1985;82:2465–2467.

181. Solvason N, Wu W, Kabra N, Wu X, Lees E, Howard M. Induction of cell cycle regulatory proteins in anti-immunoglobulin-stimulated mature B lymphocytes. *J Exp Med* 1996;184:407.

182. Tanguay D, Chiles T. Regulation of the catalytic subunit (p34PKS-J3/cdk4) for the major D-type cyclin in mature B lymphocytes. *J Immunol* 1996;156:539.

183. Reid S, Snow EC. The regulated expression of cell cycle-regulated proteins as B lymphocytes enter and progress through the G1 cell cycle stage following delivery of complete versus partial activation stimuli. *Mol Immunol* 1996;33:1139–1151.

184. Fero ML, Rivkin M, Tasch M, et al. A syndrome of multiorgan hyperplasia with features of gigantism, tumorigenesis, and female sterility in p27(Kip1)-deficient mice. *Cell* 1996;85:733–744.

185. Nakayama K, Ishida N, Shirane M, et al. Mice lacking p27(Kip1) display increased body size, multiple organ hyperplasia, retinal dysplasia, and pituitary tumors. *Cell* 1996;85:707–720.

186. Padeh S, Levitzki A, Gazit A, Mills GB, Roifman CM. Activation of phospholipase C in human B cells is dependent on tyrosine phosphorylation. *J Clin Invest* 1991;87:1114–1118.

187. Monroe JG, Kass MJ. Molecular events in B cell activation. I. Signals required to stimulate Go to G1 transition of resting B lymphocytes. *J Immunol* 1985;135:1674–1682.

188. Paul WE, Mizuguchi J, Brown M, et al. Regulation of B-lymphocyte activation, proliferation, and immunoglobulin secretion. *Cell Immunol* 1986;99:7–13.

189. Rothstein TL, Baeker TR, Miller RA, Kolber DL. Stimulation of murine B cells by the combination of calcium ionophore plus phorbol ester. *Cell Immunol* 1986;102:364–373.

190. Sigal NH, Dumont FJ. Cyclosporin A, FK-506, and rapamycin: pharmacologic probes of lymphocyte signal transduction. *Ann Rev Immunol* 1992;10:519–560.

191. Tarakhovsky A, Turner M, Schaal S, et al. Defective antigen receptor-mediated proliferation of B and T cells in the absence of Vav. *Nature* 1995;374:467–470.

192. Zhang R, Alt FW, Davidson L, Orkin SII, Swat W. Defective signalling through the T- and B cell antigen receptors in lymphoid cells lacking the vav proto-oncogene. *Nature* 1995;374:470–473.

193. Taniuchi I, Kitamura D, Maekawa Y, Fukuda T, Kishi H, Watanabe T. Antigen-receptor induced clonal expansion and deletion of lymphocytes are impaired in mice lacking HS1 protein, a substrate of the antigen-receptor-coupled tyrosine kinases. *EMBO J* 1995;14:3664–3678.

194. White MW, McConnell F, Shu GL, Morris DR, Clark EA. Activation of dense human tonsilar B cells. Induction of c-myc gene expression via two distinct signal transduction pathways. *J Immunol* 1991;146:846–853.

195. Rooney JW, Dubois PM, Sibley CH. Cross-linking of surface IgM activates NF-κB in B lymphocytes. *Eur J Immunol* 1991;21:2993–3008.

196. Liu J, Chiles TC, Sen R, Rothstein TL. Inducible nuclear expression of NF-κB in primary B cells stimulated through the surface Ig receptor. *J Immunol* 1991;146:1685–1691.

197. Lenardo M, Baltimore D. NF-κB: A pleiotropic mediator of inducible and tissue-specific gene control. *Cell* 1989;58:227–229.

198. Stancovski I, Baltimore D. NF-κB activation: The IκB kinase revealed? *Cell* 1997;91:299–302.

199. Kontgen F, Grumont RJ, Strasser A, et al. Mice lacking the c-rel proto-oncogene exhibit defects in lymphocyte proliferation, humoral immunity, and interleukin-2 expression. *Genes Dev* 1995;15:1965–1977.

200. Doi TS, Takahashi T, Taguchi O, Azuma T, Obata Y. NF-kappa B RelA-deficient lymphocytes: normal development of T cells and B cells, impaired production of IgA and IgG1 and reduced proliferative responses. *J Exp Med* 1997;185:953–961.

201. Montminy, M. Transcriptional regulation by cyclic AMP. *Ann Rev Biochem* 1997;66:807–822.

202. Amato SF, Nakajima K, Hirano T, Chiles TC. Transcriptional regulation of the junB promoter in mature B lymphocytes. Activation through a cyclic adenosine 3′,5′-monophosphate-like binding site. *J Immunol* 1996;157:146–155.

203. Maltzman J, Monroe JG. Transcriptional regulation of the Icam-1 gene in antigen receptor and phorbol ester stimulated B lymphocytes: Role for transcription factor EGR1. *J Exp Med* 1996;183:1747–1759.

204. Maltzman J, Monroe JG. A role for EGR1 in regulation of stimulus-dependent CD44 transcription in B lymphocytes. *Mol Cell Biol* 1996;16:2283–2294.

205. Chiles TC, Liu J, Rothstein TL. Crosslinking of surface Ig receptors on murine B lymphocytes stimulates the expression of nuclear tetradecanol phorbol acetate-response element-binding proteins. *J Immunol* 1991;146:1730–1735.

206. Karin M, Liu ZG, Zandi E. AP-1 function and regulation. *Curr Opin Cell Biol* 1997;9:240–246.

207. Grandori C, Eisenman RN. Myc target genes. *Trends Biochem Sci* 1997;22:177–181.

208. Davidson HW, Reid PA, Lanzavecchia A, Watts C. Processed antigen binds to

209. Dennis GJ, Mizuguchi J, McMillan V, Finkelman FD, Ohara J, Mond JJ. Comparison of the calcium requirement for the induction and maintenance of B cell class II molecule expression and for B cell proliferation stimulated by mitogens and purified growth factors. *J Immunol* 1987;138:4307–4312.

210. Ohara J, Paul W. Receptors for B-cell stimulatory factor-1 expressed on cells of haematopoietic lineage. *Nature* 1987;325:537–540.

211. Suzuki T, Cooper M. Comparison of the expression of IL-2 receptors by human T and B cells: Induction by the polyclonal mitogens, phorbol myristate acetate, and anti-μ antibody. *J Immunol* 1985;134:3111–3119.

212. Liu Y, Linsley PS. Costimulation of T-cell growth. *Curr Opin Immunol* 1992;4:265–270.

213. Bachmann M, Hengartner H, Zinkernagel R. T helper cell-independent neutralizing B cell response against vesicular stomatitis virus: Role of antigen patterns in B cell induction? *Eur J Immunol* 1995;25:3445–3451.

214. Milich D, McLachlan A. The nucleocapsid of hepatitis B virus is both a T-cell-independent and a T-cell-independent antigen. *Science* 1986;234:1398–1401.

215. Szomolanyi-Tsuda E, Welsh RM. T cell-independent antibody-mediated clearance of polyoma virus in T cell-deficient mice. *J Exp Med* 1996;183:403–411.

216. Jelinek DF, Lipsky PE. Regulation of human B lymphocyte activation, proliferation, and differentiation. *Adv Immunol* 1987;40:1–59.

217. Mond JJ, Lees A, Snapper C. T cell-independent antigens type 2. *Ann Rev Immunol* 1995;13:655–692.

218. Ahonkhai VI, Lukacs LJ, Jonas LC, Calandra GB. Clinical experience with PedvaxHIB, a conjugate vaccine of Haemophilus influenzae type b polysaccharide–Neisseria meningitidis outer membrane protein. *Vaccine* 1991;9(suppl):38–41.

219. Snapper CM, Mond JJ. A model for induction of T cell-independent humoral immunity in response to polysaccharide antigen. *J Immunol* 1996;157:2229–2233.

220. Medzhitov R, Janeway CA Jr. Innate immunity: The virtues of a nonclonal system of recognition. *Cell* 1997;91:295–296.

221. Ip YT, Levine M. Molecular genetics of Drosophila immunity. *Curr Opin Genet Dev* 1994;4:672–677.

222. Muta T, Iwanaga S. Clotting and immune defense in Limulidae. *Prog Mol Subcell Biol* 1996;15:154–189.

223. Morrison DC, Ryan JL. Bacterial endotoxins and host immune responses. *Adv Immunol* 1979;28:293–450.

224. Morrison DC, Ryan JL. Endotoxins and disease mechanisms. *Ann Rev Med* 1987;38:417–432.

225. Corbel C, Melchers F. Requirement for macrophages or for macrophage- or T-cell-derived factors in the mitogenic stimulation of murine B lymphocytes by lipopolysaccharides. *Eur J Immunol* 1983;13:528–533.

226. Ulevitch RJ, Tobias PS. Receptor-dependent mechanisms of cell stimulation by bacterial endotoxin. *Ann Rev Immunol* 1995;13:437–457.

227. Bachmann MF, Zinkernagel RM. Neutralizing antiviral B cell responses. *Ann Rev Immunol* 1997;15:235–270.

228. Dintzis HM, Dintzis RZ, Vogelstein B. Molecular determinants of immunogenicity: The immunon model of immune response. *Proc Natl Acad Sci USA* 1976;73:3671–3675.

229. Symer DE, Reim J, Dintzis RZ, Voss EW Jr, Dintzis HM. Durable elimination of high affinity, T cell-dependent antibodies by low molecular weight antigen arrays in vivo. *J Immunol* 1995;155:5608–5616.

230. Brunswick M, June CH, Finkelman FD, Dintzis HM, Inman JK, Mond JJ. Dextran conjugated anti-Ig antibody stimulates B cells by repetitive signal transduction: A model for T cell independent B cell activation. *Proc Natl Acad Sci USA* 1989;86:6724–6728.

231. Sato S, Steeber DA, Tedder TF. The CD19 signal transduction molecule is a response regulator of B-lymphocyte differentiation. *Proc Natl Acad Sci USA* 1995;92:11558–11562.

232. Allison KC, Strober W, Harriman GR. Induction of IL-5 receptors on normal B cells by cross-linking surface Ig with anti-Ig-dextran. *J Immunol* 1991;146:4197–4203.

233. Pisetsky DS. Immune activation by bacterial DNA: A new genetic code. *Immunity* 1996;5:303–310.

234. MacLennan I, Gray D. Antigen-driven selection of virgin and memory B cells. *Immunol Rev* 1986;91:61–85.

235. MacLennan I, Gray D, Kumararatne D, Bazin H. The lymphocytes of splenic marginal zones: A distinct B-cell lineage. *Immunol Today* 1982;3:305–307.

236. Snapper CM, Yamaguchi H, Moorman MA, Mond JJ. An in vitro model for T cell-independent induction of humoral immunity. A requirement for NK cells. *J Immunol* 1994;152:2884–4892.

237. Kantor AB. The development and repertoire of B-1 cells (CD5 B cells). *Immunol Today* 1991;12:389–391.

238. Kantor AD. V-gene usage and N-region insertions in B-1a, B-1b and conventional B cells. *Semin Immunol* 1996;8:29–35.

239. Stall AM, Wells SM, Lam K-P. B-1 cells: Unique origins and functions. *Semin Immunol* 1996;8:45–59.

240. Krose FGM, de Waard R, Bos NA. B-1 cells and their reactivity with the murine intestinal flora. *Semin Immunol* 1996;8:11–18.

241. Yin XM, Vitetta ES. The lineage relationship between virgin and memory B cells. *Int Immunol* 1992;4:691–698.

242. Cong YZ, Rabin E, Wortis HH. Treatment of murine CD5 B cells with anti-Ig,

but not LPS, induces surface CD5: Two B-cell activation pathways. *Int Immunol* 1991;3:467–476.

243. Cyster JG, Goodnow CC. Protein tyrosine phosphatase 1C negatively regulates antigen receptor signaling in B lymphocytes and determines thresholds for negative selection. *Immunity* 1995;2:13–24.

244. Kelsoe G, Zheng B. Sites of B-cell activation in vivo. *Curr Opin Immunol* 1993; 5:418–422.

245. Liu Y-J. Sites of B lymphocyte selection, activation, and tolerance in spleen. *J Exp Med* 1997;186:625–629.

246. Stuber E, Strober W. The T cell-B cell interaction via OX40-OX40L is necessary for the T cell-dependent humoral immune response. *J Exp Med* 1996;183: 979–989.

247. Lanzavecchia A. Receptor-mediated antigen uptake and its effect on antigen presentation to class II restricted T lymphocytes. *Ann Rev Immunol* 1990;8:773–793.

248. Davidson HW, West MA, Watts C. Endocytosis, intracellular trafficking, and processing of membrane IgG and monovalent antigen/membrane IgG complexes in B lymphocytes. *J Immunol* 1990;144:4101–4109.

249. Tony H-P, Phillips NE, Parker DC. Role of membrane immunoglobulin (Ig) crosslinking in membrane Ig-mediated, major histocompatability-restricted T cell-B cell cooperation. *J Exp Med* 1985;162:1695–1708.

250. Shaw AC, Mitchell RN, Weaver YK, Campos-Torres J, Abbas AK, Leder P. Mutations of immunoglobulin transmembrane and cytoplasmic domains: Effects on intracellular signaling and antigen presentation. *Cell* 1990;63:381–392.

251. Mitchell RN, Barnes KA, Grupp SA, et al. Intracellular targeting of antigens internalized by membrane immunoglobulin in B lymphocytes. *J Exp Med* 1995; 181:1705–1714.

252. Patel KJ, Neuberger MS. Antigen presentation by the B cell antigen receptor is driven by the α/β sheath and occurs independently of its cytoplasmic tyrosines. *Cell* 1993;74:939–946.

253. Bonnerot C, Lankar D, Hanau D, et al. Role of B cell receptor Ig alpha and Ig beta subunits in MHC class II-restricted antigen presentation. *Immunity* 1995;3: 335–347.

254. Knight AM, Lucocq JM, Prescott AR, Ponnambalam S, Watts C. Antigen endocytosis and presentation mediated by human membrane IgG1 in the absence of the Ig(alpha)/Ig(beta) dimer. *EMBO J* 1997;16:3842–3850.

255. Casten LA, Lakey EK, Jelachich ML, Margoliash E, Pierce SK. Anti-immunoglobulin augments the B-cell antigen-presentation function independently of receptor-antigen complex. *Proc Natl Acad Sci USA* 1985;82:5890–5894.

256. Lenschow DJ, Sperling AI, Cooke MP, et al. Differential up-regulation of the B7-1 and B7-2 costimulatory molecules after Ig receptor engagement by antigen. *J Immunol* 1994;153:1990–1997.

257. Kearse KP, Cassatt DR, Kaplan AM, Cohen DA. The requirement for surface Ig signaling as a prerequisite for T cell:B cell interactions. *J Immunol* 1988;140: 1770–1778.

258. Dang LH, Rock KL. Stimulation of B lymphocytes through surface Ig receptors induces LFA-1 and ICAM-1-dependent adhesion. *J Immunol* 1991;146: 3273–3279.

259. Kishimoto T, Ishizaka K. Regulation of antibody response in vitro. IX. Induction of secondary anti-hapten IgG antibody response by anti-immunoglobulin and enhancing soluble factor. *J Immunol* 1975;114:585.

260. Parker DC, Fothergill JJ, Wadsworth DC. B lymphocyte activation by insoluble anti-immunoglobulin: Induction of immunoglobulin secretion by a T cell-dependent soluble factor. *J Immunol* 1979;123:931–941.

261. Howard M, Farrar J, Hilfiker M, et al. Identification of a T cell-derived B cell growth factor distinct from interleukin 2. *J Exp Med* 1982;155:914–923.

262. Nakanishi K, Howard M, Muraguchi A, et al. Soluble factors involved in B cell differentiation: Identification of two distinct T cell-replacing factors (TRF). *J Immunol* 1983;130:2219–2224.

263. Morse L, Chen D, Franklin D, Xiong Y, Chen-Kiang S. Induction of cell cycle arrest and B cell terminal differentiation by CDK inhibitor p18(INK4c) and IL-6. *Immunity* 1997;6:47–56.

264. Turner CA Jr, Mack DH, Davis MM. Blimp-1, a novel zinc finger-containing protein that can drive the maturation of B lymphocytes into immunoglobulin-secreting cells. *Cell* 1994;77:297–306.

265. Schliephake DE, Schimpl A. Blimp-1 overcomes the block in IgM secretion in lipopolysaccharide/anti-mu F(ab′)2-co-stimulated B lymphocytes. *Eur J Immunol* 1996;26:268–271.

266. Wetzel GD. Interleukin 5 regulation of peritoneal Ly-1 B lymphocyte proliferation, differentiation, and autoantibody secretion. *Eur J Immunol* 1989;19:1701–1707.

267. Takatsu K. Interleukin-5. *Curr Opin Immunol* 1992;4:299–306.

268. Takatsu K, Takaki S, Hitoshi Y. Interleukin-5 and its receptor system: Implications in the immune system and inflammation. *Adv Immunol* 1994;57:145–190.

269. Loughnan MS, Nossal GJV. Interleukins 4 and 5 control expression of IL-2 receptor on murine B cells through independent induction of its two chains. *Nature* 1989;340:76–79.

270. Blackman M, Tigges MA, Minie ME, Koshland ME. A model system for peptide hormone action in differentiation: interleukin 2 induces a B lymphoma to transcribe the J chain gene. *Cell* 1986;47:609–617.

271. Phillips C, Klaus GGB. Soluble anti-μ monoclonal antibodies prime resting B cells to secrete immunoglobulins in response to interleukins-4 and -5. *Eur J Immunol* 1992;22:1541–1545.

272. Stein P, Dubois P, Greenblatt D, Howard M. Induction of antigen-specific proliferation in affinity-purified small B lymphocytes: Requirement for BSF-1 by type 2 but not type 1 thymus-independent antigens. *J Immunol* 1986;136:2080–2089.

273. Grupp SA, Snow EC, Harmony JAK. The phosphatidylinositol response is an early event in the physiologically relevant activation of antigen-specific B lymphocytes. *Cell Immunol* 1987;109:181–191.

274. Snow EC, Fetherston JD, Zimmer S. Induction of the c-myc protooncogene after antigen binding to hapten-specific B cells. *J Exp Med* 1986;164:944–949.

275. Myers CD, Kriz MK, Sullivan TJ, Vitetta ES. Antigen-induced changes in phospholipid metabolism in antigen-binding B lymphocytes. *J Immunol* 1987;138: 1705–1711.

276. Swain SL, Wetzel GD, Soubiran P, Dutton RW. T cell replacing factors in the B cell response to antigen. *Immunol Rev* 1982;63:111–128.

277. Leibson HJ, Gefter M, Zlotnik A, Marrack P, Kappler JW. Role of interferon in antibody producing responses. *Nature* 1984;309:799–801.

278. Jelinek DF, Splawski JB, Lipsky PE. The role of interlukin 2 and interferon-γ in human B cell activation, growth and differentiation. *Eur J Immunol* 1986;16:925.

279. Vitetta ES, Fernandez-Botran R, Myers CD, Sanders VM. Cellular interactions in the humoral immune response. *Adv Immunol* 1989;45:1–105.

280. Noelle RJ, Snow EC. Cognate interactions between helper T cells and B cells. *Immunol Today* 1990;11:361–368.

281. Foy TM, Durie FH, Noelle RJ. The expansive role of CD40 and its ligand, gp39, in immunity. *Semin Immunol* 1994;6:259–266.

282. Armitage RJ, Fanslow WC, Stockbine L, et al. Molecular and biological characterization of a murine ligand for CD40. *Nature* 1992;347:80–82.

283. Banchereau J, Bazan F, Blanchard D, et al. The CD40 antigen and its ligand. *Ann Rev Immunol* 1994;12:881–922.

284. Clark LB, Foy TM, Noelle RJ. CD40 and its ligand. *Adv Immunol* 1996;63:43–78.

285. Snapper CM, Rosas F, Moorman MA, et al. IFN-gamma is a potent inducer of Ig secretion by sort-purified murine B cells activated through the mIg, but not the CD40, signaling pathway. *Int Immunol* 1996;8:877–885.

286. Rothstein TL, Wang JK, Panka DJ, et al. Protection against Fas-dependent Th1-mediated apoptosis by antigen receptor engagement in B cells. *Nature* 1995;374: 163–165.

287. Xu J, Foy TM, Laman JD, et al. Mice deficient for the CD40 ligand. *Immunity* 1994;1:423–431.

288. Sanders VM, Fernandez-Botran R, Coffman RL, Mosmann TR, Vitetta ES. A single antigen-specific B cell can conjugate to either a type 1 or a type 2 helper T cell. *Proc Natl Acad Sci USA* 1988;85:7724–7728.

289. Kupfer A, Singer SJ. Cell biology of cytotoxic and helper T cell functions: Immunofluorescence microscopic studies of single cells and cell couples. *Ann Rev Immunol* 1989;7:309–337.

290. Poo W-J, Conrad L, Janeway CA Jr. Receptor-directed focusing of lymphokine release by helper T cells. *Nature* 1988;332:378–380.

291. Clark EA, Ledbetter JA. How B and T cells talk to each other. *Nature* 1994;367: 425–428.

292. Dustin ML, Springer TA. Role of lymphocyte adhesion receptors in transient interactions and cell locomotion. *Ann Rev Immunol* 1991;9:27–66.

293. Baluyut AR, Subbarao B. The synergistic effects of anti-IgM and monoclonal anti-Ia antibodies in induction of murine B lymphocyte activation. *J Mol Cell Immunol* 1988;1:45.

294. Cambier JC, Lehmann KR. Ia mediated signal transduction leads to proliferation of primed B cells. *J Exp Med* 1989;170:877–886.

295. Cambier JC, Newell MK, Justement LB, McGuire JC, Leach KL, Chen ZZ. Ia binding ligands and cAMP stimulate nuclear translocation of PKC in B lymphocytes. *Nature* 1987;327:629–632.

296. Pollok KE, O'Brien V, Marshall L, Olson JW, Noelle RJ, Snow EC. The development of competence in resting B cells: The induction of cyclic AMP and ornithine decarboxylase activity after direct contact between B and T helper cells. *J Immunol* 1991;146:1633–1641.

297. Lane PJL, McConnell GM, Schieven GL, Clark EA, Ledbetter JA. The role of class II molecules in human B cell activation: Association with phosphatidylinositol turnover, protein tyrosine phosphorylation and proliferation. *J Immunol* 1990;144:3684–3692.

298. Armitage RJ. Tumor necrosis factor receptor superfamily members and their ligands. *Curr Opin Immunol* 1994;6:407–413.

299. Kuhne MR, Robbins M, Hambor JE, et al. Assembly and regulation of the CD40 receptor complex in human B cells. *J Exp Med* 1997;186:337–342.

300. Xu Y, Cheng G, Baltimore D. Targeted disruption of TRAF3 leads to postnatal lethality and defective T-dependent immune responses. *Immunity* 1996;5:407–415.

301. Ishida T, Mizushima SI, Azuma S, et al. Identification of TRAF6, a novel tumor necrosis factor receptor-associated factor protein that mediates signaling from an amino-terminal domain of the CD40 cytoplasmic region. *J Biol Chem* 1996;271: 28745–28748.

302. Hasbold J, Klaus GGB. B cells from CBA/N mice do not proliferate following ligation of CD40. *Eur J Immunol* 1994;24:152–157.

303. Sakata N, Patel HR, Terada N, Aruffo A, Johnson GL, Gelfand EW. Selective activation of c-Jun kinase mitogen-activated protein kinase by CD40 on human B cells. *J Biol Chem* 1995;270:30823–30828.

304. Tooze RM, Doody GM, Fearon DT. Counterregulation by the coreceptors CD19 and CD22 of MAP kinase activation by membrane immunoglobulin. *Immunity* 1997;7:59–67.

305. Finkelman FD, Holmes J, Katona IM, et al. Lymphokine control of in vivo immunoglobulin isotype selection. *Ann Rev Immunol* 1990;8:303–333.

306. Paul WE, Seder RA. Lymphocyte responses and cytokines. *Cell* 1994;76:241–251.

307. Pistoia V. Production of cytokines by human B cells in health and disease. *Immunol Today* 1997;18:343–350.

308. Torcia M, Bracci-Laudiero L, Lucibello M, et al. Nerve growth factor is an autocrine survival factor for memory B lymphocytes. *Cell* 1996;85:345–356.

309. Swain SL, Bradley LM, Croft M, et al. Helper T-cell subsets: Phenotype, function and the role of lymphokines in regulating their development. *Immunol Rev* 1991;123:115–144.

310. Seder RA, Paul WE, Davis MM, Fazekas de St. Groth B. The presence of interleukin 4 during in vitro priming determines the lymphokine-producing potential of CD4+ T cells from T cell receptor transgenic mice. *J Exp Med* 1992;176:1091–1098.

311. Croft M, Swain SL. B cell response to T helper cell subsets. II. Both the stage of T cell differentiation and the cytokines secreted determine the extent and nature of helper activity. *J Immunol* 1991;147:3679–3689.

312. Croft M, Swain SL. B cell response to fresh and effector T helper cells. Role of cognate T-B interaction and the cytokines IL-2, IL-4, and IL-6. *J Immunol* 1991;146:4055–4064.

313. Croft M, Swain SL. Analysis of CD4+ T cells that provide contact-dependent bystander help to B cells. *J Immunol* 1992;149:3157–3165.

314. Gray D, Bergthorsdottir S, van Essen D, Wykes M, Poudrier J, Siepmann K. Observations on memory B-cell development. *Semin Immunol* 1997;9:249–254.

315. Bachmann MF, Schorle H, Kuhn R, et al. Antiviral immune responses in mice deficient for both interleukin-2 and interleukin-4. *J Virol* 1995;69:4842–4846.

316. Kopf M, Le Gros G, Coyle AJ, Kosco-Vilbois M, Brombacher F. Immune responses of IL-4, IL-5, IL-6 deficient mice. *Immunol Rev* 1995;148:45–69.

317. Huang S, Hendriks W, Althage A, et al. Immune response in mice that lack the interferon-gamma receptor. *Science* 1993;259:1742–1745.

318. Yoshida T, Ikuta K, Sugaya H, et al. Defective B-1 cell development and impaired immunity against Angiostrongylus cantonensis in IL-5R alpha-deficient mice. *Immunity* 1996;4:483–494.

319. Forster R, Mattis AE, Kremmer E, Wolf E, Brem G, Lipp M. A putative chemokine receptor, BLR1, directs B cell migration to defined lymphoid organs and specific anatomic compartments of the spleen. *Cell* 1996;87:1037–1047.

319a. Gunn MD, Ngo VN, Ansel KM, Ekland EH, Cyster JG, Williams LT. A B-cell-homing chemokine made in lymphoid follicles activates Burkitt's lymphoma receptor-1. *Nature* 1998;391:799–803.

320. Kelsoe G. Life and death in germinal centers (redux). *Immunity* 1996;4:107–111.

321. MacLennan I. Germinal centers. *Ann Rev Immunol* 1994;12:117–139.

322. Jacob J, Kelsoe G, Rajewsky K, Weiss U. Intraclonal generation of antibody mutants in germinal centres. *Nature* 1991;354:389–392.

323. Berek C, Berger A, Apel M. Maturation of the immune response in germinal centers. *Cell* 1991;67:1121–1129.

324. Wabl M, Steinberg C. Affinity maturation and class switching. *Curr Opin Immunol* 1996;8:89–92.

325. MacLennan ICM, Casamayor-Palleja M, Toellner KM, Gulbranson-Judge A, Gordon J. Memory B-cell clones and the diversity of their members. *Semin Immunol* 1997;9:229–234.

326. Shokat KM, Goodnow CC. Antigen-induced B-cell death and elimination during germinal-centre immune responses. *Nature* 1995;375:334–338.

327. Pulendran B, Kannourakis G, Nouri S, Smith KG, Nossal GJ. Soluble antigen can cause enhanced apoptosis of germinal-centre B cells. *Nature* 1995;375:331–334.

328. Han S, Zheng B, Dal Porto J, Kelsoe G. In situ studies of the primary immune response to (4-hydroxy-3-nitrophenyl)acetyl. IV. Affinity-dependent, antigen-driven B cell apoptosis in germinal centers as a mechanism for maintaining self-tolerance. *J Exp Med* 1995;182:1635–1644.

329. Smith KG, Weiss U, Rajewsky K, Nossal GJ, Tarlinton DM. Bcl-2 increases memory B cell recruitment but does not perturb selection in germinal centers. *Immunity* 1994;1:803–813.

330. Smith KG, Nossal GJ, Tarlinton DM. FAS is highly expressed in the germinal center but is not required for regulation of the B-cell response to antigen. *Proc Natl Acad Sci USA* 1995;92:11628–11632.

331. Klinman NR. The cellular origins of memory B cells. *Semin Immunol* 1997;9:241–247.

332. Merville P, Dechanet J, Desmouliere A, et al. Bcl-2+ tonsillar plasma cells are rescued from apoptosis by bone marrow fibroblasts. *J Exp Med* 1996;183:227–236.

333. Arpin C, Dechanet J, Van Kooten C, et al. Generation of memory B cells and plasma cells in vitro. *Science* 1995;268:720–722.

334. Ambrus JL Jr, Chesky L, Stephany D, McFarland P, Mostowski H, Fauci AS. Functional studies examining the subpopulation of human B lymphocytes responding to high molecular weight B cell growth factor. *J Immunol* 1990;145:3949–3955.

335. Schittek B, Rajewsky K. Maintenance of B-cell memory by long-lived cells generated from proliferating precursors. *Nature* 1990;346:749–751.

336. Nunez G, Hockenbery D, McDonnell TJ, Sorensen CM, Korsmeyer SJ. Bcl-2 maintains B cell memory. *Nature* 1991;353:71–73.

337. Strasser A, Whittingham S, Vaux DL, et al. Enforced Bcl-2 expression in B-lymphoid cells prolongs antibody responses and elicits autoimmune disease. *Proc Natl Acad Sci USA* 1991;88:8661–8665.

338. Radic MZ, Zouali M. Receptor editing, immune diversification, and self-tolerance. *Immunity* 1996;5:505–511.

339. Monroe JG. Tolerance sensitivity of immature-stage B cells. Can developmentally regulated B cell antigen receptor (BCR) signal transduction play a role? *J Immunol* 1996;156:2657–2660.

340. Carsetti R, Kohler G, Lamers MC. Transitional B cells are the target of negative selection in the B cell compartment. *J Exp Med* 1995;181:2129–2140.

341. Klinman NR. The "clonal selection hypothesis" and current concepts of B cell tolerance. *Immunity* 1996;5:189–195.

342. Nossal GJV. Cellular mechanisms of immunologic tolerance. *Ann Rev Immunol* 1983;1:33–62.

343. Goodnow CC. Transgenic mice and analysis of B-cell tolerance. *Ann Rev Immunol* 1992;10:489–518.

344. Hartley SB, Crosbie J, Brink R, Kantor AB, Basten A, Goodnow CC. Elimination from peripheral lymphoid tissues of self-reactive B lymphocytes recognizing membrane-bound antigens. *Nature* 1991;353:765–769.

345. Ho WY, Cooke MP, Goodnow CC, Davis MM. Resting and anergic B cells are defective in CD28-dependent costimulation of naive CD4+ T cells. *J Exp Med* 1994;179:1539–1549.

346. Rathmell JC, Cooke MP, Ho WY, et al. CD95 (Fas)-dependent elimination of self-reactive B cells upon interaction with CD4+ T cells. *Nature* 1995;376:181–184.

347. Rathmell JC, Townsend SE, Xu JC, Flavell RA, Goodnow CC. Expansion or elimination of B cells in vivo: dual roles for CD40- and Fas (CD95)-ligands modulated by the B cell antigen receptor. *Cell* 1996;87:319–329.

Fundamental Immunology, Fourth Edition,
edited by William E. Paul
Published by Lippincott–Raven Publishers, Philadelphia 1999.

CHAPTER 8

The Major Histocompatibility Complex

David H. Margulies

INTRODUCTION

The immune system relies on many regulatory mechanisms that govern its ability to respond to infectious agents and neoplastic tissues, but no single scheme is as much a cellular and molecular microcosm of complex biologic systems as that controlled by the major histocompatibility complex (*Mhc*). The *Mhc* is a set of linked genes, located on chromosome 6 of the human, chromosome 17 of the mouse, and chromosome 20 of the rat, that was first identified for its effects on tumor or skin transplantation and control of immune responsiveness (1,2). The *Mhc* also plays a role in the resistance to infection and in susceptibility to a number of autoimmune diseases. Indeed, the provocative early observations that indicated an *Mhc*-linked control of immune responsiveness (3–6) have been the basis of many detailed investigations over the past two decades and have culminated in a molecular understanding of the critical details of genetically encoded cellular recognition in the immune system. Although the control of transplantion and the other immune responses are the phenotypic consequences of the function of molecules encoded in the *Mhc*, understanding the *Mhc* becomes clear if we think of it in molecular and cellular terms. MHC molecules are cell surface receptors that bind antigen fragments and display them to various cells of the immune system, most importantly T cells that bear $\alpha\beta$ receptors (7–9). *Natural killer* (NK) cells also are influenced by interactions with MHC molecules (10,11), as are T cells that express $\gamma\delta$ receptors (12). In recent years, we have been fortunate to witness a transition in our knowledge from that of mysterious genetic entities with unclear mechanism but distinct immunologic function and genetic location, to that of specific molecules with known structure, biosynthetic pathway, biophysical parameters of interaction, and temporal expression that convey specific signals between and within cells, and that map precisely to defined regions of the chromosome. Thus, the study of the Mhc has also made a transition, from that of genetics and cellular immunology, to detailed molecular mechanism. In this chapter we hope to provide the reader with an opportunity to understand the basic principles unique to this encoded protein system, to explore the mechanistic details that draw from genetics, cell biology, and molecular biochemistry, and at the same time to preserve some of the historical perspective that conveys the excitement of discovery and the wonder of natural science.

Major improvements in our knowledge over the past few years are due to many converging factors: the widespread availability of inbred and recombinant mouse strains; a library of well-characterized monoclonal antibodies that detect cell surface markers specifically and potently; genomic and cDNA clones for *Mhc*-encoded proteins derived from several different species; high-resolution linkage maps based on cosmid and artificial chromosome clones; methods for the controlled expression of *Mhc* genes in transfectant cell lines and transgenic mice; knockout animals with directed mutations of particular genetic loci; expression systems for producing large amounts of homogeneous, soluble analogues of MHC molecules; and high-resolution X-ray crystallographic structures of MHC molecules and associated proteins. In addition, the availability of computer accessible databases for obtaining current information on the nucleotide and amino acid sequence, as well as the three-dimensional structures of many of these factors, makes the study of the *Mhc* particularly exciting and challenging.

D. H. Margulies. Molecular Biology Section, Laboratory of Immunology, National Institute of Allergy and Infectious Diseases, National Institutes of Health, Bethesda, MD 20892

The focus of this chapter is the *Mhc,* and in concert with contemporary understanding of structure and function, the goal will be to outline the general principles of molecular organization and function of both the genetic regions that encode MHC molecules and the functional cell surface molecules themselves.

A Note on Nomenclature

One of the most confusing topics for students of the *Mhc* has been its nomenclature. Like language, nomenclature evolves, and our attempts at standardization are inevitably incompletely successful. With new discoveries, additional complexities are recognized, and a need for greater precision undermines the simpler systems of the past. Current usage differs from species to species, journal to journal, and writer to writer; however, there are standards of which the informed scientist should be aware. For the mouse *Mhc,* these are available in several publications: *Genetic Variants and Strains of the Laboratory Mouse* (13), now in its third edition, and the Jackson Laboratory home page (http://www.informatics.jax.org/nomen/). For the human *Mhc,* there is a standard World Health Organization (WHO) nomenclature that is periodically evaluated and revised (14). The standard usage and nomenclatures for the designation of the general genetic region and some of the genes encoded therein are summarized here. The convention is that genes or genetic loci are indicated by designations in italics and the encoded protein product or phenotypic descriptions are shown in a standard font. For the genes of the human *Mhc,* this convention is often overlooked, while for those of the mouse and other species, it is frequently followed. We will attempt to make this distinction between genes and encoded proteins by use of italics, and we will also specifically clarify whether the discussion focuses on genes, genetic loci, or encoded proteins. The mouse *Mhc* is referred to as *H-2* because it was the second genetic locus involved in control of expression of erythrocyte antigens to be identified by Gorer (15,16). Now, the *Mhc* is known to consist of many loci, and the extended genetic region is referred to as the *complex;* thus, the general term used for all species is the *Mhc* or MHC (for major histocompatibility complex). (With the use of databases and computerized maps, the tendency is to eliminate the use of the hyphen, thus, *H-2* is evolving to *H2,* but we will use the more common *H-2* here). The *Mhc* in the rat is known as *RT1,* and virtually all *Mhc*s in other species are known by a variant of that used for the human, human leukocyte antigen (*HLA*). Thus, we have *ChLA* for the chimpanzee, *DLA* for the dog, *GPLA* for the guinea pig, *SLA* for the swine, *RLA* for the rabbit, and *RhLA* for the Rhesus monkey.

Because the first genes of the *Mhc* to be identified were those that encoded cell surface molecules that could be detected by antibodies or by transplantation responses, these are the ones that are referred to as *Mhc* genes. Now we know of over 400 genes that map to the human or mouse *Mhc,* and though technically they are all *Mhc* genes, the MHC molecules refer specifically to MHC-I or MHC-II molecules that are related in structure and function. Other *Mhc*-encoded molecules with distinct structure and function are referred to by their more specific names.

Particular *Mhc* genes are designated by a letter (or letters) for the locus (e.g., *H-2K, H-2D, H-2L, H-2IA* in the mouse; and *HLA-A, HLA-B, HLA-C, HLA-DR* in the human). Allelic genes (and their expressed cell surface protein products) have been denoted in the mouse by the addition of a superscript (e.g., *H-2K*b

and *H-2K*d are distinct alleles at the same locus), or in the human by the addition of a number or a letter and a number (*HLA-A2* and *HLA-A3* are alleles, as are *HLA-B8* and *HLA-B27*). Precise designation of human genes is by a nomenclature including a four-digit number following the locus (e.g., HLA-A*0101 and HLA-DRB1*0101). Clarity in understanding the human designations requires a conversion table to align the older nomenclature based on serology with the more recent DNA typing (Tables 1 and 2).

For the *Mhc* class II genes, the designation in the human is *HLA-D,* while in the mouse, *H-2IAa, H-2IAb, H-2IEa,* and *H-2IEb* are used, and frequently shortened to *IAa, IAb, IEa,* and *IEb,* respectively. *a* and *b* refer to the *a* or α (alpha) and *b* or β (beta) chain encoding genes, respectively. Current usage tends to employ the Roman letter for the gene designation, and the Greek for the encoded protein chain. The MHC-II molecules are often referred to as IA or IE, with a superscript denoting the haplotype (i.e., IAb, IAd, or IEd). Another complication that demands the precise use of gene and encoded protein names is that the number of genes in a particular homologous genetic region can differ between strain and strain or individual and individual. In the mouse, while some strains have only a single gene at the *D* locus (*H-2D*b, for instance), other strains may have as many as five genes in the homologous region [*H-2D*d, *H-2D2*d, *H-2D3*d, *H-2D4*d, and *H-L*d (17)].

An important description commonly used is *haplotype,* which refers to the linkage of particular alleles at distant loci that occur as a group on a parental chromosome (18). The concept of haplotype is important in typing the *HLA* loci in the human, where the linked *Mhc* genes of one chromosome of one parent will generally segregate as a linkage group to the children. Individual haplotypes of the *Mhc* in the mouse are referred to by a lower case letter superscript as *H-2*b, *H-2*d, or *H-2*k. Thus, the *H-2*k haplotype refers to the full set of linked genes—*H-2K*k, *H-2IA*k, *H-2IE*k, *H-2D*k— and extends to the genes of the *Q* and *T* regions as well (19). (Some haplotype designations, like *H-2*a, refer to natural recombinants and thus have some of the linked genes from one haplotype and others from another). The realization that the similar *H-2* haplotypes represented by different mouse strains have significant differences, particulary in the number and allelic identity of *Mhc* class Ib genes, has supported a proposal to refine the nomenclature (20). Table 3 is a summary of the haplotypes of common mouse strains.

In parallel with the genetic nomenclature system, a system has developed that focuses on the expressed proteins rather than just on the genes, and by its use emphasizes both structural and functional differences. The main distinction of MHC molecules is between the MHC class I (MHC-I) and MHC class II (MHC-II) molecules. [MHC class III molecules (MHC-III) have also been included in a group, but these are serum molecules that are involved in the complement system (C4) or those encoded in the genetically linked loci.] A proposal to call the region in the human that lies distal to *Mhc-III* and proximal to *Mhc-I* the *Mhc* class IV region has been made (21).

MHC-I molecules all consist of a heavy chain (also called an α chain), which is noncovalently assembled with a light chain known as β2-microglobulin (β2-m, encoded by the *B2m* gene). MHC-I molecules are subclassified into the MHC class Ia and MHC class Ib groups, distinctions made based on amino acid sequence differences as well as gene location (22). MHC-IIs are heterodimeric as well, composed of an α chain noncovalently assembled with a β

TABLE 1. *Listing of HLA class I alleles*

HLA-A		HLA-B		HLA-C		HLA-E		HLA-G	
Serology	Alleles	Serology	Alleles	Serology	Alleles	Serology	Alleles	Serology	Alleles
A1	A*0101,0102	B7	B*0702–0706	Cw1	Cw*0102,0103	—	E*0101–	—	G*01011–
A2	A*0201–0217	B8	B*0801–0803	Cw2	Cw*02021,02022		0104		0104
A3	A*0301,0302	B13	B*1301–1303	Cw3	Cw*0302–0304				
A11	A*1101–1103	B14	B*1401,1402	Cw4	Cw*0401–0403				
A23(9)	A*2301	B15	B*1501–1531	Cw5	Cw*0501				
A24(9)	A*2402–2410	B18	B*1801–1803	Cw6	Cw*0602				
A25(10)	A*2501	B27	B*2701–2710	Cw7	Cw*0701–0705				
A26(10)	A*2601–2608	B35	B*3501–3518	Cw8	Cw*0801–0803				
A29(19)	A*2901,2902	B37	B*3701–3702	—	Cw*12021–1203				
A30(19)	A*3001–3004	B38(16)	B*3801–3802	—	Cw*1301				
A31(19)	A*31012	B39(16)	B*39011–3909	—	Cw*1402,1403				
A32(19)	A*3201	B40	B*40011–4008	—	Cw*1502–1505				
A33(19)	A*3301–3303	B41	B*4101,4102	—	Cw*1601,1602				
A34(10)	A*3401,3402	B42	B*4201,4202	—	Cw*1701,1702				
A36	A*3601	B44(12)	B*4402–4407						
A43	A*4301	B45(12)	B*4501						
A66	A*6601,6602	B46	B*4601						
A68(28)	A*68011–6803	B47	B*4701						
A69(28)	A*6901	B48	B*4801,4802						
A74(19)	A*7401	B49(21)	B*4901						
—	A*8001	B50(21)	B*5001						
		B51(5)	B*5101–5107						
		B52(5)	B*52011,52012						
		B53	B*5301						
		B54(22)	B*5401						
		B55(22)	B*5501–5503						
		B56(22)	B*5601,5602						
		B57(17)	B*5701–5704						
		B58(17)	B*5801,5802						
		B59	B*5901						
		B67	B*67011,67012						
		B73	B*7301						
		B78	B*7801,7802						
		—	B*8101						
		—	B*8201						

This list summarizes the designations of the human MHC-I HLA gene products as they have been known based on serology, and as they have been assigned by nucleotide (and thus inferred amino acid) sequences. This table is taken from that of McCluskey (262). Frequently updated listings of HLA alleles as well as alignments of their sequences can be found at: http://www.icnet.uk/axp/tia. Current serologic designations are given in the "serology" column, with older corresponding numbers listed in parentheses. It is apparent that some of the most recently identified alleles (in particular, those of HLA-E and HLA-G) have not been identified serologically.

chain. The heterodimers usually consist of the assembled products of the linked genes encoding the two chains. In the mouse, the products of the *IAa* (also known as *IAα*) and *IAb* (or *IAβ*) genes assemble to form the IA heterodimer, and similarly, the products of the *IEa* (*IEα*) and *IEb* (*IEβ*) genes assemble to form IE. IA and IE are often referred to as *isotypes*. The allelic forms are usually referred to as *IAᵇ*, *IAᵈ*, or *IAᵏ*. Under some circumstances, mixed heterodimers, which can be of immunologic importance, are observed (23–27). Thus, if one is referring to a mixed heterodimer consisting of the α chain of *IEᵈ* and the β chain of *IAᵈ*, one must use the more precise but cumbersome description IAβᵈEαᵈ (IAbᵈEaᵈ). In the human, particularly in referring to MHC-II molecules, the distinctions between molecules identified by antibodies and those identified by DNA sequence typing must be made (see Tables 1 and 2). The bulk of the serologically defined differences rest with the β chain.

The Function of MHC Molecules

The major function of the molecules encoded by the *Mhc* is to facilitate the display of unique molecular fragments on the surface of cells in an arrangement that permits their recognition by immune effectors such as T-lymphocytes. The MHC-I or MHC-II molecules are those cell surface glycoproteins that actually perform the binding and recognition steps, while other genes that map to the *Mhc-I* or *Mhc-II* regions may contribute to antigen-processing and -presentation functions in other distinct ways. The MHC molecule accomplishes its major role in immune recognition by satisfying two distinct molecular functions: the binding of peptides (or in some cases nonpeptidic molecules) and the interaction with T cells, usually via the αβ T-cell receptor (TCR). The binding of peptides by an MHC-I or MHC-II molecule is the selective event that permits the cell expressing the MHC molecule (the antigen-

TABLE 2. *Listing of HLA class II alleles*

HLA-DR		HLA-DQ		HLA-DP	
Serology	Alleles	Serology	Alleles	Serology	Alleles
α-Chain					
	DRA*0101–0102		DQA1*0101–0105		DPA1*0103–0104
			DQA1*0201		DPA1*0201–0202
			DQA1*0301–0303		DPA1*0301
			DQA1*0401		DPA1*0401
			DQA1*0501–0503		
			DQA1*0601		
β-Chain					
DR1	DRB1*0101–0104	DQ5(1)	DQB1*0501–0504	DPw1	DPB1*0101
DR15(2)	DRB1*1501–1505	DQ6(1)	DQB1*0601–0611	DPw2	DPB1*0202–0202
DR16(2)	DRB1*1601–05	DQ2	DQB1*0201–0203	DPw3	DPB1*0301
DR3	DRB1*0301–0308	DQ3	DQB1*0301–0306	DPw4	DPB1*0401–0402
DR4	DRB1*0401–0423	DQ4	DQB1*0401–0402	DPw5	DPB1*0501
DR11(5)	DRB1*1101–1127			DPw6	DPB1*0601
DR12(5)	DRB1*1201–1204			—	DPB1*0801–4101
DR13(6)	DRB1*1301–1312			—	DPB1*4401–6501
DR14(6)	DRB1*1401–1425				
DR7	DRB1*0701				
DR8	DRB1*0801–0813				
DR9	DRB1*0901				
DR10	DRB1*1001				
	DRB3*0101				
DR52	DRB3*0201–0205				
	DRB3*0301				
DR53	DRB4*0101–0103				
	DRB4*01011–02N				
DR51	DRB5*0101–0105				
	DRB5*0201–0203				

Lists of HLA alleles and regular updates and aligned sequences can be assessed from the TAL Homepage at: http://www.icnet.uk/axp/tia

As illustrated by this table, the serologic assignments of HLA class II molecules do not always correlate with the DNA nomenclature. Serologic assignment of HLA-DR molecules is largely determined by the DRB1 gene product, while assignment of DQ molecules reflects serologic contributions from both DQA1 and DQB1 gene products. As new alleles of DR and DQ have been identified, the assignments have been "split." Thus, DR15 and DR16 are splits of DR2, DR11 and DR12 are splits of DR5, and so forth. The "w" designations (for HLA-C and HLA-DP) are "workshop" assignments because the serologic assignments have been imprecise.

presenting cell, APC) to sample either its own proteins (in the case of MHC-I) or the proteins ingested from the immediate extracellular environment (in the case of MHC-II). In particular, cell surface MHC class I glycoproteins gather from the cell's biosynthetic pathway fragments of proteins derived from infecting viruses, intracellular parasites, or self molecules, either normally expressed or dysregulated by tumorigenesis, and then display these molecular fragments at the cell surface (7,9,28). Here the cell-bound MHC-I–peptide complex exposed on the APC is displayed to T cells. The second characteristic of the MHC-I molecule, the ability to interact with TCR, then allows the APC bearing a particular MHC–peptide complex to engage an appropriate αβ TCR as the first step in the activation of a cellular program that might lead to cytolysis of the APC as a target and/or to the secretion of lymphokines by the T cell. The interaction with the TCR is dependent on both the peptide and the MHC molecule. As a rule, a specific TCR will not bind the MHC molecule alone or when complexed with an unrelated peptide. Some would argue that the major evolutionary basis for the development of such a system is to discriminate those cells of the host that are infected by viruses or other obligate intracellular parasites (28). Thus, a system that originally evolved for identifying cells afflicted by viruses or other intracellular parasites might then

also function to identify antigens specific to tumor cells (29). For MHC-I restricted antigens, the usual rule is that the peptides are generated in the same cell that synthesizes the MHC-I molecule. Generally speaking, these peptides derive from proteins found in the cytosol that are then degraded by the multiproteolytic proteasome complex into peptides, and the resulting peptides, transported from the cytosol to the endoplasmic reticulum with the aid of the intrinsic membrane transporter, the transporter associated with antigen processing (TAP), are then cooperatively folded into the newly synthesized MHC-I molecule (30).

Exploiting similar molecular mechanisms, MHC class II molecules bind peptides derived from the degradation of proteins ingested by MHC-II–expressing APC, and display them at the cell surface for recognition by specific T-lymphocytes. The MHC-II antigen presentation pathway is based on the initial assembly of the MHC-II αβ heterodimer with a dual function molecule, the invariant chain (Ii) that serves as a chaperone to direct the αβ heterodimer to an endosomal, acidic protein–processing location, where it encounters antigenic peptides, which also serves to protect the antigen-binding site of the MHC-II molecule so that it preferentially will be loaded with antigenic peptides in this endosomal–lysosomal location (31,32). The loading of the MHC-II mole-

TABLE 3. *Commonly used mouse Strains: H-2 haplotypes*[a]

Strain	Haplotype	H-2 complex							
		K	Ab	Aa	Eb	Ea	D	Oal	Tla
Common strains									
129/J	bc	b	b	b	b	—	b	b	f
AKR/J	k	k	k	k	k	k	k	b	b
A.SW/Sn	s	s	s	s	s	—	s	b	b
BALB/cJ	d	d	d	d	d	d	d	b	c
C3H/HeJ	k	k	k	k	k	k	k	b	b
CBA/J	k	k	k	k	k	k	k	b	b
C57BL/6	b	b	b	b	b	—	b	b	b
C57BL/10	b	b	b	b	b	—	b	b	b
C57BR	k2	k	k	k	k	k	k	a	a
DBA/2J	d	d	d	d	d	d	d	b	c
NZB/BINJ	d2	d	d	d	d	d	d	a	a
P/J	p	p	p	p	p	p	p	a	e
RIIIS/J	r	r	r	r	r	r	r	c(r)	b
SJL	s2	s	s	s	s	—	s	a	a
Congenic strains									
B10.BR	k2	k	k	k	k	k	k	a	a
B10.D2	d	d	d	d	d	d	d	b	c
B10.S	s	s	s	s	s	—	s	b	b
BALB.B	b	b	b	b	b	—	b	b	b
BALB.K	k	k	k	k	k	k	k	b	b
C3H.SW	b	b	b	b	b	—	b		
Recombinant strains									
A	a	k	k	k	k	k	d		
A.TL	t1	s	k	k	k	k	d		
B10.A	a	k	k	k	k	k	d		
B10.A(1R)	h1	k	k	k	k	k	b		
B10.A(2R)	h2	k	k	k	k	k	b		
B10.A(3R)	l3	b	b	b	b/k	k	d		
B10.A(4R)	h4	k	k	k	k/b	—	b		
B10.A(5R)	l5	b	b	b	b/k	k	d		
B10.T(6R)	y2	q	q	q	q	–	d		
B10.S(7R)	t2	s	s	s	s	—	d		
B10.S(8R)	as1	k	k	k	k/s	—	s		
B10.S(9R)	t4	s	s	s	s/k	k	d		
B10.HTT	t3	s	s	s	sd/k	k	d		

[a]A dash indicates that the gene at that locus is not expressed normally, though the precise mechanism in different strains may differ (270). Several designations, such as *bc*, *s2*, and *k2*, follow the suggestion of Lindahl (19) to clarify differences in the genotype in some of the distal MHC loci.

cule with antigenic peptide, a process dependent on the release of the Ii-derived CLIP peptide, in part dependent on the MHC-II-like molecule, HLA-DM in the human (33,34), then leads to the cell surface expression of MHC-II peptide complexes. The MHC-II–recognizing T cells then secrete lymphokines and may also be induced to proliferate. Although these cell surface MHC molecules have been named for their strong effects in tumor and tissue transplantation across genetic barriers, their molecular and cellular function is more general, and it is perhaps better to think of MHC-I or MHC-II as the names of the peptide receptor on the APC.

MHC-I and MHC-II molecules, because of differences in their protein structure and the resulting differences in the cellular compartments that they traverse from their biosynthesis to their maturation, have strong preferences for the origin of the proteins that they sample for antigen presentation (35,36). The MHC-I antigen presentation pathway is most easily thought of as an inside-out pathway by which protein fragments of molecules synthesized by the cell are delivered to and bound by the MHC-I molecule during its biosynthesis. In contrast, the MHC-II antigen presentation pathway is best more clearly visualized as an outside-in one in which ingested proteins are degraded by enzymes in the endosomal–lysosomal system and are delivered to the MHC-II molecules in that degradative compartment (37). These processes are schematically illustrated in Fig 1 and are described in more detail elsewhere in this volume. The biochemical steps involved in the production of antigen fragments from large molecules are collectively known as *antigen processing*, while those that concern the binding of antigen fragments by MHC molecules and their display at the cell surface are known as *antigen presentation*. In general, the antigen-processing and -presentation pathways have been described experimentally for peptide antigenic fragments derived from proteins, and processing is a series of events focused on identification of the dysregulated or foreign protein and its proteolytic degradation into short peptides. Presentation consists of the binding of the peptide

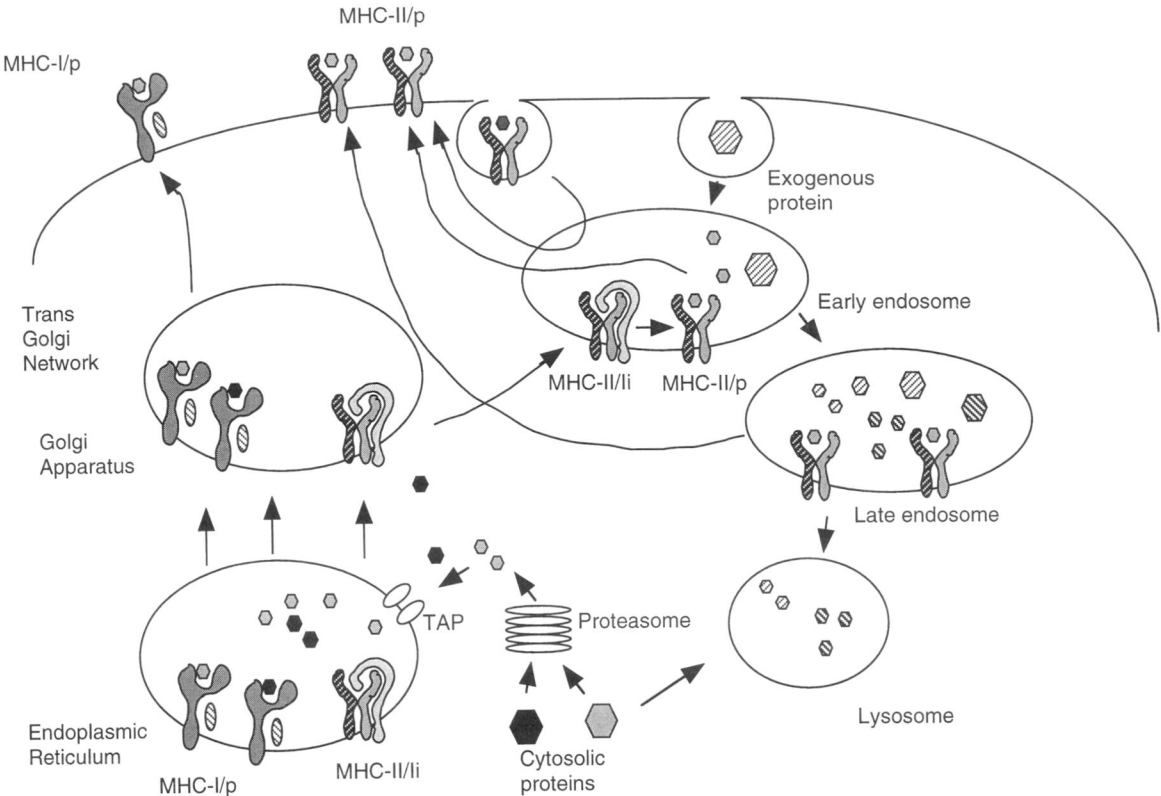

FIG. 1. Antigen processing and presentation. The major pathways of processing and presentation are shown. Cytosolic proteins (*shaded hexagons*) are degraded in proteasomes to peptide fragments that are then transported into the endoplasmic reticulum by TAP, where they assemble with MHC–I/β2-m complexes. From there they pass through the Golgi and trans Golgi network to the cell surface. Exogenous proteins (*striped hexagons*) enter the endosomal pathway, and in early or late endosomes, or lysosomes, they are progressively degraded to peptides. In early and late endosomes, MHC-II–invariant chain complexes (that have been trafficked there from the endoplasmic reticulum) are converted to MHC-II/CLIP complexes that are loaded with peptides with the catalytic aid of HLA-DM. These MHC-II–peptide complexes then go to the plasma membrane. (Adapted from refs. 37 and 146.)

fragment by the MHC-I or MHC-II molecule and the subsequent movement to the cell surface for display to the extracellular environment.

In addition to showing preference to distinct pathways of antigen presentation, the MHC-I and MHC-II molecules also show preferential restriction to T cells of the CD8- or CD4-bearing subsets. This is related to the observation that CD8 binds to the nonpolymorphic α3 domain of MHC-I molecules (38–41), while CD4 interacts with membrane proximal domains of MHC-II (42–44). The CD8 and CD4 molecules serve as coreceptors on the surface of the T-lymphocyte, providing both adhesion (avidity increase) and specific activating signals that modulate the avidity of the T cell in a time-dependent manner (45). Table 4 summarizes the similarities and differences between MHC-I and MHC-II molecules.

As high-resolution maps of the *Mhc* are developed, it has become clear that a number of molecules with function related to antigen presentation, but not necessarily the antigen-presenting molecules themselves, also map to the *Mhc*. These include the H-2M and HLA-DM molecules of the mouse and human, which are MHC-II-like in amino acid sequence, but which appear to play a catalytic role in augmenting the binding of peptides to MHC-II molecules in the acidic endosomal or lysosomal compartment of

the APC (46). The *TAP1* and *TAP2* genes encode molecules that are related to those of the ATP-binding cassette transporter family (47), which are important in the delivery of peptides generated in the cytosol to the nascent MHC-I molecule as it assembles with its light chain β2-m.

An additional function of MHC molecules that is not directly related to T-cell recognition has been recognized in recent years. This is to serve as elements for signal transduction to natural killer (NK) cells. NK cells are non-T lymphoid cells that are capable of lysing some tumor cells' targets and some cells infected with intracellular pathogens through a process known as natural killing. The expression by the target cell of MHC class I molecules can, in certain cases, protect the target from killing by the the NK effector, and target cells defective in the expression of normal MHC class I cells are susceptible to such NK-cell lysis (11,48). In some other cases, receptors on NK cells that interact with MHC-I are activated by the interaction. Studies have revealed several families of activating and inhibitory receptors in the human, rat, and mouse. These NK receptors, in addition to falling into roughly two classes of inhibitory receptors or activating receptors, also, by their structure, can be classed as either those that belong to the immunoglobulin supergene family or those that belong to the C-type lectin family (49).

TABLE 4. *Comparison of MHC-I and MHC-II molecules*

	MHC-Ia and Ib	MHC-II
Genetics	Multiple heavy-chain loci, most linked to the MHC Light-chain, $\beta2$-m is genetically unlinked.	Several heavy- and light-chain loci, α- and β-chain genes linked to each other
Tissue-specific expression	MHC-Ia, ubiquitous	MHC-II on B cells, macrophages, dendritic cells, Langerhans cells (in the mouse); in human, also found on T cells and many activated cell types
Molecular structure	Heavy-chain–light-chain form heterodimer. Obligate cell-surface molecule. Heavy chain has three extracellular domains, $\alpha1$, $\alpha2$, and $\alpha3$. $\alpha1/\alpha2$ form peptide binding site; $\alpha3$ and $\beta2$-m are Ig-like. Only heavy chain is membrane-bound, $\beta2$-m is noncovalently assembled.	α and β chains form heterodimer of four domains; $\alpha1/\beta1$ form peptide binding site; $\alpha2$ and $\beta2$ are Ig-like. Both chains are membrane-bound. Association of nascent MHC-II with invariant chain.
Site of peptide acquisition	1. In endoplasmic reticulum during biosynthesis 2. At cell surface when exposed to exogenous peptides	In endosome or lysosome where degraded products of ingested proteins are encountered; binding of peptides mediated by H-2M (in mouse) or HLA-DM (human).
Nature of peptides bound	MHC-Ia preference for 8 to 10 mers; though longer peptides can be bound. "motif" residues for particular MHC-I molecules CD1 capable of binding lipid antigens	Longer peptides are acceptable.
T-cell recognition	Primarily $CD8^+$	Primarily $CD4^+$
Associate molecules	$\beta2$-microglobulin TAP Tapasin Calnexin	Ii-invariant chain H-2M, (HLA-DM)
Alternate functions	Interaction with NK receptors As nFcR, binding Fc	Interactions with NK receptors

THE MAJOR HISTOCOMPATIBILITY COMPLEX

Mhc Genetic Maps

The MHC is an extended region of the genome that spans some 4 million basepairs (bp) on the short arm of human chromosome 6 between 6p21.31 and 6p21.32. In the mouse, the MHC occupies a central region of about 2 cM of chromosome 17 that extends from 18.0 to 20.0 cM. Although this region has not yet been contiguously physically mapped in the mouse, it is likely that it will extend for about the same distance (19). Genome mapping and sequencing have identified numerous genes in this region, many of which have functions critically related to those of the MHC class I or class II proteins, others of which have immunologically relevant functions as well. However, a large number of genes that map to this region also seem to have very little in common with immunologic function. Figure 2 shows schematically a map of some of the major genes of the human, mouse, and rat *Mhc,* which includes those that encode MHC-I and MHC-II proteins. These comparative maps are not drawn to scale and do not show every gene identified in the region. Three markers, Ke3, Bat1, and Mog serve to define the gross colinearity of the MHC of the three species (50), though there are clearly major differences between strains and individuals within a species and between the species as well. The mapping information now available for the human is more extensive than that available for the mouse, and the rat lags behind the other species. A database of the human *Mhc* is available via the World Wide Web (http://www.hgmp.mrc.ac.uk) (51). A map showing the homology of mouse chromosome 17 to the human can be found at (http://www3.ncbi.nlm.nih.gov/Homology/mouse17.html), and a YAC map of the human *Mhc*-*I* region is at (http://chimera.biotech.washington.edu/UWGC/projects/hla-I/HLAyacs.htm). One tabulation counts 212 genes in 451 loci that have been identified (51). With the continuing progress of the human genome project, we can expect that the full sequence of the 4,000 kbp of the human *Mhc* will be completed and the precise identification of open reading frames there will be made. Because of its importance as a model system, the linear sequence of the *Mhc* of the mouse should also be completed.

The human MHC map reveals clusters of genes grouped roughly into an *Mhc* class II region covering about 1,000 kb, an *Mhc* class III region, and an *Mhc* class I region (see Fig. 2). *HLA-DP* genes (*DPA* encoding the α chain, and *DPB* encoding the β chain) are proximal to the centromere on the short arm of the chromosome and are linked to the genes encoding the related HLA-DM molecule (*DMB* and *DMA*). Between these and the *DQ* genes lie *LMP* genes (for low-molecular-weight proteins (52–55)) and *TAP* (56–60) (for transporter associated with antigen-processing) genes. *LMP* and *TAP* genes encode molecules that are involved in peptide generation in the cytosol and peptide transport across the endoplasmic reticulum (ER) membrane, respectively. The *TAP* genes encode a two-chain intrinsic membrane protein that resides in the ER of all cells, and functions as an ATP-dependent transporter that pumps peptides generated in the cytosol into the lumen of the ER (47). The current view of the LMPs is that they are subunits of the multicatalytic proteolytic proteasome complex that regulate the specificity of cleavage of proteins, and thus modulate the repertoire of peptides available for MHC-I restricted antigen presentation (61, 62). An elegant description of the selective transport of cytoplasmically generated peptides by different TAP proteins in the rat demonstrates that the spectrum of MHC–peptide complexes

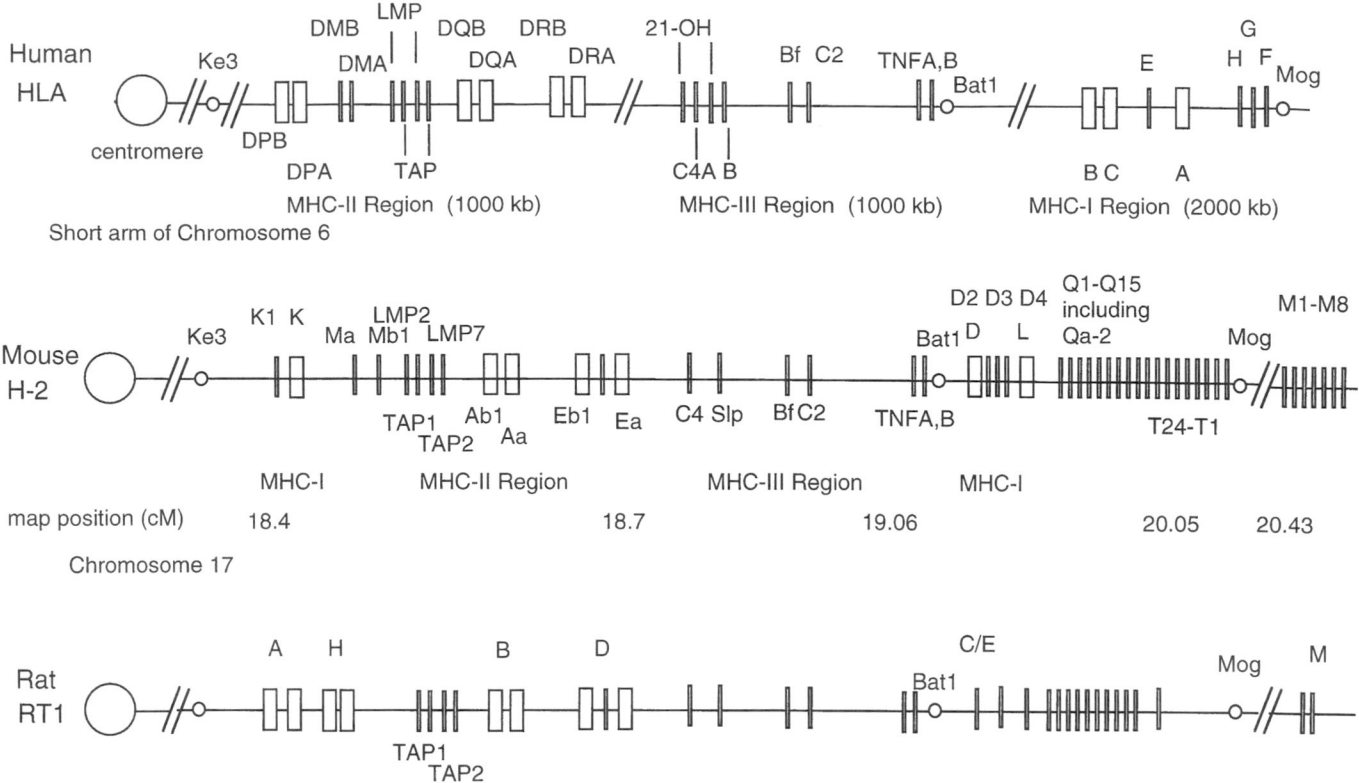

FIG. 2. Genetic maps of the *Mhc*. Comparative map of the human, mouse, and rat MHC. This schematic map is not complete, nor is it drawn to scale. It is derived from maps available on the World Wide Web (51) and those illustrations previously published (21,50,262). The centromere and major genes are indicated.

expressed at the cell surface can be significantly altered by differences in the antigen-presentation pathway (63–65). A locus in the mouse *Mhc* that controls the sets of peptides presented by a transgene-encoded HLA-B27 molecule has been identified that reveals a phenotype similar to that of variant rat *TAP* alleles (66).

The other major *Mhc-II* genes of the human are *HLA-DRA* and *HLA-DRB,* which encode the chains that form the HLA-DR molecule, a major antigen-presentation element. The *Mhc-III* region is important in immunologic terms for several reasons—the structural genes for several complement components map here, as well as the structural genes for 21-hydroxylase (67,68), an enzyme critical in the biosynthesis of glucocorticoids, a deficiency of which can lead to the genetic disease congenital adrenal hyperplasia. Also linked in the Mhc-III region are the structural genes for tumor necrosis factors A and B (TNF-A and TNF-B), which are lymphokines made by activated T cells (69,70). TNF-B is also known as lymphotoxin α.

The more distal region of the *Mhc* encodes other MHC molecules. In the human, the cluster of the major *Mhc-I* genes lies here, including the genes encoding HLA-B, HLA-C, HLA-E, and HLA-A, as well as HLA-H, HLA-G, and HLA-F. HLA-A, HLA-B, and HLA-C are the major MHC-I molecules of humans. (A summary of the serologic and genetic identification of these is in Table 1). Serologic identification of HLA-C molecules has been difficult and imprecise; however, they are particularly important in interactions with receptors on NK cells (71). The precise functions of HLA-E, HLA-F, and HLA-G are not yet clear. HLA-E shows some

similarities in amino acid sequence and in peptide-binding motif to the mouse MHC-Ib molecule Qa-1 (72,73). Some evidence now suggests antigen-presentation function of HLA-E, -F, and -G (74), and the tissue-restricted expression of HLA-G (75,76) suggests that this molecule may be involved in the mother's immunologic tolerance of the fetus. *HLA-H* (77) is a pseudogene mapping to this region and should not be confused with *HLA-HFE,* an *Mhc-Ib* gene that controls hereditary hemochromatosis and is more distantly related to the *Mhc-I* genes, but has been erroneously called *HLA-H* by some authors (78–80).

Comparison of the mouse and rat *Mhc* maps with that of the human reveals several interesting points (81,82). The proximal *Mhc* genes of the mouse and rat belong to the *Mhc-I* family, rather than to the *Mhc-II* family. This mapping has suggested that an intrachromosomal recombination event displaced some of the *Mhc-I* genes from a more distal location to the proximal site. Inspection of the current human, mouse, and rat maps clearly indicates other similarities in the relative locations of *Mhc-II, Mhc-III,* and *Mhc-I* genes. The major rat MHC-I molecule is RT1.A. Various genetic expansions and contractions are obvious as well. In particular, the mouse *Q* and *T* regions have clearly expanded the pool of *Mhc-I* genes, which are relatively few in the human and the rat. Early studies of congenic mouse strains mapped multiple genes to the *Q* and *T* regions (83–85), and evidence suggests significant differences in the number of genes of this region in different strains. The mouse has some class Ib genes that seem to be relatively unique in function to the species. In particular, the *H-2M3* gene (not to be confused with the *Mhc-II H-2Ma* and *H-2Mb* genes, which encode the homologues of the human HLA-DMA and HLA-DMB proteins), which maps distal to the *Q* and *T* regions, encodes a protein that exhibits a preference for binding peptides that have *N*-formyl amino-terminal modifications, an antigen-presentation function that may be geared to bacterial, protozoal, and mitochondrial antigens (86–90).

Mhc Polymorphism

The *Mhc*s function in immune responsiveness is also reflected in its genetic polymorphism. *Polymorphism* is the presence at any given time of a larger than expected number of genetic variants in a population. As populations change and evolve, we expect there to be genetic variants, but because of constraints on the function of some genetic markers, relatively few of these genetic variants are able to persist. We generally accept the convention that a genetic locus that exhibits more than 1% of the alleles as variant at any one time is polymorphic. A polymorphic locus or gene, then, is one that has a high frequency (not number) of genetic variants (2). A genetic locus that is relatively invariant is often referred to by the rather imprecise term *monomorphic*. HLA genes exhibit a high degree of polymorphism, and a number of different explanations have developed to explain the generation and maintenance of polymorphism. Among these is the suggested selective advantage of a pool of antigen-presenting elements that might allow the binding and presentation of antigenic peptides derived from a wide variety of environmental pathogens. Limited polymorphism would make the entire population susceptible to a chance infectious agent for which all individuals would be unable to respond, while widespread polymorphism would be expected to allow at least a proportion of the population to effectively bind and present antigens derived from invading pathogens.

The human *Mhc-I* and *Mhc-II* genes are clearly polymorphic, with many more than 50 alleles at each of the *HLA-A, HLA-B,* and *HLA-DRB* loci well identified (91). In experimental animals, it is more difficult to demonstrate polymorphism in such population genetic terms, although typing of wild mice has confirmed the impression gained from the analysis of inbred strains and mutants derived from them (92). The polymorphism of *Mhc-I* and *Mhc-II* genes, so evident in human and mouse, has also been documented in analyses of cichlid fishes, animals that diverged from the line leading to mammals at least several hundred million years ago (93,94).

Mhc Evolutionary Mechanisms

As both an extended genetic region and a group of genes with many belonging to the immunoglobulin supergene family (95,96), the *Mhc* has served as a prototype for elucidating and understanding mechanisms that contribute to the evolution of a multigene family and that add to the polymorphism that is such a dominant characteristic of the classical MHC molecules (82). The analysis of mutations in the mouse, mostly those of *Mhc-I* genes, has led to the understanding of the mechanisms that give rise to polymorphism. The mutations have been identified in mice based on screening of large numbers of animals by skin grafting of siblings. Both induced and spontaneous mutations affecting skin graft acceptance or rejection have been identified, and many of these have been mapped to the *Mhc*. Gross recombinational events have been documented

(97,98), as well as more subtle mutations, many of which are multiple amino acid substitutions in a relatively small part of the protein that seem to derive from nonreciprocal crossovers. Such nonreciprocal recombinational events that occur over short sequences are known as gene conversion because of their similarity to a phenomenon that occurs in yeast (99–105).

The mechanism of gene conversion in mice is now better understood because nucleotide sequence analysis and oligonucleotide-specific hybridization have been used not only to characterize the mutations that have occurred, but also to identify the *Mhc* genes that have been the donors of the mutant sequences. Although the precise enzymatic details are not clear, we now understand gene conversion as a genetic event that allows the copying or transposition of short sequences from a donor gene to a recipient. Some of the polymorphisms that have been identified clearly reflect point mutations (106). Table 5 summarizes the most important *H-2* mutants and the identified donor genes. In addition to such mouse mutants, a number of somatic cell variants and mutants, some due to major deletions or regulatory defects and others clearly point mutants of structural genes, have been described (107). The characterization of three mutants of the *H2K^b* gene, mutants that have a complex set of several mutations over a more extended region of DNA, suggests that no single donor gene can be identified for these mutants. An effort to identify the donor gene for the *H2K^bm3*, *H2K^bm23*, and *H2D^bm23* mutations concludes that these complex mutations must have arisen by the contribution of at least two different donor genes (108), acting either in sequence or in synergy.

TABLE 5. H-2 *mutants*

Mutant	Altered amino acids	Donor gene
K^bm1	E152A	Q10
	R155Y	
	L156Y	
K^bm3	D77S	
	A89K	
K^bm4	K173E	
	N174L	
K^bm5	F116Y	
K^bm16	F116Y	
K^bm6	F116Y	Q4
	C121R	
K^bm7	F116Y	
	C121R	
K^bm9	F116Y	Q4
	C121R	
K^bm8	F22Y	
	I23M	
	E24S	
K^bm10	T163A	K1
	V165M	
	W107S	
	K173E	
	N174L	
K^bm11	D77S	D^b
	T80N	
D^bm28	Q97W	
	S99Y	
H-2^dm1	D^d/l^d recombinant	
H-2^dm2	L^d deletion	

Amino acid substitutions and donor gene designations are summarized in refs. 102 and 2.

The *Mhc* and Transplantation

Although the early description of the genes of the *Mhc* was based on identification of loci involved in tumor and allograft rejection, and although these genes clearly play a role in these complex phenomena, a contemporary understanding of the function of *Mhc* genes in immunology requires little understanding of the rules of transplantation. The early history of transplantation is chronicled extensively in several books (1,2) and reflects the developing interest in tumor immunology and congenic mouse strains. The most extensively studied species for tumor, tissue, and organ transplantation has been the mouse, so a brief description of some relevant principles is in order. Comprehensive manuals and reviews are available (109). Propagation of a mouse strain by repeated matings of brothers and sisters leads to the establishment of an inbred strain, a group of animals that is genetically identical at all loci. More complete descriptions of the process by which brother–sister mating leads to homozygosity at all loci are given elsewhere (1,2). The probability of fixation of all loci (P_{fix}) as a function of the number of generations, n, is given by $P_{fix} = 1 - (7/8)^{n-1}$. Thus, after 5 generations of brother × sister matings, the probability of being identical all at loci is 0.414; after 10 generations, 0.7; after 15 generations, 0.85; and after 20 generations, 0.91.

Congenic mouse strains, also known as congenic-resistant or CR strains, are those derived by first crossing two inbred strains that differ in a histocompatibility phenotype (such as resistance to a transplantable tumor or ability to reject a skin graft). These are then successively back-crossed to one parental strain, and the resistance phenotype is preserved. Following at least 10 back-cross generations (N10), a point at which $(1/2)^9 = 0.002$ of the genes of the selected strain should be present, the new strain is propagated by brother × sister mating. From such breeding schemes, a number of strains critical to genetic studies of the *Mhc* have been derived. Several relevant inbred mouse strains, CR strains, are listed in Table 3, along with their *H-2* designations. Since strains maintained by brother × sister matings may reveal genetic drift as spontaneous mutations accumulate in the strain, it is crucial to keep track of the stock from which the animals were derived and the number of generations that they have been propagated without back-crossing to founder stock. This has been of particular concern in recent years as various lines of embryonic stem cells derived from different lines of strain 129 have been used for genetic manipulation (gene knockout experiments) (110) and there are clearly differences in histocompatibility (111).

The early rules of transplantation were determined by observation of the ability of either transplantable tumors or of allografts (usually from skin) to survive in a particular inbred mouse strain host. The graft rejection phenomenon is an extremely sensitive and specific bioassay that permits the discrimination of genetic differences as small as a single amino acid in an MHC protein to be detected. It has been particularly valuable in assessing spontaneous and induced mutants (see discussion above) and remains the absolute experimental discriminator of histocompatibility.

The *Mhc* and Disease

In addition to the control of transplant acceptance and immune responsiveness, it has been recognized for many years that the *Mhc* in the human plays an important role in the etiology of a number of diseases, many of which are autoimmune in nature (112,113). Several of the human diseases are associated with the *Mhc* class III genes, because some of the structural genes for enzymes involved in the adrenal steroid biosynthetic pathway (i.e., 21-hydroxylase) map to this region (114). Over 40 diseases have well-established genetic linkages to the *Mhc* (113,115), and the most important are summarized in Table 6. The precise mechanisms underlying the association of most of these diseases with the particular *Mhc* haplotypes are unknown, but several models have been proposed, including the cross-reactivity of antibodies to microorganisms with particular MHC molecules (116), and the molecular mimicry of T-cell responses to viral antigens for self antigens (117–120). The very high incidence of some diseases associated with certain *HLA* genes assists in the diagnosis as well as the counseling of patients and their families. Several of these diseases are of particular note. Since 100% of patients with narcolepsy have *HLA-DR2* [*HLA-DQB1*0602* (121,122)], a suspicion of the disease can be confirmed by HLA typing. Ankylosing spondylitis is so strongly associated with the *Mhc-I* allele *HLA-B27* and the presence of some bacterial pathogens, that it is a popular hypothesis that ankylosing spondylitis in some cases is due to the stimulation of particular T cells by HLA-B27–presented bacterial antigens. These T cells are then thought to initiate an inflammatory cascade. Particular mutant alleles of *HLA-HFE*, a human *Mhc-Ib* gene, have been strongly associated with familial hemochromatosis, an iron-overload illness (123). Although the precise relationship that these apparently mutant *HLA-HFE* alleles have with the pathogenesis of the disease is unclear, it is intriguing that mice that are homozygous for an induced defect of β2-microglobulin, and thus are likely to be defective in expression of the murine homologue of HLA-HFE, also have hemochromatosis (124,125). Thus, two lines of evidence point directly to a β2-m assembled and cell surface–expressed molecule playing a critical role in protection from iron overload. Although the number of different *HLA* class I and class II alleles that are associated with insulin-dependent diabetes mellitus clearly indicates that this relatively common disease has a complex etiology, the identification of a novel *Mhc-II* haplotype in the mutant nonobese diabetic (NOD) mouse (126–130) and the recognition that particular TCRs can mediate disease (131) suggest that a cross-reactive response to a common self or environmental antigen may play an important role in the etiology of this disease as well.

Mutations at the *H-2* Locus

Mutations at the *H-2* locus have been identified in animals screened by skin grafting in extensive experiments carried out over a 25-year period (132,133). By grafting tail skin of siblings to and from each other, spontaneous or induced mutant animals that displayed either a gain, loss, or gain plus loss transplantation phenotype were identified. Gain mutants are those that express a new transplantation antigen—thus their skin is rejected by their non-mutant siblings; loss mutants have lost a transplantation antigen—thus they recognize the skin of their siblings as foreign and reject that graft. Gain plus loss mutations give effects in both directions—they reject the skin of their siblings, and their skin is rejected by their siblings as well. In a classic series of experiments extending over an extended period of time, Melvold, Kohn, and their colleagues screened a large number of mouse progeny. Both homozygous inbred and F1 animals were examined, yielding a total of 25 *H-2* mutations identified at *K, D, L,* and *Ab* loci, and an additional 80 mutations of non–*H-2* histocompatibility genes. Although earlier studies suggested that all *H-2* genes might be hypermutable,

TABLE 6. *HLA disease associations*

Disease	Antigen	Race	Frequency[a] Patients	Frequency[a] Controls
Narcolepsy	HLA-DR2	C	1.0	0.22
		O	1.0	0.34
Ankylosing spondylitis	HLA-B27	C	0.89	0.09
		O	0.81	0.01
		N	0.58	0.04
Reiter's disease	HLA-B27	C	0.47	0.10
Insulin-dependent diabetes mellitus	HLA-B8	C	0.40	0.21
	HLA-B15	C	0.22	0.14
	HLA-DR3	C	0.52	0.22
	HLA-DR4	C	0.74	0.24
	HLA-DR2	C	0.04	0.29
	HLA-DRB1*0301	C	0.54	0.27
	HLA-DRB1*0401	C	0.59	0.25
	HLA-DQA1*0301	C	0.85	0.35
	HLA-DQB1*0302	C	0.81	0.23
Rheumatoid arthritis	HLA-DR4	C	0.68	0.25
		O	0.66	0.39
		N	0.44	0.10
Hodgkin's disease	HLA-A1	C	0.40	0.32
	HLA-DRB1*1104[b]	C	0.058	0.013
Hemochromatosis	HLA-A3	C	0.76	0.28
Psoriasis	HLA-Cw6	C	0.87	0.33
Celiac disease	HLA-DR3	C	0.79	0.26
Multiple sclerosis	HLA-DR2	C	0.59	0.26

C, Caucasian; O, Oriental; N, Black.

[a]The frequencies given are the total genotypic frequencies of all individuals with at least one copy of the disignated allele. Both homozygous and heterozygous individuals are included.

[b]In this case, the frequencies are based on allele frequencies, not genotype frequencies.

Taken from ref. 113.

a more complete retrospective evaluation of the available data suggests that with the exception only of the *H-2K*[b] gene, the spontaneous mutation rate for *H-2* genes was comparable to that for non–*H-2* genes (134). The characterization of these mutant animals, first based on peptide maps and amino acid sequences of the H-2 proteins (135–138) and later based on the nucleotide sequences of the cloned cDNAs or genes (101,102), provided some of the basic biochemical information on which later studies of structure and function and mechanism of gene evolution were based.

Expression of MHC Molecules

MHC molecules, synthesized in the ER and destined for cell surface expression, are controlled at many steps before their final disposition as receptors available for interaction with either T cells or NK cells. The MHC-I molecules should be viewed as trimers, consisting of the polymorphic heavy chain, the light chain, β2-microglobulin, and the assembled self peptide. Since there are numerous steps in the biosynthesis of the MHC-I molecule, regulatory controls can be exerted at almost every step. In addition, reflecting the continuous struggle between the immune system of the vertebrate organism, and rapidly adaptible infectious agents, a number of steps in biosynthesis and expression are inhibited by virus-encoded proteins.

The first level of control of MHC-I expression is genetic; that is, the genes for a particular chain must be present for the trimer to be expressed. This is of course most relevant for β2-microglobulin, which is the obligate light chain for the complex. Induced β2-m–defective animals (*B2m*[o/o]) (139–141) lack normal levels of MHC-I expression, though for some molecules detectable amounts are present.

The next level of MHC-I expression control is transcriptional, and interferon-γ (IFN-γ) regulation is particularly important (142). For the most part, MHC-Ia molecules are ubiquitously expressed, and the basis of the more limited tissue-specific expression of MHC-Ib molecules is only beginning to be explored (143–145). Interest in the regulation of placental HLA-E and HLA-G expression is prompted by a potential role in the mother's tolerance of the fetus.

The rest of the MHC-I biosynthetic pathway is dependent on proper generation of cytosolic peptides by the proteasome and delivery to the ER by TAP, appropriate core glycosylation in the ER, transport through the Golgi, and arrival at the plasma membrane (146). A number of persistent viruses have evolved mechanisms for subverting this pathway of expression. The herpes simplex virus encodes a protein, ICP47, that blocks the activity of the peptide transporter TAP (147–149). Two proteins encoded by the human cytomegalovirus (HCMV), US2 and US11, cause rapid protein degradation of MHC-I molecules, and another HCMV protein, US18, which has sequence similarity to MHC-I molecules, may affect normal MHC-I function by limiting β2-m availability. The precise mechanism of US18 effects remains controversial. Several viruses, including murine cytomegalovirus (150), adenovirus 2

(151), and HCMV also have genes that function in blocking the transfer of folded assembled MHC-I molecules from the ER to the Golgi.

MHC-II molecules are also susceptible to regulation at multiple steps. The clear-cut tissue dependence of MHC-II expression—MHC-II molecules are generally found on cells that have specific antigen-presentation functions, such as macrophages, dendritic cells, Langerhans' cells, thymic epithelial cells, and B cells, and can also be detected on activated T cells of the human and rat—suggests that transcriptional regulation plays an important role. Extensive studies of the promoter activities of *Mhc-II* genes have defined a number of specific transcriptional regulatory sequences (152). Considerations of differential expression of MHC-II molecules in different tissues, MHC-II deficiency diseases known as bare lymphocyte syndromes (153–156), and current views of the role of the balance of Th1 and Th2 T-lymphocyte subsets, lead to a provocative hypothesis that suggests that the contribution of MHC-II differential expression and the resulting balance of Th1- and Th2-derived lymphokines are critical in the control of autoimmune disease (157).

A unique aspect of MHC-II regulation is the need to protect its peptide-binding site from loading of self peptides in the ER, and to traffic to an acidic endosomal compartment where antigenic peptides, the products of proteolytic digestion of exogenous proteins, can be obtained. These two functions are provided by the type II membrane protein, Ii (32,158,159), that forms a nine-subunit complex [consisting of three Ii and three (αβ) MHC-II heterodimers]. The region of Ii that protects the MHC-II peptide-binding groove, CLIP, is progressively trimmed from Ii and is ultimately released from the MHC-II by the action of HLA-DM in the endosome to allow exchange for peptides generated there. The important role of Ii in regulating MHC-II expression has been emphasized by the behavior of induced mutant mice lacking normal Ii (160–162), which exhibit a profound defect in MHC-II function and expression.

STRUCTURE OF MHC MOLECULES

Since the structure of an MHC molecule reflects its function as a peptide receptor and as a TCR ligand simply and elegantly, we will systematically describe the known structures of MHC-I and MHC-II molecules and then return to a more detailed discussion of their function.

Amino Acid Sequences

Before the cloning of *Mhc* genes, the biochemical purification and amino acid sequence determination of the human MHC-I molecules, HLA-A2 and HLA-B7, and of the mouse molecule H-2K^b (163,164) indicated that the MHC molecules had similarities to immunoglobulins in their membrane proximal regions. Early concerns were to identify the differences between allelic gene products as well as the differences between MHC proteins encoded at different loci. With the cloning of cDNAs and genomic clones for MHC-I molecules (99,165–167,) and then for MHC-II molecules (168–171), the encoded amino acid sequences of a large number of MHC molecules of a number of species quickly became available. The comparison of gene and cDNA structures gave an indication of the exon–intron organization of the genes and explained the evolution of the MHC molecules as having been derived from primordial single-domain structures of a unit size of a single immunoglobulin domain (such as the light-chain β2-microglobulin), which duplicated to form the basic unit of the MHC-II chain (two extracellular domains) and the MHC-I chain (three extracellular domains) (82). This gene–exon organization is illustrated in Fig. 3. Thus, the canonical MHC-I molecule has a heavy chain that is an intrinsic type I integral membrane protein with amino-terminal domains called α1, α2, and α3; is embedded in the cell membrane by a hydrophobic transmembrane domain; and extends into the cytoplasm of the cell with a carboxyl-terminal tail. The light chain of the MHC-I molecule, β2-microglobulin, is a single-domain mole-

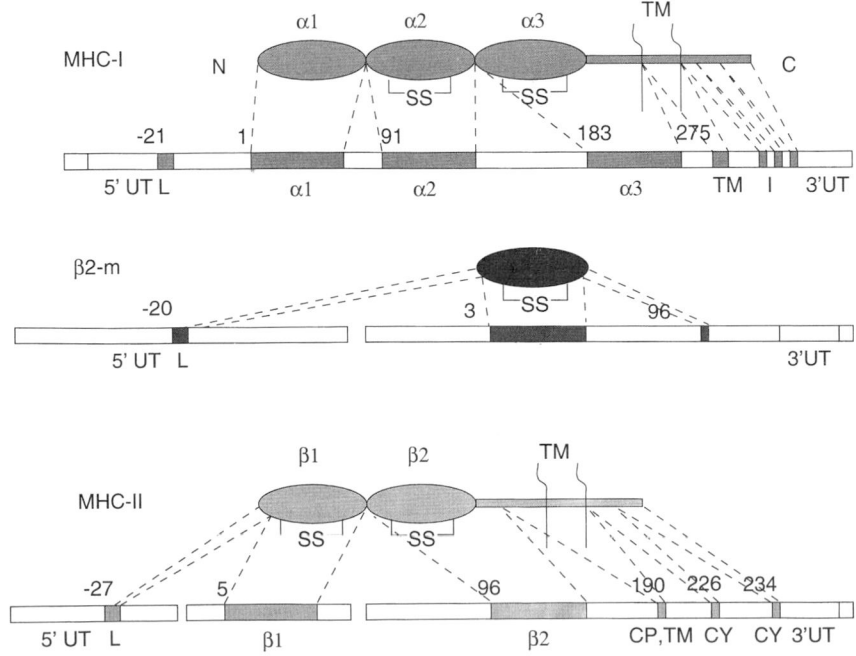

FIG. 3. Gene–exon correspondence of *Mhc* genes and proteins. Examples of MHC-I heavy chain, β2-m, and an MHC-II β chain are shown with their domains corresponding to the canonical gene structure. The proteins are shown above, and the genes below 5′-untranslated regions (5′ UT) are indicated. Disulfide bonds found within the heavy-chain α2 and α3 domains, β2-m, and both extracellular domains of the MHC-II β chain are shown. (The α1 domain of the MHC-II α chain has no disulfide). (Adapted from ref. 263.)

cule. (Indeed, several alleles of β2-m have been identified both in inbred strains and wild mouse populations (172), though it should not be considered polymorphic). The MHC-II molecule consists of two chains inserted in the membrane, an α chain and a β chain, each consisting of two major extracellular domains, α1 and α2 and β1 and β2, respectively, each linked to a transmembrane domain and cytoplasmic sequences. Thus, both MHC-I and MHC-II molecules are noncovalently assembled heterodimers consisting of four extracellular domains; the two membrane proximal domains (α3 and β2-m for MHC-I and α2 and β2 for MHC-II) of each molecule are immunogobulin-like, while the two amino-terminal domains (α1 and α2 of MHC-I and α1 and β1 of MHC-II) are not. The α1 domains of both MHC-I and MHC-II lack the intradomain disulfide bond characteristic of the other extracellular domains. The cytoplasmic domains of MHC-I molecules can be regulated by splicing and differential phosphorylation, and are likely to play a role in cell surface stability and molecular cycling into the cell (173–176). The MHC-II transmembrane and cytoplasmic domains have clear effects on the level of cell surface expression, the efficiency of antigen presentation, and the rate of lateral diffusion of the molecules in the cell membrane (177). Amino acid sequence alignments of MHC-I and MHC-II proteins, particularly of the human molecules, are available in a number of databases (http://histo.cryst.bbk.ac.uk/; http://immuno.bme.nwu.edu/).

With the realization that MHC molecules were encoded by genes with modular exon structure, a number of laboratories began to explore the structure–function relationship of MHC molecules by generating various recombinants of the encoding genes *in vitro* and analyzing the expressed proteins following transfection into suitable cell types. These early studies allowed the mapping of serologic epitopes (178,179), sites for recognition by monoclonal antibodies, and the mapping of various *Mhc*-restricted responses, such as the recognition by either allospecific or antigen-specific cytolytic T-lymphocytes (180,181). The general results of these kinds of experiments were that the membrane distal domains of the MHC molecules, the α1 and α2 domains of the MHC-I molecules, acted together to form a functional element for the recognition by T cells. A clearer understanding of the significance of these findings was obtained with the determination of the three dimensional structure of the MHC class I molecule, HLA-A2, as purified after papain cleavage from tissue culture cells (182,183).

Figure 3 shows the canonical relationship between the gene that encodes an MHC-I or MHC-II molecule and the encoded protein. For the *Mhc-I* genes, there is a single transcriptional unit (exon) that encodes the 5′ untranslated region as well as the signal peptide that denotes that the protein is destined for the lumen of the ER. This exon is spliced to the coding block for the first extracellular domain of the encoded protein, an exon of about 270 nucleotides, encoding the first domain (the α1 domain), which is about 90 amino acids in length. The third exon encodes the second extracellular domain (α2 domain), and the fourth exon, the third extracellular domain (α3). The transmembrane exon of the *Mhc-I* gene encodes the transmembrane domain of the protein, and the remainder of the gene encodes several small exons that can be alternatively spliced, that can serve as phosphorylation sites, and that may play a role in the cycling of the molecule to the cell surface.

Similarly, the *Mhc-II* genes exhibit an exon–domain correspondence, though for the MHC-II molecules, there are two extracellular domains [α1 and α2 for the α (or a) chain and β1 and β2 for the β (or b) chain, respectively] for each polypeptide chain, and both chains have transmembrane regions.

Identification of Peptides Bound by MHC Molecules

Many different lines of evidence coalesced over a period of a few years to prove that MHC molecules function by binding peptides. From functional experiments, MHC-II–restricted T-cell responses to protein antigens were shown to be dependent on peptide fragments (184). The first direct evidence of MHC–peptide interactions came from the demonstration that purified MHC-II proteins could bind synthetic peptides in a specific, saturable, and stable manner (185,186) with measurable affinity. For MHC-I molecules, the results were at first less clear, but the realization that some cell lines defective in MHC-I surface expression could be induced to express higher levels of surface MHC-I molecules by exposure to the appropriate peptides (187,188) led the way for direct measurement of MHC-I peptide binding (189).

Several laboratories were successful in developing methods for the partial purification and identification of the peptides that copurified with MHC-I molecules. One approach for identifying the peptide derived from a virus that was bound by the MHC-I molecule H-2K^b involved recovering MHC molecules from infected cells, identifying a peak of functional biologic activity in a cytotoxic T-cell assay, and the determination of the amino acid sequence of the recovered peptide by radiochemical techniques (190). Another method that was useful for identifying both viral-derived peptides as well as the motif of self peptides by particular MHC-I molecules involved first the isolation of a large amount of detergent-solubilized MHC-I with appropriate antibodies, the elution of the bound peptides, their partial purification as pools by reverse-phase high-pressure liquid chromatography, and the determination of the amino acid sequence of the bound peptides by classic Edman degradation of the peptide pools (191–193). The unpredictable and surprising result obtained from these studies of MHC-I–derived peptides was that specific amino acid residues were favored at particular positions of the sequence, depending on the MHC-I molecule from which the peptides were obtained, and that the length of the bound peptides was well defined and short, ranging from eight to ten amino acids. From such experiments, a number of peptide motifs of peptides bound to particular MHC-I molecules and allelic products were identified. Further refinements in methodology included the application of mass spectrometry to the identification of individual peptides and their sequencing (194). Alternative approaches for identifying peptide motifs include the use of soluble analogues of MHC-I molecules to ease the purification (195,196) or the use of peptide display libraries to identify those peptides that can bind the MHC (197). A summary of MHC-I peptide motifs is given in Table 7. An online database that is regularly maintained is at (http://wehih.wehi.edu.au/mhcpep/) (198,199). An algorithm that allows the prediction of candidates for MHC-I–restricted peptides based on the amino acid sequence of the protein of interest is available (http://www-bimas.dcrt.nih.gov/molbio/hla__bind/index.html) (200). The distinction between motif residues of an MHC-restricted peptide and anchor residues is an important one. *Motif* refers to those amino acid residues that are identified based on the sequences of self or antigenic peptides that have been demonstrated to bind or copurify with a particular MHC molecule. *Anchor* implies a biophysical function of the particular amino acid residue as specifically interacting with a particular part of the MHC molecule itself. Thus, the assignment of a motif residue as an anchor requires either the structural confirmation by x-ray crystallography or a comprehensive binding analysis based on a set of substituted synthetic peptides.

TABLE 7. *Peptide binding motifs for some MHC-I molecules[a]*

Positions	1	2	3	4	5	6	7	8	9
HLA-A*0101			DE						Y
HLA-A*0201		LM							V
HLA-A*0301		LM							YK
HLA-A*1101									K
HLA-A*3101		LVYF	FLYW			LFVI			R
HLA-B*0701		P							LF
HLA-B*0801			KR		KR			L or	LI
HLA-B*2702		R							FY
HLA-B*2705		R							LFK
HLA-B*5301		P							LIVMYF
H-2Kb			Y		FY			LMIV	
H-2Kd		V							IL
H-2Kk		ED							LFM
H-2Db		M			N				MIL
H-2Dd		G	P						LIF
H-2Ld		P							FLM
Qa-2							H		LIF
H-2M3	N-formyl-met								

[a]Peptide binding motifs for the indicated MHC-I molecules are shown in the single amino acid code. *Position* refers to the amino acid position of the peptide from the amino terminus. Only the most common residues are shown. These motifs are taken from the more extensive summary of ref. 271.

The identification of MHC-II–bound self or antigenic peptides by biochemical methods similar to those employed for MHC-I molecules has proved more difficult, because the MHC-II molecules do not seem to have the rigorous requirement for a defined amino-terminus or the restricted length that MHC-I molecules need. Whereas MHC-I molecules bind peptides with a particular motif residue at a specific position, resulting in the ability to identify the dominant residue at a particular step in the Edman degradation, even amidst a pool of peptides, MHC-II molecules bind peptides with ragged ends, and little information is obtained from the sequencing of pools of peptides (201–204). Identification of MHC-II peptide-binding motifs by bacteriophage display is also possible (205). In accord with the view that MHC-II molecules present peptides derived from an outside-in pathway, many of the peptides that copurify with MHC-II molecules represent molecules derived from the extracellular milieu of the medium in which the cells were grown. A summary of MHC-II peptide motifs is given in Table 8.

High-resolution Crystallographic Structures

MHC-I Molecules

A most graphic description of the relationship of form and function of the MHC molecule was made by Bjorkman and colleagues (182,183), who determined the three-dimensional structure of the human MHC-I molecule, HLA-A2, by x-ray crystallography. These molecules were purified after papain cleavage of the extracellular part of the molecule from the surface of tissue culture cells, and at the time there was not a clear appreciation either of the role of peptide in the assembly of the molecule or of the nature of the recognition of the MHC molecule by TCRs. The most important insight in the interpretation of the electron density map was that part of the density, and thus part of the structure, was due to a heterogeneous collection of peptides bound tightly by the molecule, and that this density could not be modeled based on the known amino acid sequence of HLA-A2. This is illustrated in Colorplate 1. In panel A

TABLE 8. *Peptide binding motifs for some MHC-II molecules[a]*

Positions[b]	i (P1)	i+1	i+2	i+3 (P4)	i+4	i+5 (P6)	i+6	i+7	i+8 (P9)	i+9
DRB1*0101	FYWLVI			LM		SAG			LAVI	
DRB1*0301	IYLVFM		AI	NQEDK		KIRHEQ			YLF	
DRB1*0401	YFWMVL			MALV		TSVLIM	LQMN[KR]		[DERK]	
DRB1*0405/B4*0101	Y					VT			D	
DQA1*0501/B1*0301	FYIMLV				VLIMY		FLYMVIA			VYI
IAb	NQD						P			
IAd	VILA	Q				ASG				
IAs	ITVF	TSA					HR			
IEb	Y	LV	YI					RK	RH	YF
IEd	H or	R or	R	HR	[DERK]	RK				
IEk	ILWV	Hydrophobic	Hydrophobic			ATQEN			KR	

[a]MHC-II peptide binding motifs. These are drawn from the more extensive summary of ref. 271.
[b]As indicated, the peptide positions are relative, with *i* being the amino acid residue that is thought to be situated in pocket P1, i+1, P2, and so forth.

is shown the molecular surface representation (in blue) of the top of the MHC-I molecule without the additional density of the bound peptide, while in panel B is shown the same surface representation along with the peptide assigned density (in red).

This first MHC-I structure clarified several important aspects of the mechanism by which the MHC-I molecule carries out its peptide-binding function. The amino-terminal domains (α1 and α2) of the MHC-I heavy chain form the binding site for peptide. This consists of a floor of eight strands of antiparallel β-pleated sheet, which support two α-helices, one contributed from the α1 domain and one from the α2 domain, aligned in an antiparallel orientation. The membrane proximal α3 domain has a fold similar to that of immunoglobulin domains and pairs asymmetrically with the other immunoglobulin domain of the molecule contributed by β2-m. The nature of recognition by T cells was suggested by comparing the location of those amino acid residues that had been characterized as being strong elements in T-cell recognition, residues that distinguished closely related allelic gene products and amino acid residues that had been identified as those that were responsible for the transplant rejection of the mutants of the *H-2Kᵇ* series (206). Amino acid residues of the MHC-I molecule responsible for T-cell recognition were most clearly classified into one of two categories or an overlapping set: those residues that were on the top of the molecule, exposed to solvent and available for direct interaction with the TCR, and those residues whose side chains pointed into the peptide-binding groove and might be considered crucial in the peptide-binding specificity of the particular MHC molecule. The original publications, based on a structure determined to a resolution of 3.5 Å, focused mainly on the structural outline of the mol-

ecule. The positions and numbering of the α-carbon atoms of the α1/α2 domain peptide-binding unit are shown in Fig. 4. Ribbon diagrams of HLA-A2, as seen from the side (colorplate 2A) and from the top (Colorplate 2B), indicate how the entire structure of the molecule is designed: The peptide binding site is supported by the β-sheet floor, and the floor is supported by the two immunoglobulin-like domains.

The comparison of this structure and higher resolution refinement of it with that of the closely related human MHC-I molecule, HLA-Aw68 (now known as HLA-A68, or more accurately, HLA-A*A68011; see Table 1), suggested that surface depressions in the groove of the MHC-I molecule, now known as pockets A through F, would be available for interactions with some of the side chains of the bound peptide (207,208). The amino acid side chains that contribute to these six pockets are illustrated in Colorplate 2C. These MHC-I structures were determined of molecules purified from tissue culture cells and containing a heterogeneous spectrum of self peptides. Concurrently with the structural studies, a number of laboratories developed the ability to identify the motifs of peptides bound by particular MHC-I molecules (see discussion of MHC-bound peptides above). Concomitant with the determination of the x-ray structure of the human MHC-I molecule, HLA-B*2705 (209), the motif of the peptides that were recovered from this molecule was determined, permitting the more precise modeling of the bound peptide in the cleft of the MHC-I (210). For HLA-B27, this was of particular interest, since the bound peptides had a strong overrepresentation of arginine at position 2 of the bound peptide (210), and scrutiny of HLA-B27 suggested that the amino acid residues lining the B pocket, particularly the acidic glutamic

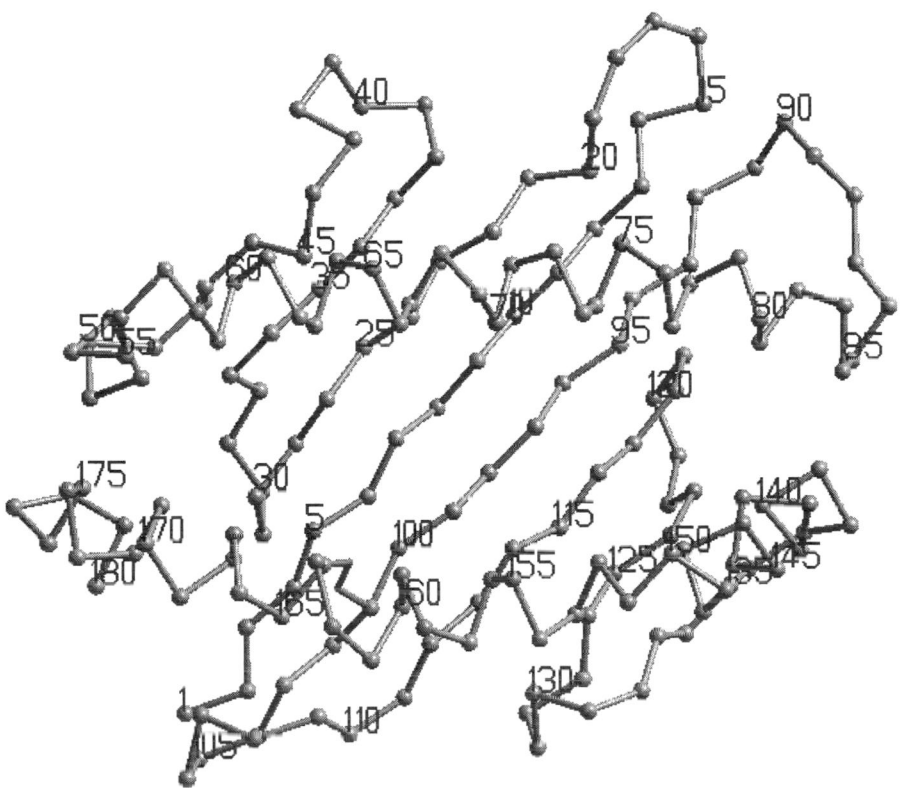

FIG. 4. Alpha-carbon backbone of the α1 and α2 domains of HLA-A2. This is the top view of protein data bank (*PDB*) file 3hla (208), displayed using SETOR (264). Residue 1 and every five residues thereafter are numbered.

acid at position 45 as well as cysteine 67, were complementary to the long, positively charged arginine side chain of the peptide amino acid at position 2 (209). These structural studies supported a view of MHC-I–peptide binding in which the side chain of the carboxyl-terminal residue of the bound peptide sits deep in the F pocket. In addition, the amino-terminal amino group forms strong hydrogen bonds with the hydroxyl groups of conserved amino acids tyrosine 59 and tyrosine 171. A hydrogen bond from the amino group of conserved tryptophan 147 to the backbone carbonyl oxygen of the penultimate peptide amino acid (usually position 8) also seems important, as do charge interactions and hydrogen bonds of the free carboxyl group at the carboxyl-terminus of the peptide with tyrosine 84, threonine 143, and lysine 146.

Other structures of MHC-I molecules were determined of complexes produced with homogeneous peptide, assembled either *in vitro* from bacterially expressed proteins with synthetic peptide (211), or exploiting MHC proteins expressed in insect cells (212). The structures determined with homogeneous peptide served to confirm the impression obtained from the structure obtained with heterogeneous self peptides. Specifically, the structures of the H-2K^b molecule complexed with peptides derived either from Sendai virus, vesicular stomatitis virus (213), or chicken ovalbumin (214) revealed that the same MHC molecule can bind peptides of different sequence and structure by virtue of their conserved motifs. Although small changes of the MHC are detectable on binding the different peptides, the main distinction in the recognition of different peptides bound by the same MHC molecule is due to the location, context, size, and charge of amino acid side chains of the peptide displayed when bound by the MHC molecule.

The most consistent rule obtained from the first x-ray structures and complemented by peptide recovery and early binding studies was that MHC-I bound peptides were required to embed the side chain of their carboxyl-terminal amino acid into the F pocket. However, with further studies, it became clear that MHC-I molecules could bind longer peptides that extended beyond the residue anchored in the F pocket (215). This was well established by the crystallographic visualization of a structure of such a complex (216).

MHC-II Structures

An initial model for the structure of an MHC-II molecule was based on the alignment of amino acid sequences and the available MHC-I three-dimensional structure (217). This model made a number of valid predictions that were borne out by the subsequent structural determination of HLA-DR1 (218). The MHC-II molecule clearly showed structural similarity to MHC-I and formed its binding groove by the juxtaposition of the α1 and β1 domains. The position of the electron density representing the heterogeneous peptide that copurified with the HLA-DR1 was identified. Colorplate 3 shows the electron density of the copurifying peptides superimposed on the van der Waals surface of the HLA-DR1 structure. In comparison to the MHC-I structure (see Colorplate 1), the peptides bound to the MHC-II molecule extend through the binding groove, rather than being anchored in it by both ends.

A comparison of the α-carbon backbone of the peptide-binding region of the MHC-I structure with that of the MHC-II structure is shown in Colorplate 4. It is remarkable that the structures are so similar, whether the binding domain is built of the α1 and α2 domains from the same chain (for MHC-I) or of the α1 and β1 domains that derive from two chains (for MHC-II). Comparative

ribbon diagrams (Colorplate 5), in which the location of the amino acid residues that are polymorphic for the human MHC-I and MHC-II chains are indicated, show that the bulk of the polymorphism derives from amino acid variability in regions that line the peptide-binding groove. This suggests that MHC polymorphism is needed to allow the MHC molecules, and as a result, the organism and its species, to respond to a changing antigenic environment.

As with MHC-I, a further understanding of the details of the interactions of peptides with the MHC-II molecule came from crystallographic studies of molecules prepared with homogeneous peptide, in the first case, HLA-DR1 complexed with an antigenic peptide derived from the hemagglutinin of influenza virus (219). Colorplate 6 shows from both top (panel A) and side (panel B) views the structure of the bound peptide superimposed on a surface representation of the HLA-DR molecule. Based on this structure, a set of pockets was designated, numbered for the peptide position that is bound. For the influenza peptide studied in this example, the major interactions were from peptide positions 1, 4, 6, 7, and 9, which are indicated in Colorplate 7. The deep P1 pocket accommodates the tyrosine (the third position of the peptide PKYVKQNTLKLAT), and the pockets indicated by 4, 6, 7, and 9 fit the Q, T, L, and L residues, respectively. The MHC-II is similar in its mode of binding to MHC-I, but reveals important differences: the lack of need for free amino and carboxyl-termini of the peptide, the binding of the peptide in a relatively extended conformation (like that of a type II polyproline helix), and a number of hydrogen bonds between conserved amino acids that line the binding-cleft and main-chain atoms of the peptide.

Among the most provocative observations from the first MHC-II structures was that the molecule was visualized as a dimer of dimers, and this moved a number of investigators to consider the possibility that activation of the T cell via its receptor might require the dimerization or multimerization of the TCR, an event thought to be dependent on the propensity of the MHC–peptide complex to self dimerize. The simple elegance of this dimer of dimers is illustrated in Colorplate 8. Several arguments support the dimerization hypothesis: the finding of a dimer of dimers in the crystals of HLA-DR that formed in several different space groups (218–220), the observation that a TCR Vα domain formed tight dimers and in its crystals formed dimers of the dimers (221), the demonstration of the ability to immunoprecipitate MHC-II dimers from B cells (222), the requirement for purified MHC-I dimers for stimulation of a T cell in an *in vitro* system (223), and the finding that MHC-II–peptide–TCR complexes could form higher order multimers in solution, as detected by quasi-elastic light scattering (224). However, a number of strong counterarguments draw this hypothesis into question. MHC-II molecules, other than HLA-DR1, that have been crystallized do not seem to form the same kind of dimer of dimers in their crystals (225). None of the MHC-I molecules that have been examined by x-ray crystallography show dimers in the same orientation as the MHC-II ones reported. A different Vα domain fails to dimerize, even at high concentration (226). The reported x-ray structures of TCR–MHC–peptide complexes (227,228) fail to show dimerization. Despite its simple elegance, then, it is likely that additional experimentation will be required to understand the topologic requirements for T-cell activation through the αβ TCR.

MHC-Ib Molecules

To this point, our description of MHC-I molecules has focused on the classical molecules, represented by HLA-A, HLA-B, and

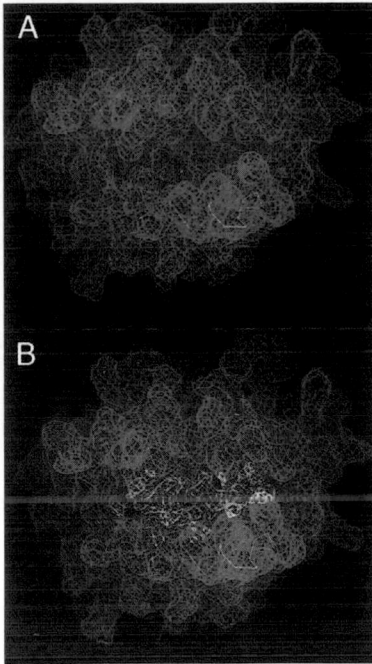

COLORPLATE 1. Electron density in the cleft of HLA-A2. **A:** A surface representation of the HLA-A2 structure is shown in comparison with the surface representation, including the electron density (**B**) that could not be accounted for by the amino acid sequence of the protein. (From ref. 183, with permission.)

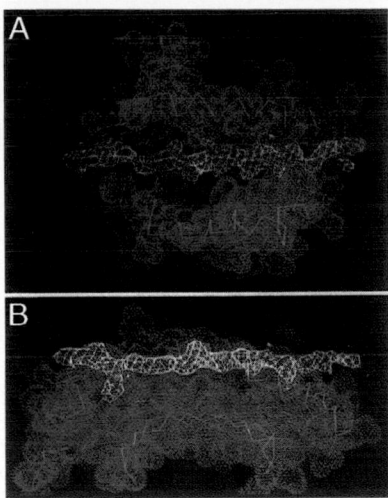

COLORPLATE 2. The location of the electron density in the cleft of HLA-DR1. **A:** A classical top view of the MHC-II–binding cleft with the α1 helix *above* and the β1 helix *below.* **B:** The orthogonal view looking at the same site from the side. The β1 helix is proximal to the bound peptide. In this illustration, the MHC-II surface is represented in *blue* and the bound peptide electron density in *red.* (From ref. 218, with permission.)

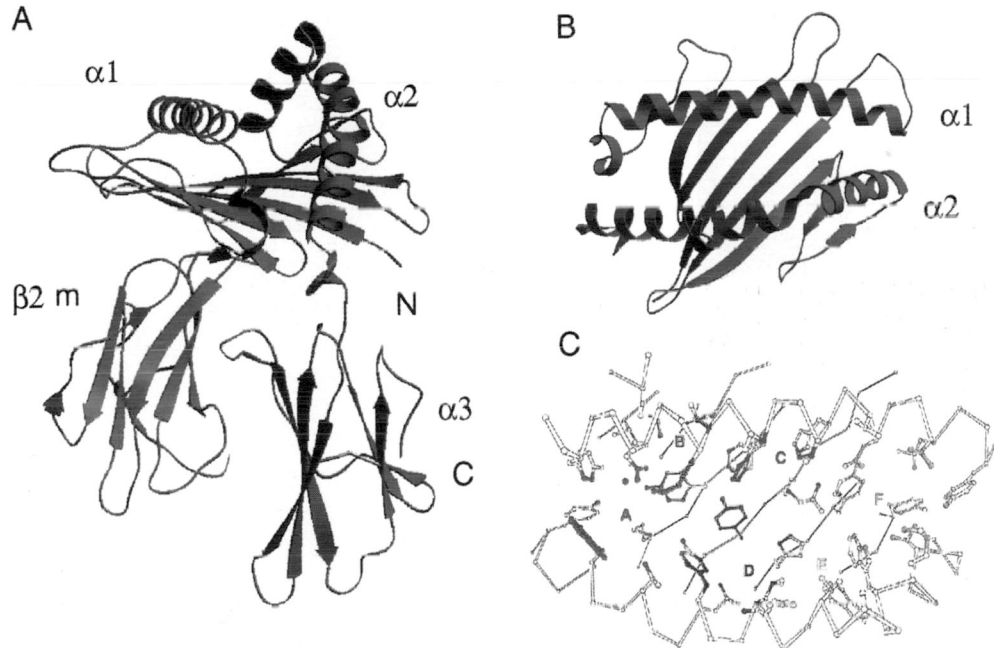

COLORPLATE 3. Color ribbon representation of HLA-A*0201. **A:** Side view. **B:** Top view. **C:** Top view with positions of pockets A through F indicated. Panels (A) and (B) of this illustration were made with SETOR (264), based on the protein data bank (PDB) coordinates of 3hla. Panel (C) of this illustration is taken directly from Saper et al. (265), with permission.

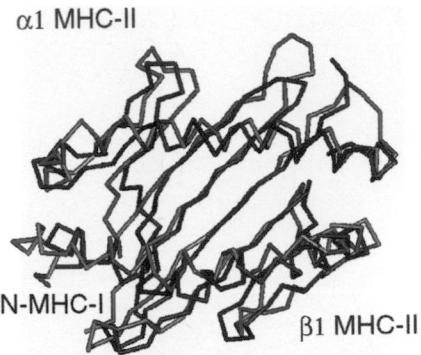

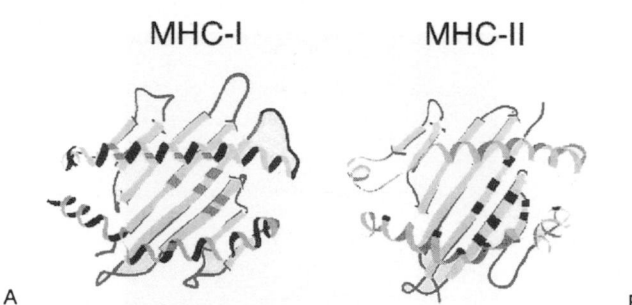

COLORPLATE 4. Superposition of the α-carbon backbones of an MHC-I and an MHC-II molecule. The α-carbon backbones of the MHC-I molecule HLA-A2 (PDB 3hla) with the MHC-II molecule HLA-DR1 (PDB 1dlh) are shown. The molecules were displayed and superposed using QUANTA 97 (Molecular Simulations, Inc.). The backbone of the MHC-I molecule is shown in *blue,* and its amino-terminus is indicated. Similarly, the backbones of the α1 and β1 domains of HLA-DR are shown in *red.* The amino-termini of both chains are shown.

COLORPLATE 5. Location of polymorphic amino acid residues in MHC-I and MHC-II molecules. **A:** The polymorphic residues of human MHC-I molecules are shown in *green,* and (**B**) the polymorphic residues of the human MHC-II molecules are shown in *red.* (From ref. 262, with permission.)

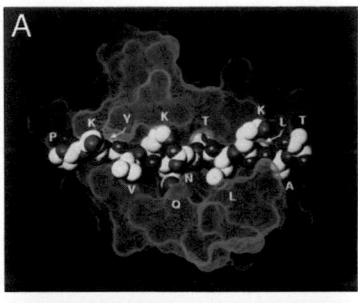

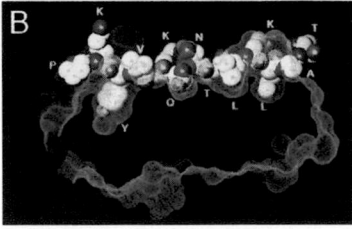

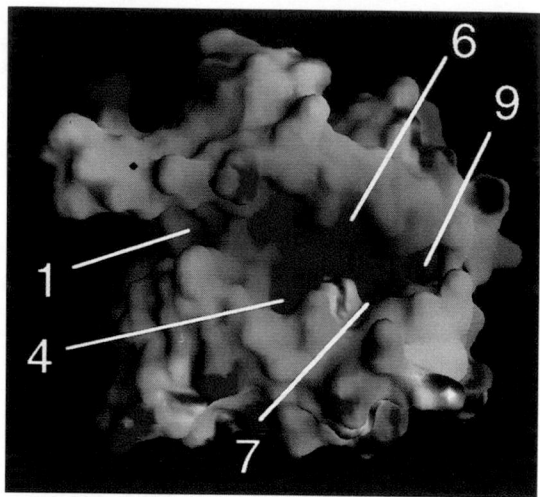

COLORPLATE 6. Location of pockets in HLA-DR1 based on the cocrystal of HLA-DR1, with a peptide derived from influenza hemagglutinin. The surface representations of the α1 and β1 domains are shown in *blue.* A space-filling model of the bound peptide, PKYVKQNTLKLAT, is also shown. Panel (**A**) shows the top view, and panel (**B**) shows the side view. (From ref. 219, with permission.)

COLORPLATE 7. Numbering of the major pockets of the binding groove of HLA-DR1, according to Stern et al. (219). The structure of HLA-DR1, PDB file 1dlh, was displayed with GRASP (266).

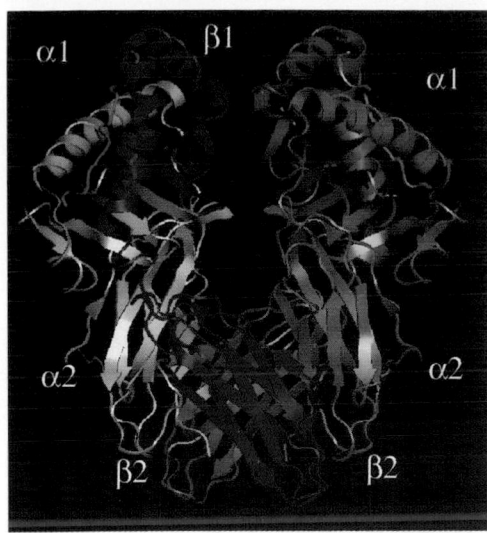

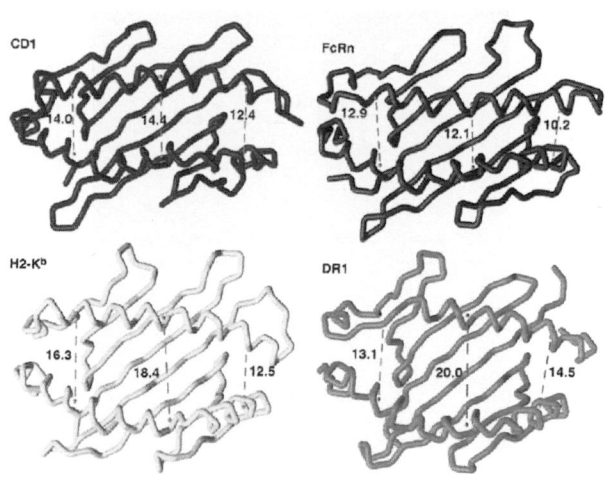

COLORPLATE 8. Ribbon diagram of HLA-DR1 (PDB file 1dlh), showing the position of the crystallographic dimer of dimers and the location of the individual domains of the protein. α chains are in *grey* and *pink,* β chains in *magenta* and *orange,* and peptide in *green* and *blue.* This illustration was composed in QUANTA 97.

COLORPLATE 9. Comparison of the α-carbon backbone tracings and size of the peptide binding cleft of MHC-I molecule H-2K[b], MHC-II molecule HLA-DR1, and the MHC-Ib molecules, CD1 and FcRn. (From ref. 235, with permission.)

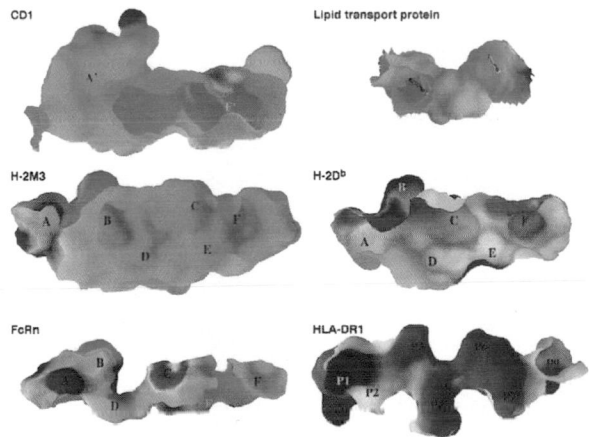

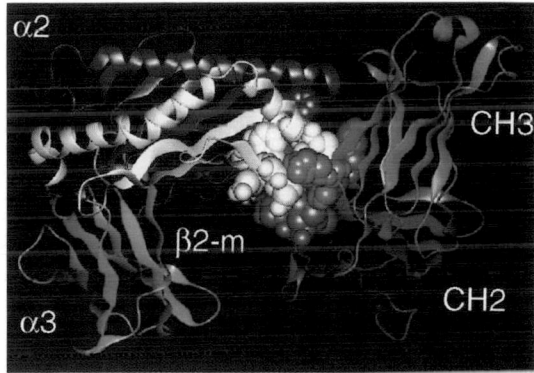

COLORPLATE 10. Shape, size, and charge of the binding groove of CD1 compared with those of several other MHC molecules and with a known lipid transport protein. Surface representation of the binding cleft is displayed with acidic regions in *red,* basic regions in *blue,* and neutral regions in *green.* (From ref. 235, with permission.)

COLORPLATE 11. Principal interactions between the MHC-Ib molecule, FcRn, and immunoglobulin Fc. Ribbon diagrams of FcRn and Fc are shown, with domains α1, α2, α3, and β2-m in *red, yellow, green,* and *purple,* respectively, and Fc (CH2 and CH3 domains) in *blue* and *light green.* The main contact residues are shown as space-filling structures (α1 domain, residue 90; α2, residues 113–119 and 131–135; β2-m, residues 1–4 and 86). (From ref. 267, with permission, based on ref. 243.)

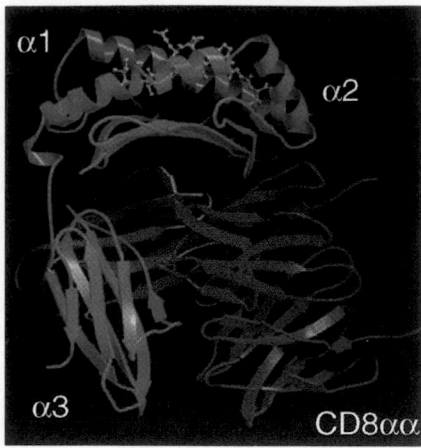

COLORPLATE 12. The interaction of the coreceptor, CD8, with the α3 domain of the MHC-I molecule. The MHC-I molecule, HLA-A2, is displayed with its α1, α2, and α3 domains labeled, bound to the CD8αα homodimer in *red* and *blue*. (From ref. 246, with permission.)

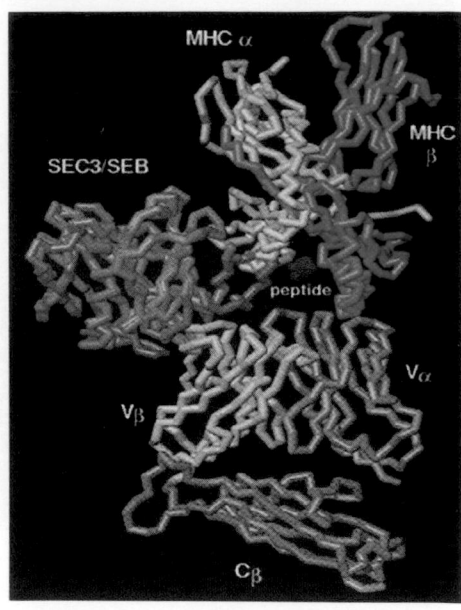

COLORPLATE 13. A model of the interaction of e superantigens SEC3 and SEB with the α1 domain of HLA-DR1, as scaffolded by the Vβ domain of the TCR. (From ref. 268, with permission.)

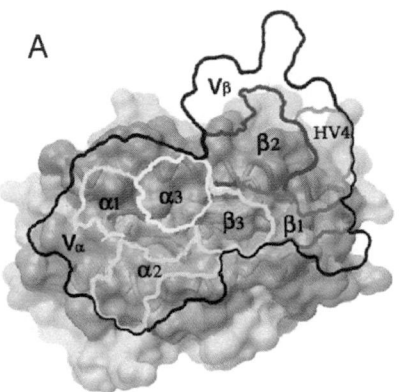

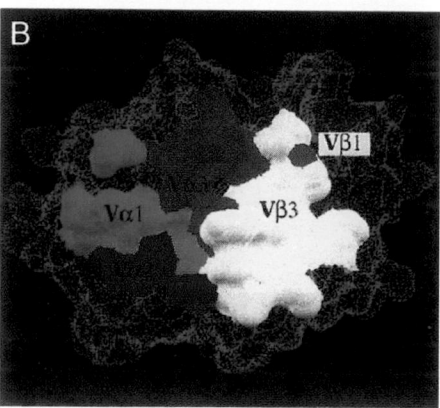

COLORPLATE 14. Footprints of TCRs visualized on their cognate MHC-I–peptide complexes. Panel (**A**) illustrates the 2C TCR complexed with H-2Kb and the dEV8 peptide. (From ref. 228, with permission.) Panel (**B**) shows the footprint of the A6 TCR complexed with HLA-A2 and the Tax peptide. (From ref. 227, with permission.)

HLA-C in the human and by H-2K, H-2D, and H-2L in the mouse. Two groups of related MHC-Ib molecules, for which three-dimensional structures have been determined, are of particular interest: the CD1 molecules (229) and H-2M3 (90). H-2M3 is of particular note because of its ability to bind and present peptide antigens that contain amino-terminal N-formyl groups. H-2M3 was originally identified as the MHC-Ib molecule that presents an endogenous peptide derived from the mitochondrially encoded protein ND1, which has been called maternally transmitted factor (MTF) (230). Thus, it was of interest to understand in structural terms how this molecule binds such N-formylated peptides (231). The crystal structure of H-2M3 complexed with an N-formylated nonamer peptide, fMYFINILTL, revealed that the structure of the A pocket, highly conserved among MHC-Ia molecules, which have tyrosine 7, tyrosine 59, tyrosine 159, tryptophan 167, and tyrosine 171, is quite different, so that it can accommodate the N-formyl group in the A pocket. In particular, H2-M3 has leucine at 167 and phenylalanine at 171, and because of the side-chain orientation of leucine 167, the A pocket is dramatically reduced in size, causing the amino-terminal nitrogen of the formylated peptide to be positioned where the peptide position 2 amino nitrogen would lie in an MHC-Ia molecule. Thus, the unique peptide selectivity of H-2M3 is explained in structural terms.

Another MHC-Ib molecule of great interest is CD1, representative of a class of MHC-I molecules that map outside of the MHC, that have limited tissue-specific expression, and that seem capable of interaction with both αβ and γδ T cells (229). In the human, CD1b and CD1c have been shown to be capable of presenting nonpeptidic mycobacterial cell wall components, such as mycolic acid–containing lipids and lipoarabinomannan lipoglycans (232,233), and a minor subset of T cells is suspected of being restricted to CD1 (234). For these reasons, the crystal structure of mouse CD1d1, which corresponds to human CD1d, was determined (235), and it revealed a classic MHC-I structure with a basic α-carbon fold quite similar to that of the MHC-Ia molecules. Consistent with its apparent biologic function of binding hydrophobic lipid-containing molecules, its binding groove is somewhat narrower and deeper than that of either MHC-Ia molecules or MHC-II molecules. The backbone configuration of the α1α2 domain structure of CD1 is shown in Colorplate 9, where it is compared with the homologous region of H-2Kb, HLA-DR1, and another MHC-Ib molecule, the FcRn, a neonatal Fc receptor. To get a three-dimensional understanding of the shape and charge distribution of the peptide-binding grooves of several examples of MHC-Ia, MHC-Ib and MHC-II molecules, Zeng et al. (235) displayed a surface representation of the binding regions with electrostatic potentials mapped to that surface (see Colorplate 10). Despite the narrowness of the entrance to the groove based on the distance between the α-helices, the CD1 binding groove, because of its depth, is the largest. The depth of the groove results from the merging of pockets to form what have been termed the A and F pockets in place of the MHC-Ia A through F pockets. This A pocket is about the size of the binding site of a nonspecific lipid-binding protein. For comparison, the groove of H-2M3, with a small charged A pocket and deep B and F pockets, is shown. An example of an MHC-Ia molecule, H-2Db (236), shows how different charge distributions occur in molecules of this group, and the depiction of HLA-DR1 reveals the depth of side-chain pockets there. The very narrow groove of FcRn (see below) lacks enough space to accommodate a peptide antigen.

Another example of an MHC-Ib molecule, noteworthy because it serves as an example of a novel function of MHC molecules, is the neonatal Fc receptor. Originally described in the rat as a molecule of the intestinal epithelium that is involved in the transport of colostral immunoglobulin from the lumen to the bloodstream (237,238), homologues in the mouse and human have also been described (239–241), and the structure of the rat molecule has been determined crystallographically (242). As suggested by the amino acid sequence similarity of the FcRn to MHC-I proteins, the three-dimensional structure revealed considerable similarity to MHC-Ia molecules (242); specifically, α1 and α2 domains have similar topology to the MHC-I molecule, although, as discussed above, what would be the peptide-binding groove in the MHC-Ia molecules is closed tightly and lacks space enough for a ligand. The most provocative feature of the molecule is observed in the lower resolution structure of the complex of the FcRn with Fc (243), which is illustrated in Colorplate 11. The FcRn has taken the MHC-I fold and diverted its function to an interaction with the Fc of the immunoglobulin. Amino acids at what would classically be considered the right-hand side of the peptide-binding groove make contact with the Fc interface that lies between CH2 and CH3 domains. In the FcRn/FcR cocrystal a network of interactions exists that suggests the possibility of interaction of molecules on two parallel membranes, such as might exist at the surface of the microvilli of the intestinal epithelial cells, where these molecules are expressed. The FcRn serves as an excellent example of similar structures in the immune system being diverted for alternate purpose. The importance of the FcRn has been underscored by the observations of differences in the serum half-life of immunoglobulin in animals that, as a result of an induced deletion of β2-m, lack the normal expression FcRn as well, and seem to metabolize serum immunoglobulin aberrantly (244).

Complexes of MHC Molecules with Ligands

Our structure–function survey will be completed by brief descriptions of the interactions of MHC-I molecules with the coreceptor CD8, putative interactions of CD4 with MHC-II, the formation of complexes of HLA-DR with superantigens, and the interaction of TCRs with MHC–peptide complexes. Each of these structural studies complements a host of biologic experiments that have led up to an appreciation of the importance of understanding the structural basis of these immune reactions.

CD8, the coreceptor on MHC-I–restricted αβ T cells, exists as a cell surface homodimer of two α chains or a heterodimer of α and β chains that plays an important role both in the activation of mature peripheral T cells as well as in the thymic development of MHC-I–restricted lymphocytes (245). This dual role seems to be related both to an adhesive function based on the interaction of CD8 with the MHC-I molecule as well as its contribution to TCR-mediated signaling. The three-dimensional structure of a complex made between the human MHC-I molecule HLA-A2 complexed with the pol peptide and a soluble recombinant form of the the human CD8αα homodimer was determined (246). This structure has offered some surprises. An extensive mutational analysis of HLA-A2 indicated that amino acid residues of both the α2 and α3 domains affected the interaction with CD8αα transfectants as assayed by cell adhesion (247). This led the authors to propose that the interaction with CD8 would promote the dimerization of the MHC-I molecules, which would be needed for T-cell activation. The three-dimensional structure, however, although it clearly shows CD8 interaction with both the α2 and α3 domains of the MHC, reveals that the CD8αα homodimer forms an antibody-like combining site that focuses on an exposed loop of the MHC-I α3 domain. This interaction is illustrated in Colorplate 12, which shows the flexible loop of residue 223–229 clamped into the CD8-combining site.

The T-cell coreceptor associated with cells restricted to MHC-II antigens, CD4, has also been the subject of detailed structural studies, in part because of its role as a receptor for attachment and entry of the human immunodeficiency virus (HIV) (248). X-ray structural studies of CD4, though not yet available in complex with MHC-II molecules, have clearly outlined the structure of this molecule as having four tandem immunoglobulin-like domains, known as D1 through D4. A structural determination of the complete extracellular portion of the molecule indicates that there is segmental flexibility between domains D2 and D3, and both crystallographic and biochemical data suggest that dimerization of cell surface CD4 occurs (249). These results have been interpreted to support a role for CD4-mediated MHC-II–dependent dimerization in facilitating TCR dimerization and signaling.

MHC-II interactions with superantigens, such as those derived from pathogenic bacteria, are the first step in the presentation of the multivalent array of the APC-bound superantigen to T cells bearing receptors of the family or class that can bind the superantigen (250). Structural analysis of crystals derived from staphylococcal enterotoxin B (SEB) complexed with HLA-DR1 (220) and from toxic shock syndrome toxin-1 (TSST-1) complexed with HLA-DR1 (251) revealed that the two toxins bind to an overlapping site, primarily on the MHC-II α chain, and indicated that the SEB site would not be expected to be influenced by the specific peptide bound by the MHC, although the TSST-1 site would. Looking at superantigen complexes made with a TCR β chain, Fields et al. (252) have developed a model of the complete complex of MHC-II/SEB/TCR. This model is shown in Colorplate 13. This illustration emphasizes how a molecule presented by the MHC, predominantly by contact with the α chain, can then interact with the TCR on the T cell.

Perhaps the most exciting of the more recent structural observations has been the solution of x-ray structures of MHC molecules complexed with both specific peptides and TCR. This has been accomplished in two systems. The mouse MHC-I molecule H-2K^b has been cocrystallized with a self peptide, dEV8, and a TCR known as 2C (228). The HLA-A2 MHC-I molecule bound to the Tax peptide has been cocrystallized with its cognate TCR, A6, derived from a cytolytic T cell (227). Both of these structures offer a first glimpse at the orientation of the TCR on the MHC–peptide complex. The footprints of the TCRs, as mapped onto their respective MHC–peptide complexes, are illustrated in Colorplate 14. Colorplate 14 shows that the complementarity-determining regions (CDRs) sit symmetrically on the MHC–peptide complexes. For the 2C/H-2K^b/dEV8 complex (see Fig. 18A), the region contacted by the CDRs of the Vα domain of the TCR lie to the left, and that contacted by the CDRs of the Vβ domain lie to the right. The regions contacted by CDR3, labeled α3 (for that contacted by CDR3 of Vα) and β3, are at the center of the bound peptide, while the regions contacted by CDR1 and CDR2 of both Vα and Vβ lie peripherally. The footprint of the A6 TCR on the HLA-A2/Tax peptide complex is somewhat different in that although the contacts from the CDRs of the Vα domain are similar to those in the other MHC/TCR complex, the contacts of the Vβ domain are due almost exclusively to the CDR3. This may in part be due to the relatively long CDR3β of this particular TCR. Clearly, additional structures of a wide variety of TCR and MHC–peptide complexes will need to be determined to appreciate the general rules.

MOLECULAR INTERACTIONS OF MHC MOLECULES

Whereas the crystal stuctures provide a vivid static illustration of the interactions of MHC molecules with their peptide, FcRn, CD8, SA, and TCR ligands, the dynamic aspects of these binding steps can be approached by a variety of biophysical methods (253). It is not the place here to consider these exhaustively, but it is important to note that affinities and kinetics of interaction of MHC–peptide complexes for TCR have been determined by several methods in a variety of systems (224,254–261). Although there are clear differences in the affinity and kinetics of binding of different TCRs for different MHC–peptide complexes, the generally consistent findings are that the affinities are low to moderate (i.e., $K_d = 5 \times 10^{-5}$ to 10^{-7} M) and are characterized by relatively rapid dissociation rates (i.e., $k_d = 10^{-1}$ to 10^{-3} sec^{-1}). Although there have been some studies attempting to correlate the affinity of particular MHC–peptide complexes for particular TCRs with the outcome of thymic selection or activation of mature T cells, these have not yet been applied widely enough to draw firm conclusions.

RECAPITULATION

This survey of the *Mhc* as a genetic region and of MHC molecules as immunologic effectors has taken us from the mouse to the human, from the gene to its encoded protein. *Mhc* genes in higher organisms represent the product of an ongoing evolutionary enterprise in which the multicellular organism struggles to combat biologic and molecular invasions from without and within, and the organism has at this stage succeeded in large part because of the success of its immune system in being able to detect and respond to such incursions. The systems encoded by the *Mhc* not only regulate the response to soluble foreign antigens presented via the MHC-II pathway, but also control reactions to viral and other intracellular infectious agents, and by the same mechanism can respond to the dysregulated protein expression that is the hallmark of malignant transformation. Though MHC-I–restricted antigen presentation used to be thought of as the prime territory of CD8-expressing T cells, it is clear that molecules of the same family regulate responses of NK cells as well, and their ability to function as Fc receptors suggests that the more distantly related members of the MHC protein family may also have alternative functions, even beyond the immune system. As we become more skilled at deciphering chemical and biologic codes, I suspect that we will learn that Nature's imagination has been more vivid than our own.

ACKNOWLEDGMENTS

This chapter is dedicated to the memory of Sergei Khilko, colleague and friend. I would like to thank the members of my laboratory, L. F. Boyd, R. Carey, D. H. Chung, M. Jelonek, K. Natarajan, D. Plaksin, and K. Polakova, for their patience during the writing of this chapter, and K. Natarajan and D. Eilat for comments on the text.

REFERENCES

1. Snell GD, Dausset J, Nathenson S. *Histocompatibility.* New York: Academic Press, 1976.
2. Klein J. *Natural history of the major histocompatibility complex.* New York: Wiley-Interscience, 1986.
3. Benacerraf B, McDevitt HO. Histocompatibility-linked immune response genes. *Science* 1972;175:273–279.
4. Shevach EM, Rosenthal AS. Function of macrophages in antigen recognition by guinea pig T lymphocytes. II. Role of the macrophage in the regulation of genetic control of the immune response. *J Exp Med* 1973;138:1213–1229.
5. Zinkernagel RM, Doherty PC. Restriction of in vitro T cell-mediated cytotoxicity in lymphocytic choriomeningitis within a syngeneic or semiallogeneic system. *Nature* 1974;248:701–702.
6. Shearer GM, Rehn TG, Garbarino CA. Cell-mediated lympholysis of trinitrophenyl-modified autologous lymphocytes. Effector cell specificity to modified cell surface components controlled by H-2K and H-2D serological regions of the murine major histocompatibility complex. *J Exp Med* 1975;141:1384–1364.
7. Germain RN, Margulies DH. The biochemistry and cell biology of antigen processing and presentation. *Annu Rev Immunol* 1993;11:403–450.
8. Germain RN. MHC-dependent antigen processing and peptide presentation: providing ligands for T lymphocyte activation. *Cell* 1994;76:287–299.
9. York IA, Rock KL. Antigen processing and presentation by the class I major histocompatibility complex. *Annu Rev Immunol* 1996;14:369–396.
10. Karre K. Natural killer cells and the MHC class I pathway of peptide presentation. *Semin Immunol* 1993;5:127–145.
11. Yokoyama WM, Daniels BF, Seaman WE, Hunziker R, Margulies DH, Smith HR. A family of murine NK cell receptors specific for target cell MHC class I molecules. *Semin Immunol* 1995;7:89–101.
12. Schild H, Mavaddat N, Litzenberger C, et al. The nature of major histocompatibility complex recognition by gamma delta T cells. *Cell* 1994;76:29–37.
13. Lyon MF, Rastan S, Brown SDM. *Genetic variants and strains of the laboratory mouse.* Oxford: Oxford University Press, 1996.
14. Bodmer JG, Marsh SG, Albert ED, et al. Nomenclature for factors of the HLA system, 1996. *Hum Immunol* 1997;53:98 128.
15. Gorer PA. The detection of antigenic differences in mouse erythroctyes by the employment of immune sera. *Br J Exp Pathol* 1936;17:42–50.
16. Gorer PA. The role of antibodies in immunity to transplanted leukemia in mice. *J Pathol Bacteriol* 1942;54:51–65.
17. Duran IW, Horton RM, Birschbach CW, Chang-Miller A, Pease LR. Structural relationships among the H-2 D-regions of murine MHC haplotypes. *J Immunol* 1989;142:288–296.
18. Ceppellini R. *Histocompatibility testing, 1967.* Copenhagen: Munksgaard, 1967: 149.
19. Yoshino M, Xiao H, Jones EP, et al. Genomic evolution of the distal Mhc class I region on mouse Chr 17. *Hereditas* 1997;127(1–2):141–148.
20. Lindahl KF. On naming H2 haplotypes: functional significance of MHC class Ib alleles. *Immunogenetics* 1997;46:53–62.
21. Gruen JR, Weissman SW. Evolving views of the major histocompatibility complex. *Blood* 1997;11:4252–5265.
22. Stroynowski I, Lindahl KF. Antigen presentation by non-classical class I molecules. *Curr Opin Immunol* 1994;6:38–44.
23. Germain RN, Quill H. Unexpected expression of a unique mixed isotype class II MIIC molecule by transfected L cells. *Nature* 1986;320:72–75.
24. Malissen B, Shastri N, Pierres M, Hood L. Cotransfer of the Ed alpha and Ad beta genes into L cells results in the surface expression of a functional mixed-isotype Ia molecule. *Proc Natl Acad Sci USA* 1986;83:3958–3962.
25. Spencer JS, Kubo RT. Mixed isotype class II antigen expression. A novel class II molecule is expressed on a murine B cell lymphoma. *J Exp Med* 1989;169: 625–640.
26. Matsunaga M, Seki K, Mineta T, Kimoto M. Antigen-reactive T cell clones restricted by mixed isotype A beta d/E alpha d class II molecules. *J Exp Med* 1990;171:577–582.
27. Natarajan K, Burstyn D, Zauderer M. Major histocompatibility complex determinants select T-cell receptor alpha chain variable region dominance in a peptide-specific response. *Proc Natl Acad Sci USA* 1992;89:8874–8878.
28. Yewdell JW, Bennink JR. Cell biology of antigen processing and presentation to major histocompatibility complex class I molecule-restricted T lymphocytes. *Adv Immunol* 1992;52:1–123.
29. Boon T, van der Bruggen P. Human tumor antigens recognized by T lymphocytes. *J Exp Med* 1996;183:725–729.
30. Heemels MT, Ploegh H. Generation, translocation, and presentation of MHC class I-restricted peptides. *Annu Rev Biochem* 1995;64:463–491.
31. Cresswell P. Antigen presentation. Getting peptides into MHC class II molecules. *Curr Biol* 1994;4:541–543.
32. Cresswell P. Invariant chain structure and MHC class II function. *Cell* 1996;84: 505–507.
33. Denzin LK, Hammond C, Cresswell P. HLA-DM interactions with intermediates in HLA-DR maturation and a role for HLA-DM in stabilizing empty HLA-DR molecules. *J Exp Med* 1996;184:2153–2165.
34. Pierre P, Denzin LK, Hammond C, et al. HLA-DM is localized to conventional and unconventional MHC class II-containing endocytic compartments. *Immunity* 1996;4:229–239.
35. Germain R. Immunology. The ins and outs of antigen processing and presentation. *Nature* 1986;322:687–689.
36. Yewdell JW, Bennink JR. The binary logic of antigen processing and presentation to T cells. *Cell* 1990;62:203–206.
37. Brodsky FM, Guagliardi LE. The cell biology of antigen processing and presentation. *Annu Rev Immunol* 1991;9:707–744.
38. Connolly JM, Potter TA, Wormstall EM, Hansen TH. The Lyt-2 molecule recognizes residues in the class I alpha 3 domain in allogeneic cytotoxic T cell responses. *J Exp Med* 1988;168:325–341.
39. Norment AM, Salter RD, Parham P, Engelhard VH, Littman DR. Cell-cell adhesion mediated by CD8 and MHC class I molecules. *Nature* 1988;336:79–81.
40. Salter RD, Norment AM, Chen BP, et al. Polymorphism in the alpha 3 domain of HLA-A molecules affects binding to CD8. *Nature* 1989;338:345–347.
41. Salter RD, Benjamin RJ, Wesley PK, et al. A binding site for the T-cell co-receptor CD8 on the alpha 3 domain of HLA-A2. *Nature* 1990;345:41–46.
42. Doyle C, Strominger JL. Interaction between CD4 and class II MHC molecules mediates cell adhesion. *Nature* 1987;330:256–259.
43. Konig R, Huang LY, Germain RN. MHC class II interaction with CD4 mediated by a region analogous to the MHC class I binding site for CD8. *Nature* 1992;356: 796–798.
44. Konig R, Shen X, Germain RN. Involvement of both major histocompatibility complex class II alpha and beta chains in CD4 function indicates a role for ordered oligomerization in T cell activation. *J Exp Med* 1995;182:779–787.
45. Luescher IF, Vivier E, Layer A, et al. CD8 modulation of T-cell antigen receptor-ligand interactions on living cytotoxic T lymphocytes. *Nature* 1995;373:353–356.
46. Sloan VS, Cameron P, Porter G, et al. Mediation by HLA-DM of dissociation of peptides from HLA-DR. *Nature* 1995;375:802–806.
47. Elliott T. Transporter associated with antigen processing. *Adv Immunol* 1997;65: 47–109.
48. Ljunggren HG, Karre K. In search of the 'missing self': MHC molecules and NK cell recognition. *Immunol Today* 1990;11:237–244.
49. Karre K. Express yourself or die: peptides, MHC molecules, and NK cells. *Science* 1995;267:978–979.
50. Rolstad B, Vaage JT, Naper C, et al. Positive and negative MHC class I recognition by rat NK cells. *Immunol Rev* 1997;155:91–104.
51. Newell WR, Trowsdale J, Beck S. MHCDB: database of the human MHC (release 2). *Immunogenetics* 1996;45:6–8.
52. Monaco JJ, McDevitt HO. H-2-linked low-molecular weight polypeptide antigens assemble into an unusual macromolecular complex. *Nature* 1984;309: 797–799.
53. Monaco JJ, McDevitt HO. The LMP antigens: a stable MHC-controlled multisubunit protein complex. *Hum Immunol* 1986;15:416–426.
54. Martinez C, Monaco J. Homology of proteasome subunits to a major histocompatibility complex-linked LMP gene. *Nature* 1991;353:664–667.
55. Monaco JJ. Genes in the MHC that may affect antigen processing. *Curr Opin Immunol* 1992;4:70–73.
56. Hill A, Ploegh H. Getting the inside out: the transporter associated with antigen processing (TAP) and the presentation of viral antigen. *Proc Natl Acad Sci USA* 1995;92:341–343.
57. Howard JC. Supply and transport of peptides presented by class I MHC molecules. *Curr Opin Immunol* 1995;7:69–76.
58. Yang Y, Sempe P, Peterson PA. Molecular mechanisms of class I major histocompatibility complex antigen processing and presentation. *Immunol Res* 1996;15:208–233.
59. Powis SJ. Major histocompatibility complex class I molecules interact with both subunits of the transporter associated with antigen processing, TAP1 and TAP2. *Eur J Immunol* 1997;27:2744–2747.
60. Spee P, Neefjes J. TAP-translocated peptides specifically bind proteins in the endoplasmic reticulum, including gp96, protein disulfide isomerase and calreticulin. *Eur J Immunol* 1997;27:2441–2449.
61. Driscoll J, Brown MG, Finley D, Monaco JJ. MHC-linked LMP gene products specifically alter peptidase activities of the proteasome. *Nature* 1993;365: 262–264.
62. Nandi D, Jiang H, Monaco JJ. Identification of MECL-1 (LMP-10) as the third IFN-gamma-inducible proteasome subunit. *J Immunol* 1996;156:2361–2364.
63. Livingstone AM, Powis SJ, Diamond AG, Butcher GW, Howard JC. A trans-acting major histocompatibility complex-linked gene whose alleles determine gain and loss changes in the antigenic structure of a classical class I molecule. *J Exp Med* 1989;170:777–795.
64. Livingstone AM, Powis SJ, Gunther E, Cramer DV, Howard JC, Butcher GW. Cim: an MHC class II-linked allelism affecting the antigenicity of a classical class I molecule for T lymphocytes. *Immunogenetics* 1991;34:157–163.
65. Powis SJ, Young LL, Joly E, et al. The rat cim effect: TAP allele-dependent changes in a class I MHC anchor motif and evidence against C-terminal trimming of peptides in the ER. *Immunity* 1996;4:159–165.
66. Simmons WA, Roopenian DC, Summerfield SG, et al. A new MHC locus that influences class I peptide presentation. *Immunity* 1997;7:641–652.
67. White PC, Chaplin DD, Weis JH, Dupont B, New MI, Seidman JG. Two steroid 21-hydroxylase genes are located in the murine S region. *Nature* 1984;312: 465–467.
68. White PC, New MI, Dupont B. HLA-linked congenital adrenal hyperplasia results from a defective gene encoding a cytochrome P 450 specific for steroid 21-hydroxylation. *Proc Natl Acad Sci USA* 1984;81:7505–7509.

69. Browning JL, Ngam-ek A, Lawton P, et al. Lymphotoxin beta, a novel member of the TNF family that forms a heteromeric complex with lymphotoxin on the cell surface. *Cell* 1993;72:847–856.

70. Lawton P, Nelson J, Tizard R, Browning JL. Characterization of the mouse lymphotoxin-beta gene. *J Immunol* 1995;154:239–246.

71. Ciccone E, Pende D, Viale O, et al. Involvement of HLA class I alleles in natural killer (NK) cell-specific functions: expression of HLA-Cw3 confers selective protection from lysis by alloreactive NK clones displaying a defined specificity (specificity 2). *J Exp Med* 1992;176:963–971.

72. Braud V, Jones EY, McMichael A. The human major histocompatibility complex class Ib molecule HLA-E binds signal sequence-derived peptides with primary anchor residues at positions 2 and 9. *Eur J Immunol* 1997;27:1164–1169.

73. Grimsley C, Ober C. Population genetic studies of HLA-E: evidence for selection. *Hum Immunol* 1997;52:33–40.

74. Le Bouteiller P, Lenfant F. Antigen-presenting function(s) of the non-classical HLA-E,-F and -G class I molecules: the beginning of a story. *Res Immunol* 1996;147:301–313.

75. Wei XH, Orr HT. Differential expression of HLA-E, HLA-F, and HLA-G transcripts in human tissue. *Hum Immunol* 1990;29:131–142.

76. Schmidt CM, Orr HT. HLA-G transgenic mice: a model for studying expression and function at the maternal/fetal interface. *Immunol Rev* 1995;147:53–65.

77. Chorney MJ, Sawada I, Gillespie GA, Srivastava R, Pan J, Weissman SM. Transcription analysis, physical mapping, and molecular characterization of a non-classical human leukocyte antigen class I gene. *Mol Cell Biol* 1990;10:243–253.

78. Feder JN, Gnirke A, Thomas W, et al. A novel MHC class I-like gene is mutated in patients with hereditary haemochromatosis. *Nat Genet* 1996;13:399–408.

79. Bodmer JG, Parham P, Albert ED, Marsh SG, Marsh SG. Putting a hold on "HLA-H". The WHO Nomenclature Committee for Factors of the HLA System [Letter; Comment]. Nomenclature for factors of the HLA System, update June 1996. *Nat Genet* 1997;15:234–235.

80. Mercier B, Mura C, Ferec C. Putting a hold on "HLA-H" [Letter; Comment]. *Nat Genet* 1997;15:234.

81. Klein J, Figueroa F. Evolution of the major histocompatibility complex. *Crit Rev Immunol* 1986;6:295–386.

82. Lawlor DA, Zemmour J, Ennis PD, Parham P. Evolution of class-I MHC genes and proteins: from natural selection to thymic selection. *Annu Rev Immunol* 1990;8:23–63.

83. Margulies D, Evans G, Flaherty L, Seidman J. H-2-like genes in the Tla region of mouse chromosome 17. *Nature* 1982;295:168–170.

84. Pease LR, Nathenson SG, Leinwand LA. Mapping class I gene sequences in the major histocompatibility complex. *Nature* 1982;298:382–385.

85. Steinmetz M, Minard K, Horvath S, et al. A molecular map of the immune response region from the major histocompatibility complex of the mouse. *Nature* 1982;300:35–42.

86. Shawar SM, Cook RG, Rodgers JR, Rich RR. Specialized functions of MHC class I molecules. I. An N-formyl peptide receptor is required for construction of the class I antigen Mta. *J Exp Med* 1990;171:897–912.

87. Kurlander R, Shawar S, Brown M, Rich R. Specialized role for a murine class I-b MHC molecule in prokaryotic host defenses. *Science* 1992;257:678–679.

88. Shawar SM, Vyas JM, Rodgers JR, Rich RR. Antigen presentation by major histocompatibility complex class I-B molecules. *Annu Rev Immunol* 1994;12:839–880.

89. Smith GP, Dabhi VM, Pamer EG, Lindahl KF. Peptide presentation by the MHC class Ib molecule, H2-M3. *Int Immunol* 1994;6:1917–1926.

90. Lindahl KF, Byers DE, Dabhi VM, et al. H-2M3, a full-service class IB histocompatibility antigen. *Annu Rev Immunol* 1997;15:851–879.

91. Parham P, Ohta T. Population biology of antigen presentation by MHC class I molecules [see comments]. *Science* 1996;272:67–74.

92. Figueroa F, Tichy H, McKenzie I, Hammerling U, Klein J. Polymorphism of lymphocyte antigens-encoding loci in wild mice. *Curr Top Microbiol Immunol* 1986;127:229–235.

93. Sultmann H, Mayer WE, Figueroa F, O'HUigin C, Klein J. Zebrafish Mhc class II alpha chain-encoding genes: polymorphism, expression, and function. *Immunogenetics* 1993;38:408–420.

94. Sato A, Klein D, Sultmann H, Figueroa F, O'HUigin C, Klein J. Class I mhc genes of cichlid fishes: identification, expression, and polymorphism. *Immunogenetics* 1997;46:63–72.

95. Hood L, Steinmetz M, Malissen B. Genes of the major histocompatibility complex of the mouse. *Annu Rev Immunol* 1983;1:529–568.

96. Williams AF. Immunoglobulin-related domains for cell surface recognition. *Nature* 1985;314:579–580.

97. Burnside SS, Hunt P, Ozato K, Sears DW. A molecular hybrid of the H-2D^d and H-2L^d genes expressed in the dm1 mutant. *Proc Natl Acad Sci USA* 1984;81:5204–5208.

98. Sun YH, Goodenow RS, Hood L. Molecular basis of the dm1 mutation in the major histocompatibility complex of the mouse: a D/L hybrid gene. *J Exp Med* 1985;162:1588–1602.

99. Evans G, Margulies D, Camerini-Otero R, Ozato K, Seidman J. Structure and expression of a mouse major histocompatibility antigen gene, H-2L^d. *Proc Natl Acad Sci USA* 1982;79:1994–1998.

100. Schulze DH, Pease LR, Geier SS, et al. Comparison of the cloned H-2Kbm1 variant gene with the H-2K^b gene shows a cluster of seven nucleotide differences. *Proc Natl Acad Sci USA* 1983;80:2007–2011.

101. Geliebter J, Zeff R, Schulze D, et al. Interaction between K^b and Q4 gene sequences generates the K^{bm6} mutation. *Mol Cell Biol* 1986;6:645–652.

102. Nathenson SG, Geliebter J, Pfaffenbach GM, Zeff RA. Murine major histocompatibility complex class-I mutants: molecular analysis and structure-function implications. *Annu Rev Immunol* 1986;4:471–502.

103. Hemmi S, Geliebter J, Zeff RA, Melvold RW, Nathenson SG. Three spontaneous H-2D^b mutants are generated by genetic micro-recombination (gene conversion) events. Impact on the H-2-restricted immune responsiveness. *J Exp Med* 1988;168:2319–2335.

104. Nathenson S, Kesari K, Sheil J, Ajitkumar P. Use of mutants to analyze regions on the H-2K^b molecule for interaction with immune receptors. *Cold Spring Harb Symp Quant Biol* 1989;54:Pt 1:521–528.

105. Hasenkrug K, Nathenson S. Nucleic acid sequences of the H-2K^s and H-2K^{sm1} genes. *Immunogenetics* 1991;34:60–61.

106. Zemmour J, Parham P. HLA class I nucleotide sequences, 1992. *Immunogenetics* 1993;37:239–250.

107. Witte T, Smolyar A, Spoerl R, et al. Major histocompatibility complex recognition by immune receptors: differences among T cell receptor versus antibody interactions with the VSV8/H-2Kb complex. *Eur J Immunol* 1997;27:227–233.

108. Yun TJ, Melvold RW, Pease LR. A complex major histocompatibility complex D locus variant generated by an unusual recombination mechanism in mice. *Proc Natl Acad Sci USA* 1997;94:1384–1389.

109. Silver LM. *Mouse genetics: concepts and applications.* New York: Oxford University Press, 1995:362.

110. Simpson EM, Linder CC, Sargent EE, Davisson MT, Mobraaten LE, Sharp JJ. Genetic variation among 129 substrains and its importance for targeted mutagenesis in mice. *Nat Genet* 1997;16:19–27.

111. Sechler JMG, Yip JC, Rosenberg AS. Cutting edge: genetic variation 129 substrains: practical consequences. *J Immunol* 1997;159:5766–5768.

112. Nepom G, Erlich H. MHC class-II molecules and autoimmunity. *Annu Rev Immunol* 1991;9:493–525.

113. Thomson G. HLA disease associations: models for the study of complex human genetic disorders. *Crit Rev Clin Lab Sci* 1995;32:183–219.

114. Wedell A. Molecular approaches for the diagnosis of 21-hydroxylase deficiency and congenital adrenal hyperplasia. *Clin Lab Med* 1996;16:125–137.

115. Tiwari JL, Terasaki PI. *HLA and disease associations.* New York: Springer-Verlag, 1985.

116. Baines M, Ebringer A. HLA and disease. *Mol Aspects Med* 1992;13:263–378.

117. Oldstone MB, McChesney MB, Oldstone MB. Virus-induced autoimmunity: molecular mimicry as a route to autoimmune disease. Virus-induced immunosuppression: infections with measles virus and human immunodeficiency virus. *J Autoimmun* 1989;2[Suppl]:187–194.

118. Wucherpfennig KW, Strominger JL. Molecular mimicry in T cell-mediated autoimmunity: viral peptides activate human T cell clones specific for myelin basic protein. *Cell* 1995;80:695–705.

119. Wucherpfennig KW, Yu B, Bhol K, et al. Structural basis for major histocompatibility complex (MHC)-linked susceptibility to autoimmunity: charged residues of a single MHC binding pocket confer selective presentation of self-peptides in pemphigus vulgaris. *Proc Natl Acad Sci USA* 1995;92:11935–11939.

120. Oldstone MB. Viruses and autoimmune diseases. *Scand J Immunol* 1997;46:320–325.

121. Mignot E, Tafti M, Dement WC, Grumet FC. Narcolepsy and immunity. *Adv Neuroimmunol* 1995;5:23–37.

122. Ellis MC, Hetisimer AH, Ruddy DA, et al. HLA class II haplotype and sequence analysis support a role for DQ in narcolepsy. *Immunogenetics* 1997;46:410–417.

123. Jouanolle AM, Fergelot P, Gandon G, Yaouanq J, Le Gall JY, David V. A candidate gene for hemochromatosis: frequency of the C282Y and H63D mutations. *Hum Genet* 1997;100:544–547.

124. Rothenberg BE, Voland JR. Beta2 knockout mice develop parenchymal iron overload: a putative role for class I genes of the major histocompatibility complex in iron metabolism. *Proc Natl Acad Sci USA* 1996;93:1529–1534.

125. Santos M, Schilham MW, Rademakers LH, Marx JJ, de Sousa M, Clevers H. Defective iron homeostasis in beta 2-microglobulin knockout mice recapitulates hereditary hemochromatosis in man. *J Exp Med* 1996;184:1975–1985.

126. Hattori M, Buse JB, Jackson RA, et al. The NOD mouse: recessive diabetogenic gene in the major histocompatibility complex. *Science* 1986;231:733–735.

127. Acha-Orbea H, McDevitt HO. The first external domain of the nonobese diabetic mouse class II I-A beta chain is unique. *Proc Natl Acad Sci USA* 1987;84:2435–2439.

128. Tochino Y. The NOD mouse as a model of type I diabetes. *Crit Rev Immunol* 1987;8:49–81.

129. Wicker LS, Miller BJ, Fischer PA, Pressey A, Peterson LB. Genetic control of diabetes and insulitis in the nonobese diabetic mouse. Pedigree analysis of a diabetic H-2nod/b heterozygote. *J Immunol* 1989;142:781–784.

130. Quartey-Papafio R, Lund T, Chandler P, et al. Aspartate at position 57 of nonobese diabetic I-A^{g7} beta-chain diminishes the spontaneous incidence of insulin-dependent diabetes mellitus. *J Immunol* 1995;154:5567–5575.

131. Tisch R, McDevitt H. Insulin-dependent diabetes mellitus. *Cell* 1996;85:291–297.

132. Kohn HI, Melvold RW. Spontaneous histocompatibility mutations detected by dermal grafts: significant changes in rate over a 10-year period in the mouse H-system. *Mutat Res* 1974;24:163–169.

133. Melvold RW, Kohn HI. Histocompatibility gene mutation rates: H-2 and non-H-2. *Mutat Res* 1975;27:415–418.

134. Melvold R, Wang K, Kohn H. Histocompatibility gene mutation rates in the mouse: a 25-year review. *Immunogenetics* 1997;47:44–54.

135. Ewenstein BM, Uehara H, Nisizawa T, Melvold RW, Kohn HI, Nathenson SG. Biochemical studies on the H-2K antigens of the MHC mutants bm3 and bm11. *Immunogenetics* 1980;11:383–395.

136. Pease LR, Ewenstein BM, McGovern D, Melvold RW, Nisizawa T, Nathenson SG. Biochemical studies on the H-2K mutant B6.C-H-2^{bm10}. *Immunogenetics* 1983;17:7–17.

137. Yamaga KM, Pfaffenbach GM, Pease LR, et al. Biochemical studies of H-2K antigens from a group of related mutants. I. Identification of a shared mutation in B6-H-2^{bm5} and B6-H-2^{bm16}. *Immunogenetics* 1983;17:19–29.

138. Yamaga KM, Pfaffenbach GM, Pease LR, et al. Biochemical studies of H-2K antigens from a group of related mutants. II. Identification of a shared mutation in B6-H-2^{bm6}, B6.C-H-2^{bm7}, and B6.C-H-2^{bm9}. *Immunogenetics* 1983;17:31–41.

139. Zijlstra M, Li E, Sajjadi F, Subramani S, Jaenisch R. Germ-line transmission of a disrupted beta 2-microglobulin gene produced by homologous recombination in embryonic stem cells. *Nature* 1989;342:435–438.

140. Koller BH, Marrack P, Kappler JW, Smithies O. Normal development of mice deficient in beta 2M, MHC class I proteins, and CD8+ T cells. *Science* 1990;248:1227–1230.

141. Zijlstra M, Bix M, Simister NE, Loring JM, Raulet DH, Jaenisch R. Beta 2-microglobulin deficient mice lack CD4-8+ cytolytic T cells. *Nature* 1990;344:742–746.

142. Boehm U, Klamp T, Groot M, Howard JC. Cellular responses to interferon-gamma. *Annu Rev Immunol* 1997;15:749–795.

143. Houlihan JM, Biro PA, Harper HM, Jenkinson HJ, Holmes CH. The human amnion is a site of MHC class Ib expression: evidence for the expression of HLA-E and HLA-G. *J Immunol* 1995;154:5665–5674.

144. McMaster MT, Librach CL, Zhou Y, et al. Human placental HLA-G expression is restricted to differentiated cytotrophoblasts. *J Immunol* 1995;154:3771–3778.

145. Le Bouteiller P, Rodriguez AM, Mallet V, Girr M, Guillaudeux T, Lenfant F. Placental expression of HLA class I genes. *Am J Reprod Immunol* 1996;35:216–225.

146. Wiertz EJHJ, Mukherjee S, Ploegh HL. Viruses use stealth technology to escape from the host immune system. *Mol Med Today* 1997;3:116–123.

147. Fruh K, Ahn K, Djaballah H, et al. A viral inhibitor of peptide transporters for antigen presentation. *Nature* 1995;375:415–418.

148. Hill A, Jugovic P, York I, et al. Herpes simplex virus turns off the TAP to evade host immunity *Nature* 1995;375:411–415.

149. Ahn K, Meyer TH, Uebel S, et al. Molecular mechanism and species specificity of TAP inhibition by herpes simplex virus ICP47. *Embo J* 1996;15:3247–3255.

150. Koszinowski UH, Reddehase MJ, Del Val M. Principles of cytomegalovirus antigen presentation in vitro and in vivo. *Semin Immunol* 1992;4:71–79.

151. Burgert HG, Kvist S. The E3/19K protein of adenovirus type 2 binds to the domains of histocompatibility antigens required for CTL recognition. *Embo J* 1987;6:2019–2026.

152. Glimcher LH, Kara CJ. Sequences and factors: a guide to MHC class-II transcription. *Annu Rev Immunol* 1992;10:13–49.

153. Rijkers GT, Roord JJ, Koning F, Kuis W, Zegers BJ. Phenotypical and functional analysis of B lymphocytes of two siblings with combined immunodeficiency and defective expression of major histocompatibility complex (MHC) class II antigens on mononuclear cells. *J Clin Immunol* 1987;7:98–106.

154. Ploeger-Marshall S, Haas A, Clement LT, et al. Interferon-induced expression of class II major histocompatibility antigens in the major histocompatibility complex (MHC) class II deficiency syndrome. *J Clin Immunol* 1988;8:285–295.

155. Hume CR, Lee JS. Congenital immunodeficiencies associated with absence of HLA class II antigens on lymphocytes result from distinct mutations in trans-acting factors. *Hum Immunol* 1989;26:288–309.

156. Mach B, MHC class II regulation—lessons from a disease. *N Engl J Med* 1995;332:120–122.

157. Guardiola J, Maffei A, Lauster R, Mitchison NA, Accolla RS, Sartoris S. Functional significance of polymorphism among MHC class II gene promoters. *Tissue Antigens* 1996;48:615–625.

158. Roche PA, Cresswell P. Invariant chain association with HLA-DR molecules inhibits immunogenic peptide binding. *Nature* 1990;345:615–618.

159. Roche PA, Marks MS, Cresswell P. Formation of a nine-subunit complex by HLA class II glycoproteins and the invariant chain. *Nature* 1991;354:392–394.

160. Bikoff EK, Huang LY, Episkopou V, van Meerwijk J, Germain RN, Robertson EJ. Defective major histocompatibility complex class II assembly, transport, peptide acquisition, and CD4+ T cell selection in mice lacking invariant chain expression. *J Exp Med* 1993;177:1699–1712.

161. Viville S, Neefjes J, Lotteau V, et al. Mice lacking the MHC class II-associated invariant chain. *Cell* 1993;72:635–648.

162. Bonnerot C, Marks MS, Cosson P, et al. Association with BiP and aggregation of class II MHC molecules synthesized in the absence of invariant chain. *Embo J* 1994;13:934–944.

163. Orr HT, Lopez de Castro JA, Parham P, Ploegh HL, Strominger JL. Comparison of amino acid sequences of two human histocompatibility antigens, HLA-A2 and HLA-B7: location of putative alloantigenic sites. *Proc Natl Acad Sci USA* 1979;76:4395–4399.

164. Coligan JE, Kindt TJ, Uehara H, Martinko J, Nathenson SG. Primary structure of a murine transplantation antigen. *Nature* 1981;291:35–39.

165. Ploegh HL, Orr HT, Strominger JL. Molecular cloning of a human histocompatibility antigen cDNA fragment. *Proc Natl Acad Sci USA* 1980;77:6081–6085.

166. Sood AK, Pereira D, Weissman SM. Isolation and partial nucleotide sequence of a cDNA clone for human histocompatibility antigen HLA-B by use of an oligodeoxynucleotide primer. *Proc Natl Acad Sci USA* 1981;78:616–620.

167. Steinmetz M, Frelinger JG, Fisher D, et al. Three cDNA clones encoding mouse transplantation antigens: homology to immunoglobulin genes. *Cell* 1981;24:125–134.

168. Choi E, McIntyre K, Germain RN, Seidman JG. Murine I-A beta chain polymorphism: nucleotide sequences of three allelic I-A beta genes. *Science* 1983;221:283–286.

169. Hood L, Steinmetz M, Goodenow R, et al. Genes of the major histocompatibility complex. *Cold Spring Harb Symp Quant Biol* 1983;47:Pt 2:1051–1065.

170. Mathis DJ, Benoist CO, Williams VEd, Kanter MR, McDevitt HO. The murine E alpha immune response gene. *Cell* 1983;32:745–754.

171. Robinson RR, Germain RN, McKean DJ, Mescher M, Seidman JG. Extensive polymorphism surrounding the murine Ia A beta chain gene. *J Immunol* 1983;131:2025–2031.

172. Robinson PJ, Steinmetz M, Moriwaki K, Lindahl KF. Beta-2 microglobulin types in mice of wild origin. *Immunogenetics* 1984;20:655–665.

173. Lew AM, Margulies DH, Maloy WL, Lillehoj EP, McCluskey J, Coligan JE. Alternative protein products with different carboxyl termini from a single class I gene, H-2^{Kb}. *Proc Natl Acad Sci USA* 1986;83:6084–6088.

174. Lew AM, McCluskey J, Maloy WL, Margulies DH, Coligan JE. Multiple class I molecules generated from single genes by alternative splicing of pre-mRNAs. *Immunol Res* 1987;6:117–132.

175. Handy DE, McCluskey J, Lew AM, Coligan JE, Margulies DH. Signals controlling alternative splicing of major histocompatibility complex H-2 class I pre-mRNA. *Immunogenetics* 1988;28:81–90.

176. Vega MA, Strominger JL. Constitutive endocytosis of HLA class I antigens requires a specific portion of the intracytoplasmic tail that shares structural features with other endocytosed molecules. *Proc Natl Acad Sci USA* 1989;86:2688–2692.

177. St-Pierre Y, Nabavi N, Ghogawala Z, Glimcher LH, Watts TH. A functional role for signal transduction via the cytoplasmic domains of MHC class II proteins. *J Immunol* 1989;143:808–812.

178. Evans G, Margulies D, Shykind B, Seidman J, Ozato K. Exon shuffling: mapping polymorphic determinants on hybrid mouse transplantation antigens. *Nature* 1982;300:755–757.

179. Bluestone JA, Foo M, Allen H, Segal D, Flavell RA. Allospecific cytolytic T lymphocytes recognize conformational determinants on hybrid mouse transplantation antigens. *J Exp Med* 1985;162:268–281.

180. Ozato K, Evans G, Margulies D, Seidman J, Levy R. The use of hybrid H-2 genes for localizing the positions of polymorphic determinants recognized by antibodies and by cytotoxic T cells. *Transplant Proc* 1983;15:2079–2076.

181. Reiss C, Evans G, Margulies D, Seidman J, Burakoff S. Allospecific and virus-specific cytolytic T lymphocytes are restricted to the N or C1 domain of H-2 antigens expressed on L cells after DNA-mediated gene transfer. *Proc Natl Acad Sci USA* 1983;80:2709–2712.

182. Bjorkman PJ, Strominger JL, Wiley DC. Crystallization and x-ray diffraction studies on the histocompatibility antigens HLA-A2 and HLA-A28 from human cell membranes. *J Mol Biol* 1985;186:205–210.

183. Bjorkman PJ, Saper MA, Samraoui B, Bennett WS, Strominger JL, Wiley DC. Structure of the human class I histocompatibility antigen, HLA-A2. *Nature* 1987;329:506–512.

184. Schwartz RH. Immune response (Ir) genes of the murine major histocompatibility complex. *Adv Immunol* 1986;38:31–201.

185. Babbitt B, Allen P, Matsueda G, Haber E, Unanue E. Binding of immunogenic peptides to Ia histocompatibility molecules. *Nature* 1985;317:359–361.

186. Buus S, Sette A, Colon S, Jenis D, Grey H. Isolation and characterization of antigen-Ia complexes involved in T cell recognition. *Cell* 1986;47:1071–1077.

187. Townsend A, Ohlén C, Bastin J, Ljunggren H, Foster L, Kärre K. Association of class I major histocompatibility heavy and light chains induced by viral peptides. *Nature* 1989;340:443–448.

188. Townsend A, Elliott T, Cerundolo V, Foster L, Barber B, Tse A. Assembly of MHC class I molecules analyzed in vitro [published erratum appears in *Cell* 1990;62(6):following 1233]. *Cell* 1990;62:285–295.

189. Boyd LF, Kozlowski S, Margulies DH. Solution binding of an antigenic peptide to a major histocompatibility complex class I molecule and the role of beta 2-microglobulin. *Proc Natl Acad Sci USA* 1992;89:2242–2246.

190. Van Bleek GM, Nathenson SG. Isolation of an endogenously processed immunodominant viral peptide from the class I H-2Kb molecule. *Nature* 1990;348:213–216.

191. Falk K, Rötzschke O, Rammensee H. Cellular peptide composition governed by major histocompatibility complex class I molecules. *Nature* 1990;348:248–251.

192. Rötzschke O, Falk K, Deres K, et al. Isolation and analysis of naturally processed viral peptides as recognized by cytotoxic T cells. *Nature* 1990;348:252–254.

193. Rammensee HG, Falk K, Rotzschke O. Peptides naturally presented by MHC class I molecules. *Annu Rev Immunol* 1993;11:213–244.

194. Hunt D, Henderson R, Shabanowitz J, et al. Characterization of peptides bound

to the class I MHC molecule HLA-A2.1 by mass spectrometry. *Science* 1992; 255:1261–1263.

195. Corr M, Boyd LF, Frankel SR, Kozlowski S, Padlan EA, Margulies DH. Endogenous peptides of a soluble major histocompatibility complex class I molecule, H-2L$_d$s: sequence motif, quantitative binding, and molecular modeling of the complex. *J Exp Med* 1992;176:1681–1692.

196. Corr M, Boyd LF, Padlan EA, Margulies DH. H-2D^d exploits a four residue peptide binding motif. *J Exp Med* 1993;178:1877–1892.

197. Gavin MA, Dere B, Grandea AGr, Hogquist KA, Bevan MJ. Major histocompatibility complex class I allele-specific peptide libraries: identification of peptides that mimic an H-Y T cell epitope. *Eur J Immunol* 1994;24:2124–2133.

198. Brusic V, Rudy G, Kyne AP, Harrison LC. MHCPEP, a database of MHC-binding peptides: update 1996. *Nucleic Acids Res* 1997;25:269–271.

199. De Groot AS, Jesdale BM, Szu E, Schafer JR, Chicz RM, Deocampo G. An interactive Web site providing major histocompatibility ligand predictions: application to HIV research. *AIDS Res Hum Retroviruses* 1997;13:529–531.

200. Parker KC, Bednarek MA, Coligan JE. Scheme for ranking potential HLA-A2 binding peptides based on independent binding of individual peptide side-chains. *J Immunol* 1994;152:163–175.

201. Rudensky A, Preston-Hurlburt P, Hong S, Barlow A, Janeway CJ. Sequence analysis of peptides bound to MHC class II molecules. *Nature* 1991;353:622–627.

202. Chicz R, Urban R, Lane W, et al. Predominant naturally processed peptides bound to HLA-DR1 are derived from MHC-related molecules and are heterogeneous in size. *Nature* 1992;358:764–768.

203. Janeway CA Jr, Mamula MJ, Rudensky A. Rules for peptide presentation by MHC class II molecules. *Int Rev Immunol* 1993;10:301–311.

204. Urban RG, Chicz RM, Vignali DA, Strominger JL. The dichotomy of peptide presentation by class I and class II MHC proteins. *Chem Immunol* 1993;57: 197–234.

205. Hammer J, Takacs B, Sinigaglia F. Identification of a motif for HLA-DR1 binding peptides using M13 display libraries. *J Exp Med* 1992;176:1007–1013.

206. Bjorkman PJ, Saper MA, Samraoui B, Bennett WS, Strominger JL, Wiley DC. The foreign antigen binding site and T cell recognition regions of class I histocompatibility antigens. *Nature* 1987;329:512–518.

207. Garrett TP, Saper MA, Bjorkman PJ, Strominger JL, Wiley DC. Specificity pockets for the side chains of peptide antigens in HLA-Aw68. *Nature* 1989;342:692–696.

208. Saper MA, Bjorkman PJ, Wiley DC. Refined structure of the human histocompatibility antigen HLA-A2 at 2.6 Å resolution. *J Mol Biol* 1991;219: 277–319.

209. Madden D, Gorga J, Strominger J, Wiley D. The structure of HLA-B27 reveals nonamer self-peptides bound in an extended conformation. *Nature* 1991;353: 321–325.

210. Jardetzky TS, Lane WS, Robinson RA, Madden DR, Wiley DC. Identification of self peptides bound to purified HLA-B27. *Nature* 1991;353:326–329.

211. Zhang W, Young AC, Imarai M, Nathenson SG, Sacchettini JC. Crystal structure of the major histocompatibility complex class I H-2K^b molecule containing a single viral peptide: implications for peptide binding and T-cell receptor recognition. *Proc Natl Acad Sci USA* 1992;89:8403–8407.

212. Fremont D, Matsumura M, Stura E, Peterson P, Wilson I. Crystal structures of two viral peptides in complex with murine MHC class I H-2K^b. *Science* 1992; 257:919–927.

213. Zhang W, Young AC, Imarai M, Nathenson SG, Sacchettini JC. Crystal structure of the major histocompatibility complex class I H-2K^b molecule containing a single viral peptide: implications for peptide binding and T-cell receptor recognition. *Proc Natl Acad Sci USA* 1992;89:8403–8407.

214. Fremont DH, Stura EA, Matsumura M, Peterson PA, Wilson IA. Crystal structure of an H-2Kb-ovalbumin peptide complex reveals the interplay of primary and secondary anchor positions in the major histocompatibility complex binding groove. *Proc Natl Acad Sci USA* 1995;92:2479–2483.

215. Joyce S, Kuzushima K, Kepecs G, Angeletti RH, Nathenson SG. Characterization of an incompletely assembled major histocompatibility class I molecule (H-2K^b) associated with unusually long peptides: implications for antigen processing and presentation. *Proc Natl Acad Sci USA* 1994;91:4145–4149.

216. Collins EJ, Garboczi DN, Wiley DC. Three-dimensional structure of a peptide extending from one end of a class I MHC binding site. *Nature* 1994;371: 626–629.

217. Brown JH, Jardetzky T, Saper MA, Samraoui B, Bjorkman PJ, Wiley DC. A hypothetical model of the foreign antigen binding site of class II histocompatibility molecules. *Nature* 1988;332:845–850.

218. Brown JH, Jardetzky TS, Gorga JC, et al. Three-dimensional structure of the human class II histocompatibility antigen HLA-DR1. *Nature* 1993;364:33–39.

219. Stern LJ, Brown JH, Jardetzky TS, et al. Crystal structure of the human class II MHC protein HLA-DR1 complexed with an influenza virus peptide. *Nature* 1994;368:215–221.

220. Jardetzky TS, Brown JH, Gorga JC, et al. Three-dimensional structure of a human class II histocompatibility molecule complexed with superantigen. *Nature* 1994;368:711–718.

221. Fields BA, Ober B, Malchiodi EL, et al. Crystal structure of the V alpha domain of a T cell antigen receptor. *Science* 1995;270:1821–1824.

222. Schafer PH, Pierce SK. Evidence for dimers of MHC class II molecules in B lymphocytes and their role in low affinity T cell responses. *Immunity* 1994;1: 699–707.

223. Abastado JP, Lone YC, Casrouge A, Boulot G, Kourilsky P. Dimerization of soluble major histocompatibility complex-peptide complexes is sufficient for activation of T cell hybridoma and induction of unresponsiveness. *J Exp Med* 1995;182:439–447.

224. Reich Z, Boniface JJ, Lyons DS, Borochov N, Wachtel EJ, Davis MM. Ligand-specific oligomerization of T-cell receptor molecules. *Nature* 1997;387: 617–620.

225. Fremont DH, Hendrickson WA, Marrack P, Kappler J. Structures of an MHC class II molecule with covalently bound single peptides. *Science* 1996;272: 1001–1004.

226. Plaksin D, Chacko S, McPhie P, Bax A, Padlan EA, Margulies DH. A T cell receptor V alpha domain expressed in bacteria: does it dimerize in solution? *J Exp Med* 1996;184:1251–1258.

227. Garboczi DN, Ghosh P, Utz U, Fan QR, Biddison WE, Wiley DC. Structure of the complex between human T-cell receptor, viral peptide and HLA-A2. *Nature* 1996;384:134–141.

228. Garcia KC, Degano M, Stanfield RL, et al. An alphabeta T cell receptor structure at 2.5 A and its orientation in the TCR-MHC complex. *Science* 1996;274:209–219.

229. Porcelli SA. The CD1 family: a third lineage of antigen-presenting molecules. *Adv Immunol* 1995;59:1–98.

230. Loveland B, Wang CR, Yonekawa H, Hermel E, Lindahl KF. Maternally transmitted histocompatibility antigen of mice: a hydrophobic peptide of a mitochondrially encoded protein. *Cell* 1990;60:971–980.

231. Wang CR, Castano AR, Peterson PA, Slaughter C, Lindahl KF, Deisenhofer J. Nonclassical binding of formylated peptide in crystal structure of the MHC class Ib molecule H2-M3. *Cell* 1995;82:655–664.

232. Beckman EM, Porcelli SA, Morita CT, Behar SM, Furlong ST, Brenner MB. Recognition of a lipid antigen by CD1-restricted alpha beta+ T cells. *Nature* 1994;372:691–694.

233. Melian A, Beckman EM, Porcelli SA, Brenner MB. Antigen presentation by CD1 and MHC-encoded class I-like molecules. *Curr Opin Immunol* 1996;8:82–88.

234. Bendelac A, Lantz O, Quimby ME, Yewdell JW, Bennink JR, Brutkiewicz RR. CD1 recognition by mouse NK1+ T lymphocytes. *Science* 1995;268:863–865.

235. Zeng Z-H, Castaño AR, Segelke B, Stura EA, Peterson PA, Wilson IA. The crystal structure of murine CD1: an MHC-like fold but with a large hydrophobic antigen binding groove. *Science* 1997;277:339–345.

236. Young AC, Zhang W, Sacchettini JC, Nathenson SG. The three-dimensional structure of H-2Db at 2.4 Å resolution: implications for antigen-determinant selection. *Cell* 1994;76:39–50.

237. Simister NE, Rees AR. Isolation and characterization of an Fc receptor from neonatal rat small intestine. *Eur J Immunol* 1985;15:733–738.

238. Simister NE, Mostov KE. Cloning and expression of the neonatal rat intestinal Fc receptor, a major histocompatibility complex class I antigen homolog. *Cold Spring Harb Symp Quant Biol* 1989;54 Pt:1:571–580.

239. Ahouse JJ, Hagerman CL, Mittal P, et al. Mouse MHC class I-like Fc receptor encoded outside the MHC. *J Immunol* 1993;151:6076–6088.

240. Simister NE. IgG Fc receptors that resemble class I major histocompatibility complex antigens. *Biochem Soc Trans* 1993;21:973–976.

241. Story CM, Mikulska JE, Simister NE. A major histocompatibility complex class I-like Fc receptor cloned from human placenta: possible role in transfer of immunoglobulin G from mother to fetus. *J Exp Med* 1994;180:2377–2381.

242. Burmeister WP, Gastinel LN, Simister NE, Blum ML, Bjorkman PJ. Crystal structure at 2.2 Å resolution of the MHC-related neonatal Fc receptor. *Nature* 1994;372:336–343.

243. Burmeister WP, Huber AH, Bjorkman PJ. Crystal structure of the complex of rat neonatal Fc receptor with Fc. *Nature* 1994;372:379–383.

244. Israel EJ, Wilsker DF, Hayes KC, Schoenfeld D, Simister NE. Increased clearance of IgG in mice that lack beta 2-microglobulin: possible protective role of FcRn. *Immunology* 1996;89:573–578.

245. Zamoyska R. The CD8 coreceptor revisited: one chain good, two chains better. *Immunity* 1994;1:243–246.

246. Gao GF, Tormo J, Gerth UC, et al. Crystal structure of the complex between human CD8αα and HLA-A2. *Nature* 1997;387:630–634.

247. Sun J, Leahy DJ, Kavathas PB. Interaction between CD8 and major histocompatibility complex (MHC) class I mediated by multiple contact surfaces that include the alpha 2 and alpha 3 domains of MHC class I. *J Exp Med* 1995;182:1275–1280.

248. Weiss A, Littman DR. Signal transduction by lymphocyte antigen receptors. *Cell* 1994;76:263–274.

249. Wu H, Kwong PD, Hendrickson WA. Dimeric association and segmental variability in the structure of human CD4. *Nature* 1997;387:527–530.

250. Herman A, Kappler JW, Marrack P, Pullen AM. Superantigens: mechanism of T-cell stimulation and role in immune responses. *Annu Rev Immunol* 1991;9: 745–772.

251. Kim J, Urban RG, Strominger JL, Wiley DC. Toxic shock syndrome toxin-1 complexed with a class II major histocompatibility molecule HLA-DR1. *Science* 1994;266:1870–1874.

252. Fields BA, Malchiodi EL, Li H, et al. Crystal structure of a T-cell receptor beta chain complexed with a superantigen. *Nature* 1996;384:188–192.

253. Fremont DH, Rees WA, Kozono H. Biophysical studies of T-cell receptors and their ligands. *Curr Opin Immunol* 1996;8:93–100.

254. Matsui K, Boniface JJ, Reay PA, Schild H, Fazekas de St. Groth B, Davis MM. Low affinity interaction of peptide-MHC complexes with T cell receptors. *Science* 1991;254:1788–1791.

255. Corr M, Slanetz AE, Boyd LF, et al. T cell receptor-MHC class I peptide interactions: affinity, kinetics, and specificity. *Science* 1994;265:946–949.

256. Matsui K, Boniface JJ, Steffner P, Reay PA, Davis MM. Kinetics of T-cell receptor binding to peptide/I-Ek complexes: correlation of the dissociation rate with T-cell responsiveness. *Proc Natl Acad Sci USA* 1994;91:12862–12866.

257. Khilko SN, Jelonek MT, Corr M, Boyd LF, Bothwell AL, Margulies DH. Measuring interactions of MHC class I molecules using surface plasmon resonance. *J Immunol Methods* 1995;183:77–94.

258. Sykulev Y, Cohen RJ, Eisen HN. The law of mass action governs antigen-stimulated cytolytic activity of CD8+ cytotoxic T lymphocytes. *Proc Natl Acad Sci USA* 1995;92:11990–11992.

259. Alam SM, Travers PJ, Wung JL, et al. T cell receptor affinity and thymocyte positive selection. *Nature* 1996;381:616–620.

260. Garcia KC, Tallquist MD, Pease LR, et al. Alphabeta T cell receptor interactions with syngeneic and allogeneic ligands: affinity measurements and crystallization. *Proc Natl Acad Sci USA* 1997;94:13838–13843.

261. Plaksin D, Polakova K, McPhie P, Margulies DH. A three-domain T cell receptor is biologically active and specifically stains cell surface MHC/peptide complexes. *J Immunol* 1997;158:2218–2227.

262. McCluskey J. *The human leucocyte antigens and clinical medicine.* Oxford: Oxford University Press, 1997:415–427.

263. Margulies D, McCluskey J. Exon shuffling: new genes from old. *Surv Immunol Res* 1985;4:146–159.

264. Evans SV. SETOR: hardware lighted three-dimensional solid model representations of macromolecules. *J Mol Graphics* 1993;11:134–138.

265. Saper MA, Bjorkman PJ, Wiley DC. Refined structure of the human histocompatibility antigen HLA-A2 at 2.6 Å resolution. *J Mol Biol* 1991;219:277–319.

266. Nicholls A, Sharp KA, Honig B. Protein folding and association: insights from the interfacial and thermodynamic properties of hydrocarbons. *Proteins* 1991;11:281–296.

267. Ravetch JV, Margulies DH. Immunology. New tricks for old molecules. *Nature* 1994;372:323–324.

268. Fields BA, Malchiodi EL, Li H, et al. Crystal structure of a T-cell receptor beta-chain complexed with a superantigen. *Nature* 1996;384:188–192.

269. Kruisbeck, AM Commonly used mouse strains. In: Coligan JE, Kruisbeek AM, Margulies DH, Shevach EM, Strober W, eds. *Current protocols in immunology.* New York: John Wiley and Sons, 1998 (*in press*).

270. Mathis DJ, Benoist C, Williams VED, Kanter M, McDevitt HO. Several mechanisms can account for defective E alpha gene expression in different mouse haplotypes. *Proc Natl Acad Sci USA* 1983;80:273–277.

271. Parker KC, Martin R. *Appendix 11. Peptide binding motifs for MHC class I and II molecules.* New York: John Wiley and Sons, 1997.

Fundamental Immunology, Fourth Edition,
edited by William E. Paul
Published by Lippincott–Raven Publishers, Philadelphia 1999.

CHAPTER 9

Antigen Processing and Presentation

Ronald N. Germain

Antigen Recognition and Immune Responses
Nonclonal Host Defense Mechanisms · Clonal Host Defense Mechanisms · Distinctive Characteristics of Antigens Stimulating B- and T-Lymphocyte Responses · Recognition of Peptide–MHC Molecule Complexes by T Lymphocytes · Why Peptides?

Historical Development of the Peptide Presentation Paradigm
Early Models for the Role of MHC Molecules in T-Cell Immunity · Early Evidence for a Single T-Cell Receptor Complex Mediating Recognition of Physically Associated Antigen–MHC Molecule Combinations · Direct Evidence for a Single T-Cell Receptor Mediating Recognition of Physical Complexes of Peptide Antigen and MHC-Encoded Molecules · Specialization of Class I and Class II MHC Molecules for Presentation of Peptides from Different Intracellular Compartments

Genetic Organization and Protein Structure of Ligand-Binding Molecules Involved in Antigen Presentation
Organization of the MHC · MHC Class I and Class II Genes and Proteins

Identification and Characteristics of Peptides Naturally Associated with Class I and Class II Molecules
Peptides Bound by Class I Molecules · Peptides Associated with Class II Molecules

Peptides as Integral Parts of MHC Class I and Class II Molecular Structure
Changes in Structure and Assembly State Accompanying Peptide Binding by Class I Molecules · Relationships Between Peptide Binding and MHC Class II Molecule Biochemical Behavior · Kinetic Aspects of MHC Molecule Interaction with Peptides

Biosynthesis and Intracellular Transport of MHC Class I and Class II Molecules
The Basic Pattern of Class I Biosynthesis · Overview of Class II Biosynthesis and Transport to the Plasma Membrane · The Intracellular Transport and Localization of Invariant Chain and MHC Class II Molecules

Sites of Peptide Generation and Association with MHC Molecules
Class I · Class II

Summary of the Conventional MHC Class I and Class II Antigen-Presentation Pathways
New Techniques for Studying Antigen Processing and Presentation
Biologic Consequences of the Peptide–MHC Molecule Focus of T-Cell Recognition
Effects of Biological Variation in Protein Structure on Immune Recognition and Response · Consequences of the Differences in Location of Peptides Effective In Loading Class I Versus Class II Molecules for Immune Defense and Vaccine Strategies · Pathogen Interference with Antigen Presentation · MHC Molecules, Peptides, and Selection and Maintenance of the T-Cell Repertoire

Conclusion
References

ANTIGEN RECOGNITION AND IMMUNE RESPONSES

Nonclonal Host Defense Mechanisms

Host resistance to invasion, colonization, tissue damage, and disease caused by microorganisms and parasites is mediated by a variety of distinct mechanisms (1). In multicellular organisms, the first line of host resistance involves physical barriers to pathogen invasion. The second line involves responses to characteristic features of invading organisms that distinguishes them as a group from the "self" characteristics of the host. Examples of

these differences are the formyl-methionine of the NH_2 terminus of prokaryotic proteins that can activate neutrophils via the F-met-leu-phe receptor, the repeating polysaccharides in the cell walls of yeast and certain bacteria that activate the alternative pathway of complement, and the double-stranded RNA genomes of viruses that induce interferon (IFN)-α and -β responses. Although initiation of this category of responses is specific for certain chemical structures, the recognition systems involved do not discriminate among different pathogens whose components include a suitable constituent, all effector cells of a given histologic type share identical receptors, and the humoral factors use monomorphic binding sites. In addition, these generic defense modalities usually do not show a permanent change once the initiator material is removed from the system; that is, there is no selective memory of the interaction.

R.N. Germain. Laboratory of Immunology, National Institute of Allergy and Infectious Diseases, National Institutes of Health, Bethesda, Maryland 20892

Clonal Host Defense Mechanisms

A distinct category of defense mechanisms is associated with the concept of specific resistance to infection and especially of adaptive immunity, which is the quantitatively and/or qualitatively greater response of an organism upon repeated exposure to the same antigen. Reactions of this type are dependent on the function of two classes of lymphocytes: the T and B cells. They involve the selective activation of a small number of lymphocytes from among a large cohort of histologically similar cells, based on specific recognition events mediated by clonally distributed cell surface receptors created by somatic gene rearrangements. It is the increase in number of such clonally activated lymphocytes, their permanent differentiation into cells with an altered responsiveness to receptor reengagement, and the prolonged presence of secreted antibodies that account for the heightened response to previously encountered antigens or the specific pathogen resistance characteristic of adaptive immunity. Thus, a central issue in immunology is understanding the molecular basis of clonal antigen recognition by B and T lymphocytes.

Distinctive Characteristics of Antigens Stimulating B- and T-Lymphocyte Responses

The responses of B lymphocytes to a broad array of chemical substances was readily understood after the identification of cell surface immunoglobulin as the B-cell antigen receptor (see Chapters 6 and 7). The well-established ability of the secreted form of such receptors (antibodies) to interact with an almost limitless array of antigen structures made it simple to see how the B cells giving rise to such antibodies could also show the appropriate broad reactivity through the use of these surface analogs of the immunoglobulin effector molecule.

When the small lymphocyte pool was recognized to consist of both B- and T-lineage cells, the nature of T-cell antigen recognition became an issue of major importance. Studies by Gell and Benacerraf dating back to the 1950s showed that denatured proteins were usually poorly reactive with antibodies elicited against the conformationally native molecule, but secondary T-cell responses giving rise to delayed-type hypersensitivity were unaffected by the same denaturation of the antigen (2). These data suggested that lymphocytes involved in delayed-type hypersensitivity responses (later found to be T cells) might not recognize native conformational determinants, as was typical of antibodies. It also was found that T-lymphocyte effector responses could not generally be evoked by numerous substances to which antibodies could be developed, for example, various polysaccharides. Only proteins or derivatized proteins seemed effective. Attempts to demonstrate direct antigen binding to T lymphocytes were largely unsuccessful, in contrast to similar studies with B cells (3), and antiimmunoglobulin reagents did not reliably react with T cells. Based on these observations, it was concluded that the immunoglobulin genes involved in producing the B-cell receptor were not used by T cells to generate their clonally distributed antigen recognition structures and that T cells recognized a form of antigen distinct from that seen by B cells.

Other differences in antigen responsiveness of B and T cells became apparent in the early 1970s. T cells required the association of antigen with other cell types in order to became activated, again consistent with the failure to demonstrate direct binding of soluble antigen. T cell–dependent responses also were found to be under the control of genes encoded in the major histocompatibility complex (MHC; see Chapter 11). Polymorphism at MHC loci controlled the ability of an animal to mount a measurable T cell–dependent immune response to certain antigens, such as synthetic polypeptides with a simple repeating structure or to proteins from a closely related species that differed by only a few residues from the animal's own equivalent molecules. This phenomenon was termed "*immune response* (IR) gene control of responsiveness" (4). This critical contribution of MHC polymorphism to antigen-specific T-cell function was noted during examination of proliferative responses to antigen (5), tests of cytotoxic killing activity (6,7), and collaboration with B lymphocytes for antibody production (8) (see Chapters 6 and 7).

Recognition of Peptide–MHC Molecule Complexes by T Lymphocytes

An explanation for all these unique aspects of T-cell antigen recognition can now be found in the concept that the ligand for the αβ immunoglobulinlike receptor of most CD4+ and CD8+ T cells (see Chapter 10) consists of a complex formed by association of a short peptide with a cell surface glycoprotein product of the polymorphic class I or class II loci of the MHC (see Chapter 8) (9). This explains the focus of T cells on protein antigens, their lack of a requirement for preserved native conformation, the need for physical interaction with another cell whose membrane contains the MHC molecule–peptide complexes, and the allele specificity of antigen responses. Allelic differences in binding of specific peptides derived from proteins differing in a limited way from self, together with tolerance to self peptides (see Chapters 11 and 20), account for IR gene regulation.

Peptide complexes with MHC class I or class II constitute the effective T-cell stimulus in a variety of situations. This includes responses within a species to the major transplantation antigens themselves (the phenomenon from which the MHC acquired its name), minor histocompatibility antigens [for some of which the relevant specific peptide is now known, e.g., H-Y (10)], microbial pathogens (fungi, bacteria, viruses, protozoa, multicellular parasites), contact sensitizing agents, allergens, and tumors.

Why Peptides?

If a pathogen manages to penetrate the physical barriers of the host and evade the clonally unspecific cellular and humoral innate defenses, there are clearly two distinct potential sites of subsequent lymphocyte-dependent effector activity. One involves the extracellular form of the organism or its products, the other the intracellular stage of the organism's life cycle, if such exists. In either case, for agents like viruses and bacteria, the ability of many pathogens to replicate at rates far in excess of possible clonal expansion of the relevant lymphoid population necessitates a host defense strategy that minimizes such pathogen numerical advantage (11). B lymphocytes have developed an amplification strategy for dealing with this problem, based on high-rate secretion of soluble forms of the cell surface immunoglobulin receptors that initiated B-cell recruitment into the host response or mutated, higher affinity analogs of these immunoglobulins generated by somatic mutation and selection during germinal center differentiation (Chapter 25). A differentiated B lymphocyte (plasma cell) can produce a large number of identical antibody molecules, only one or a few of which are needed to inactivate each viral or bacterial particle. However, this strategy is primarily effective for the extracellular phase of pathogen growth or during pathogen movement between host cells for those organisms with an intracellular growth phase (Fig. 1). In most cases, this limb of the immune system is largely blind to organisms once inside a host cell, until molecules unique to the invading species are exposed to the extracellular fluid where soluble antibody molecules or surface immunoglobulin receptors are able to make contact, although in some circumstances endocytic uptake of antibodies may lead to inhibition of viral assembly or attack organisms resident in vesicles that are functionally connected to the endocytic pathway. Thus, antibodies are highly effective in inhibiting new infection and the spread of infection, but they do so largely only after each round of intracellular replication. Viral replication and progeny formation usually is well advanced before antibodies can target an infected cell upon expression of viral components on the plasma membrane, and for nonenveloped viruses, surface expression of a target structure might not occur at all before progeny release by the infected cell. This mechanism is also ineffective against parasites with prolonged intracellular (cytosolic) residence.

Given this limitation of the B-lymphocyte/antibody limb of the immune system, it is clearly evolutionarily desirable to have a means of detecting the intracellular presence of a pathogen, whether in the cytosol or in endosomal organelles, preferably at an early time after cellular invasion before substantial replication can occur. But if no unique chemical structures are available on the surface of an infected cell for recognition by the broad immunoglobulin repertoire of B cells, how can such early recognition be accomplished? T-cell recognition of peptides bound to MHC molecules provides a solution to this problem. All living organisms contain and produce one or more unique protein species. In principle, small fragments of these proteins, even from those molecules never reaching the plasma membrane in an intact form, can be generated by proteolysis, captured by MHC molecules, and delivered to the cell surface in a multivalent array suitable for T-cell recogni-

tion. These peptides can be derived from unique proteins that are carried preformed into the infected cell with the invading organism or can come from newly synthesized proteins that constitute one of the first biochemical events of pathogen replication. Recognition of the presence of such early markers of infection can result in the elimination of pathogen replicative bursts by direct action on the infected cell, whether by increasing its resistance to pathogen survival or through sacrifice of the infected cell, preventing the production of a large number of progeny. This mechanism also provides a means of detecting organisms that maintain intracellular residence after infection and are only transiently accessible to the humoral immune system.

Peptide recognition has additional advantages as a pathogen detection strategy. Most proteins can accommodate substantial changes in the amino acid side chains exposed on the surface of the molecule without loss of function. Many fewer substitutions are possible for interior residues if protein folding patterns and activity are to be maintained. Because of this difference in the range of permitted change, the selection of organisms with genetic variations encoding altered protein surface structure readily occurs under the influence of antibodies that recognize such surface features as part of either continuous or discontinuous conformational epitopes (12). However, change in the chemical composition of core amino acid residues of a protein is less common, due to the structural constraints on side-chain packing in the interior of proteins. A peptide-based recognition system that can operate via protein fragments derived from any portion of the foreign protein, irrespective of the fragment's location in the folded molecule or the evolved function of the protein, makes it difficult to avoid the recognition system solely through changes in nonessential side chains on the protein surface.

At the same time, a peptide-specific recognition system requires a number of attributes beyond the existence of peptide-binding proteins such as class I and class II MHC molecules. First, the cell must be able to efficiently generate suitable peptide fragments from already folded proteins that might be relatively protease resis-

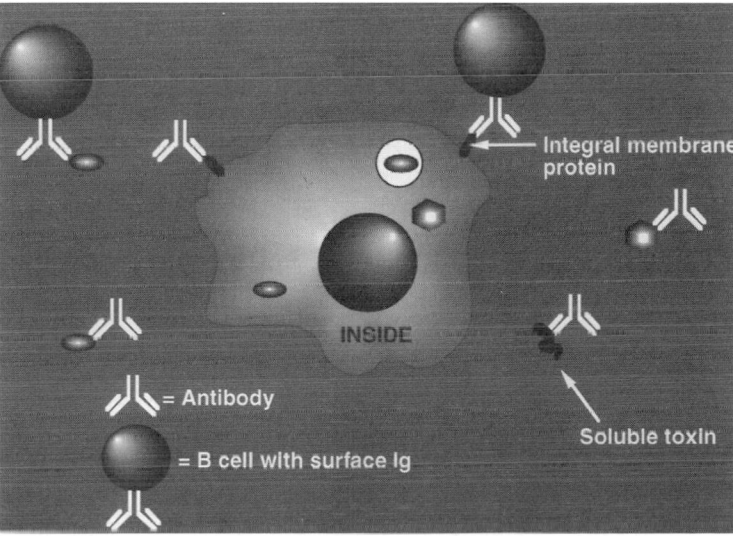

FIG. 1. Limitation of direct antigen recognition by B-cell surface immunoglobulin to extracellular ligands underlies the need to express tags from intracellular antigens on the cell surface to provide a means of stimulating adaptive immunity to intracellular pathogens.

tant and yet prevent excessive degradation of the fragments as they are generated that might prevent capture by MHC molecules. If the system is to identify cells rapidly after infection and before full replication of the pathogen, especially viruses, it must have a way to create fragments from cytosolic or nuclear proteins, which are often the products of the first genes expressed by viruses, and deliver them to the outside of the cell; that is, they must move across the membrane barrier that differentiates the topologic inside of the cell from the outside, where T-cell recognition must occur. The binding specificity of the MHC molecules must be broad enough to avoid easy evasion by pathogens through mutation and selection of noninteracting peptide sequences: this same attribute of the binding system makes it impossible to differentiate in most cases between peptides derived from self and foreign proteins. This means that the immune system must have mechanisms for establishing tolerance to self peptide–MHC molecule complexes and that cells must make sufficient MHC molecules to avoid saturation of the binding system by peptides derived from self proteins. Furthermore, when a specific T lymphocyte interacts with a cell, it must sort through all the MHC molecules on that cell's membrane to determine if some are occupied with the specific peptide for which the T-cell receptor (TCR) is specific. To make the scanning system efficient, the time devoted to this process on each potential target cell needs to be limited. Given that the larger the pool of MHC molecules on the surface, the longer it takes to scan them, it follows that maximizing the expression of useful MHC molecules on the cell surface is a desirable feature, and useful to T cells means loaded with peptide. Empty MHC molecules are a distraction for the system and would inhibit efficient recognition of MHC molecules containing foreign peptides. Thus, the cell needs mechanisms for limiting the number of empty MHC molecules that reach or reside on the cell surface. Similarly, in the case of effector cell activity in which the goal is the selective destruction of cells that are actively infected or transformed, and not the destruction of other uninfected cells, it is essential to prevent loading of the MHC molecules on the surface of uninfected cells. This also means limiting the availability of empty MHC molecules on the cell membrane that could capture free peptide from the extracellular environment, especially at sites of substantial tissue damage where such external peptides might be in significant concentration.

This chapter first reviews the historical development of this peptide presentation paradigm. It then examines how the presentation system fulfills the requirements discussed above by describing the biochemical features of MHC molecules that allow them to serve their role as presenters of protein antigen fragments to the T-cell limb of the immune system, the cell biology underlying the generation of antigenic peptides and their effective interaction with MHC molecules, and the characteristics of the recognition of the resultant complexes by T lymphocytes. New findings are described suggesting that additional specialized pathways of antigen presentation exist for both a subset of peptide ligands and for nonpeptidic moieties, each of which possess structural features that globally distinguish them from self structures. Recent data establishing that natural killer (NK) cells use MHC class I molecules to regulate their effector functions are also summarized. These latter discoveries indicate that some aspects of adaptive immune recognition are built on the type of chemical pattern discrimination between self and nonself that is also used by the innate immune system, providing a bridge between the nonclonal, generic responses of the latter and the peptide sequence–specific clonal responses characteristic of many TCR αβ CD4$^+$ and CD8$^+$ T cells.

HISTORICAL DEVELOPMENT OF THE PEPTIDE PRESENTATION PARADIGM

Early Models for the Role of MHC Molecules in T-Cell Immunity

The two phenomena of MHC-linked IR gene control of T cell–dependent immunity and of MHC-restricted recognition of antigen by T cells (see Chapters 10, 11, and 12) led to three general models for the role of MHC molecules in T-lymphocyte responses. The earliest model was that the MHC molecules themselves were the clonally distributed antigen-specific receptors of T cells (13). According to this hypothesis, the absence of the correct MHC-encoded receptor protein would deprive the animal of those T cells necessary for recognition of a particular antigen, resulting in a failure to respond. However, the bone marrow–reconstituted radiation chimera model, initially developed by von Boehmer and Sprent (14) (see Chapter 20) and applied to antigens under classical MHC-linked IR gene control, showed that such IR gene control was not inherent in the genotype of the T cell but in the genotype of the environment in which the T cell developed and was exposed to antigen (15,16). If the MHC genes encoded receptors expressed by the T cells themselves, the opposite result would have been expected; therefore, this model was abandoned, as was a variant model in which the MHC molecules served as receptors for themselves on the antigen-bearing cell (like–like recognition).

The two remaining models that competed for over a decade were the dual recognition and altered self models (17). Dual recognition held that T cells used two distinct receptors to mediate physically independent recognition of antigen and of allele-specific features of MHC molecules. Ligand binding to each class of receptor was presumed to provide unique signals to the T cell, both of which were required for activation. This would explain the need for the simultaneous presence of both antigen and the MHC-encoded proteins on the same cell but avoid the necessity for direct chemical interaction of the two entities. Because activation was postulated to require concurrent generation of two unique signals, one from each recognition event, a high concentration of one or the other ligand alone could not substitute for the presence of both. Developmental selection of the MHC-specific subset of receptors expressed by mature T cells would explain the chimera data showing environmental control of MHC restriction. The chimera data on IR gene control was more difficult to explain by this mechanism because it required some sort of functional linkage of expression of the two receptors such that certain antigen-specific receptors were not expressed when particular anti-MHC receptors were absent as a result of environmental differences during development. However, such a linkage could not be ruled out a priori and hence did not eliminate this model (18).

The alternative view was that there was a physical interaction of the protein antigen (or a fragment derived from this antigen) and the MHC molecule that created a complex recognized by a single receptor with a conjoint specificity for both components of the ligand. This model explained IR gene function by postulating that certain antigens could not associate with particular allelic forms of MHC molecules, thus preventing effective T-cell recognition (19). MHC-restricted antigen recognition could be understood by requiring a contribution of both components of the antigen–MHC molecule complex to specific binding by the combining site of a single TCR. The chimera data on the role of environment in MHC-restricted antigen recognition would follow from an influence of the MHC molecules in the host on the choice of such receptors available on the mature T cells, so that they were biased for best recognition of complexes involving antigen associated with the allelic forms of the MHC molecules present during T-cell development. The primary concern raised about this model was the requirement that a limited number of MHC molecules in each individual interact in a highly specific way with the many protein antigens to which the immune system could respond.

Early Evidence for a Single T-Cell Receptor Complex Mediating Recognition of Physically Associated Antigen–MHC Molecule Combinations

The development of continuous T-cell hybridoma lines (somatic cell hybrids between a transformed thymoma cell and nontransformed antigen-specific T cells) that maintained the antigen and MHC molecule specificity characteristic of the parent immune T cell allowed Kappler et al. (20) to perform an important test of these two competing models of T-cell recognition of antigen (Fig. 2). These investigators fused together two T-hybridomas specific for different antigens and distinct alleles of class II MHC molecules. If the dual specificity of T cells was mediated by two receptors, each with independent reactivity to physically separate antigen and MHC molecules, then a double hybridoma should not only respond to each of the parental antigen–MHC molecule combinations, but it should also show mixed responses involving the antigen reactivity of one parent and the MHC molecule specificity of the other (Fig. 2A). But this was not observed. The double hybridoma showed only the two original conjoint antigen–MHC molecule recognition properties of the parent T cells and did not gain new reactivities that represented reassortments of the individual parental antigen and MHC molecule specificities. These data indicated that either the TCRs were single physical complexes that could not undergo functionally useful cross-pairing (Fig. 2B) or the antigen and MHC molecules showed a strict allele-specific association that was necessary for stimulating the T cell (Fig. 2C).

Schwartz and colleagues, using a model system involving cytochrome c antigen, conducted an elegant series of studies that strongly argued for an important physical interaction between antigen and MHC molecules (21). They were able to identify T cells specific for pigeon cytochrome c that also responded to moth cytochrome c presented by cells bearing the $E_\alpha^k E_\beta^k$ class II molecule. These same cells responded to moth cytochrome c presented by $E_\alpha^k E_\beta^k$ but failed to respond to pigeon cytochrome presented by cells bearing this MHC molecule. These data were not readily explained by dual receptor recognition of physically independent antigen and MHC molecules. According to a straightforward dual recognition model, the response to moth cytochrome in the presence of either allele of class II molecule argued that the putative anti-MHC receptor on these T cells must be able to recognize both alleles. The ability of the cells to respond to pigeon cytochrome c on cells bearing $E_\alpha^k E_\beta^k$ showed that the putative antigen receptor on the T cell must be able to recognize this antigen. But if both an antipigeon cytochrome receptor and an independent receptor capable of $E_\alpha^k E_\beta^b$ recognition existed on the cells, then they should have responded to pigeon cytochrome on the $E_\alpha^k E_\beta^b$-bearing cells, which they did not. A better explanation of these data was that the $E_\alpha^k E_\beta^b$ molecule could interact with moth but not pigeon cytochrome for presentation of the physically associated pair to a receptor or receptors on the T cell, and that $E_\alpha^k E_\beta^k$ could interact

appropriately with both forms of cytochrome, a conjecture later proved correct (22).

Rock and Benacerraf were the first to clearly demonstrate that two antigens recognized by different T cells in association with the same allelic form of MHC class II molecule could interfere with each other's presentation (23). Such a result would not be predicted by a strict dual recognition model involving independent antigens and MHC molecule targets for the TCR, but it was readily explained by requiring a physical complex of antigen and MHC molecule for such receptor stimulation. The irrelevant antigen would then compete for such MHC molecule binding by the potentially stimulatory antigen, interfering with T-cell activation.

These two series of studies on MHC–antigen interaction unfortunately limited the value of the Kappler et al. experiment with respect to understanding the nature of the TCR because it indicated that the failure to see the emergence of new response specificities with the double hybridoma could have been due to an inability to produce new antigen–MHC pairs rather than to an absence of receptors with distinct reactivities. Nevertheless, these studies did indicate that if two separate TCRs existed, they must function only when brought together intimately by a physical complex of antigen and MHC molecule.

Direct Evidence for a Single T-Cell Receptor Mediating Recognition of Physical Complexes of Peptide Antigen and MHC-Encoded Molecules

Several groups in the early 1980s began to use fragments of whole proteins as antigens for T cells whose stimulation depended on MHC class II molecules. The ability of such fragments to serve as substitute antigens was expected from the ability of denatured proteins to elicit T cell–dependent responses. Ziegler and Unanue made the critical observations that (a) presentation of initially intact protein antigens to T cells responding in the context of MHC class II molecules was blocked by agents such as chloroquine that raised intracellular pH and inhibited the activity of acid proteases and (b) effective presentation of such intact antigens required metabolic activity on the part of the antigen-presenting cell (APC) (24). Shimonkevitz et al. then combined these findings to demonstrate that the required metabolic activity involved the breakdown of the original intact protein into smaller pieces that could be replaced by predigested protein fragments. Such fragments were able to stimulate MHC class II–restricted T cells when presented by metabolically inactive cells incapable of stimulating the same T cells in the presence of the intact form of the antigen (25). This key finding made it clear that at least CD4+ T cells were responding to smaller parts of the protein, in accord with the lack of a requirement for maintenance of native protein conformation in eliciting delayed type hypersensitivity responses mediated by this T-cell subset, and that degradation of antigen to such smaller fragments was essential to the presentation/recognition process. These results established the concept of active antigen processing as a prelude to effective antigen presentation in the context of MHC class II molecules.

The ability to bypass the metabolic machinery of living cells with antigen fragments led to the use of synthetic peptides that could serve as analogs of naturally generated T-cell antigens and hence to the possibility of directly exploring antigen–MHC molecule interactions in vitro. Despite the predictions by many biochemists that MHC molecules could not possibly be physically interacting in a stable manner with such a diversity of protein struc-

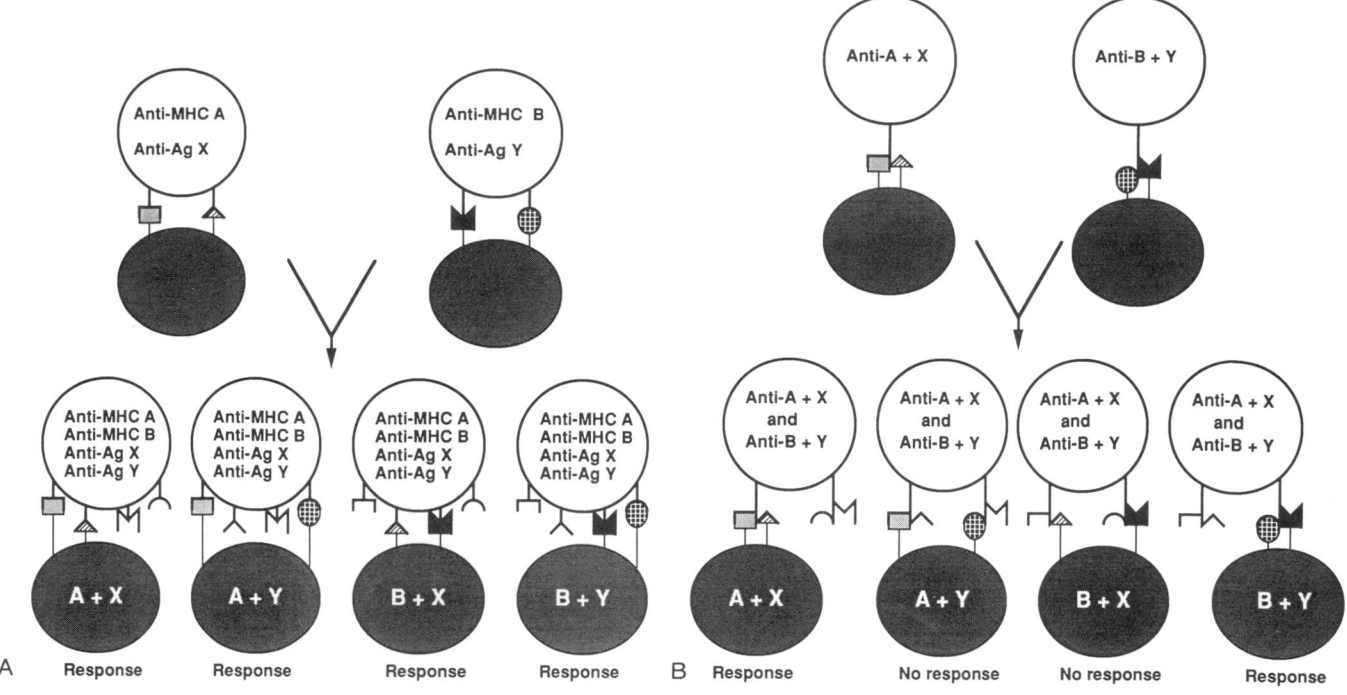

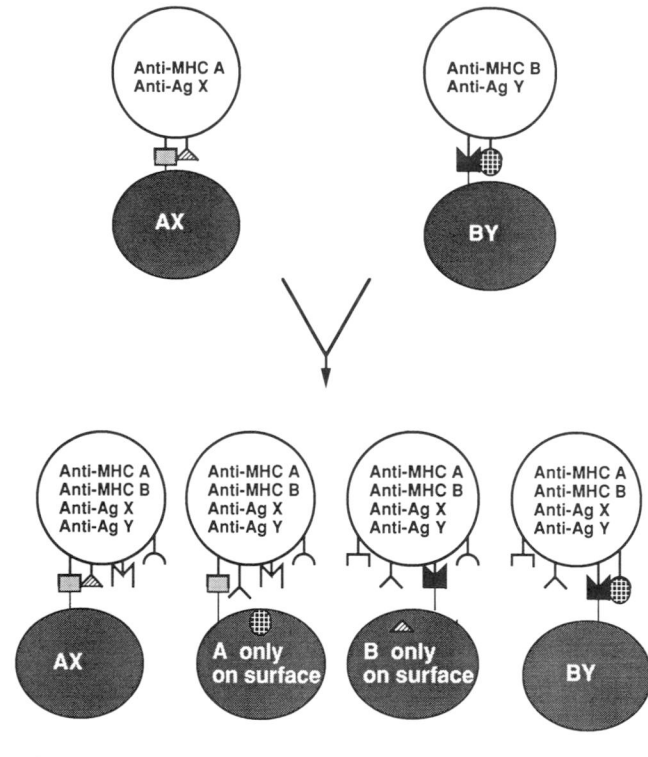

FIG. 2. T-cell hybridoma fusion test for independent recognition of antigen and MHC molecules. This figure shows a schematic representation of the experiment by Kappler et al. (20) designed to test whether T cells have receptors with independent recognition of antigen and of MHC molecules. Two T-cell hybridomas of different protein antigen specificity (X and Y) and distinct MHC restriction (to MHC A or MHC B) were fused, and the resulting hybrid–hybridomas were tested for response to each combination of antigen and MHC molecule. **A:** The results expected if the T cell possessed two separate receptors, one for antigen and one for MHC molecules, that could function in activating the T cell any time at least one antigen receptor and one MHC receptor were simultaneously occupied. Not only would the original antigen and MHC allele combinations be effective, but mixtures of the antigen specificity of one parent and the MHC specificity of the other would also work. **B:** The results expected if the T cells had only a single receptor with conjoint specificity for both the antigen and for MHC molecules. Only the original combinations of antigen and MHC allele would be stimulatory. **C:** The results expected if there were a required specific physical interaction of antigen and MHC molecule and the T cell had two independent receptors, one for antigen and one for MHC molecules, which must both be occupied to stimulate the T cell. Just as with a single TCR model, the only stimulatory combinations would be those that were seen by the original parental T hybridomas. The actual results of the experiment fit models B and C, but not model A, indicating that either there was a single receptor or there was a required and specific interaction of antigen with MHC molecules.

tures as would be needed to explain antigen recognition by T cells, Babbitt et al. used such a synthetic peptide antigen and immunoaffinity purified class II MHC molecules to show direct allele-specific binding of these isolated components (26). These results were rapidly confirmed and extended by Buus et al., who first reported on the remarkable longevity of such peptide–MHC

class II molecule complexes (27). These biochemical data confirmed the allele-specific interaction of antigen and MHC molecules predicted by the functional studies of Schwartz et al. (21) and Rock and Benacerraf (23) and established the paradigm of MHC-restricted antigen presentation as a reflection of stable association of MHC molecules with peptide antigen for recognition by T cells.

During the same time period, a series of studies also provided molecular evidence that the dual specificity of T cells for such peptide–MHC complexes was carried by a single clonally distributed receptor. First protein data and then gene cloning identified immunoglobulinlike structures (the αβ TCR) with clonal expression by T cells (see Chapter 10). Examination of variants of a single T-cell hybridoma line for rearranged genes in the α and β families and for functional antigen–MHC molecule recognition allowed Yagüe et al. to suggest that a single pair of α and β chains assembled into a single receptor structure mediating T-cell dual specificity (28). This interpretation was given molecular support by the work of two groups who used gene transfer methods to directly demonstrate that the antigen and MHC molecule fine specificity of a T cell could be transferred to an unrelated recipient T cell by genes encoding one α and one β chain that assembled into a single physical dimer (29,30).

Thus, peptide-binding experiments showed that the ligand for the TCR on class II–restricted T lymphocytes was a long-lived physical complex of peptide antigen and MHC molecule, and gene transfer studies provided evidence that this complex was recognized by a single immunoglobulinlike receptor with what appeared to be a single combining site, all in accord with the expectations of the altered self model of T-cell recognition. However, no comparable experiments using antigen fragments or peptides, or showing inhibition of presentation by agents interfering with intracellular proteolysis, existed for antigens presented by MHC class I molecules. Thus, despite the strong evidence for peptide–MHC class II complexes as the ligand for the receptor on some αβ T cells (the CD4+ subpopulation), the prevailing view was that class I molecules physically interacted with intact membrane-bound forms of viral or self proteins. Evidence seemingly consistent with this model was presented by Morrison et al., who found that influenza hemagglutinin was presented to class II–restricted T cells if it was introduced as a preformed protein into the endocytic pathway where acid-dependent proteolysis could occur, but not if it was synthesized transiently by the cell (31). Conversely, such active synthesis was necessary for class I presentation, and intact protein taken up from the outside was ineffective for recognition by class I–restricted CD8+ cytotoxic cells.

A complete shift in thinking accompanied the unexpected demonstration by Townsend et al. that the internal nucleoprotein of influenza was a common determinant for class I–restricted cytotoxic cells and that a peptide analog of a portion of the nucleoprotein could substitute for actively synthesized material (32). These data were entirely consistent with the peptide–MHC molecule model established for class II molecules. They suggested that the protein antigens recognized by class I–restricted T cells were likely to be presented as small fragments bound to class I, rather than as intact proteins expressed on the cell surface, as later biochemical studies confirmed.

Specialization of Class I and Class II MHC Molecules for Presentation of Peptides from Different Intracellular Compartments

The evidence that both class I and class II MHC molecules presented antigen as short peptides to T cells that used the same set of gene segments to produce their αβ receptors raised the question of whether the two classes of MHC molecules had distinct roles in antigen presentation. Based on the observations of Morrison et al.

concerning differential presentation of proteins acquired from outside the cell versus synthesized within it (31), and the known distinctions in effector function of CD4+ MHC class II–restricted versus CD8+ MHC class I–restricted T cells, it was proposed that each class of MHC molecule, independent of allelic differences within a class, was specialized for capturing peptides in different compartments of the cell (33). The proteins contributing peptides to these compartments would largely, but not absolutely, be divided according to their intracellular location, with those synthesized in the cell or accessing the cytosol by such means as viral fusion supplying peptides to the class I molecules and those entering the endocytic pathway from the cell surface or from outside the cell supplying peptides to class II molecules (33–35).

This hypothesis concerning MHC class-specific specialization in antigen presentation, together with the studies firmly establishing the peptide–MHC molecule complex paradigm as the general rule for recognition of antigen by αβ T cells, led to intensive investigation of the molecular basis for peptide–MHC molecule interaction, the cellular physiology of peptide generation, capture, and display, and the details of T-cell recognition of peptide–MHC complexes. Such studies have identified the peptides associated with MHC class I and class II molecules produced by living cells; yielded crystallographic images of peptide–MHC complexes, of the αβ TCR, and of peptide–MHC molecule/αβ TCR complexes; defined new genes involved in the processing and presentation of antigens; and revealed the complex patterns of intracellular transport that precede surface expression of recognizable peptide–MHC complexes. The roles of specialized nonclassical MHC molecules and of MHC-like proteins encoded outside of the MHC itself in the presentation of unique peptide and nonpeptide structures have been discovered, and alternative pathways for presentation of peptides by conventional class I and class II MHC molecules have been described. The key contributions to antigen processing made by protein degradation systems in the cytosol and in endosomal organelles and involved in many other cellular functions have been made clear. We thus now have begun to acquire a rather comprehensive understanding of this key aspect of adaptive immune recognition.

GENETIC ORGANIZATION AND PROTEIN STRUCTURE OF LIGAND-BINDING MOLECULES INVOLVED IN ANTIGEN PRESENTATION

Organization of the MHC

Detailed maps have been derived for the chromosomal regions containing the major histocompatibility complexes of the human, mouse, and rat, and less complete but informative mapping studies have been performed for other animals such as chimpanzees and miniature swine. Large-scale mapping and nucleotide sequencing is rapidly providing a complete molecular picture of the human MHC (36,37) (see Chapter 8 for a more extensive description of MHC gene organization). The MHC in each species covers several megabases of DNA. Figure 3 contains schematic maps of the MHC of the human and mouse that show the principal class I and class II genes. In addition to these genes, the MHC contains nonclassical class I genes and in the class II region, a number of genes whose products are either known or suspected to participate in the formation of antigenic peptides and their availability to the class I and

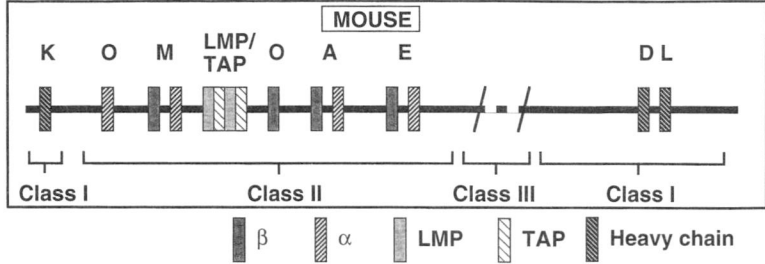

FIG. 3. Schematic map of the human and mouse MHC complexes. This diagram shows the relative position of the principal class I and class II genes of humans and mice, as well as several additional MHC-linked genes believed to be involved in antigen processing and presentation. Class Ib genes are not shown for simplicity (see Chapter 8 for additional details).

class II MHC molecules. These genes— TAP-1 and -2, LMP-2 and -7, DMα and DMβ, and DOα and DOβ—will be discussed in detail in the sections describing the cell biology of antigen processing. The MHC also contains a number of other genes encoding products with immune functions not known to be directly related to antigen processing and presentation, such as those for the fourth component of complement and for tumor necrosis factor (TNF)-α, although the role of the latter in the maturation of dendritic cells (38–40) may be considered to give this cytokine a key place in antigen presentation and, hence, a possible reason for its presence in the MHC.

MHC Class I and Class II Genes and Proteins

Class I

A large number of distinct class I loci have been identified. In humans, functional genes have been found for the HLA-A, -B, -C, -E, -F, and -G loci (41). The A and B loci show extensive intraspecies polymorphism, whereas the C locus shows less variation and the G locus little if any differences among individuals. In mice, functional, highly polymorphic proteins are encoded by the H-2K, D, and L loci. Less variable proteins are encoded by a number of the Qa and TL loci, which are considered to constitute the numerically predominant members of the class Ib or nonclassical class I family of MHC proteins (42). The products of the various class I loci show distinct tissue distributions and regulation of expression. The HLA-A, -B, and -C and H-2K, D, and L products are expressed on a wide variety of somatic cells, although to varying extents, with the highest expression being on hematopoietic cells. HLA-G is expressed by trophoblasts of the fetus (43), and Qa-2 in mice is expressed strongly on mature T lymphocytes (44). Expression of class I molecules is strongly affected by several cytokines, especially IFN-γ and TNF-α.

The products of most of these classical and nonclassical class I loci are structurally similar, consisting of a type I integral mem-

brane protein of about 45 kDa in its mature glycosylated form. This chain is designated the class I heavy chain, and it can be divided into several structural subdomains based on both biochemical properties and relationship to gene exon–intron organization (45). The most amino-terminal region is denoted α1 and the next segment α2. Each of these two domains is encoded by a single exon, and together they contain the large majority of the positions exhibiting extensive intraspecies polymorphism. The third protein domain is also encoded by a separate exon and consists of a region of limited polymorphism with substantial sequence homology to an immunoglobulin domain. One portion of this immunoglobulin-like domain includes a loop extending from residues 223 to 233 that forms part of the major binding site for the CD8 coreceptor (46,47). This exon is followed by a series of exons encoding the transmembrane region and the cytoplasmic tail. The use of several small exons to encode the cytoplasmic tail of class I molecules allows variation in function as a consequence of alternative splicing patterns that produces molecules with differing protein sequence in the cytoplasmic region.

In addition to the heavy chain, mature, surface-expressed class I molecules contain a noncovalently associated polypeptide of about 12 kDa termed β2 microglobulin (β2m). The gene encoding β2m is not located within the MHC, and it shows little allelic variation. β2m consists of a single, soluble, immunoglobulinlike domain encoded by the large second exon of the β2m gene.

Class II

Class II molecules each consist of a noncovalently associated αβ heterodimer (48). Both the α chain (33 kDa) and the β chain (29 kDa) are type I integral membrane proteins, in contrast to the membrane anchoring of only the heavy chain and not the β2m portion of the class I molecule, and there is evidence that the two transmembrane segments interact to facilitate dimer formation and stability (49). Because class II α and β genes (encoding the α and β chains of the class II molecule, respectively) are usually coordinately expressed, a single cell can contain several class II α and β chains from distinct loci and two allelic forms encoded at a single locus. In principle, this permits the assembly and expression of a large variety of class II heterodimers produced by mixing and matching the various α and β chains. In practice, however, it appears that the products of each tightly linked cluster of α- and β-chain genes have evolved to assemble best with each other, usually showing inefficient assembly with chains from other loci (48,50,51). A combination of such preferential pairing and competition for available chains gives rise to the characteristic isotypes of class II dimers observed in biochemical and serologic studies (52). The human DR locus has more than one functional β chain encoded by closely linked genes, each of which is able to pair and be expressed effectively with the single, relatively nonpolymorphic DRα chain. Similar, though less stringent, restrictions on assembly and expression apply to allelic variants at a single locus, suggesting coevolution of the polymorphic regions of coinherited α- and β-chain genes for optimal coassembly and expression (51). Despite these general rules of locus- and allele-restricted assembly and expression, some cross-pairing does occur and gives rise to mixed isotype or mixed allele dimers (53) that, even if expressed at low levels, can have important biologic functions (54).

The primary polymorphic class II molecules in the human (DRαDRβ, DPαDPβ, and DQαDQβ) and mouse (AαAβ and EαEβ) are typically expressed by a variety of hematopoietic cells such as B lymphocytes, monocytes, macrophages, and dendritic cells, as well as by numerous epithelial cells, especially in the thymus. They are absent from most other somatic cells except after exposure to certain lymphokines, most notably IFN-γ, which can induce class II expression on many cell types. Other class II dimers such as DO show a more restricted tissue distribution and lower absolute levels of surface expression (55,56).

As for class I, the protein structure of class II molecules can be correlated with the exon–intron organization of the α and β genes. Following an initial exon encoding the signal sequence and a few of the most NH$_2$-terminal residues of the mature polypeptide, the second exons of the α and β genes encode regions of approximately 90 residues each termed α1 and β1, respectively, that contain the bulk of the positions showing extensive intraspecies polymorphism. These exons are followed by third exons encoding the α2 and β2 domains that show substantial homology to immunoglobulin and only limited allelic variation. The transmembrane and intracytoplasmic regions are encoded by exons 5 and 6 (α) or 5 to 7 (β). The human DQβ genes have a defect in the splice acceptor signal for what is a functional exon 6 in the homologous mouse Aβ gene, and the corresponding middle portion of the cytoplasmic tail is absent from the DQβ protein.

Detailed Molecular Structure of MHC Molecules and the Chemistry of Peptide Binding and Presentation

In the late 1970s and early 1980s, a large number of studies examined the structure–function relationships of MHC class I and class II molecules using cells expressing wild-type or mutant forms of these molecules. In vitro mutagenesis of cloned DNA-encoding class I or class II proteins and the expression of the mutant proteins after DNA-mediated gene transfer (transfection) were extensively used as a technique to address how the different portions and even individual amino acids of these proteins contributed to peptide

bindings or T-cell recognition (57,58). These investigations resulted in the identification of specific residues affecting protein folding, assembly, surface expression, serologic reactivity, and antigen binding and presentation to T cells. The combined data from such work led to the generation of model structures for the domain organization of these proteins and, for class II, the disposition of clusters of polymorphic residues in the fully folded molecules (59). These crude but generally accurate representations were supplanted in 1987 by the first crystallographic analysis of an MHC molecule, the human HLA-A2 class I protein (see Chapter 8) (60,61). This study showed for the first time the detailed structure of an MHC molecule peptide-binding site and the location and orientation of the polymorphic residues known to play such a critical role in both peptide binding and T-cell recognition events.

A large number of refined high-resolution x-ray crystallographic structures have now been derived for both conventional class I and class II molecules of mice and humans, as well as the class I–like molecule CD1. Each represents the extracellular portion of the molecule generated by proteolytic cleavage of surface molecules from lymphoid cells, secreted as truncated soluble proteins by transfected or recombinant baculovirus-infected insect cells, or produced by bacteria. Some of the structures, notably those derived using MHC molecules recovered from lymphoid cells, contain a heterogeneous array of bound peptides, whereas others involve only single peptide species. The latter structures have shown at an atomic level the details of how individual peptides bind to MHC molecules.

The class I structures show that the α1 and α2 domains combine to form a single peptide-binding site supported by a β-pleated sheet floor containing eight strands and bounded by two α helices, one from α1 and one from α2. β2m makes contact not only with the immunoglobulinlike α3 domain but also with the β sheet floor of the α1α2 peptide-binding region. Each of the structures shows the presence of a series of pockets studding the peptide-binding groove (62–65). In some cases these pockets extended deep between the floor and helical walls of the binding domain. A similar but not identical overall distribution of pockets exists in many of the class I molecules examined to date, and these have now been designated A through F.

One of the most remarkable and satisfying features noted in the first HLA-A2 structure was that the large majority of the side chains of class I amino acids at highly polymorphic positions pointed into the peptide-binding region, where they would clearly exert a significant influence on the nature of the peptides that could be bound (61). Few such variable residues pointed up from the helical walls of the site or out and away from the peptide-binding region. These data clearly support the idea that the polymorphic nature of MHC molecules is primarily related to diversification of their peptide-binding specificities and that different alleles are meant to bind distinct sets of peptides. They also indicate that such sequence diversity in MHC molecules is not primarily selected to directly control interactions with TCRs because most of the variable side chains are buried after peptide binding and would not be accessible to the TCR. The recent crystallographic solutions of the structure of MHC class I molecule–peptide complexes bound to an αβ TCR (66,67) show substantial interaction of the TCR with MHC class I in the region surrounding the peptide, but as expected from the early data on the location of polymorphic side chains, this TCR binding primarily involves conserved features of the class I molecule. Interestingly, in the few examples of such TCR/ligand structures obtained so far, the general rotational orientation of the

TCR with respect to the MHC class I molecule is the same, suggesting that there may be a relatively conserved set of interactions between the germline V segments of the TCR α and β chains and the conserved features of the MHC molecules surrounding bound peptides. The implications of this latter finding are discussed further in the section below on T-cell recognition.

The chemistry of peptide–MHC class I molecule interaction also has been determined from these crystal structures (68). Most bound peptides are eight or nine residues long and in an extended conformation with a central kink. A critical aspect of peptide binding to class I is the direct formation of hydrogen bonds at each peptide's common NH_2-terminal amine through conserved MHC residues tyrosine 7, tyrosine 59, and tyrosine 171, as well as extensive hydrogen bonding to the common terminal carboxyl group from class I tyrosine 84, threonine 143, and lysine 146. Additional hydrogen bonds are made to the carbonyl groups of the first and penultimate amino acid residues by tyrosine 159 and tryptophan 147, respectively (64,69). Conserved bonds from invariant residues to structural components characteristic of all peptides explains how polymorphic class I molecules can each act as an effective peptide-binding protein for a wide diversity of peptide sequences (70). Because these conserved bonds play a major role in stabilizing peptide–MHC class I interaction, peptides whose N and C termini cannot effectively participate in these interactions are less likely, although not unable, to become tightly associated with class I molecules. This places a relatively strict length constraint on peptides for optimum binding to class I molecules: those substantially longer or shorter than the eight- or nine-residue optimum cannot readily make these bonds and still fit snugly in the remainder of the binding region. In those cases in which longer peptides are bound, either some residues bulge up in the center if the N and C termini are properly complexed with the conserved regions (71), or a less stable bond is made by the conserved residues near the F pocket to a carbonyl group of a peptide bond, and the remaining residues of the peptide beyond this site extend up and out of the binding site (72). Neither of these configurations results in the highest affinity binding seen with short, optimal length peptides of class I molecules, but such complexes involving long peptides may contribute to effective ligands for some TCR. The analysis of the same class I K^b molecule crystallized with either an eight-residue or nine-residue bound peptide also showed that the fine structure of a single class I molecule can vary significantly depending on the peptide bound, giving some biochemical support to the old notion of T-cell recognition as involving "altered self," in this case, the different disposition of residues in the $\alpha2$ α helix that are accessible to the TCR (63).

The second striking feature of the class I–peptide interaction shown by these studies is the contribution of allelic polymorphism to the shape and chemical character of the pockets within the binding region and the role of these features in discriminating among peptides of similar length but differing sequence for binding to the MHC class I molecule. The bulk of the polymorphic positions contribute to variations in the shape and chemical nature of the pockets within the binding domain. For example, the B pocket of HLA-A2 has a hydrophobic character well suited to binding of the leucine residue at position 2 of known HLA-A2–presented peptides. The HLA-B27 B pocket with an aspartic acid is chemically compatible with the arginines found in peptides presented by this HLA molecule. A deep C pocket in H-2K^b allows it to accommodate the preferred bulky phenylalanines or tyrosines at position 5.

One intriguing question that is only partially answered is the extent to which class Ib molecules are able to bind peptides using the chemical strategy just outlined for classical class I molecules. In at least one case, a specialized modification of the otherwise conserved structure of the class I molecule involved in binding the NH_2 terminus of peptides has been discovered. Studies of a unique cytotoxic T-cell response first identified the class Ib molecule now called H-2M3 as the presenting element for a mitochondrial peptide with a formyl-methionine on the NH_2 terminus (73). This modification is common to mitochondrial and prokaryotic proteins but is not found on eukaryotic proteins, thus constituting a general chemical distinction between self and nonself proteins. H-2M3 has phenylalanine substituting for the highly conserved tyrosine 171 found in classical class I molecules and involved in hydrogen bonding to the free NH_2 terminus of typical peptides, a change that appears to be critical to the ability of H-2M3 to accommodate an N-formyl group (74). The immunologic value of an MHC molecule specialized for presentation of N-formylated peptides can be appreciated from the finding that peptides from the intracellular bacterial pathogen *Listeria monocytogenes* are presented by H-2M3 and that cytotoxic T lymphocytes (CTLs) directed to this peptide–MHC molecule combination can be protective against disease caused by infection with this organism (75,76).

The non-MHC encoded but class I–like (heavy chain + $\beta2m$) CD1 molecule of the mouse also has been analyzed at the crystallographic level. In contrast to a typical class I molecule, the putative ligand binding domain is altered substantially. It lacks the conserved residues that would make H bonds to the free N and C termini of short peptides, the end of the groove where the A and B pockets are normally found is narrowed, and the remaining groove is extremely hydrophobic (77). These characteristics fit well with the notion that CD1 is involved in presentation primarily of non-peptide ligands with lipid components (78,79) that associate strongly with the "greasy pocket" seen in the binding domain.

A number of MHC class II molecule structures also have been solved crystallographically (80–85). The regions of the class I and class II molecules composing the peptide-binding domain and showing strong sequence homology turn out to be almost identical in main chain three-dimensional structure between the two classes. This is in agreement with mutagenesis-based structure–function studies demonstrating that changes at many homologous amino acid positions have similar effects on peptide binding and T-cell recognition in either class I or class II molecules. Like class I molecules, class II molecules possess numerous polymorphic pockets in the peptide binding domain into which the side chains of specific amino acids of bound peptides fit.

At the same time, several areas of the class II molecule whose structure could not be confidently predicted from the class I conformation turn out to have a significantly divergent organization. These differences in structure have important functional consequences. Perhaps most significantly, the highly conserved set of residues that coordinate binding to the N and C termini of short peptides interacting with class I molecules is not present in class II molecules, and changes in several residues in the regions forming the closed ends of the class I molecule peptide-binding groove make these parts of the class II molecule more open. This contributes to the lack among class II–associated peptides of the same strict length restriction observed for peptides bound to class I, and the crystal structure shows peptide residues extending beyond the ends of the binding domain of class II molecules, in contrast to class I molecules. Nevertheless, class II molecules, like class I molecules, also have features that promote generic, sequence-independent interaction with peptides. These are primarily hydrogen bonds to main chain atoms of the peptide, rather than to N and C termini, and they include a series of asparagine residues that are spaced along the two α helices, as well as conserved residues binding near the N and C termini of the portions of the peptide that lie within the binding groove. There is also a more linear, rather than kinked, structure to the peptides bound to class II molecules as compared with those bound to class I molecules (86). The spatial relationship of the α2 and β2 immunoglobulinlike domains is different than that of the corresponding β2m and α3 domains of class I molecules.

Perhaps the most unexpected feature of MHC class II molecules is the presence of dimers of class II dimers, or "superdimers," in several class II crystals, although the precise orientation of the monomers in the superdimer is distinct in the published human and mouse class II crystal structures. The physiologic significance of this self-association of class II molecules during crystallization is unknown at present but may relate to stabilizing TCR interactions necessary for activation of second messenger pathways (80,87) (see Chapters 10 and 12). The primary site controlling interaction of the class II molecule with the CD4 coreceptor has been mapped to residues 137–143 of the β2 domain, and this region is seen in the crystal structures to constitute a loop analogous to the 223–239 loop involved in binding of MHC class I molecules to CD8 (88,89). Intriguingly, a second site affecting class II–CD4 interactions has been identified in the class II α2 domain (90). This is on the opposite side of the molecule from the β2 site and is unlikely to interact with the same CD4 molecule (Fig. 4A). It comes close to the β2 site in the superdimer structure (Fig. 4B) and so might be involved

in stabilizing oligomeric structures involved in T-cell signaling upon TCR recognition of peptide–MHC class II ligands. A role for such oligomers is also suggested by the ability of CD4 to dimerize (91) and of TCR/peptide–MHC class II complexes to form higher order structures in solution (92).

Class II molecules are also involved in the presentation of non-peptide ligand to T cells. A variety of viral and microbial products have been termed "superantigens" (see Chapter 10) based on their ability to stimulate a large fraction of the total T-cell pool without regard for the clonal specificity of the individual TCRs borne by the responding cells (93). This results from the specific interaction of the superantigens with conserved portions of particular germline TCR Vβ segments (94–97). Neither the bacterial nor viral super-antigens require proteolysis to small peptides for function in T-cell stimulation, and crystallographic analysis of bacterial toxin super-antigens has shown that the putative residues involved in interaction with the TCR are brought together in the folded molecule from distant locations in the linear protein chain (98), as are the various residues involved in binding to MHC class II molecules. Functional presentation of bacterial superantigens (e.g., SEB, SEA, TSST-1) depends on physical interaction with class II molecules, and the structures of several such superantigenic toxins bound to MHC class II molecules have now been solved (82,83). SEB and TSST-1 have different footprints on the MHC class II molecule, although they both involve the α chain. As expected from functional and mutagenesis studies, the toxins bind outside the peptide binding groove, although TSST-1 drapes over the binding groove in

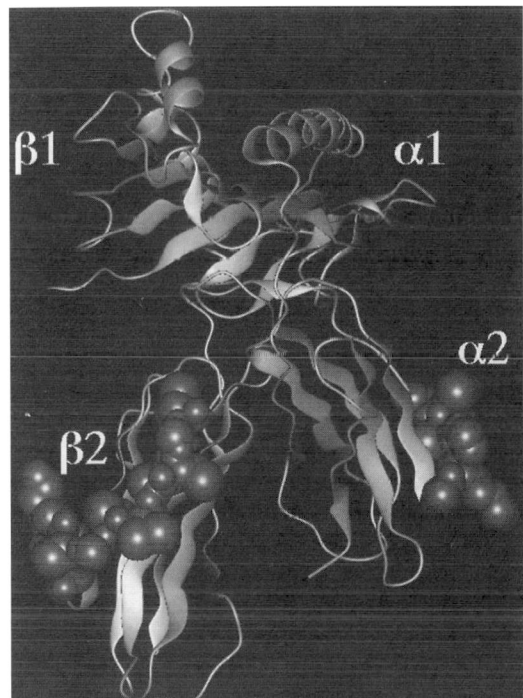 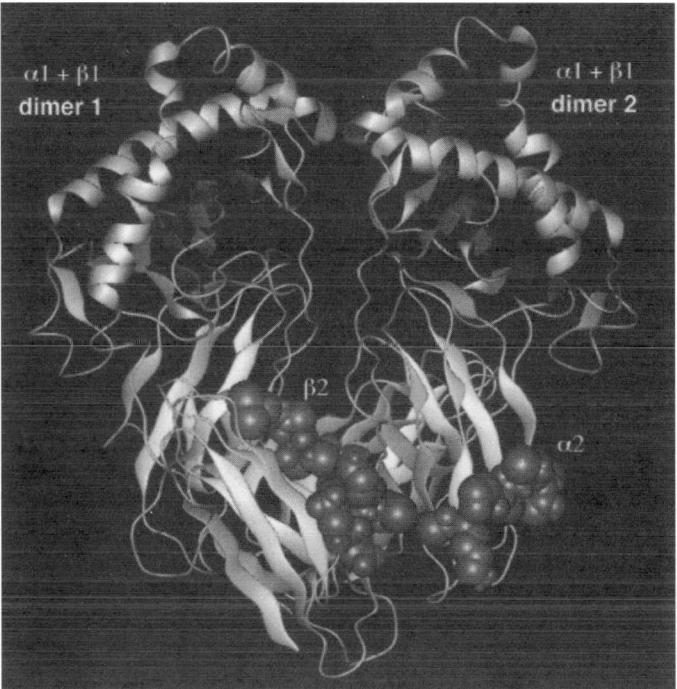

A   **B**

FIG. 4. A: Location of two sites controlling interaction of CD4 with MHC class II molecules (spherical residues in red). One site is within the β chain loop involving residues 137 to 143 (labeled β2) and is homologous to the primary CD8 interaction site with MHC class I molecules. The other is in the α2 domain of the α chain (labeled α2), positioned in a single MHC class II molecule so that it does not seem able to make contact with the same CD4 molecule as that involved in binding to the β2 site. **B:** In the view shown here, two class II αβ heterodimers (dimer 1 and dimer 2) are illustrated in the crystallographic dimer of dimers first reported by Brown et al. (80), showing that the β2 site from one class II dimer now is adjacent to the α2 site from the second class II dimer. This may indicate that the two sites are seen as a conjoint surface by a CD4 molecule, which would aid in stabilizing TCR oligomers in a signaling complex.

such a way that the side chains of bound peptides might influence the strength of association (99,100). As a result of interaction primarily outside the binding groove with these more conserved regions of the class II molecule, allelic polymorphism plays a lesser role than in presentation of peptides, although an effect of such variation can be observed. The interactions with MHC class II molecules of viral superantigens, such as the mouse mammary tumor virus-encoded *orf* proteins, have not been as extensively analyzed, but it is likely that they too interact with class II largely outside the peptide-binding groove.

Biologic Implications of the Chemical Nature of MHC Molecule–Peptide Interaction

Various biologic properties of antigen presentation to T cells can readily be understood from these new molecular insights into peptide–MHC molecule interaction and structure. In particular, the allele specificity of T-cell antigen recognition can be seen to comprise a sum of three distinct effects of MHC molecule polymorphism. One is the role of side-chain differences along the top of the α helices bordering the exposed residues of the peptide; the recent solutions of the structures of MHC class I–TCR complexes shows that MHC polymorphism in this region can directly influence the binding of the TCR. Even when allelic changes might allow some binding to still occur, alterations in the orientation of the specific combining (CDR3) region of the TCR due to the allelic substitutions could interfere with interactions with exposed peptide side chains (66,67,101,102). Thus, even if two MHC molecules bound identical peptides in the same conformation, allelic differences in these exposed regions would restrict recognition. There are not many fully exposed residues of this type with extensive variation among alleles of MHC molecules, but such differences do exist, and the partially exposed side chains of residues pointing into the binding site from the helices can participate in regulating TCR fit.

Second, there is the role of allelic differences within the binding site, especially those affecting the size and chemical characteristics of the various pockets, that regulate the ability of particular peptides to be effectively bound to a given allelic MHC product. Among all the peptides produced from a given protein antigen, allelically distinct MHC molecules tend to bind different ones. This quantitative effect of allelic differences on the binding of available peptides from a protein underlies the determinant selection principle suggested by Rosenthal (103) and Benacerraf (19) to account for both allele-restricted antigen responses and IR gene function. It is clear that a T cell specific for the exposed residues of one peptide–MHC complex would be unlikely to have a high affinity for a different peptide–MHC complex, even if the allelic MHC molecules binding the two peptides did not differ in exposed side chains. This binding and presentation of distinct peptides account at least in part for what is seen as allele-specific antigen presentation. In addition, self proteins will give rise to peptides that when complexed with MHC molecules will lead to self-tolerance in the T-cell compartment (104) (see Chapters 10 and 20). Foreign proteins that differ at only a few positions from these self proteins will give rise to only one or a few peptides differing from self and thus in principle can still be seen by available functional T cells. With such a limited number of peptides potentially available to stimulate a response, it is likely that the particular MHC alleles present in a single individual might fail to effectively bind any of these nonself peptides, giving rise to the nonresponder state. As expected from

this explanation of IR gene function, such deficits are more rarely seen with proteins differing extensively from self.

A third effect of polymorphism on T-cell responses is a qualitative one. Some changes in the binding region of the MHC molecule will not prevent the binding of certain peptides in a quantitative sense, but they will change how the peptide is bound, that is, the relationship of specific side chains to the exposed structural features of the MHC; alternatively, the binding could also alter the conformation of the MHC molecule in comparison with other MHC molecules of identical primary protein sequence associated with different peptides, as seen with the K^b molecule and a Sendai versus vesicular stomatitis virus peptide pair (63). An example of the first case is a change in a residue pointing up into the binding site from the central part of the β-strand floor. Such a residue would not be available for direct TCR interaction, but it could distort the shape of a bound peptide compared with an allelic MHC molecule with a difference only at this strand position. Both could bind the same amount of the same peptide, but the actual conformation of the surface available for interaction with the TCR could be different in a significant way (22). This emphasizes that linear amino acid sequence limits but does not fully determine the true antigenic structure of peptide antigens: this structure is only acquired after binding to the MHC molecule and is dependent on properties of the MHC protein to which binding occurs. Thus, the same peptide can be considered a different antigen when bound to two distinct MHC molecules. TCR recognition is thus not independent of conformation; it just does not depend on the conformation the antigenic peptide possessed as part of the original protein from which it was derived.

IDENTIFICATION AND CHARACTERISTICS OF PEPTIDES NATURALLY ASSOCIATED WITH CLASS I AND CLASS II MOLECULES

Major advances in our understanding of the details of peptide interactions with MHC molecules have come from the development of methods for size and sequence analysis of the peptides eluted from MHC molecules purified from living normal or infected cells (Fig. 5), as well as from in vitro binding studies involving synthetic peptides (105), combinatorial peptide libraries (106), or phage peptide display (107). These methods have permitted the determination of the lengths of naturally processed peptides, the identification of the source proteins for many of these peptides, and the discovery of preferred chemical structures in peptides binding to particular MHC allelic products. They also have allowed the rapid characterization of peptide antigens derived from a pathogen and bound to the MHC molecules of the infected cell being studied and the identification of self peptides or mutant peptides as tumor-associated antigens (108–112). The chemical characteristics of eluted peptides have provided a greater understanding of the role of the characteristic allelic polymorphism of MHC class I and class II molecules in selective antigen presentation, and knowledge of the source proteins of the bound peptides has given insight into the antigen-processing and peptide-loading pathways within the cell. The study of large numbers of variant synthetic peptides and of peptide libraries in particular has provided enough data to allow the construction of algorithms for predicting the binding strength of each peptide sequence within a protein to a particular MHC class I or class II allele and for identifying potential binding sequences in protein data bases.

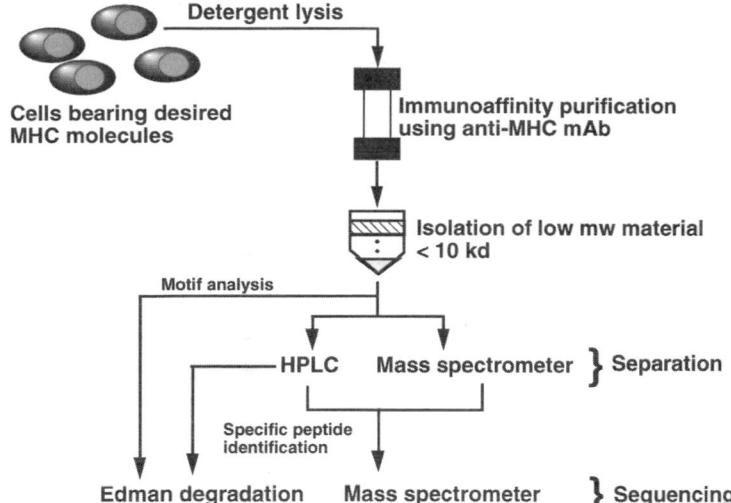

FIG. 5. Technique for elution, identification, and sequencing of MHC-associated peptides. The diagram shows how MHC molecules from a chosen cell source are obtained by detergent lysis and affinity chromatography on immobilized anti-MHC molecule monoclonal antibody. The recovered MHC molecules are denatured by treatment with acid, and the stripped peptides are separated from the larger MHC chains (and β2m in the case of class I) by filtration. Either the peptide pool is sequenced as a whole, to look for dominant motif or anchor residues at particular points in the sequence, or individual peptides are identified and isolated using HPLC with or without mass spectrometry. The individual peptides are then sequenced by Edman degradation or mass spectrometry. Motifs can be discerned in the pooled sequences from many individual peptides, and source proteins can be identified from the separate sequences. Peptides of biologic interest can be preidentified before sequencing by testing individual fractions of the HPLC separation for the ability to stimulate a specific primed T-cell population.

Peptides Bound by Class I Molecules

The known amino acid sequence of the HLA-A2 heavy chain or of β2m could not account for some portions of the electron density maps of HLA-A2 crystals (60). The location of this extra density within the presumed peptide-binding groove, in addition to the heterogeneous nature of the material, was most consistent with it representing multiple peptides that had remained associated with the class I protein throughout the immunoaffinity purification and crystallization steps. This indicated that the interaction of peptide with class I was very stable, and that it might be possible to purify class I proteins and then elute the bound peptides in suitable quantity for direct chemical analysis. The initial tests of this prediction involved functional assays of the eluted peptides. As diagrammed in Fig. 5, Rammensee and colleagues isolated large amounts of mouse MHC class I protein using monoclonal antibodies, then eluted bound peptides with acid. The eluted material with low molecular weight (<10 kDa) was subjected to separation using reversed-phase high-performance liquid chromatography (HPLC), and the HPLC fractions were then tested for their ability to sensitize cells to become targets for specific cytotoxic T cells. Discrete fractions from the HPLC gradient separation were able to sensitize the target cells, and different fractions had activity in this assay when T cells of distinct specificity were used as effector cells (113,114). These data provided clear evidence that biologically active, and presumably intact, peptides could be recovered from class I molecules after natural intracellular processing and binding and suggested that if sufficient material could be obtained, it would be possible to chemically characterize the recovered peptides. An unexpected observation was made in the course of these studies. When one looked for specific peptides usually associated with a particular class I molecule in cells synthesizing the known source proteins but lacking the relevant class I molecule, such peptides could not be found (115). Thus, the accumulation of a detectable amount of the specific short peptides found stably associated with class I molecules required those class I molecules to be present and to capture the peptide. Otherwise, such peptides appear to be degraded too rapidly to reach a steady-state level of even one to two copies per cell.

The first application of the elution approach to the identification of a specific naturally processed viral antigenic peptide did not involve direct sequencing of the eluted peptide but rather the use of the characteristic HPLC elution position of a naturally processed influenza hemagglutinin determinant to identify a synthetic peptide with identical chromatographic properties. This peptide corresponded to a nonamer within the stretch of amino acids of the hemagglutinin molecule previously shown to contain the T-cell determinant recognized by the indicator T-cell clone (116). A refinement of this approach involved the application of microsequencing to peptides eluted from isolated H-2Kb molecules of metabolically radiolabeled cells infected with vesicular stomatitis virus, which showed an octamer with tyrosines at positions 3 and 5 and leucine at position 8, corresponding to a core sequence present in synthetic peptides already known to be capable of sensitizing cells for recognition by vesicular stomatitis virus–specific, H-2Kb–restricted CTLs (117).

Several distinct methodologies subsequently have been used to gather sufficient data to identify common structural characteristics of the peptides bound to a single allele of class I molecule. Falk et al. (118) subjected pools of peptides eluted from single class I alleles to Edman degradation. Although unique sequences were not obtained from these heterogeneous mixes, particular amino acids gave very strong signals at specific positions, and the sequencing signals did not usually extend beyond position 9. The occurrence of strong signals at a given position in the sequence indicated that the NH2 termini were a fixed number of amino acids from these abundant, shared residues in each peptide. The predominant residues could be found in comparable positions in most peptides previously identified as being presented by the relevant class I molecule. This gave rise to the concept of motif or anchor amino acids important in promoting peptide binding to a particular allele of class I, and such residues identified by sequence analysis have been found to correspond to the residues whose side chains occupy the major (usually polymorphic) pockets in the class I–binding site. Thus, there is satisfying concordance between the molecular images we have of peptide–MHC class I interactions and the functional behavior of class I molecules in cells in terms of selective capture of peptides with particular chemical structures. This correspondence extends beyond the allele-specific motifs that involve binding to the polymorphic pockets of the class I–binding groove. The lack of strong sequencing signals beyond nine amino acids in the pools of eluted peptide fits well with the eight- and nine-residue length of the specific viral peptides found associated with class I molecules, and with the crystallographic picture of bound peptides with anchored N and C termini making hydrogen bonds to the conserved residues at either end of the binding groove. Other techniques also have been used to identify, characterize, and sequence large numbers of individual peptides associated with particular allelic forms of class I. In one approach, HPLC-purified single peptide peaks have been sequenced by chemical degradation. An even more powerful method has been developed involving microcapillary HPLC and electrospray ionization–tandem mass spectrometry to evaluate both the complexity of bound peptides as well as their sequences. This methodology suggested that perhaps 2,000 different peptides copurify with HLA-A2 recovered from a clonal cell source and permitted the sequencing of numerous individual peptide species (119). Used in combination with T-cell detection of antigen-containing HPLC fractions, this powerful mass spectroscopic method has permitted the identification of human tumor antigens (112).

More recently, several investigators have analyzed the binding of individual synthetic peptides of a fixed length containing variations in the amino acids at each position, or of complex peptide libraries to particular MHC class I molecules. The methods used to measure binding have involved labeled peptides and competition assays, as well as the more sophisticated method of surface plasmon resonance, which permits assessment of the kinetics of binding as well as affinity of association (120). These studies have generated a large body of quantitative data relating peptide sequence to strength of interaction with MHC class I molecules. Together with the analysis of pooled and individual sequences of peptides eluted from the class I molecules of living cells, these data have allowed the description of many motifs consisting of particular amino acids at specific positions within a peptide of a given length that together lead to optimal binding to a particular MHC class I allelic product (see Chapters 8 and 19). These findings also have been used to produce computer programs that calculate the likely strength of association of any sequence of amino acids with the MHC class I molecule whose ligand binding has been analyzed in this manner. Such algorithms take into account not only the positive contributions of the preferred residues that the crystallographic studies have shown occupy specific pockets of the MHC class I molecule, but also the negative or inhibitory effects of inappropriate residues at these or other positions in the peptide. It is now recognized that interfering effects contribute substantially to the specificity of peptide binding (121,122), and their inclusion in the algorithms has markedly improved the accuracy of the predictions made by these programs. These algorithms have proven very useful for limiting the number of synthetic peptides that need to be made to identify the amino acid sequence from within a known antigenic protein recognized by a particular T cell together with a given MHC class I molecule, although it should be noted that not all biologically relevant peptides are the best binding peptides within a protein sequence, and analysis of only the top predicted sequences can lead to failure in identification of the active antigenic peptide (123).

The isolation and sequencing of specific peptides bound to class I molecules of living cells also has allowed determination of the source proteins of many of the isolated peptides, based on homology or identity to sequences contained in DNA or protein data bases (Table 1). Of the peptides whose source protein could be unambiguously identified by this approach, most are from abun-

TABLE 1. *Sources of peptides found naturally associated with class I and class II MHC molecules*

Class I associated	Class II associated
Ribosomal protein 60S (cytosolic)	Retroviral envelope (integral membrane protein)
Heat-shock protein HSP89α (cytosolic)	MHC Class II Eα (integral membrane protein)
Heat-shock protein HSP89β (cytosolic)	Invariant chain (integral membrane protein)
Elongation factor 2 (cytosolic)	Bovine serum albumin (prevalent serum component)
Helicase (nuclear)	Apolipoprotein (prevalent serum component)
Histone H3 (nuclear)	Transferrin receptor (integral membrane protein)
Signal sequence (ER)	MHC class I heavy chain (integral membrane protein)
Leukocyte common antigen (endogenously synthesized membrane protein)	Immunoglobulin heavy chain (integral membrane protein)
Phosphoglycerate kinase (cytosolic)	Na+/K+ ATPase (integral membrane protein)

dant cytoplasmic or nuclear proteins, as expected from the general model in which such intracellular proteins serve as the major source of peptide for presentation by the class I pathway. Exceptions to this general finding in normal, and especially mutant, cell lines will be discussed in a later section.

Peptides Associated with Class II Molecules

The same methods used to analyze class I–associated peptides have been used to study the peptides naturally bound to class II molecules. Immunoaffinity-purified class II molecules have been treated with acid and the eluted peptides analyzed by Edman degradation or mass spectroscopy (124–127). Such analyses have shown that each MHC allele gives a characteristic profile of eluted peptides, consistent with the role of allelic polymorphism in determinant selection. In contrast to the situation with class I, class II bound peptides are longer and more heterogeneous in size, ranging in length from 12 to more than 24 residues. This heterogeneity is not simply the result of differing lengths for peptides derived from distinct proteins but also reflects the capture of nested peptide sets from a single protein, that is, peptides that share a core of amino acids but have different overall lengths and N and C termini. Both amino- and carboxy-terminal extensions are observed, consistent with the crystallographic findings that class II has an open structure that allows the ends of these longer peptides to extend out of the binding groove, and hence, for the central region of the long peptide to lie in the binding groove without substantial kinking.

Because class II–associated peptides with common core sequences show staggered NH2 termini, sequencing of mixed pools of eluted peptides has been somewhat less successful in identifying motifs or anchor residues, although some notable progress has still been made by this approach. One major finding arising from the pooled sequence method has been the higher than predicted frequency of detection of proline at the +2 position (128). Because many amino peptidases fail to cleave further when the +2 position of the remaining peptide sequence is proline, these data suggest that the ragged ends of class II molecule–associated peptides are generated by the action of such peptidases on longer peptide sequences already bound to MHC class II molecules, a proposition for which evidence continues to accumulate (129). However, most analysis of class II–associated peptides has involved sequencing of distinct peptide species after HPLC or mass spectroscopic isolation, with the resulting data aligned by sliding the core regions of the overlapping sequences with respect to one another. A much larger data set addressing both preferred and inhibitory residues has been generated using large numbers of individual synthetic peptides with the entire set together containing multiple substitutions at each peptide position (105,130) or using peptide libraries displayed on filamentous phage (107). Using these methods, it has been possible to identify motifs for optimal peptide binding to particular class II alleles. These generally involve only two to four residues from among a core region of seven to nine residues. The motif residues have been shown to occupy major or minor pockets in the crystallographic structure of the corresponding class II molecule.

The sources of peptides bound to class II molecules fit with the general model of class II function and the class II processing pathway, in that the predominant identifiable species are derived from proteins with ready access to the endocytic pathway (Table 1). This implies that intracellular proteins access the class II pathway inefficiently compared with the class I pathway, although some apparent exceptions have been reported. It remains to be determined whether these latter exceptional peptides are derived from cytoplasmic proteins that access the endocytic pathway from within the cell, bind to class II in early parts of the secretory pathway rather than in endosomes, or arise from the endocytic uptake of cytoplasmic proteins after cell death in the mass cultures used to provide the source of MHC class II molecules for the peptide analysis. As for class I molecules, differences are observed in the spectrum of peptides associated with class II molecules from normal and mutant cell lines with altered antigen presentation, and these will be discussed in a later section.

PEPTIDES AS INTEGRAL PARTS OF MHC CLASS I AND CLASS II MOLECULAR STRUCTURE

The visualization of peptides in class I MHC molecule crystals, the ability to nearly quantitatively recover peptides from MHC molecules even after the harsh treatments involved in affinity purification, and the very slow dissociation rates measured for MHC class II–synthetic peptide complexes all gave evidence of the tight nature of peptide–MHC molecule association. Nevertheless, until 1989, well after the MHC class I crystallographic structure was solved, MHC molecules were considered to be fully folded proteins with stable binding sites into which peptides fit. A major change in thinking accompanied the studies of Townsend and colleagues on a mutant mouse lymphoma cell (RMA-S) that synthesized normal amounts of class I heavy chains and β2m but had only low steady-state surface expression of class I molecules (131,132). Biochemical studies showed that these cells were defective in postsynthesis assembly of heavy chain–β2m complexes and in the export of class I from the endoplasmic reticulum (ER), explaining the low surface class I level. Although the RMA-S cells were deficient in presentation of antigen produced during active viral infection as might have been expected from their low class I expression, they were remarkably effective in presenting synthetic peptide. The addition of antigenic peptide

was found to increase markedly the surface expression of class I molecules in strict accord with the known ability of the class I allele to present the particular added peptide to T cells. A significant increase in stably assembled heavy chain–β2m complexes reactive with α1α2 conformation-specific antibodies could be detected in detergent lysates of such peptide-treated cells. Although this increase in assembled and properly folded class I molecules actually resulted from peptide binding after cell lysis, rather than peptide entry into the cells during culture as originally thought (133), the investigators nonetheless correctly concluded that peptide was responsible for actively promoting stable assembly of heavy chains and β2m into a class I molecule with a native conformation. They also suggested that RMA-S showed poor expression of class I due to a defect in supplying the peptides needed for such assembly of the class I heavy chains and β2m in the ER. These seminal experiments made clear that despite their contribution to our detailed understanding of the chemical basis for MHC class I binding of peptides, the analysis of static crystal structures had failed to uncover a critical dynamic aspect of the biochemical properties of MHC class I molecules essential to understanding their biology.

Changes in Structure and Assembly State Accompanying Peptide Binding by Class I Molecules

The observations made with RMA-S have provided the framework for a large number of subsequent studies that have given additional insight into the relationship among peptide, β2m, and heavy chain association in the generation of functional class I molecules expressed at the cell surface for T-cell recognition. The ability of peptides known to bind to particular class I alleles to increase surface expression on cells with high-level synthesis but low surface expression has been confirmed for numerous mouse and human molecules, using mutant cells deficient in their ability to present naturally processed antigens (134), normal cells that appear unable to provide adequate peptide to fully load certain class I alleles, such as H-2L^d (135), or embryonic cells whose differentiation state affects the peptide-loading process (136).

Inhibitors of protein export or synthesis prevent increases in surface class I upon peptide addition to cells with the RMA-S phenotype. This indicates that the primary mechanism underlying the increased expression is preservation on the cell surface of molecules that normally reach the plasma membrane and are either rapidly cleared or irreversibly denatured under physiologic conditions, rather than the induction of folding among a large steady-state cohort of nonnative, surface-resident molecules. This is consistent with the idea that the class I molecules made by such cells are unstable; even if they reach the cell membrane as heavy chain–β2m dimers, they appear to dissociate rapidly and undergo permanent denaturation. Evidence for this denaturation model comes from experiments showing that the mutant RMA-S cells have enhanced surface class I expression when cultured at room temperature (137). The molecules that accumulate on such cells are quickly lost to serologic detection after the temperature is increased to 37°C, indicating that the class I molecules accumulating on the surface at room temperature are thermally labile. Similarly, in cell lysates the class I–β2m complexes that accumulate when RMA-S cells are cultured at room temperature rapidly denature when brought to 37°C. These data support a model in which class I–β2m association is thermodynamically unstable in the absence of proper peptide binding. Association is prolonged at lower temperatures, preserving the heavy-chain structure. Increased temperature causes the rapid dissociation of the complexes and heavy-chain denaturation (class I molecule "melting").

Peptide-induced stabilization of the class I heavy chain–β2m complex is optimal with short peptides identical in length and sequence to those found naturally associated with class I isolated from intact infected cells (138). These data indicate that very efficient selection of optimal peptides occurs in the cell and that the ability of a peptide to stabilize the class I structure is an important feature in selecting peptides for presentation to T cells. This ability of class I molecules to bind preferentially short peptides of an appropriate length and composition has been demonstrated graphically in several studies by examining the peptides recovered from class I molecules after exposure to complex peptide mixtures (106). It also can be seen in the dramatic effect of serum proteases on the ability of certain long peptides to stimulate T cells: the proteases produce small quantities of properly trimmed peptides that are efficiently captured by available class I binding sites (139,140). The potency of such long peptide preparations in sensitization of target cells decreases by several orders of magnitude if the protease is removed or inactivated, due in large measure to the poor ability of such peptides to be stably bound by class I. In fact, much of the bioactivity in many synthetic peptide preparations in which the designed sequence is longer than the optimal length has been traced to low levels of contaminating short peptides (116,141).

These various observations emphasize that physiologically stable class I molecules are actually trimers of heavy chains, β2m, and peptide. As expected from this conclusion, not only is peptide an essential contributor to the establishment of a stable heavy chain–β2m interaction, but the availability of free β2m contributes to enhanced binding of peptide to the heavy chain. Thus, there is a mutual stabilization of heavy-chain interaction with peptide and

β2m upon binding of both components (142). Consistent with this, several groups have shown that free β2m substantially contributes to effective presentation of exogenously added peptides (143–145). From these and other studies using either analysis of class I molecules in cell-free lysates or on cell surfaces, the concept has emerged of equilibrium reactions among the three components of the mature class I trimer (heavy chain, β2m, and peptide) during assembly (Fig. 6). Both binary reactions involving the heavy chain (heavy chain–β2m and heavy chain–peptide) have been demonstrated, but the apparent lifetime of the binary pairs is low compared with the trimeric complex. Thus, peptide can conform class I heavy chains in the absence of β2m, but this requires high peptide concentrations and most of the resulting molecules are unstable. Conversely, high concentrations of free β2m can preserve class I heavy-chain folding, but again, the structure is relatively unstable, although clearly longer lived than most heavy chain–peptide complexes. Peptide and β2m synergize in forming a long-lived, properly folded complex (138,143,146). This has been demonstrated most dramatically in studies using fully denatured heavy chains and β2m from cells or bacteria. Development of properly folded, stable class I molecules was found to be dependent on the addition of specific peptide (147). These latter data, along with refolding studies on cell surface molecules, also establish that intracellular chaperones are not essential to proper folding and assembly, although it is likely that such proteins enhance the efficiency with which this occurs, at a minimum by preventing irreversible heavy-chain misfolding and possible aggregation before association with a suitable peptide. These results have obvious implications for our understanding of the capture of peptides by class I molecules within cells. The relationship of peptide structure to stability of the class I molecule also bears on the lifetime of exported class I (and in turn their continued availability for recognition by T cells) and the loading of class I with exogenous peptides.

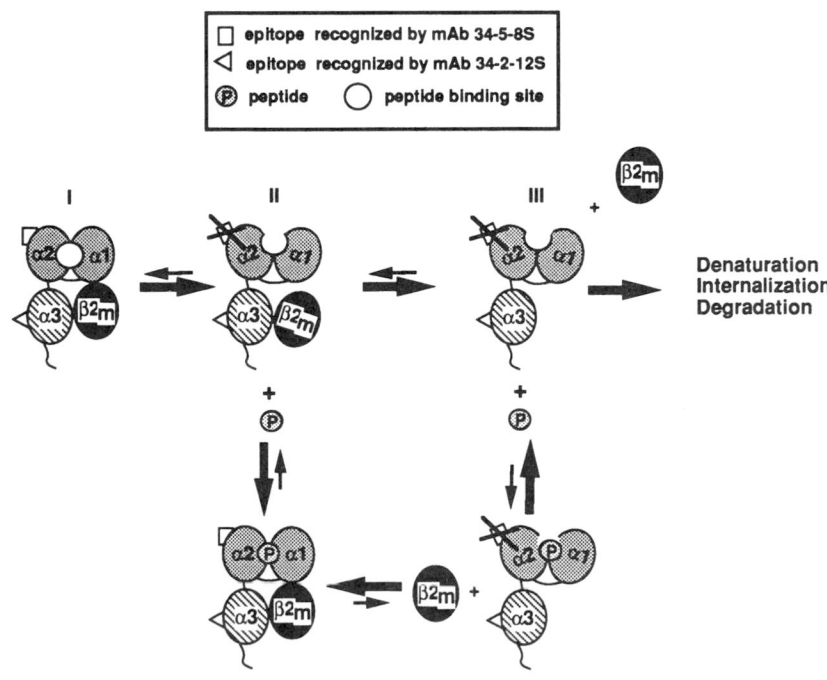

FIG. 6. Reversible equilibrium reactions among class I heavy chains, β2m, and peptide in assembly and denaturation of MHC class I complexes. The diagram shows the possible binary and ternary associations and reaction pathways among the three components of mature class I molecules. Heavy arrows indicate favored reactions, light arrows unfavored reactions. Adapted with permission (146).

Relationships Between Peptide Binding and MHC Class II Molecule Biochemical Behavior

The demonstration that peptides made a critical contribution to the assembly and structural stability of mature class I molecules raised the question of whether peptide plays a similar role in class II assembly and stability. Several groups had noted in the 1970s that isolated class II molecules remained associated as noncovalent dimers during sodium dadecyl sulfate–polyacrylamide gel electrophoresis (SDS-PAGE) if the samples were not heated before application to the gel (148,149). This indicated that, despite lacking covalent interchain bonds, the class II α and β chains were tightly associated in the mature state, much more so than class I heavy chain–β2m dimers. Mild denaturation sufficient to begin to elute peptides from the class II molecules changed this gel mobility and retarded migration without a loss of the dimer state, suggesting a partial unfolding of the molecule. Stronger denaturation resulted in molecules running as separate α and β chains upon electrophoresis (150). These data suggested a possible relationship between peptide binding and dimer stability, but these studies could not distinguish between the loss of peptide leading to the change in dimer behavior, or the denaturation of the class II molecule leading to a loss of peptide binding.

This issue was finally resolved by experiments that showed a loss of the SDS-resistant dimer structure upon acid stripping of peptide from mature class II molecules and the recovery of the stable dimer state upon addition of synthetic peptides known to bind to the class II allele under investigation (151). These in vitro results were consistent with data obtained from ex vivo studies of intracellular maturation of class II molecules. These experiments established that newly synthesized class II molecules dissociated in SDS buffer without sample heating. Several hours after synthesis, however, a variable fraction of these same dimers became SDS-denaturation resistant, but only under culture conditions known to permit peptide generation and loading (152,153). This established that, as with class I molecules, peptide contributed to the stabilization of class II dimers (Fig. 7). However, the precise nature of the contribution was different. For class II, the peptide was not needed for maintenance of chain association at physiologic temperature and pH, as it was for class I heavy chain–β2m association.

Some studies have shown that not all class II dimers that are associated with peptide possess the SDS-stable phenotype (154,155). These results may indicate that the dimer state that resists SDS dissociation results from two distinct effects of peptide. One is a contribution to dimer stability by interaction of the peptide with portions of both the α and β chains. The second component appears to involve a change in the structure of the class II αβ dimer per se that adds to the intrinsic stability of the class II molecule. As a general rule, class II molecules that have never bound peptide dissociate in the SDS gel system; dimers resistant to SDS dissociation contain peptide; however, dimers that come apart into α and β chains in such gels may nevertheless have contained peptide or another ligand occupying the peptide-binding domain (e.g., invariant chain or a fragment of this protein) before dissociation in the SDS buffer. Thus, the method is useful for establishing that peptide binding has occurred, based on the presence of stable dimers, but the absence of such dimers cannot prove a lack of peptide binding or binding site occupancy. The limitations of this assay must be remembered when evaluating the results of experiments in which this approach is used to identify the sites or extent of peptide acquisition by class II molecules within the cell.

Differences in the role played by peptide in class I versus class II MHC protein structure are apparently related in significant measure to the dissimilar domain organization of the two molecules, especially the presence of transmembrane segments in both chains of class II. These transmembrane regions have been found to contain structural motifs that promote α–β chain interaction shortly after synthesis and probably help to maintain chain association even in the absence of peptide (49). The related but distinct effects of peptide on the biochemical characteristics of class I versus class II molecules have important implications for understanding the mechanisms and sites of peptide capture by each class of MHC molecule.

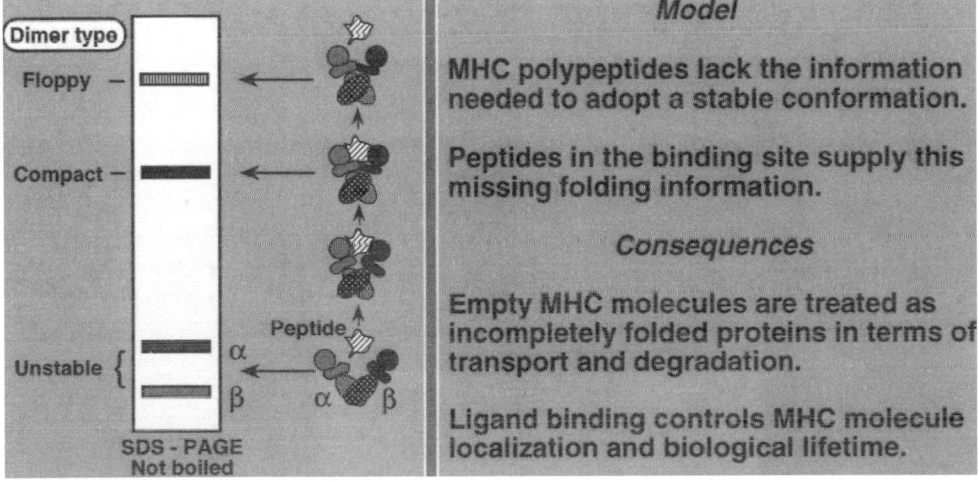

FIG. 7. Schematic representation of the relationship between class II peptide binding, structural states, and SDS PAGE behavior. An idealized image of SDS-PAGE of purified class II molecules run without sample heating and the types of MHC class II molecules giving rise to the gel bands. The text describes the functional consequences of MHC class II peptide–dependent folding.

Kinetic Aspects of MHC Molecule Interaction with Peptides

The realization that peptide does not achieve stable interaction with MHC molecules by binding to a preformed, static site, together with the recognition that most binding regions of normal, expressed MHC molecules are already tightly occupied with peptide and an appreciation of the trimolecular nature of the binding process for class I, all contributed to explaining a number of puzzling features of peptide–MHC molecule interaction observed during attempts to measure the kinetic and quantitative parameters of the association process.

Initial attempts to measure binding of labeled peptides to MHC class I molecules were largely unsuccessful, giving at best occupancy of less than 1% of the theoretical level at the end of the incubation period (156). In retrospect, these difficulties can be seen to derive primarily from the use of synthetic peptides longer than the optimal lengths that are required for effective binding to class I, in part from the high peptide occupancy of mature class I molecules expressed by normal cells, in part from the selective isolation of the most tightly associated peptide–MHC class I complexes during affinity purification, and in part from the failure to provide adequate $\beta 2m$ during the binding phase. These problems were largely solved when the empty or readily "emptied" state of class I molecules produced by cells such as RMA-S or the human cell line T2, by bacteria, or by transfected insect cells was recognized and such molecules were used for the binding reactions, when eight- to 10-residue peptides were used as probes, and, in some cases, when excess $\beta 2m$ was added to the binding reaction. Under these conditions, binding is rapid, although slower than expected for true diffusion-limited reactions. Whether this is related to the conformational flexibility of the peptide in solution, so that it is in a suitable state for binding only a fraction of the time, or to the need for the class I heavy chain to undergo a conformational change during the binding reaction, or both, has not been fully determined. Length changes in the peptide probe do not seem to make large differences in measured association rates. However, length and chemical composition of the peptide have distinct influences on the dissociation rate. Optimal peptides resembling those found associated spontaneously in the cell with a given class I molecule show the slowest dissociation rates, with some peptide–MHC class I combinations surviving for hours even at 37°C in the absence of free peptide or $\beta 2m$ (157). Longer peptides, or those with less optimal chemical compositions, dissociate rapidly with a half-life ($t_{1/2}$) often of less than 30 minutes. The rates of loss of peptide or dissociation of bound $\beta 2m$ are similar, emphasizing the interdependence of peptide and $\beta 2m$ association with heavy chains. These differences are clearly great enough to have major impact on the biologic function of the peptide–MHC complex because the shorter lived combinations would not accumulate to high levels on the cell surface, limiting T-cell recognition. In addition, these results raise the possibility that longer peptides bound to class I, then released relatively rapidly at the cell surface, give rise to empty sites that can be occupied by exogenous peptides.

Peptide binding to MHC class II molecules was more readily demonstrated, although here too the occupancy in early experiments never reached a theoretical 100%. Measurement of peptide binding to isolated class II molecules using equilibrium dialysis resulted in a calculated equilibrium constant of 1 to 2 μmol/L (26). In typical circumstances (e.g., antibody–antigen interactions), this would indicate a rapid dissociation rate for the complex. However, it was known that peptide remained functionally associated with class II–bearing cells

for days. This paradox was solved by Buus et al. (27), who found that the generation of slowly dissociating class II–peptide complexes with a half-life of more than 1 day was itself a slow process with an apparent association rate of 1 mol/L per second. Thus the equilibrium constant was a result of a combination of a very slow apparent "on" rate and an equally slow "off" rate.

Why should this be? Sadegh-Nasseri and McConnell (158) demonstrated that fast, specific peptide–class II association could occur, with a $t_{1/2}$ of approximately 2 minutes. However, the complexes that rapidly formed also rapidly dissociated, with a $t_{1/2}$ of about 10 minutes. Long-lived complexes ($t_{1/2} > 30$ hours) were produced slowly under these same conditions. These investigators concluded that the limiting step in producing long-lived complexes involved an infrequent structural transition in the MHC class II–peptide complex that was necessary for attaining the stable binding state, a conclusion entirely consistent with our current knowledge of the changes in class II biochemical behavior accompanying peptide binding. Again, however, these data did not fit with common-sense notions of the likely biology of peptide binding in cells. The slow rate of stable peptide binding seemed inconsistent with an even modestly efficient capture of processed antigen during the passage of class II to the cell surface after synthesis. Although one possible solution to the kinetic problem posed by these results is the presence of specific helper molecules that catalyze peptide loading in vivo and DM may play such a kinetic role (see below), the pioneering studies of Jensen suggested another contributing factor. He simulated passage of class II molecules through the acid environment of endosomes, in which processing of antigen for loading onto class II molecules is believed to take place. Simultaneous but not sequential exposure of class II molecules to pH in the physiologic range of 5 to 6 and to specific peptide led to dramatic increases in functional peptide presentation, which were later shown to correlate with increases in total bound peptide (159,160). Application of this approach by many investigators has shown that low pH often, though not always, accelerates peptide loading of class II, with effective association rates reduced to a few minutes from the several hours observed at neutral pH (151,161–163). Part of the effect of low pH is removal of previously bound peptide from already occupied class II molecules, an effect that complicates kinetic measurements (164) but that can be overcome through the use of functionally empty class II molecules for these measurements (163,165) under which conditions an acceleration of class II loading of certain peptides can still be observed. The augmenting effect of low pH on class II binding of peptides makes physiologic sense because this is the environment in which class II is likely to find itself when it has access to peptide produced by proteolysis in the endocytic pathway.

The distinctive chemistry underlying the generic peptide-binding capacity of MHC class I versus class II molecules may play a central role in the differences between the two molecules in the apparent rate of stable peptide binding. MHC class I molecules use conserved residues to hydrogen bond to the free N and C termini of peptides. This provides a "molecular ruler" that helps select for stable binding to optimal length peptides. This feature of class I molecules plays a key role in fostering loading of class I with peptides derived from cytosolic processing and not with short segments of proteins undergoing folding in the endoplasmic reticulum. Because these conserved binding regions can help place the peptide in the proper register with respect to the pockets of the binding groove, anchor residue entry into these pockets can be facilitated and made more efficient, helping to attain a high likelihood of successful binding upon each interaction of the peptide with the MHC class I molecule. This high success rate translates into a fast on rate with stable binding.

For MHC class II molecules, generic binding occurs via main chain atoms and not the ends of the peptide, which can protrude for varying lengths out of the binding region. This makes it difficult to guide an interacting peptide into the proper frame such that the anchor residue's side chains are aligned with the pockets into which they must fit for stable binding. Instead, most peptide–MHC class II encounters will lead to binding with few if any pockets properly occupied and with most bonds made to the main chain of the sequence without regard to alignment along the peptide groove. This will lead to rapid but unstable occupancy upon most interactions of peptides and MHC class II molecules, as observed experimentally (166). Only rarely will the binding be in the proper frame and in such an orientation that pocket occupancy can occur without dissociation and rebinding being required. Thus, the rate of successful stable binding of ligand to MHC class II, and the formation of SDS-stable complexes if the peptide is capable of inducing this change of state, will be slow because optimal alignment of the two components (peptide and MHC class II molecule) is infrequent. The rate might be facilitated by low pH due to a conformational change (167) that interferes with hydrogen bonds to main chain atoms under these conditions, eliminating the potential to form loosely bound complexes that interfere with successive attempts at proper site occupancy. This also helps to focus the binding event on pocket engagement by anchor side chains, which promotes proper alignment throughout the peptide with the class II groove. As discussed later, DM may play a related role of keeping the asparagines too far apart to make simultaneous bonds to peptide main chains, again fostering binding in pockets.

BIOSYNTHESIS AND INTRACELLULAR TRANSPORT OF MHC CLASS I AND CLASS II MOLECULES

The Basic Pattern of Class I Biosynthesis

Class I heavy chains and β2m are both type 1 proteins and enter the ER via the signal-recognition and transport apparatus. The heavy chain associates rapidly with an ER resident protein variously termed p88/calnexin (168) or Ip90 (169). This molecule is a Ca^{2+}-sensitive protein that is associated with the signal sequence dependent translocation apparatus and has been reported to interact with a variety of membrane and some secreted proteins in the ER, including components of the T-cell and immunoglobulin receptors before the assembly of a complete receptor complex suitable for transport to the cell surface (170). Calnexin's binding to the class I heavy chain appears to involve both carbohydrate recognition and structural features of the protein chain itself (171,172). With human class I molecules, this chaperone dissociates from the heavy chain upon binding of β2m (173,174), at which time another ER chaperone protein, calreticulin, associates with the class I–β2m complex (175). In cells lacking β2m, class I heavy chains remain associated in the ER with calnexin, which may contribute to the inability of cells lacking β2m to express significant quantities of class I on their surface membrane (176). However, the requirement for β2m in class I transport is not absolute. A low level of certain class I heavy chains can be detected on the surface of cells lacking β2m expression (177,178). Most or all of these molecules lack numerous serologic epitopes characteristic of the same class I expressed in association with β2m, suggesting that they are in an alternative folding state.

Following B2m binding to the heavy chain, calnexin association is lost, and the complex interacts with another ER chaperone called *calreticulin*. In addition to this association with calreticulin, the heavy chain–β2m complex also associates with an MHC-encoded molecule called tapasin (175,179). This molecule in turn appears to play a role in the association of the peptide-free class I heavy chain–β2m complex with the molecular assembly in the ER membrane responsible for providing a source of antigenic peptides (179, 180). Once occupied with peptide, calreticulin and tapasin are no longer found associated with the class I complex, which exits the ER, then moves through the Golgi stacks to the trans-Golgi network and on to the cell surface by the default secretory pathway.

Overview of Class II Biosynthesis and Transport to the Plasma Membrane

The α and β subunits of MHC class II molecules can be found associated within 2 minutes of synthesis. This assembly appears to require certain conserved features of the transmembrane regions of these polypeptides. Under physiologic circumstances, the α and β chains do not coassemble alone but do so in the presence of invariant chain (Ii) (181), which is a nonpolymorphic type II membrane glycoprotein (NH_2 terminus in the cytoplasm, COOH terminus in the ER lumen) (182,183). Ii is not a single protein but a family of proteins generated by alternative splicing in the human, but not mouse, by alternative translational initiation (184). Thus, in humans there are four primary forms of Ii, called p31, p33, p41, and p43 (some investigators refer to these species as p33, p35, p43, and p45, respectively). p31 and p33 differ by 17 residues at the NH_2 terminus in the cytoplasm as a result of differential translation initiation, as do p41 and p43. The p31 versus p41 and p33 versus p43 forms differ by an alternatively spliced exon that adds a thyroglobulinlike domain to the protein (185).

Ii rapidly forms noncovalently associated trimers in the ER, and preformed class II αβ dimers either quickly associate with these trimers or the αβ heterodimers may assemble on the trimers themselves (186,187). MHC class II chains and non-class II associated Ii are themselves bound to calnexin, an association that is lost upon assembly of class II–Ii oligomers (188,189). After assembly of the αβIi complexes, these multimeric assemblies move out of the ER and through the Golgi stacks, undergoing formation of complex N- (and for Ii, O-) linked glycans and terminal sialation (190). These events take place within 30 to 60 minutes of initial class II biosynthesis. Significant accumulations of αβIi complexes are seen in the trans-Golgi network, then in the endocytic pathway rather than on the cell surface (191), where only a small number of such complexes can be found at any point in time (192,193). These complexes reside in endocytic vesicles for several (2 to 6) hours, after which class II dimers reach the surface free of Ii. Ii is removed from class II after egress from the trans-Golgi via a process that involves sequential COOH-terminal proteolytic cleavages (194). The removal of Ii from class II can be inhibited by agents that interfere with the function of acid proteases, such as leupeptin (an inhibitor of cysteine proteases) (194) and chloroquine (195), which raises endosomal/lysosomal pH.

The Intracellular Transport and Localization of Invariant Chain and MHC Class II Molecules

The accumulation of recently synthesized class II molecules in the endocytic pathway and the obvious importance of this phase of class II intracellular transport in antigen presentation has prompted careful study of class II localization and movement within the cell.

Steady-State Distribution of Class II Molecules

In transformed B cells and in activated macrophages, class II molecules can be detected in the ER, in Golgi stacks, in the trans-Golgi region, on the plasma membrane, and in intracellular vesicles. Some of these vesicles are early endosomes (196), but most are organelles ultrastructurally and histochemically related to late endosomes and lysosomes often termed MIIC (for MHC class II compartment) (Fig. 8) (197). In immature dendritic cells, a great deal of class II is found in intracellular vesicles with much less on the surface membrane, whereas more mature dendritic cells have little intracellular class II and stable, very high plasma membrane expression. These changes are consistent with the immature dendritic cell being in a state ready for efficient processing of newly acquired antigen and the mature cell being optimized for presentation at a later time of the processed peptide–MHC molecule complexes now resident on the cell membrane (198,199). The distribution of class II is thus clearly different in cells of distinct tissue type and even varies among cells of nominally identical histologic origin according to their state of differentiation.

Steady-State Invariant Chain Distribution

The human Iip33 form is retained in the ER due to an amino acid motif in the NH2-terminal segment of its cytoplasmic tail shared with the adenovirus E19 protein that mediates ER retention. Ii is usually produced in excess of class II in normal cells, and the association of p31 or p41 with p33 or p43 in trimers and higher molecular weight aggregates may contribute to retention of the p31 and p41 forms in the ER, where they undergo degradation to smaller, NH2-terminally cleaved forms.

In contrast, when not complexed with p33 or p43, varying proportions (5% to 20%) of the p31 form of human Ii, and the p31 and p41 forms of mouse Ii move through the Golgi complex and accumulate in vesicular structures (200–202). This localization depends on signals located primarily within the 30-residue NH2-terminal cytoplasmic tail involving critical dileucine motifs (203,204), as well as an undefined contribution of the transmembrane region (205). Deletion of 15 or more residues results in accumulation on the cell surface due to the removal of these endocytic targeting signals. These same truncations increase the proportion of Ii showing acquisition of endoH-resistant glycans, suggesting that this region of Ii plays a role in retarding the exit of Ii from the ER even when the E19-related retention signal is absent. The trimeric structure of

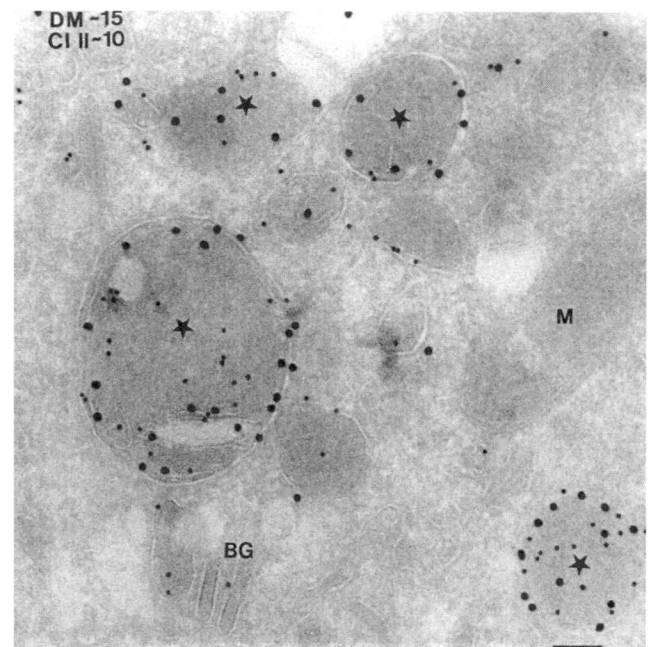

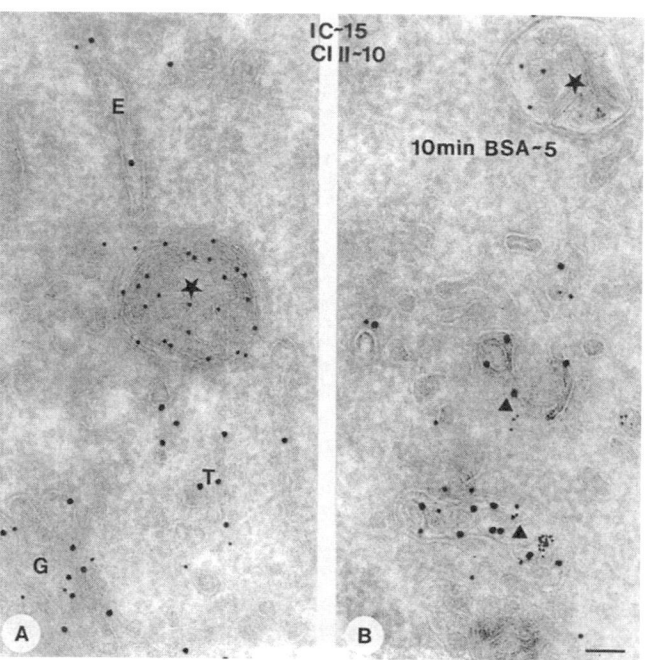

FIG. 8. A: Ultrathin cryosection of a human skin Langerhans cell, immunogold labeled for HLA-DM with 15 nm gold (DM-15) and for class II with 10 nm gold (CII-10). Several MIICs (*asterisks*) are labeled for class II, as well as for DM (primarily at the periphery). MIICs in Langerhans cells typically have electron-dense contents. BG, Birbeck granules; M, mitochondrion. Bar = 100 nm. **B:** Ultrathin cryosections of human B cells double-immunogold labeled with antibodies against the C-terminal domain of the invariant chain with 15 nm gold (IC-15) and class II with 10 nm gold (CII-10) (a). Labeling for invariant chain can be seen in the Golgi complex (G), the trans-Golgi network (T), and in the rough ER, whereas class II is primarily located in a multilaminar MIIC (*asterisk*). Note that the use of a C terminal–specific anti-invariant-chain antibody limits detection of proteolytically cleaved material in late endosomal/lysosomal organelles. (b) Before being processed for immunoelectron microscopy, the cell had endocytosed 5 nm gold particles derivatized with bovine serum albumin (BSA-5) for 10 minutes. The endocytosed BSA-gold particles are present in irregularly shaped multivesicular compartments, so-called early MIICs (*triangles*) that are strongly labeled for invariant-chain C terminus. The MIIC (*asterisk*) is only labeled for class II. Bar = 200 nm. (Images courtesy of Monique Kleijmeer and Hans. J. Geuze, Laboratory of Cell Biology, Medical School, Utrecht University, The Netherlands).

Ii also appears to contribute to the functioning of these tail signals, with two or more cytoplasmic regions functioning much more efficiently than only one tail in promoting Ii endocytic localization (206).

At high levels of Ii expression, Ii is found predominantly in an unusual cohort of intracellular vesicles (large vesicular structures [LVS] or macrosomes) (202). The most remarkable feature of these macrosomes is that they alter the rate of endocytic flow from the early endosomal sorting compartment to later endosomes and lysosomes (202,207). These findings suggest that Ii can regulate the rate of distal movement of endocytosed antigen and of newly synthesized class II–Ii complexes arriving from the trans-Golgi. The significance of these observations is unclear at present. Macrosomes may arise from the excess production of proteins (Ii) interacting with components of the endosomal transport machinery, leading to titration of a limiting factor involved in early to late endosome trafficking or maturation. Another possibility is that this effect of Ii enhances endosomal fusion and mixing so that incoming antigen and newly synthesized class II–Ii complexes will reside in the same maturing endocytic vesicle, rather than coming to occupy discrete vesicles. This might contribute to the efficiency of peptide capture by class II when antigen is limiting.

Chaperone and Transport Function of Ii Complexed with Class II

Coexpression of class II with Ii alters both the pattern of intracellular localization and the biochemistry of protein maturation of the two molecules. Although some class II leaves the ER in transfected cells lacking Ii or the cells of mice lacking a functional Ii gene, assembly of certain allelic forms of class II dimers and the egress of most class II dimers from the ER are inefficient under such circumstances (208–212). Similarly, Ii in the presence of class II moves more efficiently from the ER to Golgi, indicating that transport is mutually facilitated by class II–Ii coassembly. The effect of Ii–class II association that contributes to effective ER export of these histocompatibility molecules is the elimination of their interaction with chaperones that are known to bind to and retain misfolded or partially folded proteins in the ER (213), one such molecule being calnexin, and with their binding site–mediated association with other proteins in this same organelle (214). Recently, the transport from ER to the Golgi upon class II–Ii interaction has been found to be related to binding site occupancy of the MIIC class II molecules, in a manner analogous to the transport of fully assembled class I trimers (heavy chain, β2m, and peptide). Ii contains a segment encoded by exon 3 termed CLIP [class II–associated invariant chain-derived peptide (215)] that is associated with class II molecules expressed by cells lacking DM expression. Functional (216), serologic (217), and crystallographic studies (84) have shown that CLIP occupies the binding groove of class II molecules in a manner essentially indistinguishable from antigenic peptides (Fig. 9). The CLIP region is essential for Ii to facilitate class II transport from the ER. This led to the hypothesis that the transport function of Ii derives from the occupancy of the class II binding site by this peptide region, due to enhancement of the proper folding of class II and inhibition of class II binding to peptide sequences within proteins undergoing folding in the ER, which can occur due to the open ends of the class II binding groove. Direct evidence has shown that in the

absence of Ii, class II binds proteins in the ER (214). Furthermore, replacement of CLIP occupancy of the class II binding groove by an antigenic peptide attached covalently to the β chain's NH2 terminus leads to replacement of the chaperone function of Ii, permitting efficient class II assembly and transport from the ER through the Golgi complex in the absence of any portion of Ii (218).

The pathway of class II trafficking beyond the trans-Golgi has been studied in cells coexpressing Ii physiologically or as a result of transfection. The sialic acid residues of recently synthesized class II molecules and intact associated Ii are cleaved by neuraminidase confined to the early endocytic compartment by conjugation to transferrin (219). This implies that such recently formed complexes at least transit through early endosomes before Ii degradation and removal. Transfection experiments showed that the coexpression of Ii with class II results in the appearance of substantial amounts of class II in early as well as late endocytic compartments (202). Cell fractionation studies showed that a large fraction (more than 50% to 70%) of newly assembled class II–Ii complexes in normal activated mouse B lymphoblasts can be found within endosomes accessed by exogenous tracers within 10 minutes and containing markers of early endosomes, such as transferrin (220). Taken together, these data suggest that most class II–Ii complexes move first to early endosomes, then to late endosomes before accumulating in a prelysosomal/immature lysosome compartment distinct from terminal (dense) lysosomes. Some investigators have reported that in certain cell lines, some if not most class II–Ii complexes move directly from the trans-Golgi network to late endocytic compartments without first passing through early endosomes (197,201,221), but recent immunoelectronmicroscopic studies of human B-lymphoblastoid cells have confirmed the results obtained by fractionation of mouse cells (222), suggesting that this is the major route in most B cells.

If early endosomes are the site of class II entry into the endocytic pathway, what route do they follow to reach this compartment? Some experiments suggest movement to the cell surface, followed by rapid internalization into endosomes (193,223). Alternatively, a direct route from the trans Golgi to early endosomes without transient expression on the plasma membrane has been demonstrated for cathepsin D, which is transported in association with mannose-6-phosphate receptors (224), and αβIi complexes could follow this strictly intracellular pathway. Immunoelectron microscopy studies indicated that class II did not localize in the γ adaptin-rich regions of the trans-Golgi where mannose-6-phosphate receptors accumulate (197), but recent studies suggest that the tail of Ii can interact with adaptins involved in clathrin-coated vesicle formation (225), consistent with this as a possible transport route.

The Ii that can be observed in early endosomes is largely intact, even though significant cathepsin B activity has been observed in such vesicles (226). The possibility remains that a minor fraction of Ii is degraded at this site, freeing a cohort of class II to capture peptide and move to the cell surface. Nevertheless, the bulk of the initial C-terminal cleavage of Ii appears to occur during transport to or in later parts of the endocytic pathway, primarily late endosomes or prelysosomes, and may be mediated by cathepsins B and especially S (227), the latter of which has a unique pattern of expression, primarily in hematopoietic cells. Leupeptin inhibits late cleavage events associated with Ii removal from class II molecules, and complexes of class II with a fragment of Ii (leupeptin-

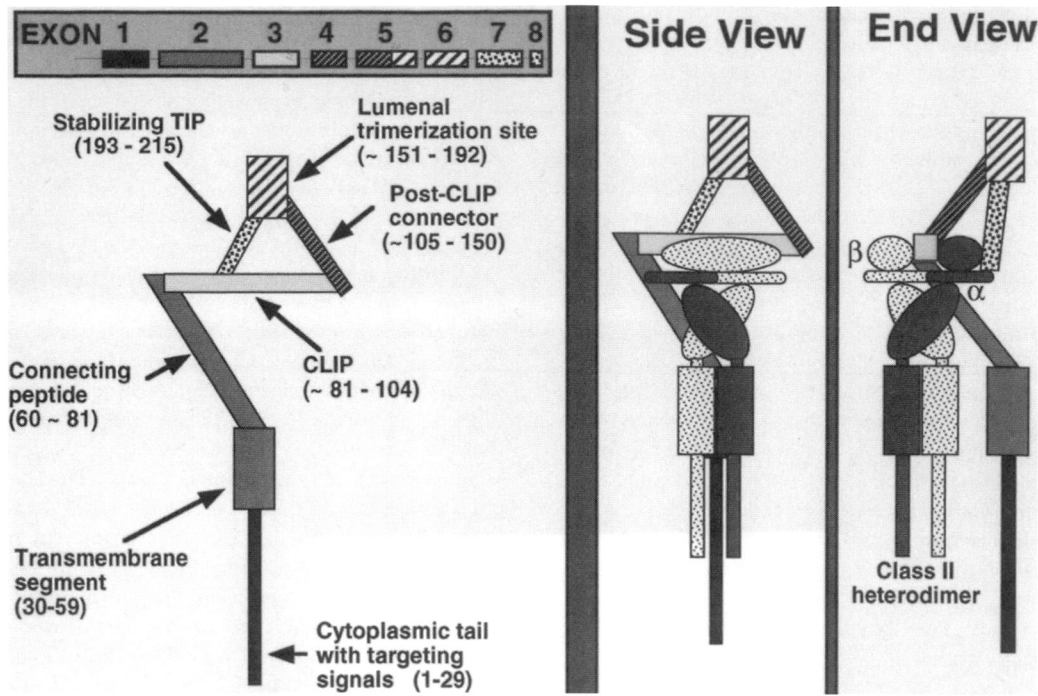

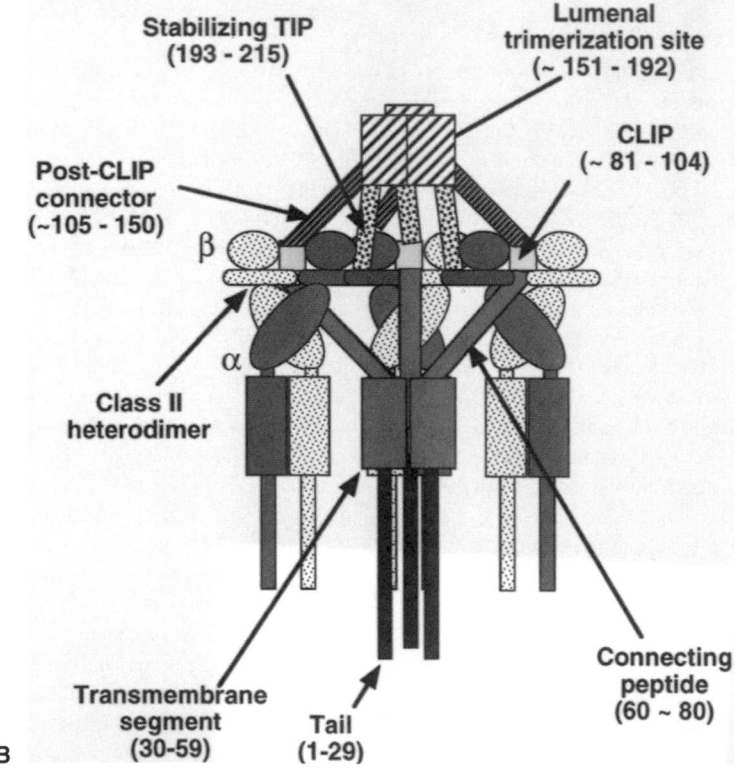

FIG. 9. Structure–function relationships of the invariant chain. **A:** The type II membrane protein orientation of Ii, the correspondence of the different segments of Ii with the intron–exon organization of the gene, the functions of the different segments of the protein, and the most likely mode of interaction between Ii and MHC class II dimers. **B:** The nonameric structure of class II–invariant chain complexes formed in the endoplasmic reticulum.

induced peptide (LIP) or small leupeptin-induced peptide [SLIP]) accumulate in cells treated with this drug. Such complexes remain trapped within the cell, accumulating in vesicles with the characteristics of late endosomes/prelysosomes (202,228,229). Thus, Ii affects not only the movement of class II within the cell from the early biosynthetic compartment to the endosomal pathway, but also the release of class II from the endosomal pathway for movement to the cell surface. This trapping function of partially degraded Ii may explain in part the site of predominant class II accumulation within cells.

Some data suggest that the p31 (p33) and p41 (p43) forms of Ii follow slightly different intracellular routes or are degraded in distinct ways. This conclusion is based on the nonidentical forms of the N-terminal proteolytic fragments of Ii associated with MHC class II in the two cases (230). These differences may arise from the capacity of the alternatively spliced exon 6b of Ii that gives rise to the p41/p43 forms to act as a protease inhibitor (231). This inhibitory function could play a role in preserving antigenic determinants from excess degradation before capture by class II binding sites, in addition to influencing the processing of the Ii chain itself.

Dissecting the pathway taken by class II free of Ii from late endocytic organelles to the plasma membrane has proved difficult. Tests for recycling back through the trans-Golgi network (TGN) do not show evidence of movement via this pathway, in distinction to the trafficking of the M6PR. There is limited evidence that some class II can be exported to the cell surface through the direct fusion of MIIC-like vesicles with the plasma membrane (232,233). Class II present in the outer membrane of such vesicles would be directly inserted in the correct orientation into the plasma membrane, whereas additional class II contained in internal vesicles within the outer MIIC membrane would be excreted into the extracellular space. It has been speculated that this latter event could allow transfer of peptide-containing class II molecules to the membranes of other cells. At present, the significance of this fusion/secretory pathway remains to be determined, and the means by which the bulk of class II molecules newly loaded with peptide reach the cell surface is still unresolved.

SITES OF PEPTIDE GENERATION AND ASSOCIATION WITH MHC MOLECULES

Class I

Transmembrane Peptide Transport and ER Lumenal Peptide Binding

Because the NH2-terminal peptide-binding region of class I is not available in the cytoplasm, due to cotranslational import of the heavy chain into the ER, the first possible site of peptide–class I association is the ER lumen. Studies with mutant cells provide data for early intracellular association of class I molecules with peptide. The presence of unstable class I heavy chain–β2m complexes in the ER of mutant cells such as RMA-S and .174 x CEM.T2 indicates a deficiency in peptide association and argues that the stable heavy chain–β2m complexes formed within 15 minutes of synthesis and present at a premedial Golgi site in normal cells result from peptide acquisition in this location. Direct evidence that the ER is the primary site of class I peptide acquisition comes from the isolation of peptides identical to those of normal surface expressed class I molecules from class I molecules confined to the ER by

engineering the class I heavy chain onto the cytoplasmic tail of the adenovirus E19 protein (234) and intracellular staining with antibody to a specific peptide-MHC class I complex, which shows the presence of such complexes within the ER (235).

Given this location for class I–peptide interaction, and the evidence from elution and sequencing that the primary source for peptides binding to class I is the pool of proteins normally residing within the cytoplasm, it is clear that either proteins considered to be exclusively cytoplasmic must at some low level enter the ER for degradation or that peptides generated in the cytosol from these proteins must cross a membrane to interact with the luminal binding domain of the class I molecule. Two closely linked genes have been identified within the class II region of the MHC encode polypeptides that have strong homology to the ABC family of transmembrane transporters (236–239). Other members of this family include the multidrug resistance (MDR) protein and a host of bacterial transporters of molecules, including sugars and small peptides. The accepted names for the genes located in the MHC are transporter associated with antigen processing (TAP)-1 and TAP-2. Transfection studies into RMA-S and human cells with mutations involving the TAP genes have established that the class I assembly and antigen presentation defects in these cells can be corrected by establishing adequate expression of these two TAP proteins (240–242). These proteins form a heterodimeric structure that resides primarily in the membrane of the ER (243,244).

Expression of TAP genes is not constitutive in all cells, and even in cells showing significant levels of TAP gene transcription in the resting state, such as in lymphocytes, activation or exposure to cytokines can increase TAP expression. Some cells, such as embryonic stem cells, lack TAP transcripts. Thus, in addition to regulation of MHC class I expression at the levels of the heavy chain and β2m protein components of the class I trimer, changes in TAP expression afford the immune system an independent means of controlling surface class I levels and antigen presentation by this route.

Human TAP proteins show allelic polymorphism, and studies in the rat have shown significant functional polymorphism of at least the TAP-2 gene (245). Structural variation in the product of this gene results in a difference in the phenotype of the product of the class I gene RT1.A. This phenotype reflects variations in the spectrum of self peptides associated with RT1.A molecules, which then affect the intracellular transport rate of this class I molecule as well as its recognition by antibodies and T cells. The demonstration of significant changes in the peptides associated with class I molecules as a consequence of polymorphism at this locus raises the possibility that variations in host response to infection and perhaps susceptibility to certain autoimmune diseases are due to such polymorphisms and not to products of the class I or class II structural genes present in the susceptible haplotype.

There is now a large body of literature establishing the peptide transport function of the TAP heterodimer and the rules governing which peptides it can bind and translocate. The most widely used method for assessing TAP function involves the use of streptolysin-O permeabilized cells with wild-type or mutant TAP subunits present in the ER membrane that are exposed to labeled peptides that contain a site for N-linked glycan addition. The binding of unlabeled peptides to TAP can be assessed by competition studies for the transport of such a labeled peptide with a glycosylation site, whereas binding and transport can be followed directly for any particular peptide by providing it with a site for labeling and carbohydrate addition. Various factors (such as adenosine triphosphate [ATP]) can be added or depleted and the temperature varied, following which the cells are solubilized in detergent and the amount of offered labeled peptide that has undergone core carbohydrate addition due to import into the ER lumen is quantitated using a lectin column to isolate only the glycosylated peptides (246,247). Using this and related methods, it has been shown directly that both TAP-1 and TAP-2 are required for formation of a competent translocation complex that moves peptides from the cytosol to the ER lumen in an ATP-dependent manner.

The transporter shows both a size and a chemical selectivity. Transport efficiency decreases for peptides substantially beyond approximately 12 residues in length, although some longer sequences can still be transported by TAP (248,249). The chemical nature of the C-terminal amino acid of the peptide plays a major role in dictating whether or not, and how well, TAP will transport a peptide (250). Remarkably, the optimal C-terminal residue varies among TAP heterodimers and matches the chemical preferences shown by the F pockets of the MHC class I molecules of the species (251,252). This provides clear evidence that TAP and the linked MHC class I proteins have coevolved for efficient cooperative activity in peptide presentation. Studies with chemical crosslinkers have identified regions of both TAP-1 and TAP-2 close to the ATP binding site as interacting directly with peptides being transported (253,254), and work is ongoing to determine the detailed mechanism by which the peptides bound to the cytoplasmic face of the ER membrane upon association with TAP are translocated into the ER lumen.

Tapasin provides a link between the nascent heavy chain–β2m complex with an available peptide binding site and TAP (175,179, 180), so that the imported peptides have an extremely high local concentration around available class I binding sites. In cells lacking tapasin, class I heavy chain–β2m–calreticulin complexes are formed that do not show the high degree of stability characteristic of peptide-occupied molecules. This observation suggests that tethering class I to the peptide transporter via tapasin might be important for the efficient loading of peptides into class I molecules, perhaps due to this concentration effect. It is also possible that tapasin regulates TAP function, so that without tapasin, peptide import via TAP might be compromised. Finally, because the class I heavy chain and β2m show some enhanced association in the presence of tapasin and also because there is an effect of binding groove polymorphism in class I association with TAP [and presumably tapasin (255)], an intriguing possibility is that a portion of tapasin directly engages the class I binding site. Because the conserved hydrogen bonding to both a free N and C terminus typical of optimal short peptide binding could not be made to this intrinsic segment of tapasin, such an interaction with the class I groove might be of low affinity (fast off-rate). However, rebinding rapidly after dissociation would be likely for this tapasin region because the two molecules are likely to be held in association through other parts of the two proteins. This would help maintain heavy chain–β2m interaction yet provide during each cycle of tapasin partial dissociation an empty site for binding of peptides entering the ER lumen via TAP. When a suitable peptide bound into the site, the stability of class I–tapasin association would be diminished because reassociation of the tapasin segment with this region of class I would be prevented. The permanent loss of this attachment site between class I and tapasin/TAP would result in the release of the loaded class I molecule to move through the secretory pathway to the cell surface. This model is a possible molecular explanation for the means by which peptide loading of class I molecules is coupled with their export from the ER. If this speculative scenario is correct, it would further emphasize the key role of regulation of MHC class I function by binding site engagement and provide an analogy to the function of invariant chain–class II molecule interaction in the ER.

Cytosolic Generation of Peptides for TAP Transport and Class I Molecule Binding

A great deal of progress also has been made in understanding how the peptide substrates for TAP transport are generated. All eukaryotic cells possess a multicatalytic protease called the proteasome (256). This molecule is a large assembly of some 16 to 20 components that is responsible for degradation of proteins in the cytosol as part of both constitutive (housekeeping) and regulated functions of the cell (256,257). Several types of proteasomes exist in the cell, differing from one another by the particular mix of subunits they contain, as well as by the presence or absence of an 11S regulatory complex. Experiments clearly show that association of peptides with newly synthesized MHC class I molecules or the presentation of antigenic peptides by MHC class I molecules is markedly diminished in cells exposed to efficient low molecular weight inhibitors of proteasome protease activity (258,259). These same inhibitors have no effect on presentation of optimal sized peptides produced in the cytosol directly following gene transfer or added exogenously to the cell. Some evidence also suggests that other cytosolic proteases, and even perhaps some ER proteases, may contribute to the generation of peptides presented by MHC class I molecules.

Two genes in the MHC, located immediately next to TAP-1 and TAP-2, encode two proteasome subunits termed LMP-2 and LMP-7. These subunits (also called delta and MB1) and another non–MHC-encoded, related protein termed MECL-1, all of which are highly IFN-γ inducible, substitute on a one-to-one basis for the LMP-9, -17, and -19 subunits found in proteasomes of nonhematopoietic cells that have not been exposed to IFN-γ (260–263). These MHC-encoded proteasome components are not essential for effective MHC class I presentation of many peptides (264,265), but they do appear to influence the specificity of proteasome cleavage (266–270), and their presence in the multicatalytic complex may favor production of peptides best suited to the MHC class I binding sites of the species. The 11S regulator of the proteasome (particularly the PA28 coactivator) also appears to contribute to generation of certain immunodominant determinants (271,272).

Many proteins degraded by proteasomes are first derivatized by the addition of a conserved polypeptide termed ubiquitin (273). There are insufficient data available to determine whether all or even most proteins giving rise to antigenic peptides suitable for TAP transport and class I binding are first subjected to ubiquitination before proteasome cleavage. Proteasomes follow certain rules with respect to the likelihood that they will degrade a protein, the best known of these being the N-end rule, which relates the cytosolic stability of a protein to the character of its N-terminal amino acid, all else about a protein being equal (274). Data have shown that the efficiency of presentation of peptides varies in accord with this rule, consistent with the involvement of proteasomes in producing the relevant peptide ligands for class I (275). This finding suggests that in recombinant vaccines intended to produce ligands for class I molecules, attention should be directed to the nature of the amino-terminal residue of the antigenic source protein, which can be manipulated by a variety of means.

Cross-Priming and the Presentation of Exogenous Antigens by Class I Molecules

It is clear that the major route for presentation by MHC class I molecules is the pathway described above involving loading of peptides imported by TAP and derived primarily from cytosolic proteins either endogenously synthesized or entering by direct fusion and penetration of the cell membrane. Nevertheless, there are well-documented cases of putatively intact antigens added to the immune system from outside the host APCs that can evoke host-restricted MHC class I–dependent responses (276,277). How does this occur?

A variety of possible explanations have been explored (Fig. 10). In some cases, the injected proteins contain a proportion of denatured or degraded molecules, either already suitable for directly binding to surface membrane class I molecules, like synthetic peptides, or able to do so after limited further degradation by serum or cell surface proteases. Thus, these examples are really equivalent to peptide sensitization of cells for class I–restricted recognition and, although of possible importance in vaccine design, do not alter our concepts of the class I processing and presentation pathway.

In some cases, intact globular proteins (278) or living cells have been used as antigens. The latter is true of several experimental models involving minor histocompatibility antigens. These experiments make clear that such minor H antigens (which we know are actually peptides containing sites of intraspecies polymorphism), when brought into a host via cells of MHC allele A, can be presented by the host's MHC allele B class I molecules (279). The injected cells could be killed by a host immune response and the released proteins of the cells degraded to external peptides, as just described for free proteins. A more intriguing possibility for these findings and those involving protein or bacterial antigens is that there are specializations of APCs that either (a) direct extracellular proteins into the conventional class I processing system, that is, bring the proteins into the cytosol even though they lack intrinsic fusion activity; (b) produce peptides in the endocytic pathway that are loaded into the small cohort of empty class I molecules present in the trans-Golgi network with which the early endocytic system communicates; or (c) recycle peptides produced in endosomes to the surface for interaction with empty MHC class I molecules on the same cell.

Several investigators have presented evidence in favor of the first possibility, although no molecular mechanism for such transport has been identified (280–282). Experiments with enzymes as model antigens have shown that a subset of macrophages or dendritic cells exposed to such material develop cytoplasmic staining that is dependent on the enzymatic activity of the antigen, suggesting the entry of undegraded protein into the cytosol from outside the cells, presumably through an endosomal mechanism (283,284). One proposal is that heat shock proteins mediate transport across the endosomal membrane, the converse of a pathway described by Dice and coworkers for movement of cytosolic proteins into endosomes for class II presentation (285,286).

Other studies have supported the second or third models, involving endosomal generation of peptides or loading of class I either within this compartment or after regurgitation of the peptide into the extracellular space (287–290). Here no special mechanism for transmembrane transport is required, and efficiency might be expected to be low. It has been speculated that this might be an effective means of ensuring class I presentation of peptides derived from organisms that reside in intracellular vesicles, so as to recruit to such parasitized cells CD8+ effectors capable of secreting IFN-γ that would enhance the infected cell's microbicidal activity. Bevan (291) has suggested that there might be a specialized set of phagocytic cells with one or the other of these properties; alternatively, the endocytic mechanism may work with released proteins rather than cells or cell fragments. A class II expressing APC that produced class I and class II molecules loaded with peptides derived from a single protein would be beneficial in at least one way. CD4 Th cells could then be activated by the class II–peptide complexes in order to provide optimal help for adjacent CD8 cells recognizing the class I–associated peptides on the same presenting cell (see Chapter 26).

Another possible pathway of exogenous antigen association with MHC class I molecules was first recognized during isolation of tumor-associated antigens suitable for CD8+ T-cell priming. Purification of tumor antigens led to the isolation of a common heat shock protein/cellular chaperone called grp96 (292). Biochemical and genetic analysis showed that this protein was unmodified from that present in untransformed host cells, yet it was able to provide tumor-specific immunity upon injection into syngeneic hosts. It now appears that this molecule, like other members of the heat shock protein family, is a peptide binding molecule, and among the peptides it binds is that corresponding to the effective class I–presented tumor-specific antigen (293). Srivastava and colleagues have suggested that this carrier protein is selectively taken up by a subset of macrophages, and the bound peptide, possibly after further trimming, enters the conventional cytosolic class I pathway and eventually binds to nascent class I–β2m complexes in the ER, which then traffic to the cell surface for T-cell recognition (294).

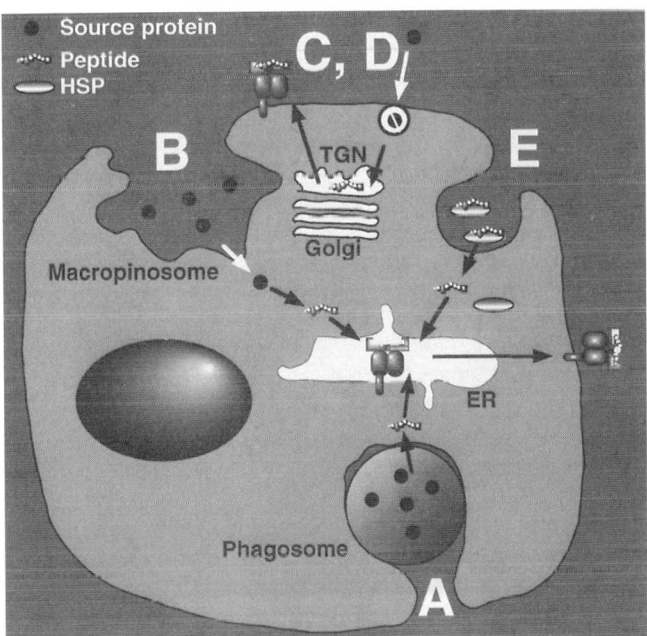

FIG. 10. Possible mechanisms by which exogenous proteins access the class I processing pathway or become associated with class I molecules. The diagram illustrates particle-facilitated entry into phagosomes and then into the cytosol, macropinocytic entry into the cytosol, regurgitation of endosomal peptides for binding to surface class I, binding of peptides to class I in the trans-Golgi network or recycling endosomes, and heat shock protein chaperoning of peptides into endosomes for delivery into the cytosol.

This area of exogenous ligand access to MHC class I molecules has become of even greater interest with the recent discovery that naked DNA can constitute an effective vaccine (295). Injection of DNA plasmids encoding all or part of candidate vaccine proteins, or skin bombardment with gold particles coated with such DNA, generates antibody along with CD4$^+$ and CD8$^+$ T-cell responses (296). Recent experiments implicate host APCs, most likely dendritic cells, as the primary cell type involved in stimulating the cellular immune response to the protein antigens produced by the injected DNA (297). In at least some cases, the DNA appears to have been taken up by or injected into only cells such as muscle, despite the involvement of hematopoietic APCs in CD8$^+$ T-cell activation. This demands a mechanism for the protein produced in the muscle cells to access the class I molecules of the hematopoietic APC, and the routes described above are likely to be involved in this process. This includes the release of antigen-associated heat shock proteins from cells at the site of DNA inoculation or particle bombardment. These data again emphasize the practical importance of this atypical pathway for class I antigen loading in vaccine circumstances.

Class II

Sites of Class II Ligand Binding

The seminal studies of Ziegler and Unanue showing a role for endocytic proteolysis in antigen presentation by MHC class II molecules (24) as well as the data of Morrison et al. (31) and others on the preferential presentation of exogenously acquired antigens by class II dimers led to the general view that MHC class II molecules interact with antigen within the endocytic pathway. The knowledge that MHC class I molecules bound their peptide ligands primarily within the lumen of the ER therefore raised the question of how MHC class II molecules, whose peptide binding site was formed in this organelle in the same lumenal orientation, avoided binding cytosol-derived peptides and retained the capacity for antigen interaction in endosomal organelles. When two groups demonstrated that the intact invariant chain interfered with peptide binding to class II molecules, a simple model became widely accepted, namely that the invariant chain kept TAP-imported, cytosol-derived peptides from binding to MHC class II molecules in the ER, preserving the distinction between the exogenous and endogenous pathways (298,299). This model was given further apparent support by the discovery that a fragment of Ii (CLIP) occupied the binding site of MHC class II molecules (84,217), accounting for the ability of Ii to interfere with MHC class II–peptide association in the ER. It was thus a substantial surprise to find that the properties of newly synthesized MHC class II molecules in the cells of invariant chain deficient mice did not agree with the predicted loading by such ER-localized peptides, but rather indicated a lack of tight association with peptides (211). This indirect result has been confirmed in transfected cells by direct analysis (300).

Given the recent data on tapasin's important contribution to MHC class I peptide binding, it is now not so surprising that invariant chain–free MHC class II molecules that are not tethered via tapasin to TAP are not efficiently occupied with cytosol-derived peptides. In addition, class II dimers do not form optimally in the absence of Ii, reducing the opportunity to bind peptides, and, even if formed, can lose peptide-binding capacity rapidly at physiologic temperatures, limiting their chance to bind peptides not immediately available at the time of dimer assembly (166,301). As reviewed above, it now seems that the occupancy of the class II binding site by CLIP relates

to effective class II folding and ER to Golgi transport, as well as to inhibition of binding to long proteins, not to short peptides. This binding to large proteins is not a problem for class I due to closed ends of the binding groove of these molecules, but this is a key property of class II molecules that has to be regulated in the secretory pathway if endosomal antigen capture is to proceed properly.

Once in the endocytic pathway, where and how do peptides become associated with MHC class II molecules? Modification of the cellular environment using drugs or temperature shifts has been used to probe the class II processing and presentation pathway. Agents that raise intracellular pH, such as chloroquine or NH$_4$Cl, usually interfere with presentation of antigen by MHC class II molecules, unless preformed peptides are used to load surface class II molecules (302). Although a decrease in the generation of processed protein antigen suitable for binding to MHC class II may be in part responsible for the effects of these agents, the published experiments have all been performed using cells coexpressing Ii. Because acid proteases are necessary for the removal of Ii from the class II–Ii complex, and such removal is necessary for both exposure of a functional class II binding site and for release from intracellular retention, assays using T cells for detection of surface membrane class II–peptide complexes cannot determine whether a lack of peptide or a failure of loading and transport or both is the explanation for the inhibitory effects of these drugs. A similar argument applies to the inhibitory effects of leupeptin. In addition to these limitations in separating proteolysis of Ii from that of antigen, such studies have not been useful in determining the specific site(s) of class II association with antigen.

More useful have been a combination of microscopic, cell fractionation, and immunochemical studies. Together these have led to general agreement on the endocytic pathway as the site of peptide–class II interaction, but there is still some disagreement concerning whether peptide loading occurs at only one or at multiple sites in this pathway and whether the classically described endosomal organelles (early endosomes, late endosomes, and lysosomes) are the sites within which functional antigen processing and antigen binding to MHC class II molecules take place. Early morphologic data were interpreted as indicating that newly synthesized class II molecules do not access all components of the endocytic pathway but are directly transported from the TGN to a specialized compartment (MIIC), where they accumulate and are loaded with incoming peptides (197,221). This hypothesis, based largely on the site of the highest steady-state level of class II molecules within the cell, is a widely accepted one that could be called the direct trafficking–unique endocytic loading site model.

Several groups have used a combination of cell fractionation and metabolic pulse-chase labeling/immunoprecipitation to further investigate this issue (Fig. 11). Density or electrophoretic approaches permit the purification of different endosomal organelles, whereas labeling and electrophoresis run under conditions allowing visualization of SDS-stable dimers allows a cohort of class II–Ii complexes to be followed after synthesis as Ii is removed and peptides are acquired (152,153). Using this technology, it has been reported that newly synthesized class II molecules localize to a unique subset of endocytic vesicles distinct from typical endosomes that also is where peptide-loaded class II dimers accumulate before expression at the cell surface (303–306). These findings support the direct trafficking–unique endocytic loading site model. At the same time, although these various studies each reported the identification of a class II–rich vesicular compartment distinct from the typical endocytic organelles, the characteristics of

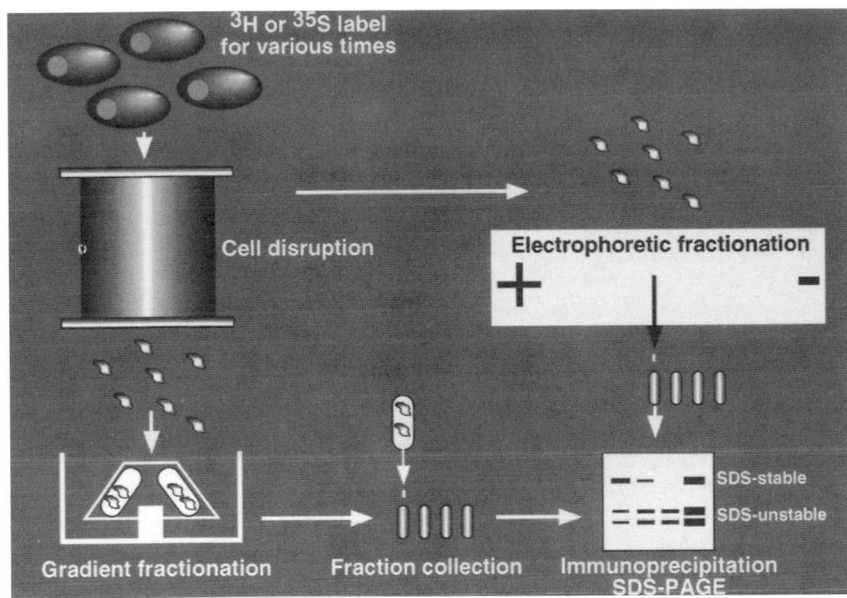

FIG. 11. Cell fractionation and SDS-PAGE analysis for determination of the site(s) of antigen binding to MHC class II molecules. The diagram illustrates density and free-flow electrophoretic fractionation of membrane-bound organelles from disrupted APCs at various times after metabolic labeling of proteins, followed by immunoprecipitation and gel electrophoretic analysis of the labeled MHC class II molecules from the organelle fractions for the presence of SDS-stable (peptide-loaded) MHC class II dimers.

these class II–containing vesicles themselves varied among these studies. For example, in the mouse A20 B-cell tumor, the compartment corresponded to some form of early endosome; in human melanoma cells and B-lymphoblastoid cells, in contrast, it had many of the characteristics of a lysosomal vesicle.

Other data are inconsistent with this simplistic model, however. Studies with nontransformed mouse B lymphoblasts using a refined cell fractionation method and an antibody whose binding to class II molecules was not blocked by intact invariant chain (a problem with the other experiments cited above) have demonstrated Ii complexes, evidence of Ii degradation, and the generation of peptide-loaded class II dimers in multiple endocytic subcompartments with the characteristics of the classic endosomal organelles (220). Because Ii prevents stable peptide–class II association, intracellular capture of peptide by class II molecules must take place after the inhibitory portion of Ii has been removed. This predicts that much of normal peptide capture occurs in later parts of the endocytic pathway, because little cleavage of intact Ii has been observed in early endosomes. In agreement with this concept, lysosomes presumably equivalent to the MIIC compartment have been found to be the site of the most readily observed antigen loading of class II molecules, but antigen binding to newly synthesized class II molecules also takes place in some earlier endocytic locations. This alternative model (sequential endosomal trafficking–multiple sites of antigen loading) is receiving increasing support from studies conducted in several laboratories. This model also seems to make biologic sense. Effective antigen processing depends on the complexity of the protein to be degraded, its complement of protease recognition sites, and its requirements for unfolding before proteolysis (307). The dissociation of Ii from MHC class II is influenced by both the protease activity within endosomes and the affinity of Ii for the different class II alleles. It thus seems reasonable that to optimize the immune system's capacity to recognize an invading organism, class II molecules would have evolved the ability to scan the endocytic pathway for antigen and capture the distinct determinants made available under differing conditions of pH and proteolytic activity. One critical concern with this proposal of a dispersed capture model is the fact that little Ii is removed during passage of newly synthesized class II complexes through early endosomes, a limitation addressed below. Recent data using an immunoelectron microscopic approach has yielded data in agreement with this sequential endosomal trafficking–multiple sites of antigen loading model (222).

A final issue is the question of whether all cells involved in class II–dependent antigen presentation process and bind antigen in the same manner and in the same intracellular compartments. Evidence is growing for substantial differences in the distribution and handling of MHC class II molecules in cells of distinct lineage, and possibly even in cells at different stages of activation. Several reports indicate that specific B-cell receptor uptake of antigen leads to presentation of certain determinants within a protein with a different efficiency compared with soluble phase uptake of the same antigen by the same cells (308). IFN-γ–activated macrophages differ from B cells and perhaps dendritic cells in which of the available determinants in a protein they most efficiently present, with a bias to the determinants within the protein core and against those superficially exposed (309,310). Dendritic cells modify the recycling rate of their class II molecules drastically upon maturation, changing the time any given molecular species spends within a given endosomal organelle, and also showing global redistribution of class II from intracellular vesicles to the plasma membrane during this differentiation process (198,199).

DM Function

The progressive proteolysis of the intact invariant chain by a series of cathepsins within the endocytic pathway results in the in situ generation of class II molecules with CLIP in their binding sites (311). For protein antigen to interact with these class II mol ecules, this binding site occupant must be removed. Several features of the endocytic environment contribute to this process. Acid pH itself promotes CLIP dissociation (312,313), but this is an inefficient process in general because cells with deletions in the class II region of the MHC produce a large number of surface-expressed class II molecules that have been shown by direct elution studies to be almost exclusively occupied by CLIP, despite the resident of these molecules in low pH endosomes for 1–3 hours (215,314). It is now clear that most CLIP removal results from the effects of a class II–like αβ heterodimer called DM, whose component chains are encoded within the MHC (315–317). This molecule has a tyrosine-based targeting motif in the β chain tail that directs the accumulation of DM within the endocytic pathway, especially in the late endosome/lysosome-like MIIC compartments (318–320). Immunoprecipitation analysis has shown that DM interacts directly with MHC class II molecules (321,322). DM appears to function like an enzyme, facilitating dissociation of ligands from the class II binding site in proportion to their intrinsic affinity, an effect that is optimized by low pH, although the extent of this pH effect varies with the class II allele (323–326). Thus, ligands with intrinsically fast dissociation rates leave the MHC class II binding site very rapidly in the presence of DM, whereas ligands with slow dissociation rates are relatively resistant to DM-induced dissociation. It is this preferential loss of ligands with modest to rapid dissociation rates at acidic pH that accounts for the ability of DM to promote removal of CLIP, which for most class II alleles has just such a modest affinity.

Because DM does not seem to directly recognize CLIP or the CLIP–class II complex uniquely, DM also seems to have a role in "editing" the ligand content of MHC class II molecules (327–329). Presumably, antigen with only modest affinity for class II is inhibited from stable binding to class II molecules within the DM-rich endosomal compartments because of the facilitated displacement of such ligands. This results in a strong bias for presentation of the best binding determinants within an antigen, a bias that can in principle be overcome by very high ligand densities within the endosome. Under such conditions, only some of the bound ligand would dissociate before the exit of the class II complexes from the processing compartment and, thus, from the influence of DM and low pH.

In B cells, DM has been shown to be associated with another class II–like heterodimer called DO (56). DO traffics to endosomal organelles and appears to require association with DM for this to take place. The functional significance of DM–DO association is still unclear, although one report suggests that DO downmodulates the activity of DM, and this has been speculated to help B cells focus their class II antigen presentation on antigens acquired in association with surface immunoglobulin rather than by fluid phase uptake (330).

Biochemical Aspects of Antigen Capture by MHC Class II Molecules

The ultimate products of endosomal processing are peptide–class II complexes expressed on the cell surface. Because most proteins entering the endosomal pathway are degraded to their constituent amino acids, short peptides are found in the eluates of purified MHC class II molecules, and the short peptides can serve as effective ligands for CD4$^+$ T cells, it is generally thought that MHC class II antigen presentation involves scavenging of late intermediates in the protein antigen degradation process. The substrates of the endosomal class II loading process detailed above are thus thought to be short peptides derived from extensively cleaved parent proteins, with only a few residues protruding from the class II binding groove subject to subsequent protease trimming. However, the actual ligands with which class II interacts within the endocytic pathway and the steps involved in producing these ligands have not been well characterized biochemically.

An important question is how class II ligand capture can occur efficiently in the highly proteolytic environment of late endosomes and lysosomes. Resistance of class II dimers to dissociation or degradation seems related to their occupancy with CLIP or antigen, so there thus must be rapid coupling of CLIP removal by DM to antigen binding, even if DM itself can help preserve the function of empty class II molecules for some time (322,331). The same argument about rapid binding would seem to apply to the antigen also because many determinants might only be available for a brief time upon protein unfolding before being internally cleaved by proteases. Conversely, other determinants may require extensive denaturation, reduction, or primary cleavages to be released from the core of highly stable, well-folded proteins (332). How can these differing sensitivities to protease attack, and the likelihood that short peptides would have a constrained life span in such an environment, be reconciled with effective antigen presentation?

Based on functional and not biochemical studies, Deng et al. proposed that antigen capture might involve the association of class II with large protein fragments just after unfolding or initial cleavages within low pH endosomes, followed by digestion that left a protected fragment in the class II binding groove (333). Some biochemical data has now been obtained that supports this view of the class II antigen capture process. Proteins complexes of 120 kDa, composed of two different MHC class II dimers bound to a single large fragment of a protein antigen, have been shown to form within the endocytic pathway of normal B lymphoblasts exposed to intact antigen (334). These data suggest that as the antigen unfolds, class II molecules from which CLIP has been removed immediately associate with the relevant determinants and protect them. This scenario implies that multiple class II molecules could bind to a single large denatured or partially cleaved protein at diverse sites. Usually, proteases would separate these bound class II–antigen complexes into single dimers with shorter ligands that might then be trimmed by N- and C-terminal peptidases to give the ragged ends typical of the short peptides eluted from mature class II molecules (129).

A clear advantage of this model over the peptide capture hypothesis is that antigenic determinants would be protected rapidly from protease attack by binding into the class II groove soon after exposure by early steps in the unfolding/cleavage process (125,127, 333). This could greatly increase the efficiency of antigen capture in late endosomal/lysosomal vesicles where competition between the action of proteases and binding to class II might otherwise favor the degradation of the antigen. This model also provides an excellent explanation for the evolution of the open ends of the class II binding groove, which would be necessary to facilitate rapid interaction with the unfolded forms of an antigen. Likewise, this would also explain the need for invariant chain protection of the class II binding site in the ER. This capacity to bind longer protein substrates does not exclude the direct binding of class II to short peptides; both mechanisms could work in parallel depending on the state of the available ligands.

Recycling Mature Class II Molecules Present a Subset of Protein Determinants

Most class II–dependent antigen presentation requires newly synthesized αβ dimers, Ii, and DM, but there are many exceptions (335–338). Different determinants even within the same protein can have distinct requirements for presentation; for example, HEL 46-61, but not four other A^k-presented peptides, requires Ii (339), and presentation of 46-61 is uniquely sensitive to inhibition of protein synthesis. It has been proposed that the existence of two distinct pathways for antigen processing and presentation by class II molecules explain these findings. One pathway would involve late endosomal/lysosomal processing and newly synthesized class II and Ii, whereas the second would involve internalization and recycling of mature surface class II molecules through early endocytic compartments.

For a long time, this latter proposal was considered suspect because of difficulties in showing recycling of mature MHC class II molecules (340). Direct evidence for these two proposed pathways has come from some recent studies. Internalization experiments have shown that wild-type HLA-DRαβ dimers are internalized from and recycle to the cell surface (193,341,342). Truncation of the cytoplasmic tail of either HLA-DR chain greatly reduces the internalization in transfected cells (343), and in the absence of Ii, the class II cytoplasmic tails were also found to be necessary for the accumulation of DR molecules in endosomal vesicles. Truncation of either class II tail differentially affects the presentation of two distinct determinants of inactivated influenza virus; class II tail truncation inhibits presentation of the hemagglutinin determinant H3, whereas the presentation of the matrix protein M1 is unaffected. These studies provided the first direct evidence for the existence of an alternative pathway for class II loading involving the recycling of surface class II molecules. Further experiments in a mouse model involving the three major different determinants within HEL presented by the $Aα^kAβ^k$ class II molecule (34-45, 46-61, and 116-129) supported and extended these human studies. Although only presentation of 46-61 is clearly dependent on new protein synthesis and Ii, all three appear to require endosomal processing for presentation. Examination of cytoplasmic tail sequences of many class II chains showed a conserved dileucine sequence preceded by an invariant glycine residue in the β-chain tail that is similar to the sequence of the membrane proximal targeting signal in Ii and was spaced a similar distance from the inner leaflet of the plasma membrane (Fig. 12). This putative dileucine

signal in the tail of the class II β chain is critical for Ii-independent presentation of HEL determinants in a superficial position in the folded protein and cannot be replaced by Ii for the presentation of HEL 116-129, although Ii can substitute for the class II tail in the presentation of HEL 34-45. This contrasts with the presentation of 46-61, for which Ii cannot be replaced by the β tail signal, nor is this signal necessary (310). Other experiments have shown a role for the MHC class II β chain cytoplasmic tail in antigen presentation in vivo (344).

These data suggest a complex pathway for the endocytic capture of distinct determinants by MHC class II molecules, with the class II tail (β chain)–dependent capture of more superficial determinants in less proteolytic, early endocytic organelles by mature recycling class II; the capture in late endosomes of partially buried determinants also by recycling class II or newly synthesized class II associated with Ii; and the efficient presentation of buried antigenic determinants primarily by newly synthesized class II molecules trafficking to lysosomelike organelles under the control of Ii (Fig. 13) (345). Such interaction of antigen with mature recycling class II molecules in early endosomes can be added to the picture derived from the study of newly synthesized class II that showed only minimal removal of Ii from the class II binding site in such locations to generate a model in which determinants can be presented by class II wherever they become available within the endocytic pathway.

Peptides and Class II Lifetime

Addition of large amounts of free whole antigen to cultured spleen cells leads to marked increases in the conversion of newly synthesized molecules to SDS-resistant dimers and up to a twofold increase in surface class II expression (152). The majority of these additional stable dimers come from class II molecules that were otherwise destined for intracellular degradation over a several hour period. Likewise, the addition to cells of a synthetic peptide with a high affinity for MHC class II leads to the prolongation of the lifetime of those class II molecules that bind that ligand, whereas the same allelic form of class II bound to a low-affinity peptide produces molecules with a short lifetime (346). These data, together with in vitro studies using purified MHC class II molecules that show a time and temperature dependent loss of ligand-binding function of empty class II molecules (166,301), argue that as for class I, peptide occupancy controls the functional lifetime of MHC class II dimers.

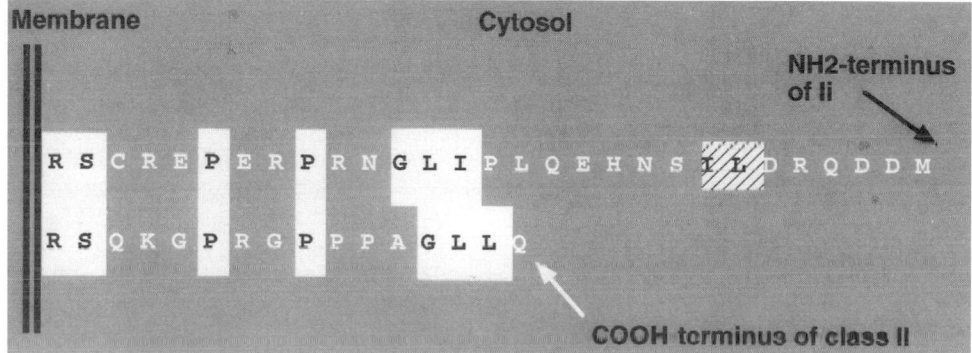

FIG. 12 Leucine-based endosomal targeting motifs in the cytoplasmic tails of invariant-chain and MHC class II β chains. The dileucine signals and a key glycine residue are indicated.

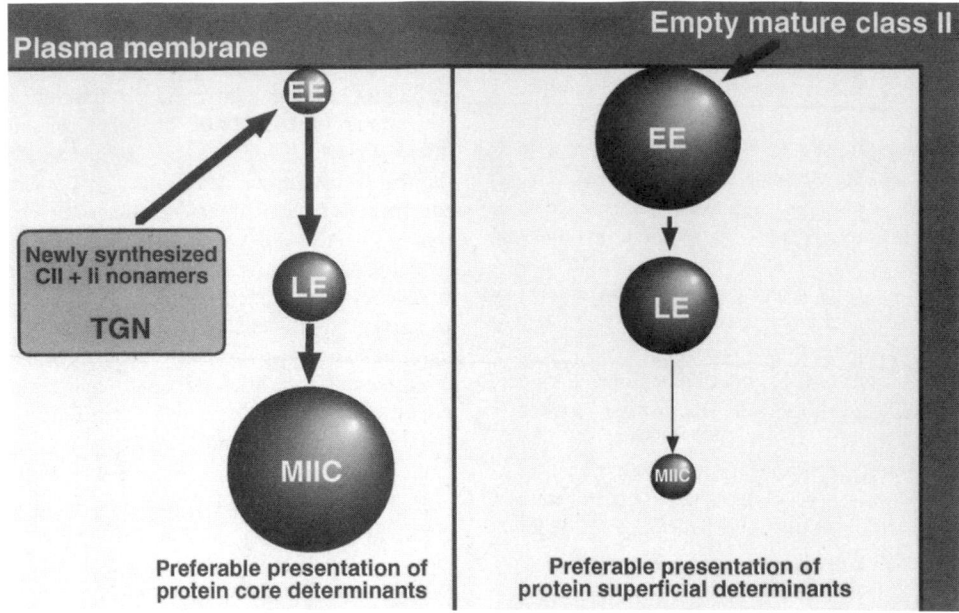

FIG. 13. A model for how the combination of an invariant-chain/newly synthesized class II molecule presentation pathway and a class II tail signal-dependent recycling pathway involving mature surface molecules allows for efficient scanning of all endosomal compartments for antigenic information. The size of the circles in each part of the diagram reflects the number of class II binding sites presumably available at the indicated location for the capture of antigen. Newly synthesized class II associated with the invariant chain shows a preference for binding determinants made available in late endosomes/lysosomes, whereas mature recycling class II molecules bind determinants preferentially in early endosomes. EE, early endosomes; LE, late endosomes; MIIC, MHC class II–rich compartments; TGN, trans-Golgi network.

The fate of class II molecules exposed to low pH in vitro with or without added peptide has shed some additional light on this issue (154). Exposure of newly synthesized class II–Ii complexes in detergent lysates to pH 5 at 37°C results in Ii dissociation and the inclusion of most of the class II in protein aggregates. If peptide able to bind to the class II molecule under study is included during the low pH treatment, more of the class II is recovered in the soluble lysate. Peptide- and Ii-free class II molecules produced in a baculovirus system tend to aggregate, and this aggregation is reversed by peptide binding (165). Thus, peptide binding seems to protect empty class II from entering into protein aggregates, consistent with its ability to preserve functional binding activity presumably as a result of preventing irreversible denaturation. This denaturation/unfolding/aggregation can account for the shorter lifetime of class II molecules occupied with rapidly dissociating peptide ligands. Class II molecules in endocytic compartments, whether still on the way to the surface after recent synthesis and release from Ii or entering endosomes from the cell surface, would face two possible fates: effective occupancy or aggregation of the empty dimers with each other or other proteins and eventual destruction in lysosomes. This mechanism would help ensure a high representation of useful (i.e., peptide-containing) class II molecules on the cell surface. The data therefore support a role of peptide in regulating not only the structure of class II molecules in vitro, but, more importantly, the fate of class II molecules within the cell, results analogous to the effect of peptide on class I.

Importance of Active Endocytic Uptake in Presentation by Class II Molecules

Fluid-phase uptake of protein will only provide antigen to the class II pathway in direct proportion to the antigen concentration in tissue fluid surrounding the cell and the volume of fluid uptake. Because the antigen concentration is often very low, especially at sites distant from a nidus of infection, large volumes of fluid would have to enter the endocytic pathway for significant amounts of antigen to pass through the processing system. This may be one strategy used by dendritic cells, which have been reported to show high constitutive levels of macropinocytosis (347). Other more specific mechanisms exist to enhance antigen uptake by presenting cells (see Chapters 6, 15, and 16). B lymphocytes use their surface immunoglobulin molecules to bind and internalize antigen. Experiments with mouse and human cells have shown that such immunoglobulin-mediated uptake can improve antigen presentation by 10^2- to 10^4-fold, based on the decrease in external antigen concentration needed for the same level of T-cell response (348,349). The ability this mechanism gives B cells to achieve effective levels of surface peptide–MHC class II complexes at very low ambient intact antigen concentrations is critical to effective focusing of helper T cells on B cells able to produce specific antibody against foreign proteins. The cytoplasmic tail of surface immunoglobulins participates in directing bound antigen to a class II processing site (350,351). Some studies suggest that molecules other than the immunoglobulin chains of the B-cell receptor, termed Igα and Igβ, also contribute to specific trafficking of antigen–surface immunoglobulin complexes to specific sites of processing or interaction with available MHC class II molecules within the endocytic organelles of B cells (352). Macrophages and dendritic cells take advantage of receptors that react with common structural features of pathogen proteins, such as exposed mannose residues that are not typically found on secreted or surface proteins of mammals, to facilitate uptake of antigen (353). This mechanism differs from surface immunoglobulin–mediated uptake by B cells in that it is not restricted to particular clones of cells among those of identical histologic type.

Similar improvements in antigen presentation can be seen with other means, whether artificial or natural, of enhancing endocytic uptake. Antigens conjugated to antibodies directed against cell surface proteins that undergo endocytosis show up to a 10^2-fold increase in presentation efficiency (354–356). Non-B cells also use an antibody-mediated mechanism to enhance antigen uptake. The FcγRIII receptor of macrophages contains a specific region contributing to the rapid endocytosis of this receptor from the cell surface; thus, cytophilic antibody bound to this receptor can augment antigen presentation by these cells (357). The region of the cytoplasmic portion of the FcγR involved in endocytic targeting in macrophages is absent from the FcγR of B cells, preventing cytophilic antibody not matching the specificity of the immunoglobulin receptor of the B cell from inappropriately augmenting presentation of irrelevant antigen.

Nonimmunoglobulin receptors can subserve the same function. Activated CD4+ human T cells expressing class II molecules are very effective presenters of soluble human immunodeficiency virus type 1 glycoprotein 120 (HIV-1 gp120), which binds to and is endocytosed in association with the CD4 molecule. CD8+ blasts of the same donor are at least 100-fold less effective at presenting gp120, due to the absence of the CD4 uptake mechanism (358). Other foreign proteins with biologic activities that depend on their binding to surface proteins of the host will also be effectively delivered to the processing machinery if such molecules are expressed by APCs. Phagocytosis improves antigen delivery at least in part by introducing a large particle usually containing many copies of particular protein molecules into a single cell at one point in time.

"Endogenous" Antigen Presentation by Class II Molecules

Although the bulk of evidence supports a specialization of class II molecules for peptide acquisition in the acidic environment of the endosomal pathway, there are nevertheless numerous observations of class II presentation of peptides derived from "endogenous" proteins (359). How can these data be accommodated by the model of the class II biosynthetic and processing pathway described above? It is useful to divide the proteins involved in such anomalous presentation into three categories: one that includes proteins known to reach the cell surface and hence to be available for endocytic entry; one that includes proteins apparently retained within the ER; and one that includes cytoplasmic proteins. Proteins in the first group are operationally "exogenous" and clearly can be processed after they reenter the cell by the standard endocytic route. The high efficiency of this pathway for membrane-anchored molecules or other proteins able to bind to such molecules is expected, based on the 10^2- to 10^4-fold increases in antigen presentation seen using ligands binding to surface immunoglobulin or cross-linked to surface proteins with substantial rates of entry into endosomes. In some experiments, putatively soluble forms of endogenously synthesized antigen have been examined and found to be efficiently presented. Cell-mixing experiments showed little or no cross-presentation. However, such experiments do not take into account the high local concentration of protein present in the immediate vicinity of the actual secretory cell itself, which would facilitate antigen uptake, the possible association of a fraction of the otherwise soluble protein product with membrane components of the producing cell that would result in rapid recycling into the

endocytic system (a route unavailable to admixed cells), or the possible direct intracellular routing of a fraction of the soluble protein from Golgi to endosomes, perhaps as part of the quality control mechanisms that might capture and route misfolded proteins to degradative compartments. Thus, for the present time, such experiments cannot be taken as firm evidence for a distinct pathway of secretory pathway processing and presentation via class II molecules, although this remains a possibility.

The second category of proteins, those imported into and then retained in the ER (e.g., by the presence of an added KDEL signal), have been used to argue strongly for a nonendosomal site of antigen processing and peptide binding to class II molecules. However, in at least some of the reported cases, the ER-localized proteins, despite being rapidly and efficiently degraded, were markedly less effective in creating a stimulatory presenting cell than the wild-type protein efficiently trafficking out of the ER (360). Thus, the situations generating more peptides gave less presentation, in some cases by several orders of magnitude, a result at odds with the ER being the relevant site of processing and peptide association with class II. Second, within the limits of the dose responses performed, proteins with the greatest "leak" out of the ER were the most potent and those that were best retained were least stimulatory. It therefore seems likely that the relevant cohort of protein was not that major fraction followed biochemically and shown to reside in the ER, but rather that small fraction that escaped this compartment, possibly moving to the endocytic pathway, where degradation and peptide loading on class II took place. Again, further study is needed to determine if presentation of peptides derived from proteins that reside mainly in the ER occurs by a novel route rather than by entry into the endocytic pathway.

The third group of antigens involves those most likely to follow a presentation pathway distinct from that for typical endocytosed proteins. Jacobson et al. first reported on the ability of a cytoplasmic antigen, the measles virus matrix protein, to be presented by MHC class II molecules (361). Subsequent work by a number of laboratories has documented class II antigen presentation of what are considered to be strictly cytoplasmic proteins. Mixing experiments ruled out trivial explanations such as bulk release and uptake from the medium into the endocytic pathway. How can these data be reconciled with the general model of class II processing and presentation? No evidence is presently available on the actual site of peptide–class II association under these conditions. Chloroquine can inhibit presentation in some cases (362,363), raising the possibility that some antigen or peptide from the antigen has reached the endosomal system for association with class II. In this case, the question is not where the peptide loads: this would be the same as for all other known ligands of class II molecules. Rather, it would be the site of peptide generation and the pathway followed by antigen or peptide to the endosomal compartment. This emphasizes that the class-specific function of MHC molecules relates primarily to their preferred site of peptide loading, which only indirectly and incompletely dictates the protein sources (exogenous/endogenous) of such peptides. Hsc70 molecules participate in moving cytoplasmic proteins or peptides into lysosomes (286) and provide one possible route for transporting such cytoplasmic antigens into the conventional class II binding environment. Another possibility is autophagy, which involves the movement of cytoplasmic components into the degradative system by vesicle formation. A more esoteric route is for peptides to be generated by the standard class I pathway and move into the ER via the TAP route presumably used by class I ligands. Such peptides could bind to class I in the ER; when this class I moved into the endocytic pathway for degradation, peptide could be released and captured by class II. This might be one explanation for the TAP dependence of presentation of a cytoplasmic minigene product that ultimately is found associated with class II and whose presentation, in contrast to class I–associated peptides, is chloroquine dependent. Nevertheless, a few experiments are difficult to explain on this basis and are likely to indicate that at least some peptides can bind to class II within the secretory pathway and be presented to T cells, although all available evidence argues against this being a particularly prevalent or effective route (364,365).

Although the mechanism of endogenous antigen presentation by class II is not fully understood in all cases, the phenomenon is important because it may play a significant role in the presentation of certain self antigens and in the immune response to particular pathogens. Understanding the route followed by antigen or peptide under these conditions might also be useful in the design of vaccine strategies.

SUMMARY OF THE CONVENTIONAL MHC CLASS I AND CLASS II ANTIGEN-PRESENTATION PATHWAYS

Although many additional features of the antigen-processing and -presentation pathways remain to be recognized and described in detail, a basic picture of the biochemical and cell biologic events involved in MHC molecule synthesis, transport, peptide acquisition, and surface expression has emerged (9,366,367) (Figs. 14 and 15). One of the major concepts arising from the intensive studies of MHC molecule structure and intracellular behavior is the critical

importance of protein-folding events and compartment-specific chaperones in the class-associated functions of MHC molecules. Misfolded or incompletely assembled proteins are usually retained in the ER by association with stress-related proteins or molecular chaperones. These chaperones are believed to participate in preventing irreversible aggregation of such molecules and in giving them an opportunity to attempt to reach a properly folded and assembled state (368). Molecules ultimately failing to fold properly are eliminated. The intracellular handling of MHC molecules can be understood if we imagine that the polypeptide chains encoded by MHC genes are functionally equivalent to protein deletion mutants. Such mutants lack the necessary information in their own primary sequence for entering a conformational state that these quality control mechanisms of the cell perceive as properly folded.

For class I molecules (Fig. 14), tapasin and calreticulin both bind to newly formed heavy chain–β2m complexes, and the association of tapasin with TAP contributes to retention of the as yet only partially stable class I dimer structure. Retention occurs in the ER until peptide has stabilized a properly folded structure and prevented continued association with both of these ER resident proteins. Apart from the hypothetical role described above for peptide interference with direct binding of a portion of tapasin to the class I groove, release of class I molecules from association with these chaperones is likely to be coordinated with the formation of a stable, conformationally correct heavy chain–β2m structure. If the affinity between empty class I heavy chains and β2m is too great and allows this to occur frequently without peptide occupancy, this would result in export of unoccupied class I molecules and inefficient endogenous peptide presentation. If the affinity of the heavy chain and β2m is too low, this imposes a requirement for too great

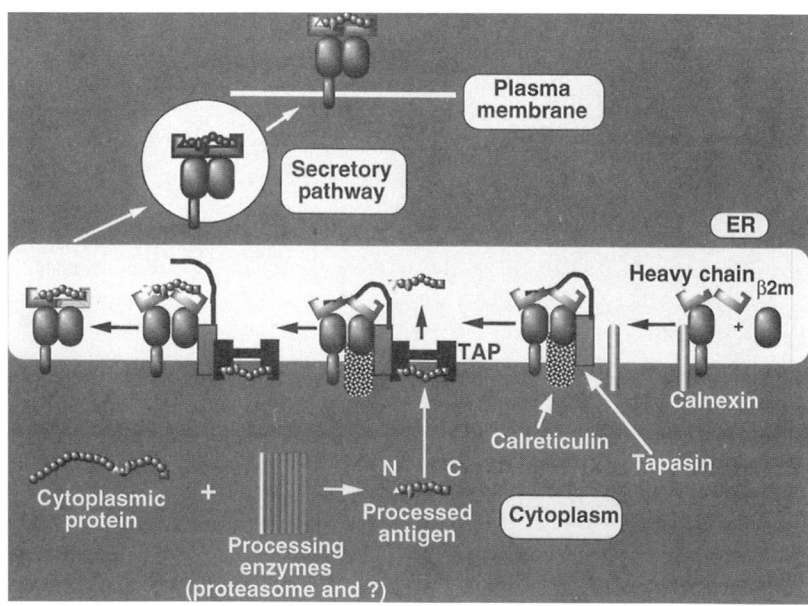

FIG. 14. Overview of class I processing and presentation pathway. The figure shows the generation of processed cytoplasmic antigen (mainly via the action of proteasomes) and its entry into the ER via the TAP complex. In the ER, class I heavy chains associated with calnexin interact with β2m, dissociating from calnexin and becoming bound to calreticulin/tapasin complexes. These class I–containing complexes associate with TAP, which transports peptides from the cytosol into the ER lumen for binding to the class I molecules. Tapasin is shown as having the capacity to transiently bind into the class I groove, preserving its structure and proving a mechanism for associating stable peptide loading with release from TAP and the ER. This complex then passes via the default secretory pathway to the cell surface, where it is available for recognition by TCRs. After some period of time depending on the affinity of the peptide and of β2m for the heavy chain, the complex dissociates and can no longer be seen by antigen-specific T cells.

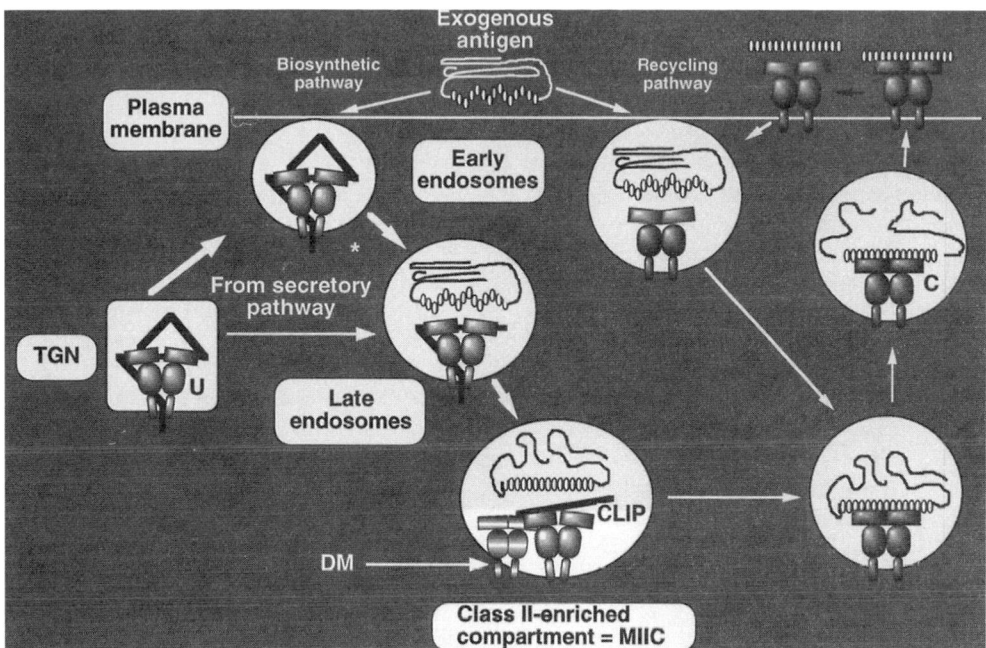

FIG. 15. Overview of the class II processing and presentation pathway. The figure shows the assembly of class II αβ dimers with invariant chain in the ER. This complex, which lacks tightly bound peptide and has CLIP in the class II binding site, is competent for exit from the ER and moves through the Golgi to the trans-Golgi network. Either from this site or after a brief stay on the cell surface, the class II–Ii complexes enter early endosomes. Here a fraction of the class II might lose Ii and gain peptide, then move to the cell surface for interaction with TCRs. Most of the class II–Ii complexes move to later endocytic locations, primarily late endosomes and prelysosomes, where the Ii is proteolytically degraded. The CLIP peptide remaining in the class II binding groove is exchanged for more stable peptide sequences contained within unfolded proteins or protein fragments. This is followed by proteolytic trimming of the bound material to the 15 to 20 residues typical of stable class II-peptide complexes. The peptide-loaded class II molecules exit this compartment and move by an uncharacterized route to the cell surface to be recognized by T cells. Mature molecules can recycle; if they have lost their peptide ligand, they can gain a new ligand, primarily in early endocytic sites. C, compact, peptide-loaded SDS-stable form of class II; U, SDS-unstable form of class II.

a contribution of peptide to the interchain association, which would in turn make the number of peptides that could be effectively presented too small. Thus, it would appear that heavy chain–β2m affinity has evolved so that in the absence of peptide there is a small proportion of heavy chains showing transient proper folding in association with β2m. This would promote escape from tapasin/calreticulin association and egress from the ER. Some chaperones move through the entire set of Golgi stacks and might recapture class I upon dissociation of the loose heavy chain–β2m complexes in these late secretory locations. Because the adaptation of the heavy chains and β2m involves intraspecies selection, trans-species heavy chain–β2 combinations that have continued to evolve apart from each other might well have too great an affinity in the peptide-free state, allowing significant transport without peptide capture. This may account for the export of most mouse class I heavy chains from TAP-deficient cells in the presence of human β2m (369).

Most class I will thus primarily exit the ER after capturing peptide. Peptides that only weakly stabilize the trimer form will contribute less to overall class I expression because they will be replaced by better binders due to exchange before class I dissociation from TAP or they will result in molecules that fail to complete their trip to the cell surface. However, those class I complexes that are poorly stabilized by peptide but still reach the surface may either reach levels able to stimulate T cells or, after peptide dissociation, give rise to most of the free class I–binding

sites that allow exogenous peptide to sensitize a target cell. The remaining molecules are associated with more optimal peptides. Once occupied by such peptides, the class I molecule is very stable. Because transport depends on this effect of peptide, surface class I expression is relatively selective for peptide-bound molecules, reducing the frequency of empty class I molecules that might interfere with recognition of useful peptide–class I complexes. On the other hand, the ability of exogenous peptide to facilitate accumulation of stable class I–β2m complexes on the surface of TAP-deficient cells indicates that there is a constant flux of dimers through the secretory pathway that are either empty or that rapidly lose a very loosely bound ligand after reaching the cell surface (132,137,370), so it appears that the editing mechanism is not extremely tight.

Thus, class I structure and its requirements for attaining a state that avoids retention by intracellular chaperones dictate its acquisition of peptides in the ER, and the biochemistry of peptide binding by class I is clearly optimized for interaction with short ligands supplied from the cytosol by TAP, rather than similar length sequences within longer polypeptide chains of the many folding proteins within the ER. Few binding sites will remain free for capturing peptides in other locations, due to the tight association of the ER peptides with most of the class I molecules transiting to the cell surface. Because many potential antigens of pathogens such as viruses would be cytoplasmic proteins, because for viruses fusing directly with the cell membrane little direct deposition of protein would occur in the endocytic pathway, and because the first proteins produced by a virus during infection are typically cytoplasmic or nuclear proteins regulating viral replication, a mechanism is required for supplying peptides derived from such proteins to the class I binding site in a topologically distinct compartment. This involves a mechanism for peptide generation in the cytosol (mainly the proteasome) and a transport apparatus for movement across the ER membrane (TAP). In this sense, the generic structure of class I dictates where it gets peptide, and additional, closely linked gene products help assure an appropriate supply of peptides in that location.

The same principles, but with important differences in the details, apply to class II (Fig. 15). MHC class II dimers do not show the same thermal instability as class I heavy chain–β2m complexes. They are nevertheless functionally sensitive to lack of binding site occupancy, and the CLIP region of Ii provides the necessary binding site occupancy for optimal dimerization and folding while keeping the class II binding site from being tightly occupied with unsuitable protein (not peptide) ligands. This combination of effects facilitates class II export from the ER. The Ii–MHC class II multimer then needs a mechanism to access peptide sequences within proteins from outside the cell that are acquired by endocytosis. Because virtually all class II leaving the ER is associated with Ii, it is reasonable to assume that the signals for movement to the endocytic pathway be in this latter molecule. Class II–Ii complexes move from the trans-Golgi network, perhaps via transient expression on the cell surface, to the endosomal pathway. They usually pass rapidly through early endosomes, where their presence may affect endosome maturation and some fractions may lose Ii and bind peptide. They then accumulate in late endosomes/prelysosomes. Most Ii is removed in this later, more acidic and proteolytically active compartment. CLIP is left in the class II binding site by the proteolytic process involved in Ii degradation, and its exchange for other ligands is facilitated by DM. These ligands are likely to be primarily stretches of sequence within large, unfolded, and incompletely degraded proteins rather than short peptides. This binding preference explains the need for the ends of the class II binding site to be open and the eventual formation of nested sets of bound peptides with differing N and C termini.

This view of MHC molecules emphasizes that the overall biochemical behavior of MHC molecules varies according to class independently of allelic polymorphism, although allelic differences influence the specific properties of each protein within this larger scheme. Such behavior strongly supports the hypothesis that the class I and class II families have evolved for different purposes defined by the intracellular environments in which they are optimized for peptide capture (33,68).

NEW TECHNIQUES FOR STUDYING ANTIGEN PROCESSING AND PRESENTATION

A number of novel methods have been introduced recently that are contributing to rapid advances in both in vitro and in vivo analysis of antigen processing and presentation by MHC class I and class II molecules. The use of combinatorial peptide libraries and phage display of peptides has been noted above in helping to produce enough information to yield useful algorithms for predicting the strength of binding of particular sequences within a source protein to a specific MHC molecule. Likewise, the appli-

cation of the most advanced methods of microchemistry, especially tandem mass spectroscopy used in concert with microcapillary electrophoresis of peptides eluted from purified MHC molecules and coanalyzed for T-cell activating potential, has produced a novel method for identification of pathogen or tumor-specific peptides involved in eliciting effector T cells. Progress also has been made in developing DNA expression approaches to cloning proteins that give rise to processed peptide bound to MHC class I or class II molecules and recognized by effector T cells specific for an infectious agent or tumor (109,371–373).

A major limitation in the past in studying the properties of a single peptide–MHC molecule species was the difficulty in producing homogeneously occupied class I or class II molecules. For MHC class I, this problem has been largely circumvented by the establishment of efficient methods for refolding recombinant forms of class I heavy chain and β2m in the presence of a specific synthetic peptide. This approach produces high yields of properly conformed class I–β2m–peptide complexes with little contamination by other peptide-occupied class I–β2m species (63,147,374). On living cells, a similar result can be achieved using TAP-deficient cells and prolonged incubation in a combination of synthetic peptide and exogenous β2m. For MHC class II, recombinant MHC class II β chains constructed to encode an antigenic peptide and a flexible linker as an NH2-terminal extension between the end of the leader sequence and the start of the wild-type sequence assemble efficiently with wild-type α chains to produce class II dimers containing just the unique covalent peptide (375). Soluble forms produced in transfected or infected cells from these chains are essentially homogeneous. In living cells, it is necessary to ensure a lack of invariant chain production because CLIP insertion in lieu of the tethered peptide occurs with significant frequency in the ER as the class II dimer forms, resulting in eventual endosomal cleavage of the attached antigenic peptide and loading of the binding site with undesired processed antigens upon CLIP removal. In the absence of such Ii competition, however, virtually homogeneous molecules filled with a single peptide can be produced and placed on the plasma membrane of presenting cells in vitro or in vivo (376). Refolding or loading of recombinant soluble class II produced in mammalian or insect cells also has yielded nearly pure class II–peptide complexes, although typically at lower yield than the covalent approach (163,165,166).

Another area of progress has been in directly identifying T cells specific for a particular peptide–MHC molecule combination among large populations of cells with diverse TCR. In the past, it was not possible to identify such antigen-specific T cells as could be done with antigen-specific B cells, using soluble antigen probes that bound tightly to specific surface receptors. The development of methods for producing homogeneously loaded class I or class II–peptide complexes, as just outlined, opened the way to the design of a strategy for such TCR-dependent staining. With the pure ligands in hand, the limiting factor became the low affinity of most TCRs for their ligands, typically in the micromolar range (377–381). Such a low affinity results in rapid dissociation of bound ligand during a wash step, making identification of the specific T cell impractical. This problem was solved by producing oligomeric forms of homogeneous peptide–MHC molecule complexes. Binding of these oligomers through multiple TCRs on the same cell membrane converts a low affinity/fast dissociating interaction into a stable, high avidity/slow dissociating complex. Using this approach with tetramers of peptide–MHC

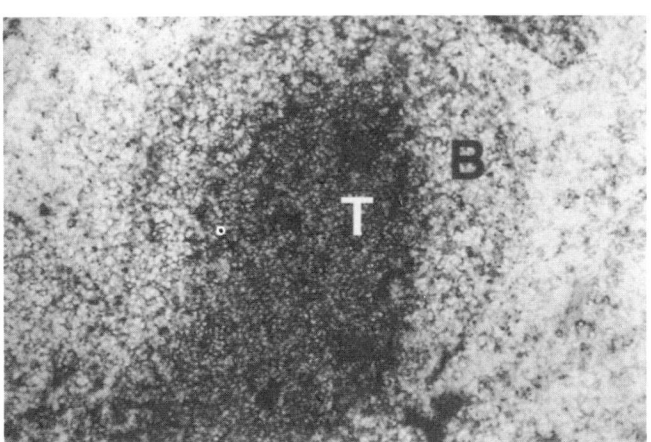

FIG. 16. Immunohistochemical detection of specific peptide–MHC class II complexes in spleens of antigen-exposed mice. Animals were injected with soluble hen egg lysozyme (HEL) a few hours before sacrifice. The spleens were removed, frozen, sectioned, and stained using a monoclonal antibody specific for the 46-61 immunodominant determinant of HEL bound to the mouse class II molecule Aα^{k}Aβ^k (B, B-cell area) as well as counterstained for the TCR complex (T, T-cell area). The image shows the presence of specific processed antigen-MHC class II complexes on nearly all B cells, irrespective of surface immunoglobulin specificity (386).

class I complexes formed through association of biotinylated ligands with streptavidin, it has been possible to directly identify HIV-reactive CTLs in the peripheral blood of HIV-infected individuals (382).

A last area of progress has been in localizing specific peptide–MHC molecule complexes within cells or on cells in tissues. Again, in the past it was only possible to trace the source protein's localization and not that of the processed peptide, or to assess processed antigen display indirectly using T cells. This prevented one from tracking individual cells bearing specific ligand within

tissues, a step necessary to understand the cell interactions during antigen presentation in vivo. It also precluded analysis of cells acquiring antigen after in vivo or in vitro administration in terms of phenotype or the amount of processed antigen displayed. Finally, this limitation made it difficult to visualize the specific sites within a cell in which peptide–MHC class I or class II complexes were formed, to track the movement of such complexes within living cells after initial formation, or to measure quantitative changes in peptide–MHC molecule formation upon manipulation of such targets as TAP or proteasomes.

Two methods have emerged that solve most of these problems. One is the engineering of soluble forms of specific TCR into oligomers, using either chimeric proteins with an immunoglobulin backbone or biotin–avidin complexing. These oligomers operate in a manner similar to the oligomers of peptide–MHC molecule complexes, turning low-affinity recognition events between the TCR binding site and the target peptide–MHC molecule ligand into high avidity interactions suitable for staining approaches such as immunohistochemistry or flow cytometry (383). Alternatively, monoclonal antibodies induced using homogeneously loaded peptide–MHC molecule complexes and carefully screened for low background against endogenous peptide–MHC molecule combinations have sufficient affinity to operate effectively in these types of procedures (235,384–388). The former method of oligomerized TCRs has been used in a more limited fashion to date, although it theoretically offers the advantage of predictable generation of the final reagent, whereas production of the desired monoclonal antibody is not assured even when the proper immunogen is used. Nevertheless, the bulk of new information on in vivo antigen presentation (Fig. 16) or the quantitative or qualitative aspects of in vitro processing (Fig. 17) has come from use of new monoclonal antibodies generated in this manner (235, 386–388). The major limitation to date of these two approaches has been the consistent finding that either TCR oligomers or monoclonal antibodies with useful affinity tend to show some binding to self peptide–MHC molecule complexes, establishing a background that sets a lower limit of sensitivity and specificity to the use of these reagents.

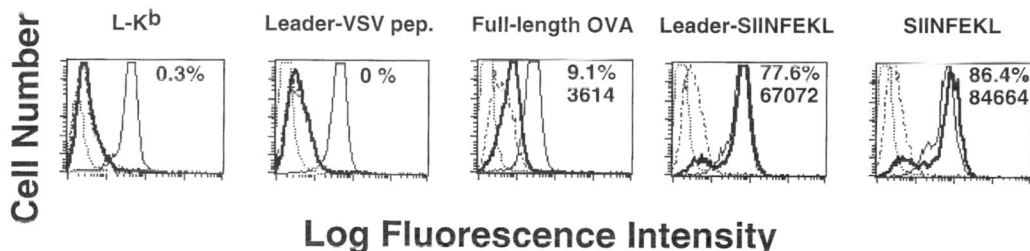

FIG. 17. Use of monoclonal antibody to a specific peptide–MHC class I complex to quantitate surface ligand density by flow cytometry. L cells expressing the mouse class I molecule K^b were infected with various vaccinia virus recombinants expressing the SIINFEKL epitope in various contexts. After several hours, cells were stained with directly fluoresceinated antibody to SIINFEKL-K^b complexes and analyzed by flow cytometry. Fluorescent standards and determination of the fluorescein to protein ratio of the labeled antibody permitted calculation of the number of specific class I–peptide complexes per cell and the percentage of total K^b molecules occupied by this peptide (shown in each panel). After infection, cells were stained with 1 μg (excess) of: thick line, FITC-labeled 25-D1.16; dot-dashed line, FITC control for 25-D1.16; thin line, FITC-antitotal K^b; dotted line, FITC control for the K^b antibody. When not all lines are visible, this indicates overlap of control and experimental stainings. Surface-expressed SIINFEKL-K^b complexes ranged from a few thousand when the intact ovalbumin source protein as produced by the virus to more than 80,000 when a sequence containing just the SIINFEKL determinant was produced (235).

BIOLOGIC CONSEQUENCES OF THE PEPTIDE–MHC MOLECULE FOCUS OF T-CELL RECOGNITION

The requirement for peptide binding to MHC class I or class II molecules before T-cell clonal recognition can occur places a number of constraints on antigen responses by T cells. It also affects the evolution of pathogens and the structure of their proteins. Furthermore, the different rules governing where peptides are acquired by class I versus class II molecules affects the strategies of pathogens seeking to evade immune elimination and vaccine developers seeking to elicit the appropriate T-cell regulatory and effector responses. Finally, it appears to dictate the need to involve MHC molecules in the selection of the functional T-cell repertoire in the thymus. The following sections discuss some of the major biologic consequences of the peptide-presentation paradigm.

Effects of Biological Variation in Protein Structure on Immune Recognition and Response

To be effectively recognized by T cells, a peptide sequence must possess at least three properties. First, it must be readily available in adequate amounts to MHC class I molecules as a short peptide or to class II as either an exposed region of protein or a peptide. Second, it must have the capacity to bind effectively (with suitable affinity) to the allelic forms of either the class I or class II MHC molecules present in the cell in which it is generated or to which it is made exogenously available. Third, once bound to an MHC molecule, it must present to the mature T cells of the individual α structure that is perceived as nonself, that is, a structure that can bind to the TCR of those T cells that have neither been deleted nor tolerized as a result of prior exposure to self peptides bound to self MHC molecules.

At present, the rules for generation of a particular peptide from a protein source are incompletely characterized for either the class I or class II pathways. Current knowledge of proteasome function indicates that this multicatalytic protease complex can cleave at a variety of residues within a protein and generate a very broad spectrum of peptides due to the presence of neutral, acidic, and basic proteases. Some recent data indicate that there are preferential sites of cleavage and that these biased cleavages change when the LMP-2, LMP-7, and MECL-1 subunits exchange for the LMP-9, -17, and -19 subunits. The 20S proteasome also appears to differ from the 26S form in functional specificity, thus influencing the peptides generated from a protein source. In at least some cases, it appears that the biologically active peptide determinant for some T cells is uniquely generated by the LMP-2/7–containing or the P28 activator–associated forms of the proteasome. The results of some experiments have suggested that alteration in the residues flanking a known antigenic peptide can significantly influence its capacity to be processed and presented (389), implying that the environment surrounding a given peptide sequence may determine if the peptide is made available for presentation (269). Other results have indicated that certain sequences within a protein that are theoretically useful determinants for class I presentation fail to be effectively presented because they are cleaved too effectively by proteosomal enzymes (390).

A similar limitation may exist in the class II pathway; the recognition sites for endopeptidases may cut within an otherwise suitable amino acid sequence for generating a class II determinant, and the rates of exopeptidase digestion may leave otherwise suitable peptides too long or too short for effective binding. These effects can be distinct in different cell types; for example, some determinants in hen egg lysozyme or insulin are not presented effectively by IFN-γ–activated macrophages but are presented well by B cells (309,310). The problem with the macrophages is a combination of too effective a proteolytic environment in endosomes and too rapid transport of antigen from early to late endosomes/lysosomes, together leading to cleavage of the antigenic sites in the protein at a faster rate than class II can bind to and protect these sites after the protein has begun to unfold. These considerations suggest that the proteins of pathogens might maintain certain functional amino acid sequences that could be effective antigenic peptides, but place them in a context that limits their availability to the presentation system by either hindering necessary cleavages that make the sequence available to MHC molecules or by favoring cleavages that destroy the site.

Once formed, antigenic peptides must bind to MHC molecules and then to TCR. The individual residues of an antigenic peptide can be broadly divided into two functional classes (21). One set of residues plays a predominant role in determining whether the peptide containing them can be recognized by unprimed or immune T cells of the host after binding to an MHC molecule. If the peptide–MHC complexes formed from the protein of a pathogen mimic self peptide–MHC complexes, these pathogen-derived complexes will typically fail to stimulate a T-cell response due to self tolerance in the T-cell compartment. In the case of a protein whose peptides do not initially have such self-mimicry properties, mutations in the gene encoding the source protein can affect one or more of these specificity-determining residues. If the new amino acid present at one of these positions is not chemically compatible with the binding sites of the TCR of T cells previously activated by recognition of this antigen, effective presentation of this determinant to such immune cells will cease, even though peptide–MHC molecule complexes may be present in quantitatively suitable amounts (391). However, unless the change leads to mimicry of a self peptide–MHC complex, changes in these epitopic residues of the peptide will usually lead to the development of a new round of responding T cells with different TCRs from those first stimulated by the original peptide–MHC complex. Thus, mutations that lead to epitopic substitutions give the pathogen a temporary advantage, and the immune system must "play catch-up." Nonetheless, continued effector responses can still occur, provided self mimicry does not occur and assuming the function of the cellular immune system is otherwise intact. In HIV-infected individuals, there is some evidence that as the CD4 compartment declines in activity, suitable help for new rounds of primary CD8⁺ T-cell responses is lost and the system no longer can keep up with the changing viral population (392). Interference with the function of existing immune T cells also can occur through sequence changes that lead to the generation of peptide–MHC molecule combinations that act as TCR antagonists of the original ligand, allowing a mutant pathogen subpopulation to protect the parent organism from immune attack by already primed cells (393,394). The epitopic residues involved in any of these events can be either those actually exposed between the helices of the binding groove and available to direct interaction with the TCR, or residues that might be buried within the binding pocket and that, when altered, affect the conformation of the bound peptide. This altered binding can change the position of the residues that are exposed, or even the shape of the MHC molecule itself, thus changing what the TCR can recognize.

A second category of residues involves those positions that control the affinity of peptide interaction with MHC molecules. If an amino acid in this category is mutated in the protein of a pathogen, the change could prevent any significant binding to the particular allelic MHC products present in the host. In this circumstance, previously primed effector cells will lose their ability to respond, and in contrast to the first instance, in which T cells specific for the new shape of the mutant peptide–MHC complexes typically arise, no new T-cell responses will ensue.

This analysis makes it clear that it is potentially much more devastating to the host if a mutation leads to the loss of MHC binding than if it leads to a loss of primed T-cell recognition. If the binding regions of MHC molecules were monomorphic, it would be relatively easy for mutations to result in a protein without sequences needed for effective MHC molecule binding because only one suitable motif would exist and its elimination would provide invisibility to the protein in question. The allelic diversification of MHC molecules, the presence of codominantly expressed, multiple loci for each class of MHC molecule, and the heterozygous nature of most individuals provide protection against such simple escape (395). The distinct chemical characteristics of the binding pockets in MHC molecules make it likely that the mutation of a key binding residue suitable for interaction with one MHC product will result in its replacement with a residue suitable for binding to another MHC product, if not in the same host, then in the susceptible population. Diversity is therefore a protection against easy mutational evasion of the peptide presentation system.

This same diversity also makes it difficult to design universally effective vaccines based on the use of single peptides. Such peptides would be unlikely to bind well enough to the different alleles of class I or class II molecules present in all members of the population for immunity to result in all vaccinated individuals, although our increased understanding of the molecular rules of peptide MHC molecule interaction have permitted the design of synthetic peptides that retain the epitopic properties of a target antigen and yet are able to bind well to a greater diversity of MHC alleles (130,396). Because primed T cells typically can be activated by lower amounts of TCR ligand than unprimed T cells (397), even for those alleles with low intrinsic affinity for the wild-type peptide that would be available during infection or from a tumor antigen, this strategy could help provide effective immunity in a wider segment of the population. Nevertheless, in general this feature of the antigen presentation system means that peptide-based vaccines will need to contain pools of peptides able to bind effectively to a majority of the most common alleles in the population, or to be formulated separately for different individuals or subpopulations possessing particular MHC types.

Identification within the proteins of a pathogen of the different peptides that bind well to distinct MHC alleles can now be accomplished in two ways. First, computer search algorithms can be used to scan protein sequences for matches between sequences in the protein and the binding motifs of the alleles in question. Identified candidate sequences can be synthesized, then tested for MHC molecule binding in vitro and for stimulation of T cells from immune individuals of the proper MHC type. This is an effective strategy when the proteins of the organism are completely characterized, as for many viruses, but is less effective [but still feasible (398)] for protozoa or more complex parasites for which only a few protein sequences are available. A second approach is direct elution of peptides from MHC molecules of infected cells or cells exposed to extracts of the organism in question. If indicator T cells are available to locate the fractions of interest after separation by various

chromatographic methods, the relevant fractions can be analyzed and sequenced. Candidate peptides can then be synthesized and tested for both binding and the capacity to stimulate the indicator T cells, to prove authenticity.

Consequences of the Differences in Location of Peptides Effective in Loading Class I Versus Class II Molecules for Immune Defense and Vaccine Strategies

Although exceptions exist in both directions, the bulk of available data indicates that class I molecules predominantly bind peptides that enter or are produced in the ER, whereas class II molecules preferentially bind those peptides entering or generated in acidic vesicles in the endosomal/lysosomal pathway. Because CD8+ and CD4+ T cells focus on class I– versus class II–associated peptides, respectively (399,400), these differences in sites of peptide binding also mean that distinct T-cell subsets and effector modalities will be stimulated by proteins giving rise to peptides entering one or the other loading compartment.

Pathogens that live in the cytoplasm will produce proteins mainly giving rise to peptides entering the ER and presented by class I molecules (401,402). This can result in stimulation of CD8+ T cells, whose effector mechanisms include cytotoxicity (death of the target cells) and secretion of cytokines such as TNF-β and IFN-γ. This is a suitable set of effector responses to such intracellular parasites, but it does not include help for antibody production; such antibodies might be useful in attacking the pathogen during any extracellular phases of its life cycle. Conversely, a parasite that resides in a modified endosome may generate peptides that could load class II molecules, if the pathologic vesicle communicates with the class II–containing segments of the endocytic pathway. However, the proteins of this pathogen may not give rise to peptides resulting in class I presentation, unless the putative endosome-to-cytosol route of exogenous antigen entry into the class I pathway or the binding of endosomally generated peptides to mature class I molecules by "regurgitation" can occur in this circumstance. This would limit effector responses to CD4+ T cells. Although antigen-specific CD4+ cytotoxic cells exist (358,403), it is unclear what their in vivo potential is. Cytokines might activate mechanisms in the host cell that would attack the pathogen (e.g., NO production), but some organisms have actually adapted to host responses of this type and use cytokines as regulators of their own biologic processes. Extracellular debris could be taken up endocytically by class II–bearing cells, then processed and presented for activation of CD4+ effector/regulatory cells, including those suitable for helping B-cell antibody production. This mechanism is especially useful against exotoxins because antibody is the only effective way of combating the biologic effects of such toxins.

In designing vaccines, it is critical to understand the influence of mode of antigen delivery on processing and presentation and to develop a clear idea of the effector activities that contribute to host defense against the organism that the vaccine is designed to combat. One area of importance and also of frequent confusion involves T cell–dependent production of antibodies to conformational determinants of protein antigens. If neutralizing antibodies would be the most efficacious defense, then efficient entry of the antigen into the endocytic pathway of professional APCs involved in activating CD4+ T cells and uptake by antigen-specific B cells that will ultimately produce the desired antibody are needed. As emphasized above, CD4$^+$ T cells and antigen-specific B cells both have receptors sensitive to the conformation of their respective ligands, but the conformation of the peptide derived from the intact antigen and bound to MHC class II molecules does not usually resemble that of the same stretch of amino acids in the native antigen. Furthermore, the relevant set of residues involved in formation of the TCR ligand may lie in a different portion of the protein (e.g., buried in the folded core) than the site seen by the B-cell receptor, which is typically on the surface.

Despite these differences, the processing and presentation pathway described above provides a straightforward and elegant way to allow two lymphoid cells with such different recognition specificities for the same antigen to effectively cooperate with each other. Protein antigen still in its native folded state will bind avidly to the surface immunoglobulin receptors of a small number of B cells, providing these B cells with a substantial advantage in antigen uptake over antigen-unspecific B cells in the same environment. These few B cells, genetically programmed to make antibody specific for the native conformational determinant involved in this antigen-binding reaction, will process the acquired antigen in the endocytic pathway to produce MHC class II–peptide complexes that are displayed at the plasma membrane. CD4$^+$ T cells, most likely already activated by the same processed form of antigen on the membrane of a dendritic cell, will move into the B-cell area of the spleen or lymph node and scan the surfaces of the B cells they contact. When these T cells locate the B cells displaying the same processed antigen as that which initially activated them, TCR recognition of the processed antigen will result in upregulation of membrane and soluble cytokine production by the CD4$^+$ cells, providing help for B-cell proliferation and differentiation. The B cells will become high-rate antibody-secreting cells, and the antibody they produce will be specific for the native antigenic determinant that was involved in capturing the protein for processing into the MHC class II–associated peptide seen by the CD4$^+$ T cells. This same general linkage of native and processed antigen recognition for B–T cooperation also subserves development of somatically mutated, higher affinity antibody because the B cells with these genetically modified immunoglobulins must retain specificity for the target antigen in order to capture, process, and present antigen to CD4$^+$ T cells, whose signals are needed for B-cell survival and differentiation (see Chapters 7 and 25).

Preexisting antibody can facilitate antigen uptake into macrophages and immature dendritic cells via Fcγ receptors that contain a specific structural specialization in the cytoplasmic tail that promotes endocytosis (357). B-cell Fcγ receptors lack this feature, which presumably prevents nonspecific antigen uptake in competition with the surface immunoglobulin that accurately reflects the specificity of the antibody eventually secreted by the B cells. B cells whose surface immunoglobulin can bind a region of the protein without making effector antibodies capable of neutralization or opsonization can compete with those B cells whose antibodies would be more useful. Some organisms have evolved specific surface characteristics that promote development of such ineffectual B-cell responses so as to avoid effective antigen uptake by the B cells more useful to the host response. Passively acquired antibody or maternal antibodies also can compete with cell-bound immunoglobulin and prevent potential effector B cells from acquiring adequate antigen to present to CD4$^+$ Th cells. Thus, vaccines designed to elicit specific neutralizing antibodies must contain components that target the proper presenting cells and avoid evoking unneeded, competing B-cell responses.

If inflammatory Th1-type responses are key to host defense, for example, against certain intracellular parasites, then targeting of antigen to class II–bearing cells that promote differentiation in this direction is needed. Because we now appreciate the central role of interleukin (IL)-12 in promoting Th1 responses by CD4$^+$ T cells (404–406), a means of ensuring the production of this cytokine by the targeted APCs is also needed. Activation of APCs so that this and other cosignals for effective and directed T-cell activation occur are the role of adjuvants. These materials, especially those containing microbial products to which the myeloid series of cells in general and dendritic cells in particular (407) are responsive, evoke the synthesis and expression of IL-12, the B7 family of CD28-costimulatory molecules, and other molecules that are needed for a T cell to translate TCR signaling into effector differentiation.

If CD8$^+$ effector cells are critical, then the administered antigen must make its way into the class I presentation pathway from outside the cell. Although the mechanism of cross-priming remains obscure, this pathway has allowed exogenously administered intact protein antigens to stimulate CD8$^+$ T-cell responses even without special means to enforce entry of the antigen into the cytosol. Available evidence indicates that this process plays a major role in the presentation of antigens expressed after DNA (297) or whole cell tumor vaccination that elicits CD8$^+$ CTL responses (408). At the same time, other data indicate that the use of vaccine delivery systems that enhance antigen access to the cytosol of the presenting cell are especially effective in providing ligands to the TCR of CD8$^+$ T cells. Various means of achieving cytosolic delivery have been reported. These include live viral vectors such as vaccinia or adenovirus (409), fusogenic liposomes (410,411), and formulations containing mild detergents (412). Peptides [modified (413) or not (414)] have been shown in some cases to be effective immunogens for CD8$^+$ T cells. The disadvantage of peptides is the concern that they might broadly sensitize host cells for the damaging effects of CTLs if used as boosters in already primed individuals, resulting in unacceptable tissue damage. There also may be limitations on stimulating effective CD8$^+$ responses without simultaneous CD4$^+$ T-cell help (415,416). In addition, serum proteases and exoproteases can rapidly degrade optimized peptides to a size that would be ineffective: it will be necessary to design the peptides to remain in or give rise to optimally immunogenic forms while under attack by such proteases.

An unresolved question is how CD4$^+$ T-cell help for CD8$^+$ T-cell responses occurs. In contrast to the clear pathway described above for linking uptake of conformationally intact antigen via B-cell surface immunoglobulin with presentation to CD4$^+$ T cells of processed antigen via MHC class II molecules of the same B cell, no such simple model can explain how two T cells, specific for different processed peptides within a single protein or even different proteins in a pathogen, interact in an antigen-specific manner. Neither T cell acquires intact antigen directly through their surface receptors, making untenable a focusing model in which the CD8$^+$ T cells would display a processed class II ligand for the CD4$^+$ T cell, in analogy to the antigen-specific B cell. The best available model, based on data from cell-mixing experiments in vivo, postulates that a single professional APC, most likely a dendritic cell, displays both the CD4$^+$ T cell-recognized MHC class II ligand and the CD8$^+$ T cell-recognized MHC class I ligand (417). The activation of both T cells in proximity to each other upon recognition of these distinct ligands on the same presenting cell's membrane would permit secreted cytokines of the CD4$^+$ cells, such as IL-2, to augment the differentiation and proliferation of the CD8$^+$ T cell. This scenario argues that optimal CD8$^+$ T-cell effector development will require methods that deliver the source antigen for class II presentation to the endocytic pathway of the same cell to which the antigen for class I presentation is delivered to the cytosol for conventional processing or endosomes for alternative pathway presentation.

Pathogen Interference with Antigen Presentation

There is little question that the immune system plays a decisive role in host defense against microbial pathogens, and it should not have come as a surprise to find that many pathogens have the ability to produce molecules that modulate the host response (418). In most cases, this involves blunting host defense mechanisms, often by manipulation of the cytokine pathways (see Chapters 21, 25, and 26). In some cases, however, this involves the paradoxical promoting of host defense, apparently to ensure host survival for a sufficient period of time so that the invading organism can reproduce and have a substantial likelihood of transmission to a new host. During the past few years, the key role played by peptide antigen presentation to CD4$^+$ and especially CD8$^+$ T cells in combating infection has been made especially clear by the discovery that many organisms have the capacity to produce molecules that interfere with crucial steps in the MHC-dependent antigen-presentation pathways that have been described in this chapter (419).

The most striking results have been obtained for viruses and MHC class I molecules. Different viruses have been shown to produce proteins that interfere with (a) peptide binding to TAP (ICP47 of herpes simplex) (420–422) or peptide translocation by TAP (US6 of human cytomegalovirus) (423,424); (b) stable insertion of the class I heavy chain into the ER membrane (US2 and US11 of human cytomegalovirus (425–427) and HIV vpu (428); (c) release of assembled class I–peptide complexes from the ER (E19 of adenovirus) (429); (d) inhibition of MHC class I heavy-chain gene transcription (adenovirus, HIV) (429,430); and (v) accelerated clearance of surface class I (HIV Nef) (431). Other data suggest that some viruses also target the MHC class II pathway; for example, Epstein-Barr virus produces a molecule that binds the human DR β chain (432).

The T-cell response to herpes simplex in humans has been found to have the unusual feature of eliciting primarily CD4$^+$ cytotoxic cells, and not stimulating much in the way of a CD8$^+$ CTL response. Cells infected with herpes simplex were found to have a defect in the stable assembly of MHC class I heavy chain–β2m dimers and the export of class I molecules to the cell surface, which later was recognized to resemble the situation in cells lacking effective peptide import into the ER as a result of mutations in TAP-1 or -2. The assembly/expression defect was used as a screen for individual viral proteins able to mediate the same effect, and ICP47 was identified as being necessary and sufficient for this disruption of the class I pathway. Further work has shown that this protein associates with the cytoplasmic portion of TAP and interferes with the ability of the transporter to stably bind peptides. This in turn prevents the peptides from being transported into the ER, thus interfering with antigen presentation. The effect is not selective for herpes-derived peptides, hence the general effect on class I assembly and transport. ICP47 reacts well with human TAP, but poorly with mouse TAP, indicating a clear evolutionary selection for function in the relevant host of the viral pathogen.

Infection of cells with human cytomegalovirus (HCMV) also leads to loss of surface MHC class I expression. As with ICP47, the US2 protein made by this virus interferes with TAP function, although at a different step in the transport process. In addition, in contrast to herpes simplex, the class I in CMV-infected cells is not merely unable to find suitable peptide partners and leave the ER in a properly assembled state. Instead, newly synthesized class I heavy chains rapidly disappear during metabolic labeling and immunoprecipitation experiments seeking to analyze the fate of MHC class I proteins made in the presence of HCMV infection. This effect has been traced to the US2 and US11 proteins of HCMV. Most remarkably, it has been found that these proteins act to dislocate the class I heavy chain from the ER membrane after it has been cotranslationally inserted into that lipid bilayer and after core glycosylation has occurred. Once in the cytosol, the class I heavy chain is deglycosylated and then degraded by the proteasome. These exciting data have not only revealed a novel mechanism by which a pathogen attempts to evade the class I presentation system (a cell unable to produce stable class I protein cannot present CMV peptides in association with MHC class I molecules), but it also has had a dramatic effect on the notion of ER protein degradation. This pathway, which was presumed to account for the degradation of misfolded proteins held in the ER by the quality control apparatus of the cell (433), is now considered to possibly reflect a variation on the US11 mode of protein degradation, involving exit of the protein from the ER lumen into the cytosol for proteosomal degradation. HIV vpu also leads to degradation of newly synthesized class I heavy chains, although the detailed mechanism by which this occurs is not yet known (428).

A third viral strategy for evading the class I presentation system is to interfere with transport of assembled class I–peptide–β2m complexes from the ER to the plasma membrane, thus inhibiting T-cell recognition without preventing the ligands from actually forming. Certain adenoviruses possess a protein called E19 that can bind to many class I heavy chains in the ER. In the cytoplasmic tail of this transmembrane protein is a sequence that has been shown to lead to retention of the protein in the ER (434). The dibasic motif identified in the E19 cytoplasmic tail has subsequently been found in the tail of other proteins that reside in the ER membrane, and transplantation of this sequence to another molecule leads to its retention in this organelle. Thus, investigation of viral interference with the class I pathway has provided new insight into fundamental cell biologic processes, as with US11.

Other categories of interference mechanisms involve either more proximal or more distal events in the class I pathway. Rather than block assembly or transport of class I ligands for the TCR after heavy-chain synthesis, some viruses attack the genes encoding the heavy chains themselves, interfering with transcription, and thus the production of the heavy chain in the first place. This strategy is known to be used by adenovirus (E19) and HIV (Tat) (435). Conversely, HIV Nef downregulates expression of class I reaching the cell surface, again limiting CD8$^+$ cell recognition (431).

In the past few years, it has become apparent that the immune system is organized to deal with these attempts by pathogens to evade recognition dependent on expression of specific peptide–MHC molecule complexes on the plasma membrane. Cells generally categorized as belonging to the innate immune system, namely NK cells, have been shown to possess two distinct sets of surface receptors. One set promotes activation of effector functions such as cytotoxicity or cytokine secretion—this includes the Fc receptors occupied by specific antibody and other receptors whose specific targets are poorly understood. The other group includes two subsets of receptors that inhibit cell activation mediated by the first group of receptors. These killer inhibitory receptors (KIRs) are either immunoglobulin superfamily molecules or members of the C-type lectin family (436). Multiple different versions of each of these receptors exist in the germline and various assortments of several members of each family are present on the surface of each NK cell (437,438). Thus, the distribution of these KIRs is neither homogeneous nor completely clonal. Most remarkably, both the immunoglobulin superfamily KIR and the C-type lectin KIR, despite their lack of structural similarity, recognize MHC class I molecules (439–442) and both mediate their inhibitory effects through recruitment of phosphatase to the site of activating receptor aggregation (443,444), preventing propagation of phosphotyrosine-dependent signals arising from the activating receptors.

The specificity of KIRs prevents NK cells from acting against cells expressing normal class I molecules. If a cell loses expression of MHC class I, however, either through a genetic change as in some tumors or via the action of the various gene products of infectious organisms, KIR signaling decreases, allowing NK activating receptors to function and promote effector activity (445). Thus, because of the similarity in function between NK cells and CD8$^+$ $\alpha\beta$ TCR-bearing T cells, the effect on the adaptive immune system of decreased MHC class I presentation mediated by pathogen defensive proteins is compensated for in terms of cytotoxicity and IFN-γ production by NK cells made active by this same loss of MHC class I expression. This mode of NK activation, as important as it is for host defense against infection and transformed cells, has a down side in clinical practice. Attempts to make allografts "invisible" to the adaptive immune system through interference with MHC molecule expression results in the enhancement of the ability of NK cells to attack the same grafts, diminishing the effectiveness of the MHC manipulation on graft survival.

MHC Molecules, Peptides, and Selection and Maintenance of the T-Cell Repertoire

The demonstration that cytotoxic T-lymphocyte–mediated lysis of target cells, that the antigen-dependent induction of proliferation of primed T cells, and that the cooperation of helper T cells with B cells in antibody responses were all controlled by MHC class I or class II allelic polymorphism was key to the development of the peptide-presentation paradigm that has been the focus of the preceding sections of this chapter. However, we still do not have a complete and well-accepted explanation of how populations of T lymphocytes become functionally restricted to recognition of antigen in the context of particular allelic forms of MHC molecules. This concluding section describes both early and more recent attempts to explain this phenomenon based on the contributions of allele-dependent selective maturation of T cells in the thymus in the absence of the specific foreign antigen–derived peptide to which the mature cell will eventually respond (see also Chapter 11), and very new results suggesting that a similar set of self-recognition events is involved in maintaining the viability of T cells in peripheral lymphoid tissues.

Evidence for an Allelic Bias in the T-Cell Repertoire

It was discovered early on that F1 animals developed at least two distinct populations of responding T cells upon immunization with large protein antigens, each recognizing antigen in the context of one or the other parental MHC type (446,447). One basis for this phe-

nomenon, involving selection of distinct peptides from the processed protein for presentation by each MHC allele, and distinct functional ligand conformations even for similar peptides bound to different MHC molecules, has been detailed above. Thus, a large part of MHC restriction involves the selective activation of mature T cells in the periphery based on the ability of their clonally distributed receptors (TCRs) to recognize particular complexes of peptide and MHC molecules whose physical formation and persistence is allele related. The involvement of these varying sets of peptide–MHC complexes in T-cell priming gives rise to the apparent MHC allele–related specificity seen during secondary challenge of the immune T cells because the same peptide–MHC molecule combination must be present for effective restimulation to occur.

Does this postmaturation effect entirely account for MHC allelic bias in T-cell responses? Put another way, could effective responses to any peptide–MHC combination be elicited from the T cells in a single individual, as long as APCs bearing the peptide–MHC complexes of interest were used for priming? This question cannot be addressed by simply allowing cells to process the test antigen, then injecting them into an animal, because of the strong allogeneic responses elicited by complexes of donor foreign MHC molecules with peptides derived from the donor's own proteins, complexes to which the recipient would not be tolerant (see Chapter 20). This alloantigen response would obscure detection of the antigen-specific response being examined. To prevent this problem, investigators used a variety of depletion techniques to purge the T-cell pool of cells with such alloreactivity, then tested the remaining cells for foreign peptide–nonself MHC recognition. The results of such experiments were mixed, with some studies showing substantial responses to antigen–nonself MHC combinations (448,449). These studies showed that self-MHC restriction is relative, not absolute. The precise meaning of this lack of absolute restriction was difficult to determine because other studies demonstrated degenerate recognition by individual T cells; that is, a single T lymphocyte could recognize and respond to self MHC plus antigen A, as well as to foreign MHC plus antigen B (450,451). Thus, even if the actual peripheral T-cell pool were in principle completely biased to see antigen with self-MHC molecules in an allele-specific manner, it might always be possible to find a response to antigen plus foreign MHC as a result of this degenerate recognition. Therefore, the existence of responses not fully self restricted did not strongly argue against the existence of a bias toward self MHC–peptide complexes in the available mature repertoire.

To investigate this issue further, several laboratories turned to radiation chimeras. These animals have been lethally irradiated, to prevent their own bone marrow from repopulating the hematopoietic system, and then given foreign bone marrow to allow blood and lymphoid regeneration. This procedure appears to destroy the thymic hematopoietic elements of the recipient while preserving function of the epithelial components. Thus, the reconstituted animals have a thymic stroma of host origin and developing T cells, as well as other hematopoietically derived thymic and peripheral components, from the donor strain. By choosing various donor–host combinations, the effects of differences in particular MHC alleles and loci on the resulting mature T-cell pool were evaluated. The most revealing of these experiments involved introducing F1 (A × B) bone marrow into either parent A or parent B irradiated recipients (452). These animals will have F1 lymphocytes and F1 APCs, but the T cells will have matured in a thymus whose nonlymphoid stromal elements are either A or B only. When given antigen after reconstitution, the antigen should be presented via both A and B allelic forms of the MHC molecules expressed by the reconstituting F1 APCs. Because of the presence of F1 hematopoietic cells in the animal and especially the thymus during T-cell differentiation, the animal is functionally tolerant to both A and B MHC haplotypes. The question posed was whether the responses that were elicited under these conditions would resemble an F1 (strong responses to antigen plus A and to antigen plus B) or whether the response would be biased to the MHC type of the thymic stromal elements. A large number of such studies were performed, and although there has been some variation in the extent of the effect, these experiments clearly support the view that the allelic form of MHC molecule present on the thymic stroma strongly biases the potential response of mature T cells. Cells developing in an A thymus give much better responses to antigen plus MHC A than to antigen plus MHC B, even though the APCs are F1. Cells developing in a B thymus give the reciprocal pattern, responding best to antigen plus MHC B. These studies strongly argue for a special role of the allelic forms of MHC molecules present in the thymus in dictating the output of functional T cells. Because the F1 → parent chimeras are equally tolerant to the hematopoietic APCs of both parents (i.e., they have deleted or inactivated those T cells that might respond to self MHC plus self peptide on such cells), it appears that the bias is the result of a positive effect of the MHC type present in the thymus, rather than the result of a negative effect of hematopoietic elements. As discussed in Chapter 11, this selection for maturation is termed positive selection, and it can clearly be documented using transgenic mice whose T cells express a single TCR. In such animals, development of mature T cells with the transgenic TCR is dependent on the expression by the thymic stroma of the proper allelic form of self MHC.

TCR Recognition of MHC Molecule Structure

How does this apparently allele-dependent selection of T cells occur, what is the role of self peptides, and how does the thymus manage to promote the maturation of T cells that it does not delete during the creation of the self-tolerant state, using the same MHC molecules to perform both the positive and negative selection processes? It is first important to consider the relationships between the genes and proteins involved in these events. TCR genes are located on different chromosomes from the genes encoding MHC molecules (see Chapters 8 and 10), and the two sets of genes assort independently during meiosis. Thus, although the TCR and MHC peptide complexes must eventually productively interact for a T-cell response to occur, the basis for any allele-specific interaction cannot be in coordinate inheritance of receptors preadapted for recognition of specific MHC alleles.

Claverie and Kourilsky (453) proposed the simple hypothesis that no direct TCR interaction with the MHC molecules took place. Under these conditions, all allelic specificity was postulated to reflect the role of MHC polymorphism in selecting the sets of bound peptides seen by the mature cells, with the differences in these sets giving rise to the allele-related recognition restrictions observed. Such a model eliminates the need for the structure of the TCR to be in any way preselected for interaction with MHC molecules, whether with respect to conserved or to variable elements. Attractive as this model is in the abstract, both mutagenesis results (454) and the crystallographic data on TCR complexes with peptide–MHC molecule ligand show that it is incorrect (66,67).

What does this fact that the TCR directly contacts MHC molecules mean for understanding the relationship between TCR

germline element structure and allelic restriction of T cells? If the only useful TCRs are those that can recognize peptide–MHC molecule ligands, then any germline TCR element that is structurally incapable of participating in the formation of a receptor with this potential will likely be lost over evolutionary time because there would be no selective pressure to maintain it as an active gene. This argues that there is some type of bias in the germline repertoire for effective fit with the MHC molecules of the species. This predicted intrinsic bias of the T-cell repertoire for effective interaction with MHC molecules even before positive selection has recently been documented experimentally (455). Two classes of models can be imagined for the nature of this intrinsic reactivity. One hypothesis suggests that certain germline TCR elements are preevolved for preferential interaction with the allelic features of MHC molecules. The other suggests that germline TCR elements, if they contribute to direct interaction with MHC molecules, do so primarily by binding to conserved, nonvariable sites. The first model would predict very strong and readily identifiable MHC allele-related biases in the germline TCR elements expressed on mature thymocytes. Some biases of this type have been reported, but they are not in any way absolute—not all TCRs with the given element are selected in the presence of the relevant MHC molecule, and other MHC molecules can select cells with TCR containing the same V segment (456–459). This is in accord with the second model, which predicts that each of the germline TCR elements can be used effectively to interact with a wide range of classes and alleles of MHC molecules, although not necessarily with equal effectiveness.

TCR CDR3 Regions, Peptide Recognition, and Allelic Polymorphism

If the germline elements do not alone play the major role in the allele-specific recognition of peptide–MHC molecule complexes that can be observed experimentally, this implies that the junctional regions must do so, and this has been well documented to be the case in both functional experiments and in the TCR-ligand crystals (66,67,460). But this function of CDR3 is observed after antigen priming of mature cells and clearly involves specific interaction with the epitopic sites of the bound peptide, not the MHC molecule itself. Thus, these data do not address the key issue of an intrinsic bias for peptide–MHC molecule recognition in the unprimed repertoire as seen in the F1 → parent chimeras. Why should an allelic bias that appears to involve both the germline and nongermline parts of the TCR be present in the T-cell repertoire even before selective T-cell activation by bound foreign peptides? Either there must be an evolutionary advantage to such skewing, or it is an inevitable consequence of the way antigen is presented to T cells, and the imposition of such a restriction on the repertoire is not sufficiently damaging to be selected against.

What could the evolutionary advantage be? Suppose a TCR effective in recognition of one peptide bound by a particular MHC molecule were more likely to recognize another, unrelated peptide bound to the same MHC molecule than it was to recognize a related peptide bound to a different MHC molecule. By filling the peripheral T-cell pool with those cells bearing TCR pretested for such a bias to peptide–self-MHC recognition, one could increase significantly the density/frequency of T cells likely to recognize a foreign peptide presented by the available allelic forms of MHC molecules. If such a bias were not introduced, many of the T cells in peripheral lymphoid tissues might be useless, thus reducing the speed and strength of a T-cell response upon infection.

There is little direct evidence that such allele-related degeneracy exists. However, it is now clear that each MHC molecule will tend to bind peptides whose solvent-exposed (epitopic) residues lie in a certain spatial relationship to the peptide-binding groove, depending on the location of the most crucial binding pockets in the MHC molecule and the anchor residues in the peptide. Given this structural bias in epitopic residue display, it is easily imagined that TCR using given germline elements that are optimized for interaction with certain conserved elements of the MHC molecule–binding region will require junctional regions of a certain length and chemistry to effectively position the CDR3 loops in the right relative position for appropriate interaction with the epitopic residues whose position varies with the allele of presenting molecule (461). Thus, selection based on suitable interaction with an epitope of a self peptide bound to self-MHC molecules could significantly increase the likelihood of high-affinity binding to a foreign peptide associated with the same allelic MHC molecule, due to the similar spatial location of the epitopic residues of the self and foreign peptides bound by the same allele of MHC molecule.

The influence of self peptide could be either to increase or to decrease effective receptor affinity for the MHC molecule. One could postulate that the germline forms of TCR α and β chains assemble into a receptor with a rather high effective affinity for MHC molecules independent of the epitopic structure of the bound peptide. Such affinity would be too high to permit on cells in the periphery because it would lead to strong autoreactivity. The CDR3 region, which distinguishes receptors containing the same germline elements, could discriminate among different bound peptides, and only T cells whose CDR3 lowered the effective affinity for MHC just the correct amount would be selected (462,463). Too little reduction would lead to negative selection; too little residual affinity would result in no effective TCR signal and nonselection. Of course, although the proper affinity range might be met by a given peptide–MHC combination, another peptide bound to the same MHC would give another result, perhaps higher or lower. To be a useful selection method, all such self peptide–MHC combinations would need to be screened. This condition will be met as long as there are not marked differences in overall peptide display on different APCs of the same physiologic type, so that interaction of a developing thymocyte with any one APC of a given type is the same as interaction with any other in the same set. This model implies that specific binding to or recognition of the self peptides associated with self-MHC molecules via the CDR3 region of the TCR is not important in most T cell–positive selection, although this region of the receptor contributes to effective selection through certain modulating effects on affinity of the germline TCR components for the allelic MHC molecules available during selection. This has been called the "plain" or "vanilla" peptide model (464) and has gained some favor with the publication of evidence for the MHC allelic bias of some germline TCR elements.

An alternative and more widely held model is that the TCR needs to increase in effective affinity over interaction with MHC alone due to recognition of the bound peptide by the CDR3 region. Too little gain would lead to nonselection, too much to negative selection, just the right amount to positive selection. This model allows the effects of presentation by a single APC to be sufficient to fully define the positive-selection phenotype for a cell, but it suffers the converse problem as the preceding model; negative selection would only be fully effective if all APCs were homogeneous

for their peptide–MHC complexes within a compartment or if the T cell scanned all APCs in the compartment, so that a critical negative selecting complex were not missed.

None of these various models stresses the role of specific MHC residues that interact directly with the TCR in such allele-biased selection. Surely any MHC residues oriented toward the plane in which the exposed epitopic residues of the bound peptide lie will have such an effect, but there are actually only a small number of highly variable residues exclusively in such positions that could be expected to have a major influence on interaction with the TCR and not affect peptide binding. Thus, such polymorphism does not appear to have been strongly selected. Furthermore, evidence exists that major effects on repertoire selection can be imposed by changes in MHC structure at sites not accessible to the TCR (465), indicating that peptide-related events have the capacity to mold the repertoire independent of changes in MHC residues involved in direct TCR contact.

Although the models discussed above have been presented in hypothetical terms, there is now a substantial body of data indicating a role for peptides in the positive selection process. Older data showed that mutations in the floor of the peptide-binding site could alter T-cell development so that some but not other responses to foreign antigens presented by the wild-type molecule are lost as a result of a failure of positive selection. More recently, fetal thymic organ cultures have been performed with thymuses from mutant animals with defects in peptide-dependent antigen presentation via MHC class I or class II molecules, and the resultant T-cell repertoire analyzed. Dramatic findings have emerged from the use of TAP or β2m-deficient animals that also express a transgenic TCR originally derived from an antigen-specific, mature CD8+ T cell. Organ culture of thymuses from such animals shows little development of mature CD8+ T cells. Addition to the culture of synthetic peptide (together with exogenous β2m in the case of the β2m mutants) can correct the selection defect to a greater or lesser extent (466–470). Additional data in support of a peptide dependency of positive selection has come from analysis of mice whose MHC molecules possess a limited diversity of bound peptides, perhaps only a single one in some cases (471–474).

Extensive work has also been done on the relationship between peptide/MHC recognition and negative selection (development of self-tolerance). A deletional basis for much of the functional tolerance noted in earlier experiments was clearly documented when monoclonal antibodies to TCR became available (475) and when mice expressing single TCR as a result of introduction of rearranged genes into the germline were developed (476). In some of these models, experimental exposure in vivo (477), in thymic organ cultures (478,479), and in cultures of dissociated thymocytes (480) to peptide known to be the ligand for the TCR in question resulted in rapid apoptotic death of the developing thymocytes bearing the cognate TCR. Thus, it is well established that occupancy of the TCR of developing T cells with ligands known to be capable of peripheral activation (agonists) can lead to induced cell death within the thymus. Comparison of the efficiency of various peptides to stimulate transgenic TCR-bearing T cells after maturation and to delete the T cells bearing these receptors in the thymus has shown that variant peptide–MHC complexes poorly able, or even unable, to stimulate the mature form of the T cell can nevertheless be effective in intrathymic deletion (468,469,479,481), in accord with the generally held view that negative selection operates at a TCR-based signaling threshold lower than that required for activation of mature T cells. This makes sense because it builds in a margin of error in the deletion/tolerance process so that minor variations in the density of self peptide–MHC complexes on thymic cells mediating negative selection do not lead to the escape to the periphery of T cells with self reactivity.

How Peptide Recognition Results in Useful T-Cell Selection

If self peptides are involved in both positive and negative selection during thymocyte differentiation, how do a proportion of the thymocytes receive a peptide–MHC dependent signal for development without also receiving a signal from the same peptide–MHC complexes for elimination/inactivation? A number of models that are not mutually exclusive have been proposed to explain this apparent paradox (see Chapter 11). They can be broadly divided into those that postulate a major role for differences in the quantity of TCR peptide–MHC complex interaction, those that relate to variation in the quality of this interaction, and those that focus on developmental variation in the response to this interaction.

The oldest model often has been mistakenly called the affinity model of thymocyte selection. This name is misleading because the actual hypothesis relates to differences in quantitative occupancy of the TCR, rather than to qualitative effects of differing affinity of the TCR for specific peptide–MHC complexes per se. This model suggests that different thresholds of intracellular signal transduction exist for distinct physiologic responses of the affected cell for which there is now accumulating evidence at least for mature T cells (482–485). The threshold for induction of further differentiation is postulated to be lower than that for induction of a death pathway. Therefore, low occupancy, due to either low numbers of relevant complexes on thymic APCs, even if the TCR has high affinity, or high numbers of complexes but low TCR affinity, would give rise to signaling that reached only the first but not the second threshold, resulting in net positive selection of such T cells.

A true affinity model would actually be a specific case of a more general model in which the quality of the interaction of the TCR with ligand changes the type of signal received by the T cell and hence its response (486). There is now abundant evidence that alternative structurally-related ligands for the same TCR can give rise to distinct responses by the T cell that cannot be readily explained to result from simple changes in overall receptor occupancy (487–489). Thus, even large amounts of a ligand that is intrinsically unable to induce programmed cell death via the TCR could act as a positive selecting element in the thymus.

The simplest form of the third general model states that during early developmental stages, occupancy of the TCR with enough peptide–MHC complexes to generate intracellular signals will result solely in progressive differentiation (positive selection), whereas such occupancy at later stages will result in death (negative selection). The useful repertoire would come from the presence of distinct sets of peptides on the APCs involved in the two stages, so that T cells selected by peptide A on the APC functioning with early thymocytes will not encounter peptide A on the APC at later times in the thymus and thus will be positively selected without undergoing deletion (490). Our understanding of the antigen-processing pathways makes it clear that two APCs producing distinct differentiation-specific proteins will have at least some nonoverlapping peptide–MHC complexes on their surface. Thus, tests of this model cannot involve searching for evidence that such distinct peptide–MHC complexes merely exist, as they must, but rather

whether such differences play the major role in defining the functional T-cell repertoire.

Some evidence has already been generated that indicates no absolute barrier to negative selection mediated by cortical epithelial cells that would be the major presenting cell to initial stages of developing thymocytes (477) or to positive selection by hematopoietic cells that would be available for interaction at later stages (491). This makes it likely that the stage-specific model just described cannot be correct in its purest form. It is nevertheless true that there seems to be a difference in the efficiency with which epithelial and hematopoietic cells mediate the two types of selection. However, this could be due either to intrinsically different responses of developing thymocytes to antigen presentation, or to differences in the quality of the signals provided by non-MHC molecule ligands on the two APC types. In the latter case, quantitative differences in presentation of the same peptides by the two APCs could give rise to net positive selection. This would occur if the signaling due to the level of peptide–MHC complex on the epithelial cell were adequate for further differentiation, but the amount of this complex on the hematopoietic cell were too low to generate adequate TCR-based signals that together with non-TCR signals led to activation of the death mechanism. This hypothesis implicates quantitative rather than qualitative differences in peptide display among presenting cell types as a critical component of the selection process in combination with additional qualitatively distinct signals provided by the presenting cells bearing the peptide–MHC complexes.

One major issue in the area of thymocyte selection continues to be the role of the structure of particular peptides in positive selection of T cells bearing a specific TCR. One set of investigators ascribes the induction of effective selection in fetal thymic organ cultures involving TAP- or β2m-deficient donors to the structural rescue of class I molecule expression by peptide-induced stabilization of the heavy chain β2m complex. Selection is presumed to require a high density of class I expression on the cell surface to compensate for the presumed low affinity of recognition postulated to be necessary for positive selection without induction of cell death. Any contributions of the epitopic residues of the peptide are considered to be of minor consequence in this model. Data that are frequently cited in support of this conclusion include the ability of a single peptide to promote differentiation of a large number of different TCR-bearing CD8$^+$ T cells in cultures performed with non-TCR transgenic thymuses (466,467) and the ability of apparently structurally unrelated peptides to all induce selection in TCR transgenic situations (492). Others argue for the central role of peptide specificity in the process, citing the substantial improvement in overall CD8$^+$ T-cell selection that occurs as the peptide occupants of the class I molecules are diversified (466,467), as well as the effect of minor changes in peptide structure on effective selection in TCR transgenic situations (469,493).

Additional data bearing on interpretations of these class I data have emerged from studies of mice bearing a predominant or only a single peptide bound to expressed MHC class II molecules, achieved through the use of covalent association with the β chain in a transgenic model (471,494) or using DM-mutant mice whose class II molecules in the H-2^b haplotype appear almost exclusively bound to CLIP (472–474). In each case, a CD4$^+$ mature T-cell pool approaching 25% of normal appears in the thymus of such animals and shows diversity in the use of TCR genetic elements. These data agree with some of the class I results from non-TCR transgenic models in which single peptides could reconstitute about 20% to 30% of the normal number of mature CD8$^+$ cells in the thymic cultures.

One problem with the view that peptide specificity plays at best a minor role in positive selection comes from considering the numbers of cells effectively selected in the thymus under physiologic circumstances. Only about 5% of the CD4$^+$CD8$^+$ precursors avoid "neglect" and undergo activation for either positive or negative selection (476). If germline V-D-J elements interacting with generic or allelic features of the expressed MHC molecules independent of the specific structure of the bound peptides accounted for effective signaling and selection, one would have imagined that this fraction would be much higher. This is because unless the unique CDR3 region of each TCR interfered with signaling by preventing engagement of the TCR with almost all of the diverse peptide-containing MHC molecules on the cell, there would be no reason why every properly assembled αβ TCR would not provide the proper signal for such activation through the germline recognition of MHC structure. One might argue that certain combinations of V-D-J segments are unable to bind properly to certain MHC alleles, but in an animal with two to four class I molecules and two to four class II molecules, a failure of 95% of the combinations to find an acceptable target is inconsistent with this model, given the presence of representatives of nearly every Vβ and Vα in the repertoire of distinct haplotypes, and no exclusions to selection of all tested Vα–Vβ combinations in such repertoires.

How can these various results and interpretations thus be reconciled? One possibility is that for most T-cell selection, the structure of specific peptides plays a role, but there is a great deal of flexibility/degeneracy in the matches that are adequate to drive effective recognition and signaling events. Thus, individual peptides at high concentration could select a substantial repertoire, through such degenerate recognition and the augmenting effects of extremely high ligand density, whereas low amounts of single peptides better matched to a given TCR, could be effective for such selection as well. In short, as would be expected of a recognition system in which there is great diversity in both the receptors and ligands, there would be substantial range of interactions that would be acceptable to the system, with affinity of ligand recognition and density of ligand offered allowing a spectrum of interactions to meet the requirements for initiating selection. This notion of multiple effective recognition patterns would be consistent with the evidence from studies of allorecognition, in which some TCRs require a particular peptide bound to the allo-MHC protein to elicit a response from a specific T cell (matching the data in some transgenic TCR models in fetal thymus organ cultures [FTOCs] showing precision of peptide selection), whereas others require one of a family of peptides (consistent with the degeneracy but not peptide structure independence seen in some TCR transgenic FTOC models), and others nearly any peptide bound to the relevant class I (consistent with the single peptide elicitation of broad repertoires under some circumstances).

As for the properties of ligands able to promote positive selection with respect to a given TCR, nearly all investigators agree that TCR with high affinity for an MHC molecule independent of the peptide occupants of that allelic form would be negatively selected due to the very high density of ligand available to the developing T cell. For TCR with high affinity for a particular peptide–MHC molecule combination rather than for just the MHC component itself, there is some evidence that very low densities of such TCR ligands can promote development without deletion (470,495). However, the T cells that mature under these conditions do not respond to this peptide–MHC molecule combination after leaving the thymus, raising the question of whether the cell bearing the TCR was able to signal in an agonist fashion through its TCR upon recognition of this ligand. Evidence

indicates that other aspects of the signaling apparatus of a T cell can modify how a TCR interprets recognition of a particular peptide–MHC molecule ligand independently of the innate affinity of the recognition process. One explanation for this is the density of CD4 or CD8 coreceptor on the cell (468,496,497). Thus, among the many precursor CD4$^+$CD8$^+$ cells bearing a transgenic TCR, only those whose coreceptor level prevents agonistlike signaling may have the capacity for effective selection without deletion. Recent data also support the possibility that unique peptides bound by MHC molecules on cortical epithelial cells but not elsewhere in the thymus can promote positive selection without deletion due to a unique signaling property of precursor thymocytes that allows limited agonist signaling without induction of cell death (B. Lucas and R. Germain, unpublished observations). If these cells do not encounter this same ligand again before full maturation in the thymus, such cells may escape the late hematopoietic negative selection that plays a major role in shaping the expressed TCR repertoire (498).

Thus, as in much of biology, competing hypotheses are often not mutually exclusive, and in the case of thymic development, there is presently every reason to believe that a combination of several of the features of competing models for the requirements promoting net positive selection contributes to the process. There is almost assuredly a difference in the peptides presented by epithelial versus thymic APCs, these cells clearly differ in cosignaling competence, and quantitative and qualitative variations in peptide–MHC molecule signaling outcomes can occur that also differ among T cells at distinct stages of maturation. The challenge will be to determine the relative roles of each of these mechanisms in establishing the useful T-cell repertoire.

Self-Peptide Presentation, Thymic Selection, and Autoimmunity

MHC molecules are not generally designed to discriminate between peptides arising from self proteins and those derived from foreign proteins. As detailed above, most of the peptides that can be eluted from MHC molecules of normal cells derive from self proteins made by the APC itself or acquired by the cell from its immediate tissue fluid or serum environment. This inability of the presentation system to perform biochemical self–nonself discrimination means that the T-cell immune system must have its own mechanisms to learn how to distinguish operationally between self peptide– and foreign peptide–MHC molecule complexes to diminish the likelihood of deleterious autoimmune reactions.

The preceding section emphasized that much of this discrimination takes place in the thymus during T-cell development, with deletion of thymocytes recognizing effectively presented self peptides, especially on hematopoietic cells that are the primary professional APC in the periphery for stimulation of mature T cells to effector activity (499). However, it is unlikely that this intrathymic screening can be absolute for those antigens present in the thymus or that it applies to those with only extrathymic, tissue-specific expression. In the thymus, self peptide–MHC molecule complexes will surely exist that occupy too few receptors to induce negative selection of thymocytes bearing cognate receptors, especially for ligands predominantly or exclusively expressed on cortical epithelial cells acting at APCs for CD4$^+$CD8$^+$ thymocytes that are protected in part from the deletion-inducing activity of agonist-type ligands (B. Lucas and R. Germain, unpublished observations). These T cells can mature and will exist in the periphery as quiescent, potentially autoreactive cells. A variety of circumstances could allow such cells to reach sufficient levels or quality of TCR occupancy to be activated, giving rise to an autoimmune response. A second category of autoreactive cells are those specific for peptides from proteins not expressed in cells within the thymus. Such differentiation-specific proteins could produce adequate peptide–MHC molecule complexes to stimulate the newly emerging T cells that did not see such complexes during thymic development. Some evidence suggests that peripheral tolerance mechanisms related to the absence of needed costimulatory signals on nonhematopoietic APCs in the body exist to inactivate these cells that would otherwise pose a threat of autoimmune disease (500,501). It is easy to imagine how certain conditions could permit such autoreactive T cells to encounter their tissue-specific ligands in the presence of unanticipated costimulation, resulting in development of pathologic autoimmunity. This type of peripheral tolerance based on absence of costimulation would obviously not be suitable for the self peptide–MHC molecule complexes on professional APCs in the periphery, which have effective levels of costimulatory counterreceptors, hence the requirement for very effective intrathymic deletion due to exposure to such APC in that location before complete T-cell maturation and export.

The quantitative nature of tolerance to self peptide–MHC complexes and the prominent role of hematopoietic cells in this process in the thymus raise the possibility that numerous cells exist in the periphery that could respond to self peptides presented in greater quantity than is characteristic of these APCs (502,503). The number of MHC molecules containing a particular peptide reflects not only the amount of the relevant protein produced by a cell but the specific physiology of the APC, the presence of competing ligands for the MHC molecules, and other factors. For example, competition for binding of class II molecules by invariant chain peptides could keep low-affinity peptides or those produced in modest amounts from reaching high levels on hematopoietic APCs. However, these same peptides, due to diminished competition or increased production,

could reach such levels on tumor cells, where they would then constitute a tumor rejection antigen. The activity of effector cells recognizing these complexes would in fact be an autoimmune response in the truest sense of the word because the peptides being presented come from unmutated self proteins (108,109,504). This concept of useful autoimmunity may hold promise for the design of effective tumor immunotherapy approaches.

The issue of self recognition versus self reactivity at a level sufficient to induce pathology becomes even more relevant with the exciting recent findings of a role for self-MHC recognition in maintenance of the peripheral T-cell pool. Several investigators have found that naive and memory CD4$^+$ or CD8$^+$ T cells die rapidly in host animals lacking class II or class I molecule expression, respectively (505–509). In one case, class II expression only on dendritic cells was adequate to promote CD4$^+$ survival (508). Taken as a whole, these findings indicate that positive selection actually continues after thymic maturation is complete. Although it has not yet been directly demonstrated, it is presumed that the self-MHC requirement involves TCR recognition and signaling, consistent with the finding that freshly isolated T cells show evidence of TCR complex phosphorylation (510). An important area for future investigation will be determining what signals are received by such putative self-recognition events, whether they differ for naive and memory cells, and how the system avoids frequently exceeding the threshold for activation to effector function, an event that could lead to autoimmune dysfunction.

CONCLUSION

This chapter has detailed the primary focus of $\alpha\beta$ receptor-bearing T cells on antigen displayed as peptides bound to cell membrane–associated polymorphic products of the major histocompatibility complex (Fig. 18). The picture of antigen processing and

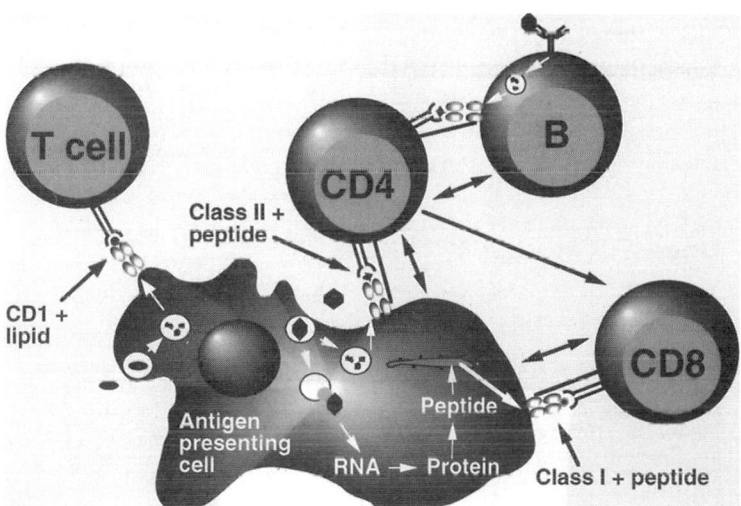

FIG. 18. Antigen presentation in adaptive immunity. An APC, possibly a dendritic cell, is shown providing class I, class II, and CD1 ligands to various T cells for recognition. The same dendritic cell is shown presenting viral antigens to CD4$^+$ and CD8$^+$ T cells. It is still unclear if this three-cell interaction occurs in vivo. After surface immunoglobulin uptake of antigen, B cell presentation of the same peptide–MHC class II complex seen on the dendritic cells is also shown, illustrating the relationship between T-cell priming via dendritic cells and cognate T–B cell collaboration for antibody production. The simultaneous contact of the CD4$^+$ T cell with the dendritic cell and the antigen specific B cell is not intended to indicate that this occurs in vivo, although the discovery of dendritic cells in germinal centers (511) suggests this possibility.

presentation drawn here may seem to many to be rather complete. We now have a detailed knowledge of the biochemistry of the class I and class II MHC molecules, both a broad and detailed understanding of the intracellular pathways that give rise to peptides able to bind to MHC molecules, of the sites of acquisition of these peptides by MHC molecules, and (except for the last step of MHC class II molecule export) of the movement of these peptide–MHC molecule complexes within the cell and to the plasma membrane. The specialization of each class of MHC molecule for acquisition of peptides in distinct intracellular compartments and from different protein sources has become clear, as has the importance of the effect of peptide binding on the intracellular handling of class I and class II molecules. The relationships of these processing and presentation pathways and of the biochemistry of peptide–MHC molecule interaction to functional T-cell recognition of antigen, thymic selection of the T-cell repertoire, autoimmunity, and vaccine effectiveness are apparent. We have identified a set of key accessory molecules that expressed together with MHC class I or class II structural proteins show good, if not yet perfect, reconstruction of the presentation pathways in heterologous cell systems. The existence of related pathways for presentation of structurally unique peptides (such as those containing a N-formyl methionine) and nonpeptide ligands (such as glycolipids by CD1) has been uncovered and the cell biology of these systems also dissected in some detail. Crystallographic images of each of the major MHC molecules in association with peptide or superantigen, of the TCR, and even of TCR complexes with specific peptide–MHC molecule ligands are now available.

But it also should be obvious that much remains to be learned. We still do not have an adequate appreciation of the rules for cleavage of ligands by the proteasome or by endosomal hydrolases that fully explains the preferential presentation of some sequences within source proteins. The in vivo presentation of specific peptides is still a largely open area. Methods for tracking cells bearing a specified peptide–MHC molecule combination have only recently been developed and are just beginning to be applied, so that we can begin to understand which cells act as the relevant APC under different conditions of antigen exposure. The molecular mechanisms controlling intracellular trafficking of proteins containing specific cytoplasmic signals are just starting to be defined, and the regulation of these systems is far from understood. Thus, although in some respects many of the mysteries that made understanding T-cell antigen recognition so fascinating to two generations of immunologists have been solved, many immunologic, cell biologic, and biochemical problems remain for investigation.

REFERENCES

1. Janeway CJ. Approaching the asymptote? Evolution and revolution in immunology. *Cold Spring Harb Symp Quant Biol* 1989;1:1–13.
2. Gell PGH, Benacerraf B. Studies on hypersensitivity. II. Delayed hypersensitivity to denatured protein in guinea pigs. *Immunology* 1959;2:64–70.
3. Unanue ER. Antigen-binding cells. I. Their idenification and role in the immune response. *J Immunol* 1971;107:1168–1174.
4. Schwartz RH. Immune response (Ir) genes of the murine major histocompatibility complex. *Adv Immunol* 1986;38:31–201.
5. Rosenthal AS, Shevach EM. Function of macrophages in antigen recognition by guinea pig T lymphocytes. I. Requirement for histocompatible macrophages and lymphocytes. *J Exp Med* 1973;138:1194–1212.
6. Zinkernagel RM, Doherty PC. Restriction of in vitro T cell-mediated cytotoxicity in lymphocytic choriomeningitis within a syngeneic or semiallogeneic system. *Nature* 1974;248:701–702.
7. Bevan MJ. The major histocompatibility complex determines susceptibility to cytotoxic T cells directed against minor histocompatibility antigens. *J Exp Med* 1975;142:1349–1364.
8. Katz DH, Hamaoka T, Dorf ME, Benacerraf B. Cell interactions between histoincompatible T and B lymphocytes. The H-2 gene complex determines successful physiologic lymphocyte interactions. *Proc Natl Acad Sci U S A* 1973;70:2624–2628.
9. Germain RN. MHC-dependent antigen processing and peptide presentation: Providing ligands for T lymphocyte activation. *Cell* 1994;76:287–299.
10. Meadows L, Wang W, den Haan JM et al. The HLA-A*0201-restricted H-Y antigen contains a posttranslationally modified cysteine that significantly affects T cell recognition. *Immunity* 1997;6:273–281.
11. Cohn M, Langman RE. The protecton: The unit of humoral immunity selected by evolution. *Immunol Rev* 1990;115:11–147.
12. Smith DB, Inglis SC. The mutation rate and variability of eukaryotic viruses: An analytical review. *J Gen Virol* 1987;68:2729–2740.
13. Benacerraf B, McDevitt HO. Histocompatibility-linked immune response genes. *Science* 1972;175:273–279.
14. von Boehmer H, Hudson L, Sprent J. Collaboration of histoincompatible T and B lymphocytes using cells from tetraparental bone marrow chimeras. *J Exp Med* 1975;142:989–997.
15. Longo DL, Schwartz RH. Gene complementation. Neither Ir-GLf gene need be present in the proliferative T cell to generate an immune response to Poly(Glu55Lys36Phe9)n. *J Exp Med* 1980;151:1452–1467.
16. Singer A, Hathcock KS, Hodes RJ. Self recognition in allogeneic radiation bone marrow chimeras. A radiation-resistant host element dictates the self specificity and immune response gene phenotype of T-helper cells. *J Exp Med* 1981;153:1286–1301.
17. Doherty PC, Blanden RV, Zinkernagel RM. Specificity of virus-immune effector T cells for H-2K or H-2D compatible interactions: Implications for H-antigen diversity. *Transplant Rev* 1976;29:89–124.
18. von Boehmer H, Haas W, Jerne NK. Major histocompatibility complex-linked immune-responsiveness is acquired by lymphocytes of low-responder mice differentiating in thymus of high-responder mice. *Proc Natl Acad Sci U S A* 1978;75:2439–2442.
19. Benacerraf B. A hypothesis to relate the specificity of T lymphocytes and the activity of I region-specific Ir genes in macrophages and B lymphocytes. *J Immunol* 1978;120:1809–1812.
20. Kappler JW, Skidmore B, White J, Marrack P. Antigen-inducible, H-2-restricted, interleukin-2-producing T cell hybridomas. Lack of independent antigen and H-2 recognition. *J Exp Med* 1981;153:1198–1214.
21. Heber-Katz E, Hansburg D, Schwartz RH. The Ia molecule of the antigen-presenting cell plays a critical role in immune response gene regulation of T cell activation. *J Mol Cell Immunol* 1983;1:3–18.
22. Racioppi L, Ronchese F, Schwartz RH, Germain RN. The molecular basis of class II MHC allelic control of T cell responses. *J Immunol* 1991;147:3718–3727.
23. Rock KL, Benacerraf B. Inhibition of antigen-specific T lymphocyte activation by structurally related Ir gene-controlled polymers. Evidence of specific competition for accessory cell antigen presentation. *J Exp Med* 1983;157:1618–1634.
24. Ziegler K, Unanue ER. Identification of a macrophage antigen-processing event required for I-region-restricted antigen presentation to T lymphocytes. *J Immunol* 1981;127:1869–1875.
25. Shimonkevitz R, Colon S, Kappler JW, Marrack P, Grey HM. Antigen recognition by H-2-restricted T cells. II. A tryptic ovalbumin peptide that substitutes for processed antigen. *J Immunol* 1984;133:2067–2074.
26. Babbitt BP, Allen PM, Matsueda G, Haber E, Unanue ER. Binding of immunogenic peptides to Ia histocompatibility molecules. *Nature* 1985;317:359–361.
27. Buus S, Sette A, Colon SM, Jenis DM, Grey HM. Isolation and characterization of antigen-Ia complexes involved in T cell recognition. *Cell* 1986;47:1071–1077.
28. Yagüe J, White J, Coleclough C, Kappler J, Palmer E, Marrack P. The T cell receptor: The alpha and beta chains define idiotype, and antigen and MHC specificity. *Cell* 1985;42:81–87.
29. Dembíc Z, Haas W, Weiss S, et al. Transfer of specificity by murine alpha and beta T-cell receptor genes. *Nature* 1986;320:232–238.
30. Saito T, Weiss A, Miller J, Norcross MA, Germain RN. Specific antigen-Ia activation of transfected human T cells expressing murine Ti ab-human T3 receptor complexes. *Nature* 1987;325:125–130.
31. Morrison LA, Lukacher AE, Braciale VL, Fan DP, Braciale TJ. Differences in antigen presentation to MHC class I-and class II-restricted influenza virus-specific cytolytic T lymphocyte clones. *J Exp Med* 1986;163:903–921.
32. Townsend AR, Gotch FM, Davey J. Cytotoxic T cells recognize fragments of the influenza nucleoprotein. *Cell* 1985;42:457–467.
33. Germain RN. The ins and outs of antigen processing and presentation. *Nature* 1986;322:687–689.
34. Long EO. Intracellular traffic and antigen processing. *Immunol Today* 1989;10:232–234.
35. Yewdell JW, Bennink JR. The binary logic of antigen processing and presentation to T cells. *Cell* 1990;62:203–206.
36. Newell WR, Trowsdale J, Beck S. MHCDB—database of the human MHC. *Immunogenetics* 1994;40:109–115.
37. Abdulla S, Alderton RP, Glynne RJ et al. DNA sequencing of the MHC class II region and the chromosome 6 sequencing effort at the Sanger Centre. *DNA Seq* 1996;7:5–7.
38. Sallusto F, Lanzavecchia A. Efficient presentation of soluble antigen by cultured human dendritic cells is maintained by granulocyte/macrophage colony-stimu-

lating factor plus interleukin 4 and downregulated by tumor necrosis factor alpha. *J Exp Med* 1994;179:1109–1118.

39. Jonuleit H, Knop J, Enk AH. Cytokines and their effects on maturation, differentiation and migration of dendritic cells. *Arch Dermatol Res* 1996;289:1–8.

40. Wang B, Kondo S, Shivji GM, Fujisawa H, Mak TW, Sauder DN. Tumour necrosis factor receptor II (p75) signalling is required for the migration of Langerhans' cells. *Immunology* 1996;88:284–288.

41. Heinrichs H, Orr HT. HLA non-A,B,C class I genes: Their structure and expression. *Immunol Res* 1990;9:265–274.

42. Klein J, Benoist C, David CS, et al. Revised nomenclature of mouse H-2 genes. *Immunogenetics* 1990;32:147–149.

43. Wei XH, Orr HT. Differential expression of HLA-E, HLA-F, and HLA-G transcripts in human tissue. *Hum Immunol* 1990;29:131–142.

44. Vernachio J, Li M, Donnenberg AD, Soloski MJ. Qa-2 expression in the adult murine thymus. A unique marker for a mature thymic subset. *J Immunol* 1989;142:48–56.

45. Hood L, Steinmetz M, Malissen B. Genes of the major histocompatibility complex of the mouse. *Annu Rev Immunol* 1983;1:529–568.

46. Salter RD, Benjamin RJ, Wesley PK, et al. A binding site for the T-cell co-receptor CD8 on the alpha 3 domain of HLA-A2. *Nature* 1990;345:41–46.

47. Gao GF, Tormo J, Gerth UC, et al. Crystal structure of the complex between human CD8alpha(alpha) and HLA- A2. *Nature* 1997;387:630–634.

48. Kaufman JF, Auffray C, Korman AJ, Shackelford DA, Strominger J. The class II molecules of the human and murine major histocompatibility complex. *Cell* 1984;36:1–13.

49. Cosson P, Bonifacino JS. Role of transmembrane domain interactions in the assembly of class II MHC molecules. *Science* 1992;258:659–662.

50. Murphy DB, Jones PP, Loken MR, McDevitt HO. Interaction between I region loci influences the expression of a cell surface Ia antigen. *Proc Natl Acad Sci U S A* 1980;77:5404–5408.

51. Germain RN, Bentley DM, Quill H. Influence of allelic polymorphism on the assembly and surface expression of class II MHC (Ia) molecules. *Cell* 1985;43:233–242.

52. Sant AJ, Germain RN. Intracellular competition for component chains determines class II MHC cell surface phenotype. *Cell* 1989;57:797–805.

53. Germain RN, Quill H. Unexpected expression of a unique mixed-isotype class II MHC molecule by transfected L-cells. *Nature* 1986;320:72–75.

54. Ruberti G, Sellins KS, Hill CM, Germain RN, Fathman CG, Livingstone A. Presentation of antigen by mixed isotype class II molecules in normal H-2^d mice. *J Exp Med* 1992;175:157–162.

55. Karlsson L, Surh CD, Sprent J, Peterson PA. A novel class II MHC molecule with unusual tissue distribution. *Nature* 1991;351:485–488.

56. Liljedahl M, Kuwana T, Fung-Leung WP, et al. HLA-DO is a lysosomal resident which requires association with HLA-DM for efficient intracellular transport. *EMBO J* 1996;15:4817–4824.

57. Germain RN, Malissen B. Analysis of the expression and function of class-II major histocompatibility complex-encoded molecules by DNA-mediated gene transfer. *Annu Rev Immunol* 1986;4:281–315.

58. Jelachich ML, Biddison WE. Class I antigen presentation. *Year Immunol* 1989;4:41–58.

59. Braunstein NS, Germain RN. I-A-restricted T cell antigen recognition. Analysis of the roles of Aa and Ab using DNA-mediated gene transfer. *J Exp Med* 1986;163:678–696.

60. Bjorkman PJ, Saper MA, Samraoui B, Bennett WS, Strominger JL, Wiley DC. Structure of the human class I histocompatibility antigen, HLA-A2. *Nature* 1987;329:506–512.

61. Bjorkman PJ, Saper MA, Samraoui B, Bennett WS, Strominger JL, Wiley DC. The foreign antigen binding site and T cell recognition regions of class I histocompatibility antigens. *Nature* 1987;329:512–518.

62. Garrett TP, Saper MA, Bjorkman PJ, Strominger JL, Wiley DC. Specificity pockets for the side chains of peptide antigens in HLA-Aw68. *Nature* 1989;342:692–696.

63. Fremont DH, Matsumura M, Stura EA, Peterson PA, Wilson IA. Crystal structures of two viral peptides in complex with murine MHC class I H-2K^b. *Science* 1992;257:919–927.

64. Matsumura M, Fremont DH, Peterson PA, Wilson IA. Emerging principles for the recognition of peptide antigens by MHC class I molecules. *Science* 1992;257:927–934.

65. Madden DR, Garboczi DN, Wiley DC. The antigenic identity of peptide-MHC complexes: A comparison of the conformations of five viral peptides presented by HLA-A2. *Cell* 1993;75:693–708.

66. Garcia KC, Degano M, Stanfield RL, et al. An αβ T cell receptor structure at 2.5 A and its orientation in the TCR-MHC complex. *Science* 1996;274:209–219.

67. Garboczi DN, Ghosh P, Utz U, Fan QR, Biddison WE, Wiley DC. Structure of the complex between human T-cell receptor, viral peptide and HLA-A2. *Nature* 1996;384:134–141.

68. Stern LJ, Wiley DC. Antigenic peptide binding by class I and class II histocompatibility proteins. *Structure* 1994;2:245–251.

69. Madden DR, Gorga JC, Strominger JL, Wiley DC. The structure of HLA-B27 reveals nonamer self-peptides bound in an extended conformation. *Nature* 1991;353:321–325.

70. Bouvier M, Wiley DC. Importance of peptide amino and carboxyl termini to the stability of MHC class I molecules. *Science* 1994;265:398–402.

71. Guo HC, Jardetzky TS, Garrett TP, Lane WS, Strominger JL, Wiley DC. Different length peptides bind to HLA-Aw68 similarly at their ends but bulge out in the middle. *Nature* 1992;360:364–366.

72. Collins EJ, Garboczi DN, Wiley DC. Three-dimensional structure of a peptide extending from one end of a class I MHC binding site. *Nature* 1994;371:626–629.

73. Fischer-Lindahl K, Hermel E, Loveland BE, Wang C-R. Maternally transmitted antigen of mice: A model transplantation antigen. *Ann Rev Immunol* 1991;9:351–372.

74. Wang CR, Lindahl KF, Deisenhofer J. Crystal structure of the MHC class Ib molecule H2-M3. *Res Immunol* 1996;147:313–321.

75. Kurlander RJ, Shawar SM, Brown ML, Rich RR. Specialized role for a murine Class-I-b MHC molecule in prokaryotic host defenses. *Science* 1992;257:678–679.

76. Pamer EG, Wang C-R, Flaherty L, Fischer-Lindahl K, Bevan MJ. H-2M3 presents a Listeria monocytogenes peptide to cytotoxic T lymphocytes. *Cell* 1992;70:215–223.

77. Zeng Z, Castao AR, Segelke BW, Stura EA, Peterson PA, Wilson IA. Crystal structure of mouse CD1: An MHC-like fold with a large hydrophobic binding groove. *Science* 1997;277:339–345.

78. Beckman EM, Porcelli SA, Morita CT, Behar SM, Furlong ST, Brenner MB. Recognition of a lipid antigen by CD1-restricted αβ$^+$ T cells. *Nature* 1994;372:691–694.

79. Sieling PA, Chatterjee D, Porcelli SA, et al. CD1-restricted T cell recognition of microbial lipoglycan antigens. *Science* 1995;269:227–230.

80. Brown JH, Jardetzky TS, Gorga JC, et al. Three-dimensional structure of the human class II histocompatibility antigen HLA-DR1. *Nature* 1993;364:33–39.

81. Stern LJ, Brown JH, Jardetzky TS, et al. Crystal structure of the human class II MHC protein HLA-DR1 complexed with an influenza virus peptide. *Nature* 1994;368:215–221.

82. Kim J, Urban RG, Strominger JL, Wiley DC. Toxic shock syndrome toxin-1 complexed with a class II major histocompatibility molecule HLA-DR1. *Science* 1994;266:1870–1874.

83. Jardetzky TS, Brown JH, Gorga JC, et al. Three-dimensional structure of a human class II histocompatibility molecule complexed with superantigen. *Nature* 1994;368:711–718.

84. Ghosh P, Amaya M, Mellins E, Wiley DC. The structure of an intermediate in class II MIIC maturation: CLIP bound to HLA-DR3. *Nature* 1995;378:457–462.

85. Fremont DH, Hendrickson WA, Marrack P, Kappler J. Structures of an MHC class II molecule with covalently bound single peptides. *Science* 1996;272:1001–1004.

86. Jardetzky TS, Brown JH, Gorga JC, et al. Crystallographic analysis of endogenous peptides associated with HLA-DR1 suggests a common, polyproline II-like conformation for bound peptides. *Proc Natl Acad Sci U S A* 1996;93:734–738.

87. Germain RN. Seeing double! *Curr Biol* 1993;3:586–589.

88. König R, Huang L-Y, Germain RN. MHC class II interaction with CD4 mediated by a region analogous to the MHC class I binding site for CD8. *Nature* 1992;356:796–798.

89. Cammarota G, Scheirle A, Takacs B, et al. Identification of a CD4 binding site on the β2 domain of HLA-DR molecules. *Nature* 1992;356:799–801.

90. König R, Shen X, Germain RN. Involvement of both MHC class II α and β chains in CD4 function indicates a role for ordered oligomerization in T cell activation. *J Exp Med* 1995;182:779–787.

91. Wu H, Kwong PD, Hendrickson WA. Dimeric association and segmental variability in the structure of human CD4. *Nature* 1997;387:527–530.

92. Reich Z, Boniface JJ, Lyons DS, Borochov N, Wachtel EJ, Davis MM. Ligand-specific oligomerization of T-cell receptor molecules. *Nature* 1997;387:617–620.

93. Herman A, Kappler JW, Marrack P, Pullen AM. Superantigens: Mechanism of T-cell stimulation and role in immune responses. *Annu Rev Immunol* 1991;9:745–772.

94. Choi YW, Herman A, DiGiusto D, Wade T, Marrack P, Kappler J. Residues of the variable region of the T-cell-receptor β-chain that interact with *S. aureus* toxin superantigens. *Nature* 1990;346:471–473.

95. Pullen AM, Wade T, Marrack P, Kappler JW. Identification of the region of T cell receptor β chain that interacts with the self-superantigen Mls-1a. *Cell* 1990;61:1365–1374.

96. Kappler J, White J, Kozono H, Clements J, Marrack P. Binding of a soluble αβ T-cell receptor to superantigen/major histocompatibility complex ligands. *Proc Natl Acad Sci U S A* 1994;91:8462–8466.

97. Fields BA, Malchiodi EL, Li H, et al. Crystal structure of a T-cell receptor β-chain complexed with a superantigen. *Nature* 1996;384:188–192.

98. Swaminathan S, Furey W, Pletcher J, Sax M. Crystal structure of staphylococcal enterotoxin B, a superantigen. *Nature* 1992;359:801–806.

99. Thibodeau J, Cloutier I, Lavoie PM, et al. Subsets of HLA-DR1 molecules defined by SEB and TSST-1 binding. *Science* 1994;266:1874–1878.

100. von Bonin A, Ehrlich S, Malcherek G, Fleischer B. Major histocompatibility complex class II-associated peptides determine the binding of the superantigen toxic shock syndrome toxin-1. *Eur J Immunol* 1995;25:2894–2898.

101. Davis MM, Bjorkman PJ. T-cell antigen receptor genes and T-cell recognition. *Nature* 1988;334:395–402.

102. Zerrahn R, Claverie JM, Prochnicka CA, Spetz ILA, Larsson EC. How important is the direct recognition of polymorphic MHC residues by TCR in the gen-

eration of the T-cell repertoire? *Cold Spring Harb Symp Quant Biol* 1989;1: 93–103.

103. Rosenthal AS. Determinant selection and macrophage function in genetic control of the immune response. *Immunol Rev* 1978;40:136–152.

104. Schwartz RH. A clonal deletion model for Ir gene control of the immune response. *Scan J Immunol* 1978;7:3–10.

105. Hammer J, Bono E, Gallazzi F, Belunis C, Nagy Z, Sinigaglia F. Precise prediction of major histocompatibility complex class II-peptide interaction based on peptide side chain scanning. *J Exp Med* 1994;180:2353–2358.

106. Schumacher TNM, Van Bleek GM, Heemels M-T, et al. Synthetic peptide libraries in the determination of T cell epitopes and peptide binding specificity of class I molecules. *Eur J Immunol* 1992;22:1405–1412.

107. Hammer J, Takacs B, Sinigaglia F. Identification of a motif for HLA-DR1 binding peptides using M13 display libraries. *J Exp Med* 1992;176:1007–1013.

108. van der Bruggen P, Traversari C, Chomez P, et al. A gene encoding an antigen recognized by cytolytic T lymphocytes on a human melanoma. *Science* 1991; 254:1643–1647.

109. Kawakami Y, Eliyahu S, Delgado CH, et al. Cloning of the gene coding for a shared human melanoma antigen recognized by autologous T cells infiltrating into tumor. *Proc Natl Acad Sci U S A* 1994;91:3515–3519.

110. Wang RF, Robbins PF, Kawakami Y, Kang XQ, Rosenberg SA. Identification of a gene encoding a melanoma tumor antigen recognized by HLA-A31-restricted tumor-infiltrating lymphocytes [erratum *J Exp Med* 1995;181:1261]. *J Exp Med* 1995;181:799–804.

111. Boon T, van der Bruggen P. Human tumor antigens recognized by T lymphocytes. *J Exp Med* 1996;183:725–729.

112. Engelhard VH. Direct identification of tumor-associated peptide antigens. *Springer Semin Immunopathol* 1996;18:171–183.

113. Rötzschke O, Falk K, Wallny HJ, Faath S, Rammensee HG. Characterization of naturally occurring minor histocompatibility peptides including H-4 and H-Y. *Science* 1990;249:283–287.

114. Wallny HJ, Rammensee HG. Identification of classical minor histocompatibility antigen as cell-derived peptide. *Nature* 1990;343:275–278.

115. Falk K, Rötzschke O, Rammensee HG. Cellular peptide composition governed by major histocompatibility complex class I molecules. *Nature* 1990;348: 248–251.

116. Rötzschke O, Falk K, Deres K, et al. Isolation and analysis of naturally processed viral peptides as recognized by cytotoxic T cells. *Nature* 1990;348:252–254.

117. Van Bleek GM, Nathenson SG. Isolation of an endogenously processed immunodominant viral peptide from the class I H-2Kb molecule. *Nature* 1990;348: 213–216.

118. Falk K, Rötzschke O, Stevanovïc S, Jung G, Rammensee HG. Allele-specific motifs revealed by sequencing of self-peptides eluted from MHC molecules. *Nature* 1991;351:290–296.

119. Hunt DF, Henderson RA, Shabanowitz J, et al. Characterization of peptides bound to the class I MHC molecule HLA-A2.1 by mass spectrometry. *Science* 1992;255:1261–1263.

120. Khilko SN, Jelonek MT, Corr M, Boyd LF, Bothwell AL, Margulies DH. Measuring interactions of MHC class I molecules using surface plasmon resonance. *J Immunol Methods* 1995;183:77–94.

121. Boehncke WH, Takeshita T, Pendleton CD, et al. The importance of dominant negative effects of amino acid side chain substitution in peptide-MHC molecule interactions and T cell recognition. *J Immunol* 1993;150:331–341.

122. Ruppert J, Sidney J, Celis E, Kubo RT, Grey HM, Sette A. Prominent role of secondary anchor residues in peptide binding to HLA-A2.1 molecules. *Cell* 1993;74:929–937.

123. Parker KC, Shields M, DiBrino M, Brooks A, Coligan JE. Peptide binding to MHC class I molecules: Implications for antigenic peptide prediction. *Immunol Res* 1995;14:34–57.

124. Rudensky A, Preston HP, Hong SC, Barlow A, Janeway CAJ. Sequence analysis of peptides bound to MHC class II molecules. *Nature* 1991;353:622–627.

125. Chicz RM, Urban RG, Lane WS, et al. Predominant naturally processed peptides bound to HLA-DR1 are derived from MHC-related molecules and are heterogeneous in size. *Nature* 1992;358:764–768.

126. Hunt DF, Michel H, Dickinson TA, et al. Peptides presented to the immune system by the murine class II major histocompatibility complex molecule I-Ad. *Science* 1992;256:1817–1820.

127. Rudensky AY, Preston-Hulbert P, Al-Ramadi B, Hong S-C, Rothbard J, Janeway CA Jr. Truncation variants of peptides isolated from MHC class II molecules suggest sequence motifs. *Nature* 1992;359:429–431.

128. Falk K, Rötzschke O, Stevanovïc S, Jung G, Rammensee HG. Pool sequencing of natural HLA-DR, DQ, and DP ligands reveals detailed peptide motifs, constraints of processing, and general rules. *Immunogenetics* 1994;39:230–242.

129. Nelson CA, Vidavsky I, Viner NJ, Gross ML, Unanue ER. Amino-terminal trimming of peptides for presentation on major histocompatibility complex class II molecules. *Proc Natl Acad Sci U S A* 1997;94:628–633.

130. Alexander J, Sidney J, Southwood S, et al. Development of high potency universal DR-restricted helper epitopes by modification of high affinity DR-blocking peptides. *Immunity* 1994;1:751–761.

131. Ljunggren HG, Pääbo S, Cochet M, Kling G, Kourilsky P, Kärre K. Molecular analysis of H-2-deficient lymphoma lines. Distinct defects in biosynthesis and association of MHC class I heavy chains and β2-microglobulin observed in cells with increased sensitivity to NK cell lysis. *J Immunol* 1989;142:2911–2917.

132. Townsend A, Öhlén C, Bastin J, Ljunggren HG, Foster L, Kärre K. Association of class I major histocompatibility heavy and light chains induced by viral peptides. *Nature* 1989;340:443–448.

133. Townsend A, Elliott T, Cerundolo V, Foster L, Barber B, Tse A. Assembly of MHC class I molecules analyzed in vitro. *Cell* 1990;62:285–295.

134. Cerundolo V, Alexander J, Anderson K et al. Presentation of viral antigen controlled by a gene in the major histocompatibility complex. *Nature* 1990;345: 449–452.

135. Lie WR, Myers NB, Gorka J, Rubocki RJ, Connolly JM, Hansen TH. Peptide ligand-induced conformation and surface expression of the Ld class I MHC molecule. *Nature* 1990;344:439–441.

136. Bikoff EK, Jaffe L, Ribaudo RK, Otten GR, Germain RN, Robertson EJ. MHC class I surface expression in embryo-derived cell lines inducible with peptide or interferon. *Nature* 1991;354:235–238.

137. Ljunggren HG, Stam NJ, Öhlén C, et al. Empty MHC class I molecules come out in the cold. *Nature* 1990;346:476–480.

138. Elliott T, Cerundolo V, Elvin J, Townsend A. Peptide-induced conformational change of the class I heavy chain. *Nature* 1991;351:402–406.

139. Sherman LA, Burke TA, Biggs JA. Extracellular processing of peptide antigens that bind class I major histocompatibility molecules. *J Exp Med* 1992;175: 1221–1226.

140. Kozlowski S, Corr M, Takeshita T, et al. Serum angiotensin-1 converting enzyme activity processes a human immunodeficiency virus 1 gp160 peptide for presentation by major histocompatibility complex class I molecules. *J Exp Med* 1992;175:1417–1422.

141. Schumacher TN, De BM, Vernie LN, et al. Peptide selection by MHC class I molecules. *Nature* 1991;350:703–706.

142. Elliott T. How do peptides associate with MHC class I molecules? *Immunol Today* 1991;12:386–388.

143. Rock KL, Rothstein LE, Gamble SR, Benacerraf B. Reassociation with β2-microglobulin is necessary for Kb class I major histocompatibility complex binding of exogenous peptides. *Proc Natl Acad Sci U S A* 1990;87:7517–7521.

144. Vitiello A, Potter TA, Sherman LA. The role of β2-microglobulin in peptide binding by class I molecules. *Science* 1990;250:1423–1426.

145. Kozlowski S, Takeshita T, Boehncke WH, et al. Excess β2 microglobulin promoting functional peptide association with purified soluble class I MHC molecules. *Nature* 1991;349:74–77.

146. Otten GR, Bikoff E, Ribaudo RK, Kozlowski S, Margulies DH, Germain RN. Peptide and β2-microglobulin regulation of cell surface MHC class-I conformation and expression. *J Immunol* 1992;148:3723–3732.

147. Silver ML, Parker KC, Wiley DC. Reconstitution by MHC-restricted peptides of HLA-A2 heavy chain with β2-microglobulin, in vitro. *Nature* 1991;350:619–622.

148. Springer TA, Kaufman JF, Siddoway LA, Mann DL, Strominger JL. Purification of HLA-linked B lymphocyte alloantigens in immunologically active form by preparative sodium dodecyl sulfate-gel electrophoresis and studies on their subunit association. *J Biol Chem* 1977;252:6201–6207.

149. Cresswell P. Human B cells alloantigens; separation from other membrane molecules by affinity chromatography. *Eur J Immunol* 1977;7:636–639.

150. Dornmair K, Rothenhäusler B, McConnell HM. Structural intermediates in the reactions of antigenic peptides with MHC molecules. *Cold Spring Harb Symp Quant Biol* 1989;1:409–416.

151. Sadegh-Nasseri S, Germain RN. A role for peptide in determining MHC class II structure. *Nature* 1991;353:167–170.

152. Germain RN, Hendrix LR. MHC class II structure, occupancy and surface expression determined by post-endoplasmic reticulum antigen binding. *Nature* 1991;353:134–139.

153. Davidson HW, Reid PA, Lanzavecchia A, Watts C. Processed antigen binds to newly synthesized MHC class II molecules in antigen-specific B lymphocytes. *Cell* 1991;67:105–116.

154. Germain RN, Rinker AG Jr. Peptide binding inhibits protein aggregation of invariant-chain free class II dimers and promotes selective cell surface expression of occupied molecules. *Nature* 1993;363:725–728.

155. Lanzavecchia A, Reid PA, Watts C. Irreversible association of peptides with class-II MHC molecules in living cells. *Nature* 1992;357:249–252.

156. Chen BP, Parham P. Direct binding of influenza peptides to class I HLA molecules. *Nature* 1989;337:743–745.

157. Cerundolo V, Elliott T, Elvin J, Bastin J, Rammensee HG, Townsend A. The binding affinity and dissociation rates of peptides for class I major histocompatibility complex molecules. *Eur J Immunol* 1991;21:2069–2075.

158. Sadegh-Nasseri S, McConnell HM. A kinetic intermediate in the reaction of an antigenic peptide and I-Ek. *Nature* 1989;337:274–276.

159. Jensen PE. Regulation of antigen presentation by acidic pH. *J Exp Med* 1990; 171:1779–1784.

160. Jensen PE. Enhanced binding of peptide antigen to purified class II major histocompatibility glycoproteins at acidic pH. *J Exp Med* 1991;174:1111–1120.

161. Harding CV, Roof RW, Allen PM, Unanue ER. Effects of pH and polysaccharides on peptide binding to class II major histocompatibility complex molecules. *Proc Natl Acad Sci U S A* 1991;88:2740–2744.

162. Sette A, Southwood S, O'Sullivan D, Gaeta FC, Sidney J, Grey HM. Effect of pH on MHC class II-peptide interactions. *J Immunol* 1992;148:844–851.

163. Reay PA, Wettstein DA, Davis MM. pH dependence and exchange of high and low responder peptides binding to a class II MHC molecule. *Embo J* 1992;11: 2829–2839.

164. Tampé R, McConnell HM. Kinetics of antigenic peptide binding to the class II major histocompatibility molecule I-Ad. *Proc Natl Acad Sci U S A* 1991;88: 4661–4665.

165. Stern LJ, Wiley DC. The human class II MHC protein HLA-DR1 assembles as empty alpha beta heterodimers in the absence of antigenic peptide. *Cell* 1992;68:465–477.

166. Sadegh-Nasseri S, Stern LJ, Wiley DC, Germain RN. MHC class II function preserved by low-affinity peptide interactions preceding stable binding. *Nature* 1994;370:647–650.

167. Boniface JJ, Lyons DS, Wettstein DA, Allbritton NL, Davis MM. Evidence for a conformational change in a class II major histocompatibility complex molecule occurring in the same pH range where antigen binding is enhanced. *J Exp Med* 1996;183:119–126.

168. Degen E, Williams DB. Participation of a novel 88-kD protein in the biogenesis of murine class I histocompatibility molecules. *J Cell Biol* 1991;112:1099–1115.

169. Hochstenbach F, David V, Watkins S, Brenner MB. Endoplasmic reticulum resident protein of 90 kilodaltons associates with the T-cell and B-cell antigen receptors and major histocompatibility complex antigens during their assembly. *Proc Natl Acad Sci U S A* 1992;89:4734–4738.

170. Hammond C, Helenius A. A chaperone with a sweet tooth. *Curr Biol* 1993;3: 884–886.

171. Zhang Q, Tector M, Salter RD. Calnexin recognizes carbohydrate and protein determinants of class I major histocompatibility complex molecules. *J Biol Chem* 1995;270:3944–3948.

172. Ware FE, Vassilakos A, Peterson PA, Jackson MR, Lehrman MA, Williams DB. The molecular chaperone calnexin binds Glc1Man9GlcNAc2 oligosaccharide as an initial step in recognizing unfolded glycoproteins. *J Biol Chem* 1995;270: 4697–4704.

173. Ortmann B, Androlewicz MJ, Cresswell P. MHC class I/β2-microglobulin complexes associate with TAP transporters before peptide binding. *Nature* 1994;368: 864–867.

174. Rajagopalan S, Brenner MB. Calnexin retains unassembled major histocompatibility complex class I free heavy chains in the endoplasmic reticulum. *J Exp Med* 1994;180:407–412.

175. Sadasivan B, Lehner PJ, Ortmann B, Spies T, Cresswell P. Roles for calreticulin and a novel glycoprotein, tapasin, in the interaction of MHC class I molecules with TAP. *Immunity* 1996;5:103–114.

176. Zamoyska R, Parnes JR. Rescue of Daudi cell HLA expression by transfection of the mouse beta 2-microglobulin gene. *J Exp Med* 1988;167:288–299.

177. Williams DB, Barber DH, Flavell RA, Allen H. Role of β2-microglobulin in the intracellular transport and surface expression of murine class I histocompatibility molecules. *J Immunol* 1989;142:2796–2806.

178. Zijlstra M, Bix M, Simister NE, Loring JM, Raulet DH, Jaenisch R. β2-microglobulin deficient mice lack CD4⁻8⁺ cytolytic T cells. *Nature* 1990;344: 742–746.

179. Ortmann B, Copeman J, Lehner PJ, et al. A critical role for tapasin in the assembly and function of MHC class I-TAP complexes. *Science* 1997;277:1306–1309.

180. Grandea AGr, Androlewicz MJ, Athwal RS, Geraghty DE, Spies T. Dependence of peptide binding by MHC class I molecules on their interaction with TAP. *Science* 1995;270:105–108.

181. Jones PP, Murphy DB, Hewgill D, McDevitt HO. Detection of a common polypeptide chain in I—A and I—E sub-region immunoprecipitates. *Mol Immunol* 1979;16:51–60.

182. Singer PA, Lauer W, Dembïc Z, et al. Structure of the murine Ia-associated invariant (Ii) chain as deduced from a cDNA clone. *EMBO J* 1984;3:873–877.

183. Strubin M, Mach B, Long EO. The complete sequence of the mRNA for the HLA-DR-associated invariant chain reveals a polypeptide with an unusual transmembrane polarity. *EMBO J* 1984;3:869–872.

184. Strubin M, Berte C, Mach B. Alternative splicing and alternative initiation of translation explain the four forms of the Ia antigen-associated invariant chain. *EMBO J* 1986;5:3483–3488.

185. Koch N, Lauer W, Habicht J, Dobberstein B. Primary structure of the gene for the murine Ia antigen-associated invariant chains (Ii). An alternatively spliced exon encodes a cysteine-rich domain highly homologous to a repetitive sequence of thyroglobulin. *EMBO J* 1987;6:1677–1683.

186. Marks MS, Blum JS, Cresswell P. Invariant chain trimers are sequestered in the rough endoplasmic reticulum in the absence of association with HLA class II antigens. *J Cell Biol* 1990;111:839–855.

187. Roche PA, Marks MS, Cresswell P. Formation of a nine-subunit complex by HLA class II glycoproteins and the invariant chain. *Nature* 1991;354:392–394.

188. Anderson KS, Cresswell P. A role for calnexin (IP90) in the assembly of class II MHC molecules. *EMBO J* 1994;13:675–682.

189. Romagnoli P, Germain RN. Inhibition of invariant chain (Ii)-calnexin interaction results in enhanced degradation of Ii but does not prevent the assembly of αβ complexes. *J Exp Med* 1995;182:2027–2036.

190. Cresswell P, Blum JS, Kelner DN, Marks MS. Biosynthesis and processing of class II histocompatibility antigens. *Crit Rev Immunol* 1987;7:31–53.

191. Neefjes JJ, Stollorz V, Peters PJ, Geuze HJ, Ploegh HL. The biosynthetic pathway of MHC class II but not class I molecules intersects the endocytic route. *Cell* 1990;61:171–183.

192. Koch N, Moldenhauer G, Hofmann WJ, Moller P. Rapid intracellular pathway gives rise to cell surface expression of the MHC class II-associated invariant chain (CD74). *J Immunol* 1991;147:2643–2651.

193. Roche PA, Teletski CL, Stang E, Bakke O, Long EO. Cell surface HLA-DR-invariant chain complexes are targeted to endosomes by rapid internalization. *Proc Natl Acad Sci U S A* 1993;90:8581–8585.

194. Blum JS, Cresswell P. Role for intracellular proteases in the processing and transport of class II HLA antigens. *Proc Natl Acad Sci U S A* 1988;85:3975–3979.

195. Nowell J, Quaranta V. Chloroquine affects biosynthesis of Ia molecules by inhibiting dissociation of invariant (gamma) chains from aα-β dimers in B cells. *J Exp Med* 1985;162:1371–1376.

196. Guagliardi LE, Koppelman B, Blum JS, Marks MS, Cresswell P, Brodsky FM. Co-localization of molecules involved in antigen processing and presentation in an early endocytic compartment. *Nature* 1990;343:133–139.

197. Peters PJ, Neefjes JJ, Oorschot V, Ploegh HL, Geuze HJ. Segregation of MHC class II molecules from MHC class I molecules in the Golgi complex for transport to lysosomal compartments. *Nature* 1991;349:669–676.

198. Cella M, Engering A, Pinet V, Pieters J, Lanzavecchia A. Inflammatory stimuli induce accumulation of MHC class II complexes on dendritic cells. *Nature* 1997;388:782–787.

199. Pierre P, Turley SJ, Gatti E, et al. Developmental regulation of MHC class II transport in mouse dendritic cells. *Nature* 1997;388:787–792.

200. Bakke O, Dobberstein B. MHC class II-associated invariant chain contains a sorting signal for endosomal compartments. *Cell* 1990;63:707–716.

201. Lotteau V, Teyton L, Peleraux A, et al. Intracellular transport of class II MHC molecules directed by invariant chain. *Nature* 1990;348:600–605.

202. Romagnoli P, Layet C, Yewdell J, Bakke O, Germain RN. Relationship between invariant chain expression and MHC Class II transport into early and late endocytic compartments. *J Exp Med* 1993;177:583–596.

203. Pieters J, Bakke O, Dobberstein B. The MHC class II-associated invariant chain contains two endosomal targeting signals within its cytoplasmic tail. *J Cell Sci* 1993;106:831–846.

204. Bremnes B, Madsen T, Gedde-Dahl M, Bakke O. An LI and ML motif in the cytoplasmic tail of the MHC-associated invariant chain mediate rapid internalization. *J Cell Sci* 1994;107:2021–2032.

205. Odorizzi CG, Trowbridge IS, Xue L, Hopkins CR, Davis CD, Collawn JF. Sorting signals in the MHC class II invariant chain cytoplasmic tail and transmembrane region determine trafficking to an endocytic processing compartment. *J Cell Biol* 1994;126:317–330.

206. Arneson LS, Miller J. Efficient endosomal localization of major histocompatibility complex class II-invariant chain complexes requires multimerization of the invariant chain targeting sequence. *J Cell Biol* 1995;129:1217–1228.

207. Gorvel JP, Escola JM, Stang E, Bakke O. Invariant chain induces a delayed transport from early to late endosomes. *J Biol Chem* 1995;270:2741–2746.

208. Layet C, Germain RN. Invariant chain promotes egress of poorly expressed, haplotype-mismatched class II major histocompatibility complex AαAβ dimers from the endoplasmic reticulum/cis-Golgi compartment. *Proc Natl Acad Sci U S A* 1991;88:2346–2350.

209. Anderson MS, Miller J. Invariant chain can function as a chaperone protein for class II major histocompatibility complex molecules. *Proc Natl Acad Sci U S A* 1992;89:2282–2286.

210. Viville S, Neefjes J, Lotteau V, et al. Mice lacking the MHC class II-associated invariant chain. *Cell* 1993;72:635–648.

211. Bikoff EK, Huang L-Y, Episkopou V, Van Meerwijk J, Germain RN, Robertson EJ. Defective major histocompatibility complex class II assembly, transport, peptide acquisition, and CD4⁺ T cell selection in mice lacking invariant chain expression. *J Exp Med* 1993;177:1699–1712.

212. Elliott EA, Drake JR, Amigorena S, et al. The invariant chain is required for intracellular transport and function of major histocompatibility complex class II molecules. *J Exp Med* 1994;179:681–694.

213. Schaiff WT, Hruska KA Jr, McCourt DW, Green M, Schwartz BD. HLA-DR associates with specific stress proteins and is retained in the endoplasmic reticulum in invariant chain negative cells. *J Exp Med* 1992;176:657–666.

214. Busch R, Cloutier I, Sékaly R-P, Hämmerling GJ. Invariant chain protects class II histocompatibility antigens from binding intact polypeptides in the endoplasmic reticulum. *EMBO J* 1996;15:418–428.

215. Riberdy JM, Newcomb JR, Surman MJ, Barbosa JA, Cresswell P. HLA-DR molecules from an antigen-processing mutant cell line are associated with invariant chain peptides. *Nature* 1992;360:474–477.

216. Romagnoli P, Germain RN. The CLIP region of invariant chain plays a critical role in regulating MHC class II folding, transport, and peptide occupancy. *J Exp Med* 1994;180:1107–1113.

217. Morkowski S, Goldrath AW, Eastman S, et al. T cell recognition of major histocompatibility complex class II complexes with invariant chain processing intermediates. *J Exp Med* 1995;182:1403–1413.

218. Zhong G, Castellino F, Romagnoli P, Germain RN. Evidence that binding site occupancy is necessary and sufficient for effective major histocompatibility complex (MHC) class II transport through the secretory pathway redefines the primary function of class II-associated invariant chain peptides (CLIP). *J Exp Med* 1996;184:2061–2066.

219. Cresswell P. Intracellular class II HLA antigens are accessible to transferrin-neuraminidase conjugates internalized by receptor-mediated endocytosis. *Proc Natl Acad Sci U S A* 1985;82:8188–8192.

220. Castellino F, Germain RN. Extensive trafficking of MHC class II invariant chain complexes in the endocytic pathway and appearance of peptide-loaded class II in multiple compartments. *Immunity* 1995;1:73–88.

221. Benaroch P, Yilla M, Raposo G, et al. How MHC class II molecules reach the endocytic pathway. *EMBO J* 1995;14:37–49.
222. Kleijmeer MJ, Morkowski S, Griffith JM, Rudensky AY, Geuze HJ. Major histocompatibility complex class II compartments in human. *J Cell Biol* 1997;139:639–649.
223. Warmerdam PA, Long EO, Roche PA. Isoforms of the invariant chain regulate transport of MHC class II molecules to antigen processing compartments. *J Cell Biol* 1996;133:281–291.
224. Ludwig T, Griffiths G, Hoflack B. Distribution of newly synthesized lysosomal enzymes in the endocytic pathway of normal rat kidney cells. *J Cell Biol* 1991;115:1561–1572.
225. Salamero J, Le Borgne R, Saudrais C, Goud B, Hoflack B. Expression of major histocompatibility complex class II molecules in HeLa cells promotes the recruitment of AP-1 Golgi-specific assembly proteins on Golgi membranes. *J Biol Chem* 1996;271:30318–30321.
226. Blum JS, Fiani ML, Stahl PD. Proteolytic cleavage of ricin A chain in endosomal vesicles. Evidence for the action of endosomal proteases at both neutral and acidic pH. *J Biol Chem* 1991;266:22091–22095.
227. Riese RJ, Wolf PR, Bromme D, et al. Essential role for cathepsin S in MHC class II-associated invariant chain processing and peptide loading. *Immunity* 1996;4:357–366.
228. Neefjes JJ, Ploegh HL. Inhibition of endosomal proteolytic activity by leupeptin blocks surface expression of MHC class II molecules and their conversion to SDS resistance alpha beta heterodimers in endosomes. *EMBO J* 1992;11:411–416.
229. Loss G Jr, Sant AJ. Invariant chain retains MHC class II molecules in the endocytic pathway. *J Immunol* 1993;150:3187–3197.
230. Fineschi B, Arneson LS, Naujokas MF, Miller J. Proteolysis of major histocompatibility complex class II-associated invariant chain is regulated by the alternatively spliced gene product, p41. *Proc Natl Acad Sci U S A* 1995;92:10257–10261.
231. Fineschi B, Sakaguchi K, Appella E, Miller J. The proteolytic environment involved in MHC class II-restricted antigen presentation can be modulated by the p41 form of invariant chain. *J Immunol* 1996;157:3211–3215.
232. Wubbolts R, Fernandez-Borja M, Oomen L, et al. Direct vesicular transport of MHC class II molecules from lysosomal structures to the cell surface. *J Cell Biol* 1996;135:611–622.
233. Raposo G, Nijman HW, Stoorvogel W, et al. B lymphocytes secrete antigen-presenting vesicles. *J Exp Med* 1996;183:1161–1172.
234. Lapham CK, Bacik I, Yewdell JW, Kane KP, Bennink JR. Class I molecules retained in the endoplasmic reticulum bind to antigenic peptides. *J Exp Med* 1993;177:1633–1641.
235. Porgador A, Yewdell JW, Deng Y, Bennink JR, Germain RN. Localization, quantitation, and in situ detection of specific peptide-MHC class I complexes using a monoclonal antibody. *Immunity* 1997;6:715–726.
236. Monaco JJ, Cho S, Attaya M. Transport protein genes in the murine MHC: Possible implications for antigen processing. *Science* 1990;250:1723–1726.
237. Deverson EV, Gow IR, Coadwell WJ, Monaco JJ, Butcher GW, Howard JC. MHC class II region encoding proteins related to the multidrug resistance family of transmembrane transporters. *Nature* 1990;348:738–741.
238. Trowsdale J, Hanson I, Mockridge I, Beck S, Townsend A, Kelly A. Sequences encoded in the class II region of the MHC related to the "ABC" superfamily of transporters. *Nature* 1990;348:741–744.
239. Spies T, Bresnahan M, Bahram S, et al. A gene in the human major histocompatibility complex class II region controlling the class I antigen presentation pathway. *Nature* 1990;348:744–747.
240. Spies T, DeMars R. Restored expression of major histocompatibility class I molecules by gene transfer of a putative peptide transporter. *Nature* 1991;351:323–324.
241. Powis SJ, Townsend AR, Deverson EV, Bastin J, Butcher GW, Howard JC. Restoration of antigen presentation to the mutant cell line RMA-S by an MHC-linked transporter. *Nature* 1991;354:528–531.
242. Spies T, Cerundolo V, Colonna M, Cresswell P, Townsend A, DeMars R. Presentation of viral antigen by MHC class I molecules is dependent on a putative peptide transporter heterodimer. *Nature* 1992;355:644–646.
243. Kelly A, Powis SH, Kerr LA, et al. Assembly and function of the two ABC transporter proteins encoded in the human major histocompatibility complex. *Nature* 1992;355:641–644.
244. Kleijmeer MJ, Kelly A, Geuze IIJ, Slot JW, Townsend A, Trowsdale J. Location of MHC-encoded transporters in the endoplasmic reticulum and cis-Golgi. *Nature* 1992;357:342–344.
245. Powis SJ, Deverson EV, Coadwell WJ, et al. Effect of polymorphism of an MHC-linked transporter on the peptides assembled in a class-I molecule. *Nature* 1992;357:211–215.
246. Neefjes JJ, Momburg F, Hämmerling GJ. Selective and ATP-dependent translocation of peptides by the MHC-encoded transporter. *Science* 1993;261:769–771.
247. Androlewicz MJ, Anderson KS, Cresswell P. Evidence that transporters associated with antigen processing translocate a major histocompatibility complex class I-binding peptide into the endoplasmic reticulum in an ATP-dependent manner. *Proc Natl Acad Sci U S A* 1993;90:9130–9134.
248. Androlewicz MJ, Cresswell P. Human transporters associated with antigen processing possess a promiscuous peptide-binding site. *Immunity* 1994;1:7–14.
249. Momburg F, Roelse J, Hämmerling GJ, Neefjes JJ. Peptide size selection by the major histocompatibility complex-encoded peptide transporter. *J Exp Med* 1994;179:1613–1623.
250. Neefjes J, Gottfried E, Roelse J, et al. Analysis of the fine specificity of rat, mouse and human TAP peptide transporters. *Eur J Immunol* 1995;25:1133–1136.
251. Momburg F, Roelse J, Howard JC, Butcher GW, Hämmerling GJ, Neefjes JJ. Selectivity of MHC-encoded peptide transporters from human, mouse and rat. *Nature* 1994;367:648–651.
252. Powis SJ, Young LL, Joly E et al. The rat cim effect: TAP allele-dependent changes in a class I MHC anchor motif and evidence against C-terminal trimming of peptides in the ER. *Immunity* 1996;4:159–165.
253. Androlewicz MJ, Ortmann B, van Endert PM, Spies T, Cresswell P. Characteristics of peptide and major histocompatibility complex class I/β2-microglobulin binding to the transporters associated with antigen processing (TAP1 and TAP2). *Proc Natl Acad Sci U S A* 1994;91:12716–12720.
254. Nijenhuis M, Schmitt S, Armandola EA, Obst R, Brunner J, Hämmerling GJ. Identification of a contact region for peptide on the TAP1 chain of the transporter associated with antigen processing. *J Immunol* 1996;156:2186–2195.
255. Neisig A, Wubbolts R, Zang X, Melief C, Neefjes J. Allele-specific differences in the interaction of MHC class I molecules with transporters associated with antigen processing. *J Immunol* 1996;156:3196–3206.
256. Peters JM. Proteasomes: Protein degradation machines of the cell. *Trends Biochem Sci* 1994;19:377–382.
257. Goldberg AL, Rock KL. Proteolysis, proteasomes and antigen presentation. *Nature* 1992;357:375–379.
258. Rock KL, Gramm C, Rothstein L, et al. Inhibitors of the proteasome block the degradation of most cell proteins and the generation of peptides presented on MHC class I molecules. *Cell* 1994;78:761–771.
259. Harding CV, France J, Song R, et al. Novel dipeptide aldehydes are proteasome inhibitors and block the MHC-I antigen-processing pathway. *J Immunol* 1995; 155:1767–1775.
260. Belich MP, Glynne RJ, Senger G, Sheer D, Trowsdale J. Proteasome components with reciprocal expression to that of the MHC- encoded LMP proteins. *Curr Biol* 1994;4:769–776.
261. Fruh K, Gossen M, Wang K, Bujard H, Peterson PA, Yang Y. Displacement of housekeeping proteasome subunits by MHC-encoded LMPs: A newly discovered mechanism for modulating the multicatalytic proteinase complex. *EMBO J* 1994; 13:3236–3244.
262. Groettrup M, Kraft R, Kostka S, Standera S, Stohwasser R, Kloetzel PM. A third interferon-gamma-induced subunit exchange in the 20S proteasome. *Eur J Immunol* 1996;26:863–869.
263. Nandi D, Jiang H, Monaco JJ. Identification of MECL-1 (LMP-10) as the third IFN-gamma-inducible proteasome subunit. *J Immunol* 1996;156:2361–2364.
264. Momburg F, Ortiz-Navarrete V, Neefjes J, et al. Proteasome subunits encoded in the major histocompatibility complex are not essential for antigen presentation. *Nature* 1992;360:174–177.
265. Yewdell J, Lapham C, Bacik I, Spies T, Bennink J. MHC-encoded proteasome subunits LMP2 and LMP7 are not required for efficient antigen presentation. *J Immunol* 1994;152:1163–1170.
266. Driscoll J, Brown MG, Finley D, Monaco JJ. MHC-linked LMP gene products specifically alter peptidase activities of the proteasome. *Nature* 1993;365: 262–264.
267. Gaczynska M, Rock KL, Goldberg AL. Gamma-interferon and expression of MHC genes regulate peptide hydrolysis by proteasomes. *Nature* 1993;365: 264–267.
268. Gaczynska M, Rock KL, Spies T, Goldberg AL. Peptidase activities of proteasomes are differentially regulated by the major histocompatibility complex-encoded genes for LMP2 and LMP7. *Proc Natl Acad Sci U S A* 1994;91: 9213–9217.
269. Eggers M, Boes-Fabian B, Ruppert T, Kloetzel PM, Koszinowski UH. The cleavage preference of the proteasome governs the yield of antigenic peptides. *J Exp Med* 1995;182:1865–1870.
270. Sibille C, Gould KG, Willard-Gallo K, et al. LMP2+ proteasomes are required for the presentation of specific antigens to cytotoxic T lymphocytes. *Curr Biol* 1995;5:923–930.
271. Groettrup M, Ruppert T, Kuehn L, et al. The interferon-gamma-inducible 11 S regulator (PA28) and the LMP2/LMP7 subunits govern the peptide production by the 20 S proteasome in vitro. *J Biol Chem* 1995;270:23808–23815.
272. Groettrup M, Soza A, Eggers M, et al. A role for the proteasome regulator PA28alpha in antigen presentation. *Nature* 1996;381:166–168.
273. Ciechanover A, Schwartz AL. The ubiquitin-mediated proteolytic pathway: Mechanisms of recognition of the proteolytic substrate and involvement in the degradation of native cellular proteins. *Faseb J* 1994;8:182–191.
274. Varshavsky A. The N-end rule. *Cold Spring Harb Symp Quant Biol* 1995;60: 461–478.
275. Grant EP, Michalek MT, Goldberg AL, Rock KL. Rate of antigen degradation by the ubiquitin-proteasome pathway influences MHC class I presentation. *J Immunol* 1995;155:3750–3758.
276. Staerz UD, Karasuyama H, Garner AM. Cytotoxic T lymphocytes against a soluble protein. *Nature* 1987;329:449–451.
277. Carbone FR, Bevan MJ. Class I-restricted processing and presentation of exogenous cell-associated antigen in vivo. *J Exp Med* 1990;171:377–387.
278. Rock KL, Gamble S, Rothstein L. Presentation of exogenous antigen with class I major histocompatibility complex molecules. *Science* 1990;249:918–921.
279. Matzinger P, Bevan MJ. Induction of H-2-restricted cytotoxic T cells: In vivo induction has the appearance of being unrestricted. *Cell Immunol* 1977;33:92–100.
280. Kovacsovics-Bankowski M, Rock KL. A phagosome-to-cytosol pathway for exogenous antigens presented on MHC class I molecules. *Science* 1995;267:243–246.

281. Reis e Sousa C, Germain RN. MHC class I presentation of peptides derived from soluble exogenous antigen by a subset of cells engaged in phagocytosis. *J Exp Med* 1995;182:841–852.

282. Shen Z, Reznikoff G, Dranoff G, Rock KL. Cloned dendritic cells can present exogenous antigens on both MHC class I and class II molecules. *J Immunol* 1997;158:2723–2730.

283. Norbury CC, Hewlett LJ, Prescott AR, Shastri N, Watts C. Class I MHC presentation of exogenous soluble antigen via macropinocytosis in bone marrow macrophages. *Immunity* 1995;3:783–791.

284. Norbury CC, Chambers BJ, Prescott AR, Ljunggren HG, Watts C. Constitutive macropinocytosis allows TAP-dependent major histocompatibility complex class I presentation of exogenous soluble antigen by bone marrow-derived dendritic cells. *Eur J Immunol* 1997;27:280–288.

285. Isenman LD, Dice JF. Secretion of intact proteins and peptide fragments by lysosomal pathways of protein degradation. *J Biol Chem* 1989;264:21591–21596.

286. Chiang HL, Terlecky SR, Plant CP, Dice JF. A role for a 70-kilodalton heat shock protein in lysosomal degradation of intracellular proteins. *Science* 1989;246: 382–385.

287. Pfeifer JD, Wick MJ, Roberts RL, Findlay K, Normark SJ, Harding CV. Phagocytic processing of bacterial antigens for class I MHC presentation to T cells. *Nature* 1993;361:359–362.

288. Harding CV, Song R. Phagocytic processing of exogenous particulate antigens by macrophages for presentation by class I MHC molecules. *J Immunol* 1994;153:4925–4933.

289. Schirmbeck R, Melber K, Reimann J. Hepatitis B virus small surface antigen particles are processed in a novel endosomal pathway for major histocompatibility complex class I-restricted epitope presentation. *Eur J Immunol* 1995;25. 1063–1070.

290. Bachmann MF, Oxenius A, Pircher H, et al. TAP1-independent loading of class I molecules by exogenous viral proteins. *Eur J Immunol* 1995;25:1739–1743.

291. Bevan MJ. Class discrimination in the world of immunology. *Nature* 1987; 325:192–194.

292. Palladino MJ, Srivastava PK, Oettgen HF, DeLeo AB. Expression of a shared tumor-specific antigen by two chemically induced BALB/c sarcomas. *Cancer Res* 1987;47:5074–5079.

293. Lammert E, Arnold D, Nijenhuis M, et al. The endoplasmic reticulum-resident stress protein gp96 binds peptides translocated by TAP. *Eur J Immunol* 1997; 27:923–927.

294. Suto R, Srivastava PK. A mechanism for the specific immunogenicity of heat shock protein-chaperoned peptides. *Science* 1995;269;1585–1588

295. Manickan E, Karem KL, Rouse BT. DNA vaccines—a modern gimmick or a boon to vaccinology?. *Crit Rev Immunol* 1997;17:139–154.

296. Fynan EF, Webster RG, Fuller DH, Haynes JR, Santoro JC, Robinson HL. DNA vaccines: Protective immunizations by parenteral, mucosal, and gene-gun inoculations. *Proc Natl Acad Sci U S A* 1993;90:11478–11482.

297. Ulmer JB, Deck RR, Dewitt CM, Donnhly JI, Liu MA. Generation of MHC class I-restricted cytotoxic T lymphocytes by expression of a viral protein in muscle cells: Antigen presentation by non-muscle cells. *Immunology* 1996;89:59–67.

298. Roche PA, Cresswell P. Invariant chain association with HLA-DR molecules inhibits immunogenic peptide binding. *Nature* 1990;345:615–618.

299. Teyton L, O'Sullivan D, Dickson PW, et al. Invariant chain distinguishes between the exogenous and endogenous antigen presentation pathways. *Nature* 1990, 348:39–44.

300. Busch R, Vturina IY, Drexler J, Momburg F, Hämmerling GJ. Poor loading of major histocompatibility complex class II molecules with endogenously synthesized short peptides in the absence of invariant chain. *Eur J Immunol* 1995; 25:48–53.

301. Mason K, McConnell HM. Short-lived complexes between myelin basic protein peptides and IAk. *Proc Natl Acad Sci U S A* 1994;91:12463–12466.

302. Harding CV, Unanue ER. Cellular mechanisms of antigen processing and the function of class I and II major histocompatibility complex molecules. *Cell Regul* 1990,1:499–509.

303. Amigorena S, Drake JR, Webster P, Mellman I. Transient accumulation of new class II MHC molecules in a novel endocytic compartment in B lymphocytes. *Nature* 1994;369:113–120.

304. Qiu Y, Xu X, Wandinger-Ness A, Dalke DP, Pierce SK. Separation of subcellular compartments containing distinct functional forms of MHC class II. *J Cell Biol* 1994;125:595–605.

305. Tulp A, Verwoerd D, Dobberstein B, Ploegh HL, Pieters J. Isolation and characterization of the intracellular MHC class II compartment. *Nature* 1994;369:120–126.

306. West MA, Lucocq JM, Watts C. Antigen processing and class II MHC peptide-loading in human B-lymphoblastoid cells. *Nature* 1994;369:147–151.

307. Sercarz EE, Lehmann PV, Ametani A, Benichou G, Miller A, Moudgil K. Dominance and crypticity of T cell antigenic determinants. *Annu Rev Immunol* 1993; 11:729–766.

308. Simitsek PD, Campbell DG, Lanzavecchia A, Fairweather N, Watts C. Modulation of antigen processing by bound antibodies can boost or suppress class II major histocompatibility complex presentation of different T cell determinants. *J Exp Med* 1995;181:1957–1963.

309. Frosch S, Bonifas U, Reske-Kunz AB. The capacity of bone marrow-derived macrophages to process bovine insulin is regulated by lymphokines. *Int Immunol* 1993;5:1551–1558.

310. Zhong G, Romagnoli P, Germain RN. Related leucine-based cytoplasmic targeting signals in invariant chain and major histocompatibility complex class II mol-

311. ecules control endocytic presentation of distinct determinants in a single protein. *J Exp Med* 1997;185:429–438.

311. Avva RR, Cresswell P. In vivo and in vitro formation and dissociation of HLA-DR complexes with invariant chain-derived peptides. *Immunity* 1994;1:763–774.

312. Urban RG, Chicz RM, Strominger JL. Selective release of some invariant chain-derived peptides from HLA-DR1 molecules at endosomal pH. *J Exp Med* 1994;180:751–755.

313. Kropshofer H, Vogt AB, Stern LJ, Hämmerling GJ. Self-release of CLIP in peptide loading of HLA-DR molecules. *Science* 1995;270:1357–1359.

314. Sette A, Ceman S, Kubo RT, et al. Invariant chain peptides in most HLA-DR molecules of an antigen-processing mutant. *Science* 1992;258:1801–1804.

315. Morris P, Shaman J, Attaya M, et al. An essential role for HLA-DM in antigen presentation by class II major histocompatibility molecules. *Nature* 1994;368:551–554.

316. Fling SP, Arp B, Pious D. HLA-DMA and -DMB genes are both required for MHC class II/peptide complex formation in antigen-presenting cells. *Nature* 1994;368:554–558.

317. Denzin LK, Robbins NF, Carboy-Newcomb C, Cresswell P. Assembly and intracellular transport of HLA-DM and correction of the class II antigen-processing defect in T2 cells. *Immunity* 1994;1:595–606.

318. Sanderson F, Kleijmeer MJ, Kelly A, et al. Accumulation of HLA-DM, a regulator of antigen presentation, in MHC class II compartments. *Science* 1994;266:1566–1569.

319. Marks MS, Roche PA, van Donsclaar E, Woodruff L, Peters PJ, Bonifacino JS. A lysosomal targeting signal in the cytoplasmic tail of the β chain directs HLA-DM to MHC class II compartments. *J Cell Biol* 1995;131:351–369.

320. Copier J, Kleijmeer MJ, Ponnambalam S, et al. Targeting signal and subcellular compartments involved in the intracellular trafficking of HLA-DMB. *J Immunol* 1996;157:1017–1027.

321. Sanderson F, Thomas C, Neefjes J, Trowsdale J. Association between HLA-DM and HLA-DR in vivo. *Immunity* 1996;4:87–96.

322. Denzin LK, Hammond C, Cresswell P. HLA-DM interactions with intermediates in HLA-DR maturation and a role for HLA-DM in stabilizing empty HLA-DR molecules. *J Exp Med* 1996;184:2153–2166.

323. Sloan VS, Cameron P, Porter G, et al. Mediation by HLA-DM of dissociation of peptides from HLA-DR. *Nature* 1995;375:802–806.

324. Denzin LK, Cresswell P. HLA-DM induces CLIP dissociation from MHC class II alpha beta dimers and facilitates peptide loading. *Cell* 1995;82:155–165.

325. Sherman MA, Weber DA, Jensen PE. DM enhances peptide binding to class II MHC by release of invariant chain-derived peptide. *Immunity* 1995;3:197–205.

326. Weber DA, Evavold BD, Jensen PE. Enhanced dissociation of HLA-DR-bound peptides in the presence of HLA-DM. *Science* 1996;274:618–620.

327. Kropshofer H, Vogt AB, Moldenhauer G, Hammer J, Blum JS, Hämmerling GJ. Editing of the HLA-DR peptide repertoire by HLA-DM. *EMBO J* 1996;15:6144–6154.

328. Katz JF, Stebbins C, Appella E, Sant AJ. Invariant chain and DM edit self-peptide presentation by major histocompatibility complex (MHC) class II molecules. *J Exp Med* 1996;184:1747–1753.

329. van Ham SM, Gruneberg U, Malcherek G, Broker I, Melms A, Trowsdale J. Human histocompatibility leukocyte antigen (HLA)-DM edits peptides presented by HLA-DR according to their ligand binding motifs. *J Exp Med* 1996;184:2019–2024.

330. Denzin LK, Sant'Angelo DB, Hammond C, Surman MJ, Cresswell P. Negative regulation by HLA-DO of MHC class II-restricted antigen processing. *Science* 1997;278:106–109.

331. Kropshofer H, Arndt SO, Moldenhauer G, Hämmerling GJ, Vogt AB. HLA-DM acts as a molecular chaperone and rescues empty HLA-DR molecules at lysosomal pH. *Immunity* 1997,6.293–302.

332. Collins DS, Unanue ER, Harding CV. Reduction of disulfide bonds within lysosomes is a key step in antigen processing. *J Immunol* 1991;147:4054–4059.

333. Deng H, Apple R, Clare-Salzler M, et al. Determinant capture as a possible mechanism of protection afforded by major histocompatibility complex class II molecules in autoimmune disease. *J Exp Med* 1993;178:1675–1680.

334. Castellino F, Zappacosta F, Coligan JE, Germain RN. (submitted for publication).

335. Nadimi F, Moreno J, Momburg F, et al. Antigen presentation of hen egg-white lysozyme but not of ribonuclease A is augmented by the major histocompatibility complex class II-associated invariant chain. *Eur J Immunol* 1991;21:1255–1263.

336. Peterson M, Miller J. Antigen presentation enhanced by the alternatively spliced invariant chain gene product p41. *Nature* 1992;357:596–598.

337. Ceman S, Sant AJ. The function of invariant chain in class II-restricted antigen presentation. *Semin Immunol* 1995;7:373–387.

338. Stebbins CC, Loss GJ, Elias CG, Chervonsky A, Sant AJ. The requirement for DM in class II-restricted antigen presentation and SDS-stable dimer formation is allele and species dependent. *J Exp Med* 1995;181:223–234.

339. Momburg F, Fuchs S, Drexler J, et al. Epitope-specific enhancement of antigen presentation by invariant chain. *J Exp Med* 1993;178:1453 1458.

340. Davis JE, Cresswell P. Lack of detectable endocytosis of B lymphocyte MHC class II antigens using an antibody-independent technique. *J Immunol* 1990;144: 990–997

341. Reid PA, Watts C. Cycling of cell-surface MHC glycoproteins through primaquine-sensitive intracellular compartments. *Nature* 1990;346:655–657.

342. Weber DA, Buck LB, Delohery TM, Agostino N, Ferris B. Class II MHC molecules are spontaneously internalized in acidic endosomes by activated B cells. *J Mol Cell Immunol* 1990;4:255–266

343. Pinet V, Vergelli M, Martin R, Bakke O, Long EO. Antigen presentation mediated by recycling of surface HLA-DR molecules. *Nature* 1995;375:603–606.

344. Smiley ST, Laufer TM, Lo D, Glimcher LH, Grusby MJ. Transgenic mice expressing MHC class II molecules with truncated A beta cytoplasmic domains reveal signaling-independent defects in antigen presentation. *Int Immunol* 1995;7:665–677.

345. Castellino F, Zhong G, Germain RN. Antigen presentation by MHC class II molecules: Invariant chain function, protein trafficking, and the molecular basis of diverse determinant capture. *Hum Immunol* 1997;54:159–169.

346. Nelson CA, Petzold SJ, Unanue ER. Peptides determine the lifespan of MHC class II molecules in the antigen-presenting cell. *Nature* 1994;371:250–252.

347. Sallusto F, Cella M, Danieli C, Lanzavecchia A. Dendritic cells use macropinocytosis and the mannose receptor to concentrate macromolecules in the major histocompatibility complex class II compartment: Downregulation by cytokines and bacterial products. *J Exp Med* 1995;182:389–400.

348. Lanzavecchia A. Antigen-specific interaction between T and B cells. *Nature* 1985;314:537–539.

349. Rock KL, Benacerraf B, Abbas AK. Antigen presentation by hapten-specific B lymphocytes. I. Role of surface immunoglobulin receptors. *J Exp Med* 1984;160:1102–1113.

350. Mitchell RN, Barnes KA, Grupp SA, et al. Intracellular targeting of antigens internalized by membrane immunoglobulin in B lymphocytes. *J Exp Med* 1995;181:1705–1714.

351. Weiser P, Muller R, Braun U, Reth M. Endosomal targeting by the cytoplasmic tail of membrane immunoglobulin. *Science* 1997;276:407–409.

352. Bonnerot C, Lankar D, Hanau D, et al. Role of B cell receptor Ig alpha and Ig beta subunits in MHC class II-restricted antigen presentation. *Immunity* 1995;3: 335–347.

353. Jiang W, Swiggard WJ, Heufler C, et al. The receptor DEC-205 expressed by dendritic cells and thymic epithelial cells is involved in antigen processing. *Nature* 1995;375:151–155.

354. Snider DP, Segal DM. Targeted antigen presentation using crosslinked antibody heteroaggregates. *J Immunol* 1987;139:1609–1616.

355. Lichtman AH, Tony HP, Parker DC, Abbas AK. Antigen presentation by hapten-specific B lymphocytes. IV. Comparative ability of B cells to present specific antigen and anti-immunoglobulin antibody. *J Immunol* 1987;138:2822–2825.

356. Casten LA, Kaumaya P, Pierce SK. Enhanced T cell responses to antigenic peptides targeted to B cell surface Ig, Ia, or class I molecules. *J Exp Med* 1988;168: 171–180.

357. Amigorena S, Salamero J, Davoust J, Fridman WH, Bonnerot C. Tyrosine-containing motif that transduces cell activation signals also determines internalization and antigen presentation via type-III receptors for IgG. *Nature* 1992;358:337–341.

358. Siliciano RF, Lawton T, Knall C, et al. Analysis of host-virus interactions in AIDS with anti-gp120 T cell clones: Effect of HIV sequence variation and a mechanism for CD4+ cell depletion. *Cell* 1988;54:561–575.

359. Long EO. Antigen processing for presentation to CD4+ T cells. *New Biol* 1992;4: 274–282.

360. Weiss S, Bogen B. MHC class II-restricted presentation of intracellular antigen. *Cell* 1991;64:767–776.

361. Jacobson S, Sekaly RP, Bellini WJ, Johnson CL, McFarland HF, Long EO. Recognition of intracellular measles virus antigens by HLA class II restricted measles virus-specific cytotoxic T lymphocytes. *Ann N Y Acad Sci* 1988;540:352–353.

362. Jin Y, Shih WK, Berkower I. Human T cell response to the surface antigen of hepatitis B virus (HBsAg). Endosomal and nonendosomal processing pathways are accessible to both endogenous and exogenous antigen. *J Exp Med* 1988;168:293–306.

363. Malnati MS, Marti M, LaVaute T et al. Processing pathways for presentation of cytosolic antigen to MHC class II-restricted T cells. *Nature* 1992;357:702–704.

364. Long EO, LaVaute T, Pinet V, Jaraquemada D. Invariant chain prevents the HLA-DR-restricted presentation of a cytosolic peptide. *J Immunol* 1994;153: 1487–1494.

365. Dodi AI, Brett S, Nordeng T, et al. The invariant chain inhibits presentation of endogenous antigens by a human fibroblast cell line. *Eur J Immunol* 1994;24:1632–1639.

366. Cresswell P. Assembly, transport, and function of MHC class II molecules. *Annu Rev Immunol* 1994;12:259–293.

367. York IA, Rock KL. Antigen processing and presentation by the class I major histocompatibility complex. *Annu Rev Immunol* 1996;14:369–396.

368. Rothman JE. Polypeptide chain binding proteins: Catalysts of protein folding and related processes in cells. *Cell* 1989;59:591–601.

369. Alexander J, Payne JA, Murray R, Frelinger JA, Cresswell P. Differential transport requirements for HLA and H-2 class I glycoproteins. *Immunogenetics* 1989;29:380–388.

370. Ortiz-Navarrete V, Hämmerling GJ. Surface appearance and instability of empty H-2 class I molecules under physiological conditions. *Proc Natl Acad Sci U S A* 1991;88:3594–3597.

371. van der Bruggen P, Traversari C, Chomez P, et al. A gene encoding an antigen recognized by cytolytic T lymphocytes on a human melanoma. *Science* 1991;254:1643–1647.

372. Karttunen J, Sanderson S, Shastri N. Detection of rare antigen-presenting cells by the lacZ T-cell activation assay suggests an expression cloning strategy for T-cell antigens. *Proc Natl Acad Sci U S A* 1992;89:6020–6024.

373. Sanderson S, Campbell DJ, Shastri N. Identification of a CD4+ T cell-stimulat-

ing antigen of pathogenic bacteria by expression cloning. *J Exp Med* 1995;182: 1751–1757.

374. Garboczi DN, Hung DT, Wiley DC. HLA-A2-peptide complexes: Refolding and crystallization of molecules expressed in *Escherichia coli* and complexed with single antigenic peptides. *Proc Natl Acad Sci U S A* 1992;89:3429–3433.

375. Kozono H, White J, Clements J, Marrack P, Kappler J. Production of soluble MHC class II proteins with covalently bound single peptides. *Nature* 1994;369:151–154.

376. Ignatowicz L, Winslow G, Bill J, Kappler J, Marrack P. Cell surface expression of class II MHC proteins bound by a single peptide. *J Immunol* 1995;154:3852–3862.

377. Matsui K, Boniface JJ, Reay PA, Schild H, Fazekas de St. Groth B, Davis MM. Low affinity interaction of peptide-MHC complexes with T cell receptors. *Science* 1991;254:1788–1791.

378. Corr M, Slanetz AE, Boyd LF, et al. T cell receptor-MHC class I peptide interactions: Affinity, kinetics, and specificity. *Science* 1994;265:946–949.

379. Matsui K, Boniface JJ, Steffner P, Reay PA, Davis MM. Kinetics of T-cell receptor binding to peptide/I-Ek complexes: Correlation of the dissociation rate with T-cell responsiveness. *Proc Natl Acad Sci U S A* 1994;91:12862–12866.

380. Alam SM, Travers PJ, Wung JL, et al. T-cell-receptor affinity and thymocyte positive selection. *Nature* 1996;381:616–620.

381. Lyons DS, Lieberman SA, Hampl J, et al. A TCR binds to antagonist ligands with lower affinities and faster dissociation rates than to agonists. *Immunity* 1996;5:53–61.

382. Altman JD, Moss PAH, Goulder PJR, et al. Phenotypic analysis of antigen-specific T lymphocytes. *Science* 1996;274:94–96.

383. Plaksin D, Polakova K, McPhie P, Margulies DH. A three-domain T cell receptor is biologically active and specifically stains cell surface MHC/peptide complexes. *J Immunol* 1997;158:2218–2227.

384. Murphy DB, Rath S, Pizzo E, et al. Monoclonal antibody detection of a major self peptide–MHC class-II complex. *J Immunol* 1992;148:3483–3491.

385. Andersen PS, Stryhn A, Hansen BE, Fugger L, Engberg J, Buus S. A recombinant antibody with the antigen-specific, major histocompatibility complex-restricted specificity of T cells. *Proc Natl Acad Sci U S A* 1996;93:1820–1824.

386. Zhong G, Reis e Sousa C, Germain RN. Antigen-unspecific B cells and lymphoid dendritic cells both show extensive surface expression of processed antigen-major histocompatibility complex class II complexes after soluble protein exposure in vivo or in vitro. *J Exp Med* 1997;186:673–682.

387. Dadaglio G, Nelson CA, Deck MB, Petzold SJ, Unanue ER. Characterization and quantitation of peptide-MHC complexes produced from hen egg lysozyme using a monoclonal antibody. *Immunity* 1997;6:727–738.

388. Zhong G, Reis e Sousa C, Germain RN. Production, specificity, and functionality of monoclonal antibodies to specific peptide:MHC class II complexes formed by active processing of exogenous protein. *Proc Natl Acad Sci U S A* 1997 (in press).

389. Eisenlohr LC, Yewdell JW, Bennink JR. Flanking sequences influence the presentation of an endogenously synthesized peptide to cytotoxic T lymphocytes. *J Exp Med* 1992;175:481–487.

390. Niedermann G, Butz S, Ihlenfeldt HG, et al. Contribution of proteasome-mediated proteolysis to the hierarchy of epitopes presented by major histocompatibility complex class I molecules. *Immunity* 1995;2:289–299.

391. Pircher H, Moskophidis D, Rohrer U, Bürki K, Hengartner H, Zinkernagel RM. Viral escape by selection of cytotoxic T cell-resistant virus variants in vivo. *Nature* 1990;346:629–633.

392. Goulder PJ, Phillips RE, Colbert RA, et al. Late escape from an immunodominant cytotoxic T-lymphocyte response associated with progression to AIDS. *Nat Med* 1997;3:212–217.

393. Klenerman P, Rowland JS, McAdam S, et al. Cytotoxic T-cell activity antagonized by naturally occurring HIV-1 Gag variants. *Nature* 1994;369:403–407.

394. Bertoletti A, Sette A, Chisari FV, et al. Natural variants of cytotoxic epitopes are T-cell receptor antagonists for antiviral cytotoxic T cells. *Nature* 1994;369:407–410.

395. Nagy ZA, Lehmann PV, Falcioni F, Muller S, Adorini L. Why peptides? Their possible role in the evolution of MHC-restricted T-cell recognition. *Immunol Today* 1989;10:132–138.

396. Lorenz RG, Tyler AN, Allen PM. Reconstruction of the immunogenic peptide RNase (43-56) by identification and transfer of the critical residues into an unrelated peptide backbone. *J Exp Med* 1989;170:203–215.

397. Alexander MA, Damico CA, Wieties KM, Hansen TH, Connolly JM. Correlation between CD8 dependency and determinant density using peptide-induced, Ld-restricted cytotoxic T lymphocytes. *J Exp Med* 1991;173:849–858.

398. Hill AVS, Elvin J, Willis AC, et al. Molecular analysis of the association of HLA-B53 and resistance to severe malaria. *Nature* 1992;360:434–439.

399. Swain SL. T cell subsets and the recognition of MHC class. *Immunol Rev* 1983;74:129–142.

400. Biddison WE, Shaw S. Possible involvement of the OKT4 molecule in T-cell recognition of class II HLA antigens. *Diagn Immunol* 1983;1:112–115.

401. Pamer EG, Harty JT, Bevan MJ. Precise prediction of a dominant class I MHC-restricted epitope of Listeria monocytogenes. *Nature* 1991;353:852–855.

402. Schafer R, Portnoy DA, Brassell SA, Paterson Y. Induction of a cellular immune response to a foreign antigen by a recombinant *Listeria monocytogenes* vaccine. *J Immunol* 1992;149:53–59.

403. Shinohara N, Watanabe M, Sachs DH, Hozumi N. Killing of antigen-reactive B cells by class II-restricted, soluble antigen-specific CD8+ cytolytic T lymphocytes. *Nature* 1988;336:481–484.

404. Seder RA, Paul WE. Acquisition of lymphokine-producing phenotype by CD4+ T cells. *Annu Rev Immunol* 1994;12:635–673.

405. Macatonia SE, Hosken NA, Litton M, et al. Dendritic cells produce IL-12 and direct the development of Th1 cells from naive CD4+ T cells. *J Immunol* 1995;154:5071–5079.

406. Hsieh CS, Macatonia SE, O'Garra A, Murphy KM. T cell genetic background determines default T helper phenotype development in vitro. *J Exp Med* 1995;181:713–721.

407. Reis e Sousa C, Hieny S, Scharton-Kersten T et al. In vivo microbial stimulation induces rapid CD40 L-independent production of Interleukin 12 by dendritic cells and their redistribution to T cell areas. *J Exp Med* 1997;186:1819–1829.

408. Huang AY, Golumbek P, Ahmadzadeh M, Jaffee E, Pardoll D, Levitsky H. Role of bone marrow-derived cells in presenting MHC class I-restricted tumor antigens. *Science* 1994;264:961–965.

409. Yewdell J, Bennink J, Smith G, Moss B. Use of recombinant vaccinia viruses to examine cytotoxic T lymphocyte recognition of individual viral proteins. *Adv Exp Med Biol* 1988;239:151–161.

410. Collins DS, Findlay K, Harding CV. Processing of exogenous liposome-encapsulated antigens in vivo generates class I MHC-restricted T cell responses. *J Immunol* 1992;148:3336–3341.

411. Reddy R, Zhou F, Nair S, Huang L, Rouse BT. In vivo cytotoxic T lymphocyte induction with soluble proteins administered in liposomes. *J Immunol* 1992;148:1585–1589.

412. Takahashi H, Takeshita T, Morein B, Putney S, Germain RN, Berzofsky JA. Induction of CD8+ cytotoxic T cells by immunization with purified HIV-1 envelope protein in ISCOMs. *Nature* 1990;344:873–875.

413. Schild H, Deres K, Wiesmüller KH, Jung G, Rammensee HG. Efficiency of peptides and lipopeptides for in vivo priming of virus-specific cytotoxic T cells. *Eur J Immunol* 1991;21:2649–2654.

414. Kast WM, Roux L, Curren J, et al. Protection against lethal Sendai virus infection by in vivo priming of virus-specific cytotoxic T lymphocytes with a free synthetic peptide. *Proc Natl Acad Sci U S A* 1991;88:2283–2287.

415. Rees MA, Rosenberg AS, Munitz TI, Singer A. In vivo induction of antigen-specific transplantation tolerance to Qa1a by exposure to alloantigen in the absence of T-cell help. *Proc Natl Acad Sci U S A* 1990;87:2765–2769.

416. Guerder S, Matzinger P. A fail-safe mechanism for maintaining self-tolerance. *J Exp Med* 1992;176:553–564.

417. Mitchison NA. Linked help in the cytotoxic T-cell response revealed by adoptive transfer. *Transplant Proc* 1983;15:2121–2124.

418. Spriggs MK. One step ahead of the game: Viral immunomodulatory molecules. *Annu Rev Immunol* 1996;14:101–130.

419. Ploegh HL. Trafficking and assembly of MHC molecules: How viruses elude the immune system. *Cold Spring Harb Symp Quant Biol* 1995;60:263–266.

420. Hill A, Jugovic P, York I, et al. Herpes simplex virus turns off the TAP to evade host immunity. *Nature* 1995;375:411–415.

421. Ahn K, Meyer TH, Uebel S, et al. Molecular mechanism and species specificity of TAP inhibition by simplex virus ICP47. *EMBO J* 1996;15:3247–3255.

422. Tomazin R, Hill AB, Jugovic P et al. Stable binding of the herpes simplex virus ICP47 protein to the binding site of TAP. *EMBO J* 1996;15:3256–3266.

423. Ahn K, Gruhler A, Galocha B, et al. The ER-luminal domain of the HCMV glycoprotein US6 inhibits peptide translocation by TAP. *Immunity* 1997;6:613–621.

424. Lehner PJ, Karttunen JT, Wilkinson GW, Cresswell P. The human cytomegalovirus US6 glycoprotein inhibits transporter associated with antigen processing-dependent peptide translocation. *Proc Natl Acad Sci U S A* 1997;94:6904–6909.

425. Wiertz EJ, Jones TR, Sun L, Bogyo M, Geuze HJ, Ploegh HL. The human cytomegalovirus US11 gene product dislocates MHC class I heavy chains from the endoplasmic reticulum to the cytosol. *Cell* 1996;84:769–779.

426. Wiertz EJ, Tortorella D, Bogyo M, et al. Sec61-mediated transfer of a membrane protein from the endoplasmic reticulum to the proteasome for destruction. *Nature* 1996;384:432–438.

427. Machold RP, Wiertz EJ, Jones TR, Ploegh HL. The HCMV gene products US11 and US2 differ in their ability to allelic forms of murine major histocompatibility complex (MHC) class heavy chains. *J Exp Med* 1997;185:363–366.

428. Kerkau T, Bacik I, Bennink JR, et al. The human immunodeficiency virus type 1 (HIV-1) Vpu protein interferes with an early step in the biosynthesis of major histocompatibility complex (MHC) class I molecules. *J Exp Med* 1997;185:1295–1305.

429. Pääbo S, Severinsson L, Andersson M, Martens I, Nilsson T, Peterson PA. Adenovirus proteins and MHC expression. *Adv Cancer Res* 1989;52:151–163.

430. Howcroft TK, Strebel K, Martin MA, Singer DS. Repression of MHC class I gene promoter activity by two-exon Tat of HIV. *Science* 1993;260:1320–1322.

431. Schwartz O, Marechal V, Le Gall S, Lemonnier F, Heard JM. Endocytosis of major histocompatibility complex class I molecules induced by the HIV-1 Nef protein. *Nat Med* 1996;2:338–342.

432. Spriggs MK, Armitage RJ, Comeau MR, et al. The extracellular domain of the Epstein-Barr virus BZLF2 protein binds the HLA-DRb chain and inhibits antigen presentation. *J Virol* 1996;70:5557–5563.

433. Klausner RD. Architectural editing: Determining the fate of newly synthesized membrane proteins. *New Biol* 1989;1:3–8.

434. Nilsson T, Jackson M, Peterson PA. Short cytoplasmic sequences serve as retention signals for transmembrane proteins in the endoplasmic reticulum. *Cell* 1989;58:707–718.

435. Howcroft TK, Palmer LA, Brown J, et al. HIV Tat represses transcription through Sp1-like elements in the promoter. *Immunity* 1995;3:127–138.

436. Long EO, Burshtyn DN, Clark WP, et al. Killer cell inhibitory receptors: Diversity, specificity, and function. *Immunol Rev* 1997;155:135–144.

437. Wagtmann N, Biassoni R, Cantoni C, et al. Molecular clones of the p58 NK cell receptor reveal immunoglobulin-related molecules with diversity in both the extra- and intracellular domains. *Immunity* 1995;2:439–449.

438. Raulet DH, Held W, Correa I, Dorfman JR, Wu MF, Corral L. Specificity, tolerance and developmental regulation of natural killer cells defined by expression of class I-specific Ly49 receptors. *Immunol Rev* 1997;155:41–52.

439. Christiansen FT, Witt CS, Ciccone E, et al. Human natural killer (NK) alloreactivity and its association with the major histocompatibility complex: Ancestral haplotypes encode particular NK-defined haplotypes. *J Exp Med* 1993;178:1033–1039.

440. Malnati MS, Peruzzi M, Parker KC, et al. Peptide specificity in the recognition of MHC class I by natural killer cell clones. *Science* 1995;267:1016–1018.

441. Rajagopalan S, Long EO. The direct binding of a p58 killer cell inhibitory receptor to human histocompatibility leukocyte antigen (HLA)-Cw4 exhibits peptide selectivity. *J Exp Med* 1997;185:1523–1528.

442. Yokoyama WM, Daniels BF, Seaman WE, Hunziker R, Margulies DH, Smith HR. A family of murine NK cell receptors specific for target cell MHC class I molecules. *Semin Immunol* 1995;7:89–101.

443. Burshtyn DN, Scharenberg AM, Wagtmann N, et al. Recruitment of tyrosine phosphatase HCP by the killer cell inhibitor receptor. *Immunity* 1996;4:77–85.

444. Nakamura MC, Niemi EC, Fisher MJ, Shultz LD, Seaman WE, Ryan JC. Mouse Ly-49A interrupts early signaling events in natural killer cell cytotoxicity and functionally associates with the SHP-1 tyrosine phosphatase. *J Exp Med* 1997;185:673–684.

445. Kärre K, Ljunggren HG, Piontek G, Kiessling R. Selective rejection of H-2-deficient lymphoma variants suggests alternative immune defence strategy. *Nature* 1986;319:675–678.

446. Kees U, Blanden RV. A single genetic element in H-2K affects mouse T cell antiviral function in poxvirus infection. *J Exp Med* 1976;143:450–455.

447. Katz DH, Katz LR, Bogowitz CA. Haplotype preference in lymphocyte differentiation. II. F1 hybrid helper T cells generated with antigen-bearing parental macrophages can cooperate with B lymphocytes of either parent. *Cell Immunol* 1979;42:124–138.

448. Thomas DW, Shevach EM. Nature of the antigenic complex recognized by T lymphocytes: Specific sensitization by antigens associated with allogeneic macrophages. *Proc Natl Acad Sci U S A* 1977;74:2104–2108.

449. Doherty PC, Bennink JR. Vaccinia specific cytotoxic T-cell responses in the context of H-2 antigens not encountered in the thymus may reflect aberrant recognition of a virus-H-2 complex. *J Exp Med* 1979;149:150–157.

450. Lemonnier F, Burakoff SJ, Germain RN, Benacerraf B. Cytolytic thymus-derived lymphocytes specific for allogeneic stimulator cells crossreact with chemically modified syngeneic cells. *Proc Natl Acad Sci U S A* 1977;74:1229–1233.

451. Hünig T, Bevan MJ. Specificity of T-cell clones illustrates altered self hypothesis. *Nature* 1981;294:460–462.

452. Schwartz RH. T-lymphocyte recognition of antigen in association with gene products of the major histocompatibility complex. *Annu Rev Immunol* 1985;3:237–261.

453. Claverie JM, Kourilsky P. The peptidic self model: A reassessment of the role of the major histocompatibility complex molecules in the restriction of the T cell response. *Ann Inst Pasteur Immunol* 1986;137D:425–442.

454. Ajitkumar P, Geier SS, Kesari KV. Evidence that multiple residues on both the alpha-helices of the class I MHC molecule are simultaneously recognized by the T cell receptor. *Cell* 1988;54:47–56.

455. Zerrahn J, Held W, Raulet DH. The MHC reactivity of the T cell repertoire prior to positive and negative selection. *Cell* 1997;88:627–636.

456. Liao NS, Maltzman J, Raulet DH. Positive selection determines T cell receptor V beta 14 gene usage by CD8+ T cells. *J Exp Med* 1989;170:135–143.

457. Jameson SC, Kaye J, Gascoigne NR. A T cell receptor V alpha region selectively expressed in CD4+ cells. *J Immunol* 1990;145:1324–1331.

458. Lucas B, Vasseur F, Penit C. Stochastic coreceptor shut-off is restricted to the CD4 lineage maturation pathway. *J Exp Med* 1995;181:1623–1633.

459. Asmuss A, Hofmann K, Hochgrebe T, Giegerich G, Hunig T, Herrmann T. Alleles of highly homologous rat T cell receptor beta-chain variable segments 8.2 and 8.4: Strain-specific expression, reactivity to. *J Immunol* 1996;157:4436–4441.

460. Sorger SB, Paterson Y, Fink PJ, Hedrick SM. T cell receptor junctional regions and the MHC molecule affect the recognition of antigenic peptides by T cell clones. *J Immunol* 1990;144:1127–1135.

461. Germain RN. Making a molecular match. *Nature* 1990;344:19–22.

462. Bogue M, Candeias S, Benoist C, Mathis D. A special repertoire of α:β T cells in neonatal mice. *EMBO J* 1991;10:3647–3654.

463. Feeney AJ. Junctional sequences of fetal T cell receptor beta chains have few N regions. *J Exp Med* 1991;174:115–124.

464. Schumacher TNM, Ploegh HL. Are MHC-Bound peptides a nuisance for positive selection? *Immunity* 1994;1:721–723.

465. Nikolic-Zugic J, Bevan MJ. Role of self-peptides in positively selecting the T-cell repertoire. *Nature* 1990;344:65–67.

466. Hogquist KA, Gavin MA, Bevan MJ. Positive selection of CD8+ T cells induced by major histocompatibility complex binding peptides in fetal thymic organ culture. *J Exp Med* 1993;177:1469–1473.

467. Ashton-Rickardt PG, Van Kaer L, Schumacher TN, Ploegh HL, Tonegawa S. Peptide contributes to the specificity of positive selection of CD8$^+$ T cells in the thymus. *Cell* 1993;73:1041–1049.

468. Jameson SC, Hogquist KA, Bevan MJ. Specificity and flexibility in thymic selection. *Nature* 1994;369:750–752.

469. Hogquist KA, Jameson SC, Heath WR, Howard JL, Bevan MJ, Carbone FR. T cell receptor antagonist peptides induce positive selection. *Cell* 1994;76:17–27.

470. Ashton-Rickardt PG, Bandeira A, Delaney JR, et al. Evidence for a differential avidity model of T cell selection in the thymus. *Cell* 1994;76:651–663.

471. Ignatowicz L, Kappler J, Marrack P. The repertoire of T cells shaped by a single MHC/peptide ligand. *Cell* 1996;84:521–529.

472. Miyazaki T, Wolf P, Tourne S, et al. Mice lacking H-2M complexes, enigmatic elements of the MHC class II peptide-loading pathway. *Cell* 1996;84:531–541

473. Martin WD, Hicks GG, Mendiratta SK, Leva HI, Ruley HE, Van Kaer L. H2-M mutant mice are defective in the peptide loading of class II molecules, antigen presentation, and T cell repertoire selection. *Cell* 1996;84:543–550.

474. Surh CD, Lee DS, Fung-Leung WP, Karlsson L, Sprent J. Thymic selection by a single MHC/peptide ligand produces a semidiverse repertoire of CD4$^+$ T cells. *Immunity* 1997;7:209–219.

475. Pullen AM, Marrack P, Kappler JW. The T-cell repertoire is heavily influenced by tolerance to polymorphic self-antigens. *Nature* 1988;335:796–801.

476. von Boehmer H, Teh HS, Kisielow P. The thymus selects the useful, neglects the useless and destroys the harmful. *Immunol Today* 1989;10:57–61.

477. Murphy KM, Heimberger AB, Loh DY. Induction by antigen of intrathymic apoptosis of CD4$^+$CD8$^+$TCRlo thymocytes in vivo. *Science* 1990;250:1720–1723.

478. Spain LM, Berg LJ. Developmental regulation of thymocyte susceptibility to deletion by "self"-peptide. *J Exp Med* 1992;176:213–223.

479. Hogquist KA, Jameson SC, Bevan MJ. Strong agonist ligands for the T cell receptor do not mediate positive selection of functional CD8$^+$ T cells. *Immunity* 1995;3:79–86.

480. Vasquez NJ, Kaye J, Hedrick SM. In vivo and in vitro clonal deletion of double-positive thymocytes. *J Exp Med* 1992;175:1307–1316.

481. Pircher H, Rohrer UH, Moskophidis D, Zinkernagel RM, Hengartner H. Lower receptor avidity required for thymic clonal deletion than for effector T-cell function. *Nature* 1991;351:482–485.

482. Racioppi L, Ronchese F, Matis LA, Germain RN. Peptide-major histocompatibility complex class II complexes with mixed agonist/antagonist properties provide evidence for ligand-related differences in T cell receptor-dependent intracellular signaling. *J Exp Med* 1993;177:1047–1060.

483. Valitutti S, Müller S, Dessing M, Lanzavecchia A. Different responses are elicited in cytotoxic T lymphocytes by different levels of T cell receptor occupancy. *J. Exp. Med.* 1996;183:1917–1921.

484. Viola A, Lanzavecchia A. T cell activation determined by T cell receptor number and tunable thresholds. *Science* 1996;273:104–106.

485. Itoh Y, Germain RN. Single cell analysis reveals regulated hierarchical T cell antigen receptor signaling thresholds and intraclonal heterogeneity for individual cytokine responses of CD4$^+$ T cells. *J Exp Med* 1997;186:757–766.

486. Mannie MD. A unified model for T cell antigen recognition and thymic selection of the T cell repertoire. *J Theor Biol* 1991;151:169–192.

487. Evavold BD, Sloan-Lancaster J, Allen PM. Tickling the TCR: Selective T-cell functions stimulated by altered peptide ligands. *Immunol Today* 1993;14:602–609.

488. Jameson SC, Bevan MJ. T cell receptor antagonists and partial agonists. *Immunity* 1995;2:1–11.

489. Madrenas J, Germain RN. Variant TCR ligands: New insights into the molecular basis of antigen-dependent signal transduction and T cell activation. *Semin Immunol* 1996;8:83–101.

490. Marrack P, Kappler J. T cells can distinguish between allogeneic major histocompatibility complex products on different cell types. *Nature* 1988;332:840–843.

491. Bix M, Raulet D. Inefficient positive selection of T cells directed by haematopoietic cells. *Nature* 1992;359:330–333.

492. Pawlowski TJ, Singleton MD, Loh DY, Berg R, Staerz UD. Permissive recognition during positive selection. *Eur J Immunol* 1996;26:851–857.

493. Sebzda E, Kundig TM, Thomson CT, et al. Mature T cell reactivity altered by peptide agonist that induces positive selection. *J Exp Med* 1996;183:1093–1104.

494. Fukui Y, Ishimoto T, Utsuyama M, et al. Positive and negative CD4$^+$ thymocyte selection by a single MHC class II/peptide ligand affected by its expression level in the thymus. *Immunity* 1997;6:401–410.

495. Sebzda E, Wallace VA, Mayer J, Yeung RS, Mak TW, Ohashi PS. Positive and negative thymocyte selection induced by different concentrations of a single peptide. *Science* 1994;263:1615–1618.

496. Mannie MD, Rosser JM, White GA. Autologous rat myelin basic protein is a partial agonist that is converted into a full antagonist upon blockade of CD4. Evidence for the integration of efficacious and nonefficacious signals during T cell antigen recognition. *J Immunol* 1995;154:2642–2654.

497. Madrenas J, Chau LA, Smith J, Bluestone JA, Germain RN. The efficiency of CD4 recruitment to ligand-engaged TCR controls the agonist/partial agonist properties of peptide-MHC molecule ligands. *J Exp Med* 1997;185:219–230.

498. van Meerwijk JPM, Marguerat S, Lees RK, Germain RN, Fowlkes BJ, MacDonald HR. Quantitative impact of thymic clonal deletion on the T cell repertoire. *J Exp Med* 1997;185:377–384.

499. Matzinger P, Guerder S. Does T-cell tolerance require a dedicated antigen-presenting cell? *Nature* 1989;338:74–76.

500. Schwartz RH. Acquisition of immunologic self-tolerance. *Cell* 1989;57:1073–1081.

501. Matzinger P. Tolerance, danger, and the extended family. *Annu Rev Immunol* 1994;12:991–1045.

502. Schild H, Rötzschke O, Kalbacher H, Rammensee HG. Limit of T cell tolerance to self proteins by peptide presentation. *Science* 1990;247:1587–1589.

503. Salemi S, Caporossi AP, Boffa L, Longobardi MG, Barnaba V. HIVgp120 activates autoreactive CD4-specific T cell responses by unveiling of hidden CD4 peptides during processing. *J Exp Med* 1995;181:2253–2257.

504. Robbins PF, el-Gamil M, Li YF, et al. Cloning of a new gene encoding an antigen recognized by melanoma-specific HLA-A24-restricted tumor-infiltrating lymphocytes. *J Immunol* 1995;154:5944–5950.

505. Takeda S, Rodewald HR, Arakawa H, Bluethmann H, Shimizu T. MHC class II molecules are not required for survival of newly generated CD4$^+$ T cells, but affect their long-term life span. *Immunity* 1996;5:217–228.

506. Tanchot C, Lemonnier FA, Perarnau B, Freitas AA, Rocha B. Differential requirements for survival and proliferation of CD8 naive or memory T cells. *Science* 1997;276:2057–2062.

507. Rooke R, Waltzinger C, Benoist C, Mathis D. Targeted complementation of MHC class II deficiency by intrathymic delivery of recombinant adenoviruses. *Immunity* 1997;7:123–134.

508. Brocker T. Survival of mature CD4 T lymphocytes is dependent on major histocompatibility complex class II-expressing dendritic cells. *J. Exp. Med.* 1997;186:1223–1232.

509. Kirberg J, Berns A, von Boehmer H. Peripheral T cell survival requires continual ligation of the T cell receptor to major histocompatibility complex-encoded molecules. *J. Exp. Med.* 1997;186:1269–1275.

510. van Oers NS, Tao W, Watts JD, Johnson P, Aebersold R, Teh HS. Constitutive tyrosine phosphorylation of the T-cell receptor (TCR) z subunit: Regulation of TCR-associated protein tyrosine kinase activity by TCR z. *Mol Cell Biol* 1993;13:5771–5780.

511. Grouard G, Durand I, Filgueira L, Banchereau J, Liu YJ. Dendritic cells capable of stimulating T cells in germinal centres. *Nature* 1996;384:364–367.

Fundamental Immunology, Fourth Edition,
edited by William E. Paul
Lippincott–Raven Publishers, Philadelphia © 1999.

CHAPTER 10

T-Cell Antigen Receptors

Mark M. Davis and Yueh-Hsiu Chien

The characteristics of T-lymphocyte recognition and the nature of T-cell antigen receptors (TCRs) have been difficult and controversial areas for immunologists. However, in the last decade and a half there has been tremendous progress in identifying the molecules and genes that govern T-cell recognition, and more recent years have seen the first concrete information on their biochemistry and structure. While TCRs share many similarities, both structurally and genetically, with B-cell antigen receptors [immunoglobulins (Ig)], they also possess a number of unique features related to their specific biologic functions.

For classically defined helper and cytotoxic T cells, the most important of these differences was suggested by the experiments of Zinkernagel and Doherty (1,2), who showed that viral antigen recognition by cytotoxic T cells was possible only with a certain major histocompatibility complex (MHC) haplotype on the infected cell. Evidence for this phenomenon of MHC-restricted recognition also had been demonstrated for helper T cells (3,4). We now know that this type of T-cell recognition involves the recognition of fragments of antigens (e.g., peptides) bound to specific MHC molecules (see Chapters 8 and 9). Since all antigens must eventually be degraded, this form of T-cell recognition seems very complementary to that of B cells, in which pathogens can escape recognition by obscuring an antibodybinding site or employing "decoy" molecules.

TCRs occur as either of two distinct heterodimers, αβ or γδ, both of which are expressed with the nonpolymorphic CD3 polypetides γ, δ, ε, ζ, and in some cases, the RNA splicing variant of ζ,η or with FcεRIγ chains. The CD3 polypeptides, especially ζ and its variants, are critical for intracellular signaling (5). The αβ TCR heterodimer-expressing cells predominate in most lymphoid compartments (90% to 95%) of humans and mice, and they are responsible for the classical helper or cytotoxic T-cell responses. In most cases, the αβ TCR ligand is a peptide antigen bound to a class I or class II MHC molecule. T cells bearing γδ TCR are less numerous than the αβ type in most cellular compartments of humans and mice. However, they make up a substantial fraction of T-lymphocytes in cows, sheep, and chickens (6). Work on the structural characteristics and specificity of γδ TCRs suggests that they may be much more like Igs than αβ TCRs in their antigen-recognition properties. In particular, they do not seem to require MHC protein or other molecules to present antigens, but instead appear to rec

M.M. Davis: Department of Microbiology and Immunology, Stanford University School of Medicine, Howard Hughes Medical Institute, Stanford, California 94305.

Y.-H. Chien: Department of Microbiology and Immunology, Stanford University School of Medicine, Stanford, California 94305.

ognize antigens directly (6). While it is not yet clear what role they play in the immune response, this is a very active area of current research, and many interesting leads are being pursued.

TCR POLYPEPTIDES

The search for the molecules responsible for T-cell recognition first focused on deriving antisera or monoclonal antibodies specific for molecules on T-cell surfaces. Ultimately, a number of groups identified "clonotypic" sera (7) or monoclonal antibodies (8–12). A number of these antibodies were able to block antigen-specific responses by the T cells they were raised against or, when coated on a surface, could activate the T cells they are specific for. They were also able to immunoprecipitate 85,000- to 90,000-MW disulfide-bonded heterodimers from different T-cell clones or hybridomas consisting of two 40,000- to 50,000-MW glycosylated subunits, referred to as α and β. Peptide mapping studies showed that there was a striking degree of polymorphism between heterodimers isolated from T cells of differing specificity, thus suggesting that these antigen-recognition molecules might be akin to Igs (13,14).

Work in parallel with these serologic studies exploited the small differences (approximately 2%) observed between B- and T-cell

gene expression (15) and isolated both a mouse (16,17) and a human (18) T cell–specific gene that had antibody-like variable (V)-, joining (J)-, and constant (C)-region sequences and could rearrange in T-lymphocytes (16). This molecule was identified as TCRβ by partial sequence analysis of immunoprecipitated materials (19). Subsequent subtractive cloning work rapidly identified two other candidate TCR cDNAs, identified as TCRα (20,21) and TCRγ (22). It was quickly established that all antigen–specific helper or cytotoxic T cell expressed TCR αβ heterodimers. Where TCRγ fit in remained a puzzle until work by Brenner et al. (23) showed that it was expressed on a small (5% to 10%) subset of peripheral T cells together with another polypeptide, TCRδ. The structure of TCRδ remained unknown until a new TCR locus was discovered within the TCRα locus, between V_α and J_α (24). Antisera raised against portions of this gene quickly showed that this was TCRδ (25–27). Formal proof that the TCR α and β subunits were sufficient to transfer antigen–MHC recognition from one T cell to another came from gene transfection experiments (28,29), and equivalent experiments have also been done with γδ TCRs (30).

As shown in Fig. 1, all TCR polypeptides have a similar primary structure, with distinct V, diversity (D) (in the case of TCR β and δ), J, and C regions exactly analogous to their Ig counterparts. They

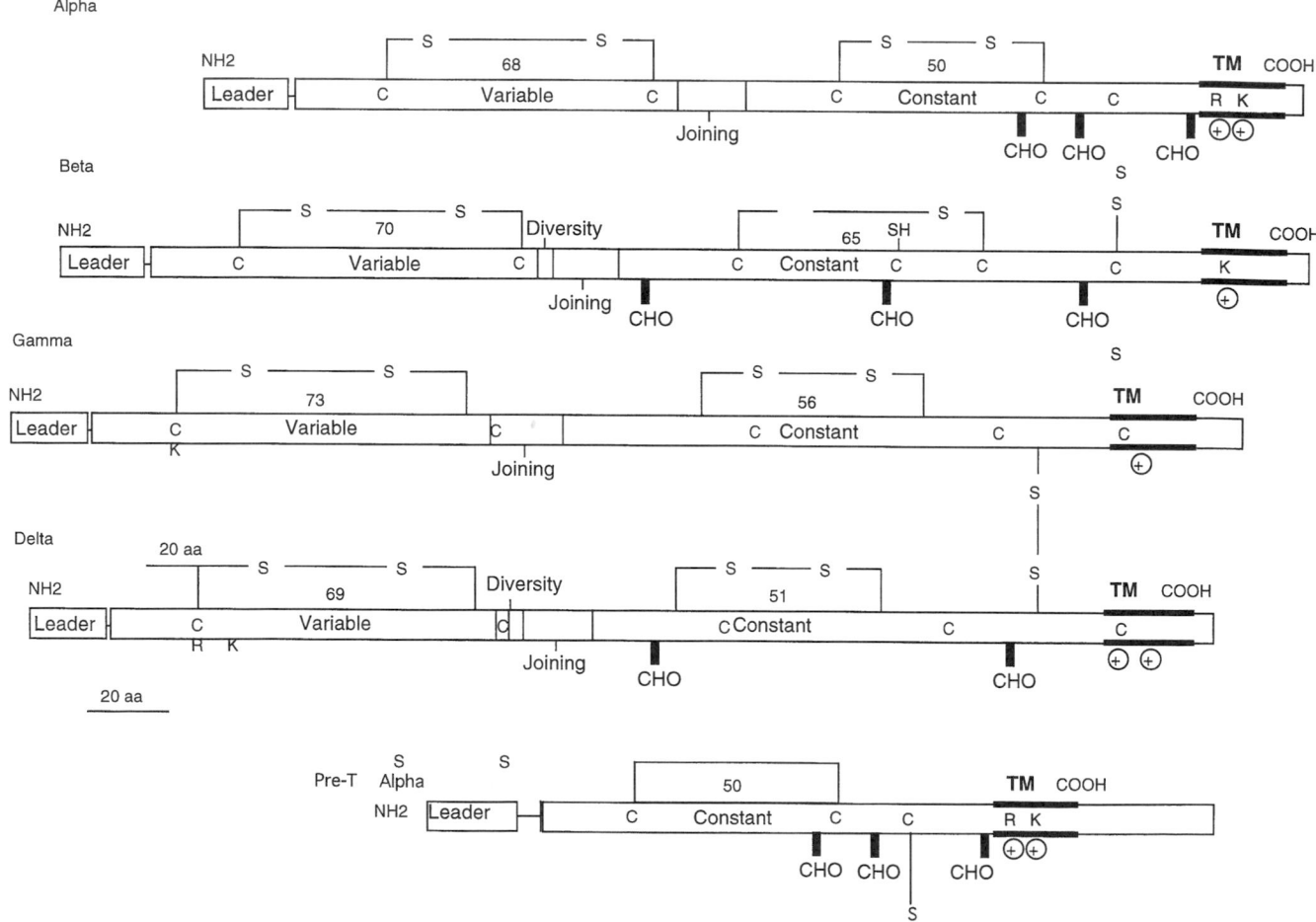

FIG. 1. Structural features of TCR and pre-T α polypeptides. Leader (L)-, variable (V)-, diversity (D)-, joining (J)-, and constant (C)- region gene segments are indicated. TM and bold horizontal lines delineate the putative transmembrane regions. CHO indicates potential carbohydrate addition sites. C and S refer to cysteine residues that form inter- and intrachain disulfide bonds. R and K indicate the positively charged amino acids (arginine and lysine, respectively) that occur in the transmembrane regions.

also share many of the amino acid residues thought to be important for the characteristic V and C domains of Ig (31). The C$_\beta$ region is particularly homologous, sharing 40% of its amino acid sequences with C$_\kappa$ and C$_\lambda$ (17,18). The TCR polypeptides all contain a single C-region domain (versus up to four for Igs), followed by a connecting peptide or hinge region, usually containing the cysteine for the disulfide linkage found joining the two chains of the heterodimer (some human TCR γδ isoforms lack this cysteine and consequently are not disulfide-linked; see ref. 32). N-linked glycosylation sites vary from two to four for each polypeptide, with no indications of O-linked sugar addition. C-terminal to the connecting peptide sequences are the hydrophobic transmembrane regions, which have no similarity to those of IgH genes, but instead have one or two positively charged residues that appear to be important for interaction with the CD3 molecules and T-cell signaling (33), perhaps through interaction with the acidic residues found in all CD3 transmembrane regions. The newest member of the TCR polypeptide family is the pre-T α chain, which serves as a chaperone for TCRβ in early thymocytes, similar to the role of λ5 in pre-B cells. It was first identified and cloned by von Boehmer and colleagues (34,35). The pre-T α chain has an interesting structure, which consists of a single Ig C region–like domain, followed by a cysteine-containing connecting peptide, a transmembrane region containing two charged residues, and an arginine and a lysine spaced identically to the location of those residues in the TCRα transmembrane region. The cysteine in the connecting peptide is

presumably what allows heterodimer formation with TCRβ, and the similarity to TCRα in the transmembrane region is most likely to accommodate the CD3 polypeptides. In both the mouse and human, the cytoplasmic tail is much longer than any of the TCR chains (37 and 120 amino acids, respectively), and the murine sequence contains two likely phosphorylation sites and sequences homologous to an SH3 domain–binding region. These are not present in the human sequence, however, and thus their functional significance is questionable (35).

TCR STRUCTURE

As discussed, the sequences of TCR polypeptides show many similarities to those of Ig; thus it has long been suggested that both heterodimers would be antibody-like in structure (37–39). These similarities include the number and spacing of specific cysteine residues within domains, which in antibodies form intrachain disulfide bonds. Also conserved are many of the inter- and intradomain contact residues, and in addition, secondary structure predictions are largely consistent with an Ig-like "β-barrel" structure. This consists of three to four antiparallel β strands on one side of the barrel facing a similar number on the other side, with a disulfide bridge (usually) connecting the two β "sheets" (sets of β strands in the same plane). A diagramatic representation of a typical V-region structure is shown in Fig 2A. All Ig V- and C-region domains have this structure, with slight variations in the number of

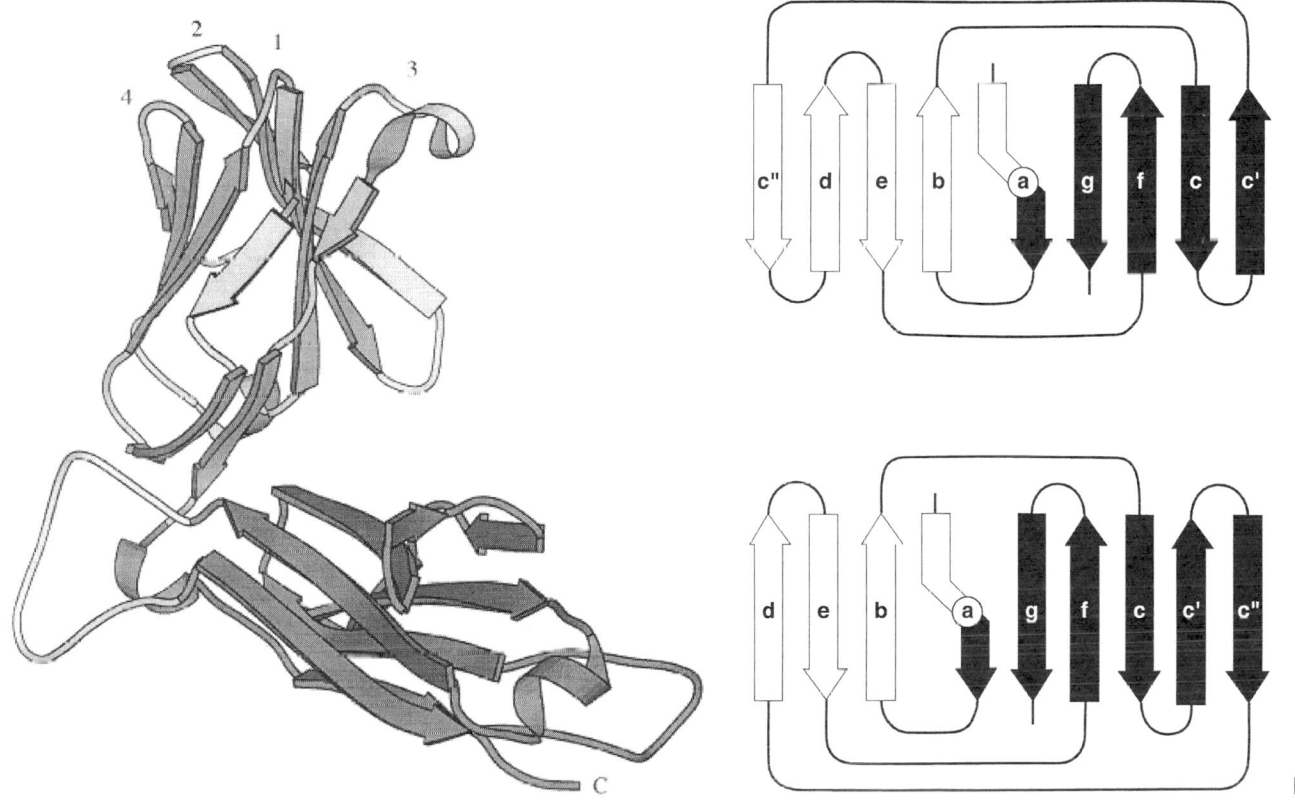

FIG. 2. TCRβ and Vα. **A:** Ribbon diagram of the first TCR crystal structures, showing the antiparallel β sheets of a Vβ Cβ polypeptide. The Vβ and Cβ domains show the classical eight and seven β-strand "barrels" characteristic of Ig V and C domains, respectively. Also shown are the positions of CDR loops 1, 2, and 3 at the end of Vβ, as well as the fourth loop, which has been implicated in superantigen interactions. **B:** A schematic of the β strands in a typical V-region domain, which contrast with the alterations found in a Vα domain.

β strands in V-region domains (by convention, including V, D, and J sequences) compared with C domains (35).

Efforts to derive x-ray crystal structures of TCR heterodimers and fragments of heterodimers have been very difficult. One reason is that it requires engineering the molecules into a soluble form. A second is that many of the TCRs are heavily glycosylated, and that it is necessary to eliminate most or all of the carbohydrate on each chain to achieve high-quality crystals. An alternative is to express soluble TCRs in insect cells, which have compact N-linked sugars, or in *E. coli,* which have none. The first successes in TCR crystallization came from the laboratory of Mariuzza and collaborators, who solved the structure of first a Vβ Cβ polypeptide (40) and then a Vα fragment (41). In general, these domains are very Ig-like, with the classical β-barrel structure in evidence in all three. At each end of the barrel in each V region-domain, there are four loops between the β sheets, three of which form the complementary-determining regions (CDRs) of Ig. The fourth loop, between the D and E strands, has been implicated in superantigen binding. The six CDR loops from the two V domains form the antigen-binding surface of Ig, and, as we will discuss shortly, TCRs as well. While the Vβ domain depicted in Fig. 2A follows the canonical V-domain β-sheet structure, Vα differs significantly in that one of the sheets has been translocated to the other half of the barrel (as schematized in Fig. 2B). This acts to remove a bulge in the side of the Vα domain, and it has been suggested that this would allow dimers of TCRs or perhaps higher order structures to assemble (41). More recently, Garcia and colleagues (43) were able to solve the structure of the Cα in the context of a complete heterodimer, and it has a remarkable variation of the classical Ig-like domain. Here there is only one half of the classical β barrel, that is, one set (or "sheet") of β strands, while the rest of the somewhat truncated domain exhibits random coils. This type of structure is unprecedented in the Ig superfamily, and it seems likely that it will be true for Cδ as well, because it has many similarities to Cα. The functional significance of such a variant structure in unknown, but it has been suggested that this incompletely formed Ig-like domain may be responsible for the observed lability of TCR α, and this may allow greater flexibility in the regulation of its expression. Another possible explanation is that this alteration may be designed to accommodate one or more of the CD3 molecules (43). Interestingly, the recently solved structure of a Vδ domain (44) shows a somewhat more V_H-like pattern, consistent with CDR3 length analyses and its apparent ligand recognition properties (see below).

With respect to complete heterodimer structures, there are now data from three αβ heterodimers (43,45,46), and they largely resemble a Fab fragment of an antibody (as shown in Colorplate 1). While many features of these structures are shared with their antibody counterparts, several unusual features are emerging that may be significant: (a) In one structure (43), four out of seven N-linked sugars diffracted to high resolution, indicating that they are not free to move very much and thus are likely to play a structural role, particularly in Cα Cδ interactions. This correlates with mutagenesis data indicating that certain Cα sugars could not be eliminated without abolishing protein expression in mammalian cells (47) and the disordered state of a Cα domain in the structure of a TCR lacking glycosylation (45). (b) There is much more contact between Vβ and somewhat more between Vα and Cα than in the equivalent regions of antibodies. (c) The geometry of the interaction of Vα and Vβ more closely resembles that of the C_H3 domains of antibodies than $V_H V_L$. (d) Between the CDR3 loops of Vα and Vβ there is a pocket

that can (and does in at least one case; see ref. 45) accommodate a large side chain from the peptide bound to an MHC. Another key question is whether any conformational change occurs in the TCR upon ligand binding. Conformational changes in the TCR or in the CD3 polypeptides in particular may hold important clues as to the mechanism of signal transduction across the membrane after TCR engagement. Studies have also indicated that TCR–peptide–MHC complexes have an inherent ability to self-associate (48), and thus it would be very interesting to know the structure of such a cluster and how it may relate to early signaling events.

THE CD3 POLYPEPTIDES

Immunoprecipitation of the TCR with antiidiotypic antibodies after solubilization with the nonionic detergent, noniodet P_{40} (NP_{40}), shows only the α- and β-chain heterodimer. However, the use of gentler detergents, such as digitonin or Triton-X100, reveals five other proteins (as reviewed in 5,49). This is shown most clearly in a form of two-dimensional gel electrophoresis, in which the first dimension is run without a reducing agent, whereas the second gel is run with one (Fig. 3). The result is that most proteins fall along a diagonal, whereas the subunits from disulfide-bonded multimeric proteins fall below the diagonal. Analysis of mouse T cells by this technique shows the two TCR subunits (α,β) running at 40,000 MW together with CD3γ (20,000), CD3δ (25,000), CD3ε (20,000), and a fourth running below the diagonal at 16,000 MW (50) (ζ) (Colorplate 1). The fact that the ε chain runs above the diagonal indicates that it migrates faster when disulfide bonds are intact than when they are broken. This in turn implies that there are intrachain disul-

NR →

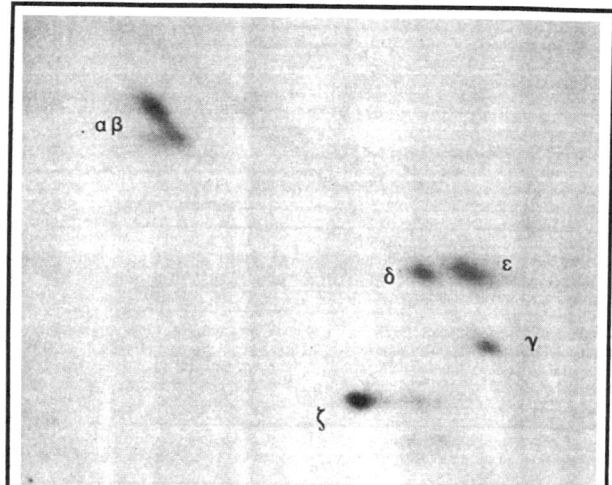

FIG. 3. TCR αβ CD3 complexes. SDS-PAGE analysis of TCR-CD3 complexes, using immunoprecipitation and the two-dimensional "diagonal" gel method of Goding (50a) T-cell hybridoma cells were surface-labeled with 125I and immunoprecipitated with an anti-TCR antibody. The first dimension was run on SDS-PAGE without reducing agents, and the second dimension included them. Molecules that are not disulfide-linked multimers cluster along a diagonal, whereas those that are, "fall off" the diagonal as their molecular weight decreases as they dissociate into their component chains. Shown here are TCR α, β, and CD3 γ, δ, ε, and ζ chains.

fide bonds that hold the molecule in a compact configuration. The migration of the ζ chain is indicative of a disulfide-bonded homodimer; however, further studies have shown that the ζ chain can be part of a heterodimer in at least two forms. In mouse T cells, the ζ chain can disulfide bond with a minor variant called the η (eta) chain (51,52). This latter chain is an alternate splicing variant of the ζ-chain gene (53). This alternatively spliced species of the ζ chain is not found in significant quantities in human T cells (54). The second type of ζ chain containing heterodimer contains the γ chain associated with the FcεRI (FcεRI γ) and FcγRIII (CD16) receptors (55,56).

With respect to overall stoichiometry, current evidence favors at least two TCR heterodimers per CD3 cluster. This is based on a number of findings, particularly the work of Terhorst and colleagues (as reviewed in ref. 5), who showed that in a T-T hybridoma, a monoclonal antibody against one TCRαβ pair could comodulate a second αβ heterodimer. In addition, sucrose gradient centrifugation of TCR/CD3 showed a predicted molecular weight of 300 kDa, more than 100 kDa larger than expected from a minimal δ subunit com-

plex (α,β,γ,δ,ε₂,ζ₂). Another study suggesting that there are least two TCRs in a given CD3 complex is a Scatchard analysis, indicating that the number of CD3ε(molecules on a T-cell surface equals the number of αβ TCRs (57–59). Finally, there is the recent report of Fernandez-Miguel et al. (60), who showed that in T cells that have two transgenic TCRβ chains, antibodies to one Vβ can immunoprecipitate the other. It was also found that they are often close enough to allow fluorescence energy transfer, meaning that the two TCRβs in a cluster are within 50 Å of each other (60). Interestingly, it appears that the TCR complexes with CD3 have either CD3γ or CD3δ but not both, and these two receptor types are expressed in different ratios in different cells. Furthermore, in cell types that express the FcεRIg chain, these two forms of the receptor can be further divided into those that contain the ζζ homodimer and those that have the ζ FcεRIg heterodimer (55,56). Thus, as shown in Fig. 4, the best evidence to date suggests a stoichiometry of the core cluster being $[\alpha\beta]_2[\gamma/\delta\varepsilon]_2[\zeta\zeta]_4$, with a number of the variations involving FcεR, as discussed above. Having two TCR heterodimers

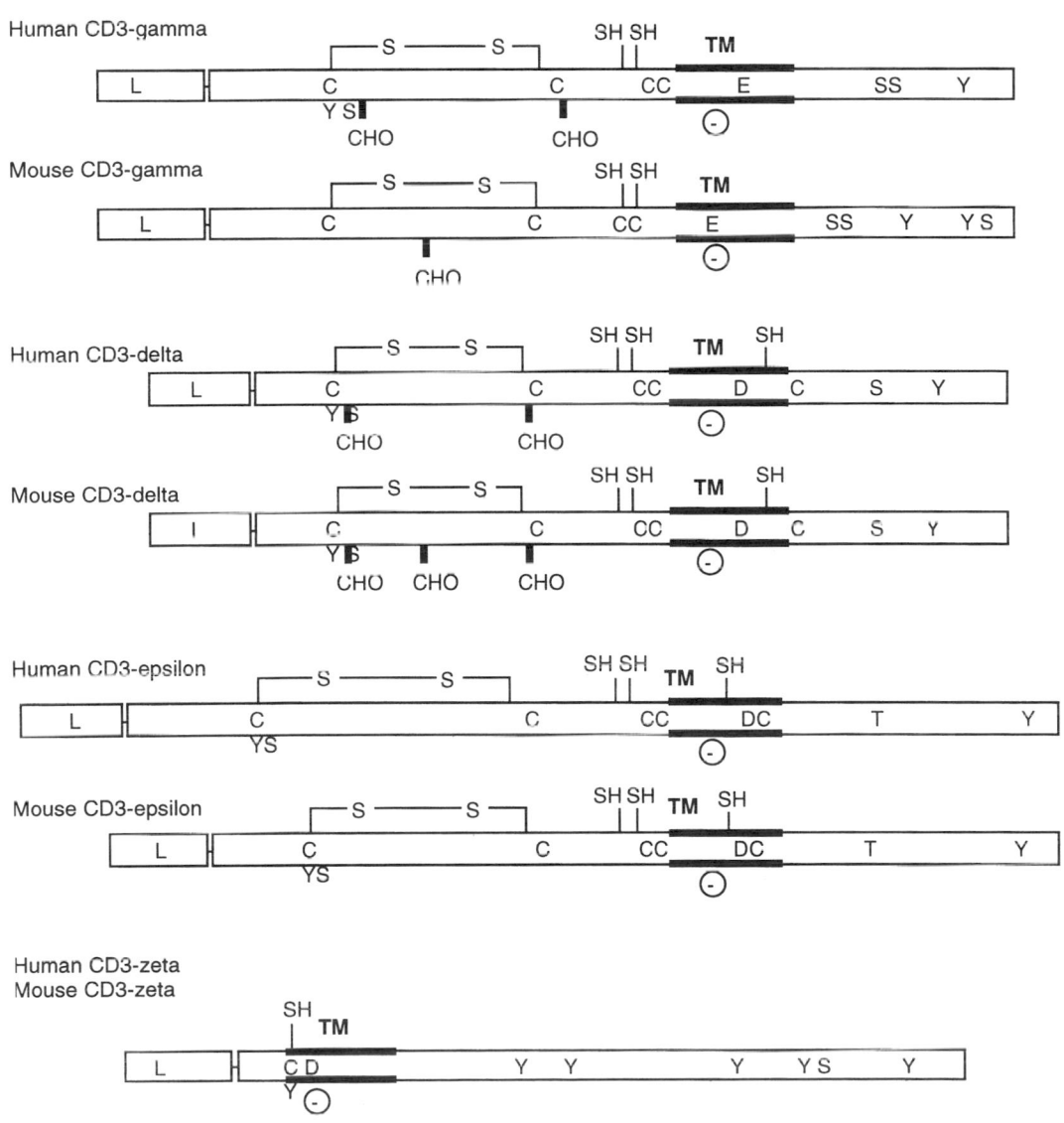

FIG. 4. Structural features of the CD3 molecules. As Fig. in 1, transmembrane regions (TM), carbohydrate addition sites (CHO), and cysteine residues (C) are indicated. In addition, negatively charged transmembrane residues (D for aspartic acid and E for glutamic acid) as well as putative phosphorylation sites are shown.

per complex is particularly interesting with respect to aggregation models of T-cell triggering through the TCR (48).

Sequence and Structure of the CD3 Polypeptides

Figure 4 illustrates the principal structural features of the γ-, δ-, ε-, and ζ-chain polypeptides as derived from gene cloning and sequencing (as reviewed in refs. 5,61). The extracellular domains of the γ, δ, and ε chains show a significant degree of similarity to one another. These domains retain the cysteines that have been shown to form intrachain disulfide bonds, and each consists of a single Ig superfamily domain. The spacing of the cysteines in these domains indicates a compact Ig fold, similar to a C-region domain. All of the extracellular domains contain a pair of closely spaced cysteines just before the predicted membrane-spanning regions, and these are likely candidates for the formation of intermolecular disulfide bonds, as described above. The extracellular domain of the ζ chain consists of only nine amino acids and contains the only cysteine, which is responsible for the disulfide linkage of the ζζ homodimer or the alternative ζ FcεRI heterodimer. In the transmembrane regions, it is particularly striking that all of the CD3 polypeptides have a conserved, negatively charged amino acid, complementary to the positive charges seen in the TCR transmembrane regions and also necessary for proper assembly (62,63).

The intracellular domains of the γ, δ, ε, and ζ chains are the intracellular signaling "domains" of the TCR heterodimer (61–64). Each of these molecules contains an amino acid sequence motif that can mediate cellular activation (65,66). In T cells that are defective in ζ-chain expression, a small but significant amount of interleukin-2 (IL-2) production can be elicited using either the superantigen, SEA, or an antibody specific for thy-1. However, the ζ chain is required for optimal stimulation by antigen, and the intracellular sequences responsible for this activation are contained within as few as 18 amino acids, with the sequence $X_2YX_2L/IX_7YX_2L/I$ (63,64). Both of the tyrosines in this sequence motif are absolutely required to mediate signal transduction since mutation

of either completely prevents the mobilization of free Ca++ or cytolytic activity. This sequence occurs three times in the ζ chain and once in each of the CD3 γ, δ, ε, and FcεRI γ chains. There are also pairs of tyrosines present in the cytoplasmic domains of the γ, δ, ε, and ζ chains (see Fig. 5). This sequence motif is also present in the mβ-1 and B29 chains associated with the (Ig) β-cell receptor, and in the FcεRI β chain (67). The tyrosines in these cytoplasmic sequences are substrates for tyrosine phosphorylation, which is one of earliest steps in T-cell signaling (68,69) and is thought to occur aberrantly in nonproductive T-cell responses (e.g., antagonism; see below). Serine phosphorylation of the CD3γ also occurs upon antigen or mitogenic stimulation of T cells (70,71) and thus may play a role as well.

Intracellular Assembly and Degradation of the TCR/CD3 Complex

The assembly of newly formed TCR α and β chains with the CD3 γ, δ, ε, and ζ chains and their intracellular fate have been studied in detail (as reviewed in refs. 5, 49, 72). Studies have focused on mutant hybridoma lines that fail to express TCR on their cell surfaces and on transfection studies using cDNA for the different chains in the receptor.

Experiments in a nonlymphoid cell system (73) have shown that TCR α can assemble with CD3 δ and ζ but not CD3 γ and ζ. In contrast, the TCR β chain can assemble with any of the CD3 chains except the ζ chain. When the ζ chain was transfected with either α- or β-chain genes, or any of the three CD3 chains, no pairwise interaction occurred. Only when all six cDNAs were cotransfected was it shown that the ζ chain could be coprecipitated with the other chains (73). Based on these data (5), a model has been proposed that suggests that the TCR α chain pairs with CD3 δ and ε chains and that the TCR β chain pairs with the CD3 γ and ε chains in the completed molecule. The ζ chain is thought join the TCR and other CD3 polypeptides in that last stage of assembly. Figure 5 shows how the CDS polypeptides are thought to interact with the two TCR heterodimers (5).

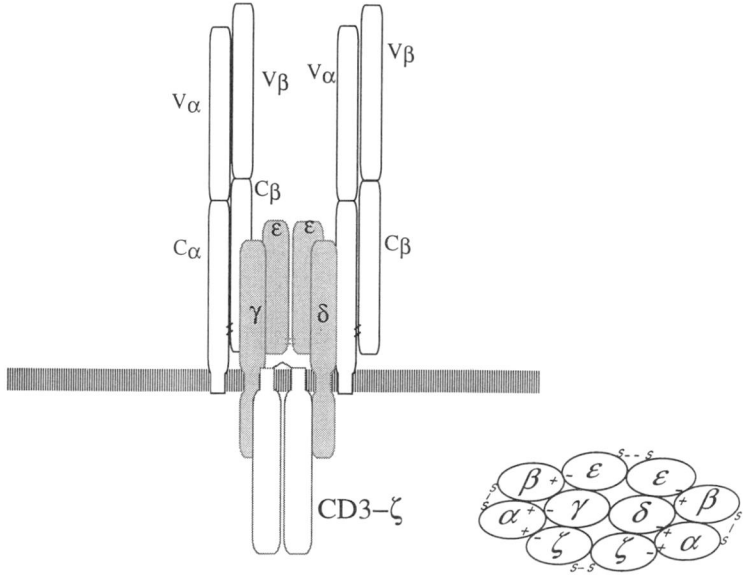

FIG. 5. A model of the TCR αβ complex. While the precise arrangement of TCR polypeptides and CD3 molecules in a given cluster is not known, the fragmentary data that exist have been schematized by Terhorst and colleagues into this working model of the complex. This model is also consistent with the data of de la Hera et al. (60), which greatly strengthens the view that there are two TCR heterodimers in each cluster. (From ref. 5)

Pulse chase experiments have shown that all six chains are assembled in the endoplasmic reticulum (ER), transported to the Golgi apparatus, and then transferred to the plasma membrane. It also appears that the amount of ζ chain is rate limiting, as it is synthesized at only 10% of the level of the other chains. This results in the vast majority of newly synthesized α, β, or CD3 components being degraded within 4 hours of their synthesis (74). The remaining nondegraded chains are long-lived and form complete TCR/CD3 complexes with the limiting ζ chain (74). TCR/CD3 lacking CD3 ζ chains migrate through the ER and Golgi intact but then are transported to and degraded in the lysosomes. A lysosome-targeting motif has been identified in the CD3 δ and γ chains and consists of a dileucine-based motif (DKQTLL) and a tyrosine-based motif (75) in the carboxy-terminal-region. Mutants lacking these sequences escape lysozomal transport and degradation when transfected into ζ chain–deficient cells (76).

Three of the components of the TCR/CD3 complex—TCRα, TCRβ, and CD3δ—are rapidly degraded in a pre-Golgi compartment (77–79), whereas γ, ε, and ζ chains are stable for hours within the ER. In the β chain, the signal for pre-Golgi proteolysis is encoded within the transmembrane region and short cytoplasmic tail. Removal of the latter amino acids from the β chain resulted in retention in the ER (80). Analysis using transfectants of individual chains or pairs of chains has shown that CD3 γ and δ chains contain ER retention signals. If these signals are removed, the chains are transported through the Golgi apparatus and rapidly degraded in the lysosomes. The immunologic significance of this pre-Golgi degradation pathway is most evident in CD4⁺CD8⁺ thymocytes, where, despite high levels of synthesis of both mRNA and protein for all the TCR, CD3, and ζ chains, surface expression is relatively low. The TCR chains in immature thymocytes seem to be selectively degraded (81). Thus, posttranslation regulation appears to be an important means of controlling the cell surface expression of TCR heterodimers.

TCR GENES

As shown in Fig. 6, TCR gene segments are organized similarly to those of Ig, and the same recombination machinery seems responsible for joining separate V and D segments to a particular J and C. This was initially indicated by the fact that the characteristic seven- and nine-nucleotide conserved sequences adjacent to the V, D, and J regions with the 12- or 23-nucleotide spacing between them, first described for Ig genes, are also present in TCRs (82,83). The most conclusive evidence of this common rearrangement mechanism has been shown by the fact that both a naturally occurring recombination-deficient mouse strain (severe combined immune deficiency, SCID; ref. 84) and mice engineered to lack recombinase-activating genes (RAG) 1 (85) or 2 (86) are unable to rearrange either TCR or Ig gene segments properly. As with Ig, if the V-region and J-region gene segments are in the same transcriptional orientation, the intervening DNA is deleted during recombination. DNA circles of such material can be observed in the thymus (87,88), the principal site of TCR recombination (see below). In the case of TCRβ (89) and TCRδ (90), there is a single V region 3' to the C in the opposite transcriptional orientation to J and C. Thus, rearrangement to these gene segments occurs via an inversion. Variable points of joining are seen along the V, D, and J gene segments as well as random nucleotide addition (N regions) in postnatal TCRs (91). The addition of several nucleotides in an inverted repeat pattern, referred to as a P-element insertion, at the V–J junction of the TCRγ chains has also been observed (92).

Organization of the TCR α/δ Locus

In humans and in mice there is a single α-chain C-region gene that is composed of four exons encoding (a) the C-region domain; (b) 16 amino acids, including the cysteine that forms the interchain disulfide bond; (c) the transmembrane and intracytoplasmic domains; and (d) the 3' untranslated region (93–95). The entire α/δ locus in humans has now been mapped (96) and spans about 1.1 MB. The mouse TCR locus appears to be similar in size. There are 50 different J-region gene segments upstream of the C region (see Fig. 6) in the murine locus (97). At least eight of the J-region gene elements are nonfunctional because of in-frame stop codons or rearrangement and splicing signals that are likely to be defective. A similar number of α-chain J regions are present in the human locus (95,96). This very large number of α-chain J regions compared to the Ig loci may indicate that the functional diversity contributed by the J segment of the TCR (which constitutes a major portion of the CDR3 loop) makes a particularly important contribution to antigen recognition (see below).

Both the murine and human Cδ, Jδ, and two Dδ gene segments are located between the Vα and Jα gene segments (24,98–100). In

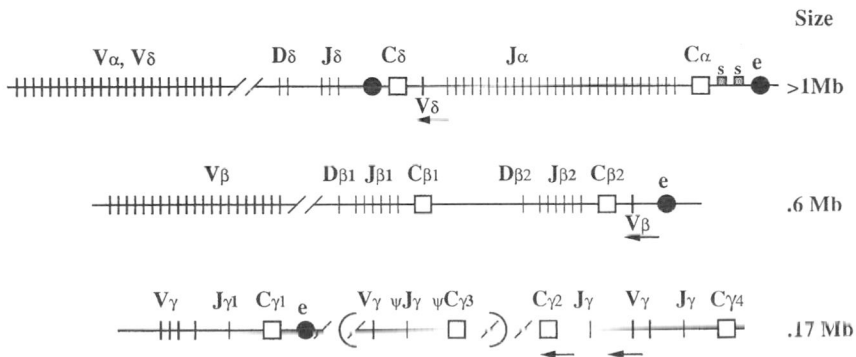

FIG. 6. TCR gene organization in mice and humans. Schematic of V, D, J, and C elements of the TCR genes. E denotes enhancers, and 3 denotes silencer elements. Transcriptional orientation is from left to right except where noted. The overall size of each locus is indicated on the right-hand side. (Adapted from ref. .)

the murine system there are two Jδ and two Dδ gene segments on the 5′ aide of Cδ (24,98), and the Cδ gene is approximately 75 kb upstream of the Cα gene, but only approximately 8 kb upstream of the most 5′ known Jα gene segments. The human organization is similar, with three Dα gene segments and two Jδ (101). Suprisingly, in both species, all of the D elements can be used in one rearranged gene, rather than alternating, as is the case with TCRβ or IgH. That is, in mice, one frequently finds Vδ, D_1, D_2, Jδ rearrangements (91) and in humans, Vδ, D_1, D_2, D_3, Jδ (101). This greatly increases the junctional or CDR3 diversity that is available, especially because of the potential for N-region addition between each gene segment. This property makes TCRδ the most diverse of any of the antigen receptors known, with approximately 10^{12} to 10^{13} different amino acid sequences in a relatively small (10- to 15-amino acid) region (91).

The location of Dδ, Jδ, and Cδ genes between Vα and Jα gene segments raises the possibility that TCR δ and α could share the same pool of V-gene segments. While there is some overlap in V-gene usage, in the murine system, four of the commonly used Vδ genes (Vδ1, Vδ2, Vδ4, Vδ5) are very different than known Vα sequences and they have not been found to associate with Cα (102). The other four Vδ gene families overlap with or are identical to Vα subfamilies (Vδ3, Vδ6, Vδ7, Vδ8 with Vα6, Vα7, Vα4, Vα11, respectively).

The mechanisms that account for the preferential usage of certain gene segments to produce δ versus α chain are not known. While some Vδ genes are located closer to the Dδ and Jδ fragments than Vα genes (such as Vδ1), other Vδ's (such as Vδ6) are rarely deleted by Vα Jα rearrangements and thus seem likely to be located 5′ of many Vα gene segments (91).

One of the Vδ gene segments, Vδ5, is located approximately 2.5 kb to the 3′ of Cδ in the opposite transcriptional orientation and rearranges by inversion (90). Despite its close proximity to Dδ Jδ gene segments, Vδ5 is not frequently found in fetal γδ T cells. Instead, the Vδ5→DJδ rearrangement predominates in adult γδ T cells.

An implicit characteristic of the α/δ gene locus is that a rearrangement of Vα to Jα deletes the entire D-J-C core of the δ-chain locus. In many αβ T cells, the α-chain locus is rearranged on both chromosomes and thus no TCR δ could be made. In most cases, this is due to Vα→Jα rearrangement, but evidence suggesting an intermediate step in the deletion of TCRδ has been reported (103). This involves rearrangements of an element termed *TEA* to a pseudo-Jα 3′ of Cδ. The rearrangement of TEA to this pseudo-Jα would eliminate the δ-chain locus in αβ T cells. Gene targeting of the TEA element resulted in normal levels of αβ and γδ T cells, but usage of the most Jα was severely restricted (104), suggesting that its function has to do with governing the accessibility of the most 5′ Jα for recombination.

Organization of the TCR β Locus

The entire human 685-kb β-chain gene locus has been completely sequenced (105), and the organization is shown in Figure 6. One interesting feature is the tandem nature of J_β–C_β in the *TCRβ* locus (106,107). This arrangement is preserved in all higher vertebrate species that have been characterized thus far (mouse, human, chicken, frog). The two C_β coding sequences are identical in the mouse and nearly so in humans and other species. Thus, it is unlikely that they represent two functionally distinct forms of C_β. However, the J_β clusters have relatively unique sequences and thus

this may be a mechanism for increasing the number of J_β gene segments. Together with the large number of Jα gene segments, there is far more combinatorial diversity (Jα × Jβ = 50 × 12 = 600) provided by J regions in αβ TCRs than in Ig.

Most of the V regions are located upstream of the J and C regions, and in the same transcriptional orientation as the D and J gene element and rearrange to the DβJβ gene via deletion. Similar to the case of Vδ5, a single Vβ gene, Vβ14, is located 3′ to C regions and in the opposite transcriptional orientation; thus, rearrangements involving Vβ14 occur via inversion (89).

In the NZW strain of mouse, there is a deletion in the β chain locus that spans from Cβ1 up to and including the Jβ2 cluster (108). In SJL, C57BR, and C57L mice, there is a deletion (77) in the V-region locus from Vδ5 to Vβ9. These mice also express a V gene, Vβ17, which is not expressed in other strains of mice. Deletion of about half of the V genes (in SJL, C57BR, and C57L mice) (109) does not seem to have any particular effect on the ability of these mice to mount immune responses, whereas mice that have deleted the $J_\beta2$ cluster show impaired responses (110).

Organization of the TCR γ Locus

The organization of the mouse γ-chain locus is shown in Fig. 6 (111,112,117). The human γ genes span about 150 kb (113–116) and are organized in a fashion similar to that of the β-chain locus with two JγCγ regions. An array of Vγ, in which at least six of the V regions are pseudogenes, are located 5′ to these JγCγ clusters, and each of the V genes are potentially capable of rearranging to any of the five J regions. The sequences of the two human Cγ regions are very similar overall and only differ significantly in the second exon. In Cγ2, this exon is duplicated two to three times, and the cysteine, which forms in the interchain disulfide bond, is absent. Thus, Cγ2-bearing human T cells have an extra large γ chain (55,000 MW) that is not disulfide bonded to its δ-chain partner (113).

The organization of the murine γ-chain genes is very different than that of the human genes in that there are three separate rearranging loci (111,112) that span about 205 kb (117). Of four murine Cγ genes, Cγ3 is apparently a pseudogene in BALB/c mice, and the Jγ3 Cγ3 region is deleted in several mouse strains, including C57BL/10. Cγ1 and Cγ2 are very similar in coding sequences. The major differences between these two genes is in the 5-amino acid deletion in the Cγ2 gene, which is located in the C II exon at the amino acid terminal of the cysteine residue used for the disulfide formation with the δ chain. The Cγ4 gene differs significantly in sequences from the other Cγ genes (with 66% overall amino acid identity). In addition, the Cγ4 sequences contain a 17-amino acid insertion (compared to Cγ1) in the C II exon located at a position similar to that of the 5-amino acid deletion of the Cγ2 gene (G. Kershard, S.M. Hedrick, unpublished results).

Each of the Cγ genes is associated with a single Jγ gene segment. The sequences of Jγ1 and Jγ2 are identical at the amino acid level, whereas Jγ4 differs from Jγ1 and Jγ2 at 9 out of 19 amino acid residues.

The murine Vγ genes usually rearrange to the Jγ Cγ gene that is most proximal and in the same transcription orientation. Thus, Vγ1.1 rearranges to Jγ4; Vγ1.2 to Jγ2; and Vγ2, Vγ3, Vγ4, Vγ5 to Jγ1. Interestingly, it appears that different Vγ genes are rearranged and expressed preferentially during γδ T-cell ontogeny and in different adult tissues as well (92,118).

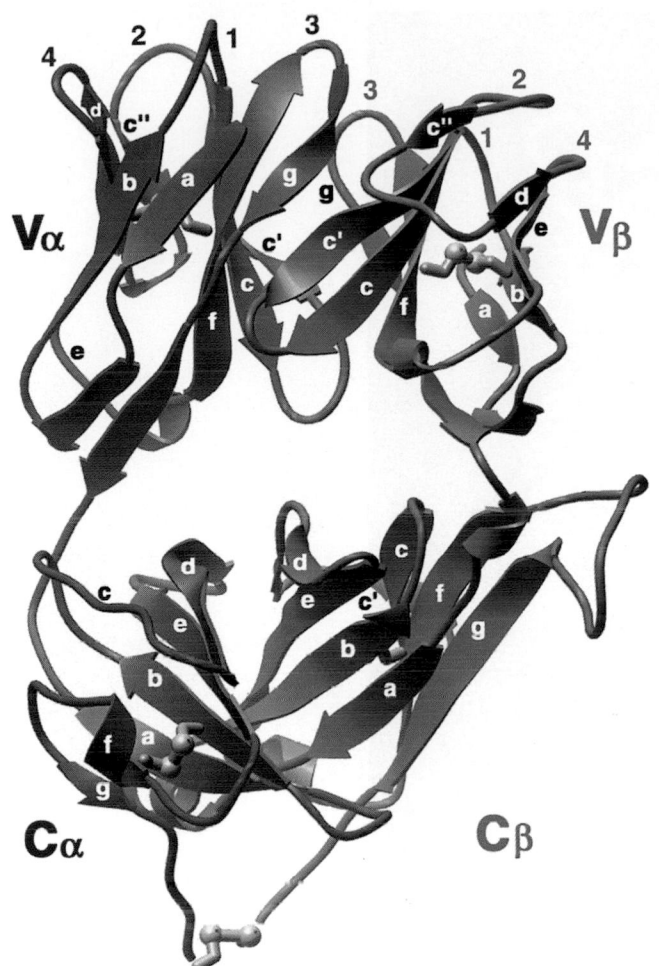

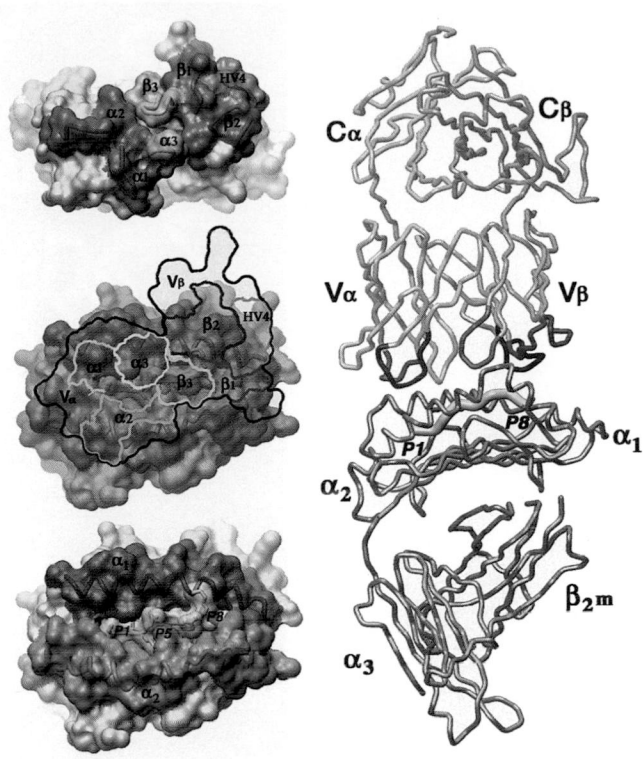

COLORPLATE 1. Complete TCR αβ structure. A ribbon diagram of the first TCR αβ heterodimer structure from Garcia et al. (43). β strands in all domains are indicated by letters and the CDR1, 2, 3 and 4 loops by numbers.

COLORPLATE 2. TCR–peptide–MHC crystal structure of a TCR–peptide–MHC complex. Key peptide anchor residues for MHC binding are indicated as P1, P5, and P8, and the TCR Vα and Vβ CDR regions are labeled as α1 (for CDR1α), α2, etc. MHC α helices are labeled α_1 α_2. (From ref. 43.)

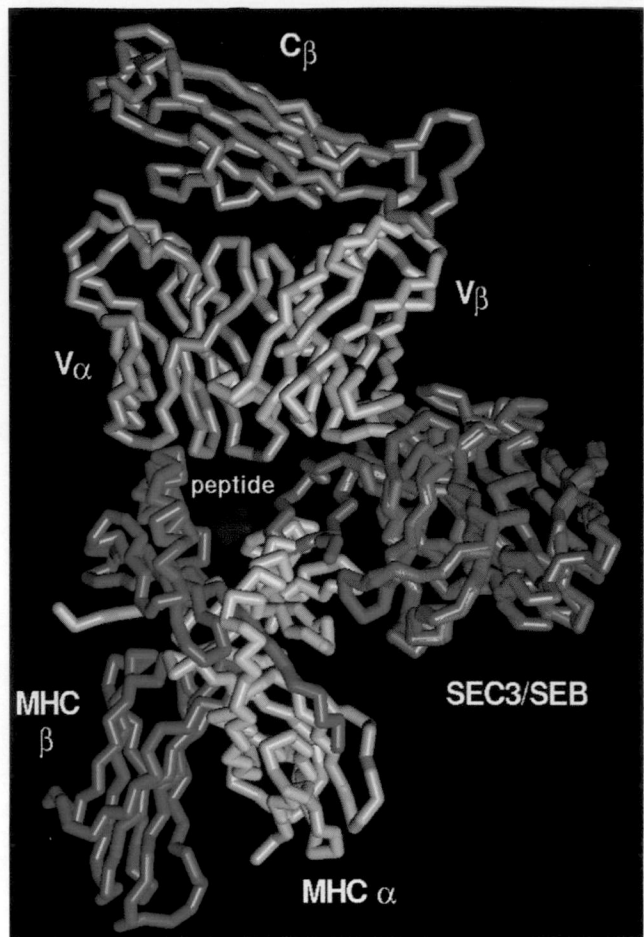

COLORPLATE 3. Crystal structure of a TCR β/Super antigen complex. Fields et al. (248) have crystallized TCR-SAg complexes and from the structure of the same superantigens with a class II MHC molecule and are able to deduce the relative spatial arrangement of the three molecules. This model suggests that TCR does not contact the MHC very strongly, consistent with the relative peptide insensitivity of SAg activation.

Transcriptional Control

Transcriptional regulation of the TCR genes has been studied extensively, with enhancer sequences first being identified in the TCRβ locus 3' of Cβ2 (119,120) and subsequently for the other TCR loci as well (reviewed in ref. 121), as indicated in Fig. 6. These TCR enhancers all share sequence similarities with each other. Some of the transcriptional factors that bind to the TCR genes are also found to regulate Ig gene expressions. Work by Sleckman and colleagues (122) has shown that the TCRα enhancer (Eα) not only is important for normal rearrangement and expression for the α chain locus, but also is required for the normal expression level of mature TCRδ transcripts (122). Also interesting is the work of Lauzurica and Krangel (124), who have shown that a human TCRδ enhancer-containing minilocus in transgenic mice is able to rearrange equally well in αβ T cells as in δ T cells, but that an Eα-containing construct was only active in αβ lineage T cells. Similar to Ig genes, promoter sequences are located 5' to the V-gene segments. Although D → Jβ rearrangement and transcription occur fairly often in B cells, and in -cell tumors (125), Vβ rearrangement and/or transcription appears highly specific to T cells. In addition to enhancers, there also appear to be "silencer" sequences 3' of Cα (126,127) and in the Cγ1 locus (128). It has been suggested that these "repressor" sites could turn off the expression of either of these genes, influencing T-cell differentiation toward either the αβ or the γδ T-cell lineage.

Chromosomal Locations and Translocations Associated with Disease

The chromosomal locations of the different TCR loci have been delineated in both mice and humans and the results are summarized in Table 1 (as reviewed in ref. 129). One significant factor in cancers of hematopoietic cells are chromosomal translocations, which result in the activation of genes that are normally turned off or the inactivation of genes that are normally turned on. Thus, B- or T-lymphocyte neoplasia is frequently associated with inter- or intrachromosomal rearrangements of Ig or TCR loci, and in some cases, both (130,131).

TABLE 1. *Chromosomal locations of T-cell receptor, Ig, and related loci in mouse and human*

	Mouse chromosome	Human chromosome
TCR-α	14	14(q11–q12)
TCR-δ	14	14(q11–q12)
IgH	12	14(qter)
TCR-β	6	7(q35)
CD4	6	12
CD8	6	2(p11)
Igκ	6	2(p12)
TCR-γ	13	7(p14)
CD3-γ	9	11(q23)
CD3-δ	9	11(q23)
CD3-ε	9	11(q23)
CD3-ζ	1	1
Thy-1	9	11(q23)
Igλ	16	22(q11.2)
MHC	17	6(p21)
Pre Tα	17	6

These translocations seemed to be mediated by the V(D)J recombinase machinery, indicating the inherent danger and need for tight regulation of this pathway. Such rearrangements are particularly common in the α/δ locus, perhaps because this locus spans the longest developmental window in terms of gene expression, with TCRδ being the first and TCRα the last gene to rearrange during T-cell ontogeny (as discussed in more detail below). In addition, the α/δ locus is in excess of 1 Mb in size, and this provides a larger target for rearrangement than either TCRβ or TCRγ. Interestingly, in humans, TCRα/δ is on the same chromosome as the IgH locus, and V_H→Jα rearrangements (by inversion) have been observed in some human tumor material (132,133). The functional significance of this is not known.

Particularly frequent is the chromosome 8–14 translocation [t(8;14) (q24;q11)], which joins the α/δ locus to the c-myc gene, analogous to the C-myc→IgH translocation in many mouse myeloma tumors and in Burkitt's lymphomas in humans (130,131). In one cell line, a rearrangement occurred between the Jα-region coding sequences and a region 3' of c-myc (134). In both B- and T-cell malignancies, the translocation of c-myc into IgH or TCR α/β appears to increase the expression of c-myc, and may be a major factor in the unregulated cell growth that characterizes cancerous cells. Other putative protooncogenes that have been found translocated into the TCR α/β locus are the LIM domain containing transcription factors Ttg-1 (135) and Ttg-2 (136,137), which are involved in neural development; the helix–loop–helix proteins Lyl-1 (138,139) and Scl (140,141), which are involved in early hematopoietic development; and the homeobox gene Hox 11 (142), which is normally active in the liver. How these particular translocations contribute to malignancy is unknown, but they presumably cause aberrations in gene expression that contribute to cell growth or escape from normal regulation. In T-cell leukemia patients infected with the HTLV-I virus, there are large numbers of similar translocations, and here it is thought that HTLV-I itself is not directly leukemogenic, but acts by causing aberrant rearrangements in the T cells that it infects, some of which become malignant.

Another disorder that exhibits frequent TCR and Ig locus translocations is ataxia telangiectasia (AT), an autosomal recessive disorder characterized by ataxia, vascular telangiectasis, immunodeficiency, increased incidence of neoplasia, and an increased sensitivity to ionizing radiation. Peripheral blood lymphocyte (PBL) cells from patients with AT have an especially high frequency of translocations involving chromosomes 7 and 14 (143). These sites correspond to the TCR γ, β, and α loci, and the Ig heavy-chain locus (144,145). Thus, it appears as though one of the characteristics of AT patients is a relatively error-prone rearrangement process that indiscriminately recombines genes that have the TCR and Ig rearrangement signals.

Allelic Exclusion

In Ig, generally only one allele of the heavy-chain locus and one of the light-chain alleles are productively rearranged and expressed, a phenomenon termed *allelic exclusion* (see Chapters 5 and 6). With respect to αβ TCR expression, current data indicate that while TCRβ exhibits allelic exclusion (146), TCRα does not (147,148) and that some mature T cells express two functional TCRα chains. As the chances of forming an in-frame joint with any antigen receptor is only one in three, the probability that a T cell would have two productively rearranged TCRα chains is only (1/3 × 1/3 = 9) or 11%. However, even when this happens, the two

TCRα chains may not form heterodimers equally well with the single TCRβ that is expressed, and thus only one heterodimer may be expressed.

Data strongly suggest an important role for the pre-TCR heterodimer (e.g., pre-Tα:TCRβ) in blocking further TCRβ rearrangement, thus ensuring allelic exclusion at that locus (149,150). In particular, pre-Tα–deficient mice had a significant increase in the number of cells with two productive TCRβ rearrangements, compared with wild-type mice (149).

Commitment to the αβ Versus the γδ Lineage

One important issue in T-cell development concerns the lineage relationship between αβ and γδ T cells; that is, what governs the differentiation of the thymic stem cells to become either αβ or γδ T cells? Two different models have been proposed. In one, which could be termed the *sequential rearrangement model* (24), the precursor cells first rearrange the γ- and δ-chain genes. Those cells that fail to make a functional TCRγ or δ would progress to the αβ lineage and attempt to rearrange the TCR β- and α-chain loci. The second is referred to as the *separate lineage model* and postulates that T cells differentiate into two lineages prior to rearrangement. One line of evidence that supports the sequential rearrangement model is a study that found that δ chains are often found rearranged on chromosomes that undergo an α-chain rearrangement (151), but a subsequent, more extensive investigation found most had unrearranged sequences (152). Further evidence in favor of the separate lineage model comes from transgenic mice bearing rearranged TCR γ- and δ-chain genes. In these mice, although all of the precursor cells expressed functional γδ genes, there are normal numbers of αβ T cells in the thymus (153). This is the opposite of what one would expect if successful γδ TCR expression blocked the rearrangement of the α and β loci. In another study of early αβ precursor thymocytes, it was found that in half of the cells, TCRδ had not rearranged at all, but the TEA transcript was being expressed (154), presumably just prior to Vα → Jα rearrangement. In mice that are defective in either αβ TCR or γδ TCR, there is no obvious effect on the development of the remaining lineage (155–157). Taken together, almost all of the data in the literature favor a separate lineage model, not sequential rearrangement.

Other Genetic Mechanisms

One important mechanism of antibody diversification that has not been reproducibly found in *TCR* genes is somatic hypermutation. In antibodies, this form of mutation typically raises the affinities of antigen-specific Ig several orders of magnitude, typically from the micromolar range (10^{-6}M) to the nanomolar (10^{-9}M) for protein antigens. We now know that most cell surface receptors that bind ligands on other cell surfaces, including TCRs', typically have affinities in the micromolar range, but they compensate for this relatively low affinity by engaging multiple receptors simultaneously (e.g., increasing the valency) and by functioning in a confined, largely two-dimensional volume (e.g., between two cells). Cells employing such receptors most likely require weak (but highly specific) interactions so that they can disengage quickly (158,159). The rapid off-rate seen with TCRs has even been postulated to amplify the effects of small numbers of ligands (i.e., the serial engagement model; see below).

There has also been no enduring evidence for a naturally secreted form of either an αβ or γδ TCR. Here again it can be argued that such a molecule would have no obvious function, as it is too low in affinity to be very useful. In the case of most TCRs, the concentration of protein would have to be very high (in the milligram per milliliter range) to achieve an effect similar to serum antibodies.

A third mechanism seen in antibodies but not in TCRs is C_H switching, which allows different Ig isotypes to maintain a given V-region specificity and associate it with different C regions, which have different properties in solution (e.g., complement fixation, basophil binding, etc.). As there is no secreted form of the TCR, it is not obvious how this would be useful.

BIOCHEMISTRY OF αβ TCR–LIGAND INTERACTIONS

Although it has long been established that T cells recognize a peptide in association with an MHC molecule, a formal biochemical demonstration that this was due to TCR binding to a peptide–MHC complex has only been possible in the last few years. Part of the difficulty in obtaining measurements of this type has been the intrinsically membrane-bound nature of MHC and TCR molecules. Another major problem is that the affinities are relatively low, with K_{ds} of 10^{-4} to 10^{-7} M, too unstable to measure by conventional means (see Fig. 7).

The problem of normally membrane-bound molecules can be circumvented by expressing soluble forms of TCR and MHC, which is also essential for structural studies (see above). For TCR, it has been solved in a variety of ways, including replacing the transmembrane regions with signal sequences for glycolipid linkage (160) expressing chains without transmembrane regions in either insect or mammalian cells (43,161), or a combination of cysteine mutagenesis and *E. coli* expression (48) has worked well. Unfortunately, no one method seems to work for all TCR heterodimers. The production of soluble forms of MHC molecule has a much longer history, starting with the enzymatic cleavage of detergent-solubilized native molecules (162) as well as some of the same methods employed for TCR, such as gpi linkage (163), *E. coli* expression and refolding (164,165), and insect cell expression of truncated molecules (166,167). One interesting variant that seems necessary for the stable expression of some class II MHC molecules in insect cells has been the addition of a covalent peptide to the N-terminus of the β chain (168).

The first measurements of TCR affinities for peptide–MHC complexes were made by Matsui et al. (169) and Weber et al. (170). Matsui and colleagues used a high concentration of soluble peptide—MHC to block the binding of a labeled anti-TCR Fab fragment to T cells specific for those complexes, obtaining a K_d value of approximately 50 μM for several different T cells and two different cytochrome peptide–I-E^k complexes (as shown in Table 1). Weber and colleagues used a soluble TCR to inhibit the recognition of a flu peptide–I-E^d complex by a T cell and obtained a K_D value of approximately 10 μM. Later experiments, using the antibody competition approach, obtained a significantly higher affinity (K_D of 0.1 μM) in an alloreactive peptide–class I MHC system (171). It may be significant that in this last system, the alloreactive peptide disassociates rapidly from the class I molecule (L^d), perhaps selecting for a higher than usual affinity TCR. While these measurements represent an important start in TCR biochemistry, they could

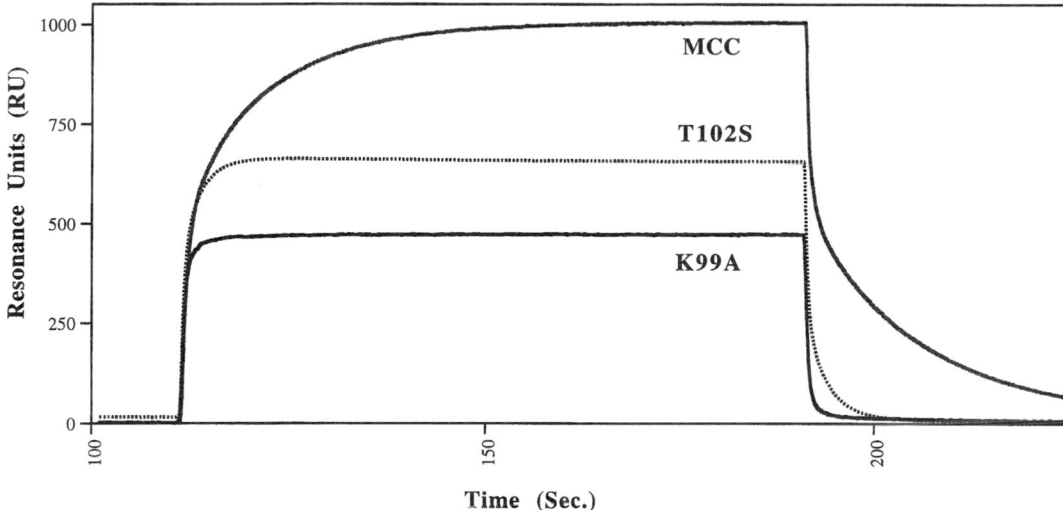

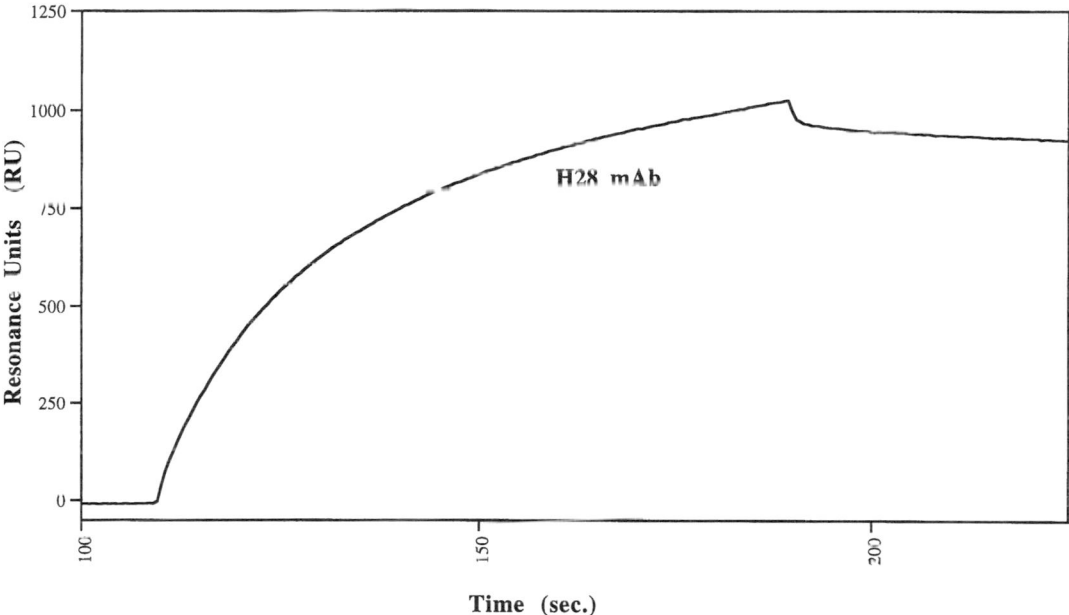

FIG. 7. TCR binding to peptide–MHC complexes. The upper profile shows a typical surface plasmon resonance analysis of the binding characteristics of a TCR specific for a cytochrome-c peptide bound to the mouse class II MHC molecule, I-EK. Here the soluble TCR is fixed to a solid support and different peptide–MHC complexes are passed over it in solution. The most robust profile represents the original peptide MCC (88–103) complexes to I-EK, a strong agonist, whereas T102s represents a weak agonist, K99, a null peptide (see also Tables 1 and 2). These profiles are compared to the lower trace in the illustration, which shows an antibody specific for Cα binding to the same TCR. Note the sharper initial phase, which is a measure of the association rate, and the very stable decay phase, which is a measure of the dissociation rate. The x-axis is the time in seconds, and the y-axis is in arbitrary resonance units. (Courtesy of D. S. Lyons.)

give no direct information about the kinetics of TCR–ligand interactions (although indirect measurements were reported in ref. 171). Fortunately, the development of surface plasmon resonance instruments, particularly the BIAcore (Pharmacia Biosensor Up alla, Sweden), with its remarkable sensitivity to weak macromolecular interactions (172), has allowed rapid progress in this area. With this technique, one component is covalently cross-linked to a surface, and then buffer containing the ligand is passed in solution over it. The binding of even approximately 5% of the surface-bound material is sufficient to cause a detectable change in the resonance state of gold electrons on the surface. This method allows the direct measurement of association and dissociation rates (i.e., kinetic parameters) and also has the advantage of being completely cell-free. Figure 7 shows the type of resonance profile obtained, con

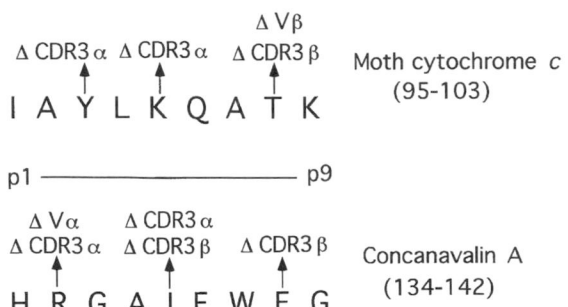

FIG. 8. Sensitivity of TCR CDR3 sequences and Vα/Vβ usage to changes in the antigen peptide. Here we summarize the data of Jorgensen et al. (199,200) and Sant'Angelo et al. (201), who immunized single-chain transgenic mice (TCRα or TCRβ) with antigenic peptides (MCC or CVA) altered at residues that influence T-cell recognition but not MHC binding. These data show that such changes invariably affect the CDR3 sequences of Vα or Vβ, or both, and that there appears to be a definite topology in which Vα governs the N-terminal region and Vβ seems more responsible for the C-terminal portion of the peptide.

trasting the weak but specific binding of a particular peptide–MHC complex in solution to a bound JCR with the binding pattern of an antibody to the same TCR. The affinity of cytochrome c/I-E^K/2B4 TCR measured with this instrument (173) matches very closely (see Table 2) with previous results obtained from cell-based measurements, definitively showing that TCR and peptide-loaded MHC molecules alone are sufficient for this interaction and also that expression in a soluble form has not altered the ability of these molecules to bind to each other. In addition to confirming some of the previous affinity measurements (174–178), the surface plasmon resonance technique has thus far been the method of choice for measuring the kinetics of TCR binding to its ligands (excepting the very highest affinity TCRs; see ref. 179). As shown in Table 2,

these measurements show that while the on-rates of TCRs binding to peptide–MHC molecules vary from very slow (1,000 M sec) to moderately fast (200,000 M sec), their off-rates fall in a relatively narrow range (0.5 to 0.01 sec^{-1}) or a $t_{1/2}$ of 1 to 60 seconds at 25°C, similar to other membrane-bound receptors that recognize membrane molecules on other cells (158,159). In the case of the class I MHC restricted TCR, 2C, this relatively fast off-rate is significantly stabilized (tenfold) if soluble CD8 is introduced (180). This same effect of CD8 stabilization had previously been seen by Renard et al. (181) in their unique cell-based TCR labeling assay. Similar BIAcore experiments using soluble CD4 have not produced comparable results (J. Hampl and J. Boniface, unpublished results), but it is always possible that there is some deficiency in the recombinant molecule compared to the native form on the cell surface. While all of the BIAcore measurements cited above were performed at 25°C due to instrument limitations, the off-rates are likely to be much faster (10 to 20 times) at 37°C (J. Boniface and Z. Reich, personal communication and ref. 181).

To what extent are we now able to predict a T-cell response based on the binding characteristic of its TCR to a ligand? One of the most intriguing discoveries concerning T-cell reactivity in recent years has been the phenomenon of altered peptide ligands. These are single amino acid variants of antigenic peptides which either change the nature or degree of the T-cell response (partial agonists) or prevent a response to a normally stimulating ligand (antagonists) (182,183). Discussions concerning the mechanism of these altered peptide responses have centered around whether they are due to some conformational phenomenon involving TCRs and/or CD3 molecules or to affinity or kinetic characteristics. With the data in hand, we can now say that most, but not all, T-cell responses correlate very well with the binding characteristics of their TCRs. In particular, Sykulev et al. (171) first noted that higher affinity peptide variants elicited more robust T-cell responses. Subsequently, Matsui et al. (173) found that in a series of three agonist peptides, increasing dissociation rates correlated with decreasing agonist

TABLE 2. *T-cell receptor–ligand binding*

	Ligand	K_D (μM)	k_{on} (M^{-1}s^{-1})	k_{off}(s^{-1})	Method	Ref.
T$_H$ cells						
5C.C7	MCC/E^k	50	—	—	anti-TCR comp.	Matsui et al. (169)
2B4	MCC/E^k	50	—	—	anti-TCR comp.	Matsui et al. (169)
2B4	MCC/E^k	30	—	—	anti-P/MHC comp.	Matsui et al. (173)
2B4	MCC/E^k	90	600	0.057	BIA1	Matsui et al. (173)
228.5	MCC 99E/E^k	50	—	—	anti-TCR comp.	Matsui et al. (169)
14.3.d	Flu H1N1/E^d	~10	—	—	sol. TCR	Weber et al. (170)
14.3.d	SEC1,2,3	5.4–18.2	>100,000	>0.1	BIA1	Malchiodi et al. (244)
HA1.7	HA/DR1	>25	—	—	BIA1	Seth et al. (175)
HA1.7	SEB	0.82	13,000	0.001	BIA1	Seth et al. (175)
T$_C$ cell						
2C	p2Ca/L^d	0.5	11,000	0.0055	anti-TCR comp.	Sykulev et al. (171)
2C	p2Ca/L^d	0.1	21,0000	0.026	BIA1	Corr et al. (174)
2C	QL9/L^d	0.065	53,000	0.003	Labeled MHC	Sykulev et al. (179)
4G3	pOV/L^b	0.65	22,000	0.02	Labeled MHC	Sykulev et al. (179)
42.12	OVA/K^b	6.5	3,135	0.02	BIA4	Alam et al. (176)
2C	p2Ca/L^d	3.3	8,300	0.027	BIA1	Garcia et al. (180)
HY	M80/D^b	23.4	6,200	0.145	BIA1	Garcia et al. (180)
HY	CD8 α/β + M80/D/^b	2.0	5,100	0.01	BIA1	Garcia et al. (180)
2C	CD8 α/β + p2Ca/L^d	0.32	1,2000	0.0038	BIA1	Garcia et al. (180)

Note: BIA1 = TCR amine coupled, BIA2 = TCR cysteine coupled, BIA3 = MHC–peptide amine coupled in competition experiment, and BIA4 = TCR coupled using H57 antibody and MHC coupled via amine chemistry.

activity. Lyons et al. (178) found that this correlation extended to antagonist peptides in the same antigen system (moth cytochrome c/E^k). They also showed that while an antagonist peptide might differ only slightly in affinity compared with the weakest agonist, its dissociation rate differed by tenfold or more (see Table 3). This data in a class II MHC restricted system is largely supported by the studies of Alam et al. in a class I MHC system (176), who also see a drop-off in affinities and an increase in off-rates (with one exception, as noted in Table 3) with antagonist versus agonist ligands. Interestingly, Al-Ramadi et al. (177) also saw one outlier in a set of related peptide–MHC ligands, suggesting that other factors (such as TCR/CD3 conformation) may also contribute agonist or antagonist affects. In the cell-based TCR labeling system of Kessler et al., a survey of related peptide ligands of varying potency also found a general, but not absolute, correlation between receptor occupancy and stimulatory ability (184). Thus, while there is a general trend toward weaker T-cell responses and faster off-rates and lower affinities, this does not seem to be an absolute rule, and thus other factors such as conformation may be important in some cases.

How might the relatively small differences in the binding characteristics of the ligands summarized in Tables 2 and 3 cause such different T cell–signaling outcomes as agonism or antagonism? As McKeithan (185) and Rabinowitz et al. (186) have noted, any multistep system such as T-cell recognition has an inherent ability to amplify small differences in signals that are received on the cell surface to much larger differences at the end of the pathway, in this case, gene transcription in the nucleus. Thus, antagonism may occur at one threshold and an agonist response at another. Alternatively, an antagonist ligand may traverse the activation pathway just far enough to use up some critical substrate, as proposed by Lyons et al. (178). Yet another possibility that has also been suggested is that some antagonists may act even earlier, by blocking TCR clustering at the cell surface (48).

Another controversy bearing on this data is the serial engagement model of Lanzavecchia and colleagues (187,188), which proposes that one way in which a small number of peptide–MHC complexes can initiate T-cell activation is by transiently binding many TCRs in a sequential fashion. Estimates based on TCR downregulation have suggested that one peptide–MHC complex could bind to as many as 200 TCR molecules in succession (187). While the dissociation rates reviewed here show that TCR binding is likely to be very transient, they do not, in fact, support the statement that more interactions are better. This is because, thus far, all improvements in TCR–peptide–MHC stability within any one system result in a more robust T-cell response rather than exhibiting a normal distribution around some optimum value.

Role of CD4 and CD8

What is the role of CD4 and CD8 with respect to the T-cell response to agonist and antagonist peptides? In the case of a T helper cell response, the presence of CD4 greatly augments the amount of cytokine produced and, in some cases, determines whether there is a response at all (as reviewed in ref. 189). Much of the effect of CD4 seems to come from the recruitment of lck to the TCR/CD3 complexes. In addition, there is also a significant positive effect, even with CD4 molecules that are unable to bind lck, and thus there appears to be an affect on TCR–ligand interaction as well. CD8 also greatly augments the response of class I MHC–specific T cells (183), and, as discussed above, CD8 stabilizes TCR–peptide–MHC complexes by approximately tenfold (see Table 2). Overall, it seems likely that each of these coreceptor molecules has two roles: to stabilize TCR–ligand interactions physically and to aid in signaling by recruiting lck. Consistent with this are data showing that the presence of CD4 can convert an antagonist peptide into a weak agonist (190,191). Data in the cytochrome system by Hampl et al. (192) puts a new twist on this by showing that while weak agonist peptides are made almost as potent as the best peptides by the presence of CD4, little or no effect is seen on antagonism.

These results suggest that CD4 engagement is not automatic and simultaneous with TCR binding, but instead is recruited later into preexisting TCR–peptide–MHC complexes (or oligomers), as suggested by Madrenas et al. (193,194). In some cases, antagonist–MHC complexes will be stable long enough for CD4 to have an effect, in which case the T cell could be stimulated, but in the antagonism experiments of Hampl et al. the TCR–ligand association does not last long enough for CD4 to affect the outcome.

TABLE 3. *Weak agonist–antagonist binding*

T cell	Ligand	Type	K_D (μM)	k_off (s⁻¹)	t_1/2	Method	Ref.
2B4	MCC/E^k	Strong agonist	90	0.057	12	BIA 1	Matsui et al. (173)
			40	0.063	11	BIA 2	Lyons et al. (178)
2B4	PCC/E^k	Agonist	80	0.09	8.0	BIA 1	Matsui et al. (173)
2B4	MCC 102S/E^k	Weak agonist	240	0.36	2.0	BIA 2	Lyons et al. (178)
2B4	MCC 102N/E^k	Weak agonist	320	0.44	1.6	BIA 2	Lyons et al. (178)
2B4	MCC 99R/E^k	Antagonist	500	4.8	0.15	BIA 2	Lyons et al. (178)
			330	—	—	BIA 3	
2B4	MCC 102G/E^k	Antagonist	1500	5.1	0.14	BIA 2	Lyons et al. (178)
			900–1200	—	—	BIA 3	
2B4	MCC 99Q/E^k	Weak antagonist	2100	—	—	BIA 3	Lyons et al. (178)
42.12	OVA/K^b	Strong agonist	6.5	0.02	24.5	BIA 4	Alam et al. (176)
42.12	OVA E1/K^b	Weak agonist	22.6	0.068	7.3	BIA 4	Alam et al. (176)
42.12	V-OVA/K^b	Antagonist	29.8	0.030	12.9	BIA 4	Alam et al. (176)
42.12	OVA R4/K^b	Antagonist	57.1	0.146	3.4	BIA 4	Alam et al. (176)
42.12	OVA K4/K^b	Null	>360	>0.2	<2.5	BIA 4	Alam et al. (176)

See Table 2 for explanation of BIAcore methods.

TOPOLOGY OF TCR–PEPTIDE–MHC INTERACTIONS

An analysis of TCR sequence diversity has shown that the vast majority of amino acid variation resides in the region between the V- and J-region gene segments, which corresponds to the CDR3 regions of antibodies (195). This has led to models in which the CDR3 loops of Vα and Vβ make the principal contacts with the antigenic peptide bound to the MHC (38,195,196). Support for such a model has come from many studies in which it has been shown that the CDR3 sequences of TCRs are important predictors of specificity (as reviewed in ref. 195), as well as from the elegant mutagenesis studies of Engel and Hedrick (197) and Katayama et al. (198), who showed that a single CDR3 point mutation could alter the specificity of a TCR (197) and also that a CDR3 transplant could confer the specificity of the donor TCR onto the recipient (198). In addition, a new approach to TCR–ligand interactions was developed by Jorgensen et al. (199,200), who made single amino acid changes at positions that affect T-cell recognition but not MHC binding in a given peptide. These variant peptides are then used to immunize mice that express either the α or β chain of a TCR that recognizes the original peptide, and the responding T cells are analyzed. Using mice transgenic for a single TCR α or β allows the resulting T cells to keep one half of the receptor constant, while allowing considerable variation in the chain that pairs with it. The results from this study and work in another system by Sant'Angelo et al. (201) are very similar in that every mutation at a TCR-sensitive residue triggered a change in the CD3 sequence of Vα, Vβ, or both, and in some cases changed the Vα or Vβ gene segment as well (as summarized in Fig. 8). One of the more striking examples of a CDR3–peptide interaction occurred

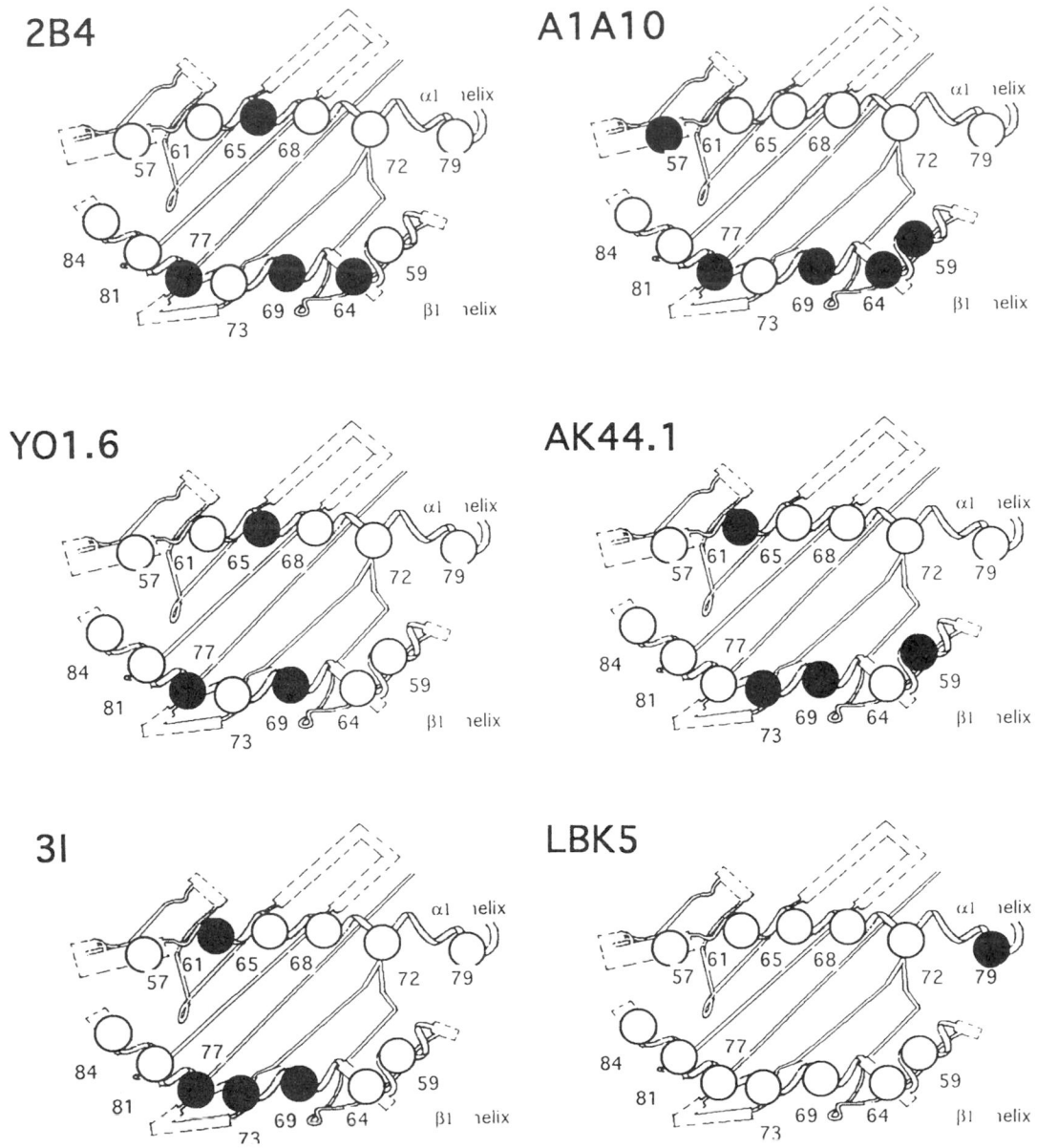

FIG. 9. A γδ TCR does not recognize the same epitope as αγ TCRs. Shown here are the effects of a panel of mutation located on the α helices of the I-EK molecule on T-cell recognition. Inhibition of recognition is denoted by a filled circle. The one γδ T cell in this survey, LBK5, does not recognize a part of the central peptide-binding groove. This is also consistent with its indifference to which peptides occupy this site (see text). (From ref. 277.)

in the cytochrome *c* system, where a Lys→Glu change in the central TCR determinant on the peptide triggered a Glu→Lys charge reversal in the Vα CDR3 loop, arguing for a direct Lys→Glu contact between the two molecules (199).

Another interesting finding was the order of Vα→Vβ preference going from the N-terminal to the C-terminal residues of the peptides. This led Jorgensen et al. (199,200) to propose a "linear" topology of TCR–peptide–MHC interaction in which the CDR3 loops of Vα and Vβ line up directly over the peptide. Sant'Angelo et al. (201) proposed an orientation of the TCR in which the CDR3 loops are perpendicular to the peptide. This was partially based on intriguing data suggesting an interaction between the CDR1 of Vα and an N-terminal residue of the peptide. A third orientation was proposed by Sun et al. (202) based on the analysis of a large number of class I MHC mutants and their effect on TCR reactivity. This produced a roughly diagonal footprint of TCRs over the MHC, compared to the two previous models. On the other hand, an extensive class II MHC mutagenesis study failed to reveal a consistent "footprint" of TCR interaction, and it furthermore found that the pattern of TCR sensitivity was remarkably labile and highly dependent on sequences in the TCR CDR3 region or the peptide (203).

This controversy has begun to be resolved by the work of Garcia et al. (43) and Garboczi et al. (45), who, nearly simultaneously, solved the crystal structures of two different TCR–peptide–class I MHC complexes. These studies show a TCR binding surface much like an antibody fitting down between the two opposite "high points" of the class I MHC α helices, in a roughly diagonal configuration. In these structures, one of which is shown in Colorplate 2, the CDR3 loops are centrally located over the peptide, but the Vα CDR1 and the Vβ CDR1 are also in a position to contact the N-terminal and C-terminal peptide residues, respectively. Such a contact between Vα CDR1 and an N-terminal residue was seen in the Garboczi structure, while that of Garcia et al. has insufficient resolution at this point. While more structures are needed, especially TCRs complexed to class II MHC-peptides, the results are sufficiently consistent with the results of the peptide-immunization and mutation experiments cited previously to indicate that all TCR–peptide–MHC complexes will have roughly the same topology. A new mutagenesis–modeling study also arrives at this same orientation (204). This oriented recognition constitutes a major departure from antibody–antigen interactions and may derive from the need to intercalate CD4/CD8 molecules during activation. The structure of a class I MHC–CD8 complex is a first step in understanding how this might be accomplished (205).

αβ TCR AND SUPERANTIGENS

One of the most interesting and unexpected areas to emerge from the study of αβ T-cell reactivities is the discovery of superantigens. Whereas a particular antigenic peptide might only be recognized by one in 100,000 or fewer T cells in a naive organism, a given superantigen might stimulate 1% to 20% of the T cells (as reviewed in refs. 206–208). As will be discussed in more detail below, the physical basis for this is that the superantigen binds to a Vβ domain of the TCR on T cells while simultaneously binding to an MHC class II molecule on an antigen-presenting cell (although not in the peptide-binding groove). This allows a single superantigen, such as SEA in Table 4, to stimulate virtually every murine T cell-bearing Vβ 1, 3, 10, 11, 12, or 17 (approximately 15% of all αβ T cells), regardless of which Vα it is paired with or which CDR3 sequence is expressed. Clearly, this is a unique class of T cell–stimulatory molecule.

The first indication of a superantigen effect was the discovery by Kappler and colleagues (209,210) of a mouse strain–specific deletion of T cells expressing a specific Vβ, which showed that this affect was due to certain alleles of the minor histocompability loci, known as Mls, whose products had the ability to stimulate specific Vβ-bearing T cells and caused the elimination of those T cells in mouse strains that carried that particular allele (211–214). Intensive efforts to clone these loci revealed that they were endogenous retroviruses of the mouse mammary tumor virus family (215–218) and that various family members bind different Vβ domains (as shown in Table 4). Meanwhile, Janeway and colleagues (220) showed that staphylococcal enterotoxins could polyclonally activate naive T cells in a Vβ-specific manner without a requirement for antigen processing. Many of these enterotoxins have been characterized extensively (221–227). Unlike the MMTV proteins, which are type II membrane proteins, the enterotoxins are secreted. Subsequently, proteins having superantigenic properties have been isolated from other bacteria [*Yersinia pseudotuberculosis* (228,229), *Streptococcus* (230), and *Mycoplasma* (231,232)]. There is also evidence of superantigen-like activities in other mammalian viruses, such as rabies (233), Epstein Barr virus (234), cytomegalovirus (235), and also in the parasites malaria falciparum (236) and *Toxoplasma gondii* (237), but the actual molecules have not been identified. Since so many pathogenic or parasitic organisms possess these molecules, apparently by convergent evolution, there must be some selective advantage, but in most cases, there is no conclusive evidence as to what this might be. The one exception is the case of MMTV superantigens, in which it has been shown that polyclonal T-cell stimulation allows the virus to much more efficiently infect the B-lymphocytes that are activated by the T cells (238–239). This may be a special case, however, and most authors have suggested that superantigens primarily serve to confuse and occupy the immune system, while the pathogen escapes specific targeting and elimination. Large doses of superantigens have also been implicated in various "shock" syndromes, such as food poisoning or toxic shock (206–208), but this is probably not their everyday purpose, as it would violate the general rule that the host and parasite should coexist.

It has also been suggested that superantigens might be involved in triggering autoimmune diseases. Here, the hypothesis is that a large number of some Vβ-bearing T cells are activated by a pathogenic superantigen and that subsequently self-reactive T cells within those activated cells are stimulated by a particular tissue antigen. While a superantigen-like predominance of particular Vβ-bearing cells has been reported in rheumatoid arthritis (240) and Kawasaki's disease (241), other investigators have not been able to confirm these reports (242). However, there has been a report of a human superantigen that, like the Mls loci, is an endogenous retrovirus that specifically stimulates Vβ7 T cells and is expressed during islet-cell infiltration in the early stages of type I diabetes (243)

While the biochemistry of superantigen binding to TCR and MHC is similar to that of TCR–peptide–MHC interactions (177,244), the topology is quite different. In particular, it has been found that Mls-1a presentation to T cells is most affected by mutations on the "outside" surface of the Vβ domain (amino acids 22, 70, 71), which do not affect peptide–MHC recognition (245,246). In contrast, CDR grafting experiments by Patten and colleagues (247) have implicated CDR1 and CDR2 of Vβ3 in bacterial superantigen reactivity. Similarly, other investigators have found differences in the way different superantigens bind to the same TCRs, but none have found any involvement of CDR3 sequences.

TABLE 4. *Vβ specificity of exogenous and endogenous superantigens*

Bacterial superantigen	Human Vβ specificity	Ref.	Murine Vβ specificity	Ref.
SEA	ND		1, 3, 10, 11, 12, 17	222, 223
SEB	3, 12, 14, 15, 17, 20	167, 168	(3), 7, 8.1, 8.3, (11), (17)	222, 226, 227
SEC$_1$	12	167	7, 8.2, 8.3, 11	222
SEC$_2$	12, 13, 14, 15, 17, 20	167, 168	8.2, 10	222
SEC$_3$	5, 12	167	(3), 7, 8.2	222
SED	5, 12	167	3, 7, (8.2), 8.3, 11, 17	222
SEE	5.1, 6.1–6.3, 8, 18	167, 168	11, 15, 17	222
TSST-1	2	167	15, 16	222
ExFT	2	168	10, 11, 15	222
Strep M	2, 4, 8	230	ND	

Endogenous proviruses	Vβ specificity	Mls type[a]	Chromosome	Ref.
Mtv-1	3	c, 4a	7	As reviewed in 207, 208
Mtv-2	14	NA	18	
Mtv-3	3, 17	c	11	
Mtv-6	3, 17	c, 3a	16	
Mtv-7	6, 7, 8.1, 9	a, 1a	1	
Mtv-8	11, 12	f, Dvbll.1	6	
Mtv-9	5, 11, 12	f, Etc-1,	12	
Mtv-11	11, 12	f, Dvbll.3	14	
Mtv-13	3	c, 2a	4	
Mtv-43	6, 7, 8.1, 9	Mls-like	ND	

Exogenous viruses	Vβ specificity	Mls type		Ref.
MMTV-C3H	14, 15	NA		216, 217
MMTV-SW	6, 7, 8.1, 9	Mls-like		221
Rabies			Suspected	233
EBV			Suspected	234
CMV			Suspected	235

Other Pathogens	Vβ specificity	Name		Ref.
Mycoplasma	h17, 6, 8.1, 8.3	MAM		231, 232
Toxoplasma gondii			Suspected	237
Malaria falciparum			Suspected	236

Vβ in parentheses are reactive with commercial but not recombinant enterotoxins (197).
NA, not applicable; ND, not determined.
[a]The nomenclature in use prior to the discovery that the phenotype was due to endogenous retroviruses.

The x-ray crystal structures of the superantigens SEC2 and SEC3, complexed with a mouse TCRβ chain, have been reported (248). Similar to the data of Patten et al. (247), these bacterial superantigens bind to CDR1 and CDR2 and somewhat to the outside of the Vβ domain. As shown in Colorplate 3, when modeled on the superantigen–MHC structures, the resulting TCR/SAg/MHC complex would displace the TCR somewhat (but not entirely) away from the MHC-binding groove (248), thus making the interaction largely insensitive to the TCR–peptide specificity, as suggested by Jorgensen et al. (200). Since this is only the first report of the structure of TCR/SAg complex, it is entirely possible that other molecules will interact differently. In particular, because the Mls antigens are structurally very different than the bacterial SAgs and in their mode of MHC binding, their mode of binding to Vβ domains is likely to be unique as well.

Why do superantigens interact only with the β chain? One possibility is that the β chain offers the only accessible "face" of the TCR, perhaps because CD4 blocks the Vα side (as suggested by antibody blocking studies). A second more exotic possibility is that superantigens have usurped a physiologically important mechanism for T-cell activation that is used only rarely. For example,

immature thymocytes express only low levels of the TCR and yet are remarkably sensitive to antigen. Perhaps there exists a cellular protein that links the TCR β-chain with an MHC molecule as an adjunct to normal binding and recognition (249).

A SECOND TYPE OF RECEPTOR: γδ-CD3

Identification of γδ T cells

Although αβ T cells were originally defined on the basis of functional characteristics, such as providing T-cell "help" or initiating cytotoxicity, γδ TCR–bearing cells were not discovered through any cellular assay or by serologic analysis, but instead were identified through gene cloning. Thus, most work on these cells has been devoted to the understanding of what they recognize and how they function within the immune system. While there has been substantial progress, these questions are still largely unresolved. We will review here some of the salient characteristics of these enigmatic cells.

γδ T cells are the first to appear in the fetal thymus fully 2 days before αβ T cells in the mouse, but in later weeks, αβ T cells quickly predominate. In both mouse and human adults, γδ T cells represent only a small fraction of thymocytes (250,251), and lymphocytes in all of the secondary lymphoid organs. However, they are found in larger numbers in the mucous membranes of a variety of tissues, such as the skin (252), small intestine (253), female reproductive tract (254), and lung (255).

One population of γδ T cells that has been studied intensively is the CD4⁻CD8⁻γδT-lymphocytes that have a dendritic morphology and are embedded in the epidermis of the skin, (252,256). These cells have been termed *dendritic epidermal cells* (DECs). Curiously, 90% of these cells express a TCR with identical Vγ and Vδ sequences (256). This has now been shown to result from the fact that most DECs are generated during days 15 to 17 of fetal life (119). At this stage in development, there is a preference for Vγ3 rearrangement and little or no terminal deoxynucleotidyl transferase expressed; consequently, N-region diversity is absent. In addition, the mechanism of gene rearrangement has been shown to be biased by nucleotide homologies between the end of the V region and the beginning (in this case) of the J region (257). Thus one could argue for a limited repertoire of γδ sequences at this stage, but to have so many identical ones so reproducibly indicates that there is either some additional recombinational mechanism other than those cited or a strong selection for this particular outcome.

As to what these DECs "see," experiments have shown that they can respond to mouse keratinocytes or to an extract of keratinocytes added directly to the DECs (258). The nature of the determinant recognized is presently unknown. Other intraepithelial lymphocytes (IELs) show distinct receptor expression as well. The γδ T cells found in the female reproductive epithelia and in the tongues of mice preferentially express Vγ4 and Vδ1 (254). In the BALB/c strain of mice, most of the TCRδ sequences are the same (259) but others are diverse. This phenomenon has not been seen in other strains.

Another population of γδ T cells that has been studied extensively is resident in the epithelium of the small intestine (253). The gut IELs consist of a population of αβ T cells and a population of γδ T cells. The function of these intestinal IELs is presently unknown. They are phenotypically CD4⁻CD8⁻ or CD4⁻CD8⁺, Unlike CD8⁺ αβ T cells, the CD8 molecules on γδ IELs express CD8 α chain but no CD8 β (260,261). IEL γδ TCRs use different Vγ and Vδ, and the CDR3 regions of both the γ and δ chains show significant diversity in both length and sequence, suggesting that they can "see" a wide variety of ligands.

What is the origin of this correlation between γδ TCR expression and anatomically different epithelia, and does it reflect an immune function? Is it the result of unique homing processes, or does it reveal some aspect of ontogeny? No concrete answers to these questions are yet at hand.

γδ T Cells Contribute to Host Immune Defense Differently Than αβ T Cells

Earlier studies showed that γδ T cells can secrete a variety of lymphokines and mount cytolytic responses, and therefore have the potential to function like αβ T cells. Their preferential localization in the epithelium also suggested that they may be responsible for a "first line of defense" (reviewed in ref. 262). This hypothesis is supported by the increase of γδ T-lymphocytes, seen early in infections, by some bacteria and a virulent Sendai virus strain, before αβ T-cell responses are observed (263,264). However, in other infection models, γδ T cells accumulate within the inflammatory

lesions late in the infection, after the virus have been cleared (reviewed in ref. 265), suggesting that they may be responding to cells that are damaged and/or stressed by the infection. Consistent with this is the demonstration that some γδ T cells can kill virus-infected cells *in vitro* but that the recognition is not virus-specific (266).

More recently, mice deficient in αβ or γδ T cells have been used to dissect the roles of these cells in the immune defense against intracellular pathogens (bacteria, protozoa, and viruses) (267–270). These T-cell deficiencies were induced by either the administration of an mAb against αβ or γδ T-lymphocytes or by disruption of a TCR gene through homologous recombination. It was found that the role(s) γδ T cells play is dependent on the types of infection. In models such as BCG and *Salmonella* infections, αβ but not γδ T cells are essential in controlling the infection. In other cases, such as in *M. tuberculosis* and *Listeria monocytogenes,* γδ T cells are able to compensate for the absence of αβ T cells. Interestingly, in *Listeria* and *Vermiformis* infections, a lack of γδ T cells does not change the pathogen load but results in a different pathology in the infected tissue (267–270). This has led to the suggestion that γδ T cells may somehow regulate immune and nonimmune cells to maintain host tissue integrity (271). This possibility is supported by data showing that certain γδ T cells can produce keratinocyte growth factor and chemokines (258) as well as regulate the development of epithelial cells (272) and influence αβ T-cell responses (273–276). It is also compatible with the analysis of γδ T-cell recognition requirements, in that these cells can mediate cellular immune functions without a requirement for antigen-processing and specialized antigen-presenting cells (reviewed in ref. 6). Therefore, they have the capacity to initiate immune responses by recognizing other lymphoid cells or damaged cells and/or tissues directly. While all of these experiments point to an unique role for γδ T cells in the immune system, γδ T-cell specificity and the exact effector functions of these cells in any pathologic situation remains undefined. It is interesting to note that the function of γδ T cells has mainly been studied in mouse and human, yet they are significantly more abundant in birds and artiodactyla (251,262). Thus, γδ T cells in these species may encompass other functions as well.

Antigen Recognition by γδ T Cells Does Not Require Processing

During the past few years, a number of studies have shown that γδ T cells have profound differences in their antigen-recognition requirements compared to αβ T cells. Some γδ T cells also seem to recognize entirely different types of antigens. More specifically, these experiments suggest that the antigens recognized by many γδ T cells do not have to be processed and presented and that they also do not have to be proteins (as reviewed in ref. 6).

Because most αβ T cells recognize protein antigens processed inside the cell and presented by MHC molecules, it was originally assumed that γδ T cells follow the same general pattern. Despite early work showing that classical MHC molecules are not involved in antigen recognition by γδ T cells, it was assumed that nonclassical MHC molecules, heat shock proteins, or as yet to be identified surface proteins might play a similar role.

During the past few years, the recognition requirements for γδ T cells have been evaluated in three model systems that allow a precise interpretation of the results. These are (a) the recognition of the mouse class II MHC molecules IE^k by the T cell clone LBK5

(277), (b) the recognition of the mouse nonclassical MHC class I molecules T10 and T22 by the T-cell clone G8 (277,278), and (c) the recognition of a herpes simplex virus glycoprotein, gI, by the T-cell clone TgI4.4 (279).

The IE^k-encoded protein has been shown to bind peptides, and the T10 and T22 molecules have been postulated to do so by virtue of the fact that they are homologous to classical MHC class I molecules. Furthermore, all three proteins listed above have the potential to be degraded into peptides and "presented" for recognition. Strikingly, in all three cases, neither peptides bound to these proteins, nor peptides derived from them, are recognized by the γδ T-cell clones. Instead, protein antigens are recognized directly without any requirement for antigen processing. An example of this is shown in Table 5, which shows the effect of temperature-sensitive endocytic compartment mutants on αβ T-cell recognition of a protein antigen versus the recognition of I-EK by LBK5 (277). Note that the endosomal mutants disrupt processing of cytochrome-c but have no effect on γδ T-cell recognition. In addition, epitope mapping with mutant IE molecules (Fig. 9) shows that amino acid residues in the α helices of the IEα and IEβ chains that affect data αβ T-cell recognition do not affect LBK5 stimulation (257).

Interestingly, T10 and the closely related T22 molecules (94% identity) were identified as the ligands of another γδ clone, KN6 (280,281). While G8 was generated by immunizing BALB/c nude mice with B10.BR spleen cells, KN6 was derived from double-negative C57BL/6 thymocytes. Thus, these nonclassical class I molecules can be considered "natural" ligands for γδ T cells. Not only does the primary structure of T10 and T22 indicate that they lack essential structural features that are important for peptide binding by classical MHC molecules (282), but results also show that T10 and β2 microglobulin expressed in *E. coli* are able to fold into stable complexes without exogenously added peptide. This folded material is fully functional in stimulating G8 (283). Thus, not only does G8 recognize T10 in the absence of peptide, but it also seems that T10 and T22 do not bind peptide.

γδ T Cells Can Be Stimulated by Nonpeptide Antigens

γδ T cells from healthy human peripheral blood and from patients with tuberculoid leprosy or rheumatoid arthritis were found to respond to heat-killed mycobacteria. The major T cell–stimulatory components in the former are not the mycobacterial heat shock proteins, but instead have been identified to be phosphate-containing, nonpeptide molecules (284–287). While the consensus is that "phosphate" is a necessary component, compounds identified from various laboratories with different mycobacteria-responsive clones

appear to be distinctive in their structures (Table 6). The nonphosphate moieties include unusual carbohydrate and phosphate moieties; a 5'-triphosphorylated thymidine or uridine substituted at its γ phosphate by an as yet to be characterized low-molecular-weight structure; isopentenyl pyrophosphate and related prenyl pyrophosphate derivatives, synthetic alkenyl and prenyl derivatives of phosphate, pyrophosphate; as well as γ-monoethyl derivatives of nucleoside and deoxynucleoside triphosphates (287). Although the relative biologic importance of these compounds remains to be determined, it is clear that a major class of stimulants are phosphate-containing nonpeptides. It is also clear that multiple phosphate-containing compounds are able to stimulate different clones with different efficacy.

An important finding is that all of these compounds can be found in both microbial and mammalian cells. Constant et al. (285) proposed that the mammalian TTP-X and UTP-X conjugate may be involved in a "salvage pathway" in DNA and RNA synthesis, and thus could be involved in a metabolic pathway related to DNA or RNA synthesis, such as cell proliferation. Such a molecule would fit with the "stress antigen" or "conserved primitive stimulus" expected for γδ T-cell ligands (262). Tanaka et al. (287) proposed that a link in the recognition of both microbial pathogens and hematopoietic tumor cells by these γδ T cells is provided by the common set of prenyl pyrophosphate intermediates, isopentenyl and related prenyl pyrophosphate derivatives. These compounds are present in normal mammalian cells as precursors in lipid metabolism for the synthesis of farnesyl pyrophosphate. In mammalian cells, the addition of farnesyl has been proposed to be a critical modification for the membrane association of the ras protein and is required for transforming activity. The observation that this γδ T-cell population accumulates in lesions caused by mycobacterial infections in humans (288,289) and is able to respond to virally and bacterially infected cells would suggest that these γδ cells respond to a class of antigens shared by a number of pathogens and transformed, damaged, or stressed cells.

Other Antigen Specificities of γδ T Cells

Even the earliest studies of γδ T-cell reactivities showed that classical MHC molecules are not the major ligands for these cells (251). While some have been found that can recognize either classical MHC or related molecules such as TL, Qa^d or CD1, the frequency of such clones derived from a mixed lymphocyte reaction is low—about 1 in 10^5—which is much lower than the frequency of αβ alloreactive generated in such reactions (1 in 10). In many cases, these γδ T cells also show a broad cross-reactivity that is not seen for most α<β alloreactive T cells, consistent with the suggestion that there is a fundamental difference between their recognition properties.

TABLE 5. *Effect of temperature-sensitive endocytic compartment mutants on αβ T-cell recognition of antigen versus recognition of I-E$_k$ by LBK-5*

	2B4 peptide (αβ)		2B4 protein (αβ)		A1A10 (αβ)		LBK5 (γδ)	
	34°C	39°C	34°C	39°C	34°C	39°C	34°C	39°C
IE^k-CHO	+++	++++	+++	++++	++	+++	++	+++
IE^k-G8.1 (end1)	+++	++++	++	0	+	0	++	+++
IE^k-25.2.2 (end2)	+++	++++	+++	+	+	0	++	+++
IE^k-G7.1 (end3)	+++	++++	++	0	+	0	++	+++

(From ref. 277.)

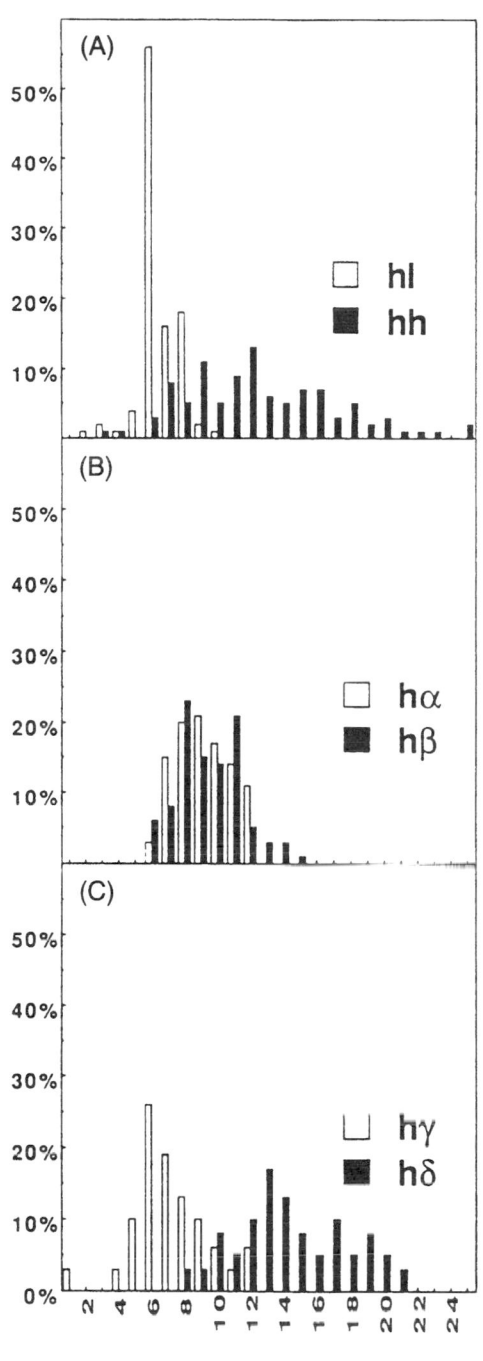

FIG. 10 A–C. CDR3 length distributions show that γδ TCRs are more antibody-like in character. These histograms show the distribution of CDR3 lengths in human antigen receptor genes, counting from the conserved cysteine in the C-terminus of the V region to the first conserved glycine in the J region (less two amino acids). (From ref. 295.)

There are also two reports in which the γδ T-cell recognition may involve a "complexed antigen" on cell surface: (a) a γδ T-cell hybridoma that responded to synthetic copolymer Glu-Tyr (GT) in the presence of stimulator cells expressing the Qa-1ʰ (but not the Qa-1ᵃ) molecule (290) and (b) a human γδ T-cell clone from the

synovial fluid of a patient with early rheumatoid arthritis responding to fragment C of tetanus toxin (TT) (291). The TT response requires the presence of cells expressing an MHC class II molecule, DRw53, and can be inhibited by an anti-DRw53 antibody. In these two cases, it is not clear whether the Glu–Tyr polymer and the TT are "processed" and if so, what kind of antigen processing is required. In addition to these specificities, γδ T cells that are responsive to mycobacterial 60-kDa heat shock protein and peptide derived from it (292), staphylococcal enterotoxin A (SEA) (293), and an Ig light chain–derived peptide in the context of the heat shock protein have also been reported (294).

CDR3 Length Distribution Analysis Shows That γδ TCRs Are More Immunoglobulin-like

In an effort to find a molecular basis for these surprising differences in γδ versus αβ T-cell recognition, Rock et al. (295) characterized the length distribution of CDR3 regions in three different immune receptor chains: Ig, αβ TCR, and γδ TCR as shown in Fig. 10. It was found that the CDR3 lengths of both α and β TCR polypeptides are nearly identical and have very constrained length distributions. In contrast, CDR3 lengths of Ig heavy chains are long and variable, while those of light chains are much shorter and more constrained. X-ray structural analysis has shown that CDR3 loops of the Ig are critical for antigen binding (36), and for the αβ TCRs, they appear to be particularly important in contacting the antigenic peptides bound to MHC molecules (45,197–201). The constraints on α and β CDR3 length may reflect this functional requirement. Surprisingly, δ chain CDR3 lengths are long and variable, but those of TCR γ chains are much shorter and constrained. In this respect, γδ TCR CDR3 length distributions are similar to those of Ig and distinct from those of αβ TCR. Thus, γδ TCRs as a group may be more "Ig-like" in their antigen-recognition properties.

In this context, the observations that the frequency of γδ T-cell clones recognizing allogeneic MHC molecules in a mixed lymphocyte reaction is very low (compared to αβ alloreactive clones) and that the majority of these clones show a high degree of cross-reactivity (seen only rarely with αβ alloreactive clones) (reviewed in ref. 6) are consistent with the proposal that γδ TCR recognition is more Ig-like, focusing on the common features shared by MHC molecules. It is noteworthy that the specificity of LBK5 (IEᵇ and IEᵏ, but not IEᵈ) is the same as two previously described anti-IE antibodies (296,297).

Along this line, human γδ T-cell clones from healthy donors that respond to mycobacteria extract have been found to express Vγ9 and Vδ2 with diverse junctional (CDR3) sequences (298). This is reminiscent of the Ig-receptor usage in naturally occurring mouse B cells that recognize phosphorylcholine. There, it was found that only very restricted Ig heavy- (VH11, VH12, or Q52) and light-chain V-gene segments are used, coupled with variable CDR3 junctional sequences (K. Seidl, Ph.D. thesis, Stanford University, 1995). In the later case, the restricted usage of the V genes may be more significant, because several hundred to a thousand VH-gene segments are available to mount an Ig response.

The suggestion that γδ TCR recognition is more Ig-like does not preclude the possibility that some γδ T cells may recognize similar or identical ligands as αβ T cells. It is clear, for example, that one can make antibodies that are specific for different subtypes of MHC molecules or even particular peptide–MHC complexes (299,300).

TABLE 6. *Nonpeptide mycobacterial antigens that stimulate human Vγ9Vδ2(Vγ2Vδ2) T cells[a]*

Name	Structure	Ref.
Phosphocarbohydrates	Unusual carbohydrates with terminal phosphorylation	Schoel et al. (284)
TUBag3	X-uridine 5'-triphosphate	J. J. Fournié, personal communication
TUBag4	X-thymidine 5'-triphosphate	Constant et al. (285)
Isopentenyl pyrophosphate	$CH_2=C(CH_3)CH_2CH_2=PP_i$	Tanaka et al. (287)

[a]All compounds have been isolated from myobacterial extracts and require some type of phosphorylation for stimulatory activity. The unknown structure "X", when phosphorylated, is the minimal active stimulatory component of the TUBag compounds. "X" is not a prenyl or alkenyl derivative (J. J. Fournié, personal communication).

As discussed earlier, by considering all elements that contribute to the variability of the junctional (CDR3) region, such as the numbers of D and J elements used, D-element reading frame, junctional diversity, and N-region nucleotide addition, it was calculated that the number of possible CDR3 sequences is greatest for γδ TCR, least for Ig (irrespective of somatic mutation), and intermediate for αβ TCR (195). This suggests that γδ T cells have the potential to recognize a wide variety of different antigens.

Mutivalence of Ligands Is Required for Activation

γδ TCR, as well as αβ TCR, needs to associate with CD3 molecules for cell surface expression. Therefore, signaling through the antigen receptor requires a multivalent form of the antigen so that the engaged receptors can be cross-linked. Cell surface molecules can be recognized as such, but soluble antigen must be rendered polyvalent. A demonstration of this requirement is that in the three cases of γδ T cells recognizing cell surface molecules—IE[k], T10/T22, and HSV gI protein—a soluble form of the protein can be recognized only when bound to plastic plates (e.g., presented in a multivalent form) (277–279). Interestingly, the stimulation of mycobacterial extract–reactive γδ T-cell clones by small phosphate-containing compounds requires cell–cell contact (see Fig. 4), and all cell types are able to induce the recognition (301,302).

The requirement for mutivalent antigens would then suggest that soluble antigens (such as the phosphate-containing compounds) must be associated with certain cell surface molecules for their recognition. It is important to know if the binding and display of soluble antigens is achieved by a variety of different molecules on the surface or by a limited set of molecules, and if they normally form part of the epitope recognized by the antigen receptors.

Although the recognition requirements discussed above are largely derived from observations with model systems, the identification of the mycobacterial antigen clearly stems from a "physiologically relevant" event. It will be interesting to determine the generality of these rules in other systems, especially pathologic ones. This should lead us to a much better definition of the role or roles of γδ T cells. This includes the identification of what γδ T cells recognize and what is the consequence of such recognition in pathologic situations.

The issue of γδ T-cell specificity is also important in the understanding of the development of these cells. While some experiments with γδ TCR transgenic mice suggest that they are both positively and negatively selected much the same way as αβ T cells, others show an entirely different mode of selection (303). Interestingly, the phosphate-containing compounds isolated from mycobacterial extracts can be found both in pathogens and in mammalian cells. Thus, they are "self" as well as "nonself". Yet γδ T cells with this specificity do not seem to have been eliminated from the normal repertoire

CDR3 DIVERSIFICATION: A GENERAL STRATEGY FOR TCR AND IMMUNOGLOBULIN COMPLEMENTARITY TO ANTIGENS?

One interesting observation that emerges from a detailed analysis of the gene rearrangements that create both TCR and Ig is how the diversity of the CDR3 loop region in one or both of the chains in a given TCR is so much greater than that available to the other CDRs. A schematic of this skewing of diversity for human Ig and for αβ and γδ TCR heterodimers is shown in Fig. 11. In the case of αβ TCRs, this concentration of diversity occurs in both Vα and Vβ CDR3 loops, and structural data (43,45) have confirmed that these loops sit largely over the center of the antigenic peptide (see previous section). While this concentration of diversity in αβ TCRs in the regions of principal contact with the many possible antigenic peptides seems reasonable, it is much harder to explain for Ig or γδ TCRs. Clearly, there must be some chemical or structural logic behind this phenomenon. A clue as to what this might be comes from the elegant studies of Cunningham and Wells (304) and Clackson and Wells (305), who systematically mutated all of the amino acids (to alanine) at the interface of human growth hormone and its receptor, as determined by x-ray crystallography. Interestingly, only one-fourth of the 30 or so mutations on either side had any effect on the binding affinity, even in cases in which the x-ray structural analysis showed that the amino acid side chains of most of the residues were buried in the other. These studies illustrate an important caveat to the interpretation of protein crystal structures— that while they are invaluable for identifying which amino acids could be important in a given interaction, they do not indicate which ones are the most important. This is presumably because the "fit" at many positions is not "exact" enough to add significant binding energy to the interaction. In this context, we (306) have proposed a new model, in which the principal antigen specificity of an Ig or TCR is derived from its most diverse CDR3 loops. In the case of antibodies, we imagine that most of the specific contacts with antigen are made by the V_H CDR3 and that the other CDRs provide opportunistic contacts that make, generally, only minor contributions to the energy of binding and specificity. Once antigen has been encountered and clonal selection activates a particular B cell, somatic mutation would then improve the binding of the CDR1s and CDR2s to convert the typically low-affinity antibodies to the higher affinity models, as observed by Berek and Milstein (307) and more recently by Patten et al. (308). This model suggests that even a single TCR or Ig V region in either a TCR or Ig locus might be able to accommodate most antigens, provided that full

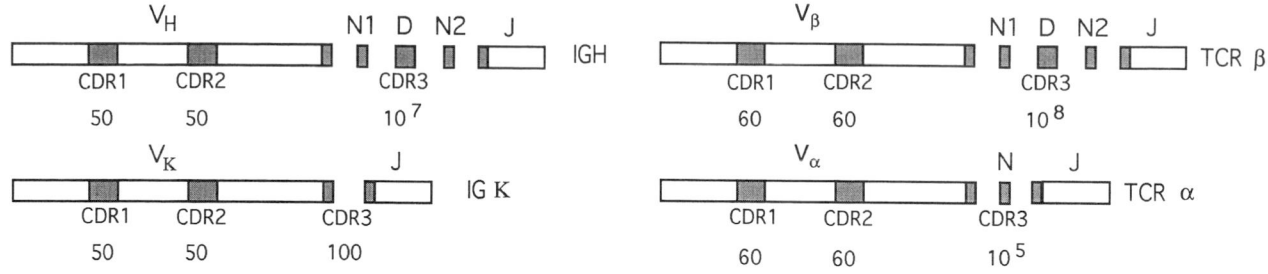

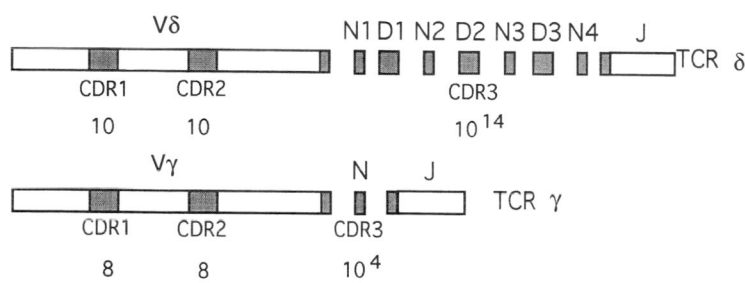

FIG. 11. Diversity "map" of immunoglobulin's and TCR's calculated potential for sequence diversity in human antigen receptor molecules. N-region addition is assumed to contribute zero to six nucleotides to the junction of each gene segment, excepting IgK chains, which seldom utilize this form of diversity. (From ref. 306.)

CDR3 diversity was possible, as has been observed by Taylor et al. (309) and in our own experiments (J. L. Xu and M. M. Davis, unpublished). With respect to αβ TCRs, we expect that most of the specificity of the interaction with a typical ligand will reside in the CDR3–peptide contacts, and here again, the CDR1 and CDR2 regions will make less important contacts. The case of γδ TCRs would be more like an antibody, only without the affinity improvements that are gained from somatic hypermutation. We have only an *ad hoc* explanation for the extremes of diversity seen in the TCRδ CDR3, which is that it has to recognize both protein surfaces and small nonpeptidic molecules with a high degree of specificity. Perhaps the lack of somatic mutation forces it to provide more diversity in the initial repertoire.

Although direct tests of this hypothesis are just beginning, it would seem to hold considerable promise as a general mechanism for antigen-receptor specificity and as an answer to an intriguing molecular genetic puzzle.

CONCLUSION

Since TCRs were first identified in the early 1980s, information about their genetics, biochemistry, structure, and function has accumulated to become almost a field unto itself. Despite this very real progress, many issues still remain unsolved: What do γδ T cells normally "see," and what function do they serve? What do superantigens actually do during the course of a normal response, and how is this of benefit to the pathogen and/or parasite? What is the structural–chemical basis of TCR specificity? What sort of rearrangements or conformational changes occur in the TCR/CD3 molecular ensemble upon ligand engagement? These and other questions should serve as a source of entertainment for many years to come.

ACKNOWLEDGMENTS

We are very grateful to Dr. Stephen Hedrick for allowing us to build so freely on his excellent previous chapters for this volume and to the Howard Hughes Medical Institute and NIH for research support. We also thank H. Li, R. Mariuzza, C. Garcia, and I. Wilson for providing the TCR structure figures and D. Lyons for preparing the artwork.

REFERENCES

1. Zinkernagel RM, Doherty PC. Immunological surveillance against altered self components by sensitized T-lymphocytes in lymphocytic choriomeningitis. *Nature* 1974;251:547.
2. Zinkernagel R, Doherty P. H-2 compatibility requirement for T-cell-mediated lysis of target cells infected with lymphocytic choriomeningitis virus: different cytotoxic T cell specificities are associated with structures from H-3K or H-2D. *J Exp Med* 1975;141:1427.
3. Shevach EM, Rosenthal AS. Function of macrophages in antigen recognition by guinea pig T lymphocytes. II. Role of the macrophage in the regulation of genetic control of the immune response. *J Exp Med* 1973;138:1213.
4. Katz DH, Hamaoka T, Benacerraf B. Cell interactions between histoincompatible T and B lymphocytes. II. Failure of physiological cooperative interactions between T and B lymphocytes from allogeneic donor strains in humoral response to hapten-protein conjugates. *J Exp Med* 1973;137:1405.
5. Terhorst C, Spits H, Stall F, Exley M. T lymphocyte signal transduction. In: Hames BD, Glover DM, eds. *Molecular immunology.* 2nd ed. Oxford: IRL Press, 1996.
6. Chien Y-H, Jores R, Crowley MP. Recognition by γ/δ T cells. *Annu Rev Immunol* 1996;14:511.
7. Infante AJ, Infante PD, Gillis S, Fathman CG. Definition of T cell idiotypes using anti-idiotype antisera produced by immunization with T cell clones. *J Exp Med* 1982;155:1100.
8. Allison JP, McIntyre BW, Bloch D. Tumor-specific antigen of murine T lymphoma defined with monoclonal antibody. *J Immunol* 1982; 129:2293.
9. Meuer SC, Fitzgerald KA, Hussey RE, Hodgdon JC, Schlossman SF, Reinherz EL. Clonotypic structures involved in antigen specific human T cell function: relationship to the T3 molecular complex. *J Exp Med* 1983;157:705.
10. Haskins K, Kubo R, White J, Pigeon M, Kappler J, Marrack P. The major histocompatibility complex-restricted antigen receptor on T cells. I. Isolation with a monoclonal antibody. *J Exp Med* 1983;157:1149.

11. Kaye J, Procelli S, Tite J, Jones B, Janeway CAJ. Both a monoclonal antibody and antisera specific for determinants unique to individual cloned helper T cell lines can substitute for antigen and antigen-presenting cells in the activation of T cells. *J Exp Med* 1983;158:836.

12. Samelson LE, Germain RN, Schwartz RH. Monoclonal antibodies against the antigen receptor on a cloned T cell hybrid. *Proc Natl Acad Sci USA* 1983;80:6972.

13. MacIntyre BW, Allison JP. Biosynthesis and processing of murine T-cell antigen receptor. *Cell* 1984;38:654.

14. Kappler J, Kubo R, Haskins K, et al. The major histocompatibility complex-restricted antigen receptor on T cells in mouse and man. V. Identification of constant and variable peptides. *Cell* 1983;35:295.

15. Davis MM, Cohen DI, Nielsen EA, DeFranco AL, Paul WE. The isolation of B and T cell-specific genes. In: Vitteta E, ed. *B and T cell tumors,* UCLA Symposia on Molecular and Cellular Biology, vol. 24. New York: Academic Press, 1982: 215.

16. Hedrick SM, Cohen DI, Nielsen EA, Davis MM. Isolation of cDNA clones encoding T cell-specific membrane-associated proteins. *Nature* 1984;308:149.

17. Hedrick SM, Nielsen EA, Kavaler J, Cohen DI, Davis MM. Sequence relationships between putative T-cell receptor polypeptides and Igs. *Nature* 1984;308: 153.

18. Yanagi Y, Yoshikai Y, Leggett K, Clark SP, Aleksander I, Mak TW. A human T cell-specific cDNA clone encodes a protein having extensive homology to immunoglobulin chains. *Nature* 1984;308:145.

19. Acuto O, Fabbi M, Smart J, et al. Purification and NH2-terminal amino acid sequencing of the beta subunit of a human T-cell antigen receptor. *Proc Natl Acad Sci USA* 1984;81:3851.

20. Chien Y, Becker DM, Lindsten T, Okamura M, Cohen DI, Davis MM. A third type of murine T-cell receptor gene. *Nature* 1984;312:31.

21. Saito H, Kranz D, Takagaki Y, Hayday A, Eisen H, Tonegawa S. A third rearranged and expressed gene in a clone of cytotoxic T lymphocytes. *Nature* 1984;312:36.33.

22. Saito H, Kranz DM, Takagaki Y, Hayday AC, Eisen HN, Tonegawa S. Complete primary structure of a heterodimeric T-cell receptor deduced from cDNA sequences. *Nature* 1984;309:757.

23. Brenner MB, McLean J, Dialynas DP, et al. Identification of a putative second T-cell receptor. *Nature* 1986;322:145.

24. Chien YH, Iwashima M, Kaplan KB, Elliott JF, Davis MM. A new T-cell receptor gene located within the alpha locus and expressed early in T-cell differentiation. *Nature* 1987;327:677.

25. Loh EY, Lanier LL, Turck CW, et al. Identification and sequence of a fourth human T cell antigen receptor chain. *Nature* 1987;330:569.

26. Born W, Miles C, White J, et al. Peptide sequences of T-cell receptor delta and gamma chains are identical to predicted Cx and gamma proteins. *Nature* 1987; 330:572.

27. Bonyhadi M, Weiss A, Tucker PW, Tigelaar RE, Allison JP. Delta is the Cx gene product in the γδ antigen receptor of dendritic epidermal cells. *Nature* 1987;330:574.

28. Dembic Z, Haas W, Weiss S, et al. Transfer of specificity by murine α and β T-cell receptor genes. *Nature* 1986;320:232.

29. Saito T, Weiss A, Miller J, Norcross MA, Germain RN. Specific antigen-Ia activation of transfected human T cells expressing murine Ti ab-human T3 receptor complexes. *Nature* 1987;325:125.

30. Havran WL, Chien YH, Allison JP. Recognition of self antigens by skin-derived T cells with invariant gamma delta antigen receptors. *Science* 1991;252:1430.

31. Novotny J, Tonegawa S, Saito H, Kranz DM, Eisen HN. Secondary, tertiary, and quaternary structure of T-cell specific immunoglobulin-like polypeptide chains. *Proc Natl Acad Sci USA* 1986;83:742.

32. Brenner MB, McLean J, Scheft H, et al. Two forms of the TCR gamma protein found on peripheral blood cytotoxic T lymphocytes. *Nature* 1987;325:689.

33. Tan L, Turner J, Weiss TM. Regions of the T cell receptor alpha and beta chains that are responsible for interactions with CD3. *J Exp Med* 1991;173:1247.

34. Groettrup M, Ungewiss K, Azogui O, et al. A novel disulfide-linked heterodimer on pre-T cells consists of the T cell receptor β chain and a 33 kDa glycoprotein. *Cell* 1993;75:283.

35. Saint-Ruf C, Ungewiss K, Groettrup M, Bruno L, Fehling HJ, von Boehmer H. Analysis and expression of a cloned pre-T cell receptor gene. *Science* 1994;206:1208.

36. Davies DR, Metzger HA. Structural basis of antibody function. *Annu Rev Immunol* 1983;1:87.

37. Novotny J, Tonegawa S, Saito H, Kranz DM, Eisen H. Secondary, tertiary, and quaternary structure of T-cell-specific immunoglobulin-like polypeptide chains. *Proc Natl Acad Sci USA* 1986;83:742.

38. Chothia C, Boswell DR, Lesk AM. An outline structure of the T cell receptor. *EMBO J* 1988;7:3745.

39. Beale D, Coadwell J. Unusual features of the T cell receptor C domains are revealed by structural comparisons with other members of the immunoglobulin superfamily. *Biochem Physiol* 1986;85:205.

40. Bentley GA, Boulot G, Karjalainen K, Mariuzza RA. Crystal structure of the beta chain of a T cell antigen receptor. *Science* 1995;267:1984–1987.

41. Fields BA, Ober B, Malchiodi EL, et al. Crystal structure of the V alpha domain of a T cell antigen receptor. *Science* 1995;270:1821–1824.

42. Bentley GA, Mariuzza RA. The structure of the T cell antigen receptor. *Annu Rev Immunol* 1996;14:563.

43. Garcia KC, Decagon M, Stanfield RL, et al. The structure of an αβ T-cell receptor at 2.5Å. *Science* 1996;274:209.

44. Li H, Lebedeva MI, Llera AS, Fields BA, Brenner MB, Mariuzza RA. Structure of the Vδ domain of a human γδ T cell antigen receptor. *Nature* 1998;391:502.

45. Garboczi DN, Ghosh P, Utz U, Fan QR, Biddison WE, Wiley DC. Structure of the complex between human T-cell receptor, viral peptide and HLA-A2. *Nature* 1996;384:134–140.

46. Housset D, Mazza G, Gregoire C, Piras C, Malissen B, Fontecilla-Camps JC. The three-dimensional structure of a T cell antigen receptor V alpha V beta heterodimer reveals a novel arrangement of the V beta domain. *EMBO J* 1997;14: 4205–4216.

47. Strong RK, Penny DM, Feldman RM, et al. Engineering and expression of a secreted murine T cell receptor with reduced N-linked glycosylation. *J Immunol* 1994;153:4111.

48. Reich Z, Boniface JJ, Lyons DS, Borochov N, Wachtel EJ, Davis MM. Ligand-specific oligomerization of T-cell receptor molecules. *Nature* 1997;387:617–620.

49. Klausner RD, Lippincott-Schwartz J, Bonifacino JS. The T cell antigen receptor: insights into organelle biology. *Annu Rev Cell Biol* 1990;6:403.

50. Samelson LE, Harford HB, Klausner RD. Identification of the components of the murine T cell antigen receptor complex. *Cell* 1985;43:223.

50a. Goding, JW. A symmetrical surface IgG on MOPC-21 plasmacytoma cells contains one membrane heavy chain and one secretory heavy chain. *J. Immunol* 1982;128:2416.

51. Orloff DG, Frank SJ, Robey FA, Weissman AM, Klausner RD. Biochemical characterization of the eta chain of the T-cell receptor. *J Biol Chem* 1989;264: 14812.

52. Jin YJ, Clayton LK, Howard FD, et al. Molecular cloning of the CD3 eta subunit identifies a CD3 zeta-related product in thymus-derived cells. *Proc Natl Acad Sci USA* 1990;87:3319.

53. Clayton LK, DAdamio L, Howard FD, et al. CD3 eta and CD3 zeta are alternatively spliced products of a common genetic locus and are transcriptionally and/or post-transcriptionally regulated during T-cell development. *Proc Natl Acad Sci USA* 1991;88:5202.

54. Rodewald HR, Arulanandam AR, Koyasu S, Reinherz EL. The high affinity Fc epsilon receptor gamma subunit (Fc epsilon RI gamma) facilitates T cell receptor expression and antigen/major histocompatibility complex-driven signaling in the absence of CD3 zeta and CD3 eta. *J Biol Chem* 1991;266:15974.

55. Orloff DG, Ra CS, Frank SJ, Klausner RD, Kinet JP. Family of disulphide-linked dimers containing the zeta and eta chains of the T-cell receptor and the gamma chain of Fc receptors. *Nature* 1990;347:189.

56. Koyasu S, DAdamio L, Arulanandam AR, Abraham S, Clayton LK, Reinherz EL. T cell receptor complexes containing Fc epsilon RI gamma homodimers in lieu of CD3 zeta and CD3 eta components: a novel isoform expressed on large granular lymphocytes. *J Exp Med* 1992;175:203.

57. Exley M, Wileman T, Mueller B, Terhorst C. Evidence for multivalent structure of T cell antigen receptor complex. *Mol Immunol* 1995;32:829.

58. Blumberg RS, Ley S, Sancho J, et al. Structure of the T-cell receptor: evidence for two CD3 epsilon subunits in the T-cell receptor-CD3 complex. *Proc Natl Acad Sci USA* 1990;87:7220.

59. Jin YJ, Koyasu S, Moingeon P, Steinbrich R, Tarr GE, Reinherz EL. A fraction of CD3 epsilon subunits exists as disulfide-linked dimers in both human and murine T lymphocytes. *J Biol Chem* 1990;265:15850.

60. Fernandez-Miguel G, Alarcón B, Iglesias A, Sanz E, de la Hera A. Multivalent structure of an αβ T cell receptor. *(submitted for publication).*

61. Clevers H, Alarcon B, Wileman T, Terhorst C. The T cell receptor/CD3 complex: a dynamic protein ensemble. *Annu Rev Immunol* 1988;6:629.

62. Cosson P, Lankford SP, Bonifacino JS, Klausner RD. Membrane protein association by potential intramembrane charge pairs. *Nature* 1991;351:414.

63. Hall C, Berhout B, Alarcon B, et al. Requirements for cell surface expression of the human TCR/CD3 complex in non-T cells. *Int Immunol* 1991;3:359.

64. Alarcon B, Ley SC, Sanchez-Madrid F, et al. The CD3-gamma and CD3-delta subunits of the T cell antigen receptor can be expressed within distinct functional TCR/CD3 complexes. *EMBO J* 1991;10:903.

65. Letourneur F, Klausner RD. Activation of T cells by a tyrosine kinase activation domain in the cytoplasmic tail of CD3 epsilon. *Science* 1992;255:79.

66. Letourneur F, Klausner RD. T-cell and basophil activation through the cytoplasmic tail of T-cell-receptor zeta family proteins. *Proc Natl Acad Sci USA* 1991;88:8905.

67. Wegener AM, Letourneur F, Hoeveler A, Brocker T, Luton F, Malissen B. The T cell receptor/CD3 complex is composed of at least two autonomous transduction modules. *Cell* 1992;68:83.

68. Romeo C, Amiot M, Seed B. Sequence requirements for induction of cytolysis by the T cell antigen/Fc receptor zeta chain. *Cell* 1992;68:889.

69. Klausner RD, Samelson LE. T cell antigen receptor activation pathways: the tyrosine kinase connection. *Cell* 1991;64:875.

70. Cantrell DA, Davies AA, Crumpton MJ. Activators of protein kinase C down-regulate and phosphorylate the T3/T-cell antigen receptor complex of human T lymphocytes. *Proc Natl Acad Sci USA* 1985;82:8158.

71. Patel MD, Samelson LE, Klausner RD. Multiple kinases and signal transduction. Phosphorylation of the T cell antigen receptor complex. *J Biol Chem* 1987;262:5831.

72. Ashwell JD, Klausner RD. Genetic and mutational analysis of the T-cell antigen receptor. *Annu Rev Immunol* 1990;8:139.

73. Manolios N, Letourneur F, Bonifacino JS, Klausner RD. Pairwise, cooperative

and inhibitory interactions describe the assembly and probable structure of the T-cell antigen receptor. *EMBO J* 1991;10:1643.

74. Minami Y, Weissman AM, Samelson LE, Klausner RD. Building a multichain receptor: synthesis, degradation and assembly of the T-cell antigen receptor. *Proc Natl Acad Sci USA* 1987;84:2688.

75. Letourneur F, Klausner RD. A novel di-leucine motif and a tyrosine-based motif independently mediate lysosomal targeting and endocytosis of CD3 chains. *Cell* 1992;69:1143.

76. Frank SJ, Niklinska BB, Orloff DG, Mercep M, Ashwell JD, Klausner RD. Structural mutations reveal a novel role for the TCR zeta chain in cell activation. *Science* 1990;249:174.

77. Chen C, Bonifacino JS, Yuan L, Klausner RD. Selective degradation of T cell antigen receptor chains retained in a pre-Golgi compartment. *J Cell Biol* 1988; 107:2149.

78. Alarcon B, Berkhout B, Breitmeyer J, Terhorst C. Assembly of the human T cell receptor-CD3 complex takes place in the endoplasmic reticulum and involves intermediary complexes between the CD3-gamma, delta, epsilon core and single T cell receptor alpha or beta chains. *J Biol Chem* 1988;263:2953.

79. Bonifacino JS, Suzuki CK, Lippincott-Schwartz J, Weissman AM, Klausner RD. Pre-golgi degradation of newly synthesized T cell antigen receptor chains: intrinsic sensitivity and the role of subunit assembly. *J Cell Biol* 1989;109:73.

80. Wileman T, Carson GR, Concino J, Ahmed A, Terhorst C. The γ and ε subunits of the CD3 complex inhibit pre-Golgi degradation of newly synthesized T cell receptors. *J Cell Biol* 1990;110:973.

81. Bonifacino JS, Suzuki CK, Klausner RD. A peptide sequence confers retention and degradation in the endoplasmic reticulum. *Science* 1990;247:79.

81a. Davis MM, Chien Y. T Cell receptors. In *Molecular Immunology*, 2ed. Glover D and Homes D, eds. 1996. Oxford: IRL Press, pp. 101–131.

82. Chien Y, Gascoigne NRJ, Kavaler J, Lee NE, Davis MM. Somatic recombination in a murine T-cell receptor gene. *Nature* 1984;309:322–326.

83. Kavaler J, Davis MM, Chien Y. Localization of a T-cell receptor diversity-region element. *Nature* 1984;310:421–423.

84. Bosma M. B and T cell leakiness in the SCID mouse mutant. *Immunodefic Rev England* 1992;3:261.

85. Mombaerts P, Iacomini J, Johnson RS, Herrup K, Tonegawa S, Papaioannou VE. RAG-1-deficient mice have no mature B and T lymphocytes. *Cell* 1992;68:869.

86. Shinkai Y, Rathbun G, Lam KP, et al. RAG-2-deficient mice lack mature lymphocytes owing to inability to initiate V(D)J rearrangement. *Cell* 1992;68:855.

87. Fujimoto S, Yamagishi H. Isolation of an excision product of T-cell receptor alpha-chain gene rearrangements. *Nature* 1987;327:242.

88. Okazaki K, Davis DD, Sakano HT. Cell receptor beta gene sequences in the circular DNA of thymocyte nuclei: direct evidence for intramolecular DNA deletion in V-D-J joining. *Cell* 1987;49:477.

89. Malissen M, McCoy C, Blanc D, et al. Direct evidence for chromosomal inversion during T-cell receptor beta-gene rearrangements. *Nature* 1986;319:28.

90. Iwashima M, Green A, Davis MM, Chien Y-H. Variable region (Vδ) gene segment most frequently utilized in adult thymocytes is 3′ of the constant region. *Proc Natl Acad Sci USA* 1988;85:8161.

91. Elliott JF, Rock EP, Patten PA, Davis MM, Chien Y. The adult T-cell receptor δ-chain is diverse and distinct from that of fetal thymocytes. *Nature* 1988;331: 627–631.

92. Heilig J3, Tonegawa S. Diversity of murine gamma genes and expression in fetal and adult T lymphocytes. *Nature* 1986;322:836.

93. Hayday AC, Diamond DJ, Tanigawa G, et al. Unusual organization and diversity of T-cell receptor alpha-chain genes. *Nature* 1985;316:828.

94. Winoto A, Mjolsness S, Hood L. Genomic organization of the genes encoding mouse T-cell receptor alpha-chain. *Nature* 1985;316:832.

95. Yoshikai Y, Clark SP, Taylor S, et al. Organization and sequences of the variable, joining and constant region genes of the human T-cell receptor alpha-chain. *Nature* 1985;316:837.

96. Boysen C, Simon MI, Hood L. Analysis of the 1.1-Mb human alpha/delta T-cell receptor locus with bacterial artificial chromosome clones. *Genome Res* 1997;4: 330.

97. Koop BF, Wilson RK, Wang K, et al. Organization, structure, and function of 95 kb of DNA spanning the murine T cell receptor Cα/Cδ region. *Genomics* 1992; 13:1209.

98. Chien Y, Iwashima M, Wettstein DA, et al. T-cell receptor δ gene rearrangements in early thymocytes. *Nature* 1987;330:722–727.

99. Band H, Hochstenbach F, McLean J, Hata S, Krangel MS, Brenner MB. Immunochemical proof that a novel rearranging gene encodes the T cell receptor δ subunit. *Science* 1987;238:682.

100. Hata S, Brenner MB, Krangel MS. Identification of putative human T cell receptor δ complementary DNA clones. *Science* 1987;238:678.

101. Hata S, Satyanarayana K, Devlin P, et al. Extensive junctional diversity of rearranged human T cell receptor δ genes. *Science* 1988;250:1541.

102. Raulet DH. The structure, function, and molecular genetics of the γ/δ T cell receptor. *Annu Rev Immunol* 1989;7:175.

103. de Villartay JP, Lewis D, Hockett R, Waldmann TA, Korsmeyer SJ, Cohen DI. Deletional rearrangement in the human T-cell receptor a-chain locus. *Proc Natl Acad Sci USA* 1987;84:8608.

104. Villey I, Caillol D, Selz F, Ferrier P, de Villartay JP. Defect in rearrangement of the most 5′ TCR-Jα (TEA) implications for TCR α locus accessibility. *Immunity* 1996;5:331.

105. Rowen L, Koop BF, Hood L. The complete 685-kilobase DNA sequence of the human beta T cell receptor locus. *Science* 1996;272:5269:1755.

106. Gascoigne NR, Chien Y, Becker DM, Kavaler J, Davis MM. Genomic organization and sequence of T-cell receptor beta-chain constant and joining-region genes. *Nature* 1984;310:387.

107. Malissen M, Minard K, Mjolsness S, et al. Mouse T cell antigen receptor: structure and organization of constant and joining gene segments encoding the beta polypeptide. *Cell* 1984;37:1101.

108. Noonan DJ, Kofler R, Singer PA, Cardenas G, Dixon FJ, Theofilopoulos AN. Delineation of a defect in T cell receptor beta genes of NZW mice predisposed to autoimmunity. *J Exp Med* 1986;163:644.

109. Chou HS, Nelson CA, Godambe SA, Chaplin DD, Loh DY. Germline organization of the murine T cell receptor beta-chain genes. *Science* 1987;238:545.

110. Woodland DL, Kotzin B, Palmer E. Functional consequences of a T cell receptor Dβ2 and Jβ2 gene segment deletion. *J Immunol* 1990;14:379.

111. Hayday AC, Saito H, Gillies SD, et al. Structure, organization, and somatic rearrangement of T cell gamma genes. *Cell* 1985;40:259.

112. Garman RD, Doherty PJ, Raulet DH. Diversity, rearrangement, and expression of murine T cell gamma genes. *Cell* 1986;45:733.

113. Lefranc MP, Forster A, Rabbitts TH. Genetic polymorphism and exon changes of the constant regions of the human T-cell rearranging gene gamma. *Proc Natl Acad Sci USA* 1986;83:9596.

114. Lefranc MP, Forster A, Baer R, Stinson MA, Rabbitts TH. Diversity and rearrangement of the human T cell rearranging gamma genes: nine germ-line variable genes belonging to two subgroups. *Cell* 1986;45:237.

115. Huck S, Dariavach P, Lefranc MP. Variable region genes in the human T-cell rearranging gamma (TRG) locus: V-J junction and homology with the mouse genes. *EMBO J* 1988;7:719.

116. Strauss WM, Quertermous T, Seidman JG. Measuring the human T cell receptor gamma-chain locus. *Science* 1987;237:1217.79.

117. Vernooij BT, Lenstra JA, Wang K, Hood L. Organization of the murine T-cell receptor gamma locus. *Genomics* 1993;3:566.

118. Havran WL, Allison JP. Developmentally ordered appearance of thymocytes expressing different T cell antigen receptors. *Nature* 1988;335:443.

119. McDougall S, Peterson CL, Calame K. A transcriptional enhancer 3′ of C β 2 in the T cell receptor β locus. *Science* 1988;241:205.

120. Krimpenfort P, de Jong R, Uematsu Y, et al. Transcription of T cell receptor β-chain genes is controlled by a down-stream regulatory element. *EMBO J* 1988;7:745.

121. Leiden JM. Transcriptional regulation of T cell receptor genes. *Annu Rev Immunol* 1993;11:539.

122. Sleckman BP, Bardon CG, Ferrini R, Davidson L, Alt FW. Function of the TCRα enhancer in αβ and γδ T cells. *Immunity* 1997;7:505.

123. Lauzurica P, Krangel MS. Temporal and lineage-specific control of T cell receptor alpha/delta gene rearrangement by T cell receptor alpha and delta enhancers. *J Exp Med* 1994;179:1913.

124. Lauzurica P, Krangel MS. Enhancer-dependent and -independent steps in the rearrangement of a human T cell receptor delta transgene. *J Exp Med* 1994; 179:43.

125. Waldmann TA, Davis MM, Bongiovanni KF, Korsmeyer SJ. Rearrangements of genes for the antigen receptor on T cells as markers of lineage and clonality in human lymphoid neoplasms. *N Engl J Med* 1985;313:776.

126. Winoto A, Baltimore D. αβ lineage-specific expression of the T cell receptor α gene by nearby silencers. *Cell* 1989;59:649.

127. Diaz P, Cado D, Winoto A. A locus control region in the T cell receptor α/δ locus. *Immunity* 1994;1:207.

128. Ishida I, Verbeek S, Bonneville M, Itohara S, Berns A, Tonegawa S. T-cell receptor γδ and γ transgenic mice suggest a role of a γ gene silencer in the generation of αβ T cells. *Proc Natl Acad Sci USA* 1990;87:3067.

129. Kronenberg M, Siu G, Hood LE, Shastri N. The molecular genetics of the T-cell antigen receptor and T-cell antigen recognition. *Annu Rev Immunol* 1986;4:529.

130. Korsmeyer SJ. Chromosomal translocations in lymphoid malignancies reveal novel proto-oncogenes. *Annu Rev Immunol* 1992;10:785.

131. Finger LR, Harvey RC, Moore RC, Showe LC, Croce CM. A common mechanism of chromosomal translocation in T- and B-cell neoplasia. *Science* 1986;234:982.

132. Baer R, Chen K-C, Smith SD, Rabbitts TH. Fusion of an immunoglobulin variable gene and a T cell receptor constant gene in the chromosome 14 inversion associated with T cell tumors. *Cell* 1986;43:705.

133. Denny CT, Yoshikai YU, Mak TW, Smith SD, Hollis GF, Kirsch IR. A chromosome 14 inversion in a T cell lymphoma is caused by site-specific recombination between immunoglobulin and T cell receptor loci. *Nature* 1986;320:549.

134. Boehm T, Greenberg JM, Buluwela L, Lavenir I, Forster A, Rabbitts TH. An unusual structure of a putative T cell oncogene which allows production of similar proteins from distinct mRNAs. *EMBO J* 1990;9:857.

135. McGuire EA, Hockett RD, Pollock KM, Bartholdi MF, O'Brien SJ, Korsmeyer SJ. The t(11;14)(p15;q11) in a T cell acute lymphoblastic leukemia cell line activates multiple transcripts, including *ltg-1*, a gene encoding a potential zinc finger protein. *Mol Cell Biol* 1989;9:2124.101.

136. Royer Pokora B, Loos U, Ludwig W-D. *Ttg-2*, a new gene encoding a cysteine-rich protein with the LIM motif is overexpressed in acute T-cell leukaemia with the t(11;14)(p13;q11). *Oncogene* 1991;6:1887.

137. Boehm T, Foroni L, Kaneko Y, Perutz MF, Rabbitts TH. The rhombotin family of cysteine-rich LIM-domain oncogenes: distinct members are involved in T-cell

translocations to human chromosomes 11p15 and 11p13. *Proc Natl Acad Sci USA* 1991;88:4367.

138. Visvader J, Begley CG, Adams JM. Differential expression of the LYL, SCL and E2A helix-loop-helix genes within the hemopoietic system. *Oncogene* 1991;6:187.

139. Begley CG, Aplan PD, Davey MP, et al. Chromosomal translocation in a human leukemic stem-cell line disrupts the T-cell antigen receptor δ-chain diversity region and results in a previously unreported fusion transcript. *Proc Natl Acad Sci USA* 1989;86:2031.

140. Chen Q, Chen J-T, Tsai L-H, et al. The tal gene undergoes chromosome translocation in T cell leukemia and potentially encodes a helix-loop-helix protein. *EMBO J* 1990;9:415.

141. Finger LR, Kagan J, Christopher G, et al. Involvement of the TCL5 gene on human chromosome 1 in T-cell leukemia and melanoma. *Proc Natl Acad Sci USA* 1989;86:5039.

142. Hatano M, Roberts CWM, Minden M, Crist WM, Korsmeyer SJ. Deregulation of a homeobox gene *HOXII,* by the t(10;14) in T cell leukemia. *Science* 1991;253:79.

143. O'Conner RD, Brown MG, Francke U. Immunologic and karyotypic studies in ataxia-telangiectasia: specificity of break points on chromosomes 7 and 14 in lymphocytes from patients and relatives. In: Bridges BA, Harnden DG, eds. *Ataxia-telangiectasia-a cellular and molecular link: Cancer, neuropathology and immune deficiency.* New York: John Wiley and Sons, 1982:259.

144. Aurias A, Dutrillaux B. Probable involvement of immunoglobulin superfamily genes in most recurrent chromosomal rearrangements from ataxia telangiectasia. *Hum Genet* 1986;72:210.

145. Lipkowitz S, Stern MH, Kirsch IR. Hybrid T cell receptor genes formed by interlocus recombination in normal and ataxia-telangiectasis lymphocytes. *J Exp Med* 1990;172:409.

146. Uematus Y, Ryser S, Dembic Z, et al. In transgenic mice the introduced functional T cell receptor beta gene prevents expression of endogenous beta genes. *Cell* 1988;52:831.

147. Padovan E, Casorati G, Dellabona P, Meyer S, Brockhaus M, Lanzavecchia A. Expression of two T cell receptor alpha chains: dual receptor T cells. *Science* 1993;262:422.

148. Malissen M, Trucy J, Jouvin-Marche E, Cazenave PA, Scollay R, Malissen B. Regulation of TCR alpha and beta gene allelic exclusion during T-cell development. *Immunol Today England* 1992;13:315.

149. Aifantis I, Buer J, von Boehmer H, Azogui H. Essential role of the pre-T cell receptor in allelic exclusion of the T cell receptor β locus. *Immunity* 1997;7:601.

150. O Shea CC, Thornell AP, Rosewell IR, Hayes B, Owen MJ. Exit of the pre-TCR from the ER/cis-golgi is necessary for signaling differentiation, proliferation, and allelic exclusion in immature thymocytes. *Immunity* 1997;7:591.

151. Takeshita S, Toda M, Yamagishi H. Excision products of T cell receptor gene support a progressive rearrangement model of the alpha/delta locus. *EMBO J* 1989;8:3261.

152. Winoto A, Baltimore D. Separate lineages of T cells expressing the alpha beta and gamma delta receptors. *Nature* 1989;338:430.

153. Dent AL, Matis LA, Hooshmand F, Widacki SM, Bluestone JA, Hedrick SM. Self-reactive gamma delta T cells are eliminated in the thymus. *Nature* 1990;343:714.

154. Wilson A, de Villartay J-P, MacDonald HR. T cell receptor δ gene rearrangement and T early α (TEA) expression in immature αβ lineage thymocytes: implications for αβ/γδ lineage commitment. *Immunity* 1996;4:37.

155. Mombaerts P, Clarke AR, Rudnicki MA, et al. Mutations in T-cell receptor genes α and β block thymocyte development at different stages. *Nature* 1992;360:225.

156. Philpott KL, Viney JL, Kay G, et al. Lymphoid development in mice congenitally lacking T cell receptor αβ-expressing cells. *Science* 1992;256:1448.

157. Itohara S, Mombaerts P, Lafaille J, et al. T cell receptor delta gene mutant mice: independent generation of alpha beta T cells and programmed rearrangements of gamma delta TCR genes. *Cell* 1993;72:337.

158. van der Merwe PA, Barclay AN. Transient intercellular adhesion: the importance of weak protein-protein interactions. *Trends Biochem Sci* 1994;19:354–358.

159. Boniface JJ, Davis MM. The affinity and kinetics of T-cell receptor binding to peptide/MHC complexes and the analysis of transient biomolecular interactions. In: Weir DM, Herzenberg LA, Blackwell C, Herzenberg LA, eds. *Handbook of Experimental Immunology,* 5th ed. Cambridge, MA: Blackwell Scientific, 1996.

160. Lin AY, Devaux B, Green A, Sagerström C, Elliott JF, Davis MM. Expression of T cell antigen receptor heterodimers in a lipid-linked form. *Science* 1990;249: 677–679.

161. Gregoire C, Lin SY, Mazza G, Rebai N, Luescher IF, Malissen B. Covalent assembly of a soluble T cell receptor-peptide-major histocompatibility class I complex. *Proc Natl Acad Sci USA* 1996;14:7184–7189.

162. Parham P, Lomen CE, Lawlor DA, et al. Nature of polymorphism in HLA-A,-B, and-C molecules. *Proc Natl Acad Sci USA* 1988;85:4005–4009.

163. Wettstein, DA, Boniface JJ, Reay PA, Schild H, Davis MM. Expression of a functional Class II MHC heterodimer in a lipid-linked form with enhanced peptide/soluble MHC complex formation at low pH. *J Exp Med* 1991;174:219–228.

164. Garboczi DN, Hung DT, Wiley DC. HLA-A2-peptide complexes: refolding and crystallization of molecules expressed in Escherichia coli and complexed with single antigenic peptides. *Proc Natl Acad Sci USA* 1992;89:3429–3433.

165. Altman JD, Reay PA, Davis MM. Formation of functional class II MHC/peptide complexes from subunits produced in *E. coli. Proc Natl Acad Sci USA* 1993;90:10330–10334.

166. Jackson MR, Song ES, Yang Y, Peterson PA. Empty and peptide-containing conformers of class I major histocompatibility complex molecules expressed in Drosophila melanogaster cells. *Proc Natl Acad Sci USA* 1992;89:12117–12121.

167. Stern LJ, Wiley DC. The human class II MHC protein HLA-DR1 assembles as empty alpha beta heterodimers in the absence of antigenic peptide. *Cell* 1992; 68:465–477.

168. Kozono H, White J, Clements J, Marrack P, Kappler J. Production of soluble MHC class II proteins with covalently bound single peptides. *Nature* 1994;369: 151-154.

169. Matsui K, Boniface JJ, Reay PA, Schild H, Fazekas de St Groth B, Davis MM. Low affinity interaction of peptide-MHC complexes with T cell receptor. *Science* 1991;254:1788–1791.

170. Weber S, Traunecker A, Oliveri F, Gerhard W, Karjalainen K. Specific low-affinity recognition of major histocompatibility complex plus peptide by soluble T-cell receptor. *Nature* 1992;356:793–796.

171. Sykulev Y, Brunmark A, Jackson M, Cohen RJ, Peterson PA, Eisen HN. Kinetics and affinity of reactions between an antigen-specific T cell receptor and peptide-MHC complexes. *Immunity* 1994;1:15–22.

172. Malmqvist M. Biospecific interaction analysis using biosensor technology. *Nature* 1993;361:186.

173. Matsui K, Boniface JJ, Steffner P, Reay PA, Davis MM. Kinetics of T cell receptor binding to peptide-MHC complexes: correlation of the dissociation rate with T cell responsiveness. *Proc Natl Acad Sci USA* 1994;91:12862–12866.

174. Corr M, Slanetz A, Boyd L, et al. T cell receptor-MHC class I peptide interactions: affinity, kinetics, and specificity. *Science* 1994;265, 946–949.

175. Seth A, Stern LJ, Ottenhoff THM, et al. Binary and ternary complexes between T-cell receptor, class II MHC and superantigen *in vitro. Nature* 1994;369: 324–327.

176. Alam SM, Travers PJ, Wung JL, et al. T cell receptor affinity and thymocyte positive selection. *Nature* 1996;381:616–620.

177. Al-Ramadi BK, Jelonek MT, Boyd LF, Margulies DH, Bothwell ALM. Lack of strict correlation of functional sensitization with the apparent affinity of MHC/peptide complexes for the TCR. *J Immunol* 1995;155:662–673.

178. Lyons DS, Lieberman SA, Hampl J, et al. T cell receptor binding to antagonist peptide/MHC complexes exhibits lower affinities and faster dissociation rates than to agonist ligands. *Immunity* 1996;5:53–61.

179. Sykulev Y, Brunmark A, Tsomides TJ, et al. High-affinity reactions between antigen-specific T-cell receptors and peptides associated with allogeneic and syngeneic major histocompatibility complex class I proteins. *Proc Natl Acad Sci USA* 1994b;91:11487–11491.

180. Garcia K, Scott C, Brunmark A, et al. CD8 enhances formation of stable T–cell receptor/ MHC class I molecule complexes. *Nature* 1996;384:577–581.

181. Renard V, Romero P, Vivier E, Malissen B, Luescher IF. CD8 beta increases CD8 coreceptor function and participation in TCR-ligand binding. *J Exp Med* 1996; 184:2439–2444.

182. Kersh GJ, Allen PM. Essential flexibility in the T-cell recognition of antigen. *Nature* 1996;380:495.

183. Jameson SC, Bevan MJ. T cell receptor antagonists and partial agonists. *Immunity* 1995;2:1.

184. Kessler BM, Bassanini P, Cerottini J-C, Luescher IF. Effects of epitope modification on T cell receptor-ligand binding and antigen recognition by seven H-2K^d-restricted cytotoxic T lymphocyte clones specific for a photoreactive peptide derivative. *J Exp Med* 1997;185:4:629.

185. McKeithan K. Kinetic proofreading in T-cell receptor signal transduction. *Proc Natl Acad Sci USA* 1995;92:5042–5046.

186. Rabinowitz JD, Beeson C, Lyons DS, Davis MM, McConnell HM. Kinetic discrimination in T cell activation. *Proc Natl Acad Sci USA* 1997;93:1401–1405.

187. Vallitutti S, Muller S, Cella M, Padovan E, Lanzavecchia A. Serial triggering of many T-cell receptors by a few peptide-MHC complexes. *Nature* 1995;375: 148–151.

188. Viola A, Lanzavecchia A. T cell activation determined by T cell receptor number and tunable threshholds. *Science* 1996;273:104–106.

189. Janeway CA Jr. The T cell receptor as a multicomponent signalling machine: CD4/CD8 coreceptors and CD45 in T cell activation. *Annu Rev Immunol* 1992; 10:645–674.

190. Mannie MD, Rosser JM, White GA. Autologous rat myelin basic protein is a partial agonist that is converted into a full antagonist upon blockade of CD4. Evidence for the integration of efficacious and nonefficacious signals during T cell antigen recognition. *J Immunol* 1995;154:2642–2654.

191. Vidal K, Hsu BL, Williams CB, Allen PM. Endogenous altered peptide ligands can affect peripheral T cell responses. *J Exp Med* 1996;183:1311–1321.

192. Hampl J, Chien Y, Davis MM. CD4 augments the response of a T cell to a agonist but not to antagonist ligands. *Immunity* 1997;7:1–20.

193. Madrenas J, Chau, LA, Smith J, Bluestone JA, Germain RN. The efficiency of CD4 recruitment to ligand-engaged TCR controls the agonist/partial agonist properties of peptide-MHC molecule ligands. *J Exp Med* 1997;185:219.

194. Madrenas J, Germain RN. Variant TCR ligands: new insights into the molecular basis of antigen-dependent signal transduction and T-cell activation. *Semin Immunol* 1996;8:83.

195. Davis MM, Bjorkman PJ. T cell antigen receptor genes and T cell recognition. *Nature* 1988;334:395.

196. Claverie JM, Prochinicka CA, Bouguelert L. Implications of a Fab-like structure for the T-cell receptor. *Immunol Today* 1989;10:10.

197. Engel I, Hedrick SM. Site-directed mutations in the VDJ junctional region of T cell recptor beta chain cause changes in antigenic peptide recognition. *Cell* 1988;54:473.

198. Katayama CD, Eidelman FJ, Duncan A, Hooshmand F, Hedrick SM. Predicted complementarity determining regions of the T cell antigen receptor determine antigen specificity. *EMBO J* 1995;14:927.

199. Jorgensen JL, Esser U, Fazekas de St Groth B, Reay PA, Davis MM. Mapping T cell receptor/peptide contacts by variant peptide immunization of single-chain transgenics. *Nature* 1992;355:224.

200. Jorgensen JL, Reay PA, Ehrich EW, Davis MM. Molecular components of T-cell recognition. *Annu Rev Immunol* 1992;10:835.

201. Sant, Angelo DB, Waterbury G, Preston-Hurlburt P, et al. The specificity and orientation of a TCR to its peptide-MHC class II ligands. *Immunity USA* 1996;4:367.

202. Sun R, Shepherd SE, Geier SS, Thomson CT, Sheil JM, Nathenson SG. Evidence that the antigen receptors of cytotoxic T lymphocytes interact with a common recognition pattern on the H-2Kb molecule. *Immunity USA* 1995;3:573.

203. Ehrich EW, Devaux B, Rock EP, Jorgensen JL, Davis MM, Chien Y. T cell receptor interaction with peptide/MHC and superantigen/MHC ligands is dominated by antigen. *J Exp Med* 1993;178:713–722.

204. Chang H-C, Smolyar A, Spoerl R, et al. Topology of T cell receptor-peptide/class I MHC interaction defined by charge reversal complementation and function analysis. *J Mol Biol* 1997;271:278.

205. Gao GF, Tormo J, Gerth UC, et al. Crystal structure of the complex between human CD8 alpha and HLA-A2. *Nature* 1997;387:630.

206. Marrack P, Kappler J. The staphylococcal enterotoxins and their relatives. *Science* 1990;248:705.

207. Herman A, Kappler JW, Marrack P, Pullen AM. Superantigens: mechanism of T-cell stimulation and role in immune responses. *Annu Rev Immunol* 1991;9:745.

208. McDonald KR, Acha-Orbea H. Superantigens of mouse mammary tumor virus. *Annu Rev Immunol* 1995;13:459.

209. Kappler JW, Wade T, White J, et al. A T cell receptor V beta segment that imparts reactivity to a class II major histocompatibility complex product. *Cell* 1987;49:263.

210. Kappler J, Roehm N, Marrack P. T cell tolerance by clonal elimination in the thymus. *Cell* 1987;49:273.

211. Kappler JW, Staerz U, White J, Marrack P. T cell receptor Vβ elements which recognize Mls-modified products of the major histocompatibility complex. *Nature* 1988;332:35.

212. MacDonald HR, Schneider R, Lees RK, et al. T-cell receptor Vβ use predicts reactivity and tolerance to Mlsa-encoded antigens. *Nature* 1988;332:40.

213. Happ MR, Woodland DL, Palmer E. A third T-cell receptor β-chain variable region gene encodes reactivity to Mls-1a gene products. *Proc Natl Acad Sci USA* 1989;86:6293.

214. Pullen AM, Marrack P, Kappler JW. The T cell repertoire is heavily influenced by tolerance to polymorphic self antigens. *Nature* 1988;335:796.

215. Woodland DL, Happ MP, Gollob KJ, Palmer E. An endogenous retrovirus mediating deletion of αβ T cells. *Nature* 1991;349:529.

216. Marrack P, Kushnir E, Kappler J. A maternally inherited superantigen encoded by a mammary tumour virus. *Nature* 1991;349:524.

217. Choi Y, Kappler JW, Marrack P. A superantigen encoded in the open reading frame of the 3′ long terminal repeat of mouse mammary tumour virus. *Nature* 1991;350:203.

218. Dyson PJ, Knight AM, Fairchild S, Simpson E, Tomonari K. Genes encoding ligands for deletion of Vβ11 T cells cosegregate with mammary tumour virus genomes. *Nature* 1991;349:531.

219. Frankel WN, Rudy C, Coffin JM, Huber BT. Linkage of Mls genes to endogenous mammary tumour viruses of inbred mice. *Nature* 1991;349:526.

220. Janeway CA, Yagi J, Conrad PJ, et al. T-cell responses to Mls and to bacterial proteins that mimic its behavior. *Immunol Rev* 1989;107:61.

221. Held W, Shakhov AN, Waanders G, et al. An exogenous mouse mammary tumor virus with properties of Mls-1a (Mtv-7). *J Exp Med* 1992;175:1623.

222. Callahan JE, Herman A, Kappler JW, Marrack P. Stimulation of B10.BR T cells with superantigenic staphylococcal toxins. *J Immunol* 1990;144:2473.

223. Takimoto H, Yoshikai Y, Kishihara K, et al. Stimulation of all T cells bearing V beta 1, V beta 3, V beta 11 and V beta 12 by staphylococcal enterotoxin A. *Eur J Immunol* 1990;20:617.

224. Kappler J, Kotzin B, Herron L, et al. V beta-specific stimulation of human T cells by staphylococcal toxins. *Science* 1989;244.811.

225. Choi YW, Kotzin B, Herron L, Callahan J, Marrack P, Kappler J. Interaction of Staphylococcus aureus toxin "superantigens" with human T cells. *Proc Natl Acad Sci USA* 1989;86:8941.

226. White J, Herman A, Pullen AM, Kubo R, Kappler JW, Marrack P. The V beta-specific superantigen staphylococcal enterotoxin B: stimulation of mature T cells and clonal deletion in neonatal mice. *Cell* 1989;56:27.

227. Yagi J, Baron J, Buxser S, Janeway CA. Bacterial proteins that mediate the association of a defined subset of T cell receptor: CD4 complexes with class II MHC. *J Immunol* 1990;144:892.

228. Stuart PM, Woodward JG. Yersinia enterocolitica produces superantigenic activity. *J Immunol* 1992;148:225.

229. Abe J, Takeda T, Watanabe Y, et al. Evidence for superantigen production by Yersinia pseudotuberculosis. *J Immunol* 1993;151:4183.

230. Tomai M, Kotb M, Majumdar G, Beachey EH. Superantigenicity of streptococcal M protein. *J Exp Med* 1990;172:359.

231. Cole BC, Kartchner DR, Wells DJ. Stimulation of mouse lymphocytes by a mitogen derived from Mycoplasma arthritidis. VII. Responsiveness is associated with expression of a product(s) of the V beta 8 gene family present on the T cell receptor alpha/beta for antigen. *J Immunol* 1989;142:4131.

232. Friedman SM, Crow MK, Tumang JR, et al. Characterization of the human T cells reactive with the Mycoplasma arthriditis-derived superantigen (MAM): generation of a monoclonal antibody against Vβ17, the T cell receptor gene product expressed by a large fraction of MAM-reactive human T cells. *J Exp Med* 1991;174:891.

233. Lafon M, Scott-Algara D, March PN, Cazenave P-A, Jouvin-Marche E. Neonatal deletion and selective expansion of mouse T cells by exposure to rabies virus nucleocapsid superantigen. *J Exp Med* 1994;180:1207.

235. Dobrescu D, Ursea B, Pope M, Asch AS, Posnett DN. Enhanced HIV-1 replication in Vβ12 T cells due to human cytomegalovirus in monocytes: evidence for a putative herpesvirus superantigen. *Cell* 1995;82:753.

236. Yao Z, Maraskovsky E, Spriggs MK, Cohen JI, Armitage RJ, Alderson MR. Herpesvirus saimiri open reading frame 14, a protein encoded by T lymphotropic herpesvirus binds to MHC class II molecules and stimulates T cell proliferation. *J Immunol* 1996;156:3260.

237. Denkers EY, Caspar P, Sher A. Toxoplasma gondii possesses a superantigen activity that selectively expands murine T cell receptor V beta 5-bearing CD8+ lymphocytes. *J Exp Med* 1994;180:985.

238. Held W, Waanders GA, Shakhov AN, Scarpellino L, Acha-Orbea H, MacDonald HR. Superantigen-induced immune stimulation amplifies mouse mammary tumor virus infection and allows virus transmission. *Cell* 1993;74:529.

239. Golovkina TV, Chervonsky A, Dudley JP, Ross SR. Transgenic mouse mammary tumor virus superantigen expression prevents viral infection. *Cell* 1992;69:637.

240. Howell MD, Diveley JP, Lundeen KA, et al. Limited T-cell receptor beta-chain heterogeneity among interleukin 2 receptor-positive synovial T cells suggests a role for superantigen in rheumatoid arthritis. *Proc Natl Acad Sci USA* 1991;88:10921.

241. Paliard X, West SG, Lafferty JA, et al. Evidence for the effects of a superantigen in rheumatoid arthritis. *Science* 1991;253:325.

242. Abe J, Kotzin BL, Jujo K, et al. Selective expansion of T cells expressing T-cell receptor variable regions V beta 2 and V beta 8 in Kawasaki disease. *Proc Natl Acad Sci USA* 1992;89:4066.

243. Conrad B, Weissmahr RN, Boni J, Arcari R, Schupbach J, Mach B. A human endogenous retroviral superantigen as candidate autoimmune gene in type I diabetes. *Cell* 1997;90:303.

244. Malchiodi EL, Eisenstein E, Fields BA, et al. Superantigen binding to a T cell receptor β chain of known three-dimensional structure. *J Exp Med* 1995;182:1.

245. Pullen AM, Wade T, Marrack P, Kapper JW. Identification of the region of T cell receptor beta chain that interacts with the self-superantigen Mls-1a. *Cell* 1990;61:1365.

246. Cazenave P-A, Marche PN, Jouvin-Marche E, et al. Vβ17 gene polymorphism in wild-derived mouse strains: two amino acid substitutions in Vβ17 region greatly alter T cell receptor specificity. *Cell* 1990;63:717.

247. Patten PA, Rock EP, Sonoda T, Fazekas de St Groth B, Davis MM. Transfer of putative CDR loops of T cell receptor V domains confers toxin reactivity, but not peptide specificity. *J Immunol* 1993;150:2281–2294.

248. Fields BA, Malchiodi EL, Li H, et al. Crystal structure of a T cell receptor beta-chain complexed with a superantigen. *Nature* 1996;384:188.

249. Hedrick SM, Eidelman FJ. T lymphocyte antigen receptors. In: Paul WE, ed. *Fundamental Immunology*, 3rd ed. New York: Raven Press, 1993:383–420.

250. Lew AM, Pardoll DM, Maloy WL, et al. Characterization of T cell receptor gamma chain expression in a subset of murine thymocytes. *Science* 1986;234:1401.

251. Haas W, Pereira P, Tonegawa S. Gamma/delta cells. *Annu Rev Immunol* 1993;11.637.

252. Sting G, Gunter KC, Tschachler E, et al. Thy-1+ dendritic epidermal cells belong to the T-cell lineage. *Proc Natl Acad Sci USA* 1987;84:2430.

253. Goodman T, Lefrancois L. Expression of the gamma-delta T-cell receptor on intestinal CD8+ intraepithelial lymphocytes. *Nature* 1988;333:855.

254. Itohara S, Farr AG, Lafaille JJ, et al. Homing of γδ thymocyte subset with homogeneous T-cell receptors to mucosal epithelia. *Nature* 1990;343:754.

255. Augustin A, Kubo RT, Sim GK. Resident pulmonary lymphocytes expressing the γ/δ T-cell receptor. *Nature* 1989;340:239.

256. Asarnow DM, Kuziel WA, Bonyhadi M, Tigelaar RE, Tucker PW, Allison J. Limited diversity of γδ antigen receptor genes of Thy-1+ dendritic epidermal cells. *Cell* 1988;55:837.

257. Feeney AJ. Predominance of VH-D-JH junctions occurring at sites of short sequence homology results in limited junctional diversity in neonatal antibodies. *J Immunol* 1992;149:222.

258. Boismenu R, Havran W. Modulation of epithelial cell growth by intraepithelial gamma delta T cells. *Science* 1994;266:1253.

259. Sim G-K, Augustine A. Dominate expression of BID, an invariant undiversified T cell receptor δ chain. *Cell* 1990;61:397.

260. De Geus B, Van den Enden M, Coolen C, Nagelkerken L, Van der Heijden P, Rosing J. Phenotype of intraepithelial lymphocytes in euthymic and athymic mice: implications for differentiation of cells bearing a CD3-associated γδ T cell receptor. *Eur J Immunol* 1990;20:291.

261. Cron RQ, Gajewski TF, Sharrow SO, Fitch FW, Matis LA, Bluestone JA. Phenotypic and functional analysis of murine CD3+, CD4-, CD8- TCR-gamma/delta-expressing peripheral T cells. *J Immunol* 1989;142:3754.

262. Allison JP, Havran WL. The immunobiology of T cells with invariant γδ antigen receptors. *Annu Rev Immunol* 1991;9:679.

263. Ohga S, Yoshokai Y, Takeda Y, Hiromatsu K, Nomoto K. Sequential appearance of γδ- and αβ-bearing T cells in the peritoneal cavity during an i.p. infection with Listeria monozytogenes. *Eur J Immunol* 1990;20:533.

264. Ferrick D, Schrenzel M, Mulvania T, Hsieh B, Ferlin W, Lepper H. Differential production of interferon-γ and interleukin-4 in response to Th1- and Th2-stimulating pathogens by γδ T cells in vivo. *Nature* 1995;373:255.

265. Kaufmann S. Bacterial and protozoal infections in genetically disrupted mice. *Curr Opin Immunol* 1994;6:518.

266. Carding S, Allan W, Kyes S, Hayday A, K B, Doherty P. Late dominance of the inflammatory process in murine influenza by gamma/delta + T cells. *J Exp Med* 1990;172:1225.

267. Hiromatsu K, Yoshikai Y, Matsuzaki, G et al. A protective role of γ/δ T cells in primary infection with Listeria monocytogenes in mice. *J Exp Med* 1992;175:49.

268. Viney J, Dianda L, Roberts S, et al. Lymphocyte proliferation in mice congenitally deficient in T-cell receptor alpha beta + cells. *Proc Natl Acad Sci USA* 1994;91:11948.

269. Mombaerts P, Arnoldi J, Russ F, Tonegawa S, Kaufmann S. Different roles of αβ and γδ T cells in immunity against an intracellular bacterial pathogen. *Nature* 1993;365:53.

270. Kaufmann S, Ladel C. Role of T cell subsets in immunity against intracellular bacteria: experimental infections of knock-out mice with Listeria monocytogenes and Mycobacterium bovis BCG. *Immunobiology* 1994;191:509.

271. Kaufmann, SHE. γ/δ and other unconventional T lymphocytes: what do they see and what do they do? *Proc Natl Acad Sci USA* 1996;93:2272.

272. Komano H, Fuijura Y, Kawaguchi M, et al. Homeostatic regulation of intestinal epithelia by intraepithelial γδ T cells. *Proc Natl Acad Sci USA* 1995;92:

273. Kaufmann S, Blum C, Yamamoto S. Crosstalk between alpha/beta T cells and gamma/delta T cells in vivo: activation of alpha/beta T-cell responses after gamma/delta T-cell modulation with the monoclonal antibody GL3. *Proc Natl Acad Sci USA* 1993;90:9620.

274. McMenamin C, Pimm C, McKersey M, Holt P. Regulation of IgE responses to inhaled antigen in mice by antigen-specific gamma delta T cells. *Science* 1994;265:1869.

275. Wen L, Roberts S, Viney J, et al. Immunoglobulin synthesis and generalized autoimmunity in mice congenitally deficient in alpha beta(+) T cells. *Nature* 1994;369:654.

276. Horner A, Jabara H, Ramesh N, Geha R. Gamma/delta T lymphocytes express CD40 ligands and induce isotype-switching in B lymphocytes. *J Exp Med* 1995;181:1239.

277. Schild H, Mavaddat N, Litzenberger C, et al. The nature of major histocompatibility complex recognition by γδ T cells. *Cell* 1994;76:29.

278. Weintraub B, Jackson M, Hedrick S. Gamma delta T cells can recognize nonclassical MHC in the absence of conventional antigenic peptides. *J Immunol* 1994;153:3051.

279. Sciammas R, Johnson R, Sperling A, et al. Unique antigen recognition by a herpesvirus-specific TCR gamma delta cell. *J Immunol* 1994;152:5392.

280. Van Kaer L, Wu M, Ichikawa Y, et al. Recognition of MHC TL gene products by gamma delta T cells. *Immunol Rev* 1991;120:89.

281. Ito K, Van Kaer L, Bonneville M, Hsu S, Murphy D, Tonegawa S. Recognition of the product of a novel MHC TL region gene (27b) by a mouse gamma delta T cell receptor. *Cell* 1990;62:549.

282. Teitell M, Cheroutre H, Panwala C, Holcombe H, Eghtesady P, Kronenberg M. Structure and function of H-2 T (Tla) region class I MHC molecules. *Crit Rev Immunol* 1994;14:1.

283. Crowley MP, Reich Z, Mavaddat N, Altman JD, Chien Y. The recognition of the nonclassical major histocompatibility complex (MHC) class I molecule, T10, by the gamma delta T cell, G8. *J Exp Med* 1997;7:1223.

284. Schoel B, Sprenger S, Kaufmann S. Phosphate is essential for stimulation of V gamma 9V delta 2 T lymphocytes by mycobacterial low molecular weight ligand. *Eur J Immunol* 1994;24:1886.

285. Constant P, Davodeau F, Peyrat M, et al. Stimulation of human gamma delta T cells by nonpeptidic mycobacterial ligands. *Science* 1994;264:267.

286. Tanaka Y, Sano S, Nieves E, et al. Nonpeptide ligands for human gamma delta T cells. *Proc Natl Acad Sci USA* 1994;91:8175.

287. Tanaka Y, Morita C, Tanaka Y, Nieves E, Brenner M, Bloom B. Natural and synthetic non-peptide antigens recognized by human gamma delta T cells. *Nature* 1995;375:155.

288. Janis EM, Kaufman SHE, Schwartz RH, Pardoll DM. Activation of γδ T cells in the primary immune response to mycobacterium tuberculosis. *Science* 1989; 244:713.

289. Modlin RL, Pirmez C, Hofman FM, et al. Lymphocytes bearing antigen-specific γδ T-cell receptors accumulate in human infectious disease lesions. *Nature* 1989; 339:544.

290. Vidovic D, Roglic M, McKune K, Guerder S, MacKay C, Dembic Z. Qa-1 restricted recognition of foreign antigen by a gamma delta T-cell hybridoma. *Nature* 1989;340:646.

291. Holoshitz J, Vila LM, Keroack BJ, McKinley DR, Baynme NK. Dual antigenic recognition by cloned human γ-δ T-cells. *J Clin Invest* 1992;89:308.

292. Born W, Hall L, Dallas A, et al. Recognition of a peptide antigen by heat shock reactive γδ T lymphocytes. *Science* 1990;249:67.

293. Loh EY, Wang M, Bartkowiak J, et al. Gene transfer studies of T-cell receptor-γ/δ recognition. Specifity for staphylococcal enterotoxin-A is conveyed by V-γ-9 alone. *J Immunol* 1994;152:3324.

294. Kim HT, Nelson EL, Clayberger C, Sanjanwala M, Sklar J, Krensky AM. Gamma delta T cell recognition of tumor Ig peptide. *J Immunol* 1995;154:1614.

295. Rock E, Sibbald P, Davis M, Chien Y. CDR3 length in antigen-specific immune receptors. *J Exp Med* 1994;179:323.

296. Lerner E, Matis L, Janeway CJ, Jones P, Schwartz R, Murphy D. Monoclonal antibody against an Ir gene product? *J Exp Med* 1980;152:1085.

297. Ozato K, Mayer N, Sachs D. Hybridoma cell lines secreting monoclonal antibodies to mouse H-2 and Ia antigens. *J Immunol* 1980;124:533.

298. Fisch P, Malkovsky M, Kovats S, et al. Recognition by human Vγ9/Vδ2 T cells of a GroEL homolog on Daudi Burkitt's lymphoma cells. *Science* 1990;250: 1269.

299. Porgador A, Yewdell JW, Deng Y, Bennink JR, Germain RN. Localization, quantitation, and in situ detection of specific peptide-MHC class I complexes using a monoclonal antibody. *Immunity* 1997;6:715.

300. Dafaglio G, Nelson CA, Deck BM, Petzold SJ, Unanue ER. Characterization and quantitation of peptide-MHC complexes produced from hen egg lysozyme using a monoclonal antibody. *Immunity* 1997;6:727.

301. Lang F, Peyrat M, Constant P, et al. Early activation of human Vγ9Vδ2 T cell broad cytotoxicity and TNF production by nonpeptidic mycobacterial ligands. *J Immunol* 1995;154:5986.

302. Morita CT, Beckman EM, Bukaurki JF, et al. Direction presentation of nonpeptide prenyl pyrophosphate antigens to human γδ T cells. *Immunity* 1995;3:495.

303. Iwashima M, Green A, Bonyhadi M, Davis M, Allison J, Chien Y. Expression of a fetal γδ T-cell receptor in adult mice triggers a non-MHC-linked form of selective depletion. *Int Immunol* 1991;3:385.

304. Cunningham BC, Wells JA. Comparison of a structural and a functional epitope. *J Mol Biol* 1993;234:554.

305. Clackson T, Wells JA. A hot spot of binding energy in a hormone-receptor interface. *Science* 1995;267:383.

306. Davis MM, Chien Y, Arden B. The logic of immune recognition: correlating the genetics of antigen receptors with their function. *Proc Natl Acad Sci USA (submitted)*.

307. Berek C, Milstein C. The dynamic nature of the antibody repertoire. *Immunol Rev* 1988;105:5.

308. Patten PA, Gray NS, Yang PL, et al. The immunological evolution of catalysis. *Science* 1996;271:1078.

309. Taylor LD, Carmack CE, Huszar D, et al. Human immunoglobulin transgenes undergo rearrangement, somatic mutation and class switching in mice that lack endogenous IgM. *Int Immunol* 1994;6:579.

Fundamental Immunology, Fourth Edition,
edited by William E. Paul
Lippincott–Raven Publishers, Philadelphia © 1999.

CHAPTER 11

T-Lymphocyte Differentiation and Biology

Christophe Benoist and Diane Mathis

Key Elements of T-Lymphocyte Biology
T Cells Are Responsible for Cellular Immunity, in Its Diverse Manifestations · T Cells Recognize Antigen by Means of a Highly Variable Cell Surface Receptor · α:β T Cells Recognize Antigens as Peptide Fragments Bound to Major Histocompatibility Complex Class I and II Molecules · Most T Cells Are Produced in the Thymus but Some Are Not · Naive α:β T Cells Circulate Through Secondary Lymphoid Organs until They Encounter Antigen · There Are Two Major Lineages of T Cells (Each Subdivided) and Some Minor Ones

Important Tools and Techniques: Old and New
Cell Surface Markers · Polyclonal Mitogens and Superantigens · T-Cell Clones and Hybridomas · Fetal Thymic Organ Cultures · Radiation Bone Marrow Chimeras · Transgenic Mice · Gene-Targeted Mice

T-Cell Signaling

The Thymus: What It Is and What It Does
The Thymus of a Young Adult Mouse: Stromal Cells · The Thymus of a Young Adult Mouse: Thymocytes · The Pathway of T-Cell Differentiation · The Generation of T Cells Through Ontogeny

Important Events in the Life of a Thymocyte
Commitment to the T-Cell Lineage · TCR Gene Rearrangement · Pre-TCR mediated Selection · The α.β/γ:δ Split · Positive Selection: Generating a Self MHC–Restricted Repertoire · Negative Selection: Producing a Self-Tolerant Repertoire

Peripheral Circulation of T-Lymphocytes
Circuits · Adhesive Interactions

T-Cell Responses

T-Cell Effector Functions
B-Cell Help · Stimulation of Inflammation · Cytolysis · γ:δ Cells · Nonconventional T Cells · Regulation

T-Lymphocyte Memory

T-Cell Homeostasis and Life Span

Conclusions and Perspectives

References

T-lymphocytes are the most diverse and versatile of the immune system players. They circulate through the blood and lymphatic vessels, and populate the classical lymphoid organs such as the thymus, spleen, and lymph nodes, but they also can be found in large numbers at less expected sites, including the skin, gut, and liver. They are known to perform a variety of functions—killing unwanted cells, controlling the activities of immune system collaborators, secreting regulatory molecules—and the properties of certain of the less characterized subsets hint that other functions may await discovery. Thus, the goal of this chapter, to provide an overview of the properties and activities of T cells, is a difficult one. We will begin by preparing the stage: outlining some of the cardinal features of T-cell biology and briefly describing certain of the techniques and tools that have been crucial in their elucidation. Most of the points raised in this introductory material are more extensively addressed in other chapters or later in this one.

KEY ELEMENTS OF T-LYMPHOCYTE BIOLOGY

T Cells Are Responsible for Cellular Immunity, in Its Diverse Manifestations

Higher organisms can make both innate and adaptive immune responses when challenged with a foreign antigen. The adaptive response has two major arms: humoral immunity, which is mediated by antibodies secreted by B-lymphocytes, and cellular immunity, the domain of T-lymphocytes. The cellular arm is responsible for many of the immune reactions we commonly study, such as cell-mediated lympholysis (CML), delayed-type hypersensitivity (DTH), allograft rejection, and graft-versus-host (GVH) disease; it is also a major element in many autoimmune reactions.

Cellular immunity encompasses a wide array of cellular responses and cell–cell interactions. T cells are known to directly kill target cells, to provide "help" for such killers, to activate other immune system cells (like macrophages), to help B cells make an antibody response, to downmodulate the activities of various

C. Benoist and D. Mathis: Department of Immunology, Institut de Génétique et de Biologie Moléculaire et Cellulaire, 67400 Strasbourg, France.

immune system cells, and to secrete cytokines, chemokines, and other mediators. These diverse activities are often the domain of distinct types of T cells. Thus, for example, one hears of killer versus helper subsets (based on the primary effector function), of type 1 and type 2 helper classes (defined by cytokine secretion profiles), or of naive versus activated versus memory populations (based on their experience with antigen). Often the distinct T-cell types can be distinguished on the basis of their expression of particular cell surface markers, a classic example being display of the CD4 molecule and lack of expression of CD8 by the major helper cell subset, and the inverse pattern by the major subset of killers.

For a more elaborate introduction to cellular immunity, see Chapter 1.

T Cells Recognize Antigen by Means of a Highly Variable Cell Surface Receptor

A T-lymphocyte is provoked to activity when it recognizes a particular antigen via receptors displayed on its surface. T-cell receptors (TCRs) have many structural and functional analogies with the receptors on B cells, the immunoglobulins (Igs). Like the situation with B cells, the T-cell compartment as a whole can respond to billions of different antigens, but each individual cell is normally responsive only to a single antigen or, due to cross-reactivity, a limited number. This is because TCRs are tremendously diverse molecules, but each T cell usually displays only one molecular species at the surface.

TCR diversity is generated by many of the same mechanisms as those responsible for Ig diversification. Each TCR has two highly variable chains, either α and β or γ and δ, all members of the Ig superfamily (Fig. 1). Extensive sequence variability is achieved by the rearrangement of scattered gene segments; for example, for the murine β gene, one of about 25 variable (V) segments, one of two diversity (D) stretches, and one of 12 joining (J) segments are juxtaposed in the genome, and their common

transcript is spliced to those from the constant (C) region exons. In most cases, rearrangement of the different segments is essentially random, but there are exceptions, notably with γ:δ TCRs. Additional diversity arises from enzymatic additions and subtractions of nucleotides coincident with the joining of the different segments. Finally, variability is enhanced by the pairing of different α with β or γ with δ chains; again this is largely random, although not for certain γ:δ or for particular species of α:β TCRs (described below). So far, there is no indisputable evidence of TCR genes in functional T cells having undergone somatic hypermutation as is characteristic of Ig genes in responding B cells. This, coupled with the relatively limited number of V segments, means that most TCR diversity is concentrated in one stretch, the complementary determining region (CDR)-3.

Expression of a single species of TCR at the cell surface is achieved by two poorly understood processes called isotypic and allelic exclusion. Isotypic exclusion ensures that only α:β or only γ:δ chains are expressed on any one T cell, implying a choice of one lineage at the expense of the other. The result of allelic exclusion is that the product of the rearranged locus of only one of the chromosome pairs is expressed on any given T cell. As will be described below, neither isotypic nor allelic exclusion is an entirely faultless process.

None of the variable chains of the TCR has an extensive cytoplasmic tail that could function in signaling ligand engagement to the interior of the cell. Rather, this is performed by a complex of invariable chains called CD3, composed of two ε, one γ and δ, and two ζ-like chains (Fig. 1). A significant portion of each of these chains is intracytoplasmic and can potentially interact with signal-transducing molecules. It is possible that the different CD3 elements combine to form more than one signaling module that can transmit qualitatively different signals. The CD3 complex is also crucial for the intracellular transport of the variable TCR chains and their efficient display at the cell surface.

The TCR on α:β cells is almost always associated with one of two coreceptors at the cell surface, either CD4 or CD8 (Fig. 1). These molecules bind to a constant portion of the antigenic ligand (detailed in the next section), and both have cytoplasmic tails that bind the signal-transducing molecule p56 lck. The coreceptors are thought to increase the avidity of the interaction with ligand or to enhance signaling upon ligand engagement. Although CD4 and CD8 seem to have similar functions, they have distinct structures. Most γ:δ cells do not express a coreceptor.

Signaling through the TCR, in association with the CD4 or CD8 coreceptor, is not alone sufficient to stimulate a naive T cell to proliferate and secrete effector cytokines. A second, costimulatory, signal is also required. This is classically provided through engagement of the CD28 molecule on the T cell by the B7-1 and B7-2 molecules expressed on "professional" antigen-presenting cells (APCs) such as B cells, macrophages, and dendritic cells (Fig. 1). B7-1/2 engagement of a CD28 homologue called CTLA-4 also may provide costimulation under certain circumstances, especially once the response has been initiated, but more probably it exerts a negative influence. Not only does signaling through the TCR in the absence of a costimulatory signal not result in stimulation of the naive T cell, it actually induces a state of nonresponsiveness, called anergy, whereby the cell is no longer capable of responding productively even when provided with both stimulatory and costimulatory signals.

More detail on TCR structure can be found in Chapter 10, and on costimulation in Chapter 13.

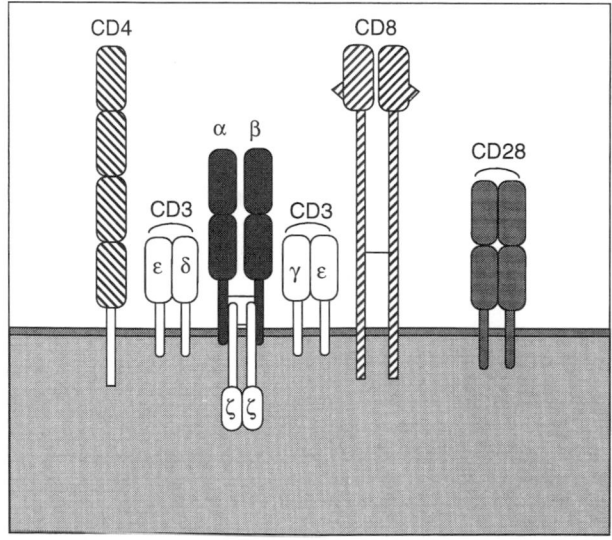

FIG. 1. The α:β TCR and associated molecules. Shown schematically are the α:β TCR, the various CD3 subunits, the CD4 and CD8 coreceptors, and the costimulatory molecule, CD28. The structure of CD3 is not known definitively; the current consensus is illustrated.

α:β T Cells Recognize Antigens as Peptide Fragments Bound to Major Histocompatibility Complex Class I and II Molecules

Unlike B cells, an α:β T cell can recognize an antigen only in association with one of the molecules encoded within the major histocompatibility complex (MHC), and then only if it is the appropriate allelic variant. This phenomenon, called MHC restriction, intrigued immunologists after its discovery in the 1970s, but its molecular basis became clear only gradually over the next 20 years, thanks largely to the cloning and sequencing of MHC genes and x-ray crystallographic analysis of the proteins they encode.

As mentioned above, mature α:β T cells can be divided into two major subsets according to whether they express the CD4 or CD8 coreceptor molecule. CD4+ and CD8+ cells differ in their primary effector function, in the class of MHC molecule they recognize antigens associated with, and in the types of antigen they monitor.

CD8+ α:β T cells are primarily responsible for the elimination of target cells via direct killing, e.g., cells infected by viruses or those expressing tumor-specific neoantigens. A CD8+ cell responds when its receptor recognizes a particular MHC class I molecule with a particular antigen associated (Fig. 2). The classical class I molecules are expressed throughout the body on essentially all cell types. They are composed of a heavy, or α, chain and a light chain, β2 microglobulin (β2μ), which is not encoded in the MHC. The membrane-distal α1 and α2 domains are highly polymorphic, whereas α3 is less polymorphic and has an Ig-like structure; β2μ also has an Ig-like structure and is essentially invariable in sequence. X-ray crystallographic studies have shown that most of the polymorphic residues contribute to the walls and floor of a cleft whose dimensions would accomodate a short peptide. Indeed, it is possible to load the "empty" class I molecules expressed on certain mutant cells with synthetic peptides in vitro, and to elute a heterogeneous set of peptides from the class I molecules displayed on the surface of normal cells. Peptides that can bind to class I molecules are usually eight to 10 amino acids long and have defined sequence motifs that vary with the particular class I isotype and allele to which they are binding, reflecting structural pockets in the cleft. These peptides are generated mostly from proteins synthesized within the target cell, primarily those residing in the cytoplasm. Proteosomes chop the cytosolic proteins into peptide

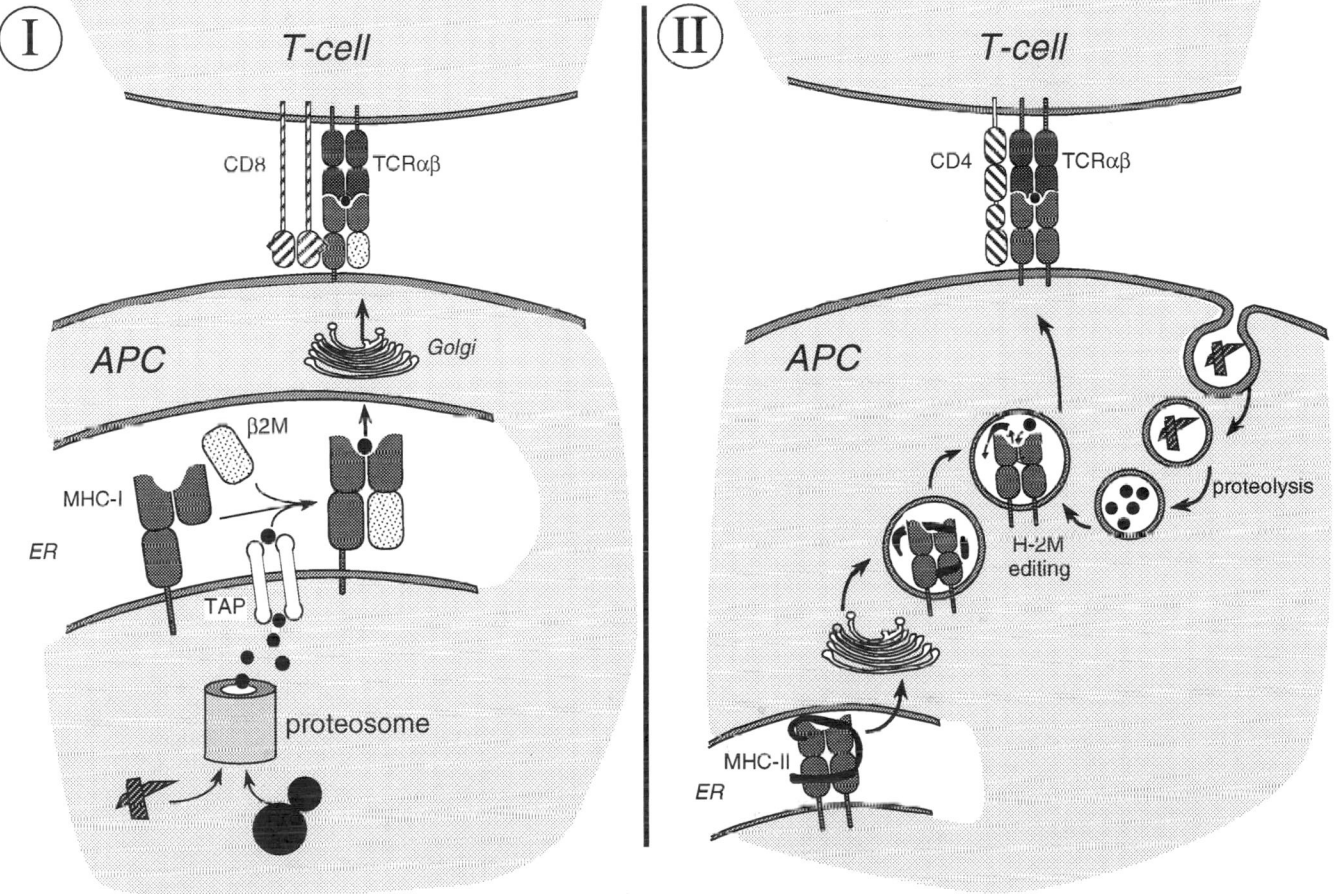

DOI 117

FIG. 2. MHC class I– and class–II restricted antigen presentation. To the left is illustrated the assembly of a peptide-loaded MHC class I molecule and its recognition by an α:β TCR on a CD8+ T cell. Peptides are derived from cytosolic proteins by proteosomal degradation and are carried into the lumen of the ER by the TAP transporter. To the right, assembly of a peptide-loaded class II molecule and its recognition by the TCR on a CD4+ T cell is schematized. The molecule shown associated with the class II dimer in the ER is the invariant chain. By the time the complex reaches the endosomal compartments, only a short fragment of it, called CLIP, is bound in the class II cleft. By a process involving the H-2M molecule, CLIP is replaced by peptides derived from proteins in the endosomes.

fragments, which are actively translocated into the lumen of the endoplasmic reticulum (ER) with the help of the transporter associated with antigen processing (TAP) molecule. In the ER, the peptide fragments bind to class I heavy- and light-chain dimers, conferring stability. The peptide–class I complexes follow the typical transport pathway to the cell surface, where they can be recognized by the receptor on CD8+ cells, the variable TCR chains focusing on the peptide and polymorphic residues contributing to the class I cleft, and the CD8 molecule binding to a constant stretch of sequence in the class I α3 domain.

CD4+ α:β T cells, on the other hand, primarily function by regulating other immune system cells, either by direct cell–cell contact or by secreting mediators. CD4+ cells respond when their TCRs see an antigen bound to an MHC class II molecule found on a limited set of cells in the body, particularly professional APCs, including B cells, macrophages, and dendritic cells (Fig. 2). Class II molecules are made up of an α and a β chain, once again members of the Ig superfamily. As for MHC class I molecules, the two membrane-distal domains, α1 and β1, are the most polymorphic, and the allelically variable residues are major components of a peptide-binding cleft. Recent x-ray crystallographic data showed that class I and class II molecules have a similar overall structure but that the latter has a shallower cleft, more open at the ends. Consequently, class II molecules can bind more extended peptides, usually about 13 to 15 amino acids long, but sometimes far longer; another consequence seems to be that the sequence motifs in class II molecules are less stringent, perhaps reflecting slippage within the groove. Peptides that bind to class II molecules are generated in the endosomal pathway either from endogenously synthesized proteins or from proteins or pathogens internalized from the surrounding milieu. After their synthesis in the ER, class II α and β chains combine with the invariant chain (Ii), which has the dual function of preventing the binding of peptides residing in the ER and of targeting the complex to the endosomal compartments. By an active process, heterogeneous peptides generated by vesicular proteases replace the invariant chain, now just a fragment, and then the peptide–class II complexes are exported by an unknown mechanism to the cell surface, where they can be recognized by CD4+ T cells. The variable TCR chains recognize the antigenic peptide and polymorphic region around the class II cleft, whereas the CD4 coreceptor binds to constant stretches along the class II α2 and β2 domains.

Thus, the immune system has evolved an effective means via the CD8+ cell/class I–restricted peptide, CD4+ cell/class II–restricted peptide dichotomy of bringing together antigens delivered by different routes and the effector cells most appropriate for eliminating them (Fig. 2).

γ:δ T cells also can recognize MHC class I and II molecules, but this is not a requirement. No peptide antigen has been identified so far; rather, a heterogeneous group of small phosphate-containing nonpeptide molecules. The interaction between the γ:δ TCR and its ligands appears to be quite different from α:β TCR recognition of peptide–MHC complexes, the former being more reminiscent of an antibody–antigen interaction.

For more information on the generation and recognition of TCR ligands, see Chapters 8 and 9.

Most T Cells Are Produced in the Thymus but Some Are Not

The thymus is the primary organ for producing T cells. Located in the upper thorax, it has two major components: stromal cells of different types and T-lymphocytes, also called thymocytes, at diverse stages of differentiation. The stromal cells include epithelial cells, macrophages, and dendritic cells and are organized into discrete architectural and functional regions. They produce a variety of soluble mediators and express MHC class I and II molecules, upon which the thymocytes are educated. T cells enter the thymus as poorly defined progenitors still capable of engendering a few other lymphoid lineages; they exit as mature cells that can respond to a multitude of foreign antigens presented in the context of the individual's self-MHC molecules but usually not to self antigens presented by self-MHC molecules. In between, an elaborate program of differentiation unfolds; in addition, massive proliferation and sorting occur such that only a small percentage of the cells produced in the thymus ever exits to the periphery. Important events that take place during this time include the following:

- The decision to become a T cell rather than, for example, a natural killer (NK) or dendritic cell
- Rearrangement of the TCR genes in order to generate a functional receptor
- The decision to become an α:β versus a γ:δ cell
- The decision to become a class I–restricted CD8+ or a class II–restricted CD4+ cell
- Shaping of the repertoire toward recognition of foreign antigens in association with self-MHC molecules (self-MHC restriction; positive selection)
- Purging of the repertoire to eliminate or inactivate most cells reactive to self antigens presented by self-MHC molecules (self tolerance; negative selection)

Some T cells also can be produced extrathymically. The best example of this is a larger population of cells residing in the intestine—intraepithelial lymphocytes (IELs)—thought to be produced in situ. Few, if any, of these cells are released into the circulation in normal animals, at least in mice.

Differentiation of T cells inside and outside the thymus is covered in more detail later in this chapter, as well as in Chapter 14.

Naive α:β T Cells Circulate Through Secondary Lymphoid Organs until They Encounter Antigen

After emerging from the thymus, most α:β T-lymphocytes enter a pool of cells that monitor the body for foreign antigens. The naive T-cell pool consists of small resting cells that have a long life span: months in mice, years in humans. These cells continuously recirculate from the bloodstream to central lymphatic vessels via the spleen, lymph nodes, and Peyer's patches. These secondary lymphoid organs have an intricate architecture that promotes the interaction between passing T cells and professional APCs. Macrophages and B cells present most of the particulate and soluble antigens filtered from the blood; mature dendritic cells present antigens that they captured as immature cells in nearby tissues or surfaces, prompting their differentiation and migration to the regional lymphoid organs.

If a given T cell meets its cognate antigen on a professional APC in a secondary lymphoid organ, it is retained, becomes activated, and proliferates, and its progeny differentiate. This process, called priming, results in a number of phenotypic alterations: changes in activation requirements and sensitivity, secretion of effector cytokines, expression of other effector functions, alterations in migratory properties, changes in life span. T cells primed in the peripheral lymphoid organs can migrate to the original site(s) of antigen exposure, for example, epithelial and mucosal surfaces and sites of inflammation. There they can be restimulated by cognate antigen and consequently express effector functions such as cytotoxicity and cytokine secretion.

Most activated cells become short-lived effector cells, but a proportion of them enters a long-lived "memory" T-cell pool. Memory T cells respond more rapidly to antigen challenge, at lower concentrations and in the absence of costimulation.

The activities of $\alpha{:}\beta$ T cells in the periphery, both before and after antigen challenge, are addressed later in this chapter, as well as in Chapters 26 and 31.

There Are Two Major Lineages of T Cells (Each Subdivided) and Some Minor Ones

Two major lineages of T-lymphocytes have been delineated on the basis of the gene segments that encode their TCRs. $\alpha{:}\beta$ T cells are responsible for most of the immune responses we presently study; $\gamma{:}\delta$ T cells can respond to antigenic challenge, although this has mostly been demonstrated under artificial experimental conditions. Besides the receptor chains they express, $\alpha{:}\beta$ and $\gamma{:}\delta$ lymphocytes have a number of distinct properties:

1. The timing of their appearance in ontogeny
2. Their pathway of differentiation in the thymus
3. Their distribution in the body
4. Their profile of diversity
5. The types of antigens they respond to and the manner in which they recognize them
6. The effector functions they perform

The two major T-cell lineages can be further subdivided. As mentioned above, most $\alpha.\beta$ T cells fall into two subpopulations, either the CD4 or CD8 coreceptor. These are commonly referred to as conventional T cells, and much of this chapter is devoted to their generation and behavior. Both subpopulations can be further split on the basis of the cytokines they produce, although this was first, and remains best, established for CD4$^+$ helpers. T helper (Th)1 cells secrete proinflammatory cytokines (interferon [IFN]-γ, cytokines of the tumor necrosis factor [TNF] family), whereas Th2 cells produce cytokines that generally stimulate Ig responses (interleukin [IL]-4, -5, -6, -9, and -10). These biases tend to be self-reinforcing: IL 10 represses Th1 cell activity; IL-4 stimulates and IFN-γ inhibits Th2 cells. It is not clear whether the Th1/Th2 distinction corresponds to a simple dichotomy or rather to two extreme poles, between which intermediate patterns of cytokine production can be found; in addition, there is mounting evidence for other helper classes. Nonetheless, the distinctions in effector capacity can have profound consequences on the ability of an animal to respond to microbiologic aggressions, depending on the particular pathogen. Whether a response is predominantly type 1 or type 2 is established in the first days and appears to depend on the dose of antigen, the local cytokine balance, and the type of APC.

$\gamma{:}\delta$ T cells as a group are composed of several distinct subpopulations, which appear at discrete times during ontogeny, express particular TCR chains, and have distinct tissue localizations. Some $\gamma{:}\delta$ cells with diverse TCR repertoires are found in the usual lymphoid organs and in the gut; others, which express essentially invariant receptors, are found only in external epithelia of the skin (DEC cells), the lung, or various mucosa (tongue, reproductive tract). Their generation and function are discussed at several points throughout the remainder of this chapter.

Some minor T-lymphocyte lineages also have been described, and certain of them are attracting increasing interest. Chief among these is a population of T cells expressing some markers usually found on NK cells, therefore termed NK-T cells. Most murine NK-T cells display only a limited subset of the possible TCR Vβ segments and an essentially monomorphic TCR α chain; the human equivalents express a homologous α chain with little variability. NK-T cells appear to follow an atypical pathway of differentiation in the thymus, and some may be produced extrathymically. Both their selection in the thymus and their activation in the periphery depend on nonclassical class I molecules, in particular CD-1. The function of NK-T cells is presently unknown but may be related to an unusual profile of cytokine secretion.

Nonconventional, especially $\gamma{:}\delta$, T cells are discussed at several points throughout the remainder of this chapter.

IMPORTANT TOOLS AND TECHNIQUES: OLD AND NEW

Throughout the years, a number of tools and techniques have been critical for studies on T-lymphocyte differentiation and biology. Certain of them have permitted a "quantum leap" in our understanding of important issues. Some are unique to the field of immunology, but most were perspicaciously adapted from other domains. The most significant are discussed in this section.

Cell Surface Markers

T-lymphocytes display hundreds of different proteins at the cell surface. The expression of certain of them changes with the state of maturation or varies in cells with different functions. Such proteins can be used as markers for particular T-cell differentiation stages or T effector classes after "tagging" with a specific antibody, now routinely a monoclonal antibody (mAb). Alone or in combination, mAbs against cell surface markers can be used to visualize a subset of T cells, purify it, deplete it, or block it. The most sophisticated visualization and purification of T-cell subsets is presently performed using a flow cytometer to detect as many as six fluorescent mAb-tagged markers.

Table 1 lists some of the cell surface markers commonly used in studies on T-lymphocytes.

Polyclonal Mitogens and Superantigens

T cells reactive to any particular antigen normally constitute only a minute fraction of the repertoire. Thus, it is extremely difficult to monitor their behavior upon activation and to elucidate any biochemical changes that might take place. This problem has been circumvented by using reagents that stimulate a much larger fraction of the T-cell repertoire. One class consists of the polyclonal mitogens, such as phytohemagglutinin and concanavalin A, which induce mitosis in almost all T cells by a mechanism that is independent of the variable TCR chains. They have been widely used in in vitro studies of the T-cell activation process. A second class comprises the superantigens (sAgs), including certain bacterial endotoxins and products of endogenous retrovirus genomes (1). Superantigens, at extremely low doses, stimulate large numbers of T cells by forming a bridge between a region outside CDR 3 on a subset of Vβ chains and an area on MHC class II molecules that is mostly exterior to the cleft. T cells respond to sAgs in a manner that is sim-

TABLE 1. *T-cell surface markers*

CD name	Distribution on T cells	Function	Other names
CD1a,b,c,d	Cortical thymocytes	MHC class I–like molecule	
CD2	Most thymocytes and T cells	Adhesion molecule; binds CD58 (LFA-3).	LFA-2
CD3	Thymocytes and T cells	Part of the TCR complex	
CD4	Thymocyte subsets, helper and inflammatory T cells	TCR co-receptor for MHC class II molecules	L3T4
CD5	Thymocytes and T cells	T cell activation; binds to CD72	Ly1
CD7	Thymocytes and T cells	Unknown	
CD8	Thymocyte subsets, cytotoxic T cells	TCR co-receptor for MHC class I molecules	Lyt2,3
CD11a	Broad distribution	Adhesion molecule; binds to CD54 (ICAM-1), ICAM-2 and ICAM-3	LFA-1
CD25	Immature thymocytes, activated T cells	IL-2 receptor subunit	Tac, IL-2Rα
CD28	Thymocytes and T cells	Positive regulation of T cell activation; ligand for B7-1 and B7-2	
CD44	Thymocyte subsets, activated T cells	Adhesion; binds hyaluronic acid	Pgp-1
CD45	Thymocytes and T-cell subsets	Tyrosine phosphatase; augments signaling through the TCR; multiple isoforms result from alternative splicing	LCA, B220
CD49d	Thymocytes	α4- integrin; binds fibronectin, Mad CAM-1, VCAM-1	VLA-4
CD54	Broad distribution	Adhesion molecule, binds CD11A/CD18 integrin (LFA-1) and CD11b/CD18 integrin (Mac-1)	ICAM-1
CD58	Broad distribution	Adhesion molecule; binds CD2	LFA-3
CD62L	T cells, mostly naive	Mediates rolling interactions with endothelium; binds CD34, GlyCAM	LAM-1, L-selectin, LECAM-1
CD90	Thymocytes and T cells (mouse); prothymocytes (human)	Unknown	Thy-1
CD95	Uncertain; activated T cells	Induces apoptosis; binds Fas-L	Apo-1, Fas
CD117	Immature thymocytes	Stem cell factor (SCF) receptor	c-kit
CD119	Mature T cells	IFN-γ receptor subunit	IFN-γR
CD124	Mature T cells	IL-4 receptor subunit	Il-4Rα
CD127	Immature thymocytes, mature T cells	Il-7 receptor subunit	Il-7Rα
CD152	Activated T cells	Negative regulator of T-cell activation; ligand for B7-1 and B7-2	CTLA-4
CD154	Activated T cells, mostly CD4+	T cell help; ligand for CD40	CD40-L
	Activated T cells	Ligand for CD95	Fas-L

ilar, but not identical, to that by which they react to peptide antigens. sAgs have been particularly useful for studies on negative selection in the thymus and periphery, but also have been used in a number of in vitro contexts.

T-Cell Clones and Hybridomas

It is possible to establish long-term lines of T cells reactive to a single antigen by plating primed cells in vitro and restimulating them at regular intervals. A clone of T cells displaying a single TCR can then be derived by limiting dilution. T-cell clones are good tools because they can maintain antigen specificity over long periods and because their behavior upon antigen stimulation is easily assayed and seems to reflect that of antigen-stimulated T cells in vivo. However, they can be tedious to maintain and slow to grow.

T-cell hybridomas, on the other hand, are quite simple to generate and propagate. Hybridomas are produced by fusing a population of antigen-stimulated T cells with a T-cell lymphoma line (a lymphoma that does not express the variable TCR chains); they are subsequently cloned by limiting dilution. Growth of hybridomas is conveniently antigen independent and rapid, and they respond to antigen stimulation by secreting easily assayed cytokines. Unfortu-

nately, hybridomas can be genetically unstable, and their phenotype and behavior upon stimulation is influenced by the genome of the lymphoma fusion partner. They are also unsuitable for in vivo transfer studies.

Because of their many advantages (and despite their disadvantages), much of what we know about T-lymphocyte specificity and effector function derives from experiments that have used T-cell clones or hybridomas expressing a single TCR specificity (2).

Fetal Thymic Organ Cultures

A thymus removed from a mouse embryo before the 14th day of fetal development contains epithelial stromal cells and only immature thymocytes. However, if it is cultured in vitro under the appropriate conditions, the immature thymocytes will differentiate fairly normally along the usual pathways, and fully mature T cells will eventually emerge (3). Fetal thymus organ cultures (FTOCs) have revealed much important information about thymocyte differentiation.

One often-used variation of the standard FTOC is a chimeric system where the immature thymocytes in the excised thymus are destroyed by irradiation or treatment with 2-deoxyguanosine and replaced with precursor cells from another individual. Another is a disaggregation–reaggregation system, whereby cells of the excised organ are dispersed by enzyme treatment, depleted of certain components or supplemented with extraneous constituents, and then permitted to aggregate into a thymuslike organ in culture (4).

Radiation Bone Marrow Chimeras

If an animal is treated with the appropriate dose of ionizing radiation from an x-ray or γ-ray source, essentially all cells of hematopoietic origin are destroyed, but the epithelial stromal cells in the primary and secondary lymphoid organs remain and are functional. It is possible to transfer hematopoietic stem cells (usually obtained from the bone marrow) from one animal into a different irradiated individual and thereby generate a chimera whose hematopoietic cells, including all lymphocyte populations, are essentially only of donor origin (Fig. 3). It is also possible to transfer donor cells derived from more than one animal into a single host to produce a mixed bone marrow chimera. Radiation bone marrow chimeras have been exploited extensively in studies on T-cell repertoire selection, particularly for elucidating the principles of MHC restriction, as discussed below.

More recently, a variant strategy has become popular, aimed at avoiding irradiation-induced damage to host cells of non-hematopoietic origin, which has been suspected in several studies. Hematopoietic stem cells are transferred into unirradiated or only lightly irradiated hosts congenitally lacking hematopoietic (or just lymphoid) cells because of a natural or engineered mutation: most commonly mice bearing the severe combined immunodeficiency (SCID) mutation or a null mutation in one of the recombination activator genes (RAGs). The SCID mouse also has been used as a host for human lymphoid organ fragments (including some stem cells), permitting the reconstitution of certain aspects of the human immune system (5).

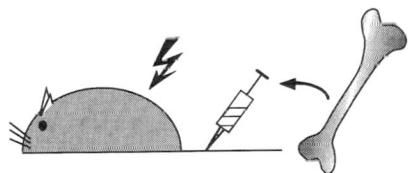

Host	Donor
	Stem cells
	↳ T lymphocytes
	↳ B lymphocytes
MØ, DC	
Epithelia (cortex, medulla, extra-thymic)	

FIG. 3. Construction of a radiation bone marrow chimera. Irradiation of a mouse destroys hematopoietic cells but not epithelial stromal cells in the primary or secondary lymphoid organs. Injection of bone marrow cells from another mouse containing hematopoietic stem cells leads to a chimeric animal after 1 or 2 months: lymphocytes derived from the donor, APCs from both the donor and host (macrophages can be quite radioresistant), and epithelial cells from the host (MØ, macrophages, DC, dendritic cells).

Transgenic Mice

It is now routine practice to insert extraneous genetic material into the genome of a mouse by transgenesis (6). Cloned DNA fragments are injected into a fertilized egg, which is then implanted into the uterus of a foster mother. Among her offspring are a few carrying the injected DNA stably integrated into the genome, and these can be used as founders to propagate a transgenic line. At present, it is not possible to control the site of DNA integration or the number of fragments incorporated, resulting in some variation in the levels and precise patterns of transgene expression in lines derived from different founders. Nevertheless, transgenic mice have been put to good use to dissect gene regulatory elements, to target protein expression to a particular cell type, to evaluate the effect of overexpression or misexpression of a protein, or to inhibit a protein via synthesis of a dominant-negative mutant.

TCR transgenic mice have proven particularly valuable for studies on T-cell differentiation, most notably for experiments aimed at elucidating the positive and negative selection processes (7). If already rearranged TCR α and β genes are inserted into the mouse genome, allelic exclusion of the endogenous TCR loci takes place so that the T-cell repertoire is highly skewed for the transgene-encoded specificity. Thus, instead of the usual one in 10^4 to 10^6, a given specificity can represent as much as 1%, 10%, or more than 90% of the repertoire, depending on the efficiency of allelic exclusion at the endogenous TCR loci. A monoclonal mouse can be generated by introducing into the TCR transgenic line an SCID or RAG mutation that abrogates endogenous TCR gene rearrangement (8).

The most recent advances in transgenesis technology have adapted prokaryotic transcriptional regulatory systems to permit controllable expression of transgenes (both the level and timing of expression). So far, most success has been achieved with a tetracycline-regulatable system, adapting elements of the tet operon from *Escherichia coli* (9,10).

Gene-Targeted Mice

Techniques for targeting a deletion, insertion, or substitution to a specific locus in the genome of a mouse also have become routine, although they remain time consuming (11). First, the desired mutation of the chosen gene is introduced into undifferentiated embryonic stem (ES) cells via homologous recombination between the gene residing in the cells' genome and a targeting vector containing an engineered variant of it. Next, ES cells carrying the mutation are injected into a blastocyst, which is then reimplanted into the uterus of a foster mother; the ES cells are potentially capable of giving rise to all cell lineages, including the germline. Offspring carrying the modified locus in the germline in a heterozygous state are propagated and mated to produce animals with the homozygous mutation. Mice carrying targeted mutations of specific genes are now important tools in all areas of immunology, often permitting cleaner experiments and novel approaches (12). However, the possibility of functional redundancy of certain gene products and long-term phenotypic adaptations to certain mutations must always be borne in mind.

Mutations, especially in the null form, are often lethal at a stage of mouse development that is too early to permit an assessment of the immune system. Nevertheless, certain aspects of immune system development and function can be studied in chimeras constructed by injecting ES cells bearing a homozygous null mutation into RAG-deficient, instead of the standard, blastocysts (13). In mice lacking RAG products, B- and T-lymphocyte differentiation is cleanly arrested at a very immature stage due to the inability to make Igs and TCRs. In the chimeras, then, nonlymphoid cells are of both ES cell and blastocyst origin, permitting the animal to survive, but all lymphocytes that progress beyond the RAG block derive from the ES cells and thus carry the mutation of interest.

More recent advances in gene-targeting technology have exploited elements of prokaryotic site-specific recombination systems, most notably the cre-loxP system from the bacteriophage P1, to permit spatial and temporal control of the engineered mutation (14,15). This approach usually requires two mouse lines: in one, the targeted locus is flanked by sequences containing the specific recognition site (loxP) of the recombinase; in a second line, the recombinase (cre) is synthesized in a cell type–specific or inducible fashion, usually as a transgene but sometimes after insertion into a chosen locus; crossing the two lines together results in controlled deletion or modification of the target gene (9,16,17). An alternative strategy is to express in the second line a fusion between cre and a steroid hormone ligand-binding domain, thus rendering cre activity hormone regulatable (18).

T-CELL SIGNALING

Recognition of a peptide–MHC complex is the key event for many aspects of T-cell physiology. Engagement of the TCR prompts it to cluster in concert with a group of other surface proteins (19); a signal is then relayed to the cell nucleus, provoking modifications in the transcription program. The complexities of signal transduction in T cells will be outlined below as they are crucial to an understanding of T-cell differentiation.

A central concept is that signaling through the TCR is a highly variable and adaptable process (20,21); it can lead to any one of several outcomes when triggered by peptide–MHC ligands for which the TCR has only fine differences in affinity/avidity (22,23). In early thymocytes, TCR engagement may result in further differentiation, but also in apoptosis; in mature T cells, it can lead to proliferation or to anergy. Thus, the signal transduction systems must be able to amplify small differences in TCR ligands, such as variations in their thermodynamic characteristics or in the conformational changes they impose on the TCR. TCR signaling does not behave as an on/off switch but as a high-gain transistor. It is powerful, though, in that a hundred or more genes may be activated as a result (24). These properties are achieved by a transduction system that branches out quickly along several parallel pathways (e.g., Ca^{2+}, protein kinase C [PKC], ras). However, there is extensive cross-talk between the signaling pathways, and they can converge in part on the same families of transcription factors. Finally, another central notion is that, like most biologic processes, signal transduction from the TCR is based on a cascade of phosphorylations that can have positive or negative consequences depending on their context.

Figure 4 schematizes the concentric shock waves of signal that radiate from the TCR after engagement. It is probably fair to state that our global grasp of the pathways and their integration decreases with the distance from the TCR. At the very center are the immunoreceptor tyrosine-phophorylated activation motifs (ITAMs) located in the cytoplasmic tails of the CD3 subunits. Their consensus sequence, YXXL/I(X6–8)YXXL/I, is also found in other activation molecules, such as the Ig transduction complex. ITAMs are the focus of the activation event, undergoing phosphorylation

that in turn creates binding sites for the SH2 domains of several downstream factors. Although analogous in structure and largely interchangeable, each ITAM in the complex may not relay quite the same signal, and it is here that differential handling of the signal begins. The next level is that of the protein tyrosine kinases (PTKs), whose interplay is reasonably well understood (25,26). They comprise the src family kinases (the lck/fyn pair). Lck is brought into the signaling complex via its association with the cytoplasmic tails of the CD4 and CD8 co-receptors, and phosphorylates ITAMs; the ZAP70/syk pair, whose SH2 domains bind phosphorylated ITAMs, are then phosphorylated by lck/fyn kinases (and autophosphorylate when juxtaposed). These sets of kinases are essential for signaling, and although there is some internal redundancy within each pair, at least one member is absolutely required at all steps of T-cell differentiation (27–30). At this level of the signal transduction cascade, dampening influences are already found: the csk kinase phosphorylates the regulatory tyrosines of lck/fyn, thus inhibiting their activity (31). This phosphate is removed by the phophatase activity of CD45, which thus acts to enhance TCR signaling (32). Several regulatory phosphatases (e.g., SHP-1, SHP-2) dampen ZAP-70 phosphorylation and consequently TCR-induced activation (33–35).

After the PTKs comes a set of adaptor molecules which serve to connect the tyrosine phosphorylation events with the main downstream pathways. These mainly consist of SH2/SH3 domains, and most are not specific to T cells. Their connections are quite difficult to decipher: grb2, for example, is the classical relay to the ras pathway through the Sos adaptor, yet it also can interact with the Shc, LAT, cbl, or SLP76 adaptors (21,36). It is also difficult to assign unique adaptors to any of the main signaling pathways that are found downstream. Many of these are essential to T-cell physiology, and it is presumably their combinatorial recruitment that relays differential TCR signaling.

The main pathways that adaptor factors feed into are also those commonly involved in signal transduction in a variety of systems, from yeast to mammals. 1) Phospholipase C (PLC)-γ1 is recruited to the cell membrane and cleaves phospholipids to generate inositol 1,4,5 triphosphate (IP3) and diacylglycerol (DG). IP3 induces the release of Ca^{2+} from intracellular stores (the classical immediate signal in T-cell activation readouts), which activates several calcium-dependent enzymes (CaMK, calcineurin) impacting directly on transcription factors. The best studied example is the calcineurin pathway that results in release, dephosphorylation, and nuclear translocation of NF-AT (37). DG stimulates the PKC family; here again, this large family of enzymes with different biochemical properties has a varied impact on T-cell physiology—both a positive one by activating mitogen-response transcription factors and a negative one via cross-talk with PKA (19,38–40). 2) The GTP-binding proteins ras and rac/rho are at the apex of a cascade of serine/threonine kinases (MAPKKKs activating MAPKKs, activating MAPKs). There are many such S/T kinases at each level, which are differentially triggered by ras- or rac/rho-derived signals (36). They eventually impact on gene expression and cell cycle by phosphorylating transcription or cell-cycle-control factors. 3) Phosphoinositide 3-kinase (PI3K) is activated. Its phospholipiel products activate several other kinases (PKC, the S/T cascade), particularly PKB (or c-akt), which has antiapoptotic properties through interaction with the bcl family (41,42). As was the case at higher levels, there is substantial cross-talk between these pathways (e.g., Ca^{2+} affects the activity of the calcium-sensitive PKC isoforms, PI3K affects PKC).

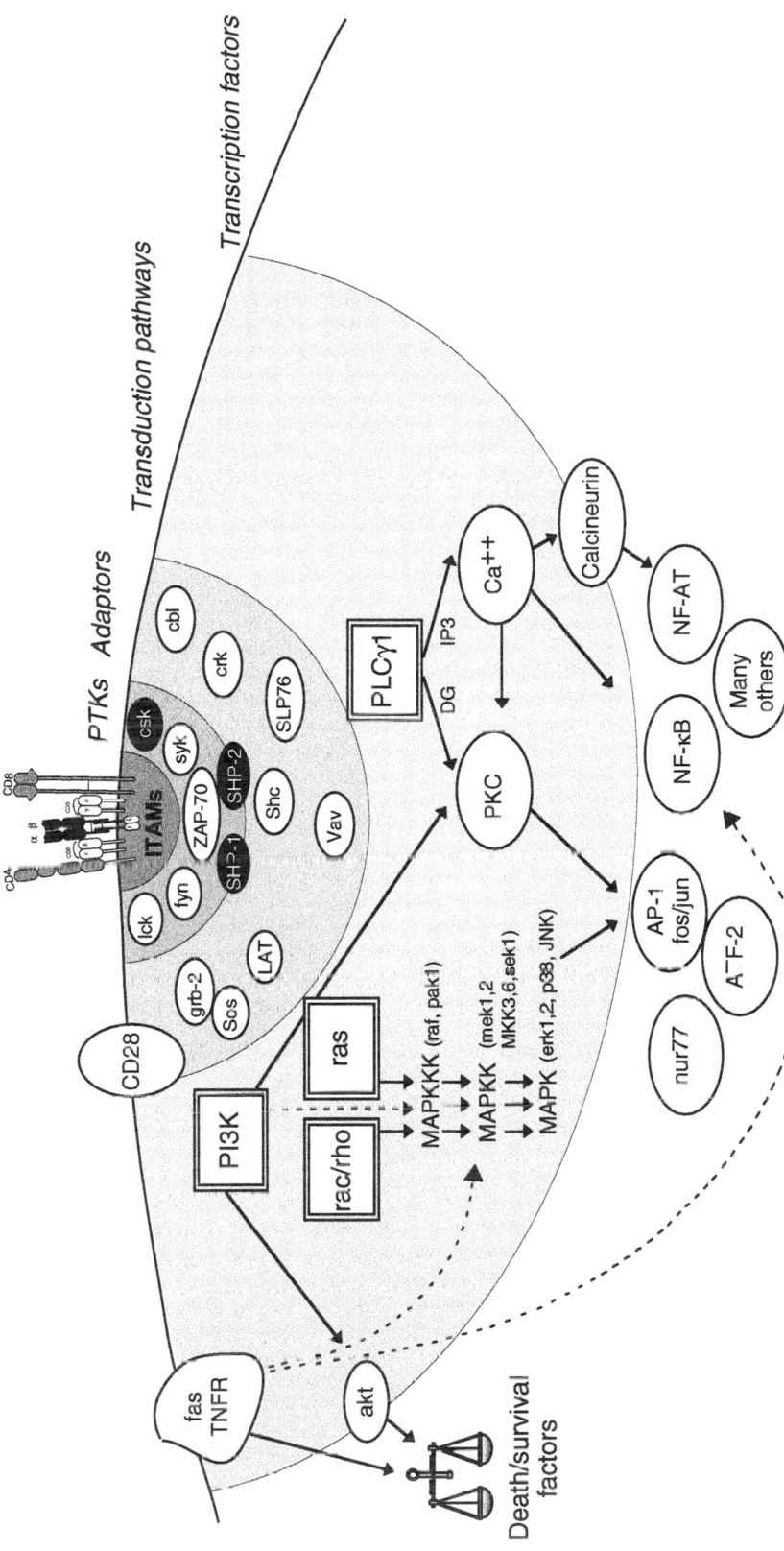

FIG. 4. Signal transduction in T cells: from the TCR to gene control. A schematic representation of the players involved in relaying the activation signal that derives from engagement of the TCR by cognate MHC–peptide complexes. At the apex of the signaling cascades are the ITAM motifs of the intracellular portion of CD3 chains, which are the focus of phosphorylation by several tyrosine-kinases; negative control at this level is confered by several phosphatases or kinases (*black symbols*). The various adaptor molecules of the next circle (lnk, grb-2, Shc, etc.), in succession or in combination, transduce the tyrosine phosphorylation signals to the main activation pathways: the S/T kinase cascades downstream from the ras or rac/rho G-proteins (shown here as generic MAPKKK, MAPKK, and MAPK factors, but which include several distinct phosphorylation cascades triggered by the different inputs), phosphoinositol metabolism through PI-3-kinase or phospholipase-C (*squares*). These pathways terminate by activating transcription factors by a variety of means: induced synthesis, activation through phosphorylation, derepression, proteolytic activation, induced translocation to the nucleus. Concomitant signaling to the protein families that control cell death and survival is a so indicated.

At the level of transcription factors themselves, it is even harder to draw a comprehensive picture of the interplay between activators that respond to TCR triggering and T-lineage–specific transcription factors expressed at particular stages of T-cell differentiation. Few T-lymphocyte–specific promoters have been studied in much detail, the best example being the IL-2 enhancer–promoter complex (24). The activation pathways outlined above converge on generic activation factors such as the fos/jun (AP1), ATF, NF-AT, and NF-kB families. Together (heterodimer formation between such factors being a common feature) they generate the responses to TCR engagement: entry into the cell cycle, apoptosis, cytokine gene expression, and activation or repression of differentiation stage-specific genes. Several T cell–specific transcription factors have been described (43,44). A few have been demonstrated in knockout experiments to be specifically required for different events related to T-cell physiology (e.g., Tcf-1, LKLF, IRF-1, Ets-1) (45–48), but at present an integrated view of T cell–specific transcription is beyond our reach.

Of course, the intricacies of TCR-promoted responses are only a fraction of the signals a T cell must integrate. Its fate also will be determined by ligand binding through cytokine receptors, whose signals are primarily mediated through the JAK/STAT chain (49) or through the tangled death signaling pathways initiated by the TNFR/Fas surface molecules (50,51).

A much more detailed treatment of T-cell activation and all aspects of signaling can be found in Chapter 12.

THE THYMUS: WHAT IT IS AND WHAT IT DOES

Most T-lymphocytes that circulate via the blood and lymph and populate the spleen and lymph nodes are produced in the thymus. The thymus is found in the upper thorax of vertebrate animals, resting on the heart and extending into the base of the neck. It is bilaterally symmetrical, composed of two discreet lobes that join at the midline. It consists primarily of T cells at various stages of differentiation (thymocytes) and a heterogeneous set of supporting cells (forming the stroma).

That the thymus is a major producer of lymphocytes was first established in the early 1960s when neonatally thymectomized mice were found to have a reduction in lymphocyte numbers and deficient immune capabilities—for example, they were unable to clear viral infections or reject skin grafts (52). An association between the lack of a thymus and defective lymphocyte pools and immune responses also was noted for children with the DiGeorge syndrome (53). That the thymus generates only some lymphocytes—T cells—was recognized soon thereafter, as was the fundamental division of immune system labor between T and B cells, initially through experiments on chickens (54).

Our understanding of the intricacies of the thymus and of the details of thymocyte differentiation has increased enormously over the past decade, largely through studies on the mouse. Thus, we would like to begin this section with an instructive snapshot: a description of the steady-state thymus in a young adult mouse, first the stromal cell and then the thymocyte component. We will then provide a more dynamic view by tracking the pathway of T-cell differentiation in the young adult, as well as by following the development of the thymus and differentiation of thymocytes through ontogeny. Information on the thymus in humans and in evolutionarily more primitive species will be integrated when of particular interest.

The Thymus of a Young Adult Mouse: Stromal Cells

The thymic lobes of a young mouse are surrounded by a capsule of connective tissue, which repeatedly invaginates to form septae demarcating numerous lobules, each filled with stroma and thymocytes (Fig. 5). The stromal cells are very heterogeneous, as assessed by morphologic criteria and by patterns of staining with a panel of mAbs (55–57). Most prominent is an extensive network of epithelial cells of diverse types. Interspersed within this network are some mesenchymal cells, mainly fibroblasts, and a number of hematopoietic cells, primarily macrophages and dendritic cells (more precisely, interdigitating cells). Some B cells, mostly of the B-1 class, are also present, but these are concentrated at the ends of the septae.

The stromal cells segregate into three architecturally and, as we shall see later, functionally distinct regions (Fig. 5). Above all, these regions can be distinguished according to their most dominant stromal cell types. From the exterior to the interior: the subcapsular zone is characterized by baskets of epithelial reticular cells, the cortex by a network of spider-shaped and sheetlike epithelial cells, and the medulla by a network of stubby epithelial cells and numerous dendritic cells. The less prominent stromal cell types are also differentially distributed between the three regions—

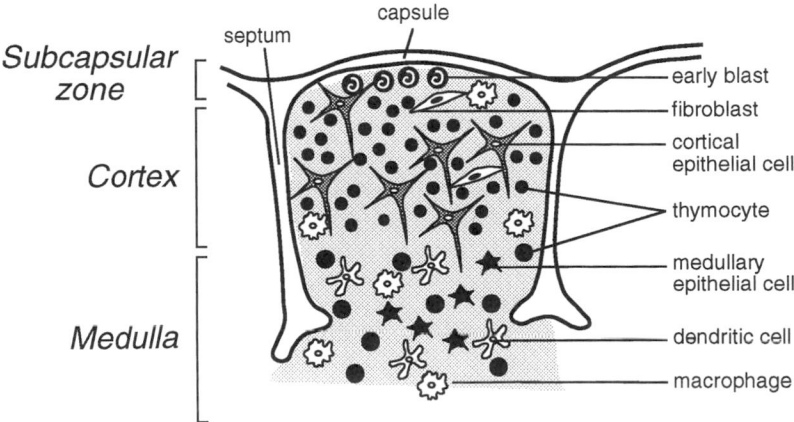

FIG. 5. Thymus organization. A thymus section through a single lobule is shown. The different forms of stromal cells are indicated: cortical and medullary epithelial cells, dendritic cells, macrophages, and fibroblasts. Some of these, such as medullary epithelial cells, actually comprise distinct cell types (56). The maturation of thymocytes from blasts in the subcapsular zone, to small resting cells in the cortex, to larger medullary cells is also illustrated.

fibroblasts primarily in the cortex, macrophages throughout the cortex and medulla, and B cells at the junction between the cortex and medulla. Reflecting their different cell-type compositions, the three stromal regions show distinct patterns of staining for MHC molecules: weak staining in the subcapsular zone, a reticular pattern in the cortex (due to the epithelial cell network), and a confluent staining pattern in the medulla (due mainly to dendritic cells and a subset of epithelial cells).

A stromal component that is undoubtedly important but that has been neglected until quite recently is the extracellular matrix (ECM) (57,58). It consists of certain of the collagens, glucosaminoglycans, and glycoproteins such as fibronectin and laminin, secreted by epithelial cells and fibroblasts.

It should be kept in mind that although stromal cells and thymocytes are the major components of the thymus, they are not the only ones. Connective tissue, nervous tissue, blood vessels, lymphatic vessels, even primitive muscle cells have all been found in the thymus and should be considered when contemplating its activities.

The Thymus of a Young Adult Mouse: Thymocytes

The thymus of a young mouse contains a few hundred million thymocytes. These include undifferentiated progenitors, fully differentiated T cells of various types, and all of the intermediate maturational stages. The different types of thymocytes can be identified by their profiles of surface marker expression (59). Most commonly, one sees profiles of CD4 versus CD8 expression, as in the cytofluorimetric analysis presented in Fig. 6. Four major populations are evident:

- CD4⁻CD8⁻ (double-negative [DN]) cells constitute about 5% of thymocytes. This is a very heterogeneous population that can be subdivided at a first level on the basis of TCR expression. A minor subpopulation displays the γ:δ TCR and contains the more mature thymocytes of the γ:δ lineage; another displays the α:β

TCR, and its origin and fate are a mystery, except that it includes the precursors of NK-T cells. The major subpopulation of DN cells (two thirds of the total) expresses neither the α:β nor the γ:δ receptor and is therefore often called the triple-negative (TN; CD4⁻CD8⁻TCR/CD3⁻) subpopulation. It can be further split into four components according to expression of the CD44 and CD25 molecules. Some important differences characterizing cells of the CD44⁺25⁻, CD44⁺25⁺, CD44^{lo}25⁺, and CD44⁻25⁻ subsets are the rearrangement status of their TCR-β genes, whether they express the β chain at the cell surface, the proportion of dividing cells, their dependence on mesenchymal cells (60), and their response to or dependence on various cytokines (61).

- CD4⁺CD8⁺ (double-positive [DP]) cells make up the large majority of thymocytes (about 80%). They have rearranged TCR-α and -β genes, and most express at least low levels of the α:β TCR/CD3 complex on the surface. Most DPs are small resting cells, but there is a significant proportion of dividing blasts. The DP population contains most of the apoptotic cells present in the thymus (62) and is particularly sensitive to death-inducing agents such as the glucocorticoids.

- CD4⁺8⁻ and CD4⁻8⁺ (single-positive [SP]) cells together constitute about 15% of thymocytes; the ratio of the two subpopulations varies in different mouse strains and in individual humans, under genetic control (63,64). Both SP subpopulations can be subdivided on the basis of TCR expression: a minor, immature fraction (ISP) expresses only low levels of CD3 and no detectable α:β or γ:δ TCR; the major, mature, fraction displays high levels of α:β TCR in association with CD3. In humans, the immature component is more prominent in the CD4⁺8⁻ than the CD4⁻8⁺ compartment (65), whereas the reverse is true in most mice, although there is some strain-to-strain variation (66). The majority of ISP cells are dividing blasts; although most of the mature cells are in the resting state, it is possible to detect a few in division. The mature component includes cells with variable expression levels of several cell surface markers, e.g., heat stable antigen (HSA), the receptor for peanut agglutinin (PNAr), and the activation molecule CD69. This is paralleled by variable degrees of immunocompetence. The SP compartment includes a small fraction of cells that have returned to the thymus after activation in the periphery (67).

The Pathway of T-Cell Differentiation

The last two sections provided a snapshot of T-cell differentiation—a frozen image of the steady-state thymus in a young adult mouse. Converting this to a more dynamic view has proven very challenging because of the multiplicity and interconnectedness of the events that take place, and because of the convoluted routes thymocytes sometimes follow. Early attempts to construct a pathway of T-cell differentiation were content with following a logical sequence of surface marker turn-on and turn-off, but this approach often resulted in errors. Now it is clear that one must evaluate experimentally, for each thymocyte subset, what cells can give rise to it and what cells it can engender. This can be done by purifying a defined subset and monitoring its behavior after introduction into an FTOC system or, even better, after injection directly into the thymus of an appropriate host. Another useful approach is to label dividing cells with nucleotide precursors (³H-thymidine [TdR] or bromodeoxyuridine [BrdU]) and to watch the flow of label into different thymocyte subsets with time. Using such strategies, the following

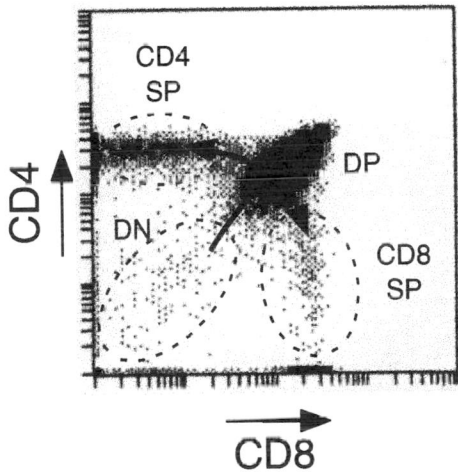

FIG. 6. A typical cytofluorimetric analysis of thymocytes. Thymocytes from a 6-week-old mouse are stained with mAbs specific for CD4 and CD8. The mAbs were labeled with two different fluorescent compounds allowing simultaneous detection of the two coreceptors. The four major thymocyte populations are delineated: DN, DP, CD4 SP, and CD8 SP. The major flow of T cell differentiation is indicated by arrows: DN → DP → CD4 SP or CD8 SP. Courtesy of M. Correia-Neves.

rather detailed, but still incomplete, pathway of T-cell differentiation has been elaborated over the past several years (59) (Fig. 7).

The first stage is entry of T-cell progenitors into the thymus. In many ways, this is the step we understand the least. It is known that T cells ultimately derive from hematopoietic stem cells, produced primarily in the fetal liver and the adult bone marrow. Still unclear are just how the progenitors enter the thymus and precisely what their degree of commitment is. In irradiated adult mice, precursors were seen to enter through venules in the medulla and at the corticomedullary junction (68), but it is not known whether this applies to unmanipulated mice as well. As a population, the progenitors can give rise to NK cells, B-lymphocytes, and dendritic cells in addition to T-lymphocytes; not surprisingly, then, the TCR genes of these early T-cell precursors are in the germline state.

The TN stage is rich in important differentiation events, including the commitment to become a T cell, the onset of TCR gene rearrangements, positive selection to continue maturation, and the decision to become an α:β versus a γ:δ T cell. As alluded to above, the TN subpopulation can be split into four components on the basis of CD44 and CD25 expression. The CD44+25− subset is the most immature, including a fraction of cells that display low levels of CD4 and are thought to comprise the earliest intrathymic T-cell progenitors (69,70). CD44+25− cells can give rise to NK, B, dendritic, and T cells and have unrearranged TCR genes. Few are dividing. This changes abruptly in the ensuing CD44+25+ subset,

which is in rapid division under the influence of cytokines such as c-kit and IL-7 (71). CD44+25+ cells can still engender dendritic, but not NK or B, cells and still have germline TCR genes. Rearrangements are first detected in the CD44lo25+ subset of the β, γ and δ genes, but not of the α genes; at least some of the CD3 subunits are also in evidence (72–74). This subset cannot give rise to non–T-lymphocyte classes and is an important control point for the T lineage. Some CD44lo25+ cells manage to express functional γδ TCRs at the surface and split off to engender the γδ cell lineage. Some, on the other hand, display a functional TCR β chain at the surface, in association with a nonvariable pre-TCR α (pTα) chain and some of the CD3 subunits (to form a pre-TCR) and these will continue along the pathway to become α:β cells. However, the majority follow neither route and soon die. CD44lo25+ cells are mostly in the resting state. Passage to the next stage, the CD44−25− subset, is accompanied by the turn-off of TCR gene rearrangement and the onset of rapid cell division. CD44−25− cells gradually begin to express CD4 and CD8 molecules and to open their TCR-α loci for rearrangement.

The ISP stage is poorly understood. Murine CD4−8+ cells will spontaneously convert to CD4+8+ cells upon culture in suspension in vitro, so it could be that the existence of ISP cells just reflects differential kinetics of CD4 and CD8 expression at the cell surface. However, some engineered mouse strains have a block (or pause) in thymocyte differentiation at the ISP stage (45,75).

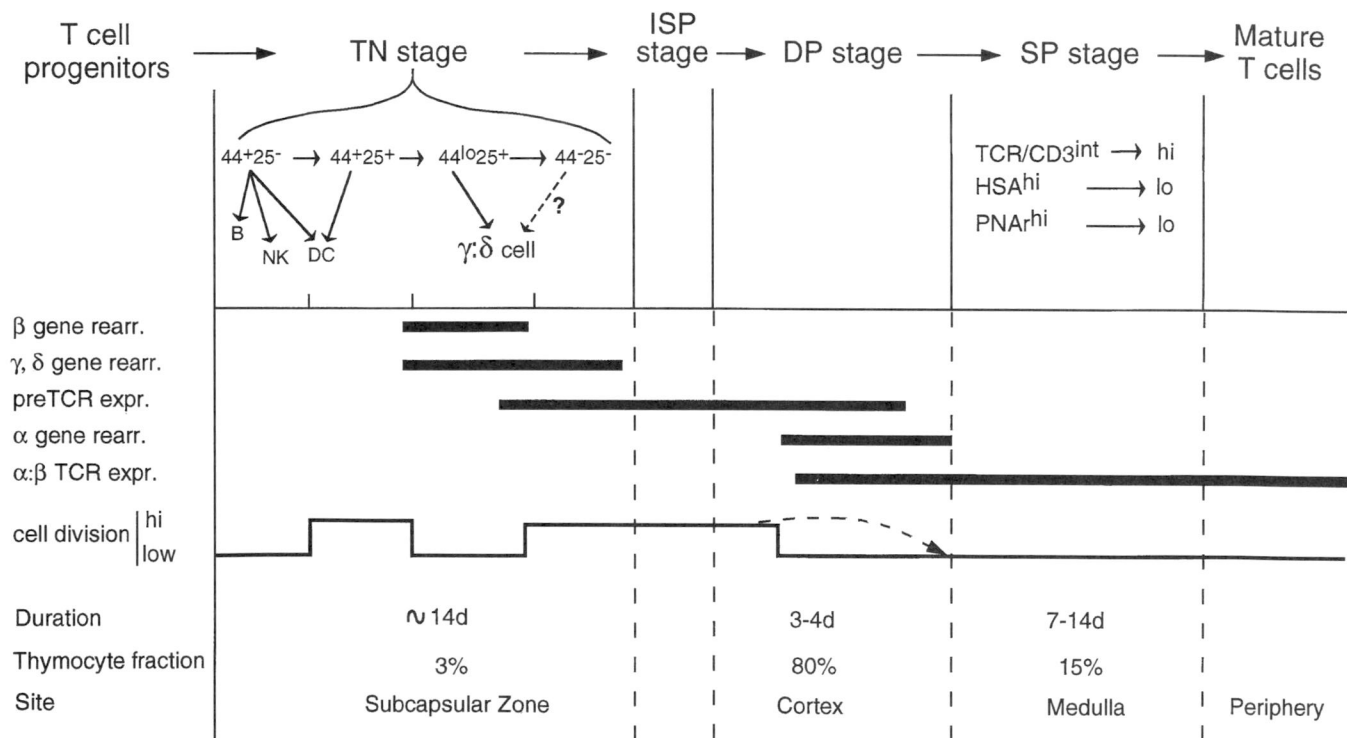

FIG. 7. The pathway of α:β T-cell differentiation in the thymus. From top to bottom: the major thymocyte transitions; blow-ups of particular stages showing, to the left, CD44/25 splits of the TN stage and their precursor potential and, to the right, surface marker evolution during the SP stage; status of complete TCR gene rearrangements and expression of TCR complexes at the cell surface; degree of cell division; average time spent at the various stages; fraction that the different stages make of total thymocytes; and anatomic location in which cells of the different stages reside. The dashed arrow with a question mark reflects the observation that CD44−25− cells can give rise to γ:δ T cells (242) but that it is not known whether these cells lost CD25 before or after commitment to the γ:δ lineage and whether they are precisely the same CD44−25− cells that can give rise to the α:β T cells. The other dashed arrow reflects the finding, still somewhat controversial, that some blasting DP cells can directly engender SP cells (286).

The DP stage is another that is rich in important differentiation events: successive TCR-α gene rearrangements, positive selection to impose self-MHC restriction, the decision to become a CD4$^+$ versus a CD8$^+$ cell, and negative selection to inflict self-tolerance. As a result of these events, the DP subset undergoes heavy attrition, more than 95% of the cells never completing maturation. Most die because they fail to be positively selected (62). A DP cell will succumb to apoptosis within 3 or 4 days after generation unless it expresses a TCR that can interact with one of the MHC molecules displayed on stromal cells. Success is signaled by upregulation of the α:β TCR/CD3 complex and downregulation of one of the coreceptors. Depending on whether the TCR interacts with a class I or II molecule, the DP cell will become either a CD4$^-$8$^+$ or a CD4$^+$8$^-$ SP cell. The precise pathway followed during the DP to SP transition remains controversial, but it appears to be rather convoluted, and perhaps not parallel for cells destined to join the two mature compartments. Some DP cells die by a process called clonal deletion because the TCR they begin to express reacts too strongly with thymic self antigens bound to MHC molecules on stromal cells.

The SP stage is the final phase of thymocyte maturation. Thymocytes enter this stage as unreactive CD3^{int}HSA^{hi}PNA^{hi} cells and end up as fully competent CD3^{hi}HSA^{lo}PNA^{lo} cells; the details of this progression are unknown. As SP cells encounter new self antigens presented by the MHC molecules displayed on new stromal cell types, they undergo further negative selection by clonal deletion, although this may be limited to the least mature members of the subset (76). Fully mature SP cells are exported from the thymus via blood and lymph vessels at the corticomedullary junction by an unknown mechanism that is dependent on a Gi protein and is therefore an active process (77). After export, some further maturation takes place, as evidenced by the evolution of surface marker expression and functional competence (78,79).

T-cell differentiation in the thymus is thus a complicated affair. It is also a long one (80). It has been estimated that it takes about 14 days to complete the TN stage (80), 3 to 4 days for the DP (81,82), and 7 to 14 days for the SP (83–85). The last value is rather intriguing: a thymocyte spends about one third of its time as a final-stage SP cell; what is it doing?

The different stages of thymocyte differentiation take place in distinct regions of the thymus. The subcapsular zone contains the DN cells, housing the majority of thymocytes undergoing rapid division. Most of the DP cells are found in the cortex, in close apposition to the epithelial cell network. The medulla contains only SP cells. The thymocytes depend on the stromal cells for contacts and for soluble mediators, good examples being that survival of CD44$^+$ cells does not occur in the absence of mesenchymal cells (60) and the DP to SP transition in the absence of cortical epithelial cells (86). But the stromal cells also depend on the thymocytes because the cortex is aberrant in mice lacking cells beyond the CD44$^+$25$^-$ stages (87), and a normal medulla does not develop in animals lacking SP cells (55,88).

Little information is so far available about thymocyte movement to, within, and from the thymus, about soluble attractants or stromal cell surface ligands, and the corresponding receptors on thymocytes that might govern these processes. Recent studies have implicated α4-integrin in the release of T-cell progenitors from the bone marrow to seed the adult thymus (89), and α4/α5-integrin interactions with fibronectin appear to be involved in the movement of thymocytes from the cortex to the medulla (90). But we still have a lot to learn on this topic.

This description has focused on the differentiation pathway leading to mature α:β T cells. The point of divergence for the γ:δ lineage was indicated, but the remaining stages along this pathway were not described because we know almost nothing about them. We are also ignorant of the route(s) to become members of the α:β TCR-expressing DN subpopulation and the route(s) these cells take upon further maturation.

The Generation of T Cells Through Ontogeny

Another dynamic view of thymocyte differentiation comes from monitoring how it evolves during the lifetime of a mouse. This has the advantage that the whole process is starting off de novo so that one can follow relatively synchronous cohorts of cells undergoing a defined sequence of events. However, this approach is not so easy in the mouse because many critical processes occur before birth, forcing one to work with a series of staged fetuses or with culture systems that permit continued maturation in vitro. It is an even more problematic strategy in humans because more of the crucial processes take place before birth, the neonatal and pubertal human thymuses being much the same. Nonetheless, the ontogenetic approach has been quite successful and has revealed some important facets of T-cell differentiation.

Ontogeny of Thymus Development

In the mouse, development of the thymus begins on about the ninth day of fetal life (fd9), signaled by invagination of the ectoderm of the third branchial cleft and the endoderm of the third or fourth pharyngeal pouch (57). Progressively, the two ingrowing embryonic layers come into contact, the ectoderm surrounds the endoderm, and, at about fd11, the invaginations close to form a thymic rudiment, or anlage. It has been commonly held that both the ectodermal and endodermal layers are required for normal thymus development, the former giving rise to the epithelial cells in the cortex and the latter to the medullary epithelial cells. This conviction is based largely on old morphologic studies of the nude mouse strain, which concluded that the lack of a thymus was the result of faulty growth of the ectodermal layer (91). However, a contradictory view came from grafting experiments with birds, in which pharyngeal endoderm engendered a normal thymus as long as mesenchyme was also present (92). Recently, the target of the nude mutation was identified as the gene encoding a transcription factor (winged-helix nude [WHN]) (93), and more sophisticated analyses of thymus development in nude mice have been performed (94,95). The thymus anlage still develops in the absence of whn, but it appears to be filled with primitive epithelial cells that do not specialize and segregate into subregions.

Mesenchyme plays an important inductive as well as structural role during thymus development (96). Migration and expansion of mesenchymal cells derived from the neural crest is associated with the ectodermal and endodermal invaginations, and the developing organ becomes surrounded by mesenchymal cells, initially of neural crest and later of mesodermal origin (97). Experimental ablation of embryonic neural crest cells results in thymic dysgenesis (98). Recently, studies on mice bearing an engineered mutation of one of the Hox genes (Hoxa-3) has implicated this transcription factor in the process by which mesenchymal cells influence thymus development—either their ability to induce differentiation in surrounding cells or their own intrinsic capacity to differentiate (99),

Interestingly, the phenotype of the Hoxa-3 knock-out strain appears very similar to that of human patients with the DiGeorge syndrome (100).

The thymus anlage is eventually permeated by blood vessels associated with mesoderm-derived mesenchyme. The vessels deliver a variety of cells of hematopoetic origin, including, above all, lymphoid cell progenitors that will give rise to thymocytes, as well as some NK, B, and dendritic cells; also included are macrophages and/or their precursors. All ingredients are now in place. At this stage, the organ is not yet differentiated into subcapsular, cortical, and medullary regions; instead, there is a dominant cortex broken by small islands of medullary tissue. A distinct medulla appears just before birth, at the time when mature α:β T cells emerge, an observation highly reminiscent of recent findings on knock-out mice. Those lacking mature T cells (e.g., strains with RAG or MHC deficiencies) have only a poorly developed thymus (55,88). The subcapsular zone is not evident until about a week after birth (56); it is not yet known whether this explains why neonatal thymuses are more permeable to invasion by circulating peripheral cells (101) and how this might be related to the greater susceptibility of neonatal mice to tolerance induction.

In short, the development of the thymus is a complex process, depending on cells of diverse embryonic origin. The early stages rely critically on epithelial–mesenchymal cell interactions and the later on cross-talk between epithelial and lymphoid cells.

Ontogeny of Thymocyte Differentiation

T-cell progenitors first enter the thymus on fd11, from the yolk sac or fetal liver, via the bloodstream (102,103). They proliferate extensively but undergo only limited differentiation, such that on fd14 essentially all are still at the TN stage. Initially, differentiation along the γ:δ pathway predominates, giving rise to waves of specialized T cells expressing essentially homogeneous TCRs (the Vγ5+ and Vγ6+ subsets). But some thymocytes also start down the long and convoluted α:β pathway. Complete VDJ rearrangements at the TCR-β locus are first detectable on fd14 to 15, and CD4 and CD8 are displayed on the cell surface from fd15 to 16. Over the next few days, cells at the DP stage become the dominant population. Fully functional SP cells are first demonstrable on fd18 to 19, the CD8+ subset lagging behind its CD4+ counterpart by about a day. At birth, on fd20, the thymus resembles that of an adult in many aspects, but there are still differences in several details.

Many investigators have assumed that the pathway of T-cell differentiation in the adult thymus can be directly extrapolated from the unfolding of thymocyte maturation during fetal ontogeny. Certainly, studies on fetal systems have brought important information that is often applicable to the adult. However, differences in the differentiation processes at the two life stages increasingly confront us. Early examples were mostly at the cellular level: stem cells originating from different sites and with very different potentials for engendering particular T-cell populations (notably Vγ5+ cells) seed fetal and adult thymuses (104); fetal thymocytes divide much more prolifically, continuing even into the most mature stages (105); fetal thymocyte differentiation is faster than that of adult thymocytes; the relative production of CD4+ and CD8+ cells differs in the two cases (106); and fetal thymocytes are less pruned by negative selection (107). About the same time, it was found that the fetal TCR repertoire is much more restricted than that of the adult, both for α:β and γ:δ T cells (108). Programmed V segment usage,

prevalent homology-directed recombination, and the delayed expression of terminal deoxynucleotidyl transferase (TdT) all play a role in this restriction. In recent years, knock-out mice have provided several examples of differences at the molecular level: a differential dependence on transcription factors [Ikaros (109) and TCF-1 (45)], signaling molecules [Rho (110)], cytokines (IL-7), and adhesion molecules [α4-integrin (89)]. Thus, we must always keep in mind that thymocyte maturation in the fetal thymus may not be the perfect exemplar for that in the adult.

The export of T cells from the thymus is maximum in young adults. With increasing age, starting at 3 months in mice, the thymus begins to shrink and export dwindles (111). This process, called thymic involution, is more or less extreme in different animal species, and is reversible in some cases (112). The mechanism of thymic involution, and its raison d'être, are unknown at this time. Given their interdependence, the primary defect could be in either the stromal cell or thymocyte compartments.

IMPORTANT EVENTS IN THE LIFE OF A THYMOCYTE

So far, our treatment of T-cell differentiation has been essentially descriptive. We would now like to take a more integrative tack, focusing on six critical events that take place during thymocyte maturation. Each of these has received much attention over the past several years, and significant progress in resolving the outstanding issues has been made, stimulated by technologic innovations such as transgenic and gene-targeted mice, novel in vitro systems, and analysis of minute numbers of cells. However, it will become clear from reading this section that for each event many points remain in contention.

Commitment to the T-Cell Lineage

The earliest events of T-cell differentiation are perhaps the foggiest. One would like to know where T-cell progenitors come from, how they are attracted to the thymus, by what route(s) they enter, what their state of commitment is, and, if pluripotential, when and how they make a lasting commitment. Most of these questions have not yet been answered satisfactorily (102,103).

T-lymphocytes, like all lymphoid cells, ultimately derive from hematopoietic stem cells. The hematopoietic organ that gives rise to thymocyte progenitors varies through mouse development—primarily the liver during fetal life and bone marrow thereafter. Progenitors arising from the two sources have different properties, notably their capacity to engender the homogeneous populations of γδ cells that appear early in development (104). By what means the progenitors reach the thymus using what ligands and what receptors is largely unknown. Several molecules have been implicated, and some remain viable candidates (89,113), but controversy has arisen because of several cases where opposing conclusions issued from experiments based on mAb blocking and those using knock-out mouse strains. Perhaps one exception is α4-integrin that is required for T-precursors to emerge from adult bone marrow but, interestingly, is dispensable for the seeding and effective functioning of the fetal thymus (89). Also unclear is precisely how the progenitors enter the thymus. In recovering irradiated mice, new immigrants are seen in large venules in the medulla and at the corticomedullary junction (68), but it is unclear whether this also applies to unmanipulated animals and at all stages of development.

A recent study on birds demonstrated infused precursors entering by both trans-capsular and corticomedullary routes (114).

The issue of T-progenitor commitment can be viewed from both ends—whether lymphocyte-restricted or T-committed cells can be found in fetal liver and adult bone marrow, and whether uncommitted cells show up in the thymus. So far, the answer to the first question seems to be probably and probably not. Cells with some of the properties that one would expect from a lymphocyte-restricted population were detected in fetal liver (115). These cells exhibited T- and B-progenitor activity, had an appropriate constellation of cell-surface markers, and synthesized transcripts for $pT\alpha$ and the pre-B cell receptor chain VpreB. However, the population also could give rise to some nonlymphoid cells, particularly those of the myeloid lineage. Whether the lymphoid and myeloid progenitor activity derive from a single cell is not known. In addition, it is not clear whether the T and B potential resided in the same cells or just in the same population. TCR gene rearrangements, which would argue for T commitment, are essentially undetectable in the fetal liver (115,116). As concerns the bone marrow, a population of cells with properties in between those of hematopoietic stem cells and the most immature thymocytes has been identified (117) and germline transcripts of TCR genes detected (118,119), but there has been no clear evidence of TCR gene rearrangements. Thus, at the moment, it seems there might be lymphocyte-restricted progenitors in the hematopoietic organs subserving the thymus, but there are probably not T-committed precursors. The inverse question of whether uncommitted progenitors appear in the thymus also has an equivocal answer at this point. Cells from fd12 thymuses are able to give rise to both lymphoid and nonlymphoid (mainly myeloid) cells (120,121). In contrast, older animals (121) and adults (69,70,122,123) have very little myeloid (and other nonlymphoid) progenitor activity. Thus, it remains possible that some quite uncommitted progenitors reside in the thymus, although one must keep in mind the usual caveat that we are not sure that all of the different precursor activities can be attributed to a single cell.

A final point regarding this issue is that it can be instructive to look, not just at the ends, but also in the middle. Hoping to catch progenitors on their way to the thymus, some investigators have evaluated the precursor potential of fetal blood cells. Both pluripotent and T-restricted progenitors have been demonstrated (124–127).

Thus, at present, we are not sure about the state of commitment of progenitors entering the thymus. However, it seems clear, at least at the population level, that there are precursors for NK (128), B (70,120,123,129,130), and dendritic (131) cells. In fact, in humans, a common progenitor for T and NK cells has been demonstrated at the single-cell level (132). These precursors are all present at the CD44$^+$25$^-$ TN stage, but only those engendering dendritic cells persist to the next, CD44$^+$25$^+$, stage (129,130). One step later, only T-cell precursors are found. The simplest, but not only, interpretation of these results is that final commitment to the T-cell lineage occurs at the CD44^{lo}25$^+$ TN stage, coincident with TCR gene rearrangement.

The heavily caveated conclusions presented above are quite unsatisfying. Certainly, these are difficult issues to address given the rarity and complexity of the populations involved. Fortunately, gene-targeted mice have recently opened a new avenue of investigation. Abrogating the synthesis of certain transcription factors has had some revealing effects (133). Targeted mutation of the gene for PU.1, a member of the ets family, resulted in a defect in the lymphoid and myeloid, but not other hematopoietic, lineages (134),

whereas a dominant-negative mutation that shuts off Ikaros and related zinc-finger proteins blocked lymphoid, but not myeloid, cell differentiation (132,135). Strikingly, another mutation of the PU.1 gene (136) and a simple null mutation of the Ikaros gene (109,135) were permissive for the differentiation of adult, but not fetal, T cells. Defects in the production of some types of $\gamma\delta$ T cells, NK cells, and dendritic cells were also observed in these latter mutants. Finally, inactivation of the gene for GATA-3, another zinc-finger protein, resulted in a normal complement of hematopoietic cells, with the sole exception of T cells, which were incapable of progressing beyond the initial stage of thymocyte maturation (136). It is hoped that these and additional transcription factor gene mutations will finally resolve the many outstanding issues concerning commitment of progenitors to the T lineage.

TCR Gene Rearrangement

It is not known how tightly rearrangement of the TCR loci is linked to an uncommitted thymocyte's decision to become a T cell; at the very least, it confirms the choice. TCR gene rearrangement is also a critical element in the α:β versus γ:δ and CD4$^+$ versus CD8$^+$ lineage decisions.

Mechanics

The mechanics of rearrangement for the four TCR loci are basically like those of the Ig genes (137). For TCR-β (Fig. 8A), one of the Dβ segments is first juxtaposed to one of the several Jβ segments; actually, the two Dβ segments on one chromosome can rearrange essentially simultaneously as can the two Dβ segments on the other chromosome, allowing four possible Dβ-Jβ combinations. Subsequently a β segment is juxtaposed to one of the Dβ-Jβ fusions; given the four possible Dβ-Jβ combinations, there are four chances to achieve a productive Vβ-Dβ-Jβ rearrangement. The rearranged stretch is joined to the constant stretch, and the constant exons are attached via RNA splicing. For TCR-α (Fig. 8B), only V and J segments are involved, but significant diversity is still generated due to the large number of possible Vα and Jα segments. The TCR-δ gene segments are embedded within the TCR-α locus (Fig. 8B). TCR-δ has an enormous potential for diversity, the greatest for any of the TCR loci, because two Dδ segments can join together at a single rearranged locus, and because both Vα and Vδ segments can be used in assembling a TCR-δ gene. In this case, the V and D segments are joined first, then the J segment is added on. The location of the TCR-δ locus between the Vα and Jα segments means that it is deleted upon TCR-α locus rearrangement. For TCR-γ (Fig. 8C), there are four separate rearranging loci (three functional), each with its own V and J segments, but no D segments. TCR-γ is the TCR locus with the least potential for diversity.

For all of the TCR genes, additional diversity is created at the rearranged junctions by two processes. The enzyme TdT adds nucleotides in a template-independent manner to generate what is called N-region diversity (138,139). In the mouse, TdT is not expressed in the thymus until after birth (140); in humans, expression is also delayed, although given the relatively precocious state of the thymus in human neonates, N-region diversity is detected in T cells produced before birth (141). The second means of creating diversity at the junctions is exonuclease-mediated deletion of nucleotides.

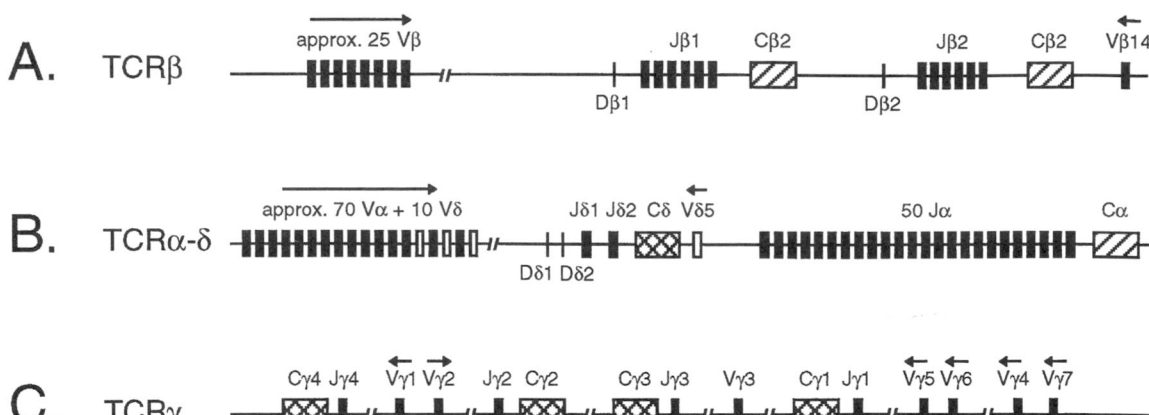

FIG. 8 A–C. TCR gene organization. Thick solid bars represent variable and junctional segments, except for the Vγ segments which are shown as thick open bars. Thin solid bars represent diversity segments, and stippled rectangles represent constant segments. The direction of transcription is indicated by arrows above the different maps. The Cγ3 segment is a pseudogene. Additional Jβ1 and Jβ2 segments (Jβ1.7, Jβ2.7) have been left out because they are nonfunctional. The γ gene nomenclature is that of Heilig and Tonegawa (534).

The enzymology of TCR (and Ig) gene rearrangement is understood only sketchily, but one gets the impression that the current rapid movement in this field will soon provide a detailed picture. Lymphocyte-specific molecules, such as the two RAG products, as well as ubiquitously expressed proteins, like the catalytic and Ku subunits of DNA-dependent protein kinase, both play a role. This has been clearly indicated in studies on mutant mice (142–147) and has been confirmed with powerful in vitro recombination systems (148).

Control During Thymus Development

Rearrangements of the different TCR loci do not occur randomly during thymus development, but follow a highly programmed sequence (149). In the mouse, the first mature T cells to emerge display predominantly γ:δ receptors. Initially, a wave of cells expresses essentially a single receptor: a Vγ5Jγ1Cγ1 chain paired with a Vδ1Dδ2Jδ2 chain, neither with significant N-region diversity. These begin to appear on fd14, are dominant until fd17, and begin to decline by fd18. The homogenous Vγ5+ cells home to the epidermis, constituting an enigmatic population of dendritic epidermal cells (DECs). A second wave of γ:δ cells, expressing a homogeneous Vγ6Jγ1Cγ1 chain paired with the same δ chain, lags a few days behind. These home to the epithelial layers of the reproductive tract and the tongue. They begin to decline at birth, replaced by a population of γ:δ cells that express heterogeneous receptors (Vγ segments 1, 2, 4, and 7 with ample N-region diversity) and populate the thymus, spleen, and other lymphoid organs. Also around birth, α:β T cells begin to gain prominence, eventually representing more than 95% of thymocytes. After birth, T cells are no longer produced in waves, but continuously.

The factors controlling these different thymocyte waves, with their characteristic patterns of TCR gene rearrangements, are only poorly understood. On the cellular level, it has been suggested that different T-cell progenitor populations have a different proclivity for engendering the different T-cell populations. For example, there is evidence that in order for DECs to be generated, the progenitors must come from fetal liver rather than adult bone marrow and must

mature in a fetal, not adult, thymus (104). On the molecular level, there are indications that differential rearrangement of the various TCR-γ loci reflects variable accessibility to the recombination machinery due to variations in chromatin structure (150). The homogeneity of the receptors displayed in the first two thymocyte waves no doubt reflects the delayed onset of TdT expression, resulting in the absence of N-region diversity, but also somehow promoting more homogeneous joints at sites of short stretches of sequence homology (homology-directed recombination) (138, 139).

We do not yet know whether similar waves characterize the development of the T-cell repertoire in humans. γ:δ cells are numerous in the lymphoid organs of adult humans, and a particular receptor composed of a Vγ9+ chain paired with a Vδ2+ chain is quite prominent in peripheral blood, but it is not known when these cells first arise (151).

Control During T-Cell Differentiation

Rearrangement of the TCR loci is also highly regulated during T-cell differentiation (152). The first complete rearrangements occur at the TN stage, in the CD44lo25+ subset, where rearrangements of the TCR-β, -γ, and -δ genes can all be detected. As discussed in detail later in this chapter, if a functional γ:δ receptor is assembled at the surface, the cell proceeds along the pathway to become a mature γ:δ cell; if a functional β chain is produced, it assembles with pTα and the CD3 subunits, appearance of this preTCR complex at the cell surface signaling a halt to further TCR-β gene rearrangement and allowing differentiation along the α:β pathway. Allelic exclusion at the β locus is very efficient in TCR-β transgenic mice (153), but in unmanipulated animals, particularly humans, it may not be 100% effective (154,155). At the DP stage, rearrangements at the TCR-α locus start being detectable. Multiple rearrangements can occur in a single cell, involving both chromosomes as well as successive V-J joinings on a single chromosome (156). V-J rearrangement at the TCR-α locus results in deletion of the TCR-δ gene segments, so that once both α loci have rearranged, the thymocyte is irreversibly confirmed in its decision to become an α:β cell. TCR-α locus rearrangement is not shut off, even when a functional α:β receptor is assembled at the surface, but rather coincident with positive selection if the receptor can recognize a self-MHC molecule (157). Thus, allelic exclusion at the TCR-α locus does not really occur; as a consequence, mature T cells can display more than one α:β receptor (158–160). Nevertheless, there is almost always a functional exclusion because one of the receptors may assemble much more efficiently than the other, and because cells have little chance of expressing two receptors that can interact with a self-MHC molecule (160–162).

Little is known about the molecular mechanism(s) controlling the turn-on and turn-off of TCR gene rearrangement during differentiation (163,164). Certainly control of RAG transcription and of RAG product expression plays a central role. It has been suggested that the IL-7 dependence of early steps in thymocyte differentiation reflects direct control of RAG transcription (165,166), but this remains controversial (167). RAG products are expressed before and during the CD44^lo25+ TN stage with its active TCR-β, -γ, and -δ gene rearrangement; the RAG-2 product is rapidly degraded concomitant with expression of the pre-TCR, passage to the CD44−25− stage and onset of cell division (168); transcription of RAG-1 and -2 is also turned off (169). A second peak of RAG-1 and -2 transcription occurs at the DP stage (169) and is terminated upon successful positive selection (157,170,171). However, control of RAG expression cannot explain locus-specific rearrangement.

Another important factor seems to be variable accessibility of the different TCR loci to the recombination machinery, a reflection of their chromatin structure (172). Accessibility has been correlated with lineage-specific and stage-specific transcription of the loci before rearrangement, under the dictates of transcriptional control elements located within each locus. However, even though removal or addition of enhancer elements can have a strong effect on recombination in transgenic or knock-out systems (173–179), the correlation between rearrangements and transcription is not absolute. In the case of the TCR-γ enhancer, effects on rearrangement have been attributed to individual binding sites of transcription factors (178,179), but these could have an additional role in the recruitment of the recombination apparatus.

The mechanisms whereby rearrangement of TCR genes are permanently shut off as a reflection of isotypic exclusion remain to be defined, but probably also involve control of accessibility to the rearrangement apparatus. Some of the initial events are beginning to be clarified, but we are still ignorant of the downstream processes.

Pre–TCR-mediated Selection

It is only during the past several years that we have become aware of an important quality-control point at the TN stage of thymocyte differentiation, marked by the transition of CD44^lo25+ to CD44−25− cells (103). This control point has a close analog in the B-cell differentiation pathway (180).

The first real hint of a TCR-controlled transition in early thymocyte differentiation was the observation that introduction of rearranged TCR-α/β transgenes into SCID mice leads to the generation of fully mature T cells, overcoming a block at the TN-to-DP transition (8). Even more intriguing was the finding that a rearranged TCR-β transgene alone can partially surmount the obstacle, allowing progression to the DP but not the SP stage (181). The block has since been more precisely localized to the

CD44^lo25+ stage and has been found, with varying degrees of severity, in several mouse strains bearing null or dominant negative mutations of genes encoding structural or signaling components of the α:β TCR/CD3 complex: the RAG (142,143), TCR-β (182), CD3-ε, -γ, and -ζ (183–187), p56 lck (188,189), CD45 (190,191), ZAP-70/Syk (192), rho (110,193) and MEK-1 (194) genes. Certain drugs also interfere with thymocyte differentiation specifically at this point: tyrosine kinase inhibitors (195), cyclic adenosine monophosphate analogs (196), and the immunosuppressant deoxyspergualin (197). The block can be lifted by introduction of a TCR-β transgene (181,198), by introduction of a constitutively activate p56lck (199,200) or p21ras (201) transgene, or by engagement of CD3-ε with an mAb (72–74).

An early goal was to characterize the cell surface complex responsible for exerting this control, but this may have been only partially realized. The importance of the TCR-β chain was recognized from the beginning (181,182,198,202), and biochemical studies soon implicated at least some of the CD3 subunits (202,203). The role of individual CD3 subunits was controversial for some time, but more recent knock-out experiments have argued for the involvement of CD3-ε, -γ, and -ζ (183–187), but not δ (204). Biochemical studies also led to the identification of a partner for the TCR-β chain: an invariant polypeptide termed pTα (205,206). The gene for pTα was cloned, revealing that it is a type 1 transmembrane protein with a single, Ig-like, extracellular domain (206). Knock out of the pTa gene resulted in a phenotype much like that of animals lacking the TCR-β chain (207). As illustrated in Fig. 9, there may be another subunit yet to come: if one takes the analogous pre-B cell receptor as a model, there appears to be a missing Ig domain, the analog of VpreB. The human pTα chain also has been described. It is basically the same in overall structure, but the cytoplasmic tail is quite different (208), and its expression peaks a little later in thymocyte differentiation, at the ISP stage (209).

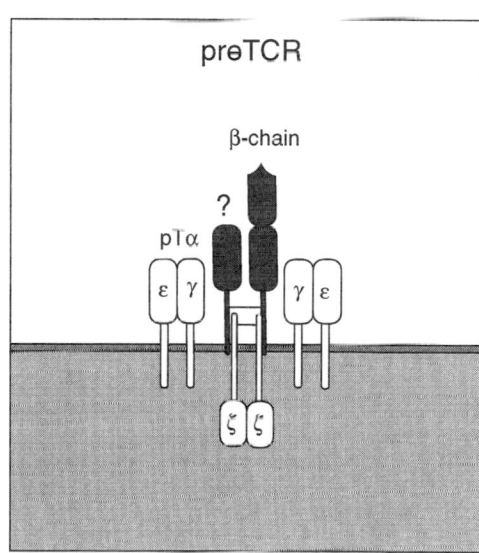

FIG. 9. The pre-TCR. The question mark represents a possible additional pre-TCR subunit suggested by analogy with the pre-BCR and by the unpaired Ig-like domain in the β chain (a rare occurrence in the Ig superfamily). The structure of CD3 is not definitively known; shown here is a synthesis from results on knock-out animals, as detailed in the text.

Information on the mechanism by which the pre-TCR exerts its control is scant. It is not known whether this receptor needs to engage a particular ligand or whether its mere assembly in the cell membrane is sufficient. Exit from the ER is required, but the Vβ exon is dispensable (210,211). It is also not clear how the signal is transduced. The TCR-β chain has almost no cytoplasmic tail, and although pTα has a tail that potentially could bind signaling molecules, its sequence is not conserved (208) and it is dispensable (200). The fact that the pre-TCR, but not the α:β TCR, can function in thymocyte generation independently of CD3-δ (204) hints that signal transduction by the two receptor complexes could differ, and the differential effect of certain drugs on early and late maturation events (197,212,213) supports this notion. p56 lck is somehow involved in signaling (188,189,199,200), but it is not clear whether this is through a direct interaction with the pre-TCR. The ras pathway also has been implicated (110,193,194,201).

Precisely what processes does the pre-TCR regulate, and to what end? Transition from the CD44^{lo}25$^+$ to CD44$^-$25$^-$ stage is accompanied by several important events: allelic exclusion at the TCR-β locus, enrichment for cells with functional TCR-β rearrangements (β selection) (168,214,215), onset of rapid cell division, eventual expression of the CD4 and CD8 coreceptors, and promotion of TCR-α gene rearrangement. Although there has been some debate, it is now clear that pTα, and hence the pre-TCR, plays an important role in promoting shut-down of further rearrangements at the TCR-β locus (216–218). The pre-TCR must be present for efficient expansion of cells beyond the CD44^{lo}25$^+$ stage (182,207), and it may actually signal the onset of cell division (168,219). Not surprisingly, then, the pre-TCR needs to be expressed to have a healthy CD4$^+$8$^+$ population (142,143,182,183,207), but it is not clear whether this reflects a true block in differentiation or just the aforementioned inhibition of expansion. The α:β and γ:δ TCRs can replace the pre-TCR in this role, but this is inefficient except in gene-manipulated animals (182,207,220–222). In addition, many experimental interventions without obvious link to the pre-TCR, such as γ irradiation (223,224) or mutation of p53 (225,226), can lead to conversion of TN to DP cells, but again only a small DP population usually emerges. Finally, the pre-TCR promotes the onset of TCR-α gene rearrangement, although this can still happen at a low level in its absence (182,183,222).

Considering its strong influence on these various processes, it would appear that the pre-TCR functions primarily as a quality-control monitor. If rearrangement at the TCR-β locus results in a functional β chain, it assembles with other receptor components at the cell surface; display of the pre-TCR somehow signals shut-down of further TCR-β gene rearrangements and probably proliferation, multiplying the number of cells expressing the particular β chain; differentiation proceeds, resulting in the induction of TCR-α gene rearrangements. If, on the other hand, rearrangement at the TCR-β locus (and TCR-γ and -δ loci) is not successful, the cell dies via apoptosis (219,227). In short, the pre-TCR mediates positive selection of cells expressing a functional β chain and optimizes their opportunity to assemble a functional α:β TCR.

The α:β/γ:δ Split

Two very different classes of T cells populate the periphery of an animal: α:β and γ:δ cells, defined according to the antigen-specific receptor chains they express. Both ultimately derive from hematopoietic stem cells and are produced in the thymus as well as

a few extrathymic sites. When and how does a maturing T-cell progenitor decide to become one or the other? Early in ontogeny, the decision is so biased that it amounts to essentially no choice at all: production of the earliest waves of T cells appears to be programmed at the level of the stem cell to engender primarily γ:δ cells expressing first a homogeneous Vγ5$^+$, then an equally invariant Vγ6$^+$, receptor (104,149,228). Later, however, members of both T-cell classes displaying heterogeneous TCRs are generated, and even though production is heavily skewed toward α:β cells, a choice has to be made.

Three basic models have been proposed to explain the α:β/γ:δ split (Fig. 10). The first, the independent model, contends that the two types of T cells derive from independent progenitors. Certainly, both are ultimately derived from hematopoietic stem cells, but either there is stem cell heterogeneity or the two lineages split off very early, perhaps even before entering the thymus. The sequential model proposes, on the other hand, that the two types of cell have a common percursor: the maturing thymocyte first attempts to be a γ:δ cell, but if it is unsuccessful at producing functional rearrangements at the TCR-γ and -δ loci, it then tries to be an α:β cell. This order, rather than the reverse, is suggested by the fact that mature γ:δ cells emerge before α:β cells during ontogeny. The competitive

1. Independent

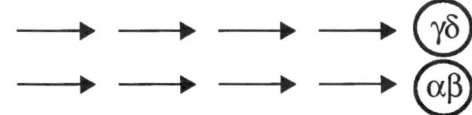

2. Sequential

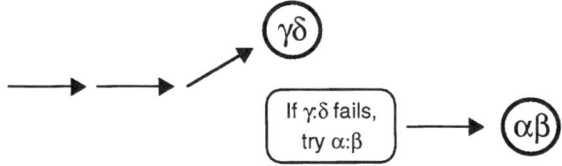

3. Competitive

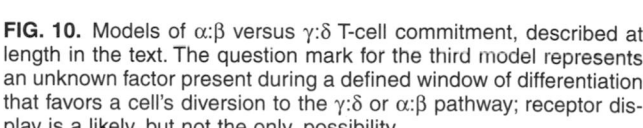

FIG. 10. Models of α:β versus γ:δ T-cell commitment, described at length in the text. The question mark for the third model represents an unknown factor present during a defined window of differentiation that favors a cell's diversion to the γ:δ or α:β pathway; receptor display is a likely, but not the only, possibility.

model also postulates a common precursor: during a certain window of thymocyte differentiation, both types of cells can be generated, some molecular parameter, most likely receptor display, determining for each progenitor whether it will become a γ:δ or an α:β cell.

Early attempts at distinguishing the three models exploited the fact that the TCR-δ gene segments are entirely embedded within the TCR-α locus and are excised as circles upon successful α gene rearrangement. Thus, it would be incompatible with the first model but not the second and third to find extrachromosomal circles with rearranged δ segments in mature α:β T cells. Unfortunately, conflicting results were obtained on this point (229–232). Another approach was to analyze the T-cell repertoires of TCR transgenic mice. α:β TCR transgenes should not influence the production of γ:δ cells, and vice versa, according to the first model, but not the other two. However, once again, contradictory results have been reported (233–236).

The best distinction between the different models has come only recently with a series of analyses on the rearranged TCR genes in α:β versus γ:δ T cells. First, it was shown that mature and maturing α:β cells have rearranged γ and δ genes that are impoverished in in-frame sequences (237–239). This observation implies that cells with functional γ and δ rearrangements split off from the α:β pathway, and would thus be incompatible with the independent model. Second, it was found that γ:δ cells have in-frame β gene and even some (predominantly out-of-frame) α gene rearrangements (215,238,240,241). Moreover, transfer experiments indicate that γ:δ cells can be produced from thymocytes as late as the latest TN stage, after TCR-mediated positive selection for continued maturation along the α:β pathway (242). These findings render the sequential model too simple an explanation and are the basis for the present popularity of the competitive model.

A possible scenario may proceed as follows: β, γ, and δ rearrangements all begin at the onset of the CD44^{lo}25$^+$ stage; if a functional β chain is produced and assembles with pTα to form a pre-TCR complex, the cell is selected to continue along the α:β pathway; if a functional γ:δ TCR is made, the cell usually proceeds down the γ:δ pathway. The former is probably the most frequent simply because it entails fewer rearrangement events, but irreversible commitment to the α:β lineage may not take place until both TCR-α loci have rearranged and the δ gene segments have been excised. Thus, a functional γ:δ receptor may be produced before, coincident with, or perhaps even after a functional β chain. We do not know what nudges the cell along the γ:δ pathway, maybe even after it is on its way to becoming an α:β cell. Indeed, it is not even clear whether the real role of the TCR is to determine lineage or just to confirm it. It seems that there is no equivalent γ:δ pre-TCR complex, certainly not one that incorporates pTα (207); however, there is some positive selection for cells with functional γ:δ rearrangements at the CD44^{lo}25$^+$ to CD44$^-$25$^-$ transition (243). A role for locus-specific transcriptional control elements in determining or confirming the α:β/γ:δ choice has been suggested (234,235,244,245), as has a role for the Notch gene product (246), but at present both require corroborative evidence.

Positive Selection: Generating a Self MHC–Restricted Repertoire

The role of the thymus in selecting the T-cell repertoire has been one of the most fascinating and controversial issues in immunology over the past 20 years. Fascinating, because it constitutes a situation unique in developmental biology, where the developing organ must adapt to genetic variability (germline polymorphism for the MHC, somatic diversity for the TCR) rather than merely follow a program preordained in the organism's homeotic genes; also, the system must select for the potential to recognize a ligand (the antigen–MHC complex), which will only be encountered at a later stage, if ever. Controversial, because the field has always prompted speculation and heated debate. Even though the dust has settled on most of the early polemics (e.g., the very existence of positive selection in the thymus), basic cellular and genetic mechanisms are still the topic of lively exchanges.

It is now generally accepted that positive selection promotes the differentiation step whereby an immature, short-lived, DP thymocyte escapes from programmed cell death and becomes an end-stage, long-lived, SP cell—a process that is mediated by an interaction between the TCR on the thymocyte and MHC molecules on thymic stroma. The selection process is rigorous, sparing only a small fraction of the DP population. Positive selection also coincides with lineage commitment, the decision to become a CD4 or CD8 SP cell, as a function of the class of MHC molecule the TCR can interact with.

Thymic selection has a built-in paradox: both positive selection and negative selection (tolerance induction) involve interactions between the TCR and peptide–MHC complexes on thymic stromal cells. Any coherent view of thymic education must integrate the two processes.

Whether and Why Positive Selection?

The concept of positive selection was developed over the past 20 years from results of experiments using a variety of approaches. The concept originated from the necessity of explaining the self-MHC restriction of T-cell function (247). Within a few years, studies involving tetraparental mice or bone marrow chimeras showed that restriction did not correspond to a necessary matching between the MHC genotypes of T cells and APCs, but instead the potential for T cells to react varied according to the environment in which they matured (248,249). A theoretical framework for this notion came with the concept of adaptative differentiation (250), firm support eventually being provided by the seminal F1 → parent chimera experiments (251): the capacity to lyse A or B targets was imposed by the MHC type of the host in which A × B F1 T cells had differentiated (Fig. 11, top). That the thymus was the site of this education to self (rather than peripheral tissues) was quickly demonstrated by thymus transfer experiments (252–255) (Fig. 11, bottom). Matters rested there for a few years, the concept of positive selection being energetically questioned by some on the basis of discordant results and potential artefacts, such as possible interference by suppressor cells or allogenic responses, molding of the repertoire by peripheral rather than thymic influences, etc. (256). Further supportive evidence came with the observation that particular MHC class II molecules could enhance the frequency of mature T cells expressing particular Vβ regions (257,258), and from the finding that blockade of MHC molecules in F1 mice by allele-specific mAbs inhibited the appearance of helper or cytotoxic T cells restricted by the blocked allele, but not by the other (259,260).

However, it was the construction of TCR transgenic mice that provided the definitive evidence for positive selection. In such

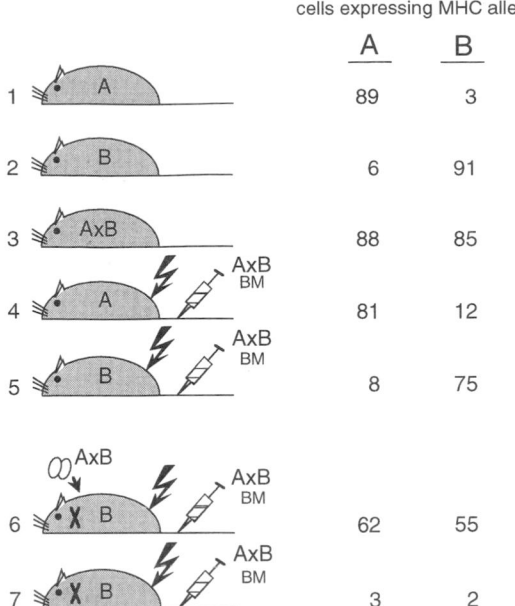

Percent lysis of ^{51}Cr-labeled
cells expressing MHC alleles

	A	B
1	89	3
2	6	91
3	88	85
4	81	12
5	8	75
6	62	55
7	3	2

FIG. 11. Restriction by self-MHC alleles is acquired in the thymus. An idealized experiment is depicted, a composite of seminal experiments by Bevan, Zinkernagel, and colleagues (251–253), which first demonstrated the importance of thymic selection of the MHC-restricted repertoire. These experiments examine the capacity of various mice to lyse targets cells of A or B genotypes (bearing viral or minor histocompatibility antigens, both of which elicit strong CTL responses after in vivo priming). Lines 1–3: the basic MHC restriction of the response; T cells primed in a given strain are only able to lyse targets of the same MHC haplotype, but can lyse both targets if originating from F1 mice. Lines 4 and 5: the host H-2 antigens determine immune responsiveness; lethally irradiated mice are reconstituted with bone marrow precursors from F1 mice (depleted of mature T cells); the T cells that develop from these precursors can only lyse targets that match the MHC alleles of the host, even though they themselves carry both MHC haplotypes. These results were the clearest demonstration of the fact that the repertoire is molded to match the MHC of the host, or adaptive differentiation (interestingly, though, they were interpreted at first in the context of Jerne's then dominant, but quite wrong, theory of somatic mutations of TCR genes). These results did not indicate which host component is responsible for this effect. This point was established by the thymus grafts (lines 6 and 7): F1 bone marrow into parent B chimeras, similar to line 5 except that the hosts were thymectomized and grafted with F1 thymus before bone marrow reconstitution; in this instance, T cells responsive to antigen in the context of both MHC alleles can be selected. The control of line 7, in which the thymic graft did not take and no responses are detected, ensures that the response does require the thymic graft.

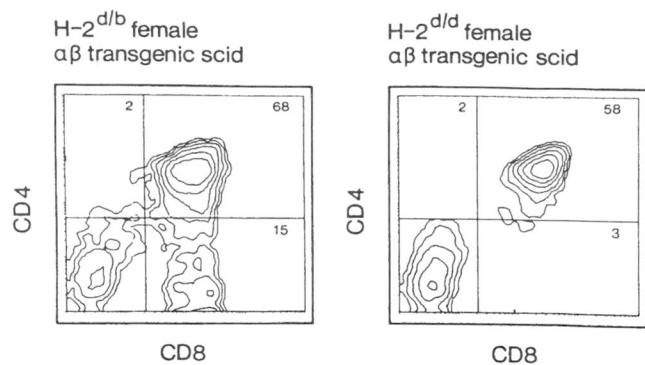

FIG. 12. Thymic positive selection demonstrated in TCR transgenic mice. In this classical experiment, transgenic mice were constructed that express, on the vast majority of their thymocytes, a single TCR restricted by class I molecules of the H-2^b MHC haplotype. Thymi from transgenic mice carrying different MHC alleles were analyzed by cytofluorimetry after staining for CD4 and CD8. In H-2^b–positive mice (left panel), there is a strong bias of maturation toward the CD4$^-$CD8$^+$ compartment (compare with the normal profile shown in Fig. 6), indicating that thymocyte maturation largely correlates with the restriction specificity of the receptor. In the absence of H-2^b molecules (right panel), selection is absent, and thymocytes remain trapped in the immature double-positive population. Reproduced with permission from Teh et al. (261).

mice, large numbers of lymphocytes expressing the receptor derived from a T-cell clone of known antigen specificity and MHC restriction are generated, and their behavior as a function of the environment in which they mature can be readily tracked. The critical conclusion from these studies was that full maturation of T cells displaying the transgene-encoded TCR was only observed when the mice expressed the MHC allele corresponding to the original T-cell clone (261–265). In the absence of the correct MHC allele, immature DP cells failed to mature to SPs (Fig. 12). This differential was clearest when the TCR transgenes were crossed onto SCID or RAG-deficient genetic backgrounds, where no rearrangement of endogenously encoded TCR-α genes is possible,

meaning that all differentiation must be mediated by the transgene-encoded receptor. Importantly, positive selection was dominant in the F1 situation (262,263) and, even more importantly, was induced by simple introduction of the selecting MHC molecule via transgenesis (264), ruling out that negative selection was responsible for the observed phenotypes.

The other important conclusion from these studies was that the phenotype of the resulting SP cells matched the restriction of the receptor: transgenics expressing MHC class I–restricted TCRs gave rise to CD8$^+$ cells, whereas those displaying class II–restricted receptors generated CD4$^+$ cells. These findings imply that the class of MHC molecule engaged during the positive selection process somehow conditions the program of gene transcription induced in the differentiating cell. This decision-making process will be discussed below.

The strong arguments on the basis of results from TCR transgenic mice were further reinforced by results from gene-targeted animals. The striking finding was that the absence of MHC class I molecules precluded the development of CD8$^+$ cells in the thymus (266,267), whereas the CD4$^+$ compartments were absent in mice devoid of class II molecules (Fig. 13) (268,269). As expected, radiation chimera experiments with these mutant animals indicated that the MHC molecules on the radioresistant thymic stroma were the dominant elements mediating selection (270,271), a conclusion solidified by complementation of the MHC class II deficit by transgenes with compartmentalized class II gene expression (272).

Why positive selection? In hindsight, it seems obvious that such a process needs to exist. Unlike B-cell receptors, which recognize antigen directly and for which any conformationally stable surface Ig is potentially useful against the world of antigenic epitopes, the TCR sees antigen in a manner that mandates a degree of compatibility with the MHC molecules of the animal. The TCR/MHC fit is problematic because the MHC molecules come in several classes, isotypes, and alleles within the species, and the scramble of genetic

T-Lymphocyte Differentiation and Biology / 387

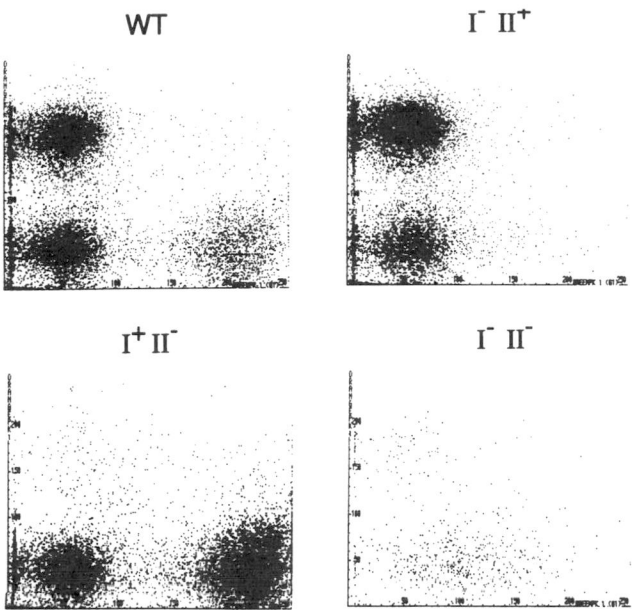

FIG. 13. Positive selection evidenced in MHC-deficient mice. The mice analyzed here are deficient for MHC class I (β2m knock-out), or class II (Aβ knock-out) or both. The panels represent lymph node T cells stained with anti-CD4 and -CD8 reagents. Note that CD8+ cells are missing in the absence of class I, and conversely that CD4+ cells do not appear without class II; both are missing in the double-deficient mouse (the very few cells left represent selection on alternate MHC-like molecules). Courtesy of S. Chan.

elements encoding the TCR cannot be expected to spontaneously match any or all of them. Some degree of selection must thus sift out those "useful" cells (273) whose TCR can accomodate the individual's MHC molecules and whose coreceptor matches the class of MHC molecules it is restricted by. Nonetheless, thymic selection is a highly wasteful process. Of the enormous numbers of DPs that are generated, only a minute proportion (approximately 3% in a normal mouse) matures and is exported to the periphery. This is largely due to failure of positive selection (62), although some cells are also lost due to negative selection (274–276). There is also a degree of competition involved: in TCR transgenic mice expressing a receptor that should allow all cells to mature, only a small proportion actually do (82). This inefficiency may reflect a limited number of stromal niches available for fostering positive selection (277).

One should be aware that the picture of positive selection painted here is an idealized one. The outcome of chimeric and transgenic mouse experiments has not always been "black-and-white." Some of the early radiation chimeras showed some response restricted by the MHC allele absent from the thymic stroma; this has been reproduced in some of the TCR transgenics, where an MHC allele different from the selecting one could also promote positive selection (278). In addition, some TCR transgenic mice exhibit only inefficient positive selection, even in the presence of the supposedly selecting MHC molecule (279); in others, the CD4/CD8 bias is far from absolute, a small number of bona fide CD8+ cells maturing in some of the transgenics expressing a class II restricted TCR (280,281) Thus, one should consider that the allele specificity of TCR/MHC interactions is not absolute (which explains why incompatible bone marrow grafts can suc-

ceed). But given what we know today, there is not really any reason to think that strict specificity should exist: the MHC surfaces in contact with the TCR show only limited allelic variation, in contrast to the extensive polymorphism in the peptide-binding groove; in addition, it has been reported that a significant proportion of MHC class I–restricted receptors on CD8+ cells can also react with class II–restricted antigens when CD4 is artificially introduced (282). It may be useful to consider positive selection in probabilistic terms—a given level of TCR–MHC interaction results in a finite probability for the cell to be selected into the CD4+ or CD8+ pathway, or of being negatively selected. Given the enormous numbers of cells in lymphoid populations, even improbable events will be represented. Finally, it is possible that the positive selection process initiated in the thymus is continued in the periphery, as the continued TCR–MHC engagement required for T-cell survival (283).

Cellular Pathways

The early events of thymocyte differentiation and expansion result in a large cohort of DPs, each expressing a functional TCR-β chain. TCR-α gene rearrangement takes place within this population, with the potential for multiple, successive attempts at making a productive rearrangement. Surface expression of a functional α:β TCR marks the entry of a DP cell into the process of positive selection, permitting a chosen few to mature into SP cells. However, most DPs fail at this stage. The life span of a DP cell is on the order of 3 to 4 days, selected cells appearing in the mature SP compartment 3 days after becoming DPs (82), and nonselected cells succumbing to apoptosis, which is visible in the cortex (62). Positive selection is a differentiative event, without proliferation; the overrepresentation of mature thymocytes often induced by TCR transgenes in the presence of the selecting MHC molecule does not result from a preferential expansion by cell division, but rather from an increased differentiative flow of cells into the compartment (82).

TCR expression at the cell surface is the basic requirement for selection. Both early (still cycling) large DPs and small resting DPs can undergo selection, although it is possible that only particular DP subsets may be selected, a point of some debate (284–286). Although earlier effects can be detected, one of the more notable changes accompanying selection is upregulation of TCR levels at the surface (287). This differential display before and after selection corresponds to a developmentally regulated, posttranslational control of TCR-α chains more than to an increase of a gene transcription (288). Beyond this early stage, many phenotypic modifications take place (Table 2). The most dramatic, and probably the most important functionally, is a shut-down of one of the two coreceptors. As discussed below, this event occurs rather late in the process and may be temporally complex, with sequential shutdown and reexpression phases. For CD4, it has been shown that its turn-off corresponds to the influence of an intronic silencer element, inactive in DPs but active in CD8 SPs (289,290). Some of the other changes appear to be acknowledgments of the fact that assembly of a functional α:β TCR has taken place, i.e., shutdown of genes involved in TCR gene rearrangement, such as the RAG or TdT genes (140,157,170,291). Others correspond to increased surface expression of proteins usually found on activated mature T cells (CD44, CD69), likely reflecting new signal transduction through the TCR (292). Yet others correspond to the acquisition of

TABLE 2. *Phenotypic changes induced by positive selection*

CD4 ⎫ CD8 ⎭	Early, slight surface reduction of both; later, complete shut off of one
TCRαβ ⎫ CD3 ⎭	Very early, strong increase in surface protein (not mRNA)
RAG ⎫ TdT ⎭	Shut off
Bcl2	↑
CD69 ⎫ CD44 ⎭	Turned on, not all cells, CD4SP > CD8SP
CD5	↑
CD28	↑
MHC-I	↑
HSA	↓
PNAr	↓ Progressive decrease, absent in fully mature SPs

surface molecules necessary for mature T cells (such as the CD28 costimulator, CD5, CD45, or MHC class I molecules) or to modified expression of proteins of unknown function (HSA, PNAr). Finally, an important shift occurs in the intracellular proteins of the Bcl-2 family of apoptosis regulators. Bcl-2 is expressed at very low levels in DPs and is markedly induced after positive selection (293,294). This induction correlates with loss of the exquisite sensitivity of DPs to many inducers of apoptosis (radiation, glucocorticoids, high-affinity TCR cross-linking by antibodies). It is thus tempting to hypothesize that the rescue from apoptosis that marks positive selection is due to this increased expression of antiapoptotic factors. One should not be oversimplistic, though, because apoptosis in DP cells is complex, with positive or negative interferences between the death pathways induced by various agents (295); these are not all affected by Bcl-2 (294,296–298).

Some of the changes in gene transcription patterns that appear to correlate with positive selection are already detectable in bone fide DP cells—CD69 is induced, and RAG and TdT gene expression is already lower in CD3^int DPs on the selecting, but not the nonselecting, background (170,292). Interruption of TCR/MHC contacts inhibits the progression of selection, with reinduction of RAG expression (299,300). Additionally, chimeric disaggregation–reaggregation FTOCs have shown that developing thymocytes do not scan the cortical epithelial network in search of an appropriate ligand, but rather remain faithfully bound to a single cell or small group of cells (277,301). Thus, it is important to think of positive selection as a long continuous process, during which the signal is sustained over a period of many hours, rather than the short hits (of less than an hour) that one usually associates with activation of mature T cells by antigen.

Positive selection also induces an important modification in cellular localization: selected cells migrate out of the cortex and into the medulla. It is not yet clear at what stage of selection this takes place, or what the molecular mechanisms of this migration might be (58,90).

Lineage commitment at the time of positive selection has been the subject of much interest and controversy in the past few years. At the time of selection, the cell has a four-way choice: death by neglect, life as a CD4+ cell, life as a CD8+ cell, or death by negative selection. The critical question is how the match is made between the class of MHC molecule that restricts the TCR and the type of mature cell the thymocyte becomes. An answer to this question at the cellular level is important because it conditions our

understanding of gene control processes during positive selection. Unfortunately, the answer is rather muddled at present. One of the problems is that understanding the cellular pathways of lineage commitment requires being able to "catch" transitional intermediates. However, these have been difficult to apprehend. Some investigators have relied on educated (but ultimately questionable) guesses, others on direct experimentation, but unfortunately by strategies that require engagement of cell surface receptors and so are liable to modify the behavior of the cells.

The simple symmetry of the differentiative choice (CD4 versus CD8 shut-down) may be deceptive, and the cellular transitions that generate CD4 and CD8 SPs are probably not identical either in time [CD4 SPs are generated faster (302)] or in route [CD8 SPs appear to arrive via convoluted circuits (303)]. The body of existing data is not compatible with models of commitment proposed earlier (Fig. 14): lineage is not instructed by the coreceptor signal received at the time of the TCR engagement; the basic stochastic model is also essentially wrong (see legend to Fig. 14). A few facts are clear:

- A TCR–MHC signal is essential; nothing happens in its absence.
- Coreceptor input is important, but can be dispensed with.
- Mismatched commitment (class II–restricted CD8 SPs, and vice versa) can occur for both lineages.
- Levels of coreceptors at the cell surface are not necessarily good indicators of lineage commitment.
- Lineage commitment is more complex than a simple two-way split (i.e., there is more than one way to become a CD8 SP).

One view is compatible with most of the data. Cells start differentiating in a manner that is not directly dependent on the nature of the coengaged coreceptor, but rather is dependent on other influences such as the physicochemical characteristics of the TCR–MHC signal [intensity, kinetic parameters, avidity (281)] or other microenvironmental influences [e.g., cell survival* or "fate switch" gene products (293,294,304)]. Secondarily, the validity of the cell's choice is verified, and only those cells that have maintained expression of the coreceptor that matches the TCR's restriction molecule can complete the maturation process and be exported from the thymus.

Site of

An important issue has been the nature of the cells that display self-MHC molecules to the differentiating thymocytes during positive selection. The question is whether there is a distinct type of positively selecting cell, one whose primary function is to present MHC molecules to DPs for sampling. Any such specialized cell type could have a distinct mode of protein processing and express a particular complement of costimulatory/adhesion molecules more conducive to survival than to death.

Several arguments support the notion that cortical epithelial cells play a special role in positive selection—both intuitive, because the DPs undergoing selection are enmeshed within the cortical epithelium network, and experimental, derived from several lines of evidence. First, healthy T-cell populations could be generated when nude mice were grafted with thymic rudiments depleted

---

*One of the oddest observations in this respect is perhaps that the absence of Fas (due to the lpr mutation) allows T-cell maturation in SCID mice, with a bias toward CD8+ cells (536).

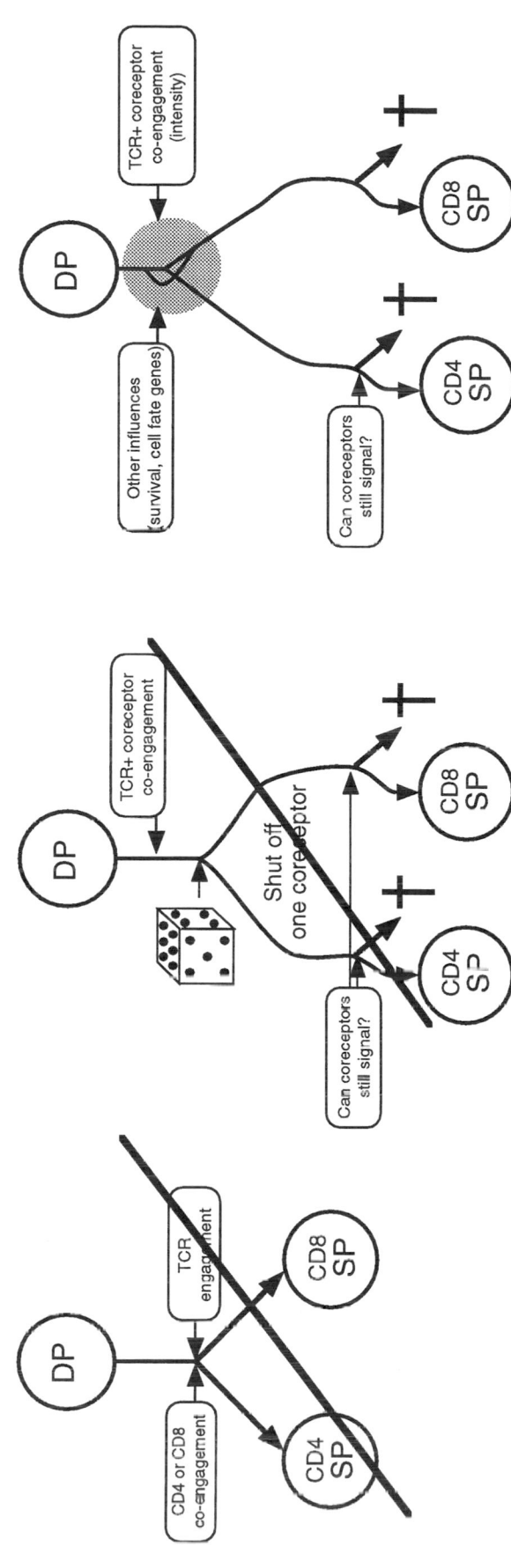

FIG. 14. Models of lineage commitment during positive selection. Depicted here are three different explanations of the cellular and molecular decision-making processes that lead T cells to commit to either the CD4+ or the CD8+ lineages during positive selection. In the first model, direct perception of the class of MHC molecules that engages the TCR (most readily by recognition of which coreceptor is engaged concomitantly) channels differentiation along one of the pathways. Although an early favorite, this model is in disfavor because mismatched differentiation can be readily demonstrated and rescued by forced co-receptor expression through a transgene, and because differentiation of mature cells can take place in co-receptor knock-out mice, if with reduced efficiency. These data, and the description of mismatched selection intermediates, supported the second model, which proposes that the early events of positive selection lead to commitment in an essentially random manner, but that the validity of the choice made by individual cells is confirmed secondarily after expression of one of the co-receptors is shut off; only those cells that keep the co-receptor matched to their TCR's specificity can survive. The stochastic aspect of the lineage choice, perhaps inherently unpalatable ("God does not play dice with either the Universe or positive selection") was also disproved by several observations: varying the affinity/avidity of the TCR/MHC interaction can induce different flows of differentiation, and cell survival or fate genes can also alter the balance of early commitment events. The third model incorporates these inductive influences on lineage choice, as well as the demonstration that commitment (at least to the CD8 lineage) can follow several routes, with apparent fluctuations in coreceptor expression.

of hematopoietic components or with fd10 thymus rudiments (before any colonization by hematopoietic precursors) (305,306). Second, positive selection in transgenic mice with compartmentalized MHC gene expression requires display of the selecting molecule on the cortical epithelium (272). Finally, only thymic epithelial cells could promote positive selection in disaggregation–reaggregation FTOCs (307). Given their likely role in positive selection, it is interesting that cortical epithelial cells appear to have antigen-processing pathways that differ markedly from those of dendritic cells or macrophages, characterized in particular by a defect in the ability to process exogenous proteins (308–310).

There are, however, a few discordant observations. For example, in reciprocal bone marrow chimeras between wild-type and MHC-deficient mice, positive selection by MHC class II molecules strictly followed the genotype of the radioresistant stroma (271); in contrast, class I–expressing hematopoietic cells had a clear capacity to positively select $CD8^+$ cells, although efficiency was substantially lower than with class I–positive epithelium (270). This dichotomy between class I– and class II–restricted selection is reminiscent of some older observations in radiation chimeras (311,312). In another set of experiments, positive selection was induced in MHC-deficient mice by intrathymic injection of cells expressing MHC molecules; the type of injected cell mattered little, and even fibroblast lines were active in this context (313–315). However, it was not possible to rule out transfer of MHC molecules, or three-cell interactions, in these protocols; nevertheless, these results did bring a note of caution to the preeminent position of the cortical epithelial cell. Overall, it is probable that the latter does indeed play a dominant role in positive selection, if only because it is the main MHC-positive cell type in the cortex and because of its tight anatomic connections with developing thymocytes. This role does not imply a unique set of peptides or surface phenotypic properties.

Ligands

Another issue is the exact nature of the MHC ligand involved in positive selection. In the thymus, as elsewhere, MHC molecules are loaded with peptides processed from self proteins. The question is whether there is any role for these peptides in positive selection and how any such involvement might relate to their stimulation of mature T cells. As illustrated in Fig. 15, it is conceivable that the TCRs on maturing thymocytes interact with MHC molecules carrying essentially any peptide, a specific subset of peptides, or a single peptide. Conceptually, the question traces back to the old one/two receptor debates (316): Are there regions of the TCR solely preoccupied with MHC contact and others only engaged by peptide, and what is the importance of either for positive selection? More generally, the eventual answer will have profound implications for the distinction between positive and negative selection in the thymus, and the role of self reactivity in shaping the repertoire.

This issue, which may not yet be entirely resolved, has been the focus of imaginative experimental strategies over the past decade. One elegant approach was the addition of peptides to FTOCs derived from mouse strains carrying mutations that interfere with peptide loading or surface display of MHC class I molecules (TAP, β2μ). Such experiments were most revealing when adapted to monitor the ability of various peptides to select cells displaying a single transgene-encoded TCR (317). An important conclusion from these studies was that peptides do play a specific role in pos-

1. Structural stabilization

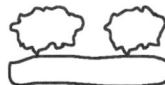
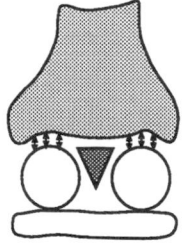

2. Not getting in the way

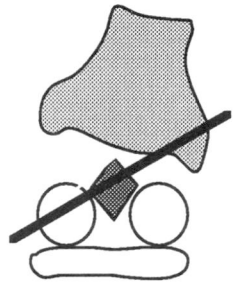
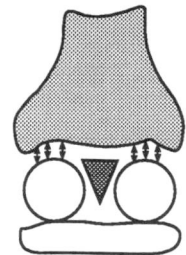

3. Direct recognition

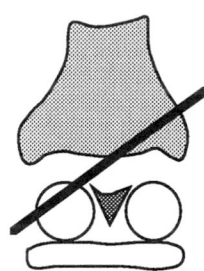
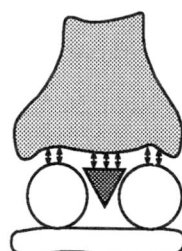

FIG. 15. Possible roles of peptidic ligands during positive selection. These cartoons depict possible interpretations of the role of MHC-bound peptides during positive selection. In panel 1, peptides merely serve a structural role, stabilizing the MHC molecule; this interpretation has been ruled out by many observations demonstrating a specific influence of peptide sequence on selection efficiency. In panel 2, the peptide does not positively contribute to the efficiency of selection, but the system only seeks to avoid TCR–peptide steric hindrance, TCR–MHC interactions driving the process. In panel 3, peptide plays a positive role, TCR–peptide contacts contributing significantly to the energetic balance of the tripartite interaction. Models 2 and 3 are quite difficult to distinguish experimentally, although data on the specificity of selection might favor interpretation 3.

itive selection, their ability to promote maturation going beyond mere stabilization of the MHC molecule (318,319). Later, the question was turned around, asking what receptors could be selected in mice engineered to express a single peptide–MHC complex, or in mice displaying a broad range of peptides but supplemented with particular single peptides (320).

Collectively, the experiments on ligands have permitted the conclusion that peptides partake in the specificity of positive selection, but with a large degree of degeneracy and promiscuity. The main points may be summarized as follows:

- There is no unequivocal relationship between a single TCR and a single peptide. MHC molecules carrying essentially a sole peptide are able to select a wide repertoire of T cells—perhaps as many as 20% to 50% of the normal amount (274,319,321–323). Conversely, the selection of a given TCR can be promoted by several peptides.

- Selection can be effected by MHC molecules loaded with peptides structurally and functionally related to the antigenic peptide able to stimulate mature cells. It was initially thought that antagonist analogs (variants incapable of stimulating the mature T cell, but able to prevent its stimulation by agonists) were best, an attractive notion because it provided a possible escape from the positive/negative selection conundrum (324). However, this did not prove to be generally applicable, and in several in vitro or in vivo systems there was no correlation between antagonist and selecting ability. Indeed, it was found that a peptide that stimulates a given mature T cell also can promote its selection (325 327). Clearly, then, positive selection yields a repertoire that has a significant component of self reactivity, at least until negative selection is allowed to take its toll. Overall, that peptides able to promote selection ranged from neutral to fully stimulatory for mature T cells is not directly compatible with simple affinity/avidity models of selection, and leave open the possibility that elements of peptide recognition other than basic thermodynamic parameters may have an influence (328).

- On the other hand, this similarity between selecting and antigenic peptide is not essential: selection could be enhanced by peptides unrelated in structure or apparent stimulatory capacity to the final antigenic peptide (327,329,330); conversely, single peptides could select broad repertoires of T cells with no particular reactivity toward analogs of the selecting peptide (274,275).

- This promiscuity of selection is probably a reflection of the general mode of TCR binding to its target and parallels that observed with the stimulation of mature T cells (331,332). In the crystallographic structures of TCR–peptide/MHC complexes, many amino acids of the TCR CDR3 loop that contact variable positions of the MHC molecules also contact peptide (333). Positive selection, while evaluating the general compatibility of the TCR with the MHC molecule, cannot but be influenced by bound self peptides

Signaling: The Positive/Negative Selection Paradox

TCR–MHC interaction is at the root of positive selection. It also directs negative selection. How then can the two be reconciled? The easiest way out of this dilemma is to propose that affinity/avidity differences condition the outcome of selection—high avidity interaction leading to apoptosis, lower avidity interactions provoking it to mature (334). The level of affinity/avidity could provoke differential responses either as a reflection of the degree of TCR/CD3 aggregation (e.g., high cross-linking leading to more ZAP-70 autophosphorylation) or through a time element, such as the duration of the Ca^{2+} flux (335). This notion has received some experimental support: for example, the finding that agonist or antagonist peptides can induce positive selection at low doses in FTOCs but provoke clonal elimination at higher concentrations (324 326). However, the outcome of FTOC experiments was often less straightforward (336,337); peptides that induce positive selec-

tion in vivo can have a wide range of effects later on in mature T cells (fully agonistic, antagonistic, or no detectable effect), and it seems difficult to resolve the dilemma purely on affinity considerations.* It has also been proposed that the signals leading to positive and negative selection differ in the nature of conformational changes imposed on the TCR by the chemistry of the peptide ligand (317,328); this notion has yet to receive direct support.

It is implicit in both models that a different signal must emanate from the TCR during positive and negative selection. Indeed, some evidence to this effect has been obtained. As might be expected (Fig. 4), the PTKs at the apex of the signaling cascades are necessary for all TCR-mediated signals, as made clear from the effects of ZAP-70 or lck gene inactivations (28,188). On the other hand, the ras pathway is important for positive selection signals but seems largely dispensable for negative selection, demonstrated by expressing dominant-negative mutants of ras or downstream kinases in transgenic mice (338,339). Signals through the calcineurin pathway, blocked by cyclosporine A, also seem more essential for positive than for negative selection (212,340). One potential caveat is that these differences could be quantitative, rather than qualitative, and may only reflect more robust signal transduction during negative signals (either pathway alone being sufficient for negative selection).

Negative Selection: Producing a Self-Tolerant Repertoire

Negative selection in the thymus is the first (and principal) screen for establishing self tolerance in the T-lymphocyte repertoire. Most of the common tissue antigens are encountered there, as are soluble proteins (as well as some proteins often erroneously relegated purely to specialized organs, e.g., insulin and myelin basic protein). Imparting tolerance to these self antigens early during the differentiation of T cells, before these have a chance to wreak havoc in specialized organs, is thus the second side of repertoire selection in the thymus. However, negative selection in the thymus is not foolproof, particularly for strictly extrathymic antigens; nor should it be absolute because a repertoire completely free of reactivity to self might well be devoid of reactivity to anything. The peptidic self that matters for T cells is only a minor fraction of the genomic self, limited by accessibility to processing pathways, by the specificities of proteolytic enzymes, by structural constraints on peptide binding to MHC molecules, and by quantitative requirements for a critical mass of antigen to initiate an effective response.

It has long been obvious that the most efficient way to deal with autoreactivity is to delete it (341). However, for a long time, clonal deletion was difficult to visualize, prompting alternative hypotheses such as suppression. Direct evidence for deletion first came from studies on tolerance to sAgs and from the analysis of self-reactive TCR transgenic mice. A classic study was the analysis of the frequency of CD4+ T cells expressing the Vβ17 region, which confers reactivity to endogenous mtv sAgs presented by the class II E molecule, and can be detected with a Vβ17-specific mAb. Significantly fewer Vβ17+ cells were found in E+ than in E mice

---

*There is also a built-in paradox for avidity models, in that the DP cell subject to positive selection is precisely that which expresses the lowest amount of TCR and should thus be the least sensitive to subliminal levels of signals.

(Fig. 16) (342). This applied to peripheral T cells and to the mature (TCR^{hi}) thymocyte pool but not to DPs, indicating that immature Vβ17$^+$ cells did exist in E$^+$ mice, but were somehow eliminated before maturity. This basic observation was reproduced in a number of Vβ:sAg combinations (343). The second clear proof of the principle of clonal deletion came from experiments on transgenic mice expressing a TCR reactive to the male-specific H-Y antigen. Deletion of the clonotype-expressing thymocytes was evident in male mice displaying the relevant MHC molecule (344). Similar observations were made in a variety of TCR transgenic mouse strains, with many forms of antigen and different restricting molecules (263,345–348). It is also possible to mimick thymocyte clonal deletion in vitro in suspension cultures or in FTOC systems (349,350).

Clonal deletion is an extremely sensitive process. Weakly agonistic antigens, or alloantigenic MHC variants that cannot stimulate mature T cells, are nevertheless capable of inducing deletion (351).

After some controversy, it is now clear that negative selection by clonal deletion can take place at various points along the differentiation pathway. For sAgs, it is mainly a late process, with deletion of TCR^{hi} thymocytes but little effect on DPs (342). With most peptide antigens derived from self proteins, deletion is earlier, a major reduction in DP cell numbers being observed; some peptide-specific TCR transgenics do exhibit late deletion, though, only affecting SP pools (348). It is only late in the maturation process that T cells become resistant to clonal deletion (76). The point of deletion is probably governed by which thymic compartment expresses a given antigen. TCR affinity also may play a role; given the different receptor levels expressed by DP and SP cells, higher affinity receptors may go first.

Not surprisingly, then, many stromal cell types are able to induce clonal deletion. Hematopoietic cells in the medulla (DCs in particular) may be particularly efficient because of their expression of costimulatory molecules (352), but epithelial components and even antigen carried on T cells themselves can induce clonal deletion (353–356). As mentioned above, the nature of the cell presenting the deleting antigen and its anatomic location both have a strong influence on the differentiative stage at which deletion is induced (353).

Apoptosis is the generic death mechanism responsible for negative selection in the thymus (59). It can be strikingly visualized by TUNEL histology, as in the sAg-mediated deletion illustrated in Fig. 17 (62). Interestingly, this study also showed that apoptotic cells in the thymus are cleared by macrophages extremely rapidly, apparently through interactions with scavenger receptors (357); this solves the old puzzle of why standard histologic stains of the thymus never showed the graveyard one would have expected of an organ in which 50 million cells die every day. The molecular pathways resulting in death after TCR triggering by self antigen are still unknown. A reasonable hypothesis (358,359) would be that TCR engagement leads to enhanced cell surface expression of members of the TNFR family [perhaps via the transcription factor nur77 as an intermediate (360,361)]; binding of the corresponding ligands by these receptors would then precipitate death. However, at present there is no TNFR family member that can unequivocally be assigned such a role. CD30/CD30L interactions might be involved because CD30-deficient animals seemed to have defects in negative selection (362). Fas was initially cleared of suspicion, in large part because of the phenotypes of Fas-deficient *lpr* mutants; however, more recent data seem to suggest that Fas may play a distinct, if nonessential, role (363). Further complications arise because new TNFR cousins whose expression patterns are consistent with a role in negative selection (DR3/WSL-1/TRAMP, DR4, CAR1) have recently been identified (359).

The global impact of clonal deletion on the exported repertoire is important. Given the diversity of self peptides that are presented in the thymus, one might expect that many of the self MHC–restricted T cells that pass the test of positive selection will run into trouble from negative selection. Indeed, with a surprising degree of concordance, three estimations performed with independent experimental approaches indicated that two thirds of the cells that are positively selected on self MHC in the cortex are subsequently deleted by a full array of self peptides expressed on medullary cells (274,275,364).

Clonal deletion is not the only way for the immune system to deal with unwanted self reactivity. Some cells that are functionally unreactive to self can be exported, either because they do not express the coreceptor needed for reactivity or because expression of a second TCR-α chain dilutes clonotypic reactivity (348, 365–367). Induction of anergy also has been reported, although it has been less well documented in the thymus than in peripheral tolerance induction (368–371), as have dominant tolerance (suppression) mechanisms (372).

Mouse	H-2	IE α:β	KJ23a		KJI6	
			% T cells Staining	% of KJ23a$^+$ Parent	% T cells Staining	% of KJI6$^+$ Parent
B10 x SJA	b/s	None	2.5±0.3(5)	(bar)	9.2±0.6(3)	(bar)
AKR x SWR	k/q	k:k	0.8±0.1(9)	(bar)	8.6±0.1(5)	(bar)
BALB/c x SJA	d/s	d:d,d:s	0.2±0.1(4)	(bar)	14.0±0.6(3)	(bar)
B10.S(7R) x SWR	t2/q	None	4.5±0.1(3)	(bar)	7.7±0.2(3)	(bar)
B10.HTT x SWR	t3/q	k:s	1.2±0.1(3)	(bar)	8.0±0.1(3)	(bar)
B10.TL x SWR	t1/q	k:k	1.1±0.2(3)	(bar)	8.3±0.1(3)	(bar)
B10.Q x (AKR x SWR)F1	q/q k/q	None k:k	5.5±0.1(4) 1.0±0.1(4)	(bar) (bar)	8.6±0.2(4) 7.9±0.1(14)	(bar) (bar)

FIG. 16. Tolerance by clonal deletion induced by MHC molecules. In this first demonstration of clonal deletion in the thymus (342), the percentage of T cells expressing Vβ17a, measured in several mouse strains by flow cytometry with the KJ23a mAb, was shown to correlate with the presence or absence of the MHC class II E molecule. The frequency of cells expressing Vβ8 (KJ16 staining) is shown as a standard. That the E molecule induces the deletion was supported by an accompanying paper showing that the Vβ17a region confers a particular reactivity to E, and was quickly confirmed by crosses with mice expressing E from a single transgene. In hindsight, the interpretation was not exactly correct: Vβ17a is actually reactive to endogenous superantigens, whose presentation requires E. Reproduced with permission from Kappler et al. (342).

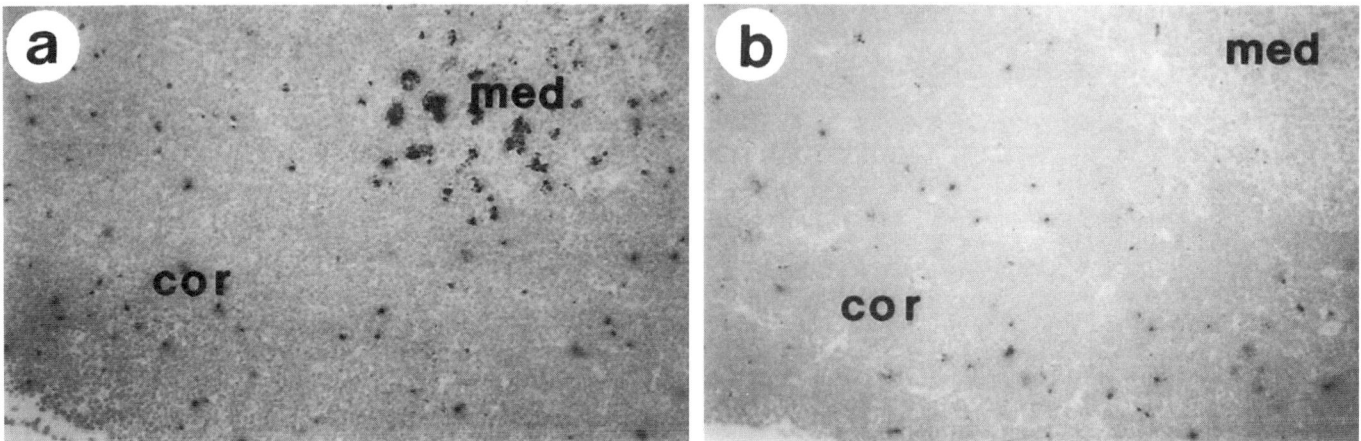

FIG. 17. Death by apoptosis induced by negative selection or by absence of positive selection. Apoptotic cells are detected by the TUNEL technique on thymic sections of transgenic mice expressing a TCR Vβ region whose deletion is induced by an endogenous superantigen presented by the MHC class II E molecule (62). In the E-positive thymus (**a**), apoptotic cells are seen scattered in the cortex, corresponding to death by lack of positive selection, and in the medulla (super antigen-induced apoptosis). The latter is missing in the E-negative thymus (**b**), cortical apoptosis is still present, but superantigen-induced apoptosis is now clearly visible in the medulla.

PERIPHERAL CIRCULATION OF T-LYMPHOCYTES

Circuits

After their export from the thymus, T cells colonize the peripheral lymphoid organs—not in a static manner, but by continuously recirculating between them. This constant circulation, via the bloodstream and the lymphatic vessels, allows lymphocytes of the relevant specificity to access antigen trapped in lymphoid organs, wherever it may enter the body: antigens breaching outer body barriers are ferried to the lymph nodes (LNs) or Peyer's patches (PPs), whereas blood-borne antigens are trapped in the spleen.

In the circuit schematized in Fig. 18, T cells leave the bloodstream to enter an LN through a particular endothelial cell lining called a *high endothelial venule* (HEV). After binding via specific receptors and adhesion molecules, they pass between these endothelial cells by diapedesis and enter the principal T-cell area of the LN, the paracortex. It is in this area that they may encounter a relevant antigen presented by the numerous dendritic cells found there, which have themselves entered the node through an afferant lymphatic vessel after collecting antigen in the outer tissues. If the T cell finds nothing exciting there, it migrates to the medullary regions of the LN and exits through an efferent lymphatic vessel. These lymphatics drain into other LNs in a chain, ultimately converging in the thoracic duct. This terminal lymphatic vessel empties into the venous bloodstream in the left subclaviar vein. From

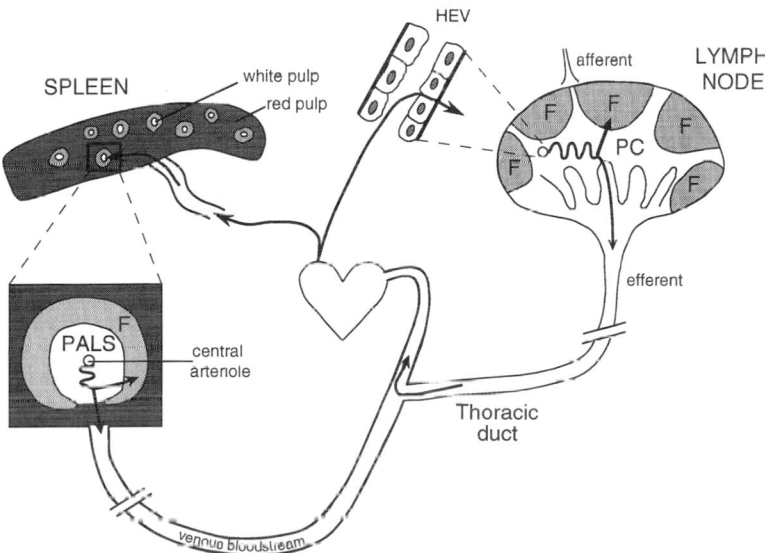

FIG. 18. A schematic representation of T-lymphocyte circulation. T cells enter the lymph node through afferent lymphatics that drain the tissues or by extravasation from the blood through the particular endothelium of HEVs, and home to the paracortex (PC). From there they can migrate to B-cell follicles and germinal centers (F), or away from the lymph node through efferent lymphatics. The latter ultimately converge into the thoracic duct, which empties into the venous bloodstream. T cells arrive in the spleen and congregate in the PALS, the central area of the splenic white pulp islands. From there, they can either migrate into B cell follicular areas if activated, or exit and recirculate through the blood stream.

the bloodstream, T-lymphocytes can then return to other LNs, but many are retained in the spleen.

Unlike LNs, the spleen benefits from a large and direct blood supply. T cells enter via the red pulp and migrate rapidly into the white pulp or may enter the white pulp directly through central arterioles. In any case, they again congregate in a particular area, the periarteriolar lymphoid sheath (PALS), the splenic equivalent of the LN paracortex, also populated by dendritic cells. In the absence of a productive encounter with the relevant antigen, T cells leave the spleen by moving into the red pulp, and from there back into the venous circulation. Overall, the circuit takes several hours, with a particularly long transit through the spleen (6 hours or so). It is estimated that naive T-lymphocytes accomplish the entire circuit once or twice a day.

A number of factors can interrupt or reroute this regular circulation pattern. Upon encounter with antigen-presenting dendritic cells in the lymphoid organ's T areas, antigen-reactive T cells are temporally sequestered there. This was originally demonstrated by introduction of antigen intravenously: in the two days after injection, antigen-reactive cells were undetectable in the thoracic duct (373). Eventually they emerge from the T areas. Some are now routed toward the B-cell follicles and the germinal centers, where they provide specific helper function, whereas others return to the general circulation but with significantly altered homing properties. The capacity to extravasate through HEVs is reduced, but the lymphocytes can now bind and migrate across flat endothelia normally impermeable to naive cells. Consequently, they can access extralymphoid sites: skin, pulmonary interstitium, intestinal connective spaces, joints, etc. Furthermore, although naive T cells have a fairly homogeneous circulation pattern, the circulation of activated cells is heterogeneous, characterized by restricted and tissue-selective homing patterns (374,375). These homing specificities tend to correlate with the location of the primary activation (376), which makes physiologic sense: a pathogen initially encountered in the PPs is more likely to be met again in the gut than in the skin. They also vary with the phenotypic properties of the T cells. For example, only Th1 cells make the carbohydrate ligands that allow them to interact with endothelial E- and P-selectins at sites of inflammation (377).

Adhesive Interactions

The differential recruitment of T cells from the vasculature is mediated by specific homing receptors on the lymphocytes, which interact with addressins on the endothelia. These interactions are molecularly complex, in that they involve multiple receptors and ligands from several protein families, members of which can be expressed on either the lymphocytes or the endothelia. The interactions can be separated into distinct steps, according to a multistep model of vascular extravasation that was originally proposed for neutrophils (374,375,378). Initially there is a rolling stage, in which the lymphocyte "rolls" along the endothelium, slowed down from its normal unimpeded flow by multiple transient, fast-on and fast-off, molecular interactions. Many of these correspond to the recognition of carbohydrate ligands by selectin molecules (L-selectin, or CD62L, being the primary player in the homing of naive cells to HEV). The rolling stage is followed by stable arrest of the T cell, mediated primarily by integrin engagement. This step involves a transient and reversible conformational change of the integrin molecules, necessary for tight binding, seemingly the

result of a G protein–mediated signaling event (possibly through a chemokine receptor) (375,379). The last stage is the actual transmigration of the lymphocyte between the endothelial cells.

It was originally thought that distinct molecular entities might mediate the different stages of lymphocyte–endothelial cell interactions as well as dictate the tissue-specific homing patterns. But now it is understood that particular adhesion molecules can play a role at several steps of the process: α4-integrins, for example, can participate in initial tethering of the lymphocyte as well as in firm contact between the lymphoid and endothelial cells, when analyzed under conditions of physiologic hydrodynamic shear (380,381). In addition, a given adhesion molecule can be involved in the initial recognition of different tissues (e.g., α4β7 integrin and various mucosa). Hence, it is the combination of adhesion molecules that confers tissue specificity to the process rather than the unique effect of any particular one. Beyond their mere presence at or absence from the cell surface, adhesion molecules are modulated by two additional features. First, conformational changes affect their activity: the paradigm here is LFA-1 (αLβ2 integrin), which undergoes a conformational change upon integrin signalling at the early phases of adhesion, acquiring much higher affinity for its ligands, ICAM-1 and -2 (382). Second, the clear topographic partitioning of adhesion molecules on the cell surface critically influences their mode of operation: L-selectin and α4β7 integrin are found exclusively on the tips of microvilli, in a position essential for interacting quickly with the endothelium during the rolling phases (383); in contrast, the β2 integrins involved in leukocyte immobilization are excluded from the microvilli, rather being concentrated on the planar area of the cell membrane (384).

Several stroma-derived chemokines of the CC and CxC families also play a role in promoting lymphocyte homing (385). By binding to the extracellular matrix, these molecules create a solid-phase gradient that can guide cells to the site of aggression. Several of the chemokines (such as IP10) have chemotactic activity that is preferential for lymphocytes over other monocytes. Correspondingly, several chemokine receptors are expressed more particularly on T cells (some acting as coreceptors for HIV infection of human CD4+ cells) (385). Display of these receptors at the surface is modulated by activation, upregulated by IL-2 but downregulated by TCR and CD28 engagement. Because of the complexity of the chemokine and chemokine receptor gene families, their interplay in directing T-cell homing and their role in the various phases of the process have yet to be fully grasped.

T-CELL RESPONSES

The study of in vivo T-lymphocyte responses to antigen was long hampered by the low frequency of T cells responsive to any given antigenic stimulus. The impossibility of tracking antigen-specific T-lymphocytes, other than by detecting their functional manifestations, restricted studies of T-cell activation to the in vitro analysis of polyclonal responses to lectin mitogens, or to frequency analysis of alloreactive responses. Newly developed tools lifted this limitation several years ago, and now three experimental systems allow one to directly follow T-cell responses in vivo: introduction of viral or bacterial sAgs, which stimulate essentially all T cells expressing a particular Vβ region (386–388), injection of peptide antigens that elicit a response with a largely invariant TCR Vα/Vβ combination (389,390), and manipulation of mice that express a rearranged TCR transgene, which can be followed with appropriate clonotype-specific reagents, either in the transgenics themselves or as mixed chimeras (391,392).

From its vantage point in the lymph node paracortex or the spleen PALS, the naive T cell is in a prime location for encountering antigen. The latter can be delivered either directly from the bloodstream or by dendritic cells that pick up material in peripheral tissues and ferry it to the lymph nodes. Upon antigen encounter, the initial phase of the response consists of a trapping and sequestering of the reactive T cells (Fig. 19), causing them to discontinue lymph/blood recirculation and to remain in situ. One set of experiments indicated that, within 24 hours after injection, antigen-specific T cells become undectable in the recirculating pools of the thoracic duct and other secondary lymphoid organs (373). Indeed, this property was exploited in classical experiments to eliminate alloreactive cells: by reconstituting alymphoid A-type hosts with B-type lymphocytes, A-reactive T cells were specifically purged from the circulating thoracic duct population (393).

Next follows an activation and proliferation phase, which lasts approximately 1 week. This is signaled by profound alterations in the cell surface expression of activation and adhesion molecules (increased CD25, CD69, CD40-L, Fas-L, and CD44, and decreased CD62L and CD45R expression). Some of these changes are necessary for cell-cycle progression, whereas others release the T cells from sequestration and allow them to disseminate through other lymphoid organs and peripheral tissues. Activated antigen-specific T cells also migrate into the adjoining germinal centers where they progressively accumulate (394) and there deliver help to relevant B cells. Activation is accompanied by the onset of cytokine synthesis, IL-2, -3, -4, IFN-γ, etc., progressively more biased toward the Th1 or Th2 phenotypes within the first few days (395,396). The extent of local expansion during this phase can be impressive: from 100- to 5,000-fold in some systems (389,391,397). Expansion is accompanied by clonal selection of cells with particular receptors in

some, but not all, responses. For example, during the response to the immunodominant peptide from moth cytochrome c, the distribution of TCR sequences dovetails with time toward the canonical Vα11/Vβ3 sequences best suited for recognition (389); however, such clonal selection was not observed with other antigens (390). At the end of a few days, this initial phase of the response generates effector T cells: fully armed CD8+ cytotoxic T-lymphocytes (CTLs) capable of direct target lysis, polarized CD4+ effectors secreting copious amounts of cytokines.

There soon follows a contraction phase that can be as dramatic as the expansion that preceded it, most of the activated CD4+ or CD8+ T cells undergoing apoptosis. This phenomenon, globally referred to as activation-induced cell death (AICD), encompasses several distinct death processes. AICD was first noted in T-hybridomas, many of which die within 24 hours of stimulation (398). It also was observed in vivo after systemic stimulation by bacterial sAgs or peptide antigens (386–388,399). AICD represents a heightened sensitivity of recently stimulated cells to apoptosis induced by TCR cross-linking, linked to the cell cycle (400); on the other hand, AICD also can eliminate T cells immediately at the time of initial stimulation, particularly in virally infected individuals (401,402). In its most extreme form, clonal exhaustion, AICD can lead to the complete elimination of all antigen-reactive cells, and is thus probably at the root of the long-recognized phenomenon of high-dose tolerance (403,404).

In the most direct form of AICD, TCR signaling activates several early-response transcription factors, such as NF-ATp, TDAG51, and members of the nur77 family of orphan receptors (358,359). These most likely act by inducing the expression of members of the NGF/TNF receptor (TNFR) family. Among these, the Fas molecule has been most strongly implicated (405), and it may be significant that, although both Fas and Fas-L expression are induced on T cells early on during the activation process, T-lymphocytes seem sensitive to Fas-triggered apoptosis only after several days (406) [indeed, Fas triggering can even be stimulatory to T cells in some instances (407)]. Fas is unlikely to be the only conduit of AICD, however; other members of the TNFR family may transduce death signals in this context, as has been demonstrated for TNFR itself (408). Growth factor (IL-2) deprivation is also a likely mechanism, particularly in the waning phases of the response, when intercrine help is limited (409). In addition, it has been shown that activated T cells express N-glycan ligands for the galectin-1 lectin, which is expressed by thymic and lymph node stromal cells and can provoke T-cell apoptosis (410). Finally, an important element of AICD may be the homing of activated T cells to tissue compartments particularly prone to cell death: germinal centers (394) or the lymphocyte graveyard in the liver (411).

Teleologically, there are several reasons why AICD is a good idea. It clears away effector T cells, which are dangerous to keep around because of the immunopathology they tend to cause. It resets the immune system to respond to the next challenge. And, finally, a responsive system in which contraction follows expansion, on a cell-autonomous basis, deals neatly with the problem of overexpansion and has a built-in control loop. Such a system can dispense with clonotype- or antigen-specific regulation.

AICD is not the only means to abort a response. Responder T cells also may be subject to anergy. This phenomenon was first documented in vitro under suboptimal conditions of stimulation (412–414) and was later shown more specifically to be induced by antagonist peptides or by TCR engagement in the absence of proper costimulation (415,416). Cells in this state do show some

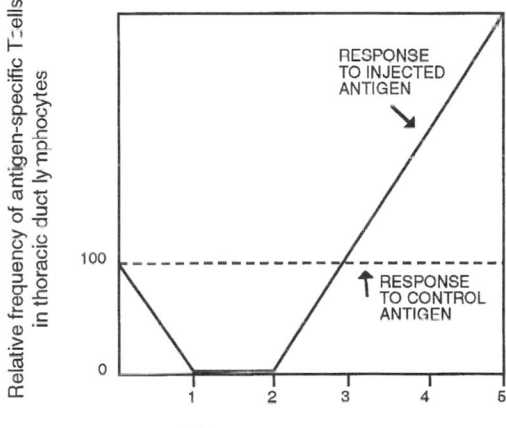

FIG. 19. Selective sequestration of T-lymphocytes exposed to antigen. Antigen administered intravenously lodges predominantly in the spleen and is taken up by APCs. Antigen-specific T cells perfusing the spleen recognize antigen and temporarily cease their normal pattern of blood-to-lymph recirculation (days 1 and 2). During this period, thoracic duct lymphocytes show no reactivity to the injected antigen. The T cells sequestered in the spleen proliferate extensively, and high numbers of their progeny reenter the circulation after about 3 days. Adapted with permission from Sprent (535).

reactivity to antigen: detectable Ca^{2+} increase, size increase, secretion of some cytokines such as IL-3 or IL-4, but no production of IL-2 or cell cycling (417). They are also more sensitive to AICD (418). Several deficiencies in signal transduction pathways correlate with this anergic state (419): a deficiency in the src family kinases (420), as well as a block in the ras transduction pathway (421,422). A negative transcriptional regulator of the IL-2 gene also has been implicated (423). It is not absolutely clear whether (or which) in vivo states correlate with these in vitro observations. More often, inappropriate stimulation by transgenic expression of MHC molecules on non-professional APCs seems to result in T populations with downmodulated TCRs, or co-receptors (424); cells surviving a massive sAg stimulation in vivo were also nonresponsive to further stimulation (399,425); finally, TCR transgenic mice tolerized by peripheral administration of antigen were also shown to be in an anergic state, through a mechanism which may depend on CTLA-4 engagement (392,426).

AICD and anergy also can be viewed in the more general context of a T cell's options after antigen encounter: activation and expansion, or anergy, or apoptosis. Several parameters enter into the choice:

1. The antigen dose and the affinity of the TCR for its ligand (suboptimal stimulation or antagonism leading preferentially to anergy)
2. The extent of coincidental costimulation and thus the nature of the APC (strong costimulator expression by the APC favoring activation)
3. The nature and amounts of cytokines in the local milieu, which can be costimulatory, support T-cell growth, or, conversely, promote AICD

The overall outcome is that antigen will lead to vigorous T-cell responses when encountered in the context of inflammation or stress, whereas anergy or death dominate in more isolated encounters with antigen on nonprofessional APCs. This dichotomy is essential to the induction of tolerance to self antigens expressed exclusively in the peripheral tissues, and is at the root of self/nonself discrimination in this context.

T-CELL EFFECTOR FUNCTIONS

The effector functions of fully stimulated T cells will only be sketched out here as they are detailed in other sections of this volume. T-cell expansion and differentiation in the first 3 or 4 days of the T-cell response leads to the generation of armed effector cells. The functions of these cells appear at first glance to be diverse and quite unrelated: killing of virally infected cells and helping B cells to proliferate and differentiate betray different "care and compassion" on the T cell's part. Yet there are many unifying elements in these diverse activities so that, in the end, they are quite similar mechanistically:

- Responsible cell. Effector activity lies in large granular lymphocytes generated within a few days after the initial challenge, and characterized by a very short life span.
- Time scale. Effector function is immediate. The TCR on the effector cell must recognize peptide–MHC complexes on the target cell to unleash the signal, with a response time on the order of seconds or minutes versus the hours or days necessary for induction of a resting T cell to secrete IL-2. The effector cell is then quickly released from the target and can turn to others.

- Sensitivity. Recognition by armed effectors is much more sensitive than that by naive cells, the former responding to far lower concentrations of peptide–MHC complexes. Although adhesion molecules are necessary to facilitate the process, it is no longer dependent on costimulation.
- Target. Much as a T cell can only recognize antigen presented by another cell, its effector functions are also exerted on cells, not on free antigen: e.g., on B cells, macrophages, or virally infected cells. Note, however, that armed effector T cells are able to kill directly some fungal or parasitic cells (427).
- Mediators. Two types of molecular mediators are used by effector T cells after TCR triggering: (a) membrane-bound molecules trigger a specific ligand on the target cell—strikingly, the cell surface molecules on the T cell all belong to the TNF family of proteins, whereas the receptors on the targets are all related to the TNFR; (b) soluble mediators are released, complementing the action of contact-dependent mediators. In both cases, the message is directed. The engaged TCR molecules cluster together with adhesion and coreceptor molecules within a small area of cell–cell contact (428). This clustering leads to focused release of exocytic granules, the activatory or lytic mediators thereby being "squirted" directly at the target cell. It also tends to focus, even if to a lesser extent, the engagement of cell surface receptor-ligand pairs. This directed mediator action restricts the effects to the relevant targets, with only limited action on bystander cells. Interestingly, the molecular mediators can have pleiotropic (even opposing) effects. The prototype here is TNF-α, which can induce apoptosis of the target cell or, in contrast, activate it, according to the dominant mode of signaling in the target cell [through FADD and the caspase family versus TRAF2 and NF-κB (429)].

B-Cell Help

The capacity to help B cells proliferate and produce specific antibody may be the most elaborate form of T-effector function (430). It is one that rests mainly with $CD4^+$ cells, particularly the Th2 subset. MHC class II molecules are an obligate conduit, as shown originally by the MHC restriction of T-B interactions (431,432), and formally confirmed by the absence of antibody responses in MHC class II–deficient animals (268). The specificity of the interaction was long a puzzle: how could a T cell know which B cell to help? Ever since the pioneering hapten-carrier experiments (433), it has been recognized that help requires the recognition of physically linked epitopes by T- and B-lymphocytes. Despite highly creative interpretations, this phenomenon was not really understandable before the molecular basis of antigen recognition by T cells became clear and before the seminal discoveries on the peculiarities of antigen presentation by B cells (434–437). The following paradigm is now generally accepted: the T cell is initially activated by antigen presented by professional APCs (primarily dendritic cells) and differentiates into an armed helper; it then delivers help primarily to those B cells that can present the same epitope; specificity of the T-B interaction stems from the huge increase in the efficiency of presentation by B cells when antigen is internalized through the surface Ig receptor, which allows much more efficient antigen uptake than nonspecific endocytic mechanisms, particularly inefficient in B cells (434). Thus, in effect, only those B cells whose Ig receptor can bind the same antigen [through a distinct epitope (438)] will process it and present the relevant peptide to activated T cells, and thereby receive effective help.

The CD40/CD40-L pair is the dominant, if not exclusive, molecular conduit for cell–cell interaction during the help process (439). CD40-L is induced upon activation of CD4$^+$ T cells by professional APCs. It can then engage CD40 on B cells, provoking activation and proliferation. This pair's unique role has been evidenced by the absence of antibody responses and germinal centers in patients (hyperIgM syndrome) or knock-out mice deficient in CD40 or CD40-L (440–446). It has long been debated whether T-cell help through cell–cell contact could trigger resting B cells to proliferation and Ig secretion in the absence of concomitant activation through the B cell's antigen receptor (447). It is now clear that engagement of CD40 on naive B cells can, alone, activate them, although stimulation through the surface Ig receptor does provide synergistic activation signals. One might argue that the primary function of sIg engagement may be to immobilize the B cells in contact with T cells in the PALS or the LN paracortex, where they may be fully activated by T cells (448).

Many of the cytokines produced by T cells influence B-cell differentiation. IL-2 enhances B-cell growth and Ig secretion. IL-4 also synergizes with signaling through CD40 to promote B-cell proliferation, but its more characteristic effect is to bias Ig class-switching, promoting a switch to the IgG1 and IgE isotypes by opening the constant region loci to transcription (449,450). In contrast, IFN-γ enhances switching to the IgG2a, and TGF-β to the IgG2b and IgA, isotypes. In mucosal tissues, IL-5 enhances IgA secretion by cells with an already switched IgA locus (451). Lymphokine secretion, particularly that of IL-4, is highly focused toward the antigen-presenting B cell (452,453).

In short, T-cell help for antibody responses is paradigmatic of T-effector functions, in that triggering is antigen specific (for both cells) and MHC restricted, but effector functions are nonspecific and nonrestricted.

Stimulation of Inflammation

This is the Th1 side of things (454). In its most immediate form, it entails the stimulation of antigen-bearing macrophages to increase their bactericidal, cytocidal, and inflammatory capacities (455), but these effectors T cells can also have direct toxic activity against parasitic or fungal organisms (427). They also induce the classical manifestations of DTH, the local reaction provoked by trans- or subcutaneous exposure of an individual to antigen:inflammation, cellular infiltration, and eventually dermatitis. When the antigen challenge persists and cannot be cleared (as with some bacterial infections), the DTH response progresses to organized granuloma formation. These phenomena are predominantly due to CD4$^+$ T cells for the classical DTH induced by protein antigens, and to CD8$^+$ cells for viral antigens or hapten-induced contact sensitivity.

The soluble mediators in this instance are mainly IFN-γ, granulocyte/macrophage colony stimulating factor (GM-CSF), lymphotoxin (TNF-β), and TNF-α, whereas the contact-dependent signal stems from membrane-bound forms of TNF. TNF and IFN-γ signals synergize in inducing an activated state in the macrophage: increased MHC molecule expression, bactericidal activity through phagosome fusion, and nitric oxide oxygen radical production. These mediators also have an important effect on the vascular endothelium early in the response, leading to increased expression of adhesion and homing molecules. These are essential for recruiting additional blood-borne leukocytes to the site of inflammation.

Cytolysis

One of the major functions of the T-cell compartment is to monitor somatic cells for infection by intracellular viruses and bacteria, as well as for oncogenic mutations, although immune responses in antitumor defenses may only be of secondary importance, compared with intracellular tumor suppressors. Being intracellular, these antigens cannot be detected directly, but only as indirect disturbances on the membrane of the afflicted cell (basically as MHC-bound peptides). Being intracellular, such antigens cannot be selectively destroyed or inactivated as they would be by antibodies in the extracellular milieu; the only resource is to destroy the entire affected cell. This takes place not through an active killing mechanism, but by suggesting suicide in a manner the target cell cannot refuse: induction of apoptosis.

CD8$^+$ cells are the major players in recognition of virally infected or allogeneic targets. Armed CD8$^+$ CTLs are generated 5 days after stimulation and kill target cells bearing cognate peptides associated with MHC class I molecules in a very rapid and dynamic fashion (456). Induction of apoptosis in the target cell is by two main mechanisms. First, death can be by exocytic release of cytotoxic granules that contain perforin and granzymes. The former is a pore-forming protein that, upon multimerization, opens a membrane-spanning pore in the target cell (457). The latter are proteases of the caspase family, which feed into the protease cascade of the common apoptosis pathway (458). Although the interconnection between granzymes and perforin is not fully established, one plausible scenario is that perforin-induced pores provoke apoptosis by eliciting a strong Ca$^+$ flux in the target cell while allowing entry of granzymes. Second, death also can be by direct cell-cell signaling, through the engagement of the Fas molecule on target cells by Fas-L on the effector T cell. Experiments combining perforin knock-out mice with Fas-deficient lpr mutants have shown convincingly that these two pathways account for essentially all of the cytotoxic activity of CD8$^+$ cells (459). The relative importance of the two depends largely on the level of Fas expressed by the target cell: lysis of fibroblasts is wholly dependent on perforin, that of Fas-positive hematopoietic cells less so.

CTL activity in CD4$^+$ effectors has been less extensively studied. It is primarily the privilege of Th1-type CD4$^+$ cells. The presence of perforin and granzymes in cytolytic CD4$^+$ T-cell clones has been reported (460), as has that of Fas-L (461). Which is the dominant killing mechanism in this instance is not clear, and may vary with the circumstances of T-cell priming and antigenic specificity (462,463).

γ:δ Cells

The function of γ:δ T cells is still somewhat nebulous (464). They do have demonstrable importance in the response to microbiologic infections (465–467). However, it has become increasingly evident that γ:δ cells, as a group, differ considerably from classical α:β cells. First, γ:δ cells can recognize nonpeptidic antigens (468–470) in a manner that is fundamentally different from how α:β cells see their antigens, without need for processing and presentation by an MHC-like molecule (471,172). In addition, the effector functions of γ:δ cells are probably quite distinct if one considers the intraepithelial populations with homogeneous receptors (Vγ5$^+$ DEC in the skin, Vγ6$^+$ intramucosal cells) and those with diverse receptors in the gut or lymphoid organs. DECs may represent a prototype for quasi-monoclonal T-cell populations (473). They express an essentially invariant repertoire generated during fetal ontogeny. Assuming a dendritic morphology, they are regularly interspersed within the epidermis, in contact with the keratinocytes. They appear to be selectively activated by a product of "stressed" keratinocytes. One hypothesis is that DECs are a frontline defense against pathogens in the skin, one that reacts when keratinocytes come under attack, initiating an inflammatory response by the secretion of Th1-like cytokines, and recruiting conventional lymphocytes by the secretion of lymphotactin, a T cell–produced chemokine that is a powerful lymphocyte attractant (474,475). It also has been suggested that intraepithelial γ:δ cells support the growth of epithelial tissues by secreting epithelial growth factors (476,477), particularly during regeneration after wounding. The diverse γ:δ cells of the gut and lymphoid organs have more conventional effector activities, comparable with those of α:β cells: cytotoxicity (478,479), help to B cells through IL-4 and CD40-L (480,481), and activation of macrophages through IFN-γ (464). Their ability to recognize antigen directly, without processing or presentation, is consistent with a role as front-line defense against pathogens.

Nonconventional T Cells

Even more enigmatic is the minor population of persistently activated α:β CD4$^+$ T cells restricted not by MHC class II molecules, but rather by nonclassical class I molecules such as CD1 and TL (482,483). A proportion of these cells uses an invariant Vα14Jα28 receptor and expresses surface markers characteristic of conventional NK cells (and are thus referred to as NK-T cells), but this is not true for all of them. Despite generating much interest (484), the role of these cells remains unclear; several properties specifically attributed to them (e.g., quick cytokine release after polyclonal stimulation, expression of NK cell markers) are also shared by activated T cells and may be a mere consequence of their activation state. Elimination of the CD1 molecule in knock-out mice strongly reduced the NK-T compartment but did not lead to detectable perturbations of immune function, except under artificial conditions (485,486).

Regulation

Are there T cells whose primary function is to regulate the activity of other lymphocytes? If one leaves out the B-cell helper or macrophage stimulatory functions described above, the answer to this question is still very much open. The immunocosmologies of the 1970s, based on creative interpretation in the absence of reliable biochemistry or genetics, have largely fallen into disfavor, taking with them the arcane circuits of suppressor cells, helper factors, and antiidiotypic networks. As a backlash, the very concept of regulatory or suppressor T cells has been endowed with a negative connotation (487,488). Much of the phenomenology attributed to antigen- or idiotype-specific regulatory cells can now be ascribed to geographically specific application of nonspecific effector activities-biasing effects of nonspecific cytokines (IL-4 will favor a Th2 response, and thus appear to suppress the Th1 response evaluated in a DTH assay); preferential enhancement of class-switching to

particular isotypes by particular cytokines (rather than direct isotype recognition by isotype-specific T helper cells); targeted help from a T cell toward a B cell presenting a particular peptide as a consequence of its surface Ig specificity (rather than antigen-specific helper factors or idiotype-specific help). It has also become clear that the immune system possesses cell-autonomous control systems to limit the extent of an immune response: AICD, negative signaling mediated, for example, by CTLA-4 (489), and cell death through cytokine deprivation. An interesting new development in this regard is the finding that activated T cells express, and can be bridled through, killer inhibitory receptors that bind MHC class I molecules and control NK activity (490,491). These forms of autonomous ergotypic regulation can largely stand in for previously postulated idiotypic regulatory circuits based on feedback cell–cell interactions. Despite these considerations, there are still a number of observations that may imply the existence of specific regulatory cells, yet to be formally characterized (492–494). Immunoregulation is one area of immunology that still has, at this writing, many veils.

T-LYMPHOCYTE MEMORY

The nature, and in fact the very existence, of T-cell memory has been a contentious issue (495–498). Its goals and mechanisms must be somewhat different from those of B-cell memory because of the inherently more cross-reactive nature of antigen recognition by TCRs; and because affinity maturation of TCRs by somatic mutation, if it exists at all (499), is very limited, so that there is little incentive to preserve cells expressing a particularly valuable receptor pain-stakingly derived by sequential somatic mutation events. Thus, T-cell memory can rely only on clonal expansion and selection of pools of antigen-specific cells expressing high-affinity receptors, and on phenotypic changes rendering memory cells more quickly or efficiently responsive to secondary stimulation.

It is difficult to designate memory T cells as a discrete class; indeed, their characterization often has been muddled by indiscriminate use of cell surface markers as specific identifiers, even though the same proteins are also expressed by short-term activated and effector cells. The potential for antigen persistence in immunized or infected individuals, leading to chronic low-level stimulation, also complicates the designation of true memory (by definition independent of antigen). Other possible complications are artefacts linked to the experimental systems used to study memory cells (e.g., cellular expansion in reconstituted lymphocyte-deficient mice, unsuspected irradiation-induced damage). That said, memory phenomena do exist in the T-lymphocyte compartment, and increased precursor frequencies can be demonstrated long after exposure to real-life antigens (500).

Despite these pitfalls, a plausible scenario may be sketched (Fig. 20). Upon activation of naive T cells, a number of distinctive phenotypic changes take place and persist, although heterogenously, in effector and memory populations: de novo or increased expression of CD44, Ly6C, α4β1-integrin and LFA1, and downregulation of CD62L and of the large alternatively spliced forms of CD45 (CD45RA, CD45RB). These phenotypic alterations are not necessarily universal, being prone to variation with the conditions of antigen stimulation (496,498). Some of these changes result in modified trafficking pathways (374), enhanced reactivity to antigen, and independence of coreceptor signals (392,501–506). Within the ensemble of antigen-experienced cells, effectors can be

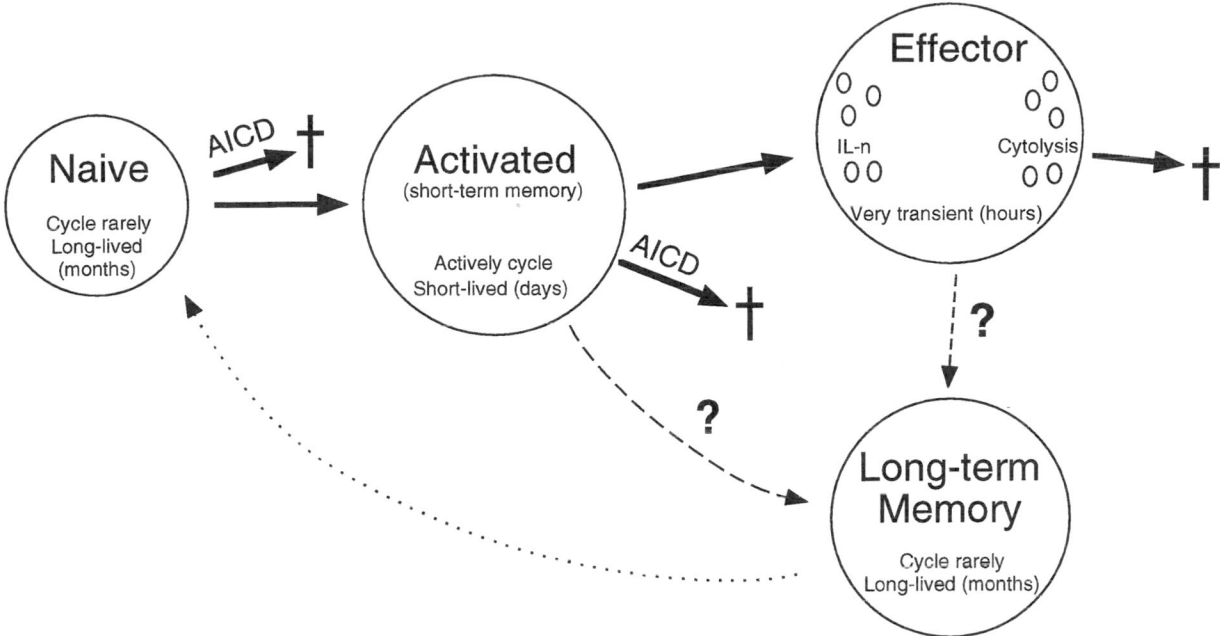

FIG. 20. Pathways of memory formation. A plausible scheme of the different states of T cells, as a consequence of exposure to cognate antigen. The fully naive T cell at left is activated by antigen, if not provoked to suicide in AICD. The activated cells proliferate extensively, but require continued stimulation or cytokine exposure for persistence. Terminal differentiation into fully active effector cells results in the capacity to secrete large amounts of cytokines (IL-n) or to induce immediate target cell lysis (through perforin/granzyme or fas-mediated killing). It is not known from whence the long-term memory populations (resting cells at higher precursor frequencies than in the naive individual) originate.

distinguished from activated or memory cells by the immediacy of their action: direct lysis of targets by effector CD8[+] CTLs and secretion of cytokines by CD4[+] helpers. In contrast, activated or memory cells require prior TCR-mediated activation, albeit short, to induce these functions.

Although the dichotomy of memory cells represented in Fig. 20 may be overly simplistic, several traits clearly distinguish short-term from long-term memory populations. Short-term memory reflects large cohorts of T cells that are amplified in the days and weeks that follow antigen stimulation to reach very high frequencies of antigen-specific cells (one in 100 or greater). These cells cycle frequently. Their trafficking pathways, as a consequence of the changes in surface expression of homing and adhesion molecules, are quite different from those of naive cells: instead of a circumscribed blood to lymph node recirculation mediated by binding to HEV, these cells can patrol nonlymphoid tissues (374,495), and are thus a major factor in early resistance to pathogens invading nonlymphoid organs (495). This short-term memory population has a rather finite life span (507) and is dependent on antigen for persistence (508,509). Several of these characteristics are quite different in long-term memory cells. These are very long lived (on the order of months to decades), but are present only at low frequencies (one in 10,000 to one in 100,000 (500). Long-term memory cells cycle very slowly, similar to naive T cells (510,511). They show at least some degree of reversion of the changes in cell surface markers mentioned above (397,506,512); for example, they have largely lost their tissue-homing capabilities (495). Protection by long-term memory cells thus requires antigen presentation in the lymphoid organs, so that their role in early protection against

agression in nonlymphoid tissues is limited. It has been shown that these long-lived cells may preserve the Th1/Th2 polarization that dominated during their inception (513). They can also maintain a memory of the initial site of their antigen encounter with antigen, evidenced as a preferential bias in circulation routes (514). Their persistence has now been convincingly shown to be independent of antigen, at least for CD8[+] cells (505,515–517), the original controversies most likely attributable to differences in experimental systems, certain of which followed short-term memory/activated cells that require antigen for high-level maintenance (508,509). What allows long-lived memory populations to persist, in contrast to the disapparance of the majority of antigen-reactive cells? Perhaps they survive because of a cell-intrinsic program of high-level expression of antiapoptotic molecules (e.g., the Bcl family), although this persistence also may require occasional TCR "tickling," as for naive cells. Stimulation by cross-reactive antigens (518) probably plays a role to some extent, and memory cells could be particularly sensitive to nonspecific activation through costimulatory molecules or cytokines.

The lineage relationships between these different types of antigen-experienced cells are essentially unknown. Do long-term memory cells differentiate from effector cells that are rescued from death? Do they differentiate from short-term activated cells in an active process? Or do they merely represent leftovers? It could be that long-term memory cells are generated primarily in the late phases of the immune response, when antigen becomes scarce and only those cells with higher affinity receptors are triggered, in a manner not conducive to activation-linked apoptosis. A degree of affinity maturation at the population level might thus be achieved in the memory T compartment, not through receptor mutation but merely by retaining the most apt cells.

T-CELL HOMEOSTASIS AND LIFE SPAN

Leukocyte populations, particularly T-lymphocytes, face a difficult task in maintaining homeostasis. As unanchored circulating cells, their population size cannot simply be constrained by an organ's physical limits as would be that of liver cells, for example. Yet such a control is essential for cells that respond to antigen recognition by proliferating, to keep them from filling up all vascular and extravascular spaces. Furthermore, leukocytes differ from most mammalian cells, which are sensitive to anoikis [death by the absence of attachement, a process that can be prevented by activation of signaling pathways or overexpression of antiapoptotic factors (519–521)]. How is this basic biologic feature addressed by T-lymphocytes that are constantly recirculating? This second difference may only be apparent: B cells excluded from follicular niches also die quickly (522). Hence, one could imagine that T cells receive and compete for survival signals from stromal cells in the PALS and paracortex.

Additionally, the immune system must be able to maintain a cohort of naive cells, potentially responsive to new antigens encountered late in the life of the individual, without becoming wholly occupied by expanded memory populations. Thus, a balance between naive and memory cell pools needs to be preserved (523).

The size of the T-lymphocyte compartments at steady state is governed (as is any compartment) by a balance between the input and output of cells. Input corresponds to the flow of naive cells exported from the thymus, but also to the expanded numbers generated by cell division in response to antigen-specific triggering and nonspecific bystander stimulation. For classical α:β T-cell populations, the input of naive cells from the thymus is maximal in young individuals and then wanes as the thymus involutes; in adults (at 8 months of age in mice or 40 years in humans), thymic cellularity and output is only 10% of its maximum (524). Although this contribution is not insignificant, the steady-state T-cell populations in an adult organism are mainly controlled by a balance between cell death due to neglect or AICD on the one hand, and pool expansion from cell division on the other. Extensive expansion can be observed when mice devoid of T-lymphocytes are reconstituted with mature T cells (525,526); it is less pronounced in normal individuals, but it still appears that peripheral expansion plays a role in reshaping the postthymic repertoires: for example, in most TCR transgenic mice, the proportion of T cells that express an endogenously encoded TCR chain due to escape from allelic exclusion is substantially greater in the peripheral populations than in compartments of mature thymic cells.

T-lymphocyte homeostasis is best understood in terms of competition for survival. Competition may be for soluble factors like cytokines or for cell-surface ligands displayed on stromal cells, or a combination of the two, cytokines being most efficiently received when the T cell is in close contact with the stromal cell. These elements define the basic niche, whose availability controls cell numbers. Total T-cell numbers, which can vary between individuals or with time, will be set (a) by the level of these extrinsic cues and (b) by the response of the T-cell population to these cues. Thus, there is a degree of flexibility in homeostatic control, which is manifest during infections or when mutations perturb the lymphocyte's response to extracellular signals. Note also that the lymphocyte populations also shape the size of their own niches. An illustrative example can be found with mice lacking mature thymocytes (SCID, RAG-deficient, MHC-deficient) in which the medullary stroma of the thymus remains but a small rudiment (55). These environmental size controls can be applied in a very discriminatory manner. For example, CD8+ T cell numbers increase to replace the missing CD4+ cells in MHC class II–deficient mice; but γδ or B cells do not expand in compensation, even when a complete MHC deficiency eliminates the classical α:β T-cell compartment. Similarly, T-lymphocytes do not expand to fill B-lymphocyte areas in B cell–deficient animals.

The population kinetics of naive and memory T-cell populations have been examined by tracer studies (usually by labeling proliferating cells with ³H-TdR or BrdU) in normal mice, in alymphoid animals reconstituted with normal T cells, or in TCR transgenic animals that allow one to follow the fate of cells expressing a single specificity; in humans, this been done mainly by following the persistence of radiation-induced chromosomal aberrations (510,526–528). These experiments have shown that the bulk of naive T cells persist for long periods of time in a quiescent state (months to years), with only rare cycling events. Memory cells (with the caveats on their identification mentioned above) contain a more actively cycling component with a short life span, but also some long-lived noncycling cells. To bolster the long life of these populations, cytokines such as IL-2, -4, and-7 may deliver survival signals (529) and the low-level cycling in the absence of TCR stimulation may be driven by type-I IFNs (530).

Interestingly, activated T-lymphocytes express tolemerase, as do self-renewable germline and hematopoietic stem cells (531). This ribonucleoprotein enzyme is normally absent from somatic cells, whose chromosomes shorten and become less stable with successive divisions. Does telomerase facilitate the long-term stability of T-cell populations?

Most recently, it has become apparent that peripheral T cells require some form of TCR–MHC engagement. In the absence of MHC molecules, or with an inappropriate allele, naive T cells have abbreviated life spans in the peripheral lymphoid organs (85,532,533). This also applies to memory cells, although the specificity of the interaction appears less fastidious in this case (533). It has been hypothesized that signals similar to those involved in thymic positive selection are required in order to "tickle" T cells out of terminal boredom.

CONCLUSIONS AND PERSPECTIVES

Some of the major challenges of T-lymphocyte biology have been met. We now know how a T cell sees foreign antigens, how a diversity of antigen receptors is generated, what the receptor on the cell surface actually looks like, how it recognizes peptides bound to MHC molecules on APCs, and how the APCs produce these peptides from antigenic proteins. Critical coreceptors, costimulatory molecules, and adhesion molecules located on the T-cell surface have been molecularly characterized, as has a growing number of signaling molecules residing within. We also know the fundamentals of how T cells are generated—how many, when, where, and by what pathways—and how they are enriched for those recognizing foreign antigens bound to self-MHC molecules and purged of those reactive to self antigens associated with self-MHC molecules. Finally, in recent years, we have constructed a molecular image of how T cells perform their diverse functions: help via secreted cytokines and cell–cell interactions mediated by receptor–ligand pairs such as CD40–CD40-L, and killing via perforin, granzymes, and Fas–Fas-L interactions.

Yet, important challenges remain to be tackled. Many of these entail progressing from an essentially descriptive to a more integrative view. For example, we need to learn how variant signals delivered through the antigen receptor and other surface molecules are channeled within the cell and collated to provoke divergent phenotypic changes. We must move beyond defining intricate pathways of T-cell differentiation to dissecting the mechanisms by which survival and lineage choices are made, which will ultimately require translating cell/cell interactions into protein–protein or protein–DNA interactions. And, now that we have a more precise image of how T cells exert their functions, the next step is to understand how the various functional capabilities are regulated, elucidating how the timbre of a response is set, and how it can be amplified, diversified, or dampened.

The remaining challenges, being of a more integrative bent, stand to be more difficult to tackle, but probably even more stimulating.

REFERENCES

1. Moller G(ed). Superantigens. Immunol Rev 1993; 131:
2. Fathman CG, Frelinger JG. T-lymphocyte clones. Ann Rev Immunol 1983;1: 633–655.
3. Jenkinson EJ, Owen JJ. T-cell differentiation in thymus organ cultures. Semin Immunol 1990;2:51–58.
4. Jenkinson EJ, Anderson G. Fetal thymic organ cultures. Curr Opin Immunol 1994;6:293–297.
5. McCune JM. Development and applications of the SCID-hu mouse model. Semin Immunol 1996;8:187–196.
6. Jaenisch R. Transgenic animals. Science 1988;240:1468–1474.
7. von Boehmer H. Developmental biology of T cells in T-cell receptor transgenic mice. Annu Rev Immunol 1990;8:531–556.
8. Scott B, Bluthmann H, Teh HS, von Boehmer H. The generation of mature T cells requires interaction of the alpha beta T-cell receptor with major histocompatibility antigens. Nature 1989;338:591–593.
9. Kistner A, Gossen M, Zimmermann F, et al. Doxycycline-mediated, quantitative and tissue-specific control of gene expression in transgenic mice. Proc Natl Acad Sci USA 1996;93:10933–10938.
10. Shockett PE, Schatz DG. Diverse strategies for tetracycline-regulated inducible gene expression. Proc Natl Acad Sci USA 1996;93:5173–5176.
11. Melton DW. Gene targeting in the mouse. Bioessays 1994;16:633–638.
12. Pfeffer K, Mak TW. Lymphocyte ontogeny and activation in gene targeted mutant mice. Annu Rev Immunol 1994;12:367–411.
13. Chen J, Shinkai Y, Young F, Alt FW. Probing immune functions in RAG-deficient mice. Curr Opin Immunol 1994;6:313–319.
14. Jiang R, Gridley T. Gene targeting: Things go better with Cre. Curr Biol 1997;7: R321–R323.
15. Gu H, Zou YR, Rajewsky K. Independent control of immunoglobulin switch recombination at individual switch regions evidenced through Cre-loxP-mediated gene targeting. Cell 1993;73:1155–1164.
16. Gu H, Marth JD, Orban PC, Mossmann H, Rajewsky K. Deletion of a DNA polymerase beta gene segment in T cells using cell type-specific gene targeting. Science 1994;265:103–106.
17. Kuhn R, Schwenk F, Aguet M, Rajewsky K. Inducible gene targeting in mice. Science 1995;269:1427–1429.
18. Feil R, Brocard J, Mascrez B, Le Meur M, Metzger D, Chambon P. Ligand-activated site-specific recombination in mice. Proc Natl Acad Sci USA 1996;93: 10887–10890.
19. Monks CR, Kupfer H, Tamir I, Barlow A, Kupfer A. Selective modulation of protein kinase C-theta during T-cell activation. Nature 1997;385:83–86.
20. Kersh GJ, Allen PM. Essential flexibility in the T-cell recognition of antigen. Nature 1996;380:495–498.
21. Alberola-Ila J, Takaki S, Kerner JD, Perlmutter RM. Differential signaling by lymphocyte antigen receptors. Annu Rev Immunol 1997;15:125–154.
22. Lyons DS, Lieberman SA, Hampl J, et al. A TCR binds to antagonist ligands with lower affinities and faster dissociation rates than to agonists. Immunity 1996;5: 53–61.
23. Alam SM, Travers PJ, Wung JL, et al. T cell receptor affinity and thymocyte positive selection. Nature 1996;381:616–620.
24. Ullman KS, Northrop JP, Verweij CL, Crabtree GR. Transmission of signals from the T lymphocyte antigen receptor to the genes responsible for cell proliferation and immune function: The missing link. Annu Rev Immunol 1990;8: 421–452.
25. Bolen JB, Brugge JS. Leukocyte protein tyrosine kinases: Potential targets for drug discovery. Annu Rev Immunol 1997;15:371–404.
26. Qian D, Weiss A. T cell antigen receptor signal transduction. Curr Opin Cell Biol 1997;9:205–212.
27. Arpaia E, Shahar M, Dadi H, Cohen A, Roifman CM. Defective T cell receptor signaling and CD8+ thymic selection in humans lacking zap-70 kinase. Cell 1994;76:947–958.
28. Chan AC, Kadlecek TA, Elder ME, et al. ZAP-70 deficiency in an autosomal recessive form of severe combined immunodeficiency. Science 1994;264: 1599–1601.
29. van Oers NS, Lowin-Kropf B, Finlay D, Connolly K, Weiss A. Alpha beta T cell development is abolished in mice lacking both Lck and Fyn protein tyrosine kinases. Immunity 1996;5:429–436.
30. Negishi I, Motoyama N, Nakayama K-I, et al. Essential role for ZAP-70 in both positive and negative selection of thymocytes. Nature 1995;376:435–438.
31. Nada S, Yagi T, Takeda H, et al. Constitutive activation of Src family kinases in mouse embryos that lack Csk. Cell 1993;73:1125–1135.
32. Trowbridge IS, Thomas ML. CD45: An emerging role as a protein tyrosine phosphatase required for lymphocyte activation and development. Annu Rev Immunol 1994;12:85–116.
33. Shultz LD, Schweitzer PA, Rajan TV, et al. Mutations at the murine motheaten locus are within the hematopoietic cell protein-tyrosine phosphatase (Hcph) gene. Cell 1993;73:1445–1454.
34. Plas DR, Johnson R, Pingel JT, et al. Direct regulation of ZAP-70 by SHP-1 in T cell antigen receptor signaling. Science 1996;272:1173–1176.
35. Marengere LE, Waterhouse P, Duncan GS, Mittrucker HW, Feng GS, Mak TW. Regulation of T cell receptor signaling by tyrosine phosphatase SYP association with CTLA-4. Science 1996;272:1170–1173.
36. Cantrell D. T cell antigen receptor signal transduction pathways. Annu Rev Immunol 1996;14:259–274.
37. Rao A, Luo C, Hogan PG. Transcription factors of the NFAT family: Regulation and function. Annu Rev Immunol 1997;15:707–747.
38. Genot EM, Parker PJ, Cantrell DA. Analysis of the role of protein kinase C-alpha, -epsilon, and -zeta in T cell activation. J Biol Chem 1995;270:9833–9839.
39. Ohoka Y, Kuwata T, Asada A, Zhao Y, Mukai M, Iwata M. Regulation of thymocyte lineage commitment by the level of classical protein kinase C activity. J Immunol 1997;158:5707–5716.
40. Leitges M, Schmedt C, Guinamard R, et al. Immunodeficiency in protein kinase c beta-deficient mice. Science 1996;273:788–791.
41. Datta SR, Dudek H, Tao X, et al. Akt phosphorylation of BAD couples survival signals to the cell-intrinsic death machinery. Cell 1997;91:231–241.
42. Ward SG, June CH, Olive D. PI 3-kinase: A pivotal pathway in T-cell activation? Immunol Today 1996;17:187–197.
43. Leiden JM, Thompson CB. Transcriptional regulation of T-cell genes during T-cell development. Curr Opin Immunol 1994;6:231–237.
44. Fitzsimmons D, Hagman J. Regulation of gene expression at early stages of B-cell and T-cell differentiation. Curr Opin Immunol 1996;8:166–174.
45. Verbeek S, Izon D, Hofhuis F, et al. An HMG box containing T-cell factor required for thymocyte differentiation. Nature 1995;374:70–74.
46. Kuo CT, Veselits ML, Leiden JM. LKLF: A transcriptional regulator of single-positive T cell quiescence and survival. Science 1997;277:1986–1989.
47. Matsuyama T, Kimura T, Kitagawa M, et al. Targeted disruption of IRF-1 or IRF-2 results in abnormal type I IFN gene induction and aberrant lymphocyte development. Cell 1993;75:83–97.
48. Muthusamy N, Barton K, Leiden JM. Defective activation and survival of T cells lacking the Ets-1 transcription factor. Nature 1995;377:639–642.
49. Darnell JE. STATs and gene regulation. Science 1997;277:1630–1635.
50. Fraser A, Evan G. A license to kill. Cell 1996;85:781–784.
51. Vaux DL, Strasser A. The molecular biology of apoptosis. Proc Natl Acad Sci USA 1996;93:2239–2244.
52. Miller JFAP. Immunological function of the thymus. Lancet 1961;2:748–749.
53. DiGeorge AM. Congenital absence of the thymus and its immunological consequences: concurrence with congenital hypothyroidism. Birth Defects 1997;4: 116–120.
54. Warner NL, Szenberg A, Burnet FM. The immunological role of different lymphoid organs in the chicken. I. Dissociation of immunological responsiveness. Aust J Exp Biol Med Sci 1962;40:373–388.
55. van Ewijk W. T-cell differentiation is influenced by thymic microenvironments. Annu Rev Immunol 1991;9:591–615.
56. Boyd RL, Tucek CL, Godfrey DI, et al. The thymic microenvironment. Immunol Today 1993;14:445–459.
57. Anderson G, Moore NC, Owen JJ, Jenkinson EJ. Cellular interactions in thymocyte development. Annu Rev Immunol 1996;14:73–99.
58. Savino W, Villa-Verde DMS, Lannes-Vieira J. Extracellular matrix proteins in intrathymic T-cell migration and differentiation? Immunol Today 1993;14: 150–161.
59. Kisielow P, von Boehmer H. Development and selection of T cells: Facts and puzzles. Adv Immunol 1995;58:87–209.
60. Anderson G, Anderson KL, Tchilian EZ, Owen JJ, Jenkinson EJ. Fibroblast dependency during early thymocyte development maps to the CD25+ CD44+

stage and involves interactions with fibroblast matrix molecules. *Eur J Immunol* 1997;27:1200–1206.

61. Zuniga-Pflucker JC, Di J, Lenardo MJ. Requirement for TNF-alpha and IL-1 alpha in fetal thymocyte commitment and differentiation. *Science* 1995;268:1906–1909.

62. Surh CD, Sprent J. T-cell apoptosis detected in situ during positive and negative selection in the thymus. *Nature* 1994;372:100–103.

63. Kraal G, Weissman IL, Butcher EC. Genetic control of T-cell subset representation in inbred mice. *Immunogenetics* 1983;18:585–592.

64. Amadori A, Zamarchi R, De Silvestro G, et al. Genetic control of the CD4/CD8 T-cell ratio in humans. *Nature Med* 1997;1:1279–1283.

65. Kraft DL, Weissman IL, Waller EK. Differentiation of CD3⁻4⁻8⁻ human fetal thymocytes in vivo: characterization of a CD3⁻4⁺8⁻ intermediate. *J Exp Med* 1993;178:265–277.

66. Hugo P, Waanders GA, Scollay R, Petrie HT, Boyd RL. Characterization of immature CD4⁺CD8⁻CD3⁻ thymocytes. *Eur J Immunol* 1991;21:835–838.

67. Agus DB, Surh CD, Sprent J. Reentry of T cells to the adult thymus is restricted to activated T cells. *J Exp Med* 1991;173:1039–1046.

68. Ceredig R, Schreyer M. Immunohistochemical localization of host and donor-derived cells in the regenerating thymus of radiation bone marrow chimeras. *Thymus* 1984;6:15–26.

69. Wu L, Scollay R, Egerton M, Pearse M, Spangrude GJ, Shortman K. CD4 expressed on earliest T-lineage precursor cells in the adult murine thymus. *Nature* 1991;349:71–74.

70. Wu L, Antica M, Johnson GR, Scollay R, Shortman K. Developmental potential of the earliest precursor cells from the adult mouse thymus. *J Exp Med* 1991;174:1617–1627.

71. Rodewald HR, Ogawa M, Haller C, Waskow C, Di Santo JP. Pro-thymocyte expansion by c-kit and the common cytokine receptor gamma chain is essential for repertoire formation. *Immunity* 1997;6:265–272.

72. Levelt CN, Ehrfeld A, Eichmann K. Regulation of thymocyte development through CD3. I. Timepoint of ligation of CD3 epsilon determines clonal deletion or induction of developmental program. *J Exp Med* 1993;177:707–716.

73. Shinkai Y, Alt FW. CD3e-mediated signals rescue the development of CD4⁺CD8⁺ thymocytes in RAG-2⁻/⁻ mice in the absence of TCR β chain expression. *Int Immunol* 1994;6:995–1001.

74. Jacobs H, Vandeputte D, Tolkamp L, de Vries E, Borst J, Berns A. CD3 components at the surface of pro-T cells can mediate pre-T cell development in vivo. *Eur J Immunol* 1994;24:934–939.

75. Miyazaki T. Two distinct steps during thymocyte maturation from CD4⁻CD8⁻ to CD4⁺CD8⁺ distinguished in the early growth response (Egr)-1 transgenic mice with a recombinase-activating gene-deficient (RAG)-2⁻/⁻ background. *J Exp Med* 1997;186:877–885.

76. Kishimoto H, Sprent J. Negative selection in the thymus includes semimature T cells. *J Exp Med* 1997;185:263–271.

77. Chaffin KE, Perlmutter RM. A pertussis toxin-sensitive process controls thymocyte emigration. *Eur J Immunol* 1991;21:2565–2573.

78. Stutman O. Intrathymic and extrathymic T cell maturation. *Immunol Rev* 1978;42:138–184.

79. Kelly KA, Scollay R. Analysis of recent thymic emigrants with subset- and maturity-related markers. *Int Immunol* 1990;2:419–425.

80. Shortman K, Egerton M, Spangrude GJ, Scollay R. The generation and fate of thymocytes. *Semin Immunol* 1990;2:3–12.

81. Egerton M, Scollay R, Shortman K. Kinetics of mature T-cell development in the thymus. *Proc Natl Acad Sci USA* 1990;87:2579–2582.

82. Huesmann M, Scott B, Kisielow P, von Boehmer H. Kinetics and efficacy of positive selection in the thymus of normal and T cell receptor transgenic mice. *Cell* 1991;66:533–540.

83. Scollay R, Godfrey DI. Thymic emigration: Conveyor belts or lucky dips? *Immunol Today* 1995;16:268–264.

84. Tough DF, Sprent J. Thymic emigration—a reply. *Immunol Today* 1995;16:273.

85. Rooke R, Waltzinger C, Benoist C, Mathis D. Targeted complementation of MHC class II deficiency by intrathymic delivery of recombinant adenoviruses. *Immunity* 1997;7:123–134.

86. Anderson G, Jenkinson EJ, Moore NC, Owen JJ. MHC class II-positive epithelium and mesenchyme cells are both required for T-cell development in the thymus. *Nature* 1993;362:70–73.

87. Hollander GA, Wang B, Nichogiannopoulou A, et al. Developmental control point in induction of thymic cortex regulated by a subpopulation of prothymocytes. *Nature* 1995;373:350–353.

88. Ritter MA, Boyd RL. Development in the thymus: It takes two to tango. *Immunol Today* 1993;14:462–469.

89. Arroyo AG, Yang JT, Rayburn H, Hynes RO. Differential requirements for alpha4 integrins during fetal and adult hematopoiesis. *Cell* 1996;85:997–1008.

90. Crisa L, Cirulli V, Ellisman MH, Ishii JK, Elices MJ, Salomon DR. Cell adhesion and migration are regulated at distinct stages of thymic T cell development: The roles of fibronectin, VLA4, and VLA5. *J Exp Med* 1996;184:215–228.

91. Cordier AC, Haumont SM. Development of thymus, parathyroids, and ultimobranchial bodies in NMRI and nude mice. *Am J Anat* 1980;157:227–263.

92. Le Douarin N, Bussonnet C, Chaumont F. Etude des capacités de différentiation et du rôle morphogène de l'endoderme pharyngier chez l'embryon d'oiseau. *Ann Embryol Morphog* 1968;1:29–37.

93. Nehls M, Pfeifer D, Schorpp M, Hedrich H, Boehm T. New member of the winged-helix protein family disrupted in mouse and rat nude mutations. *Nature* 1994;372:103–107.

94. Blackburn CC, Augustine CL, Li R, et al. The nu gene acts cell-autonomously and is required for differentiation of thymic epithelial progenitors. *Proc Natl Acad Sci USA* 1996;93:5742–5746.

95. Nehls M, Kyewski B, Messerle M, et al. Two genetically separable steps in the differentiation of thymic epithelium. *Science* 1996;272:886–889.

96. Auerbach R. Mrphogenetic interactions in the development of the mouse thymus gland. *Dev Biol* 1997;2:271–285.

97. Le Lièvre CS, Le Douarin NM. Mesenchyme derivatives of the neural crest: Analysis of chimeric quail and chick embryos. *J Embryol Exp Morphol* 1975;34:125–136.

98. Bockman DE, Kirby ML. Dependence of thymus development on derivatives of the neural crest. *Science* 1984;223:498–500.

99. Manley NR, Capecchi MR. The role of Hoxa-3 in mouse thymus and thyroid development. *Development* 1995;121:1989–2003.

100. Greenberg F. DiGeorge syndrome: An historical review of clinical and cytogenetic features. *J Med Genet* 1993;30:803–806.

101. Surh CD, Sprent J, Webb SR. Exclusion of circulating T cells from the thymus does not apply in the neonatal period. *J Exp Med* 1993;177:379–385.

102. Shortman K, Wu L. Early T lymphocyte progenitors. *Annu Rev Immunol* 1996;14:29–47.

103. Rodewald H-R, Fehling HJ. Molecular and cellular events in early thymocyte development. *Adv Immunol* 1997 (in press).

104. Ikuta K, Kina T, MacNeil I, et al. A developmental switch in thymic lymphocyte maturation potential occurs at the level of hematopoietic stem cells. *Cell* 1990;62:863–874.

105. Ceredig R. Intrathymic proliferation of perinatal mouse alpha beta and gamma delta T cell receptor-expressing mature T cells. *Int Immunol* 1990;2:859–867.

106. Adkins B. Developmental regulation of the intrathymic T cell precursor population. *J Immunol* 1991;146:1387–1393.

107. Schneider R, Lees RK, Pedrazzini T, Zinkernagel RM, Hengartner H, MacDonald HR. Postnatal disappearance of self-reactive (V beta 6+) cells from the thymus of Mlsa mice. Implications for T cell development and autoimmunity. *J Exp Med* 1989;169:2149–2158.

108. Benoist C, Mathis D. Generation of the alpha beta T-cell repertoire. *Curr Opin Immunol* 1992;4:156–161.

109. Wang JH, Nichogiannopoulou A, Wu L, et al. Selective defects in the development of the fetal and adult lymphoid system in mice with an Ikaros null mutation. *Immunity* 1996;5:537–549.

110. Galandrini R, Henning SW, Cantrell DA. Different functions of the GTPase rho in prothymocytes and late pre-T cells. *Immunity* 1997;7:163–174.

111. Scollay RG, Butcher EC, Weissman IL. Thymus cell migration. Quantitative aspects of cellular traffic from the thymus to the periphery in mice. *Eur J Immunol* 1980;10:210–218.

112. Shivatcheva TM, Hadjioloff AI. Adaptive seasonal involution of the ground squirrel thymus. *Thymus* 1987;10:251–255.

113. Aurrand-Lions M, Galland F, Bazin H, Zakharyev VM, Imhof BA, Naquet P. Vanin-1, a novel GPI-linked perivascular molecule involved in thymus homing. *Immunity* 1996;5:391–405.

114. Dunon D, Courtois D, Vainio O, et al. Ontogeny of the immune system: γ/δ and α/β T cells migrate from thymus to the periphery in alternating waves. *J Exp Med* 1997;186:977–988.

115. Sagara S, Sugaya K, Tokoro Y, et al. B220 expression by T lymphoid progenitor cells in mouse fetal liver. *J Immunol* 1997;158:666–676.

116. Rodewald HR. Pathways from hematopoietic stem cells to thymocytes. *Curr Opin Immunol* 1995;7:176–187.

117. Antica M, Wu L, Shortman K, Scollay R. Thymic stem cells in mouse bone marrow. *Blood* 1994;84:111–117.

118. Wang TG, Lybarger L, Soloff R, Dempsey D, Chervenak R. Pre-thymic transcription of TCR genes by adult murine bone marrow cells. *Mol Immunol* 1996;33:957–964.

119. Soloff RS, Wang TG, Lybarger L, Dempsey D, Chervenak R. Transcription of the TCR-beta locus initiates in adult murine bone marrow. *J Immunol* 1995;154:3888–3901.

120. Peault B, Khazaal I, Weissman IL. In vitro development of B cells and macrophages from early mouse fetal thymocytes. *Eur J Immunol* 1994;24:781–784.

121. Hattori N, Kawamoto H, Katsura Y. Isolation of the most immature population of murine fetal thymocytes that includes progenitors capable of generating T, B, and myeloid cells. *J Exp Med* 1996;184:1901–1908.

122. Papiernik M, Lepault F, Pontoux C. Synergistic effect of colony-stimulating factors and IL-2 on prothymocyte proliferation linked to the maturation of macrophage/dendritic cells within L3T4-Lyt-2-Ia-Mac- cells. *J Immunol* 1988;140:1431–1434.

123. Matsuzaki Y, Gyotoku J, Ogawa M, et al. Characterization of c-kit positive intrathymic stem cells that are restricted to lymphoid differentiation. *J Exp Med* 1993;178:1283–1292.

124. Rodewald HR, Kretzschmar K, Takeda S, Hohl C, Dessing M. Identification of pro-thymocytes in murine fetal blood: T lineage commitment can precede thymus colonization. *EMBO J* 1994;13:4229–4240.

125. Rodewald HR, Dessing M, Dvorak AM, Galli SJ. Identification of a committed precursor for the mast cell lineage. *Science* 1996;271:818–822.

126. Marcos MA, Morales-Alcelay S, Godin IE, Dieterlen-Lievre F, Copin SG, Gaspar ML. Antigenic phenotype and gene expression pattern of lymphohemopoietic progenitors during early mouse ontogeny. J Immunol 1997;158:2627–2637.

127. Delassus S, Cumano A. Circulation of hematopoietic progenitors in the mouse embryo. Immunity 1996;4:97–106.

128. Lanier LL, Spits H, Phillips JH. The developmental relationship between NK cells and T cells. Immunol Today 1992;13:392–395.

129. Moore TA, Zlotnik A. T-cell lineage commitment and cytokine responses of thymic progenitors. Blood 1995;86:1850–1860.

130. Wu L, Li CL, Shortman K. Thymic dendritic cell precursors: Relationship to the T lymphocyte lineage and phenotype of the dendritic cell progeny. J Exp Med 1996;184:903–911.

131. Ardavin C, Wu L, Li CL, Shortman K. Thymic dendritic cells and T cells develop simultaneously in the thymus from a common precursor population. Nature 1993;362:761–763.

132. Sanchez MJ, Muench MO, Roncarolo MG, Lanier LL, Phillips JH. Identification of a common T/natural killer cell progenitor in human fetal thymus. J Exp Med 1994;180:569–576.

133. Georgopoulos K. Transcription factors required for lymphoid lineage commitment. Curr Opin Immunol 1997;9:222–227.

134. Scott EW, Simon MC, Anastasi J, Singh H. Requirement of transcription factor PU.1 in the development of multiple hematopoietic lineages. Science 1994;265:1573–1577.

135. Wu L, Nichogiannopoulou A, Shortman K, Georgopoulos K. Cell-autonomous defects in dendritic cell populations of ikaros mutant mice point to a developmental relationship with the lymphoid lineage. Immunity 1997;7:483–492.

136. McKercher SR, Torbett BE, Anderson KL, et al. Targeted disruption of the PU.1 gene results in multiple hematopoietic abnormalities. EMBO J 1996;15:5647–5658.

137. Schatz DG. V(D)J recombination moves in vitro. Semin Immunol 1997;9:149–159.

138. Gilfillan S, Dierich A, Lemeur M, Benoist C, Mathis D. Mice lacking TdT: Mature animals with an immature lymphocyte repertoire. Science 1993;261:1175–1178.

139. Komori T, Okada A, Stewart V, Alt FW. Lack of N regions in antigen receptor variable region genes of TdT-deficient lymphocytes. Science 1993;261:1171–1175.

140. Bogue M, Gilfillan S, Benoist C, Mathis D. Regulation of N region diversity in antigen receptors through thymocyte differentiation and thymus ontogeny. Proc Natl Acad Sci USA 1992;89:11011–11015.

141. George JF Jr, Schroeder HW Jr. Developmental regulation of D beta reading frame and junctional diversity in T cell receptor-beta transcripts from human thymus. J Immunol 1992;148:1230–1239.

142. Mombaerts P, Iacomini J, Johnson RS, Herrup K, Tonegawa S, Papaioannou VE. RAG-1-deficient mice have no mature B and T lymphocytes. Cell 1992;68:869–877.

143. Shinkai Y, Rathbun G, Lam K-P, et al. RAG-2 deficient mice lack mature lymphocytes owing to inability to initiate V(D)J rearrangement. Cell 1992;68:855–867.

144. Kirchgessner CU, Patil CK, Evans JW, et al. DNA-dependent kinase (p350) as a candidate gene for the murine SCID defect. Science 1995;267:1178–1183.

145. Miller RD, Hogg J, Ozaki JH, Gell D, Jackson SP, Riblet R. Gene for the catalytic subunit of mouse DNA-dependent protein kinase maps to the scid locus. Proc Natl Acad Sci USA 1995;92:10792–10795.

146. Zhu C, Bogue MA, Lim DS, Hasty P, Roth DB. Ku86-deficient mice exhibit severe combined immunodeficiency and defective processing of V(D)J recombination intermediates. Cell 1996;86:379–389.

147. Nussenzweig A, Chen C, da Costa Soares V, et al. Requirement for Ku80 in growth and immunoglobulin V(D)J recombination. Nature 1996;382:551–555.

148. van Gent DC, McBlane JF, Ramsden DA, Sadofsky MJ, Hesse JE, Gellert M. Initiation of V(D)J recombination in a cell-free system. Cell 1995;81:925–934.

149. Allison JP, Havran WL. The immunobiology of T cells with invariant gamma delta antigen receptors. Annu Rev Immunol 1991;9:679–705.

150. Goldman JP, Spencer DM, Raulet DH. Ordered rearrangement of variable region genes of the T cell receptor gamma locus correlates with transcription of the unrearranged genes. J Exp Med 1993;177:729–739.

151. Kaufmann SH. gamma/delta and other unconventional T lymphocytes: What do they see and what do they do? Proc Natl Acad Sci USA 1996;93:2272–2279.

152. Willerford DM, Swat W, Alt FW. Developmental regulation of V(D)J recombination and lymphocyte differentiation. Curr Opin Genet Dev 1996;6:603–609.

153. Uematsu Y, Ryser S, Dembic Z, et al. In transgenic mice the introduced functional T cell receptor beta gene prevents expression of endogenous beta genes. Cell 1988;52:831–841.

154. Padovan E, Giachino C, Cella M, Valitutti S, Acuto O, Lanzavecchia A. Normal T lymphocytes can express two different T cell receptor beta chains: Implications for the mechanism of allelic exclusion. J Exp Med 1995;181:1587–1591.

155. Davodeau F, Peyrat M-A, Romagné F, et al. Dual T cell receptor beta chain expression on human T lymphocytes. J Exp Med 1995;181:1391–1398.

156. Malissen M, Trucy J, Jouvin-Marche E, Cazenave P-A, Scollay R. Regulation of TCR alpha and beta gene allelic exclusion during T-cell development. Immunol Today 1992;13:315–322.

157. Borgulya P, Kishi H, Uematsu Y, von Boehmer H. Exclusion and inclusion of α and β T cell receptor alleles. Cell 1992;69:529–537.

158. Padovan E, Casorati G, Dellabona P, Meyer S, Brockhaus M, Lanzavecchia A. Expression of two T cell receptor alpha chain: Dual receptor T cells. Science 1993;262:422–424.

159. Heath WR, Miller JFA. Expression of two alpha chains on the surface of T cells in T cell receptor transgenic mice. J Exp Med 1993;178:1807–1811.

160. Heath WR, Carbone FR, Bertolino P, Kelly J, Cose S, Miller JFA. Expression of two T cell receptor alpha chains on the surface of normal murine T cells. Eur J Immunol 1995;25:1617–1623.

161. Alam SM, Crispe IN, Gascoigne NR. Allelic exclusion of mouse T cell receptor alpha chains occurs at the time of thymocyte TCR up-regulation. Immunity 1995;3:449–458.

162. Hardardottir F, Baron JL, Janeway CA Jr. T cells with two functional antigen-specific receptors. Proc Natl Acad Sci USA 1995;92:354–358.

163. Sleckman BP, Gorman JR, Alt FW. Accessibility control of antigen-receptor variable-region gene assembly: Role of cis-acting elements. Annu Rev Immunol 1996;14:459–481.

164. Schlissel MS, Stanhope-Baker P. Accessibility and the developmental regulation of V(D)J recombination. Semin Immunol 1997;9:161–170.

165. Muegge K, Vila MP, Durum SK. Interleukin-7: A cofactor for V(D)J rearrangement of the T cell receptor beta gene. Science 1993;261:93–95.

166. Crompton T, Outram SV, Buckland J, Owen MJ. A transgenic T cell receptor restores thymocyte differentiation in interleukin-7 receptor alpha chain-deficient mice. Eur J Immunol 1997;27:100–104.

167. Candeias S, Muegge K, Durum SK. IL-7 receptor and VDJ recombination: Trophic versus mechanistic actions. Immunity 1997;6:501–508.

168. Hoffman ES, Passoni L, Crompton T, et al. Productive T-cell receptor beta-chain gene rearrangement: Coincident regulation of cell cycle and clonality during development in vivo. Genes Dev 1996;10:948–962.

169. Wilson A, Held W, MacDonald HR. Two waves of recombinase gene expression in developing thymocytes. J Exp Med 1994;179:1355–1360.

170. Brandle D, Muller C, Rulicke T, Hengartner H, Pircher H. Engagement of the T-cell receptor during positive selection in the thymus down-regulates RAG-1 expression. Proc Natl Acad Sci USA 1992;89:9529–9533.

171. Kouskoff V, Vonesch JL, Benoist C, Mathis D. The influence of positive selection on RAG expression in thymocytes. Eur J Immunol 1995;25:54–58.

172. Stanhope-Baker P, Hudson KM, Shaffer AL, Constantinescu A, Schlissel MS. Cell type-specific chromatin structure determines the targeting of V(D)J recombinase activity in vitro. Cell 1996;85:887–897.

173. Bories JC, Demengeot J, Davidson L, Alt FW. Gene-targeted deletion and replacement mutations of the T-cell receptor beta-chain enhancer: The role of enhancer elements in controlling V(D)J recombination accessibility. Proc Natl Acad Sci USA 1996;93:7871–7876.

174. Bouvier G, Watrin F, Naspetti M, Verthuy C, Naquet P, Ferrier P. Deletion of the mouse T-cell receptor beta gene enhancer blocks alphabeta T-cell development. Proc Natl Acad Sci USA 1996;93:7877–7881.

175. Capone M, Watrin F, Fernex C, et al. TCR beta and TCR alpha gene enhancers confer tissue- and stage-specificity on V(D)J recombination events. EMBO J 1993;12:4335–4346.

176. Lauzurica P, Krangel MS. Enhancer-dependent and -independent steps in the rearrangement of a human T cell receptor delta transgene. J Exp Med 1994;179:43–55.

177. Lauzurica P, Krangel MS. Temporal and lineage-specific control of T cell receptor alpha/delta gene rearrangement by T cell receptor alpha and delta enhancers. J Exp Med 1994;179:1913–1921.

178. Hernandez-Munain C, Lauzurica P, Krangel MS. Regulation of T cell receptor delta gene rearrangement by c-Myb. J Exp Med 1996;183:289–293.

179. Lauzurica P, Zhong XP, Krangel MS, Roberts JL. Regulation of T cell receptor delta gene rearrangement by CBF/PEBP2. J Exp Med 1997;185:1193–1201.

180. Borst J, Jacobs H, Brouns G. Composition and function of T-cell receptor and B-cell receptor complexes on precursor lymphocytes. Curr Opin Immunol 1996;8:181–190.

181. Kishi H, Borgulya P, Scott B, et al. Surface expression of the beta T cell receptor (TCR) chain in the absence of other TCR or CD3 proteins on immature T cells. EMBO J 1991;10:93–100.

182. Mombaerts P, Clarke AR, Rudnicki MA, et al. Mutations in T-cell antigen receptor genes alpha and beta block thymocyte development at different stages. Nature 1992;360:225–231.

183. Malissen M, Gillet A, Ardouin L, et al. Altered T cell development in mice with a targeted mutation of the CD3-epsilon gene. EMBO J 1995;14:4641–4653.

184. Malissen M, Gillet A, Rocha B, et al. T cell development in mice lacking the CD3-zeta/eta gene. EMBO J 1993;12:4347–4355.

185. Liu CP, Ueda R, She J, et al. Abnormal T cell development in CD3-zeta−/− mutant mice and identification of a novel T cell population in the intestine. EMBO J 1993;12:4863–4875.

186. Love PE, Shores EW, Johnson MD, et al. T cell development in mice that lack the zeta chain of the T cell antigen receptor complex. Science 1993;261:918–921.

187. Ohno H, Aoe T, Taki S, et al. Developmental and functional impairment of T cells in mice lacking CD3 zeta chains. EMBO J 1993;12:4357–4366.

188. Molina TJ, Kishihara K, Siderovski DP, et al. Profound block in thymocyte development in mice lacking p56lck. Nature 1992;357:161–164.

189. Levin SD, Anderson SJ, Forbush KA, Perlmutter RM. A dominant-negative transgene defines a role for p56lck in thymopoiesis. EMBO J 1993;12:1671–1680.

190. Kishihara K, Penninger J, Wallace VA, et al. Normal B lymphocyte development but impaired T cell maturation in CD45-exon 6 protein tyrosine phosphatase-deficient mice. *Cell* 1993;74:143–156.

191. Byth KF, Conroy LA, Howlett S, et al. CD45-null transgenic mice reveal a positive regulatory role for CD45 in early thymocyte development, in the selection of CD4-CD8- thymocytes, and B cell maturation. *J Exp Med* 1996;183:1707–1718.

192. Cheng AM, Negishi I, Anderson SJ, et al. The syk and ZAP-70 SH2-containing tyrosine kinases are implicated in pre-T cell receptor signaling. *Proc Natl Acad Sci USA* 1997;94:9797–9801.

193. Henning SW, Galandrini R, Hall A, Cantrell DA. The GTPase Rho has a critical regulatory role in thymus development. *EMBO J* 1997;16:2397–2407.

194. Crompton T, Gilmour KC, Owen MJ. The MAP kinase pathway controls differentiation from double-negative to double-positive thymocyte. *Cell* 1996;86:243–251.

195. Takahama Y, Hasegawa T, Itohara S, Ball EL, Sheard MA, Hashimoto Y. Entry of CD4-CD8- immature thymocytes into the CD4/CD8 developmental pathway is controlled by tyrosine kinase signals that can be provided through TCR components. *Int Immunol* 1994;6:1505–1514.

196. Lalli E, Sassone-Corsi P, Ceredig R. Block of T lymphocyte differentiation by activation of the cAMP-dependent signal transduction pathway. *EMBO J* 1996;15:528–537.

197. Wang B, Benoist C, Mathis D. The immunosuppressant 1,5-deoxyspergualin reveals commonality between preT and preB cell differentiation. *J Exp Med* 1996;183:2427–2436.

198. Shinkai Y, Koyasu S, Nakayama K, et al. Restoration of T cell development in RAG-2-deficient mice by functional TCR transgenes. *Science* 1993;259:822–825.

199. Mombaerts P, Anderson SJ, Perlmutter RM, Mak TW, Tonegawa S. An activated lck transgene promotes thymocyte development in RAG-1 mutant mice. *Immunity* 1994;1:261–267.

200. Fehling HJ, Iriatni BM, Krotkova A, et al. Restoration of thymopoiesis in pTa$^{-/-}$ mice by anti-CD3e antibody treatment or with transgenes encoding activated Lck or tailless pTa. *Immunity* 1997;6:703–714.

201. Swat W, Shinkai Y, Cheng HL, Davidson L, Alt FW. Activated Ras signals differentiation and expansion of CD4$^+$8$^+$ thymocytes. *Proc Natl Acad Sci USA* 1996;93:4683–4687.

202. Groettrup M, Baron A, Griffiths G, Palacios R, von Boehmer H. T cell receptor (TCR) β chain homodimers on the surface of immature but not mature α, γ, δ chain deficient T cell lines. *EMBO J* 1992;11:2735–2746.

203. Punt JA, Kubo RT, Saito T, et al. Surface expression of a T cell receptor beta (TCR-beta) chain in the absence of TCR-alpha, -delta, and -gamma proteins. *J Exp Med* 1991;174:775–783.

204. Dave VP, Cao Z, Browne C, et al. CD3 delta deficiency arrests development of the alpha beta but not the gamma delta T cell lineage. *EMBO J* 1997;16:1360–1370.

205. Groettrup M, Ungewiss K, Azogui O, et al. A novel disulfide-linked heterodimer on Pre-T cells consists of the T cell receptor β chain and a 33 kd glycoprotein. *Cell* 1993;75:283–294.

206. Saint-Ruf C, Ungewiss K, Groettrup M, Bruno L, Fehling HJ, von Boehmer H. Analysis and expression of a cloned pre-T cell receptor gene. *Science* 1994;266:1208–1212.

207. Fehling J, Krotkova A, Saint-Ruf C, von Boehmer H. Crucial role of the pre-T-cell receptor a gene in development of αβ but not γδ T cells. *Nature* 1995;375:795–798.

208. Del Porto P, Bruno L, Mattei MG, von Boehmer H, Saint-Ruf C. Cloning and comparative analysis of the human pre-T-cell receptor alpha-chain gene. *Proc Natl Acad Sci USA* 1995;92:12105–12109.

209. Ramiro AR, Trigueros C, Marquez C, San Millan JL, Toribio ML. Regulation of pre-T cell receptor (pT alpha-TCR beta) gene expression during human thymic development. *J Exp Med* 1996;184:519–530.

210. Krimpenfort P, Ossendorp F, Borst J, Melief C, Berns A. T cell depletion in transgenic mice carrying a mutant gene for TCR-beta. *Nature* 1989;341:742–746.

211. Jacobs H, Iacomini J, van de Ven M, Tonegawa S, Berns A. Domains of the TCR beta-chain required for early thymocyte development. *J Exp Med* 1996;184:1833–1843.

212. Gao EK, Lo D, Cheney R, Kanagawa O, Sprent J. Abnormal differentiation of thymocytes in mice treated with cyclosporin A. *Nature* 1988;336:176–179.

213. Jenkins MK, Schwartz RH, Pardoll DM. Effects of cyclosporine A on T cell development and clonal deletion. *Science* 1988;241:1655–1658.

214. Mallick CA, Dudley EC, Viney JL, Owen MJ, Hayday AC. Rearrangement and diversity of T cell receptor beta chain genes in thymocytes: A critical role for the beta chain in development. *Cell* 1993;73:513–519.

215. Dudley EC, Petrie HT, Shah LM, Owen MJ, Hayday AC. T cell receptor beta chain gene rearrangement and selection during thymocyte development in adult mice. *Immunity* 1994;1:83–93.

216. Xu Y, Davidson L, Alt FW, Baltimore D. Function of the pre-T-cell receptor alpha chain in T-cell development and allelic exclusion at the T-cell receptor beta locus. *Proc Natl Acad Sci USA* 1996;93:2169–2173.

217. Krotkova A, von Boehmer H, Fehling HJ. Allelic exclusion in pTa$^{-/-}$ mice: No evidence for cell surface expression of two different TCRβ chains but less efficient inhibition of endogenous β-rearrangements in the presence of a TCRβ transgene. *J Exp Med* 1997;186:767–775.

218. Aifantis I, Buer J, von Boehmer H, Azogui O. Essential role of the pre-T cell receptor in allelic exclusion of the T cell receptor β locus. *Immunity* 1997;7:601–607.

219. Falk I, Biro J, Kohler H, Eichmann K. Proliferation kinetics associated with T cell receptor-beta chain selection of fetal murine thymocytes. *J Exp Med* 1996;184:2327–2339.

220. Bruno L, Fehling HJ, von Boehmer H. The alpha beta T cell receptor can replace the gamma delta receptor in the development of gamma delta lineage cells. *Immunity* 1996;5:343–352.

221. Kersh GJ, Hooshmand FF, Hedrick SM. Efficient maturation of alpha beta lineage thymocytes to the CD4$^+$CD8$^+$ stage in the absence of TCR-beta rearrangement. *J Immunol* 1995;154:5706–5714.

222. Buer J, Aifantis I, Di Santo JP, Fehling HJ, von Boehmer H. Role of different T cell receptors in the development of pre-T cells. *J Exp Med* 1997;185:1541–1547.

223. Zuniga-Pflucker JC, Jiang D, Schwartzberg PL, Lenardo MJ. Sublethal gamma-radiation induces differentiation of CD4$^-$/CD8$^-$ into CD4$^+$/CD8$^+$ thymocytes without T cell receptor beta rearrangement in recombinase activation gene 2$^{-/-}$ mice. *J Exp Med* 1994;180:1517–1521.

224. Guidos CJ, Williams CJ, Wu GE, Paige CJ, Danska JS. Development of CD4$^+$CD8$^+$ thymocytes in RAG-deficient mice through a T cell receptor beta chain-independent pathway. *J Exp Med* 1995;181:1187–1195.

225. Mombaerts P, Terhorst C, Jacks T, Tonegawa S, Sancho J. Characterization of immature thymocyte lines derived from T-cell receptor or recombination activating gene 1 and p53 double mutant mice. *Proc Natl Acad Sci USA* 1995;92:7420–7424.

226. Jiang D, Lenardo MJ, Zuniga-Pflucker C. p53 prevents maturation to the CD4$^+$CD8$^+$ stage of thymocyte differentiation in the absence of T cell receptor rearrangement. *J Exp Med* 1996;183:1923–1928.

227. Pérrit C, Lucas B, Vasseur T. Cell expansion and growth arrest phases during the transition from precursor (CD4$^-$8$^-$) to immature (CD4$^-$8$^+$) thymocytes in normal and genetically modified mice. *J Immunol* 1995;154:5103–5113.

228. Haas W, Pereira P, Tonegawa S. Gamma/delta cells. *Annu Rev Immunol* 1993;11:637–685.

229. Okazaki K, Sakano H. Thymocyte circular DNA excised from T cell receptor alpha-delta gene complex. *EMBO J* 1988;7:1669–1674.

230. Winoto A, Baltimore D. Separate lineages of T cells expressing the alpha beta and gamma delta receptors. *Nature* 1989;338:430–432.

231. Takeshita S, Toda M, Yamagishi H. Excision products of the T cell receptor gene support a progressive rearrangement model of the alpha/delta locus. *EMBO J* 1989;8:3261–3270.

232. Nakajima PB, Menetski JP, Roth DB, Gellert M, Bosma MJ. V-D-J rearrangements at the T cell receptor delta locus in mouse thymocytes of the alpha beta lineage. *Immunity* 1995;3:609–621.

233. Ishida I, Verbeek S, Bonneville M, Itohara S, Berns A, Tonegawa S. T-cell receptor gamma delta and gamma transgenic mice suggest a role of a gamma gene silencer in the generation of alpha beta T cells. *Proc Natl Acad Sci USA* 1990;87:3067–3071.

234. Bonneville M, Ishida I, Mombaerts P, et al. Blockage of alpha beta T-cell development by TCR gamma delta transgenes. *Nature* 1989;342:931–934.

235. Sim GK, Olsson C, Augustin A. Commitment and maintenance of the alpha beta and gamma delta T cell lineages. *J Immunol* 1995;154:5821–5831.

236. Dent AL, Matis LA, Hooshmand F, Widacki SM, Bluestone JA, Hedrick SM. Self-reactive gamma delta T cells are eliminated in the thymus. *Nature* 1990;343:714–719.

237. Livak F, Petrie HT, Crispe IN, Schatz DG. In-frame TCR delta gene rearrangements play a critical role in the alpha beta/gamma delta T cell lineage decision. *Immunity* 1995;2:617–627.

238. Dudley EC, Girardi M, Owen MJ, Hayday AC. Alpha beta and gamma delta T cells can share a late common precursor. *Curr Biol* 1995;5:659–669.

239. Kang J, Baker J, Raulet DH. Evidence that productive rearrangements of TCR gamma genes influence the commitment of progenitor cells to differentiate into alpha beta or gamma delta T cells. *Eur J Immunol* 1995;25:2706–2709.

240. Burtrum DB, Kim S, Dudley EC, Hayday AC, Petrie HT. TCR gene recombination and alpha beta-gamma delta lineage divergence: Productive TCR-beta rearrangement is neither exclusive nor preclusive of gamma delta cell development. *J Immunol* 1996;157:4293–4296.

241. Mertsching E, Wilson A, MacDonald HR, Ceredig R. T cell receptor alpha gene rearrangement and transcription in adult thymic gamma delta cells. *Eur J Immunol* 1997;27:389–396.

242. Petrie HT, Scollay R, Shortman K. Commitment to the T cell receptor-alpha beta or-gamma delta lineages can occur just prior to the onset of CD4 and CD8 expression among immature thymocytes. *Eur J Immunol* 1992;22:2185–2188.

243. Passoni L, Hoffman ES, Kim S, et al. Intrathymic δ selection events in γδ cell development. *Immunity* 1997;7:83–95.

244. Shutter J, Cain JA, Ledbetter S, Rogers MD, Hockett RD Jr. A delta T-cell receptor deleting element transgenic reporter construct is rearranged in alpha beta but not gamma delta T-cell lineages. *Mol Cell Biol* 1995;15:7022–7031.

245. Diaz P, Cado D, Winoto A. A locus control region in the T cell receptor alpha/delta locus. *Immunity* 1994;1:207–217.

246. Washburn T, Schweighoffer E, Gridley T, et al. Notch activity influences the ab versus δγ T cell lineage decision. *Cell* 1997;88:833–843.

247. Zinkernagel RM, Doherty PC. The discovery of MHC restriction. *Immunol Today* 1997;18.

248. Bechtol KB, Freed JH, Herzenberg LA, McDevitt HO. Genetic control of the antibody response to TGAL in C3H–CWB tetraparental mice. *J Exp Med* 1974;140:1660–1675.

249. von Boehmer H, Hudson L, Sprent J. Collaboration of histoincompatible T- and B-lymphocytes using cells from tetraparental bone marrow chimeras. *J Exp Med* 1975;142:989–997.

250. Katz DH. The role of the histocompatibility gene complex in lymphocyte differentiation. Cold Spring Harbor Symposium on Quantitative Biology 1976;40:611–624.

251. Bevan M. In a radiation chimaera, host H-2 antigens determine immune responsiveness of donor cytotoxic cells. *Nature* 1997;269:417–418.

252. Zinkernagel RM, Callahan GN, Klein J, Dennert G. Cytotoxic T cells learn specificity for self H-2 during diffentiation in the thymus. *Nature* 1978;271:251–253.

253. Fink PJ, Bevan MJ. H-2 antigens of the thymus determine lymphocyte specificity. *J Exp Med* 1978;148:766–774.

254. von Boehmer H, Haas W, Jerne NK. Major histocompatibility complex-linked immune-responsiveness is acquired by lymphocytes of low-responder mice differentiating in thymus of high-responder mice. *Proc Natl Acad Sci USA* 1978;75:2439–2442.

255. Kappler JW, Marrack P. The role of H-2 linked genes in helper T cell function IV. Importance of T-cell genotype and host environment in I region and Ir gene expression. *J Exp Med* 1978;148:1510–1516.

256. Singer A. Experimentation and thymic selection. *J Immunol* 1988;140:2481–2483.

257. MacDonald HR, Lees RK, Schneider R, Zinkernagel RM, Hengartner H. Positive selection of CD4$^+$ thymocytes controlled by MHC class II gene products. *Nature* 1988;336:471–473.

258. Blackman MA, Marrack P, Kappler J. Influence of the major histocompatibility complex on positive thymic selection of V beta 17a$^+$ T cells. *Science* 1989;244:214–217.

259. Marrack P, Kushnir E, Born W, McDuffie M, Kappler J. The development of helper T cell precursors in mouse thymus. *J Immunol* 1988;140:2508–2514.

260. Marusic-Galesic S, Longo DL, Kruisbeek AM. Preferential differentiation of T cell receptor specificities based on the MHC glycoproteins encountered during development. Evidence for positive selection. *J Exp Med* 1989;169:1619–1630.

261. Teh HS, Kisielow P, Scott B, et al. Thymic major histocompatibility complex antigens and the alpha beta T-cell receptor determine the CD4/CD8 phenotype of T cells. *Nature* 1988;335:229–233.

262. Kisielow P, Teh HS, Bluthmann H, von Boehmer H. Positive selection of antigen-specific T cells in thymus by restricting MHC molecules. *Nature* 1988;335:730–733.

263. Sha WC, Nelson CA, Newberry RD, Kranz DM, Russell JH, Loh DY. Positive and negative selection of an antigen receptor on T cells in transgenic mice. *Nature* 1988;336:73–76.

264. Berg LJ, Pullen AM, Fazekas de St. Groth B, Mathis D, Benoist C, Davis MM. Antigen/MHC-specific T cells are preferentially exported from the thymus in the presence of their MHC ligand. *Cell* 1989;58:1035–1046.

265. Kaye J, Hsu ML, Sauron ME, Jameson SC, Gascoigne NR, Hedrick SM. Selective development of CD4$^+$ T cells in transgenic mice expressing a class II MHC-restricted antigen receptor. *Nature* 1989;341:746–749.

266. Zijlstra M, Bix M, Simister NE, Loring JM, Raulet DH, Jaenisch R. β2-microglobulin deficient mice lack CD4$^-$8$^+$ cytolytic T cells. *Nature* 1990;344:742–746.

267. Koller BH, Marrack P, Kappler JW, Smithies O. Normal development of mice deficient in β2M, MHC class I proteins, and CD8$^+$ T cells. *Science* 1990;248:1227–1229.

268. Cosgrove D, Gray D, Dierich A, et al. Mice lacking MHC class II molecules. *Cell* 1991;66:1051–1066.

269. Grusby MJ, Johnson RS, Papaioannou VE, Glimcher LH. Depletion of CD4$^+$ T cells in major histocompatibility complex class II-deficient mice. *Science* 1991;253:1417–1420.

270. Bix M, Raulet D. Inefficient positive selection of T cells directed by haematopoietic cells. *Nature* 1992;359:330–333.

271. Markowitz JS, Auchincloss H Jr, Grusby MJ, Glimcher LH. Class II-positive hematopoietic cells cannot mediate positive selection of CD4$^+$ T lymphocytes in class II-deficient mice. *Proc Natl Acad Sci USA* 1993;90:2779–2783.

272. Cosgrove D, Chan SH, Waltzinger C, Benoist C, Mathis D. The thymic compartment responsible for positive selection of CD4$^+$ T cells. *Int Immunol* 1992;4:707–710.

273. von Boehmer H, Teh HS, Kisielow P. The thymus selects the useful, neglects the useless and destroys the harmful. *Immunol Today* 1989;10:57–61.

274. Ignatowicz L, Kappler J, Marrack P. The repertoire of T cells shaped by a single MHC/peptide ligand. *Cell* 1996;84:521–529.

275. Tourne S, Miyazaki T, Oxenius A, et al. Selection of a broad repertoire of CD4$^+$ T cells in H-2Ma$^{-/-}$ mice. *Immunity* 1997;7:187–195.

276. Surh CD, Lee D S, Fung-Leung W-P, Karlsson L, Sprent J. Thymic selection by a single MHC/peptide ligand produces a semidiverse repertoire of CD4$^+$ T cells. *Immunity* 1997;7:209–219.

277. Merkenschlager M, Benoist C, Mathis D. Evidence for a single-niche model of positive selection. *Proc Natl Acad Sci USA* 1994;91:11694–11698.

278. Kaye J, Vasquez NJ, Hedrick SM. Involvement of the same region of the T cell antigen receptor in thymic selection and foreign peptide recognition. *J Immunol* 1992;148:3342–3353.

279. Bogen B, Gleditsch L, Weiss S, Dembic Z. Weak positive selection of transgenic T cell receptor-bearing thymocytes: Importance of major histocompatibility complex class II, T cell receptor and CD4 surface molecule densities. *Eur J Immunol* 1992;22:703–709.

280. Kirberg J, Baron A, Jakob S, Rolink A, Karjalainen K, von Boehmer H. Thymic selection of CD8$^+$ single positive cells with a class II major histocompatibility complex-restricted receptor. *J Exp Med* 1994;180:25–34.

281. Matechak EO, Killeen N, Hedrick SM, Fowlkes BJ. MHC class II-specific T cells can develop in the CD8 lineage when CD4 is absent. *Immunity* 1996;4:337–347.

282. Robey E, Ramsdell F, Elliott J, et al. Expression of CD4 in transgenic mice alters the specificity of CD8 cells for allogeneic major histocompatibility complex. *Proc Natl Acad Sci USA* 1991;88:608–612.

283. Speiser DE, Stubi U, Zinkernagel RM. Extrathymic positive selection of alpha beta T-cell precursors in nude mice. *Nature* 1992;355:170–172.

284. Lundberg K, Shortman K. Small cortical thymocytes are subject to positive selection. *J Exp Med* 1994;179:1475–1483.

285. Swat W, von Boehmer H, Kisielow P. Small CD4$^+$8$^+$ TCRlow thymocytes contain precursors of mature T cells. *Eur J Immunol* 1994;24:1010–1012.

286. Akashi K, Weissman IL. The c-kit$^+$ maturation pathway in mouse thymic T cell development: Lineages and selection. *Immunity* 1996;5:147–161.

287. Shortman K, Vremec D, Egerton M. The kinetics of T cell antigen receptor expression by subgroups of CD4$^+$8$^+$ thymocytes: delineation of CD4$^+$8$^+$3(2+) thymocytes as post-selection intermediates leading to mature T cells. *J Exp Med* 1991;173:323–332.

288. Kearse KP, Roberts JL, Munitz TI, Wiest DL, Nakayama T, Singer A. Developmental regulation of alpha beta T cell antigen receptor expression results from differential stability of nascent TCR alpha proteins within the endoplasmic reticulum of immature and mature T cells. *EMBO J* 1994;13:4504–4514.

289. Sawada S, Scarborough JD, Killeen N, Littman DR. A lineage-specific transcriptional silencer regulates CD4 gene expression during T lymphocyte development. *Cell* 1994;77:917–929.

290. Siu G, Wurster AL, Duncan DD, Soliman TM, Hedrick SM. A transcriptional silencer controls the developmental expression of the CD4 gene. *EMBO J* 1994;13:3570–3579.

291. Turka LA, Schatz DG, Oettinger MA, et al. Thymocyte expression of RAG-1 and RAG-2: Termination by T cell receptor cross-linking. *Science* 1991;253:778–781.

292. Swat W, Dessing M, von Boehmer H, Kisielow P. CD69 expression during selection and maturation of CD4$^+$8$^+$ thymocytes. *Eur J Immunol* 1993;23:739–746.

293. Linette GP, Grusby MJ, Hedrick SM, Hansen TH, Glimcher LH, Korsmeyer SJ. Bcl-2 is upregulated at the CD4$^+$ CD8$^+$ stage during positive selection and promotes thymocyte differentiation at several control points. *Immunity* 1994;1:197–205.

294. Tao W, Teh SJ, Melhado I, Jirik F, Korsmeyer SJ, Teh HS. The T cell receptor repertoire of CD4$^-$8$^+$ thymocytes is altered by overexpression of the BCL-2 protooncogene in the thymus. *J Exp Med* 1994;179:145–153.

295. Zacharchuk CM, Mercep M, Chakraborti PK, Simons SS Jr, Ashwell JD. Programmed T lymphocyte death. Cell activation- and steroid-induced pathways are mutually antagonistic. *J Immunol* 1990;145:4037–4045.

296. Sentman CL, Shutter JR, Hockenbery D, Kanagawa O, Korsmeyer SJ. bcl-2 inhibits multiple forms of apoptosis but not negative selection in thymocytes. *Cell* 1991;67:879–888.

297. Strasser A, Harris AW, Cory S. bcl-2 transgene inhibits T cell death and perturbs thymic self-censorship. *Cell* 1991;67:889–899.

298. Strasser A, Harris AW, Huang DC, Krammer PH, Cory S. Bcl-2 and Fas/APO-1 regulate distinct pathways to lymphocyte apoptosis. *EMBO J* 1995;14:6136–6147.

299. Brandle D, Muller S, Muller C, Hengartner H, Pircher H. Regulation of RAG-1 and CD69 expression in the thymus during positive and negative selection. *Eur J Immunol* 1994;24:145–151.

300. Wilkinson RW, Anderson G, Owen JJ, Jenkinson EJ. Positive selection of thymocytes involves sustained interactions with the thymic microenvironment. *J Immunol* 1995;155:5234–5240.

301. Merkenschlager M. Tracing interactions of thymocytes with individual stromal cell partners. *Eur J Immunol* 1996;26:892–896.

302. Lucas B, Vasseur F, Penit C. Normal sequence of phenotypic transitions in one cohort of 5-bromo-2′-deoxyuridine-pulse-labeled thymocytes. *J Immunol* 1993;151:4574–4582.

303. Lundberg K, Heath X, Kontgen F, Carbone FR, Shortman K. Intermediate steps in positive selection: Differentiation of CD4$^+$8^{int} TCR^{int} thymocytes into CD4$^-$8$^+$ TCR^{hi} thymocytes. *J Exp Med* 1995;181:1643–1651.

304. Robey E, Chang D, Itano A, et al. An activated form of Notch influences the choice between CD4 and CD8 T cell lineages. *Cell* 1996;87:483–492.

305. Lo D, Sprent J. Identity of cells that imprint H-2-restricted T-cell specificity in the thymus. *Nature* 1986;319:672–675.

306. Khazaal I, Salaun J, Coltey M, Calman F, Le Douarin N. Restoration of T-cell function in nude mice by grafting the epitheliomesenchymal thymic rudiment from 10-day-old euthymic embryos. *Cell Differ Dev* 1989;26:211–220.

307. Anderson G, Owen JJ, Moore NC, Jenkinson EJ. Thymic epithelial cells provide unique signals for positive selection of CD4$^+$CD8$^+$ thymocytes in vitro. *J Exp Med* 1994;179:2027–2031.

308. Lorenz RG, Allen PM. Thymic cortical epithelial cells lack full capacity for antigen presentation. *Nature* 1989;340:557–559.

309. Kasai M, Hirokawa K, Kajino K, et al. Difference in antigen presentation pathways between cortical and medullary thymic epithelial cells. *Eur J Immunol* 1996;26:2101–2107.

310. Oukka M, Andre P, Turmel P, et al. Selectivity of the major histocompatibility complex class II presentation pathway of cortical thymic epithelial cell lines. *Eur J Immunol* 1997;27:855–859.

311. Bradley SM, Kruisbeek AM, Singer A. Cytotoxic T lymphocyte responses in allogeneic radiation bone marrow chimeras. The chimeric host strictly dictates the self-repertoire of Ia-restricted T cells but not H-2K/D-restricted T cells. *J Exp Med* 1982;156:1650–1664.

312. Kast WM, Voordouw AC, Leupers T, Visser JW, Melief CJ. Thymic immune response gene function in radiation chimeras reconstituted with purified hemopoietic stem cells. *Eur J Immunol* 1987;17:471–475.

313. Vukmanovic S, Grandea AG, Faas SJ, Knowles BB, Bevan MJ. Positive selection of T-lymphocytes induced by intrathymic injection of a thymic epithelial cell line. *Nature* 1992;359:729–732.

314. Pawlowski T, Elliott JD, Loh DY, Staerz UD. Positive selection of T lymphocytes on fibroblasts. *Nature* 1993;364:642–645.

315. Hugo P, Kappler JW, McCormack JE, Marrack P. Fibroblasts can induce thymocyte positive selection in vivo. *Proc Natl Acad Sci USA* 1993;90:10335–10339.

316. Zinkernagel RM, Callahan GN, Althage A, Cooper S, Klein PA, Klein J. On the thymus in the differentiation of "H-2 self-recognition" by T cells: Evidence for dual recognition? *J Exp Med* 1978;147:882–896.

317. Jameson SC, Hogquist KA, Bevan MJ. Positive selection of thymocytes. *Annu Rev Immunol* 1995;13:93–126.

318. Hogquist KA, Gavin MA, Bevan MJ. Positive selection of CD8+ T cells induced by major histocompatibility complex binding peptides in fetal thymic organ culture. *J Exp Med* 1993;177:1469–1473.

319. Ashton-Rickardt PG, van Kaer L, Schumacher TNM, Ploegh HL, Tonegawa S. Peptide contributes to the specificity of positive selection of CD8+ T cells in the thymus. *Cell* 1993;73:1041–1049.

320. Benoist C, Mathis D. Positive selection of T cells: Fastidious or promiscuous? *Curr Opin Immunol* 1997;9:245–249.

321. Miyazaki T, Wolf P, Tourne S, et al. Mice lacking H-2M complexes, enigmatic elements of the MHC class II peptide-loading pathway. *Cell* 1996;84:531–541.

322. Martin WD, Hicks GG, Mendiratta SK, Leva HI, Ruley HE, van Kaer L. H2-M mutant mice are defective in the peptide loading of class II molecules, antigen presentation, and T cell repertoire selection. *Cell* 1996;84:543–550.

323. Fung-Leung WP, Surh CD, Liljedahl M, et al. Antigen presentation and T cell development in H2-M-deficient mice. *Science* 1996;271:1278–1281.

324. Hogquist KA, Jameson SC, Heath WR, Howard JL, Bevan MJ, Carbone FR. T cell receptor antagonist peptides induce positive selection. *Cell* 1994;76:17–27.

325. Ashton-Rickardt PG, Bandeira A, Delaney JR, et al. Evidence for a differential avidity model of T cell selection in the thymus. *Cell* 1994;76:651–663.

326. Sebzda E, Wallace VA, Mayer J, Yeung RSM, Mak TW, Ohashi PS. Positive and negative thymocyte selection induced by different concentrations of a single peptide. *Science* 1994;263:1615–1618.

327. Nakano N, Rooke R, Benoist C, Mathis D. Positive selection of T cells induced by viral delivery of neopeptides to the thymus. *Science* 1997;275:678–683.

328. Janeway CA Jr, Dianzani U, Portoles P, et al. Cross-linking and conformational change in T-cell receptors: Role in activation and in repertoire selection. *Cold Spring Harb Symp Quant Biol* 1989;54(Pt 2):657–666.

329. Pawlowski TJ, Singleton MD, Loh DY, Berg R, Staerz UD. Permissive recognition during positive selection. *Eur J Immunol* 1996;26:851–857.

330. Hogquist KA, Tomlinson AJ, Kieper WC, et al. Identification of a naturally occurring ligand for thymic positive selection. *Immunity* 1997;6:389–399.

331. Evavold BD, Sloan-Lancaster J, Wilson KJ, Rothbard JB, Allen PM. Specific T cell recognition of minimally homologous peptides: Evidence for multiple endogenous ligands. *Immunity* 1995;2:655–663.

332. Wucherpfennig KW, Strominger JL. Molecular mimicry in T cell-mediated autoimmunity: viral peptides activate human T cell clones specific for myelin basic protein. *Cell* 1995;80:695–705.

333. Garboczi DN, Ghosh P, Utz U, Fan QR, Biddison WE, Wiley DC. Structure of the complex between human T-cell receptor, viral peptide and HLA-A2. *Nature* 1996;384:134–141.

334. Sprent J, Lo D, Gao EK, Ron Y. T cell selection in the thymus. *Immunol Rev* 1988;101:173–190.

335. Valitutti S, Müller S, Dessing M, Lanzavecchia A. Different responses are elicited in cytotoxic T lymphocytes by different levels of T cell receptor occupancy. *J Exp Med* 1996;183:1917–1921.

336. Hogquist KA, Jameson SC, Bevan MJ. Strong agonist ligands for the T cell receptor do not mediate positive selection of functional CD8+ T cells. *Immunity* 1995;3:79–86.

337. Sebzda E, Kundig TM, Thomson CT, et al. Mature T cell reactivity altered by peptide agonist that induces positive selection. *J Exp Med* 1996;183:1093–1104.

338. Swan KA, Alberola-Ila J, Gross JA, et al. Involvement of p21ras distinguishes positive and negative selection in thymocytes. *EMBO J* 1995;14:276–285.

339. Alberola-Ila J, Hogquist KA, Swan KA, Bevan MJ, Perlmutter RM. Positive and negative selection invoke distinct signaling pathways. *J Exp Med* 1996;184:9–18.

340. Anderson G, Anderson KL, Conroy LA, et al. Intracellular signaling events during positive and negative selection of CD4+CD8+ thymocytes in vitro. *J Immunol* 1995;154:3636–3643.

341. Lederberg J. Genes and antibodies. *Science* 1959;129:1649–1652.

342. Kappler JW, Roehm N, Marrack P. T cell tolerance by clonal elimination in the thymus. *Cell* 1987;49:273–280.

343. Herman A, Kappler JW, Marrack P, Pullen AM. Superantigens: Mechanism of T-cell stimulation and role in immune responses. *Annu Rev Immunol* 1991;9:745–772.

344. Kisielow P, Bluthmann H, Staerz UD, Steinmetz M, von Boehmer H. Tolerance in T-cell-receptor transgenic mice involves deletion of nonmature CD4+8+ thymocytes. *Nature* 1988;333:742–746.

345. Pircher H, Burki K, Lang R, Hengartner H, Zinkernagel RM. Tolerance induction in double specific T-cell receptor transgenic mice varies with antigen. *Nature* 1989;342:559–561.

346. Murphy KM, Heimberger AB, Loh DY. Induction by antigen of intrathymic apoptosis of CD4+CD8+TCRlo thymocytes in vivo. *Science* 1990;250:1720–1723.

347. Berg LJ, de St. Groth BF, Pullen AM, Davis MM. Phenotypic differences between alpha beta versus beta T-cell receptor transgenic mice undergoing negative selection. *Nature* 1989;340:559–562.

348. Zal T, Volkmann A, Stockinger B. Mechanisms of tolerance induction in major histocompatibility complex class II-restricted T cells specific for a blood-borne self-antigen. *J Exp Med* 1994;180:2089–2099.

349. Swat W, Ignatowicz L, von Boehmer H, Kisielow P. Clonal deletion of immature CD4+8+ thymocytes in suspension culture by extrathymic antigen-presenting cells. *Nature* 1991;351:150–153.

350. Spain LM, Berg LJ. Developmental regulation of thymocyte susceptibility to deletion by "self"-peptide. *J Exp Med* 1992;176:213–223.

351. Pircher H, Rohrer UH, Moskophidis D, Zinkernagel RM, Hengartner H. Lower receptor avidity required for thymic clonal deletion than for effector T-cell function. *Nature* 1991;351:482–485.

352. Kishimoto H, Cai Z, Brunmark A, Jackson MR, Peterson PA, Sprent J. Differing roles for B7 and intercellular adhesion molecule-1 in negative selection of thymocytes. *J Exp Med* 1996;184:531–537.

353. Speiser DE, Pircher H, Ohashi PS, Kyburz D, Hengartner H, Zinkernagel RM. Clonal deletion induced by either radioresistant thymic host cells or lymphohemopoietic donor cells at different stages of class I-restricted T cell ontogeny. *J Exp Med* 1992;175:1277–1283.

354. Oukka M, Colucci-Guyon E, Tran PL, et al. CD4 T cell tolerance to nuclear proteins induced by medullary thymic epithelium. *Immunity* 1996;4:545–553.

355. Hoffmann MW, Allison J, Miller JF. Tolerance induction by thymic medullary epithelium. *Proc Natl Acad Sci USA* 1992;89:2526–2530.

356. Schonrich G, Strauss G, Muller KP, et al. Distinct requirements of positive and negative selection for selecting cell type and CD8 interaction. *J Immunol* 1993;151:4098–4105.

357. Platt N, Suzuki H, Kurihara Y, Kodama T, Gordon S. Role for the class A macrophage scavenger receptor in the phagocytosis of apoptotic thymocytes in vitro. *Proc Natl Acad Sci USA* 1996;93:12456–12460.

358. Wong B, Choi Y. Pathways leading to cell death in T cells. *Curr Opin Immunol* 1997;9:358–364.

359. Winoto A. Cell death in the regulation of immune responses. *Curr Opin Immunol* 1997;9:365–370.

360. Zhou T, Cheng J, Yang P, et al. Inhibition of Nur77/Nurr1 leads to inefficient clonal deletion of self-reactive T cells. *J Exp Med* 1996;183:1879–1892.

361. Cheng LE, Chan FK, Cado D, Winoto A. Functional redundancy of the Nur77 and Nor-1 orphan steroid receptors in T-cell apoptosis. *EMBO J* 1997;16:1865–1875.

362. Amakawa R, Hakem A, Kundig TM, et al. Impaired negative selection of T cells in Hodgkin's disease antigen CD30-deficient mice. *Cell* 1996;84:551–562.

363. Castro JE, Listman JA, Jacobson BA, et al. Fas modulation of apoptosis during negative selection of thymocytes. *Immunity* 1996;5:617–627.

364. van Meerwijk JPM, Marguerat S, Lees RK, Germain RN, Fowlkes BJ, MacDonald HR. Quantitative impact of thymic clonal deletion on the T cell repertoire. *J Exp Med* 1997;185:377–383.

365. Hammerling GJ, Schonrich G, Momburg F, et al. Non-deletional mechanisms of peripheral and central tolerance: Studies with transgenic mice with tissue-specific expression of a foreign MHC class I antigen. *Immunol Rev* 1991;122:47–67.

366. Husbands SD, Schonrich G, Arnold B, et al. Expression of major histocompatibility complex class I antigens at low levels in the thymus induces T cell tolerance via a non-deletional mechanism. *Eur J Immunol* 1992;22:2655–2661.

367. Blichfeldt E, Munthe LA, Rotnes JS, Bogen B. Dual T cell receptor T cells have a decreased sensitivity to physiological ligands due to reduced density of each T cell receptor. *Eur J Immunol* 1996;26:2876–2884.

368. Blackman MA, Gerhard-Burgert H, Woodland DL, Palmer E, Kappler JW, Marrack P. A role for clonal inactivation in T cell tolerance to Mls-1a. *Nature* 1990;345:540–542.

369. Ramsdell F, Fowlkes BJ. Clonal deletion versus clonal anergy: the role of the thymus in inducing self tolerance. *Science* 1990;248:1342–1348.

370. Schonrich G, Momburg F, Hammerling GJ, Arnold B. Anergy induced by thymic medullary epithelium. *Eur J Immunol* 1992;22:1687–1691.

371. Antonia SJ, Geiger T, Miller J, Flavell RA. Mechanisms of immune tolerance induction through the thymic expression of a peripheral tissue-specific protein. *Int Immunol* 1995;7:715–725.

372. Le Douarin N, Corbel C, Bandeira A, et al. Evidence for a thymus-dependent

form of tolerance that is not based on elimination or anergy of reactive T cells. *Immunol Rev* 1996;149:35–53.

373. Sprent J, Miller JFAP, Mitchell GF. Antigen-induced selective recruitment of circulating lymphocytes. *Cell Immunol* 1971;2:171–181.

374. Mackay CR. Homing of naive, memory and effector lymphocytes. *Curr Opin Immunol* 1993;5:423–427.

375. Butcher EC, Picker LJ. Lymphocyte homing and homeostasis. *Science* 1996;272: 60–66.

376. Gowans JL, Knight EJ. The route of recirculation of lymphocytes in the rat. *Proc R Soc Lond [Biol]* 1964;159:257–282.

377. Austrup F, Vestweber D, Borges E, et al. P- and E-selectin mediate recruitment of T-helper-1 but not T-helper-2 cells into inflammed tissues. *Nature* 1997;385: 81–83.

378. Butcher EC. Leukocyte-endothelial cell recognition: Three (or more) steps to specificity and diversity. *Cell* 1991;67:1033–1036.

379. Mackay C. Lymphocyte migration. A new spin on lymphocyte homing. *Curr Biol* 1995;5:733–736.

380. Berlin C, Bargatze RF, Campbell JJ, et al. alpha 4 integrins mediate lymphocyte attachment and rolling under physiologic flow. *Cell* 1995;80:413–422.

381. Bargatze RF, Jutila MA, Butcher EC. Distinct roles of L-selectin and integrins alpha 4 beta 7 and LFA-1 in lymphocyte homing to Peyer's patch-HEV in situ: The multistep model confirmed and refined. *Immunity* 1995;3:99–108.

382. Lub M, van Kooyk Y, Figdor CG. Ins and outs of LFA-1. *Immunol Today* 1995; 16:479–483.

383. von Andrian UH, Hasslen SR, Nelson RD, Erlandsen SL, Butcher EC. A central role for microvillous receptor presentation in leukocyte adhesion under flow. *Cell* 1995;82:989–999.

384. Erlandsen SL, Hasslen SR, Nelson RD. Detection and spatial distribution of the beta 2 integrin (Mac-1) and L-selectin (LECAM-1) adherence receptors on human neutrophils by high-resolution field emission SEM. *J Histochem Cytochem* 1993;41:327–333.

385. Baggiolini M, Dewald B, Moser B. Human chemokines: An update. *Annu Rev Immunol* 1997;15:675–705.

386. Webb S, Morris C, Sprent J. Extrathymic tolerance of mature T cells: Clonal elimination as a consequence of immunity. *Cell* 1990;63:1249–1256.

387. Kawabe Y, Ochi A. Programmed cell death and extrathymic reduction of Vbeta8+ CD4+ T cells in mice tolerant to Staphylococcus aureus enterotoxin B. *Nature* 1991;349:245–248.

388. Choi Y, Lafferty JA, Clements JR, et al. Selective expansion of T cells expressing V beta 2 in toxic shock syndrome. *J Exp Med* 1990;172:981–984.

389. McHeyzer-Williams M, Davis MM. Antigen-specific development of primary and memory T-cells in vivo. *Science* 1995;268:106–111.

390. Maryanski JL, Jongeneel CV, Bucher P, Casanova JL, Walker PR. Single-cell PCR analysis of TCR repertoires selected by antigen in vivo: a high magnitude CD8 response is comprised of very few clones. *Immunity* 1996;4:47–55.

391. Rocha B, von Boehmer H. Peripheral selection of the T cell repertoire. *Science* 1991;251:1225–1228.

392. Kearney ER, Pape KA, Loh DY, Jenkins MK. Visualization of peptide-specific T cell immunity and peripheral tolerance induction in vivo. *Immunity* 1994;1: 327–339.

393. Sprent J, von Boehmer H. Helper function of T cells depleted of alloantigen-reactive lymphocytes by filtration through irradiated F1 hybrid recipients. I. Failure to collaborate with allogeneic B cells in a secondary response to sheep erythrocytes measured in vivo. *J Exp Med* 1976;144:617–621.

394. Kelsoe G. The germinal center: A crucible for lymphocyte selection. *Semin Immunol* 1996;8:179–184.

395. Nakamura T, Kamogawa Y, Bottomly K, Flavell RA. Polarization of IL-4- and IFN-gamma-producing CD4+ T cells following activation of naive CD4+ T cells. J Immunol 1997;158:1085–1094.

396. Hsieh CS, Heimberger AB, Gold JS, O'Garra A, Murphy KM. Differential regulation of T helper phenotype development by interleukins 4 and 10 in an alpha beta T-cell-receptor transgenic system. *Proc Natl Acad Sci USA* 1992;89: 6065–6069.

397. Zimmermann C, Brduscha-Reim K, Blaser C, Zinkernagel RM, Pircher H. Visualization, characterization, and turover of CD8+ memory T cells in virus-infected hosts. *J Exp Med* 1996;183:1367–1375.

398. Ucker DS, Ashwell JD, Nickas G. Activation-driven T cell death. I. Requirements for de novo transcription and translation and association with genome fragmentation. *J Immunol* 1989;143.3461–3469.

399. MacDonald HR, Baschieri S, Lees RK. Clonal expansion precedes anergy and death of V beta 8+ peripheral T cells responding to staphylococcal enterotoxin B in vivo. *Eur J Immunol* 1991;21:1963–1966.

400. Lenardo MJ. Introduction: The molecular regulation of lymphocyte apoptosis. *Semin Immunol* 1997;9:1–5.

401. Green DR, Scott DW. Activation-induced apoptosis in lymphocytes. *Curr Opin Immunol* 1994;6:476–487.

402. Marrack P, Hugo P, McCormack J, Kappler J. Death and T cells. *Immunol Rev* 1993;133:119–129.

403. Dixon FJ, Maurer PH. Immunologic unresponsiveness induced by protein antigens. *J Exp Med* 1955;101:245–250.

404. Moskophidis D, Lechner F, Pircher H, Zinkernagel RM. Virus persistence in acutely infected immunocompetent mice by exhaustion of antiviral cytotoxic effector T cells. *Nature* 1993;362:758–761.

405. Russell JH, Rush B, Weaver C, Wang R. Mature T cells of autoimmune lpr/lpr mice have a defect in antigen-stimulated suicide. *Proc Natl Acad Sci USA* 1993;90:4409–4413.

406. Klas C, Debatin KM, Jonker RR, Krammer PH. Activation interferes with the APO-1 pathway in mature human T cells. *Int Immunol* 1993;5:625–630.

407. Alderson MR, Armitage RJ, Maraskovsky E, et al. Fas transduces activation signals in normal human T lymphocytes. *J Exp Med* 1993;178:2231–2235.

408. Zheng L, Fisher G, Miller RE, Peschon J, Lynch DH, Lenardo MJ. Induction of apoptosis in mature T cells by tumour necrosis factor. *Nature* 1995;377: 348–351.

409. Kirberg J, Bruno L, von Boehmer H. CD4+8− helps prevent rapid deletion of CD8+ cells after a transient response to antigen. *Eur J Immunol* 1993;23: 1963–1967.

410. Perillo NL, Pace KE, Seilhamer JJ, Baum LG. Apoptosis of T cells mediated by galectin-1. *Nature* 1995;378:736–739.

411. Huang L, Soldevila G, Leeker M, Flavell R, Crispe IN. The liver eliminates T cells undergoing antigen-triggered apoptosis in vivo. *Immunity* 1994;1:741–749.

412. Lamb JR, Skidmore BJ, Green N, Chiller JM, Feldmann M. Induction of tolerance in influenza virus-immune T lymphocyte clones with synthetic peptides of influenza hemagglutinin. *J Exp Med* 1983;157:1434–1447.

413. Jenkins MK, Schwartz RH. Antigen presentation by chemically modified splenocytes induces antigen-specific T cell unresponsiveness in vitro and in vivo. *J Exp Med* 1987;165:302–319.

414. Quill H, Schwartz RH. Stimulation of normal inducer T cell clones with antigen presented by purified Ia molecules in planar lipid membranes: specific induction of a long-lived state of proliferative nonresponsiveness. *J Immunol* 1987;138: 3704–3712.

415. Sloan-Lancaster J, Evavold BD, Allen PM. Induction of T-cell anergy by altered T-cell-receptor ligand on live antigen-presenting cells. *Nature* 1993;363: 156–159.

416. Schwartz RH. A cell culture model for T lymphocyte clonal anergy. *Science* 1990;248:1349–1356.

417. Kang SM, Beverly B, Tran AC, Brorson K, Schwartz RH, Lenardo MJ. Transactivation by AP-1 is a molecular target of T cell clonal anergy. *Science* 1992;257: 1134–1138.

418. Miethke T, Vabulas R, Bittlingmaier R, Heeg K, Wagner H. Mechanisms of peripheral T cell deletion: Anergized T cells are Fas resistant but undergo proliferation-associated apoptosis. *Eur J Immunol* 1996;26:1459–1467.

419. Schwartz RH. T cell clonal anergy. *Curr Opin Immunol* 1997;9:351–357.

420. Bhandoola A, Cho EA, Yui K, Saragovi HU, Greene MI, Quill H. Reduced CD3-mediated protein tyrosine phosphorylation in anergic CD4+ and CD8+ T cells. *J Immunol* 1993;151:2355–2367.

421. Fields PE, Gajewski TF, Fitch FW. Blocked Ras activation in anergic CD4+ T cells. *Science* 1996;271:1276–1278.

422. Li W, Whaley CD, Mondino A, Mueller DL. Blocked signal transduction to the ERK and JNK protein kinases in anergic CD4+ T cells. *Science* 1996;271: 1272–1276.

423. Becker JC, Brabletz T, Kirchner T, Conrad CT, Brocker EB, Reisfeld RA. Negative transcriptional regulation in anergic T cells. *Proc Natl Acad Sci USA* 1995; 92:2375–2378.

424. Arnold B, Schonrich G, Hammerling GJ. Multiple levels of peripheral tolerance. *Immunol Today* 1992;14:12–14.

425. Rammensee HG, Kroschewski R, Frangoulis B. Clonal anergy induced in mature V beta 6+ T lymphocytes on immunizing Mls-1b mice with Mls-1a expressing cells. *Nature* 1989;339:541–544.

426. Perez VL, Parijs LV, Biuckians A, Zheng XX, Strom TB, Abbas AK. Induction of peripheral T cell tolerance in vivo requires CTLA-4 engagement. *Immunity* 1997;6:411–417.

427. Levitz SM, Mathews HL, Murphy JW. Direct antimicrobial activity of T cells. *Immunol Today* 1995;16:387–391.

428. Shaw AS, Dustin ML. Making the T cell receptor go the distance: Review a topological view of T cell activation. *Immunity* 1997;6:361–369.

429. Nagata S. Apoptosis by death factor. *Cell* 1997;88:355–365.

430. Parker DC. T cell-dependent B cell activation. *Annu Rev Immunol* 1993;11: 331–360.

431. Kindred B, Shreffler DC. H-2 dependence of co-operation between T and B cells in vivo. *J Immunol* 1972;109:940–943.

432. Katz DH, Chiorazzi N, McDonald J, Katz LR. Cell interactions between histoincompatible T and B lymphocytes. Cooperative response between lymphocytes are controlled by genes in the I region of H-2 complex. *J Exp Med* 1975;141: 263–266.

433. Mitchison NA. The carrier effect in the secondary response to hapten-protein conjugates. *Eur J Immunol* 1971;1:18–21.

434. Chesnut RW, Grey HM. Studies on the capacity of B cells to serve as antigen-presenting cells. *J Immunol* 1981;126:1075–1079.

435. Rock KL, Benacerraf B, Abbas AK. Antigen presentation by hapten-specific B lymphocytes. I. Role of surface immunoglobulin receptors. *J Exp Med* 1984;160: 1102–1113.

436. Tony HP, Phillips NE, Parker DC. Role of membrane immunoglobulin (Ig) crosslinking in membrane Ig-mediated, major histocompatibility-restricted T cell-B cell cooperation. *J Exp Med* 1985;162:1695–1708.

437. Lanzavecchia A. Antigen-specific interaction between T and B cells. *Nature* 1985;314:537–539.

438. Simitsek PD, Campbell DG, Lanzavecchia A, Fairweather N, Watts C. Modulation of antigen processing by bound antibodies can boost or suppress class II major histocompatibility complex presentation of different T cell determinants. *J Exp Med* 1995;181:1957–1963.

439. Foy TM, Aruffo A, Bajorath J, Buhlmann JE, Noelle RJ. Immune regulation by CD40 and its ligand GP39. *Annu Rev Immunol* 1996;14:591–617.

440. Allen RC, Armitage RJ, Conley ME, et al. CD40 ligand gene defects responsible for X-linked hyper-IgM syndrome. *Science* 1993;259:990–993.

441. Korthauer U, Graf D, Mages HW, et al. Defective expression of T-cell CD40 ligand causes X-linked immunodeficiency with hyper-IgM. *Nature* 1993;361:539–541.

442. Di Santo JP, Bonnefoy JY, Gauchat JF, Fischer A, de Saint Basile G. CD40 ligand mutations in x-linked immunodeficiency with hyper-IgM. *Nature* 1993;361:541–543.

443. Aruffo A, Farrington M, Hollenbaugh D, et al. The CD40 ligand, gp39, is defective in activated T cells from patients with X-linked hyper-IgM syndrome. *Cell* 1993;72:291–300.

444. Renshaw BR, Fanslow WC, Armitage RJ, et al. Humoral immune responses in CD40 ligand-deficient mice. *J Exp Med* 1994;180:1889–1900.

445. Xu J, Foy TM, Laman JD, et al. Mice deficient for the CD40 ligand. *Immunity* 1994;1:423–431.

446. Kawabe T, Naka T, Yoshida K, et al. The immune responses in CD40-deficient mice: Impaired immunoglobulin class switching and germinal center formation. *Immunity* 1994;1:167–178.

447. Coutinho A. The theory of the "One nonspecific signal" model for B cell activation. *Transplant Rev* 1975;23:49–65.

448. Fulcher DA, Lyons AB, Korn SL, et al. The fate of self-reactive B cells depends primarily on the degree of antigen receptor engagement and availability of T cell help. *J Exp Med* 1996;183:2313–2328.

449. Kepron MR, Chen YW, Uhr JW, Vitetta ES. IL-4 induces the specific rearrangement of gamma 1 genes on the expressed and unexpressed chromosomes of lipopolysaccharide-activated normal murine B cells. *J Immunol* 1989;143:334–339.

450. Rothman P, Li SC, Gorham B, Glimcher L, Alt F, Boothby M. Identification of a conserved lipopolysaccharide-plus-interleukin-4-responsive element located at the promoter of germ line epsilon transcripts. *Mol Cell Biol* 1991;11:5551–5561.

451. Takatsu K. Interleukin-5. *Curr Opin Immunol* 1992;4:299–306.

452. Poo WJ, Conrad L, Janeway CA Jr. Receptor-directed focusing of lymphokine release by helper T cells. *Nature* 1988;332:378–380.

453. Kupfer A, Mosmann TR, Kupfer H. Polarized expression of cytokines in cell conjugates of helper T cells and splenic B cells. *Proc Natl Acad Sci USA* 1991;88:775–779.

454. Cher DJ, Mosmann TR. Two types of murine helper T cell clone. II. Delayed-type hypersensitivity is mediated by TH1 clones. *J Immunol* 1987;138:3688–3694.

455. Kaufmann SH. Immunity to intracellular bacteria. *Annu Rev Immunol* 1993;11:129–163.

456. Poenie M, Tsien RY, Schmitt-Verhulst AM. Sequential activation and lethal hit measured by [Ca^{2+}]i in individual cytolytic T cells and targets. *EMBO J* 1987;6:2223–2232.

457. Liu CC, Walsh CM, Young JD. Perforin: Structure and function. *Immunol Today* 1995;16:194–201.

458. Darmon AJ, Nicholson DW, Bleackley RC. Activation of the apoptotic protease CPP32 by cytotoxic T-cell-derived granzyme B. *Nature* 1995;377:446–448.

459. Kagi D, Ledermann B, Burki K, Zinkernagel RM, Hengartner H. Molecular mechanisms of lymphocyte-mediated cytotoxicity and their role in immunological protection and pathogenesis in vivo. *Annu Rev Immunol* 1996;14:207–232.

460. Yasukawa M, Utsunomiya Y, Inoue Y, Kimura N, Fujita S. Monoclonal proliferation of CD4$^+$ large granular lymphocytes with cytolytic activity. *Br J Haematol* 1995;91:419–420.

461. Ramsdell F, Seaman MS, Miller RE, Picha KS, Kennedy MK, Lynch DH. Differential ability of Th1 and Th2 T cells to express Fas ligand an to undergo activation-induced cell death. *Int Immunol* 1994;6:1545–1553.

462. Stalder T, Hahn S, Erb P. Fas antigen is the major target molecule for CD4$^+$ T cell-mediated cytotoxicity. *J Immunol* 1994;152:1127–1133.

463. Williams NS, Engelhard VH. Identification of a population of CD4$^+$ CTL that utilizes a perforin- rather than a Fas ligand-dependent cytotoxic mechanism. *J Immunol* 1996;156:153–159.

464. Bluestone JA, Khattri R, Sciammas R, Sperling AI. TCR gamma delta cells: A specialized T-cell subset in the immune system. *Ann Rev Cell Dev Biol* 1995;11:307–353.

465. Mombaerts P, Arnoldi J, Russ F, Tonegawa S, Kaufmann SH. Different roles of alpha beta and gamma delta T cells in immunity against an intracellular bacterial pathogen. *Nature* 1993;365:53–56.

466. Ladel CH, Blum C, Dreher A, Reifenberg K, Kaufmann SH. Protective role of gamma/delta T cells and alpha/beta T cells in tuberculosis. *Eur J Immunol* 1995;25:2877–2881.

467. Hiromatsu K, Yoshikai Y, Matsuzaki G, et al. A protective role of gamma/delta T cells in primary infection with *Listeria monocytogenes* in mice. *J Exp Med* 1992;175:49–56.

468. Pfeffer K, Schoel B, Gulle H, Kaufmann SH, Wagner H. Primary responses of human T cells to mycobacteria: A frequent set of gamma/delta T cells are stimulated by protease-resistant ligands. *Eur J Immunol* 1990;20:1175–1179.

469. Tanaka Y, Sano S, Nieves E, et al. Nonpeptide ligands for human gamma delta T cells. *Proc Natl Acad Sci USA* 1994;91:8175–8179.

470. Constant P, Davodeau F, Peyrat MA, et al. Stimulation of human gamma delta T cells by nonpeptidic mycobacterial ligands. *Science* 1994;264:267–270.

471. Schild H, Mavaddat N, Litzenberger C, et al. The nature of major histocompatibility complex recognition by gamma delta T cells. *Cell* 1994;76:29–37.

472. Weintraub BC, Jackson MR, Hedrick SM. Gamma delta T cells can recognize nonclassical MHC in the absence of conventional antigenic peptides. *J Immunol* 1994;153:3051–3058.

473. Boismenu R, Hobbs MV, Boullier S, Havran WL. Molecular and cellular biology of dendritic epidermal T cells. *Immunology* 1996;8:323–331.

474. Kelner GS, Kennedy J, Bacon KB, et al. Lymphotactin: A cytokine that represents a new class of chemokine. *Science* 1994;266:1395–1399.

475. Boismenu R, Feng L, Xia YY, Chang JC, Havran WL. Chemokine expression by intraepithelial gamma delta T cells. Implications for the recruitment of inflammatory cells to damaged epithelia. *J Immunol* 1996;157:985–992.

476. Boismenu R, Havran WL. Modulation of epithelial cell growth by intraepithelial gamma delta T cells. *Science* 1994;266:1253–1255.

477. Komano H, Fujiura Y, Kawaguchi M, et al. Homeostatic regulation of intestinal epithelia by intraepithelial gamma delta T cells. *Proc Natl Acad Sci USA* 1995;92:6147–6151.

478. Moingeon P, Jitsukawa S, Faure F, et al. A gamma-chain complex forms a functional receptor on cloned human lymphocytes with natural killer-like activity. *Nature* 1987;325:723–726.

479. Cron RQ, Gajewski TF, Sharrow SO, Fitch FW, Matis LA, Bluestone JA. Phenotypic and functional analysis of murine CD3$^+$, CD4$^-$, CD8$^-$ TCR-gamma delta-expressing peripheral T cells. *J Immunol* 1989;142:3754–3762.

480. Horner AA, Jabara H, Ramesh N, Geha RS. Gamma/delta T lymphocytes express CD40 ligand and induce isotype switching in B lymphocytes. *J Exp Med* 1995;181:1239–1244.

481. Wen L, Pao W, Wong FS, et al. Germinal center formation, immunoglobulin class switching, and autoantibody production driven by "non alpha/beta" T cells. *J Exp Med* 1996;183:2271–2282.

482. Bendelac A, Lantz O, Quimby ME, Yewdell JW, Bennink JR, Brutkiewicz RR. CD1 recognition by mouse NK1$^+$ T lymphocytes. *Science* 1995;268:863–865.

483. Cardell S, Tangri S, Chan S, Kronenberg M, Benoist C, Mathis D. CD1-restricted CD4$^+$ T cells in major histocompatibility complex class II-deficient mice. *J Exp Med* 1995;182:993–1004.

484. Bendelac A, Rivera MN, Park S-H, Roark JH. Mouse CD1-specific NK1 T cells: Development, specificity, and function. *Ann Rev Immunol* 1997;15:535–562.

485. Chen Y-H, Chiu NM, Mandal M, Wang N, Wang C-R. Impaired NK1- T cell development and early Il-4 production in CD1-deficient mice. *Immunity* 1997;6:459–467.

486. Mendiratta SK, Martin WD, Hong S, Boesteanu A, Joyce S, van Kaer L. CD1d1 mutant mice are deficient in natural T cells that promptly produce IL-4. *Immunity* 1997;6:469–477.

487. Green DR, Webb DR. Saying the "S" word in public. *Immunol Today* 1993;14:523–525.

488. Bloom BR, Salgame P, Diamond B. Revisiting and revising suppressor T cells. *Immunol Today* 1992;13:131–136.

489. Allison JP, Krummel MF. The yin and yang of T cell costimulation. *Science* 1995;270:932–933.

490. Ferrini S, Cambiaggi A, Meazza R, et al. T cell clones expressing the natural killer cell-related p58 receptor molecule display heterogeneity in phenotypic properties and p58 function. *Eur J Immunol* 1994;24:2294–2298.

491. Phillips JH, Gumperz JE, Parham P, Lanier LL. Superantigen-dependent, cell-mediated cytotoxicity inhibited by MHC class I receptors on T lymphocytes. *Science* 1995;268:403–405.

492. Powrie F. T cells in inflammatory bowel disease: Protective and pathogenic roles. *Immunity* 1995;3:171–174.

493. Offner H, Hashim GA, Vandenbark AA. T cell receptor peptide therapy triggers autoregulation of experimental encephalomyelitis. *Science* 1991;251:430–432.

494. Qin S, Cobbold SP, Pope H, et al. "Infectious" transplantation tolerance. *Science* 1993;259:974–977.

495. Zinkernagel RM, Bachmann MF, Kundig TM, Oehen S, Pirchet H, Hengartner H. On immunological memory. *Annu Rev Immunol* 1996;14:333–367.

496. Gray D. Immunological memory. *Annu Rev Immunol* 1993;11:49–77.

497. Ahmed R, Gray D. Immunological memory and protective immunity: Understanding their relation. *Science* 1996;272:54–60.

498. Sprent J. Immunological memory. *Curr Opin Immunol* 1997;9:371–379.

499. Zheng B, Xue W, Kelsoe G. Locus-specific somatic hypermutation in germinal centre T cells. *Nature* 1994;372:556–559.

500. Demkowicz WE Jr, Littaua RA, Wang J, Ennis FA. Human cytotoxic T-cell memory: Long-lived responses to vaccinia virus. *J Virol* 1996;70:2627–2631.

501. Sanders ME, Makgoba MW, June CH, Young HA, Shaw S. Enhanced responsiveness of human memory T cells to CD2 and CD3 receptor-mediated activation. *Eur J Immunol* 1989;19:803–808.

502. Byrne JA, Butler JL, Cooper MD. Differential activation requirements for virgin and memory T cells. *J Immunol* 1988;141:3249–3257.

503. Croft M, Bradley LM, Swain SL. Naive versus memory CD4 T cell response to antigen. Memory cells are less dependent on accessory cell costimulation and can respond to many antigen-presenting cell types including resting B cells. *J Immunol* 1994;152:2675–2685.

504. Farber DL, Luqman M, Acuto O, Bottomly K. Control of memory CD4 T cell activation: MHC class II molecules on APCs and CD4 ligation inhibit memory but not naive CD4 T cells. *Immunity* 1995;2:249–259.

505. Bruno L, Kirberg J, von Boehmer H. On the cellular basis of immunological T cell memory. *Immunity* 1995;2:37–43.

506. Pihlgren M, Dubois PM, Tomkowiak M, Sjögren T, Marvel J. Resting memory CD8+ T cells are hyperreactive to antigenic challenge in vitro. *J Exp Med* 1996;184:2141–2151.

507. Roost HP, Charan S, Zinkernagel RM. Analysis of the kinetics of antiviral memory T help in vivo: Characterization of short lived cross-reactive T help. *Eur J Immunol* 1990;20:2547–2554.

508. Gray D, Matzinger P. T cell memory is short-lived in the absence of antigen. *J Exp Med* 1991;174:969–974.

509. Oehen S, Waldner H, Kundig TM, Hengartner H, Zinkernagel RM. Antivirally protective cytotoxic T cell memory to lymphocytic choriomeningitis virus is governed by persisting antigen. *J Exp Med* 1992;176:1273–1281.

510. Tough DF, Sprent J. Turnover of naive- and memory-phenotype T cells. *J Exp Med* 1994;179:1127–1135.

511. Bruno L, von Boehmer H, Kirberg J. Cell division in the compartment of naive and memory T lymphocytes. *Eur J Immunol* 1996;26:3179–3184.

512. Bunce C, Bell EB. CD45RC isoforms define two types of CD4 memory T cells, one of which depends on persisting antigen. *J Exp Med* 1997;185:767–776.

513. Swain SL. Generation and in vivo persistence of polarized Th1 and Th2 memory cells. *Immunity* 1994;1:543–552.

514. Gallichan WS, Rosenthal KL. Long-lived cytotoxic T lymphocyte memory in mucosal tissues after mucosal but not systemic immunization. *J Exp Med* 1996;184:1879–1890.

515. Hou S, Hyland L, Ryan KW, Portner A, Doherty PC. Virus-specific CD8+ T-cell memory determined by clonal burst size. *Nature* 1994;369:652–654.

516. Lau LL, Jamieson BD, Somasundaram T, Ahmed R. Cytotoxic T-cell memory without antigen. *Nature* 1994;369:648–652.

517. Mullbacher A. The long-term maintenance of cytotoxic T cell memory does not require persistence of antigen. *J Exp Med* 1994;179:317–321.

518. Selin LK, Nahill SR, Welsh RM. Cross-reactivities in memory cytotoxic T lymphocyte recognition of heterologous viruses. *J Exp Med* 1994;179:1933–1943.

519. Frisch SM, Francis H. Disruption of epithelial cell-matrix interactions induces apoptosis. *J Cell Biol* 1994;124:619–626.

520. Ruoslahti E, Reed JC. Anchorage dependence, integrins, and apoptosis. *Cell* 1994;77:477–478.

521. Raff MC. Social controls on cell survival and cell death. *Nature* 1992;356:397–400.

522. Cyster JG, Hartley SB, Goodnow CC. Competition for follicular niches excludes self-reactive cells from the recirculating B-cell repertoire. *Nature* 1994;371:389–395.

523. Tanchot C, Rocha B. The peripheral T cell repertoire: Independent homeostatic regulation of virgin and activated CD8+ T cell pools. *Eur J Immunol* 1995;25:2127–2136.

524. George AJ, Ritter MA. Thymic involution with ageing: Obsolescence or good housekeeping? *Immunol Today* 1996;17:267–272.

525. Rocha B, Dautigny N, Pereira P. Peripheral T lymphocytes: Expansion potential and homeostatic regulation of pool sizes and CD4/CD8 ratios in vivo. *Eur J Immunol* 1989;19:905–911.

526. Sprent J, Schaefer M, Hurd M, Surh CD, Ron Y. Mature murine B and T cells transferred to SCID mice can survive indefinitely and many maintain a virgin phenotype. *J Exp Med* 1991;174:717–728.

527. von Boehmer H, Hafen K. The life span of naive alpha/beta T cells in secondary lymphoid organs. *J Exp Med* 1993;177:891–896.

528. Mclean AR, Michie CA. In vivo estimates of division and death rates of human T lymphocytes. *Proc Natl Acad Sci USA* 1995;92:3707–3711.

529. Boise LH, Minn AJ, June CH, Lindsten T, Thompson CB. Growth factors can enhance lymphocyte survival without committing the cell to undergo cell division. *Proc Natl Acad Sci USA* 1995;92:5491–5495.

530. Tough DF, Borrow P, Sprent J. Induction of bystander T cell proliferation by viruses and type I interferon in vivo. *Science* 1996;272:1947–1950.

531. Hiyama K, Hirai Y, Kyoizumi S, et al. Activation of telomerase in human lymphocytes and hematopoietic progenitor cells. *J Immunol* 1995;155:3711–3715.

532. Takeda S, Rodewald HR, Arakawa H, Bluethmann H, Shimizu T. MHC class II molecules are not required for survival of newly generated CD4+ T cells, but affect their long-term life span. *Immunity* 1996;5:217–228.

533. Tanchot C, Lemonnier FA, Pérarnau B, Freitas AA, Rocha B. Differential requirements for survival and proliferation of CD8 naïve or memory T cells. *Science* 1997;276:2057–2058.

534. Heilig JS, Tonegawa S. Diversity of murine gamma genes and expression in fetal and adult T lymphocytes. *Nature* 1986;322:836–839.

535. Sprent J. Role of H-2 gene products in the function of T helper cells from normal and chimeric mice in vivo. *Immunol Rev* 1978;42:108–137.

536. Yasutomo K, Maeda K, Hisaeda H, Good RA, Kuroda Y, Himeno K. The Fas-deficient SCID mouse exhibits the development of T cells in the thymus. *J Immunol* 1997;158:4729–4733.

Fundamental Immunology, Fourth Edition,
edited by William E. Paul
Lippincott–Raven Publishers, Philadelphia © 1999.

CHAPTER 12

T-Lymphocyte Activation

Arthur Weiss

Experimental Models Used to Study T-Cell Activation
   Responding T Cells and Antigen-presenting Cells • Stimuli: Complex Antigens and Peptides • Stimuli: Superantigens • Stimuli: Lectins • Stimuli: Monoclonal Antibodies • Pharmacologic Agents
Requirements for the Initiation of T-Cell Activation
   Primary Signal Required for T-Cell Activation: Requirement or Dependency for TCR Involvement • CD4 and CD8 Coreceptors Contribute to the Primary Activation Signal • Accessory Molecules Increase the Avidity of the T Cell–APC Interaction • A Costimulatory Signal Is Required for T-Cell Activation
Signal Transduction by the T-Cell Antigen Receptor
   Complex Structure of the TCR and Its Signal Transduction Function • TCR ITAMs Interact with Cytoplasmic Protein Tyrosine Kinases • Src PTKs Involved in TCR Signal Transduction • Function of SH2 Domains in Signal Transduction Pathways • The Protein Tyrosine Phosphatase CD45 Plays a Critical Role in TCR Signal Transduction • Consequences of TCR-mediated PTK Activation
The Consequences of Early Signal Transduction Events
   Early Biochemical Events • Cellular Responses • Gene-activation Events
The Regulation of T-Cell Proliferation
   Role of IL-2 • Other Mechanisms Regulating T-Cell Growth
Terminating T-CELL Responses
T-Cell Inactivation
Conclusion
References

The immune system has evolved to provide a flexible and dynamic mechanism to respond specifically to a wide variety of antigens. For a response to occur following antigen challenge, antigen not only must be recognized by antigen-specific lymphocytes, but such recognition must be translated into signal transduction events that are responsible for the initiation of cellular responses. T-lymphocytes, together with B-lymphocytes, represent the two antigen-specific components of the cellular immune system. The activation of resting T cells is critical to most immune responses and allows these cells to exert their regulatory or effector capabilities. During activation, these relatively quiescent T cells in the G_0 stage of the cell cycle undergo complex changes resulting in cell differentiation and proliferation.

Since each T cell expresses T-cell antigen receptors (TCRs) of a single antigen specificity, only a small subset of T cells is activated by any particular antigen (clonal selection). This results in the clonal expansion of antigen-reactive T cells, which acquire differentiated functional capacities. However, the activation of T-lymphocytes is actually a consequence of multiple ligand–receptor interactions that occur at the interface of the T cell and an antigen-presenting cell (APC). In sum, these interactions initiate intracellular biochemical events within the T cell that culminate in cellular responses.

It is clear that a large number of different cell surface molecules on the T-lymphocyte and the APC, only some of which are depicted in Fig. 1, may participate in the complex cell–cell interaction that occurs during antigen presentation. In view of the specificity of T-cell responses, antigen-induced T-lymphocyte activation must be directed by TCR. The ligand for the TCR is a short peptide antigen fragment, derived by proteolysis from a larger molecule, which is bound to a syngeneic major histocompatibility complex (MHC) molecule (see Chapters 8 and 9). The antigen receptor is a multichain structure derived from at least six genes (Fig. 2). On most T cells, it contains at least one disulfide-linked Ti α/β heterodimer responsible for antigen recognition (see Chapter 10). A small subset of T cells, which may preferentially play a role in immune responses in epithelial tissues, recognizes antigen with a Ti $\gamma\delta$ heterodimer. The Ti $\alpha\beta$ or Ti $\gamma\delta$ heterodimer is noncovalently associated with invariant chains derived from the ζ and CD3 γ, δ, and ε genes that are responsible for coupling the receptor to intracellular signal transduction components (1–3) (see below).

Antigen-induced stimulation of the TCR delivers the primary signal in initiating activation. In naive resting T cells, stimulation of the TCR alone is insufficient to induce proliferative responses by purified resting G_0 T cells, but it may be sufficient to induce

A. Weiss: Department of Medicine, Howard Hughes Medical Institute, University of California, San Francisco, San Francisco, CA 94143.

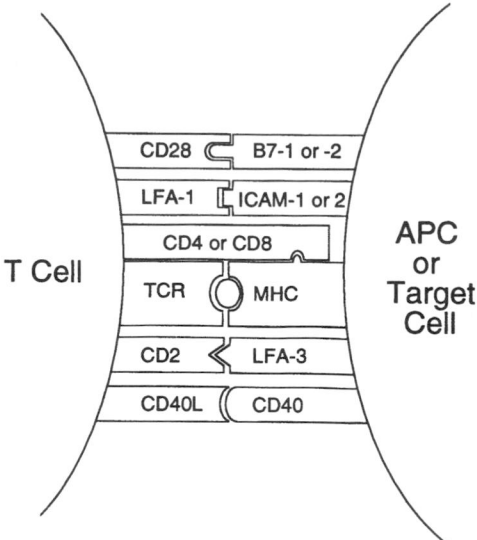

FIG. 1. Schematic representation of some of the ligand–receptor interactions that occur during the interaction of a T cell with an antigen-presenting cell (*APC*) or target cell.

activation of more differentiated T-cell populations or to induce a state of unresponsiveness, termed *anergy* (reviewed in ref. 4). Other cell surface molecules expressed on T cells, by binding to their respective ligands, play a role in antigen-specific activation by functioning as accessory molecules in the initial antigen-specific events occurring between an APC and a T cell. These accessory molecules may contribute to the initiation of cellular

activation by (a) functioning as adhesion molecules, strengthening the interaction between the T cell and APC (i.e., LFA-1 and CD2); (b) modifying the transmembrane signal initiated via the antigen receptor (i.e., CD4 and CD8); and/or (c) initiating their own trans-membrane-signaling events, distinct from those of the TCR, which are necessary for cellular responses [i.e., CD28 and the interleukin-1 receptor (IL-1R)]. These latter signal transduction events are responsible for the requisite second signal, or costimulatory signal, required to activate resting T cells. A more detailed discussion of the structure and function of some of these accessory molecules is presented in Chapter 13.

The interaction of the TCR with its ligand, or the costimulatory receptor with its ligand, initiates cellular activation by inducing signals that result in the formation of intracellular biochemical mediators called *second messengers*. These second messengers can function as biochemical signals that initiate or influence cellular response pathways. In resting T cells, such signals affect the regulation of specific receptive genes that become transcriptionally active or inactive. In differentiated effector T cells, such signals can initiate the activation of the cytolytic mechanism, a stimulus-coupled secretory response in which exocytosis of previously synthesized and packaged proteins involved in the cytolytic apparatus occurs.

During the process of T-cell activation, there are early responses occurring within minutes or hours after the initiation of signal transduction, while others may only occur days after the stimulating event. The early cellular responses may be the result of TCR- or other receptor-mediated signal transduction, directly or indirectly. During the early phase of T-cell activation, T cells undergo enormous changes, characterized by protein phosphorylation, membrane lipid changes, ion fluxes, cyclic nucleotide alterations, increased or decreased RNA synthesis of constitutive and

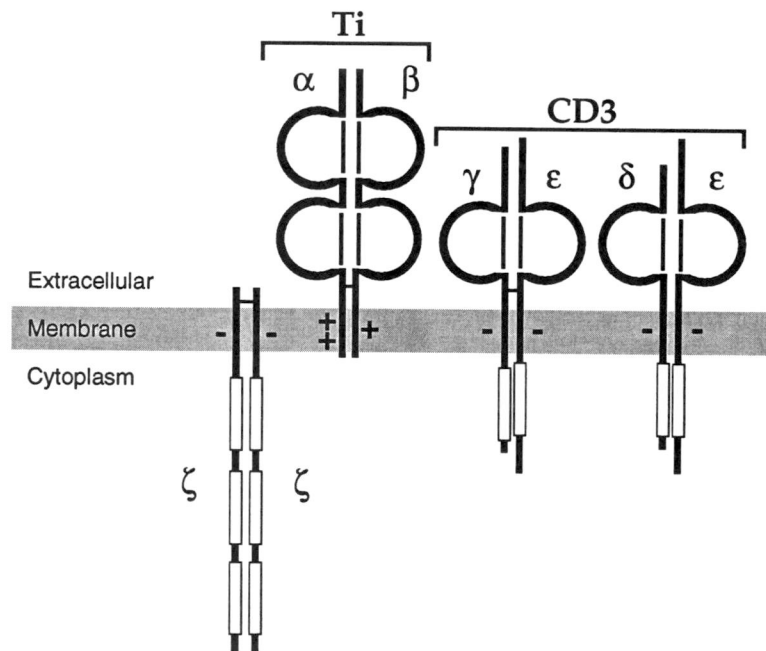

FIG. 2. T-cell antigen receptor. Illustrated schematically is the antigen-binding subunit comprised of an α/β heterodimer, Ti, and the associated invariant CD3 and ζ chains. Acidic (–) and basic (+) residues located within the plasma membrane are indicated. The *open rectangular boxes* indicate motifs (see Fig. 3) within the cytoplasmic domains that interact with cytoplasmic protein tyrosine kinases.

newly activated gene products, and cell volume increases (blast transformation). The later cellular responses, such as proliferation, generally result from a complex cascade of gene activation events and the coordinated sequential influence of the products of these genes. For instance, stimulation of the TCR can drive a resting G_0 T cell into G_1, where it expresses lymphokine receptors, but further progression through the cell cycle requires the action of growth factors such as IL-2 or IL-4 to act on their respective receptors (5,6). The process of T-cell activation represents a contingent cascade of events in which each event is dependent on the expression of the previous components (7). Ultimately, activation of the resting T-lymphocyte may be manifested in a variety ways but includes the expression of new cell surface molecules, secretion of a host of lymphokines, cell proliferation, cellular differentiation, and even programmed cell death (apoptosis). All or only some of these events might be manifested by activated T cells and dominate a particular response.

EXPERIMENTAL MODELS USED TO STUDY T-CELL ACTIVATION

A great deal of interest has focused on the requirements for the induction of T-cell activation. This has primarily concerned the initial cellular and molecular interactions involved in the stimulation of resting, previously unstimulated (naive) T cells by antigen. However, a number of features of antigen-induced activation of T-lymphocytes have hampered such analyses. First, study of the interaction of the T cell with antigen, as it is presented on an APC, involves a cell–cell interaction. This interaction is extremely difficult to study due to the complexities of the stimulating ligand and the TCR. In addition, there are uncertainties regarding the diverse intermolecular ligand–receptor binding events involving other plasma membrane proteins that may occur during this cell–cell interaction (see Fig. 1). Second, the frequency of antigen-specific responding T cells for any given antigen is exceedingly low, representing tenths to hundredths of a percent of unselected T cells. Third, the responding T-cell populations are heterogeneous, representing an ever-increasing mixture of subpopulations of T cells. Each T-cell subpopulation may have different requirements for activation or may respond in a different manner. Moreover, from tissues or blood, these T-cell populations are isolated and mixed together with non-T cells that are difficult to remove completely. These non-T cells may play distinct roles in the initiation of the response. Fourth, the source of responding T cells influences the requirements for activation; freshly isolated naive G_0 T cells have activation requirements that are more stringent than propagated T cell lines, clones, or hybridomas. Fifth, the resulting response may not reflect the response to the initial stimulus, but instead may result from a response to products (e.g., lymphokines) of another responding cell population. Finally, these inherent ambiguities have been confounded by the various parameters used to assess T-cell activation experimentally. These parameters include (a) early signal transduction events, such as protein tyrosine phosphorylation or an increase in cytoplasmic free calcium ($[Ca^{2+}]_i$), that do not necessarily lead to a cellular response; (b) expression of new cell surface activation antigens, including the a chain (CD25) of the IL-2 receptor (IL-2R), the transferrin receptor, class II MHC molecules on human T cells, and CD69, a molecule with as yet unknown function; (c) production of lymphokines, such as IL-2 or IL-4; (d) cell proliferation; and (e) cytolytic activity.

Responding T Cells and Antigen-presenting Cells

In an effort to circumvent the inherent difficulties in studying the complex interactions that occur during antigen-induced T-cell activation, model systems have been developed to simplify the interacting cells as well as the stimulating ligands. T-cell populations that are used include T-cell clones, hybridomas, or leukemic lines. The major advantages of the use of such models are that they represent homogeneous clonal cell populations that can be obtained in large numbers and have well-characterized antigen receptors and responses. However, it is precisely these characteristics, as well as the immortality and other differentiated features, that may not permit extrapolation of all results to responses of resting naive T cells. To avoid these problems, investigators have relied on purified fractionated preparations of T cells derived from more complex mixtures of cells. The major shortcomings of such studies, as discussed, are the difficulties in the isolation procedures and the compromises that are made in the purity of the cell populations obtained. The development of transgenic mice containing T cells that express TCRs of a single specificity has greatly facilitated such studies.

The most commonly used models of APCs have been B-cell lines or adherent cells isolated from peripheral blood mononuclear cells or spleen cells. More emphasis is being placed on studies of dendritic cells, since these cells appear to be the most potent APCs (see Chapters 9 and 16). Differences in the abilities of these cell populations to present and/or process antigen is well documented (8). This should be considered in questions of how APCs participate in the processes that lead to T-cell activation. Additional differences in APC function relate to the ability of some, but not all, cells to provide a costimulatory signal (9,10). In addition, a variety of tumor lines and lymphoblasts have served as target cells to present antigen to cytolytically active T cells. The use of planar lipid membranes or lipid-coated beads that have been reconstituted with limited numbers of purified proteins to stimulate T-cell clones and hybridomas represents an attempt to further simplify the ligands on the APC, as well as to eliminate the need for intact cell systems (11,12). Immobilization at high concentration of such molecules is probably required to achieve a sufficiently high avidity, since the affinities in solution of the TCR to MHC-bound peptide or accessory molecules with their ligands are so low, generally in the micromolar range (reviewed in ref. 13).

Through the use of gene transfer studies in cell lines or transgenic mice, as well as mice made deficient in expression of an ever-increasing number of molecules by homologous recombination, the role of surface molecules in T-cell activation is being explored. By expressing such molecules on the surface of a variety of functional T cells or APCs, which do not normally express them, new cellular models to test the function of these molecules have been developed. T cells or APCs that develop in mice in which a particular gene has been inactivated have provided important insights into the requirements for T-cell activation. Examining the function of transfected mutant or hybrid molecules is a further sophistication of this approach and underscores the power of such genetic analyses.

Stimuli: Complex Antigens and Peptides

Early studies of T-cell activation examined the responses of heterogeneous cell populations to complex cellular or soluble antigens. As efforts evolved to simplify the nature of the responding cell, so too have efforts to simplify the stimulating antigen.

Alloantigens expressed on cells have received a great deal of attention, because they represent a class of antigens for which the precursor frequency of antigen-responsive T cells is high enough to permit measurable responses following a primary antigen stimulus. Although allogeneic cells with many antigenic differences are often used, more recent studies have relied on cells expressing transfected cloned allogeneic molecules or the development of transgenic mice whose T cells express an allo-specific TCR. Further sophistication of this sort of analysis has included the use of transfected chimeric allogeneic molecules (14).

The study of responses to alloantigens has suffered from the necessity of using cells with the antigen expressed as an integral plasma membrane molecule. In such analyses, the contribution of other cell surface molecules or of processing of alloantigens to the activation events is largely undefined. Planar lipid membranes or lipid-coated beads have been reconstituted with purified preparations of MHC molecules to address such ambiguities (11,15). Soluble synthetic peptides derived from the primary sequence of alloantigens or other cellular proteins can be used as agonists or antagonists in sensitizing cells or purified MHC molecules (16). Such approaches with peptides have allowed the type of flexible manipulation of alloantigens that has existed for soluble antigens by permitting the use of MHC molecules containing homogeneous peptides.

The other major type of antigen stimulation that is widely used relies on well-defined soluble proteins presented by APCs. A major limitation in using such soluble antigens is the low frequency of antigen-responsive T cells in the spleen, lymph node, or blood and the resultant difficulty in studying primary responses. However, the study of responses to soluble antigens has been greatly facilitated by the availability of homogenous antigen-responsive T-cell clones, hybridomas, or T cells from TCR transgenic mice. Synthetic peptides prepared from the deduced sequence of more complex antigens are now widely used. It has been possible to obtain near-pure preparations of class I MHC molecule–peptide complexes by taking advantage of cells deficient in peptide transporters (17). Under these circumstances, synthetic peptides rescue the expression of unstable MHC molecules. The ability to load MHC molecules on APCs with uniform preparations of peptides offers real advantages in studying the biochemical events involved in T-cell activation.

Stimuli: Superantigens

A unique group of bacterial and viral products, including bacterial enterotoxins, can activate large numbers of T cells and has been termed *superantigens* (see Chapters 9 and 41). These superantigens stimulate T cells due to their abilities to interact with TCR Vβ framework regions outside of the peptide–MHC binding site (18,19). As a consequence, 5% to 20% of T cells may be stimulated by some of these superantigens. The *in vivo* effects of such massive T-cell stimulation often results in disease (i.e., toxic shock syndrome and food poisoning in humans) (18). Unlike conventional peptide antigens, which are bound to the antigen-binding groove in MHC molecules, superantigens interact with MHC molecules outside of the peptide-binding groove and do not require antigen processing. Although such superantigens may have dire consequences for the host *in vivo,* as activators of large numbers of T cells, they have been quite useful for *in vitro* studies, because their mode of T-cell stimulation seems similar, though perhaps not identical, to conventional antigens (20–23).

Stimuli: Lectins

A number of different reagents have been used to substitute for the stimulating antigen–MHC molecule. Many of these stimuli represent reagents that can polyclonally activate T cells, thereby eliminating the difficulties encountered in studying small numbers of antigen-specific responding cells within complex polyclonal T-cell populations. Among these reagents are several lectins, plant-derived proteins that bind various carbohydrate groups (24). These lectins, phytohemagglutinin (PHA), concanavallin A (Con A), and pokeweed mitogen (PWM), were among the first recognized polyclonal activators of T cells (25). Because they can induce the proliferative responses, they are among a class of reagents termed *mitogens*. They bind to a number of glycoproteins expressed on the plasma membrane of a variety cells in addition to T cells. Con A and PHA are selective T-cell mitogens when compared with their effects on B cells, whereas PWM is a T- and B-cell mitogen (24). The relative mitogenic selectivity of lectins is not dependent on their binding specificity for particular cell populations but, rather, reflects the heterogeneity in the carbohydrate groups expressed on different glycoproteins of various cells. Their mitogenic effects for T cells are felt to depend on their ability to bind and cross-link relevant receptors involved in physiologic T-cell activation. Studies with PHA and Con A suggest that these lectins can bind to component chains of the TCR (26) and that their ability to activate T cells is dependent on the expression and function of the TCR (27). However, it should be emphasized that their effects represent the summation of the effects of the binding of these lectins to a large number of distinct molecules, in addition to the TCR. Despite such heterogenous interactions, stimulation of naive T cells or resting T-cell clones with Con A still requires a costimulatory signal (28).

Stimuli: Monoclonal Antibodies

A major advance in the study of T-cell activation came from the use of monoclonal antibodies (mAbs) as specific probes to study the role of distinct T-cell surface molecules. These mAbs have been used as agonists or antagonists to mimic or interrupt the intermolecular interactions that occur between the T cell and APC or target cell. Among these are mAbs reactive with either the Ti or the CD3 subunits of the TCR. These mAbs have been used to mimic the agonist effects of antigenic peptide–MHC or interrupt the binding of antigenic peptide–MHC to the TCR. Additional mAbs reactive with other T-cell surface molecules have been used in a large number of experimental models to address whether other T-cell or APC surface molecules may participate in T-cell activation. A variation on this theme has come from the use of immunoglobulin (Ig) fusion proteins linked to the extracellular domains of molecules expressed on the T cell or APC. This allows for a more physiologic interaction than may be obtained using mAbs. These approaches have led to the identification of a large number of T-cell and APC surface molecules that participate directly in initiating T-cell activation or may serve to modify the process of activation.

A degree of caution, however, must be exercised in the interpretation of studies that rely solely on mAbs or fusion proteins. It should be apparent that the binding of these reagents may not truly mimic the physiologic ligand-binding event with respect to epitope specificity, avidity, or valency. The non–antigen-binding portions of mAbs may influence the effects of the mAb used; notably, this has been well documented for anti-CD3 mAbs in which immobilization of these mAbs via the Fc receptor to adherent cells contained in cultures is critical for their mitogenic effects for T cells (29). The agonist or antagonist effects of mAbs may not completely mimic or interrupt the effects of the physiologic ligand but may have effects of their own. Confusion regarding the role of the physiologic receptor may thus arise; for instance, in the case of CD2, agonist as well as antagonist effects of mAbs reactive with this receptor have been observed, depending on the experimental model and specific mAb used (30–32). In addition, the extensive cross-linking of all of the molecules reactive with a particular mAb is not a situation likely to be mimicked by physiologic ligands for such cell surface molecules. Despite these cautionary notes, the use of mAbs has proven invaluable in approaching the problem of studying the complex intermolecular events that may occur between the T cell and APC during the initiation of T-cell activation.

Pharmacologic Agents

Pharmacologic agents that can mimic or inhibit some of the intracellular events associated with T-cell activation have been used as probes to address the importance of these events in initiating cellular activation responses. Notably, the calcium ionophores A23187 and ionomycin, which increase cytoplasmic free calcium $[Ca^{2+}]_i$, and phorbol esters, which activate protein kinase C (PKC), can act synergistically to induce many of the gene-activation events and proliferation responses observed during T-cell activation (33,34). The use of these reagents to mimic some of the events associated with ligands that bind to the TCR has been of considerable value in understanding the signal transduction function of the TCR (see below).

A large number of pharmacologic agents have been used as inhibitors of particular intracellular events or as agents that prevent certain cellular responses. Some of the more commonly used inhibitors are listed in Table 1. The targets of such inhibitors are diverse and often ill defined. However, under some circumstances, these inhibitors are enormously helpful in assessing the contribution of a particular target in cellular responses. Notably, the inhibitors of protein tyrosine kinases (PTKs), genestein and her-

TABLE 1. *Inhibitors used to study T-cell activation*

Inhibitor	Target
Neomycin	Phosphatidylinositol turnover
Lithium	Inositol phosphate phosphatase
H7	Protein kinase C
Sphingosine	Protein kinase C
Staurosporine	Protein kinase C
Genestein	Tyrosine kinase
Herbimycin A	Tyrosine kinase
Tyrphostin	Tyrosine kinase
Vanadate	Tyrosine phosphatase
Phenylarsine oxide	Tyrosine phosphatase (?)
EDTA	Ca^{2+} and Mg^{2+}
EGTA	Ca^{2+}
Dimethylamiloride	Na^+/H^+ antiporter
Glucocorticoids	Glucocorticoid receptor; diverse effects
Cyclosporin A	Calcineurin
FK506	Calcineurin
Rapamycin	mTor
Wortmannin	Phosphatidylinositol 3-kinase
LY294002	Phosphatidylinositol 3-kinase

bimycin A, were among the first clues that PTKs regulated the phosphatidylinositol (PI) pathway in T cells (35,36).

Some inhibitors of T-cell activation have found great utility in clinical medicine, such as cyclosporin A (CsA), FK506, rapamycin, and glucocorticoids. *In vitro* studies with of the mechanism of action of CsA and Fk506 have provided remarkable insights into previously unrecognized molecular components of the TCR-regulated signal transduction pathway (see below and Chapter 36).

The use of inhibitors in the study of T-cell activation depends upon their specificity and low toxicity. Unfortunately, in practice, few of these inhibitors have the required exquisite specificity and low toxicity. Nonetheless, through the use of several different pharmacologic inhibitors and agonists, much can be learned about the processes and events involved in T-cell activation.

Although each experimental model has its ambiguities and limitations, a great deal has been learned from such experimental approaches. These model systems provide the basis for much of the discussion in this and subsequent chapters on cell surface molecules and events involved in T-cell activation.

REQUIREMENTS FOR THE INITIATION OF T-CELL ACTIVATION

Antigen-specific T-cell activation is initiated during an extraordinarily complex cell–cell interaction. Antigenic peptides bound to MHC molecules on APCs are recognized by T cells bearing antigen-specific TCRs. However, a large number of molecules, some of which are depicted in Fig. 1, also participate in the response. The TCR and other cell surface molecules contribute to the initiation of T-cell activation by inducing signal transduction events and by contributing to the overall avidity of the T cell–APC interaction. Considerable evidence has accumulated to suggest that at least one molecule, a costimulatory receptor, must initiate signal transduction events distinct from the TCR in order to initiate IL-2 secretion and induce a proliferative response in naive T cells.

Primary Signal Required for T-Cell Activation: Requirement or Dependency for TCR Involvement

Clearly, central to antigen activation of the T cell is the TCR. Stimulation of the TCR delivers the primary signal required for the activation of resting T cells. However, under appropriate conditions, stimulation of several other distinct cell surface molecules is able to mimic this function of the TCR. Among those that have been most extensively studied CD2, CD28, and, in the murine system, Thy-1 and Ly-6 can all induce signal transduction events similar to those initiated by the TCR (reviewed in refs. 37,38). With the exceptions of CD2 (39) and CD28 (9), the physiologic ligands of these other cell surface molecules are as yet unidentified. Therefore, the physiologic significance of signal transduction events leading to T-cell activation via these molecules is not known. In general, for the non-TCR molecules to mediate such a primary activation signal, their extensive cross-linking, usually with mAbs, is required. Such a requirement is not likely to be met by physiologic ligands. Nor is it clear, when the ligand may be expressed fairly broadly, as is the case for CD2 ligands, how activation via these molecules would be regulated in a manner that would be beneficial to the host. Some of these molecules may have other more important functions, including to increase the avidity of the T-cell–APC interaction or to mediate other distinct signal transduction events, as has been demonstrated for CD28 (10). Moreover, the dependency of these non-TCR molecules on the expression and functional competency of the TCR to initiate a primary activation signal suggests the pathways by which these molecules induce a primary signal must converge with the TCR-regulated pathway (40–43). Thus, in some way, perhaps through a direct or indirect physical interaction that results from extensive cross-linking, the TCR appears to be responsible for the signal transduction events attributed to this group of molecules. This is consistent with the demonstration that the TCR ζ chain participates in and is required for CD2-mediated signaling events (44).

The TCR has two functions in the antigen-induced activation of T cells. First, it must bind the specific peptide–MHC molecule complex on the surface of an APC. Second, this binding event must be converted into a transmembrane signal transduction event in which cytoplasmic signaling machinery is activated that can regulate subsequent cellular responses (see below for a detailed discussion of TCR signal transduction). It is clear from gene transfer studies that the TCR α/β heterodimer contains all of the information necessary for the recognition of the antigen peptide–MHC molecule. However, how peptide–MHC binding to the α/β heterodimer induces signal transduction by the associated CD3 and ζ chains of the TCR is not fully understood. This has become an increasing area of interest because distinct or minimally altered peptides [altered peptide ligands (APL)] bound to the same MHC molecule can induce distinct signal transduction events by the TCR (45–47). The analyses of the effects of the APLs on TCR signal transduction have been hampered by the complexity of the ligand (i.e., peptide–MHC molecule) and by the fact that this interaction occurs during a complex cell–cell interaction that involves many other molecules on the T cell and APC. Differences in signal transduction have been attributed to differences in the allosteric conformation of the TCR during peptide–MHC recognition, to differences in the interaction of the TCR with accessory molecules, as well as to distinct on–off rates involved in these intermolecular interactions (48,49).

Efforts to study signal transduction by the TCR alone have also taken advantage of mAbs that react with distinct chains of the TCR. Monoclonal antibodies reactive with clone-specific variable or constant determinants of the α/β heterodimer as well as CD3 have been used as agonists to initiate T cell activation (reviewed in ref. 37). Under appropriate conditions, which usually require immobilization to a solid support or binding to an Fc receptor on adherent cells, these mAbs can induce resting T cells to secrete lymphokines [such as IL-2 and interferon-γ, (IFNγ)], to express a number of new cell surface molecules (including the high-affinity IL-2R and CD69), and to proliferate. Such mAbs also have been used to activate T-cell clones and tumor lines to produce lymphokines and to induce the cytolytic mechanism by differentiated cytolytic T-lymphocytes (CTLs). Interestingly, mAbs reactive with the TCR αβ heterodimer differ in their ability to function as agonists (50,51). In addition, stimulation of the receptor with mAbs that selectively react with either Ti or CD3 components may differ in their functional effects (52). These observations, together with studies of chimeric TCRs (discussed below), suggest that structurally distinct domains and components of the TCR may have distinct signal transduction functions.

The very low concentrations of peptide–MHC complexes or of mAbs required for activation suggest that occupancy of relatively few receptors, perhaps less than a few hundred, is sufficient to initiate T-cell activation (53–57). This is consistent with the relatively few relevant antigenic peptides that are likely to be associated with MHC molecules on the surface of an APC. An alternate possibility has emerged from more recent studies that relates the relatively low affinity–short half-life of the TCR–peptide–MHC interaction. Some experimental evidence suggests that relatively large numbers of TCRs may be serially engaged by the few specific peptide/MHC complexes on an APC, resulting in signal transduction by large number of TCRs that are engaged for relatively short periods of time before they are internalized (58). However, when mAbs are used, it is clear that engagement of only a few TCRs is sufficient to generate a signal that can result in T-cell activation.

Monoclonal antibodies reactive with either CD3 or the α/β Ti can also function as antagonists to inhibit the antigen-specific interaction between T cells and APC or target cells. The ability of these mAbs to function as either agonists or antagonists in a particular experimental model probably depends on the conditions under which they are used. Immobilization of anti-TCR mAbs usually results in an agonist effect, but this is not always necessary for an agonist effect. Such immobilization may prevent receptor internalization and enhance receptor cross-linking. Soluble anti-TCR mAbs have generally been used in experiments in which antagonist effects are observed.

In a similar manner, though less frequently, purified MHC molecules that have been pulsed with peptides have been used to stimulate T cells. Usually, any induced response requires immobilization of these molecules to plastic surfaces, within lipid bilayers, or on some other matrix (11,12). Successful activation with such purified molecules is usually seen only with hybridomas or some T-cell clones. Primary resting T cells, even if derived from TCR transgenic mice, have additional requirements for activation (59). The signal transduction events induced by such purified peptide–MHC complexes and anti-TCR mAbs are similar but may not be identical.

Superantigens such as staphylococcal enterotoxins or Mls antigens, molecules encoded by endogenous mouse mammary tumor virus genomes, have also been used to induce a primary signal via the TCR (reviewed in ref. 18). Responses to these superantigens are dependent on their interaction with class II MHC molecules on APCs and TCRs derived from appropriate Vβ-gene segments (as discussed above). Interestingly, stimulation with such antigens has variable outcomes. In some cases, polyclonal T-cell proliferative and lymphokine responses are observed. However, subsequent clonal deletion and anergy have also been observed (60). The reasons for the diversity in the responses are likely to depend on whether such superantigens are presented to T cells in the setting of an inflammatory response (61). This is likely not to reflect a special property of responses to superantigen, although it may be more easily recognized due to the large number of responsive T cells, as similar deletion of conventional antigen responsive T cells occurs in the absence of concomitant inflammation (62). There is some controversy regarding whether the signal transduction events observed with superantigens are identical to those induced by antigen or mAbs (20,21,23,63,64). Nevertheless, these bacterial and viral products have proven to be potent reagents in stimulating the TCR and valuable probes for the new insights they have provided.

Engagement of the TCR by ligand is not sufficient for the full activation of T cells. However, before considering other signals required for T-cell activation, the requirements for activation via the TCR must be defined in terms of the parameters of activation examined and the cell population being stimulated. For instance, expression of CD25 (the α chain of the IL-2R) can be induced on naive resting T cells in the absence of a demonstrable proliferative response by stimulating the TCR alone (65,66). In contrast, the production of the lymphokine IL-2 by these cells is more stringently regulated and requires additional stimuli provided by costimulatory receptors (see below). Hence, a T-cell proliferative response is more likely to be limited by IL-2 production than by IL-2R expression.

Antigen or mAb-induced IL-2 production and proliferative responses by resting G_0 T cells are dependent on several functions by the APC that influence the delivery of the primary signal. Some functions have been delineated by using anti-TCR mAbs. One function appears to involve the immobilization of the mAb via its Fc domain to Fc receptors on the APC (29,67). This function of the APC can be bypassed by stimulating the T cell with anti-TCR mAbs that have been bound to Sepharose beads or to a plastic culture dish. The immobilized mAb may be analogous to the cell-bound peptide–MHC complex when it is presented to a T cell. This suggests that the formation of a high local concentration or of a cross-linked array of TCRs by antigenic peptide–MHC molecules or mAbs may be important to initiate activation. Such multimerization of ligands will also serve to increase their effective valency and avidity. Alternatively, stimulation with immobilized rather than soluble ligands may serve to prevent TCR internalization and thus potentiate the duration and magnitude of the stimulus.

CD4 and CD8 Coreceptors Contribute to the Primary Activation Signal

The CD4 and CD8 molecules are expressed on and define the two major subsets of mature $\alpha\beta$ TCR–bearing T cells (see Chapter 11). They bind to nonpolymorphic regions of class II and class I MHC molecules, respectively. In general, CD4 cells are involved in T helper–cell function and are involved in host responses to antigens that are processed via the endocytic pathway. In contrast, CD8 T cells give rise to cytolytic effector cells and recognize peptides that are derived from the endogenous biosynthetic pathway (68). The coreceptors function in concert with the TCR during antigen recognition to increase the sensitivity of TCR responsiveness to antigen and contribute to the primary activation stimulus delivered by the TCR.

CD4 and CD8 are integral membrane glycoproteins whose structures have been studied extensively (69). The extracellular domain of CD4 consists of four Ig domains joined in tandem. The two more membrane-distal or N-terminal domains interact with the $\beta2$ domain of class II MHC molecules, whereas the more membrane-proximal two Ig domains may play a role in homooligomerization (70). The N-terminal two Ig domains also are involved in the interaction with the envelope glycoprotein gp120 of the human immunodeficiency virus (HIV). CD8 on TCR $\alpha\beta$-expressing T cells is a heterodimer of an α and a β chain, but can be expressed as an $\alpha\alpha$ homodimer on TCR $\gamma\delta$-bearing T cells. The N-terminal Ig domain of the α chain binds to the $\alpha3$ domain of class I MHC molecules (71, 72). It is not clear whether the CD8 β chain, which cannot be expressed independently of the CD8 α chain, can bind class I MHC molecules (73). The binding of CD4 and CD8 to MHC molecules is a relatively low-affinity interaction, in the micromolar range. However, the ability of these coreceptors to interact with regions of the MHC molecule not involved with peptide recognition allows for the simultaneous binding of the TCR and coreceptor to a single peptide–MHC molecule. This can lead to the enhanced stability of the tetrameric complex (74,75). Hence, it is not surprising that many, though not all, functional interactions of TCRs with antigen are dependent on appropriate CD4 or CD8 coreceptor engagement. The antigen responses that are coreceptor-independent frequently involve memory responses and may involve T cells with TCRs that have been selected for higher affinity.

Whereas the CD4 and CD8 coreceptors can contribute to the formation of a more stable interaction of the TCR with the peptide–MHC complex, they also communicate with intracellular signal transduction events through the interaction of their intracellular domains with the cytoplasmic PTK Lck. A more detailed discussion of the function of Lck in TCR signaling pathways will follow. Here, we will focus on its role in coreceptor function.

Both coreceptors interact noncovalently with the N-terminal unique region of Lck via paired cysteine residues (76,77). The interaction of Lck with CD4 is of higher affinity than with CD8 (78). Some evidence suggests that the differences in the interaction of the coreceptors with Lck lead to distinct signal transduction events (79,80). This model may explain the distinct developmental outcomes that occur during positive selection in the thymus as well as the distinct functions of the resultant CD4 and CD8 subsets of mature T cells.

Coligation of the TCR with either coreceptor can markedly enhance signal transduction by the TCR (81,82). The contribution of Lck to CD4 and CD8 coreceptor function is important but not essential for effective TCR signaling function during development or at high antigen concentrations. The function of Lck in thymic development can be overcome, presumably by higher levels of coreceptor engagement (83). The role of Lck may be twofold: A kinase-independent function of Lck has been identified that may be able to deliver or strengthen the interaction of the coreceptor with the TCR–peptide–MHC complex (84). In fact, the strength of binding of CD4 or CD8 to MHC molecules may be regulated by TCR signal transduction events that influence the localization or interactions of Lck to cytoskeletal components (85) or to the stimulated TCR (86,87). This may lead to the formation and stabilization of the tetrameric complex. A second function is mediated by the kinase domain, which the coreceptor delivers to the stimulated TCR complex (82,88). In this case, the kinase domain of Lck may function by phosphorylating critical substrates (see below). These two functions probably act in concert, rather than independently, to increase the overall sensitivity of the TCR for antigen recognition.

Independent engagement of the coreceptors can lead to a signal that inhibits T-cell activation. Whereas the binding of CD4 and CD8 to MHC molecules has been demonstrated in cells that massively overexpress these molecules (89,90), these interactions probably occur normally only during simultaneous TCR recognition of peptide–MHC molecule. However, experimental ligation of CD4 with anti-CD4 mAbs primes T cells for apoptosis when the TCR is subsequently stimulated (91). In vivo, this may be relevant to interactions of the HIV envelope glycoprotein gp120 with CD4, where apoptosis results if the TCR is subsequently engaged (92). The mechanisms underlying these inhibitory events have not been determined.

In most primary immune responses, the involvement of CD4 or CD8 is required. Thus, in general, mAbs reactive with either CD4 or CD8 can block the responses of the appropriate subset of cells to antigens during primary but not secondary immune responses. However, the dependency of an individual T cell on the involvement of CD4 or CD8 is highly clone-dependent. In the case of CD4, its contribution to the antigen response depends not only on its extracellular domain that interacts with MHC class II molecules, but also on the sequences in its cytoplasmic domain that interact with Lck (93). This suggests critical roles for domains of these molecules that bind to MHC molecules and for the domains responsible for the redistribution of the Lck PTK. It is also clear from such studies that requirement for the interaction of CD4 or CD8 with an MHC molecule during antigen recognition requires that these molecules interact with the same MHC molecule that is presenting peptide to the TCR. This has at least two functions: First, it serves to increase the overall avidity of the antigen-recognition complex. Second, it serves to deliver Lck into the close proximity to the TCR that is being stimulated by antigen, potentially allowing Lck to regulate this interaction.

Accessory Molecules Increase the Avidity of the T-Cell–APC Interaction

Several nonantigen-dependent molecular interactions have been identified that serve to increase the overall avidity of the interaction of T cells with APCs and may help to organize the complex intercellular interaction. These include the LFA-1 (CD11a/CD18) with ICAM-1 (CD54) or ICAM-2 (CD102) (13,94); CD2 with LFA-3 (CD58) or CD59 (95); and CD4 with MHC class II or CD8 with MHC class I (96). Whereas the TCR may dictate the specificity of the recognition event, these antigen-independent molecular interactions serve in a permissive manner to facilitate the interaction of the T cell with the APC.

The affinity of the TCR for the specific peptide–MHC complex is believed to be relatively low, on the order of 10^{-5} M (97). For this reason, and because nonspecific cell conjugates have been observed between T cells and potential APCs, it has been proposed that the initial encounter of a T cell with a potential APC may not be due to antigen-specific recognition (13,98). A nonspecific T cell–APC conjugate may form initially and be mediated, in part, by the molecular interactions listed above. Such nonantigen-specific adhesion between a T cell and an APC may permit the TCR to survey peptide–MHC molecules and, if engaged by sufficient specific complexes, to initiate signal transduction events. These signal transduction events not only can lead to the activation of biochemical pathways responsible for T-cell activation, but also can increase the avidity of several of these accessory molecule pairs. Such a TCR-mediated increase in avidity has been observed for interactions of LFA-1 with ICAM-1 (99); CD2 with LFA-3 (100); and CD8 with class I MHC molecules (12,85). This increase in avidity serves to further stabilize the interaction between the T cell and APC and promotes the activation of the T cell by prolonging signal transduction. If the TCR does not encounter its specific peptide antigen during the initial interaction, signal transduction events that contribute to the increased avidity of the accessory molecules are not induced. This permits the disengagement of the T cell and APC from a low-avidity interaction and allows the T cell to move on to interactions with other potential APCs. The functions of these accessory molecules are discussed in further detail in Chapter 13.

A Costimulatory Signal Is Required for T-Cell Activation

As is clear, the molecules expressed in an APC provide many functions for the initiation of T-cell activation. In addition to peptide presentation and the adhesion functions, molecules on or secreted by the APC induce additional signal transduction events necessary for T-cell activation. This latter function is termed a *costimulatory function* or *signal* (101). The function of costimulation is to ensure that

the antigenic peptide recognized is a non-self peptide. This is accomplished by requiring that the resting T cell is only activated by peptide antigens presented by dedicated APCs, such as dendritic cells, macrophages, or activated B cells. These dedicated APCs constitutively express or are induced by inflammatory stimuli to express ligands for costimulatory receptors on T cells.

The costimulatory function has been revealed primarily in studies involving the response of resting G_0 T cells or resting T-cell clones of the Th1 type that have been depleted of APCs contained in the adherent cell population. Purified resting T cells fail to produce IL-2 or proliferate in response to mitogenic lectins, immobilized anti-TCR mAbs, or antigen-pulsed fixed APCs (fixed APCs cannot provide a costimulatory signal), but they are induced to express IL-2Rs and will proliferate if exogenous IL-2 is provided (65,66,101,102). In contrast, T-cell hybridomas and cytolytic T-cell clones will frequently produce IL-2 and/or proliferate in response to immobilized anti-TCR mAbs, antigen-pulsed fixed APCs alone, or even lipid membranes reconstituted with peptide–MHC molecules (11,15,103), whereas such stimulation of T helper–cell clones may fail to induce IL-2 production or proliferation and can induce an unresponsive state (4). This state of unresponsiveness will be discussed later in this chapter and in Chapters 13 and 20. The critical event necessary to avoid the anergic state is the response to IL-2 (104). In most cases, this will reflect the production of IL-2 by the same T cell. The variable dependency of some T-cell clones and hybridomas on a costimulatory signal may reflect the state of differentiation of these cells. T-cell clones already express high-affinity IL-2Rs, transferrin receptors, and, in the case of human clones, class II MHC molecules, characteristics not shared by resting naive T cells. Thus, these observations suggest that the activation of resting naive T cells and, in some cases, T helper–cell clones requires two independent signals for IL-2 production, proliferation and differentiation. One signal is provided by the TCR. The other signal is provided by a soluble factor or by cell surface molecules on the APC that interact with molecules on the T cell.

One molecule that functions as a costimulatory receptor on T cells is CD28 (reviewed in ref. 10). The function of CD28 is discussed in detail in Chapter 13. Briefly, CD28 is a disulfide-linked homodimer of 44-kD glycoprotein monomers. It is expressed on most T cells, but in the human approximately 50% of CD8 T cells do not express CD28. CD28 has two well-characterized ligands, B7-1 (CD80) and B7-2 (CD86), that are expressed on potent APCs, including activated B cells, activated macrophages, and dendritic cells. Costimulatory function can be provided by anti-CD28 mAbs, soluble B7-Ig fusion proteins, or cells expressing B7 molecules (105–108). Interruption of the CD28–B7 interaction can block costimulatory function and prevent T-cell activation *in vitro* or *in vivo* (107,109–111), highlighting the importance of this interaction. Moreover, mice made deficient in CD28 or B7-1 and B7-2 have markedly impaired immune responses (112,113).

A critical event necessary for costimulatory function is the induction or upregulation of B7 molecules on the surface of APCs, particularly when B cells function as APCs. Studies suggest that this involves the sequential stimulation of the TCR on the interacting T cells and CD40 on the antigen-presenting B cell (Fig. 3) (114,115). During this interaction, stimulation of the TCR on a resting T cell results in the induced expression of gp39, the CD40 ligand (CD40L), a membrane-bound member of the tumor necrosis family (116). This, in turn, allows for the stimulation of CD40 on the B cell which induces upregulation of B7-1 and B7-2, which can then stimulate CD28. Inflammatory mediators, such as lipopolysaccharide

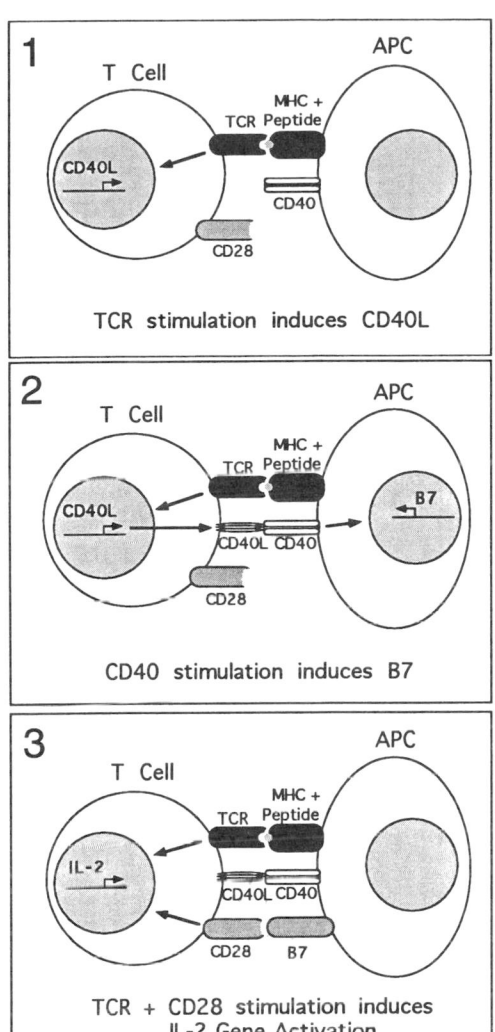

FIG. 3. Interactions between a T cell and APC that lead to IL-2 production. The sequential interactions of the TCR with peptide antigen–MHC complex lead to the induced expression of CD40L on the T cell, which interacts with CD40 on the APC. This induces the expression of B7 molecules on the APC, which can then stimulate CD28, the costimulatory receptor on the T cell. The two signals induced by the TCR and CD28 lead to IL-2 gene expression.

have been identified (123–126). The biochemical signals induced by CD28 stimulation that are responsible for its costimulatory function remain ill defined. Several distinct events have been identified and will be described below and in Chapter 13.

Despite the importance of the interaction of CD28 with B7 molecules, blockade of the interactions or deficiency of the interaction in mice that do not express CD28 or B7 molecules does not always result in an anergic state. Indeed, CD28-deficient mice can mount a significant immune response to some pathogens (112,127). These results suggest that other molecules may provide similar, though perhaps not identical, costimulatory functions. Of the other molecules on or secreted by the APCs, heat-stable antigen (128) and IL-1 have received the greatest attention. Although it is quite clear that recombinant IL-1 can mimic a second stimulus provided by APC in some cell systems (66,129,130), many have failed to detect this accessory function of IL-1 (28,131). The failure of IL-1 to provide this accessory function may relate to the distribution of IL-1Rs on T cells. A high degree of variability in the number of IL-1Rs on T-cell subsets has been reported (132,133). Alternatively, the effects of IL-1 may be quite indirect. For instance, IL-1 can upregulate the expression of B7 (134). The intracellular events initiated by or modified by the binding of IL-1 to its receptor have not been well characterized. However, the cytoplasmic domain of IL-1 is homologous to the cytoplasmic domain of *Drosophila* Toll. Recently, the mammalian Toll homologue was identified and is expressed on lymphoid cells (135). Interestingly, stimulation of all three of these molecules activates nuclear factor (NF-κB) transcription factors (136). It is likely that stimulation of these receptors will lead to activation of the IκB kinase (137). The activation of NF-κB is likely to play a role in inducing the transcriptional activation of B7 genes.

Other reagents and mAbs against other cell surface molecules have produced second signals required for T-cell lymphokine production and proliferation. In some systems, IL-6 alone or in combination with IL-1 can provide a costimulatory signal (138). Finally, a second signal can be provided by pharmacologic reagents, namely phorbol esters that activate PKC isozymes (65,139). The mechanism by which phorbol esters provide a costimulatory signal is not clear, because TCR stimulation should activate PKC (see below). It seems likely that there are many ways to provide a second signal that can lead to T-cell activation. These signals may not necessarily be qualitatively equivalent and may not functionally activate the same T-cell populations.

SIGNAL TRANSDUCTION BY THE T-CELL ANTIGEN RECEPTOR

Complex Structure of the TCR and Its Signal Transduction Function

The TCR contains a Ti αβ or Ti γδ heterodimer that is responsible for peptide antigen–MHC molecule recognition. These Ti subunits are transported to the plasma membrane in an obligatory association with as many as six other invariant proteins derived from four genes, although the precise stoichiometry of the chains within the TCR complex is uncertain (1,3,140). Among the associated proteins are those composing the CD3 complex. CD3 consists of three homologous noncovalently linked transmembrane proteins: γ, δ and ε. The CD3 genes are closely linked and are presumed to have arisen via gene duplication (1). Within each TCR

(LPS), have also been shown to upregulate B7-1 and B7-2 expression (117), ensuring that costimulatory function will be provided at sites of inflammation. This allows for the initial response of the innate immune response to recruit the adaptive immune response. Such a complex scheme has probably evolved to ensure that T cells are activated only under appropriate circumstances.

The mechanism by which CD28, which does not have intrinsic enzymatic activity, mediates signals responsible for costimulation remains elusive. The signals responsible for IL-2 production have been studied most intensively, though CD28 regulates the production of several other T cell-derived lymphokines (118,119). CD28 signals regulate the transcriptional activity of the IL-2 gene (discussed below) and its posttranscriptional regulation (120,121). The cytoplasmic tail of CD28 is sufficient to mediate the signals required for costimulation of IL-2 gene transcription and production of the lymphokine (122), and residues critical for this function

complex, there appear to be two copies of CD3 ε that associate with either δ or γ to form dimers, but γ and δ cannot associate with each other (141–143). In addition, the TCR contains a disulfide-linked homo- or heterodimer containing the ζ chain, which has little overall structural homology to the CD3 chains. The predominant form of the TCR contains ζζ homodimers. On some CTLs, ζ forms disulfide-linked dimers with the γ-chain of the high-affinity IgE Fc receptor (144). The γ chain gene is closely linked to ζ and exhibits structural homology to ζ, particularly in the transmembrane domain. The function of such complexity in TCR structure is still not known, but it may allow for diversification of the signal transduction functions of the receptor.

The function of the Ti heterodimer is in ligand (peptide–MHC molecule) recognition, but the scant five residues in the cytoplasmic domains of the α and β chains do not contain sufficient information to couple to intracellular signal transduction machinery. Instead, the signal transduction function of the TCR complex is conveyed by the associated CD3 and ζ subunits. Initial clues to this function came from studies using mAbs reactive with extracellular domains of the CD3 complex that were able to mimic the effects of antigen by inducing many of the manifestations of T-cell activation (56,57). When the structural features of the CD3 and ζ chains are compared to the Ti chains, it is clear that although the cytoplasmic domains of the CD3 and ζ chains do not encode an intrinsic enzymatic activity, they are sufficiently large (40 to 113 residues) and more likely to interact with cytoplasmic signal transduction molecules.

Studies with chimeric molecules that included the cytoplasmic domain of ζ, CD3 ε, or related molecules provided evidence for this signal transduction function. Earlier studies had revealed that the regions surrounding and including the transmembrane domains of the TCR component contain the information necessary for the assembly of the TCR subunits (142,145). This permitted the development of a strategy in which the functions of the cytoplasmic domains of the individual chains of the TCR could be studied in isolation. Chimeric molecules were constructed in which the extracellular and, importantly, the transmembrane domains of CD4, CD8, CD16, or the IL-2R α chain (which can be expressed independently of the TCR) were fused to the cytoplasmic domains of either the TCR ζ, CD3 ε or IgE Fc receptor γ chains (146–148). These chimeric molecules could be expressed independently of endogenous TCR chains in T-cell lines or clones or in basophil lines. Stimulation of these chimeras induced early signal transduction events and later manifestations of T-cell activation, such as lymphokine secretion and cytolytic activity, associated with stimulation of the intact oligomeric TCR. Thus, the TCR ζ and CD3 chains both can couple the ligand-binding subunit of the TCR to intracellular signal transduction mechanisms. This is consistent with TCR reconstitution studies of a T-cell hybridoma, which suggested that CD3 and ζ chains could function as independent signal transduction modules (149).

The apparent paradoxical redundancy of function of the CD3 and ζ subunits is explained by the recognition of a common sequence motif contained in the cytoplasmic domains of the non–ligand binding subunits of many hematopoietic cell receptors involved in antigen recognition (150). This motif termed the *immunoreceptor tyrosine-based activation motif* (ITAM), based on conservation of the consensus sequence **(D/E)XXYXXLX$_{(6-8)}$ YXXL**, is triplicated within the cytoplasmic domain of the ζ chain and is contained as a single copy in the cytoplasmic domains of each of the CD3 chains (Fig. 4). This motif is also contained in the β and γ chains of the IgE Fc receptor and the Igα and Igβ chains

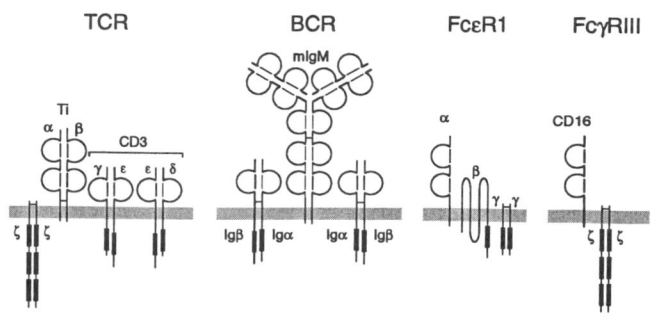

ITAMs
(Immunoreceptor Tyrosine-Based Activation Motif)

```
hζ1        N Q L Y N E L N L G R R E E - Y D V L
hζ2        E G L Y N E L Q K D K M A E A Y S E I
hζ3        D G L Y Q G L S T A T K D T - Y D A L

hCD3γ      D Q L Y Q P L K D R E D D Q - Y S H L
hCD3ε      N P D Y E P I R K G Q R D L - Y S G L
hCD3δ      D Q V Y Q P L R D R D D A Q - Y S H L

rIgE FcR γ  D A V Y T G L N T R N Q E T - Y E T L
rIgE FcR β  D R L Y E E L - H V Y S P I - Y S A L

mIg α      E N L Y E G L N L D D C S M - Y E D I
mIg β      D H T Y E G L N I D Q T A T - Y E D I

BLV gp30   D S D Y Q A L L P S A P E I - Y S H L
EBV LMP-2  H S D Y Q P L G T Q D Q S L - Y L G L
SIV Nef    G D L Y E R L L R A R G E T - Y G R L

Consensus  D/E - - Y - - L - - - - - - - - Y - - L
```

FIG. 4. ITAMs in receptors involved in antigen recognition.

associated with the membrane Ig antigen receptor on B cells (see Chapters 7 and 35 and Fig. 4). The observations made with TCR chimeric receptors have been extended to other invariant chains of receptors associated with oligomeric receptors expressed on B cells (the B-cell antigen receptor) and mast cells (the high-affinity IgE Fc receptor). Chimeric receptors containing only a single copy of most, but perhaps not all, ITAMs are sufficient to induce the early and late events associated with stimulation of the intact oligomeric TCR (148,151,152). The β chain of the IgE Fc receptor, which is the only ITAM with a six-residue spacer, appears to function as an amplifier rather than as an independently functioning unit (153). Mutagenesis of the ITAM sequences has demonstrated the importance of the tyrosine and leucine residues in ITAM signaling function. It is not surprising that the ITAMs may have similar functions within distinct receptors because the exon–intron organization of the various ITAMs is conserved, suggesting a common evolutionary precursor (149).

The multiplicity of the ITAMs within the TCR is a striking feature of the receptor that is likely to have functional consequences. Although the precise stoichiometry of the chains composing the TCR is not clear, if one assumes the most common model of receptor structure (see Figs. 2 and 4), then a single TCR complex contains ten copies of this motif. The redundancy of this motif within the receptor allows a single TCR to interact with and activate multiple copies of the same signal transduction component. This can lead to amplification of signal transduction by a single ligand-binding event (152), thereby increasing the sensitivity of the TCR (154). Alternatively, the motifs contain sufficiently distinct sequences to allow them to interact with distinct intracellular signal transduction molecules, permitting diversification of the signal transduction events (155,156). Thus, it is possible that selective involvement of ITAMs following TCR stimulation can lead to distinct cellular responses (46,157,158).

It is not surprising that viruses that target lymphocytes have acquired ITAM sequences that aid them in their pathogenic mechanisms. At least three viruses have ITAM sequences that can couple to intracellular signaling mechanisms in lymphocytes and have been shown to play important roles in pathology. The bovine leukemia virus envelope glycoprotein gp130 contains an ITAM sequence. This virus, which transforms B cells in ruminants, depends on the ITAM sequence for infection and for high viral titers (159). The Epstein-Barr virus latent membrane protein 2 (LMP2) plays an important role in maintaining viral latency in transformed B cells. The ITAM in LMP2 is thought to act as a cellular decoy to prevent cytoplasmic signaling proteins from interacting with the stimulated B-cell antigen receptor ITAMs (160). An unusual isolate of the simian immunodeficiency virus (SIV) causes fulminant infection of resting T cell, in contrast to the chronic and latent infection observed with most SIV isolates. The highly unusual behavior of this virus has been mapped to two mutations in the viral Nef protein that create an ITAM sequence (161). Thus, these viral ITAM sequences appear to have taken advantage of the function of the ITAM present in the TCR or other antigen receptors in order to interact with intracellular signaling molecules involved in lymphocyte activation.

The CD3 chains may serve an additional regulatory function within the TCR. The human CD3 γ and δ chains are phosphorylated on serine residues in response to events that lead to PKC activation (see below) (162,163). This has been associated with diminished TCR signal transduction function. Thus, this may represent a feedback regulatory mechanism leading to receptor desensitization.

The mechanism by which the Ti chains transmit ligand occupancy to the CD3 and ζ subunits remains poorly understood. The ability to stimulate simple single- or double-chain chimeric receptors containing ζ or CD3 ε cytoplasmic domains with mAbs is most consistent with a cross-linking or dimerization model. However, the complex structure of the receptor and the varying sensitivity of Ti and CD3 to stimulation by mAbs suggests that allosteric changes could play a role in receptor activation (52,164). The varying ability of peptide ligands with similar affinities to induce distinct signaling events also favors an allosteric model, though differences in kinetic parameters could also explain such differences (49). Finally, the CD3 and ζ chains may also serve a "docking" function to permit other cell surface molecules, such as CD2, CD4, or CD8, to interact with the TCR in forming a properly assembled receptor complex. This latter function is consistent with observed stable or induced associations of the TCR with CD4 (49,165). Such

a docking function is also consistent with the observed requirement for a functional TCR or ζ chain–containing chimera in CD2-mediated signal transduction (44).

TCR ITAMs Interact with Cytoplasmic Protein Tyrosine Kinases

Stimulation of the TCR by peptide antigen–MHC molecules or by agonist anti-TCR mAbs must induce intracellular biochemical events in order to initiate a cellular response. A number of intracellular biochemical changes occur during the first few seconds to minutes after stimulation of the TCR. These include protein phosphorylation, increases in cytoplasmic free calcium $[Ca^{2+}]_i$, changes in pH, and changes in cyclic nucleotides. The primary sequences of the TCR component chains do not encode proteins with intrinsic enzymatic activity. Instead, the TCR ITAMs couple the TCR to intracellular enzymes.

The most rapid event associated with TCR stimulation is the induced phosphorylation of several proteins on tyrosine residues (166,167). Notably, among these phosphorylated substrates are the ITAMs of the TCR ζ and CD3 chains (168–170). Such tyrosine phosphorylation can be observed within seconds of TCR stimulation and persists for hours (146,166,167). Inhibitors of PTKs can inhibit most if not all of the later events associated with TCR stimulation (35,36). Since the ITAMs contain all of the information necessary for TCR signal transduction function, it seemed likely that the ITAMs regulate the function of PTKs. Two families of cytoplasmic PTKs, the Src and Syk families, interact directly with TCR ITAMs in a sequential and highly coordinated manner (64,171). Members of these two families of PTKs have been shown to play critical roles in TCR signaling function.

Src PTKs Involved in TCR Signal Transduction

Lck and Fyn are the major Src family PTKs expressed in T cells. Both have been implicated in interactions with ITAMs and in TCR signal transduction. Prior to reviewing the specific role of each of these kinases, the overall common structural features (Fig. 5) and the functions of the domains of these PTKs will be discussed.

The Src kinases vary from approximately 50 to 60 kDa (172). At the N-terminus of each of these kinases, at position 2, is a glycine residue that is myristoylated. This allows for membrane attachment. Some of the Src kinases, including Lck, are also palmitoylated at one or two cysteine residues contained within the first ten residues, and this modification may be dynamically regulated (173,174). This further facilitates membrane localization, particularly the plasma membrane. Within the N-terminal, 40 to 70

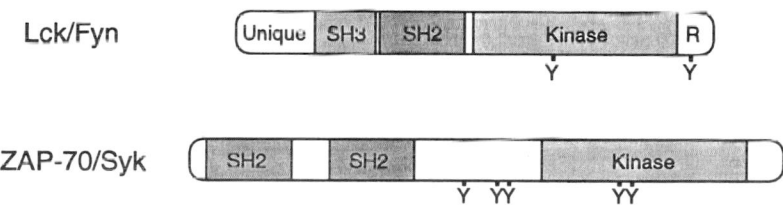

FIG. 5. PTKs involved in TCR signal transduction. Shown are schematic representations of the Lck/Fyn and Syk/ZAP-70 PTKs. The unique, SH3, SH2, kinase, and regulatory domains are indicated. Also shown are the two sites of phosphorylation in Lck/Fyn and some of the sites in Syk/ZAP-70.

residues are also the most distinguishing sequences among this family that probably play important roles in the unique functions and interactions of each of these kinases. The unique region is followed by the Src homology 3 (SH3) domain, which consists of approximately 60 residues. The SH3 domain is involved in directing protein–protein interactions by binding in a sequence specific context to residues contained in proline-rich regions. The SH3 domain is followed by a 100-amino acid structural domain, the SH2 domain. The SH2 domain also is involved in protein–protein interactions by binding to phosphorylated tyrosine residues contained in a particular sequence-specific context.

The SH2 domain is followed by the catalytic domain, the kinase domain. The crystal structure of the activated Lck kinase domain has been solved and, like other kinase domains, it is a two-lobed structure consisting of approximately 250 residues (175). Like most kinases, the catalytic activity of the kinase is regulated by an activation loop. Within the activation loop of the Src family is a single tyrosine residue that regulates kinase activity. Phosphorylation of this tyrosine residue activates catalytic function by relocalization of the activation loop, allowing for substrate access to the catalytic site.

At the C-terminus of the Src kinases is the regulatory domain. This short region contains the second well-characterized tyrosine phosphorylation site in Src kinases. Phosphorylation of this tyrosine results in the inactivation of the kinase. The crystal structure of two Src family kinases, Hck and Src, which are phosphorylated at this position, have been solved and are remarkably similar (176,177). The structure reveals that in the inactive phosphorylated state, the kinase is in a closed conformation, in which the C-terminal–negative regulatory phosphorylated tyrosine interacts with the SH2 domain of the same molecule, and that the SH3 domain interacts, in a previously unanticipated manner, with a proline-containing spacer sequence contained between the SH2 and kinase domain. These interactions prevent the kinase domain from assuming an active conformation. Thus, activation of the kinase requires the dephosphorylation of the C-terminal tyrosine residue and phosphorylation of the tyrosine in the activation loop.

The Fyn PTK

Several lines of evidence have implicated the Fyn PTK in TCR signal transduction. Fyn is a 59-kDa protein and is expressed ubiquitously but at particularly high levels in the brain and hematopoietic system. Two isoforms of Fyn exist that are differentially expressed in hematopoietic cells or the brain (178). The molecular basis for these two forms of Fyn is the tissue-specific alternative splicing of two homologous but nonidentical copies of exon 7 that encode a portion of the kinase domain. Overexpression of either of the two forms of Fyn in an antigen-specific T-cell hybridoma can have different functional consequences (179). Whereas both forms of Fyn-enhanced anti-TCR mAb increases in protein tyrosine phosphorylation, only the Fyn isoform expressed in hematopoietic cells augmented antigen-induced IL-2 production. Thus, the two forms of Fyn may serve distinct functions, possibly by interacting with distinct intracellular signal transduction molecules.

The interaction of Fyn with the TCR has been difficult to study. Fyn can be coimmunoprecipitated with the TCR complex, albeit at low stoichiometry, if mild detergents are used to solubilize the complex (180). Fyn protein has also been reported to colocalize with the TCR when TCR capping is induced by anti-CD3 mAb, consistent with either a direct or indirect association (181). A specific association between Fyn and ζ, CD3 γ, or CD3 ε fusion proteins could be detected in a sensitive heterologous expression system (182). This interaction mapped to the ten most N-terminal residues of Fyn (which also encode the residues responsible for membrane localization) and sequences within ITAMs, though no single residue seemed critical in the interaction. These observations must be tempered by localization studies in which Fyn protein is primarily detected in regions around the microtubule organizing complex, and it was only detected at the plasma membrane when it was overexpressed (183). Thus, these biochemical and cellular studies suggest the possibility of an indirect as well as direct association of Fyn with the TCR.

The functional importance of the interaction of Fyn with the TCR has been addressed in a variety of biochemical and genetic approaches. Stimulation of the TCR induces an increase in Fyn PTK activity, which is associated with an increase in tyrosine phosphorylation of Fyn-associated proteins (184,185). Expression of activated versions of both isoforms of Fyn in a T-cell hybridoma results in heightened TCR signal transduction (179). The activated version of Fyn here refers to a protein in which the C-terminal–negative regulatory tyrosine has been mutated. Similar effects have been observed with other activated Src family members (186,187), so that this effect may not reveal a function specific to Fyn. An alternative approach has been to express increased levels of normal Fyn as a transgene within the T-cell lineage. This resulted in heightened responses to TCR responsiveness, whereas mice expressing a kinase-deficient mutant of Fyn had diminished TCR signal transduction capability (188). Surprisingly, disruption of the *fyn* gene by homologous recombination resulted in a relatively restricted deficiency in signal transduction function. Mature single-positive thymocytes (CD4$^+$ or CD8$^+$) had a rather striking impairment in TCR signal transduction, whereas double-positive (CD4$^+$CD8$^+$) and mature T-peripheral T cells had a more modest decrease in TCR signal transduction capacity (189,190). These experiments with the mice containing the disrupted *fyn* gene suggest a potential role for Fyn in TCR signal transduction that is developmentally restricted to a specific stage in T-cell development. The loss of *fyn*, however, did not appear to have untoward consequences on thymic development, suggesting the possibility of compensatory mechanisms involving other PTKs that may have redundant function. Indeed, results discussed below suggest an important role for the Lck kinase.

Although redundancy among Src family members may be observed in developmental studies in which selective pressures in the developing populations of cells are brought to bear, it is likely that each Src kinase may have specific functions as well, particularly involving the unique N-terminal domains of the PTKs. A unique functional role for Fyn has been revealed in studies of the Pyk2 kinase, which is homologous to the focal adhesion kinase (191). Although the function for Pyk2 is not yet understood, its phosphorylation and catalytic activity is regulated by TCR signal transduction (192). However, in Fyn-deficient mice, Pyk2 is neither activated nor phosphorylated. These results suggest that Fyn is required to couple the TCR to Pyk2. Thus, the failure to activate Pyk2 may contribute to some of the functional defects seen in Fyn-deficient mice.

The Lck PTK

Lck, a 56-kD Src family PTK, plays a critical role in TCR signal transduction. It is expressed predominantly in T cells. Lck associates with CD4 and CD8 via interactions that involve cysteine residues present in the cytoplasmic domains of the coreceptors and within the unique N-terminal domain of Lck (76,77,193,194). Although not all of Lck is associated with either CD4 or CD8, the stoichiometry is relatively high. This direct interaction of Lck with the coreceptors CD4 and CD8 positions it to play an important functional role in TCR signal transduction during antigen recognition.

The demonstrated role of CD4 and CD8 as coreceptors with the TCR during peptide–MHC interactions supports an important functional role for Lck during TCR signal transduction (68). Cross-linking of the TCR together with CD4, but not separately, with mAbs markedly enhances TCR-mediated signal transduction (81). This suggests a model in which the coreceptors CD4 and CD8 function not only to increase avidity of the TCR with the antigen peptide–MHC complex, but also to colocalize Lck with the signaling apparatus contained within the cytoplasmic domains of the TCR. This model has been supported by work involving a CD4-dependent antigen-specific T-cell hybridoma. Antigen-induced IL-2 production by this hybridoma was reconstituted by wild-type CD4, but not by mutants of CD4, which could not associate with Lck (93). Thus, Lck appears to play a critical role during CD4- and CD8-dependent TCR signal transduction.

A function for Lck in TCR-mediated signal transduction, independent of its association with CD4 or CD8, is suggested by a variety of observations. Some T-cell clones or hybridomas can respond to antigen in the absence of CD4 or CD8 expression. CD4 and CD8 participation in antigen recognition is generally less important in secondary immune responses. Expression of activated Lck within a class II MHC–restricted IL-2–secreting T-cell hybridoma that failed to express CD4 still markedly increased the sensitivity of this cell to antigen (187). At least an indirect interaction of Lck with the TCR is implied by experiments in which the expression of CD4 in a CD4⁻ T-cell clone could inhibit the ability of anti-TCR mAbs from activating this cell through the TCR by apparently sequestering Lck away from the TCR (195). Moreover, Lck can be detected in immunoprecipitates of TCR components, though it is not clear whether the interaction is direct (86,196–198). The mechanism by which Lck might directly interact with TCR components has not been defined, although it is properly positioned at the plasma membrane to interact with TCR components (183). Thus, Lck can contribute to TCR signal transduction through CD4/CD8-dependent and -independent mechanisms.

A critical role for Lck in TCR signal transduction is evident from genetic studies of mice and cell lines deficient in Lck function. TCR induction of protein tyrosine phosphorylation as well as downstream events are markedly impaired in Lck-deficient T cells (199–202). Moreover, a critical role for Lck in thymic development, which likely involves its function within the pre-TCR and mature TCR signaling pathways, is well illustrated by the profound, but incomplete, arrest in thymic development in mice in which the *lck* gene has been disrupted by homologous recombination (200). The major defect appears to occur at an early developmental checkpoint, the CD4⁻/CD8⁻ to CD4⁺/CD8⁺ transition, where the pre-TCR mediates a signal to indicate that the TCR β chain has been functionally rearranged and expressed on the cell surface (see Chapter 11). A complete block is observed at this developmental checkpoint in mice lacking both Lck and Fyn (203,204). Since no developmental defect is observed in the Fyn-deficient mice, these results suggest that Lck plays the major role in pre-TCR signaling function, but that Fyn can partially compensate for its loss.

The activation of Lck catalytic activity following TCR stimulation can be detected (205). In addition, a twofold to fourfold increase in Lck kinase activity can also be detected following cross linking of the CD4 molecule (206). Activation of the PTK activity is associated with phosphorylation of a tyrosine residue (Y394) within the activa-

tion loop of the kinase domain, a characteristic site of autophosphorylation of activated Src-family members (82). This is presumed to allow access of the substrate to the catalytic site. It is noteworthy that although cross-linking of CD4 increases Lck catalytic activity, the characteristic increase in cellular tyrosine phosphoproteins associated with TCR stimulation is not observed (81). Therefore, Lck represents a critically important PTK involved in TCR signal transduction, but it is not likely be the only PTK involved.

Syk-Family PTKs Associate with Stimulated TCR

The Syk family of PTKs, consisting of only Syk and ZAP-70, plays an important role in TCR signal transduction (207). ZAP-70 is expressed exclusively in T cells and natural killer (NK) cells (208). It was first identified as a 70-kDa TCR ζ-associated tyrosine phosphoprotein in immunoprecipitates isolated from TCR-stimulated cells (209). Syk is 72 kDa and is more broadly expressed within the hematopoietic lineage (210). However, within the T-cell lineage, it is expressed early in thymic ontogeny and is downregulated in mature T cells, except for the γδ lineage, where it appears to be expressed in greater abundance (211,212). Both of these kinases have similar functions within signaling pathways mediated by receptors of cells of the hematopoietic lineages. They associate with doubly phosphorylated ITAMs and are inducibly phosphorylated following TCR stimulation.

The overall structure of ZAP-70 and Syk is similar. They each have two N-terminal SH2 domains and a more C-terminal catalytic domain (see Fig. 5). It is now well recognized that the ZAP-70 SH2 domains bind in tandem to a single doubly phosphorylated ITAM with relatively high affinity (10 to 30 nM) (64,213,214). This affinity is substantially higher than is seen with isolated SH2 domains, which bind with micromolar affinities (215). The structure of the two ZAP-70 SH2 domains bound to a single doubly phosphorylated TCR ζ ITAM has been solved by x-ray crystallography (216). The phospho-ITAM has an extended structure, and the more C-terminal SH2 (SH2C) domain has a typical structure and binds to the more N-terminal pYXXL sequences in the ITAM. In contrast, the N-terminal SH2 domain (SH2N) is atypical. It is an incomplete SH2 domain. The SH2N phosphotyrosine-binding (PTB) pocket is only completed when it is brought into close apposition to SH2C. The close relationship between SH2N and SH2C, when bound to the doubly phosphorylated ITAM, emphasizes the importance of the critical spacing between the YXXL groups of the ITAM. Greater or less than the seven or eight residues would probably not permit appropriate binding to occur. The other interesting feature revealed from the structure is the formation of a coiled–coiled loop in interdomain A, which separates the SH2 domains. The function of interdomain A is not clear, though it may help to stabilize the structure. Based on studies of Syk, phosphorylation of this loop could regulate the binding of the SH2 domains to a phospho-ITAM (217). The structure of the Syk SH2 domains is likely to be similar.

The ZAP-70 SH2 and kinase domains are separated by approximately 65 residues, composing interdomain B. This domain is believed to play a regulatory function. Y292, within interdomain B, is an *in vivo* autophosphorylation site in ZAP-70 (218), and its phosphorylation inhibits ZAP-70 function (219–221). There are also other potential sites of phosphorylation within interdomain B in ZAP-70, Y315 and Y319. The homologous sites in Syk have been shown to be *in vitro* autophosphorylation sites (222). These sites may serve a positive regulatory function by recruiting substrates to ZAP-70. Y315 is important for ZAP-70 function and for the phosphorylation of the protooncogene Vav (see below). However, deletion of interdomain B has a net positive effect on ZAP-70 function, suggesting that the region has an overall negative regulatory function (220).

The catalytic domains of ZAP-70 and Syk are typical of PTK domains. TCR stimulation increases the catalytic activities of both of these kinases. Their catalytic activities are regulated by phosphorylation of residues contained within their putative activation loops. Phosphorylation of Y493 in the activation loop of ZAP-70 and the homologous residue in Syk, Y519, increases kinase activity (223–225). In contrast, Y492 in ZAP-70 has a negative regulatory function (219,221,223). These two residues within the same activation loop may be sequentially phosphorylated in a dynamic feedback regulatory circuit (223). Interestingly, the intrinsic catalytic activity of Syk is greater than that of ZAP (226). Based on expression studies of mutant forms of ZAP-70 and Syk in cell lines and a natural mutation of ZAP-70 in mice (64,224,227,228), the catalytic activities of ZAP-70 and Syk are critical for their function.

The functional importance of ZAP-70 and Syk in T cells has been established from natural and experimental genetic models. A human severe combined immunodeficiency (SCID) syndrome, characterized by defective TCR signal transduction and developmental abnormalities in the T-cell lineage, results from ZAP-70 mutations (229–231). In these SCID patients, only mature CD4+ T cells are detectable, but these T cells have defective TCR signal transduction. In mice deficient in ZAP-70 protein or with a kinase-defective ZAP-70 protein (228,232), thymocyte development is blocked at the CD4+/CD8+ stage, a time when signal transduction by the mature TCR is required for positive selection. The ability to bypass the developmental checkpoint mediated by the pre-TCR may reflect compensation by the Syk kinase, which is expressed at higher levels earlier in thymocyte development (211). Differences between the phenotypes of humans and mice deficient in ZAP-70 remain unexplained, but could reflect differences in Syk expression (233). The normal function of Syk in the T-cell lineage is best revealed by mice made deficient in Syk expression by gene targeting. In these mice, the predominant defect in T cells is the failure of epithelial T cells expressing the γδ TCR to develop. Collectively, these results suggest that this family of kinases plays an important role in TCR signal transduction and that these kinases may be able to play some redundant and some unique functions.

Interaction of Src and Syk PTKs

The Src and Syk kinases interact with TCR in a highly coordinated and sequential manner. In cell lines or T cells cultured *in vitro*, TCR ITAMs are inducibly phosphorylated following receptor stimulation. In *ex vivo* thymocytes or T cells, the TCR ζ ITAMs are constitutively phosphorylated, though CD3 ITAMs are inducibly phosphorylated (234). Both the inducible and constitutive phosphorylation of the ITAMs appears to be principally mediated by Lck (64,202). ZAP-70 or Syk bind to the doubly phosphorylated ITAMs. Once bound, they can be activated in the stimulated TCR complex by phosphorylation of their activation loops. Phosphorylation of Y493, the critical residue in the ZAP-70 activation loop, is thought to be mediated by Lck (64,218,223). In contrast, Syk may be able to autophosphorylate and activate its kinase activity upon ITAM binding (235). Indeed, it appears that Syk may be less dependent on Src kinases in T cells for its activation (236,237). However, in *ex vivo* thymocytes and T cells, receptor stimulation is required for the inducible phosphorylation of ZAP-70 or Syk, which are constitutively associated with the TCR ζ chain (202). ITAM-bound Syk or ZAP-70 in the stimulated TCR complex forms a stable complex with Lck via the Lck SH2 domain (86,87). This likely leads to a further increase in PTK activity and substrate phosphorylation.

These studies suggest important interactions between Lck- and Syk-family PTKs that may occur during T-cell responses to antigen. One model that may account for the interaction of Lck and ZAP-70 is depicted in Fig. 6. During the recognition of peptide

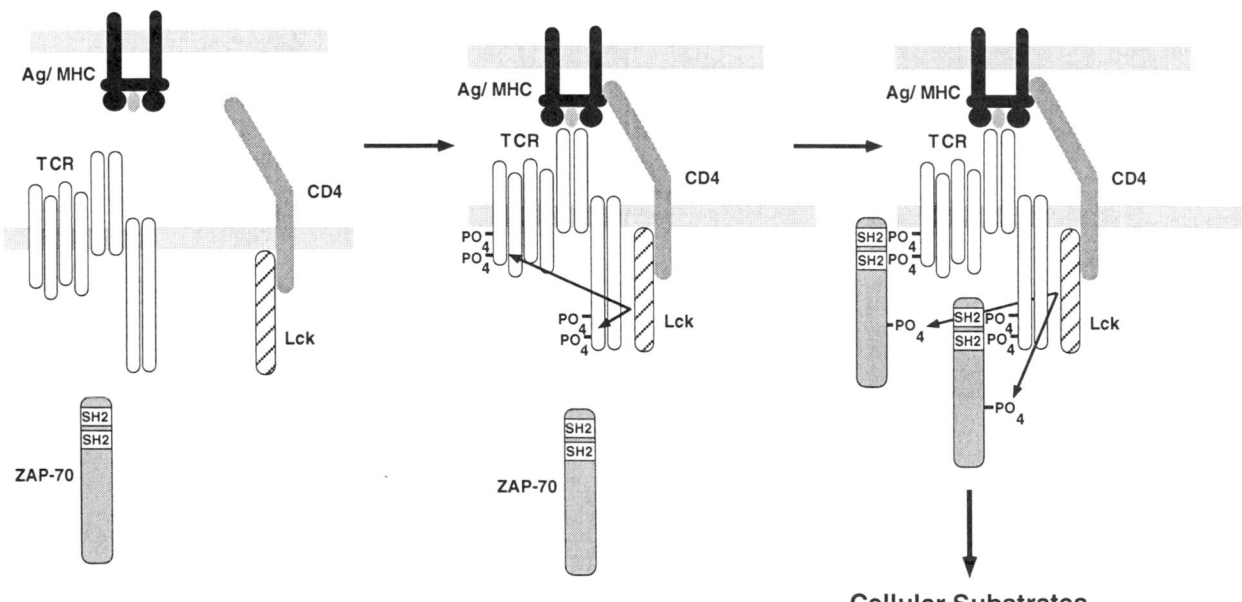

FIG. 6. A speculative model of the interaction of Lck and ZAP-70 during antigen recognition by a CD4+ T cell. During TCR and CD4 engagement of an MHC class II molecule, Lck is brought into close proximity with the TCR cytoplasmic domain and phosphorylates CD3 and ζ chains. ZAP-70 is recruited to the tyrosine phosphorylated CD3 and ζ chains via its SH2 domains, which allows Lck to transphosphorylate and thereby activate ZAP-70.

antigen bound to class II MHC molecules, colocalization of the TCR and CD4 occurs. This recruits Lck into close proximity with the cytoplasmic domains of the TCR chains containing ITAMs. This could result in phosphorylation of tyrosine residues within the ITAMs. *In vivo*, perhaps this results only in CD3 phosphorylation. Such tyrosine phosphorylation of ITAMs allows for the recruitment of ZAP-70 or Syk. Such colocalization of ZAP-70 and/or Syk with Lck facilitates the interaction and transphosphorylation–activation of these kinases. A similar model may apply to the recognition of peptides bound to class I MHC molecules by CD8+ cells. However, this model does not account for the mechanism by which the TCR can induce signal transduction events independent of CD4 or CD8. In these situations, cytoplasmic Lck which is not bound to CD4 or CD8, may be recruited to the TCR complex through oligomerization of the ITAMs. The net result of these interactions is the coordinated activation of these kinases leading to the tyrosine phosphorylation of downstream effector molecules and substrates that represent critical regulators in signaling pathways.

Function of SH2 Domains in Signal Transduction Pathways

The activation of the catalytic function of cytoplasmic PTKs by the TCR has several consequences, not the least of which is the use of tyrosine phosphorylation to facilitate protein–protein interactions. Considerable progress was made toward understanding how proteins in PTK or protein tyrosine phosphatase (PTPase) signal transduction pathways interact with the recognition that sequences containing phosphotyrosine residues can bind to SH2 domains (215). SH2 domains are homologous sequences consisting of approximately 100 residues that are present in a variety of molecules that have been implicated in signal transduction pathways involving protein tyrosine phosphorylation. Some of the proteins implicated in TCR signal transduction pathways that contain SH2 domains are listed in Table 2.

TABLE 2. *Protein with Src homology-2 domains that may be associated with T cell-activation*

Protein tyrosine kinases
  Fyn
  Lck
  Syk
  ZAP-70
  Csk
  Itk
Protein tyrosine phosphatases
  SHP-1
  SHP-2
Proteins with enzymatic functions
  Phospholipase C γ1 (PLC γ1)
  Phosphatidylinositol 3′-kinase (PI 3-kinase), p85 subunit
Adaptors and Regulators
  GTPase activating protein (GAP)
  SOS
  Vav
  Slp-76
  Shc
  Nck
  Grb2
  Crk

Isolated SH2 domains can interact independently with phosphoproteins or phosphopeptides with micromolar affinities. It has been possible to demonstrate specificity in these interactions, which depends on the sequences that surround the phosphotyrosine residue (215,238,239). The structural basis for this specificity and for the interaction with phosphotyrosine is evident from the three-dimensional structure of SH2 domains (240,241). Each SH2 domain contains a binding pocket for phosphotyrosine, but sequences surrounding the binding pocket influence this interaction. Thus, the ability of this structural domain to recognize sequences surrounding phosphotyrosine can define the specificity of the interactions that occur among proteins in a signal transduction pathway.

SH2 domains may serve multiple functions. First, they can be responsible for recruiting signal transduction molecules to activated PTKs. Activated PTKs often contain sites of auto- or transphosphorylation, which may represent the sites to which downstream signal transduction components bind via SH2 domains. For instance, the Vav SH2 domain binds to phospho-Y315 in ZAP-70, and this binding event is required for the tyrosine phosphorylation and function of Vav (242). Second, they may protect tyrosine-phosphorylated sites from the action of PTPases, thereby prolonging the effects of tyrosine phosphorylation (243). Third, they may permit the recruitment of kinases or phosphatases to potential substrates or sites of action. PTKs of the Src and Syk families all contain SH2 domains (82,207), as do at least two cytosolic tyrosine phosphatases (244). Fourth, SH2 domains may play important regulatory functions to enhance or inhibit enzymatic functions. For instance, the negative regulatory site of tyrosine phosphorylation in Src-family PTKs interacts with the SH2 domain contained within these molecules to inhibit kinase activity (82,176,177). Thus, SH2 domains can play a variety of distinct roles by interacting with phosphotyrosine residues within proteins in a signal transduction pathway.

It is important to recognize that SH2 domains are not the only structural domains that bind phosphotyrosine and that other structural domains may contribute to protein–protein interactions within a signaling pathway. For instance, PTB domains bind to tyrosine phosphorylated residues (245,246). The specificities of the PTB domain may be more limited. Many other modular domains that bind to residues other than phosphotyrosine contribute to the interactions observed in signaling pathways. These include the SH3, PH, WW, WD40, and PDZ domains. The SH2 domain is frequently found in tandem with one or more SH3 domains. As discussed, SH3 domains bind to sequences rich in proline residues, so that no covalent posttranslational modification is necessary for the interaction of SH3 domains with their targets. However, allosteric changes in the target sequence may be critical. The SH2 and SH3 domains of different molecules vary in sequence sufficiently to impart specificity in their binding events. The affinities of the SH2 and SH3 domains for their peptide ligands are only in the low micromolar range, and for SH2 domains this affinity is only 20- to 50-fold greater than for isolated phosphotyrosine. However, by using pairs or combinations of these protein modules, a much higher degree of specificity and affinity may be achieved in these protein–protein interactions.

The Protein Tyrosine Phosphatase CD45 Plays a Critical Role in TCR Signal Transduction

Protein phosphorylation can be regulated by stimulating PTKs, but it can also be induced by inhibiting PTPases. Many PTPases are expressed in T cells. CD45 (leukocyte common antigen or T200) and PTPase α (or LRP) are transmembrane tyrosine phosphatases (247–249). Many cytosolic PTPases (including T-cell phosphatase, PEP, SHP-1 and-2, and low-molecular-weight phosphatase) are expressed in T cells (249,250). Although all of these PTPases may contribute to TCR signal transduction, the role of CD45 is best understood.

CD45 represents a family of transmembrane PTPases consisting of various isoforms that are derived by the alternative splicing of exons four through six (247). All of the isoforms contain two tandem 300-amino acid domains that are homologous with other PTPases (249). Only the first domain has catalytic activity (251,252), but its activity depends on the second domain.

CD45 proteins are expressed at high levels on all cells of the hematopoietic lineage except mature erythrocytes. The individual CD45 isoforms, 180 to 220 kD, are expressed differentially in a tissue- and activation-specific manner. On T cells, these isoforms have been used to distinguish helper T-cell subsets (253) and resting or activated T cells (254,255). For instance, activated T cells express only the 180-kD isoform (CD45RO) in which the products of exons 4, 5, and 6 are excluded. The highly regulated expression of the various isoforms suggests that the extracellular domain has a specific function. This notion is supported by the ability of individual isoforms to differentially reconstitute CD45 function in an antigen-specific hybridoma (256). The ligands for the various isoforms, if they exist, have not been established. Both stimulatory and inhibitory effects of mAbs reactive with the various CD45 isoforms have been observed. Some investigators have suggested that CD45 isoforms differentially interact with other molecules, such as CD4, on the same cell (257). Independent of ligand interactions, distinct roles have been proposed for CD45 isoforms, based on the size and charge differences of the isoforms, that influence the ability of T cells to interact with APCs (13). However, studies with a chimeric molecule in which the extracellular and transmembrane domains of the epidermal growth factor receptor were substituted for those of CD45 suggest that ligand-induced dimerization may inhibit CD45 function (258).

A function for CD45 has emerged from genetic studies in which mutant T-cell lines or mice, deficient in CD45 expression, have been isolated. Loss of CD45 expression in most T-cell lines and clones is associated with a selective loss in TCR signal transduc-

tion function, including the ability of the TCR to induce increases in tyrosine phosphoproteins (259–262). Similarly, a developmental arrest and an impairment in TCR function are found in mice made deficient in CD45 by gene targeting (263, 264). The loss of this major membrane PTPase is not associated with a general increase in tyrosine phosphoproteins. Since the initial signal transduction event associated with TCR stimulation is activation of a PTK, CD45 appears to play a selective role in regulating the ability of the TCR to activate the PTK pathway.

Studies with CD45-deficient cells suggest that one target of this PTPase is the negative regulatory site of Lck, and this has led to the model of Lck regulation shown in Fig. 7. CD45 can dephosphorylate this site in vitro, resulting in the activation of Lck (265). This site in Lck, Y505, is hyperphosphorylated in CD45-deficient T-cell lines (266–268). The homologous site in Fyn is also be affected, but to a lesser extent. The mechanism by which this site of phosphorylation inhibits kinase function was revealed when the structure of the inactive kinase was solved by x-ray crystallography (176,177). When phosphorylated at the C-terminus, the SH2 domain binds to this site in an intramolecular interaction, and the SH3 domain contributes to the inactive conformation by binding to a proline helix encoded by sequences between the SH2 and kinase domains. As a result of these interactions, the kinase domain is kept in an inactive state. The tyrosine associated with negative regulation of kinase function is phosphorylated by a ubiquitous PTK, termed *Csk*, which shares some homology with Src PTKs (82). Thus, CD45 may serve to dephosphorylate the negative regulatory site in Lck (or other Src members) *in vivo* and allow the kinase to become activated and participate during TCR signal transduction. The hyperphosphorylated form of Lck in CD45-deficient cells would be blocked from participation in TCR signal transduction events. Thus, a complex and likely very dynamic relationship between Src PTKs and PTPases exists that influences the ability of the TCR to induce signal transduction events.

Consequences of TCR-mediated PTK Activation

TCR-mediated induction of PTK activity results in the tyrosine phosphorylation of a large number of cellular proteins, in addition to the component chains of the TCR as well as the Src- and Syk-family kinases. Some of the many proteins that are inducibly phosphorylated following TCR stimulation are listed in Table 3. To a

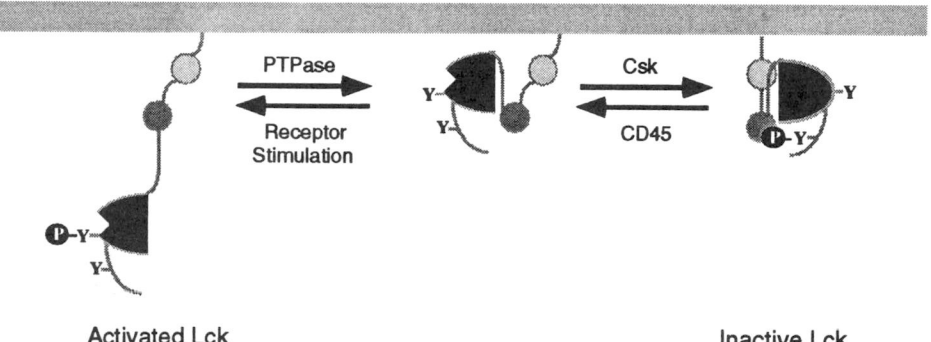

FIG. 7. Dynamic regulation of Lck. A schematic representation of the regulation of the two phosphorylation sites of Lck. Csk phosphorylates Lck at the C-terminal negative regulatory site, driving the kinase into the "closed" inactive state. CD45 dephosphorylates this site, opening the kinase and allowing it to be activated by receptor stimulation. Receptor stimulation leads to the phosphorylation of the tyrosine in the activation loop, increasing kinase activity. An as yet unidentified PTPase dephosphorylates the activation loop, thereby decreasing kinase activity.

TABLE 3. *Some of the proteins that are tyrosine phosphorylated following TCR stimulation*

TCR subunits
  CD3 δ, ε, γ
  ζ
Protein tyrosine kinases
  Itk
  Lyn
  Lck
  MAPKs
  Pyk2
  Syk
  ZAP-70
Proteins with enzymatic function
  Phospholipase C γ1 (PLC γ1)
Others
  Cbl
  CD5
  CD6
  Ezrin
  LAT
  Shc
  Slap-130
  Slp-76
  Shc
  α Tubulin
  Valosin containing protein
  Vav

great extent, the function of the phosphorylation of these proteins is not understood. Some of the proteins (i.e., Grb2, Shc, and Slp-76) have no intrinsic enzymatic activity but instead function as adaptors, by using SH2 and/or SH3 domains, to couple the TCR to important intracellular pathways. Others have well-characterized enzymatic activities, such as phospholipase C γ1 (PLCγ1), Itk, and mitogen-activated protein kinase (MAPK), that are influenced by tyrosine phosphorylation. Still many others do not have a well-defined function in TCR signal transduction pathways.

Activation of the Phosphatidylinositol Second-messenger Pathway

One of the best characterized of TCR-induced tyrosine phosphoproteins is PLCγ1. The precise mechanism by which TCR stimulation leads to PLCγ1 tyrosine phosphorylation and activation is not well understood. PLCγ1 is normally a cytoplasmic enzyme (269). A fraction of it probably translocates to the membrane as the result of the interaction of its SH2 domains with tyrosine-phosphorylated residues on Syk, ZAP-70 or an adaptor protein. PLCγ1 has been shown to interact via its SH2 domains with Y348 and Y352 residues in interdomain B of Syk in B cells (270), although a similar interaction has not been observed in T cells. The best candidate for an adaptor protein that could couple PLCγ1 to the TCR signaling pathway is a recently identified TCR-induced tyrosine phosphoprotein of 36 kDa, LAT, which interacts with PLCγ1 and Grb2 (271a), an adaptor involved in the Ras pathway (see below). Since LAT is exclusively found in the particulate fraction, it could help to localize PLCγ1 to the plasma membrane. Once localized to the plasma membrane, PLCγ1 would be in position to be phosphorylated by any of the TCR-regulated kinases, resulting in its acti-

vation. PLCγ1 is not phosphorylated or activated in Lck-deficient or ZAP-70–deficient T cells (228,230,272). Interestingly, deficiency of Btk, the Itk homologue expressed in B cells, results in the failure to activate PLC (273). By analogy, Itk could play an important role in T cells. Since phosphorylation of PLCγ1 in T cells occurs on several tyrosine residues and this is associated with the activation of its catalytic function (274), multiple PTKs could directly or indirectly contribute to its activation via events involved in recruitment or phosphorylation of the enzyme.

PLCγ1 is only one of several enzymes with PLC activity. Activation of PLC enzymes results in the generation of second messengers of the PI pathway. The contribution of the PI pathway to T-cell activation has been well studied. Early studies with calcium ionophores and certain phorbol esters demonstrated that these reagents synergize in inducing lymphokine secretion, IL 2R expression, T-cell proliferation, and the activation of the cytolytic mechanism of CTL (reviewed in ref. 37). Moreover, these reagents could induce lymphokine secretion in mutant cell lines that failed to express the TCR (33,40), suggesting that these pharmacologic reagents mimicked important signals downstream of the TCR. Since calcium ionophores induce an increase in cytoplasmic free calcium ($[Ca^{2+}]_i$) and agonist phorbol esters activate the serine–threonine kinase, PKC (275), this led to the notion that the TCR may function to initiate T-cell activation by a signal transduction mechanism that involves similar events.

The development of calcium-sensitive fluorescent dyes (i.e., quin 2, indo 1, and fura 2) that can be used to monitor changes in $[Ca^{2+}]_i$ in small cells such as lymphocytes permitted the test of this hypothesis (276). These changes can be monitored in bulk populations within a spectrofluorimeter, within subsets of cells in a flow cytometer, or within individual cells with sensitive microscopic techniques. Indeed, increases in $[Ca^{2+}]_i$ from basal levels of approximately 100 nM to greater than 1.0 μM are induced within seconds to minutes and may be sustained for hours following stimulation of the TCR (33,277,278). Similarly, a rapid and sustained activation of PKC is observed following TCR stimulation (279, 280). The agonist effects of calcium ionophores and phorbol esters suggest that the observed increase in $[Ca^{2+}]_i$ and activation of pkC induced by stimulation of the TCR are physiologically important intracellular events.

An increase in $[Ca^{2+}]_i$ and activation of PKC are characteristic events that result from a common receptor-mediated signal transduction pathway, the PI pathway. The key regulatory event in the PI pathway involves the hydrolysis of a relatively rare membrane phospholipid called phosphatidylinositol 4,5-bisphosphate (PIP₂) (281). TCR stimulation activates the PI pathway through the tyrosine phosphorylation of PLCγ1 (272,274). Activation of this enzyme is associated with its cleavage of the phosphodiester linkage of PIP₂, resulting in the formation of inositol 1,4,5-trisphosphate (1,4,5-IP₃) and 1,2-diacylglycerol (DG) (Fig. 8). These molecules, in turn, function as intracellular "second messengers" to induce an increase in $[Ca^{2+}]_i$ and activation of PKC, respectively. Within seconds following stimulation of the TCR by antigen or anti-TCR mAb, a substantial increase in 1,4,5-IP₃ and the immediate metabolite of DG, phosphatidic acid, are observed (282). Second-messenger generation has been shown to continue as long as occupancy of the receptor persists (27).

Function of Second Messengers of the PI Pathway

The role of 1,4,5-IP₃ in increasing intracellular calcium has been studied intensively. This water-soluble sugar has a specific intracel-

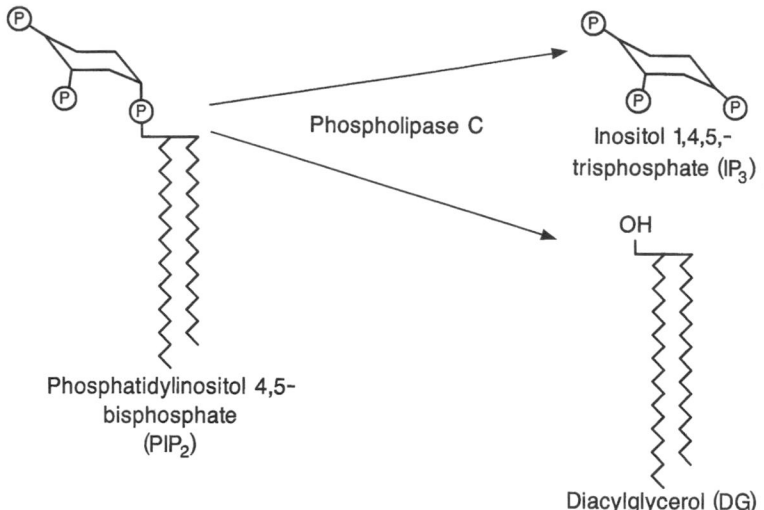

FIG. 8. The structure of phosphatidylinositol 4,5-bisphosphate (PIP₂) and the products of its hydrolysis by phospholipase C.

lular receptor that regulates the mobilization of $[Ca^{2+}]_i$ from intracellular Ca^{2+} stores associated with the endoplasmic reticulum (283,284). The release of intracellular stores of Ca^{2+} by 1,4,5-IP₃ can account for most of the initial increase in $[Ca^{2+}]_i$ that occurs during the first minute or two following TCR stimulation (282). However, at the cell population level, stimulation of the TCR induces increases in $[Ca^{2+}]_i$ that persist for several hours (27,285). At the level of individual cells, patch clamp and image analyses indicate that the sustained increase observed at the population level following TCR stimulation with various types of ligands reflects the summation of asynchronous oscillatory increases of $[Ca^{2+}]_i$ in individual cells (47, 286). Both the sustained $[Ca^{2+}]_i$ increase and the persistence of oscillations require a transmembrane flux of calcium from the outside of the cell to the inside. The persistent response is necessary for certain cellular responses, notably the initiation of IL-2 gene transcription (27,285,287). The mechanism responsible for the regulation of the transmembrane flux of Ca^{2+} in T cells involves a non–voltage-gated Ca^{2+} channel that is regulated by an unidentified mediator released when intracellular stores are depleted (288,289). Once the intracellular stores are refilled from transmembrane fluxes of Ca^{2+}, the plasma membrane channel closes. This type of regulation of calcium currents is termed *capacitative calcium entry*. High levels of $[Ca^{2+}]_i$ appear to have a negative influence on transmembrane calcium currents (288,290). This negative feedback could account for the observed oscillations and function to keep $[Ca^{2+}]_i$ within the required relatively narrow physiologic range.

The potential contribution of inositol phosphates to events involved in cell activation is raised to an increased level of complexity by the various forms of inositol phospholipids, the large number of distinct inositol phosphate isomers, and the numerous enzymes that regulate these compounds (reviewed in ref. 291). The possibility that each of these phospholipid or inositol phosphate isomers, as well as other forms not depicted, might regulate some intracellular event illustrates how receptors coupled to the PI pathway may exert effects on a number of intracellular events.

One set of the inositol phosphate lipid metabolites deserves special mention, those formed by the action of PI3-kinase. This enzyme consists of two components, a p85 subunit, which serves as an adaptor and regulatory subunit and a catalytic p110 subunit (292). This enzyme is activated through stimulation of a number of receptors, including the TCR, CD28, and the IL-2R (122,293–296). Activation of PI3-kinase leads to the generation of several inositol phospholipids, including PI 3-P, PI 3,4-P₂ and PI 3,4,5-P₃. The activity of PI3-kinase can be blocked by two inhibitors, wortmannin and LY294002. These inhibitors help to define the importance of PI3-kinase and its metabolites in receptor-mediated signaling events. These phospholipids and their inositol phosphate metabolites generated through the activation of PI3-kinase have been implicated in a number of important functions, including receptor endocytosis, cytoskeletal rearrangements, cell proliferation, and apoptosis (292).

The other hydrolysis product of PIP₂ is DG. DG is also a potent "second messenger" that regulates a family of serine–threonine kinases, consisting of the PKC isozymes (297). DG activates PKC isozymes by increasing the affinity of this kinase for phospholipid. Many of the isozymes are also Ca^{2+}-dependent, so that activation occurs through the synergistic actions of DG and Ca^{2+} at physiologic $[Ca^{2+}]_i$ levels. Activation of PKC isozymes has been observed in cells following TCR stimulation (279,280,298,299). Likewise, phorbol esters are also potent activators of PKC, explaining the ability of these reagents to synergize with calcium ionophores, together mimicking the effects of anti-TCR mAb.

PKC represents a family of closely related enzymes that share structural features and requirements for Ca^{2+}, phospholipid and DG (297). All identified forms can be activated by agonist phorbol esters but differ in their calcium sensitivities. Many, but not all, of the isozymes are expressed in T cells. Of those expressed, evidence is strongest for the importance of the PKC α, β, and θ isozymes (298,299). At least some T-cell responses, including IL-2 production, can occur in the absence of PKC β (300). Redundant function among some isozymes seems likely, because expression of a constitutively active form of PKC β could induce IL-2 transcriptional activity in the presence of calcium ionophore stimulation only (301). It still remains possible, however, that distinct isozymes may have overlapping as well distinct functions in T cells. A specific function for PKC θ is suggested by its specific localization at the interface of the T cell and APC (302). It is the only PKC isozyme that relocalizes during an antigen-specific interaction.

The activation of PKC may be influenced in several ways. First, metabolism of DG to phosphatidic acid by DG-kinase will serve to limit the availability of DG. Second, a calcium-activated protease, calpain, can cleave PKC *in vitro* into a cytosolic constitutively active 50-kD enzyme that is Ca^{2+} and phospholipid independent (303). Whether calpain activity contributes to the activation or modification of PKC in T cells is not known. Third, the nature of the stimulating ligand may influence the observed activation of PKC. Stimulation of T cells with immobilized anti-CD3 mAb induces more prolonged translocation of PKC activity to the plasma membrane than does the same mAb used in soluble form, probably the result of more sustained PIP_2 turnover (279,304). Such sustained activation of PKC is important for subsequent T-cell proliferative responses (280). Thus, the activation and regulation of PKC may be more complex than first appreciated. One can expect that differences in the regulation of these intracellular events will have an impact on the cellular responses observed.

Consequences of Increases in $[Ca^{2+}]_i$ and Activation of PKC

The synergistic effects of increases in $[Ca^{2+}]_i$ and activation of PKC must be explained by the impact of these intracellular events on subsequent signaling pathways. Although the details of the events leading from increases in $[Ca^{2+}]_i$ and activation of PKC to cellular responses are not known, considerable progress has been made. A model outlining and encompassing these events leading from the TCR to the transcriptional activation of the IL-2 gene is depicted in Fig. 9. The increase in $[Ca^{2+}]_i$ influences calmodulin-dependent events, including the activation of calcineurin (PP2B) and Ca^{2+}/calmodulin-dependent kinase (CAM-kinase).

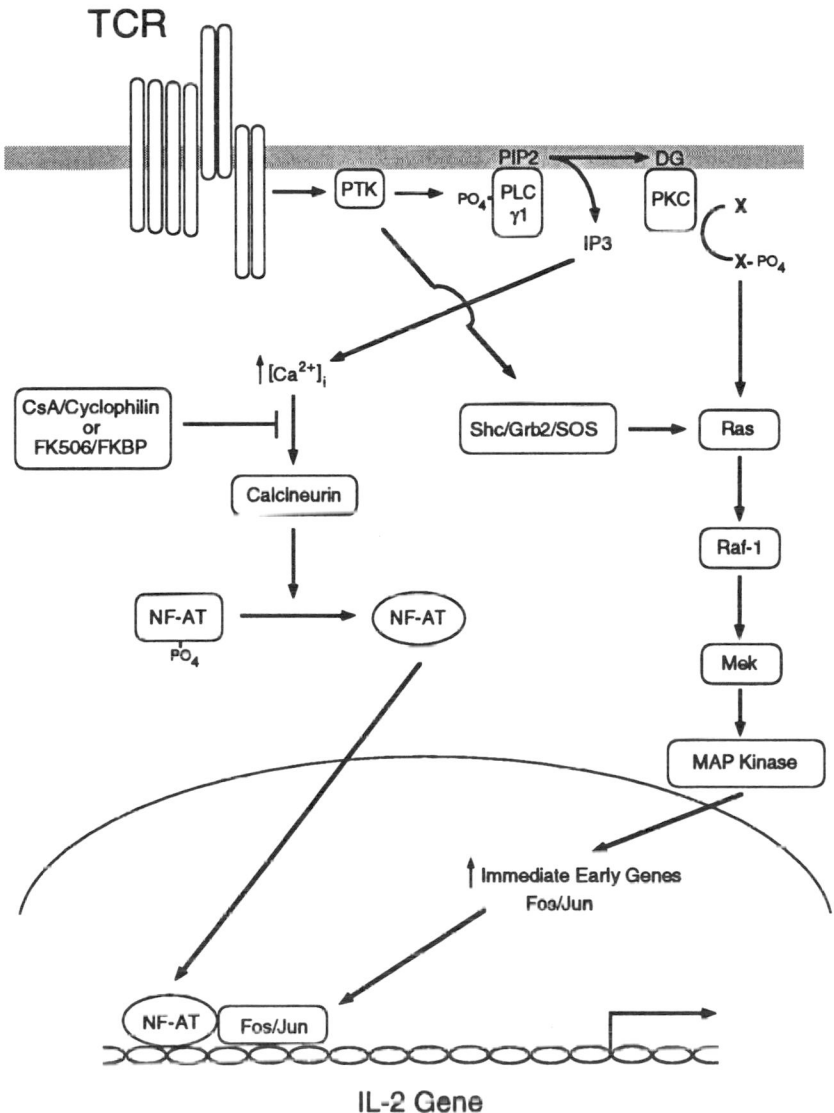

FIG. 9. Model of TCR-mediated signal transduction leading to lymphokine (IL-2) gene transcription. Note that the *arrows* between the protein components do not necessarily reflect direct interactions.

A critical role for the Ca^{2+}/calmodulin-dependent serine–threonine phosphatase calcineurin is now well established. Calcineurin is the molecular target for the immunosuppressives CsA and FK506, drugs that have revolutionized clinical organ transplantation (reviewed in ref. 305). CsA and FK506 form molecular complexes with their cellular receptors, cyclophilin and FKBP, respectively. It is these molecular complexes, not the isolated drugs, that inhibit the phosphatase function of calcineurin (306). Calcineurin is expressed ubiquitously but is expressed at only low levels in T-lymphocytes. This probably accounts for the relative specificity of the immunosuppressive drugs in targeting T-cell function.

A critical function for calcineurin has been established in the regulation of IL-2 gene expression (7). One target of calcineurin involves a protein(s) called *nuclear factor of activated T cells,* (NF-AT), which is involved in the transcriptional regulation of many lymphokine genes, including IL-2 (307). NF-AT constitutes a family of cytoplasmic phosphoproteins that translocate to the nucleus in response to calcium increases (287,308). This translocation is a critical regulatory event, because enforced nuclear localization of NF-AT activates its transcriptional function (287). Calcineurin phosphatase activity is critical for the activity of NF-AT transcriptional reporter constructs (309,310). Moreover, calcineurin can dephosphorylate NF-AT (311). This dephosphorylation is likely to reveal an NF-AT nuclear localization site that allows for its translocation. Thus, calcineurin activation, resulting from an increase in $[Ca^{2+}]_i$, leads to the dephosphorylation and activation of a key transcriptional factor involved in lymphokine gene expression (see below).

Another enzyme that is responsive to increases in $[Ca^{2+}]_i$ is the multifunctional Ca^{2+}/calmodulin-dependent kinase (CAM-kinase). This kinase is activated following TCR stimulation. Activation of CAM-kinase alone appears to have a negative regulatory influence on IL-2 gene expression (312). This is consistent with the ability of calcium ionophores, when used alone, to induce anergy in T cells (28).

The relevant substrates of PKC are of considerable interest. A number of proteins are phosphorylated on serine or threonine residues as a result of PKC activation following treatment of T cells with phorbol esters or following TCR stimulation. Among these are the human CD3 γ and δ chains (162), the murine CD3 δ and CD3 ε chains (313), CD4 (314), the transferrin receptor, the IL-2R, and HLA class I heavy chains (315). Some of these proteins are not direct substrates of PKC, and the functional significance of these phosphorylations is not yet clear. However, the activity of PKC in T cells is of considerable interest and importance to T-cell responses, as discussed below.

Activation of the Ras Pathway

Stimulation of T cells with phorbol esters or with TCR ligands induces the rapid activation of the protooncogene Ras (316). Ras is a 21-kDa peripheral membrane protein and is one of many related proteins that can bind and hydrolyze guanine nucleoside triphosphate (GTP). Ras is activated in the GTP-bound state and is inactive in the GDP-bound state. Its guanosine triphosphatase (GTPase) activity is regulated by interactions with guanine nucleotide exchange proteins, such as Sos, and GTPase-activating proteins (GAPs) (Fig. 10) (reviewed in refs. 317,318).

Activation of Ras by the TCR is the result of both PKC-dependent and PKC-independent mechanisms (319). How PKC activa-

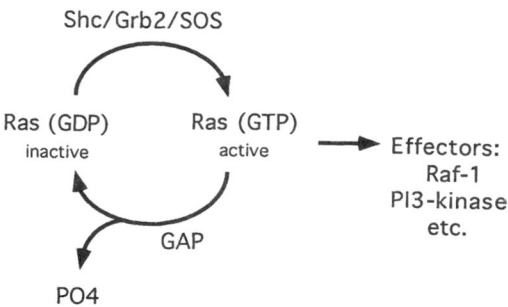

FIG. 10. Regulation of the Ras GTPase.

tion leads to Ras activation remains unclear. Initial studies suggested that the activation of Ras in T cells following phorbol ester addition or TCR stimulation occurs as the result of inhibition of GAP activity (320). GAP is weakly tyrosine phosphorylated following TCR stimulation and associates with an induced 62-kDa tyrosine phosphoprotein that has been recently cloned (299). The involvement of this complex in Ras activation in T cells remains to be established. However, more recent studies have implicated the involvement of a guanine nucleotide exchange protein, Sos, as the means by which Ras function is predominantly regulated. A number of genetic and biochemical studies have implicated the coupling protein Grb2, which binds to the guanine nucleotide exchange protein Sos, in Ras regulation (318). Grb2 is an adaptor protein, consisting of an SH2 domain flanked on each side by SH3 domains. In TCR-stimulated cells, the SH2 domain of Grb2 binds to LAT (271a,321), a phosphoprotein that also binds to PLCγ1, as well as to another adaptor protein called Shc (322). Shc has been reported to be inducibly tyrosine phosphorylated and to bind to tyrosine-phosphorylated residues in the TCR ζ chain (323). The SH3 domains of Grb2 bind to proline-rich regions in Sos. Thus, TCR stimulation may activate Ras via the recruitment of a Grb2/Sos complex to tyrosine phosphorylated Shc bound to the TCR or to membrane-associated LAT. The membrane-associated Sos molecule can then activate Ras by inducing nucleotide exchange.

Ras has multiple downstream effectors, including Raf, PI3-kinase, and other GTP-binding proteins, including Rac and Cdc42 (324,325). The function of the Ras-Raf interaction is best characterized and has been shown to be important in TCR signaling function leading to IL-2 gene activation (299,326). Ras interacts directly with the serine–threonine kinase Raf-1. Raf-1 is activated in T cells following TCR stimulation or PKC activation with phorbol esters (327). Raf-1 can regulate the activation of a dual-specific tyrosine–serine threonine kinase, MEK, that in turn activates MAPKs (328,329). In T cells, the activation of MAPKs has also been associated with PKC activation (330). This complex kinase cascade can function to regulate nuclear events involved in the growth and differentiation of a variety of cells.

The activation of Ras contributes to the transcriptional activation of the IL-2 gene (299). Expression of an activated form of Ras, which has reduced capacity to hydrolyze GTP, can substitute, in part, for phorbol esters in synergizing with calcium ionophores to induce transcription driven by the IL-2 upstream regulatory region or a multimer of the NF-AT site (326,331). Moreover, dominant-negative mutants of Ras or Raf inhibit TCR-induced IL-2 transcription (326,332). Activated-Ras is likely to be involved in the induction of the anisomycin-sensitive and calcium-independent nuclear component of NF-AT, AP-1, which is a heterodimer composed of Fos and Jun-related proteins (333–335). Expression of the Fos is highly dependent on the activation of MAPKs. Thus, the integration of distinct branches of the TCR-induced signaling pathway, those mediating increases in $[Ca^{2+}]_i$ and those mediating activation of Ras, result in the activation of distinct transcriptional factors that coordinately regulate IL-2 gene expression (see Fig. 9).

Other PTK-regulated Events

As indicated in Table 3, a large number of proteins are inducibly phosphorylated following TCR stimulation. The foregoing discussion focused on only a limited number of these proteins. The functions of the other proteins inducibly phosphorylated by the TCR-regulated PTKs is largely unknown, but they are likely to be important in T-cell activation. In this regard, two induced phosphoproteins, Vav and Slp-76, deserve some further discussion.

Vav is a 95-kDa protein with multiple modular domains involved in signaling function that is expressed exclusively in cells of the hematopoietic lineage and trophoblast cells (reviewed in ref. 336). It is inducibly phosphorylated following TCR stimulation (337,338). The importance of Vav in TCR function is highlighted by the impaired T-cell development that occurs in the absence of Vav expression (339,340). The T cells that do develop have an ill-defined TCR signal transduction, leading to IL-2 gene expression. Moreover, overexpression of Vav leads to constitutive and enhanced TCR-induced IL-2 gene expression (341). These studies indicate that Vav plays an important role in TCR signal transduction pathways.

The mechanism by which Vav contributes to TCR signal transduction pathways is not clear. Deletion of its N-terminal 65 residues results in an oncogenic protein in fibroblasts (342), but overexpression of oncogenic Vav fails to recapitulate the activating effects of the wild-type protein in T cells (341), suggesting an important function for this domain. Its guanine nucleotide exchange domain is specific for Rac, Rho, and Cdc42 (343), GTP-binding proteins that have been implicated in actin cytoskeletal rearrangements. This guanine nucleotide exchange activity can activated by its in vitro tyrosine phosphorylation by Lck. The role of the actin cytoskeleton in TCR signaling function is not clear. However, as discussed below, actin polymerization occurs in T cells adjacent to sites of T cell–APC interactions (344). It is possible that the organization of actin cytoskeletal components helps to organize components in the TCR signal transduction pathway.

The Vav SH2 domain plays an important role in interactions with at least two proteins. The SH2 domain binds directly to tyrosine-phosphorylated ZAP-70, and the binding function of the SH2 domain is required for Vav tyrosine phosphorylation (242,345). The SH2 sequence was predicted to have specificity for Y315 in ZAP-70, and this site has been shown to be required for interactions with Vav and for ZAP-70 function in TCR signaling pathways (242). The SH2 domain of Vav also binds to tyrosine-phosphorylated Slp-76, an adaptor protein that is exclusively expressed in cells of the hematopoietic lineage. Like Vav, overexpression of Slp-76 potentiates TCR signals, leading to NF-AT activation (346). Moreover, the importance of the interaction between Vav and Slp-76 is suggested by the ability of these two proteins to synergize in activating NF-AT in overexpression studies (347). These studies suggest that the complex of Vav and Slp-76 plays an important role in the TCR signal transduction pathways, and this may involve the actin cytoskeleton.

THE CONSEQUENCES OF EARLY SIGNAL TRANSDUCTION EVENTS

Early Biochemical Events

As a consequence of signal transduction events initiated by the TCR, and presumably by other accessory receptors, a cascade of intracellular biochemical changes occur that contribute to the events that lead to a demonstrable cellular response. Among these early biochemical events are protein phosphorylation and activation of a variety of kinases (as discussed above), cytoplasmic alkalinization, fluxes in ions, and changes in levels of cyclic nucleotides. Such events are not confined to the T cell but have been widely observed in receptor-mediated activation of many cell types. They are likely to be important, through mechanisms that have yet to be elucidated, in regulating later cellular responses.

Changes in pH

One mechanism whereby intracellular functions may be influenced and could be envisioned to initiate a cellular response is by altering the cytoplasmic ionic milieu, specifically cytoplasmic pH. Changes in pH can have profound effects on the activities of enzymes. Cellular alkalinization is known to occur during receptor-initiated PIP_2 hydrolysis in many cell types (348). An increase in pH has been demonstrated in T-cell lines and thymocytes following lectin stimulation or TCR stimulation by mAb (349,350). This appears to be the result of an increased activity of the plasma membrane Na^+/H^+ antiporter. Evidence suggests that this effect may be regulated by PIP_2 hydrolysis because both a dependency on extracellular calcium and the ability of pkC-activating phorbol esters to mimic the effect of lectins and TCR mAb have been reported (349,350).

Fluxes in Cyclic Nucleotides

Changes in the cyclic nucleotides, cyclic adenosine monophosphate (cAMP) and cyclic guanosine monophosphate (cGMP), regulate cellular functions in a variety of cell types. Changes in cyclic nucleotides in T-lymphocyte mitogenic responses received considerable attention in early work on T-cell activation. Following mitogenic lectin stimulation of T cells, a rise followed by a fall in cAMP levels was thought to be important in T-cell proliferative responses (351). An increase in cAMP levels has been reported following stimulation of a T-cell line with anti-CD3 mAb (352). Inhibitory effects of high levels of cAMP on T-cell proliferative responses are well documented (353, 354). High cAMP levels inhibit T-cell proliferative responses by blocking IL-2 production but not by inhibiting the effects of IL-2 on its receptor (355). The mechanism for this inhibitory effect of cAMP on T-cell responses is somewhat controversial, although it is likely to involve the action of cAMP-dependent protein kinase. Inhibition of PIP_2 hydrolysis by cAMP in T cells has been observed by some (356), but not all, investigators (357). Another target for cAMP-dependent kinase is the Raf-1 kinase, which can be inactivated by serine phosphorylation (358). Inhibition of either of these events would have a negative effect. Since T cells express a variety of receptors that can induce an increase in cAMP, including β-adrenergic receptors, it is likely that T-cell function may be influenced by immunologic and nonimmunologic mediators.

An increase in cGMP has also been observed following mitogenic lectin stimulation of T cells (359). The physiologic function of these cGMP increases is yet to be established.

Changes in Membrane Potential

Like other cells, T cells have an electrochemical gradient of ions across their plasma membranes. This gradient is established by the unequal distribution of ions on the two sides of the plasma membrane and is responsible for a resting negative electrical potential of approximately −70 mV. This negative resting potential influences the tendency of charged ions to cross the plasma membrane down their concentration gradients. However, the ability of ions such as Na^+, K^+, Cl^- and Ca^{2+} to cross the plasma membrane is limited by the permeability of the plasma membrane to each of these ions. Events that result in changes in the membrane permeability of a particular ion, which can be receptor-mediated, will change the membrane potential. In addition, rapid changes in membrane permeability, such as channel opening, will establish a diffusion potential as long as the channel remains open and the ionic gradient persists. Thus, receptor-signal transduction may influence changes in the plasma membrane permeability to certain ions. These changes in permeability may be manifested as changes in the membrane potential.

Transient hyperpolarization (i.e., a more negative potential) followed later by depolarization (i.e., more positive potential) of T cells after lectin stimulation has been appreciated for many years (360). Using sensitive patch clamping techniques, voltage-gated potassium channels have been shown to be a major ion-gated channels in T cells (361). Heterogeneity of these potassium channels has been observed in murine T cells and thymocytes of various phenotypes (362). Three types of K^+ channels have been detected—n, n′, and l—although only n channels are present in human T cells. The functional significance of this heterogeneity is not clear. The gating properties of these channels change following the addition of T-cell mitogens, but it is not clear whether these channels can be regulated directly by T-cell surface molecules as a result of ligand–receptor interactions. Extracellular Ca^{2+} does not pass through these channels. The observed transient hyperpolarization response appears to be regulated by the increase in $[Ca^{2+}]_i$ (363). The mechanism explaining the later depolarization is not well understood. The relatively delayed changes in membrane potential depolarization observed in T-cell mitogenic responses would suggest that these channels are regulated indirectly by membrane receptor–associated signal transduction. The importance of the activity of these channels has been suggested by the ability of K^+ channel blockers to inhibit T cell proliferative responses (364, 365). Blockade of K^+ channels with charybdotoxin appears to influence the extent of Ca^{2+} increase that is achieved following TCR stimulation. This does not appear to be an effect mediated on classic voltage-gated Ca^{2+} channels. Further work on understanding the functions of K^+ channels is required.

Cellular Responses

Cytoskeletal Changes

The redistribution and reorientation of cytoskeletal elements in T cells has been studied during the interactions between helper T cell clones and APCs, as well as cytolytic T-lymphocytes (CTLs) and their targets (344). A specific antigen-dependent reorientation of the microtubule organizing center (MTOC) in the T helper cell and CTL towards the cell with which either interacts occurs. This reorientation of the MTOC does not occur in the APC or target cell. In addition, redistribution of some (i.e., talin and F-actin) but not all (i.e., α-actinin) actin cytoskeletal proteins to the region of the T cell that is in contact with the APC or target cell occurs in antigen-specific interacting pairs of cells.

Since antigen-specific interactions are required for the polarization of the cytoskeleton, it is likely that TCR-mediated signal transduction may play a role in these processes. Studies suggest that a TCR ITAM is required as are the TCR-regulated PTKs (366a). The ITAM could serve as the focal point to orient the redirected cytoskeleton. Although the activation of Ras does not appear to be required for these events, another GTP-binding protein, Cdc42, has been implicated in the polarization of T cells (366b). Since the guanine nucleotide exchange function of Vav can regulate the activation of Cdc42 (343), it is tempting to speculate that the interaction of Vav with ZAP-70 and Vav tyrosine phosphorylation, with resultant activation of its GEF function for *rho*-family GTPases, could serve to reorient the T-cell cytoskeleton. It is also interesting that α-tubulin is tyrosine phosphorylated following TCR stimulation and that tyrosine-phosphorylated tubulin is found in the depolymerized fraction of cellular tubulin (367). This suggests that the tyrosine phosphorylation of tubulin might play a role in the polarization of the MTOC. Polarization of the cytoskeleton in T cells also depends on calcium (368). Myosin light-chain kinase, which can regulate cytoskeletal structure, is activated by elevations in $[Ca^{2+}]_i$ (369). These observations suggest complex mechanisms function to reorient the T-cell cytoskeleton to achieve properly oriented and localized T-cell responses.

An attractive notion for a functional consequence of this reorientation is the directional secretion of prepackaged or newly synthesized secretory products. In the case of the CTL, this could represent the focused secretion of cytolytic components (see below and Chapter 31) toward only the relevant antigen-bearing target cell. In the case of the helper T cell, newly synthesized lymphokines important in macrophage activation or B-cell differentiation–proliferation could be envisioned to be targeted toward the relevant APC. For the B cell that presents antigen to the T cell, this might serve to limit the effects of such lymphokines to antigen-specific B cells.

Activation of the Cytolytic Mechanism

The initiation of the lytic process occurs during the complex cell–cell interaction between receptors on the CTL and ligands on the target cell. TCR-initiated signal transduction events contribute to the activation of the cytolytic mechanism. In keeping with this notion is the observation that in most instances extracellular Ca^{2+} is necessary for target cell lysis, but not for the binding of the CTL to its target (reviewed in ref. 370). Moreover, calcium ionophores and phorbol esters synergize in inducing the lysis of bystander cells by CTL in an antigen-independent manner (371). Increases in $[Ca^{2+}]_i$ in CTL interacting with specific targets have been observed at the single-cell level (372). Collectively, these observations strongly suggest that stimulation of the TCR on a CTL by target-cell antigens initiates transmembrane signaling events, including PIP_2 hydrolysis. The resultant increase in $[Ca^{2+}]_i$ and/or the activation of PKC leads to activation of a cytolytic mechanism.

Two cytolytic mechanisms are activated by TCR signaling events. These two mechanisms are discussed in detail in Chapter 31. Briefly, one mechanism involves the secretion of prepackaged cytolytic granules that contain perforin and serine esterase enzymes called *granzymes* (370). Perforin is a calcium-dependent pore-forming protein that contributes to the osmotic destruction of the target cell. Granzymes help to initiate the apoptotic pathway in target cells. Secretion of these granules can be induced by the reagents that mimic TCR-initiated PIP_2 hydrolysis, phorbol esters and calcium ionophores. The activation of this cytolytic mechanism by the TCR-induced signal transduction events involving PIP_2 hydrolysis is consistent with the stimulus–secretion coupling mechanism that is observed in platelets, neutrophils, and mast cells which use similar receptor-mediated signal transduction mechanisms. In fact, it has been possible to transfer perforin and granzymes into mast-cell granules and induce these cells to kill sensitized target cells (373). In the case of the CTL, linking the reorientation of the cytoskeletal elements, particularly the MTOC, serves to focus the stimulus–secretion of the cytolytic granules toward the relevant target and prevent non–antigen-specific bystander cell lysis (368). In contrast, the bystander lysis that is observed when calcium ionophores and phorbol esters are used to stimulate lysis is likely to represent a situation in which cell surface receptors play no role, with resultant secretion of lytic granules in a nonfocused manner (371).

A second mechanism is used by CTL to induce target -cell destruction. This involves the Fas system (see Chapters 22 and 30). Fas is a member of the tumor necrosis factor receptor family. Sequences in its cytoplasmic domain are responsible for interacting with proteins that can initiate the apoptotic pathway and destruction of the target cell. Only Fas-expressing target cells are sensitive to this cytolytic mechanism. For T cells to mediate destruction of target cells via the Fas system, they must be induced to express the Fas ligand (Apo-1), a member of the tumor necrosis factor family (374). Fas ligand expression is transcriptionally induced by TCR signal transduction events and involves the activation of the NF-AT transcription factor. Thus, TCR signal transduction events regulate two very distinct mechanisms that contribute to target-cell destruction by CTLs.

Gene-activation Events

As a result of receptor-mediated signal transduction events in T cells, stimuli at the plasma membrane induce a set of specifically responsive genes to become transcriptionally active. These transcriptional events are responsible for the differentiation and proliferation of the stimulated T cells. Considerable progress has been made in our understanding of how cytoplasmic signal transduction pathways lead to the activation of key transcription factors.

It has become increasingly clear that receptor-mediated signal transduction events leading to the proliferation and acquisition of differentiated functions by the T cell are not the result of a single wave of gene-activation events. Instead, these are likely to result from a regulated cascade of sequential gene-activation events that may be conditionally regulated. Hence, following initial signal transduction events that lead to the transcriptional activation of a certain set of genes, the products of this first wave of activated genes may contribute to the transcriptional activation of a second set of targeted genes, and so on. At some point, there is commitment to the final response (measured as differentiation or prolifer-

ation), although there is substantial evidence that T-cell responses are not quantal.

An appreciation of this type of cascade is readily apparent if one considers the activation of the IL-2 gene and its receptor, IL-2R. Transcription of these genes begin during the first few hours of T-cell stimulation (reviewed in refs. 7, 307). The transcriptional activation of the IL-2 gene itself is dependent on protein synthesis, and this reflects the requirement for the translation of the product(s) of a gene(s) needed for the initiation of IL-2 transcription (308). Once produced, the binding of IL-2 to its receptor initiates distinct signal transduction events that result in a cascade of events involved in regulating cell growth. This is manifested many hours to days later as a proliferative response. For such a cascade of gene activation events to function, the activation of the initial set of responsive genes must be tightly regulated. Otherwise, uncontrolled proliferation or differentiation might ensue.

Early Gene-activation Events

The transcriptional activation of some genes is readily apparent in T cells within minutes of certain activating stimuli (7,307). This set of "immediate early activation genes" represents a relatively large number of newly expressed genes, whose expression is not dependent on protein synthesis. Hence, the immediate early genes represent the first in a cascade of genes induced during T-cell activation. The ability of inhibitors of protein synthesis to prevent subsequent IL-2 gene transcriptional activation suggests that at least one of the products of these early activation genes influences IL-2 gene regulation (27,375). Thus, one or more members of this set of genes may contribute to the appearance of nuclear proteins that bind to or influence important regulatory sequences of the IL-2 gene (see below). Advances in this area permit a more complete understanding of the regulation of these immediate early activation genes and their functions in the ensuing waves of gene activation that occur during T-cell responses.

Two protoonocogenes, *c-myc* and *c-fos*, encode nuclear proteins that are immediate early genes involved in transcriptional regulation (376,377). They serve as useful models to study the set of immediate early activation genes. The long-sought function of c-myc in cell growth remains ill defined, but it can bind DNA; forms complexes with other nuclear proteins, including Max; and can regulate transcription (378,379). C-fos forms a dimer with another protein, called c-jun, to form the transcriptional complex, AP-1 (377). Whereas the appearance of c-myc and c-fos mRNA is not restricted to T cells, these genes are among the first to become transcriptionally active following stimulation of the TCR on resting T cells. Transcripts for both c-myc and c-fos are readily detectable within 5 to 10 minutes of stimulation by PHA, or with mAbs reactive with the TCR or CD2 (380,381). In studies to examine the requirements for the transcriptional activation of c-myc and c-fos in T cells, an increase in either $[Ca^{2+}]_i$ or activation of PKC alone could induce their expression (382). However, synergy between these two events is evident from the combined effects of calcium ionophores and phorbol esters. Protein synthesis is not required for the transcriptional activation of either c-myc or c-fos in T cells, indicating that the transcription of these genes is directly regulated by the biochemical events that result from receptor-mediated signal transduction. MAPK family members, including Jun N terminal kinase (Jnk) and Erk kinases, which are activated in T cells in response to antigen receptor signals together with phorbol esters or costimulatory signals, have been directly implicated in regulating c-fos transcription by the phosphorylation of transcription factors such as the ternary response and serum response factors that bind to the c-fos promoter (377).

The products of such early activation genes, together with the effects of ongoing signal transduction events, initiate the next wave of gene activation. Indeed, several products of early activation genes have been implicated in the regulation of IL-2 gene expression, including those composing the AP-1 complex (333,383). Interestingly, persistent signal transduction is required for the transcriptional activation of the IL-2 gene, even after the appearance of transcripts of the early activation genes. Although there are several possible explanations for this, the posttranslational modification of products of the early activation genes may be required for their functions. Indeed, the posttranslational phosphorylation of c-fos and c-jun by Jnk and an ill-defined c-fos kinase is required for AP-1 transcriptional activity (377,384,385). Thus, a well-coordinated cascade of events involving signal transduction events and gene activation serves to regulate subsequent waves of gene activation that ultimately induce in T-cell proliferative responses.

Activation of Lymphokine Genes

Many of the prominent manifestations of T-cell activation are mediated by one of the many T cell–derived, secreted soluble proteins, termed *lymphokines*. These lymphokines exert a great diversity of effects on many cell types and tissues. In resting T cells, the production of lymphokines results from the transcriptional activation of the genes that encode them. Individual T cells produce different sets of lymphokines in response to the similar stimuli. While the distinct patterns of lymphokines may reflect the profiles of lymphokines secreted by the two major subsets of helper T cells (Th1 and Th2; see Chapter 26), the molecular basis for the heterogeneity in expression of these inducible genes within distinct subsets is only partially understood. Differences in tissue-specific expression of regulatory factors certainly account for some of these differences in expression. For instance, persistence in the transcriptional factor GATA-3 is associated with the Th2 phenotype (386). Selective expression of the c-Maf transcription factor in the presence of NIP45, a recently identified NF-AT–binding protein, as well as NF-AT, is also associated with the tissue-specific transcriptional activation of the IL-4 gene (387,388). The determinants involved in the tissue-specific expression of GATA-3 and c-Maf are not clear. IL-4 is a major determinant in Th2 subset commitment. Therefore, signaling pathways from the IL-4 receptor may influence the specific expression of c-Maf and/or GATA-3. Alternatively, INF-γ and IL-12 are the lymphokines that predominantly

drive T cells to commit to the Th1 phenotype. These lymphokines could positively influence another set of transcriptional factors or negatively influence the expression of GATA-3 and/or c-Maf. Alternatively, there may be differences in the transmembrane signals generated by cell surface receptors or cytoplasmic proteins expressed in different T cell subsets or when T cells engage different receptors on distinct populations of APCs. Such events could contribute to the differences in the menu of lymphokine genes that becomes transcriptionally active. The varied manifestations of T-cell activation may reflect the summation of the effects of the products of the lymphokine genes that become transcriptionally active. A detailed discussion of the effects of the various lymphokines that are expressed during the course of T-cell activation is presented in a subsequent chapter (Chapter 26).

Since substantial progress has been made in understanding the mechanisms involved in the transcriptional regulation of the IL-2 gene, the following discussion focuses on its regulation. It is likely that the general principles that hold for the regulation of the IL-2 gene will also apply to the transcriptional regulation of other lymphokine genes. As discussed, signaling pathways emanating from the TCR that are regulated by protein tyrosine phosphorylation are required for the transcriptional activation of the IL-2 gene.

Genomic DNA sequences involved in the regulation of the IL-2 gene were initially identified by their increased sensitivity to DNAase I digestion (389). More detailed analyses of the regulation of the IL-2 gene demonstrated that a 275-bp segment upstream of the transcription initiation site contains most of the sequences that regulate its transcriptional activation (7). This region is responsive to the synergistic actions of stimuli that increase $[Ca^{2+}]_i$ and induce the activation of PKC or Ras (326,390). From kinetic analyses and the ability of inhibitors of protein synthesis to block the transcriptional activation of IL-2, it is clear that products of immediate early genes are necessary for this activation (7). The involvement of c-Fos in many of the AP-1 sites offers at least a partial explanation for this requirement.

DNAse "footprint" analyses, assays with transcriptional reporter constructs, and electromobility shift analyses have demonstrated that there are several distinct nuclear protein–binding sites within this region are responsive to TCR-derived and CD28-derived signal transduction events (7,391) (Fig. 11). The proteins that bind to this region contribute to the transcriptional activation, as well as to the suppression of transcription of the IL-2 gene. TCR signal transduction events influence the binding and/or activity of at least six nuclear complexes, depicted in Fig. 11. All of these sites are required to coordinately respond to TCR-derived signal transduction events.

The NF-IL2A site binds Oct-1, a homeodomain transcription factor. The activity of this factor is regulated by a protein complex,

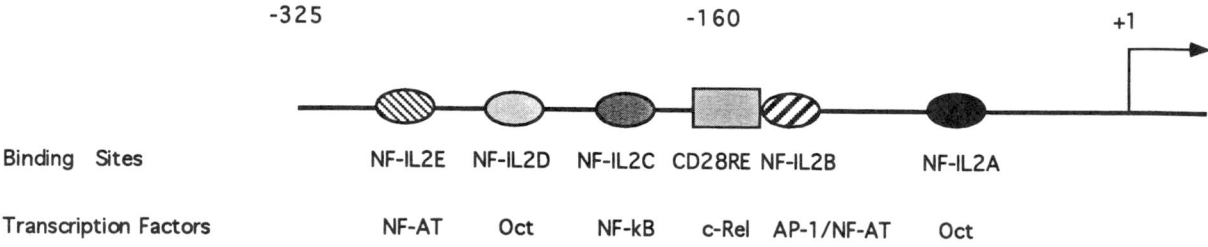

FIG. 11. IL-2 gene upstream (5′) regulatory regions with TCR- (*ovals*) and CD28-responsive elements (*rectangle*) indicated.

termed *OAP*, that contains a *jun*-family member that associates with Oct-1 only after stimulation (383,392). The complex NF-IL2B site, which binds AP-1 or related proteins and the NF-AT transcription factor, appears to be a major site of PKC responsiveness (393,394). The failure to activate AP-1 proteins that bind to this site has also been implicated in anergic T cells (395). This is consistent with the impaired activation of MAPKs and Jnk proteins in anergic T cells (396,397) and the roles of MAPKs and Jnk in regulating AP-1 function. The NF-IL2C site has been reported to bind several distinct transcription factors including NF-κB and AP-3. However, the contribution of this site to the inducibility of the IL-2 gene has been questioned (393,398). The NF-IL2D site is another Oct-binding site. It has not been studied in detail.

At least two sites bind NF-AT transcription factors within the IL-2 regulatory region: the proximal NF-AT site adjacent to the NF-IL2B site and the NF-IL2E site (7,307,391). The DNA-binding and -activation domain of the NF-AT family of proteins is homologous to the Rel-family of transcription factors. The favored DNA-binding site for NF-AT resembles Rel-binding sites. The NF-AT–binding sites in the IL-2 gene are actually composite transcriptional elements that bind proteins derived from one of the four NF-AT proteins in conjunction with AP-1 protein complexes. Binding of the entire protein complex is required for function. These sites can be multimerized to create transcriptional reporter constructs, which have been very useful in studying T-cell activation. The signals required for NF-AT translocation to the nucleus, where it can interact with a nuclear AP-1 complex that has been activated through the actions of MAPKs, Jnks, and Frk, were discussed above.

Stimulation of CD28 can also regulate lymphokine gene transcription, if TCR-derived signals are also provided (119,121). As discussed above, the proximal signal transduction events regulated by CD28 that influence lymphokine gene expression are not known, although they are CsA- and FK506-insensitive. In the presence of TCR signals or calcium ionophore plus phorbol esters, CD28 stimulation induces a nuclear factor that binds to homologous sequence element, the CD28RE, contained in multiple lymphokine genes, including IL-2, INF-γ, GM-CSF, and IL-3 (119). These sites are responsible for the effects of CD28 signals upon transcription of these genes and may, in part, be responsible for the costimulatory effects of CD28. The CD28RE has been reported to bind a number of *rel* family transcription factors as well as NF-AT (399–401). The CD28RE site in the IL-2 gene is adjacent to the neighboring NF-IL2B site that binds AP-1. Studies have suggested that this site functions as a composite element to bind c-Rel and AP-1 (402,403). In this regard, it is noteworthy that T cells from c-Rel–deficient mice fail to produce IL-2 unless they are stimulated with calcium ionophore and phorbol ester (404). This site appears to be a site of signal integration, where requirements for both TCR and CD28 signals are required for c-Rel and AP-1 activation.

Although transcriptional regulation represents a major mechanism for controlling lymphokine production, posttranscriptional regulation also represents an important mechanism. Most lymphokine transcripts, including IL-2, contain an AU-rich 3' untranslated sequence that confers instability to these mRNAs (405). Stimulation of T cells with phorbol esters or CD28 ligands has been reported to stabilize lymphokine mRNA (120,405,406). These observations on the transcriptional and posttranscriptional regulation of lymphokine genes suggest that complex regulatory mechanisms govern the expression of these important regulatory molecules.

Expression of New Cell Surface Molecules

A number of cell surface molecules appear on the surface of the T cell during the events associated with their activation, differentiation, and proliferation. These include lymphokine receptors (i.e., CD25, the α chain of the IL-2R) (6,407); nutrient receptors (i.e., the transferrin receptor and insulin receptor) (380); class II MHC antigens on human T cells, but not on murine T cells (408); and other cell surface molecules, the functions of which are largely unknown (i.e., CD69 and 4F2) (409,410). These proteins may subserve different roles in the growth, differentiation, and function of T cells following activation. The kinetics of the appearance of some of these proteins differ, with some appearing within minutes to hours after stimulation (i.e., CD25 and CD69) and others appearing only days (i.e., VLA-2) following T-cell activation. As the appearance of most of these proteins is transcriptionally regulated, different mechanisms of transcriptional regulation must be operative.

In addition to the appearance of new cell surface molecules, new antigenic epitopes on existing cell surface proteins indicate a different mechanism of functionally regulating certain receptors. For instance, concomitant with T-cell activation, a new antigenic epitope on the CD2 molecule (T11₃ epitope) is detected, which is probably the result of an allosteric change (31,38). Another mechanism responsible for the expression of new epitopes involves the regulated alternative splicing of exons, as in the case of CD45. Activated T cells and some helper T-cell subsets express a distinct 180-kDa isoform of CD45, CD45RO, which lacks the products of exons 4, 5, and 6. This is in contrast to the 200 to 210 CD45RA or CD45RB isoforms, which include some of these exons that are expressed on resting T cells. This is the result of regulated alternative splicing of exons that encode a portion of the extracellular domain (247,411). It is tempting to speculate that such regulated splicing may affect the ligand-binding function of CD45.

A detailed analysis of the regulation of all of the cell surface proteins induced during T-cell activation is beyond the scope of this chapter. However, a brief discussion of CD25, the α chain of the human IL-2R, a 55-kDa glycoprotein recognized by the anti-Tac mAb, is instructive (6). Expression of the IL-2R α chain is transcriptionally regulated. It is not expressed in resting G₀ T cells. The finding of at least three distinct sites of transcription initiation under different conditions that induce expression suggests that different modes of T-cell activation may influence distinct regulatory sequences flanking these sequences (412). Regulatory sequences responsive to certain stimuli involved in the activation of T cells have been identified in the upstream flanking regions of the IL-2R α-chain gene (413). NF-κB appears to play a critical role in regulating the gene. The post-translational regulation of NF-κB function via IκB phosphorylation and degradation is the predominant means by which NF-κB is regulated (136). The recent identification of the IκB kinase that is responsible for the phosphorylation event that leads to IκB ubiquitination and degradation is likely to provide new inroads toward studying the regulation of expression of the IL-2R α chain (137).

The regulation of expression of the IL-2R α chain differs from the regulation of its ligand, IL-2: (a) Reagents that activate PKC only are sufficient and more potent than those that increase $[Ca^{2+}]_i$ only to induce IL-2R α-chain gene expression (414). (b) IL-2 itself upregulates the expression of the IL-2R α chain via a transcriptional mechanism (413). This can, in part, account for the synergistic effects observed with reagents that increase $[Ca^{2+}]_i$ and activate

PKC, that is, the resulting IL-2 upregulates IL-2R α-chain expression. (c) The induction of IL-2R α-chain expression by PMA is not inhibitable by CsA (416), a potent inhibitor of IL-2 expression (417). (d) Finally, the expression of extremely high levels of IL-2R α-chain expression on HTLV-1–transformed human T-cell lines in the absence of IL-2 production suggests another distinct mechanism of IL-2R α-chain regulation (412,413). Hence, the regulation of this lymphokine receptor chain is not as stringently regulated as the lymphokine itself. This allows for the recruitment of IL-2R–expressing cells at sites of immune responses where other cells are producing IL-2, a paracrine effect. Since cells that have been previously activated continue to express low levels of IL-2R α chains, this would be a particularly attractive means by which the recruitment of memory T cells into an immune response might be facilitated. This paracrine effect is also the most widely accepted explanation for the synergy observed between CD4+ IL-2 producing cells and CD8+ CTL precursors that do not generally produce abundant quantities of IL-2. It is clear that the regulation of the IL-2R α-chain during T-cell activation is complex. It is likely that many other cell surface receptors expressed during the activation of T cells have equally complex but distinct mechanisms of regulation.

THE REGULATION OF T-CELL PROLIFERATION

One of the most important events during a primary immune response is the proliferation of clones of antigen-specific T cells. Since the frequency of antigen-specific precursor T cells is low in any given peripheral lymphoid tissue of an unimmunized animal, the expansion of the pool of antigen-reactive effector cells and of memory cells is critical for an effective specific immune response and for the development of long-lived specific immunity. For such clonal expansion to occur, the proliferative response must be highly regulated and limited mainly to those cells reactive with the stimulating antigen. This is accomplished by tightly regulating the production of certain lymphokines, which function as growth factors, and by regulating the expression of the receptors for these lymphokines, as described above.

Role of IL-2

The interaction of IL-2 with its receptor plays an important role in regulating antigen-induced T-cell proliferation (418–420). Once T cells are stimulated to secrete IL-2, the soluble lymphokine can interact with the very same cell that produced this growth factor (an autocrine effect), or it can interact with any other cell that expresses IL-2R (a paracrine effect) (see Fig. 12). Hence, antigen-activated T cells that produce IL-2 can (a) promote their own clonal expansion, (b) promote the proliferation of other T cells that are activated by the same or a related specific antigen but can not produce IL-2 (i.e., CD8+ cells), (c) promote the expansion of previously stimulated cells that express low levels of high-affinity IL-2Rs (i.e., memory T cells), and (d) promote the proliferation of non-T cells that express IL-2Rs (i.e., B cells or NK cells). In addition to its growth-promoting effects on various cell populations, IL-2 can influence the development of various differentiated functional activities (discussed in Chapter 21).

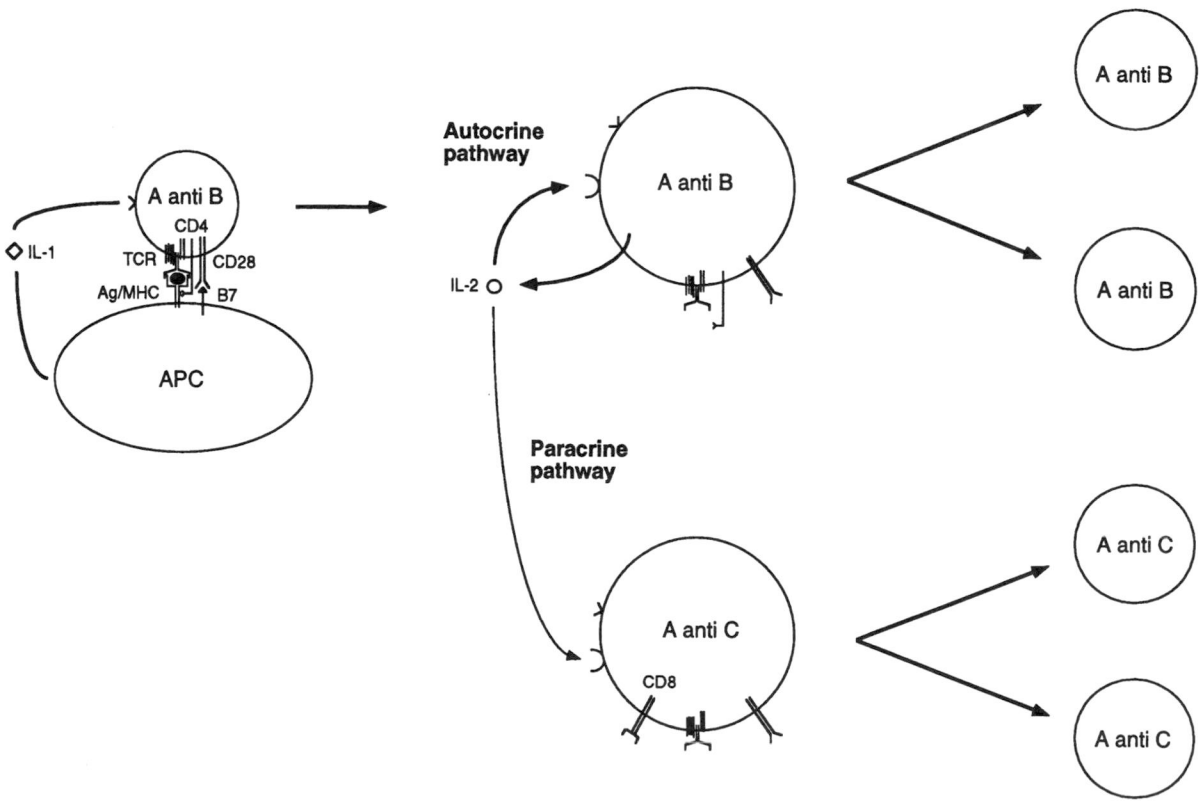

FIG. 12. Model of autocrine and paracrine pathways of T-cell proliferation.

Stimulation of the TCR induces naive T cells to progress from the G_0 to the G_1 stage of the cell cycle and to express high-affinity IL-2Rs (5,419). The function of IL-2 is to promote further progression through the cell cycle. The ability of IL-2 to induce cell cycle progression, from G_1 through S, G_2, and M, depends on the binding of IL-2 to its high-affinity receptor. Although IL-2 may not be the only lymphokine that can induce T-cell proliferation, the importance of IL-2 in promoting such cell cycle progression in peripheral T cells is underscored by the decreased proliferative response to mitogenic and antigen stimulation of T cells from mice in which the IL-2 has been disrupted by homologous recombination (421,422). Hence, the binding of IL-2 to its receptor and the ensuing signal transduction events play central roles in most immune responses.

At least three different binding affinities for the IL-2R have been detected on T cells (Fig. 13). The molecular basis for this heterogeneity in binding reflects the fact that there are three proteins that can contribute to the binding of IL-2 by the high-affinity receptor (407,419). CD25, the IL-2R α chain, is a 55-kD integral membrane glycoprotein that has an affinity constant (K_D) of 10^{-8} M (423). This low-affinity form of the IL-2R comprises the most abundant form of the IL-2R expressed on activated T cells and human T-cell leukemia virus—transformed lines. However, it is not expressed on resting T cells. It is also expressed on some early CD4$^-$/CD8$^-$ thymocytes. The IL-2R β chain, a 70-kD glycoprotein, binds IL-2 with intermediate affinity (K_D of approximately 10^{-9} M) when it is expressed on T cells (424), but is unable to bind IL-2 when expressed on fibroblasts (425). The latter result was clarified when a third component of the IL-2R was identified (426). The IL-2R γ chain is a 64-kD integral membrane protein. It does not bind IL-2 itself, but will reconstitute an intermediate-affinity binding site when coexpressed with the β chain in fibroblasts. The β and γ chains of the IL-2R are members of a family of cytokine receptors that have related structural features in their extracellular domains (427). Neither the β nor γ chain alone binds IL-2, but together they reconstitute the intermediate-affinity IL-2R that is detected at low levels on naive T cells, NK cells, and B cells. The high-affinity form of the IL-2R is dependent on all three chains, although a mol-

ecular complex of all three chains is difficult to detect biochemically. This may be due to the fact that the interaction between these chains is induced by IL-2 binding and the tetramolecular complex may be quite transient. Remarkable features of the IL-2R relate to its strikingly different IL-2 association and dissociation rates (428,429). Rapid on- and rapid off-rates are characteristic of the α chain, whereas IL-2 binding to the β chain (and presumably the γ chain) is characterized by slow on- and slow off-rates. The high-affinity receptor has rapid binding properties but IL-2 dissociates from it rather slowly. Hence, the high-affinity IL-2–binding site appears to result from the combined characteristics of the α, β, and γ chains.

Following stimulation of T cells with lectins or anti-TCR mAbs, the high-affinity receptor and the low-affinity receptor are expressed at a ratio of 1:10 on the cell surface. The number of β chains (and perhaps γ chains) appears to be limiting in the expression of the high-affinity receptor. It is only the high-affinity IL-2R that is thought to be able to bind IL-2 at physiologic concentrations, to internalize it, and to initiate T cell proliferation. However, at high concentrations of IL-2, the intermediate-affinity IL-2R, but not low-affinity receptor, appears to be able to induce T-cell proliferation.

The importance of the various chains of the IL-2R system has been most definitively established from studies of a human disease and from mice whose genes have been disrupted by homologous recombination. Mutations in the IL-2R γ chain are responsible for most cases of X-linked severe combined immunodeficiency syndrome (XSCID) (430). A similar phenotype has been observed in mice deficient in the γ chain (431). However, the phenotype of patients and mice deficient in the γ chain is more severe than would have been anticipated from studies of IL-2–deficient mice (421,422). This is explained by the fact that the γ chain is actually a component of several other lymphokine receptors, including the receptors for IL-4, IL-7, IL-9, and IL-15 (407). These lymphokines play critical roles in T- and B-cell development. Mice deficient in the α or β chains of the IL-2R have also been derived (432,433). In each case, the surprising outcome is a severely disregulated immune system with many of manifestations of autoimmunity. These results are not simply explained, but they do emphasize the importance of the IL-2/IL-2R system in maintaining normal homeostasis and regulation within the immune system.

The binding of IL-2 to the high- or intermediate-affinity forms of the receptor must initiate transmembrane signals in order to induce the events that promote the progression of T cells through the cell cycle. Such signal transduction events must also account for other effects of IL-2, such as the upregulation of transcription of the IL-2R α chain. The IL-2 R α chain has a relatively short cytoplasmic domain, and it appears that its main function is to increase the sensitivity of the receptor by increasing its binding affinity for IL-2. It is the β and γ chains that are responsible for the signal transduction function of the receptor. Studies with chimeric molecules containing the cytoplasmic domains of β and γ established that the signaling function of the receptor is initiated by the heterodimerization of the cytoplasmic domains of these two subunits (434,435). The cytoplasmic domains of these chains do not encode enzymatic activity. Instead, they interact with cytoplasmic proteins to initiate the signals required for the proliferative and differentiation responses.

The β and γ chains of the IL-2R share a signal transduction mechanism, involving the cytoplasmic Jak family of PTKs and signal transducers and activators of transcription (STAT) family of transcription factors, with other members of the cytokine receptor fam-

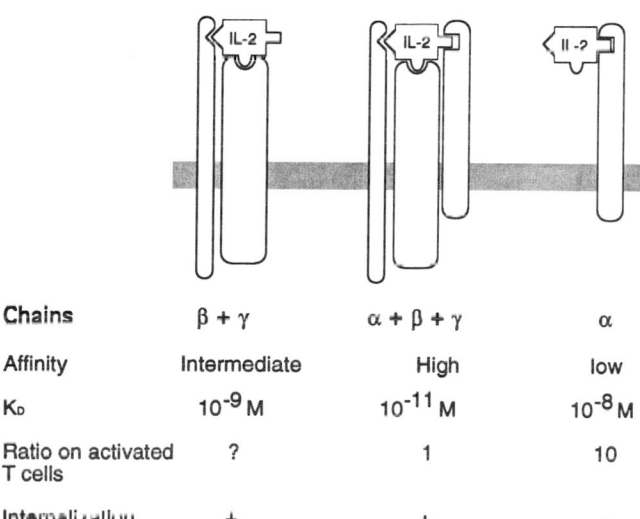

Chains	β + γ	α + β + γ	α
Affinity	Intermediate	High	low
K_D	10^{-9} M	10^{-11} M	10^{-8} M
Ratio on activated T cells	?	1	10
Internalization	+	+	-

FIG. 13. Various forms of the IL-2R. Neither the β nor the γ chain alone has detectable IL-2–binding capacity.

ily, which is discussed in detail in Chapter 21 (also reviewed in refs. 436,437). Briefly, the β and γ chains, through conserved regions that are adjacent to the plasma membrane, specifically interact with the Jak1 and Jak3 PTKs, respectively (438). The importance of Jak3 in this interaction has been established by the SCID syndrome that results in patients harboring Jak3 mutations or in mice in which the Jak3 gene has been disrupted (439,440). Dimerization of the β and γ chains leads to dimerization and activation of the associated Jak1 and Jak3 PTKs. This induces the phosphorylation mainly of associated STAT5 proteins. It is not clear how STAT proteins associate with the Jaks or receptor chains, though tyrosine phosphorylation of specific sites within the IL-2R β chain appears to be important for STAT5 phosphorylation (441). Thus, Jaks may phosphorylate cytokine receptor subunits to recruit the STAT5 to the stimulated receptor–Jak complex, where they are then phosphorylated by the PTKs. The tyrosine-phosphorylated STAT proteins then homo- or heterodimerize through the binding of their SH2 domains to a tyrosine-phosphorylated residue on their partner STAT. This induces the STATs to translocate to the nucleus, perhaps by revealing cryptic nuclear localization sequences. The nuclear-translocated STAT dimers bind to specific DNA target sequences and contribute to the transcriptional activation of target genes. Although the specific STAT-regulated target genes responsible for cell proliferation have not been identified, several genes relevant to growth control are induced by IL-2R stimulation, including c-myc, c-fos, c-jun and bcl-2 (419,436). The integrated actions of these and other target genes are likely to contribute to the overall cellular response.

Several other events have been associated with signal transduction by the IL-2R. In addition to the activation of the Jak–STAT system, stimulation of the IL-2R has been reported to activate other PTKs, namely Lck, Lyn and Syk (442–444). The Src kinases are thought to interact directly with the acidic region and Syk with the serine-rich region within the IL-2R β chain. These interactions have been correlated with the activation of Fos/Jun and Myc pathways, respectively (419,444). However, mice deficient in Lck and/or Fyn or in the Syk PTKs still have functional IL-2Rs (200,203,445,446). This suggests that other pathways may be able to subserve the functions associated with these interactions.

In addition to the associated PTKs, the tyrosine-phosphorylated IL-2R β chain interacts with two other molecules of interest, Shc and PI3-kinase (296,407,447). As mentioned, Shc functions as an adaptor to link the Ras pathway components to activated receptor systems. Ras is rapidly activated following IL-2R stimulation (316). The interaction of Shc with Y338 in the β chain of the IL-2R and the requirement for phosphorylation of this residue for c-fos transcriptional activation suggest that the interaction of Shc with the IL-2R β chain is functionally important (441). The SH2 domains of the p85 subunit of PI3-kinase also interact with tyrosine-phosphorylated residues of the β chain. This interaction is associated with activation of PI3-kinase function. The role of PI3-kinase in the control of cell growth is rapidly evolving, and multiple downstream pathways have been implicated (292). However, one downstream effector of PI3-kinase appears to be Akt (also known as PKB), a serine–threonine kinase. A function for Akt in blocking apoptosis has been described (448). It is tempting to speculate that at least one function of IL-2R–mediated activation of PI3-kinase is to block T-cell apoptosis during T-cell proliferative responses to a specific antigen.

Rapamycin is an immunosuppressive agent that has been used to probe the IL-2/IL-2R pathway (reviewed in ref. 449). It binds to the same cellular receptor as FK506, FKBP, and it is the

drug–receptor complex that mediates inhibition of T-cell function. However, unlike FK506, rapamycin does not inhibit the induction of IL-2, nor is its target calcineurin. Instead, it inhibits IL-2–driven T-cell proliferative responses by blocking the function of another enzyme, called mTOR (for mamalian target of rapamycin; also called FRAP, for FKBP12-rapamycin–associated protein). mTOR is a member of a larger family of proteins with PI-kinase domains. Efforts to identify mTOR targets through the use of rapamycin have focused on three targets that could be involved in the G_1 to S transition that is blocked by rapamycin. Ribosomal p70 S6 kinase activity is blocked by rapamycin, and mTOR has been implicated as an upstream regulator of p70 S6 kinase (450). Although the activation of p70 S6 kinase is universally observed in mitogenic responses, its specific requirement for S-phase entry is not established. Protein translational control may be under the control of mTOR through its phosphorylation of PHAS-1, the eukaryotic initiation factor (eIF)-4E–binding protein (451). Rapamycin blocks the mTOR-mediated phosphorylation of PHAS-1. This leads to blockade of the participation of eIF-4E in protein translation initiation, a critical step for G_1 progression. Finally, the effects of rapamycin have also been linked to cell-cycle control via its action on Kip-1, an inhibitor of the G_1 cyclin-cdks (452). Rapamycin blocks the downregulation of Kip-1 that is induced by IL-2 (453). How mTOR might prevent the downregulation of Kip-1 remains to be determined. Thus, while much remains to be clarified, the effects of rapamycin on mTor are likely to reveal important regulatory events involved in the proliferative responses of T cells.

Other Mechanisms Regulating T-Cell Growth

Although IL-2–driven T-cell proliferation has been widely considered to be the major mechanism responsible for T-cell growth, under some circumstances, T-cell proliferation can occur independently of IL-2. For instance, murine T-cell cytolytic clones can proliferate in response to anti-TCR mAb in the absence of detectable IL-2 (454), as can resting human T cells (455). Most importantly, the preservation of some proliferative responses in IL-2–deficient mice supports a role for mechanisms that can bypass IL-2–driven T-cell proliferation. Under these circumstances, limited T-cell proliferation may result from stimulation of the TCR itself, but sustained proliferation is likely to be dependent on growth factors.

It is most likely that IL-2–independent T-cell proliferation is the result of the actions of other lymphokines that can support the proliferative responses of T cells. IL-4 and IL-15 are the most likely to function as T-cell growth factors in the absence of IL-2. A detailed discussion of these lymphokines will be provided in Chapters 21 and 26. The contribution of other lymphokines to T-cell growth needs to be considered because different populations of T cells may undergo expansion. Hence, if IL-4 production predominates in a particular T-cell response, as it does in response to parasites and allergens, one may observe T-cell proliferation, but this proliferation may be restricted only to certain subsets of T cells (i.e., Th2 T-cell clones). The converse holds true for responses dominated by IL-2 production. Whether a growth factor is necessary in all cases of T-cell proliferation also remains an unanswered question. It is likely that more sustained T cell proliferative responses and recruitment of T cells will occur in instances in which T-cell growth factors such as IL-2, IL-4, or IL-15 are produced.

TERMINATING T-CELL RESPONSES

An uncontrolled or unending T-cell response would be devastating to the host. Relatively little is known about how the level of T-cell responses is regulated or how the responses are terminated. Exhaustion or elimination of a stimulating antigen may lead to termination of the input signal, but what determines when the response must end? Some regulatory mechanisms are known to exist. This is an area of research that is just evolving. However, it is useful to mention a few of the identified mechanisms that are likely to play important roles.

Of the signal transduction mechanisms that are induced during antigen recognition, most involve tyrosine or serine–threonine phosphorylation events. The PTKs and serine–threonine kinases exist in equilibrium with PTPases and serine–threonine phosphatases. The phosphatases themselves may be regulated through activation by phosphorylation or relocalization to substrates. PTPases with SH2 domains, such as SHP-1 and SHP-2, can be activated by their own tyrosine phosphorylation and can be targeted to relevant substrates via their SH2 domains (244). Mice deficient in SHP-1 have a lethal disease characterized by an overly active inflammatory system and have hyperresponsive Src kinase activities in their thymocytes (456,457).

A noteworthy example involves CTLA-4, which has been reported to interact with the SHP-2 PTPase (458). CTLA-4 is a transmembrane molecule that is homologous to CD28 (117). It is upregulated during T-cell activation. Mice deficient in CTLA-4 have a massive lymphoproliferative syndrome early in life, which appears to result from the unchecked polyclonal activation of T cells (459). Thus, CTLA-4 may serve in a negative-feedback loop to autoregulate T-cell responses, once initiated, by recruiting the SHP-2 PTPase to the plasma membrane, where it can act on relevant substrates associated with the TCR complex.

Csk, as mentioned previously, is a PTK that phosphorylates the negative regulatory sites in Src kinases, such as Lck. Although Csk is not regulated by its phosphorylation, its regulatory function depends on its SH2 and SH3 domains, which may serve to target it to its substrate after an immune response has been initiated (82). Studies suggest a model in which the tyrosine phosphatase PEP may serve to target Csk to the activated TCR complex to suppress the function of activated Lck and/or Fyn (460).

Lymphokines are extremely potent biologic mediators. Overproduction, such as occurs during food poisoning or toxic shock syndrome due to staphylococcal enterotoxins, can have devastating consequences on the host. Therefore, most lymphokines tend to be produced only transiently during an immune response. One mechanism to ensure their transient production is through the AU-rich 3′ untranslated region present in most lymphokines (405). This AU-rich region confers instability on the mRNAs encoding lymphokines, ensuring only a transient production of these potent mediators.

The final example of a mechanism that may contribute to the termination of T-cell activation during an immune response involves apoptosis. During the activation of antigen-responsive lymphocytes, the Fas ligand is upregulated on responsive T cells (62). In fact, expression of the Fas ligand gene is regulated by the same TCR signals that regulate lymphokine responses (461). In the absence of appropriate inflammatory signals, the expansion of antigen responsive T cells is followed by elimination of the activated T cells via apoptosis of Fas and Fas ligand–expressing T cells (61). As yet ill defined inflammatory cytokines or other signals of inflammation can prevent apoptosis of antigen-responsive T cells,

thus perpetuating an immune response in an inflammatory setting. The failure of this system can have dire consequences, as evidenced from the lymphoproliferative syndomes that result in humans with Fas mutations and in mice lacking functional Fas (*lpr* mice) or Fas ligand (*gld* mice) (374,462).

The termination and regulation of the immune response is as important as its initiation. The appropriate level of an immune response is critically important for the host. The regulatory systems involved in terminating the response are likely to be at least as complex as the systems that have evolved to initiate it.

T-CELL INACTIVATION

Stimulation of T cells, under certain *in vivo* conditions as well as certain *in vitro* culture conditions, with reagents that normally function as agonists can lead to a long-lived state in which they are unresponsive to subsequent TCR stimulation (101). This state of unresponsiveness has been termed *anergy*. The unresponsive state has been induced in T-cell clones stimulated with mitogens, antigen, altered peptide ligands, anti-TCR mAb, and lymphokines. These experimental models may be relevant to understanding certain forms of tolerance, particularly to peripheral (extrathymic) antigens, as well as in understanding how the outcomes of immune responses may differ as a result of different types of antigenic challenge.

Several factors appear to influence the ability of stimuli to induce unresponsiveness rather than activation of T-cell clones. A critical factor toward the induction of the unresponsive state is the nature of the responding cell. Unresponsiveness has only been induced in helper T-cell clones of the Th1 subtype (463,464). Under similar conditions, unresponsiveness could not be induced in cytolytic T-cell clones (465). Similar states of unresponsiveness have not been induced in T-cell hybridomas or leukemic lines. However, anergy has been induced by antigen injection in naive mice (466).

The nature and the context of the stimulus are critical factors in the induction of unresponsiveness. Antigen presented on the surface of fixed APCs or on planar lipid membranes reconstituted only with class II MHC molecules induces a long-lived state of unresponsiveness to subsequent antigenic challenge in antigen-specific murine helper T-cell clones, but not hybridomas, as measured by proliferative responses or IL-2 production (166,467). Inactivation is not complete and refers mainly to the proliferative response because suboptimal IFN-γ and IL-3 are produced in response to subsequent antigen challenge. Moreover, the proliferative response can be restored by exogenous IL-2 (28). The principle defect during the induction of the anergic state appears to be the reception of a TCR-derived signal, which involves a rise in $[Ca^{2+}]_i$, in the absence of a subsequent IL-2 stimulus (101,104).

The failure to produce IL-2 in most of these models is due to the failure of the T cell to receive a costimulatory signal. The preponderance of evidence suggests that the interaction of CD28 with either B7-1 or B7-2 is responsible for the costimulatory signal, as discussed earlier (reviewed in ref. 117). However, blockade of the CD28–B7 interaction only occasionally results in the induction of the anergic state (107,112,127,468). This suggests that there may be other costimulatory pathways that can lead to IL-2 production. Alternatively, under some circumstances of very potent TCR stimuli, it may be possible to induce IL-2 production in the absence of costimulation. This is consistent with the observations that CD28-deficient mice can still make some immune responses (112,127).

Altered-peptide ligands can also induce an anergic state in the presence of appropriate costimulatory signals (45). This may result from an inadequate TCR signal, perhaps due to ineffective TCR ζ-chain phosphorylation and ZAP-70 activation (46). It is clear, however, that it is the failure to produce and respond to IL-2 that is the most important determinant of whether anergy is induced (104).

The establishment and characterization of the unresponsive state has received considerable attention. Induction of the unresponsive state requires protein synthesis, suggesting that a newly synthesized protein may be required for the maintenance of the unresponsive state. Studies suggest a defect in Ras activation, with resulting defects in MAPK and Jnk activation following the stimulation of the TCR in anergized T cells (396,397). The failure to activate Ras and these kinases helps to explain previous results that demonstrated diminished AP-1 activity in an anergized T-cell clone (395). The failure to activate Ras, however, remains to be explained.

CONCLUSION

The activation of T-lymphocytes is a complex process that results in cell growth and differentiation. Examples of the major events involved are presented in Table 4. T-cell activation is initiated by ligand–receptor interactions that occur at the interface of the T cell and APC or target cell. The TCR plays a prominent role in this interaction, but other molecules on the T cell and APC also contribute to the ultimate activation of the T cell. Stimulation of the TCR induces a highly ordered sequence of tyrosine phosphorylation events that are orchestrated by PTKs and are regulated by other PTKs and PTPases. These phosphorylation events lead to signaling pathways that activate a variety of enzymes and induce a multitude of protein interactions. Second messengers are produced, and ion fluxes occur. Cascades of these signaling events determine the T-cell response. In some cases, effector functions are activated. In others, expression of a variety of genes is induced, which contributes to the clonal expansion and differentiation of appropriate antigen-specific T cells. In still others, where signaling events are inadequate, a state of unresponsiveness ensues. Future studies promise to unravel some of the complexities of the events that occur in signaling pathways that lead from the membrane to the nucleus. The activation of the T cell has proven to be a unique system for sampling and exploring the complex mechanisms regulating cell growth and differentiation.

TABLE 4. *Major events involved in T-cell activation*

Event	Example
Cell–cell interaction	T cell–APC
	CTL–Target Cell
Receptor-ligand binding	TCR-Antigen/MHC
Transmembrane signal transduction	Activation of Lck
Generation of second messengers	1,4,5-IP_3 and DG
Second messenger effects	Ca^{2+} mobilization
	Protein kinase C activation
Biochemical pathways	Phosphatidylinositol pathway
	Ras pathway
Cellular events	MTOC reorganization
	Secretion of cytolytic granules
Early gene activation	c-*myc*, c-*fos*
Intermediate gene activation	Lymphokines, lymphokine receptors, nutrient receptors
Late gene activation	Genes involved in cell proliferation 4F2, VLA-2

REFERENCES

1. Clevers H, Alarcon B, Willeman T, Terhorst C. The T cell receptor/CD3 complex: a dynamic protein ensemble. *Annu Rev Immunol* 1988;6:629–662.
2. Ashwell JD, Klausner RD. Genetic and mutational analysis of the T cell antigen receptor. *Annu Rev Immunol* 1990;8:139–168.
3. Weiss A. Molecular and genetic insights into T cell antigen receptor structure and function. *Annu Rev Genet* 1991;25:487–510.
4. Schwartz RH. Costimulation of T lymphocytes: the role of CD28, CTLA-4, and B7/BB1 in interleukin-2 production and immunotherapy. *Cell* 1992;71:1065–1068.
5. Smith KA. Interleukin-2: inception, impact, and implications. *Science* 1986;240:1169–1176.
6. Waldmann TA. The IL-2/IL-2 receptor system: A target for rational immune intervention. *Immunol Today* 1993;14:264–270.
7. Crabtree GR, Clipstone NA. Signal transmission between the plasma membrane and nucleus of T lymphocytes. *Annu Rev Biochem* 1994;63:1045–1083.
8. Marrack P, Kappler J. T cells can distinguish between allogeneic major histocompatibility complex products on different cell types. *Nature* 1988;332:840–843.
9. Linsley PS, Ledbetter JA. The role of the CD28 receptor during T cell responses to antigen. *Annu Rev Immunol* 1993;11:191–212.
10. June CH, Bluestone JA, Nadler LM, Thompson CB. The B7 and CD28 receptor families. *Immunol Today* 1994;15:321–331.
11. Watts TH, Brian AA, Kappler JW, Marrack P, McConnell H. Antigen presentation by supported planar membranes containing affinity-purified I-Ad *Proc Natl Acad Sci USA* 1984;81:7564–7568.
12. O'Rourke AM, Rogers J, Mescher MF. Activated CD8 binding to class I protein mediated by the T-cell receptor results in signalling. *Nature* 1990;346:187–189.
13. Shaw AS, Dustin ML. Making the T cell receptor go the distance: a topological view of T cell activation. *Immunity* 1997;6:361–369.
14. Ronchese F, Schwartz RH, Germain RN. Functionally distinct subsites on a class II major histocompatibility complex molecule. *Nature* 1987;329:254–256.
15. Goldstein SAN, Mescher MF. Cytotoxic T cell activation by class I protein on cell size artificial membranes: antigen density and Lyt-2/3 function. *J Immunol* 1987;138:2034–2043.
16. Clayberger C, Parham P, Rothbard J, Ludwig DS, Schoolnik GK, Krensky AM. HLA-A2 peptides can regulate cytolysis by human allogeneic T lymphocytes. *Nature* 1987;330:763–765.
17. York I, Rock KL. Antigen processing and presentation by the class I major histocompatibility complex. *Annu Rev Immunol* 1996;14:369–396.
18. Herman A, Kappler JW, Marrack P, Pullen AM. Superantigens: mechanism of T-cell stimulation and role in immune responses. *Annu Rev Immunol* 1991;9:745–772.
19. Fields BA, Malchiodi EL, Li H, et al. Crystal structure of a T-cell receptor β-chain complexed with a superantigen. *Nature* 1996;384:188–192.
20. Fraser JD, Newton ME, Weiss A. CD28 and T cell antigen receptor signal transduction coordinately regulate interleukin 2 gene expression in response to superantigen stimulation. *J Exp Med* 1992;175:1131–1134.
21. O'Rourke AM, Mescher MF, Webb SR. Activation of polyphosphoinositide hydrolysis in T cells by H-2 alloantigen but not MLS determinants. *Science* 1990;249:171–174.
22. Yamasaki S, Tachibana M, Shinohara N, Iwashima M. Lck-independent triggering of T-cell antigen receptor signal transduction by staphylococcal enterotoxin. *J Biol Chem* 1997;272:14787–14791.
23. Liu H, Lampe MA, Iregui MV, Cantor H. Conventional antigen and superantigen may be coupled to distinct and cooperative T-cell activation pathways. *Proc Natl Acad Sci USA* 1991;88:8705–8709.
24. Sharon N. Lectin receptors as lymphocyte surface markers. *Adv Immunol* 1983;34:213–298.
25. Nowell PC. Phytohemagglutinin: an initiator of mitosis in cultures of normal human leukocytes. *Cancer Res* 1960;20:462–466.
26. Kanellopoulos JM, De Petris S, Leca G, Crumpton MJ. The mitogenic lectin from Phaseolus vulgaris does not recognize the T3 antigen of human T lymphocytes. *Eur J Immunol* 1985;15:478–486.
27. Weiss A, Shields R, Newton M, Manger B, Imboden J. Ligand-receptor interactions required for commitment to the activation of the interleukin 2 gene. *J Immunol* 1987;138:2169–2176.
28. Mueller DL, Jenkins MK, Schwartz RH. Clonal expansion vs functional inactivation. *Annu Rev Immunol* 1989;7:445–480.
29. Tax WJM, Hermes FFM, Willems RW, Capel PJA, Koene RAP. Fc receptors for mouse IgG1 on human monocytes: Polymorphism and its role in antibody-induced T cell proliferation. *J Immunol* 1984;133:1185–1189.
30. Palacios R, Martinez-Maza O. Is the E receptor on human T lymphocytes a "negative signal receptor"? *J Immunol* 1982;129:2479–2485.

31. Meuer SC, Hussey RE, Fabbi M, et al. An alternative pathway of T-cell activation: a functional role of the 50 kd T11 sheep erythrocyte receptor protein. *Cell* 1984;36:897–906.
32. Yang SY, Chouaib S, Dupont B. A common pathway for T lymphocyte activation involving both the CD3-Ti complex and CD2 erythrocyte receptor determinants. *J Immunol* 1986;137:1097–1100.
33. Weiss A, Imboden J, Shoback D, Stobo J. Role of T3 surface molecules in human T-cell activation: T3-dependent activation results in an increase in cytoplasmic free calcium. *Proc Natl Acad Sci USA* 1984;81:4169–4173.
34. Truneh A, Albert F, Golstein P, Schmitt-Verhulst AM. Early steps of lymphocyte activation bypassed by synergy between calcium ionophores and phorbol ester. *Nature* 1985;313:318–320.
35. Mustelin T, Coggeshall KM, Isakov N, Altman A. T cell antigen receptor-mediated activation of phospholipase C requires tyrosine phosphorylation. *Science* 1990;247:1584–1587.
36. June CH, Fletcher MC, Ledbetter JA, et al. Inhibition of tyrosine phosphorylation prevents T cell receptor-mediated signal transduction. *Proc Natl Acad Sci USA* 1990;87:7722–7726.
37. Weiss A, Imboden JB. Cell surface molecules and early events involved in human T lymphocyte activation. *Adv Immunol* 1987;41:1–38.
38. Bierer BE, Sleckman BP, Ratnofsky SE, Burakoff SJ. The biological roles of CD2, CD4, and CD8 in T-cell activation. *Immuno Rev* 1989;7:579–599.
39. Dustin ML, Sanders ME, Shaw S, Springer TA. Purified lymphocyte function-associated antigen 3 binds to CD2 and mediates T lymphocyte adhesion. *J Exp Med* 1987;165:677–692.
40. Schmitt-Verhulst AM, Guimezanes A, Boyer C, et al. Pleiotropic loss of activation pathways in a T-cell receptor a-chain deletion variant of a cytolytic T-cell clone. *Nature* 1987;325:628–631.
41. Gunter KC, Germain RN, Kroczek R, A., et al. Thy-1-mediated T-cell activation requires co-expression of CD3/Ti complex. *Nature* 1987;326:505–507.
42. Breitmeyer JB, Daley JF, Levine HF, Schlossman SF. The T11 (CD2) molecule functionally linked to the T3/Ti T cell receptor in the majority of T cells. *J Immunol* 1987;139:2899–2905.
43. Bockenstedt LK, Goldsmith MA, Dustin M, Olive D, Springer TA, Weiss A. The CD2 ligand LFA-3 activates T cells but depends on the expression and function of the antigen receptor. *J Immunol* 1988;141:1904–1911.
44. Howard FD, Moingeon P, Moebius U, et al. The CD3ζ cytoplasmic domain mediates CD2-induced T cell activation. *J Exp Med* 1992;176:139–145.
45. Sloan-Lancaster J, Evavold BE, Allen P. Induction of T-cell anergy by altered T-cell-receptor ligand on live antigen-presenting cells. *Nature* 1993;363:156–159.
46. Sloan-Lancaster J, Shaw AS, Rothbard JB, Allen PM. Partial T cell signaling: altered phospho-zeta and lack of zap70 recruitment in APL-induced T cell anergy. *Cell* 1994;79:913–922.
47. Rabinowitz JD, Beeson C, Wulfing C, et al. Altered T cell receptor ligands trigger a subset of early T cell signals. *Immunity* 1996;5:125–135.
48. Lyons DS, Lieberman SA, Hampl J, et al. A TCR binds to antagonist ligands with lower affinities and faster dissociation rates than to agonists. *Immunity* 1996;5:53–61.
49. Madrenas J, Germain R. Variant TCR ligands: new insights into the molecular basis of antigen-dependent signal transduction and T cell activation. *Semin Immunol* 1996;8:83–101.
50. Lanier LL, Ruitenberg JJ, Allison JP, Weiss A. Distinct epitopes on the T cell antigen receptor of HPB-ALL tumor cells identified by monoclonal antibodies. *J Immunol* 1986;137:2286–2292.
51. Rojo JM, Janeway J, CA. The biological activity of anti-T cell receptor antibodies is determined by the epitope recognized. *J Immunol* 1988;140:1081–1088.
52. Finkel TH, Cambier JC, Kubo RT, Born WK, Marrack P, Kappler JW. The thymus has two functionally distinct populations of immature ab+ T cells: one population is deleted by ligation of abTCR. *Cell* 1989;58:1047–1054.
53. Demotz S, Grey HM, Sette A. The minimal number of class II MHC-antigen complexes needed for T cell activation. *Science* 1990;249:1028–1030.
54. Harding CV, Unanue E. Quantitation of antigen-presenting cell MHC class II/peptide complexes necessary for T-cell stimulation. *Nature* 1990;346:574–576.
55. Christinick ER, Luscher MA, Barber BH, Williams DB. Peptide binding to class I MHC on living cells and quantitation of complexes required for CTL lysis. *Nature* 1991;352:67–70.
56. Chang TW, Kung PC, Gingras SP, Goldstein G. Does OKT3 monoclonal antibody react with an antigen-recognition structure on human T cells? *Proc Natl Acad Sci USA* 1981;78:1805–1809.
57. Van Wauwe JP, De Mey JR, Goosens JG. OKT3: a monoclonal anti-human T lymphocyte antibody with potent mitogenic properties. *J Immunol* 1980;124:2708–2713.
58. Valitutti S, Muller S, Cella M, Padovan E, Lanzavecchia A. Serial triggering of many T-cell receptors by a few peptide-MHC complexes. *Nature* 1995;375:148–151.
59. Sagerstrom CG, Kerr EM, Allison JP, Davis MM. Activation and differentiation requirements of primary T cells *in vitro*. *Proc Natl Acad Sci USA* 1993;90:8987–8991.
60. Webb S, Morris C, Sprent J. Extrathymic tolerance of mature T cells: Clonal elimination as a consequence of immunity. *Cell* 1990;63:1249–1256.
61. Vella AT, McCormack JE, Linsley PS, Kappler JW, Marrack P. Lipopolysaccharide interferes with the induction of peripheral T cell death. *Immunity* 1995;2:261–270.
62. van Parijs L, Abbas A. Role of Fas-mediated cell death in the regulation of immune responses. *Curr Opin Immunol* 1996;8:355–361.
63. Chatila T, Wood N, Parsonnet J, Geha RS. Toxic shock syndrome toxin-1 induces inositol phospholipid turnover, protein kinase C translocation, and calcium mobilization in human T cells. *J Immunol* 1988;140:1250–1256.
64. Iwashima M, Irving BA, van Oers NSC, Chan AC, Weiss A. Sequential interactions of the TCR with two distinct cytoplasmic tyrosine kinases. *Science* 1994;263:1136–1139.
65. Hara T, Fu SM. Human cell activation: I. Monocyte-independent activation and proliferation induced by anti-T3 monoclonal antibodies in the presence of tumor promoter 12-o-Tetradecanoyl Phorbol-13-acetate. *J Exp Med* 1985;161:641–656.
66. Williams JM, Deloria D, Hansen JA, et al. The events of primary T cell activation can be staged by use of sepharose-bound anti-T3 (64.1) monoclonal antibody and purified interleukin 1. *J Immunol* 1985;135:2249–2255.
67. Ceuppens JL, Bloemmen FJ, Van Wauwe JP. T cell unresponsiveness to the mitogenic activity of OKT3 antibody results from a deficiency of monocyte Fcg receptors for murine IgG2α and inability to cross-link the T3-Ti complex. *J Immunol* 1985;135:3882–3886.
68. Janeway CA Jr. The T cell receptor as a multicomponent signalling machine: CD4/CD8 coreceptors and CD45 in T cell activation. *Annu Rev Immunol* 1992;10:645–674.
69. Leahy DJ. A structural view of CD4 and CD8. *FASEB J* 1995;9:17–25.
70. Sakihama T, Smolyar A, Reinherz EL. Oligomerization of CD4 is required for stable binding to class II major histocompatibility complex proteins but not for interaction with human immunodeficiency virus gp120. *Proc Natl Acad Sci USA* 1995;92:6444–6448.
71. Salter RD, Norment AM, Chen BJ, et al. Polymorphism in the a2 domain of HLA-A molecules affects binding to CD8. *Nature* 1989;338:345–347.
72. Gao GF, Tormo J, Gerth UC, et al. Crystal structure of the complex between human CD8αα and HLA-A2. *Nature* 1997;387:630–634.
73. Zamoyska R. The CD8 coreceptor revisted: one chain good, two chains better. *Immunity* 1994;1:243–246.
74. Luescher IF, Vivier E, Layer A, et al. CD8 modulation of T-cell antigen receptor-ligand interactions on living cytotoxic T lymphocytes. *Nature* 1995;373:353–356.
75. Garcia KC, Scott CA, Brunmark A, et al. CD8 enhances formation of stable T-cell receptor/MHC class I molecule complexes [see comments]. *Nature* 1996;384:577–581.
76. Shaw AS, Amrein KE, Hammond C, Stern DF, Sefton BM, Rose JK. The lck protein tyrosine kinase interacts with the cytoplasmic tail of the CD4 glycoprotein through its unique amino terminal domain. *Cell* 1989;59:627–636.
77. Turner JM, Brodsky MH, Irving BA, Levin SD, Perlmutter RM, Littman DR. Interaction of the unique N terminal region of tyrosine kinase p56lck with cytoplasmic domains of CD4 and CD8 mediated by cysteine motifs. *Cell* 1990;60:755–765.
78. Wiest DL, Yuan L, Jefferson J, et al. Regulation of T cell receptor expression in immature CD4+CD8+ thymocytes by p56lck tyrosine kinase: basis for differential signaling by CD4 and CD8 in immature thymocytes expressing both coreceptor molecules. *J Exp Med* 1993;170:1701–1712.
79. Itano A, Salmon P, Kioussis D, Tolaini M, Corbella P, Robey E. The cytoplasmic domain of CD4 promotes the development of CD4 lineage T cells. *J Exp Med* 1996;183:731.
80. Robey E, Fowlkes BJ. Selective events in T cell development. *Annu Rev Immunol* 1994;12:675–705.
81. Ledbetter JA, Gilliland LK, Schieven GA. The interaction of CD4 with CD3/Ti regulates tyrosine phosphorylation of substrates during T cell activation. *Semin Immunology* 1990;2:99–106.
82. Chow LML, Veillette A. The Src and Csk families of tyrosine protein kinases in hemopoietic cells. *Semin Immunol* 1995;7:207–226.
83. Killeen N, Littman DR. Helper T-cell development in the absence of CD4-p56lck association. *Nature* 1993;364:729–732.
84. Xu H, Littman DR. A kinase-independent function of lck in potentiating antigen-specific T cell activation. *Cell* 1993;74:633–644.
85. O'Rourke AM, Mescher MF. Cytotoxic T-lymphocyte activation involves a cascade of signaling and adhesion events. *Nature* 1992;358:253–255.
86. Thome M, Duplay P, Guttinger M, Acuto O. Syk and ZAP-70 mediate recruitment of p56lck/CD4 to the activated T cell receptor/CD3/ζ complex. *J Exp Med* 1995;181:1997–2006.
87. Straus DB, Chan AC, Patai B, Weiss A. SH2 domain function is essential for the role of the Lck tyrosine kinase in T cell receptor signal transduction. *J Biol Chem* 1996;271:9976–9981.
88. Lee-Fruman KK, Collins TL, Burakoff SJ. Role of the Lck Src homology 2 and 3 domains in protein tyrosine phosphorylation. *J Biol Chem* 1996;271:25003–25010.
89. Doyle C, Strominger JL. Interaction between CD4 and class II MHC molecules mediates cell adhesion. *Nature* 1988;330:256–258.
90. Norment AM, Salter RD, Parham P, Engelhard VH, Littman DR. Cell-cell adhesion mediated by CD8 and MHC class I molecules. *Nature* 1988;336:79–81.
91. Newell MK, Haughn LJ, Maroun CR, Julius MH. Death of mature T cells by separate ligation of CD4 and the T-cell receptor for antigen. *Nature* 1990;347:286–289.
92. Banda NK, Bernier J, Kurahara DK, et al. Crosslinking CD4 by human immunodeficiency virus gp120 primes T cells for activation-induced apoptosis. *J Exp Med* 1992;176:1099–1106.
93. Glaichenhaus N, Shastri N, Littman DR, Turner JM. Requirement for association of p56lck with CD4 in antigen-specific signal transduction in T cells. *Cell* 1991;64:511–520.
94. Dustin ML, Springer TA. Role of lymphocyte adhesion receptors in transient interactions and cell locomotion. *Annu Rev Immunol* 1991;9:27–68.

95. Davis SJ, van der Merwe PA. The structure and ligand interactions of CD2: Implications for T cell function. *Immunol Today* 1996;17:177–187.

96. Janeway CA. The co-receptor function of CD4. *Semin Immunol* 1991;3:153–160.

97. Matsui K, Boniface JJ, Reay PA, Schild H, Fazekas De St. Groth B, Davis MM. Low affinity interaction of peptide-MHC complexes with T cell receptors. *Science* 1991;254:1788–1791.

98. Shimizu Y, van Seventer G, Horgan KJ, Shaw S. Roles of adhesion molecules in T-cell recognition: fundamental similarities between four integrins on resting human T cells (LFA-1, VLA-4, VLA-5, VLA-6) in expression, binding, and costimulation. *Immunol Rev* 1990;114:109–143.

99. Dustin ML, Springer TA. T-cell receptor cross-linking transiently stimulates adhesiveness through LFA-1. *Nature* 1989;341:619–624.

100. Hahn WC, Burakoff SJ, Bierer BE. Signal transduction pathways involved in T cell receptor-induced regulation of CD2 avidity for CD58. *J Immunol* 1993;150:2607–2619.

101. Schwartz RH. T cell clonal anergy. *Curr Opin Immunol* 1997;9:351–357.

102. Jenkins MK, Pardoll DM, Mizuguchi J, Chused TM, Schwartz RH. Molecular events in the induction of a nonresponsive state in interleukin 2-producing helper T-lymphocyte clones. *Proc Natl Acad Sci USA* 1987;84:5409–5413.

103. Shimonkevitz R, Kappler J, Marrack P, Grey H. Antigen recognition by H-2-restricted T cells. *J Exp Med* 1983;158:303–316.

104. Madrenas J, Schwartz RH, Germain RN. Interleukin 2 production, not the pattern of early T-cell antigen receptor-dependent tyrosine phosphorylation, controls anergy induction by both agonists and partial agonists. *Proc Natl Acad Sci USA* 1996;93:9736–9741.

105. Ledbetter JA, Martin PJ, Spooner CE, et al. Antibodies to Tp67 and Tp44 augment and sustain proliferative responses of activated T cells. *J Immunol* 1985;135:2331–2336.

106. Weiss A, Manger B, Imboden J. Synergy between the T3/antigen receptor complex and Tp44 in the activation of human T cells. *J Immunol* 1986;137:819–825.

107. Harding FA, McArthur JG, Gross JA, Raulet DH, Allison JP. CD28-mediated signalling co-stimulates murine T cells and prevents induction of anergy of T-cell clones. *Nature* 1992;356:607–609.

108. Linsley PS, Brady W, Grosmaire L, Aruffo A, Damle NK, Ledbetter JA. Binding of the B cell activation antigen B7 to CD28 costimulates T cell proliferation and interleukin 2 mRNA accumulation. *J Exp Med* 1991;173:721–730.

109. Linsley PS, Brady W, Urnes M, Grosmaire LS, Damle NK, Ledbetter JA. CTLA-4 is a second receptor for the B cell activation antigen B7. *J Exp Med* 1991;174:561–569.

110. Linsley PS, Wallace PM, Johnson J, et al. Immunosuppression in vivo by a soluble form of the CTLA-4 T cell activation moleucle. *Science* 1992;257:792–795.

111. Lenschow DJ, Zeng Y, Thisthwaite JR, et al. Long-term survival of xenogeneic pancreatic islet grafts induced by CTLA4lg. *Science* 1992;257:789–792.

112. Shahinian A, Pfeffer K, Lee KP, et al. Differential T cell costimulatory requirements in CD28-deficient mice. *Science* 1993;261:609–612.

113. Borriello F, Sethna MP, Boyd SD, et al. B7-1 and B7-2 have overlapping, critical roles in immunoglobulin class switching and germinal center formation. *Immunity* 1997;6:303–313.

114. Grewal IS, Foellmer HG, Grewal KD, et al. Requirement for CD40 ligand in costimulation induction, T cell activation, and experimental allergic encephalomyelitis. *Science* 1996;273:1864–1867.

115. Yang Y, Wilson JM. CD40 Ligand-dependent T cell activation: requirement of B7-CD28 signaling through CD40. *Science* 1996;273:1862–1864.

116. Foy TM, Aruffo A, Bajorath J, Buhlmann JE, Noelle RJ. Immune regulation by CD40 and its ligand GP39. *Annu Rev Immunol* 1996;14:591–617.

117. Lenschow DJ, Walunas TL, Bluestone JA. CD28/B7 system of T cell costimulation. *Annu Rev Immunol* 1996;14:233–258.

118. Thompson CG, Lindstein T, Ledbetter JA, et al. CD28 activation pathway regulates the production of multiple T-cell-derived lymphokines/cytokines. *Proc Natl Acad Sci USA* 1989;86:1333–1337.

119. Fraser JD, Weiss A. Regulation of T cell lymphokine transcription by the accessory molecule CD28. *Mol Cell Biol* 1992;12:4357–4363.

120. Lindsten T, June CH, Ledbetter JA, Stella G, Thompson CB. Regulation of lymphokine messenger RNA stability by a surface-mediated T cell activation pathway. *Science* 1989;244:339–342.

121. Fraser JD, Irving BA, Crabtree GR, Weiss A. Regulation of interleukin-2 gene enhancer activity by the T cell accessory molecule CD28. *Science* 1991;251:313–316.

122. Stein PH, Fraser JD, Weiss A. The cytoplasmic domain of CD28 is both necessary and sufficient for costimulation of interleukin-2 secretion and association with phosphatidylinosital 3'-kinase. *Mol Cell Biol* 1994;14:3392–3402.

123. Crooks MEC, Littman DR, Carter RH, Fearon DT, Weiss A, Stein PH. CD28-mediated costimulation in the absence of phosphatidylinositol 3-kinase association and activation. *Mol Cell Biol* 1995;15:6820–6828.

124. Truitt KE, Shi J, Gibson S, Segal LG, Mills GB, Imboden JB. CD28 delivers costimulatory signals independently of its association with phosphatidylinositol 3-kinase. *J Immunol* 1995;155:4702–4710.

125. Cai Y-C, Cefai D, Schneider H, Raab M, Nabavi N, Rudd CE. Selective CD28pYMNM mutations implicate phosphatidylinositol 3-kinase in CD86-CD28-mediated costimulation. *Immunity* 1995;3:417–426.

126. Pages F, Ragueneau M, Rottapel R, et al. Binding of phosphatidyl-inositol-3-OH kinase to CD28 is required for T-cell signalling. *Nature* 1994;369:327–329.

127. Kundig TM, Shahinian A, Kawai K, et al. Duration of TCR stimulation determines costimulatory requirement of T cells. *Immunity* 1996;5:41–52.

128. Liu Y, Jones B, Aruffo A, Sullivan KM, Linsley PS, Janeway CA. Heat-stable antigen is a costimulatory molecule for CD4 T cell growth. *J Exp Med* 1992;175:437–445.

129. Kaye J, Janeway CA Jr. The Fab fragment of a directly activating monoclonal antibody that precipitates a disulfide-linked heterodimer from a helper T cell clone blocks activation by either allogeneic Ia or antigen and self-Ia. *J Exp Med* 1984;159:1397–1412.

130. Abraham RT, Ho SN, Barna TJ, McKean DJ. Transmembrane signaling during interleukin 1-dependent T cell activation: interactions of signal 1- and signal 2-type mediators with the phosphoinositide-dependent signal transduction mechanism. *J Biol Chem* 1987;262:2719–2728.

131. Bekoff M, Kubo R, Grey HM. Activation requirements for normal T cells: accessory cell-dependent and-independent stimulation by anti-receptor antibodies. *J Immunol* 1986;137:1411–1419.

132. Dower SK, Kronheim SR, March CJ, et al. Detection and characterization of high affinity plasma membrane receptors for human interleukin 1. *J Exp Med* 1985;162:501–515.

133. Lowenthal JW, MacDonald HR. Binding and internalization of interleukin 1 by T cells. *J Exp Med* 1986;164:1060–1074.

134. Furue M, Chang CH, Tamaki K. Interleukin-1 but not tumour necrosis factor alpha synergistically upregulates the granulocyte-macrophage colony-stimulating factor-induced B7-1 expression of murine Langerhans cells. *Br J Dermatol* 1996;135:194–198.

135. Medzhitov R, Preston-Hurlburt P, Janeway CA, Jr. A human homologue of the Drosophila Toll protein signals activation of adaptive immunity [see comments]. *Nature* 1997;388:394–397.

136. Baeuerle PA, Henkel T. Function and activation of NF-kB in the immune system. *Annu Rev Immunol* 1994;12:141–179.

137. DiDonato JA, Hayakawa M, Rothwarf DM, Zandi E, Karin M. A cytokine-responsive IkappaB kinase that activates the transcription factor NF-kappaB [see comments]. *Nature* 1997;388:548–554.

138. Van Snick J. Interleukin-6: an overview. *Annu Rev Immunol* 1990;8:253–278.

139. Weiss A, Wiskocil R, Stobo JD. The role of T3 surface molecules in the activation of human T cells: a two stimulus requirement for IL-2 production reflects events occurring at a pre-translational level. *J Immunol* 1984;133:123–128.

140. Frank SJ, Samelson LE, Klausner RD. The structure and signalling functions of the invariant T cell receptor components. *Semin Immunol* 1990;2:89–97.

141. Blumberg R, Ley S, Sancho J, et al. Structure of the T-cell antigen receptor: evidence for two CD3 ε subunits in the T-cell receptor-CD3 complex. *Proc Natl Acad Sci USA* 1990;87:7220–7224.

142. Manolios N, Letourneur F, Bonifacino JS, Klausner RD. Pairwise, cooperative and inhibitory interactions describe the assembly and probable structure of the T-cell antigen receptor. *EMBO J* 1991;10:1643–1651.

143. Kearse KP, Roberts JL, Singer A. TCRα-CD3δε association is the initial step in αβ dimer formation in murine T cells and is limiting in immature CD4+CD8+ thymocytes. *Immunity* 1995;2:391–399.

144. Orloff DG, Ra C, Frank SJ, Klausner RD, Kinet J-P. Family of disulphide-linked dimers containing ζ and η chains of the T-cell receptor and the γ chain of Fc receptors. *Nature* 1990;347:189–191.

145. Tan L, Turner J, Weiss A. Regions of the T cell antigen receptor α and β chains that are responsible for interactions with CD3. *J Exp Med* 1991;173:1247–1256.

146. Irving B, Weiss A. The cytoplasmic domain of the T cell receptor ζ chain is sufficient to couple to receptor-associated signal transduction pathways. *Cell* 1991;64:891–901.

147. Romeo C, Seed B. Cellular immunity to HIV activated by CD4 fused to T cell or Fc receptor polypeptides. *Cell* 1991;64:1037–1046.

148. Letourneur F, Klausner RD. Activation of T cells by a tyrosine kinase activation domain in the cytoplasmic tail of CD3ε. *Science* 1992;255:79–82.

149. Wegener A-MK, Letourneur F, Hoeveler A, Brocker T, Luton F, Malissen B. The T cell receptor/CD3 complex is composed of at least two autonomous transduction modules. *Cell* 1992;68:83–95.

150. Reth M. Antigen receptor tail clue. *Nature* 1989;338:383–384.

151. Romeo C, Amiot M, Seed B. Sequence requirements for induction of cytolysis by the T cell antigen/Fc receptor ζ chain. *Cell* 1992;68:889–897.

152. Irving BA, Chan AC, Weiss A. Functional characterization of a signal transducing motif present in the T cell receptor ζ chain. *J Exp Med* 1993;177:1093–1103.

153. Lin S, Cicala C, Scharenberg AM, Kinet J-P. The FceR1b subunit functions as an amplifier of FceR1γ-mediated cell activation signals. *Cell* 1996;85:985–995.

154. Shores EW, Tran T, Grinberg A, Sommers CL, Shen H, Love PE. Role of the multiple T cell receptor (TCR)-ζ chain signaling motifs in selection of the T cell repertoire. *J Exp Med* 1997;185:893–900.

155. Letourneur F, Klausner RD. T-cell and basophil activation through the cytoplasmic tail of T-cell-receptor ζ family proteins. *Proc Natl Acad Sci USA* 1991;88:8905–8909.

156. Osman N, Turner H, Lucas S, Reif K, Cantrell DA. The protein interactions of the immunoglobulin receptor family tyrosine-based activation motifs present in the T cell receptor ζ subunits and the CD3γ,δ and ε chains. *Eur J Immunol* 1996;26:1063–1068.

157. Rozdzial MM, Malissen B, Finkel TH. Tyrosine-phosphorylated T cell receptor ζ chain associates with the actin cytoskeleton upon activation of mature T lymphocytes. *Immunity* 1995;3:623–633.

158. Combadière B, Freedman M, Chen L, Shores EW, Love P, Lenardo MJ. Qualitative and quantitative contributions of the T cell receptor zeta chain to mature T cell apoptosis. *J Exp Med* 1996;183:2109–2117.

159. Willems L, Gatot JS, Mammerickx M, et al. The YXXL signalling motifs of the bovine leukemia virus transmembrane protein are required for in vivo infection and maintenance of high viral loads. *J Virol* 1995;69:4137–4141.

160. Miller CL, Burkhardt AL, Lee JH, et al. Integral membrane protein 2 of Epstein-Barr virus regulates reactivation from latency through dominant negative effects on protein-tyrosine kinases. *Immunity* 1995;2.

161. Du Z, Lang SM, Sasseville VG, et al. Identification of a nef allele that causes lymphocyte activations and acute disease in macaque monkeys. *Cell* 1995;82:665–674.

162. Cantrell DA, Davies AA, Crumpton MJ. Activators of protein kinase C down-regulate and phosphorylate the T3/T-cell antigen receptor complex of human T lymphocytes. *Proc Natl Acad Sci USA* 1985;82:8158–8162.

163. Dietrich J, Hou X, Wegener AM, Pedersen LO, Odum N, Geisler C. Molecular characterization of the di-leucine-based internalization motif of the T cell receptor. *J Biol Chem* 1996;271:11441–11448.

164. Goldsmith MA, Weiss A. Isolation and characterization of a T-lymphocyte somatic mutant with altered signal transduction by the antigen receptor. *Proc Natl Acad Sci USA* 1987;84:6879–6883.

165. Dianzani U, Shaw A, Al-Ramadi BK, Kubo RT, Janeway CA Jr. Physical association of CD4 with the T cell receptor. *J Immunol* 1992;148:678–688.

166. Hsi ED, Siegel JN, Minami Y, Luong ET, Klausner RD, Samelson LE. T cell activation induces rapid tyrosine phosphorylation of a limited number of cellular substrates. *J Biol Chem* 1989;264:10836–10842.

167. June CH, Fletcher MC, Ledbetter JA, Samelson LE. Increases in tyrosine phosphorylation are detectable before phospholipase C activation after T cell receptor stimulation. *J Immunol* 1990;144:1591–1599.

168. Samelson LE, Patel MD, Weissman AM, Harford JB, Klausner RD. Antigen activation of murine T cells induces tyrosine phosphorylation of a polypeptide associated with the T cell antigen receptor. *Cell* 1986;46:1083–1090.

169. Baniyash M, Garcia-Morales P, Luong E, Samelson LE, Klausner RD. The T cell antigen receptor ζ chain is tyrosine phosphorylated upon activation. *J Biol Chem* 1988;263:18225–18230.

170. Qian D, Griswold-Prenner I, Rosner MR, Fitch FW. Multiple components of the T cell antigen receptor complex become tyrosine-phosphorylated upon activation. *J Biol Chem* 1993;268:4488–4493.

171. Weiss A. T cell antigen receptor signal transduction: a tale of tails and cytoplasmic protein-tyrosine kinases. *Cell* 1993;73:209–212.

172. Brown MT, Cooper JA. Regulation, substrates and functions of src. *Biochim Biophys Acta* 1996;1287:121–149.

173. Yurchak LK, Sefton BM. Palmitoylation of either Cys-3 or Cys-5 is required for the biological activity of the Lck tyrosine protein kinase. *Mol Cell Biol* 1995;15:6914–6922.

174. Shenoy-Scaria AM, Gauen LKT, Kwong J, Shaw AS, Lublin DM. Palmitoylation of an amino-terminal cysteine motif of protein tyrosine kinases p56lck and p59fyn mediates interactions with glycosyl-phosphatidylinositol-anchored protein. *Mol Cell Biol* 1993;13:6385–6392.

175. Yamaguchi H, Hendrickson WA. Structural basis for activation of human lymphocyte kinase Lck upon tyrosine phosphorylation. *Nature* 1996;384:484–489.

176. Sicheri F, Moarefi I, Kuriyan J. Crystal structure of the Src family tyrosine kinase Hck. *Nature* 1997;385:602–609.

177. Xu W, Harrison SC, Eck MJ. Three-dimensional structure of the tyrosine kinase c-Src. *Nature* 1997;385:595–602.

178. Cooke MP, Perlmutter RM. Expression of a novel form of the fyn proto-oncogene in hematopoietic cells. *New Biologist* 1989;1:66–74.

179. Davidson D, Chow LML, Fournel M, Veillette A. Differential regulation of T cell antigen responsiveness by isoforms of the src-related tyrosine protein kinase p59fyn. *J Exp Med* 1992;175:1483–1492.

180. Samelson LE, Phillips AF, Luong ET, Klausner RD. Association of the fyn protein-tyrosine kinase with the T-cell antigen receptor. *Proc Natl Acad Sci USA* 1990;87:4358–4362.

181. Gassmann M, Amrein KE, Flint NA, Schraven B, Burn P. Identification of a signaling complex involving CD2, ζ chain and p59fyn in T lymphocytes. *Eur J Immunol* 1994;24:139–144.

182. Gauen LKT, Kong A-NT, Samelson LE, Shaw AS. p59fyn tyrosine kinase associates with multiple T-cell receptor subunits through its unique amino-terminal domain. *Mol Cell Biol* 1992;12:5438–5446.

183. Ley SC, Marsh M, Bebbington CR, Proudfoot K, Jordan P. Distinct intracellular localization of Lck and Fyn protein tyrosine kinases in human T lymphocytes. *J Cell Biol* 1994;125:639–649.

184. Tsyganov AY, Broker BM, Fargnoli J, Ledbetter JA, Bolen JB. Activation of tyrosine kinase p60fyn following T cell antigen receptor cross-linking. *J Biol Chem* 1992;267:18259–18262.

185. Tsyganov AY, Spana C, Rowley RB, Penhallow RC, Burkardt AL, Bolen JS. Activation-dependent tyrosine phosphorylation of Fyn-associated proteins in T lymphocytes. *J Biol Chem* 1994;269:7792–7800.

186. O'Shea JJ, Ashwell JD, Bailey TL, Cross SL, Samelson LE, Klausner RD. Expression of v-src in a murine T-cell hybridoma results in constitutive T-cell receptor phosphorylation and interleukin 2 production. *Proc Natl Acad Sci USA* 1991;88:1741–1745.

187. Abraham N, Miceli MC, Parnes JR, Veillette A. Enhancement of T-cell responsiveness by the lymphocyte-specific tyrosine protein kinase p56lck. *Nature* 1991;350:62–66.

188. Cooke MP, Abraham KM, Forbush KA, Perlmutter RM. Regulation of T cell receptor signaling by a src family protein-tyrosine kinase (p59fyn). *Cell* 1991;65:281–292.

189. Appleby MW, Gross JA, Cooke MP, Levin SD, Qian X, Perlmutter RM. Defective T cell receptor signaling in mice lacking the thymic isoform of p59fyn. *Cell* 1992;70:751–763.

190. Stein PL, Lee H-M, Rich S, Soriano P. pp59fyn mutant mice display differential signaling in thymocytes and peripheral T cells. *Cell* 1992;70:741–750.

191. Lev S, Moreno H, Martinez R, et al. Protein tyrosine kinase PYK2 involved in Ca^{2+}-induced regulation of ion channel and MAP kinase functions. *Nature* 1995;376:737–745.

192. Qian D, Lev S, van Oers NSC, Dikic I, Schlessinger J, Weiss A. Tyrosine phosphorylation of Pyk2 is selectively regulated by Fyn during TCR signaling. *J Exp Med* 1997;185:1253–1259.

193. Rudd CE, Trevillyan JM, Dasgupta JD, Wong LL, Schlossman SF. The CD4 receptor is complexed in detergent lysates to a protein-tyrosine kinase (pp58) from human T lymphocytes. *Proc Natl Acad Sci USA* 1988;85:5190–5194.

194. Veillette A, Bookman MA, Horak EM, Bolen JB. The CD4 and CD8 T cell surface antigens are associated with the internal membrane tyrosine-protein kinase p56lck. *Cell* 1988;55:301–308.

195. Haughn L, Gratton S, Caron L, Sekaly R-P, Veillette A, Julius M. Association of tyrosine kinase p56lck with CD4 inhibits the induction of growth through the T-cell receptor. *Nature* 1992;358:328–331.

196. Beyers AD, Spruyt LL, Williams AF. Molecular associations between the T-lymphocyte antigen receptor complex and the surface antigens CD2, CD4, or CD8 and CD5. *Proc Natl Acad Sci USA* 1992;89:2945–2949.

197. Burgess KE, Odysseos AD, Zalvan C, et al. Biochemical identification of a direct physical interaction between the CD4:p56lck and Ti(TCR)/CD3 complexes. *Eur J Immunol* 1991;21:1663–1668.

198. Straus DB, Weiss A. The CD3 chains of the T cell antigen receptor associate with the ZAP-70 tyrosine kinase and are tyrosine phosphorylated after receptor stimulation. *J Exp Med* 1993;178:1523–1530.

199. Straus D, Weiss A. Genetic evidence for the involvement of the Lck tyrosine kinase in signal transduction throught the T cell antigen receptor. *Cell* 1992;70:585–593.

200. Molina TJ, Kishihara K, Siderovski DP, et al. Profound block in thymocyte development in mice lacking p56lck. *Nature* 1992;357:161–164.

201. Karnitz L, Sutor SL, Torigoe T, et al. Effects of p56lck on the growth and cytolytic effector function of an interleukin-2-dependent cytotoxic T-cell line. *Mol Cell Biol* 1992;12:4521–4530.

202. van Oers NSC, Killeen N, Weiss A. Lck regulates the tyrosine phosphorylation of the T cell receptor subunits and ZAP-70 in murine thymocytes. *J Exp Med* 1996;183:1053–1062.

203. van Oers NSC, Lowin-Kropf B, Finlay D, Connolly K, Weiss A. ab T cell development is abolished in mice lacking both Lck and Fyn protein tyrosine kinases. *Immunity* 1996;5:429–436.

204. Groves T, Smiley P, Cooke MP, Forbush K, Perlmutter RM, Guidos CJ. Fyn can partially substitute for Lck in T lymphocyte development. *Immunity* 1996;5:417–428.

205. Danielian S, Alcover A, Polissard L, et al. Both T cell receptor (TcR)-CD3 complex and CD2 increase the tyrosine kinase activity of p56lck. CD2 can mediate TcR-independent and CD45-dependent activation of p56lck. *Eur J Immunol* 1992;22:2915–2921.

206. Veillette A, Bookman MA, Horak EM, Samelson LE, Bolen JB. Signal transduction through the CD4 receptor involves the activation of the internal membrane tyrosine-protein kinase p56lck. *Nature* 1989;338:257–259.

207. van Oers NSC, Weiss A. The Syk/ZAP-70 protein tyrosine kinase connection to antigen receptor signalling processes. *Semin Immunol* 1995;7:227–236.

208. Chan AC, Iwashima M, Turck CW, Weiss A. ZAP-70: A 70kD protein tyrosine kinase that associates with the TCR ζ chain. *Cell* 1992;71:649–662.

209. Chan AC, Irving BA, Fraser JD, Weiss A. The ζ-chain is associated with a tyrosine kinase and upon T cell antigen receptor stimulation associates with ZAP-70, a 70 kilodalton tyrosine phosphoprotein. *Proc Natl Acad Sci USA* 1991;88:9166–9170.

210. Taniguchi T, Kobayashi T, Kondo J, et al. Molecular cloning of a porcine gene syk that encodes a 72-kDa protein-tyrosine kinase showing high susceptibility to proteolysis. *J Biol Chem* 1991;266:15790–15796.

211. Chan AC, van Oers NSC, Tran A, et al. Differential expression of ZAP-70 and Syk protein tyrosine kinases, and the role of this family of protein tyrosine kinases in T cell antigen receptor signaling. *J Immunol* 1994;152:4758–4766.

212. Mallick-Wood CA, Pao W, Cheng AM, et al. Disruption of epithelial gd T cell repertoires by mutation of the Syk tyrosine kinase. *Proc Natl Acad Sci USA* 1996;93:9701–9705.

213. Wange RL, Malek SN, Desiderio S, Samelson LE. Tandem SH2 domains of ZAP-70 bind to T cell antigen receptor z and CD3e from activated Jurkat T cells. *J Biol Chem* 1993;268:19797–19801.

214. Bu J-Y, Shaw AS, Chan AC. Analysis of the interaction of ZAP-70 and syk protein-tyrosine kinases with the T-cell antigen receptor by plasmon resonance. *Proc Natl Acad Sci USA* 1995;92:5106–5110.

215. Pawson T, Schlessinger J SH2 and SH3 domains. *Curr Biol* 1993;3:434–442.

216. Hatada MH, Lu X, Laird ER, et al. Molecular basis for interaction of the protein tyrosine kinase ZAP-70 with the T cell receptor. *Nature* 1995;377:32–38.

217. Keshvara LM, Isaacson C, Harrison ML, Geahlen RL. Syk activation and dissociation from the B-cell antigen receptor is mediated by phosphorylation of tyrosine 130. *J Biol Chem* 1997;272:10377–10381.

218. Watts JD, Affolter M, Krebs DL, Wange RL, Samelson LE, Aebersold R. Identification by electrospray ionization mass spectrometry of the sites of tyrosine

phosphorylation induced in activated Jurkat T cells on the protein tyrosine kinase ZAP-70. *J Biol Chem* 1994;269:29520–29529.

219. Kong G, Dalton M, Wardenburg JB, Straus D, Kurosaki T, Chan AC. Distinct tyrosine phosphorylation sites in ZAP-70 mediate activation and negative regulation of antigen receptor function. *Mol Cell Biol* 1996;16:5026–5035.

220. Zhao Q, Weiss A. Enhancement of lymphocyte responsiveness by a gain-of-function mutation of ZAP-70. *Mol Cell Biol* 1996;16:6765–6774.

221. Wange RL, Guitian R, Isakov N, Watts JD, Aebersold R, Samelson LE. Activating and inhibitory mutations in adjacent tyrosines in the kinase domain of ZAP-70. *J Biol Chem* 1995;270:18730–18733.

222. Furlong MT, Mahrenholz AM, Kim KH, Ashendel CL, Harrison ML, Geahlen RL. Identification of the major sites of autophosphorylation of the murine protein-tyrosine kinase Syk. *Biochim Biophys Acta* 1997;1355:177–190.

223. Chan AC, Dalton M, Johnson R, et al. Activation of ZAP-70 kinase activity by phosphorylation of tyrosine 493 is required for lymphocyte antigen receptor function. *EMBO J* 1995;14:2499–2508.

224. Kurosaki T, Johnson SA, Pao L, Sada K, Yamamura H, Cambier JC. Role of the Syk autophosphorylation site and SH2 domains in B cell antigen receptor signaling. *J Exp Med* 1995;182:1815–1823.

225. Chan AC, Shaw AS. Regulation of antigen receptor signal transduction by protein tyrosine kinases. *Curr Opin Immunol* 1996;8:394–401.

226. Latour S, Chow LML, Veillette A. Differential intrinsic enzymatic activity of Syk and Zap-70 protein-tyrosine kinases. *J Biol Chem* 1996;271:22782–22790.

227. Kong G-H, Bu J-Y, Kurosaki T, Shaw AS, Chan AC. Reconstitution of Syk function by the ZAP-70 protein tyrosine kinase. *Immunity* 1995;2:485–492.

228. Wiest DL, Ashe JM, Howcroft TK, et al. A spontaneously arising mutation in the DLAARN motif of murine ZAP-70 abrogates kinase activity and arrests thymocyte development. *Immunity* 1997;6:663–671.

229. Arpaia E, Shahar M, Dadi H, Cohen A, Roifman CM. Defective T cell receptor signaling and CD8+ thymic selection in humans lacking ZAP-70 kinase. *Cell* 1994;76:947–958.

230. Chan AC, Kadlecek TA, Elder ME, et al. ZAP-70 deficiency in an autosomal recessive form of severe combined immunodeficiency. *Science* 1994;264:1599–1601.

231. Elder ME, Lin D, Clever J, et al. Human severe combined immunodeficiency due to a defect in ZAP-70, a T-cell tyrosine kinase. *Science* 1994;264:1596–1599.

232. Negishi I, Motoyama N, Nakayama K-I, et al. Essential role for ZAP-70 in both positive and negative selection of thymocytes. *Nature* 1995;376:435–438.

233. Gelfand EW, Weinberg K, Mazer BD, Kadlecek TA, Weiss A. Absence of ZAP-70 prevents signaling through the antigen receptor on peripheral blood T cells but not thymocytes. *J Exp Med* 1995;182:1057–1066.

234. van Oers NSC, Tao W, Watts JD, Johnson P, Aebersold R, Teh H-S. Constitutive tyrosine phosphorylation of the T cell receptor (TCR) ζ subunit: regulation of TCR-associated protein kinase activity by TCR ζ. *Mol Cell Bio* 1993;13:5771–5780.

235. Shiue L, Zoller MJ, Brugge JS. Syk is activated by phosphotyrosine-containing peptides representing the tyrosine-based activation motifs of the high affinity receptor for IgE. *J Biol Chem* 1995;270:10498–10502.

236. Kolanus W, Romeo C, Seed B. T cell activation by clustered tyrosine kinases. *Cell* 1993;74:171–183.

237. Chu DH, Spits H, Peyron J-F, Rowley RB, Bolen JB, Weiss A. The Syk protein tyrosine kinase can function independently of CD45 and Lck in T cell antigen receptor signaling. *EMBO J* 1996;15:6251–6261.

238. Fantl WJ, Escobedo JA, Martin GA, et al. Distinct phosphotyrosines on a growth factor receptor bind to specific molecules that mediate different signaling pathways. *Cell* 1992;69:413–423.

239. Songyang Z, Shoelson SE, Chaudhuri M, et al. SH2 domains recognize specific phosphopeptide sequences. *Cell* 1993;72:767–778.

240. Overduin M, Rios CB, Mayer BJ, Baltimore D, Cowburn D. Three-dimensional solution structure of the src homology 2 domain of c-abl. *Cell* 1992;70:697–704.

241. Eck MJ, Shoelson SE, Harrison SC. Recognition of a high-affinity phosphotyrosyl peptide by the Src homology-2 domain of p56[lck]. *Nature* 1993;362:87–91.

242. Wu J, Zhao Q, Kurosaki T, Weiss A. The Vav binding site (Y315) in ZAP-70 is critical for antigen receptor-mediated signal transduction. *J Exp Med* 1997;185:1877–1882.

243. Rotin D, Margolis B, Mohammadi M, et al. SH2 domains prevent tyrosine dephosphorylation of the EGF receptor, identification of Tyr992 as the high affinity binding site for SH2 domains of phospholipase Cg. *EMBO J* 1992;11:559–567.

244. Charbonneau H, Tonks NK. 1002 protein phosphates. *Annu Rev Cell Biol* 1992;8:463–493.

245. Kavanaugh WM, Turck CW, Williams LT. PTB domain binding to signaling proteins through a sequence motif containing phosphotyrosine. *Science* 1995;268:1177–1179.

246. van der Geer P, Pawson T. The PTB domain: a new protein module implicated in signal transduction. *Trends Biochem Sci* 1995;20:277–280.

247. Trowbridge IS, Thomas ML. CD45: an emerging role as a protein tyrosine phosphatase required for lymphocyte activation and development. *Annu Rev Immunol* 1994;12:85–116.

248. Sap J, D'Eustachio P, Givol D, Schlessinger J. Cloning and expression of a widely expressed receptor tyrosine phosphatase. *Proc Natl Acad Sci USA* 1990;87:6112–6116.

249. Fischer EH, Charbonneau H, Tonks NK. Protein tyrosine phosphatases: a diverse family of intracellular and transmembrane enzymes. *Science* 1991;253:401–406.

250. Thomas ML. Positive and negative regulation of leukocyte activation by protein tyrosine phosphatases. *Semin Immunol* 1995;7:279–288.

251. Johnson P, Ostergaard HL, Wasden C, Trowbridge IS. Mutational analysis of CD45: a leukocyte-specific protein tyrosine phosphatase. *J Biol Chem* 1992;12:8035–8041.

252. Desai DM, Sap J, Silvennoinen O, Schlessinger J, Weiss A. The catalytic activity of the CD45 membrane proximal phosphatase domain is required for TCR signaling and regulation. *EMBO J* 1994;13:4002–4010.

253. Bottomly K, Luqman M, Greenbaum L, et al. A monoclonal antibody to murine CD45R distinguishes CD4 T cell populations that produce different cytokines. *Eur J Immunol* 1989;19:617–623.

254. Byrne JA, Butler JL, Cooper MD. Differential activation requirements for virgin and memory T cells. *J Immunol* 1988;141:3249–3257.

255. Akbar AN, Terry L, Timms A, Beverley PCL, Janossy G. Loss of CD45R and gain of UCHL1 reactivity is a feature of primed T cells. *J Immunol* 1988;140:2171–2178.

256. Novak TJ, Farber D, Leitenberg D, Hong SC, Johnson P, Bottomly K. Isoforms of the transmembrane tyrosine phosphatase CD45 differentially affect T cell recognition. *Immunity* 1994;1:109–119.

257. Leitenberg D, Novak TJ, Farber D, Smith BR, Bottomly K. The extracellular domain of CD45 controls association with the CD4-T cell receptor complex and the response to antigen-specific stimulation. *J Exp Med* 1996;183:249–259.

258. Desai DM, Sap J, Schlessinger J, Weiss A. Ligand-mediated negative regulation of a chimeric transmembrane receptor tyrosine phosphatase. *Cell* 1993;73:541–554.

259. Pingel JT, Thomas ML. Evidence that the leukocyte-common antigen is required for antigen-induced T lymphocyte proliferation. *Cell* 1989;58:1055–1065.

260. Koretzky GA, Picus J, Thomas ML, Weiss A. Tyrosine phosphatase CD45 is essential for coupling T cell antigen receptor to the phosphatidylinositol pathway. *Nature* 1990;346:66–68.

261. Koretzky G, Picus J, Schultz T, Weiss A. Tyrosine phosphatase CD45 is required for both T cell antigen receptor and CD2 mediated activation of a protein tyrosine kinase and interleukin 2 production. *Proc Natl Acad Sci USA* 1991;88:2037–2041.

262. Weaver CT, Pingel JT, Nelson JO, Thomas ML. CD8+ T-cell clones deficient in the expression of the CD45 protein tyrosine phosphatase have impaired responses to T-cell receptor stimuli. *Mol Cell Biol* 1991;11:4415–4422.

263. Byth KF, Conroy LA, Howlett S, et al. CD45-Null transgenic mice reveal a positive regulatory role for CD45 in early thymocyte development, in the selection of CD4+CD8+ thymocytes, and in B cell maturation. *J Exp Med* 1996;183:1707–1718.

264. Kishihara K, Penninger J, Wallace VA, et al. Normal B lymphocyte development but impaired T cell maturation in CD45-Exon6 protein tyrosine phosphatase-deficient mice. *Cell* 1993;74:143–156.

265. Mustelin T, Coggeshall KM, Altman A. Rapid activation of the T-cell tyrosine protein kinase pp56[lck] by the CD45 phosphotyrosine phosphatase. *Proc Natl Acad Sci USA* 1989;86:6302–6306.

266. McFarland EDC, Hurley TR, Pingel JT, Sefton BM, Shaw A, Thomas ML. Correlation between Src family member regulation by the protein-tyrosine-phosphatase CD45 and transmembrane signaling through the T-cell receptor. *Proc Natl Acad Sci USA* 1993;90:1402–1406.

267. Ostergaard HL, Shackelford DA, Hurley TR, et al. Expression of CD45 alters phosphorylation of the lck—encoded tyrosine protein kinase in murine lymphoma T-cell lines. *Proc Natl Acad Sci USA* 1989;86:8959–8963.

268. Sieh M, Bolen JB, Weiss A. CD45 specifically modulates binding of Lck to a phosphopeptide encompassing the negative regulatory tyrosine of Lck. *EMBO J* 1993;12:315–322.

269. Todderud G, Wahl MJ, Rhee SG, Carpenter G. Stimulation of phospholipase C-g1 membrane association by epidermal growth factor. *Science* 1990;249:296–298.

270. Law CL, Chandran KA, Sidorenko SP, Clark EA. Phospholipase C-gamma 1 interacts with conserved phosphotyrosyl residues in the linker region of Syk and is a substrate for Syk. *Mol Cell Biol* 1996;16:1305–1315.

271. Sieh M, Batzer A, Schlessinger J, Weiss A. GRB2 and phospholipase C-γl associate with a 36- to 38-kilodalton phosphotyrosine protein after T-cell receptor stimulation. *Mol Cell Biol* 1994;14:4435–4442.

271a.Zhang W, Sloan-Lancaster J, Kitchen J, et al. LAT: The ZAP-70 tyrosine kinase substrate that links T cell receptor to cellular activation. *Cell* 1998;92:83–92.

272. Weiss A, Koretzky G, Schatzman R, Kadlecek T. Stimulation of the T cell antigen receptor induces tyrosine phosphorylation of phospholipase C γl. *Proc Natl Acad Sci USA* 1991;88:5484–5488.

273. Takata M, Kurosaki T. A role for Bruton's tyrosine kinase in B cell antigen receptor-mediated activation of phospholipase C-γ2. *J Exp Med* 1996;184:31–40.

274. Park DJ, Rho HW, Rhee SG. CD3 stimulation causes phosphorylation of phospholipase C-γl on serine and tyrosine residues in a human T cell line. *Proc Natl Acad Sci USA* 1991;88:5453–5456.

275. Nishizuka Y. The molecular heterogeneity of protein kinase C and its implications for cellular regulation. *Nature* 1988;334:661–665.

276. Grynkiewicz G, Poenie M, Tsien RY. A new generation of Ca++ indicators with greatly improved fluorescent properties. *J Biol Chem* 1985;260:3440–3448.

277. Oettgen HC, Terhorst C, Cantley LC, Rosoff PM. Stimulation of the T3-T cell receptor complex induces a membrane-potential-sensitive calcium influx. *Cell* 1985;40:583–590.

278. Rabinovitch PS, June CH, Grossman A, Ledbetter JA. Heterogeneity among T cells in intracellular free calcium responses after mitogen stimulation with PHA or anti-CD3, simultaneous use of indo-1 and immunofluorescence with flow cytometry. *J Immunol* 1986;137:952–961.

279. Manger B, Weiss A, Imboden J, Laing T, Stobo J. The role of protein kinase C in

transmembrane signaling by the T cell receptor complex: effects of stimulation with soluble or immobilized T3 antibodies. *J Immunol* 1987;139:395–407.

280. Berry N, Ase K, Kishimoto A, Nishizuka Y. Activation of resting human T cells requires prolonged stimulation of protein kinase C. *Proc Natl Acad Sci USA* 1990;87:2294–2298.

281. Berridge MJ, Irvine RF. Inositol phosphates and cell signalling. *Nature* 1989;341:197–205.

282. Imboden JB, Stobo JD. Transmembrane signalling by the T cell antigen receptor: perturbation of the T3-antigen receptor complex generates inositol phosphates and releases calcium ions from intracellular stores. *J Exp Med* 1985;161:446–456.

283. Furuichi T, Yoshikawa S, Miyawaki A, Wada K, Maeda N, Mikoshiba K. Primary structure and functional expression of the inositol 1,4,5-trisphosphate-binding protein P400. *Nature* 1989;342:32–38.

284. Sugawara H, Kurosaki M, Takata M, Kurosaki T. Genetic evidence for involvement of type 1, type 2 and type 3 inositol 1,4,5-trisphosphate receptors in signal transduction through the B-cell antigen receptor. *EMBO J* 1997;16:3078–3088.

285. Goldsmith M, Weiss A. Early signal transduction by the antigen receptor without commitment to T cell activation. *Science* 1988;240:1029–1031.

286. Lewis RS, Cahalan MD. Mitogen-induced oscillations of cytosolic Ca^{2+} and membrane Ca^{2+} current in human leukemic T cells. *Cell Reg* 1989;1:99–112.

287. Timmerman LA, Clipstone NA, Ho SN, Northrop JP, Crabtree GR. Rapid shuttling of NF-AT in discrimination of Ca^{2+} signals and immunosuppression. *Nature* 1996;383:837–840.

288. Putney JW, Bird GSJ. The signal for capacitative calcium entry. *Cell* 1993;75:199–201.

289. Randriamampita C, Tsien RY. Emptying of intracellular Ca^{2+} stores releases a novel small messenger that stimulates Ca^{2+} influx. *Nature* 1993;364:809–814.

290. Gardner P. Patch clamp studies of lymphocyte activation. *Annu Rev Immunol* 1990;8:231–252.

291. Majerus PW, Ross TS, Cunningham TW, Caldwell KK, Jefferson AB, Bansal VS. Recent insights in phosphatidylinositol signaling. *Cell* 1990;63:459–465.

292. Toker A, Cantley LC. Signaling through the lipid products of phosphatidylinositide-3-OH kinase. *Nature* 1997;387:673–676.

293. Ward SG, Westwick J, Hall ND, Sansom DM. Ligation of CD28 receptor by B7 induces formation of D-3 phosphoinositides in T lymphocytes independently of T cell receptor/CD3 activation. *Eur J Immunol* 1993;23:2572–2577.

294. Ward SG, Reif K, Ley S, Fry MJ, Waterfield MD, Cantrell DA. Regulation of phosphoinositide kinases in T cells. *J Biol Chem* 1992;267:23862–23869.

295. Truitt KE, Hicks CM, Imboden JB. Stimulation of CD28 triggers an association between CD28 and phosphatidylinositol 3-kinase in Jurkat T cells. *J Exp Med* 1994;179:1071–1076.

296. Truitt KE, Mills GB, Turck CW, Imboden JB. SH2-dependent association of phosphatidylinositol 3'-kinase 85-kD regulatory subunit with the interleukin-2 receptor b chain. *J Biol Chem* 1994;269:5937–5943.

297. Nishizuka Y. Protein kinase C and lipid signaling for sustained cellular responses. *FASEB J* 1995;9:484–496.

298. Genot EM, Parker PJ, Cantrell DA. Analysis of the role of protein kinase C-α,-ε, and-ζ in T cell activation. *J Biol Chem* 1995;270:9833–9839.

299. Cantrell D. T cell antigen receptor signal transduction pathways. *Annu Rev Immunol* 1996;14:259–274.

300. Koretzky GA, Wahi MM, Newton ME, Weiss A. Heterogeneity of protein kinase C isoenzyme gene expression in human T cell lines: Protein kinase C-β is not required for several T cell functions. *J Immunol* 1989;143:1692–1695.

301. Muramatsu M, Kaibuchi K, Arai K. A protein kinase C cDNA without the regulatory domain is active after transfection in vivo in the absence of phorbol ester. *Mol Cell Biol* 1989;9:831–836.

302. Monks CR, Kupfer H, Tamir I, Barlow A, Kupfer A. Selective modulation of protein kinase C-theta during T-cell activation. *Nature* 1997;385:83–86.

303. Melloni E, Pontremoli S, Michetti M, et al. Binding of protein kinase C to neutrophil membranes in the presence of Ca^{2+} and its activation by a Ca^{2+} requiring proteinase. *Proc Natl Acad Sci USA* 1985;82:6435–6439.

304. Graber M, Bockenstedt LK, Weiss A. Signalling via the inositol phospholipid pathway by the T cell antigen receptor is limited by receptor number. *J Immunol* 1991;146:2935–2943.

305. Schreiber SL, Crabtree GR. The mechanism of action of cyclosporin A and FK506. *Immunol Today* 1992;13:136–142.

306. Liu J, Farmer JD, Lane WS, Friedman J, Weissman I, Schreiber SL. Calcineurin is a common target of cyclophilin-cyclosporin A and FKBP-FK506 complexes. *Cell* 1991;66:807–815.

307. Rao A, Luo C, Hogan PG. Transcription factors of the NFAT family: regulation and function. *Annu Rev Immunol* 1997;15:707–747.

308. Flanagan WM, Corthesy B, Bram RJ, Crabtree GR. Nuclear association of a T-cell transcription factor blocked by FK-506 and cyclosporin A. *Nature* 1991;352:803–807.

309. Clipstone NA, Crabtree GR. Identification of calcineurin as a key signalling enzyme in T-lymphocyte activation. *Nature* 1992;357:695–697.

310. O'Keefe SJ, Tamura J, Kincaid RL, Tocci MJ, O'Neil EA. FK-506- and CsA-sensitive activation of the interleukin-2 promoter by calcineurin. *Nature* 1992;357:692–694.

311. Jain J, McCaffrey PG, Miner Z, et al. The T-cell transcription factor $NFAT_p$ is a substrate for calcineurin and interacts with Fos and Jun. *Nature* 1993;365:352–355.

312. Nghiem P, Ollick T, Gardner P, Schulman H. Interleukin-2 transcriptional block by multifunctional Ca^{2+}/calmodulin kinase. *Nature* 1994;371:347–350.

313. Samelson LE, Harford JB, Klausner RD. Identification of the components of the murine T cell antigen receptor complex. *Cell* 1985;43:223–231.

314. Acres RB, Conlon PJ, Mochizuki DY, Gallis B. Rapid phosphorylation and modulation of the T4 antigen on cloned helper T cells induced by phorbol myristate acetate or antigen. *J Biol Chem* 1986;261:16210–16214.

315. Shackelford DA, Trowbridge IS. Identification of lymphocyte integral membrane protein as substrates for protein kinase C. *J Biol Chem* 1986;261:8334–8341.

316. Downward J, Graves J, Cantrell D. The regulation and function of p21ras in T cells. *Immunol Today* 1992;13.89–92.

317. Polakis P, McCormick F. Structural requirements for the interaction of p21ras with GAP, exchange factors, and its biological effector target. *J Biol Chem* 1993;268:9157–9160.

318. Schlessinger J. How receptor tyrosine kinases activate Ras. *TIBS* 1993;18:273–275.

319. Izquierdo M, Downward J, Graves JD, Cantrell DA. Role of protein kinase C in T-cell antigen receptor regulation of p21ras: evidence that two p21ras regulatory pathways coexist in T cells. *Mol Cell Biol* 1992;12:3305–3312.

320. Downward J, Graves JD, Warne PH, Rayter S, Cantrell DA. Stimulation of p21ras upon T-cell activation. *Nature* 1990;346:719–723.

321. Buday L, Egan SE, Rodriguez Viciana P, Cantrell DA, Downward J. A complex of Grb2 adaptor protein, Sos exchange factor, and a 36-kDa membrane-bound tyrosine phosphoprotein is implicated in ras activation in T cells. *J Biol Chem* 1994;269:9019–9023.

322. Ravichandran K, Lorenz U, Shoelson SE, Burakoff SJ. Interaction of Shc with Grb2 regulates association of Grb2 with mSOS. *Mol Cell Biol* 1995;15:593–600.

323. Ravichandran KS, Lee KK, Songyang A, Cantley LC, Burn P, Burakoff SJ. Interaction of Shc with the ζ chain of the T cell receptor upon T cell activation. *Science* 1993;262:902–905.

324. McCormick F, Wittinghofer A. Interactions between Ras proteins and their effectors. *Curr Opin Biotechnol* 1996;7:449–456.

325. Rodriguez-Viciana P, Warne PH, Khwaja A, et al. Role of phosphoinositide 3-OH kinase in cell transformation and control of the actin cytoskeleton by Ras. *Cell* 1997;89:457–467.

326. Rayter SI, Woodrow M, Lucas SC, Cantrell DA, Downward J. p21ras mediates control of IL-2 gene promoter function in T cell activation. *EMBO J* 1992;11:4549–4556.

327. Siegel JN, Klausner RD, Rapp UR, Samelson LE. T cell antigen receptor engagement stimulates c-raf phosphorylation and induces c-raf-associated kinase activity via a protein kinase C-dependent pathway. *J Biol Chem* 1990;265:18472–18480.

328. Howe LR, Leevers SJ, Gomez N, Nakielny S, Cohen P, Marshall CJ. Activation of MAP kinase pathway by the protein kinase raf. *Cell* 1992;71:335–342.

329. Davis R. The mitogen-activated protein kinase signal transduction pathway. *J Biol Chem* 1993;20:14553–14556.

330. Nel AE, Hanekom C, Rheeder A, et al. Stimulation of map-2 kinase activity in T lymphocytes by anti-CD3 or anti-Ti monoclonal antibody is partially dependent on protein kinase C. *J Immunol* 1990;144:2683–2689.

331. Woodrow MA, Rayter S, Downward J, Cantrell D. p21ras function is important for T cell antigen receptor and protein kinase C regulation of nuclear factor of activated T cells. *J Immunol* 1993;150:3853–3861.

332. Owaki H, Varma R, Gillis B, et al. Raf-1 is required for T cell IL2 production. *EMBO J* 1993;12:4367–4373.

333. Jain J, McCaffrey PG, Valge Archer VE, Rao A. Nuclear factor of activated T cells contains Fos and Jun. *Nature* 1992;356:801–804.

334. Boise LH, Petryniak B, Mao X, et al. The NFAT-1 DNA binding complex in activated T cells contains Fra-1 and JunB. *Mol Cell Biol* 1993;13:1911–1919.

335. Northrup JP, Ullman KS, Crabtree GR. Characterization of the nuclear and cytoplasmic components of the lymphoid-specific nuclear factor of activated T cells (NF AT) complex. *J Biol Chem* 1993;268:2917–2923.

336. Bustelo XR. The VAV family of signal transduction molecules. *Crit Rev Oncog* 1996;7:65–88.

337. Bustelo XR, Ledbetter JA, Barbacid M. Product of vav proto-oncogene defines a new class of tyrosine protein kinase substrates. *Nature* 1992;356:68–71.

338. Margolis B, Hu P, Katzav S, et al. Tyrosine phosphorylation of vav proto-oncogene product containing SH2 domain and transcription factor motifs. *Nature* 1992;356:71–74.

339. Tarakhovsky A, Turner M, Schaal S, et al. Defective antigen receptor-mediated proliferation of B and T cells in the absence of Vav. *Nature* 1995;374:467–470.

340. Fischer K-D, Zmuldzinas A, Gardner S, Barbacid M, Bernstein A, Guidos C. Defective T-cell receptor signalling and positive selection of Vav-deficient CD4+CD8+ thymocytes. *Nature* 1995;374:474–477.

341. Wu J, Katzav S, Weiss A. A functional T-cell receptor signaling pathway is required for p95vav activity. *Mol Cell Biol* 1995;15:4337–4346.

342. Katzav S, Cleveland JL, Heslop HE, Pulido D. Loss of the amino-terminal helix-loop-helix domain of the vav proto-oncogene activates its transforming potential. *Mol Cell Biol* 1991;11:1912–1920.

343. Han J, Das B, Wei W, et al. Lck regulates Vav activation of members of the Rho family of GTPases. *Mol Cell Biol* 1997;17:1346–1353.

344. Kupfer A, Singer SJ. Cell biology of cytotoxic and helper T cell functions: immunofluorescence microscopic studies of single cells and cell couples. *Annu Rev Immunol* 1989;7:309–337.

345. Katzav S, Sutherland M, Packham G, Yi T, Weiss A. The protein tyrosine kinase ZAP-70 can associate with the SH2 domain of proto-Vav. *J Biol Chem* 1994;269:32579–32585.

346. Motto DG, Ross EE, Wu J, Hendricks-Taylor LR, Koretzky GA. Implication of

the GRB2-associated phosphoprotein SLP-76 in TCR-mediated IL-2 production. *J Exp Med* 1996;183:1937–1943.

347. Wu J, Motto DG, Koretzky GA, Weiss A. Vav and SLP-76 interact and functionally cooperate in IL-2 gene activation. *Immunity* 1996;4:593–602.

348. Grinstein S, Goetz-Smith JD, Stewart D, Beresford BJ, Mellors A. Protein phosphorylation during activation of Na+/H+ exchange by phorbol esters and by osmotic shrinking. *J Biol Chem* 1986;261:8009–8016.

349. Grinstein S, Goetz JD, Rothstein A. 22Na+ fluxes in thymic lymphocytes: II. Amiloride-sensitive Na+/H+ exchange pathway reversibility of transport and asymmetry of the modifier site. *J Gen Physiol* 1984;84:585–600.

350. Rosoff PM, Cantley LC. Stimulation of the T3-T cell receptor-associated Ca2+ influx enhances the activity of the Na+/H++ exchanger in a leukemic human T cell line. *J Biol Chem* 1985;260:14053–14059.

351. Wang T, Sheppard JR, Foker JE. The rise and fall of cAMP required for onset of lymphocyte DNA synthesis. *Science* 1978;201:155–157.

352. Ledbetter JA, Parsons M, Martin PJ, Hansen JA, Rabinovitch PS, June CH. Antibody binding to CD5 (Tp67) and Tp44 cell surface molecules: effects of cyclic nucleotides, cytoplasmic free calcium and cAMP-mediated suppression. *J Immunol* 1986;137:3299–3305.

353. Mills AJT, Forrest GA, Pious DA. Cyclic AMP-dependent regulation of mitosis in human lymphoid cells. *Exp Cell Res* 1974;83:335–343.

354. Smith JW, Steiner AL, Newberry WM, Parker CW. Cyclic AMP in human lymphocytes. Alterations after PHA stimulation. *J Clin Invest* 1971;50:432–441.

355. Novogrodsky A, Patya M, Rubin AL, Stenzel KH. Agents that increase cellular cAMP inhibit production of interleukin-2, but not its activity. *Biochem Biophys Res Commun* 1983;114:93–98.

356. Patel MD, Samelson LE, Klausner RD. Multiple kinases and signal transduction. *J Biol Chem* 1987;262:5831–5838.

357. Imboden JB, Shoback DM, Pattison G, Stobo JD. Cholera toxin inhibits the T-cell antigen receptor-mediated increases in inositol trisphosphate and cytoplasmic free calcium. *Proc Natl Acad Sci USA* 1986;83:5673–5677.

358. Cook SJ, McCormick F. Inhibition of cAMP of Ras-dependent activation of raf. *Science* 1993;262:1069–1072.

359. Atkinson JP, Kelley JP, Weiss A, Wedner HJ, Parker CW. Enhanced intracellular cGMP concentrations and lectin-induced lymphocyte transformation. *J Immunol* 1978;121:2282–2291.

360. Tsien RY, Pozzan T, Rink T. T cell mitogens cause early changes in cytoplasmic free Ca2+ and membrane potential in lymphocytes. *Nature* 1982;295:68–71.

361. DeCoursey TE, Chandy KG, Gupta S, Cahalan MD. Voltage-gated K+ channel in human T lymphocytes: a role in mitogenesis? *Nature* 1984;307:465–468.

362. Lewis RS, Cahalan MD. Subset-specific expression of potassium channels in developing murine T lymphocytes. *Science* 1988;239:771–775.

363. Gray LS, Gnarra JR, Russell JH, Engelhard VH. The role of K+ in the regulation of the increase in intracellular Ca2+ mediated by the T lymphocyte antigen receptor. *Cell* 1987;50:119–127.

364. Chandy KG, DeCoursey TE, Cahalan MD, McLaughlin C, Gupta S. Voltage-gated potassium channels are required for human T lymphocyte activation. *J Exp Med* 1984;160:369–385.

365. Lin CS, Boltz RC, Blake JT, et al. Voltage-gated potassium channels regulate calcium-dependent pathways involved in human T lymphocyte activation. *J Exp Med* 1993;177:637–645.

366a.Lowin-Kropf B, Shapiro VS, Weiss A. Cytoskeletal polarization of T cells is regulated by an immunoreceptor tyrosine-based activation motif-dependent mechanism. *J Cell Biol* 1998;140:861–871.

366b.Stowers L, Yelon D, Berg LJ, Chant J. Regulation of the polarization of T cells toward antigen-presenting cells by Ras-related GTPase CDC42. *Proc Natl Acad Sci USA* 1995;92:5027–5031.

367. Ley SC, Verbi W, Pappin DJC, Druker B, Davies AA, Crumpton MJ. Tyrosine phosphorylation of a tubulin in human T lymphocytes. *Eur J Immunol* 1994;24:99–106.

368. Kupfer A, Singer SJ, Dennert G. On the mechanism of unidirectional killing in mixtures of two cytotoxic lymphocytes. *J Exp Med* 1986;163:489–498.

369. Means AR, Dedman JR. Calmodulin-an intracellular calcium receptor. *Nature* 1980;285:73–77.

370. Berke G. The binding and lysis of target cells by cytotoxic lymphocytes: molecular and cellular aspects. *Annu Rev Immunol* 1994;12:735–773.

371. Lancki DW, Weiss A, Fitch FW. Requirements for triggering of lysis by cytolytic T lymphocyte clones. *J Immunol* 1987;138:3646–3653.

372. Poenie M, Tsien RY, Schmitt-Verhulst A-M. Sequential activation and lethal hit measured by [Ca2+]i in individual cytolytic T cells and targets. *EMBO J* 1987;6:2223–2232.

373. Shiver JW, Su L, Henkart PA. Cytotoxicity with target DNA breakdown by rat basophilic leukemia cells expressing both cytolysin and granzyme A. *Cell* 1992;71:315–322.

374. Nagata S, Golstein P. The Fas death factor. *Science* 1995;267:1449–1456.

375. Shaw J-P, Utz PJ, Durand DB, Toole JJ, Emmel EA, Crabtree GR. Identification of a putative regulator or early T cell activation genes. *Science* 1988;241:202–205.

376. Lewin B. Oncogenic conversion by regulatory changes in transcription factors. *Cell* 1991;64:303–312.

377. Karin M, Liu Z, Zandi E. AP-1 function and regulation. *Curr Opin Cell Biol* 1997;9:240–246.

378. Blackwell T, K., Kretzner L, Blackwood EM, Eisenman RN, Weintraub H. Sequence-specific DNA binding by the c-myc protein. *Science* 1990;250:1149–1151.

379. Prendergast GC, Lawe D, Ziff EB. Association of myn, the murine homologue of max, with c-myc stimulates methylation-sensitive DNA binding and ras cotransformation. *Cell* 1991;65:395–407.

380. Reed JC, Alpers JD, Nowell PC, Hoover RG. Sequential expression of protooncogenes during lectin-stimulated mitogenesis of normal human lymphocytes. *Proc Natl Acad Sci USA* 1986;83:3982–3986.

381. Ship MA, Reinherz E. Differential expression of nuclear proto-oncogenes in T cells triggered with mitogenic and nonmitogenic T3 and T11 activation signals. *J Immunol* 1987;139:2143–2148.

382. Grausz JD, Fradelizi D, Dautry F, Monier R, Lehn P. Modulation of c-fos and c-myc mRNA levels in normal human lymphocytes by calcium ionophore A23187 and phorbol ester. *Eur J Immunol* 1986;16:1217–1221.

383. Ullman KS, Northrup JP, Admon A, Crabtree GR. Jun family members are controlled by a calcium-regulated, cyclosporin A-sensitive signaling pathway in activated T lymphocytes. *Genes Dev* 1993;7:188–196.

384. Derijard B, Hibi M, Wu I-H, et al. JNK1: A protein kinase stimulated by UV light and Ha-Ras that binds and phosphorylates the c-Jun activation domain. *Cell* 1994;76:1025–1037.

385. Deng T, Karin M. c-Fos transcriptional activity stimulated by H-Ras-activated protein kinase distinct from JNK and ERK. *Nature* 1994;371:171–175.

386. Zheng W-P, Flavell RA. The transcription factor GATA-3 is necessary and sufficient for Th2 cytokine gene expression in CD4 T cells. *Cell* 1997;89:587–596.

387. Hodge MR, Chun HJ, Rengarajan J, Alt A, Lieberson R, Glimscher LH. NF-AT-driven interleukin-4 transcription potentiated by NIP45. *Science* 1996;274:1903–1905.

388. Ho I-C, Hodge MR, Rooney JW, Glimscher LH. The proto-oncogene c-maf is responsible for tissue-specific expression of interleukin-4. *Cell* 1996;85:973–983.

389. Siebenlist U, Durand DB, Bressler P, et al. Promoter region of interleukin-2 gene undergoes chromatin structure changes and confers inducibility on chloramphenicol acetyltransferase gene during activation of T cells. *Mol Cell Biol* 1986;6:3042–3049.

390. Durand DB, Shaw J-P, Bush MR, Replogle RE, Gelagaje R, Crabtree GR. Characterization of antigen receptor response elements within the interleukin-2 enhancer. *Mol Cell Biol* 1988;8:1715–1724.

391. Serfling E, Avots A, Neumann M. The architecture of the interleukin-2 promoter: a reflection of T lymphocyte activation. *Biochim Biophys Acta* 1995;1263:181–200.

392. Ullman KS, Flanagan WM, Edwards CA, Crabtree GR. Activation of early gene expression in T lymphocytes by Oct-1 and inducible protein, OAP40. *Science* 1991;254:558–562.

393. Jain J, Valge-Archer VE, Sinskey AJ, Rao A. The AP-1 site at-150 bp, but not the NF-kB site, is likely to represent the major target of protein kinase C in the interleukin 2 promoter. *J Immunol* 1992;175:853–862.

394. Jain J, Valge-Archer VE, Rao A. Analysis of the AP-1 sites in the IL-2 promoter. *J Immunol* 1992;148:1240–1250.

395. Kang S-M, Beverly B, Tran A-C, Brorson K, Schwartz RH, Lenardo MJ. Transactivation by AP-1 is a molecular target of T cell clonal anergy. *Science* 1992;257:1134–1138.

396. Li W, Whaley CD, Mondino A, Mueller DL. Blocked signal transduction to the ERK and JNK protein kinases in anergic CD4+ T cells. *Science* 1996;271:1272–1276.

397. Fields PE, Gajewski TF, Fitch FW. Blocked Ras activation in anergic CD4+ T cells. *Science* 1996;271:1276–1278.

398. Ullman KS, Northrop JP, Verweij CL, Crabtree GR. Transmission of signals from the T lymphocyte antigen receptor to the genes responsible for cell proliferation and immune function: the missing link. *Annu Rev Immunol* 1990;8:421–452.

399. Lai J-H, Horvath G, Subleski J, Bruder J, Ghosh P, Tan T-H. RelA is a potent transcriptional activator of the CD28 response element within the interleukin 2 promoter. *Mol Cell Biol* 1995;15:4260–4271.

400. Ghosh P, Tan T-H, Rice NR, Sica A, Young HA. The interleukin 2 CD28-responsive complex contains at least three members of the NFkB family: c-Rel, p50 , and p65. *Proc Natl Acad Sci USA* 1993;90:1696–1700.

401. Rooney JW, Sun YL, Glimcher LH, Hoey T. Novel NFAT sites that mediate activation of the interleukin-2 promoter in response to T-cell receptor stimulation. *Mol Cell Biol* 1995;15:6299–6310.

402. Shapiro VS, Truitt KE, Imboden JB, Weiss A. CD28 mediates transcriptional upregulation of the interleukin-2 (IL-2) promoter through a composite element containing the CD28RE and NF-IL-2B AP-1 sites. *Mol Cell Biol* 1997;17:4051–4058.

403. McGuire KL, Iacobelli M. Involvement of Rel, Fos, and Jun proteins in binding activity to the IL-2 promoter CD28 response element/AP-1 sequence in human T cells. *J Immunol* 1997;159:1319–1327.

404. Kontgen F, Grumont RJ, Strasser A, et al. Mice lacking the c-rel proto-oncogene exhibit defects in lymphocyte proliferation, humoral immunity, and interleukin-2 expression. *Genes Dev* 1995;9:1965–1977.

405. Shaw G, Kamen R. A conserved AU sequence from the 3' untranslated region of GM-CSF mRNA mediates selective mRNA degradation. *Cell* 1986;46:659–667.

406. Umlauf SW, Beverly B, Lantz O, Schwartz RH. Regulation of interleukin 2 gene expression by CD28 costimulation in mouse T-cell clones: both nuclear and cytoplasmic RNAs are regulated with complex kinetics. *Mol Cell Biol* 1995;15:3197–3205.

407. Sugamura K, Asao H, Kondo M, et al. The interleukin-2 receptor g chain: its role in the multiple cytokine receptor complexes and T cell development in XSCID. *Annu Rev Immunol* 1996;14:179–205.

408. Ko HS, Fu SM, Winchester RJ, Yu DTY, Kunkel HG. Ia determinants on stimulated human T lymphocytes: occurrence on mitogen- and antigen-activated cells. *J Exp Med* 1979;150:246–257.

409. Lanier LL, Buck DW, Rhodes L, et al. Interleukin 2 activation of natural killer cells rapidly induces the expression and phosphorylation of the Leu-23 activation antigen. *J Exp Med* 1988;167:1572–1585.

410. Haynes BF, Hemler ME, Mann DL, et al. Characterization of a monoclonal antibody (4F2) that binds to human monocytes and to a subset of activated lymphocytes. *J Immunol* 1981;126:1409–1414.

411. Rothstein DM, Saito H, Streuli M, Schlossman SF, Morimoto C. The alternative splicing of the CD45 tyrosine phosphatase is controlled by negative regulatory trans-acting splicing factors. *J Biol Chem* 1992;267:7139–7147.

412. Bohnlein E, Lowenthal JW, Siekevitz M, Ballard DW, Franza BR, Greene WC. The same inducible nuclear proteins regulate mitogen activation of both the interleukin-2 receptor-alpha gene and type 1 HIV. *Cell* 1988;53:827–836.

413. Cross SL, Feinberg MB, Wolf JB, Holbrook NJ, Wong-Staal F, Leonard WJ. Regulation of the human interleukin-2 receptor α chain promoter: activation of a nonfunctional promoter by the transactivator gene of HTLV-1.*Cell* 1987;49:47–56.

414. Leonard WJ, Kronke M, Peffer NJ, Depper JM, Green WC. Interleukin 2 receptor gene expression in normal human T lymphocytes. *Proc Natl Acad Sci USA* 1985;82:6281–6285.

415. Smith KA, Cantrell DA. Interleukin 2 regulates its own receptors. *Proc Natl Acad Sci USA* 1985;82:864–868.

416. Yamamoto Y, Ohmura T, Fujimoto K, Onoue K. Interleukin 2 mRNA induction in human lymphocytes: analysis of the synergistic effect of a calcium ionophore A23187 and a phorbol ester. *J Immunol* 1985;15:1204–1208.

417. Schreiber SL. Immunophilin-sensitive protein phosphatase action in cell signaling pathways. *Cell* 1992;70:365–368.

418. Waldmann T. The interleukin-2 receptor. *J Biol Chem* 1991;266:2681–2684.

419. Taniguchi T, Minami Y. The IL-2/IL-2 receptor system: a current overview. *Cell* 1993;73:5–8.

420. Horak I, Lohler J, Ma A, Smith K. Interleukin-2 deficient mice: a new model to study autoimmunity and self tolerance. *Immunol Rev* 1995;148:35–44.

421. Schorle H, Holtshke T, Hunig T, Schimpl A, Horak I. Development and function of T cells in mice rendered interleukin-2 deficient by gene targetting. *Nature* 1991;352.621–624.

422. Kundig TM, Schorle H, Bachmann MF, Hengartner H, Zinkernagel RM, Horak I. Immune responses in interleukin-2-deficient mice. *Science* 1993;262:1059–1061.

423. Leonard WJ, Depper JM, Crabtree GR, et al. Molecular cloning and expression of cDNAs for the human interleukin-2 receptor. *Nature* 1984;311:626–631.

424. Hatakeyama M, Tsudo M, Minamoto S, et al. Interleukin-2 receptor β chain gene: Generation of three receptor forms by cloned human α and β chain cDNA's. *Science* 1989;244:551–556.

425. Tsudo M, Karasuyama H, Kitamura F, et al. The IL-2 receptor β-chain (p70): Ligand binding ability of the cDNA-encoding membrane and secreted forms. *J Immunol* 1990;145:599–606.

426. Takeshita T, Asao H, Ohtani K, et al. Cloning of the γ chain of the human IL-2 receptor. *Science* 1992;257:379–382.

427. Bazan JF. Structural design and molecular evolution of a cytokine receptor superfamily. *Proc Natl Acad Sci USA* 1990;87:6934–6938.

428. Lowenthal JW, Greene WC. Contrasting interleukin 2 binding properties of the α (p55) and β (p70) protein subunits of the human high-affinity interleukin 2 receptor. *J Exp Med* 1987;166:1156–1161.

429. Matsuoka M, Takeshita T, Ishii N, Nakamura M, Ohkubo T, Sugamura K. Kinetic study of interleukin-2 binding on the reconstituted interleukin-2 receptor complexes including the human γ-chain. *Eur J Immunol* 1993;23:2472–2476.

430. Noguchi M, Yi H, Rosenblatt HM, et al. Interleukin-2 receptor γ chain mutation results in X-linked severe combined immunodeficiency in humans. *Cell* 1993;73:147–157.

431. Disanto JP, Muller W, Guy-Grand D, Fischer A, Rajewsky K. Lymphoid development in mice with a targeted deletion of the interleukin-2 receptor gamma chain. *Proc Natl Acad Sci USA* 1995;92:377–381.

432. Willerford DM, Chen J, Ferry JA, Davidson L, Ma A, Alt FW. Interleukin-2 receptor alpha chain regulates the size and content of the peripheral lymphoid compartment. *Immunity* 1995;3:521–530.

433. Suzuki H, Kundig TM, Furlonger C, et al. Deregulated T cell activation and autoimmunity in mice lacking interleukin-2 receptor beta. *Science* 1995;268:1472–1476.

434. Nakamura Y, Russell SM, Mess SA, et al. Heterodimerization of the IL-2 receptor β- and γ-chain cytoplasmic domains is required for signalling. *Nature* 1994;369:330–333.

435. Nelson BH, Lord JD, Greenberg PD. Cytoplasmic domains of the interleukin-2 receptor β and γ chains mediate the signal for T-cell proliferation. *Nature* 1994;369:333–336.

436. Ihle JN, Witthuhn BA, Quelle FW, Yamamoto K, Silvennoinen O. Signaling through the hematopoietic cytokine receptors. *Annu Rev Immunol* 1995;13:369–398.

437. O'Shea JJ. Jaks, STATs, cytokine signal transduction, and immunoregulation: are we there yet? *Immunity* 1997;7:1–11.

438. Miyazaki T, Kawahara A, Fujii H, et al. Functional activation of Jak1 and Jak3 by selective association with IL-2 receptor subunits. *Science* 1994;266:1045–1047.

439. Thomis DC, Gurniak CB, Tivol E, Sharpe AH, Berg LJ. Defects in B lymphocyte maturation and T lymphocyte activation in mice lacking Jak3. *Science* 1995;270:794–797.

440. Russell SM, Tayebi N, Nakajima H, et al. Mutation of Jak3 in a patient with SCID: essential role of Jak3 in lymphoid development. *Science* 1995;270:797–800.

441. Gaffen SL, Lai SY, Ha M, et al. Distinct tyrosine residues within the interleukin-2 receptor β chain drive signal transduction specificity, redundancy and diversity. *J Biol Chem* 1996;271:221381–21390.

442. Hatakeyama M, Kono T, Kobayashi N, et al. Interaction of the IL-2 receptor with the src-Family kinase p56lck: Identification of novel intermolecular association. *Science* 1991;252:1523–1528.

443. Horak ID, Gress RE, Lucas PJ, Horak EM, Waldmann TA, Bolen JB. T-lymphocyte interleukin 2-dependent tryosine protein kinase signal transduction involves the activation of p56lck. *Proc Natl Acad Sci USA* 1991;88:1996–2000.

444. Minami Y, Nakagawa Y, Kawahara A, et al. Protein tyrosine kinase Syk is associated with and activated by the IL-2 receptor: Possible link with the c-myc induction pathway. *Immunity* 1995;2:89–100.

445. Turner M, Mee PJ, Costello PS, et al. Perinatal lethality and blocked B-cell development in mice lacking the tyrosine kinase Syk. *Nature* 1995;378:298–302.

446. Cheng AM, Rowley B, Pao W, Hayday A, Bolen JB, Pawson T. Syk tyrosine kinase required for mouse viability and B-cell development. *Nature* 1995;378:303–306.

447. Ravichandran KS, Burakoff SJ. The adaptor protein shc interacts with the interleukin-2 (IL-2) receptor upon IL-2 stimulation. *J Biol Chem* 1994;269:1599–1602.

448. Dudek H, Datta SR, Franke TF, et al. Regulation of neuronal survival by the serine-threonine protein kinase Akt. *Science* 1997;275:661–665.

449. Abraham RT, Wiedeerrecht GJ. Immunopharmacology of rapamycin. *Annu Rev Immunol* 1996;14:483–510.

450. Brown E, Beal PA, Keith CT, Chen J, Shin T, Schreiber S. Control of p70 S6 kinase by kinase activity of FRAP. *Nature* 1995;377:441–446.

451. Brunn GJ, Hudson CC, Sekulic A, et al. Phosphorylation of the translational repressor PHAS-1 by the mammalian target of rapamycin. *Science* 1997;277:99–101.

452. Scherr CJ, Roberts JM. Inhibitors of mammalian G1 cyclin-dependent kinases. *Genes Devel* 1995;9:1149–1163.

453. Nourse J, Firpo E, Flanagan W, et al. Interleukin-2 mediated elimination of the p27Kip1 cyclin-dependent kinase inhibitor prevented by rapamycin. *Nature* 1994;372:570–573.

454. Moldwin RL, Lancki DW, Herold KC, Fitch FW. An antigen receptor-driven interleukin 2-independent pathway for proliferation of murine cytolytic T lymphocyte clones. *J Exp Med* 1986;163:1566–1582.

455. Laing TJ, Weiss A. IL-2 independent proliferation in human T cells. *J Immunol* 1988;140:1056–1062.

456. Schultz LD, Sidman CL. Genetically determined murine models of immunodeficiency. *Annu Rev Immunol* 1987;5:367–404.

457. Lorenz U, Ravichandran KS, Burakoff SJ. Lack of SHPTP1 results in src-family kinase hyperactivation and thymocyte hyperresponsiveness. *Proc Natl Acad Sci USA* 1996;93:9624–9629.

458. Marengere LEM, Waterhouse P, Duncan GS, Mittrucker H-W, Feng G-S, Mak TW. Regulation of T cell receptor signaling by tyrosine phosphatase SYP association with CTLA-4. *Science* 1996;272:1170–1173.

459. Waterhouse P, Penninger JM, Timms E, et al. Lymphoproliferative disorders with early lethality in mice deficient in Ctla-4. *Science* 1995;270:985–988.

460. Cloutier J-F, Veillette A. Association of inhibitory tyrosine protein kinase p50csk with protein tyrosine phosphatase PEP in T cells and other hemopoietic cells. *EMBO J* 1996;15:4909–4918.

461. Latinis KM, Carr LL, Peterson EJ, Norian LA, Eliason SL, Koretzky GA. Regulation of CD95 (Fas) ligand expression by TCR-mediated signaling events. *J Immunol* 1997;158:4602–4611.

462. Fisher GH, Rosenberg FJ, Straus SE, et al. Dominant interfering Fas gene mutations impair apoptosis in a human autoimmune lymphoproliferative syndrome. *Cell* 1995;81:935–946.

463. Wilde DB, Fitch FW. Antigen-reactive cloned helper T cells. I. Unresponsiveness to antigenic restimulation develops after stimulation of cloned helper T cells. *J Immunol* 1984;132:1632–1638.

464. Williams ME, Shea CM, Lichtman AH, Abbas AK. Antigen receptor-mediated anergy in resting T lymphocytes and T cell clones: correlation with lymphokine secretion patterns. *J Immunol* 1992;149:1921–1926.

465. Nau GJ, Moldwin RL, Lancki DW, Kim D-K, Fitch FW. Inhibition of IL 2-driven proliferation of murine T lymphocyte clones by supraoptimal levels of immobilized anti-T cell receptor monoclonal antibody. *J Immunol* 1987;139:114–122.

466. Jenkins MK, Schwartz RH. Antigen presentation by chemically modified splenocytes induces antigen-specific T cell unresponsiveness *in vitro* and *in vivo*. *J Exp Med* 1987;165:302–319.

467. Quill H, Schwartz RH. Stimulation of normal inducer T cell clones with antigen presented by purified Ia molecules in planar lipid membranes: Specific induction of a long-lived state of proliferative nonresponsiveness. *J Immunol* 1987;138:3704–3712.

468. Lin H, Bolling SF, Linsley PS, et al. Long-term acceptance of major histocompatibility complex mismatched cardiac allografts induced by CTLA4Ig plus donor-specific transfusion. *J Exp Med* 1993;178:1801–1806.

Fundamental Immunology, Fourth Edition,
edited by William E. Paul
Lippincott–Raven Publishers, Philadelphia © 1999.

CHAPTER 13

Accessory Molecules

Jeffrey A. Bluestone, Roli Khattri, and Gijs A. van Seventer

HISTORICAL PERSPECTIVE

In the early 1980s, Dr. Richard Gershon of Yale University was famous for starting his lectures with a series of four histology slides that portrayed the various lymphocyte subsets of the immune system. First, he would show a picture of a single lymphocyte stained with hematoxylin and eosin (H&E). The title on the slide read, "This is a helper T cell." This slide was followed by several additional H&E stained images representing a cytolytic T cell, suppressor T cell, and B cell. All the pictures were identical: each round lymphocyte had a smooth surface, a dark blue nucleus, and a small ring of pale uncluttered cytoplasm The different lymphocytes could be distinguished only by the written title on each slide. The point of this myopic view of the lymphocyte was that H&E pictures alone could not anticipate the enormous complexity of the cell function or the hundreds of unique cell surface proteins, glycoproteins, and glycolipids expressed on the cell membrane that distinguish each lymphocyte subset and stage in lymphocyte differentiation.

Historically, the absence of serologic tools to detect individual cell types led experimental immunologists to rely on anatomic location and chromosomal markers to distinguish the various lymphocyte subsets (i.e., the antibody-producing B cell from the thymically-derived T cell). The study of cell surface accessory molecules started with the simple goal of developing serologic reagents that could distinguish these lymphocyte subsets. The

development of the lymphocyte-specific antisera completely changed the field of immunology (1). These antisera were used to define unique markers or flags that could distinguish and separate the different lymphocyte subsets based on expression of so-called cell differentiation antigens. Antisera against cell surface proteins, such as anti–Ly-1 and anti–Ly-2, were instrumental in distinguishing helper T cells from cytolytic T cells. Initially, polyclonal anti-Thy-1 antibodies were used to isolate purified murine T-cell populations, and antitheta antisera made against thymocytes were the first to define T cells in humans (2). With the development of monoclonal antibody (mAb) technology, there was an explosion of reagents that identified individual cell surface molecules expressed in unique patterns on different lymphocyte subsets. In 1996, the Sixth International Leukocyte Culture Conference officially designated over 160 individual cell surface molecules on the surface of resting and activated lymphocytes (3). The genes encoding all these cell surface molecules have been cloned, and the serologic epitopes have been defined by multiple mAbs. In order to define this broad array of cell surface molecules, the cluster of differentiation (CD) nomenclature was developed by the International Leukocyte Workshop.

Although the identification of the CD molecules was critical for immunophenotyping and descriptive analyses, defining the function of these cell surface molecules on individual lymphocytes became the real challenge. It is important to keep in mind that the T-cell receptor (TCR) complex represents less than 1% of the cell surface protein on a T-lymphocyte. Thus, increased emphasis on the study of cell differentiation molecules as functional elements of the lymphocyte became equally important. Initially, it was pre-

---

J. A. Bluestone, R. Khattri, and G. A. van Seventer: Ben May Institute for Cancer Research, University of Chicago, Chicago, Illinois 60637.

sumed that these cell surface structures would facilitate and complement antigen recognition and signaling by the antigen receptor on the lymphocyte. However, the investigations quickly determined that the role of the accessory molecules was far more complex.

In the past decade, sophisticated molecular and biochemical tools have accelerated and enhanced our ability to study accessory molecules. This chapter will not be a superficial survey of the over 100 molecules expressed on T cells at various stages of activation and differentiation. Instead, general paradigms will be discussed with selected focus on several cell surface proteins that mediate essential T-cell functions and represent the major elements of the cascade of events that regulate T-cell function.

OVERVIEW: THE FUNCTION OF ACCESSORY MOLECULES ON T CELLS

Exposure of the body to a foreign antigen leads to a cascade of events that results in the sequential induction of pathogen processing and presentation followed by effector cell activation. The foreign antigen (such as a virus or bacteria) enters the body where antigen-presenting cells (APCs) in the peripheral tissues, such as Langerhans' cells and other dendritic cells, pick up antigen and migrate through the efferent lymphatics to the secondary lymphoid tissues to present the major histocompatibility complex (MHC)-bound pathogen-derived peptides. T cells are constantly circulating through the blood, monitoring draining lymph nodes to explore for the presence of foreign substances. The circulating T cells adhere to specialized high endothelial venules (HEVs), after which they extravasate and transmigrate into the underlying secondary lymphoid tissues. Cell surface glycolipids, called selectins, and soluble factors, called chemokines, provide important homing functions to maximize the trafficking of the T cells to the site of the APCs bearing the foreign antigen.

The T cells enter the secondary lymphoid tissues where they scan the APCs for the presence of antigenic peptides in the grooves of the MHC molecules. This initial scanning process requires intimate cell–cell contact, which is provided through binding of adhesion molecules expressed on the cell surface of both the T cells and the APCs. If no specific recognition occurs, then the T cell disengages and moves on in search of another APC with which to repeat this scanning process. When antigen-specific recognition does occur, the T cell receives specific activation signals through its TCR/CD3 complex, which results in a further strengthening and prolongation of the adhesive interaction between T cells and APCs. Thus, adhesion molecules are important in both the antigen-independent and antigen-dependent binding of the T cells to the APCs. Subsequent to the initial antigen-driven process, secondary, so-called costimulatory interactions provide essential signals that lower the threshold for antigen-dependent signal transduction, promote clonal expansion, maintain sustained cell survival, and initiate T-cell differentiation into the effector cells that mediate inflammatory, cytolytic, and humoral responses.

Each stage in this immune response is controlled by specific accessory molecules that regulate homing, TCR interactions, adhesion, and costimulation on the T cells. The dynamic interactions of these molecules determine the efficiency and effectiveness of the immune reaction complementing the specificity generated by TCR recognition with essential immune system architecture and amplification processes.

T-CELL COSTIMULATION

General Aspects

In the late 1950s, Burnet published his landmark paper describing the clonal selection theory (4). His hypothesis was based on the observation that antibodies produced by each individual did not react to self molecules. The clonal selection theory hypothesized that maturing B cells and, similarly, T cells would be exposed to the vast majority of self antigens during development in order to eliminate self-reactive clones rendering the individual self tolerant. For T cells, self tolerance is initiated by processes manifested centrally in the thymus by clonal deletion during T-cell development (see Chapter 11). However, not all self antigens are expressed in or traffic to the thymus. Therefore, the body sustains tolerance to tissue-specific self proteins uniquely expressed extrathymically or induced during organ development, cell death, or viral infection by a number of peripheral processes that prevent potentially autoreactive immune responses from arising in the adult animal. A two-signal activation model, a concept first introduced by Bretscher and Cohn in the 1970s for B cell activation (5), has provided a mechanism for the maintenance of peripheral tolerance. The model proposed that B cells engage two separate structures on APCs, both of which required the B cell to become effectively activated. The first interaction is initiated by the recognition of antigen by the B-cell receptor (surface immunoglobulin [Ig]). This signal 1 initiates the activation cascade but causes clonal paralysis unless a second cell surface structure, the so-called costimulatory molecules were ligated during a temporally restricted period. These studies in the B-cell compartment laid the groundwork for a similar two-signal hypothesis by Kevin Lafferty for the T cell-compartment. He noted that, like B cells, T cells required both antigen recognition (signal 1) as well as some other signal from an APC (signal 2) in order to become fully activated (6). The best APCs for an allogeneic transplant reaction were hematopoietically derived cells (i.e., dendritic cells, macrophages, and activated B cells); thus, Lafferty proposed that these cells possessed the necessary costimulatory signal to fully activate the T cell. In a seminal set of experiments performed using allogeneic thyroid organs, Lafferty and Talmage demonstrated that removal of the bone marrow–derived APCs by in vitro culture for several days eliminated the costimulatory ability of the graft leading to permanent graft acceptance.

The concept of T cell costimulation, now generally accepted, had led to a field of study that has resulted in over 1,000 publications since 1991 focusing on the identification of cell surface accessory molecules capable of providing costimulatory signals to T cells. To date, over 20 molecules (including the integrins, CD2, HSA, CD44, CD40L, CD43, 4-1BB, CD30, OX40, and CD28) have been shown to augment the T cell's proliferative response to antigenic stimuli and promote T-cell activation (Fig. 1). However, the mechanism by which each molecule functions is distinct, ranging from those molecules that simply enhance adhesion to those that deliver essential biochemical signals to the T cell that complement those delivered via the TCR complex. In this section, we will focus on two major classes of costimulation. The first, represented by the CD28/B7 pathway, provides the major costimulus on resting naive and memory T cells. The second, illustrated by the tumor necrosis factor receptor (TNF-R) family members—CD40L, CD30, and 4-1BB—are activation-induced costimulatory receptors that extend and enhance T-cell expansion, promote T-cell differentiation, and mediate collaborative interactions between T cells and B cells.

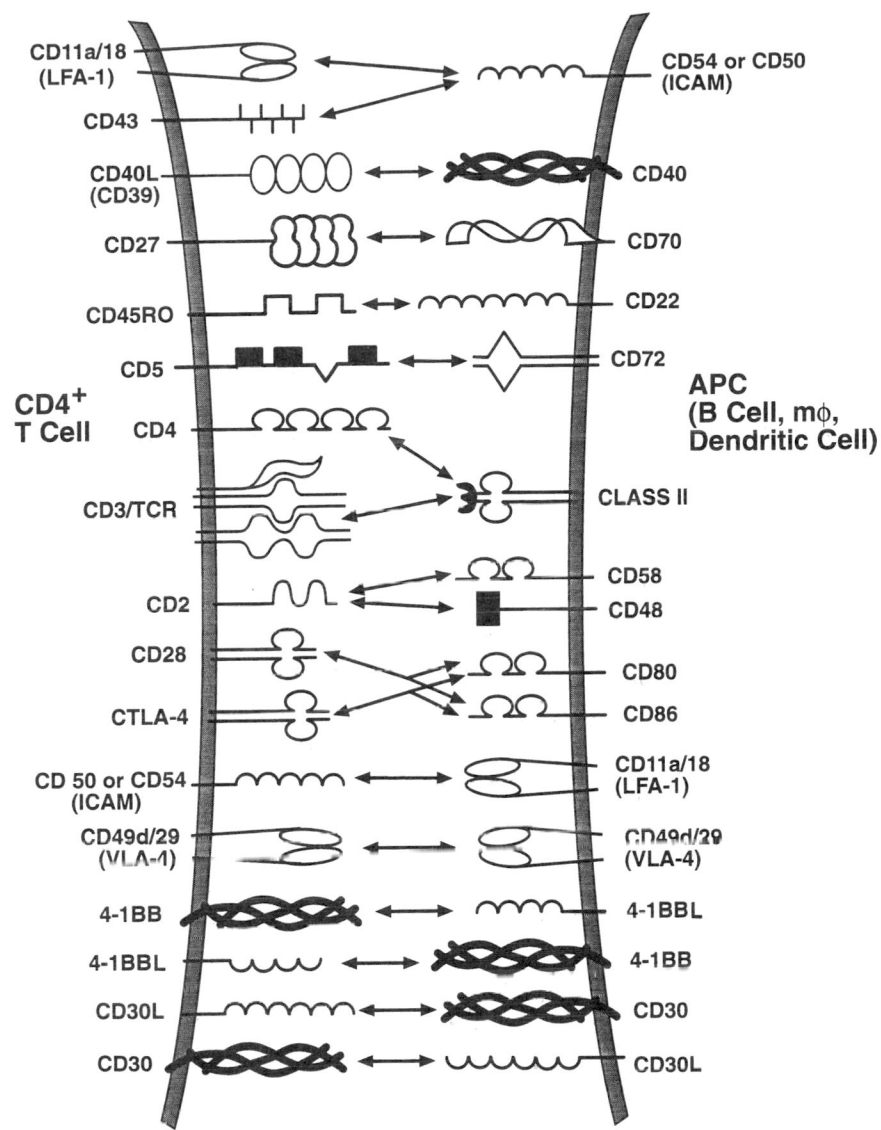

CD4+ T Cell

CD11a/18 (LFA-1)
CD43
CD40L (CD39)
CD27
CD45RO
CD5
CD4
CD3/TCR
CD2
CD28
CTLA-4
CD 50 or CD54 (ICAM)
CD49d/29 (VLA-4)
4-1BB
4-1BBL
CD30L
CD30

APC (B Cell, mφ, Dendritic Cell)

CD54 or CD50 (ICAM)
CD40
CD70
CD22
CD72
CLASS II
CD58
CD48
CD80
CD86
CD11a/18 (LFA-1)
CD49d/29 (VLA-4)
4-1BBL
4-1BB
CD30
CD30L

FIG. 1. Selected examples of accessory molecule pairs between CD4+ T cells and APCs. The schematics structures are representative but not a genuine reflection of the individual structures.

Characteristics of CD28, CTLA-4, CD80, and CD86

The importance of the CD28/B7 pathway in T-cell costimulation has become increasingly clear in the past 10 years. In 1987, Jenkins and colleagues demonstrated that Th1 clones encountering nominal antigen–MHC complexes in the absence of appropriate costimulatory signals were rendered functionally inactive (7). Upon restimulation, these anergic T cells failed to proliferate and produce lymphokines, most prominently interleukin (IL)-2. The induction of anergy is reversed during the initial activation event by either the addition of exogenous IL-2 or, more importantly, by ligation of the CD28 cell surface glycoprotein either with anti-CD28 mAbs or its ligands, B7-1(CD80) and B7-2(CD86) (8). In fact, exposure of purified resting CD4+ T-lymphocytes to a TCR stimulus such as immobilized anti-CD3 mAbs together with B7-1 or B7-2 is sufficient to drive IL-2 production and T-cell proliferation (9). Thus, the CD28/B7 pathway has emerged as the dominant costimulatory pathway on resting naive and memory T cells.

CD28

The CD28 molecule is a cell surface glycoprotein expressed predominantly on T cells and developing thymocytes (8,10). Under normal circumstances, 50% of human CD8+ T cells and virtually all human CD4+ T cells, as well as all murine T cells, express CD28. A percentage of plasma cells and natural killer (NK) cells express CD28, although the function of the glycoprotein on these differentiated lymphocyte populations remains unclear. The gene for the CD28 molecule is located on chromosome 2q33 in humans (11) and chromosome 1 in mice (12). The gene is organized into 4 exons. Exon 1 encodes the leader sequence; exon 2, the extracellular Ig V region-like domain; and exons 3 and 4, the transmembrane and cytoplasmic domains, respectively. Human CD28 is expressed as a 44-kDa type I receptor glycoprotein, composed of a 134 amino acid extracellular domain, a 27 amino acid hydrophobic transmembrane domain, and a 41 amino acid cytoplasmic tail (13). The extracellular domain shows structural homology to the Ig variable (V)-region domains with a predicted sheet sandwich and three complementarity determining region (CDR) loops. This IgV-like domain is followed by a 16–amino acid stretch that contains a cysteine residue involved in homodimerization, although CD28 also exists as a monomeric glycoprotein on the T-cell surface, particularly on chicken T cells (14). A comparison of the amino acid sequences of the human, rodent, bovine, and avian forms of CD28 demonstrated significant homology (67% between mouse and human). This high level of conservation supports an important and evolutionarily conserved role for CD28 in T-cell function. There is an especially high homology within the ligand binding site (a hexapeptide stretch, MYPPPY, in the CDR3 region). Interestingly, although the methionine has been exchanged for a leucine in bovine CD28, its ability to bind human B7-2 is retained, suggesting that the MYPPPY motif is not immutable (15).

Finally, it is worth noting that although CD28 is constitutively expressed on the majority of T cells, its expression is dynamic. CD28 expression increases transiently after T-cell activation and then decreases after its engagement with its ligand, B7. This reduction in CD28 expression results in a decreased ability of the T cell to mobilize intracellular stores of calcium, a critical component to effective T-cell signaling (16).

Cytotoxic T-Lymphocyte Antigen-4

Cytotoxic T-lymphocyte antigen-4 (CTLA-4), a structural homolog of CD28 (30% homologous), was discovered in a complementary DNA library of T cell–specific, activation-induced genes (17). CTLA-4 is expressed on activated CD4$^+$ and CD8$^+$ T cells at levels 10- to 100-fold less than CD28 but binds to both B7-1 and B7-2 with a 20- to 50-fold higher dissociation constant (K_d) relative to CD28 (18–22). The gene for CTLA-4 is closely linked to CD28 and has a similar intron/exon organization with single extracellular IgV-like domain, a transmembrane region, and a cytoplasmic domain (14,21,23). The CTLA-4 protein is expressed as a type I receptor glycoprotein (33 to 45 kDa), with a similar ligand binding domain centered around the MYPPPY binding site (8,20,24). CTLA-4 can be expressed on the cell surface as both a monomer and homodimer but does not dimerize with CD28. It should be noted that dimeric CTLA-4 can bind two B7-2 molecules providing for a potential to cross-link and signal through either of the B7 molecules (25). Finally, there is 100% conservation in the 36 amino acid sequence of the cytoplasmic domain of the human, bovine, and mouse CTLA-4 molecules, but only an approximately 30% homology with the cytoplasmic domain of CD28, suggesting a distinct but important preservation of signaling function.

There are other distinct differences between CD28 and CTLA-4. Although CD28 is constitutively expressed on the majority of resting human and murine T cells, CTLA-4 is expressed only after T-cell activation, with peak expression after 48 to 72 hours (18,20). Although CTLA-4 glycoprotein is expressed on the surface of both activated CD4$^+$ and CD8$^+$ T cells, the majority of the protein remains intracellular (26,27). This intracellular localization of the CTLA-4 glycoprotein is a direct consequence of the presence of an internalization localization motif (TTGVYVKMPPT) within the cytoplasmic domain that causes rapid endocytosis (26). The ligation of the CD28 molecule is essential for maximal CTLA-4 expression. CD28-deficient T cells do not efficiently upregulate CTLA-4 messenger RNA (mRNA) after activation unless exogenous IL-2 is added (27). Anti-CD28 mAbs accelerate the kinetics of CTLA-4 mRNA accumulation among human peripheral blood lymphocytes, whereas upregulation of CTLA-4 in response to antigen is blocked by CD28 antagonists (28). Thus, there appears to be a coordinated relationship between CD28 and CTLA-4 expression and function.

B7-1 (CD80) and B7-2 (CD86)

The first ligand to be identified for CD28 was the B-cell activation molecule, B7 or BB-1 (B7-1/CD80) (29), based on the ability of CD28-transfected CHO cells to bind to a lymphoblastoid cell line. This binding was inhibited by antibodies reactive with a previously identified B-cell activation marker, B7 (CD80). The expression of B7-1 is quite diverse, ranging from activated B cells and T cells, dendritic cells, Langerhans' cells, activated monocytes, certain endothelial cells and a variety of tumor lines. The human and murine B7-1 genes are members of the Ig superfamily. Exon 1 encodes the signal peptide; exons 2 and 3 encode the extracellular IgV-like and Ig constant region (C)-like domains; exon 4 encodes the transmembrane domain; and exon 5 encodes the cytoplasmic tail (30). The B7-1 genes have been localized to chromosomes 3 and 16 in the human and mouse, respectively (31,32). While studying B7-1, several groups noted that certain cell types that bound soluble or membrane-bound forms of CD28 and CTLA-4 did not react with B7-1–specific mAbs, including activated B cells from B7-1–deficient knock-out (KO) mice (33,34). These observations led to the identification and eventual cloning of a second B7 family member, B7-2 (CD86) (35). The overall structure of B7-2 is very similar to B7-1 although the two genes share only limited sequence homology (about 25%), especially in the intracytoplasmic tail. The homology is highest near sequences required for the formation of the Ig domains and CD28/CTLA-4 binding sites. Both B7-1 and B7-2 interact with CTLA-4 with 20- to 50-fold higher affinity than to CD28, but B7-2 dissociates more rapidly from CTLA-4 Ig than B7-1 (22). In fact, the fine specificity of the B7-1 and B7-2 interaction with CTLA-4 is different. A single amino acid mutation in the MYPPPY motif of CTLA-4 completely abolished B7-2 binding, while retaining B7-1 reactivity (36).

The B7-1 and B7-2 molecules not only interact differently with their counter receptors, but the regulation of their expression is distinct. Both molecules are found on activated APCs; however, after B-cell activation, for example, B7-2 levels increase much more rapidly than do B7-1 levels. The upregulation of B7-2 occurs within 6 hours of stimulation, with maximal levels of expression achieved after 18 to 24 hours (37). In contrast, the increase in B7-1 expression is not detected until 24 hours poststimulation and does not reach maximal levels until 48 to 72 hours later. Furthermore, activated B cells and dendritic cells express quantitatively higher levels of B7-2 than B7-1 (38), and B7-2 has been shown to be the major functional CD28 ligand on human dendritic cells (39). It should be noted that B7-1 and B7-2 are expressed on both rodent and human T cells as well. B7-2 is constitutively expressed on resting T cells, especially memory T cells, but decreases after T-cell activation, whereas B7-1, absent from resting T cells, is induced after T-cell signaling (40). The functional role of these molecules on T cells is unclear. However, B7-1 has been shown to be phosphorylated after T-cell activation; B7-2 is alternatively glycosylated on human T cells, leading to selective binding to CTLA-4; and blockade of B7 molecules results in increased T-cell proliferation and cytokine production.

Cell surface molecules modulate B7-1 and B7-2 expression. MHC class II molecules and CD40 cross-linking upregulates both B7-1 and B7-2. The cross-linking of surface Ig with anti-Ig or antigen rapidly induces B7-2 on the B-cell surface, transforming a resting B cell into a fully competent APC (37) but does not induce detectable levels of B7-1 (41). Cytokines such as IL-4 and interferon (IFN)-γ also have been shown to dramatically increase the expression of B7-2 while having little or no effect on B7-1 expression. Other signals downregulate B7-1 and B7-2 expression. The engagement of the Fc receptor decreases the expression of both B7-1 and B7-2 on monocytes that have been activated with either IFN-γ or granulocyte-macrophage colony-stimulating factor (GM-CSF) (42,43). IL-10 blocks both B7-1 and B7-2 upregulation on peritoneal macrophages and downregulates B7-2, but not B7-1, on human dendritic cells, suggesting that the immunosuppressive properties of IL-10 may, in part, be a result of its regulation of CD28/CTLA-4 ligands (44). The ability of various cell surface molecules and cytokines to regulate both qualitatively and quantitatively the levels and temporal expression of B7-1 and B7-2 may result in distinct effects during the course of an immune response.

Role of CD28 and CTLA-4 Pathways in T-Cell Development

Early studies demonstrated that CD28 is highly expressed on thymocytes including both the immature CD4+CD8+ cells and mature CD4+ and CD8+ T-cell subsets. The high expression of CD28 on these thymocytes suggested that CD28/B7 interactions may be critical for T-cell development. Indeed a role for CD28 in thymus ontogeny was suggested by studies showing that anti-CD28 mAbs prevented apoptosis of immature thymocytes (45). Although groups have shown that mAb-mediated cross-linking of CD28 inhibited T-cell development by increasing apoptosis among the CD4+CD8+ immature thymocytes (46), the addition of CD28 antagonists had no effect on the negative selection of autoreactive cells in a class II–specific TCR transgenic mouse, or in the deletion of T cells reactive with endogenous superantigens (47). Consistent with these observations, negative and positive selection of normal and TCR transgenic T cells could not be distinguished between wild-type and CD28−/− mice, including TCR transgenics expressing class I– and class II–restricted TCR γδ or TCR-αβ transgenes. However, CD28+ T cells do have a selective survival advantage in mice reconstituted with a mixture of CD28+ and CD28−/− bone marrow (48). Therefore, although CD28 and CTLA-4 are not essential for development, they may play a subtle role in thymocyte differentiation. The role of CTLA-4 in thymic selection also has been controversial. Original studies in the CTLA-4 KO mice suggested a potential role for CTLA-4 in thymic selection. Thymuses from 2- to 3-week-old animals had a dramatically increased number of CD4+ and CD8+ mature thymocytes (49). However, recent studies by Allison and colleagues suggest that these cells are lymphocytes present in surrounding parathymic lymph nodes enlarged due to the uncontrolled lymphoproliferation observed in these animals (50).

CD28 and CTLA-4 Function

Ligation of CD28 in the presence of TCR engagement has been shown to have multiple functional consequences in T cells. The earliest studies showed that CD28-mediated T-cell costimulation regulated cytokine production and proliferation in both CD4+ and CD8+ lymphocytes. CD28 engagement induced up to a 100-fold increase in IL-2 production, whereas T cells from the CD28 mice produce less than one tenth the amount of IL-2 after activation (51,52). In addition, the production of other cytokines, such as IL-4, IL-5, IL-13, IFN-γ, TNF-α, and GM-CSF, also increases after CD28 engagement (8,53). The CD28-mediated increases in cytokine production reflect both an increased level of gene transcription and mRNA stability (54,55). CD28 costimulation has been shown to enhance the expression of IL-2 receptor α, β, and γ chains (56) and increase IL-4 responsiveness due to an increase in production of IL-1 (57). One major consequence of CD28-mediated regulation of cytokines has been the observation that stimulation of Th1 T-cell clones in the presence of CD28 antagonists inhibits proliferation, blocks IL-2 production, and causes cells to become anergic (8). These anergic T cells can be rescued from this nonfunctional state by CD28-mediated costimulation or by the addition of exogenous IL-2. Thus, it has been suggested that the major role for CD28 costimulation in T-cell activation is the regulation of growth factors that control T-cell function.

The CD28-dependent induction of anergy has been largely restricted to Th1 T-cell clones. Resting naive or memory T cells, or for that matter Th2 clones, do not become anergic after TCR-mediated activation in the absence of CD28 costimulation. However, the responses of these cell subsets are suppressed, suggesting that there exists other important, CD28-mediated effects on T cells (58). The study of the CD28 KO mice and the use of a CTLA-4 Ig in primary T-cell cultures provided the first hints that CD28 engagement may regulate multiple T-cell functions other than anergy induction. First, CD28-mediated costimulation of resting T cells has been shown to regulate the threshold of T-cell responses. In the presence of an effective CD28 signal, the degree of TCR engagement required for effective T cell activation is reduced significantly (59). CD28 signal transduction also synergizes with TCR engagement to enhance the survival of lymphocytes activated in response to antigenic challenge (60). CD28 costimulation induces bcl-xL, an intracellular factor (see Chapter 23) essential for long-term survival of activated T cells. This function of CD28 cannot be mimicked by the addition of cytokines. Second, there is a fundamental role for CD28 in the differentiation of Th1/Th2 subsets. In the absence of CD28 signaling, T cells activated with TCR-specific stimuli are biased toward a Th1 phenotype. IFN-γ, but no IL-4, was produced by activated CD28 KO T cells or when CD28/B7 interactions were blocked with CTLA-4 Ig (53,61). In contrast, increasing CD28 costimulation promotes both IL-4 and IL-5 production (61). Finally, CD28 appears to be essential for the differentiation of CD8+ T cells into cytolytic effectors. In both human and murine systems, stimulation of purified CD8+ T cells with B7-1 transfectants promotes the development of cytolytic T cells (62). In fact, the addition of potent costimulation obviates the requirement for help from CD4+ T cells due to increased IL-2 production by the activated CD8+ T cells. Taken together, these data suggest that CD28/B7 interactions play multiple roles during an immune response, including, under certain circumstances, ablation of the immune response leading to tolerance, alteration of the Th1/Th2 balance, and regulation of cytolytic effector activity.

Although CD28 is clearly a costimulatory molecule, the function of CTLA-4 remains controversial. Several studies examining the role of CTLA-4 in in vitro proliferative responses suggest that CTLA-4, like CD28, functions as a costimulatory molecule on activated T cells (63,64). However, other functional studies in both the murine and human systems have suggested that CTLA-4 can deliver downregulatory signals to activated T cells. The blockade of CTLA-4/B7 interactions in vitro increased T-cell proliferation and cytokine production (28,65). Furthermore, cross-linking of the CTLA-4 molecule with mAbs resulted in the blockade of critical cell cycle progression factors and inhibition of IL-2 receptor expression (66). Most importantly, CTLA-4 KO mice exhibit a profound spontaneous autoimmune disease. At 2 to 3 weeks of age, the CTLA-4 KO mice manifest a massive lymphoproliferative disorder and develop an apparent autoimmune myocarditis and pancreatitis that is uniformly fatal within 4 to 5 weeks (49). Finally, it is interesting to note that one of the genetic loci linked to susceptibility to the human autoimmune diseases Graves disease and insulin-dependent diabetes mellitus has been CTLA-4 (67).

Biochemical Basis of CD28 and CTLA-4 Function

One of the hallmarks of CD28-mediated T-cell costimulation is the concept that CD28 signaling is TCR independent and downstream from early activation events. This is supported by the observations that the signals delivered by CD28 to the T cell can be spatially and temporally separated from TCR signaling. For the most part, the biochemical events induced after CD28 engagement are similar to those seen by TCR cross-linking (57). Phosphatidylinositol 3-kinase associates with the CD28 cytoplasmic domain upon CD28 ligation (67). Similarly, CD28 binds to the GRB-2–SOS complex, recruits LAT(p36), and initiates downstream signaling via the Ras pathway of T-cell activation (57,68). Finally, CD28 cross-linking enhances various biochemical events triggered by TCR-mediated signaling, including the activation of PLC-γ^1, p56^{lck}, and Raf-1 kinase, as well as inducing the influx of Ca^{2+} and generation of phosphoinositides.

Among the biochemical pathways that appear to be uniquely regulated by CD28 is the activation of cJun, an important transcription factor that regulates the IL-2 gene. cJun phosphorylation requires a calcium signal delivered via TCR ligation and the CD28-mediated activation of jun-specific kinases, JNK1 and JNK2 (69). The interaction of CD28 with either B7-1 or B7-2 can activate JNK (70). This is consistent with the finding that CD28 costimulation enhances transactivation mediated by AP-1. Interestingly, a block in the ras/JNK signaling pathway is responsible for the inability of anergic T cells to respond to antigenic challenge, and the inability to activate the Ras pathway in anergic T cells correlates with a failure to activate the mitogen-activated protein kinases, Erk-1, and Erk-2 (71,72). Blockade of CD28/B7 also results in a failure to activate the AP-1 transcription factor complex. This suggests a plausible mechanism for the inability to initiate IL-2 gene transcription after T cells enter the anergic state. Another target of CD28 costimulation is NF-κB. After CD28-mediated costimulation, IκB, an NF-κB inhibitor, is degraded, allowing NF-κB to act on early T-cell activation genes such as IL-2 (73). Finally, itk, an src-related tyrosine kinase, becomes phosphorylated and associates with CD28 within minutes after CD28 engagement (74). There is increased anti-CD28–induced T-cell proliferation in itk KO mice, consistent with an important role for itk in the regulation of CD28 function (Dan Littman, personal communication). Together the biochemical studies suggest that there are both independent and cross-connections in the CD28/B7 and TCR signaling pathways.

The biochemical basis for CTLA-4-mediated control of immune responses has not been fully characterized. There is an almost 100% conservation of the intracytoplasmic domains of mouse, bovine, rat, and human CTLA-4. This degree of homology along with the presence of several potential sites for phosphorylation and association with certain signaling molecules suggests an important role for CTLA-4 signaling in the regulation of both the TCR and CD28 signaling pathways. The CTLA-4 molecule distributes into the TCR activation cap, providing an opportunity for CTLA-4 to act proximal to the TCR signaling pathway (75). Furthermore, T cells isolated from CTLA-4 KO mice exhibit enhanced activity of p56lck and p59fyn tyrosine kinases, as well as hyperphosphorylation of TCR signaling molecules such as shc and ZAP-70 (76).

A mechanism for CTLA-4 modification of the TCR complex and CD28 signaling events recently was proposed. CTLA-4 interacts with the phosphotyrosine phosphatase SHP-2 (76). This phosphatase associates with the CTLA-4 molecule through an SH2–phosphotyrosine interaction, mapping to the YVKM amino acid sequence of CTLA-4, also found to be the site of PI-3 kinase interaction. Moreover, this phosphatase has been shown to dephosphorylate TCR–CD28 activation complex associated phosphoproteins. There is a second tyrosine-based motif (YFIP) present in the cytoplasmic tail of CTLA-4 that may be the binding site of other phosphotyrosine-binding proteins important for T-cell signal transduction. Based on these data, it is tempting to speculate that, under some conditions, CTLA-4 may function to negatively signal activated T cells by translocating into the TCR–CD28 activation complex, where it would either dephosphorylate critical signaling components of the T-cell activation cascade due to its association with SHP-2 or compete for critical signaling molecules (such as PI-3 kinase or other phosphotyrosine-binding proteins) that are essential downstream substrates for signal transduction. Finally, because CTLA-4 has a higher avidity for the B7-1 and B7-2 molecules than does CD28, it also may compete with CD28 for ligand binding and terminate CD28 signaling. Thus, CTLA-4 may affect TCR–CD28 mediated signal transduction by competing for the CD28 costimulatory ligands (66).

Role of B7-1 and B7-2 in CD28 and CTLA-4 Function

In vitro studies using gene transfectants demonstrated that B7-1 and B7-2 can interact with CD28 to costimulate both antigen- and mitogen-driven T-cell proliferation and IL-2 production (77). Similarly, overexpression of either B7-1 or B7-2 on different tissues in vivo, including tumors and pancreatic cells, resulted in potent costimulation and subsequent augmentation of immunity. In fact, transduction of B7 directly into established tumors using virally mediated gene therapy induced an active immune response resulting in tumor regression and long-term tumor-specific immunity (78). These findings suggest that ectopic expression of either B7-1 or B7-2 on cells can provide a sufficient costimulatory signal to initiate a potent immune response.

It has been much more difficult to demonstrate that B7-1 functions on normal APCs to costimulate T cells. Anti–B7-1 mAbs have minimal effect on primary mixed lymphocyte reactions, and B7-1–deficient mice respond normally to foreign antigens in vitro and in vivo (58,79). In contrast, blockade of B7-2 engagement profoundly effects CD28-mediated T-cell costimulation. Anti–B7-2 mAbs block allograft rejection, the development of autoimmune disease, initiation of antiviral responses, and antibody responses to soluble antigens (58). Moreover, B7-2 KO mice are selectively defective in mediating primary humoral responses to soluble antigens (79). Collectively, these results indicate that B7-2, not B7-1, is the primary costimulatory molecule responsible for initiating T cell responses and providing cognate help for B cells. The dominance of B7-2 in these situations may be due to a unique capacity of B7-2 to costimulate naive T-cell populations. However, this seems unlikely because, as noted above, B7-1 transfectants costimulate naive T cells as effectively as B7-2–transfected cells. Alternatively, it is likely that anatomic and temporal differences in B7-2 expression on naturally occurring APC populations result in the predominant role for this CD28 ligand. Unlike B7-1, B7-2 is constitutively expressed on some dendritic cells and B cells and is rapidly upregulated on a subset of APCs during inflammatory responses (38).

Under certain conditions, however, B7-1 can provide an important costimulatory function in vivo. In a model of experimental autoimmune encephalitis (EAE), blockade of B7-1 during clinical remission can ameliorate central nervous system histopathology and clinical relapses. The anti–B7-1 mAbs had no effect on the T cells specific for the immunizing epitope but blocked the recruitment of T cells into the lesion that were potentially reactive against distinct autoantigens. This blockade of so-called epitope spreading (80) by anti–B7-1 mAbs was related to the selective upregulation of B7-1, but not B7-2, on hematopoietic cells during the initial clinical episode in response to inflammatory cytokines. This fits with recent studies of B7-1/B7-2 double-KO mice and anti-B7 antibody therapy, which suggested that blockade of both costimulatory ligands completely blocked primary T-cell responses (58) and fits with multiple studies in humans demonstrating the upregulation of B7-1 during chronic inflammatory reactions. Thus, B7-2 appears to dominate in the initiation of both inflammatory and humoral responses, whereas B7-1 appears to play a more important role in some chronic inflammatory responses. There may be differences in B7-1 and B7-2 function due to intrinsic differences in the two molecules as well. Under certain circumstances, B7-1 appears to be selectively involved in stimulating inflammatory responses, whereas costimulation by B7-2 preferentially promotes humoral responses (81). For instance, although mAbs to B7-1 inhibit the development of Th1-mediated murine EAE, anti–B7-2 mAb therapy made the disease worse, reflecting the fact that stimulation of T cells by cells expressing B7-1 as opposed to B7-2 led to the expansion of Th1 rather than Th2 T cells. These findings could be due to the distinct binding domains and kinetics of CD28 binding of B7-1 and B7-2, resulting in distinct signaling events that bias T-cell activation and subsequent Th1/Th2 differentiation. Further studies will be required to determine the precise roles of B7-1 and B7-2 in the regulation of immune responses in different normal and disease settings. Finally, it is interesting to note that the late phase of the immune response, regulated by CTLA-4, is coincident with the upregulation of B7-1 on a variety of APCs and T cells. These results suggest a potential link between CTLA-4 signaling and B7-1 engagement late in immune responses and may explain the disease-exacerbating effects of anti–B7-1 therapy in several autoimmune models (37,80).

Other Costimulatory Pathways

Several lines of evidence suggest that other costimulatory molecules may substitute or complement CD28/B7 interactions. The blockade of CD28-mediated signals does not fully inhibit primary T cell response. T cells isolated from CD28-deficient mice proliferate in response to alloantigen, nominal antigen, and anti-CD3 mAbs. In fact, CD28-deficient animals can clear some viral infections and reject foreign tissue grafts (82). During the course of an immune response, it appears that CD28 costimulation may take on a diminished role. Secondary reactions are less inhibited by blockade of signals through CD28, and the CD28 molecule is less able to transmit a costimulatory signal. These results suggest that other molecules provide essential signals to the activated T cells. Over

the past few years, a growing number of cell surface molecules have been shown to provide costimulatory signals to activated T cells. A description of all these molecules would make the scope of this chapter unreasonable; however, several reviews have been referenced as guides to the field (58,83,84). Instead, the focus of this section will be on one class of accessory proteins, members of the TNF-R and TNF families (Fig. 2). These molecules, which include TNF-R family members CD30, CD40, 4-1BB, CD27, Fas, and OX40 and TNF family members TNF-α, TNF-β, CD30L, CD40L, 4-1BBL, and FasL, have been shown to be important regulators of T-cell responses. Many members of the TNF-R superfamily function to regulate either cell growth or cell death. For instance, Fas and TNF-R ligation on activated T cells typically results in the activation of a biochemical cascade of caspases that lead to apoptosis. However, under certain circumstances, these same cell surface molecules activate downstream signals that promote cell survival and proliferation. The differences in activity of these molecules relates to the complicated structures of their intracytoplasmic domains that contain both death effector domains and amino acid motifs that bind TNF-R–associated factors (TRAFs) and promote NF-κB activation (see Chapter 23). Other members of the TNF-R superfamily, such as CD40, CD30, and 4-1BB, lack the intracellular domains that lead to the death effector pathways and thus promote selectively costimulatory pathways in T and B cells, leading to increased cell survival, cell cycle progression, and regulation of Th1/Th2 development (83,84). Thus, these accessory molecules represent a new class of costimulators that play an important role in regulating activated lymphocyte function.

CD40L–CD40 interactions are primarily involved in the generation of primary and secondary antibody responses and B cell memory. Ligation of CD40 on B-lymphocytes signals increases homotypic B-cell aggregation, B-cell proliferation, Ig secretion, and Ig class switching. Moreover, CD40L/CD40 ligation during CD4+ T cell–monocyte interactions promotes iNOS, IL-1, IL-6, and GM-CSF production in the monocyte; CD4+ T cell–macrophage and–dendritic cell interactions induce IL-12 and enhance the intracellular killing of pathogens; and CD4+ T cell–endothelial cell interactions promote adhesion molecule expression and lymphocyte extravasation during an immune response (83).

CD40 is a 40- to 45-kDa integral membrane protein predominantly expressed on immature and mature B cells, follicular dendritic cells, bone marrow derived dendritic cells, thymic epithelium, endothelial cells, and activated macrophages. There have been reports of CD40 expression on T cells, although its functional role on these cells is unclear. The CD40 glycoprotein contains four homologous repeating cysteine-rich extracellular domains (45 amino acids each), characteristic motifs of TNF-R family members. Recent efforts to elucidate the biochemical basis of CD40-mediated B-cell signaling pathways have identified members of the TRAF protein family associated with the cytoplasmic tail of CD40. CD40 cross-linking acts intracellularly to multimerize members of the TRAF family of second messengers (specifically TRAF-2 and TRAF-3) that induce gene transcription via the NF-κB family as well as AP-1 and NF-AT complexes (85). The association of TRAF family members with the cytoplasmic tail of CD40 modulates protein tyrosine kinase and tyrosine phosphatase activities that effect the cell cycle, and cdk genes (86) and upregulates the survival factors bcl-2 and bcl-xL to protect B cells from apoptosis.

The CD40 ligand (CD40L, also called glycoprotein [gp]39) molecule is expressed on activated CD4+ and some CD8+ T cells, monocytes, NK cells, human mast cells, and basophils (83). It is

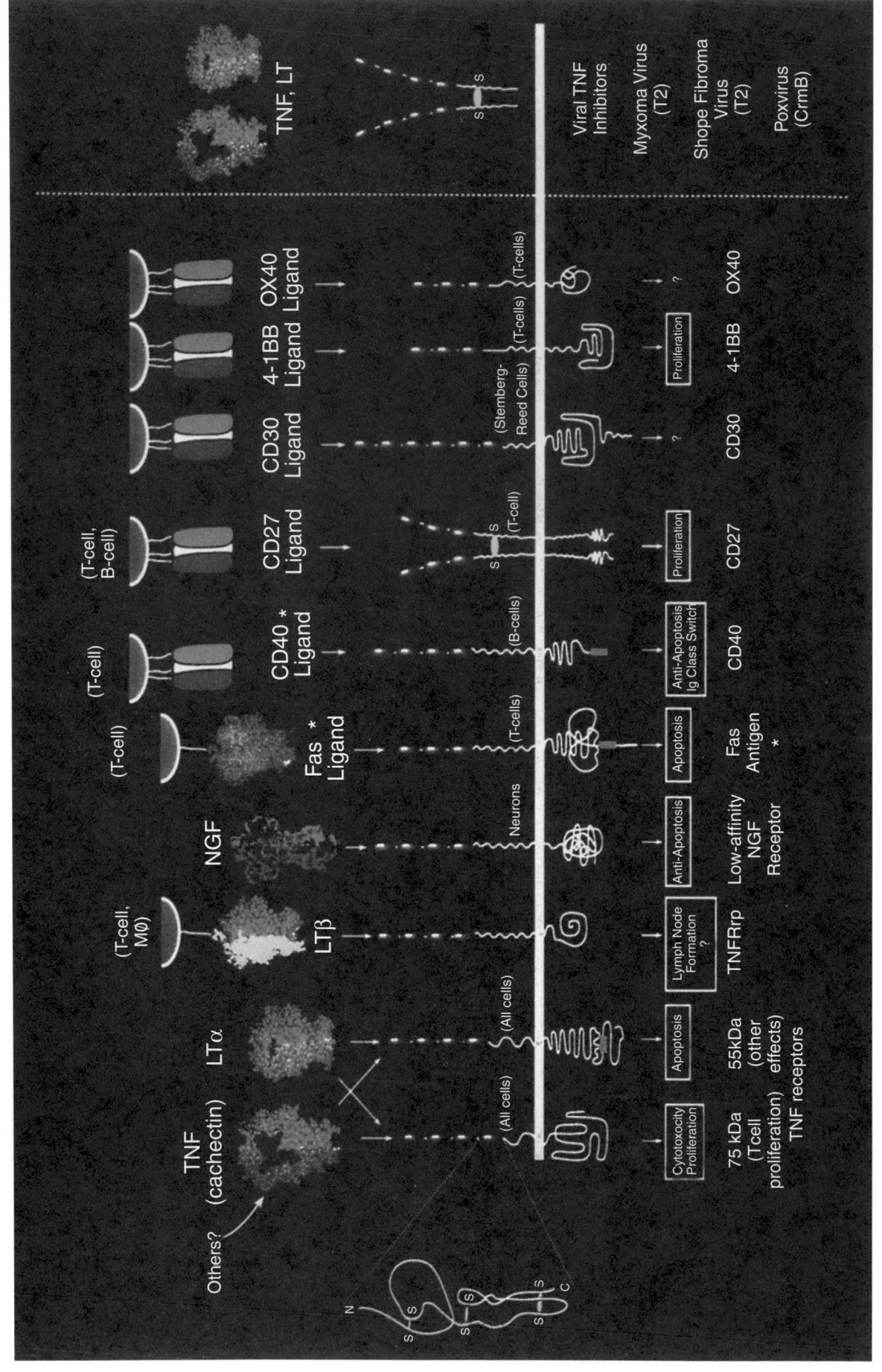

FIG. 2. Structural depiction of members of the TNF and TNF-R family members. In some cases, crystallographic structures, molecular weight, and functional attributes are listed. Asterisks refer to proteins with natural mutations that cause disease.

a type II integral membrane protein with sequence homology to TNF and a predicted tertiary structure similar to that of the TNF trimer. Thus, it has the capacity to multimerize CD40 upon ligation. CD40L is rapidly induced on CD4$^+$ T cells and a subset of CD8$^+$ T cells within 4 to 6 hours after activation, peaks in expression at 24 hours, and decreases over time. In vivo intravenous injection of antigen results in somewhat slower kinetics with maximal frequency of CD40L$^+$ cells at 3 to 4 days after T-dependent antigen administration. The CD40L$^+$ T cells localize to the mantle and centrocytic zones of lymphoid follicles and the periarteriolar regions of the spleen in close proximity to CD40$^+$ B cells. Initial studies showed that CD40L is essential in signaling B cells through its interaction with CD40. Furthermore, crosslinking CD40L on human CD4$^+$ cells generates a costimulatory signal that upregulates IL-4 (87) and intercellular adhesion molecule (ICAM)-1 (88). Functional studies have shown that in vivo treatment of mice with anti-CD40L mAbs abolishes antibody responses and prevents autoimmunity in several different animal models (83).

Perhaps the most important aspect of CD40L–CD40 function is its interrelationship with the CD28 costimulatory pathway. After CD28/B7-dependent CD40L upregulation, CD40L–CD40 interactions signal APCs to upregulate both B7-1 and B7-2, which in turn enhances the costimulatory activity of the B cells, macrophages, and dendritic cells. Thus, CD28/B7 and CD40–CD40L interactions synergize to initiate and amplify T cell–dependent immune responses (89,90). This is most apparent in the CD40L KO mice that have defects in Th1-type immune responses, including defects in antiviral immunity and impaired memory CD8$^+$ T-cell responses (90). These animals have been shown to have defective alloantigen responses that can be reconstituted after upregulation of B7-1. In fact, in one model of autoimmunity, the Th1 deficiency was reversed by injecting constitutive B7-1–expressing B cells into the CD40L-deficient animals. Thus, the CD28/B7 and CD40L–CD40 costimulatory pathways are interrelated and synergistic. This is most apparent in a variety of studies demonstrating the synergistic ability of CD40 and CD28 antagonists in vivo to block murine models of autoimmune diseases, organ graft rejection, allergic contact dermatitis, and antibody production (83,91) (Fig. 3).

CD30–CD30L and 4-1BB–4-1BBL cell surface receptor pairs have gained recent prominence as inducible costimulatory molecules that regulate cell proliferation and promote T-cell differentiation (84). CD30 was first identified as a serologic marker on Reed-Sternberg cells present in patients with Hodgkin's disease and a subset of non-Hodgkin's lymphomas, including Burkitt's lymphoma and Epstein-Barr virus (EBV)-transformed B cells (92). The association of CD30 with lymphoid malignancies serves as a useful marker for malignant cells in the lymphoid system. However, increased awareness of the expression of this cell surface protein on activated normal cells suggested an important role in immune function. The human and murine genes encoding CD30 were cloned and shown to be members of the TNF-R family. The gene encodes a highly glycosylated, 120-kDa surface antigen. The CD30 molecule is expressed on a variety of activated cells, including T cells, B cells, and APCs, and is regulated by cytokines such as IL-4 (93). Signaling through the CD30 cell surface receptor enhances Ig secretion of EBV-immortalized lymphoblastoid cell lines and proliferation of activated T cells. However, CD30 induces apoptosis in certain tumor lines (see Chapter 23). The CD30 extracellular domain contains cysteine-rich motifs

like other members of the family, although it is more highly glycosylated and divergent from other family members. The CD30 internal domain is 188 amino acids long and has potential phosphorylation sites for serine/threonine kinases as well as tyrosine kinases. Several groups have shown that like CD40 and other members of the family, the intracellular domain of CD30 binds several of the TRAF proteins (TRAF-1, TRAF-2, and TRAF-3) that mediate release of intracellular calcium and inactivate NF-κB after CD30 cross-linking. This is particularly relevant to human immunodeficiency virus (HIV), in which CD30 ligation has been shown to increase replication and transcription of the virus (94,95).

4-1BB is expressed on activated CD4$^+$ and CD8$^+$ T cells as both a 30-kDa monomer and 55-kDa homodimer. Peak expression occurs at 6 days poststimulation, can be augmented by the addition of cytokines such as IL-2 and IL-4, and is largely restricted to CD45RO$^+$ T cells. Crosslinking 4-1BB can costimulate T-cell proliferation and IL-2 production in the presence of suboptimal TCR signaling. The intracytoplasmic tail of 4-1BB contains a Cys-Arg-Cys-Pro sequence that has been shown to be a binding site for p56^{lck}. Under certain circumstances, 4-1BB costimulation can initiate T-cell proliferation in a CD28-independent manner. Ligation of 4-1BB induces proliferation of T cells isolated from CD28-deficient mice, and a combination of both CD28 and 4-1BB antagonists is most effective in blocking allogeneic mixed lymphocyte reactions (96,97).

CD30L and 4-1BBL are type II membrane proteins whose C termini (receptor binding portion) are homologous to other members of the TNF cytokine family. Either CD30L, or 4-1BBL, or both glycoproteins are expressed on a variety of activated cells, including T cells, B cells, myeloid cells, macrophages, and dendritic cells. CD30L is more highly glycosylated than other family members, perhaps reflecting the structural divergence of the CD30 molecule. Ligation of CD30L on T-cell tumor lines induces a rapid tyrosine phosphorylation of ERK and phosphorylation of the ERK substrate, myelin basic protein. Both CD30L and 4-1BBL induce proliferation of T cells in the presence of TCR cross-linking, and CD30L can induce apoptosis in CD30$^+$ tumor lines. Cross-linking of the CD30L molecule triggers increased production of the chemokine IL-8, induces oxidative bursts, and augments IL-6 production (95,96).

Functionally, CD30 has been implicated in T cell development because disruption of the CD30 gene results in hypercellularity in the thymus and impairs negative selection under some circumstances (97). However, the most interesting aspect of CD30–CD30L and 4-1BB–4-1BBL interactions is their apparent association with Th1–Th2 differentiation (98). Although CD30 has been found to have costimulatory properties on antigen-activated cells of both Th1 and Th2 phenotypes, CD30 is preferentially expressed on CD4$^+$ and CD8$^+$ T-cell clones that produce IL-4 and IL-5, Th2-type cytokines (98). Furthermore, there is an inverse relationship between CD30 expression and IFN-γ expression. Finally, costimulation through the CD30 molecules selectively activates IL-4 production in T cells. In contrast, 4-1BB is more highly expressed on T cells of the Th1 phenotype, and 4-1BB–mediated T-cell activation coincides with Th1 differentiation, especially when combined with CD28 costimulation (97). Thus, 4-1BB and CD30 may be selectively expressed on distinct T-cell subsets, and costimulation via these inducible costimulatory molecules may direct T-cell differentiation into Th1 and Th2 type T cells, respectively (Fig. 3).

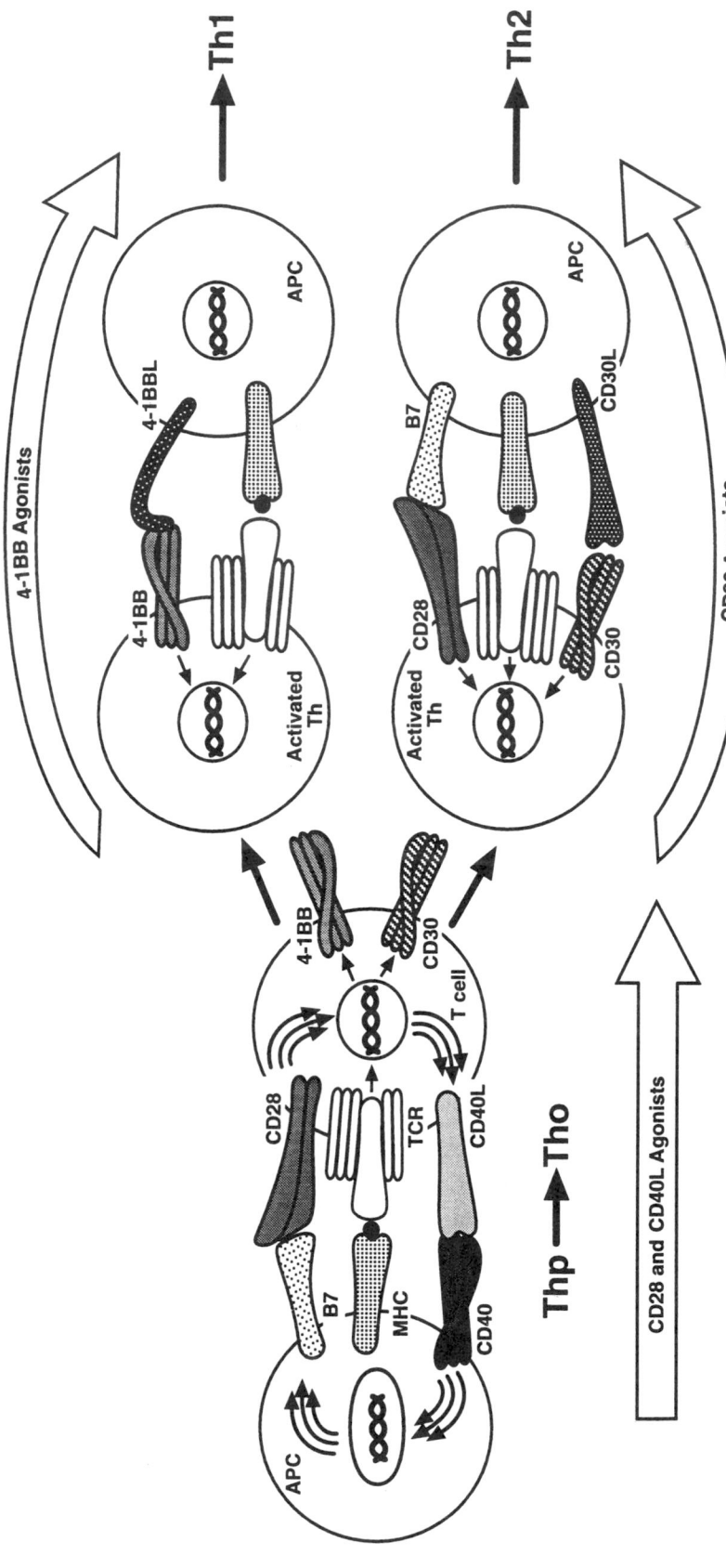

FIG. 3. Model depicting the interrelationships of costimulatory molecules in T-cell activation and differentiation. CD28/B7 and CD40L–CD40 interactions synergize to regulate early activation and differentiation events, whereas members of the TNF-R family regulate subsequent steps in the process.

In Vivo Function of the Costimulatory Pathways

The importance of CD28/B7 interactions in vivo was illustrated first in allograft and xenograft transplant models in which CTLA-4 Ig treatment led to long-term graft survival and, in many cases, induced donor-specific tolerance (37). Similarly, CTLA-4 Ig treatment reduced the morbidity and lethality associated with allogeneic graft-versus-host disease (GVHD) and blocked a variety of autoimmune diseases (37). The effects of CTLA-4 Ig therapy, however, were dependent on the strain combinations used in the studies, the species, and the dosing regimen. Recent efforts to augment the effectiveness of CTLA-4 Ig by combining with other immunosuppressive regimens has been more successful. For instance, CTLA-4 Ig treatment accompanied by donor-specific peripheral blood or bone marrow transfusions leads to donor-specific tolerance in situations in which CTLA-4 Ig alone prolongs graft survival only transiently. The blockade of CD28/B7 and LFA-1–ICAM-1 interactions are more effective than CTLA-4 Ig alone at preventing GVHD-induced lethality (99). Treatment of mice with CTLA-4 Ig and suboptimal doses of cyclosporine A at the time of transplantation prolongs graft survival beyond that of CTLA-4 Ig alone (100). Most dramatically combined CTLA-4 Ig and anti-CD40L antibody therapy results in indefinite skin graft survival in mice (101). The mechanism by which CTLA-4 Ig promotes graft acceptance has been controversial. In addition to its effects on cell survival and anergy induction, some studies have shown that long-term graft acceptance is associated with the skewing of the immune response toward the Th2 phenotype (100). However, it is uncertain whether the effects are a direct consequence of the CTLA-4 Ig treatment or indirectly associated with the long-term presence of the graft in the animals.

The humoral response is also profoundly inhibited by CTLA-4 Ig therapy. Primary antibody responses to soluble proteins such as KLH or cell-bound antigens such as sheep red blood cells are totally blocked by CTLA-4 Ig therapy that also reduces secondary and tertiary responses to the nominal antigen. In addition, the small amount of antibodies produced in this setting have a low affinity for the immunizing antigen because CD28 blockade suppresses somatic hypermutation (102,103). These results are consistent with the important role of CD28 in regulating Th2 development, and agrees with the profound decrease in germinal center formation noted in the CD28 KO and CTLA-4 Ig transgenic mice (51,58,61). In these animals, the basal Ig levels are only 20% of that observed in normal mice, with a dramatic decrease in the levels of IgG1 and IgG2b, whereas the levels of Th1-type IgG2a isotype antibodies were increased as compared with normal mice. T cell–dependent antibody production to antigens are defective in CD28 KO mice. Normal levels of anti-VSV antibodies of the IgM class (a T-independent response) were produced in response to a primary challenge, whereas no T-dependent IgG antibodies were produced in these mice. Therefore, blockade of the CD28/B7 interactions results in a profound defect in T-dependent B-cell responses to antigen in vivo.

Lastly, CD28 blockade affects the clinical course of several murine autoimmune disease models, including those that are either Th1-type responses (nonobese diabetic mice and EAE) or Th2-type response (glomerular nephritis and murine lupus), although the time course of the treatment is quite critical (37). In the murine model for systemic lupus erythematosus (SLE), NZB/NZW F1 mice (B/W) spontaneously develop a lupuslike autoimmune disease characterized by the production of autoantibodies to self molecules such as double-stranded DNA. The treatment of these mice with murine CTLA-4 Ig before the detection of autoantibodies significantly inhibited autoantibody production and disease progression, even after cessation of treatment. In a relapsing model of EAE, CTLA-4 Ig treatment during antigen priming blocked the development of clinical disease. Similarly, treatment of NOD mice with CTLA-4 Ig blocks diabetes when administered relatively late after birth. However, in both EAE and NOD mice, early therapy actually exacerbates the disease (37,80). This emphasizes the complicated regulation of autoimmunity by T-cell costimulation but also supports its potential for clinical application.

The multiple consequences of CD40L–CD40 signaling are most apparent in vivo. CD40–CD40L interactions are critical for Th-dependent antibody responses because the injection of mice with CD40 agonists, such as CD40L Ig or anti-CD40 mAbs, promotes B-cell apoptosis in germinal centers, prevents B-cell differentiation, and suppresses antibody-mediated autoimmunity manifested in murine models of lupus nephritis and oophoritis. Other Th1-mediated immune responses are also affected by CD40L–CD40 blockade, including the generation of allospecific CTL responses, collagen-induced arthritis, and experimental autoimmune encephalitis (83, 90). Most strikingly, CD40 KO and CD40L KO mice, as well as humans that express X-linked mutations in the CD40L gene, express a hyper-IgM syndrome manifested as a selective defect in their ability to generate germinal centers, produce IgG1 responses, and develop memory B cells. Thus, the CD40–CD40L interaction is critical for promoting humoral immune responses. Finally, studies are just starting to get underway examining the in vivo affects of antagonists against other costimulatory pathways.

CTLA-4 acts in an opposite role to regulate immunity in vivo. Treatment of mice with antagonists of CTLA-4 binding, such as Fab fragments of anti-CTLA-4 mAbs, increased T-cell proliferation and cytokine production, enhanced T cell responses to nominal antigen, intensified superantigen-mediated toxicity, and augmented antitumor activity (66,104). Moreover, blockade of CTLA-4 in vivo concomitantly with tolerogenic antigen prevented clonal inactivation of T cells. These results suggest that CTLA-4–mediated downregulation of T-cell function may be a normal consequence of antigen-driven T-cell expansion and contraction observed during the natural course of an antigen-specific T-cell response. Finally, in a number of murine models of autoimmune disease, such as the relapsing/remitting form of EAE, blockade of CTLA-4/B7 interactions promotes disease onset and exacerbates disease progression (66). The CTLA-4 KO mouse exhibits a profound spontaneous autoimmune disease. At 2 to 3 weeks of age the CTLA-4 KO mice manifest a massive lymphoproliferative disorder and develop an apparent autoimmune myocarditis and pancreatitis that is uniformly fatal within 4 to 5 weeks.

Summary

In summary, T-cell activation is a multistep process wherein CD28/B7 interactions act closely with TCR signaling to initiate clonal expansion by reducing the threshold for TCR signaling, promoting cell cycle progression, protecting cells from apoptosis, and initiating T-cell differentiation along the Th1 Th2 pathways. These effects on the immune response depend on antigen dose,

APC function, cytokine milieu, and level of costimulation. Early in the immune response, under conditions of low antigen density, CD28 ligation is essential and largely dependent on B7-2–mediated costimulation. As the immune response progresses, both B7-1 and B7-2 are upregulated, resulting in increased costimulatory signals that promote T-cell expansion and cytokine production and may skew the T-cell response toward the Th2 phenotype. Thus, any reagent or situation that reduces costimulation during this response promotes Th1 responses. High levels of costimulation coupled with high TCR occupancy may, in fact, downregulate immune responses. This effect may occur due to the extensive signaling via the TCR and CD28, which would explain high zone tolerance or clonal exhaustion. Alternatively, hyperstimulation may substantially upregulate CTLA-4 on the activated T cells. Because the ligation of CTLA-4 can inhibit immune responses, the interactions of CTLA-4 with either B7-1 or B7-2 may further amplify the suppression observed under these conditions. CD40–CD40L interactions amplify these early events by triggering APCs to upregulate the CD28 ligands B7-1 and B7-2. These early activation events induce the expression of a series of inducible costimulatory receptors, exemplified by CD30 and 4-1BB, that promote effector cell differentiation. However, all of the family members modulate distinct costimulatory pathways through their ability to associate with specific TRAF family members and subgroups of the TRAF-adaptor proteins. Together these costimulatory pathways control both the initiation and differentiation of the immune response (Fig. 3).

TCR CORECEPTOR MOLECULES: CD2 AND CD45

General Aspects

The TCR is the primary antigen recognition and signaling structure on T cells. However, effective T-cell activation not only depends on TCR ligation, but on interactions of a number of associated cell surface proteins on lymphocytes that do not directly contribute to the specificity of the antigen recognition but play a critical role as coreceptors in activation. These cell surface molecules can enhance the avidity of the TCR complex or contribute to the activation by providing essential cell–cell interactions and biochemical signaling in association with the TCR. These cell surface signaling molecules are distinguished from integrins and costimulatory molecules such as CD28 by the dependency on TCR expression for their signaling function. The prototype coreceptor molecules are the CD4 and CD8 molecules that are described in detail in Chapter 11. In this section, the structural and immunologic characteristics of two other well-studied molecules, CD2 and CD45, are summarized.

Characteristics of CD2

CD2 (also referred to as T11, Leu 5, and LFA-2, the sheep red blood cell [SRBC] receptor) is a 45- to 55-kDa glycoprotein expressed on all mature human T cells and thymocytes, most NK cells, and a small proportion (9% to 12%) of bone marrow cells (105,106). CD2 homologs are expressed on thymocytes and peripheral T cells in rodents but also on B cells in the mouse and macrophages in rats (107,108). The gene for human CD2 has been mapped to the pericentric loci on human chromosome 1p13 and the equivalent loci on mouse chromosome 3 (109). The human gene encodes a polypeptide of 360 amino acids, whereas mouse CD2 is 322 amino acids in length (110). Sequence comparisons combined with nuclear magnetic resonance analysis and crystallographic studies have shown that CD2 has two protein domains that belong to the Ig superfamily, a linker between the two domains and a stalk. Domain 1 is made of an antiparallel β barrel formed by two β-pleated sheets, a structure similar to other members of the Ig superfamily.

Sheep red blood cell rosetting was classically used to purify human T cells from the mononuclear cell populations. This purification protocol took advantage of unique cell surface structures on human T cells that bound to the SRBCs. An analysis of a panel of mAbs showed that CD2 was the SRBC receptor as anti-CD2 mAbs inhibited E-rosetting. Epitope mapping of the CD2 binding sites have defined three regions: region I composed of 13 amino acids surrounding amino acid 48, region II composed of 13 amino acids surrounding amino acid 95, and region III surrounding amino acids 140 to 142. Epitope loss mutants of region I and II are defective in T-cell rosetting and binding to CD58 (111,112). The epitope defined by region III (CD2R [T$_{11.3}$]) is localized to the flexible CD2 linker region between domain 1 and the membrane-proximal extracellular domain 2, and antibodies to this region do not affect binding to CD58 (112–114). The CD2R epitope expressed weakly on resting T cells and expressed after activation of T cells is dependent on posttranslational changes in conformation. The expression of CD2R epitope is accompanied by redistribution and clustering of CD2 to the region of cell–cell contact. CD2 has several ligands. It binds two homologous glycoproteins—CD58 (LFA-3) in humans and CD48 in rodents—both of which are expressed widely on hematopoietic and non-hematopoietic cells (109,115–120). The affinity for CD2 binding to CD48 (K_d = 60 to 90 μmol/L) is much lower than the affinity of CD2–CD58 (K_d = 10 to 20 μmol/L) interaction (109,121). CD58 maps to human chromosome 1p13 and CD48 to the distal end of chromosome 1, 1q21-23. In addition, CD2's ligands, CD58 and CD48, have a very similar structure; they belong to a subfamily within the Ig superfamily that has an N-terminal V-set domain (domains with sequence and structural similarity to Ig variable domains) and a C-terminal C2-set domain (domains with sequence and structural similarity to the Ig constant domain) and a conserved pattern of disulfide bonds (Fig. 4). Both CD2 ligands, CD48 and an isoform of CD58, are expressed as glycophosphatidylinositol (GPI) anchored membrane proteins. This type of membrane association provides for high lateral mobility to enhance CD2–ligand interactions.

The affinity of CD2 for its ligand CD58 is dependent on activation signals via the TCR complex (106,115,122). Signaling through the TCR leads to modifications in the cytoplasmic tail of CD2, leading to an increase in the avidity of the extracellular portion of CD2 for its ligands (inside-out signaling). The increased avidity can be inhibited by tyrosine kinase inhibitors or induced by elevating intracellular levels of cyclic adenosine monophosphate (cAMP). The upregulation of CD2 avidity requires the asparagine residue in the carboxy terminus of CD2 (106,115,122). These results suggest a central role for CD2–CD58 interaction in enhancing T cell responses via potentiating T-cell contact with APCs.

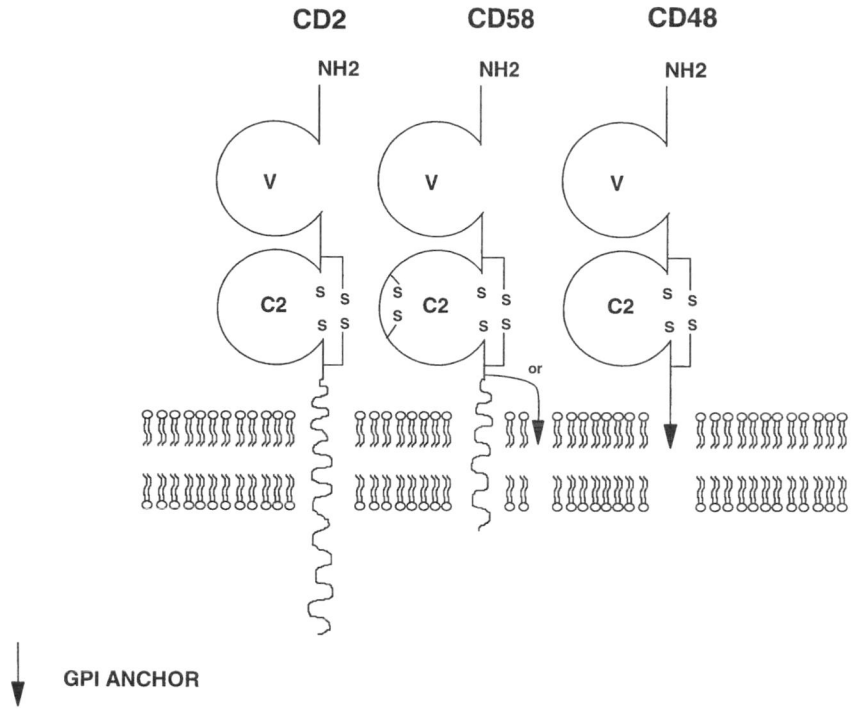

FIG. 4. CD2 and its ligands CD58 and CD48 are depicted as members of a subfamily within the immunoglobulin superfamily. They contain the N-terminal V-set domain (a domain with sequence and structural similarity to the Ig variable domains), C-terminal C2-set domain (a domain with sequence and structural similarity to the Ig constant domain), and a conserved pattern of disulfide bonds. Both CD2 ligands, CD48, and an isoform of CD58 are also expressed as GPI-anchored membrane proteins

CD2 Function

CD2 interaction with its ligands promotes adhesion between T cells and the APCs contributing to the overall avidity of TCR binding. Anti-CD2 mAbs, soluble CD2 ligands, and antibodies to CD2 ligands can inhibit antigen-specific and nonspecific conjugate formation, thus inhibiting T-cell proliferation, cytokine secretion, and cytotoxicity (105). As stated above, the regulation of CD2 avidity by TCR-mediated activation events is important for CD2 function. Thus, there is a synergistic effect in combining CD2 and TCR signals because activation through each enhances the function of the other. Additionally, because the extracellular portions of the TCR and CD2 have similar dimensions (approximately 75 Å), the CD2 interaction with its ligands creates an optimal distance for TCR–antigen/MHC interaction to occur. Finally, the association of CD2 with the TCR complex helps to aggregate the TCR in the regions of cell–cell contact, allowing the stabilization of low-affinity TCR/MHC interactions.

In addition to enhancing T-cell adhesion, signaling through CD2 contributes to T-cell activation, both through antigen-dependent as well as antigen-independent pathways (123,124). Signaling via the CD2 molecule with natural ligand and mAbs can enhance IL-2 production in an adhesion-independent manner, although mAb-mediated activation of T cells through CD2 requires pairs of mAbs (113). The mAb pairs must include antibodies to the CD2R region (113,125) or a combination of anti-CD2 antibody with PMA. Besides enhancing T-cell function, signals through CD2 may play a role in downregulating T-cell responses by induction of anergy and apoptosis. T cells activated with a mitogenic pair of anti-CD2 mAbs

and IL-2 are susceptible to Fas-independent apoptosis when stimulated with a third CD2-specific mAb that recognizes an epitope distinct from the two mitogenic antibodies (126). Induction of apoptosis was restricted to activated T cells (126). Furthermore, blocking both CD2–CD58 and LFA-1–ICAM-1 interaction during primary alloantigen stimulation can result in antigen-specific anergy (127). Similar observations have been made in vivo, where treatment of mice with nondepleting anti-CD2 led to T-cell unresponsiveness to antigenic stimulation (127). Finally, CD2 is involved in the regulation of cytokine production by T cells. Stimulation via the CD2 pathway can skew the cytokine profile toward a Th2-like phenotype. Stimulation of CD4+ memory T cells with LFA-3, but not ICAM-1, induced high levels of IL-5 (128), and stimulation of T-cell clones with a combination of anti-CD2 and anti-CD28 mAbs enhanced the production of IL-1, IL-2, IL-4, IL-6, CSF-1, IL-10, TNF-α and IFN-γ secretion (129–133) beyond the levels observed with a combination of anti-CD3 and anti-CD28 mAbs. CD2–CD58 interactions regulate T-cell differentiation by altering the T-cell responsiveness to IL-12. Blockade of CD2–CD58 or promotion of CD2–CD48 interactions inhibited T-cell responsiveness to IL-12 (134). Thus, in addition to contributing to T-cell adhesion and enhancing T-cell activation, CD2 interactions with its ligands regulate the differentiation of Th1 and Th2 cells.

Studies examining the role of CD2 in vivo have shown that administration of anti-CD2 or anti-CD48 mAbs inhibited T-cell responses such as development of cytotoxic T cells and delayed-type hypersensitivity (127,135–137). Anti-CD2 mAb treatment has been shown to be efficacious in blocking graft rejection in a series of organ transplant models. The graft survival was accompanied by donor-specific tolerance. Similar observations have been made in heart allograft models using CD2 KO mice expressing the human CD2 transgene and in baboon models (138–140). However, in one clinical trial anti-CD2 treatment combined with anti–LFA-1 has yielded mixed results in bone marrow transplantation for immunodeficiency and leukemias in humans (141). Similar suppressive effects have been observed after the administration of anti-CD2 antibody in models of autoimmune disease. Administration of anti-CD2 mAb given at the time of onset of experimental autoimmune neuritis in rats dramatically inhibited the progression of disease and prevented the worsening of disease if given later in the disease process. In addition, cells from allergic patients, patients with Omenns's syndrome, and patients with severe fungal infections produced higher levels of IL-4 in response to anti-CD2 and anti-CD28 stimulation in vitro (142). These observations combined with the effect of anti-CD2 antibody on inhibiting T-cell responsiveness to IL-12 has led to the hypothesis that engagement of CD2 in all these models inhibits T-cell adhesion and leads to the selective suppression of Th1 cytokine production. This would explain the immunosuppressive effect of anti-CD2 antibody in transplant and Th1-mediated autoimmunity and the exacerbating effect in Th2-mediated autoimmunity.

Biochemical Basis of CD2 Function

Initial observations that antibodies to CD2 can stimulate T cells led to the suggestion that CD2 provided an alternative pathway for T-cell activation in contrast to the classical pathway mediated through CD3–TCR. However, CD2 has been shown to associate with the TCR–CD3 complex, and the activation of T cells through CD2 requires TCR–CD3 expression, specifically the expression of the CD3 ζ chain (115,143). In fact, CD2 cross-linking does not signal in CD3$^-$ mutant cell lines or TCR-modulated resting T cells. Thus, the pathways of CD2 signaling are thought to be tightly linked with those characterized for the TCR signaling complex. In this regard, like TCR cross-linking, signaling through CD2 activates p56^{lck} and PLC-γ-1 and induces calcium influx and cAMP production (106,113,115). CD2-dependent T-cell signaling requires the presence of the cytoplasmic tail of CD2 (106), although it is not required for CD58 (LFA-3) binding. Recent studies with chimeric proteins in which the CD2 transmembrane and cytoplasmic domains were either deleted or exchanged with similar domains from CD4, CD28, or CD58 showed that the cytoplasmic domain of CD2 was required for the interaction with the TCR–CD3 chain. However, the cytoplasmic deletion mutants of CD2 retained their interaction with CD45, indicating that the extracellular domain of CD2 was largely responsible for interaction with CD45. The cytoplasmic domain of CD2 is highly conserved (71% to 84% nucleotide homology), and the most conserved regions are rich in prolines. Proline-rich regions are known to bind to src homology 3 (SH3) domains. The SH3 domain of p56lck binds to the proline-rich regions in the cytoplasmic domain of CD2. Other signaling molecules, such as p59^{fyn} and PI-3 kinase, known to associate with CD2, also may interact via their SH3 domains with the proline-rich region of CD2. In summary, the CD2 interaction with its ligands increases the strength of T-cell binding, and signaling through the cytoplasmic domain of CD2 enhances the T-cell signal.

Characteristics of CD45

CD45 (also known as the leukocyte common antigen, Ly-5, T200, and B220 for the B cell form) is a membrane-bound tyrosine phosphatase present on all hematopoietic cells. The CD45 gene (located on chromosome 1 in mice and humans [1q32]), is encoded by 33 exons, of which exons 3 to 15 encode the extracellular domains, exon 16 encodes the transmembrane domain, and exons 17 to 32 encode the intracytoplasmic domain. The extracellular domain of CD45 has an N terminus containing several O-linked carbohydrate attachment sites and a cysteine-rich region. The multiple exons, combined with the differential glycosylation, results in the expression of many different isoforms of CD45 expressed in a cell-specific manner, wherein the different isoforms of CD45 have variable extracellular domains and a constant intracellular domain. Eight different isoforms of CD45, generated by alternative splicing of the extracellular domain of exons 4, 5, and 6 (also known as exons A, B, and C) (144,145), dramatically effect the size and degree of the O-linked carbohydrates on the various isoforms. The O-linked carbohydrate regions are highly charged and form rigid rods. Thus, the variable usage of exons changes the length of the extracellular domain from 28 to 51 nm. The different isoforms of CD45 are recognized by mAbs specific for splicing and glycosylation-dependent epitopes (145). The antibodies that recognize restricted epitopes are designated as CD45R specific. Thus, CD45RA-specific mAbs recognize a CD45 isoform dependent on exon 4, whereas CD45RB and CD45RC-specific mAbs are dependent on the isoforms using exons 5 and 6, respectively. The CD45 isoform expressed in the absence of exons 4, 5, and 6 is recognized by CD45RO-specific mAbs (Fig. 5).

The expression of CD45 isoforms is complex. The earliest developing B cells and TCR$^-$CD4$^-$CD8$^-$ thymocytes express the largest molecular form of CD45, termed CD45R/B220. This form of the protein is highly glycosylated and includes all the exons. Upon stimulation, the immature thymocytes switch to the low molecular weight CD45RO isoform. As the thymocytes continue to mature and migrate to the medullary region and periphery, the higher molecular weight (CD45RA, CD45RB, and CD45RC) isoforms appear but are dynamic, with the relative amounts of each changing with activation. In humans, the CD45RA isoform, detected by the 2H4 mAb, identifies the naive T-cell subset. These T cells proliferate in response to mitogens but are unable to secrete the cytokines that promote the development of IgG-secreting B cells. After in vitro and in vivo stimulation, the memory/activated CD4$^+$ T cells express the CD45RO isoform. The CD45RO$^+$ T cell population has lower responses to mitogens but provides help to B cells for IgG secretion. Similar changes are observed in rodents, although the precise exon usage differs. Antibodies specific for CD45RA do not react with murine CD4$^+$ T cells; instead, naive and memory CD4$^+$ T cells in rodents are distinguished based on CD45RB and CD45RC expression. Naive CD4$^+$ T cells in mice have a CD45RB^{hi} phenotype, which is downregulated to the CD45RB^{lo} phenotype after antigen exposure. Murine T cells also express the CD45R/B220 isoform after activation. In rats, high levels of CD45RC expression defines the naive T-cell population that is downregulated after antigen priming. CD8$^+$ murine T cells and B cells express multiple CD45 isoforms (CD45R/B220 expressed on mature murine B cells); however, their correlation with function is less clear. There have been reports of changes in CD45 expression in autoimmune as well as inflammatory disease conditions, such as decreased expression of CD45 in certain leukemias and lymphomas and the presence of CD45R autoantibodies in systemic lupus erythematosus (145). The significance of these changes may reflect changes in lymphocyte populations rather than a direct role for CD45 in disease progression. Little information is currently available on the ligand for CD45, although observations that anti-CD45 antibodies

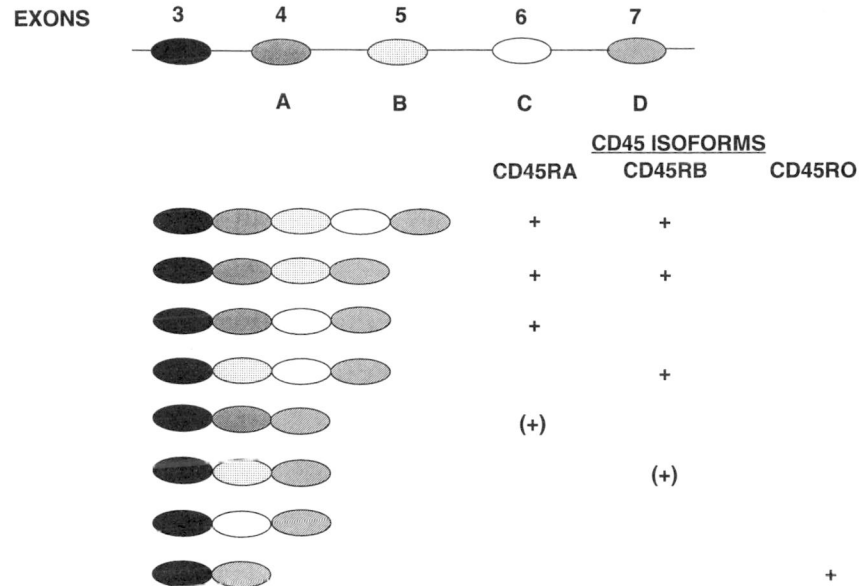

FIG. 5. The CD45 extracellular domain is encoded by several exons. Exons 4, 5, and 6 (or A, B, and C) are variably expressed in different isoforms. These different isoforms of CD45 are recognized by mAbs specific for splicing as well as glycosylation-dependent epitopes. The antibodies that recognize restricted epitopes are designated as CD45R specific. Thus, CD45RA-specific mAbs recognize a CD45 isoform dependent on exon 4, CD45RB mAbs recognize the isoform dependent on exon 5, CD45RC mAbs recognize the isoform dependent on exon 6, and the CD45 isoform expressed in the absence of exon 4, 5, and 6 is recognized by CD45RO-specific mAbs.

can modulate lymphocyte responses in vitro suggest that CD45-ligand interactions might regulate T-cell function. In fact, the highly conserved pattern of usage of the exons encoding the extracellular domains of CD45 molecule as well as the tightly regulated expression of different isoforms used by functionally distinct lymphoid and myeloid subsets suggest that the extracellular portion of the cell surface glycoprotein is important for CD45 function. Some studies have suggested that CD45 may interact with lectins or other glycoproteins on the cell surface. For example, the B-cell glycoprotein CD22, and the serum-mannan binding protein (S-MBP), a calcium-dependent C-type lectin involved in innate immunity, have been reported to interact with the carbohydrate moiety on CD45 (146,147). S-MBP binds specifically to the high mannose type or hybrid type of N-linked oligosaccharides present on CD45RO isoform expressed on the immature thymocytes with the $CD4^+CD8^+CD3^{lo}$ phenotype. In this regard, studies have shown selective association and activation of different isoforms of CD45 with the TCR. However, it should be emphasized that the extracellular portion of the CD45 molecule is not essential for its function. The defective TCR responses observed in CD45-deficient lymphoma lines (see below) can be rescued with CD45 chimeric proteins that retain only the CD45 cytoplasmic domain (148).

Role of CD45 in Development

The direct involvement of CD45 in T-cell development was shown in CD45 KO mice (149,150). In these mice there was a significant inhibition in transition from $CD4^-CD8^-$ thymocytes to $CD4^+CD8^+$ thymocytes and in the transition from $CD4^+CD8^+$ thymocytes to $CD4^+$ and $CD8^+$ thymocytes that finally resulted in a dramatically reduced number (5% to 10%) of mature peripheral T

cells. The few $CD4^+CD8^+$ cells present in these mice were less sensitive than wild-type T cells to apoptotic signals induced in response to TCR stimulation in vitro, but were more susceptible to apoptosis in the absence of any stimulation. This has led to the speculation that the CD45 molecules play a critical role in various stages of T-cell development and may influence both positive and negative selection by altering the threshold for TCR stimulation. As a result, CD45-deficient cells would require a much stronger signal for both positive and negative selection. Thus, $CD4^+CD8^+$ thymocytes interacting with positively selecting low-affinity peptides would die due to lack of effective signaling, whereas those effectively selected would be less susceptible to apoptosis in response to a negatively selecting TCR stimulation.

CD45 Function

Early studies showed that cells lacking CD45 were severely impaired in their functional responses. Moreover, the simultaneous cross-linking of CD45 and the antigen receptor blocked calcium mobilization (151). Finally, in vivo treatment of mice with anti-CD45 mAb inhibited T cell–dependent antibody responses to antigen (152). Together these functional studies suggested that CD45 might provide an essential role in lymphocyte activation. Direct biochemical evidence that CD45 was critical for antigen-specific T-cell responses came from studies using CD45-deficient cell lines. These mutant cell lines were found to be defective in most TCR-mediated signaling events, such as the tyrosine phosphorylation of proximal signaling components, phosphoinositol generation, calcium influx, protein kinase C activation, and IL-2 secretion (145,149). Whereas the role of CD45 extracellular domains still needs to be resolved, CD45 cytoplasmic phosphatase domain has been shown to be required and sufficient to restore normal signaling in CD45⁻ cell lines. These studies have been confirmed in CD45 exon-6 KO mice, which develop few peripheral T cells that are largely unresponsive to TCR stimulation (150). However, the T cells from CD45-deficient mice proliferate normally to phorbol ester and calcium ionophore stimulation, suggesting that the defect in signaling in these cells was proximal to the TCR activation. Similar results have been observed in B cells. Normal B-cell responses to antigen receptor stimulation are inhibited by the addition of mAb to CD45, and the simultaneous cross-linking of CD45 and the antigen receptor blocks calcium mobilization. In vivo injection of anti-CD45 mAb specific for the B-cell epitope into mice inhibited the T cell–dependent antibody response to antigen (145,152). These observations were confirmed by studies in CD45-deficient mice in which the B cells had defective responses to stimulation with B-cell receptor–specific antibodies. The CD45⁻ B cells were defective in calcium mobilization, activation of phospholipase C, mitogen-activated protein kinase (MAPK), and p21^{ras} activation in response to antigen receptor stimulation. However, the B-cell response to CD40-mediated signals are not affected in CD45 null mice, and CD45-deficient B cells responded normally to T cell–independent B cell responses to viral antigen (153). These results suggest that BCR and CD40 signals are sufficiently intact to promote B-cell responses in the absence of CD45 in the presence of a strong primary stimulus.

The individual functional roles of the distinct isoforms of CD45 is not well defined. However, a sequence comparison of CD45 extracellular domains in vertebrates indicates that the three extracellular domains are highly conserved. Moreover, T-cell subsets expressing different isoforms have different functions. The CD4⁺ CD45RA T cells (naive T cells) proliferate well in response to mitogens and provide sufficient help for inducing IgE secretion by B cells, but are poor inducers of IgG synthesis. In contrast, CD45RO T cells (memory T cells) respond poorly to mitogens and support IgG but not IgE responses. Recent studies suggest that the CD45 isoform plays a critical role in these distinct functions. T cells transfected with the lower molecular weight isoforms of CD45 responded better to antigen stimulation than did T cells expressing the higher molecular weight forms. The magnitude of the response to antigen correlated with the ability of the CD45 isoform to coassociate with CD4. Because the coassociation of CD45 with CD4 did not require the cytoplasmic domain of CD45, the external domains are essential for mediating this activity (154). Support for a differential role of CD45 isoforms also comes from studies showing that only certain isoforms of CD45 are involved in the regulation of cytokine secretion. Cross-linking of CD45 by an mAb that recognizes an epitope common to all CD45 isoforms induced TNF-α, TNF-β, IL-2, and IL-3 gene expression. This effect was specific to one epitope because mAbs recognizing other epitopes did not induce any significant increase in cytokine expression.

Because CD45 has a critical role in T-cell activation, it has become an attractive *in vivo* target for regulating T cells. Antibodies to CD45 are an effective treatment in preventing rejection of renal transplants in several different small animal models. Two injections of anti-CD45RB after a renal allograft resulted in prolonged allograft survival and normal renal function in mice (155). Treatment with the anti-CD45RB mAb also has been shown to reverse acute renal graft rejection. This immunosuppressive effect was epitope specific because a purified antiserum against CD45 and a pan-CD45 mAb were ineffective in prolonging graft survival. Initial studies have been performed in humans. Pretreatment of human renal allografts with a rat anti-CD45 mAb correlated with a lower incidence of rejection (156). Therefore, the in vitro observations of a critical role for CD45 in T-cell activation are supported by the in vivo studies in which modulating CD45 activity with antibodies is sufficient to prevent T-cell activation.

Biochemical Basis of CD45 Function

As mentioned above, CD45 is a membrane-bound tyrosine phosphatase. Tyrosine phosphatases play essential roles in regulating immune responses. For the most part, phosphatases have been thought to downregulate lymphocyte function by dephosphorylating the critical biochemical mediators (such as p56^{lck}, ZAP-70, CD3ζ, or p59^{fyn}) proximal to TCR signaling. For instance, both intracellular phosphotyrosine phosphatases (PTPs), PTP-1C and PTP-1D, function to downregulate B-cell signaling either by directly affecting BCR signal transduction or regulating Fc receptor function. In contrast, CD45 is a critical component of TCR signaling because modulating CD45 function before TCR stimulation leads to uncoupling of the TCR from intracellular calcium mobilization and activation of Ca^{2+}/calmodulin-activated kinase. CD45 influences TCR-mediated upregulation of the tyrosine kinase activity of p56^{lck} and p59^{fyn} by regulating the phosphorylation of the negative regulatory tyrosine at the C terminus of these src family kinases (Tyr-505 in p56^{lck} and Tyr-528 in p59^{fyn}) (144,145,149). Cells deficient in CD45 have increased tyrosine phosphorylation of the negative-regulatory tyrosine correlating with lower src kinase activity. In addition, p56^{lck} is hyperphosphorylated at Tyr-394 in CD45-deficient cell lines and purified intracellular portion of CD45-dephosphorylated p56^{lck} at position Tyr-394 in vitro. This indicates that CD45 can fine tune the activity of p56^{lck} by determining the balance of tyrosine phosphorylation on the activation versus the inhibition sites. In fact, there exists a direct interaction between the amino-terminal and SH2 domains of p56^{lck} with the cytoplasmic domain of CD45. In some instances, CD45-deficient cell lines can signal through their TCR. Interestingly, the TCR signal transduction in these cells is linked to the syk rather than ZAP-70 tyrosine kinase. This signaling pathway appears to be independent of CD45 and p56^{lck}. Finally, CD45 may also directly regulate the tyrosine phosphorylation of some of the other molecules involved in TCR signaling. Transfection of the largest CD45 (ABC) isoform in Jurkat cells enhanced TCR-mediated tyrosine phosphorylation, association of SLP-76 with the GNEF and, Vav, as well as IL-2 production. Interestingly, transmission of the smallest CD45 isoform, CD45RO, was not as efficient in upregulating T-cell signaling in this system.

As with T cells, CD45-deficient B cells also expressed altered proximal signaling. The positive autophosphorylation site of the src family kinase, lyn, was hyperphosphorylated, whereas the C-terminal negative regulatory tyrosine was underphosphorylated, consistent with a role for CD45-mediated regulation in B cells. Thus, similar to T cells, the receptor-associated src family kinase, lyn, is a potential substrate for CD45 in B cells. Therefore, CD45 regulates T-cell as well as B-cell receptor signaling by upregulating the tyrosine kinase activity of the src family kinases associated with these receptors.

Summary

Accessory molecules, such as CD2 and CD45, contribute to T cell activation both by enhancing the affinity of T-cell interaction with APCs and by signaling through their intracellular domains. Although CD2 has been shown to interact with CD48 and CD58, CD45 ligands have yet to be defined. However, because the expression of different isoforms of CD45 is tightly regulated during T-cell maturation and activation, it is likely that CD45 interaction with molecules either on T cells or on apposing cells regulates lymphocyte activation. Both CD2 and CD45 intracellular domains have signaling capacities. The intracellular domain of CD45 has tyrosine phosphatase activity that plays a crucial role in initiation of the T-cell receptor signaling cascade by positively regulating the src family kinase activity. Although CD2 does not directly contribute to TCR signaling, CD2 signaling is dependent on TCR expression. The intracellular tail of CD2 is coupled to signaling pathways similar to TCR; thus, CD2 signals may further enhance T-cell activation. Current experimental evidence strongly suggests that in vivo activation of T cells involves a complex regulation of activation via the TCR and the multiple accessory molecules, such as CD2 and CD45, expressed on the cell surface.

REGULATION OF T-CELL ADHESION: INTEGRINS

General Aspects

Among the first functionally important accessory molecules identified on the T-cell surface were the leukocyte function–associated (LFA) antigens, including LFA-1, LFA-2, and LFA-3. mAbs against these surface antigens blocked antigen-specific T-cell proliferation and prevented cytotoxic T cell–mediated cytotoxicity (157). Interestingly, all three LFA antigens were identified as adhesion molecules involved in cell–cell contact between T cells and other cells. The most broadly expressed LFA antigen on leukocytes is LFA-1, a member of a large family of structurally related adhesion molecules, the integrin supergene family. The other two, LFA-2 and LFA-3, are both members of the Ig supergene family that forms the receptor/ligand pair, CD2(LFA-2)/CD58(LFA-3), involved in coreceptor and adhesion pathways. The fact that adhesion molecules were among the first functionally defined accessory molecules on T cells emphasizes the important role of this subset of accessory molecules in promoting critical T-cell signal-transducing events through both their adhesive interactions with apposing cells and the surrounding extracellular matrix (ECM).

It is now clear that members of the integrin superfamily are important in multiple aspects of T-cell activation. Evidence accumulated in the early to mid-1980s suggested that interactions involving LFA-1 were the major contributing adhesive forces between T cells, B cells, and macrophages (158–160). A concept evolved suggesting that T cells initiate antigen-independent adhesive interactions with apposing cells to scan the surface for specific antigen, followed by even stronger antigen-dependent adhesive interactions that would allow for specific activation of T-cell proliferation, cytokine production, or the delivery of a lethal hit to the target cell (161,162).

Characteristics of Integrin Supergene Family

The integrin supergene family members are expressed on virtually every cell type in the body and are involved in both cell–cell contact and interactions of cells with the ECM (163,164). Integrins are important for many different physiologic processes, including embryogenesis, thrombosis, wound healing, tumorigenesis and immune responses. The integrin supergene family consists of a number of cell surface $\alpha\beta$ heterodimers. The α and β chains are type I transmembrane glycoproteins with a single hydrophobic transmembrane domain, a short cytoplasmic tail, and an extracellular domain that associates noncovalently to form the heterodimer. Both the α and β chains are required for cell surface expression. Most integrins are involved in attachment to ECM components, but an increasing number also can bind to ligands expressed on the cell surface. Sixteen α chains and eight β chains have been described (Fig. 6). The consensus nomenclature most often used to describe a specific heterodimer is to specify the α and β chain that makes up the heterodimer. The α chains are indicated with numbers or letters, α_{1-9}, α_{IIb}, α_V, α_E, α_M, α_L, α_X and α_D. The β chains are identified by numbers, β_{1-8}. The α chains that pair with β_2 are all located on human chromosome 16 (α_L, α_M, α_x, and α_D) (165,166), whereas β_2 itself is encoded on chromosome 21 (165). Loci for other integrin chains are found scattered throughout the genome, with major clusters on chromosomes 2, 12 and 17, with α_4 and α_v both on chromosome 2 (167,168) and β_1 on chromosome 10 (169). The α and β chains can combine in different heterodimers to form multiple shared and unique specificities (Fig. 7). In general, the α chains can only pair with one specific β chain, whereas the β chains can pair with various α chains. For instance, the β_2 chain can pair with the α_L, α_M, α_X, and α_D chains (Fig. 6). In addition, different $\alpha\beta$ heterodimers can sometimes share the same ligand, as is the case with $\alpha_L\beta_2$ and $\alpha_M\beta_2$, which both bind to ICAM-1. Although more than one integrin heterodimer can bind to the same ligand, integrin heterodimers often bind to nonoverlapping sites, suggesting that multimeric complexes consisting of different integrin heterodimers may form with the same ligand. The affinities of an integrin receptor for its ligands can vary significantly; thus, physiologic relevance of an expressed receptor often depends on the localization and level of expression of the ligand.

The integrin α chains are comprised of an extracellular portion that contains seven repeating domains. The overall structural homology among α chains is only 20% to 30%, with the least homology between the short cytoplasmic regions (170). The three or four most carboxyl-terminal extracellular domains have sequences very homologous to the "EF hand–like" domain of the calcium and magnesium binding proteins troponin C, calmodulin, and parvalbumin (Fig. 8). Integrin binding function is tightly regulated by divalent cations, which may explain the importance of the EF hand domain of the molecule because it is thought to have divalent cation-binding capabilities (171). A partial crystal structure of the extracellular domain of α_M showed that it consists of a row of six β-pleated sheets surrounded by seven α helixes (172). This crystal structure revealed the existence of an inserted sequence of amino acids, the I domain, that contains the metal ion (Mg^{2+})-dependent adhesion binding site (MIDAS). Only those α chains that make up the β_2 subfamily and the α_1, α_2, and α_E chains contain such an I domain (Fig. 8) (171). Recently, a computer model of the three-dimensional structure of integrin α chains predicted that they fold into a β-propeller domain, consisting of seven four-stranded β-sheets arranged in a torus around a pseudosymmetry axis. In this model, the I domain with the Mg^{2+}-binding MIDAS sequence is shown tethered to the top of the β propeller, whereas the Ca^{2+}-binding EF domains are on the lower face of the β propeller. The β chains are more homologous than the α chains (e.g., β_1 and β_2 have 44% homology) yet they are equally restricted in

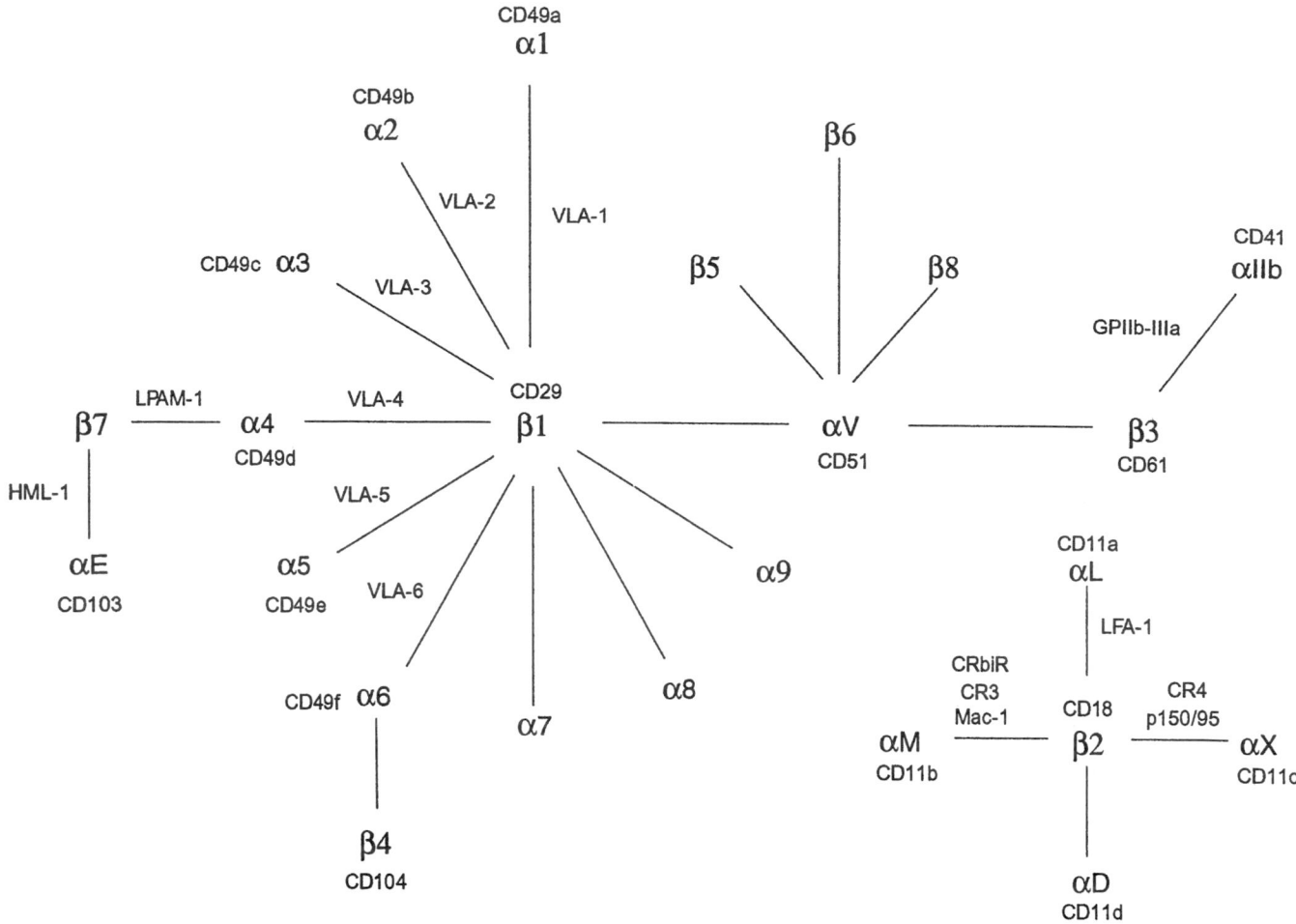

FIG. 6. Overview of known heterodimers formed by α and β chains of the integrin supergene family.

their binding specificities (170). Interestingly, the β_1, β_2, and β_3 chains share a similar MIDAS-like sequence that when mutated results in loss of integrin–ligand binding capability (173,174). These results are consistent with other structural studies that indicate that the amino-terminal domains of the integrin α and β chains combine to form the functional ligand-binding site.

In the immune system, the most important integrins, those of the β_1, β_2, and β_7 subfamilies, participate in T-cell migration and provide stimulatory signals for T-cell proliferation and effector functions (Fig. 6). The β_2 integrin subfamily (or leukointegrins) is the most functionally heterogeneous subfamily of integrins and has a tissue expression pattern restricted to leukocytes (175). Members of this family bind various cell surface molecules, ECM proteins, and certain soluble blood components. The subfamily consists of the $\alpha_L\beta_2$ (LFA-1), $\alpha_M\beta_2$ (Mac-1), $\alpha_X\beta_2$ (p150/95), and $\alpha_D\beta_2$ heterodimers. $\alpha_L\beta_2$ is constitutively expressed on all lymphoid and most myeloid lineages, increases on T cells after activation, and remains elevated (approximately twofold) on memory/effector T cells. By comparison, the expression of $\alpha_M\beta_2$ and $\alpha_X\beta_2$ glycoproteins is restricted to monocytes, macrophages, neutrophils, and granulocytes, and only a subpopulation of lymphocytes. Only a

subset of CD4$^+$ and CD8$^+$ CTL clones, as well as murine dendritic cells, express $\alpha_X\beta_2$ (170,176), whereas $\alpha_M\beta_2$ appears to be a marker of memory T cells because its expression increases with age and is correlated with high expression of IL-4 and IFN-γ (177). Finally, a novel leukointegrin, $\alpha_D\beta_2$, is expressed at low levels on a subset of T cells, monocytes, granulocytes, and macrophages, including the foamy macrophages that have been implicated in the generation of fulminant atherosclerotic lesions (178,179).

The ligands for the β_2 subfamily integrins are diverse and include various members of the Ig supergene family (Fig. 9). The predominant and highest affinity ligand for $\alpha_L\beta_2$ is ICAM-1, an extensively glycosylated cell surface protein. ICAM-1 contains five Ig-like domains, the amino-terminal domain providing the main binding site for $\alpha_L\beta_2$ (175). Other $\alpha_L\beta_2$ ligands include ICAM-2, which contains only two extracellular Ig domains homologous to the first two Ig domains of ICAM-1 (35%) (180), and ICAM-3, which contains five extracellular Ig-like domains homologous to those of ICAM-1 (48%) (181,182). There are murine homologs of only ICAM-1 and ICAM-2, but not ICAM-3 (180–182). ICAM-1 is expressed on activated T cells, B cells, macrophages, and dendritic cells. It is induced on vascular endothelial cells and fibroblasts by the proinflammatory

Integrin receptors	Ligands	
	Extracellular Matrix Proteins	*Cell Surface Proteins*
β₁ Subfamily		
α₁β₁ (CD49a/CD29)	Collagen, Laminin	
α₂β₁ (CD49b/CD29)	Collagen, Laminin	
α₃β₁ (CD49c/CD29)	Collagen, Laminin, Fibronectin (RGD)	
α₄β₁ (CD49d/CD29)	Fibronectin (CS-1)	VCAM-1 (CD106), MAdCAM-1
α₅β₁ (CD49e/CD29)	Fibronectin (RGD),	
α₆β₁ (CD49f/CD29)	Laminin	
αᵥβ₁ (CD51/CD29)	Fibronectin (RGD), Vitronectin (RGD)	
β₂ Subfamily		
αLβ₂ (CD11a/CD18)		ICAM-1 (CD54), ICAM-2 (CD102), ICAM-3 (CD50) Telencephalin
αMβ₂ (CD11b/CD18)	C3bi, Factor X, Fibrinogen	ICAM-1
αXβ₂ (CD11c/CD18)	C3bi, Fibrinogen	ICAM-1?
αDβ₂ (CD11d/CD18)		ICAM-3
β₃ Subfamily		
αᵥβ₃ (CD61/CD51)	Vitronectin (RGD), Fibronectin (RGD), von Willebrand factor, Fibrinogen, Laminin, Thrombospondin, Osteopontin	PECAM-1 (CD31)
β₄ Subfamily		
α₆β₄ (CD49f/CD104)	Laminin	
β₇ Subfamily		
α₄β₇ (CD49d/CD?)	Fibronectin (CS-1)	MAdCAM-1, VCAM-1
αEβ₇ (CD103/CD?)		E-Cadherin

FIG. 7. Integrin heterodimers expressed on leukocytes and their ligands.

cytokines IL-1, IFN-γ, and TNF-α. By comparison, ICAM-2 is constitutively expressed on endothelium, T cells, and monocytes and is not upregulated by cytokines, whereas ICAM-3 expression is restricted to cells of the hematopoietic lineage (lymphocytes, monocytes, and dendritic cells) and is absent on resting or activated endothelium. Recently, a novel human αLβ₂ ligand, telencephalin, has been cloned (183,184). Telencephalin is an Ig superfamily member with nine Ig-like domains (Fig. 9) and is expressed in the central nervous system. It has a high homology with ICAM-1 (50%) and ICAM-3 (55%) in the amino-terminal first five domains. The clustered chromosomal location for ICAM-1, ICAM-3, and telencephalin on human chromosome 19 (184), and that of their corre-

sponding α chains receptors (αL, αM, αD) on chromosome 16, suggests that these integrin ligands are derived from gene duplication events. Finally, ICAM-1 also can bind αMβ₂, although its binding site for Mac-1 is located in the third Ig-like domain (185). αDβ₂ also can bind ICAM-3 (178), whereas αXβ₂ binds ICAM-1 (186), the C3bi complement component, fibrinogen, and lipopolysaccharide (187). Finally, αMβ₂ also binds C3bi, fibrinogen, and the clotting component factor X (175) (Fig. 7)

The β₁ integrin subfamily (previously known as the very late activation [VLA] antigens) (188) are expressed widely on many tissue types and bind almost exclusively to the ECM (Fig. 7) (163,175). The binding of these integrins to ECM proteins gener-

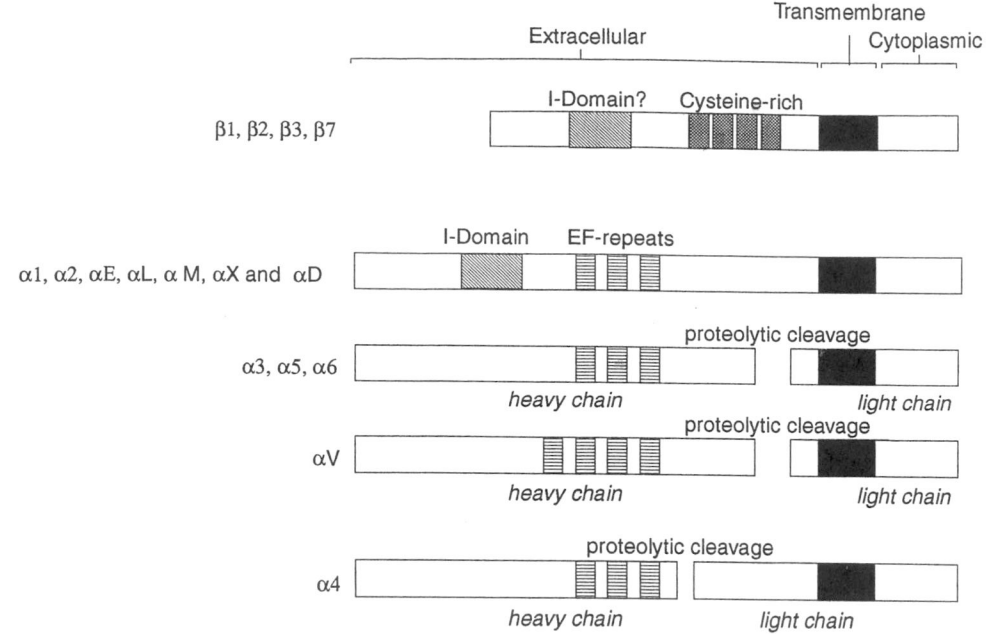

FIG. 8. Generalized integrin structure of integrins expressed on leukocytes.

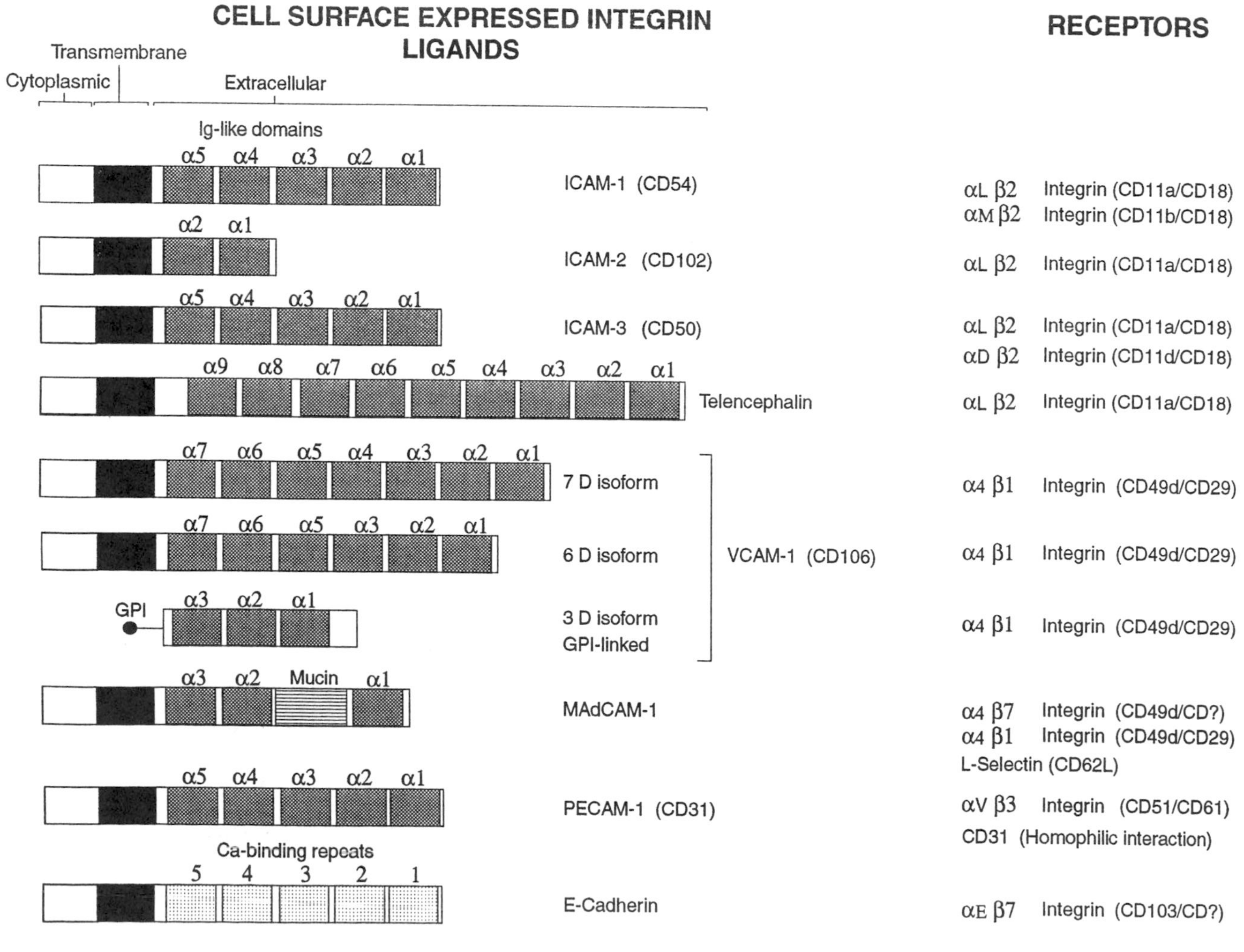

CELL SURFACE EXPRESSED INTEGRIN LIGANDS

RECEPTORS

FIG. 9. Generalized structure of cell surface expressed ligands for leukocyte integrins.

ally occurs via a direct recognition of the specific peptide sequence Arg-Gly-Asp (RGD) shared between fibronectin and vitronectin. However, $\alpha_4\beta_1$ also can bind to fibronectin via an alternative amino acid sequence, EILDV, encoded in the CS-1 site and formed as a consequence of alternative splicing (163). The $\alpha_4\beta_1$ heterodimer is the only β_1 integrin subfamily member that binds both an ECM protein, fibronectin, and a cell surface molecule, vascular cell adhesion molecule-1 (VCAM-1) (189,190) (Fig. 9). VCAM-1 is a member of the Ig supergene family located on chromosome 1 in humans (191). The $\alpha_4\beta_1$ ligand exists in several forms, including a seven Ig-like domain form, an alternatively spliced six Ig-like domain form, and an inflammation-specific phosphatidyl inositol-anchored truncated form expressed on mouse cells (175,192) (Fig. 9). The $\alpha_4\beta_1$ binding to VCAM-1 is predominantly via the recognition of the first amino-terminal Ig-like domain, but also involves the homologous fourth Ig-like domain (193). Thus, binding of $\alpha_4\beta_1$ integrin to fibronectin and VCAM-1 takes place through functionally distinct sites on the integrin heterodimer (194). A homophilic interaction can occur through direct interaction of two α_4 molecules (either $\alpha_4\beta_1$ or $\alpha_4\beta_7$) expressed on apposing cells (195).

Most β_1-associated α chains undergo posttranslational modifications (Fig. 8). The α_3, α_5, α_6, and α_V chains are cut by a proteolytic process in the extracellular domain close to the transmembrane domain, but remain connected and expressed on the cell surface through their disulfide linkage to the β_1 chain. The α_4 chains undergo proteolytic cleavage in a region closer to the EF hand domains (196). Cleavage of these α chains into two fragments takes place soon after association with the β_1 chain (170).

Lymphocyte expression of β_1 integrin subfamily members is correlated with the state of differentiation of the lymphocyte. Naive T cells express low levels of the $\alpha_4\beta_1$ heterodimer. In contrast, activated T cells and resting memory T cells express high levels of $\alpha_4\beta_1$ and other β_1 subfamily members, including $\alpha_3\beta_1$, $\alpha_5\beta_1$, and $\alpha_6\beta_1$ (197). In fact, prolonged in vitro stimulation (7 to 14 days) can lead to $\alpha_1\beta_1$ and $\alpha_2\beta_1$ expression as well (198). B cells and monocytes express varying levels of these β_1 integrins (170). The ECM ligands for the β_1 family are widely expressed throughout the body, whereas VCAM-1, which has a more limited expression pattern, is restricted to inflamed endothelium, follicular dendritic cells, certain macrophages in spleen and thymus, fibroblastlike synoviocytes, bone marrow, and stroma (170). IL-4 and certain inflammatory cytokines such as TNF-α, IFN-γ, and IL-1 induce VCAM-1 expression on endothelium, suggesting that this ligand for $\alpha_4\beta_1$ may predominate at local sites of inflammation.

The β_7 integrin subfamily is involved in T-cell homing to Peyer's patches, the secondary lymphoid tissue lining the intestinal tract (175,199). The β_7 (previously β_p) chain pairs with two different α chains, α_4 and α_E. The $\alpha_4\beta_7$ integrin, also known as the lymphocyte Peyer's patch adhesion molecule-1 (LPAM-1), functions as a gut homing receptor (200) and binds with high affinity to the mucosal addressin cell adhesion molecule-1 (MAdCAM-1) (201). Integrin $\alpha_4\beta_7$ also can interact with lower affinity to the more widely expressed fibronectin and VCAM-1 molecules (202). The gene for the MAdCAM-1 or mucosal vascular addressin transmembrane glycoprotein is located on human chromosome 10 (203). Its extracellular portion is composed of three Ig-like domains and a highly glycosylated mucinlike domain rich in serine/threonine residues. The amino-terminal two Ig-like domains have homology with ICAM-1 and VCAM-1, whereas the third Ig-like domain is similar to the Cα2 domain of IgA. The mucinlike sequence is located between the second and third Ig-like domain (204) (Fig. 9). In the

postcapillary HEVs of the Peyer's patch, this mucinlike region of MAdCAM-1 can be decorated with a carbohydrate moiety that is a functional ligand for L-selectin (205), a member of the selectin family of cell surface–expressed adhesion molecules with a lectin-like domain. MAdCAM-1 has alternatively spliced transcripts that effect the mucinlike domain, which may prevent expression of the L-selectin ligand outside the HEV (203).

The expression of MAdCAM-1 changes during development. In newborn mice, MAdCAM-1 is expressed on the HEV of all lymph nodes, but in adult mice, MAdCAM-1 is not expressed at all in the peripheral lymph nodes but is instead localized to the HEV of Peyer's patches, gut-associated lamina propria, and the vessels of lactating breasts (206). The proinflammatory cytokines TNF-α and IL-1 induce MAdCAM-1 on murine endothelial cells (207). All naive T cells and B cells express integrin $\alpha_4\beta_7$, which allows them to circulate through the Peyer's patches. However, only a subpopulation of effector/memory T cells maintain integrin $\alpha_4\beta_7$ expression and thus have the capacity to enter noninflamed gut-associated lamina propria. Integrin $\alpha_4\beta_7$ is downregulated under certain conditions, such as in vitro T-cell activation with the superantigen staphylococcal enterotoxin A (208). Presently it is not clear what mechanisms regulate the expression of integrin $\alpha_4\beta_7$ during normal immune responses in vivo.

The other α chain that can pair with β_7 is α_E, also known as α_{IEL} or α_{290}. The $\alpha_E\beta_7$ heterodimer is expressed on intraepithelial lymphocytes (IELs) present in the gut mucosa (209) and binds to E-cadherin expressed on mucosal epithelial cells (210) (Fig. 9). Transforming growth factor (TGF)-β upregulates the expression of α_E in vitro (211), and the presence of high levels of TGF-β in the gut-associated mucosa is thought to be the stimulus for expression of this integrin on IELs. Although the integrin $\alpha_4\beta_7$ functions as a genuine gut homing receptor, the integrin $\alpha_E\beta_7$ integrin functions more as a retention receptor to localize IELs to the gut epithelium after they have extravasated from the blood and entered the gut-associated lamina propria.

Finally, although the β_1, β_2, and β_7 integrin subfamilies are the major immunologically relevant integrin subfamilies, other integrins can play critical roles in the immune system. The vitronectin receptor $\alpha_V\beta_3$ is expressed on $\gamma\delta$ T cells and can provide the costimulation necessary for proliferation (212). $\alpha_V\beta_3$ also can bind platelet endothelium cellular adhesion molecule-1 (PECAM-1), also known as CD31 (213), an Ig supergene family member expressed on various cell types including T cells and endothelium (Fig. 9). Another integrin subfamily member, the laminin receptor ($\alpha_6\beta_4$), may play a role in thymocyte development because its expression is regulated on early murine thymocyte populations (214).

Integrin Function

T-cell migration into tissues requires T-cell binding to and extravasation through endothelium (175,199,215), an integrin-dependent process. Current models propose that chemokines deliver the critical biochemical signals that promote endothelial binding through the upregulation of integrin avidity on the T cell (216–218). Chemokines, released either by inflamed endothelium or underlying tissues, can be bound by proteoglycans expressed on the lumenal side of the endothelium (219) or interact directly with the endothelial cell surface, like the recently described membrane-bound chemokine fractalkine (220). As cells pass along the endothelium, they adhere weakly via the selectins and α_4 integrin. This rolling phase allows T cells expressing appropriate chemokine receptors to bind to the endothelium-bound or -expressed chemokines. The chemokine receptors transduce signals leading to rapid upregulation of integrin avidity. The increased avidity of the integrins ($\alpha_4\beta_1$, $\alpha_4\beta_7$, and β_2) results in the arrest of cell migration, strong adhesion, and cell spreading. After this chemokine-induced adhesion, the T-lymphocytes transmigrate into the tissue, where they participate in the inflammatory response. This process of extravasation is dependent on CD31 (221), which can bind to CD31 or $\alpha_v\beta_3$ expressed on T cells and endothelium (Fig. 10).

Integrin-mediated events are also critical for T cells that participate in immune surveillance. As resting T cells circulate through the blood, they adhere specifically to the specialized endothelium of the postcapillary venules of secondary lymphoid organs or HEVs and extravasate from the bloodstream into the underlying secondary lymphoid tissues. Homing receptors, in this case the peripheral lymph node receptor L-selectin, bind to specific carbohydrate moieties on tissue-bound proteoglycans called mucins. At least two HEV-specific L-selectin ligands or peripheral lymph node addressins are expressed in the peripheral lymph node, the glycosylated cellular adhesion molecule-1 (GlyCAM-1), and a specifically glycosylated form of CD34 (222,223). In gut mucosal areas, the HEVs express an L-selectin ligand present on the mucin domain of MAdCAM-1 (205). The expression of MAdCAM-1 in Peyer's patch HEVs allows for efficient binding through both L-selectin and $\alpha_4\beta_7$ integrin, both of which are expressed on naive T cells. L-selectin binding to GlyCAM-1 in vitro upregulates β_2 integrin-mediated binding by inducing high-affinity receptors, without affecting the level of integrin expression (224). This mechanism may facilitate resting naive T cell binding and migration into secondary lymphoid organs without the need of chemokines. This is important because T-cell expression of most chemokine receptors

requires prior T-cell activation. Thus, L-selectin–initiated integrin binding specifically may facilitate adhesion or migration of naive T cells, whereas memory/effector T cells may use chemokine-induced integrin adhesion.

Regulation of Integrin Function

The migratory properties of T cells critical to the initiation and progression of an immune response depend directly on the adhesive properties of the adhesion and homing receptors expressed. However, this essential attribute raises a problem. How do the adhesion molecules regulate their binding activity to allow both the attachment as well as detachment characteristics required for transmigration into and out of the inflamed endothelium and draining lymph nodes? Lymphocytes have solved this problem by tightly regulating the affinity and avidity of integrin receptors. Integrin binding can be regulated by activation-induced conformational changes in the extracellular domains of the integrins that transform a low-affinity receptor to a high-affinity receptor (225,226). These conformational changes are dependent on the presence of specific divalent cations, which are bound by the extracellular domains of integrins. Replacement of bound Ca^{2+} with Mg^{2+} for β_2 integrins or Mn^{2+} for β_1 integrins results in increased receptor affinity for their ligands (227). Recently activated effector/memory T cells express higher levels of activated $\alpha_L\beta_2$ molecules, as measured by conformation-specific reporter mAbs (228). Stimulation of T cells with either antigen-dependent or antigen-independent signals increases integrin affinity. MAb cross-linking of CD3 leads to a rapid but transient increase in $\alpha_L\beta_2$-mediated ICAM-1 binding to apposing cells or ECM proteins (229,230). Antigen-independent signals regulate integrin-

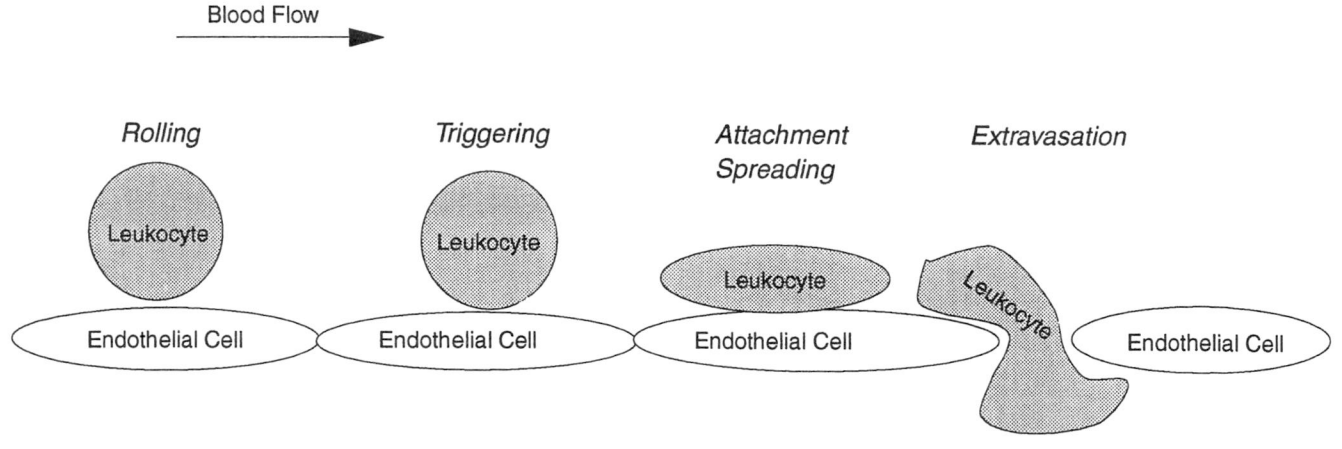

FIG. 10. Multistep model of leukocyte adhesion and migration out of blood.

mediated affinity on lymphocytes (231–233). Cross-linking ICAM-3 or CD28 on resting T cells results in increased affinity of the $\alpha_L\beta_2$ receptor (231,234). Thus, integrin binding is highly regulated by TCR-dependent and -independent events that promote cell adhesion and enhance the activation of the T cells both before and during antigen engagement. Finally, the overall avidity of the receptor–ligand interaction can be regulated by receptor reorganization without altering the affinity of the individual receptor (235). For instance, PMA-induced increases in integrin binding to ICAM-1 or fibronectin are a consequence of cytoskeletal rearrangements that increase overall integrin avidity and induce cell spreading but do not lead to high-affinity integrin receptor (236,237). This change in avidity can occur through mechanisms that allow for increases in lateral mobility (238) and recruitment of receptors to the area of contact or stronger association of the cytoplasmic domain of the receptor with cytoskeletal components.

Interestingly, chemokine-induced upregulation of integrin avidity can occur by affecting both integrin affinity and avidity. Chemokine binding to their receptors, the seven-transmembrane domain containing G protein–coupled molecules, regulates β_1 and β_2 integrin-mediated binding to VCAM-1, fibronectin, and ICAM-1 through an actin-dependent mechanism that does not involve conformational changes in the extracellular domains of the integrin receptor (216–218). Similar effects are observed in chemokine-induced $\alpha_4\beta_1$ binding to VCAM-1 by eosinophils (239). By comparison, the chemokines can induce high-affinity integrin receptors through induction of conformational changes as observed when eosinophil-expressed $\alpha_M\beta_2$ binds to ICAM-1 after chemokine exposure (239).

Inside-Out/Outside-In Signaling

Activation-induced changes in integrin binding are due to intracellular biochemical signals that alter extracellular conformation. This inside-out signaling of the integrin receptor is distinguished from the integrin-mediated signaling that occurs as a consequence of extracellular ligand binding, outside-in signaling. The nature of the intracellular signals involved in the inside-out activation of integrin binding are still unclear, but both serine/threonine and tyrosine phosphorylation of the cytoplasmic tail are critical regulators of signaling leading to increased avidity of the integrin for its ligand. A conserved motif (NPXY) in the cytoplasmic domains of most integrins has been identified as another important site regulating integrin binding induced by PMA (240). The α_L chain of $\alpha_L\beta_2$ is constitutively serine/threonine phosphorylated, whereas the β_2 chain is serine/threonine phosphorylated only upon PMA activation, suggesting a direct or indirect role for protein kinase C. However, the role of these posttranslational modifications of the integrins is unclear. Although deletion mutant studies of the β_2 chain have shown that a carboxy-terminal stretch of five amino acids, including three contiguous threonines (Thr 758-760), are crucial for PMA-induced binding of β_2 to ICAM-1, the amino-terminal 28 amino acids of the cytoplasmic domain can be eliminated. Moreover, the elimination of carboxy-terminal five–amino acid sequence does not alter receptor affinity, as determined by a conformation-specific mAb, but prevents postreceptor events required for binding (241). Similarly, although PMA stimulation of T cells induced phosphorylation of Ser 756 in the β_2 chain, this phosphorylation is not required for induction of PMA-induced β_2 binding to ICAM-1

(242). However, CD2- and CD28-induced β_1 integrin binding is blocked by Wortmannin, a PI-3-kinase inhibitor (243–244), suggesting that activation of this kinase can be critical for inducing integrin binding, and chemokine receptor-mediated signaling has been shown to involve the Rho family of small guanosine triphosphate (GTP)-binding proteins (245).

Recently a family of cytoplasmic proteins has been described, termed cytohesins (246) or integrin regulating proteins (IRPs), one of which specifically regulates ligand adhesion of the β_2 integrin via its interaction with the cytoplasmic domain. The IRPs interact with the integrin chains through a domain, termed Sec-7, which regulates the increased adhesion. The Sec-7 domains are homologous to a yeast protein that controls Golgi transport and can function as a GTP exchange factor for small GTPases of the ARF family. Interestingly, the Sec7 domain of one of the IRPs also has GTP exchange factor activity. In addition, these proteins contain a Pleckstrin homology domain, and in two cytohesin family members binds PtdIns(3,4,5)P$_3$ (247), linking their function with PI-3 kinase. Thus, this new class of intracellular molecules has the ability to both bind and regulate integrin function as well as function as adaptor molecules that bridge the integrins to important intracellular biochemical pathways.

The inside-out signaling of integrin molecules is regulated by both cell surface and intracellular protein interactions. For example, the CD47 molecule, also known as the integrin-associated protein (IAP), is a transmembrane molecule with a single extracellular Ig-like domain that forms a calcium channel for integrin-mediated Ca^{2+} influx that regulates many $\alpha_V\beta_3$ integrin–ligand binding functions. Similarly, antibody cross-linking of the tetraspan CD9 protein, which associates with β_3 and β_1 integrins, can influence integrin-binding activity on B cells (248). Four other tetraspan family members—CD81, CD82, CD63, and CD53—have been found associated with $\alpha_4\beta_1$ (249). The plasminogen activator receptor (uPA-R) is associated with $\alpha_L\beta_2$ and $\alpha_M\beta_2$ (250, 251). Finally, $\alpha_M\beta_2$ can bind through a lectinlike site in α_M to the FcRIIIβ (CD16) (252). Together these, and undoubtably other, cell surface molecular interactions regulate the early events in integrin binding and signal transduction.

Finally, although much attention has been focused on the upregulation of integrin-binding function via intracellular signals, equally important are the biochemical events that downregulate integrin binding to allow for detachment or de-adhesion of T cells from the ECM or apposing cell. Preliminary insights into these processes have come from studies showing that $\alpha_L\beta_2$-mediated binding to ICAM-1 was downregulated by increasing the intracellular levels of cAMP (229), which promotes cAMP-dependent kinase (PKA) activity. This kinase has been shown to break down actin filaments, resulting in dissociation of $\alpha_L\beta_2$ from the cytoskeleton and decreasing the overall avidity of the integrin–ligand interaction (253). Furthermore, the high-affinity conformation of integrins can be altered by the small GTP-binding protein H-Ras and its effector kinase Raf-1. This reduction in high-affinity integrin binding correlated with activation of the ^{E}RK/MAP kinase pathway (254), suggesting that the Ras-linked MAP kinase pathway may mediate a negative feedback loop in integrin function.

As discussed above, both the antigen dependent and antigen-independent conjugates between T cells and apposing cells can be blocked with anti-$\alpha_L\beta_2$ mAbs (161,162). These results were interpreted as demonstrating that this adhesion pathway functioned predominantly as glue that brings cells together. However, it has become increasingly clear that integrin binding initiates critical intracellular signaling events as well. T-cell proliferative responses are enhanced when membrane-bound or immobilized soluble ICAM-1 cross-links $\alpha_L\beta_2$ in the presence of TCR signals (255,256). In fact, a number of integrin ligands—including ICAM-2, ICAM-3, and the β_2 integrin ligands VCAM-1, fibronectin, and laminin—can provide T-cell costimulation in this setting (257–260). This enhanced T-cell responsiveness is not simply a consequence of increased adhesion (261). Integrins can transduce signals upon ligand interaction, which can result in T-cell costimulation, leading to both cell proliferation and cytokine secretion. ICAM-1– and VCAM-1–mediated costimulation induced secretion of various cytokines, such as IL-2, IL-4, and IFN-γ (261), although unlike both CD28/B7-1 and CD2/LFA-3 costimulation, ICAM-1 and VCAM-1 ligation do not stimulate activated T cells or induce the survival signals essential for rescue of the T cells from activation-induced apoptosis (262). In addition, ICAM-1– and VCAM-1–mediated T-cell activation induced increased CD28 responsiveness in T cells (263,264). β_1-integrin–mediated signals can rescue some nonlymphoid cells from apoptosis (265,266), and engagement of the vitronectin receptor $\alpha_V\beta_3$ can costimulate $\gamma\delta$ T cell clones (213). However, integrin-mediated T-cell activation is not limited to T-cell costimulatory signals. Antigen-independent integrin activation of T cells can occur via $\alpha_4\beta_1$ binding to VCAM-1, which induces secretion of a 72-kDa gelatinase on the surface of T cells (267). T cell–secreted metalloproteases, such as gelatinase, are thought to facilitate extravasation through the basement membrane of endothelium (268).

The precise signal transduction pathways that are used for T-cell integrin-mediated signaling have yet to be fully elucidated. T-cell binding to immobilized fibronectin or anti-β_1 integrin mAb induces multiple signaling events, including the tyrosine phosphorylation of PLC-γ_1, pp59^{FYN}, pp56^{LCK}, pp125^{FAK}, MAP kinase (269), the cytoskeletal protein paxillin (270), and pp105^{CAS-L} (271), as well as induction of the DNA-binding protein AP-1 (272). Cross-linking of $\alpha_L\beta_2$ on T cells by mAbs or coimmobilized anti-CD3 mAbs and ICAM-1 induced prolonged tyrosine phosphorylation of PLC-γ_1 (273), PIP$_2$ hydrolysis, and a sustained increase in intracellular Ca^{2+} (274,275). Similar $\alpha_L\beta_2$ integrin cross-linking with VCAM-1 did not induce PLC-γ1 tyrosine phosphorylation, suggesting unique regulation of the integrins depending on their ligand binding (273). The cytoplasmic domain of the integrin β_2 chain binds the cytoskeletal protein filamin (276), whereas the β_1 integrin subunit has been reported to bind talin, α-actinin and a serine/threonine kinase, integrin-linked kinase (p59^{ILK}) (277,278). In vitro, the nonreceptor tyrosine kinase focal adhesion kinase (pp125^{FAK}) can bind to GST-fusion proteins containing a consensus sequence present in the cytoplasmic domains of β_1, β_2, and β_3 integrins (279). The importance of β_1 chain signaling linking to FAK is illustrated by functional studies demonstrating that T-cell binding to fibronectin or VCAM-1 strongly synergizes with anti-CD3 mAb to initiate β_1 integrin-mediated tyrosine phosphorylation of FAK (280). The linking of β_1 to FAK is particularly crucial to integrin-mediated signaling because FAK not only functions as a docking protein for cytoskeletal molecules like talin (281) and paxillin (270), but is also associated with other effector pathways such as PI-3 kinase and Ras. In fact, in fibroblasts, the binding of β_1 chains to fibronectin results in autophosphorylation of tyrosine-397 of FAK, which leads to binding of the nonreceptor tyrosine kinase, pp60^{src}, which upon binding can transphosphorylate FAK on tyrosine-925, allowing FAK to bind Grb-2 and Sos (282). These bio-chemical events may initiate Grb-2 or Sos activation of Ras, which leads to cell growth and differentiation. Alternatively, PI-3 kinase can bind through the same autophosphorylated tyrosine-397 in FAK (283), resulting in alterations in cytoskeletal reorganization and cell motility. Together these results suggest that FAK is crucial in regulating outside-in signaling for β_1 integrins in T cells.

The Importance of the Integrin Pathways *In Vivo*

The physiologic importance of integrins for various immune functions is best illustrated in individuals lacking expression of specific integrin chains either due to naturally occurring mutations or through genetic engineering. In humans, a rare autosomal-recessive disorder, leukocyte adhesion deficiency type 1 (LAD-1), originates from the lack or deficient expression of the β_2 integrin chain, which affects $\alpha_L\beta_2$, $\alpha_M\beta_2$, $\alpha_X\beta_2$, and $\alpha_D\beta_2$ expression (284). These individuals suffer from recurrent bacterial and fungal infections and impaired wound healing. This disorder affects leukocyte binding to endothelium, chemotaxis, and phagocytosis. Although T-cell functions are suboptimal, LAD-1 patients do clear viral infections, suggesting that other adhesion pathways, such as $\alpha_4\beta_1$/VCAM-1, may compensate for some of the β_2 integrin functions on T cells. These studies have been confirmed using genetically engineered $\alpha_L\beta_2$-deficient mice. α_L KO mice display normal CTL responses against viruses but fail to reject immunogenic tumors (285,286). A similar capacity to generate effective antiviral immune responses was observed in mice deficient for both $\alpha_L\beta_2$ and ICAM-1 (287). ICAM-1–deficient mice are further resistant to septic shock (288) and renal or cerebral ischemic reperfusion injury (289,290). Interestingly, these mice fail to show superantigen-induced proliferation of CD4$^+$ T cells (291). Unfortunately, β_1 integrin– or VCAM-1–deficient embryos are not viable (292–295) due to a defective development of the embryonic and extraembryonic circulatory systems (294,295). However, β_1 integrin–null embryonic stem cells have been used to generate chimeric mice. Under these conditions, both T- and B-cell development is compromised in vivo due to a lack of homing of hematopoietic stem cells from the yolk sac tissue to the fetal liver (296). The β_7-null chimeric mice have validated the critical importance of β_7 integrins for gut-associated immune responses. These integrin-deficient animals are totally devoid of gut-associated lymphoid tissue (GALT) (297). The α_4-null chimeric mice are also devoid of GALT due to a lack of $\alpha_4\beta_7$ integrin expression and in addition have a major defect in T- and B-cell development (298). B-cell differentiation is blocked before the pro-B cell stage, whereas T-cell numbers and phenotype, although normal in blood and secondary lymphoid organs, are abnormal in Peyer's patches. In addition, there is a precipitous decrease in T-cell numbers, and the thymus involutes more rapidly with age in these α_4-deficient mice compared with wild-type mice. Thus, the use of the mutant mice confirms an essential role for these molecules in lymphocyte development and homing.

The studies summarized above have given important impetus to therapeutic application of integrin antagonists in a variety of clinical settings, and clinical trials are currently under evaluation. Antibodies directed at $\alpha_L\beta_2$ and ICAM-1 have been used in transplant models to suppress graft rejection with the goal to prevent leukocyte migration into the graft and cell contact–mediated damage to the transplant. Treatment with specific mAbs has been shown to enhance survival of renal (299) and islet allografts (300) just by pretreating the graft tissue with anti–ICAM-1 mAb. In fact, in a rat cardiac transplant model, a short treatment with a combination of anti-$\alpha_L\beta_2$ and anti–ICAM-1 mAbs (301) or anti-α_4 and anti–VCAM-1 mAbs prevented rejection and rendered the recipient tolerant for an extended period (302). The therapeutic effects of antagonists of integrin binding has also been explored in various autoimmune diseases. Blocking of $\alpha_4\beta_1$ or VCAM-1 prevents adoptive transfer of EAE (303). Interestingly, in the same model, antibodies against the chemokine MIP-1α, but not MCP-1, prevent adoptive transfer of the EAE (304), suggesting that $\alpha_4\beta_1$-mediated binding to the capillary endothelial cells lining the brain is regulated through this chemokine.

The physiologic importance of integrins is not limited to immune cell functions. Many pathogenic organisms specifically use integrins or their ligands for their pathogenesis. In viruses, the I domain of the integrin $\alpha_2\beta_1$ has been shown to be a receptor for echovirus 1 (305). More then 90% of all human rhinoviruses, the cause of the common cold, specifically use the integrin ligand ICAM-1 as a receptor (306,307). In fact, soluble ICAM-1 has been shown in experimental models to be an effective inhibitor of rhinovirus infections (308,309). The protozoal parasite *Plasmodium falciparum* causes malaria and infects erythrocytes as part of its life cycle. Infected erythrocytes bind to various adhesion molecules on endothelium (310), and recently the *Plasmodium falciparum* erythrocyte membrane protein-1 was identified as a receptor that binds to the adhesion molecules, CD34 and ICAM-1, as well as to thrombospondin (311). Binding of infected erythrocytes to ICAM-1 on activated endothelium of brain vessels is thought to be the cause for the often fatal form of cerebral malaria (312). Bacteria also infect cells through integrin binding. Invasin, a *Yersina pseudotuberculosis*–derived membrane protein binds to $\alpha_4\beta_1$ integrins and can even trigger T-cell costimulatory signals (313). Another bacterial membrane protein, intimin, expressed on enteropathogenic *Escherichia coli,* can bind to both $\alpha_4\beta_1$ and $\alpha_4\beta_7$ integrins (314).

Summary

One of the most important functional characteristics of T cells is their capacity to migrate freely throughout the whole body yet undergo intimate cell–cell contacts, either brief or prolonged, depending on the nature of the cell the T-lymphocyte encounters. This process requires a complex regulation of molecular interactions to allow for adhesion and de-adhesion of the cells. Integrins are cell surface–expressed heterodimers that are critically involved in both these antigen-independent and -dependent adhesive interactions of T cells with apposing cells and ECM. Specifically, the T cell–expressed integrins $\alpha_L\beta_2$, $\alpha_4\beta_1$, and $\alpha_4\beta_7$ are directly involved in homing and extravasation into tissue. $\alpha_L\beta_2$ and, possibly, $\alpha_4\beta_1$ play a major role in T-cell interaction with APCs. Integrin receptor binding to ligands is rapidly upregulated by cellular activation or inside-out signaling, which include signals from chemokine receptors, TCR/CD3 complex, and various accessory molecules. The increased integrin receptor binding can be affected by upregulating the integrin receptor affinity through conformational changes in the extracellular portion of the heterodimer or by increasing the overall avidity by altering postreceptor ligand binding events, resulting in cell spreading. In addition, integrins can transduce signals upon binding to their ligands in an outside-in fashion. Finally, the importance of the integrins has been clearly shown in organ transplantation and in vivo models of infectious and autoimmune diseases, prompting the potential use of integrin antagonists in the clinical setting.

REFERENCES

1. Cantor H, Boyse EA. Functional subclasses of T-lymphocytes bearing different Ly antigens. I. The generation of functionally distinct T-cell subclasses is a differentiative process independent of antigen. *J Exp Med* 1975;141:1376–1389.
2. Boumsell L, Bernard A, Coppin H, et al. Human T cell differentiation antigens and correlation of their expression with various markers of T cell maturation. *J Immunol* 1979;123:2063–2067.
3. CD Antigens 1996. *Immunol Today* 1997;18:100–101.
4. Burnet FM. *The Clonal Selection Theory of Immunity.* Nashville, TN: Vanderbilt University Press, 1959.
5. Bretscher P, Cohn M. A theory of self-nonself discrimination. *Science* 1970; 169:1042–1049.
6. Lafferty KJ, Gill RG. The maintenance of self-tolerance. *Immunol Cell Biol* 1993;71:209–214.
7. Jenkins MK, Pardoll DM, Mizuguchi J, Quill H, Schwartz RH. T-cell unresponsiveness in vivo and in vitro. Fine specificity of induction and molecular characterization of the unresponsive state. *Immunol Rev* 1987;95:113–135.
8. June CH, Bluestone JA, Nadler LM, Thompson CB. The B7 and CD28 receptor families. *Immunol Today* 1994;15:321–331.
9. Linsley PS, Brady W, Grosmaire L, Aruffo A, Damle NK, Ledbetter JA. Binding of the B cell activation antigen B7 to CD28 costimulates T cell proliferation and interleukin 2 mRNA accumulation. *J Exp Med* 1991;173:721–730.
10. Gross JA, Callas, E, Allison, JP. Identification and distribution of the costimulatory receptor CD28 in the mouse. *J Immunol* 1992;149:380–388.
11. Lafage-Pochitaloff M, Costello R, Couez D, et al. Human CD28 and CTLA-4 Ig superfamily genes are located on chromosome 2 at bands q33-q34. *Immunogenetics* 1990;31:198–201.
12. Howard TA, Rochell JM, Seldin MF. CD28 and CTLA-4, two related members of the Ig supergene family, are tightly linked on proximal mouse chromosome 1. *Immunogenetics* 1991;33:74–76.
13. Lee KP, Taylor C, Petryniak B, Turka LA, June CH, Thompson CB. The genomic organization of the CD28 gene. Implications for the regulation of CD28 mRNA expression and heterogeneity. *J Immunol* 1990;145:344–352.
14. Lindsten T, Lee KP, Harris ES, et al. Characterization of CTLA-4 structure and expression on human T cells. *J Immunol* 1993;151:3489–3499.
15. Parsons KR, Young JR, Collins BA, Howard CJ. Cattle CTLA-4, CD28 and chicken CD28 bind CD86: MYPPPY is not conserved in cattle CD28. *Immunogenetics* 1996;43:388–391.
16. Linsley PS, Bradshaw J, Urnes M, Grosmaire L, Ledbetter JA. CD28 engagement by B7/BB-1 induces transient down-regulation of CD28 synthesis and prolonged unresponsiveness to CD28 signaling. *J Immunol* 1993;150:3161–3169.
17. Brunet JF, Denizot F, Luciani MF, et al. A new member of the immunoglobulin superfamily—CTLA-4. *Nature* 1987;328:267–270.
18. Linsley PS, Brady W, Urnes M, Grosmaire LS, Damle NK, Ledbetter JA. CTLA-4 is a second receptor for the B cell activation antigen B7. *J Exp Med* 1991;174: 561–569.
19. Walunas TL, Lenschow DJ, Bakker CY, et al. CTLA-4 can function as a negative regulator of T cell activation. *Immunity* 1994;1:405–413.
20. Lindsten T, Lee KP, Harris ES, et al. Characterization of CTLA-4 structure and expression on human T cells. *J Immunol* 1993;151:3489–3499.
21. Harper K, Balzano C, Rouvier E, Mattëi MG, Luciani MF, Golstein P. CTLA-4 and CD28 activated lymphocyte molecules are closely related in both mouse and human as to sequence, message expression, gene structure, and chromosomal location. *J Immunol* 1991;147:1037–1044.
22. Linsley PS, Greene JL, Brady W, Bajorath J, Ledbetter JA, Peach R. Human B7-1 (CD80) and B7-2 (CD86) bind with similar avidities but distinct kinetics to CD28 and CTLA-4 receptors. *Immunity* 1994;1:793–801.
23. Dariavach P, Mattëi MG, Golstein P, Lefranc MP. Human Ig superfamily CTLA-4 gene: Chromosomal localization and identity of protein sequence between murine and human CTLA-4 cytoplasmic domains. *Eur J Immunol* 1988;18:1901–1905.
24. Linsley PS, Greene JL, Tan P, et al. Coexpression and functional cooperation of CTLA-4 and CD28 on activated T lymphocytes. *J Exp Med* 1992;176:1595–1604.
25. Linsley J, Nadler SG, Bajorath J, et al. Binding stoichiometry of the cytotoxic T lymphocyte-associated molecule-4 (CTLA-4). A disulfide-linked homodimer binds two CD86 molecules. *J Biol Chem* 1995;270:15417–15424.
26. Shiratori T, Miyatake S, Ohno H, et al. Tyrosine phosphorylation controls internalization of CTLA-4 by regulating its interaction with clathrin-associated adaptor complex AP-2. *Immunity* 1997;6:583–589.
27. Alegre ML, Noel PJ, Eisfelder BJ, et al. Regulation of surface and intracellular expression of CTLA4 on mouse T cells. *J Immunol* 1996;157:4762–4770.
28. Walunas TL, Bakker CY, Bluestone JA. CTLA-4 ligation blocks CD28-dependent T cell activation. *J Exp Med* 1996;183:2541–2550.
29. Linsley PS, Clark EA, Ledbetter JA. T-cell antigen CD28 mediates adhesion with B cells by interacting with activation antigen B7/BB-1. *Proc Natl Acad Sci U S A* 1990;87:5031–5035.
30. Freeman GJ, Gray GS, Gimmi CD, et al. Structure, expression, and T cell cos-

timulatory activity of the murine homologue of the human B lymphocyte activation antigen B7. *J Exp Med* 1991;174:625–631.

31. Freeman GJ, Disteche, CM, Gribben JG, et al. The gene for B7, a costimulatory signal for T-cell activation, maps to chromosomal region 3q13.3-3q21. *Blood* 1992;79:489–494.

32. Fernandez-Ruiz E, Somoza C, Sanchez-Madrid F, Lanier LL. CD28/CTLA-4 ligands: The gene encoding CD86 (B70/B7.2) maps to the same region as CD80 (B7/B7.1) gene in human chromosome 3q13-q23. *Eur J Immunol* 1995;25:1453–1456.

33. Lenschow DJ, Su GH-T, Zuckerman LA, et al. Expression and functional significance of an additional ligand for CTLA-4. *Proc Natl Acad Sci U S A* 1993;90:11054–11058.

34. Freeman GJ, Gribben JG, Boussiotis VA, et al. Cloning of B7-2: A CTLA-4 counter-receptor that costimulates human T cell proliferation. *Science* 1993;262:909–911.

35. Azuma MD, Ito H, Yagita K, et al. B70 antigen is a second ligand for CTLA-4 and CD28. *Nature* 1993;366:76–78.

36. Truneh A, Reddy M, Ryan P, Lyn SD. Differential recognition by CD28 of its cognate counter receptors CD80 (B7.1) and CD86 (B7.2): Analysis by site-directed mutagenesis. *Mol Immunol* 1996;33:321–334.

37. Lenschow DJ, Walunas TL, Bluestone JA. CD28/B7 System of T cell costimulation. *Annu Rev Immunol* 1996;14:233–258.

38. Inaba K, Witmer-Pack M, Inaba M, Hathcock KS, et al. The tissue distribution of the B7-2 costimulator in mice: Abundant expression on dendritic cells in situ and during maturation in vitro. *J Exp Med* 1994;180:1849–1860.

39. Caux C, Vanbervliet B, Massacrier C, et al. B70/B7-2 is identical to CD86 and is the major functional ligand for CD28 expressed on human dendritic cells. *J Exp Med* 1994;180:1841–1847.

40. Prabhu Das MR, Zamvil SS, Borriello F, Weiner HL, Sharpe AH, Kuchroo VK. Reciprocal expression of costimulatory molecules, B7-1 and B7-2, on murine T cells following activation. *Eur J Immunol* 1995;25:207–211.

41. Freeman GJ, Freedman AS, Segil JM, Lee G, Whitman JF, Nadler LM. B7, a new member of the Ig superfamily with unique expression on activated and neoplastic B cells. *J Immunol* 1989;143:2714–2722.

42. Stack RM, Lenschow DJ, Gray GS, Bluestone JA, Fitch FW. IL-4 treatment of small splenic B cells induces costimulatory molecules B7-1 and B7-2. *J Immunol* 1994;152:5723–5733.

43. Barcy SM, Wettendorff O, Leo J, et al. FcR cross-linking on monocytes results in impaired T cell stimulatory capacity. *Int Immunol* 1995;7:179–189.

44. Ozawa H, Aiba S, Nakagawa S, Tagami H. Interferon-gamma and interleukin-10 inhibit antigen presentation by Langerhans cells for T helper type 1 cells by suppressing their CD80 (B7-1) expression. *Eur J Immunol* 1996;26:648–652.

45. Groux H, Torpier G, Monte D, Mouton Y, Capron A, Amieson JC. Activation-induced by apoptosis in CD4- cells from human immunodeficiency virus-infected asymptomatic individuals. *J Exp Med* 1992;175:331–340.

46. Punt JA, Osborne BA, Takahama Y, Sharrow SO, Singer A. Negative selection of CD4+CD8+ thymocytes by T cell receptor-induced apoptosis requires a costimulatory signal that can be provided by CD28. *J Exp Med* 1994;179:709–713.

47. Amsen D, Kruisbeek AM. CD28-B7 interactions function to co-stimulate clonal deletion of double-positive thymocytes. *Int Immunol* 1996;8:1927–1936.

48. Walunas TL, Sperling AI, Khattri R, Thompson CB, Bluestone JA. CD28 expression is not essential for positive and negative selection of thymocytes or peripheral T cell tolerance. *J Immunol* 1996;156:1006–1013.

49. Tivol EA, Borriello F, Schweitzer AN, Lynch WP, Bluestone JA, Sharpe AH. Loss of CTLA-4 leads to massive lymphoproliferation and fatal multiorgan tissue destruction, revealing a critical negative regulatory role of CTLA-4. *Immunity* 1995;3:541–547.

50. Chambers CA, Cado D, Truong T, Allison JP. Thymocyte development is normal in CTLA-4-deficient mice. *Proc Natl Acad Sci* 1997;94:9296–9301.

51. Shahinian AK, Pfeffer K, Lee TM, et al. Differential T cell costimulatory requirements in CD28-deficient mice. *Science* 1993;261:609–612.

52. Green JM, Noel PJ, Sperling AI, et al. Absence of B7-dependent responses in CD28-deficient mice. *Immunity* 1994;1:501–508.

53. Seder RA, Germain RN, Linsley PS, Paul WE. CD28-mediated costimulation of interleukin 2 (IL-2) production plays a critical role in T cell priming for IL-4 and interferon gamma production. *J Exp Med* 1994;179:299–304.

54. Fraser JD, Irving BA, Crabtree GR, Weiss A. Regulation of interleukin-2 gene enhancer activity by the T cell accessory molecule CD28. *Science* 1991;251:313–316.

55. Lindsten T, June CH, Ledbetter JA, Stella G, Thompson CB. Regulation of lymphokine messenger RNA stability by a surface-mediated T cell activation pathway. *Science* 1989;244:339–342.

56. Cerdan C, Martin Y, Couroul M, Mawas C, Birg F, Olive D. CD28 costimulation up-regulates long-term IL-2R beta expression in human T cells through combined transcriptional and post-transcriptional regulation. *J Immunol* 1995;154:1007–1013.

57. Ward SG. CD28: a signaling perspective. *Biochem J* 1996;318:361–377.

58. Sperling AI, Bluestone JA. The complexities of T cell co-stimulation: CD28 and beyond. *Immunol Rev* 1996;153:155–182.

59. Muraille E, DeBecker G, Bakkus M, et al. Co-stimulation lowers the threshold for activation of naive T cells by bacterial superantigens. *Int Immunol* 1995;7:295–304.

60. Sperling AI, Auger JA, Ehst BD, Rulifson IC, Thompson CB, Bluestone JA. CD28/B7 interactions deliver a unique signal to naive T cells that regulates cell survival but not early proliferation. *J Immunol* 1996;157:3909–3917.

61. Rulifson IC, Sperling AI, Fields PE, Fitch FW, Bluestone JA. CD28 co-stimulation promotes the production of Th2 cytokines. *J Immunol* 1997;158:658–665.

62. Warnier G, Duffour MT, Uyttenhove C, et al. Induction of a cytolytic T-cell response in mice with a recombinant adenovirus coding for tumor antigen P815A. *Int J Cancer* 1996;67:303–310.

63. Linsley PS, Greene JL, Tan P, et al. Coexpression and functional cooperation of CTLA-4 and CD28 on activated T lymphocytes. *J Exp Med* 1992;176:1595–1604.

64. Wu Y, Guo Y, Huang A, Zheng P, Liu Y. CTLA-4-B7 interaction is sufficient to costimulate T cell clonal expansion. *J Exp Med* 1997;185:1327–1335.

65. Krummel MF, Allison JP. CD28 and CTLA-4 deliver opposing signals which regulate the response of T cells to stimulation. *J Exp Med* 1995;182:459–65.

66. Bluestone JA. Commentary: Is CTLA-4 a master switch for peripheral T cell tolerance? *J Immunol* 1997;158:1989–1993.

67. Donner H, Rau H, Walfish PG, et al. CTLA4 alanine-17 confers genetic susceptibility to Graves' disease and to type 1 diabetes mellitus. *J Clin Endocrinol Metab* 1997;82:143–146.

68. Raab M, Cai Y-C, Bunnell SC, Heyeck SD, Berg LJ, Rudd CE. p56Lck and p59Fyn regulate CD28 binding to phosphatidylinositol 3-kinase, growth factor receptor-bound protein GRB-2, and T cell-specific protein-tyrosine kinase ITK: Implications for T-cell costimulation. *Proc Natl Acad Sci U S A* 1995;92:8891–8895.

69. Su B, Jacinto E, Hibi M, Kallunki T, Karin M, Ben-Neriah Y. JNK is involved in signal integration during costimulation of T lymphocytes. *Cell* 1994;77:727–736.

70. Nunes JA, Battifora M, Woodgett JR, Truneh A, Olive D, Cantrell DA. CD28 signal transduction pathways. A comparison of B7-1 and B7-2 regulation of the MAP kinases: ERK2 and JUN kinases. *Mol Immunol* 1996;33:63–70.

71. Li W, Whaley CD, Mondino A, Mueller DL. Blocked signal transduction to the ERK and JNK protein kinases in anergic CD4+ T cells. *Science* 1996;271:1272–1276.

72. Fields PE, Gajewski TF, Fitch FW. Blocked Ras activation in anergic CD4+ T cells. *Science* 1996;71:1276–1278.

73. Lai JH, Horvath G, Li Y, Tan TH. Mechanisms of enhanced nuclear translocation of the transcription factors c-Rel and NF-kappa B by CD28 costimulation in human T lymphocytes. *Ann NY Acad Sci* 1995;766:220–223.

74. August A, Gibson S, Kawakami Y, Kawakami T, Mills GB, Dupont B. CD28 is associated with and induces the immediate tyrosine phosphorylation and activation of the Tec family kinase ITK/EMT in the human Jurkat leukemic T-cell line. *Proc Natl Acad Sci U S A* 1994;91:9347–9351.

75. Linsley PS, Bradshaw J, Greene J, Peach R, Bennett KL, Mittler RS. Intracellular trafficking of CTLA-4 and focal localization towards sites of TCR engagement. *Immunity* 1996;4:535–543.

76. Waterhouse P, Marengere LE, Mittrucker HW, Mak TW. CTLA-4, a negative regulator of T-lymphocyte activation. *Immunol Rev* 1996;153:183–207.

77. Lanier LL, O'Fallon S, Somoza C, et al. CD80 (B7) and CD86 (B70) provide similar costimulatory signals for T cell proliferation, cytokine production, and generation of CTL. *J Immunol* 1995;154:97–105.

78. Yang G, Hellstrom KE, Hellstrom I, Chen L. Antitumor immunity elicited by tumor cells transfected with B7-2, a second ligand for CD28/CTLA-4 costimulatory molecules. *J Immunol* 1995;154:2794–2800.

79. Borriello F, Sethna MP, Boyd SD, et al. B7-1 and B7-2 have overlapping, critical roles in immunoglobulin class switching and germinal center formation. *Immunity* 1997;6:303–313.

80. Bluestone JA, Miller S. The yin/yang of CD28 T-cell costimulation in autoimmunity. In: Bancherau J, Dodet B, Schwartz R, Trannoy E, eds. *Immune Tolerance*. Paris: Elsevier, 1996:105–113.

81. Kuchroo VK, Das MP, Brown JA, et al. B7-1 and B7-2 costimulatory molecules activate differentially the Th1/Th2 developmental pathways: Application to autoimmune disease therapy. *Cell* 1995;80:707–718.

82. Kawai K, Shahinian A, Mak TW, Ohashi PS. Skin allograft rejection in CD28-deficient mice. *Transplantation* 1996;61:352–355.

83. Foy TM, Aruffo A, Bajorath J, Buhlmann JE, Noelle RJ. Immune regulation by CD40 and its ligand GP39. *Annu Rev Immunol* 1996;14:591–617.

84. Romagnani S. Role for CD30 antigen in human T helper 2-type responses. *Ciba Found Symp* 1995;195:55–62.

85. Kehry MR. CD40-mediated signaling in B cells balancing cell survival, growth, and death. *J Immunol* 1996;156:2345–2348.

86. Ishida T, Kobayashi N, Tojo T, Ishida S, Yamamoto T, Inoue J. CD40 signaling-mediated induction of Bcl-XL, Cdk4, and Cdk6. Implication of their cooperation in selective B cell growth. *J Immunol* 1995;155:5527–5535.

87. Blotta MH, Marshall JD, DeKruyff RH, Umetsu DT. Cross-linking of the CD40 ligand on human CD4+ T lymphocytes generates a costimulatory signal that up-regulates IL-4 synthesis. *J Immunol* 1996;156:3133–3140.

88. Barrett TB, Shu G, Clark EA. CD40 signaling activates CD11a/CD18 (LFA-1)-mediated adhesion in B cells. *J Immunol* 1991;151:1722–1726.

89. Ding L, Green JM, Thompson CB, Shevach EM. B7/CD28-dependent and -independent induction of CD40 ligand expression. *J Immunol* 1995;155:5124–5132.

90. Grewal IS, Flavell RA. The role of CD40 ligand in costimulation and T-cell activation. *Immunol Rev* 1996;153:85–106.

91. Hollander GA, Castiglia E, Kulbacki R, et al. Induction of alloantigen-specific tolerance by B cells from CD40-deficient mice. *Proc Natl Acad Sci U S A* 1996;93:4994–4998.

92. Smith CA, Gruss H-J, Davis T, et al. CD30 antigen, a marker for Hodgkin's lymphoma, is a receptor whose ligand defines an emerging family of cytokines with homology to TNF. *Cell* 1993;73:1349–1360.

93. Bowen MA, Lee RK, Miragliotta G, Nam SY, Podack ER. Structure and expres-

sion of murine CD30 and its role in cytokine production. *J Immunol* 1996;156: 442–449.

94. Duckett CS, Gedrich RW, Gilfillan C, Thompson CB. Induction of nuclear factor B by the CD30 receptor is mediated by TRAF1 and TRAF2. *Mol Cell Biol* 1997;17:1535–1542.

95. Del Prete G, Maggi E, Pizzolo G, Romagnani S. CD30, Th2 cytokines and HIV infection: A complex and fascinating link. *Immunol Today* 1995;16:76–80.

96. Hurtado JC, Kim SH, Pollok KE, Lee ZH, Kwon BS. Potential role of 4-1BB in T cell activation. Comparison with the costimulatory molecule CD28. *J Immunol* 1995;155:3360–3367.

97. Kim Y-J, Kim SH, Kwon BS. Human 4-1BB (CD137) signal regulates CD28 costimulation to promote type I cytokines. *Eur J Immunol* 1998;28:881–890.

98. Romagnani S. Th1 and Th2 in human diseases. *Clin Immunol Immunopathol* 1996;80:225–235.

99. Blazar BR, Taylor PA, Panoskaltsis-Mortari A, Gray GS, Vallera DA. Co-blockade of the LFA1-ICAM and CD28/CTLA4:B7 pathways is a highly effective means of preventing acute lethal graft-versus-host disease induced by fully major histocompatibility complex-disparate donor grafts. *Blood* 1995;85:2607–2618.

100. Judge TA, Tang A, Turka LA. Immunosuppression through blockade of CD28:B7-mediated costimulatory signals. *Immunol Res* 1996;15:38–49.

101. Larsen CP, Elwood ET, Alexander DZ, et al. Long-term acceptance of skin and cardiac allografts after blocking CD40 and CD28 pathways. *Nature* 1996;381: 434–438.

102. Ferguson SE, Han S, Kelsoe G, Thompson CB. CD28 is required for germinal center formation. *J Immunol* 1996;156:4576–4581.

103. Hathcock KS, Laszlo G, Pucillo C, Linsley P, Hodes RJ. Comparative analysis of B7-1 and B7-2 costimulatory ligands: Expression and function. *J Exp Med* 1994; 180:631–640.

104. Leach DR, Krummel MF, Allison JP. Enhancement of antitumor immunity by CTLA-4 blockade. *Science* 1996;271:1734–1736.

105. Bierer BE, Sleckman BP, Ratnofsky SE, Burakoff SJ. The biologic roles of CD2, CD4, and CD8 in T-cell activation. *Annu Rev Immunol* 1989;7:579–599.

106. Collins TL, Hahn WC, Bierer BE, Burakoff SJ. CD4, CD8 and CD2 in T cell adhesion and signaling. *Curr Top Microbiol Immunol* 1993;184:223–233.

107. Yagita H, Nakamura T, Asakawa J, et al. CD2 expression in murine B cell lineage. *Int Immunol* 1989;1:94–98.

108. Williams AF, Barclay AN, Clark SJ, Paterson DJ, Willis AC. Similarities in sequences and cellular expression between rat CD2 and CD4 antigens. *J Exp Med* 1987;165:368–380.

109. Davis SJ, van der Merwe PA. The structure and ligand interactions of CD2: Implications for T cell function. *Immunol Today* 1996;17:177–187.

110. Seed B, Aruffo A. Molecular cloning of the CD2 antigen, the T-cell erythrocyte receptor, by a rapid immunoselection procedure. *Proc Natl Acad Sci U S A* 1987; 84:3365–3369.

111. Peterson A, Seed B. Monoclonal antibody and ligand binding sites of the T cell erythrocyte receptor (CD2). *Nature* 1987;329:842–846.

112. Bernard A, Knowles RW, Naito K, et al. A unique epitope on the CD2 molecule defined by the monoclonal antibody 9-1: Epitope-specific modulation of the E-rosette receptor and effects on T-cell functions. *Hum Immunol* 1986; 17:388–405.

113. Meuer SC, Hussey RE, Fabbi M, et al. An alternative pathway of T-cell activation: A functional role for the 50 kd T11 sheep erythrocyte receptor protein. *Cell* 1984;36:897–906.

114. Li J, Smolyar A, Sunder-Plassmann R, Reinherz EL. Ligand-induced conformational change within the CD2 ectodomain accompanies receptor clustering: Implication for molecular lattice formation. *J Mol Biol* 1996;263:209–226.

115. Collins TL, Kassner PD, Bierer BE, Burakoff SJ. Adhesion receptors in lymphocyte activation. *Curr Biol* 1994;6:385–393.

116. Selvaraj P, Plunkett ML, Dustin M, Sanders ME, Shaw S, Springer TA. The T lymphocyte glycoprotein CD2 binds the cell surface ligand LFA-3. *Nature* 1987;326:400–403.

117. Shaw S, Luce GE, Quinones R, Gress RE, Springer TA, Sanders ME. Two antigen-independent adhesion pathways used by human cytotoxic T-cell clones. *Nature* 1986;323:262–264.

118. Takai Y, Reed ML, Burakoff SJ, Herrmann SH. Direct evidence for a receptor-ligand interaction between the T-cell surface antigen CD2 and lymphocyte-function-associated antigen 3. *Proc Natl Acad Sci U S A* 1987;84:6864–6868.

119. Kato K, Koyanagi M, Okada H, et al. CD48 is a counter-receptor for mouse CD2 and is involved in T cell activation. *J Exp Med* 1992;176:1241–1249.

120. van der Merwe PA, McPherson DC, Brown MH, et al. The NH2-terminal domain of rat CD2 binds rat CD48 with a low affinity and binding does not require glycosylation of CD2. *Eur J Immunol* 1993;23:1373–1377.

121. Dustin ML, Sanders ME, Shaw S, Springer TA. Purified lymphocyte function-associated antigen 3 binds to CD2 and mediates T lymphocyte adhesion. *J Exp Med* 1987;165:677–692.

122. Hahn WC, Rosenstein Y, Calvo V, Burakoff SJ, Bierer BE. A distinct cytoplasmic domain of CD2 regulates ligand avidity and T-cell responsiveness to antigen. *Proc Natl Acad Sci U S A* 1992;89:7179–7183.

123. Krensky AM, Sanchez-Madrid F, Robbins E, et al. The functional significance, distribution, and structure of LFA-1, LFA-2, and LFA-3: Cell surface antigens associated with CTL-target interactions. *J Immunol* 1983;131:611–616.

124. Palacios R, Martinez-Maza O. Is the E receptor on human T lymphocytes a "negative" signal receptor"? *J Immunol* 1982;129:2479–2485.

125. Bernard A, Knowles RW, Naito K, et al. A unique epitope on the CD2 molecule defined by the monoclonal antibody 9-1: Epitope-specific modulation of the E-rosette receptor and effects on T-cell functions. *Hum Immunol* 1986;17: 388–405.

126. Mollereau B, Deckert M, Deas O, et al. CD2-induced apoptosis in activated human peripheral T cells: A Fas-independent pathway that requires early protein tyrosine phosphorylation. *J Immunol* 1996;156:3184–3190.

127. Guckel B, Berek C, Lutz M, Altevogt P, Schirmacher V, Dyewski BA. Anti-CD2 antibodies induce T cell unresponsiveness in vivo. *J Exp Med* 1991;174:957–967.

128. Semnani RT, Nutman TB, Hochman P, Shaw S, van Seventer GA. Costimulation by purified intercellular adhesion molecule 1 and lymphocyte function-associated antigen 3 induces distinct proliferation, cytokine and cell surface antigen profiles in human naive and memory CD4+ T cells. *J Exp Med* 1994;180:2125–2135.

129. Cerdan C, Martin Y, Brailly H, et al. IL-1 alpha is produced by T lymphocytes activated via the CD2 plus CD28 pathways. *J Immunol* 1991;146:560–564.

130. Cerdan C, Razanajaona D, et al. Contributions of the CD2 and CD28 T lymphocyte activation pathways to the regulation of the expression of the colony-stimulating factor (CSF-1) gene. *J Immunol* 1992;149:373–379.

131. Santi, AG, Campanero MR, Alonso JL, Sanchez-Madrid F. Regulation of tumor necrosis factor (TNF)-α synthesis and TNF receptors expression in T lymphocytes through the CD2 activation pathway. *Eur J Immunol* 1992;22:1253–1259.

132. Van der Pouw-Kraan T, Van Kooten C, Rensink I, Aarden L. Interleukin (IL)-4 production by human T cells: Differential regulation of IL-4 vs. IL-2 production. *Eur J Immunol* 1992;22:1237–1241.

133. Valentine H, Groux H, Gelin C, Chretien I, Bernard A. Modulation of lymphokine release and cytolytic activities by activating peripheral blood lymphocytes via CD2. *J Immunol* 1990;144.875–882.

134. Gollob JA, Ritz J. CD2-CD58 interaction and the control of T-cell interleukin-12 responsiveness. Adhesion molecules link innate and acquired immunity. *Ann NY Acad Sci* 1996;795:71–81.

135. Qin L, Chavin KD, Lin J, Yagita H, Bromberg JS. Anti-CD2 receptor and anti-CD2 ligand (CD48) antibodies synergize to prolong allograft survival. *J Exp Med* 1994;179:341–346.

136. Chavin KD, Qin L, Lin, J, Woodward et al. Anti-CD48 (murine CD2 ligand) mAbs suppress cell mediated immunity in vivo. *Int Immunol* 1994;6:701–709.

137. Chavin KD, Qin L, Yon R, Lin J, Yagita H, Bromberg JS. Anti-CD2 mAbs suppress cytotoxic lymphocyte activity by the generation of Th2 suppressor cells and receptor blockade. *J Immunol* 1994;152:3729–3739.

138. Woodward JE, Qin L, Chavin KD, et al. Blockade of multiple costimulatory receptors induces hyporesponsiveness: Inhibition of CD2 plus CD28 pathways. *Transplantation* 1996;62:1011–1018.

139. Kapur S, Khanna A, Sharma VK, Li B, Suthanthiran M. CD2 antigen targeting reduces intragraft expression of mRNA-encoding granzyme B and IL-10 and induces tolerance. *Transplantation* 1996;62:249–255.

140. Kaplon RJ, Hochman PS, Michler RE, et al. Short course single agent therapy with an LFA-3-IgG1 fusion protein prolongs primate cardiac allograft survival. *Transplantation* 1996;61:356–363.

141. Cavazzana-Calvo M, Bordigoni P, Michel G, et al. A phase II trial of partially incompatible bone marrow transplantation for high-risk acute lymphoblastic leukaemia in children: Prevention of graft rejection with anti-LFA-1 and anti-CD2 antibodies. Societe Francaise de Greffe de Moelle Osseuse. *Br J Hematol* 1996;93:131–138.

142. Holter W, Schwarz M, Cerwenka A, Knapp W. The role of CD2 as a regulator of human T-cell cytokine production. *Immunol Rev* 1996;153:107–122.

143. Beyers AD, Spruyt LL, Williams AF. Molecular associations between the T-lymphocyte antigen receptor complex and the surface antigens CD2, CD4, or CD8 and CD5. *Proc Natl Acad Sci U S A* 1992;89:2945–2949.

144. Janeway CA Jr. The T cell receptor as a multicomponent signalling machine: CD4/CD8 coreceptors and CD45 in T cell activation. *Annu Rev Immunol* 1992; 10:645–674.

145. Trowbridge IS, Thomas ML. CD45: An emerging role as a protein tyrosine phosphatase required for lymphocyte activation and development. *Annu Rev Immunol* 1994;12:85–116.

146. Stamenkovic I, Sgroi D, Aruffo A, Sy MS, Anderson T. The B lymphocyte adhesion molecule CD22 interacts with leukocyte common antigen CD45RO on T cells and α2-6 sialyltransferase, CD75, on B cell. *Cell* 1991;66:1133–1144.

147. Uemura K, Yokota Y, Kozutsumi Y, Kawasaki T. A unique CD45 glycoform recognized by the serum mannan-binding protein in immature thymocytes. *J Biol Chem* 1996;271:4581–4584.

148. Hovis RR, Donovan JA, Musci MA, et al. Rescue of signaling by a chimeric protein containing the cytoplasmic domain of CD45. *Science* 1993;260:544–546.

149. Frearson JA, Alexander DR. Protein tyrosine phosphatase in T-cell development, apoptosis and signalling. *Immunol Today* 1996;17:385–391.

150. Kishihara K, Penninger J, Wallace VA, et al. Normal B lymphocyte development but impaired T cell maturation in CD45-exon6 protein tyrosine phosphatase-deficient mice. *Cell* 1993;74:143–156.

151. Justement LB, Brown VK, Lin J. Regulation of B-cell activation by CD45: A question of mechanism. *Immunol Today* 1994;15:399–405.

152. Domiati-Saad R, Ogle EW, Justement LB. Administration of anti-CD45 mAb specific for a B cell-restricted epitope abrogates the B cell response to a T-dependent antigen in vivo. *J Immunol* 1993;151:5936–5947.

153. Byth KF, Conroy LA, Howlett S, et al. CD45-null transgenic mice reveal a positive regulatory role for CD45 in early thymocyte development, in the selection of CD4+CD8- thymocytes, and B cell maturation. *J Exp Med* 1996;183: 1707–1718.

154. Novak TJ, Farber D, Leitenberg D, Hong SC, Johnson P, Bottomly K. Isoforms of the transmembrane tyrosine phosphatase CD45 differentially affect T cell recognition. *Immunity* 1994;1:109–119.

155. Lazarovits AI, Poppema S, Zhang Z, et al. Prevention and reversal of renal allograft rejection by antibody against CD45RB. *Nature* 1996;380:717–720.

156. Goldberg LC, Bradley JA, Connolly J, et al. Anti-CD45 monoclonal antibody perfusion of human renal allografts prior to transplantation. A safety and immunohistological study. CD45 Study Group. *Transplantation* 1995;59:1285–1293.

157. Springer TA, Dustin ML, Kishimoto TK, Marlin SD. The lymphocyte function associated LFA-1, CD2, and LFA-3 molecules: Cell adhesion receptors of the immune system. *Annu Rev Immunol* 1987;5:223–252.

158. Martz E. LFA-1 and other accessory molecules functioning in adhesions of T and B lymphocytes. *Hum Immunol* 1987;18:3–37.

159. Sanders VM, Snyder JM, Uhr JW, Vitetta ES. Characterization of the physical interaction between antigen-specific B and T cells. *J Immunol* 1986;137: 2395–2404.

160. Golde WT, Kappler JW, Greenstein J, Malissen B, Hood L, Marrack P. Major histocompatibility complex-restricted antigen receptor on T cells. VIII. Role of the LFA-1 molecules. *J Exp Med* 1985;161:635–640.

161. Spits H, an Schooten W, Keizer G, et al. Alloantigen recognition is preceded by nonspecific adhesion of cytotoxic T cells and target cells. *Science* 1986;232: 403–405.

162. Shaw S, Luce GE. The lymphocyte function-associated antigen (LFA)-1 and CD2/LFA-3 pathways of antigen-independent human T cell adhesion. *J Immunol* 1987;139:1037–1045.

163. Shimizu Y, Shaw S. Lymphocyte interactions with extracellular matrix. *FASEB J* 1991;5:2292–2299.

164. Hynes RO. Integrins: A family of cell surface receptors. *Cell* 1987;48:549–554.

165. Corbi AL, Larson RS, Kishimoto TK, Springer TA, Morton CC. Chromosomal location of the genes encoding the leukocyte adhesion receptors LFA-1, Mac-1 and p150,95. Identification of a gene cluster involved in cell adhesion. *J Exp Med* 1988;167:1597–1607.

166. Wong DA, Davis EM, LeBeau M, Springer TA. Cloning and chromosomal localization of a novel gene-encoding a human beta 2-integrin alpha subunit. *Gene* 1996;171:291–294.

167. Fernandez-Ruiz E, Pardo-Manuel de Villena F, Rubio MA, Corbi AL, Rodriguez de Cordoba S, Sanchez-Madrid F. Mapping of the human VLA-alpha 4 gene to chromosome 2q31-q32. *Eur J Immunol* 1992;22:587–590.

168. Fernandez-Ruiz E, Pardo-Manuel de Villena F, Rodriguez de Cordoba S, Sanchez-Madrid F. Regional localization of the human vitronectin receptor alpha subunit gene (VNRA) to chromosome 2q31→q32. *Cytogenet Cell Genet* 1993;62:26–28.

169. Wu JS, Giuffra LA, Goodfellow PJ, et al. The beta subunit locus of the human fibronectin receptor: DNA restriction fragment length polymorphism and linkage mapping studies. *Hum Genet* 1989;83:383–390.

170. Shevach EM. Accessory molecules. In: Paul WE, ed. *Fundamental Immunology*, 3rd ed. New York: Raven, 1992:531–575.

171. Stewart M, Thiel M, Hogg N. Leukocyte integrins. *Curr Opin Cell Biol* 1995; 7:690–696.

172. Lee JO, Rieu P, Arnaout MA, Liddington R. Crystal stucture of the a-domain from the a-subunit of the integrin CR3 (CD11b/CD18). *Cell* 1995;80:631–638.

173. Loftus JC, Smith JW, Ginsberg MH. Integrin-mediated cell adhesion: The extracellular face. *J Biol Chem* 1994;269:25235–25238.

174. Bajt ML, Goodman T, MacGuire SL. Mutation of a ligand binding domain of 3 integrin. *J Biol Chem* 1994;269:20913–20919.

175. Springer TA. Traffic signals for lymphocyte recirculation and leukocyte emigration: The multistep paradigm. *Cell* 1994;76:301–314.

176. Metlay JP, Witmer-Pack MD, Agger R, Crowley MT, DeSales L, Steinman RM. The distinct leukocyte integrins of mouse spleen dendritic cells as identified with hamster monoclonal antibodies. *J Exp Med* 1990;171:1753–1771.

177. Hoshino T, Yamada A, Honda J, et al. Tissue-specific distribution and age-dependent increase of human CD11b- T cells. *J Immunol* 1993;151:2237–2246.

178. Van der Vieren M, Le Trong H, Wood CL, et al. A novel leukointegrin, αdβ2, binds preferentially to ICAM-3. *Immunity* 1995;3:683–690.

179. Dalinenko DM, Rossitto PV, Van der Vieren M, et al. A novel canine leukointegrin, alphadbeta2, is expressed by specific macrophage subpopulations in tissue and in a minor CD8+ lymphocyte subpopulation in pheripheral blood. *J Immunol* 1995;155:35–44.

180. de Fougerolles AR, Stacker SA, Schwarting R, Springer TA. Characterization of ICAM-2 and evidence for a third counter-receptor for LFA-1. *J Exp Med* 1991;174:253–267.

181. de Fougerolles AR, Springer TA. Intercellular adhesion molecule 3, a third adhesion counter-receptor for lymphocyte function-associated molecule 1 on resting lymphocytes. *J Exp Med* 1992;175:185–190.

182. Fawcett J, Holness CLL, Needham LA, et al. Molecular cloning of ICAM-3, a third ligand for LFA-1, constitutively expressed on resting leukocytes. *Nature* 1992;360:481–488.

183. Tian L, Yoshihara Y, Mizuno T, Mori K, Gahmberg CG. The neuronal glycoprotein telencephalin is a cellular ligand for the CD11a/CD18 leukocyte integrin. *J Immunol* 1997;158:928–936.

184. Mizuno T, Yoshihara Y, Inazawa J, Kagamiyama H, Mori K. cDNA cloning and chromosomal localization of the human telencephalin and its distinctive interaction with lymphocyte function-associated antigen-1. *J Biol Chem* 1997;272: 1156–1163.

185. Diamond MS, Staunton DE, Marlin SD, Springer TA. Binding of the integrin Mac-1 (CD11b/CD18) to the third immunoglobulin-like domain of ICAM-1 (CD54) and its regulation by glycosylation. *Cell* 1991;65:961–971.

186. Blackford J, Reid HW, Pappin DJC, Bowers FS, Wilkinson JM. A monoclonal antibody, 3/22, to rabbit CD11c which induces homotypic T cell aggregation: Evidence that ICAM-1 is a ligand for CD11c/CD18. *Eur J Immunol* 1996;26: 525–531.

187. Ingalls RR, Gollenbock DT. CD11c/CD18, a transmembrane signaling receptor for lipopolysaccharide. *J Exp Med* 1995;181:1473–1479.

188. Hemler ME. VLA proteins in the integrin family: Structures, functions, and their role on leukocytes. *Annu Rev Immunol* 1990;8:365–400.

189. Osborn L, Hession C, Tizard R, et al. Direct cloning of vascular cell adhesion molecule 1, a cytokine-induced endothelial protein that binds to lymphocytes. *Cell* 1989;59:1203–1211.

190. Pepinsky B, Hession C, Chen L, et al. Structure/function studies on vascular cell adhesion molecule-1. *J Biol Chem* 1992;267:17820–17826.

191. Cybulsky MI, Fries JW, Williams AJ, et al. Gene structure, chromosomal location, and basis for alternative mRNA splicing of the human VCAM1 gene. *Proc Natl Acad Sci U S A* 1991;88:7859–7863.

192. Moy P, Lobb R, Tizard R, et al. Cloning of an inflammatory-specific phosphatidyl inosotol-linked form of murine vascular cell adhesion molecule-1. *J Biol Chem* 1993;268:8835–8841.

193. Vonderheide RH, Tedder TF, Springer TA, Staunton DE. Residues within a conserved amino acid motif of domains 1 and 4 of VCAM-1 are required for binding of VLA-4. *J Cell Biol* 1994;125:215–222.

194. Elices MJ, Osborn L, Tanaka Y, et al. VCAM-1 on activated endothelium interacts with the leukocyte integrin VLA-4 at a site distinct from the VLA-4/fibronectin binding site. *Cell* 1990;60:577–584.

195. Altevogt P, Hubbe M, Ruppert M, et al. The α4 integrin chain is a ligand for α4β7 and α4β1. *J Exp Med* 1995;182:345–355.

196. Teixido J, Parker CM, Kassner PD, Hemler ME. Functional and structural analysis of VLA-4 integrin α4 subunit cleavage. *J Biol Chem* 1992;267:1786–1791.

197. Shimizu Y, van Seventer GA, Horgan KJ, Shaw S. Costimulation of proliferative responses of resting CD4- T cells by the interaction of VLA-4 and VLA-5 with fibronectin or VLA-6 with laminin. *J Immunol* 1990;145:59–67.

198. Hemler ME, Jacobson JG, Brenner MB, Mann D, Strominger JL. VLA-1: A T cell surface antigen which defines a novel late stage of human T cell activation. *Eur J Immunol* 1985;15:502–508.

199. Butcher EC, Picker LJ. Lymphocyte homing and homeostasis. *Science* 1996;272: 60–66.

200. Hu MCT, Crowe DT, Weissman IL, Holzmann B. Cloning and expression of mouse integrin beta p(beta 7): A functional role in Peyer's patch-specific lymphocyte homing. *Proc Natl Acad Sci U S A* 1992;89:8254–8258.

201. Berlin C, Berg EL, Briskin MJ, et al. Alpha4 beta7 integrin mediates lymphocyte binding to the mucosal vascular addressin MadCAM-1. *Cell* 1993;74:185–195.

202. Andrew DP, Berlin C, Honda S, et al. Distinct but overlapping epitopes are involved in alpha 4 beta 7-mediated adhesion to vascular cell adhesion molecule-1, mucosal addressin-1, fibronectin, and lymphocyte aggregation. *J Immunol* 1994;153:3847–3861.

203. Sampaio SO, Li X, Takeuchi M, et al. Organization, regulatory sequences, and alternatively spliced transcripts of the mucosal addressin cell adhesion molecule-1 (MAdCAM-1) gene. *J Immunol* 1995;155:2477–2486.

204. Briskin MJ, McEvoy LM, Butcher EC. MadCAM-1 has homology to immunoglobulin and mucin-like adhesion receptors and to IgA1. *Nature* 1993; 363:461–464.

205. Berg EL, McEvoy LM, Berlin C, Bargatze RF, Butcher EC. L-selectin-mediated lymphocyte rolling on MadCAM-1. *Nature* 1993;366:695–698.

206. Mebius RE, Streeter PR, Michie S, Butcher EC, Weissman IL. A developmental switch in lymphocyte homing receptor and endothelial vascular addressin expression regulates lymphocyte homing and permits CD4+ CD3- cells to colonize lymph nodes. *Proc Natl Acad Sci U S A* 1996;93:11019–11024.

207. Sikorski EE, Hallmann R, Berg EL, Butcher EC. The Peyer's patch high endothelial receptor for lymphocytes, the mucosal vascular addressin, is induced on a murine endothelial cell line by tumor necrosis factor-alpha and IL-1. *J Immunol* 1993;151:5239–5250.

208. Hernandez-Caselles T, Martinez-Esparza M, Lazarovits AI, Aparicio P. Specific regulation of VLA-4 and alpha 4 beta 7 integrin expression on human activated T lymphocytes. *J Immunol* 1996;156:3668–3677.

209. Cepek KL, Parker CM, Madara JL, Brenner MB. Integrin αEβ7 mediates adhesion of T lymphocytes to epithelial cells. *J Immunol* 1993;150:3459–3470.

210. Cepek KL, Shaw SK, Parker CM. Adhesion between epithelial cells and T lymphocytes mediated by E-Cadherin and the αEβ7 integrin. *Nature* 1994;372:190–193.

211. Kilshaw PJ, Murant SJ. Expression and regulation of beta 7 (beta p) integrins on mouse lymphocytes:relevance to mucosal immune system. *Eur J Immunol* 1991; 21:2591–2597.

212. Halvorson MJ, Coligan JE, Sturmhofel K. The vitronectin receptor (alpha V beta 3) as an example for the role of integrins in T lymphocyte stimulation. *Immunol Res* 1996;15:16–29.

213. Piali L, Hammel P, Uherek C, et al. CD31/PECAM-1 is a ligand for αvβ3 integrin involved in adhesion of leukocytes to endothelium. *J Cell Biol* 1995;130:451–460.

214. Wadsworth S, Halvorson MJ, Coligan JE. Developmentally regulated expression of the beta 4 integrin on immature mouse thymocytes. *J Immunol* 1992;149: 421–428.

215. Dunon D, Piali L, Imhof BA. To stick or not to stick: the new leukocyte homing paradigm. *Curr Opin Cell Biol* 1996;8:714–723.

216. Tanaka Y, Adams DH, Hubscher S, Hirano H, Siebenlist U, Shaw S. T-cell adhesion induced by proteoglycan-immobilized cytokine MIP-1b. *Nature* 1993;361:79–82.

217. Lloyd AR, Oppenheim JJ, Kelvin DJ, Taub DD. Chemokines regulate T cell adherence to recombinant adhesion molecules and extracellular matrix proteins. *J Immunol* 1996;156:932–938.

218. Carr MW, Alon R, Springer TA. The C-C chemokine MCP-1 differentially modulates the avidity of beta 1 and beta 2 integrins on T lymphocytes. *Immunity* 1996;4:179–187.

219. Tanaka Y, Adams DH, Shaw S. Proteoglycans on endothelial cells present adhesion-inducing cytokines to leukocytes. *Immunol Today* 1993;14:111–114.

220. Bazan JF, Bacon KB, Hardiman G, et al. A new class of membrane-bound chemokine with Cx3C motif. *Nature* 1997;385:640–645.

221. Wakelin MW, Sanz MJ, Dewar A, et al. An anti-platelet-endothelial cell adhesion molecule-1 antibody inhibits leukocyte extravasation from mesenteric microvessels in vivo by blocking the passage through the basement membrane. *J Exp Med* 1996;184:229–239.

222. Lasky LA, Singer MS, Dowbenko D, et al. An endothelial ligand for L-selectin is a novel mucin-like molecule. *Cell* 1992;69:927–938.

223. Baumhueter S, Singer MS, Henzel W, et al. Binding of L-selectin to the vascular sialomucin CD34. *Science* 1993;262:436–438.

224. Hwang ST, Singer MS, Giblin PA, et al. GlyCAM-1, a physiological ligand for L-selectin activates 2 integrin on naive peripheral lymphocytes. *J Exp Med* 1996;184:1343–1348.

225. Dransfield I, Cabanas C, Craig A, Hogg N. Divalent cation regulation of the function of the leukocyte integrin LFA-1. *J Cell Biol* 1992;116:219–226.

226. van Kooyk Y, Weder P, Hogervorst F, et al. Activation of LFA-1 through a Ca2(+)-dependent epitope stimulates lymphocyte adhesion. *J Cell Biol* 1991;112:345–354.

227. Shimizu Y, Mobley JL. Distinct divalent cation requirements for integrin-mediated CD4+ T lymphocyte adhesion to ICAM-1, fibronectin, VCAM-1, and invasin. *J Immunol* 1993;151:4106–4115.

228. Picker LJ, Treer JR, Nguyen M, Terstappen LW, Hogg N, Yednock T. Coordinate expression of beta 1 and beta 2 integrin "activation" epitopes during T cell responses in secondary lymphoid tissue. *Eur J Immunol* 1993;23:2751–2757.

229. Dustin ML, Springer TA. T-cell receptor crosslinking transiently stimulates adhesiveness through LFA-1. *Nature* 1989;341:619–624.

230. Shimizu Y, van Seventer GA, Horgan KJ, Shaw S. Regulated expression and binding of three VLA (beta 1) integrin receptors on T cells. *Nature* 1990;345:250–253.

231. Campanero MR, del Pozo MA, Arroyo AG, et al. ICAM-3 interacts with LFA-1 and regulates the LFA-1/ICAM-1 cell adhesion pathway. *J Cell Biol* 1993;123:1007–1016.

232. Shimizu Y, van Seventer GA, Ennis E, Newman W, Horgan KJ, Shaw S. Crosslinking of the T cell-specific accessory molecules CD7 and CD28 modulates T cell adhesion. *J Exp Med* 1992;175:577–582.

233. van Kooyk Y, van de Wiel-van Kemenade P, Weder P, Kuijpers TW, Figdor CG. Enhancement of LFA-1-mediated cell adhesion by triggering through CD2 or CD3 on T lymphocytes. *Nature* 1989;342:811–813.

234. Turcovski-Corrales SM, Fenton RG, Peltz G, Taub DD, CD28·B7 interactions promote adhesion. *Eur J Immunol* 1995;25:3087–3093.

235. Stewart M, Hogg N. Regulation of leukocyte integrin function: Affinity vs. avidity. *J Cell Biochem* 1996;61:554–561.

236. Faull RJ, Kovach NL, Harlan JM, Ginsberg MH. Stimulation of integrin-mediated adhesion of T lymphocytes and monocytes: Two mechanisms with divergent biological consequences. *J Exp Med* 1994;179:1307–1317.

237. Stewart MP, Cabanas C, Hogg N. T cell adhesion to intercellular adhesion molecule-1 (ICAM-1) is controlled by cell spreading and the activation of integrin LFA-1. *J Immunol* 1996;156:1810–1817.

238. Kucik DF, Dustin ML, Miller JM, Brown EJ. Adhesion-activating phorbol ester increases the mobility of leukocyte integrin LFA-1 in cultured lymphocytes. *J Clin Invest* 1996;97:2139–2144.

239. Weber C, Katayama J, Springer TA. Differential regulation of beta 1 and beta 2 integrin avidity by chemoattractants in eosinophils. *Proc Natl Acad Sci U S A* 1996;93:10939–10944.

240. O'Toole TE, Ylanne J, Culley BM. Regulation of integrin affinity states through an NPXY motif in the b-subunit: sites required for binding to intercellular adhesion molecule 1 and the phorbol-ester-stimulated phsophorylation site. *J Biol Chem* 1995;270:8553–8558.

241. Peter K, O'Toole TE. Modulation of cell adhesion by changes in the αLβ2 (LFA-1, CD11a/CD18) cytoplasmic domain/cytoskeleton interaction. *J Exp Med* 1995;181:315–326.

242. Hibbs ML, Jakes S, Stacker SA, Wallace RW, Springer TA. The cytoplasmic domain of the integrin lymphocyte function-associated antigen 1 beta subunit: Sites required for binding to intercellular adhesion molecule 1 and the phorbol exter-stimulated phosphorylation site. *J Exp Med* 1991;174:1227–1238.

243. Shimizu Y, Mobley JL, Finkelstein LD, Chan AS. A role for phosphatidylinositol 3-kinase in the regulation of beta 1 integrin activity by the CD2 antigen. *J Cell Biol* 1995;131:1867–1880.

244. Zell T, Hunt SW 3rd, Mobley JL, Finkelstein LD, Shimizu Y. CD28-mediated up-regulation of beta 1-integrin adhesion involves phosphatidylinositol 3-kinase. *J Immunol* 1996;156:883–886.

245. Laudanna C, Campbell JJ, Butcher EC. Role of Rho in chemoattractant-activated leukocyte adhesion through integrins. *Science* 1996;271:981–983.

246. Kolanus W, Nagel W, Schiller B, et al. AlphaL beta 2 integrin/LFA-1 binding to ICAM-1 induced by cytohesin-1, a cytoplasmic regulatory molecule. *Cell* 1996;86:233–242.

247. Klarlund JK, Guilherme A, Holik JJ, et al. A human exchange factor for ARF contains sec7- and pleckstrin-homology domains. *Nature* 1996;384:481–484.

248. Masellis-Smith A, Shaw ARE. CD9 regulated adhesion. Anti-CD9 monoclonal antibody induce pre-B cell adhesion to bone marrow fibroblasts through de novo recognition of fibronectin. *J Immunol* 1994;152:4630–4640.

249. Mannion BA, Berditchevski F, Kraeft SK, Chen LB, Hemler ME. Transmembrane-4 superfamily proteins CD81 (TAPA-1), CD82, CD63, and CD53 specifically associated with integrin alpha 4 beta 1 (CD49d/CD29). *J Immunol* 1996;157:2039–2047.

250. Xue W, Kindzelskii AL, Todd RF, Petty HR. Physical association of complement receptor type 3 and urokinase-type plasminogen activator receptor in neutrophil membranes. *J Immunol* 1990;152:4630–4640.

251. Bohuslav J, Horesji V, Hansmann C, et al. Urokinase palsminogen activator receptor, b2-integrins, and src-kinases within a single receptor complex of human monocytes. *J Exp Med* 1995;181:1381–1390.

252. Stockl J, Majdic O, Pickl WF, et al. Granulocyte activation via a binding site near the C-terminal region of complement receptor type 3 α-chain (CD11b) potentially involved in transmemebranc complex formation with glycosylphosphatidylinositol-anchored FcγRIIIB (CD16) molecules. *J Immunol* 1995;154:5452–5463.

253. Rovere P, Inverardi L, Bender JR, Pardi R. Feedback modulation of ligand-engaged αL/β2 leucyte integrin (LFA-1) by cyclic AMP-dependent protein kinase. *J Immunol* 1996;156:2273–2279.

254. Hughes PE, Ranch MW, Pfaff M, et al. Suppression of integrin activation: A novel function of a Ras/Raf-initiated MAP kinase pathway. *Cell* 1997;88:521–530.

255. Altmann DM, Hogg N, Trowsdale J, Wilkinson D. Cotransfection of ICAM-1 and HLA-DR reconstitutes human antigen-presenting cell function in mouse L cells. *Nature* 1989;338:512–524.

256. van Seventer GA, Shimizu Y, Horgan KJ, Shaw S. The LFA-1 ligand ICAM-1 provides an important costimulatory signal for T cell receptor-mediated activation of resting T cells. *J Immunol* 1990;144:4579–4586.

257. Damle NK, Klussman K, Aruffo A. Intercellular adhesion molecule-2, a second counter-receptor for CD11a/CD18 (leukocyte function-associated antigen-1), provides a costimulatory signal for T-cell receptor-initiated activation of human T cells. *J Immunol* 1992;148:665–671.

258. Hernandez-Caselles T, Rubio G, Campanero MR, et al. ICAM-3, the third LFA-1 counterreceptor, is a co-stimulatory molecule for both resting and activated T lymphocytes. *Eur J Immunol* 1993;23:2799–2806.

259. Davis LS, Oppenheim-marks N, Bednarczyk JL, McIntyre BW, Lipsky PE. Fibronectin promotes proliferation of naive and memory T cells by signaling through both the VLA-4 and VLA-5 integrin molecules. *J Immunol* 1990;145:785–793.

260. Nojima Y, Humphries MJ, Mould AP, et al. VLA-4 mediates CD3-dependent CD4+ T cell activation via the CS1 alternately spliced domain of fibronectin. *J Exp Med* 1990;172:1185–1192.

261. van Seventer GA, Newman W, Shimizu, Y, et al. Analysis of T cell stimulation by superantigen plus histocompatibility complex class II molecules or by CD3 monoclonal antibody: costimulation by purified adhesion ligands VCAM-1, ICAM-1, but not ELAM-1. *J Exp Med* 1991;174:901–913.

262. Damle NK, Klussman K, Leytze G, et al. Costimulation with integrin ligands interacellular adhesion molecule-1 or vascular cell adhesion molecule-1 augments activation-induced death of antigen-specific CD4+ T lymphocytes. *J Immunol* 1993;151:2368–2379.

263. Damle NK, Klussman K, Leytze G, et al. Costimulation via vascular cell adhesion molecule-1 induces in T cells increased responsiveness to the CD28 counter-receptor B7. *Cell Immunol* 1993;148:144–156.

264. Damle NK, Klussman K, Linsley PS, Aruffo A, Ledbetter JA. Differential regulatory effects of intercellular adhesion molecule-1 on costimulation by the CD28 counter-receptor B7. *J Immunol* 1992;149:2541–2548.

265. Boudrea N, Sympson CJ, Werb Z, Bissel MJ. Supression of ICE and apoptosis in mammary epithelial cells by extracellular matrix. *Science* 1995;267:891–893.

266. Zhang Z, Vuori K, Reed JC, Ruoslahti E. The α5β1 integrin supports survival of cells on fibronectin and upregulates Bcl-2 expression. *Proc Natl Acad Sci U S A* 1995;92:6161–6165.

267. Romanic AM, Madri JA. The induction of 72 kD gelatinase in T cells upon adhesion to endothelial cells is VCAM-1 dependent. *J Cell Biol* 1994;125:1165–1178.

268. Leppert D, Waubant E, Galardy R, Bunnett NW, Hauser SL. T cell gelatinases mediate basement membrane transmigration in vitro. *J Immunol* 1995;154:4379–4389.

269. Sato T, Tachibana K, Nojima Y, D Avirro N, Morimoto C. Role of the VLA-4 molecule in T cell costimulation. Identification of the tyrosine phosphorylation pattern induced by the ligation of VLA-4. *J Immunol* 1995;155:2938–2947.

270. Tachibana K, Sato T, D'Avirro N, Morimoto C. Direct association of pp125FAK with paxillin, the focal adhesion-targeting mechanism of pp125FAK. *J Exp Med* 1995;182:1089–1099.

271. Minegishi M, Tachibana K, Sato T, Iwata S, Nojima Y, Morimoto C. Structure and function of Cas-L, a 105 kD Crk associated substrate-related protein that is involved in beta 1 integrin-mediated signaling in lymphocytes. *J Exp Med* 1996;184:1365–1375.

272. Yamada A, Nikaido T, Nojima Y, Schlossman SF, Morimoto C. Activation of human CD4 T lymphocytes. Interaction of fibronectin with VLA-5 receptor on CD4 cells induces the AP-1 transcription factor. *J Immunol* 1991;146:53–56.

274. Wacholz MC, Patel SS, Lipsky PE. Leukocyte function-associated antigen 1 is an activation molecule for human cells. *J Exp Med* 1989;170:431–448.

275. van Seventer GA, Bonvini E, Yamada H, et al. Costimulation of TCR/CD3-mediated activation of resting human CD4+ T-cells by LFA-1 ligand ICAM-1 involves prolonged inositol phospholipid hydrolysis and sustained increase of intracellular Ca²⁺ levels. *J Immunol* 1992;149:3872–3880.

276. Sharma CP, Ezzell RM, Arnaout MA. Direct interaction of filamin (ABP280) with the β2 integrin subunit CD18. *J Immunol* 1995;154:3461–3470.

277. Hannigan GE, Leung-Hagestein C, Fitz-Gibbon L, et al. Regulation of cell adhesion and anchorage-dependent growth by a new β1-integrin-linked protein kinase. *Nature* 1996;379:91–96.

278. Dedhar S, Hannigan GE. Integrin cytoplasmic interactions and bidirectional transmembrane signalling. Curr Opin Cell Biol 1996;8:657–669.

279. Schaller MD, Otey CA, Hildebrand JD, Parsons JT. Focal adhesion kinase and paxillin bind to peptides mimicking β integrin cytoplasmic domains. *J Cell Biol* 1995;130:1181–1187.

280. Maguire JE, Danahey KM, Burkly LC, van Seventer GA. T cell receptor- and beta 1 integrin-mediated signals synergize to induce tyrosine phosphorylation of focal adhesion kinase (pp125FAK) in human T cells. *J Exp Med* 1995;182:2079–2090.

281. Chen HC, Appeddu PA, Parsons JT, Hildebrand JD, Schaller MD, Guan JL. Interaction of focal adhesion kinase with cytoskeletal protein talin. *J Biol Chem* 1995;270:16995–16999.

282. Schaepfer DD, Hanks SK, Hunter T, van der Geer P. Integrin-mediated signal transduction linked to Ras pathway by GRB2 binding to focal adhesion kinase. *Nature* 1994;372:786–791.

283. Chen HC, Appenddu PA, Isoda H, Guan JL. Phosphorylation of tyrosine 397 in focal adhesion kinase is required for binding phosphatidylinositol 3-kinase. *J Biol Chem* 1996;271:26329–26334.

284. Anderson DC, Springer TA. Leukocyte adhesion deficiency: An inherited defect in the Mac-1, LFA-1, and p150,95 glycoproteins. *Annu Rev Med* 1987;38:175–194.

285. Shier P, Otulakowski G, Ngo K, et al. Impaired immune responses towards alloantigens and tumor cells but normal thymic selection in mice deficient in the beta2 integrin leukocyte function-associated antigen-1. *J Immunol* 1996;157: 5375–5386.

286. Schmits R, Kundig TM, Baker DM, et al. LFA-1-deficient mice show normal CTL responses to virus but fail to reject immunogenic tumor. *J Exp Med* 1996; 183:1415–1426.

287. Christensen JP, Marker O, Thomsen AR. T-cell-mediated immunity to lymphocytic choriomeningitis virus in beta2-integrin (CD18)- and ICAM-1 (CD54)-deficient mice. *J Virol* 1996;70:8997–9002.

288. Xu H, Gonzalo JA, St Pierre Y, et al. Leukocytosis and resistance to septic shock in intercellular adhesion molecule 1-deficient mice. *J Exp Med* 180:95–109.

289. Kelly KJ, Williams WW Jr, Colvin RB, et al. Intercellular adhesion molecule-1-deficient mice are protected against ischemic renal injury. *J Clin Invest* 1996; 97:1056–1063.

290. Soriano SG, Lipton SA, Wang YF, et al. Intercellular adhesion molecule-1-deficient mice are less susceptible to cerebral ischemia-reperfusion injury. *Ann Neurol* 1996;39:618–624.,

291. Gonzalo JA, Martinez C, Springer TA, Gutierrez-Ramos JC. ICAM-1 is required for T cell proliferation but not for anergy or apoptosis induced by *Staphylococcus aureus* enterotoxin B in vivo. *Int Immunol* 1995;7:1691–1698.

292. Fassler R, Meyer M. Consequences of lack of β1 integrin gene expression in mice. *Genes Dev* 1995;9:1896–1908.

293. Stephens LE, Sutherland Ae, Klimanskaya IV, et al. Deletion of β1 integrins in mice results in inner cell mass failure and peri-implantation. *Genes Dev* 1995;9: 1883–1895.

294. Kwee L, Baldwin HS, Shen HM, et al. Defective development of the embryonic and extraembryonic circulatory systems in vascular cell adhesion molecule (VCAM-1) deficient mice. *Development* 1995;121:489–503.

295. Gurtner GC, Davis V, Li H, McCoy MJ, Sharpe A, Cybulsky MI. Targeted disruption of the murine VCAM1 gene: Essential role of VCAM-1 in chorioallantoic fusion and placentation. *Genes Dev* 1995;9:1–14.

296. Hirsch E, Iglesias A, Potocnik AJ, Hartmann U, Fassler R. Impaired migration but not differentiation of haematopoietic stem cells in the absence of β1 integrins. *Nature* 1996;380:171–175.

297. Wagner N, Loehler J, Kunkel EJ, et al. Essential role for β7 integrins in the formation of gut associated lymphoid tissue. *Nature* 1996;382–370.

298. Arroyo AG, Yang JT, Rayburn H, Hynes RO. Differential requirements for α4 integrins during fetal and adult hematopoiesis. *Cell* 1996;85:997–1008.

299. Cosimi AB, Conti D, Delmonico FL, et al. In vivo effects of monoclonal antibody to ICAM-1 (CD54) in nonhuman primates with renal allografts. *J Immunol* 1990;144:4604–4612.

300. Zeng Y, Torres MA, Thistlethwaite JR Jr, Montag A, Bluestone JA. Prolongation of human pancreatic islet xenografts by pretreatment of islets with anti-human ICAM-1 monoclonal antibody. *Transplant Proc* 1994;26:1120.

301. Isobe M, Yagita H, Okumura K, Ihara A. Specific acceptance of cardiac allograft after treatment with anti-ICAM-1 and anti-LFA-1. *Science* 1992;255:1125–1127.

302. Isobe M, Suzuki J, Yagita H, et al. Immunosuppression to cardiac allografts and soluble antigens by anti-vascular cellular adhesion molecule-1 and anti-very late antigen-4 monoclonal antibodies. *J Immunol* 1994;153:5810–5818.

303. Yednock TA, Cannon C, Fritz L, Sanchez-Madrid F, Steinman L, Karin N. Prevention of experimental allergic encephalomyelitis by antibodies against α4β1 integrin. *Nature* 1992;356:63–66.

304. Karpus WJ, Lukacs NW, McRae BL, Strieter RM, Kunkel SL, Miller SM. An important role for chemokine macrophage inflammatory protein-1a in the pathogenesis of the T cell-mediated autoimmune disease, experimental autoimmune encephalomyelitis. *J Immunol* 1995;155:5003–5010.

305. King SL, Cunningham JA, Finberg RW, Bergelson JM. Echovirus 1 interaction with the isolated VLA-2 I domain. *J Virol* 1995;69:3237–3239.

306. Staunton DE, Merluzzi VJ, Rothlein R, Barton R, Marlin SD, Springer TA. A cell adhesion molecule, ICAM-1, is the major surface receptor for rhinovirus. *Cell* 1989;56:849–853.

307. Greve JM, Davis G, Meyer AM, et al. The major human rhinovirus receptor is ICAM-1. *Cell* 1989;56:839–847.

308. Marlin SD, Staunton DE, Springer TA, et al. A soluble form of intercellular adhesion molecule-1 inhibits rhinovirus infection. *Nature* 1990;344:70–72.

309. Martin S, Casasnovas JM, Staunton DE, Springer TA. Efficient neutralization and disruption of rhinovirus by chimeric ICAM-1/immunoglobulin molecules. *J Virol* 1993;67:3561–3568.

310. Pasloske BL, Howard RJ. Malaria, the red cell, and the endothelium. *Ann Rev Med* 1994;5:283–295.

311. Baruch DI, Gormely JA, Ma C, Howard RJ, Pasloske BL. Plasmodium falciparum erythrocyte membrane protein 1 is a parasitized erythrocyte receptor for adherence to CD36, thrombospondin, and intercellular adhesion molecule 1. *Proc Natl Acad Sci U S A* 1996;93:3497–3502.

312. Rudin W, Eugster HP, Bordmann G, et al. Resistance to cerebral malaria in tumor necrosis factor-alpha/beta-deficient mice is associated with a reduction of intercellular adhesion molecule-1 up-regulation and T helper type 1 response. *Am J Pathol* 1997;150:257–266.

313. Ennis E, Isberg RR, Shimizu Y. Very late antigen 4-dependent adhesion and costimulation of resting human T cells by the bacterial beta 1 integrin ligand invasin. *J Exp Med* 1993;177:207–212.

314. Frankel G, Lider O, Hershkoviz R, et al. The cell-binding domain of intimin from entreopathogenic *Escherichia coli* binds to beta 1 integrins. *J Biol Chem* 1996; 271:20359–20364.

Fundamental Immunology, Fourth Edition,
edited by William E. Paul
Lippincott–Raven Publishers, Philadelphia © 1999.

CHAPTER 14

Lymphoid Tissues and Organs

Louis J. Picker and Mark H. Siegelman

The evolutionary development of the mammalian antigen-specific immune system—in which an individual immunocyte recognizes only a minute subset of all potential antigenic determinants—markedly increased the efficiency of host defense by allowing increasingly powerful immune effector mechanisms to be selectively targeted on foreign invaders. However, this advance introduced significant logistical problems in the detection of invading pathogens that were not apparent with less sophisticated, non-antigen–specific host-defense mechanisms (innate or nonadaptive host-defense mechanisms; for example, phagocytes). In a non–antigen-specific system, individual components are capable of responding to a wide variety of insults, and antimicrobial processes can often be initiated by any subset of the whole population that localizes at the inciting stimulus. In contrast, the functional components of an antigen-specific system are not interchangeable: The overall immunocyte population is split into an extraordinarily large number of distinct clones, each of which responds only in the presence of its specific antigen. Indeed, the potential diversity of the immunoglobulin repertoire in the mouse (approximately 10^{11} combinations) (1) is several orders of magnitude higher than the total number of B cells per mouse at any given time ($< 10^9$). These clones often require not only their specific antigen for triggering, but also complex interactions with both antigen-specific and nonspecific accessory populations. Thus, given these premises, it would appear that the immune system's ability to respond to a wide spectrum of potential antigens would depend on the continual representation of all immunocyte clones and accessory cell types at all potential sites of antigen deposition—a daunting, if not impossible, proposition, given the huge surface area of the cutaneous and mucosal environmental interfaces and the limited number of lymphocytes specific for any given antigen! Moreover, whereas innate immune mechanisms are triggered by many of the fundamentally

distinct molecular components of microorganisms as compared to mammalian cells (e.g., bacterial cell wall components such as lipopolysaccharide), antigen-specific immunity can be triggered by myriad small molecular epitopes, potentially including epitopes shared by both pathogen and host. Avoidance of self-reactivity thus becomes a much more serious consideration with antigen-specific as opposed to innate immune mechanisms.

These considerations suggest that while the basic unit of the immune system is the individual antigen-specific lymphocyte clone, successful host defense must require that activity of these clones be subject to a high degree of systemic coordination so as to ensure consistent, efficacious responses to foreign antigens, no matter the portal of antigen entry, and at the same time, avoiding reactivity to normal host tissues. At the systemic level, an antigen-specific immune system is faced with three distinct and complex tasks. First, it must provide microenvironment(s) that can efficiently support the production of a population of clonally diverse lymphocytes (capable of distinguishing a huge spectrum of potential foreign antigens from self components) from pluripotent, nonfunctional precursors. Second, it must bring together antigen and those rare, mature lymphocytes bearing appropriate antigen receptors in specialized microenvironment(s) (containing requisite accessory cells) that will support and regulate the subsequent antigen-driven clonal expansion and differentiation of the responding cells. Finally, it must disperse the resulting effector and memory lymphocyte populations to those sites in the body where they can do the most good in eliminating acute invasion, and in surveying the body's tissues for the future return of the same invaders.

The mammalian immune system has met these requirements by compartmentalizing the principal functions of the immune system into discrete organs and tissues in the body, and then functionally unifying these compartments via an elaborate system of targeted lymphocyte trafficking and recirculation. The purpose of this chapter is therefore threefold: (a) to explore the systemic physiology of the immune system, including the structure, function, and interde-

L. J. Picker and M. H. Siegelman: Department of Pathology, University of Texas Southwestern Medical Center, Dallas, TX 75235-9072.

pendence of the various lymphoid tissues of the body (primary vs. secondary vs. tertiary) and their associated microenvironments; (b) to elucidate what is known regarding the cellular and molecular mechanisms that underlie the efficient operation of these specialized lymphoid microenvironments and the homing process that connects these various sites; and (c) to emphasize the importance of viewing the immune system at a systemic level, for only when viewed in this manner can the immune system's role in host defense be fully appreciated.

COMPARTMENTALIZATION OF THE IMMUNE SYSTEM

From an immunologic perspective, the various tissues of the body can be functionally divided into primary, secondary, and tertiary lymphoid organs. *Primary lymphoid tissues* represent those sites that contain microenvironments capable of supporting the production of functionally mature (albeit naive) T and B cells from nonfunctional progenitors. Key events that occur in these sites include the concomitant development of (a) antigen-recognition capability, as determined by rearrangement of antigen-receptor genes [immunoglobulin (Ig) and T-cell receptors (TCRs)], expression of these receptors, and selection of cells with functionally "appropriate" receptors; (b) the necessary cellular apparatus (cell surface molecules and associated signal transduction pathways) required (in addition to antigen receptors) to interact with accessory populations and allow differentiation into functionally disparate memory–effector cell populations; and (c) homing capability—the ability to recirculate and localize in the proper microenvironment in the periphery. *Secondary lymphoid tissues* represent those sites in which naive lymphocytes and exogenous antigen are brought together for the first time. These tissues are designed and situated so as to funnel antigen derived from essentially any site of entry into highly organized lymphoid microenvironments capable of driving the antigen-dependent activation and differentiation of naive (also known as virgin) T and B cells into expanded effector and memory populations. Antigen-receptor repertoire selection also occurs in these sites, deleting or inactivating autoreactive cells that "escaped" the selection process during primary lymphogenesis. Finally, *tertiary lymphoid tissues* comprise the immune effector sites of the body, sites in which memory–effector lymphocytes manifest immunologic responses such as immunoglobulin secretion, cytotoxicity, delayed-type hypersensitivity, or immunoregulation. These sites, the "battlefield" on which the immune system defends the tissues from microbial invasion, can be interpreted to include essentially all tissues of the body; however, the quantitatively most important of these sites are those tissues with direct contact with the "external" environment, primarily the skin and mucosal lining of the gastrointestinal, pulmonary, and genitourinary tracts.

Certain tissues are classically designated primary, secondary, or tertiary lymphoid tissues, because in the best-studied mammalian species—the mouse and the human—their constitutive immunologic function focuses on one of these three broad roles. Such tissues include the thymus and bone marrow (primary lymphoid tissues), lymph nodes, Peyer's patches, and spleen (secondary lymphoid tissues), and skin and mucosal lamina propria (tertiary lymphoid tissues). However, it is important to note that the site of occurrence of primary, secondary, or tertiary lymphoid tissue function is highly dependent on species and physiologic circumstances, and it is possible for a single tissue or organ to encompass more than one functional designation. For example, effector responses represent the pre-

dominant, characteristic immune activity in tertiary lymphoid tissues, but, of course, such responses can and do occur in primary and secondary lymphoid tissues. In this regard, the quintessential primary lymphoid tissue—the bone marrow—is a major site of plasma-cell redistribution (2–4), and it is thus a key B-lineage effector organ. In mice and human, intestinal Peyer's patches principally function as secondary lymphoid tissues (see below), whereas in other species, notably sheep, they play a major role in B-lymphogenesis (5,6), a primary lymphoid tissue function. Even in the same species, the functional designation of a given site can vary. For example, in situations of prolonged chronic inflammation, tertiary sites such as the skin can transform into secondary lymphoid tissues with all their characteristic structural elements (7). Thus, understanding of lymphoid tissue physiology requires an appreciation for the component parts of these tissues that confer a specific functional potential. Each lymphoid tissue is organized into discrete microenvironments characterized by a distinct complement of lymphocyte subsets and accessory/stromal cells, and it is the distribution and regulation of these microenvironments that determines overall function. It should be emphasized that neither the lymphoid nor stromal elements comprising these specialized microenvironments exist independently of the other. Indeed, as will be made clear, these disparate elements, as well as associated differentiated epithelium, have a complex, interacting relationship in which all elements contribute to the differentiated, specialized immune function of the mature tissue.

Primary Lymphoid Tissues: Sites of Lymphogenesis

In many ways, the production of functionally mature lymphocytes from immature precursors resembles that of their hematopoietic cousins: the erythroid, myeloid, and megakaryocytic lineages. All of these lineages arise from a common, self-renewing hematopoietic stem cell that primarily resides (except for early fetal life) in the bone marrow, and all undergo regulated, coordinate changes in gene expression that lead to the specialized form and function of the mature cell (8–12). However, the heterogeneity of the mature lymphocyte—in terms of antigen specificity, means of recognizing antigen (i.e., as free antigen or in the context of self histocompatability antigens), and ultimate function (e.g., antibody production vs. cell-mediated cytolysis vs. lymphokine production)—poses unique challenges in the production of these cells. Among hematopoietic lineages, only the lymphocyte must couple lineage-specific differentiation with the construction of a vast, heterogeneous primary antigen-receptor repertiore from germline components, and then, as appropriate for the lymphocyte lineage, modify this repertoire in line with future function.

Since, in most instances, T cells play the major role in the initiation and regulation of immune responses and thus bear the major burden in distinguishing self from nonself, the requirement for stringent tailoring of the primary antigen-receptor repertoire is most applicable to this subset. Indeed, the demands on the T-cell recognition process has led to the evolutionary development of the thymus, a highly specialized primary lymphoid tissue whose primary function is creation of a mature, virgin T-cell population with an "appropriate" antigen-receptor repertoire, one that is capable of recognizing foreign, but not self, determinants in the context of self major histocompatibility (MHC) antigens. Thus, the great majority of early T-lineage precursors are programmed to leave the bone marrow and migrate to the thymus for their "special education" through both positive and negative selection. Evidence for a clonal selection process for the primary B-lineage repertoire also exists, but to date, is less compelling than that for T cells. Indeed, the B-lineage repertoire normally includes clones bearing antigen receptors with self-reactivity (13). There is some bias in immunoglobulin V-region utilization among peripheral B cells (13), but it is unclear whether this bias results from genetic mechanisms (i.e., preferential recombination) or from an as yet poorly defined clonal selection process (14). In any case, it is likely that B-lineage "primary education" is less stringent than that of T cells, perhaps explaining why the bone marrow has the capacity to support the entire sequence of B-lineage maturation from pluripotent stem cell to virgin B cell. It should be noted, however, that while the primary T-cell repertoire is *not* thought to be modified by exposure to antigen [i.e., antigen exposure does not generally result in genetic changes in T-cell antigen receptors (15,16)], this is not true for B cells. As will be discussed in detail, antigen exposure in the peripheral immune system induces profound changes in the structure and function of the B-cell repertoire.

Bone Marrow: Structure and Function

The bone marrow, primarily contained within the cylindrical cavities of the long bones and the interstices of the spongy bone within vertebral bodies, sternum, ribs, flat bones of the cranium, and pelvis, accounts for about 5% of total body mass in the adult human. It is the major hematopoietic organ in most mammalian species, and is critically involved in the production of all formed blood elements in postnatal life. Because of the evanescent nature of most of these elements, the bone marrow is a particularly dynamic organ system, constantly monitoring the need for differentiated hematolymphoid cells and providing them in accordance with these needs. The remarkable span of cell types and differentiation supported by the bone marrow microenvironment is testament to its unique, variegated, and pivotal role in hematopoiesis, lymphopoiesis, and immune responsiveness.

The marrow is a richly cellular tissue, composed of blood cell precursors from stem cells through to mature cells of all hematopoietic cell types (with the exception of T cells; see below), as well as macrophages, reticular and stromal cells, and an "adjustable" amount of adipose tissue (17). Because it is bounded by bone, the marrow is strictly delimited in its maximum expansibility, and therefore in its maximum size under conditions of physiologic stress. However, the space occupied by adipose tissue (which may be as high as 50% to 70% in adult humans) reflects a reserve that may be called upon for additional hematopoiesis when extra demand exists. The bone marrow space is perfused by arteries, which penetrate the bone and empty directly into venous sinuses, which are an elaborate interconnecting array of vascular spaces that eventually coalesce to form larger veins. The hematopoietic compartment of the marrow is contained within the irregular cords of intervening tissue that are given scaffolding by the so-called bone marrow stroma —a specialized admixture of reticular stromal cells, macrophages, adipocytes, and their associated extracellular matrix that contributes to the mechanical support of the crowded hematopoietic cells, as well as to the provision of inductive interactions and factors required for the differentiation of these cells. Hematopoietic elements are arranged in a nonrandom fashion within the marrow cavity, with early precursors usually situated in the region adjacent to the bony endosteum and the more mature elements projecting more centrally into the marrow cavity. Separate lineages tend to be disposed in charac-

teristic patterns with respect to the venous sinuses, but the products are all delivered to these sinuses in order to access the periphery (there are no lymphatics in the bone marrow).

The Origin of Lymphoid as Well as All Other Hematologic Cells Is from a Common Precursor Hematopoietic Stem Cell

To maintain hematopoietic function throughout the life of the organism, the putative pluripotent hematopoietic stem cell (HSC) would be expected to have the capacity to (a) self-renew, (b) differentiate along a number of alternate pathways (multilineage differentiation), and (c) in animal models, rescue lethally irradiated animals from hematopoietic death and reconstitute all hematopoietic lineages in a long-term fashion. HSCs comprise a population that migrates extensively during development before taking up permanent residence within the bone marrow. In the mouse, embryonic hematopoiesis begins at day 7.5 gestation both within the yolk sac blood islands, and within the embryo in certain paraaortic regions. Stem cells from both of these sites apparently migrate to the liver to take up temporary residence from about day 11 through day 15 of gestation (third trimester in the human), before emigration to their final resting place in the bone marrow.

The earliest experiments suggesting both the existence of such a multipotent cell and the vital role of stromal microenvironments in determining terminal differentiation came from studies based on injection of bone marrow cells into lethally irradiated hosts at limiting dilution (18–22). The analysis of individual splenic colonies resulting from these injections (including their chromosomal markers) revealed that cells of multiple lineages could derive from a single cell, thereby confirming the existence of a multipotent hematopoietic precursor. In addition, the bone marrow cells responsible for forming these colonies could be shown to be spatially distributed in long bones, with decreasing numbers from the bony (endosteal) surface of the marrow cavity inward toward the axis (23). Moreover, these colonies contained cells with the capacity for the continued generation of more clonogenic splenic hematopoietic colonies upon reinjection (fulfilling the requirement of self-renewal), and could prevent hematopoietic death in lethally irradiated mice as well (24). By cytologic criteria, it appeared that lymphoid cell precursors were also included in the progeny of these clonogenic cells (22). Therefore, without having isolated the entity, the presence of a pluripotent HSC that gives rise to all hematolymphoid circulating cells could be deduced.

Early HSC enrichment studies used physical cell-separation techniques such as velocity and equilibrium centrifugation to isolate cellular subpopulations containing stem-cell activities (25,26). However, definitive HSC purification and characterization did not become possible until the development of more refined cell-separation techniques based on the use of monoclonal antibodies against cell surface molecules (8–10,27–29). In the mouse, HSCs are contained within a population that is Thy-1^{lo}, Ly-6A/E$^+$, c-kit$^+$, and negative for a number of lineage-specific markers of myelomonocytic, lymphoid, or erythroid type (Lin$^-$). Such cells are present in murine bone marrow at a frequency of 1 in 1,000 to 1 in 2,000 (8). Analysis of the more differentiated products of these precursors was facilitated by the development of *in vitro* bone marrow stromal culture systems, which were able to partially replicate the bone marrow microenvironment and thus support either myeloid (30,31) or B-lymphoid (32) differentiation. More recently, cloned stromal cell lines from these mixtures have been isolated that permit preferential long-term differentiation to predominantly myeloid (33) and/or preB-lymphoid lineages (34–36). As few as potentially a single one of these putative HSCs has been shown to demonstrate multilineage differentiation and reconstitution of all hematolymphoid lineages (37,38). However, there is some suggestion that long-term reconstitution activity is separable from radioprotective and splenic colony-forming activity (CFU-S) (39–42). This is an important distinction, because long-term repopulation represents a critical determinant of true HSC activity. A further subdivision of the Thy-1^{lo}, Lin$^-$, Ly-6A/E$^+$ population has been made using the mitochondrial dye Rh-123, thought to preferentially accumulate in the mitochondria of metabolically active cells, and thus the Rh-123^{lo} subset contains the predominant self-renewing and long-term hematopoietic reconstituting activity, as compared to the Rh-123^{hi} population (37,43). Therefore, it appears that the isolation to homogeneity of murine HSCs is indeed approaching.

Remarkable progress toward the isolation of HSCs has also been made in the human, despite the limitation that the human "model" has had to rely heavily on *in vitro* measures of hematopoietic function. It was initially recognized that the presence of the cell surface marker CD34 in the human correlated with bone marrow progenitors, which *in vitro* demonstrated a high proliferative response to hematopoietic cytokines (44,45). Subsequently, investigators developed human stromal cell culture systems that permitted the outgrowth of the myeloid and erythroid lineages from these primitive progenitors cells (46–48). The differentiation potential of the CD34$^+$ progenitor population has been broadened to include development into B- and T-cell lymphoid lineages as well, using an *in vivo* immunodeficient mouse system [severe combined immunodeficiency (SCID) mice] (49–51). The potential for *in vivo* reconstitution by CD34$^+$ cells has also been demonstrated in lethally irradiated baboons (52) and in human patients (53). Thus, CD34 has become a primary marker for HSC in clinical transplantation (54). It has also become possible to phenotypically distinguish long-term renewing, multipotent human HSCs (CD34$^+$/CD38$^-$) from those committed to one or another lineage (CD34$^+$/CD38$^+$) (10,55). The rapid developments in the understanding of human HSCs have had, and will continue to have, a profound impact on therapeutic approaches to a broad spectrum of both genetic and malignant human diseases.

The Bone Marrow Microenvironment: Molecular Demonstration of a Putative Stem-Cell Factor and Its Ligand Highlights the Crucial Role of the Microenvironment

On arrival in the bone marrow, HSCs are presumed to settle as nests in their proper microenvironmental niches, which are neither physically nor biochemically well characterized. An amalgam of nurturing stromal cells, reticular cells, endothelial cells, fat cells, and macrophages, combined with the supporting extracellular matrix components, supply the requirements for HSC maintenance and self-renewal. While the complexities of these requirements remain largely mysterious, there is evidence that cell surface adhesive interactions play a role (see below). Adhesion receptors may also contribute to the migration of embryonic HSC from yolk sac to fetal liver, as this appears dependent on a β1 integrin (56). Thus, adhesive interactions form one element with a significant influence on hematopoietic development.

The critical interplay of the marrow microenvironment and HSCs has been elegantly illustrated by studies that defined the molecular lesions of two mutant mouse strains with defective hematopoiesis. These two mutant mouse strains, one resulting from mutation at the white spotting (W) locus on chromosome 5 and the other from mutation at the steel (Sl) locus on chromosome 10, display similar defects in the development of the reproductive system, melanocyte production, and hematopoietic function (macrocytic anemia and increased radiation sensitivity). Transplantation studies indicated that the defect for W phenotype was at the level of HSCs, whereas the Sl phenotype resulted from a defective microenvironment for the support of HSCs (57–59). The initial breakthrough was the determination that the W locus encoded the protooncogene c-kit, a member of a family of cell surface receptors with tyrosine kinase activity (60,61). Because of the complementary relationship between Sl and W, it was quite plausible that the gene product of Sl [stem-cell factor (SCF)] might represent the ligand for c-kit, and this has indeed been confirmed by several groups (62–68). The c-kit ligand is produced by bone marrow stroma cells, may be found in both membrane-bound and soluble forms, and has been demonstrated to (a) have mast cell growth factor activity (63,64,67), (b) act in concert with other cytokines to stimulate hematopoietic colony formation *in vitro* (64,66–68), (c) partially correct the characteristic macrocytic anemia and mast-cell deficiencies of the Sl-deficient mouse after *in vivo* administration (62), (d) stimulate hematopoiesis in primates (69) and mice (70,71), and (e) rescue mice from the hematopoietic consequences of lethal irradiation by increasing progenitor HSC when administered prior to treatment (72,73). The definition of the c-kit/c-kit ligand interaction represents one of the first inroads into the understanding of the dynamic relationship between hematopoietic cells and marrow stromal elements at the molecular level. This example forms a paradigm that has provided significant impetus to the quest to understand hematopoiesis in molecular detail, and to isolate cytokines or combinations of factors that will permit selective growth and proliferation of HSCs. In this regard, a c-kit homologue, flk-2 (which is enriched in populations of pluripotent stem cells), has been identified and has been shown to have a role in lymphohematopoiesis (74,75). In addition, the transcriptional coactivator core binding protein beta (CBFB) has been shown by targeted disruption to result in defective liver hematopoiesis (76,77), further expanding the genre of molecules participating in the intricate process of hematopoietic cell development.

B-Lymphopoiesis in the Bone Marrow

In vertebrates, humoral immunity results from the antibody-producing cells of the immune system, cells of B-lymphocyte origin. Mature B cells are uniquely defined by their clonally expressed antigen receptor (surface Ig), made up of a tetramer composed of two heavy (H) and two light (L) chains. These cells originate primarily in the bone marrow in adult mammals, a process that is antigen-independent, spanning development from HSC to naive cell surface Ig–bearing B cell, or "virgin" B cell. Encounter with antigen occurs predominantly after migration to the peripheral lymphoid organs, at which point, proliferation is induced and progeny are able to differentiate into plasma cells, the terminally differentiated, Ig-secreting effector cells of the humoral immune response, as well as memory B cells (see below). While the bone marrow can be home to many of these stages, both generative and effector, we will restrict our consideration in this section to the marrow's role in supporting early B-lineage development—prior to the advent of the circulating virgin B cell. We will also focus our attention on conventional B cells; the relatively independent lineage of B cell, the B-1 or Ly-1$^+$ B cell, will be considered in a later section of this chapter.

During early embryogenesis, the site of B-lymphocyte development migrates from the placenta and embryonic blood, to fetal liver and then to spleen (78) before finally settling in the bone marrow. In most mammals that have been studied, the bone marrow remains the primary site of continuous B-cell differentiation from precursor (pre) B cells (79–81). In murine bone marrow, B-lineage cells represent about 30% of the nucleated cells (82). It is within this organ that large numbers of immature B cells are generated throughout life from a small number of B lineage–committed progenitors. However, well-documented non–bone marrow sites of B-cell generation exist in other species—the primary site of B-lymphogenesis in chickens is the bursa of Fabricius (83), and in fetal and neonatal sheep, B cells are generated in ileal Peyer's patches (6).

The progression of B-cell maturation is usually gauged by two criteria: (a) the expression of B lineage–restricted cell surface antigens or intracellular proteins and (b) the status of the Ig genes, from rearrangement of Ig gene DNA segments (V, D, and J), sequential cytoplasmic expression of H and L chains, assembly within the cell, and expression on the cell surface. The first stage of B-cell development is characterized by the upregulation of certain "early" B-lineage surface antigens (such as CD19, CD34, and CD10) in the human (84–87) and B220 and CD43 (S7) antigens in the mouse (88,89), and also, the machinery required to effect Ig-gene recombination, exemplified by the recombination-activating genes RAG-1 and RAG-2 (90,91). Subsequently, early progenitor cells first rearrange DNA segments (V, D, J, and C) (92) to form a contiguous gene encoding the H chain μ of IgM. The general progression of rearrangements within a B cell follows a sequence of D$_H$ segments joining to J$_H$ segments, followed by V$_H$ to D$_H$J$_H$, then L-chain rearrangements of V$_κ$ to J$_κ$, and then V$_λ$ to J$_λ$. While the V-gene segments are being assembled, there is also transient and precisely regulated activation of the terminal deoxynucleotidyl transferase (TdT) gene, which contributes to the diversity of Ig genes by inserting nucleotides (N regions) at the ends of certain of these gene segments so that when they join, the amino acid sequence of the final antibody is modified from the germline in a way that potentially alters or generates new binding specificities (93–95). Coordinate with Ig gene rearrangements, maturing B cells display a stereotyped pattern of cell surface antigen expression, ultimately leading to the mature, virgin B-cell phenotype (84,88).

Classically, B-cell precursors (defined by the expression of B lineage–restricted surface antigens) had been subdivided into progenitor (pro)-B cells, pre-B cells, and mature, virgin B cells based on their expression of no Ig, cytoplasmic μ H chains or complete surface Ig, respectively. This classification has required redefinition since the discovery of pre-B cell–specific genes, which encode proteins related to Ig chains and reside on chromosome 16 in the mouse (with other λ genes). The products of these genes, called λ5 or omega (in the human) and V$_{preB}$, associate noncovalently with each other, forming a primitive L-chain analogue. The λ5 product associates by disulfide linkage with μ H chains in pre-B cells, thereby allowing expression on the cell surface (96–101). Homologous genes and cell surface protein products have also been identified in humans and other mammals (102–105). Although first identified on pre-B-cell lines, cell surface Ig containing these "surrogate" L-chain-like molecules have been demonstrated in certain compartments of pre-

B cells in normal mouse bone marrow (106–108). Some studies have suggested the existence of other surrogate Ig gene products as well (109,110), some of which are potentially expressed on the cell surface (111); more recently, surrogate L chains have been shown to be associated with a complex of glycoproteins that include a gp130 prior to μ gene expression (112). In addition to the obvious implications these surrogate Ig polypeptides have for the control of B-lineage differentiation (discussed below), the existence of these novel structures suggests a redefinition of the B-lineage differentiation paradigm—namely, the separation of B-lineage maturation into successive stages based on the appearance of different surrogate Ig on the cell surface of B-lineage precursors, followed by the replacement of surrogate Ig with mature κ or λ L chain–bearing Ig (Fig. 1). Obviously, adoption of such a paradigm will first require further characterization of the diversity of these surrogate Ig and their natural ligands and the determination of their patterns of expression with progressive differentiation.

The in situ maturation of B-lineage precursors in the bone marrow has been described as progressing vectorily, with the most immature pro-B cells occupying microenvironments adjacent to the bone endosteum and their more differentiated progeny extending centripetally into the marrow cavity (see Fig. 1). The more mature, centrally located B-lineage precursors are often identified in intimate association with macrophages, and finally are found clustered within the central venous sinusoids undergoing final maturation prior to export to the periphery (113–115). Therefore, in essence, the radially organized maturation pathway for B cells is similar to other hematopoietic lineages (see above). B-precursor maturation is dependent on and closely regulated by interaction with bone marrow stromal cells, including signaling via both cell–cell contact and soluble factors (32,34,116–121). The importance of cell contact is evidenced by a number of adhesion systems, which have been suggested to functionally participate in the interaction between stromal and lymphoid cells, including fibronectin (122), the proteoglycan link member CD44 and one of its ligands, hyaluronate (123,124), the integrin molecule VLA-4 (α4β1) (125) on lymphoid progenitors and its ligand on stromal cells VCAM-1 (126), neural cell adhesion molecules (127), and the membrane proteoglycan syndecan (128). A role in both B- and T-cell development for α4 integrin has been further confirmed by targeted disruption of this locus (129). A variety of short-range growth factors are elaborated by stromal cells, and interleukin-7 (IL-7) in particular has been shown to be required for the maintenance and proliferative expansion of certain pro- and pre-B cell–differentiation stages (130–134). Another stromal cell–derived cytokine, IL-11, has been implicated in the growth stimulation of plasmacytoma cell lines, B-cell differentiation, and megakaryocyte growth (135), and the stromal-derived factor insulin-like growth factor 1 (IGF-1) can also regulate pro-B-cell growth (136). Finally, c-kit is expressed on early pre-B cells, and its interactions with c-kit ligand on bone marrow stromal cells also appear to influence B-lymphopoiesis (137,138).

An important aspect of B-lineage differentiation is the extent of precursor deletion that occurs during this process. B-lymphocytes are continually generated throughout life at a rate of approximately 5×10^7 each day in the adult mouse, yet less than 25% survive to enter the periphery (139–141). In the ileal Peyer's patches of the sheep, which, as mentioned earlier, are primary sites of B-cell genesis in this species, more than 95% of cells undergo cell death by the process of apoptosis (see below, discussion of thymus) (142,143). Extensive attrition of B-lymphocytes by apoptosis is

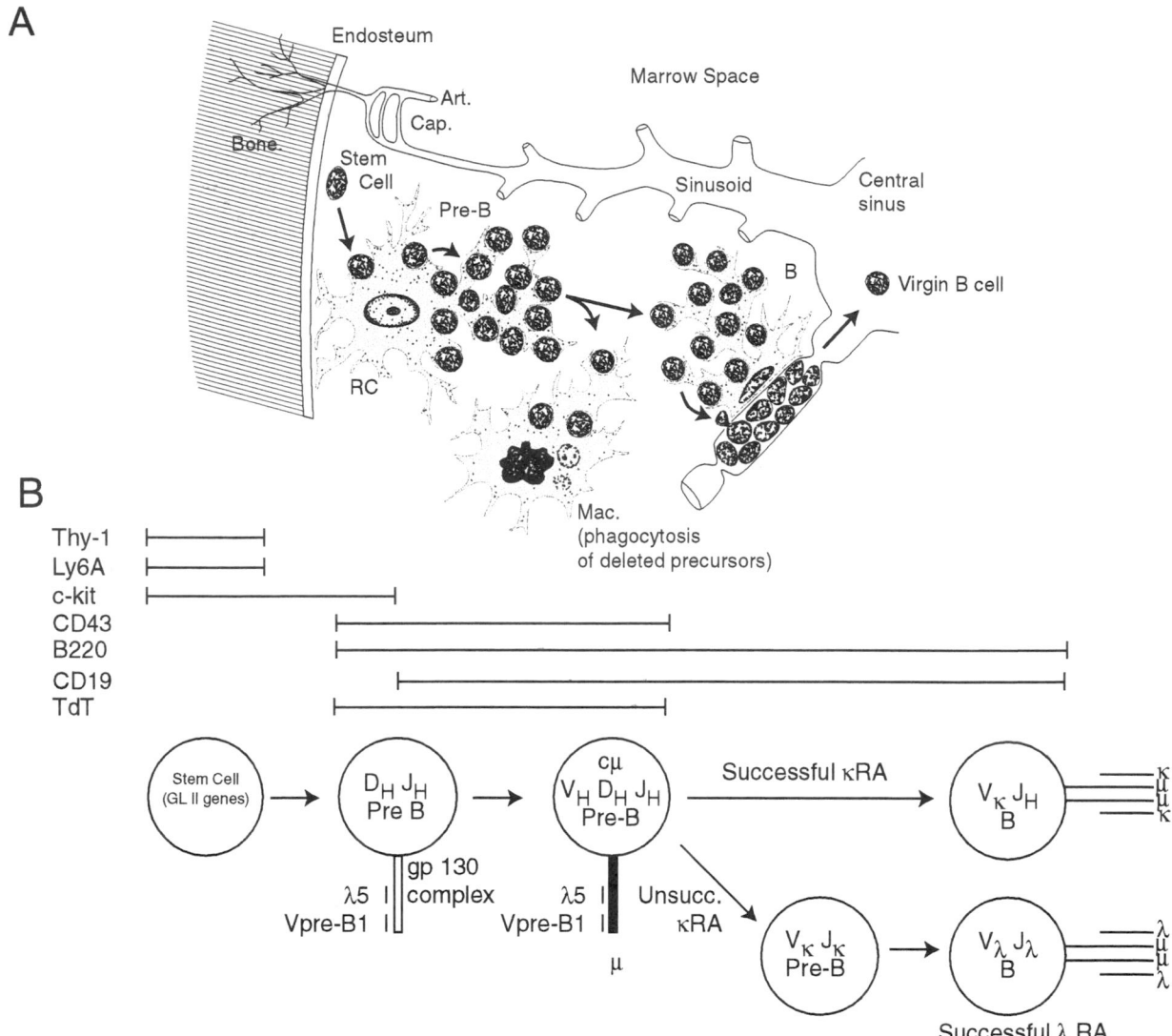

FIG. 1. B-cell generation in the bone marrow. **A:** Representation of B-cell maturation within the bone marrow cavity. Development is depicted as progressing from the endosteal (inner) surface of bone toward the center of the marrow space, where final mature products are emptied into sinusoids, which converge into a central venous sinus and from there exit to the periphery. Sequential arrows (left to right) schematize passage of B-cell progenitors through maturational stages. A stem cell is shown at left near the bony surface. Close association with nearby stromal reticular cells (*RC*) supports differentiation along the B-lineage pathway. Only a fraction of cells successfully place productively rearranged Ig gene products appropriately in the plasma membrane. Therefore, most cells are abortive and are scavenged and removed by resident macrophages (*Mac.*). Surviving maturing B cells continue to be nurtured by supportive stromal cells through the final stages of development, whereupon mature "virgin" B cells enter the circulation via a network of sinusoids. (Adapted from ref. 115, with permission.) **B:** B-cell markers during differentiation in the bone marrow. Three general aspects of B-cell maturation in the mouse are shown: (1) Expression pattern of maturation-dependent (non-Ig) markers (top)—Thy-1, Ly6A, c-kit, CD43, CD19, and B220 are all cell surface markers present during portions of B-cell differentiation from stem cells; TdT (terminal deoxynucleotidyl transferase) is an enzyme expressed intracellularly during the period of heavy-chain gene rearrangement (*bars* reflect periods of expression). (2) Ig gene rearrangement pattern—stem cells containing Ig genes in germline (*GL*) configuration are shown to progress to pre-B cells, which successively rearrange heavy-chain variable-region segments followed by κ or λ light-chain rearrangements (*RA*) before mature surface Ig (sIg) is expressed on the membrane. Light chains are shown to rearrange sequentially as κ, followed by λ, when κ rearrangement is unsuccessful. (3) Expression pattern of surrogate Ig—cell surface expression of λ_5 and V_{preB} (together forming "surrogate" light chain) appears during the pre-B stage, initially apparently in association with a glycoprotein complex, and then with a mature μ chain (see text).

also found in the chicken bursa of Fabricius (143). In the bone marrow of most mammals, presumably close interaction with macrophages en route to central sinusoids serves to cull out defective, inappropriate, or potentially harmful B cells. Much of this loss has been attributed to the deletion of precursors with inappropriate Ig gene rearrangements, as the process of rearrangement is imprecise and frequently results in the production of defective Ig proteins that cannot be properly assembled or placed on the cell surface. It is unclear whether any of this loss can be attributed to an environmental check against self specificities to eliminate autoreactivities, a mechanism that certainly exists for T cells in the thymus (see below). However, there is some evidence for the elimination (144, 145–147) or functional inactivation (anergy induction) (148–150) of autoreactive B cells during development (see below).

The rapid and active selection of B cells expressing functional Ig rearrangements and intact surface Ig is mediated by signals that are incompletely understood. It is possible that microenvironmental signals transmitted through intact surface Ig are required to maintain viability and appropriate differentiation of maturing B-lineage precursors. Early in differentiation, intact μ chain associated with surrogate light (SL) chains may transmit such putative signals; later in differentiation, mature Ig might subserve this function. Such signals may also feed back to inhibit the recombinational machinery once a functional Ig product appears on the cell surface, thereby ensuring that only one functional Ig is produced per B-cell clone. In support of this, there is considerable evidence from transgenic models that membrane-bound (surface) Ig is required for pre-B-cell survival, and acts to suppress further endogenous H- and L-chain gene rearrangements (151–154). There is also evidence to suggest that (a) crosslinking of cell surface SL chain/μ, and even SL chain in the absence of μ (155), can transduce Ca^{2+} release and tyrosine phosphorylation signals (155–157); and (b) targeted disruption of the λ5 gene results in B cell–deficient mice in which B-cell development in the bone marrow is arrested at the pre-B-cell stage (158). Thus, SL chains may play roles in signaling both allelic exclusion of a second H-chain locus and the proliferative expansion of pre-B cells to the preBII stage (159). Finally, the Ig-associated signal transduction molecules mb-1 (Igα) and B29 (Igβ) (160–164) (which are thought to be functionally analogous to the T-cell receptor–associated CD3 molecule) are able to mediate signal transduction and internalization of bound antigen for presentation in pre-B-cell lines and early B-lineage cells (157,165,166), and this may be in association with surrogate Ig. Taken together, these findings support a critical functional role for mature or surrogate Ig in B-lineage development. However, it should be acknowledged that little is known about the putative natural ligands for these pre-B Igs or the physiologic circumstances under which these putative ligands may act.

Both during the process of B-cell development in bone marrow and later in the periphery, the B-cell repertoire is screened against autoreactivity. The mechanisms for achieving this screen may be analogous to those utilized by T cells (see thymus section), although the inherent differences in T- and B-cell antigen recognition (e.g., the requirement for MHC in T-cell recognition) and function would suggest that the requirement for and stringency of B-cell selection is likely less that than for T cells. Clonal deletion of autoantibody-bearing B cells has been shown to occur, and appears to proceed in two stages: an early developmental arrest followed by death (146,167, 168). Moreover, elimination can occur peripherally as well as centrally (169,170). B-cell tolerance has also been shown to be achieved through the induction of an unresponsive state, or anergy (145,149, 150,171) Another more recently described mechanism for adjusting

the B-cell receptor repertoire has been designated "receptor editing." Studies primarily using mice transgenic for Ig molecules with specificity for autoantigens have shown that there is suppression of the autoreactive transgenic L chain in favor of endogenous L chains, which alters the specificity of the resulting antibody so that self-reactivity is eluded (172–175). The differential choice of an alternate L chain may be mediated either by a different V-region rearrangement to the same L-chain constant locus or simply by pairing of an H chain to an unrelated L chain such that a nonautoreactive L chain displaces the autoreactive one. While there have been some suggestions that the B-cell repertoire may be ligand-selected (176), only of late has evidence begun to emerge that positive selection, the encouragement of the development of useful antibody specificities based on the recognition of self antigens (see section on thymus, below), may occur during B-lymphopoiesis (177–179). However, a role for positive selection during affinity maturation of B cells in the periphery (e.g., germinal centers) appears more apparent (see section on secondary lymphoid tissues).

T-Lymphopoiesis in the Bone Marrow

We will discuss shortly the enormous influence that the thymus has in the nurturing, development, and maturation of T-cells. However, thymopoiesis operates on a marrow-derived stem cell (180), and the question arises as to whether the "prothymocyte" seeding the thymus has undergone T-lineage differentiation and commitment in the marrow before thymic localization. Evidence from in vitro systems has suggested that such precommitment may occur. The bone marrow of both athymic (nude) and normal mice has been found to contain an intrinsic population expressing low levels of the TCR-associated complex CD3. These cells, when cultured with particular growth factors, could be shown to differentiate into cells of more mature T-cell phenotype (181). Some surface markers, such as those recognized by the ER-MP-12 (182) and Joro 75 (183) antibodies, may delineate bone marrow populations with preferential thymus-repopulating activities. Similarly, human bone marrow cells bearing an early T-cell marker, CD7, were shown to display a significant capacity to generate T-cell clones when cultured in limiting dilution, accompanied by the sequential expression of mature T cell–specific markers on their surface (184). Moreover, studies employing high-resolution multiparameter flow cytometry have revealed a subpopulation of bone marrow stem cells that shows a striking phenotypic similarity to the earliest thymocytes, including the coexpression of the stem-cell marker CD34 with T lineage–restricted markers such as CD2, CD7, and cytoplasmic CD3 (11). In addition, it has been reported that a subpopulation of bone marrow cells defined by a set of three cell surface markers has been isolated that reconstitute T- but not B-cell development following transfer into SCID mice in vivo (185). More recently, a T cell–progenitor cell has been found in murine fetal blood, characterized as Thy-1+, c-kit^{lo} and CD3⁻ (186), further suggesting committment prior to thymic colonization. In addition, a CD4+CD3⁻ precursor with partially rearranged TCR β chain and expressing RAG-1, which are capable of developing into phenotypically mature T cells, has been identified in adult human blood, which may represent either a thymic precursor or an extrathymic developmental pathway (187). Taken together, these findings suggest some degree of commitment to the T lineage in the bone marrow. However, the observations that purified HSCs appear able to directly colonize an irradiated thymus (8,188), and that the thymus contains CD34⁺ precursors and can yield myeloerythroid as well as B-cell precursors under certain circumstances (37,188–191), sustain the possibility that multipotent HSCs may lodge in the thymus and contribute to the production of maturing thymocytes. However, these data should be interpreted cautiously, as the capability of primitive "uncommitted" HSCs to reconstitute thymus under experimental conditions does not necessarily imply that this is the type of precursor *normally* responsible for this function.

The possible existence of a distinct common progenitor to both B and T lineages has also been an item of considerable interest and debate. Experiments using retroviral markers to follow lineages of cells suggested that B and T cells shared a common precursor with myeloid cells (192). Reconstitution studies at limiting dilution in irradiated SCID mice from cells in long-term bone marrow cultures indicated that both B- and T-cell function could be transferred, and it was suggested that a single precursor for the generation of both B and T cells existed (193). More recently, targeted disruption of genes in mice, particularly those that may regulate transcriptional events, has shed further light on this issue. It has been shown that loss of the *Ikaros* gene, encoding a zinc finger DNA-binding protein restricted to hematolymphoid tissues, results in the complete failure of the development of even the earliest precursors of B-, T-, and natural killer (NK)-cell lineages, while leaving myeloid and erythroid lineages intact (194). Inactivation of E2A (195,196) or Pax-5 (197) results in the developmental arrest of pro-B cells at the CD43$^+$ stage. Finally, there is recent evidence in both mouse and human of a phenotypically discrete progenitor cell subset that generates lymphoid, but not myeloid, precursors. In the human, a CD34^{hi} Lin$^-$CD10$^+$ bone marrow population appears to exclusively contain progenitors of B, T, NK, and dendritic cells (198). In the mouse, an analogous population displays a Lin$^-$, IL = 7R$^+$, Thy = 1$^-$, Sca $-$ 1^{10}, c = kit^{10} phenotype (198a). Thus supporting evidence continues to accumulate that suggests the existence of an exclusive panlymphoid precursor.

Some progress is also being made in the understanding of the mechanism of homing of T-cell precursors to the thymus. Characterization of this process has been made difficult primarily due to the relatively minute numbers of cells involved. Similar to other tissue-specific localization of circulating cells, precursors must first encounter the thymic microvasculature, adhere, and extravasate. It is unclear whether specific adhesion molecules contribute to this specialized homing pathway. The widely expressed proteoglycan-link family member CD44 has been shown to be expressed on early thymic precursors and to potentially subserve a thymic homing function (199), and a novel cell surface glycoprotein, designated Vanin-1, has been implicated in adhesion of bone marrow cells to thymic microvessels in sections and in being required for long-term thymic regeneration (200).

Thymus: A Specialized Microenvironment Supporting T-Lymphopoiesis

The thymus was generally thought to be immunologically irrelevant until definitive neonatal thymectomy experiments by Miller (201) demonstrated the contrary. We now understand that the thymus is the primary site of T-lymphopoiesis, and, among its most important immunologic roles, must (a) receive T-cell progenitors; (b) serve as the primary maturational, educational, and culling center for developing T-lymphocytes; and (c) coordinate the release of competent T-cells to the periphery. Thymocyte maturation involves a complex series of interactions of incoming lymphoid progenitors with nonlymphoid cellular elements as the lymphoid cells traverse the diverse microenvironments contained within the thymic architecture. Along the way, survivors of this process undergo an ordered sequence of inductive and instructive events leading to the expression of an array of lineage-restricted genes, particularly the rearrangement and cell surface expression of TCR genes (γ, δ, α, and β). The result of this sojourn is a mature, virgin T cell that has an antigen-receptor specificity finely honed to recognize foreign antigen in the context of self-MHC gene products, while largely precluding autoimmunity. It is these events that we will attempt to place in the context of the thymic architecture in this section.

Anatomy of the Thymus

The thymus is a median pyramid-shaped organ in the superior mediastinum just dorsal to the sternum. It consists of bilaterally symmetrical halves (lobes), which meet in the midline. The base of the organ rests on the pericardial surface, with extension of each of the lobes superiorly into the root of the neck. Thymic development occurs early, relative to other lymphoid organs, and the maximum relative weight of the thymus is attained at birth, though absolute growth continues until about puberty, with a maximal weight of 30 to 40 g achieved in the human (202). Thereafter, the thymus undergoes progressive involution, until, in the adult, it is largely replaced by adipose tissue, which may contain some residual islands of potentially functional lymphoepithelial elements (17).

Investing the thymus is a thin connective-tissue capsule, which invaginates repeatedly into the organ as connective-tissue septae to subdivide the thymic lobes into lobules. These septae also carry the blood vessels, efferent lymphatics, and innervation. The thymus has no clear afferent lymphatics. Each lobule is divided into two fundamental layers, a peripheral lymphocyte-dense region, the *cortex*, and a central, more epithelial-rich region, the *medulla* (Figs. 2 and 3). In addition, a separate thin *subcapsular zone* is also recognized, a layer thought to give residence to the most recent and immature thymic immigrants. Efferent lymphatics form at the corticomedullary junction (CMJ), which is the depth, during fetal development, to which the in-growing septae extend, widen, and end. The CMJ is also the point at which vessels leave the septae to penetrate into cortex and medulla. The blunted widened ends of the septae form the perivascular spaces, which serve as sites of exchange of cells and solutes between perithymic stroma and the periphery. These perivascular spaces contain myeloid cells, plasma cells, and mast cells, and are the residence of much of the thymic B-cell population, which can take the form of scattered individual cells, lymphoid follicles, or even active germinal centers (203). This region is clearly separated from thymic parenchyma by an epithelial barrier (204), suggesting that exchange between these regions is restricted (see below).

Embryologically, the thymus is distinct from other lymphoid organs in that the stroma develops primarily from epithelial cells. The thymic epithelial rudiment in humans is widely recognized to form from (a) endoderm of the third pharyngeal pouch, (b) ectoderm of the corresponding branchial clefts, and (c) stromal cells of the associated mesenchyme from the pharyngeal arch; the latter in turn derives from neural crest. Interaction between two types of epithelium (e.g., endoderm and ectoderm) appears necessary for the development of proper thymic structure, as illustrated in

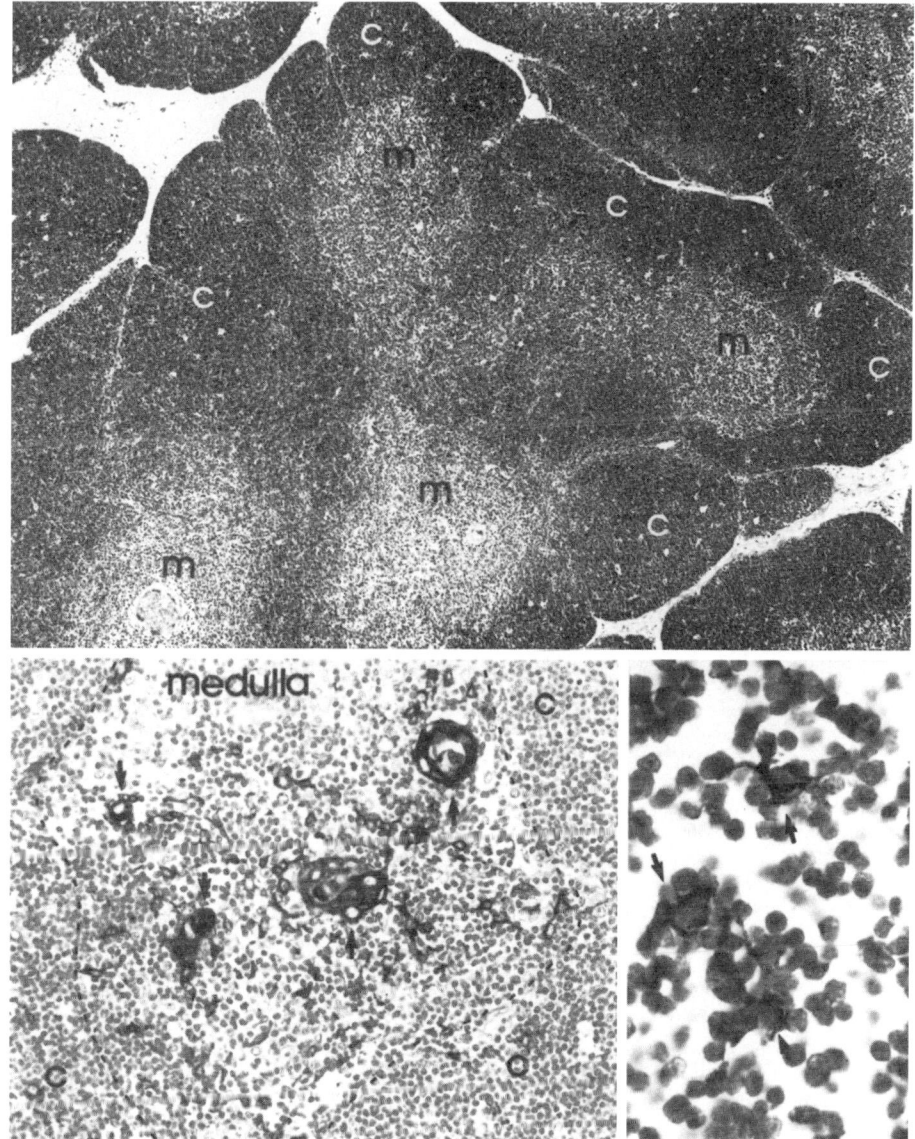

FIG. 2. Architecture of the thymus. **Top:** Low-power view of a human thymic lobule, showing the relationship of the more darkly staining cortex (*c*) to the pale staining medulla (*m*). Delicate connective tissue septa separate the polyhedral thymic lobules from each other and provide a route for the thymic vascular supply (H&E stain). **Bottom, left:** A higher power view of a human thymus immunostained for cytokeratins expressed by medullary epithelial cells [a dotted line delineates the medulla from the adjacent cortex (*c*)]. Note that the darkly stained medullary epithelial cells exist both as roughly spherical structures, called Hassall's corpuscles (*arrows*), and as dispersed single cells with fusiform to stellate shapes. **Bottom, right:** The same thymus immunostained for cytokeratins expressed by cortical thymic epithelial cells reveals the dendritic shape of those cells (darkly stained cells, delineated by *arrows*), as well as their intimate association with maturing thymocytes (the thymocytes appear to cluster along the dendritic epithelial cell processes).

the development of the nude mouse embryo, wherein ectoderm of the third cleft involutes after day 11.5, with the result that further development of the endoderm is halted and the thymus never becomes lymphoid (205). Extirpation experiments have likewise shown neural crest necessary for proper thymic development (206), and the resulting defects are recapitulated in certain human clinical syndromes, such as DiGeorge and Pierre Robin (see Chapter 13). Therefore, proper interaction between different types of epithelium and neural crest derivatives is necessary for normal thymic development.

Circulating lymphoid cells begin to colonize the epithelial thymic rudiment before the organ is vascularized. In avian and murine models, influx of lymphoid cells occurs as cyclic waves of progenitor cells at programmed times of embryonic development, leading to self-perpetuating and differentiating populations of T-lymphocytes (207–210). More recent evidence suggests that this pattern extends into early postnatal life in the mouse as well (211). The incoming pre-thymic cells first derive from the earliest hematopoietic centers, yolk sac and paraaortic foci (212,213), then fetal liver, and postnatally from the bone marrow (180).

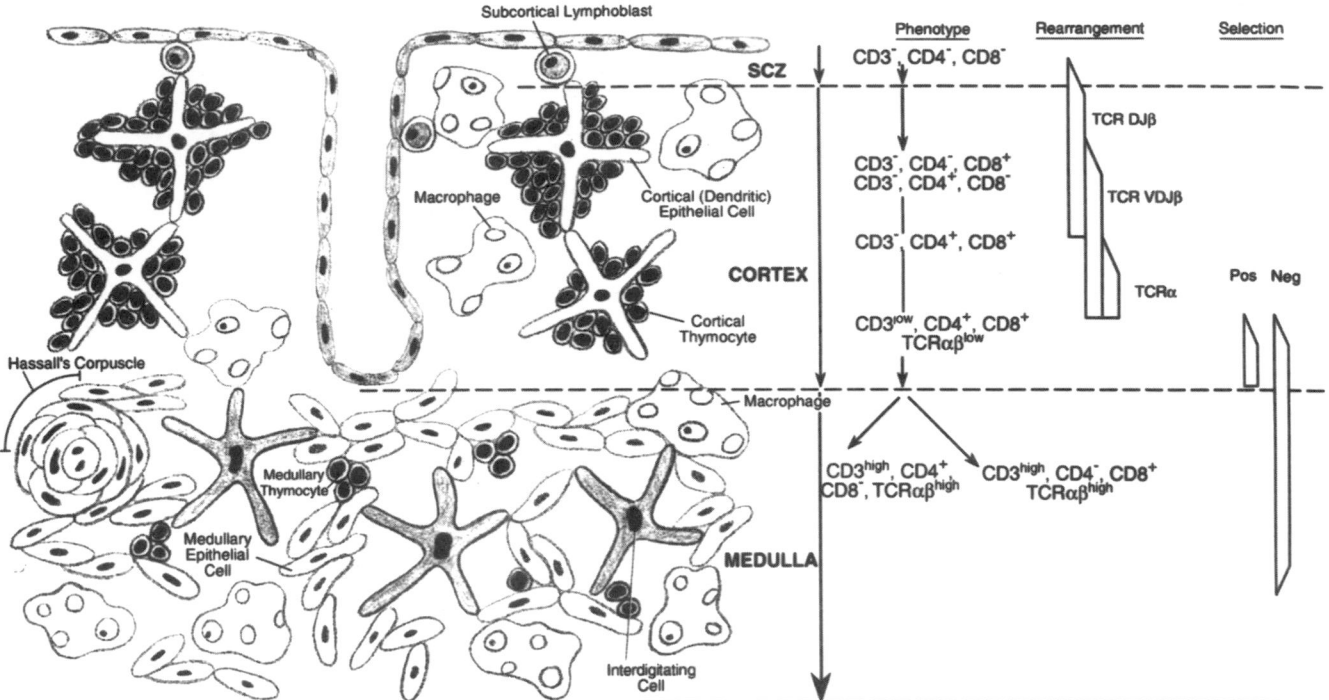

FIG. 3. T-lineage lymphoid development in the thymic microenvironment. **Left:** Diagram of thymic architecture. The three major compartments shown are the subcapsular zone (*SCZ*), cortex, and medulla. A layer of cortical epithelium is seen to line the surface of the thymus. Connective tissue septae extend into the thymus (epithelial layer underneath is shown to invaginate) to end at the junction of the cortex and medulla. The septae cordon the thymus into lobules; a portion of two are depicted here. Subcortical T lymphoblasts are shown in the SCZ, the first layer, where these very immature cells predominantly localize. The layer subjacent to this is the cortex, containing a rich admixture of cells, including macrophages, and a dense population of cortical thymocytes in close contact with the dendritic processes of epithelial cells, an important interaction for their maturation. The deepest layer of the thymus is the medulla, which has a much larger component of epithelial cells, generally morphologically regular and rounded to fusiform, in distinction to the elaborate processes of epithelium in the cortex. It also contains macrophages, interdigitating (dendritic) cells, and a scattered population of medullary thymocytes. **Right:** Approximations of events related to cell surface phenotype, TCR-gene rearrangements, and selection are given to correspond to portions of thymic architecture as thymocyte maturation proceeds from SCZ to medulla (see text for details).

Thymic Epithelial Microenvironment

The pivotal role of the thymic epithelium in determining thymocyte fate is overwhelming; therefore, its composition will be given substantial consideration here. The mature thymus contains morphologically distinct types of epithelium (214,215), and the regions occupied by these types are also associated with differing populations of thymocytes (see below) (see Fig. 3). Proceeding from the periphery of the thymus inward, subcapsular–perivascular epithelium is first encountered. This epithelium lines the inner surface of the capsule of the organ and all perivascular spaces as a flattened sheath on the basal lamina, and it forms a tight and complete investment of the thymus, separating intrathymic space proper from surrounding vascularized mesenchyme. Vascular investment by subcapsular epithelium persists all the way to the level of the capillaries. This layer was proposed to form the basis for the alleged thymic–blood barrier (216,217), which was thought to insulate the thymic cortex (but not medulla) from exposure to circulating antigens. The stringency of this putative barrier was called into question with the discovery that antigens are indeed found to enter the thymic cortex through the transcapsular route (218–220). In addition, antigens can be carried by monocyte–macrophages

and/or dendritic (interdigitating) cells from the periphery and gain access to the thymic cortex by normal pathways of cellular traffic (221–223). Therefore, not only are thymocytes exposed to the intrinsic self antigens borne by cells in the thymus, but they also are potentially bathed by foreign antigens from the periphery. Cortical epithelial cells are those that are often seen in intimate contact with cortical thymocytes. Indeed, thymocytes are often seen either entwined in the cytoplasmic processes of these epithelial cells, or frankly engulfed within them individually or in groups (the latter as large lymphoepithelial complexes; see Fig. 2). Distinct epithelial cells are found in the medulla and at the CMJ. These are also found in close association with thymocytes, which are present at a much lower density compared with the cortex. It has been reported that the embryonic origin of medullary epithelium is distinct from that of the cortex (224). Medullary epithelium in adult murine thymus has been subdivided into two phenotypic subsets based on the expression of classical and atypical MHC-related molecules (225), and a subset of medullary epithelial cells with potential functional consequences (see below) has been identified on the basis of its expression of a fucosylated moiety, which binds the *Ulex europeus* agglutinin lectin, UEA-1 (226). This morphologically distinct type of medullary epithelium has dendritic as opposed to "spatulate" morphology and high levels of MHC class II. Yet another type of epithelial cells forms the prominent medullary (restricted) structures known as *Hassall's corpuscles,* the most identifiable light microscopic structures of the thymus (see Fig. 2). The primordia of Hassall's corpuscles are seen as separate small tubular clusters composed of epithelial cells at about the tenth week in the human fetus (227). In fully developed Hassall's corpuscles, the epithelial cells are concentrically arranged in an onion-like appearance, are highly keratinized, and share antigenic properties with ectodermal epithelium (228–231). While distinctive, the functional role of these structures remains unknown, although their association with cell debris and products of cell death has resulted in speculation that they serve as thymocyte graveyards.

It is the cortical epithelial cells that are thought to represent thymic nurse cells (TNCs), identified *in vitro* in the mouse (232). Moreover, it was shown that TNCs isolated from human thymus bear MHC surface structures (233), and that these structures are actually synthesized by the epithelial cells (234). Because MHC molecules are key to the development of the T cell–recognition repertoire (235–240), this is clearly of functional import, since the intimate association of lymphocyte and epithelium appears to reflect a site at which T-lymphocytes acquire MHC-restricted recognition potential and are selected to distinguish self from non-self (see below). Thymic epithelium is also capable of elaborating its own complement of cytokines, including IL-1, IL-3, IL-6, IL-7, leukocyte inhibitory factor (LIF), and GM-CSF (241–244). This epithelial source of cytokines undoubtedly participates in the existing dynamic interplay of cytokines (245) and likely acts in a coordinated and sequential fashion to control passage of precursor thymocytes through stages of development in the thymus. Moreover, thymic epithelial cells display cell surface adhesion molecules such as LFA-3 and ICAM-1, known to be complementary to ligands on the thymocyte cell surface (CD2 and LFA-1, respectively). These adhesion molecule–ligand pairs likely mediate the adhesive association between these cell types and may also function in transducing activation signals, presumably along with appropriate costimulatory molecules operative during thymocyte development as well (246,247).

Finally, the thymus has also been recognized as a producer of peptide hormones (248–251) and chemotactic peptides (252,253). Many have been shown to be synthesized by thymic epithelial cells, and some (e.g., thymulin) to be produced exclusively by these cells (249). The precise physiologic functions of these thymic hormones remain unclear, although a variety of roles—including induction of stem-cell differentiation to prothymocytes, induction of T-cell surface markers, activation, and enhancement of effector function—have been proposed. Observations have brought to light a potential role of some peptides in the development of extrathymic T cells. Administration of the neuropeptide thyrotropin-releasing hormone to neonatally thymectomized mice has been reported to support the development of gut intraepithelial T cells (254), and overexpression of the IL-6 relative oncostatin M leads to the accumulation of mature T cells in the periphery of athymic nu/nu mice (255).

Nonlymphoid Bone Marrow–derived Elements

Monocytes and dendritic cell precursors [the latter being a distinct marrow-derived lineage of professional accessory (antigen-presenting) cells described in detail below; (256,257)] presumably enter the thymus along with thymocyte progenitors and differenti-

ate there into conventional macrophages (which localize primarily in the cortex and particularly at the CMJ) and interdigitating cells (which predominate in the medulla (258); see Fig. 3), respectively. Thymic interdigitating cells are remarkable for an irregular network of cytoplasmic projections and processes, which extend among epithelial and lymphoid cells. The latter can often be seen to be fully enveloped by these projections. In the human, these cells have been shown to be largely MHC class II–positive and to be effective antigen-presenting cells *in vitro* (259). As discussed below, these cells likely participate in the selection of the T-cell antigen receptor repertoire. In the cortex, macrophages have been demonstrated to form rosette-like structures with surrounding thymocytes. The functions of macrophages in the thymus may be quite varied. Since they are potent phagocytes and, as described below, the overwhelming majority of thymocytes are thought to die in the thymus, they may be associated with removal of these nonsurviving cells. Indeed, degenerating lymphoid cells can be identified in phagocytic vacuoles of thymic macrophages. Alternatively, macrophages are capable of a wide array of cytokine production, some of which may participate in the various differentiative stages of T-cell ontogeny and proliferation (245). Finally, like the interdigitating cells, macrophages express MHC antigens and can function as antigen-presenting cells in the immune system, suggesting the possiblity that, through the processes of positive and negative selection (see below), they participate in the shaping of the peripheral T-cell antigen receptor repertoire.

A final nonlymphoid cellular participant within the thymus is the myoid cell, an unusual muscle cell of uncertain function, which is found scattered and in clusters predominantly in the medulla and derives from neural crest (260). The cells contain myofilaments, though not in orderly array, and show immunoreactivity for actin, desmin, striated muscle myosin, and cell surface acetylcholine receptor. These specialized cells have been thought to potentially be involved in the pathogenesis of myasthenia gravis, and they have been shown, under some circumstances, to differentiate into striated muscle cells (261).

Overview of Thymus Architecture and Function

The thymus consists of three distinct phenotypic and maturational compartments: (a) the subcapsular zone, which appears to be the site of entrance of progenitors from the bone marrow and the location of the most primitive lymphoblasts; (b) the subjacent cortex, densely packed with the lymphoblasts small lymphocyte progeny, which are closely entwined with the elaborate processes of cortical epithelial cells undergoing MHC-based selection and enormous attrition, and (c) the medulla, containing blunt-ended spatulate epithelium, giving residence to scattered surviving medium-sized lymphocytes, which undergo the final selection and maturational processes prior to export to the periphery. We will attempt to place, to the extent current knowledge permits, the maturational stages of lymphocyte development in the context of the thymic compartments. To do so, we must first consider the phenotypic maturational stages of T-lineage precursors and the flux of cells through these stages within the thymus.

As discussed, the nature of the prothymocyte, which seeds the thymus from the bone marrow, is somewhat controversial, although the evidence points to the acquisition of at least some T lineage characteristics prior to the bone marrow-to-thymus migration step. In the mouse, the putative prothymocyte has been characterized to express particular levels of numerous markers, including Thy-1, heat-stable antigen (HSA), Pgp-1, H-2, Sca-1 (Ly-6-A/E), and more recently, low levels of CD4 (262–265). These cells have all TCR genes in the germline state (265). The functional significance of these markers on thymocyte precursors remains uncertain. It seems clear that CD4 does not have a central functional role early in T-cell development, since mice homozygously disrupted at this locus have no apparent defects at these early stages (266). In the human, putative thymocyte precursors express a unique signature of markers, including CD7, CD2, CD34, and cytoplasmic CD3 (11,267,268). Due to the relatively small numbers of cells entering the adult thymus, precise points of entry are difficult to define. In the mouse, progenitors have been shown to enter through large venules in the medulla and at the CMJ (269). It has also been shown that cycling cells in the regenerating mouse thymus are first located at the CMJ and then in the subcapsular region (270).

The stages of T-cell development are generally monitored by a combination of assessing the status of TCR genes and an assortment of cell surface markers. The earliest thymocytes are blast cells that closely resemble the putative prothymocyte population, bearing some T-lineage markers (Thy-1 and very early low levels of CD4 in the mouse; CD7/CD2/CD5/cytoplasmic CD3 in the human), but then lacking surface expression of CD4 (this marker is rapidly lost from the earliest immigrants), CD8, and CD3. This population, frequently referred to as the CD4/CD5 double-negative (DN) or the CD3/CD4/CD8 triple-negative (TN) thymocyte subset (11,267,268,271–279), makes up about 1% to 3% of the total thymocyte population (see Fig. 3). These cells begin to rearrange their γ, δ, β (β locus first) even at the DN stage (263,280) (extensively by the end of the DN maturation stage) to give two broad and likely separate T-cell populations: (a) the γδ TCR–bearing T-cells (281, 282), which may remain DN (or later acquire CD8 only) and may leave the thymus early to undergo further differentiation in tertiary sites (see section on tertiary lymphoid tissues), and (b) the more mainstream pathway, which proceeds to a CD4$^+$/CD8$^+$ [double-positive (DP)] stage and ultimately TCR αβ-bearing CD4$^+$ or CD8$^+$ [single-positive (SP)] T cells. These choices are governed by complex and incompletely understood biochemical and gene regulatory mechanisms. The DN stage of differentiation is characterized by a signficant expansion of the original thymus-seeding prothymocyte population. In experiments that followed the early differentiation of thymocytes after direct injection of multipotent stem cells into irradiated mouse thymus, there was 50-fold expansion and a long time delay before significant transition to the Thy-1^{high} DN phenotype, which was followed in turn by a roughly tenfold expansion prior to transitioning to the DP stage (188).

DN cells appear to transiently pass through either a CD4$^-$/CD8$^+$ or CD4$^+$/CD8$^-$ intermediary stage to the CD4$^+$/CD8$^+$ DP phenotype, depending on the species or mouse strain being examined (11, 283–289). A crucial regulatory point in progression to the DP stage appears to be the successful rearrangement of the β chain, which occurs prior to any rearrangement of the α chain (290–292). Perhaps in quite analogous fashion to the λ5 and VpreB genes in early B-cell development (see above), it has further been established that TCR β chains are initially expressed on developing thymocytes in association with a nonpolymorphic 33-kDa glycoprotein, designated pre-TCRα or pTα, which is presumed to serve as a surrogate for the α chain (293–295) and to regulate the survival and/or expansion of developing thymocytes before the final α chain is selected. Final allelic exclusion of the α chain is thought to occur at the time of

positive selection (see below) (296). The overwhelming number of thymocytes (85% to 90%) have a DP phenotype, and these are the predominant residents of the cell-dense thymic cortex. However, this is by no means a homogenous population. Progressive maturation within the DP subset is evidenced by the stereotyped up- and/or downregulation of a wide variety of other differentiation markers (11). While all of these markers undoubtedly have functional signficance, the maturational change that is most germane to the development of the T cell–recognition repertoire is the continuation of the TCR-gene rearrangements initiated in the DN stage, ultimately leading to the coordinate appearance of TCR and CD3 on the DP thymocyte's cell surface. The DP population is nevertheless equally divided among those that do and those that do not express the αβ TCR. As will be discussed in detail, cell surface expression of TCR is an obvious prerequisite for the processes of positive and negative selection (i.e., the determination of the survivors of this rigorous screening process).

About 25% of the DP population are large dividing blast cells, while the remaining 75% are small nondividing G$_0$ progeny of these cells (297,298). Even though the cells at this stage may be in their last few cell divisions before elimination or full maturation (full transit time for the DP stage is about 3 days on average), because they result from the previous many rounds of expansion of less mature cells, they account for the large bulk of cells dividing within the thymus (298–300). They are also the most dynamic bulk thymic population, with about one-third being replaced per day. From the end of the DN stage to the end of the DP stage, there is an approximate 50-fold expansion in the mouse, representing about 5×10^7 cells per day. After selection (see below), the final product of the DP cells is the mature SP cells (bearing either CD4 or CD8), and these are produced and exported to the periphery at about 1 to 2×10^6 cells per day.

The fate of the major population of DP cells has long been an issue of controversy in immunology. DP cells isolated from the intrathymic compartment are functionally defective by numerous criteria (301), and they are not generally found among thymic emigrants to lymphoid organs (302). It has generally been thought that the vast overproduction of thymocytes at this stage (over that required to replenish the peripheral T-cell pool) necessitates the intrathymic death of upwards of 97% of thymocytes (303,304). However, it had been difficult to reconcile this with the minimal extent of intrathymic cell death observed histologically (305). The recognition of apoptosis as a mechanism for cell death (306, 307) has ameliorated these concerns. *Apoptosis* is defined as programmed cell death that is not accompanied by necrosis. It is characterized by cytoplasmic blebbing and activation of endogenous endonucleases that cleave DNA into oligonucleosomal fragments (seen as ladder-like bands experimentally on separation gels), as a result of which chromatin and nuclei become condensed. Apoptosis is dependent on RNA and protein synthesis by the dying cell. Affected cells are then phagocytosed by macrophages. Although the mechanism for the signaling of apoptosis is unclear, described elevations in intracellular calcium concentrations in cells bearing anti-self receptors *in vivo* may reflect activation signals leading to intrathymic death (308). Apoptotic thymocytes and cell debris within macrophages can indeed be found in the thymus (reviewed in ref. 309), and intrathymic death is also supported by kinetic arguments (304). More recently, further direct evidence for intrathymic apoptosis has been provided using methods for detecting cells with DNA strand breaks in thymus sections. Apoptotic cells could thus be directly seen engulfed within macrophages

(310). *In vitro* and *in vivo* evidence in model systems has also supported the relevance of apoptosis (311–313). For instance, mice transgenic for a TCR specific for a particular peptide contain thymocytes that progress from the immature to the mature phenotype, and administration of the peptide antigen to these mice results in a rapid deletion through apoptosis of the immature CD4$^+$/CD8$^+$/TCR^{lo} thymocytes (313). Mice transgenic for the protooncogene bcl-2 (antagonizes apoptosis) show disturbances in thymic apoptosis [with concommitant alterations in T-cell maturation and development (314,315)], and this molecule does appear to be upregulated at the DP stage of thymocyte development (316). The apoptosis-inducing surface molecule, FAS, has also been implicated in thymocyte deletion (317,318), but neither bcl-2 nor FAS function (319,320) can completely explain negative selection, which can occur without (FAS) or in spite of (bcl-2) the participation of these molecules. Finally, although most lines of evidence support the predominance of *intrathymic* death, it cannot be entirely excluded that T cells destined to be eliminated are exported and rapidly scavenged by liver, spleen, or intestine (321). Although the mechanism or mechanisms mediating cell loss remain incompletely defined, this "cytodeletion" is clearly a primary means by which the TCR repertoire is adjusted.

As DP thymocytes mature, they gradually lose expression of either CD4 or CD8 [producing SP (CD4$^+$ *or* CD8$^+$) thymocytes], increase their surface expression of CD3 and TCR, and adjust their expression of other antigens (e.g., homing receptors) to that seen on naive, peripheral T cells (11). This DP-to-SP transition is thought to be accompanied by the progressive translocation of the maturing thymocytes from cortex to medulla. The CMJ displays a particular concentration of dendritic cells and macrophages, which are aligned in a downstreaming, lacy network perpendicular to the thymic capsule. This network possibly forms a negative selective barrier (see below), which must be "survived" for terminal thymocyte differentiation to occur. This survival has been shown to be associated with the upregulation of cell surface markers, as well as such anti-apoptotic molecules as bcl-2 (316). Presumably, the 10% to 15% of SP, CD3^{high} thymocytes (which largely reside in the medulla) result from this final culling process. Only within the last few years have clues begun to emerge as to the mechanism of this crucial migration step of developing thymocytes from cortex to medulla. It has been reported that interaction of the integrins VLA-4 and VLA-5 on thymocytes with fibronectin on thymic stroma may participate in this process (322). The turnover time of medullary thymocytes is much larger (12 to 16 days) than the preceding DP stage in the cortex (299,300,323). Although changes within the medulla are subtle in comparison to those undergone in the cortex, some degree of medullary maturation apparently does occur with respect to both TCR triggerability and cell surface markers (324–326). Furthermore, although medullary thymocytes can be distinguished from mature peripheral T cells on the basis of size, buoyant density, and surface antigens (327), evidence indicates that these cells have acquired most, if not all, of the properties of mature T-lymphocytes. For example, it has been shown that the vast majority of recent migrants from the thymus are phenotypically mature in that the markers expressed are similar to peripheral T cells and medullary thymocytes, and quite disparate from cortical thymocytes (327). It is, however, also likely that some recent thymic migrants undergo some final phenotypic changes in the periphery (328). The process whereby medullary thymocytes are selected for export to the periphery is not well characterized, but several potential mechanisms exist, including a final proliferative step within the medulla (329–331). Mature thymocytes probably leave

the thymus at the CMJ through high-walled postcapillary venules, through thickened double-walled capillaries of transcapsular arteries, or through lymphatics (332). The latter originate at the CMJ, and the perivascular spaces that form in this region are often seen filled with lymphocytes (333,334).

It is important to note that phenotypically mature and even antigen-activated peripheral T cells migrate into the thymus, localizing in the medulla and forming at least some of the SP pool present there (335–338). The role of these thymic-homing peripheral T cells is unclear, but it is possible they represent a means by which peripheral immune responses can feed back and modulate T-lymphopoiesis. It is also notable that in mice in which the TCR α chain gene has been disrupted, with the consequence that αβ TCR surface expression is muted (339), and in SCID mice in which recombinational defects have the same effect (340), thymus architecture is modified to exclude development of a distinct medulla. Moreover, relatively normal achitecture can be restored in the SCID thymus on introduction of TCR$^+$ cells (341), and the dependence on expression of both α and β TCR chains has been reinforced in systems expressing transgenic TCRs, in which reconstitution of proper thymic architecture absolutely depends on full assembly of the TCR complex (342). These observations again punctuate the mutual and maleable relationship between lymphoid cell development and the development of lymphoid organs.

Thymic Shaping of the T-Cell Antigen Receptor Repertoire: Positive and Negative Selection

The critical immunologic function of the thymus—indeed, its likely reason for evolutionary development—is to provide for the creation of a repertoire of TCRs that is capable of recognizing and responding to myriad foreign antigens in the context of self MHC, but not self antigen alone. This goal is achieved primarily by a systematic rescue of appropriate thymocytes from programmed cell death based on a theme of self-recognition, and the release of these cells into the periphery to serve as self-tolerant T cells. The recombinatorial events that lead to the formation of diverse TCRs, while perhaps not entirely random [i.e., there is evidence for biases in Vα to Jα as well as Vβ to Jβ joining throughout ontogeny (343–347)], are governed by complex biochemical and genetic regulatory mechanisms that are independent of the set of self antigens—MHC or otherwise—expressed within the organism. These genetic mechanisms lead to the production of a large set of potential TCRs (presumably including structural motifs that range from having no affinity for self-MHC antigens to those with avid binding) from which the final functional TCR repertoire is selected. Somatic genetic alterations, so important in the final tailoring of the memory B-cell antigen receptor repertoire (see below), does not occur substantially for TCR genes (348–350), indicating that the shaping of the TCR repertoire is likely a more "pure" selection process. The role of the thymus is thus twofold: First, it must select from the original TCR pool those receptors that have at least some recognition of self MHC (so-called positive selection), and, second, it must eliminate from this "provisional" pool those receptors with so much reactivity with self MHC that their release into the peripheral immune system would result in autoimmunity (so-called negative selection). Appropriate receptors for the final repertoire would therefore include all those TCR with "poor" or "mediocre" recognition of self MHC—that group of TCR with the potential for high-efficiency recognition of self MHC "slightly" modified by the presence of foreign peptide within the peptide binding groove of self MHC (351,352).

In essence, the thymus can be considered a site of TCR "evolution," the key role of which is to provide a microenvironment that gives a profound survival advantage to those thymocyte clones that possess "appropriate" TCRs (leaving those with "inappropriate" specificities to be deleted via apoptosis or other mechanisms). Obviously, before a cell can be selected on the basis of its TCR specificity, it must first have rearranged its TCR genes (both mature α and β) and expressed on the surface the resulting unique receptor structure. From our previous discussion, this prerequisite is not met until well into the DP stage of thymocyte development. Selection is therefore thought to be normally confined to a fairly short interval corresponding roughly to the DP stage following the cessation of proliferation, perhaps extending through the early SP stage in the medulla (see Fig. 3) (286,353–357). This, then, broadly frames the difficult problem of immunologic selection in the thymus—operation on a discrete, thus far indivisible subpopulation of thymocytes that traverses through these crucial events very quickly.

Positive Selection: The Preservation of Thymocyte Clones with Some Self-MHC Reactivity

Positive selection of thymocytes is critically dependent on the appropriate engagement of their TCR with cells of the thymic microenvironment presenting MHC class I and II (235,238,239, 358–361), presumably in association with endogenous peptides. The fundamental question of how the final T-cell specificity for foreign antigens results from selection, presumably entirely on self molecules, within the thymus remains an enigma; nevertheless, the outcome of this process is the "skewing" of the T-cell repertoire to recognize foreign antigen (after cellular processing) in bimolecular complex with self MHC. CD4$^+$ cells result from interaction with class II antigens, and CD8$^+$ cells from interaction with class I antigen (362–366). Both classes of MHC molecules are present on dendritic *epithelial* cells of the thymic cortex (367), as well as on bone marrow–derived macrophages and dendritic cells. The intimate contact of cortical thymocytes with epithelial cells morphologically (thymocytes can be seen completely enveloped in epithelial membrane; see Fig. 2), including immunohistochemical studies showing capping of receptors on developing thymocytes at contact points with epithelium (suggesting TCR–ligand interactions) (368), as well as the relative resistance of positive selection to irradiation and deoxyguanosine, which eliminate bone marrow–derived elements (240,276,369,370), suggested a critical role for the cortical epithelial cell in this fundamental interaction. This conclusion was elegantly supported in experiments using mice that express transgenes for a specific TCR heterodimer recognizing a particular class II MHC antigen *as well as* a transgene for the appropriate MHC antigen, the latter of which is engineered to be specifically expressed in various thymic compartments. This was achieved by manipulating promoter sequences so that expression is directed to restricted types of cells that localize exclusively or predominantly in one compartment (371,372). Only when MHC expression included cortical thymic epithelium could positive selection be effected in a number of transgenic systems (365,366,373). Direct evidence for the capacity of a thymic epithelial cell line to induce positive selection *in vivo* has also been provided (374). Further confirmation of the importance of cortical epithelium in positive, but not negative, selection has come from relB-deficient mice, which have an abnormal thymus that does not contain medullary epithelium (indeed, no medullary structures

are present) or dendritic cells (375), yet positive selection proceeds unabated. Thus, thymic cortical epithelium appears not only necessary, but also perhaps sufficient for positive selection.

Although a consensus appears to have formed favoring the role of the cortical epithelial cell in positive selection, alternative views have been presented. Perhaps deriving appeal from the fact that bone marrow–derived cells have a key role as antigen-presenting cells in triggering immune responses in the periphery, evidence has also been presented that supports a role for radiation-resistant bone marrow–derived cells, such as macrophages and dendritic cells, in positive selection; these cells have also been noted to have thymocytes clustered on them (376,377). Moreover, in a mouse model disrupted for the β2 microglobulin gene, and thus incapable of expressing class I MHC antigens, transplanted hematopoietic cells (i.e., bone marrow–derived cells) were shown to have clear, although reduced, capacity for positive selection in a class I antigen–dependent system (378). In addition, fibroblast cell lines injected intrathymically have also been shown to induce positive selection (379,380). Thus, while under certain experimental conditions, nonepithelial elements are able to induce positive selection, the thymic epithelial cell is likely to be the primary, if not exclusive, promoter of this activity physiologically.

Primary factors (variables) that likely influence positive selection are (a) affinity for the selecting ligand as determined by TCR density, ligand density, and binding constants; (b) alterations in thymocyte activation states and/or signal transduction machinery and its linkage to TCR engagement during development (381,382); and (c) differences in thymic stromal cell populations, which may contain pools of disparate peptides for presentation on MHC molecules (383). Extensive evidence has accumulated in support of a differential avidity model, whereby low-avidity TCR interactions lead to positive selection, and high-avidity interactions lead to negative selection (reviewed in ref. 384). We can extrapolate to suggest that interaction with MHC of proper avidity provides a protective signal for developing lymphocytes whose default course is toward apoptosis and elimination. Experimental evidence supports such an assertion. For example, in one of the early transgenic models, a TCR from a clone of an H-2^b mouse reactive with a class I molecule (H-2L^d) could only give rise to peripheral T cells (primarily of CD8 type) bearing the TCR transgene if the transgene is backcrossed onto the original H-2^b background (363); that is, survival of thymocytes bearing this TCR depends on proper interaction with the original MHC molecules on which the TCR was selected; absence of this presenting MHC results in the loss of cells bearing the TCR. Similarly, in an independent model, selection of the transgenic αβTCR recognizing the male specific H-Y antigen in conjunction with H-2D^b requires this MHC background for transgenic TCR$^+$ cells to reach the periphery in significant numbers, that is, for positive selection to occur (this occurs only in female mice, in which H-Y is not expressed) (362,364,385). While these results applied to TCR and antigens restricted by class I MHC, similar results were obtained utilizing TCRs obtained from MHC class II–restricted clones (365,386).

Another technologic advance that has furthered our understanding of positive selection has been that of targeted gene disruption. Loss of the β2 microglobulin gene, required for cell surface class I MHC expression, resulted in the absence of CD8$^+$ mature T cells in the periphery (387,388). Similarly, creation of class II–negative mice has demonstrated its requirement for the generation of mature CD4 T cells in the periphery (389,390). Absence of class II–associated invariant chain, which enables proper antigen loading and translocation to the endoplasmic reticulum, results in reduced class II surface expression and consequent decreased CD4$^+$ T cells (391), and, similarly, disruption of the transporter protein associated with antigen presentation (TAP-1) results in decreased class I expression and concomitant lack of positive selection and circulating CD8 T cells (392). Experiments have also addressed the role of receptor rearrangement. A mechanism that provides for more diversity in antigen binding by the TCR is supplied by addition of nucleotides at VDJ or VJ junctures, and this is mediated by terminal deoxynucleotidyl transferase (TdT). Absence of this gene paradoxically *increases* the efficiency of positive selection from the DP pool, suggesting that the unmodified germline configuration of TCR chains may have a more focused theme of self-recognition than when modified by TdT (393,394).

The fundamental interplay of TCR with peptides within the antigen-binding pocket of MHC molecules, which harbors either self or foreign peptides, has been demonstrated in experiments exploiting MHC variants that are discrete and limited (395–399). Slight structural alteration of residues within the antigen-binding pocket can abrogate positive selection of the TCR repertoire as well as peptide binding. Since T cells are educated within the thymic environment, presumably on MHC in complex with self peptides, it is reasonable that foreign antigen recognition might result from prior selection of TCR on MHC presenting mimicking self peptides. This suggestion is evidenced by similar requirements found for the amino acid residues within the antigen-binding pocket in MHC for positive selection as for recognition of an ovalbumin (foreign) peptide (397). Experiments in transgenic models, one addressing TCR recognition of I-E^b (400) and another based on recognition of H-2K^b and its mutants (401), have also elegantly supported the role of the peptide-binding regions of MHC molecules in positive selection, and positive selection of CD4 SP cells has been shown to depend on endogenously derived peptides as well (402,403). Additional analysis of TCR transgenic thymocyte development *in vitro* in fetal thymic organ culture (FTOC) of MHC-deficient mice has further emphasized the crucial influence of peptides and the peptide–MHC density on molding the T-cell repertoire and on positive and negative selection (404–409). The precise rules governing the interactions leading to these developmental choices, however, remain to be fully clarified.

In addition to TCR and MHC molecules, there is also thought to be an influence provided by the CD4 and CD8 coreceptor molecules in the selection process (410,411). Experiments in which the genes for CD8 and CD4 have been disrupted by homologous recombination have demonstrated the discrete functional roles these molecules have in the development of helper cells for CD4 and cytotoxic T cells for CD8 (266,412–415). However, the actual signals mediating the downregulation of one of the coreceptors in transition from the DP stage remain obscure. Finally, data have also suggested that components of the signal transduction machinery may be differentially brought to bear during positive and negative selection (416–426).

Negative Selection: Elimination of TCR with Deleterious Self-reactivity

Self-tolerance, the inability of an organism to mount a productive immune response against its own cells, is a fundamental mandate of the immune system. Although there is clear evidence that T-lineage tolerance can, in some instances, be generated in the peripheral immune system (427–429), the most compelling body of evidence suggests that this task is primarily implemented in the thymus. Thus, while the thymus grants a survival advantage to thymocyte clones with some self reactivity (positive selection), those

clones interacting too strongly with MHC and self peptides must be eliminated (clonal deletion) or at least inactivated (clonal anergy or paralysis). While this discussion will focus primarily on deletional mechanisms of negative selection, we should, at the outset, acknowledge that well-characterized nondeletional pathways also exist, such as anergy (430,431), downregulation of coreceptor molecules (432,433), or raising of T cell–activation thresholds (434).

Initial observations of restricted Vβ usage in recognition of particular self antigens permitted some of the first systematic examinations of these processes, particularly those supporting the existence of clonal deletion (435–438). In these model systems, specific antigen-reactive cells could be monitored by virtue of their preferential expression and high representation of certain TCR β variable (Vβ) domains, generally reactive with Mls or I-E determinants, and detectable and quantifiable with specific Vβ antibodies. Loss of peripheral T cells bearing these particular Vβ domains was shown to correlate with expression of these self components in the thymus. For example, I-E recognizing Vβ17a-bearing cells could be selectively eliminated from the peripheral T-cell and mature thymocyte pools of mice expressing I-E, but they were present in expected numbers in the immature DP thymocyte population of such animals. This suggested that tolerance induction could occur in the thymus at the time immature thymocytes are selected to move into the mature thymocyte pool, and the critical junction was formed in the DP stage. Furthermore, since Vβ17a-positive (low-density) cells could be identified in the thymic cortex, but not in the medulla, it suggested that the medulla or CMJ was the site of negative selection. The key participation of the medulla in negative selection has also been suggested by studies showing that mice with I-A expression restricted to thymic cortical cells and relB-deficient mice, which lack thymic medullary structures (including both dendritic cells and the UEA-1 medullary epithelial cells; see below) show deficiencies in negative selection (375,470).

The advent of TCR transgenic mice (designed to have potentially self-reactive TCRs) provided additional experimental support for the operational clonal deletion in the thymus (432,439–445). However, it should be cautioned that, insofar as the timing and level of expression of TCR contribute to normal selection mechanisms, transgenic models (generally with distinctly nonphysiologic regulation of TCR expression) have the potential of distorting certain outcomes (particularly the timing of these processes). For example, in one H-Y antigen-specific TCR transgenic model (444), it was shown that clonal deletion could occur *prior* to the DP stage. While these results are interesting, in that they provide evidence that CD4 or CD8 expression may *not* be an obligate requirement for negative selection, they should not be construed to imply that negative selection normally occurs at this stage, as the transgenic TCR is prematurely expressed. Models based on affinity arguments generally have suggested that negative selection would occur relatively late (271), since TCR expression increases with maturation, and it is the high-affinity interactions that would lead to elimination. Direct intrathymic transfer of normal DP blasts has suggested that negative selection indeed occurs only after cells have been positively selected to SP pathways (446). Supporting this, in one system using TCR β-chain-only transgenics (allowing for the normal rearrangement of endogenous α to be a prerequisite for cell surface TCR expression), mature SP peripheral T cells were diminished (deleted), but DP cells were much less affected (441). However, the demonstration of the inhibition of deletion of CD8 SP T cells by anti-CD4 suggests that negative selection can also occur at the DP stage (447,448), and in another αβ TCR transgenic model, in which the transgenic receptor displayed specificity for *both* lymphocytic choriomeningitis virus antigen in the context of H-2 and Mls[a], the results suggested that the maturational stage at which autoreactive T-cells are deleted varies over a wide spectrum, depending on the antigen in the thymus serving as the self antigen (442,445). Finally, there is evidence indicating that a spectrum of small DP thymocytes, both the less mature TCR[low] and the more mature TCR[high] cells, can be deleted through apoptosis (449,450). Taken together, these observations suggest that microenvironmental structures mediating negative selection do not necessarily exclusively operate on a single thymocyte differentiative stage. The relative difficulty in pinpointing a discrete timepoint for negative selection may reflect a general requirement for environmental checks at more than one stage to optimize the stringency at which autoreactive cells are prevented from escaping into the periphery (see below).

A significant body of evidence suggests that the critical cell in the thymus with which the thymocyte must interact to undergo negative selection is a bone marrow–derived cell in the form of a macrophage or dendritic (interdigitating) cell. A number of studies in a variety of systems have shown that implantation of allogeneic thymuses resulted in tolerance to graft alloantigens, but not if they were depleted of hematolymphoid cells (451–454). T-cell tolerance also was shown to appear coordinately with the entry of donor hematolymphoid cells into host thymuses of animals given tolerizing doses of semiallogeneic cells at birth (455). Studies using bone marrow chimeras have also implicated a relatively radio-resistant, presumably bone marrow–derived cell in deletion (456–458). Purified dendritic cells have been shown *in vitro* to tolerize T cells in thymic organ culture (459), and in a transgenic model *in vivo,* dendritic cell expression of I-E was shown to drive negative but not positive selection (460). Therefore, bone marrow–derived cells— perhaps macrophages, but more likely dendritic cells—seem to be a major and potent component of negative selection (see ref. 461 for review). This role makes teleologic sense in that (as discussed below) the dendritic cell is the primary accessory–antigen-presenting cell supporting antigen activation of naive T cells in the periphery; thus, it would be of paramount importance to delete from the mature, naive T cell–repertoire cells capable of responding to self peptides normally associated with dendritic cell MHC molecules. In other words, it is of particular importance that dendritic-cell "self" is ignored by mature T cells, since dendritic cell–associated foreign peptides are the primary trigger of peripheral immune responses.

The mechanism for the predilection for a bone marrow–derived cell in negative selection remains unclear, although increased MHC antigen density on these cells, specialized accessory molecules, and particular tolerogenic peptides presented by these cells have all been suggested (462). The extremely high efficiency of deletion has been illustrated in one interpretation of an experiment in transgenic mice expressing I-E on only relatively few bone marrow–derived cells in the thymic medulla, where deletion of T cells bearing Vβ17a is as complete as in normal animals (372). The potential role of the accessory–costimulatory molecules ICAM-1 and B7.1 has been explored (463). Using a model of MHC class I–transfected *Drosophila* cells that were cotransfected with ICAM-1 and/or B7.1 as antigen-presenting cells, it was shown that expression of B7.1 or both molecules caused apoptosis of particular TCR transgenic DP thymocytes, while expresssion of ICAM-1 alone inhibited apoptosis. This observation is quite suggestive, as the distribution of these molecules in the thymus places B7.1 and ICAM-

1 together in the thymic medulla on both epithelial and bone marrow–derived cells, and ICAM-1 but not B7.1 on cortical epithelium, where positive selection occurs (464–466). Thus, it must be considered that not only TCR interaction with peptide–MHC, but also the *sum* of interactions of a T cell with its microenvironment, including coreceptor, adhesion, costimulatory, and extracellular matrix molecules, contribute to the final selection process.

In contrast to positive selection, early studies indicated that thymic epithelial cells were unable to induce deletion of particular TCR Vβ–expressing thymocytes (467). However, it should be noted that in several studies, thymic *medullary* epithelium has been shown to potentially induce *anergy* (though not always deletion) in differentiating T cells specific for peptide, or minor and, to some extent, MHC antigens (453,457,468,469); for example, I-E[+] thymic epithelium could delete I-E-specific T-cells when chimeric for I-E[-] bone marrow (371,439). The medullary epithelial cell shares many common features with bone marrow-derived dendritic cells, including dendritic morphology, high level of class II expression, constitutive B7 expression, and expression of the NF-kB transcription factor relB (464,471), and it has been implicated in negative selection of superantigen-specific T cells in transgenic models when I-E is selectively expressed on the UEA-1 medullary epithelium (465,472). It has been suggested that thymocyte–self interactions on thymic epithelial cells generally result in nondeletional tolerance, whereas these interactions on hematopoietic cells result in deletion (427,428,474). Given the vital task of the immune system to avert autoimmunity, it should not be surprising that negative selection can apparently occur at more than one thymocyte stage, by more than one cell type, and by more than one mechanism (442,445,475). Such a system would have multiple "checks" to ensure against the unleashing of T-cell clones with potentially pathogenic autoreactivity (271).

As the technology for removing and cloning thymic stromal cell populations has advanced, detailed and systematic analysis of the phenomena observed in complex biologic models can be anticipated. For example, a thymic stromal cell–clonal cell line was developed as a model for clonal deletion (476). When KLH-I-E–specific T helper clones were cultured on these cells in the absence of KLH, proliferation resulted, but when KLH was included and presumably presented by the stromal cell, complete inhibition of growth occurred, and this depended on the proper MHC molecule expression as well as a cytokine elaborated by the stromal cell, thymic stroma–derived T-cell growth factor (TSTGF). More recently, thymic epithelial cells lines have also been developed, and these have been shown *in vivo* and *in vitro* to induce positive and/or negative selection of T cells (477–479)

Secondary Lymphoid Tissues: Sites of Immune Sensitization and the Virgin to Memory–Effector Cell Conversion

The unique and, indeed, defining function of secondary lymphoid tissue is the initiation of immune responses: the bringing together of antigen and naive lymphocytes in highly organized, lymphoid microenvironments that support the antigen-specific clonal expansion of these cells and their differentiation into memory–effector subsets. This function is reflected by certain structural elements of secondary lymphoid tissues that are held in common to all such sites. First, all secondary lymphoid tissues display specialized mechanisms by which antigen or antigen-bearing accessory cells are collected from their "assigned" territory (i.e., associated nonlymphoid tissues that represent portals of antigen entry into the body), and which transport this antigen to the appropriate lymphoid microenvironment. Second, all of these tissues display specialized vascular adaptations designed to recruit lymphocytes, particularily *naive* lymphocytes, from the blood. Finally, all secondary lymphoid tissues display a unique juxtaposition of distinct lymphoid microenvironments, the so-called T-cell and B-cell zones. As we will see below, these terms are somewhat misnamed because critical B-cell functions occur in T zones, and vice versa. Nevertheless, these designations define two distinct but interacting microenvironments that characterize secondary lymphoid tissue function.

The final differentiated form of these common elements varies among the different types of secondary lymphoid tissue—lymph node versus mucosa-associated lymphoid tissue (e.g., Peyer's patch, appendix) versus spleen—as the final structure also reflects the specialized missions of each of these tissue types. Lymph nodes are the termination point of afferent lymphatics that drain lymph (extracellular fluid) from most tissues of the body, collecting antigen from sites of deposition within these tissues. The spleen filters the blood, collecting antigens that have been introduced into the vascular system. The mucosa-associated lymphoid tissues, of which the Peyer's patch represents the paradigm, comprise lymphoid tissues specialized for the collection of antigen across mucosal epithelia.

Secondary Lymphoid Tissues: Structure and Organization

Since antigen collection and lymphocyte recruitment are defining functions of secondary lymphoid tissues, it is useful to explore the structure of these tissues in relation to the vascular system that is critically involved in these functions. Lymph nodes are integral components of the lymphatic vasculature, a system of thin-walled, specialized vessels that originate as fine, anastomosing capillary channels in the extracellular space (17). Lymphatic capillaries are blind-ended and are freely permeable to fluid and particulate matter, including lymphocytes and accessory cells. Anchoring filaments connecting the lymphatic endothelium to adjacent collagen bundles serve as "guy wires" to keep these channels open, even in the face of the increasing extracelluar fluid pressure that occurs with ongoing immune–inflammatory responses. Lymphatic capillaries are widely distributed, but they are most numerous beneath the skin and the mucosa of the gastrointestinal, respiratory, and genitourinary tracts, sites that likely account for the majority of collected lymph. Lymphatics are not found in the central nervous system, the eye globe, or those parts of the spleen, liver, and bone marrow that are supplied by venous sinusoids. The ramifying lymphatic capillaries eventually collect into larger lymphatic vessels (the afferent lymphatics), which then converge toward and empty into regional lymph nodes. Each lymph node or group of lymph nodes thus serves a distinct region of the body defined by the afferent lymphatics.

Lymph nodes are ovoid (bean-shaped), encapsulated structures that cluster in groups at particular sites, usually those associated with vascular junctions, such as the axillary, inguinal, and cervical regions, or the intestinal mesentery (17,480). Characteristically, multiple afferent (in-coming) lymphatic vessels empty into the convex aspect of the node, opposite from the so-called lymph node hilum, which serves as the entry point for nodal arteries and an exit

point for both nodal veins and the efferent (out-going) lymphatics (Fig. 4, top). Efferent lymphatics (containing filtered lymph and lymphocytes) continue up the body, converging into larger lymphatic vessels and more central lymph nodes until, ultimately, they all converge into a single lymphatic vessel, the thoracic duct. The thoracic duct empties into one of the great veins supplying blood to the heart, thereby returning the lymph and its cellular inhabitants (primarily recirculating lymphocytes; see below) back into the bloodstream.

Within the lymph node (see Fig. 4), the afferent lymphatics open into the subcapsular, or marginal, sinus, a slitlike opening separating the fibrous capsule of the node from the underlying highly organized lymphoid tissue, the nodal cortex. Lymphocytes may be found in the subcapsular sinus, but macrophages, dendritic cells, and poorly defined stromal cells usually comprise the major cell types in this location. In general, lymph and particulate material (including cells) flowing into the subcapsular sinus must pass through the dense lymphocyte infiltrates of the cortex via ill-defined radial sinuses prior to reaching the central part of the node, or medulla. The medulla consists of branching partitions of stromal cells and fibers, separated by (medullary) sinuses that are rich in macrophages and plasma cells. These sinuses eventually coalesce into the efferent lymphatic vessel. Thus, it is clear that with this anatomic arrangement, lymph-borne antigens derived from distant tissues sites are subject to obligate contact with the immune system as they filter through the nodal cortex. Lymphocytes, particularly naive lymphocytes, are also continuously passing through the cortex. Naive lymphocytes enter lymph nodes via unique postcapillary venules in the T zone of the cortex (the so-called paracortex) that are uniquely defined by this function (Figs. 4 and 5). These specialized venules have a plump, cuboidal endothelium that gives them their name—the high endothelial venules (HEVs) (481). HEVs display particular adhesion molecules that interact with counterreceptors (homing receptors) on the lymphocyte surface and serve to recruit circulating lymphocytes (again, particularly naive lymphocytes) into the paracortex with high efficiency. Some memory–effector lymphocytes also extravasate into nodal cortex via HEVs, but can, because of their ability to extravasate in tertiary sites, also access lymph node via the afferent lymph. The dense lymphoid infiltrate of the nodal cortex tends to obscure a lattice of collagen fibrils and associated extracellular matrix components, which serves as scaffolding for the lymphocytes, supporting their further migration to specialized micorenvironments within the lymph node or to the efferent lymphatics. Interestingly, this lattice radiates from HEVs to the subcapsular sinus and has been shown to serve as a conduit for the rapid transport of soluble factors from afferent lymph to the HEVs (482). Such factors may regulate the lymphocyte recruitment activity of the HEVs in response to inflammatory–immune stimuli in the tissues. The physiology and molecular basis of lymphocyte homing are described in more detail in a subsequent section.

The cortex can be broadly divided into two structural and functional regions: the aforementioned T and B zones (481,483) (see Figs. 4 and 5). In lymph node, the B zones, as their name implies, consists of predominantly (but not exclusively) B-lymphocytes arranged in distinct nodules, or follicles. Non–B-cell components of the follicles include a scaffolding of so-called follicular dendritic reticulum cells (FDCs), specialized macrophages (tingible body macrophages), and a minority of T cells, predominantly CD4$^+$ memory–effector cells (see below). These follicles can be morphologically subdivided into two categories, designated primary and sec-

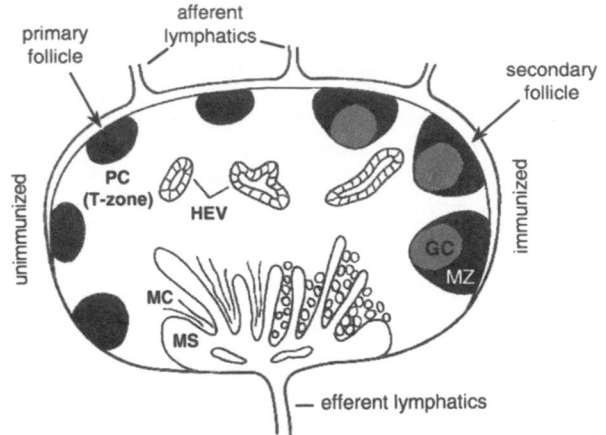

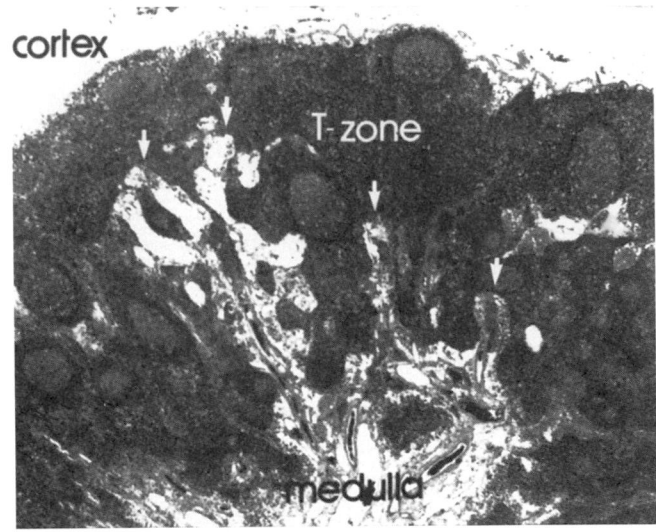

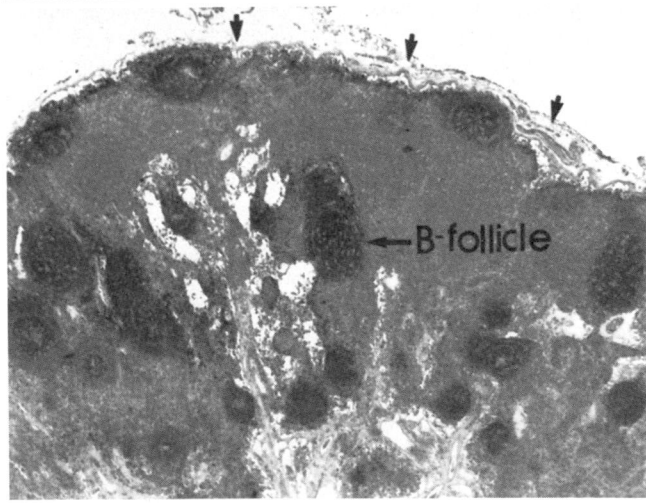

FIG. 4. Architecture of the lymph node I. **Top:** Schematic representation of lymph node structure. Afferent (incoming) lymphatic vessels empty into the convex aspect of the lymph node adjacent to the lymph node cortex. This cortex consists of the predominantly B-lineage lymphoid follicles and the predominantly T-lineage paracortex (*PC;* also called the T zone). In a resting (unimmunized) lymph node, primary follicles (*left*), composed of resting B cells, are the predominant lymphoid follicle. However, following immunization, secondary follicles (*right*), composed of activated germinal center (*GC*) B cells surrounded by resting mantle-zone (*MZ*) B cells, predominate. Within the paracortex are the specialized high endothelial venules (*HEVs*) that function in lymphocyte (particularly naive lymphocyte) recruitment. The lymph node medulla consists of alternating medullary cords (*MC*), which in an immunized lymph node are typically filled with plasma cells (**right**), and medullary sinuses (*MSs*), which coalesce to form the outgoing "efferent" lymphatic vessels. **Middle and Bottom:** Serial sections of an antigen-stimulated human lymph node stained with H&E (middle) or immunostained with a B lineage–specific monoclonal antibody (*bottom*). *White arrows* in the H&E-stained section delineate dilated medullary sinuses that, in this example, extend well up into the cortex. Within the medulla, these dilated sinuses join to form large efferent lymphatic vessels. Dilated veins (containing dark-appearing erythrocytes) can also be observed in this region. Note the numerous B-lineage follicles dispersed throughout the cortex. The *dark arrows* in the lower photomicrograph indicate the fibrous lymph node capsule, directly underneath which is a slitlike space that corresponds to the marginal (or subcapsular) sinus. Afferent lymphatics (which are not visible in these sections) empty into this sinus. Antigens present in the afferent lymph must percolate through the lymphocyte-rich cortex before entering the medullary sinuses and efferent lymphatics.

ondary follicles (see Fig. 5). The former is composed of small, resting B cells associated with a loose network of FDC processes, whereas the latter contains an inner region of activated B cells associated with a relatively dense network of FDCs and scattered tingible body macrophages (the germinal center), surrounded by a rim of resting B cells and loose FDCs identical to those in primary follicles (the mantle zone). Characteristically, these structures are located in

the upper cortex immediately subjacent to the subcapsular sinus, but they may be present anywhere in the cortex. The number of follicles in a given lymph node and the relative percentage of primary versus secondary follicles is highly dependent on the immune status of the lymph node in question. Resting lymph nodes (those with little or no immunogen influx) may have only a few scattered primary follicles, whereas immunized lymph nodes may have an expanded cortex

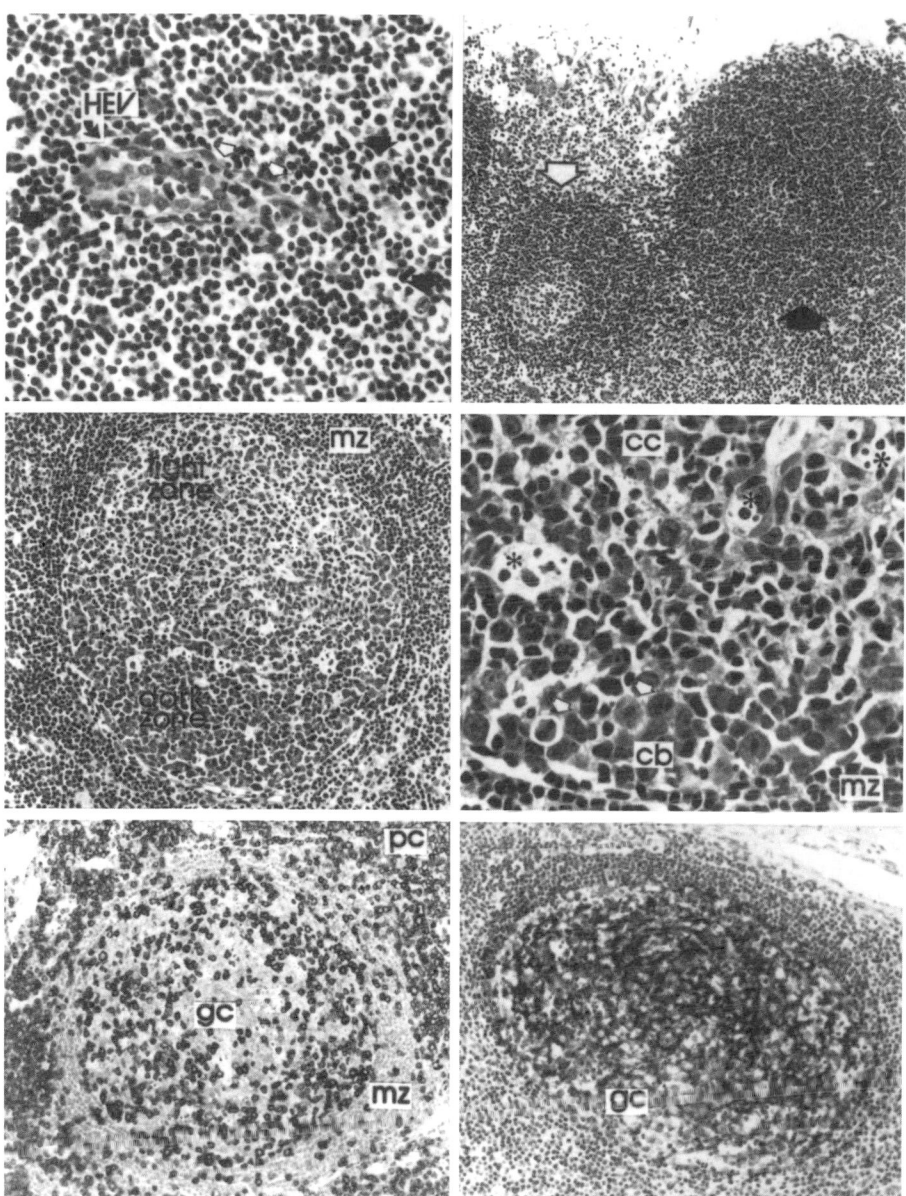

FIG. 5. Architecture of the lymph node II. **Top, left:** Close-up view of the paracortex of an antigen-stimulated human lymph node (H&E-stained) showing a high endothelial venule (*HEV*) with transmigrating lymphocytes (*small white arrows;* note the small, dark-staining lymphocyte nuclei within the endothelium or between the endothelium and perivascular spindle cells). Most of the paracortical cells are small resting lymphocytes (predominantly T cells), but occasional lymphoid blasts (*large dark arrows,* most likely T blasts) are also observed. **Top, right:** Subcapsular cortex, containing a primary B-cell follicle (*dark arrow*), and an adjacent early germinal center (*white arrow*) in which primary follicle B cells (now forming a mantle zone) are pushed apart by proliferating germinal center blasts. These germinal center cells have not yet polarized into light and dark zones that characterize the mature germinal center (H&E stain). **Middle, left:** A mature germinal center surrounded by a somewhat attenuated mantle zone (*mz*). Polarization into a centroblast-containing dark zone and a centrocyte-containing light zone is easily discerned (H&E stain). **Middle, right:** A higher power view of the same germinal center, showing the interface between the dark and light zones. Centroblasts (*cb*) are uniformly large cells with round nuclei containing open chromatin and prominent nucleoli. Nearly all of these cells are cycling, and numerous mitotic figures are present (*white arrows*). Centrocytes (*cc*) are more variably sized B cells that have irregular, often "cleaved" nuclei with condensed chromatin and absent or relatively inconspicuous nucleoli. These cells arise from the proliferating centroblasts but are not thought to proliferate themselves. Just inside the light zone, at the light zone–dark zone border, numerous tingible body macrophages (*) are seen. These cells contain the phagocytosed remains of apoptotic centrocytes. **Bottom, left:** A germinal center immunostained with a T cell–specific monoclonal antibody. Although a minority population, darkly stained T cells (almost all CD4+/CD45RA-/RO+ memory–effector, class II MHC–restricted helper cells) are not infrequent within the germinal center (*gc*), they are, however, relatively fewer in the mantle zone (*mz*). The paracortex (*pc*) contains a great majority of T cells, which, in contrast to the germinal center, are an admixture of memory–effector versus naive and CD4+ versus CD8+ T cells. **Bottom, right:** A germinal center immunostained with a follicular dendritic cell (*FDC*)–specific monoclonal antibody. The darkly stained dendritic processes of the FDC are clearly apparent in this photomicrograph.

nearly filled with secondary follicles. Between the follicles lies the paracortex, with its predominance of T-cells (CD4$^+$ T cells usually about threefold more numerous than the CD8$^+$ subset), and characteristic HEVs. The paracortex is also rich in a type of dendritic cell (distinct from the FDC mentioned above), termed *interdigitating cells*, after the manner in which their dendritic processes insinuate between adjacent lymphocytes. The functional interrelationship of these microenvironments in the manifestation of cellular and humoral immune responses is described in detail below.

The structural organization of the mucosa-associated secondary lymphoid tissues varies somewhat from site to site, but overall these tissues are highly analogous to each other and to lymph node (17,484,485). The major differences between these sites and lymph node concern the mechanism by which these lymphoid tissues are exposed to antigen: In mucosal secondary lymphoid tissues, antigen influx occurs across a mucosal epithelium, rather than through afferent lymph. Secondary lymphoid tissue may be associated with virtually any organ containing a mucosal surface in contact with the outside world, including the gastrointestinal, pulmonary, and genitourinary tracts. However, the relative distribution of these structures is highly species-dependent. For example, in humans, about 1,000 individual Peyer's patch structures (small intestinal secondary lymphoid tissues) are concentrated in the terminal ileum. In contrast, mice and rats display 2 to 11 relatively larger Peyer's patches that are uniformly distributed throughout the small intestine, and in pigs, coalescent Peyer's patches comprise nearly all of the surface epithelium in the distal 100 cm of ileum (486). Similarly, bronchus-associated secondary lymphoid tissue is a prominent, constitutive lymphoid tissue in rabbits, but not in humans (487). This heterogeneity likely results from species-specific differences in environmental conditions that dictate the usual kind and location of antigen to which the body is exposed (e.g., the character and distribution of normal intestinal flora). The size and distribution of mucosa-associated secondary lymphoid tissues is also dependent on the individual organism's history of antigen exposure. As mentioned above, chronic inflammatory stimuli can lead to the *de novo* appearance of otherwise typical secondary lymphoid tissue structures in mucosal, as well as nonmucosal, sites.

The secondary lymphoid tissue within mucosal organs is usually situated within the lamina propria, the highly vascularized connective tissue immediately subjacent to the mucosal epithelium, but may extend into deeper layers (17). Like the lymph node, these tissues demonstrate clearly demarcated B follicles surrounded by a T zone analogous to lymph node paracortex (Fig. 6), including the presence of HEVs. These structures clearly differentiate mucosa-associated secondary lymphoid tissue from normal or recently inflamed lamina propria (tertiary lymphoid tissue; see below), which have lymphoid components (predominantly effector elements) arrayed in a diffuse pattern without morphologically obvious organization. The mucosal epithelium overlying these secondary lymphoid sites appears to be specially modified for immune function, specifically the uptake and transport of luminal antigens across the epithelium. In the small intestinal Peyer's patch, these specialized epithelial cells, designated M cells (microfold cells; after the characteristic morphology of their luminal surface), have been reported to be capable of transporting particles ranging in size from proteins to intact microorganisms from the lumen to the underlying lymphoid tissue (486). Plexuses of lymphatic capillaries surround mucosal secondary lymphoid tissues and serve to transport lymphocytes and accessory cells, as well as antigen, to draining lymph nodes and, ultimately, the thoracic duct.

The largest lymphoid tissue of the body is the spleen, accounting for about 25% of the body's lymphocytes (488). Blood flow through the spleen is immense relative to its size: This 100- to 150-g organ in humans (< 0.3% of body weight) receives about 200 to 300 mL per minute (about 5% of cardiac output) (489). The bulk of this blood flow percolates through the splenic red pulp—that part of the spleen that functions as a general filter, removing particulate matter and damaged erythrocytes from the circulation (17,490,491). However, this blood flow also supplies the other, more immunologic compartment of the spleen with both antigen and lymphocytes. This compartment, the white pulp [accounting for about 15% of the splenic parenchyma in humans (490)], is the splenic version of secondary lymphoid tissue, and constitutes the major initiator of immune responses against blood-borne antigens (492,493). Like the other secondary lymphoid tissues discussed previously, the white pulp is segregated into B and T zones organized around their supply of antigen and lymphocytes. This organization, however, is somewhat modified from lymph node and Peyer's patch and therefore warrants separate description (17,490, 493,494) (Fig. 7).

The splenic artery enters the spleen at its hilum and immediately branches into smaller trabecular arteries, which in turn branch into even smaller central arteries. These central arteries course through the splenic parenchyma, eventually branching into penicilliary arterioles, which empty into the red pulp. Investing the central arteries and penicilliary arterioles is a concentric cuff of lymphocytes, the great majority of which are T cells. These cuffs, termed the *periarterial lymphatic sheaths* (PALS), constitute the T zones of the spleen. Periodically, usually at arterial branch points, B-lineage lymphoid follicles, either primary or secondary, appear as outgrowths of the PALS. These follicles are structurally identical to their counterparts in other secondary lymphoid tissues. Surrounding the primary follicle or mantle zone of the secondary follicle (and the PALS in rodents) is the marginal zone. Although not unique to the spleen, this lymphoid compartment is uniquely prominent and constitutively present in this organ (see below). The marginal zone contains both B and T cells (usually a majority of the former; see Fig. 7) and is thought to be the site in which splenic B and T cells initially encounter blood-borne antigens (493). Indeed, the marginal zone appears to be a primary site of entry of both B and T lymphocytes into the white pulp. The spleen lacks HEVs, but it is thought that specialized marginal zone sinuses (which are supplied by small arteriolar branches of the central arteries) subserve an analogous function to the HEVs in other secondary lymphoid sites (490). The marginal zone has also been reported to be a localization site for at least some of the memory B cells generated during a primary immune response (495,496) (see below). Marginal zones are not morphologically conspicuous components of secondary lymphoid tissues other than spleen; however, there is evidence to suggest that B-cell regions analogous to the marginal zone can be detected in both lymph node and mucosa-associated secondary lymphoid tissues, especially under conditions of immune activation (497,498).

Secondary Lymphoid Tissue Function: Production of Memory–Effector Lymphocytes

Newly produced lymphocytes, exported to the peripheral immune system from primary lymphoid tissues, are capable of recognizing and initiating an immune response to their cognate antigen, but effector responses to such primary immunizations are slow and less effective than those that are observed after reimmunization (secondary

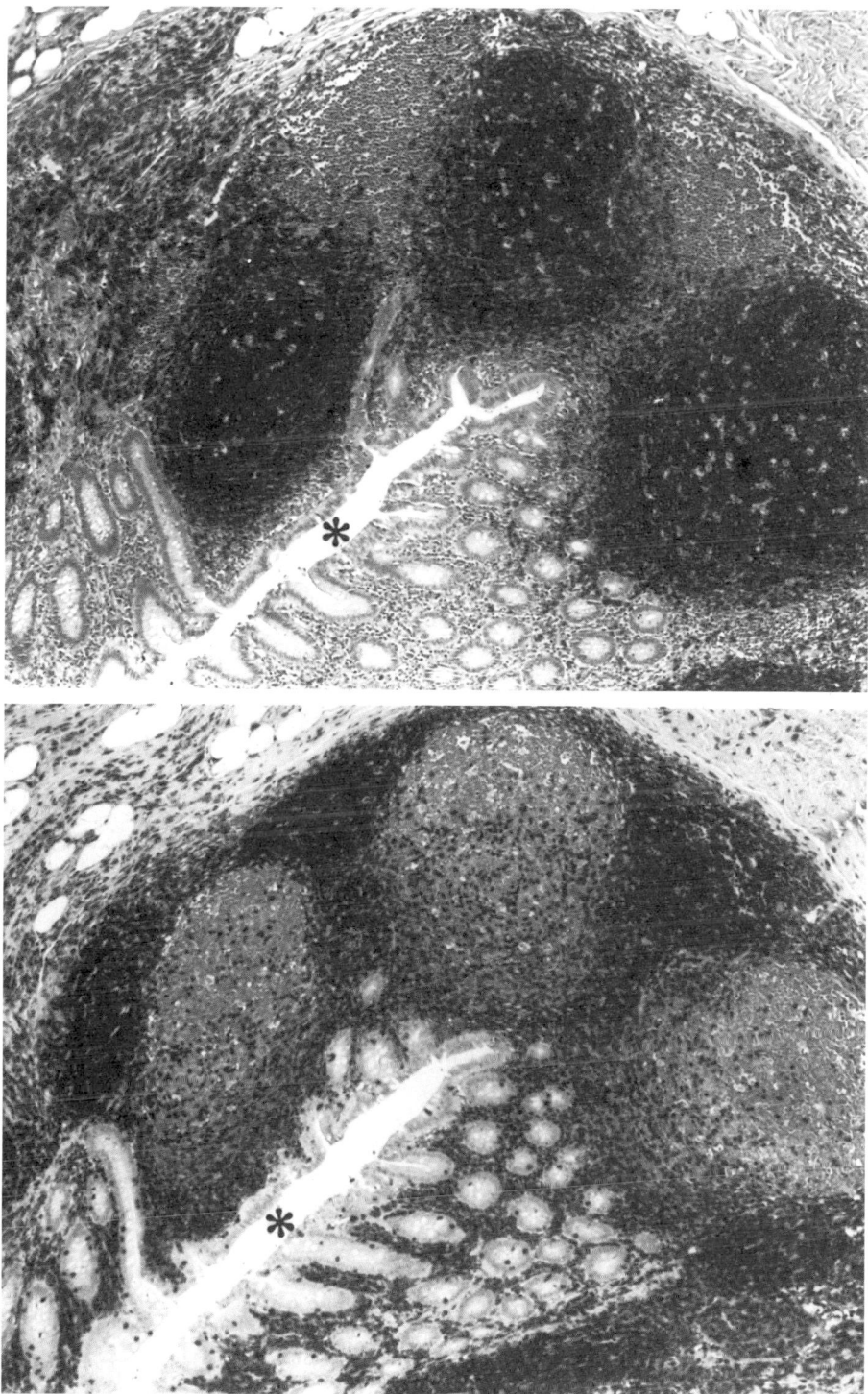

FIG. 6. Architecture of mucosa-associated secondary lymphoid tissues. A human appendix immunostained with B lineage–specific (**top**) versus T lineage–specific (**bottom**) monoclonal antibodies (the *asterisk* represents the appendiceal lumen; note the appendiceal epithelium and glands) demonstrates the juxtaposition of B-lineage (almost exclusively secondary follicles in the continually antigen-exposed appendix) and T-lineage zones that characterize secondary lymphoid tissues. HEVs are present in the T zone of this tissue but are not apparent at the low magnification shown.

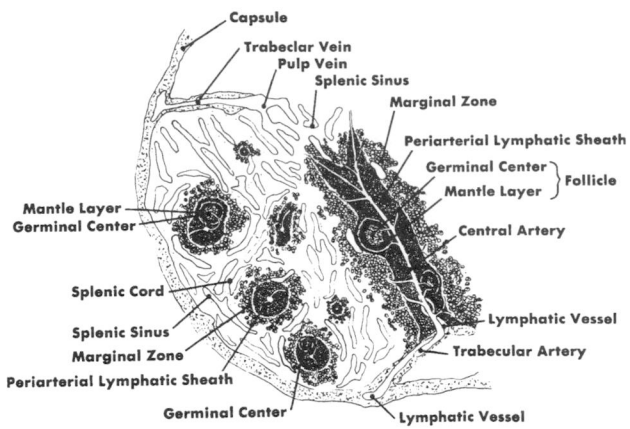

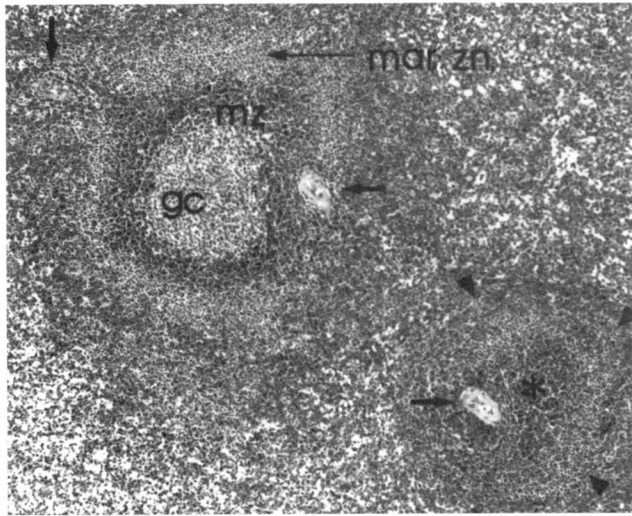

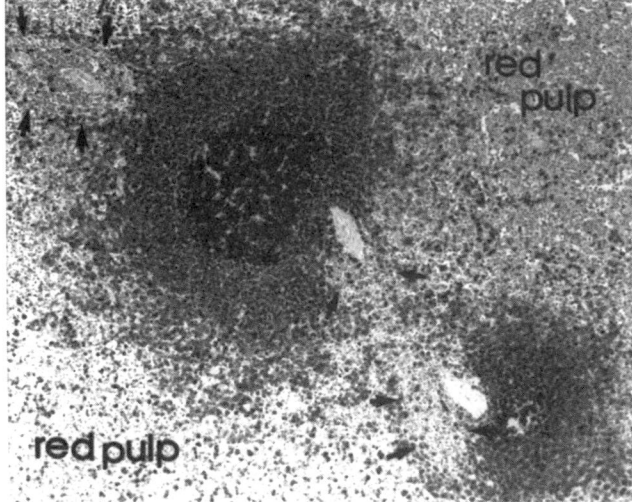

FIG. 7. Architecture of the spleen. **Top:** Schematic representation of the spleen (From Weiss L, Tavassoli M. Anatomic hazards to the passage of erythrocytes through the spleen. *Semin Hematol* 7:372, 1970, with permission). **Middle and Bottom:** Serial sections of an antigen-stimulated human spleen stained with H&E (middle) or immunostained with a B lineage–specific monoclonal antibody (**bottom**). Three penicilliary arterioles (*small arrows,* middle panel) with adjacent white pulp are shown. The periarteriolar lymphatic sheaths—the splenic T zones—are best seen in the lower photomicrograph, where they stand out in negative relief (*small arrows*) against the darkly stained B-cell areas. The B-cell area between the uppermost and middle arterioles demonstrates the classic arrangement of a germinal center (*gc*) within its mantle zone (*mz*), which is, in turn, within the marginal zone (*marg. zn.*). In the white pulp adjacent to the lowermost arteriole, the cut of the section misses the germinal center, revealing only the mantle zone (*) and surrounding marginal zone (*arrowheads*).

immunization) with the same antigen. This enhanced response to subsequent encounters with the same antigen has been termed a *memory response,* and it is demonstrable for both B cell– and T cell–mediated processes (15). As will be described below, the available data indicate that while the cellular and molecular basis of memory responses differs between the B and T lineages, it is clear that for both lineages, the enhanced vigor and effectiveness of secondary

responses has two components: (a) a quantitative component reflecting an increased population of lymphocytes specific for the immunizing antigen, and (b) of likely more importance, a qualitative component reflecting antigen-driven differentiation of the naive lymphocytes to specially adapted memory–effector cells. (The effector cell of the B lineage—the plasma cell—is easily distinguishable from the small memory B cell or memory B blast; memory and effector T-cell populations are, to the best of our knowledge, largely overlapping on the cellular level, leading to the combined designation of memory–effector.) For T-lymphocytes, both the proliferative and differentiative components of the naive- (or virgin) T-cell-to-memory–effector T-cell transition occur in the T zones of secondary lymphoid tissues and involve epigenetic changes in (a) activation apparatus, (b) effector machinery (including the ability to secrete cytokines or mediate cellular lysis), and (c) homing capabilities (see below), but not, for the vast majority of T cells, in their antigen-recognition capability [i.e., there generally do not appear to be postthymic changes in the TCR repertoire (15,16,499,500)]. For B-lymphocytes, the naive-to-memory–effector transition is even more profound, involving their differentiation into distinct memory and effector subsets (plasma cells), as well alterations in the genetic structure of their antigen receptor–effector molecules (immunoglobulins) that increase its affinity for antigen (so-called affinity maturation) as well as its effector capability (i.e., the Ig class switch to functionally specialized isotypes). As will be described in detail, peripheral B-cell maturation initiates in the T zones of secondary lymphoid tissues, but then translocates to the specialized microenvironment of the germinal center.

T-Cell Differentiation in Secondary Lymphoid Tissues

As was the case with T- or B-cell maturation in primary lymphoid tissues (described previously), analysis of the differentiative changes that occur during the naive-to-memory–effector transition in secondary lymphoid tissues has been greatly facilitated by the development of functional criteria and phenotypic markers, which correlate with a given T cell's maturational status. In mature human immune systems, peripheral T cells, both CD4$^+$ and CD8$^+$, can be separated into two major subsets—naive versus memory–effector—by a constellation of correlated functional and phenotypic features, including (a) activation requirements, (b) effector function (e.g., cytokine synthesis), (c) homing behavior, (d) adhesion function, and (e) cell surface phenotype. The putative naive subset, which predominates in immature (i.e., neonatal) immune systems (Fig. 8) and resembles the most mature thymocytes (501–503), demonstrates (a) little or no response to recall antigens (502, 504–506); (b) little or no ability to produce effector cytokines such as interferon-γ (IFN-γ) or IL-4 (507–512); (c) high costimulatory requirements for TCR-mediated activation (513–515); (d) inefficient maturation into MHC-restricted cytotoxic T cells (516,517); (e) efficient in vivo localization in secondary lymphoid tissues but not tertiary sites (518–521); (f) relatively low susceptibility to apoptosis (522,523) and, corresponding to these functional characteristics, (g) a predominance of the high-molecular-weight (low-activity) RA isoforms of the CD45 protein tyrosine phosphatase (524–531); (h) uniform low expression of many general adhesion molecules, such as CD11a/CD18 (LFA-1), CD54 (ICAM-1), CD2, CD58 (LFA-3), and CD44, the apoptosis-triggering molecule CD95/FAS (523), and the tertiary site (skin)–selective homing receptor CLA (501,502,524,531–534); (i) uniform high expression of the peripheral lymph node homing receptor L-selectin and the costimulatory molecule CD27 (501,535,536); and (j) uniform moderate expression of the Peyer's patch homing receptor α4β7 integrin (531,537).

In contrast, the memory–effector subset, which contains the vast majority of cells capable of responding to recall antigens and can be generated in vitro from the aforementioned naive subset following appropriate activation (509,526,538), predominantly expresses the

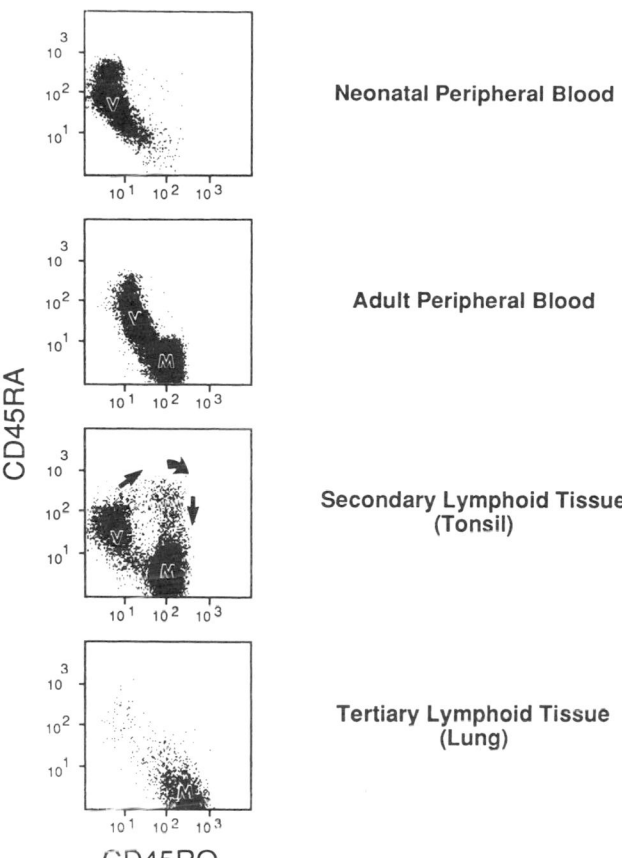

FIG. 8. The distribution of the CD45RA$^+$/RO$^{-\text{ to low}}$ virgin (*v*) versus the CD45RA$^-$/RO^{high} memory–effector (*m*) T-cell subsets in human blood and lymphoid tissues, as demonstrated by multiparameter (three-color) flow cytometry (CD3, CD45RA, and CD45RO). The cells shown (each black dot represents a single cell) were gated on the CD3$^+$ population within these specimens and are thus pure T cells. In keeping with their relative immunologic experiences, T cells from neonatal peripheral blood are essentially all of the virgin subset, whereas adult peripheral blood T cells show a roughly equal admixture of both virgin and memory–effector cells. Both subsets are represented in (postnatal) secondary lymphoid tissues such as the tonsil, but in addition, a CD45RA$^+$/RO$^+$ transitional subset is observed. Both in vitro and in vivo, stimulated virgin T cells "mature" through intermediate stages in the direction of the arrows as they convert to the memory–effector phenotype (526). The vast majority (usually 90% to 95%) of T cells within tertiary sites, such as the pulmonary T cells shown here, have the memory–effector phenotype. (Note: CD8$^+$ memory T cells with an "inverted" CD45RA$^+$/RO^{low} phenotype are negligible in these profiles.)

low-molecular-weight (high-activity) RO CD45 isoform (although some putative memory CD8$^+$ T cells are CD45RA expressing; see below) and shows efficient effector function (production of effector cytokines, cytotoxicity), increased CD95/FAS expression, and increased susceptibility to apoptosis, high levels of CD11a/CD18 and the other general adhesion molecules listed above, and heterogenous expression of the L-selectin, α4β7 integrin, and CD27 (same references as above). Most significantly, memory–effector cells differ from their phenotypically and functionally homogeneous naive predecessors by their extraordinary functional heterogeneity (see Figs. 9 and 16). As will be discussed in more detail, the overall

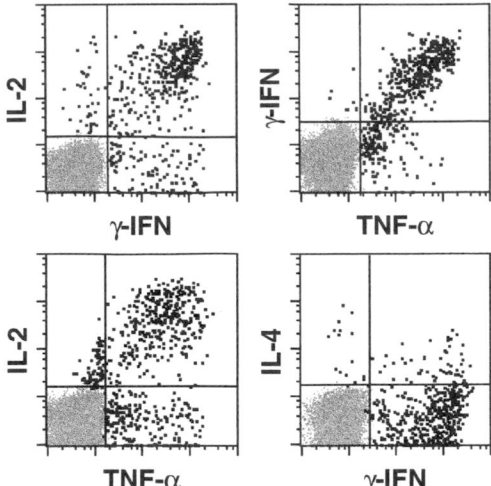

FIG. 9. Memory T cells are heterogenous with respect to the cytokines they are capable of producing upon stimulation with specific antigen. Here, the response of CD4+ memory T cells to cytomegalovirus is shown using flow cytometric evaluation of cytokine synthesis in cytomegalovirus-stimulated, secretion-inhibited T cells (secretion inhibition retains synthesized cytokine inside the cells so that it can be specifically stained). Each *black* or *gray dot* represents a CD4+ T cell (45,000 total are shown), with the *enlarged, black dots* representing the responding fraction. Note that while the majority of responding cells simultaneously produce γ-IFN, TNF-α, and IL-2, there are subsets of responding cells producing these cytokines and IL-4 in virtually all possible combinations. Such cytokine profiles would be expected to vary for each type of antigen; for example, T cells responding to an allergen in an allergic individual would likely show a much higher proportion of IL-4 production among the responding cells.

memory–effector T-cell population is composed of myriad subsets with distinct functional potential, including heterogeneity in such key functional attributes as homing–migratory behavior, cytokine synthesis–secretion capabilities, and possibly their activation thresholds. The TCR repertoire of the memory–effector subset is antigen-selected [(500); see below] but, with rare exceptions (539), is not structurally changed during the naive-to-memory–effector transition (in contrast to B cells) and is therefore a subset of the original thymus-selected naive T-cell repertoire.

The specific markers of memory–effector T-cell differentiation described above largely apply to the human, but it is clear that an analogous naive–memory T-cell dichotomy exists in animal, particularly rodent, models as well (540). The phenotypic definition of these subsets in the mouse and rat remains somewhat less well defined than in the human because of (a) the fewer (relative to the human system) markers available and (b) species-specific differences in the regulation of many markers that have been examined. For example, although rodents produce CD45 isoforms similar to those produced by humans, the regulation of these isoforms relative to T-cell maturation and function appears to differ from that of humans (541,542); thus, care must be taken with any *detailed* cross-species extrapolation of naive-to-memory–effector marker paradigms. For any species, it should be noted that the differentiation between naive and memory–effector T cells cannot be made reliably on the basis of only one or two phenotypic markers, but must rest on the composite phenotype of the cells in question. For example, it has been widely assumed that expression of the RA and RO isoforms of CD45 always differentiates naive and mem-

ory–effector T cells, respectively, in the human. While this remains generally true for CD4+ T cells, data indicate that a significant proportion of CD8+ memory T cells may reverse their expression of these isoforms (e.g., assume a CD45RA+/RO− phenotype), yet retain other phenotypic and functional characteristics of memory cells (531,543–545).

The existence of memory–effector lymphocyte functional heterogeneity was first demonstrated, although not widely appreciated, in studies of lymphocyte homing in the 1970s and early 1980s (7,520,546). These studies demonstrated that certain lymphoid subsets, now classifiable as memory–effector subsets (both T and B lineage), exhibit differential migration to mucosal versus peripheral sites upon intravenous injection. More work has confirmed these early studies, indicating that both homing receptor expression and homing behavior (to both secondary and tertiary sites) are highly heterogenous among memory–effector T cells (see the section on homing, below). However, widespread appreciation of memory T-cell functional specialization awaited the discovery of cytokine synthesis heterogeneity among these cells in the late 1980s (547). The first studies described distinct cytokine synthesis–secretion patterns among various cloned murine CD4+ T cells. Two general patterns were observed: (a) the TH1 pattern, characterized by IL-2, IFN-γ, and TNF-β production; and (b) the TH2 pattern, characterized by IL-4, IL-5, IL-6, IL-10 (and later IL-13) production (548,549). The physiologic relevance of these TH1 and TH2 clones was suggested by the demonstration of polarized TH1- and TH2-like cytokine responses in different *in vivo* situations that often correlated with immune protection against different infectious agents (547,550, 551). Analogous, although not identical, patterns of cytokine expression were demonstrated with human CD4+ T-cell clones, and cytokine polarization was also documented in human inflammatory or hypersensitivity sites *in vivo* (552–558). More recently, the availability of multiparameter flow cytometric techniques that can simultaneously assess production of multiple cytokines in single, freshly isolated, short-term activated memory–effector T cells has revealed considerably more complexity in cytokine-secretion patterns than suggested by the TH1/TH2 paradigm [(506,511,559); see Fig. 9]. These studies indicate that although there are definitely preferred or predominant patterns of cytokine synthesis, at least a small proportion of cells manifesting virtually all possible patterns of cytokine synthesis (e.g., combinations of the various cytokines) could be detected within the overall CD4+ memory–effector T-cell population, a finding suggesting that regulation of the synthesis of each cytokine is potentially independent. Finally, it should be noted that studies have indicated that cytokine synthesis is a critical effector function of CD8+ T cells as well [playing a key role, for example, in the control of many noncytopathic viruses (560,561)], and that cytokine synthesis heterogeneity analogous to that observed in CD4+ memory–effector T cells is also exhibited by the CD8+ memory–effector population (562–564).

Taken together, these data indicate a critical differentiative pathway, starting with naive, functionally limited T cells and leading to functionally heterogeneous memory–effector T cells that have both potent effector capabilities and the capacity to migrate to extralymphoid sites of inflammation. Since naive T cells localize predominantly, if not exclusively, in secondary lymphoid tissues, it follows that the naive-to-memory–effector differentiation pathway occurs (or at least initiates; see below) in these sites. In keeping with this, phenotypic and functional transitions between naive and memory–effector T cells have been observed in secondary lymphoid tissues in both mice and humans (500,526,565) and, essentially, only in these sites (see Fig. 8). Moreover, if naive T-cell migration to lymph node is significantly blocked (e.g., in the L-selectin knock-out mouse), topically applied antigens cannot sensitize for a cutaneous T cell–mediated hypersensitivity reaction, despite clear evidence that the T cells are otherwise capable of differentiating into appropriate effector cells (566).

This naive-to-memory–effector differentiative pathway differs from that occurring in primary lymphoid tissues in that it is *antigen driven.* In the absence of antigen, the naive T-cell subset is thought to comprise a stable population of long-lived cells, which are thought to continuously migrate between the various secondary lymphoid tissues (329,518,567). Once they encounter their cognate antigen associated with appropriate antigen-presenting cells, naive T cells are activated and are simultaneously induced to proliferate

and undergo the coordinate phenotypic and functional changes associated with the naive-to-memory–effector transition (Fig. 10). The microenvironmental conditions presiding over this naive-cell activation differentially regulate the naive-to-memory–effector differentiation process, generating the memory–effector T-cell functional heterogeneity discussed above (520,521,547). It is clear that signals delivered to the activated naive T cell by specific cytokines or by cell–substrate or cell–cell adhesion events (the latter often referred to as costimulation) determine patterns of homing-receptor expression, cytokine synthesis capabilities, and, perhaps, activation threshold–costimulatory requirements of the resultant memory T cells. For example, the cytokine IL-12 promotes the differentiation of memory–effector T cells that produce high levels of IFN-γ upon restimulation, whereas IL-4 promotes the differentia-

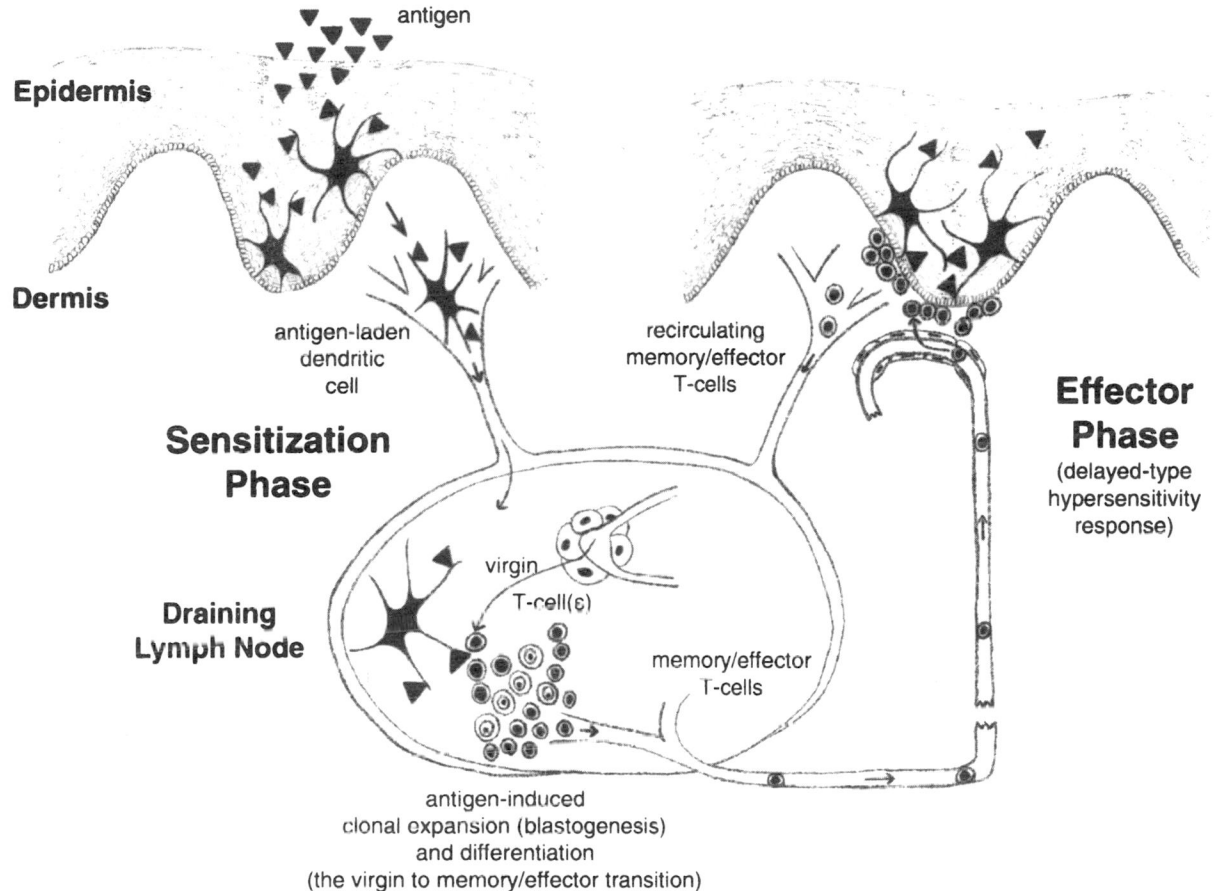

FIG. 10. The production of T-cell immune effector responses requires the cooperative function of both secondary and tertiary lymphoid sites. The elicitation of a delayed-typed hypersensitivity response to an epidermally applied (contact) antigen is illustrated. Epidermal dendritic cells take up antigen and transport it to draining lymph nodes, where it is presented to antigen-specific virgin (naive) T cells (which have entered the lymph node via high endothelial venules). Historically, these mobile dendritic cells have been given different names depending, on their location—in the skin, they are called Langerhans' cells; in the lymph, veiled cells; and in the T zone of the lymph node, interdigitating cells—but these are indeed the same cells at different stages of their functional lives. Under the influence of the lymph node microenvironment, antigen-stimulated virgin (naive) T cells are induced to proliferate and to undergo maturation changes, such as the gain of complex effector capabilities and the ability to selectively migrate to tertiary sites—the virgin to memory–effector transition. These memory–effector T cells can then migrate to the skin and, via production of cytokines or direct contact with other cell types, elicit the inflammatory changes that characterize the delayed-type hypersensitivity response. It should be noted that extravasation into the cutaneous inflammatory site is not antigen-restricted; any memory–effector cell with appropriate homing receptors can be recruited, and the antigen-specific memory effector T cells (upon whose function the response depends) are a small minority of the overall T-cell infiltrate.

tion of T cells that preferentially produce IL-4 (568,569) (see Chapter 26). This coordinate regulation of memory–effector T-cell function is complex and remains incompletely characterized, but it is thought that extralymphoid (tertiary) tissues within the region of the body subserved by a particular secondary lymphoid tissue (e.g., tissues within the lymphatic bed of a particular regional lymph node) can contribute regulatory elements (either soluble or cellular) that influence the functional potential of memory–effector T cells generated within that lymphoid tissue. For example, naive T cells responding to a cutaneous virus in skin-draining lymph nodes might be directed by that particular microenvironment to develop into memory–effector cells that home back to skin (329), and have the capacity to secrete a functionally appropriate (e.g., antiviral) cytokine such as IFN-γ. Such a system would allow local microenvironments to precisely tailor the nature of immune effector responses in accord with local conditions.

The physiologic basis of the unique ability of secondary lymphoid tissue T zones to mediate naive T-cell activation and differentiation is incompletely understood, but one possible explanation is the simultaneous presence of both naive T cells (which selectively migrate to these sites; see below) and a uniquely capable accessory cell population required for naive T-cell activation. Activation of both the naive and memory–effector subsets depends on recognition of antigen in the context of self MHC, either class I MHC for the CD8$^+$ T-cell subset or class II MHC for the CD4$^+$ subset. Essentially all cell types express class I MHC, and a wide variety of cell types express or can be induced to express class II MHC, but not all of these cell types have equivalent ability to appropriately process and present cognate antigen to T cells, particularly naive T cells. One cell type that stands out in this regard is the dendritic cell, a lineage or related group of lineages (570) of bone marrow–derived accessory cells characterized by their shape, lack of adherence to tissue culture surfaces and phagocytic function, high expression of MHC products, and most importantly, a unique ability to initiate T-cell responses in unprimed immune systems (256).

In a variety of *in vitro* and *in vivo* assays of accessory cell function (particularly those involving naive T cells), dendritic cells consistently demonstrate a 1 to 2 order of magnitude greater efficiency than other putative accessory cell types (571–576). For example, after *in vitro* pulsing with a protein antigen, the injection of as few as 10^5 dendritic cells effectively sensitized CD4$^+$ T cells in draining lymph node, whereas ten times as many spleen cells (predominantly B cells) or peritoneal macrophages had little or no effect (573). The basis of the potent antigen-presenting function exhibited by dendritic cells may relate to their high levels of MHC products, including both I-A and I-E in the mouse and HLA-DP,-DQ, and -DR in the human, or their (inducible) high expression of a wide of variety of cell adhesion molecules known to participate in and/or amplify T-cell activation (256,576–578), including β2 integrins, ICAM-1 (CD54; ligand for T cell LFA-1), LFA-3 (CD58; ligand for T-cell CD2), and B7-1/B7-2 (CD80/CD86; both ligands for the T-cell costimulatory molecule CD28). Dendritic cells have also been proposed to have a unique ability to capture and process antigens and then retain them for long periods in an immunogenic form (256,528,579,580). Indeed, the *in vivo* distribution and migratory properties of dendritic cells strongly support the hypothesis that these cells are highly specialized for the capture and transport of foreign antigen (256). Dendritic cells are found in blood, T zones of secondary lymphoid tissues (where they have been designated "interdigitating cells"), afferent lymph (the so-called veiled cell), skin (the Langerhans cell), and virtually all other tertiary lymphoid tissues where they have been sought (lung, gastrointestinal tract, liver, cardiac muscle). (As indicated in the section on the thymus, they are also present in this primary lymphoid tissue, where they play a critical role in the shaping of the TCR repertoire.) In studies using the fluorochrome FITC as a contact antigen, the epidermal Langerhans cell has been directly observed to collect the topically applied fluorochrome antigen and transport it, via afferent lymph, to the T zones of draining lymph nodes, where antigen-specific T responses are then initiated (579,581) (see Fig. 10). It is significant that freshly isolated antigen-exposed Langerhans cells from the skin are effective at stimulating antigen-primed, memory–effector T cells, but *not* naive T cells. However, short-term *in vitro* culture of the same antigen-exposed Langerhans cells results in the development of potent naive T cell–priming capabilities (582). Moreover, fresh Langerhans cells are far superior to cultured Langerhans cells in their ability to process native protein antigens (583). Taken together, these results suggest that while the dendritic cells in tertiary tissues are specialized for the uptake and processing of antigen, the special ability of these cells to initiate immune responses (i.e., activate naive T cells) develops as tertiary tissue dendritic cells migrate to secondary lymphoid tissue. The observation that ablation of afferent lymphatics prevents naive T-cell sensitization (584) illustrates the critical importance of the migrating, antigen-carrying dendritic cell in the initiation of immune responses. A similar role for dendritic cells in collecting antigen from the lung and intestines and then sensitizing naive T cells in regional secondary lymphoid tissues has also been demonstrated (585,586), and antigen-carrying dendritic cells in the blood have also been shown to either home to T-dependent areas of the splenic white pulp [where they appear as typical interdigitating cells and initiate splenic immune responses (587)], or to liver and then to liver-draining lymph nodes (588). Thus, these data implicate the dendritic cell as a critical link in the afferent limb of the immune response, serving as antigen-capture (and -processing) cells in the tissues, antigen transport cells in the blood and lymph, and finally antigen-presenting cells in the T zones of secondary lymphoid tissues. Dendritic cells can also function as antigen-presenting cells to memory–effector T cells in effector sites (582–584), but it is likely that other less specialized MHC-bearing accessory cells can serve in this capacity as well.

Newly produced memory–effector T cells leave their secondary lymphoid tissue of origin via the efferent lymph, ultimately to enter the blood and then to continuously migrate through tissues for which they possess appropriate homing receptors (see Fig. 10). This migration is markedly increased to tissues in which an inflammatory response is developing, and once within such tissues, encounter with specific antigen will lead to the rapid (e.g., within hours), activation of the memory cell's preprogrammed effector response. Memory T cells are known to have a heightened susceptibility to programmed cell death (apoptosis), and it is now thought that many, if not most, memory cells responding to antigen in effector sites perform their particular effector function and then die by this process (589–593). Some memory cells will survive, however, and even proliferate, ultimately to reenter the recirculating memory–effector pool. Importantly, these cells may also continue the differentiation process initiated during the first antigen encounter (e.g., the naive-to-memory–effector transition). Depending on the local array of cytokine and costimulatory signals, these memory cells may modify (or have reinforced) their original functional capabilities (520,521,569).

The long-term fate of these memory–effector T cells is less well understood. It is clear that memory T-cell responses to antigen can occur years, even decades, after antigen exposure (15), but the parameters governing the maintenance of T-cell memory, including such parameters as memory–effector T-cell lifespan and turnover, the dependence or independence of memory on continued antigen stimulation, and the stability of memory–effector T-cell phenotypes, are controversial. Studies have suggested a model of memory-cell homeostasis that may help resolve these controversies (506,521,594,595). This model proposes that the homeostasis of immunologic memory to any given antigen is dependent on the ability of the memory–effector lymphocyte(s) reactive with that antigen to compete for survival with similar cells reactive with other antigens (clonotype competition). These clones compete for access to specialized microenvironments and for the trophic or regulatory factors they provide, and their ability to compete determines the balance between cell survival, expansion, differentiation, and death. The protective niches for memory T cells are both finite and limited in their capacity to provide viability support. Thus, like in the childhood game of musical chairs, those cells "caught" outside of the appropriate niche die, particularly those encountering antigen or other activating stimuli in nonsupportive microenvironments. When supportive niches are overcrowded, competition for access is increased, and cell death will occur until a balance between cell number and supportive factors is again achieved. Conversely, when a niche is empty, the available survival factors would support the viability of most or all cells reseeding the locale until the niche is repopulated and competition is resumed. Such survival factors might include trophic signals mediated through cytokines or adhesion molecule ligation, as well as blocking factors that interfere with death-promoting signals. Indeed, it is likely that the temporal "integration" of a complex combination of microenvironmental signals determines the ultimate fate of any given memory cell.

Since the overall numbers of memory T cells appears to be relatively constant throughout most of adult life (540,596), this model implies that as new memory cells are produced from naive precursors or are expanded from preexistent memory cells, their entry into the recirculating pool involves loss of unrelated memory cells. Thus, immunologic events seemingly unrelated to a particular antigen-specific clone can impact on the homeostasis of that clone. Indeed, ultimately, it is possible that T-cell memory to a particular antigen may be lost entirely if memory T cells reactive with that antigen are "outcompeted" by memory cells arising in or expanded by subsequent antigen encounters. Antigen availability in the tissues is one of the most potent (usually positive) influences on clonal survival, and thus, the number and extent of disparate antigen encounters subsequent to any given antigen will greatly influence the homeostasis of the T cells responding to that first antigen. Whether continued access to antigen is *required* for the survival of memory T cells specific for that antigen may differ from individual to individual based on the nature and frequency of other antigen encounters—in individuals with lower overall antigen exposure, the requirement for the continued presence of a given antigen for the maintenance of memory to that antigen may be less, since competition for memory-cell survival would be less intense. Interestingly, in HIV disease, a situation in which antigen encounters are frequent and protective niches are likely decreased due to viral-mediated damage, clonal representation within the memory T-cell population can change dramatically, with selective preservation or expansion of CD4+ memory cells reactive with ubiquitous patho-

gens, such as cytomegalovirus, at the expense of memory to less pervasive pathogens, such as the mumps virus (506).

This model can be extended to provide for the establishment of tolerance to self antigens that are not present during thymic selection. For example, memory cells arising in response to a self antigen expressed by cutaneous keratinocytes (or arising to a foreign antigen, but cross-reactive with this putative self antigen) would be noncompetitive for long-term survival; such cells would migrate to skin and likely encounter this antigen in a nonsupportive microenvironment (e.g., on non–antigen-presenting cell types, without appropriate costimulation or cytokine support) and, as a consequence, undergo "peripheral" deletion via apoptosis (597).

B-Cell Differentiation in Secondary Lymphoid Tissues

In many respects, the maturational pathways followed by conventional T and B cells in secondary lymphoid tissues are highly analogous. Both lineages release naive cells into the periphery in a functionally inefficient, albeit antigen-receptive, state; both lineages have their initial contact with antigen in secondary lymphoid tissues, and both lineages require antigen-induced maturational changes at these sites for the production of efficient effectors. However, given the relatively specific primary function of the B lineage—that of producing and maintaining levels of Ig—it is not surprising that this lineage has deviated from the T-cell model in several key respects.

Perhaps the most significant difference between the maturation of B- and T-lineage immune responses is the mechanism by which their respective antigen-receptor repertoires are altered for enhanced function. As discussed, the central role of the T cell in the overall regulation of immune responses, and the peculiarities of T-cell antigen recognition (i.e., the requirement for antigen recognition in the context of self MHC), dictate that, for the most part, the T-cell antigen-receptor repertoire is shaped in the thymus, a primary lymphoid tissue, and is independent of exogenous antigen. The maturational changes induced by initial antigen contact in secondary lymphoid tissues are largely restricted to effector and homing mechanisms, and thus, the memory–effector T-cell repertoire represents an essentially unmodified subset of the virgin repertoire—those clones that have happened to encounter antigen. In contrast, the B lineage recognizes antigen directly with antigen receptors that double as effector molecules, and has the major function of producing, as quickly as possible, Ig with as high as possible affinity for antigen and functional (effector) efficiency. This antigen-recognition mechanism and unique functional mission have led to a complex, multilayered system of antigen-induced B-cell differentiation in secondary lymphoid tissues, which involves, for most antigens, *the genetic modification and selection of antigen receptors (Ig) based on antigen affinity* (15,598–601). Thus, unlike T cells, B cells are subject to an antigen-dependent *mutation* and *selection* process in secondary lymphoid tissue that is designed to increase the affinity and functional efficiency of the memory Ig repertoire (15,16). As with T-lineage repertoire selection in the thymus, B-lineage repertoire selection is a closely regulated process that is functionally linked with a specialized microenvironment—the germinal center (598–605).

The double functional imperatives of response rapidity and response efficiency (i.e., the relative affinity and functional efficiency of the secreted Ig) has led to a two-tiered system of (conventional) B-cell maturation in secondary lymphoid tissues. The initial phase (the first 3 to 4 days) of a primary antibody response (i.e., an antibody response to a new, not previously encountered, antigen) involves the rapid conversion of naive B cells into relatively short-lived plasma cells that produce genetically unmodified (relatively low-affinity) Ig, largely of the IgM isotype (598,599,604,606–609). While this initial antibody response represents only the early phase of a B-lineage response to most protein antigens (antigens that require T-cell help to activate B cells—so-called T-dependent antigens), for a variety of carbohydrate antigens that activate B cells in the absence of T-cell help (so called T-independent antigens), it may be the only response observed. These initial responses are thought to be critical in holding microbial invaders at bay during the initial stages of infection [see also the discussion of (unconventional) B-1 (Ly-1⁺) B cells, below], but they may be inadequate for complete elimination of the infectious agent or for prevention of reinfection. Fortunately, for T-dependent antigens, initial antigen contact gives rise to a second phase of antibody response that may become manifest later during the course of the serum antibody response to the initial immunization or infection (usually after days 4 to 5) or, in some instances, only after reimmunization (reinfection) with the same antigen. This second phase gives rise to (a) long-lived plasma cells that produce high-affinity (genetically modified) and high-titer, predominantly non-IgM (mostly IgG or IgA, with some IgE) antibody, and (b) memory B cells capable of differentiation into similar plasma cells in subsequent exposures to antigen (598,599,609,610). Both the high affinity of these second-phase antibody variable regions and the linkage of these variable regions with diverse, functionally specialized and efficient non-IgM constant regions combine with the high-antibody titers generated during late-phase responses to eradicate those infectious agents susceptible to humoral immunity (15). The presence of previously modified (primed) memory B cells accounts for the characteristic rapid increase in high-affinity serum Ig in secondary or later immunizations (611) that serves to prevent reinfection with many microorganisms.

Studies of peripheral B-cell function in rodent models suggest the following sequence of events in the genesis of humoral immune response to a conventional (T-dependent) antigen (Fig. 11) (2,7,598, 599,601,604,606–609,612,613). Recirculating naive, surface IgD⁺, IgM⁺ B cells enter secondary lymphoid tissues via HEVs or, in the spleen, marginal zone sinuses. In the absence of their specific antigen, these cells traverse the T zone (or marginal zone) and migrate to either primary follicles or the mantle zones of secondary follicles (resting B cells are excluded from the germinal center part of secondary follicles). Periodically, it is thought that these cells leave the primary follicle or mantle zone, reenter the circulation (either via the efferent lymph and thoracic duct or the red pulp of the spleen), and then recirculate to another primary follicle or mantle zone within secondary lymphoid tissue. It is likely that these cells continuously recirculate among secondary lymphoid sites until they either die or encounter their specific antigen while traversing the T zone (or marginal zone) of one of these sites (see section on lymphocyte homing).

The presence of antigen, either free antigen or antigen associated with interdigitating cells [not, however, antigen–antibody complexes (612)], interrupts this recirculation for those virgin B cells with the appropriate antigen specificity. These antigen-stimulated virgin B cells undergo a blastogenic response, forming the so-called primary (T-zone) B blasts (604,606,607). Many of these cells differentiate into relatively short-lived plasma cells that subsequently localize in the medullary cords of the lymph node or in the outer PALS and red pulp of the spleen. Although class switching can occur in these "extrafollicular" B blasts (604), the majority of these plasma cells produce IgM with unmodified (low-affinity) variable regions (598,599,604,606–609). These cells account for the classic "pri-

mary" IgM response mentioned earlier (that is observed in the serum the first 3 to 4 days following immunization). As intimated above, not all primary B blasts undergo this differentiation route. In the presence of T-cell help, some will continue their journey to primary follicles, where they will proliferate in response to antigen–antibody complexes on the surface of follicular DRC (598,599,605,614,615) (see below). These proliferating blasts will push apart the resting B cells of the primary follicle and ultimately form a classic secondary follicle in which the progeny of the primary B blasts form the germinal center and the original primary follicle becomes the mantle zone (see Fig. 5). Since individual (mature) germinal centers have been demonstrated to be oligoclonal, containing the progeny from one to three primary B blasts (604,607,616), there appears to be a limited window of time in which primary B blasts can enter a given germinal center and contribute to its formation; thereafter, both resting B cells and primary B blasts are excluded by unknown mechanisms. The factors that influence the primary B blast's decision point—between differentiating into a primary plasma cell or going on to form a germinal center—are largely unknown. It has been proposed that the B cells differentiating along these two pathways represent distinct lineages that are preprogrammed for differentiation in only one direction (617). However, data indicating a close structural relationship between the Ig genes of primary B blasts and B cells in adjacent germinal centers, while not ruling out this dual lineage hypothesis, suggest that primary and secondary B blasts arise from a common pool (604).

In the initial stages of germinal center formation, the follicle-colonizing B blasts proliferate extremely rapidly, with doubling times on the order of 6 to 7 hours (618). As these cells fill the follicular dendritic cell (FDC) network, they undergo a maturational change that dramatically alters the appearance of the germinal center (598,605). At one pole of the mature germinal center, the B cells continue to rapidly proliferate and retain blast morphology (note mitotic figures in Fig. 5, middle panels). These cells, called centroblasts, form the so-called dark zone of the germinal center, which is usually oriented opposite to the subcapsular sinus in lymph nodes and opposite to the mucosal surface in mucosa-associated secondary lymphoid tissues. The other pole of the germinal center—the light zone—is predominantly composed of centrocytes, a morphologically distinct B-cell type characterized by irregular, often cleaved nuclei and more condensed chromatin. DNA-labeling studies indicate that centrocytes do not themselves proliferate but, instead, arise continuously from the proliferating centroblast population (607,619). Within the light zone, close to the border with the dark zone, are situated tingible body macrophages filled with phagocytosed remains of centrocytes that have undergone a programmed cell death (apoptosis). Surviving centrocytes give rise to plasmablasts and plasma cells as well as to memory B blasts and small memory B cells. In general, these latter populations are morphologically rather inconspicuous components of the germinal center as, concomitant with their differentiation to these cell types, they migrate from the germinal center to take up residence elsewhere (see below). In the absence of further antigen injection, this germinal center structure is maintained for about 3 weeks following immunization [or longer, depending on the nature of the inciting antigen (620)], whereupon the germinal centers begin to decrease in size and ultimately lose their distinctive polarized morphology. However, as discussed below, clusters of follicular DRC (bearing the original antigen in the form of immune complex) and secondary (memory) B blasts are thought to persist for long periods after immunization, perhaps years.

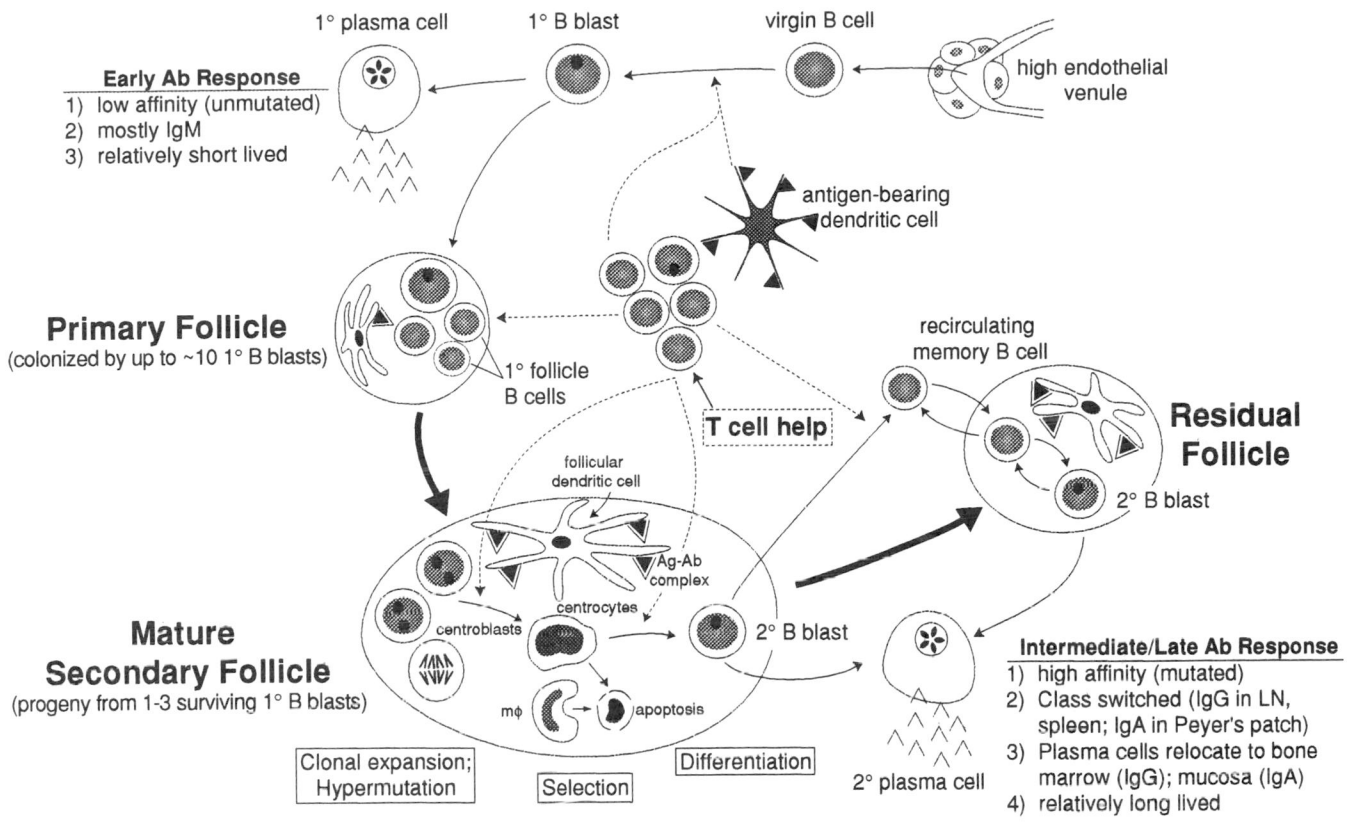

FIG. 11. A model of B-cell maturation in secondary lymphoid tissue. The schematic shown is for the B-cell response to a new, T-dependent antigen to which T-cell help is not limiting. This diagram demonstrates what is thought to occur in lymph node or mucosa-associated secondary lymphoid tissue, but with minor alterations (i. e., the entrance of virgin B cells via HEVs rather than marginal zone sinuses) is equally applicable to spleen. The sequence of events depicted in this schematic are described in detail in the text. Please note that the events shown are for the first exposure to a given antigen, although the response to reexposure to the same antigen can be extrapolated easily from this model—reimmunization would result in massive stimulation of the memory B cells (illustrated in the lower right quadrant of the diagram) and their differentiation into secondary plasma cells. Thus, the secondary antibody response is functionally equivalent to the intermediate–late phase of the primary response (high affinity–class switched) but, because of the "preformed" B cell–memory population, is much more rapid.

Centroblasts and centrocytes can be distinguished from each other and from their naive B-cell precursors and their memory B-cell and plasma cell progeny by a number of phenotypic features (621–624). For example, in the human, both centroblasts and centrocytes—but not resting naive B cells or B memory cells—express CD10 and moderately high levels of CD38, with the centroblasts expressing CD77 and the centrocytes lacking this marker. Naive B cells are IgD+/IgM+, whereas surface Ig is considerably downregulated on centroblasts. Non-IgD surface Ig is reexpressed on centrocytes and is often "switched" to non-IgM isotypes (IgG, IgA). Developing memory B cells downregulate germinal center cell markers (CD10/CD38/CD77) but can be differentiated from naive B cells by their lack of IgD. In contrast, plasma cells further upregulate CD38 but downregulate CD20 [which is present on all the other subsets; (3)], and switch from surface Ig to predominantly cytoplasmic (secretory-phenotype) Ig expression.

Thus, three major stages of differentiation characterize the mature germinal center: (a) the rapidly proliferating, surface Ig^low centroblast; (b) the nonproliferating (often dying), surface Ig+ centrocyte; and (c) the memory and effector (plasma) cell progeny of

the surviving centrocytes. The functional implications of these stages begin to become clear upon consideration that the primary function of germinal centers is thought to be the creation of an Ig repertoire that is of higher affinity for the eliciting antigen than is coded for by germline Ig gene sequences. Antigen-binding studies of primary versus secondary (postgerminal center) response antibodies indicate that a tenfold increase in affinity can develop in as little as two weeks (599,608). Comparison of Ig gene sequences from pre- and postgerminal center B cells reveals that secondary-response antibodies differ structurally from those of the primary response by virtue of specific point mutations within the antigen-binding domain (599,600,609,625). Indeed, detailed analysis of germinal center cell Ig sequences suggests that a new mutation will be introduced into the variable region of the antibody gene in nearly every division cycle [mutation rate of 10^-3 per base pair per generation (599)]. Since these mutations are random and, therefore, in most cases, will either reduce or have no impact on Ig affinity, the occurrence of affinity maturation (i.e., the production of Ig with higher affinity) would require the germinal center to have in place a mechanism by which those few cells bearing mutations resulting in higher antigen affinity could be positively selected and ultimately induced to differentiate into small memory B cells or plasma cells.

Thus, on a functional level, germinal center physiology can be conceptually divided into a four-step maturational process that closely correlates with the three morphologic–phenotypic stages described above: (a) clonal expansion (primary germinal center blasts and centroblasts), (b) Ig gene hypermutation (centroblasts), (c) clonal selection (primarily centrocytes; see below), and (d) re-differentiation to memory or effector (plasma) cells. The first two steps provide an expanded repertoire of modified antigen-specific Ig genes. The third step chooses those that are "improvements," and the fourth step "reconfigures" the improved clones into a form that is conducive to effector and/or memory function. The process of Ig class switching, which also determines final effector function, occurs in parallel with, but independent of, these three stages (604,626,627). Operationally, the four steps outlined here may be considered to occur consecutively, with two possible exceptions. First, data suggest that some "selection" may actually precede somatic hypermutation, culling primary B blasts with marginal Ig affinity for antigen. For example, it is thought that while perhaps ten primary B blasts might originally colonize a given germinal center, these clones are usually winnowed down to one to three by antigen selection prior to hypermutation initiation (likely driven by the dramatic drop in surface Ig by centroblasts) (499,628,629). Second, it is possible that centrocytes and centroblasts may cycle back and forth multiple times prior to final memory–effector differentiation (499,630), allowing clones to undergo more than one episode of hypermutation and selection before final differentiation to memory B or plasma cells.

The primary impetus for all of these processes is antigen, which initiates the clonal expansion and hypermutation of the primary blasts and centroblasts, serves as the primary selection criterion for the positive selection of centrocytes, and stimulates specific T cells to provide necessary signals for all aspects of these processes (598,599,601,614,631). It is important to note that while free antigen drives extrafollicular B-cell responses, including the recruitment of naive B cells into germinal centers, the form of antigen that operates within the germinal center is an immune complex. This distinction is highly significant for three reasons. Remember first that germinal centers form and operate long after the onset of (primary-response) antibody production. If germinal centers were to require free antigen for operation, the complexing of free antigen by the primary IgM response would bring them to a halt, thereby preventing the induction of memory cells and long-lived (high-affinity) plasma cells. Second, it is thought that competition between the (relatively low-affinity) antibody forming the immune complex and the mutated Ig on centrocytes drives the affinity maturation selection process. Centrocytes appear to be committed to death by apoptosis unless they receive positive signals through their surface Ig (605,631,632). Thus, centrocyte survival (selection) would require a cell surface Ig receptor that, by virtue of higher affinity, can out-compete the antibody in the original immune complex. As higher and higher affinity antibody is produced during the evolution of an immune response, high-affinity immune complexes will replace those of lower affinity, and thus make the centrocyte selection process even more restrictive. Finally, it should be noted that data indicate that free antigen actually induces germinal center cell apoptosis (169,633). This phenomenon has been proposed to be a mechanism by which potentially autoreactive B cells, generated during the hypermuta-

tion process, might be eliminated prior to their differentiation into memory B or plasma cells.

The differentiation process of germinal center cells is critically dependent on the function of the FDC. These cells display a heterogeneous phenotype (605,634) and have a controversial ontogenetic origin, possibly derived from either precursor stromal cells in each tissue or alternatively from bone marrow progenitors (635–637). They are not apparently related to the antigen-presenting T-zone dendritic cells described above, but interestingly, they appear to require functional T- and B-lymphoid compartments for their differentiation (638). FDCs are by no means just an inert scaffolding for germinal center B and T cells. First and foremost, these cells are highly adapted to serve as reservoirs of the antigen–antibody complexes that, as discussed above, drive the differentiation process (639). Most FDCs bear receptors for both Ig (Fc receptors) and complement component 3 (which, as a result of their intrinsic complement-activating activity, is frequently bound to the immune complex and therefore serves as an alternative mechanism by which to "trap" these molecules) and have been demonstrated to be coated with both IgM and IgG in vivo (640). FDCs are thought to be able to sequester antigen in an immunogenic form for long periods—perhaps years—making it available for the restimulation of memory cells and the maintenance of the serum antibody levels (639). These cells have been demonstrated to shed particles of membrane-associated immune complexes (called iccosomes) that can be taken up by germinal center B cells or dendritic cells and appropriately presented to antigen-specific memory–effector (helper) T cells within the follicle (641,642). DRCs express a variety of cell adhesion molecules (such as ICAM-1 and VCAM-1; ligands for the lymphocyte β2- and α4 integrins, respectively) that mediate adherence of the different germinal center B-cell subsets (615,643,644) and likely serve to maintain these subsets in the appropriate microenvironments. Finally, these cells (along with T cells; see below) are thought to express both cell surface signaling molecules and cytokines that (in addition to antigen) help maintain germinal center cell viability (i.e., prevent apoptosis) and regulate the differentiation process. Indeed, in vitro culture studies have demonstrated that germinal center B cells in physical contact with FDCs are relatively protected from apoptosis, in comparison to B cells excluded from this contact (645,646).

FDCs are not the only regulators of germinal center function. As described, germinal centers contain a distinct subset of class II MHC–restricted (CD4$^+$), memory–effector (CD45RA$^-$/RO$^+$) T cells (527,647,648), and a variety of studies indicate that germinal center formation is critically dependent on the presence of antigen- (or carrier-) specific T cells (598,605,615,644,649). These antigen-specific T cells appear to originate in the T zones of the secondary lymphoid tissue and to migrate into the nascent germinal center along with primary B-cell blasts (650,651). Within the germinal center, these T cells may be activated by antigen presented to them by either the B cells themselves or a unique subset of dentritic cells (distinct from FDCs and analogous to interdigitating cells) that have been shown to exist in this location (652). A wide variety of cytokines, many of which are produced by memory–effector T cells, have been shown to influence germinal center cell viability, proliferation, and differentiation, including class switching and terminal differentiation (601). For example, IL-4 has been implicated in promoting the isotype switching to the IgG1 and IgE isotypes, IFN-γ to IgG2a, and transforming growth factor-β to IgA (653–656). IL-5 and IL-6 have been implicated in the induction of plasma-cell differentiation and the resultant increase in Ig secretion

(656–660), and IL-10 (which may derive from T cells or the B cells themselves) has been shown to prevent germinal center B-cell death (661).

T-cell surface molecules also play a critical role in regulation of germinal center cell survival and differentiation. Perhaps the best-studied example of such regulatory T-cell molecules is CD40L, an activation-induced 33-kDa glycoprotein belonging to the TNF gene family. Its ligand is CD40, a 40-kDa member of the TNF-receptor gene family that is expressed on B cells (including germinal center cells), dendritic cells, activated macrophages, and FDCs (662–665). CD40L/CD40 interactions are required for germinal center formation, as germinal centers (and their associated functions in humoral immunity, as described above) are absent in humans or mice genetically lacking CD40L (e.g., either the human X-linked hyper IgM immunodeficiency syndrome or CD40L-/- knock-out mice). Moreover, treatment of normal mice treated with a blocking anti-CD40L antibody causes germinal centers to abruptly disappear. CD40L/CD40 interactions have been proposed to function at several levels during the germinal center reaction, including (a) induction of the critical costimulatory molecules CD80/CD86 (CD28 ligands) on antigen-presenting cells (either B cells or dendritic cells) that are required for T-cell activation, (b) stimulation of germinal center B-cell proliferation–differentiation, (c) stimulation of isotype switching, (d) rescue of germinal center B cells from apoptosis, and (e) initiation of differentiation of germinal center cells into small memory B cells (or if CD40L/CD40 interactions are terminated, shunting germinal center cell differentiation toward plasma cells) (601, 632,662–671).

These findings underscore the complexity of the germinal center microenvironment in which myriad molecular interactions are simultaneously occurring and are often directing multiple physiologic processes. This complexity is further highlighted by the finding that germinal centers in distinct tissues can regulate B-lineage memory–effector differentiation differently. The best example of such local, microenvironmental regulation of germinal centers is the functional dichotomy between mucosa- and non–mucosa-associated lymphoid tissues. Mucosa-associated lymphoid tissues, such as the Peyer's patch, are characterized by a high degree of switching to the IgA (secretory) isotype (672–676). Moreover, IgA-producing plasma cells produced at these sites migrate selectively to mucosal effector sites such as the intestinal lamina propria (7,546,677–679,762,763). [In contrast, peripheral lymph node and spleen are characterized by the production of IgG-secreting plasma cells, which migrate selectively to bone marrow, the site in which much of the body's IgG is produced (2,4,680)]. A variety of lines of evidence implicate local T cells and/or DRCs in the differential regulation of isotype switch and homing receptor expression (681–684), but it is likely that the ultimate arbitrators of this differential response are the differentiated epithelial and/or mesenchymal cells associated with the various secondary lymphoid sites (either within the lymphoid tissue itself or within the lymphatic bed of the lymphoid tissue). "Factors" produced by (or associated with) these cells may directly influence activated B cells or may serve to create a milieu that differentially supports the recruitment and/or differentiation of functionally specific T-cell or accessory-cell subtypes. Our understanding of these molecular events is truly in its infancy, but it is clear from the few tantalizing known examples of cytokine and adhesion molecule regulation of germinal center function that this specialized "local" microenvironment regulates the tempo and

outcome of secondary B-cell differentiation, just as described above for secondary T-cell differentiation.

The functional product of germinal centers is plasma cells that migrate to intestinal lamina propria or bone marrow and produce high-affinity Ig. Bone marrow cells can be quite long-lived (685,685a), but long-time maintenance of serum antibody levels suggest that these plasma cells must be renewed in some manner, long after the overt germinal center cell reaction has dissipated. As indicated above, FDCs at the site of the original germinal center can sequester antigen for long periods, and it is thought that this antigen maintains a small population of antigen-specific secondary blasts that can differentiate into additional plasma cells. These secondary blasts are likely in equilibrium with recirculating, small memory B cells, which when exposed to FDC-associated antigen (immune complex), transform into proliferating secondary blasts and then into either plasma cells or additional small memory B cells. Thus, B-cell memory has three components: 1) small recirculating memory B cells, 2) FDC-associated secondary blasts, and 3) long-lived plasma cells (4,599,686). Periodic restimulation with Ag is thought to be important for maintenance of the memory B-cell subset (687), but may not be required for long-lived plasma cells (685a).

Reimmunization of an animal with antigen (secondary immunization) results in the transient presence of free antigen (not immune complexes), which induces a rapid and massive differentiation of small memory cells into secondary blasts and plasma cells (598,610). The affinity of this secondary-response antibody reflects the mutation and selection that occurred during the original germinal center response (611). The issue of whether memory B cells can reinitiate the affinity-maturation process upon secondary of later immunizations is controversial, but it is clear that antibody affinity can increase with each successive round of antigen administration (601,602,611,688–690). Thus, either memory cells can undergo further rounds of somatic hypermutation and selection, or new naive B cells recruited into germinal centers with each subsequent antigen exposure must improve on the affinity of the previous memory response to survive the germinal center selection process (e.g., because they have to compete with high-affinity antibody for selection) (598,602).

Considered as a whole, it is clear the development and homeostasis of B-lineage responses has the same competitive elements as proposed above for the T lineage. Data suggest that naive B-cell entry into the recirculating pool is competitive (691,692), with for example, B cells reactive with self antigens being competitively excluded from primary follicles and left to die in the T zones (692). Clearly, as described, germinal center B-cell development is competitive, with only the very fittest surviving to become memory–effector cells. Less is known about the biology of memory B cells, but it is likely that these cells, like their T-cell brethren, must compete for their continued existence.

Tertiary Lymphoid Tissues: Sites of Effector Responses

The tertiary lymphoid tissues comprise all tissues of the body whose primary immunologic function is in the collection of antigen or the completion of immune effector responses. Since any tissue of the body can be a site of microbial colonization or other process requiring an immune response, it is clear that this designation would apply to essentially all tissues of the body, including, in certain pathophysiologic circumstances, classical primary or secondary lymphoid tissues. For the sake of this discussion, however, the term *tertiary lymphoid tissue* will be used to indicate sites traditionally thought of as extralymphoid, tissues with either absent or relatively small lymphoid components under normal circumstances, but which have the capability to rapidly import appropriate lymphoid and accessory populations after appropriate inflammatory "provocation."

Obviously, it is beyond the scope of this chapter to discuss in any detail the diverse histology of the myriad tertiary lymphoid tissues. However, from an immunologic perspective, this complex structure can be simplified into two compartments: (a) a vascularized connective tissue (composed of fibroblasts, histiocytes–macrophages, mast cells, and both blood and lymphatic vascular channels embedded in extracellular matrix) that is in some fashion adjacent to (b) the differentiated parenchymal cells (e.g., epithelial cells, muscle cells, nerves cells, etc.) that make up a given organ or tissue. The former compartment provides the route of lymphocyte recruitment into the tissues (and egress via lymphatics), frequently serves as a primary immunologic–inflammatory "battleground," and also plays a major role in the tissue repair that follows immune effector responses (693). The differentiated parenchymal cells of the latter compartment are not merely passive observers of these responses, but, as will be discussed below, can directly participate in the immunologic interactions leading to a productive effector response.

The most immunologically active tertiary lymphoid sites are clearly those that interface directly with the external environment—primarily the skin and the various mucosal epithelia of the gastrointestinal, pulmonary, and genitourinary tracts—and these sites serve as a paradigm for tertiary tissues as a whole. Structurally, these sites are highly analogous to each other, being composed of an epithelium—a keratinizing, stratified squamous epithelium in the case of the skin, and either a columnar, squamous, or transitional epithelium in the case of mucosal tissues—and an underlying vascularized connective tissue—the dermis versus the lamina propria (or pulmonary interstitium) (Fig. 12) (17). With a few exceptions (discussed below), the great preponderance of the lymphoid components present in these (and other) tertiary lymphoid tissues (both constitutively and under conditions of inflammation) are *memory–effector* populations (525,527–530), including CD45RA$^-$/RO$^+$ T cells, NK cells, and plasma cells (see Fig. 12; nonlymphoid effector populations, such as mononuclear phagocytes, are usually present as well). Importantly, only those subsets appropriate for a particular site or pathophysiologic process are efficiently recruited to that site. For example, intestinal lamina propria appears to selectively import plasma-cell precursors (especially IgA expressers) and a distinct subset of memory–effector T cells (7,501,674,694–696). Skin, on the other hand, generally recruits a different subset of memory–effector T cells, but (usually) fewer plasma cells or plasma cell precursors (7,695,697–699). (The physiologic and molecular basis of this differential recruitment is discussed below.)

Given the obvious importance of lymphoid effector function in tertiary tissues, it is surprising that we have so limited an understanding of these processes. Part of the problem lies in the fact that only recently has it been widely appreciated that the nonlymphoid elements of these tertiary tissues, particularly the epithelial cells, interact extensively with the lymphoid components in a manner that is not often adequately recapitulated in *in vitro* models of effector function. This point has been most convincingly demonstrated in the skin. With appropriate stimuli, both the epithelial cell

of the skin—the keratinocyte—and other cutaneous nonlymphoid elements (Langerhans cells, melanocytes, dermal fibroblasts and endothelial cells) synthesize and secrete a large variety of immunomodulatory cytokines (700–704). Keratinocytes alone have been demonstrated to produce IL-1 (α and β), -3, -6, -8, -10; TGF-α and -β; TNF-α; G and GM colony–stimulating factors; and monocyte chemotactic and activating factor (MCAF); and this is likely an incomplete list (700–704). Many of these factors play a role in the recruitment of memory–effector T cells. For example, IL-1 is a powerful inducer of the endothelial cell adhesion molecule E-selectin, (705), which selectively recruits a distinct skin-associated subset of memory–effector T cells (706). However, they also impact directly on the effector function of recruited T cells and monocytes. Moreover, T-cell cytokines can directly influence keratinocyte physiology, including growth, differentiation, factor secretion, and adhesion molecule expression (702,703,707). The ability of the (memory–effector) T-cell cytokine IFN-γ to induce the expression of class II MHC and ICAM-1 on keratinocytes (both mediating direct cell-to-cell binding–signaling between T cells and keratinocytes), as well as keratinocyte secretion of TGF-α (a powerful autocrine growth factor for keratinocytes), is but one of many examples of the complex functional interactions between the lymphoid and nonlymphoid elements of tertiary tissues (707,708). Although our understanding of these interactions is limited, the available data strongly suggest that (a) the mounting of an effective immune–inflammatory response to any pathologic stimulus is critically dependent on functional cooperation between lymphoid and nonlymphoid cell types, and (b) the character of the "fixed" nonlymphoid cell types in any given tissue (e.g., keratinocytes vs. intestinal epithelial cells) influences both the nature of the hematolymphoid cell types recruited to that site as well as the functional response of these cells once they are present.

The foregoing discussion provides a model of the immune system in which effector responses are mediated by lymphocytes that have undergone at least two prior differentiative processes: the initial development of naive cells in primary lymphoid tissues, followed by a secondary (antigen-induced) differentiation to memory–effector cells in secondary lymphoid tissue. While the available evidence suggests that this pathway characterizes the physiology of most lymphocytes ("conventional" lymphocytes) in the body, there are at least two lymphocyte subsets that deviate from this general pattern. These include (a) the B-1 B-cell subset (formerly known as the Ly-1$^+$ or CD5$^+$ B-cell subset) and (b) the unusual TCR-$\gamma\delta$ T-cell subsets that reside in epithelia. Although these subsets display antigen receptor–initiated immune function (qualifying them as true immunocytes), their overall characteristics suggest that they are the modern versions of an evolutionarily more primitive class of immunocyte—functional intermediates between the "innate" immune system (macrophages, NK cells, nonimmune antimicrobial plasma proteins, etc.) and the "adaptive" immune systems (conventional lymphocytes). These subsets appear to leave the primary lymphoid tissues at a very early stage of development, with subsequent maturation and function in distinct tertiary tissue microenvironments (omitting the intermediate differentiative step in secondary lymphoid tissues that characterizes conventional lymphocyte subsets).

The B-1 B-cell subset (found in both mouse and human, but primarily characterized in the former system) was initially defined by expression of the Ly-1 (CD5) antigen, although it is now thought that some members of this subset can lack this marker (709–714). However, B-1 B cells as a group can be recognized by their unique sig-

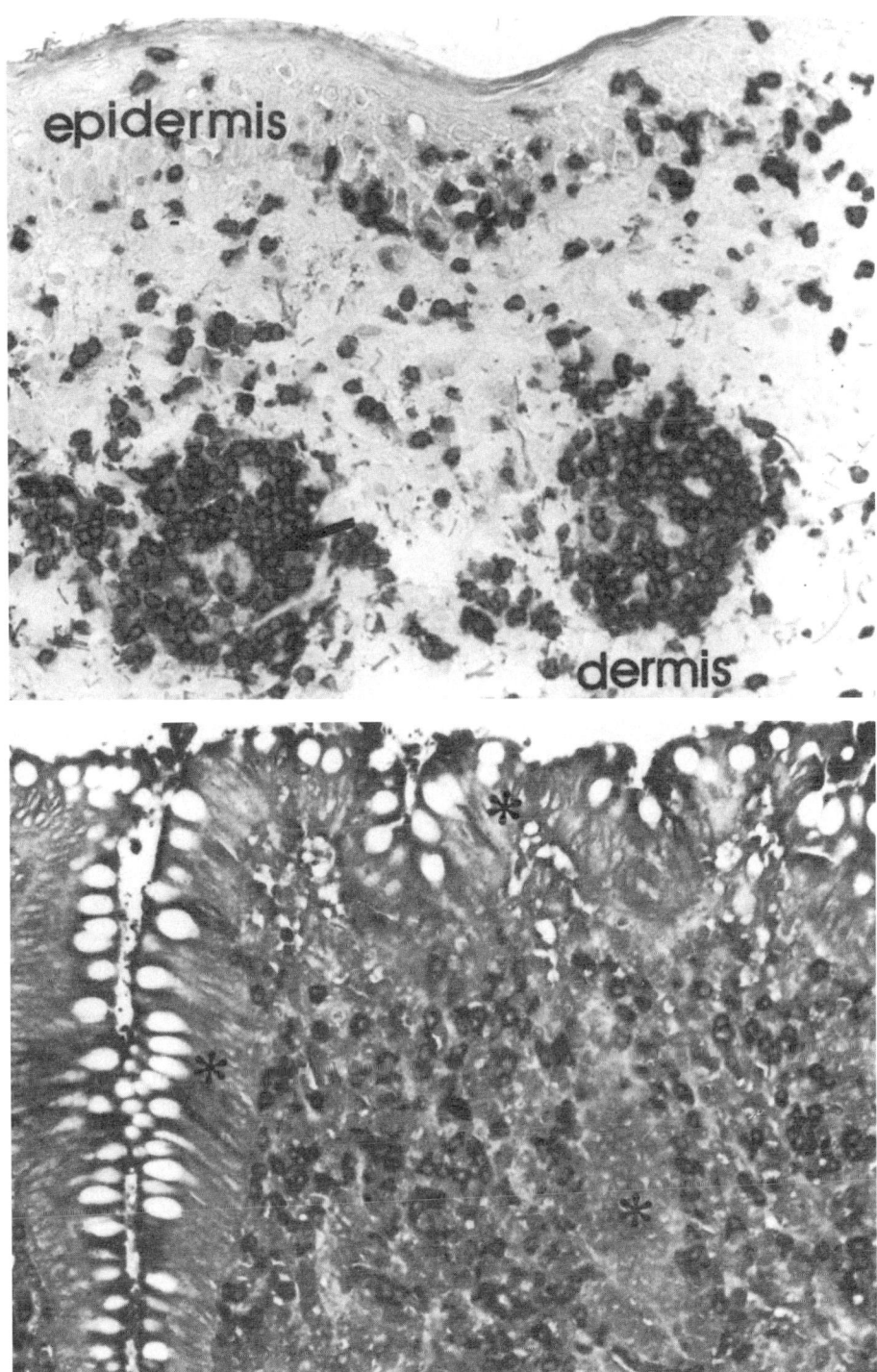

FIG. 12. Examples of tertiary lymphoid tissues. **Top:** Inflamed skin (a delayed-type hypersensitivity response to a topically applied antigen) immunostained with a T cell–specific monoclonal antibody. Note the extensive accumulation of T cells in the superficial dermis adjacent to the activated postcapillary venules (seen in negative image; *arrow*) through which they have recently extravasated. Some T cells specifically migrate from these perivascular clusters to the epidermis. The vast majority of T cells (usually > 95%) within skin or any other tertiary site are members of the memory–effector subset. **Bottom:** Inflamed colonic lamina propria (*asterisks* delineate the surface and glandular epithelial cells) immunostained with a monoclonal antibody specific for κ light chains. The cells with darkly stained cytoplasm represent plasma cells producing a κ-containing Ig. Many of the negatively stained cells in the lamina propria are λ-expressing plasma cells, although memory–effector T cells are present as well.

nature of other B-cell surface markers, including (relative to conventional B cells) high levels of IgM and low levels of IgD, and by their possession of a distinct Ig gene repertoire (less diverse than that of conventional B cells). B-1 B-cell populations arise from what are believed to be distinct progenitor cells that are present in embryonal–fetal splanchnopleura, omentum, liver, and perhaps bone marrow, but not adult bone marrow. During fetal life, B-1 B-cells comprise the major B-lineage subset in the spleen. However, with the development of conventional B cells, their numbers in the spleen dramatically decrease to adult levels of less than 1% to 2%. This subset is not found to any significant degree in the other secondary lymphoid tissues of adult mice. Instead, B-1 cells occur in high frequencies in the body (peritoneal–pleural) cavities of normal animals, where they constitute a stable, self-replenishing population. These cells do not appear to play a major role in the humoral response (both primary and secondary) to conventional T-dependent antigens. Their functional role may be in the "spontaneous" production of polyreactive, low-affinity antibodies, including antibodies reactive with self-determinants (715). The physiologic function of these broadly reactive antibodies is unknown, but it has been suggested that by virtue of their "generic" reactivity with a broad spectrum of microorganisms and their constitutive presence in serum, these antibodies may be able to combat a variety of infections prior to the development of the primary antibody response (714,715). Thus, they may constitute the humoral immune system's first line of defense against primary infections. Most of these polyreactive antibodies are of the IgM isotype; however, isotype switching to both IgG and IgA has been reported (716). Indeed, the B-1 lineage has been suggested to produce a significant proportion of the IgA-secreting plasma cells in intestinal lamina propria (717).

T cells bearing γδ TCRs comprise a heterogeneous population of cells, including, perhaps, T cells with a physiology that parallels that of the predominant (conventional) αβ subset. However, some γδ T-cell subsets display a unique physiology. In the mouse, specific γδ T-cell subsets, each characterized by a specific invariant TCR, leave primary lymphoid tissues at discrete times during fetal development and proceed to directly seed the epithelium of a specific tertiary site [insinuating themselves between epithelial cells so as to become "intraepithelial" lymphocytes (718)]. For example, T cells bearing invariant Vγ3-TCRs peak in the day-17 fetal thymus prior to seeding the skin and developing into the intraepithelial dendritic epidermal T-cell subset; Vγ2-bearing T cells peak a day later in thymic development and seed the female reproductive tract. These subsets are thought to leave the thymus at a relatively immature stage and then continue their development in the tertiary site (719). Indeed, some (if not all) of the intraepithelial γδ T cells of the intestine (predominantly Vγ5-expressing, although there is considerably more TCR variability in this population than in the γδ subsets of skin and reproductive epithelium) appear to skip intrathymic maturation altogether, developing entirely in the intestinal mucosa (720,721). These subsets do not appear in secondary lymphoid tissues, and their development in tertiary sites is thought to be independent of exogenous antigen. Discrete, invariant, intraepithelial γδ T-cell subsets have not been demonstrated in the human (722), but γδ T cells do comprise a substantial percentage of epithelia-associated T cells in the human, particularly in the gastrointestinal tract (723). The exact immunologic role or roles of γδ T cells is obscure, and multiple functions have been proposed. In mouse skin, Vγ3 T cells appear to respond to a keratinocyte stress-induced antigen, and thus may function as sentinels, manifesting a general response to tissue insult (724). This *in situ* non–pathogen-specific response may serve as an initial line of

host defense prior to the recruitment of conventional antigen-specific effector mechanisms. Other γδ T cells appear to respond to nonpeptide molecules that are unique to particular pathogens. For example, human Vγ2/Vδ2 T cells, a major γδ T-cell subset in humans, respond uniformly to isopentenyl pyrophosphate and related compounds (725), which are natural products from mycobacteria, and these cells may play a key role in the initial immune response against these pathogens.

LYMPHOCYTE HOMING AND RECIRCULATION

Lymphocyte homing and recirculation comprises the physiologic processes by which lymphocytes seek out and localize to particular tissues and to specific microenvironments therein (7,521,546). These mechanisms play a major part in the development and maintenance of these specialized microenvironments, and they are critical for the dispersal and targeting of naive and memory lymphocyte populations that are required for effective immune surveillance. Figure 13 describes the homing behavior and localization patterns of (conventional) naive and memory T and B cells, summarizing all the concepts described in detail in previous sections of this chapter. The key role of lymphocyte homing in the overall operation of the immune system becomes apparent on consideration of the homing events required during the lifetime of a typical T cell, for example, a cell destined to initiate a delayed hypersensitivity response in the skin. Minimally, this hypothetical T cell would have had to translocate (a) from bone marrow to thymus during its ontogeny; (b) from thymus to peripheral lymph node for sensitization, and finally (c) from lymph node to skin for initiation of the delayed hypersensitivity response (steps 2 and 3, illustrated in Fig. 10). With regard to the second and third trips, it is evident that effective immune surveillance would require this and other lymphocytes to continuously patrol potential sites of antigen deposition. Indeed, physiologic evidence indicates that most subsets of mature lymphocytes are in continuous motion, recirculating through the tissues, using the blood and lymph as conduits. An individual lymphocyte may make a complete circuit—blood to tissue to lymph to blood—as often as one to two times per day (726). Moreover, physiologic and, more recently, molecular data indicate that lymphocyte subsets show remarkable tissue specificity in their homing characteristics, with the homing behavior of a given subset seemingly matched to the physiologic potential of that subset.

Conventional, naive B- and T-lymphocytes, exported to the periphery from the primary lymphoid tissues, localize preferentially in organized secondary lymphoid organs (7,521,546), which are, as discussed above, "designed" for the sensitization of these cells. In general, such lymphocytes migrate poorly, if at all, to tertiary sites, even under conditions of inflammation. Their migratory properties appear to be determined ontogenetically as a function of their class (i.e., T vs. B cell; CD4+ vs. CD8+ T cell), but within a class, they show roughly equivalent migration to the different secondary sites. Naive lymphocytes probably traffic continuously between the different secondary lymphoid organs until they die or respond to their cognate antigen (7,727). (As discussed, there are exceptions to this general pattern, however, including the unconventional B-1 (Ly-1/CD5+) B-cell subset and the unique subsets of the γδ T cells with invariant TCRs.)

Memory and effector lymphocytes, generated in secondary lymphoid tissues in response to antigen and then exported back into the

Lymphoid tissues

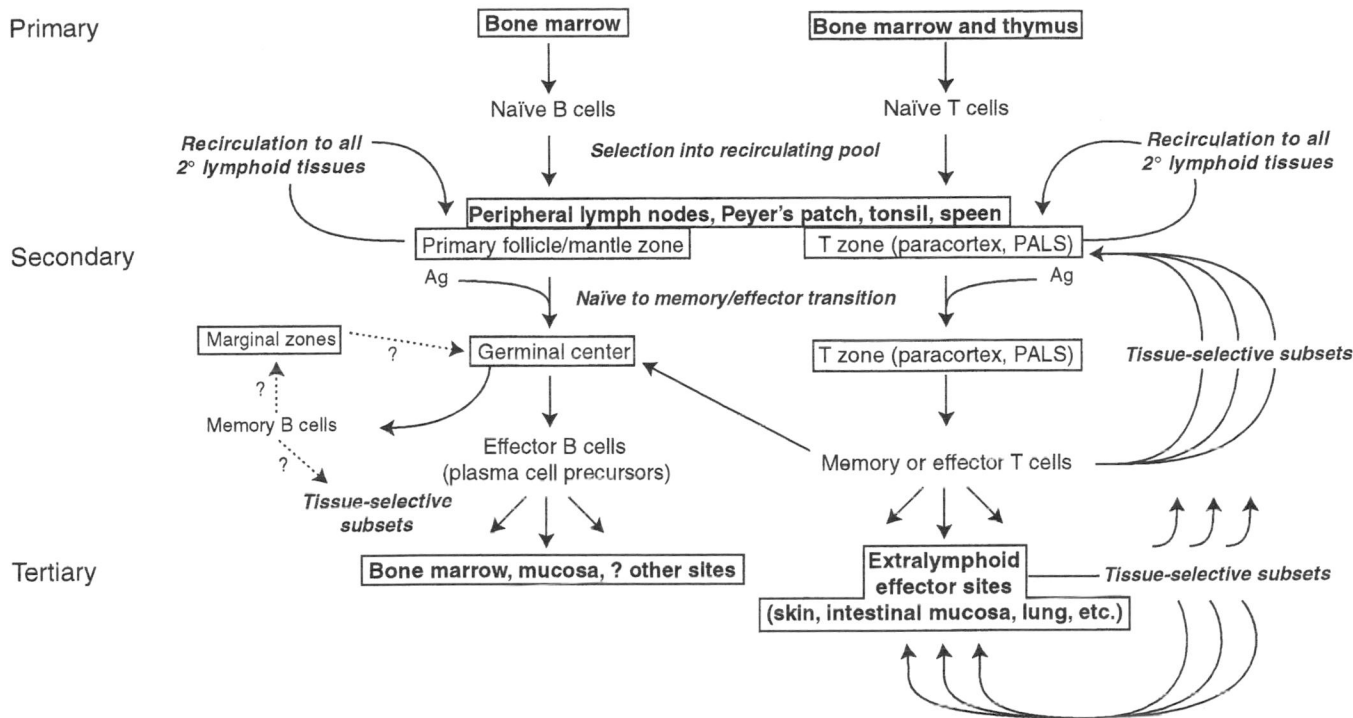

FIG. 13. Summary of the homing–migration patterns of conventional B- and T-lymphocytes. (From ref. 521, with permission.)

circulation, display migratory properties that are very different than those of naive cells (7,519,521). First, in keeping with their role in mediating effector responses, these cells, as a group, traffic effectively to tertiary lymphoid tissues such as skin or intestinal lamina propria, particularly when these tissues are inflamed. Second, differentiation into the memory–effector subset is accompanied by the heterogeneous development of *tissue selectivity* in migratory potential. In other words, the memory–effector population is composed of multiple subsets that have diverse, often tissue-restricted homing capability (including, for example, memory–effector T cells that preferentially home to the skin vs. mucosal sites or vice versa). Indeed, memory–effector lymphocytes have been shown to preferentially migrate back to the region of the body in which they were first activated. For example, naive T cells initially activated in Peyer's patch preferentially return to mucosal secondary or tertiary lymphoid tissues, whereas, otherwise similar T cells activated in peripheral lymph node preferentially recirculate back to lymph node and associated tertiary sites, such as the skin. The tissue-selective homing properties of memory and effector cell subsets are thought to enhance the efficiency of the immune system by targeting immune surveillance and effector responses to tissues most similar to those where the antigen initially entered the body (e.g., in ensuring that mucosal antigens elicit a secretory IgA antibody response and that IgA-secreting effector cells are generally distributed to mucosal epithelia), and they might also be important in reducing opportunities for autoimmune cross-reactions with tissue components from unrelated tissues.

The physiology of lymphocyte homing–recirculation is largely determined by the differential regulation of lymphocyte adhesion

and de-adhesion. Lymphocytes have an extraordinary ability to finely regulate their adhesive properties throughout their lifespan (728), and essentially all of these myriad adhesive events have some impact on a given lymphocyte's recirculatory potential. However, while lymphocyte adhesion to tissue components plays a crucial role in determining the tendency of a given lymphocyte subset to recirculate (by regulating the ability of that cell type to pass through a particular tissue, appear in the lymph, and return to the circulation), the adhesive interaction that is central to the regulation of lymphocyte homing is that between blood-borne lymphocytes and postcapillary venular endothelium (7). Lymphocyte binding to endothelium is a requisite first step in the process of extravasation, and this interaction—mediated by lymphocyte homing receptors, endothelial ligands for these homing receptors, and activating factors and their lymphocyte counterreceptors (see below)—largely determines the extravasation potential of lymphocytes at various tissue sites. It should be emphasized that the specificity of the homing process is independent of antigen; that is, there is no support for the notion that the ability of a lymphocyte to extravasate in a given tissue is influenced by the presence or absence of its cognate antigen. Indeed, the vast majority of lymphocytes recruited to a given site (e.g., in a delayed hypersensitivity reaction) is not specific for whatever antigen was used to elicit an immune reaction in that site (729). The presence of antigen can, however, influence the retention of antigen-specific lymphocytes in particular sites (Fig 14). Antigen stimulation initiates the functional activation of various adhesive systems on lymphocytes, which serve to (temporarily) tether antigen-specific

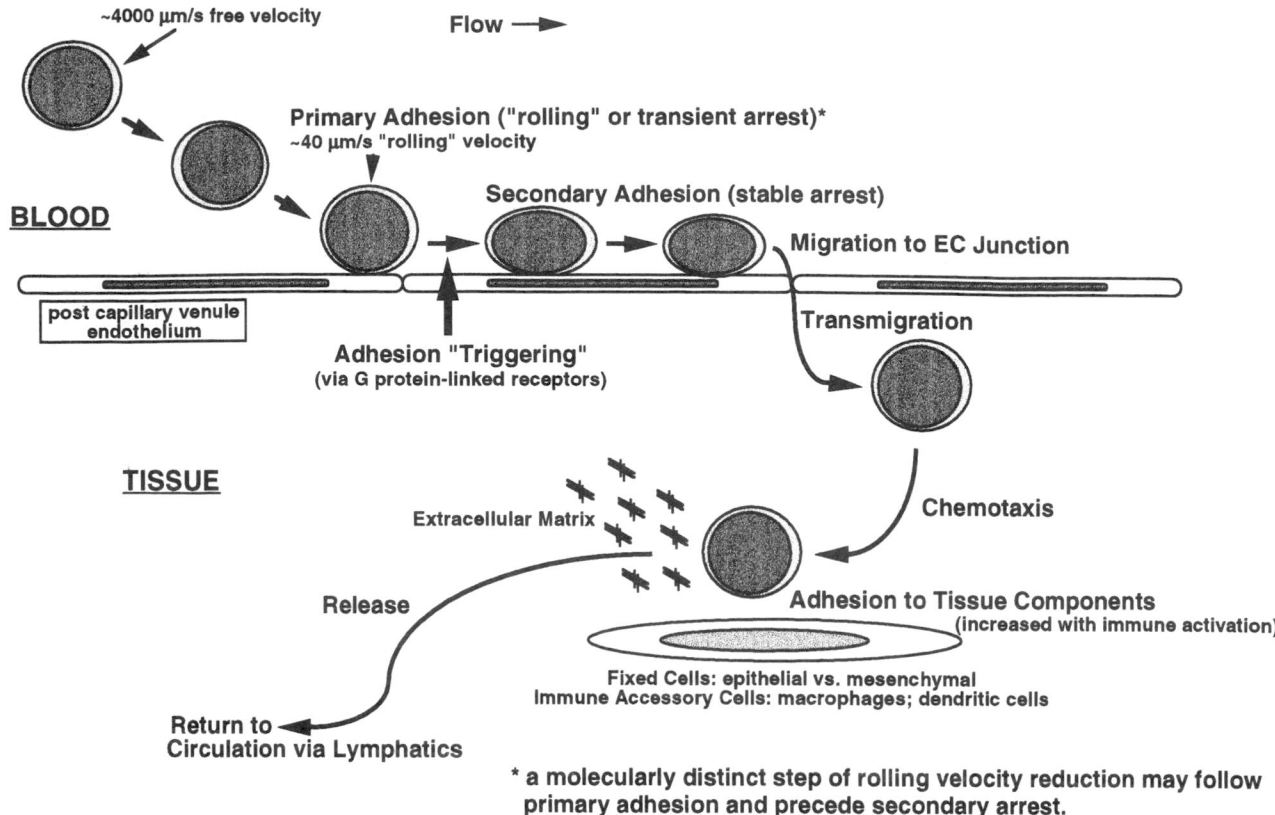

FIG. 14. The multistep model of leukocyte extravasation. Free-flowing lymphocytes are thought to use primary, acti-vation-independent receptors to initially interact with regulated counterreceptors on endothelium. This initial adhe-sion is unstable under shear and is therefore transient unless the cell receives a second activating signal originating from the endothelial cell or surrounding tissues. Activation results in the participation of secondary activation-depen-dent adhesion systems. Secondary adhesion is stable under shear and leads to lymphocyte arrest on the endothe-lial surface and then transmigration across the vessel wall into the tissues. In some instances, a molecularly distinct step of rolling velocity reduction may be required for intravascular arrest to occur. Thus, successful extravasation requires leukocyte and endothelial expression of two or more reciprocal adhesion molecule–ligand pairs and the availability of leukocyte-type–specific activating factors, all of which may be differentially regulated to ensure extrava-sation specificity. Once in the tissues, lymphocytes migrate to specific micorenvironments under the influence of chemotactic and haptotactic gradients. This migration and microenvironmental retention is mediated through the fine control of adhesion and deadhesion with both cellular and matrix componets of the tissues. The duration of time a particular lymphocyte remains in the tissues will depend on its array of adhesion molecules, their activation state (which in turn will depend on the activation state of the lymphocyte), and the availabilty of ligands for these mole-cules within the tissue.

cells to local tissue components and thereby delay their appear-ance in the efferent lymph (546).

Adhesion of blood-borne lymphocytes to endothelium at sites of extravasation occurs under flow and in the face of high shear stresses [up to 30 dynes/cm² in postcapillary venules, (730)]. Stud-ies demonstrate that evolution has confronted this physical chal-lenge by making lymphocyte (indeed, all leukocyte) extravasation a multistep process, in which initial interaction under flow and sub-sequent binding stabilization can be mediated by independent, spe-cialized adhesion pathways (731–733). Four distinct, major steps in the extravasation process have been defined: (a) primary adhesion, (b) leukocyte activation, (c) secondary adhesion, and (d) transmi-gration–chemotaxis (see Fig. 14).

Primary adhesion is the initial recognition and attachment of free-flowing leukocytes to appropriate endothelium—either the special-ized endothelium of high endothelial venules or suitably activated endothelium in (inflamed) tertiary effector sites. In this first step,

constitutively functional lymphocyte homing receptors interact with their regulated vascular ligands under conditions of high blood flow. This primary adhesion can involve separable contact formation (tethering) with loose rolling along the vessel wall, and molecularly distinct mechanisms for slowing rolling velocity (734). In other sit-uations, it can involve a transient, immediate arrest without dis-cernible rolling (735). Strikingly, receptors that mediate initial cell contact under shear tend to be highly concentrated for presentation to the endothelium on the tips of lymphocyte microvilli (the sites of initial cell–cell contact under flow), which dramatically enhances the efficiency of attachment under physiologic shear (736). Primary adhesion slows the transit of lymphocytes by a factor of several hundred or more, thus allowing sufficient time for the lymphocyte to sample the vessel for soluble or endothelial surface proadhesive factors. Importantly, this interaction is rapidly reversible, and lym-phocytes are released back into the circulation unless secondary adhesion mechanisms are brought into play.

The prototypic primary homing receptor is L-selectin, a C-type lectin with affinity for sulfated, fucosylated carbohydrate determinants displayed by specialized postcapillary venules, especially the HEVs in peripheral lymph nodes (737,738), where these carbohydrate ligands are presented by a number of glycoproteins composing the peripheral lymph node addressin (PNAd; Table 1) (739). L-selectin is concentrated on microvilli and displays a rapid on-rate, allowing extremely efficient contact initiation under high shear. It also has a rapid off-rate, resulting in a loose, even rolling of interacting cells under physiologic flow. Subsets of lymphocytes

TABLE 1. *Molecules Involved in Lymphocyte-Endothelial Cell Recognition and Lymphocyte Homing*

Molecular family	Proposed primary function in lymphocyte homing
Selectins	
L-selectin (LECAM-1, Mel-14, LAM-1 Ags)	The prototypic primary "activation-independent" homing receptor. It has been called the "peripheral lymph node homing receptor" based on its critical role in mediating lymphocyte homing to this site; it also facilitates naive lymphocyte homing to Peyer's patch, and memory lymphocyte (subset) homing to some tertiary sites (peripheral > mucosal). In lymph node and tertiary sites, L-selectin recognizes sialylated oligosaccharide determinants on the peripheral lymph node vascular addressin (PNAd). In Peyer's patch, appropriate oligosaccharides are presented by MAdCAM-1.
E-selectin (ELAM-1)	Inflammation-induced endothelial adhesion molecule, which in the setting of chronic inflammation is selectively expressed in the skin (i.e., is a skin vascular addressin-mediating primary adhesion). Recognizes the cutaneous lymphocyte antigen, CLA.
P-selectin (GMP-140)	Supports T-cell primary adhesion *in vitro*; *in vivo* role is unknown. Recognizes oligosaccharides associated with PSGL-1.
Oligosaccharide ligands for the selectins	
Peripheral node addressin (PNAd; gylcans)	Selectively expressed on peripheral lymph node HEV; contains the sialylated carbohydrate ligand for L-selectin and multiple protein cores (including CD34). Appears to be inducible late in the course of chronic inflammation in many tertiary sites. In Peyer's patch, MAdCAM-1 itself can be decorated with the appropriate carbohydrates and serve as an L-selectin ligand (see below).
CLA (cutaneous lymphocyte-associated antigen)	Skin-selective lymphocyte homing receptor. Sialylated oligosaccharide ligand for E-selectin [protein core(s) not defined], expressed on a skin-associated subset of memory-effector T cells.
PSGL-1 (P-selectin glycoprotein ligand-1)	Protein core that is associated with oligosaccharide ligands for P-selectin. Physiologic role in lymphocyte homing remains undefined.
Integrins	
β2-class (CD18)	
αLβ2 (LFA-1)	ICAM-1 and -2 are the endothelial ligands. LFA-1 is the prototypic, activation-dependent secondary adhesion molecule.
α4-class (CD49d)	
α4β1 (VLA-4)	VCAM-1 is the predominant endothelial ligand. Also recognizes fibronectin. Currently thought to participate in memory lymphocyte (subset) homing to sites of chronic inflammation, potentially functioning in primary adhesion, rolling velocity reduction, and secondary adhesion.
α4β7	MAdCAM-1 is the predominant endothelial ligand. Serves as a mucosal homing receptor, playing a critical role in naive lymphocyte homing to Peyer's patch, and memory lymphocyte (subset) homing to nonpulmonary, mucosal tertiary sites; functions in primary adhesion, rolling velocity reduction, and secondary adhesion.
Ig Superfamily	
ICAM-1,-2 (intercellular adhesion molecule-1, -2)	Widely expressed endothelial ligand for LFA-1; ICAM-1 is upregulated with inflammation, but ICAM-2 is constitutively expressed. Functions in secondary adhesion and transmigration.
VCAM-1 (vascular cell adhesion molecule-1)	Endothelial ligand for α4β1. Inflammation induced. *In vivo* distribution is incompletely characterized, but expression is heterogeneous, suggesting the possibility of tissue- or microenvironment-selective function.
MAdCAM-1 (mucosal addressin)	Endothelial adhesion molecule selectively expressed on mucosal HEV and lamina propria vessels. Binds mucosa-homing lymphoid subsets through interactions with α4β7 (α4βp). In Peyer's patch, but not lamina propria, it is decorated with L-selectin ligands to facilitate naive lymphocyte homing to this site.
Proteoglycan-cartilage-link protein	
CD44 (HCAM, Pgp-1)	Predominant endothelial ligand is hyaluronate; mediates primary adhesion of activated (by not resting) lymphocytes, likely participating in the homing of memory-effector blasts to sites of inflammation.
Other	
VAP-1 (vascular adhesion, protein-1)	Constitutively expressed by peripheral lymph node HEV, and widely upregulated on inflamed venules; lymphocyte ligand and physiologic roles remain undefined.

can also manifest primary adhesion on vascular E- and P-selectins, on VCAM-1 and MAdCAM-1 (Ig-family vascular ligands for the lymphocyte $\alpha 4$ homing receptors $\alpha 4\beta 1$ and $\alpha 4\beta 7$), and on hyaluronate via a CD44-mediated mechanism (735,740–742). CD44 is unique in that it is constitutively inactive, prior cell activation (involving protein kinase C) for 6 or more hours being required for its activity (742). The $\alpha 4$ integrins, like the selectins, are constitutively active, but their function can be dramatically enhanced by lymphocyte activation, and these adhesion molecules thus can participate in both primary and secondary interactions with endothelium (734,735,741) (see below). The vascular selectins E- and P-selectin and, especially, the $\alpha 4$ integrins characteristically mediate much slower rolling than does L-selectin. This is an important distinction, because, in some situations, rolling through L-selectin is so loose that the participation of $\alpha 4$ integrins or other mechanisms to slow rolling velocity is required as a "bridging" event for subsequent lymphocyte activation and secondary adhesion (see below).

The second step of the extravasation process, lymphocyte "activation," is the least well characterized in molecular terms. It is clear that activation of secondary adhesion (e.g., integrin activation; see below) can occur during *in situ* lymphocyte–endothelial cell interactions as rapidly as 2 to 3 seconds after primary adhesion, and that triggering through G protein–linked receptors plays a critical role in those instances examined (743). When G-protein signaling is inhibited (with pertussis toxin, for example), lymphocytes interact with endothelium, manifesting an exclusively rolling phentoype, but stable (integrin-mediated) endothelial binding is prevented, and, consequently, extravasation does not occur. Seven-span serpentine receptors for the large and diverse *chemokine* family of chemoattractants signal through pertussis toxin–sensitive G proteins and, in neutrophils and transfected lymphocytes, can trigger integrin activation in seconds. Moreover, adhesion triggered through these chemoattractant receptors reverses spontaneously within minutes, allowing arrested cells to revert to a rolling phenotype under flow (thus ensuring reversibility of adhesion *in vivo*, unless followed by diapedesis). Thus, there was a great deal of initial excitement about possible involvement of the diverse chemokine family in the activation step of the lymphocyte extravasation process. This excitement was dampened, at least for conventional chemokines, by the increasing realization that the response of resting lymphocytes to known soluble chemokines at physiologic concentrations is too weak or too slow to produce a sufficiently robust proadhesive response to these agents in the timeframe of the extravasation process (521,744,745). However, a number of recently discovered soluble chemokines (SDF-1, 6-C-Kine, MIP-3α, and MIP-3β) have been shown to induce arrest of rolling lymphocytes under flow conditions (746). Moreover, a novel membrane-bound chemokine has been identified. Preliminary data indicate that this CX$_3$C chemokine is strongly expressed by activated human endothelial cells and promotes strong adhesion of leukocytes, including T cells (746a).

The third step in lymphocyte extravasation—activation-dependent stable arrest—must be mediated by adhesion molecules that are constitutively inactive or active with low avidity, but that can be triggered within seconds to mediate strong shear-resistant adhesion. To date, only the heterodimeric integrins, including the $\alpha 4$ integrins $\alpha 4\beta 1$ and $\alpha 4\beta 7$ and the $\beta 2$ integrins LFA-1 ($\alpha L\beta 2$, CD11a/CD18) and MAC-1 ($\alpha M\beta 2$, CD11b/CD18), have been conclusively shown to participate in this function (731–733). Interestingly, unlike the $\alpha 4$ integrins (736), $\beta 2$ integrins are found on the planar cell body of leukocytes and are largely excluded from microvilli (747). This exclusion from sites of first cell contact may explain in part the inability of $\beta 2$ integrins, even when preactivated, to initiate adhesion under flow (735). Activation-dependent stable arrest is followed by diapedesis, the final step in the extravasation process. The same $\beta 2$ and $\alpha 4$ integrins involved in secondary adhesion are also thought to participate in this migration through the vessel wall.

A critical implication of this multistep process is that the specificity of lymphocyte extravasation can be determined at any one or combination of these steps, since successful recruitment requires all to be accomplished. Lymphocyte homing is thus controlled by an algorithm involving a series of "yes" (continue to the next step) or "no" (return to blood) decisions. Since homing can be regulated at any or all of the decision points, diversity and specificity are thus provided for through a mechanism of combinatorial association of the receptor–ligand pairs available at each step. Such a process allows the specificity of recruitment to greatly exceed that of any of the individual steps (731). As a consequence, highly successful and specialized adhesion receptors, such as the L-selectin or LFA-1, can be (and are) utilized in multiple, independently regulated trafficking pathways. Table 1 lists key molecular "players" identified to date, each involved in their own distinct, if overlapping, settings of physiologic homing. Figure 15 illustrates how the cooperative, sequential activity of adhesion receptors can yield tissue-specific homing (521). For example, as mentioned above, naive lymphocytes must be able to extravasate in all secondary lymphoid tissues (including Peyer's patch), while at the same time be generally prevented from extravasating in extralymphoid (effector) sites. *In situ* studies of exteriorized mouse Peyer's patches indicate that naive lymphocyte homing to this site is acheived by the sequential engagement of L-selectin to initiate contact, $\alpha 4\beta 7$ to slow rolling, and LFA-1 in conjunction with $\alpha 4\beta 7$ to mediate activation-dependent arrest (734). L-selectin dominates contact initiation because naive lymphocytes display only relatively low levels and activity of $\alpha 4\beta 7$. On the other hand, L-selectin rolling on Peyer's patch HEVs (which express only low levels of L-selectin ligand) is too fast to allow direct engagement of LFA-1, thus necessitating involvement of $\alpha 4\beta 7$. The additional requirement for LFA-1 for arrest may reflect the relatively low levels of $\alpha 4\beta 7$ on naive cells. The $\alpha 4\beta 7$ endothelial ligand MAdCAM-1 is not expressed by peripheral lymph node HEVs, where naive cells also home, but because peripheral lymph node HEVs display uniquely high levels of L-selectin ligands, L-selectin–mediated rolling may be slow enough to allow direct conversion to LFA-1–mediated arrest. Importantly, $\alpha 4\beta 7$ levels (and activity) on naive cells are insufficient to promote their direct binding to the MAdCAM-1$^+$, L-selectin ligand$^-$ venules in the intestinal lamina propria (an extralymphoid effector site). As mentioned extensively above, memory T cells are heterogenous with respect to homing receptor expression, with, for example, distinct populations lacking or expressing (often high) levels of $\alpha 4\beta 7$, CLA, and L-selectin (Fig. 16). Depending on the pattern of expression of these homing receptors, memory cells either will or will not efficiently extravasate into various tissues, all which display distinct patterns of (inducible) homing receptor ligands on their postcapillary endothelium. As illustrated in Fig. 15, $\alpha 4\beta 7^{high}$/CLA$^-$ memory T cells will extravasate efficiently into intestinal lamina propria but not inflamed skin, whereas the converse is true for $\alpha 4\beta 7^-$/CLA$^+$ memory T cells. Taken together, these examples illustrate the mechanisms by which the immune system ensures that naive lymphocytes have access to both mucosal and peripheral secondary lymphoid tissue, but not to tertiary (effector) sites, and that memory T

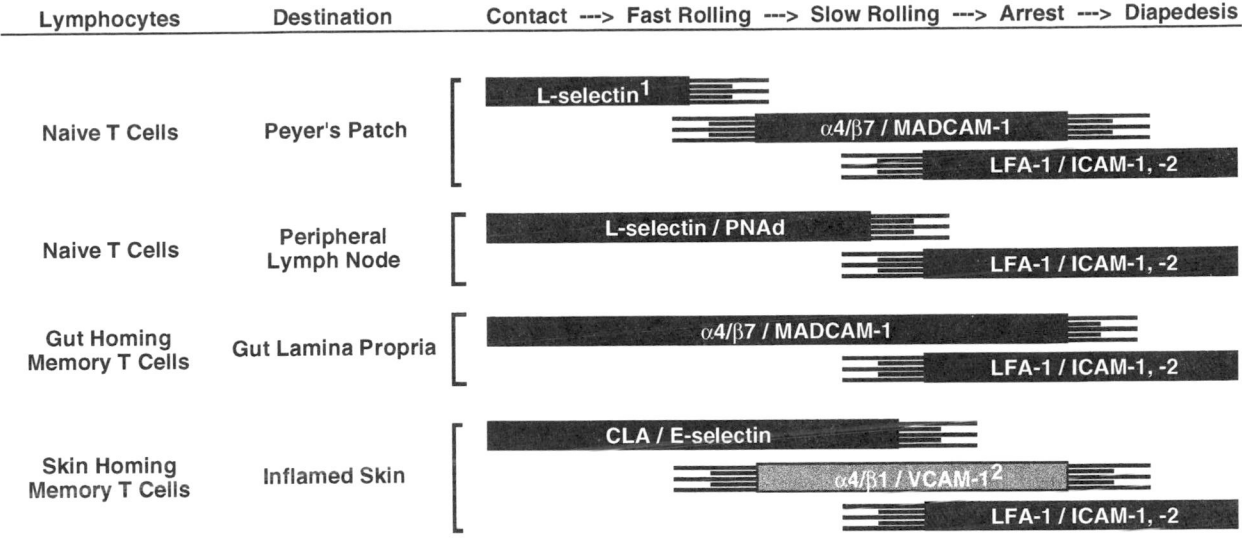

Lymphocytes	Destination	Contact ---> Fast Rolling ---> Slow Rolling ---> Arrest ---> Diapedesis
Naive T Cells	Peyer's Patch	L-selectin[1] / α4/β7 / MADCAM-1 / LFA-1 / ICAM-1, -2
Naive T Cells	Peripheral Lymph Node	L-selectin / PNAd / LFA-1 / ICAM-1, -2
Gut Homing Memory T Cells	Gut Lamina Propria	α4/β7 / MADCAM-1 / LFA-1 / ICAM-1, -2
Skin Homing Memory T Cells	Inflamed Skin	CLA / E-selectin / α4/β1 / VCAM-1[2] / LFA-1 / ICAM-1, -2

[1] In Peyer's Patch, L-selectin binds to MADCAM-1-associated carbohydrates

[2] α4β1 / VCAM-1 "bridging" is not required on CLA (bright) memory T cells.

FIG. 15. Lymphocyte extravasation—contact, rolling, rolling velocity reduction, arrest, and diapedesis—in different vascular beds depends on the sequential, overlapping utilization of different homing receptor–endothelial ligand pairs. The pathways shown are the best characterized to date, but they likely represent only a minority of those available for use in the targeting of various lymphocyte subsets to different tissue sites. (Adapted from ref. 521, with permission.) It is important to emphasize that qualitative and quantitative regulation of both the lymphocyte homing receptors and their counterreceptors on endothelium is crucial to specificity control. Activating factors are also thought to play a key role in specificity control, but they are not shown in this illustration. Note that with these pathways, naive cells can extravasate in both peripheral lymph node and Peyer's patch (secondary lymphoid tissues), but not in skin or gut lamina propria (tertiary sites). Memory cells extravasate efficiently in either gut or skin (usually not both), depending on their expression pattern of the relevant homing receptors (see Fig. 16 as well).

cells can be differentially targeted to distinct tertiary sites. Thus, by varying the expression levels of key homing receptors and their endothelial counterreceptors and by allowing some of these adhesion systems to work cooperatively in sequence, the immune system can construct many specific homing pathways using a relatively few distinct molecular components.

Once recruited into tissues, lymphocytes disperse into specialized microenvironmental domains. These would include the histologically discrete structures (e.g., primary B-cell follicles, germinal centers, marginal zones and T-cell zones of secondary lymphoid tissues, the epithelium of tertiary sites), as well as less discrete microenvironments that would comprise dispersed, specialized stromal elements in tertiary sites. Just as mechanisms of tissue-selective trafficking permit segregation and specialization of immune responses at the systemic level, microenvironmental homing permits specialization of local stromal–accessory components into domains capable of supporting the complex cellular interactions required for immune responses.

Very little is known about the molecular basis of this "microenvironmental" homing, but the available evidence suggests some common themes. First, targeted homing within tissues, like recruitment from the blood, is likely combinatorially determined by overlapping regulatory, adhesion, and migratory events. Each microenvironmental domain would be characterized by a unique, organized display of adhesive ligands and regulatory factors—both within the domain itself and leading to it from the microvasculature—such that sequential chemotactic or haptotactic and contact guidance mechanisms can guide appropriate lymphocytes to that site. Second, as in the extrava-

sation process, adhesion regulation is fundamental to the control of microenvironmental homing. In some instances, microenvironments may upregulate new lymphocyte adhesive elements such as the TGF-β1 inducible αeβ7 integrin, which targets lymphocytes to intraepithelial sites by binding to E-cadherin (748). In other instances, constitutively expressed adhesion molecules (including many of those associated with extravasation) may be involved; for example, α4 integrins mediate germinal center B-cell binding to VCAM-1⁺ antigen-presenting FDCs in germinal centers (643,644). Importantly, the adhesive function of lymphocyte integrins and other adhesion receptors, such as CD44, can be regulated by signaling through many cell surface receptors, including not only chemoattractant receptors, but also adhesion receptors themselves, Fc receptors, and a number of Ig-family members, including the T- and B-cell antigen receptors themselves and their associated costimulatory molecules (749–752). Indeed, as lymphocytes migrate to a given site, they must continuously integrate proadhesive and potentially antiadhesive signals from diverse cell surface receptors that may be engaged coordinately in complex in vivo environments.

Several classes of soluble factors and their receptors have been functionally implicated in the regulation of lymphocyte locomotion, including a variety of cytokines and growth factors [IL-2, IL-10, IL-15, TGF-β1, hepatocyte growth factor, among others (753–757)]. However, the chemokines, a large family of structurally related polypeptides that bind a family of homologous G protein–associated seven transmembrane–spanning (serpentine) receptors, have, because of their diversity, widespread tissue expression and chemotactic specificity for functionally distinct

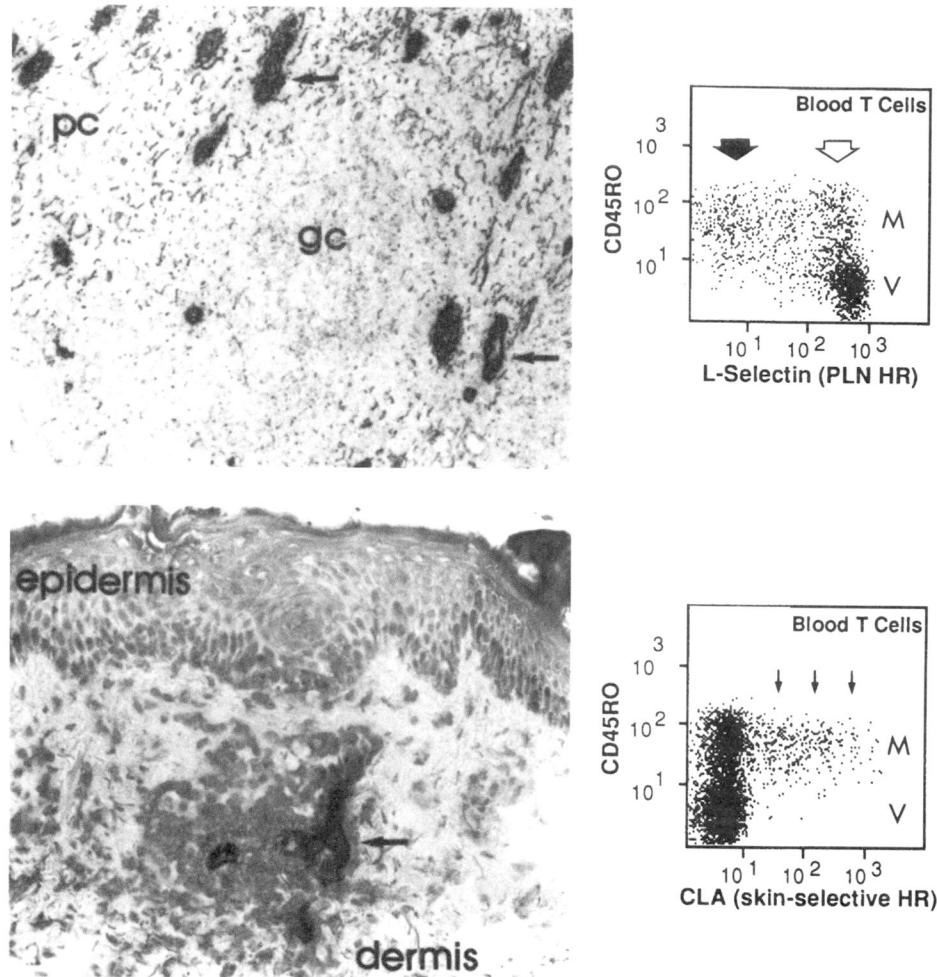

FIG. 16. Differential expression of homing receptors and their endothelial ligands: peripheral lymph node versus skin. **Top, left:** Immunostaining of an antigen-stimulated human peripheral lymph node (*PLN*), demonstrating the expression of the PLN addressin (*PNAd*) on PLN HEVs (*arrows; gc,* germinal center; *pc,* paracortex; some dendritic staining of uncertain significance is also apparent in the paracortex). PNAd is the endothelial cell ligand for L-selectin, which functions as a primary peripheral lymph node homing receptor. **Bottom, left:** Immunostaining of inflamed human skin (a delayed-type hypersensitivity response is shown) demonstrating the intense expression of E-selectin on postcapillary venules (*arrow*) within the superficial dermis. Note that the stained venules are associated with pale gray mononuclear cells that represent a memory–effector T-cell infiltrate. In the setting of chronic inflammation, E-selectin is selectively expressed on cutaneous venules as opposed to the great majority of other tertiary sites. In keeping with this, the T-cell E-selectin ligand (*CLA*) is present on essentially all memory–effector T cells in inflamed skin, but few of those in extracutaneous inflammatory sites (537 697). **Right panels:** The pattern of expression of L-selectin and CLA on peripheral blood T cells (as demonstrated by three-color flow cytometry) is in keeping with their role in mediating tissue-selective homing to secondary (PLN) and tertiary (skin) lymphoid sites, respectively. As explained in the legend for Fig. 8, the cells shown are gated on CD3 and are thus pure T cells (each *black dot* equals one T cell); CD45RO expression differentiates the virgin (*V;* CD45RO⁻) and memory–effector (*M;* CD45RO⁺) T-cell subsets. **Top, right:** In keeping with the ability of the virgin T-cell subset to extravasate relatively homogeneously in PLN, essentially all CD45RO⁻ T cells in peripheral blood are L-selectin⁺. In contrast, memory–effector T cells are known to be heterogeneous in homing capability, with some cells migrating preferentially to peripheral sites and others to mucosal sites, and this heterogeneity is reflected by the bimodal expression of L-selectin by the CD45RO⁺ T-cell subset (*closed* versus *open arrows*). **Bottom, right:** Virgin T cells do not extravasate with any degree of efficiency into inflamed skin, and the CD45RO⁻ (virgin) T-cell subset in peripheral blood lacks the skin-selective homing receptor CLA. CLA is exclusively expressed by the subset of CD45RO⁺ memory–effector T cells (*arrows*) that efficiently migrates to skin.

lymphocyte subsets, received particular attention (521,744,745,758). Many chemokines and chemokine receptors are induced or modulated during inflammation, rendering them strong candidates for regulating altered lymphocyte targeting during immune and inflammatory responses. Chemokines can also bind and be presented by glycosaminoglycans, suggesting that haptotactic responses to substrate or cell-bound chemokines may be as or more important than classical chemotaxis (759–761). Moreover, different glycosaminoglycans display binding selectivity for different chemokines, adding another level of control.

Lymphocyte homing should not be considered an isolated lymphocyte function. Homing-related interactions are seamlessly integrated into the overall interaction of the lymphocyte with its environment, and thus participate directly in the control of both lymphocyte function and lifespan. For example, the adhesive and chemotactic interactions involved in directing lymphocyte migration likely also provide signals that regulate cell activation or programmed cell death. Moreover, homing mechanisms play a critical role in the process of clonal competition that, as decribed above, is integral to the regulation of the peripheral immune repertoire. These mechanisms provides the "stirring" by which the overall repertoire of a given lymphocyte subset is repeatedly exposed to the culling effect of niche competition. Finally, it should be emphasized once again that the microenvironments in turn feed back to regulate homing: Signals received from the microenvironments, especially at the time of cellular activation, regulate expression and activity of adhesion–homing–chemoattractant receptors, and thereby repeatedly program the migratory behavior of each lymphocyte.

CONCLUSIONS

In this era of astounding progress in the molecular and cell biology of the lymphocyte function, it is easy to forget that our appreciation of immunity at the systemic level is still in its formative stages. Modern immunology still has only limited awareness of the myriad, complex series of physiologic events that constitute either protective or pathologic immune responses *in vivo*. In this chapter, we have attempted to outline some of what is known about the organization of the immune system *in vivo*, particularly emphasizing the functional consequences of this organization. The basic lesson from this discourse is twofold: First, immunity is a systemic phenomenon; all immune responses require the coordinated function of spatially distinct compartments of the immune system. Second, immunocyte function cannot be studied in isolation, divorced from the regulatory influences of their normal microenvironments; the normal, *in vivo* physiology of the immune system is inexorably linked to its physical structure and organization, including the critical functional contribution of nonhematolymphoid cell types. The challenge for the future, therefore, is to interpret the rapidly evolving data base on lymphocyte cell and molecular biology within the context of systemic immune physiology. Only by assessing the molecular and cellular relationships between the lymphocyte and its microenvironment(s) can a true appreciation for the operation of the immune system be obtained.

ACKNOWLEDGMENTS

We would like to thank Robin Arndt for secretarial assistance, and Benita Stewart for photography and graphics. Special gratitude is extended to Dr. Jane Bardwell for her outstanding artwork in Figs. 3, 10, and 11.

REFERENCES

1. Davis MM, Bjorkman PJ. T-cell antigen receptor genes and T-cell recognition. *Nature* 1988;334:395.
2. Tew JG, DiLosa RM, Burton GF, et al. Germinal centers and antibody production in bone marrow. *Immunol Rev* 1992;126:99.
3. Terstappen LWMM, Johnson S, Segers-Nolten MJ, Loken MR. Identification and characterization of plasma cells in normal human bone marrow by high-resolution flow cytometry. *Blood* 1990;76:1739.
4. Bachmann MF, Kundig TM, Odermatt B, Hengartner H, Zinkernagel RM. Free recirculation of memory B cells versus antigen-dependent differentiation to antibody-forming cells. *J Immunol* 1994;153:3386.
5. Reynolds JD, Kennedy L, Peppard J, Pabst R. Ileal Peyer's patch emigrants are predominantly B cells and travel to all lymphoid tissues in sheep. *Eur J Immunol* 1991;21:283.
6. Reynaud CA, Mackay CR, Muller RG, Weill JC. Somatic generation of diversity in a mammalian primary lymphoid organ: the sheep ileal Peyer's patches. *Cell* 1991;64:995.
7. Picker LJ, Butcher EC. Physiological and molecular mechanisms of lymphocyte homing. *Annu Rev Immunol* 1992;10:561.
8. Spangrude GJ, Heimfeld S, Weissman IL. Purification and characterization of mouse hematopoietic stem cells. *Science* 1988;241:58.
9. Huang S, Terstappen LWMM. Formation of both hematopoietic microenvironment and hematopoietic stem cells from single human bone marrow stem cells. *Nature* 1992;360:745.
10. Terstappen LWMM, Huang S, Safford M, Lansdorp PM, Loken MR. Sequential generation of hematopoietic colonies derived from single nonlineage-committed CD34+CD38− progenitor cells. *Blood* 1991;77:1218.
11. Terstappen LW, Huang S, Picker LJ. Flow cytometric assessment of human T-cell differentiation in thymus and bone marrow. *Blood* 1992;79:666.
12. Loken MR, Shah VO, Dattilio KL, Civin CI. Flow cytometric analysis of human bone marrow. II. Normal B lymphocyte development. *Blood* 1987;70:1316.
13. Stewart AK, Huang C, Long AA, Stollar BD, Schwartz RS. VH-gene representation in autoantibodies reflects the normal human B-cell repertoire. *Immunol Rev* 1992;128:101.
14. Gu H, Tarlinton D, Muller W, Rajewsky K, Forster I. Most peripheral B cells in mice are ligand selected. *J Exp Med* 1991;173:1357.
15. Vitetta ES, Berton MT, Burger C, Kepron M, Lee WT, Yin X-M. Memory B and T cells. *Annu Rev Immunol* 1991;9:193.
16. Cochet M, Pannetier C, Regnault A, Darche S, Leclerc C, Kourilsky P. Molecular detection and *in vivo* analysis of the specific T cell response to a protein antigen. *Eur J Immunol* 1992;22:2639.
17. Weiss L. *Cell and tissue biology: a textbook of histology.* Baltimore: Urban and Schwarzenberg, 1988.
18. Trentin JJ. Influence of hematopoietic organ stroma (hematopoietic inductive microenvironments) on stem cell differentiation. In: Gorden AS, ed. *Regulation of hematopoiesis.* New York: Appleton-Century, 1970:161.
19. Till JE, McCulloch EA. A direct measurement of the radiation sensitivity of normal mouse bone marrow cells. *Radiat Res* 1961;14:213.
20. Wolf NS, Trentin JJ. Hemopoietic colony studies. V. Effect of hemopoietic organ stroma on differentiation of pluripotent stem cells. *J Exp Med* 1968;127:205.
21. Abramson S, Miller RG, Phillips RA. The identification in adult bone marrow of pluripotent and restricted stem cells of the myeloid and lymphoid systems. *J Exp Med* 1977;145:1567.
22. Wu AM, Till JE, Siminovitch L, McCulloch EA. Cytological evidence for a relationship between normal hematopoietic colony-forming cells and cells of the lymphoid system. *J Exp Med* 1968;127:455.
23. Lord BI, Testa NG, Hendry JH. The relative spatial distributions of CFUs and CFUc in the normal mouse femur. *Blood* 1975;46:65.
24. Siminovitch L, McCulloch EA, Till JE. The distribution of colony-forming cells among spleen colonies. *J Cell Comp Physiol* 1963;62:327.
25. Worton RG, McCulloch EA, Till JE. Physical separation of hemopoietic stem cells from cells forming colonies in culture. *J Cell Physiol* 1969;74:171.
26. Worton RG, McCulloch EA, Till JE. Physical separation of hemopoietic stem cells differing in their capacity for self-renewal. *J Exp Med* 1969;130:91.
27. Bertoncello I, Hodgson GS, Bradley TR. Multiparameter analysis of transplantable hemopoietic stem cells: I. The separation and enrichment of stem cells homing to marrow and spleen on the basis of rhodamine-123 fluorescence. *Exp Hematol* 1985;13:999.
28. Visser JW, Bauman JG, Mulder AH, Eliason JF, de Leeuw AM. Isolation of murine pluripotent hemopoietic stem cells. *J Exp Med* 1984;159:1576.
29. Ploemacher RE, Brons NH. Isolation of hemopoietic stem cell subsets from murine bone marrow: I. Radioprotective ability of purified cell suspensions differing in the proportion of day-7 and day-12 CFU-S. *Exp Hematol* 1988;16:21.
30. Dexter TM, Allen TD, Lajtha LG. Conditions controlling the proliferation of haemopoietic stem cells in vitro. *J Cell Physiol* 1977;91:335.
31. Dexter TM, Allen TD, Lajtha NG, Krizsa F, Testa NG, Moore MAS. In vitro analysis of self-renewal and commitment of hematopoietic stem cells. In: Clarkson B, Marks PA, Till JE, eds. *Differentiation of normal and neoplastic hematopoietic cells.* Cold Spring Harbor Laboratory, NY: 1978:63.
32. Whitlock CA, Witte ON. Long-term culture of B lymphocytes and their precursors from murine bone marrow. *Proc Natl Acad Sci USA* 1982;79:3608.
33. Zipori D, Duksin D, Tamir M, Argaman A, Toledo J, Malik Z. Cultured mouse marrow stromal cell lines. II. Distinct subtypes differing in morphology, collagen types, myelopoietic factors, and leukemic cell growth modulating activities. *J Cell Physiol* 1985;122:81.
34. Whitlock CA, Tidmarsh GF, Muller SC, Weissman IL. Bone marrow stromal cell lines with lymphopoietic activity express high levels of a pre-B neoplasia-associated molecule. *Cell* 1987;48:1009.
35. Hunt P, Robertson D, Weiss D, Rennick D, Lee F, Witte ON. A single bone marrow-derived stromal cell type supports the in vitro growth of early lymphoid and myeloid cells. *Cell* 1987;48:997.
36. Dorshkind K, Johnson A, Collins L, Keller GM, Phillips RA. Generation of puri-

fied stromal cell cultures that support lymphoid and myeloid precursors. *J Immunol Methods* 1986;89:37.

37. Spangrude GJ, Johnson GR. Resting and activated subsets of mouse multipotent hematopoietic stem cells. *Proc Natl Acad Sci USA* 1990;87:7433.

38. Smith LG, Weissman IL, Heimfeld S. Clonal analysis of hematopoietic stem-cell differentiation in vivo. *Proc Natl Acad Sci USA* 1991;88:2788.

39. Kiefer F, Wagner EF, Keller G. Fractionation of mouse bone marrow by adherence separates primitive hematopoietic stem cells from in vitro colony-forming cells and spleen colony-forming cells. *Blood* 1991;78:2577.

40. Ploemacher RE, Brons RH. Separation of CFU-S from primitive cells responsible for reconstitution of the bone marrow hemopoietic stem cell compartment following irradiation: evidence for a pre-CFU-S cell. *Exp Hematol* 1989;17:263.

41. Jones RJ, Celano P, Sharkis SJ, Sensenbrenner LL. Two phases of engraftment established by serial bone marrow transplantation in mice. *Blood* 1989;73:397.

42. Jones RJ, Wagner JE, Celano P, Zicha MS, Sharkis SJ. Separation of pluripotent haematopoietic stem cells from spleen colony-forming cells [see comments]. *Nature* 1990;347:188.

43. Spangrude GJ, Brooks DM, Tumas DB. Long-term repopulation of irradiated mice with limiting numbers of purified hematopoietic stem cells: in vivo expansion of stem cell phenotype but not function. *Blood* 1995;85:1006.

44. Andrews RG, Singer JW, Bernstein ID. Monoclonal antibody 12-8 recognizes a 115-kd molecule present on both unipotent and multipotent hematopoietic colony-forming cells and their precursors. *Blood* 1986;67:842.

45. Strauss LC, Rowley SD, La Russa VF, Sharkis SJ, Stuart RK, Civin CI. Antigenic analysis of hematopoiesis. V. Characterization of My-10 antigen expression by normal lymphohematopoietic progenitor cells. *Exp Hematol* 1986;14:878.

46. Andrews RG, Singer JW, Bernstein ID. Human hematopoietic precursors in long-term culture: single CD34+ cells that lack detectable T cell, B cell, and myeloid cell antigens produce multiple colony-forming cells when cultured with marrow stromal cells. *J Exp Med* 1990;172:355.

47. Sutherland HJ, Lansdorp PM, Henkelman DH, Eaves AC, Eaves CJ. Functional characterization of individual human hematopoietic stem cells cultured at limiting dilution on supportive marrow stromal layers. *Proc Natl Acad Sci USA* 1990;87:3584.

48. Sutherland HJ, Eaves CJ, Eaves AC, Dragowska W, Lansdorp PM. Characterization and partial purification of human marrow cells capable of initiating long-term hematopoiesis in vitro. *Blood* 1989;74:1563.

49. McCune JM, Namikawa R, Kaneshima H, Shultz LD, Lieberman M, Weissman IL. The SCID-hu mouse: murine model for the analysis of human hematolymphoid differentiation and function. *Science* 1988;241:1632.

50. Peault B, Weissman IL, Baum C, McCune JM, Tsukamoto A. Lymphoid reconstitution of the human fetal thymus in SCID mice with CD34+ precursor cells. *J Exp Med* 1991;174:1283.

51. Baum CM, Weissman IL, Tsukamoto AS, Buckle AM, Peault B. Isolation of a candidate human hematopoietic stem-cell population. *Proc Natl Acad Sci USA* 1992;89:2804.

52. Berenson RJ, Andrews RG, Bensinger WI, et al. Antigen CD34+ marrow cells engraft lethally irradiated baboons. *J Clin Invest* 1988;81:951.

53. Berenson RJ, Bensinger WI, Hill RS, et al. Engraftment after infusion of CD34+ marrow cells in patients with breast cancer or neuroblastoma. *Blood* 1991;77:1717.

54. Collins RJ. CD34+ selected cells in clinical transplantation [review, 45 refs]. *Stem Cells* 1994;12:577.

55. Civin CI, Almeida PG, Lee MJ, Olweus J, Terstappen LW, Zanjani ED. Sustained, retransplantable, multilineage engraftment of highly purified adult human bone marrow stem cells in vivo. *Blood* 1996;88:4102.

56. Hirsch E, Iglesias A, Potocnik AJ, Hartmann U, Fassler R. Impaired migration but not differentiation of haematopoietic stem cells in the absence of beta1 integrins. *Nature* 1996;380:171.

57. McCulloch EA, Siminovitch L, Till JE. Spleen-colony formation in anemic mice of genotype WW^v. *Science* 1964;144:844.

58. McCulloch EA, Siminovitch L, Till JE, Russell ES, Bernstein SE. The cellular basis of the genetically determined hemopoietic defect in anemic mice of genotype Sl/Sld. *Blood* 1965;26:399.

59. Russell ES. Hereditary anemias of the mouse: a review for geneticists. *Adv Genet* 1979;20:357.

60. Chabot B, Stephenson DA, Chapman VM, P. Besmer P, Bernstein A. The proto-oncogene c-kit encoding a transmembrane tyrosine kinase receptor maps to the mouse W locus. *Nature* 1988;335:88.

61. Geissler EN, Ryan MA, Housman DE. The dominant-white spotting (W) locus of the mouse encodes the c-kit proto-oncogene. *Cell* 1988;55:185.

62. Zsebo KM, Williams DA, Geissler EN, et al. Stem cell factor is encoded at the Sl locus of the mouse and is the ligand for the c-kit tyrosine kinase receptor. *Cell* 1990;63:213.

63. Williams DE, Eisenman J, Baird A, et al. Identification of a ligand for the c-kit proto-oncogene. *Cell* 1990;63:167.

64. Huang E, Nocka K, Beier DR, et al. The hematopoietic growth factor KL is encoded by the Sl locus and is the ligand of the c-kit receptor, the gene product of the W locus. *Cell* 1990;63:225.

65. Copeland NG, Gilbert DJ, Cho BC, et al. Mast cell growth factor maps near the steel locus on mouse chromosome 10 and is deleted in a number of steel alleles. *Cell* 1990;63:175.

66. Zsebo KM, Wypych J, McNiece IK, et al. Identification, purification, and biological characterization of hematopoietic stem cell factor from buffalo rat liver–conditioned medium. *Cell* 1990;63:195.

67. Anderson DM, Lyman SD, Baird A, et al. Molecular cloning of mast cell growth factor, a hematopoietin that is active in both membrane bound and soluble forms [published erratum appears in *Cell* 1990 Nov 30;63(5):following 1112]. *Cell* 1990;63:235.

68. Martin FH, Suggs SV, Langley KE, et al. Primary structure and functional expression of rat and human stem cell factor DNAs. *Cell* 1990;63:203.

69. Andrews RG, Knitter GH, Bartelmez SH, et al. Recombinant human stem cell factor, a c-kit ligand, stimulates hematopoiesis in primates. *Blood* 1991;78:1975.

70. Ulich TR, del Castillo CJ, McNiece IK, et al. Stem cell factor in combination with granulocyte colony-stimulating factor (CSF) or granulocyte-macrophage CSF synergistically increases granulopoiesis in vivo. *Blood* 1991;78:1954.

71. Molineux G, Migdalska A, Szmitkowski M, Zsebo K, Dexter TM. The effects on hematopoiesis of recombinant stem cell factor (ligand for c-kit) administered in vivo to mice either alone or in combination with granulocyte colony-stimulating factor. *Blood* 1991;78:961.

72. Zsebo KM, Smith KA, Hartley CA, et al. Radioprotection of mice by recombinant rat stem cell factor. *Proc Natl Acad Sci USA* 1992;89:9464.

73. Harrison DE, Zsebo KM, Astle CM. Splenic primitive hematopoietic stem cell (PHSC) activity is enhanced by steel factor because of PHSC proliferation. *Blood* 1994;83:3146.

74. Matthews W, Jordan CT, Wiegand GW, Pardoll D, Lemischka IR. A receptor tyrosine kinase specific to hematopoietic stem and progenitor cell-enriched populations. *Cell* 1991;65:1143.

75. Mackarehtschian K, Hardin JD, Moore KA, Boast S, Goff SP, Lemischka IR. Targeted disruption of the flk2/flt3 gene leads to deficiencies in primitive hematopoietic progenitors. *Immunity* 1995;3:147.

76. Sasaki K, Yagi H, Bronson RT, et al. Absence of fetal liver hematopoiesis in mice deficient in transcriptional coactivator core binding factor beta. *Proc Natl Acad Sci USA* 1996;93:12359.

77. Castilla LH, Wijmenga C, Wang Q, et al. Failure of embryonic hematopoiesis and lethal hemorrhages in mouse embryos heterozygous for a knocked-in leukemia gene CBFB-MYH11. *Cell* 1996;87:687.

78. Melchers F. Three waves of B lymphocyte development during embryonic development in the mouse. *INSERM Symp* 1979;10:281.

79. Yoshida Y, Osmond DG. Identity and proliferation of small lymphocyte precursors in cultures of lymphocyte-rich fractions of guinea pig bone marrow. *Blood* 1971;37:73.

80. Osmond DG, Nossal G. Differentiation of lymphocytes in mouse bone marrow. II. Kinetics of maturation and renewal of antiglobulin-binding cells studied by double labeling. *Cell Immunol* 1974;13:132.

81. Osmond DG. Population dynamics of bone marrow B lymphocytes. *Immunol Rev* 1986;93:103.

82. Kincade PW, Lee G, Pietrangeli CE, Hayashi S, Gimble JM. Cells and molecules that regulate B lymphopoiesis in bone marrow. *Annu Rev Immunol* 1989;7:111.

83. Cooper MD, Raymond DA, Peterson RD, South MA, Good RA. The functions of the thymus system and the bursa system in the chicken. *J Exp Med* 1966;123:75.

84. Loken MR, Shah VO, Hollander Z, Civin CI. Flow cytometric analysis of normal B lymphoid development. *Pathol Immunopathol Res* 1988;7:357.

85. Bancherau J, Rousset F. Human B lymphocytes: phenotype, proliferation, and differentiation. *Adv Immunol* 1992;52:125.

86. LeBien TW, Wormann B, Villablanca JG, et al. Multiparameter flow cytometric analysis of human fetal bone marrow B cells. *Leukemia* 1990;4:354.

87. Burrows PD, Cooper MD. B-cell development in man. *Curr Opin Immunol* 1993;5:201.

88. Hardy RR, Carmack CE, Shinton SA, Kemp JD, Hayakawa K. Resolution and characterization of pro-B and pre-pro-B cell stages in normal mouse bone marrow. *J Exp Med* 1991;173:1213.

89. Li YS, K. Hayakawa K, Hardy RR. The regulated expression of B lineage associated genes during B cell differentiation in bone marrow and fetal liver. *J Exp Med* 1993;178:951.

90. Oettinger MA, Schatz DG, Gorka C, Baltimore D. RAG-1 and RAG-2, adjacent genes that synergistically activate V(D)J recombination. *Science* 1990;248:1517.

91. Schatz DG, Oettinger MA, Baltimore D. The V(D)J recombination activating gene, RAG-1. *Cell* 1989;59:1035.

92. Tonegawa S. Somatic generation of antibody diversity. *Nature* 1983;302:575.

93. Desiderio SV, Yancopoulos GD, Paskind M, et al. Insertion of N regions into heavy-chain genes is correlated with expression of terminal deoxytransferase in B cells. *Nature* 1984;311:752.

94. Tillinghast JP, Russell JH, Fields LE, Loh DY. Protein kinase C regulation of terminal deoxynucleotidyl transferase. *J Immunol* 1989;143:2378.

95. Kunkel TA, Gopinathan KP, Dube DK, Snow ET, Loeb LA. Rearrangements of DNA mediated by terminal transferase. *Proc Natl Acad Sci USA* 1986;83:1867.

96. Kudo A, Melchers F. A second gene, VpreB in the lambda 5 locus of the mouse, which appears to be selectively expressed in pre-B lymphocytes. *EMBO J* 1987;6:2267.

97. Kudo A, Pravtcheva D, Sakaguchi N, Ruddle FH, Melchers F. Localization of the murine lambda 5 gene on chromosome 16. *Genomics* 1987;1:277.

98. Pillai S, Baltimore D. Formation of disulphide-linked mu 2 omega 2 tetramers in pre-B cells by the 18K omega-immunoglobulin light chain. *Nature* 1987;329:172.

99. Sakaguchi N, Melchers F. Lambda 5, a new light-chain-related locus selectively expressed in pre-B lymphocytes. *Nature* 1986;324:579.

100. Rolink A, Melchers F. Molecular and cellular origins of B lymphocyte diversity. *Cell* 1991;66:1081.

101. Tsubata T, Reth M. The products of pre-B cell-specific genes (lambda 5 and VpreB) and the immunoglobulin mu chain form a complex that is transported onto the cell surface. *J Exp Med* 1990;172:973.

102. Bossy D, Milili M, Zucman J, Thomas G, Fougereau M, Schiff C. Organization and expression of the lambda-like genes that contribute to the mu-psi light chain complex in human pre-B cells. *Int Immunol* 1991;3:1081.

103. Bauer SR, Kudo A, Melchers F. Structure and pre-B lymphocyte restricted expression of the VpreB in humans and conservation of its structure in other mammalian species. *EMBO J* 1988;7:111.

104. Schiff C, Bensmana M, Guglielmi P, Milili M, Lefranc MP, Fougereau M. The immunoglobulin lambda-like gene cluster (14.1, 16.1 and F lambda 1) contains gene(s) selectively expressed in pre-B cells and is the human counterpart of the mouse lambda 5 gene. *Int Immunol* 1990;2:201.

105. Kerr WG, Cooper MD, Feng L, Burrows PD, Hendershot LM. Mu heavy chains can associate with a pseudo-light chain complex (psi L) in human pre-B cell lines. *Int Immunol* 1989;1:355.

106. Nishimoto N, Kubagawa H, Ohno T, Gartland GL, Stankovic AK, Cooper MD. Normal pre-B cells express a receptor complex of mu heavy chains and surrogate light-chain proteins. *Proc Natl Acad Sci USA* 1991;88:6284.

107. Cherayil BJ, Pillai S. The omega/lambda 5 surrogate immunoglobulin light chain is expressed on the surface of transitional B lymphocytes in murine bone marrow. *J Exp Med* 1991;173:111.

108. Karasuyama H, Rolink A, Shinkai Y, Young F, Alt FW, Melchers F. The expression of Vpre-B/lambda 5 surrogate light chain in early bone marrow precursor B cells of normal and B cell-deficient mutant mice. *Cell* 1994;77:133.

109. Yancopoulos GD, Alt FW. Developmentally controlled and tissue-specific expression of unrearranged VH gene segments. *Cell* 1985;40:271.

110. Reth MG, Alt FW. Novel immunoglobulin heavy chains are produced from DJH gene segment rearrangements in lymphoid cells. *Nature* 1984;312:418.

111. Tsubata T, Tsubata R, Reth M. Cell surface expression of the short immunoglobulin mu chain (D mu protein) in murine pre-B cells is differently regulated from that of the intact mu chain. *Eur J Immunol* 1991;21:1359.

112. Karasuyama H, Rolink A, Melchers F. A complex of glycoproteins is associated with VpreB/lambda 5 surrogate light chain on the surface of mu heavy chain-negative early precursor B cell lines. *J Exp Med* 1993;178:469.

113. Hermans MH, Hartsuiker H, Opstelten D. An in situ study of B-lymphocytopoiesis in rat bone marrow. Topographical arrangement of terminal deoxynucleotidyl transferase-positive cells and pre-B cells. *J Immunol* 1989;142:67.

114. Osmond DG, Kim N, Manoukian R, Phillips RA, Rico VS, Jacobsen K. Dynamics and localization of early B-lymphocyte precursor cells (pro-B cells) in the bone marrow of scid mice. *Blood* 1992;79:1695.

115. Jacobsen K, Osmond DG. Microenvironmental organization and stromal cell associations of B lymphocyte precursor cells in mouse bone marrow. *Eur J Immunol* 1990;20:2395.

116. Dorshkind K, Witte ON. Long-term murine hemopoietic cultures as model systems for analysis of B lymphocyte differentiation. *Curr Top Microbiol Immunol* 1987;135:23.

117. Kincade PW. Experimental models for understanding B lymphocyte formation *Adv Immunol* 1987;41:181.

118. Collins LS, Dorshkind K. A stromal cell line from myeloid long-term bone marrow cultures can support myelopoiesis and B lymphopoiesis. *J Immunol* 1987;138:1082.

119. Dorshkind K. In vitro differentiation of B lymphocytes from primitive hemopoietic precursors present in long-term bone marrow cultures. *J Immunol* 1986;136:422.

120. Pietrangeli CE, Hayashi S, Kincade PW. Stromal cell lines which support lymphocyte growth: characterization, sensitivity to radiation and responsiveness to growth factors. *Eur J Immunol* 1988;18:863.

121. Landreth KS, Dorshkind K. Pre-B cell generation potentiated by soluble factors from a bone marrow stromal cell line. *J Immunol* 1988;140:845.

122. Bernardi P, Patel VP, Lodish HF. Lymphoid precursor cells adhere to two different sites on fibronectin. *J Cell Biol* 1987;105:489.

123. Miyake K, Underhill CB, Lesley J, Kincade PW. Hyaluronate can function as a cell adhesion molecule and CD44 participates in hyaluronate recognition. *J Exp Med* 1990;172:69.

124. Miyake K, Medina KL, Hayashi S, Ono S, Hamaoka T, Kincade PW. Monoclonal antibodies to Pgp-1/CD44 block lympho-hemopoiesis in long-term bone marrow cultures. *J Exp Med* 1990;171:477.

125. Miyake K, Weissman IL, Greenberger JS, Kincade PW. Evidence for a role of the integrin VLA-4 in lympho-hemopoiesis. *J Exp Med* 1991;173:599.

126. Miyake K, Medina K, Ishihara K, Kimoto M, Auerbach R, Kincade PW. A VCAM-like adhesion molecule on murine bone marrow stromal cells mediates binding of lymphocyte precursors in culture. *J Cell Biol* 1991;114:557.

127. Thomas PS, Pietrangeli CE, Hayashi S, et al. Demonstration of neural cell adhesion molecules on stromal cells that support lymphopoiesis. *Leukemia* 1988;2:171.

128. Sanderson RD, Sneed TD, Young LA, Sullivan GL, Lander AD. Adhesion of B lymphoid (MPC-11) cells to type I collagen is mediated by integral membrane proteoglycan, syndecan. *J Immunol* 1992;148:3902.

129. Arroyo AG, Yang JT, Rayburn H, Hynes RO. Differential requirements for alpha4 integrins during fetal and adult hematopoiesis. *Cell* 1996;85:997.

130. Namen AE, Lupton S, Hjerrild K, et al. Stimulation of B-cell progenitors by cloned murine interleukin-7. *Nature* 1988;333:571.

131. Sudo T, Ito M, Ogawa Y, et al. Interleukin 7 production and function in stromal cell-dependent B cell development. *J Exp Med* 1989;170:333.

132. Hayashi S, Kunisada T, Ogawa M, et al. Stepwise progression of B lineage differentiation supported by interleukin 7 and other stromal cell molecules. *J Exp Med* 1990;171:1683.

133. Rolink A, Kudo A, Karasuyama H, Kikuchi Y, Melchers F. Long-term proliferating early pre B cell lines and clones with the potential to develop to surface Ig-positive, mitogen reactive B cells in vitro and in vivo. *EMBO J* 1991;10:327.

134. Billips LG, Petitte D, Dorshkind K, Narayanan R, Chiu CP, Landreth KS. Differential roles of stromal cells, interleukin-7, and kit-ligand in the regulation of B lymphopoiesis. *Blood* 1992;79:1185.

135. Paul SR, Bennett F, Calvetti JA, et al. Molecular cloning of a cDNA encoding interleukin 11, a stromal cell-derived lymphopoietic and hematopoietic cytokine. *Proc Natl Acad Sci USA* 1990;87:7512.

136. Landreth KS, Narayanan R, Dorshkind K. Insulin-like growth factor-I regulates pro-B cell differentiation. *Blood* 1992;80:1207.

137. Rolink A, Streb M, Nishikawa S, Melchers F. The c-kit-encoded tyrosine kinase regulates the proliferation of early pre-B cells. *Eur J Immunol* 1991;21:2609.

138. Ogawa M, Matsuzaki Y, Nishikawa S, et al. Expression and function of c-kit in hemopoietic progenitor cells. *J Exp Med* 1991;174:63.

139. Deenen GJ, Van Balen I, Opstelten D. In rat B lymphocyte genesis sixty percent is lost from the bone marrow at the transition of nondividing pre-B cell to sIgM+ B lymphocyte, the stage of Ig light chain gene expression. *Eur J Immunol* 1990;20:557.

140. Park YH, Osmond DG. Dynamics of early B lymphocyte precursor cells in mouse bone marrow: proliferation of cells containing terminal deoxynucleotidyl transferase. *Eur J Immunol* 1989;19:2139.

141. Osmond DG. B cell development in the bone marrow. *Semin Immunol* 1990;2:173.

142. Reynolds JD. Evidence of extensive lymphocyte death in sheep Peyer's patches. I. A comparison of lymphocyte production and export. *J Immunol* 1986;136:2005.

143. Motyka B, Reynolds JD. Apoptosis is associated with the extensive B cell death in the sheep ileal Peyer's patch and the chicken bursa of Fabricius: a possible role in B cell selection. *Eur J Immunol* 1991;21:1951.

144. Brombacher F, Kohler G, Eibel H. B cell tolerance in mice transgenic for anti-CD8 immunoglobulin mu chain. *J Exp Med* 1991;174:1335.

145. Hartley SB, Crosbie J, Brink R, Kantor AB, Basten A, Goodnow CC. Elimination from peripheral lymphoid tissues of self-reactive B lymphocytes recognizing membrane-bound antigens. *Nature* 1991;353:765.

146. Nemazee DA, Burki K. Clonal deletion of B lymphocytes in a transgenic mouse bearing anti-MHC class I antibody genes. *Nature* 1989;337:562.

147. Russell DM, Dembic Z, Morahan G, Miller JF, Burki K, Nemazee D. Peripheral deletion of self-reactive B cells. *Nature* 1991;354:308.

148. Erikson J, Radic MZ, Camper SA, Hardy RR, Carmack C, Weigert M. Expression of anti-DNA immunoglobulin transgenes in non-autoimmune mice. *Nature* 1991;349:331.

149. Goodnow CC, Crosbie J, Adelstein S, et al. Altered immunoglobulin expression and functional silencing of self-reactive B lymphocytes in transgenic mice. *Nature* 1988;334:676.

150. Goodnow CC, Crosbie J, Jorgensen H, Brink RA, Basten A. Induction of self-tolerance in mature peripheral B lymphocytes [see comments]. *Nature* 1989;342:385.

151. Gu H, Zou YR, Rajewsky K. Independent control of immunoglobulin switch recombination at individual switch regions evidenced through Cre-loxP mediated gene targeting. *Cell* 1993;73:1155.

152. Kitamura D, Roes J, Kuhn R, Rajewsky K. A B cell-deficient mouse by targeted disruption of the membrane exon of the immunoglobulin mu chain gene. *Nature* 1991;350:423.

153. Kitamura D, Rajewsky K. Targeted disruption of mu chain membrane exon causes loss of heavy-chain allelic exclusion. *Nature* 1992;356:154.

154. Storb U, Engler P, Manz J, et al. Expression of immunoglobulin genes in transgenic mice and transfected cells. *Ann NY Acad Sci* 1988;546:51.

155. Misener V, Downey GP, Jongstra J. The immunoglobulin light chain related protein lambda 5 is expressed on the surface of mouse pre-B cell lines and can function as a signal transducing molecule. *Int Immunol* 1991;3:1129.

156. Takemori T, Mizuguchi J, Miyazoe I, et al. Two types of mu chain complexes are expressed during differentiation from pre-B to mature B cell. *EMBO J* 1990;9:2493.

157. Nomura J, Matsuo T, Kubota E, Kimoto M, Sakaguchi N. Signal transmission through the B cell-specific MB-1 molecule at the pre-B cell stage. *Int Immunol* 1991;3:117.

158. Kitamura D, Kudo A, Schaal S, Muller W, Melchers F, Rajewsky K. A critical role of lambda 5 protein in B cell development. *Cell* 1992;69:823.

159. Melchers F, Rolink A, Grawunder U, et al. Positive and negative selection events during B lymphopoiesis [review, 119 refs]. *Curr Opin Immunol* 1995;7:214.

160. Sakaguchi N, Kashiwamura S, Kimoto M, Thalmann P, Melchers F. B lympho-

cyte lineage-restricted expression of mb-1, a gene with CD3-like structural properties. *EMBO J* 1988;7:3457.

161. Hombach J, Leclercq L, Radbruch A, Rajewsky K, Reth M. A novel 34-kd protein co-isolated with the IgM molecule in surface IgM-expressing cells. *EMBO J* 1988;7:3451.

162. Kashiwamura S, Koyama T, Matsuo T, Steinmetz M, Kimoto M, Sakaguchi N. Structure of the murine mb-1 gene encoding a putative sIgM-associated molecule. *J Immunol* 1990;145:337.

163. Hombach J, Tsubata T, Leclercq L, Stappert H, Reth M. Molecular components of the B-cell antigen receptor complex of the IgM class. *Nature* 1990;343:760.

164. Hombach J, Lottspeich F, Reth M. Identification of the genes encoding the IgM-alpha and Ig-beta components of the IgM antigen receptor complex by amino-terminal sequencing. *Eur J Immunol* 1990;20:2795.

165. Matsuo T, Nomura J, Kuwahara K, et al. Cross-linking of B cell receptor-related MB-1 molecule induces protein tyrosine phosphorylation in early B lineage cells. *J Immunol* 1993;150:3766.

166. Igarashi H, Kuwahara K, Nomura J, et al. B cell Ag receptor mediates different types of signals in the protein kinase activity between immature B cell and mature B cell. *J Immunol* 1994;153:2381.

167. Nemazee D, Buerki K. Clonal deletion of autoreactive B lymphocytes in bone marrow chimeras. *Proc Natl Acad Sci USA* 1989;86:8039.

168. Hartley SB, Cooke MP, Fulcher DA, et al. Elimination of self-reactive B lymphocytes proceeds in two stages: arrested development and cell death. *Cell* 1993;72:325.

169. Shokat KM, Goodnow CC. Antigen-induced B-cell death and elimination during germinal-centre immune responses. *Nature* 1995;375:334.

170. Chen C, Nagy Z, Radic MZ, et al. The site and stage of anti-DNA B-cell deletion. *Nature* 1995;373:252.

171. Nossal GJ, Pike BL. Clonal anergy: persistence in tolerant mice of antigen-binding B lymphocytes incapable of responding to antigen or mitogen. *Proc Natl Acad Sci USA* 1980;77:1602.

172. Gay D, Saunders T, Camper S, Weigert M. Receptor editing: an approach by autoreactive B cells to escape tolerance. *J Exp Med* 1993;177:999.

173. Radic MZ, Erikson J, Litwin S, Weigert M. B lymphocytes may escape tolerance by revising their antigen receptors. *J Exp Med* 1993;177:1165.

174. Tiegs SL, Russell DM, Nemazee D. Receptor editing in self-reactive bone marrow B cells. *J Exp Med* 1993;177:1009.

175. Lang J, Jackson M, Teyton L, Brunmark A, Kane K, Nemazee D. B cells are exquisitely sensitive to central tolerance and receptor editing induced by ultralow affinity, membrane-bound antigen. *J Exp Med* 1996;184:1685.

176. Gu H, Tarlinton D, Muller W, Rajewsky K, Forster I. Most peripheral B cells in mice are ligand selected. *J Exp Med* 1991;173:1357.

177. Pospisil R, Fitts MG, Mage RG. CD5 is a potential selecting ligand for B cell surface immunoglobulin framework region sequences. *J Exp Med* 1996;184:1279.

178. Cyster JG, Healy JI, Kishihara K, Mak TW, Thomas ML, Goodnow CC. Regulation of B-lymphocyte negative and positive selection by tyrosine phosphatase CD45. *Nature* 1996;381:325.

179. Pospisil R, Young CG, Mage RG. Preferential expansion and survival of B lymphocytes based on VH framework 1 and framework 3 expression: "positive" selection in appendix of normal and VH-mutant rabbits. *Proc Natl Acad Sci USA* 1995;92:6961.

180. Le Douarin NM, Dieterlen-Lièvre F, Oliver PD. Ontogeny of primary lymphoid organs and lymphoid stem cells. *Am J Anat* 1984;170:261.

181. Benveniste P, Chadwick BS, Miller RG. Development of T cells in vitro from precursors in mouse bone marrow. *Cell Immunol* 1990;127:92.

182. Slieker WA, van der Loo JC, de Rijk-de Bruijn R, et al. ER-MP12 antigen, a new cell surface marker on mouse bone marrow cells with thymus-repopulating ability: II. Thymus-homing ability and phenotypic characterization of ER-MP12-positive bone marrow cells. *Int Immunol* 1993;5:1099.

183. Golunski E, Palacios R. Fetal liver and bone marrow JORO 75+ lymphocyte progenitors are precursors of CD4+8– TCR/CD3– early thymocytes. *J Exp Med* 1994;179:721.

184. Bertho JM, Mossalayi MD, Dalloul AH, Mouterde G, Debre P. Isolation of an early T-cell precursor (CFU-TL) from human bone marrow. *Blood* 1990;75:1064.

185. Palacios R, Samaridis J, Thorpe D, Leu T. Identification and characterization of pro-T lymphocytes and lineage-uncommitted lymphocyte precursors from mice with three novel surface markers. *J Exp Med* 1990;172:219.

186. Rodewald HR, Kretzschmar K, Takeda S, Hohl C, Dessing M. Identification of pro-thymocytes in murine fetal blood: T lineage commitment can precede thymus colonization. *EMBO J* 1994;13:4229.

187. Bruno L, Res P, Dessing M, Cella M, Spits H. Identification of a committed T cell precursor population in adult human peripheral blood. *J Exp Med* 1997;185:875.

188. Spangrude GJ, Scollay R. Differentiation of hematopoietic stem cells in irradiated mouse thymic lobes. Kinetics and phenotype of progeny. *J Immunol* 1990;145:3661.

189. Kurtzberg J, Denning SM, Nycum LM, Singer KH, Haynes BF. Immature human thymocytes can be driven to differentiate into nonlymphoid lineages by cytokines from thymic epithelial cells. *Proc Natl Acad Sci USA* 1989;86:7575.

190. Marquez C, Trigueros C, Fernandez E, Toribio ML. The development of T and non-T cell lineages from CD34+ human thymic precursors can be traced by the differential expression of CD44. *J Exp Med* 1995;181:475.

191. Matsuzaki Y, Gyotoku J, Ogawa M, et al. Characterization of c-kit positive intrathymic stem cells that are restricted to lymphoid differentiation. *J Exp Med* 1993;178:1283.

192. Keller G, Paige C, Gilboa E, Wagner EF. Expression of a foreign gene in myeloid and lymphoid cells derived from multipotent haematopoietic precursors. *Nature* 1985;318:149.

193. Fulop GM, Phillips RA. Use of scid mice to identify and quantitate lymphoid-restricted stem cells in long-term bone marrow cultures. *Blood* 1989;74:1537.

194. Georgopoulos K, Bigby M, Wang JH, et al. The Ikaros gene is required for the development of all lymphoid lineages. *Cell* 1994;79:143.

195. Zhuang Y, Soriano P, Weintraub H. The helix-loop-helix gene E2A is required for B cell formation. *Cell* 1994;79:875.

196. Bain G, Maandag EC, Izon DJ, et al. E2A proteins are required for proper B cell development and initiation of immunoglobulin gene rearrangements [see comments]. *Cell* 1994;79:885.

197. Urbanek P, Wang ZQ, Fetka I, Wagner EF, Busslinger M. Complete block of early B cell differentiation and altered patterning of the posterior midbrain in mice lacking Pax5/BSAP. *Cell* 1994;79:901.

198. Galy A, Travis M, Cen D, Chen B. Human T, B, natural killer, and dendritic cells arise from a common bone marrow progenitor cell subset. *Immunity* 1995;3:459.

198a. Kondo M, Weissman IL, Alaski K. Identification of clonogenic common lymphoid progenitors in mouse bone marrow. *Cell* 1997;91:661.

199. Wu L, Kincade PW, Shortman K. The CD44 expressed on the earliest intrathymic precursor population functions as a thymus homing molecule but does not bind to hyaluronate. *Immunol Lett* 1993;38:69.

200. Aurrand-lions M, Galland F, Bazin H, Zakharyev VM, Imhof BA, Naquet P. Vanin-1, a novel gpi-linked perivascular molecule involved in thymus homing. *Immunity* 1996;5:391.

201. Miller JFAP. Immunological function of the thymus. *Lancet* 1961;2:748.

202. Steinmann GG. Changes in the human thymus during aging. *Curr Top Pathol* 1986;75:43.

203. Middleton G. The incidence of follicular structures in the human thymus at autopsy. *Aust J Biol Med Sci* 1967;45:189.

204. Levine G, Bearman R. Electron microscopy of the human thymus. In: Johannessen J, ed. *Electron microscopy in human medicine.* New York: McGraw-Hill, 1980:5.

205. Cordier AC, Haumont SM. Development of thymus, parathyroids, and ultimo-branchial bodies in NMRI and nude mice. *Am J Anat* 1980;157:227.

206. Bockman DE, Kirby ML. Neural crest interactions in the development of the immune system. *J Immunol* 1985;135:766.

207. Jotereau FV, Le Douarin NM. Demonstration of a cyclic renewal of the lymphocyte precursor cells in the quail thymus during embryonic and perinatal life. *J Immunol* 1982;129:1869.

208. Fontaine PJ, Calman FM, Kaplan C, Le Douarin NM. Seeding of the 10-day mouse embryo thymic rudiment by lymphocyte precursors in vitro. *J Immunol* 1981;126:2310.

209. Le Douarin N. The microenvironment of T and B lymphocyte differentiation in avian embryos. *Curr Top Dev Biol* 1986;20:291.

210. Chen CH, Sowder JT, Lahti JM, Cihak J, Losch U, Cooper MD. TCR3: a third T-cell receptor in the chicken. *Proc Natl Acad Sci USA* 1989;86:2351.

211. Morin C, Jotereau F, Augustin A. Patterns of responsiveness of T-cell lines and thymocytes reveal waves of specific activity in the post-natal murine thymus. *Int Immunol* 1992;4:1091.

212. Moore MA, Owen JJ. Experimental studies on the development of the thymus. *J Exp Med* 1967;126:715.

213. Owen JJ, Ritter MA. Tissue interaction in the development of thymus lymphocytes. *J Exp Med* 1969;129:431.

214. van de Wijngaert FP, Kendall MD, Schuurman HJ, Rademakers LH, Kater L. Heterogeneity of epithelial cells in the human thymus. An ultrastructural study. *Cell Tissue Res* 1984;237:227.

215. von Gaudecker B. Functional histology of the human thymus. *Anat Embryol* 1991;183:1.

216. Marshall AH, White RG. The immunological reactivity of the thymus. *Br J Exp Pathol* 1961;42:379.

217. Raviola E, Karnovsky MJ. Evidence for a blood-thymus barrier using electron-opaque tracers. *J Exp Med* 1972;136:466.

218. Sainte-Marie G. Antigen penetration into the thymus. *J Immunol* 1963;91:840.

219. Nieuwenhuis P, Stet RJ, Wagenaar JP, Wubbena AS, Kampinga J, Karrenbeld A. The transcapsular route: a new way for (self-) antigens to by-pass the blood-thymus barrier? *Immunol Today* 1988;9:372.

220. Stet RJ, Wagenaar HJ, Nieuwenhuis P. Thymus localization of monoclonal antibodies circumventing the blood-thymus barrier. *Scand J Immunol* 1987;25:441.

221. Eggli P, Schaffner T, Gerber HA, Hess MW, Cottier H. Accessibility of thymic cortical lymphocytes to particles translocated from the peritoneal cavity to parathymic lymph nodes. *Thymus* 1986;8:129.

222. Hess MW, Mueller C, Schaffner T, Gerber HA, Eggli P, Cottier H. Thymic lymphopoiesis: protected from, or influenced by, external stimulation? *Ann NY Acad Sci* 1985;459:14.

223. Koelsch E. Migration of macrophages carrying antigen into the thymus. *Experientia* 1968;24:951.

224. Owen JJ, Jenkinson EJ. Embryology of the lymphoid system. [review, 143 refs]. *Prog Allergy* 1981;29:1.

225. Surh CD, Gao EK, Kosaka H, et al. Two subsets of epithelial cells in the thymic medulla. *J Exp Med* 1992;176:495.

226. Farr AG, Anderson SK. Epithelial heterogeneity in the murine thymus: fucose-specific lectins bind medullary epithelial cells. *J Immunol* 1985;134:2971.

227. Shier KJ. The thymus according to Schambacher: medullary ducts and reticular epithelium of thymus and thymomas. *Cancer* 1981;48:1183.

228. Gnezditskaya EV, Beletskaya LV. Immunofluorescence study of keratin of Hassell's corpuscles and epidermis of the human skin. *Bull Exp Biol Med* 1974;77:431.

229. Takigawa M, Imamura S, Ofuji S. Demonstration of epidermis-specific heteroantigens in thymic epithelial cells. *Int Arch Allergy Appl Immunol* 1977;55:58.

230. Beletskaya LV, Gnesditskaya EV. Detection of squamous epithelial intercellular substance antigen(s) in Hassall's corpuscles of human and animal thymus. *Scand J Immunol* 1980;12:93.

231. Lobach DF, Scearce RM, Haynes BF. The human thymic microenvironment. Phenotypic characterization of Hassell's bodies with the use of monoclonal antibodies. *J Immunol* 1985;134:250.

232. Wekerle H, Ketelsen UP, Ernst M. Thymic nurse cells. Lymphoepithelial cell complexes in murine thymuses: morphological and serological characterization. *J Exp Med* 1980;151:925.

233. Ritter MA, Sauvage CA, Cotmore SF. The human thymus microenvironment: in vivo identification of thymic nurse cells and other antigenically-distinct subpopulations of epithelial cells. *Immunology* 1981;44:439.

234. Rouse RV, Ezine S, Weissman IL. Expression of major histocompatibility complex antigens in the thymuses of chimeric mice. *Transplantation* 1985;40:422.

235. Zinkernagel RM, Callahan GN, Althage A, Cooper S, Klein PA, Klein J. On the thymus in the differentiation of "H-2 self-recognition" by T cells: evidence for dual recognition? *J Exp Med* 1978;147:882.

236. Zinkernagel RM, Althage A, Cooper S, et al. Ir-genes in H-2 regulate generation of anti-viral cytotoxic T cells. Mapping to K or D and dominance of unresponsiveness. *J Exp Med* 1978;148:592.

237. Zinkernagel RM. Thymus and lymphohemopoietic cells: their role in T cell maturation in selection of T cells' H-2-restriction-specificity and in H-2 linked Ir gene control. *Immunol Rev* 1978;42:224.

238. Zinkernagel RM, Callahan GN, Althage A, Cooper S, Streilein JW, Klein J. The lymphoreticular system in triggering virus plus self-specific cytotoxic T cells: evidence for T help. *J Exp Med* 1978;147:897.

239. Zinkernagel RM, Callahan GN, Klein J, Dennert G. Cytotoxic T cells learn specificity for self H-2 during differentiation in the thymus. *Nature* 1978;271:251.

240. Bevan MJ. In a radiation chimaera, host H-2 antigens determine immune responsiveness of donor cytotoxic cells. *Nature* 1977;269:417.

241. Haynes BF, Denning SM, Le PT, Singer KH. Human intrathymic T cell differentiation. *Semin Immunol* 1990;2:67.

242. Dalloul AH, Arock M, Fourcade C, et al. Human thymic epithelial cells produce interleukin-3. *Blood* 1991;77:69.

243. Le PT, Lazorick S, Whichard LP, et al. Human thymic epithelial cells produce IL-6, granulocyte-monocyte-CSF, and leukemia inhibitory factor. *J Immunol* 1990;145:3310.

244. Fujiwara H, Ogata M, Mizushima Y, Tatsumi Y, Takai Y, Hamaoka T. Proliferation and differentiation of immature thymocytes induced by a thymic stromal cell clone. *Thymus* 1990;16:159.

245. Carding SR, Hayday AC, Bottomly K. Cytokines in T-cell development. *Immunol Today* 1991;12:239.

246. Singer KH, Denning SM, Whichard LP, Haynes BF. Thymocyte LFA-1 and thymic epithelial cell ICAM-1 molecules mediate binding of activated human thymocytes to thymic epithelial cells. *J Immunol* 1990;144:2931.

247. Haynes BF, Telen MJ, Hale LP, Denning SM. CD44—a molecule involved in leukocyte adherence and T-cell activation [published erratum appears in *Immunol Today* 1990 Mar;11(3):80] *Immunol Today* 1989;10:423.

248. Safieh B, Kendall MD. Methods for assaying thymic hormones. *Thymus Update* 1988;1:117.

249. Dardenne M, Bach JF. Functional biology of thymic hormones. *Thymus Update* 1988;1:101.

250. Kendall MD. Functional anatomy of the thymic microenvironment. *J Anat* 1991;177:1.

251. Kinoshita Y, Hato F. Cellular and molecular effects of thymic epithelial cells on thymocytes during differentiation and maturation. *Int Rev Cytol* 1994;156:159.

252. Dargemont C, Dunon D, Deugnier MA, et al. Thymotaxin, a chemotactic protein, is identical to beta 2-microglobulin. *Science* 1989;246:803.

253. Imhof BA, Deugnier MA, Girault JM, et al. Thymotaxin: a thymic epithelial peptide chemotactic for T-cell precursors [published erratum appears in *Proc Natl Acad Sci USA* 1989 Mar;86(6):1992]. *Proc Natl Acad Sci USA* 1988;85:7699.

254. Wang J, Klein JR. Thymus-neuroendocrine interactions in extrathymic T cell development. *Science* 1994;265:1860.

255. Clegg CH, Rulffes JT, Wallace PM, Haugen HS. Regulation of an extrathymic T-cell development pathway by oncostatin. *Nature* 1996;384:261.

256. Steinman RM. The dendritic cell system and its role in immunogenicity. *Annu Rev Immunol* 1991;9:271.

257. Wu L, Li CL, Shortman K. Thymic dendritic cell precursors—relationship to the T lymphocyte lineage and phenotype of the dendritic cell progeny. *J Exp Med* 1996;184:903.

258. Kaiserling E, Stein H, Muller HH. Interdigitating reticulum cells in the human thymus. *Cell Tissue Res* 1974;155:47.

259. Beller DI, Unanue ER. IA antigens and antigen-presenting function of thymic macrophages. *J Immunol* 1980;124:1433.

260. Nakamura H, Ayer, LeLievre C. Neural crest and thymic myoid cells. *Curr Top Dev Biol* 1986;20:111.

261. Spuler S, Marx A, Kirchner T, Hohlfeld R, Wekerle H. Myogenesis in thymic transplants in the severe combined immunodeficient mouse model of myasthenia gravis. Differentiation of thymic myoid cells into striated muscle cells. *Am J Pathol* 1994;145:766.

262. Pearse M, Gallagher P, Wilson A, et al. Molecular characterization of T-cell antigen receptor expression by subsets of CD4- CD8- murine thymocytes. *Proc Natl Acad Sci USA* 1988;85:6082.

263. Pearse M, Wu L, Egerton M, Wilson A, Shortman K, Scollay R. A murine early thymocyte developmental sequence is marked by transient expression of the interleukin 2 receptor. *Proc Natl Acad Sci USA* 1989;86:1614.

264. Scollay R, Wilson A, D'Amico A, et al. Developmental status and reconstitution potential of subpopulations of murine thymocytes. *Immunol Rev* 1988;104:81.

265. Wu L, Scollay R, Egerton M, Pearse M, Spangrude GJ, Shortman K. CD4 expressed on earliest T-lineage precursor cells in the adult murine thymus. *Nature* 1991;349:71.

266. Rahemtulla A, Fung Leung WP, Schilham MW, et al. Normal development and function of CD8+ cells but markedly decreased helper cell activity in mice lacking CD4. *Nature* 1991;353:180.

267. Campana D, Janossy G, Coustan SE, et al. The expression of T cell receptor-associated proteins during T cell ontogeny in man. *J Immunol* 1989;142:57.

268. Haynes BF, Martin ME, Kay HH, Kurtzberg J. Early events in human T cell ontogeny. Phenotypic characterization and immunohistologic localization of T cell precursors in early human fetal tissues [published erratum appears in *J Exp Med* 1989 Feb 1;169(2):603]. *J Exp Med* 1988;168:1061.

269. Ceredig R, Schreyer M. Immunohistological location of host and donor derived cells in the regenerating thymus of radiation bone marrow chimeras. *Thymus* 1984;6:15.

270. Penit C, Vasseur F. Sequential events in thymocyte differentiation and thymus regeneration revealed by a combination of bromodeoxyuridine DNA labeling and antimitotic drug treatment. *J Immunol* 1988;140:3315.

271. Sprent J, Webb SR. Function and specificity of T cell subsets in the mouse. *Adv Immunol* 1987;41:39.

272. Adkins B, Mueller C, Okada CY, Reichert RA, Weissman IL, Spangrude GJ. Early events in T-cell maturation. *Annu Rev Immunol* 1987;5:325.

273. Scollay R, Jacobs S, Jerabek L, Butcher E, Weissman I. T cell maturation: thymocyte and thymus migrant subpopulations defined with monoclonal antibodies to MHC region antigens. *J Immunol* 1980;124.2845.

274. Fowlkes BJ, Pardoll DM. Molecular and cellular events of T cell development. *Adv Immunol* 1989;44:207.

275. Crispe IN, Moore MW, Husmann LA, Smith L, Bevan MJ, Shimonkevitz RP. Differentiation potential of subsets of CD4-8- thymocytes. *Nature* 1987;329:336.

276. Kingston R, Jenkinson EJ, Owen JJ. A single stem cell can recolonize an embryonic thymus, producing phenotypically distinct T-cell populations. *Nature* 1985;317:811.

277. Civin CI, Banquerigo ML, Strauss LC, Loken MR. Antigenic analysis of hematopoiesis. VI. Flow cytometric characterization of My-10-positive progenitor cells in normal human bone marrow. *Exp Hematol* 1987;15:10.

278. van Dongen JJ, Hooijkaas H, Comans-Bitter M, et al. Human bone marrow cells positive for terminal deoxynucleotidyl transferase (TdT), HLA-DR, and a T cell marker may represent prothymocytes. *J Immunol* 1985;135.3144.

279. Lobach DF, Hensley LL, Ho W, Haynes BF. Human T cell antigen expression during the early stages of fetal thymic maturation. *J Immunol* 1985;135:1752.

280. Godfrey DI, Zlotnik A. Control points in early T-cell development [review, 69 refs] *Immunol Today* 1993;14:547.

281. van Dongen JJ, Comans-Bitter WM, Wolvers TI, Borst J. Development of human T lymphocytes and their thymus-dependency. *Thymus* 1990;16:207.

282. Winoto A, Baltimore D. Separate lineages of T cells expressing the alpha beta and gamma delta receptors. *Nature* 1989;338:430.

283. MacDonald HR, Budd RC, Howe RC. A CD3- subset of CD4-8+ thymocytes: a rapidly cycling intermediate in the generation of CD4+8+ cells. *Eur J Immunol* 1988;18:519.

284. Paterson DJ, Williams AF. An intermediate cell in thymocyte differentiation that expresses CD8 but not CD4 antigen. *J Exp Med* 1987;166:1603.

285. Nikolic-Zugic J, Bevan MJ. Thymocytes expressing CD8 differentiate into CD4+ cells following intrathymic injection. *Proc Natl Acad Sci USA* 1988;85:8633.

286. Guidos CJ, Weissman IL, Adkins B. Intrathymic maturation of murine T lymphocytes from CD8+ precursors. *Proc Natl Acad Sci USA* 1989;86:7542.

287. Hugo P, Waanders GA, Scollay R, Shortman K, Boyd RL. Ontogeny of a novel CD4+CD8-CD3- thymocyte subpopulation: a comparison with CD4- CD8+ CD3- thymocytes. *Int Immunol* 1990;2:209.

288. Matsumoto K, Yoshikai Y, Moroi Y, Asano T, Ando T, Nomoto K. Two differential pathways from double-negative to double-positive thymocytes. *Immunology* 1991;72:20.

289. Hugo P, Waanders GA, Scollay R, Petrie HT, Boyd RL. Characterization of immature CD4+CD8-CD3- thymocytes. *Eur J Immunol* 1991;21:835.

290. Shinkai Y, Koyasu S, Nakayama K, et al. Restoration of T cell development in RAG-2-deficient mice by functional TCR transgenes. *Science* 1993;259:822.

291. Mombaerts P, Clarke AR, Rudnicki MA, et al. Mutations in T-cell antigen receptor genes alpha and beta block thymocyte development at different stages [published erratum appears in *Nature* 1992 Dec 3;360(6403):491]. *Nature* 1992;360:225.

292. Kishi H, Borgulya P, Scott B, et al. Surface expression of the beta T cell receptor (TCR) chain in the absence of other TCR or CD3 proteins on immature T cells. *EMBO J* 1991;10:93.

293. Groettru M, Ungewiss K, Azogu O, et al. A novel disulfide-linked heterodimer on pre-T cells consists of the T cell receptor beta chain and a 33 kd glycoprotein. *Cell* 1993;75:283.

294. Groettrup M, von Boehmer H. A role for a pre-T-cell receptor in T-cell development [review, 46 refs]. *Immunol Today* 1993;14:610.

295. Saint Ruf C, Ungewiss K, Groettrup M, Bruno L, Fehling HJ, von Boehmer H. Analysis and expression of a cloned pre-T cell receptor gene. *Science* 1994;266:1208.

296. Alam SM, Crispe IN, Gascoigne NRJ. Allelic exclusion of mouse T cell receptor alpha chains occurs at the time of thymocyte TCR up-regulation. *Immunity* 1995;3:449.

297. Borum K. Cell kinetics in mouse thymus studied by simultaneous use of 3H-thymidine and colchicine. *Cell Tissue Kinet* 1973;6:545.

298. Bryant B. Renewal and fate in the mammalian thymus: mechanisms and inferences of thymocytokinetics. *Eur J Immunol* 1972;2:38.

299. Egerton M, Scollay R, Shortman K. Kinetics of mature T-cell development in the thymus. *Proc Natl Acad Sci USA* 1990;87:2579.

300. Huesmann M, Scott B, Kisielow P, von Boehmer H. Kinetics and efficacy of positive selection in the thymus of normal and T cell receptor transgenic mice. *Cell* 1991;66:533.

301. Rothenberg EV, McGuire KL, Boyer PD. Molecular indices of functional competence in developing T cells. *Immunol Rev* 1988;104:29.

302. Scollay R, Bartlett P, Shortman K. T cell development in the adult murine thymus: changes in the expression of the surface antigens Ly2, L3T4 and B2A2 during development from early precursor cells to emigrants. *Immunol Rev* 1984;82:79.

303. Metcalf D. The nature and regulation of lymphopoiesis in normal and neoplastic thymus. In: Wolstenholme GWE, Porter R, eds. *The thymus: experimental and clinical studies, CIBA Foundation Symposium.* London: Churchill, 1966:242.

304. Shortman K, Egerton M, Spangrude GJ, Scollay R. The generation and fate of thymocytes. *Semin Immunol* 1990;2:3.

305. Poste ME, Olson IA. An investigation of the sites of mitotic activity in the guinea-pig thymus using autoradiography and colcemid-induced mitotic arrest. *Immunology* 1973;24:691.

306. Kerr JF, Wyllie AH, Currie AR. Apoptosis: a basic biological phenomenon with wide-ranging implications in tissue kinetics. *Br J Cancer* 1972;26:239.

307. Wyllie AH, Kerr JF, Currie AR. Cell death: the significance of apoptosis. *Int Rev Cytol* 1980;68:251.

308. Nakayama T, Ueda Y, Yamada H, Shores EW, Singer A, June CH. In vivo calcium elevations in thymocytes with T cell receptors that are specific for self ligands. *Science* 1992;257:96.

309. Kendall MD. The cell biology of cell death in the thymus. *Thymus Update* 1990;3:47.

310. Surh CD, Sprent J. T-cell apoptosis detected in situ during positive and negative selection in the thymus. *Nature* 1994;372:100.

311. Smith CA, Williams GT, Kingston R, Jenkinson EJ, Owen JJ. Antibodies to CD3/T-cell receptor complex induce death by apoptosis in immature T cells in thymic cultures. *Nature* 1989;337:181.

312. Jenkinson EJ, Kingston R, Smith CA, Williams GT, Owen JJ. Antigen-induced apoptosis in developing T cells: a mechanism for negative selection of the T cell receptor repertoire. *Eur J Immunol* 1989;19:2175.

313. Murphy KM, Heimberger AB, Loh DY. Induction by antigen of intrathymic apoptosis of CD4+CD8+TCRlo thymocytes in vivo. *Science* 1990;250:1720.

314. Strasser A, Harris AW, Cory S. bcl-2 transgene inhibits T cell death and perturbs thymic self-censorship. *Cell* 1991;67:889.

315. Sentman CL, Shutter JR, Hockenbery D, Kanagawa O, Korsmeyer SJ. bcl-2 inhibits multiple forms of apoptosis but not negative selection in thymocytes. *Cell* 1991;67:879.

316. Linette GP, Grusby MJ, Hedrick SM, Hansen TH, Glimcher LH, Korsmeyer SJ. Bcl-2 is upregulated at the CD4(+)CD8(+) stage during positive selection and promotes thymocyte differentiation at several control points. *Immunity* 1994;1:197.

317. Ogasawara J, Suda T, Nagata S. Selective apoptosis of CD4(+)CD8(+) thymocytes by the anti-Fas antibody. *J Exp Med* 1995;181:485.

318. Castro JE, Listman JA, Jacobson BA, et al. Fas modulation of apoptosis during negative selection of thymocytes. *Immunity* 1996;5:617.

319. Watanabe FR, Brannan CI, Copeland NG, Jenkins NA, Nagata S. Lymphoproliferation disorder in mice explained by defects in Fas antigen that mediates apoptosis. *Nature* 1992;356:314.

320. Sidman CL, Marshall JD, Von Boehmer H. Transgenic T cell receptor interactions in the lymphoproliferative and autoimmune syndromes of lpr and gld mutant mice. *Eur J Immunol* 1992;22:499.

321. Joel DD, Chanana AD, Cottier H, Cronkite EP, Laissue JA. Fate of thymocytes: studies with 125I-iododeoxyuridine and 3H-thymidine in mice. *Cell Tissue Kinet* 1977;10:57.

322. Crisa L, Cirulli V, Ellisman MH, Ishii JK, Elices MJ, Salomon DR. Cell adhesion and migration are regulated at distinct stages of thymic T cell development: the roles of fibronectin, VLA4, and VLA5. *J Exp Med* 1996;184:215.

323. Lucas B, Vasseur F, Penit C. Production, selection, and maturation of thymocytes with high surface density of TCR. *J Immunol* 1994;153:53.

324. Fischer M, MacNeil I, Suda T, Cupp JE, Shortman K, Zlotnik A. Cytokine production by mature and immature thymocytes. *J Immunol* 1991;146:3452.

325. Bendelac A, Schwartz RH. CD4+ and CD8+ T cells acquire specific lymphokine secretion potentials during thymic maturation. *Nature* 1991;353:68.

326. Nikolic-Zugic J. Phenotypic and functional stages in the intrathymic development of alpha beta T cells. *Immunol Today* 1991;12:65.

327. Scollay R. Thymus cell migration: cells migrating from thymus to peripheral lymphoid organs have a "mature" phenotype. *J Immunol* 1982;128:1566.

328. Kelly KA, Scollay R. Analysis of recent thymic emigrants with subset- and maturity-related markers. *Int Immunol* 1990;2:419.

329. Tough DF, Sprent J. Turnover of naive- and memory-phenotype T cells. *J Exp Med* 1994;179:1127.

330. Scollay R, Godfrey DI. Thymic emigration: conveyor belts or lucky dips? *Immunol Today* 1995;16:268.

331. Lo D, Reilly CR, Burkly LC, Dekoning J, Laufer TM, Glimcher LH. Thymic stromal cell specialization and the T-cell receptor repertoire. *Immunol Res* 1997;16:3.

332. Clark SL. The thymus in mice of strain 129/J studied with the electron microscope. *Am J Anat* 1961;112:1.

333. Kato S. Intralobular lymphatic vessels and their relationship to blood vessels in the mouse thymus. Light- and electron-microscopic study. *Cell Tissue Res* 1988;253:181.

334. Kendall MD. The morphology of perivascular spaces in the thymus. *Thymus* 1989;13:157.

335. Naparstek Y, Holoshitz J, Eisenstein S, et al. Effector T lymphocyte line cells migrate to the thymus and persist there. *Nature* 1982;300:262.

336. Michie SA, Rouse RV. Traffic of mature lymphocytes into the mouse thymus. *Thymus* 1989;13:141.

337. Surh CD, Sprent J, Webb SR. Exclusion of circulating T cells from the thymus does not apply in the neonatal period. *J Exp Med* 1993;177:379.

338. Agus DB, Surh CD, Sprent J. Reentry of T cells to the adult thymus is restricted to activated T cells. *J Exp Med* 1991;173:1039.

339. Philpott KL, Viney JL, Kay G, et al. Lymphoid development in mice congenitally lacking T cell receptor alpha beta-expressing cells. *Science* 1992;256:1448.

340. Custer RP, Bosma GC, Bosma MJ. Severe combined immunodeficiency (SCID) in the mouse. Pathology, reconstitution, neoplasms. *Am J Pathol* 1985;120:464.

341. Shores EW, Van Ewijk W, Singer A. Disorganization and restoration of thymic medullary epithelial cells in T cell receptor-negative scid mice: evidence that receptor-bearing lymphocytes influence maturation of the thymic microenvironment. *Eur J Immunol* 1991;21:1657.

342. Shores EW, Vanewijk W, Singer A. Maturation of medullary thymic epithelium requires thymocytes expressing fully assembled CD3-TCR complexes. *Int Immunol* 1994;6:1393.

343. Candeias S, Waltzinger C, Benoist C, Mathis D. The V beta 17+ T cell repertoire: skewed J beta usage after thymic selection; dissimilar CDR3s in CD4+ versus CD8+ cells. *J Exp Med* 1991;174:989.

344. Roth ME, Holman PO, Kranz DM. Nonrandom use of J alpha gene segments. Influence of V alpha and J alpha gene location. *J Immunol* 1991;147:1075.

345. Thompson SD, Pelkonen J, Hurwitz JL. First T cell receptor alpha gene rearrangements during T cell ontogeny skew to the 5' region of the J alpha locus. *J Immunol* 1990;145:2347.

346. Hurwitz JL, Samaridis J, Pelkonen J. Immature and advanced patterns of T cell receptor gene rearrangement among lymphocytes in splenic culture. *J Immunol* 1989;142:2533.

347. Roth ME, Lacy MJ, McNeil LK, Kranz DM. Selection of variable-joining region combinations in the alpha chain of the T cell receptor [published erratum appears in *Science* 1989 Sep 8;245(4922):245]. *Science* 1988;241:1354.

348. Patten P, Yokota T, Rothbard J, Chien Y, Arai K, Davis MM. Structure, expression and divergence of T-cell receptor beta-chain variable regions. *Nature* 1984;312:40.

349. Behlke MA, Spinella DG, Chou HS, Sha W, Hartl DL, Loh DY. T-cell receptor beta-chain expression: dependence on relatively few variable region genes. *Science* 1985;229:566.

350. Fink PJ, Matis LA, McElligott DL, Bookman M, Hedrick SM. Correlations between T-cell specificity and the structure of the antigen receptor. *Nature* 1986;321:219.

351. Bjorkman PJ, Saper MA, Samraoui B, Bennett WS, Strominger JL, Wiley DC. Structure of the human class I histocompatibility antigen, HLA-A2. *Nature* 1987;329:506.

352. Bjorkman PJ, Saper MA, Samraoui B, Bennett WS, Strominger JL, Wiley DC. The foreign antigen binding site and T cell recognition regions of class I histocompatibility antigens. *Nature* 1987;329:512.

353. Hunig T, Wallny HJ, Hartley JK, Lawetsky A, Tiefenthaler G. A monoclonal antibody to a constant determinant of the rat T cell antigen receptor that induces T cell activation. Differential reactivity with subsets of immature and mature T lymphocytes. *J Exp Med* 1989;169:73.

354. Kinnon C, Diamond RA, Rothenberg EV. Activation of T cell antigen receptor alpha- and beta-chain genes in the thymus: implications for the lineages of developing cortical thymocytes. *J Immunol* 1986;137:4010.

355. Jenkinson EJ, Kingston R, Owen JJ. Importance of IL-2 receptors in intra-thymic generation of cells expressing T-cell receptors. *Nature* 1987;329:160.

356. Ewing T, Egerton M, Wilson A, Scollay R, Shortman K. Subpopulations of CD4-CD8- murine thymocytes: differences in proliferation rate in vivo and proliferative responses in vitro. *Eur J Immunol* 1988;18:261.

357. Kishimoto H, Sprent J. Negative selection in the thymus includes semimature T cells. *J Exp Med* 1997;185:263.

358. Fink PJ, Bevan MJ. H-2 antigens of the thymus determine lymphocyte specificity. *J Exp Med* 1978;148:766.

359. Kruisbeek AM, Fultz MJ, Sharrow SO, Singer A, Mond JJ. Early development of the T cell repertoire. In vivo treatment of neonatal mice with anti-Ia antibodies interferes with differentiation of I-restricted T cells but not K/D-restricted T cells. *J Exp Med* 1983;157:1932.

360. McDuffie M, Born W, Marrack P, Kappler J. The role of the T-cell receptor in thymocyte maturation: effects in vivo of anti-receptor antibody. *Proc Natl Acad Sci USA* 1986;83:8728.

361. Marusic-Galesic S, Stephany DA, Longo DL, Kruisbeek AM. Development of CD4-CD8+ cytotoxic T cells requires interactions with class I MHC determinants. *Nature* 1988;333:180.

362. Teh HS, Kisielow P, Scott B, et al. Thymic major histocompatibility complex antigens and the alpha beta T-cell receptor determine the CD4/CD8 phenotype of T cells. *Nature* 1988;335:229.

363. Sha WC, Nelson CA, Newberry RD, Kranz DM, Russell JH, Loh DY. Selective expression of an antigen receptor on CD8-bearing T lymphocytes in transgenic mice. *Nature* 1988;335:271.

364. Kisielow P, Teh HS, Bluthmann H, von Boehmer H. Positive selection of antigen-specific T cells in thymus by restricting MHC molecules. *Nature* 1988;335:730.

365. Berg LJ, Pullen AM, Fazekas DS, et al. Antigen/MHC-specific T cells are preferentially exported from the thymus in the presence of their MHC ligand. *Cell* 1989;58:1035.

366. Bill J, Palmer E. Positive selection of CD4+ T cells mediated by MHC class II-bearing stromal cell in the thymic cortex. *Nature* 1989;341:649.

367. Van Ewijk W, Rouse RV, Weissman IL. Distribution of H-2 microenvironments in the mouse thymus. Immunoelectron microscopic identification of I-A and H-2K bearing cells. *J Histochem Cytochem* 1988;28:1089.

368. Farr AG, Anderson SK, Marrack P, Kappler J. Expression of antigen-specific, major histocompatibility complex-restricted receptors by cortical and medullary thymocytes in situ. *Cell* 1985;43:543.

369. Ron Y, Lo D, Sprent J. T cell specificity in twice-irradiated F1–parent bone marrow chimeras: failure to detect a role for immigrant marrow-derived cells in imprinting intrathymic H-2 restriction. *J Immunol* 1986;137:1764.

370. Lo D, Sprent J. Identity of cells that imprint H-2-restricted T-cell specificity in the thymus. *Nature* 1986;319:672.

371. Widera G, Burkly LC, Pinkert CA, et al. Transgenic mice selectively lacking MHC class II (I-E) antigen expression on B cells: an in vivo approach to investigate Ia gene function. *Cell* 1987;51:175.

372. van Ewijk W, Ron Y, Monaco J, et al. Compartmentalization of MHC class II gene expression in transgenic mice. *Cell* 1988;53:357.

373. Benoist C, Mathis D. Positive selection of the T cell repertoire: where and when does it occur? *Cell* 1989;58:1027.

374. Vukmanovic S, Grandea AG III, Faas SJ, Knowles BB, Bevan MJ. Positive selection of T lymphocytes induced by intrathymic injection of a thymic epithelial cell line. *Nature* 1992;359:729.

375. Dekoning J, Dimolfetto L, Reilly C, Wei Q, Havran WL, Lo D. Thymic cortical epithelium is sufficient for the development of mature T cells in relb-deficient mice. *J Immunol* 1997;158:2558.

376. Kyewski BA, Rouse RV, Kaplan HS. Thymocyte rosettes: multicellular complexes of lymphocytes and bone marrow-derived stromal cells in the mouse thymus. *Proc Natl Acad Sci USA* 1982;79:5646.

377. Longo DL, Schwartz RH. T-cell specificity for H-2 and Ir gene phenotype correlates with the phenotype of thymic antigen-presenting cells. *Nature* 1980;287:44.

378. Bix M, Raulet D. Inefficient positive selection of T cells directed by haematopoietic cells. *Nature* 1992;359:330.

379. Pawlowski T, Elliott JD, Loh DY, Staerz UD. Positive selection of T lymphocytes on fibroblasts. *Nature* 1993;364:642.

380. Hugo P, Kappler JW, McCormack JE, Marrack P. Fibroblasts can induce thymocyte positive selection in vivo. *Proc Natl Acad Sci USA* 1993;90:10335.

381. Finkel TH, Cambier JC, Kubo RT, Born WK, Marrack P, Kappler JW. The thymus has two functionally distinct populations of immature alpha beta + T cells: one population is deleted by ligation of alpha beta TCR. *Cell* 1989;58:1047.

382. Finkel TH, Kubo RT, Cambier JC. T-cell development and transmembrane signaling: changing biological responses through an unchanging receptor. *Immunol Today* 1991;12:79.

383. Marrack P, Kappler J. T cells can distinguish between allogeneic major histocompatibility complex products on different cell types. *Nature* 1988;332:840.

384. Jameson SC, Hogquist KA, Bevan MJ. Positive selection of thymocytes. *Annu Rev Immunol* 1995;13:93.

385. Scott B, Bluthmann H, Teh HS, von Boehmer H. The generation of mature T cells requires interaction of the alpha beta T-cell receptor with major histocompatibility antigens. *Nature* 1989;338:591.

386. Kaye J, Hsu ML, Sarvon ME, Jameson SC, Gascoigne NR, Hedrick SM. Selective development of CD4+ T cells in transgenic mice expressing a class II MHC-restricted antigen receptor. *Nature* 1989;341:746.

387. Zijlstra M, Bix M, Simister NE, Loring JM, Raulet DH, Jaenisch R. Beta 2-microglobulin deficient mice lack CD4-8+ cytolytic T cells [see comments]. *Nature* 1990;344:742.

388. Koller BH, Marrack P, Kappler JW, Smithies O. Normal development of mice deficient in beta 2M, MHC class I proteins, and CD8+ T cells. *Science* 1990;248:1227.

389. Cosgrove D, Gray D, Dierich A, et al. Mice lacking MHC class II molecules. *Cell* 1991;66:1051.

390. Grusby MJ, Johnson RS, Papaioannou VE, Glimcher LH. Depletion of CD4+ T

391. cells in major histocompatibility complex class II-deficient mice. *Science* 1991;253:1417.

391. Viville S, Neefjes J, Lotteau V, et al. Mice lacking the MHC class II-associated invariant chain. *Cell* 1993;72:635.

392. Van Kaer L, Ashton RP, Ploegh HL, Tonegawa S. TAP1 mutant mice are deficient in antigen presentation, surface class I molecules, and CD4-8+ T cells. *Cell* 1992;71:1205.

393. Gilfillan S, Waltzinger C, Benoist C, Mathis D. More efficient positive selection of thymocytes in mice lacking terminal deoxynucleotidyl transferase. *Int Immunol* 1994;6:1681.

394. Gilfillan S, Dierich A, Lemeur M, Benoist C, Mathis D. Mice lacking TdT: mature animals with an immature lymphocyte repertoire [published erratum appears in Science 1993 Dec 24;262(5142):1957]. *Science* 1993;261:1175.

395. Garrett TP, Saper MA, Bjorkman PJ, Strominger JL, Wiley DC. Specificity pockets for the side chains of peptide antigens in HLA-Aw68. *Nature* 1989;342:692.

396. Nikolic-Zugic J, Carbone FR. Peptide presentation by class-I major histocompatibility complex molecules. *Immunol Res* 1991;10:54.

397. Nikolic-Zugic J, Bevan MJ. Role of self-peptides in positively selecting the T-cell repertoire [see comments]. *Nature* 1990;344:65.

398. Jacobs H, Von DH, Melief CJ, Berns A. Mutations in the major histocompatibility complex class I antigen-presenting groove affect both negative and positive selection of T cells. *Eur J Immunol* 1990;20:2333.

399. Sha WC, Nelson CA, Newberry RD, et al. Positive selection of transgenic receptor-bearing thymocytes by Kb antigen is altered by Kb mutations that involve peptide binding. *Proc Natl Acad Sci USA* 1990;87:6186.

400. Berg LJ, Frank GD, Davis MM. The effects of MHC gene dosage and allelic variation on T cell receptor selection. *Cell* 1990;60:1043.

401. Sha WC, Nelson CA, Newberry RD, et al. Positive selection of transgenic receptor-bearing thymocytes by Kb antigen is altered by Kb mutations that involve peptide binding. *Proc Natl Acad Sci USA* 1990;87:6186.

402. Hsu BL, Evavold BD, Allen PM. Modulation of T cell development by an endogenous altered peptide ligand. *J Exp Med* 1995;181:805.

403. Tourne S, Nakano N, Viville S, Benoist C, Mathis D. The influence of invariant chain on the positive selection of single T cell receptor specificities. *Eur J Immunol* 1995;25:1851.

404. Ashton-Rickardt PG, Van KL, Schumacher TN, Ploegh HL, Tonegawa S. Peptide contributes to the specificity of positive selection of CD8+ T cells in the thymus. *Cell* 1993;73:1041.

405. Hogquist KA, Gavin MA, Bevan MJ. Positive selection of CD8+ T cells induced by major histocompatibility complex binding peptides in fetal thymic organ culture. *J Exp Med* 1993;177:1469.

406. Sebzda E, Wallace VA, Mayer J, Yeung RS, Mak TW, Ohashi PS. Positive and negative thymocyte selection induced by different concentrations of a single peptide. *Science* 1994;263:1615.

407. Sebzda E, Kundig TM, Thomson CT, et al. Mature T cell reactivity altered by peptide agonist that induces positive selection. *J Exp Med* 1996;183:1093.

408. Hogquist KA, Jameson SC, Heath WR, Howard JL, Bevan MJ, Carbone FR. T cell receptor antagonist peptides induce positive selection. *Cell* 1994;76:17.

409. Ashton-Rickardt PG, Bandeira A, Delaney JR, et al. Evidence for a differential avidity model of T cell selection in the thymus [see comments]. *Cell* 1994;76:651.

410. von Boehmer H, Teh HS, Kisielow P. The thymus selects the useful, neglects the useless and destroys the harmful. *Immunol Today* 1989;10:57.

411. Loh DY. Molecular requirements for cell fate determination during T-lymphocyte development. *New Biologist* 1991;3:924.

412. Fung-Leung WP, Schilham MW, Rahemtulla A, et al. CD8 is needed for development of cytotoxic T but not helper T cells. *Cell* 1991;65:443.

413. Killeen N, Sawada S, Littman DR. Regulated expression of human CD4 rescues helper T cell development in mice lacking expression of endogenous CD4. *EMBO J* 1993;12:1547.

414. Crooks ME, Littman DR. Disruption of T lymphocyte positive and negative selection in mice lacking the CD8 beta chain. *Immunity* 1994;1:277.

415. Fung-Leung WP, Kundig TM, Ngo K, et al. Reduced thymic maturation but normal effector function of CD8+ T cells in CD8 beta gene-targeted mice. *J Exp Med* 1994;180:959.

416. Arpaia E, Shahar M, Dadi H, Cohen A, Roifman CM. Defective T cell receptor signaling and CD8+ thymic selection in humans lacking zap-70 kinase. *Cell* 1994;76:947.

417. Swan KA, Alberola IJ, Gross JA, et al. Involvement of p21ras distinguishes positive and negative selection in thymocytes. *EMBO J* 1995;14:276.

418. Wang CR, Hashimoto K, Kubo S, et al. T cell receptor-mediated signaling events in CD4+CD8+ thymocytes undergoing thymic selection: requirement of calcineurin activation for thymic positive selection but not negative selection. *J Exp Med* 1995;181:927.

419. Gelfand EW, Weinberg K, Mazer BD, Kadlecck TA, Weiss A. Absence of ZAP-70 prevents signaling through the antigen receptor on peripheral blood T cells but not on thymocytes. *J Exp Med* 1995;182:1057.

420. Anderson G, Anderson KL, Conroy LA, et al. Intracellular signaling events during positive and negative selection of CD4+CD8+ thymocytes in vitro. *J Immunol* 1995;154:3636.

421. Alberola-Ila J, Forbush KA, Seger R, Krebs EG, Perlmutter RM. Selective requirement for MAP kinase activation in thymocyte differentiation. *Nature* 1995;373:620.

422. Negishi I, Motoyama N, Nakayama K, et al. Essential role for ZAP-70 in both positive and negative selection of thymocytes. *Nature* 1995;376:435.

423. Elder ME, Lin D, Clever J, et al. Human severe combined immunodeficiency due to a defect in ZAP-70, a T cell tyrosine kinase. *Science* 1994;264:1596.

424. Chan AC, Kadlecek TA, Elder ME, et al. ZAP-70 deficiency in an autosomal recessive form of severe combined immunodeficiency. *Science* 1994;264:1599.

425. Fischer KD, Zmuidzinas A, Gardner S, Barbacid M, Bernstein A, Guidos C. Defective T-cell receptor signalling and positive selection of Vav-deficient CD4(+) CD8(+) thymocytes. *Nature* 1995;374:474.

426. Zhang R, Alt FW, Davidson L, Orkin SH, Swat W. Defective signalling through the T and B-cell antigen receptors in lymphoid cells lacking the vav proto-oncogene. *Nature* 1995;374:470.

427. Hammerling GJ, Schonrich G, Momburg F, et al. Non-deletional mechanisms of peripheral and central tolerance: studies with transgenic mice with tissue-specific expression of a foreign MHC class I antigen. *Immunol Rev* 1991;122:47.

428. Jones LA, Chin LT, Kruisbeek AM. Acquisition of self-tolerance in T cells is achieved by different mechanisms, operating both inside and outside the thymus. *Thymus* 1990;16:195.

429. Webb S, Morris C, Sprent J. Extrathymic tolerance of mature T cells: clonal elimination as a consequence of immunity. *Cell* 1990;63:1249.

430. Ramsdell F, Fowlkes BJ. Clonal deletion versus clonal anergy: the role of the thymus in inducing self tolerance. *Science* 1990;248:1342.

431. Schonrich G, Kalinke U, Momburg F, et al. Down-regulation of T cell receptors on self-reactive T cells as a novel mechanism for extrathymic tolerance induction. *Cell* 1991;65:293.

432. Kisielow P, Bluthmann H, Staerz UD, Steinmetz M, von Boehmer H. Tolerance in T-cell-receptor transgenic mice involves deletion of nonmature CD4+8+ thymocytes. *Nature* 1988;333:742.

433. Jameson SC, Hogquist KA, Bevan MJ. Specificity and flexibility in thymic selection. *Nature* 1994;369:750.

434. Kawai K, Ohashi PS. Immunological function of a defined T-cell population tolerized to low-affinity self antigens [published erratum appears in *Nature* 1995 Nov 23;378(6555):419]. *Nature* 1995;374:68.

435. Kappler JW, Roehm N, Marrack P. T cell tolerance by clonal elimination in the thymus. *Cell* 1987;49:273.

436. Kappler JW, Staerz U, White J, Marrack PC. Self-tolerance eliminates T cells specific for Mls-modified products of the major histocompatibility complex. *Nature* 1988;332:35.

437. MacDonald HR, Schneider R, Lees RK, et al. T-cell receptor V beta use predicts reactivity and tolerance to Mlsa-encoded antigens. *Nature* 1988;332:40.

438. MacDonald HR, Pedrazzini T, Schneider R, Louis JA, Zinkernagel RM, Hengartner H. Intrathymic elimination of Mlsa-reactive (V beta 6+) cells during neonatal tolerance induction to Mlsa-encoded antigens. *J Exp Med* 1988;167:2005.

439. Gao EK, Lo D, Sprent J. Strong T cell tolerance in parent–F1 bone marrow chimeras prepared with supralethal irradiation. Evidence for clonal deletion and anergy. *J Exp Med* 1990;171:1101.

440. Bill J, Palmer E. Positive selection of CD4+ T cells mediated by MHC class II-bearing stromal cell in the thymic cortex. *Nature* 1989;341:649.

441. Berg LJ, de St Groth BF, Pullen AM, Davis MM. Phenotypic differences between alpha beta versus beta T-cell receptor transgenic mice undergoing negative selection. *Nature* 1989;340:559.

442. Pircher H, Burki K, Lang R, Hengartner H, Zinkernagel RM. Tolerance induction in double specific T-cell receptor transgenic mice varies with antigen. *Nature* 1989;342:559.

443. Sha WC, Nelson CA, Newberry RD, Kranz DM, Russell JH, Loh DY. Positive and negative selection of an antigen receptor on T cells in transgenic mice. *Nature* 1988;336:73.

444. Takahama Y, Shores EW, Singer A. Negative selection of precursor thymocytes before their differentiation into CD4+CD8+ cells. *Science* 1992;258:653.

445. Ohashi PS, Pircher H, Burki K, Zinkernagel RM, Hengartner H. Distinct sequence of negative or positive selection implied by thymocyte T-cell receptor densities. *Nature* 1990;346:861.

446. Guidos CJ, Danska JS, Fathman CG, Weissman IL. T cell receptor-mediated negative selection of autoreactive T lymphocyte precursors occurs after commitment to the CD4 or CD8 lineages. *J Exp Med* 1990;172:835.

447. Fowlkes BJ, Schwartz RH, Pardoll DM. Deletion of self-reactive thymocytes occurs at a CD4+8+ precursor stage. *Nature* 1988;334:620.

448. MacDonald HR, Hengartner H, Pedrazzini T. Intrathymic deletion of self-reactive cells prevented by neonatal anti-CD4 antibody treatment. *Nature* 1988;335:174.

449. Swat W, Ignatowicz L, von Boehmer H, Kisielow P. Clonal deletion of immature CD4+8+ thymocytes in suspension culture by extrathymic antigen-presenting cells. *Nature* 1991;351:150.

450. Swat W, Ignatowicz L, Kisielow P. Detection of apoptosis of immature CD4+8+ thymocytes by flow cytometry. *J Immunol Methods* 1991;137:79.

451. Schuurman HJ, Vaessen LM, Vos JG, et al. Implantation of cultured thymic fragments in congenitally athymic nude rats: ignorance of thymic epithelial haplotype in generation of alloreactivity. *J Immunol* 1986;137:2440.

452. Von Boehmer H, Schubiger K. Thymocytes appear to ignore class I major histocompatibility complex antigens expressed on thymus epithelial cells. *Eur J Immunol* 1984;14:1048.

453. von Boehmer H, Hafen K. Minor but not major histocompatibility antigens of thymus epithelium tolerize precursors of cytolytic T cells. *Nature* 1986;320:626.

454. Jenkinson EJ, Jhittay P, Kingston R, Owen JJ. Studies of the role of the thymic environment in the induction of tolerance to MHC antigens. *Transplantation* 1985;39:331.

455. Morrissey PJ, Sharrow SO, Kohno Y, Berzofsky JA, Singer A. Correlation of intrathymic tolerance with intrathymic chimerism in neonatally tolerized mice. *Transplantation* 1985;40:68.

456. Speiser DE, Lees RK, Hengartner H, Zinkernagel RM, MacDonald HR. Positive and negative selection of T cell receptor V beta domains controlled by distinct cell populations in the thymus. *J Exp Med* 1989;170:2165.

457. Speiser DE, Schneider R, Hengartner H, MacDonald HR, Zinkernagel RM. Clonal deletion of self-reactive T cells in irradiation bone marrow chimeras and neonatally tolerant mice. Evidence for intercellular transfer of Mlsa. *J Exp Med* 1989;170:595.

458. Roberts JL, Sharrow SO, Singer A. Clonal deletion and clonal anergy in the thymus induced by cellular elements with different radiation sensitivities. *J Exp Med* 1990;171:935.

459. Matzinger P, Guerder S. Does T-cell tolerance require a dedicated antigen-presenting cell? *Nature* 1989;338:74.

460. Brocker T, Riedinger M, Karjalainen K. Targeted expression of major histocompatibility complex (MHC) class II molecules demonstrates that dendritic cells can induce negative but not positive selection of thymocytes in vivo. *J Exp Med* 1997;185:541.

461. Robey E, Fowlkes BJ. Selective events in T cell development. *Annu Rev Immunol* 1994;12:675.

462. Marrack P, Kappler J. The T-cell repertoire for antigen and MHC. *Immunol Today* 1988;9:308.

463. Kishimoto H, Cai Z, Brunmark A, Jackson MR, Peterson PA, Sprent J. Differing roles for B7 and intercellular adhesion molecule-1 in negative selection of thymocytes [see comments]. *J Exp Med* 1996;184:531.

464. Nelson AJ, Hosier S, Brady W, Linsley PS, Farr AG. Medullary thymic epithelium expresses a ligand for CTLA4 in situ and in vitro. *J Immunol* 1993;151:2453.

465. Degermann S, Surh CD, Glimcher LH, Sprent J, Lo D. B7 expression on thymic medullary epithelium correlates with epithelium-mediated deletion of V beta 5+ thymocytes. *J Immunol* 1994;152:3254.

466. Prieto J, Takei F, Gendelman R, Christenson B, Biberfeld P, Patarroyo M. MALA-2, mouse homologue of human adhesion molecule ICAM-1 (CD54). *Eur J Immunol* 1989;19:1551.

467. Marrack P, Lo D, Brinster R, et al. The effect of thymus environment on T cell development and tolerance. *Cell* 1988;53:627.

468. Hoffmann MW, Allison J, Miller JF. Tolerance induction by thymic medullary epithelium. *Proc Natl Acad Sci USA* 1992;89:2526.

469. Salaun J, Bandeira A, Khazaal I, et al. Thymic epithelium tolerizes for histocompatibility antigens. *Science* 1990

470. Laufer TM, Dekoning J, Markowitz JS, Lo D, Glimcher LH. Unopposed positive selection and autoreactivity in mice expressing class II MHC only on thymic cortex. *Nature* 1996;383:81.

471. Burkly L, Hession C, Ogata L, et al. Expression of relB is required for the development of thymic medulla and dendritic cells. *Nature* 1995;373:531.

472. Burkly LC, Degermann S, Longley J, et al. Clonal deletion of V beta 5+ T cells by transgenic I-E restricted to thymic medullary epithelium. *J Immunol* 1993;151:3954.

473. Bonomo A, Matzinger P. Thymus epithelium induces tissue-specific tolerance. *J Exp Med* 1993;177:1153.

474. Carlow DA, Teh SJ, Teh HS. Altered thymocyte development resulting from expressing a deleting ligand on selecting thymic epithelium. *J Immunol* 1992;148:2988.

475. Douek DC, Corley K, Zal T, Mellor A, Dyson PJ, Altmann DM. Negative selection by endogenous antigen and superantigen occurs at multiple thymic sites. *Int Immunol* 1996;8:1413.

476. Kosaka H, Ogata M, Hikita I, et al. Model for clonal elimination in the thymus. *Proc Natl Acad Sci USA* 1989;86:3773.

477. Vukmanovic S, Jameson SC, Bevan MJ. A thymic epithelial cell line induces both positive and negative selection in the thymus. *Int Immunol* 1994;6:239.

478. Hugo P, Kappler JW, Godfrey DI, Marrack PC. Thymic epithelial cell lines that mediate positive selection can also induce thymocyte clonal deletion. *J Immunol* 1994;152:1022.

479. Vukmanovic S, Grandea AG, Faas SJ, Knowles BB, Bevan MJ. Positive selection of T-lymphocytes induced by intrathymic injection of a thymic epithelial cell line. *Nature* 1992;359:729.

480. Wright DH, Isaacson PG. The normal lymph node and spleen. In: *Biopsy pathology of the lymphoreticular system*, Gottlieb LS, Neville AM, Walker F, eds. Baltimore: Williams & Wilkins, 1983.

481. Rouse RV, Reichert RA, Gallatin WM, Weissman IL, Butcher EC. Localization of lymphocyte subpopulations in peripheral lymphoid organs: directed lymphocyte migration and segregation into specific microenvironments. *Am J Anat* 1984;170:391.

482. Ebnet K, Kaldjian EP, Anderson AO, Shaw S. Orchestrated information transfer underlying leukocyte endothelial interactions. *Annu Rev Immunol* 1996;14:155.

483. Davies AJ, Carter RL, Leuchars E, Wallis V. The morphology of immune reactions in normal, thymectomized and reconstituted mice. II. The response to oxazolone. *Immunology* 1969;17:111.

484. Sminia T, van der Brugge-Gamelkoorn GJ, Jeurissen SH. Structure and function of bronchus-associated lymphoid tissue (BALT). *Crit Rev Immunol* 1989;9:119.

485. Kuper CF, Koornstra PJ, Hameleers DMH, Duijvestijn AM, van Breda PJC, Sminia T. The role of nasopharyngeal lymphoid tissue. *Immunol Today* 1992;13: 219.

486. Owen RL, Ermak TH. Structural specializations for antigen uptake and processing in the digestive tract. *Springer Semin Immunopathol* 1990;12:139.

487. Pabst R. Is BALT a major component of the human lung immune system? *Immunol Today* 1992;13:119.

488. Brown AR. Immunological functions of splenic B-lymphocytes. *Crit Rev Immunol* 1992;11:395.

489. Koyama K. Hemodynamics of the spleen in Banti's syndrome. *Tohoku J Exp Med* 1967;93:199.

490. Pabst R. The role of the spleen in lymphocyte migration. In: Husband AJ, ed. *Migration and homing of lymphoid cells*. Boca Raton: CRC Press, 1988:63.

491. Wolf BC, Neiman RS. *Major problems in pathology*. Bennington JL, ed. Philadelphia: WB Saunders, 1989.

492. Van Rooijen N. The humoral immune response in the spleen. *Res Immunol* 1991; 142:328.

493. Van den Eertwegh AJM, Boersma WJA, Claassen E. Immunological functions and *in vivo* cell-cell interactions of T cells in the spleen. *Crit Rev Immunol* 1992; 11:337.

494. Timens W. The human spleen and the immune system: not just another lymphoid organ. *Res Immunol* 1991;142:316.

495. Y. J. Liu YJ, S. Oldfield S, I. C. MacLennan IC. Memory B cells in T cell-dependent antibody responses colonize the splenic marginal zones. *Eur J Immunol* 1988;18:355.

496. Dunn-Walters DK, Isaacson PG, Spencer J. Analysis of mutations in immunoglobulin heavy chain variable region genes of microdissected marginal zone (MGZ) B cells suggests that the MGZ of human spleen is a reservoir of memory B cells. *J Exp Med* 1995;182:559.

497. van den Oord JJ, de Wolf-Peeters C, Desmet VJ. The marginal zone in the human reactive lymph node. *Am J Clin Pathol* 1986;86:475.

498. Spencer J, Finn T, Pulford KA, Mason DY, Isaacson PG. The human gut contains a novel population of B lymphocytes which resemble marginal zone cells. *Clin Exp Immunol* 1985;62:607.

499. Kelsoe G. Life and death in germinal centers (redux). *Immunity* 1996;4:107.

500. McHeyzer-Williams MG, Davis MM. Antigen-specific development of primary and memory T cells in vivo. *Science* 1995;268:106.

501. Picker LJ, Terstappen LWMM, Rott LS, Streeter PR, Stein H, Butcher EC. Differential expression of homing-associated adhesion molecules by T-cell subsets in man. *J Immunol* 1990;145:3247.

502. Sanders ME, Makagoba MW, Sharrow SO, et al. Human memory T lymphocytes express increased levels of three cell adhesion molecules (LFA-3, CD2, and LFA-1) and three other molecules (UCHL1, CDw29, and Pgp-1) and have enhanced IFN-g production. *J Immunol* 1988;140:1401.

503. Vanhecke D, Leclercq G, Plum J, Vandekerckhove B. Characterization of distinct stages during the differentiation of human CD69+CD3+ thymocytes and identification of thymic emigrants. *J Immunol* 1995;155:1862.

504. Plebanski M, Sauders M, Burtles SS, Crowe S, Hooper DC. Primary and secondary human *in vitro* T-cell responses to soluble antigens are mediated by subsets bearing different CD45 isoforms. *Immunology* 1992;75:86.

505. Merkenschlager M, Terry L, Edwards R, Beverly PCL. Limiting dilution analysis of proliferative responses in human lymphocyte populations defined by the monoclonal antibody UCHL1:Implications for differential CD45 expression in T cell memory formation. *Eur J Immunol* 1988;18:1653.

506. Waldrop SL, Pitcher CJ, Peterson DM, Maino VC, Picker LJ. Determination of antigen-specific memory/effector CD4 cell frequencies by flow cytometry. *J Clin Invest* 1997;99:1739.

507. Salmon M, Kitas GD, Bacon PA. Production of lymphokine mRNA by CD45R+ and CD45R- helper T cells from human peripheral blood and by human CD4+ T cell clones. *J Immunol* 1989;143:907.

508. Kasahara Y, Miyawaki T, Kato K, et al. Role of interleukin 6 for differential responsiveness of naive and memory CD4+T cells in CD2-mediated activation. *J Exp Med* 1990;172:1419.

509. Kristensson K, Borrebaeck CAK, Carlsson R. Human CD4+T cells expressing CD45RA acquire the lymphokine gene expression of CD45RO+T-helper cells after activation *in vitro*. *Immunology* 1992;76:103.

510. Holter W, Majdic O, Kalthoff FS, Knapp W. Regulation of interleukin-4 production in human mononuclear cells. *Eur J Immunol* 1992;22:2765.

511. Picker LJ, Singh MK, Zdraveski Z, et al. Direct demonstration of cytokine synthesis heterogencity among human memory/effector T cells by flow cytometry. *Blood* 1995;86:1408.

512. Constant S, Zain M, West J, Pasqualini T, Ranney P, Bottomly K. Are primed CD4+ T lymphocytes different from unprimed cells? *Eur J Immunol* 1994;24: 1073.

513. Damle NK, Klussman K, Linsley PS, Aruffo A. Differential costimulatory effects of adhesion molecules B7, ICAM-1, LFA-3, and VCAM-1 on resting and antigen-primed CD4+T lymphocytes. *J Immunol* 1992;148:1985.

514. Schwinzer R, Siefken R, Franklin RA, Saloga J, Wonigeit K, Gelfand EW. Human CD45RA+ and CD45RO+ T cells exhibit similar CD3/T cell receptor-mediated transmembrane signaling capacities but differ in response to co-stimulatory signals. *Eur J Immunol* 1994;24:1391.

515. Luqman M, Bottomly K. Activation requirements for CD4+ T cells differing in CD45R expression. *J Immunol* 1992;149:2300.

516. de Jong R, Brouwer M, Miedema F, van Lier RAW. Human CD8 T lymphocytes

517. Schlunck T, Schraut W, Riethmüller G, Ziegler-Heitbrock HWL. Inverse relationship of CA2+ mobilization and cell proliferation in CD8+ memory and virgin T cells. *Eur J Immunol* 1990;20:1957.

518. Picker LJ, Butcher EC. Physiological and molecular mechanisms of lymphocyte homing. *Annu Rev Immunol* 1992;10:561.

519. C. R. Mackay. Migration pathways and immunologic memory among T lymphocytes. *Semin Immunol* 1992;4:51.

520. Picker LJ. Control of lymphocyte homing. *Curr Opin Immunol* 1994;6:394.

521. Butcher EC, Picker LJ. Lymphocyte homing and homeostasis. *Science* 1996;272: 60.

522. Akbar AN, Borthwick N, Salmon M, et al. The significance of low bcl-2 expression by CD45RO T cells in normal individuals and patients with acute viral infections. The role of apoptosis in T cell memory. *J Exp Med* 1993;178:427.

523. Salmon M, Pilling D, Borthwick NJ, et al. The progressive differentiation of primed T cells is associated with an increasing susceptibility to apoptosis. *Eur J Immunol* 1994;24:892.

524. Pitzalis C, Kingsley G, Haskard D, Panayi G. The preferential accumulation of helper-inducer T lymphocytes in inflammatory lesions: evidence for regulation by selective endothelial and homotypic adhesion. *Eur J Immunol* 1988;18:1397.

525. Pitzalis C, Kingsley GH, Covelli M, Meliconi AM, Panayi GS. Selective migration of the human helper-inducer memory T cell subset: confirmation by *in vivo* cellular kinetic studies. *Eur J Immunol* 1991;21:369.

526. Picker L, Treer JR, Ferguson-Darnell B, Collins PA, Buck D, Terstappen LW. Control of lymphocyte recirculation in man. I. Differential regulation of the peripheral lymph node homing receptor I -selection on T cells during the virgin to memory cell transition. *J Immunol* 1993;150:1105.

527. Janossy G, Bofill M, Rowe D, Muir J, Beverley PC. The tissue distribution of T lymphocytes expressing different CD45 polypeptides. *Immunology* 1989;66:517.

528. Marathias KP, Preffer FI, Pinto C, Kradin RL. Most human pulmonary infiltrating lymphocytes display the surface immune phenotype and functional responses of sensitized T cell. *Am J Respir Cell Mol Biol* 1991;5:470.

529. Zeitz M, Schieferdecker HL, James SP, Riecken EO. Special functional features of T-lymphocyte subpopulations in the effector compartment of the intestinal mucosa and their relation to mucosal transformation. *Digestion* 1990;46:280.

530. Volpes R, van den Oord JJ, Desmet VJ. Memory T cells represent the predominant lymphocyte subset in acute and chronic liver inflammation. *Hepatology* 1991;13:826.

531. Collins RH, Sackler RH, Pitcher CJ, et al. Immune reconstitution with donor-derived memory/effector T cells after orthotopic liver transplantation. *Exp Hematol* 1997;25:147.

532. Shimizu Y, Van Seventer GA, Horgan KJ, Shaw S. Regulated expression and binding of three VLA (b1) integrin receptors on T cells. *Nature* 1990;345:250.

533. Shimizu Y, Newman W, Gopal TV, et al. Four molecular pathways of T cell adhesion to endothelial cells: roles of LFA-1, VCAM-1, and ELAM-1 and changes in pathway hierarchy under different activation conditions. *J Cell Biol* 1991;113: 1203.

534. Buckle AM, Hogg N. Human memory T cells express intercellular adhesion molecule-1 which can be increased by interleukin 2 and interferon-g. *Eur J Immunol* 1990;20:337.

535. Hintzen RQ, de Jong R, Lens SM, Brouwer M, Baars P. Regulation of CD27 expression on subsets of mature T-lymphocytes. *J Immunol* 1993;151:2426.

536. Baars PA, Maurice MM, Rep M, Hooibrink R, van Lier A. Heterogeneity of the circulating human CD4+ T cell population. Further evidence that the CD4+CD45RA-CD27- T cell subset contains specialized primed T cells. *J Immunol* 1995;154:17.

537. Picker LJ, Martin RJ, Trumble A, et al. Differential expression of lymphocyte homing receptors by human memory/effector T cells in pulmonary versus cutaneous immune effector sites. *Eur J Immunol* 1994;24:1269.

538. Akbar AN, Terry L, Timms A, Beverly PCL, Janossy G. Loss of CD45R and gain of UCHL1 reactivity is a feature of primed T cells. *J Immunol* 1988;140:2171.

539. Zheng B, Xue W, Kelsoe G. Locus-specific somatic hypermutation in germinal centre T cells. *Nature* 1994;372:556.

540. Sprent J, Tough DF. Lymphocyte life-span and memory. *Science* 1994;265:1395.

541. Rogers PR, Pilapil S, Hayakawa K, Romain PL, Parker DC. CD45 alternative exon expression in murine and human CD4 T cell subsets. *J Immunol* 1992; 148:4054.

542. Sparshott SM, Bell EB, Sarawar SR. CD45R CD4 T cell subset-reconstituted nude rats: subset-dependent survival of recipients and bi-directional isoform switching. *Eur J Immunol* 1991;21:993.

543. Rabin RL, Roederer M, Maldonado Y, Petru A, Herzenberg LA, Herzenberg LA. Altered representation of naive and memory CD8 T cell subsets in HIV-infected children. *J Clin Invest* 1995;95:2054.

544. Roederer M, Dubs JG, Anderson MT, Raju PA, Herzenberg LA. CD8 naive T cell counts decrease progressively in HIV-infected adults. *J Clin Invest* 1995;95: 2061.

545. Okumura M, Fujii Y, Inada K, Nakahara K, Matsuda H. Both CD45RA+ and CD45RA- subpopulations of CD8+ T cells contain cells with high levels of lymphocyte function-associated antigen-1 expression, a phenotype of primed T cells. *J Immunol* 1993;150:429.

546. Butcher EC. The regulation of lymphocyte traffic. *Curr Top Microbiol Immunol* 1986;128:85.

547. Paul WE, Seder RA. Lymphocyte responses and cytokines. *Cell* 1994;76:241.

548. Mosmann TR, Coffman RL. TH1 and TH2 cells: different patterns of lymphokine secretion lead to different functional properties. *Annu Rev Immunol* 1989;7:145.

549. Street NE, Mosmann TR. Functional diversity of T lymphocytes due to secretion of different cytokine patterns. *FASEB J* 1991;5:171.

550. Sher A, Coffman RL. Regulation of immunity to parasites by T cells and T cell-derived cytokines [review, 133 refs]. *Annu Rev Immunol* 1992;10:385.

551. Locksley RM. Th2 cells: help for helminths. *J Exp Med* 1994;179:1405.

552. Romagnani S, Del Prete G, Maggi E, et al. Human Th1 and Th2 Subsets. *Int Arch Allergy Immunol* 1992;99:242.

553. Romagnani S. Regulation of the development of type 2 T-helper cells in allergy. *Curr Opin Immunol* 1994;6:838.

554. King CL, Mahanty S, Kumaraswami V, et al. Cytokine control of parasite-specific anergy in human lymphatic filariasis. Preferential induction of a regulatory T helper type 2 lymphocyte subset. *J Clin Invest* 1993;92:1667.

555. Orme IM, Roberts AD, Griffin JP, Abrams JS. Cytokine secretion by CD4 T lymphocytes acquired in response to Mycobacterium tuberculosis infection. *J Immunol* 1993;151:518.

556. Pirmez C, Yamamura M, Uyemura K, Paes-Oliveira M, Conceicao-Silva F, Modlin RL. Cytokine patterns in the pathogenesis of human leishmaniasis [see comments]. *J Clin Invest* 1993;91:1390.

557. elGhazali GE, Paulie S, Andersson G, et al. Number of interleukin-4- and interferon-gamma-secreting human T cells reactive with tetanus toxoid and the mycobacterial antigen PPD or phytohemagglutinin: distinct response profiles depending on the type of antigen used for activation. *Eur J Immunol* 1993;23:2740.

558. Hamid Q, Boguniewicz M, Leung DY. Differential in situ cytokine gene expression in acute versus chronic atopic dermatitis. *J Clin Invest* 1994;94:870.

559. Kelso A. Th1 and Th2 subsets: paradigms lost? *Immunol Today* 1995;16:374.

560. Guidotti LG, Chisari FV. To kill or to cure: options in host defense against viral infection [review, 58 refs]. *Curr Opin Immunol* 1996;8:478.

561. Kagi D, Hengartner H. Different roles for cytotoxic T cells in the control of infections with cytopathic versus noncytopathic viruses. *Curr Opin Immunol* 1996;8:472.

562. Seder RA, Boulay JL, Finkelman F, et al. CD8+ T cells can be primed in vitro to produce IL-4. *J Immunol* 1992;148:1652.

563. Kelso A, Troutt AB, Maraskovsky E, et al. Heterogeneity in lymphokine profiles of CD4+ and CD8+ T cells and clones activated in vivo and in vitro. *Immunol Rev* 1991;123:85.

564. Croft M, Carter L, Swain SL, Dutton RW. Generation of polarized antigen-specific CD8 effector populations: reciprocal action of interleukin (IL)-4 and IL-12 in promoting type 2 versus type 1 cytokine profiles. *J Exp Med* 1994;180:1715.

565. Rogers WO, Weaver CT, Kraus LA, Li JM, Li LF, Bucy RP. Visualization of antigen-specific T cell activation and cytokine expression in vivo. *J Immunol* 1997;158:649.

566. Catalina MD, Carroll MC, Arizpe H, Takashima A, Estess P, Siegelman MH. The route of antigen entry determines the requirement for l-selectin during immune responses. *J Exp Med* 1996;184:2341.

567. Sprent J, Schaefer M, Hurd M, Surh CD, Ron Y. Mature murine B and T cells transferred to SCID mice can survive indefinitely and many maintain a virgin phenotype. *J Exp Med* 1991;174:717.

568. Openshaw P, Murphy EE, Hosken NA, et al. Heterogeneity of intracellular cytokine synthesis at the single-cell level in polarized T helper 1 and T helper 2 populations. *J Exp Med* 1995;182:1357.

569. Sornasse T, Larenas PV, Davis KA, de Vries JE, Yssel H. Differentiation and stability of T helper 1 and 2 cells derived from naive human neonatal CD4+ T cells, analyzed at the single-cell level. *J Exp Med* 1996;184:473.

570. Caux C, Vanbervliet B, Massacrier C, et al. CD34+ hematopoietic progenitors from human cord blood differentiate along two independent dendritic cell pathways in response to GM-CSF+TNF alpha. *J Exp Med* 1996;184:695.

571. Freudenthal PS, Steinman RM. The distinct surface of human blood dendritic cells, as observed after an improved isolation method. *Proc Natl Acad Sci USA* 1990;87:7698.

572. Crowley M, Inaba K, Steinman RM. Dendritic cells are the principal cells in mouse spleen bearing immunogenic fragments of foreign proteins. *J Exp Med* 1990;172:383.

573. Inaba K, Metlay JP, Crowley MT, Steinman RM. Dendritic cells pulsed with protein antigens in vitro can prime antigen-specific, MHC-restricted T cells in situ [published erratum appears in *J Exp Med* 1990 Oct 1;172(4):1275]. *J Exp Med* 1990;172:631.

574. Boog CJ, Boes J, Melief CJ. Role of dendritic cells in the regulation of class I restricted cytotoxic T lymphocyte responses. *J Immunol* 1988;140:3331.

575. Sprent J, Schaefer M. Antigen-presenting cells for unprimed T cells. *Immunol Today* 1989;10:17.

576. Cassell DJ, Schwartz RH. A quantitative analysis of antigen-presenting cell function: activated B cells stimulate naive CD4 T cells but are inferior to dendritic cells in providing costimulation. *J Exp Med* 1994;180:1829.

577. Larsen CP, Ritchie SC, Pearson TC, Linsley PS, Lowry RP. Functional expression of the costimulatory molecule, B7/BB1, on murine dendritic cell populations. *J Exp Med* 1992;176:1215.

578. Teunissen MB, Rongen HA, Bos JD. Function of adhesion molecules lymphocyte function-associated antigen-3 and intercellular adhesion molecule-1 on human epidermal Langerhans cells in antigen-specific T cell activation. *J Immunol* 1994;152:3400.

579. Cumberbatch M, Kimber I. Phenotypic characteristics of antigen-bearing cells in the draining lymph nodes of contact sensitized mice. *Immunology* 1990;71:404.

580. Bujdoso R, Hopkins J, Dutia BM, Young P, McConnell I. Characterization of sheep afferent lymph dendritic cells and their role in antigen carriage. *J Exp Med* 1989;170:1285.

581. Macatonia SE, Knight SC, Edwards AJ, Griffiths S, Fryer P. Localization of antigen on lymph node dendritic cells after exposure to the contact sensitizer fluorescein isothiocyanate. Functional and morphological studies. *J Exp Med* 1987;166:1654.

582. Dai R, Grammer SF, Streilein JW. Fresh and cultured Langerhans cells display differential capacities to activate hapten-specific T cells. *J Immunol* 1993;150:59.

583. Streilein JW, Grammer SF. *In vitro* evidence that Langerhans cells can adopt two functionally distinct forms capable of antigen presentation to T lymphocytes. *J Immunol* 1989;143:3925.

584. Bergstresser PR. Sensitization and elicitation of inflammation in contact dermatitis. In: Norns D, ed. *Immunologic mechanisms in cutaneous disease*. New York: Marcel Dekker Inc, 1988:220.

585. Xia W, Pinto CE, Kradin RL. The antigen-presenting activities of Ia+ dendritic cells shift dynamically from lung to lymph node after an airway challenge with soluble antigen. *J Exp Med* 1995;181:1275.

586. Liu LM, MacPherson GG. Antigen acquisition by dendritic cells: intestinal dendritic cells acquire antigen administered orally and can prime naive T cells in vivo. *J Exp Med* 1993;177:1299.

587. Austyn JM, Kupiec WJ, Hankins DF, Morris PJ. Migration patterns of dendritic cells in the mouse. Homing to T cell-dependent areas of spleen, and binding within marginal zone. *J Exp Med* 1988;167:646.

588. Kudo S, Matsuno K, Ezaki T, Ogawa M. A novel migration pathway for rat dendritic cells from the blood: hepatic sinusoids-lymph translocation. *J Exp Med* 1997;185:777.

589. Akbar AN, Salmon M, Savill J, Janossy G. A possible role for bcl-2 in regulating T-cell memory—a `balancing act' between cell death and survival. *Immunol Today* 1993;14:526.

590. Osborne BA. Apoptosis and the maintenance of homoeostasis in the immune system. *Curr Opin Immunol* 1996;8:245.

591. Doherty PC, Topham DJ, Tripp RA. Establishment and persistence of virus-specific CD4(+) and CD8(+) T cell memory. *Immunol Rev* 1996;150:23.

592. Kabelitz D, Pohl T, Pechhold K. Activation-induced cell death (apoptosis) of mature peripheral T lymphocytes. *Immunol Today* 1993;14:338.

593. Russell JH. Activation-induced death of mature T cells in the regulation of immune responses. *Curr Opin Immunol* 1995;7:382.

594. Freitas AA, Agenes F, Coutinho GC. Cellular competition modulates survival and selection of CD8(+) T cells. *Eur J Immunol* 1996;26:2640.

595. Selin LK, Vergilis K, Welsh RM, Nahill SR. Reduction of otherwise remarkably stable virus-specific cytotoxic T lymphocyte memory by heterologous viral infections. *J Exp Med* 1996;183:2489.

596. Franceschi C, Monti D, Sansoni P, Cossarizza A. The immunology of exceptional individuals: the lesson of centenarians [see comments]. *Immunol Today* 1995;16:12.

597. Matzinger P. Tolerance, danger, and the extended family. *Annu Rev Immunol* 1994;12:991.

598. MacLennan IC, Liu YJ, Johnson GD. Maturation and dispersal of B-cell clones during T cell-dependent antibody responses. *Immunol Rev* 1992;126:143.

599. Berek C. The development of B cells and the B-cell repertoire in the microenvironment of the germinal center. *Immunol Rev* 1992;126:5.

600. Nossal GJV. The molecular and cellular basis of affinity maturation in the antibody response. *Cell* 1992;68:1.

601. Tsiagbe VK, Inghirami G, Thorbecke GJ. The physiology of germinal centers. *Crit Rev Immunol* 1996;16:381.

602. Berek C, Jarvis JM, Milstein C. Activation of memory and virgin B cell clones in hyperimmune animals. *Eur J Immunol* 1987;17:1121.

603. Coico RF, Bhogal BS, Thorbecke GJ. Relationship of germinal centers in lymphoid tissue to immunologic memory. VI. Transfer of B cell memory with lymph node cells fractionated according to their receptors for peanut agglutinin. *J Immunol* 1983;131:2254.

604. Jacob J, Kelsoe G. In situ studies of the primary immune response to (4-hydroxy-3-nitrophenyl)acetyl. II. A common clonal origin for periarteriolar lymphoid sheath-associated foci and germinal centers. *J Exp Med* 1992;176:679.

605. Liu YJ, Johnson GD, Gordon J, MacLennan IC. Germinal centers in T-cell-dependent antibody responses. *Immunol Today* 1992;13:17.

606. Jacob J, Kassir R, Kelsoe G. In situ studies of the primary immune response to (4-hydroxy-3-nitrophenyl)acetyl. I. The architecture and dynamics of responding cell populations. *J Exp Med* 1991;173:1165.

607. Liu YJ, Zhang J, Lane PJ, Chan EY, MacLennan IC. Sites of specific B cell activation in primary and secondary responses to T cell-dependent and T cell-independent antigens [published erratum appears in *Eur J Immunol* 1992 Feb;22(2):615]. *Eur J Immunol* 1991;21:2951.

608. Huchet R, Feldmann M. Studies on antibody affinity in mice. *Eur J Immunol* 1973;3:49.

609. Siekevitz M, Kocks C, Rajewsky K, Dildrop R. Analysis of somatic mutation and class switching in naive and memory B cells generating adoptive primary and secondary responses. *Cell* 1987;48:757.

610. van Rooijen N. Direct intrafollicular differentiation of memory B cells into plasma cells. *Immunol Today* 1990;11:154.

611. Weiss U, Rajewsky K. The repertoire of somatic antibody mutants accumulating

in the memory compartment after primary immunization is restricted through affinity maturation and mirrors that expressed in the secondary response. *J Exp Med* 1990;172:1681.

612. Gray D. Recruitment of virgin B cells into an immune response is restricted to activation outside lymphoid follicles. *Immunology* 1988;65:73.

613. Seijen HG, Bun JC, Wubbena AS, Lohlefink KG. The germinal center precursor cell is surface mu and delta positive. *Adv Exp Med Biol* 1988;237:233.

614. Leanderson T, Kallberg E, Gray D. Expansion, selection and mutation of antigen-specific B cells in germinal centers. *Immunol Rev* 1992;126:47.

615. Kosco MH, Gray D. Signals involved in germinal center reactions. *Immunol Rev* 1992;126:63.

616. Kroese FG, Wubbena AS, Seijen HG, Nieuwenhuis P. Germinal centers develop oligoclonally. *Eur J Immunol* 1987;17:1069.

617. Linton PJ, Decker DJ, Klinman NR. Primary antibody forming cells and secondary B cells are generated from separate precursor cell subpopulations. *Cell* 1989;59:1049.

618. Zhang J, MacLennan IC, Liu YJ, Lane PJ. Is rapid proliferation in B centroblasts linked to somatic mutation in memory B cell clones? *Immunol Lett* 1988;18:297.

619. Fliedner TM, Kress M, Cronkite EP, Robertson JS. Cell proliferation in germinal centers of the rat spleen. *Ann NY Acad Sci* 1964;113:578.

620. Bachmann MF, Odermatt B, Hengartner H, Zinkernagel RM. Induction of long-lived germinal centers associated with persisting antigen after viral infection. *J Exp Med* 1996;183:2259.

621. Pascual V, Liu YJ, Magalski A, de Bouteiller O, Bancereau J, Capra JD. Analysis of somatic mutation in five B cell subsets of human tonsil. *J Exp Med* 1994; 180:329.

622. Liu Y-J, Bancereau J. The paths and molecular controls of peripheral B-cell development. *Immunologist* 1996;4:55.

623. Hardie DL, Johnson GD, Khan M, MacLennan IC. Quantitative analysis of molecules which distinguish functional compartments within germinal centers. *Eur J Immunol* 1993;23:997.

624. Klein U, Kuppers R, Rajewsky K. Human IgM+IgD+ B cells, the major B cell subset in the peripheral blood, express V kappa genes with no or little somatic mutation throughout life. *Eur J Immunol* 1993;23:3272.

625. Griffiths GM, Berek C, Kaartinen M, Milstein C. Somatic mutation and the maturation of immune response to 2-phenyl oxazolone. *Nature* 1984;312:271.

626. Shan H, Shlomchik M, Weigert M. Heavy-chain class switch does not terminate somatic mutation. *J Exp Med* 1990;172:531.

627. Manser T. Evolution of antibody structure during the immune response. The differentiative potential of a single B lymphocyte. *J Exp Med* 1989;170:1211.

628. Ziegner M, Steinhauser G, Berek C. Development of antibody diversity in single germinal centers: selective expansion of high-affinity variants. *Eur J Immunol* 1994;24:2393.

629. McHeyzer-Williams MG, McLean MJ, Lalor PA, Nossal GJ. Antigen-driven B cell differentiation in vivo. *J Exp Med* 1993;178:295.

630. Kepler TB, Perelson AS. Cyclic re entry of germinal center B cells and the efficiency of affinity maturation [review]. *Immunol Today* 1993;14:412.

631. Liu YJ, Joshua DE, Williams GT, Smith CA, Gordon J, MacLennan IC. Mechanism of antigen-driven selection in germinal centres. *Nature* 1989;342:929.

632. Liu YJ, Mason DY, Johnson GD, et al. Germinal center cells express bcl-2 protein after activation by signals which prevent their entry into apoptosis. *Eur J Immunol* 1991;21:1905.

633. Pulendran B, Kannourakis G, Nouri S, Smith KG, Nossal GJ. Soluble antigen can cause enhanced apoptosis of germinal-centre B cells. *Nature* 1995;375:331.

634. Tew JG, Kosco MH, Burton GF, Szakal AK. Follicular dendritic cells as accessory cells. *Immunol Rev* 1990;117:185.

635. Humphrey JH, Grennan D, Sundaram V. The origin of follicular dendritic cells in the mouse and the mechanism of trapping of immune complexes on them. *Eur J Immunol* 1984;14:859.

636. Kapasi ZF, Kosco-Vilbois MH, Shultz LD, Tew JG, Szakal AK. Cellular origin of follicular dendritic cells. *In Vivo Immunol* 1994 231.

637. Clark EA, Grabstein KH, Gown AM, et al. Activation of B lymphocyte maturation by a human follicular dendritic cell line, FDC-1. *J Immunol* 1995;155:545.

638. Kapasi ZF, Burton GF, Shultz LD, Tew JG, Szakal AK. Induction of functional follicular dendritic cell development in severe combined immunodeficiency mice. Influence of B and T cells. *J Immunol* 1993;150:2648.

639. Mandel TE, Phipps RP, Abbot A, Tew JG. The follicular dendritic cell: long term antigen retention during immunity. *Immunol Rev* 1980;53:29.

640. Petrasch S, Perez-Alvarez C, Schmitz J, Kosco M, Brittinger G. Antigenic phenotyping of human follicular dendritic cells isolated from nonmalignant and malignant lymphatic tissue. *Eur J Immunol* 1990;20:1013.

641. Szakal AK, Kosco MH, Tew JG. A novel in vivo follicular dendritic cell-dependent iccosome-mediated mechanism for delivery of antigen to antigen-processing cells. *J Immunol* 1988;140:341.

642. Kosco MH, Szakal AK, Tew JG. In vivo obtained antigen presented by germinal center B cells to T cells in vitro. *J Immunol* 1988;140:354.

643. Koopman G, Parmentier HK, Schuurman HJ, Newman W, Meijer CJ, Pals ST. Adhesion of human B cells to follicular dendritic cells involves both the lymphocyte function-associated antigen 1/intercellular adhesion molecule 1 and very late antigen 4/vascular cell adhesion molecule 1 pathways. *J Exp Med* 1991;173:1297.

644. Kosco MH, Pflugfelder E, Gray D. Follicular dendritic cell-dependent adhesion and proliferation of B cells in vitro. *J Immunol* 1992;148:2331.

645. Koopman G, Keehnen RM, Lindhout E, et al. Adhesion through the LFA-1 (CD11a/CD18) ICAM-1 (CD54) and the VLA-4 (CD49d)-VCAM-1 (CD106)

646. Lindhout E, Mevissen ML, Kwekkeboom J, Tager JM, de Groot C. Direct evidence that human follicular dendritic cells (FDC) rescue germinal centre B cells from death by apoptosis. *Clin Exp Immunol* 1993;91:330.

647. Poppema S, Bhan AK, Reinherz EL, McCluskey RT, Schlossman SF. Distribution of T cell subsets in human lymph nodes. *J Exp Med* 1981;153:30.

648. Bowen MB, Butch AW, Parvin CA, Levine A, Nahm MH. Germinal center T cells are distinct helper-inducer T cells. *Hum Immunol* 1991;31:67.

649. Vonderheide RH, Hunt SV. Does the availability of either B cells or CD4+ cells limit germinal centre formation? *Immunology* 1990;69:487.

650. Zheng B, Han SH, Kelsoe G. T helper cells in murine germinal centers are antigen-specific emigrants that downregulate thy-1. *J Exp Med* 1996;184:1083.

651. Fuller KA, Kanagawa O, Nahm MH. T cells within germinal centers are specific for the immunizing antigen. *J Immunol* 1993;151:4505.

652. Grouard G, Durand I, Filgueira L, Bancereau J, Liu YJ. Dendritic cells capable of stimulating T cells in germinal centres. *Nature* 1996;384:364.

653. Snapper CM, Paul WE. Interferon-gamma and B cell stimulatory factor-1 reciprocally regulate Ig isotype production. *Science* 1987;236:944.

654. Lebman DA, Lee FD, Coffman RL. Mechanism for transforming growth factor beta and IL-2 enhancement of IgA expression in lipopolysaccharide-stimulated B cell cultures. *J Immunol* 1990;144:952.

655. Islam KB, Nilsson L, Sideras P, Hammarstrom L, Smith CI. TGF-beta 1 induces germ-line transcripts of both IgA subclasses in human B lymphocytes. *Int Immunol* 1991;3:1099.

656. Sonoda E, Matsumoto R, Hitoshi Y, et al. Transforming growth factor beta induces IgA production and acts additively with interleukin 5 for IgA production. *J Exp Med* 1989;170:1415.

657. Harriman GR, Kunimoto DY, Elliott JF, Paetkau V, Strober W. The role of IL-5 in IgA B cell differentiation. *J Immunol* 1988;140:3033.

658. Schoenbeck S, McKenzie DT, Kagnoff MF. Interleukin 5 is a differentiation factor for IgA B cells. *Eur J Immunol* 1989;19:965.

659. Beagley KW, Eldridge JH, Kiyono H, et al. Recombinant murine IL-5 induces high rate IgA synthesis in cycling IgA-positive Peyer's patch B cells. *J Immunol* 1988;141:2035.

660. Akira S, Hirano T, Taga T, Kishimoto T. Biology of multifunctional cytokines: IL6 and related molecules (IL1 and TNF). *FASEB J* 1990;4:2860.

661. Levy Y, Brouet JC. Interleukin-10 prevents spontaneous death of germinal center B cells by induction of the bcl-2 protein. *J Clin Invest* 1994;93:424.

662. Durie FH, Foy TM, Masters SR, Laman JD, Noelle RJ. The role of CD40 in the regulation of humoral and cell-mediated immunity. *Immunol Today* 1994;15:403.

663. Stout RD, Suttles J. The many-roles of CD40 in cell-mediated inflammatory responses. *Immunol Today* 1996;17:487.

664. Grewal IS, Flavell RA. A central role of CD40 ligand in the regulation of CD4(+) T-cell responses. *Immunol Today* 1996;17:410.

665. Noelle RJ. CD40 and its ligand in host defense. *Immunity* 1996;4:415.

666. Liu YJ, Cairns JA, Holder MJ, et al. Recombinant 25-kDa CD23 and interleukin 1 alpha promote the survival of germinal center B cells: evidence for bifurcation in the development of centrocytes rescued from apoptosis. *Eur J Immunol* 1991; 21:1107.

667. Han S, Hathcock K, Zheng B, Kepler TB, Hodes R, Kelsoe G. Cellular interaction in germinal centers. Roles of CD40 ligand and B7-2 in established germinal centers. *J Immunol* 1995;155:556.

668. Lederman S, Yellin MJ, Cleary AM, et al. T-BAM/CD40-L on helper T lymphocytes augments lymphokine-induced B cell Ig isotype switch recombination and rescues B cells from programmed cell death. *J Immunol* 1994;152:2163.

669. Galibert L, Burdin N, de Saint-Vis B, et al. CD40 and B cell antigen receptor dual triggering of resting B lymphocytes turns on a partial germinal center phenotype. *J Exp Med* 1996;183:77.

670. Parry SL, Hasbold J, Holman M, Klaus GG. Hypercross linking surface IgM or IgD receptors on mature B cells induces apoptosis that is reversed by costimulation with IL-4 and anti-CD40. *J Immunol* 1994;152:2821.

671. Arpin C, Dechanet J, Van Kooten C, et al. Generation of memory B cells and plasma cells in vitro. *Science* 1995;268:720.

672. Craig SW, Cebra JJ. Peyer's patches: an enriched source of precursors for IgA-producing immunocytes in the rabbit. *J Exp Med* 1971;134:188.

673. Weinstein PD, Cebra JJ. The preference for switching to IgA expression by Peyer's patch germinal center B cells is likely due to the intrinsic influence of their microenvironment. *J Immunol* 1991;147:4126.

674. Brandtzaeg P, Bjerke K. Immunomorphological characteristics of human Peyer's patches. *Digestion* 1990;2:262.

675. Butcher EC, Rouse RV, Coffman RL, Nottenburg CN, Hardy RR, Weissman IL. Surface phenotype of Peyer's patch germinal center cells: implications for the role of germinal centers in B cell differentiation. *J Immunol* 1982;129:2698.

676. Weinstein PD, Schweitzer PA, Cebra TJ, Cebra JJ. Molecular genetic features reflecting the preference for isotype switching to IgA expression by Peyer's patch germinal center B cells. *Int Immunol* 1991;3:1253.

677. Husband AJ. Kinetics of extravasation and redistribution of IgA-specific antibody-containing cells in the intestine. *J Immunol* 1982;128:1355.

678. McDermott MR, Bienenstock J. Evidence for a common mucosal immunologic system. I. Migration of B immunoblasts into intestinal, respiratory, and genital tissues. *J Immunol* 1979;122:1892.

679. Quiding-Jarbrink M, Lakew M, Nordstrom I, et al. Human circulating specific antibody-forming cells after systemic and mucosal immunizations: differential

homing commitments and cell surface differentiation markers. *Eur J Immunol* 1995;25:322.

680. Dilosa RM, Maeda K, Masuda A, Szakal AK, Tew JG. Germinal center B cells and antibody production in the bone marrow. *J Immunol* 1991;146:4071.

681. Kawanishi H, Saltzman LE, Strober W. Mechanisms regulating IgA class-specific immunoglobulin production in murine gut-associated lymphoid tissues. I. T cells derived from Peyer's patches that switch sIgM B cells to sIgA B cells in vitro. *J Exp Med* 1983;157:433.

682. Benson EB, Strober W. Regulation of IgA secretion by T cell clones derived from the human gastrointestinal tract. *J Immunol* 1988;140:1874.

683. Spalding DM, Griffin JA. Different pathways of differentiation of pre-B cell lines are induced by dendritic cells and T cells from different lymphoid tissues. *Cell* 1986;44:507.

684. Mega J, McGhee JR, Kiyono H. Cytokine- and Ig-producing T cells in mucosal effector tissues: analysis of IL-5- and IFN-gamma-producing T cells, T cell receptor expression, and IgA plasma cells from mouse salivary gland-associated tissues. *J Immunol* 1992;148:2030.

685. MacLennan IC, Gray D. Antigen-driven selection of virgin and memory B cells. *Immunol Rev* 1986;91:61.

685a. Slifka MK, Antia R, Whitmire JK, Ahmed R. Humoral immunity due to long-lived plasma cells. *Immunity* 1998;8:363.

686. Kraal G, Weissman IL, Butcher EC. Memory B cells express a phenotype consistent with migratory competence after secondary but not short-term primary immunization. *Cell Immunol* 1988;115:78.

687. Gray D, Skarvall H. B-cell memory is short-lived in the absence of antigen. *Nature* 1988;336:70.

688. Dell CL, Lu YX, Claflin JL. Molecular analysis of clonal stability and longevity in B cell memory. *J Immunol* 1989;143:3364.

689. McHeyzer-Williams MG, Nossal GJ, Lalor PA. Molecular characterization of single memory B cells. *Nature* 1991;350:502.

690. Rada C, Gupta SK, Gherardi E, Milstein C. Mutation and selection during the secondary response to 2-phenyloxazolone. *Proc Natl Acad Sci USA* 1991;88:5508.

691. Freitas AA, Rosado MM, Viale AC, Grandien A. The role of cellular competition in B cell survival and selection of B cell repertoires. *Eur J Immunol* 1995;25:1729.

692. Cyster JG, Hartley SB, Goodnow CC. Competition for follicular niches excludes self-reactive cells from the recirculating B-cell repertoire. *Nature* 1994;371:389.

693. Cotran RS, Kumar V, Robbins SL. Inflammation and repair. In: *Pathologic basis of disease*. Cotran RS, Kumar V, Robbins SL, eds. Philadelphia: WB Saunders, 1989.

694. Berg M, Murakawa Y, Camerini D, James SP. Lamina propria lymphoyctes are derived from circulating cells that lack the Leu-8 lymph node homing receptor. *Gastroenterology* 1991;101:90.

695. Mackay CR, Marston WL, Dudler L, Spertini O, Tedder TF, Hein WR. Tissue-specific migration pathways by phenotypically distinct subpopulations of memory T cells. *Eur J Immunol* 1992;22:887.

696. Weisz-Carrington P, Emancipator S, Kelemen PR. Specific attachment of mesenteric IgA lymphoblasts to specialized endothelium of intestinal mucosa lamina propria capillaries. *Cell Immunol* 1991;132:494.

697. Picker LJ, Michie SA, Rott LS, Butcher EC. A unique phenotype of skin-associated lymphocytes in humans: preferential expression of the HECA-452 epitope by benign and malignant T-cells at cutaneous sites. *Am J Pathol* 1990;136:1053.

698. Picker LJ, Treer JR, Ferguson-Darnell B, Collins PA, Buck D, Terstappen LWMM. Control of lymphocyte recirculation in man: I. Differential regulation of the peripheral lymph node homing receptor L-selectin on T cells during the virgin to memory cell transition. *J Immunol* 1993; 152:1105.

699. Smolle J. Mononuclear cell patterns in the skin. An immunohistological and morphometrical analysis. *Am J Dermatopathol* 1988;10:36.

700. Ansel J, Perry P, Brown J, et al. Cytokine modulation of keratinocyte cytokines. *J Invest Dermatol* 1990;94:101.

701. Luger TA, Schwarz T. Evidence for an epidermal cytokine network. *J Invest Dermatol* 1990;95:100.

702. McKenzie RC, Sauder DN. The role of keratinocyte cytokines in inflammation and immunity. *J Invest Dermatol* 1990;95:105.

703. Kupper TS. Immune and inflammatory processes in cutaneous tissues. Mechanisms and speculations. *J Clin Invest* 1990;86:1783.

704. Enk AH, Katz SI. Identification and induction of keratinocyte-derived IL-10. *J Immunol* 1992;149:92.

705. Groves RW, Ross E, Barker JNWN, Ross JS, Camp RDR, MacDonald DM. Effect of *in vivo* interleukin-1 on adhesion molecule expression in normal human skin. *J Invest Dermatol* 1992;98:384.

706. Picker LJ, Kishimoto TK, Smith CW, Warnock RA, Butcher EC. ELAM-1 is an adhesion molecule for skin-homing T cells. *Nature* 1991;349:796.

707. Nickoloff BJ, Griffiths CEM, Barker JNWN. The role of adhesion molecules, chemotactic factors, and cytokines in inflammatory and neoplastic skin disease—1990 update. *J Invest Dermatol* 1990;94:151.

708. Barker JNWN, Mitra RS, Griffiths CEM, Dixit VM, Nickoloff BJ. Hypothesis: keratinocytes as initiators of inflammation. A unifying explanation for the diverse array of environmental stimuli which produce cutaneous inflammation. *Lancet* 1991;337:211.

709. Kantor AB. The development and repertoire of B-1 cells (CD5 B cells). *Immunol Today* 1991;12:389.

710. Hardy RR, Hayakawa K. Development and physiology of Ly-1 B and its human homolog, Leu-1 B. *Immunol Rev* 1986;93:53.

711. Herzenberg LA, Stall AM, Lalor PA, et al. The Ly-1 B cell lineage. *Immunol Rev* 1986;93:81.

712. Hayakawa K, Hardy RR. Normal, autoimmune, and malignant CD5+ B cells: the Ly-1 B lineage? *Annu Rev Immunol* 1988;6:197.

713. Kantor AB, Herzenberg LA. Origin of murine B cell lineages [review, 158 refs]. *Annu Rev Immunol* 1993;11:501.

714. Tarakhovsky A. Bar mitzvah for B-1 cells: how will they grow up? *J Exp Med* 1997;185:981.

715. Casali P, Notkins AL. CD5+ B lymphocytes, polyreactive antibodies and the human B-cell repertoire. *Immunol Today* 1989;10:364.

716. Casali P, Notkins AL. Probing the human B-cell repertoire with EBV: polyreactive antibodies and CD5+ B lymphocytes. *Annu Rev Immunol* 1989;7:513.

717. Kroese FG, Butcher EC, Stall AM, Lalor PA, Adams S, Herzenberg LA. Many of the IgA producing plasma cells in murine gut are derived from self-replenishing precursors in the peritoneal cavity. *Int Immunol* 1989;1:75.

718. Allison JP, Havran WL. The immunobiology of T cells with invariant γδ antigen receptors. *Annu Rev Immunol* 1991;9:679.

719. Elbe A, Kilgus O, Strohal R, Payer E, Schreiber S, Stingl G. Fetal skin: a site of dendritic epidermal T cell development. *J Immunol* 1992;149:1694.

720. Lefrancois L, LeCorre R, Mayo J, Bluestone JA, Goodman T. Extrathymic selection of TCR gd+ T cells by class II major histocompatibility complex molecules. *Cell* 1990;63:333.

721. Guy-Grand D, Cerf-Bensussan N, Malissen B, Malassis-Seris M, Briottet C, Vassalli P. Two gut intraepithelial CD8+ lymphocyte populations with different T cell receptors: a role for the gut epithelium in T cell differentiation. *J Exp Med* 1991;173:471.

722. Foster CA, Yokozeki H, Rappersberger K, et al. Human epidermal T cells predominately belong to the lineage expressing α/β T cell receptor. *J Exp Med* 1990;171:997.

723. Groh V, Porcelli S, Fabbi M, et al. Human lymphocytes bearing T cell receptor gamma/delta are phenotypically diverse and evenly distributed throughout the lymphoid system. *J Exp Med* 1989;169:1277.

724. Boismenu R, Havran WL. An innate view of γδ T cells. *Curr Opin Immunol* 1997;9:57.

725. Tanaka Y, Morita CT, Tanaka Y, Nieves E, Brenner MB, Bloom BR. Natural and synthetic non-peptide antigens recognized by human gamma delta T cells. *Nature* 1995;375:155.

726. Smith ME, Ford WL. The recirculating pool of the rat: a systematic description of the migratory behavior of recirculating lymphocytes. *Immunology* 1983;49:83.

727. Sprent J, Schaefer M, Hurd M, Surh CD, Ron Y. Mature murine B and T cells transferred to SCID mice can survive indefinitely and many maintain a virgin phenotype. *J Exp Med* 1991;174:717.

728. Springer TA. Adhesion receptors of the immune system. *Nature* 1990;346:426.

729. Kalish RS, Johnson KL. Enrichment and function of urushiol (poison ivy)-specific T lymphocytes in lesions of allergic contact dermatitis to urushiol. *J Immunol* 1990;145:3706.

730. Firrell JC, Lipowsky HH. Leukocyte margination and deformation in mesenteric venules of rat. *Am J Physiol* 1989;256:H1667.

731. Butcher EC. Leukocyte-endothelial cell recognition: three (or more) steps to specificity and diversity. *Cell* 1991;67:1033.

732. Springer TA. Traffic signals on endothelium for lymphocyte recirculation and leukocyte emigration. *Annu Rev Physiol* 1995;57:827.

733. Imhof BA, Dunon D. Leukocyte migration and adhesion. *Adv Immunol* 1995;58:345.

734. Bargatze RF, Jutila MA, Butcher EC. Distinct roles of L-selectin and integrins alpha 4 beta 7 and LFA-1 in lymphocyte homing to Peyer's patch-HEV in situ: the multistep model confirmed and refined. *Immunity* 1995;3:99.

735. Jones DA, McIntire LV, Smith CW, Picker LJ. A two-step adhesion cascade for T cell/endothelial cell interactions under flow conditions. *J Clin Invest* 1994;94:2443.

736. von Andrian UH, Hasslen SR, Nelson RD, Erlandsen SL, Butcher EC. A central role for microvillous receptor presentation in leukocyte adhesion under flow. *Cell* 1995;82:989.

737. Gallatin WM, Weissman IL, Butcher EC. A cell-surface molecule involved in organ-specific homing of lymphocytes. *Nature* 1983;304:30.

738. Siegelman MH, Checn IC, Weissman IL. The mouse lymph node homing receptor is identical with the lymphocyte cell surface marker Ly-22: role of the EGF domain in endothelilal binding. *Cell* 1990;61:611.

739. Kansas GS. Selectins and their ligands: current concepts and controversies. *Blood* 1996;88:3259.

740. Alon R, Rossiter H, Wang X, Springer TA, Kupper TS. Distinct cell surface ligands mediate T lymphocyte attachment and rolling on P and E selectin under physiological flow. *J Cell Biol* 1994;127:1485.

741. Berlin C, Bargatze RF, Campbell JJ, et al. Alpha 4 integrins mediate lymphocyte attachment and rolling under physiologic flow. *Cell* 1995;80:413.

742. DeGrendele HC, Estess P, Picker LJ, Siegelman MH. CD44 and its ligand hyaluronate mediate rolling under physiologic flow: a novel lymphocyte-endothelial cell primary adhesion pathway. *J Exp Med* 1996;183:1119.

743. Bargatze RF, Butcher EC. Rapid G protein-regulated activation event involved in lymphocyte binding to high endothelial venules. *J Exp Med* 1993;178:367.

744. Mackay CR. Chemokine receptors and T cell chemotaxis. *J Exp Med* 1996;184: 799.

745. Carr MW, Alon R, Springer TA. The C-C chemokine MCP-1 differentially modulates the avidity of beta 1 and beta 2 integrins on T lymphocytes. *Immunity* 1996;4:179.

746a.Bazan JF, Bacon KB, Hardiman G, et al. A new class of membrane bound chemokine with CX3C motif. *Nature* 1997;385:640.

746b.Campbell JJ, Hendrick J, Zlotnik A, Siani MA, Thompson DA, Butcher EC. Chemokines and the arrest of lymphoid under flow conditions. *Science* 1998;279:381.

747. Erlandsen SL, Hasslen SR, Nelson RD. Detection and spatial distribution of the beta 2 integrin (Mac-1) and L-selectin (LECAM-1) adherence receptors on human neutrophils by high-resolution field emission SEM. *J Histochem Cytochem* 1993;41:327.

748. Cepek KL, Parker CM, Madara JL, Brenner MB. Integrin alpha E beta 7 mediates adhesion of T lymphocytes to epithelial cells. *J Immunol* 1993;150:3459.

749. Kansas GS, Tedder TF. Transmembrane signals generated through MHC class II, CD19, CD20, CD39, and CD40 antigens induce LFA-1-dependent and independent adhesion in human B cells through a tyrosine kinase-dependent pathway. *J Immunol* 1991;147:4094.

750. Hynes RO. Integrins: versatility, modulation, and signaling in cell adhesion. *Cell* 1992;69:11.

751. Tanaka Y, Shaw S. T cell adhesion cascades: general considerations and illustration with CD31. *Adv Exp Med Biol* 1992;323:157.

752. Lesley J, Howes N, Perschl A, Hyman R. Hyaluronan binding function of CD44 is transiently activated on T cells during an in vivo immune response. *J Exp Med* 1994;180:383.

753. Jinquan T, Larsen CG, Gesser B, Matsushima K, Thestrup-Pedersen K. Human IL-10 is a chemoattractant for CD8+ T lymphocytes and an inhibitor of IL-8-induced CD4+ T lymphocyte migration. *J Immunol* 1993;151:4545.

754. Jinquan T, Deleuran B, Gesser B, et al. Regulation of human T lymphocyte chemotasix in vitro by T-cell derived cytokines IL-2, IFN-g, IL-4, IL-10, and IL-13[1]. *J Immunol* 1995;154:3742.

755. Adams DH, Hathaway M, Shaw J, Burnett D, Eliase E, Strain AJ. Transforming growth factor-b induces human T lymphocyte migration in vitro. *J Immunol* 1991; 147:609.

756. Adams DH, Harvath L, Bottaro DP, et al. Hepatocyte growth factor and macrophage inflammatory protein 1 beta: structurally distinct cytokines that induce rapid cytoskeletal changes and subset-preferential migration in T cells. *Proc Natl Acad Sci USA* 1994;91:7144.

757. Wikinson PC, Liew FY. Chemoattraction of human blood T lymphocytes by interleukin-15. *J Exp Med* 1995;181:1255.

758. Forster R, Mattis AE, Kremmer E, Wolf E, Brem G, Lipp M. A putative chemokine receptor, BLR1, directs B cell migration to defined lymphoid organs and specific anatomic compartments of the spleen. *Cell* 1996;87:1037.

759. Gilat D, Hershkoviz R, Mekori YA, Vlodavsky I, Lider O. Regulation of adhesion of CD4+ T lymphocytes to intact or heparinase-treated subendothelial extracellular matrix by diffusible or anchored RANTES and MIP-1 beta. *J Immunol* 1994;153:4899.

760. Witt DP, Lander AD. Differential binding of chemokines to glycosaminoglycan subpopulations. *Curr Biol* 1994;4:394.

761. Tanaka Y, Adams DH, Shaw S. Proteoglycans on endothelial cells present adhesion-inducing cytokines to leukocytes. *Immunol Today* 1993;14:111.

762. Kantele A, Kantele JM, Savilahti E, et al. Homing potentials of circulating lymphocytes in humans depend on the site of activation—oral, but not parenteral, typhoid vaccination induces circulating antibody-secreting cells that bear homing receptors directing them to the gut. *J Immunol* 1997;158:574.

763. Quiding-Javbrink M, Nordstom I, Granstrom G, et al. Differential expression of tissue-specific adhesion molecules on human circulating antibody-forming cells after systemic, enteric, and nasal immunizations. *J Clin Invest* 1997;99:1281.

Fundamental Immunology, Fourth Edition,
edited by William E. Paul
Lippincott–Raven Publishers, Philadelphia © 1999.

CHAPTER 15

Macrophages and the Immune Response

Siamon Gordon

Macrophages represent a family of mononuclear leukocytes that are widely distributed throughout the body, within and outside lympho-hematopoietic organs. They vary considerably in life span and phenotype, depending on their origin and local microenvironment. Mature macrophages are highly phagocytic, relatively long-lived cells, adaptable in their biosynthetic responses to antigens and microbial stimuli. The functions of macrophages within tissues are homeostatic, regulating the local and systemic milieu through diverse plasma membrane receptors and varied secretory products. They react to, and themselves generate, signals that influence growth, differentiation, and death of other cells, recognizing and engulfing senescent and abnormal cells. These activities contribute substantially to recognition and defense functions against invading microorganisms, foreign particulates, and other immunogens. Innate immune functions of macrophages complement their contributions to acquired humoral and cellular immunity, in which they regulate activation of T- and B-lymphocytes; this is achieved in part through their specialized derivatives, dendritic cells (DCs) of myeloid origin. Macrophages, with or without DC, process and present antigen, produce chemokines and cytokines such as interleukin (IL)-1, IL-6, IL-12, IL-18, tumor necrosis factor (TNF)-α, and IL-10, and phagocytose apoptotic and necrotic cells. Acting directly or under the influence of other immune cells, macrophages capture extra- and intracellular pathogens, eliminate invaders, and deliver them to appropriate subcompartments of lymphoid organs. As key regulators of the specific as well as natural immune response, macrophages boost as well as limit induction and effector mechanisms of the specific immune response by positive and negative feedback.

The properties and roles of DCs are described in detail in the chapter by Steinman elsewhere in this volume. Here we focus on other members of the macrophages lineage, consider their inter-

relationship, and outline specialized properties that underlie their roles in the execution and regulation of immune responses.

SOME LANDMARKS IN THE STUDY OF MACROPHAGES

Our understanding of macrophages developed in parallel with the growth of immunology as an experimental science. Metchnikoff, a comparative developmental zoologist, is widely credited for his recognition of phagocytosis as a fundamental host defense mechanism of primitive, as well as highly developed, multicellular organisms. He clearly stated the link between capture of infectious microorganisms by the spleen and subsequent appearance of reactive substances (antibodies) in the blood, although mistakenly ascribing their production to the phagocytes themselves. The importance of systemic clearance of particles by macrophages, especially Kupffer cells in the liver and other endothelial cells, was hallowed in the term *reticuloendothelial system* (RES). Although rejected by influential investigators in the field in favor of the term *mononuclear phagocyte system* (MPS), the proposal that sinus-lining macrophages in the liver and elsewhere share common properties with selected endothelial cells is worth preserving. Earlier studies by Florey and his students, including Gowans, established that circulating monocytes give rise to tissue macrophages. Van Furth and his colleagues investigated the life history of macrophages by kinetic labeling methods; subsequently, the development of membrane antigen markers facilitated a more precise definition of specialized macrophage subpopulations in tissues such as the brain. The appearance and potential importance of macrophages during development also became evident as a result of sensitive immunocytochemical methods. Morphologic and functional studies by Humphrey and many others drew attention to striking diversity among macrophagelike cells in secondary lymphoid organs, especially within the marginal zone of the spleen,

S. Gordon: Sir William Dunn School of Pathology, University of Oxford, Oxford, OX1 3RE, United Kingdom.

where complex particulates and polysaccharides are captured from the circulation.

The era of modern cell biology impinged on macrophage studies following the studies of Cohn, Hirsch, and their colleagues. Their work touched on many aspects of cell structure and function, including phagocytosis (the zipper mechanism of Silverstein), fluid- and receptor-mediated endocytosis, secretion, and antimicrobial resistance. Isolation and in vitro culture systems became available for cells from mice and humans, especially after the identification of specific growth and differentiation factors such as colony stimulating factor (CSF)-1 (M-CSF). It is perhaps fitting that the earliest known natural knock out (KO) of macrophages, the osteopetrotic mouse (op/op), should implicate this molecule. Cell lines retaining some, but not all, features of mature macrophages have been useful for many biochemical and cellular studies.

The role of macrophages as antigen-processing cells (APCs) able to initiate adaptive immune responses had false trails (immunogenic RNA was thought to be involved at one time) and encompassed early genetic strategies. Macrophages from the Biozzi strain of mice selected for high antisheep erythrocyte antibody responses displayed enhanced degradative properties; adherent cells from defined guinea pig strains were shown to play an important role in Ia (major histocompatibility complex [MHC])-restricted antiinsulin responses. For many years the APC functions of adherent cells were highly controversial as promoted by Unanue, who concentrated on intracellular processing by macrophages, and Steinman, who discovered the specialized role of dendritic cells in antigen presentation to naive T-lymphocytes. The importance of macrophages as effector cells in immunity to intracellular pathogens such as *Mycobacterium tuberculosis* was recognized early by Lurie and Dannenberg. Mackaness made use of *Listeria monocytogenes* and Bacillé calmette guerin (BCG) infection in experimental models and developed the concept of macrophage activation as an antigen-dependent, but immunologically nonspecific, enhancement of antimicrobial resistance. The subsequent delineation of T-lymphocyte subsets and characterization of interferon (IFN)-γ as the major lymphokine involved in macrophage activation, including MHC II induction, merged with increasing knowledge of the role of reactive oxygen and, later, nitrogen metabolites as cytotoxic agents. The role of virus-infected macrophages as MHC I–restricted targets for antigen-specific CD8$^+$ killer cells was part of the initial characterization of this phenomenon by Zinkernagel and Doherty. D'Arcy Hart was an early investigator of the intracellular interactions between macrophages and invaders of the vacuolar system, especially mycobacteria, which survive within macrophages by evading host resistance mechanisms. Mouse breeding studies by several groups defined a common genetic locus involved in resistance to BCG, *Leishmania,* and *Salmonella* organisms. The host phenotype was shown to depend on expression in macrophages and, many years later, the gene (called for natural resistance-associated membrane protein [N-ramp]) was identified by positional cloning by Skamene, Gross, and their colleagues.

This brief survey concludes with the identification of macrophages as key target cells for infection, as well as dissemination and persistence of human immunodeficiency virus (HIV), which is tropic for macrophages by virtue of their expression of CD4 and chemokine coreceptors. Although macrophages had been implicated by earlier workers such as Mims as important in antiviral resistance generally, their role in this regard was neglected before the emergence of HIV as a major pathogen.

Many molecules have been identified as important in macrophage functions in immunity and serve as valuable markers to study their properties in mice and humans. These include Fc and complement receptors, important in opsonic phagocytosis, killing, and immunoregulation; nonopsonic lectin receptors, such as the mannose receptor (MR); and secretory products such as lysozyme, neutral proteinases, TNF-α, chemokines, and many other cytokines. A range of membrane antigens expressed by human and rodent mononuclear phagocytes has been characterized and reagents made available for further study of macrophages in normal and diseased states. Recently, the role of DNA-binding transcription factors including members of the NF-κB and ETS (Pu-1) families has received increased attention in the study of differential gene expression by macrophages. Gene inactivation has confirmed the important role of many of these molecules within the intact host, although little use has yet been made of cell-specific KO animals to uncover the role of macrophages in immunologic processes. Naturally occurring inborn errors in humans such as the leukocyte adhesion deficiency syndrome and chronic granulomatous disease have contributed to the analysis of important leukocyte functions, including those of macrophages, in host resistance to infection. The validity of murine KO models for human genetic deficiencies has been confirmed for key molecules involved in macrophage activation, such as IFN-γ and IL-12. Others will undoubtedly follow.

PROPERTIES OF MACROPHAGES AND THEIR RELATIONSHIP TO IMMUNE FUNCTIONS

Introduction

Macrophages participate in the production, mobilization, activation, and regulation of all immune effector cells. They interact reciprocally with other cells while their own properties are modified to perform specialized immunologic functions. As a result of cell surface, autocrine, and paracrine interactions, macrophages display marked heterogeneity in phenotype, a source of interest and considerable confusion to the investigator. Increasing knowledge of cellular and molecular properties of macrophages bears strongly on our understanding of their role in the immune response. I will review these briefly, with emphasis on functional significance, and draw attention to unresolved and controversial issues.

Growth and Differentiation: Life History and Turnover

In contrast with T- and B-lymphocytes, monocytes from blood give rise to terminally differentiated macrophages that cannot recirculate or reinitiate DNA replication except in a limited way; DCs may represent specialized migratory derivatives of mononuclear cells. Unlike other granulocytic cells, macrophages can be long lived and retain the ability to synthesize RNA and protein to a marked extent, even when in a relatively quiescent state, as resident cells. These are distributed throughout the tissues of the body and constitute a possible alarm-response system, but also mediate poorly understood trophic functions. After inflammatory and immune stimuli, many more monocytes can be recruited to local sites and give rise to elicited or immunologically activated macrophages with altered surface, secretory, and cytotoxic properties. The origins of macrophages from precursors are well known: from yolk sac (and possibly earlier progenitors), migrating to fetal liver, then spleen and bone marrow, before and after birth. In the fetus, mature macrophages proliferate actively during tissue remodeling in developing organs. In the normal adult, tissue macrophage do not self-renew extensively except in specialized microenvironments such as the lung or pituitary; after injury, there can be considerable further replication at local sites of inflammation. Growth and differentiation are tightly regulated by specific growth factors (e.g., IL-3, CSF-1, granulocyte-macrophage [GM]-CSF, IL-4, and IL-13) and inhibitors (e.g., IFN-α/β, transforming growth factor [TGF]-β, leukemia inhibitory factor (LIF), which vary considerably in their potency and selectivity. These processes are modulated by interactions with adjacent stromal and other cells (e.g., through c-kit–ligand and Flt-3–ligand interactions). The growth response of the target cell to an extrinsic stimulus decreases progressively and markedly (from 10^8 or more to 10^0) during differentiation from stem cell to committed precursor to monoblast, monocyte, and macrophage, yet even the most terminally differentiated macrophages such as microglial cells can be reactivated to a limited extent by local stimuli. Elicited/activated macrophages respond more vigorously than resident macrophages to growth stimuli in vivo and in vitro, but the molecular basis for their enhanced proliferation is unknown.

Although the general picture of blood monocyte to tissue macrophage differentiation has been clear for some time, as a result of parabiosis, adoptive transfer, and irradiation-reconstitution experiments, there are still major unsolved issues. Are all monocytes equivalent or is there heterogencity in the circulating mononuclear cell pool corresponding with the ultimate tissue localization of their progeny? Our present understanding of DCs and osteoclast differentiation is compatible with a relatively simple model (Fig. 1) in which major macrophage populations in tissues can be characterized by selected antigen markers such as F4/80 (Emr1, a member of a new family of EGF-TM7 molecules) and macrosialin (CD68), a pan-macrophage endosomal glycoprotein related to the lysosome-associated membrane protein (LAMP) family. The DCs of myeloid origin (see Chapter 16) can be viewed as products of Langerhans-type cells in nonlymphoid organs such as skin and airway epithelium, which undergo further differentiation and migrate to secondary lymphoid organs in response to an antigenic stimulus. Circulating precursors of DCs and recirculating progeny are also present in the mononuclear fraction of blood in small numbers and already may be marked for distribution to peripheral sites as Langerhans' cells. Circulating precursors for osteoclasts are less defined and differentiate into mononucleate cells in bone and cartilage, where they fuse to form multinucleate bone-resorbing osteoclasts. Local stromal cells, growth factors such as CSF-1, steroids (vitamin D metabolites) and hormones (e.g., calcitonin for which osteoclasts express receptors), all contribute to local maturation. Recently, it has been found that osteoprotegerin, a naturally occurring secreted protein with homology to members of the TNF receptor family, interacts with TRANCE, a TNF-related protein, to regulate osteoclast differentiation and activation in vitro and in vivo.

Antigen markers such as CD34 on progenitors and CD14 on monocytes, and the use of multichannel fluorescence-activated cell sorting (FACS) analysis make it possible to isolate minor leukocyte populations and study their progeny. The mononuclear fraction of blood may contain precursors of other tissue cells, including fibrocytes, thought to be hematopoietic yet able to synthesize matrix proteins such as collagen, and some endothelial

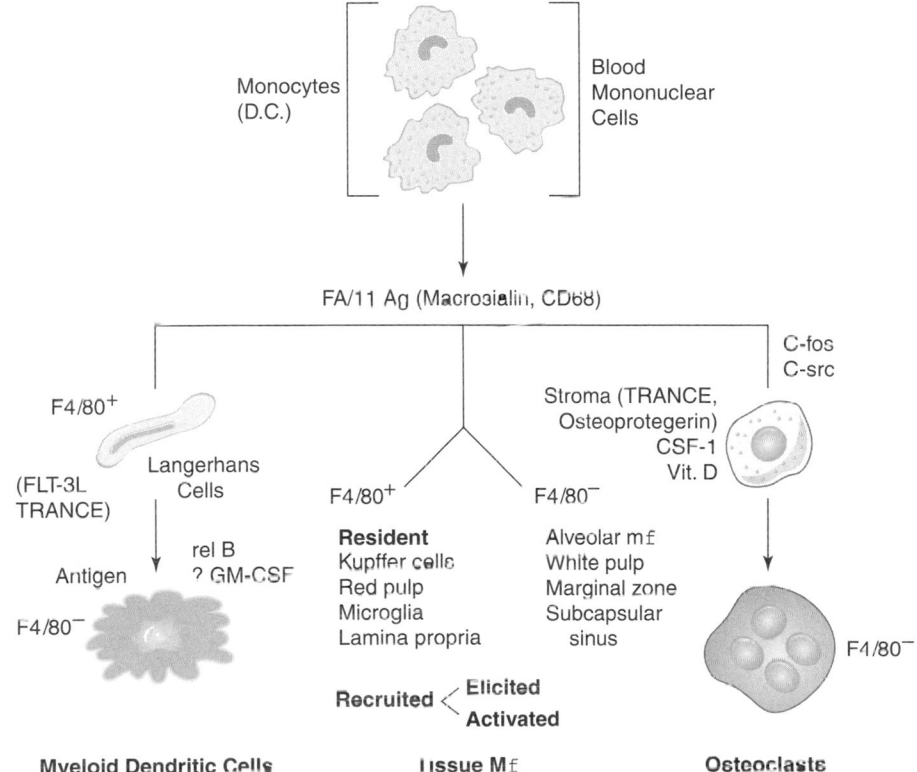

FIG. 1. Differentiation of mononuclear phagocytes, based on antigen markers FA-11 (macrosialin, murine CD68) and F4/80.

cells. Perhaps the mysterious follicular dendritic cells (FDCs), with mixed hematopoietic and mesenchymal properties, fall into this category.

The large-scale production of immature and mature DC-like cells from bulk monocytes in cytokine-supplemented culture systems (IL-4, GM-CSF, TNF-α) has revolutionized the study of these specialized APCs (see Chapter 16). Individually, the same cytokines give rise to macrophage-like cells, and early during in vitro differentiation the cellular phenotype is reversible. Later, when mature DCs with high MHC II, APC function, and other characteristic markers are formed, differentiation is irreversible. This process is independent of cell division, although earlier progenitors in bone marrow and G-CSF–mobilized blood mononuclear cells can be stimulated to multiply, as well as differentiate, in vitro. These examples of terminal differentiation observed with DCs and osteoclasts may extend to other specialized, more obvious macrophage-like cells. Mature macrophages can be derived by growth and differentiation in steroid-supplemented media in Dexter-type long-term bone marrow cultures, which contain stromal fibroblasts and hematopoietic elements. These macrophages express adhesion molecules responsible for divalent cation-dependent cluster formation with erythroblasts (EbRs). This receptor, possibly related to vascular cell adhesion molecule (VCAM), cannot be induced on terminally differentiated peritoneal macrophages if they are placed in the same culture system. This contrasts sharply with the ready adaptation of many tissue macrophages to conventional cell culture conditions, when the cells often adopt a common, standard phenotype. Therefore, irreversible stages of macrophage differentiation may occur in specialized microenvironments in vitro or in vivo.

Little is known about determinants of macrophage longevity and turnover. Growth factors such as CSF-1 enhance macrophage survival and prevent induction of an apoptotic program. The expression of Fas-L and Fas on macrophages has been studied less thoroughly than that on lymphocytes; they and other members of the TNF and its receptor family may play a major role in determining macrophage survival, especially in induced populations, where cell turnover is markedly enhanced. Tissue macrophages vary greatly in their life span, from days to months. Apart from inflammatory stimuli, local and systemic environmental factors such as salt loading and hormones, including estrogen, are known to influence macrophage turnover.

Tissue Distribution and Phenotypic Heterogeneity of Resident Macrophages in Lymphoid and Nonlymphoid Organs

The use of the F4/80 plasma membrane antigen made it possible to detect mature macrophages in developing and adult murine tissues and define their anatomic relationship to other cells in endothelium, epithelium, and connective tissue, as well as the nervous system. Subsequently, other membrane antigens (e.g, macrosialin and sialoadhesin) were identified as useful markers for macrophages in situ (Table 1). Macrophage subpopulations in different tissues display considerable heterogeneity in expressing these and selected receptor antigens (complement receptor type 3 (CR3) and class A scavenger receptor [SR-A]), drawing attention to mechanisms of homing, emigration, and local adaptation to particular microenvironments. From the viewpoint of immune responses, a few aspects deserve comment.

Fetal Liver and Bone Marrow

Mature macrophages form an integral part of the hematopoietic microenvironment and play a key role in the production, differentiation, and destruction of all hematopoietic cells. The fetal liver is a major site of definitive erythropoiesis from mid-gestation. The bone marrow becomes active in the production of hematopoietic cells from shortly before birth, and macrophages are a prominent component of the hematopoietic stroma throughout adult life. Mature stromal macrophages in fetal liver and adult bone marrow express nonphagocytic adhesion molecules such as sialoadhesin, an immunoglobulin (Ig) superfamily sialic acid binding lectin

TABLE 1. *Differentiation Antigens Used To Study Murine Macrophage Herogeneity*

Antibody	Antigen	Structure	Ligands	Cellular expression	Function	Comment
F4/80	F4/80 (EMR1)	EGF, TM7	?	Mature macrophages, absent T areas	?	Useful marker development, CNS
FA-11	Macrosialin (CD68)	Mucin, Lamp	OX-LDL	Pan macrophages, DCs	Late endosomal	Glycoforms regulated by inflammation and phagocytosis
5C6	CR3 (CD11b, CD18)	β2 Integrin	IC3B, ICAM	Monocytes, Microglia, PMNS, NK Cells	Phagocytosis, adhesion	Important in inflammatory recruitment, PMN apoptosis
2F8	SR-A (I,II)	Collagenous, type II glycoprotein, isoforms differ, cysteine-rich domain	Polyanions, LTA, LPS, modified proteins, β amyloid	Macrophages, sinusoidal endothelium	Adhesion, endocytosis, phagocytosis of apoptotic cells and bacteria	Protects host against LPS-induced shock, promotes atherosclerosis
SER-4 3D6	Sialoadhesin (Siglec 1)	Ig superfamily	Sialyl glycoconjugates (e.g., CD43)	Subsets, tissue macrophages	Lectin	Strongly expressed marginal zone metallophils in spleen and subcapsular sinus of lymph nodes

(Table 1), and the EbR referred to above, which is also involved in adhesion of developing myeloid and possibly lymphoid cells (Fig. 2). VLA-4 (very late antigen) has been implicated as a ligand for EbR. Ligands for sialoadhesin include CD43 on developing granulocytes and on lymphocyte subpopulations. Sialoadhesin clusters at sites of contact between stromal macrophages and myeloid, but not erythroid cells. Chemokines can induce polarized expression of adhesion molecules such as intercellular adhesion molecules (ICAMs) and CD43 in leukocytes, but the significance of altered ligand distribution for interactions between macrophages and bound hematopoietic cells is unknown. Adhesion of immature cells to stromal macrophages may play a role in regulating their intermediate stages of development before release into the blood stream, whereas fibroblasts in the stroma associate with earlier progenitors, as well as with macrophages. Discarded nuclei of mammalian erythroid cells are rapidly engulfed by stromal macrophages, but the receptors involved in their binding and phagocytosis are unknown. Macrophages also phagocytose apoptotic hematopoietic cells generated in bone marrow, including large numbers of myeloid and B cells. We still know little about the plasma membrane molecules and cytokine signals operating within this complex milieu, but it is clear that stromal macrophages constitute a neglected constituent within the hematopoietic microenvironment.

Thymus

Apart from their remarkable capacity to remove apoptotic thymocytes, the possible role of macrophages in positive and negative selection of thymocytes has been almost totally overlooked; more attention has been devoted to local DCs, which may derive from lymphoid, rather than myeloid, precursors. Mature macrophages with specialized properties are present in the cortex and medulla. Clusters of viable thymocytes and macrophages can be isolated from the thymus of young animals by collagenase digestion and adherence to a substratum (Fig. 2). The nonphagocytic adhesion receptors responsible for cluster formation are more highly expressed by thymic than other macrophages, but their nature is unknown (N. Platt, unpublished observations). These macrophages also express MHC class II antigens and other receptors such as SR-A, which contributes to phagocytosis of apoptotic thymocytes. Other markers such as the F4/80 antigen are poorly expressed in situ but can be readily detected after cell isolation. A striking difference between thymic and several other

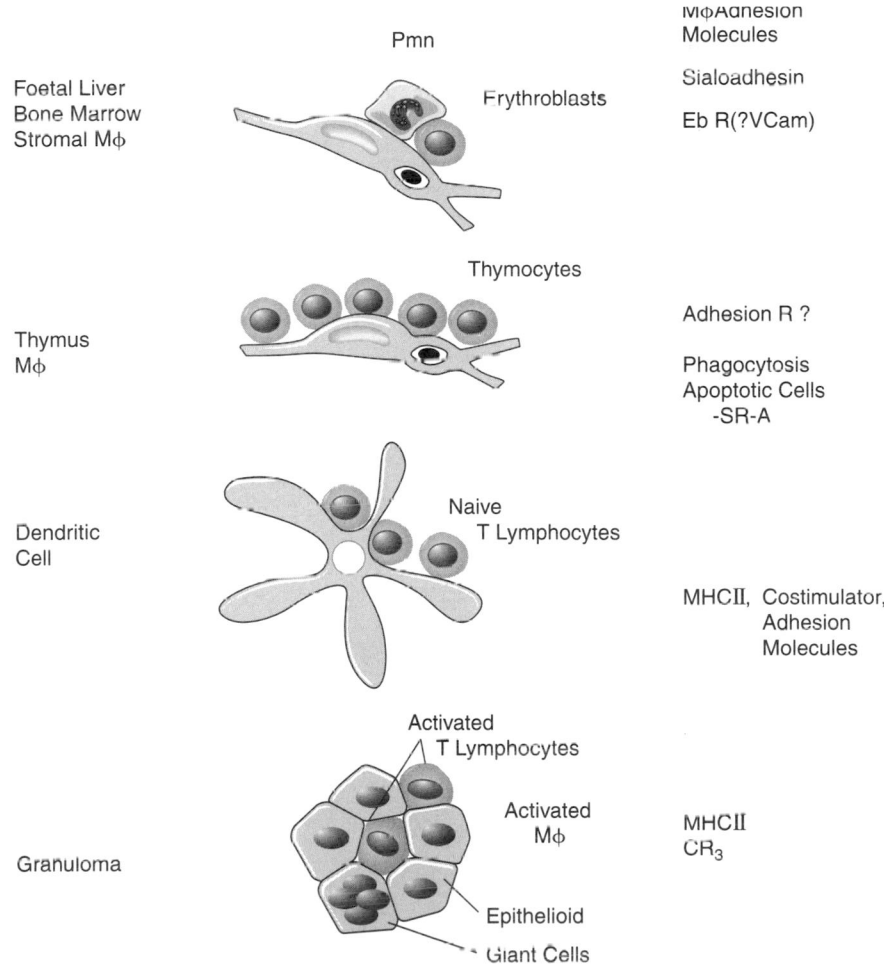

FIG. 2. Associations of tissue macrophages with other hematopoietic cells, to illustrate variations on a common theme.

tissue macrophage subpopulations is their independence of CSF-1; the CSF-1–deficient op/op mouse lacks osteoclasts and some macrophage populations (including monocytes, peritoneal cells, and Kupffer cells), but contains normal numbers of thymic macrophages, as well as DCs and selected macrophages in other sites. Factors involved in constitutive recruitment of thymic macrophages are unknown. After the death of thymocytes induced by ionizing radiation or glucocorticoids, intensely phagocytic macrophages appear in large numbers; it is not known what proportion arises locally and by recruitment.

Spleen

From the viewpoint of the macrophages, the spleen is perhaps the most complex organ in the body. It contributes to hematopoiesis, which persists postnatally in some species or can be induced by increased demand, and to the turnover of all blood elements at the end of their natural life span. In addition, the spleen filters a substantial proportion of total cardiac output, captures particulate and other antigenic materials from the blood stream, and plays an important role in natural and acquired humoral and cellular immunity. The organ is rich in subpopulations of macrophages that differ in microanatomic localization, phenotype, life history,

and functions (Fig. 3). Macrophages are central to antigen capture, degradation, transport, and presentation to T- and B-lymphocytes and contribute substantially to antimicrobial resistance. Because other hematopoietic and secondary lymphoid organs can replace many of these functions after maturation of the immune system, the unique properties of the spleen have been recognized primarily in the immature host and in immune responses to complex polysaccharides. Splenectomy in the adult renders the host susceptible to infection by pathogenic bacteria such as pneumococci, which contain saccharide-rich capsular antigens; the marginal zone of the spleen in particular may play an essential role in this aspect of host resistance.

The properties of macrophages in the unstimulated mature mouse spleen are very different according to their localization in red or white pulp, as well as in the marginal zone. Macrophages are intimately associated with the specialized vasculature. Species differences in splenic anatomy are well recognized, but macrophages display broadly common features in humans and rodent, where studied. Subpopulations of macrophages, DCs (myeloid and lymphoid in origin), and cells with mixed phenotypes have been characterized by in situ analysis with antigen markers, toxic liposome depletion studies, various immunization and infection protocols, and, recently, cytokine and receptor gene KO models in the mouse.

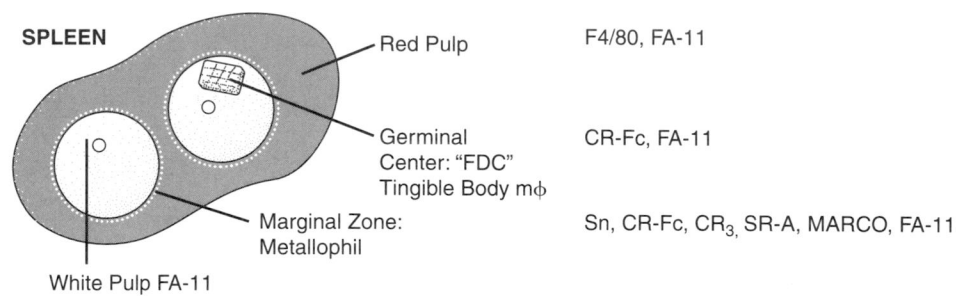

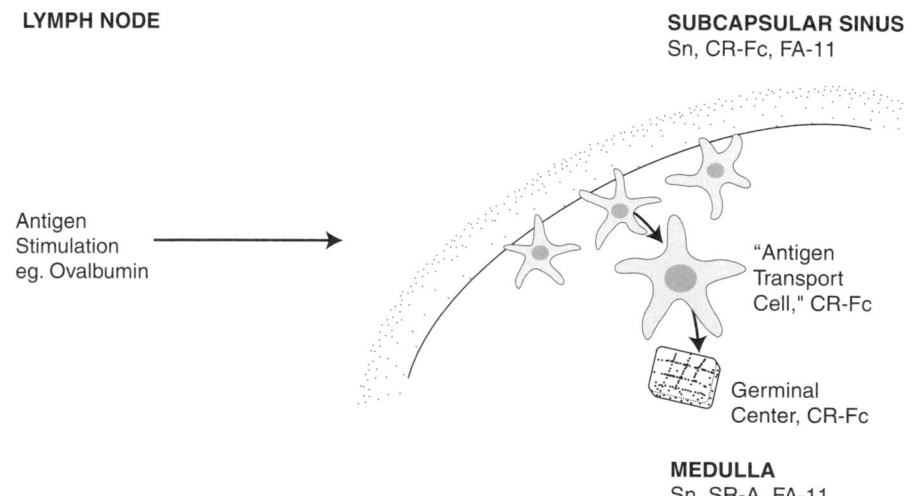

FIG. 3. Microheterogeneity of macrophages in spleen, resting, and antigen-stimulated lymph nodes. See text for markers and details.

The results raise questions about the dynamics and molecular basis of cell production, recruitment, differentiation, emigration, and death within each distinct splenic microenvironment. Cell isolation methods are still primitive in correlating in vitro properties with those of macrophage subpopulations in vivo and provide an important challenge for the future. Detailed aspects of splenic architecture, DC origin and function, and T- and B-lymphocyte induction and differentiation are described elsewhere in this volume. I shall highlight some features of macrophages in the normal and immunoreactive organ.

Marginal Zone Macrophages

The marginal zone of the spleen consists of a complex mixture of resident cells (reticular and other fibroblasts, endothelium), macrophages, DCs, and lymphoid cells, including subpopulations of B-lymphocytes. It constitutes an important interface with the circulation, which delivers cells, particulates, or soluble molecules directly into the marginal sinus or via the red pulp. Resident macrophages are present as specialized metallophilic cells in the inner marginal zone, and other macrophages are found in the outer zone; the latter may be more phagocytic. Sialoadhesin is very strongly expressed by the marginal metallophils, compared with only weak expression in red pulp and its virtual absence in the white pulp (Table 1). Sialoadhesin-positive cells appear in this zone 2 to 4 weeks postnatally in the mouse as the white pulp forms. Liposomes containing clodronate, a cytotoxic drug, can be delivered systemically and deplete sialoadhesin-positive cells and other macrophages; recovery of different macrophage subpopulations in the spleen occurs at different times, and this procedure has been used to correlate their reappearance with distinct immunologic functions. Marginal zone macrophages lack F4/80 but express CR3, which is absent on red pulp macrophages. Marginal zone macrophages express other phagocytic receptors, such as SR-A, which is more widely present on tissue macrophages, as well as macrophage receptor collagenous domain (MARCO), a distinct collagenous scavenger receptor that is almost exclusively present on these macrophages. The structures and possible role of these pattern-recognition receptors in uptake of microbes will be discussed below. Recent studies have shown that a macrophage lectin, the MR, which has not been localized in situ, may be involved in transfer of mannosylated ligands to the site of an immune response in the white pulp. The MR contains a highly conserved cysteine-rich domain, not directly involved in mannosyl recognition, that reacts strongly with a ligand on marginal metallophilic macrophages, possibly sialoadhesin itself; this has been demonstrated with a chimeric probe of the cysteine-rich domain of the MR and human Fc (CR-Fc) and by immunochemical analysis of tissue sections and spleen ligands. After immunization this probe additionally labels undefined cells in the FDC network of germinal centers, as well as tingible body macrophages. It is possible that marginal zone macrophages can be induced to migrate into white pulp; alternatively, they may shed complexes of soluble MR–glycoprotein ligand for transfer to other CR-Fc+ cells, which may be other resident or newly recruited mononuclear cells. Finally, the marginal metallophilic macrophage population depends on CSF-1 for its appearance and on members of the TNF receptor family, as shown with op/op and experimentally produced KO mice.

White Pulp Macrophages

The F4/80 antigen is strikingly absent on murine white pulp macrophages that express FA-11 (macrosialin), the murine homolog of CD68. Actively phagocytic macrophages express this intracellular glycoprotein in abundance, compared with DCs. After uptake of a foreign particle (e.g., sheep erythrocytes) or an infectious agent (e.g. BCG, Plasmodium yoellii), white pulp macrophages become more prominent, although it is not known whether there is migration of cells into the white pulp or transfer of phagocytosed material and reactivation of previous resident macrophages. Tingible body macrophages appear to be involved in uptake and digestion of apoptotic B-lymphocytes.

Red Pulp Macrophages

These express F4/80 antigen strongly and in the mouse include stromal-type macrophages involved in hematopoiesis. Extensive phagocytosis of senescent erythrocytes results in accumulation of bile pigments and ferritin. The role of various phagocytic receptors in clearance of host cells and pathogens by red pulp macrophages requires further study.

There is no evidence that macrophages, other than interdigitating DCs, associate directly with CD4+ T-lymphocytes in the normal spleen. After infection by BCG, for example, or by other microorganisms such as Salmonella, there is massive recruitment and local production of macrophages, many of which associate with T-lymphocytes. Newly formed granulomata often appear first in the marginal zone. Infections spread into the white and red pulp and granulomata become confluent, obscuring or disrupting the underlying architecture of the spleen. The possible role of activated macrophages in T-cell apoptosis and clearance in the spleen has not been defined.

Lymph Nodes

As illustrated in Fig. 3, F4/80 ag is relatively poorly expressed in lymph nodes, but many macrosialin (CD68)-positive cells are present. The subcapsular sinus is analogous to the marginal zone and contains strongly sialoadhesin-positive cells; this is the site where afferent lymph enters, containing antigen and migrating DCs derived from Langerhans' cells. The medulla contains sialoadhesin-positive, CD68+ macrophages that also express high levels of SR-A. As in the spleen marginal zone, subcapsular sinus macrophages are strongly labeled by the CR-Fc probe. After primary or secondary immunization, the staining pattern moves deeper into the cortex and eventually becomes concentrated in germinal centers. The kinetics of this process strongly suggest a transport process by macrophage-related cells resembling the antigen transport cells described previously. CR-Fc+ cells can be isolated by digestion of lymph nodes and form clusters with CR-Fc- lymphocytes. Adoptive transfer has shown that FACS-isolated CR-Fc+ cells resemble DCs in their ability to home to T-cell areas; under these conditions there is no homing to germinal centers (M. Kosco-Vilbois and L. Martinez-Pomares, unpublished observations). Overall, there is considerable heterogeneity in the population of migratory APCs involved in antigen capture, transport, and delivery to T and B cells, and it may turn out that specialized tissue macrophages as well as myeloid-type DCs can migrate in response to immunologic stimuli, especially of a particulate nature.

Peyer's Patches

Although not studied thoroughly, the macrophages in Peyer's patches resemble the CD68$^+$ F4/80$^-$ cells described in the spleen and white pulp, as well as in other T cell–rich areas. They are well placed to interact with gut-derived antigens and pathogens taken up via specialized epithelial M cells in the dome, as well as transfer antigens to afferent lymphatics. These macrophages are distinct from abundant F4/80$^+$ cells in the lamina propria found all the way down the gastrointestinal tract and may play a role in the induction of mucosal immunity.

Nonlymphoid Organs

Regional F4/80$^+$ and CD68$^+$ macrophages are well described in liver (Kupffer cells), dermis, neuroendocrine and reproductive organs, and serosal cavities where they are able to react to systemic and local stimuli. In the lung, alveolar macrophages are strongly CD68$^+$ but only weakly F4/80$^+$ and are distinct from interstitial macrophages and intraepithelial DCs. Additionally, resident macrophages are found throughout connective tissue and within the interstitium of organs, including the heart, kidney, and pancreas. These cells vary greatly depending on their local microenvironment (e.g., in the central nervous system microglia within the neuropil differ strikingly from macrophages in the meninges or choroid plexus). Perivascular macrophages in the brain can be distinguished from resident microglia by their expression of endocytic receptors (e.g., the SR-A) and of MHC I and II antigens. Microglia are highly ramified, terminally differentiated cells of monocytic origin, and many macrophages markers are downregulated; their phenotype is influenced by the blood–brain barrier, normally absent in circumventricular organs, and disrupted by inflammatory stimuli. Microglia can be reactivated by local lipopolysaccharide (LPS) and neurocytotoxins and are then difficult to distinguish from newly recruited monocytes that acquire microglial features once they enter the parenchyma of the brain. Resting microglia are unusual among many tissue macrophages in that they constitutively express high levels of CR3 and respond to CR3 ligands, such as monoclonal antibodies (mAbs), by induced DNA synthesis and apoptosis. Natural ligands for CR3 in the CNS are not defined.

Enhanced Recruitment of Monocytes by Inflammatory and Immune Stimuli: Activation In Vivo

In response to local tissue and vascular changes, partly induced by resident macrophages during (re)activation by inflammatory and immunologic stimuli, monocytes are recruited from marrow pools and blood in increased numbers; they diapedese and differentiate into macrophages with altered effector functions as they enter the tissues. These macrophages are classified as elicited when cells are generated in the absence of IFN-γ and as immunologically activated after exposure to IFN-γ. Enhanced recruitment also can involve that of other myeloid or lymphoid cells; selectiv-

ity of the cellular response depends on the nature of the evoking stimulus (immunogenic or not), the chemokines produced, and the receptors expressed by different leukocytes. Macrophages and other cells produce a range of different chemokines and express multiple seven-transmembrane, G protein–coupled chemokine receptors. The chemokines also can act in the marrow compartment, especially if anchored to matrix and glycosaminoglycans, and may display other growth regulatory functions. Locally bound or soluble chemokines induce the surface expression and activity of adhesion molecules on circulating white cells, as well as directing their migration through and beyond endothelium. Feedback mechanisms from the periphery to central stores and within the marrow stroma may depend on cytokines and growth factors such as macrophage inflammatory protein 1a (MIP1a) and granulocyte macrophage-CSF (GM-CSF), which inhibit or enhance monocyte production, respectively. The adhesion molecules involved in the recruitment of monocytes, originally defined by studies in humans with inborn errors and by use of inhibitory antibodies in experimental animal models, overlap with those of polymorphonuclear cells (PMNs) and lymphocytes and include L-selectin, β$_2$ integrins, especially CR3, and CD31, an Ig superfamily molecule; additional monocyte adhesion molecules for activated endothelium include CD44, VCAM, β$_1$ integrins, and newly described receptors. The mechanisms of constitutive entry of monocytes into developing and adult tissues, in the absence of an inflammatory stimulus, are unknown.

The migration and differentiation of newly recruited monocytes once they have left the circulation are poorly understood. They are able to enter all tissues, undergoing alterations in membrane molecules and secretory potential under the influence of cytokines and surface interactions with endothelial cells, leukocytes, and other local cells. Phenotypic changes mentioned below have been characterized by a range of in vitro and in vivo studies. Well-studied examples include murine peritoneal macrophages: resident, elicited by thioglycollate broth or biogel polyacrylamide beads, and immunologically activated by BCG infection. The latter provides a useful model of granuloma formation in solid organs but does not fully mimic the human counterpart associated with *M. tuberculosis* infection. Granuloma macrophages vary in their turnover and immune effector functions and display considerable heterogeneity; lesions contain recently recruited monocytes, mature epithelioid macrophages (described as secretory cells), and Langhans' giant cells. Interactions with T-lymphocytes, other myeloid cells, DCs, fibroblasts, and microorganisms yield a dynamic assembly of cells as the granuloma evolves, heals, and resolves (Fig. 2). Apoptosis and necrosis of macrophages and other cells contribute to the balance of continued recruitment and local proliferation. The emigration of macrophages rather than DCs from sites of inflammation is less evident, although it has become clear that elicited macrophages within the peritoneal cavity, for example, migrate actively to draining lymph nodes.

Gene KO models have confirmed the role of molecules previously implicated in recruitment, activation, and granuloma formation. These include the adhesion molecules listed above, their ligands, such as ICAM-1, and key cytokines such as IFN-γ, IL-12, and TNF-α, as well as their receptors. Antimicrobial resistance and macrophage cytotoxicity resulting from production of reactive oxygen and nitrogen metabolites are now accessible to study in knock-outs of the phagocyte oxidase and inducible nitric oxide synthase (i-NOS). Knock-outs of membrane molecules of immunologic interest expressed by macrophages and other cells

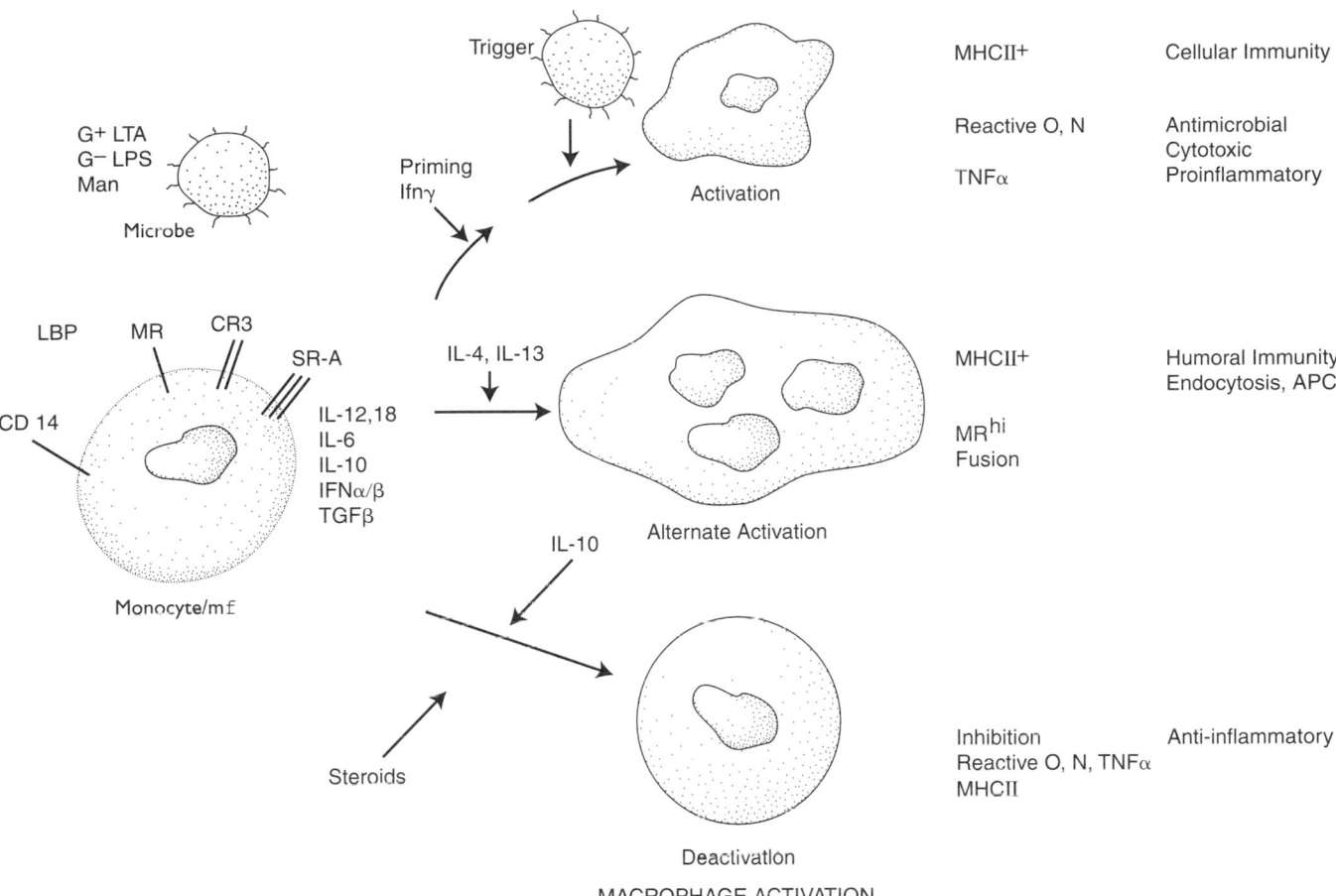

FIG. 4. Macrophage activation. Role of microbial stimuli and cytokines.

include MHC class I and II, CD4, and CD40L, other accessory molecules such as B7-1 and B7-2, and the macrophage-restricted intracellular molecule N-ramp.

The potential for Th1- and Th2-type regulation of macrophages demonstrated in vitro, and discussed below, can result in highly complex, often coexistent, heterogeneity of macrophage phenotype in situ (Fig. 4). Although almost all granuloma macrophages express lysozyme, only minor subpopulations express cytokines such as IL-1β, IL-6, and TNF-α. Through their production of IL-12, IFN-γ–inducing factor (IL-18), IL-10, and TGF-β, macrophages and other sources achieve a balance between activation and deactivation of macrophages in vivo.

Apart from the local interactions outlined, macrophages regulate systemic host reactions to immune and infectious stimuli by producing circulating cytokines such as IL-6, as well as arachidonate- and other lipid-derived metabolites. These act on neural and endocrine centers, crossing the blood–brain barrier, or are generated locally by reactive microglia and macrophages. Glucocorticosteroids are powerful immunomodulators and form part of a regulatory network that may involve macrophages through circulating mediators such as migration inhibition factor. Macrophages also contain potent enzymes involved in steroid biosynthesis and catabolism.

Although the immunologic relevance of macrophage-induced responses may seem evident, many aspects remain unclear. For example, do macrophages actively destroy activated T-lymphocytes, thus contributing to regulation of immune responses and peripheral tolerance, or are macrophages only passive removers of dying cells? Do macrophages contribute to recruitment, differentiation, and death of DCs at sites of inflammation before their migration to secondary lymphoid organs? Do adjuvant-stimulated macrophages interact with B-lymphocytes, directing their migration into germinal centres? Are interactions of activated macrophages with antibody and complement, through different Fc and complement receptors, implicated in fine tuning humoral responses? Are activated macrophages themselves cytocidal for infected host cells, and to what extent do they in turn provide targets for attack by natural killer (NK) cells and cytotoxic T-lymphocytes? Study of a range of experimental models and disease processes in vivo should yield new insights, as well as extend and confirm mechanisms already defined in vitro.

Phagocytic Recognition and Intracellular Infection

The initiation and localization of an immune response depend on recognition by macrophages and other cells of particulate agents or soluble proteins that are foreign or modified self. Phagocytic and endocytic recognition by macrophages and DCs depends on opsonic (mainly antibody and complement) and nonopsonic pattern recognition receptors that interact with a range of related ligands. Innate and acquired responses are thus interlinked. Different FcRs are involved in uptake and destruction of targets as well as in negative regulation of effector functions. Complement receptors are also heterogeneous. CR3 interacts with C_3-derived ligands formed by activation of the classical or alternate pathways and mediate phagocytosis, cell migration, and activation. Other ligands include ICAM. CR3 functions are modulated by fibronectin via integrins, other adhesion molecules, and inflammatory stimuli. FcR ligation and cross-linking activates tyrosine kinases such as syk, which are essential for phagocytosis. CR3 signaling is less defined and may not trigger a respiratory burst or arachidonate release, unlike FcR, thus favoring pathogen entry. Antibody-mediated uptake targets an organism or soluble antigen to a different, degradative compartment and usually results in its neutralization and destruction, although enhancement of infection also can occur in macrophages. For example, flavivirus infection in the presence of specific antibody can result in the Dengue hemorrhagic shock syndrome. Immune complexes, with or without complement, localize antigens to FDC and other FcR+ CR+ cells. Macrophages themselves can produce all components of the complement cascade in significant amounts at local sites, which may be less accessible to circulating proteins made by hepatocytes.

Nonopsonic receptors reacting directly with ligands on microorganisms include CR3, lectins (especially the MR), and the scavenger receptors SR-A and MARCO (Fig. 4). MRs are present on macrophages, DCs, and sinusoidal endothelium. They mediate phagocytosis and endocytosis, including macropinocytosis, and structurally resemble another multilectin (Dec 205) present on DCs as well as tissue macrophages and epithelial cells in the thymus; carbohydrate recognition by the latter has not been demonstrated. The MR has eight C-type lectin domains, homologous to the mannose binding protein (MBP) a circulating hepatocyte-derived acute-phase reactant. MBP contains a single lectin domain per polypeptide, which oligomerizes like other collectins to achieve multivalent interactions and activate complement via associated serine proteases. MR expression on macrophages is selectively down- and upregulated by IFN-γ and IL-4/13, respectively. The possible role of the cysteine-rich domain in transport of immunogenic glycopeptides within secondary lymphoid organs has been noted.

The SR-A mediates endocytosis of modified proteins (e.g., acetylated lipoproteins) and selected polyanions, such as LPS and lipoteichoic acid. In addition, it can serve as an adhesion molecule and contributes to phagocytic clearance of apoptotic thymocytes and Gram-negative as well as Gram-positive bacteria. CD36 (thrombospondin receptor), vitronectin receptors, and CD44 also have been implicated in the uptake of senescent PMNs by macrophages. A role for macrophage SR-A in immune induction has not been demonstrated, but studies in SR-A KO mice have shown an important inhibitory role in limiting TNF-α production by immunologically activated macrophages. Wild-type, BCG-primed mice produce granulomata rich in SR-A+ macrophages; SR-A KO mice restrict growth of this organism and form normal granulomata containing activated MHC II+ macrophages; upon additional challenge with LPS, the KO mice die about 10 times more readily than do wild-type animals. TNF-α levels in the circulation increase markedly because of unopposed triggering via CD14, a receptor for the LPS-binding protein, and contribute to septic shock because blocking anti-TNF mAb protects these mice.

Naturally occurring microbial ligands for these nonopsonic receptors are still poorly defined; individual receptors mediate microbial binding and uptake of microorganisms, although each contributes only part of total binding. Particle uptake involves the cytoskeleton, bulk membrane flow, and remodeling, as well as multiple plasma membrane receptors. Phagosome formation and maturation resemble endocytic uptake, initiating macrophage vesicle trafficking and recirculation, fusion with lysosomes, acidification, ion fluxes, and digestion. GTP-binding proteins and complex signaling cascades play an important role in these dynamic events. A key issue that needs to be resolved is how cell and receptor functions are modulated so that microbial phagocytosis or invasion induce inflammatory responses, unlike the uptake of apoptotic cells. The MHC II biosynthesis and subcellular localization and proteolytic processing of peptide antigens in vacuolar and cytosolic compartments of APCs are discussed elsewhere in this volume (see Chapter 9). Cytokines—especially IL-4/13, IL-10, and IFN-γ—influence endocytosis via MR-dependent and -independent pathways, and selectively alter vesiule dynamics.

Pathogens vary in using macrophage plasma membrane molecules for entry and modify the composition of the resultant phagosome membrane. Mycobacteria, for example, use a range of mechanisms to evade killing by macrophages, including delayed maturation of phagosomes and inhibition of fusion with lysosomes and acidification. *Listeria monocytogenes* escapes into the cytosol by disruption of the phagosome membrane, whereas *Leishmania* multiplies in phagolysosomes. Humoral (antibody and complement) and cellular (IFN-γ) mechanisms overcome parasitization of macrophages by diversion to lysosomes, or induce killing via O/N-dependent (oxygen/nitrogen) and other mechanisms.

Major unsolved questions remain concerning phagocytosis, intracellular infection, and immune responses. How do particulate antigens and microbial agents induce T-cell responses, and what are the relative contributions to this process of macrophages, DCs, and highly and minimally efficient phagocytes? What determines the balance between total antigen degradation and loading of MHC molecules? What interactions take place between intracellular pathogens and host macrophages, especially in regard to nutritional requirements of the organism? What is the role of pathogen-derived secretory products in the vacuolar milieu, in recruitment of organelles such as endoplasmic reticulum and mitochondria and in effects on host cell biosynthesis? What are the intracellular killing mechanisms and how can organisms survive, or become latent, within macrophages? Finally, what specific receptor-mediated signals induce the secretion of macrophage molecules such as IL-12 that direct the resultant specific immune response?

Gene Expression and Secretion

After surface and endocytic stimulation, the mature macrophage can secrete a large range of high and low molecular weight products. These include enzymes involved in antimicrobial resistance (lysozyme), neutral proteinases and arachidonate metabolites that contribute to inflammation and tissue repair, cytokines such as IL-1 and TNF-α that modulate the activities of other leukocytes and endothelium, and reactive oxygen and nitrogen intermediates implicated in host defense. Proinflammatory cytokines account for part of the effects of immune adjuvants in promoting, broadening, and sustaining humoral responses. The ability to release these products depends on the prior history of the macrophage; whether resident, recruited, or activated (primed), its encounters with microbial wall products, including LPS, and exposure to cytokines and other immunomodulatory molecules in its immediate environment. Ligation of specific receptors induces various signaling pathways and is able to alter gene expression in the macrophage selectively. Transcription factors such as the NF-κB and Pu-1 families contribute to macrophage-restricted or activation-dependent changes in gene expression. Product expression depends further on translational regulation, posttranslational modification such as proteolytic processing, and coexpression of inhibitors such as IL-10. Messenger RNA turnover varies greatly for different products, due to the presence or absence of specific 3′ instability sequences. Many macrophage products are labile and act close to the cell surface; overproduction results in tissue catabolism and systemic effects associated with widespread infection or chronic inflammation, often as a result of an immunologically driven disease process.

Although most bioactivities have been defined in vitro, there is evidence that expression of macrophage secretory activities may be quite different in situ; lysozyme production is characteristic of all macrophages in culture but is downregulated on most resident cells in vivo and depends on induction by immune or phagocytic stimuli. 5′ promoter sequences of human lysozyme transgenes have been used to target tissue- and macrophage activation–specific expression of a reporter molecule in vivo. The promoters of other macrophage-restricted molecules may, in due course, make it possible to direct macrophage biosynthetic activities precisely, to boost or inhibit immune responses.

Modulation of Macrophage Activation In Vitro

Our understanding of macrophage activation derives from studies of induction of the MHC II antigen; of effector functions such as proteinase, TNF-α, reactive oxygen intermediates, and reactive nitrogen intermediates release; of expression of membrane receptors such as MR; and of resistance to infectious agents (e.g., mycobacteria, Listeria, Candida, and HIV). Generalizations can be made, but it must be remembered that organisms vary considerably in their ability to evade or survive macrophage restriction mechanisms and interact with macrophages in individual ways.

Figure 4 illustrates various pathways of macrophage activation that result from microbial, cellular, and cytokine interactions. Knowledge is based mainly on in vitro experiments and in vivo challenge of selected animal models. Analysis of the actions of individual cytokines (IFN-γ, IL-10, and IL 4/13) on defined macrophage targets (murine peritoneal macrophages and human monocyte-derived macrophages) reveals three characteristic and distinctive in vitro phenotypes across a spectrum of activation. IFN-γ and its own production and amplification via IL-12 or IGIF (IL-18) play a central role in MHC II induction, enhanced antimicrobial resistance, and proinflammatory cytokine production, characteristic of Th1-type responses. Conversely, IL-10 suppresses markers of activation, while inducing selective expression of other macrophage genes. The identification of a comparable link between macrophages/APCs and the induction of Th2-type responses has proved elusive. IL-4 and IL-13 have closely overlapping functions and induce an alternative activation phenotype in macrophages consistent with increased APC function and humoral responses. Although in this chapter I shall not enter the debate regarding polarized Th1 and Th2-type responses, it is possible to categorize, by use of the markers described, analogous M1- and M2-type macrophage phenotypes. It is also important to distinguish modulation of macrophage immunologic properties by IL-4 and IL-13 from marked deactivation and inhibition of proinflammatory and cytotoxic functions by IL-10. The interplay of cytokines derived from macrophages themselves, from activated T- and B-lymphocytes, and from other cells (NK and endothelial cells) results in reciprocal positive or negative interactions and time-dependent changes in activating and inhibitory signals. Some predictions from in vitro studies can be extended to the intact host. For example, IFN-

γ and IL-12 deficiency results in the inability to restrict opportunistic organisms in murine models and in humans, and i-NOS is important for resistance to a range of infectious agents. IL-10 deficiency, on the other hand, results in overactive Th1-dependent inflammation (e.g., in the gut). IL-4 deficiency by itself has little effect on macrophage phenotype in vivo because IL-13 mimics many of its actions. These cytokines share a common receptor subunit, and it will be interesting to study macrophages from KO mice that lack the ability to respond to both IL-4 and IL-13.

The above analysis is oversimplified. Combinations of cytokines, in vitro, have different effects on macrophages than the sum of the parts. For example, the combination of IL-4 and GM-CSF induces differentiation of human monocytes into immature DCs, whereas each alone induces cells with distinctive macrophage properties. Furthermore, a particular Th2-type cytokine such as IL-10 can display radically different effects on antimicrobial (i-NOS–dependent) killing, which is markedly suppressed, and anti-HIV activities of macrophages, which are enhanced. Although IFN-γ and IL-4 have opposing actions on MR expression and phagocytosis of yeasts, in combination they synergize to enhance uptake markedly. Other combinations of cytokines, such as IFN-$\alpha\beta$ and IFN-γ, can antagonize each other, presumably by competition for signaling pathways. Although extrapolations with predictive value can be made in some situations, a great deal remains to be discovered about macrophage behavior in complex immune environments in vivo.

CONCLUSIONS AND SOME REMAINING ISSUES

Macrophages influence and respond to all other cells involved in immunity, in both the afferent and efferent limbs. Many of the molecules that mediate particular functions are now defined, but their roles within the macrophages and in intercellular interactions are often poorly understood. Macrophages developed during the evolution of multicellular organisms before the immunologically specific, clonotypic responses of B- and T-lymphocytes emerged. Macrophages themselves diversified in parallel with T-helper lymphocytes, generating DCs as specialized APCs for naive T-lymphocytes, and yielding a range of effector cell phenotypes in response to diverse activated T cells, both CD4$^+$ and CD8$^+$. Macrophages and their derivatives cluster with differentiating hematopoietic cells in fetal liver and bone marrow, with developing thymocytes, with naive CD4$^+$ T-lymphocytes and antigen during immune induction, and with activated T cells and microbial pathogens in granuloma formation (Fig. 2). In addition, they associate with antigen-stimulated B-lymphocytes during cell expansion, diversification, and apoptosis. A major challenge will be to define the role of specific and accessory surface molecules by which macrophages discriminate between live and dying cells and to uncover the intrinsic and extrinsic factors that control macrophage activities within these diverse immune cell interactions.

Our understanding of the multiple roles of macrophages and DCs in immunoregulation is also evolving as we better appreciate their specializations and adaptations. Central issues in the immunobiology of macrophages remain obscure and interesting for further investigation:

1. Macrophages display broad functions in homeostasis, beyond host defense and immunity, which may be special instances of a more general role in preserving host integrity, comparable

with that of the central nervous system and endocrine system. Their dispersion, plasticity, and responsiveness raise obvious questions for the biologist. In particular, what are their roles in development and in trophic interactions within different organs?

2. The macrophage lies at the heart of the classic immunologic question of recognition of altered or nonself, especially of particulates. What are the actual ligands recognized by the diverse range of plasma membrane receptors capable of direct discrimination and what determines whether uptake of a target is immunologically silent or productive? How can this information be harnessed to vaccine development?

3. Once activated, macrophages change their ability to recognize and destroy targets, directly or in concert with antibody, complement, and other less defined opsonins. Can macrophages directly kill virus-infected and other immunologically activated cells? If so, do they use MHC matching, even in a limited way, and do they contribute to tolerance and, by implication, autoimmunity by failure to perform a suppressive function?

4. A special case in which macrophages are present in large numbers at a site of failure to respond immunologically is the fetoplacental unit. CSF-1 is produced locally at high levels; does this deactivate macrophages or make them switch to perform a trophic role? Do tumors that are rich in macrophages adopt a similar strategy?

5. Although macrophages express a large number of genes involved in household functions and share expression of others with a limited range of cell types, they also express highly restricted molecules responsible for unique functions. Can these be harnessed for macrophage-specific gene targeting at selected microanatomic sites to deliver functionally precise signals at predetermined times? Techniques are becoming available to realize at least part of this scenario and should provide new insights into the multiple roles of the macrophages in immunity.

ACKNOWLEDGMENT

I thank the members of my laboratory for discussions and Christine Holt for preparing the manuscript. Research in the author's laboratory is supported by grants from the Medical Research Council, UK, the Wellcome Trust, Arthritis and Rheumatism Research Council, the British Heart Foundation, the Histiocytosis Association of America, and GlaxoWellcome plc.

SUGGESTED READING

Books

Beelen RHJ. The macrophage: Basic and clinical aspects. *Immunobiology* 1996;195: 401–664.

Gordon S. The myeloid system. In: Herzenberg LA, Weir DM, Herzenberg LA, Blackwell C, eds. *Weir's Handbook of Experimental Immunology,* 5th ed. Vol. IV. The Integrated Immune System. Boston: Blackwell Scientific, 1997:153–175.

Karnovsky MC, Bolis L, eds. *Phagocytosis—Past and Future.* New York: Academic, 1982.

Lewis C, McGee JOD, eds. *The Macrophage.* Oxford, England: IRL Press, 1992.

Metchnikoff E. *Immunity in Infective Disease.* Translated by Binnie FG. Cambridge, England. Cambridge University Press, 1905.

Mims CA. *The Pathogenesis of Infectious Disease,* 2nd ed. London: Academic, 1982.

Phagocytosis. *Trends Cell Biol* 1995;15:85–142.

Tauber AI, Chernyak L. *Metchnikoff and the Origins of Immunology. From Metaphor to Theory.* Oxford, England: Oxford University Press, 1991.

Van Furth R, ed. *Mononuclear Phagocytes. Biology of Monocytes and Macrophages.* Dordrect, The Netherlands: Kluwer, 1992. (Also see earlier volumes of Leiden Conferences).

Zembala M, Asherson GL, eds. *Human Monocytes.* London: Academic, 1989.

Zwilling BS, Eisenstein, eds. *Macrophage-Pathogen Interactions.* New York: Marcel Dekker, 1994.

Selected Reviews

Bach EA, Aguet M, Schreiber RD. The IFNγ receptor: A paradigm for cytokine receptor signalling. *Ann Rev Imunol* 1997;15:563–591.

Bacon KB, Schall TJ. Chemokines as mediators of allergic inflammation. *Int Arch Allergy Immunol* 1996;109:97–109.

Clarke S, Gordon S. Myeloid-specific gene expression. *J Leukoc Biol* 1998; 63:153–168.

Crocker PR, Hartnell A, Munday J, Nath D. The potential role of sialoadhesin as a macrophage recognition molecule in health and disease. *Glycoconjugate J* 1997;14: 601–609.

Daeron M. Fc receptor biology. *Ann Rev Immunol* 1997;15:203–234.

Gordon S. Mononuclear phagocyte system and tissue homeostasis. In: *Oxford Textbook of Medicine.* Oxford, England: Oxford University Press, 1995:84–95.

Gordon S. My favourite cell: The macrophage. *Bioessays* 1995;17:977–986.

Gordon S. Overview: The myeloid system. In: Herzenberg LA, Weir DM, Herzenberg LA, Blackwell C, eds. *Weir's Handbook of Experimental Immunology,* 5th ed. Vol. IV. The Integrated Immune System. Chapter 153. Cambridge, MA: Blackwell Science, 1997:1–9.

Gordon S. Macrophage activation. In: *Encyclopaedia of Immunology,* 2nd ed. San Diego: Academic, 1998 (in press).

Gordon S, Clarke S, Greaves D, Doyle A. Molecular immunobiology of macrophages: Recent progress. *Curr Opin Immunol* 1995;7:24–33.

Gordon S, Hughes DA. Macrophages and their origins: Heterogeneity in relation to tissue microenvironment. In: Lipscomb M, Russell S, eds. *Lung Macrophages and Dendritic Cells.* New York: Marcel Dekker, 1997:3–31.

Gordon S, Keshav S, Stein M. BCG-induced granuloma formation in murine tissues. *Immunobiology* 1994;191:369–377.

Gordon S, Lawson L, Rabinowitz S, Crocker PR, Morris L, Perry VH. Antigen markers of macrophage differentiation in murine tissues. In: Russell S, Gordon S, eds. *Macrophage Biology and Activation (Current Topics in Microbiology and Immunology).* Vol. 181. Berlin: Springer-Verlag, 1992:1–37.

Greenberg S, Silverstein SC. Phagocytosis. In: Paul W, ed. *Fundamental Immunology,* 3rd ed. New York: Raven, 1993:941–964.

Kraal G. Cells in the marginal zone of the spleen. *Int Rev Cytol* 1992;132:31–74.

MacMicking J, Xie Q-w, Nathan C. Nitric oxide and macrophage function. *Ann Rev Immunol* 1997;15:323–350.

Mahoney JA, Gordon S. Macrophage receptors and innate immunity. *Biochemist* 1998;20:12–16.

McKnight AJ, Gordon S. EGF-TM7: A novel subfamily of seven-transmembrane-region leukocyte cell-surface molecules. *Immunol Today* 1996;17:283–287.

McKnight AJ, Gordon S. Membrane molecules as markers of murine macrophage differentiation. *Adv Immunol* 1998;68:271–314.

Medzhitov R, Janeway CA Jr. Innate immunity: impact on the adaptive immune response. *Curr Opin Immunol* 1997;9:4–9.

Pearson AM. Scavenger receptors in innate immunity. *Curr Opin Immunol* 1996;8: 20–28.

Perry VH, Andersson P-B, Gordon S. Macrophages and inflammation in the central nervous system. *Trends Neurosci* 1993;16:268–273.

Pontow SE, Kery V, Stahl PD. Mannose receptor. *Int Rev Cytol* 1992;137B:221–244.

Ravetch JV. Fc receptors. *Curr Opin Immunol* 1997;9:121–125.

Rollins B. Chemokines. *Blood* 1997;90:909–928.

Steinman RM, Moberg CL. Zanvil Alexander Cohn 1926–1993. An appreciation of the physician-scientist. The macrophage in cell biology and resistance to infectious disease. *J Exp Med* 1994;179:1–30.

Trinchieri G. Cytokines acting on or secreted by MØ during intraclulular infection (IL-10, IL-12, IFNγ). *Curr Opin Immunol* 1997;9:17–23.

Wiktor-Jedrzejczak W, Gordon S. Cytokine regulation of the MØ system using the colony stimulating factor-1 deficient op/op mouse. *Physiol Rev* 1996;76:927–947.

Selected Papers

Andersson P-B, Perry VH, Gordon S. The acute inflammatory response to lipopolysaccharide in CNS parenchyma differs from that in other body tissues. *Neuroscience* 1992;48:169–186.

Bell MD, Lopez-Gonzalez R, Lawson LJ, et al. Upregulation of the macrophage scavenger receptor in response to different forms of injury in the CNS. *J Neurocytol* 1994;23:605–613.

Clarke S, Greaves DR, Chung L-P, Tree P, Gordon S. The human lysozyme promoter directs reporter gene expression to activated myelomonocytic cells in transgenic mice. *Proc Natl Acad Sci U S A* 1996;93:1434–1438.

Crocker PR, Mucklow S, Bouckson V, et al. Sialoadhesin, a macrophage-specific adhesion molecule for haemopoietic cells with 17 immunoglobulin-like domains. *EMBO J* 1994;13:4490–4503.

Crowley MT, Costello PS, Fitzer-Attas CJ, et al. A critical role for Syk in signal transduction and phagocytosis mediated by Fcg receptors on macrophages. *J Exp Med* 1997;186:1027–1039.

Dalton DK, Pitts-Meek S, Keshav S, Figari IS, Bardley A, Stewart TA. Multiple defects of immune cell function in mice with disrupted interferon-γ genes. *Science* 1993;259:1739–1742.

Doyle AG, Herbein G, Montaner LJ, et al. Interleukin 13 alters the activation state of murine macrophages in vitro: Comparison with interleukin-4 and interferon γ. *Eur J Immunol* 1994;24:1441–1445.

Fraser IP, Hughes DA, Gordon S. Divalent cation-independent macrophage adhesion inhibited by monoclonal antibody to murine scavenger receptor. *Nature* 1993;364: 343–346.

Gruenheid S, Pinner E, Desjardins M, Gros P. Natural resistance to infection with intracellular pathogens: The Nramp1 protein is recruited to the membrane of the phagosome. *J Exp Med* 1997;185:717–730.

Havell EA. Production of tumor necrosis factor during murine listeriosis. *J Immunol* 1987;139:4225–4231.

Haworth R, Platt N, Keshav S, et al. The macrophage scavenger receptor type A (SR-A) is expressed by activated macrophages and protects the host against lethal endotoxic shock. *J Exp Med* 1997;186:1431–1439.

Haziot A, Ferrero E, Kontgen F, et al. Resistance to endotoxin shock and reduced dissemination of gram-negative bacteria in CD14-deficient mice. *Immunity* 1996;4: 407–414.

Holness CL, da Silva RP, Fawcett J, Gordon S, Simmons DL. Macrosialin, a mouse macrophage restricted glycoprotein, is a member of the lamp/lgp family. *J Biol Chem* 1993;268:9661–9666.

Hutchings P, Rosen H, O'Reilly L, Simpson E, Gordon S, Cooke A. Transfer of diabetes in mice prevented by blockade of adhesion-promoting receptor on macrophages. *Nature* 1990;348:639–642.

Keshav S, Chung L-P, Milon G, Gordon S. Lysozyme is an inducible marker of macrophage activation in murine tissues as demonstrated by in situ hybridization. *J Exp Med* 1991;174:1049–1058.

Kindler V, Sappino A-P, Grau GE, Piguet P-F, Vassalli P. The inducing role of tumor necrosis factor in the development of bactericidal granulomas during BCG infection. *Cell* 1989;56:731–740.

Lee S-H, Starkey P, Gordon S. Quantitative analysis of total macrophage content in adult mouse tissues. Immunochemical studies with monoclonal antibody F4/80. *J Exp Med* 1985;161:475–489.

Martinez-Pomares L, Kosco-Vilbois M, Darley E, Tree P, Herren S, Bonnefoy J-Y, Gordon S. Fc chimeric protein containing the cysteine-rich domain of the murine mannose receptor binds to macrophages from splenic marginal zone and lymph node subcapsular sinus, and to germinal centres. *J Exp Med* 1996;184:1927–1937.

McWilliam A, Tree P, Gordon S. Interleukin-4 regulates induction of sialoadhesin, the macrophage sialic acid specific receptor. *Proc Natl Acad Sci U S A* 1992;89: 10522–10526.

Morris L, Crocker PR, Gordon S. Murine foetal liver macrophages bind developing erythroblasts by a divalent cation-dependent haemagglutinin. *J Cell Biol* 1988;106: 649–656.

Morris L, Graham CF, Gordon S. Macrophages in haemopoietic and other tissues of the developing mouse detected by monoclonal antibody F4/80. *Development* 1991; 112:517–526.

Platt N, Suzuki H, Kurihara Y, Kodama T, Gordon S. Role for the class A macrophage scavenger receptor in the phagocytosis of apoptotic thymocytes. *Proc Natl Acad Sci U S A* 1996;93:12456–12460.

Rabinowitz S, Gordon S. Macrosialin, a macrophage-restricted membrane sialoprotein differentially glycosylated in response to inflammatory stimuli. *J Exp Med* 1991; 174:827–836.

Reid DM, Perry VH, Andersson P-B, Gordon S. Mitosis and apoptosis of microglia in vivo induced by an anti-CR3 monoclonal antibody which crossed the blood-brain barrier. *Neuroscience* 1994;56:529–533.

Ren Y, Silverstein RL, Allen J, Savill J. CD36 gene transfer confers capacity for phagocytosis of cells undergoing apoptosis. *J Exp Med* 1995;181:1857–1862.

Stein M, Keshav S, Harris N, Gordon S. IL-4 potently enhances murine macrophage mannose receptor activity: A marker of alternative immune macrophage activation. *J Exp Med* 1992;176:287–293.

Witmer-Pack MD, Hughes D, Schuler G, et al. Identification of macrophages and dendritic cells in the osteopetrotic [op/op] mouse. *J Cell Sci* 1993;104:1021–1029.

Fundamental Immunology, Fourth Edition,
edited by William E. Paul
Lippincott–Raven Publishers, Philadelphia © 1999.

CHAPTER 16

Dendritic Cells

Ralph M. Steinman

THE IMPORTANCE OF ACCESSORY CELLS OR PROFESSIONAL ANTIGEN-PRESENTING CELLS

The major histocompatibility complex (MHC) and antigen presentation have been on the center stage of immunology for decades. The MHC was identified as a gene complex encoding the major transplantation antigens for T cell–mediated graft rejection.

R.M. Steinman: Laboratory of Cellular Physiology and Immunology, Rockefeller University, New York, New York 10021-6399.

An intense research effort then proved that MHC products bind peptides that are processed from proteins, both foreign and self antigens. These MHC–peptide complexes are then presented to, or recognized by, the clonotypic T-cell receptor (TCR), so that either immunity or tolerance can begin.

This chapter addresses antigen presentation at another level that may best be termed immune responsiveness. The immune system contains a distinct group of antigen-presenting cells (APCs), called dendritic cells (DCs), that are specialized to capture antigens and initiate T-cell immunity. An emerging body of literature suggests that DCs also can induce T-cell tolerance.

DCs were discovered in an attempt to understand what were initially called accessory cells. Before T cells were discovered to recognize antigenic fragments presented on MHC products, immunologists were trying to generate immunity in tissue culture. This was surprisingly difficult because clonal selection theory stated that antigens should simply select and expand responsive lymphocytes. However, when attempts were made to stimulate purified lymphocytes with antigens and even mitogens, additional accessory cells were required. The two main systems for studying accessory cells were the primary antibody response by mouse splenocytes (1) and the recall response to protein antigens by cells from primed guinea pigs (2,3) and humans (4,5).

Several distinct areas of research evolved to pursue the accessory cell phenomenon (Table 1). In addition to processing antigens to peptides that are presented on MHC products (signal 1), accessory cells express a plethora of second signals that mediate T-cell binding and costimulation. Most of these are membrane glycoproteins such as intracellular adhesion molecules (ICAMs; CD50, CD54, CD102), lymphocyte function associated antigens (LFAs) (CD2, CD11a, CD58), and B7s (CD80, CD86). The term "professional APC" is now used to denote cells that have both antigen-presenting and accessory (costimulatory) functions.

There proved to be many different types of accessory cells, and the type determined the quality and quantity of the immune response. DCs are unusually potent, especially for initiating T-cell responses. Once activated, T cells interact efficiently with other APCs. B cells are the only APCs that produce antibody upon presentation to T cells, and macrophages can increase antimicrobial activity. So all these cells can present antigens, but the character of the immune response depends on the type of APC.

Accessory cells have been pursued most in tissue culture, but current emphasis is on function *in vivo* in animals and in humans. Function takes place in several steps: an afferent limb, in which antigens that are deposited in different parts of the body are either scavenged for destruction or processed for presentation to lymphocytes; a central limb, where lymphocytes, usually in lymphoid organs, are selected to expand clonally and differentiate (make antibodies, lymphokines, and cytolysins); and an efferent limb, where the activated lymphocytes and APCs work together to perform effector functions that eliminate antigens wherever the latter have gained entry. Accessory cell research now impinges significantly on the study of disease states and on the differences between the induction of tolerance and immunity *in vivo*.

We will use the term "antigen presentation" to describe all the events that are required to express MHC–peptide complexes at cell surfaces. DCs express a host of additional or accessory properties that enhance T-cell responses, particularly in the setting of whole animals. This chapter considers some of the main concepts of DC function, how these concepts developed, and current understanding of the tissue distribution and development of DCs.

TABLE 1. *Areas of accessory cell research*

Mechanisms of antigen presentation: uptake, processing, MHC–peptide complex formation
Adhesion and costimulatory molecules for inducing immunity
Different types of accessory cells
Antigen presentation *in vivo* and in disease states
Pathways for immune tolerance

DISTINCT DENDRITIC CELLS IN LYMPHOID CELL SUSPENSIONS: INITIAL IDENTIFICATION

Approaches to Enriching and Depleting Accessory Cells in Mouse Spleen Suspensions

The early model to study accessory cell function was the primary antibody response in cultures of mouse splenocytes (1). Sheep red blood cells were the antigen, but hapten–carrier conjugates were also used. Several experimental approaches indicated that, in addition to B and T cells, another population, called accessory cells, was needed to generate antibody-secreting cells. The first involved adherence to glass and later plastic, where the accessory cells were adherent and the lymphocytes nonadherent (6). A second approach involved flotation on dense media such as bovine serum albumin (BSA), where the accessory cells had a low buoyant density and the responding lymphocytes a high density (7). A third method used columns packed with materials to which the accessory cells adhered. Sephadex G10 allowed both B and T cells to pass through (8), and nylon wool allowed T cells to pass (9). Plastic adherent accessory cells were then added back to the cells that emerged from the G10 or nylon wool columns.

These approaches were all empirical because functional assays would determine if one had enriched or depleted accessory cells. Because of the adherence property, the accessory cells were presumed to be macrophages. Adherence, however, is not a specific property of macrophages but is exhibited by most cell types, including fibroblasts, endothelial cells, and even B cells. The best source for accessory cells was the adherent fraction of mouse splenocytes. However, a standard source of mouse macrophages, the peritoneal cavity, was typically inactive in supporting antibody responses and often suppressive, even at modest doses.

Identification of DCs as a Distinct and Active Cell Type in Accessory Populations

Because of the weak or absent function of peritoneal macrophages as accessory cells for the antibody response, and because cell biologic studies showed that antigens were thoroughly degraded in macrophages (10,11), an examination of adherent mouse splenocytes was begun. These were found to be heterogeneous. Only a fraction were phagocytes, defined by the main criteria that were then available, i.e., active uptake of particles, especially immune complexes and antibody coated red blood cells, and an abundance of lysosomes and esterases (12,13).

The other major, plastic-adherent cell was a cell that had not been seen before, and we termed it "dendritic cell" (12,13). DCs had unusual cell and nuclear shapes, and continually formed and retracted processes. Unlike macrophages (Fig. 1), DCs had scarce lysosomes, lacked Fc receptors, and were poorly endocytic *in vivo* and *in vitro* (13,14). DCs were bone marrow derived, independent of T cells (present in nude mice), did not respond to either B- or T-cell mitogens, and had limited viability in culture (15). Nonphagocytic cells with a similar appearance to isolated DCs were evident in sections of mouse spleen, primarily in the lymphocyte-rich white pulp rather than the macrophage-rich red pulp (12). Less than 1% of splenocytes were DCs, but they could be enriched 10- to 20-fold by flotation on dense BSA (13,14,16).

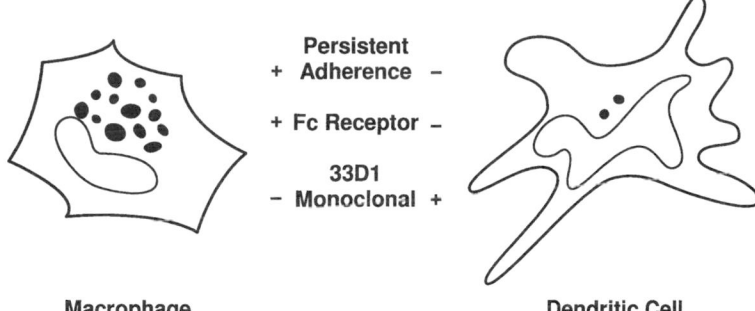

Persistent
+ Adherence −

+ Fc Receptor −

33D1
− Monoclonal +

Macrophage   **Dendritic Cell**

FIG. 1. Features used initially to distinguish mouse spleen macrophages from DCs.

Three independent approaches were used to prepare highly enriched populations of macrophages and DCs (Fig. 1). By each approach, the DCs were found to be the active accessory cells for the antibody response (17–20), whereas macrophages were inactive or suppressive (21). After overnight culture, DCs could be separated from macrophages either as the Fc receptor negative or nonadherent fraction (14) (Fig. 1). Later a DC-specific monoclonal antibody (mAb) called 33D1 was prepared (22). When 33D1 and complement selectively depleted the trace DC component from fresh spleen, the antibody response plummeted (18); small numbers of DCs, purified by means other than the 33D1 antibody, restored the response.*

In retrospect, the early approaches that were used to enrich and deplete accessory cells can all be explained at the level of DC content. It is preferable to identify DCs directly because some populations of DCs may not even exhibit transient adherence [e.g., DCs in most organs of rats (23) or DCs in afferent lymph of all species (24,25)], and others may not have a low buoyant density [e.g., some immature DCs (26,27)]. A useful approach is to examine a cell population for DCs, both before and after culture. The cells are best spun onto slides with a cytocentrifuge. This special centrifuge sediments and dries the cells as a spot on a slide. One looks for large, irregularly shaped cells with abundant MHC II and other DC traits (Fig. 2).

High Expression of Ia Antigens or MHC Class II Products on DCs

In several functional assays, immunologists were eliminating accessory cells with anti–MHC II antibodies and complement (originally termed "anti-Ia" for "MHC I region associated," where "I" encoded immune response or Ir genes). In retrospect, anti–MHC II antibodies could not define the responsible cell type, but instead defined the MHC products that were required on any APC to present antigen to CD4⁺ T cells. DCs were enriched as cells with distinctive morphology and surface properties and were subsequently found to react vigorously (immunofluorescence and

complement cytotoxicity) with alloantisera and new monoclonals to MHC II (14,28). In quantitative binding studies, MHC II products were abundant on DCs, much higher than the prototype MHC II–positive cells, B-lymphocytes (28). Most macrophages in the peritoneal cavity and spleen of mice proved to be MHC II negative (14). The cells only became MHC II positive when exposed to lymphokines *in vitro* (most likely to interferon [IFN]-γ) (29,30) or when elicited during a cell-mediated immune response *in vivo*, e.g., after administration of mycobacteria such as bacille Calmette-Guerin (BCG) (31).

Function of MHC II on DCs in the MLR: The Difference Between Antigen-Presenting Cells and Accessory or Costimulatory Cells

The observation that DCs had high levels of MHC II required proof that these gene products were functional. MHC II products were known to be the major antigens for stimulation of T-cell proliferation in the primary mixed leukocyte reaction or MLR.† When DCs were tested as MLR stimulators (32,33), the findings were quite surprising given the prior belief that any cell that expressed MHC II (such as B cells) could stimulate an MLR. First, the DCs were unusually potent stimulators and could be used in roughly 100 times smaller numbers than bulk leukocytes. Second, other MHC II positive cells, including B cells and macrophages, were weak or inactive (29,32,33). Potency in MLR stimulation is still the most convenient assay for demonstrating the function of mature DCs, and both CD4⁺ helper and CD8⁺ killer responses are induced (34,35).

These MLR findings provided the first clues to the physiologic role of DCs in initiating T cell–dependent immunity. Antigen presentation alone was necessary but not sufficient to initiate a response by resting T cells *in vitro*. B cells and macrophages presented allo-MHC, as detected with alloantibodies or activated T cells, but lacked the accessory or costimulatory functions that were expressed by DCs to initiate the primary MLR.

---

*33D1 has had considerable utility, but it also has shortcomings. The antigen recognized by 33D1 has yet to be identified, and the monoclonal reacts with a major subset of DCs from mouse spleen but not other sources. Expression of the antigen is weak, so that 33D1 does not give strong staining in fluorescence-activated cell sorting (FACS) analysis, nor is binding of 33D1 detectable in tissue sections.

---

†The MLR was originally used in tissue typing for transplantation to identify incompatibility between a potential graft donor or stimulator, and graft recipient or responder. When donor and recipient differ at the MHC, stimulator cells from the donor induce proliferation and cytolysis from T cells of the recipients. MLR originally stood for "mixed lymphocyte reaction," but when it was found that lymphocytes were poor MLR stimulators, it was renamed "mixed leukocyte reaction."

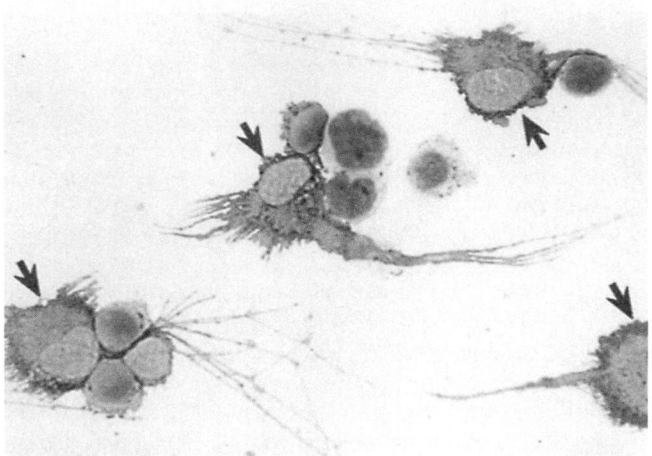

FIG. 2. Cytospin preparations of DCs that are stained for MHC class II products. Shown here are lymph node cells enriched by virtue of a low buoyant density. The unusual shape of the DCs (*arrows*) on cytospins is best evident when the surface is stained, here for MHC II.

FUNCTIONS OF DENDRITIC CELLS: EARLY STUDIES OF "NATURE'S ADJUVANT"

Immunologists for decades have used a number of different artificial substances, termed adjuvants, to enhance the immune response to an antigen. Oils in complete Freund's adjuvant and colloidal aluminum salts (alum) are among the most widely used. Once the trace subset of DCs could be enriched from lymphoid cell suspensions, it was apparent that these APCs could prime T cells in the absence of any other adjuvant. Three new features emerged from the initial functional studies (Table 2) and indicated that DCs were acting as nature's adjuvant.

Potency

Splenic DCs were unusually potent in a number of MHC-restricted, T-cell stimulation assays, including the MLR (29,32,33), the MHC I–restricted killer cell response to hapten-modified cells (31), the MHC II–restricted syngeneic MLR (36), and MHC II–mediated presentation of protein antigens, including those under Ir gene control (37,38). Splenic DCs were 30 to 300 times more effective than the irradiated bulk splenocytes that were generally used as accessory cells.

Comparably potent DCs were identified in many mammals. An early example was the plastic adherent population from human blood. This contained a small DC subset that actively stimulated

TABLE 2. *Functional features of dendritic cells*

Potency
  Small numbers of DCs pulsed with low doses of antigen
    stimulate strong T-cell responses.
Primary responses
  Naive and quiescent T cells can be activated with antigens on
    DCs.
Physiology
  CD4+ T helpers and CD8+ T killers are primed *in vivo*.

the MLR and proliferation to antigens (24,39–41). DCs were also isolated from human tonsil (42). When enriched from rat lymphoid tissues, DCs were strong accessory cells for the MLR and a T-cell mitogenesis assay termed oxidative mitogenesis. In this assay, either the DCs or the T cells were oxidized with sodium periodate, or with neuraminidase followed by galactose oxidase. The aldehyde groups formed Schiff bases with lysine ε-NH_2 groups, leading to cross-linking and T-cell activation. When either oxidized DCs or T cells were mixed with the other cell type, extensive proliferation ensued, even with 1% or fewer DCs (23,43). One difference between rat and mouse DCs [as well as potent APCs for oxidative mitogenesis (44)] is that rat DCs did not have a transient plastic adherence phase and were therefore easier to distinguish from macrophages.

Priming

The initial studies of DCs indicated that these APCs could prime naive T cells. Once activated by DCs, T cells efficiently interacted with other APCs in either the antibody response or the MLR (20,45). In the antibody response, DCs could prime helper T cells that were specific for carrier proteins such as keyhole limpet hemocyanin (KLH) and human serum albumin (HSA). The primed T-helpers could then interact with hapten-specific B cells, in the apparent absence of DCs, to stimulate the antibody response (20). The interaction between the primed T helpers and B cells was both antigen-dependent and MHC-restricted (Fig. 3).

Therefore, both DCs and B cells functioned as APCs in the antibody response, presenting proteins in an MHC-restricted fashion to T cells. However, DCs were indispensable for initiating the response. This was also true in the MLR. T cells did not respond to unstimulated B cells, but after activation to allogeneic MHC products on DCs, the T-cell blasts now responded vigorously to the B cells and reciprocally caused B cells to proliferate and make antibody (45). Therefore, T-cell responses developed in two phases: an afferent limb in which priming was induced by DCs, and an efferent limb in which helper-dependent, antibody formation required B cells as the APCs.

T-cell priming *in vitro* occurred in discrete cell clusters that could be isolated and shown to contain most of the DCs and responding lymphocytes in the culture. Clusters were noted in the primary antibody response (19), the MLR (34,36,39,45–47), and responses to protein antigens and superantigens (48,49). At the time of the early experiments with DCs, the soluble macrophage product interleukin (IL)-1 was thought to be an essential lymphocyte-activating factor. However, neutralizing antibodies to IL-1 did not block the capacity of DCs to activate lymphocytes in clusters (50). Exogenous IL-1 could amplify responses at the level of the DC rather than the T cell (51,52). However, IL-1 was produced during the secondary MHC-restricted interaction between macrophages and activated T cells, but not during the primary response (50,53).

Formally, the T cells that were being primed by DCs in these initial studies might not have been truly naive because the cells could have been primed by cross-reacting antigens in the environment. More recent studies have confirmed priming of naive cells, where the latter are defined by high CD62L, low CD44, or low CD45 activation isoforms (54–56). These experiments are facilitated by TCR-transgenic mice in which most T cells recognize a single MHC–peptide complex.

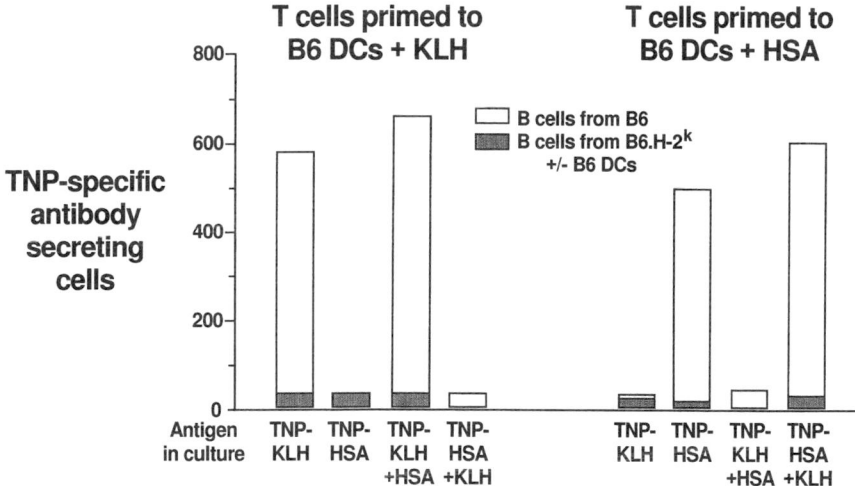

FIG. 3. Carrier-specific helper T cells, primed by DCs in vitro, interact with hapten-specific B cells in an antigen-dependent and MHC-restricted fashion (20). The experiment is conducted in two stages: first carrier-specific helper cells (specific for either HSA or KLH) are primed with DCs pulsed with the corresponding protein. Then the primed T-helpers are mixed with B cells (in the absence of DCs) to elicit the formation of hapten-specific, antibody-secreting cells. Note that the T-helpers only help B cells of the appropriate MHC (here $H-2^b$) and when hapten and carrier are linked.

Physiology *In Vivo*

DCs also function as efficient APCs *in vivo*. This was shown initially in models of graft rejection, in which a small number of allogeneic DCs could trigger the rejection of kidney (57) and endocrine (58,59) grafts. The grafts were otherwise accepted because of the prior depletion of what were called passenger leukocytes but were most likely resident DCs. A reinfusion of DCs from the graft donor, but not B cells and macrophages, elicited rejection (57).

DCs that had been pulsed with protein antigens could prime mice in a genetically restricted fashion (60). If DCs were pulsed *ex vivo* with proteins and readministered into the foot pads, $CD4^+$ T cells were primed in the draining lymph nodes. Much larger numbers of peritoneal macrophages and B cells were inactive. The injected DCs primed T cells directly and did not simply transport antigen for presentation by host APCs. This was shown by the fact that priming was restricted to the MHC alleles of the immunizing DCs (Fig. 4). In this experiment, F1 mice ($H-2^d \times H-2^k$) were primed with DCs from either parental strain. F1 mice have separate T cells that are restricted to antigen presented on $H-2^d$ or $H-2^k$. If $H-2^d$ DCs were priming F1 T cells directly, only the $H-2^d$ restricted clones should be primed, whereas if $H-2^k$ DCs were the immuno-

gen, the primed T cells should only respond to $H-2^k$ APCs. This was indeed observed, so DCs mediated the genetic restriction of a primary immune response *in vivo*.

The *in vivo* priming capacity of DCs has now been documented in several $CD4^+$ (61–64) and $CD8^+$ (65–70) T-cell responses in rodents and possibly humans (71). Therefore, DCs can function *in vivo* without other adjuvants. One wonders if standard adjuvants can enhance immunity by increasing the access of antigens to DCs, or the numbers and function of DCs.

DISTRIBUTION OF DENDRITIC CELLS *IN VIVO* (INTERDIGITATING CELLS, LANGERHANS' CELLS, VEILED CELLS, INTERSTITIAL DENDRITIC CELLS): A DISTINCT SYSTEM OF ANTIGEN-PRESENTING CELLS

The concept of DCs as nature's adjuvant is supported by many features *in vivo*. DCs are distributed in a way that maximizes antigen capture and, subsequently, the binding and activation of specific T cells.

Peripheral Lymphoid Organs as Sites for Generating Immunity

Lymphoid organs, both peripheral and mucosal, are the sites where primary immune responses develop, including the stimulation of helper, killer, and antibody-forming cells. The lymphoid organ that is activated is the one that drains the site where antigens have been deposited, e.g., skin, lung, intestine, blood. The anatomy of lymphoid organs is specialized in three ways to initiate immunity (Fig. 5).

First, there are pathways whereby antigens gain access to the organ. As diagrammed at the top of Fig. 5, access to the spleen is via the blood, to peripheral lymph nodes via afferent lymph, and to mucosal lymphoid organs via special antigen-transporting M cells (72–74).

Second, B- and T-lymphocytes traffic continuously through lymphoid organs, facilitating access to antigen. The lymphocytes seg-

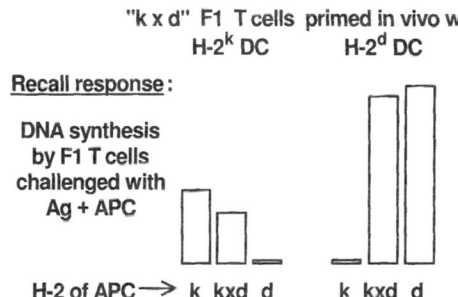

FIG. 4. DCs prime $CD4^+$ T cells in vivo in a genetically restricted manner. F1 T cells were primed with antigen-pulsed DCs from either parent, and then rechallenged *in vitro* with F1 and parental DCs. The MHC of the priming DC is seen to control the genetic restriction of the primed F1 T cells.

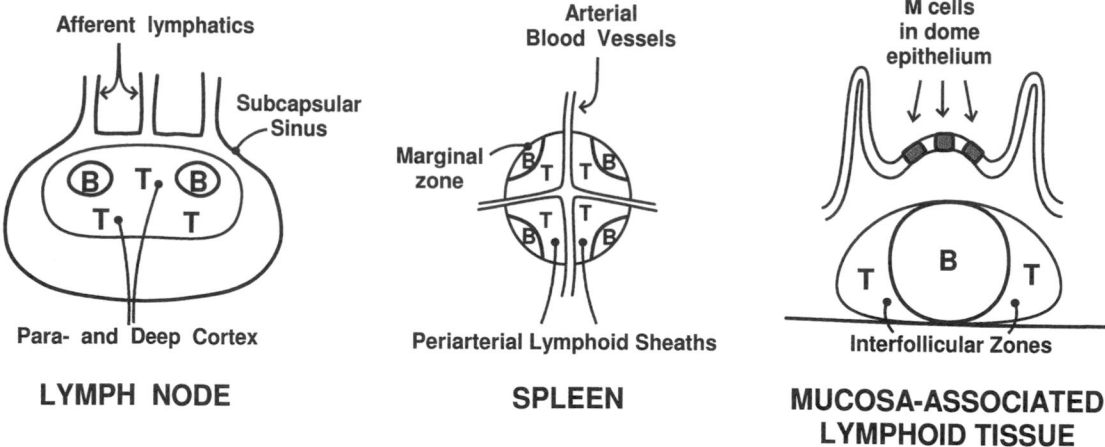

FIG. 5. Pathways for antigen access (*top*) to the three main types of peripheral lymphoid organs: lymph node, spleen, and mucosa-associated lymphoid tissue or MALT. These organs have discrete B-cell areas or follicles, and discrete T-cell areas that are given different names in each organ (*bottom*).

regate into separate regions, B-cell areas (or follicles), and T-cell areas. T-cell areas are called periarterial lymphoid sheaths in the spleen, deep and paracortical regions in the lymph nodes, and inter-follicular zones in mucosal-associated lymphoid tissue (MALT) such as Peyer's patches (Fig. 5).

Third, lymphoid organs are a rich source of specialized APCs that can select lymphocytes trafficking through the B- and T-cell areas. Antigen-processing DCs are abundant in the T-cell areas, where they are also called interdigitating cells (IDCs). B-cell areas are enriched in another type of cell called the follicular dendritic cell (FDC) (75,76). FDCs are likely to be stromal or fibroblast cells because they do not express the CD45 molecule that is found on all leukocytes (77) and because they share properties with fibroblasts in culture (78). FDCs retain native antigens as immune complexes for presentation to B cells (79–81). Therefore, apart from a coincidence in nomenclature, FDCs bear little relation to DCs, which are marrow-derived leukocytes that present processed antigens to T cells.

family member, CD83 (96), and two intracellular proteins called p55 (97) and S-100 (98–100). In the mouse, a set of useful markers, which remain uncharacterized at the molecular level, are antigens in intracellular granules. These are recognized by mAbs MIDC-8 (101), M342 (102), and 2A1 (103). CD68 is an endosomal marker that results in abundant anti-CD68 staining of macrophages, but only a perinuclear spot of stain in IDCs and isolated mature DCs (104). Other molecules that are expressed by IDCs are the integrin CD11c (105,106) and a lectinlike receptor for antigen uptake, originally called NLDC-145 (107) and later DEC-205 (108).

As will be discussed in the section on tolerance below, information is developing that there may be more than one origin for IDCs in the T-cell area. One, called myeloid or nonlymphoid, includes DCs that immigrate into the T-cell area with antigen from the periphery to initiate immunity. The other more resident lymphoid DC population may specialize in immune regulation and peripheral tolerance.

Interdigitating Cells in the T-Cell Areas of Peripheral Lymphoid Organs

Interdigitating cells, first described in a Ph.D. thesis (82), are large cells that extend numerous processes between the T cells (83). The cytologic features of IDCs are similar to those of DCs (84), but many descriptions of IDCs liken them to macrophages (85–90). Like DCs, IDCs lack numerous phagosomes and lysosomes, showing only a perinuclear spot of lysosomal acid phosphatase by cytochemistry, and IDCs do not actively internalize endocytic tracers *in vivo* (85,91–93). In contrast, macrophages contain abundant phagosomes and acid phosphatase and are actively endocytic *in vivo*.

A number of antigenic markers, detected with mAbs, show the similarity between IDCs in the T-cell areas and isolated mature DCs (94) (Fig. 6) (95). For human lymphoid organs, some markers that are expressed at high levels are an immunoglobulin (Ig) gene

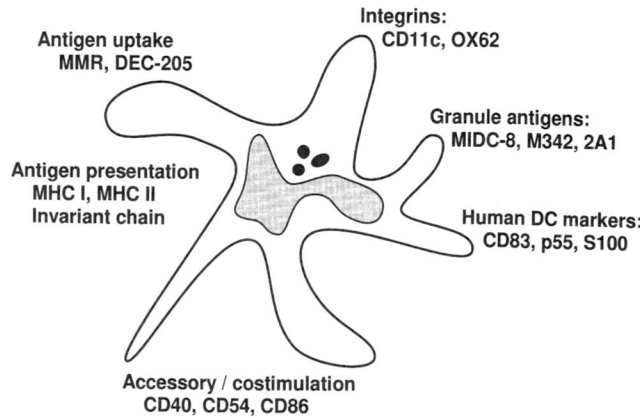

FIG. 6. Markers that are shared between mature DCs and the IDCs in sections of lymphoid organs.

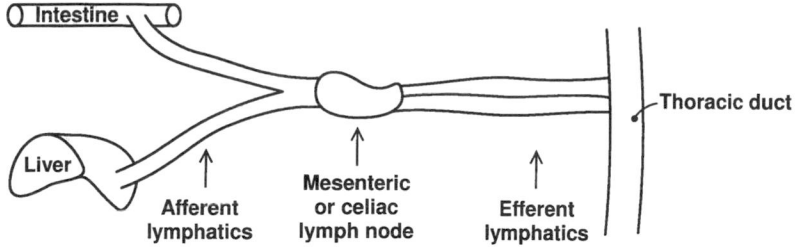

FIG. 7. A method to access pseudoafferent lymph DCs. When lymph nodes are removed, the afferent lymphatics anastomose with efferent lymphatics and empty directly into the thoracic duct. The latter can be cannulated in a small animal like the rat, providing access to afferent lymph DCs or veiled cells.

Veiled Cells in Afferent Lymphatics

Infectious agents and other antigens use afferent lymphatics to gain access to the draining lymph node (Fig. 5).* Typical DCs are also found in afferent lymphatics, e.g., from rabbits (24,109), guinea pigs (110), sheep (111), and humans (112,113). These large cells have motile processes, also called veils because of their sheet-like appearance. In rats, veiled cells are identified within pseudoafferent lymph (25,114,115). The rat lymphatics are too narrow to cannulate, but the thoracic duct is accessible and can be made to contain afferent lymph. To do so, the mesenteric or celiac lymph nodes are surgically removed. When the afferent lymphatics that drain the intestine and liver reanastomose to efferent lymphatics, afferent lymph flows into the thoracic duct (Fig. 7).

In all these sites, veiled cells exhibit typical functional features of DCs (24,25,109,110,115). The cells neither bind antibody-coated red cells nor internalize particulates and are nonadherent both at the time of isolation and during culture. When antigens are administered to an animal, the lymph DCs that drain the injection site carry the antigen in a form that is immunogenic for T cells (61,111). Veiled cells are potent accessory cells for the MLR and mitogen responses (25,109).

The cells in efferent and afferent lymphatics differ. Efferent lymphatics lack DCs, and the T cells include many naive lymphocytes that continually recirculate through the lymphoid tissues, from blood to efferent lymphatics. Afferent lymphatics have substantial numbers of DCs, whereas the T cells have a memory phenotype (116). Some of the DCs form tight conjugates with the T cells in lymph (110,113,117,118), but the physiologic role for these conjugates is not known. One possibility is that the conjugates selectively traffic into B-cell areas, because there is recent evidence that DCs enter germinal centers, presumably to stimulate helper T cells there (119).

Epidermal Langerhans' Cells

As a medical student, Paul Langerhans had described a peculiar subset of cells in skin that were named after him (120,121). The nature of these Langerhans' cells (LCs) was obscure until they were shown to be bone marrow derived (122) and to express features of white blood cells or leukocytes, like Fc receptors (123) and MHC II (124–126). LCs were identified as the active cells in epidermis for presenting antigen to primed T cells (127).

When mouse LCs were studied in cultured epidermal suspensions, they developed all the features of DCs (128,129). In fresh suspensions, LCs differed from mature DCs because there were low levels of surface MHC II and such features as Fc receptors, nonspecific esterase, and an antigen called F4/80. Within 1 to 3 days of culture, MHC II rose to very high levels, and the other traits decreased or disappeared (Fig. 8). The cells became larger and more dendritic in shape and were always nonadherent. Even if one added macrophage colony-stimulating factor (M-CSF), development into macrophages did not occur (130). MLR stimulatory activity increased 10 to 30-fold in culture, so that LCs were even more potent than splenic DCs in activating T cells. Thus, freshly isolated LCs were immature but committed to mature into DCs. Maturation, to be discussed below, also takes place with human LCs (131,132) and in vivo.

Relationship Between Langerhans' Cells, Veiled Cells, and Interdigitating Cells

A link between LCs and veiled cells became apparent in morphologic studies of contact allergy. After the application of contact allergens, the afferent lymphatics in skin contained many LCs (133,134). The LCs were identified by electron microscopy, using

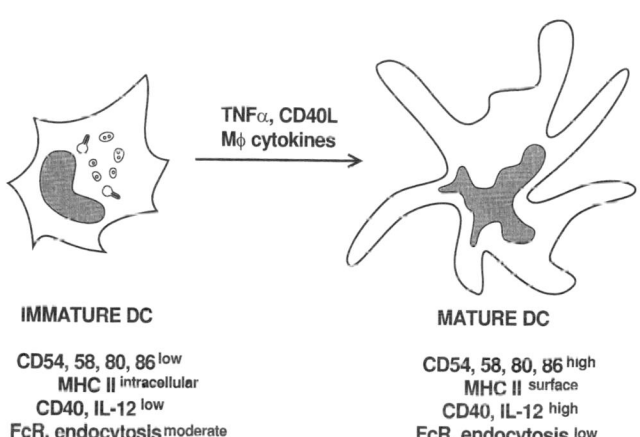

IMMATURE DC

CD54, 58, 80, 86 low
MHC II intracellular
CD40, IL-12 low
FcR, endocytosis moderate

MATURE DC

CD54, 58, 80, 86 high
MHC II surface
CD40, IL-12 high
FcR, endocytosis low

FIG. 8. Some of the changes in epidermal LCs during culture. Not shown here is the fact that T-cell stimulatory function increases by at least 10- to 30-fold.

---

*Afferent lymphatics are important at all times for retrieving lymph, the fluid that is always escaping blood capillaries as a protein-rich transudate. Tissues would swell with lymph if afferent lymphatics did not retrieve this transudate and return it to the blood stream via lymph nodes, efferent lymphatics, and the thoracic duct. In fact, when lymphatics are severed or obstructed, as can occur after surgery for tumors, the corresponding part of the body swells or develops lymphedema.

the Birbeck granule as a marker. These granules have the appearance of a tennis racket in which the racket is a membrane-bound vacuole and the handle is formed by the tight approximation of the membranes to enclose a rigid striated structure (Fig. 9) (135). Although more needs to be learned about the function of Birbeck granules, they express an antigen recognized by the Lag-1 monoclonal antibody (136), acquire endocytic tracers (137), and are acidic (138).

The destination of LCs, after entry into the lymph, was then ascribed to the morphologically similar IDC compartment in the T-cell areas (139–141). However, only in rare instances do IDCs contain Birbeck granules, although this does occur when lymph nodes enlarge in allergic states, i.e., allergic lymphadenitis (142,143). Likewise, the CD1a antigen that is found on immature LCs within the epidermis is only infrequently found on IDCs. Most likely, the LCs mature as they migrate to the T-cell areas, and the phenotype changes much as it does *in vitro*. Nevertheless, IDCs probably have other origins than LCs because IDCs are found in the T-cell areas of all peripheral and mucosal lymphoid tissues, not just those that drain the skin.

A related demonstration of the link between DCs in the skin and lymphoid organs involved the use of contact allergens that were also fluorescent, e.g., fluorescein isothiocyanate (FITC). Within 8 to 24 hours of applying FITC to the skin, FITC-labeled DCs were found in suspensions of draining lymph node cells (144–147). FITC-modified DCs adoptively transferred contact sensitivity to naive recipients (148).

The importance of the afferent lymphatics during cell-mediated immunity had been appreciated long ago, when it was noted that priming to skin transplants (149) and contact allergens (150) was blocked by lymphatic ablation. A traffic of immunogenic DCs from skin via the afferent lymphatics now seems the most likely explanation for these findings.

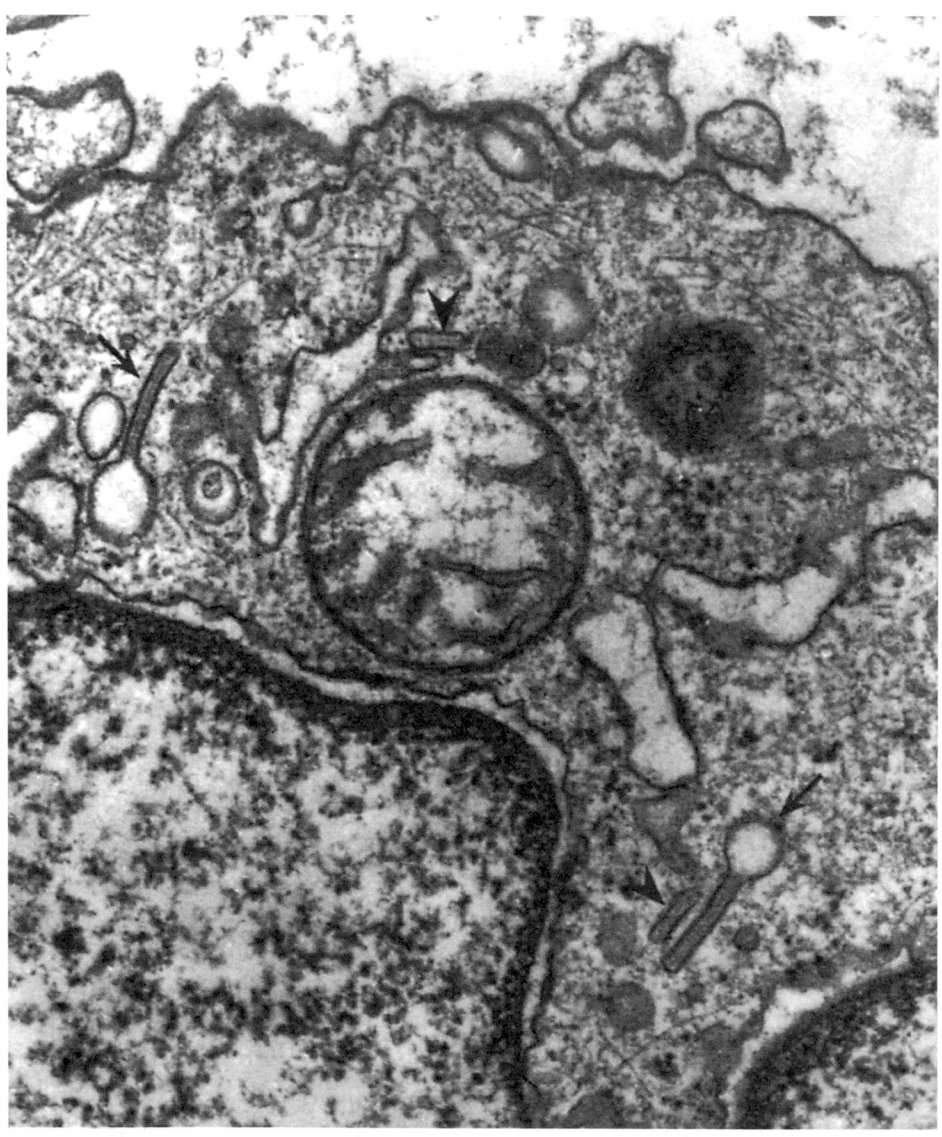

FIG. 9. Electron micrograph (courtesy of Drs. G. Schuler and N. Romani) from an LC, which is similar to DCs in other sites except for the content of Birbeck granules. Two each of the complete (*arrow*) and partial (*arrowhead*) tennis racket–shaped granule are evident here. Birbeck granules are more abundant in fresh rather than cultured epidermal suspensions.

DCs at Other Body Surfaces

Cells that are similar to epidermal LCs are found in all stratified squamous epithelia such as the vagina, cervix, anus, pharynx, and esophagus. In other epithelia, as in the airways of the lung (151–156), the intestine (157), and the iris and ciliary body (158,159), DCs may lie within the epithelium but maintain ready contact with the subepithelial space. To visualize this, it is important to section tangentially through the epithelium and then stain for a marker like MHC class II. The identification of DCs within intestinal epithelium is a recent observation (157) because prior studies have emphasized their presence in the underlying lamina propria (160–162).

Mucosal lymphoid tissues are lymphoid organs that are found at most body surfaces other than skin, especially the gut. In the small intestine, they are called Peyer's patches, and in the nasopharynx, they comprise the adenoids and palatine tonsils of Waldeyer's ring. There are numerous DCs just beneath the epithelium of these mucosal lymphoid organs (163–165). Because this epithelium also contains specialized transporting M cells (72–74), antigens and infectious agents can move from the gut lumen or the pharynx directly into a network of DCs. These DCs may be more mature than at other body surfaces, given the potential influx of DC activators such as lipopolysaccharide (LPS) from gut microorganisms.

There is relatively little information on the life span or turnover rates of DCs in these different compartments. The life span of LCs in the epidermis is very long [half-life of at least 1 month (122)], but very short in the airway [half-life of 2 to 3 days (166)].

Interstitial DCs

Most organs except the brain have MHC II–rich DCs within the interstitial spaces that are drained by afferent lymphatics (167–169). One example is the heart, where both DCs and macrophages can be identified in the spaces between muscle fibers (167,170). The DCs have more abundant MHC II products but less lysosomal hydrolases than macrophages and are more sensitive to ablative treatments such as cyclophosphamide and ionizing irradiation. During the rejection of cardiac allografts, T cells can be observed to be in contact with DCs (171). DCs have been isolated from the heart and kidney, although the procedure is demanding. When this is done, a short period of culture is required for maturation into strongly stimulatory DCs (172). Another more accessible depot of interstitial DCs is the dermis (173,174).

Migration of DCs Into and Out of Nonlymphoid Organs

The migratory potential of cutaneous DCs, especially during contact allergy, has been summarized above. Many other nonlymphoid populations of DCs are known to migrate to the T-cell areas. When hearts are transplanted, graft-derived DCs migrate via the blood to the recipient's spleen (175). Intestinal DCs enter the mesenteric lymph (25,176). Liver DCs are located in the portal triads (106) and along the sinusoids (177,178), where they express the OX62 DC marker (179) that is not found on liver macrophages (Kupffer cells). Liver DCs migrate into hepatic lymph and then to the celiac lymph nodes (115). To delineate this migratory capacity, DCs from mesenteric (176) and hepatic (178) lymph, as well as spleen (180,181), have been reinfused into animals. Within a day, the DCs home to the T-cell areas of the draining lymph node. Homing allows the DCs to sample and select antigen-reactive T cells from the recirculating stream, a recirculation that is essential for primary responses (182).

The entry of DCs into nonlymphoid tissues from the blood is also being outlined. DCs can move from blood into liver, using the macrophages or Kupffer cells as guideposts (178). When a number of different inflammatory stimuli are aerosolized into rat lungs, there is a striking and short-lived mobilization of DCs that is as rapid as the neutrophil response (154). These DCs do not enter the airway, in contrast to alveolar macrophages, but presumably patrol the airway epithelium for antigens before moving to the mediastinal lymph nodes.

A DC System of Antigen-Presenting Cells

Mature DCs from different tissues, as described in this section, have been given different names (Fig. 10), but they share several properties. These features include (a) unusual shape and motility, (b) a lack of macrophage and lymphocyte markers (including Fc receptors and plastic adherence), (c) high expression of surface MHC II and costimulatory molecules, and (d) potent T-cell stimulatory activity. In many cases, the typical features of DCs develop only after a short maturation period in culture.

Mature DCs are an end stage of differentiation and do not convert into either macrophages or lymphocytes. Given their distinctive and shared properties, and the many instances in which DCs in

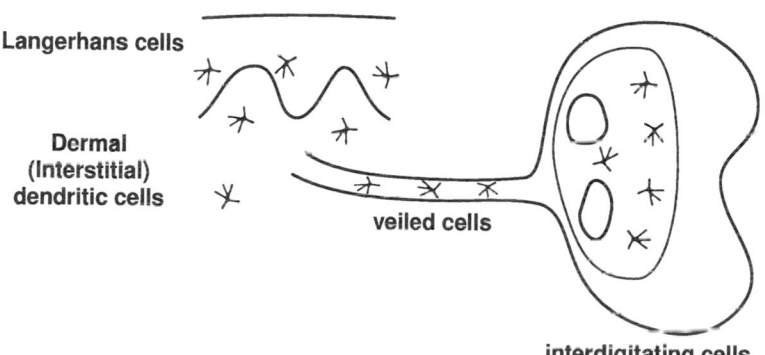

FIG. 10. A system of stellate, antigen presenting DCs where the cells from different compartments are given different names but share fundamental features in terms of morphology, phenotype, origin, and function.

one compartment migrate to another, the DCs in Fig. 10 can be considered as a distinct lineage and system (140,141,183,184).

ANTIGEN CAPTURE BY DENDRITIC CELLS *IN VIVO*

Visualizing the DC–T Cell Interaction *In Vivo*

Immunologists have identified methods to visualize the T cells that are responding *in situ* during the early steps of immunity. If cytokine messenger RNA (mRNA) production is followed by *in situ* hybridization, both IL-2 and IFN-γ mRNA producing cells are identified at the junctions of B- and T-cell areas (185). During a response to superantigen, T cells bearing the appropriate TCR variable (V) elements accumulate next to DCs in the T-cell areas (186). In the early stages of an immune response to allogeneic DCs, the proliferating T cells are also in direct contact with the injected DCs (178). When TCR-transgenic T cells are transferred into naive recipients, and the latter are challenged with the corresponding antigen in adjuvant, the antigen-specific T cells accumulate in the T-cell areas, after which some move into the B-cell follicles (187). More recently, antigen-pulsed DCs and TCR-transgenic T cells have been labeled with different fluorochromes and injected into naive mice without any adjuvant. The results of these experiments have shown that DCs cluster large numbers of antigen-specific T cells in the T-cell areas (188).

Evidence for Efficient Antigen Processing by DCs *In Vivo*

Another approach to demonstrating antigen processing *in vivo* is to administer an antigen to an animal (mice, rats, and sheep have been used) and then isolate different subsets of APCs. DCs are the major cell type transporting the antigen in an immunogenic form for T cells (61,111,189–193), as tested by using the DCs to stimulate T cells that have been immunized to that antigen. Such functional readouts, in which T cells respond to antigens on APCs, reflect both the presence of an MHC-peptide complex as well as costimulatory molecules. In a recent study, IDCs were successfully isolated from lymph nodes and shown to express high levels of signal 1 and 2 (194). Signal 1 was quantified with the Y-Ae antibody, which recognizes a complex of a self peptide presented on I-A^b (195,196). DCs express the highest levels of the Y-Ae epitope as well as CD40/54/86 costimulators *in vivo*, although B cells are clearly positive for signals 1 and 2 as well (194).

Functions of High Levels of Signal 1, MHC–Peptide Complexes on DCs

It is often assumed that DCs better activate naive T cells by expressing high levels of MHC–peptide complexes. However, high levels of signal 1 are not essential for priming by DCs. This has been found for low levels of superantigens presented on MHC II (56) and anti-CD3 molecules on Fc receptors (197). A few hundred molecules of TCR ligand per DC suffices to activate a T cell. This is probably the case for peptides on MHC I because nonreplicating virions are presented well by DCs to CD8$^+$ T cells (198).

What other functions might be mediated by the high levels of MHC products on DCs if these are not essential for T-cell activation? First, high levels of MHC II would facilitate by mass action the capture of peptides at low protein concentrations, which is evident with DCs (199). Second, high levels of MHC products might allow DCs to retain immunogens over long periods and help generate memory.

MATURATION OF DENDRITIC CELLS: A CONTROL POINT FOR INITIATING IMMUNITY

Given that DCs with high levels of MHC products could be isolated from several different tissues, it was first assumed that these APCs were constitutively able to initiate immunity *in vivo*. Upon further examination, it became evident that DCs were often in an immature state in which the cells were poised to capture and process antigens and then would develop the accessory functions that were needed to stimulate T cells. Maturation can be driven by the antigen itself, by cytokines, and by interaction with T cells.

Changes that Occur During the Maturation of DCs

Accessory cells must perform two sets of functions to stimulate T cells: one is the processing and presentation of antigens on MHC products, and the other involves the expression of a large number of membrane-bound glycoproteins that mediate T-cell binding and activation. These functions develop sequentially during DC maturation (200–205). Immature DCs capture and process intact antigens, and synthesize MHC II at high rates, yet lack optimal accessory function, whereas mature DCs downregulate antigen capture and MHC biosynthesis but are powerful stimulators of quiescent T cells.

During maturation, DCs also change their capacity to produce and to respond to cytokines. For example, mature DCs secrete high levels of IL-12 (206,207), which enhances formation of Th1 type helper and killer cells. Mature DCs also are resistant to the suppressive effects of IL-10 (208). IL-10 can block T-cell proliferation and IFN-γ production, the latter most likely because IL-10 dampens IL-12 production (208–212). IL-10 also can induce apoptosis in developing DCs, a process that is overcome by the addition of tumor necrosis factor (TNF)-α or CD40L (213).

The DCs that reside within nonlymphoid organs are immature, i.e., not fully potent to prime T cells. The levels of surface MHC products are 10-fold or more lower than mature DCs, and certain accessories such as CD40, CD54, and CD86 are expressed at low levels or not at all (103,214–217). With immature human DCs, markers such as CD83 (96) and p55 (97) are lacking, and with mouse DCs the granule antigens recognized by MIDC-8 (101), M342 (102), and 2A1 (103) are missing. T-cell stimulatory activity, and most of the properties shown in Figs. 6 and 8, develop only after a short period in culture or after application of an appropriate stimulus *in vivo*. Given the capacity of DCs to prime T cells, the maturation of DCs from immature precursors provides an important control point in the initiation of immunity.

There are several instances in which DCs mature in culture. The first to be recognized was the cultured epidermal LC (128). Granulocyte-macrophage (GM)-CSF is an important cytokine for promoting viability and maturation of LCs (130,218). Other tissues that are known to contain similarly immature DCs include rat lung (219), mouse spleen (220), and human blood (27,221,222). The immature DCs seem committed to mature into DCs in culture rather than other cell types, and for example do not give rise to macrophages when stimulated with M-CSF (130,220).

Control of DC Maturation *In Vivo*

Two of the best known stimuli for DC maturation are CD40 ligand and TNF-α (223–227). TNF-α has an important effect on the terminal maturation of DCs from marrow and monocyte progenitors (199,204,228). Immature DCs also may undergo terminal maturation during their interaction with T cells (229,230), most likely via the CD40L expressed on activated T cells (216,223). Thus, the simplest current view of the control of DC maturation is that it requires signaling through TNF-type receptors, or their associated signal-transducing pathways.

Signaling via TNF receptors and CD40 activates the NF-κB/rel family of transcription factors. NF-κB controls the activity of many immune and inflammatory genes (231). NF-κB/rel proteins are particularly abundant in DCs (rel A or p65, rel B, rel C, p50, p52), with rel B and p50 showing the most activity in electromobility shift assays with consensus oligonucleotide sequences (232). Evidence that NF-κB/rel is active in DCs *in situ* derives from genetically altered mice. RelB knock-out mice have a deficit of thymic DCs (233,234). Transgenic mice also have been constructed in which the human immunodeficiency virus (HIV)-1 promoter drives the herpes thymidine kinase gene. The HIV-1 promoter contains important NF-κB sites that should be activated in DCs, whereas the thymidine kinase makes cells sensitive to the toxic thymidine analog ganciclovir, so DCs are selectively killed when these transgenic mice are given the drug (235). Furthermore, the chicken v-rel oncogene skews marrow development toward DCs (236).

Another pathway that is activated via the TNF receptor involves the metabolism of sphingolipids to produce ceramide. Ceramide can mediate DC maturation, particularly the downregulation of antigen uptake mechanisms (237).

Mature DCs are terminally differentiated and typically short lived. For example, mature DCs are abundant as veiled cells in afferent lymph, but do not emerge into efferent lymph. Presumably the DCs that enter lymph nodes die, unless they encounter cognate T cells. The life span of DCs can be prolonged by fibroblasts that are transfected with CD40L (216). Mature DCs express high levels of CD40, whereas activated T cells express CD40L. Therefore, a successful T-DC interaction in lymph nodes should lead to prolonged survival of DCs via CD40.

Coupling of Maturation and Migration *In Vivo*

DC maturation has been documented *in vivo*, where in addition it is evident that the DCs begin to migrate to identify the appropriate specific T cell. When skin is transplanted, even to a syngeneic recipient, the epidermal LCs within hours begin to increase expression of MHC II (238) and CD86 (239). Simultaneously the maturing LCs begin to enter the lymph, forming cords of DCs in the dermal lymphatics (238,239). Similar events occur in explant cultures of skin (238,240–242). The DCs migrate from the lymphatics into the culture medium, where they express high levels of MHC II and CD86, as well as the DC-restricted markers p55 and CD83. When contact allergens are applied, skin DCs also begin to enlarge, upregulate MHC II, and emigrate (243). It appears that migration and maturation do not take place if the applied chemicals are nonsensitizing, i.e., do not lead to T-cell immunity or contact allergy (244). Therefore, two of the most powerful stimuli of cell-mediated immunity, skin transplants and contact allergens, are associated with the maturation and migration of antigen-bearing DCs.

The controls for migration *in vivo* are not worked out. An intravenous injection of LPS induces the maturation and migration of skin LCs in mice (245) and intestinal DCs in rats (246). DCs at the periphery of the T-cell areas in mouse spleen are immature (220), and an injection of LPS causes their maturation and movement into the T-cell areas (247). For many cell types, LPS is a powerful stimulus for the production of chemokines and cytokines, like TNF-α, an important factor for DC maturation *in vivo* (246). The cytokine requirements for maturation are likely to be complex, e.g., multiple cytokines are needed during the terminal maturation of blood monocytes into DCs (248–250). This mixture of cytokines is currently obtained by stimulating monocytes with immune complexes and collecting the conditioned medium.

In addition to cytokines, other polypeptides must be considered in analyzing the control of DC maturation and migration *in vivo*. Two groups of candidate polypeptides interact with 7-transmembrane–spanning, G protein–coupled receptors. One group are the chemokines. DCs have receptors for chemokines that are now being studied in the context of chemotaxis (251) and infection with HIV-1 (252). A chemokine receptor (CCR6) for MIP-3α, has been described to be expressed primarily on DCs (253). DCs also may produce chemokines, with some products being DC restricted or "dendrokines" that can attract naive T cells (254). A second group of polypeptides that interact with 7-transmembrane–spanning, G protein–coupled receptors are usually associated with endocrine and metabolic functions. Polypeptides such as calcitonin gene–related peptide may influence DC function and are present in nerve terminals that make contact with epidermal LCs (255).

Maturation from Proliferating CD34⁺ Progenitors

The paucity of the primary populations of immature DCs *in vivo* has limited their study. Recently more abundant populations of developing DCs have become available. These include both proliferating and nonproliferating precursors.

Extensive proliferation of DC progenitors has been described in mouse blood (256) and marrow (103,257), and from human CD34⁺ cells in blood (224,258–260) and marrow (226). GM-CSF and TNF-α are the cytokines that are currently emphasized for the development of DCs. Under some culture conditions, these cytokines may not drive the full maturation of DCs, in that the final steps might be mediated by the T cell itself after antigen presentation (229), e.g., through the CD40–CD40L interaction (216,223). Other factors such as c-kit ligand and flt3 ligand can sustain more primitive progenitors of DCs *in vitro* and thereby increase the yield of DCs severalfold from cultured progenitors (261,262).

M-CSF supports monocyte/macrophage development but has no apparent effect on maturing DCs (103,130,227). Mature DCs lack surface receptors for M-CSF (249,263). Osteopetrotic mice, which are genetically deficient in M-CSF, lack monocytes and select pools of macrophages, yet contain many populations of DCs (264,265).

In suspension cultures of developing DCs, the proliferating cells form aggregates that have a distinctive appearance (Fig. 11) relative to the macrophage and granulocyte aggregates that are also present. Granulocytes grow as round cells in aggregates that do not attach to the culture vessel. Macrophages grow as more flattened cells in dispersed but firmly adherent colonies. DCs grow in aggregates that attach to the underlying stroma and are covered with veiled or dendritic protrusions

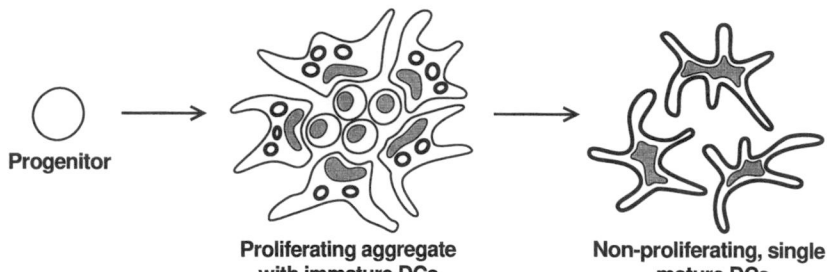

FIG. 11. Development and maturation of DCs from proliferating progenitors. Proliferation (high ³H-thymidine labeling index) occurs in distinctive aggregates in which the DCs have an immature phenotype. One manifestation are the large numbers of intracellular, MHC II⁺ vacuoles or MIICs. Nonproliferating mature DCs, with high levels of surface MHC II, are released from the aggregates.

The cells in proliferating DC aggregates are immature, having low levels of surface MHC II and CD86, but both molecules are abundant on the surface of nonproliferating DCs that emerge from the aggregate. In addition, the phenotype of DCs changes in other ways during maturation (266). Bundles of microtubules become prominent, whereas actin cables or stress fibers disappear (267). In mice, the antigens recognized by monoclonals MIDC-8, M342, and 2A1 are expressed. The endocytic apparatus and turnover of MHC II molecules change dramatically (268) (Fig. 11).

As will be discussed in the section on tolerance, there now appears to be more than one pathway of DC development from proliferating progenitors. These are being termed myeloid and lymphoid. Myeloid DC development uses GM-CSF *in vitro,* and the progeny express markers that are shared with phagocytes such as CD11b and CD33. Lymphoid DC development can use IL-3 but not GM-CSF (269), and the progeny can lack CD11b and CD33. The cytokine flt-3L dramatically expands both lymphoid and myeloid DCs *in vivo* (270).

DC Lines

The different systems for generating DCs from proliferating progenitors allow DCs to grow for weeks in the case of mouse marrow and, as recently described, more than 1 year for mouse spleen (267). Such systems might be used to transform DCs at different stages of development and provide corresponding cell lines, as is now being reported (271–274).

Maturation from Nonproliferating, Monocyte Progenitors

Immature, nonproliferating DCs are not abundant in most tissues, but more numerous blood monocytes can now be used to study many aspects of DC maturation. Current methods require the addition of a complex set of cytokines and prolonged culture to induce monocytes to become DCs (Fig. 12). The monocytes first are cultured for a week in a mixture of GM-CSF and either IL-4 or IL-13 (199,275). At this point the cells are more immunostimulatory than monocytes but still do not have the high levels of surface MHC II and CD86 that characterize mature DCs. The GM-CSF/IL-4 cells have abundant CD68, as is typical of macrophages, and lack several markers of mature DCs in blood and skin [CD83 (96), p55 (97), and CD25 (248)]. The cells revert back to macrophages upon cytokine removal (248,249).

To bring about stable and full DC differentiation, the GM-CSF– and IL-4–treated immature DCs are exposed to a mixture of cytokines from stimulated monocytes (Fig. 12). It is known that monocytes release large amounts of cytokines (e.g., IL-1, IL-6, TNF-α, IFN-α, IL-12) when stimulated via Fc receptors. No one cytokine is responsible for DC maturation, and it is possible that a combination is required to induce the many different features of DCs (250).

The terms "monocyte" and "macrophage" are often used interchangeably, but this is probably no longer appropriate. Monocytes can give rise to either macrophages or DCs under distinct cytokine-driven conditions *in vitro.* An analogous bipotential intermediate develops from CD34⁺ cells in bone marrow (227) and cord blood (225).

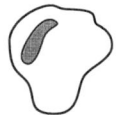 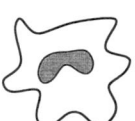 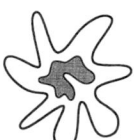

PRECURSOR

HLA-DR ˡᵒʷ
CD86 ˡᵒʷ
p55, CD83 ˡᵒʷ
CD1a ˡᵒʷ
CD68 ʰⁱᵍʰ
CD25 ˡᵒʷ

IMMATURE DC

HLA-DR ᵐᵒᵈᵉʳᵃᵗᵉ
CD86 ᵐᵒᵈᵉʳᵃᵗᵉ
p55, CD83 ˡᵒʷ
CD1a ʰⁱᵍʰ
CD68 ʰⁱᵍʰ
CD25 ˡᵒʷ

MATURE DC

HLA-DR ʰⁱᵍʰ
CD86 ʰⁱᵍʰ
p55, CD83 ʰⁱᵍʰ
CD1a ˡᵒʷ
CD68 ˢᵖᵒᵗ
CD25 ʰⁱᵍʰ

FIG. 12. Cytokine-driven differentiation of human monocytes into mature DCs.

The *in vivo* counterparts of the maturation of monocytes to DCs *in vitro,* and for the production of the requisite monocyte conditioned medium and IL-4 (or IL-13), are not clear. Possibly this is the pathway used for the production of DCs that are continually entering the spleen and afferent lymph.

MECHANISM OF DENDRITIC CELL FUNCTION: ANTIGEN UPTAKE, PROCESSING, AND PRESENTATION

It was for many years puzzling that DCs were such potent stimulators of T-cell responses and yet they displayed so little of the endocytic activity that is required for presentation on MHC II (276). This is because antigen uptake and T-cell stimulation are separable in time in DC biology. Immature DCs are quite specialized for antigen uptake and processing, as are mature DCs for retention of MHC–peptide complexes.

Particle Uptake

A distinguishing feature of mature DCs is their inability to endocytose particulates. This is not the case for immature DCs. Particles such as yeasts are taken up by freshly isolated LCs (277), whereas BCG organisms are phagocytosed by DCs proliferating in marrow aggregates (278). Marrow-derived DCs can present bacterial peptides on both MHC I and II products (279).

The best example of particle uptake *in vivo* by DCs involves the precursors to veiled cells in hepatic lymph. Veiled cells do not internalize particles if challenged *in vitro* (24,25,115). However, if latex is given intravenously, DCs that line liver sinusoids internalize some of the beads before entering the lymph (210). The DCs then migrate with their particles to the T-cell areas of celiac nodes (178). Therefore, immature DCs likely capture particulates, including infectious agents, and then move into the lymph or blood. The extent of phagocytosis is not large, but massive uptake is not needed to present sufficient peptides for T-cell recognition. Extensive phagocytosis for purposes of scavenging and antimicrobial function is primarily a feature of phagocytes.

Another *in vivo* example is *Leishmania* organisms within dermal DCs as well as DCs in the T-cell areas of the draining lymph node (280). A migration of parasite-bearing DCs from dermis to lymph node should lead to T-cell immunity to *Leishmania* antigens. However, the life cycle of *Leishmania* and other organisms in DCs is not worked out. Can DCs support microbial growth, and do DCs have antimicrobial mechanisms? Some DCs lack the inducible nitric oxide synthase that is important in killing many organisms (281).

Multilectin Receptors

It has always been thought that antigen-nonspecific cells such as DCs had to internalize soluble or particulate antigens by nonspecific or bulk mechanisms. More efficient mechanisms of uptake are now recognized. For example, DCs express two different multilectin receptors for endocytic uptake. The receptors are termed the macrophage mannose receptor (MMR) (204) and DEC-205 (282,283), and have eight and 10 contiguous C-type lectin domains, respectively. Normally C-type lectin domains recognize glycans. The MMR clearly binds mannosylated BSA (284), but ligands have not been defined yet for DEC-205.

Both MMR (284) and DEC-205 (283) mediate adsorptive endocytosis via coated pits. Bound ligands (for DEC-205, antibodies to the receptor are used as artificial ligands) can be presented 100 times more efficiently to T cells than nonbound ligands (204,283). In other words, multilectin receptors on DCs may function to enhance antigen presentation in an analogous fashion to the role of surface Ig in presentation by B cells (285). FITC–dextran is a commonly used tracer for fluid phase or bulk pinocytosis, but DCs internalize FITC–dextran via the MMR (204).

Fc Receptors

Immature DCs, like freshly isolated epidermal LCs and GM-CSF– and IL-4–treated blood monocytes, express low levels of FcγR that can function in the presentation of immune complexes (199). The receptors are downregulated during DC maturation. FcεR1 also have been found on DCs from skin (286,287) and blood (288), and these can enhance presentation in the presence of IgE antibodies (288).

Macropinocytosis

Large, 0.25- to 1.0-μm pinocytic vesicles develop transiently in cells that are stimulated with growth factors, e.g., macrophages treated with M-CSF and fibroblasts with epidermal growth factor. In DCs that are stimulated with GM-CSF and IL-4, macropinocytic activity takes place at high levels but continuously (204). This allows DCs to sample large volumes of extracellular fluid and to present very low levels of protein solutes efficiently (204,276).

MHC II Compartments (MIICs and CIIVs)

MHC II molecules have been localized to intracellular vacuoles in APCs (289). DCs in skin, spleen, and blood (222,290,291) are particularly rich in these MIICs. In the electron microscope, MIICs have either a multivesicular or multilaminar appearance, and by immunolabeling contain HLA-DM, cathepsin, and lysosome-associated membrane proteins (CD107a,b) (289,292). MIICs are endosomal compartments in which peptides that are derived from exogenous antigens likely gain access to newly synthesized MHC II and lysosomal products that are emerging from the rough endoplasm reticulum (RER) and Golgi. The MHC II–peptide complexes then traffic to the cell surface for presentation to T cells.

MIICs are found in immature DCs, e.g., in proliferating marrow-derived aggregates, in fresh spleen suspensions, and in epidermis *in situ* (268). MIICs seem more abundant in immature DCs than in any other cell type. As DCs mature, MHC II molecules traffic to the cell surface, and this occurs in CIIVs (268), which are nonlysosomal MHC II–rich vacuoles (293,294). Within 12 hours, immature DCs with many intracellular MIICs convert to mature DCs with very high levels of MHC II on the surface and few lysosomes in the perinuclear region. The same set of events, i.e., lysosomal MIICs giving rise to nonlysosomal CIIVs and then high levels of surface MHC II, also takes place when DCs mature *in situ* within the epidermis (268). In parallel, the degradation rate or turnover of MHC II changes from rapid in immature DCs to very slow on mature cells (268).

MHC II–peptide complexes are stable on mature DCs. Direct measurements for an MHC II–tetanus toxoid peptide showed a half-life of more than 100 hours (295). Also, it is possible to pulse immature DCs with a protein and wait several days before adding the DCs to antigen-specific T cells (201,268). Yet antigen-presenting activity does not decay, and can even increase, whereas decay of T cell–stimulating activity is rapid when other APCs are cultured after being pulsed with antigen (296).

GM-CSF– and IL-4–treated, immature, human blood DCs contain large numbers of MIICs (204). These cytokine-treated cells seem frozen in a state capable of high antigen capture and abundant MIICs. After additional stimuli, such as LPS, TNF-α, or CD40L, the cells mature, losing the MIICs but now expressing high levels of surface MHC II products (204).

From the perspective of lineage differentiation during hematopoiesis, it is of interest that in GM-CSF–stimulated mouse bone marrow cultures, two distinct lineages of mononuclear cells grow alongside each other. There are colonies of firmly adherent macrophages with very little MHC II but abundant lysosomes, and aggregates of loosely adherent DCs with unusually high levels of MHC II in MIICs. In other words, in the same cultures one is generating cells with endocytic systems that are specialized for long-term scavenging, extensive degradation, and antimicrobial function (MHC II–poor terminal lysosomes in macrophages) or for long-lived presentation of peptides (endosomal recycling compartments, MIICs, and CIIVs in DCs).

Presentation of Viruses on MHC Class I

DCs are potent stimulators of CD8+ T-cell responses to hapten-modified cells (31), allo-MHC (34,35,297), viruses (298–301), and tumors (65–69). For human CD8+ T cells, the studies on the presentation of influenza virus are probably the most detailed (198,302,303) (Table 3). Most individuals have been exposed to influenza and have primed CD8+ T cells. When autologous T cells are challenged with influenza-pulsed DCs, strong proliferative and cytotoxic T lymphocyte (CTL) responses develop within a week. This is a noteworthy result because in the absence of enriched DCs, it is necessary to repeatedly stimulate the T cells or to add IL-2 to expand memory CD8+ T cells and develop good CTL responses.

The standard route for viral antigen presentation is for peptides to be cleaved by proteasomes from newly synthesized proteins, followed by the transporter associated with antigen processing (TAP)-mediated translocation into the endoplasmic reticulum. Influenza infection of DCs is accompanied by new viral protein synthesis because the infected cells can be stained with mAbs to viral gene products, such as nucleoprotein, hemagglutinin, and the nonstructural protein NS1 (302). Influenza also infects monocytes, but the latter quickly undergo apoptosis, within 5 hours of infection (304).

TABLE 3. *Features of human CTL responses to influenza-pulsed dendritic cells*

Strong CD4+ and CD8+ CTL responses develop.
CD8+ CTL responses need not require the presence of CD4+ helper cells.
CD8+ T cells proliferate actively.
Cytokines and chemokines are made by the responding CD8+ T cells.
Nonreplicating influenza is efficiently presentd by DCs.
Exogenous IL-12 amplifies the CTL and cytokine responses, when the latter are weak.

Strikingly, DCs can present nonreplicating influenza as well as replicating virus to autologous CD8+ T cells (198). The virus is inactivated by heating at 56°C for 30 minutes or by ultraviolet light. These treatments do not inactivate the hemagglutinating or hemolytic activity of the virus. As a result, the early stages of virus uptake are probably intact. The hemagglutinin of the viral envelope should mediate binding to surface sialic acid residues, internalization in coated vesicles, delivery to acidic endosomes, and fusion with the endosomal membrane to deliver the ribonucleoprotein into the cytoplasm. When the fusogenic activity of the hemagglutinin is inactivated by treatment at pH 5, antigen presentation is markedly inhibited.

Therefore, DCs may be such efficient APCs that delivery of virion proteins, or synthesis of relatively small amounts of viral protein in a nonproductive infection, sufficiently charges MHC I with peptides. *In vivo,* one might not detect active viral infection of DCs, yet the cells may still be presenting noninfectious virus to CD8+ T cells. This finding also has implications for the future immunotherapeutic use of DCs, modified with genes or proteins, to generate killer cell responses *in vivo*. High-level gene expression in DCs may not be essential for these approaches to succeed.

Exogenous and Cross-Priming Pathways for Presentation on MHC I

There is evidence that cellular and protein antigens can be presented on MHC I even though the antigens have no obvious mechanism for accessing the cytoplasmic processing and transport machinery (proteasomes and TAPs). This kind of presentation has been called the exogenous pathway. It became evident in the phenomenon of cross-priming in which minor histocompatibility antigens (305) and later tumor antigens (306) were found to be presented not on the injected cells but on host APCs. How could these noninfectious, cellular antigens gain access to the cytoplasm to be processed? Also, the protein ovalbumin could be presented on MHC I molecules of APCs (307), especially when delivered as a protein–particle conjugate (308). The term "exogenous pathway" implies that antigens (proteins, proteins bound to particles, and minor histocompatibility and tumor antigens on other cells) do not have to gain access to the cytoplasm. However, more recent studies have indicated a requirement for proteasomes (272) and the classical TAP transporter (309), at least in some instances of cross priming.

Some populations of DCs, such as cells from mouse spleen, are not active in presenting exogenous proteins on MHC I (310,311). More recent studies show an active cross-priming pathway in which DCs process antigens from apoptotic cells (312). This finding is critical because it allows DCs to capture and present antigens from virus-infected, malignant, and transplanted cells that typically lack the accessory functions for stimulating immunity *in vivo*.

MECHANISMS OF DENDRITIC CELL FUNCTION: ACCESSORY OR COSTIMULATORY MOLECULES

It is remarkable how many molecular couples have been defined that mediate interactions between APCs and T cells. Some of the best known are ICAMs interacting with LFA-1, LFA-3 with CD2, and B7s with CD28 and CTLA-4. ICAMs, LFAs, and B7s are expressed by DCs, and at high levels (215,217,313–315). These molecular couples contribute to an optimal DC–T cell interaction. For example, blocking CD2, CD11a, or CD28 individually reduces the MLR between DCs and T cells by 50% to 70%, and blocking at least two reduces the MLR by more than 90% (217,315). As mentioned above, high levels of signal 1 are not required for DCs to prime T cells. This must reflect the high content of accessory molecules on DCs because the number of interactions between MHC–peptide and the TCR that is required to stimulate a T cell is decreased in the presence of costimulators (316).

There are differences between the expression of membrane-bound accessories on DCs relative to other APCs. The levels on DCs can be much higher, especially ICAM-1–CD54 and B7-2–CD86. Regulatory controls also may differ. Immature DCs rapidly upregulate expression of several molecules (CD40, CD54, CD58, CD80, and CD86) within a day of culture. Macrophages and B cells require additional stimuli, such as LPS or anti-Ig, and even then the upregulation is far less prominent than on DCs.

What is the consequence of having so many accessory molecules for T cells? More information is needed on the behavior of cells from animals with genetic deletions in these molecules, as well as the associated signal transduction pathways. For example, APCs that are genetically deficient in either CD80 or CD86 can prime T cells to make IFN-γ and IL-4, but priming is less efficient when cell numbers or antigen doses are decreased (317).

Accessory molecules might be most critical during immunity *in situ*, a situation that differs considerably from standard *in vitro* models. Physiologic immunity involves low levels of MHC–peptide and not artificially high levels of signal 1 in experiments that use anti-CD3 antibodies. The T cell is naive or quiescent *in vivo*, whereas *in vitro*, activated T-T hybridomas and clones are most often used. *In vivo*, the T cells and APCs initially are in different parts of the body and moving, rather than juxtaposed in cultures.

The remarkable feature of T-cell activation is that the antigen-specific signal (i.e., MHC–peptide complexes on APCs) is ostensibly very weak (318–320). How do T cells ever find and respond to APCs when the ligand (MHC–peptide) is (a) scarce, a few hundred molecules or less per cell, (b) membrane-bound rather than soluble, and (c) recognized with low affinity? It is known that mature DCs can bind T cells loosely but in an antigen-independent fashion. This may provide the opportunity for small amounts of MHC-peptide to be recognized (321,322). The molecular mechanisms for the initial loose DC–T cell interaction need to be worked out. A recent proposal is that CD2 on the T cell interacts with LFA-3/CD58 or CD48 on the DC, and this is followed by an interaction between CD43 on the T cell and MHC I on the DC (323).

Current thinking of the steps in the DC–T cell interaction is as follows: molecules like CD2 and CD43 first help T cells bind loosely to DCs, antigen is recognized and the TCR begins to signal, integrins are activated to bind ICAMs and solidify the cell–cell interaction (324), then other costimulators such as B7–CD28 and CD40–CD40L successively come into play. In other words, the many molecular couples function in a cascade to optimize the APC–T cell interaction. The molecular dialogue is two way, activating not only the growth and production of lymphokines and cytolysins by T cells, but also signaling the DC, e.g., through CD40 (216).

DENDRITIC CELLS AND T CELL–MEDIATED IMMUNITY

Instead of considering T cells in generic terms, we now consider DC function in the setting of several different types of T-cell responses. T-cell priming is emphasized, but it should be kept in mind that DCs seem designed to retain high levels of MHC–peptide complexes for long periods on the cell surface (see section on DC maturation). This could be important in the development and maintenance of T-cell memory.

The Helper T-Cell Response and Production of IL-12

IL-12 is one of the critical cytokines that skews the function of helper T cells to Th1 and elicits IFN-γ production from NK cells. IL-12 in concert with antigen-bearing DCs also amplifies the antigen-specific CTL response *in vitro* (303). Both macrophages and DCs can make the active heterodimer of IL-12, but B cells probably do not. The interaction of macrophages with microorganisms or LPS can induce IL-12 (325), but for DCs, T cells seem to be the major stimulus (326,327). IL-12 production by DCs proceeds best via CD40, and the amount of secreted IL-12 is unusually high (206,207).

There are two important features of IL-12 production by DCs. The first is that mature DCs are most active, in part because mature DCs express high levels of the required CD40. The second is that it is not necessary for DCs to be presenting antigen to the T cell. T cells that express CD40L, either during activation or memory, can directly stimulate DCs to make IL-12 in the absence of the cognate antigen for that T cell (207). When memory T cells traffic through tissues and lymph, they may chronically induce IL-12 from DCs that they encounter, given that DC–memory T cell binding is quite easy to demonstrate (240,328).

When naive T cells are responding to antigens on DCs, CD40L will be expressed and signal the DCs via CD40 to make IL-12. This in turn will lead to skewing of the T-cell phenotype to Th1, with high-level IFN-γ production (206,207,326,327,329). Th1 development therefore seems to be the default pathway during DC presentation of antigen. B cells in contrast are not known to make IL-12, so it is unlikely that a B cell can skew the response toward Th1.

However, if IL-4 is present during DC function, then the T cell can be skewed toward the Th2 pathway (54). Possible sources of IL-4 are T cells that are primed with IL-6 from APCs such as B cells or macrophages (330) (DCs are not known to make significant amounts of IL-6), NK1.1+ T cells, and basophils and mast cells.

The CD8+ Cytolytic or Killer Cell Response

Prior sections have summarized the capacity of DCs to induce CD8+ T-cell responses *in vivo* and to present viral antigens on MHC I molecules. The DC is an unusual APC in that it efficiently presents antigens on both MHC I and II products, and clusters both helper and killer T cells within the same microenvironment, thereby optimizing the CTL response (331).

An important unknown is to determine if pathogens and tumors can gain access to the MHC class I molecules of DCs *in vivo*. There may only be a select group of viruses that can synthesize viral proteins in DCs, e.g., influenza (302,332), measles (333,334), tick borne encephalitis (335), and HIV-1/simian immunodeficiency virus (SIV) (328,336,337). However it is possible that many bacteria and enveloped viruses have the capacity to enter DCs, not replicate, but charge MHC class I with sufficient peptides for successful presentation. DCs also may acquire peptides derived from apoptotic cells (e.g., virus-infected cells and tumor cells) via the exogenous pathway (312).

Contact Allergy

The strength of the immune response to contact allergens may be ascribed to the capacity of these chemicals to bind to DCs and induce their maturation and migration into afferent lymph. The T-cell response is complex, however. The main effector cell is a CD8$^+$ Th1 cell (338,339). A CD4$^+$ Th2-type regulatory cell is also induced. This is surprising because LCs can make IL-12 and should therefore skew the response to a Th1 type. When small amounts of contact allergens are used to induce tolerance (340), the tolerance is mediated by Th2-type CD8$^+$ cells. The complexity of the T-cell response to contact allergens may result from the function of keratinocytes, which can produce an array of cytokine products.

T-Dependent Antibody Formation

The standard view of DC function has been that these cells activate CD4$^+$ T helpers, which then interact directly with B cells to provide help. However, recent findings open up a role for direct DC–B cell interaction after the DC has been activated through the CD40–CD40L couple. The signal to CD40 on DCs has been provided in vitro using fibroblasts transfected with CD40L or with anti-CD40 antibodies. The activated DCs then enhance IgM production (341) and can switch naive IgD$^+$ cells to become IgA secretors (342).

T cell–dependent B-cell responses are also coming under direct study in situ. Early in the antibody response, the antibody-secreting cells appear in an extrafollicular position at the T cell–B cell junction (343). This finding parallels in vitro experiments in which DCs first activate T-helper cells, which then drive the primary B-cell response within discrete aggregates of the three cell types (19,20). In these aggregates, DCs may enhance B-cell responses in concert with two T cell–derived signals, CD40L and IL-2 (341,344). Later in the antibody response, germinal centers develop, and there, B cells undergo somatic mutation and affinity maturation. The germinal center reaction can be driven by T cells. It had always been assumed that B cells were the major APCs, but a population of germinal center DCs has been found with much stronger T-cell stimulatory function than germinal center B cells (119).

T Cells at Mucosal Surfaces

Mucosal immunology is important from the perspectives of vaccines, inflammatory diseases, and oral tolerance. DCs need to be considered in these contexts, but with the anatomy in mind. DCs are found in two types of tissue within mucosal surfaces such as lung and intestine, i.e., the majority of the mucosal surface that is involved in transport and exchange with the outside world, and the MALT.

The bulk of the DCs that are isolated from mucosal surfaces, such as lung and intestine, are immature. Does this mean that the DCs are actively suppressed in situ? In the lung (219,345) and

intestine (346), macrophages can suppress DC function, and macrophages are most abundant at these body surfaces (347,348). Several macrophage and epithelial products are candidates, e.g., IL-10, prostaglandins, and nitric oxide. Such suppression is considered valuable because proteins are constantly present in the airway and gut lumen, and the presence of mature DCs could then lead to chronic inflammation and allergy at these important mucosal surfaces.

DCs in MALT are found in the subepithelial or lymphoepithelial regions beneath antigen-transporting M cells (163–165) and the interfollicular zones (T-cell areas)(349,350). There is still little direct study of these DCs in terms of phenotype and function immediately upon isolation or in vivo. However, it is likely that these DCs pick up antigens that are administered into the gut and then migrate into mesenteric lymph (61). The intriguing point is that even though DCs in mesenteric lymph can prime naive mice to the associated intestinal-derived antigens, it is not evident that priming to gut or airway proteins is occurring normally in vivo. The DCs that one isolates from lymph, when injected into a nonmucosal site (61), may escape some important regulatory mechanism that operates at mucosal surfaces.

DENDRITIC CELLS AND T-CELL TOLERANCE

Studies on the role of DCs in immune regulation and the induction of tolerance are intensifying. Mucosal immunology is one such area, as mentioned above. What follows is speculative in many parts but indicates some additional avenues of research.

Central or Thymic Tolerance

The thymic medulla contains many bone marrow–derived DCs (351,352). These were first recognized as IDCs with the electron microscope. Subsequently, DCs were isolated from thymus and shown to be similar to other DCs in morphology, phenotype, and function (189,353–355). Current mAbs that react with DCs and that primarily stain thymic medulla (Fig. 13) are the N418 mAb to mouse CD11c (102,105), as well as two antibodies that see antigens within endocytic vacuoles of DCs (M342 and 2A1) (102,103). MHC and costimulatory molecules are most abundant on medullary DCs (215) (Fig. 13).

Bone marrow–derived cells mediate negative selection or clonal elimination in the thymus, especially to self antigens that are expressed there. DCs are likely to be the active APCs. If foreign or allogeneic splenic DCs are added to fetal thymic organ cultures, the T cells that develop therein are selectively tolerant to the MHC of the added DCs (356). If DCs bearing a superantigen are injected into an adult thymus, they mediate deletion or anergy of the T cells that express the superantigen reactive V elements (357,358). DCs are more effective than cortical epithelium in deleting superantigen reactive T cells in thymic reaggregation cultures (359). DCs are the most effective cells for presenting the self serum protein, complement component C5, in a way that deletes reactive thymocytes in vitro (360). Both medullary and cortical epithelial cells also have the potential to mediate negative selection (361).

A new approach to evaluating the role of DCs in self tolerance is to target the expression of antigens to DCs as transgenes. In the mouse, CD11c is expressed at high levels on DCs. Recently, a CD11c promoter element has been identified that primarily targets the expression of an I-E transgene to DCs (362). Tolerance to I-E

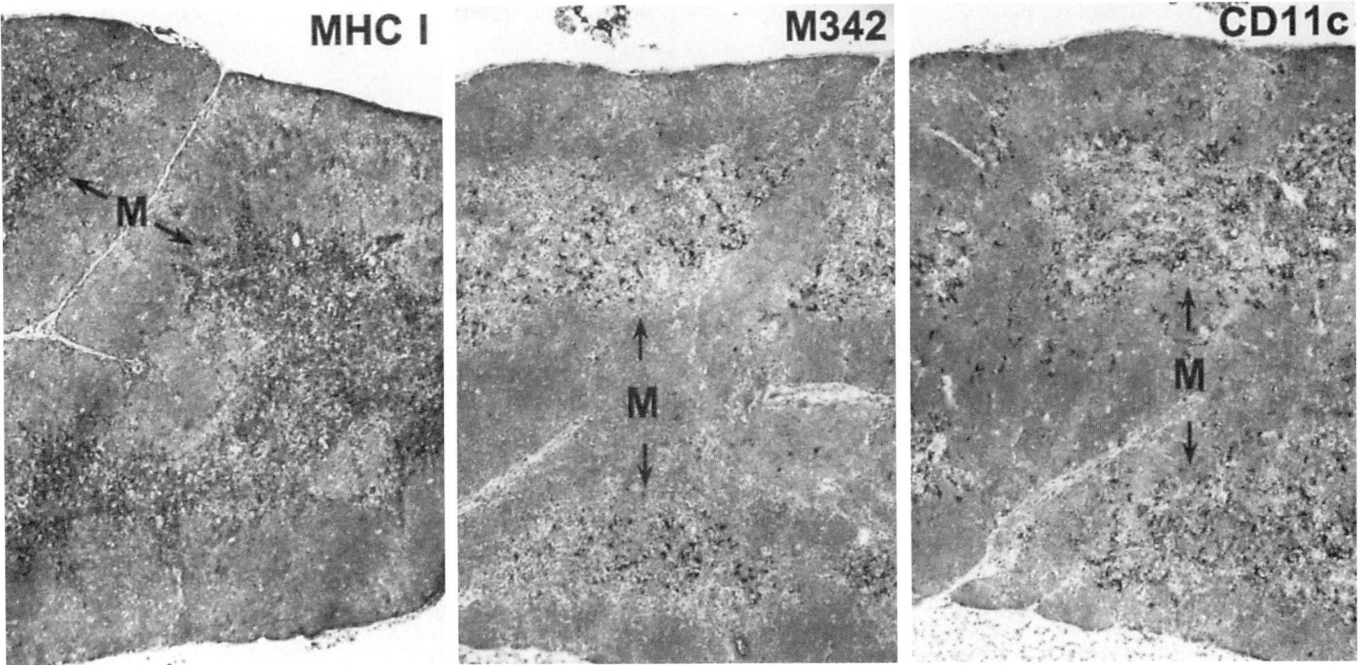

FIG. 13. Mouse thymus stained for CD11c integrin (*right*), the M342 endosomal antigen (*middle*), and MHC class I (*left*). The DC restricted markers CD11c and M342 are primarily expressed in the medulla (M, *arrows*), where MHC products (both class I and II) also are the most abundant.

ensues, indicating that DCs are sufficient to mediate efficient neg-ative selection *in vivo*. The reciprocal is that autoimmunity devel-ops if transgenic mice are constructed in which MHC II products are expressed only by epithelial cells and not by marrow-derived APCs (363).

In vivo, thymic DCs appear specialized to effect negative selec-tion (a) being located in the medulla (Fig. 13), where positively selected thymocytes leave the cortex, (b) having special lectins that may capture self antigens in low amounts, and (c) expressing mol-ecules such as B7-2 (215), CD40 (216) and fas-L (364), which may enhance the efficacy of negative selection.

Peripheral Tolerance

Because many self antigens may not have a means to access the thymus, self tolerance via negative selection in the thymus would not take place. Can tolerance to these self antigens develop in the periph-ery, and via DCs? A clue comes from the observation that DCs are potent APCs for the male or H-Y transplantation antigen (365), yet H-Y–reactive T cells do not cause an inflammatory or rejection response when injected into male mice (366). Likewise, superanti-gens are presented by DCs *in vivo* (186), yet the injection of a super-antigen into mice leads to immunity followed by tolerance.

Peripheral tolerance may occur by different means. An important pathway, especially for CD4+ T cells (367), involves the apoptotic death of lymphocytes that have begun to respond to antigen and express fas (368,369). There is evidence that some DCs express active fas-L, and that these DCs may have an immunoregulatory role (364).

Functional assays indicate that DCs from lymphoid organs can stimulate T cells specific for the self protein, β2-microglobulin

(191). Recently it has been found that the IDCs in the T-cell area express the highest levels of a particular MIIC–self peptide com-plex, detected with an mAb called Y-Ae (194). Self antigens from a peripheral tissue, such as the insulin-secreting cells of the pan-creatic islets of Langerhans, are presented by APCs in lymph nodes that drain the pancreas (370). Therefore, it is likely that DCs are presenting self antigens *in vivo,* and recent studies show that APCs in lymph nodes are tolerogenic for self antigens (371).

Are There Separate Myeloid and Lymphoid Pathways for DC Development, and Do These Function in Immunity and Tolerance Respectively?

There now appear to be several pathways for generating mature DCs. In all cases, the progeny are large cells with the properties summarized in Fig. 6, but each pathway may have important dif-ferences in origin, phenotype, and function. Recently, the possibil-ity has been raised that select subsets of DCs are designed to induce tolerance rather than immunity.

There are two immunizing types of DCs that are currently con-sidered as myeloid, meaning that the cells are responsive to GM-CSF and the progeny express some surface markers in common with phagocytes (macrophages and granulocytes), especially CD11b and CD33. Starting with CD34+ progenitors from human cord blood (225), one pathway yields cells that are identical to epi-dermal LCs. The progeny express Birbeck granules, LAG-1 (136), CD1a antigens, and E-cadherin (372). E-cadherin may be impor-tant for positioning LCs in the epidermis. The other myeloid path-way, which may take place in the production of dermal and other interstitial DCs, proceeds through a CD14+ intermediate, and the progeny express markers such as CD2, CD9, CD36, and factor XIII transglutaminase (225). In this pathway, there is a CD14$^+$ bipotential intermediate that can give rise to macrophages or DCs depending on the cytokines (M-CSF vs. GM-CSF, respectively) (225,227). This CD14$^+$ bipotential intermediate is reminiscent of the nonproliferating monocyte progenitor to DCs in human blood. However, the latter cell requires an exposure to IL-4 to develop into DCs, yet these cytokines are not being added to the cultures of CD34$^+$ cells that are generating myeloid DCs.

Functional differences have been noted for the two myeloid pathways. The LC pathway exhibits much less endocytic activity via the macrophage mannose receptor. The CD14$^+$ pathway has greater and more long lasting endocytic activity, and much greater expression of nonspecific esterases. Of greater interest is that the CD14$^+$ cells exclusively bind immune complexes and amplify primary B-cell responses in concert with IL-2 and CD40L (344). This suggests that CD14$^+$-derived DCs can play a selective role in T-dependent antibody responses *in vivo,* e.g., by driving the extrafollicular primary antibody response and by transporting immune complexes to the germinal center.

These two myeloid pathways may derive from separate populations of CD34$^+$ progenitors in colony assays (262). CD34$^+$ cells also have been divided into two fractions on the basis of a cutaneous lymphocyte antigen (CLA). CLA$^+$ progenitors are the source of epidermal LCs, whereas CLA$^-$ cells yield DCs that lack Birbeck granules and LAG-1 (373). It is also possible that the LC pathway of development is critically dependent on TGF-β (374) given the fact that TGF-β1 knock-out mice have a selective deficit in LCs (375).

Another pathway of DC development is called lymphoid. The term reflects two features: that these DCs may share a precursor with T cells (376,377) and that the cells lack myeloid markers but may express lymphoid ones like CD8 (378). Lymphoid DCs have recently been described to express high levels of surface fas-L and to induce apoptosis of antigen-specific CD4$^+$ T cells (364).

It is now possible to generate DCs from thymic precursors that express low levels of CD4 (269). Development is not influenced by GM-CSF but uses IL-3, IL-1 and TNF-α. A likely CD4$^+$ intermediate has also been identified in human tonsil and blood (379). This cell has a peculiar morphology, resembling plasma cells, and differentiates with IL-3 into lymphoid-type DCs with little or no CD13 and CD33.

What might these pathways mean in functional terms? Perhaps the DC system has two levels, one for immunity and one for tolerance, that represent progeny of myeloid and lymphoid pathways, respectively. Immunity uses DCs that are present in most nonlymphoid organs and the circulation (blood, lymph, and marginal zone of spleen). Stimuli like TNF-α, LPS, and CD40L activate these cells, which acquire foreign antigen and T-cell stimulatory activity (maturation) and migrate to lymphoid organs to select recirculating clones of antigen-specific T cells. Tolerance, both central and peripheral, may use DCs that express high levels of surface fas-L and perhaps other members of the TNF family. As a result, responding T cells are deleted.

DENDRITIC CELLS IN CLINICAL IMMUNOLOGY

Several clinical areas, to be considered below, are known to involve T cells. Yet research in these areas usually emphasizes antigens and T cells, to the exclusion of specific accessory cells that are pivotal in terms of the quality and quantity of immune responses. What follows are some examples where the study of DCs is either ongoing or might prove fruitful.

Transplantation

Initially there was enthusiasm for deleting DCs from grafts, as a way of eliminating the most potent known stimulus of the recipient's T cells. For small endocrine grafts in mice, treatment with anti-DC antibody and complement led to survival across an MHC barrier (58,59). This is problematic for larger grafts because graft peptides can be presented by host DCs via the indirect or cross-priming pathway of allorecognition (57). When host DCs populate the graft, there will be presentation of graft peptides and chronic inflammation (delayed-type hypersensitivity).

If DCs can induce peripheral tolerance, e.g., by expressing fas-L, it could prove valuable to chimerize graft recipients with tolerogenic donor DCs. A graft, particularly one with hematopoietic potential (e.g., a hepatic graft), can be the source for donor-derived microchimerism. This has been proposed to induce long-term graft acceptance (380–382).

Contact Allergy

One approach to these allergies is to try to block DC function in the skin because DC maturation and migration occur after application of contact allergens (243,244,383). Enhanced local IL-10 production may block the maturation of immunostimulatory DCs (208,209). There is a report that IL-10–treated DCs are tolerogenic for contact allergens *in vivo* (384). IL-10 also can have direct tolerizing effects on T cells (385) and can block cutaneous inflammation (386).

Autoimmunity

Several human diseases, e.g., juvenile diabetes mellitus, psoriasis, certain arthritidies, and multiple sclerosis, are likely to have a major autoimmune component. DCs are abundant in the synovial exudates of rheumatoid arthritis (387,388). DCs from the dermis of psoriatic skin stimulate autologous T cells (389). However, direct evidence for joint- or skin-reactive T cells has not been obtained. For example, glutamic acid decarboxylase (GAD) is a critical autoantigen in the nonobese diabetes mouse model of juvenile diabetes (390,391), but there still are no systems in which one can show GAD reactivity in bulk T cells from diabetics. Perhaps the use of more abundant and potent DCs in these assays would allow the detection of autoreactive T cells.

Vaccination

It is important to develop noninfectious and subunit vaccines that elicit strong T cell–mediated immunity. Vaccine design has yet to emphasize targeting and manipulation of specialized cells such as DCs and FDCs. Vaccine targeting to potent DCs should be advantageous, given the capacity of these APCs to secrete large amounts of IL-12 and to act as natural adjuvants for CTLs and T-dependent antibody production. Maturing DCs might be targeted to take up antigens and then be mobilized as strong immunostimulatory cells.

One approach is to capitalize on the fact that GM-CSF has many potentiating effects on DCs, sustaining viability and maturation (130,218), mobilizing DCs to tissues (392), and mediating expansion from progenitors (103,224,256). GM-CSF has been engineered in such a way to enhance immune responses to proteins and tumor cells (393–395).

Genetic immunization with naked or plasmid DNA, so-called DNA vaccines, have the capacity to prime B cells, T-helpers, and CTLs, even though the DNA is primarily expressed in nonprofessional APCs such as muscle cells. However, it has now been shown that bone marrow–derived APCs present the product of the injected DNA (396–398), and there is recent evidence that DCs in particular can carry the injected DNA, capture proteins from muscle cells, and present DNA-encoded peptides to T cells (399,400).

Tumor Immunotherapy

Immunologists are encouraged by the identification of tumor-reactive T cells, e.g., in the setting of melanoma. However, to date the T cells are clones and lines that have been expanded in culture. There is little evidence that comparable T cells are being expanded and activated in the patient, so, for example, expanded CTL precursor frequencies have not been detected to melanoma or other tumor antigens. A critical barrier to immunogenicity may be the lack of access of tumor antigens to effective APCs, although there have been reports of DCs internalizing foreign cells (312,401). Ways possibly could be devised to make tumor antigens more accessible to the MHC molecules of DCs, especially MHC I. Another perspective is the proposal that tumors can secrete cytokines, such as vascular endothelial growth factor, that block the maturation of DCs within a tumor (402).

The observed lack of detectable tumor-specific immune responses in humans provides a strong impetus to use autologous DCs in active immunotherapy. The DCs would be expanded from progenitors ex vivo, charged with tumor antigens, and reinfused (403,404). Many approaches are underway to genetically modify DCs with antigens encoded by viral and nonviral vectors (273,405–407). DCs also might be used to vaccinate humans at the time that a primary tumor is resected. Then an immune response could be available to act on metastases that are not detectable at the time the primary tumor is identified.

Viral Pathogenesis: Measles and HIV-1

Measles infection has long been known to be associated with reduced T-cell responsiveness. Recent papers describe the capacity of measles to infect DCs, to induce syncytia that are analogous to Warthin-Finkeldey giant cells in mucosal epithelium, and to suppress both IL-12 production and T-cell stimulatory function (333,334).

DCs have always been of interest in the setting of HIV-1. DCs express the CD4 receptor for HIV-1 (27,408) as well as essential chemokine coreceptors for viral entry (252). DCs interact closely and for days with CD4+ T cells that are responding to antigens and superantigens (39,47,48,409). These activated CD4+ T cells are the major known site for cytopathic infection with HIV-1 (410,411). Therefore, DCs can provide a major route for capturing HIV-1 and transmitting the virus to T cells for a cytopathic infection (412–414).

However, it has been difficult to identify productively infected cells in the T-cell areas of lymphoid tissues (415,416), where DCs should be interacting with T cells. For this reason, attention is turning to the body surfaces that are sites for HIV-1 access during sexual transmission. Some evidence exists that DCs in the genital mucosa are an early site for HIV-1 (417–420) and SIV (420,421) transmission. The number of maturing DCs relative to T cells is quite large at these surfaces and in draining afferent lymph. Recent studies indicate that DCs and T cells, when isolated from body surfaces, provide a naturally permissive environment for HIV-1 and SIV replication (328,336). In other words, stimuli such as mitogens, fetal calf serum, and IL-2 need not be added for the mucosal leukocytes to support active replication of HIV-1 and SIV.

In mucosal lymphoid tissues, relatively large numbers of DCs and lymphocytes are found where antigens gain access to the lymphoid organ. Because lymphocytes (and DCs) are so numerous within or below these epithelia, the term "lymphoepithelium" is often used. There is evidence that lymphoepithelia, particularly in oral lymphoid organs, are sites where DCs are actively infected with HIV-1 (164,165).

A critical aspect of HIV-1 infection is that DCs could be potent APCs for HIV-1–specific, CD8+ T cells. These might kill infected cells or secrete chemokines that block infection (422–424). A battleground must exist in patients because HIV-1 replicates actively for many years, yet the levels of plasma viremia can remain steady and the patients clinically asymptomatic for long periods (425,426). Noninfectious virus and apoptotic, infected cells are both abundant in patients. The potential of DCs to present these to CD8+ T cells may explain the observed resistance. Therefore, HIV-1 infection may be a battle in which DCs, especially those at mucosal surfaces, control both armies: replication via CD4+ T cells and resistance via CD8+ T cells.

CONCLUSION

Dendritic cells, specialized APCs for T-lymphocytes, initiate CD4+ and CD8+ responses, especially in vivo. Their distinctive features and functions became apparent by preparing enriched populations from lymphoid tissues, blood, and afferent lymph. It was found that DCs were potent accessory cells for primary antibody responses and the primary MLR in vitro. After priming by DCs, the activated T cells interacted with other APCs.

DCs arise from immature cells, typically in nonlymphoid tissues, where they can capture antigens. Immature antigen-capturing DCs, typified by epidermal LCs, have abundant MHC II–rich, intracellular compartments or MIICs. Upon maturation, which can be triggered by TNF-α and by CD40 ligand, the lysosomal MIICs move to the cell surface, and costimulatory molecules are upregulated (CD40, CD54, CD58, CD80, and CC86). Mature T-cell stimulatory DCs express very high levels of stable, surface MHC products. These motile, nonadherent cells have high levels of all members of the NF-κB/rel family of transcriptional control proteins, make large amounts of IL-12, and resist the suppressive effects of IL-10.

DCs comprise a system of APCs designed to capture antigens at sites of antigen entry and then migrate to identify cognate T cells, especially in the T-cell areas of peripheral lymphoid organs. Members of the DC system include LCs of the epidermis and other stratified squamous epithelia; DCs at mucosal surfaces, within the respiratory and gut lining as well as the subepithelial region of mucosal lymphoid tissues; interstitial DCs in heart and kidney, but not brain parenchyma; veiled cells in afferent lymph and blood; and IDCs of the thymic medulla and T-cell areas of lymphoid tissue. While sharing many properties, some of these different DCs may develop from different progenitors and have different functions as noted below.

Large numbers of DCs, derived by stimulating precursors with cytokines, are now available, making cell biologic and molecular studies more feasible. Recent examples include the identification of C-type lectin receptors for antigen presentation, and DC-restricted chemokines and chemokine receptors.

The physiologic capacities of DCs continue to provide many surprises. For B-cell responses, DCs have been identified in germinal centers, and *in vitro*, a subset of DCs can interact directly with CD40-activated B cells to drive isotype switching and IgG/IgA secretion. For MHC I–restricted, CD8[+] CTL responses, DCs can present peptides that are derived from nonreplicating virus, bacteria, and apoptotic cells. For helper cells, DCs can prime either Th1 or Th2 responses, the latter if exogenous IL-4 is present. DCs have a major role in negative selection in the thymus, and a subset is now being implicated in peripheral tolerance as well. DCs are the subject of clinical studies, including new approaches to vaccination against infectious agents and tumors, and to the pathogenesis of viral infections such as measles and HIV-1.

REFERENCES

1. Mishell RI, Dutton RW. Immunization of dissociated spleen cell cultures from normal mice. *J Exp Med* 1967;126:423–442.
2. Rosenthal AS, Shevach EM. Function of macrophages in antigen recognition by guinea pig T lymphocytes. I. Requirements for histocompatible macrophages and lymphocytes. *J Exp Med* 1973;138:1194–1212.
3. Shevach EM, Rosenthal AS. Function of macrophages in antigen recognition by guinea pig T lymphocytes. II. Role of the macrophage in the regulation of genetic control of the immune response. *J Exp Med* 1973;138:1213–1229.
4. Seeger RC, Oppenheim JJ. Synergistic interaction of macrophages and lymphocytes in antigen-induced transformation of lymphocytes. *J Exp Med* 1970;132:44–62.
5. Cline MJ, Swett VC. The interaction of human monocytes and lymphocytes. *J Exp Med* 1968;128:1309–1325.
6. Mosier DE. A requirement for two cell types for antibody formation in vitro. *Science* 1967;158:1573–1575.
7. Shortman K, Diener E, Russell P, Armstrong WD. The role of non-lymphoid accessory cells in the immune response to different antigens. *J Exp Med* 1970;131:461–482.
8. Ly IA, Mishell RI. Separation of mouse spleen cells by passage through columns of sephadex G-10. *J Immunol Methods* 1974;5:239–247.
9. Julius MH, Simpson E, Herzenberg LA. A rapid method for the isolation of functional thymus derived murine lymphocytes. *Eur J Immunol* 1973;3:645–649.
10. Steinman RM, Cohn ZA. The interaction of soluble horseradish peroxidase with mouse peritoneal macrophages in vitro. *J Cell Biol* 1972;55:186–204.
11. Steinman RM, Cohn ZA. The interaction of particulate horseradish peroxidase (HRP)-anti HRP immune complexes with mouse peritoneal macrophages *in vitro*. *J Cell Biol* 1972;55:616–634.
12. Steinman RM, Cohn ZA. Identification of a novel cell type in peripheral lymphoid organs of mice. I. Morphology, quantitation, tissue distribution. *J Exp Med* 1973;137:1142–1162.
13. Steinman RM, Cohn ZA. Identification of a novel cell type in peripheral lymphoid organs of mice. II. Functional properties in vitro. *J Exp Med* 1974;139:380–397.
14. Steinman RM, Kaplan G, Witmer MD, Cohn ZA. Identification of a novel cell type in peripheral lymphoid organs of mice. V. Purification of spleen dendritic cells, new surface markers, and maintenance in vitro. *J Exp Med* 1979;149:1–16.
15. Steinman RM, Lustig DS, Cohn ZA. Identification of a novel cell type in peripheral lymphoid organs of mice. III. Functional properties in vivo. *J Exp Med* 1974;139:1431–1445.
16. Swiggard WJ, Nonacs RM, Witmer-Pack MD, Inaba K, Steinman RM. Enrichment of dendritic cells by plastic adherence and EA rosetting. In: Coligan JE, Kruisbeek AM, Margulies DH, Shevach EM, Strober W, eds. *Current Protocols in Immunology*, 2nd ed. New York: Greene and Wiley-Interscience, 1992: 3.7.1–3.7.11.
17. Inaba K, Nakano K, Muramatsu S. Cellular synergy in the manifestation of accessory cell activity for in vitro antibody response. *J Immunol* 1981;127: 453–461.
18. Inaba K, Steinman RM, Van Voorhis WC, Muramatsu S. Dendritic cells are critical accessory cells for thymus-dependent antibody responses in mouse and man. *Proc Natl Acad Sci U S A* 1983;80:6041–6045.
19. Inaba K, Witmer MD, Steinman RM. Clustering of dendritic cells, helper T lymphocytes, and histocompatible B cells, during primary antibody responses in vitro. *J Exp Med* 1984;160:858–876.
20. Inaba K, Steinman RM. Protein-specific helper T lymphocyte formation initiated by dendritic cells. *Science* 1985;229:475–479.
21. Komatsubara S, Hirayama Y, Inaba K, et al. Role of macrophages as modulators but not as autonomous accessory cells in primary antibody response. *Cell Immunol* 1985;95:288–296.
22. Nussenzweig MC, Steinman RM, Witmer MD, Gutchinov B. A monoclonal antibody specific for mouse dendritic cells. *Proc Natl Acad Sci U S A* 1982;79: 161–165.
23. Klinkert WEF, Labadie JH, Bowers WE. Accessory and stimulating properties of dendritic cells and macrophages isolated from various rat tissues. *J Exp Med* 1982;156:1–19.
24. Kelly RH, Balfour BM, Armstrong JA, Griffiths S. Functional anatomy of lymph nodes. II. Peripheral lymph-borne mononuclear cells. *Anat Rec* 1978;190:5–21.
25. Pugh CW, MacPherson GG, Steer HW. Characterization of nonlymphoid cells derived from rat peripheral lymph. *J Exp Med* 1983;157:1758–1779.
26. Young JW, Steinman RM. Accessory cell requirements for the mixed leukocyte reaction and polyclonal mitogens, as studied with a new technique for enriching blood dendritic cells. *Cell Immunol* 1988;111:167–182.
27. O'Doherty U, Steinman RM, Peng M, et al. Dendritic cells freshly isolated from human blood express CD4 and mature into typical immunostimulatory dendritic cells after culture in monocyte-conditioned medium. *J Exp Med* 1993;178: 1067–1078.
28. Nussenzweig MC, Steinman RM, Unkeless JC, Witmer MD, Gutchinov B, Cohn ZA. Studies of the cell surface of mouse dendritic cells and other leukocytes. *J Exp Med* 1981;154:168–187.
29. Steinman RM, Nogueira N, Witmer MD, Tydings JD, Mellman IS. Lymphokine enhances the expression and synthesis of Ia antigen on cultured mouse peritoneal macrophages. *J Exp Med* 1980;152:1248–1261.
30. Steeg PS, Moore RN, Oppenheim JJ. Regulation of murine macrophage Ia-antigen expression by products of activated spleen cells. *J Exp Med* 1980;152: 1734–1744.
31. Nussenzweig MC, Steinman RM, Gutchinov B, Cohn ZA. Dendritic cells are accessory cells for the development of anti-trinitrophenyl cytotoxic T lymphocytes. *J Exp Med* 1980;152:1070–1084.
32. Steinman RM, Witmer MD. Lymphoid dendritic cells are potent stimulators of the primary mixed leukocyte reaction in mice. *Proc Natl Acad Sci U S A* 1978; 75:5132–5136.
33. Steinman RM, Gutchinov B, Witmer MD, Nussenzweig MC. Dendritic cells are the principal stimulators of the primary mixed leukocyte reaction in mice. *J Exp Med* 1983;157:613–627.
34. Inaba K, Young JW, Steinman RM. Direct activation of CD8[+] cytotoxic T lymphocytes by dendritic cells. *J Exp Med* 1987;166:182–194.
35. Boog CJP, Boes J, Melief CJM. Stimulation with dendritic cells decreases or obviates the CD4[+] helper cell requirement in cytotoxic T lymphocyte responses. *Eur J Immunol* 1988;18:219–223.
36. Nussenzweig MC, Steinman RM. Contributions of dendritic cells to stimulation of the murine syngeneic mixed leukocyte reaction. *J Exp Med* 1980;151: 1196–1212.
37. Sunshine GH, Gold DP, Wortis HH, Marrack P, Kappler JW. Mouse spleen dendritic cells present soluble antigens to antigen-specific T cell hybridomas. *J Exp Med* 1983;158:1745–1750.
38. Sunshine GH, Katz DR, Feldmann M. Dendritic cells induce T cell proliferation to synthetic antigens under Ir gene control. *J Exp Med* 1980;152:1817–1822.
39. Flechner ER, Freudenthal PS, Kaplan G, Steinman RM. Antigen-specific T lymphocytes efficiently cluster with dendritic cells in the human primary mixed-leukocyte reaction. *Cell Immunol* 1988;111:183–195.
40. Kuntz-Crow M, Kunkel HG. Human dendritic cells: Major stimulators of the autologous and allogeneic mixed leukocyte reactions. *Clin Exp Immunol* 1982; 49:338–346.
41. Van Voorhis WC, Valinsky J, Hoffman E, Luban J, Hair LS, Steinman RM. Relative efficacy of human monocytes and dendritic cells as accessory cells for T cell replication. *J Exp Med* 1983;158:174–191.
42. Hart DN, McKenzie JL. Isolation and characterization of human tonsil dendritic cells. *J Exp Med* 1988;168:157–170.
43. Klinkert WEF, Labadie JH, O'Brien JP, Beyer CF, Bowers WE. Rat dendritic cells function as accessory cells and control the production of a soluble factor required for mitogen responses of T lymphocytes. *Proc Natl Acad Sci U S A* 1978;77:5414–5418.
44. Austyn JM, Steinman RM, Weinstein DE, Granelli-Piperno A, Palladino MA. Dendritic cells initiate a two-stage mechanism for T lymphocyte proliferation. *J Exp Med* 1983;157:1101–1115.
45. Inaba K, Steinman RM. Resting and sensitized T lymphocytes exhibit distinct stimulatory (antigen-presenting cell) requirements for growth and lymphokine release. *J Exp Med* 1984;160:1717–1735.
46. Green J, Jotte R. Interactions between T helper cells and dendritic cells during the rat mixed leukocyte reaction. *J Exp Med* 1985;162:1546–1560.
47. Pancholi P, Steinman RM, Bhardwaj N. An approach to isolating T cell lines that

react to antigens presented on the surface of dendritic cells. *Clin Exp Immunol* 1991;85:349–356.

48. Pancholi P, Steinman RM, Bhardwaj N. Dendritic cells efficiently immunoselect mycobacterial-reactive T cells in human blood, including clonable antigen-reactive precursors. *Immunology* 1992;76:217–224.

49. Bhardwaj N, Hodtsev AS, Nisanian A, et al. Human T cell responses to *Mycoplasma arthritidis* derived superantigen (MAM). *Infect Immun* 1994;62:135–144.

50. Bhardwaj N, Lau LL, Friedman SM, Crow MK, Steinman RM. Interleukin 1 production during accessory cell–dependent mitogenesis of T lymphocytes. *J Exp Med* 1989;169:1121–1136.

51. Koide SL, Inaba K, Steinman RM. Interleukin-1 enhances T-dependent immune responses by amplifying the function of dendritic cells. *J Exp Med* 1987;165:515–530.

52. Inaba K, Witmer-Pack MD, Inaba M, Muramatsu S, Steinman RM. The function of Ia$^+$ dendritic cells, and Ia$^-$ dendritic cell precursors, in thymocyte mitogenesis to lectin and lectin plus IL-1. *J Exp Med* 1988;167:149–162.

53. Koide S, Steinman RM. Induction of interleukin-1α mRNA during the antigen-dependent interaction of sensitized T lymphoblasts with macrophages. *J Exp Med* 1988;168:409–416.

54. Seder RA, Paul WE, Davis MM, Fazekas de St. Groth B. The presence of interleukin 4 during in vitro priming determines the lymphokine-producing potential of CD4$^+$ T cells from T cell receptor transgenic mice. *J Exp Med* 1992;176:1091–1098.

55. Croft M, Duncan DD, Swain SL. Response of naive antigen-specific CD4$^+$ T cells in vitro: Characteristics and antigen-presenting cell requirements. *J Exp Med* 1992;176:1431–1437.

56. Bhardwaj N, Young JW, Nisanian AJ, Baggers J, Steinman RM. Small amounts of superantigen, when presented on dendritic cells, are sufficient to initiate T cell responses. *J Exp Med* 1993;178:633–642.

57. Lechler RI, Batchelor JR. Restoration of immunogenicity to passenger cell–depleted kidney allografts by the addition of donor strain dendritic cells. *J Exp Med* 1982;155:31–41.

58. Faustman DL, Steinman RM, Gebel HM, Hauptfeld V, Davie JM, Lacy PE. Prevention of rejection of murine islet allografts by pretreatment with anti-dendritic cell antibody. *Proc Natl Acad Sci U S A* 1984;81:3864–3868.

59. Iwai H, Kuma S-I, Inaba MM, et al. Acceptance of murine thyroid allografts by pretreatment of anti-Ia antibody or anti-dendritic cell antibody in vitro. *Transplantation* 1989;47:45–49.

60. Inaba K, Metlay JP, Crowley MT, Steinman RM. Dendritic cells pulsed with protein antigens in vitro can prime antigen-specific, MHC-restricted T cells in situ. *J Exp Med* 1990;172:631–640.

61. Liu LM, MacPherson GG. Antigen acquisition by dendritic cells: Intestinal dendritic cells acquire antigen administered orally and can prime naive T cells in vivo. *J Exp Med* 1993;177:1299–1307.

62. Sornasse T, Flamand V, DeBecker G, et al. Antigen-pulsed dendritic cells can efficiently induce an antibody response in vivo. *J Exp Med* 1992;175:15–21.

63. Havenith CEG, Breedijk AJ, Betjes MGH, Calame W, Beelen RHJ, Hoefsmit ECM. T cell priming in situ by intratracheally instilled antigen-pulsed dendritic cells. *Am J Respir Cell Mol Biol* 1993;8:319–324.

64. Flamand V, Sornasse T, Thielemans K, et al. Murine dendritic cells pulsed in vitro with tumor antigen induce tumor resistance in vivo. *Eur J Immunol* 1994;24:605–610.

65. Porgador A, Gilboa E. Bone marrow generated dendritic cells pulsed with a class I restricted peptide are potent inducers of cytotoxic T lymphocytes. *J Exp Med* 1995;182:255–260.

66. Zitvogel L, Mayordomo JI, Tjandrawan T, et al. Therapy of murine tumors with tumor peptide pulsed dendritic cells: Dependence on T-cells, B7 costimulation, and Th1-associated cytokines. *J Exp Med* 1996;183:87–97.

67. Celluzzi CM, Mayordomo JI, Storkus WJ, Lotze MT, Falo LD Jr. Peptide-pulsed dendritic cells induce antigen-specific, CTL-mediated protective tumor immunity. *J Exp Med* 1996;183:283–287.

68. Paglia P, Chiodoni C, Rodolfo M, Colombo MP. Murine dendritic cells loaded in vitro with soluble protein prime CTL against tumor antigen in vivo. *J Exp Med* 1996;183:317–322.

69. Mayordomo JI, Zorina T, Storkus WJ, et al. Bone marrow–derived dendritic cells pulsed with synthetic tumour peptides elicit protective and therapeutic antitumour immunity. *Nature Med* 1995;1:1297–1302.

70. Boczkowski D, Nair SK, Snyder D, Gilboa E. Dendritic cells pulsed with RNA are potent antigen-presenting cells in vitro and in vivo. *J Exp Med* 1996;184:465–472.

71. Hsu FJ, Benike C, Fagnoni F, et al. Vaccination of patients with B-cell lymphoma using autologous antigen-pulsed dendritic cells. *Nature Med* 1996;2:52–58.

72. Frey A, Giannasca KT, Weltzin R, et al. Role of the glycocalyx in regulating access of microparticles to apical plasma membranes of intestinal epithelial cells: Implications for microbial attachment and oral vaccine targeting. *J Exp Med* 1996;184:1045–1059.

73. Neutra MR, Pringault E, Kraehenbuhl J-P. Antigen sampling across epithelial barriers and induction of mucosal immune responses. *Ann Rev Immunol* 1996;14:275–300.

74. Neutra MR, Frey A, Kraehenbuh J-P. Epithelial M cells: Gateways for mucosal infection and immunization. *Cell* 1996;86:345–348.

75. Mandel TE, Phipps RP, Abbot A, Tew JG. The follicular dendritic cell: Long term antigen retention during immunity. *Immunol Rev* 1980;53:29–59.

76. Liu Y-J, Grouard G, de Bouteiller O, Banchereau J. Follicular dendritic cells and germinal centers. *Int Rev Cytol* 1996;166:139–179.

77. Schriever F, Freedman AS, Freeman G, Messner E, Daley J, Nadler LM. Isolated human follicular dendritic cells display a unique antigenic phenotype. *J Exp Med* 1989;169:2043–2058.

78. Lindhout E, Lakeman A, Mevissen MLCM, de Groot C. Functionally active Epstein-Barr Virus-transformed follicular dendritic cell-like cell lines. *J Exp Med* 1994;179:1173–1184.

79. Nossal GJV, Abbot A, Mitchell J, Lummus Z. Antigen in immunity. XV. Ultrastructural features of antigen capture in primary and secondary lymphoid follicles. *J Exp Med* 1968;127:277–296.

80. Chen LL, Frank AM, Adams JC, Steinman RM. Distribution of horseradish peroxidase (HRP)-anti HRP immune complexes in mouse spleen, with special reference to follicular dendritic cells. *J Cell Biol* 1978;79:184–199.

81. Szakal AK, Kosco MH, Tew JG. Microanatomy of lymphoid tissue during humoral immune responses: Structure function relationships. *Annu Rev Immunol* 1989;7:91–109.

82. Veldman JE. Histophysiology and electron microscopy of the immune response. Groningen, 1970, PhD thesis.

83. Veldman JE, Kaiserling E. Interdigitating cells. In: Carr I, Daems WT, eds. *The Reticuloendothelial System: Morphology.* New York: Plenum, 1980:381–416.

84. Steinman RM, Adams JC, Cohn ZA. Identification of a novel cell type in peripheral lymphoid organs of mice. IV. Identification and distribution in mouse spleen. *J Exp Med* 1975;141:804–820.

85. Veerman AJP. On the interdigitating cells in the thymus-dependent area of the rat spleen: A relation between the mononuclear phagocyte system and T-lymphocytes. *Cell Tissue Res* 1974;148:247–257.

86. Veerman AJP, Van Ewijk W. White pulp compartments in the spleen of rats and mice. A light and electron microscopical study of lymphoid and non-lymphoid cell types in T- and B-areas. *Cell Tissue Res* 1974;156:417–441.

87. Kaiserling E, Lennert K. Interdigitating reticulum cell in the human lymph node. A specific cell of the thymus dependent region. *Virchows Arch [B]* 1974;16:51–61.

88. Van Ewijk W, Verzijden JHM, Kwast TM, Van Der Luijex-Meijer SWM. Reconstruction of the thymus dependent area in the spleen of lethally irradiated mice. A light and electron microscopic study of the T-cell microenvironment. *Cell Tissue Res* 1974;149:43–60.

89. Hoefsmit EC. Mononuclear phagocytes, retriculum cells and dendritic cells in lymphoid tissues. In: van Furth R, ed. *Mononuclear Phagocytes in Immunity, Infection and Pathology.* Oxford: Blackwell Scientific, 1975:129–146.

90. Fossum S. The architecture of rat lymph nodes. I. Combined light and electron microscopy of lymph node cell types. *Anat Embryol* 1983;167:229

91. Eikelenboom P. Characterization of non-lymphoid cells in the white pulp of the mouse spleen: An in vivo and in vitro study. *Cell Tissue Res* 1978;195:445–460.

92. Dijkstra CD. Characterization of nonlymphoid cells in rat spleen, with special reference to strongly Ia-positive branched cells in T-cell areas. *J Reticuloendothel Soc* 1982;32:167–178.

93. Fossum S. The architecture of rat lymph nodes. IV. Distribution of ferritin and colloidal carbon in the draining lymph nodes after foot-pad injection. *Scand J Immunol* 1980;12:433–441.

94. Witmer MD, Steinman RM. The anatomy of peripheral lymphoid organs with emphasis on accessory cells: Light microscopic, immunocytochemical studies of mouse spleen, lymph node and Peyer's patch. *Am J Anat* 1984;170:465–481.

95. Steinman RM, Pack M, Inaba K. Dendritic cells in the T cell areas of lymphoid organs. *Immunol Rev* 1997;156:25–37.

96. Zhou L-J, Tedder TF. Human blood dendritic cells selectively express CD83, a member of the immunoglobulin superfamily. *J Immunol* 1995;154:3821–3835.

97. Mosialos G, Birkenbach M, Ayehunie S, et al. Circulating human dendritic cells differentially express high levels of a 55-kd actin-bundling protein. *Am J Pathol* 1996;148:593–600.

98. Takahashi K, Isobe T, Ohtsuki Y, Sonobe H, Takeda I, Akagi T. Immunohistochemical localization and distribution of S-100 proteins in the human lymphoreticular system. *Am J Pathol* 1984;116:497–503.

99. Takahashi K, Yamaguchi H, Ishizeki J, Nakajima T, Nakazata Y. Immunohistochemical and immunoelectron microscopic localization of S-100 protein in the interdigitating reticulum cells of the human lymph node. *Virchows Arch [B]* 1981;37:125–135.

100. Shiro BC, Siegal GP. The use of monoclonal antibodies to S100 protein in diagnostic immunochemistry. In: Wick MR, Siegal GP, eds. *Monoclonal Antibodies in Diagnostic Immunohistochemistry.* New York: Marcel Dekker, 1990:455–503.

101. Breel M, Mebius RE, Kraal G. Dendritic cells of the mouse recognized by two monoclonal antibodies. *Eur J Immunol* 1987;17:1555–1559.

102. Agger R, Witmer-Pack M, Romani N, et al. Two populations of splenic dendritic cells detected with M342, a new monoclonal to an intracellular antigen of interdigitating dendritic cells and some B lymphocytes. *J Leukoc Biol* 1992;52:34–42.

103. Inaba K, Inaba M, Romani N, et al. Generation of large numbers of dendritic cells from mouse bone marrow cultures supplemented with granulocyte/macrophage colony-stimulating factor. *J Exp Med* 1992;176:1693–1702.

104. Rabinowitz SS, Gordon S. Macrosialin, a macrophage-restricted membrane sialoprotein differentially glycosylated in response to inflammatory stimuli. *J Exp Med* 1991;174:827–836.

105. Metlay JP, Witmer-Pack MD, Agger R, Crowley MT, Lawless D, Steinman RM.

The distinct leukocyte integrins of mouse spleen dendritic cells as identified with new hamster monoclonal antibodies. *J Exp Med* 1990;171:1753–1771.

106. Witmer-Pack MD, Crowley MT, Inaba K, Steinman RM. Macrophages, but not dendritic cells, accumulate colloidal carbon following administration in situ. *J Cell Sci* 1993;105:965–973.

107. Kraal G, Breel M, Janse M, Bruin G. Langerhans cells, veiled cells, and interdigitating cells in the mouse recognized by a monoclonal antibody. *J Exp Med* 1986;163:981–997.

108. Witmer-Pack MD, Swiggard WJ, Mirza A, Steinman RM. Tissue distribution of the DEC-205 protein that is detected by the monoclonal antibody NLDC-145. II. Expression in situ in lymphoid and nonlymphoid tissues. *Cell Immunol* 1995; 163:157–162.

109. Knight SC, Balfour BM, O'Brien J, Buttifant L, Sumerska T, Clark J. Role of veiled cells in lymphocyte activation. *Eur J Immunol* 1982;12:1057–1060.

110. Drexhage HA, Mullink H, de Groot J, Clarke J, Balfour BM. A study of cells present in peripheral lymph of pigs with special reference to a type of cell resembling the Langerhans cells. *Cell Tissue Res* 1979;202:407–430.

111. Bujdoso R, Hopkins J, Dutia BM, Young P, McConnell I. Characterization of sheep afferent lymph dendritic cells and their role in antigen carriage. *J Exp Med* 1989;170:1285–1302.

112. Spry CJF, Pflug AJ, Janossy G, Humphrey JH. Large mononuclear (veiled) cells with "Ia-like" membrane antigens in human afferent lymph. *Clin Exp Immunol* 1980;39:750

113. Brand CU, Hunziker T, Gerber HA, Schaffner T, Limat A, Braathen LR. Rosettes of Langerhans cells and activated T cells in human skin lymph derived from irritant contact dermatitis. In: Banchereau J, Schmitt D, eds. *Advances in Experimental Medicine and Biology.* New York: Plenum, 1995:527–529.

114. Mayrhofer G, Holt PG, Papadimitriou JM. Functional characteristics of the veiled cells in afferent lymph from the rat intestine. *Immunology* 1986;58: 379–387.

115. Matsuno K, Kudo S, Ezaki T, Miyakawa K. Isolation of dendritic cells in the rat liver lymph. *Transplantation* 1995;60:765–768.

116. Mackay CR, Marston WL, Dudler L. Naive and memory T cells show distinct pathways of lymphocyte recirculation. *J Exp Med* 1990;171:801–818.

117. Mackay CR, Hein WR, Brown MH, Matzinger P. Unusual expression of CD2 in sheep: Implications for T cell interactions. *Eur J Immunol* 1989;18:1681–1688.

118. Galkowska H, Olszewski WL. Spontaneous cluster formation of dendritic (veiled) cells and lymphocytes from skin lymph obtained from dogs with chronic lymphedema. *Lymphology* 1992;25:106–113.

119. Grouard G, Durand I, Filgueira L, Banchereau J, Liu Y-J. Dendritic cells capable of stimulating T cells in germinal centres. *Nature* 1996;384:364–367.

120. Wolff K. The fascinating story that began in 1868. In: Schuler G, ed. *Epidermal Langerhans Cells.* Boca Raton, FL: CRC Press, 1991:1–21.

121. Wolff K. The Langerhans cell. *Curr Prob Dermatol* 1972;4:79–145.

122. Katz SI, Tamaki K, Sachs DH. Epidermal Langerhans cells are derived from cells originating in bone marrow. *Nature* 1979;282:324–326.

123. Stingl G, Wolff-Schreiner EC, Pichler WJ, Gschnait F, Knapp W. Epidermal Langerhans cells bear Fc and C3 receptors. *Nature* 1977;268:245–246.

124. Tamaki K, Stingl G, Gullino M, Sachs DH, Katz SI. Ia antigens in mouse skin are predominantly expressed on Langerhans cells. *J Immunol* 1979;123: 784–787.

125. Rowden G, Lewis MG, Sullivan AK. Ia antigen expression on human epidermal Langerhans cells. *Nature* 1977;268:247–248.

126. Klareskog L, Malmnas-Tjernlund U, Forsum U, Peterson PA. Epidermal Langerhans cells express Ia antigens. *Nature* 1977;268:248–250.

127. Stingl G, Katz SI, Clements L, Green I, Shevach EM. Immunologic functions of Ia-bearing epidermal Langerhans cells. *J Immunol* 1978;121:2005–2013.

128. Schuler G, Steinman RM. Murine epidermal Langerhans cells mature into potent immunostimulatory dendritic cells in vitro. *J Exp Med* 1985;161:526–546.

129. Inaba K, Schuler G, Witmer MD, Valinsky J, Atassi B, Steinman RM. The immunologic properties of purified Langerhans cells: Distinct requirements for the stimulation of unprimed and sensitized T lymphocytes. *J Exp Med* 1986;164:605–613.

130. Witmer-Pack MD, Olivier W, Valinsky J, Schuler G, Steinman RM. Granulocyte/macrophage colony-stimulating factor is essential for the viability and function of cultured murine epidermal Langerhans cells. *J Exp Med* 1987;166: 1484–1498.

131. Teunissen MBM, Wormmeester J, Krieg SR, et al. Human epidermal Langerhans cells undergo profound morphologic and phenotypical changes during in vitro culture. *J Invest Dermatol* 1990;94:166–173.

132. Romani N, Lenz A, Glassel H, et al. Cultured human Langerhans cells resemble lymphoid dendritic cells in phenotype and function. *J Invest Dermatol* 1989;93: 600–609.

133. Silberberg-Sinakin I, Thorbecke GJ, Baer RL, Rosenthal SA, Berezowsky V. Antigen-bearing Langerhans cells in skin, dermal lymphatics and in lymph nodes. *Cell Immunol* 1976;25:137–151.

134. Lens JW, Drexhage HA, Benson W, Balfour BM. A study of cells present in lymph draining from a contact allergic reaction in pigs sensitized to DNFB. *Immunology* 1983;49:415–422.

135. Steinman RM, Schuler G, Romani N, Kaplan G. Dendritic cells. In: Zucker-Franklin D, Greaves MF, Grossi CE, Marmont AM, eds. *Atlas of Blood Cells: Function and Pathology,* 2nd ed. Philadelphia, PA: Lea & Febiger, 1988: 359–377.

136. Kashihara M, Ueda M, Horiguchi Y, Furukawa F, Hanaoka M, Imamura S. A monoclonal antibody specifically reactive to human Langerhans cells. *J Invest Dermatol* 1986;87:602–607.

137. Hanau D, Fabre M, Schmitt DA, et al. Human epidermal Langerhans cells internalize by receptor-mediated endocytosis T6 (CD1″NA1/34) surface antigen. Birbeck granules are involved in the intracellular traffic of the T6 antigen. *J Invest Dermatol* 1987;89:172–177.

138. Stossel H, Koch F, Kampgen E, et al. Disappearance of certain acidic organelles (endosomes and Langerhans cell granules) accompanies loss of antigen processing capacity upon culture of epidermal Langerhans cells. *J Exp Med* 1990;172: 1471–1482.

139. Hoefsmit ECM, Duijvestijn AM, Kamperdijk WA. Relation between Langerhans cells, veiled cells, and interdigitating cells. *Immunobiology* 1982;161:255–265.

140. Steinman RM, Nussenzweig MC. Dendritic cells: Features and functions. *Immunol Rev* 1980;53:127–147.

141. Tew JG, Thorbecke J, Steinman RM. Dendritic cells in the immune response: Characteristics and recommended nomenclature. *J Reticuloendothel Soc* 1982; 31:371–380.

142. van den Oord JJ, De Wolf-Peeters C, de Vos R, Desmet VJ. The paracortical area in dermatopathic lymphadenitis and other reactive conditions of the lymph node. *Virchows Arch [B]* 1984;45:289–299.

143. Rausch E, Kaiserling E, Goos M. Langerhans cells and interdigitating reticulum cells in the thymus-dependent region in human dermatopathic lymphadenitis. *Virchows Arch [B]* 1977;25:327–343.

144. Macatonia SE, Knight SC, Edwards AJ, Griffiths S, Fryer P. Localization of antigen on lymph node dendritic cells after exposure to the contact sensitizer fluorescein isothiocyanate. *J Exp Med* 1987;166:1654–1667.

145. Kripke ML, Munn CG, Jeevan A, Tang J-M, Bucana C. Evidence that cutaneous antigen-presenting cells migrate to regional lymph nodes during contact sensitization. *J Immunol* 1990;145:2833–2838.

146. van Wilsem EJG, Breve J, Kleijmeer M, Kraal G. Antigen-bearing Langerhans cells in skin draining lymph nodes: Phenotype and kinetics of migration. *J Invest Dermatol* 1994;103:217–220.

147. Cumberbatch M, Kimber I. Phenotypic characteristics of antigen-bearing cells in the draining lymph nodes of contact sensitized mice. *Immunology* 1990;71: 404–410.

148. Macatonia SE, Edwards AJ, Knight SC. Dendritic cells and the initiation of contact sensitivity to fluorescein isothiocyanate. *Immunology* 1986;59:509–514.

149. Barker CF, Billingham RE. The role of afferent lymphatics in the rejection of skin homografts. *J Exp Med* 1968;128:197–221.

150. Frey JR, Wenk P. Experimental studies on the pathogenesis of contact eczema in the guinea pig. *Int Arch Allergy Appl Immunol* 1957;11:81–100.

151. Schon-Hegrad MA, Oliver J, McMenamin PG, Holt PG. Studies on the density, distribution, and surface phenotype of intraepithelial class II major histocompatability complex antigen (Ia)-bearing dendritic cells (DC) in the conducting airways. *J Exp Med* 1991;173:1345–1356.

152. Holt PG, Schon-Hegrad MA, Oliver J. MHC class II antigen-bearing dendritic cells in pulmonary tissues of the rat. Regulation of antigen presentation activity by endogenous macrophage populations. *J Exp Med* 1987;167:262–274.

153. Holt PG, Schon-Hegrad MA, Oliver J, Holt BJ, McMenamin PG. A contiguous network of dendritic antigen presenting cells within the respiratory epithelium. *Int Arch Allergy Appl Immunol* 1990;91:155–159.

154. McWilliam AS, Nelson D, Thomas JA, Holt PG. Rapid dendritic cell recruitment is a hallmark of the acute inflammatory response at mucosal surfaces. *J Exp Med* 1994;179:1331–1336.

155. Sertl K, Takemura T, Tschachler E, Ferrans VJ, Kaliner MA, Shevach EM. Dendritic cells with antigen-presenting capability reside in airway epithelium, lung parenchyma, and visceral pleura. *J Exp Med* 1986;163:436–451.

156. Pollard AM, Lipscomb MF. Characterization of murine lung dendritic cells: Similarities to Langerhans cells and thymic dendritic cells. *J Exp Med* 1990;172: 159–168.

157. Maric I, Holt PG, Perdue MH, Bienenstock J. Class II MHC antigen (Ia)-bearing dendritic cells in the epithelium of the rat intestine. *J Immunol* 1996;156: 1408–1414.

158. McMenamin PG, Holthouse I, Holt PG. Class II major histocompatibility complex (Ia) antigen-bearing dendritic cells within the iris and ciliary body of the rat eye: Distribution, phenotype and relation to retinal microglia. *Immunology* 1992;77:385–393.

159. Steptoe RJ, Holt PG, McMenamin PG. Functional studies of major histocompatibility class II-positive dendritic cells and resident tissue macrophages isolated from the rat iris. *Immunology* 1995;85:630–637.

160. Pavli P, Hume DA, Van de Pol E, Doe WF. Dendritic cells, the main antigen-presenting cells of the human colonic lamina propria. *Immunology* 1993;78: 132–141.

161. Mayrhofer G, Pugh CW, Barclay AN. The distribution, ontogeny and origin in the rat of Ia-positive cells with dendritic morphology and of Ia antigen in epithelia, with special reference to the intestine. *Eur J Immunol* 1983;13:112–122.

162. Pavli P, Mawell L, Van de Pol E, Doe WF. Distribution of human colonic dendritic cells and macrophages. *Clin Exp Immunol* 1996;104:124–132.

163. Kelsall BL, Strober W. Distinct populations of dendritic cells are present in the subepithelial dome and T cell regions of the murine Peyer's patch. *J Exp Med* 1996;183:237–247.

164. Frankel SS, Wenig BM, Burke AP, Mannan P, Thompson LDR, Abbondanzo SL,

et al. Replication of HIV-1 in dendritic cell-derived syncytia at the mucosal surface of the adenoid. *Science* 1996;272:115–117.

165. Frankel SS, Tenner-Racz K, Racz P, et al. Active replication of HIV-1 in the lymphoepithelial surface of the tonsil. *Am J Pathol* 1997;151:89–96.

166. Holt PG, Haining S, Nelson DJ, Sedgwick JD. Origin and steady-state turnover of class II MHC-bearing dendritic cells in the epithelium of the conducting airways. *J Immunol* 1994;153:256–261.

167. Hart DNJ, Fabre JW. Demonstration and characterization of Ia-positive dendritic cells in the interstitial connective tissues of rat heart and other tissues, but not brain. *J Exp Med* 1981;154:347–361.

168. Prickett TCR, McKenzie JL, Hart DNJ. Characterization of interstitial dendritic cells in human liver. *Transplantation* 1988;46:754–761.

169. Daar A, Fuggle S, Hart DNJ, et al. Demonstration and phenotypic characterization of HLA-DR positive interstitial dendritic cells widely distributed in human connective tissues. *Transplantation* 1983;15:311–315.

170. Spencer SC, Fabre JW. Characterization of the tissue macrophage and the interstitial dendritic cell as distinct leukocytes normally resident in the connective tissue of rat heart. *J Exp Med* 1990;171:1841–1851.

171. Forbes RDC, Parfrey NA, Gomersall M, Darden AG, Guttmann RD. Dendritic cell–lymphoid cell aggregation and major histocompatibility antigen expression during rat cardiac allograft rejection. *J Exp Med* 1986;164:1239–1258.

172. Austyn JM, Hankins DF, Larsen CP, Morris PJ, Rao AS, Roake JA. Isolation and characterization of dendritic cells from mouse heart and kidney. *J Immunol* 1994;152:2401–2410.

173. Lenz A, Heine M, Schuler G, Romani N. Human and murine dermis contain dendritic cells: Isolation by means of a novel method and phenotypical and functional characterization. *J Clin Invest* 1993;92:2587–2596.

174. Nestle FO, Zheng X-G, Thompson CB, Turka LA, Nickoloff BJ. Characterization of dermal dendritic cells obtained from normal human skin reveals phenotypic and functionally distinctive subsets. *J Immunol* 1993;151:6535–6545.

175. Larsen CP, Morris PJ, Austyn JM. Migration of dendritic leukocytes from cardiac allografts into host spleens: A novel pathway for initiation of rejection. *J Exp Med* 1990;171:307–314.

176. Fossum S. Lymph-borne dendritic leucocytes do not recirculate, but enter the lymph node paracortex to become interdigitating cells. *Scand J Immunol* 1989;27:97–105.

177. Matsuno K, Ezaki T, Kudo S, Uehara Y. A life stage of particle-laden rat dendritic cells in vivo: Their terminal division, active phagocytosis and translocation from the liver to hepatic lymph. *J Exp Med* 1996;183:1865–1878.

178. Kudo S, Matsuno K, Ezaki T, Ogawa M. A novel migration pathway for rat dendritic cells from the blood: Hepatic sinusoids-lymph translocation. *J Exp Med* 1997;185:777–784.

179. Brenan M, Puklavec M. The MRC OX-62 antigen: A useful marker in the purification of rat veiled cells with the biochemical properties of an integrin. *J Exp Med* 1992;175:1457–1465.

180. Kupiec-Weglinski JW, Austyn JM, Morris PJ. Migration patterns of dendritic cells in the mouse. Traffic from the blood, and T cell-dependent and -independent entry to lymphoid tissues. *J Exp Med* 1988;167:632–645.

181. Austyn JM, Kupiec-Weglinski JW, Hankins DF, Morris PJ. Migration patterns of dendritic cells in the mouse. Homing to T cell–dependent areas of spleen, and binding within marginal zone. *J Exp Med* 1988;167:646–651.

182. Bradley LM, Watson SR, Swain SL. Entry of naive CD4 T cells into peripheral lymph nodes requires L-selectin. *J Exp Med* 1994;180:2401–2406.

183. Steinman RM. The dendritic cell system and its role in immunogenicity. *Annu Rev Immunol* 1991;9:271–296.

184. Young JW, Steinman RM. The hematopoietic development of dendritic cells: A distinct pathway for myeloid differentiation. *Stem Cells* 1996;14:376–387.

185. Rogers WO, Weaver CT, Kraus LA, Li J, Li L, Bucy RP. Visualization of antigen-specific T cell activation and cytokine expression in vivo. *J Immunol* 1997;158:649–657.

186. Luther SA, Gulbranson-Judge A, Acha-Orbea H, MacLennan ICM. Viral superantigen drives extrafollicular and follicular B differentiation leading to virus-specific antibody production. *J Exp Med* 1997;185:551–562.

187. Kearney ER, Pape KA, Loh DY, Jenkins MK. Visualization of peptide-specific T cell immunity and peripheral tolerance induction in vivo. *Immunology* 1994;1:327–339.

188. Ingulli E, Mondino A, Khoruts A, Jenkins MK. In vivo detection of dendritic cell antigen presentation to CD4+ T cells. *J Exp Med* 1997;185:2133–2141.

189. Kyewski BA, Fathman CG, Rouse RV. Intrathymic presentation of circulating non-MHC antigens by medullary dendritic cells. An antigen-dependent microenviroment for T cell differentiation. *J Exp Med* 1986;163:231–246.

190. Crowley M, Inaba K, Steinman RM. Dendritic cells are the principal cells in mouse spleen bearing immunogenic fragments of foreign proteins. *J Exp Med* 1990;172:383–386.

191. Guery J C, Adorini L. Dendritic cells are the most efficient in presenting endogenous naturally processed self-epitopes to class II–restricted T cells. *J Immunol* 1995;154:536–544.

192. Xia W, Pinto CE, Kradin RL. The antigen-presenting activities of Ia+ dendritic cells shift dynamically from lung to lymph node after an airway challenge with soluble antigen. *J Exp Med* 1995;181:1275–1283.

193. Guery J-C, Ria F, Adorini L. Dendritic cells but not B cells present antigenic complexes to class II–restricted T cells after administration of protein in adjuvant. *J Exp Med* 1996;183:751–757.

194. Inaba K, Paek M, Inaba M, Sakuta H, Isdell F, Steinman RM. High levels of an

MHC II- self peptide complex on dendritic cells from lymph node. 1997; *J Exp Med* 1997;186:665–672.

195. Murphy DB, Rath S, Pizzo E, Rudensky AY, George A, Larson JK, et al. Monoclonal antibody detection of a major self peptide. *J Immunol* 1992;148:3483–3491.

196. Rudensky AY, Rath S, Preston-Hurlburt P, Murphy DB, Janeway CA Jr. On the complexity of self. *Nature* 1991;353:660–662.

197. Romani N, Inaba K, Pure E, Crowley M, Witmer-Pack M, Steinman RM. A small number of anti-CD3 molecules on dendritic cells stimulate DNA synthesis in mouse T lymphocytes. *J Exp Med* 1989;169:1153–1168.

198. Bender A, Bui LK, Feldman MAV, Larsson M, Bhardwaj N. Inactivated influenza virus, when presented on dendritic cells, elicits human CD8+ cytolytic T cell responses. *J Exp Med* 1995;182:1663–1671.

199. Sallusto F, Lanzavecchia A. Efficient presentation of soluble antigen by cultured human dendritic cells is maintained by granulocyte/macrophage colony-stimulating factor plus interleukin 4 and downregulated by tumor necrosis factor α. *J Exp Med* 1994;179:1109–1118.

200. Romani N, Koide S, Crowley M, et al. Presentation of exogenous protein antigens by dendritic cells to T cell clones: Intact protein is presented best by immature, epidermal Langerhans cells. *J Exp Med* 1989;169:1169–1178.

201. Pure E, Inaba K, Crowley MT, et al. Antigen processing by epidermal Langerhans cells correlates with the level of biosynthesis of major histocompatibility complex class II molecules and expression of invariant chain. *J Exp Med* 1990;172:1459–1469.

202. Kampgen E, Koch N, Koch F, et al. Class II major histocompatibility complex molecules of murine dendritic cells: Synthesis, sialylation of invariant chain, and antigen processing capacity are down-regulated upon culture. *Proc Natl Acad Sci U S A* 1991;88:3014–3018.

203. Koch F, Trockenbacher B, Kampgen E, et al. Antigen processing in populations of mature murine dendritic cells is caused by subsets of incompletely matured cells. *J Immunol* 1995;155:93–100.

204. Sallusto F, Lanzavecchia A. Dendritic cells use macropinocytosis and the mannose receptor to concentrate antigen in the MHC class II compartment. Downregulation by cytokines and bacterial products. *J Exp Med* 1995;182:389–400.

205. Streilein JW, Grammer SF. In vitro evidence that Langerhans cells can adopt two functionally distinct forms capable of antigen presentation to T lymphocytes. *J Immunol* 1989;143:3925–3933.

206. Cella M, Scheidegger D, Palmer-Lehmann K, Lane P, Lanzavecchia A, Alber G. Ligation of CD40 on dendritic cells triggers production of high levels of interleukin-12 and enhances T cell stimulatory capacity: T-T help via APC activation. *J Exp Med* 1996;184:747–752.

207. Koch F, Stanzl U, Jennewien P, et al. High level IL-12 production by murine dendritic cells: Upregulation via MHC class II and CD40 molecules and downregulation by IL-4 and IL-10. *J Exp Med* 1996;184:741–747.

208. Enk AH, Angeloni VL, Udey MC, Katz SI. Inhibition of Langerhans cell antigen-presenting function by IL-10. *J Immunol* 1993;151:2390–2398.

209. Peguet-Navarro J, Moulon C, Caux C, Dalbiez-Gauthier C, Banchereau J, Schmitt D. Interleukin-10 inhibits the primary allogeneic T cell response to human epidermal Langerhans cells. *Eur J Immunol* 1994;24:884–891.

210. Macatonia SE, Doherty TM, Knight SC, O'Garra A. Differential effect of IL-10 on dendritic cell-induced T cell proliferation and IFN-gamma production. *J Immunol* 1993;150:3755–3765.

211. Caux C, Massacrier C, Vanbervliet B, Barthelemy C, Liu Y-J, Banchereau J. Interleukin 10 inhibits T cell alloreaction induced by human dendritic cells. *Int Immunol* 1994;6:1177–1185.

212. Buelens C, Verhasselt V, De Groote D, Thielemans K, Goldman M, Willems F. IL-10 prevents the generation of dendritic cells from peripheral blood mononuclear cells cultured with interleukin-4 and granulocyte/macrophage-colony-stimulating factor. *Eur J Immunol* 1997;27:756–762.

213. Ludewig B, Graf D, Gelderblom HR, Becker Y, Kroczek RA, Pauli G. Spontaneous apoptosis of dendritic cells is efficiently inhibited by TRAP (CD40-ligand) and TNF-α, but strongly enhanced by interleukin-10. *Eur J Immunol* 1995;25:1943–1950.

214. Larsen CP, Ritchie SC, Pearson TC, Linsley PS, Lowry RP. Functional expression of the costimulatory molecule, B7/BB1, on murine dendritic cell populations. *J Exp Med* 1992;176:1215–1220.

215. Inaba K, Witmer-Pack M, Inaba M, et al. The tissue distribution of the B7-2 costimulator in mice: Abundant expression on dendritic cells in situ and during maturation in vitro. *J Exp Med* 1994;180:1849–1860.

216. Caux C, Massacrier C, Vanbervliet B, et al. Activation of human dendritic cells through CD40 cross-linking. *J Exp Med* 1994;180:1263–1272.

217. Caux C, Vanbervliet B, Massacrier C, et al. B70/B7-2 is identical to CD86 and is the major functional ligand for CD28 expressed on human dendritic cells. *J Exp Med* 1994;180:1841–1847.

218. Heufler C, Koch F, Schuler G. Granulocyte/macrophage colony-stimulating factor and interleukin 1 mediate the maturation of murine epidermal Langerhans cells into potent immunostimulatory dendritic cells. *J Exp Med* 1988;167:700–705.

219. Bilyk N, Holt PG. Inhibition of the immunosuppressive activity of resident pulmonary alveolar macrophages by granulocyte/macrophage colony-stimulating factor. *J Exp Med* 1993;177:1773–1777.

220. Crowley MT, Inaba K, Witmer-Pack MD, Gezelter S, Steinman RM. Use of the fluorescence activated cell sorter to enrich dendritic cells from mouse spleen. *J Immunol Methods* 1990;133:55–66.

221. O'Doherty U, Peng M, Gezelter S, et al. Human blood contains two subsets of dendritic cells, one immunologically mature, and the other immature. *Immunology* 1994;82:487–493.

222. Nijman HW, Kleijmeer MJ, Ossevoort MA, et al. Antigen capture and MHC class II compartments of freshly isolated and cultured human blood dendritic cells. *J Exp Med* 1995;182:163–174.

223. Flores-Romo L, Bjorck P, Duvert V, Van Kooten C, Saeland S, Banchereau J. CD40 ligation on human CD34- hematopoietic progenitors induces their proliferation and differentiation into functional dendritic cells. *J Exp Med* 1997;185:341–349.

224. Caux C, Dezutter-Dambuyant C, Schmitt D, Banchereau J. GM-CSF and TNF-α cooperate in the generation of dendritic Langerhans cells. *Nature* 1992;360:258–261.

225. Caux C, Vanbervliet B, Massacrier C, et al. CD34+ hematopoietic progenitors from human cord blood differentiate along two independent dendritic cell pathways in response to GM-CSF+ TNF α. *J Exp Med* 1996;184:695–706.

226. Szabolcs P, Moore MAS, Young JW. Expansion of immunostimulatory dendritic cells among the myeloid progeny of human CD34+ bone marrow precursors cultured with c-kit ligand, granulocyte-macrophage colony-stimulating factor, and TNF-α. *J Immunol* 1995;154:5851–5861.

227. Szabolcs P, Avigan D, Gezelter S, et al. Dendritic cells and macrophages can mature independently from a human bone marrow-derived, post-CFU intermediate. *Blood* 1996;87:4520–4530.

228. Yamaguchi Y, Tsumura H, Miwa M, Inaba K. Contrasting effects of TGF 1 and TNFα on the development of dendritic cells from progenitors in mouse bone marrow. *Stem Cells* 1997;15:144–153.

229. Kitajima T, Caceres-Dittmar G, Tapia FJ, Jester J, Bergstresser PR, Takashima A. T cell-mediated terminal maturation of dendritic cells. *J Immunol* 1996;157:2340–2347.

230. Kitajima T, Arizumi K, Bergstresser PR, Takashima A. A novel mechanism of glucocorticoid-induced immune suppression: The inhibition of T cell–mediated terminal maturation of a murine dendritic cell line. *J Clin Invest* 1996;98:142–147.

231. Baldwin AS Jr. The NF-kB and IkB proteins: New discoveries and insights. *Annu Rev Immunol* 1996;14:649–681.

232. Granelli-Piperno A, Pope M, Inaba K, Steinman RM. Coexpression of REL and SP1 transcription factors in HIV-1 induced, dendritic cell–T cell syncytia. *Proc Natl Acad Sci U S A* 1995;92:10944–10948.

233. Weih F, Carrasco D, Durham SK, et al. Multiorgan inflammation and hematopoietic abnormalities in mice with a targeted disruption of RelB, a member of the NF-kB/Rel family. *Cell* 1995;80:331–340.

234. Burkly L, Hession C, Ogata L, et al. Expression of relB is required for the development of thymic medulla and dendritic cells. *Nature* 1995;373:531–536.

235. Salomon B, Lores P, Pioche C, Racz P, Jami J, Klatzmann D. Conditional ablation of dendritic cells in transgenic mice. *J Immunol* 1994;152:537–548.

236. Boehmelt G, Madruga J, Dorfler P, et al. Dendritic cell progenitor is transformed by a conditional v-Rel estrogen receptor fusion protein v-RelER. *Cell* 1995;80:341–352.

237. Sallusto F, Nicolo C, De Maria R, Corinti S, Testi R. Ceramide inhibits antigen uptake and presentation by dendritic cells. *J Exp Med* 1996;184:2411–2416.

238. Larsen CP, Steinman RM, Witmer-Pack M, Hankins DF, Morris PJ, Austyn JM. Migration and maturation of Langerhans cells in skin transplants and explants. *J Exp Med* 1990;172:1483–1493.

239. Larsen CP, Ritchie SC, Hendrix R, et al. Regulation of immunostimulatory function and costimulatory molecule (B7-1 and B7-2) expression on murine dendritic cells. *J Immunol* 1994;152:5208–5219.

240. Pope M, Betjes MGH, Hirmand H, Hoffman L, Steinman RM. Both dendritic cells and memory T lymphocytes emigrate from organ cultures of human skin and form distinctive dendritic–T cell conjugates. *J Invest Dermatol* 1995;104:11–18.

241. Richters CD, Hoekstra MJ, van Baare J, du Pont JS, Hoefsmit ECM, Kamperdijk EWA. Isolation and characterization of migratory human skin dendritic cells. *Clin Exp Immunol* 1994;98:330–337.

242. Lukas M, Stoessel H, Hefel L, et al. Human cutaneous dendritic cells migrate through dermal lymphatic vessels in a skin organ culture model. *J Invest Dermatol* 1996;106:1293–1299.

243. Enk AH, Angeloni VL, Udey SI. An essential role for Langerhans cell-derived IL-1 beta in the initiation of primary immune responses in skin. *J Immunol* 1993;150:3698–3704.

244. Weinlich G, Sepp N, Koch F, Schuler G, Romani N. Evidence that Langerhans cells rapidly disappear from the epidermis in response to contact sensitizers but not to tolerogens/nonsensitizers. *Arch Dermatol Res* 1989;281:556.

245. Roake JA, Rao AS, Morris PJ, Larsen CP, Hankins DF, Austyn JM. Dendritic cell loss from non-lymphoid tissues following systemic administration of lipopolysaccharide, tumour necrosis factor, and interleukin-1. *J Exp Med* 1995;181:2237–2248.

246. MacPherson GG, Jenkins CD, Stein MJ, Edwards C. Endotoxin-mediated dendritic cell release from the intestine: Characterization of released dendritic cells and TNF dependence. *J Immunol* 1995;154:1317–1322.

247. De Smedt T, Pajak B, Muraille E, et al. Regulation of dendritic cell numbers and maturation by lipopolysaccharide in vivo. *J Exp Med* 1996;184:1413–1424.

248. Bender A, Sapp M, Schuler G, Steinman RM, Bhardwaj N. Improved methods for the generation of dendritic cells from nonproliferating progenitors in human blood. *J Immunol Methods* 1996;196:121–135.

249. Romani N, Reider D, Heuer M, et al. Generation of mature dendritic cells from human blood: An improved method with special regard to clinical applicability. *J Immunol Methods* 1996;196:137–151.

250. Reddy A, Sapp M, Feldman M, Subklewe M, Bhardwaj N. A monocyte conditioned medium is more effective than defined cytokines in mediating the terminal maturation of human dendritic cells. *Blood* 1997;90:3640–3646.

251. Sozzani S, Sallusto F, Luini W, et al. Migration of dendritic cells in response to formyl peptides, C5a, and a distinct set of chemokines. *J Immunol* 1995;155:3292–3295.

252. Granelli-Piperno A, Moser B, Pope M, et al. Efficient interaction of HIV-1 with purified dendritic cells via multiple chemokine coreceptors. *J Exp Med* 1996;184:2433–2438.

253. Greaves DR, Wang W, Dairaghi DJ, et al. CCR6, a CC chemokine receptor which interacts with MIP-3α and is highly expressed in human dendritic cells. 1997 (submitted for publication).

254. Adema GJ, Hartgers F, Verstraten R, et al. DC-CK1, a dendritic cell specific C-C chemokine highly expressed in tonsils preferentially attracts naive T cells. *Nature* 1997 (in press).

255. Hosoi J, Murphy GF, Egan CL, et al. Regulation of Langerhans cell function by nerves containing calcitonin gene-related peptide. *Nature* 1993;363:159–162.

256. Inaba K, Steinman RM, Witmer-Pack M, Aya H, Inaba M, Sudo T, et al. Identification of proliferating dendritic cell precursors in mouse blood. *J Exp Med* 1992;175:1157–1167.

257. Scheicher C, Mehlig M, Zecher R, Reske K. Dendritic cells from mouse bone marrow: In vitro differentiation using low doses of recombinant granulocyte-macrophage colony-stimulating factor. *J Immunol Methods* 1992;154:253–264.

258. Mackensen A, Herbst B, Kohler G, et al. Delineation of the dendritic cell lineage by generating large numbers of Birbeck granule-positive Langerhans cells from human peripheral blood progenitor cells in vitro. *Blood* 1995;86:2699–2707.

259. Santiago-Schwartz F, Belilos E, Diamond B, Carsons SE. TNF in combination with GM-CSF enhances the differentiation of neonatal cord blood stem cells into dendritic cells and macrophages. *J Leukoc Biol* 1992;52:274–281.

260. Strunk D, Rappersberger K, Egger C, et al. Generation of human dendritic cells/Langerhans cells from circulating CD34+ hematopoietic progenitor cells. *Blood* 1996;87:1292–1302.

261. Rosenzwajg M, Camus S, Guigon M, Gluckman JC. The influence of interleukin (IL)-4, IL-13 and Flt3 ligand on human dendritic cell differentiation from cord blood CD34+ progenitors. *Exp Hematol* 1998;26:63–72.

262. Young JW, Szabolcs P, Moore MAS. Identification of dendritic cell colony-forming units among normal CD34+ bone marrow progenitors that are expanded by c-kit-ligand and yield pure dendritic cell colonies in the presence of granulocyte/macrophage colony-stimulating factor and tumor necrosis factor α. *J Exp Med* 1995;182:1111–1120.

263. Kampgen E, Koch F, Heufler C, et al. Understanding the dendritic cell lineage through a study of cytokine receptors. *J Exp Med* 1994;179:1767–1776.

264. Witmer-Pack MD, Hughes D, Schuler G, et al. Identification of macrophages and dendritic cells in the osteopetrotic (op/op) mouse. *J Cell Sci* 1993;104:1021–1029.

265. Takahashi K, Naito M, Shultz LD, Hayashi S, Nishikawa S. Differentiation of dendritic cell populations in macrophage colony-stimulating factor-deficient mice homozygous for the osteopetrosis (op) mutation. *J Leukoc Biol* 1993;53:19–28.

266. Winzler C, Rovere P, Rescigno M, et al. Maturation stages of mouse dendritic cells in growth factor-dependent long-term cultures. *J Exp Med* 1997;185:317–328.

267. Paglia P, Girolomoni G, Robbiati F, Granucci F, Ricciardi-Castagnoli P. Immortalized dendritic cell line fully competent in antigen presentation initiates primary T cell responses in vivo. *J Exp Med* 1993;178:1893–1901.

268. Pierre P, Turley SJ, Gatti E, et al. Developmental regulation of MHC class II transport in mouse dendritic cells. *Nature* 1997;388:787–792.

269. Saunders D, Lucas K, Ismaili J, et al. Dendritic cell development in culture from thymic precursor cells in the absence of granulocyte/macrophage colony-stimulating factor. *J Exp Med* 1996;184:2185–2196.

270. Maraskovsky E, Brasel K, Teepe M, et al. Dramatic increase in the numbers of functionally mature dendritic cells in Flt3 ligand-treated mice: Multiple dendritic cell subpopulations identified. *J Exp Med* 1996;184:1953–1962.

271. Lutz MB, Granucci F, Winzler C, et al. Retroviral immortalization of phagocytic and dendritic cell clones as a tool to investigate functional heterogeneity. *J Immunol Methods* 1994;174:269–279.

272. Shen Z, Reznikoff G, Droanoff G, Rock KL. Cloned dendritic cells can present exogenous antigens on both MHC class I and class II molecules. *J Immunol* 1997;158:2723–2730.

273. Brossart P, Goldrath AW, Butz EA, Martin S, Bevan MJ. Virus-mediated delivery of antigenic epitopes into dendritic cells as a means to induce CTL. *J Immunol* 1997;158:3270–3276.

274. Volkmann A, Neefjes J, Stockinger B. A conditionally immortalized dendritic cell line which differentiates in contact with T cells or T-cell derived cytokines. *Eur J Immunol* 1997;26:2565–2572.

275. Romani N, Gruner S, Brang D, et al. Proliferating dendritic cell progenitors in human blood. *J Exp Med* 1994;180:83–93.

276. Steinman RM, Swanson J. Commentary. The endocytic activity of dendritic cells. *J Exp Med* 1995;181:283–288.

277. Reis e Sousa C, Stahl PD, Austyn JM. Phagocytosis of antigens by Langerhans cells in vitro. *J Exp Med* 1993;178:509–519.

278. Inaba K, Inaba M, Naito M, Steinman RM. Dendritic cell progenitors phagocytose particulates, including *Bacillus* Calmette-Guerin organisms, and sensitize mice to mycobacterial antigens in vivo. *J Exp Med* 1993;178:479–488.

279. Svensson M, Stockinger B, Wick MJ. Bone marrow-derived dendritic cells can process bacteria for MHC-I and MHC-II presentation to T cells. *J Immunol* 1997;158:4229–4236.

280. Moll H, Fuchs H, Blank C, Rollinghoff M. Langerhans cells transport *Leishmania major* from the infected skin to the draining lymph node for presentation to antigen-specific T cells. *Eur J Immunol* 1993;23:1595–1601.

281. Blank C, Bogdan C, Bauer C, Erb K, Moll H. Murine epidermal Langerhans cells do not express inducible nitric oxide synthase. *Eur J Immunol* 1996;26:792–796.

282. Swiggard WJ, Mirza A, Nussenzweig MC, Steinman RM. DEC-205, a 205 kDa protein abundant on mouse dendritic cells and thymic epithelium that is detected by the monoclonal antibody NLDC-145: Purification, characterization and N-terminal amino acid sequence. *Cell Immunol* 1995;165:302–311.

283. Jiang W, Swiggard WJ, Heufler C, et al. The receptor DEC-205 expressed by dendritic cells and thymic epithelial cells is involved in antigen processing. *Nature* 1995;375:151–155.

284. Stahl P, Schlesinger PH, Sigardson E, Rodman JS, Lee YC. Receptor-mediated pinocytosis of mannose glycoconjugates by macrophages: Characterization and evidence for receptor recycling. *Cell* 1980;19:207–215.

285. Lanzavecchia A. Antigen-specific interaction between T and B cells. *Nature* 1985;314:537–539.

286. Bieber T, de la Salle H, Wollenberg A, et al. Human epidermal Langerhans cells express the high affinity receptor for immunoglobulin E (Fcε). *J Exp Med* 1992;175:1285–1290.

287. Wang B, Rieger A, Kilgus O, et al. Epidermal Langerhans cells from normal human skin bind monomeric IgE via FcεRI. *J Exp Med* 1992;175:1353–1365.

288. Maurer D, Fiebiger E, Ebner C, et al. Peripheral blood dendritic cells express FcεRI as a complex composed of FcεRIα- and FcεR1 gamma-chains and can use this receptor for IgE-mediated allergen presentation. *J Immunol* 1996;157:607–616.

289. Peters PJ, Neefjes JJ, Oorschot V, Ploegh HL, Geuze HJ. Segregation of MHC class II molecules from MHC class I molecules in the Golgi complex for transport to lysosomal compartments. *Nature* 1991;349:669–676.

290. Kleijmeer MJ, Oorschot VMJ, Geuze HJ. Human resident Langerhans cells display a lysosomal compartment enriched in MHC class II. *J Invest Dermatol* 1994;103:516–523.

291. Kleijmeer MJ, Ossevoort MA, Van Veen CJH, et al. MHC class II compartments and the kinetics of antigen presentation in activated mouse spleen dendritic cells. *J Immunol* 1995;154:5715–5724.

292. Sanderson F, Kleijmeer MJ, Kelly A, et al. Accumulation of HLA-DM, a regulator of antigen presentation, in MHC class II compartments. *Science* 1994;266:1566–1569.

293. Amigorena S, Drake JR, Webster P, Mellman I. Transient accumulation of new class II MHC molecules in a novel endocytic compartment in B lymphocytes. *Nature* 1994;369:113–120.

294. Tulp A, Verwoerd D, Dobberstein B, Ploegh HL, Pieters J. Isolation and characterization of the intracellular MHC class II compartment. *Nature* 1994;369:120–126.

295. Cella M, Engering A, Pinet V, Pieters J, Lanzavecchia A. Inflammatory stimuli induce accumulation of MHC class II complexes on dendritic cells. *Nature* 1997;388:782–787.

296. Harding CV, Roof RW, Unanue ER. Turnover of Ia-peptide complexes is facilitated in viable antigen-presenting cells: Biosynthetic turnover of Ia vs. peptide exchange. *Proc Natl Acad Sci U S A* 1990;86:4230–4234.

297. Young JW, Steinman RM. Dendritic cells stimulate primary human cytolytic lymphocyte responses in the absence of CD4+ helper T cells. *J Exp Med* 1990;171:1315–1332.

298. Macatonia SE, Taylor PM, Knight SD, Askonas BA. Primary stimulation by dendritic cells induces anti-viral proliferative and cytotoxic T cell responses in vitro. *J Exp Med* 1989;169:1255–1264.

299. Nonacs R, Humborg C, Tam JP, Steinman RM. Mechanisms of mouse spleen dendritic cell function in the generation of influenza-specific, cytolytic T lymphocytes. *J Exp Med* 1992;176:519–529.

300. Kast WM, Boog CJP, Roep BO, Voordouw AC, Melief CJM. Failure or success in the restoration of virus-specific cytotoxic T lymphocyte response defects by dendritic cells. *J Immunol* 1988;140:3186–3193.

301. Hengel H, Lindner M, Wagner H, Heeg K. Frequency of herpes simplex virus-specific murine cytotoxic T lymphocyte precursors in mitogen- and antigen-driven primary in vitro T cell responses. *J Immunol* 1987;139:4196–4202.

302. Bhardwaj N, Bender A, Gonzalez N, Bui LK, Garrett MC, Steinman RM. Influenza virus-infected dendritic cells stimulate strong proliferative and cytolytic responses from human CD8+ T cells. *J Clin Invest* 1994;94:797–807.

303. Bhardwaj N, Seder RA, Reddy A, Feldman MV. IL-12 in conjunction with dendritic cells enhances anti-viral, CD8+ CTL responses in vitro. *J Clin Invest* 1996;98:715–722.

304. Fesq H, Bacher M, Nain M, Gemsa D. Programmed cell death (apoptosis) in human monocytes infected by influenza virus. *Immunobiology* 1994;190:175–182.

305. Bevan MJ. Cross-priming for a secondary cytotoxic response to minor H antigens with H-2 congenic cells which do not cross-react in the cytotoxic assay. *J Exp Med* 1976;143:1283–1288.

306. Huang AYC, Golumbek P, Ahmadzadeh M, Jaffee E, Pardoll D, Levitsky H. Role of bone marrow-derived cells in presenting MHC class I-restricted tumor antigens. *Science* 1994;264:961–965.

307. Carbone FR, Bevan MJ. Class I–restricted processing and presentation of exogenous cell–associated antigen in vivo. *J Exp Med* 1990;171:377–387.

308. Kovacsovics-Bankowski M, Rock KL. A phagosome-to-cytosol pathway for exogenous antigens presented on MHC class I molecules. *Science* 1995;267:243–246.

309. Huang AYC, Bruce AT, Pardoll DM, Levitsky HI. In vivo cross-priming of MHC class I–restricted antigens requires the TAP transporter. *Immunology* 1996;4:349–355.

310. Brumeanu TD, Swiggard WJ, Steinman RM, Bona CA, Zaghouani H. Efficient loading of identical peptide onto class II molecules by antigenized immunoglobulin and PR8 virus. *J Exp Med* 1993;178:1795–1799.

311. Reis e Sousa C, Germain RN. Major histocompatibility complex class I presentation of peptides derived from soluble exogenous antigen by a subset of cells engaged in phagocytosis. *J Exp Med* 1995;182:841–851.

312. Albert M, Sauter B, Bhardwaj N. Dendritic cells acquire antigens apoptotic cells and induce class I-restricted CTLS. *Nature* 1998;392:86–89.

313. Freudenthal PS, Steinman RM. The distinct surface of human blood dendritic cells, as observed after an improved isolation method. *Proc Natl Acad Sci U S A* 1990;87:7698–7702.

314. Pinchuk LM, Polacino PS, Agy MB, Klaus SJ, Clark EA. The role of CD40 and CD80 accessory cell molecules in dendritic cell–dependent HIV-1 infection. *Immunology* 1994;1:317–325.

315. Young JW, Koulova L, Soergel SA, Clark EA, Steinman RM, Dupont B. The B7/BB1 antigen provides one of several costimulatory signals for the activation of CD4+ T lymphocytes by human blood dendritic cells in vitro. *J Clin Invest* 1992;90:229–237.

316. Viola A, Lanzavecchia A. T cell activation determined by T cell receptor number and tunable thresholds. *Science* 1996;273:104–106.

317. Schweitzer AN, Borriello F, Wong RCK, Abbas AK, Sharpe AH. Role of costimulators in T cell differentiation. *J Immunol* 1997;158:2713–2722.

318. Demotz S, Grey HM, Sette A. The minimal number of class II MHC-antigen complexes needed for T cell activation. *Science* 1990;249.1028–1030.

319. Harding CV, Unanue ER. Quantitation of antigen-presenting cell MHC class II/peptide complexes necessary for T-cell stimulation. *Nature* 1990;346:574–576.

320. Christinck ER, Luscher MA, Barber BH, Williams DB. Peptide binding to class I MHC on living cells and quantitation of complexes required for CTL lysis. *Nature* 1991;352:67–70.

321. Inaba K, Steinman RM. Accessory cell–T lymphocyte interactions: Antigen dependent and independent clustering. *J Exp Med* 1986;163:247–261.

322. Inaba K, Romani N, Steinman RM. An antigen-independent contact mechanism as an early step in T-cell–proliferative responses to dendritic cells. *J Exp Med* 1989;170:527–542.

323. Stockl J, Majdic O, Kohl P, Pickl WF, Menzel JE, Knapp W. Leukosialin (CD43)–major histocompatibility class I molecule interactions involved in spontaneous T cell conjugate formation. *J Exp Med* 1996;184:1769–1779.

324. Dustin ML, Springer TA. T-cell receptor cross-linking transiently stimulates adhesiveness through LFA-1. *Nature* 1989;341:619–624.

325. Hsieh C-S, Macatonia SE, Tripp CS, Wolf SF, O'Garra A, Murphys KM. Development of Th1 CD4+ T cells through IL-12 produced by *Listeria*-induced macrophages. *Science* 1993;260:547–549.

326. Macatonia SE, Hosken NA, Litton M, et al. Dendritic cells produce IL-12 and direct the development of Th1 cells from naive CD4+ T cells. *J Immunol* 1995;154:5071–5079.

327. Heufler C, Koch F, Stanzl U, et al. Interleukin-12 is produced by dendritic cells and mediates T helper 1 development as well as interferon-gamma production by T helper 1 cells. *Eur J Immunol* 1996;26:659–668.

328. Pope M, Betjes MGH, Romani N, et al. Conjugates of dendritic cells and memory T lymphocytes from skin facilitate productive infection with HIV-1. *Cell* 1994;78:389–398.

329. Ohshima Y, Delespesse G. T cell–derived IL-4 and dendritic cell–derived IL-12 regulate the lymphokine-producing phenotype of alloantigen-primed naive human CD4 T cells. *J Immunol* 1997;158:629–636.

330. Rincon M, Anguita J, Nakamura T, Fikrig E, Flavell RA. Interleukin (IL)-6 directs the differentiation of IL-4 producing CD4+ T cells. *J Exp Med* 1997;185:461–469.

331. Stuhler G, Schlossman SF. Antigen organization regulates cluster formation and induction of cytotoxic T lymphocytes by helper T cell subsets. *Proc Natl Acad Sci U S A* 1997;94:622–627.

332. Bender A, Albert M, Reddy A, Feldman M, Sauter B, Kaplan G, Hellmann W, Bhardwaj N. The distinctive features of influenza virus infection of dendritic cells. *Immunobiology* 1997;198:64–79.

333. Grosjean I, Caux C, Bella C, et al. Measles virus infects human dendritic cells and blocks their allostimulatory properties for CD4+ T cells. *J Exp Med* 1997;186:801–812.

334. Fugier-Vivier I, Servet-Delprat C, Rivailler P, Rissoan M C, Liu Y-J, Rabourdin-Combe C. Measles virus suppresses cell-mediated immunity by interfering with the survival and functions of DC and T cells. 1997 (submitted for publication).

335. Labuda M, Austyn JM, Zuffova E, et al. Importance of localized skin infection in tick-borne encephalitis virus transmission. *Virology* 1996;219:357–366.

336. Pope M, Elmore D, Ho D, Marx P. Dendritic cell–T cell mixtures, isolated from the skin and mucosae of macaques, support the replication of SIV. *AIDS Res Hum Retrovir* 1997;13:819–827.

337. Pope M, Gezelter S, Gallo N, Hoffman L, Steinman RM. Low levels of HIV-1 in cutaneous dendritic cells initiate a productive infection upon binding to memory CD4+ T cells. *J Exp Med* 1995;182:2045–2056.

338. Xu H, Dilulio NA, Fairchild RL. T cell populations primed by hapten sensitization in contact sensitivity are distinguished by polarized patterns of cytokine production: Interferon gamma-producing (Tc1) effector CD8+ T cells and interleukin (II) 4/II-10–producing (Th2) negative regulatory CD4+ T cells. *J Exp Med* 1996;183:1001–1012.

339. Gocinski B, Tigelaar R. Roles of CD4+ and CD8+ T cells in murine contact sensitivity revealed by in vivo monoclonal antibody depletion. *J Immunol* 1990;144:4121–4128.

340. Steinbrink K, Sorg C, Macher E. Low zone tolerance to contact allergens in mice: A functional role for CD8+ T helper type 2 cells. *J Exp Med* 1996;183:759–768.

341. Dubois B, Vanbervliet B, Fayette J, et al. Dendritic cells enhance growth and differentiation of CD40-activated B lymphocytes. *J Exp Med* 1997;185:941–951.

342. Fayette J, Dubois B, Vandenabelle S, et al. Human dendritic cells skew isotype switching of CD40-activated naive B cells towards IgA1 and IgA2. *J Exp Med* 1997;185:1909–1918.

343. Liu Y-J, Zhang J, Lane PJL, Chan EY-T, Maclennan ICM. Sites of specific B cell activation in primary and secondary responses to T cell–dependent and T cell–independent antigens. *Eur J Immunol* 1991;21:2951–2962.

344. Caux C, Massacrier C, Vanbervliet B, et al. CD34+ hematopoietic progenitors from human cord blood differentiate along two independent dendritic cell pathways in response to GM-CSF-TNF α. II. Functional analysis. *Blood* 1997;90:1458–1470.

345. Holt PG, Oliver J, Bilyk N, et al. Downregulation of the antigen presenting cell function(s) of pulmonary dendritic cells in vivo by resident alveolar macrophages. *J Exp Med* 1993;177:397–407.

346. Pavli P, Woodhams CE, Doe WF, Hume DA. Isolation and characterization of antigen-presenting dendritic cells from the mouse intestinal lamina propria. *Immunology* 1990;70:40–47.

347. Hume DA, Robinson AP, MacPherson GG, Gordon S. The mononuclear phagocyte system of the mouse defined by immunohistochemical localization of antigen F4/80. Relationship between macrophages, Langerhans cells, reticular cells, and dendritic cells in lymphoid and hematopoietic organs. *J Exp Med* 1983;158:1522–1536.

348. Lee S-H, Starkey PM, Gordon S. Quantitative analysis of total macrophage content in adult mouse tissues. *J Exp Med* 1985;161:475–489.

349. Wilders MM, Sminia T, Plesch BEC, Drexhage HA, Welte-Vreden EF, Meuwissen SGM. Large mononuclear Ia-positive veiled cells in Peyer's patches. II. Localization in rat Peyer's patches. *Immunology* 1983;48:461–467.

350. Wilders MM, Drexhage HA, Weltevreden EF, Mullink H, Duijvestijn A, Meuwissen SGM. Large mononuclear Ia-positive veiled cells in Peyer's patches. I. Isolation and characterization in rat, guinea-pig and pig. *Immunology* 1983;48:453–460.

351. Barclay AN, Mayrhofer G. Bone marrow origin of Ia-positive cells in the medulla of rat thymus. *J Exp Med* 1981;153:1666–1671.

352. Guillemot FP, Oliver PD, Peault BM, LeDourain NM. Cells expressing Ia antigen in the avian thymus. *J Exp Med* 1984;160:1803–1819.

353. Wong TW, Klinkert WEF, Bowers WE. Immunological properties of thymus cell subpopulations: Rat dendritic cells are potent accessory cells and stimulators in a mixed leukocyte culture. *Immunobiology* 1982;160:413–423.

354. Crowley M, Inaba K, Witmer-Pack M, Steinman RM. The cell surface of mouse dendritic cells: FACS analyses of dendritic cells from different tissues including thymus. *Cell Immunol* 1989;118:108–125.

355. Beaulieu S, Landry D, Bergeron D, Cohen EA, Montplaisir S. An improved method for purifying human thymic dendritic cells. *J Immunol Methods* 1995;180:225–236.

356. Matzinger P, Guerder S. Does T-cell tolerance require a dedicated antigen-presenting cell? *Nature* 1989;338:74–76.

357. Inaba M, Inaba K, Hosono M, Kumamoto T, Ishida T, Muramatsu S, et al. Distinct mechanisms of neonatal tolerance induced by dendritic cells and thymic B cells. *J Exp Med* 1991;173:549–559.

358. Mazda O, Watanabe Y, Gyotoku J-I, Katsura Y. Requirement of dendritic cells and B cells in the clonal deletion of Mls-reactive T cells in the thymus. *J Exp Med* 1991;173:539–547.

359. Jenkinson EJ, Anderson G, Owen JJT. Studies on T cell maturation on defined thymic stromal cell populations in vitro. *J Exp Med* 1992;176:845–853.

360. Zal T, Volkmann A, Stockinger B. Mechanisms of tolerance induction in major histocompatibility complex class II-restricted T cells specific for a blood-borne self-antigen. *J Exp Med* 1994;180:2089–2099.

361. Volkmann A, Zal T, Stockinger B. Antigen-presenting cells in thymus that can negatively select MHC class II–restricted T cells recognizing a circulating self antigen. *J Immunol* 1997;158:693–706.

362. Brocker T, Karjalainen K. Targeted expression of MHC class II molecules demonstrates that dendritic cells can induce negative but no positive selection of thymocytes in vivo. *J Exp Med* 1997;185:541–550.

363. Laufer TM, DeKoning J, Markowitz JS, Lo D, Glimcher LH. Unopposed positive selection and autoreactivity in mice expressing class II MHC only on thymic cortex. *Nature* 1996;383:81–85.

364. Suss G, Shortman K. A subclass of dendritic cells kills CD4 T cells via Fas/Fas-ligand induced apoptosis. *J Exp Med* 1996;183:1789–1796.

365. Boog CJP, Kast WM, Timmers HTM, Boes J, De Waal LP, Melief CJM. Abolition of specific immune response defect by immunization with dendritic cells. *Nature* 1985;318:59–62.

366. Rocha B, von Boehmer H. Peripheral selection of the T cell repertoire. *Science* 1991;251:1225–1228.

367. Zheng L, Fisher G, Miller RE, Peschon J, Lynch DH, Lenardo MJ. Induction of apoptosis in mature T cells by tumor necrosis factor. *Nature* 1995;377:348–351.

368. Singer GG, Abbas AK. The Fas antigen is involved in peripheral but not thymic deletion of T lymphocytes in T cell receptor transgenic mice. *Immunology* 1996;1:365–371.

369. Parijs LV, Ibraghimov A, Abbas AK. The roles of costimulation and fas in T cell apoptosis and peripheral tolerance. *Immunology* 1996;4:321–328.

370. Kurts C, Heath WR, Carbone FR, Allison J, Miller JFAP, Kosaka H. Constitutive class I-restricted exogenous presentation of self antigens in vivo. *J Exp Med* 1996;184:923–930.

371. Kurts C, Kosaka H, Carbone FR, Miller JFAP, Heath WR. Class I–restricted cross-presentation of exogenous self antigens leads to deletion of autoreactive CD8+ T cells. *J Exp Med* 1997;186:239–245.

372. Tang A, Amagai M, Granger LG, Stanley JR, Udey MC. Adhesion of epidermal Langerhans cells to keratinocytes mediated by E-cadherin. *Nature* 1993;361:82–85.

373. Strunk D, Egger C, Leitner G, Hanau D, Stingl G. A skin homing molecule defines the Langerhans cells progenitor in human peripheral blood. *J Exp Med* 1997;185:1131–1136.

374. Strobl H, Riedl E, Scheinecker C, Bello-Fernandez C, Pickl WF, Rappersberger K, et al. TGF-β1 promotes in vitro development of dendritic cells from CD34+ hemopoietic progenitors. *J Immunol* 1996;157:1499–1507.

375. Borkowski TA, Letterio JJ, Farr AG, Udey MC. A role for endogenous transforming growth factor 1 in Langerhans cell biology: The skin of transforming growth factor 1 null mice is devoid of epidermal Langerhans cells. *J Exp Med* 1996;184:2417–2422.

376. Ardavin C, Wu L, Li C, Shortman K. Thymic dendritic cells and T cells develop simultaneously in the thymus from a common precursor population. *Nature* 1993;362:761–763.

377. Wu L, Li C-L, Shortman K. Thymic dendritic cell precursors: Relationship to the T lymphocyte lineage and phenotype of the dendritic cell progeny. *J Exp Med* 1996;184:903–911.

378. Vremec D, Zorbas M, Scollay R, et al. The surface phenotype of dendritic cells purified from mouse thymus and spleen: Investigation of the CD8 expression by a subpopulation of dendritic cells. *J Exp Med* 1992;176:47–58.

379. Grouard G, Rissoan M-C, Filgueira L, Durand I, Banchereau J, Liu Y-J. The enigmatic plasmacytoid T cells develop into dendritic cells with IL-3 and CD40-ligand. *J Exp Med* 1997;185:1101–1111.

380. Starzl TE, Demetris AJ, Trucco M, et al. Chimerism and donor specific nonreactivity 27 to 29 years after kidney allotransplantation. *Transplantation* 1993;55:1272–1277.

381. Qian S, Demetris AJ, Murase N, Rao AS, Fung JJ, Starzl TE. Murine liver allograft transplantation: Tolerance and donor cell chimerism. *Hepatology* 1994;19:916–924.

382. Starzl TE, Demetris AJ, Murase N, Thomson AW, Trucco M, Ricordi C. Cell chimerism permitted by immunosuppressive drugs is the basis of organ transplant acceptance and tolerance. *Immunol Today* 1993;14:326–332.

383. Enk A, Katz SI. Early molecular events in the induction phase contact sensitivity. *Proc Natl Acad Sci U S A* 1992;89:1398–1402.

384. Enk AH, Saloga J, Becker D, Mohamadzadeh M, Knop J. Induction of hapten-specific tolerance by interleukin-10 in vivo. *J Exp Med* 1994;179:1397–1402.

385. Growx H, Bigler M, de Vries JE, Roncarolo M-G. Interleukin-10 induces a long-term antigen-specific anergic state in human CD4+ T cells. *J Exp Med* 1996;184:19–29.

386. Berg DJ, Leach MW, Kuhn R, et al. Interleukin 10 but not interleukin 4 is a natural suppressant of cutaneous inflammatory responses. *J Exp Med* 1995;182:99–108.

387. Thomas R, Davis LS, Lipsky PE. Rheumatoid synovium is enriched in mature antigen-presenting dendritic cells. *J Immunol* 1994;152:2613–2623.

388. Zvaifler NJ, Steinman RM, Kaplan G, Lau LL, Rivelis M. Identification of immunostimulatory dendritic cells in the synovial effusions of patients with rheumatoid arthritis. *J Clin Invest* 1985;76:789–800.

389. Nestle FO, Turka LA, Nickoloff BJ. Characterization of dermal dendritic cells in psoriasis. Autostimulation of T lymphocytes and induction of Th1 type cytokines. *J Clin Invest* 1994.

390. Kaufman DL, Clare-Salzler M, Tian J, et al. Spontaneous loss of T-cell tolerance to glutamic acid decarboxylase in murine insulin-dependent diabetes. *Nature* 1993;366:69–72.

391. Tisch R, Yang X-Y, Singer SM, Libiau RS, Fugger L, McDevitt HO. Immune response to glutamic acid decarboxylase correlates with insulitis in non-obese diabetic mice. *Nature* 1993;366:72–75.

392. Kaplan G, Walsh G, Guido LS, et al. Novel responses of human skin to intradermal recombinant granulocyte/macrophage-colony-stimulating factor: Langerhans cell recruitment, keratinocyte growth, and enhanced wound healing. *J Exp Med* 1992;175:1717–1728.

393. Tao M-H, Levy R. Idiotype/granulocyte-macrophage colony-stimulating factor fusion protein as a vaccine for B-cell lymphoma. *Nature* 1993;362:755–758.

394. Dranoff G, Jaffee E, Lazenby A, et al. Vaccination with irradiated tumor cells engineered to secrete murine granulocyte-macrophate colony-stimulating factor stimulates potent, specific, and long-lasting anti-tumor immunity. *Proc Natl Acad Sci U S A* 1993;90:3539–3543.

395. Pardoll DM. Paracrine cytokine adjuvants in cancer immunotherapy. *Annu Rev Immunol* 1995;13:399–415.

396. Doe B, Selby M, Barnett S, Baenziger J, Walker CM. Induction of cytotoxic T lymphocytes by intramuscular immunization with plasmid DNA is facilitated by bone marrow-derived cells. *Proc Natl Acad Sci U S A* 1996;93:8578–8583.

397. Corr M, Lee DJ, Carson DA, Tighe H. Gene vaccination with naked plasmid DNA: Mechanism of CTL priming. *J Exp Med* 1996;184:1555–1560.

398. Ulmer JB, Deck RR, DeWitt CM, Donnelly JJ, Liu MA. Generation of MHC class I–restricted T lymphocytes by expression of a viral protein in muscle cells: Antigen presentation by non-muscle cells. *Immunology* 1996;89:59–67.

399. Condon C, Watkins SC, Celluzzi CM, Thompson K, Falo Jr. DNA-based immunization by in vivo transfection of dendritic cells. *Nature Med* 1996;2:1122–1128.

400. Casares S, Inaba K, Brumeanu T, Steinman RM, Bona CA. Antigen presentation by dendritic cells following immunization with DNA encoding a class II–restricted viral epitope. *J Exp Med* 1997;186:1481–1486.

401. Fossum S, Rolstad B. The roles of interdigitating cells and natural killer cells in the rapid rejection of allogeneic lymphocytes. *Eur J Immunol* 1986;16:440–450.

402. Gabrilovich DI, Chen HI, Girgis KR, et al. Production of vascular endothelial growth factor by human tumors inhibits the functional maturation of dendritic cells. *Nature Med* 1996;2:1096–1103.

403. Steinman RM. Dendritic cells and immune-based therapies. *Exp Hematol* 1996;24:859–862.

404. Mayordomo JI, Zorina T, Storkus WJ, et al. Bone marrow–derived dendritic cells serve as potent adjuvants for peptide-based antitumor vaccines. *Stem Cells* 1997;15:94–103.

405. Bronte V, Carroll MW, Goletz TJW, et al. Antigen expression by dendritic cells correlates with the therapeutic effectiveness of a model recombinant poxvirus tumor vaccine. *Proc Natl Acad Sci U S A* 1997;94:3183–3188.

406. Alijagic S, Moller P, Artuc M, Jurgovsky K, Czarnetzki BM, Schadendorf D. Dendritic cells generated from peripheral blood transfected with human tyrosinase induce specific T cell activation. *Eur J Immunol* 1995;25:3100

407. Szabolcs P, Gallardo HF, Ciocon D, Sadelain M, Young JW. Retrovirally transduced human dendritic cells express a normal phenotype and potent T cell stimulatory capacity. *Blood* 1997;90:2160–2167.

408. Wood GS, Warner NL, Warnke RA. Anti–Leu-3/T4 antibodies react with cells of monocyte/macrophage and Langerhans lineage. *J Immunol* 1983;131:212–216.

409. Bhardwaj N, Friedman SM, Cole BC, Nisanian AJ. Dendritic cells are potent antigen-presenting cells for microbial superantigens. *J Exp Med* 1992;175:267–273.

410. Leonard R, Zagury D, Desportes I, Bernard J, Zacury J-F, Gallo RC. Cytopathic effect of human immunodeficiency virus in T4 cells is linked to the last stage of virus infection. *Proc Natl Acad Sci U S A* 1988;85:3570–3574.

411. Klatzmann D, Barré-Sinoussi F, Nugeyre MT, et al. Selective tropism of lymphadenopathy associated virus (LAV) for helper-inducer T lymphocytes. *Science* 1984;225:59–63.

412. Cameron PU, Freudenthal PS, Barker JM, Gezelter S, Inaba K, Steinman RM. Dendritic cells exposed to human immunodeficiency virus type-1 transmit a vigorous cytopathic infection to CD4+ T cells. *Science* 1992;257:383–387.

413. Cameron PU, Pope M, Gezelter S, Steinman RM. Infection and apoptotic cell death of CD4+ T cells during an immune response to HIV-1 pulsed dendritic cells. *AIDS Res Hum Retrovir* 1994;10:61–71.

414. Weissman D, Barker TD, Fauci AS. The efficiency of acute infection of CD4+ T cells is markedly enhanced in the setting of antigen-specific immune activation. *J Exp Med* 1996;183:687–692.

415. Tenner Racz K, Racz P, Schmidt H, et al. Immunohistochemical, electron microscopic and in situ hybridization evidence for the involvement of lymphatics in the spread of HIV-1. *AIDS* 1988;2:299–309.

416. Cameron PU, Dawkins RL, Armstrong JA, Bonifacio E. Western blot profiles, lymph node ultrastructure and viral expression in HIV-infected patients: A correlative study. *Clin Exp Immunol* 1987;68:465–478.

417. Pomerantz RJ, de la Monte SM, Donegan SP, et al. Human immunodeficiency virus (HIV) infection of the uterine cervix. *Ann Intern Med* 1988;108:321–327.

418. Nuovo GJ, Forde A, MacConnell P, Fahrenwald R. In situ detection of PCR-amplified HIV-1 nucleic acids and tumour necrosis factor cDNA in cervical tissues. *Am J Pathol* 1993;143:40–48.

419. Miller CJ, Alexander NJ, Vogel P, Anderson J, Marx PA. Mechanism of genital transmission of SIV: A hypothesis based on transmission studies and the location of SIV in the genital tract of chronically infected female rhesus macaques. *J Med Primatol* 1992;21:64–68.

420. Spira AI, Marx PA, Patterson BK, et al. Cellular targets of infection and route of viral dissemination following an intravaginal inoculation of SIV into rhesus macaques. *J Exp Med* 1996;183:215–225.

421. Miller CJ, Alexander NJ, Sutjipto S, et al. Genital mucosal transmission of simian immunodeficiency virus: Animal model for heterosexual transmission of human immunodeficiency virus. *J Virol* 1989;63:4277–4284.

422. Koup RA, Safrit JT, Yunzhen C, et al. Temporal association of cellular immune responses with the initial control of viremia in primary human immunodeficiency virus type 1 syndrome. *J Virol* 1994;68:4650–4655.

423. Borrow P, Lewicki H, Hanh BH, Shaw GM, Oldstone MB. Virus-specific CD8+ cytotoxic T-lymphocyte activity associated with control of viremia in primary human immunodeficiency virus type 1 infection. *J Virol* 1994;68:6103–6110.

424. Cocchi F, DeVico AL, Garzino-Demo A, Arya SK, Gallo RC, Lusso P. Identification of RANTES, MIP-1 α and MIP-1 β as the major HIV-suppressive factors produced by CD8+ T cells. *Science* 1996;270:1811–1816.

425. Ho DD, Neumann AU, Perelson AS, Chen W, Leonard JM, Markowitz M. Rapid turnover of plasma virions and CD4 lymphocytes in HIV-1 infection. *Nature* 1995;373:123–126.

426. Wei X, Ghosh SK, Taylor ME, Johnson VA, Emini EA, Deutsch P, et al. Viral dynamics in human immunodeficiency virus type 1 infection. *Nature* 1995;373:117–122.

Fundamental Immunology, Fourth Edition,
edited by William E. Paul
Lippincott–Raven Publishers, Philadelphia © 1999.

CHAPTER 17

Natural Killer Cells

Wayne M. Yokoyama

Definition of NK Cells
NK-Cell Recognition of Targets
The NK Gene Complex
Role of NK Cells in Host Defense and Immunoregulation
NK Cells and Maternal–Fetal Interactions
NK-Cell Development
Clinical Relevance of NK Cells
Acknowledgment
References

Natural killer (NK) cells belong to the lymphoid lineage and therefore should be considered as the third major lymphocyte population. Initial studies of NK cells concentrated on their ability to kill tumor cells, but like other lymphocytes, NK cells are now appreciated as having a broader role in host defense against invading pathogens, especially in the earliest phases of host immune responses. They also regulate the subsequent development of specific immunity through cytokine secretion. Consistent with their apparent role in innate host immune responses, phylogenetic studies have demonstrated that many vertebrates, including fish, possess cells that display spontaneous cytotoxicity against certain targets (1). Noncytotoxic histocompatibility reactions reminiscent of NK-cell specificity have even been described in a type of marine sponge (2), suggesting that the NK-cell system evolved before the specific immune system. In this chapter, the salient features and biology of these important lymphocytes will be reviewed. We will define NK cells by comparing them to T cells and lymphokine-activated killer (LAK) cells, summarize current efforts to understand their target recognition systems with particular emphasis on their major histocompatibility complex (MHC) class I–specific receptors, describe the NK gene complex, discuss the role of NK cells in biologic responses, and consider the current status of NK-cell development, before concluding with remarks on the clinical relevance of NK cells.

DEFINITION OF NK CELLS

The initial definitions of NK cells stemmed from their capacity to spontaneously kill certain tumor targets (3–6). This natural killing ability did not require prior deliberate immunization of the host with the target cells, and the current assay to detect natural killing is notable for its simplicity. Most often an NK-sensitive target is labeled by incubation with sodium [^{51}Cr] chromate; the radiolabel is trapped intracellularly, and free ^{51}Cr is washed from the cells (7). The prototypical NK-sensitive tumor target for mouse NK cells is yeast artificial chromosome (YAC)-1, a thymoma derived from Moloney virus–infected A strain mice. For human NK cells, the standard tumor target is K562, a cell line derived from an erythroleukemic lineage. In microtiter plates, a constant number of radiolabeled targets is incubated either alone (spontaneous), with detergent (maximum), or with varying numbers of effector cells (experimental). The latter is expressed as effector-to-target ratios (E:T). Ratios of less than 10:1 frequently produce maximal killing by enriched, activated NK cells, whereas unfractionated, freshly isolated peripheral blood or splenocyte preparations require ratios of more than 100:1. Although a small amount of label is released spontaneously, much larger amounts are released into the supernatant when membrane integrity is disrupted by the killing process that is mediated by the exocytosis of lysosomal granules containing a pore-forming protein (perforin), serine proteases (granzymes), and other enzymes. The released label is not reused. After a 4-hour incubation, cell-free supernatants are harvested and radioactivity determined in a gamma counter. Assay variations include target labeling with fluorescent dyes and measuring target

W. M. Yokoyama: Howard Hughes Medical Institute, Rheumatology Division, Department of Medicine, Washington University School of Medicine, St. Louis, Missouri 63110.

cell lysis by release of the dye into the supernatant with a fluorescent microplate reader. Alternatively, the release of granule enzymes can be determined by conversion of an appropriate substrate. In most experiments, the data are represented according to a standard formula:

$$\% \text{ Specific Cytotoxicity} = 100 \times \left[\frac{(\text{Experimental cpm} - \text{spontaneous cpm})}{(\text{Maximum cpm} - \text{spontaneous cpm})} \right]$$

Morphologically, NK cells are usually large lymphocytes containing azurophilic granules (8). This description was formerly used to define NK cells and served as the basis for separation of NK cells by density gradient centrifugation (9). However, the large granular lymphocyte (LGL) morphology is not invariably associated with natural killing because small, agranular lymphocytes may demonstrate similar cytolytic activity (10). Moreover, the description is not specific because activated cytotoxic T-lymphocytes (CTLs) can display the LGL morphology (11). It is thus not surprising that density gradient separation results in relatively poor enrichment of NK cells. Thus, the LGL characteristic was once synonymous with NK cells but has since fallen out of favor.

Recent studies have provided strong evidence that NK cells belong to the lymphocyte lineage (discussed in detail below). NK cells more closely resemble T cells than B cells because neither T nor NK cells express surface immunoglobulin (sIg), and they share expression of many cell surface molecules and functional attributes, including effector mechanisms (Table 1). Indeed, before the molecular description of T cells (i.e., as cells that express the T-cell receptor [TCR]–CD3 complex), NK cells were frequently confused with T cells. Because detailed examination has shown that T and NK cells constitute distinct lymphocyte lineages, it is first useful to compare and contrast these two lymphocyte populations before concluding with a definition of NK cells.

NK Cells Versus T Cells

Several cell surface molecules are expressed by both NK and T cells (Table 1) (12,13), and their similar lytic capacities result in difficulty in distinguishing between these two populations. Under certain conditions, even cloned CTL lines otherwise demonstrating exquisite specificity for an allo-MHC class I molecule, for example, may kill a broader panel of targets, including NK-sensitive tar-

TABLE 1. *Similarities and pertinent differences between NK and T cells*

	NK cells	MHC class I–restricted CD8+ T cells
General		
Large granular lymphocyte morphology	Usually	+ (activated)
Presence in athymic or recombinase-deficient rodents	+	–
Cell surface molecules		
TCR/CD3 complex	–	+
Cytoplasmic CD3 components	+	+
CD2	+	+
CD3ζ (surface)	+	+
FcεRIγ	+	+
CD5	–	+
CD8	Sometimes	+
CD11a (LFA-1α)	+	+
CD11b (Mac-1α)	+	–
CD11c (p150α)	+	+
CD16	+ (FcγRIIIA)	– (except early thymocytes)
CD18 (β2 integrin)	+	+
CD28	+	+
CD45 (B220 in mouse)	+	–
CD56 (human)	+ (human)	–
CD57 (human)	+ (human)	+/–
CD69	+ (activated)	+ (activated)
CD94 (human)	+	+/–
NKG2 (human)	+	–
Heat stable antigen (J11d) (rodent)	-	+ (immature)
IL-2Rβ	+ (constitutive)	+ (activated)
2B4 (mouse)	+	+ (activated)
NKR-P1 (rodent)	+	Small subset
Ly-49 (rodent)	+ (overlapping subsets)	Small subset
Asialo-GM₁ (rodent)	+	+/–
KIR (p58, NKB1/p70, NKAT, p140) (human)	+	Small subset
gp49B1 (mouse)	+	–
Functions		
Cytokine production	+	+
Target lysis (granule exocytosis, Fas)	+	+
MHC class I recognition	+	+
Effect of MHC class I on target on killing	Inhibit	Required

gets such as YAC-1 or K562 (11,14,15). This promiscuous cytotoxicity (also known as non–MHC-restricted killing) of CTLs resembles natural killing and is indicative of the similarities between NK cells and T cells.

Although the biochemical pathways for NK-cell activation are not well understood, both NK and T cells appear to kill targets by similar mechanisms (16). NK cells and CTLs contain cytotoxic granules with similar components, such as perforin, a complement component-related molecule, and granzymes (serine proteases). Both cell types release their granule components upon activation, whereby Ca^{2+}-dependent polymerization of perforin results in perforation of the target cell plasma membrane through which granzymes enter and mediate apoptosis. Consistent with this granule exocytosis model and the requirement for both molecules in inducing target lysis and apoptosis, recent studies have demonstrated that CTL and NK-cell lytic activity was abolished in mice with a targeted null mutation in either the perforin or granzyme B gene (17–20). Although perforin is a single molecular entity, the granzymes constitute a family of related molecules that are selectively expressed in CTLs or NK cells, implying more complexity than is currently appreciated (21). CTLs also may induce perforin-independent target cell apoptotic changes by expressing Fas ligand that can trigger apoptosis when it binds and cross-links Fas on the target (22). Recent evidence suggests that activated NK cells also can express Fas ligand that can induce apoptosis by Fas-expressing targets (23–26). However, the relative contribution of this pathway to natural killing of typical NK-sensitive targets has not been elucidated. Nevertheless, NK cells and T cells use similar mechanisms for inducing target cell lysis.

NK cells also produce cytokines that are similarly produced and secreted by T cells (27). NK cells are major producers of interferon (IFN)-γ, tumor necrosis factor (TNF)-α, and the hematopoietic colony stimulating factors (CSFs) granulocyte-macrophage (GM)-CSF and interleukin (IL)-3. These cytokines may be released when NK cells are exposed to cells (i.e., tumor targets and cytokines such as IL-2 and IL-12) or by ligation of cell surface receptors (i.e., FcγRIII) (27). Also, NK and T cells express receptors for multiple cytokines, especially IL-2, IL-12, and TNF-α that may influence their function.

Despite these similarities and the resultant confusion, mature NK cells are not T cells (Table 1) (28). NK cells do not require a thymus for development and are normal in athymic nude mice. NK cells do not express the T-cell antigen receptor (TCR) on the cell surface. Indeed, NK cells do not produce mature transcripts for TCR chains and do not rearrange TCR genes (29,30). Mice with the *scid* mutation or targeted mutations in the RAG-1 and RAG-2 genes lack TCR gene rearrangements and mature T cells but possess NK cells with apparently normal function (31–34). Full functional expression of the TCR requires coexpression of the CD3 complex, composed of the CD3 δ, γ, ε, and ζ polypeptide chains (35). Several CD3 components may be found in the cytoplasm of NK cells, particularly immature NK cells, but they are not displayed on the cell surface (36). NK cells may express the CD3 ζ chain, but it is expressed on the cell surface in association with the transmembrane form of the CD16 (FcγRIIIA in humans) molecule instead of the TCR–CD3 complex (37,38). [However, CD16 is more commonly associated with homodimers of the γ chain of the high-affinity Fc receptor for IgE (FcεRI) (39)]. Thus, NK cells do not require a normal thymus or recombinase machinery for development and do not express the TCR-CD3 complex on their plasma membranes, clearly distinguishing NK from T cells.

Several other lymphoid cell surface molecules are absent on NK cells. The CD5 (Ly-1) molecule is found on almost all T cells but not on NK cells (13,28). Although subsets of thymocytes and mature T cells may express CD1, CD4, and the heat-stable antigen (HSA, recognized by monoclonal antibody [mAb] J11d), NK cells express neither these molecules nor sIg, CD19, MHC class II, nor other molecules that are expressed by B cells. Conversely, NK cells express B220, an isoform of mouse CD45 (CD45R), which is often used as a B cell–specific marker, suggesting that CD19 rather than B220 is more reliable as an indicator of the B-cell lineage (40).

Human NK cells selectively express several molecules that are useful markers, such as CD56. Although it is also found on neural tissues and some tumors, CD56 is not expressed by other hematopoietic cells or lymphocytes (less than 5% of peripheral blood T cells) (41–43). This 140-kDa molecule is derived from alternative splicing of the gene encoding neural cell adhesion molecule (NCAM) involved in nervous system development and cell–cell interactions (44,45). CD56 is composed of five Ig-like and two fibronectin type III domains, and may be involved in adhesion between NK cells and their targets (46), but this function is controversial. Curiously, mouse CD56 is not reliable as an NK-cell specific marker, suggesting that its functional role on NK cells is not conserved. The CD57 (HNK-1, Leu-7) determinant is less useful in discriminating NK cells from other cells even though it was originally thought to be NK cell specific (12,13). Although it is present on most NK cells, it is also expressed by significant numbers of T and B cells, as well as monocytes. Like CD56, CD57 is expressed on neural tissues but is less well understood. Thus, CD56 is particularly useful as a pan–NK-cell marker in humans.

A relatively specific human and mouse NK-cell surface molecule is the CD16 (FcγRIII) molecule. Although CD16 is expressed on neutrophils and macrophages, it is not expressed by other lymphocytes (47,48), except in the earliest stages of thymocyte development (49). The CD16 molecule is responsible for antibody-dependent cellular cytotoxicity (ADCC) and is discussed in greater detail below.

The murine NK1.1, Ly-49, and 2B4 molecules; human killer inhibitory receptors (KIRs, also known as p58, NKB1, p70, p140, p50, and NKAT); and CD94 and NKG2 molecules are selectively and constitutively expressed by NK cells. Although these molecules are also expressed by small subsets of T cells, they are relatively NK cell specific, especially when conventional TCR–CD3+ T cells are excluded. They appear to play important roles in NK-cell specificity because of their functional activity in natural killing, as discussed in greater detail below. The NK1.1 (NKR-P1C) molecule is especially important as a marker on mouse NK cells in the C57BL strains (28). In fluorescence-activated cell sorting (FACS) experiments, the NK1.1+ fraction contained all of the natural killing activity in the spleen (50). In vivo administration of the anti-NK1.1 mAb PK136 [HB-191 from the American Type Culture Collection (ATCC)] abrogated natural killing but did not affect humoral or T cell–mediated immune responses (51). Unfortunately, the readily available mAb PK136 recognizes an epitope on NK1.1 that is confined to C57BL/6, C57BL/10, and a few other strains (Table 2). It does not recognize the NK1.1 allele in other strains such as BALB/c (52). However NK1.1+ congenic strains such as BALB-B6-*Cmv1r* now exist in which the C57BL/6 allele of NK1.1 has been transferred to the BALB/c background (Table 2). Recently, the mAb DX5 has been produced, which recognizes a molecule that is coexpressed on CD3– NK1.1+ cells (J.H. Phillips, L.L. Lanier, personal communication). In addition, the antigen is

TABLE 2. *Strain reactivity of mAb PK136*

NK1.1+ strains	NK1.1− strains
C57BL/6 and congenic strains	A/J
C57BL/10 and congenic strains	AKR/J
C57BR/cdJ	BALB/c and congenic strains
C58/J	C3HeB/FeJ
CE/J	DBA/2J
NZB/B1NJ	NOD/LtJ
NZW/LacJ	129/J
ST/bJ	
BALB.B6-*Cmv1ʳ*	

Adapted with permission from Koo and Peppard (52), which was based on elimination of natural killing by antibody and complement treatment. Expression was confirmed and extended by flow cytometry on IL-2–activated NK cells (unpublished observations, A.H. Idris and W.M. Yokoyama). Expression on NK cells from SJL/J and C57L/J is controversial. MAb PK136 reactivity generally corresponds to consolidation of inbred strains belonging to the four different RFLP variants identified by a MusNKR-P1 cDNA probe (125) into two groups.

expressed on small populations of splenocytes in NK1.1⁻ strains, consistent with identification of NK cells in all strains. Although the molecule recognized by this mAb and its function remain unknown, this mAb appears to be NK cell specific and may prove to be useful in identifying NK cells, especially in mouse strains that do not express the NK1.1 epitope. It may also be useful for depletion of NK cells. Nevertheless, the NK1.1 molecule is currently the most specific serologic marker of CD3⁻ NK cells in strains that express the epitope.

The glycolipid determinant asialo-GM1 is expressed by most if not all murine NK cells and a subpopulation of T cells (53–55). Although the functional significance of this molecule is unknown, polyclonal rabbit anti–asialo-GM₁ is frequently used to deplete NK cells in vitro and in vivo. In more recent studies, the anti-NK1.1 mAb PK136 has succeeded anti–asialo-GM₁ for this purpose because of the availability of a defined mAb and its more restricted reactivity with NK cells (28,50–52). However, because mAb PK136 can only be used in mice expressing the allelic form of the NK1.1 antigen (Table 2) (52), anti–asialo-GM₁ remains a useful agent to deplete NK cells in other strains.

Finally, in an important functional distinction with CD8⁺ MHC class I–restricted T cells, NK cells do not require the presence of MHC class I molecules on their targets for lysis. Indeed, NK cells kill more efficiently when their targets lack MHC class I expression. This phenomenon is also significant because it is a focus of current research into the molecular basis for natural killing and is described in greater detail in a later section of this chapter.

NK Cells and LAK Cells

Both NK cells and T cells display enhanced target killing upon exposure to cytokines. Natural killing of tumor targets can be enhanced in vitro by treating NK cells with IFN-α/β or γ (5,6,56). A similar phenomenon occurs in vivo when mice are injected with polyinosinic-polycytidylic acid (poly I:C) or bacterial preparations, such as heat-killed *Corynebacterium parvum* or BCG, that trigger the production of the IFNs that in turn stimulate NK-cell activity. In a related observation, low concentrations of IL-2 also can enhance NK-cell cytolytic activity after a brief (overnight or less) in vitro exposure. Interestingly, some of these agents also may acti-

vate cloned T-cell lines to display a similar phenotype (15) related to promiscuous killing. The basis for enhanced killing has not been established, although cell proliferation appears not to be required.

Significant cellular proliferation and the generation of LAK cells occur when human or rodent lymphocytes are exposed to high concentrations of IL-2 (800 to 1,000 U/mL) in vitro (57–60). Although the majority of these cells are TCR–CD3 NK cells, TCR–CD3⁺ T cells also contribute to the stimulated population, another demonstration of the similarities between NK and T cells. To distinguish NK cells within this population and to minimize confusion, the lymphokine-activated CD3⁻ NK cells are sometimes more precisely termed "IL-2–activated NK cells." In addition to the typical NK-sensitive targets, the activated NK cells kill a broader panel of targets, including those that are generally resistant to freshly isolated NK cells, such as the murine P815 mastocytoma cell line and freshly explanted tumors. Why the IL-2–activated NK or T cells have enhanced killing potential is not known, but the activated cells do express additional receptors that can deliver stimulatory signals. Such receptors include mouse Ly-6 and CD69 and rat gp42, which are not expressed on the resting cells (61,62), raising the possibility that these activation molecules may be responsible for this broader specificity. Alternatively, enhanced killing could be due to molecules such as Fas ligand CD80 and CD54 (intracellular adhesion molecule [ICAM]-1) on targets and their appropriate counterreceptors on the effector cells (63,64).

Although NK and T cells are similar with regard to the capacity to respond to certain cytokines and the expression of cytokine receptors (27), there are important differences, especially in IL-2 responses. The IL-2 receptor (IL-2R) has been well characterized and is composed of three chains: α (p55), which binds IL-2 with low affinity, and the β (p75) and γ (p64) chains, which bind IL-2 with even lower affinity (65). These chains can be potentially associated with each other in every pair combination, but only the intermediate-affinity βγ receptor (dissociation constant [K_d] approximately ~1nM) and the high-affinity αβγ receptor (K_d ~approximately 10 pM) are capable of signaling. Resting NK cells constitutively express the IL-2Rβ chain and low levels of IL-2Rγ. Upon activation, they may upregulate α- and γ-chain expression (65). The ability of resting NK cells to proliferate in response to high concentrations of IL-2 (1,000 U/mL) is apparently due to an intermediate affinity IL-2 receptor βγ that is preferentially expressed with an excess of β chains (65,66). In contrast, resting T cells generally do not express any functional IL-2 receptors except for the γ chain at low levels, and most T cells do not respond to high concentrations of IL-2. These data demonstrate that receptors for a given cytokine may be differentially displayed, with functional consequences on NK and T cells.

The response of NK cells to high concentrations of IL-2, however, may not represent a physiologically important phenomenon. It is unknown whether such high concentrations of IL-2 can be achieved, even locally, to allow NK-cell maturation or to drive expansion during an immune response. Furthermore, NK cells tend to be early participants in immune responses, whereas the prime reservoir of IL-2 is the activated T cell that produces it somewhat later. Because NK cells are apparently normal in mice with a targeted mutation in the IL-2 gene or the IL-2Rα chain (67,68), IL-2 itself does not seem to be required for normal NK-cell development.

Despite these incongruities, NK cells are deficient in mice with a mutation in either the IL-2Rβ or IL-2Rγ chain (69–71). The discrepancies may be best understood when considering that the IL-2Rγ chain is used by receptors for other cytokines, including IL-4,

IL-7, IL-9, and IL-15 (72). In this context, it is termed the common γ subunit (γc). Although IL-4, IL-7, and IL-9 are not known to stimulate NK-cell proliferation, the recent discovery of IL-15 and its receptor (73,74) provides a compelling explanation for the findings with IL-2Rβ and γc. IL-15 does not have sequence homology with IL-2, but it has a similar short-chain four α helix bundle arrangement and two conserved intrachain disulfide linkages. Like IL-2, IL-15 can bind and stimulate cells through the IL-2Rβγ complex. However, it does not bind to IL-2Rα but instead appears to utilize a unique IL-15Rα chain to form a high-affinity complex with IL-2Rβγ (74,75). The IL-15Rα chain does not directly participate in IL-15R signaling. Its distribution is widespread and has been documented on numerous cell and tissue lineages, including NK cells. These studies suggest that NK cells may be (high-dose) IL-2 activated through IL-2Rβγ, which may be expressed in association with the IL-15Rα chain as part of an IL-15 receptor signaling complex. Moreover, a physiologic role of IL-15 in NK-cell development is directly supported by studies demonstrating that NK cells can develop from bone marrow precursors that are cultivated in IL-15 in vitro (76,77). One interpretation of these results is that the NK-cell defect in the IL-2Rβ and γc-deficient mice is due to an inability to respond to IL-15, a hypothesis that is readily testable. Therefore, IL-15 may prove to be extremely important in NK-cell development and NK cell–mediated effects.

A Molecular Definition of NK Cells?

NK cells therefore clearly resemble T cells and are apparently derived from a common progenitor cell. However, the accumulated data indicate that NK cells form a lymphocyte lineage that can be distinguished from other cells. Although this lineage separation can be made according to differential expression of certain cell surface molecules, the NK cell is still defined by function and by exclusion. These lymphocytes spontaneously lyse certain tumor cells, and, unlike other lymphocytes, NK cells do not express sIg or the TCR–CD3 complex and generally do not require MHC class I expression on targets for lysis. Therefore, the best working definition is that an NK cell is an sIg⁻, TCR–CD3⁻ lymphocyte that can mediate natural killing against targets that may lack MHC class I expression.

In the mouse, CD3⁻ NK cells frequently can be identified by surface expression of NK1.1 (in appropriate strains) and FcγRII/III (CD16), whereas in humans, NK cells generally express the CD16 and CD56 molecules. This identification, however, is imprecise. A precise definition of NK cells will require molecular characterization of their recognition systems and determination of the molecular basis for specificity in natural killing.

It is noteworthy that T cells historically were defined by a similarly awkward functional definition (thymus-derived, sIg⁻ lymphocytes responsible for cell-mediated immunity) just over 10 years ago (78). With the molecular definition of the TCR and coexpressed CD3 molecules, immunologists can now define a T cell as a cell that expresses the TCR–CD3 complex (79). The availability of molecular probes and mAbs directed against this complex provides precise definition even in pathologic tissue sections, without the need for functional analysis (cell-mediated immunity, thymus dependence). Similarly, a molecular definition will permit unequivocal identification of NK cells to define their role in normal immune responses and pathologic settings. Such a definition will require knowledge of the molecular basis for NK cell function, such as the receptors used in recognition of their targets.

NK-CELL RECOGNITION OF TARGETS

Early leads to a molecular understanding of NK-cell recognition of susceptible targets were confounded by an inability to distinguish TCR–CD3⁻ NK cells and TCR–CD3⁺ T cells. Whereas initial studies suggested that natural killing was unrelated to MHC molecules on targets, the recent substantial progress in understanding NK-cell recognition began with ascertaining the role of MHC class I molecules in natural killing.

Target Cell MHC Class I Molecules and Susceptibility to NK Cells: The "Missing-Self" Hypothesis

The NK cell, in contrast to the MHC class I–restricted CTL, does not require target cell expression of MHC class I molecules for cytotoxic effector function (Fig. 1). Kärre and colleagues demonstrated that MHC class I–deficient tumors remained susceptible to in vivo rejection, apparently mediated by NK cells (80). Subsequent analysis showed that target cell expression of MHC class I molecules appeared to have a protective effect against NK cell–mediated lysis in vitro. Preincubation of targets with IFN-γ provided relative protection against natural killing; this was attributed to enhanced MHC class I expression (81). However, other IFN-γ–mediated effects could not be excluded, and other groups found that transfected MHC class I molecules did not confer protection. Thus, the MHC class I effect on natural killing was controversial for some time.

Several groups, however, observed that MHC class I–expressing parental targets were resistant to natural killing, whereas mutants selected for absence of MHC class I expression became susceptible (Fig. 1). The parental (resistant) phenotype could be restored by reconstitution of MHC class I expression by transfected expression of molecules to correct the defect, such as β2 microglobulin (β2m) (82), or more recently with transporter associated with processing (TAP) (83,84). These studies provided definitive evidence that MHC class I expression by target cells can confer resistance to natural killing.

Studies using mice with a targeted mutation in the β2m gene corroborated the in vitro findings (85,86). Because normal expres-

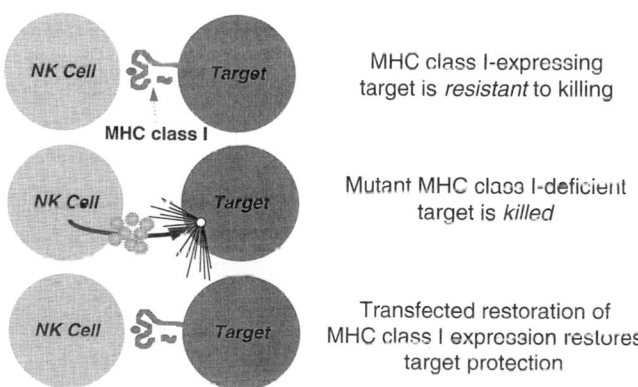

FIG. 1. MHC class I expression and susceptibility to natural killing. The parental target expressing MHC class I is generally resistant to killing. Mutants selected for absence of MHC class I expression become susceptible to killing. Resistance is restored upon correction of the expression defect, such as by transfection of cDNA encoding β2m (82).

sion of MHC class I heavy chains requires coexpression of β2m, these mice fail to express MHC class I molecules normally. Lymphoblasts from these mice are susceptible to lysis by normal NK cells. Moreover, when bone marrow from these mice was transplanted into otherwise syngeneic animals, the β2m–/– cells were rejected by the recipient (86,87). NK cells mediated this effect because injection of the anti-NK1.1 mAb abrogated rejection. This resembled hybrid resistance whereby irradiated F₁ hybrid mice reject parental bone marrow transplants (88). Hybrid resistance is mediated by host NK cells and is regulated by parental determinants that are genetically linked to the MHC region, possibly the MHC class I region, H-2D (89). One interpretation of specificity in this system is that the recipient NK cells can detect an absence of the full complement of expressed MHC determinants on the transplanted donor cells. Because parental (donor) grafts do not express the complete MHC class I repertoire expressed by the F₁ hybrid cells (which also coexpress MHC class I molecules inherited from the other parent), the parental stem cells are therefore susceptible to F₁ NK cells and are rejected. (However, other interpretations are possible.) Thus, in several distinct NK-cell recognition systems, the target cell expression of certain MHC class I molecules appears to correlate with resistance to natural killing.

Despite the aforementioned experiments showing a clear role for MHC class I molecules, several inconsistencies were noted. There is significant variability in capacity of specific MHC class I molecules to protect targets from natural killing (90). For example, transfection of H-2Kᵇ into an H-2Kᵇ loss murine hepatoma cell line did not confer resistance to natural killing by murine NK cells (91). On the other hand, several but not all transfected HLA class I molecules could protect an NK-sensitive, MHC class I–deficient cell from killing by bulk populations of human NK cells (92). The protective effect was ultimately narrowed to a residue (amino acid 74) in the α1 helix. Although some of these differences were due to experimental systems, it became apparent that NK cells recognize specific MHC class I alleles and that a specific MHC class I molecule may influence killing by only those NK cells that bear the appropriate receptors. In addition, when NK cells were grown in a manner exploiting differences in a polymorphic site of human leukocyte antigen (HLA)-C alleles, NK-cell specificity for certain HLA-C but not other HLA molecules could be demonstrated (93). This suggests that in vitro culture conditions could influence the specificity of the NK cells. Indeed, analysis of a large panel of apparently randomly selected and polyclonally activated NK-cell clones showed that human NK-cell reactivity is extremely complex, and the specificities of individual clones toward specific MHC class I alleles were difficult to easily assign to specific MHC class I alleles (94). Finally, there may be cell-specific resistance (or susceptibility) that is independent of MHC class I expression. Nevertheless, the general concept that MHC class I molecules inhibit natural killing is supported by an abundance of current information, involving human and murine NK cells in vitro and in vivo, and using different targets.

NK cells, therefore, have a different relationship to target cell MHC class I molecules than do the MHC class I-restricted CTLs. Strictly speaking, NK-cell lysis is non–MHC restricted, at least as far as MHC restriction is precisely defined for cloned T cells with an antigen-presenting cell requirement involving specific self-MHC molecules presenting a given peptide antigen (95). However, the frequently used term "non–MHC-restricted" (and its synonyms) is a poor description of the role of MHC class I in natural killing because it implies that MHC plays no role in NK-cell lysis.

Avoidance of the term "non–MHC-restricted killing" will minimize confusion concerning the relationship of target cell MHC class I molecules with NK-cell specificity and eliminate any preconceived notions about how this process operates.

The generally opposite requirements of NK and T cells for target cell MHC class I expression may be physiologically important. Several pathogens, including herpes viruses, possess mechanisms that prevent the normal expression of MHC class I molecules on infected cells, providing means to avoid MHC class I–restricted T cells (96–98). Moreover, tumorigenesis is frequently associated with alterations in MHC molecules—either mutation in structural genes or decreased expression—again leading to escape from T-cell surveillance (99–101). In either case, however, the MHC class I–deficient cells should become more susceptible to natural killing.

As initially observed and discussed by Kärre, the inherent function of NK cells thus differs from that of T cells (102). He proposed that although T cells are triggered by detection of "foreign" epitopes, NK cells are equipped to detect the absence of self epitopes. The "missing-self" hypothesis suggests that NK cells are responsible for surveying tissues for normal expression of MHC class I molecules that are usually ubiquitously expressed and that chronically inhibit NK-cell activity. If MHC class I molecules are downregulated or mutated, NK cells are released from this inhibition and the target is lysed. The host therefore may be endowed with two (T and NK cells) components of a fail-safe system, with opposing requirements for self MHC class I peptide expression. This system should eliminate pathologic processes that might otherwise evade immune responses by any alteration of MHC class I expression (either increased to avoid NK cells or decreased to avoid T cells). The missing-self hypothesis has provided a teleologic explanation for MHC class I–associated resistance, creating a framework for understanding NK-cell recognition. Several predictions of the hypothesis have been supported by studies of NK-cell receptors.

Models of MHC Class I Protection

The MHC class I–associated resistance to natural killing has provided a basis for models to explain not only resistance but also natural killing. One possibility suggested that MHC class I molecules may prevent an NK-cell activation receptor from engaging its putative target cell ligand. This target interference or masking model predicted that a single NK-cell receptor activates natural killing when it engages its putative target cell ligand (102). MHC class I molecules mask the putative target cell ligand and block its recognition by the NK-cell receptor. Although this hypothesis was initially favored because it was the simplest and the initial data did not contradict it, enthusiasm waned for several reasons. Upon exposure of NK cells to their sensitive targets, biochemical events, such as Ca²⁺ influx and inositol phosphate metabolism, are triggered (103). When NK cells are exposed to targets that are rendered resistant because of MHC class I, these early biochemical events were still triggered (104), suggesting that MHC class I molecules do not block the initial phases of target recognition. Alternatively, the effector inhibition model suggested that NK cells may be inhibited from natural killing by an NK-cell receptor that binds MHC class I on the target and delivers negative signals overriding a default pathway of activation (102). As a modification of this hypothesis, it has been suggested that NK cells express two different receptors for target cell ligands (105,106). In this two-receptor model, one receptor would be capable of interacting with a target cell ligand for activation whereas another receptor would bind target cell MHC class I molecules and inhibit activation by negative signaling (Fig. 2). Although the first two hypotheses have not been refuted, collectively the data strongly support the two-receptor model.

Activation Receptors

Upon activation by sensitive targets, NK cells display biochemical events such as Ca^{2+} flux and inositol phosphate turnover (103), leading presumably to granule exocytosis, cytokine secretion, and possibly to transcription of genes for cytokines, cytokine receptors, and granule components. These phenomena, however, have been difficult to demonstrate when NK cells are activated by targets, perhaps due to relatively weak stimulation or activation of only a subset of the effector cell population. In any event, the process has been poorly characterized to date. Additionally, NK cells can be activated to kill targets by better characterized mechanisms, including ADCC, (antibody-induced) redirected lysis, and lectin-facilitated killing, all of which appear to mimic physiologic NK-cell activation. Although the initial steps of activation (engagement of cell surface molecule) may be distinct because these pathways are not known to be physically associated with each other on the cell surface, the outcome of target killing appears to result from a final common pathway involving granule exocytosis. As the molecular basis for natural killing specificity and activation pathways become clearer, it will become possible to more precisely delineate the relationship between them.

There is yet to be a consensus on the NK-cell receptor that would be the defining counterpart of the TCR–CD3 complex and the B-cell receptor (BCR) on T and B cells, respectively. Despite intense investigation, the approaches and methodologies that yielded the molecular definition of the TCR have not yet been fully successful in unraveling the complexities of NK-cell target recognition. For example, subtractive hybridization has met with only limited success (107). Functional NK-cell tumors are rare (103). Attempts to block natural killing with mAbs against the NK cell generally have not been successful. In contrast, the ability to induce specific stimulation of NK cells through mAbs has proven to be extremely useful in identifying candidate activation receptors and in studying NK-cell activation. Several molecules have been characterized through this general approach (Table 3).

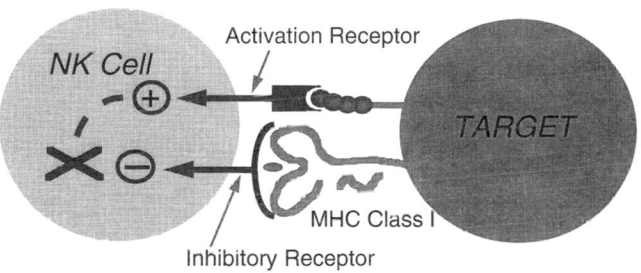

FIG. 2. A two-receptor model for natural killing. This model predicts that NK cells express two types of receptors, one for activation, presumably upon interaction with a target cell ligand. Another receptor interacts with target cell MHC class I molecules then delivers an inhibitory signal that disrupts signaling through the activation receptor.

TABLE 3. *Putative activation receptors on NK cells*

Molecule	Ligand
CD16 (FcγRIII)	Fc of IgG
NKR-P1 (NK1.1)	Carbohydrates?
LAG-3	?
2B4	?
NK-TR1	?
CD2	LFA-3
CD69	?
Ly-6	?
gp42	?
p50	MHC class I
Ly-49D	MHC class I (?)

Perhaps the best defined activation receptor is the FcγRIII (CD16) molecule, through which NK cells mediate ADCC against targets coated with IgG (108,109). Unlike other Fcγ receptor-bearing effector cells, NK cells are unique because they express only one of the known Fcγ receptors, FcγRIII, which binds the Fc portion of IgG with low affinity (48). Although recent studies suggest that NK cells may express receptors for other Ig isotypes (110), such receptors have not yet been molecularly characterized. Human NK cells express only one (huFcγRIIIA) of the two FcγRIII isoforms (48). The huFcγRIIIA molecule possesses the identical extracellular domain as the huFcγRIIIB molecule, but huFcγRIIIA is a transmembrane molecule whereas huFcγRIIIB is linked to the cell membrane via phosphatidylinositol and is expressed by neutrophils. In mice, only one FcγRIII (transmembrane) isoform is present (111), and it displays 95% sequence conservation with muFcγRII. The widely used mAb reactive with muFcγRIII, mAb 2.4G2 (ATCC HB 197), also reacts with muFcγRII (111).

The transmembrane huFcγRIIIA and muFcγRIII molecules are physically associated with the ζ chain of the TCR–CD3 complex or, more commonly, with the γ chain of the high-affinity IgE receptor (FcεRI) (39). Either associated chain is required for optimal cell surface expression of huFcγRIIIA and muFcγRIII molecules and coupling to intracellular signal transduction pathways. After cross-linking, the receptor activates biochemical events that are reminiscent of T-cell activation, including Ca^{2+} flux, metabolism of inositol phosphates, and activation of p56lck, phospholipase-Cg1, phosphatidylinositol 3-kinase, and transcription factors such as NFAT (112–116). Moreover, CD16 stimulation leads to increased transcription of cytokine genes (IFN-γ, TNF-α), receptors (IL-2Rα), and granule components (perforin, granzymes) as well as proliferation (when accompanied by an appropriate growth factor such as IL-2). Finally, NK-cell activation through CD16 leads to granule exocytosis and target killing. NK cells therefore mediate ADCC against sensitized targets and are generally activated upon cross-linking of FcγRIII.

In the laboratory, the ADCC assay is performed in essentially the same manner as the natural killing assay. The target should be relatively insensitive to spontaneous lysis by the NK cell but susceptible in the presence of an antibody that is directed to an antigen on the surface of the target. When a target is used for which there are no convenient antigens, or specific antibodies, the target could be haptenized with trinitrophenyl (TNP) groups and an anti-TNP mAb will mediate ADCC (117). If mouse antitarget mAbs are used, the mAb must be of an isotype that can bind to the CD16 molecule. There are species differences in CD16 binding to mouse IgG isotypes; mouse IgG3 binds human CD16 the most efficiently (3 > 2a

> 2b >> 1), whereas it binds mouse CD16 with the lowest affinity (2b > 2a > 1 >> 3) (48). If necessary, a rabbit antimouse Ig polyclonal antibody could be added to the mouse Ig-coated targets to mediate ADCC because rabbit IgG generally binds strongly to both human and mouse CD16. Alternatively, a polyclonal antiserum could be raised against the target cell for use in this assay. To demonstrate that the antibody induces killing by an ADCC mechanism, cytolysis should be dependent on the anti–target cell antibody and its Fc, and/or the FcγRIII receptor on the NK cell. Blockade of FcγRIII on the NK cell can be accomplished with protein A or G or anti-FcγRIII mAbs. However, if the target also expresses Fc receptors, Fab or F(ab')₂ fragments of anti-FcγRIII mAbs must be used because anti-FcγRIII can trigger through CD16 in a process termed "reverse ADCC" or "redirected lysis."

In vivo, ADCC may be useful in host defense against pathogens if antibodies are bound to their surface or to the surface of infected cells, leading to killing of the pathogen or infected cell, respectively. Inasmuch as CD16 triggers cytokine release and cytokine receptor expression, CD16 also may modulate subsequent immune responses or prepare NK cells to respond to cytokines. However, NK cells generally participate early in an immune response that contrasts with the delay required for isotype switching to IgG production. These discordant kinetics make unclear the role of ADCC in NK-cell responses in vivo.

Nevertheless, ADCC appears to be remarkably similar to natural killing and is important for the characterization of NK-cell activation pathways. However, CD16 is not required for NK-cell target recognition because CD16⁻CD3⁻ lymphocytes can still mediate natural killing (47). Moreover, CD3ζ is phosphorylated upon ligation of CD16 but not when NK cells are exposed to NK-sensitive targets. In addition, Wortmannin, a relatively selective inhibitor of phosphatidylinositol 3-kinase, blocked CD16 stimulation but not natural killing (118,119). These data strongly suggested that ADCC and natural killing use distinct proximal signaling pathways. Although it is possible that NK-cell stimulation with target cells may be much weaker than stimulation with deliberate cross-linking of CD16 with mAbs, further investigation of the γ chain of Fc receptors has shown that it is more commonly associated with CD16 on NK cells. A targeted mutation of the γ chain abrogated ADCC but not natural killing (108). Thus, despite the capacity of CD16 to activate NK cells and serve as a model for NK-cell activation, CD16 is not responsible for natural killing.

NK cells also can be activated to kill targets when a plant lectin such as concanavalin A (ConA) is added to the cytotoxicity assays. Related to this lectin-facilitated lysis phenomenon, recent studies, particularly of mouse NK cells, have made extensive use of lymphoblast targets derived from ConA-activated spleen cell preparations (120). Because the lectin is not routinely depleted (with its specific monosaccharide, α-methyl mannoside), it is possible that the natural killing of the ConA-stimulated lymphoblast targets may be due to lectin-facilitated killing. Nevertheless, these effects presumably mimic natural killing and other NK-cell activation processes in the same way that lectin-induced activation of T cells mimics TCR–CD3 stimulation. Like T-cell activation via lectins, the molecules involved in lectin-facilitated lysis by NK cells have not been clearly defined.

In the redirected lysis assay (121), by contrast, the molecules involved in NK-cell activation are often defined at the molecular level. Several mAbs can activate NK cells in this assay (Table 3), highlighting a relatively unique functional property of the recognized molecules because activation does not occur when most NK-cell surface molecules are cross-linked by specific mAbs. The redirected lysis assay is performed in a manner analogous to the ADCC assay. In the redirected lysis assay, however, the antibody binds in the opposite orientation than in ADCC (Fig. 3). The antibody reacts specifically with the NK-cell surface molecule, and its Fc portion binds to a target cell Fc receptor that is required, apparently for bridging and cross-linking effects (121). The antibody generally does not induce lysis of a target that does not express Fc receptors. In addition, prevention of antibody binding to the target cell Fc receptor inhibits redirected lysis and may be accomplished using F(ab')₂ fragments generated by pepsin cleavage. In such preparations, intact IgG and Fc fragments should be removed by protein A-sepharose chromatography, and antibody specificity should be demonstrably intact. Alternatively, IgG binding to target cell Fcγ receptor may be prevented by saturating the Fc region of the activating antibody with addition of protein A or G. If anti–target cell Fcγ receptor antibodies are used for blockade, Fc regions must be removed to prevent inadvertent activation of the ADCC phenomenon via Fc engagement of CD16 on the NK cell. Thus, when properly controlled, the redirected lysis assay has been extremely useful in identifying cell surface molecules that activate NK-cell activity.

First identified in redirected lysis assays, the original rat NKR-P1 molecule appeared to be expressed by all NK cells as a disul-

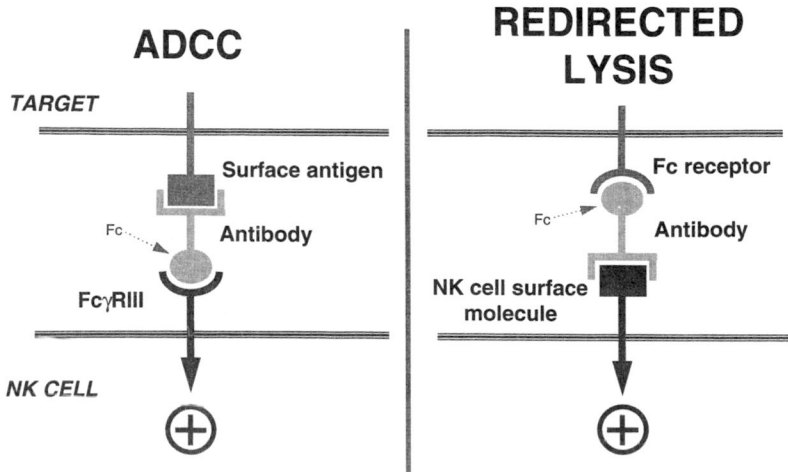

FIG. 3. Schematic comparison of ADCC and redirected lysis. Note that the antibody is in opposite orientation with respect to the NK cell.

fide-linked homodimer (60 kDa) with 30-kDa subunits (122). This expression is relatively selective, although NKR-P1 molecules are expressed by a subset of α/β T cells known as the NK1$^+$ T cell (123) (described in detail below). NKR-P1 is now known to belong to a family of molecules encoded by distinct genes displaying allelic polymorphism (124–126). The deduced molecules are type II integral membrane proteins (external carboxyl terminus) with a domain that is homologous to the C-type lectin superfamily (127). Although rat NKR-P1 isoforms have not been described in the literature, there are at least three NKR-P1 genes in mice, termed MusNKR-P1A, B, and C, with significant nucleotide homology (106). The NK1.1 molecule is encoded by MusNKR-P1C in C57BL/6 mice (126). Transcripts for all three isoforms are readily detected in Northern blots of bulk and cloned NK-cell populations (124,125,128). This suggests that individual NK cells can express multiple members of the NKR-P1 family simultaneously, but this has yet to be proven at the protein level because of a lack of appropriate serologic reagents. The C57BL/6 and BALB/c allelic forms of these genes differ from each other by 1% to 10%, correlating with known differences in restriction fragment length polymorphic (RFLP) variations detected by Southern blot analysis of genomic DNA (124,125,129). There are also strain differences in expression of these molecules with markedly lower expression on BALB/c NK cells (129). Finally, the genes encoding the mouse NKR-P1 molecules are clustered in a region of chromosome 6, termed the *NK gene complex* (NKC) (106,125).

Several studies indicated that rodent NKR-P1 molecules may activate NK cells. As mentioned, mAbs directed against the NKR-P1 molecules can trigger both freshly isolated and IL-2–activated NK cells to lyse targets in the redirected lysis assay (61,122). Moreover, anti–NKR-P1 mAbs stimulate events similar to those found after exposure of NK cells to their sensitive targets, such as inositol phosphate metabolism, Ca^{2+} flux, and granule exocytosis (122,130). Importantly, an NKR-P1 loss mutant of the rat RNK-16 cell line fails to kill certain targets even though it kills others, including YAC-1 (131). Transfection of rat NKR-P1A restored the capacity of the mutant to kill the normally sensitive IC-21 targets, consistent with the hypothesis that NKR-P1A is an NK cell activation receptor that is specific for determinants on the IC-21 target cell. Inasmuch as NKR-P1 molecules are homologous to C-type lectins, and several members of this superfamily bind to carbohydrate determinants in a Ca^{2+}-dependent manner, the ligand for NKR-P1A is presumed to be a carbohydrate. However, its precise nature is not yet known, and the downstream signaling events have not been dissected. Nevertheless, NKR-P1A was one of the first NK-cell activation receptors to be defined in natural killing of targets.

A universal acceptance of the role of NKR-P1 molecules in natural killing is prevented by several discrepancies. First, mAbs against rodent NKR-P1 molecules do not block natural killing of susceptible targets. However, this may be explained by the expression of more than one NKR-P1 family member on a single NK cell (105,106). If these molecules have overlapping specificities and the anti–NKR-P1 mAbs block only one NKR-P1 family member, the others still may be capable of activating the NK cell. Another explanation is that the antirodent NKR-P1 mAbs may be predominantly activating. The human form of NKR-P1 has been identified by complementary DNA (cDNA) cloning, but the antihuman NKR-P1 mAb conversely does not activate NK cells (132). Instead, the mAb blocks natural killing of a murine target. Second, the NKR-P1 loss mutant of RNK-16 retained the ability to kill several

targets (131). Finally, BALB/c mice possess allelic forms of the NKR-P1 genes but express them at very low levels or not at all (129). Although BALB/c NK cells can mediate natural killing against YAC-1 targets, this corroborates the observation that the NKR-P1 loss mutant can still kill YAC-1. One interpretation of these discrepant data is that NK cells use other receptors, perhaps yet to be defined isoforms of NKR-P1 or other receptors in recognition and activation of natural killing. Importantly, these results also strongly suggest that NK cells may have several different receptors for natural killing, which together could provide a polyclonal population of NK cells with the capacity to kill a panel of different targets. Nevertheless, the available data strongly support a role for NKR-P1 as an activation receptor responsible for natural killing of at least some targets.

Other candidate activation molecules include the mouse 2B4 molecule (133). It is a type I integral membrane protein that is a member of the Ig superfamily and is homologous to CD48 and CD58 (LFA-3) (134). Expression of the molecule can be correlated with spontaneous cytotoxic activity of freshly isolated spleen cells and IL-2–activated NK and T cells. The anti-2B4 mAb recognizes an allelic determinant in the same strain distribution as NK-cell reactivity with the anti-NK1.1 mAb PK136. However, 2B4 is not linked to the NKC on chromosome 6 and instead is encoded on mouse chromosome 1. Importantly, anti-2B4 enhanced killing of several targets, but apparently this was not Fc receptor dependent, suggesting that the redirected lysis mechanism was not involved and that anti-2B4 might directly activate. Alternatively, anti-2B4 mAb may block an inhibitory interaction. An understanding of its role will be aided by identification of its ligand.

Another activation molecule is LAG-3, which is highly related to CD4 in its structure. It is a type I integral membrane protein and a member of the Ig superfamily with an Ig V region–like domain and three Ig C2 region–like domains (135). Its gene colocalizes with, but is distinct from, the CD4 gene on mouse chromosome 6 (136). LAG-3 is expressed on activated T and NK cells but not on resting lymphocytes. Although there is evidence that it can bind MHC class II like CD4 (135), a null mutation in mouse LAG-3 resulted in a defect in natural killing by poly I:C-activated NK cells (137), consistent with a possible function as an activation receptor capable of target recognition. However, as with CD4 on an MHC class II–restricted T cell, LAG-3 could be a coreceptor for a putative activation receptor. These issues should be resolved by further analysis.

The NK-TR1 molecule was identified on human NK cells by Ortaldo and colleagues (138–140). In a series of studies, they first produced an mAb against K562 that blocked natural killing. Subsequently, they developed a rabbit antiidiotype antiserum against the mAb that reacted with 80-, 110-, and 150-kDa molecules on most CD56$^+$ lymphocytes and blocked binding of LGLs to targets. F(ab')$_2$ fragments of the antiserum blocked killing but could also trigger granule exocytosis and IFN-γ production. The anti-Id antiserum was used to clone a cDNA that encodes a 150-kDa molecule with several hydrophobic regions and a domain homologous to cyclophilin with apparent species conservation. When antisense constructs to NK-TR1 were expressed in a rat NK-cell line, natural killing was diminished; this could be correlated to the efficiency at which the antisense transcripts were produced. However, ADCC was not affected. Recent studies have extended these observations into human and mouse NK cells (141). These studies suggest that the NK-TR1 molecule may play a significant role in signal transduction during natural killing but not ADCC. Subsequent detailed analysis should provide insight into the role of this molecule in NK-cell function.

Several other NK cell–expressed molecules can activate cytolysis. Of these, the best characterized are the CD2, mouse CD69 and Ly-6, and rat gp42 molecules. Anti-CD2 mAbs can induce CD3⁻ NK cells to lyse targets in the redirected lysis assay (142), but CD2⁻ NK cells can still mediate natural killing (12). Similarly, mAbs against mouse CD69 and Ly-6 and rat gp42 can trigger killing (61,62). (A polyclonal anti-Ig is required for the rat anti–Ly-6 mAb to induce this effect.) CD69 is encoded in the NK gene complex and is structurally related to other NKC receptors, including NKR-P1 and Ly-49. Interestingly, CD69 expression is not confined to NK cells, and it is functionally active on a large variety of hematopoietic cells when cross-linked by anti-CD69 mAbs. Ly-6 belongs to a large family of small (15 to 18 kDa) glycosyl phosphatidylinositol (GPI) anchored molecules that can activate lymphocytes when cross-linked (143). Rat glycoprotein (gp)42 was originally identified on IL-2–activated NK cells and the rat RNK-16 NK-cell line (62). It consists of two Ig-like domains and is also GPI anchored. Anti-gp42 can activate RNK-16 but not IL-2–activated NK cells. However, the antibodies directed against CD69, Ly-6, and gp42 molecules do not trigger resting NK cells because these molecules are not expressed on freshly isolated NK cells and are expressed only after activation through other pathways. Because freshly isolated NK cells are still capable of natural killing, CD69, Ly-6, and gp42 therefore are not involved in triggering natural killing. Although their physiologic role is unknown, their activation potential, coupled with the observation that IL-2–activated NK cells can kill a broader panel of targets than freshly isolated NK cells, suggest that these molecules may contribute to this phenotype.

Emerging information on NK-cell MHC class I–specific receptors has shown that not all of these receptors are inhibitory, as described in detail below. Several examples have been described whereby the receptors have similar external domains to MHC class I–specific receptors but lack the cytoplasmic motifs that are involved in inhibition. For example, in humans, the KIRs were initially described as p58 molecules that inhibit NK-cell killing upon recognition of HLA class I molecules on targets. Interestingly, the p50 molecules contain truncations in their cytoplasmic domains when compared with the otherwise highly related p58 KIRs (144,145). Cross-linking of p50 molecules with either anti-p50 mAbs or MHC class I ligands appear to costimulate NK-cell or T-cell activation, respectively (146). Similarly, in mice, the Ly-49D and Ly-49H molecules possess cytoplasmic domains that differ from inhibitory receptors such as Ly-49A, but their external domains are much more closely related to the rest of the Ly-49 family (147). Recent studies indicate that anti–Ly-49D mAb can activate NK cells by direct cross-linking (148), although it is not clear if its presumed MHC class I ligands could trigger activation. These results suggest that one aspect of NK-cell activation may be direct stimulation (or costimulation) by MHC class I. Indeed, one illustration of this possibility is the description of rat NK-cell alloreactivity, which suggests a role for allo-MHC class I in stimulation, rather than inhibition (149).

The role of accessory molecules in NK-cell activation has been difficult to address without knowledge of the NK-cell (activation) receptor. It is currently unclear as to which molecule might be the primary trigger, analogous to the TCR, and which would play more of an accessory role. Nevertheless, NK-cell function is likely to be dependent on adhesion molecules, such as LFA-1, and molecules that modulate biochemical activation, such as CD45 (63,150–153). However, the roles of other molecules such as CD28 and CD44 on NK cells, and B7-1 on targets, remain somewhat difficult to integrate into current knowledge of NK-cell activation, even though they may prove to be very important as costimulatory molecules or play other roles (154–158).

Clearly, NK cells can be triggered through several different receptors, and it is likely that a susceptible target interacts with NK cells through multiple different receptors simultaneously. In view of these observations, some investigators support the hypothesis that activation results from signals through one or more receptors that are not necessarily NK cell specific and might be generally classified as adhesion molecules, such as CD2, integrins (LFA-1), or costimulatory molecules, including CD28 (159). Ligand binding to any one of these molecules could potentially stimulate NK cells, implying that no one receptor system is specifically involved in natural killing. On the other hand, NKR-P1 is an example of an activation receptor that fulfills an apparent recognition and activation role in natural killing and is relatively NK cell specific. Yet, NKR-P1 does not account for all natural killing; other NK cell–specific activation receptors await identification.

Inhibitory NK-Cell Receptors Specific for MHC Class I Molecules

MHC class I inhibitory receptors on NK cells have either of two general structures (160) (Fig. 4): (a) C-type lectin-like receptors that are disulfide-linked type II integral membrane proteins (extracytoplasmic carboxyl terminus). All known molecules of this type are encoded in the NK gene complex and were first described in mice. (b) Ig superfamily receptors that are type I integral membrane proteins. These molecules are encoded in a different genetic locus and were first described in humans. Ongoing studies indicate that both types of receptors are expressed on mouse and human NK cells; their relationship to each other is under intense investigation. Inasmuch as more is known about the lectin-like receptors in mice and the Ig-like receptors in humans, our discussion of these receptors will begin with description of these respective receptors before integrating information on the less well-known reciprocal receptors.

Mouse NK-Cell Receptors for MHC Class I

The Ly-49A cell surface molecule was the first inhibitory MHC class I–specific receptor on NK cells to be described at the molecular level (161). Ly-49A shares unusual structural features with NKR-P1, including cell surface expression as a disulfide-linked homodimer (44-kDa subunits), type II integral membrane orientation, and C-type lectin superfamily homology (Fig. 4). Previously termed Ly-49, it is now appreciated that the Ly-49A molecule belongs to a family of highly related molecules and that the Ly-49 and NKR-P1 families of molecules are encoded by distinct, genetically linked loci in the NK gene complex on mouse chromosome 6 (106,147,162). In contrast to NKR-P1 which is on all NK cells, Ly-49A is expressed only on a distinct subpopulation (20%) of NK cells in C57BL/6 mice, and the function of Ly-49A appears to be opposite to that of the NKR-P1 molecules.

Several lines of evidence support the hypothesis that Ly-49A is an MHC class I–specific receptor:

1. In vitro functional analysis. The Ly-49A⁺ NK-cell subset could not lyse targets expressing MHC class I molecules of H-2ᵈ and

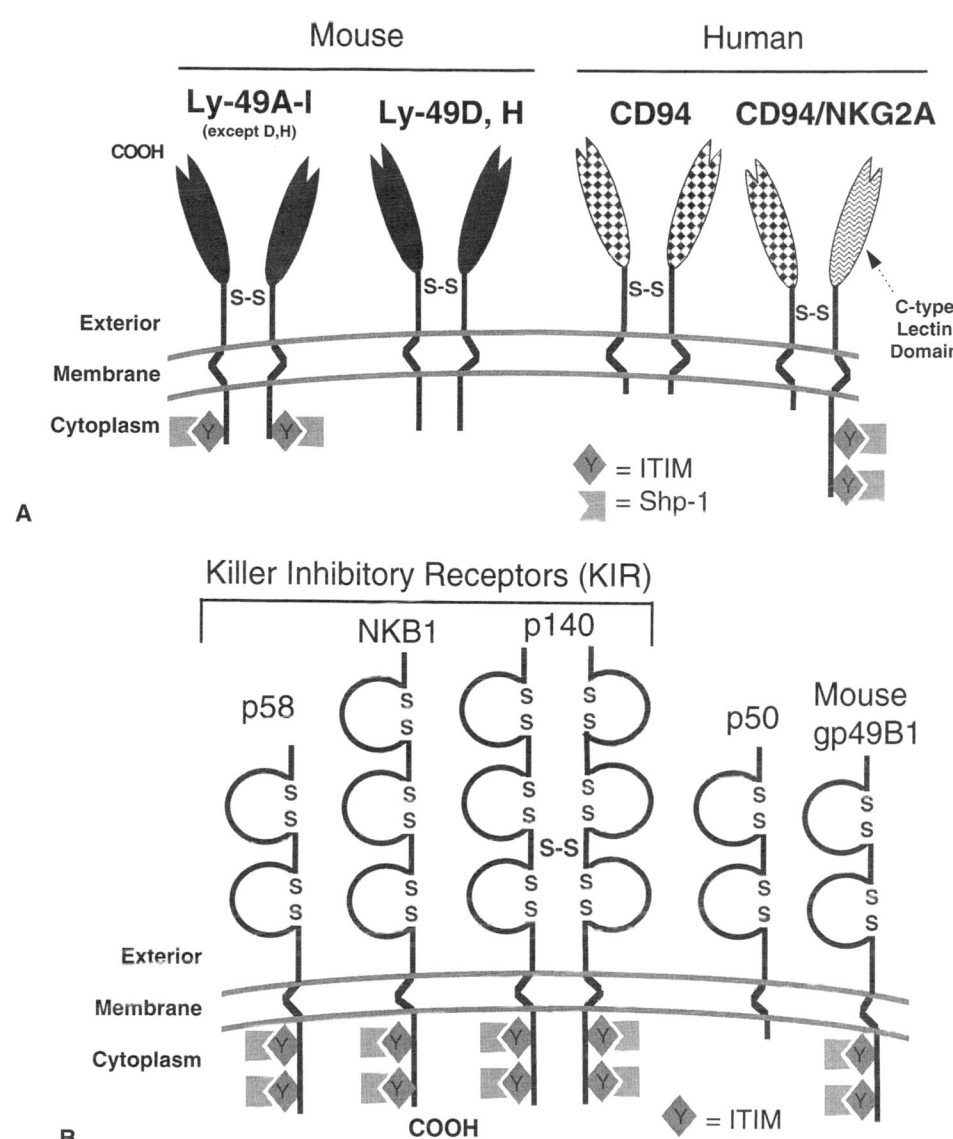

FIG. 4. MHC class I–specific receptors on NK cells. Recent evidence supports the hypothesis that mouse and human NK cells express two structural types of receptors that are specific for MHC class I molecules. These molecules provide NK cell specificity by directly interacting with MHC class I molecules on targets and modulating NK cell activity. One type of NK-cell receptors (**A**), first identified in mice, consists of lectin-like, type II transmembrane proteins that form disulfide-linked dimers. In the mouse, Ly-49 molecules form homodimers capable of binding H-2 class I molecules, irrespective of bound peptide, and deliver inhibitory signals. Ly-49D and H have different cytoplasmic domains and charged residues in transmembrane domains, and are capable of activating. Human CD94 has a small cytoplasmic domain and forms homodimers or heterodimers with NKG2 molecules to provide activation or inhibitory signals depending on whether the NKG2 molecule contains an ITIM, such as NKG2A. Mouse Ly-49 and human CD94 and NKG2 appear to be distinct receptors. The other type of receptor (**B**), first identified in humans, consist of Ig superfamily, type I integral membrane proteins with two or three Ig domains and can confer specificity for HLA-A, -B, and -C by binding to a region on the α1 helix of MHC class I. The p140 receptor is a disulfide-linked dimer. Otherwise, all are expressed as monomers. The HLA specificity appears to be influenced by bound peptides, suggesting direct contact between KIR and the peptide as well as HLA class I. A related molecule, gp49B1, is expressed on mouse NK cells. Three general types of cytoplasmic domains have been found in both lectin and Ig-SF receptors. The inhibitory receptors contain ITIM sequences. Molecules that appear to be truncated (p50), have charged residues in transmembrane domains, or alternate cytoplasmic domains (Ly-49D and Ly-49H) may stimulate NK cells, perhaps through associated signaling molecules. At the present time, it appears that all of these receptors are expressed on overlapping subsets of NK cells; an individual NK cell can express multiple receptors of either type.

H-2^k haplotypes (163–165). Transfected expression of H-2D^d rendered a susceptible target resistant to natural killing, and to ADCC by Ly-49A$^+$ NK cells (163–165). Yet the transfected target and other H-2^d or H-2^k targets remained susceptible to lysis by Ly-49A NK cells

2. Cell binding analysis. Chinese hamster ovary (CHO) cells expressing transfected Ly-49A at high levels by DNA amplification bound to targets expressing transfected H-2D^d (166). Binding only occurred when the CHO cell and the target expressed Ly-49A and its ligand, H-2D^d, respectively, by trans-

fection. Similar results were obtained in experiments using tumor cell lines constitutively expressing Ly-49A and immobilized, immunopurified MHC class I molecules (167).

3. In vivo expression analysis. As detected by two-color flow cytometry on NK1.1$^+$ cells with the anti–Ly-49A mAb A1, the level of Ly-49A expressed per NK cell was downregulated only in MHC congenic and H-2D^d-transgenic mice expressing H-2D^d or H-2D^k (168). This appeared to be due to an extracellular interaction between Ly-49A and host MHC class I because bone marrow chimeric studies demonstrated that Ly-49A expression on donor C57BL/10 (H-2b) NK cells (usually expressing normal levels of Ly-49A) was downregulated when developing in B10.A (H-2D^d) recipients (169). This was not due to negative selection because the same percentage of Ly-49A$^+$ NK cells was present and Ly-49A (as in Ly-49A$^-$) expression was restored upon in vitro cultivation (170). However, in vivo interaction with MHC class I appears to alter NK-cell activity as detailed in the NK-cell development section below.

4. Antibody blocking studies. F(ab')$_2$ fragments of mAb directed against either Ly-49A or the $\alpha1/\alpha2$ (but not the $\alpha3$ domain) of H-2D^d could reverse resistance in killing experiments (permitted lysis) and blocked adhesion in the cell binding assay (163,164,166).

5. Gene transfer analysis. Expression of a Ly-49A transgene under control of an MHC class I promoter resulted in uniform expression of Ly-49A on all NK cells (as well as other tissues) (171). Bulk populations of the transgenic NK cells were specifically inhibited by H-2D^d, whereas wild-type NK cells were not. Because most wild-type NK cells are Ly-49A (as in Ly-49A$^-$) and are not inhibited by H-2D^d, this result indicates that the genetic transfer of Ly-49A conferred the functional effect. Moreover, transfection of the Ly-49A cDNA into the RNK-16 rat NK cell line conferred an inability to lyse targets expressing H-2D^d (172). Limited studies also indicate that Ly-49A recognizes H-2D^k, as evidenced by parallel studies in killing experiments and in vivo expression analysis. Therefore, Ly-49A is an MHC class I–specific receptor for H-2D^d and H-2D^k.

The molecular interaction between Ly-49A and H-2D^d has been further characterized. Anti–Ly-49 mAbs that block interaction with MHC class I appear to bind to the putative carbohydrate recognition domain (CRD) (173). In addition, it appears that this region and a membrane-proximal 19–amino acid domain is required for interaction with MHC class I. This is consistent with conclusions based on alignment of Ly-49 molecules with the CRD of C-type lectins, indicating that the membrane-proximal region is like a stalk supporting the distal CRD. With regard to sites on MHC class I, it now appears that Ly-49A specifically engages the peptide-binding domains of the H-2D^d molecule (161). The anti-H-2D^d mAb blocking studies mentioned above support this model. Additionally, Ly-49A expression was downregulated in B10.D2^{dm1} mice (168) that express the dm1 chimeric molecule composed of the $\alpha1$ and amino-terminal half of the $\alpha2$ domain of H-2D^d with the remainder of the molecule derived from H-2L^d. Because H-2L^d did not react with Ly-49A in the killing or binding experiments, this localizes the Ly-49A binding site on H-2D^d to this region of the peptide-binding domain. Therefore, the interaction of Ly-49A with MHC class I appears to be analogous to TCR recognition of MHC class I molecules rather than the binding of CD8 molecules to the relatively invariant $\alpha3$ domains of MHC class I molecules (95).

The nature of the Ly-49A interaction with H-2D^d, however, appears to be fundamentally different from TCR–MHC class I interactions because the former appears to be independent of peptide. Correa and Raulet used several synthetic peptides (174) corresponding to H-2D^d-associated peptides previously determined by immunopurification and sequencing (175). When exogenously supplied to TAP-deficient cells containing transfected H-2D^d, these peptides stabilized H-2D^d expression and conferred resistance to killing by Ly-49A$^+$ NK cells. Analysis of natural peptides associated with H-2D^d demonstrated that there was no particular peptide fraction that enhanced protection. Moreover, Orihuela et al. showed that alanine-substituted peptides containing only the required H-2D^d anchor motifs could stabilize H-2D^d and confer resistance to killing by Ly-49A$^+$ NK cells (176). Conversely, exogenous $\beta2m$ could stabilize H-2D^d expression in the "empty" configuration and did not confer resistance. Finally, an mAb that is relatively specific for a peptide-induced conformation on H-2D^d was the only mAb capable of blocking the interaction between Ly-49A and H-2D^d. Thus, Ly-49A binds to a peptide-induced conformational determinant on H-2D^d but does not appear to bind peptides directly.

These studies on Ly-49A support basic tenets of the missing-self hypothesis (102). Regardless of peptide bound, H-2D^d molecules should interact with Ly-49A. If H-2D^d is mutated in the $\alpha1/\alpha2$ domains, peptide binding is altered or lost, or MHC class I expression is downregulated by any mechanism, Ly-49A should no longer bind and will not provide an inhibitory signal. Consequently, the target should become susceptible to lysis by those NK cells expressing Ly-49A. On the other hand, if a pathogen-encoded peptide is present without alteration in H-2D^d expression, the target will continue to be protected from lysis by Ly-49A$^+$ NK cells but should be susceptible to lysis by antigen-specific H-2D^d-restricted T cells.

If Ly-49A is important in dictating the MHC class I specificity of an NK cell, what determines the specificity of Ly-49A$^-$ NK cells? The extreme polygenism and polymorphism (multiple genes, multiple alleles) of MHC class I molecules also suggests that MHC class I receptors on NK cells should be similarly diverse. Although there is no evidence for physical rearrangements of the Ly-49 genes, diversity of the Ly-49 family exists at several levels (multiple genes, multiple alleles, alternative splicing). Nine distinct Ly-49 molecules (Ly-49A through Ly-49I) have been identified in C57BL/6 mice (147,162,177). In addition, the Ly-49 family differs among strains; thus, each gene may have multiple alleles. The Ly-49A cDNA identifies at least five different RFLP variants among common laboratory mouse strains (178). At least two allelic forms of Ly-49A and Ly-49C have been reported, and there are several Ly-49A alleles that correspond to the RFLP groups (179,180). Moreover, Ly-49 alleles may be subject to allelic exclusion (179) (covered in the NK-cell development section below). Finally, there is evidence for alternative splicing of the Ly-49 genes. The Ly-49G group contains at least two expressed sequences that differ by deletion or insertion of colinear exonic DNA segments (147), and the Ly-49D and Ly-49H transcripts also appear to be alternatively spliced (181). Thus, the Ly-49 family consists of a small but diverse repertoire of molecules.

Studies of Ly-49C/I and Ly-49G2 demonstrate similar properties to Ly-49A, providing support for a general role for the Ly-49 family in determining the specificity of NK cells. The mAb SW5E6 reacts with a disulfide-linked homodimer (54-kDa subunits) present on approximately 40% of NK cells in C57BL/6 mice (182). Initial cDNA cloning and expression analysis suggested that this mAb reacts with Ly-49C and that 5E6+ NK cells are specifically inhibited by H-2K^b (183). However, it was recently noted that mAb 5E6 is also reactive with Ly-49I, complicating previous analysis (184). The mAb 4LO3311, reactive with an antigen previously known as NK2.1, appears to be specific for Ly-49C and does not react with Ly-49I. Although a reevaluation of the specificity of Ly-49C and Ly-49I is required, the properties of these molecules resemble Ly-49A. The LGL-1 antigen is recognized by rat mAb 4D11 that reacts with a subset of murine NK cells (185) and is expressed as a disulfide-linked homodimer (87 kDa nonreduced, 40 kDa reduced) that is difficult to reduce with 2-mercaptoethanol (186). When a cDNA encoding the LGL-1 molecule was isolated from a CB.17-scid NK-cell library, it was found to be most closely related to the Ly-49G sequences from C57BL/6 mice and may represent a BALB/c allelic form of Ly-49G2 (187). The LGL-1 molecule appears to be an inhibitory receptor with specificity for H-2D^d and H-2L^d. Paradoxically, however, either anti–H-2D^d or anti–H-2L^d specific mAb alone can permit lysis of H-2^d targets (bearing both H-2D^d and H-2L^d) by Ly-49G2+ NK cells when either MHC class I ligand should have continued to provide a negative signal to the Ly-49G2+ NK cells despite blockade of recognition of the other. The data suggest that Ly-49G2 may recognize both molecules simultaneously. Regardless, available data suggest that members of the Ly-49 family, other than Ly-49A, are MHC class I-specific inhibitory receptors.

An evaluation of carbohydrate specificities of Ly-49 molecules was prompted by their structural relatedness to the C-type lectin superfamily that can bind carbohydrate determinants in a Ca^{2+}-dependent manner (127). Moreover, anti–Ly-49 mAbs that block interaction with MHC class I appear to bind to the putative carbohydrate recognition domain (173). In addition, it appears that this region and a membrane-proximal 19–amino acid domain is required for interaction with MHC class I. Indeed, Ly-49A binds complex polysaccharides; this is partially inhibited by cation chelation (188). Similar reports have been presented for Ly-49C/I (189). This suggests that Ly-49 molecules may bind to the carbohydrate determinant on MHC class I ligands. Because Asn-linked glycosylation sites are conserved among MHC class I molecules and the associated carbohydrates appear to be relatively uniform (190), this may provide a basis for Ly-49 specificities. However, the binding of Ly-49 molecules to the carbohydrate residues on MHC class I has not been directly shown. Importantly, C-type lectins may have both carbohydrate and noncarbohydrate ligands that bind to the same C-type lectin domain. For example, CD23 binds the Fc region of IgE (FcεRII) with low affinity and independent of glycosidic residues on IgE (191). Yet, CD23 specifically binds carbohydrate determinants on CD21 (192). Thus, further analysis of the carbohydrate binding of Ly-49 receptors is required, and it may be possible to block its interaction with MHC class I with exogenously added sugars regardless of whether its binding to MHC class I is carbohydrate dependent or not.

Finally, despite the general concept that MHC class I molecules inhibit NK cells, not all Ly-49 family members are inhibitory receptors. Although most contain a cytoplasmic region with a single immunoreceptor tyrosine-based inhibitory motif (ITIM) that has been implicated in negative signaling (described in detail below), Ly-49D and Ly-49H do not (147). The ligands for Ly-49D and Ly-49H are not known, but it would not be surprising if these receptors interact with MHC molecules and directly activate or costimulate NK-cell function. In support of this, an anti–Ly-49D specific mAb appears to directly stimulate NK-cell activation

(148). Moreover, rat NK-cell alloreactivity to MHC appears to be mediated by activating receptors that map to the Ly49 cluster (193). Future investigation of the Ly-49 receptors will be aided by development of serologic tools to discriminate between the individual members.

Human NK-Cell MHC Class I–Specific Receptors

A series of studies (194) on human NK-cell clones showed that the mAbs GL183 and EB6 identify serologically distinct 55-kDa or 58-kDa molecules, initially termed p58, with several features. First, they are selectively expressed by overlapping NK-cell subsets. Second, the expression of these molecules correlated with the expression of certain MHC class I alleles on targets. Third, a target susceptible to a given NK-cell clone bearing p58 molecules reactive with either mAb was made resistant by transfection of cDNAs encoding certain HLA-C molecules. Fourth, the resistant, HLA-C–transfected targets could be lysed in the presence of the appropriate anti-p58 mAbs. The mAb effect occurred with F(ab')₂ fragments, suggesting that the interaction between p58 and an HLA class I molecule on the target cell is mediating the inhibition. Thus, the p58 molecules display features consistent with a role as inhibitory human NK-cell receptors specific for MHC class I, analogous to the Ly-49A system that was being studied in parallel as described above.

Interestingly, other studies noted that NK-cell specificity could be skewed when the NK cells were grown in the presence of cells bearing allo-MHC determinants (195,196). This specificity correlated with reactivities that mapped to paired residues at positions 77 and 80 in the α1 domain of HLA-C. All known HLA-C molecules could be divided into two groups, one with Asn77-Lys80 (HLA-Cw2, -Cw4, -Cw5, and Cw6) and the other with Ser77-Asn80 (HLA-Cw1, -Cw3, -Cw7, and -Cw8). Indeed, transfection analysis showed that p58 specificity for HLA-C molecules was related to expression of the EB6 epitope for the former (specificity 1) whereas the latter was related to the GL183 epitope (specificity 2) on the NK-cell clones (195,197,198). Thus, human NK-cell receptors for HLA-C showed promiscuous specificity that was dependent on residues 77 and 80.

The NKB1 (p70) molecule is similar to the p58 molecules with regard to subset expression, and correlation of expression on NK-cell clones to specificity for HLA class I (159,199). In contrast to p58 molecules, however, NKB1 has a distinct molecular weight (70 kDa) and specificity for HLA-B. The NKB1+ clones were specifically inhibited by targets expressing transfected HLA-Bw4 molecules, and the anti-NKB1 mAb reversed the inhibition. Analysis of informative HLA-B alleles showed that this specificity was conferred by a region in the α1 domain that overlaps the area on HLA-C that is recognized by the p58 molecules (200). Moreover, absence of the N-linked glycosylation site (residue 86) in HLA-Bw4 did not change reactivity, demonstrating that carbohydrates are not required for NKB1 interaction with HLA-Bw4. Finally, HLA-A3– and -A11–specific receptors have properties similar to those of p58 and NKB1 except that they appear to be disulfide-linked dimers (p140) (201), whereas others have found that a monomeric HLA-A3–specific receptor resembling NKB1 (202). Thus, at the current time, representative alleles of all classical HLA class I loci are capable of inhibiting NK cells through p58/NKB1/p140 receptors, although it is not yet known if there are receptors reactive with each of the classical HLA class I alleles.

When the cDNAs for the p58 and NKB1 molecules, now collectively called KIRs (203), were cloned, they were surprisingly found to encode type I integral membrane proteins with Ig-like domains (204–206), rather than features similar to the Ly-49 family (Fig. 4). Subsequently, multiple cDNAs were identified and found to encode two major classes of receptors, composed of either two or three C2-type Ig-SF domains (159,194,196,207–211). The p58 molecules contain two Ig domains, whereas NKB1 (p70) possesses three Ig domains and the p140 molecules are composed of disulfide-linked monomers of the three Ig domain-type receptors. The KIR extracellular domains are homologous to human Fcα receptor and mouse gp49, a mast cell–specific molecule. Also contained in the extracellular domain are histidine-rich regions containing Zn^{2+}-binding motifs. Although these domains have been shown to bind Zn^{2+}, current data suggest that Zn^{2+} binding is not required for interaction with HLA class I (207). Most importantly, both types of KIR molecules possessed relatively long cytoplasmic domains (76 or 84 amino acids) containing two ITIM sequences that can recruit mediators capable of inhibiting cellular activation.

Subsequent analysis has provided unequivocal evidence that the KIR molecules are inhibitory HLA class I–specific receptors:

1. KIRs bind directly to HLA class I. Soluble p58-Fc fusion proteins bind to cells expressing the appropriate transfected HLA class I alleles (212,213). In addition, a soluble p58 molecule containing only the extracellular domain was shown to bind specifically to its HLA-C ligand in solution as shown by native gel electrophoresis (214).
2. Gene transfer of KIR. Vaccinia constructs containing KIR cDNAs were transiently expressed in human NK-cell clones; specificity and inhibitory function were transferred (212). Thus, KIR molecules are clearly MHC class I specific inhibitory receptors on NK cells.

Recent studies have demonstrated that residue 80 on the HLA molecule is more significant in KIR interaction than residue 77 (215–218). However, the KIR footprint on the HLA-C molecule encompasses a larger area with significant influence from residues 73, 76, and 90. Interestingly, empty HLA class I molecules can be recognized (217), but other studies indicate that KIR molecules appear to be influenced by peptides bound to the HLA molecule (219). The latter may be related to previous observations indicating bulk human NK-cell specificity for a single residue in a side pocket of HLA class I binding cleft (92). Moreover, detailed analysis with a transfection system involving a single KIR molecule supports a role for bound peptides (220). Further analysis may be required to determine if there are recognition differences among the various KIR molecules.

Molecular cloning of the KIR family also led to the identification of two domain NK-cell receptors (also known as p50) with truncated cytoplasmic domains (39 residues) that lack the ITIM (144,221) (Fig. 4). Yet, these molecules contain extracellular domains that are highly related to the extracellular domains of the KIR molecules. These molecules activate NK cells when stimulated by anti-p58 mAbs in the redirected lysis assay. Also, studies of T-cell clones that constitutively express p50 demonstrate that p50 molecules are costimulatory with concomitant activation through the TCR–CD3 complex (146). Although the role of these molecules in NK-cell activation is being evaluated, available data suggest that p50 molecules may be costimulatory receptors rather than direct activators of NK cells.

There are currently more than 20 known KIR sequences that encode polypeptides with 66% to 99% identity (159,194,196, 207–211). The relationship between the various cloned cDNAs for the KIR family of molecules is still under investigation. It is not yet clear which are allelic variants, separate gene products, or alternatively spliced forms. The relationship of these receptors to the MHC haplotype of any given individual remains to be elucidated although serologic expression of NKB1 appears unrelated to HLA haplotype (222). Nevertheless, the molecular cloning of human KIR provided significant insight into MHC class I activation and inhibitory receptors.

The discrepancy between the structures of the human KIR molecules and the Ly-49 family led to speculation that humans and mice evolved structurally distinct receptor systems to deal with missing self (223). However, it is now clear that mouse IL-2–activated NK cells express gp49B1, a type I integral membrane protein with two Ig-like domains (224,225). The gp49 molecules, now recognized as a family of three proteins, were first characterized as mast cell–specific molecules. gp49A is a monomeric transmembrane molecule without a cytoplasmic ITIM, whereas gp49B1 is an alternatively spliced product of a gene that also encodes an apparently soluble molecule (gp49B2) that is truncated proximal to the transmembrane domain (226,227). Although it has not been established that gp49B1 interacts with MHC class I and it may not represent the murine homolog of KIR molecules, gp49B1 contains an ITIM in its cytoplasmic tail that can inhibit NK-cell activity (225). In mast cells, mAb-induced cross-linking of gp49B1 inhibits activation through FcεRI (228). Thus, mouse IL-2–activated NK cells express molecules that belong to both major families of inhibitory receptors.

Reciprocally, there is also evidence that human NK cells can express lectin-like receptors. Human NK-cell clones were identified that could be inhibited by HLA class I molecules but in a p58-independent manner (229). When mAbs were produced that permitted lysis of a resistant target, these mAbs reacted with CD94, previously known to modulate NK-cell activity. CD94 is variably expressed on human NK cells (230). Immunoprecipitation analysis of ^{125}I-labeled cells showed mAb reactivity with a disulfide-linked dimer (70 kDa NR, 43 kDa R) that was previously termed Kp43. The expression of CD94 on some NK-cell clones could be correlated with the protective effect of target cell HLA-B7 molecules (229). Transfection of C1R targets with HLA-B7 protected the target from lysis by CD94^High NK-cell clones. Lysis was restored by intact anti-CD94 mAb or its F(ab′)₂ fragments, consistent with the recognition of HLA-B7 by CD94 and subsequent inhibition of cytotoxicity. In contrast, for other NK cells, CD94 engagement appeared to activate NK-cell activity (231). Thus, functional analysis of CD94 showed opposing results (activation or inhibition by specific MHC class I), depending on the NK-cell clone.

Expression cloning with anti-CD94 mAbs yielded a cDNA encoding a type II integral membrane protein with external C-type lectin domains, distantly related to NKR-P1 and Ly-49 (232). Curiously, CD94 contains a short cytoplasmic domain (seven amino acids), suggesting that it must be associated with another component to mediate its functional activity. Furthermore, anti-CD94 mAbs immunoprecipitated molecules that were not detectable from ^{125}I-labeled CD94 transfectants, despite easily detectable expression on FACS analysis with the same mAbs (233,234). When a polyclonal antiserum was made against CD94, it detected a 27-kDa species on Western blots that was not visualized in immunoprecipitates from ^{125}I-labeled NK-cell clones, suggesting that this species did not label with [125]I. Yet the anti-CD94 mAbs reacted with a 43-kDa molecule in lysates from ^{125}I-labeled NK-cell clones (233). Subsequently, the 43-kDa molecule was found to be NKG2A; it is therefore the 43-kDa molecule previously identified as Kp43 (235,236). Therefore, CD94 forms a heterodimer with NKG2A providing explanations for otherwise discrepant functional and biochemical studies.

NKG2A belongs to a small family of highly related molecules that are type II integral membrane proteins with external C-type lectin domains (237), distantly related to NKR-P1, Ly-49, and CD94. These molecules were previously identified by subtractive hybridization and are relatively NK cell specific. NKG2A and NKG2B may be alternatively spliced products of the same gene, whereas NKG2C and NKG2D are products of different genes. Although NKG2A contains an ITIM, the other known NKG2 molecules do not, possibly indicating that these molecules are involved in other NK-cell functions such as activation. In this regard, previous studies suggested that NKG2C could recognize structures on tumor targets (238). Although the CD94 molecule apparently can be expressed as a homodimer, the relevance of this molecule is presently unknown. Conversely, NKG2 molecules appear to be expressed only when complexed with another molecule such as CD94 to form CD94–NKG2 heterodimers. The specificities of these molecules are just beginning to be unraveled (239), but it seems likely that specificity and function of the heterodimers will depend on the NKG2 partner chain in the dimer. Whether CD94 can associate with other partners is not known. Therefore, human NK cells also express C-type lectin receptors (159,194,240).

Among the C-type lectin receptors, there are several notable differences between human CD94–NKG2A receptors and mouse Ly-49. First, CD94–NKG2A molecules are heterodimers, whereas Ly-49 molecules have only been described as homodimers (173,241). Second, no Ly-49 family member has been described with as short a cytoplasmic domain as CD94. Third, CD94 appears to have minimal polymorphism and may be expressed on every human NK cell, possibly as an invariant partner chain, whereas studies to date indicate that Ly-49 molecules are polymorphic and individual Ly-49 family members are expressed on overlapping subsets of NK cells. Finally, the CD94 and NKG2 molecules do not appear to be strict homologs of Ly-49. There is only distant relatedness by sequence alignment, suggesting that these molecules comprise distinct gene families. Thus, humans and mice may express both CD94–NKG2 and Ly-49 receptors, a topic of future investigation.

Although the relationship between the C-type lectin receptors and Ig-superfamily receptors has not been clearly elucidated, there may be differences among them that extend beyond their obvious structural differences. The Ly-49A molecule binds its MHC class I ligand without regard to the MHC-associated peptide (174,176), whereas KIR molecules can have peptide specificity (219,220). Evaluation of these features for the other receptors is presumably in progress.

The functional outcome (i.e., activation or inhibition) of an NK-cell target interaction appears to be dependent on the NK-cell receptors (for either activation or inhibition) and the ligands for these receptors on the target. Importantly, many of these receptors are coexpressed on individual NK cells. Unlike the BCR and TCR, there has yet to be described an NK-cell receptor that is expressed on an individual NK cell to the exclusion of other receptors. However, research in the field of NK-cell receptors is still in its early stages. Much more work is required to determine the existence of other receptors, the specific properties of the known receptors, the

relationship of these receptors to each other, and the relative contribution of each receptor to the overall specificity of individual NK cells. It is not yet clear, for example, if the two structural types of receptors could be coreceptors for each other, analogous to CD8 and TCR on the MHC class I–restricted T cell (242). Finally, the role of other accessory molecules, such as adhesion molecules and costimulatory molecules, is currently unknown with respect to these receptors. Significant progress is anticipated in this rapidly moving field.

Biochemical Mechanism of Inhibition by NK-Cell Receptors

Engagement of the Ly-49A molecule significantly influences NK-cell specificity in distinct assays of NK cytolytic function such as natural killing and ADCC; redirected lysis using anti-CD69, Ly-6, or NK1.1; and lectin-facilitated lysis (163–165). Because these activation pathways are not physically associated on the cell surface, these results suggested that Ly-49A is an inhibitory receptor. Recently, studies of Ly-49A transgenic T cells indicate inhibition of T-cell alloreactivity by Ly-49A engagement (171). Similar inhibitory effects were found with engagement of the human KIR molecules on NK cells (159,194,196,207,210,240). Moreover, KIR engagement inhibits activation through the TCR on T cells that constitutively express KIR molecules (243). Finally, early analysis of activation events in MHC class I–inhibited NK cells showed differences in signaling (244). Thus, inhibitory effects appeared to dominate over activation events, and this was thought to be secondary to negative signaling by the MHC class I–specific receptors.

Significant insight into the inhibitory mechanism was provided by studies showing that the ITIM, present in the cytoplasmic domain of CD22 and FcγRIIB and consisting of the sequence ψxYxxL (where ψ = hydrophobic), is phosphorylated upon receptor cross-linking (245,246). This leads to recruitment of the tyrosine phosphatase (SHP-1), which can antagonize the activation of tyrosine kinases by dephosphorylating a phosphorylated activation molecule. A human KIR molecule has two ITIMs separated by 24 residues. Each ITIM can be phosphorylated upon cross-linking (or tyrosine phosphatase inhibition) and can directly bind SHP-1 (247–249). In contrast, Ly-49A has only one ITIM per chain, but Ly-49 molecules are normally expressed as homodimers. Although phosphorylation of Ly-49A has only been shown to date with pervanadate (tyrosine phosphatase inhibitor) treatment, phosphopeptides representing the ITIM of Ly-49A can bind SHP-1, and engagement of Ly-49A recruits SHP-1 (172,250). In addition, the critical role of the tyrosine in the Ly-49A ITIM has been demonstrated (172). However, in mast cells, the ITIM also can bind the SH2 domain–containing inositol polyphosphate 5-phosphatase that regulates inositol phosphate metabolism (251). At the current time, the role of this enzyme in the inhibitory signaling cascade in NK cells is unknown. Nevertheless, available data strongly support an inhibitory mechanism consisting of receptor cross-linking followed by ITIM phosphorylation, and recruitment of SHP-1, and that this mechanism operates with both types of inhibitory receptors.

In studies of KIR transfectants of the human T-cell Jurkat cell line, the KIR ITIM appears to be phosphorylated by the p56[lck] tyrosine kinase (252). Although NK cells do express p56[lck], it is not yet known if this is the mechanism whereby NK cells phosphorylate all of their inhibitory receptors. The downstream mediators of the inhibitory effect are not well understood because the activation pathways in natural killing have yet to be described in detail. Nevertheless, recent studies have suggested that one major phosphoprotein differentially phosphorylated upon KIR cross-linking is pp36, which appears to be an adapter molecule that interacts with Grb2 and the phospholipase PLCγ1 (252,253). In NK cells exposed to sensitive targets, pp36 is phosphorylated; this is blocked by KIR engagement of an MHC class I ligand on the target. Moreover, a similar phosphoprotein is detected upon cross-linking of CD16 (254), providing a convenient explanation for inhibition of ADCC by MHC class I receptors. Further insight in this field will come from a dissection of the inhibitory as well as activation pathways in NK cells.

THE NK GENE COMPLEX

The NKC was first defined by the genetic linkage of the NKR-P1 and Ly-49 gene families after studies demonstrating linkage of *Ly49* to the locus controlling NK1.1 expression (178,255). By virtue of linkage to the unrelated *Prp* locus, these genes were localized to distal mouse chromosome 6 (125,178). Initial genetic mapping data were provided by strain distribution profiles in recombinant inbred mice of RFLP variants. The tight linkage was confirmed by analysis of large backcross panels, indicating less than 0.1 centiMorgan (cM) distance between *Nkrp1* and *Ly49* (256,257). Because the mouse genome is estimated to be more than 1,500 cM, the linkage between these genes seemed unlikely to be fortuitous. Although the gene families encode proteins that share several unusual features (selective NK-cell expression, disulfide-linked dimer, type II transmembrane orientation, external C-type lectin superfamily homology, polymorphism, functionally active in determining NK-cell specificity), there is no nucleotide homology between families. In addition, mapping studies indicated recombination between these loci, demonstrating separation by genetic linkage analysis. Thus, the Ly-49 and NKR-P1 families are highly related but are encoded by distinct loci; genetic linkage suggested that this genomic region may be relevant to NK-cell function.

The importance of the NKC is highlighted by its identification in mice, rats, and humans (Fig. 5). The mouse NKC lies in the midst of a chromosomal region with conservation in the linkage order of several genetic loci, indicating that the human syntenic region should be chromosome 12p13 because of the location of the human homolog of *Prp* (106,125). Subsequent localization of the human NKR-P1 and CD69 genes provided validation of this location (132,258). The similarities between the NKR-P1 and Ly-49 families also suggested that there may be additional molecules encoded within the NKC that have relevance to NK-cell function and that are structurally related. These predictions have been supported by the finding that the CD94 and NKG2 molecules (not yet identified in the mouse and thought to be distinct from Ly-49) are encoded within the human NKC (232,259,260) (Fig. 6). This may provide a means to identify mouse CD94 and NKG2 that have resisted cross-hybridization methods.

The CD69 gene is also encoded within the human and mouse NKC (258,261). Although CD69 is usually absent on resting hematopoietic cells, mitogens, such as phorbol ester and anti-CD3, induce the very rapid expression of CD69 transcripts and protein (258,261–263). The CD69 polypeptide is expressed as a disulfide-linked dimer with 28- and 32-kDa subunits. The deglycosylated peptides have identical migration on sodium dodecyl sulfate polyacrylamide gel electrophoresis (SDS-PAGE), suggesting that it is expressed as a disulfide-linked homodimer of monomers with varying degrees of glycosylation. Although the putative ligand for CD69 has not yet been identified, anti-CD69 mAb triggers several events in diverse cells, including T-cell proliferation and platelet activation (264). In the redirected lysis assay, cytolytic activity by IL-2–activated NK cells also can be triggered by anti-CD69 (61). Recent cloning of a cDNA encoding CD69 showed that it is a type II integral membrane protein belonging to the C-type lectin superfamily with approximately 20% to 25% homology to Ly-49 and NKR-P1 (258,265,266), indicating that the NKC is not restricted to genes that encode NK cell–specific molecules. CD69 differs from Ly-49 and NKR-P1 molecules by absence of a stalk domain in CD69. This has been reiterated in studies of the activation-induced C-type lectin (AICL) molecule (267). It is another type II transmembrane molecule with external C-type lectin domain that is most homologous to CD69 in sequence (35% amino acid identity), overall structure (no external stalk), and expression on hematopoietic cells that is induced upon activation. Although its function is not known, it resembles CD94 in the virtual absence (seven residues) of a cytoplasmic domain. Thus, the NKC encodes type II transmembrane C-type lectin-like molecules whose expression may be more widespread than just NK cells.

Recently, two high-resolution genetic linkage maps of the NKC were produced by analysis of large panels of backcross mice, and a physical map was produced by evaluation of YACs (257,268,269). The maps are in general agreement, validate previous genetic linkage assignments, and can be oriented to each other (Fig. 6). Based on a contig of overlapping nonchimeric YACs, and verified by multiple coverage, the 2.1-megabase physical map indicates separate clustering of the *Nkrp1* family and the *Ly49* family in two distinct regions (269). All of the known mouse NKC genes can be accounted for except Ly-49B, which lies telomeric to the *Ly49* cluster (270). Interestingly, the nonpolymorphic CD69 gene lies between *Nkrp1* and *Ly49*, despite the extensive polygenism and allelic polymorphism of both flanking gene clusters. Moreover, the NKC covers a considerable physical distance, occupying more than 1 megabase between *Nkrp1* and *Ly49*, and may extend beyond this region to encompass the murine homologs of human CD94 and NKG2.

MOUSE	RAT	HUMAN	
Ly49	rLy49	?	**Type II C-type lectin Disulfide-linked dimer**
Nkrp1	rNkrp1	NKRP1	
?	?	CD94	
?	rNkg2	NKG2	
Cd69	?	CD69	
?	?	AICL	
Cmv1	?	?	**Functionally defined**
Rmp1	?	?	
Chok	?	?	
?	Nka	?	

FIG. 5. The NKC is conserved between mouse, rat, and human genomes and contains other NK cell genes and loci.

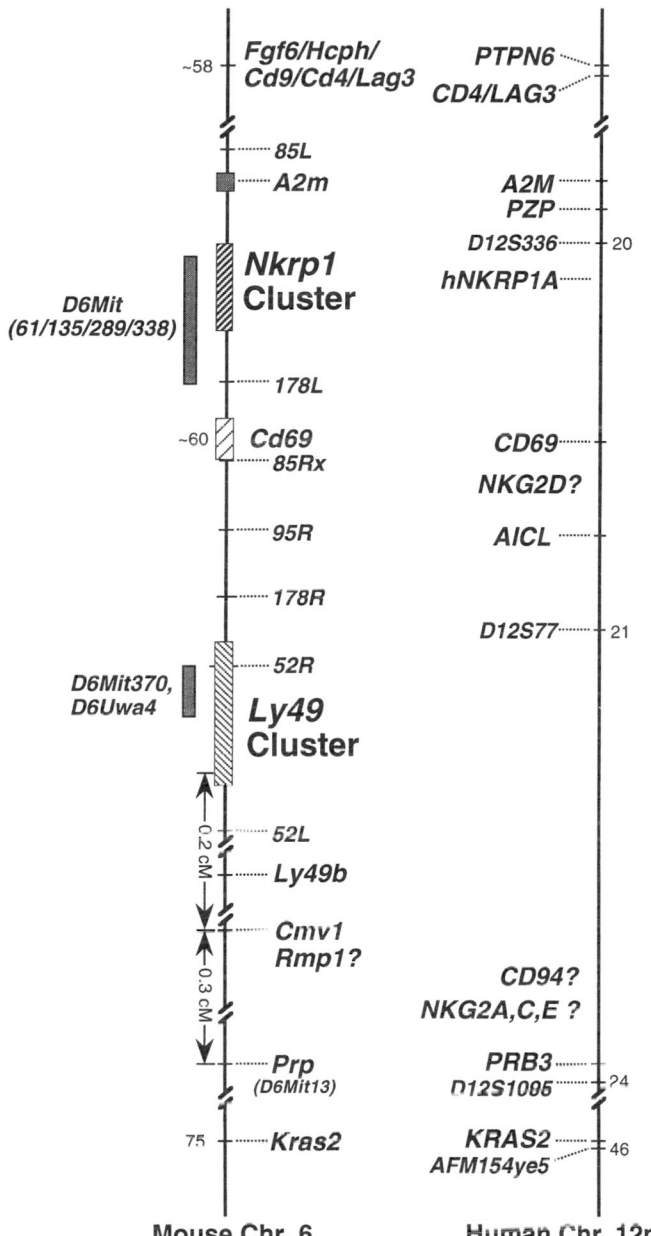

FIG. 6. Composite maps of the mouse (chromosome 6) and human (chromosome 12p) NKC. The chromosomal linkage groups (centromere-*Hcph/Cd4/Lag3*-*A2m*-*Cd69*-*Prp*-*Kras2*-telomere) and (telomere-*PTPN6*-*CD4/LAG3*-*A2M*-*CD69*-*PRB3*-*KRAS2*-centromere) facilitated alignment of the mouse and human genomic regions, respectively. However, the chromosomal orientation of the mouse interval is inverted with respect to the human. Physically mapped mouse NKC genes are shown (*shaded boxes*). The physical distance between the *Nkrp1* and *Ly49* clusters in mice is approximately 1 megabase. Additionally, the *Ly49* gene order within the *Ly49* cluster region has been determined (centromere-*Ly49e*-*Ly49d/f*-*Ly49h*-*Ly49g*-*Ly49c*-*Ly49a*-telomere) and is not shown. A genetic position for mouse *Cmv1*, determined by recombination frequencies between the indicated loci, is shown. Human NKC genes that have been precisely mapped are indicated with chromosome ticks. NKC genes that have not been precisely mapped but whose positions have been inferred by comparison of rodent and human NKCs are indicated by absence of chromosome ticks. Precise locations of other NKC-linked genes within this genomic region are not known (?). Sequence tagged site (STS) markers for the mouse and human chromosomes are also shown. Genetic map units measured in centiMorgans are indicated.

Although it has been proposed that the LAG-3 gene should be included in the NKC (137), it is genetically located in a much more distant region. Interestingly, the *Hcph* gene encoding SHP-1 is also in a nearby region, but its considerable distance currently precludes formal consideration as an NKC gene. Nevertheless, because both encode structurally distinct molecules, this raises the possibility that the NKC, like the MHC, may contain genes for molecules that are functionally related but structurally distinct (270). For example, in addition to antigen presentation (MHC) molecules, the MHC contains genes for antigen processing, peptide transport, and MHC assembly (271). In a similar way, the NKC may encode structurally distinct molecules that are important in NK-cell activity. The linked *A2m* gene encoding α2 macroglobulin and other NKC genes may be relevant in this regard.

The significance of the NKC to NK-cell function is also indicated by NK cell–mediated phenotypic traits that have been mapped to this genetic region. Genetically determined resistance to murine cytomegalovirus (MCMV) is under multigenic control with contributions from MHC and non-MHC loci. The only defined non-MHC locus, *Cmv1*, contributes to resistance to otherwise lethal MCMV infection (272). In this model, resistance is manifested by markedly lower viral replication in the spleen in resistant strains (C57BL/6) when compared to susceptible mice (BALB/c). NK cells appear to mediate resistance to MCMV because elimination of NK cells with anti-NK1.1 or anti–asialo-GM₁ antibodies abrogates resistance (273,274). Interestingly, however, *Cmv1* does not control MCMV in the liver, suggesting that NK-cell effects are tissue specific (275). Scalzo and colleagues initially localized *Cmv1* to distal chromosome 6 with linkage to the NKC (256,272). Recent mapping studies on large backcross panels support tight linkage to *Ly49* and recombination with *Nkrp1*, suggesting that *Cmv1* may encode a molecule on NK cells that is responsible for recognition of MCMV-infected cells or MCMV itself (257,268). Although the gene product may be structurally related to other members of the NKC, it is not yet clear if *Cmv1* encodes an activation or inhibitory molecule. With regard to the latter, herpes viruses contain open reading frames that encode MHC class I–like molecules (276,277) that could engage MHC class I–specific receptors and inhibit NK-cell function. Identification of the *Cmv1* gene product should provide a major advance in understanding of the role of NK cells in viral resistance.

Also localizing to the NKC is *Rmp1*, a locus encoding allelic differences in capacity of inbred mice to resist mousepox (ectromelia) in a manner that is highly reminiscent of *Cmv1* (278). Its relationship to *Cmv1* is not known. It could be identical to *Cmv1* or a tightly linked and highly related but distinct gene. In rats, NK cell–mediated allospecificity for MHC class I molecules also maps to the NKC near *Ly49*. Surprisingly, this gene, termed *Nka*, appears to encode differences that may be due to MHC-induced activation of NK cells rather than inhibition (149,193,279). This may be relevant to the capacity of certain mouse Ly-49 molecules to apparently activate NK cells (148). Finally, C57BL/6 and BALB/c NK cells have an intrinsic difference in ability to kill CHO cells even though they have equivalent capacity to kill many other tumor targets. The phenotype maps to a genetic locus, termed *Chok*, that is linked to the NKC (280). Thus, further analysis of the NKC will be revealing for not only the genes that are known (*Nkrp1*, *Ly49*, *Cd69*, *NKG2*, and *CD94*) but also for genes (*Cmv1*, *Rmp1*, *Nka*, and *Chok*) that encode phenotypic traits mediated by NK cells.

ROLE OF NK CELLS IN HOST DEFENSE AND IMMUNOREGULATION

NK Cells and Tumor Surveillance

An abundant body of literature supports the role of NK cells in resisting tumor growth and metastasis but in general, these studies utilize adoptive transfer of tumors (5). In addition, LAK cells, composed primarily of IL-2–activated TCR–CD3 NK cells, have been infused into patients with cancers refractory to conventional therapy (281). Several cases of complete remission were reported, but the treatment required intravenous administration of high doses of recombinant human IL-2 that has significant toxicity. Nevertheless, this form of immunotherapy shows some promise for effective cancer treatment.

In experimental protocols involving adoptive transfer of tumor cells into mice, NK cells appeared to eliminate more than 90% of tumor cells within the first 24 hours (282). This can be directly correlated with the level of NK-cell activity in various mouse strains as assessed in vitro with natural killing assays against the tumors. Inhibition of NK-cell activity or NK-cell depletion with antibodies abrogated tumor rejection. Also, if the cytolytic machinery of NK cells is rendered impotent by targeted mutation, tumor rejection is markedly diminished in vivo. For example, the perforin-deficient mice are unable to clear tumors (283). On the other hand, augmentation of NK-cell activity with various agents including poly I:C and *C. parvum* increases the capacity of the hosts to eliminate tumors (282). Further evaluation with experimental systems demonstrating selective NK-cell effects will build on these observations, particularly with regard to prevention of tumors.

Although inbred mice have been noted to have variability in intrinsic NK-cell activity, the genetic basis for the differences have not been fully explored. However, the development of a mouse congenic for the NKC may be useful in this regard (284). In addition, there are currently several mouse strains that are useful in analysis of NK-cell function in vivo. Mice with defects in V(D)J recombination (*scid*, RAG-1–/–, RAG-2–/–) do not have T cells that can confuse analysis, and NK cells occupy a larger percentage of the spleen (32–34). In comparison with these recombination-defective mice, several mouse strains may be useful because of defects in NK and T-cell development due to overexpression of human CD3ε (285) or human FcεRIγ (286), or a null mutation in IL-2Rβ chain (69). The beige (*bg*) mouse possesses a mutation that affects NK-cell killing capacity, but the defect is in a putative lysosomal transport protein that affects the granules of many different cell types, such that the defect is not NK cell specific (287–289). Thus, although there are no mice available with specific NK-cell deficiencies, several strains are useful in evaluating NK-cell function in vivo.

Several assays of in vivo tumor clearance are available. Tumor inoculi can be followed by monitoring long-term animal survival or lesion size if subcutaneously administered. However, T-cell immune responses may affect tumor survival, even in syngeneic hosts due to the presence of tumor specific peptides. Radiolabeled tumor cells can be followed by the lung clearance assay in which the radioactivity of the lung is an index of tumor burden. Because this assay can be performed at 4 to 48 hours after tumor inoculation, it can provide an index that is relatively confined to NK-cell responses in an unimmunized host.

In vitro natural killing assays of tumor sensitivity to NK cells may not precisely correlate with in vivo rejection of tumors (282).

Not infrequently, tumors that are relatively resistant in vitro are susceptible in vivo. One possible explanation is the relative sensitivities of the assays, although it is possible that NK cells are more efficient in vivo. Another explanation is that tumors change during cultivation in vitro; some investigators passage their tumor targets in vivo to avoid tissue culture–induced states. However, most assays of NK cells involve YAC-1 or K562 targets that are cultivated in vitro.

NK Cells and Host Defense Against Pathogenic Organisms

The role of NK cells in host defense to pathogens is highlighted by a patient with a selective deficiency in human NK cells (290). In her peripheral blood there were normal numbers of B and T cells but no detectable CD56+ cells. In vitro functional analysis demonstrated normal B and T cell responses, but there was no natural killing by her peripheral blood and it could not be stimulated by IFN. Her clinical course was dominated by frequent, recurrent episodes with uncontrolled blood-borne infections with multiple bacteria and herpes viruses, including varicella, cytomegalovirus, and herpes simplex, normally only a mucosal pathogen. In other case reports, the NK cell–deficient patients did not have a dramatic clinical course but did have problems with recurrent viral infections or clinical manifestations that have been associated with virus infections (291,292). Finally, the NK-cell compartment does not appear to be fully developed at birth as indicated by lower natural killing by cord blood lymphocytes and corroborated by studies on the ontogeny of splenic NKR-P1 expression in rodents (293,294). Interestingly, in the classic TORCH syndrome, birth defects and severe fetal anomalies are associated with maternal *Toxoplasma,* rubella, cytomegalovirus, and herpes virus infections (295). Because NK cells are generally active against these organisms, the relative immaturity of NK cells during the neonatal period may be clinically relevant. Interestingly, therefore, diminished NK-cell activity is associated with susceptibility to infection.

Abnormal NK-cell activity has been reported in patients infected with human immunodeficiency virus type 1 (HIV-1) (296). NK cells can be infected with human herpes virus 6, which induces cytopathic changes and de novo expression of CD4, a cellular receptor for HIV-1, which is not normally expressed by NK cells (297). This renders NK cells susceptible to infection by HIV-1, abrogating natural immunity. This finding provides a reasonable explanation for significantly diminished NK activity in patients with acquired immunodeficiency syndrome (AIDS) and may be another reason for opportunistic infections with organisms against which NK cells are active.

In experimental models, NK cells are significant in infections with several viruses, including eradication of MCMV as described above. However, NK cells are not effective against all viruses. For example, they have a less significant role in immune defense against influenza and lymphocytic choriomeningitis virus, even though infection can stimulate NK-cell activity (298). It is not yet known why NK cells are effective against certain pathogens and not others, but there is some evidence to suspect that there may be tissue-specific differences in dominant immune responses. Moreover, the mechanism by which NK cells mediate their antiviral effects are not clearly understood. NK cells also have activity against several other pathogens, including both Gram-negative and Gram-positive bacteria (e.g., *Listeria monocytogenes*) (299). They also have been reported to have activity against *Mycobacterium* species, fungi such as *Cryptococcus,* and protozoan parasites including *Leishmania* and *Toxoplasma.*

It should be emphasized that the NK-cell response is consistent with its perceived role in the innate immune system in tumor models and complements the specific, adaptive immune response. NK-cell activity does not require prior exposure to the pathogen or in vivo clonal expansion, in contrast to the amplified response by cells in the specific effector arm of the immune system (B and T cells). Amplification by clonal expansion requires significant time, usually days to weeks. By then a host may succumb to certain pathogenic infections. During this period, NK cells can provide an early defense system. In support of this, when antibodies are given for in vivo elimination of NK cells, the antibodies must be administered either before or within 48 hours after viral inoculation to demonstrate immune susceptibility to MCMV infection (274,300). If antibody injection is delayed, the mice remain resistant, suggesting that the NK-cell effect occurs within the first 48 hours of viral infection.

NK cells, however, are not static participants in host defense because NK cells accumulate at sites of viral replication (301,302). In addition, recent studies demonstrate a significant expansion of NK cells after repeated exposure to nonvirulent *T. gondii* in mice with a targeted mutation in β2m (303). This is associated with NK cell–mediated resistance to virulent infection. Although the predominant mechanism for this accumulation (recruitment by migration, in situ proliferation, or both) has not been elucidated, it raises the possibility that NK-cell activity can be enhanced by immunization.

Immunoregulation of NK Cells

In addition to cytotoxicity involving natural killing and ADCC that were discussed previously, NK cells produce and respond to cytokines. The pivotal role of NK-cell cytokine production in regulating specific immune responses is best demonstrated by studies examining in vivo NK-cell responses to infection and influences on T cells (299,304). Helper T cells differentiate into functional subsets, Th1 and Th2, based on their cytokine production profiles (305). Th1 cells contribute to cell-mediated immunity by producing IL-2 and IFN-γ, whereas Th2 cells secrete IL-4, IL-5, and IL-10, which regulate humoral immune responses, including Ig isotype production. In resistant hosts, the protective T-cell response to various intracellular organisms, such as *Leishmania major,* is predominantly regulated by IFN-γ, a pleiotropic cytokine that significantly influences the differentiation of naive T cells into the Th1 subset (304,306). Although IFN-γ is also produced by Th1 cells, the importance of IFN-γ from NK cells is emphasized in the timing of its production (307). Although Th1 cells produce IFN-γ several days to weeks after acute experimental challenge with pathogens, NK cells produce detectable IFN-γ within 2 days after acute infection. Thus, the characteristic early NK-cell response in host responses, e.g., IFN-γ production, appears to be a major determinant in regulating the T-cell response to intracellular pathogens.

What stimulates NK cells to produce IFN-γ? The major factor appears to be IL-12, also known as NK stimulatory factor. It is a disulfide-linked heterodimer composed of 35-kDa and 40-kDa chains derived from two separate genes (308). IL-12 is produced by B cells and by phagocytic cells, such as macrophages and neutrophils, in response to ingestion of intracellular organisms, and exposure to bacterial endotoxin. Upon infection with *Leishmania major* or *Listeria monocytogenes* (309,310), for example, host

macrophages produce IL-12, a potent inducer of IFN-γ production by NK cells in vivo and in vitro. TNF-α can augment IL-12–induced IFN-γ production, but TNF-α alone is not stimulatory (309). Importantly, this series of events appear to provide protection even in *scid* mice that lack mature T and B cells. Similar studies have been reported in mice infected with MCMV that can be controlled primarily by NK cells (311,312). Interestingly, IFN-γ control of MCMV is primarily manifested in the liver, whereas NK cell–mediated cytotoxicity predominated in the spleen, suggesting organ-specific differences in NK-cell effector mechanisms (275). In these systems, however, it remains unknown whether direct NK-cell activation by noncytokine factors is also involved. On the other hand, the NK-cell response to IL-12 can be inhibited by other cytokines. The monocyte-produced cytokine, IL-10 (also produced by Th2 cells), inhibits IFN-γ production by both murine and human NK cells (309). Finally, the IL-12 receptors on NK cells have not yet been characterized, although recent studies demonstrate that two chains (IL-12Rβ1 and IL-12Rβ2) are required for IL-12 stimulation of T cells and are differentially regulated (313). Nevertheless, NK-cell production of IFN-γ appears to be important in regulating subsequent immune responses and is itself positively and negatively regulated by other cytokines.

NK cells can regulate other components of the specific immune system. Presumably through IFN-γ, for example, NK cells are capable of regulating Ig secretion by inducing Th1 cells that promote IgG2a and IgG3 class switching (314,315). NK cells apparently produce other cytokines, including IL-1β, IL-3, IL-6, TGF-β, TNF-α, TNF-β, GM-CSF, and macrophage CSF (M-CSF), that regulate other components of the immune system (27,316–321). It must be cautioned, however, that production of certain cytokines have been generally detected in experiments using heterogeneous populations of lymphocytes enriched for NK cells. The difficulty in excluding T cells in these enriched NK-cell preparations raises the possibility that some of these cytokines may be secreted by contaminating cells. One experimental model to avoid this problem uses *scid* mice that do not have mature T cells but have normal NK-cell function (309). It also will be informative to examine cloned NK-cell lines for cytokine production. In this regard, there is no evidence (as yet) that NK cells can be divided into immunoregulatory subsets based on cytokine production, as have T-helper cells. Nevertheless, it is clear that NK cells have the potential to significantly influence immune responses.

Conversely, differentiation to the Th2 phenotype appears to be regulated by IL-4, produced by a cell early in an immune response. Interestingly, this cell appears to resemble NK cells at several levels but is a TCR–CD3+ T cell (123). In mice, the NK1+ T cell expresses an invariant Vα14–Jα281 TCR chain usually in combination with Vβ8, Vβ2, or Vβ7 chains. A similar T-cell population has been described in humans. Like mouse NK cells, NK1+ T cells express molecules that are otherwise NK cell selective such as NK1.1 and the Ly-49 family of molecules. Despite expression of CD4, however, these T cells are CD1 restricted and require CD1 expression for development in contrast to NK cells (322,323). Similar to the counterpart NK cells that produce IFN-γ early in the immune response that can drive differentiation of T-helper cells to the Th1 phenotype, NK1+ T cells may induce differentiation to the Th2 phenotype by the early production of IL-4 in response to TCR engagement (324,325). Although the role of NK1.1 and inhibitory influence of Ly-49 molecules have been less well studied, further examination of these cells may reveal a closer relationship to NK cells than is currently appreciated.

NK-Cell Regulation of Hematopoiesis: Hybrid Resistance

NK cells regulate the ability of bone marrow grafts to repopulate irradiated recipients. For example, NK cells in otherwise syngeneic irradiated mice reject the bone marrow grafts from β2m-deficient mice (86,87). This provides a clear-cut example and insight into a related phenomenon, termed hybrid resistance (88). In this transplantation model that violates the classical laws of solid tissue transplantation, irradiated F_1 hybrid mice reject bone marrow donated by either inbred parent. That hybrid resistance is mediated by host NK cells (326) is supported by studies demonstrating that *scid* mice exhibit the phenomenon, and elimination of NK cells by administration of anti–NK cell antibodies abrogates rejection of parental bone marrow (327,328). The process appears to involve specific recognition of parental determinants encoded in a locus linked to the H-2D region (89). Investigations of a C57BL/6 mouse transgenic for H-2D^d and the dm1 chimeric mouse strongly suggest that the parental determinant can be an MHC class I molecule such as H-2D^d itself (329,330).

Several observations, however, seemed to indicate that other parental determinants, termed hematopoietic histocompatiblity-1 (Hh-1), are involved in hybrid resistance (88). Extensive studies of MHC-congenic mice demonstrated that the specificity of rejection could not be grouped according to conventional MHC class I haplotypes of donor or recipient. Moreover, there is significant overlap between the specificities. Although analyses of MHC recombinant mice indicated that putative Hh-1 genes could be separated from the H-2D subregion and reside in a more centromeric region (89), this is based on a small number of recombinant mice in which it is not clear that the H-2D gene is intact. To further complicate the analysis of hybrid resistance, rat NK cells have allospecificity for MHC molecules that appears to be due to activation rather than inhibitory receptors (149,193,279). Therefore, the issue of hybrid resistance has been extremely difficult to understand.

As another approach to characterize NK-cell specificity for these parental determinants, mAbs were produced to identify NK cells that mediate rejection of specific donor marrow (182). Injection of the anti–Ly-49C/I specific mAb SW5E6 abrogated rejection of bone marrow cells expressing H-2^d but not H-2^b, suggesting that Ly-49 molecules may be involved in specificity of hybrid resistance. Furthermore, transgenic expression of Ly-49A prevented rejection of H-2^d bone marrow grafts in an allogeneic transplantation system (171). These observations provide an additional complication because previous analyses of parental determinants were performed without knowledge of the specificities of the putative receptors (89). In the case of Ly-49 molecules, this consideration may be significant because these receptors have promiscuous specificity, involving MHC class I molecules that would not have been grouped otherwise, such as H-2D^d and H-2D^k but not H-2D^b for Ly-49A (331,332). Furthermore, it is not yet known if the different allelic forms of individual Ly-49 family members have different specificities. Nevertheless, the Ly-49 family is implicated in the specificity of NK cells in hybrid resistance.

Recent studies tend to support the interpretation that hybrid resistance is due to missing self. The specificity of Ly-49C/I was investigated using an in vitro model of hybrid resistance. In this analysis, IL-2–activated NK cells are used in a killing assay against ConA-stimulated lymphoblasts (120). Although it is possible that this killing represents lectin-facilitated killing, the assay has been useful in determining the specificity of NK cells for MHC class I.

The Bennett and Kumar group has determined that 5E6$^+$ NK cells from F_1 hybrid mice kill H-2^d but not H-2^b lymphoblasts, consistent with the in vivo rejection data using mAb SW5E6 administration (182,183). However, in light of the new data indicating that this mAb recognizes two Ly-49 molecules (Ly-49C and Ly-49I), further specificity analysis will be required (184). Nevertheless, hybrid resistance appears to be explained by the in vivo reactivity of NK cells against bone marrow precursors that do not express the full complement of MHC class I molecules expressed in the host.

The mechanism of rejection is not clearly understood. NK cells could directly kill stem cells in a manner consistent with natural killing (88,333). However, granzyme B is not required for hybrid resistance even though it is required for natural killing (334,335). Moreover, perforin and Fas-mediated cytotoxicity are apparently not involved in a related experimental model, rejection of allogeneic bone marrow grafts (336), suggesting that the NK-cell influence on bone marrow engraftment is not due to direct cytolysis of stem cells. Alternatively, NK cells may indirectly affect hematopoiesis by production of cytokines, such as CSFs, that influence the growth and differentiation of hematopoietic cells (319,320). In support of a role for cytokines, treatment with granulocyte CSF abrogates hybrid resistance (337), but the mechanism for protection is unclear. Thus, further evaluation of hybrid resistance is necessary.

Therefore, the ability of NK cells to modulate bone marrow engraftment represents an important experimental system for dissection of NK-cell specificity and recognition. It is also an area of obvious clinical importance with the wider acceptance of bone marrow transplantation for treatment of human disease.

NK CELLS AND MATERNAL–FETAL INTERACTIONS

One emerging area of interest is the circumstantial evidence of a role for NK cells in maternal–fetal interactions (338). Several observations are related.

NK cells accumulate in the uterus, near the fetal trophoblast layer, in all mammalian species examined thus far (339). Initially described as granulated metrial gland cells, they are now recognized as maternal and bone marrow–derived NK cells. The cells display typical NK-cell markers and appear to be activated because of the expression of activation markers such as CD69. Functional analysis suggest that these cells behave like conventional NK cells.

The nonclassical MHC class I molecule, HLA-G, is expressed on extravillous trophoblasts (340). In contrast, other MHC class I or II molecules are not expressed there. Although a murine ortholog has not been identified, recently an MHC class Ib molecule has been described with selective expression in the mouse blastocyst and placenta, suggesting that it might be a functional analog of HLA-G (341). Although HLA-G can bind peptides and possibly present antigen to HLA-G–restricted T cells (342–344), HLA-G expression also can inhibit human NK cells via interaction with KIRs, CD94–NKG2A, or other undefined molecules (343,345–348). Interestingly, HLA-G appears to completely inhibit natural killing by polyclonal NK-cell populations from many different donors (348). This raises the possibility that fetal trophoblast expression of HLA-G molecules inhibits maternal NK cells, providing protection from rejection. On the other hand, mice with MHC class I deficiencies due to targeted mutations in the β2m or TAP genes apparently show normal development (349,350). However, HLA-G expression may not have the same requirements for assembly and transport to the cell surface as classical MHC class I molecules; HLA-G can be expressed on cells that lack TAP expression (351). Moreover, alternatively spliced HLA-G transcripts have been described (352) that encode soluble molecules with apparent functional activity. Therefore, sudies of NK cells and HLA-G may be relevant to maternal tolerance to the fetus.

NK-CELL DEVELOPMENT

Several model systems demonstrated that NK cells are bone marrow derived (353,354). Early studies on bone marrow chimeric mice indicated that transplanted bone marrow cells from mice with low or high splenic NK-cell activity could transfer the respective activity regardless of the intrinsic capability of the irradiated host (355). The bone-seeking radioisotope, strontium 89, selectively ablates the bone marrow and affects NK-cell activity (356), apparently because of the capacity of other hematopoietic elements to develop in splenic foci (357). Similar findings have been reported in mice treated with estradiol, which affects bone marrow development, and congenitally osteopetrotic mice (358). More recently, NK cells have been shown to develop from hematopoietic stem cells; transfer of small numbers of these precursors gives rise to donor-originated hematopoietic lineages and NK cells in the host (359,360). Importantly, myeloid progenitors and NK-cell progenitors appeared to be distinct.

Although the subsequent lymphocyte lineage separation is not clearly understood, studies of the *Ikaros* gene has provided evidence that this gene is pivotally involved in the initiation of lymphocyte lineage differentiation. *Ikaros* encodes a family of zinc finger transcription factors that belong to the Krüppel family of DNA-binding proteins and that are selectively expressed in lymphocytes (361). Targeted mutation in this gene by homologous recombination resulted in complete deficiency of B, T, and NK cells (362). Importantly, because the mice were developmentally normal and all other hematopoietic lineages appeared intact, this strongly suggests that NK cells are derived from lymphocyte precursors.

Inasmuch as NK cells more closely resemble T cells than B cells, it is not surprising that NK and T cells may arise from an immediate common progenitor cell. However, NK cells are apparently normal in mice with mutations in the recombinase machinery, i.e., *scid* and targeted mutations in RAG-1 or RAG-2 (32–34). NK cells are also apparently normal in athymic nude mice (294), demonstrating that a functional thymus is not required for NK-cell development. Yet, in day 14.5 fetal thymus, a subpopulation of cells expresses FcγRIII that is normally not expressed on T cells (49). These FcγRIII+ cells did not express NK1.1 in vivo but did so upon in vitro cultivation. The cells did not have evidence for TCR gene rearrangements and displayed natural killing capacity against YAC-1 targets that resembled adult peripheral NK cells. Interestingly, intrathymic transfer of these cells resulted in T- and NK-cell development of donor origin. Although these experiments have not yet been repeated with cloned populations of cells, these technically difficult studies have been supported by in vitro analysis of the development of human NK cells that can develop from a CD56+CD5− subpopulation of CD3−CD4−CD8− (triple negative, TN) fetal thymocytes when placed in murine fetal thymic organ cultures (FTOCs) (363). NK cells develop from a population of CD34Bright TN cells, whereas only T cells developed from CD34Dim

cells under identical conditions. Furthermore, similar results were obtained in analysis of the in vitro effects of IL-2 and IL-15 on IL-2Rβ chain–expressing, TCR–CD3− cells in fetal murine thymocyte cultures (364). Such thymocytes appear to differentiate into TCR–CD3+ cells when transferred to alymphoid thymic lobes, whereas culture in cell suspension with IL-15 resulted in TCR–CD3 NK-cell development. High concentrations of IL-2 or IL-15 supported preferential development of NK cells. These studies strongly support the thesis that NK and T cells share a common progenitor cell immediately before terminal lineage separation.

Several additional lines of evidence support the existence of a bipotential T- and NK-cell progenitor stage. In early development, both NK cells and T cells appear to originate from hematopoietic progenitors in the developing fetal liver. Human fetal liver contains cells that resemble mature NK cells and lack surface expression of CD3 components (36). These cells display an NK-like killing profile, NK-cell surface molecules, and germline configuration of TCR genes. Yet, these cells resemble mature T cells because they express CD3γ, δ, and ε components in their cytoplasm, suggesting that once the TCR genes have been productively rearranged, they may be readily expressible on the cell surface. In contrast, adult human NK cells express only cytoplasmic CD3ε, perhaps due to selective loss of the other CD3 components (365). Similar cells have recently been reported in mice (366). Fetal liver precursors may migrate to the thymus where they appear to still have potential to develop into either T cells or NK cells (49,367–369). Moreover, granzyme gene expression can be detected in most immature (fetal) mouse thymocytes, whereas granzymes are usually only detected in mature cytotoxic lymphocytes (370). Finally, the transgenic overexpression of the human CD3ε gene results in selective deficiency in both T and NK development, consistent with the expression of CD3 components in the NK/T-cell progenitor (285). However, CD3ε expression is not required for NK-cell development because NK cells appear normal in mice with a CD3ε targeted mutation (371). Consistent results have been reported in studies of transgenes that overexpress the γ chain of FcεRI (286). Taken together, the available data strongly support a close developmental relationship between NK and T cells.

The role of adhesion receptors in NK-cell development requires further examination. Nevertheless, in studies of bone marrow chimeric mice, Mac-1 (αM, β1 integrin) expression is not generally found on donor bone marrow cells that express NK1.1 but can be shown to be expressed on splenic NK cells (372). In in vitro experiments, Mac-1+ bone marrow cells respond to IL-2 and produce cytolytic NK cells (373). Thus, integrins such as Mac-1 may either mark a developmental stage or be involved in homing of NK cells to tissue sites.

The role of cytokines in NK-cell development is also still under investigation. Although NK cells can proliferate in high concentrations of IL-2 in vitro, targeted mutations in either IL-2 or IL-2Rα chain appear not to affect NK-cell development (67,68). On the other hand, targeted mutation in either IL-2Rβ or IL-2Rγ (γc) results in NK-cell deficiency as well as other defects in the immune system (69–71). However, the IL-7 receptor uses similar components, yet IL-7Rα–deficient mice have normal NK cells (374). One explanation for these observations points to IL-15 because it uses the IL-2Rβ and IL-2Rγ chains as components in a signaling receptor (73,74). Indeed, murine and human NK cells can be derived from bone marrow cells or fetal thymocytes cultivated in vitro with IL-15 (76,77,364). Disruption of the downstream pathway of IL-2R signaling should result in NK-cell defects as well. For example, JAK1 and JAK3 are Janus family tyrosine kinases involved in IL-2 receptor signaling. Disruption of JAK3 results in NK-cell deficiency (among other defects) (375), but NK-cell development in other signal transduction–defective mice has not been fully evaluated.

NK cells clearly respond to other cytokines, but these responses may be primarily during effector responses rather than during development. Disruption of such cytokines (IL-12) or cytokine pathways (IL-12R or STAT4, JAK2, Tyk2) might not result in any developmental NK-cell defect and instead affect effector function. However, recent studies indicate that IL-12 can induce the development of human NKR-P1A$^+$ CD56$^-$ progenitor cells into typical NKR-P1A$^+$ CD56$^-$ NK cells (376). Thus, further analysis is required to provide details on the role of cytokines in NK-cell development.

With regard to NK-cell development and expression of NK-cell receptors, the NKR-P1 molecule is useful in analysis of NK-cell ontogeny in rodents. Although the anti-NK1.1 (MusNKR-P1C) mAb PK136 does not stain tissue sections, NK1.1 expression by flow cytometry has been detected in putative precursor cells from fetal thymus (49). Studies of splenic NKR-P1 expression show an age-related increase in percentage of positive cells from birth until several weeks of age in rats (294), confirming that neonatal animals do not have fully functional NK cells at birth, as indicated by clinical susceptibility to infections and lowered natural killing in cord blood (293,295).

In terms of the developmental expression of Ly-49 molecules, they are expressed on murine NK cells that develop in bone marrow cultures exposed to IL-15 (76). Interestingly, however, murine NK cells that develop in vitro from fetal sources often do not express any member of the Ly-49 family (366,377), consistent with previous observations that murine NK cell clones derived by other methods also have this phenotype (128). Among several different explanations, the currently favored hypothesis is that the NK cells that do not express any Ly-49 member may represent immature cells that are better capable of in vitro growth. This interpretation is supported by the in vivo observations that expression of Ly-49 molecules is a relatively late maturation event in ontogeny (378). Studies of other NK-cell receptors are apparently underway and should yield interesting results because these molecules define NK-cell specificity.

MHC class I molecules appear to influence NK-cell development. With respect to Ly-49 expression, there is clear evidence that these molecules interact with their MHC class I ligands in vivo (168,169). In H-2D^d or H-2D^k mice, the expression of Ly-49A is downregulated, but Ly-49A$^+$ cells are not deleted unlike the negative selection of T cells that bear self-reactive TCRs. One functional consequence of Ly-49 engagement in vivo is the observation that Ly-49A$^+$ NK cells from mice expressing its ligand appear to have alterations in their sensitivity to their ligands (170,379–381). However, current methodologies require isolation of specific NK cells by positive selection with mAbs directed against Ly-49 molecules. Because such mAbs may block interaction between the Ly-49 molecule and its ligand, functional assessment of freshly isolated NK cells is not feasible unless the cells are grown in vitro; this might affect NK-cell activity that may not correspond to the situation in vivo. Nevertheless, the MHC haplotype appears to affect the repertoire of Ly-49 molecules that are expressed (382).

There may be an allelic exclusion process that regulates the expression of the alternate allele for each Ly-49 molecule, such that an individual NK cell appears to express only one allele for any given Ly-49 molecule (179). However, a stochastic process has not been excluded whereby NK cells expressing both alleles for a given Ly-49 molecule may occur by chance and such dual expressing cells may be extremely difficult to find. Some of these issues will be addressable with transgenic mice expressing Ly-49 molecules on large percentages of NK cells.

On the other hand, there is some evidence for a tolerance mechanism that is independent of MHC class I. Although β2m-deficient bone marrow is rejected by otherwise syngeneic normal NK cells (86,87), NK cells from β2m-deficient mice are tolerant to β2m-deficient bone marrow and cannot reject allogeneic bone marrow (85). This may be due to the reduced activity of the β2m-deficient NK cells, which are less potent against YAC-1 targets in vitro. Similar findings have been reported for TAP-deficient mice (383). The basis for tolerance of the NK cells in MHC class I–deficient mice is not fully understood but could be related to differences in activation receptors.

Finally, some caution is needed in the evaluation of NK-cell development. Until a consensus on the molecular definition of an NK cell is reached, it is necessary to rely on markers (CD56, NK1.1) and exclude T cells. However, in immature NK-cell populations, there could be discordant regulation of the expression of cell surface markers otherwise thought to be NK cell specific. Moreover, TCR–CD3$^-$ but committed T-cell precursors could easily be confused with NK cells. Clearly, the development of new molecular and serologic tools to faithfully and specifically identify NK cells and their precursors will be extremely helpful.

CLINICAL RELEVANCE OF NK CELLS

Discussed previously are the issues of tumor surveillance and possible usefulness of NK cells in immunotherapy, role in host defense against infections, bone marrow transplantation, and immunoregulation. In contrast to NK-cell deficiencies, there are several other clinical settings in which expansion of NK cells are important. Recently, an NK-cell lymphoma has been characterized (384). Particularly prevalent in Asia, the tumors are frequently present in an unusual location—the sinuses or nasal tract. Characteristically, the tumor cells do not express surface CD3 and have unrearranged germline TCR genes, but NK-cell markers such as CD56 are usually found. Interestingly, the majority of these tumors are associated with antecedent Epstein-Barr virus infections. Patients also may have concurrent cutaneous vasculitis. In an apparently unrelated disorder, several patients have been described with an NK-cell lymphocytosis (385). These patients may have an associated red blood cell aplasia, neutropenia with sepsis, and vasculitis, suggesting an autoimmune disease. Finally, patients with immune thrombocytopenic purpura have increased numbers of circulating NK cells (386). Thus, several clinical syndromes have been described where there is an increased number of NK cells, both malignant and nonmalignant polyclonal expansions.

NK cells also may play a role in the pathogenesis of autoimmune disorders. In early rheumatoid arthritis, cells infiltrating the synovium have been found to express granzymes but not T-cell markers (387), suggesting that NK cells are involved in early immune response to a putative etiologic agent or may initiate or sustain an autoimmune state in which T cells have documented involvement. In patients with the rare inclusion body myositis syndrome associated with immunodeficiency, an NK-cell infiltrate into striated muscle has been described (388). In mouse models of autoimmune disease, NK cells appear to influence the development of disease (389,390). Finally, NK cells have been implicated in acute graft-versus-host disease, either clinically or in experimental models (391,392). Collectively, these studies indicate that NK cells may play a significant role in clinical disease. Further understanding will be significantly aided by development of a molecular definition of NK cells.

ACKNOWLEDGMENT

I thank past and current members of my laboratory and our collaborators for their continued interest in dissecting the molecular basis for natural killing. I also thank Mike Brown, Jon Heusel, Tony Scalzo, Hamish Smith, and Larry Wang for their comments on this chapter. Thanks also to Mike Brown for producing Figure 6. Investigations in the author's laboratory are supported by the National Institutes of Health, the Barnes-Jewish Hospital Research Foundation, the Monsanto-Washington University research agreement, and the Howard Hughes Medical Institute.

REFERENCES

1. Savary CA, Lotzova E. Phylogeny and ontogeny of NK cells. In: Lotzova E, Herberman RB, eds. *Immunobiology of Natural Killer Cells.* Vol. 1. Boca Raton, FL: CRC Press, 1986:45–60.
2. Humphreys T, Reinherz EL. Invertebrate immune recognition, natural immunity and the evolution of positive selection. *Immunol Today* 1994;15:316–320.
3. Kiessling R, Klein E, Wigzell H. Natural killer cells in the mouse. I. Cytotoxic cells with specificity for mouse Moloney leukemia cells: Specificity and distribution according to genotype. *Eur J Immunol* 1975;5:112.
4. Herberman RB, Nunn ME, Lavrin DH. Natural cytotoxic reactivity of mouse lymphoid cells against syngeneic and allogeneic tumors. I. Distribution of reactivity and specificity. *Int J Cancer* 1975;16:216.
5. Herberman R. *NK Cells and Other Natural Effector Cells.* New York: Academic, 1982.
6. Trinchieri G. Biology of natural killer cells. *Adv Immunol* 1989;47:187–376.
7. Brunner KT, Mauel J, Cerottini JC, Chapuis B. Quantitative assay of the lytic action of immune lymphoid cells on ^{51}Cr-labelled allogeneic target cells in vitro: Inhibition by isoantibody and by drugs. *Immunology* 1968;14:181.
8. Timonen T, Ortaldo J, Herberman RB. Characteristics of human large granular lymphocytes and relationship to natural killer and K cells. *J Exp Med* 1981; 153:569.
9. Timonen T, Saksela E. Isolation of human NK cells by density gradient centrifugation. *J Immunol Methods* 1980;36:285.
10. Inverardi L, Witson JC, Fuad SA, Winkler-Pickett RT, Ortaldo JR, Bach FH. CD3 negative "small agranular lymphocytes" are natural killer cells. *J Immunol* 1991;146:4048–4052.
11. Shortman K, Wilson A, Scollay R, Chen WF. Development of large granular lymphocytes with anomalous, non-specific cytotoxicity in clones derived from Ly 2+ T cells. *Proc Natl Acad Sci U S A* 1983;80:2728.
12. Lanier LL, Phillips JH. A map of the cell surface antigens expressed on resting and activated human natural killer cells. In: Reiherz EL, ed. *Leukocyte Typing II.* Vol 3. New York: Springer-Verlag, 1986:165–180.
13. Barclay AN, Birkeland ML, Brown MH, et al. *The Leucocyte Antigen Factsbook.* London: Academic, 1993.
14. Shuskik C, Cohen IR, Schwartz RS, Lathan-Griffin E, Waksal SD. T lymphocytes with promiscuous cytotoxicity. *Nature* 1976;263:699.
15. Brooks CG, Holscher M, Urdal D. Natural killer activity in cloned cytotoxic T lymphocytes: Regulation by interleukin 2, interferon, and specific antigen. *J Immunol* 1985;135:1145–1152.
16. Berke G. The binding and lysis of target cells by cytotoxic lymphocytes: Molecular and cellular aspects [Review]. *Annu Rev Immunol* 1994;12:735–73.
17. Lowin B, Beermann F, Schmidt A, Tschopp J. A null mutation in the perforin gene impairs cytolytic T lymphocyte- and natural killer cell–mediated cytotoxicity. *Proc Natl Acad Sci U S A* 1994;91:11571–5.
18. Kojima H, Shinohara N, Hanaoka S, et al. Two distinct pathways of specific killing revealed by perforin mutant cytotoxic T lymphocytes. *Immunity* 1994;1: 357–364.
19. Kagi D, Ledermann B, Burki K, et al. Cytotoxicity mediated by T cells and natural killer cells is greatly impaired in perforin-deficient mice. *Nature* 1994;369: 31–7.
20. Heusel JW, Wesselschmidt RL, Shresta S, Russell JH, Ley TJ. Cytotoxic lymphocytes require granzyme B for the rapid induction of DNA fragmentation and apoptosis in allogeneic target cells. *Cell* 1994;76:977–987.

21. Shresta S, Heusel JW, Macivor DM, Wesselschmidt RL, Russell JH, Ley TJ. Granzyme B plays a critical role in cytotoxic lymphocyte-induced apoptosis [Review]. *Immunol Rev* 1995;146:211–221.
22. Henkart PA. Lymphocyte-mediated cytotoxicity: Two pathways and multiple effector molecules. *Immunity* 1994;1:343–346.
23. Montel AH, Bochan MR, Hobbs JA, Lynch DH, Brahmi Z. Fas involvement in cytotoxicity mediated by human NK cells. *Cell Immunol* 1995;166:236–246.
24. Arase H, Arase N, Saito T. Fas-mediated cytotoxicity by freshly isolated natural killer cells. *J Exp Med* 1995;181:1235–1238.
25. Lee RK, Spielman J, Zhao DY, Olsen KJ, Podack ER. Perforin, Fas ligand, and tumor necrosis factor are the major cytotoxic molecules used by lymphokine-activated killer cells. *J Immunol* 1996;157:1919–1925.
26. Oshimi Y, Oda S, Honda Y, Nagata S, Miyazaki S. Involvement of Fas ligand and Fas-mediated pathway in the cytotoxicity of human natural killer cells. *J Immunol* 1996;157:2909–2915.
27. Perussia B. Lymphokine-activated killer cells, natural killer cells and cytokines [Review]. *Curr Opin Immunol* 1991;3:49–55.
28. Lanier LL, Phillips JH, Hackett J Jr, Tutt M, Kumar V. Natural killer cells: Definition of a cell type rather than a function [errata *J Immunol* 1987;138:996 and 1987;138:2745]. *J Immunol* 1986;137:2735–9.
29. Ritz J, Campen TJ, Schmidt RE, et al. Analysis of T-cell receptor gene rearrangement and expression in human natural killer clones. *Science* 1985;228:1540.
30. Lanier LL, Cwirla S, Federspiel N, Phillips JH. Human natural killer cells isolated from peripheral blood do not rearrange T cell receptor β chain genes. *J Exp Med* 1986;163:209.
31. Dorshkind K, Pollack SB, Bosma MJ, Phillips RA. Natural killer (NK) cells are present in mice with severe combined immunodeficiency (scid). *J Immunol* 1985;134:3798.
32. Hackett J Jr, Bosma GC, Bosma MJ, Bennett M, Kumar V. Transplantable progenitors of natural killer cells are distinct from those of T and B lymphocytes. *Proc Natl Acad Sci U S A* 1986;83:3427–3431.
33. Mombaerts P, Iacomini J, Johnson RS, Herrup K, Tonegawa S, Papaioannou VE. RAG-1-deficient mice have no mature B and T lymphocytes. *Cell* 1992;68: 869–877.
34. Shinkai Y, Rathbun G, Lam K-P, et al. Rag-2–deficient mice lack mature lymphocytes owing to inability to initiate V(D)J rearrangement. *Cell* 1992;68:855–867.
35. Ashwell JD, Klausner RD. Genetic and mutational analysis of the T-cell antigen receptor. *Annu Rev Immunol* 1990;8:139–168.
36. Phillips JH, Hori T, Nagler A, Spits H, Lanier LL. Ontogeny of human natural killer (NK) cells: Fetal NK cells mediate cytolytic function and express cytoplasmic CD3 epsilon, delta proteins. *J Exp Med* 1992;175:1055–66.
37. Anderson P, Caligiuri M, Ritz J, Schlossman SF. CD3-negative natural killer cells express zeta TCR as part of a novel molecular complex. *Nature* 1989;341: 159.
38. Lanier LL, Yu G, Phillips JH. Co-association of CD3 zeta with a receptor (CD16) for IgG Fc on human natural killer cells. *Nature* 1989;342:803–805.
39. Letourneur O, Kennedy IC, Brini AT, Ortaldo JR, O'Shea JJ, Kinet JP. Characterization of the family of dimers associated with Fc receptors (Fc epsilon RI and Fc gamma RIII). *J Immunol* 1991;147:2652–6.
40. Rolink A, ten Boekel E, Melchers F, Fearon DT, Krop I, Andersson J. A subpopulation of B220+ cells in murine bone marrow does not express CD19 and contains natural killer cell progenitors. *J Exp Med* 1996;183:187–194.
41. Hercend T, Griffin JD, Bensussan A, et al. Generation of monoclonal antibodies to a human natural killer clone: Characterization of two natural killer associated antigens, NKH1A and NKH2, expressed on subsets of large granular lymphocytes. *J Clin Invest* 1985;75:932.
42. Lanier LL, Le AM, Civin CI, Loken MR, Phillips JH. The relationship of CD16 (Leu-11) and Leu-19 (NKH-1) antigen expression on human peripheral blood NK cells and cytotoxic T lymphocytes. *J Immunol* 1986;136:4480.
43. Lanier LL, Testi R, Bindl J, Phillips JH. Identity of Leu-19 (CD56) leukocyte differentiation antigen and neural cell adhesion molecule. *J Exp Med* 1989;169: 2233.
44. Cunningham BA, Hemperly JJ, Murray BA, Prediger EA, Brackenbury R, Edelman GM. Neural cell adhesion molecule: Structure, immunoglobulin-like domains, cell surface modulation, and alternative RNA splicing. *Science* 1987; 236:799.
45. Rutishauser U, Acheson A, Hall AK, Mann DM, Sunshine J. The neural cell adhesion molecule (NCAM) as a regulator of cell-cell interactions. *Science* 1988;240:53.
46. Nitta T, Yagita H, Sato K, Okumura K. Involvement of CD56 (NKH1/Leu-19 antigen) as an adhesion molecule in natural killer–target cell interactions. *J Exp Med* 1989;170:1757.
47. Lanier LL, Ruitenberg JJ, Phillips JH. Functional and biochemical analysis of CD16 antigen on natural killer cells and granulocytes. *J Immunol* 1988;136: 3478–3485.
48. Ravetch JV, Kinet JP. Fc receptors. *Annu Rev Immunol* 1991;9:457–491.
49. Rodewald HR, Moingeon P, Lucich JL, Dosiou C, Lopez P, Reinherz EL. A population of early fetal thymocytes expressing Fc gamma RII/III contains precursors of T lymphocytes and natural killer cells. *Cell* 1992;69:139–50.
50. Hackett T Jr, Tutt M, Lipscomb M, Bennett M, Koo G, Kumar V. Origin and differentiation of natural killer cells. II. Functional and morphologic studies of purified NK-1.1 cells. *J Immunol* 1986;136:3124–31.
51. Seaman WE, Sleisenger M, Eriksson E, Koo GC. Depletion of natural killer cells

in mice by monoclonal antibody to NK-1.1. Reduction in host defense against malignancy without loss of cellular or humoral immunity. *J Immunol* 1987;138:4539–4544.

52. Koo GC, Peppard JR. Establishment of monoclonal anti-Nk-1.1 antibody. *Hybridoma* 1984;3:301–303.

53. Kasai M, Iwamori M, Nagai Y, Okumura K, Tada T. A glycolipid on the surface of mouse natural killer cells. *Eur J Immunol* 1980;10:175–180.

54. Young WW Jr, Hakomori SI, Durdik JM, Henney CS. Identification of ganglio-N-tetraosylceramide as a new cell surface marker for murine natural killer (NK) cells. *J Immunol* 1980;124:199–201.

55. Suttles J, Schwarting GA, Stout RD. Flow cytometric analysis reveals the presence of asialo GM1 on the surface membrane of alloimmune cytotoxic T lymphocytes. *J Immunol* 1986;136:1586–1591.

56. Reynolds CW, Wiltrout RH. *Functions of the Natural Immune System*. New York: Plenum, 1989.

57. Grimm EA, Mazumder A, Zhang HZ, Rosenberg SA. Lymphokine-activated killer cell phenomenon. Lysis of natural killer–resistant fresh solid tumor cells by interleukin 2–activated autologous human peripheral blood lymphocytes. *J Exp Med* 1982;155:1823–1841.

58. Trinchieri G, Matsumoto-Kobayashi M, Clark SC, Seehra J, London L, Perussia B. Response of resting human peripheral blood natural killer cells to interleukin 2. *J Exp Med* 1984;160:1147–1169.

59. Phillips JH, Lanier LL. Dissection of the lymphokine-activated killer phenomenon. Relative contribution of peripheral blood natural killer cells and T lymphocytes to cytolysis. *J Exp Med* 1986;164:814–825.

60. Ortaldo JR, Mason A, Overton R. Lymphokine-activated killer cells. Analysis of progenitors and effectors. *J Exp Med* 1986;164:1193–1205.

61. Karlhofer FM, Yokoyama WM. Stimulation of murine natural killer (NK) cells by a monoclonal antibody specific for the NK1.1 antigen. IL-2–activated NK cells possess additional specific stimulation pathways. *J Immunol* 1991;146:3662–3673.

62. Seaman WE, Niemi EC, Stark MR, Goldfien RD, Pollock AS, Imboden JB. Molecular cloning of gp42, a cell-surface molecule that is selectively induced on rat natural killer cells by interleukin 2: Glycolipid membrane anchoring and capacity for transmembrane signaling. *J Exp Med* 1991;173:251–260.

63. Umehara H, Takashima A, Minami Y, Bloom ET. Signal transduction via phosphorylated adhesion molecule, LFA-1 beta (CD18), is increased by culture of natural killer cells with IL-2 in the generation of lymphokine-activated killer cells. *Int Immunol* 1993;5:19–27.

64. Nishio M, Spielman J, Lee RK, Nelson DL, Podack ER. CD80 (B7.1) and CD54 (intracellular adhesion molecule-1) induce target cell susceptibility to promiscuous cytotoxic T cell lysis. *J Immunol* 1996;157:4347–4353.

65. Taniguchi T, Minami Y. Minireview: The IL-2/IL-2 receptor system: A current overview. *Cell* 1993;73:5–8.

66. Nakarai T, Robertson MJ, Streuli M, et al. Interleukin 2 receptor γ chain expression on resting and activated lymphoid cells. *J Exp Med* 1994;180:241–251.

67. Schorle H, Holtschke T, Hunig T, Schimpl A, Horak I. Development and function of T cells in mice rendered interleukin-2 deficient by gene targeting. *Nature* 1991;352:621–4.

68. Willerford DM, Chen J, Ferry JA, Davidson L, Ma A, Alt FW. Interleukin-2 receptor alpha chain regulates the size and content of the peripheral lymphoid compartment. *Immunity* 1995;3:521–530.

69. Suzuki H, Duncan GS, Takimoto H, Mak TW. Abnormal development of intestinal intraepithelial lymphocytes and peripheral natural killer cells in mice lacking the IL-2 receptor beta chain. *J Exp Med* 1997;185:499–505.

70. DiSanto JP, Muller W, Guy-Grand D, Fischer A, Rajewsky K. Lymphoid development in mice with a targeted deletion of the interleukin 2 receptor gamma chain. *Proc Natl Acad Sci U S A* 1995;92:377–381.

71. Cao X, Shores EW, Hu-Li J, et al. Defective lymphoid development in mice lacking expression of the common cytokine receptor gamma chain. *Immunity* 1995;2:223–238.

72. Sugamura K, Asao H, Kondo M, et al. The interleukin-2 receptor gamma chain: Its role in the multiple cytokine receptor complexes and T cell development in XSCID [Review]. *Annu Rev Immunol* 1996;14:179–205.

73. Cosman D, Kumaki S, Ahdieh M, et al. Interleukin 15 and its receptor. *Ciba Found Symp* 1995;195:221–233.

74. Tagaya Y, Bamford RN, DeFilippis AP, Waldmann TA. IL-15: A pleiotropic cytokine with diverse receptor/signaling pathways whose expression is controlled at multiple levels [Review]. *Immunity* 1996;4:329–336.

75. Giri JG, Kumaki S, Ahdieh M, et al. Identification and cloning of a novel IL-15 binding protein that is structurally related to the alpha chain of the IL-2 receptor. *EMBO J* 1995;14:3654–3663.

76. Puzanov IJ, Bennett M, Kumar V. IL-15 can substitute for the marrow microenvironment in the differentiation of natural killer cells. *J Immunol* 1996;157:4282–4285.

77. Mrozek E, Anderson P, Caligiuri MA. Role of interleukin-15 in the development of human CD56+ natural killer cells from CD34+ hematopoietic progenitor cells. *Blood* 1996;87:2632–2640.

78. Paul WE. *Fundamental Immunology*. New York: Raven, 1984.

79. Paul WE. *Fundamental Immunology*, 3rd ed. New York: Raven, 1993.

80. Kärre K, Ljunggren H-G, Piontek G, Kiessling R. Selective rejection of H-2–deficient lymphoma variants suggests alternative immune defence strategy. *Nature* 1986;319:675–678.

81. Piontek GE, Taniguchi K, Ljuggren HG, et al. YAC-1 MHC class I variants reveal an association between decreased NK sensitivity and increased H-2 expression after interferon treatment or in vivo passage. *J Immunol* 1985;135:4281–4288.

82. Quillet A, Presse F, Marchiol-Fournigault C, et al. Increased resistance to non-MHC–restricted cytotoxicity related to HLA A,B expression. Direct demonstration using beta 2-microglobulin–transfected Daudi cells. *J Immunol* 1988;141:17–20.

83. Franksson L, George E, Powis S, Butcher G, Howard J, Kärre K. Tumorigenicity conferred to lymphoma mutant by major histocompatibility complex–encoded transporter gene. *J Exp Med* 1993;177:201–205.

84. Salcedo M, Momburg F, Hammerling GJ, Ljunggren HG. Resistance to natural killer cell lysis conferred by TAP1/2 genes in human antigen-processing mutant cells. *J Immunol* 1994;152:1702–1708.

85. Liao NS, Bix M, Zijlstra M, Jaenisch R, Raulet D. MHC class I deficiency: Ssusceptibility to natural killer (NK) cells and impaired NK activity. *Science* 1991;253:199–202.

86. Hoglund P, Ohlen C, Carbone E, et al. Recognition of beta 2-microglobulin–negative (beta 2m⁻) T-cell blasts by natural killer cells from normal but not from beta 2m⁻ mice: Nonresponsiveness controlled by beta 2m⁻ bone marrow in chimeric mice. *Proc Natl Acad Sci U S A* 1991;88:10332–10336.

87. Bix M, Liao NS, Zijlstra M, Loring J, Jaenisch R, Raulet D. Rejection of class I MHC–deficient haemopoietic cells by irradiated MHC-matched mice. *Nature* 1991;349:329–331.

88. Yu YYL, Kumar V, Bennett M. Murine natural killer cells and marrow graft rejection. *Annu Rev Immunol* 1992;10:189–213.

89. Rembecki RM, Kumar V, David CS, Bennett M. Bone marrow cell transplants involving intra-H-2 recombinant inbred mouse strains. Evidence that hemopoietic histocompatibility-1 (Hh-1) genes are distinct from H-2D or H-2L. *J Immunol* 1988;141:2253–2260.

90. Ljunggren HG, Kärre K. In search of the "missing self": MHC molecules and NK cell recognition [Review]. *Immunol Today* 1990;11:237–244.

91. Nishimura MI, Stroynowski I, Hood L, Ostrand-Rosenberg S. H-2Kb antigen expression has no effect on natural killer susceptibility and tumorigenicity of a murine hepatoma. *J Immunol* 1988;141:4403.

92. Storkus WJ, Salter RD, Alexander J, et al. Class I–induced resistance to natural killing: Identification of nonpermissive residues in HLA-A2. *Proc Natl Acad Sci U S A* 1991;88:5989–5992.

93. Colonna M, Brooks EG, Falco M, Ferrara GB, Strominger JL. Generation of allospecific natural killer cells by stimulation across a polymorphism of HLA-C. *Science* 1993;260:1121–1124.

94. Litwin V, Gumperz J, Parham P, Phillips JH, Lanier LL. Specificity of HLA class I antigen recognition by human NK clones: Evidence for clonal heterogeneity, protection by self and non-self alleles, and influence of the target cell type. *J Exp Med* 1993;178:1321–36.

95. Jorgensen JL, Reay PA, Ehrici EW, Davis MM. Molecular components of T-cell recognition. *Annu Rev Immunol* 1992;10:835–873.

96. Burgert HG, Maryanski JL, Kvist S. "E3/19K" protein of adenovirus type 2 inhibits lysis of cytolytic T lymphocytes by blocking cell-surface expression of histocompatibility class I antigens. *Proc Natl Acad Sci USA* 1987;84:1356–1360.

97. Browne H, Smith G, Beck S, Minson T. A complex between the MHC class I homologue encoded by human cytomegalovirus and beta 2 microglobulin. *Nature* 1990;347:770.

98. Howcroft TK, Strebel K, Martin MA, Singer DS. Repression of MHC class I gene promoter activity by two-exon tat of HIV. *Science* 1993;260:1320–1322.

99. Holtkamp B, Cramer M, Rajewsky K. Somatic variation of H-2Kk expression and structure in a T-cell lymphoma: Instability, stabilization, high production and structural mutation. *EMBO J* 1983;2:1943–1951.

100. Gattoni-Celli S, Kirsch K, Timpane R, Isselbacher KJ. Beta 2-microglobulin gene is mutated in a human colon cancer cell line (HCT) deficient in the expression of HLA class I antigens on the cell surface. *Cancer Res* 1992;52:1201–1204.

101. Korkolopoulou P, Kaklamanis L, Pezzella F, Harris AL, Gatter KC. Loss of antigen-presenting molecules (MHC class I and TAP-1) in lung cancer. *Br J Cancer* 1996;73:148–153.

102. Kärre K. Role of target histocompatibility antigens in regulation of natural killer activity: A reevaluation and a hypothesis. In: Herberman RB, Callewaert DM, eds. *Mechanisms of Cytotoxicity by NK cells*. Orlando: Academic, 1985:81–103.

103. Seaman WE, Eriksson E, Dobrow R, Imboden JB. Inositol trisphosphate is generated by a rat natural killer cell tumor in response to target cells or to crosslinked monoclonal antibody OX-34: Possible signaling role for the OX-34 determinant during activation by target cells. *Proc Natl Acad Sci USA* 1987;84:4239–4243.

104. Kaufman DS, Schoon RA, Leibson PJ. MHC class I expression on tumor targets inhibits natural killer cell-mediated cytotoxicity without interfering with target recognition. *J Immunol* 1993;150:1429–1436.

105. Yokoyama WM. Recognition structures on natural killer cells [Review]. *Curr Opin Immunol* 1993;5:67–73.

106. Yokoyama WM, Seaman WE. The Ly-49 and NKR-P1 gene families encoding lectin-like receptors on natural killer cells: The NK gene complex [Review]. *Annu Rev Immunol* 1993;11:613–635.

107. Houchins JP, Yabe T, McSherry C, Miyokawa N, Bach FH. Isolation and characterization of NK cell or NK/T cell-specific cDNA clones. *J Mol Cell Immunol* 1990;4:295–304.

108. Takai T, Li M, Sylvestre D, Clynes R, Ravetch JV. FcR gamma chain deletion results in pleiotrophic effector cell defects. *Cell* 1994;76:519–529.

109. Hazenbos WLW, Gessner JE, Hofhuis FMA, et al. Impaired IgG-dependent anaphylaxis and arthus reaction in Fc-gamma-RIII (CD16) deficient mice. *Immunity* 1996;5:181–188.

110. Rabinowich H, Manciulea M, Metes D, et al. Physical and functional association of Fc mu receptor on human natural killer cells with the zeta- and Fc epsilon RI gamma-chains and with src family protein tyrosine kinases. *J Immunol* 1996;157:1485–1491.

111. Perussia B, Tutt MM, Qiu WQ, et al. Murine natural killer cells express functional Fc gamma receptor II encoded by the Fc gamma R alpha gene. *J Exp Med* 1989;170:73–86.

112. Anegon I, Cuturi MC, Trinchieri G, Perussia B. Interaction of Fc receptor (CD16) ligands induces transcription of interleukin 2 receptor (CD25) and lymphokine genes and expression of their products in human natural killer cells. *J Exp Med* 1988;167:452–472.

113. Cassatella MA, Anegon I, Cuturi MC, Griskey P, Trinchieri G, Perussia B. Fc gamma R(CD16) interaction with ligand induces Ca²⁺ mobilization and phosphoinositide turnover in human natural killer cells. Role of Ca²⁺ in Fc gamma R(CD16)-induced transcription and expression of lymphokine genes. *J Exp Med* 1989;169:549–567.

114. Azzoni L, Kamoun M, Salcedo TW, Kanakaraj P, Perussia B. Stimulation of Fc gamma RIIIA results in phospholipase C-gamma 1 tyrosine phosphorylation and p56lck activation. *J Exp Med* 1992;176:1745–1750.

115. Kanakaraj P, Duckworth B, Azzoni L, Kamoun M, Cantley LC, Perussia B. Phosphatidylinositol-3 kinase activation induced upon Fc gamma RIIIA-ligand interaction. *J Exp Med* 1994;179:551–558.

116. Aramburu J, Azzoni L, Rao A, Perussia B. Activation and expression of the nuclear factors of activated T cells, NFATp and NFATc, in human natural killer cells: Regulation upon CD16 ligand binding. *J Exp Med* 1995;182:801–810.

117. Wunderlich J, Shearer G. Unit 3.11. Induction and measurement of cytotoxic T lymphocyte activity. In: Coligan JE, Kruisbeek AM, Margulies DH, Shevach EM, Strober W, eds. *Current Protocols in Immunology.* New York: Greene Publishing, 1993.

118. Vivier E, Morin P, O'Brien C, Druker B, Schlossman SF, Anderson P. Tyrosine phosphorylation of the Fc gamma RIII(CD16): Zeta complex in human natural killer cells. Induction by antibody-dependent cytotoxicity but not by natural killing. *J Immunol* 1991;146:206–210.

119. Bonnema JD, Karnitz LM, Schoon RA, Abraham RT, Leibson PJ. Fc receptor stimulation of phosphatidylinositol 3-kinase in natural killer cells is associated with protein kinase C–independent granule release and cell-mediated cytotoxicity. *J Exp Med* 1994;180:1427–1435.

120. Chadwick BS, Miller RG. Hybrid resistance in vitro. Possible role of both class I MHC and self peptides in determining the level of target cell sensitivity. *J Immunol* 1992;148:2307–2313.

121. Leo O, Sachs DH, Samelson LE, et al. Identification of monoclonal antibodies specific for the T cell receptor complex by Fc receptor-mediated CTL lysis. *J Immunol* 1986;137:3874–3880.

122. Chambers WH, Vujanovic NL, DeLeo AB, Olszowy MW, Herberman RB, Iierodt JC. Monoclonal antibody to a triggering structure expressed on rat natural killer cells and adherent lymphokine-activated killer cells. *J Exp Med* 1989;169:1373–1389.

123. Bendelac A. Mouse NK1⁺ T cells [Review]. *Curr Opin Immunol* 1995;7:367–374.

124. Giorda R, Trucco M. Mouse NKR-P1. A family of genes selectively coexpressed in adherent lymphokine-activated killer cells. *J Immunol* 1991;147:1701–1708.

125. Yokoyama WM, Ryan JC, Hunter JJ, Smith HR, Stark M, Seaman WE. cDNA cloning of mouse NKR-P1 and genetic linkage with LY-49. Identification of a natural killer cell gene complex on mouse chromosome 6. *J Immunol* 1991;147:3229–3236.

126. Ryan JC, Turck J, Niemi EC, Yokoyama WM, Seaman WE. Molecular cloning of the NK1.1 antigen, a member of the NKR-P1 family of natural killer cell activation molecules. *J Immunol* 1992;149:1631–1635.

127. Drickamer K. Ca²⁺-dependent carbohydrate-recognition domains in animal proteins. *Curr Opin Struct Biol* 1993;3:393–400.

128. Karlhofer FM, Orihuela MM, Yokoyama WM. Ly-49-independent natural killer (NK) cell specificity revealed by NK cell clones derived from p53-deficient mice. *J Exp Med* 1995;181:1785–1795.

129. Giorda R, Weisberg EP, IP TK, Trucco M. Genomic structure and strain-specific expression of the natural killer cell receptor NKR-P1. *J Immunol* 1992;149:1957–1963.

130. Ryan JC, Niemi EC, Goldfien RD, Hiserodt JC, Seaman WE. NKR-P1, an activating molecule on rat natural killer cells, stimulates phosphoinositide turnover and a rise in intracellular calcium. *J Immunol* 1991;147:3244–3250.

131. Ryan JC, Niemi EC, Nakamura MC, Seaman WE. NKR-P1A is a target-specific receptor that activates natural killer cell cytotoxicity. *J Exp Med* 1995;181:1911–1915.

132. Lanier LL, Chang C, Phillips JH. Human NKR-P1A. A disulfide-linked homodimer of the C-type lectin superfamily expressed by a subset of NK and T lymphocytes. *J Immunol* 1994;153:2417–2428.

133. Mathew PA, Garni-Wagner BA, Land K, et al. Cloning and characterization of the 2B4 gene encoding a molecule associated with non-MHC-restricted killing mediated by activated natural killer cells and T cells. *J Immunol* 1993;151:5328–5337.

134. Garni-Wagner BA, Purohit A, Mathew PA, Bennett M, Kumar V. A novel function-associated molecule related to non–MHC-restricted cytotoxicity mediated by activated natural killer cells and T cells. *J Immunol* 1993;151:60–70.

135. Baixeras E, Huard B, Miossec C, et al. Characterization of the lymphocyte activation gene 3-encoded protein. A new ligand for human leukocyte antigen class II antigens. *J Exp Med* 1992;176:327–337.

136. Triebel F, Jitsukawa S, Baixeras E, et al. LAG-3, a novel lymphocyte activation gene closely related to CD4. *J Exp Med* 1990;171:1393–1405.

137. Miyazaki T, Dierich A, Benoist C, Mathis D. Independent modes of natural killing distinguished in mice lacking Lag3. *Science* 1996;272:405–408.

138. Frey JL, Bino T, Kantor RRS, et al. Mechanism of target cell recognition by natural killer cells: Characterization of a novel triggering molecule restricted to CD3⁻ large granular lymphocytes. *J Exp Med* 1991;174:1527–1536.

139. Anderson SK, Gallinger S, Roder J, Frey J, Young HA, Ortaldo JR. A cyclophilin-related protein involved in the function of natural killer cells. *Proc Natl Acad Sci U S A* 1993;90:542–546.

140. Giardina SL, Anderson SK, Sayers TJ, et al. Selective loss of NK cytotoxicity in antisense NK-TR1 rat LGL cell lines. Abrogation of antibody-independent tumor and virus-infected target cell killing. *J Immunol* 1995;154:80–87.

141. Ortaldo JR, Mason AT, Mason LH, Winklerpickett RT, Gosselin P, Anderson SK. Selective inhibition of human and mouse natural killer tumor recognition using retroviral antisense in primary natural killer cells—involvement with MHC class I killer cell inhibitory receptors. *J Immunol* 1997;158:1262–1267.

142. Siliciano RF, Pratt JC, Schmidt RE, Ritz J, Reinherz EL. Activation of cytolytic T lymphocyte and natural killer cell function through the T11 sheep erythrocyte binding protein. *Nature* 1985;317:428–430.

143. Gumley TP, McKenzie IF, Sandrin MS. Tissue expression, structure and function of the murine Ly-6 family of molecules [Review]. *Immunol Cell Biol* 1995;73:277–296.

144. Biassoni R, Cantoni C, Falco M, et al. The human leukocyte antigen (HLA)-C-specific "activatory" or "inhibitory" natural killer cell receptors display highly homologous extracellular domains but differ in their transmembrane and intracytoplasmic portions. *J Exp Med* 1996;183:645–650.

145. Bottino C, Sivori S, Vitale M, et al. A novel surface molecule homologous to the p58/p50 family of receptors is selectively expressed on a subset of human natural killer cells and induces both triggering of cell functions and proliferation. *Eur J Immunol* 1996;26:1816–1824.

146. Mandelboim O, Davis DM, Reyburn HT, et al. Enhancement of class II–restricted T cell responses by costimulatory NK receptors for class I MHC proteins. *Science* 1996;274:2097–2100.

147. Smith HRC, Karlhofer FM, Yokoyama WM. The Ly-49 multigene family expressed by IL-2–activated natural killer cells. *J Immunol* 1994;153:1068–1079.

148. Mason LH, Anderson SK, Yokoyama WM, Smith HRC, Winklerpickett R, Ortaldo JR. The Ly-49D receptor activates murine natural killer cells. *J Exp Med* 1996;184:2119–2128.

149. Vaage JT, Naper C, Lovik G, et al. Control of rat natural killer cell-mediated allorecognition by a major histocompatibility complex region encoding nonclassical class I antigens. *J Exp Med* 1994;180:641–651.

150. Melero I, Balboa MA, Alonso JL, et al. Signaling through the LFA-1 leucocyte integrin actively regulates intercellular adhesion and tumor necrosis factor-alpha production in natural killer cells. *Eur J Immunol* 1993;23:1859–1865.

151. Bell GM, Dethloff GM, Imboden JB. CD45-negative mutants of a rat natural killer cell line fail to lyse tumor target cells. *J Immunol* 1993;151:3646–3653.

152. Liu JH, Wei S, Blanchard DK, Djeu JY. Restoration of lytic function in a human natural killer cell line by gene transfection. *Cell Immunol* 1994;156:24–35.

153. Helander TS, Carpen O, Turunen O, Kovanen PE, Vaheri A, Timonen T. ICAM-2 redistributed by ezrin as a target for killer cells. *Nature* 1996;382:265–268.

154. Nandi D, Gross JA, Allison JP. CD28-mediated costimulation is necessary for optimal proliferation of murine NK cells. *J Immunol* 1994;152:3361–3369.

155. Galandrini R, De Maria R, Piccoli M, Frati L, Santoni A. CD44 triggering enhances human NK cell cytotoxic functions. *J Immunol* 1994;153:4399–4407.

156. Wu TC, Huang AY, Jaffee EM, Levitsky HI, Pardoll DM. A reassessment of the role of B7-1 expression in tumor rejection. *J Exp Med* 1995;182:1415–1421.

157. Yeh KY, Pulaski BA, Woods ML, et al. B7-1 enhances natural killer cell-mediated cytotoxicity and inhibits tumor growth of a poorly immunogenic murine carcinoma. *Cell Immunol* 1995;165:217–224.

158. Chambers BJ, Salcedo M, Ljunggren HG. Triggering of natural killer cells by the costimulatory molecule CD80 (B7-1). *Immunity* 1996;5:311–317.

159. Lanier LL, Corliss B, Phillips JH. Arousal and inhibition of human NK cells [Review]. *Immunol Rev* 1997;155:145–154.

160. Yokoyama WM. Natural killer cells. Right-side up and up-side-down NK-cell receptors [Review]. *Curr Biol* 1995;5:982–985.

161. Yokoyama WM, Daniels BF, Seaman WE, Hunziker R, Margulies DH, Smith HR. A family of murine NK cell receptors specific for target cell MHC class I molecules [Review]. *Semin Immunol* 1995;7:89–101.

162. Wong S, Freeman JD, Kelleher C, Mager D, Takei F. Ly 49 multigene family. New members of a superfamily of type II membrane proteins with lectin-like domains. *J Immunol* 1991;147:1417.

163. Karlhofer FM, Ribaudo RK, Yokoyama WM. MHC class I alloantigen specificity of Ly-49⁺ IL-2–activated natural killer cells. *Nature* 1992;358:66–70.

164. Karlhofer FM, Ribaudo RK, Yokoyama WM. The interaction of Ly-49 with H-2Dd globally inactivates natural killer cell cytolytic activity. *Trans Assoc Am Physicians* 1992;105:72–85.

165. Correa I, Corral L, Raulet DH. Multiple natural killer cell–activating signals are inhibited by major histocompatibility complex class I expression in target cells. *Eur J Immunol* 1994;24:1323–1331.

166. Daniels BF, Karlhofer FM, Seaman WE, Yokoyama WM. A natural killer cell receptor specific for a major histocompatibility complex class I molecule. *J Exp Med* 1994;180:687–692.

167. Kane KP. Ly-49 mediates EL4 lymphoma adhesion to isolated class I major histocompatibility complex molecules. *J Exp Med* 1994;179:1011–1015.

168. Karlhofer FM, Hunziker R, Reichlin A, Margulies DH, Yokoyama WM. Host MHC class I molecules modulate in vivo expression of a NK cell receptor. *J Immunol* 1994;153:2407–2416.

169. Sykes M, Harty MW, Karlhofer FM, Pearson DA, Szot G, Yokoyama W. Hematopoietic cells and radioresistant host elements influence natural killer cell differentiation. *J Exp Med* 1993;178:223–229.

170. Olsson MY, Kärre K, Sentman CL. Altered phenotype and function of natural killer cells expressing the major histocompatibility complex receptor Ly-49 in mice transgenic for its ligand. *Proc Natl Acad Sci U S A* 1995;92:1649–1653.

171. Held W, Cado D, Raulet DH. Transgenic expression of the Ly49A natural killer cell receptor confers class I major histocompatibility complex (MHC)-specific inhibition and prevents bone marrow allograft rejection. *J Exp Med* 1996;184:2037–2041.

172. Nakamura MC, Niemi EC, Fisher MJ, Shultz LD, Seaman WE, Ryan JC. Mouse Ly-49A interrupts early signaling events in natural killer cell cytotoxicity and functionally associates with the Shp-1 tyrosine phosphatase. *J Exp Med* 1997;185:673–684.

173. Brennan J, Mahon G, Mager DL, Jefferies WA, Takei F. Recognition of class I major histocompatibility complex molecules by Ly-49: Specificities and domain interactions. *J Exp Med* 1996;183:1553–1559.

174. Correa I, Raulet DH. Binding of diverse peptides to MHC class I molecules inhibits target cell lysis by activated natural killer cells. *Immunity* 1995;2:61–71.

175. Corr M, Boyd LF, Padlan EA, Margulies DH. H-2Dd exploits a four residue peptide binding motif. *J Exp Med* 1993;178:1877–1892.

176. Orihuela M, Margulies DH, Yokoyama WM. The NK cell receptor Ly-49A recognizes a peptide-induced conformational determinant on its MHC class I ligand. *Proc Natl Acad Sci U S A* 1996;93:11792–11797.

177. Brennan J, Mager D, Jefferies W, Takei F. Expression of different members of the Ly-49 gene family defines distinct natural killer cell subsets and cell adhesion properties. *J Exp Med* 1994;180:2287–2295.

178. Yokoyama WM, Kehn PJ, Cohen DI, Shevach EM. Chromosomal location of the Ly-49 (A1, YE1/48) multigene family. Genetic association with the NK 1.1 antigen. *J Immunol* 1990;145:2353–2358.

179. Held W, Roland J, Raulet DH. Allelic exclusion of Ly49-family genes encoding class I MHC-specific receptors on NK cells. *Nature* 1995;376:355–358.

180. Sundback J, Kärre K, Sentman CL. Cloning of minimally divergent allelic forms of the natural killer (NK) receptor LY-49C, differentially controlled by host genes in the MHC and NK gene complexes. *J Immunol* 1996;157:3936–3942.

181. Silver ET, Elliott JF, Kane KP. Alternatively spliced LY-49D and H transcripts are found in IL-2-activated NK cells. *Immunol Today* 1996;44:14–17.

182. Sentman CL, Hackett J Jr, Kumar V, Bennett M. Identification of a subset of murine natural killer cells that mediates rejection of Hh-1d but not Hh-1b bone marrow grafts. *J Exp Med* 1989;170:191–202.

183. Yu YY, George T, Dorfman JR, Roland J, Kumar V, Bennett M. The role of Ly49A and 5E6(Ly49C) molecules in hybrid resistance mediated by murine natural killer cells against normal T cell blasts. *Immunity* 1996;4:67–76.

184. Brennan J, Lemieux S, Freeman JD, Mager DL, Takei F. Heterogeneity among LY-49c natural killer (NK) cells—characterization of highly related receptors with differing functions and expression patterns. *J Exp Med* 1996;184:2085–2090.

185. Mason L, Giardina SL, Hecht T, Ortaldo J, Mathieson BJ. LGL-1: A non-polymorphic antigen expressed on a major population of mouse natural killer cells. *J Immunol* 1988;140:4403–4412.

186. Mason LH, Yagita H, Ortaldo JR. LGL-1: A potential triggering molecule on murine NK cells. *J Leukoc Biol* 1994;55:362–370.

187. Mason LH, Ortaldo JR, Young HA, Kumar V, Bennett M, Anderson SK. Cloning and functional characteristics of murine large granular lymphocyte-1: A member of the Ly-49 gene family (Ly-49G2). *J Exp Med* 1995;182:293–303.

188. Daniels BF, Nakamura MC, Rosen SD, Yokoyama WM, Seaman WE. Ly-49A, a receptor for H-2Dd, has a functional carbohydrate recognition domain. *Immunity* 1994;1:785–792.

189. Brennan J, Takei F, Wong S, Mager DL. Carbohydrate recognition by a natural killer cell receptor, Ly-49C. *J Biol Chem* 1995;270:9691–9694.

190. Barber LD, Patel TP, Percival L, et al. Unusual uniformity of the N-linked oligosaccharides of HLA-A, -B, and -C glycoproteins. *J Immunol* 1996;156:3275–3284.

191. Vercelli D, Helm B, Marsh P, Padlan E, Geha RS, Gould H. The B-cell binding site on human immunoglobulin E. *Nature* 1989;338:649–651.

192. Aubry JP, Pochon S, Graber P, Jansen KU, Bonnefoy JY. CD21 is a ligand for CD23 and regulates IgE production. *Nature* 1992;358:505–507.

193. Dissen E, Ryan JC, Seaman WE, Fossum S. An autosomal dominant locus, Nka, mapping to the Ly-49 region of a rat natural killer (NK) gene complex, controls NK cell lysis of allogeneic lymphocytes. *J Exp Med* 1996;183:2197–2207.

194. Moretta A, Biassoni R, Bottino C, et al. Major histocompatibility complex class I-specific receptors on human natural killer and T lymphocytes [Review]. *Immunol Rev* 1997;155:105–117.

195. Colonna M, Borsellino G, Falco M, Ferrara GB, Strominger JL. HLA-C is the inhibitory ligand that determines dominant resistance to lysis by NK1- and NK2-specific natural killer cells. *Proc Natl Acad Sci U S A* 1993;90:12000–12004.

196. Colonna M. Specificity and function of immunoglobulin superfamily NK cell inhibitory and stimulatory receptors [Review]. *Immunol Rev* 1997;155:127–133.

197. Ciccone E, Pende D, Viale O, et al. Involvement of HLA class I alleles in natural killer (NK) cell-specific functions: Expression of HLA-Cw3 confers selective protection from lysis by alloreactive NK clones displaying a defined specificity (specificity 2). *J Exp Med* 1992;176:963.

198. Moretta A, Vitale M, Bottino C, et al. P58 molecules as putative receptors for major histocompatibility complex (MHC) class I molecules in human natural killer (NK) cells. Anti-p58 antibodies reconstitute lysis of MHC class I-protected cells in NK clones displaying different specificities. *J Exp Med* 1993;178:597–604.

199. Litwin V, Gumperz J, Parham P, Phillips JH, Lanier LL. NKB1: A natural killer cell receptor involved in the recognition of polymorphic HLA-B molecules. *J Exp Med* 1994;180:537–543.

200. Gumperz JE, Litwin V, Phillips JH, Lanier LL, Parham P. The Bw4 public epitope of HLA-B molecules confers reactivity with natural killer cell clones that express NKB1, a putative HLA receptor. *J Exp Med* 1995;181:1133–1144.

201. Pende D, Biassoni R, Cantoni C, et al. The natural killer cell receptor specific for HLA-A allotypes: A novel member of the p58/p70 family of inhibitory receptors that is characterized by three immunoglobulin-like domains and is expressed as a 140-kD disulphide-linked dimer. *J Exp Med* 1996;184:505–518.

202. Dohring C, Scheidegger D, Samaridis J, Cella M, Colonna M. A human killer inhibitory receptor specific for HLA-A. *J Immunol* 1996;156:3098–3101.

203. Long EO, Colonna M, Lanier LL. Inhibitory MHC class I receptors on NK and T cells: A standard nomenclature [Letter]. *Immunol Today* 1996;17:100.

204. Wagtmann N, Biassoni R, Cantoni C, et al. Molecular clones of the p58 NK receptor reveal immunoglobulin-related molecules with diversity in both the extra- and intracellular domains. *Immunity* 1995;2:439–449.

205. Colonna M, Samaridis J. Cloning of immunoglobulin-superfamily members associated with HLA-C and HLA-B recognition by human natural killer cells. *Science* 1995;268:367–368.

206. D'Andrea A, Chang C, Franz-Bacon K, McClanahan T, Phillips JH, Lanier LL. Molecular cloning of NKB1. A natural killer cell receptor for HLA-B allotypes. *J Immunol* 1995;155:2306–2310.

207. Long EO, Burshtyn DN, Clark WP, et al. Killer cell inhibitory receptors—diversity, specificity, and function [Review]. *Immunol Rev* 1997;155:135–144.

208. Salter RD, Chan HW, Tadikamalla R, Lawlor DA. Domain organization and sequence relationship of killer cell inhibitory receptors [Review]. *Immunol Rev* 1997;155:175–182.

209. Selvakumar A, Steffens U, Dupont B. Polymorphism and domain variability of human killer cell inhibitory receptors [Review]. *Immunol Rev* 1997;155:183–196.

210. Valiante NM, Lienert K, Shilling HG, Smits BJ, Parham P. Killer cell receptors—keeping pace with MHC class I evolution [Review]. *Immunol Rev* 1997;155:155–164.

211. Renard V, Cambiaggi A, Vely F, et al. Transduction of cytotoxic signals in natural killer cells—a general model of fine tuning between activatory and inhibitory pathways in lymphocytes [Review]. *Immunol Rev* 1997;155:205–221.

212. Wagtmann N, Rajagopalan S, Winter CC, Peruzzi M, Long EO. Killer cell inhibitory receptors specific for HLA-C and HLA-B identified by direct binding and by functional transfer. *Immunity* 1995;3:801–809.

213. Dohring C, Colonna M. Human natural killer cell inhibitory receptors bind to HLA class I molecules. *Eur J Immunol* 1996;26:365–369.

214. Fan QOR, Garboczi DN, Winter CC, Wagtmann N, Long EO, Wiley DC. Direct binding of a soluble natural killer cell inhibitory receptor to a soluble human leukocyte-Cw4 class I major histocompatibility complex molecule. *Proc Natl Acad Sci U S A* 1996;93:7178–7183.

215. Cella M, Longo A, Ferrara GB, Strominger JL, Colonna M. NK3-specific natural killer cells are selectively inhibited by Bw4-positive HLA alleles with isoleucine 80. *J Exp Med* 1994;180:1235–1242.

216. Luque I, Solana R, Galiani MD, et al. Threonine 80 on HLA-B27 confers protection against lysis by a group of natural killer clones. *Eur J Immunol* 1996;26:1974–1977.

217. Mandelboim O, Reyburn HT, Valesgomez M, et al. Protection from lysis by natural killer cells of group 1 and 2 specificity is mediated by residue 80 in human histocompatibility leukocyte antigen C alleles and also occurs with empty major histocompatibility complex molecules. *J Exp Med* 1996;184:913–922.

218. Mandelboim O, Reyburn HT, Sheu EG, et al. The binding site of NK receptors on HLA-C molecules. *Immunity* 1997;6:341–350.

219. Malnati MS, Peruzzi M, Parker KC, et al. Peptide specificity in the recognition of MHC class I by natural killer cell clones. *Science* 1995;267:1016–1018.

220. Peruzzi M, Wagtmann N, Long EO. A p70 killer cell inhibitory receptor specific for several HLA-B allotypes discriminates among peptides bound to HLA-B-asterisk-2705. *J Exp Med* 1996;184:1585–1590.

221. Moretta A, Sivori S, Vitale M, et al. Existence of both inhibitory (p58) and activatory (p50) receptors for HLA-C molecules in human natural killer cells. *J Exp Med* 1995;182:875–884.

222. Gumperz JE, Valiante NM, Parham P, Lanier LL, Tyan D. Heterogeneous phenotypes of expression of the NKB1 natural killer cell class I receptor among individuals of different human histocompatibility leukocyte antigens types appear genetically regulated, but not linked to major histocompatibililty complex haplotype. *J Exp Med* 1996;183:1817–1827.

223. Gumperz JE, Parham P. The enigma of the natural killer cell [Review]. *Nature* 1995;378:245–248.

224. Wang LL, Mehta IK, Leblanc PA, Yokoyama WM. Cutting edge: Mouse natural killer cells express GP49b1, a structural homologue of human killer inhibitory receptors. *J Immunol* 1997;158:13–17.

225. Rojo S, Burshtyn DN, Long EO, Wagtmann N. Type I transmembrane receptor with inhibitory function in mouse mast cells and NK cells. *J Immunol* 1997;158:9–12.

226. Arm JP, Gurish MF, Reynolds DS, et al. Molecular cloning of gp49, a cell-surface antigen that is preferentially expressed by mouse mast cell progenitors and is a new member of the immunoglobulin superfamily. *J Biol Chem* 1991;266:15966–15973.

227. Castells MC, Wu X, Arm JP, Austen KF, Katz HR. Cloning of the gp49B gene of the immunoglobulin superfamily and demonstration that one of its two products is an early-expressed mast cell surface protein originally described as gp49. *J Biol Chem* 1994;269:8393–8401.

228. Katz HR, Vivier E, Castells MC, McCormick MJ, Chambers JM, Austen KF. Mouse mast cell gp49B1 contains two immunoreceptor tyrosine-based inhibition motifs and suppresses mast cell activation when coligated with the high-affinity Fc receptor for IgE. *Proc Natl Acad Sci U S A* 1996;93:10809–10814.

229. Moretta A, Vitale M, Sivori S, et al. Human natural killer cell receptors for HLA-class I molecules. Evidence that the Kp43 (CD94) molecule functions as receptor for HLA-B alleles. *J Exp Med* 1994;180:545–555.

230. Aramburu J, Balboa MA, Izquierdo M, Lopez-Botet M. A novel functional cell surface dimer (Kp43) expressed by natural killer cells and gamma/delta TCR+ T lymphocytes. II. Modulation of natural killer cell cytotoxicity by anti-Kp43 monoclonal antibody. *J Immunol* 1991;147:714–721.

231. Brumbaugh KM, Perezvillar JJ, Dick CJ, Schoon RA, Lopezbotet M, Leibson PJ. Clonotypic differences in signaling from CD94 (KP43) on NK cells lead to divergent cellular responses. *J Immunol* 1996;157:2804–2812.

232. Chang C, Rodriguez A, Carretero M, Lopez-Botet M, Phillips JH, Lanier LL. Molecular characterization of human CD94: A type II membrane glycoprotein related to the C-type lectin superfamily. *Eur J Immunol* 1995;25:2433–2437.

233. Phillips JH, Chang CW, Mattson J, Gumperz JE, Parham P, Lanier LL. CD94 and a novel associated protein (94ap) form a NK cell receptor involved in the recognition of HLA-A, HLA-B, and HLA-C allotypes. *Immunity* 1996;5:163–172.

234. Perez-Villar JJ, Carretero M, Navarro F, et al. Biochemical and serologic evidence for the existence of functionally distinct forms of the CD94 NK cell receptor. *J Immunol* 1996;157:5367–5374.

235. Lazetic S, Chang C, Houchins JP, Lanier LL, Phillips JH. Human natural killer cell receptors involved in MHC class I recognition are disulfide-linked heterodimers of CD94 and NKG2 subunits. *J Immunol* 1996;157:4741–4745.

236. Carretero M, Cantoni C, Bellon T, et al. The CD94 and NKG2-A C-type lectins covalently assemble to form a natural killer cell inhibitory receptor for HLA class I molecules. *Eur J Immunol* 1997;27:563–567.

237. Houchins JP, Yabe T, McSherry C, Bach FH. DNA sequence analysis of NKG2, a family of related cDNA clones encoding type II integral membrane proteins on human natural killer cells. *J Exp Med* 1991;173:1017–1020.

238. Duchler M, Offterdinger M, Holzmuller H, et al. NKG2-C is a receptor on human natural killer cells that recognizes structures on K562 target cells. *Eur J Immunol* 1995;25:2923–2931.

239. Sivori S, Vitale M, Bottino C, et al. CD94 functions as a natural killer cell inhibitory receptor for different HLA class I alleles—identification of the inhibitory form of CD94 by the use of novel monoclonal antibodies. *Eur J Immunol* 1996;26:2487–2492.

240. Lopez-Botet M, Perezvillar JJ, Carretero M, et al. Structure and function of the CD94 C type lectin receptor complex involved in recognition of HLA class I molecules [Review]. *Immunol Rev* 1997;155:165–174.

241. Yokoyama WM, Jacobs LB, Kanagawa O, Shevach EM, Cohen DI. A murine T lymphocyte antigen belongs to a supergene family of type II integral membrane proteins. *J Immunol* 1989;143:1379–1386.

242. Janeway CA Jr. The T cell receptor as a multicomponent signalling machine: CD4/CD8 coreceptors and CD45 in T cell activation. *Annu Rev Immunol* 1992;10:645–674.

243. Phillips JH, Gumperz JE, Parham P, Lanier LL. Superantigen-dependent, cell-mediated cytotoxicity inhibited by MHC class I receptors on T lymphocytes. *Science* 1995;268:403–405.

244. Kaufman DS, Schoon RA, Robertson MJ, Leibson PJ. Inhibition of selective signaling events in natural killer cells recognizing major histocompatibility complex class I. *Proc Natl Acad Sci U S A* 1995;92:6484–6488.

245. D'Ambrosio D, Hippen KL, Minskoff SA, et al. Recruitment and activation of PTP1C in negative regulation of antigen receptor signaling by FcγRIIB1. *Science* 1995;268:293–297.

246. Campbell MA, Klinman NR. Phosphotyrosine-dependent association between CD22 and protein tyrosine phosphatase 1C. *Eur J Immunol* 1995;25:1573–1579.

247. Burshtyn DN, Scharenberg AM, Wagtmann N, et al. Recruitment of tyrosine phosphatase HCP by the killer cell inhibitor receptor. *Immunity* 1996;4:77–85.

248. Campbell KS, Dessing M, Lopez-Botet M, Cella M, Colonna M. Tyrosine phosphorylation of a human killer inhibitory receptor recruits protein tyrosine phosphatase 1C. *J Exp Med* 1996;184:93–100.

249. Fry AM, Lanier LL, Weiss A. Phosphotyrosines in the killer cell inhibitory receptor motif of NKB1 are required for negative signaling and for association with protein tyrosine phosphatase 1C. *J Exp Med* 1996;184:295–300.

250. Olcese L, Lang P, Vely F, et al. Human and mouse killer-cell inhibitory receptors recruit PTP1C and PTP1D protein tyrosine phosphatases. *J Immunol* 1996;156:4531–4534.

251. Ono M, Bolland S, Tempst P, Ravetch JV. Role of the inositol phosphatase SHIP in negative regulation of the immune system by the receptor Fc(gamma)RIIB. *Nature* 1996;383:263–266.

252. Binstadt BA, Brumbaugh KM, Dick CJ, et al. Sequential involvement of LCK and SHP-1 with MHC-recognizing receptors on NK cells inhibits FcR-initiated tyrosine kinase activation. *Immunity* 1996;5:629–638.

253. Valiante NM, Phillips JH, Lanier LL, Parham P. Killer cell inhibitory receptor recognition of human leukocyte antigen (HLA) class I blocks formation of a PP36/PLC-gamma signaling complex in human natural killer (NK) cells. *J Exp Med* 1996;184:2243–2250.

254. Galandrini R, Palmieri G, Piccoli M, Frati L, Santoni A. CD16-mediated p21ras activation is associated with Shc and p36 tyrosine phosphorylation and their binding with Grb2 in human natural killer cells. *J Exp Med* 1996;183:179–186.

255. Sentman CL, Hackett J Jr, Moore TA, Tutt MM, Bennett M, Kumar V. Pan natural killer cell monoclonal antibodies and their relationship to the NK1.1 antigen. *Hybridoma* 1989;8:605–614.

256. Scalzo AA, Lyons PA, Fitzgerald NA, Forbes CA, Yokoyama WM, Shellam GR. Genetic mapping of Cmv1 in the region of mouse chromosome 6 encoding the NK gene complex-associated loci Ly49 and musNKR-P1. *Genomics* 1995;27:435–441.

257. Forbes CA, Brown MG, Cho R, Shellam GR, Yokoyama WM, Scalzo AA. The Cmv1 host resistance locus is closely linked to the Ly49 multigene family within the natural killer cell gene complex (NKC) on mouse chromosome 6. *Genomics* 1997;41:406–413.

258. Lopez Cabrera M, Santis AG, Fernandez-Ruiz E, et al. Molecular cloning, expression, and chromosomal localization of the human earliest lymphocyte activation antigen AIM/CD69, a new member of the C-type animal lectin superfamily of signal-transmitting receptors. *J Exp Med* 1993;178:537–547.

259. Yabe T, McSherry C, Bach FH, et al. A multigene family on human chromosome 12 encodes natural killer-cell lectins. *Immunogenetics* 1993;37:455–460.

260. Plougastel B, Jones T, Trowsdale J. Genomic structure, chromosome location, and alternative splicing of the human NKG2A gene. *Immunogenetics* 1996;44:286–291.

261. Ziegler SF, Levin SD, Johnson L, et al. The mouse CD69 gene. Structure, expression, and mapping to the NK gene complex. *J Immunol* 1994;152:1228–1236.

262. Hara T, Jung LKL, Bjorndahl JM, Fu SM. Human T cell activation. III. Rapid induction of a phosphorylated 28 kD/32 kD disulfide-linked early activation antigen (EA 1) by 12-o-teradecanoyl phorbol-13-acetate, mitogens, and antigens. *J Exp Med* 1986;164:1988–2005.

263. Yokoyama WM, Koning F, Kehn PJ, et al. Characterization of a cell surface-expressed disulfide-linked dimer involved in murine T cell activation. *J Immunol* 1988;141:369–376.

264. Testi R, D'Ambrosio D, De Maria R, Santoni A. The CD69 receptor: a multipurpose cell-surface trigger for hematopoietic cells [Review]. *Immunol Today* 1994;15:479–483.

265. Hamann J, Fiebig H, Strauss M. Expression cloning of the early activation antigen CD69, a type II integral membrane protein with a C-type lectin domain. *J Immunol* 1993;150:4920–4927.

266. Ziegler SF, Ramsdell F, Hjerrild KA, et al. Molecular characterization of the early activation antigen CD69: A type II membrane glycoprotein related to a family of natural killer cell activation antigens. *Eur J Immunol* 1993;23:1643–1648.

267. Hamann J, Montgomery KT, Lau S, Kucherlapati R, van Lier RAW. AICL: A new activation-induced antigen encoded by the human NK gene complex. *Immunogenetics* 1997;45:295–300.

268. Depatie C, Muise E, Lepage P, Gros P, Vidal SM. High-resolution linkage map in the proximity of the host resistance locus CMV1. *Genomics* 1997;39:154–163.

269. Brown MG, Fulmek S, Matsumoto K, et al. A 2 megabase YAC contig and physical map of the natural killer gene complex on mouse chromosome 6. *Genomics* 1997;42:16–25.

270. Brown MG, Scalzo AA, Matsumoto K, Yokoyama WM. The natural killer gene complex—a genetic basis for understanding natural killer cell function and innate immunity [Review]. *Immunol Rev* 1997;155:53–65.

271. York IA, Rock KL. Antigen processing and presentation by the class I major histocompatibility complex [Review]. *Annu Rev Immunol* 1996;14:369–396.

272. Scalzo AA, Fitzgerald NA, Simmons A, La Vista AB, Shellam GR. Cmv-1, a genetic locus that controls murine cytomegalovirus replication in the spleen. *J Exp Med* 1990;171:1469–1483.

273. Shanley JD. In vivo administration of monoclonal antibody to the NK 1.1 antigen of natural killer cells: Effect on acute murine cytomegalovirus infection. *J Med Virol* 1990;30:58–60.

274. Scalzo AA, Fitzgerald NA, Wallace CR, et al. The effect of the Cmv-1 resistance gene, which is linked to the natural killer cell gene complex, is mediated by natural killer cells. *J Immunol* 1992;149:581–589.

275. Tay CH, Welsh RM. Distinct organ-dependent mechanisms for the control of murine cytomegalovirus infection by natural killer cells. *J Virol* 1997;71: 267–275.

276. Beck S, Barrell BG. Human cytomegalovirus encodes a glycoprotein homologous to MHC class-I antigens. *Nature* 1988;331:269–272.

277. Rawlinson WD, Farrell HE, Barrell BG. Analysis of the complete DNA sequence of murine cytomegalovirus. *J Virol* 1996;70:8833–8849.

278. Delano ML, Brownstein DG. Innate resistance to lethal mousepox is genetically linked to the NK gene complex on chromosome 6 and correlates with early restriction of virus replication by cells with an NK phenotype. *J Virol* 1995;69: 5875–5877.

279. Rolstad B, Vaage JT, Naper C, et al. Positive and negative MHC class I recognition by rat NK cells [Review]. *Immunol Rev* 1997;155:91–104.

280. Idris AH, Scalzo AA, Yokoyama WM. A genetic locus controlling tumor killing maps to the NKC [Abstract]. *J Allergy Clin Immunol* 1997;99(suppl):256.

281. Rosenberg SA, Lotze MT, Muul LM, et al. Observations on the systemic administration of autologous lymphokine-activated killer cells and recombinant interleukin-2 to patients with metastatic cancer. *N Engl J Med* 1985;313:1485–92.

282. Herberman RB, Gorelik E. Role of the natural immune system in control of primary tumors and metastasis. In: Reynolds CW, Wiltrout RH, eds. *Functions of the Natural Immune System.* New York: Plenum, 1989:3–37.

283. van den Broek MF, Kagi D, Zinkernagel RM, Hengartner H. Perforin dependence of natural killer cell–mediated tumor control in vivo. *Eur J Immunol* 1995;25:3514–3516.

284. Scalzo AA, Lyons PA, Fitzgerald NA, Forbes CA, Shellam GR. Establishment of the BALB.B6-Cmv-1r strain: A mouse strain congenic for the Cmv-1 resistance gene and the natural killer cell gene complex on mouse chromosome 6. *Immunogenetics* 1995;41:148–151.

285. Wang B, Biron C, She J, et al. A block in both early T lymphocyte and natural killer cell development in transgenic mice with high-copy numbers of the human CD3E gene. *Proc Natl Acad Sci U S A* 1994;91:9402–9406.

286. Flamand V, Shores EW, Tran T, et al. Delayed maturation of CD4⁻ CD8⁻ Fc gamma RII/III⁺ T and natural killer cell precursors in Fc epsilon RI gamma transgenic mice. *J Exp Med* 1996;184:1725–1735.

287. Barbosa MD, Nguyen QA, Tchernev VT, et al. Identification of the homologous beige and Chediak-Higashi syndrome genes. *Nature* 1996;382:262–265.

288. Kingsmore SF, Barbosa MD, Tchernev VT, et al. Positional cloning of the Chediak-Higashi syndrome gene: Genetic mapping of the beige locus on mouse chromosome 13. *J Invest Med* 1996;44:454–461.

289. Perou CM, Moore KJ, Nagle DL, et al. Identification of the murine beige gene by YAC complementation and positional cloning. *Nat Genet* 1996;13:303–308.

290. Biron CA, Byron KS, Sullivan JL. Severe herpesvirus infections in an adolescent without natural killer cells. *N Engl J Med* 1989;320:1731–1735.

291. Ballas ZK, Turner JM, Turner DA, Goetzman EA, Kemp JD. A patient with simultaneous absence of "classical" natural killer cells (CD3⁻, CD16⁺ and NKH1⁺) and expansion of CD3⁺, CD4⁻, CD8⁻, NKH1⁺ subset. *J Allergy Clin Immunol* 1990;85:453–459.

292. Jawahar S, Moody C, Chan M, Finberg R, Geha R, Chatila T. Natural Killer (NK) cell deficiency associated with an epitope-deficient Fc receptor type IIIA (CD16-II). *Clin Exp Immunol* 1996;103:408–413.

293. Seki H, Ueno Y, Taga K, Matsuda A, Miyawaki T, Taniguchi N. Mode of in vitro augmentation of natural killer cell activity by recombinant human interleukin 2: A comparative study of Leu-11⁺ and Leu-11⁻ cell populations in cord blood and adult peripheral blood. *J Immunol* 1985;135:2351–2356.

294. Cook JL, Ikle DN, Routes BA. Natural killer cell ontogeny in the athymic rat. Relationship between functional maturation and acquired resistance to E1A oncogene-expressing sarcoma cells. *J Immunol* 1995;155:5512–5518.

295. Greenough A. The TORCH screen and intrauterine infections [Review]. *Arch Dis Child* 1994;70:F163–165.

296. Rook AH, Masur H, Lane HC, et al. Interleukin-2 enhances the depressed natural killer and cytomegalovirus-specific cytotoxic activities of lymphocytes from patients with the acquired immune deficiency syndrome. *J Clin Invest* 1983;72: 398–403.

297. Lusso P, Malnati MS, Garzino-Demo A, Crowley RW, Long EO, Gallo RC. Infection of natural killer cells by human herpesvirus 6. *Nature* 1993;362: 458–462.

298. Welsh RM, Tay CH, Varga SM, Odonnell CL, Vergilis KL, Selin LK. Lymphocyte-dependent natural immunity to virus infections mediated by both natural killer cells and memory T cells. *Semin Virol* 1996;7:95–102.

299. Bancroft GJ. The role of natural killer cells in innate resistance to infection [Review]. *Curr Opin Immunol* 1993;5:503–510.

300. Bukowski JF, Woda BA, Welsh RM. Pathogenesis of murine cytomegalovirus infection in natural killer cell-depleted mice. *J Virol* 1984;52:119–128.

301. Biron CA, Turgiss LR, Welsh RM. Increase in NK cell number and turnover rate during acute viral infection. *J Immunol* 1983;131:1539–1545.

302. Natuk RJ, Welsh RM. Accumulation and chemotaxis of natural killer/large granular lymphocytes at sites of virus replication. *J Immunol* 1987;138:877–883.

303. Denkers EY, Gazzinelli RT, Martin D, Sher A. Emergence of NK1.1⁺ cells as effectors of IFN-gamma dependent immunity to *Toxoplasma gondii* in MHC class I–deficient mice. *J Exp Med* 1993;178:1465–1472.

304. Locksley RM. Interleukin 12 in host defense against microbial pathogens [Comment]. *Proc Natl Acad Sci U S A* 1993;90:5879–5880.

305. Mosmann TR, Coffman RL. Heterogeneity of cytokine secretion patterns and functions of helper T cells. *Adv Immunol* 1989;46:111.

306. Trinchieri G. Interleukin-12 and its role in the generation of Th1 cells. *Immunol Today* 1993;14:335–338.

307. Scharton TM, Scott P. Natural killer cells are a source of interferon gamma that drives differentiation of CD4⁺ T cell subsets and induces early resistance to *Leishmania* major in mice. *J Exp Med* 1993;178:567–577.

308. Trinchieri G. Interleukin-12: A proinflammatory cytokine with immunoregulatory functions that bridge innate resistance and antigen-specific adaptive immunity [Review]. *Annu Rev Immunol* 1995;13:251–276.

309. Tripp CS, Wolf SF, Unanue ER. Interleukin 12 and tumor necrosis factor alpha are costimulators of interferon gamma production by natural killer cells in severe combined immunodeficiency mice with listeriosis, and interleukin 10 is a physiologic antagonist. *Proc Natl Acad Sci U S A* 1993;90:3725–3729.

310. Tripp CS, Gately MK, Hakimi J, Ling P, Unanue ER. Neutralization of IL-12 decreases resistance to Listeria in SCID and C.B-17 mice. Reversal by IFN-gamma. *J Immunol* 1994;152:1883–1887.

311. Orange JS, Wang B, Terhorst C, Biron CA. Requirement for natural killer cell-produced interferon gamma in defense against murine cytomegalovirus infection and enhancement of this defense pathway by interleukin 12 administration. *J Exp Med* 1995;182:1045–1056.

312. Orange JS, Biron CA. Characterization of early IL-12, IFN-alphabeta, and TNF effects on antiviral state and NK cell responses during murine cytomegalovirus infection. *J Immunol* 1996;156:4746–4756.

313. Szabo SJ, Dighe AS, Gubler U, Murphy KM. Regulation of the interleukin (IL)-12Rbeta2 subunit expression in developing T helper 1 (Th1) and Th2 cells. *J Exp Med* 1997;185:817–824.

314. Michael A, Hackett JJ, Bennett M, Kumar V, Yuan D. Regulation of B lymphocytes by natural killer cells. Role of IFN-g. *J Immunol* 1989;142:1095–1101.

315. Snapper CM, Yamaguchi H, Moorman MA, Mond JJ. An in vitro model for T cell-independent induction of humoral immunity. A requirement for NK cells. *J Immunol* 1994;152:4884–4892.

316. Robertson MJ, Ritz J. Biology and clinical relevance of human natural killer cells. *Blood* 1990;76:2421.

317. Peters PM, Ortaldo JR, Shalaby MR, et al. Natural killer-sensitive targets stimulate production of TNF-α but not TNF-β (lymphotoxin) by highly purified human peripheral blood large granular lymphocytes. *J Immunol* 1986;137:2592.

318. Paya CV, Kenmotsu N, Schoon RA, Leibson PJ. Tumor necrosis factor and lymphotoxin secretion by human natural killer cells leads to antiviral cytotoxicity. *J Immunol* 1988;141:1989.

319. Cuturi MC, Anegon I, Sherman F, et al. Production of hematopoietic colony stimulating factors by human natural killer cells. *J Exp Med* 1989; 169:569.

320. Pistoia V, Zupo S, Corcione A, et al. Production of colony-stimulating activity by human natural killer cells: Analysis of the conditions that influence the release and detection of colony stimulating activity. *Blood* 1989;74:156.

321. Vitolo D, Vujanovic NL, Rabinowich H, Schlesinger M, Herberman RB, Whiteside TL. Rapid IL-2-induced adherence of human natural killer cells. Expression of mRNA for cytokines and IL-2 receptors in adherent NK cells. *J Immunol* 1993;151:1926–1937.

322. Bendelac A, Lantz O, Quimby ME, Yewdell JW, Bennink JR, Brutkiewicz RR. CD1 recognition by mouse NK1+ T lymphocytes. *Science* 1995;268:863–865.

323. Bendelac A. Positive selection of mouse NK1+ T cells by CD1-expressing cortical thymocytes. *J Exp Med* 1995;182:2091–2096.

324. Yoshimoto T, Bendelac A, Hu-Li J, Paul WE. Defective IgE production by SJL mice is linked to the absence of CD4⁺, NK1.1⁺ T cells that promptly produce interleukin 4. *Proc Natl Acad Sci U S A* 1995;92:11931–11934.

325. Yoshimoto T, Bendelac A, Watson C, Hu-Li J, Paul WE. Role of NK1.1⁺ T cells in a TH2 response and in immunoglobulin E production. *Science* 1995;270: 1845–1847.

326. Bordignon C, Daley JP, Nakamura I. Hematopoietic histoincompatibility reactions by NK cells in vitro: Model for genetic resistance to marrow grafts. *Science* 1985;230:1398–1401.

327. Murphy WJ, Kumar V, Bennett M. Rejection of bone marrow allografts by mice with severe combined immune deficiency (SCID). Evidence that natural killer cells can mediate the specificity of marrow graft rejection. *J Exp Med* 1987;165: 1212–1217.

328. Sentman CL, Kumar V, Koo G, Bennett M. Effector cell expression of NK1.1, a murine natural killer cell–specific molecule, and ability of mice to reject bone marrow allografts. *J Immunol* 1989;142:1847–1853.

329. Öhlén C, Kling G, Hoglund P, et al. Prevention of allogeneic bone marrow graft rejection by H-2 transgene in donor mice. *Science* 1989;246:666–668.

330. Milisauskas VK, Nakamura I. The ability of H-2Dd molecule to affect natural resistance to hemopoietic allografts is an intrinsic property shared by Ddm1 but not Ld. *Eur J Immunol* 1994;24:336–342.

331. Yokoyama WM. Commentary. Hybrid resistance and the Ly-49 family of natural killer cell receptors. *J Exp Med* 1995;182:273–277.

332. Zheng WP, Kiura K, Milisauskas VK, Denardin E, Nakamura I. Murine NK cell allospecificity-1 is defined by inhibitory ligands. *J Immunol* 1996;156:4651–4655.

333. Bellone G, Valiante NM, Viale O, Ciccone E, Moretta L, Trinchieri G. Regulation of hematopoiesis in vitro by alloreactive natural killer cell clones. *J Exp Med* 1993;177:1117–1125.

334. Graubert TA, Russell JH, Ley TJ. The role of granzyme B in murine models of acute graft-versus-host disease and graft rejection. *Blood* 1996;87:1232–1237.

335. Shresta S, MacIvor DM, Heusel JW, Russell JH, Ley TJ. Natural killer and lymphokine-activated killer cells require granzyme B for the rapid induction of apoptosis in susceptible target cells. *Proc Natl Acad Sci U S A* 1995;92: 5679–5683.

336. Baker M, Podack ER, Levy RB. Fas and perforin cytotoxic pathways are not the major effector mechanisms in allogeneic resistance to bone marrow. *Ann N Y Acad Sci* 1995;770:368–369.

337. Iizuka K, Kaneko H, Yamada T, Kimura H, Kokai Y, Fujimoto J. Host F1 mice pretreated with granulocyte colony-stimulating factor accept parental bone marrow grafts in hybrid resistance system. *Blood* 1997;89:1446–1451.

338. Yokoyama WM. Commentary. The mother-child union: The case of missing-self and protection of the fetus. *Proc Natl Acad Sci U S A* 1997;94:5998–6000.

339. Croy BA. Granulated metrial gland cells: Hypotheses concerning possible functions during murine gestation [Review]. *J Reprod Immunol* 1994;27:85–94.

340. Schmidt CM, Orr HT. Maternal/fetal interactions: The role of the MHC class I molecule HLA-G [Review]. *Crit Rev Immunol* 1993;13:207–224.

341. Sipes SL, Medaglia MV, Stabley DL, et al. A new major histocompatibility complex class I b gene expressed in the mouse blastocyst and placenta. *Immunogenetics* 1996;45:108–120.

342. Shawar SM, Vyas JM, Rodgers JR, Rich RR. Antigen presentation by major histocompatibility complex class I-B molecules [Review]. *Annu Rev Immunol* 1994;12:839–880.

343. Diehl M, Munz C, Keilholz W, et al. Nonclassical HLA-G molecules are classical peptide presenters. *Curr Biol* 1996;6:305–314.

344. Schust DJ, Hill AB, Ploegh HL. Herpes simplex virus blocks intracellular transport of HLA-G in placentally derived human cells. *J Immunol* 1996;157: 3375–3380.

345. Pazmany L, Mandelboim O, Valesgomez M, Davis DM, Reyburn HT, Strominger JL. Protection from natural killer cell-mediated lysis by HLA-G expression on target cells. *Science* 1996;274:792–795.

346. Munz C, Holmes N, King A, et al. Human histocompatibility leukocyte antigen (HLA)-G molecules inhibit NKAT3 expressing natural killer cells. *J Exp Med* 1997;185:385–391.

347. Soderstrom K, Corliss B, Lanier LL, Phillips JH. CD94/NKG2 is the predominant inhibitory receptor involved in recognition of HLA-G by decidual and peripheral blood NK cells. *J Immunol* 1997;159:1072–1075.

348. Rouas-Freiss N, Marchal RE, Kirszenbaum M, Dausset J, Carosella ED. The alpha1 domain of HLA-G1 and HLA-G2 inhibits cytotoxicity induced by natural killer cells. Is HLA-G the public ligand for natural killer cell inhibitory receptors? *Proc Natl Acad Sci U S A* 1997;94:5249–5254.

349. Zijlstra M, Bix M, Simister NE, Loring JM, Raulet DH, Jaenisch R. Beta 2-microglobulin deficient mice lack CD4-8¹ cytolytic T cells. *Nature* 1990;344: 742–746.

350. Van Kaer L, Ashton-Rickardt PG, Ploegh HL, Tonegawa S. TAP1 mutant mice are deficient in antigen presentation, surface class I molecules, and CD4-8⁺ T cells. *Cell* 1992;71:1205–1214.

351. Lee N, Malacko AR, Ishitani A, et al. The membrane-bound and soluble forms of HLA-G bind identical sets of endogenous peptides but differ with respect to TAP association. *Immunity* 1995;3:591–600.

352. Ishitani A, Geraghty DE. Alternative splicing of HLA-G transcripts yields proteins with primary structures resembling both class I and class II antigens. *Proc Natl Acad Sci U S A* 1992;89:3947–3951.

353. Spits H, Lanier LL, Phillips JH. Development of human T and natural killer cells [Review]. *Blood* 1995;85:2654–2670.

354. Moore TA, Bennett M, Kumar V. Murine natural killer cell differentiation—past, present, and future. *Immunol Res* 1996;15:151–162.

355. Haller O, Kiessling R, Orn A, Wigzell H. Generation of natural killer cells: An autonomous function of the bone marrow. *J Exp Med* 1977;145:1411–1416.

356. Haller O, Wigzell H. Suppression of natural killer cell activity with radioactive strontium: Effector cells are marrow dependent. *J Immunol* 1977;118:1503–1506.

357. Kumar V, Ben-Ezra J, Bennett M, Sonnenfeld G. Natural killer cells in mice treated with 89strontium: Normal target-binding cell numbers but inability to kill even after interferon administration. *J Immunol* 1979;123:1832–1838.

358. Seaman WE, Gindhart TD, Greenspan JS, Blackman MA, Talal N. Natural killer cells, bone, and the bone marrow: Studies in estrogen-treated mice and in congenitally osteopetrotic (mi/mi) mice. *J Immunol* 1979;122:2541–2547.

359. Hackett J Jr, Bennett M, Kumar V. Origin and differentiation of natural killer cells. I. Characteristics of a transplantable NK cell precursor. *J Immunol* 1985; 134:3731–3738.

360. Moore T, Bennett M, Kumar V. Transplantable NK cell progenitors in murine bone marrow. *J Immunol* 1995;154:1653–1663.

361. Molnar A, Georgopoulos K. The Ikaros gene encodes a family of functionally diverse zinc finger DNA-binding proteins. *Mol Cell Biol* 1994;14:8292–8303.

362. Georgopoulos K, Bigby M, Wang JH, et al. The Ikaros gene is required for the development of all lymphoid lineages. *Cell* 1994;79:143–156.

363. Sanchez MJ, Muench MO, Roncarolo MG, Lanier LL, Phillips JH. Identification of a common T/natural killer cell progenitor in human fetal thymus. *J Exp Med* 1994;180:569–576.

364. Leclercq G, Debacker V, de Smedt M, Plum J. Differential effects of interleukin 15 and interleukin-2 on differentiation of bipotential T/natural killer progenitor cells. *J Exp Med* 1996;184:325–336.

365. Lanier LL, Chang C, Spits H, Phillips JH. Expression of cytoplasmic CD3 epsilon proteins in activated human adult natural killer (NK) cells and CD3 gamma, delta, epsilon complexes in fetal NK cells. Implications for the relationship of NK and T lymphocytes. *J Immunol* 1992;149:1876–1880.

366. Manoussaka M, Georgiou A, Rossiter B, et al. Phenotypic and functional characterization of long-lived NK cell lines of different maturational status obtained from mouse fetal liver. *J Immunol* 1997;158:112–119.

367. Skinner M, Le Gros G, Marbrook J, Watson JD. Development of fetal thymocytes in organ cultures. Effect of interleukin 2. *J Exp Med* 1987;165:1481–1493.

368. Skinner M, Marbrook J. Effect of interleukin 2 on fetal thymocytes in organ cultures: Generation of lymphokine-activated killer cells. *Cell Immunol* 1988;112: 104–111.

369. Plum J, Koning F, Leclercq G, Tison B, De Smedt M. Expansion of large granular lymphocytes in IL-2–driven 14-day-old fetal thymocytes in organ culture. *J Immunol* 1990;144:3710–3717.

370. Ebnet K, Levelt CN, Tran TT, Eichmann K, Simon MM. Transcription of granzyme A and B genes is differentially regulated during lymphoid ontogeny. *J Exp Med* 1995;181:755–763.

371. Renard V, Ardouin L, Malissen M, et al. Normal development and function of natural killer cells in CD3 epsilon delta 5/delta 5 mutant mice. *Proc Natl Acad Sci U S A* 1995;92:7545–7549.

372. Miller SC. The development of natural killer (NK) cells from Thy-1loLin-Sca-1⁺ stem cells: Acquisition by NK cells in vivo of the homing receptor MEL-14 and the integrin Mac-1. *Immunobiology* 1994;190:385–398.

373. Migliorati G, Moraca R, Nicoletti I, Riccardi C. IL-2–dependent generation of natural killer cells from bone marrow: Role of MAC-1⁻, NK1-1⁻ precursors. *Cell Immunol* 1992;141:323–331.

374. He YW, Malek TR. Interleukin-7 receptor alpha is essential for the development of gamma delta + T cells, but not natural killer cells. *J Exp Med* 1996;184: 289–293.

375. Park SY, Saijo K, Takahashi T, et al. Developmental defects of lymphoid cells in Jak3 kinase-deficient mice. *Immunity* 1995;3:771–782.

376. Bennett IM, Zatsepina O, Zamai L, Azzoni L, Mikheeva T, Perussia B. Definition of a natural killer NKR-PLA(+)/CD56(-)/CD16(-) functionally immature human NK cell subset that differentiates in vitro in the presence of interleukin 12. *J Exp Med* 1996;184:1845–1856.

377. Brooks CG, Georgiou A, Jordan RK. The majority of immature fetal thymocytes can be induced to proliferate to IL-2 and differentiate into cells indistinguishable from mature natural killer cells. *J Immunol* 1993;151:6645–6656.

378. Dorfman JR, Raulet DH. Developmental expression of Ly49 receptors on murine natural killer cells [Abstract]. *J Allergy Clin Immunol* 1997;99(suppl):256.

379. Sentman CL, Olsson MY, Kärre K. Missing self recognition by natural killer cells in MHC class I transgenic mice. A "receptor calibration" model for how effector cells adapt to self [Review]. *Semin Immunol* 1995;7:109–119.

380. Hoglund P, Sundback J, Olssonalheim MY, et al. Host MHC class I gene control of NK-cell specificity in the mouse [Review]. *Immunol Rev* 1997;155:11–28.

381. Dorfman JR, Raulet DH. Major histocompatibility complex genes determine natural killer cell tolerance. *Eur J Immunol* 1996;26:151–155.

382. Held W, Dorfman JR, Wu MF, Raulet DH. Major histocompatibility complex class I dependent skewing of the natural killer cell LY49 receptor repertoire. *Eur J Immunol* 1996;26:2286–2292.

383. Ljunggren HG, Van Kaer L, Ploegh HL, Tonegawa S. Altered natural killer cell repertoire in Tap-1 mutant mice. *Proc Natl Acad Sci U S A* 1994;91:6520–6524.

384. Jaffe ES, Chan JK, Su IJ, et al. Report of the Workshop on Nasal and Related Extranodal Angiocentric T/Natural Killer Cell Lymphomas. Definitions, differential diagnosis, and epidemiology. *Am J Surg Pathol* 1996;20:103–111.

385. Tefferi A, Li CY, Witzig TE, Dhodapkar MV, Okuno SH, Phyliky RL. Chronic natural killer cell lymphocytosis: A descriptive clinical study. *Blood* 1994;84: 2721–2725.

386. Garcia-Suarez J, Prieto A, Reyes E, et al. Persistent lymphocytosis of natural killer cells in autoimmune thrombocytopenic purpura (ATP) patients after splenectomy. *Br J Haematol* 1995;89:653–655.

387. Tak PP, Kummer JA, Hack CE, et al. Granzyme-positive cytotoxic cells are specifically increased in early rheumatoid synovial tissue. *Arthritis Rheum* 1994; 37:1735–1743.

388. Dalakas MC, Illa I. Common variable immunodeficiency and inclusion body myositis: A distinct myopathy mediated by natural killer cells. *Ann Neurol* 1995;37:806–810.

389. Takeda K, Dennert G. The development of autoimmunity in C57BL/6 lpr mice correlates with the disappearance of natural killer type 1-positive cells: Evidence for their suppressive action on bone marrow stem cell proliferation, B cell immunoglobulin secretion, and autoimmune symptoms. *J Exp Med* 1993;177: 155–164.

390. Harada M, Lin T, Kurosawa S, et al. Natural killer cells inhibit the development of autoantibody production in (C57BL/6 x DBA/2) F1 hybrid mice injected with DBA/2 spleen cells. *Cell Immunol* 1995;161:42–49.

391. Acevedo A, Aramburu J, Lopez J, Fernandez-Herrera J, Fernandez-Ranada JM, Lopez-Botet M. Identification of natural killer (NK) cells in lesions of human cutaneous graft-versus-host disease: Expression of a novel NK-associated surface antigen (Kp43) in mononuclear infiltrates. *J Invest Dermatol* 1991;97:659–666.

392. Muluk SC, Hakim FT, Shearer GM. Murine cytomegalovirus infection can enhance hybrid resistance through modulation of host natural killer activity. *J Immunol* 1990;145:1113–1119.

Fundamental Immunology, Fourth Edition,
edited by William E. Paul
Lippincott–Raven Publishers, Philadelphia © 1999.

CHAPTER 18

Origin and Evolution of the Vertebrate Immune System

Louis Du Pasquier and Martin Flajnik

All living organisms are exposed to pathogens and parasites from early in their development, yet they preserve their individuality displaying various types of immunity. Whether these different forms of immunity share the same principles of foreign recognition and are phylogenetically related to one another has been a major preoccupation of many evolutionary biologists and immunologists. Certainly all the elements of the vertebrate immune system are not present throughout the animal kingdom but it ought to be possible to trace the origin of many of them in other phyla. To achieve similar defense functions, various phyla will exploit different strategies, resulting in analogies (convergences) as well as in homologies. Moreover, when the survival of the individual is at stake, nature will rarely allocate this function to a single mechanism. In principle, a convenient immune system could work if it recognized foreign invaders either with a defense mechanism that is inhibited by self but is activated in the absence of self, or with a repertoire of specific receptors depleted of antiself activity. In fact, the vertebrate immune system uses both strategies and the molecules involved in each are sometimes the same, or belong to the same family. In evolution both systems may not have always coexisted, and a comparative study will help define the relationship between them.

In the following sketch the characteristics of an adaptive immune system are italicized.

During ontogeny the adaptive immune system accumulates a population of *lymphocytes* that are each equipped with unique surface receptors able to recognize biologic, nonself material in cognate interactions. Any cell recognizing an epitope proliferates and differentiates (*clonal selection*). After *signal transduction*, following the stimulation of several receptors by *cytokines* or by-products of innate immunity, the cell's progeny acquires *effector functions* (i.e., killing or secretion of antibody).

The antigen-specific receptors, *immunoglobulin* (Ig) and *T-cell receptor* (TCR), are dimers of polypeptide chains made of Ig domains. Their antigen specificity is acquired by a somatic process of gene *rearrangement* that constructs the variable part of the molecule, which interacts with the epitope. Complex *selection* processes check the specificity of the receptor expressed on the surface by means of the *major histocompatibility complex* (MHC) class I and II molecules presenting peptides and, in principle, spare only the cells whose receptors cannot react to self in the periphery. When in action, the system mounts an immune response characterized by *specificity* and *memory*. The development and unfolding of responses to antigens in the adaptive immune system is a clear case of somatic evolution during ontogeny and during the immune response; the cells are subjected to the same laws of mutation and Darwinian selection as are individuals of a species. The immune system of vertebrates also exploits innate immunity, sometimes involving receptors that do not rearrange somatically, the nature of which might help elucidate the origin of the specific adaptive immune system.

Comparisons across phyla and classes may not only give an idea of the history of the immune system but, by distinguishing what has been conserved from what has varied, they will tell more about what is essential and what is accessory in the human immune system.

L. Du Pasquier: Basel Institute for Immunology, CH-4005 Basel, Switzerland.

M. Flajnik: Department of Microbiology and Immunology, University of Maryland, Baltimore, Maryland 21201-1559.

ORIGIN OF THE ELEMENTS OF THE IMMUNE SYSTEM

Generalities

To study its evolution we can only compare the immune system in representatives of various taxa and detect analogies and homologies. Unfortunately, the species studied today are the rare survivors of a much more diversified and potentially richer fauna. Most species survive 1 to 2 million years on average. There are fewer groups of higher taxonomic rank now than in the past. It is as if, morphologically, very distinctive groups of animals forming as many phyla appeared rapidly during the early phase of evolution, most of which disappeared because they failed to diversify (1). If evolution proceeds "by experimentation and then by standardization" (2), so does the immune system.

Living organisms must prevent invasion or destruction by parasites and compete for resources with members of their own species. The possibility of fusion or contamination with cells from one's own species still exists in many marine metazoa (e.g., Porifera, Cnidaria, or tunicates) but has practically disappeared in vertebrates. Ancient polymorphism–recognition mechanisms might have been turned inward in vertebrates and led to the evolution of cell–cell interactions in the immune system.

Origin of Macrophages, Leukocytes, and Lymphocytes

Hematopoietic cells originate from mesoderm. It seems logical to call for possible ancestors in phyla where one can find a true mesoderm (Fig. 1). A true mesoderm derived from embryonic cells initially associated with the entoderm defines the triploblastic metazoa (3). The discovery of a GATA factor in *Drosophila* involved in hematopoiesis (such as GATA 1,2,3 in vertebrates), implies that some aspects of the molecular mechanisms underlying hematopoiesis are indeed shared between deuterostomes and protostomes (4).

The macrophage function is ancient and of course devoted to the whole animal in protozoa and to bone marrow–derived cells in mammals. Coiling phagocytosis, in which pseudopods whirl around the body of the microorganism, is shared by hemocytes from invertebrate and mammalian macrophages but not by the protozoan *Amoeba* (5). Circulating monocytes of mammals and some hemocytes from some invertebrates are both involved in innate immunity. In some instances, conservation of molecules expressed in macrophages from different organisms has been shown. Among those, the scavenger receptor (SRC) family is involved at the surface of cells in recognizing nonself ligands (6). Intercellular nitric oxide (NO) is involved with various aspects of mammalian physiology, ranging from vasodilation to macrophage killing, and this is conserved among triploblastic metazoa (7). A macrophage receptor (croquemort) for apoptotic cells has been isolated in *Drosophila*. It is a member of the CD36 family and mediates removal of apoptotic cells by macrophages. Thus, the primordial function of "macrophages may have been in tissue modeling and that their adapted role is in host defense" (8).

Involved in cell-mediated transplantation immunity in annelids and nemertines, the lymphocytelike cells, which appeared first in coelomates, have been thought of as primitive T cells. In the same classes of animals, stimulation of coelomocytes by concanavalin A (ConA), phytohemagglutinin (PHA), and lipopolysaccharide (LPS) did not distinguish lineages (9–12). Echinoderm and urochordate lymphocytelike cells participate in graft rejection and in natural killing; in urochordates they appear to respond to PHA (13,14).

So far none of the invertebrate leukocytes seem to express Ig superfamily (Igsf) members with a variable (V) domain that could look like an ancestor for Ig or TCR. Amalgam (15) is the only candidate whose expression is restricted to mesoderm, even if like fasciclin and lachesin it is used in cells of the nervous system (16). Igsf members such as twitchin can be found in muscle cells (also of mesodermic origin). It would be interesting to determine whether an exchange of promoter motifs in evolution has occurred across cell lineage, resulting in the lymphocyte specialization of genes originally expressed in other tissues.

Does Recognition of Polymorphism Involve Similar Mechanisms in All Phyla?

This section addresses histocompatibility reactions in invertebrates, investigations for specific memory, and determination of cell types involved in the effector function. It was assumed that specific memory in graft rejection reactions is an indication of a specific amplification of clones of effector cells carrying receptors recognizing nonself. This approach leaves us with ambiguous answers (Fig. 1, Table 1). Although allorecognition is encountered in most phyla, specific memory is difficult to demonstrate unequivocally outside gnathostomes. Thus, clonal selection—expansion of a small cell population expressing a somatically acquired receptor—does not operate in all systems of allorecognition.

Porifera

Cellular surface polymorphic determinants prevent sponges of the same species from forming a single colony (1,2).

There are at least two categories of allograft rejections in Porifera: barrier formation and cytotoxicity (17,18). No memory could be demonstrated in either sort (19). Cytotoxicity is associated with infiltration of the grafted tissues by archaeocytes, whereas barrier formation is linked to collencyte-mediated rejections (17,20,21).

In the marine sponge *Microciona prolifera*, immediate and specific recognition could perhaps be analog to that of natural killer (NK) cells encountering their target (18). Species-specific cell adhesion in *Microciona* is mediated by a multimolecular complex (aggregation factor). Chemical deglycosylation showed one component accounting for nearly 90% of the total protein. The amino acid sequence of this component (35 kDa) shares homology with the Na^+-Ca^{2+} exchanger protein. Sponge cell adhesion might be based on the assembly of multiple small glycosylated protein subunits (22). In *Callyspongia diffusa* (23), aggregates obtained after mixing cells from different individuals are killed by cytotoxic reactions mediated by the gray cells. To explain their results, the authors favor a model of a positive selection for self recognition during sponge immunocyte development. Claims have been made that a polymorphism exists in the Ig C2 domain of a tyrosine kinase receptor in *Geodia*. It would be interesting to correlate this polymorphism with transplantation reactions (24).

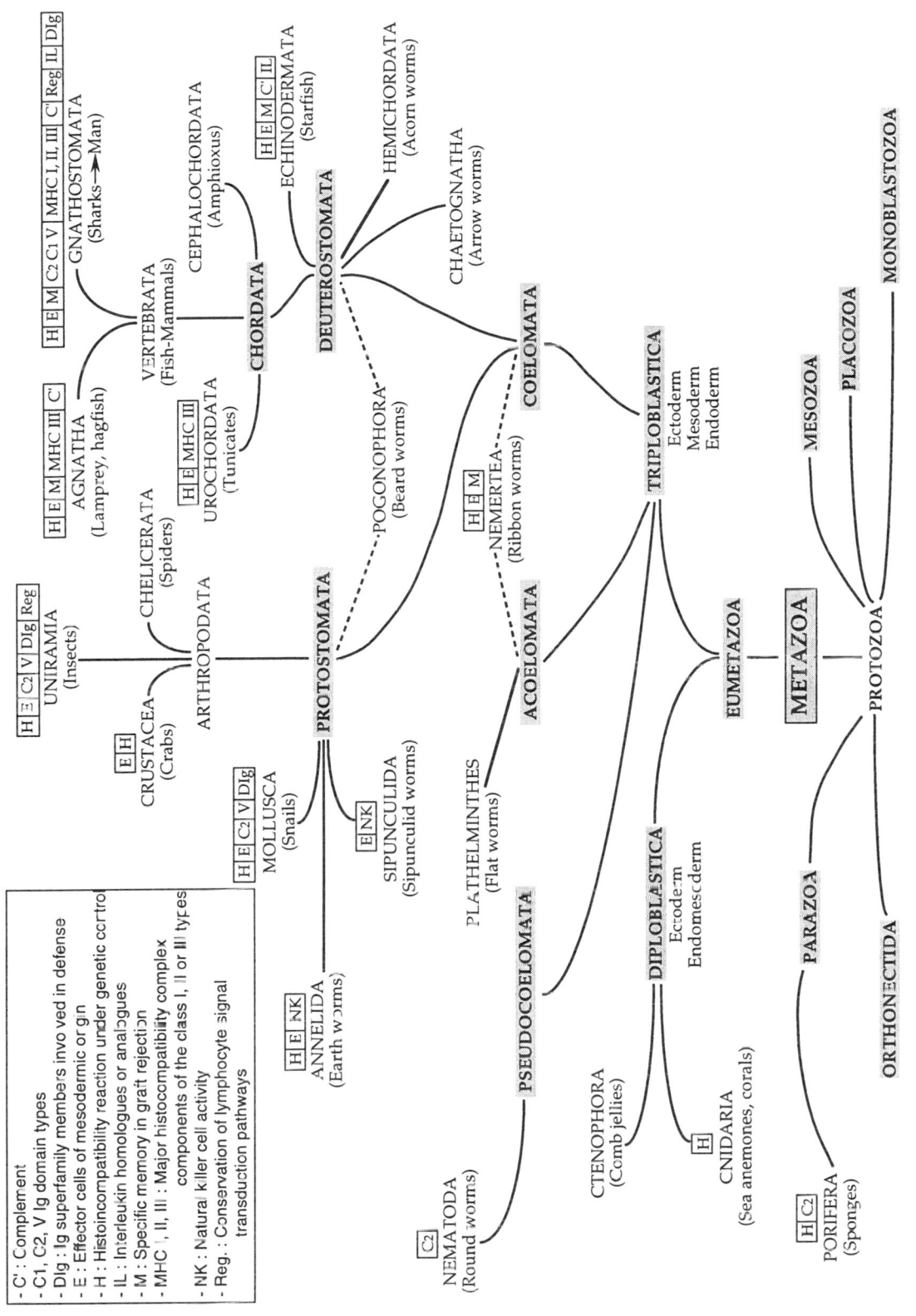

FIG. 1. Elements of the immune system in the animal kingdom.

TABLE 1. *Specific memory in histocompatibility reactions throughout the animal kingdom*

| Phylum or class | Host species | Allo or xeno combination | Rejection times in days | | | Comments | Refs. |
			First set	Second set (3rd set)	Third party		
Porifera	*Callyspongia*	Allo	7–11	3.8–7.2	4.6–6.8	Specific memory	17
	Hymeniacidon	Allo	5.2–11.1	7–9.8	5.4–12.25	No memory	20
	Ephudatia	Allo				No memory	19
Cnidaria	*Montipora*	Allo	19.2–25.3	11.6–14.4	18.4–28.5	Specific memory	27
	Eunicella	Allo				No memory in in vitro killing assays	30
	Anthopleura	Allo				No memory	28
Nemertea	*Lineus*	Xeno	14–16	6.8–9.8	12.3–18	Specific memory	36
Annelida	*Lumbricus*	Xeno	7–60 (17.8)	4–32 (15.7)	5–81 (43)	Specific memory (20∞C)	51, 52
	Eisenia	Xeno	66.30 ± 20.4	67.0 ± 22.6	ND	No specific memory (15∞C)	47–50
						In both cases, second graft applied 5 days after the first. Conflicting results, also in allotransplantations	
Arthropoda	*Periplaneta*	Allo	7	3.5	7	Specific memory (subcuticular tissue)	42
	Periplaneta	Allo				No specific memory (cuticle transfer)	39,40
Echinodermata	*Cucumaria*	Allo	165	43	ND	Memory?	
	Dermasterias	Allo	213	44	44 > n > 300	Specific memory	54
	Lytechinus	Allo	38	12	12	Memory without specificity	55
Tunicata	*Styela*	Allo	38.2 ± 5.9	22 ± 2.6	30	Specific memory	14
	Botryllus	Allo	13–53	7–62	ND	No memory	
			32–95	9–72	ND	No memory	67
Vertebrata	Agnatha (*Eptatretus*)	Allo	71.9	28	19–85	Specific memory	547
	Gnathostomata (*Xenopus*)	Allo	30.9 ± 5.1	18.6 ± 1.9	35 ± 7.8	Specific memory	476

Cnidaria

Allorecognition, xenorecognition, and killing mechanisms have been demonstrated in both Hydrozoa (four species) and Anthozoa (at least 70 species) (25–27). The effector mechanisms range from contact avoidance involving remote sensing, to barrier formation, or usage of nematocysts. Specific memory has not been demonstrated unequivocally (Table 1) (27–30). Reported with some variations in *Montipora verrucosa* (Anthozoans) memory was not evident in *Eunicella* (30). Sea anemones activate their acrorraghia (nematocyst-bearing vesicles in the collar region) more rapidly after repeated histocompatible contacts, but no specific memory has been demonstrated (28,29).

In *Hydractinia* (hydrozoans) allorecognition is under the control of one polymorphic gene, the six alleles of which trigger different strengths of reactivities (31,32). In family studies it looked as if one haplotypic difference could trigger a visible reaction of incompatibility (33). A hierarchy of dominance among strains was later established based on degrees of stolon overgrowth (hyperplasy) (34). During breeding some autodestructive mutants were isolated. Is the self destruction due to a mutation in the recognition structures or in the recognized epitopes? The authors of this discovery favor a germline-encoded program rather than a somatic mechanism to account for self tolerance (35).

Nemertea

These triploblastic worms (Fig. 1) are now considered as Coelomates (Protostomata). *Lineus* does not reject allografts and even some xenografts (*Lineus ruber–Lineus viridis*) heal without rejection. When it occurs, rejection seems to be due to specific recognition, with memory and recruitment of specialized cells (Table 1) (36,37). Immunocompetent cells come from the intestinal segment close to the esophagus. Antecerebral ends from *Lineus ruber*

donors were grafted onto chimeric worms previously constructed with an anterior part of *Lineus lacteus* and the intestinal segment of *Lineus sanguineus*. In such a case, the rejection is identical to that of the *Lineus ruber–Lineus sanguineus* combination. If the intestinal segment remains from *Lineus lacteus*, the rejection is typical of a *Lineus ruber–Lineus lacteus* combination (38). The removal of the immunocyte-producing area in the intestinal segments leads to impairment of graft rejection (38).

Arthropoda

Allogeneic recognition is not universal in insects, and in certain combinations of species even xenogeneic recognition is lacking (39). The cockroach *Periplaneta americana* does not normally reject *Blatta orientalis* grafts. However, if immunized with an implant from an incompatible species (*Blaberus craniifer*), they will reject grafts from the otherwise compatible *Blatta orientalis* (39). In other words, by somehow altering its threshold for recognition, the host immune system was activated to recognize as nonself an otherwise acceptable tissue (40). However, in *Periplaneta americana*, incompatibility has been reported between members of the same species (41). Quick reactions were observed (7 days), and indices of specific memory (42) would support the existence of specific recognition of nonself in Arthropoda.

Mollusca

Due to technical difficulties, transplantation experiments have led to inconclusive results. Molluscs seem to lack the ability to reject allografts [studies conducted in lammellibranches and cephalopods have been reviewed elsewhere (43,44)]. However, encapsulation of xeno- or alloimplants (ganglia or tentacles) has been observed in the gastropod *Planorbarius corneus* (45). The work done on molluscs did not permit speculation about relationships with other invertebrate immune systems and *a fortiori* with vertebrates until recently, when a molecule consisting of five domains of the C2 type of the Igsf was discovered in *Lymnaea* and seems to be involved in reactions against parasites in the mollusc defense molecule (MDM) (46). Reaction against parasites in another snail, *Biomphalaria glabrata*, also involves molecules sharing similarities with the Igsf. Fibrinogen-related proteins (FREP) acting as lectins can precipitate parasite-derived proteins. They possess at their N-terminus a domain resembling Ig V domains (47).

Annelida and Sipunculida

In this phylum there is debate as to whether incompatibility is due to immune phenomena or improper healing with a lack of vascularization and innervation (48–50). Body wall allografts are rejected when the specimens come from different geographic origins. The rejection is mediated by cells (coelomocytes) of mesodermic origin coming from splanchnopleura (51). Because allosponses were usually weak, most authors (Table 1) investigated the response to xenografts (48,52,53). However, like in vertebrates, xenograft rejection could be due to mechanisms quite different from those controlling allograft rejection. Grafts are attacked by mesoderm-derived phagocytic and/or killer leukocytes. The large cells (10 to 30 μm in diameter) adhering to and apparently destroying the graft have been called macrophages or neutrophilic or granulocytic coelomocytes and are rich in acid phosphatase and lysosomes. Proliferation of small cells also has been observed (9,10).

When leukocytes of *Sipunculus* are mixed with xenogeneic or allogeneic erythrocytes, cytolysis of up to 40% of the target cells occurs within 4 to 6 hours (11). This spontaneous activity of cells accompanied by synthesis of polypeptides demands contact between the effector and the target and resembles that of NK cells (11). The effector cells resemble vertebrate small lymphocytes. This type of killing mechanism is considered primitive and may be an example of a primordial system of immune surveyance.

Echinodermata

The echinoderms are of particular interest because of their relatedness to the vertebrates. Three species of echinoderms are able to reject allografts: holothurid, starfish, and sea urchins (13) (summary in Table 1). The most convincing data with evidence of specific immune memory comes from starfish (*Dermasterias imbricata*) (54) (Table 1). Clear-cut evidence for specific memory is, nevertheless, not found in all cases. The sea urchin, *Lytechinus pictus* (55), rejects allografts with a speed somewhat proportional to the degree of relatedness of the partners, but without a specific second-set response. Third-party grafts were rejected at the same time as the specific second-set grafts. In *Dermasterias*, the effector cells and coelomocytes do not respond *in vitro* to PHA and pokeweed mitogen, but significant stimulation has been observed with LPS or ConA (13). Sea urchin phagocytes isolated from the coelomic fluid kill allogenic cells *in vitro* (56).

Urochordates

In urochordates *Botryllus primigenus* or *shlosseri* (colonial tunicates), the histocompatibility reactions governed by the fusion (fu/HC) locus are complex (57,58). During colony fusion, the so-called compatible one-haplotype combinations do in fact exhibit some cellular reactivity, although less visible (59). The lack of reaction between individuals with one haplotype in common could reflect thresholds and gene dose effects. Resorptions between individuals differing at one polymorphic allele of the Fu/HC locus (58,60–62) depend on several other genetic loci. Heterozygous animals will resorb the homozygous animals. The two events—fusion/nonfusion on one hand and resorption on the other hand—could depend on different recognition steps, the first being self recognition, the second nonself recognition (63). Interestingly, the pattern of fusion in a family is predictive of the pattern of fertilization (57). Eggs from an AB (A and B representing alleles at the histocompatibility locus) individual cannot be fertilized by A or B sperm. This was taken as possible evidence of self recognition between a product on sperm and a product on egg envelopes.

Buss suggested that this histocompatibility was selected in evolution in order to limit germ cell parasitism (64). Indeed, either in the laboratory or in natural populations of *Botryllus schlosseri*, somatic and germ cell parasitism in chimeras has been demonstrated (57,65). As expected, fused *Botryllus* organisms have higher frequencies of germ cell parasitism than nonfused ones. This is consistent with the idea that polymorphism at the fusion locus would limit the germ cell chimerism.

Styela (a solitary form) showed signs of specific memory (14) and an involvement in the response of cells comparable with lymphocytes (66). Hemocytes from the solitary urochordate *Styela clava* can effect allogeneic cytotoxicity *in vitro* depending on cell contact. No such memory was found in *Botryllus* (67).

Conclusion

The recognition and effector mechanisms underlying quasi-ubiquitous allorecognition have not yet been elucidated in most cases. Many of the studied models, particularly allorecognition in colonial ascidians, are more complex than was originally believed and remain unexplained. From the study of allorecoginition, no obvious functional similarities except the existence of allopolymorphism recognition have been discovered. Neither is it clear whether any of the invertebrate models are homologous to allorecognition responses of vertebrates.

Conservation of Signaling Pathways in Defense Reactions

Insects and crustaceans resist microorganisms via at least three main pathways (cellular, melanization, and humoral) (68–72), some of which share elements with vertebrates at the level of the control of gene expression.

The Insect Cellular Immunity

Insect hemocytes of mesodermic origin encapsulate or phagocytose foreign particles (73). In *Drosophila* larvae, those cells are found in the so-called lymph glands where they form two subpopulations. Five percent to 10% of them participate in the prophenoloxydase pathway (melanization). The more abundant plasmacytes are capable of phagocytosis and synthesis of antibacterial peptides. After penetration of a foreign particle, these cells differentiate into large flat cells (lamellocytes) that encapsulate parasites. A member of the Igsf, hemolin is released in the hemolymph of the giant silk moth *Hyalophora cecropia* after injection of bacteria. It is one of the first components to bind to bacterial surfaces, taking part in a protein complex formation that is likely to initiate immune responses (74). Hemolin stimulates phagocytic activity, which in turn can be enhanced by LPS. Hemolin affects tyrosine phosphorylation of hemocyte proteins, which suggests that it is involved in the regulation of cellular immune responses via a pathway that includes PKC activation and protein tyrosine phosphorylation (75).

The Insect Humoral Immunity

Many antibacterial and antifungal peptides are secreted rapidly from the fat bodies after infection and have been characterized in various species of insects (cecropins, diptericin, drosocine, insect defensins, metchnikovin, attacin (all antibacterial), or drosomycin (antifungus) (76,77). We want to focus only on the features by which their induction resembles that of some vertebrate proteins. Potential transcription factor binding sites similar to those found in mammals are conserved in the 5' regions of some the above-mentioned insect genes. An interleukin (IL)-6 response element and two putative LPS response elements have been reported in the 5' region of the cecropin genes in the silk moth (78). The fat body contains at least three different nuclear proteins inducible by bacteria that bind to the 5'-untranslated region, suggesting that these proteins may be involved in cecropin B expression.

The introduction of a pathogen in *Drosophila* (fungus, bacteria) leads to the activation of proteases that cleave a precursor and generates Spätzle, an extracellular ligand of a receptor called Toll, the intracellular part of which is homologous to the IL-1 receptor cytoplasmic tail of mammals. The signaling pathway involves Nf-κB (79) (Fig. 2). A human homolog of the Toll protein has been discovered and it activates the expression of inflammatory cytokine genes via the Nf-κB pathway (80). κB motifs are necessary in *Drosophila* (and other dipterians) (81,82) for the induction of antibacterial genes. The promoters of *Drosophila* cecropin genes also possess GATA sites in association with κB motifs, a feature also observed in mammalian genes involved in immunity such as IL-6 and IL-3 (83). In mammals these motifs are recognized by the transcription factor Nf-κB, composed of two subunits belonging to the Rel family. In *Drosophila*, Dorsal, the Rel family member involved in the formation of the dorsoventral axis during embryogenesis (84), is also reexpressed during an immune response (79).

A mutation affecting the production of antibacterial peptides, *imd*, has been discovered. In mutants no DNA–protein complex has been detected with the κB motif, confirming the importance of the Nf-κB pathway. However, the gene for drosomycin, an antifungus peptide, remains inducible in the mutant. Thus, at least two regulatory pathways govern the humoral response (Fig. 2) (79). The specific role of the pathogen in the induction of one or the other pathway remains to be determined.

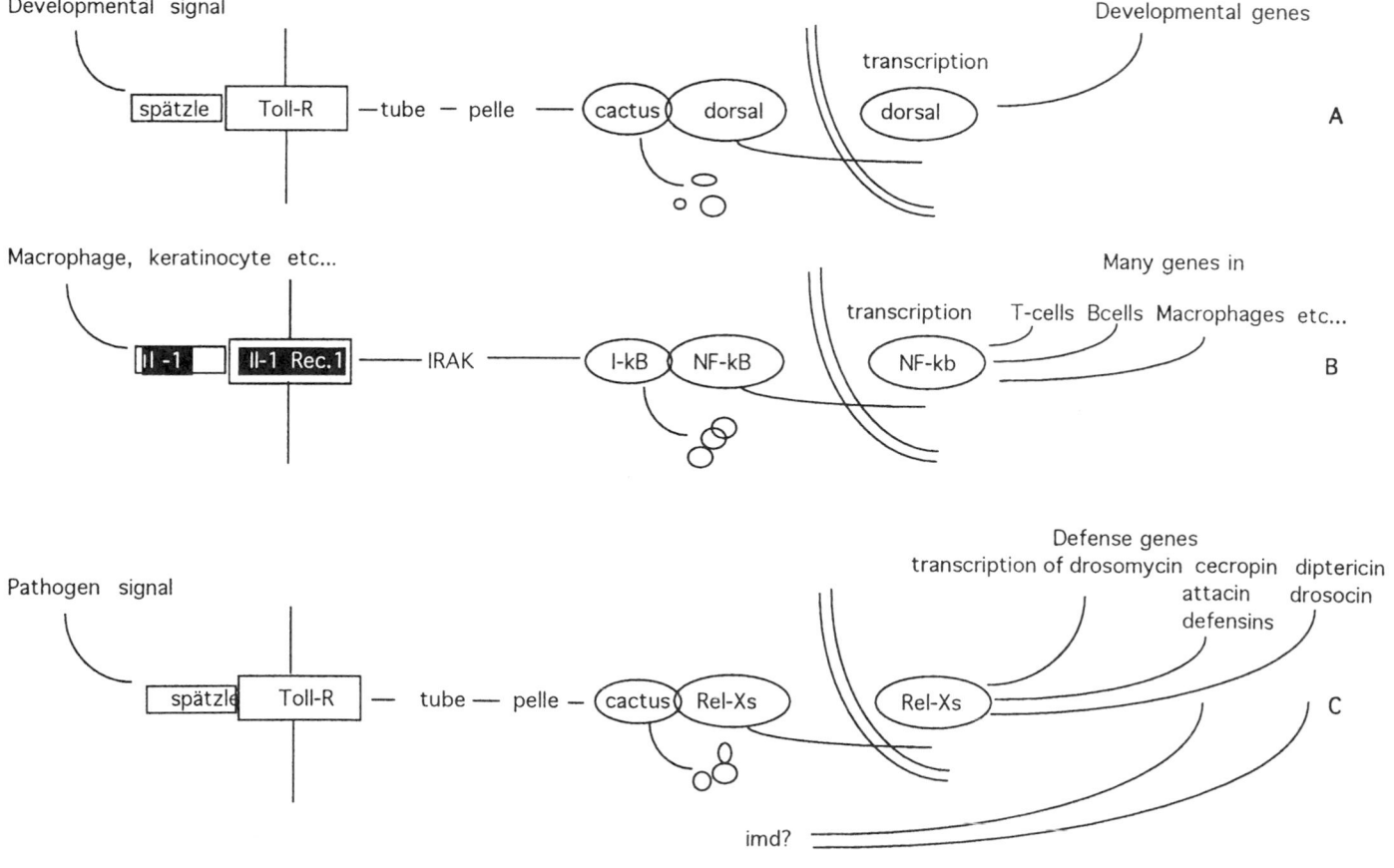

FIG. 2. Conservation of signaling pathways in defense and development.

The inhibition of the translocation to the nucleus of Nf-κB by the equivalent of I-κB in the cytoplasm is well conserved. In the case of mammals, IL-1 binding to lymphocyte through the IL-1 receptor induces the cytoplasmic dissociation of I-κB from Nf-κB (85); in the case of the dorsoventral differentiation in *Drosophila*, binding of Spätzle to the transmembrane receptor Toll initiates a cascade that leads to the dissociation of Cactus from Dorsal. In the immune response of *Drosophila*, Toll signals in the same way via Dorsal-related Rel proteins.

Plant Disease Resistance

The similarity in the signalling cascade extends even to plant disease resistance (86). The N gene from tobacco encodes a cytoplasmic protein that shares similarities in sequence with the signaling domains of Toll and IL-1 receptors, and signals via a Toll-like cascade leading to a defense response (87). Similarly in tomatoes, PTO, a homolog of the IRAK gene, is necessary for defense (88,89). In *Arabidopsis*, NPR1 is a homolog of Cactus and is necessary for responses to various pathogens (90). As stated by Wilson et al. (86) "the implications of an ancient regulatory cascade uniting insects, mammals and plants are far reaching, especially considering that the last common ancestor of these diverse groups was probably unicellular."

Origin of Immunoglobulins and T-Cell Receptors

Looking for Igsf C Domains Across the Animal Kingdom

In vertebrates, many extracellular lymphocyte receptors are built from Ig domains, but some NK-cell receptors that recognize MHC proteins are made up of either Ig domains or C-type lectins (91–93).

The Ig domain consists of a sandwich of two β-pleated sheets each made of antiparallel β strands of five to 10 amino acids, usually with a very conserved disulfide bridge between strands B and F. Some molecules from prokaryotes such as Pap D and other bacterial proteins (94–96) harbor Ig domains. Thus, a divergent evolution of the Igsf from a common ancient bacterial ancestor is a distinct possibility, although one cannot formally exclude the possibility that such domains were acquired horizontally from eukaryotes.

The existence of Igsf proteins in several phyla, including Parazoa (97) (Figs. 1 and 3), suggests that the Ig domain duplicated before the split between acoelomates and coelomates. In no case, however, do genes encoding these Ig superfamily members rearrange outside vertebrates. Among invertebrate Igsf members there are unexpected features, such as the intracellular myosin-binding protein twitchin, a cytoplasmic molecule of the nematode *Caenorhabditis elegans* (98). Some secreted molecules can be involved in immune responses: the previously mentioned hemolin (four C2 domains), MDM (46) (five C2 domains), the FREPs [fibrinogen related but harboring one V-like Ig domain (47)], and peroxidasin [containing among others four C2 Ig domains (99)].

Igsf domains are classified into two major categories: constant (C) and variable (V) (100,101). The C domain can be divided into three categories:

1. The primitive C2 type encountered in many membrane proteins in all phyla is made of eight strands organized in two β-pleated sheets. The loop interconnecting those strands varies

and is implicated in different sorts of binding (102). C2-type domains have V-type patterns in the β strand E-F region.
2. The C1 type with seven strands only is much more restricted in distribution and not found outside of MHC/TCR/Ig/tapasin, which are elements of the vertebrate adaptive immune system (103,104).
3. Many molecules classified as C2 should be reexamined to determine whether, like telokin or axonin, they resemble the intermediary (I) set that combines more features of the V frame across the whole domain and some of C1 (105).

V Domains in Invertebrate Phyla

The V domain, which confers specificity to Ig and TCR, has an extra strand and a loop, which can help provide specificity in the interaction with ligands. Figure 4 compares the various V domains mentioned in this section.

The many types of binding capacities of the Ig domains involve different portions of the molecule (102). V domains are recognizable in two insect GPI-anchored molecules– lachesin (16) and amalgam (15)—with the same V-C2-C2 organization. They could have the same features as an ancestral receptor type transmitted to deuterostomes. DTRK, a *Drosophila* tyrosine kinase receptor, also has two extracellular V domains, one of them truncated (106). V domains also can be associated with domains other than Ig C2 in invertebrates; the snail FREP hemolymph molecules, which precipitated parasite proteins, have one V domain at the distal end and correspond to a multigene family (five to 10 genes) (47). In C2 domains, loops between B and C strands, or between C' and E, are similar to complementarity determining region (CDR) loops of V domains and could mediate ligand interactions.

Two scenarios could explain the involvement of V domains in an adaptive immune system where the receptor subunit is usually a heterodimer (107,108). 1) Variability (either germline after duplication, or somatic after rearrangement or somatic mutation) preceded dimerization. 2) Dimerization (homodimerization) occurred first as a result of pressures on the receptor to interact more firmly with the ligands for affinity of binding, and the V domains became variable afterward.

V Domains and Monomeric Receptors

Perhaps some modern molecules have retained primitive characteristics such as nonrearranging V domains as well as that of C2 domains (107,109). Such molecules might be at the crossroad between adhesion molecules and specific receptors and could help us define what was the primordial receptor.

In arthropods and vertebrates, several molecules include V domains do not rearrange somatically (amalgam, lachesin, V , the genes of which C2–C2 from insects and CD2, CD86, CD80, CD58, hCAR,B7 from mammals, all V–C2). These molecules are all apparently monomers and may or may not be involved in the immune system of the given species. They have either no intron (amalgam) or a split V organization [CD4 (110), Muc 18 (111)], but no separation of the G strand into a rearrangeable J segment. Amalgam, secreted by cells of mesodermic cells, and lachesin of ectoderm origin, are made of one V domain and two C2 domains and are not integral membrane proteins. Both participate in the genesis of the nervous system. Tactile, an integral membrane protein on mammalian T cells, is most similar to amalgam and lachesin (112).

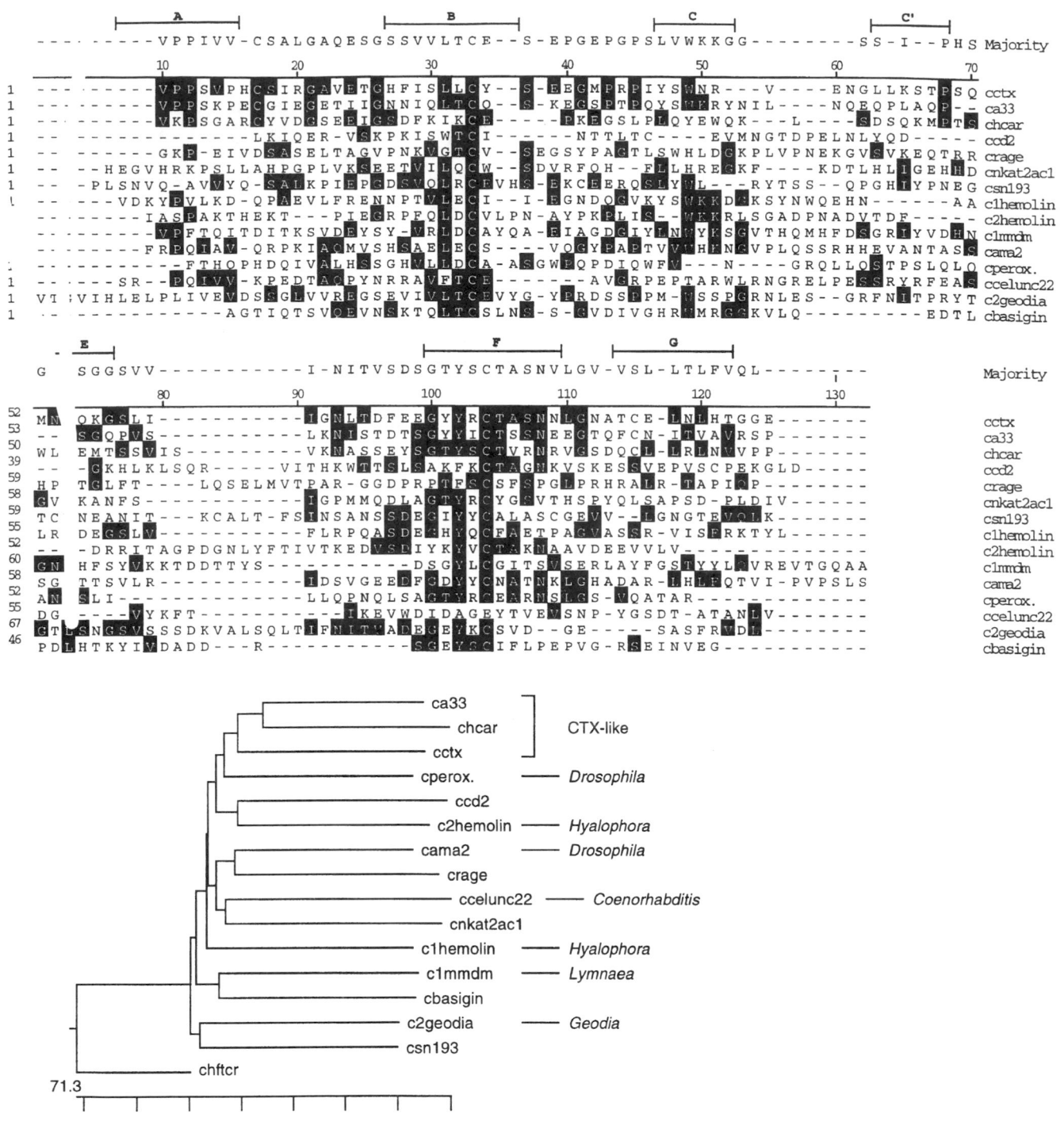

FIG. 3. Alignments and phylogenetic tree based on amino acid sequences of Ig C domains across the animal kingdom. The scale measures the distance between sequences. Units indicate the number of substitution events. The length of each pair of branches represents the distance between sequence pairs (Lasergene program). CTX, cortical thymocyte marker of *Xenopus* (115); CA33, a human homolog of CTX (117); CD2, V-C2 receptor, ligand of CD48; hcar, coxsackie virus receptor, another homolog of CTX in humans (582); cnkat2a c1, an NK cell killer inhibitor receptor (583); c RAGE, receptor for advanced glycosylation end product (121); c basigin, CD147, a surface molecule of hematopietic and epithelial cells (584); C1 and 2 hemolin, two domains from hemolin, a soluble molecule from the silkworm involved in humoral immunity (74); C ama 2, second constant domain of amalgam, an adhesion molecule from *Drosophila* (15); C perox, one of the c2 domains of peroxidasin, a molecule involved in defense and development in *Drosophila* (99); celunc22, a C2 domain from twitchin, an Igsf member–binding myosin in *Coenorhabditis elegans* (98); mdm, first C2 domain of MDM, the mollusc defense molecule from *Lymnaea* species (46); C2 geodia, the external C2 domain from a sponge tyrosine kinase receptor (23,585); ChftcR, shark TCR β chain (C1 domain given as an out group) (162). When no reference is given, see Barclay AN et al., eds. *The leucocyte antigen,* 2nd ed. Facts book series. London: Academic Press, 1997.

V Domains and Dimeric Receptors

No dimeric receptors using nonrearranging Ig V domains have been discovered outside vertebrates so far. In vertebrates, BG (113,114), CD28, cd8, [(V) × 2], CTX (115), ChT1 (116), A33 (117), and CTH (118) [(V-C2) × 2] correspond to this description, and their monomeric subunit includes a V domain associated with a C2 domain, never a C1. Such molecules could be barely modified progenies of the early lymphocyte receptors. In TCR Ig domains, the G strand encoded by the J segment of each partner of the dimer (Vα-Vβ Vγ-Vδ V_H-V_L), is characterized by the presence of a diglycine bulge that induces a "twist." This orients the side chains of some amino acids of the G strand toward the inside of the interface between the two partners, creating the so-called triple-layer packing of Igsf domains. This packing results in optimal spacing of the six CDR loops in the antigen-combining site (119). In CTX, CTH, and Cht1, the exon-intron organization of this putatively dimeric molecule (118,120) is similar to that of the receptor for advanced glycosylation end-products (RAGE) (121), which is again a nondimeric V-C2-C2, but an integral membrane protein. As in CTX, its V domain gene is characterized by a type 0 splice junction. This is rare and found only in the V domain of RAGE, CTX homologs, and Basigin. RAGE, with a nonrearranging V domain and no diglycine bulge, forms a monomer but could have a common ancestor with CTX-like molecules. RAGE recognizes heavily glycosilated aged proteins, effects a surveillance function (122), and is expressed by cells of the hematopoietic lineage (123). It could resemble the receptors present in early vertebrates when the rearranging machinery was introduced (109).

The Origin of the Rearranging Machinery

Most models propose that the generation of somatically rearranging receptors occurred abruptly in evolution via the generation of the RAG machinery made of two lymphocyte-specific proteins, RAG-1 and RAG-2 (124). Unique to gnathostomes, RAG genes have so far been isolated in four classes of vertebrates: chondrichthyes (125), Teleostei (126–128), amphibians (129), and mammals. Both RAG-1 and RAG-2 show strong conservation. In each case the genes are closely linked and in opposite orientation on the chromosome. Homologies have been found in certain parts of RAG 1 and RAG-2 with bacterial recombinases. Other relationships include yeast RAD-16, a molecule involved in DNA repair, and other genes involved in the regulation of gene expression (such as rpt-1r) (130). The close relationship to a prokaryotic protein (130) has suggested that vertebrates acquired this machinery by horizontal transfer and transposition from bacteria. Indeed, the genetic organization of the RAG locus has some transposon characteristics: the recombination signal sequences are reminiscent of sequences involved in targeting excision of transposons (108).

Origin of the MHC

Emergence of the MHC

No MHC genes have been cloned from animals in vertebrate classes older than cartilaginous fish. Class I, class II, inducible proteasome elements Imp 2 (131) and 7 (132,133), and the transporter

associated with antigen processing (TAP) all have been found in gnathostomes (Table 2), but not one has been isolated from the last two extant agnathan species, lamprey and hagfish. Thus, like Ig and TCR, MHC seems to have arisen abruptly in evolution. There are three possibilities to explain Ig/TCR/MHC absence in agnathans: (a) they had not yet emerged at the time of the appearance of cyclostomes; (b) the genes have been lost, perhaps because of the unusual life-styles (parasitic, saprophytic) of the extant species; or (c) the genes have diverged so far as to preclude their isolation by conventional methods (132).

The favored MHC precursor remains the fusion/rejection locus of tunicates, which seems similar in its genetic regulation to several other invertebrate models. Recognition of polymorphic self markers turns off the rejection cascade in this system (57,58), and this phenomenon mimics the recognition/signal transduction system of NK cells, which use a battery of receptors to block innate killing in the presence of self MHC (58,134,135). In mouse and human NK cells the class I α helix in the peptide-binding region (PBR) itself seems to be recognized (136), rather than a peptide–MHC complex like that recognized by *bona fide* TCR; thus the allogeneic response in *Botryllus* may be considered analogous to NK-cell but not T-cell allorecognition (137). It must be kept in mind that other sorts of polymorphic marker recognition have been at least partially elucidated (138), and these are not directed by MHC-like molecules.

A common feature of the invertebrate or vertebrate Igsf molecules encoded by nonrearranging genes is the presence of V, I, or C2 domains and never of C1 domains. C1 domains are restricted to Ig, TCR, MHC, and tapasin (103,104). Among surface receptors, Ig, TCR, and MHC are known to interact with other molecules either on the same cell surface like CD79 α and β coreceptors on B cells or CD3 components on T cells, or on the surface of another cell (CD8-CD4). Interestingly, these interactions take place in the C1 domain precisely in regions where C1 and C2 differ. The coreceptors of TCR and Ig provide essential systems of transduction that were perhaps a major evolutionary requirement in using a somatically rearranged receptor (139). For this reason, it is possible that C1 evolved first in the antigen-specific receptor and later was introduced by exon shuffling into the future class I and II genes (115). Alternatively, the C1 domain was part of a primordial class I/II molecule and given to the receptor. Under any scenario the evolutionary histories of molecules using C1 domains are probably closely linked.

Origins of the Peptide-Binding Region

The evolutionary derivation of the MHC peptide-binding domain remains enigmatic. The PBR could be derived from Igsf domains. Igsf domains and the class I α2 and class II β1 peptide-binding domains have similar sizes, the same phase of exon/intron splice sites, and disulfide bridges of about the same size (140). However, the topology of the β strands differs in the two families, and of course there are no similar helices in any Igsf domain. Perhaps then the PBR has been derived from another gene family (141), and MHC class I and II proteins are chimeras of this other unidentified gene family (for PBR) and the Igsf (membrane-proximal C1 domains). Heat shock protein (HSP)70 family members bind to short peptides in an extended conformation (142); they also show low sequence similarity with class I (141), and HSP70 genes

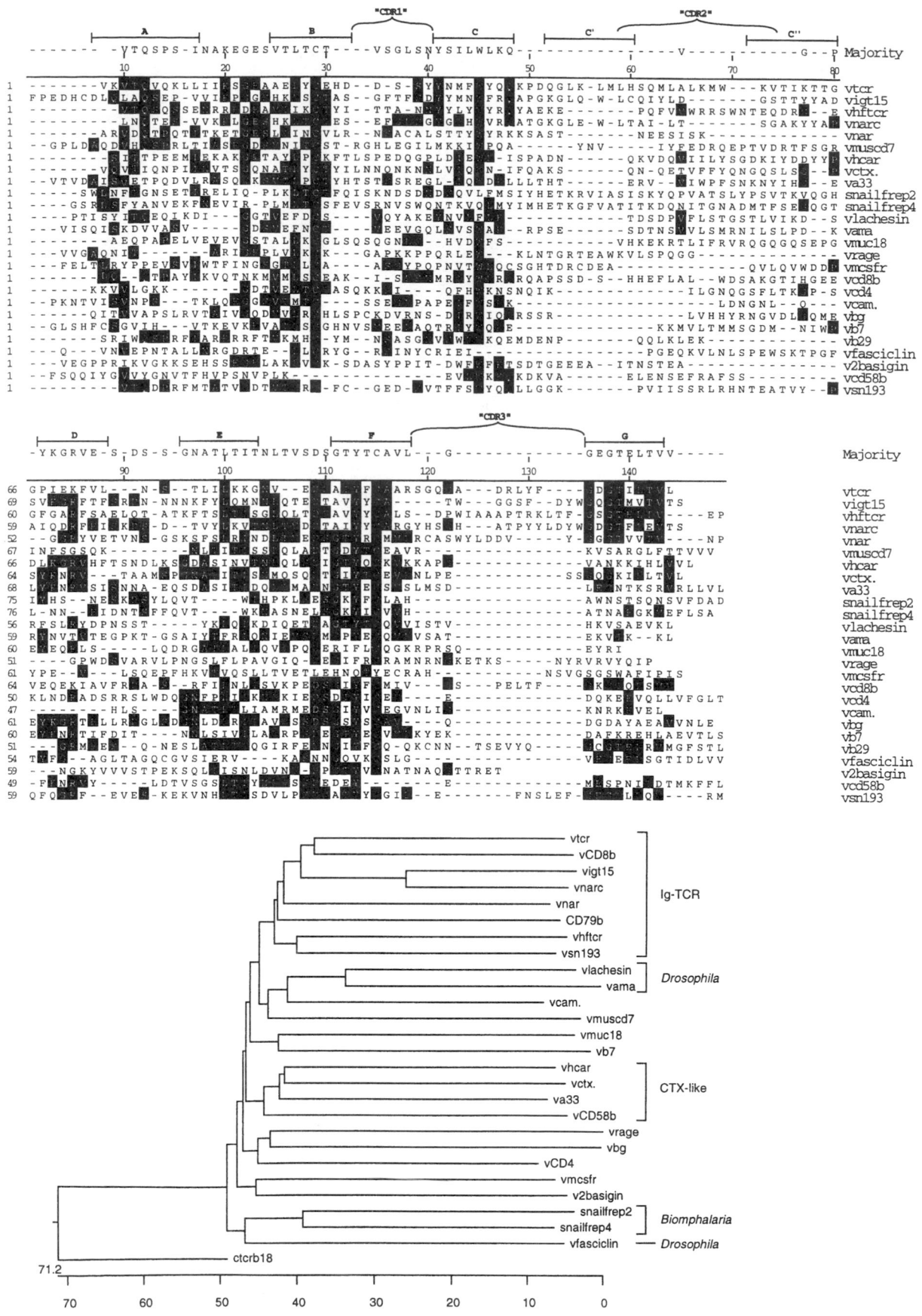

FIG. 4. Alignments and phylogenetic trees of V domains from various phyla with a special emphasis on the invertebrate Ig V domains. The scale indicates the relative genetic distance. Units indicate the number of substitution events. The length of each pair of branches represents the distance between sequence pairs (Lasergene program). V TCR, *Xenopus laevis* TCR Vβ domain (166); V Igt15, *Xenopus laevis* Ig H-chain V domain (393); V isf TCR, *Heterodontus francisci* Vβ TCR domain (162); Vnarc,: *Ginglymostoma cirratum* V domain of Ig NARC (Ig W) (188); Vnar, *Ginglymostoma cirratum* V domain of the NAR (195); Vmuscd7, V domain of mouse CD7 receptor; V car (582), CTX (111), and Va33 (117), V domains of human and amphibian members of the CTX family (see also Fig. 3 for their C domain); snail frep 2 and 4, mollusc V domains from two molecules involved in antiparasite reactions (47); V lachesin, adhesion molecule of *Drosophila* species; V ama, adhesion molecule of *Drosophila* species (15); V muc18, a V-V-C2-C2-C2 type molecule involved in melanoma growth control in humans (111); V rage, V domain of the receptor for advanced glycosylation end product (121); VM-csfr, colony-stimulating factor expressed on monocytes macrophages; V CD8 or CD, V domain of the CD8 and CD4 coreceptors; Vcam, VCAM; Vbg, BG antigen encoded in the chicken MHC, expressed on red cell thrombocytes and B and T cells (114); Vb7, B7-2 now called CD864; Vb29, coreceptor of the IgM B-cell receptor CD79 b; V fasciclin, molecules from insect involved in the growth of neurones (586); Vbasigin, adhesion molecule expressed in early embryos; Vcd58, a V-C2 type receptor of mammals, ligand of CD2; Vcd58 b, V domain of the lymphocyte receptor CD58; Vsn-193, anterior V domain of an unidentified teleost fish molecule isolated with TCR primers (155); cTCRb18, reference constant region domain of the *Xenopus* TCR beta receptor (166); snail FREP, fibrinogen-related molecule involved in antiparasite defense in the mollusc *Biomphalaria*.

map to MHC in several vertebrates (143–145). For these reasons it was suggested that HSP70 might have donated the ancestral PBR (141,146). Moreover, functional data have implicated HSP in a variety of developmental and immune functions (147). Nuclear magnetic resonance and crystallography, however, do not support a close resemblance of the HSP70 and MHC PBRs. There is a floor of β strands in the HSP70 PBR and peptides are bound there in an extended configuration, but the strands are not contiguous as in MHC; in fact, the topology is similar to that found in Igsf domains (148,149). The search for the origin of the PBR continues.

Conclusion

Analogies and homologies among elements of the immune system show that there is no clear barrier between invertebrates and vertebrates. The only machinery that seems missing in invertebrate phyla and perhaps in jawless fish is the rearranging machinery that permits the somatic generation of the B-cell and T-cell receptor and clonal selection.

The assembly of the various elements of the vertebrate immune system seems to be linked to this "invention." Indeed, it created a

TABLE 2. *MHC structure and function in vertebrates*

	Functional aspects	Genes and molecules identified
Agnatha Cyclostomata	Graft rejection (547) is chronic	Complement C3 (262,410,414,415) [C3 is on one of the MHC paralogues in human (chr. 19, Fig. 15)]
Gnathostomata Chondrichthyes	No MLR; graft rejection is chronic (433)	Class IIα (548), class IIβ (334) Class I cDNA (335,549)
Osteichthyes Teleostei	MLR; graft rejection (440,441,550); antigen presentation (451,452); intracellular antigen processing (553); histocompatibility required for T–B collaboration (551)	Class IIα (343,540), class IIβ (140,346,552–554), class Ia (390,391,555,556), and class Ib (140,391,400,552,557) cDNA and genomic from many species (zebrafish, carp, trout, salmon, cichlid, bass), β2m cDNA from carp (399), zebrafish (553), and trout (400,401)
Amphibia Anura	MLR; GVH; CTL; graft rejection; T–B collaboration is MHC-restricted; class Ia absent in tadpoles; role in T-cell education; split tolerance (476,558); polymorphism Class II on adult T cells absent on larval T cells	Class IIα (559,560), class IIβ (559–561), class Ia (352,562) genes and proteins identified. Class Ib cDNA (392). β2m-like molecules coprecipitates with class I protein (367,368,562), other proteins associate with class Ia on erythrocytes (563), C4, Bf in MHC (385–387)
Urodela	MLR weak; developmental regulation of expression (336); low proliferation; chronic graft rejection (564); class I ubiquitous (339)	Class Ia (337) and class I Ib (338) DNA; class II and class I proteins immunoprecipitated with cross-reactive xenoantisera (565)
Reptilia Lacertilia	MLR; GVH; CTL (566–568); graft rejection, but not formally linked to an MHC	Class Ia cDNAs (154). Class I, class II, and b2m-like proteins immunoprecipitated with cross-reactive xenoantisera (565)
Aves Galliformes	MLR; GVH; T–B collaboration; graft rejection; GVH; split tolerance (569); MHC restriction of T–B collaboration; polymorphism (113,570)	Class Ia (350,388), class IIβ (388), class IIα (571), and β2m (350) cDNA and proteins identified. Cosmid clones encompassing majority of MHC and Rfpy locus (388,572,573). B–G molecule cDNA and genes (336,365,574–576)
Mammalia Rodentia	All parameters defined originally here (see Chapters 8 and 12)	

Abbreviations: MHC, major histocompatibility complex; MLR, mixed lymphocyte reaction; CTL, cytoxic T-lymphocyte; GVH, graft versus host; C3, C4-complement components.

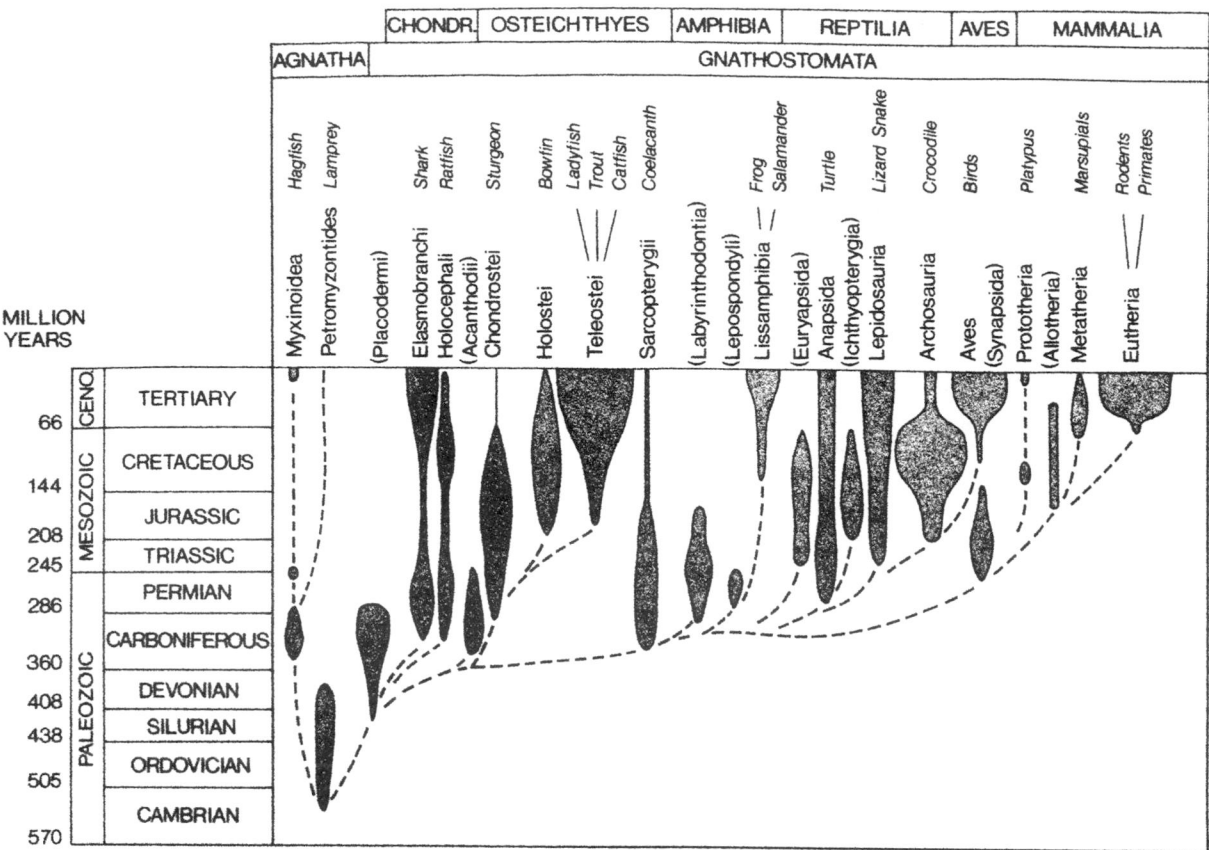

FIG. 5. The various classes of vertebrates through evolution. Note the number of extinct classes.

situation demanding selection in order to avoid autoimmunity. Therefore MHC I and II were bound to coevolve with TCR. We shall see that among vertebrates (Fig. 5) the essential architecture of the immune system as we know it in mammals is well preserved, with some minor variations.

THE IMMUNE SYSTEM OF VERTEBRATES

T-Cell Receptor

Few biochemical data are available across vertebrates, except in birds where the two types of TCR have been identified with monoclonal antibodies (mAbs) (150). Most comparative knowledge of TCR is derived from TCR gene sequences; therefore, not much is known about T-cell functions in phylogeny (see Table 2). No class switching has been observed in any class.

The genes for the two types of TCR, the αβ heterodimer (which accounts for all of the known antigen-specific regulatory and effector functions) and the γδ heterodimer [which recognize the antigens perhaps without processing in an Ig-like manner and could play an immunoregulatory role in various infections (151–153)] have existed since the early vertebrates. More precisely, complementary DNA (cDNA) sequences isolated by polymerase chain reaction (PCR) with short minimally degenerate oligonucleotides primers (154–156) from the skate, *Raja eglante-*

ria (a primitive gnathostome), produced genes homologous to the mammalian α, β, γ, and δ TCR. So far attempts to recover similar sequences from jawless vertebrates or invertebrates have failed.

Constant Region α

Comparison of the available constant regions of the α and β chains across the classes of vertebrates is presented in Φιγ. 6. The α chain from chondrichthyes (156), Teleostei (157; Wilson EMBL Y58505), amphibians (158), and avian species (159) is poorly conserved. The structure of the Cα Igsf domain itself is problematic. Among vertebrate TCR α chains, strands A, B, and C are relatively easy to identify, as are E and F, even though they are much shorter than in mammals. D seems to be missing. The overall lack of conservation of the extracellular domain sequences and its short length in birds and teleost fish (especially in the connecting peptide region) suggest that the coreceptor could have a structure rather different from the conventional CD3 complex components (157,158).

The transmembrane region, and the cytoplasmic tail, are the most conserved parts of the molecule. Like Cβ, the Cα transmembrane segment in all species studied so far shows a CART motif (160). The amino acids belonging to this motif form a surface of interaction necessary for association with the CD3 complex and

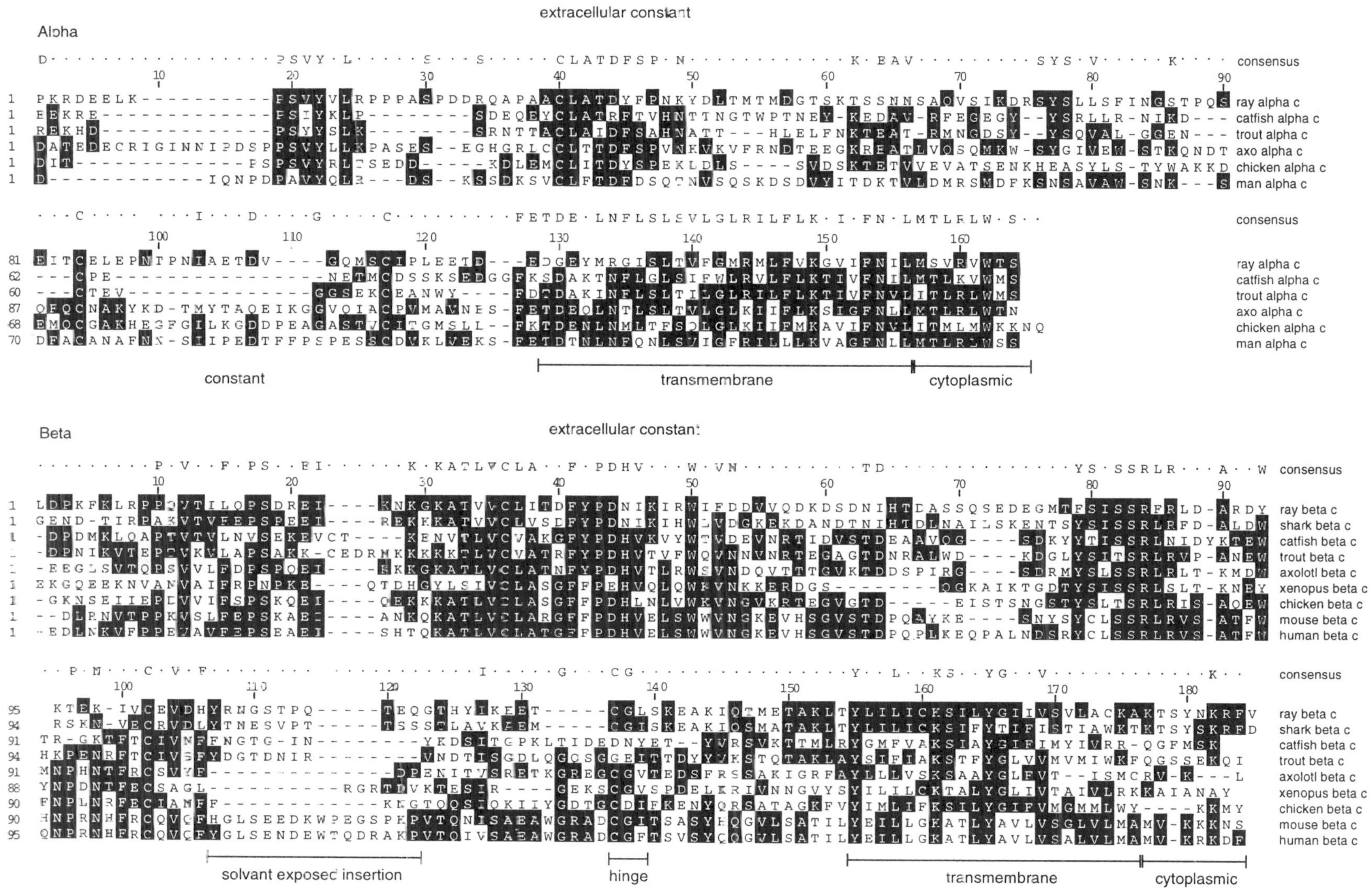

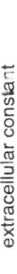

FIG. 6. Alignment of TCR-α and -β sequences in vertebrates. 1. α chain. Notice the poor conservation among the classes, but the rather good conservation in the transmembrane where the CART motifs can be found. 2. β chain. Notice the better conservation of the β sequences not only in the cystein flanking regions but in the area of segments 80 to 90, important for dimerization. The solvent exposed insertion seems to be missing in all vertebrates but mammals.

signal transduction. Outside this region, the other face with the residues IKL could be conserved for an interaction with other components of the CD3 complex. The cytoplasmic region is remarkably conserved among teleosts, birds, and mammals.

Constant Region β

TCR β genes have been sequenced in four species of cartilaginous and bony fish [horned shark (161,162), trout (163), salmon (164), catfish (Wilson 1995 EMBL U58509 U58508)] and two species of amphibians [axolotl (165), Xenopus (166)].

In addition to the typical Ig domain features, there exist several conserved regions among vertebrate TCR-β chains, especially at positions 81 to 86, that might be involved in the dimerization of the TCR (167). The CART motif in the transmembrane region is also well conserved (Fig. 6). There are also some remarkable differences. For instance, the solvent-exposed segment 98–120 in mammals is missing in all nonmammalian vertebrates. Glycosylation sites are absent from the Xenopus TCR-β constant region. The number of Cβ genes can vary. In mammals and axolotls, Cβ genes are in duplicates or quadruplicates. The horned shark seems to have more C genes than the skate, but even more Ig genes. Trout genes have not been numbered, the data being compatible either with three or fewer Cβ genes without polymorphism. There seems to be only one Cβ gene in chickens (168) and in Xenopus laevis, even though it is a pseudotetraploid species. In more polyploid forms, only the pseudooctoploid X. amieti showed evidence for two loci (166). The axolotl, which unlike most vertebrates has four Cβ genes, seems to have four DJCβ clusters that use the same collection of Vβ genes (169).

Diversity of Vα

Perhaps because T-cell recognition involves both peptide and class I or II molecules, the TCR V region may have been selected for different properties versus those of Ig; indeed, TCR V regions are much less similar to each other than are Ig V regions (170). This holds true across vertebrates. Four Vα families have been identified among six cDNA clones in the skate, six Vα families have been identified in the trout (157), and three Vα families have been identified in the channel catfish (Wilson 1995 EMBL U62043 U58507 U58506). In the axolotl, five Vα and at least 14 Jα segments were identified (158). All these sequences match mammalian Vα sequences relatively well. All α loci seem to have many J segments; 32 different trout Jα segments have been sequenced, a number much higher than for β (157). Is this high number preserved to compensate for the absence of D in the locus? More likely, the absence of D and the large numbers of J and V would favor the usage of secondary rearrangements and receptor editing. In Vα segments unlike Vβ segments, the size of the CDR3 region is surprisingly conserved. This size seems to be mandatory for the TCR/MHC–peptide interaction (171).

Diversity of Vβ

Among cold-blooded vertebrates, the large number of Vβ families, A is a conserved feature. At least seven distinct TCR Vβ families have been isolated in the horned shark (Heterodontus), where, like Ig, the TCR genes seem to be organized in clusters: four to six

in Raja (161), at least four in the trout (one with limited amino acid sequence similarity to the human Vβ 20 family); 11 in Xenopus (166), and 13 in Ambystoma (165,167).

The D segment GGGACAGGGG (Dβ of mammalian and chicken) is encountered throughout all vertebrate classes, alone or in conjunction with other Dβ. D segments usually show selection for glycines, suggesting that some of the D region residues contribute to CDR3 flexibility. There are 10 Jβ in the trout (163) and, including alleles, at least 11 in Xenopus (166).

In axolotls (165,167,172) Vβ can be classified into nine categories each with 75% or more nucleotide identity. Because only only 35 Vβ were cloned, there are likely to be more Vβ families. All Vβ are canonical. Several are more related to some mammalian Vβ genes, e.g., human Vβ13 and Vβ20 segments and their murine Vβ8 and Vβ14 homologs. N nucleotides were present in approximately 40% and 73% of the β-chain VDJ junctions in 2.5-month-old larvae and 10- to 25-month old animals, respectively. In axolotls and Xenopus, approximately 30% of the β-chain cDNAs were defectively rearranged. Many of the axolotl TCR-β CDR3 genes are the same in animals of different origins. This has not been observed in Xenopus (166).

The γδ Receptor

cDNA sequences from the chondrichthyes Raja eglanteria exhibit significant identity with prototypic γ and δ TCR genes with extensive V-region diversity, putative D segments in δ, and varying degrees of junctional diversity (156).

In the chicken, γδ cells were identified long ago (150). Transcripts were detected by probing Northern blots of thymus, spleen, and a γδ T-cell line, but not in B or αβ T-cell lines. Three V γ subfamilies, three J γ gene segments, and one C γ gene were identified in the avian TCR-γ locus. All V γ subfamilies participate in rearrangement during the first wave of thymocyte development. The γ repertoire diversifies from embryonic day 10 onward, and involves random V-J γ recombination, nuclease activity, and P- and N-nucleotides (173). The mouse and human γδ repertoires are much less diverse than the αβ. In ruminants and chickens, the two repertoires are less disparate, and there seems to be ligand-mediated selection of γδ cells during ontogeny (174). In sheep, where γδ TCR diversity is thymus dependent and follows a developmentally regulated sequence, no invariant γδ TCRs are found (175).

CD3 Complex

Elements of a CD3 complex have been isolated in only two non-mammalian classes: birds (176) and amphibians (177). In Xenopus species, one CD3 clone was homologous to both mammalian and avian CD3 γ and δ chains. It is encoded by five exons, a structure resembling the mammalian CD3 δ gene rather than the seven-exon CD3 γ gene. Because there was no evidence for a γ-like related gene, the one cloned represents an ancestral form of the mammalian CD3 γ and δ genes. Similarly, a chicken cDNA clone encoding a CD3 chain was difficult to assign to γ or δ. Perhaps this gene derived from an ancestral form of the CD3 γ and δ genes (178). The gene motifs of the cytoplasmic domain of the CD3 ε gene are important for signal transduction are highly conserved in the chicken. Among vertebrates, some residues in all CD3 chains are also highly conserved (176–179).

Immunoglobulins and Antibodies

A typical Ig molecule is composed of four polypeptide chains, two heavy [H] and two light [L] joined into a macromolecular complex via several disulfide bonds. Each chain is composed of a linear combination of Ig domains.

Ig H Chains: Constant Region

Agnatha

No Ig-like molecule has been isolated from the serum of hagfish or lampreys. Were Ig and TCR invented in a class of vertebrates now extinct (e.g., the placoderms, which are more primitive than chondrichthyes but more advanced than agnathans [Fig. 7])? Do cyclostomes have a typical vertebrate immune system?

Gnathostomata

The sequences of Ig H chain constant region genes do not appear to be well conserved in evolution. Insertions or deletions in loop segments occur more often in C than in V genes (180).

Primitive gnathostomes illustrate well the principle "diversify first then standardize." Indeed, chondrichthyes have a fairly large number of newly found Ig isotypes; homologs of those should be sought in other classes.

IgM. All features responsible for the Ig fold are preserved in all gnathostomes (181,182). The μ heavy (H) chain consists of four C1 and one V domain. H chains are associated with each other and with L chains by means of disulfide bridges, and IgM subunits form pentamers in all classes but teleost fish, where they form tetramers (183). Fluorescence depolarization suggests that the sites of flexibility and the relative amplitudes of motion are not the same in mammals and sharks (184). In all species, IgM is heavily glycosylated (reviews in refs. 185 [protein] and 186–188 [DNA]). C_H4 is best conserved, especially in the C-terminal region. There are several μ-specific residues in each of the four C_H domains among vertebrates (186), which suggests a continuous line of evolution of the vertebrate μ chain. The μ-transmembrane domains are well conserved among sharks, mammals, and amphibians (189), but the process by which the membrane version of the Ig molecule is assembled varies. In all classes except Teleostei, the transmembrane fragment is encoded by a separate exon that uses an alternative splicing site, usually located about 30 bp from the end of C_H4. In teleost fish, splicing takes place at the end of C_H3, and the C_H4 domain is missing in the membrane form (190–192). In the holostean fish there are motifs in C_H4 that could serve as cryptic splice donor sites for the production of messenger RNA (mRNA) encoding the membrane-bound form of the μ mRNA; in the bowfin there is another potential cryptic splice donor site in C_H3 (193,194).

New Antigen Receptor. New antigen receptor (NAR), a new dimer found in the serum of the nurse shark and so far restricted to chondrichthyes, is made of two H chains that each contains a variable domain generated by rearrangement and five constant C1 domains (195). Its constant region domains are not closely related to C domains of other Ig H chains. NAR was originally found in the serum but probably functions as a receptor because a transmembrane form exists, as revealed by cDNA and cell-surface staining with NAR-specific antibodies. The binding properties may resemble those of a fraction of the camelidae Ig, i.e., they bind the antigen in a monovalent fashion through a single V region. In phylogenetic trees, the NAR V domain clusters with human Vγ TCR domains. A molecule with similar characteristics also has been reported in lungfish (196).

Ig NARC (188) or Ig W (125). Isolated from sharks, cDNAs for the mature protein of this isotype encode an amino-terminal V domain followed by six C1 type constant domains and ending in a C-terminal tail typical of secreted Ig. The two amino-terminal C domains are orthologous to the IgX isotype of the skate, and the last four domains are homologous to NAR. Ig NARC H domains predicted from cDNA sequences are likely to associate with L chains, which was verified biochemically. V and C segments are likely to be in a cluster-type organization, like IgM.

IgX or IgR. First discovered as a second class of Ig protein in *Raja kenojei* (197,198), this H-chain non-μ isotype of Raja Ig genes designated as X-type (not to be confused with *Xenopus* IgX) was detected by screening a spleen cDNA library with homologous Raja V_H- and C_H1-specific probes complementing the respective regions of the μ-like isotype. The constant region of the X-type Ig H chain gene consists of two characteristic Ig domains and an unusual cysteine-rich carboxy-terminal segment (199). The distal part of the molecule seems to be encoded by duplicates of Ig NARC genes (188). IgX-producing cells do not produce IgM, but early in ontogeny double producers were observed (200). Figure 7 shows the possible relationships among the four above-mentioned isotypes.

IgD Homologs. Previously found only in primates and rodents, IgD was thought to be a recently evolved Ig. However, a novel form of Ig from a teleost fish (*Ictalurus punctatus*) is homologous in part to the δ H chain (201). It seems to be present also in lungfish (196). In addition to alternative secretory or membrane-associated C termini, this chimeric molecule contains a rearranged V domain, C_H1 of μ, and seven C domains encoded by a δ homolog. Like δ, this gene is immediately downstream of μ, has separate terminal exons for the secretory and membrane forms, and is coexpressed with μ in some but not all B cells. Larger but less flexible than IgD (no hinge region in the fish molecule), the fish molecule may not be an analog of IgD.

Other Isotypes Related to IgG, IgE, IgA, and Switch. Many isotypes consist of four constant domains: IgY and IgX in *Xenopus* species (202–205), the non-μ isotypes of *Rana* species (206), IgY of axolotls (207,208), and IgA or IgY of birds (209). In *Xenopus* species, IgY is thymus dependent; IgM and IgX are not, although thymectomy affects specific IgM antibody production (210,211). IgM and IgX plasma cells are abundant in the gut; IgY is not. In the axolotl, IgM is present in the serum early in the development and represents the bulk of specific antibody synthesis after antigenic challenge. Axolotl IgY occurs late in development and is relatively insensitive to immunization. From 1 month after hatching to the seventh month, IgY is present in the gut epithelium, associated to a secretory component. IgY progressively disappears from the gut and is undetectable in the serum of 9-month-old animals. Axolotl IgY, like *Xenopus* IgX, could be the physiologic counterpart of mammalian IgA (212). The membrane forms (mIg) of *Xenopus* Ig isotypes IgX and IgY are not homologous to any mammalian non-μ Ig isotype and are most similar to mIgM (189,213). The transmembrane and the cytoplasmic domains of mIgY share residues with avian mIgY and mammalian mIgG and mIgE, suggesting that the modern isotypes might share a common ancestor with amphibian mIgY. Although the sequence similarity between the membrane exons of avian mIgY and mammalian mIgG and mIgE is striking, the overall similarity with mIgY is very low

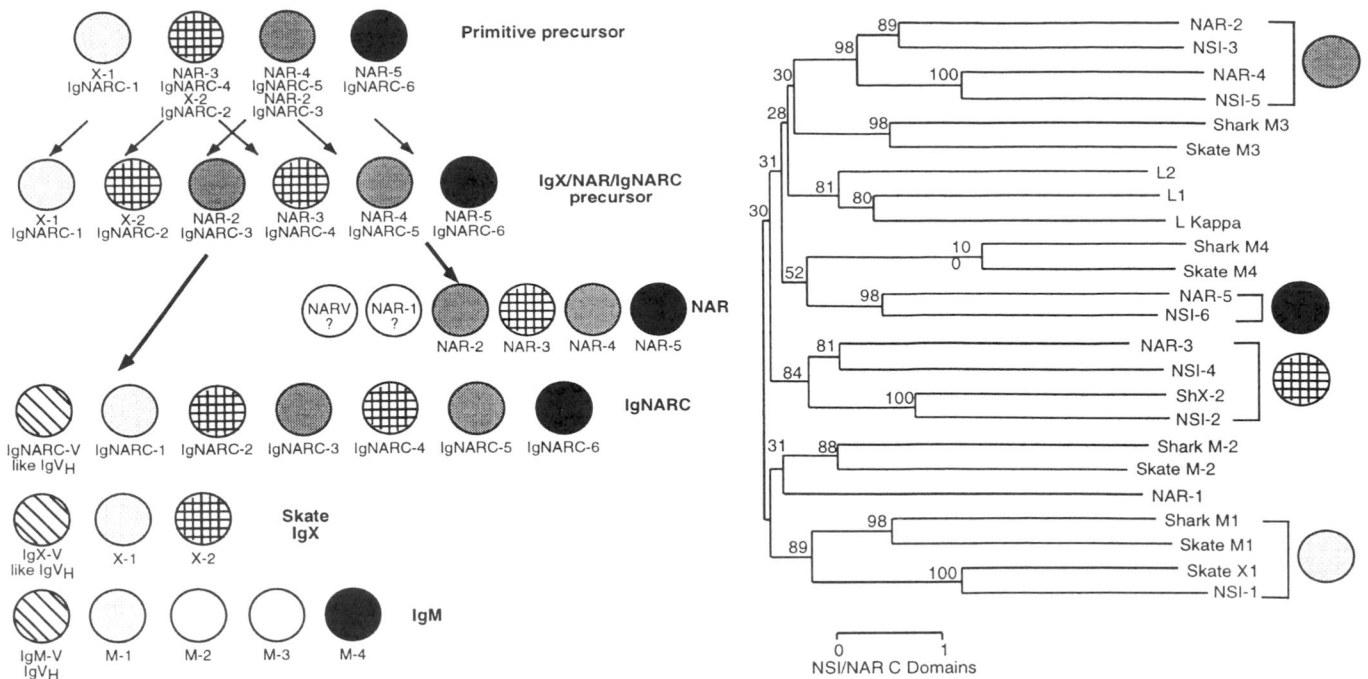

FIG. 7. A possible evolutionary progression from a primitive Ig to IgM. The relationships among Ig, NAR, and NARC are based on sequence comparisons. The amino-terminal three domains of Ig NARC (VC1C2) are homologous to IgX and the carboxy-terminal four domains are homologous to the last four NAR domains. The X1 and NAR5 domains are also homologous to IgM C1 and C4. The thin arrows indicate duplications. The thick arrows designate descent of the entire NAR and Ig NARC molecules from a common ancestor. The phylogenetic tree is a neighbor joining tree of C domains from the same various antigen receptors. It shows that IgNARC is a recent homolog of NAR and the likely ortholog of IgX. Modified from Greenberg et al (188).

Thus, the genes giving rise to *Xenopus* mIgY and those eventually leading to avian mIgY and mammalian mIgG and mIgE must have diverged at the level of the primitive amphibians or before (204,213).

Among vertebrates, H-chain class switch has now been detected in anuran amphibians (214). The *Xenopus* switchμ (Sμ) region (5 kb, for position see Fig. 8) contains 23 repeats approximately 150 bp long consisting of shorter internal repeats and palindromes, such as AGCT, as in mammals. In cells expressing IgX, the μ gene has been deleted and Sμ and Sχ are joined. Sχ is not homologous to Sμ and contains TGCA palindromes. Both Sμ and Sχ are AT rich and not GC rich, as in mammals. Recombination usually occurs at positions (microsites) where a single-stranded DNA folding program predicts the transition from a stem to a loop structure. This feature, conserved in mammalian switch junctions, points to the involvement of microsites during the determination of the recombination breakpoint. The recombinogenic nature of the S regions is therefore linked to the structure rather than to its base composition, the repetitive occurrence of palindromes being essential in creating many microsites.

Heavy Chains: Variable Region

A rearranged V_H gene consists of a leader (encoded by a split exon) followed by four framework regions and three CDRs. Canonical V_H CDR1 nucleotide sequences are conserved in all jawed vertebrates (215). The only salient germline difference is the lack of conserved octamers and TATA box in the 5' region of sharks (Fig. 8). In all species a complete Ig V gene is assembled by joining germline V, D, and J elements. In chondrichthyes, large numbers (probably over 100) of clusters are obvious for the H chain (216). For NAR there are only four V regions per haploid genome (195), and only a few NARC V genes are detected on nurse shark Southern blots (188). In Teleostei seven V_H families have been characterized in the catfish, and each contains up to seven to 10 genes, most of them with open reading frames (217). In the trout, 11 V_H families have been identified (218,219). The genus *Xenopus* has at least 11 families, three of which ($V_{H\,1-3}$) contain 20 to 30 members per haploid genome and from 10% to 30% pseudogenes. The other families are smaller (one to eight), so the total number of usable V_H elements is around 90 to 100 (220–222). Reptiles have very large pools of V_H segments (223). In the turtle *Pseudemys scripta*, four families, with a total of 700 V_H elements per haploid genome, have a frequency of only five pseudogenes out of 34 (224,225). Similarly, at least 125 genes homologue of the mouse V_H S107 were detected by hybridization another species of turtle *Chelydra serpentina*. In no cold-blooded vertebrate does the number of V_H segments seem to limit the diversity of the antibody repertoire. Among birds, chickens have about 80 V_H segments, all pseudogenes but one (226), as will be discussed later.

D Segments

In chondrichthyes, which have Ig genes organized in clusters, there are only one or two D segments per cluster and these clusters

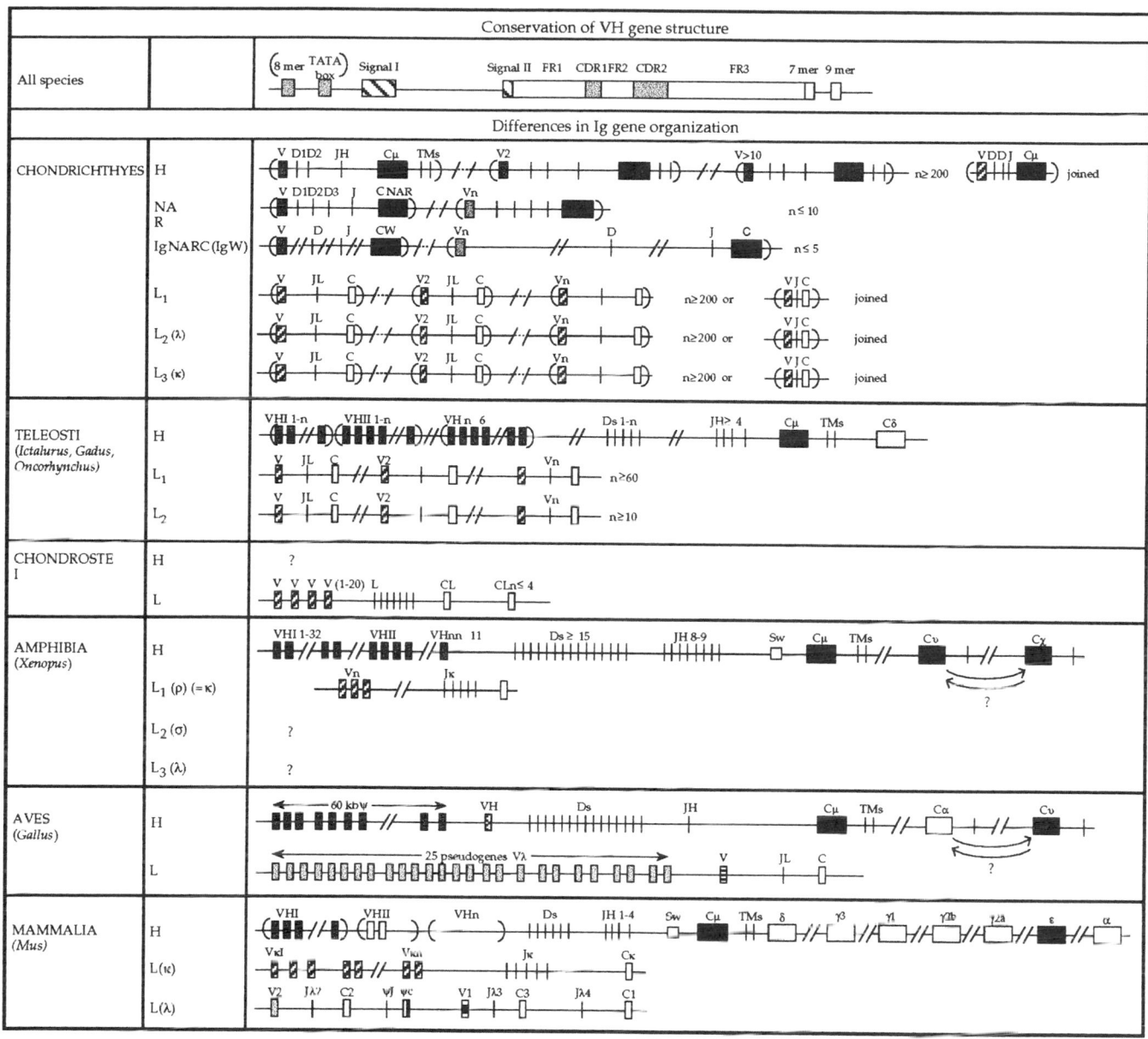

FIG. 8. Immunoglobulin genes organization in the various classes of vertebrates. FR, framework; 7mer and 9mer, heptamer and nonamer; TM, transmembrane domain. For references, see text.

are duplicates of each other with minor variations (Fig. 10) (216). Multiplicity therefore does not necessarily mean diversity. In teleosts, amphibians, and reptiles, in which the organization of the H chain locus is similar to that of mammals, the number of D segments deduced from cDNA ranges from 10 to 16. Two germline D segments have been identified in *Xenopus* species (227), and their recombination signal sequence (RSS) follow the expected rules defined in mammals. In birds, DH segments amount to 15 and are similar to each other (226).

There seem to be several reasons to keep D segments throughout evolution. One is structural. D will increase the diversity and sometimes the lengths of CDR3. Increasing the length may influence the combining site. In NAR, the length and the composition of CDR3 can fulfill a special tertiary structure requirement; a D-encoded Cys forms a bond with a Cys in Fr? and stabilizes a loop likely to be

involved in the antigen binding of this unusual monomeric receptor. In this case three different D segments contribute to CDR3.

The other reason has to do with rearrangement (107). In a heterodimer (H-LIg or αβTCR or γδTCR), only one of the V loci (VH, Vβ, or Vδ) has a D segment. If the pressure to keep the D segment was solely to increase diversity, it is likely that in some species the two chains of one receptor would have acquired the D segment. Strikingly the chain with the D segment is the one that rearranges first in both Ig and TCR (see Chapters 6, 10, and 11). This suggests that some molecular constraint is linked to the rearrangement mechanism. In fact, after VDJ rearrangement, no further arrangement is possible because the remaining unrearranged V and J segments have incompatible spacers [unless cryptic nonamers are used, which occurs in some cases (127)]. Thus, after rearrangement of the H or the β chain, when pre-B or pre-T cells that have successfully rearranged H or β proliferate, the locus is locked, which might allow time for the second locus to rearrange without losing the first one because of secondary rearrangement.

An exception to this rule would be that TCR γ rearranges before δ, but the γ locus allows few rearrangements, and δ is located inside the α locus.

[In summary, D may have been selected to allow the generation of a great diversity by N addition.] This could have been the driving force for D evolution if a receptor working as a monomer without a light chain, such as NAR, was the primordial receptor. If this receptor was a dimer, then the selective pressure for evolving a D segment was perhaps to "lock the locus."

J Segments

In chondrichthyes, multiplicity of J segments (for the same reasons as for D segments) does not necessarily mean diversity. In the channel catfish, nine J_H segments tightly cluster within 2.2 kb. Strong sequence homology and the unified length of the repeated sequences indicate that segments J_H3 to J_H7 probably arose by unequal crossing over. Each J_H segment seems functional, and junctional diversity is prominent in CDR3. The characteristic structure and organization of J_H segments in higher vertebrates therefore may have evolved early in vertebrate phylogeny (228). In *Xenopus* species, depending on the species, eight or nine J_H segments can be found. One is a pseudogene. Some of the J_H spacers contain pseudononamers that allow direct joining of a V segment (227). In the turtle *Pseudemys*, at least 16 J_H segments have been identified with characteristic RSS that differ from one to the other. Only one is a pseudogene (224,225). In birds only one J_H segment is present (226).

Evolution of V_H Genes

The V_H and V_L genes represent one of the most complex receptor gene systems to have evolved in vertebrates. One of the central questions is how do antibody V genes diversify in the CDR during evolution while they are subject to the forces of homogenization operating in multigene families (229) and in the absence of strong selection. V_H families arose before mammalian radiation and have since been conserved, which reflects selection for protein sequences. The conserved regions are localized on a solvent-exposed face of the H chain, at some distance from the antibody combining site. A family-specific region also was identified within the RSS (230).

In a phylogenetic tree the vertebrate V_H genes cluster into groups A, B, C, D, and E (Fig. 9) (231). All V_H genes from cartilaginous fish, such as sharks and skates, belong to the monophyletic group E; bony fish V_H genes cluster in group D. By contrast, group C includes some fish V_H genes as well as V_H genes from amphibians, reptiles, birds, and mammals. Group A and B genes are all composed of genes from mammals and amphibians. Another phylogenetic analysis classifies mammalian V_H genes in three clans (I, II, and III) that have coexisted in the genome for more than 400 million years. Having diverged from various functional genes, V_H pseudogenes have evolved much faster (231). There is little indication that the V_H gene families have been subject to concerted evolution that would homogenize member genes, as was suggested by the results of other studies based on the conservation of species-specific residues (232). It has been debated whether Ig V genes could be under direct positive selection or not because these genes

hypermutate somatically (233). However, several structural features (e.g., codon bias) and the discovery of a high replacement/silent ratio in the nucleotide substitution of the CDR region argue for positive selection during evolution (130,234).

In summary, vertebrates seem to conserve a large germline repertoire of V regions over long evolutionary periods. The birds look like an exception with a reduced germline repertoire, but as will be discussed below, gene conversion might compensate for this situation (235).

Light Chains

Three types of L chains have been cloned in chondrichthyes (236–238). Type 1 is the ancestral group and resembles *Xenopus* σ chains; type 2 resembles more λ chains of birds, *Xenopus*, and mammals. The type 2 light chain gene family is present in two orders of elasmobranchs, *Heterodontus* species, a galeomorph, and *Raja erinacea* a batoid, suggesting its presence throughout the cartilaginous types of fish; type 3 is more like κ. The κ-λ dichotomy is therefore very ancient (236), and intermediates that could explain the history are lacking.

Multiple L chains (molecular weight [MW] 22 to 26 kDa) are detected in fish Igs and are likely to reflect isotype diversity. In some species mAbs recognize various L-chain classes like the F and G [isotypes] of the catfish (239), and *Gadus* L1 chains are homologs of the chondrichthyes type 3 (κ-like) (240,241). In trout, two isotypes have been described, and the isotype L2 is more similar to the chondrichthyes L1-type and *Xenopus* σ chains (242).

In *Xenopus* L chains, ρ (κ-like), σ, and λ genes have been isolated (243–245). Only one C gene has been found in the ρ locus, and it corresponds to the most abundant L chain. Its RSS are of the κ type, and the five J segments are very similar to one another (246). The locus is deleted as κ is in mammals when the other isotype genes are rearranged (247). Monoclonal antibody studies also suggested the existence of three isotypes with MW of 25, 27, and 29 kDa, respectively, with highly heterogenous 2D gel patterns and a preferential association of some L chain isotype with IgY H chain (248). Southern hybridization with genomic DNA from different animals showed the V_L and C_L sequences to be both diverse and polymorphic. The third Ig L chain gene isotype in *X. laevis* predicted from these studies has been cloned and is related to mammalian λ genes. The locus consists of six distinct V_L families (245). In the σ locus the J segment has an unusual replacement of the diglycine bulge by two serines (244). The *Rana* major L chain type has an unusual disulfide intrachain bridge that is apparently responsible for the absence of covalent association of H and L chains in this species (249,250).

Two types of L chain have been identified in reptiles (251). Chickens and turkeys have only been shown to express one type of L chain architecture (Fig. 8), and the mode of usage of the locus may be responsible for this situation. Nonproductive rearrangements are not seen on the nonexpressed allele that could have generated a strong pressure to generate good joins. Such a system could have rendered the second L chain locus superfluous (236). As for the single L chain, the single chicken J segment is related to the peculiar mode of rearrangement used by birds (see next section) (252).

In mammals (see Chapters 5 and 6), L chain isotype expression varies widely; rats and mice express over 95% κ chains, whereas ruminants express mainly λ chains (253).

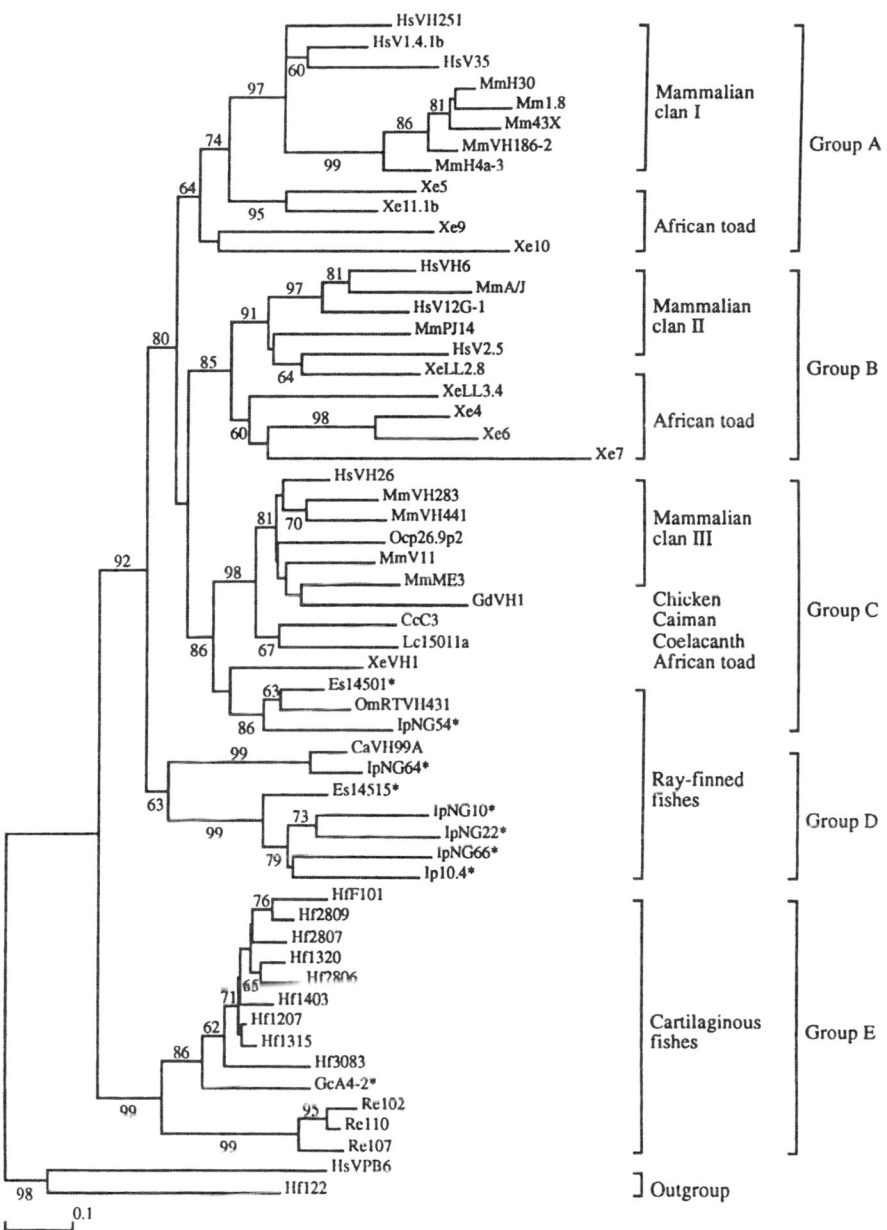

FIG. 9. Phylogenetic tree of 55 V$_H$ and two VL (outgroup) genes. The number given to each interior branch is the probability at which the branch length is different from the confidence probability. Reprinted with permission (227).

J Chain

Normal mouse IgM is synthesized as hexamers in the absence of J chain and as pentamers in its presence (254). Because some *Xenopus* studies had suggested the existence of Ig hexamers (255,256, it was of interest to look at the conservation of J chain and of putative cysteins able to form disulfide bonds with it. Homologs of the mammalian J chains have been discovered in *Rana* (257) and *Xenopus* (258) species. Sequence similarity with mammals is about 55% to 60%. The highest level of expression was detected in the intestine. Most likely the isotype that forms hexamers naturally is IgX because its H-chain gene has a stop codon before the Cys of CH4 that would be able to react with the J chain (205).

The Ig Genes Are Organized and Are Used in Different Ways in Different Species

Gene Organization

In all vertebrate species, Ig genes are build up by rearranging DNA segments scattered on the chromosome. Allelic exclusion also has been observed in cold-blooded vertebrates (259).

Among chondrichthyes, the shark (*Heterodontus francisci*) Ig H-chain gene complex consists of perhaps hundreds of clusters, each consisting of V, D, J, and C elements (260); the elements rearrange exclusively within one cluster. Although there is N diversity and sometimes two D segments are used, potential diversity must be less than in mammals. Little is known about Ig expression in *Het-*

erodontus, and the lack of the otherwise highly conserved octamer is an interesting puzzle. It seems to be replaced by a TCR-like promoter (261). The special constitution of the shark locus suggests an exclusion mechanism similar to that of mouse λ locus, where several CLs also lie on the same chromosome.

Bony fish, frogs, and mammals have very similar architectures of their Ig H locus (182,262,263). Multiple families of V$_H$ genes, each consisting of many apparently functional elements (one to 30 per family), are separated from a smaller number of genomic D and J elements. The possibility of combinatorial rearrangement clearly enables more diversification than is possible with the cluster type organization of the shark H locus.

L-chain gene organization is more variable. In elasmobranchs, the organization is the same (i.e., in clusters) as for the H-chain locus without the D segment. The prototypic chondrichthyes Ig light chain type I isolated from *Heterodontus francisci* has a clustered organization in which V, J, and C are closely linked. Germline-joined (prerearranged) genes, described originally in the H-chain genes of cartilaginous fish, also occur in L-chain genes (237). In bony fish the L-chain cluster type resembles that of sharks (183,240) and mammalian λ chain (Fig. 8). In chrondrosteans (sturgeon), the L-chain organization is like that of mammalian κ chain, which suggests that the clustered organizations seen in teleosts and chondrichthyes arose independently from each other (264). In *Xenopus* species (265) there seem to be multiple Vρ segments, presumably derived from one family, five J segments, and a single C gene segment (244,246).

Under certain circumstances a single gene can encode different forms of Ig, as in the duck IgY locus after alternative splicing (266) or in the camel (267). It has been suggested that the two avian IgY short and long forms could correspond to functional equivalent of both IgE and IgG (204,261).

B-Cell Differentiation

Progression of rearrangement during B-cell development can follow different rules in different vertebrates.

In *Xenopus* species (265) at 22°C, rearrangement starts on day 5 after fertilization for the V$_H$ locus, and within 9 days all V$_H$ are used. V$_H$1 starts first, followed by V$_H$3. V$_H$ segments 2, 6, 9, and 10 start rearranging on days 9 to 10; V$_H$ segments 5, 7, 8, and 11 rearrange on day 13.

V$_L$ rearrangement has been followed for the ρ and σ loci; ρ is the first to rearrange on day 7, i.e., 2 days after V$_H$, a situation similar to that found in mammals. During this early phase, the cells are present in the liver, where their number increases from 0 to 500. Pre-B cells can be detected before L-chain rearrangement in 5-day-old larvae (268). Later in life, rearrangement seems to stop around metamorphosis as suggested by the low incidence of pre-B cells and by the reexpression of RAG during the second histogenesis of the lymphoid system. RAG is expressed in adults, as found by Northern blotting and by the isolation of DNA excision circles (269), landmarks of ongoing rearrangements.

Until day 12, no lymphoid organ except the thymus is visible. The spleen appears on day 12 and with it the ability to respond to an antigen (270). Until this time no selection occurs as suggested by the ratio of out-of-frame/in-frame rearrangement (2:1). After day 12 this ratio becomes 1:1, i.e., the rearrangements have been selected. cDNA sequences on days 10 to 12 (when the number of B cells increases from 80 to 500) are not redundant, as if there were

no clonal selection and as if each sequence were represented by one cell. In juvenile frogs, RAG-1 and RAG-2 are highly expressed in thymus, less in liver and spleen, and even less in kidneys. In adults, the thymus and bone marrow are the principal sites of expression of both genes (129). The expression in the bone marrow together with the detection of DNA rearrangement circles (269) suggests that rearrangement is going on throughout life and is not restricted to an early period, as in birds. Tadpole rearrangements are characterized by a lack of N diversity, as in mammals (227), and short CDR3 (271), which may account for the differences in antibody repertoires and response between larvae and adults (270,272).

In birds during the embryonic period, prebursal stem cells that will give rise to B cells colonize the bursal follicles (about 10^4 follicles). They give rise inside each follicle to a population of surface IgM$^+$ cells. Three weeks after hatching, bursal cells go to the periphery and B cells can no longer be generated from a multipotent stem cell (273). Thus, only 2 × 10^4 productive rearrangements occur in the life of the chicken. Ig genes rearrange during a restricted period of time, probably during the early phase (around days 8 to 9 of incubation) of the colonization of the bursa of Fabricius. This establishes a pool of committed IgM$^+$ stem cells, ensuring the renewal of the B-cell pool during the whole life. Even though the general Ig locus architecture is similar to that of frogs and mammals, only one rearrangement is possible because there is only one functional V$_L$ or V$_H$ segment on each allele. Diversity is created during bursal ontogeny through a hyperconversion mechanism in which a pool of pseudogenes (25 ψL and approximately 80 ψH) act as donors and the unique rearranged gene acts as an acceptor (226,252,274,275). In the H chain the situation is more complex because there are multiple D elements (226). During ontogeny the selection of productive rearrangements parallels the selection of a single D reading frame, suggesting that the reason for so many is to favor D–D junction. This provides long stretches of DNA to be further diversified by gene conversion. The hyperconversion mechanism also affects D segments because the majority of donor pseudogenes are fused VD segments (226). In nonmammalian species no homologs of the pre-B receptor genes V-preB and lambda-5 has been isolated (see Chapter 6 for their usage in mammals).

Within mammals repertoire diversity can be reached by different mechanisms. In the rabbit H locus, as in the chicken, a single V$_H$ rearrangement is at the origin of most peripheral B cells, and during development in the appendix this rearrangement is diversified by gene conversion using upstream segments as donors (276). In ruminants, ileal Peyer's patches (IPP) are a bursalike primary B-cell organ. Even though bursa and sheep IPPs show morphologic similarities, the mechanisms generating diversity are different: conversion in the chicken and hypermutations in sheep (277). As data accumulate, grouping becomes possible in the function of the mode of B-cell development. Rabbits, cattle, swine, and chickens, unlike fish, amphibians, reptiles, and most mammals, have a single V$_H$ family, of which only a few members (or sometimes only one) are functional. The former group uses gene conversion in hind-gut follicles early in life (rather than bone marrow throughout life) to diversify their antibody repertoire. They also appear to lack IgD; thus, IgD might serve some purpose in repertoire development in some groups of mammals and not others (278). It would be interesting to study the generation of diversity in fish, where an IgD homolog has been found (86).

In conclusion, the potential repertoire of Ig combining sites is enormous in all gnathostomes. Not all species or all gene families use combinatorial joining because the Ig gene architecture does not permit it, but all species assemble V, D, and J gene segments to generate their functional Ig genes during B-cell ontogeny, and the imprecision of this assembly creates great somatic diversity. The coevolution of the lymphoid cell compartment with the Ig gene locus is fascinating. It is likely that some duplication and polyploidization, which are thought to have occurred in several speciation events, may have caused problems for lymphocytes. For example, what if the number of lymphocytes is too small to express the potential diversity of a freshly polyploidized V_H locus? This is not a far-fetched question; in the frog, for instance, polyploid individuals (e.g., *X. ruwenzoriensis*) are smaller and have fewer lymphocytes than their diploid counterparts (279). Polyploidy is not restricted to amphibians, for two independent IgM loci exist in the Atlantic salmon (280), a quasi-tetraploid species.

The Actual Level of Antibody Diversity During an Immune Response: Somatic Mutation

The potential diversity always exceeds the number of lymphocytes that could express it. Therefore, one must distinguish potential from actual repertoires.

Antibody diversity of nonmammalian vertebrates is low and has been studied mostly by indirect methods based on structural studies, affinity measurements during the immune response, enumeration of antigen-binding bands determined by isoelectrofocusing (IEF), and idiotype analysis. Maturation of antibody responses that occurs in mammals has been interpreted as the consequence of selection of B-cell clones capable of producing antibodies of higher affinity than that of those initially selected. Thus, maturation implies substantial antibody heterogeneity.

Agnatha

Hagfish and lampreys mount humoral responses to sheep red blood cells (SRBCs), keyhole limpet hemocyanin (KLH), bacteriophage, *Brucella*, and human RBCs (185). For anti–group A streptococcal antigens, hagfish antibodies recognize predominantly the rhamnose, whereas mammals recognize mainly the N-acetylglucosamine (281). This antibody turned out to be the complement component C3 (262). The C3 alternative pathway was known in cyclostomes from earlier studies (see complement section) (282, 283), but it is not clear whether agnathas have Ig at all. However, they do have lymphocytes and plasma cells (284–286).

Gnathostomata

Chondrichthyes

Immunized with 2-furyloxazolone–*Brucella* or p-azobenzenearsonate, the shark *Heterodontus francisci* mounts a low-affinity antibody response, which varies little among the individuals tested and which does not increase in affinity after immunization (287,288). This suggests a low-antibody heterogeneity in the species; variation of the L chains isolated from individuals is limited, with the major bands having identical isoelectric points (289). Another species of shark, *Ginglymostoma cirratum*, immunized with heat-killed streptococcal A variant vaccine, produces antibodies that among six outbred individuals have very different L-chain gel electrophoresis patterns. However, as in *Heterodontus*, the

L-chain diversity does not increase with time after immunization. In *Ginglymostoma* species, the heterogeneity of ligand binding involves intramolecular heterogeneity at the conformational level, meaning perhaps that one molecule could have dual specificities (184,290). This heterogeneity should perhaps be considered again in view of the organization of the IgM locus of this species, for which nothing is known about isotype exclusion. Perhaps chimeric molecules are made.

The unique V gene family of cartilaginous fish has 100 to 200 members (216,291). Such homogeneity in a large number of V genes hindered somatic mutation studies until a single unique reference V_H germline gene was found in the shark (292). Mutations in this gene were slightly more frequent than those in *Xenopus* species. Putative somatic mutations also were found in the expressed germline-joined V_L genes of another cartilaginous fish, the skate (293), but the conventional, rearranging V segments are used more frequently (294). Mutation rates could not be calculated, and no correlation with an immune response was attempted. The frequency and type of mutations (see *Xenopus*) were nevertheless indicative of somatic hypermutation. Thus, somatic mutation preceded diversity obtained by combinatorial association of gene segments (292).

Because in NAR there is a single V family with only four genes, it was possible to analyze somatic mutation, but as in the shark IgM study, random cDNAs were studied. The frequency of mutations is about 10 times that of *Xenopus* species and horned shark Ig, and much higher than in most studies in mammals. It is difficult to establish a pattern for the mutations due to their high frequency and because they are often contiguous. A few cDNAs contain short sequence stretches that may have been derived from other germline loci or alleles, suggesting that NAR genes undergo conversion. It is not known whether NAR genes diversify to generate a preimmune repertoire or whether they mutate in response to the antigen (195).

Teleostei

The antidinitrophenyl (anti-DNP) response of the carp consists of IgM antibodies distributed from pH 4 to 6.4 in IEF. The number of IEF antigen-binding bands per individual is small (up to 23), and there is little variation from one outbred individual to another (288,295–297). There are high levels of natural antibody to nitrophenylacetate (NP) (298), but they are of low affinity. They can represent 11% of the total Ig content. As a rule, little affinity maturation has been detected in fish, although some changes in fine specificities have been noticed in the trout (299). The mild increase in trout anti-TNP antibody affinity is attributed to selection of either minor preexisting populations or somatic mutants (300). In self-fertilized or gynogenetic trout (301), restricting genetic heterogeneity reduced the variability of response between individuals even more. In the catfish, peripheral blood leukocytes gave strong primary and secondary responses, not only *in vivo* but also *in vitro*, to thymus-dependent and -independent antigens (302). Affinity measurements by equilibrium dialysis were on the order of 2.0×10^6 M^{-1} for the anti-TNP antibodies (303). L chain usage can vary during the course of a response; antibody produced very early (1 to 2 weeks) after primary immunization contained approximately 20% of G L chains, approximately 90% of antibody produced later (3 weeks) were of the F isotype (304). Large levels of natural antibodies often have been reported, and in some cases these are correlated with resistance to virus infection (305) or furonculosis (306,307). A large amount of literature deals with vaccination attempts (see *Dev Biol Stand* 90, 1997 dealing with this issue). The availability of catfish B-cell, macrophage, and T-cell lines should help study antibody production *in vitro* and its regulation (308).

Amphibia

Urodeles express a restricted repertoire of antibodies peaking at 40 days, all of the IgM class, even though the serum also contains IgY (309). They do not respond well to thymus-dependent antigens, which may be due to lack of T-cell help. Anuran larvae can respond specifically (with only 10^6 lymphocytes) to many antigens, and a modest maturation of the IgM anti-DNP response was demonstrated. The number of different anti-DNP antibodies may not exceed 40, versus 500 in mammals. In secondary responses, the peak of the response is about 10-fold higher and is reached in 2 weeks instead of 3 weeks. There are no major changes in affinity, and spectrotypes are stable with time (310). In *Xenopus* species (311), protein sequence heterogeneity is low. Anti-DNP, or even nonimmune Ig pools, yields easily interpretable sequences for the first 16 N-terminal residues of both H- and L-chain V regions. cDNA sequences from *Xenopus* species challenged this view by showing that a huge heterogeneity of sequences could be detected in these animals (312,313). Isogenic *Xenopus* species produce rather homogenous antibodies to DNP, xenogenic RBCs, or phosphorylcholine with identical or similar IEF spectrotypes and idiotypes, whereas outbred individuals differ. Both IEF spectrotypes and idiotypes are inheritable, suggesting that diversity is due essentially to the expression of germline genes without a major contribution of somatic mutations (314,315). Thus, somatic mutations have been followed during the course of an antigen-specific immune response at the peak of the modest affinity maturation (313,316) in larvae and adults. The V_H genes, like their mammalian homologs, contain sequence motifs (A/G G C/T A/T) reported to target hypermutation (220,317). Of the 32 members of the V_H1 family (318) (involved in the anti-DNP response), expression of only five was amplified, indicating that immunization was being monitored. Only a small number of mutations were detected (average 1.6 mutations per gene, range 1 to 5). There was not a strong preference for mutations in CDR1 and 2, and virtually none was detected in CDR3 (313). Although the frequency of mutations was lower than in mammalian B cells, quantitative differences are equalized when one considers mutation rates. Taking the generation time of a lymphoid tumor cell line as a basis (319), the rate of somatic mutation appears to be quite similar to that found in mammals. The estimated rates—2.5×10^{-4} to 4.1×10^{-5}/bp/cell generation (average 1.5×10^{-4}/bp/cell generation)—are only four to seven times lower than the highest levels reported in hyperimmunized mice. Thus, there does not appear to be a shortage of variants, and the reasons for the low heterogeneity and poor-affinity maturation seems to be due to less than optimal selection of the mutants. Indeed because of a relatively low ratio of replacement to silent mutations in the CDRs and a very high ratio of GC to AT base pairs altered by mutation (not seen in properly selected mammalian somatic mutants), it was argued that there is no effective mechanism for selecting mutants, which in turn might be related to the absence of germinal centers in *Xenopus* species. The GC bias was also found in the shark (269,320).

In summary, if one put together the data from hypermutation, cDNA heterogeneity, and spectrotype dominance, perhaps we could find some correlations. In the absence of refined modes of selection, the late developing clones are "computed out" by the germline antibodies generated earlier.

Reptiles, Birds, and Mammals

Lack of an increase in affinity and homogeneity of IEF patterns suggests low heterogeneity in reptiles (321,322). Sequence data and L-chain patterns on two-dimensional gel electrophoresis showed less heterogeneity in chickens than in mice (323,324). The poor increase in affinity of chicken anti-DNP and antifluorescein antibodies [10^4-fold less than that of the rabbit (325)] again indicates a lower heterogeneity. Not many changes occur after immunization, even if one waits 1 year after several injections (325–327). A restricted population of high-affinity antibodies was found only after usage of Freund's complete adjuvant. Ongoing hyperconversion in germinal centers and somatic mutation in Ig genes have now been reported after immunization (328).

In the rabbit, maturation is conspicuous. Either hypermutation diversifies further the repertoire generated by conversion, or conversion itself goes on during the course of the immune response (329). It is not inconceivable that the relatively poor affinity maturation of the chicken response is due to a balance between gene conversion (likely to cause a loss of binding) and the somatic mutations (likely to provide at least some variants fitting the antigen better). Indeed, conversion over large segments of DNA does not seem to be a strategy ideal for the fine tuning of an immune response. The same argument should in fact apply to the rabbit, where maturation is conspicuous in the presence of gene conversion and hypermutation (329). The difference may be due to the relative contribution of each mechanism during deverification. Within mammals, big variations may be observed—from marsupials without secondary responses (330) to eutherian species with 1,000-fold increases in affinity, but the basis for them has not been established (269).

In conclusion, although all vertebrates have a large potential for generating diverse antibody, only the warm-blooded vertebrates and perhaps only some mammals exploit this possibility fully. The reasons are not obvious. Perhaps the pressures on the immune system of cold-blooded vertebrates have been less intense due to a stronger innate immunity and the architecture of their lymphoid system is not optimal for selecting somatic mutants.

The MHC

MHC and T-Cell Functions in Vertebrates

T cells distinguish self from nonself through the presentation of small peptides bound to MHC class I and class II molecules, i.e., MHC restriction (331,332). The genetic restriction of T cell–antigen-presenting cell (APC) collaboration, processing of antigen by professional APCs, and T-cell education in the thymus described in mice hold true for most vertebrate classes (Table 2). No MHC-regulated T-cell responses have been so far reported in cartilaginous fish, but the identification of polymorphic class I and II (333–335) and rearranging TCR genes (161) strongly suggests that functional analyses will reveal MHC restriction of at least some adaptive responses. Similarly, urodele amphibians are notorious for their poor immune responses, and biochemical evidence suggests that MHC polymorphism is low in the axolotl (Table 2) (309,336). However, because class I and class II genes have been isolated only recently

(337,338) in this species, we must await confirmation. In fact preliminary analyses of class I sequences suggests a much greater heterogeneity than would be expected from the earlier data (339).

High-Sequence Divergence Yet Strong Structural Similarity

The three-dimensional organizations of class I (340) and class II (341) are essentially the same. The two membrane-distal domains form a PBR composed of two antiparallel α helices resting on a floor of eight β strands, and the two membrane-proximal domains are Igsf C1. Although sequence identity of class I and class II genes among vertebrate taxa is low, the four extracellular domain organization and other conserved features are likely to be found in the ancestral gene (147,342). In class I molecules there are disulfide bridges in the PBR α2 and Igsf α3 domains and in Igsf β2 microglobulin (β2m), but not in the PBR α1 domain (343,344) (Fig. 10). The Igsf membrane-prox-

imal α2 and β2 domains of class II have the canonical disulfide bonds, and the β1 domain, which is homologous to class I α2, also has an intradomain disulfide bridge. The class II α1 domain, like class I α1, lacks a disulfide bond except in bony fish (343) a feature shared with class II DM molecules (344,345), which are as old as the *bona fide* class II genes (Fig. 11). The exon/intron structure of class I and class II extracellular domains is also well conserved, but one group of teleosts has recently acquired an intron in the exon encoding the Igsf β2 domain (346).

Other conserved features of class I genes (Fig. 10 and Table 2) include a glycosylation site on the loop between the α1 and α2 domains (shared with class II α chains), a Tyr, and one to three Ser in the cytoplasmic regions that can be phosphorylated in mammals (347,348), as well as several stabilizing ionic bonds. Class II with its two TM regions differs from class I with only one; conserved residues in the class II α and β transmembrane/cytoplasmic regions probably facilitate dimerization (349) (Fig. 10). In summary, because sequence similarity is very low among MHC and

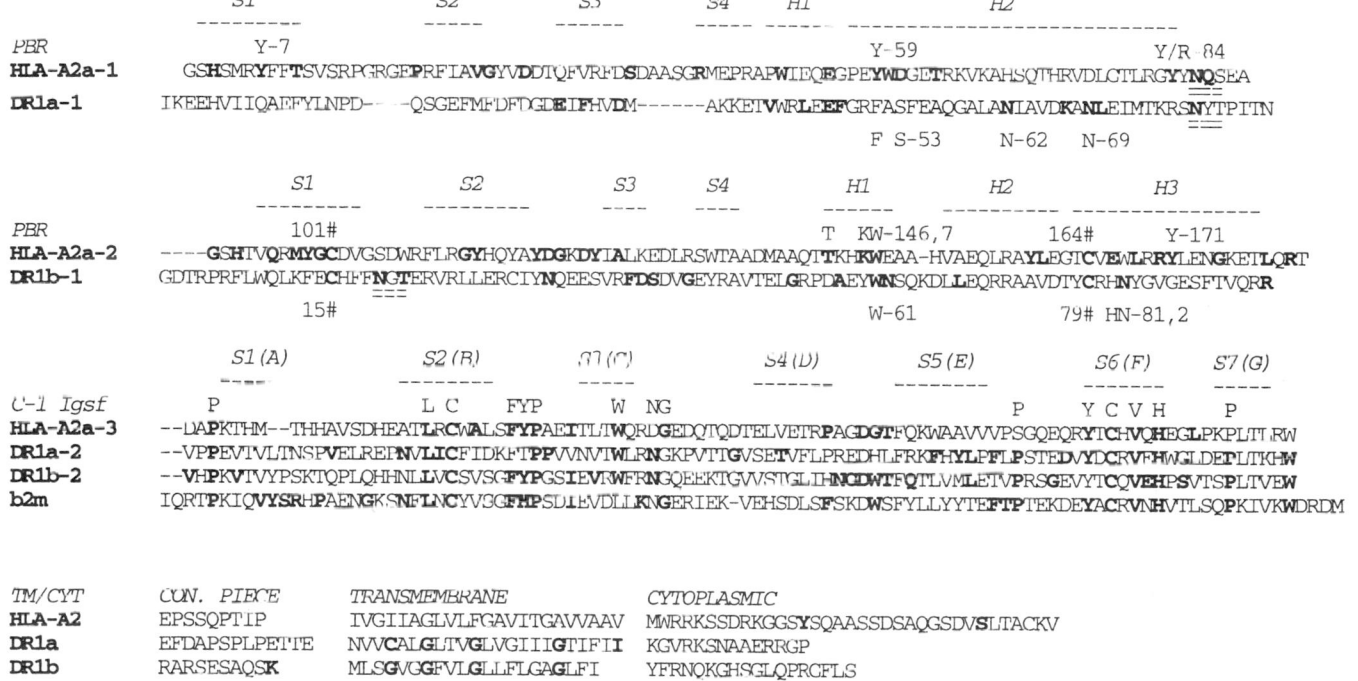

FIG. 10. Residues conserved in classical class I and class II molecules in all vertebrates. Displayed are sequences of HLA-A2 and DR1 for which crystal structures exist for the extracellular domains (340,341). Bold and shadowed amino acids indicate that the residue is found in the majority of sequences of classical class I and class II from members of all vertebrate classes or all but one vertebrate class (see legend to Table 2 for sequences used). Residues above the alignments for class I PBR a-1 and a-2 (Y-7, Y-59, Y/R-84, T-123, K-146, W-147, Y-171; note that Y-84 is invariant in mammals and is instead R in all other vertebrates) and below the alignments in class II PBR a-1 and b-1 (Fa-53, Sa-55, Na-62, Na-69, Wb-61, Hb-78, Nb-82) are nonpolymorphic residues that bind to main-chain atoms of acquired peptides (341,351,587). For the Ig domains, residues above the alignment are conserved in all C1-set domains (100) and are found in at least two of four sequences. Note that β2m has only been found in mammals (397), birds (350), and teleosts (399–401). Double-underlined residues are conserved glycosylation sites. Strands (S) and helices (H) are shown for the PBR domains and strands (S) for the Igsf domains. For the functions of the blackened residues in the PBR and transmembrane/cytoplasmic regions, see Table 0. Analysis of sequences was first performed elsewhere (342).

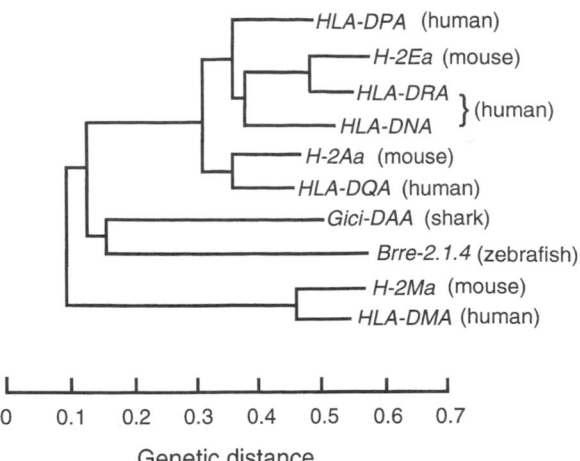

FIG. 11. Phylogenetic tree of class II a-2 domains of various species and DM molecules of mice and humans. Notice that the mammalian DM molecules branch off near the root of the tree, suggesting that they arose early in the evolution of class II molecules. Reprinted with permission from Kasahara et al. (147), from which references to sequences can be obtained.

other immune system genes in different taxa, the conserved features are likely to be important for the function and maintenance of structure.

Classical and Nonclassical Class I and Class II

Class Ia (classical) and class Ib (nonclassical) genes are found in all of the major groups of jawed vertebrates. Class Ia genes are defined by their ubiquitous expression, their presence in the MHC proper, and by high polymorphism (342,350). In addition, class Ia proteins almost always have eight conserved residues at both ends of the PBR; they interact with main chain atoms of bound peptides and constrain their size to eight to nine residues (351) (Fig. 10 and Table 3); this feature serves well in distinguishing class Ia from class Ib in amphibians and fish (352). Thus, tight binding of peptides, a likely source of conformational changes in class I, allowing transport through the ER and cell surface expression, is an evolutionarily conserved trait.

Thus far the class Ia/class Ib distinction holds true for all taxa: one to three polymorphic class Ia genes are expressed ubiquitously in all species; other, minimally polymorphic or monomorphic (class Ib) genes can be expressed in a tissue-specific fashion (342). Why have class Ib genes been perpetuated (353,354)? In mammals the function of class Ib genes such as CD1 (355,356) and M3 (357) differs or complements that of class Ia. It is also likely that class Ib genes are maintained as a reservoir of presenting molecules as they are in New World monkeys (358). Because class I molecules are unstable during biosynthesis, they can be molded to serve new functions in immune responses and perhaps even in homeostasis. For example, the neonatal Fc receptor (Fcγrt) is involved in binding and transporting of IgG molecules across epithelia (359,360), and zinc a-2 glycoprotein (AZGP1) is believed to function in zinc transport (361). Was the original MHC function not linked to antigen presentation? The molecules with functions other than presentation described to date appear to be evolutionarily derived from presenting molecules (147,362) (Fig. 12).

Class II molecules also have practically invariant residues that bind to main-chain atoms of peptides, but these are in the center of the groove (341) (Fig. 10 and Table 1). Thus, tight binding to main-chain peptide atoms occurs in the center of the class II PBR,

TABLE 3. *Function of class I/II residues in PBR and TM/Cyt that are conserved in evolution*

	Class	Residue
Salt bonds	Class I	R44-DE61; E56-RK170 (closes one end of the groove); H93-D119; E166
	Class II	Da27 (salt bond to Ha3 in many species)
Glycosylation sites	Class I	Q87
	Class II	Nb19; Tb21
	Both	N86/Na78
Disulfide bonds	Both	C101/Cb15–C164/Cb79
Tums	Class I	P20; G26; G112; G120; G175
	Class II	Gb45; Gb54
Peptide	Class I	Y7 (N-term); V25; Y59 (N-term); Y/R-84 (C-term); D119; T143 (C-term); K146 (C-term); W147 (N-term); Y159; Y171 (N-term)
	Class II	Na62; Na69; Nb82
	Both	W147/Wb61
Cysoplasmic class I*		Y-320 (exon 6 mouse, human); S-335 (exon 7)
Transmembrane class II		Ca195, Ga198, Ga202, Ga209, Kb198, Gb202, Gb205, Gb209, Gb216
PBR interaction with Ig-like domains	Class I	T10; Y27; V25; D29; Q96; Q115; G120; D122
	Class II	Ea30
	Both	D119/Nb33; L179/Rb93
Unassigned	Class I	S38, W51, W60, D61, T64, Q87, G91, Q96, M98, Y99, G100, Y113, Y118, D121, FY122, A125, L160, L168, L179, R181
	Class II	Fa32, Da35, Va42, La45, DEa47, Fa48, Ka67, La70, DNb41, Sb42, Ab58, Nb62, Lb68

Residues are numbered according to HLA-A2 (340) and DR1 α and β (341). Sequences used to detect conserved residues are classical (or presumed classical) class I and class II molecules from mouse, human (e.g., see refs. 331 and 350), bird (350,388,577), amphibian (337,352,561,578), reptile (154), teleost (343,390,391,399–401,552–556,579–581), and cartilaginous fish (333–335,549). To be included, the residue had to be either invariant or found in the majority of sequences in all vertebrate classes except one.

Modified from ref. 342, with permission.

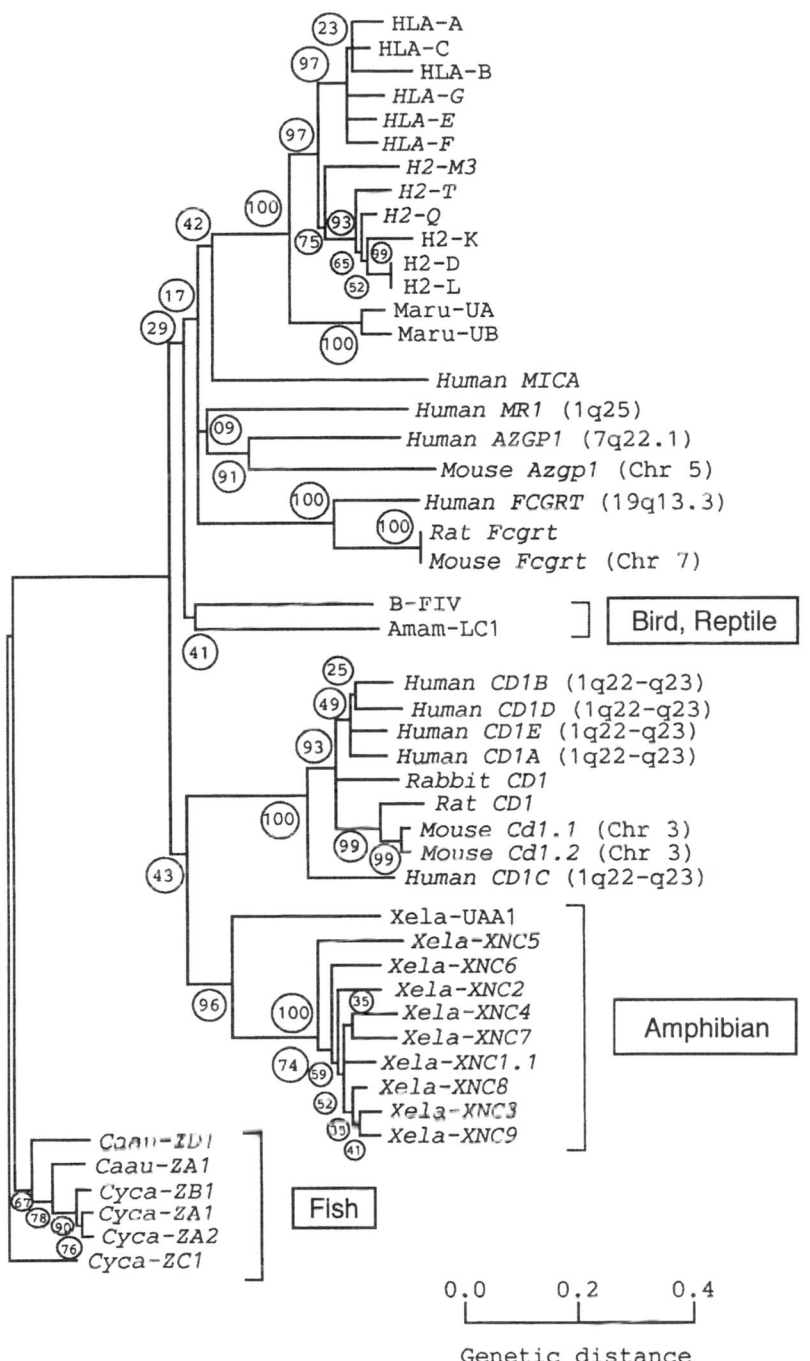

FIG. 12. Phylogenetic tree of classical (normal type) and nonclassical (italics) class I a-3 domains from various species. Note the following: (a) classical class I genes, even among mammals, are not orthologous; (b) some non-classical genes are recently derived from the same ancestor as the classical genes within a taxon, e.g., H2-M3 and H-2K,D,L, and Xela-UAA1 and XNC genes; (c) other mammalian nonclassical genes emerged from class I ancestors before the appearance of mammals, e.g., Fcyrt and CD1. Note that in this latter case, none of the class I genes except MICA are linked to the MHC proper. Reprinted with permission from Kasahara et al. (362), from which references can be obtained. (Genetic distance corresponds to the number of amino acid replacements per site).

and peptides are free to protrude from both ends. The only non-classical class II molecules so far identified are the previously mentioned DM molecules that lack these residues (344,345). DM molecules so far have been cloned only from mammalian species, but they are likely to be present in all species with canonical class II molecules.

Polymorphism of MHC Genes

In all vertebrate species MHC is the most polymorphic genetic region known, both in number of alleles and diversity among alleles (331). Besides the evolutionarily conserved PBR residues (Fig. 10 and Table 3) those that bind to acquired peptides are the most diverse. These residues are under positive selection; i.e. in almost every classical class I and II gene so far analyzed, nonsynonymous substitutions are more frequent than synonymous in codons specifying the residues (363,364). Variation in the MHC among taxa has been classically derived via mutation, gene conversion, and recombination followed by selection (147,331). This is quite different from the Ig locus, where major variations are found in gene organization and diversity generation among different species.

Disease Associations

Although it is assumed that the MHC polymorphism is important for protection against a range of pathogens (331,336) and that this acted as a driving force in evolution, it has been difficult to prove that any particular allele confers resistance/susceptibility to any virus or bacterium. In chickens, however, there are convincing associations of disease with MHC. For instance animals with the B21 haplotype show as much as 95% survival when infected with Marek's virus, and other haplotypes show varying levels of resistance (364). Because there is an inverse correlation with expression of class I and resistance to the virus, NK cells rather than T cells would seem to provide protection (134,336,365). Disease association studies in other models of commercial interest (such as fish) also could be fruitful.

Ontogeny of Expression

In mammals and birds, class II expression precedes class I during embryogenesis (331,366). The same is true in *Xenopus* species, where immunocompetent larvae express high levels of class II on APCs such as B cells, but only express no or low levels of class Ia molecules until metamorphosis (367,368). Expression of the immune proteasome element lmp7 and all class Ib isotypes is also very low. Interestingly, larval skin and gut, organs with epithelia in contact with the environment, appear to coexpress class I (transcripts) and class II. It is thought that this expression adds immune protection during larval life but that expression of class I should be limited to organs that undergo massive destruction and remodeling at metamorphosis. Class II molecules also change their distribution after metamorphosis and are highly expressed by unstimulated T cells (369,370). Axolotl class II molecules are also regulated differentially during ontogeny, being expressed in young animals on B cells and then expanding to all hematopoietic cells, including erythrocytes later in life (371). Changes in MHC expression are not correlated with cryptic metamorphosis in axolotls, but class II expression by erythrocytes is correlated to the switch from larval to adult globins. Class I transcripts isolated so far are expressed early in ontogeny, from hatching onward (339).

Carp class I and class II transcripts are detected in embryos 1 day after fertilization and reach a plateau at day 14. However, the suspected class Ia protein does not appear until week 13, whereas $\beta 2m$ can be detected several weeks earlier. It was suggested that another class I molecule is expressed during early development of the carp hematopoietic system (372).

Significance of Linkage

Because class I and class II proteins are structurally similar, it is no surprise that their genes are linked. But why are the structurally

unrelated class I processing genes, including the proteasome components lmp2 and lmp7 and the TAP genes, also found in the MHC in mammals (373–376) (Fig. 13)? There are two possible scenarios: primordial linkage of processing and presenting genes in the MHC or later recruitment of either the processing/presenting genes into a primordial MHC (143). Based on the presence of similar clusters of MHC genes on paralogous chromosomal regions in humans and mice, Kasahara et al. have suggested that ancestors of class I, class II, proteasome, transporter, and class III genes were already linked before the emergence of the adaptive immune system (377,378) (Figs. 14 and 15). Indeed, some of the genes in this cluster are linked in *Drosophila* and *Coenorhabditis elegans* (379,380) and other genes such as Igsf members of the CTX family *sensu lato* are close to several of these paralogs (381). One or perhaps two genome duplications around the time of the origin of vertebrates as proposed by Ohno (382) may have provided the raw material from which the immune system genes were assembled. Neither Ig/TCR/MHC nor lmp/TAP could be isolated from hagfish nor lampreys, and all of these genes as well as the Zn $\alpha 2$ glycoprotein could have emerged after the second round of duplications (383). Because class I genes are found on two or three of the clusters (Fig. 16), class I–like molecules may have preceded class II in evolution. Indeed, NK-like recognition of a class I molecule encoded in the ancestral linkage group may have been at the origin of the adaptive immune system (134). However, none of these receptors carries an Ig V domain that would make it look like an ancestral immune receptor.

In birds (336,365), bony fish (383), and perhaps amphibians (384), unlike in mammals, the lmp and TAP genes are linked to class I genes, not to class II (Fig. 15). This result is most striking in zebrafish because class I/lmp/TAP and class II are found on different chromosomes. Previous models suggested that the class III region, referred to as "the region of unrelated loci" (331), was inserted into the MHC rather late evolution, but factor B, C4, and HSP70 are all in the *Xenopus* MHC (144,385–387), thus extending the association of class I, II, and III to the common ancestor of mammals and amphibians 300,000 to 350,000 years ago. Again, if Kasahara's interpretation is correct (377,378), it is expected that the physical association of ancestral class I, II, and III genes predated the emergence of gnathostomes, and such affiliations in amphibians are not surprising. Taken together, the data suggest that the nonlinkage of class I and class II (and perhaps class III) in teleosts is a derived character. Linkage studies in cartilaginous fish should be informative on this point.

The chicken MHC, the B complex (336,365), is on a microchromosome, and intron sizes and intergenic distances are both quite small (Fig. 13). In fact, chicken class I genes were discovered because they were found on the same cosmid clones as class IIβ genes (388). Thus far, class Ia, class II (including DM), and TAP genes are in the MHC, but there is no evidence for proteasome genes, and almost all class III genes have been deleted except for a fragment of C4. Although most class III genes will likely be found on other chromosomes (389), lmp2/7 could be absent from the genome. Indeed, peptides bound to chicken class I molecules sometimes end in glutamic or aspartic acid, which are rare after proteolysis by mammalian proteasomes containing lmp2 and lmp7 (365). To explain the correlation of diseases with particular haplotypes, Kaufman proposed that the chicken has a minimal essential MHC composed of only those genes absolutely required to remain there.

In summary, in all nonmammalian species studied, classical class I genes map closely to the TAP and lmp genes, suggesting

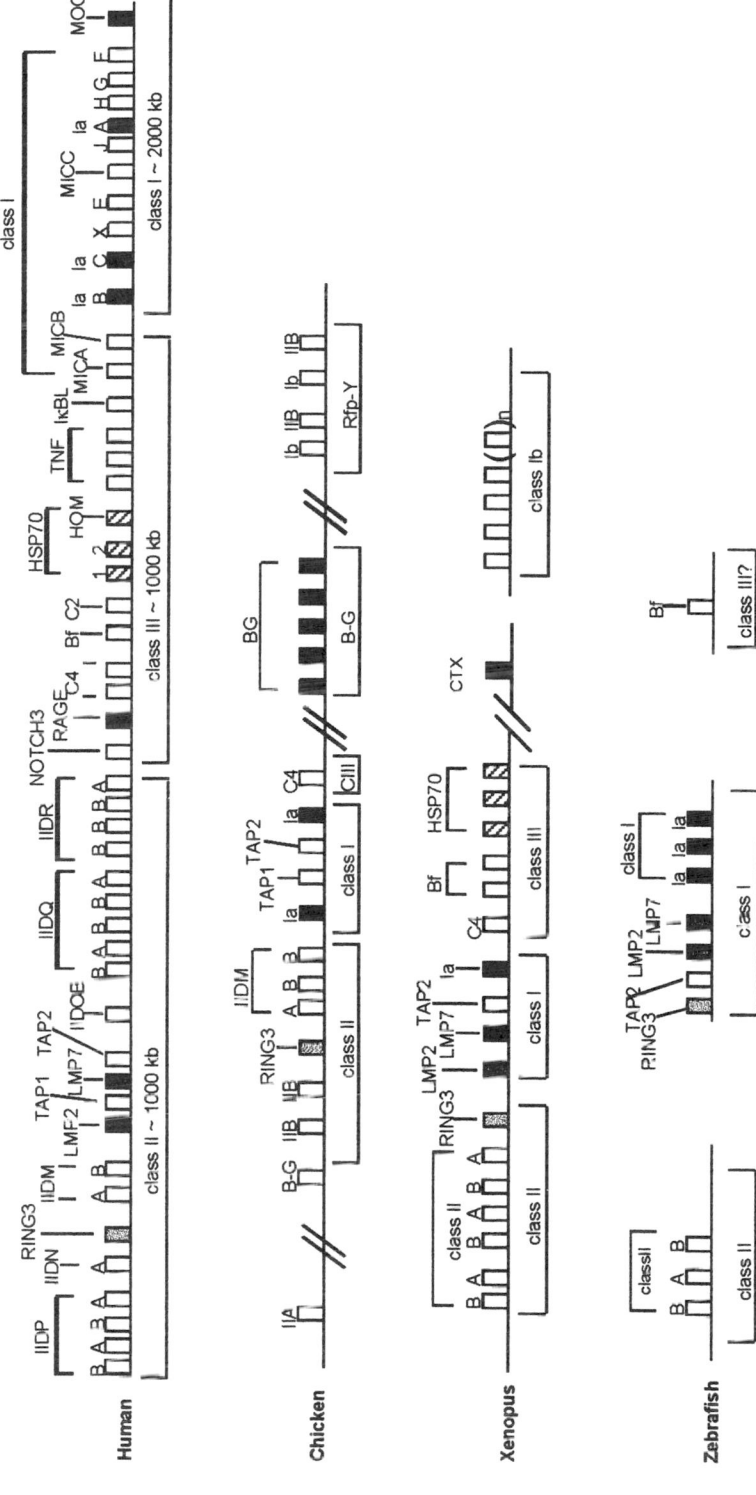

FIG. 13. MHC linkage maps of human, chicken, *Xenopus* species, and zebrafish. Distances between the genes are not to scale, but the relative order of the genes is as displayed except for *Xenopus* species, for which the order and even the potential "regions" are not well known. Only genes that are discussed in the text are displayed for all species. Large slash marks in the chicken MHC indicate linkage on the same chromosome but not in the same clusters. Separation of clusters in *Xenopus* species and zebrafish indicates nonlinkage of the indicated regions. Black boxes and boxes with forward slashes denote highly and poorly expressed class Ia genes, respectively. Maps were taken from Trowsdale [human (336,365,579)], Kaufman [chicken (143)], Flajnik [*Xenopus* species (382)], and Klein

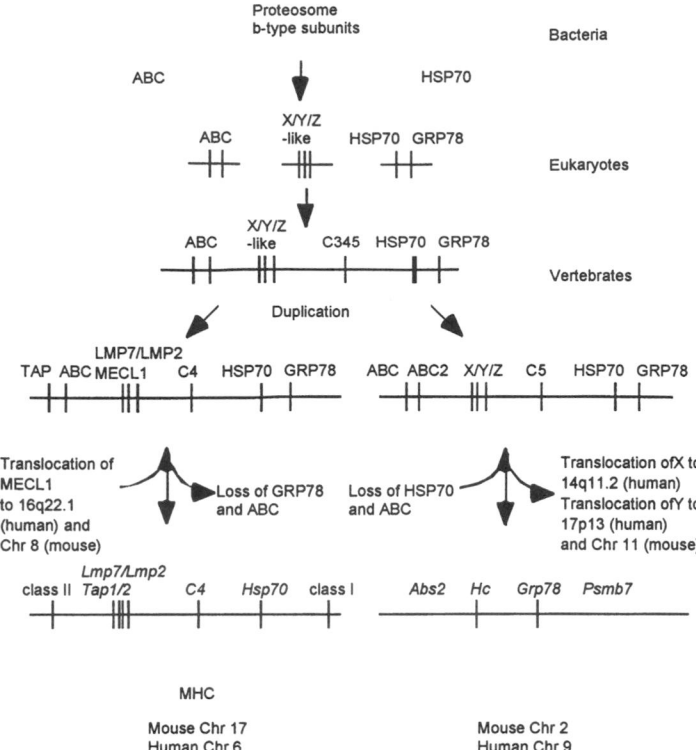

FIG. 14. Model of Kasahara et al. (378) for emergence of the MHC through block duplication. Genes not described earlier or in the text: MECL1, third immune proteasome element that is not linked to the MHC (592); X, Y, Z, constitutive forms of immune proteasome elements lmp2, MECL1, and ?, respectively (378); ABC, generic molecule related to the ATP-binding cassette multidrug-resistant proteins of which TAP is a member; GRP78, constitutive form of HSP70 that resides in the ER (591). Reprinted with permission.

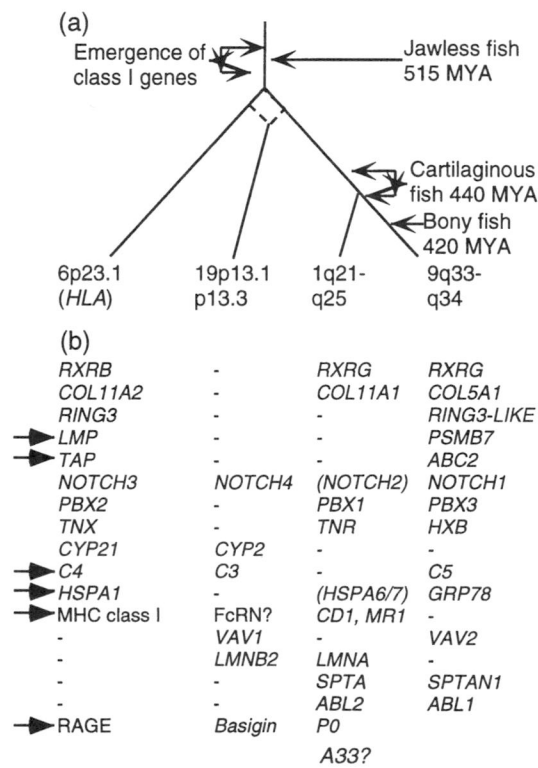

FIG. 15. Proposed timing of duplication events giving rise to paralogs with MHC-like linkage groups. Arrows denote molecules discussed extensively in the text. FcRN is on 19q, hence the ?. Reprinted with permission from Kasahara et al. (377) and modified with data from Chrétien et al. (118).

that the processing and presenting genes were in an original cluster (147,383). Although teleosts underwent an explosive adaptive radiation 100,000 years ago, there are deep lineages of class I genes in all species (390,391). In mammals the class I region is not closely linked to lmp/TAP and is very unstable (147,383). The same class I instability extends to non-MHC linked class Ib genes in *Xenopus* species (362,392,393).

Selection for a Few Expressed Class I and Class II Genes

Only a few lamical class I and class II genes are conserved in the genome, typically one to three per haplotype, with highest expression of one gene (394). In polyploid species of *Xenopus* ranging from 2n to 12n the number of detectable class I and class II genes is kept stable (one for class I, two or three for class II/haploid genome) (279,395). The silencing of MHC genes is not immediate nor compulsory for survival because laboratory-bred polyploids express multiple MHCs (395). Opposing selecting forces such as determinant density (i.e., the number of presenting molecules displaying any particular peptide) and tolerance (i.e. requiring T cells to become tolerant to all class I/II alleles in association with all self-peptides) (279,396) are believed to contribute to the stable low number of expressed MHC genes throughout evolution.

Conservation of structural features of class I and class II and in the expression of particular numbers of genes should not imply that the MHC is stable over evolutionary time. Although class Ia genes among diverse species share certain traits, the genes are not orthologous even among related taxa (50) (Fig. 14). Class II is more stable, but again orthologous genes are difficult to detect among vertebrates (147). Perhaps in the race against pathogens the number of class I and class II genes greatly expand and contract over evolutionary time in order to promote diversity in the few expressed genes. Nevertheless, the previously described canonical features have been selected and remain instrumental to MHC function, such as interaction with peptides and with TCR (394).

β2 Microglobulin

β2m was the second Igsf molecule ever to be identified, originally found at high levels in the urine of patients with kidney disease (397). It associates with almost all class I molecules (except, apparently, with human MIC proteins) (398). Besides mammals, β2m has been cloned from teleost fish [carp (399), trout (400), zebrafish (401)] and avian species [chickens and turkeys (350)]. In all cases examined, the β2m gene is not in the MHC and is a single-copy gene in all species except trout, in which it has undergone multiple duplications (400). β2m is expressed by the thymus and could perhaps act as a chemoattractant for pre-T cells (402), but β2m knock-out mice have normal thymocyte numbers (403).

The Complement

The complement system provides a vital nonadaptive immune function and plays an important role in the regulation of adaptive responses (404). Thus, evolutionary studies might tell what were the most primordial and perhaps vital functions of this system (405,406). Three major functions of complement are (a) coating pathogens to promote uptake by phagocytes (opsonization); (b) initiation of inflammatory responses by stimulating smooth muscle contraction, vasodilation, and chemoattraction of leukocytes; and (c) lysis of pathogens by perforating their membranes (Fig. 16) (see Chapter 29).

At the heart of complement is C3, the only known immune recognition molecule to date capable of covalent association (via a thiol ester bond) with biologic surfaces. C3, probably the most promiscuous protein yet discovered, interacts with at least 20 other proteins, including proteases, opsonic receptors, complement acti-

vators, and inhibitors and has a nonspecific recognition function (407). C3 forms the intersection where the alternative, classical, and lectin pathways of complement activation meet. C3 bound to surfaces associates with the protease factor-B (Bf), which is then itself cleaved by factor D, leading to the splitting of many C3 molecules in an amplification loop (Fig. 16). The covalently attached product C3b is an opsonin, perhaps the primordial active product of the system. Consistent with this idea, both C3 and Bf cDNAs have been cloned from the sea urchin, an echinoderm with no adaptive immune system defined by Ig/TCR/MHC (408,409). There is also no evidence for a lytic pathway before cartilaginous fish, suggesting that the opsonic pathway is primordial (410).

Another nonadaptive recognition system, the lectin pathway, also appears to have arisen early in evolution. The mannose-binding lectin (MBL) is functionally similar to IgM in that it binds, on its own, to surface carbohydrates of pathogens and acts as an opsonin (411). MBL is analog to the C1q with its high-avidity binding to surfaces by multiple interaction sites through globular C-terminal domains, but apparently it is not homologous to C1q. Similar to C1q, which associates with the serine proteases C1r and C1s, proteases called MASP (MBL-associated serine proteases) physically interact with MBL and not only activate the classical pathway of complement by splitting of C4 and C2 (the same function as C1s), but also seem capable of cleaving C3 and thus completely bypassing the classical pathway (Fig. 16). MASP-1 and -2 are homologs of C1r and C1s, but the sequence similarity is too low to determine the exact phylogenetic relationships among the four proteins (412). MBL and MASP have been identified in tunicates (413) and thus, like C3, clearly predate the emergence of the adaptive immune system.

C3 and MBL are vital players in the immediate innate immune response in vertebrates. Whether or not invertebrate MBL and C3 function in the same way as in their backboned cousins, it is likely that their basic functions evolved early, at least in a deuterostome ancestor. The next steps will be to determine whether similar complement receptors, which are important not only in phagocytosis but also in the alerting of other defense systems of pathogenic invasion,

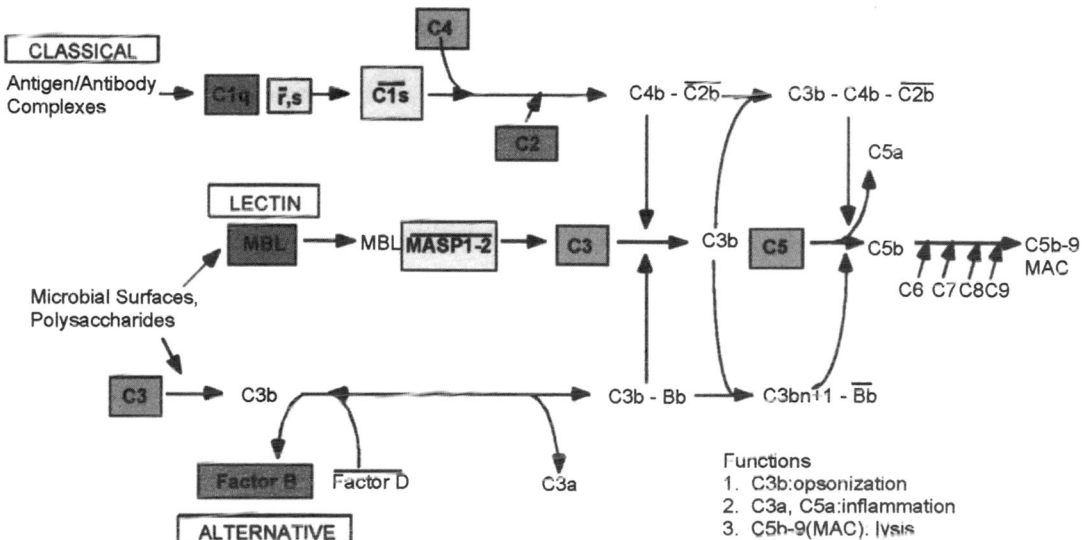

FIG. 16. Diagrammatic representation of the three major pathways of immune recognition that lead to complement fixation. Boxes with similar notations indicate analogy (C1q:MBL) or homology (C1s:MASP1,2; C2:Bf; C3, C4, C5). Modified with permission from Lambris (591).

are present in cold-blooded vertebrates (404). It also will be of interest to isolate these molecules from some protostome species.

Hagfish and lamprey C3-like genes were thought to be an ancestral C3/C4 gene because the sequence predicts two processing sites (leading to a three-chain molecule), like C4, but a C3-like properdin-binding site is clearly present (262,410,414). However, the hagfish protein is composed of only two chains of 115 and 72 kDa, like all other *bona fide* C3 molecules (415). Moreover the sea urchin C3 sequence predicts only two chains (one proteolytic processing site), as in the higher vertebrate C3 version. Teleosts can express several C3 isotypes, suggesting that in animals displaying low diversity in their antibody responses, the nonadaptive immune system may be more heterogeneous (416).

The classical pathway, which is initiated by antibody–antigen complexes, together with Ig and other markers of the adaptive immune system makes its first appearance in cartilaginous fish (417). We note, however, that MBL can activate this complement pathway in mammals. Nevertheless, C4 and C2 genes have not been detected in invertebrates or jawless fish; again, we note that C2-homolog Bf functions in both the classical and alternative pathways in a teleost [rainbow trout (418)].

The lytic pathway, with the formation of the membrane attack complex (MAC) initiated by the cleavage of C5 into C5a and C5b, also seems to be absent in the taxa older than cartilaginous fish (405,410). Perhaps opsonization and perhaps the induction of inflammatory responses were the primordial functions of the lectin/complement pathways.

Homologies

C3, C4, C5, and α macroglobulin (α2m) are homologous proteins. The protease inhibitor α2m in invertebrate and vertebrate seems to be the oldest (419,420). α2m, C3, and C4 have internal thioester sites, whereas C5 does not. The first divergence probably occurred between α2m and C3, with C5 and C4 diverging later (421). Consistent with Ohno's vertebrate polyploidization scheme is the fact that C3, C4, and C5 genes are located on three of the four previously described paralogous clusters in mammals (333,378) (Fig. 15). Such a scenario is consistent with a lack of the true classical and lytic pathways in phyla older than cartilaginous fish. α2m is found in an immune gene complex called the NK complex in mice (422); there seems, however, to be no paralogous relationship between the MHC and NK complex.

The divergence of Bf/C2 from a common ancestor within the *bona fide* MHC is more recent, perhaps after the emergence of teleost fish but before the appearance of amphibians (385). As mentioned, the late appearance of C2 does not necessarily demonstrate that the classical pathway appeared late in vertebrate evolution because Bf can perform double duty in trout (416).

Cells and Organs of the Vertebrate Immune System (Figure 17 on page 640)

Lymphocytes of Agnatha

Because lampreys can reject allografts, they might have T cells, but it is questionable whether the agnathans have a thymus at all. Lymphocyte-like cells in the muscle–velum complex and lymphoid accumulations in the branchial region have sometimes been interpreted as a thymus equivalent, but they resemble more the satellite cells of the skeletal muscle or structures of the pharyngeal epithelium functioning as blood-filtering lymphohematopoietic organs (423). Although morphologically identifiable lymphocytes appear in the blood and the lymphohematopoietic gut and pronephros, lampreys do not possess true lymphoid organs. The spleen is also considered to be absent in hagfish, where the main lymphopoietic organs are the kidneys and the intestine in the lamina propria (424). Blood cells of the hagfish *Eptatretus burgeri* are generated in the hematopoietic nests that develop around intestinal veins established primarily for transport of absorbed nutrients. In ammocoetes (the larval form of lampreys) of *Entosphenus reissneri,* blood cells and small lymphocytes are generated in the typhlosole, closely associated with venous sinusoids developing around the longitudinal mesenteric artery (425). After the disappearance of the typhlosole at metamorphosis, the major lymphohematopoietic organ becomes the fat column (supraneural body), where plasma cells are found (284–286). The liver and the intestinal epithelium of the hagfish also contain infiltrated lymphocytes. Another important site is the gut-associated lymphoid tissue (GALT), with cellular aggregations along the intestinal submucosa and pharynx.

After allografting larval lampreys, heavy infiltration by host leukocytes is visible in the graft's melanophores, adipose layers, and muscles. Melanophores are destroyed within 20 to 60 days (the mean survival time is 36 ± 12 days). From 10 to 60 days after grafting, polymorphonuclear leukocytes (PMNs) and eosinophilic granulocytes predominated, but macrophages were not observed at any stage examined. Plasma cells occurred occasionally at 40 to 60 days, but small lymphocytes were rarely found. Thus, PMNs, but not lymphocytes, seem to be the major effectors in allograft rejection (426). Electron microscopy on the typhlosole of ammocoetes hyperimmunized with SRBCs showed (a) erythroid cells, (b) granulocytes (the predominant cell type) with a lobed nucleus and membrane-bounded granules of various sizes; (c) macrophages possessing primary and secondary lysosomes and long lamellipodia; (d) lymphocytes with a large nucleocytoplasmic ratio with microvilli able to form rosettes; and (e) plasma cells possessing highly extended cisternae of rough endoplasmic reticulum suggestive of an involvment in immune responses (427).

Lymphocytes of Gnathostomata (320,428,429)

Chondrichthyes

Cartilaginous fish are the first in evolution to possess a thymus originating from pharyngeal pouches. (As in mammals, it shows a distinct cortex medulla structure [the reader is referred to a study of 22 species (430)] where lyososomal enzymes, characteristics of stage-specific thymocyte maturation, have been identified, and terminal deoxyribonucleotidyl transferase [TdT] has been detected in thymocytes with cross-reacting antisera [430].) Responsiveness to T-cell mitogens has been demonstrated, but no MLR could be initiated. GALT is also important in elasmobranchs, with the Leydig's organ and the spiral valve being the best examples. The spleen and epigonal organ (associated with the gonads) are lymphopoietic as well as erythropoietic. These organs produce mainly granulocytes, lymphocytes, and plasma cells. Lymphocytes can form nodules in the epigonal organ (431). Macrophage–lymphocyte clusters in the brain of dogfish seem to be established only after specific stimulation that prevents foreign materials from entering the parenchyme (432).

During *S. canicula* development, the liver is the first tissue to contain Ig+ cells at 2 months, followed by the interstitial kidney at 3 months. The thymus, spleen, and Leydig's organ appear at 4 months, and the epigonal and gut-associated lymphomyeloid tissues are the last tissues to differentiate. The hematopoietic/lymphoid nature of the kidney and thymus disappears after hatching, whereas the other lymphomyeloid tissues persist through adult life. At hatching when embryos are exposed to water-borne antigens, the structural development of the lymphomyeloid tissues is well advanced (401).

Teleostei (433,434)

The general organization of lymphoid tissues and organs in teleost fish is not dramatically different from that of chondrichthyes. As in other vertebrates, the teleost thymus gland originates from the pharyngeal pouch and can be uni-, bi-, or trilobate, depending on the species. It is the first organ to become lymphoid, and its structure may differ from species to species. The cortex–medulla architecture is not as precise in some species as in the amphibian, but the duality of the compartment is well visible, at least in the trout (435) and the sea bass (436). The spleen contains the basic elements seen in mammals—blood vessels, red pulp, and white pulp—but the distinction between red and white pulp is less obvious (the white pulp being poorly developed). In the spleen the ellipsoids, which are actually the terminal capillaries, have a thin endothelial layer surrounded by fibrous reticulum and an accumulation of cells, mainly macrophages. Lymphocyte accumulations are often seen in their vicinity, especially during the immune responses. They are thought to be primitive germinal centers that are *sensu stricto* absent in fish. Red pulp is rich in melanomacrophage centers, groups of pigment-containing cells at the bifurcations of larger blood vessels. These seem to play a role in regulating the immune response (437). The other main lymphoid organ is the head kidney.

Lymphocyte heterogeneity (435) resembling that of mammals exists in the trout (438). Thymus cells respond exclusively to T mitogens (ConA), lymphocytes in the kidney respond exclusively to B mitogens (LPS), and spleen cells respond to both. Peripheral blood leukocytes can be activated in MLR in the trout (439), carp (440), and catfish (441). Their T-cell functions seem to be highly temperature sensitive (442). In sea bass, functional T cells monitored with mAbs appear among thymocytes 30 days after hatching. Similar cells appear on day 45 in the gut mucosa, spleen, and kidneys. B cells are detected by day 80 (443). Thymectomy of young mouth breeders (*Tilapia*) impairs allograft and antibody response (444). During an immune response, plaque-forming cells can be detected in the thymus (445) similar to studies in mammals after an intrathymic injection (446). Antibody-forming cells can be found in the spleen or head kidney of many species (445,447). Only T cells (surface Ig) were able to respond in MLR, whereas the T cells, B cells, and macrophages could stimulate (442,448), which suggests that they all express the equivalent of MHC class II molecules. In addition, some mAbs (449) react with a distinct mucosal T-cell population and could identify the homolog of the γδ T cells frequent in various mammalian epithelia. Low temperatures inhibit MLR by affecting T cells. For antibody production *in vitro* to a thymus-dependent hapten-carrier immunogen, macrophages, T cells, and B cells are necessary, whereas for a thymus-independent antigen, only macrophages and B cells are required. These experiments provide the strongest evidence for T cells, B cells, and accessory cells in this class of vertebrate (302,450,451). Antigen processing

and presentation has been demonstrated for B-lymphocytes and monocytes in the catfish (452,453).

Nonspecific cytotoxic cells (NCCs) in teleost fish are analogous to human NK cells (454–457). They lyse spontaneously a variety of transformed human cell lines. Monoclonal antibodies inhibit their lytic activity of the fish NK-like cells. The NK cell molecule is dimeric but distinct from antigen receptors on T cells. Thus, this molecule appears to be a candidate NK-cell antigen receptor (458). Cytotoxic cells isolated from the head kidney and peripheral blood of the channel catfish appear to represent distinct subpopulations of effector cells. One lyses xenogeneic NK-cell targets, whereas the other preferentially lyses allogeneic cells. A third class of cytotoxic effectors responsible for killing virus-infected allogeneic and autologous cells also has been identified (459).

Amphibia (460,461)

Anurans

The first organ to become lymphopoietic, the thymus develops from the dorsal epithelium of the visceral pouches (the number of the pouches involved varies with species). It is colonized from days 6 to 7 onward by precursors coming from the lateral plate and ventral mesoderm through the head mesenchyme. These precursors proliferate *in situ* as the epithelium begins expressing MHC class II molecules but not the classical MHC class I molecules. By day 8 the cortex–medulla architecture begins to resemble that of other vertebrates (460). Amphibians possess a spleen with red and white pulp (463), GALT, and many nodules (but no lymph nodes), with lymphopoietic activity in the kidney, liver, mesentery, and gills. The general morphology of lymphoid organs varies greatly according to species and changes with the season (464,465). In *Xenopus* species the splenic white pulp is delineated by a boundary layer, and the central arteriole of the white pulp follicle terminates in the red pulp perifollicular area, which is a thymus-dependent zone. The spleen lacks true germinal centers. In *Bufo calamita*, colloidal carbon particles injected via the lymph sac are trapped by free macrophages in the red pulp, which then move through the marginal zone to the white pulp. Giant, ramified, nonphagocytic cells that appear in both white and red pulp have been proposed as putative dendritic cells (466). *Xenopus* bone marrow that appeared not to be a major lymphoid organ from histologic observation (467) turned out to have RAG activity (129). It will be necessary to evaluate whether the complete series of events leading to lymphocyte production takes place in the bone marrow or only rearrangements in preB- and preT-lymphocytes.

Thymectomy (reviewed in 460) decreases or abolishes allograft rejection capacity, MLR and PHA responsiveness, IgY antibody synthesis, and all antibody responses to classic thymus-dependent antigens. MLR reactivity matures before the ability to mount IgY responses in primary responses (468). Thymectomy at 7 days of age delays allograft rejection and abrogates IgY responses, whereas later in life it abrogates only the antibody response (460). Thymectomy performed later greatly affects the pool of peripheral T cells (469), as monitored with various mAbs against XTLA.1 (470), CD5 (471), and CD8 (369). The extrathymic development of T cells seems to be excluded in this species because a proper early thymectomy results in the complete absence of T cells. However cells with some T cell markers can be detected in those animals, and it would be interesting to see whether they might correspond to NK T cells (462).

In *Xenopus* species, thymocytes help and induce the graft-versus-host (GVH) reaction only poorly, whereas splenic T cells are good helpers and strong GVH inducers. The thymus contains some IgM-producing B cells and memory cells ready to switch to IgY synthesis. *In vitro* response is downregulated by thymus cells (472,473). Nitrosomethylurea (NMU) eliminates T cells and thereby abrogates alloreactivity. However, rejection of xenografts is not abolished, as if it were controlled by a thymus-independent mechanism (474). *Xenopus* B cells respond *in vitro* to low doses of B-cell mitogens—not by proliferation, but rather by Ig synthesis. They also respond to phorbol myristate acetate (475). Reports of LPS propagation were attributed to a contaminant in the preparation (476).

In *in vitro* chromium 51 release assays, NK cells were detected in *Xenopus* species (477). Splenocyte effectors from early thymectomized 1-year-old frogs lyse spontaneously allogeneic thymus tumor cell lines that lack MHC antigen expression (319,478). This ability is increased after the injection of the tumor cells, or after treating the splenocytes *in vitro* with mitogens. This suggests lymphokine activation of the killers. Spontaneous killers also have been identified in *Rana* species (479).

Few lineage-restricted surface glycoproteins have been characterized in amphibians. Nevertheless, the following homologs have been identified by mAbs and, in some cases, gene isolation: CD5 (471), CD8 (369), CD45 (480), XTLA.1 (470), and CTX (115).

Urodeles

In urodeles the embryo initially produces five pairs of thymus buds, the first two of which disappear. This results in a three-lobe thymus in *Ambystoma*, but in *Pleurodeles* and *Triturus* it forms one lobe. No cortex or medulla can be distinguished. The general appearance resembles the cortical zone of a mammalian or anuran thymus (481). There are at least three types of stromal epithelial cells. There is no lymphopoietic bone marrow in the axolotl, and hematopoeisis takes place in the spleen and in the peripheral layer of the liver (482). The spleen is not clearly divided into white and red pulp.

Lymphocytes of *Ambystoma* proliferate *in vitro* with diverse mitogenic agents. In larval or adult axolotls, a population of B cells is specifically stimulated by LPS, a B-cell mitogen in mammals (483). In the presence of LPS, axolotl B-cells can synthesize and secrete both isotypes of IgM and IgY. T-cell responses to mitogens or allogeneic determinants are allegedly poor, but adult (older than 10 months) splenocytes and thymocytes respond well to PHA when the medium is supplemented with 0.25% bovine serum albumin, instead of 1% fetal bovine serum (484). The activated cells are T-lymphocytes, as shown by depletion experiments *in vitro* with mAbs, and *in vivo* with thymectomy. Some specific markers have been detected on axolotl T cells (485,486). Axolotl lymphocytes, like mammalian lymphocytes, proliferate *in vitro* when stimulated by staphylococcal enterotoxins A and B (SEA and SEB superantigens) (483). In apodans and urodeles the spleen resembles that of fish and shows distinct white and red pulp.

Reptilia

In all reptile studies, thymic cortex and medulla are clearly separated. The spleen has well-defined white and red pulp regions, but T- and B-cell zones have not been delineated with precision, unlike in *Xenopus* species. In *Chrysemys scripta*, the parenchyma of the spleen shows a definite demarcation into a red and white pulp. The white pulp is composed of two lymphoid compartments: lymphoid tissue surrounds both central arterioles and thick layers of reticular tissue called ellipsoids. Even after paratyphoid vaccine injection, germinal centers are not found in the spleen. The red pulp of the spleen is composed of a system of venous sinuses and cords (487). In *Python reticulatus* dendritic cells involved in immune complex trapping have been identified and could be the precursors of mammalian follicular dendritic cells (488). GALT develops later than the spleen during development and appears to be a secondary lymphoid organ; it does not seem to contain the equivalent of the bursa of Fabricius (428). There have been several reports of lymph node–like structures, especially in snakes (*Elaphe*) and lizards (*Gehyra*) (489).

Reptiles, the evolutionary precursors of both birds and mammals, are a pivotal group, but unfortunately the functional heterogeneity of reptile lymphocytes is poorly documented. There seems to be T- and B-lymphocyte heterogeneity because an antithymocyte antiserum altered some T cell–dependent functions in the viviparous lizard *Chalcides ocellatus*. Embryonic thymocytes responded in two-way MLR at all stages (490), but their response to ConA first detected at stages 36 to 37 (490) increases gradually during successive stages and then declines at birth. In the alligator (*Alligator mississippiensis*), after glass-wool filtration, nonadherent peripheral blood lymphocytes responded to PHA and not to LPS, whereas adherent cells could be stimulated by LPS, results analogous to those obtained in mammals. In reptiles, cell populations undergo huge seasonal variations (429,491).

Aves (492,493)

The thymus, which develops in chickens from the third and fourth pharyngeal pouches, consists of two sets of seven lobes. Cortex and medulla are obvious. The organ becomes lymphoid around day 11 of incubation.

The spleen architecture is less differentiated than in mammals. It has no lymphopoietic role during embryogenesis. It contains germinal centers (so far not reported in more primitive species) and T-dependent areas near the periarteriolar lymphatic sheath. B cells are concentrated in the follicles with germinal centers and in the periellipsoid lymphocyte sheaths that surround capillaries. Plasma cells are located in the red pulp. $\gamma\delta$ TCR$^+$ T-lymphocytes are chiefly concentrated in the sinusoid, whereas $\alpha\beta^+$ lymphocytes fill the periarteriolar lymphocyte sheaths. IgM$^+$ B cells can be detected in the spleen from day 12 of incubation. During ontogeny the number of B cells increases rapidly after hatching (494). Lymph nodes seem to be present in water and shore birds but are lacking in the chicken.

The bursa of Fabricius is in birds a special organ for the production of B-lymphocytes. It is a temporary lymphoid organ that arises at day 5 of development and involutes 4 weeks later (see B-cell differentiation). Rabbit appendix has been proposed as a candidate bursa equivalent in mammals (495).

The T-B heterogeneity is obviously well defined in birds. Indeed, the "B" in B-cell stands for Bursa. The effects of thymectomy—T- and B-cell collaboration and generation of MHC-restricted helper and killer cells—are very similar to those of other warm-blooded vertebrates, such as mammals.

Differentiation of Lymphocytes

Lymphocytes are the specialized effector cells of the immune system. Many molecules and mechanisms are expressed only in this category of cells (e.g., RAG, TdT). To understand the evolution of the immune system, we must not only understand the origin of the receptor molecules and their pathways of gene interaction, but also their restriction of expression to certain cell lineages during evolution. Lymphoid cells originate from embryonic ventro- and dorsolateral mesoderm, and lineages are specified by stepwise activation of various transcription factors. The mechanism that controls early lineage determination from hematopoietic stem cell to lymphocyte involves master regulatory factors. In addition, highly lymphocyte-specific genes are activated in B- and T-lymphocytes, e.g., RAG-1, RAG-2 recombinatory enzymes, and TdT. Later in B cells, the expression of Ig requires control of transcription and involves enhancers. During the response, another B-lymphocyte enzymatic mechanism, the switch recombinase complex, enables H chain class switch.

Master Regulatory Factors

A candidate for the master factor is Ikaros, which contributes to lineage restriction in mammals. This gene is conserved in mammals, birds, amphibians, and teleosts (496,497). In mammals, alternate splicing of Ikaros generates six isoforms, the expression of which is conserved in birds and mammals. In the trout, another isoform was isolated. In all species studied to date except for polyploid *Xenopus* species there seem to be only one Ikaros locus (497).

Other transcription factors such as T-cell factor 1 and GATA 3 (T-lymphocyte specific) are well conserved among warm-blooded vertebrates and amphibians (498).

The nude gene *whn* is required in mice for the keratinization of the hair shaft and the differentiation of the epithelial thymus. *whn* homologs exist in humans, bony and cartilaginous fish, cyclostomes, and the cephalochordate *Amphioxus*. All share at least 80% amino acid identity in the DNA-binding domain. Given the absence of thymus in cephalochordates and agnathans, it is likely that changes in the control region of the gene were at the origin of their new functions in gnathostomes (499).

RAG

In mammals, RAG-1 and RAG-2 are two closely linked genes that are essential for V(D)J rearrangement in B and T cells. Because rearrangement was obvious from the most primitive chondrichthyes to mammals, it was no surprise that RAG-1 and RAG-2 homologs have been identified in all these classes of vertebrates (125,126,128,129,500).

No RAG homologs have been isolated from Agnathans, consistent with the absence of antibody and TCR. The teleost RAG-1 gene, unlike the mammalian one, contains a 666-bp intron in the trout and two in the zebrafish (126,500,501). Otherwise, the RAG-1 entire sequence is at least 78% identical to RAG-1 in other species and 89% from positions 417 to 1042. The RAG-2 gene is 75% identical to the RAG-2 gene of other species. Like in mammals, the RAG-2 gene is close to RAG-1 and in reverse orientation. The untranslated region between the two genes increases in size from teleost to mammals. Both RAG-1 and RAG-2 are expressed exclusively in lymphocytes from 10 days postfertilization in the trout and from day 4 in zebrafish.

In *Xenopus* species, the two genes are also in opposite transcriptional orientation, separated by 6 kb. *Xenopus* RAG-1 is 71% similar to that of warm-blooded vertebrates and 88% between positions 392 and 1012. RAG-1 and RAG-2 expression was detected in the thymus, liver, spleen, and even at a lower level in the kidneys. In adults, thymus and bone marrow are the principal sites of expression (129). This suggests that rearrangement proceeds throughout life.

TdT

Terminal deoxyribonucleotidyl transferase is a polymerase that adds nontemplated nucleotides to the 3′ ends of DNA strands during the rearrangement process, which results in the so-called N diversity between the V-D and D-J junctions of Ig and TCR genes.

N diversity has been detected in all species that rearrange, and TdT from various species of vertebrates from teleosts to amphibians and birds shows good structural conservation (126,500,502,503). It is highly expressed in the thymus and kidneys of the trout as soon as 20 days after fertilization. Together with RAG-1 TdT expression, it helps define the trout primary lymphoid tissues (127). Anti-TdT antibodies also scored positive cells in elasmobranch thymus (430).

Trout and *Xenopus* TdT amino acid sequences share over 50% identity with human, mouse, and bovine sequences. *Xenopus* TdT mRNA was found in the thymus but not in the spleen, kidney, intestines, or liver. During ontogeny, TdT appears in significant amounts in the thymus of tadpoles at metamorphic climax. The emergence of TdT only late in development correlates with the paucity of N-region addition in larval Ig H-chain sequences. In the chicken, TdT RNA is only expressed in the thymus, and not in the bone marrow or in the bursa of Fabricius before or after hatching. TdT is therefore most likely involved in N-region addition in chicken T-cell receptor genes, but not in Ig genes (503).

Enhancers

In contrast to mammals, no enhancer was observed in the major intron of the H-chain catfish locus. An activity was identified in the 3′ region of the μ gene that included the TM2 exon. B-lineage specific, the catfish enhancer is not localized in a small core region, but contains multiple, dispersed elements rich in octamer and μ E5-related motifs (504). Five variants of the consensus octamer (ATGCAAAT) are functional. Species differences in the strengths of the variant octamer motifs were evident, and in catfish B cells ATGTAAAT [also found ahead of many *Xenopus* V$_{H}$ genes (220)] is more active than the consensus octamer. Thus, the relative functional contributions of IgH enhancer motifs have changed significantly during vertebrate evolution (505). However the regulatory elements of the Ig locus from mouse induce a tissue-specific expression in transgenic trouts (506).

In summary, the organization of the lymphoid tissues is perhaps the only element of the immune system that shows a complexification that can be superimposed on the vertebrate phylogenetic tree. The absence of thymus and spleen is correlated to the absence of a rearranging receptor family in Cyclostomes. When the bone marrow is present, it is not necessarily a major lymphopoietic organ. Cellular organization in the spleen varies among vertebrates. For instance, germinal centers with follicular dendritic cells are not visible in poikilothermic vertebrates. In their absence, only the conserved structure surrounding the central arterioles ensures a very low flow rate, permitting some selection. NK cells, identified in most classes of vertebrates (457), do not need the activity of RAG-1 and RAG-2 (507). They do not kill cells expressing MHC molecules because of the action of the MHC recognition via specific inhibitory receptors (508).

Cytokines

Many cytokines and their receptors, like most molecules of the immune system, tend to evolve rapidly. It has not been a simple task to isolate their genes and proteins (509). Cytokine activities can be detected in supernatants of stimulated T cells, macrophages, and fibroblasts. Several cytokines, including interferons (IFNs), interleukins (IL-1, IL-2), and transforming growth factor (TGF)-β, have been identified in birds, amphibians, and fish. Although cytokines with vertebrate counterparts are likely to be present in invertebrates, no gene has been cloned that leaves a large gap in our knowledge of cytokine evolution.

Interleukin-1

IL-1 is normally assayed in supernatants from LPS-stimulated phagocytes by determining whether thymocytes are stimulated to proliferate when one adds suboptimal concentrations of T-cell mitogens. Coelomic fluid or freeze-thawed extracts of coelomocytes from an echinoderm (starfish) contain a 30-kDa IL-1–like protein that costimulated mammalian thymocyte and fibroblast proliferation (510). In addition, an mAb specific for human IL-1R bound in flow cytometry to starfish axial organ cells and may recognize an IL-1R homolog. IL-1–like activities also have been detected in tunicates (511), mussels (512), and snails (513). The ease by which these activities have been identified is consistent with the many functions of IL-1 in vertebrates, as well as its conservation (514). However, we should reserve judgment before concluding that *bona fide* IL-1 is responsible for the seemingly homologous functions in invertebrates.

In teleost fish, IL-1–like factors from supernatants of LPS-treated fish monocytes, or even mammalian IL-1 in supernatants from macrophage cell lines, can substitute for accessory cells in T-cell proliferation assays. Two forms of the IL-1–like protein are present in catfish supernatants: a 70-kDa polymer that also may be associated with other proteins stimulates catfish but not mouse cells, and the 15-kDa monomer shows the opposite activity (515). IL-1b has been cloned from rainbow trout (516). Identity with the mammalian IL-1b gene ranges from 47% to 57% (identity between mammalian IL-1a and IL-1b is about 25%) and expression is upregulated after LPS simulation of trout leukocytes.

Amphibian and avian LPS-stimulated leukocyte supernatants contain IL-1–like activity (517,518). Cloned chicken IL-1R has 61% identity to the mouse homolog but is most similar (76%) in the cytoplasmic domains (519). In addition, there are four blocks of high similarity to the cytoplasmic tail of the *Drosophila* Toll protein, further cementing a homologous relationship of the IL-1R and Toll (Fig. 2) (79,520).

In summary, it seems as if IL-1 and its receptor are phylogenetically conserved: (a) the molecules readily stimulate cells across species barriers; (b) cross-reactions of antisera to mammalian IL-1 on proteins of other species occurs often; and (c) there is a relative high similarity of IL-1 and IL-1R genes between divergent species. Thus, IL-1 and IL-1–like proteins might bridge immune responses of vertebrates and invertebrates.

Interleukin-2

Costimulation assays of thymocytes, as described for IL-1, and perpetuation of T cell lines with stimulated T-cell supernatants are performed to detect IL-2 or T-cell growth factor activities. Unlike IL-1, IL-2–like factors generally stimulate cells only from the same species. The report that mAb specific for human IL-2 and IL-2R bind to starfish axial organ cells (521) therefore must be considered with caution. Biochemical analyses of the starfish molecules recognized by these mAbs are obviously required.

From fish to birds, stimulated T-cell supernatants costimulate thymocyte proliferation or can maintain the growth of T-cell blasts (522–524). A candidate IL-2R in chicken was identified by an mAb recognizing a 50-kDa molecule only on stimulated T-cells (525). This mAb blocks costimulation by IL2-like molecules in chicken T-cell supernatants and also reduces the capacity of T-cell blasts to absorb IL-2–like activity from supernatants.

In summary, similar phenomena described in mammals for IL-2 and IL-2R seem to exist in all jawed vertebrates. Future studies will lead not only to an understanding of IL-2 evolution at the structural level, but also an understanding of seasonal changes in T-cell stimulation in reptiles (526), differential capacity of larval and adult amphibian T cells to produce or respond to T-cell growth factors (527), and hyperstimulation of T cells in the mutant obese chicken strain (528).

Interferons

Type I IFN is expressed in leukocytes (IFN-α) and virus-infected fibroblasts (IFN-β) and induces inhibition of viral replication in neighboring cells. In contrast, type II (formerly IFN-γ or immune IFN) is synthesized by activated T cells, activates macrophages, and upregulates class I, class II, lmp, and TAP (529).

IFN has not been detected in invertebrates, but an IFN consensus response element (GAAANN) is found in the promoter of the antibacterial diptericin gene in *Drosophila* (530). This sequence binds to a 45-kDa protein cross-reacting with an antiserum specific for mouse IFN regulatory factor I that seems to be specifically expressed in immune tissues such as fat bodies and leukocytes.

Antiviral activity is detected in supernatants from virally infected fish fibroblasts, epithelial cell lines, and leukocytes (509,531). All of the biochemical properties of mammalian type I IFN (e.g., acid-stable, temperature-resistant) are present in these fish supernatants, and the putative IFN reduces viral cytopathic effects in homologous cell lines infected with virus. *In vivo*, passive transfer of serum from virally infected fish protects naive fish from acute viral pathogenesis (532). Similar activities have been detected in tortoises (533). In chickens there are up to 10 type I IFN genes (534). Sequence identity to human type I IFN ranges from 25% to 80% with the apparent functional gene having highest similarity.

Type II or immune IFN has been more difficult to detect in lower vertebrates. In trout, a macrophage activating factor (MAF) has been isolated from ConA-stimulated purified T cells (535). It induces macrophage phagocytosis, spreading, respiratory burst, and nitric oxide production. Whether MAF is identical to type II

IFN is unclear. Chicken type II IFN, as a T-cell product with potent macrophage activation properties (536), has been cloned. The gene is 35% identical to human type II IFN and only 15% identical to chicken type I IFN (537). Recombinant chicken IFN stimulates nitric oxide production and class II expression by macrophages.

Transforming Growth Factor Beta

TGF-β forms a large family best known for its capacity to suppress adaptive immune responses across species (538). TGF-β, like IL-1, inhibits macrophage activation in trout (539) and growth of T-cell lines in *Xenopus* species (540). Trout TGF-β, most similar to mammalian TGF-β1 and -β5 (62% to 66% identity), is expressed in lymphoid tissues and brain, but not in the liver (509). Two forms of TGF-β have been isolated in *Xenopus* species, both of which act on embryonic ectoderm to induce mesoderm. Recombinant *Xenopus* TGF-β, like the mammalian form, also can inhibit IL-2–like dependent growth of splenic blasts (540).

The isolation of nonmammalian cytokines and cytokine receptor genes has lagged behind molecular characterization of antigen receptors and MHC (509). Nevertheless, cytokine assay systems in many species and certain disease states in fish, amphibians, and birds suggest that the majority of vital mammalian cytokines will be found in other vertebrates. One major question is, which cytokines are specific for the adaptive immune system and which will be involved in defense in all living things? For example, if type II IFN and IL2 can be found only in animals with a definitive T-cell arm of the immune system, we would expect other cytokines central to the adaptive system, such as IL-4 and IL-12, to be limited to the vertebrates (541). Is the relative conservation of cytokine sequences negatively correlated with their presence in phylogeny? This seems to be the case for type I IFN and IL-1 on the one hand and type II IFN and IL-2 on the other.

GENERAL CONCLUSIONS

Recent advances in comparative immunology have made obvious some bridges between vertebrates and the other phyla, and perhaps even with plants. Families of receptors and soluble effector molecules and control of gene expression pathways can be shared to some extent among diverse phyla. With the presence in invertebrates of Igsf members, recognition of foreignness could be achieved in some protostomes via interactions close to those of modern vertebrates Ig or TCR, i.e., via recognition of nonself and not by homophilic interaction or by recognition of self.

Several scenarios could account for the genesis of the vertebrate immune systems all centered around the introduction of the somatic rearrangement machinery. If one accepts that variation precedes selection, one could envision that somatic variability of the receptor was introduced in a TCR ancestor when the MHC backbone did not yet contain class I and II. They were recruited there for an obvious selection purpose. Why in this region rather than anywhere else in the genome? Perhaps because the receptor ancestor that received the possibility to rearrange somatically was in the primordial MHC region. The presence of similar Igsf members in MHC is consistent with that view (Fig. 13).

Alternatively, class I and II, like peptide–receptor interactions, were already encoded there, and the system tolerated the introduction of somatic rearrangement into a precursor receptor. However,

some structural aspects let us think that the first hypothesis is correct. MHC and somatically rearranging receptors share the usage of C1 Ig domains, and those are present only in species that rearrange somatically. If the MHC was truly ancient, it should use the more primitive C2 type of Ig domain encountered in all primitive IgsF members. It is conceivable that a signaling molecule associated with an antigen receptor did come first, and the C1 exon was transferred to pre-MHC.

The discovery of C′ in Echinoderm leaves open the possibility that a B-cell type of immunity developed first.

In vertebrates, with the introduction of somatic rearrangement and the exploitation of somatic mutations, nature seems to have favored to waste cells inside the individual rather than to waste the individual. This attitude is probably modulated as a function of the value of each individual within a species. Indeed, the utmost refinement in exploiting somatic hypermutation is seen in warm-blooded vertebrates (small progenies, individual value high) and not in amphibians or fish (large progenies, individual value low). Indeed the main adaptive value of the immune system of gnathostomes is to confer to each individual not a finished system but a potential capable of generating somatically a repertoire of receptors. This potential exceeds by far the expression capacity of the organism even in species that do not use combinatorial joining. Therefore, a fraction of the immune system may not be under selection at the level of the gene product. This does not mean that this portion of the genome does not evolve due to the intrinsic properties of DNA (transpositions, translocations, unequal crossing over, gene conversion).

With the progress of gene mapping and the actualization of Ohno's conceptions of the evolution by gene duplication, many new insights have been gained regarding the evolution of linkage groups, the most prominent of which is the MHC. The discovery of MHC paralogous regions, with or without class I and class II genes, has led to new stimulating models on the evolution of this region. Paralogies are also visible for Ig and TCR genes (542). During gnathostome evolution, all of the elements (RAG Ig TCR MHC) of the mammalian immune system were present from its inception. The number and the organization of genes may have varied, but not their principle of utilization. One element has varied more than others: the lymphoid tissue itself. Its architecture evolution parallels that of vertebrates and may have played a pivotal role in the exploitation of the molecular machinery.

Surprises may come when one finally learns more about agnathans. For the time being, only the alternate pathway of complement and lymphocytes have been identified there. An efficient mechanism of defense, the complement is used and even duplicated in some vertebrate species, which increases the diversity of its recognition capacities.

Until now we considered mainly the mechanisms creating repertoire diversity, but there is also a strong pressure to limit it: that to avoid autoimmunity. It is not surprising that mechanisms of negative selection have been conserved, ensuring self tolerance. The importance of tolerance is so great that it is likely that several mechanisms contribute to it. Moreover, at the peripheral level, from fish to mammals, there are ways of ignoring autoimmunity in its final phase, stopping the genesis of cytotoxic T-lymphocytes or ignoring autoantibodies (543).

The adaptive immune system clearly entertains relationships with the innate immune system. The study of these relationships through evolution could be the subject of another chapter (see section on insect immunity) (544–546).

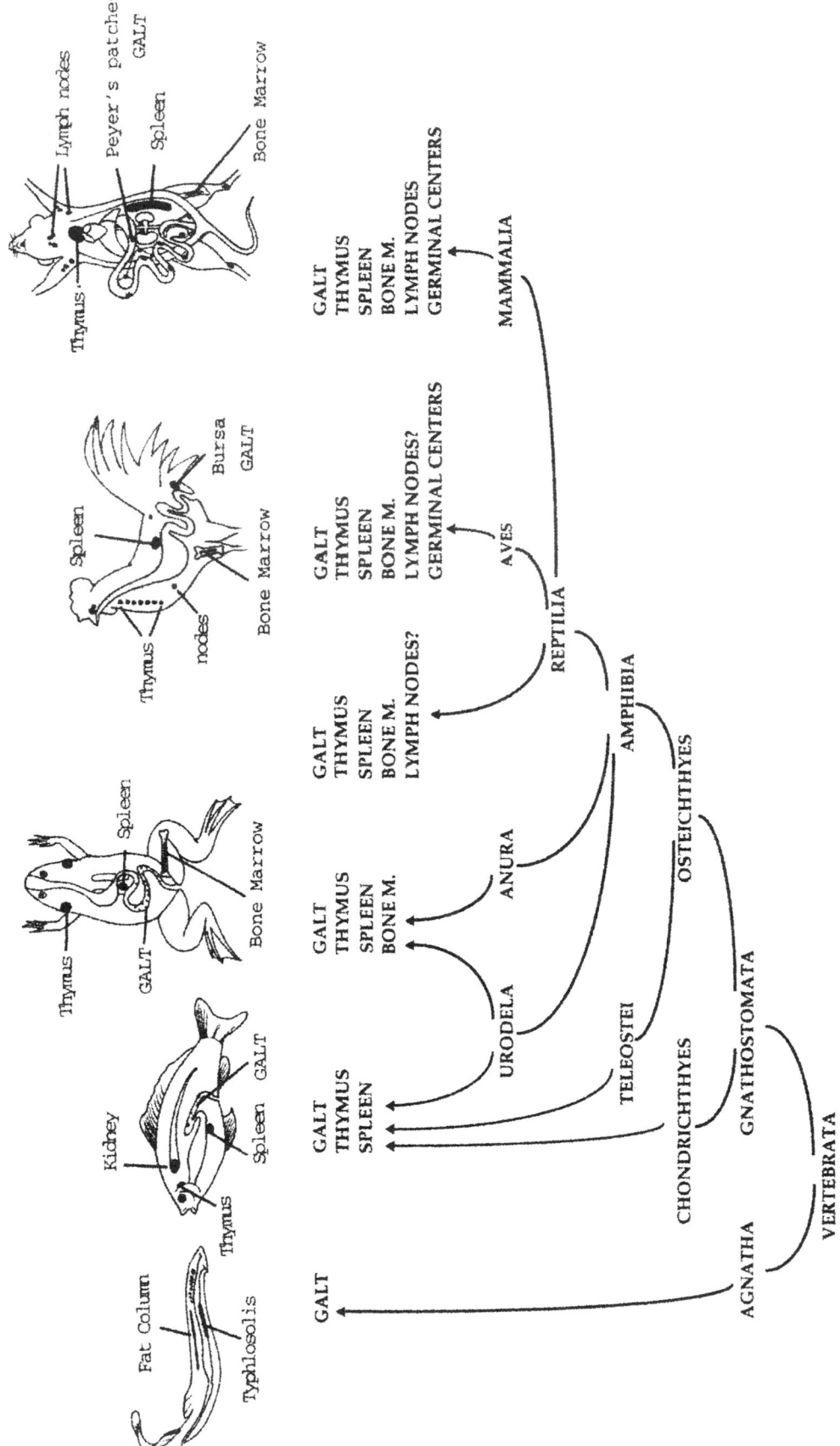

FIG. 17. Evolution of the lymphoid systems. BM, bone marrow; L. node, lymph node.

These considerations should not mask the interest of analyzing the DNA and amino acid sequence of each element. This will continue to help characterize the essential parts of the molecules and their evolution. If it is relatively easy to understand the meaning of sequence conservation and variations, it is more difficult to grasp that of qualitative variations in organization or principle of function. Perhaps one should consider these variations with some detachment, remembering that comparative studies give us only a snapshot in evolutionary history and that many of them are probably transitory, due to expansions and contractions of the genome, submitted for their maintenance or their elimination as well to the laws of selection as to those of chance.

ACKNOWLEDGMENTS

We thank Jim Kaufman and Jan Klein for allowing us to use unpublished material, as well as John Lambris and Chris Secombes for discussions on the phylogeny of complement and cytokines. We thank Charley Steinberg for computer programs, discussions, and help in the preparation of the manuscript. We thank Erika Meier and John Hansen for critically reading the manuscript. We thank Cynthia Geiger and Allan Brouwer for expert editorial assistance. The Basel Institute for Immunology was founded and is supported by F. Hoffmann-La Roche Ltd., Basel, Switzerland.

REFERENCES

1. Sepkoski Jr JJ, Bambach RJ, Raup DM, Valentine JW. Phanerozoic marine diversity and the fossil record. *Nature* 1981;293:435–437.
2. Gould SJ. *The Flamingo Smile*. London: Penguin, 1985.
3. Brusca RC, Brusca GJ. *Invertebrates*. Sunderland, Massachusettts: Sinauer Associates, 1990.
4. Rehorn KP, Thelen H, Michelson A, Reuter R. A molecular aspect of hematopoiesis and endoderm development common to vertebrates and *Drosophila. Dev Suppl* 1996;122.4023–4031.
5. Rittig MG, Kuhn KH, Dechant CA, et al. Phagocytes from both vertebrate and invertebrate species use 'coiling' phagocytosis. *Dev Comp Immunol* 1996;20: 393–406.
6. Pearson AM. Scavenger receptors in innate immunity. *Curr Opin Immunol* 1996; 8:20–28.
7. Ottaviani E, Franceschi C. The invertebrate phagocytic immunocyte: clues to a common evolution of immune and neuroendocrine systems. *Immunol Today* 1997;18.169–174.
8. Franc NC, Dimarcq JL, Lagueux M, Hoffmann J, Ezekowitz RA. Croquemort, a novel *Drosophila* hemocyte/macrophage receptor that recognizes apoptotic Cells. *Immunity* 1996;4:431–443.
9. Valembois P, Roch P. Identification par autoradiographie des leucocytes stimulés à la suite de plaies ou de greffes chez un ver de terre. *Biol Cell* 1977;28:81–82.
10. Cooper EL. Earthworm coelomocytes: Role in understanding the evolution of Cellular immunity. I. Formation of monolayers and cytotoxicity. In: Reh˘ AOcek D, Blaskovic D, Hink WF, eds. *Proceedings of the III International Colloquium on Invertebrate Tissue Culture*, Bratislavia: Publishing House of the Slovak Academy of Sciences, 1973;381–404.
11. Boieldieu D, Valembois P. Natural cytotoxicity of sipunculid leukocytes on allogeneic and xenogeneic erythrocytes. *Dev Comp Immunol* 1977;1:207–216.
12. Roch P, Valembois P, Du Pasquier L. Response of earthworm leukocytes to concanavalin A and transplantation antigens. *Adv Exp Med Biol* 1975;64:45–54.
13. Karp RD, Coffaro KA. Cellular defense systems of the Echinodermata. In: Cohen N, Sigel MM, eds. *The Reticuloendothelial System Vol. 3, Phylogeny and Ontogeny*, New York: Plenum, 1982, 257 282.
14. Raftos DA, Tait NN, Briscoe DA. Allograft rejection and alloimmune memory in the solitary urochordate, *Styela plicata*. *Dev Comp Immunol* 1987;11:343–351.
15. Seeger MA, Haffley L, Kaufman TC. Characterization of amalgam: a member of the immunoglobulin superfamily from *Drosophila*. *Cell* 1988;55:589–600.
16. Karlstrom RO, Wilder LP, Bastiani MJ. Lachesin: an immunoglobulin superfamily protein whose expression correlates with neurogenesis in grasshopper embryos. *Development* 1993;118:509–522.
17. Smith LC, Hildemann WH. Allograft rejection, autograft fusion and inflammatory responses to injury in *Callyspongia diffusa* (Porifera; Demospongia). *Proc R Soc Lond B Biol Sci* 1986;226.445–464.
18. Humphreys T, Reinherz EL. Invertebrate immune recognition, natural immunity and the evolution of positive selection. *Immunol Today* 1994;15:316–320.
19. van de Vyver G. Second set allograft rejection in two sponge species and the problem of an alloimmune memory. In: Manning MJ, ed. Phylogeny of immunological memory, Amsterdam: Elsevier North-Holland Biomedical Press, 1980, 15–21.
20. Smith LC, Hildemann WH. Alloimmune memory is absent in Hymeniacidon sinapium, a marine sponge. *J Immunol* 1984;133:2351–2355.
21. Smith LC, Hildemann WH. Allogeneic Cell interactions during graft rejection in Callyspongia diffusa (Porifera, Demospongia); a study with monoclonal antibodies. *Proc Soc Lond B Biol Sci* 1986;226:465–477.
22. Fernandez-Busquets X, Kammerer RA, Burger MM. A 35-kDa protein is the basic unit of the core from the 2 x 10(4)-kDa aggregation factor responsible for species-specific Cell adhesion in the marine sponge Microciona prolifera. J Biol Chem 1996;271:23558–23565.
23. Yin C, Humphreys T. Acute cytotoxic allogeneic histocompatibility reactions involving gray Cells in the marine sponge, Callyspongia diffusa. *Biol Bull* 1996; 191:159–167.
24. Pancer Z, Gershon H, Rinkevich B. Polymorphism in the immunoglobulin-like domains of the receptor tyrosine kinase from the sponge Geodia cydonium. *Cell Adhes Commun* 1996;4:327–339.
25. Leddy SV, Green DR. Historecognition in the Cnidaria. In: Warr GW, Cohen N, eds. *Phylogenesis of Immune Functions*, CRC Press, 1991, 103–116.
26. Neigel JE, Avise JC. Clonal diversity and population structure in a reef-building coral, Acropora cervicornis: self-recognition analysis and demographic interpretation. *Evolution* 1983;37:437–453.
27. Hildemann WH, Raison RL, Cheung G, Hull CJ, Akaka L, Okamoto J. Immunological specificity and memory in a scleractinian coral. *Nature* 1977;270: 219–223.
28. Lubbock R. Clone-specific Cellular recognition in a sea anemone. *Proc Natl Acad Sci USA* 1980;77:6667–6669.
29. Bigger CH. Interspecific and intraspecific acrorhagial aggressive behavior among sea anemones; a recognition of self and nonself. *Biol Bull* 1980;159: 117–134.
30. Theodor J. Distinction between "self" and "nonself" in lower vertebrates. *Nature* 1970;227:690–692.
31. Hauenschild C. Genetische und Entwicklungs-physiologische Untersuchungen über Intersexualität und Gewebeverträglichkeits-Eigenschaft bei Hydroidpolypen *Hydractinia echinata Flemm*. (Hydroz. Bourgainvill.). *Roux Arch Entwicklungsmechanik* 1954;147:1–41.
32. Hauenschild C. Über die Vererbung einer Gewebeverträglichkeits-Eigenschaft bei dem Hydroidpolypen *Hydractinia echinata Flemm*. (Hydroz. Bourgainvill.). *Z Naturforsch* 1956;11:132–183.
33. Du Pasquier L. The genetic control of histocompability reactions: phylogenetic aspects *Arch Biol* (Brussels) 1974;85:91–103.
34. Ivker FB. A hierarchy of histo-incompatibility in *Hydractinia echinata, Biol Bull* 1972;143:162–174.
35. Buss LW, Moore JL, Green DR. Autoreactivity and self tolerance in an invertebrate. *Nature* 1985;313:400–402.
36. Langlet C, Bierne J. Immune characteristics of graft rejection in nemerteans of the genus Lineus. *Eur J Immunol* 1982;12:705–708.
37. Langlet C, Bierne J. Immunocompetent Cells are responsible for rejection of incompatible xenogeneic grafts in Lineus (Invertebrata, Nermertea). *Transplantation* 1982;34:8–12.
38. Langlet C, Bierne J. Immunocompetent Cells requisite for graft rejection in Lineus (Invertebrata, Nemertea). *Dev Comp Immunol* 1984;8:547 557.
39. Lackie M. Transplantation, the limits of recognition. In: Gupta AP, ed. *Haemocytic and Humoral Immunity in Arthropods*, London: Wiley, 1986, 191–223.
40. Dularay B, Lackie AM. The effect of biotic and abiotic implants on the recognition of Blatta orientalis cuticular transplants by the cockraoch Periplanata americana. *Dev Comp Immunol* 1987;11:60–77.
41. George JF, Karp RD, Rheins LA. Primary integumentary xenograft reactivity in the american cockroach, *Periplaneta americana*. *Transplantation* 1984;37: 478–484.
42. Hartman RS, Karp RD. Short-term immunologic memory in the allograft response of the American cockroach. *Transplantation* 1989;47:920–.
43. Fletcher TC, Cooper-Willis CA. The Cellular defense systems of the Mollusca. In: Cohen N, Sigel MM, eds. *The Reticuloendothelial System*, Vol. 3, Phylogeny and Ontogeny, New York: Plenum, 1983, 141–166.
44. Sima P, Vetvicka V. Evolution of immune reactions. *Crit Rev Immunol* 1993;13: 83–113.
45. Ottaviani E, Vergine C. Allo-implant in the freshwater snail Planorbarius corneus (Li) (gastropoda, Pulmonata) I. Histological and histochemical study. *Zool Jb Physiol* 1990;94:261–267.
46. Hoek RM, Smit AB, Frings H, Vink JM, de Jong-Brink M, Geraerts WPM. A new Ig-superfamily member, molluscan defence (MDM) from Lymnaca stagnalis, is down-regulated during parasitosis. *Eur J Immunol* 1996;26:939–944.
47. Adema CM, Hertel LA, Miller RD, Loker ES. A family of fibrinogen-related proteins that precipitates parasite-derived molecules is produced by an invertebrate after infection. *Proc Natl Acad Sci USA* 1997;94.8691–8696.
48. Cooper EL. *Comparative Immunology*. Englewood Cliffs, N.J.: Prentice-Hall, 1976.
49. Parry MJ. Survival of body wall autographs, allografts, and Xenografts in the earthworm Eisenia foetida. *J Invert Path* 1978;31:383–388.
50. Dale RP. The basis of graft rejection in the earth worms Lumbricus vervestris and Eisenia foetida. *J Invest Pathol* 1978;32:264–272.

51. Valembois P, Roch P, Boiledieu D. Cellular defence systems of the Platy-helminthes, Nemertea, Sipunculida and Annelida. In: Cohen N, Sigel M, eds. *The Reticuloendothelial System*. Phylogeny and Ontogeny, vol. 3 New York: Plenum, 1982, 89–139.

52. Duprat P. Etude des homogreffes de paroi du corps chez le Lombricien *Eisenia foetida* SAv. Aspects histologiques et immunitaires de la prise de l'acception ou du refus des greffons. Doctoral thesis in Natural Sciences, University of Bordeaux, France.

53. Cooper EL. Specific tissue graft rejection in earthworms. *Science* 1969;166:1414–1415.

54. Karp RD, Hildemann WH. Specific allograft reactivity in the sea star *Dermasterias imbricata*. *Transplantation* 1976;22:44–439.

55. Coffaro KA, Hinegardner RT. Immune response in the sea urchin *Lytechinus pictus*. *Science* 1977;197:1389–1390.

56. Bertheussen K. The cytotoxic reaction in allogeneic mixtures of echinoid phagocytes. *Exp Cell Res* 1979;120:373–381.

57. Oka H, Watanabe H. Colony specificity in compound ascidians as tested by fusion experiments (a preliminary report). *Proc Jpn Acad Sci* 1957;33:657–658.

58. Scofield VL, Schlumberger JM, West LA, Weissman IC. Protochordate allorecognition controlled by a MHC-like gene complex. *Nature* 1982;295:499–500.

59. Tanaka K. Allogeneic distinction in *Botryllus primigenus* and other colonial ascidians. *Adv Exp Biol Med* 1975;64:115–124.

60. Sabbadin A. La basi genetiche della capacita di fusione para colonie *Botryllus scholsseri* (Ascidiacea). *Red Accad Nag Lincei* 1962;32:1031–1038.

61. Sabbadin A, Astovci C. Chimeras and histocompatibility in the colonial ascidian *Botryllus schlosseri*. *Dev Comp Immunol* 1988;12:734–742.

62. Rinkevich B, Weissman IL. Incidents of rejection and indifference in Fu/HC incompatible protochordate colonies. *J Exp Zool* 1992;263:105–111.

63. Weissman IL, Saito Y, Rinkevich B. Allorecognition histocompatibility in a protochordate species: is the relationship to MHC somatic or structural? *Immunol Rev* 1990;113:227–241.

64. Buss LW. Somatic Cell parasitism and the evolution of somatic tissue compatibility. *Proc Natl Acad Sci USA* 1982;79:5337–5340.

65. Stoner DS, Weissman IL. Somatic and germ Cell parasitism in a colonial ascidian: possible role for a highly polymorphic allorecognition system. *Proc Natl Acad Sci USA* 1996;93:15254–15259.

66. Raftos DA, Cooper EL. Proliferation of lymphocyte-like cells from the solitary tunicate, styela clava, in response to allogeneic stimuli. *J Exp Zool* 1991;260:391–400.

67. Rinkevich B, Weissman IL. Failure to find alloimmune memory in the resorption phenomenon of *Botryllus* cytomictical chimera. *Eur J Immunol* 1990;20:1775–1779.

68. Hoffmann JA. Innate immunity of insects. *Curr Opin Immunol* 1995;7:4–10.

69. Gillespie JP, Kanost MR, Trenczek T. Biological mediators of insect immunity. *Biological mediators of insect immunity* 1997;42:611–643.

70. Soderhall K, Cerenius L, Johansson MW. The prophenoloxidase activating system and its role in invertebrate defence. The prophenoloxidase activating system and its role in invertebrate defence 1994;712:155–161.

71. Soderhall K, Thornqvist PO. Crustacean immunity—a short review. *Crustacean immunity—a short review* 1997;90:45–51.

72. Johansson MW, Soderhall K. The prophenoloxidase activating system and associated proteins in invertebrates. *Prog Mol Sub Cell Biol* 1996;15:46–66.

73. Rizki TM, Rizki RM. The cellular defense syatem of *Drosophila melanogaster*. In: King RC, Akai H, eds. *Insect ultrastructure*, vol 2. Plenum, 1984, 579–604.

74. Sun SC, Lindstrom I, Boman HG, Faye I, Schmidt O. Hemolin: an insect-immune protein belonging to the immunoglobulin superfamily. *Science* 1990;250:1729–1732.

75. Lanz-Mendoza H, Bettencourt R, Fabbri M, Faye I. Regulation of the insect immune response: the effect of hemolin on cellular immune mechanisms. *Cell Immunol* 1996;169:47–54.

76. Boman H. Peptide antibiotics and their role in innate immunity. *Annu Rev Immunol* 1995;13:61–92.

77. Hoffmann JA, Janeway CA, Natori S, eds. *Phylogenetic Perspectives in Immunity: The Insect Host Defense*. Austin: R.G Landes Company, 1994.

78. Taniai K, Kadono-Okuda K, Kato Y, et al. Structure of two cecropin B-encoding genes and bacteria-inducible DNA-binding proteins which bind to the 5'-upstream regulatory region in the silkworm, *Bombyx mori*. *Gene* 1995;163:215–219.

79. Lemaitre B, Nicolas E, Michaut L, Reichhart JM, Hoffmann JA. The dorsoventral regulatory gene cassette spätzle/Toll/cactus controls the potent antifungal response in *Drosophila* adults. *Cell* 1996;86:973–983.

80. Medzhitov R, Preston-Hurlburt P, Janeway CAJ. A human homologue of the *Drosophila* Toll protein signals activation of adaptive immunity. *Nature* 1997;388:394–397.

81. Sun SC, Lindstrom I, Lee JY, Faye I. Structure and expression of the attacin genes in *Hyalophora cecropia*. *Eur J Biochem* 1991;196:247–254.

82. Hultmark D, Engstrom A, Andersson K, Steiner H, Bennich H, Boman HG. Insect immunity. Attacins, a family of antibacterial proteins from *Hyalophora cecropia*. *EMBO J* 1983;2:571–576.

83. Kadalayil L, Petersen UM, Engstrom Y. Adjacent GATA and kappa B-like motifs regulate the expression of a *Drosophila* immune gene. *Nucleic Acids Res* 1997;25:1233–1239.

84. Steward R. Dorsal, an embryonic polarity gene in *Drosophila*, is homologous to the vertebrate proto-oncogene, c-rel. *Science* 1987;238:692–694.

85. Baeuerle PA, Henkel T. Function and activation of NF-kappa B in the immune system. *Annu Rev Immunol* 1994;12:141–179.

86. Wilson I, Vogel J, Somerville S. Signalling pathways: a common theme in plants and animals? *Curr Biol* 1997;7:r175–r178.

87. Whitham S, Dinesh-Kumar SP, Choi D, Hehl R, Corr C, Baker B. The product of the tobacco mosaic virus resistance gene N: similarity to toll and the interleukin-1 receptor. *Cell* 1994;78:1101–1115.

88. Tang X, Frederick RD, Zhou J, Halterman DA, Jia Y, Martin GB. Initiation of plant disease resistance by physical Interaction of AvrPto and Pto kinase. *Science* 1996;274:2060–2063.

89. Zhou J, Tang X, Martin GB. The Pto kinase conferring resistance to tomato bacteria speck disease interacts with proteins that bind a cis-element of pathogenesis-related genes. *EMBO J* 1997;16:3207–3218.

90. Cao H, Glazebrook J, Clarke JD, Volko S, Dong X. The Arabidopsis NPR1 gene that controls systemic acquired resistance encodes a novel protein containing ankyrin repeats. *Cell* 1997;88:57–63.

91. Moretta A, Bottino C, Vitale M, Pende D, Biassoni R, Mingari MC, Moretta L. Receptors for HLA class-I molecules in human natural killer Cells. *Annu Rev Immunol* 1996;14:619–648.

92. Lanier L. Natural killer Cells: from no receptors to too many. *Immunity* 1997;6:371–378.

93. Carretero M, Cantoni C, Bellon T, et al. The CD94 and NKG2-A C-type lectins covalently assemble to form a natural killer cell inhibitory receptor for HLA class I molecules. *Eur J Immunol* 1997;27:563–567.

94. Holmgren A, Branden CI. Crystal structure of chaperone protein PapD reveals an immunoglobulin fold. *Nature* 1989;342:248–251.

95. Holmgren A, Kuehn MJ, Branden CI, Hultgren SJ. Conserved immunoglobulin-like features in a family of periplasmic pilus chaperones in bacteria. *EMBO Journal* 1992;11:1617–1622.

96. Bateman A, Eddy SR, Chothia C. Members of the immunoglobulin superfamily in bacteria. *Protein Sci* 1996;5:1939–1941.

97. Muller WE, Muller IM, Gamulin V. On the monophyletic evolution of the metazoa. *Braz J Med Biol Res* 1994;27:2083–2096.

98. Benian GM, Kiff JE, Neckelmann N, Moermann DG, Waterston RH. Sequence of an unusually large protein implicated in regulation of myosin activity in c elegans. *Nature* 1989;342:45–50.

99. Nelson RE, Fessler LI, Takagi Y, et al. Peroxidasin: a novel enzyme-matrix protein of *Drosophila* development. *EMBO J* 1994;13:3438–3447.

100. Williams AF, Barclay AN. The immunoglobulin superfamily domains for Cell-surface recognition. *Ann Rev Immunol* 1988;6:381.

101. Barclay AN, Brown MH, Law SKA, McKnight AJ, Tomlinson MG, van der Merwe PA. *The leucocyte antigen facts book*. London, San Diego: Academic Press, 1997.

102. Bork P, Holm L, Sander C. The immunoglobulin fold. Structural classification, sequence patterns and common core. *J Mol Biol* 1994;242:309–320.

103. Li S, Sjogren HO, Hellman U, Pettersson RF, P. W. Cloning and functional characterization of a subunit of the transporter associated with antigen processing. *Proc Natl Acad Sci USA* 1997;94:8708–8713.

104. Ortmann B, Copeman J, Lehner PJ, et al. A critical role for tapasin in the assembly and function of multimeric MHC class I-TAP complexes. *Science* 1997;277:1306–1309.

105. Harpaz Y, Chothia C. Many of the immunoglobulin superfamily domains in Cell adhesion molecules and surface receptors belong to a new structural set which is close to that containing variable domains. *J Mol Biol* 1994;238:528–539.

106. Pulido D, Campuzano S, Koda T, Modolell J, Barbacid M. Dtrk, a *Drosophila* gene related to the trk family of neurotrophin receptors, encodes a novel class of neural Cell adhesion molecule. *EMBO J* 1992;11:391–404.

107. Du Pasquier L, Chrétien I. CTX, a new lymphocyte receptor in Xenopus and the early evolution of Ig domains. *Res Immunol* 1996;147:218–226.

108. Thompson C. New insights into V(D)J recombination and its role in the evolution of the immune system. *Immunity* 1995;3:531–539.

109. Du Pasquier L, Chrétien I. Why is CTX all the RAGE? *Res Immunol* 1996;147:261–266.

110. Littman DR, Gettner SN. Unusual intron in the immunoglobulin domain of the newly isolated murine CD4 (L3T4) gene. *Nature* 1987;325:453–455.

111. Sers C, Kirsch K, Rothbacher U, Riethmuller G, Johnson JP. Genomic organization of the melanoma-associated glycoprotein MUC18: implications for the evolution of the immunoglobulin domains. *Proc Natl Acad Sci USA* 1993;90:8514–8518.

112. Wang PL, O'Farrell S, Clayberger C, Krensky AM. Identification and molecular cloning of tactile. A novel human T Cell activation antigen that is a member of the Ig gene superfamily. *J Immunol* 1992;148:2600–2608.

113. Miller MM, Goto R, Young S, Chirivella J, Hawke D, Miyada CG. Immunoglobulin variable-region-like domains of diverse sequence within the major histocompatibility complex of the chicken. *Proc Natl Acad Sci USA* 1991;88:4377–4381.

114. Kaufman J, Skjoedt K, Salomonsen J. The B-G multigene family of the chicken major histocompatibility complex. *Crit Rev Immunol* 1991;11:113–143.

115. Chrètien I, Robert J, Marcuz A, Garcia-Sanz JA, Courtet M, Du Pasquier L. CTX, a novel molecule specifically expressed on the surface of cortical thymocytes in Xenopus. *Eur J Immunol* 1996;26:780–791.

116. Katevuo K, Goebel T, Boyd RL, Dunon D, Koskinen R, Imhof B, Vainio O.

Chicken thymocyte antigen, Cht1, is a new member of the igsf and is involved in T Cell differertiation. *Dev Comp Immunol* 1997;21:240.

117. Heath JK, White SJ, Johnstone CN, et al. The human A33 antigen is a transmembrane glycoprotein and a novel member of the immunoglobulin superfamily. *Proc Natl Acad* 1997;94:469–474.

118. Chrètien I, Courtet M, Marcuz A, Katevuo K, Vainio O, Du Pasquier L. The Xenopus CTX thymocyte receptor defines a new family of receptors conserved and duplicated during the evolution of vertebrates. 1998:in preparation.

119. Chothia C, Novotny J, Bruccoleri R, Karplus M. Domain association in immunoglobulin molecules. The packing of variable domains. *J Mol Biol* 1985; 186:651–663.

120. Robert J, Chrètien I, Guiet C, Du Pasquier L. Cross-linking CTX, a novel thymocyte-specific molecule, inhibits the growth of lymphoid tumor Cells in Xenopus. *Mol Immunol* 1997;34:133–143.

121. Neeper M, Schmidt AM, Brett J, et al. Cloning and expression of a Cell surface receptor for advanced glycosylation end products of proteins. *J Biol Chem* 1992; 267.

122. Vlassara H, Valinsky J, Brownlee M, Cerami C, Nishimoto S, Cerami A. Advanced glycosylation endproducts on erythrocyteCellsurface induce receptor-mediated phagocytosis by macrophages. A model for turnover of aging Cells. *J Exp Med* 1987;166:539–549.

123. Imani F, Horii Y, Suthanthiran M, et al. Advanced glycosylation endproduct-specific receptors on human and rat T-lymphocytes mediate synthesis of interferon gamma: role in tissue remodeling. *J Exp Med* 1993;178:2165–2172.

124. Marchalonis JJ, Schluter SF. On the relevance of invertebrate recognition and defence mechanisms to the emergence of the immune response of vertebrates. *Scand J Immunol* 1990;32:13–20.

125. Bernstein RM, Schluter SF, Bernstein H, Marchalonis JJ. Primordial emergence of the recombination activating gene 1 (RAG1): sequence of the complete shark gene indicates homology to microbial integrases. *Proc Natl Acad Sci USA* 1996; 93:9454–9459.

126. Hansen JD, Kaattari SL. The recombination activating gene 2 (RAG2) of the rainbow trout *Oncorhynchus mykiss*. *Immunogenetics* 1996;44:204–211.

127. Hansen JD. Characterization of rainbow trout terminal deoxynucleotidyl transferase structure and expression. TdT and RAG1 co-expression defines the trout primary lymphoid tissues. *Immunogenetics* 1997 in press.

128. Greenhalgh P, Steiner LA. Recombination activating gene 1 (Rag1) in zebrafish and shark. *Immunogenetics* 1995;41:54–55.

129. Greenhalgh P, Olesen CE, Steiner LA. Characterization and expression of recombination activating genes (RAG-1 and RAG-2) in *Xenopus laevis*. *J Immunol* 1993;151:3100–3110.

130. Hughes AL, Yeager M. Molecular evolution of the vertebrate immune system. *BioEssays* 1997;19:777–786.

131. Nonaka M, Namikawa-Yamada C, Sasaki M, Salter-Cid L, Flajnik MF. Evolution of proteasome subunits delta and LMP2: complementary DNA cloning and linkage analysis with MHC in lower vertebrates. *J Immunol* 1997;159: 734–740.

132. Kandil E, Namikawa C, Nonaka M, et al. Isolation of low molecular mass polypeptide complementary DNA clones from primitive vertebrates. Implications for the origin of MHC class I restricted antigen presentation. *J Immunol* 1996;156:4245–4253.

133. Namikawa C, Salter-Cid L, Flajnik MF, Kato Y, Nonaka M, Sasaki M. Isolation of *Xenopus* LMP-7 homologues. Striking allelic diversity and linkage to MHC. *J Immunol* 1995;155:1964–1971.

134. Karre K, Ljunggren HG, Piontek G, Kiessling R. Selective rejection of H-2-deficient lymphoma variants suggests alternative immune defence strategy. *Nature* 1986;319:675–678.

135. Karre K. How to recognize a foreign submarine. *Immunol Rev* 1997;155:5–9.

136. Reyburn H, Mandelboim O, Vales-Gomez M, Sheu EG, Pazmany L, Davis DM, Strominger JL. Human NK. Cells: their ligands, receptors and functions. *Immunol Rev* 1997;155:119–125.

137. Matzinger P, Bevan MJ. Hypothesis: why do so many lymphocytes respond to major histocompatibility antigens? *Cell Immunol* 1977;29:1–5.

138. Kao TH, McCubbin AG. How flowering plants discriminate between self and non-self pollen to prevent inbreeding. *Proc Natl Acad Sci USA* 1996;93: 12059–12065.

139. Medzhitov R, Janeway CA, Jr. On the semantics of immune recognition. *Res Immunol* 1996;147:208–214.

140. Hashimoto K, Nakanishi T, Kurosawa Y. Isolation of carp genes encoding major histocompatibility complex antigens. *Proc Natl Acad Sci USA* 1990;87: 6863–6867.

141. Flajnik MF, Canel C, Kramer J, Kasahara M. Which came first, MHC class I or class II? *Immunogenetics* 1991;33:295–300.

142. Flynn GC, Pohl J, Flocco MT, Rothman JE. Peptide-binding specificity of the molecular chaperone BiP. *Nature* 1991;353:726–730.

143. Trowsdale J. "Both man & bird & beast": comparative organization of MHC genes. *Immunogenetics* 1995;41:1–17.

144. Salter-Cid L, Kasahara M, Flajnik MF. Hsp70 genes are linked to the Xenopus major histocompatibility complex. *Immunogenetics* 1994;39:1–7.

145. Sargent CA, Dunham I, Trowsdale J, Campbell RD. Human major histocompatibility complex contains genes for the major heat shock protein HSP70. *Proc Natl Acad Sci USA* 1989;86:1968–1972.

146. Rippmann F, Taylor WR, Rothbard JB, Green NM. A hypothetical model for the

147. Kasahara M, Flajnik MF, Ishibashi T, Natori T. Evolution of the major histocompatibility complex: a current overview. *Transplant Immunol* 1995;3:1–20.

148. Morshauser RC, Wang H, Flynn GC, Zuiderweg ER. The peptide-binding domain of the chaperone protein Hsc70 has an unusual secondary structure topology. *Biochemistry* 1995;34:6261–6266.

149. Zhu X, Zhao X, Burkholder WF, et al. Structural analysis of substrate binding by the molecular chaperone DnaK. *Science* 1996;272:1606–1614.

150. George JF, Cooper MD. Gamma/delta T Cells and alpha/beta T Cells differ in their developmental patterns of receptor expression and modulation requirements. *Eur J Immunol* 1990;20:2177–2181.

151. Rzepczyk CM, Anderson K, Stamatiou S, et al. Gamma delta T Cells: their immunobiology and role in malaria infections. *Int J Parasitol* 1997;27:191–200.

152. De Libero G. Sentinel function of broadly reactive human gamma delta T Cells. *Immunol Today* 1997;18:22–26.

153. Chien YH, Jores R, Crowley MP. Recognition by gamma/delta T Cells. *Annu Rev Immunol* 1996;14:511–532.

154. Grossberger D, Parham P. Reptilian class I major histocompatibility complex genes reveal conserved elements in class I structure. *Immunogenetics* 1992;36: 166–174.

155. Rast JP, Haire RN, Litman RT, Pross S, Litman GW. Identification and characterisation of T-Cell antigen receptor-related genes in phylogenetically diverse vertebrate species. *Immunogenetics* 1995;42:204–212.

156. Rast JP, Anderson MK, Strong SJ, Luer C, Litman RT, Litman GW. Alpha, beta, gamma, and delta T-Cell antigen receptor genes arose early in vertebrate phylogeny. *Immunity* 1997;6:1–11.

157. Partula S, de Guerra A, Fellah JS, Charlemagne J. Structure and diversity of the TCR alpha-chain in a teleost fish. *J Immunol* 1996;157:207–212.

158. Fellah JS, Kerfourn F, Dumay AM, Aubet G, Charlemagne J. Structure and diversity of the T-cell receptor alpha chain in the Mexican axolotl. *Immunogenetics* 1997;45:235–241.

159. Göbel TWF, Chen C-L, Lahti J, et al. Identification of T-cell receptor a-chain genes in the chicken. *Proc Natl Acad Sci USA* 1994;91:7856–7860.

160. Campbell KS, Bäckström T, Tiefenthaler G, Palmer E. CART: a conserved antigen receptor transmembrane motif. *Seminars in Immunol* 1994;6:393–410.

161. Rast JP, Litman GW. T-cell receptor gene homologs are present in the most primitive jawed vertebrates. *Proc Natl Acad Sci USA* 1994;91:9248–9252.

162. Hawke NA, Rast JP, Litman GW. Extensive diversity of transcribed TCR-b in a phylogenetically primitive vertebrate. *J Immunol* 1996;156:2458–2464.

163. Partula S, de Guerra A, Fellah JS, Charlemagne J. Structure and diversity of the T-cell antigen receptor beta-chain in a teleost fish. *J Immunol* 1995;155:699–706.

164. Hordvik I, Jacob ALJ, Charlemagne J, Endresen C. Cloning of T-cell antigen receptor beta chain cDNAs from Atlantic salmon (Salmo salar). *Immunogenetics* 1996;45:9–14.

165. Fellah JS, Kerfourn F, Guillet F, Charlemagne J. Conserved structure of amphibian T-cell antigen receptor b chain. *Proc Natl Acad Sci USA* 1993;90:6811–6814.

166. Chrètien I, Marcuz A, Fellah J, Charlemagne J, Du Pasquier L. The T-cell receptor beta genes of *Xenopus*. *Eur J Immunol* 1997;27:763–761.

167. Arnaud J, Huchenq A, Vernhes MC, et al. The interchain disulfide bond between TCR alpha beta heterodimers on human T cells is not required for TCR-CD3 membrane expression and signal transduction. *Int Immunol* 1997;9: 615–626.

168. Tjoelker L, Carlson LM, Lee K, et al. Evolutionary conservation of antigen recognition: the chicken T-cell receptor beta chain. *Proc Natl Acad Sci USA* 1990;87:7856–7860.

169. Kerfourn F, Charlemagne J, Fellah JS. The structure, rearrangement, and ontogenic expression of Db and Jb gene segments of the mexican axolotl T-cell antigen receptor beta chain (TCRB). *Immunogenetics* 1996;44:275–285.

170. Davis MM, Patten P. Evolutionary features of T-cell antigen-receptor genes. In: Schulze GKDH, ed. *Evolution and Vertebrate Immunity*, Austin: University of Texas Press, 1987, 201–211.

171. Davis MM, Bjorkman PJ. T-Cell antigen receptor genes and T-Cell recognition [published erratum appears in *Nature* Oct. 20, 1988;335(6192):744]. *Nature* 1988;334:395–402.

172. Fellah JS, Kerfourn F, Charlemagne J. Evolution of TCellreceptor genes. Extensive diversity of Vb families in the Mexican Axolotl. *J Immunol* 1994;153: 4539–4545.

173. Six A RJ, McCormack WT, Dunon D, Courtois D, Li Y, Chen CH, Cooper MD. Characterization of avian T-cell receptor gamma genes. *Proc Natl Acad Sci USA* 1996;93:15329–15334.

174. Hein WR, Dudler L. Divergent evolution of T-cell repertoires: extensive diversity and developmentally regulated expression of the sheep gamma delta T cell receptor. *EMBO J* 1993;12.715–724.

175. Cahill RN, Kimpton WG, Washington EA, Walker ID. Origin and development of the gamma delta T-cell system in sheep: a critical role for the thymus in the generation of TcR diversity and tissue tropism. *Semin Immunol* 1996;8:351–360.

176. Göbel TW, Fluri M. Identification and analysis of the chicken CD3e gene. *Eur J Immunol* 1997;27:194–198.

177. Dzialo RC, Cooper MD. An amphibian CD3 homologue of the mammalian CD3 g and d genes. *Eur J Immunol* 1997;27:1640–1647.

178. Bernot A, Auffray C. Primary structure and ontogeny of an avian CD3 transcript. *Proc Natl Acad Sci USA* 1991;88:2550–2554.

179. Göbel TW, Chen CL, Shrimpf J, et al. Characterization of avian natural killer Cells and their intra Cellular CD3 protein complex. *Eur J Immunol* 1994;24: 1685–1691.

180. Hsu E. The variation in immunoglobulin heavy chain constant regions in evolution. *Semin Immunol* 1994;6:383–391.

181. Atwell JC, Marchalonis JJ. Phylogenetic emergence of immunoglobulin classes distinct from IgM. *J Immunogenet* 1975;1:367–391.

182. Hsu E, Steiner LA. Primary structure of immunoglobulin through evolution. *Curr Op Struct Biol* 1992;2:422–431.

183. Wilson MR, Warr G. Fish immunoglobulin and the genes that encode them. *Ann Rev Fish Dis* 1992:in press.

184. Shankey TV, Clem LW. Phylogeny of immunoglobulin structure and function. VIII. Intermolecular heterogeneity of shark 19S IgM antibodies to pneumococcal polysaccharide. *Mol Immunol* 1980;17:365–375.

185. Litman GW, Marchalonis JJ. Evolution of antibodies. In: Ruben LB, Gershwin ME, eds. *Immune Regulation*, New York: Marcel Dekker Inc., 1982, 29–60.

186. Fellah JS, Wiles MV, Charlemagne J, Schwager J. Evolution of vertebrate IgM: complete amino-acid sequence of the constant region of *Ambystoma mexicanum* g chain deduced from cDNA sequence. *Eur J Immunol* 1992;22:2595–2601.

187. Schwager J, Mikoryak CA, Steiner LA. Amino acid sequence of heavy chains from *Xenopus laevis* IgM deduced from cDNA sequences: implicaiton for evolution of immunoglobulin domains. *Proc Natl Acad Sci USA* 1988;85: 2245–2249.

188. Greenberg AS, Hughes Al, Avila D, McKinney CE, Flajnik MF. A novel "chimeric" antibody class in cartilaginous fish: IgM may not be the primordial immunoglobulin. *Eur J Immunol* 1996;26:1123–1129.

189. Du Pasquier L, Schwager J. Evolutions of the Immune System. In: Melchers F, et al., ed. *Progress in Immunology*; Proceedings of the 7th International Congress of Immunology Berlin 1989, vol VII Berlin, Heidelberg, New York, London, Paris, Tokyo, Hong Kong: Springer-Verlag, 1989, 1246–1255.

190. Wilson MR, Marcuz A, van Ginkel F, et al. The immunoglobulin M heavy chain constant region gene of the channel catfish, *Ictalurus punctatus*: an unusual mRNA splice pattern produces the membrane form of the molecule. *Nucl Acids Res* 1990;18:5227–5233.

191. Lee MA, Bengtén A, Daggfeldt A, Rytting A-S, Pilström L. Characterization of rainbow trout cDNAs encoding a secreted and membrane-bound Ig heavy chain and the genomic intron upstream of the first constant exon. *Mol Immunol* 1993; 30:641–648.

192. Bengtén E, Leanderson T, Pilstrom L. Immunoglobulin heavy chain cDNA from the teleost atlantic cod (*Gadus morhua* L): Nucleotide sequences of secretory and membrane form show an unusual splicing pattern. *Eur J Immunol* 1991;21: 3027–3033.

193. Wilson MR, van Ravenstein E, Miller NW, Clem LW, Middleton DL, Warr GW. cDNA sequences and organization of IgM heavy chain genes in two Holostean fish. *Dev Comp Immunol*, 1995;19:153–164.

194. Wilson MR, Ross DA, Miller NW, Clem LW, Middleton DL, Warr GW. Alternate pre-mRNA processing pathways in the production of membrane IgM heavy chains in holostean fish. *Dev Comp Immunol* 1995;19:165–177.

195. Greenberg AS, Avila D, Hughes M, Hughes A, McKinney EC, Flajnik MF. A new antigen receptor gene family that undergoes rearrangement and extensive somatic diversification in sharks. *Nature* 1995;374:168–173.

196. Ota T, Rast JP, Litman GW, Amemiya CT. Lungfish immunoglobulins and their evolutionary implications. *Dev Comp Immunol* 1997;21:159.

197. Kobayashi K, Tomonaga S, Kajii T. A second class of immunoglobulin other than IgM present in the serum of a cartilaginous fish, the skate, Raja kenojei: isolation and characterization. *Mol Immunol* 1984;21:397–404.

198. Kobayashi K, Tomonaga S. The second immunoglobulin class is commonly present in cartilaginous fish belonging to the order Rajiformes. *Mol Immunol* 1988; 25:115–120.

199. Harding FA, Amemiya CT, Litman RT, Cohen N, Litman GT. Two distinct immunoglobulin heavy chain isotypes in a primitive, cartilaginous fish, *Raja erinacea*. *Nucl Acids Res* 1990;18:6369–6376.

200. Kobayashi K, Tomonaga S, Teshima K, Kajii T. Ontogenic studies on the appearance of two classes of immunoglobulin-forming cells in the spleen of the Aleutian skate, *Bathyraja aleutica*, a cartilaginous fish. *Eur J Immunol* 1985;15:952–956.

201. Wilson M, Bengtén E, Miller NW, Clem LW, Du Pasquier L, Warr GW. A novel chimeric Ig heavy chain from a teleost fish shares similarities to IgD. *Proc Natl Acad Sci USA* 1997;94:4593–4597.

202. Hsu E, Flajnik MF, Du Pasquier L. A third immunoglobulin class in amphibians. *J Immunol* 1985;135:1998–2004.

203. Schwager J, Hadji-Azimi I. Mitogen-induced B-cell differentiation in *Xenopus laevis*. *Differentiation* 1984;27:182–188.

204. Amemiya CT, Haire RN, Litman GW. Nucleotide sequence of a cDNA encoding a third distinct *Xenopus* immunoglobulin heavy chain isotype. *Nucleic Acids Res* 1989;17:5388.

205. Haire RN, Shamblott MJ, Amemiya CT, Litman GW. A second *Xenopus* immunoglobulin heavy chain constant region isotype gene. *Nucleic Acids Res* 1989;17:1776.

206. Steiner LA, Mikoryak CA, Lopes AD, Green C. Immunoglobulins in ranid frogs and tadpoles. *Adv Exp Biol Med* 1975;64:173–183.

207. Warr GW, Ruben LN, Edwards BJ. Evidence for low molecular weight antibodies in the serum of a urodele amphibian, *Ambystoma mexicanum*. *Immunol Lett* 1988;4:99–102.

208. Fellah JS, Charlemagne J. Characterization of IgY-like low molecular weight immunoglobulin class inthe mexican axolotl. *Mol Immunol* 1988;25:1377–1386.

209. Warr GW, Magor KE, Higgins DA. IgY: clues to the origins of modern antibodies. *Immunol Today* 1995;16:392–398.

210. Du Pasquier L, Horton JD. Restoration of antibody responsiveness in early thymectomized *Xenopus* by implantation of major histocompatibility complex–mismatched larval thymus. *Eur J Immunol* 1982;12:546–551.

211. Mussman R, Du Pasquier L, Hsu E. Is Xenopus IgX an analog of IgA? *Eur J Immunol* 1996;26:2823–2830.

212. Fellah JS, Iscaki S, Vaerman JP, Charlemagne J. Transient developmental expression of IgY and secretory component like protein in the gut of the axolotl (*Ambystoma mexicanum*). *Dev Immunol* 1992;2:181–190.

213. Mussmann R, Wilson M, Marcuz A, Courtet M, Du Pasquier L. Membrane exon sequences of the three *Xenopus* Ig classes explain the evolutionary origin of mammalian isotypes. *Eur J Immunol* 1996;26.

214. Mussmann R, Courtet M, Schwager J, Du Pasquier L. Microsites for immunoglobulin class switching from *Xenopus* to mammals. *Eur J Immunol* 1997;27:2610–2619.

215. Hsu E. Canonical VH CDR1 nucleotide sequences are conserved in all jawed vertebrates. *Int Immunol* 1996;8:847–854.

216. Kokubu F, Litman R, Shamblott MJ, Hinds K, Litman GW. Diverse organization of immunoglobulin VH gene loci in a primitive vertebrate. *EMBO J* 1988;7: 3413–3422.

217. Ventura-Holman T, Ghaffari SH, Lobb CJ. Characterization of a seventh family of immunoglobulin heavy chain VH gene segments in the channel catfish, *Ictalurus punctatus*. *Eur J Immunogenet* 1996;23:7–14.

218. Roman T, Charlemagne J. The immunoglobulin repertoire of the rainbow trout (*Oncorhynchus mykiss*): definition of nine IgH-V families. *Immunogenetics* 1994;40:210–216.

219. Roman T, Andersson E, Bengten E, et al. Unified nomenclature of Ig VH genes in rainbow trout (*Oncorhynchus mykiss*): definition of eleven VH families. *Immunogenetics* 1996;43:325–326.

220. Schwager J, Bürckert N, Courtet M, Du Pasquier L. Genetic basis of the antibody repertoire in Xenopus: analysis of the VH diversity. *EMBO J* 1989;8:2989–3001.

221. Hsu E, Schwager J, Alt FW. Evolution of immunoglobulin genes: VH families in the amphibian Xenopus. *Proc Natl Acad Sci USA* 1989;86:8010–8014.

222. Haire RN, Amemiya CT, Suzuki D, Litman GW. Eleven distinct VH gene families and additional patterns of sequence variation suggest a high degree of immunoglobulin gene complexity in a lower vertebrate, *Xenopus laevis*. *J Exp Med* 1990;171:1721–1737.

223. Litman GW, Murphy K, Berger L, Litman R, Hinds K, Erickson BW. Complete nucleotide sequences of three VH genes in caiman, a phylogenetically ancient reptile: evolutionary diversification in coding segments and variation in the structure and organization of recombination elements. *Proc Natl Acad Sci USA* 1985;82:844–848.

224. Turchin A, Hsu E. The generation of antibody diversity in the turtle. *J Immunol* 1996;156:3797–3805.

225. Desravines S, Zhang M., Hsu E. 1997, extensive immunoglobulin Vh and Jh diversity in the turtle. *J Immunol* 1997 (in press).

226. Reynaud C-A, Dahan A, Anquez V, Weill J-C. Somatic hyperconversion diversifies the single VH gene of the chicken with a high incidence in the D region. *Cell* 1989;59:171–183.

227. Schwager J, Bürckert N, Courtet M, Du Pasquier L. The ontogeny of diversification at the immunoglobulin heavy chain locus in Xenopus. *EMBO J* 1991;10: 2461–2470.

228. Hayman JR, Ghaffari SH, Lobb CJ. Heavy chain joining region segments of the channel catfish. Genomic organization and phylogenetic implications. *J Immunol* 1993;151:3587–3596.

229. Andersson E, Tormanen V, Matsunaga T. Evolution of a VH gene family in low vertebrates. *Int Immunol* 1991;3:527–533.

230. Schroeder HWJ, Hillson JL, Perlmutter RM. Structure and evolution of mammalian VH families. *Intl Immunol* 1990;2:41–50.

231. Ota T, Nei M. Divergent evolution and evolution by the birth-and-death process in the immunoglobulin VH gene family. *Mol Biol Evol* 1994;11:469–482.

232. Andersson E, Matsunaga T. Evolution of immunoglobulin heavy chain variable region genes: a VH family can last for 150–200 million years or longer. *Immunogenetics* 1995;41:18–28.

233. Rothenfluh HS, Blanden RV, Steele EJ. Evolution of V genes: DNA sequence structure of functional germline genes and pseudogenes. *Immunogenetics* 1995; 42:159–171.

234. Tanaka T, Nei M. Positive darwinian selection observed at the variable-region genes of immunoglobulins. Mol Biol Evol 1989;6:447–459.

235. Ota T, Nei M. Evolution of immunoglobulin VH pseudogenes in chickens. *Mol Biol Evol* 1995;12:94–102.

236. Greenberg AS, Steiner L, Kasahara M, Flajnik MF. Isolation of a shark immunoglobulin light chain cDNA clone encoding a protein resembling mammalian kappa light chains: implications for the evolution of light chains. *Proc Natl Acad Sci USA* 1993;90:10603–10607.

237. Rast JP, Anderson MK, Ota T, et al. Immunoglobulin light chain class multiplicity and alternative organizational forms in early vertebrate phylogeny. *Immunogenetics* 1994;40:83–99.

238. Hohman VS, Schluter SF, Marchalonis JJ. Complete sequence of a cDNA clone specifying sandbar shark immunoglobulin light chain: gene organization and

implications for the evolution of light chains. *Proc Natl Acad Sci USA* 1992;89: 276–280.

239. Lobb CJ, Olson MO, Clem LW. Immunologlobulin light chain classes in a teleost fish. *J Immunol* 1984;132:1917–1923.

240. Daggfeldt A, Bengtén E, Pilström L. A cluster type organization of the loci of the immunoglobulin light chain in Atlantic cod (*Gadus morhua L.*) and rainbow trout (*Oncorhynchus mykiss Walbaum*) indicated by nucleotide sequences of cDNAs and hybridization analysis. *Immunogenetics* 1993;38:199–209.

241. Ghaffari SH, J. LC. Structure and genomic organization of immunoglobulin light chain in the channel catfish. An unusual genomic organizational pattern of segmental genes. *J Immunol* 1993;151:6900–6912.

242. Partula S, Schwager J, Timmusk S, Pilström L, Charlemagne J. A second immunoglobulin light chain isotype in the rainbow trout. *Immunogenetics* 1996; 45:44–51.

243. Zezza DJ, Mikoryak CA, Schwager J, Steiner LA. Sequence of C region of L chains from *Xenopus laevis* Ig. *J Immunol* 1991;146:4041–4047.

244. Schwager J, Bürckert N, Schwager M, Wilson NM. Evolution of immunoglobulin light chain genes: analysis of *Xenopus* Ig L isotypes and their contribution to antibody diversity. *EMBO J* 1991;3:505–511.

245. Haire RN, Ota T, Rast JP, et al. A third Ig light chain gene isotype in *Xenopus laevis* consists of six distinct VL families and is related to mammalian l genes. *J Immunol* 1996;157:1544–1550.

246. Stewart SE, Du Pasquier L, Steiner LA. Diversity of expressed V and J regions of immunoglobulin light chains in *Xenopus laevis*. *Eur J Immunol* 1993;23:1980–1986.

247. Du Pasquier L, Courtet M, Robert J. A *Xenopus* lymphoid tumor Cell line with complete Ig genes rearrangements and T-cell characteristics. *Mol Immunol* 1995; 32:583–593.

248. Hsu E, Lefkovits I, Flajnik M, Du Pasquier L. Light chain heterogenicity in the amphibian *Xenopus*. *Mol Immunol* 1991;28:985 994.

249. Mikoryak CA, Steiner LA. Noncovalent association of heavy and light chains in *Rana catesbeiana* immunoglobulins. *J Immunol* 1984;133:376–383.

250. Mikoryak CA, Steiner LA. Amino acid sequence of the constant region of immunoglobulin light chains from *Rana catesbeiana*. *Mol Immunol* 1988;25: 695–703.

251. Saluk PH, Krauss J, Clem LW. The presence of two antigenetically distant light chains (k and l?) in alligator immunoglobulins. *Proc Soc Exp Biol Med* 1970; 133:365–369.

252. Reynaud C-A, Anquez V, Dahan A, Weill J-C. A single rearrangement event generates most of the chicken immunoglobulin light chain diversity. *Cell* 1985;40: 283–291.

253. Grant JA, Sanders B, Hood L. Partial amino acid sequences of chicken and turkey immunoglobulin light chains. Homology with mammalian lambda chains. *Biochemistry* 1971;10:3123–3132.

254. Fazel S, Wiersma EJ, Shulman MJ. Interplay of J chain and disulfide bonding in assembly of polymeric IgM. *Int Immunol* 1997;9:1149–1158.

255. Parkhouse RME, Askonas BA, Dourmashkin RR. Electron microscopic studies of mouse immunoglobulin M; structure and reconstitution following reduction. *Immunology* 1970;18:575–584.

256. Hadji-Azimi I. Anuran immunoglobulins. A review. *Dev Comp Immunol* 1979;3: 233–243.

257. Mikoryak CA, Margolies MN, Steiner LA. J chain in Rana catesbeiana high molecular weight Ig. *J Immunol* 1988;140:4279–4285.

258. Hohman V, Willett CE, Stewart SE, Steiner LA. Sequence analysis and expression patterns of J chain in *Xenopus laevis*. *Dev Comp Imm* 1997;21:200.

259. Du Pasquier L, Hsu E. Immunoglobulin expression in diploid and polyploid interspecies hybrid of *Xenopus*: evidence for allelic exclusion. *Eur J Immunol* 1983;13:585–590.

260. Hinds KR, Litman GW. Major reorganization of immunoglobulin VH segmental elements during vertebrate evolution. *Nature* 1986;320:546–549.

261. Litman GW, Rast JP, Hulst MA, et al. Evolutionary origins of immunoglobulin gene diversity. In: Gergely J, ed. *Progress in Immunology*, vol VIII Hungary: Springer-Verlag, 1993, 107–114.

262. Ishiguro H, Kobayashi K, Suzuki M, Titani K, Tomonaga S, Kurosawa Y. Isolation of a hagfish gene that encodes a complement component. *EMBO J* 1992;11: 829–837.

263. Schwager J, Grossberger D, Du Pasquier L. Organization and rearrangement of immunoglobulin M genes in the amphibian *Xenopus*. *EMBO J* 1988;7: 2409–2415.

264. Lundqvist M, Bengten E, Stromberg S, Pilström L. Ig light chain gene in the siberian sturgeon (*Acipenser baeri*). *J Immunol* 1996;157:2031–2038.

265. Mussmann R. B-cell development in the amphibian *Xenopus*, University of Basel, 1996.

266. Magor KE, Higgins DA, Middleton DL, Warr GW. One gene encodes the heavy chains for three different forms of IgY in the duck. *J Immunol* 1994;153: 5549–5555.

267. Hamers-Casterman C, Atarhouch T, Muyldermans S, et al. Naturally occurring antibodies devoid of light chains. *Nature* 1993;363:446–448.

268. Hadji-Azimi I, Schwager J, Thiébaud C. B-lymphocyte differentiation in Xenopus laevis larvae. *Dev Biol* 1982;90:253–258.

269. Du Pasquier L, Wilson M, Greenberg A, Flajnik MF. Somatic mutation in ectothermic vertebrates In: Kelsoe G, Flajnik MF, eds. *Curr Top Microbiol Immunol*, vol 229 Heidelberg: Springer, 1997, 199–216.

270. Hsu E, Du Pasquier L. Ontogeny of the immune system in *Xenopus*. I. Larval immune response. *Differentiation* 1984;28:109–115.

271. Desravines S, Hsu E. Measuring CDR3 length variability in individuals during ontogeny. *J Immunol* Methods 1994;168:219–225.

272. Hsu E, Du Pasquier L. Ontogeny of the immune system in Xenopus II. Antibody repertoire differences between larvae and adults. *Differentiation* 1984;28:116–122.

273. Reynaud CA, Dahan A, Weill JC. A gene conversion program during the ontogenesis of chicken B cells. *Trends Genet* 1987;3:248–251.

274. Weill J-C, Reynaud C-A. Early B-cell development in chickens, sheep and rabbits. *Curr Op Immunol* 1992;4:177–180.

275. Weill J-C, Reynaud C-A. The chicken BCellcompartment. *Science* 1987;238: 1094–1098.

276. Becker ES, Knight KL. Diversification of immunoglobulin heavy chain VDJ genes: evidence for somatic gene conversion in rabbits. *Cell* 1990;63:987–997.

277. Reynaud C-A, Mackay C, Müller RG, Weill JC. Somatic generation of diversity in a mammalian primary lymphoid organ: the sheep ileal Peyer's patches. *Cell* 1991;64:995–1005.

278. Butler JE, Sun J, Kacskovics I, Brown WR, Navarro P. The VH and CH immunoglobulin genes of swine: implications for repertoire development. *Vet Immunol Immunopathol* 1996;54:7–17.

279. Kobel HR, Du Pasquier L. Genetics of polyploid *Xenopus*. *Tr Genet* 1986;12: 310–315.

280. Hordvik I, Voie AM, Glette J, Male R, Endresen C. Cloning and sequence analysis of two isotypic IgM heavy chain genes from Atlantic salmon, *Salmo salar L.* *Eur J Immunol* 1992;22:2957–2962.

281. Raison RL, Hull CJ, Hildemann WH. Production and specificity of antibodies to strptococci in the Pacific hagfish *Eptatretus stoutii*. *Dev Comp Immunol* 1978; 2:253–262.

282. Nonaka M, Fujii T, Kaidoh T, et al. Purification of a lamprey complement protein homologous to the third component of the mammalian complement system. *J Immunol* 1984;133:3242–3249.

283. Fujii T, Nakamura T, Sekizawa A, Tomonaga S. Isolation and characterization of a protein from hagfish serum that is homologous to the third component of the mammalian complement system. *J Immunol* 1992;148:117–123.

284. Hagen M, Filosa MF, Youson JH. Immunocytochemical localization of antibody-producing cells in adult lamprey. *Immunol Letters* 1983;6:87–92.

285. Zapata A, F'84nge R, Mattisson A, Villena A. Plasma Cells in adult Atlantic hagfish, *Myxine glutinosa*. *Cell Tissue Res* 1984;235:691–693.

286. Zapata A, Ardavin CF, Gomariz RP, Leceta J. Plasma Cells in the ammocoete of *Petromyzon marinus*. *Cell Tissue Res* 1981;221:203–208.

287. Makel'84 O, Litman GW. Lack of heterogeneity in anti-hapten antibodies of a phylogenetically primitive shark. *Nature* 1980;287:639–640.

288. Litman GW, Scheffel C, Makelä O. Immunoglobulin diversity in the phylogenetically primitive shark *Heterodontus francisci*. Comparison of fine specificity in hapten binding by antibody to p-azobenzenearsonate. *Immunol Lett* 1980;1: 213–215.

289. Kehoe JM, Sharon J, Gerber-Jenson B, Litman GW. The structure of immunoglobulin variable regions in the horned shark, *Heterodontus francisci*. *Immunogenetics* 1979;7:35–40.

290. Clem LW, McLean WE, Shankey V. Quantitative and qualitative aspects of the antibody library of sharks. *Adv Exp Med Biol* 1975;64:231–249.

291. Kokubu F, Hinds K, Litman R, Shamblott MJ, Litman GW. Extensive families of constant region genes in a phylogenetically primitive vertebrate indicate an additional level of immunoglobulin complexity. *Proc Natl Acad Sci USA* 1987;84: 5868–5872.

292. Hinds-Frey KR, Nishikata H, Litman RT, Litman GW. Somatic variation precedes extensive diversification of germline sequences and combinatorial joining in the evolution of immunoglobulin heavy chain diversity. *J Exp Med* 1993;178: 815–824.

293. Anderson M, Amemiya C, Luer C, et al. Complete genomic sequence and patterns of transcription of a member of an unusual family of closely related, chromosomally dispersed Ig gene clusters in Raja. *Int Immunol* 1994;6:1661–1670.

294. Rast J, Amemiya CT, Litman RT, Strong S, Litman GW. The immunoglobulin heavy chain genes of a modern representative of a major independent lineage of the cartilaginous fish provide insight into the evolution of rearranging immune receptor genes. *Immunogenetics* 1997:in press.

295. Machulla HKG, Richter RF, Ambrosius H. Study of antibody heterogeneity of carp (Cyprinus carpio, L). The idiotypic specificity of anti-DNP antibodies. *Immunol Lett* 1980;1:329–334.

296. Richter RF, Ambrosius H. Antibodies of IgM-type produced in carp (Cyprinus carpio, L.). *Eur J Immunol* 1979;9:578–580.

297. Vilain C, Wetzel MC, Du Pasquier L, Charlemagne J. Structural and functional analysis of spontaneous anti-nitrophenyl antibodies in three cyprinid fish species: carp (*Cyprinus carpio*), goldfish (*Carassius auratus*) and tench (*Tinca tinca*). *Dev Comp Immunol* 1984;8:611–622.

298. Wetzel MC, Charlemagne J. Antibody diversity in fish. Isoelectrofocalisation study of individually-purified specific antibodies in three teleost fish species: tench, carp and goldfish. *Dev Comp Immunol* 1985;9:261–270.

299. Arkoosh MR, Kaattari SL. Development of immunological memory in rainbow trout (*Oncorhynchus mykiss*). I. An immunochemical and Cellular analysis of the B cell response. *Dev Comp Immunol* 1991;15:279–293.

300. Zhang H, Khor, TW, Evans D A, and Kaattari, S.L. Characterization of affinity maturation in trout. *Dev Comp Immunol* 1997;21:100.

301. Cossarini-Dunier M, Desvaux FX, Dorson M. Variability in humoral responses to DNP-KLH of rainbow trout (*Salmo gairdneri*). Comparison of antibody kinetics and immunoglobulin spectrotypes between normal trouts and trouts obtained by gynogeneis or self fertilization. *Dev Comp Immunol* 1986;10:207–217.

302. Clem LW, Miller NW, Bly JE. Evolution of lymphocyte subpopulations, their interactions and temperature sensitivities. In: Warr G, Cohen N, eds. *Phylogenesis of immune functions*, Boca Raton FL: CRC Press, 1991, 191–213.

303. von Ginkel FW, Miller NW, Lobb CJ, Clem LW. Characterization of anti-hapten antibodies generated in vitro by channel catfish peripheral blood lymphocytes. *Dev Comp Immunol* 1992;16:139–154.

304. Lobb CJ. Preferential expression of catfish light chain immunoglobulin isotypes in anti-dinitrophenyl antibodies. *J Immunogenet* 1986;13:19–28.

305. Gonzalez R. Natural anti-TNP antibodies from rainbow trout interfere with viral infection in vitro. *Res Immunol* 1989;140:675–684.

306. Michel C, Gonzalez R, Bonjour E, Avrameas S. A concurrent increasing of natural antibodies and enhancement of resistance to furunculosis in rainbow trout. *Ann Rech Vet* 1990;21:211–218.

307. Magnadottir B, Gudmundsdottir S, Gudmundsdottir BK. Study of the humoral response of Atlantic salmon (*Salmo salar L.*), naturally infected with *Aeromonas salmonicida* ssp. achromogenes. *Vet Immunol Immunopathol* 1995; 49:127–142.

308. Miller NW, Rycyzyn MA, Wilson MR, Warr GW, Naftel JP, Clem LW. Development and characterization of channel catfish long term BCelllines. *J Immunol* 1994;152:2180–2189.

309. Charlemagne J. Antibody diversity in amphibians. Non-inbred axolotls used the same unique heavy chain and a limited number of light chains for their anti-2,4-dinitrophenyl antibody responses. *Eur J Immunol* 1987;17:421–424.

310. Du Pasquier L. Antibody diversity in lower vertebrates—why is it so restricted? *Nature* 1982;296:311–313.

311. Brandt DC, Griessen M, Du Pasquier L, Jaton JC. Antibody diversity in amphibians: evidence for the inheritance of idiotypic specificities in isogenic *Xenopus*. *Eur J Immunol* 1980;10:731–736.

312. Du Pasquier L, Schwager J. Immunoglobulin genes and B cell development in amphibians. *Adv Exp Med Biol* 1991;292:1–9.

313. Wilson M, Hsu E, Marcuz A, Courtet M, Du Pasquier L, Steinberg C. What limits affinity maturation of antibodies in *Xenopus*—the rate of somatic mutation or the ability to select mutants? *EMBO J* 1992;11:4337–4347.

314. Wabl MR, Du Pasquier L. Antibody patterns in genetically identical frogs. *Nature* 1976;264:642–644.

315. Du Pasquier L, Wabl MR. Antibody diversity in amphibians: inheritance of isoelectric focusing antibody patterns in isogenic frogs. *Eur J Immunol* 1978;8: 428–433.

316. Wilson M, Marcuz A, Du Pasquier L. Somatic mutations during an immune response in *Xenopus* tadpoles. *Dev Immunol* 1995;4:227–234.

317. Wagner SD, Milstein C, Neuberger MS. Codon bias targets mutation. *Nature* 1995;376:732.

318. Wilson M, Marcuz A, Courtet M, Du Pasquier L. Sequences of C m and the VH1 family in LG7, a clonable strain of *Xenopus*, homozygous for the immunoglobulin loci. *Dev Immunol* 1992;3:13–24.

319. Du Pasquier L, Robert J. In vitro growth of thymic tumor Cell lines from *Xenopus*. *Dev Immunol* 1992;2:295–307.

320. Du Pasquier L. Phylogeny of B-cell development. *Curr Opin Immunol* 1993;5: 185–193.

321. Grey HM. Phylogeny of the immune response. Studies on some physical, chemical and serologic characteristics of antibody produced in the turtle. *J Immunol* 1963;91:819–825.

322. Ivanyi J, Moreno C. Isoelectric spectra of antibodies in chicken following recovery from immunological tolerance or bursectomy. In: Solomon J, Horton JD, eds. *Developmental Immunology*, Amsterdam: Elsevier/North-Holland, 1977.

323. Kubo RT, Rosenblum IY, Benedict AA. The unblocked N-terminal sequence of chicken IgG l-like light chains. *J Immunol* 1970;105:534–536.

324. Wasserman RL, Kehoe JM, Capra JD. The VH III subgroup of immunoglobulin heavy chains: phylogenetically associated residues in several avian species. *J Immunol* 1974;113:954–957.

325. Voss EW, Watt RH. Comparison of the microenvironment of chicken and rabbit antibody active site. *Adv Exp Med Biol* 1977;88:391–401.

326. Yamaga K, Benedict AA. Class, amounts and affinities of anti-dinitrophenyl antibodies in chickens. I. Comparison of 7S and 17S antibodies of equal affinity by intravenous injection of antigen. *J Immunol* 1975;115:750–758.

327. Yamaga K, Benedict AA. Class, amounts, and affinities of anti-dinitrophenyl antibodies in chickens. II. Production of a restricted population of high affinity 7S antibodies by injection of antigen emulsified in adjuvant. *J Immunol* 1975; 115:759–764.

328. Arakawa H, Furusawa S, Ekino S, Yamagishi H. Immunoglobulin gene hyperconversion ongoing in chicken splenic germinal centers. *EMBO J* 1996;15: 2540–2546.

329. Weinstein PD, Anderson AO, Mage RG. Rabbit IgH sequences in appendix germinal centers: VH diversification by gene conversion-like and hypermutation mechanisms. *Immunity* 1994;1:647–659.

330. Croix DA, Samples NK, Vandeberg JL, Stone WH. Immune response of a marsupial (*Monodelphis domestica*) to sheep red blood cells. *Dev Comp Immunol* 1989;13:73–78.

331. Klein J. Natural history of the histocompatibility complex. New York: John Wiley & Sons, 1986.

332. Zinkernagel RM, Doherty PC. Restriction of in vitro T cell-mediated cytotoxicity in lymphocytic choriomeningitis within a syngeneic or semiallogeneic system. *Nature* 1974;248:701–702.

333. Kasahara M, McKinney EC, Flajnik MF, Ishibashi T. The evolutionary origin of the major histocompatibility complex: polymorphism of class II alpha chain genes in the cartilaginous fish. *Eur J Immunol* 1993;23:2160–2165.

334. Bartl S, Weissman IL. Isolation and characterization of major histocompatibility complex class IIB genes from the nurse shark. *Proc Natl Acad Sci USA* 1994;91: 262–266.

335. Bartl S, Baish M.A, Flajnik MF, Ohta Y. Identification of class I genes in cartilaginous fish, the most ancient group of vertebrates displaying an adaptive immune system. 1997: *J Immunol* 159: 6097–6104 .

336. Kaufman J, Volk H, Wallny HJ. A "minimal essential Mhc" and an "unrecognized Mhc": two extremes in selection for polymorphism. *Immunol Rev* 1995; 143:63–88.

337. Sammut B, Laurens V, Tournefier A. Isolation of Mhc class I cDNAs from the axolotl *Ambystoma mexicanum*. *Immunogenetics* 1997;45:285–294.

338. Sammut B, Calin-Laurens V, Tournefier A. Evolution of the MHC: Isolation of Class II chain cDNAS from the urodele Ambystoma mexicanum. Abstracts 9th Int Cong Immunol San Francisco 1995.

339. Sammut B. *Caractérisation des gènes de classe I du complexe majeur d'histocompatibilité de deux Amphibiens urodèles du genre ambystoma*, Ambystoma mexicanum *et* Ambystoma tigrinum, Université de Bourgogne, Dijon, 1997.

340. Bjorkman PJ, Saper MA, Samraoui B, Bennett WS, Strominger JL, Wiley DC. Structure of the human class I histocompatibility antigen, HLA-A2. *Nature* 1987;329:506–512.

341. Brown JH, Jardetzky TS, Gorga JC, et al. Three-dimensional structure of the human class II histocompatibility antigen HLA-DR1. *Nature* 1993;364:33–39.

342. Kaufman J, Salomonsen J, Flajnik M. Evolutionary conservation of MHC class I and class II molecules—different yet the same. *Semin Immunol* 1994;6: 411–424.

343. Sultmann H, Mayer WE, Figueroa F, O'Huigin C, Klein J. Zebrafish Mhc class II alpha chain-encoding genes: polymorphism, expression, and function. *Immunogenetics* 1993;38:408–420.

344. Kelly AP, Monaco JJ, Cho SG, Trowsdale J. A new human HLA class II-related locus, DM. *Nature* 1991;353:571–573.

345. Cho SG, Attaya M, Monaco JJ. New class II-like genes in the murine MHC. *Nature* 1991;353:573–576.

346. Figueroa F, Ono H, Tichy H, O'Huigin C, Klein J. Evidence for insertion of a new intron into an Mhc gene of perch-like fish. *Proc R Soc Lond B Biol Sci* 1995;259:325–330.

347. Guild BC, Erikson RL, Strominger JL. HLA-A2 and HLA-B7 antigens are phosphorylated in vitro by rous sarcoma virus kinase (pp60v-src) at a tyrosine residue encoded in a highly conserved exon of the intra cellular domain. *Proc Natl Acad Sci USA* 1983;80:2894–2898.

348. Guild BC, Strominger JL. Human and murine class I MHC antigens share conserved serine 335, the site of HLA phosphorylation in vivo. *J Biol Chem* 1984; 259:9235–9240.

349. Cosson P, Bonifacino JS. Role of transmembrane domain interactions in the assembly of class II MHC molecules. *Science* 1992;258:659–662.

350. Kaufman J, Anderson R, Avila D, et al. Different features of the MHC class I heterodimer have evolved at different rates. *J Immunol* 1992;148:1532–1546.

351. Madden DR, Gorga JC, Strominger JL, Wiley DC. The structure of HLA-B27 reveals nonamer self-peptides bound in an extended conformation. *Nature* 1991; 353:321–325.

352. Shum BP, Avila D, Du Pasquier L, Kasahara M, Flajnik MF. Isolation of a classical MHC class I cDNA from an amphibian. Evidence for only one class I locus in the *Xenopus* MHC. *J Immunol* 1993;151:5376–5386.

353. Parham P. The rise and fall of great class I genes. *Semin Immunol* 1994;6: 373–382.

354. Klein J, O'Huigin C. The conundrum of nonclassical major histocompatibility complex genes. *Proc Natl Acad Sci USA* 1994;91:6251–6252.

355. Calabi F, Milstein C. A novel family of human major histocompatibility complex-related genes not mapping to chromosome 6. *Nature* 1986;323:540–543.

356. Por Celli S, Morita CT, Brenner MB. CD1b restricts the response of human CD4-8- T lymphocytes to a microbial antigen. *Nature* 1992;360:593–597.

357. Wang CR, Loveland BE, Lindahl KF. H-2M3 encodes the MHC class I molecule presenting the maternally transmitted antigen of the mouse. *Cell* 1991;66: 335–345.

358. Watkins DI, Chen ZW, Hughes AL, Evans MG, Tedder TF, Letvin NL. Evolution of the MHC class I genes of a New World primate from ancestral homologues of human non-classical genes. *Nature* 1990;346:60–63.

359. Simister NE, Mostov KE. An Fc receptor structurally related to MHC class I antigens. *Nature* 1989;337:184–187.

360. Burmeister WP, Gastinel LN, Simister NE, Blum ML, Bjorkman PJ. Crystal structure at 2.2 Å resolution of the MHC-related neonatal Fc receptor. *Nature* 1994;372:336–343.

361. Araki T, Gejyo F, Takagaki K, et al. Complete amino acid sequence of human plasma Zn-alpha 2-glycoprotein and its homology to histocompatibility antigens. *Proc Natl Acad Sci USA* 1988;85:679–683.

362. Kasahara M, Kandil E, Salter-Cid L, Flajnik MF. Origin and evolution of the

class I gene family: why are some of the mammalian class I genes encoded outside the major histocompatibility complex? *Res Immunol* 1996;147:278–285.

363. Hughes AL, Nei M. Pattern of nucleotide substitution at major histocompatibility complex class I loci reveals overdominant selection. *Nature* 1988;335:167–170.

364. Plachy J, Pink JR, Hala K. Biology of the chicken MHC (B complex). *Crit Rev Immunol* 1992;12:47–79.

365. Kaufman J, Wallny HJ. Chicken MHC molecules, disease resistance and the evolutionary origin of birds. *Curr Top Microbiol Immunol* 1996;212:129–141.

366. Jaffe L, Robertson EJ, Bikoff EK. Distinct patterns of expression of MHC class I and beta 2-microglobulin transcripts at early stages of mouse development. *J Immunol* 1991;147:2740–2749.

367. Flajnik MF, Kaufman JF, Hsu E, Manes M, Parisot R, Du Pasquier L. Major histocompatibility complex-encoded class I molecules are absent in immunologically competent *Xenopus* before metamorphosis. *J Immunol* 1986;137:3891–3899.

368. Flajnik MF, Du Pasquier L. MHC class I antigens as surface markers of adult erythrocytes during the metamorphosis of *Xenopus*. *Dev Biol* 1988;128:198–206.

369. Du Pasquier L, Flajnik MF. Expression of MHC class II antigens during *Xenopus* development. *Dev Immunol* 1990;1:85–95.

370. Rollins-Smith L, Blair P. The expression of class II major histocompatibility complex antigens on adult T Cells in *Xenopus* is metamorphosis dependent. *Dev Immunol* 1990;1:97–104.

371. Kaufman J, Skjoedt K, Salomonsen J. The MHC molecules of nonmammalian vertebrates. *Immunol Rev* 1990;113:83–117.

372. Rodrigues PNS, van Maanen A, Taverne-Thiele A, Rombout JHMW, Egberts E, Stet JM. Cell surface expression of MHC class I and 2-microglobulin in carp (*Cyprinus carpio L.*) lymphoid tissues during ontogeny. *Dev Immunol* in press.

373. Monaco JJ, McDevitt HO. Identification of a fourth class of proteins linked to the murine major histocompatibility complex. *Proc Natl Acad Sci USA* 1982;79:3001–3005.

374. Brown MG, Driscoll J, Monaco JJ. Structural and serological similarity of MHC-linked LMP and proteasome (multicatalytic proteinase) complexes. *Nature* 1991;353:355–357.

375. Deverson EV, Gow IR, Coadwell WJ, Monaco JJ, Butcher GW, Howard JC. MHC class II region encoding proteins related to the multidrug resistance family of transmembrane transporters. *Nature* 1990;348:738–741.

376. Trowsdale J, Hanson I, Mockridge I, Beck S, Townsend A, Kelly A. Sequences encoded in the class II region of the MHC related to the 'ABC' superfamily of transporters. *Nature* 1990;348:741–744.

377. Kasahara M, Nakaya J, Satta Y, Takahata N. Chromosomal duplication and the emergence of the adaptive immune system, *Trends Genet* 1997;13:90–92.

378. Kasahara M, Hayashi M, Tanaka K, Inoko H, Sugaya K, Ikemura T, Ishibashi T. Chromosomal localization of the proteasome Z subunit gene reveals an ancient chromosomal duplication involving the major histocompatibility complex. *Proc Natl Acad Sci USA* 1996;93:9096–9101.

379. Trachtulec Z, Hamvas RM, Forejt J, Lehrach HR, Vincek V, Klein J. Linkage of TATA-binding protein and proteasome subunit C5 genes in mice and humans reveals synteny conserved between mammals and invertebrates. *Genomics* 1997;44:1–7.

380. Spring J. Vertebrate evolution by interspecific hybridisation—are we polyploid? *FEBS Lett* 1997;400:2–8.

381. Du Pasquier L, Courtet M, Chrétien I. Conservation and variation in CTX gene organization and duplication from amphibians to mammals. 1998:in preparation.

382. Ohno S. *Evolution by gene duplication.* New York: Springer, 1970.

383. Nonaka M, Namikawa C, Kato Y, Sasaki M, Salter-Cid L, Flajnik MF. Major histocompatibility complex gene mapping in the amphibian *Xenopus* implies a primordial organization. *Proc Natl Acad Sci USA* 1997;94:5789–5791.

384. Bingulac-Popovic J, Figueroa F, Sato A, et al. Mapping of mhc class I and class II regions to different linkage groups in the zebrafish, *Danio rerio. Immunogenetics* 1997;46:129–134.

385. Kato Y, Salter-Cid L, Flajnik MF, et al. Isolation of the *Xenopus* complement factor B complementary DNA and linkage of the gene to the frog MHC. *J Immunol* 1994;153:4546–4554.

386. Nakamura T, Sekizawa A, Fujii T, Katagiri C. Cosegregation of the polymorphic C4 with the MHC in the frog *Xenopus laevis. Immunogenetics* 1986;23:181–186.

387. Mo R, Kato Y, Nonaka M, Nakayama K, Takahashi M. Fourth component of Xenopus laevis complement: cDNA cloning and linkage analysis of the frog MHC. *Immunogenetics* 1996;43:360–369.

388. Guillemot F, Billault A, Pourquie O, et al. A molecular map of the chicken major histocompatibility complex: the class II beta genes are closely linked to the class I genes and the nucleolar organizer. *EMBO J* 1988;7:2775–2785.

389. Koch C. A genetic polymorphism of the complement component factor B in chickens not linked to the major histocompatibility complex (MHC). *Immunogenetics* 1986;23:364–367.

390. Hansen JD, Strassburger P, Du Pasquier L. Conservation of an alpha 2 domain within the teleostean world, MHC class I from the rainbow trout Oncorhynchus mykiss. *Dev Comp Immunol* 1996;20:417–425.

391. van Erp SH, Egberts E, Stet RJ. Evidence for multiple distinct major histocompatibility complex class I lineages in teleostean fish. *Eur J Immunogenet* 1996;23:371–381.

392. Flajnik MF, Kasahara M, Shum BP, Salter-Cid L, Taylor E, Du Pasquier L. A novel type of class I gene organization in vertebrates: a large family on non-

MHC-linked class I genes is expressed at the RNA level in the amphibian *Xenopus. EMBO J* 1993;12:4385–4396.

393. Du Pasquier L, Flajnik. unpublished.

394. Klein J, Ono H, Klein D, O'Huigin C. The accordion model of MHC evolution. In: Gergely J, Petranyi G, eds. *Progress in Immunology*, Heidelberg: Springer-Verlag, 1993, 137–143.

395. Du Pasquier L, Miggiano VC, Kobel HR, Fischberg M. The genetic control of histocompatibility reactions in natural and laboratory-made polyploid individuals of the clawed toad *Xenopus. Immunogenetics* 1977;5:129–141.

396. Bevan MJ. High determinant density may explain the phenomenon of alloreactivity. *Immunology Today* 1984;5:128–130.

397. Cunningham BA, Berggard I. Structure, evolution and significance of beta2-microglobulin. *Transplant Rev* 1974;21:3–14.

398. Bahram S, Bresnahan M, Geraghty DE, Spies T. A second lineage of mammalian major histocompatibility complex class I genes. *Proc Natl Acad Sci USA* 1994;91:6259–6263.

399. Dixon B, Stet RJ, van Erp SH, Pohajdak B. Characterization of beta 2-microglobulin transcripts from two teleost species. *Immunogenetics* 1993;38:27–34.

400. Shum BP, Azumi K, Zhang S, et al. Unexpected beta 2-microglobulin sequence diversity in individual rainbow trout. *Proc Natl Acad Sci USA* 1996;93:2779–2784.

401. Ono H, Figueroa F, O'Huigin C, Klein J. Cloning of the beta 2-microglobulin gene in the zebrafish. *Immunogenetics* 1993;38:1–10.

402. Dargemont C, Dunon D, Deugnier MA, et al. Thymotaxin, a chemotactic protein, is identical to beta 2-microglobulin. *Science* 1989;246:803–806.

403. Zijlstra M, Bix M, Simister NE, Loring JM, Raulet DH, Jaenisch R. Beta 2-microglobulin deficient mice lack CD4-8+ cytolytic T cells. *Nature* 1990;344:742–746.

404. Fearon DT, Carter RH. The CD19/CR2/TAPA-1 complex of B lymphocytes: linking natural to acquired immunity. *Annu Rev Immunol* 1995;13:127–149.

405. Lambris JD, Mavroidis M, Sunyer JO. Phylogeny of third component of complement, C3. In: Erdei A, ed. *New Aspects of Complement Structure and Function*, 1994, 15–34.

406. Dodds AW. Molecular and phylogenic aspects of the complement system. In: Hoffmann JA, Janeway CA, Jr., Natori S, eds. *Phylogenic perspectives in immunity: the insect host defense*, Austin: R. G. Landes Company, 1994, 143–155.

407. Kinoshita T. Biology of complement: the overture. *Immunol Today* 1991;12:291–295.

408. Smith LC, Chang L, Britten RJ, Davidson EH, Sea urchin genes expressed in activated coelomocytes are identified by expressed sequence tags. Complement homologues and other putative immune response genes suggest immune system homology within the deuterostomes. *J Immunol* 1996;156:593–602.

409. Smith CL. Sea urchin coelomocytes specifically express a C3 complement component and a complement receptor or regulatory protein. *Devel Comp Immunol* 1997;21:143.

410. Nonaka M, Takahashi M. Complete complementary DNA sequence of the third component of complement of lamprey. Implication for the evolution of thioester containing proteins. *J Immunol* 1992;148:3290–3295.

411. Turner MW. Mannose-binding lectin: the pluripotent molecule of the innate immune system. *Immunol Today* 1996;17:532–540.

412. Thiel S, Vorup-Jensen T, Stover CM, et al. A second serine protease associated with mannan binding lectin that activates complement. *Nature* 1997;386:506–510.

413. Ji X, Azumi K, Sasaki M, Nonaka M. Ancient origin of the complement lectin pathway revealed by molecular cloning of mannan binding protein-associated serine protease from a urochordate, the Japanese ascidian, *Halocynthia roretzi. Proc Natl Acad Sci USA* 1997;94:6340–6345.

414. Hanley PJ, Hook JW, Raftos DA, Gooley AA, Trent R, Raison RL. Hagfish humoral defense protein exhibits structural and functional homology with mammalian complement components. *Proc Natl Acad Sci USA* 1992;89:7910–7914.

415. Fujii T, Hook JW, Remedios ND, Raison RL. Complement like protein form hagfish is homologous to the third component of the mammalian complement system. *Devel Comp Immunol* 1997;21:149.

416. Sunyer JO, Zarkadis IK, Sahu A, Lambris JD. Multiple forms of complement C3 in trout that differ in binding to complement activators. *Proc Natl Acad Sci USA* 1996;93:8546–8551.

417. Jensen JA, Festa E, Smith DS, Cayer M. The complement system of the nurse shark: hemolytic and comparative characteristics. *Science* 1981;214:566–569.

418. Sunyer OJ, Zarkadis, I., Lambris, J.D. Structural and functional characterization of Bf/C2 complement molecules in teleost fish. *Dev Comp Immunol* 1997;21:147.

419. Armstrong PB, Quigley JP. Limulus alpha 2-macroglobulin. First evidence in an invertebrate for a protein containing an internal thiol ester bond. *Biochem J* 1987;248:703–707.

420. Farries TC, Atkinson JP. Evolution of the complement system. *Immunol Today* 1991;12:295–300.

421. Hughes AL. Phylogeny of the C3/C4/C5 complement-component gene family indicates that C5 diverged first. *Mol Biol Evol* 1994;11:417–425.

422. Brown MG, Scalzo AA, Matsumoto K, Yokoyama WM. The natural killer gene complex: a genetic basis for understanding natural killer cell function and innate immunity. *Immunol Rev* 1997;155:53–65.

423. Zapata A. Phylogeny of the fish immune system. *Bull Inst Pasteur* 1983;81:165–186.

424. Tomonaga S, Hirokame T, Awaka K. The primitive spleen of the hagfish. *Zool Mag* 1973;82:215–219.
425. Tanaka Y, Saito Y, Gotoh H. Vascular architecture and intestinal hematopoietic nests of two cyclostomes, Eptatretus burgeri and ammoncoetes of Entosphenus reissneri: a comparative morphological study. *J Morphol* 1981;170:71–93.
426. Fujii T, Hayakawa I. A histological and electron-microscopic study of the cell-types involved in rejection of skin allografts in ammocoetes. *Cell Tissue Res* 1983;231:301–312.
427. Fujii T. Electron microscopy of the leucocytes of the typhlosole in ammocoetes, with special attention to the antibody-producing cells. *J Morphol* 1982;173:87–100.
428. Cohen N. Phylogenetic emergence of lymphoid tissues and cell. In: Marchalonis JJ, ed. *The lymphocyte structure and function* Part I, New York: Marcus Dekker, 1977, 149–202.
429. Zapata AG, Varas A, Torroba M. Seasonal variations in the immune system of lower vertebrates. *Immunol Today* 1992;13:142–147.
430. Luer CA, Walsh CJ, Bodine AB, Wyffels JT, Scott TR. The elasmobranch thymus: anatomocal histological, and preliminary functional characterization. *J Exp Zool* 1995;273:342–345.
431. Fange R, Pulsford A. Structural studies on lymphomyeloid tissues of the dogfish, *Scyliorhinus canicula L. Cell Tissue Res* 1983;230:337–351.
432. Torroba M, Chiba A, Vicente A, et al. Macrophage-lymphocyteCellclusters in the hypothalamic ventricle of some elasmobranch fish: ultrastructural analysis and possible functional significance. Anat Rec 1995;242:400–410.
433. McCumber LJ, Sigel MM, Trauger RJ, Cuchens MA. RES structure and function of the fishes. In: Cohen N, Sigel MM, eds. *The Reticuloendothelial System: Phylogeny and Ontogeny*, vol. 3. New York: Plenum Press, 1982, 393–422.
434. Van Muiswinkel WB, Lamers CH, Rombout JH. Structural and functional aspects of the spleen in bony fish. *Res Immunol* 1991;142:362–366.
435. Chilmonczyk S. The thymus in fish:development and possible function in the immune response. *Ann Rev of Fish Diseases* 1992;2:181–200.
436. Romano N, Abelli L, Mastrolia L, Scapigliati G. Immunocytochemical detection and cytomorphology of lymphocyte subpopulations in a teleost fish Dicentrarchus labrax. *Cell Tissue Res* 1997;289:163–171.
437. Ardavin CF, Zapata A. Ultrastructure and changes during metamorphosis of the lympho-hemopoietic tissue of the larval anadromous sea lamprey Petromyzon marinus. *Devel Comp Immunol* 1987;11:79–93.
438. Estepa A, Coll JM. Mitogen-induced proliferation of trout kidney leucocytes by one-step culture in fibrin clots. *Vet Immunol Immunopathol* 1992;32:165–177.
439. Kaastrup P, Nielsen B, Hoerlyck V, Simonsen M. Mixed lymphocyte reactions (MLR) in rainbow trout (*Salmo gairdneri*) sibling. *Dev Comp Immunol* 1988;12:801–808.
440. Caspi RR, Avtalion RR. The mixed leukocyte reaction (MLR) in carp: bidirectional and undirectional MLR responses. *Dev Comp Immunol* 1984;8:631–637.
441. Miller NW, Deuter A, Clem LW. Phylogeny of lymphocyte heterogeneity: the Cellular requirements for the mixed leucocyte reaction with channel catfish. *Immunol* 1986;59:123–128.
442. Bly JE, Clem LW. Temperature and teleost immune functions. *Fish and Shellfish Immunol* 1992:159–171.
443. Scapigliati G, Mazzini M, Mastrolia L, Romano N, Abelli L. Production and characterisation of a monoclonal antibody against the thymocytes of the sea bass Dicentrarchus labrax (L.) (Teleostei, Percicthydae). *Fish & Shellfish Immunol* 1995;5:393–405.
444. Sailendri K. Studies in the development of lymphoid organs and immune responses in the teleost Tilapia mossambica. PhD thesis, Madurai University, India, 1973.
445. Sailendri K, Muthukkaruppan VR. The immune response of the teleost, Tilapia mossambica to soluble and cellular antigens. *J Exp Zool* 1975;191:371–382.
446. Blau JN, Waksman BH. Immunological responses following injections of antigens in Freund's adjuvant into thymus and other tissues. *Immunology* 1964;191:371–382.
447. Smith AM, Potter M, Merchant ER. Antibody forming cells in the pronephros of the teleost Lepomis macrochirus. *J Immunol* 1967;99:876–882.
448. De Luca D, Wilson M, Warr GW. Lymphocyte heterogeneity in the trout, Salmo gairdneri, defined with monoclonal antibodies to IgM. *Eur J Immunol* 1983;13:551–555.
449. Rombout JH. The gut-associated lymphoid tissue (GALT) of carp (*Cyprinuscarpio L.*): an immunocytochemical analysis. *Dev Comp Immunol* 1993;17:55–66.
450. Miller NW, Clem LW. Temperature-mediated processes in Teleost immunity: differential effects of temperature on catfish in vitro antibody responses to thymus-dependent and thymus-independent antigens. *J Immunol* 1984;133:2356–2359.
451. Vallejo AN, Miller NW, Clem LW. Antigen processing and presentation in teleost immune responses. *Annu Rev Fish Dis* 1992;2:73–89.
452. Vallejo AN, Miller NW, Jorgensen T, Clem LW. Phylogeny of immune recognition: antigen processing/presentation in channel catfish immune responses to hemocyanins. *Cell Immunol* 1990;130:364–377.
453. Vallejo AN, Miller NW, Clem LW. Phylogeny of immune recognition: processing and presentation of structurally defined proteins in channel catfish immune responses. *Dev Immunol* 1991;1:137–148.
454. Hinuma S, Abo T, Kumagai K, Hata W. The potent activity of freshwater fish kidney Cells in cell killing. I. Characterization and species distinction f cytotoxicity. *Dev Comp Immunol* 1980;4:653–666.

455. Moody CE, Serreze DV, Reno PW. Non-specific cytotoxic activity of teleost leukocytes. *Dev Comp Immunol* 1985;9:51–64.
456. Graves SS, Evans DL, Cobb D, Dawe DL. Nonspecific cytotoxic Cells in fish (Ictalurus puntatus) I. Optimum reqirement for target cell lysis. *Dev Comp Immunol* 1983;8:293–302.
457. Evans DL, McKinney C. Phylogeny of cytotoxic Cells. In: Warr GW, Cohen N, eds. *Phylogenesis of Immune Functions*, CRC Press, 1991, 215–240.
458. Harris DT, Jaso-Friedmann L, Devlin RB, Koren HS, Evans DL. Identification of an evolutionarily conserved, function-associated molecule on human natural killer cells. *Proc Natl Acad Sci USA* 1991;88:3009–3013.
459. Hogan RJ, Stuge TB, Clem LW, Miller NW, Chinchar VG. Anti-viral cytotoxic Cells in the channel catfish (*Ictalurus punctatus*). *Dev Comp Immunol* 1996;20:115–127.
460. Manning J, Horton JD. RES structure and function of the amphibia. In: Cohen N, Sigel MM, eds. *The Reticuloendothelial System: Phylogeny and Ontogeny*, vol. 3. New York: Plenum, 1982, 423–459.
461. Manning MJ. Histological organization of the spleen: implications for immune functions in amphibians. *Res Immunol* 1991;142:355–359.
462. Horton JD, Horton TL, Ritchie P. Immune system of *Xenopus*: T cell biology. In: Tinsley RC, H.R.Kobel, eds. *The Biology of* Xenopus, Oxford: Clarendon Press, 1996.
463. Alvarez R. An ultrastructural study of the spleen of the ranid frog Rana perezi. *J Morphol* 1990;204:25–32.
464. Miodonski AJ, Bigaj J, Mika J, Plytycz B. Season-specific thymic architecture in the frog, *Rana temporaria*. *Dev Comp Immunol* 1996;20:129–137.
465. Plytycz B, Mika J, Bigaj J. Age-dependent changes in thymuses in the european common frog, *Rana temporaria*. *J Exp Zool* 1995;273:451–460.
466. Garcia Barrutia MS, Leceta J, Fonfria J, Garrido E, Zapata A. Non-lymphoid cells of the anuran spleen: an ultrastructural study in the natterjack, *Bufo calamita*. *Am J Anat* 1983;167:83–94.
467. Hadji Azimi I, Coosemans V, Canicatti C. Atlas of adult *Xenopus* laevis laevis hematology. *Dev Comp Immunol* 1987;11:807–874.
468. Flajnik MF, Hsu E, Kaufman JF, Du Pasquier L. Changes in the immune system during metamorphosis of *Xenopus*. *Immunol Today* 1987;8:58–64.
469. Gravenor I, Horton TL, Ritchie P, Flint E, Horton JD. Ontogeny and thymus-dependence of T cell surface antigens in *Xenopus*: flow cytometric studies on monoclonal antibody-stained thymus and spleen. *Dev Comp Immunol* 1995;19:507–523.
470. Nagata S. A cell surface marker of thymus dependent lymphocytes in *Xenopus* laevis is identifiable by mouse monoclonal antibody. *Eur J Immunol* 1985;15:837–841.
471. Jurgens JB, Gartland LA, Du Pasquier L, Horton JD, Göbel TW, Cooper MD. Identification of a candidate CD5 homologue in the amphibian *Xenopus laevis*. *J Immunol* 1995;155:4218–4023.
472. Hsu E, Julius MH, Du Pasquier L. Effector and regulator functions of splenic and thymic lymphocytes in the clawed toad *Xenopus*. *Ann Immunol* 1983;3:277–292.
473. Blomberg B, Bernard CC, Du Pasquier L. In vitro evidence for T-B lymphocyte collaboration in the clawed toad, *Xenopus*. *Eur J Immunol* 1980;10:869–876.
474. James HS, Knowles KR, Clothier R, Groves CJ, Balls M. Effects of early thymectomy or exposure to N-methyl-N-nitrosaurea on immune responses in *Xenopus laevis*. In: Vago C, Matz G, eds. Comptes rendus du 1er colloque international de pathologie des reptiles et des amphibiens, Angers: University of Angers, 1982, 157–162.
475. Hsu E, Leanderson T, Franklin RM. Mitogenic effects of phorbol myristate acetate (PMA) on amphibian cells. *Ann Inst Pasteur Immunol* 1985;136d:105–118.
476. Du Pasquier L, Schwager J, Flajnik MF. The immune system of *Xenopus*. *Annu Rev Immunol* 1989;7:251–275.
477. Horton TL, Ritchie P, Watson MD, Horton JD. NK-like activity against allogeneic tumour cells demonstrated in the spleen of control and thymectomized *Xenopus*. *Immunol Cell Biol* 1996;74:365–373.
478. Robert J, Guiet C, Du Pasquier L. Lymphoid tumors of *Xenopus* laevis with different capacities for growth in larvae and adults. *Dev Immunol* 1994;3:297–307.
479. Klempau AE, Cooper EL. T-lymphocyte and B-lymphocyte dichtomy in anuran amphibians. III. Assessment and identification of inducible killer T lymphocytes (IKTL) and spontaneous killer T lymphocytes (SKTL). *Dev Comp Immunol* 1984;8:649–661.
480. Barritt LC, Turpen JB. Characterization of lineage restricted forms of a *Xenopus* CD45 homologue. *Dev Comp Immunol* 1995;19:525–536.
481. Tournefier A, Lesourd, M., Gounon, P. The axolotl thymus: Cell types of the microenvironment. *Cell Tissue Res* 1990;262:387–396.
482. Jordan H, Speidel,C.C. Studies on lymphocytes. granulocytopoiesis in the Salamander with special references to the monophyletic theory of blood Cell origin. *Am J Anat* 1924;33:485–505.
483. Salvadori F, Tournefier A. Activation by mitogens and superantigens of axolotl lymphocytes: functional characterization and ontogenic study. *Immunology* 1996;88:586–592.
484. Koniski AD, Cohen N. Reproducible proliferative responses of salamander (*Ambystoma mexicanum*) lymphocytes cultured with mitogens in serum-free medium. *Dev Comp Immunol* 1992;16:441–451.
485. Kerfourn F, Guillet F, Charlemagne J, Tournefier A. T- Cell-specific membrane antigens in the mexican axolotl (urodele amphibian). *Dev Immunol* 1992;2:237–248.

486. Kerfourn F, Guillet F, Charlemagne J, Tournefier A. Characterization of a multimeric polypeptide complex on the surface of thymus-derived cells in the mexican axolotl. *Scand J Immunol* 1993;38:381–387.

487. Kroese FG, van Rooijen N. The architecture of the spleen of the Red-eared Slider, *Chrysemys scripta elegans* (Reptilia, Testudines). *J Morphol* 1982;173: 279–284.

488. Kroese FG, Leceta J, Dopp EA, Herraez MP, Nieuwenhuis P, Zapata A. Dendritic immune complex trapping cells in the spleen of the snake, *Python reticulatus*. *Dev Comp Immunol* 1985;9:641–652.

489. Muthukkaruppan VR, Borysenko M, E. Ridi R. RES structure and function of the reptile. In: Cohen N, Sigel MM, eds. *The Reticuloendothelial System: Phylogeny and Ontogeny*, vol. 3. New York: Plenum, 1982, 461–508.

490. el Deeb S, Saad AH. Ontogeny of con A responsiveness and mixed leucocyte reactivity in the lizard, Chalcides o Cellatus. *Dev Comp Immunol* 1987;11:595–604.

491. El Ridi R, Zada S, Afifi A, et al. Cyclic changes in the differentiation of lymphoid cells in reptiles. *Cell Differ* 1988;24:1–8.

492. Glick B. RES structure and function of the aves. In: Cochen N, Sigel MM, eds. *The Reticuloendothelial System* vol. 3: Phylogeny and Ontogeny, vol. 3. New York: Plenum, 1983, 509–540.

493. Le Douarin N. The microenvironment of T and B lymphocyte differentiation in avian embryos. *Curr Top Dev Biol* 1986;20:291–313.

494. Jeurissen SH. Structure and function of the chicken spleen. *Res Immunol* 1991; 142:352–355.

495. Weinstein PD, Mage RG, Anderson AO. The appendix functions as a mammalian bursal equivalent in the developing rabbit. *Adv Exp Med Biol* 1994;249:253.

496. Liippo J, Lassila O. Avian Ikaros gene is expressed early in embryogenesis. *Eur J Immunol* 1997;27:1853–1857.

497. Hansen JD, Strassburger, P. Du Pasquier, L. Conservation of a master switch gene during vertebrate evolution: isolation and characterization of Ikaros from teleost and amphibian species. *Eur J Immunol* 1997;27:3049–3058.

498. Zon LI, Mather C, Burgess S, Bolce ME, Harland RM, Orkin SH. Expression of GATA-binding proteins during embryonic development in *Xenopus laevis*. *Proc Natl Acad Sci USA* 1991;88:10642–10646.

499. Schlake T, Schorpp M, Nehls M, Boehm T. The nude gene encodes a sequence-specific DNA binding protein with homologs in organisms that lack an anticipatory immune system. *Proc Natl Acad Sci USA* 1997;94:3842–3847.

500. Hansen JD, Kaattari SL. The recombination activating gene 1 (RAG1) of rainbow trout (*Oncorhynchus mykiss*): cloning, expression, and phylogenetic analysis. *Immunogenetics* 1995;42:188–195.

501. Willett CE, Cherry JJ, Steiner LA. Characterization and expression of the recombination activating genes (rag1 and rag2) of zebrafish. *Immunogenetics* 1997;45: 394–404

502. Lee A, Hsu F. Isolation and characterization of the *Xenopus* terminal deoxynucleotidyl transferase. *J Immunol* 1994;152:4500–4507.

503. Yang B, Gathy KN, Coleman MS. T-cell specific avian TdT: characterization of the cDNA and recombinant enzyme. *Nucleic Acids Res* 1995;23:2041–2048.

504. Magor BG, Wilson MR, Miller NW, Clem LW, Middleton DL, Warr GW. An Ig heavy chain enhancer of the channel catfish Ictalurus punctatus: evolutionary conservation of function but not structure. *J Immunol* 1994;153:5556–5563.

505. Magor BG, Ross DA, Middleton DL, Warr GW. Functional motifs in the IgH enhancer of the channel catfish. *Immunogenetics* 1997;46:192–198.

506. Michard-Vanhèe C, Chourrout D, Strömberg S, Thuvander A, Pilström L. Lymphocyte expression in transgenic trout by mouse immunoglobulin promoter/enhancer. *Immunogenetics* 1994;40:1–8

507. Alt FW, Oltz EM, Young F, Gorman J, Taccioli G, Chen J. VDJ recombination. *Immunol Today* 1992;13:306–314.

508. Colonna M. Specificity and function of immunoglobulin superfamily NKCellinhibitory and stimulatory receptors. *Immunol Rev* 1997;155:127–133.

509. Secombes CJ. Phylogeny of Cytokines. *Cytokine Handbook*, 3rd ed., 1998.

510. Beck G, Habicht GS. Isolation and characterization of a primitive interleukin-1-like protein from an invertebrate, *Asterias forbesi*. *Proc Natl Acad Sci USA* 1986; 83:7429–7433.

511. Beck G, Vasta GR, Marchalonis JJ, Habicht GS. Characterization of interleukin-1 activity in tunicates. *Comp Biochem Physiol B* 1989;92:93–98.

512. Hughes TK, Jr., Smith EM, Barnett JA, Charles R, Stefano GB. LPS stimulated invertebrate hemocytes: a role for immunoreactive TNF and IL-1. *Dev Comp Immunol* 1991;15:117–122.

513. Granath WO, Jr., Connors VA, Tarleton RL. Interleukin 1 activity in haemolymph from strains of the snail *Biomphalaria glabrata* varying in susceptibility to the human blood fluke, *Schistosoma mansoni*: presence, differential expression, and biological function. *Cytokine* 1994;6:21–27.

514. Beck G, Habicht GS. Primitive cytokines: harbingers of vertebrate defense. *Immunol Today* 1991;12:180–183.

515. Clem LW, Miller NW, Bly JE. Evolution of lymphocyte subpopulations, their interactions and temperature sensitivities. In: Warr GW, Cohen N, eds. *Phylogenesis of Immune Functions*, CRC press, 1991, 241–268.

516. Zou J, Cunningham C, Secombes CJ. Rainbow trout recombinant interleukin 1b: expression, renaturation and determination of the biological activities. *Devel Comp Immunol* 27 1997:192.

517. Watkins D, Parsons SC, Cohen N. A factor with interleukin-1-like activity is produced by peritoneal Cells from the frog, *Xenopus laevis*. *Immunology* 1981;62: 669–673.

518. Hayari Y, Schauenstein K, Globerson A. Avian lymphokines, II: interleukin-1

519. Guida S, Heguy A, Melli M. The chicken IL-1 receptor: differential evolution of the cytoplasmic and extra cellular domains. *Gene* 1992;111:239–243.

520. Schneider DS, Hudson KL, Lin TY, Anderson KV. Dominant and recessive mutations define functional domains of toll, a transmembrane protein required for dorsal-ventral polarity in the *Drosophila* embryo. *Genes Dev* 1991;5:797–807.

521. Legac E, Vaugier GL, Bousquet F, Bajclan M, Leclerc M. Primitive cytokines and cytokine receptors in invertebrates: the sea star *Asterias rubens* as a model of study. *Scand J Immunol* 1996;44:375–380.

522. Caspi RR, Avtalion RR. Evidence for the existence of an IL-2-like lymphocyte growth promoting factor in a bony fish, *Cyprinus carpio*. *Dev Comp Immunol* 1984;8:51–60.

523. Watkins D, Cohen N. Mitogen-activated *Xenopus laevis* lymphocytes produce a T-cell growth factor. *Immunology* 1987;62:119–125.

524. El Ridi R, Wahby AF, Saad AH, Soliman MA. Concanavalin A responsiveness and interleukin 2 production in the snake *Spalerosophis diadema*. *Immunobiology* 1987;174:177–189.

525. Schauenstein K, Kromer G, Hala K, Bock G, Wick G. Chicken-activated-T-lymphocyte-antigen (CATLA) recognized by monoclonal antibody INN-CH 16 represents the IL-2 receptor. *Dev Comp Immunol* 1988;12:823–831.

526. Hussein MF, Badir N, El Ridi R, Akef M. Lymphoid tissue of the snake, *Spalerosophis diadema*, in the different seasons. *Dev Comp Immunol* 1979;3: 77–88.

527. Haynes L, Cohen N. Further characterization of an interleukin-2-like cytokine produced by *Xenopus laevis* T lymphocytes. *Dev Immunol* 1993;3:231–238.

528. Kroemer G, Gastinel LN, Neu N, Auffray C, Wick G. How many genes code for organ-specific autoimmunity? *Autoimmunity* 1990;6:215–233.

529. Boehm U, Klamp T, Groot M, Howard JC. Cellular responses to interferon-gamma. *Annu Rev Immunol* 1997;15:749–795.

530. Georgel P, Kappler C, Langley E, et al. Drosophila immunity. A sequence homologous to mammalian interferon consensus response element enhances the activity of the diptericin promoter. *Nucleic Acids Res* 1995;23:1140–1145.

531. Rogel-Gaillard C, Chilmonczyk S, de Kinkelin P. in vitro induction of interferon-like activity from rainbow trout leucocytes stimulated by Egtved virus. *Fish & Shellfish Immunol* 1993;3:383–394.

532. De Kinkelin P, Dorson M, Hatenberger-Baudouy AM. Interferon synthesis in trout and carp after viral infection. *Dev Comp Immunol* 1982;2:167–174.

533. Mathews JH, Vorndam AV. Interferon-mediated persistent infection of Saint Louis encephalitis virus in a reptilian cell line. *J Gen Virol* 1982;61:177–186.

534. Sick C, Schultz U, Staeheli P. A family of genes coding for two serologically distinct chicken interferons. *J Biol Chem* 1996;271:7635–7639.

535. Graham S, Secombes CJ. The production of a macrophage-activating factor from rainbow trout *Salmo gairdneri* leucocytes. *Immunology* 1988;65:293–297.

536. Lowenthal JW, Digby MR, York JJ. Production of interferon-gamma by chicken T cells. *J Interferon Cytokine Res* 1995;15:933–938.

537. Digby MR, Lowenthal JW. Cloning and expression of the chicken interferon-gamma gene. *J Interferon Cytokine Res* 1995;15:939–945.

538. Jang SI, Hardie LJ, Secombes CJ. Effects of transforming growth factor beta 1 on rainbow trout *Oncorhynchus mykiss* macrophage respiratory burst activity. *Dev Comp Immunol* 1994;18:315–323.

539. Jang SI, Hardie LJ, Secombes CJ. Elevation of rainbow trout *Oncorhynchus mykiss* macrophage respiratory burst activity with macrophage-derived supernatants. *J Leukoc Biol* 1995;57:943–947.

540. Haynes L, Cohen N. Transforming growth factor beta (TGF beta) is produced by and influences the proliferative response of *Xenopus laevis* lymphocytes. *Dev Immunol* 1993;3:223–230.

541. O'Shea JJ. Jaks, STATs, cytokine signal transduction, and immunoregulation: are we there yet? *Immunity* 1997;7:1–11.

542. Lundin L. Evolution of the vertebrate genome as reflected in paralogous chromosomal regions in man and the mouse mouse. *Genomics* 1993;16:1–19.

543. Flajnik M, Du Pasquier L. T- Cell differentiation in lower vertebrates. Progress in immunology 1989;7:274–281.

544. Medzhitov R, Janeway CA, Jr. Innate immunity: impact on the adaptive immune response. *Curr Opin Immunol* 1997;9:4–9.

545. Vasta GR, Ahmed H, Fink NE, et al. Animal lectins as self/non-self recognition molecules. Biochemical and genetic approaches to understanding their biological roles and evolution. *Ann NY Acad Sci* 1994;712:55–73.

546. Ezekowitz RAB, Hoffmann JA. Innate immunity. *Curr Opin Immunol* 1996;8:1–2.

547. Hildemann WH, Thoenes GH. Immunological responses of Pacific hagfish. I. Skin transplantation immunity. *Transplantation* 1969;7:506–521.

548. Kasahara M, Vasquez M, Sato K, Chruchill-McKinney E, Flajnik MF. Evolution of the major histocompatibility complex: isolation of class II A cDNA clones from the cartilaginous fish. *Proc Natl Acad Sci USA* 1992;89:6688–6692.

549. Okamura K, Ototake M, Nakanishi T, Kurosawa Y, Hashimoto K. The most primitive vertebrates with jaws possess highly polymorphic class I genes comparable to those of human. *Immunity* 1997;7:777–787.

550. Hildemann WH. Tissue transplantation immunity in the goldfish. *Immunology* 1958;1:46–53.

551. Miller NW, Sizemore RC, Clem LW. Phylogeny of lymphocyte heterogeneity: the Cellular requirements for in vitro antibody responses of channel leukocytes. *J Immunol* 1985;134:2884–2888.

552. Dixon B, van Erp SH, Rodrigues PN, Egberts E, Stet RJ. Fish major histocompatibility complex genes: an expansion. *Dev Comp Immunol* 1995;19: 109–133.

553. Klein D, Ono H, O'Huigin C, Vincek V, Goldschmidt T, Klein J. Extensive MHC variability in cichlid fishes of Lake Malawi. *Nature* 1993;364:330–334.

554. Hordvik I, Grimholt U, Fosse VM, Lie O, Endresen C. Cloning and sequence analysis of cDNAs encoding the MHC class II beta chain in Atlantic salmon (*Salmo salar*). *Immunogenetics* 1993;37:437–441.

555. Takeuchi H, Figueroa F, O'Huigin C, Klein J. Cloning and characterization of class I Mhc genes of the zebrafish, *Brachydanio rerio*. *Immunogenetics* 1995;42: 77–84.

556. Grimholt U, Hordvik I, Fosse VM, Olsaker I, Endresen C, Lie O. Molecular cloning of major histocompatibility complex class I cDNAs from Atlantic salmon (*Salmo salar*). *Immunogenetics* 1993;37:469–473.

557. Betz UA, Mayer WE, Klein J. Major histocompatibility complex class I genes of the coelacanth *Latimeria chalumnae*. *Proc Natl Acad Sci USA* 1994;91: 11065–11069.

558. Flajnik MF, Du Pasquier L. The major histocompatibility complex of frogs. *Immunol Rev* 1990;113:47–63.

559. Flajnik MF, Ferrone S, Cohen N, Du Pasquier L. Evolution of the MHC : antigenicity and unusual tissue distribution of *Xenopus* (frog) class II molecules. *Mol Immunol* 1990;27:451–462.

560. Kaufman JF, Flajnik MF, Du Pasquier L, Riegert P. *Xenopus* MHC class II molecules. I. Identification and structural characterization. *J Immunol* 1985;134: 3248–3257.

561. Sato K, Flajnik MF, Du Pasquier L, Katagiri M, Kasahara M. Evolution of the MHC: isolation of class II beta-chain cDNA clones from the amphibian *Xenopus laevis*. *J Immunol* 1993;150:2831–2843.

562. Flajnik MF, Kaufman JF, Riegert P, Du Pasquier L. Identification of class I major histocompatibility complex encoded molecules in the amphibian *Xenopus*. *Immunogenetics* 1984;20:433–442.

563. Flajnik MF, Taylor E, Canel C, Grossberger D, Du Pasquier L. Reagent specific for MHC I antigens of *Xenopus*. *Amer Zool* 1991;31:580–591.

564. Cohen N. Salamanders and the evolution of the major histocompatibility complex. In: Marchalonis JJ, Cohen J, eds. *Current topics in immunology*, vol 9 New York: Plenum Press, 1980, 109–140.

565. Kaufman J, Ferrone S, Flajnik M, Kilb M, Volk H, Parisot R. MHC-like molecules in some nonmammalian vertebrates can be detected by some cross-reactive monoclonal antibodies. *J Immunol* 1990;144:2273–2280.

566. Farag MA, el Ridi R. Mixed leucocyte reaction (MLR) in the snake *Psammophis sibilans*. *Immunology* 1985;55:173-181.

567. Farag MA. A contribution to the study of the major histocompatibility complex in snakes. PhD thesis, University of Cairo, Egypt, 1987.

568. Farag MA, el Ridi R. Functional markers of the major histocompatibility gene complex of snakes. *Eur J Immunol* 1990;20:2029-2033.

569. Houssaint E, Torano A, Ivanyi J. Split tolerance induced by chick embryo thymic epithelium allografted to embryonic recipients. *J Immunol* 1986;136:3155-3159.

570. Toivanen A, Toivanen P. Histocompatibility response for cellular cooperation in the chicken: generation of germinal centers. *J Immunol* 1977;118:431-436.

571. Kaufman J. unpublished.

572. Miller MM, Goto R, Bernot A, et al. Two Mhc class I and two Mhc class II genes map to the chicken Rfp-Y system outside the B complex. *Proc Natl Acad Sci USA* 1994;91:4397–4401.

573. Juul-Madsen HR, Zoorob R, Auffray C, Skjodt K, Hedemand JE. New chicken Rfp-Y haplotypes on the basis of MHC class II RFLP and MLC analyses. *Immunogenetics* 1997;45:345–352.

574. Briles WE, McGibbons WH, Irwin MR. On multiple alleles affecting cellular antigens in the chicken. *Genetics* 1950;35:633–652.

575. Goto R, Miyada CG, Young S, et al. Isolation of a cDNA clone from the B-G subregion of the chicken histocompatibility (B) complex. *Immunogenetics* 1988; 27:102–109.

576. Kaufman J, Salomonsen J. B-G: we know what it is, but what does it do? *Immunol Today* 1992;13:1–3.

577. Kaufman J. Personal communication.

578. Liu Y and Flajnik MF. Unpublished.

579. Hardee JJ, Godwin U, Benedetto R, McConnell TJ. Major histocompatibility complex class II A gene polymorphism in the striped bass. *Immunogenetics* 1995;41:229–238.

580. Klein J, Figueroa F, Klein D, Sato A, O'hUigin C. Major histocompatibility complex genes in the study of fish phylogeny. In: Kocher TD, Stepien CA, eds. *Molecular Systematics of Fishes*, San Diego, California: Academic Press, 1997, 271–283.

581. Ono H, O'HUigin C, Vincek V, Stet RJ, Figueroa F, Klein J. New beta chain-encoding Mhc class II genes in the carp. *Immunogenetics* 1993;38:146–149.

582. Tomko RP, Xu R, Philipson L. HCAR and MCAR: the human and mouse Cellular receptors for subgroup C adenoviruses and group B coxsackieviruses. *Proc Natl Acad Sci USA* 1997;94:3352–3356.

583. Dohring C, Samaridis J, Colonna M. Alternatively spliced forms of human killer inhibitory receptors. *Immunogenetics* 1996;44:227–230.

584. Miyauchi T, Kanekura T, Yamaoka A, Ozawa M, Miyazawa S, Muramatsu T. Basigin, a new, broadly distributed member of the immunoglobulin superfamily, has strong homology with both the immunoglobulin V domain and the beta-chain of major histocompatibility complex class II antigen. *J Biochem Tokyo* 1990;107:316–323.

585. Schacke H, Rinkevich B, Gamulin V, Müller IM, Müller WE. Immunoglobulin-like domain is present in the extra cellular part of the receptor tyrosine kinase from the marine sponge *Geodia cydonium*. *J Mol Recognit* 1994;7:273–276.

586. Patel NH, Snow PM, Goodman CS. Characterization and cloning of fasciclin III: a glycoprotein expressed on a subset of neurons and axon pathways in *Drosophila*. *Cell* 1987;48:975–988.

587. Saper MA, Bjorkman PJ, Wiley DC. Refined structure of the human histocompatibility antigen HLA-A2 at 2.6 Å resolution. *J Mol Biol* 1991;219: 277–319.

588. Takami K, Zaleska-Rutczynska Z, Figueroa F, Klein J. Linkage of LMP, TAP and Ring 3 with MHC class I rather than class II genes in the zebrafish. *J Immunol* 1997;159:6052–6060.

589. Hisamatsu H, Shimbara N, Saito Y, et al. Newly identified pair of proteasomal subunits regulated reciprocally by interferon gamma. *J Exp Med* 1996;183: 1807–1816.

590. Haas IG, Wabl M. Immunoglobulin heavy chain binding protein. *Nature* 1983; 306:387–389.

591. Lambris J. personal communication.

Fundamental Immunology, Fourth Edition,
edited by William E. Paul
Published by Lippincott–Raven Publishers, Philadelphia 1999.

CHAPTER 19

Immunogenicity and Antigen Structure

Jay A. Berzofsky and Ira J. Berkower

THE NATURE OF ANTIGENIC DETERMINANTS RECOGNIZED BY ANTIBODIES

Haptens

In the antigen–antibody binding reaction, the antibody-binding site is often unable to accommodate the entire antigen. The part of the antigen that is the target of antibody binding is called an antigenic determinant, and there may be one or more antigenic determinants per molecule. To study antibody specificity, we need to have antibodies against single antigenic determinants. Small functional groups that correspond to a single antigenic determinant are called haptens. For example, these may be organic compounds, such as trinitrophenyl (TNP) or benzene arsonate, a mono- or oligosaccharide such as glucose or lactose, or an oligopeptide such as pentalysine. Although these haptens can bind to antibody, immunization with them usually will not provoke an antibody response, with some exceptions (1). Immunogenicity often can be achieved by covalently attaching haptens to a larger molecule, called the carrier. The carrier is immunogenic in its own right, and immunization with the hapten–carrier conjugate elicits an antibody response to both hapten and carrier. However, the antibodies specific for hapten can be studied by equilibrium dialysis using pure hapten (without carrier) or by immunoprecipitation using hapten coupled to a different (and non–cross-reacting) carrier, or by inhibition of precipitation with free hapten.

This technique was pioneered by Landsteiner (2) and helped to elucidate the exquisite specificity of antibodies for antigenic determinants. For instance, the relative binding affinity of antibodies

prepared against succinic acid–serum protein conjugates shows marked specificity for the maleic acid analog, which is in the cis configuration, as compared to the fumaric acid (trans) form (3). Presumably, the immunogenic form of succinic acid corresponds to the cis form (3). This ability of antibodies to distinguish cis from trans configurations was reemphasized in later studies measuring relative affinities of antibodies to maleic and fumaric acid conjugates (4) (Table 1A). Table 1B shows the specificity of antibodies prepared against p-azobenzene arsonate coupled to bovine gamma globulin (5). Because the hapten is coupled through the p-azo group to aromatic amino acids of the carrier, haptens containing bulky substitutions in the para position would most resemble the immunizing antigen. In fact, p-methyl–substituted benzene arsonate has a higher binding affinity than unsubstituted benzene arsonate. However, methyl substitution elsewhere in the benzene ring reduces affinity, presumably due to interference with the way hapten fits into the antibody-binding site. Thus, methyl substitutions can have positive or negative effects on binding energy, depending on where the substitution occurs. Table 1C shows the specificity of antilactose antibodies for lactose versus cellobiose (6). These disaccharides differ only by the orientation of the hydroxyl attached to C4 of the first sugar either above or below the hexose ring. The three examples in this table, as well as many others (1), show the marked specificity of antibodies for cis–trans, ortho–meta–para, and stereoisomeric forms of the antigenic determinant.

Comparative binding studies of haptens have been able to demonstrate antibody specificity despite the marked heterogeneity of antibodies. Unlike the antibodies against a multideterminant antigen, the population of antibodies specific for a single hapten determinant is a relatively restricted population, due to the shared structural constraints necessary for hapten to fit within the antibody-combining site. However, the specificity of an antiserum depends on the collective specificities of the entire population of antibodies, which are determined by the structures of the various antibody-binding sites. When studying the cross-reactions of hap-

J. A. Berzofsky: Molecular Immunogenetics and Vaccine Research Section, Metabolism Branch, National Cancer Institute, National Institutes of Health, Bethesda, Maryland 20892.

I. J. Berkower: Laboratory of Immunoregulation, Office of Vaccines, Center for Biologics, Food and Drug Administration, Bethesda, Maryland 20892.

TABLE 1. *Exquisite specificity of anti-hapten antibodies*

Hapten	Structure	K_{ral} of antibody specific for	
A.		Maleic (cis)	Fumaric (trans)
Maleanilate		1.0	<0.01
Fumaranilate		<0.01	1.0
B.		Parasubstituted benzene arsonate	
Benzene arsonate		1.0	
o-Methyl benzene arsonate		0.2	
m-Methyl benzene arsonate		0.8	
p-Methyl benzene arsonate		1.9	
C.		Lactose	
Lactose	β gal (1 → 4) glu	1.00	
Cellobiose	β glu (1 → 4) glu	0.0025	

Part A from ref. 4; part B from ref. 5; and part C from ref. 6, with permission.

ten analogs, some haptens bind all antibodies, but with reduced K_A. Other hapten analogs reach a plateau of binding because they fit some antibody-combining sites quite well but not others (see discussion of cross-reactivity in Chapter 4). Antibodies raised in different animals may show different cross-reactivities with related haptens. Even within a single animal, antibody affinity and specificity are known to increase over time after immunization under certain conditions (7). Thus, any statements about the cross-reactivity of two haptens reflect both structural differences between the haptens that affect antigen–antibody fit and the diversity of antibody-binding sites present in a given antiserum.

Carbohydrate Antigens

The antigenic determinants of a number of biologically important substances consist of carbohydrates. These often occur as glycolipids or glycoproteins. Examples of the former include bacterial cell wall antigens and the major blood group antigens, whereas the latter group includes "minor" blood group antigens such as Rh. In addition, a number of spontaneously arising myeloma proteins have been found to show carbohydrate specificity, possibly reflecting the fact that carbohydrates are common environmental antigens. In the days before hybridoma technology, these carbohydrate-specific myeloma proteins provided an important model for studying the reaction of antigen with a monoclonal antibody.

Empirically, the predominant antigenic determinants of polysaccharides often consist of short oligosaccharides (one to five sugars long) at the nonreducing end of the polymer chain (8). This situation is analogous to a hapten consisting of several sugar residues linked to a large nonantigenic polysaccharide backbone. The remainder of the polysaccharide is important for immunogenicity, just as the carrier molecule was important for haptens. In addition, branch points in the polysaccharide structure allow for multiple antigenic determinants to be attached to the same macromolecule. This is important for immunoprecipitation by lattice formation, as discussed in Chapter 4. Several examples illustrating structural studies of oligosaccharide antigens are given later.

The technique used most widely to analyze the antigenic determinants of polysaccharides is called hapten inhibition (8). In this method, the precipitation reaction between antigen and antibody is inhibited by adding short oligosaccharides. These oligosaccharides are large enough to bind with the same affinity and specificity as the polysaccharide, but because they are monomeric, no precipitate forms. As more inhibitor is added, fewer antibody-combining sites remain available for precipitation. Using antiserum specific for a single antigenic determinant, it is often possible to block precipitation completely with a short oligosaccharide corresponding to the nonreducing end of the polysaccharide chain. Besides showing the "immunodominance" of the nonreducing end of the chain, this result also shows that the structure of the antigenic determinant of polysaccharides depends on the sequence of carbohydrates and their linkage, rather than their conformation. For inhibition by hapten to be complete, the antigen–antibody system studied must be made specific for a single antigenic determinant. For optimal sensitivity, the equivalence point of antigen and antibody should be used.

We illustrate the types of carbohydrate antigens encountered by examining three classic examples in more detail: the salmonella O antigens, the blood group antigens, and dextrans that bind to myeloma proteins.

Immunochemistry of Salmonella O Antigens

The antigenic diversity among numerous salmonella species resides in the structural differences of the lipopolysaccharide (LPS) component of the outer membrane (9). These molecules are the main target for antisalmonella antibodies. The polysaccharide moiety contains the antigenic determinant, whereas the lipid moiety is responsible for endotoxin effects. The chemical structure of LPS can be divided into three regions (Fig. 1). Region I contains the antigenic O specific polysaccharide, usually made up of repeated oligosaccharide units, which vary widely among different strains. Region II contains an oligosaccharide "common core" shared among many different strains. Failure to synthesize region II oligosaccharide or to couple completed region I polysaccharide to the growing region II core results in R (rough) mutants, which have "rough" colony morphology and lack the O antigen. Region III is the lipid part, called lipid A, which is shared among all salmonellae and serves to anchor LPS on the outer membrane. Early immunologic attempts to classify the O antigens of different salmonellae showed a large number of cross-reactions between different strains. These were detected by preparing antiserum to one strain of salmonella and using it to agglutinate bacteria of a second strain. Each cross-reacting determinant was assigned a number, and each strain was characterized by a series of O antigen determinants (in aggregate, the serotype of the strain) based on its pattern of cross-reactivity. Each strain was classified within a group, based on sharing a strong O determinant. For example, group A strains share determinant 2, whereas group B strains share determinant 4 (Table 2). However, within a group, each strain possesses additional O deter-

A. Core Oligosaccharide Structure (Region II)

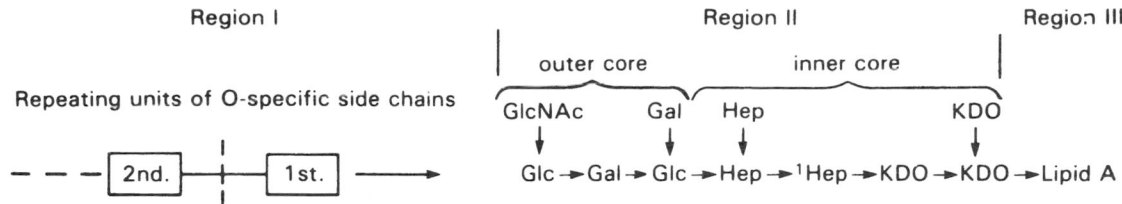

B. Oligosaccharide Antigens (Region I)

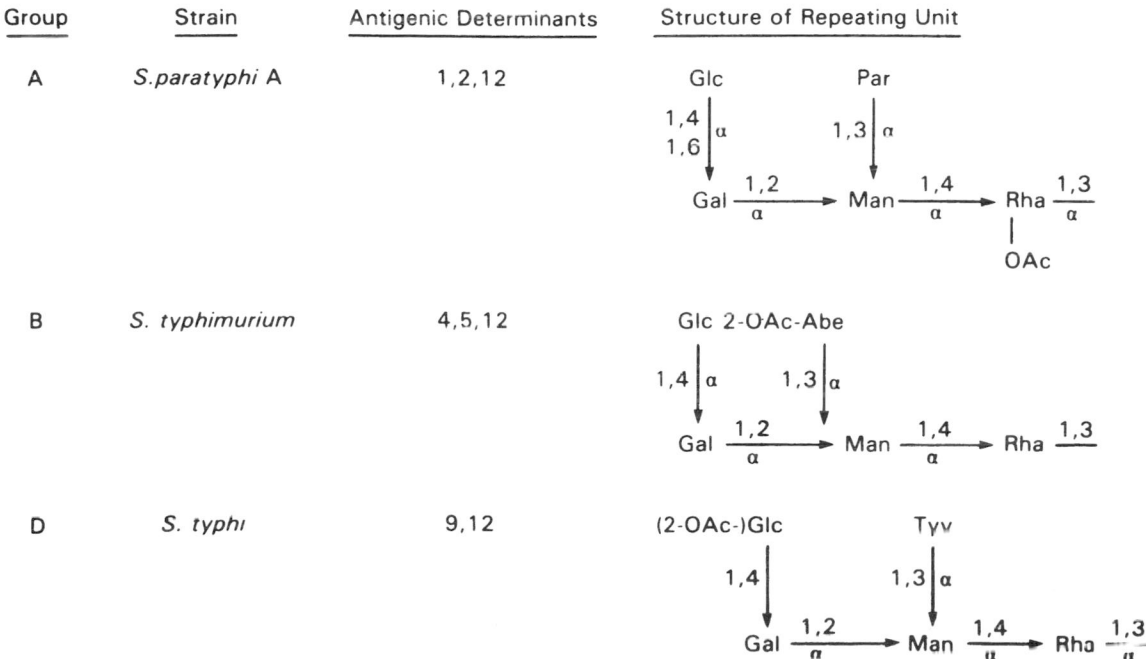

FIG. 1. Structure of salmonella lipopolysaccharide. Region I contains the unique O-antigen determinants, which consist of repeating units of oligosaccharides. These are attached to lipid moiety through the core polysaccharide. Three examples of oligosaccharide units are shown (9). Part A adapted with permission (8); part B based on the data of Jann and Westphal (9).

minants, which serve to differentiate it from other members of that group. Thus, determinant 2 coexists with determinants 1 and 12 on *Salmonella paratyphi A*. This problem of cross-reactivity based on sharing of a subset of antigenic determinants is commonly encountered in complex antigen–antibody systems. The problem may be simplified by making antibodies monospecific for individual antigenic determinants. To do this, antibodies are absorbed to remove irrelevant specificities, or cross-reactive strains are chosen that share only a single determinant with the immunizing strain. The reaction of each determinant with its specific antibody can be thought of as an antigen–antibody system. Thus, for the strains shown in Table 2, antiserum to *Salmonella typhi* (containing anti-9 and anti-12 antibodies) may be absorbed with *S. paratyphi A* to remove anti-12, leaving a reagent specific for antigen 9 (Table 2). Alternatively, the unabsorbed antiserum may be used to study the system antigen 12–anti-12 by allowing it to agglutinate *S. paratyphi B*, which shares only antigen 12 with the immunogen. Because the other determinants on *S. paratyphi B* were absent from the immunizing strain, the antiserum contains no antibodies to them.

Once the antigen–antibody reaction is made specific for a single determinant, a variety of oligosaccharides can be added to test for hapten inhibition. Since the O antigens contain repeating oligosaccharide units, it is often possible to obtain model oligosaccharides by mild chemical or enzymatic degradation of the LPS polysaccharide

TABLE 2. *Salmonella Q antigen serotyping*

Salmonella strain	Sero group	O antigenic determinants
S. paratyphi A	A	1, 2, 12
S. paratyphi B	B	1, 4, 5, 12
S. typhi	D	9, 12

Antiserum	Absorbed	Tested on	Single determinant measured
Anti-S. typhi	—	S. paratyphi B	12
Anti-S. typhi	S. paratyphi A	S. typhi	9

Reprinted with permission (8).

TABLE 3. *Analysis of salmonella O-antigen structure by hapten inhibition*

Maximum inhibition by hapten (%)	Antigen system	
	1.anti-1	19.anti-19
D-Glu	—	0
Me-α-D-Glu	35	10
α-D-Glu(1 → 6)-D-Gal	80	25
Glu.Gal.Man	80	70
Glu.Gal.Man.L-Rham	>70	>70
Deduced structure	α-D-Glu(1 → 6)-D-Gal	D-Glu-D-Gal-D-Man-L-Rham

Reprinted with permission (8).

itself. Once the most inhibitory oligosaccharide is found, its chemical structure is determined. Alternatively, a variety of synthetic mono-, di-, tri-, and oligosaccharides are tested for hapten inhibition of precipitation. For example, as shown in Table 3, antigen 1–anti-1 antibody precipitation is inhibited by methyl-α-D-glucoside. Therefore, various disaccharides incorporating this structure were tested, of which α-D-Glu(1 → 6)D-Gal was the most inhibitory. Then various trisaccharides incorporating this sequence were tested. The results indicate the sequence and size of the determinant recognized by anti-1 antibodies to be a disaccharide with the above structure. The test sequences can be guessed by analyzing the oligosaccharide breakdown products of the lipopolysaccharide, which include tetramers of D-Glu-D-Gal-D-Man-L-Rham. The results in Table 3 also suggest that the difference between determinants 1 and 19 is the length of oligosaccharide recognized by antibodies specific for each determinant. This hypothesis is supported by the observation that determinant 1 is found in some strains with, and in other strains without, determinant 19, whereas determinant 19 is always found with determinant 1. As shown in Table 3, determinant 19 requires the full tetrasaccharide for maximal hapten inhibition, including the sequence coding for determinant 1. Besides identifying the antigenic structures, these results indicate that there is variation in the size of different antigenic determinants of polysaccharides.

Genetic studies of the effect of phage lysogeny on salmonella polysaccharide antigens (10) have shown that sequential chemical modifications at the nonreducing end of the polysaccharide can cause stepwise changes in serotype (Table 4). Thus, phage E15 converts *Salmonella anatum* O antigen from determinants 3,10 to 3,15, whereas subsequent lysogeny with phage E34 converts the O antigen to determinant 34. Hapten inhibition studies show completely different patterns for all three O antigens. The first lysogeny removes the terminal acetylation of galactose and changes the disaccharide bond from α(1 → 6) to β(1 → 6). This removes determinant 10, while adding determinant 15. The subsequent lysogeny uses β-D-Gal as an acceptor for an additional D-Glu. This removes O antigen determinant 15 and adds determinant 34. In each case, removing an acetyl group and changing the first disaccharide linkage, or adding an additional sugar, changes the O antigen determinant, because the terminal sugar is immunodominant. The biochemical alteration induced by the phage is presumably due to the production of a glycosyltransferase adding the new sugar. This enzyme may be encoded by a phage gene or by a derepressed endogenous bacterial gene.

Blood Group Antigens

The major blood group antigens A and B were originally detected by the ability of serum from individuals lacking either determinant to agglutinate red blood cells bearing them (8,11–13). In addition, group O individuals have an H antigenic determinant that is not detectable on A- or B-type red blood cells, and individuals in all three groups may have additional determinants such as the Lewis (Le) antigens. Although the ABH and Le antigenic determinants are found on a carbohydrate moiety, the carbohydrate may

TABLE 4. *Stepwise changes in serotype of* S. anatum *due to phage lysogeny represents successive alterations at the nonreducing end*

Hapten concentration causing 50% inhibition (mM)	Antigen–antibody system tested		
	10.anti-10	15.anti-15	34.anti-34
AcO-Gal Man L-Rham	0.013	ND	ND
Gal-Man L-Rham	>1.6	0.005	0.16
Gal-Man	—[a]	0.027	≥0.2
Man L-Rham	—[a]	0.083	≥0.2
Glu-Gal-Man	—[a]	0.027	0.05
Glu-Gal	—[a]	1.0	0.10
Deduced structure			
Antigen 10	AcO-Galα(1 → 6)Manα(1 → 4) L-Rham		
Phage E15 ↓			
Antigen 15	Galβ(1 → 6)Manα(1 → 4) L-Rham		
Phage E34 ↓			
Antigen 34	α-D-Gluα(1 → 4)Galβ(1 → 6) Man		

Reprinted with permission (10).
ND, not done.
[a]No inhibition at any concentration tested

occur in a variety of biochemical forms. On cell surfaces, they are either glycolipids that are synthesized within the cell (AB and H antigens) or glycoproteins taken up from serum (Lewis antigens). In mucinous secretions, such as saliva, they occur as glycoproteins. Milk, ovarian cyst fluid, and gastric mucosa are a source of soluble oligosaccharides containing blood group reactivity. In addition, these antigens occur frequently in other species, including about half of the bacteria in the normal flora of the gut (11). This widespread occurrence may account for the ubiquitous anti-AB reactivity of human sera, even in people never previously exposed to human blood group substances through transfusion or pregnancy.

The immunochemistry of these antigens was simplified greatly by the fact that antigenic oligosaccharides could be used for hapten inhibition studies. Group A oligosaccharides, for example, would inhibit the agglutination of group A red blood cells by anti-A antibodies. They could also inhibit the immunoprecipitation of

group A–bearing glycoproteins by anti-A antibodies. Because the oligosaccharides are monomeric, their reaction with antibody does not form a precipitate but does block an antibody-combining site.

The inhibitory oligosaccharides from cyst fluid were purified and found to contain d-galactose, l-fucose, N-acetyl galactosamine, and N-acetylglucosamine. The most inhibitory oligosaccharides for each antigen are indicated in Fig. 2. As seen in Fig. 2, the ABH and Le antigens all share a common oligosaccharide core sequence, and the antigens appear to differ from each other by the sequential addition of individual sugars at the end or at branch points. Besides hapten inhibition, other biochemical data support this relationship among the different determinants. Enzymatic digestion of A, B, or H antigens yields a common core oligosaccharide from each. This product cross-reacts with antiserum specific for pneumococcal polysaccharide type XIV, which contains structural elements shared with blood group determinants, as

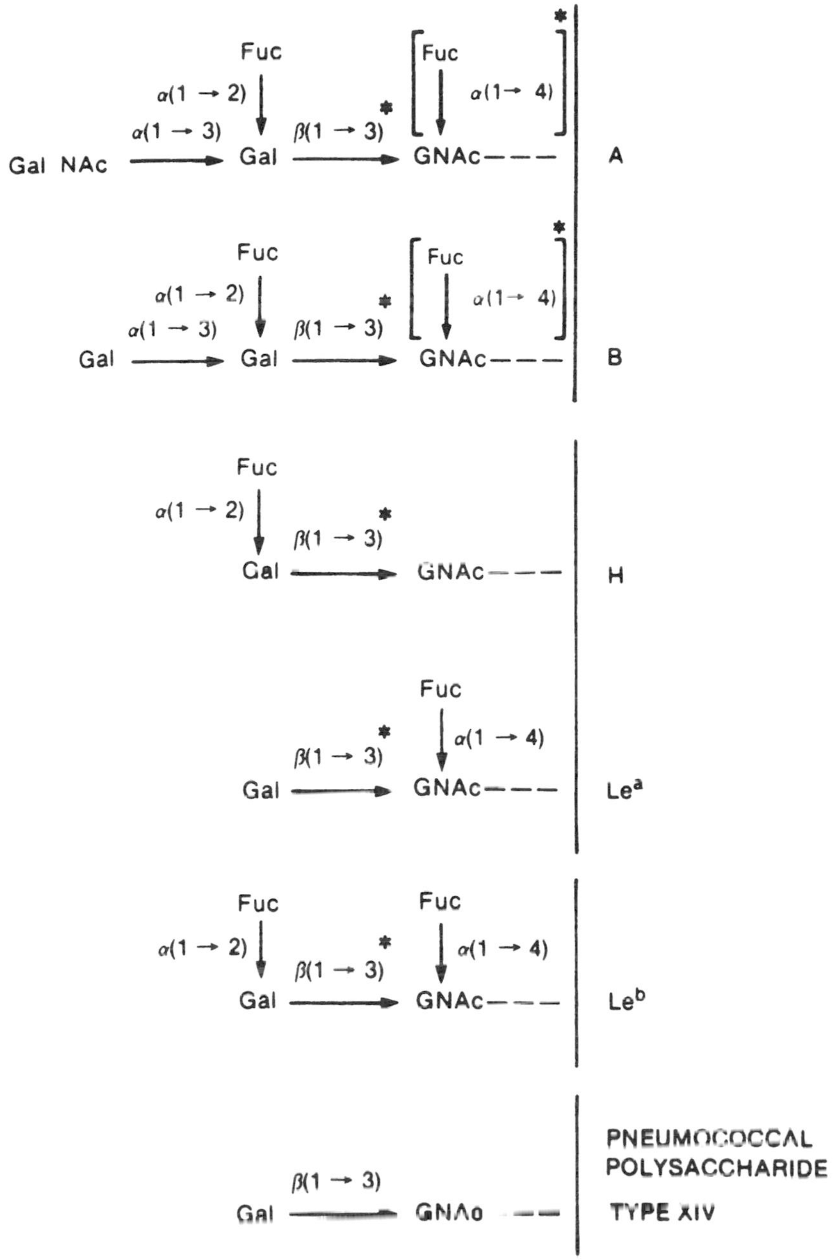

FIG. 2. Oligosaccharide chain specificity. Structure of the ABH and Le blood group antigens, as determined by hapten inhibition studies (8,12). There are two variants of each of these determinants. In type 1, the Gal-GNAc linkage is β(1 → 3), whereas in type 2, the Gal–GNAc linkage is β(1 → 4). In addition, there is heterogeneity in the A and B antigens with respect to the presence of the Le fucose attached to the GNAc. In the molecules that contain the extra fucose, when the Gal-GNAc linkage is β(1 → 3) (type 1), the fucose must be linked α(1 → 4), whereas the type 2 molecules, with the β(1 → 4) Gal-GNAc linkage, contain α(1 → 3)–linked fucose. The asterisks indicate the sites of this variability in linkage.

shown at the bottom of Fig. 2. In addition, this structure, known as precursor substance, has been isolated from ovarian cyst fluid.

Starting from precursor substance, the H determinant results from the addition of l-fucose to galactose, whereas the Le^a determinant results from the addition of l-fucose to N-acetylglucosamine, and Le^b from the addition of l-fucose to both sugars. Addition of N-acetylgalactosamine to H substance produces the A determinant, whereas addition of galactose produces the B determinant, in each case blocking reactivity of the H determinant.

The genetics of ABH and Le antigens is explained by this sequential addition of sugars via glycosyltransferases. The allelic nature of the AB antigens is explained by the addition of N-acetylgalactosamine, galactose, or nothing to the H antigen. The rare inherited trait of inability to synthesize the H determinants from precursor substance (Bombay phenotype) also blocks the expression of A and B antigens because the A and B transferases lack an acceptor substrate. However, the appearance of the Lewis^a antigen (Le^a) on red cells is independent of H antigen synthesis. Its structure, shown in Fig. 2, can be derived directly from precursor substance without going through an H antigen intermediate. Comparing different individuals, the appearance of Le^a antigen on red blood cells correlates with its presence in saliva because the Le^a antigen is not an intrinsic membrane component but must be absorbed from serum glycoproteins, which, in turn, depend on secretion. In addition to the independent synthetic pathway, the secretion of Le^a antigen is also independent of the secretory process for ABH antigens. Therefore, salivary nonsecretors of ABH antigens (which occur in 20% of individuals) may still secrete Le^a antigen if they have the fucosyl transferase encoded by the Le gene. In contrast, salivary secretors of ABH may produce Le^b antigen through the action of the H antigen–specific fucosyl transferase on the Le^a antigen followed by secretion via the secretory system for ABH antigens. Because it becomes the substrate for additional biochemical steps, Le^a antigen secretion is reduced, and it is usually undetectable on red blood cells of ABH (and Le^b) secretors. Conversely, Le^b is present only in ABH secretors.

Dextran-Binding Myeloma Proteins

Because polysaccharides are common environmental antigens, it is not surprising that randomly induced myeloma proteins were frequently found to have carbohydrate specificities. Careful studies of these monoclonal antibodies support the clonal expansion model of antibody diversity: heterogeneous antisera behave as the sum of many individual clones of antibody with respect to affinity and specificity. The IgA kappa myeloma proteins W3129 and W3434 were both found to be specific for dextrans containing α-glu (1 → 6)glu bonds (13). Hapten inhibition with a series of mono- or oligosaccharides of increasing chain length indicated that the percentage of binding energy derived from the reaction with one glucose was 75%, two glucoses 95%, three 95% to 98%, and four 100%. This suggests that most binding energy between antidextran antibodies and dextran derives from the terminal monosaccharide, and that oligosaccharides of four to six residues in length commonly fill the antibody-combining site. Human antidextran antisera behaved similarly, with tetrasaccharides contributing 95% of the binding energy. These experiments provided the first measure of the size of an antigenic determinant: four to six residues (14,15). In addition, as was observed for antisera, binding affinity of myeloma proteins was highly sensitive to modifications of the terminal sugar and highly specific for α(1 → 6) versus α(1 → 3) glycosidic bonds. However, modification of the third or fourth sugar of an oligosaccharide had relatively less effect on hapten inhibition of either myeloma protein or of antisera reacting with dextran.

Studies with additional dextran-binding myeloma proteins (16) showed that not all antipolysaccharide monoclonal antibodies are specific for the nonreducing end, as exemplified by QUPC 52. Competitive inhibition with mono- and oligosaccharides showed that less than 5% of binding energy derived from mono- or disaccharides, 72% from trisaccharides, 88% from tetrasaccharides, and 100% from hexasaccharides, in marked contrast to other myeloma proteins. A second distinctive property of myeloma protein QUPC 52 was its ability to precipitate unbranched dextran with a chain length of 200 residues. Because the unbranched dextran has only one nonreducing end, and because the myeloma protein has only one specificity, lattice formation by binding to the nonreducing ends is impossible, and precipitation must be explained by binding some other determinant. Therefore, QUPC 52 appears to be specific for internal oligosaccharide units with a chain length of three to seven residues. W3129 is specific for end determinants and will not precipitate unbranched dextran chains. Antibodies precipitating linear dextran also were detected in six antidextran human sera, comprising 48% to 90% of the total antibodies to branched chain dextran. Thus, antidextrans can be divided into those specific for terminal oligosaccharides and those specific for internal oligosaccharides; monoclonal examples of both types are available, and both types are present in human immune serum. Cisar et al. (16) speculated as to the different topology of the binding sites of W3129 or QUPC 52 necessary for terminal or internal oligosaccharide specificity. Both terminal and internal oligosaccharides have nearly identical chemical structures, differing at a single C–OH or glycoside bond. Perhaps the terminal oligosaccharide specificity of W3129 is due to the shape of the antibody-combining site, a cavity into which only the end can fit, whereas the internal oligosaccharide-binding site of QUPC 52 could be a surface groove in the antibody, which would allow the rest of the polymer to protrude at both ends. A more definitive answer depends on x-ray crystallographic studies of the combining sites of monoclonal antibodies with precisely defined specificity, performed with antigen occupying the binding site.

With the advent of hybridoma technology, it became possible to produce monoclonal antibodies of any desired specificity. Immunizing mice with nearly linear dextran (the preferred antigen of QUPC 52), followed by fusion and screening (with linear dextran) for dextran-binding antibodies, yielded 12 hybridomas (17), all with specificity similar to QUPC 52. Oligosaccharide inhibition of all 12 monoclonals showed considerable increments in affinity up to hexasaccharides, with little affinity for disaccharides and only 49% to 77% of binding energy derived from trisaccharides (18). Second, all 12 monoclonals had internal α(1 → 6) dextran specificity because they could all precipitate linear dextran. Third, nine of 11 BALB/c monoclonals shared cross-reactive idiotype with QUPC 52, whereas none shared idiotype with W3129 (19). These data support the hypothesis that different antibodies with similar specificity and similar groove-type sites may be derived from the same family of germline V$_H$ genes bearing the QUPC 52 idiotype (19).

The large number of environmental carbohydrate antigens and the high degree of specificity of antibodies elicited in response to each carbohydrate antigen suggest that a tremendous diversity of antibody molecules must be available, from which some antibodies can be selected for every possible antigenic structure. In order to regulate such a diverse system, a network theory has been proposed, in which antibodies are themselves recognized as antigenic (see Chapters 3 and 4) (20), and the response to streptococcal polysaccharide is a leading example in which antiidiotypic antibodies can be shown to regulate the response to antigen (21).

Recent studies of a series of 17 monoclonal anti-$\alpha(1 \rightarrow 6)$ dextran hybridomas (22,23) have investigated whether the binding sites of closely related antibodies would be derived from a small number of variable region genes, for both heavy and light chains, or whether antibodies of the same specificity could derive from variable region genes with highly divergent sequences. Each monoclonal had a groove-type site that could hold six or seven sugar residues (with one exception), based on inhibition of immunoprecipitation by oligosaccharides of different lengths. Thus, unlike monoclonals to haptenated proteins, the precise epitope could be well characterized and was generally quite similar among the entire series.

Studies of the V_k sequences showed that only three V_k groups were used in these hybridomas. Use of each V_k group correlated with the particular antigen used to immunize the animals, whether linear dextran or short oligosaccharides, so that 10 of the monoclonals from mice immunized the same way all used the same V_k.

In contrast, the 17 V_H chains were derived from at least five different germline genes from three distinct V_H gene families (24). The two most frequently used germline V_H genes were found in seven and five monoclonals, respectively, with minor variations explainable by somatic mutations. Once again, V_H gene usage correlated with the size of the antigen used to immunize, although the length of each complementarity determining region (CDR) did not correlate with the size of the groove-type binding site. The remarkable finding is that very different V_H chains (about 50% homologous) can combine with the same V_k to produce antibody-binding sites with nearly the same size, shape, antigen specificity, and affinity. A similar phenomenon also can occur when different V_H sequences combine with different V_k sequences to produce antibodies with very similar properties. This is a result of the fact that dextran binding depends on the antigen fitting into the groove and interacting favorably with the residues forming the sides and bottom of the groove. The results indicate that divergent variable region sequences, both in and out of the complementarity-determining regions, can be folded to form similar binding site contours, which result in similar immunochemical characteristics. Similar results have been reported in other antigen–antibody systems, such as phenyloxazolone (25).

More recently, these studies were expanded to include 34 groove-type monoclonal anti-$\alpha(1 \rightarrow 6)$ dextran-binding hybridomas (26), of which 10 used heavy-chain $V_H19.1.2$ and 11 used $V_H9.14.7$. Starting with different V_H genes, these two families of monoclonals provide an experiment of nature concerning the ability of each V_H gene to combine with different light-chain V_k and J_k genes, as well as heavy-chain D and J_H genes to produce a groove-shaped binding site of a given specificity. In each of these 21 monoclonals, the same light-chain V_k-Ox1 gene was used, but the V_H19 family used a single J_k sequence exclusively (J_k2), whereas the V_H9 family included all four of the active J_k segments (J_k1, 2, 4, and 5). Similarly, the heavy-chain J_H sequences of the V_H19 family were all of a single type (J_H3), whereas those of the VH9 family included three types (J_H1, 2, and 3). A single D region was used by both families (DFL16.1), but the junctional sequences between V_H–D and D–J_H were different, with the V_H19 using minimal substitutions, and the V_H9 allowing more variability in junctional sequences, depending on the size of the J_H gene with which it was joining. Although the amino acid sequences of

these two V_H genes are 73% identical, they use markedly different strategies to arrive at the same groove-type binding site with nearly identical size and specificity. The results suggest that the two heavy-chain variable regions, perhaps due to their conformation, may place different structural constraints on which minigene components can successfully contribute to forming a particular site. Two different strategies for generating antibody specificity are apparent, even though the same V_k and D minigenes were used by both families. For the V_H19 family, point mutations in the CDR2 generated the $\alpha(1 \rightarrow 6)$ dextran specificity, whereas the rest of the structure was held constant. For the V_H9 family, a wide variety of J_H, J_k, and V_H–D and D–J_H sequences were used to generate the groove-type site. These two blueprints for constructing a binding site also may reflect distinct cellular pathways for generating antibody diversity.

Protein and Polypeptide Antigenic Determinants

Like the proteins themselves, the antigenic determinants of proteins consist of amino acid residues in a particular three-dimensional array. The residues that make contact with complementary residues in the antibody-combining site are called contact residues. To make contact, of course, these residues must be exposed on the surface of the protein, not buried in the hydrophobic core. Since the complementarity-determining residues in the hypervariable regions of antibodies have been found to span as much as 30 to 40 Å × 15 to 20 Å × 10 Å (D.R. Davies, personal communication), these contact residues comprising the antigenic determinant may cover a significant area of protein surface, as now measured in a few cases by x-ray crystallography of antibody–protein antigen complexes (27–30). From another point of view, the size of the combining sites has been estimated using simple synthetic oligopeptides of increasing length, such as oligolysine. In this case, a series of elegant studies (31–33) suggested that the maximum length of chain a combining site could accommodate was six to eight residues, corresponding closely to that found earlier for oligosaccharides (14,15), discussed previously.

Several types of interactions contribute to the binding energy. Many of the amino acid residues exposed to solvent on the surface of a protein antigen will be hydrophilic. These are likely to interact with antibody contact residues via polar interactions. For instance, an anionic glutamic acid carboxyl group may bind to a complementary cationic lysine amino group on the antibody, or vice versa; or a glutamine amide side chain may form a hydrogen bond with the antibody. However, hydrophobic interactions also can play a major role. Proteins cannot exist in aqueous solution as stable monomers with too many hydrophobic residues on their surface. Those hydrophobic residues that are on the surface can contribute to binding to antibody for exactly the same reason. When a hydrophobic residue in a protein antigenic determinant or, similarly, in a carbohydrate determinant (8), interacts with a corresponding hydrophobic residue in the antibody-combining site, the water molecules previously in contact with each of them are excluded. The result is a significant stabilization of the interaction. A thorough review of these aspects of the chemistry of antigen–antibody binding is provided elsewhere (34).

Mapping Epitopes: Conformation Versus Sequence

The other component that defines a protein antigenic determinant, besides the amino acid residues involved, is the way these residues are arrayed in three dimensions. Because the residues are on the surface of a protein, we can also think of this component as the topography of the antigenic determinant. Sela (35) divided protein antigenic determinants into two categories, sequential and conformational, depending on whether the primary sequence or the three-dimensional conformation appeared to contribute the most to binding. On the other hand, because the antibody-combining site has a preferred topography in the native antibody, it would seem *a priori* that some conformations of a particular polypeptide sequence would produce a better fit than others and therefore would be energetically favored in binding. Thus, conformation or topography must always play some role in the structure of an antigenic determinant.

Moreover, when one looks at the surface of a protein in a space-filling model, one cannot ascertain the direction of the backbone or the positions of the helices (contrast Figs. 3 and 4) (36–40). It is hard to recognize whether two residues that are side by side on the surface are adjacent on the polypeptide backbone or whether they come from different parts of the sequence and are brought together by the folding of the molecule. If a protein maintains its native conformation when an antibody binds, then it must similarly be hard for the antibody to discriminate between residues that are covalently connected directly and those connected only through a great deal of intervening polypeptide. Thus, the probability that an antigenic determinant on a native globular protein consists of only a consecutive sequence of amino acids in the primary structure is likely to be rather small. Even if most of the determinant were a continuous sequence, other nearby residues would probably play a role as well. Only if the protein were cleaved into fragments before the antibodies were made would there be any reason to favor connected sequences.

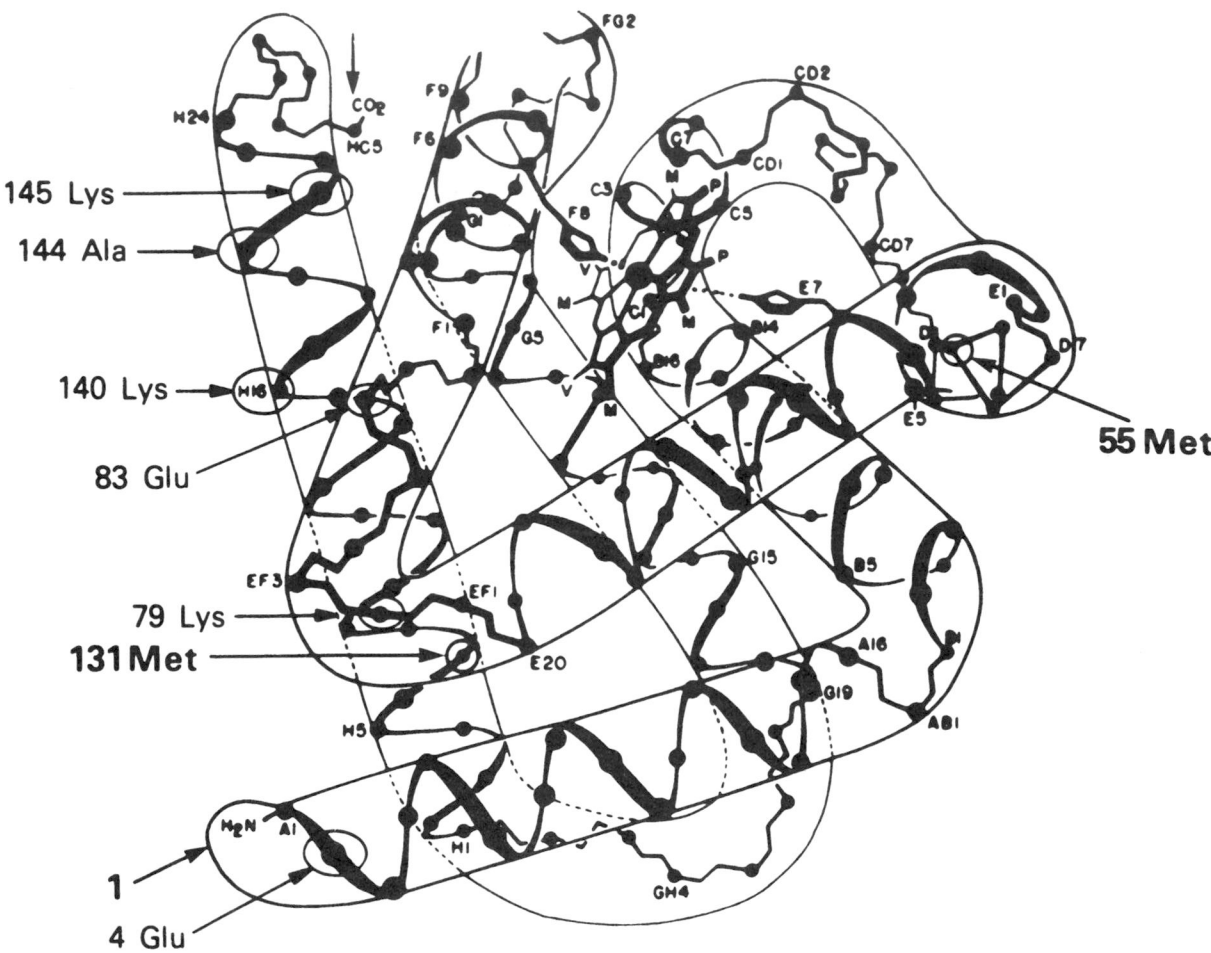

FIG. 3. Artist's representation of the polypeptide backbone of sperm whale myoglobin in its native three-dimensional conformation. The α helices are labeled A through H from the amino terminal to the carboxyl terminal. Side chains are omitted, except for the two histidine rings (F8 and E7) involved with the heme iron. Methionines at positions 55 and 131 are the sites of cleavage by cyanogen bromide (CNBr), allowing myoglobin to be cleaved into three fragments. Most of the helicity and other features of the native conformation are lost when the molecule is cleaved. A less drastic change in conformation is produced by removal of the heme to form apomyoglobin because the heme interacts with several helices and stabilizes their positions relative to one another. The other labeled residues (4 Glu, 79 Lys, 83 Glu, 140 Lys, 144 Ala, and 145 Lys) are residues that have been found to be involved in antigenic determinants recognized by monoclonal antibodies (36). Note that cleavage by CNBr separates Lys 79 from Glu 4 and separates Glu 83 from Ala 144 and Lys 145. The sequential determinant of Koketsu and Atassi (37) (residues 15 to 22) is located at the elbow, lower right, from the end of the A helix to the beginning of the B helix. Adapted with permission (38).

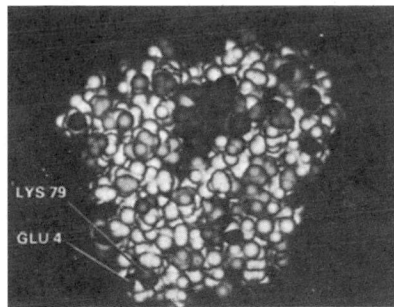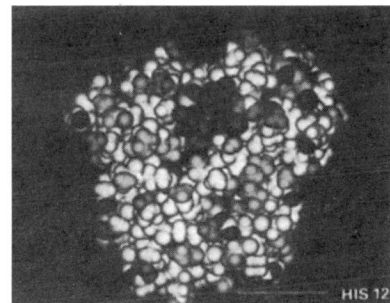

FIG. 4. Stereoscopic views of a computer-generated space-filling molecular model of sperm whale myoglobin, based on the Takano (39) x-ray diffraction coordinates. This orientation, which corresponds to that in Fig. 3, is arbitrarily designated the front view. The computer method has been described by Feldmann et al. (40). The heme and aromatic carbons are shaded darkest, followed by carboxyl oxygens, then other oxygens, then primary amino groups, then other nitrogens, and finally side chains of aliphatic residues. The backbone and the side chains of non-aliphatic residues, except for the functional groups, are shown in white. Note that the direction of the helices is not apparent on the surface, in contrast to the backbone drawing in Fig. 3. The residues Glu 4, Lys 79, and His 12 are believed to be part of a topographic antigenic determinant recognized by a monoclonal antibody to myoglobin (36). This stereo pair can be viewed in three dimensions using an inexpensive stereoviewer such as the stereoscopes sold by Abrams Instrument Corp., Lansing, MI, or Hubbard Scientific Co., Northbrook, IL. Adapted with permission (36).

This concept was analyzed and confirmed quantitatively by Barlow et al. (41), who examined the atoms lying within spheres of different radii from a given surface atom on a protein. As the radius increases, the probability that all the atoms within the sphere will be from the same continuous segment of protein sequence decreases rapidly. Correspondingly, the fraction of surface atoms that would be located at the center of a sphere containing only residues from the same continuous segment decreases dramatically as the radius of the sphere increases. For instance, for lysozyme, with a radius of 8 Å, fewer than 10% of the surface residues would lie in such a "continuous patch" of surface. These are primarily in regions that protrude from the surface. With a radius of 10 Å, almost none of the surface residues fall in the center of a continuous patch. Thus, for a contact area of about 20 × 25 Å, as found for

a lysozyme–antibody complex analyzed by x-ray crystallography, none of the antigenic sites could be completely continuous segmental sites (Fig. 5).

Antigenic sites consisting of amino acid residues that are widely separated in the primary protein sequence but brought together on the surface of the protein by the way it folds in its native conformation have been called "assembled topographic" sites (42,43) because they are assembled from different parts of the sequence and exist only in the surface topography of the native molecule. By contrast, the sites that consist of only a single continuous segment of protein sequence have been called "segmental" antigenic sites (42,43).

In contrast to T-cell recognition of "processed" fragments retaining only primary and secondary structures, the evidence is over-

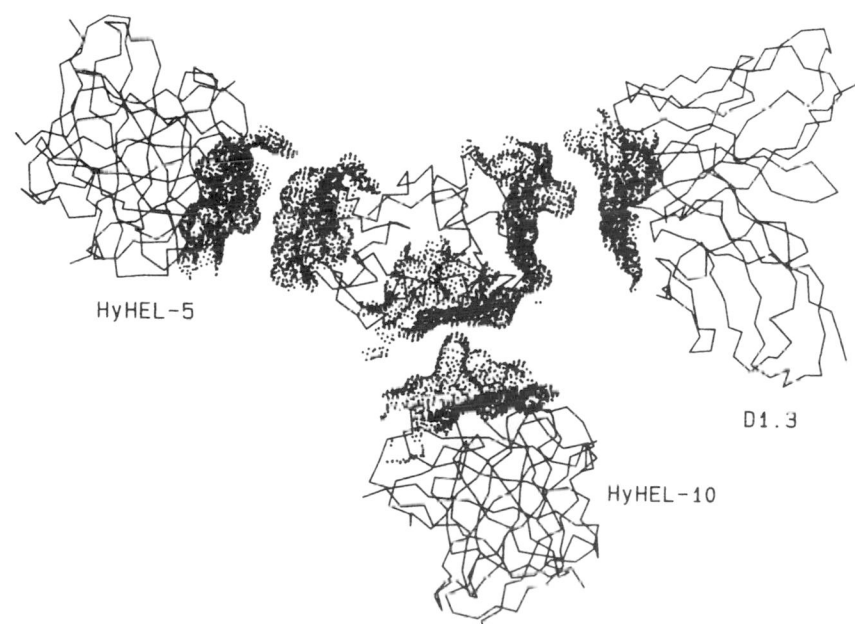

HyHEL-5

HyHEL-10

D1.3

FIG. 5. Assembled topographic sites of lysozyme illustrated by the footprints of three nonoverlapping monoclonal antibodies. Shown are the alpha carbon backbones of lysozyme in the center and the Fv portions of three antilysozyme monoclonal antibodies, D1.3, HyHEL-5, and HyHEL-10. The footprints of the antibodies on lysozyme and lysozyme on the antibodies, i.e., their interacting surfaces, are shown by a dotted representation. Note that the three antibodies each contact more than one continuous loop of lysozyme and so define assembled topographic sites. Reproduced with permission (30).

whelming that most antibodies are made against the native conformation when the native protein is used as immunogen. For instance, antibodies to native staphylococcal nuclease were found to have about a 5,000-fold higher affinity for the native protein than for the corresponding polypeptide on which they were isolated (by binding to the peptide attached to sepharose) (44). An even more dramatic example is that demonstrated by Crumpton (45) for antibodies to native myoglobin or to apomyoglobin. Antibodies to native ferric myoglobin produced a brown precipitate with myoglobin, an indication that the heme was still in the protein in what was, at least approximately, its native environment. Such antibodies did not bind well to the apomyoglobin, which, without the heme, has a slightly altered conformation. On the other hand, antibodies to the apomyoglobin, when mixed with native (brown) myoglobin, produced a white precipitate. These antibodies so strongly favored the conformation of apomyoglobin, from which the heme was excluded, that they trapped those molecules that vibrated toward that conformation and pulled the equilibrium state over to the apo form. One could almost say that the antibodies "squeezed" the heme out of the myoglobin. Looked at thermodynamically, it is clear that the conformational preference of the antibody for the apo versus native forms, in terms of free energy, had to be greater than the free energy of binding of the heme to myoglobin. Thus, in general, antibodies are made that are very specific for the conformation of the protein used as immunogen.

A number of methods have been used to identify the antigenic determinants bound by particular antibodies made against a protein. Binding to cleavage fragments and short synthetic peptides from the protein sequence has been the most widely used approach. The synthetic peptides may be made by conventional solid-phase peptide synthesis (46) or by methods designed to make large numbers of peptides for screening. In one such method, multiple peptides are made simultaneously in separate polypropylene mesh "tea-bags" that can be put through the common steps in the sequence together and separated only for the different amino acid coupling steps (47). In another method, the peptides are synthesized on the tips of plastic pins inserted in the wells of 96-well microtiter plates in such a way that these can then be used for solid-phase binding assays of antibodies without ever cleaving the peptide off the plastic support (48). These two methods especially lend themselves to studying multiple variants of the natural sequence to identify the residues critical for antibody binding. Usually, the longer the peptides, the more that specificity can be confidently determined because short peptides of only six to eight amino acid residues often manifest nonspecific binding (49). If the synthetic peptides correspond to segments of the protein antigen sequence, as is most common, then the use of peptides is limited to identifying the structures bound by antibodies specific for segmental antigenic sites.

To identify assembled topographic sites, more complex approaches have been necessary. The earliest was the use of natural variants of the protein antigen with known amino acid substitutions, where such evolutionary variants exist (42). Thus, substitution of different amino acids in proteins in the native conformation can be examined. The use of this method, which is illustrated later, is limited to studying the function of amino acids that vary among homologous proteins, that is, those that are polymorphic. It may now be extended to other residues by use of site-directed mutagenesis. A second method is to use the antibody that binds to the native protein to protect the antigenic site from modification (50) or proteolytic degradation (51). A related but less sensitive approach makes use of competition with other antibodies (52–54).

A third approach, taking advantage of the capability of producing thousands of peptides on a solid-phase surface for direct binding assays (48), is to study binding of a monoclonal antibody to every possible combination of six amino acids (48). If the assembled topographic site can be mimicked by a combination of six amino acids not corresponding to any continuous segment of the protein sequence but structurally resembling a part of the surface, then one can produce a "mimotope" defining the specificity of that antibody (48).

Myoglobin also serves as a good model protein antigen for studying the range of variation of antigenic determinants from those that are more sequential in nature to those that do not even exist without the native conformation of the protein (Fig. 3). A good example of the first, more segmental type of determinant is that consisting of residues 15 to 22 in the amino terminal portion of the molecule. Crumpton and Wilkinson (55) first discovered that the chymotryptic cleavage fragment consisting of residues 15 to 29 had antigenic activity for antibodies raised to either native or apomyoglobin. Synthetic peptides corresponding to the shorter sequence 15 to 22 were then found by two groups (37,56) to bind antibodies made to native sperm whale myoglobin, even though the synthetic peptides were only seven to eight residues long. Peptides of this length do not spend much time (in solution) in a conformation corresponding to that of the native protein. On the other hand, these synthetic peptides had a several hundred-fold lower affinity for the antibodies than did the native protein. Thus, even if most of the determinant was included in the consecutive sequence 15 to 22, the antibodies were still much more specific for the native conformation of this sequence than for the random conformation peptide. Moreover, there was no evidence to exclude the participation of other residues, nearby on the surface of myoglobin but not in this sequence, in the antigenic determinant (57–60).*

A good example of the importance of secondary structure is the case of the loop peptide (residues 64 to 80) of hen egg-white lysozyme (61). This loop in the protein sequence is created by the disulfide linkage between cysteine residues 64 and 80 and has been shown to be a major antigenic determinant for antibodies to lysozyme (61). The isolated peptide 60 to 83, containing the loop, binds antibodies with high affinity, but opening of the loop by cleavage of the disulfide bond destroys most of the antigenic activity for antilysozyme antibodies (61).

At the other end of the range of conformational requirements are those determinants involving residues far apart in the primary sequences that are brought close together on the surface of the native molecule by its folding in three dimensions. Myoglobin also provides a good example of these determinants, which are called assembled topographic determinants (42,43). Of six monoclonal antibodies to sperm whale myoglobin studied by Berzofsky et al. (36,62), none bound to any of the three cyanogen bromide cleavage fragments of myoglobin that together span the whole sequence of the molecule. Therefore these monoclonal antibodies (all with affinities between 2×10^8 and 2×10^9 M^{-1}) were all highly specific

*This is the only segmental antigenic determinant of myoglobin that has clearly been confirmed by more than one independent group of investigators. Crumpton and Wilkinson (55) measured antigenic activity for a chymotryptic fragment 147 to 153 that overlaps one of the other reported sequential determinants (57). However, two of the other reported sequential determinants (57), corresponding to residues 56 to 62 and 94 to 100, have not been reproducible when tested with other antisera, even raised in the same species (58). For related studies, the reader is referred to other sources (59,60).

for the native conformation. These were studied by comparing the relative affinities for a series of native myoglobins from different species with the known amino acid sequences of these myoglobins. With the myoglobins available, this approach allowed the definition of some of the residues involved in binding to three of these antibodies. The striking result was that two of these three monoclonal antibodies were found to recognize topographic determinants, as defined previously. One recognized a determinant including Glu 4 and Lys 79, which are on the A helix and E–F corner of the myoglobin molecule but come within about 2 Å of each other to form a salt bridge in the native molecule (Fig. 4). The other antibody recognized a determinant involving Glu 83 in the E–F corner, and Ala 144 and Lys 145 on the H helix of the myoglobin molecule (Fig. 3). Again, these are far apart in the primary sequence but are brought within 12 Å of each other by the folding of the molecule in its native conformation. Similar examples recently have been reported for monoclonal antibodies to human myoglobin (63) and to lysozyme (30,52). Other examples of such conformation-dependent antigenic determinants have been suggested using conventional antisera to such proteins as insulin (64), hemoglobin (65), tobacco mosaic virus (66), and cytochrome c (67). Moreover, the crystallographic structures of lysozyme–antibody (27,29,30) and neuraminidase antibody (28) complexes show clearly that, in both cases, the epitope bound is an assembled topographic site. In the case of the three monoclonal antibodies binding to nonoverlapping sites of lysozyme (Fig. 5), it is clear that the footprints of all three antibody-combining sites cover more than one loop of polypeptide chain and thus each encompasses an assembled topographic site (30). This result beautifully illustrates the concept that the majority of antibody-combining sites must interact with more than a continuous loop of polypeptide chain and thus must define assembled topographic sites (41).

How frequent are antibodies specific for topographic determinants compared with those that bind consecutive sequences when conventional antisera are examined? This question was studied by Lando et al (68), who passed goat, sheep, and rabbit antisera to sperm whale myoglobin over columns of sepharose-coupled cyanogen bromide cleavage fragments of myoglobin, together spanning the whole sequence. The antisera were passed sequentially, and repeatedly, over each of the three columns until no more antibodies could be removed. Nevertheless, 30% to 40% of the antibodies originally present in each serum remained after this treatment. These antibodies still bound to the native myoglobin molecule with high affinity but did not bind to any of the fragments in solution by radioimmunoassay. Thus, in four of four antimyoglobin sera tested, 60% to 70% of the antibodies could bind peptides and 30% to 40% could bind only native-conformation intact protein.

On the basis of studies such as these, it has been suggested that much of the surface of a protein molecule may be antigenic (42,69) but that the surface can be divided up into antigenic domains (36,59,60,63). Each of these domains consists of many overlapping determinants recognized by different antibodies.

An additional interesting point can be made from the above studies about the topography of protein antigenic determinants. If one examines the topographic determinant consisting of sperm whale myoglobin residues 83, 144, and 145, shown in Fig. 3, they are on both lips of a deep crevice or concavity in the protein surface. It is possible, although not yet demonstrated, that a complementary protuberance in the antibody combining site actually inserts into this cavity. From the studies of myeloma proteins that bind small hap-

tens or carbohydrates, we are accustomed to think of the antigen being engulfed by a cavity or crevice on the antibody (70). However, for globular protein antigens binding to globular protein antibodies, the situation is more structurally symmetrical (and antigen–antibody binding is also thermodynamically symmetrical). Thus, it is just as possible for a convexity on the antibody to insert into a concavity on the antigen as it is for the more conventional model to occur of a convexity on the antigen inserting into a concavity on the antibody. Now that monoclonal antibodies specific for protein antigens are available, we may encounter both types of cases. The determinant depicted in Fig. 3 might be such a case. In three published crystal structures of protein antigen–antibody complexes, the contact surfaces were broad, with local complementary pairs of concave and convex regions in both directions (27–30). However, when we limit ourselves to antigenic sites defined with short peptides, which tend to identify sites that protrude from the surface of the antigen (41,71), we are likely to see a bias toward situations in which the antigen is convex and the antibody surface concave.

Further information on the subjects discussed in this section is available in the reviews by Sela (35), Crumpton (45), Reichlin (72), Kabat (70), Benjamin et al. (42), Berzofsky (43), Getzoff et al. (34), and Davies et al. (30).

Conformational Equilibria of Protein and Peptide Antigenic Determinants

We have already referred to the fact that antibodies to a native protein have higher affinity for the native conformation than for other conformations of fragments or denatured molecules. Similarly, antibodies raised against fragments or denatured molecules generally have higher affinities for these forms than for the native conformation. In this section we discuss possible mechanisms for these affinity differences and explore how these can be used to advantage to study the conformational equilibria of proteins and peptides.

There are several possible mechanisms to explain why an antibody specific for a native protein will bind a peptide fragment in random conformation with lower affinity. Of course, the peptide may not contain all the contact residues of the antigenic determinant, so that the binding energy would be lower. However, for cases in which all the residues in the determinant are present in the peptide, several mechanisms still remain. First, the affinity may be lower because the topography of the residues in the peptide may not produce as complementary a fit in the antibody-combining site as the native conformation would. Second, it is possible that the apparent affinity is reduced because only a small fraction of the peptide molecules are in a nativelike conformation at any time. This model assumes that the antibody binds only those peptide molecules that are in the native conformation. Because the concentration of these is lower than the total peptide concentration by a factor that corresponds to the conformational equilibrium constant of the peptide, the apparent affinity is also lower by this factor. This model is analogous to an allosteric model. A third, intermediate hypothesis would suggest that initial binding of the peptide in a nonnative conformation occurs with submaximal complementarity and is followed by an intramolecular conformational change in the peptide to achieve energy minimization by assuming a nativelike conformation. This third hypothesis corresponds to an induced fit model. The loss of affinity is due to the energy required to change the conformation of the peptide, which in turn corresponds to the conformational equilibrium constant in the second hypothesis. To some extent these models could be distinguished kinetically because the first hypothesis predicts a faster "on" rate and a faster "off" rate than does the second hypothesis (73).

Although not the only way to explain the data, the second hypothesis is useful because it provides a method to estimate the conformational equilibria of proteins and peptides (44,74). The method assumes the second hypothesis, which can be expressed as follows:

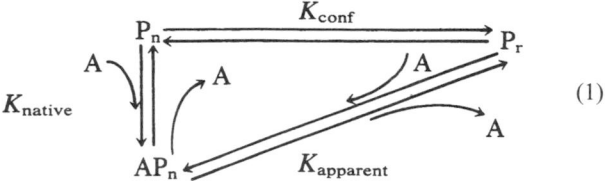

$$(1)$$

where A is antibody, P_n is native peptide, and P_r is random conformation peptide, so that

$$K_{apparent} = K_{conf}K_{native} \qquad (2)$$

Thus, the ratio of the apparent association constant for peptide to the measured association constant for the native molecule should give the conformational equilibrium constant of the peptide. Note the implicit assumption that the total peptide concentration can be approximated by $[P_r]$. This will generally be true because most peptide fragments of proteins demonstrate little native conformation; that is, $K_{conf} = [P_n]/[P_r]$ is much less than 1. Also, note that if the first hypothesis (or third) occurs to some extent, this method will overestimate K_{conf}. On the other hand, if the affinity for the peptide is lower because it lacks some of the contact residues of the determinant, this method will underestimate K_{conf} (by assuming that all the affinity difference is due to conformation). To some extent, the two errors may partially cancel out. When this method was used to determine the K_{conf} for a peptide staphylococcal nuclease, a value of 2×10^{-4} was obtained (44). Similarly, when antibodies raised to a peptide fragment were used, it was possible to estimate the fraction of time the native nuclease spends in nonnative conformations (74). In this case, the K_{conf} was found to be about 3,000-fold in favor of the native conformation.

Antipeptide Antibodies that Bind to Native Proteins at a Specific Site

In light of the conformational differences between native proteins and peptides and the observed K_{conf} effects shown by antibodies to native proteins when tested on the corresponding peptides, it was somewhat surprising to find that antibodies to synthetic peptides show extensive cross-reactions with native proteins (75,76). These two types of cross-reactions can be thought of as working in opposite directions: the binding of antiprotein antibodies to the peptide is inefficient, whereas the binding of antipeptide antibodies to the protein is quite efficient and commonly observed. This finding is quite useful because automated solid-phase peptide synthesis has become readily available. This has been particularly useful in three areas: exploitation of protein sequences deduced by recombinant DNA methods, preparation of site-specific antibodies, and the attempt to focus the immune response on a single protein site that is biologically important but may not be particularly immunogenic. This section focuses on the explanation of the cross-reaction, uses of the cross-reaction, and the potential limitations with regard to immunogenicity.

The basic assumption is that antibodies raised against peptides in an unfolded structure will bind the corresponding site on proteins folded into the native structure (76). This is not immediately obvious because antibody binding to antigen is the direct result of the antigen fitting into the binding site. Affinity is the direct consequence of "goodness of fit" between antibody and antigen, whereas antibody specificity is due to the inability of other antigens to occupy the same site. How then can the antipeptide antibodies overcome the effect of K_{conf} and still bind native proteins with good affinity and specificity? The whole process depends on the antibody-binding site forming a three-dimensional space and the antigen filling it in an energetically favorable way.

Because the peptides are randomly folded, they rarely occupy the native conformation, so they are not likely to elicit antibodies against a conformation they do not maintain. If the antibodies are specific for a denatured structure, then, like the myoglobin molecules that were denatured to apomyoglobin by antibody binding (45), the cross-reaction may depend on the native protein's ability to assume different conformational states. If the native protein is quite rigid, then the possibility of its assuming a random conformation is quite small; but if it is a flexible three-dimensional spring, then local unfolding and refolding may occur all the time. Local unfolding of protein segments may permit the immunologic cross-reaction with antipeptide antibodies because a flexible segment could assume many of the same conformations as the randomly folded peptide (76).

In contrast, the proteins' ability to crystallize (a feature that allows the study of their structure by x-ray crystallography) has long been taken as evidence of protein rigidity (77). In addition, the existence of discrete functional states of allosteric enzymes (78) provides additional evidence of stable structural states of a protein. Finally, the fact that antibodies can distinguish native from denatured forms of intact proteins is well known for proteins such as myoglobin (45).

However, protein crystals are a somewhat artificial situation because the formation of the crystal lattice imposes order on the components, each of which occupies a local energy minimum at the expense of considerable loss of randomness (entropy). Thus, the crystal structure may have artificial rigidity that exceeds the actual rigidity of protein molecules in solution. On the contrary, we may attribute some of the considerable difficulty in crystallizing proteins to disorder within the native conformation. Second, allosterism may be explained by two distinct conformations that are discrete without being particularly rigid. Finally, the ability to generate antiprotein antibodies that are conformation specific does not rule out the existence of antipeptide antibodies that are not. All antibodies are probably specific for some conformation of the antigen, but this need not be the crystallographic native conformation in order to achieve a significant affinity for those proteins or protein segments that have a "loose" native conformation.

Antipeptide antibodies have proved to be very powerful reagents when combined with recombinant DNA methods of gene sequencing (76,79). From the DNA sequence, the protein sequence is predicted. A synthetic peptide is constructed, coupled to a suitable carrier molecule, and used to immunize animals. The resulting polyclonal antibodies can be detected with a peptide-coated enzyme-linked immunosorbent assay (ELISA) plate (see Chapter 4). They are used to immunoprecipitate the native protein from a ^{35}S-labeled cell lysate and thus confirm expression of the gene product in these cells. The antipeptide antibodies also can be used to isolate the previously unidentified gene product of a new gene.

The site-specific antibodies are also useful in detecting posttranslational processing because they bind all precursors and products that contain the site. In addition, because the antibodies bind only to the site corresponding to the peptide, they are useful in probing structure–function relationships. They can be used to block the binding of a substrate to an enzyme or the binding of a virus to its cellular receptor.

Immunogenicity of Proteins and Peptides

Up to this point, we have considered the ability of antibodies to react with proteins or peptides as antigens. However, immunogenicity refers to the ability of these compounds to elicit antibodies after immunization. In principle, nearly the entire surface of a globular protein should be able to elicit antibodies, particularly when we allow for both topographic and segmental specific antibodies (42). However, several factors limit the immunogenicity of different regions of proteins, and these have been categorized as those that are intrinsic to protein structure itself versus those extrinsic to the antigen that are related to the responder and vary from one animal or species to another (43). In addition, we consider the special case of peptide immunogenicity as it applies to vaccine development.

Studies of intrinsic factors began by immunizing animals with native proteins and analyzing the antibodies that resulted. With polyclonal antisera, it is necessary to compare the relative amounts of antibodies directed at each site or class of sites: immunodominant sites are the ones that elicit the most antibodies. Monoclonal antibodies advanced our ability to study the immunogenicity of discrete sites. The features of protein structure that may explain these results include surface accessibility of the site, hydrophilicity, flexibility, and proximity to a site recognized by helper T cells.

When the x-ray crystallographic structure and antigenic structure are known for the same protein, it is not surprising to find that a series of monoclonal antibodies binding to a molecule such as influenza neuraminidase choose an overlapping pattern of sites at the exposed head of the protein (80). The stalk of neuraminidase was not immunogenic, apparently because it was almost entirely covered by carbohydrate.

Beyond such things as carbohydrate, which may sterically interfere with antibody binding to protein, accessibility on the surface is clearly a *sine qua non* for an antigenic determinant to be bound by an antibody specific for the native conformation, without any requirement for unfolding of the structure (43). Several measures of such accessibility have been suggested. All these require knowledge of the x-ray crystallographic three-dimensional structure. Some have measured accessibility to solvent by rolling a sphere with the radius of a water molecule over the surface of a protein (81,82). Others have suggested that accessibility to water is not the best measure of accessibility to antibody and have demonstrated a better correlation by rolling a sphere with the radius of an antibody-combining domain (83). Another approach to predicting antigenic sites on the basis of accessibility is to examine the degree of protrusion from the surface of the protein (71). This was done by modeling the body of the protein as an ellipsoid and examining which amino acid residues remain outside ellipsoids of increasing dimensions. The most protruding residues were found to be part of antigenic sites bound by antibodies, but usually these sites had been identified by using short synthetic peptides and so were segmental in nature. As noted above, for an antigenic site to be contained completely within a single continuous segment of protein

sequence, the site is likely to have to protrude from the surface; otherwise, residues from other parts of the sequence would fall within the area contacting the antibody (41).

Because the three-dimensional structure of most proteins is not known, other ways of predicting surface exposure have been proposed for the vast majority of antigens. For example, hydrophilic sites tend to be found on the water-exposed surface of proteins and could be favored targets for antibodies. Thus hydrophilicity has been proposed as a second indication of immunogenicity (84–86). This model has been used to analyze 12 proteins with known antigenic sites: the most hydrophilic site of each protein was indeed one of the antigenic sites. However, among the limitations are the facts that a significant fraction of surface residues can be nonpolar (81,82) and that several important examples of hydrophobic and aromatic amino acids involved in the antigenic sites are known (35,66,87,88). Specificity of antibody binding likely depends on the complementarity of surfaces for hydrogen bonding and polar bonding as well as van der Waals contacts (89), whereas hydrophobic interactions and the exclusion of water from the interacting surfaces of proteins may contribute a large but nonspecific component to the energy of binding (89).

A third factor that may play a role in immunogenicity of protein epitopes is mobility. Measurement of mobility in the native protein is largely dependent on the availability of a high-resolution crystal structure, so its applicability is limited to only a small subset of proteins. Furthermore, it has been studied only for antibodies specific for segmental antigenic sites; therefore it may not apply to the large fraction of antibodies to assembled topographic sites. Studies of mobility have taken two directions. The case of antipeptide antibodies has already been discussed, in which antibodies made to peptides corresponding to more mobile segments of the native protein were more likely to bind to the native protein (76,90). This is not considered just a consequence of the fact that more mobile segments are likely to be those on the surface and therefore more exposed, because in the case of myohemerythrin (which was used as a model), two regions of the native protein that were equally exposed but less mobile did not bind nearly as well to the corresponding antipeptide antibodies (91). However, as is clear from the earlier discussion, this result applies to antibodies made against short peptides and therefore is not directly relevant to immunogenicity of parts of the native protein. Rather, it concerns the cross-reactivity of antipeptide antibodies with the native protein and therefore is of considerable practical importance for the purposes outlined in the section on antipeptide antibodies.

Studies in the other direction—that is, of antibodies raised against native proteins—would be by definition more relevant to the question of immunogenicity of parts of the native protein. Westhof et al. (92) used a series of hexapeptides to determine the specificity of antibodies raised against native tobacco mosaic virus protein and found that six of the seven peptides that bound antibodies to native protein corresponded to peaks of high mobility in the native protein. The correlation was better than could be accounted for just by accessibility, because three peptides that corresponded to exposed regions of only average mobility did not bind antibodies to the native protein. However, when longer peptides—on the order of 20 amino acid residues—were used as probes, it was found that antibodies were present in the same antisera that bound to less mobile regions of the protein (93). They simply had not been detected with the short hexapeptides with less conformational stability. Thus, it was not that the more mobile regions were necessarily more immunogenic but rather that antibodies to these were more easily detected with short peptides as probes. A similar good correlation of antigenic sites with mobile regions of the native protein in the case of myoglobin (92) also may be attributed to the fact that seven of the nine sites were defined with short peptides of six to eight residues (57). Again, this result becomes a statement about cross-reactivity between peptides and native protein rather than about the immunogenicity of the native protein. For reviews, see Van Regenmortel (94) and Getzoff et al. (34).

To address the role of mobility in immunogenicity, an attempt was made to quantitate the relative fraction of antibodies specific for different sites on the antigen myohemerythrin (95). The premise was that, although the entire surface of the protein may be immunogenic, certain regions may elicit significantly more antibodies than others and therefore may be considered immunodominant or at least more immunogenic. Because this study was performed with short synthetic peptides from six to 14 residues long based on the protein sequence, it was limited to the subset of antibodies specific for segmental antigenic sites. Among these, it was clear that the most immunogenic sites were in regions of the surface that were most mobile, convex in shape, and often of negative electrostatic potential. The role of these parameters has been reviewed (34).

These results have important practical and theoretical implications. First, to use peptides to fractionate antiprotein antisera by affinity chromatography, peptides corresponding to more mobile segments of the native protein should be chosen when possible. If the crystal structure is not known, it may be possible to use peptides from amino or carboxyl termini or from exon–intron boundaries because these are more likely to be mobile (90). Second, these results may explain how a large but finite repertoire of antibody-producing B cells can respond to any antigen in nature or even artificial antigens never encountered in nature. Protein segments that are more flexible may be able to bind by induced fit in an antibody-combining site that is not perfectly complementary to the average native structure (34,43). Indeed, evidence from the crystal structure of antigen–antibody complexes (96–98) suggests that mobility in the antibody-combining site as well as in the antigen may allow both reactants to adopt more complementary conformations on binding to each other, that is, a two-way induced fit. A very nice example comes from the study of antibodies to myohemerythrin (97), in which the data suggested that initial binding of exposed side chains of the antigen to the antibody promoted local displacements that allowed exposure and binding of other, previously buried residues. The role of these critical amino acid side chains that are buried in the native crystal structure appeared to be one of contact residues with the antibody-combining site rather than one of stabilization of a particular conformation. The only way this could occur would be for such residues to become exposed during the course of an induced fit conformational change in the antigen (34,97). In a second very clear example of induced fit, the contribution of antibody mobility to peptide binding was demonstrated for a monoclonal antibody to peptide 75 to 110 of influenza hemagglutinin, which was crystallized with or without peptide in the binding site and analyzed by x-ray crystallography for evidence of an induced fit (98). Despite flexibility of the peptide, the antibody-binding site probably could not accommodate the peptide without a conformational change in the third complementarity determining region (CDR3) of the heavy chain, in which an asparagine residue of the antibody was rotated out of the way to allow a tyrosine residue of the peptide to fit in the binding pocket of the antibody (98).

With regard to host-limited factors, immunogenicity is certainly limited by self tolerance. Thus, the repertoire of potential antigenic sites on mammalian protein antigens such as myoglobin or cytochrome c can be thought of as greatly simplified by the sharing of numerous amino acids with the endogenous myoglobin or cytochrome of the host. For mouse, guanaco, or horse cytochrome c injected into rabbits, each of the differences between the immunogen and rabbit cytochrome c is seen as an immunogenic site on a background of immunologically silent residues (42,67,99). In another example, antibodies to beef myoglobin were made in various species (100). Rabbit and dog antibodies bound almost equally well to beef or sheep myoglobin. However, sheep antibodies bound beef but not sheep myoglobin, even though these two myoglobins differ by just six amino acids. Thus, the sheep immune system was able to screen out those clones that would be autoreactive with sheep myoglobin.

Ir genes of the host also play an important role in regulating the ability of an individual to make antibodies to a specific antigen (101). These antigen-specific immunoregulatory genes are among the major histocompatibility complex (MHC) genes that code for transplantation antigens. Structural mutations, gene transfer experiments, and biochemical studies (101) all indicate that Ir genes are actually the structural genes for MHC antigens. The mechanism of action of the MHC antigens works through their effect on helper T cells (described later). Briefly, T cells can respond to a protein antigen only when a fragment of the protein is bound to an MHC antigen, forming a compound antigen. T cells must be activated before they can help B cells respond to antigen by both expanding the appropriate clones of antigen specific B cells and differentiating the expanded clones into antibody-secreting plasma cells. There appear to be constraints on which B cells a T cell of a given specificity can help (102,103), a process called T–B reciprocity (104). Thus, if Ir genes control helper T-cell specificity, they will in turn limit which B cells are activated and thus which antibodies are made.

The immunogenicity of peptide antigens is also limited by intrinsic and extrinsic factors. Intrinsic features such as hydrophilicity and surface accessibility are not a problem, until we consider the cross-reaction of the elicited antibodies on the native protein. Bigger problems are the host-related factors extrinsic to the structure of the peptide. With less structure to go on, each small peptide must presumably contain some nonself structural feature in order to overcome self tolerance. In addition, the same peptide must contain antigenic sites that can be recognized by helper T cells as well as by B cells. When no T-cell site is present, three approaches may be helpful: graft on a T-cell site; couple the peptide to a carrier protein; or overcome T-cell nonresponsiveness to the available structure with various immunologic agents, such as interleukin (IL)-2.

An example of a biologically relevant but poorly immunogenic peptide is the asparagine–alanine–asparagine–proline (NANP) repeat unit of the circumsporozoite (CS) protein of malaria sporozoites. Studies with malaria parasites have shown that infection by the sporozoite form produced in the mosquito can be blocked by prior immunization with irradiated, killed sporozoites (105). A monoclonal antibody to CS protein can mimic the effect in murine malaria, and this antibody is specific for the repeat unit of the CS protein (106). Thus, it would be desirable to make a malaria vaccine of the repeat unit of *Plasmodium falciparum* (NANP)$_n$. However, only mice of one MHC type (H-2^b) of all mouse strains tested were able to respond to (NANP)$_n$ (107,108). One approach to overcome this limitation is to couple (NANP)_n to a site recognizable by T cells, perhaps a carrier protein such as tetanus toxoid (109). In human trials, this conjugate was weakly immunogenic and only partially protective. Moreover, because helper T cells produced by this approach are specific for the unrelated carrier, a secondary or memory response would not be expected to be elicited by the pathogen itself.

Another choice might be to identify a T cell site on the CS protein itself and couple the two synthetic peptides together to make one complete immunogen. The result with one such site, called Th2R, was to increase the range of responding mouse MHC types by one to include H-2^k as well as H-2^b (110). This approach has the potential advantage of inducing a state of immunity that could be boosted by natural exposure to the sporozoite antigen. Because CS-specific T and B cells are both elicited by the vaccine, natural exposure to the antigen could help maintain the level of immunity during the entire period of exposure.

Another strategy to improve the immunogenicity of peptide vaccines is to stimulate the T- and B-cell responses artificially by adding IL-2 to the vaccine. Results with myoglobin indicate that genetic nonresponsiveness can be overcome by appropriate doses of IL-2 (111). The same effect was found for peptides derived from malaria proteins (112; and K. Akaji, D.T. Liu, and I.J. Berkower, unpublished results). It is not yet clear whether this effect is based on immunizing T cells or whether low T-cell responsiveness is overcome by a direct effect on B cells. In the former case, active immunity could result once specific T- and B-cell clones are expanded, even in individuals who would otherwise be nonresponders.

One of the most important possible uses of peptide antigens is as synthetic vaccines. However, even though it is possible to elicit with synthetic peptides antiinfluenza antibodies to nearly every part of the influenza hemagglutinin (75), antibodies that neutralize viral infectivity have not been elicited by immunization with synthetic peptides. This may reflect the fact that antibody binding by itself often does not result in virus inactivation. Viral inactivation occurs only when antibody interferes with one of the steps in the life cycle of the virus, including binding to its cell surface receptor, internalization, and virus uncoating within the cell. Apparently, antibodies can bind to most of the exposed surface of the virus without affecting these functions. Only those antibodies that bind to certain "neutralizing" sites can inactivate the virus. In addition, as in the case of the VP1 coat protein of poliovirus, certain neutralizing sites are found only on the native protein and not on the heat-denatured protein (113). Thus, not only the site but also the conformation that is bound by the antibodies may be important for the antibody to inactivate the virus. These sites often may be assembled topographic sites not mimicked by peptide segments of the sequence. Perhaps binding of an antibody to such an assembled site can alter the relative positions of the component subsites so as to induce an allosteric neutralizing effect. Alternatively, antibodies to such an assembled site may prevent a conformational change necessary for activity of the viral protein.

One method of mapping neutralizing sites is based on the use of neutralizing monoclonal antibodies. The virus is grown in the presence of neutralizing concentrations of the monoclonal antibody, and virus mutants are selected for the ability to overcome antibody inhibition. These are sequenced, revealing the mutation that permits "escape" by altering the antigenic site for that antibody. This method has been used to map the neutralizing sites of influenza hemagglutinin (114) as well as poliovirus capsid protein VP1

(115). The influenza escaping mutations are clustered to form an assembled topographic site, with mutations distant from each other in the primary sequence of hemagglutinin but brought together by the three-dimensional folding of the native protein. At first it was thought that neutralization was the result of steric hindrance of the hemagglutinin binding site for the cell surface receptor of the virus (116). However, similar work with poliovirus has shown that neutralizing antibodies that bind to assembled topographic sites may inactivate the virus at less than stoichiometric amounts, when at least half of the sites are unbound by antibody (117). The neutralizing antibodies all cause a conformational change in the virus, which is reflected in a change in the isoelectric point of the particles from pH 7 to pH 4 (115,118). Antibodies that bind without neutralizing do not cause this shift. Thus, an alternative explanation for the mechanism of antibody-mediated neutralization is the triggering of the virus to self destruct. Perhaps the reason that neutralizing sites are clustered near receptor-binding sites is that occupation of such sites by antibody mimics events normally caused by binding to the cellular receptor, causing the virus to prematurely trigger its cell entry mechanisms. However, in order to transmit a physiologic signal, the antibody may need to bind viral capsid proteins in the native conformation (especially assembled topographic sites), which antipeptide antibodies may fail to do. Antibodies of this specificity are similar to the viral receptors on the cell surface, some of which have been cloned and expressed without their transmembrane sequences as soluble proteins. The soluble recombinant receptors for poliovirus (119) and human immunodeficiency virus (HIV)-1 (120–122) exhibit high-affinity binding to the virus and potent neutralizing activity in vitro. The HIV-1 receptor, CD4, has been combined with the human immunoglobulin heavy chain in a hybrid protein CD4–Ig (123), which spontaneously assembles into dimers and resembles a monoclonal antibody, in which the binding site is the same as the receptor-binding site for HIV-1. In these recombinant constructs, high-affinity binding depends on the native conformation of the viral envelope glycoprotein (gp)120.

For HIV-1, two types of neutralizing antibodies have been identified. The first type binds a continuous or segmental determinant, the V3 loop sequence between amino acids 296 and 331 of gp120 (124–126). Antipeptide antibodies against this site can neutralize the virus (124). However, because this site is located in a highly variable region of the envelope, these antibodies tend to neutralize a limited range of viral variants. A second type of neutralizing antibody binds at or near the CD4 receptor-binding site of gp120 (127–129). These neutralizing antibodies, which are commonly found in the sera of infected patients, are specific for a broad range of HIV-1 variants, possibly due to conserved sequences around the CD4 binding site (130). Because the shared neutralizing determinant is an assembled topographic site, dependent on the native conformation of the protein (131), a prospective gp120 vaccine would need to be in the native conformation to be able to elicit these antibodies.

ANTIGENIC DETERMINANTS RECOGNIZED BY T CELLS

Mapping Antigenic Structures

Studies of T-cell specificity for antigen were motivated by the fact that the immune response to protein antigens is regulated at the T-cell level. A hapten, not immunogenic by itself, will elicit antibodies only when coupled to a protein that elicits a T-cell response in that animal. This ability of the protein component of the conjugate to confer immunogenicity on the hapten has been termed the "carrier effect." Recognition of the carrier by specific helper T cells induces the B cells to make antibodies. Thus, the factors contributing to a good T-cell response appear to control the B cell response as well.

Nonresponder animals display an antigen-specific failure to respond to a protein antigen, both for T cells and antibody responses. The high responder phenotype for each antigen is a genetically inheritable, usually dominant trait. Using inbred strains of mice, the genes controlling the immune response were found to be tightly linked to the MHC genes (101,132). MHC-linked immune responsiveness has been shown to depend on the T-cell recognition of antigen in association with MHC antigens of the antigen-presenting cell (APC) (discussed later; see also Chapters 8 and 9). The recognition of antigen in association with MHC molecules of the B cell is necessary for carrier-specific T cells to expand and provide helper signals to B cells, which results in clonal expansion and maturation of the B cells into antibody-producing cells.

In contrast to the range of antigens recognized by antibodies, the repertoire recognized by helper and cytotoxic T cells appears to be limited largely to protein and peptide antigens, although exceptions such as the small molecule tyrosine–azobenzene arsonate (133) exist. This limitation is not fully understood but may relate to the requirement for binding of antigens within a groove of the MHC molecule (see below).

If the antigenic determinants on proteins recognized by T cells could be identified, then it would be possible to better understand immunogenicity, to explain immune-response genes, and perhaps even to enhance the antibody response to one part of a biologically relevant antigen by altering the T-cell response for another part of the antigen.

Polyclonal T-Cell Response

Significant progress in understanding T-cell specificity was made possible by focusing on T-cell proliferation *in vitro*. Proliferation of antigen-specific cells in culture mimics the positive selection via clonal expansion of antigen-specific clones that occurs *in vivo*. The proliferative response depends on only two cells: the antigen-specific T cell and an APC, usually a macrophage, dendritic cell, or B cell. The growth of T cells in culture is measured in terms of the incorporation of [^{3}H] thymidine into newly formed DNA. Under appropriate conditions, thymidine incorporation increases with antigen concentration. This assay permits the substitution of different APCs and is highly useful in defining the MHC and antigen-processing requirements of the APCs.

Using primarily this assay, several different approaches have been taken to mapping T-cell epitopes. First, comparison of sequences of stimulatory and nonstimulatory naturally occurring variants of the native protein has been used to identify positions in the protein sequence at which substitutions could affect T-cell cross-reactivity. For example, homologous proteins from different species with known amino acid substitutions may be used. Usually, this approach has led to correct localization of the antigenic site in the protein (134–136), but the possibility of long-range effects on antigen processing must be borne in mind (see the section on Antigen Processing). Also, this approach is limited in that it can focus on the correct region of the molecule but cannot

define the boundaries of the site or identify all the critical residues because it is limited to testing those positions in the sequence at which amino acid substitutions occur in natural variants. Site-directed mutagenesis may therefore expand the capabilities of this approach. A second approach is to use short peptide segments of the protein sequence, taking advantage of the fact that T cells specific for soluble protein antigens appear to see only segmental antigenic sites, not assembled topographic ones (101,137–141) (see the sections on Antigen Processing and Prediction of T-Cell Epitopes). These may be produced by chemical or enzymatic cleavage of the natural protein (139–147), solid-phase peptide synthesis (146,148–151), or recombinant DNA methodology using expression of cloned genes or gene fragments (152). In the case of class I MHC molecule–restricted cytotoxic T cells, viral gene deletion mutants expressing only part of the gene product also have been used (153–155).

For example, the T-cell response to sperm whale myoglobin was analyzed in mice of two high-responder MHC types, H-2^s and H-2^d. When H-2^s mice were immunized with sperm whale myoglobin, the T cells responded in culture to sperm whale myoglobin and about half of the 12 additional mammalian myoglobins tested (135), but they did not respond to several other whale myoglobins or to horse myoglobin (Table 5). Conversely, when mice were immunized to horse myoglobin, they responded to horse myoglobin, and the pattern of myoglobin cross-reactivity was the reciprocal of that seen in T cells from animals immunized with sperm whale myoglobin: each myoglobin that stimulated these T cells did not stimulate sperm whale–immune T cells and *vice versa*. The response to the cross-stimulatory myoglobins was as strong as to the myoglobin used to immunize the mice. This suggested that a few shared amino acid residues formed an immunodominant epitope that was essential for T-cell activation and that most substitutions had no effect on the dominant epitope. Comparing those amino acid residues that were conserved in the stimulatory myoglobins with those that were substituted in the nonstimulatory myoglobins showed that substitutions at a single residue could explain the pattern observed. All myoglobins that cross-stimulated sperm whale–immune T cells had Glu at position 109, whereas all the cross-stimulated horse-immune T cells had Asp at 109. No member of one group could stimulate T cells from donors immunized with a myoglobin of the other group. This suggested that an immunodominant epitope recognized by T cells was centered on position 109, regardless of which amino acid was substituted. This mapping was confirmed by use of a synthetic peptide 102 to 118, which stimulated the T cells (150,156). The T cells elicited by a myoglobin of either group could readily distinguish between Asp or Glu at this position. Similar results were obtained with cytochrome c, where the predominant site recognized by T cells was localized with sequence variants to the region around residue 100 at the carboxyl end of cytochrome c (134). Furthermore, the response to cytochrome c peptide 81 to 104 was as great as the response to the whole molecule. This indicated that a 24–amino acid peptide contained an entire antigenic site recognized by T cells. Subsequent studies with synthetic peptides indicated that the T cells could distinguish between peptides with Lys or Gln at position 99, although both were immunogenic with the same MHC molecule (157–159). This residue determined T-cell memory and specificity and so presumably was interacting with the T-cell receptor (TCR). A similar conclusion could be drawn for residue 109 of myoglobin. However, this type of analysis must be used with caution. When multiple substitutions at position 109 were examined for

TABLE 5. *Proliferation of B10.S T cells immune to myoglobin*

			T cells immune to	
Stimulating myoglobin	Residue number		Equine	Sperm whale

```
                                          1 | 1 1 1 1 1
                  1 1 2 2 2 3 3 4 6 6 7     0 | 1 2 3 4 5
              1 4 9 2 5 1 7 8 4 5 5 6 7 4   9 | 8 2 2 0 1
```

Stimulating myoglobin	Residue sequence		Equine	Sperm whale
1. Equine	G D Q N G I E V T G K T V G	D | K N T N F	11,580	72
2. Bovine	A V N T	— | S	11,305	ND
3. Sei whale	V L A V D I K N T	— | R D N K	20,922	1,205
4. Minke whale	V L A V D I K N T	— | R E N K	13,604	3,694
5. Goosebeaked whale	E L H A L I K H T	— | R D K	10,373	1,500[a]
6. Dog	I L K N N T	— | D K	6,863	610[a]
7. California sea lion	L L K K T	E | D K	683	6,869
8. Harbor seal	L L K S N T	E | E K	3,132	9,592
9. Killer whale	L L D I K N T A	E | R E N K	2,568	16,745
10. Dall porpoise	E L L D K N T A	E | R E N K	1,759	7,653
11. Sperm whale	V E L H A V D I K S R V T A	E | R D N K Y	3,500	18,593
Medium control			1,164	611

ND, not done.

[a]Normalized results from a second experiment.

T-cell recognition and MHC binding, residue 109 was found to affect both functions (160). The ultimate use of synthetic peptides to analyze the segmental sites of a protein that are recognized by T cells was to synthesize a complete set of peptides, each staggered by just one amino acid from the previous peptide, corresponding to the entire sequence of hen egg lysozyme (HEL) (161). Around each immunodominant site, a cluster of several stimulatory peptides was found. The minimum core sequence consisted of just those residues shared by all antigenic peptides within a cluster, whereas the full extent of sequences spanning all stimulatory peptides within the same cluster defined the determinant envelope. These two ways of defining an antigenic site differ, and one interpretation is that each core sequence corresponds to an MHC binding site, whereas the determinant envelope includes the many ways for T cells to recognize the same peptide bound to the MHC.

In each case, the polyclonal T-cell response could be mapped to a single predominant antigenic site. These results are consistent with the idea that each protein antigen has a limited number of immunodominant sites (possibly one) recognized by T cells in association with MHC molecules of the high responder type. If none of the antigenic sites could associate with MHC molecules on the APCs, then the strain would be a low responder to that antigen. The antigen would be unable to stimulate T cells, resulting in little or no immunogenicity.

Monoclonal T Cells

Further progress in mapping T-cell sites depended on the analysis of cloned T-cell lines. These were either antigen-specific T-cell lines made by the method of Kimoto and Fathman (162) or T-cell hybridomas made by the method of Kappler and co-workers (163). In the former method, T cells are allowed to proliferate in response to antigen and APCs, rested, and then restimulated again. After stimulation, the blasts can be cloned by limiting dilution and grown from a single cell in the presence of IL-2. The antigen specificity of the line is confirmed in the standard proliferation assay using antigen and APCs. In the second method, enriched populations of antigen-specific T cells are fused with a drug-sensitive T-cell tumor, and the fused cells are selected for their ability to grow in the presence of the drug. Then the antigen specificity of each fused cell line must be determined. The key to determining this in a tumor line is that antigen-specific stimulation of a T-cell hybridoma results in release of IL-2 even though proliferation is constitutive. T cells produced by either method are useful in defining epitopes, measuring their MHC associations, and studying antigen-processing requirements.

Monoclonal T cells may be useful in identifying which of the many proteins from a pathogen are important for T-cell responses. For instance, Young and Lamb (164) have developed a way to screen proteins separated by sodium dodecyl sulfate (SDS)–polyacrylamide gel electrophoresis and blotted onto nitrocellulose for stimulation of T-cell clones and have used this to identify antigens of *Mycobacterium tuberculosis* (165). Mustafa et al. (166) have even used T-cell clones to screen recombinant DNA expression libraries to identify relevant antigens of *M leprae*. Use of T cells to map epitopes has been important in defining tumor antigens (167–172).

These findings can be generalized to characterize a large number of epitopes recognized by T cells from a number of protein antigens (Table 6) (173–188). In each case, the entire site is contained on a short peptide. MHC class I–restricted antigens also follow this rule (189), even when the protein antigen is normally expressed on the surface of infected cells. This applies to viral glycoproteins, such as influenza hemagglutinin, that are recognized by cytolytic T cells after antigen processing (190) (see section on Antigen Processing below).

Sequential Steps that Focus the T-cell Response on Immunodominant Determinants

In contrast to antibodies that bind all over the surface of a native protein (42) (see section on Protein and Polypeptide Antigenic Determinants), it has been observed that T cells elicited by immunization with the native protein tend to be focused on one or a few immunodominant sites (191,192). This is true whether one deals with model mammalian or avian proteins such as cytochrome c (140), myoglobin (139,141), lysozyme (143,176,193,194), insulin

TABLE 6. *Examples of immunodominant T-cell epitopes recognized in association with class II MHC molecules*

Protein	T-cell antigenic sites (reference)	Amphipathic segments
Sperm whale myoglobin	69–78 (139)	64–78
	102–118 (150)	99–117
	132–145 (146)	128–145
Pigeon cytochrome c	93–104 (149)	92–103
Beef cytochrome c	11–25 (183)	9–29
	66–80 (184)	58–78
Influenza	109–119 (177)	97–120
Hemagglutinin	130–140 (178)	—
A/PR/8/34	302–313 (178 & 179)	291–314
Pork insulin	B 5–16 (148)	4–16
	A 4–14 (180)	1–21
Chicken lysozyme	46–61 (176)	—
	74–86 (175)	72–86
	81–96 (175)	86–102
	109–119 (136)	—
Chicken ovalbumin	323–339 (144)	329–346
Foot and mouth virus VP1	141–160 (182)	148–165
Hepatitis B virus		
Pre-S	120–132 (181)	121–135
Major surface antigen	38–52 (185)	36–49
	95–109 (185)	—
	140–154 (185)	—
λ Repressor protein CI	12–26 (186)	8–25
Rabies virus-spike glycoprotein precursor	32–44 (187)	29–46

Adapted with permission (188).

(148,180), and ovalbumin (144), or with bacterial, viral, and parasitic proteins from pathogens, such as influenza hemagglutinin (178) or nucleoprotein (189), staphylococcal nuclease (195), or malarial circumsporozoite protein (110,196). Because the latter category of proteins shares no obvious homology to mammalian proteins, the immunodominance of a few sites cannot be attributed simply to tolerance for the rest of the protein because of self-tolerance to homologous host proteins. Moreover, immunodominance is not simply the preemption of the response by a single clone of predominant T cells, because it has been observed that immunodominant sites tend to be the focus for a polyclonal response of a number of distinct T-cell clones recognizing overlapping subsites within the antigenic site or having different sensitivities to substitutions of amino acids within the site (143,144,149,150,161,175,176,197).

Immunodominant antigenic sites appear to be qualitatively different from other sites. For example, in the case of myoglobin, when the number of clones responding to different epitopes after immunization with native protein was quantitated by limiting dilution, it was observed that the bulk of the response to the whole protein in association with the high-responder class II MHC molecules was focused on a single site within residues 102 to 118 (156) (Fig. 6). There were T cells specific for other epitopes, but their numbers never reached the same level as those specific for the immunodominant site. Moreover, when T cells (from the same immunization of F1 hybrid mice) specific for the protein associated with the low-responder class II MHC molecules were compared with those discussed above, the response to nonimmunodominant sites was quantitatively similar to that for the same sites restricted to the high-responder MHC. The major difference was the absence of a response specific for the immunodominant site in association with the low-responder MHC (Fig. 6). Similar results were found for two different high-responder

and two different low-responder MHC haplotypes (156). Thus Ir gene–controlled high or low responsiveness could be accounted for by the presence or absence of a response to this immunodominant site, even though all haplotypes responded to some antigenic sites. Why didn't the response to the other sites compensate for the lack of response to the immunodominant site in the low responders? It appears that there is something special about the immunodominant site. The greater frequency of T cells specific for the immunodominant site may in part be attributed to the large number of ways this site can be recognized by different T-cell clones, as mentioned above, but this only pushes the problem back one level. Why is an immunodominant site the focus for so many different T-cell clones? Because the answer cannot depend on any particular T cell, it must depend on other factors, primarily involved in the steps in antigen processing and presentation by MHC molecules.

It also has been observed that some peptides may be immunogenic themselves, but the T-cell response they elicit is specific only for the peptide and does not cross-react with the native protein (198–200). Conversely, not all peptides that are immunogenic themselves will correspond to immunogenic sites when the native protein is used as immunogen (198–200). These are called cryptic determinants (200). The reasons for these differences may involve the way the native protein is processed to produce fragments distinct from but including or overlapping the synthetic peptides used in experiments, and also the competition among sites within the protein for binding to the same MHC molecules, as discussed further in a later section. To understand these factors that determine dominance or crypticity, one must understand the steps through which an antigen must go before it can stimulate a T-cell response.

Unlike B cells, T-cell recognition of antigen depends on the function of another cell, the APC (201). Antigen must pass through a

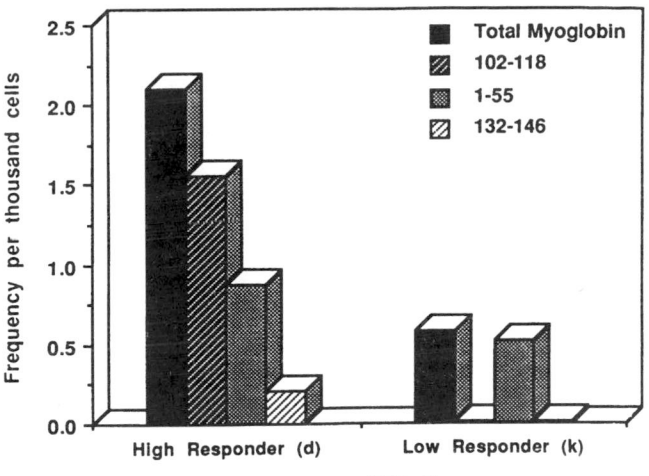

FIG. 6. Frequency of high- and low-responder MHC-restricted T cells in F1 hybrid. High responsiveness may be accounted for by the response to a single immunodominant epitope. Lymph node T cells from [low-responder (H-2^k) × high-responder (H-2^d)]F1 hybrid mice immunized with whole myoglobin were plated at different limiting dilutions in microtiter wells with either high-responder or low-responder presenting cells and myoglobin as antigen. The cells growing in each well were tested for responsiveness to whole myoglobin and to various peptide epitopes of myoglobin. The frequency of T cells of each specificity and MHC restriction was calculated from Poisson statistics and is plotted on the ordinate. Most of the difference in T-cell frequency between high- and low-responder restriction types (solid bars) can be accounted for by the presence of T cells responding to the immunodominant site at residues 102 to 118, accounting for more than two thirds of the high-responder myoglobin specific T cells, in contrast to the absence of such T cells restricted to the low-responder MHC type. Based on the data of Kojima et al. (156).

number of intracellular compartments and survive processing and transport steps before it can be effectively presented to T cells. After antigen synthesis in the cell (as in a virally infected cell) or antigen uptake via phagocytosis, pinocytosis, or, in some cases, receptor-mediated endocytosis, the subsequent steps include: (a) partial degradation (processing) into discrete antigenic fragments that can be recognized by T cells; (b) transport of these fragments into a cellular compartment where MHC binding can occur; (c) MHC binding and assembly of a stable peptide–MHC complex; and (d) recognition of that peptide–MHC complex by the expressed T-cell repertoire. At each step, a potential antigenic determinant runs the risk of being lost from the process, for example, by excessive degradation or failure to meet the binding requirements needed for transport to the next step. Only those peptides that surmount the four selective hurdles will prove to be antigenic for T cells. We will now consider each step in detail for its contribution to the strength and specificity of the T-cell response to protein antigens.

Antigen Processing

Processing of Antigen for T Cells Restricted to Class II MHC Molecules

It has long been known that T-cell responses such as delayed hypersensitivity *in vivo* or T-cell proliferation *in vitro* to exogenous proteins can be stimulated not only by the native protein but

also by denatured protein (137) and fragments of native protein (180). Indeed, this feature, along with the requirement for recognition in association with class II MHC molecules, distinguishes T- from B-cell responses. In a number of cases, the site recognized by cloned T cells has been located to a discrete synthetic peptide corresponding to a segment of the primary sequence of the protein. Examples include insulin (148,180), cytochrome c (149), lysozyme (143,175), and myoglobin (139,146,150). In each case, the stimulatory peptide must contain all the information required for antigen presentation and T-cell stimulation. The native protein conformation is lacking, although some antigenic peptides may be long enough to have significant secondary structure (alpha helicity or beta sheet) (202–205). The lack of conformational specificity does not indicate a lack of TCR specificity. Rather, it results from antigen processing into peptide fragments that destroys conformational differences before binding the TCR. One way to accomplish this is via antigen processing, which involves the partial degradation of a protein antigen into peptide fragments (Fig. 7). The primary sequence of antigenic peptides serves as the common molecular signal that is recognized by T cells responding to either native or denatured antigen.

Evidence of processing came from the fact that a single protein antigen could stimulate T cells to different epitopes, each specific for a different MHC antigen. For example, when a series of myoglobin-specific T-cell clones were tested for both antigen specificity and MHC restriction, six clones were specific for a site centering on amino acid Glu 109, and all six recognized the antigen in association with I-A^d. Nine additional T-cell clones were specific for a second epitope centered on Lys 140 and were restricted to a different MHC antigen, I-E^d. Thus, the antigen behaved as if it were split up into distinct epitopes, each with its own ability to bind MHC (173).

That T cells recognize processed antigen was demonstrated by the fact that inhibitors of processing can block antigen presentation. Early experiments by Ziegler and Unanue (206) showed that processing depends on intracellular degradative endosomes, because drugs such as chloroquine and NH$_4$Cl, which raise endosomal pH and inhibit acid-dependent proteases, could block the process. However, prior degradation of proteins into peptide fragments allows them to trigger T cells even in the presence of these inhibitors of processing (207). For example, T-cell clone 14.5 recognizes the Lys 140 site of myoglobin equally well on the antigenic peptide (residues 132 to 153), as on the native protein (Fig. 8). The difference between these two forms of antigen is brought out by the presence of processing inhibitors. Leupeptin, for example, inhibits lysosomal proteases and blocks the T-cell responses to native myoglobin but not to peptide 132 to 153. Thus, native myoglobin cannot stimulate T cells without further processing, whereas the peptide requires little or no additional processing (208).

Why is antigen processing necessary? For class II MHC molecules, experiments suggest that antigen processing may uncover functional sites that are buried in the native protein structure. For example, a form of intact myoglobin that has been partially unfolded through chemical modification can behave like a myoglobin peptide and can be presented by APC even in the presence of enough protease inhibitor or chloroquine to completely block the presentation of native myoglobin (208). Denatured lysozyme also could be presented without processing to one T-cell clone (145). This result suggests that the requirement for processing may simply be a steric requirement, that is, to uncover the two sites

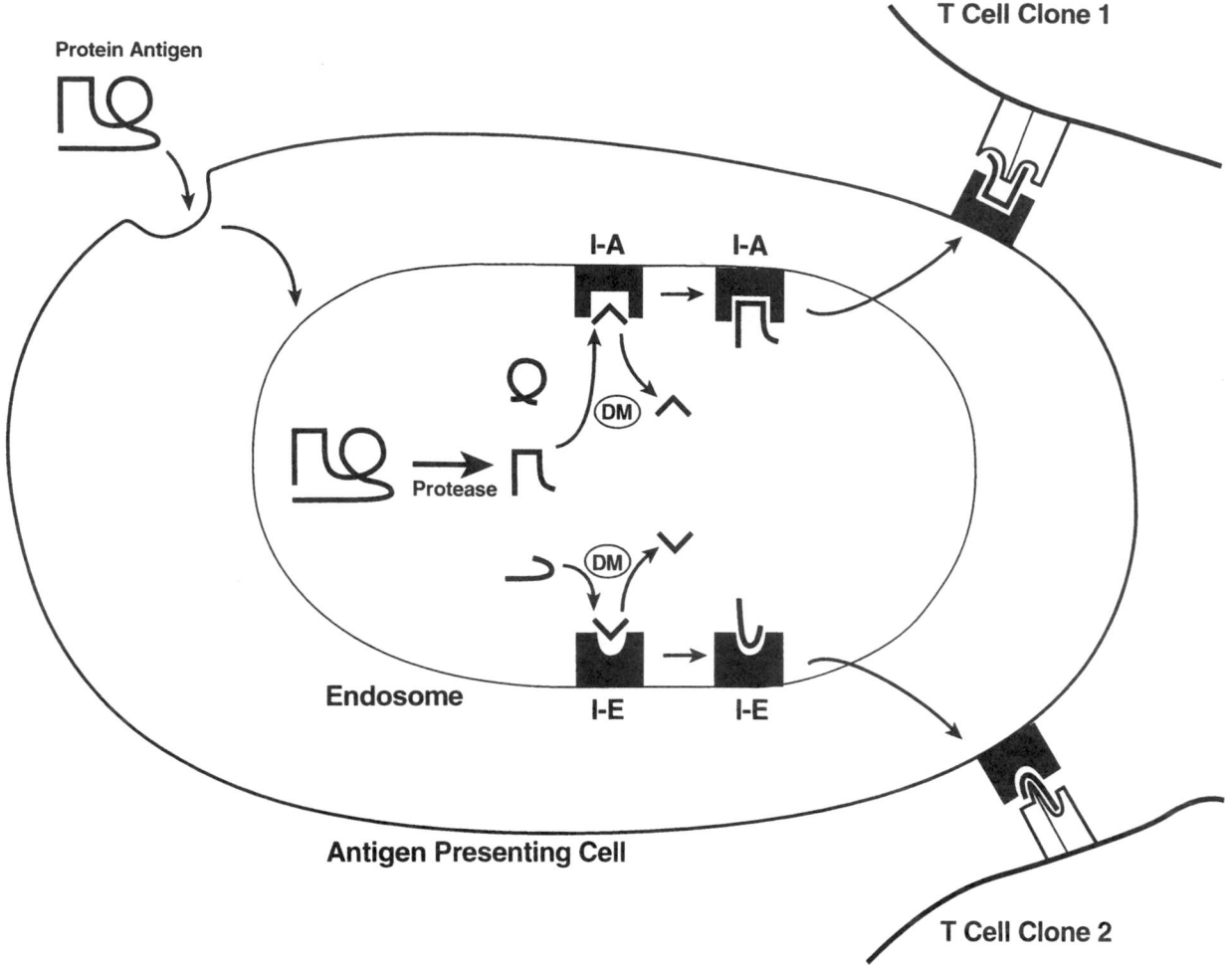

FIG. 7. Steps in antigen presentation by class II MHC molecules. Soluble antigen enters the presenting cell by phagocytosis, pinocytosis, or receptor-mediated endocytosis. It is partially degraded to peptide fragments by acid-dependent proteases in endosomes. Antigenic peptides associate with MHC class II molecules (I-A or I-E in the mouse) to form an antigenic complex that is transported to the cell surface. Before an MHC class II molecule can bind the peptide, it must release the CLIP peptide fragment of invariant chain from the binding groove, which is catalyzed by HLA-DM. Binding of T-cell receptors to the peptide–MHC complex triggers T-cell proliferation, resulting in clonal expansion of antigen-specific T cells.

needed to form the trimolecular complex between antigen and MHC and between antigen and TCR. Thus, unfolding may be sufficient without proteolysis, and proteolysis may simply accomplish an unfolding analogous to Alexander's approach to the Gordian knot.

The importance of antigen unfolding for T-cell recognition and the ability of unfolding to bypass the need for antigen processing apply not only to small proteins the size of myoglobin and lysozyme but also to a range of sizes from small peptides to extremely large proteins. At one extreme, Lee et al. (209) found that even fibrinogen, of molecular weight 340 kDa, does not need to be processed if the epitope recognized is on the carboxy-terminal portion of the α chain, which is naturally unfolded in the native molecule. At the other extreme, even a small peptide of only 18 amino acid residues, apamin, requires processing unless the two disulfide bonds that hold it in the native conformation are cleaved

artificially to allow unfolding (210). Therefore, large size does not mandate processing, and small size does not necessarily obviate the need for processing, at least for class II presentation. The common feature throughout the size range seems to be the need for unfolding. This evidence, taken together with the earlier data on unfolding of myoglobin and lysozyme, strongly supports the conclusion that unfolding, rather than size reduction, is the primary goal of antigen processing and that either antigen presentation by MHC molecules or TCR recognition frequently requires exposure of residues not normally exposed on the surface of the native protein. This conclusion is supported by recent studies of peptides eluted from class II MHC molecules, and the crystal structures of class II MHC–peptide complexes, which show that longer peptides can bind with both ends extending beyond the two ends of the MHC groove (211–213) (see section on Antigen Interaction with MHC Molecules below).

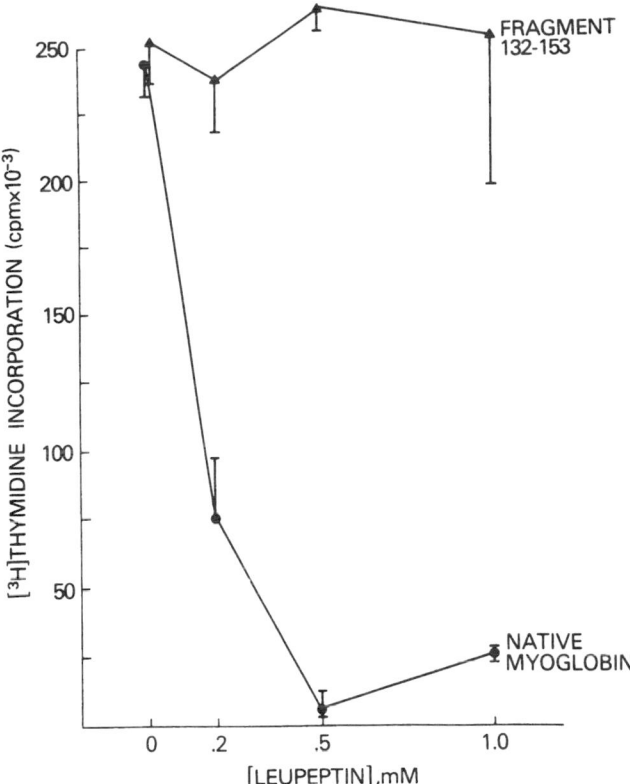

FIG. 8. Inhibition of antigen presentation by the protease inhibitor leupeptin: differential effect on presentation of the same epitope of native myoglobin or peptide 132 to 153 to the same monoclonal T-cell population. Splenic cells from nonimmunized B10.D2 mice, as a source of APCs, were incubated with leupeptin at the concentration indicated for 15 minutes before and during exposure to 2 μ native myoglobin or 1 μ peptide fragment, washed, irradiated, and cultured at 400,000 cells/well with 10,000 T cells of clone 14.5; thymidine incorporation was measured after 4 days of culture (208).

Processing of Antigen for T Cells Restricted to Class I MHC Molecules

In contrast to class II–restricted T cells, it was widely assumed that class I–restricted T cells, such as cytolytic T cells (CTLs) specific for virus-infected cells, responded mainly to unprocessed viral glycoproteins expressed on the surface of infected cells. For example, this appeared to be the case for influenza virus, where the hemagglutinin was detected on the cell surface and where CTLs specific for the hemagglutinin were demonstrated. However, converse examples began to appear at about the same time that antigen processing was demonstrated for class II–restricted T cells. For example, influenza nucleoprotein (NP) was also found to be a major target antigen for influenza-specific CTLs, even though NP remains in the nucleus of infected cells and none is detectable on the cell surface (214). This led to speculation that antigen presentation in association with class I molecules also may depend on some form of antigen processing.

Using the cloned NP gene to transfect L cells, Townsend et al. (153) showed that the NP protein could be manipulated in various ways and still function as a good target for CTLs, even though NP lacks a leader sequence to direct it to the cell surface. In addition, using a series of truncated constructs of the NP gene, they showed

that CTLs lyse cells expressing NP fragment 1 to 386 but not those expressing NP fragment 1 to 327, so the antigenic site must lie between residues 327 and 386 (153). This was confirmed when they showed that target cells that take up synthetic NP peptide 366 to 379 were lysed by NP-specific CTLs (189). This constitutes evidence that antigen presented in association with class I molecules requires processing into antigenic fragments. Also, the demonstration that synthetic peptides could sensitize targets for CTLs introduced a powerful tool for mapping and studying CTL epitopes.

In light of the results with NP, additional experiments were performed with hemagglutinin to determine whether surface expression of the intact glycoprotein was really necessary for class I–restricted CTL recognition. Removal of the leader sequence from the hemagglutinin gene inserted into vaccinia virus results in a protein antigen that is expressed within infected cells but lacks the signals for transport to the cell surface. Nevertheless, target cells expressing leader-negative hemagglutinin were lysed equally well as those with surface hemagglutinin (190). Similar conclusions were drawn from anchor-negative mutants (215). Thus, even for hemagglutinin, surface expression of native antigen is not required for antigenicity, implying that it is the processed antigen that stimulates a T-cell response. Indeed, recent studies of HIV-1 gp160 genes with or without a leader sequence suggest that removal of the leader sequence can increase the amount of protein that is retained in the cytosol and is available for processing and presentation through the class I MHC processing pathway (216). The explanation may be that the signal peptide results in cotranslational translocation of the growing peptide chain into the endoplasmic reticulum (ER), whereas proteins without a signal peptide are synthesized and remain in the cytosol, where they are accessible to the processing machinery of the class I pathway.

The antigen-processing pathway leading to class I presentation is quite different from the endosomal pathway leading to class II presentation. Unlike endosomal processing, the nonendosomal pathway is insensitive to chloroquine, NH$_4$Cl, and leupeptin. In some cases, different forms of the same antigen can be processed exclusively by one pathway or the other. For example, in one study, ultraviolet (UV)-inactivated influenza virus was processed by the endosomal pathway, whereas live virus was not (217). Cells exposed to UV-inactivated virus were recognized only by class II–restricted CTLs, whereas cells exposed to live virus were recognized by class I–restricted CTLs. A model was proposed in which endogenous synthesis of viral proteins led to nonendosomal processing, and the resultant peptides were displayed on the cell surface with class I MHC molecules. This pathway would be inaccessible to exogenous proteins, accounting for their failure to be presented with class I antigens (217). In effect, the processing pathway would determine the class restriction.

For this simple model to hold, each step in a processing pathway would have to be tightly linked, so that no crossing of pathways could occur. Given that antigen can come from either endogenous synthesis or uptake of exogenous proteins, that two processing pathways, nonendosomal and endosomal, are available, and two classes of MHC molecules are capable of binding peptides, theoretically up to eight combinations might be possible. The simple model allows for just two combinations out of the eight: exogenous antigen degraded to peptides in endosomes, leading to peptides binding to class II, or endogenously synthesized antigen degraded nonendosomally and the resultant peptides binding to class I molecules. Over time, at least four additional combinations have appeared, which may be thought of as alternative paths leading into or out of the two processing systems, although the simple model still describes the major pathways of antigen processing.

First, exogenous antigens such as those from UV-inactivated influenza virus can enter the nonendosomal pathway for presentation with class I molecules when the viral neuraminidase is inhibited (218), perhaps due to increased antigen binding and entry into cells. This effect is accentuated at acid pH (219), under conditions that activate the membrane fusion activity of influenza hemagglutinin (220) and allow virus to penetrate directly across the plasma membrane. Thus, direct entry of virus into the cytoplasm enables exogenous antigen to enter the nonendosomal processing pathway leading to MHC class I association. Similarly, experiments with hepatitis B surface antigen (HBsAg)-specific human T-cell clones (221) have shown that exogenous HBsAg particles can gain access to nonendosomal processing, which may contribute to the potency of HBsAg vaccine. Another example showing that entry into the cytoplasm is sufficient to direct antigen into the nonendosomal pathway was the uptake of ovalbumin under hyperosmotic conditions, followed by reducing the osmolality and lysing the pinocytotic vesicles into the cytoplasm. These cells presented ovalbumin fragments with class I molecules to CD8$^+$ CTLs (222). As shown in these three cases, entry to the nonendosomal pathway depends on gaining access to the cytoplasm, not on where a protein was synthesized.

In a second combination, endogenously synthesized antigen can enter endosomal processing for presentation with class II. Endogenously synthesized HBsAg can be processed by the endosomal pathway and recognized by CD4$^+$ T-cell clones in association with MHC class II (221). Similarly, Weiss and Bogen have shown that endogenously synthesized lamda light chains can be recognized by class II–restricted T cells (223,224), and Eisenlohr and Hackett made a similar finding for recognition of influenza neuraminidase by a class II–restricted T-cell hybridoma (225). In some of these cases, endosomal processing might be explained as the reentry into endosomes of antigens expressed on the cell surface. However, Polydefkis et al. (226) reported that endogenous gp160 of HIV-1 is recognized in its nonsecreted form by class II–restricted T cells, but not in its processed and secreted form. Similarly, Jaraquemada et al. (227) reported the class II–associated recognition of endogenously synthesized nonsecreted influenza virus M1 matrix protein after endosomal processing. In some cases, the endogenous antigen was expressed by cells infected with a recombinant vaccinia virus containing the appropriate gene (228), and the possibility of exogenous antigen contaminating the viral preparation was excluded by using purified virus and by showing that UV inactivation of the virus blocked antigen presentation by the infected cells.

A third and somewhat more controversial new combination is that of exogenous proteins processed by the nonendosomal processing pathway and then presented by MHC class II. For example, Nuchtern et al. (219) have studied class II–restricted CTL lines that recognize antigenic fragments of influenza matrix protein after nonendosomal processing, as shown by sensitivity to brefeldin A (an inhibitor of Golgi traffic) and resistance to chloroquine. Similarly, Jacobson et al. (229) reported class II–restricted CTLs against measles virus proteins that were chloroquine insensitive, and Y. Jin and I.J. Berkower (unpublished results) have found several class II–restricted T-cell clones that recognize exogenous HBsAg after nonendosomal processing (chloroquine and leupeptin insensitive). It should be noted that the only difference between this third combination and the classical pathway for exogenous antigen presented by class II MHC molecules is the resistance in each case

of the processing to chloroquine inhibition. A possible fourth new combination, in which endogenously expressed HBsAg was presented with class II after nonendosomal processing, was also observed for the same HBsAg-specific T-cell clones. Given these many exceptions, a new paradigm may be needed to explain antigen entry and exit from the two processing systems and the subsequent presentation of peptides by classes I and II. Cytoplasmic entry, rather than endogenous protein synthesis, is the common denominator for nonendosomal processing. Endocytosis of exogenous proteins favors endosomal processing, although some antigens may escape endosomes and proceed to nonendosomal processing. Special signals on viral proteins, such as membrane fusion peptides used by the virus to escape from endosomes, may affect localization and processing. After processing, various cellular proteins play an important role in directing the peptide products toward class I or II, based on entry into cellular compartments where MHC binding sites are accessible to peptides.

It is apparent that despite the evidence for cross-talk between the class I and class II antigen-processing pathways, there are good teleologic reasons for the pathways to be kept separate. Class I MHC molecules present antigen to CD8$^+$ T cells, which are usually cytotoxic, and provide immune surveillance to destroy cells producing inappropriate proteins endogenously, such as viral proteins in a virus-infected cell or mutant proteins or other tumor antigens in a cancer cell. In contrast, class II molecules present antigen to CD4$^+$ T cells, which generally activate the cells with which they interact, such as a B cell to make antibody or a macrophage to activate its cytolytic machinery. It would not benefit the organism if a B cell, which had been waiting all its life to encounter the antigen for which it expressed specific immunoglobulin, finally encountered that antigen only to present it to a CTL and be killed, rather than to a helper T cell to be activated. Similarly, it would be counterproductive for a virus-infected cell to present viral antigens to a helper T cell and thereby become activated to produce more virus, instead of being killed by a CTL. It is this dichotomy that may explain the evolution of two distinct classes of MHC molecules and correspondingly two distinct pathways of antigen processing to provide for both needs for sampling foreign antigens but keeping them separate.

Interestingly, the MHC itself encodes near the class II region two proteins, known as LMP-2 and LMP-7 for "low molecular weight protein," that contribute to the cytosolic processing machinery, specifically the proteasome. These LMPs assemble with about 14 others to form a high molecular weight complex of about 580 kDa. Due to MHC-linked polymorphism of these two LMPs, polyclonal anti-MHC sera bind LMP-2 and LMP-7 and precipitate the entire complex of MHC-linked and nonlinked proteins (230). This complex was described by Tanaka et al. (231,232) and Arrigo and co-workers (233), who found a 650-kDa particle associated with the ER in the cytosol, which had five distinct protease activities located at distinct sites. The proteasome is a barrel-shaped structure, with the protease activities arrayed on the inner surface, and unfolded proteins are believed to enter the barrel at one end, leaving as peptides at the other end. The different proteases cut preferentially after aromatic or branched-chain amino acids (chymotrypticlike activity), branched-chain amino acids (primarily aliphatic), basic amino acids (trypsin-like activity), acidic residues (glutamate preferring), or small neutral amino acid residues (234,235). Protease activity is increased against misfolded proteins, such as senescent proteins or viral proteins produced during infection, and proteins synthesized with artificial amino acids are particularly susceptible to degradation by proteasomes. The products of protease digestion are peptides, including 9-mers, of just the right size for MHC binding. The chymotryptic and trypsinlike activities may be particularly important for antigenic peptides because many peptides that naturally bind MHC end in hydrophobic or basic residues (236).

The LMP proteins and proteasome are closely related, since antiserum against the LMP complex and antiserum against the proteasome cross-reacted with the same complex (237), although the extent of precipitation varied, depending on which antiserum was used. All LMP complexes contain proteasome proteins, but only 5% to 10% of proteasomes contain LMP-2 and LMP-7.

The proteasome is the major processing machinery of the nonendosomal processing pathway. This is shown by the effect of proteasome inhibitors on MHC class I assembly and antigen presentation and by the effect of LMP-2 and LMP-7 mutations on antigen processing. A family of proteasome inhibitors have been described (234,235,238) that consist of short peptides, three to four amino acids in length, ending in an aldehyde, such as Ac-Leu Leu norLeu-al, carbobenzoxy-Leu Leu norVal-al (235), or nonpeptides such as lactacystin (239). Although the peptides appear to be directed primarily at the chymotrypsinlike protease activity, such as false substrates, they in fact inhibit all three types of protease activity. Presumably by occupying the catalytic site of one protease, they block the aqueous channel of the proteasome and prevent further processing by the others as well. Alternatively, it may be that proteasomal degradation is processive, requiring an ordered progression from one site to the next, or coordinated to cleave simultaneously at different sites, so that inhibiting one blocks all.

By inhibiting antigen processing, these inhibitors induce a phenotype of reduced expression of MHC class I and inability to present antigen to class I restricted CTL (235). The MHC class I heavy chains remain in the ER, as shown by failure to become resistant to endoglycosidase H (240), which occurs in the Golgi. They are also unable to form stable complexes with β2 microglobulin, due to a lack of peptides. These effects are specific for the protease function because the inhibitors do not block presentation of synthetic peptides, which also rescue MHC class I expression, and because inhibition is reversible when inhibitor is removed. These results suggests that proteasomes are the primary supplier of antigenic peptides for class I because other pathways are unable to compensate. However, it is also possible that the inhibitors could block other potential processing enzymes as well. One alternative processing pathway is provided by signal peptidase. As signal peptides are cleaved from proteins entering the ER, these hydrophobic peptides can bind MHC class I (241). Particularly for MHC molecules such as human leukocyte antigen (HLA)-A2, which prefer hydrophobic sequences, this peptidase can be an important source of antigenic peptides that are independent of proteasomes and TAP-1 and -2 transport (transporter associated with antigen processing; see section on Transport below), because they are formed inside the ER.

The function of LMP-2 and LMP-7 are not yet certain, but they do shift the preference of proteasomes for cleaving after certain sequences, resulting in the production of different peptide fragments (242–244). Proteasomes lacking LMP-2 through mutation or gene knock-out have the same affinity, but decreased cleavage rate, for sequences ending in hydrophobic or basic amino acids. The effect is specific for these proteolytic sites because the activity against sequences containing acidic amino acids actually increased (243). Despite the shift in specific peptides released, the

overall level of MHC class I expression was reduced only slightly in LMP-7 knock-outs (244) and not at all in the LMP-2 knock-outs. However, presentation of specific epitopes of the male H-Y antigen or of influenza nucleoprotein was reduced by three- to fivefold in these knock-outs.

Another protein associated with proteasomes is PA28, which assembles into 11s structures (245). Like LMP-2 and 7 (242), PA28 is inducible by interferon gamma, and its induction causes a shift in proteasome function that may lead to the production of different antigenic peptides. For example, synthetic substrates were designed to test the ability of proteasomes to generate authentic MHC binding peptides. These substrates contained the MHC binding ligand flanked by the natural sequence as found in the original protein.

To generate the MHC binding ligand, the proteasome would have to cleave the substrate twice (246). By itself, the 20s proteasome was able to produce singly cleaved fragments, but with added PA28, doubly cut peptides were generated preferentially. Thus, PA28 favored the production of antigenic peptides, possibly by keeping the peptide in the proteasome until processing was complete. Alternatively, PA28 may coordinate the proteolytic activity of two adjacent sites to generate doubly cut peptides of just the right length (eight to nine mers) to fit in the MHC groove. The distance between these nearby sites would determine the size of the peptides produced.

The specificity of this proteasomal processing system determines the first step in winnowing the number of protein segments that can become CTL epitopes by selectively producing some peptide fragments in abundance and destroying others. Thus, it is probably not just coincidental that the C-terminal residues produced by proteasomal cleavage often serve as anchor residues for binding class I MHC molecules, or that the lengths of peptides produced are optimal for class I MHC binding (242,247).

Influence of Antigen Processing on the Expressed T-Cell Repertoire

Several lines of evidence indicate that antigen processing plays a critical role in determining which potential antigenic sites are recognized and therefore what part of the potential T-cell repertoire is expressed upon immunization with a protein antigen. Because the T cell does not see the native antigen but only the products of antigen processing, it is not unreasonable that the nature of these products would at least partly determine which potential epitopes could be recognized by T cells.

One line of evidence that processing plays a major role in T-cell repertoire expression came from comparisons that were made of the immunogenicity of peptide versus native molecule in the cases of myoglobin (198) or lysozyme (199). In the case of myoglobin, a site of equine myoglobin (residues 102 to 118) that did not elicit a response when H-2^k mice were immunized with native myoglobin nevertheless was found to be immunogenic when the mice were immunized with the peptide (198). Thus, the low responsiveness to this site in mice immunized with the native myoglobin was not due to either of the classical mechanisms of Ir gene defects, namely, a hole in the T-cell repertoire or a failure of the site to interact with MHC molecules of that strain. However, the peptide-immune T cells responded only poorly to native equine myoglobin in vitro. Thus, the peptide and the native molecule did not cross-react well in either direction. The problem was not simply a failure to process the native molecule to produce this epitope, because (H-2^k × H-2^a)F1-presenting cells could present this epitope to H-2^s T cells when given native myoglobin but could not present it to H-2^k T cells. Also, because the same results applied to individual T-cell clones, which should not be contaminated with suppressor cells, the failure to respond to the native molecule was apparently not due to suppressor cells induced by the native molecule. Similar observations were made for the response to peptide 74 to 96 of hen lysozyme in B10.A mice (199). The peptide, not the native molecule, induced T cells specific for this site, and these T cells did not cross-react with the native molecule. With the above alternative mechanisms excluded, we are left with the conclusion that an appropriate peptide was produced but it differed from the synthetic peptide in such a way that a hindering site outside the minimal antigenic site interfered with presentation by presenting cells of certain MHC types.

Further evidence consistent with this mechanism came from the work of Shastri et al. (248), who found that different epitopes within the 74 to 96 region of lysozyme were immunodominant in H-2^b mice when different forms of the immunogen were used. With native hen lysozyme as immunogen, the T cells specific for this region all responded to the 74 to 90 fragment but not to the 81 to 96 fragment, whereas with the cyanogen bromide fragment 13 to 105 as immunogen, the T cells that were elicited responded to the 81 to 96 fragment but not to the 74 to 90 fragment. If the tryptic fragment 74 to 96 was used for immunization, both sets of T cells were elicited.

Another line of evidence came from fine specificity studies of individual T-cell clones. Shastri et al. (249) observed that H-2^b T-cell clones specific for hen lysozymes were about 100-fold more sensitive to ring-necked pheasant lysozyme than to hen lysozyme. Nevertheless, they were equally sensitive to the cyanogen bromide cleavage fragments containing the antigenic sites from both lysozymes. Thus, regions outside the minimal antigenic site removable by cyanogen bromide cleavage presumably interfered with presentation or recognition of the corresponding site in hen lysozyme or with processing of the native molecule to produce these sites. Similarly, it was observed that a T-cell clone specific for sperm whale myoglobin, not equine myoglobin, responded equally well to the minimal epitope synthetic peptides from the two species (198). Here, too, residues outside the actual site must be distinguishing equine from sperm whale myoglobin. It is possible that equine myoglobin is processed differently from sperm whale myoglobin, so that the fragment containing the site is poorly produced. However, experiments using F1-presenting cells that can clearly produce this epitope for presentation to other T cells proved that the problem was not a failure to produce the appropriate fragment from hen lysozyme (199) or equine myoglobin (198). Thus, these cases provide evidence that a structure outside the minimal site can hinder presentation in association with a particular MHC molecule.

Such a hindering structure was elegantly identified in a study by Grewal et al. (250) comparing HEL peptides presented by strains C57BL/6 and C3H.SW that share H-2^b but differ in non-MHC genes. After immunization with whole lysozyme, a strong T-cell response was seen to peptide 46 to 61 in C3H.SW mice but not at all in C57BL/6 mice. Because the F1 hybrids of these two strains responded, the lack of response in one strain was not due to a hole in the T-cell repertoire produced by self tolerance. It was found that peptide 46 to 60 bound directly to the I-A^b class II MHC molecule, whereas 46 to 61 did not, indicating that the C-terminal Arg at position 61 hindered binding. Evidently, a non–MHC-linked difference in antigen processing allowed this Arg to be cleaved off the 46 to 61 peptide in C3H.SW mice, in which the peptide was dominant,

but not in C57BL/6 mice, in which the peptide was cryptic. This difference in processing actually led to a nonresponsiveness of spleen cells to HEL immunized intraperitoneally in these mice, due to lack of response to the dominant 46 to 61 determinant.

Even a small peptide that does not need processing may nevertheless be processed, and that processing may affect its interaction with MHC molecules. Fox et al. (251) found that substitution of a tyrosine for isoleucine at position 95 of cytochrome c peptide 93 to 103 enhanced presentation with Eβ^b but diminished presentation with Eβ^k when live APCs were used but not when the APCs were fixed and could not process antigen. Therefore, the tyrosine residue was not directly interacting with the different MHC molecule but was affecting the way the peptide was processed, which in turn affected MHC interaction.

Besides the mechanisms suggested above, Gammon et al. (199) and Sercarz et al. (252) have proposed the possibility of competition between different MHC-binding structures (agretopes) within the same processed fragment. If a partially unfolded fragment first binds to MHC by one such site already exposed, further processing may stop, and other potential binding sites for MHC may never become accessible for binding. Such competition also could occur between different MHC molecules on the same presenting cell (199). For instance, BALB/c mice, expressing both A^d and E^d, produce a response to hen lysozyme specific for fragment 108 to 120, not for fragment 13 to 35 (199), and this response is restricted to E^d. However, B10.GD mice that express only A^d respond well to fragment 13 to 35 when immunized with lysozyme. BALB/c mice clearly express an A^d molecule, so the failure to present this 13 to 35 epitope may be due to competition from E^d, which may preempt by binding the 108 to 120 site with higher affinity and preventing the 13 to 35 site from binding to A^d. Competition between different peptides binding to the same MHC molecule could also occur.

All these results, taken together, indicate that antigen processing not only facilitates interaction of the antigenic site with the MHC molecule or the TCR but also influences the specificity of these interactions and in turn the specificity of the elicited T-cell repertoire.

Transport into a Cellular Compartment Where MHC Binding Can Occur

The second hurdle a potential epitope must surmount is to be transported into the cellular compartment for loading onto MHC molecules. These compartments are different for class I and class II molecules, as noted earlier.

Transport Pathways Leading to MHC Class I Presentation

Important information on how processing for presentation by class I MHC molecules could occur has been obtained by studies of mutant cell lines with low level expression of MHC class I, including the mutant murine line RMA-S (253) and human B-cell lines 721.174 and 721.134 (254). The class I heavy chains are synthesized, but they remain trapped in the ER, without proper glycosylation and not associated with β2 microglobulin, or they reach the cell surface in an unstable complex with β2 microglobulin, only to be degraded rapidly. As shown by Townsend et al. (255), these cells fail to present endogenously expressed viral antigens by class I for CTL recognition. However, both of these functions—MHC expression and CTL recognition—can be rescued by incubation with class I binding peptides.

Genetic analysis of these mutants revealed homozygous large or small deletions of part of the MHC class II region near the DR locus, demonstrating that a function coded in the class II region controls cell surface expression and function of class I proteins. Molecular cloning of DNA from this region showed at least 12 new genes, of which two, called TAP-1 and TAP-2, showed a typical sequence for transporter proteins (256–258), whereas two others, LMP-2 and LMP-7, were part of the proteasomal processing machinery. The TAP genes code for two 70-kDa proteins characterized by six-membrane spanning domains and a cytoplasmic ATP binding domain and sequence homology to other peptide transport proteins such as Opp D in salmonella and the multidrug-resistant protein and the cystic fibrosis transporter in humans. Their function is to transport processed peptides from the cytosol to the ER. Once in this compartment, peptides are handed off by TAP to newly formed MHC class I molecules and stabilize a tri-molecular complex with β2 microglobulin. This complex is then transported to the cell surface, where antigen presentation occurs. Without the peptide transporters, empty dimers of MHC class I with β2 microglobulin form, but these are unstable. Excess free peptide would rescue MHC class I by stabilizing the few short-lived empty complexes that reach the surface, as shown by Townsend et al. (255) and Schumacher et al. (259). Even uninfected cells need a supply of MHC-binding self peptides to produce stable MHC class I complexes and maintain normal levels of MHC on their surface. The function of the TAP proteins was demonstrated by reconstituting mutant cells with the cloned genes for each transport protein. Transfection with TAP-2 restores the antigen-presenting ability of RMA-S (260), whereas transfection with TAP-1 restores it for 721.134 (261). Mutant 721.174, with both TAP-1 and TAP-2 deleted, cannot be returned to normal antigen presentation with either TAP gene alone. The TAP-1 and TAP-2 proteins appear to be physically associated in a heterodimer because antipeptide antibodies specific for either protein will coprecipitate both (261,262).

In an infected cell, as soon as viral proteins are made, peptide fragments generated by the proteasome become available to the TAP-1 and TAP-2 transporter proteins (Fig. 9). These transport the peptide fragments into the ER for association with newly formed MHC class I molecules, which would carry them to the cell surface for antigen presentation, all within 30 minutes. Indeed, the finding of a physical association between TAP and the nascent class I heavy chain/β2 microglobulin complex suggests that the peptide may be directly handed off from TAP to the new MHC molecule without being free in solution (263,264). Thus, MHC-linked genes coding for proteolysis, peptide transport, and presentation at the cell surface have been identified. In effect, the MHC now appears to encode a complex system of multiple elements devoted to the rapid display of foreign protein determinants on the surface of an infected cell. By continuously sampling the output of the protein synthesizing machinery, this system permits rapid identification and destruction of infected cells by CTL before infectious virus can be released.

Because the TAP proteins form the link between the nonendosomal processing compartment (the cytosol) and the ER, they play an important role in MHC function. If they are highly efficient, transporting most of the peptides produced, nonendosomal processing will be tightly coupled to class I. If less efficient, some of the

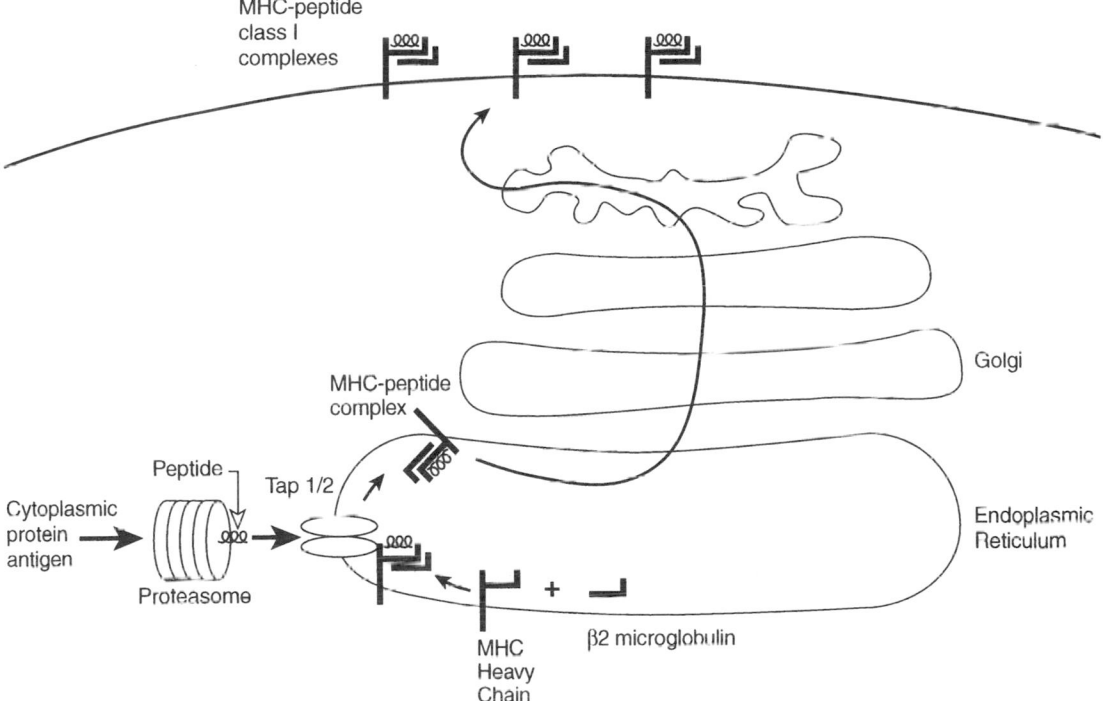

FIG. 9. Cytoplasmic antigen processing pathway leading to MHC class I presentation. Cytoplasmic antigen is degraded to fragments in the proteasome, which are transported into the endoplasmic reticulum by the TAP transporter. Peptide supplied by TAP forms a stable complex with MHC class I heavy chains and β2 microglobulin, and the complex is transported through the Golgi, where it achieves mature glycosylation, and out to the cell surface for presentation to class I–restricted T cells.

nonendosomal peptides may be available for class II binding. Conversely, if they are highly selective, then some cytosolic peptides may fail to enter the ER for presentation with class I, but if they are promiscuous, then some peptides may be transported that were better off not presented, such as those leading to autoimmunity.

The idea that other proteins may control accessibility of MHC class I binding sites for peptides originally came from the observation that two rat strains with the same MHC type (RT1.Aᵃ) were nevertheless not histocompatible, and CTLs could recognize the difference between them (265). The difference, called a *cim* effect, for "class I modification," occurred because different peptides were binding the same MHC in the two strains (266,267). The rat has two alleles for a peptide transporter supplying peptides to MHC. The one called TAP2A has peptide specificity matching that of RT1.Aᵃ and delivers a broad set of peptides for MHC binding. The other transporter allele, called TAP2B, supplies a different set of peptides that are discordant with RT1.Aᵃ, so MHC binding is slow, and fewer types of peptides are bound. Although RT1.Aᵃ would prefer to bind peptides with Arg at position 9, it has to settle for peptides with hydrophobic termini as provided by TAP2B (268), thereby accounting for the apparent histocompatibility difference. Thus, the specificity of TAP transport was shown to provide a selective step in narrowing the potential repertoire of CTL epitopes.

To measure TAP specificity in other species, a transportable peptide bearing an N-linked glycosylation site was added to cells permeabilized by treatment with streptolysin. If the peptide was transported by TAP, it would enter the ER and cis Golgi, where it would be glycosylated (269–271). The extent of glycosylation served as a measure of TAP function. When competitor peptides were added as well, TAP-mediated transport of the reporter peptide decreased, indicating saturation of peptide binding sites. In this way, a series of related peptides could be tested for the ability to compete for TAP binding and transport in order to identify the requirements for TAP binding and transport.

TAP binding and transport depended strongly on peptide length (271,272). Mouse TAP was shown to have a strong preference for peptides of nine residues or longer (272). For human TAP, peptides less than than seven amino acids long were not transported, regardless of sequence (271). Peptides eight to 11 amino acids long were almost all transported, with some variation in binding affinities depending on sequence. Peptides 14 to 21 amino acids in length were transported selectively, whereas those more than 24 amino acids in length were almost never transported intact. Thus, human TAP transport selected against peptides less than 7 or more than 24 amino acids in length, regardless of sequence.

Although TAP can and must transport a wide variety of peptides, it may still have preferences for which peptides are transported most efficiently and which MHC types are provided with the peptides they need. For example, a self peptide that naturally binds HLA B27 was modified slightly to produce an N-linded glycosylation site, resulting in the sequence RRYQNSTEL (271). Using the glycosylation of this peptide to measure transport, saturation of TAP by homologous peptides occurred with a 50% inhibitory concentration of less than 1 μ. Other peptides with unrelated sequences also inhibited, often with equally high affinity. Not only did natural HLA-binding peptides compete, but so did peptide variants lacking the MHC binding motif at positions 2 and 9. Similarly, the N- and C-terminal residues could be substituted with Ala, with no effect on transport, and nearly the entire sequence could be substituted with other amino acids without causing a significant change in transport. Clearly, peptides binding different MHC types were transported by

the same TAP protein, and even peptides that bound mouse MHC were transported by human TAP. In another example, using rat TAP proteins, peptides with Pro at position 2, 6, or 9 were found to be poor competitors for transport of a reference peptide (270).

In another approach, using a baculovirus system overexpressing TAP proteins in microsomes, the affinity of TAP binding was determined for a wide variety of synthetic peptides, allowing mapping of the important residues (273,274). Unlike MHC class I, there were no anchor positions at which a specific amino acid was required. However, there were several positions where substituting the wrong amino acid caused a marked reduction in TAP binding. In a typical MHC class I binding 9-mer, the strongest substitution effects were observed at position 9 (P9), followed by substitutions at P2 and P3, followed by P1. At the carboxy-terminal P9 position, the preferred residues were Tyr and Phe (as well as Arg and Lys), whereas Glu was worst, causing a 3-log reduction in binding. Similarly, substituting Pro at P2 caused a 1.5- to 2-log reduction in binding, as compared with preferred residues Arg, Val, and Ile. TAP preferences such as these would selectively transport some peptides more than others from cytoplasm to the ER.

Interestingly, these preferred residues are many of the same ones forming the MHC class I binding motifs (P2 and P9). However, since the MHC binding motifs differ from each other, it is not possible for TAP preferences to match them all. For example, the TAP preference for Arg at P2 and Phe, Tyr, Leu, Arg, or Lys at P9 overlaps with the binding motif of HLA-B27 and may favor the transport of peptide ligands for this MHC type. Remarkably, the variant B*2709, which does not prefer Tyr or Phe at P9, is not associated with autoimmune disease as in the more common form of HLA-B27. In contrast, HLA-B7 requires a Pro at P2, which greatly decreases TAP binding. Similarly, some peptides binding HLA-A2 have hydrophobic residues unfavorable for TAP binding, suggesting suboptimal compatibility between TAP and the most common HLA class I allele. Measurements with a series of naturally presented peptides from HLA-A2 and B27 indicated 240-fold higher affinity of TAP, on average, for the B27 peptides than for those from A2, and some of the A2 peptides did not bind TAP at all (van Endert, personal communication). How are these low-affinity peptides delivered to MHC? One suggestion is that peptide ligands for HLA-A2 and B7 may be transported as a larger precursor peptide containing the correct amino acids, which are then trimmed off to fit the MHC groove. Alternatively, some of these peptides may derive from signal peptides and enter the ER in a TAP-independent manner. The significance of selective peptide transport may be to limit immunity to self peptides. If the match between HLA-B27 and TAP specificity is too good, it may contribute to the increased incidence of autoimmune disease associated with HLA-B27 (273).

The importance of TAP proteins to antiviral immunity is shown by the fact that certain herpes viruses have targeted TAP-1 function as a way to interfere with antigen presentation to CD8⁺ CTLs. Once cells are infected with herpes simplex virus (HSV-1) or cytomegalovirus (CMV) (275,276), expression of new MHC class I molecules on the cell surface is reduced greatly, and they become unable to present viral or other antigens with MHC class I (277–279). These cells have the typical phenotype of cells, such as the TAP defective mutants, which are unable to transport antigenic peptides into the ER: normal MHC class I heavy-chain synthesis, but failure to assemble stable complexes with β2 microglobulin and trapping in the ER. Because they do not pass through the Golgi, these MHC molecules fail to acquire mature oligosaccharides, which can be easily demonstrated as failure to become resistant to endoglycosidase H. The infected cells cannot present HSV-1 antigens to CTLs, and they are also blocked in presentation of other viral antigens, such as CMV or alloantigens, to CTLs specific for them. The HSV viral protein causing the block, called ICP47, is an immediate early viral protein, 12 kDa in size, which acts alone (277) by binding to TAP and inhibiting its function.

As a way to evade immune surveillance, this strategy could contribute to viral persistence in chronic infection and viral activation in recurrent disease, as frequently occurs with HSV-1 and -2. A chronically infected patient should have plenty of virus-specific CTLs available to prevent or limit recurrences. However, by turning off antigen presentation, HSV may be able to reactivate without triggering an immune response. These findings also raise the possibility of making a live attenuated HSV vaccine (such as ICP47 defective) that would be more immunogenic than natural infection, because antigen presentation would remain intact.

An exception to this pattern is found in flaviviruses, such as dengue fever and Japanese encephalitis virus, which increase, rather than decrease, MHC expression by bypassing the TAP-1/2 pathway to supply additional peptides for MHC binding in the ER (280). In this case, virally enhanced antigen presentation, although not used to hide the virus, may contribute to cytopathology by increasing cytolysis of infected cells and possibly even by overcoming self tolerance.

Transport Pathways Leading to MHC Class II Presentation

Unlike the class I pathway, which delivers peptides to MHC, the MHC class II pathway transports MHC molecules to the endosomal compartment, where antigenic peptides are produced. During transport, the peptide binding groove must be kept free of endogenous peptides. The cell uses one protein, called invariant chain (and its processed fragment CLIP), to block the binding site until needed, and another protein, HLA-DM, to facilitate release of CLIP peptides and their exchange for antigenic peptides as they become available.

MHC class II molecules assemble in the ER, where alpha and beta chains form a complex with the invariant chain (281–283). The invariant chain binds MIIC and blocks the peptide binding groove, so endogenous peptides transported into the ER, for example by TAP, cannot bind (282,284–289). The complex of alpha, beta, and invariant chains, consisting of nine polypeptide chains in all (290), is transported via the Golgi and directed by signals on the invariant chain into endosome/lysosome-like vesicles called MHC class II compartments. The compartments contain acid-activated proteases capable of digesting foreign proteins into antigenic peptides. In addition, they degrade the invariant chain to a fragment called CLIP, corresponding to amino acids 80 to 103. As long as CLIP remains in the binding groove, antigenic peptides cannot bind, so the rate of CLIP release limits the capacity of MHC to take up antigenic peptides.

Peptide loading can be measured by its effect on MHC structure. When an MHC class II molecule binds a peptide, it changes conformation, and certain monoclonal antibodies are specific for the peptide-bound conformation (291). Also, the alpha–beta complex becomes more stable after peptide binding, which can be detected by running the MHC on an SDS gel without boiling. The peptide bound form runs on gels as a large alpha–beta dimer, whereas MHC without peptides (but still bound to CLIP) is unstable under

these conditions and falls apart to give alpha and beta chain monomers on SDS gels (292).

Mutant cell lines have been generated with a deletion between HLA-DP and HLA-DQ genes on chromosome 6 (291,293–295). These cells express normal levels of MHC class II structural proteins, HLA-DQ and DR, but fail to present protein antigens (295). Some of their class II MHC proteins appear on the cell surface, but more are retained in the MHC class II compartments. Biochemically, they still contain CLIP peptides (296), rather than peptide antigens, and they have not achieved the conformation (291) or SDS stability of peptide-binding MHC class II complexes (297). The defect was discovered to be due to loss of either of the two chains of a newly described class II molecule, HLA-DM, and the phenotype can be corrected by adding back the missing gene (298). In the presence of normal HLA-DM, MHC releases CLIP and binds antigenic peptides for presentation to T cells.

In vitro studies with purified MHC class II molecules and biotin-labeled peptides have shown that HLA-DM can accelerate loading of exogenous peptides into HLA-DR binding sites (299,300). For example, loading of myelin basic protein fragment 90 to 102 was accomplished in 9 minutes with HLA-DM versus 60 minutes without it (Table 7). Other peptides were also loaded at the same rate, suggesting that the rate-limiting step was the same for each: removal of CLIP peptides to expose the peptide binding sites on HLA-DR. The kinetic effect was optimal between pH 4.5 and 5.8, which is typical of the endosomal/lysosomal compartment where HLA-DM operates. HLA-DM did not affect the affinity, as measured by half maximal binding, but it had a marked effect on the kinetics of binding.

Conversely, when biotinylated peptides were allowed to saturate HLA-DR binding sites overnight, and then free peptides were removed, the off rate could be measured over time (299,300). As shown in Table 7 (299), the off rate for different peptides could be compared in the absence or presence of HLA-DM. The half-life for CLIP peptides was reduced from 11 hours to 20 minutes by adding HLA-DM. This could explain the enhanced loading of all other peptides because they must wait for CLIP to come off. In the case of antigenic peptides, myelin basic protein 90 to 112 was released 80-fold faster in the presence of DM than in its absence. However, another peptide, influenza hemagglutinin 307 to 319, was not

TABLE 7. *Effect of HLA-DM on peptide on rates and off rates for binding to HLA-DR1*

Peptide	HLA-DM	Halflife for binding	Halflife for release
CLIP (80–103)	–	60 min	11 hr
	+	9 min	0.3 hr
MBP (90–102)	–	62 min	86 hr
	+	9 min	1 hr
HA (307–319)	–	67 min	144 hr
	+	10 min	144 hr

Adapted from the data of Sloan et al. (299). The on (association) and off (dissociation) rates of biotinylated peptide from purified soluble HLA-DR1 were measured by fluorescence assay, in the presence or absence of HLA-DM. The on rates of all three peptides are increased similarly in the presence of DM and probably reflect the rate-limiting dissociation of the bound CLIP fragment of the invariant chain. In contrast, once the peptides are bound, the off rates differ due to differences in affinity. Thus, HLA-DM catalyzes release of more weakly binding peptides and allows stable binding of higher affinity peptides. In effect, this is an editing function of HLA-DM.

affected at all. The differential effect on these antigenic peptides suggests that HLA-DM can serve a potential role in editing which peptides stay on MHC long enough to be presented and which are removed (299). By releasing MBP preferentially and not the HA peptide, HLA-DM would favor the stable MHC binding and presentation of HA peptides over MBP peptides. The affinity of each peptide is determined by the fit between peptide and MHC groove, not by HLA-DM. However, DM can amplify the impact of the difference in affinity (i.e., signal-to-noise ratio), by facilitating release of low-affinity peptides and allowing the high-affinity ones to remain. This editing function could have an important effect on which peptides get presented and elicit a T-cell response and which do not. HLA-DM could contribute to immunodominance of a peptide binding MHC with high affinity by releasing its lower affinity competitors. Alternatively, HLA-DM could contribute to self tolerance by releasing self peptides of low affinity before they could stimulate self-reactive T cells.

MHC Binding and Assembly of a Stable Peptide–MHC Complex

Antigen Interaction with MHC Molecules

Perhaps the most selective step a potential antigenic site must pass is to bind with sufficiently high affinity to an appropriate MHC molecule.

The response of T cells to antigens on APCs or target cells provided a number of hints that antigen interacts directly with MHC molecules of the APCs. First, inheritable genes coding for immune responsiveness to a specific antigen are tightly linked to the inheritance of genes for MHC-encoded cell surface molecules (101, 132). Second, it became apparent that T-cell recognition of antigen is the step at which MHC restriction occurs (101,140,180,301). For example, in vitro T-cell responses to small protein and polypeptide antigens were found to parallel in vivo responses controlled by Ir genes, and T cells were exquisitely sensitive to differences in MHC antigens of the APC in all their antigen recognition functions. This discovery was an important advance because it became possible to separate the MHC of the T cell from that of the APC. The T-cell response to antigenic determinants on each chain of insulin depended on the MHC antigens of the APC. This was particularly apparent when (A × B)F1 T cells responded to antigen presented by APCs of either the A or B parental MHC type (180,302). Neither parental APC stimulated an allogeneic response, and the response to antigen was as much limited by the MHC of the APC as by the T-cell specificity. This ability of the APC to limit what could be presented to the T cells was termed "determinant selection" (180,302). It became obvious that even in a single (A × B)F1 animal, distinct sets of antigen-specific T cells exist that respond to each antigenic determinant only in association with MHC type A or type B (303).

Experiments on the fine specificity of antigen-specific T-cell clones suggested that the MHC of the APC could influence the T-cell response in more subtle ways than just allowing or inhibiting it. Determinant selection implied that a given processed peptide should contain both a site for MHC interaction and a distinct functional site for TCR binding. The logical consequence of this is that different peptides processed from the same protein could have different MHC restrictions, due to different MHC association sites on each, consistent with the independent Ir gene control of the response to each antigenic determinant on the same protein (142).

For example, T-cell clones specific for myoglobin responded to multiple antigenic determinants on different peptide fragments of myoglobin (173): those specific for one of the epitopes were always restricted to I-A, whereas those specific for the other were always restricted to I-E. The simplest interpretation was that each antigenic peptide contained an Ia association site for interacting with I-A or I-E. At the level of Ir genes, mouse strains lacking a functional I-E molecule could respond to one of the sites only, and those with neither I-A nor I-E molecules capable of binding to any myoglobin peptide would be low responders to myoglobin.

Evidence for a discrete MHC association site on peptide antigens came from studies with pigeon cytochrome c. The murine T-cell response to pigeon cytochrome c and its carboxy-terminal peptide (81–104) depends on the I-E molecules of the APCs (140). However, distinct structural sites on the synthetic peptide antigen appear to constitute two functional sites: an epitope site for binding to the TCR and an "agretope" (for "antigen-restriction-tope") site for interacting with the MHC molecule of the APC (140,157–159). Amino acid substitutions for Lys at position 99 on the peptide destroyed the ability to stimulate T-cell clones specific for the peptide, whereas the difference between Ala and a deletion at position 103 determined T-cell stimulation in association with some MHC antigens but not others, independent of the T-cell fine specificity. In addition, immunizing with the peptides substituted at position 99 elicited new T-cell clones that responded to the substituted peptide but not the original and showed the same pattern of genetic restriction, correlated with the residue at position 103, as the clones specific for the original peptide. These results implied that the substitutions at position 99 had not affected the MHC association site but independently altered the antigen subsite that interacts directly with the TCR. In contrast, position 103 was a likely subsite for MHC interaction, without altering the TCR binding site. This interpretation is summarized in a model in Fig. 10.

It remained to be shown that MHC molecules without any other cell surface protein were sufficient for presentation of processed peptide antigens. This was shown in two ways. First, Watts et al. (304) showed that glass slides coated with lipid containing purified I-A molecules could present an ovalbumin peptide to an ovalbumin-specific T-cell hybridoma. This result meant that no other special

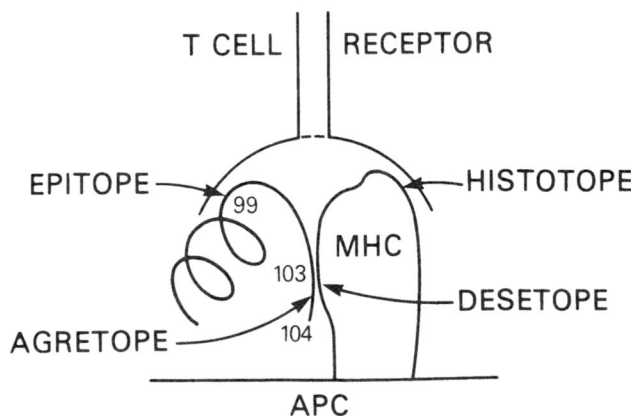

FIG. 10. A trimolecular complex type of model showing the interaction of antigen, the MHC-encoded product on the APC, and the receptor on the T cell. The antigen shown is pigeon cytochrome c fragment 81 to 104. Residues 99 and 103 or 104 are highlighted because of evidence suggesting that for this antigen they might be part of the epitope and agretope, respectively. Reprinted with permission (157).

steps were required other than antigen processing and MHC association. Likewise, Walden et al. (305) specifically stimulated T-cell hybridomas with liposomes containing nothing but antigen and MHC molecules. Second, Norcross et al. (306) transformed mouse L cells with the genes for the I-A α and β chains and converted the fibroblasts (which do not express their own class II molecules) into I-A–expressing cells. These cells were able to present several antigens to I-A–restricted T-cell clones and hybridomas (306), and similar I-E transfectants presented to I-E–restricted T cells (173). Thus, whatever processing enzymes are required are already present in fibroblasts, and the only additional requirement for antigen-presenting function is the expression of I-A or I-E antigens.

The planar membrane technique has been applied to determine the minimum number of MHC–antigen complexes per APC necessary to induce T-cell activation (307). After pulsing the presenting cells with antigen, the cells were studied for antigen-presenting activity, and some of the cells were lysed to produce a purified fraction containing MHC charged with antigenic peptides. These MHC–peptide complexes were used to reconstitute planar membranes, and their potency was compared with a reference MHC preparation pulsed with a high peptide concentration *in vitro* and presumed to be fully loaded. In this way, the relative peptide occupancy of MHC binding sites corresponding to any level of antigen presentation could be determined. For B cells and macrophages, the threshold of antigen loading necessary for triggering T cells was 0.2% of I-E^d molecules occupied by peptide, corresponding to about 200 MHC–peptide complexes per presenting cell. For artificial presenting cells, such as L cells transfected with I-E^d, the threshold was 23 times greater, or 4.6% of MHC occupied by peptide. Similarly, when MHC–peptide binding was measured directly, using radiolabeled peptide to determine the minimum level of MHC–peptide complexes required for T-cell triggering, B cells were capable of presenting antigen with as few as 200 to 300 MHC–peptide complexes per cell (308). A similar number of peptide–MHC class I molecule complexes was reported to be required on a cell for recognition by CD8$^+$ cytotoxic T cells (309). These results explain how newly generated peptide antigens can compete with all the rest of cellular antigens, because a low level of MHC occupancy is sufficient. In addition, this threshold of presentation may explain how multivalent protein antigens, such as viral particles, with 100 to 200 protein copies each, can be over 10^3-fold more immunogenic than the corresponding monomers (310). Subsequent studies titrating peptide and recombinant soluble class I MHC molecules on plastic suggested that interaction of three to five specific peptide–MHC complexes was sufficient to trigger the T cell (311,312). Because more than 10 T cells can rosette around one APC, this result is consistent with a need for a few hundred complexes per APC, not all interacting with the same T cell.

Biochemical evidence for the direct association between processed peptide and MHC molecules was based first on competition between peptides for antigen presentation (186,313–316) and then more directly on equilibrium dialysis (317), molecular sieve chromatography (318), or affinity labeling (319). Equilibrium dialysis was performed by incubating detergent-solubilized class II molecules with fluoresceinated or radioactive antigenic peptides, followed by dialysis against a large volume of buffer. In the absence of binding by class II molecules, the labeled peptide would distribute itself equally between the inside and outside of the dialysis chamber. However, when the appropriate class II molecules were added to the chamber, extra peptide molecules were retained inside it due to formation of a complex too large to diffuse across

the semipermeable membrane. In this way, direct binding of antigen and MHC was shown, and an affinity constant was determined (317,318).

A second approach was to form the antigen–MHC complex over 48 hours, followed by rapid passage over a Sephadex G50 sizing column. The bound peptide was excluded from the column because it is the size of class II molecules (about 58 kDa), whereas free peptide was usually included in the column because it is only approximately 2 kDa (Fig. 11) (318). Competitive binding showed that different peptide antigens with the same MHC restriction bind to the same site on the MHC class II molecule (320,321). For example, Table 8 shows the results with peptide antigens that are known to be presented with I-A or I-E antigens of the d or k haplotype. We observe that Ova peptide 323 to 339, which is presented with I-A^d, also binds well to purified I-A^d, whereas nonradioactive peptide competes for the antigen binding sites of the I-A^d molecule. Similarly, the other I-A^d-restricted peptide, myoglobin 106 to 118, competes with Ova 323 to 339 for the same site. However, myoglobin

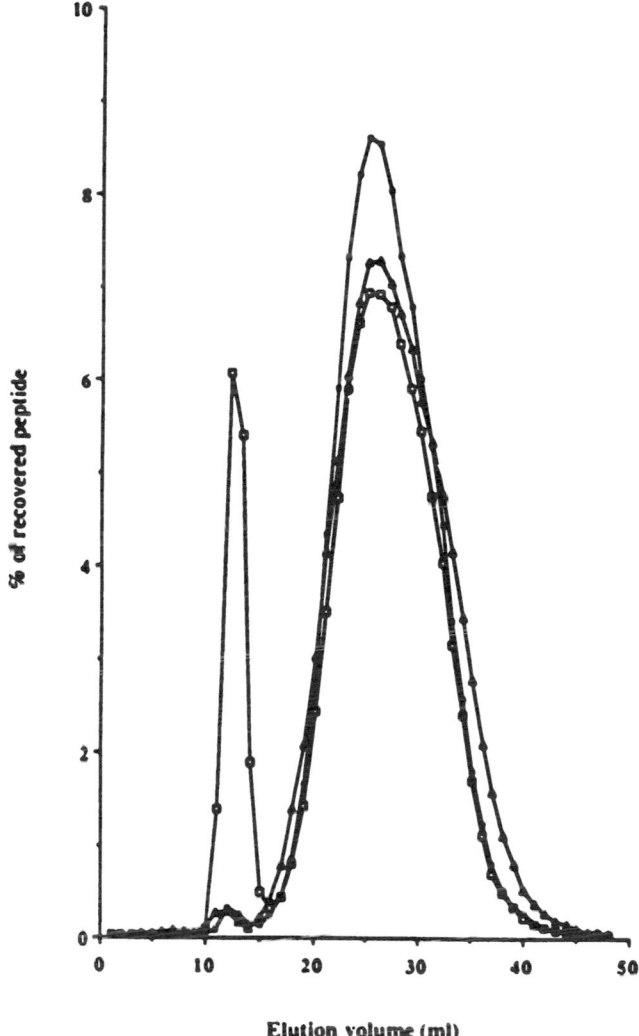

FIG. 11. Gel filtration of OVA323–339/Ia complexes. Purified I-A^d and I-E^d (or gelatin) in detergent solution was incubated for 2 days at room temperature with [^{125}I]OVA323 339 and subsequently passed over a Sephadex G50 column. The elution volume was collected in 1-ml fractions and counted for radioactivity. Reprinted with permission (318).

TABLE 8. *Correlation between MHC restriction and binding to MHC molecules*

Competitor peptide		Ova + A^d	Myo + E^d	HEL + A^k	Cyto + E^k
Ova	323–339	++++	–	++	+
Myo	106–118	++++	–	++	+/–
Myo	132–153	–	++++	–	++
HEL	46–61	+	+	++++	+
Cytochrome *c*	88–104	++	+/–	++	++++

Data from Buus et al. (321).

132 to 153, which is not restricted to I-A^d, does not compete for it but does compete for its own restriction element, I-E^d. Similarly, pigeon cytochrome c competes best for its restriction element I-E^k rather than I-A^k or I-E^d, which do not present cytochrome. Conversely, recombinant Eβ genes have been used to map separate sites on a class II MHC molecule for binding to peptide antigen and to the TCR (322).

Using these two biochemical methods, it has been possible to explain major losses of peptide antigenicity resulting from amino acid substitutions in terms of their adverse effect on epitope or agretope function. For example, the response of each of two oval-bumin-specific T-cell clones was mapped to peptide 325 to 335 by using a nested set of synthetic peptides. Five substitutions were made for each amino acid in this segment, and the resulting 55 different peptides were each tested for the ability to stimulate the clone (323). Presumably, those peptides that failed to stimulate could be defective at an epitope or an agretope functional site. In fact, only two amino acids (Val 327 and Ala 332) were essential for MHC interaction, and changes at either of these sites resulted in a loss of antigenicity for the clone. Seven other amino acids were critical for T-cell stimulation but did not affect MHC binding. Thus, these must be part of the functional epitope. Interestingly, certain substitutions for His 328, Ala 330, and Glu 333 had effects on MHC binding, whereas others had effects on T-cell stimulation without affecting MHC binding. These amino acids might participate in both agretope and epitope functional sites, or, alternatively, the substitutions may affect the conformation of the peptide as it binds, thus indirectly affecting T-cell recognition (324). The fact that substitutions at nine of 11 amino acids could be tolerated without affecting MHC binding is consistent with the determinant selection hypothesis in that multiple antigenic peptides are capable of interacting with the same antigen binding site on the MHC molecule.

Similarly, by using a T-cell clone specific for peptide 52 to 61 of HEL, substitutions at each amino acid were analyzed for the ability to bind to I-A^k and stimulate the clone (325). Four of 11 amino acid residues were silent, whereas substitutions at three positions resulted in reduced binding to I-A^k. Substitutions at the remaining three positions resulted in decreased T-cell stimulation without affecting MHC association. The epitope was very sensitive to substitutions, even conservative ones such as changing Leu 56 to Ile, norLeu, or Val. The results in both of these studies confirmed by competitive binding that the MHC molecule contains a single saturable site for peptide binding. This site must be capable of binding a broad range of antigenic peptides. It may be through binding the MHC molecule that antigenic peptides become oriented and folded into an ordered structure that is recognizable by the TCR.

Interestingly, one of the first antigenic structures for T cells to be studied in this way was not a peptide at all but rather the small molecule tyrosine–azobenzenearsonate (Tyr-ABA) (133). This molecule provides one of the exceptions to the rule that T cells recognize only peptide antigens, not carbohydrates or haptens. Indeed, other haptens such as trinitrophenyl may bind MHC molecules only when attached to a peptide that binds (326). Nevertheless, the Tyr-ABA structure seems to have some features in common with those discussed below for peptides. It was studied with a series of organic analogs in a classic type of structure–function study. The portion of the structure mapped as the epitope recognized by the TCR was identified to be a combination of the arsonate anionic group and the amino acid zwitterion (NH^{+3}, COO$^-$) of the tyrosine moiety. The component mapped as the moiety interacting with the class II MHC molecule was the planar structure consisting of the two aromatic rings of the tyrosine and the benzenearsonate, linked by the azo linkage. Thus, this nonpeptide antigenic structure is amphipathic. In this case, the planar aromatic ring structure could interact with some of the aromatic side chains, which have been found to abound within the floor of the peptide-binding groove of the MHC molecule (212,213,327–332). Therefore, although a full set of general principles explaining the specificity of antigen presentation and T-cell recognition has not yet emerged, it is studies such as these, combined with complementary structural studies characterizing the antigen-interacting portions of MHC molecules (176,212,213,322,327–334) (see Chapters 8 and 9) and of TCRs (335–341) (see Chapter 10) that will ultimately lead to an understanding of these principles.

One observation that came out of this type of structure–function study was that a single peptide can bind to a class II MHC molecule in more than one way, and thus be seen by different T cells in different orientations or conformations (324,342). This conclusion derived from studying a series of peptides with single amino acid substitutions for recognition by two different T-cell clones with the same class II molecule, and competition by inactive peptides with the wild-type peptide for binding to the MHC molecule. Several residues appeared paradoxically to reverse their roles reciprocally for binding the TCR versus binding the MHC molecule when assessed with the two different T-cell clones (324). The implication is that one cannot define a unique portion of the peptide that always binds to the MHC molecule, independent of the T cell that is responding, but rather this role may be played by different residues when the peptide is seen by different T cells.

The same conclusion can be reached from an entirely different type of study, in which mutations are introduced into the MHC molecule. Mutations in the floor of the peptide-binding groove, which cannot directly interact with the TCR, can differentially affect recognition of a peptide by one clone and not another (343–345). In a particularly thoroughly studied case, it was clear that the quantitative level of peptide binding was not affected by the mutation, but rather the change in the floor of the groove imposed an altered conformation on the peptide that differentially affected recognition by different T cells (345). If indeed the TCR cannot detect the mutation in the MHC molecule except indirectly by its effect on the peptide conformation, then one is forced to conclude that different T cells have preferences for different conformations of the same peptide bound to (what appears to the T cell as) the same MHC molecule.

Another general observation to come from this type of study is that substitution of amino acids often affects presentation by MHC and recognition by T cells through introduction of dominant negative interactions or interfering groups, whereas only a few residues are actually essential for peptide binding (346). Both for class II binding (346–349) and for class I MHC binding (350), most residues can be replaced with Ala or sometimes Pro without losing MHC binding, as long as a few critical residues are retained. Of course, T-cell recognition may require retention of other residues. If many of the amino acid side chains are not necessary for binding to the MHC molecule, then one might expect side chains of noncritical amino acids to have a profound effect in certain cases only by interfering with binding, either directly or through an effect on conformation. That is exactly what was observed for a helper epitope from the HIV-1 envelope protein when a heteroclitic peptide—that is, one that stimulated the T cells at much lower concentrations than required of the wild-type peptide—was obtained by replacing a negatively charged Glu with Ala or with Gln, which has the same size but no charge (346). An Asp, negatively charged but smaller, behaved like the Glu. Thus this residue was not necessary for binding to the class II MHC molecule, but a negatively charged side chain interfered with binding to the MHC molecule as measured by competition studies. These results have important implications for the chemistry of peptide–MHC interaction and for the design of more potent synthetic vaccines. Information about residues that interfere with binding has allowed the refinement of sequence motifs for peptides binding to MHC molecules to permit more reliable prediction of binding (351).

This observation also provides a novel approach to make more potent vaccines by epitope enhancement, the process of modifying the internal sequence of epitopes to make them more potent, for example, by increasing affinity for an MHC molecule, or more capable of inducing more broadly cross-reactive T cells specific for multiple strains of a virus (352–355). Proof of principle that this approach can make more potent peptide vaccines has recently been obtained (355). The modified enhanced helper T cell epitope from the HIV-1 envelope protein described above (346), with Ala substituted for Glu, was shown to be immunogenic at 10- to 100-fold lower doses for *in vivo* immunization than the wild-type HIV-1 peptide to induce a T-cell proliferative response specific for the wild-type peptide. Furthermore, when a peptide vaccine construct using this helper epitope coupled to a CTL epitope (356–358) was modified with the same Glu-to-Ala substitution, it was more potent at inducing CD8+ CTLs specific for the CTL epitope than was the original vaccine construct and induced 33-fold more CTL lytic units (Fig. 12) (355). The increased potency of the vaccine construct was shown to be due to improved interaction with the class II MHC molecule presenting the helper epitope, rather than some nonspecific effect such as peptide stability, by demonstration of class II MHC-linkage of the effect using congenic strains of mice expressing the same class I MHC molecule to present the CTL epitope and the same background genes, but differing in class II MHC molecules. The control strain class II molecule presented both modified and wild-type helper peptides equally well and showed no difference in potency of the two vaccine constructs (355). Thus, class II–restricted help makes an enormous difference in induction

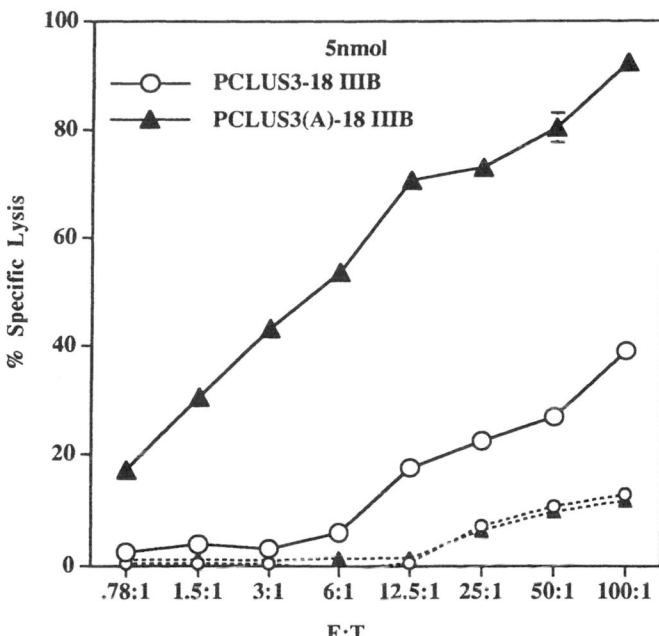

FIG. 12. Enhancement of immunogenicity of a peptide vaccine for induction of class I MHC-restricted CTLs by modification of the class II MHC-binding portion to increase CD4+ T-cell help. Peptide vaccine PCLUS3-18 IIIB contains a class II MHC binding helper region, consisting of a cluster of overlapping determinants from the HIV-1 envelope protein gp160, and a class I MHC-binding CTL epitope, P18 IIIB. Modification of the helper epitope to remove an adverse negative charge by replacement of a Glu with an Ala residue was shown to increase binding to the class II MHC molecule (346). Here introduction of the same modification of the helper epitope, to produce PCLUS3(A)-18IIIB, is shown to greatly increase immunogenicity *in vivo* for induction of CTL to the class I–binding P18IIIB portion. Immunization of A.AL mice with 5 nmol of either vaccine construct subcutaneously in montanide ISA 51 adjuvant, and stimulation of resulting spleen cells with P18IIIB for 1 week in culture, resulted in 33-fold more lytic units for lysing targets coated with P18IIIB when mice were immunized with the modified second-generation vaccine than when they were immunized with the original construct with the natural sequence. Thus, class II–restricted CD4+ T-cell help has a major impact on induction of class I–restricted CTLs, and this process of epitope enhancement can be used to make vaccines more potent than the natural viral antigens. Targets: BALB/c 3T3 fibroblasts with P18IIIB (*solid lines*) or no peptide (*dashed lines*). Modified with permission (355).

of class I–restricted CTLs, and epitope enhancement can allow construction of more potent vaccines. Other examples of enhancement of immunogenicity by modification of the sequence of viral or tumor peptides have been found as well (359,360).

In the case of class I MHC molecules, results defining sequence binding motifs generalize the conclusion that only a few critical anchor residues determine the specificity of binding to the MHC molecule (Table 9) (236,350,361–365). These motifs were defined by a detailed study of one peptide–MHC system (363), by sequencing the mixture of natural peptides eluted from a class I MHC molecule and finding that at certain positions in the sequence the same residue was shared by most of the peptides (361), and by separating and sequencing individual natural peptides eluted from a class I molecule and finding a conserved residue at certain positions (362). The latter two studies also made the important observation that the natural peptides eluted from class I MHC molecules were

TABLE 9. *Examples of motifs for peptides binding to class I and II MHC molecules*

MHC molecule	1	2	3	4	5	6	7	8	9
Class I									
H-2K[d]		Y							I,L,V
H-2D[b]					N				M,I
H-2K[b]					F,Y			L,M	
H-2L[d]		P			(phil K,R)				M,L,F
H-2D[d]		G	P		K,R				L
H-2K[k]		E						I	
HLA-A2.1		L,M							V
HLA-A3		L	(F)						Y,K
HLA-B27	K,R G	R	I,Y, F,W						K,R
Class II									
DRB1*0101	Y,V, L,F, I,A			L,A		A,G			L,A
DRB1*0301	L,I F,M V			D		K,R E,Q			Y,L F
DRB1*0401 (DR4Dw4)	F,Y W			no R,K		N,S T,Q ali	pol chg		pol ali K
DRB1*0402 (DR4Dw10)	V,I, L,M		no	D,E		N,Q, S,T K	R,K H,N Q,P		pol ali H
DRB1*1501 (DR2b)	L,V, I			F,Y I			I,L V,M F		
DQA1*0501 DQB1*0301	F,Y, I,M L,V				V,L I,M Y		Y,F M,L, V,I		

pol, polar; chg, charged; ali, aliphatic; phil, hydrophilic.
Data from references 236, 350, and 361–365.

all about the same length, eight or nine residues, and this was confirmed for a much larger collection of peptides eluted from HLA-A2 and analyzed by tandem mass spectrometry (364). This finding was consistent with other studies demonstrating that a minimal nonapeptide was many orders of magnitude more potent than longer peptides in presentation by class I molecules to T cells (366, 367). This conservation of length was critical to the success of the approach of sequencing mixtures of peptides eluted from a class I molecule (361), because such a method requires that the conserved anchor residues all be at the same distance from the N terminus. Sequencing by Edman degradation is done sequentially from the amino terminus. In a mixture of many unrelated peptides, at most positions one would expect to find close to 20 different amino acids, with no single one standing out, and that is exactly what was found at most positions in the mixture. The fact that Falk et al. (361) could find a single amino acid at certain positions, however, such as a Tyr at position 2 in peptides eluted from K[d], implies not only that most or all of the peptides bound to K[d] had a Tyr that could be aligned, but also that the peptides were already aligned as bound to the MHC molecule, with each one having just one residue N terminal to the Tyr. This result implies that the position of the N-terminal residue is fixed in the MHC molcule, even if its side chain can vary, and suggests that the processed peptides must be trimmed to size, so that nothing hangs out of the MHC groove, at least at the N terminus. It is this fact that has made the identifica-

tion of motifs for binding to class I molecules much more straightforward than finding motifs for binding class II molecules.

This conclusion has not only been confirmed but also explained by the x-ray crystallographic data on class I peptide–MHC complexes (330–332). It appears that both the N-terminal α amino group and the C-terminal carboxyl group are fixed in pockets at either end of the MHC groove, independent of what amino acids are occupying those positions, and that the rest of the peptide spans these fixed points in a more or less extended conformation. The minimum length that can span the distance between these pockets is eight residues, but nine or 10 residues can be accommodated with a slight bulge or β turn in the middle of the peptide, explaining the narrow restriction on length. Between these ends, one or two pockets in the groove can accommodate the side chain of an amino acid, usually either at position 2 binding in the B pocket, or at position 5 binding in the C pocket, depending on the particular MHC molecule. An additional side chain of the C-terminal residue can be accommodated in a pocket at the end of the groove. These residues that fit into pockets correspond exactly to the anchor residues, at positions 2 or 5, and 8 or 9, defined by the sequence motifs, and appear to be the primary determinants of specificity for peptide binding because the rest of the interactions are largely with peptide backbone atoms, including the α amino and carboxyl groups, and therefore do not contribute to sequence specificity. This finding can explain both the breadth of peptides that can bind to a single MHC molecule, because most of the binding involves only backbone atoms common to all peptides, and the exquisite specificity of binding is determined by the anchor residues that account for the Ir gene control of responsiveness.

In contrast, when natural self peptides were eluted from class II MHC molecules (211,368), the lengths were much more variable, ranging from 13 to 18 residues, and several variants of the same peptide were found with different lengths of extra sequence at one end or the other (ragged ends). This finding suggested that both ends of the peptide-binding groove of class II MHC molecules are open, in contrast to class I, so that additional lengths of peptide can hang out either side, and trimming does not have to be precise. However, a corollary is that the peptides eluted from class II molecules would not be expected to be naturally aligned in a motif, and that was indeed what was found. Although a moderately conserved motif was found in some of the peptides eluted from the murine class II molecule I-A^d, consistent with the motif defined earlier based on known antigenic peptides binding to I-A^d (369), the motif was neither so clearly defined nor so highly conserved as in the class I case and required human manipulation to align the sequences to identify a motif (368). Subsequently, a number of motifs for peptides binding to human class II MHC molecules have been defined (236,370–375). The crystal structure of a peptide bound to a human class II MHC molecule, DR1, showed that indeed the ends of the groove are open and the peptide can extend beyond the groove in both directions (212,213,376). The backbone amide nitrogen and carbonyl groups provide the conserved portions that bind, instead of the termini that are fixed in the class I groove, and anchor residues fitting into defined MIIC pockets provide the specificity as in the case of class I molecules and account for the binding motifs.

T-Cell Receptor Recognition

The last hurdle that a potential antigenic determinant must surmount is recognition by a TCR within the repertoire of the individual responding. This repertoire may be limited by the availability of combinations of V, D, and J genes in the genome that can combine to form an appropriate receptor, given the lack of somatic hypermutation in TCRs in contrast to antibodies (337,377), and then by self tolerance, as mediated by thymic or peripheral negative selection, or by limits on the repertoire that is positively selected in the thymus on existing self peptide–MHC complexes. The available repertoire also may be influenced by prior exposure to cross-reactive antigens. In general, however, it has been hard to find holes in the repertoire (378). Furthermore, when TCR repertoires of mice and humans were compared for peptides presented by HLA-A2.1, they seemed to be capable of seeing the same spectrum of peptides (379). Eleven peptides from hepatitis C virus (HCV) proteins, each of which had a motif for binding to HLA-A2.1, were tested for recognition by CTLs from HLA-A2.1 transgenic mice and human HLA-A2.1–positive patients infected with HCV. The same four peptides that were recognized by the T cells from the mice were the ones recognized by the human T cells, whereas the others were not recognized well by either murine or human T cells. The selection of which peptides were recognized seemed to be determined by binding to the HLA-A2.1 molecule, rather than by the availability of T cells. Thus, despite the differences in TCR genes in mice and humans, the repertoires are plastic enough that if a peptide passes the other three hurdles of processing, transport, and binding to

MHC molecules, T cells can be elicited to respond to it in either species (379).

On the other hand, evidence exists that MHC binding is not the whole story. Schaeffer et al. (380) examined 14 overlapping peptides covering the sequence of staphylococcal nuclease with different class II MHC molecules, constituting 54 different peptide-MHC combinations. Clearly, MHC binding plays a major role because 12 of 13 immunogenic peptides were high or intermediate binders to MHC molecules, whereas only one of 37 poor binders were immunogenic. Of high-affinity binders, five of five peptides were immunogenic. However, for intermediate-affinity MHC-binding peptides, only seven of 12 were immunogenic. Thus, MHC binding alone is not sufficient to ensure immunogenicity. The T-cell repertoire was one factor suggested that might limit the spectrum of immunogenic peptides.

Indeed, examples for selection at the level of the TCR repertoire exist. A particularly elegant example described by Moudgil et al. (381) is one in which a peptide (46 to 61) of mouse lysozyme presented by I-A^k is recognized by T cells from CBA/J and B10.A mice, expressing I-A^k and I-E^k, but not by T cells from B10.A(4R) mice expressing only I-A^k, even though the APCs from B10.A(4R) mice can present the peptide to T cells from the other strains. T cells from the B10.A(4R) mice can respond to variant 46 to 61 peptides in which the C-terminal Arg is replaced by Ala, Leu, Phe, Asn, or Lys, indicating that the C-terminal Arg is hindering recognition, but not binding by I-A^k, and in this case, not processing because the B10.A(4R) APCs can present the peptide. It appears that the hindrance interferes with recognition by TCRs available in B10.A(4R) mice, but not TCRs available in B10.A or CBA/J mice, or in (B10.A(4R) × CBA/J)F1 mice. Because the B10.A mice are congenic with the B10.A(4R) mice, the difference is not one of non–MHC-linked genes such as TCR structural genes or non-MHC self antigens producing self tolerance. Furthermore, because the F1 mice respond, the difference is not due to a hole in the repertoire produced by a self-antigen of the B10.A(4R) mice. It was concluded that the CBA/J and B10.A mice contain an additional repertoire, positively selected on I-E^k or possibly an H-2D/L class I molecule in which these strains differ, that can recognize the 46 to 61 peptide despite the hindering Arg at the C-terminus. An alternative related explanation is that strains that express I-E^k or D^k or D^d/L^d have an additional repertoire of TCRs positively selected on I-A^k presenting self peptides from processing of these other MHC molecules in the thymus. This latter explanation has the advantage that the repertoire is positively selected on I-A^k, rather than I-E^k or a class I molecule, so it is more likely to recognize other peptides presented by I-A^k. This example illustrates a case in point that subtle differences in TCR, presumably caused in this case by positive selection, can lead to responsiveness or nonresponsiveness to a determinant that has already passed all of the three earlier hurdles of processing, transport, and MHC binding.

Epitope Mapping

Precise mapping of antigenic sites recognized by T cells was made possible by the fact that T cells would respond to peptide fragments of the antigen when they contain a complete antigenic determinant. A series of overlapping peptides can be used to walk along the protein sequence and find the antigenic site. Then, by truncating the peptide at either end, the minimum antigenic peptide can be determined. For example, in the case of myoglobin, a critical amino acid residue, such as Glu 109 or Lys 140, was found by comparing the sequences of stimulatory and nonstimulatory myoglobin variants and large CNBr cleavage fragments (174), and then a series of truncated peptides containing the critical residue was synthesized with different overlapping lengths at either end (146,150). Because solid-phase peptide synthesis starts from a fixed carboxyl end and proceeds toward the amino end, it can be stopped at various positions to produce a nested series of peptides that vary in length at the amino end. Each peptide is then tested in the proliferation assay. In this way, it was found that two of the Glu 109–specific T-cell clones responded to synthetic peptides 102 to 118 and 106 to 118 but not to peptide 109 to 118 (150). One clone responded to peptide 108 to 118, whereas the other did not. Thus, the amino end of the peptide recognized by one clone was Ser 108, whereas the other clone required Phe 106 and/or Ile 107. Similar fine specificity differences have been observed with T-cell clones specific for the peptides 52 to 61 and 74 to 96 of HEL (143,175,176), the peptide 323 to 339 of chicken ovalbumin (144), and the peptide 81 to 104 of pigeon cytochrome c (149); the epitopes recognized by several T-cell clones overlap but are distinct. In addition, nine T-cell clones recognized a second T-cell determinant in myoglobin located around Lys 140, and each one responded to the cyanogen bromide cleavage fragment 132 to 153 (173). Further studies with a nested series of synthetic peptides (peptide 135 to 146 versus 136 to 146 versus 137 to 146, etc., in Fig. 13) showed that the stimulatory sequence is contained in peptide 136 to 146, whereas additional studies with peptides trimmed at the carboxyl end with carboxypeptidases B and A showed that Lys 145 is necessary, but Tyr 146 is not, although it contributes to antigenic potency (146). What these studies and others demonstrated about epitopes recognized by T cells is that they are segmental determinants, contained on synthetic peptides consisting of no more than

about 12 to 17 amino acid residues for class II or eight to 10 residues for class I. Within this size, they must contain all the information necessary to survive processing within the APC, associate with the MHC antigen, and bind to the TCR.

Mapping by Amino Acid Substitution and Effects of Altered Peptide Ligands

Once an antigenic peptide is identified, the next step is to map key amino acid residues by making a series of variant peptides, each of which differs from the native sequence by a single amino acid substitution (as described in the section MHC binding). One approach, called an alanine scan, substitutes Ala for the natural amino acid at each position in the peptide, or uses Ser or Gly to replace naturally occurring Ala. Ala is used because the side chain is only a methyl group, so it replaces whatever functional side chain is present with the smallest one other than that of Gly, which is not used because of its effects on conformation. Thus, one can ask whether loss of the naturally occurring side chain affects function, without the introduction of a new side chain that might itself affect function. Generally, each peptide will have several amino acids where Ala substitution destroys antigenicity. Some of these correspond to contact residues for the TCR, whereas others are contact residues for MHC. In many cases, the MHC binding residues can be determined by testing the substituted peptides in a competitive MHC binding assay (discussed above). The amino acid substitutions that knock out T-cell proliferation but not MHC binding are presumed to be in the epitope recognized by the TCR directly, and these can be studied with additional substitutions. For example, this technique was used to compare the residues interacting with the MHC molecule or TCR when the same HIV-1 V3 loop peptide P18 (residues 308 to 322) was presented by three different MHC molecules, a human class I molecule, a mouse class I molecule, and a mouse class II molecule (Fig. 14) (382,383). Interestingly, there was a striking concordance of function of several of the residues as presented by all three MHC molecules (Fig. 14). For example, Pro and Phe interacted with the MHC in all three cases, and the same Val interacted with the TCR in all three cases. Also, the same Arg in the middle of the peptide interacted with both the mouse class I and the mouse class II molecules, and the C-terminal Ile was an anchor residue for both human and murine class I molecules (382,383).

T-cell receptors may distinguish different chemical classes of amino acid side chains. An example of structural differences between amino acid side chains recognized by the TCR comes from an analysis of non–cross-reactive CTLs that distinguish homologous peptides from the V3 loop of different strains of HIV-1 envelope protein. The residue at position 8 in the minimal determinant was identified as a key epitopic TCR contact residue in both strain IIIB, which has a Val at this position, and strain MN, which has a Tyr at this position (382,384,385). CTLs specific for strain IIIB do not recognize the MN sequence, but will recognize peptides identical to MN except for the substitution of any aliphatic amino acid at that position, such as Val, Leu, or Ile (354). In contrast, CTLs specific for the MN strain do not recognize the IIIB sequence, but will recognize the IIIB peptide if the Val at this position is replaced by a Tyr (384). Moreover, they will see any MN variant in which the Tyr is replaced by another aromatic amino acid, such as Phe, Trp, or His (354). Thus, the two non–cross-reactive TCRs see similar peptides but discriminate strongly between pep-

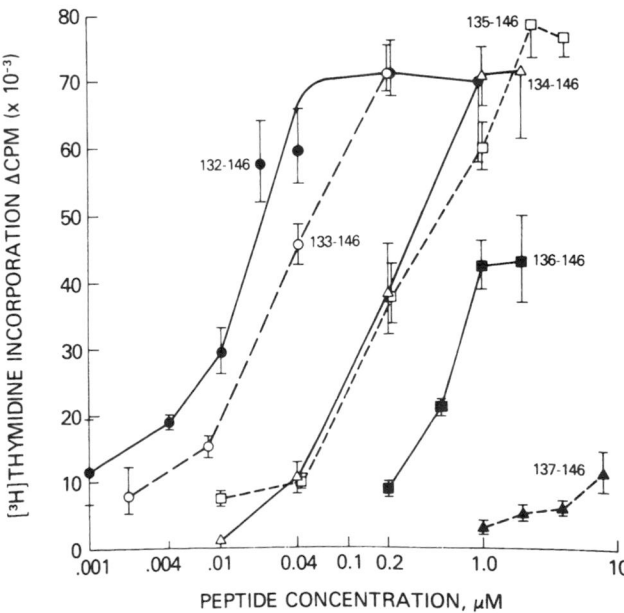

FIG. 13. Proliferative response of T-cell clone 14.5 to a series of synthetic peptides that correspond to the sequence 132 to 146 of sperm whale myoglobin. Comparison of the response to peptides that differ by a single amino acid residue at the amino end shows that Lys 133 is important for potency but is not critical for antigenicity; Glu 136 is critical for antigenicity. Background proliferation was 5561 cpm. Reprinted with permission (146).

HLA-A2

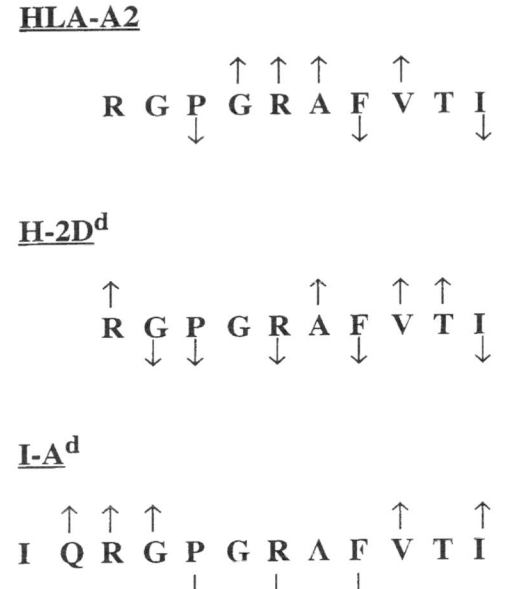

H-2Dᵈ

I-Aᵈ

FIG. 14. Comparison of the MHC-interacting (agretopic) and TCR-interacting (epitopic) residues of the same HIV-1 envelope V3 loop peptide as it is presented by human class I, murine class I, and murine class II MHC molecules to CD8⁺ CTLs and CD4⁺ helper T cells. Shown is the sequence of the optimal binding portion of peptide P18 IIIB from the HIV-1 envelope protein V3 loop for each MHC molecule, in single-letter amino acid code. Arrows pointing up indicate residues determined to interact with the TCR, and arrows pointing down indicate residues determined to interact with the MHC molecule. Mapping of residue function for binding to the human class I MHC molecule HLA-A2.1 has been described elsewhere (383), as has binding to the murine class I molecule H-2Dᵈ and the murine class II molecule I-Aᵈ (382). Note the common use of Pro and Phe for binding all three MHC molecules, and the use of the key Val residue for binding all the T-cell receptors. Also, the murine MHC molecules both use the central Arg residue as a contact residue, whereas both class I molecules use the C-terminal Ile residue as an anchor residue. Thus, there is a surprising degree of concordance.

tides with amino acids with aliphatic versus aromatic side chains. On the other hand, they do not distinguish strongly among different aliphatic residues or among different aromatic residues. In each category, however, the least active is the bulkiest member of the category, Ile and Trp, respectively, suggesting that these residues must fit into a pocket of limited size in the TCR.

The interaction of peptide ligand with TCR can be studied by introducing single substitutions of conservative amino acids at these contact residues, such as Glu for Asp, Ser for Thr, or Gln for Asn. The TCR readily distinguishes among peptides with these minor differences at a single residue, and the results have been revealing. Depending on affinity for the TCR, closely related (altered) peptides can elicit very different responses in T cells. Thus, although a substituted peptide may be very weak or nonstimulatory by itself, it may still act as a partial agonist, or even a strong antagonist of an ongoing T-cell response. Antagonistic peptides can be demonstrated by pulsing APCs with native peptide antigen first, so that one is not measuring competition for binding to MHC molecules, followed by pulsing with a 10-fold or greater excess of the antagonist, before adding T cells. In the case of influenza hemagglutinin peptide 307 to 319 presented with HLA DR1, peptide analogs such as Gln substituted for Asn 313 inhibited the proliferation of a human T-cell clone, even though they did not

stimulate the clone. Anergy was not induced, and the antagonist peptide had to be present throughout the culture to inhibit the response (386,387). Thus, lack of antagonist activity is another feature of the interaction between peptide (in complex with MHC molecule) and TCR that is required for the peptide to be a stimulatory antigenic determinant.

Partial agonists were first demonstrated using T-cell clones specific for an allelic form of mouse hemoglobin. These T cells were from CE/J mice, which express the Hbˢ allele of mouse hemoglobin, after immunization with the Hbᵈ allele. The minimum antigenic peptide corresponds to amino acids 67 to 76 of the Hbᵈ sequence and differs from Hbˢ at positions 72, 73, and 76 (388). Peptides substituted at each residue from amino acid 69 to 76 were tested for T-cell proliferation and cytokine release. Some substitutions eliminated proliferation but not IL-4 production, and these peptides are considered partial agonists (Fig. 15) (389). All but one of these peptides bound MHC with sufficient affinity to compete in a binding assay (390) and stimulate T cells. Similar alteration of cytokine profile by altering the peptide ligand can be seen in other systems (387,391,392).

For one of the Hb 64 to 76 specific T-cell clones, PL.17, substitutions at amino acids 70, 72, 73, or 76 reduced antigenic potency by 1,000-fold or more, even though conservative amino acids were

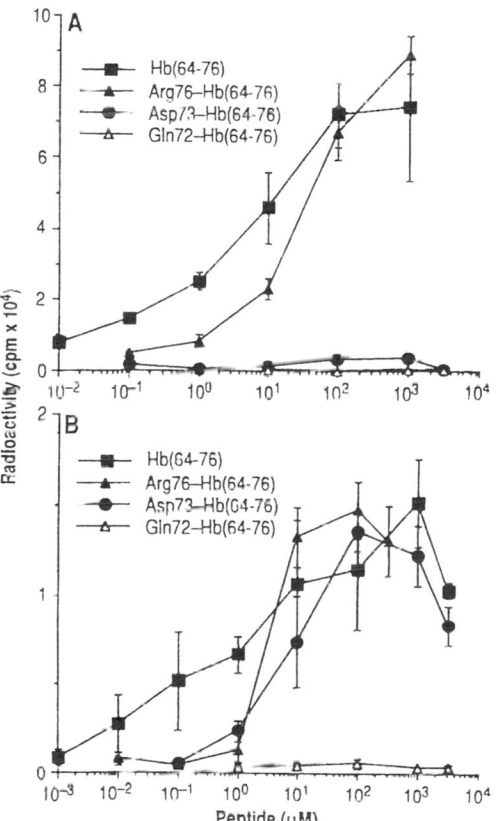

FIG. 15. Differential effect of altered peptide ligands on the response to peptide 64 to 76 from hemoglobin. **A:** Proliferative response of a T-cell line incubated with APCs and the natural Hb (64 to 76) peptide or with peptides substituted at positions 72, 73, or 76. **B:** IL-4 release by the T-cell line under the same conditions. The peptide substituted with Asp for Glu at position 73 is unable to induce T-cell proliferation, but it can still induce production of IL-4, so it is a partial agonist. In contrast, substitution of Gln for Asn at position 72 knocks out both responses equally. Modified with permission (389).

substituted. At position 72, substitution of Gln for Asn resulted in complete loss of antigenicity, as measured by T-cell proliferation or cytokine release. However, although substitution of Ser for Ala 70 prevented T-cell stimulation in both assays, there was clearly some response to this peptide because it induced expression of the IL-2 receptor (393). In addition, once T cells were exposed to the Ser 70 peptide, they became unresponsive to subsequent exposure to the natural Hb^d peptide. This phenomenon closely resembled T-cell anergy, which can be induced by presenting native peptide on chemically fixed APCs (394). In both cases, the anergic T cells failed to proliferate on subsequent challenge with native antigen plus APCs, and anergy persisted for a week or more.

The Ser 70 substitution alters a contact residue of the peptide for the TCR of clone PL.17 and affects its affinity. Other T-cell clones, however, can respond to this peptide presented on the same MHC molecule ($I-E^k$). Other Hb^d peptides substituted at this position, such as Met and Gly 70, also induced anergy but not proliferation, whereas nonconservative substitutions such as Phe, Asn, Asp, and His 70 induced neither (395).

Another well-studied example is influenza hemagglutinin peptide 306 to 318 as presented on human HLA-DR1. Based on the known crystal structure of the peptide-MHC complex (212), amino acid substitutions could be targeted to contact residues for the TCR at positions 307, 309, 310, 312, 315, and 318 (396). At each position, nonconservative substitutions often rendered the peptide inactive, whereas conservative substitutions at several sites either gave full antigenicity, or gave progressively lower stimulatory activity, down to 1,000-fold less than native peptide, while retaining the ability to induce anergy. For example, substituting His or Gly for Lys 307 gave 1,000-fold reduced stimulation of T-cell proliferation, but full ability to induce tolerance. Similarly, substituting His for Lys 315 gave complete loss of stimulation, but nearly full anergy-inducing activity. As before, induction of the IL-2 receptor (CD25) was a sign of T-cell activation by these altered peptide ligands, even when they did not induce proliferation. These peptides differ from the peptide antagonists described above because the antagonists do not induce interleukin receptors or secretion and they do not cause long-lasting tolerance. Overall, a number of altered peptide ligands have now been identified that, in appropriate complexes with MHC molecules, induce anergy or act as antagonists of the TCR and block activation by agonist ligands by delivering an abortive signal (387).

Several methods have been found to anergize T cells to a specific antigen for up to a week, and all have the common theme of delivering a partial signal via the TCR, resulting in tolerance rather than stimulation. The first method was to expose the T cells to peptide plus APCs treated with the carbodiimide crosslinker ECDI (394). This treatment may prevent accessory molecules on the presenting cell from interacting with the TCR complex, or costimulatory signals from contributing to T-cell activation. The second method was to present peptide on presenting cells with mutated I-E molecules (397,398). The third method was to use altered peptide ligands that act as TCR antagonists as described above (387,395,396). The final method was to block CD4 function with a monoclonal antibody, which would delay the recruitment of CD4 to the engaged TCR (399). Because generation of a complete stimulatory signal requires the interaction of TCR and accessory molecules, modifications that affect either component can block signaling. An altered peptide ligand, with decreased affinity for the TCR, may form an unstable complex, which cannot stay together long enough to recruit accessory molecules and generate a com-plete signal (399,400). Altered peptide ligands with low affinity for the TCR can also act as partial agonists that can compete with optimal agonists and reduce T-cell stimulation based on a similar mechanism (short dwell time of peptide–MHC complex on the TCR) (160).

Abnormal TCR signaling can be demonstrated by following the activity of protein kinases. Normal signaling produces phosphorylation of TCR subunits, such as ζ chain, as well as phosphorylation and activation of receptor-associated tyrosine kinases, such as ZAP-70. These kinases generate the downstream signal needed for T-cell activation. However, in each case studied, partial antigen signaling resulted in ζ chain phosphorylation without phosphorylation or activation of ZAP-70 (395,398,399), so downstream activation did not occur. This abnormal pattern occurred regardless of the method of anergy induction.

Partial signaling may be important for T-cell survival during negative selection in the thymus or in maintaining peripheral tolerance. By treating self antigens as if they were altered ligands presented in the thymus, T cells could use anergy induction as a successful strategy for avoiding clonal deletion. Similarly, peripheral tolerance may be an important mechanism for preventing autoimmune disease. Immunotherapy with altered peptide ligands could be envisioned as a way to block an ongoing response or induce tolerance to a specific antigen. This could be potentially useful in suppressing undesirable immune responses, such as to allergens, to synovium in arthritis, or to foreign MHC antigens in allograft rejection. However, a potential pitfall is that different T cells recognize the same peptide differently, so a peptide that is seen as an altered peptide ligand by some T cell clones may be seen as a complete antigen by others. In addition, the choice of peptide would vary with MHC type. To be effective, an altered peptide ligand should antagonize or anergize polyclonal T cells and should work with each patient's MHC type.

Prediction of T-Cell Epitopes

As just discussed, T cells recognize protein antigens only on the surface of another cell, and only after processing, which involves either cleavage into small fragments or at least unfolding. This fact leads to the ironic situation that T-cell recognition of antigens, which is more complex than antibody recognition due to the ternary complex needed between TCR, antigen, and MHC molecule, may actually be focused on simpler structures than those seen by most antibodies specific for native protein antigens. In contrast to the assembled topographic antigenic sites seen by many antibodies (42,43), T cells specific for processed antigens are limited to seeing short segments of continuous sequence (138,193). Therefore, the tertiary structure of the protein plays little if any role in the structure of the epitope recognized by T cells, although it may play a more distant role in determining the way the protein is processed and therefore indirectly influence which epitopes are available for T-cell recognition, as discussed previously. However, the structure of the T-cell antigenic site itself must be limited to primary (sequence) and secondary structure, the latter depending only on local rather than long-range interactions. This limitation greatly simplifies the problem of identifying structural properties important to T-cell recognition, because one can deal with sequence information, which can now be obtained from DNA without having a purified protein, and with the secondary structure implicit therein without having to obtain an x-ray crystallographic three-dimensional structure of the native protein, a much more difficult task.

These features have greatly facilitated the structural analysis of antigenic sites recognized by T cells by allowing the use of short synthetic peptides and recombinant fragments that do not retain the native structure of the protein. The comparative ease of producing overlapping and truncated peptides and sequence variants, combined with the limitation of the search for salient features to primary and secondary structure, has led to a major surge in efforts to identify properties that will be useful in predicting the location of antigenic sites.

Because the key feature necessary for a peptide to be recognized by T cells is its ability to bind to an MHC molecule, most approaches for predicting T-cell epitopes are based on predicting binding to MHC molecules. These approaches, which have been reviewed recently (401,402), can be divided into those that focus on specific individual MHC molecules one at a time, such as motif-based methods, and those that look for general structural properties of peptide sequences. We shall discuss first the methods based on general properties, and then those directed to individual MHC molecules.

The first structural feature of amino acid sequences found associated with T-cell epitopes that remains in use today is helical amphipathicity (188,203,204,403,404). Although this property is associated with helicity, which was identified earlier in association with the immunodominant site of pigeon cytochrome c (149,202, 205), it is statistically significant independent of the tendency to form a helix (204). Because the x-ray crystallographic structures of both MHC class I (330–332,405) and class II molecules (212,406) have consistently shown peptides to be bound in extended, not alpha-helical conformation, helicity per se has been abandoned as an associated structural feature of T-cell epitopes. However, as discussed below, other explanations of amphipathic structures have been discovered that do not require the peptide to be bound to the MHC molecule as an alpha helix. Amphipathicity is the property of having hydrophobic and hydrophilic regions separated in space. It was observed that both of the immunodominant T-cell epitopes for myoglobin corresponded to amphipathic helices (146,150). To see whether this observation was peculiar to myoglobin, which has a high helical content, or whether it was true of immunodominant T-cell antigenic sites in other proteins as well, DeLisi and Berzofsky (203) developed an algorithm to search for segments of protein sequence that could fold as amphipathic helices. The approach was based on the idea that, because hydrophilicity is the negative of hydrophobicity, the hydrophobicity of the amino acids in the sequence must oscillate as one goes around an amphipathic helix. For the hydrophobic residues to line up on one side and the hydrophilic residues on the other, the periodicity of this oscillation must be approximately the same as the structural periodicity of the helix (Fig. 16). For an alpha helix, this is 100 degrees per turn (360 degrees per 3.6 residues per turn) and for a 3_{10} helix, this is 120 degrees per turn (360 degrees per three residues per turn).

A microcomputer program implementing this analysis was published (404). Subsequently, Margalit et al. (188) optimized the original approach (203) by comparing a number of related algorithms and found that, for short segments, a least-squares best fit to a sinusoidal function (407) was more effective than the Fourier transform. This algorithm correctly identified 18 of the 23 immunodominant helper T-cell antigenic sites seen in association with class II MHC molecules from the 12 proteins in an expanded database ($p < 0.001$) (188) (Table 6). Indeed, when newly discovered helper T-cell determinants were included to expand the data base to twice and then four times its original size, the correlation remained

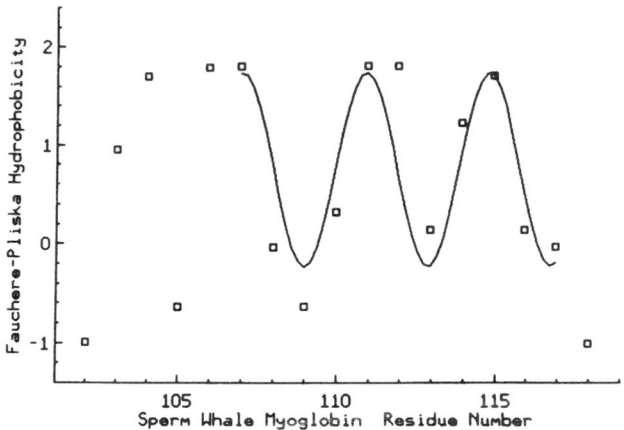

FIG. 16. Plot of hydrophobicity of each amino acid in sperm whale myoglobin 102 to 118, according to the scale of Fauchère and Pliska (468), as a function of amino acid sequence, showing least-squares fit of a sinusoidal function to the sequence of hydrophobicities from 107 to 117. Reprinted with permission (141).

highly significant, and the fraction of sites predicted remained relatively stable (34 of 48 sites = 71%, $p < 0.003$; 61 of 92 sites = 66%, $p < 0.001$) (408,409). However, it is clear that a sizable fraction of determinants do not have this property.

At the time of the initial studies, very few peptides presented by class I MHC molecules to CD8+ CTLs had been identified. However, subsequent analysis of 51 peptides presented by class I molecules indicated that 33 (65%) could fold as amphipathic helices ($p = 0.05$) J. L. Cornette, H. Margalit, C. DeLisi, J.A. Berzofsky, unpublished results). Moreover, seven of 11 natural endogenous peptides eluted from HLA-B27 by Jardetzky et al. (362) had this property, compared with two of 11 or three of 11 for control sets of peptides ($p = 0.02$) (409). Thus, it appears that a similar fraction of sites presented by class I MHC molecules also can fold as amphipathic helices. A primary sequence pattern found in a substantial number of T-cell epitopes by Rothbard and Taylor was consistent with one turn of an amphipathic helix (410). Also, another approach, called the strip-of-the-helix algorithm, which searches for helices with a hydrophobic strip down one face, also found a correlation between amphipathic helices and determinants presented by both class II and class I MHC molecules (403,411).

Recent studies have provided at least two explanations, not mutually exclusive, for this correlation in the absence of helical structures found in the peptides bound to MHC molecules (412). First, crystal structures of peptides bound to class II MHC molecules have found that the peptides are bound in an extended conformation, but with a 130 degree twist like that of a type II polyproline helix (212,406). The first such structure, that of an influenza peptide bound to HLA DR1 (212), was actually quite amphipathic because of this twist. Although the 130 degree twist is distinct from that of an alpha helix, it gives a periodicity similar enough that the algorithms used to detected such periodicity for amphipathic helices would pick up this signal. Second, it was observed that spacing of the anchor residues in the motifs for peptides binding to class I and II MHC molecules was consistent with the spacing of turns of an alpha helix, for example, at positions 2 and 9 (seven residues apart like two turns of a helix) or at positions 5 and 9 (spaced like one turn of a helix) (412). Because the anchor residues are most often hydrophobic, this pattern resulted in an amphipathic periodicity pattern like that of an amphipathic alpha helix for just the anchor residues alone, seen in the majority of motifs (412). Thus, if the other residues have a random pattern, the anchor residue spacing alone, which is enforced by the spacing of the pockets in the MHC molecules that bind these anchor residues, will produce the amphipathic helical signal, even though the peptide is bound in an extended conformation. This amphipathic helical periodicity has held up as a correlate for peptides defined as T-cell epitopes (412), and has continued to be a useful predictive tool for identifying potential epitopes, successful in a number of studies, when one does not want to focus on individual MHC alleles.

Other approaches to predicting T-cell epitopes are generally based on sequences found to bind to specific MHC molecules (401,402). The simplest approach is to apply standard sequence search algorithms to known protein sequences to locate motifs for peptides binding to particular MHC molecules, using collections of motifs identified in the literature (236), as described above. This approach showed early success for epitopes in proteins from *Listeria monocytogenes* (413) and malaria (414), but it also became apparent that only about 30% of sequences bearing motifs actually bound to the corresponding MHC molecules (413,415,416). This discrepancy may relate to adverse interactions created by nonanchor residues (346,351,417) and could be overcome to some extent by generating extended motifs taking into account the role of each residue in the sequence (351). These adverse interactions can be determined by examining peptides with different amino acid substitutions (346,351) or by comparing sets of peptides known to bind to a given MHC molecule with those known not to bind, and testing for patterns of chemical features (such as charge, hydrophobicity, hydrogen-bonding potential, size, etc.) at different positions associated with binding or not binding (417).

To determine whether one could locate regions of proteins with high densities of motifs for binding multiple MHC molecules, Meister et al. developed the algorithm Epimer, which determined the density of motifs per length of sequence (418). A surprising result was that the motifs were not uniformly distributed, but clustered. Thus, there were segments of proteins relatively devoid of motifs, and others containing a high density of overlapping motifs in a short segment. This clustering may reflect the fact that many motifs are related, and that the same anchor residues are shared by several motifs, perhaps because MHC molecules are also related and their variable segments that define some of the binding pockets are sometimes exchanged by gene conversion events (419). In the case of HIV, the densities of motifs for class I MHC binding were anomalous at both the low and high ends of the spectrum (420). Clustering at the high end may be due to anchor sharing and showed no correlation with conserved or variable regions of the sequence. However, at the low end, long stretches with low motif density occurred preferentially in variable regions, suggesting that the virus was mutating to escape the CTL immune system (420). This clustering may be useful in vaccine development because identification of sequences containing overlapping motifs for multiple MHC molecules may define promiscuously presented peptides that would elicit responses in a broad segment of the population (418).

Another type of MHC allele-specific approach is the use of matrices defining the positive or negative contribution of each amino acid possible at each position in the sequence toward binding to an MHC molecule. A positive or negative value is assigned to each of the 20 possible amino acids that can occur at each posi-

tion in a peptide sequence, and these are summed to give the estimated potential of that peptide for binding. The values in the matrix are derived from either experimental binding studies using peptide panels with single positions substituted with each possible amino acid (375,421–423), or from comparisons of peptides known to bind in a compilation of the literature, if the number known is sufficiently large (402,424). Davenport et al. (425,426) also developed a motif method based on Edman degradation sequencing of pooled peptides eluted from MHC molecules. All of these methods have had some success in predicting peptides binding to particular MHC molecules (402), but they all require the assumption that each position in a peptide must be acting independently of its neighbors, which is a reasonable first approximation, but exceptions are likely to be found. The more experimental data that goes into generating the matrix, the more reliable the predictions. Therefore, the predictive success may be greater for some of the more common HLA molecules for which more data exist. This matrix approach has been used for both class I and class II MHC molecules.

A potentially very useful observation is the finding that HLA class I molecules can be grouped into families (HLA supertypes) that share similar binding motifs (374,421,427,428). The broader motifs that encompass several MHC molecules have been called supermotifs. For example, HLA-A*0301, A*1101, A*3101, A*3401, A*6601, A*6801, and A*7401 all fall into the HLA-A3 superfamily (427). A peptide that carried this supermotif should be active in a broader range of individuals than one which was presented by a single HLA molecule. Moreover, because several HLA supertypes have been defined, it should be possible to design a vaccine effective in a large fraction of the population with only a limited number of well-selected antigenic determinants.

Another approach for predicting peptides that bind to MHC molecules is based on free energy calculations of peptides docked into the groove of a known MHC structure, for which the crystallographic coordinates are known, or on structural modeling of the MHC molecule by homologous extension from another MHC molecule, when the crystal structure is not known, followed by peptide docking calculations (429,430). It is important to use free energy rather than energy because the latter alone cannot find the most stable orientation of a side chain and cannot correctly rank order different side chains at the same position. For example, for HLA-A2.1, which preferentially binds peptides with a Leu at position 2 binding in the B pocket, the standard CHARMm energy procedure predicts a charged Lys at position 2, whereas a newer free energy model, which allows for evaluating solvation free energy, correctly predicts the hydrophobic Leu (429). This approach correctly predicts the structure of several known peptide–MHC complexes when starting with the crystal structure of a different complex, in each case to within 1.2 to 1.6 Å all-atom root mean square deviation (430). Using this structural modeling can allow one to extend motifs to nonanchor positions for cases where only anchor residue motifs are known and can allow one to predict new motifs for MHC molecules whose motifs have not yet been determined.

Another approach to predicting MHC binding sequences uses a technique called threading that has been developed for predicting peptide secondary structure, based on threading a sequence through a series of known secondary structures and calculating the energies of each structure. Altuvia et al. (431) showed that threading could be applied to peptides in the groove of MHC molecules because when several peptides that bind to the same MHC molecule are compared crystallographically, the conformation of the peptides is fairly similar, as for example in several peptides crystallized bound to HLA-A2.1 (405). In testing the threading approach, Altuvia et al. (431) showed that known antigenic peptides are highly ranked among all peptides in a given protein sequence, and the rank order of peptides that had been compared by competitive binding studies could be correctly predicted. The advantage of this approach is that it is independent of known binding motifs and can identify peptides that bind despite lack of the common motif for the MHC molecule in question. It can also be used to rank a set of peptides all containing a known motif.

Finally, artificial neural networks (ANNs) can be trained on a set of peptides that bind to a given MHC molecule to recognize patterns present in binding peptides (432). When the predictions of the ANNs are tested, the results can be used to further train the ANNs to improve the predictive capability in an iterative fashion.

As all these methods are further developed and refined, they promise to allow accurate prediction of peptides that will bind to different MHC molecules and thus allow the design of vaccines without empirical binding studies until the end of the process. Although current methods are not yet fully adequate to bypass experimental binding studies, the problem of prediction of binding to well-characterized MHC molecules appears to be ultimately surmountable. In the meantime, these methods can potentially narrow the search and save considerable time and expense in identifying appropriate peptides. Localization of clusters of adjacent or overlapping binding sequences in a short segment of protein sequence also can be useful for selecting sequences that will be broadly recognized.

RELATIONSHIP BETWEEN HELPER T-CELL EPITOPES AND B-CELL EPITOPES ON A COMPLEX PROTEIN ANTIGEN

We have seen that the factors that determine the location of antigenic sites for T cells and for B cells, with the possible exception of self tolerance, are largely different. Indeed, if B cells (with their surface antibody) bind sites that tend to be especially exposed or protruding—sites that are also more accessible and susceptible to proteolytic enzymes involved in processing—then there is reason to think that T cells may have a lower probability of being able to recognize these same sites, which may be more likely to be destroyed during processing. Certainly, assembled topographic sites are going to be destroyed during processing. On the other hand, there are examples in which T cells and antibodies seem to see the same, or very closely overlapping, sites on a protein (36,146,173,433–435), although fine specificity analysis usually indicates that the antibody and T-cell fine specificities are not identical. The question posed here is whether, besides such structural features that T- and B-cell epitopes may or may not have in common, there are any functional or regulatory factors in T cell–B cell cooperation that would produce a relationship between helper T-cell specificity and B-cell specificity in the response to a given protein antigen.

The first evidence that helper T cells might influence the specificity of the antibodies produced came from studies of Ir gene control of antibody specificity. A number of studies showed that Ir genes, which appeared to act through effects of T-cell help, could influence the specificity of antibodies produced to a given antigen (142,436–443). An apparent exception was the case of insulin in the guinea pig (444). It is easy to envision how Ir genes, which

encode MHC molecules that present antigen to T cells, can influence which epitopes of a given protein can be presented to T cells by presenting cells of a given MHC type or how MHC products could influence the T cell repertoire of a given individual. But it is harder to imagine how Ir genes could determine which epitopes of a protein elicit antibodies, when such antibodies are generally not MHC restricted. One explanation suggested was that the Ir genes first select which helper T cells are activated, and these in turn influence which B cells, specific for particular epitopes, could be activated (104). Because, for cognate help, the B cell has to present the antigen in association with an MHC molecule to the helper T cell, the Ir gene control of antibody specificity must operate at least partly at this step by selecting which helper T cell can be activated by and help a given B cell. An example is the case of F1 hybrid T cells helping parental B cells of one or the other haplotype. Conversely, if the helper T cell selects a subset of B cells to be activated on the basis of their antibody specificity, then there is a reciprocal interaction between T and B cells influencing each other's specificity. Therefore, this hypothesis was called T–B reciprocity (104). Steric constraints on the epitopes that could be used by helper T cells to help a B cell specific for another particular epitope of the same protein were also proposed by Sercarz et al. (445).

The first attempts to test these ideas involved limiting the fine specificity of helper T cells to one or a few epitopes and then determining the effect on the specificities of antibodies produced in response to the whole molecule. Cecka et al. (446) accomplished this by inducing T-cell tolerance to certain epitopes of lysozyme by tolerizing rabbits to cross-reacting lysozymes. Others (102,447,448) used T cells from animals immune to peptide fragments of the protein. In each case, the limitation on the helper T-cell specificity repertoire influenced the repertoire of antibodies produced. An apparent exception was the case of T cells and B cells specific for a decapeptide epitope of tobacco mosaic virus protein, although in this case the selection was largely among T cells and B cells with different fine specificities for the same epitope rather than for different epitopes (449).

At a time when antigen was thought to serve as a direct bridge between the B-cell receptor (immunoglobulin) and the TCR, one explanation suggested for these constraints was steric hindrance (104,445). For the antibody, TCR, and MHC to bind simultaneously to the intact protein, the sites they bound in relation to each other were subject to steric constraints. However, it has become apparent that T cells recognize antigen on B cells as on other APCs, not in its intact form but after processing and association with an MHC molecule (450–452). Indeed, these and other studies (453–457) indicated that one purpose of the B-cell surface immunoglobulin was to take up the specific antigen with high affinity, but that the antigen was then internalized by receptor-mediated endocytosis and processed like any other antigen. Therefore, another explanation was proposed: the surface immunoglobulin, which acts as the receptor to mediate endocytosis, sterically influences the rate at which different parts of the antigen are processed because what the B cell is processing is not free antigen but a monoclonal antibody–antigen immune complex (104) (Fig. 17). This concept presupposes that many antibody–antigen complexes are stable near pH 6 in the endosome and that what matters is the kinetics of production of large fragments, rather than the products of complete digestion, when both the antigen and the antibody may be degraded to single amino acids. Such protection from proteolysis of antigen epitopes by bound antibody can be demonstrated at least in vitro (51). More recently, the effect of antigen-specific B-cell

A

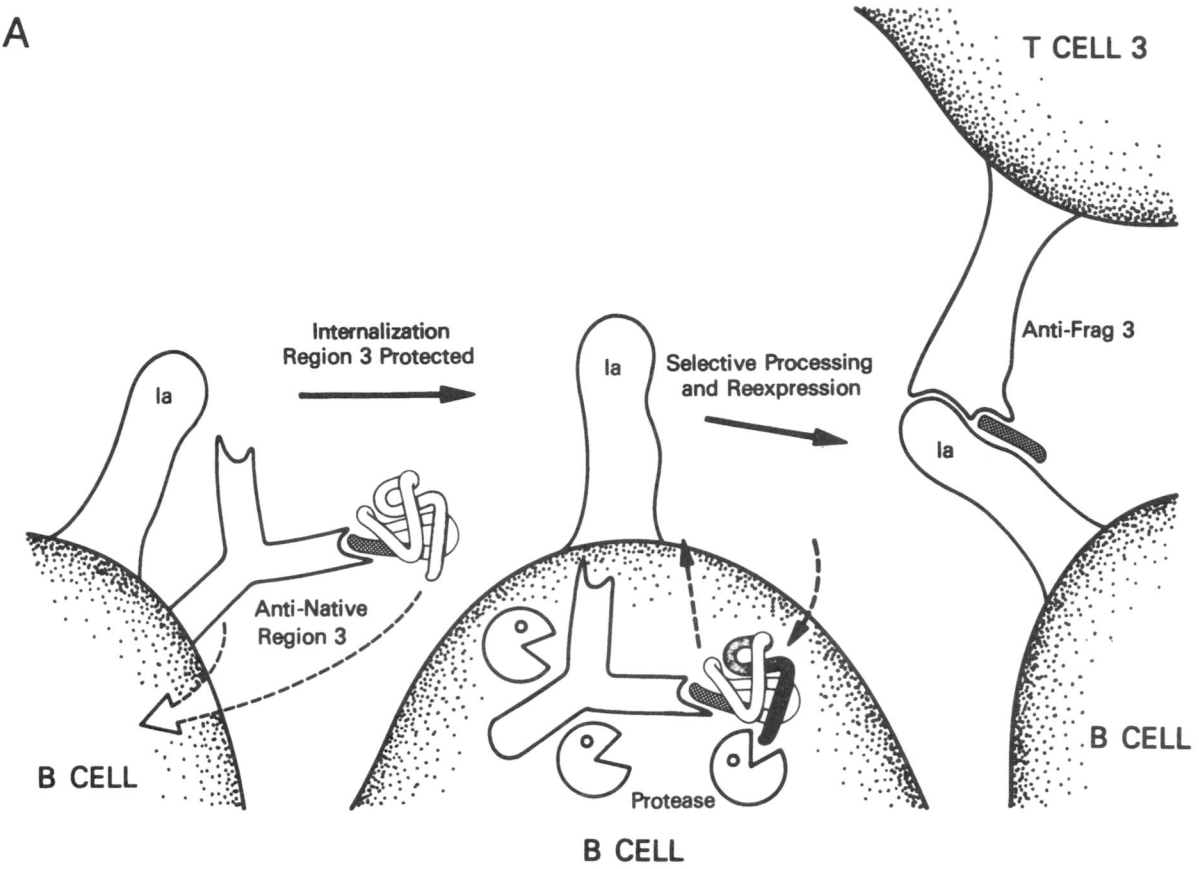

B

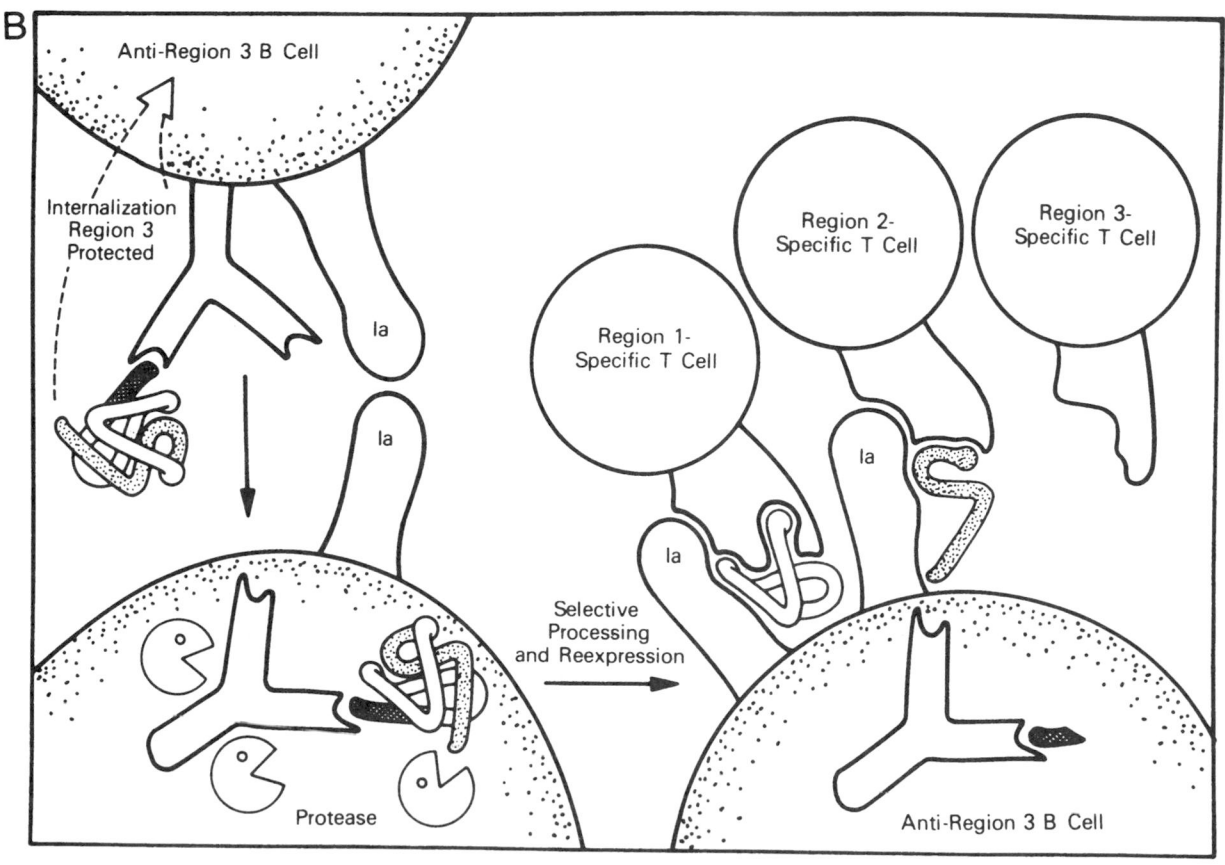

surface immunoglobulin on the fragments produced by proteolytic processing of antigen was elegantly demonstrated by Davidson and Watts (458). They demonstrated that the pattern of fragmentation of tetanus toxoid, as measured by SDS–polyacrylamide gel electrophoresis, produced during processing by B-lymphoblastoid clones specific for tetanus toxoid, varied among B-cell clones depending on their specificity for different epitopes within the antigen. Binding to the antibody also may influence which fragments are shuttled to the surface and which are shunted into true lysosomes for total degradation. Thus, different B cells bearing different surface immunoglobulin would preferentially process the antigen differently to put more of some potential fragments than others on their surface, in contrast to nonspecific presenting cells that would process the antigen indifferently. By this mechanism, it is proposed that B cell specificity leads to selective antigen presentation to helper T cells and therefore to selective help from T cells specific for some epitopes more than from T cells specific for others (104).

To test this hypothesis from the B-cell point of view, Ozaki and Berzofsky (103) made populations of B cells effectively monoclonal for purposes of antigen presentation (but not secretion) by coating polyclonal B cells with a conjugate of monoclonal antimyoglobin coupled to anti-IgM antibodies. They found that B cells coated with one such conjugate presented myoglobin less well to one myoglobin-specific T-cell clone than to others. B cells coated with other conjugates presented myoglobin to this clone equally well as to other clones. Therefore, the limitation on myoglobin presentation by this B-cell population to this particular T-cell clone depended on the specificity of both the monoclonal antibody coating the B cell and the receptor of the T-cell clone. It happened in this case that both the monoclonal antibody and the T-cell clone were specific for the same or closely overlapping epitopes. Therefore, it appears that the site bound by the B-cell surface immunoglobulin is less well presented to T cells. This finding is also consistent with a recent study of chimeric proteins in which one or more copies of an ovalbumin helper T-cell determinant were inserted in different positions (459). Although the position of the ovalbumin determinants did not affect the antibody response to an amino-terminal site from the heat-stable enterotoxin from *Escherichia coli*, the position did matter for antibody production to the carboxyl-terminal determinant of the chimeric protein derived from insulinlike growth factor I. An ovalbumin determinant inserted distal to the carboxyl-terminal antibody epitope was much more effective in providing help than one inserted adjacent to the same epitope, when both constructs were used as immunogens, even though both constructs elicited similar levels of ovalbumin-specific T-cell proliferation in the presence of nonspecific presenting cells *in vitro*, as a control for nonspecific effects of flanking residues on processing and presentation of the helper T-cell determinants. However, circumstantial evidence from the Ir gene studies mentioned previously suggests that T cells may preferentially help

B cells that bind with some degree of proximity to the T-cell epitope because there was a correlation between T-cell and antibody specificity for large fragments of protein antigens under Ir gene control (101,104,142,439,440,443). Therefore, antibodies may have both positive and negative selective effects on processing. Further studies on presentation of β-galactosidase–monoclonal antibody complexes by nonspecific APCs suggest similar conclusions (460,461). Presumably, the conjugates are taken up via Fc receptors on the presenting cells and processed differentially according to the site bound by the antibody, so that they are presented differentially to different T-cell clones. Thus, non-B presenting cells can be made to mimic specific B presenting cells. This also suggests that circulating antibody may have a role in the selection of which T cells are activated in a subsequent exposure to antigen.

The issue of whether bound antibody enhanced or suppressed presentation of specific determinants to T cells was explored further by Watts and Lanzavecchia and their coworkers (462,463). They first found that the tetanus toxoid–specific Epstein-Barr virus–transformed human B-cell clone 11.3 failed to present the tetanus toxoid epitope 1174 to 1189 to specific T cells, whereas it presented another epitope, 947 to 967, as well as other B cells, and another B-cell clone presented the 1174 to 1189 epitope well. Moreover, the free immunoglobulin from the 11.3 clone also inhibited presentation of this epitope to T cells at the same time that it enhanced presentation of other epitopes by Fc receptor–facilitated uptake and endocytosis (462). They subsequently found that the same 11.3 B cell and antibody actually enhanced presentation of another epitope of tetanus toxoid, 1273 to 1284, by about 10-fold, even though both epitopes were within the footprint of the antibody, as determined by protection from proteolytic digestion (463). The enhancement also could be mediated by free antibody as well as Fab fragments thereof, indicating that the mechanism did not involve Fc receptor–facilitated uptake. Furthermore, the 11.3 antibody had no effect on presentation of another determinant in the same tetanus toxoid C fragment, 947 to 967, that was not within the footprint of the antibody, and another antibody to the C fragment did not enhance presentation of 1273 to 1284. The authors concluded that the same antibody or surface immunoglobulin can protect two determinants from proteolysis, but sterically hinder the binding of one to class II MHC molecules while facilitating the binding of the other (463). The facilitation simply may involve protection from degradation, or also may involve stabilization of a certain conformation. This antibody-mediated enhancement of presentation of selected epitopes to helper T cells can greatly lower the threshold for induction of a T-cell response and may thereby elicit responses to otherwise subdominant epitopes. It also can contribute to epitope spreading, for example, in autoimmune disease, in which an initial response to one dominant determinant leads to a subsequent response to other subdominant determinants, perhaps by helping for antibody production which in turn facilitates presentation of the other determinants.

FIG. 17. Antigen presentation by B cells: positive (**A**) or negative (**B**) selection. A B cell specific for region 3 of a particular antigen internalizes the antigen molecule with the region 3 protected by an antibody against the region. The part of the antigen under the influence of the antibody is protected from proteolytic enzymes (selective processing). In positive selection (**A**), that part is preferentially reexpressed and presented. In negative selection (**B**), the reexpression of that part takes much longer or is much more limited than that for the other parts of the antigen, which are free from the influence of the antibody. Therefore, such a B cell can present any part of the antigen, except the one bound to the antibody (region 3), to the relevant helper T cells (selective presentation). Part A reprinted with permission (104); part B reprinted with permission (103).

Taken together, these results support the concept of T–B reciprocity in which helper T cells and B cells each influence the specificity of the other's expressed repertoire (104). This mechanism also may provide an explanation for some of the cases in which Ir genes have been found to control antibody idiotype (464,465), although certain cases would require another explanation (466). Although we do not yet know all the constraints on the relationships between T- and B-cell epitopes and therefore cannot yet use this information in a predictive way, these relationships probably play a significant role in regulating the fine specificity of immune response of both arms of the immune system. Therefore, they also will be of importance in the design of synthetic or recombinant fragment vaccines that incorporate both T- and B-cell epitopes to elicit an antibody response.

REFERENCES

1. Goodman JW. Antigenic determinants and antibody combining sites. In: Sela M, ed. *The antigens.* New York: Academic Press, 1975:127–187.
2. Landsteiner K. *The specificity of serological reactions.* Cambridge, MA: Harvard University Press, 1945.
3. Landsteiner K, Van der Scheer J. Serological studies on azoproteins. Antigens containing azo components with aliphatic side chains. *J Exp Med* 1934;59:751–768.
4. Pressman D, Grossberg AL. *The structural basis of antibody specificity.* New York: Benjamin, 1968.
5. Pressman D, Siegel M, Hall LAR. The closeness of fit of antibenzoate antibodies about haptens and the orientation of the haptens in combination. *J Am Chem Soc* 1954;76:6336–6341.
6. Karush F. The interaction of purified anti–β-lactoside antibody with haptens. *J Am Chem Soc* 1957;79:3380–3384.
7. Eisen HN, Siskind GW. Variations in affinities of antibodies during the immune response. *Biochemistry* 1964;3:996–1008.
8. Kabat EA. *Structural concepts in immunology and immunochemistry,* 2nd ed. New York: Holt. Rinehart & Winston, 1976.
9. Jann K, Westphal O. Microbial polysaccharides. In: Sela M, ed. *The antigens.* New York: Academic Press, 1975:1–125.
10. Uchida T, Robbins PW, Luria SE. Analysis of the serologic determinant groups of the Salmonella E-group O-antigens. *Biochemistry* 1963;2:663–668.
11. Springer GF. Blood group and Forssman antigenic determinants shared between microbes and mammalian cells. In: Kallos P, Waksman BH, eds. *Progress in allergy.* Basel, Switzerland: Karger, 1971:9–77.
12. Marcus DM. The ABO and Lewis blood-group system. Immunochemistry, genetics, and relation to human disease. *N Engl J Med* 1969;280:994–1006.
13. Watkins WM. Biochemistry and genetics of the ABO, Lewis, and P blood group systems. *Adv Hum Genet* 1980;10:1–136.
14. Kabat EA. The upper limit for the size of the human antidextran combining site. *J Immunol* 1960;84:82–85.
15. Kabat EA. The nature of an antigenic determinant. *J Immunol* 1966;97:1–11.
16. Cisar J, Kabat EA, Dorner MM, Liao J. Binding properties of immunoglobulin combining sites specific for terminal or nonterminal antigenic determinants in dextran. *J Exp Med* 1975;142:435–459.
17. Sharon J, Kabat EA, Morrison SL. Studies on mouse hybridomas secreting IgM or IgA antibodies to α(1→6)-linked dextran. *Mol Immunol* 1981;18:831–846.
18. Sharon J, Kabat EA, Liao J, Potter M. Immunochemical characterization of binding sites of hybridoma antibodies specific for α(1→6) linked dextran. *Mol Immunol* 1982;19:375–388.
19. Sharon J, D'Hoostelaere L, Potter M, Kabat EA, Morrison SL. A cross-reactive idiotype, QUPC 52 IdX, present on most but not all anti-α(1→6) dextran-specific IgM and IgA hybridoma antibodies with combining sites of different sizes. *J Immunol* 1982;128:498–500.
20. Jerne NK. Towards a network theory of the immune system. *Ann Immunol Inst Pasteur* 1974;125C:373–389.
21. Eichmann K. Expression and function of idiotypes on lymphocytes. *Adv Immunol* 1978;26:195–254.
22. Sikder SK, Akolkar PN, Kaladas PM, Morrison SL, Kabat EA. Sequences of variable regions of hybridoma antibodies to α(1→6) dextran in BALB/c and C57BL/6 mice. *J Immunol* 1985;135:4215–4221.
23. Akolkar PN, Sikder SK, Bhattacharya SB, et al. Different V_L and V_H germline genes are used to produce similar combining sites with specificity for α(1→6) dextrans. *J Immunol* 1987;138:4472–4479.
24. Brodeur PM, Riblet R. The immunoglobulin heavy chain variable region (Igh-v) locus in the mouse. I. One-hundred Igh-v genes comprise seven families of homologous genes. *Eur J Immunol* 1984;14:922–930.
25. Griffiths GM, Berek C, Kaartinen M, Milstein C. Somatic mutation and the maturation of immune response to 2-phenxyloxazolone. *Nature* 1984;14:271–275.
26. Wang D, Chen H-T, Liao J, et al. Two families of monoclonal antibodies to α(1-

27. 6)dextran, V_H19.1.2. and V_H9.14.7, show distinct patterns of J_K and J_H minigene usage and amino acid substitutions in CDR3. *J Immunol* 1990;145:3002–3010.
28. Amit AG, Mariuzza RA, Phillips SEV, Poljak RJ. Three-dimensional structure of an antigen–antibody complex at 2.8 Å resolution. *Science* 1986;233:747–758.
28. Colman PM, Laver WG, Varghese JN, et al. Three-dimensional structure of a complex of antibody with influenza virus neuraminidase. *Nature* 1987;326:358–363.
29. Sheriff S, Silverton EW, Padlan EA, et al. Three-dimensional structure of an antibody–antigen complex. *Proc Natl Acad Sci U S A* 1987;84:8075–8079.
30. Davies DR, Padlan EA. Antibody–antigen complexes. *Annu Rev Biochem* 1990;59:439–473.
31. Schlossman SF, Yaron A, Ben-Efraim S, Sober HA. Immunogenicity of a series of α,N-DNP-L-lysines. *Biochemistry* 1965;4:1638–1645.
32. Schlossman SF, Levine H. Desensitization to delayed hypersensitivity reactions. With special reference to the requirement for an immunogenic molecule. *J Immunol* 1967;99:111–114.
33. Van Vunakis H, Kaplan J, Lehrer H, Levine L. Immunogenicity of polylysine and polyornithine when complexed to phosphorylated bovine serum albumin. *Immunochemistry* 1966;3:393–402.
34. Getzoff ED, Tainer JA, Lerner RA, Geysen HM. The chemistry and mechanisms of antibody binding to protein antigens. *Adv Immunol* 1988;43:1–98.
35. Sela M. Antigenicity: some molecular aspects. *Science* 1969;166:1365–1374.
36. Berzofsky JA, Buckenmeyer GK, Hicks G, Gurd FRN, Feldmann RJ, Minna J. Topographic antigenic determinants recognized by monoclonal antibodies to sperm whale myoglobin. *J Biol Chem* 1982;257:3189–3198.
37. Koketsu J, Atassi MZ. Immunochemistry of sperm-whale myoglobin-XVI: accurate delineation of the single region in sequence 1-55 by immunochemical studies of synthetic peptides. Some conclusions concerning antigenic structures of proteins. *Immunochemistry* 1974;11:1–8.
38. Dickerson RE. X-ray analysis and protein structure. In: Neurath H, ed. *The proteins,* 2nd ed. New York: Academic Press, 1964:603–778.
39. Takano T. Structure of myoglobin refined at 2.0 Å resolution. I. Crystallographic refinement of metmyoglobin from sperm whale. *J Mol Biol* 1977;110:537–568.
40. Feldmann RJ, Bing DH, Furie BC, Furie B. Interactive computer surface graphics approach to the study of the active site of bovine trypsin. *Proc Natl Acad Sci U S A* 1978;75:5409–5412.
41. Barlow DJ, Edwards MS, Thornton JM. Continuous and discontinuous protein antigenic determinants. *Nature* 1986;322:747–748.
42. Benjamin DC, Berzofsky JA, East IJ, et al. The antigenic structure of proteins: a reappraisal. *Annu Rev Immunol* 1984;2:67–101.
43. Berzofsky JA. Intrinsic and extrinsic factors in protein antigenic structure. *Science* 1985;229:932–940.
44. Sachs DH, Schechter AN, Eastlake A, Anfinsen CB. An immunological approach to the conformational equilibria of polypeptides. *Proc Natl Acad Sci U S A* 1972;69:3790–3794.
45. Crumpton MJ. Protein antigen: the molecular bases of antigenicity and immunogenicity. In: Sela M, ed. *The antigens.* New York: Academic Press, 1974:1–79.
46. Merrifield RB. Automated synthesis of peptides. *Science* 1965;150:178–185.
47. Houghten RA. General method for the rapid solid–phase synthesis of large numbers of peptides: specificity of antigen–antibody interaction at the level of individual amino acids. *Proc Natl Acad Sci U S A* 1985;82:5131–5135.
48. Geysen HM, Rodda SJ, Mason TJ, Tribbick G, Schoofs PG. Strategies for epitope analysis using peptide synthesis. *J Immunol Methods* 1987;102:259–274.
49. Shi P-T, Riehm JP, Todd PEE, Leach SJ. The antigenicity of myoglobin-related peptides synthesised on polyacrylamide and polystyrene resin supports. *Mol Immunol* 1984;21:489–496.
50. Burnens A, Demotz S, Corradin G, Binz H, Bosshard HR. Epitope mapping by chemical modification of free and antibody-bound protein antigen. *Science* 1987;235:780–783.
51. Jemmerson R, Paterson Y. Mapping epitopes on a protein antigen by the proteolysis of antigen–antibody complexes. *Science* 1986;232:1001–1004.
52. Smith-Gill SJ, Wilson AC, Potter M, Prager EM, Feldmann RJ, Mainhart CR. Mapping the antigenic epitope for a monoclonal antibody against lysozyme. *J Immunol* 1982;128:314–322.
53. Kohno Y, Berkower I, Minna J, Berzofsky JA. Idiotypes of anti-myoglobin antibodies: shared idiotypes among monoclonal antibodies to distinct determinants of sperm whale myoglobin. *J Immunol* 1982;128:1742–1748.
54. Streicher HZ, Cuttitta F, Buckenmeyer GK, Kawamura H, Minna J, Berzofsky JA. Mapping the idiotopes of a monoclonal anti-idiotypic antibodies: detection of a common idiotope. *J Immunol* 1986;136:1007–1014.
55. Crumpton MJ, Wilkinson JM. The immunological activity of some of the chymotryptic peptides of sperm-whale myoglobin. *Biochem J* 1965;94:545–556.
56. Smith JA, Hurrell JGR, Leach SJ. A novel method for delineating antigenic determinants: peptide synthesis and radioimmunoassay using the same solid support. *Immunochemistry* 1977;14:565–568.
57. Atassi MZ. Antigenic structure of myoglobin: the complete immunochemical anatomy of a protein and conclusions relating to antigenic structures of proteins. *Immunochemistry* 1975;12:423–438.
58. Berzofsky JA, Buckenmeyer GK, Hicks G, et al. Topographic antigenic determinants detected by monoclonal antibodies to myoglobin. In: Celada F, Sercarz E, Shumaker V, eds. *Protein conformation as immunological signal.* New York: Plenum Press, 1983:165–180.
59. Hurrell JGR, Smith JA, Todd PE, Leach SJ. Cross-reactivity between mam-

malian myoglobins: linear vs. spatial antigenic determinants. *Immunochemistry* 1977;14:283–288.

60. East IJ, Todd PE, Leach SJ. On topographic antigenic determinants in myoglobins. *Mol Immunol* 1980;17:519–525.

61. Maron E, Shiozawa C, Arnon R, Sela M. Chemical and immunological characterization of a unique antigenic region in lysozyme. *Biochemistry* 1971;10: 763–771.

62. Berzofsky JA, Hicks G, Fedorko J, Minna J. Properties of monoclonal antibodies specific for determinants of a protein antigen, myoglobin. *J Biol Chem* 1980; 255:11188–11191.

63. East IJ, Hurrell JGR, Todd PE, Leach SJ. Antigenic specificity of monoclonal antibodies to human myoglobin. *J Biol Chem* 1982;257:3199–3202.

64. Arquilla ER, Bromer WW, Mercola D. Immunology conformation and biological activity of insulin. *Diabetes* 1969;18:193–205.

65. Lau HKF, Reichlin M, Noble RW. Preparation of antibodies that bind to HbF but not to the isolated α and γ subunits. *Fed Proc* 1975;34:975.

66. Benjamini E, Shimizu M, Yound JD, Leung CY. Immunochemical studies on the tobacco mosaic virus protein. VII. The binding of octanoylated peptides of the tobacco mosaic virus protein with antibodies to the whole protein. *Biochemistry* 1968;7:1261–1264.

67. Urbanski GJ, Margoliash E. Topographic determinants on cytochrome c. I. The complete antigenic structures of rabbit, mouse, and guanaco cytochromes c in rabbits and mice. *J Immunol* 1977;118:1170–1180.

68. Lando G, Berzofsky JA, Reichlin M. Antigenic structure of sperm whale myoglobin. I. Partition of specificities between antibodies reactive with peptides and native protein. *J Immunol* 1982;129:206–211.

69. White TJ, Ibrahimi IM, Wilson AC. Evolutionary substitutions and the antigenic structure of globular proteins. *Nature* 1978;274:92–94.

70. Kabat EA. The structural basis of antibody complementarity. *Adv Protein Chem* 1978;32:1–76.

71. Thornton JM, Edwards MS, Taylor WR, Barlow DJ. Location of "continuous" antigenic determinants in protruding regions of proteins. *EMBO J* 1986;5:409–413.

72. Reichlin M. Amino acid substitution and the antigenicity of globular proteins. *Adv Immunol* 1975;20:71–123.

73. Berzofsky JA, Schechter AN. The concepts of crossreactivity and specificity in immunology. *Mol Immunol* 1981;18:751–763.

74. Furie B, Schechter AN, Sachs DH, Anfinsen CB. An immunological approach to the conformational equilibria of staphylococcal nuclease. *J Mol Biol* 1975;92: 497–506.

75. Green N, Alexander H, Wilson A, et al. Immunogenic structure of the influenza virus hemagglutinin. *Cell* 1982;28:477–487.

76. Lerner R. Antibodies of predetermined specificity in biology and medicine. *Adv Immunol* 1984;36:1–44.

77. Perutz MF. Hemoglobin structure and respiratory transport. *Sci Am* 1978;239: 92–125.

78. Monod J, Wyman J, Changeux J-P. On the nature of allosteric transitions: a plausible model. *J Mol Biol* 1965;12:88–118.

79. Papkoff J, Lai MH-T, Hunter T, Verma IM. Analysis of transforming gene products from Moloney murine sarcoma virus. *Cell* 1981;27:109–119.

80. Colman PM, Varghese JN, Laver WG. Structure of the catalytic and antigenic sites in influenza virus neuraminidase. *Nature* 1983;303:41–44.

81. Lee B, Richards FM. The interpretation of protein structures: estimation of static accessibility. *J Mol Biol* 1971;55:379–400.

82. Connolly ML. Solvent-accessible surfaces of proteins and nucleic acids. *Science* 1983;221:709–713.

83. Novotny J, Handschumacher M, Haber E, et al. Antigenic determinants in proteins coincide with surface regions accessible to large probes (antibody domains). *Proc Natl Acad Sci U S A* 1986;83:226–230.

84. Hopp TP, Woods KR. Prediction of protein antigenic determinants from amino acid sequences. *Proc Natl Acad Sci U S A* 1981;78:3824–3828.

85. Fraga S. Theoretical prediction of protein antigenic determinants from amino acid sequences. *Can J Chem* 1982;60:2606–2610.

86. Hopp TP. Protein surface analysis: methods for identifying antigenic determinants and other interaction sites. *J Immunol Methods* 1986;88:1–18.

87. Leach SJ. How antigenic are antigenic peptides? *Biopolymers* 1983;22:425–440.

88. Todd PEE, East IJ, Leach SJ. The immunogenicity and antigenicity of proteins. *Trends Biochem Sci* 1982;7:212–216.

89. Chothia C, Janin J. Principles of protein–protein recognition. *Nature* 1975;256: 705–708.

90. Tainer JA, Getzoff ED, Paterson Y, Olson AJ, Lerner RA. The atomic mobility component of protein antigenicity. *Annu Rev Immunol* 1985;3:501–535.

91. Tainer JA, Getzoff ED, Alexander H, et al. The reactivity of anti-peptide antibodies is a function of the atomic mobility of sites in a protein. *Nature* 1984;312: 127–133.

92. Westhof E, Altschuh D, Moras D, et al. Correlation between segmental mobility and the location of antigenic determinants in proteins. *Nature* 1984;311:123–126.

93. Al Moudallal Z, Briand JP, Van Regenmortel MHV. A major part of the polypeptide chain of tobacco mosaic virus protein is antigenic. *EMBO J* 1985;4: 1231–1235.

94. Van Regenmortel MHV. Antigenic cross-reactivity between proteins and peptides: new insights and applications. *Trends Biochem Sci* 1987;12:237–240.

95. Geysen HM, Tainer JA, Rodda SJ, et al. Chemistry of antibody binding to a protein. *Science* 1987;235:1184–1190.

96. Edmundson AB, Ely KR, Herron JN. A search for site-filling ligands in the Meg Bence-Jones dimer: crystal binding studies of fluorescent compounds. *Mol Immunol* 1984;21:561–576.

97. Getzoff ED, Geysen HM, Rodda SJ, Alexander H, Tainer JA, Lerner RA. Mechanisms of antibody binding to a protein. *Science* 1987;235:1191–1196.

98. Gahm S-J, Fowlkes BJ, Jameson SC, et al. Profound alteration in an αβ T-cell antigen receptor repertoire due to polymorphism in the first complementarity-determining region of the β chain. *Proc Natl Acad Sci USA* 1991;88: 10267–10271.

99. Jemmerson R, Margoliash E. Topographic antigenic determinants on cytochrome c. Immunoadsorbent separation of rabbit antibody populations directed against horse cytochrome c. *J Biol Chem* 1979;254:12706–12716.

100. Cooper HM, East IJ, Todd PEE, Leach SJ. Antibody response to myoglobins: effect of host species. *Mol Immunol* 1984;21:479–487.

101. Berzofsky JA. Ir genes: antigen-specific genetic regulation of the immune response. In: Sela M, ed. *The antigens*. New York: Academic Press, 1987:1–146.

102. Manca F, Kunkl A, Fenoglio D, Fowler A, Sercarz E, Celada F. Constraints in T-B cooperation related to epitope topology on *E. coli* β-galactosidase. I. The fine specificity of T cells dictates the fine specificity of antibodies directed to conformation-dependent determinants. *Eur J Immunol* 1985;15:345–350.

103. Ozaki S, Berzofsky JA. Antibody conjugates mimic specific B cell presentation of antigen: relationship between T and B cell specificity. *J Immunol* 1987;138: 4133–4142.

104. Berzofsky JA. T-B reciprocity: an Ia-restricted epitope-specific circuit regulating T cell- B cell interaction and antibody specificity. *Surv Immunol Res* 1983;2: 223–229.

105. Nussenzweig RS, Nussenzweig V. Development of sporozoite vaccines. *Philos Trans R Soc Lond [Biol]* 1984;307:117.

106. Potocnjak P, Yoshida N, Nussenzweig RS, Nussenzweig V. Monovalent fragments (Fab) of monoclonal antibodies to a sporozoite surface antigen (Pb44) protect mice against malarial infection. *J Exp Med* 1980;151:1504.

107. Good MF, Berzofsky JA, Maloy WL, et al. Genetic control of the immune response in mice to a *Plasmodium falciparum* sporozoite vaccine: widespread non-responsiveness to a single malaria T epitope in highly repetitive vaccine. *J Exp Med* 1986;164:655–660.

108. Del Giudice G, Cooper JA, Merino J, et al. The antibody response in mice to carrier-free synthetic polymers of *Plasmodium falciparum* circumsporozoite repetitive epitope is I-A^b-restricted: possible implications for malaria vaccines. *J Immunol* 1986;137:2952–2955.

109. Herrington DA, Clyde DF, Losonsky G, et al. Safety and immunogenicity in man of a synthetic peptide malaria vaccine against *Plasmodium falciparum* sporozoites. *Nature* 1987;328:257–259.

110. Good MF, Maloy WL, Lunde MN, et al. Construction of a synthetic immunogen: use of a new T-helper epitope on malaria circumsporozoite protein. *Science* 1987;235:1059–1062.

111. Kawamura H, Rosenberg SA, Berzofsky JA. Immunization with antigen and interleukin-2 in vivo overcomes Ir genetic low responsiveness. *J Exp Med* 1985; 162:381–386.

112. Good MF, Pombo D, Lunde MN, et al. Recombinant human interleukin-2 (IL-2) overcomes genetic nonresponsiveness to malaria sporozoite peptides. Correlation of effect with biological activity of IL-2. *J Immunol* 1988;141:972–977.

113. Le Bouvier GL. The D → C change in poliovirus particles. *Br J Exp Pathol* 1959;40:605–620.

114. Gerhard W, Yewdell JW, Frankel ME, Webster RG. Antigenic structure of influenza virus hemagglutinin defined by hybridoma antibodies. *Nature* 1981; 290:713–717.

115. Emini EA, Kao S-Y, Lewis AJ, Crainic R, Wimmer E. Functional basis of poliovirus neutralization determined with mono-specific neutralizing antibodies. *J Virol* 1983;46:466–474.

116. Wiley DC, Wilson EA, Skehel JJ. Structural identification of the antibody-binding sites of Hong Kong influenza haemagglutinin and their involvement in antigenic variation. *Nature* 1981;289:373–378.

117. Icenogle J, Shiwen H, Duke G, Gilbert S, Rueckert R, Anderegg J. Neutralization of poliovirus by a monoclonal antibody: kinetics and stoichiometry. *Virology* 1983;127:412–425.

118. Mandel B. Interaction of viruses with neutralizing antibodies. In: Fraenkel-Conrat H, Wagner RR, eds. *Comprehensive virology 15: viral–host interactions*. New York: Plenum Press, 1979.

119. Kaplan G, Freistadt MS, Racaniello VR. Neutralization of poliovirus by cell receptors expressed in insect cells. *J Virol* 1990;64:4697–4702.

120. Smith DH, Byrn RA, Marsters SA, Gregory T, Groopman JE, Capon DJ. Blocking of HIV-1 infectivity by a soluble, secreted form of the CD4 antigen. *Science* 1987;238:1704–1707.

121. Fisher RA, Bertonis JM, Meier W, et al. HIV infection is blocked in vitro by recombinant soluble CD4. *Nature* 1988;331:76–78.

122. Hussey RE, Richardson NE, Kowalski M, et al. A soluble CD4 protein selectively inhibits HIV replication and syncytium formation. *Nature* 1988;331: 78–81.

123. Capon DJ, Chamow SM, Mordenti J, et al. Designing CD4 immunoadhesins for AIDS therapy. *Nature* 1989;337:525–531.

124. Palker TJ, Clark ME, Langlois AJ, et al. Type-specific neutralization of the human immunodeficiency virus with antibodies to env-encoded synthetic peptides. *Proc Natl Acad Sci U S A* 1988;85:1932–1936.

125. Rusche JR, Javaherian K, McDanal C, et al. Antibodies that inhibit fusion of HIV infected cells bind a 24 amino acid sequence of the viral envelope, gp120. *Proc Natl Acad Sci U S A* 1988;85:3198–3202.

126. Goudsmit J, Debouck C, Meloen RH, et al. Human immunodeficiency virus type 1 neutralization epitope with conserved architecture elicits early type-specific antibodies in experimentally infected chimpanzees. *Proc Natl Acad Sci U S A* 1988;85:4478–4482.

127. Kang C-Y, Nara P, Chamat S, et al. Evidence for non–V3-specific neutralizing antibodies that interfere with gp120/CD4 binding in human immunodeficiency virus 1–infected humans. *Proc Natl Acad Sci U S A* 1991;88:6171–6175.

128. Berkower I, Murphy D, Smith CC, Smith GE. A predominant group-specific neutralizing epitope of human immunodeficiency virus type 1 maps to residues 342 to 511 of the envelope glycoprotein gp120. *J Virol* 1991;65:5983–5990.

129. Thali M, Olshevsky U, Furman C, Gabuzda D, Posner M, Sodroski J. Character-ization of a discontinuous human immunodeficiency virus type 1 gp120 epitope recognized by a broadly reactive neutralizing human monoclonal antibody. *J Virol* 1991;65:6188–6193.

130. Berkower I, Smith GE, Giri C, Murphy D. Human immunodeficiency virus-1: predominance of a group-specific neutralizing epitope that persists despite genetic variation. *J Exp Med* 1989;170:1681–1695.

131. Steimer KS, Scandella CJ, Skiles PV, Haigwood NL. Neutralization of divergent HIV-1 isolates by conformation-dependent human antibodies to Gp120. *Science* 1991;254:105–108.

132. Benacerraf B, McDevitt HO. Histocompatibility-linked immune response genes. *Science* 1972;175:273–279.

133. Godfrey WL, Lewis GK, Goodman JW. The anatomy of an antigen molecule: functional subregions of L-tyrosine-p-azobenzenearsonate. *Mol Immunol* 1984; 21:969–978.

134. Solinger AM, Ultee ME, Margoliash E, Schwartz RH. The T-lymphocyte response to cytochrome c. I. Demonstration of a T-cell heteroclitic proliferative response and identification of a topographic antigenic determinant on pigeon cytochrome c whose immune recognition requires two complementing major histocompatibility complex–linked immune response genes. *J Exp Med* 1979; 150:830–848.

135. Berkower I, Buckenmeyer GK, Gurd FRN, Berzofsky JA. A possible immun-odominant epitope recognized by murine T lymphocytes immune to different myoglobins. *Proc Natl Acad Sci U S A* 1982;79:4723–4727.

136. Katz ME, Maizels RM, Wicker L, Miller A, Sercarz EE. Immunological focus-ing by the mouse major histocompatibility complex: mouse strains confronted with distantly related lysozymes confine their attention to very few epitopes. *Eur J Immunol* 1982;12:535–540.

137. Gell PGH, Benacerraf B. Studies on hypersensitivity II Delayed hypersensitivity to denatured proteins in guinea pigs. *Immunology* 1959;2:64–70.

138. Berzofsky JA. The nature and role of antigen processing in T cell activation. In: Cruse JM, Lewis RE Jr, eds. *The Year in Immunology 1984–1985.* Basel: Karger, 1985:18–24.

139. Livingstone A, Fathman CG. The structure of T cell epitopes. *Annu Rev Immunol* 1987;5:477–501.

140. Schwartz RH. T-lymphocyte recognition of antigen in association with gene products of the major histocompatibility complex. *Annu Rev Immunol* 1985;3: 237–261.

141. Berzofsky JA, Cease KB, Cornette JL, et al. Protein antigenic structures recog-nized by T cells: potential applications to vaccine design. *Immunol Rev* 1987;98: 9–52.

142. Berzofsky JA, Richman LK, Killion DJ. Distinct H-2–linked Ir genes control both antibody and T cell responses to different determinants on the same anti-gen, myoglobin. *Proc Natl Acad Sci U S A* 1979;76:4046–4050.

143. Manca F, Clarke JA, Miller A, Sercarz EE, Shastri N. A limited region within hen egg-white lysozyme serves as the focus for a diversity of T cell clones. *J Immunol* 1984;133:2075–2078.

144. Shimonkevitz R, Colon S, Kappler JW, Marrack P, Grey H. Antigen recognition by H-2–restricted T cells. II. A tryptic ovalbumin peptide that substitutes for processed antigen. *J Immunol* 1984;133:2067–2074.

145. Allen PM, Unanue ER. Differential requirements for antigen processing by macrophages for lysozyme-specific T cell hybridomas. *J Immunol* 1984;132: 1077–1079.

146. Berkower I, Buckenmeyer GK, Berzofsky JA. Molecular mapping of a histo-compatibility-restricted immunodominant T cell epitope with synthetic and natural peptides: implications for antigenic structure. *J Immunol* 1986;136: 2498–2503.

147. Kurokohchi K, Akatsuka T, Pendleton CD, et al. Use of recombinant protein to identify a motif-negative human CTL epitope presented by HLA-A2 in the hepatitis C virus NS3 region. *J Virol* 1996;70:232–240.

148. Thomas JW, Danho W, Bullesbach E, Fohles J, Rosenthal AS. Immune response gene control of determinant selection. III. Polypeptide fragments of insulin are differentially recognized by T but not by B cells in insulin immune guinea pigs. *J Immunol* 1981;126:1095–1100.

149. Schwartz RH, Fox BS, Fraga E, Chen C, Singh B. The T lymphocyte response to cytochrome c. V. Determination of the minimal peptide size required for stimu-lation of T cell clones and assessment of the contribution of each residue beyond this size to antigenic potency. *J Immunol* 1985;135:2598–2608.

150. Cease KB, Berkower I, York-Jolley J, Berzofsky JA. T cell clones specific for an amphipathic alpha helical region of sperm whale myoglobin show differing fine

151. Kurata A, Palker TJ, Streilein RD, Scearce RM, Haynes BF, Berzofsky JA. Immunodominant sites of human T-cell lymphotropic virus type 1 envelope pro-tein for murine helper T cells. *J Immunol* 1989;143:2024–2030.

152. Lamb JR, Ivanyi J, Rees ADM, et al. Mapping of T cell epitopes using recombi-nant antigens and synthetic peptides. *EMBO J* 1987;6:1245–1249.

153. Townsend ARM, Gotch FM, Davey J. Cytotoxic T cells recognize fragments of the influenza nucleoprotein. *Cell* 1985;42:457–467.

154. Walker BD, Flexner C, Birch-Limberger K, et al. Long-term culture and fine specificity of human cytotoxic T lymphocyte clones reactive with human immunodeficiency virus type 1. *Proc Natl Acad Sci U S A* 1989;86:9514–9518.

155. Hosmalin A, Clerici M, Houghten R, et al. An epitope in HIV-1 reverse tran-scriptase recognized by both mouse and human CTL. *Proc Natl Acad Sci U S A* 1990;87:2344–2348.

156. Kojima M, Cease KB, Buckenmeyer GK, Berzofsky JA. Limiting dilution com-parison of the repertoires of high and low responder MHC-restricted T cells. *J Exp Med* 1988;167:1100–1113.

157. Heber-Katz E, Hansburg D, Schwartz RH. The Ia molecule of the antigen-pre-senting cell plays a critical role in immune response gene regulation of T cell activation. *J Mol Cell Immunol* 1983;1:3–14.

158. Matis LA, Longo DL, Hedrick SM, Hannum C, Margoliash E, Schwartz RH. Clonal analysis of the major histocompatibility complex restriction and the fine specificity of antigen recognition in the T cell proliferative response to cytochrome c. *J Immunol* 1983;130:1527–1535.

159. Hansburg D, Heber-Katz E, Fairwell T, Appella E. Major histocompatibility complex–controlled antigen presenting cell–expressed specificity of T cell anti-gen recognition. *J Exp Med* 1983;158:25–39.

160. England RE, Kullberg MC, Cornette JL, Berzofsky JA. Molecular analysis of a heteroclitic T-cell response to the immunodominant epitope of sperm whale myoglobin: implications for peptide partial agonists. *J Immunol* 1995;155: 4295–4306.

161. Gammon G, Geysen HM, Apple RJ, et al. T cell determinant structure: cores and determinant envelopes in three mouse major histocompatibility complex haplo-types. *J Exp Med* 1991;173:609–617.

162. Kimoto M, Fathman CG. Antigen-reactive T cell clones I transcomplementing hybrid I-A–region gene products function effectively in antigen presentation. *J Exp Med* 1980;152:759–770.

163. Kappler JW, Skidmore B, White J, Marrack P. Antigen-inducible H-2–restricted interleukin-2–producing T cell hybridomas. Lack of independent antigen and H-2 recognition. *J Exp Med* 1981;153:1198–1214.

164. Young DB, Lamb JR. T lymphocytes respond to solid-phase antigen: a novel approach to the molecular analysis of cellular immunity. *Immunology* 1986;59: 167–171.

165. Lamb JR, Young DB. A novel approach to the identification of T-cell epitopes in *Mycobacterium tuberculosis* using human T-lymphocyte clones. *Immunology* 1987;60:1–5.

166. Mustafa AS, Gill HK, Nerland A, et al. Human T-cell clones recognize a major M. Leprae protein antigen expressed in *E. coli. Nature* 1986;319:63–66.

167. De Plaen E, Lurquin C, Van Pel A, et al. Immunogenic (tum−) variants of mouse tumor P815: cloning of the gene of tum− antigen P91A and identification of the tum− mutation. *Proc Natl Acad Sci U S A* 1988;85:2274–2278.

168. Van der Bruggen P, Traversari C, Chomez P, et al. A gene encoding an antigen recognized by cytolytic T lymphocytes on a human melanoma. *Science* 1991; 254:1643–1647.

169. Guilloux Y, Lucas S, Brichard VG, et al. A peptide recognized by human cytolytic T lymphocytes on HLA-A2 melanomas is encoded by an intron sequence of the N-acetylglucosaminyltransferase B gene. *J Exp Med* 1996;183: 1173–1183.

170. Kawakami Y, Eliyahu S, Delgado CH, et al. Cloning of the gene coding for a shared human melanoma antigen recognized by autologous T cells infiltrating into tumor. *Proc Natl Acad Sci U S A* 1994;91:3515–3519.

171. Robbins PF, El-Gamil M, Li YF, et al. A mutated b-catenin gene encodes a melanoma-specific antigen recognized by tumor infiltrating lymphocytes. *J Exp Med* 1996;183:1185–1192.

172. Wang R-F, Parkhurst MR, Kawakami Y, Robbins PF, Rosenberg SA. Utilization of an alternative open reading frame of a normal gene in generating a novel human cancer antigen. *J Exp Med* 1996;183:1131–1140.

173. Berkower I, Kawamura H, Matis LA, Berzofsky JA. T cell clones to two major T cell epitopes of myoglobin: effect of I-A/I-E restriction on epitope dominance. *J Immunol* 1985;135:2628–2634.

174. Berkower I, Matis LA, Buckenmeyer GK, Gurd FRN, Longo DL, Berzofsky JA. Identification of distinct predominant epitopes recognized by myoglobin-spe-cific T cells under control of different Ir genes and characterization of represen-tative T-cell clones. *J Immunol* 1984;132:1370–1378.

175. Shastri N, Oki A, Miller A, Sercarz EE. Distinct recognition phenotypes exist for T cell clones specific for small peptide regions of proteins. Implications for the mechanisms underlying major histocompatibility complex–restricted antigen recognition and clonal deletion models of immune response gene defects. *J Exp Med* 1985;162:332–345.

176. Allen PM, McKean DJ, Beck BN, Sheffield J, Glimcher LH. Direct evidence that a class II molecule and a simple globular protein generate multiple determinants. *J Exp Med* 1985;162:1264–1274.

specificities for synthetic peptides: a multideterminant/single structure interpretation of immunodominance. *J Exp Med* 1986;164:1779–1784.

177. Hackett CJ, Dietzschold B, Gerhard W, et al. Influenza virus site recognized by a murine helper T cell specific for H1 strains. *J Exp Med* 1983;158:294–302.

178. Hurwitz JL, Heber-Katz E, Hackett CJ, Gerhard WJ. Characterization of the murine TH response to influenza virus hemagglutinin: evidence for three major specificities. *J Immunol* 1984;133:3371–3377.

179. Lamb JR, Eckels DD, Lake P, Woody JN, Green N. Human T cell clones recognize chemically synthesized peptides of influenza hemagglutinin. *Nature* 1982; 300:66–69.

180. Rosenthal AS. Determinant selection and macrophage function in genetic control of the immune response. *Immunol Rev* 1978;40:136–152.

181. Milich DR, McLachlan A, Chisari FV, Thornton GB. Nonoverlapping T and B cell determinants on an hepatitis B surface antigen pre-S(2) region synthetic peptide. *J Exp Med* 1986;164:532–547.

182. Francis MJ, Fry CM, Rowlands DJ, et al. Immunological priming with synthetic peptides of foot and mouth disease virus. *J Gen Virol* 1985;66:2347–2352.

183. Corradin GP, Juillerat MA, Vita C, Engers HD. Fine specificity of a BALB/c T cell clone directed against beef apo cytochrome c. *J Mol Immunol* 1983;20: 763–768.

184. Corradin GP, Wallace CJA, Proudfoot AEI, Baumhuter S. Murine T cell response specific for cytochrome c. In: Sercarz EE, Berzofsky JA, eds. *The immunogenicity of protein antigens: repertoire and regulation.* Boca Raton, FL: CRC Press, 1987:43–48.

185. Milich DR, Peterson DL, Leroux-Roels GG, Lerner RA, Chisari FV. Genetic regulation of the immune response to hepatitis B surface antigen (HBsAg). VI. Fine specificity. *J Immunol* 1985;134:4203–4211.

186. Guillet J-G, Lai M-Z, Briner TJ, Smith JA, Gefter ML. Interaction of peptide antigens and class II major histocompatibility complex antigens. *Nature* 1986; 324:260–262.

187. Macfarlan RI, Dietzschold B, Wiktor TJ, et al. T cell responses to cleaved rabies virus glycoprotein and to synthetic peptides. *J Immunol* 1984;133:2748–2752.

188. Margalit H, Spouge JL, Cornette JL, Cease K, DeLisi C, Berzofsky JA. Prediction of immunodominant helper T-cell antigenic sites from the primary sequence. *J Immunol* 1987;138:2213–2229.

189. Townsend ARM, Rothbard J, Gotch FM, Bahadur G, Wraith D, McMichael AJ. The epitopes of influenza nucleoprotein recognized by cytotoxic T lymphocytes can be defined with short synthetic peptides. *Cell* 1986;44:959–968.

190. Townsend ARM, Bastin J, Gould K, Brownlee GG. Cytotoxic T lymphocytes recognize influenza haemagglutinin that lacks a signal sequence. *Nature* 1986; 324:575–577.

191. Berzofsky JA. Structural features of protein antigenic sites recognized by helper T cells: What makes a site immunodominant? In: Cruse JM, Lewis RE Jr, eds. *The year in immunology 1985–1986.* Basel, Switzerland: Karger, 1986:28–38.

192. Berzofsky JA. Immunodominance in T lymphocyte recognition. *Immunol Lett* 1988;18:83–92.

193. Allen PM. Antigen processing at the molecular level. *Immunol Today* 1987;8: 270–273.

194. Goodman JW, Sercarz EE. The complexity of structures involved in T-cell activation. *Annu Rev Immunol* 1983;1:465–498.

195. Finnegan A, Smith MA, Smith JA, Berzofsky JA, Sachs DH, Hodes RJ. The T cell repertoire for recognition of a phylogenetically distant protein antigen: peptide specificity and MHC restriction of staphylococcal nuclease specific T cell clones. *J Exp Med* 1986;164:897–910.

196. Good MF, Pombo D, Quakyi IA, et al. Human T cell recognition of the circumsporozoite protein of *Plasmodium falciparum.* Immunodominant T cell domains map to the polymorphic regions of the molecule. *Proc Natl Acad Sci U S A* 1988; 85:1199–1203.

197. Nanda NK, Arzoo KK, Geysen HM, Sette A, Sercarz EE. Recognition of multiple peptide cores by a single T cell receptor. *J Exp Med* 1995;182:531–539.

198. Brett SJ, Cease KB, Berzofsky JA. Influences of antigen processing on the expression of the T cell repertoire: evidence for MHC specific hindering structures on the products of processing. *J Exp Med* 1988;168:357–373.

199. Gammon G, Shastri N, Cogswell J, et al. The choice of T-cell epitopes utilized on a protein antigen depends on multiple factors distant from as well as at the determinant site. *Immunol Rev* 1987;98:53–73.

200. Sercarz EE, Lehmann PV, Ametani A, Benichou G, Miller A, Moudgil K. Dominance and crypticity of T cell antigenic determinants. *Annu Rev Immunol* 1993; 11:729–766.

201. Unanue ER. Antigen-presenting function of the macrophage. *Annu Rev Immunol* 1984;2:395–428.

202. Pincus M, Gerewitz F, Schwartz RH, Scheraga HA. Correlation between the conformation of cytochrome c peptides and their stimulatory activity in a T-lymphocyte proliferation assay. *Proc Natl Acad Sci USA* 1983;80:3297–3300.

203. DeLisi C, Berzofsky JA. T cell antigenic sites tend to be amphipathic structures. *Proc Natl Acad Sci U S A* 1985;82:7048–7052.

204. Spouge JL, Guy HR, Cornette JL, et al. Strong conformational propensities enhance T-cell antigenicity. *J Immunol* 1987;138:204–212.

205. Carbone FR, Fox BS, Schwartz RH, Paterson Y. The use of hydrophobic a-helix-defined peptides in delineating the T cell determinant for pigeon cytochrome c. *J Immunol* 1987;138:1838–1844.

206. Ziegler HK, Unanue ER. Decrease in macrophage antigen catabolism caused by ammonia and chloroquine is associated with inhibition of antigen presentation to T cells. *Proc Natl Acad Sci U S A* 1982;79:175–178.

207. Shimonkevitz R, Kappler J, Marrack P, Grey H. Antigen recognition by H-2 restricted T cells. I. Cell free antigen processing. *J Exp Med* 1983;158:303–316.

208. Streicher HZ, Berkower IJ, Busch M, Gurd FRN, Berzofsky JA. Antigen conformation determines processing requirements for T-cell activation. *Proc Natl Acad Sci USA* 1984;81:6831–6835.

209. Lee P, Matsueda GR, Allen PM. T cell recognition of fibrinogen. A determinant on the Aa-chain does not require processing. *J Immunol* 1988;140:1063–1068.

210. Régnier-Vigouroux A, Ayeb ME, Defendini M-L, Granier C, Pierres M. Processing by accessory cells for presentation to murine T cells of apamin, a disulfide-bonded 18 amino acid peptide. *J Immunol* 1988;140:1069–1075.

211. Rudensky AY, Preston-Hurlburt P, Hong S-C, Barlow A, Janeway CA Jr. Sequence analysis of peptides bound to MHC class II molecules. *Nature* 1991; 353:622–627.

212. Stern LJ, Brown JH, Jardetzky TS, et al. Crystal structure of the human class II MHC protein HLA-DR1 complexed with an influenza virus peptide. *Nature* 1994;368:215–221.

213. Stern LJ, Wiley DC. Antigenic peptide binding by class I and class II histocompatibility proteins. *Structure* 1994;2:245–251.

214. Townsend ARM, Skehel JJ. The influenza A virus nucleoprotein gene controls the induction of both subtype specific and crossreactive cytotoxic T cells. *J Exp Med* 1984;160:552–563.

215. Braciale TJ, Braciale VL, Winkler M, et al. On the role of the transmembrane anchor sequence of influenza hemagglutinin in target cell recognition by class I MHC-restricted hemagglutinin-specific cytolytic T lymphocytes. *J Exp Med* 1987;166:678–692.

216. Tobery T, Siliciano RF. Targeting of HIV-1 antigens for rapid intracellular degradation enhances cytotoxic T lymphocytes (CTL) recognition and the induction of de novo CTL responses in vivo after immunization. *J Exp Med* 1997;185:909–920.

217. Morrison LA, Lukacher AE, Braciale VL, Fan DP, Braciale TJ. Differences in antigen presentation to MHC class I and class II-restricted influenza virus specific cytolytic T lymphocyte clones. *J Exp Med* 1986;163:903–921.

218. Yewdell JW, Bennink JR, Hosaka Y. Cells process exogenous proteins for recognition by cytotoxic T lymphocytes. *Science* 1988;239:637–640.

219. Nuchtern JG, Biddison WE, Klausner RD. Class II MHC molecules can use the endogenous pathway of antigen presentation. *Nature* 1990;343:74–76.

220. Matlin KS, Reggio H, Helenius A, Simons K. Infectious entry pathway of influenza virus in a canine kidney cell line. *J Cell Biol* 1981;91:601–613.

221. Jin Y, Shih JW-K, Berkower IJ. Human T cell response to HBsAg: endosomal and nonendosomal processing pathways are accessible to both endogenous and exogenous antigen. *J Exp Med* 1988;168:293–306.

222. Moore MW, Carbone FR, Bevan MJ. Introduction of soluble protein into the class I pathway of antigen processing and presentation. *Cell* 1988;54:777–785.

223. Weiss S, Bogen B. B-lymphoma cells process and present their endogenous immunoglobulin to major histocompatibility complex–restricted T cells. *Proc Natl Acad Sci U S A* 1989;86:282–286.

224. Weiss S, Bogen B. MHC class II–restricted presentation of intracellular antigen. *Cell* 1991;64:767–776.

225. Eisenlohr LC, Hackett CJ. Class II major histocompatibility complex–restricted T cells specific for a virion structural protein that do not recognize exogenous influenza virus. Evidence that presentation of labile T cell determinants is favored by endogenous antigen synthesis. *J Exp Med* 1989;169:921–931.

226. Polydefkis M, Koenig S, Flexner C, et al. Anchor sequence–dependent endogenous processing of human immunodeficiency virus 1 envelope glycoprotein gp160 for CD4+ T cell recognition. *J Exp Med* 1990;171:875–887.

227. Jaraquemada D, Marti M, Long EO. An endogenous processing pathway in vaccinia virus infected cells for presentation of cytoplasmic antigens to class II–restricted T cells. *J Exp Med* 1990;172:947–954.

228. Smith GL, Mackett M, Moss B. Infectious vaccinia virus recombinants that express hepatitis B virus surface antigen. *Nature* 1983;302:490–495.

229. Jacobson S, Sekaly RP, Jacobson CL, McFarland HF, Long EO. HLA class II–restricted presentation of cytoplasmic measles virus antigens to cytotoxic T cells. *J Virol* 1989;63:1756–1762.

230. Monaco JJ, McDevitt HO. Identification of a fourth class of proteins linked to the murine major histocompatibility complex. *Proc Natl Acad Sci U S A* 1982; 79:3001–3005.

231. Tanaka K, Ii K, Ichihara A, Waxman L, Goldberg AL. A high molecular weight protease in the cytosol of rat liver. I. Purification, enzymological properties, and tissue distribution. *J Biol Chem* 1986;261:15197–15203.

232. Tanaka K, Yoshimura T, Ichihara A, Kameyama K, Takagi T. A high molecular weight protease in the cytosol of rat liver. II. Properties of the purified enzyme. *J Biol Chem* 1986;261:15204–15207.

233. Arrigo A-P, Tanaka K, Goldberg AL, Welch WJ. Identity of the 19S "prosome" particle with the large multifunctional protease complex of mammalian cells (the proteasome). *Nature* 1992;331:192–194.

234. Vinitsky A, Antón LC, Snyder HL, Orlowski M, Bennink JR, Yewdell JW. The generation of MHC class I–associated peptides is only partially inhibited by proteasome inhibitors. Involvement of nonproteasomal cytosolic proteases in antigen processing? *J Immunol* 1997;159:554–564.

235. Rock KL, Gramm C, Rothstein L, et al. Inhibitors of the proteasome block the degradation of most cell proteins and the generation of peptides presented on MHC class I molecules. *Cell* 1994;78:761–771.

236. Rammensee H-G, Friede T, Stevanovic S. MHC ligands and peptide motifs: first listing. *Immunogenetics* 1995;41:178–228.

237. Brown MG, Driscoll J, Monaco JJ. Structural and serological similarity of MHC-linked LMP and proteasome (multicatalytic proteinase) complexes. *Nature* 1991; 353:355–357.

238. Vinitsky A, Cardozo C, Sepp-Lorenzino L, Michaud C, Orlowski M. Inhibition of the proteolytic activity of the multicatalytic proteinase complex (proteasome) by substrate-related peptidyl aldehydes. *J Biol Chem* 1994;269:29860–29866.

239. Fenteany G, Standaert RF, Lane WS, Choi S, Corey EJ, Schreiber SL. Inhibition of proteasome activities and subunit-specific amino-terminal threonine modification by lactacystin. *Science* 1995;268:726–731.

240. Hughes EA, Ortmann B, Surman M, Cresswell P. The protease inhibitor, N-Acetyl-L-Leucyl-L-Leucyl-L-Norleucinal, decreases the pool of major histocompatibility complex class I–binding peptides and inhibits peptide trimming in the endoplasmic reticulum. *J Exp Med* 1996;183:1569–1578.

241. Henderson RA, Michel H, Sakaguchi K, et al. HLA-A2.1–associated peptides from a mutant cell line: a second pathway of antigen presentation. *Science* 1992; 255:1264–1266.

242. Gaczynska M, Rock KL, Goldberg AL. γ-Interferon and expression of MHC genes regulate peptide hydrolysis by proteasomes. *Nature* 1993;365:264–267.

243. Van Kaer L, Ashton-Rickardt PG, Eichelberger M, et al. Altered peptidase and viral-specific T cell response in LMP2 mutant mice. *Immunity* 1994;1: 533–541.

244. Fehling HJ, Swat W, Laplace C, et al. MHC class I expression in mice lacking the proteasome subunit LMP-7. *Science* 1994;265:1234–1237.

245. Dubiel W, Pratt G, Ferrell K, Rechsteiner M. Purification of an 11 S regulator of the multicatalytic protease. *J Biol Chem* 1992;267:22369–22377.

246. Dick TP, Ruppert T, Groettrup M, et al. Coordinated dual cleavages induced by the proteasome regulator PA28 lead to dominant MHC ligands. *Cell* 1996;86: 253–262.

247. Goldberg AL, Rock KL. Proteolysis, proteasomes and antigen presentation. *Nature* 1992;357:375–379.

248. Shastri N, Gammon G, Horvath S, Miller A, Sercarz EE. The choice between two distinct T cell determinants within a 23 amino acid region of lysozyme depends upon structure of the immunogen. *J Immunol* 1986;137:911–915.

249. Shastri N, Miller A, Sercarz EE. Amino acid residues distinct from the determinant region can profoundly affect activation of T cell clones by related antigens. *J Immunol* 1986;136:371–376.

250. Grewal IS, Moudgil KD, Sercarz EE. Hindrance of binding to class II major histocompatibility complex molecules by a single amino acid residue contiguous to a determinant leads to crypticity of the determinant as well as lack of response to the protein antigen. *Proc Natl Acad Sci U S A* 1995;92:1779–1783.

251. Fox BS, Carbone FR, Germain RN, Paterson Y, Schwartz RH. Processing of a minimal antigenic peptide alters its interaction with MHC molecules. *Nature* 1988;331:538–540.

252. Sercarz E, Wilbur S, Sadegh-Nasseri S, et al. The molecular context of a determinant influences its dominant expression in a T cell response hierarchy through "fine processing." In: Cinader B, Miller RG, eds. *Progress in immunology VI.* New York: Academic Press, 1986:227–237.

253. Kärre K, Ljunggren H-G, Piontek G, Kiessling R. Selective rejection of H-2–deficient lymphoma variants suggests alternative immune defence strategy. *Nature* 1986;319:675–678.

254. DeMars R, Rudersdorf R, Chang C, et al. Mutations that impair a posttranscriptional step in expression of HLA-A and -B antigens. *Proc Natl Acad Sci U S A* 1985;82:8183–8187.

255. Townsend A, Öhlén C, Bastin J, Ljunggren H-G, Foster L, Kärre K. Association of class I major histocompatibility heavy and light chains induced by viral peptides. *Nature* 1989;340:443–448.

256. Monaco JJ, Cho S, Attaya M. Transport protein genes in the murine MHC: possible implications for antigen processing. *Science* 1990;250:1723–1726.

257. Deverson EV, Gow IR, Coadwell WJ, Monaco JJ, Butcher GW, Howard JC. MHC class II region encoding proteins related to the multidrug resistance family of transmembrane transporters. *Nature* 1990;348:738–741.

258. Trowsdale J, Hanson I, Mockridge I, Beck S, Townsend A, Kelly A. Sequences encoded in the class II region of the MHC related to the "ABC" superfamily of transporters. *Nature* 1990;348:741–743.

259. Schumacher TNM, Heemels M-T, Neefjes JJ, Kast WM, Melief CJM, Ploegh HL. Direct binding of peptide to empty MHC class I molecules on intact cells and in vitro. *Cell* 1990;62:563–567.

260. Attaya M, Jameson S, Martinez CK, et al. Ham-2 corrects the class I antigen-processing defect in RMA-S cells. *Nature* 1992;355:647–649.

261. Spies T, Cerundolo V, Colonna M, Cresswell P, Townsend A, DeMars R. Presentation of viral antigen by MHC class I molecules is dependent on a putative peptide transporter heterodimer. *Nature* 1992;355:644–646.

262. Kelly A, Powis SH, Kerr L-A, et al. Assembly and function of the two ABC transporter proteins encoded in the human major histocompatibility complex. *Nature* 1992;355:641–644.

263. Ortmann B, Androlewicz MJ, Cresswell P. MHC class I/β2-microglobulin complexes associate with TAP transporters before peptide binding. *Nature* 1994;368: 864–867.

264. Suh W-K, Cohen-Doyle MF, Fruh K, Wang K, Peterson PA, Williams DB. Interaction of MHC class I molecules with the transporter associated with antigen processing. *Science* 1994;264:1322–1326.

265. Livingstone AM, Powis SJ, Diamond AG, Butcher GW, Howard JC. A trans-acting major histocompatibility complex–linked gene whose alleles determine gain

266. and loss changes in the antigenic structure of a classical class I molecule. *J Exp Med* 1989;170:777–795.

266. Livingstone AM, Powis SJ, Günther E, Cramer DV, Howard JC, Butcher GW. Cim: an MHC class II–linked allelism affecting the antigenicity of a classical class I molecule for T lymphocytes. *Immunogenetics* 1991;34:157–163.

267. Powis SJ, Deverson EV, Coadwell WJ, et al. Effect of polymorphism of an MHC-linked transporter on the peptides assembled in a class I molecule. *Nature* 1992; 357:211–215.

268. Powis SJ, Young LL, Joly E, et al. The rat cim effect: TAP allele–dependent changes in a class I MHC anchor motif and evidence against C-terminal trimming of peptides in the ER. *Immunity* 1996;4:159–165.

269. Neefjes JJ, Momburg F, Hämmerling GJ. Selective and ATP-dependent translocation of peptides by the MHC-encoded transporter. *Science* 1993;261: 769–771.

270. Neefjes J, Gottfried E, Roelse J, et al. Analysis of the fine specificity of rat, mouse and human TAP peptide transporters. *Eur J Immunol* 1995;25: 1133–1136.

271. Androlewicz MJ, Cresswell P. Human transporters associated with antigen processing possess a promiscuous peptide-binding site. *Immunity* 1994;1:7–14.

272. Schumacher TNM, Kantesaria DV, Heemels M-T, et al. Peptide length and sequence specificity of the mouse TAP1/TAP2 translocator. *J Exp Med* 1994; 179:533–540.

273. van Endert PM, Riganelli D, Greco G, et al. The peptide-binding motif for the human transporter associated with antigen processing. *J Exp Med* 1995;182: 1883–1895.

274. van Endert PM. Peptide selection for presentation by HLA class I: a role for the human transporter associated with antigen processing? *Immunol Res* 1996; 15:265–279.

275. Del Val M, Hengel H, Häcker H, et al. Cytomegalovirus prevents antigen presentation by blocking the transport of peptide-loaded major histocompatibility complex class I molecules into the medial-Golgi compartment. *J Exp Med* 1992; 176:729–738.

276. Beersma MFC, Bijlmakers MJE, Ploegh HL. Human cytomegalovirus downregulates HLA class I expression by reducing the stability of class I H chains. *J Immunol* 1993;151:4455–4464.

277. York IA, Roop C, Andrews DW, Riddell SR, Graham FL, Johnson DC. A cytosolic herpes simplex virus protein inhibits antigen presentation to CD8+ T lymphocytes. *Cell* 1994;77:525–535.

278. Früh K, Ahn K, Djaballah H, et al. A viral inhibitor of peptide transporters for antigen presentation. *Nature* 1995;375:415–418.

279. Hill A, Jugovic P, York I, et al. Herpes simplex virus turns off the TAP to evade host immunity. *Nature* 1995;375:411–415.

280. Müllbacher A, Lobigs M. Up-regulation of MHC class I by flavivirus-induced peptide translocation into the endoplasmic reticulum. *Immunity* 1995;3:207–214.

281. Stockinger B, Pessara U, Lin RH, Habicht J, Grez M, Koch N. A role for Ia-associated invariant chains in antigen processing and presentation. *Cell* 1989;56: 683–689.

282. Brodsky FM, Guagliardi LE. The cell biology of antigen processing and presentation. *Annu Rev Immunol* 1991;9:707–744.

283. Germain RN, Margulies DH. The biochemistry and cell biology of antigen processing and presentation. *Annu Rev Immunol* 1993;11:403–450.

284. Elliot WL, Stille CJ, Thomas LJ, Humphreys RE. An hypothesis on the binding of an amphipathic, a helical sequence in Ii to the desetope of class II antigens. *J Immunol* 1987;138:2949–2952.

285. Roche PA, Cresswell P. Invariant chain association with HLA-DR molecules inhibits immunogenic peptide binding. *Nature* 1990;345:615–618.

286. Teyton L, O'Sullivan D, Dickson PW, et al. Invariant chain distinguishes betweeen the exogenous and endogenous antigen presentation pathways. *Nature* 1990;348:39–44.

287. Roche PA, Cresswell P. Proteolysis of the class II–associated invariant chain generates a peptide binding site in intracellular HLA-DR molecules. *Proc Natl Acad Sci U S A* 1991;88:3150–3154.

288. Bodmer H, Viville S, Benoist C, Mathis D. Diversity of endogenous epitopes bound to MHC class II molecules limited by invariant chain. *Science* 1994;263: 1284–1286.

289. Long EO, LaVaute T, Pinet V, Jaraquemada D. Invariant chain prevents the HLA-DR–restricted presentation of a cytosolic peptide. *J Immunol* 1994;153: 1487–1494.

290. Roche PA, Marks MS, Cresswell P. Formation of a nine-subunit complex by HLA class II glycoproteins and the invariant chain. *Nature* 1991;354:392–394.

291. Fling SP, Arp B, Pious D. HLA-DMA and DMB genes are both required for MHC class II/peptide complex formation in antigen-presenting cells. *Nature* 1994;368:554–558.

292. Sadegh-Nasseri S, Stern LJ, Wiley DC, Germain RN. MHC class II function preserved by low-affinity peptide interactions preceding stable binding. *Nature* 1994;370:647–650.

293. Mellins E, Kempin S, Smith L, Monji T, Pious D. A gene required for class II–restricted antigen presentation maps to the major histocompatibility complex. *J Exp Med* 1991;174:1607–1615.

294. Riberdy JM, Newcomb JR, Surman MJ, Barbosa JA, Cresswell P. HLA-DR molecules from an antigen-processing mutant cell line are associated with invariant chain peptides. *Nature* 1992;360:474–477.

295. Morris P, Shaman J, Attaya M, et al. An essential role for HLA-DM in antigen

presentation by class II major histocompatibility molecules. *Nature* 1994;368: 551–554.

296. Sette A, Ceman S, Kubo RT, et al. Invariant chain of peptides in most HLA-DR molecules of an antigen-processing mutant. *Science* 1992;258: 1801–1804.

297. Denzin LK, Cresswell P. HLA-DM induces CLIP dissociation from MHC class II αβ dimers and facilitates peptide loading. *Cell* 1995;82:155–165.

298. Denzin LK, Robbins NF, Carboy-Newcome C, Cresswell P. Assembly and intracellular transport of HLA-DM and correction of the class II antigen-processing defect in T2 cells. *Immunity* 1994;1:595–606.

299. Sloan VS, Cameron P, Porter G, et al. Mediation by HLA-DM of dissociation of peptides from HLA-DR. *Nature* 1995;375:802–806.

300. Sherman MA, Weber DA, Jensen PE. DM enhances peptide binding to class II MHC by release of invariant chain–derived peptide. *Immunity* 1995;3:197–205.

301. Benacerraf B. A hypothesis to relate the specificity of T lymphocytes and the activity of I region–specific Ir genes in macrophages and B lymphocytes. *J Immunol* 1978;120:1809–1812.

302. Rosenthal AS, Barcinski MA, Blake JT. Determinant selection is a macrophage-dependent immune response gene function. *Nature* 1977;267:156–158.

303. Paul WE, Shevach EM, Pickeral S, Thomas DW, Rosenthal AS. Independent populations of primed F1 guinea pig T-lymphocytes respond to antigen-pulsed parental peritoneal exudate cells. *J Exp Med* 1977;145:618–630.

304. Watts TH, Brian AA, Kappler JW, Marrack P, McConnell HM. Antigen presentation by supported planar membranes containing affinity-purified I-A^d. *Proc Natl Acad Sci U S A* 1984;81:7564–7568.

305. Walden P, Nagy ZA, Klein J. Induction of regulatory T-lymphocyte responses by liposomes carrying major histocompatibility complex molecules and foreign antigen. *Nature* 1985;315:327–329.

306. Norcross MA, Bentley DM, Margulies DH, Germain RN. Membrane Ia expression and antigen-presenting accessory cell function of L cells transfected with class II major histocompatibility genes. *J Exp Med* 1984;160:1316–1337.

307. Demotz S, Grey HM, Sette A. The minimal number of class II MHC–antigen complexes needed for T cell activation. *Science* 1990;249:1028–1030.

308. Harding CV, Unanue ER. Quantitation of antigen-presenting cell MHC class II/peptide complexes necessary for T-cell stimulation. *Nature* 1990;346: 574–576.

309. Christinck ER, Luscher MA, Barber BH, Williams DB. Peptide binding to class I MHC on living cells and quantitation of complexes required for CTL lysis. *Nature* 1991;352:67–70.

310. Cabral GA, Marciano-Cabral F, Funk GA, et al. Cellular and humoral immunity in guinea pigs to two major polypeptides derived from hepatitis B surface antigen. *J Gen Virol* 1978;38:339–350.

311. Takeshita T, Kozlowski S, England RD, et al. Role of conserved regions of class I MHC molecules in the activation of CD8+ CTL by peptide and purified cell-free class I molecules. *Int Immunol* 1993;5:1129–1138.

312. Brower RC, England R, Takeshita T, et al. Minimal requirements for peptide mediated activation of CD8+ CTL. *Mol Immunol* 1994;31:1285–1293.

313. Werdelin O. Chemically related antigens compete for presentation by accessory cells to T cells. *J Immunol* 1982;129:1883–1891.

314. Rock KL, Benacerraf B. Inhibition of antigen-specific T lymphocyte activation by structurally related Ir gene–controlled polymers. Evidence of specific competition for accessory cell antigen presentation. *J Exp Med* 1983;157: 1618–1634.

315. Rock KL, Benacerraf B. Inhibition of antigen-specific T lymphocyte activation by structurally related Ir gene–controlled polymers II: competitive inhibition of I-E. *J Exp Med* 1984;160:1864–1879.

316. Guillet J-G, Lai M-Z, Briner TJ, et al. Immunological self, nonself discrimination. *Science* 1987;235:865–870.

317. Babbitt BP, Allen PM, Matsueda G, Haber E, Unanue ER. The binding of immunogenic peptides to Ia histocompatibility molecules. *Nature* 1985;317: 359–361.

318. Buus S, Sette A, Colon SM, Jenis DM, Grey HM. Isolation and characterization of antigen–Ia complexes involved in T cell recognition. *Cell* 1986;47:1071–1077.

319. Phillips ML, Yip CC, Shevach EM, Delovitch TL. Photoaffinity labeling demonstrates binding between Ia molecules and nominal antigen on antigen-presenting cells. *Proc Natl Acad Sci U S A* 1986;83:5634–5638.

320. Babbitt BP, Matsueda G, Haber E, Unanue ER, Allen PM. Antigenic competition at the level of peptide-Ia binding. *Proc Natl Acad Sci U S A* 1986;83:4509–4513.

321. Buus S, Sette A, Colon SM, Miles C, Grey HM. The relation between major histocompatibility complex (MHC) restriction and the capacity of Ia to bind immunogenic peptides. *Science* 1987;235:1353–1358.

322. Ronchese F, Schwartz RH, Germain RN. Functionally distinct subsites on a class II major histocompatibility complex molecule. *Nature* 1987;329:254–256.

323. Sette A, Buus S, Colon S, Smith JA, Miles C, Grey HM. Structural characteristics of an antigen required for its interaction with Ia and recognition by T cells. *Nature* 1987;328:395–399.

324. Kurata A, Berzofsky JA. Analysis of peptide residues interacting with MHC molecule or T-cell receptor: can a peptide bind in more than one way to the same MHC molecule? *J Immunol* 1990;144:4526–4535.

325. Allen PM, Matsueda GR, Evans RJ, Dunbar JB Jr, Marshall GR, Unanue ER. Identification of the T-cell and Ia contact residues of a T-cell antigenic epitope. *Nature* 1987;327:713–717.

326. Ortmann B, Martin S, von Bonin A, Schiltz E, Hoschützky H, Weltzien HU. Synthetic peptides anchor T cell–specific TNP epitopes to MHC antigens. *J Immunol* 1992;148:1445–1450.

327. Brown JH, Jardetzky T, Saper MA, Samraoui B, Bjorkman PJ, Wiley DC. A hypothetical model of the foreign antigen binding site of Class II histocompatibility molecules. *Nature* 1988;332:845–850.

328. Bjorkman PJ, Saper MA, Samraoui B, Bennett WS, Strominger JL, Wiley DC. Structure of the human class I histocompatibility antigen HLA-A2. *Nature* 1987; 329:506–512.

329. Bjorkman PJ, Saper MA, Samraoui B, Bennett WS, Strominger JL, Wiley DC. The foreign antigen binding site and T cell recognition regions of class I histocompatibility antigens. *Nature* 1987;329:512–518.

330. Madden DR, Gorga JC, Strominger JL, Wiley DC. The structure of HLA-B27 reveals nonamer self-peptides bound in an extended conformation. *Nature* 1991; 353:321–325.

331. Matsumura M, Fremont DH, Peterson PA, Wilson IA. Emerging principles for the recognition of peptide antigens by MHC class I molecules. *Science* 1992; 257:927–934.

332. Fremont DH, Matsumura M, Stura EA, Peterson PA, Wilson IA. Crystal structures of two viral peptides in complex with murine MHC class I H-2K^b. *Science* 1992;257:919–927.

333. Germain RN, Ashwell JD, Lechler RI, et al. "Exon-shuffling" maps control of antibody and T-cell-recognition sites to the NH2 terminal domain of the class II major histocompatibility polypeptide Abeta. *Proc Natl Acad Sci U S A* 1985;82: 2940–2944.

334. Glimcher LH. T cells recognize multiple determinants on a single class II molecule, some of which depend on tertiary conformation. In: Sercarz EE, Berzofsky JA, eds. *Immunogenicity of protein antigens: repertoires and regulation.* Boca Raton, FL: CRC Press, 1987:131–138.

335. Haskins K, Kappler J, Marrack P. The major histocompatibility complex–restricted antigen receptor on T cells. *Annu Rev Immunol* 1984;2:51–66.

336. Meuer SC, Acuto O, Hercend T, Schlossman SF, Reinherz EL. The human T-cell receptor. *Annu Rev Immunol* 1984;2:23–50.

337. Davis MM. Molecular genetics of the T cell-receptor beta chain. *Annu Rev Immunol* 1985;3:537–560.

338. Kronenberg M, Siu G, Hood LE, Shastri N. The molecular genetics of the T-cell antigen receptor and T-cell antigen recognition. *Annu Rev Immunol* 1986;4: 529–591.

339. Vasmatzis G, Cornette J, Sezerman U, DeLisi C. TcR recognition of the MHC–peptide dimer: structural properties of a ternary complex. *J Mol Biol* 1996; 261:72–89.

340. Garcia KC, Degano M, Stanfield RL, et al. An αβ T cell receptor structure at 2.5 Å and its orientation in the TCR–MHC complex. *Science* 1996;274:209–219.

341. Garboczi DN, Ghosh P, Utz U, Fan QR, Biddison WE, Wiley DC. Structure of the complex between human T-cell receptor, viral peptide and HLA-A2. *Nature* 1996;384:134–141.

342. Bhayani H, Paterson Y. Analysis of peptide binding patterns in different major histocompatibility complex/T cell receptor complexes using pigeon cytochrome c-specific T cell hybridomas. Evidence that a single peptide binds major histocompatibility complex in different conformations. *J Exp Med* 1989;170: 1609–1625.

343. Brett SJ, McKean D, York-Jolley J, Berzofsky JA. Antigen presentation to specific T cells by Ia molecules selectively altered by site-directed mutagenesis. *Int Immunol* 1989;1:130–140.

344. McMichael AJ, Gotch FM, Santos-Aguado J, Strominger JL. Effect of mutations and variations of HLA-A2 on recognition of a virus peptide epitope by cytotoxic T lymphocytes. *Proc Natl Acad Sci U S A* 1988;85:9194–9198.

345. Racioppi L, Ronchese F, Schwartz RH, Germain RN. The molecular basis of class II MHC allelic control of T cell responses. *J Immunol* 1991;147: 3718–3727.

346. Boehncke W-H, Takeshita T, Pendleton CD, et al. The importance of dominant negative effects of amino acids side chain substitution in peptide–MHC molecule interactions and T cell recognition. *J Immunol* 1993;150:331–341.

347. Rothbard JB, Busch R, Howland K, et al. Structural analysis of a peptide–HLA class II complex: identification of critical interactions for its formation and recognition by T cell receptor. *Int Immunol* 1989;1:479–486

348. Jardetzky TS, Gorga JC, Busch R, Rothbard J, Strominger JL, Wiley DC. Peptide binding to HLA-DR1: a peptide with most residues substituted to alanine retains MHC binding. *EMBO J* 1990;9:1797–1803.

349. Rothbard JB, Busch R, Bal V, Trowsdale J, Lechler RI, Lamb JR. Reversal of HLA restriction by a point mutation in an antigenic peptide. *Int Immunol* 1989;1: 487–495.

350. Maryanski JL, Verdini AS, Weber PC, Salemme FR, Corradin G. Competitor analogs for defined T cell antigens: peptides incorporating a putative binding motif and polyproline or polyglycine spacers. *Cell* 1990;60:63–72.

351. Ruppert J, Sidney J, Celis E, Kubo RT, Grey HM, Sette A. Prominent role of secondary anchor residues in peptide binding to HLA-A2.1 molecules. *Cell* 1993; 74:929–937.

352. Berzofsky JA. Epitope selection and design of synthetic vaccines: molecular approaches to enhancing immunogenicity and crossreactivity of engineered vaccines. *Ann N Y Acad Sci* 1993;690:256–264.

353. Berzofsky JA. Designing peptide vaccines to broaden recognition and enhance potency. *Ann N Y Acad Sci* 1995;754:161–168.

354. Takahashi H, Nakagawa Y, Pendleton CD, et al. Induction of broadly cross-reac-

tive cytotoxic T cells recognizing an HIV-1 envelope determinant. *Science* 1992; 255:333–336.

355. Ahlers JD, Takeshita T, Pendleton CD, Berzofsky JA. Enhanced immunogenicity of HIV-1 vaccine construct by modification of the native peptide sequence. *Proc Natl Acad Sci U S A* 1997;94:10856–10861.

356. Ahlers JD, Dunlop N, Pendleton CD, Newman M, Nara PL, Berzofsky JA. Candidate HIV type1 multideterminant cluster peptide-P18MN vaccine constructs elicit type1 helper T cells, cytotoxic T cells, and neutralizing antibody, all using the same adjuvant immunization. *AIDS Res Hum Retrovir* 1996;12:259–272.

357. Shirai M, Pendleton CD, Ahlers J, Takeshita T, Newman M, Berzofsky JA. Helper-CTL determinant linkage required for priming of anti-HIV CD8+ CTL in vivo with peptide vaccine constructs. *J Immunol* 1994;152:549–556.

358. Ahlers JD, Dunlop N, Alling DW, Nara PL, Berzofsky JA. Cytokine-in-adjuvant steering of the immune response phenotype to HIV-1 vaccine constructs: GM-CSF and TNFα synergize with IL-12 to enhance induction of CTL. *J Immunol* 1997;158:3947–3958.

359. Pogue RR, Eron J, Frelinger JA, Matsui M. Amino-terminal alteration of the HLA-A*0201-restricted human immunodeficiency virus pol peptide increases complex stability and in vitro immunogenicity. *Proc Natl Acad Sci U S A* 1995; 92:8166–8170.

360. Parkhurst MR, Salgaller ML, Southwood S, et al. Improved induction of melanoma-reactive CTL with peptides from the melanoma antigen gp100 modified at HLA-A*0201-binding residues. *J Immunol* 1996;157:2539–2548.

361. Falk K, Rötzschke O, Stevanovic S, Jung G, Rammensee H-G. Allele-specific motifs revealed by sequencing of self-peptides eluted from MHC molecules. *Nature* 1991;351:290–296.

362. Jardetzky TS, Lane WS, Robinson RA, Madden DR, Wiley DC. Identification of self peptides bound to purified HLA-B27. *Nature* 1991;353:326–329.

363. Romero P, Corradin G, Luescher IF, Maryanski JL. H-2Kᵈ–restricted antigenic peptides share a simple binding motif. *J Exp Med* 1991;174:603–612.

364. Hunt DF, Henderson RA, Shabanowitz J, et al. Characterization of peptides bound to the class I MHC molecule HLA-A2.1 by mass spectrometry. *Science* 1992;255:1261–1263.

365. Corr M, Boyd LF, Padlan EA, Margulies DH. H-2Dᵈ exploits a four residue peptide binding motif. *J Exp Med* 1993;178:1877–1892.

366. Schumacher TNM, De Bruijn MLH, Vernie LN, et al. Peptide selection by MHC class I molecules. *Nature* 1991;350:703–706.

367. Tsomides TJ, Walker BD, Eisen HN. An optimal viral peptide recognized by CD8+ T cells binds very tightly to the restricting class I major histocompatibility complex protein on intact cells but not to the purified class I protein. *Proc Natl Acad Sci U S A* 1991;88:11276–11280.

368. Hunt DF, Michel H, Dickinson TA, et al. Peptides presented to the immune system by the murine class II major histocompatibility complex molecule I-Aᵈ. *Science* 1992;256:1817–1820.

369. Sette A, Buus S, Appella E, et al. Prediction of major histocompatibility complex binding regions of protein antigens by sequence pattern analysis. *Proc Natl Acad Sci U S A* 1989;86:3296–3300.

370. Chicz RM, Urban RG, Gorga JC, Vignali DAA, Lane WS, Strominger JL. Specificity and promiscuity among naturally processed peptides bound to HLA-DR alleles. *J Exp Med* 1993;178:27–47.

371. Chicz RM, Urban RG, Lane WS, et al. Predominant naturally processed peptides bound to HLA-DR1 are derived from MHC-related molecules and are heterogeneous in size. *Nature* 1992;358:764–768.

372. Hammer J, Takacs B, Sinigaglia F. Identification of a motif for HLA-DR1 binding peptides using M13 display libraries. *J Exp Med* 1992;176:1007–1013.

373. Hammer J, Valsasnini P, Tolba K, et al. Promiscuous and allele-specific anchors in HLA-DR–binding peptides. *Cell* 1993;74:197–203.

374. Sinigaglia F, Hammer J. Motifs and supermotifs for MHC class II binding peptides. *J Exp Med* 1995;181:449–451.

375. Marshall KW, Wilson KJ, Liang J, Woods A, Zaller D, Rothbard JB. Prediction of peptide affinity to HLA DRB1*0401. *J Immunol* 1995;154:5927–5933.

376. Jardetzky TS, Brown JH, Gorga JC, et al. Three-dimensional structure of a human class II histocompatibility molecule complexed with superantigen. *Nature* 1994;368:711–718.

377. Davis MM, Bjorkman PJ. T-cell antigen receptor genes and T-cell recognition. *Nature* 1988;334:395–402.

378. Ogasawara K, Maloy WL, Schwartz RH. Failure to find holes in the T cell repertoire. *Nature* 1987;325:450.

379. Shirai M, Arichi T, Nishioka M, et al. CTL responses of HLA-A2.1–transgenic mice specific for hepatitis C viral peptides predict epitopes for CTL of humans carrying HLA-A2.1. *J Immunol* 1995;154:2733–2742.

380. Schaeffer EB, Sette A, Johnson DL, et al. Relative contribution of "determinant selection" and "holes in the T-cell repertoire" to T-cell responses. *Proc Natl Acad Sci U S A* 1989;86:4649–4653.

381. Moudgil KD, Grewal IS, Jensen PE, Sercarz EE. Unresponsiveness to a self-peptide of mouse lysozyme owing to hindrance of T cell receptor-major histocompatibility complex/peptide interaction caused by flanking epitopic residues. *J Exp Med* 1996;183:535–546.

382. Takeshita T, Takahashi H, Kozlowski S, et al. Molecular analysis of the same HIV peptide functionally binding to both a class I and a class II MHC molecule. *J Immunol* 1995;154:1973–1986.

383. Alexander-Miller MA, Parker KC, Tsukui T, Pendleton CD, Coligan JE, Berzofsky JA. Molecular analysis of presentation by HLA-A2.1 of a promiscuously binding V3 loop peptide from the HIV-1 envelope protein to human CTL. *Int Immunol* 1996;8:641–649.

384. Takahashi H, Merli S, Putney SD, et al. A single amino acid interchange yields reciprocal CTL specificities for HIV gp160. *Science* 1989;246:118–121.

385. Takahashi H, Houghten R, Putney SD, et al. Structural requirements for class-I MHC molecule-mediated antigen presentation and cytotoxic T-cell recognition of an immunodominant determinant of the HIV envelope protein. *J Exp Med* 1989;170:2023–2035.

386. De Magistris MT, Alexander J, Coggeshall M, et al. Antigen analog-major histocompatibility complexes act as antagonists of the T cell receptor. *Cell* 1992;68: 625–634.

387. Sette A, Alexander J, Ruppert J, et al. Antigen analogs/MHC complexes as specific T cell receptor antagonists. *Annu Rev Immunol* 1994;12:413–431.

388. Lorenz RG, Allen PM. Direct evidence for functional self-protein/Ia-molecule complexes in vivo. *Proc Natl Acad Sci U S A* 1988;85:5220–5223.

389. Evavold BD, Allen PM. Separation of IL-4 production from Th cell proliferation by an altered T cell receptor ligand. *Science* 1991;252:1308–1310.

390. Evavold BD, Williams SG, Hsu BL, Buus S, Allen PM. Complete dissection of the Hb(64-76) determinant using Th1, Th2 clones and T cell hybridomas. *J Immunol* 1992;148:347–353.

391. Pfeiffer C, Stein J, Southwood S, Ketelaar H, Sette A, Bottomly K. Altered peptide ligands can control CD4 T lymphocyte differentiation in vivo. *J Exp Med* 1995;181:1569–1574.

392. Chaturvedi P, Yu Q, Southwood S, Sette A, Singh B. Peptide analogs with different affinities for MHC alter the cytokine profile of T helper cells. *Int Immunol* 1996;8:745–755.

393. Sloan-Lancaster J, Evavold BD, Allen PM. Induction of T-cell anergy by altered T-cell-receptor ligand on live antigen-presenting cells. *Nature* 1993;363:156–159.

394. Mueller DL, Jenkins MK, Schwartz RH. Clonal expansion versus functional clonal inactivation: a costimulatory signalling pathway determines the outcome of T cell antigen receptor occupancy. *Annu Rev Immunol* 1989;7:445–480.

395. Sloan-Lancaster J, Shaw AS, Rothbard JB, Allen PM. Partial T cell signaling: altered phospho-ζ and lack of Zap70 recruitment in APL-induced T cell anergy. *Cell* 1994;79:913–922.

396. Tsitoura DC, Holter W, Cerwenka A, Gelder CM, Lamb JR. Induction of anergy in human T helper 0 cells by stimulation with altered T cell antigen receptor ligands. *J Immunol* 1996;156:2801–2808.

397. Racioppi L, Ronchese F, Matis LA, Germain RN. Peptide–major histocompatibility complex class II complexes with mixed agonist/antagonist properties provide evidence for ligand-related differences in T cell receptor–dependent intracellular signaling. *J Exp Med* 1993;177:1047–1060.

398. Madrenas J, Wange RL, Wang JL, Isakov N, Samelson LE, Germain RN. ζ phosphorylation without ZAP-70 activation induced by TCR antagonists or partial agonists. *Science* 1995;267:515–518.

399. Madrenas J, Chau LA, Smith J, Bluestone JA, Germain RN. The efficiency of CD4 recruitment to ligand-engaged TCR controls the agonist/partial agonist properties of peptide–MHC molecule ligands. *J Exp Med* 1997;185:219–229.

400. McKeithan TW. Kinetic proofreading in T-cell receptor signal transduction. *Proc Natl Acad Sci U S A* 1995;92:5042–5046.

401. DeGroot AS, Meister GE, Cornette JL, Margalit H, DeLisi C, Berzofsky JA. Computer prediction of T-cell epitopes. In: Levine MM, Woodrow GC, Kaper JB, Cobon GS, eds. *New generation vaccines,* 2nd ed. New York: Marcel Dekker, 1997:127–138.

402. DeGroot AS, Jesdale BM, Berzofsky JA. Prediction and determination of MHC ligands and T cell epitopes. In: Kaufmann SHE, Kabelitz D, eds. *Immunological methods in microbiology.* London: Academic Press, 1998:79–106.

403. Stille CJ, Thomas LJ, Reyes VE, Humphreys RE. Hydrophobic strip-of-helix algorithm for selection of T cell–presented peptides. *Mol Immunol* 1987;24: 1021–1027.

404. Sette A, Doria G, Adorini L. A microcomputer program for hydrophilicity and amphipathicity analysis of protein antigens. *Mol Immunol* 1986;23:807–810.

405. Madden DR, Garboczi DN, Wiley DC. The antigenic identity of peptide–MHC complexes: a comparison of the conformations of five viral peptides presented by HLA-A2. *Cell* 1993;75:693–708.

406. Ghosh P, Amaya M, Mellins E, Wiley DC. The structure of an intermediate in class II MHC maturation: CLIP bound to HLA-DR3. *Nature* 1995;378:457–462.

407. Cornette JL, Cease KB, Margalit H, Spouge JL, Berzofsky JA, DeLisi C. Hydrophobicity scales and computational techniques for detecting amphipathic structures in proteins. *J Mol Biol* 1987;195:659–686.

408. Cornette JL, Margalit H, DeLisi C, Berzofsky JA. Concepts and methods in the identification of T cell epitopes and their use in the construction of synthetic vaccines. *Methods Enzymol* 1989;178:611–634.

409. Cornette JL, Margalit H, DeLisi C, Berzofsky JA. The amphipathic helix as a structural feature involved in T-cell recognition. In: Epand RM, ed. *The amphipathic helix.* Boca Raton, FL: CRC Press, 1993:333–346.

410. Rothbard JB, Taylor WR. A sequence pattern common to T cell epitopes. *EMBO J* 1988;7:93–100.

411. Reyes VE, Chin LT, Humphreys RE. Selection of class I MHC-restricted peptides with the strip-of-helix hydrophobicity algorithm. *Mol Immunol* 1988;25: 867–871.

412. Cornette JL, Margalit H, Berzofsky JA, DeLisi C. Periodic variation in side-chain polarities of T-cell antigenic peptides correlates with their structure and activity. *Proc Natl Acad Sci USA* 1995;92:8368–8372.

413. Pamer EG, Harty JT, Bevan MJ. Precise prediction of a dominant class I MHC-restricted epitope of *Listeria monocytogenes*. *Nature* 1991;353:852–855.

414. Hill AVS, Elvin J, Willis AC, et al. Molecular analysis of the association of HLA-B53 and resistance to severe malaria. *Nature* 1992;360:434–439.

415. Lipford GB, Hoffman M, Wagner H, Heeg K. Primary in vivo responses to ovalbumin: probing the predictive value of the K^b binding motif. *J Immunol* 1993; 150:1212–1222.

416. Nijman HW, Houbiers JGA, Vierboom MPM, et al. Identification of peptide sequences that potentially trigger HLA-A2.1–restricted cytotoxic T lymphocytes. *Eur J Immunol* 1993;23:1215–1219.

417. Altuvia Y, Berzofsky JA, Rosenfeld R, Margalit H. Sequence features that correlate with MHC restriction. *Mol Immunol* 1994;31:1–19.

418. Meister GE, Roberts CGP, Berzofsky JA, DeGroot AS. Two novel T cell epitope prediction algorithms based on MHC-binding motifs; comparison of predicted and published epitopes from *Mycobacterium tuberculosis* and HIV protein sequences. *Vaccine* 1995;13:581–591.

419. Kaufman JF, Auffray C, Korman AJ, Shackelford DA, Strominger J. The class II molecules of the human and murine major histocompatibility complex. *Cell* 1984;36:1–13.

420. Zhang C, Cornette JL, Berzofsky JA, DeLisi C. The organization of human leukocyte antigen class I epitopes in HIV genome products: implications for HIV evolution and vaccine design. *Vaccine* 1997;

421. Hammer J, Bono E, Gallazzi F, Belunis C, Nagy Z, Sinigaglia F. Precise prediction of major histocompatibility complex class II–peptide interaction based on peptide side chain scanning. *J Exp Med* 1994;180:2353–2358.

422. Parker DC, Bednarek MA, Coligan JE. Scheme for ranking potential HLA-A2 binding peptides based on independent binding of individual peptide side-chains. *J Immunol* 1994;152:163–175.

423. Fleckenstein B, Kalbacher H, Muller CP, et al. New ligands binding to the human leukocyte antigen class II molecule DRB1*0101 based on the activity pattern of an undecapeptide library. *Eur J Biochem* 1996;240:71–77.

424. Jesdale BM, Mullen L, Meisell J, Marznello M, Deocampo G, De Groot AS. Epimatrix and epimer, tools for HIV research. In: *Vaccines*. Cold Spring Harbor Laboratory Press, 1997.

425. Davenport MP, Ho Shon IAP, Hill AVS. An empirical method for the prediction of T-cell epitopes. *Immunogenetics* 1995;42:392–397.

426. Davenport MP, Godkin A, Friede T, et al. A distinctive peptide binding motif for HLA-DRB1*0407, an HLA-DR4 subtype not associated with rheumatoid arthritis. *Immunogenetics* 1997;45:229–232.

427. Sidney J, Grey HM, Southwood S, et al. Definition of an HLA-A3–like supermotif demonstrates the overlapping peptide-binding repertoires of common HLA molecules. *Hum Immunol* 1996;45:79–93.

428. Kropshofer H, Max H, Halder T, Kalbus M, Muller CA, Kalbacher H. Self-peptides from four HLA-DR alleles share hydrophobic anchor residues near the NH_2-terminal including proline as a stop signal for trimming. *J Immunol* 1993; 151:4732–4742.

429. Vajda S, Weng Z, Rosenfeld R, DeLisi C. Effect of conformational flexibility and solvation on receptor-ligand binding free energics. *Biochemistry* 1994;33: 13977–13988.

430. Sezerman U, Vajda S, DeLisi C. Free energy mapping of class I MHC molecules and structural determination of bound peptides. *Protein Sci* 1996;5:1272–1281.

431. Altuvia Y, Schueler O, Margalit H. Ranking potential binding peptides to MHC molecules by a computational threading approach. *J Mol Biol* 1995;249:244–250.

432. Brusic V, Rudy G, Harrison LC. Prediction of MHC binding peptides using artificial neural networks. In: Stonier RJ, Yu XS, eds. *Complex systems mechanism of adaptation*. Amsterdam: IOS Press, 1994:253–260.

433. Takahashi H, Cohen J, Hosmalin A, et al. An immunodominant epitope of the HIV gp160 envelope glycoprotein recognized by class I MHC molecule–restricted murine cytotoxic T lymphocytes. *Proc Natl Acad Sci U S A* 1988;85:3105–3109.

434. Langton BC, Mackewicz CE, Wan AM, Andria ML, Benjamini E. Structural features of an antigen required for cellular interactions and for T-cell activation in an MHC-restricted response. *J Immunol* 1988;141:447–456.

435. Thomas DB, Skehel JJ, Mills KHG, Graham CM. A single amino acid substitution in influenza haemagglutinin abrogates recognition by a monoclonal antibody and a spectrum of subtype-specific L3T4+ T cell clones. *Eur J Immunol* 1987;17:133–136.

436. Mozes E, McDevitt HO, Jaton J-C, Sela M. The nature of the antigenic determinant in genetic control of antibody response. *J Exp Med* 1969;130:493–504.

437. Mozes E, McDevitt HO, Jaton J-C, Sela M. The genetic control of antibody specificity. *J Exp Med* 1969;130:1263–1278.

438. Bluestein HG, Green I, Maurer PH, Benacerraf B. Specific immune response genes of the guinea pig. V: Influence of the GA and GT immune response genes on the specificity of cellular and humoral immune responses to a terpolymer of L-glutamic acid, L-alanine, and L-tyrosine. *J Exp Med* 1972;135:98–109.

439. Berzofsky JA, Schechter AN, Shearer GM, Sachs DH. Genetic control of the immune response to staphylococcal nuclease III. Time course and correlation between the response to native nuclease and the response to its polypeptide fragments. *J Exp Med* 1977;145:111–112.

440. Berzofsky JA, Schechter AN, Shearer GM, Sachs DH. Genetic control of the immune response to staphylococcal nuclease IV. H-2–linked control of the relative proportions of antibodies produced to different determinants of native nuclease. *J Exp Med* 1977;145:123–145.

441. Campos-Neto A, Levine H, Schlossman SJ. T cell regulation of specific B cell responses. *J Immunol* 1978;121:2235–2240.

442. Campos-Neto A, Levine H, Schlossman SJ. Immune response gene control of antibody specificity. *Cell Immunol* 1982;69:128–137.

443. Kohno Y, Berzofsky JA. Genetic control of the immune response to myoglobin. V. Antibody production in vitro is macrophage and T cell–dependent and is under control of two determinant-specific Ir genes. *J Immunol* 1982;128:2458–2464.

444. Barcinski MA, Rosenthal AS. Immune response gene control of determinant selection. I. Intramolecular mapping of the immunogenic sites on insulin recognized by guinea pig T and B cells. *J Exp Med* 1977;145:726–742.

445. Sercarz E, Cecka JM, Kipp D, Miller A. The steering function of T cells in expression of the antibody repertoire directed against multideterminant protein antigen. *Ann Immunol Inst Pasteur* 1977;128:599.

446. Cecka JM, Stratton JA, Miller A, Sercarz EE. Structural aspects of immune recognition of lysozymes. III. T cell specificity restriction and its consequences for antibody specificity. *Eur J Immunol* 1976;6:639–646.

447. Ferguson TA, Peters T Jr, Reed R, Pesce A, Michael JG. Immunoregulatory properties of antigenic fragments from bovine serum albumin. *Cell Immunol* 1983;78:1–12.

448. Kawamura H, Berkower I, Glover C, Berzofsky J. Helper T cell epitope specificity regulates B cell (antibody) specificity. *J Cell Biochem* 1984;8A:211.

449. Benjamini E, Wan AM, Langton BC, Andria ML. Induction of immunity by model synthetic vaccines derived from tobacco mosaic virus protein. In: Dreesman GR, Bronson JG, Kennedy R, eds. *High technology route to virus vaccines*. Washington, DC: American Society of Microbiology, 1985:30–42.

450. Chesnut RW, Colon SM, Grey HM. Antigen presentation by normal B cells B cell tumors and macrophages: functional biochemical comparison. *J Immunol* 1982;128:1764–1768.

451. Chesnut RW, Colon SM, Grey HM. Requirements for the processing of antigen by antigen-presenting cells. I. Functional comparison of B cell tumors and macrophages. *J Immunol* 1982;129:2382–2388.

452. Lanzavecchia A. Antigen-specific interaction between T cells and B cells. *Nature* 1985;314:537–539.

453. Chesnut RW, Grey HM. Studies on the capacity of B cells to serve as antigen-presenting cells. *J Immunol* 1981;126:1075–1079.

454. Malynn BA, Wortis HH. Role of antigen-specific B cells in the induction of SRBC-specific T cell proliferation. *J Immunol* 1984;132:2253–2258.

455. Rock KL, Benacerraf B, Abbas AK. Antigen presentation by hapten-specific B lymphocytes I Role of surface immunoglobulin receptors. *J Exp Med* 1984;160: 1102–1113.

456. Tony H-P, Parker DC. Major histocompatibility complex–restricted polyclonal B cell responses resulting form helper T cell recognition of antiimmunoglobulin presented by small B lymphocytes. *J Exp Med* 1985;161:223–241.

457. Kawamura H, Berzofsky JA. Enhancement of antigenic potency in vitro and immunogenicity in vivo by coupling the antigen to anti-immunoglobulin. *J Immunol* 1986;136:58–65.

458. Davidson HW, Watts C. Epitope-directed processing of specific antigen by B lymphocytes. *J Cell Biol* 1989;109:85–92.

459. Löwenadler B, Lycke N, Svanholm C, Svennerholm A-M, Krook K, Gidlund M. T and B cell responses to chimeric proteins containing heterologous T helper epitopes inserted at different positions. *Mol Immunol* 1992;29: 1185–1190.

460. Manca F, Fenoglio D, Kunkl A, Cambiaggi C, Sasso M, Celada F. Differential activation of T cell clones stimulated by macrophages exposed to antigen complexed with monoclonal antibodies. A possible influence of paratope specificity on the mode of antigen processing. *J Immunol* 1988;140:2893–2898.

461. Manca F, Fenoglio D, Li Pira G, Kunkl A, Celada F. Effect of antigen/antibody ratio on macrophage uptake, processing, and presentation to T cells of antigen complexed with polyclonal antibodies. *J Exp Med* 1991;173:37–48.

462. Watts C, Lanzavecchia A. Suppressive effect of antibody on processing of T cell epitopes. *J Exp Med* 1993;178:1459–1463.

463. Simitsek PD, Campbell DG, Lanzavecchia A, Fairweather N, Watts C. Modulation of antigen processing by bound antibodies can boost or suppress class II major histocompatibility complex presentation of different T cell determinants. *J Exp Med* 1995;181:1957–1963.

464. Bekoff MC, Levine H, Schlossman SF. T cell and Ir gene regulation of expression of a cross-reactive idiotype. *J Immunol* 1982;129:1173–1180.

465. Kawamura H, Kohno Y, Busch M, Gurd FRN, Berzofsky JA. A major anti-myoglobin idiotype. influence of H-2–linked Ir genes on idiotype expression. *J Exp Med* 1984;160:659–678.

466. Babu UM, Maurer PH. The expression of anti-poly (L-Glu60 L-Phe40) idiotypic determinants dictated by the gene products in the major histocompatibility complex (H-2). *J Immunol* 1981;154:649–658.

467. Germain RN. The ins and outs of antigen processing and presentation. *Nature* 1986;322:687–689.

468. Fauchère JL, Pliska V. Hydrophobic parameters q of amino-acid side chains from the partitioning of N-acetyl-amino-acid amides. *Eur J Med Chem* 1983;18: 369–374.

Fundamental Immunology, Fourth Edition,
edited by William E. Paul
Published by Lippincott–Raven Publishers, Philadelphia 1999.

CHAPTER 20

Immunological Tolerance

Ronald H. Schwartz

At the turn of the century, Ehrlich and Morgenroth (1) observed that goats they had injected with red blood cells from another goat always made hemolytic antibodies directed against the immunizing cells, but these antisera never reacted against the recipients' own red blood cells. Furthermore, they deliberately immunized a goat with its own red blood cells and also observed that no antibody response was elicited. They coined the latin phrase *horror autotoxicus* to describe this situation. To them, the term meant that the animals avoided self-destructive responses, although it has often been interpreted by others to mean a failure to make any immune responses against self components. In fact, in a footnote in their paper (1), they made clear the distinction between autoreactivity and autoimmune disease when they discussed the experiments of Metalinikoff, who found that guinea pigs injected with their own sperm made cytotoxic antibodies against these cells. Because the

antibodies did not kill the sperm in vivo (e.g., the animals remained fertile), Ehrlich and Morgenroth deemed the antibodies not to be autotoxic.

In this chapter on immunologic tolerance, I would like to keep this same perspective. Hence, I define *tolerance* as a physiologic state in which the immune system does not react destructively against the components of an organism that harbors it or against antigens that are introduced to it. Destructive responses are prevented by a variety of mechanisms that operate during development of the immune system *and* during the generation of each immune response. Pharmacologic manipulations are not included. This broad view allows one to consider immunoregulation as part of the tolerance process.

TOLERANCE IS AN ADAPTIVE PROCESS

Why didn't the goats make antibodies against their own red blood cells? The first observations that shed light on this issue

R.H. Schwartz: Laboratory of Cellular and Molecular Immunology, National Institute of Allergy and Infectious Diseases, National Institutes of Health, Bethesda, Maryland 20892-0420.

were made by Owen (2) on dizygotic bovine twins and quintuplets. He analyzed the surface antigens of red blood cells from these cattle with alloantisera of the type raised by Ehrlich in goats and showed that each offspring possessed all of the antigens found in the parents, even though some of these determinants were not expressed by both parents. In the quintuplets, this seemed highly unlikely to result from codominant heterozygosity, as the outbred parents would have had to be homozygous at multiple genetic loci. Instead, he was able to show in cytotoxicity assays that the offspring were chimeric; that is, their blood contained a mixture of cells with different phenotypes. Based on the earlier work of Lillie (3), who had suggested that dizygotic cattle could exchange products through anastomoses of the blood vessels in their two placentas, Owen postulated that hemopoietic stem cells from each sibling migrated to the bone marrow of the others to create a stable chimeric state that persisted after the sibs were separated at birth. Because the chimerism of the antigenically disparate cells was not disturbed by an immune response, he described this state of peaceful coexistence as one of tolerance. The observations suggested that a foreign substance could be either reacted against or tolerated by an immune system, depending on when the antigen was presented to it. The observations also suggested that there was no fundamental distinction between self molecules (encoded by the host's genome) and foreign molecules in their ability to induce a tolerant state.

Burnet and Fenner (4) were strongly influenced by Owen's observations, as well as those of Traub (5), who demonstrated that a carrier state for the lymphocytic choriomeningitis virus (LCMV) could be induced in mice by natural exposure to this virus *in utero* or during the neonatal period. Their interpretation of both results was that the developing immune system was malleable and that if a foreign substance were introduced early enough, it would induce tolerance rather than immunity. The first experimental data to support this hypothesis were generated by Billingham et al. (6). They injected cell suspensions from mixed tissues of mouse strain A into neonatal or fetal mice of strain B

and showed that as adults the strain-B mice could accept skin grafts from a strain-A mouse, although they would rapidly reject skin grafts from a third-party strain-C mouse. The concept derived from this work, that tolerance was an acquired state, was confirmed by Hašek (7), who experimentally reproduced the observations of Owen by parabiosis of chick embryos. After separation at birth, the adult birds could not make an antibody response against their partner's red blood cells (Ehrlich's experiment) and could not reject each other's skin grafts (Medawar's experiment). Burnet subsequently gave a theoretical framework to all of these results in his clonal selection theory, in which he postulated that clones of lymphocytes with receptors on their surface specific for molecules present during the development of the immune system would be selectively eliminated by a deletion process (8) (Fig. 1).

Consistent with the idea that the immune system learns to be tolerant during its development was the subsequent experiment of Triplett (9). He removed the pituitary anlage from tree frog larvae and let them differentiate under the skin of other larvae. When the tadpoles went through metamorphosis, he gave back to the adult frogs their own pituitaries and found that the animals rejected the autografts. Partial hypophysectomized animals did not reject the grafts, which argued that the rejection was not caused by the acquisition of new antigens, through either abnormal differentiation or carry-over of the temporary host's tissues. Thus, tolerance, even to self antigens, appears to be an acquired state, requiring the presence of the antigen to induce it.

The adaptive nature of tolerance is a fundamental property of the immune system. Given the task of the system, which is to recognize and respond to unexpected molecules using the random structural diversity generated from rearranging T- and B-cell antigen-receptor genes, there is no way to genetically program it to know what molecules will lead to self-destructive responses. Instead, a series of steps must be undertaken somatically during which the environment is sampled and the system fine-tuned to avoid its own destruction. The nature of these steps in both the

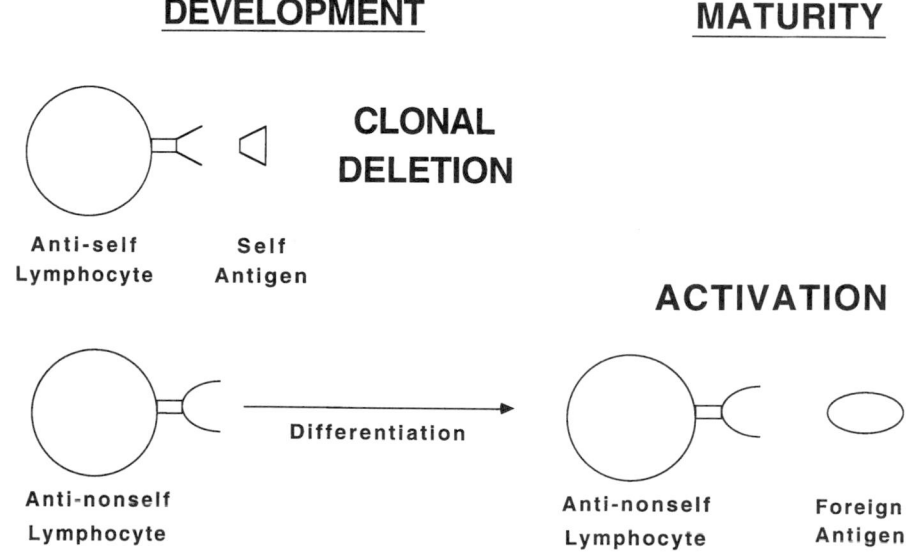

FIG. 1. Burnet's clonal selection model. Developing lymphocytes are deleted if they encounter a self antigen for which they are specific. After differentiation, nondeleted cells are now activatable on encounter with foreign antigens.

mature and developing immune system will be the principal focus of this chapter.

NEGATIVE SELECTION DURING T-CELL DEVELOPMENT

The first demonstration of clonal deletion was published by Kappler et al. (10). They used a monoclonal antibody against the variable region of a T-cell receptor (TCR) beta chain (anti-Vβ17a) to follow the fate of T cells expressing this chain. In mice expressing an E molecule encoded by MHC class II genes, Vβ17-bearing cells were eliminated. This process was later shown to be related to expression of an endogenous superantigen (the ORF gene product of mouse mammary tumor viruses 6, 8, or 9) (Mtv-6/8/9), which is capable of interacting with both Vβ17 and the E molecule (11). When E$^+$ and E$^-$ strains were crossed, the resulting F$_1$ animals also showed a deleted phenotype. This elimination process was shown to take place in the thymus. Cells expressing Vβ17 were found in only slightly reduced numbers in the immature CD4$^+$8$^+$ TCR low population, but were greatly depleted among the more mature single-positive (CD4$^+$8$^-$ and CD4$^-$8$^+$) thymocytes. The possibility that the cells had simply downregulated their receptors was subsequently ruled out by showing that Vβ17 mRNA was also absent in mature T-cell populations. The actual deletion of the cells, however, was not observed until much later by other investigators (12) (see the section on the biochemical events in thymocyte clonal deletion). Similar observations were made by MacDonald et al. (13) for Vβ6$^+$ T cells. Subsequent studies (14,15) demonstrated that the deletion was occurring at the late double-positive stage when TCR expression is high and the CD4 and CD8 coreceptors have begun to downmodulate.

These observations were extended by Kisielow et al. (16) to a more conventional antigen system, the male-specific antigen H-Y. They took advantage of an alpha–beta TCR (TCRαβ$^+$) transgenic mouse developed by Blüthmann et al. (17) to follow the fate of a large cohort of T cells expressing the same anti-H-Y receptor, either in females, which do not express the antigen (controls), or in males, which do. The male mice had a thymus of greatly reduced size (10% of normal) and a tremendous reduction in the percentage of double-positive thymocytes. Similar observations were made by Sha et al. (18) using a transgenic mouse carrying genes encoding a TCRαβ$^+$ receptor specific for a major histocompatibility complex (MHC) class I alloantigen. These mice also deleted T cells bearing the receptor at the double-positive stage when they were crossed to mice expressing the alloantigen. Thus, the basic model postulated by Burnet appears to be correct for the standard TCRαβ$^+$ cell; that is, immature T cells encountering their antigen during development are clonally deleted (see Fig. 1). This process is referred to as negative selection.

In addition to TCRαβ$^+$ thymocytes, TCRγδ$^+$ cells can undergo negative selection in the thymus. A transgenic mouse expressing a γδ receptor specific for an MHC class Ib molecule that it did not have contained predominantly CD4$^-$8$^-$ T cells bearing this γδ receptor in the thymus and a major subpopulation of these cells in the spleen (19). When the mouse was crossed to a strain expressing the MHC class Ib molecule, cells bearing the transgenic receptor were not found in either the thymus or the spleen. Thus, in the presence of the antigen, the cells appeared to be clonally deleted. Similarly, the CD4$^-$8$^-$ and CD4$^+$8$^-$ TCRαβ$^+$ subpopulations expressing the NK1.1 and Ly6c markers, which are part of a separate T-cell lineage, appear

to be susceptible to negative selection in the thymus (20–22). In strains harboring the Mtv-7 or Mtv-6/8/9 mouse mammary tumor viruses, V β11- and V β17-bearing CD4$^-$8$^-$, Ly 6c$^+$ T cells were significantly reduced in number when MHC class II E molecules were also expressed. For the CD4$^+$8$^-$, NK1.1$^+$ T cells, forced expression of a CD8 transgene resulted in their deletion, presumably due to increased avidity for self antigens. Finally, in the intestine, the intraepithelial lymphocyte population was shown to be depleted of Vβ11$^+$ and Vβ6$^+$ cells in Mtv-7$^+$ strains expressing MHC class II E molecules (23). From these results we can generalize that all T cells are susceptible to the process of negative selection.

Stages of T-Cell Development at Which Negative Selection Occurs

The experiments involving tolerance to the H-Y antigen suggested that clonal deletion takes place at the early double-positive stage, whereas the experiments involving tolerance to superantigens suggested that clonal deletion takes place at the transition from the double-positive to the single-positive stage. It has been suggested that the early deletion seen in transgenic mice is a consequence of their premature expression of high levels of TCRs (14) and represents a different process, akin to maturational arrest (24). However, one transgenic mouse carrying a receptor specific for both a viral antigen and an Mtv-7–encoded superantigen deleted the double-positive cells when the mice carried the virus, but deleted only the single-positive cells when the mice were mated to animals expressing the Mtv-7 superantigen (25). Thus, it is likely that the nature of the antigen and where and how it is expressed for antigen presentation determine the stage at which the cells are deleted. Whether positive selection must take place as a necessary maturational step prior to negative selection is still not clear.

Evidence that clonal deletion can occur at the single-positive stage of T-cell development is also compelling. MacDonald and Lees (26) showed that Mtv-7 superantigen–reactive CD4$^+$8$^-$ thymocytes disappear within the first few days of life. In vitro culture of these cells demonstrated that this was not just migration out of the thymus, but an active death process that could be inhibited by low temperature, cycloheximide, or actinomycin D. In vivo experiments with a superantigen and an anti-TCR monoclonal antibody (27,28) have suggested that it is the earliest heat stable antigen (HSA) high CD4$^+$8$^-$ cells that are being deleted. Overall, it thus appears that thymocytes are susceptible to negative selection from the time that they first express their TCRs until the time they are fully mature single-positive T cells.

Antigen-presenting Cells for Negative Selection

Which cells are involved in presenting antigen for clonal deletion in the thymus has long been a point of contention. Consensus exists that bone marrow–derived cells play an important role, based initially on experiments with radiation-induced bone marrow chimeras (29). (A × B)F$_1$ bone marrow transferred into a lethally irradiated strain-B recipient results in tolerance to both strain-A and strain-B peptide–MHC complexes, as measured in a mixed leukocyte culture (Table 1). In the Vβ17 model, the T cells were deleted when the E molecules were expressed only on the donor-derived bone marrow cells (30), thus showing that these cells are sufficient for negative selection. The most likely bone marrow–derived cell responsible for inducing deletion is the den-

TABLE 1. *Tolerance in radiation-induced bone marrow chimeras*

Chimeras (BM → x-rayed host)	Thymic dendritic cells	Thymic epithelial cells	Mixed leukocyte response to
$(A \times B)F_1 \rightarrow P_B$	A and B	B only	Neither A nor B
$P_B \rightarrow (A \times B)F_1$	B only	A and B	A not B

BM → x-rayed host, bone marrow stem cells transferred into lethally irradiated mice.

dritic cell, because donor-derived dendritic cells repopulate an irradiated thymus quickly (31) and because allogeneic dendritic cells from the spleen introduced into a thymic organ culture can induce tolerance to the alloantigens, as measured in a cytotoxic T-lymphocyte (CTL) assay (32). Thus, a professional antigen-presenting cell (APC) capable of activating peripheral T cells tolerizes thymocytes. Subsequent experiments with thymocyte suspensions from TCR transgenic mice showed directly that splenic APCs could induce deletion of CD4$^+$8$^+$ T cells (33). These two observations suggest that it is the developmental stage of the T cell that determines the negative outcome of antigen presentation in the thymus, rather than a thymus-specific APC.

The role of thymic stromal (nonhematopoietic) cells in negative selection has been more controversial. Initial experiments (34) with parental B bone marrow into (A × B)F$_1$-irradiated hosts revealed alloreactivity against strain-A APC (see Table 1). Similarly, deoxyguanosine-treated fetal thymuses (depleted of hematopoietic cells), when grafted into allogeneic nude mice, produced T cells that reacted in a mixed leukocyte response (MLR) (35) and cell-mediated lympholysis (CML) (36) against the alloantigens of the thymus donor. The initial conclusion from these and other studies was that thymic stromal cells could not induce negative selection. A careful examination of the experiments, however, reveals that some negative effects did take place. For example, alloreactivity in the MLRs was often quantitatively diminished (37) and the nude mice did not reject their thymus grafts. Subsequent experiments with TCR transgenic animals revealed strong evidence for thymic stromal cell–mediated deletion. Transfer of TCR-transgenic bone marrow cells from a nondeleting strain into a virus-infected irradiated host, expressing on its stromal cells the MHC molecule required for virus-specific deletion, led to massive elimination of the cells in the thymus at the double-positive stage (38). Furthermore, grafts of allogeneic thymic anlagen (epitheliomesenchymal rudiment) induced tolerance to subsequent skin grafts (39), although not to allogeneic spleen-cell stimulation in an *in vitro* interleukin-2 (IL-2) production assay. The same result was also observed in the frog when the anterior portion of an embryo (containing the anlagen of the thymic stromal cells) was fused to the posterior portion of an allogeneic embryo containing the anlagen of the hematopoietic cells (40): The chimeras accepted skin grafts from frogs of the same MHC type as the thymus, but displayed an *in vitro* MLR against spleen cells of that MHC type. Thus, thymic stromal cells clearly can present antigens and induce negative selection, but perhaps not as completely as dendritic cells.

How does one account for the failure to completely induce tolerance by thymic stromal cell antigen presentation? One likely possibility is that the tolerance is tissue-specific, that is, only for those peptides expressed by the stromal cells (41). Hence, MLR and CML assays, in which splenic dendritic cells do the presenting, will stimulate T cells specific for those hematopoietic cell–derived peptides not expressed by the thymic stromal cells (41). When a

second whole thymus graft is given, only the hematopoietic cells are rejected, not the stromal cells. The fate of other tissue grafts depends on how much peptide overlap there is between the thymus and those grafts. This explanation, however, is not sufficient to explain the absence of clonal deletion by endogenous viral superantigens. For the most part, these molecules stimulate regardless of what peptides are bound to the MHC molecules. The failure to delete is not due to inaccessibility of the superantigens to the thymic stroma, because experiments in tissue culture, involving reconstitution of deoxyguanosine-treated thymic stromal cells with fresh T cells and dendritic cells, showed that addition of the superantigen staphylococcal enterotoxin B (SEB) could rapidly induce full deletion of Vβ8$^+$ T cells (with which SEB reacts) only in the presence of dendritic cells, even though SEB was shown to bind to the epithelial cell MHC class II molecules (42). Cultures lacking dendritic cells, however, did demonstrate deletion on prolonged exposure to SEB. The reason for the inefficiency of stromal cell presentation is unknown. It could relate to the nature or level of the cell adhesion molecules they express, their level of MHC molecule expression, differences in antigen processing (for endogenous viral superantigens, this could involve proteases at the cell surface), or the absence of costimulatory molecules. Nonetheless, in one TCR transgenic model, superantigen-induced deletion clearly took place at the double-positive stage (43), while antigen-induced deletion took place at that point only when it was highly expressed as a transgene (44). For the same antigen transgenic, however, deletion occurred at the single-positive stage, when a TCR transgenic of lower avidity for the antigen was used (44). These results suggest that, although stromal cells are less efficient at antigen presentation, they can effectively induce T-cell deletion, depending on the affinity of the particular TCR and the density of the peptide–MHC complexes that it recognizes. To some extent, this blurs the distinction between the two mechanisms, tissue-specific tolerance and inefficient antigen presentation, because many thymic stromal cell–specific self peptides will be present in large amounts, while peptides from other tissues usually will not.

The particular thymic stromal cell types involved in the tolerance process have been studied using transgenic mice expressing MHC molecules under the control of tissue-specific promoters. Targeting of a class I MHC molecule to the medullary epithelium with a keratin IV promoter (45) or an aberrantly expressed Eμ promoter (46) resulted in tolerance. As expected, the tolerance was tissue-specific (split); that is, the animals accepted skin grafts but manifested a CTL response *in vitro* in the presence of IL-2 (46). Thus, medullary epithelial cells seem capable of inducing tolerance. The data on targeting class II MHC molecules to the cortical epithelium have been contradictory. Mouse I-E–encoded molecules were reported to induce tolerance, as defined by the loss of an MLR (30) and in one case, the deletion of Vβ17$^+$ cells (47). In contrast, mouse I-A–encoded molecules expressed in cortical epithelium were reported to leave a strong MLR and therefore not

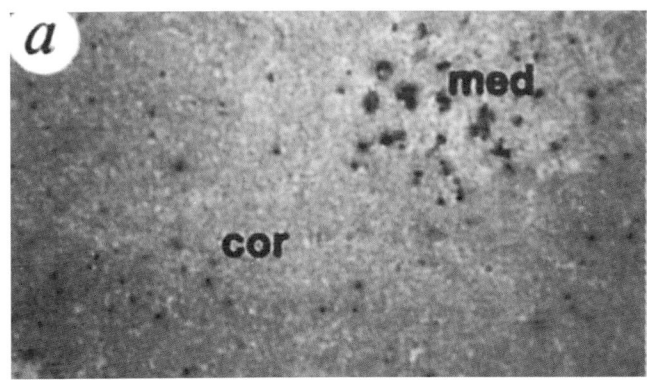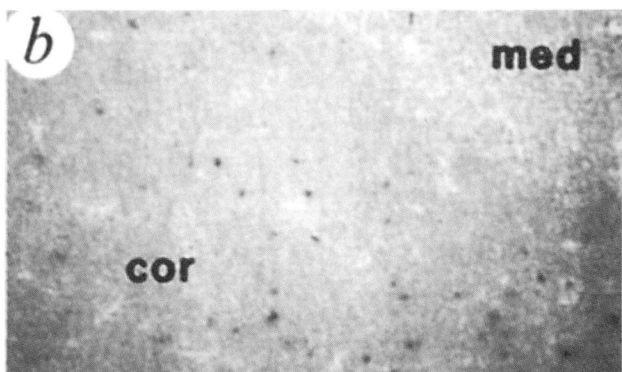

FIG. 2 a and **b.** T-cell apoptosis in the thymus. **(A)** Staining of apoptotic cells inside of macrophages by terminal deoxynucleotidyl transferase–mediated dUTP-biotin nick end-labeling (TUNEL assay). MED, medulla; COR, cortex. **(B)** The medullary spots are absent in mice lacking MHC class II E molecules, supporting the notion that they represent cells undergoing negative selection. (From ref. 12, with permission.)

to induce tolerance (48). The latter observation is the expected result, as the mice should be tolerant only to thymic cortical epithelial antigens. Unfortunately, thymic grafting experiments were not carried out to prove this. The negative MLR with the I-E–encoded molecules might come about because class II E molecule differences do not stimulate strong MLRs, and thus tolerance to just the shared stromal and dendritic cell peptides might be sufficient to reduce this weak MLR to background levels.

Finally, a few reports in the literature suggest that even developing T cells can present antigen for tolerance induction (49). In these experiments, lethally irradiated syngeneic bone marrow–reconstituted mice were injected intrathymically with purified Thy1⁺ CD4⁻8⁻ T cells that were haploidentical to the host [(A × B)F₁ T cells into an A host]. Assay of host cells 50 days later showed specific tolerance to "B" class I alloantigens of parent B as measured in a CTL response. This effect was not due to contaminating dendritic cells, because the host cells were not tolerant to MHC "B" class II alloantigens in an MLR. Note that mouse T cells do not express class II molecules, whereas dendritic cells do. Thus, the injected T cells appeared capable of inducing tolerance. A similar conclusion was reached from in vitro experiments using purified CD4⁻8⁺ thymocytes from a TCR transgenic mouse (50). These cells were killed when exposed to the peptide for which they were specific, presumably by recognizing peptide–MHC class I complexes on the surface of other T cells in the culture. This result suggests that T cells can directly induce clonal deletion of immature thymocytes. Overall, these experiments suggest that any cell type that can display antigen on its surface is capable of inducing negative selection in the thymus (51).

The Biochemical Events in Thymocyte Clonal Deletion

The fact that all types of APCs induce tolerance in thymocytes indicates that the T cells at this stage of their development are tolerizable only. Burnet (8), as well as Lederberg (52), postulated that this occurs by signaling through the antigen-specific receptor followed by cell death. Histologic examination of the thymus does not reveal much evidence for ongoing cell death; yet kinetic labeling studies have demonstrated that more than 95% of the cells generated in the thymus die there (53). Experiments using a sensitive assay to detect DNA strand breaks have shown that macrophages contain the debris of thymocytes that have died by apoptosis (Fig

2). In a TCR Vβ5 transgenic mouse expressing MHC class II E molecules and an endogenous Vβ5-reactive superantigen, the medulla of the thymus was found to contain aggregates of apoptotic cells that were engulfed by MAC3⁺ macrophages (12).

While a consensus now exists that thymocytes die by apoptosis during negative selection, the molecular mechanisms responsible for inducing apoptosis are not fully known. Multiple experiments in vitro have shown that cross-linking the TCRs on isolated double-positive thymocytes is not sufficient to induce cell death (54,55); but several studies have suggested that adding anti-CD28 plus anti-TCR antibodies will cause their demise (28,55). The CD28 knockout mouse, however, has no problem with negative selection (56), suggesting that CD28 is not the only receptor capable of facilitating this process. In vivo, CD28 may only be involved in late-stage deletion, as its ligand, B7, is expressed in the medulla, but not in the cortex (57).

The molecular pathways that lead to apoptosis following TCR engagement are also not clear. Mutations in the Fas and Fas ligand molecules have no effect on negative selection (58). Similarly, null mutations in the tumor necrosis factor (TNF) and TNF-receptor molecules are without effect (59). Only gene targeting of the CD30 molecule, a member of the TNF/NGF cytokine receptor family, has been reported to influence negative selection (60). This mutation increased thymocyte number twofold and impaired anti-CD3–induced death of thymocytes in vitro. However, when crossed to either a TCRαβ or a TCRγδ transgenic mouse bearing a strong negative selecting ligand, deletion was only partially reduced (mostly that seen at the double-positive stage), and the emerging peripheral T cells functioned normally (i.e., they were not autoreactive). Deletion by endogenous superantigens was unaffected. These results suggest that CD30 may be only one of several molecular pathways capable of mediating apoptosis in thymocytes.

Activation Versus Tolerance Thresholds

After T cells complete their maturation in the thymus, they are capable of responding to a foreign antigen when the concentration of peptide–MHC complexes derived from that antigen reaches a certain critical threshold for activation. The relationship between this threshold and the concentration of intact antigen depends on processing and presentation requirements, in addition to the intrinsic affinity of the TCR for the peptide–MHC complex. An important question is the relationship between this threshold for activation and the one involved in negative selection. If a self antigen presented in the thymus induces clonal deletion in only a subset of T cells, what happens if that antigen is expressed in peripheral tissues in increased amounts during tissue destruction in an inflammatory response? Will T-cell clones with low affinity for the self peptide–MHC complexes now become activated? This usually is not the case; that is, trauma rarely leads to autoimmunity. The question is, why?

Early observations on endogenous viral superantigens suggested that T cells bearing certain Vβ could be deleted *in vivo* if the mice carried the Mtv, but that these same cells could not be stimulated *in vitro* to give a T cell–proliferative response by APCs expressing that Mtv (61). This suggested that tolerance induction was more easily achieved than activation, although a large part of this difference stemmed from the difference between *in vivo* and *in vitro* assay systems (62). The use of thymic organ cultures and TCR transgenic mice allowed a more quantititive analysis of the problem. Deletion of TCR^hi Vβ8+ cells by SEB in thymic organ culture was shown to occur at concentrations that were 30- to 100-fold lower than those required to activate mature CD4+ cells to proliferate (63). A similar but less dramatic result was observed for antigen-specific, transgenic CD4+8+ thymocytes (64); these were deleted by concentrations of peptide in suspension culture that were not adequate to stimulate IL-2 production or proliferation from adult transgenic lymph node T cells. The quantitation in this system was quite reliable, as the same APC was used in each *in vitro* assay.

For T-cell help generated in thymic organ cultures, exposure to the liver F protein during *in vitro* culture induced tolerance at a tenfold lower concentration than that required for proliferation of mature T cells (65). Finally, variant lymphocyte choriomeningitis viruses (LCMVs) were compared for their ability to elicit antiviral responses in TCR transgenic mice and for their ability to induce neonatal tolerance in these mice (66). One viral variant could not activate a CTL response or be cleared by the animal over a 1,000-fold range of viral challenge doses; yet it was capable of inducing a partial deletion (30% to 40%) of transgenic TCR+CD8+ T cells in the thymus after neonatal tolerization. Another LCMV variant that gave poor activation *in vivo* induced complete tolerance by thymic deletion. Thus, all the experiments suggest that the concentration threshold required for tolerance induction of immature T cells is lower than the threshold required by the mature T cell for activation. The biochemical basis for the difference in thresholds has not yet been elucidated.

Coreceptor and Receptor Downmodulation

In the male H-Y–specific TCR transgenic, the thymus is one-tenth normal size, and very few CD8+4− cells expressing the transgenic receptor are found (16). In the periphery, however, such cells are readily seen, but their level of expression of CD8 is consistently lower than normal. Interestingly, when the H-Y transgenic mouse was crossed to a transgenic mouse that constitutively expresses CD8, the T cells expressing low levels of endogenous CD8 disappeared from both the thymus and the periphery (67). Thus, either the increased CD8 levels during selection or an inability to down-regulate the CD8 transgene caused a complete deletion in the thymus. The low level of CD8, when it occurs, seems to be a stable phenotype, because the peripheral cells retain this level after activation and proliferation (68). Also of interest is the observation that T cells can exist with different levels of CD8, depending on the strength of the negative selection pressure (68).

Another type of escape from negative selection can result when the level of the TCR is lowered. This occurs in TCR transgenic

mice through rearrangement and expression of endogenous α-chain genes (69). In those cases in which the second α chain can pair with the transgenic β chain, the T cell expresses, to varying degrees, two receptors on the cell surface. This lowers the surface level of the transgenic TCR, which can allow the T cell to escape negative selection. Interestingly, many normal T cells also express two receptors (70,71). Thus, these observations could have relevance for the development of autoimmune disease (see the section on the breaking of tolerance).

NEGATIVE SELECTION DURING B-CELL DEVELOPMENT

Is There Negative Selection in the B-Cell Compartment?

The introduction of fluorescein-tagged and radiolabeled antigens in the late 1960s allowed, for the first time, the quantitation of antigen-binding cells. Most of the cells detected were B cells, as defined by the expression of surface immunoglobulin (Ig). When this technique was applied to tolerant animals, whether natural or acquired, the surprising observation was made that the animals had antigen-binding cells specific for the tolerogen. For example, cells binding thyroglobulin were observed repeatedly in human peripheral blood, whereas cells specific for human serum albumin were not (72). This suggested that tolerance did not always involve deletion of clones, as postulated by Burnet (8). Furthermore, when adult B cells were stimulated with polyclonal activators such as the lipopolysaccharide (LPS) from *E. coli*, some of them differentiated into IgM-secreting plasma cells whose antibodies reacted against self components (73). Such autoantibody-forming cells were then found without LPS stimulation in normal (74,75) and germ-free mice (76) as well as in humans (77).

Evidence subsequently showed that negative selection for certain self antigens existed only in the T-cell compartment and not in the B-cell compartment. The first example was for the F protein from liver, which exists in two allelic forms (differing only by a single amino acid). Mouse strains expressing the right MHC haplotype (responders) could make an antibody response against the allelic product of F that they did not express (78,79). The antibodies elicited, however, reacted equally well with both forms of the F protein. These experiments were subsequently interpreted as implying the absence of T cells specific for the self peptide derived from the polymorphic region of the protein and the presence of T cells with reactivity to the nonself peptide encoded by the other allele, as well as no negative selection at the B-cell level. A second example was observed for IgE, which is nonimmunogenic on its own but elicits a strong antibody response in syngeneic mice when coupled to a foreign carrier protein (80). Finally, a similar conclusion was reached for the fifth component of complement (C5) (81). In this case, one mutant subline (o) of the mouse B10.D2 strain does not produce C5 and is therefore not tolerant to this protein. Transfer into irradiated nontolerant (B10.D2/o) recipients of T cells from this mouse, along with B cells from the nonmutant (and therefore tolerant) subline (B10.D2/n), allowed production of an antibody response after immunization with C5 in Freund's complete adjuvant (CFA) (Table 2). Transfer of the cell mixture into an irradiated tolerant (B10.D2/n) mouse also resulted in an antibody response. In this case, the antigenic challenge came from the normal circulating levels of C5 in that mouse, and the response was measured as a decrease in C5 levels 12 days after transfer. This experiment defines a case in which the B cells from a tolerant animal were capable of

TABLE 2. *Some tolerant animals have not undergone B cell–negative selection*

Source of T cells	Source of B cells	Irradiated recipient	Antibody response
Nontolerant	Tolerant	Nontolerant	Yes
Tolerant	Tolerant	Nontolerant	No
Nontolerant	Tolerant	Tolerant	Yes
Tolerant	Tolerant	Tolerant	No

Data are a schematic summary of the experiments in ref. 81.

responding to a physiologic concentration of the self antigen in the presence of T cells from a nontolerant animal.

This series of experiments led many investigators to question whether negative selection existed at all in the B-cell compartment. Yet several lines of evidence suggest that it must exist, at least to some degree. First, immunization to produce xeno- and alloantisera almost always yields antibodies that are specific for the foreign protein and that crossreact poorly if at all with the animal's own protein counterpart (82–84). This is true for cell surface proteins, such as MHC molecules, as well as soluble protein antigens, such as hemoglobin. The absence of antibodies against the self proteins is not simply due to absorption by antigen in the animal, because hybridomas derived from these mice show the same preference for the foreign antigen (84,85). Second, the presence of antigen-binding cells and LPS-elicited IgM antibodies that react with self proteins in *in vitro* assays could be explained by low-affinity interactions that are not functionally relevant, that is, not adequate to lead to activation of the B cell in a physiologic situation. Thus tolerance in the B-cell compartment might affect only high-affinity clones.

Evidence in favor of this point of view comes from the studies of Tsubata et al. (86), who generated a series of IgM-secreting hybridomas making anti–single-stranded DNA antibody. LPS-activated bone marrow pre-B cells and mature splenic B cells from B6 mice yielded a similar percentage of these anti-DNA hybridomas; however, only 2% of the mature B-cell antibodies were of high affinity, while 17% of the pre-B-cell antibodies were of high affinity. These results suggest that some self-reactive cells are purged from the B-cell repertoire during the transition from the pre-B cell to mature B cell stage and that these B cells have, on average, a higher affinity for the antigen. The mechanism(s) of this purging was not clear from these experiments. Addressing this issue required the development of Ig receptor transgenic mice in order to provide an appropriate experimental tool to follow the fate of individual B cells during this transition.

Mechanisms of Negative Selection in the Bone Marrow

The first direct demonstration of negative selection at the B-cell level was made by Nemazee and Bürki (87). They constructed a transgenic mouse expressing an IgM B-cell receptor (BCR) specific for the MHC class I molecules K^k and D^k. On the neutral MHC^d background, 25% to 50% of splenic B cells (B220$^+$, IgM$^+$) expressed this receptor, and IgM antibody of this specificity was expressed in the serum. When crossed to an MHC^k mouse, however, both the peripheral B cells and the antibody disappeared. The site of negative selection appeared to be the bone marrow, as no transgenic receptor–bearing cells were detected in the spleen. In the bone marrow, IgM and receptor idiotype levels were low to undetectable, but B220 expression was normal. This suggested that

the tolerance process might involve the downmodulation (patching, capping, and internalization) of the Ig receptor after antigen encounter. This is consistent with much earlier studies (88,89), which showed that treatment of bone marrow or fetal liver B cells with high concentrations of anti-IgM antibody caused the permanent disappearance of Ig from the surface of the cell.

There is uniform agreement that sufficient engagement of the Ig receptor on immature B cells (B220$^+$, IgD$^-$, CD23$^-$) can lead to a state of maturational arrest (90,91). BCR transgenic bone marrow cells placed in culture with membrane-bound antigen or anti-kappa antibody downregulate their receptors and remain alive. If the cells come from double transgenic animals expressing the BCR and the relevant antigen, then the *in vivo* arrested cells persist in culture in the presence of antigen. Interestingly, they come out of this state in the absence of antigen and differentiate into more mature B cells (B220^{hi}, IgD$^+$, CD23$^+$) (90). Thus, the maturational arrest is reversible.

What is the function of this maturational arrest? Two groups have presented evidence suggesting that the B cells undergo a change in their Ig light chains, a process they call "receptor editing" (91–94). BCR transgenic bone marrow cells arrested at the IgD$^-$, CD23$^-$ stage increase the level of their RAG enzymes and undergo endogenous light-chain gene rearrangements when stimulated with an anti-kappa-chain antibody. Similar results were observed *in vivo* when the BCR transgenic B cells encountered their cognate antigen. Also, immature B cells from normal mice showed an increased percentage of lambda-bearing cells (without undergoing cell division) following stimulation with an anti-kappa antibody. The results suggest that feedback inhibition of light-chain gene rearrangements by a productively rearranged receptor (allelic exclusion) does not take place, and that the immature B cell can modify its receptor by light-chain exchange in order to escape silencing when it encounters self antigens in the bone marrow.

What happens to the B cell if light-chain replacement fails to shift its specificity sufficiently away from autoreactivity? This situation is probably best mimicked by stimulating immature B cells with anti-Ig (88,89). In these studies, removal of the antibody did not reveal reexpression of surface Ig, suggesting that the maturational arrest may be followed by cell death. This was demonstrated directly by Norvell et al. (95), who showed that isolated immature B cells from the bone marrow undergo apoptosis when stimulated with high levels of anti-Ig. This observation is consistent with earlier *in vivo* experiments in which anti-μ antibodies, given to chickens (96) or mice (97) from birth, completely eliminated all B cells in the animal. In the BCR transgenic mice, exposure to the antigen during development also results in a depleted peripheral B-cell pool—at least in early adulthood, before the receptor-editing process has a chance to accumulate sufficient escapees to populate the periphery (87,98). All of these results are consistent with B-cell turnover studies, which have shown that only 10% of the produced B cells ever leave the bone marrow (99). Thus, the bone marrow compartment has two mechanisms for dealing with autoreactive cells: One is a receptor selection process that allows cell survival following encounter with self antigens at an immature stage of development by exchange of light chains; the second is a clonal deletion process by apoptosis, which ensues if the receptor is repeatedly occupied over a sufficient period of time without relief from receptor editing.

Antigen Characteristics Required for Negative Selection of B Cells

Insights into what characteristics of self-reactive B cells and of the autoantigen determine which B cells will be deleted can be inferred from early studies on B cell–tolerance induction to foreign antigens. Using the *in vivo* limiting dilution splenic focus assay to study B-cell tolerance, Metcalf and Klinman (100) first demonstrated that if immature hapten-specific B cells (neonatal spleen or Ig⁻ bone marrow cells) were exposed for 24 hours to the hapten in the absence of T-cell help, they become unresponsive to subsequent stimulation by the hapten in the presence of T-cell help. To induce tolerance in this system, the antigen had to be multivalent. DNP_4 ovalbumin was tolerogenic for DNP-specific B cells, but DNP_1 papain was not. This observation suggests that signaling through the Ig receptor requires cross-linking in order to induce tolerance. Thus the MHC^k class I antigen in the BCR transgenic experiments described earlier, which is a transmembrane glycoprotein and therefore displayed on cell surfaces in a multimeric array, makes an excellent tolerogen. In contrast, when the BCR transgenic was crossed to a different transgenic mouse expressing a soluble form of the MHC K^k molecule, no deletion of the B cells was observed (101). Although it is difficult to compare the levels of Ig receptor occupancy in these two models, the observations suggest that only self antigens that can be presented to the B cell in a multivalent form will be tolerogenic. Consistent with this idea that surface-displayed antigens are good tolerogens is the general finding that many of the natural autoreactive B cells and antibodies are specific for intracellular molecules (76,102,103); only a few have been identified that react with cell surface proteins (104,105). Finally, observations on two more recently described Ig-receptor transgenic mice are also consistent with the idea that B cells specific for cell surface molecules are negatively selected, whereas B cells specific for intracellular polymers are not. A transgenic with an Ig receptor specific for a determinant on the surface of red blood cells negatively selected many of its B cells (106), whereas a transgenic with an Ig receptor specific for single-stranded DNA did not (107). Interestingly, in the latter system, if only an Ig heavy-chain transgenic was created, allowing pairing with multiple light chains to generate both anti–double-stranded and anti–single-stranded DNA antibodies, only B cells with anti–single-stranded DNA reactivity were found (108). The absence of B cells with specificity for double-stranded DNA has been observed in normal mice (109–111) and is possibly caused by the stability of oligonucleosomes released from dying cells (112), which might allow multimeric display of the antigen to developing B cells.

Tolerance to secreted self antigens is a more complex issue. From the *in vitro* experiments of Metcalf and Klinman (100) it is clear that to induce B-cell tolerance, a molecule must not only be multivalent, but also be present at a high enough concentration, and react with the Ig receptor with a high enough affinity. The importance of concentration has been confirmed *in vivo* in a series of transgenic mice that express hen eggwhite lysozyme at different circulating levels (113). When the serum concentration was greater than 10^{-10} M, the animals were tolerant, even if they were immunized in CFA with lysozyme coupled to a foreign carrier to provide T-cell help. The tolerance manifested itself as a markedly decreased plaque-forming cell response consisting only of low-affinity B cells. Below 10^{-10} M, the animals were still tolerant at the T-cell level, but they could now make a normal high-affinity antibody response if given T-cell help. This model of natural tolerance is consistent with the original experiments of Chiller et al. (114), which were done with foreign antigens, and supports the notion that antigen concentration determines the situations in which only the T-cell compartment is unresponsive. Why the thresholds for B- and T-cell negative selection should be different is not understood.

The absolute concentrations required to tolerize a particular set of B cells will obviously vary with the nature of the antigen. In the case of the C5 molecule discussed earlier (81), a circulating antigen concentration of 5×10^{-7} M was not adequate to induce tolerance, whereas in the case of lysozyme, 10^{-10} M was. It should be noted, however, that the actual form of the antigen that induces the tolerance is not necessarily the free protein. For example, some evidence suggests that the tolerogenic form of lysozyme might be molecules bound to a high-molecular-weight serum protein, a modification that presumably gives lysozyme its tolerogenic efficacy by making it multivalent (115). When lysozyme was engineered to be expressed as a membrane-bound protein under the control of an MHC class I promoter, it led to negative selection of B cells in the bone marrow of a lysozyme-specific Ig-receptor transgenic mouse (98). Under these conditions, lysozyme is presented as a multimeric antigen at high local concentrations in the bone marrow.

Immature B Cells Are Not Tolerizable Only

T cells in the thymus presented with antigens on splenic dendritic cells are tolerized, consistent with the predictions of the clonal selection model. In contrast, when immature B cells were exposed to antigen in the presence of T-cell help, they made an antibody response (100,116). In these experiments, surface Ig⁻ bone marrow or neonatal spleen cells were transferred at limiting dilution to keyhole limpet hemocyanin (KLH) carrier–primed irradiated recipients. As the naive B cells matured in splenic focus cultures *in vitro*, presentation of the DNP hapten coupled to KLH led to an IgM antibody response. In contrast, if the hapten were presented on another carrier (DNP-HGG), to which the T cells were not primed, then there was no antibody made to DNP. The antigen was recognized, however, because an initial 24-hour exposure to DNP-HGG prevented the antibody response to DNP-KLH. This showed that the developing immature B cells were tolerized to the hapten in the absence of T-cell help. Thus, the same B cells could be activated or tolerized, depending on the presence of helper T cells.

Consistent with these observations are *in vitro* studies in which immature surface IgM⁺, IgD⁻ bone marrow–derived B cells were stimulated with anti-IgM antibodies (95). When the anti-μ was given alone, the B cells died by apoptosis, but if IL-4 was also added to the cultures, the apoptosis was prevented and the B cells proliferated. IL-4 is one of the known cytokines to participate in T-cell help. At a molecular level, the anti-IgM induced cyclin-dependent kinase (cdk)-4 and its regulatory subunit cyclin D2, which only allowed the cell to go from G0 to G1. With the addition of IL-4, however, the expression of cyclin E and cdk-2 was also induced, and this allowed the cell to transit into the S phase of the cell cycle (117). Thus, these experiments support the idea that tolerizable immature B cells can be rescued by T-cell help.

These observations are inconsistent with the clonal selection ideas proposed by Burnet (8), but they fit nicely with the general model for B-cell activation originally proposed by Bretscher and Cohn (118) (Fig. 3). In an attempt to explain why immune responses require the recognition of two different determinants on the antigen (119) and how the same antigen could both tolerize and immunize when given at different doses (120), Bretscher and Cohn first suggested that antibody forming cells must be tolerizable when stimulated through their antigen-specific receptor (this was referred to as signal one), but activated if they also received a second signal (referred to as signal two). This second signal was also postulated to be antigen-specific, and both antigenic determinants

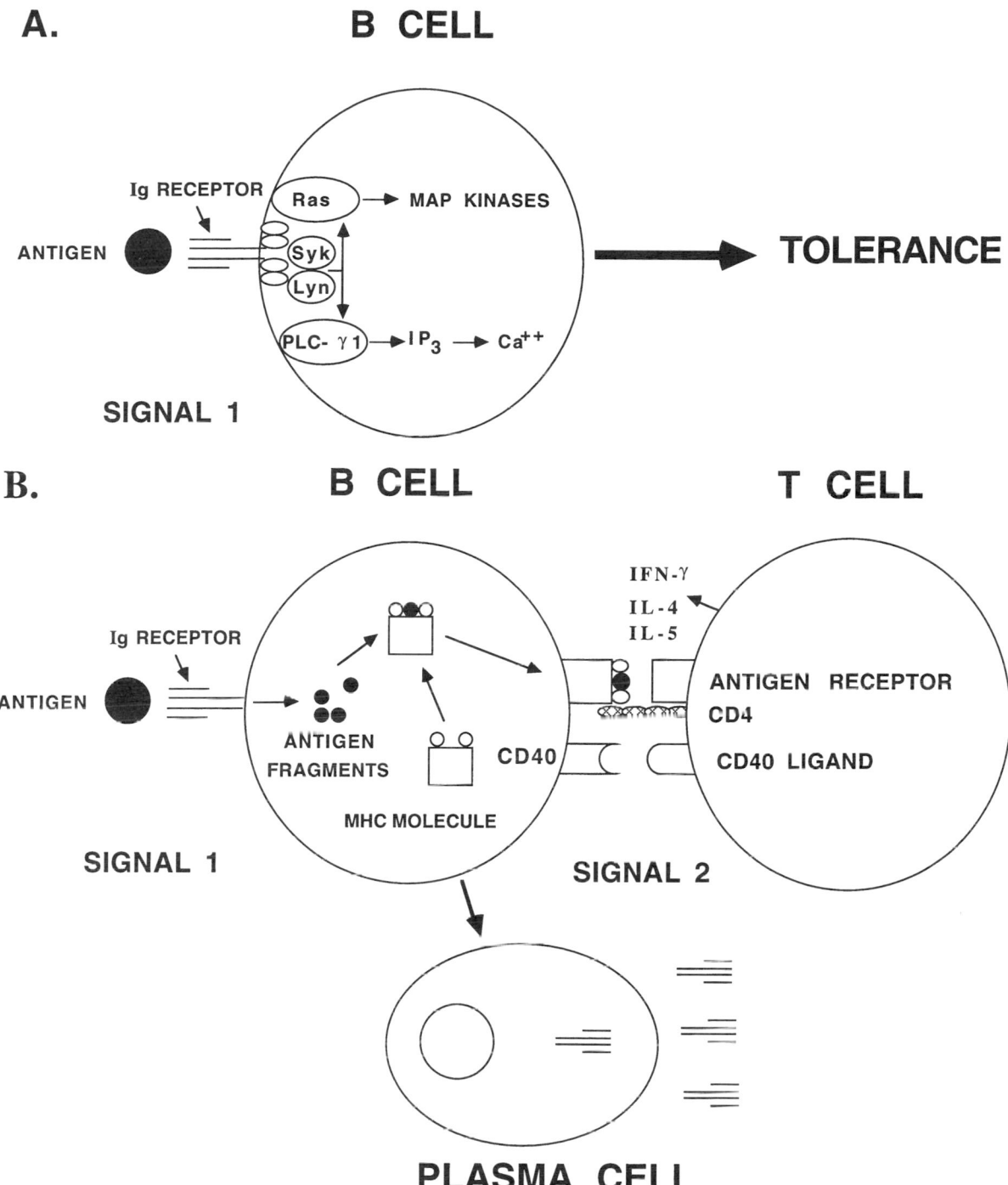

FIG. 3. A modern version of the Bretscher-Cohn two-signal model for B-cell activation. **A:** Antigen binding to the Ig receptor transduces the first signal into the B cell through the tyrosine kinases Syk and Lyn. This leads to activation of the small GTP-binding protein Ras and stimulation of the mitogen-activated protein (MAP) kinases, as well as phosphorylation of phospholipase (PLC)-γ1, which generates inositol-1,4,5-trisphosphate (IP_3) and a rise in intracellular calcium (Ca^{2+}). This signal given alone is proposed to tolerize the cell. **B:** Internalization of the bound Ig receptors brings the antigen into the cell, where it is fragmented by endosomal proteases. Some of the peptides formed bind to MHC class II molecules and are brought back out to the surface for presentation to T cells. Recognition of these peptide–MHC complexes by the T-cell antigen–specific receptor activates the T cell both to express CD40 ligand, which signals the B cell through CD40, and to secrete the lymphokines IL-4 and IL-5 for Th2 cells, or IFN-γ for Th1 cells. When the B cell receives these second signals, it proliferates and some of its progeny differentiate into plasma cells. In this model, signals 1 and 2 must synergize in order to activate the B cell. Signal 2 alone does nothing.

were required to be linked together on the same molecule. In the original model, the second signal was delivered by antibody from another B cell via an antigen bridge. With the subsequent discovery of T-lymphocytes, the second signal became help from T cells specific for the same antigen (see Fig. 3). In today's way of thinking, the B cell binds the antigen via its Ig receptor, which transduces the first signal into the cell via activation of tyrosine kinases, such as syk and lyn. The receptor–antigen complex is then internalized, the antigen processed, and peptide–MHC complexes displayed on the B-cell surface. If T cells exist with receptors that can recognize these peptide–MHC complexes, then the ensuing T cell–B cell interaction provides the second signals in the form of a CD40 ligand–CD40 interaction and the release of stimulatory cytokines such as IL-4 and IL-5 or IFN-γ. In this framework then, antigen stimulation of B cells in the absence of T-cell help leads to tolerance, while stimulation in the presence of antigen-specific T-cell help leads to proliferation and differentiation. Based on the experiments described above, it appears that these rules govern the response to antigens by immature B cells.

NATURAL KILLER CELL TOLERANCE

Natural killer (NK) cells, which arise in both the bone marrow and the thymus, were originally thought to be part of the nonadaptive immune system. Early studies on their role in bone marrow transplant rejection, however, suggested that the cells might have specificity for MHC gene products and that an adaptive tolerance process could take place (121–123) (see Chapter 17). It has taken a long time to gain insight into the workings of this system, but the past few years have produced great progress with the identification and

cloning of many of the receptor molecules involved in the recognition and regulation process (124). Each NK cell has receptors (such as the IL-2 receptor and the F_c receptor) that can activate the cell to kill. In addition, each cell expresses one or more inhibitory receptors, which, if engaged, inhibit the cell from killing. There are two general families of inhibitory receptors, both of which recognize MHC class I molecules. One set belongs to the Ig superfamily and recognizes MHC class I molecules in a nonallelic manner, while the other set belongs to the C-type lectin superfamily and recognizes specific allelic products of MHC class I molecules. Chapter 17 provides a detailed discussion of NK cells and their receptors. Here we are only concerned with how these cells are tolerized.

Several experiments suggest that tolerance in the NK population is mediated by molecular adaptation within the cell rather than by a negative cellular selection process. The first set of experiments involved creating MHC class I transgenic or knock-out mice to vary the level of expression of these proteins, and then examining the mice for their level of expression of the NK inhibitory receptors that are specific for those particular MHC molecules (125–130). The system involving the Ly49A receptor specific for the murine allele D^d is the best characterized. Creation of a B6 transgenic mouse expressing the ligand D^d results in an NK population with cells expressing the Ly49A receptor at low levels. These NK cells kill target cells that lack D^d as well as targets from a β2M knock-out mouse, a mutation that prevents most (but not all) class I MHC expression. When the D^d transgenic was crossed to the β2M knock-out mouse, the expression of D^d decreased dramatically, while the expression of the Ly49A receptors increased (131). The NK cells from this mouse could no longer kill β2M negative targets, although they retained the ability to kill D^d negative targets.

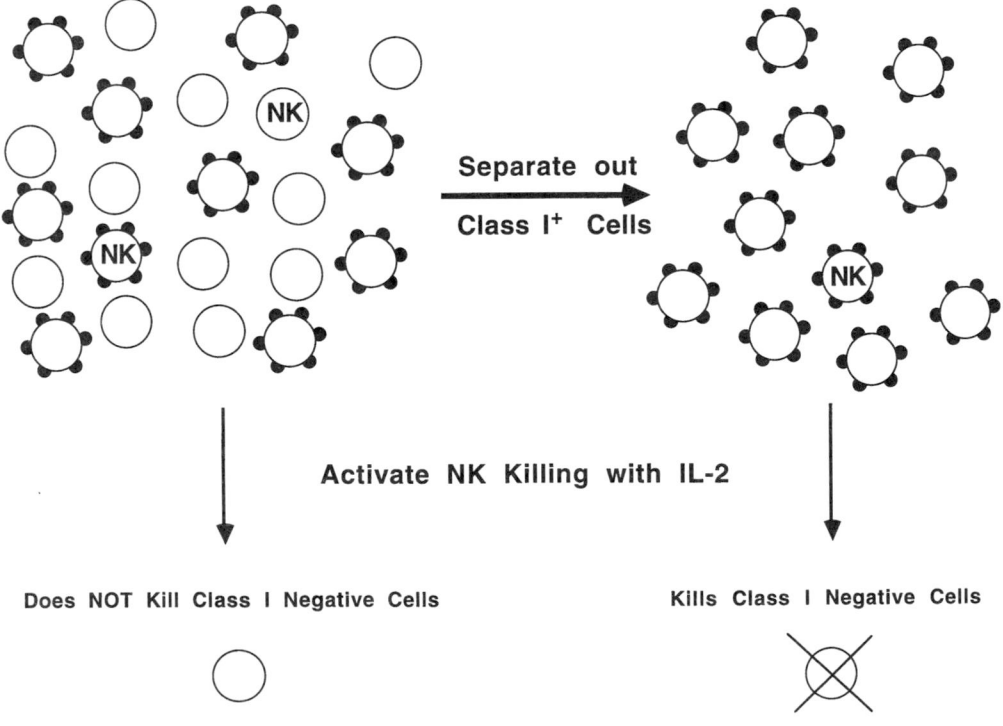

FIG. 4. NK cells from an MHC class I mosaic mouse are adaptable in their ability to kill class I–negative targets. The mosaic mouse contains a mixture of MHC class I–positive and –negative cells of all types, which on activation with IL-2 do not show NK killing activity against class I–negative targets. In contrast, separation of the class I–positive cells followed by activation reveals NK killing of such targets. (This illustration is based on experiments in ref. 133.)

Thus, it appeared from this inverse correlation as if the level of Ly 49A inhibitory receptors were being titrated against the level of D^d. In a different experiment, manipulation of the Ly49A receptor was examined in B6 transgenic mice by expressing it under the control of an MHC class I promoter (132). This places the receptor on all of the NK cells instead of on just 20% of them, as is seen in normal B6 mice. These transgenic mice were found to be tolerant of D^d grafted bone marrow and tumor cells, even though they had not been exposed to D^d during development. Both of these experiments suggest that the distribution and density of inhibitory receptors on NK cells play key roles in the tolerance process.

The second set of experiments took advantage of a mosaic mouse that was created in a transgene experiment attempting to express in B6 mice a D^d/L^d hybrid molecule recognized by Ly49A (133). In one of the founder lines, it was observed that 10% to 80% of the cells in each of the offspring expressed the D^d/L^d molecule at normal levels, while the remaining cells expressed none (Fig. 4). In contrast to the conventional D^d transgenic mouse described above, the NK-cell population from this animal did not kill targets lacking D^d; that is, they were tolerant. Interestingly, if the two NK-cell subtypes (D^d/L^d positive and D^d/L^d negative) in the population were separated and activated independently in culture with IL-2, the D^d/L^d-positive cells acquired the ability to kill D^d-negative targets. In contrast, if the cells were stimulated as a mixture, no killing ability was gained. These results suggest that NK cells capable of killing D^d targets had not been previously eliminated from this population by a clonal deletion process. Rather, the cells had somehow adjusted to their surroundings and were capable of readjusting.

Overall, these observations suggest that NK cells adapt to their environment (become tolerant), possibly by adjusting their inhibitory receptor levels (and probably other molecules) to prevent them from destroying neighboring cells in the host. Knowing how they learn in a mosaic animal to functionally adjust to the level of the lowest MHC class I–expressing cells will be critical to our understanding of how this tolerance process works. The mechanism appears to be more complicated than CD8 downmodulation in T cells or receptor editing in B cells. Nonetheless, from a tolerance point of view, all of these mechanisms could be viewed as receptor modulation, a form of adaptation that is functionally distinct from the cellular deletion process envisioned in the original clonal selection theory.

TOLERANCE TO PERIPHERAL ANTIGENS

At the completion of development, T and B cells emerge from the primary lymphoid organs and enter the recirculating pool of peripheral lymphocytes. One of the first things these naive cells encounter in their fully mature state are antigens from various nonlymphoid organs that are not expressed in the thymus. In this section, we will discuss whether these antigens are recognized by the immune system, whether the antigens are only expressed in the peripheral tissues, and whether the immune system is tolerant to them.

Tissue-specific Peptide Antigens

When Medawar was asked if he could distinguish dizygotic from monozygotic bovine twins, he was certain this could be done by skin grafting; however, when Anderson et al, (134) attempted to test this, they found that most of the time (7/8), skin grafts exchanged between dizygotic twins were not rejected. This surprising result led Medawar to conclude that skin does not contain any unique trans-

TABLE 3. *Tissue-specific antigens in mice*

Donor Cells			
BM and spleen	Epidermal	X-rayed host	Rejection of A-strain skin graft
$(A \times B6)F_1$	None	B6	43% at 100 days
$(A \times B6)F_1$	A 5×10^6 ip at days 0, 50, 85	B6	0% at 100 days 63% at 300 days

Bone marrow (BM) and spleen cells from $(A \times B)F1$ mice were injected into lethally irradiated B6 mice with or without injection of A epidermal cells Strain-A skin grafts were performed and monitored for rejection.

plantation antigens, that is, none other than those found on the hematopoietic cells for which the twins were chimeric (6). Thus, the concept emerged that blood cells tolerize for all tissues.

The first challenge to this intellectual framework came from the studies of Billingham and Brent (135) on neonatal tolerance in mice. They found that B6 newborns injected with A spleen cells were not tolerant of A skin grafts. Boyse et al. (136) corroborated this finding in radiation-induced $(A \times B6)F_1 \rightarrow B6$ bone marrow chimeras, where they were able to show that the recipient contained $(A \times B6)F_1$ hematopoietic cells but still rejected A skin (Table 3). Tolerance could be induced, however, if A-strain epidermal cells were injected along with the F_1 bone marrow (137). They concluded that there must be a skin-specific transplantation antigen (Sk) expressed by A and not by B6 mice. Subsequent studies showed that two genes controlled the expression of this antigen(s) (138) and that Sk antigens could be identified in other strain combinations (139). These studies thus appeared at odds with the original Medawar results.

A resolution of the contradiction was achieved by Emery and McCullagh (140). They repeated the experiments of Anderson et al. with a small technical modification. In the original experiments, skin grafts were prepared from the ears of the donor and placed on the back (whithers) of the recipient. Instead, Emery and McCullagh exchanged flank skin grafts. In this case, all dizygotic twins rejected their sib's graft. Repeating the technique of Anderson et al., they confirmed that many animals did not reject under these conditions (in their hands, 50%). Thus, cattle also have skin-specific antigens.

The failure to elicit a rejection with ear skin grafts most likely relates to the "strength" of antigen presentation (e.g., the density of Langerhans' cells), which has been shown in mice to vary in different areas of skin (141). Although Anderson et al. demonstrated that their ear skin grafts were antigenic across a complete MHC genetic disparity (i.e., outbred cattle), differences in skin-specific antigens between dizygotic twins is a situation in which the two immune systems are tolerant to all processed peptides derived from proteins of hematopoietic cells, but not to peptides derived from proteins unique to the skin. In the cases in which the gene encoding a skin protein exists in two allelic forms, the potential exists for peptides to be expressed by the graft tissue that are not present in the host's skin. To elicit an immune response, such peptides have to be able to bind (one each) to the MHC class I and class II molecules, perhaps explaining why two genes "control" the expression of the Sk antigen. These three constraints—(a) requirement for allelic polymorphism, (b) requirement for peptide binding to MHC molecules (Ir gene control), and (c) tolerance to minor histocompatibility antigens that are also expressed by hematopoietic cells—explain why not all mouse-strain combinations reveal an immune response to skin-specific antigens. Outbred animals, such as cattle, however, should show this reactivity more frequently because of greater diversity in the genes encoding their skin-specific proteins.

The concept of tissue-specific antigens is not unique to skin. The experiment of Triplett (9), demonstrating that immunologic tolerance is an acquired state, showed that frog pituitary also expresses tissue-specific antigens. Because an attempt to confirm that study for pituitary, thyroid, and eye in other species of frog failed (142), McCullagh (143) readdressed the issue using the thyroid of fetal lambs. At 54 days of gestation, the lamb's immune system has not yet developed and the animal will accept allografts of adult skin. When the thyroid gland was removed at that time, implanted into a nude mouse for 5 to 9 weeks, and then reimplanted subcutaneously into the same lamb, autoimmune thyroiditis developed. Partial thyroidectomized lambs did not get the disease, which argues that the immune response was specific for thyroid antigens and not any xenogeneic mouse tissue. These observations demonstrate that the immune system normally learns to become tolerant of other self tissues and that it has mechanisms for dealing with the problem of tolerance to antigens that are only synthesized in peripheral nonlymphoid tissues.

Can Delivery of Antigens to the Thymus Account for Peripheral Tolerance?

The existence of tissue-specific antigens creates a problem for the immune system, because the primary mechanism for induction of tolerance in the T-cell compartment is by clonal deletion in the thymus. One possible solution to this problem is for these antigens to also be expressed in the thymus. For example, myelin basic protein, a constituent of the myelin sheath made by oligodendrocytes in the brain, is also expressed at low levels in the embryonic thymus (144). Other antigens, such as glutamic acid decarboxylase (GAD) from the β cells of the pancreas, have not been found there, even with reverse-transcriptase polymerase chain reaction (RT-PCR) technology. In addition, certain self antigens may only appear after the immune system is fully developed, for example, in breast tissue at the onset of puberty.

Another possible solution is that all molecules not expressed in the thymus are brought there. It has been speculated that dendritic cells could pick up peripheral antigens and bring them back to the thymus for tolerance induction (32). However, veiled dendritic cells (activated Langerhans' cells migrating from tissues to lymph nodes) are found only in afferent lymph (145) and have never been demonstrated to migrate to the thymus. Finally, it is possible that circulating proteins and their fragments derived from the turnover of peripheral tissues could travel to the medulla of the thymus. It has been shown that exogenous antigens injected intravenously can be processed by thymic dendritic cells and presented on MHC class II molecules in a form that stimulates T-cell clones to proliferate (146). For peptides presented by MHC class I molecules, however, which largely derive from cytoplasmic proteins, this pathway would be far less efficient at providing peripheral antigens for tolerance induction. Nonetheless, experiments were done to test the idea of movement of peripheral antigens to the thymus by expressing MHC class I and II molecules in peripheral tissues, using tissue-specific promoters. In contrast to soluble proteins, these MHC molecules must remain intact in order to present their tissue-specific peptides. Thus, if processed by dendritic cells for presentation in the thymus, they would not tolerize T cells that are specific for the peptide–MHC complexes expressed in the peripheral tissue.

The first transgenic model of this type expressed the MHC class II E molecule either in β cells of the pancreas under the control of the rat insulin promoter (147) or in acinar cells of the pancreas under the control of the elastase promotor (148). These animals were tolerant of the E molecule in an MLR, although they failed to delete certain Vβ-expressing T cells that are normally deleted when this E molecule is expressed in the thymus. Some of the cells expressing those Vβ were unresponsive when stimulated in culture with anti-Vβ antibodies immobilized on a plate (149). The possibility that the tolerance was induced by low-level expression of the E molecule in the thymus was eliminated with nontransgenic thymus grafts into adult thymectomized, lethally irradiated and bone marrow–reconstituted (AT×BM) transgenic mice (148). Under these conditions, the T cells mature in a thymic environment that does not endogenously express the transgene. These mice were also tolerant, which argues in favor of a peripheral tolerance mechanism. Subsequent experiments with A-molecule transgenics expressed in the same tissue under either the insulin (150,151) or elastase (152) promoter gave a slightly different result. These mice were not tolerant in a mixed lymphocyte culture, but they did not reject the tissue. The most likely explanation for these observations is that the tolerance was specific only for peptides presented by the beta or acinar cells. Consistent with this hypothesis is the observation that injection of allogeneic spleen cells (the APC in the MLR) into the transgenic mouse did not induce tissue rejection (150).

A similar series of experiments have been done with class I MHC molecules expressed in a variety of peripheral tissues. Morahan et al. (153) used a transgenic mouse expressing the class I molecule K^b under the control of the zinc-inducible metallothionein promoter, which allowed the protein to be expressed in the liver, kidney, and exocrine pancreas. The transgenic mice appeared tolerant to K^b, even after induction with zinc, immunization with K^b-expressing splenocytes, or treatment with cyclophosphamide or exogenous interleukins. The mice also did not reject K^b-expressing skin grafts. Nonetheless, CTLs specific for K^b could be generated in vitro. In another model (154,155) the nonclassical class Ib MHC molecule Q10 was utilized. This molecule is synthesized exclusively in the liver as a secreted protein. A transgenic mouse was constructed in which the α3, transmembrane, and cytoplasmic domains of a classical class I MHC molecule, L^d, were attached to the α1 and α2 domains of Q10 to create a membrane-bound hybrid MHC class I molecule (Q10/L) that was only expressed in the liver. The transgenic mice showed no evidence of hepatic inflammation, even if immunized with spleen cells expressing L^d. Surprisingly, these same spleen cells could stimulate a CTL response in vitro, and the responding transgenic killer cells showed cross-reactive lysis against targets expressing the hybrid Q10/L molecule. The magnitude of this CTL response, however, was significantly lower than that obtained from nontransgenic mice, and in vivo immunization failed to elicit the cross-reactive CTLs. Thus, a critical subset of anti-Q10/L CTL precursors appeared to be tolerant in vivo. Transfer of the T cells to sublethally irradiated, thymectomized, nontransgenic recipients for 3 weeks failed to reverse the diminished CTL response assayed in vitro. This suggested that the tolerance was not due to a reversible process and might involve deletion. Overall, these results demonstrate that T-lymphocytes emerging from the thymus can encounter peptide–MHC complexes in the peripheral tissues for the first time and be rendered tolerant.

B-Cell Peripheral Tolerance

B-cell tolerance to peripheral antigens also has been examined with a receptor transgenic mouse specific for the K^b MHC class I molecule (156). This BCR transgenic mouse was crossed to an MHC transgenic mouse expressing K^b in the liver, pancreas, and kidney, under the control of a metallothionein promoter (153). The double transgenic offspring had only a few transgenic receptor–positive B cells in the spleen and lymph node, although there were large numbers in the bone marrow. Because the number of $B220^+$ cells was also greatly reduced in the peripheral lymphoid tissues and because no mRNA encoding the transgenic receptor could be detected, it was concluded that the B cells had been deleted. Thus, B-cell recognition of K^b in certain peripheral tissues, even with very low affinity in this particular case, resulted in tolerance.

The mechanism of this tolerance is most easily explained by the Bretscher and Cohn model. Because the T cells are tolerized to K^b (as discussed above), the B cells would encounter K^b in the absence of T-cell help, thus receiving signal 1 in the absence of signal 2. Not all investigators, however, accept this model for tolerance induction of mature B cells, as will be detailed in the following sections.

TOLERANCE INDUCTION IN MATURE B CELLS: MECHANISMS

The ability of both mature T- and B-cell populations to become tolerant to peripheral self antigens suggests that similar mechanisms must exist for inducing tolerance to foreign antigens. The earliest work in this area was performed by Felton and colleagues (157). They studied the immunogenicity of polysaccharides from *Pneumococcus pneumoniae* and found that doses of 0.5 mg paralyzed the immune system such that subsequent infection with the bacterium often led to death of the animal. The major immunologic effect appeared to be an inhibition of the antibody response to an optimal dose (0.5 µg) of the polysaccharide. This paralysis was specific for the particular polysaccharide used, was induced in adult animals, and lasted for a long time, presumably because of the poor degradability of the molecules. Although Felton was sure that the effect was on antibody-forming cells, it was difficult at the time to rule out a masking of the antibody response by adsorption on the persisting antigen.

In the 1950s, a number of investigators extended these observations to protein antigens by showing that high doses of protein would paralyze the immune system and prevent it from making an antibody response to a subsequent immunogenic dose of the antigen (158,159). Because this tolerance induction was rapid, it was assumed to be a direct effect on mature lymphoid cells. These experiments reinforced the paradoxical notion that antigens could both activate and inactivate the immune system, depending on the administered dose (120). A critical experiment, which first pointed toward a way out of this paradox by having more than one signal be required to activate a lymphocyte, was performed by Dresser (159). He discovered that protein antigens could be tolerogenic in adult animals in reasonably low doses, if the preparation were spun in an ultracentrifuge to remove protein aggregates prior to injection (Table 4). Interestingly, this same preparation was immunogenic if administered in CFA. Dresser concluded that paralysis ensued when lymphocytes recognized the deaggregated antigen alone, but that if this were accompanied by a second component, which he termed *adjuvanticity*, then an antibody response was made. Adjuvanticity could have simply been reaggregation of the antigen or

TABLE 4. *First evidence for a two-signal model in which the second signal is not antigen-specific*

Form of the first antigen	Form of the second antigen	Antibody response
Aggregated	None	Yes
Deaggregated	None	No
Deaggregated	Aggregated	No
Deaggregated plus adjuvant	None	Yes

When injected alone, deaggregated antigens induce tolerance, but when injected in adjuvant, they induce immunity.

mediated by the mycobacterial components in the adjuvant. Presciently, Frei et al. (160) interpreted adjuvanticity as stimulation of antigen uptake by macrophages, which then converted the antigen to an immunogenic form. Unfortunately, the molecular ideas at the time (that the immunogenic form was antigen bound to RNA) did not turn out to be correct, and the macrophage activation idea was generally abandoned.

Subsequently, the Bretscher and Cohn model (see Fig.3) was proposed to explain the antigen dose paradox as well as the requirement for two antigenic determinants to stimulate an immune response (hapten-carrier–linked recognition). It also helped to explain how mature B cells could somatically mutate to increase the affinity of their Ig receptors without endangering the host by generating anti-self receptors. If only the BCR acquired an anti-self receptor and the T cell did not, then the B cell would be inactivated by receiving signal 1 alone. Support for their model initially came from the experiments of Havas (161) and Golan and Borel (162). They immunized mice with the hapten DNP coupled to the self protein mouse IgG and found that the animals became tolerant to the hapten; that is, they failed to make an antibody response to the hapten when subsequently immunized with it coupled to a foreign protein carrier. Katz and colleagues (163–165) (in an extension of the polysaccharide experiments of Felton) used hapten coupled to poorly degradable synthetic D amino acid copolymers and showed that guinea pig B cells were directly affected, even if they had been primed. Also, the degradable L form of the copolymer could induce tolerance to the hapten if given to a strain of guinea pig that was a T-cell nonresponder to the carrier. In each of these cases, the antigen used was not immunogenic for T cells because the animal either was tolerant to the carrier protein (mouse Ig) or could not recognize it because of problems in antigen processing (D copolymer) and/or MHC molecule binding (copolymer peptides). Thus, the absence of T-cell help elicited by the second antigenic determinant (signal 2) resulted in tolerance.

Receptor Blockade

Initially, it was thought that the B-cell unresponsiveness induced in these models might be due to receptor blockade by poorly degradable antigens that were stuck to the B-cell surface. Diener and Paetkau (166) were the first to discover that antigen given to adult animals in tolerogenic doses could persist on the surface of lymphocytes. Such cells with bound antigen were also observed in the hapten IgG model of Aldo-Benson and Borel (167). Only tolerogenic conjugates such as $DNP_{12} IgG_1$ produced these cells, not closely related nontolerogenic conjugates such as $DNP_{52} IgG_3$. At high doses of tolerogen, the cells persisted for weeks, as did the tolerance, and when the tolerance waned, the cell-bound antigen was no longer detected. Culturing the cells *in vitro* allowed the antigen to be shed and the tolerance to disappear on adoptive transfer (168,169).

Physical properties of the antigen, such as size (170–172) and hapten density (173), were shown to be important variables in receptor blockade. In a rigorous series of experiments, Dintzis et al. (174,175) made linear polymers of acrylamide of various lengths, coupled with haptens at various densities, and found that large polymers with high hapten density were immunogenic, whereas small polymers with low hapten density were not. The latter, however, could block activation by the former. These results were interpreted as the need for BCRs to be clustered into complexes of ten to 15 receptors each in order to signal the cell. The small polymers with low hapten density could not achieve this configuration, but they were able to tie up receptors in nonproductive complexes and therefore block activation by the larger polymers. This model provides one molecular mechanism for a receptor blockade.

Another mechanism emerged from the comparison of DNP_{12} IgG_1 with DNP_{52} IgG_3. The class of antibody turned out to be the critical variable in determining the outcome (176). TNP_{11} IgG_1 induced tolerance, while $TNP_{11}IgG_3$ was immunogenic. Furthermore, removal of the Fc portion of the antibody from human gamma-globulin to make $TNP_{10}F(ab')_2$ created an immunogen out of a tolerogen. These results suggested that engagement of the Fc receptor on B cells might be responsible for the tolerance (177). More recent studies have shown that signaling through the BCR can be inhibited if Fc receptors are simultaneously engaged in the the same complex, most typically brought about by the binding of antigen–antibody complexes (178).

Early studies had demonstrated that some forms of tolerance induced in adult B cells could be reversed by trypsination of the cells to remove bound antigen and the receptors, followed by receptor reexpression (179). Unresponsiveness in these cases was likely to be caused by receptor blockade without signaling. Tolerance induced by other antigens, however, could not be reversed by simply removing the surface molecules, indicating a requirement for active metabolic processes during induction (180). For example, the D copolymers induced unresponsiveness at 37°C, even if the B cells were subsequently trypsinized to clear the bound Ig receptors from the cell surface. In contrast, exposure of the cells to antigen at 4°C did not induce tolerance. The low temperature presumably prevented the necessary signaling to the cell required for tolerance. Even this tolerant state, however, was subsequently reported to be reversible in the splenic focus assay following extensive washing and exposure to excess T-cell help (181). In several other systems, stimulation with mitogens such as LPS was also reported to reverse B-cell tolerance (182,183). These observations suggested that there might exist a stable but reversible unresponsive state for mature B cells.

B-Cell Anergy and Death

Not all models of B-cell tolerance in adults revealed receptor blockade, although the B cells were still unresponsive to antigen (169,183,184). Because the total number of B cells capable of binding labeled antigen was not diminished, the tolerant state was referred to as clonal anergy rather than clonal deletion or abortion (184). This was difficult to prove, however, because in a normal mouse, only 1% to 3% of the antigen-binding cells (assayed at limiting dilution) were responsive to antigen or produced specific antibodies when stimulated with LPS. Thus, a small fraction of functionally important cells could have been deleted, but their absence may not have been detected amid the mass of low-affinity antigen-binding cells. Subsequent limiting dilution experiments, with a more

potent mitogenic mixture of dextran sulfate and LPS as a stimulant, revealed that some tolerized B cells could be stimulated to differentiate into antibody-forming cells when the BCR was bypassed (183). This reversal suggested that at least a portion of the cells had been rendered functionally unresponsive (anergized) rather than deleted.

A much clearer picture of the nature of B-cell anergy became possible with the introduction of BCR transgenic mice (185). A transgenic animal was created, expressing on its B cells a high-affinity receptor (both IgM and IgD) specific for hen eggwhite lysozyme. About 90% of the B cells in this mouse expressed the transgenic receptor. When this BCR transgenic was crossed with a second transgenic mouse constitutively expressing the lysozyme antigen, the double transgenic offspring still expressed large numbers of transgenic, lysozyme-binding B cells in their spleens and lymph nodes. On immunization with lysozyme, these B cells failed to make an antibody or plaque-forming cell response. Because the failure to respond could have been caused by tolerance at the level of the T cells, spleen cells from these animals were transferred to irradiated nontransgenic recipients along with spleen cells from mice primed to horse or sheep red blood cells (RBCs) as a source of T-cell help. The recipients were then boosted with lysozyme–RBC conjugates. Compared with control BCR transgenics, the B cells from double transgenics made a ten- to 100-fold lower plaque-forming cell response. Thus, although the B cells had not been deleted, they appeared to be functionally hyporesponsive. Such an intrinsic, functionally unresponsive state has become the definition of *anergy*.

The most striking characteristic of this anergic state was a 90% reduction of IgM on the surface of the B cells, resulting from a block in IgM transport from the endoplasmic reticulum to the Golgi (186). IgD levels were normal, as were other surface markers, such as B220 and J11d. The cells were also still capable of binding lysozyme and, the antigen could be detected on the surface of B220$^+$ cells freshly isolated from both the bone marrow and the spleen, giving the appearance of receptor blockade. Interestingly, when the BCR transgenic was crossed to a different lysozyme transgenic, which expressed tenfold lower levels of circulating antigen, the B cells were found not to be tolerant, and no decrease in surface IgM was noted (187). If these animals were fed zinc in their drinking water, induction of the metallothionein promoter of the lysozyme transgene enhanced the circulating concentrations of lysozyme by 70-fold over a 4-day period. During this time, membrane IgM gradually decreased on the surface of all the transgenic BCR–bearing B cells, eventually reaching the low levels found in the initial double transgenic mice described above. These cells appeared to have been tolerized, as they failed to respond well to lysozyme–RBC conjugates when adoptively transferred into irradiated mice along with horse RBC–primed helper T cells. Similar results were observed when B cells from the Ig-receptor transgenic mice were transferred into a lysozyme transgenic mouse expressing high levels of circulating antigen. Thus, the anergic state could be induced in mature adult B cells within 4 days.

The block in anergic B-cell activation appears to be entirely at the level of the Ig receptor, as activation for proliferation through CD40 or by LPS is unaffected in the absence of antigen (188,189). The Ig-signaling block impairs the normal upregulation of the B7 costimulatory molecules (190). Biochemically, the block is at the earliest events in signal transduction, as tyrosine kinase activation is greatly reduced (191). This results in diminished calcium oscillations and a failure to activate the transcription factor NF-κB as well as the Jun N-terminal kinase (JNK) pathway (192). In contrast, activation of the NF-AT transcription factor and stimulation through the extracellular–signal regulated kinase (ERK) pathway is normal.

The anergic state can be reversed in culture by stimulation with LPS (189). The B cells fully reexpress surface IgM by 2 days, and after 3 days their antibody production increases. Interestingly, if antigen was included in the culture along with LPS, the B cells' ability to secrete antibody remained inhibited, even though they proliferated just as well during the treatment. This suggests that BCR occupancy by antigen is the critical signal for maintaining the state as well as inducing it.

The fate of anergic B cells *in vivo* was examined by bromodeoxyuridine-labeling studies to determine the turnover of the cells (193). In contrast to normal mature B cells, which have a half-life of 4 to 5 weeks, anergic B cells were found to last for only 3 to 4 days. The rate of entry of B cells into the mature pool was similar for the two groups, suggesting that anergic B cells died more quickly. This result, however, occurred only in the presence of antigen. If the anergic B cells were adoptively transferred into irradiated, antigen-free recipients, the cells survived as long as normal B cells (189,194). Interestingly, their IgM levels returned to normal after 5 to 10 days, but when challenged with antigen, they still did not respond. Thus, decreased IgM serves as a marker for anergic cells, but it is not an essential component of the unresponsiveness.

Surprisingly, the fate of these anergic cells in response to antigen and T-cell help turned out to be cell death (195) (Fig. 5). Nontolerant B cells from the BCR single transgenic mice proliferated and made antibodies against lysozyme when stimulated with antigen in the presence of CD4+ T cells from a lysozyme-specific TCR transgenic. In contrast, if the B cells came from a double transgenic, where they had been exposed from early development to sol-

uble circulating lysozyme, these anergic B cells underwent cell death by apoptosis in response to the same stimulus. Death was prevented on a CD95-deficient (lpr) background, suggesting that the Fas/Fas ligand pathway was essential for the killing. Subsequent studies demonstrated that the CD40 receptor also had to be engaged in order to get cell death, as signaling through CD40 was required to upregulate Fas expression on anergic B cells (196) (see Fig. 5). Normal transgenic B cells did not die under the same circumstances and in fact required both CD40 ligation and FAS expression for optimal clonal expansion and antibody production. If BCR occupancy by antigen was bypassed, by pulsing the B cells with the peptide recognized by T cells, then even nontolerized B cells were killed. Thus, signaling through the BCR is critical for determining the outcome of helper T cell–B cell interactions, and, presumably, anergic B cells die because of their block in BCR signaling.

These results suggest that for mature B cells, signal 2 alone (as might occur in certain bystander situations) is tolerogenic. This is still consistent with the original Bretscher and Cohn model, which only predicted that signals 1 and 2 were both required for activation, but never made any prediction about signal 2 alone. Overall, it would appear that B-cell anergy is a transient state that normally leads to death of the B cell by persistent receptor occupancy in the absence of T-cell help. The receptor blockade experiments, however, suggest that if the antigen is removed soon enough (certainly within the first 24 hours) and T-cell help is provided, the B cells can be rescued from death and instead activated. Whether a fully anergic B cell can be rescued for a useful purpose by any physiologic signals akin to LPS remains to be determined.

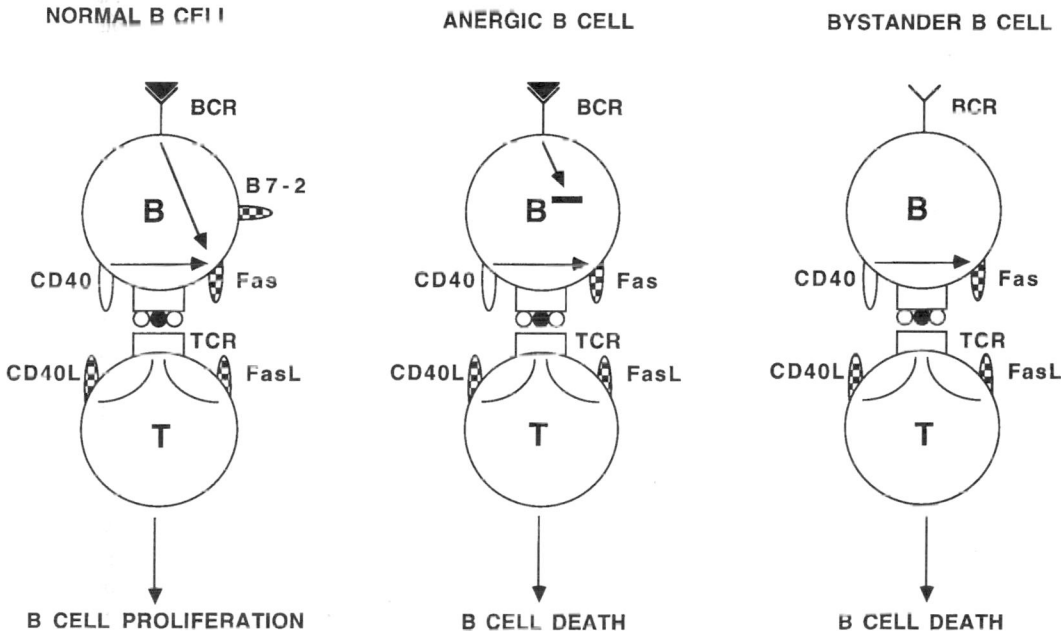

FIG. 5. The outcome of B-cell activation, proliferation or death, is determined by BCR signaling during or prior to T-cell help. B-cell presentation of antigen to T cells leads to expression of CD40 ligand and Fas ligand by the T cell. CD40L then stimulates the B cell through CD40 to express Fas and B7-2, which then allows the B cell to be signaled by FasL. In the presence of antigen signaling through the BCR, the Fas signal synergizes with the CD40 signal to enhance B-cell proliferation. In contrast, in the absence of an antigen-specific signal (bystander B cell), or if this signal is blocked (anergic B cell), the outcome of Fas signaling is apoptotic cell death, possibly because B7 is not induced. The *checkered symbols* represent molecules whose expression is induced. (This figure is based on experiments in ref. 196.)

Memory B Cells

Once a B cell has been activated and divides, some of its progeny terminally differentiate into antibody-forming cells and die (197). This process is retarded in *lpr* and *gld* mice because of genetic defects in the Fas or Fas ligand molecules required for cell death (198). These mice get an antibody-mediated autoimmune disease similar to lupus erythematosis in humans (199). B-cell death is also impaired in bcl-2 transgenic lines of mice, which express the bcl-2 protein at high levels in the B-cell lineage (200). These mice get B-cell lymphomas (201) as well as autoimmunity (202). Based on these indirect experiments, it is assumed that apoptotic cell death is a normal part of the B-cell response to foreign antigens and that this is, at least in part, Fas/FasL mediated. The observations also suggest that Fas-dependent death helps maintain self-tolerance by deleting peripheral B cells that have generated autoreactive receptors.

A fraction of the activated B cells also migrate to germinal centers, where they undergo the process of somatic hypermutation (203). There may also exist an independent subset of HSA^{lo} B cells that migrates into the germinal center (204). In both cases, these B cells first remove the BCR from their surface, undergo several rounds of division, and then reexpress mutated Ig receptors (205). The cells then undergo a negative selection process similar to immature B cells. The antigen is provided from antigen–antibody complexes on follicular dendritic cells (206). Survival requires the receptor to be of high enough affinity to out-compete the already circulating antibody and allow B-cell uptake and processing of antigen for display of peptides to primed helper T cells (203), which have also moved into the germinal centers (207). If the B cell receives T-cell help, it survives and is stimulated to undergo another round of expansion and differentiation. If T-cell help is not received, the B cells can become anergized or die by apoptosis (208,209). Apoptotic cell death was demonstrated by giving large amounts of soluble antigen at the time of optimal germinal center formation. The antigen was either selected to lack the critical T-cell determinant required for help or deaggregated by ultracentrifugation (in the manner of Dresser) to reduce APC processing for T-cell activation. In each case, the high-affinity B cells, located in both the germinal centers and the nearby lymphoid zones rich in T cells, underwent apoptosis rather than the affinity maturation seen with T-cell help. Thus, as for immature B cells, signaling of mature B cells in the absence of T-cell help resulted in tolerization, consistent with the Bretscher and Cohn model.

Thymic-independent Antigens

All of the experiments described so far suggest that activation and tolerance of mature B cells follow the general scheme of Bretscher and Cohn. There exists, however, a class of antigens that appear to be able to elicit antibody responses in a T cell–independent (TI) manner (210). They are divided into two categories. TI-1 antigens represent haptens coupled to B-cell mitogens such as LPS (211). LPS bypasses the need for T-cell help and fully activates B cells to proliferate and differentiate into antibody-forming cells, including Ig class switching. Under limiting conditions, TI-1 antigens can be targeted to specific B cells via high-affinity binding to Ig receptors that are specific for the hapten. Presumably, the response to TI-1 antigens represents a special adaptation to bypass the need for T-cell help in the face of unique bacterial products that signal signs of infection.

The TI-2 antigens represent a more puzzling class of molecules (212). These are not mitogenic for B cells and consist of large-mol-ecular-weight polymers such as polysaccharides composed of repeating antigenic determinants (175,213). They are usually poorly degradable and often capable of activating complement via the alternative pathway (214). They mostly stimulate mature B cells and often do not elicit responses in neonates or CBA/N mice (215) [which have a genetic defect (*xid*) in their *btk* kinase]. Several models have been put forth to explain how these antigens work. First, B cells primed to environmental antigens may already be in an activated state (216). Such "large" B cells, already in the G1 phase of the cell cycle, may read out Ig receptor occupancy by TI-2 antigens as a positive rather than a negative signal. Second, when the B cell is resting in Go, factors in addition to the TI-2 antigen are often required to get a response. For example, cytokines from T cells, such as IL-2 and IL-5, augment secretory responses to TI-2 antigens (217) and prevent B-cell clonal deletion in certain model systems (218). Complement components such as C3d, which are activated by some TI-2 antigens, can bind to CR2 (CD21) receptors on B cells and greatly enhance antibody responses by lowering the threshold for signaling through the Ig receptor (219). Even cytokines produced by the B cells themselves may play a role if the antigen stimulates their production. For example, TNFα production by B cells has been shown to be involved in the B-cell proliferation stimulated by anti-Ig (220). Finally, IL-2–activated NK cells have been shown to augment Ig secretion induced by TI-2 antigens by an unkown mechanism (221).

A third possibility is that the repetitive array of antigenic determinants on TI-2 antigens engages the B-cell Ig receptor in a unique way, which signals for activation instead of anergy or cell death. In the immune response to vesicular stomatitis virus (VSV), the early IgM-neutralizing antibody to the glycoprotein (G) on the virus was elicited in a T helper cell–independent manner. In contrast, immunization with VSV-G–infected cells, which do not present an ordered lattice structure of the protein, led to an antibody response that was largely T cell–dependent (222). A search for cryptic second signals brought in by the viral particle failed to reveal any polyclonal B-cell stimulation, involvement of complement or TNF molecules, or activation of NK cells (223). Thus, the authors concluded that the rigid paracrystalline structure of the virus particle, with its determinant spacing of 5 to 10 nm, could activate rather than tolerize the B cell.

A final possibility is that the responding B cells represent a discrete subpopulaton of cells that does not follow the Bretscher-Cohn rules. The response to some TI-2 antigens has been localized to the marginal zone in the spleen, where the responding B cells are CD23$^-$, IgM^{bright}, IgD ^{dull} (224). This is the surface phenotype of the B-1 (CD5$^+$) B-cell subpopulation (225). These cells are absent in the CBA/N mouse, which fails to respond to TI-2 antigens. Also, B-1 cells are largely responsible for the low-affinity IgM autoreactive antibodies in normal mice and humans (discussed earlier). This subset is resistant to tolerization by anti-Ig *in vitro* (226) and may not need to be under two-signal control because the B cells do not undergo somatic hypermutation (227). Unfortunately, purified B-1 cells do not respond to the TI-2 antigen TNP-Ficoll in tissue culture (228), suggesting that maybe one or more of the other properties mentioned above is also required for their response.

Overall, the results suggest that the B-cell immune system does have way(s) to respond directly to certain special antigens in the absence of cognate T-cell help. Preservation of this direct and perhaps more primitive type of immune response suggests that it is still necessary sometimes to make a quick antibody response (probably germline-encoded) to neutralize certain rapidly multiplying infectious agents (229). Tolerance of the B cells that make these antibodies is possibly mediated by the receptor-blockade mechanisms discussed earlier.

TOLERANCE INDUCTION IN MATURE T CELLS: MECHANISMS

The two-signal model of Bretscher and Cohn (see Fig. 3) requires that lymphocytes receive two different antigen-specific signals in order to be activated. The experiments of Dresser (see Table 4), however, suggested that, under some circumstances *in vivo,* the second signal (e.g., CFA) could be non–antigen-specific. Subsequent observations made with murine CD4+ Th1 clones supported this idea (230). Activation of these cells to proliferate requires live APCs. When the APCs were chemically treated with fixatives such as paraformaldehyde and used to present peptide (processed) antigens, the T cells did not proliferate (231). Instead, by 24 hours they had entered a new state, in which they failed to proliferate or make IL-2 when restimulated with normal APC and antigen. The T cells were alive, as they could proliferate in response to added IL-2. This unresponsive state lasted for at least 2 weeks in tissue culture. Simultaneous studies using planer lipid membranes composed of MHC class II molecules spread out on a plastic surface and pulsed with peptide antigen induced the same state (232). This suggested that TCR occupancy was all that was required to induce the state; that is, an antigen-specific signal 1 alone was inhibitory for the cell.

Although these observations fit with the Bretscher and Cohn model, subsequent reconstitution experiments to identify the second signal did not. Addition of untreated, allogeneic APC (which could not present the peptide) to chemically fixed syngeneic APC and peptide prevented the induction of the unresponsive state (233). It also reconstituted the initial proliferative response. This suggested that the fixed cells were presenting antigen properly but that the fixation prevented other signals from being delivered by the APC. Addition of the allogeneic APCs allowed these second signals to be delivered in *trans,* although the process was relatively inefficient, requiring a 100-fold higher antigen concentration to achieve a comparable proliferative response. No soluble cytokines were ever effective in substituting for the allogeneic APC, and biochemical studies on signal transduction showed that the costimulatory signals were independent of those generated by TCR occupancy (234). Subsequent studies demonstrated that for the IL-2 production required for T-cell proliferation, CD28 is the receptor that receives the costimulatory signal, while the ligand on the APC is either B7-1 (CD80) or B7-2 (CD86) (235–238). Thus, the second signal is clearly not directly antigen-specific, nor does it originate from an antigen-specific cell. In fact, the activation of CD4+ T cells is more akin to a model originally proposed by Lafferty and Cunningham (239), in which TCR occupancy leads to a

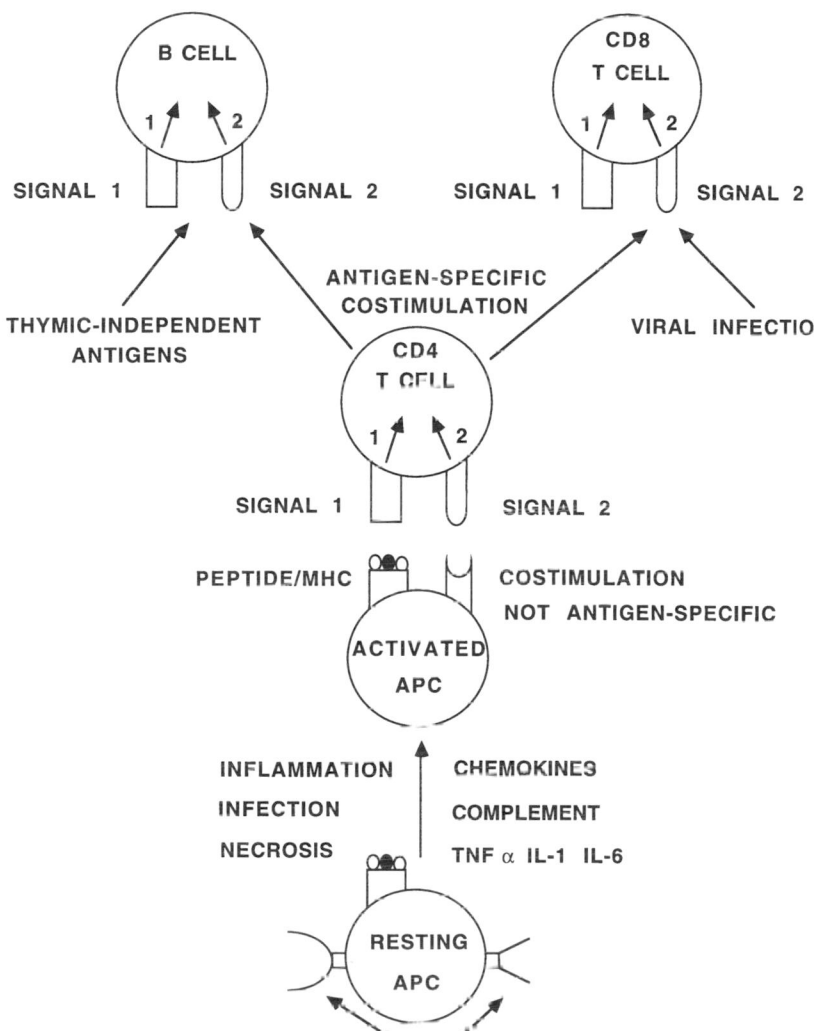

FIG. 6. An integration of antigen-specific and non–antigen-specific forms of costimulation. Resting antigen-presenting cells (*APCs*) are activated by bacterial products or inflammatory stimuli (cytokines, chemokines, complement activation) to become competent to deliver a non–antigen-specific costimulatory signal(s). The activated APC can now present peptide–MHC molecule complexes to CD4+ helper T cells. Once activated, the CD4+ T cells provide help to B cells or CD8+ T cells. This interaction can be viewed as an antigen-specific form of costimulation. It can be bypassed by thymic-independent antigens or viruses, which do not seem to require CD4+ T-cell help.

cross-linking of MHC class II molecules on the APC surface, which in turn induces the expression of a generic costimulatory molecule on the APC required as the second signal for T-cell activation. Currently, the evidence suggests that TCR signaling upregulates CD40 ligand on the T cell that stimulates the APC through CD40 to express B7-2, which in turn costimulates the T cell through CD28 (Fig. 5). Note, however, that this model places the induction of costimulation under the control of the antigen-specific receptor, which would mean that signal 1 alone is positive. To preserve a two-signal model would require that costimulation be turned on by another mechanism.

It is important to realize that in this type of model, in which the second signal is not antigen-specific, one needs to rethink the importance of self–nonself discrimination in the induction of tolerance, because the APC has no obvious way to tell whether it is presenting a self or a foreign antigen. The first person to confront this problem was Janeway (240,241), who proposed that costimulation was actually the switch that controlled whether the organism made an immune response. In this scenario, the B7/CD28 interaction was a later event, requiring something other than TCR occupancy to turn it on. Janeway postulated that the switch was controlled by receptors and stimulants that were part of the innate or nonadaptive immune system. Their job was to initially detect the invasion of infectious pathogens by recognizing unique chemical markers on such organisms. For bacteria, this would involve recognition of molecules such as LPS, formylated methionine–containing peptides, and unmethylated CpG sequences in their DNA. For viruses, this would involve detection of double-stranded RNA and the production and release of IFN-α or -β. The receptors could be positioned on the professional APCs such that their signaling would directly turn on the costimulation pathway. Alternatively, the receptors could be located on other cells, which would then release secondary mediators (such as chemokines, TNFα, IL-1, and IL-6) and indirectly activate the APCs. In fact, any of the arms of the innate immune system that can be triggered by the pathogen, such as activation of the alternative pathway of complement, could contribute to this process. Thus, this theory for the first time suggested a necessary link between the adaptive and nonadaptive immune responses.

These concepts were generalized by Matzinger (242) to incorporate all forms of adaptive immune responses. She postulated that graft rejection, which usually does not involve exposure to infectious agents, could also only be initiated by "danger" signals, which turn on the ability of the APCs to deliver costimulation. In this case, it would be the response to injury initiated by necrotic cell death that transmitted the inductive signal. Although molecularly still undefined, this pathway completes the linkage to primitive defense mechanisms by including injury along with infection as a way to switch on the adaptive immune response. Thus, it is the context in which the antigen is seen that determines whether an immune response will be made.

Figure 6 summarizes these ideas and attempts to integrate them with the Bretscher and Cohn model for B-cell activation. Injury or infection turns on the innate immune response by an inflammatory process that activates the costimulatory pathways of the APC in a non–antigen-specific way. Any antigens from the environment displayed as peptide–MHC complexes on these APCs are then presented to the T-cell population in an immunogenic form. T cells specific for self peptides on these professional APCs have largely been deleted in the thymus. CD4$^+$ T cells specific for all other peptides will be activated. Once activated, they can help B cells and

CD8$^+$ cytotoxic T cells proliferate and differentiate into effector cells. Although the actual molecular second signals delivered by helper T cells are not antigen-specific, the cell interactions that trigger them involve an antigen-specific recognition event, and thus they meet the Bretscher and Cohn requirement for two antigen-specific signals for activation. Exceptions to this scheme, also shown in Fig. 6, will be discussed later.

Activation-induced Cell Death (Homeostasis and Clonal Exhaustion)

The frequency of responding T cells in an MLR is quite high, ranging from 2% to 5% of the CD4$^+$ T-cell population (243). Proliferation following priming does not increase this frequency (244), suggesting that many of the dividing cells must die. Sprent and Miller (245,246) followed the fate of the reactive cells in this assay by isolating 4-day blasts from the thoracic duct of F$_1$ mice injected with parental cells, labeling the cells and transferring them back to syngeneic parental hosts. These cells homed to the spleen and intestine, and then most of them disappeared, appearing to die *in situ* and be degraded by macrophages or be excreted into the lumen of the gut over a 2-week period. Only a few survived to become memory cells that were capable of responding more rapidly.

Modern studies on the fate of T cells stimulated with superantigens have confirmed these early findings with alloreactive T cells. Injection of spleen cells expressing Mtv-7 into mice lacking Mtv-7 (247), or injection of staphylococcal enterotoxin B (SEB) into strains expressing Vβ8 and/or Vβ3 T cells (248), results in an initial expansion of the reactive T cells followed by extensive death via apoptosis. This is not simply a phenomenon observed with superantigens, as transfer into male nude mice of spleen cells from a transgenic female mouse expressing the TCR$\alpha\beta$ anti–H-Y receptor resulted in a similar expansion and disappearance of CD8$^+$ T cells (249). The general pattern of response to all of these stimuli is shown in Fig. 7.

The biochemical pathway responsible for signaling the cell to die is initiated mainly via a FAS–Fas ligand interaction (250), although TNF and its receptor have also been implicated (251). The initial TCR stimulation induces Fas ligand expression. This trimer is cleaved from the cell surface and can interact with Fas, which is constitutively expressed on either the same cell or neighboring cells (252). During the first few days after stimulation, the activated T cell is resistant to cell death, possibly because the T-cell stimulation also increases the synthesis of bcl-2 family members such as bcl-X$_L$ (253). When the latter decay, the cell becomes vulnerable to Fas-mediated death. The cell can be protected from such death if there are T-cell growth hormones, such as IL-2 or IL-4, in the environment (254,255) or if the expression of Fas ligand also decays. If restimulated through the antigen receptor, the cell is killed by a rapid reexpression of the Fas ligand (the "propriocidal" effect) (255). Other cells die simply when the IL-2 is withdrawn (254).

The balance between expansion and death is a subtle one, and all of the quantitative parameters that influence the cell's fate are not fully understood. Importantly, costimulation through CD28/B7 interactions is thought to play a critical role. This signal increases Bcl-X$_L$ (252) and possibly other bcl-2 family members in the T cell, as well as greatly amplifying the production of IL-2 (by both stabilizing the mRNA and increasing gene transcription) (256,257). All of these CD28 effects would protect the cell from death. Thus, the two-signal idea that an antigen-specific first signal

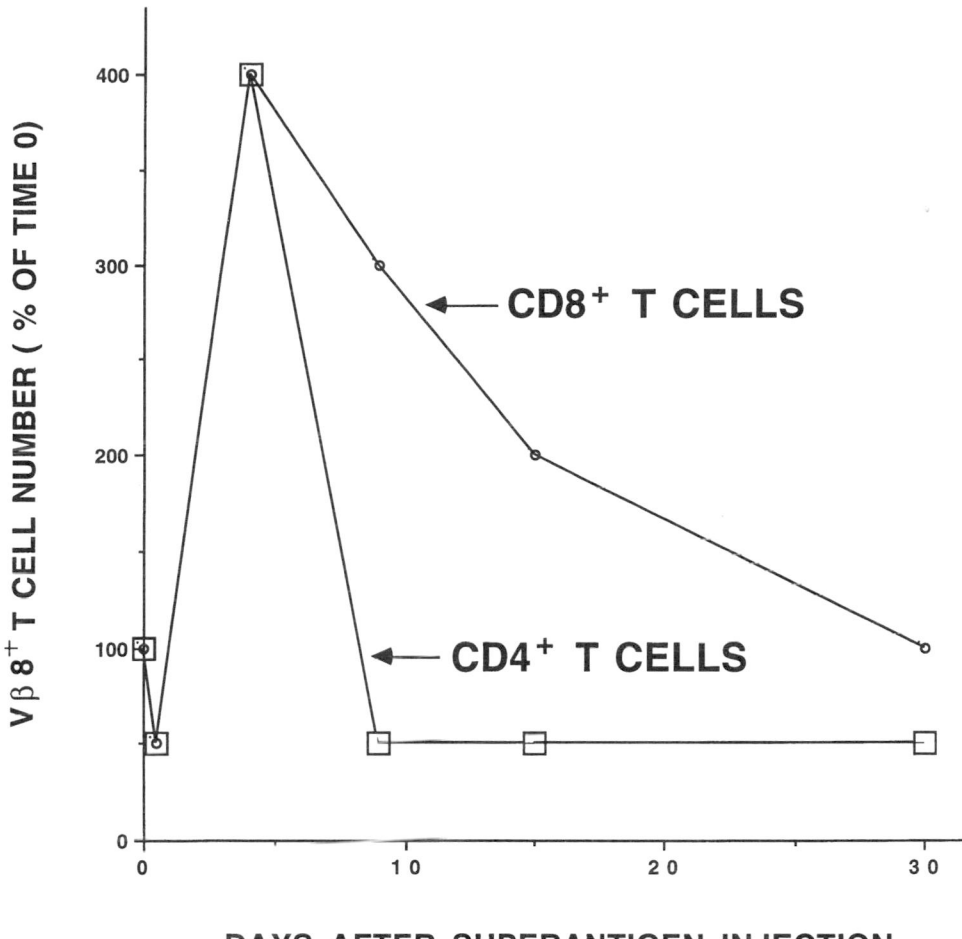

DAYS AFTER SUPERANTIGEN INJECTION

FIG. 7. The general pattern of *in vivo* responses of CD4+ and CD8+ T cells to superantigen stimulation. The response of Vβ8+ T cells to staphylococcal enterotoxin B is shown as a model. The response occurs in three phases. During the first 12 hours, the massive release of cytokines can result in significant cell death in the stimulated cells. In the second phase, the remaining stimulated cells divide, increasing four- to eightfold over a period of 4 days. In the third phase, CD4+ T cells die off rapidly, but leave a residue of cells that appear to be anergized. CD8+ T cells, in contrast, slowly decrease in number, returning to normal levels after 30 days.

leads to the death of the T cell, while the addition of a second CD28 signal would lead to its activation fits with these observations. There is still contention, however, as to what constitutes a first signal, as some experiments with naive T cells suggest that receptor occupancy by peptide–MHC complexes alone is not adequate to signal the cell (258). Furthermore, in the propriocidal effect, CD28 signaling does not protect against the Fas ligand–mediated death induced by TCR reengagement (259). *In vivo*, only LPS or proinflammatory cytokines such as IL-1 and TNFα could prevent the cell death seen following superantigen injection (260,261); CD28 and B7 were ineffective. Finally, in many of the *in vivo* experiments, only the CD4+ T cells die rapidly at day 4 following SEB injection, while the CD8+ T cells do not (262). Thus, a completely different explanation for CD4+ T-cell depletion has been proposed by Jiang and colleagues (262), who removed CD8+ T cells from the mice prior to SEB injection by treatment with anti-CD8 antibody. This manipulation prevented the rapid loss of CD4+ T cells at day 4. They postulated that the activated CD8+ T cells normally kill off the activated CD4+ T cells by a perforin- and granzyme-mediated cytotoxicity mechanism.

One of the most interesting aspects of these observations is that more than 90% of T cells responding to antigen or superantigen die. This is best understood in the context of homeostatic regulation of the immune system, rather than antigen-specific tolerance per se. There is only so much space in the body for lymphocytes, and room must be maintained for the influx of new naive cells from the thymus, as well as the preservation of memory T cells, for an extended period of time. Transfer of splenic T cells into nude mice showed that the cells could expand (presumably in response to environmental antigens) only until a critical cell number is reached (approximately 2×10^8 cells per mouse) (263–265). Surprisingly, memory T cells and naive T cells were independently regulated; that is, each subpopulation did not influence the expansion of the other (266). Their half-lives were also controlled in different manners, as naive T cells were dependent on TCR recognition of self MHC molecules for survival, whereas memory T cells were not (267). In the immune response to a virus, the frequency of the responding antigen-specific cells increases dramatically over an 8-day period, up to a frequency of 10% of the total CD8+ T cells in the spleen (268). As these cells begin to effectively eliminate the virus, however, their frequency drops, and in the memory phase of the response, it becomes only 1/300 to 1/1000 of the total CD8[+] pool. In transgenic models, where the fate of the cells can be followed, the CD8[+] T cells die by apoptosis (269). Thus, homeostasis is maintained by allowing most of the generated new cells to die once the antigen is cleared.

Homeostasis per se is not a tolerance mechanism, but when pushed to an extreme by experimental manipulation or overwhelming infection, it can end up inducing such a state. Infection with low numbers of LCMV particles elicits a CTL response that clears the virus. Administration of large numbers of particles, however, results in an abortive response, followed by a tolerant state in which the virus persists (270). This phenomenon has been called clonal exhaustion and has been shown to result from clonal deletion of the antigen-specific CD8[+] T cells using TCR transgenic mice (270).

T-Cell Clonal Anergy

Following the death of CD4[+] T cells in mice given SEB or Mtv7[+] spleen cells, there remains a population of Vβ8[+] CD4[+] T cells that fails to proliferate on restimulation with SEB (271,272) (see Fig. 7). These cells stay in this functionally unresponsive state for weeks, especially if the animal has been thymectomized. In the H-Y transgenic model, the residual CD8[+] T cells are also unresponsive (249). This only occurs when the cells are kept in an environment in which the male antigen they recognize is highly expressed (e.g., on transfer into male nude mice) (273). If the cells are removed from this environment and parked in a female nude mouse, the CD8[+] T cells recover their function (274). Dependence of CD4[+] T-cell unresponsiveness on the persistence of antigen has also been reported (275). The unresponsive state for both CD4[+] and CD8[+] T cells has been called anergy because it shows some resem-

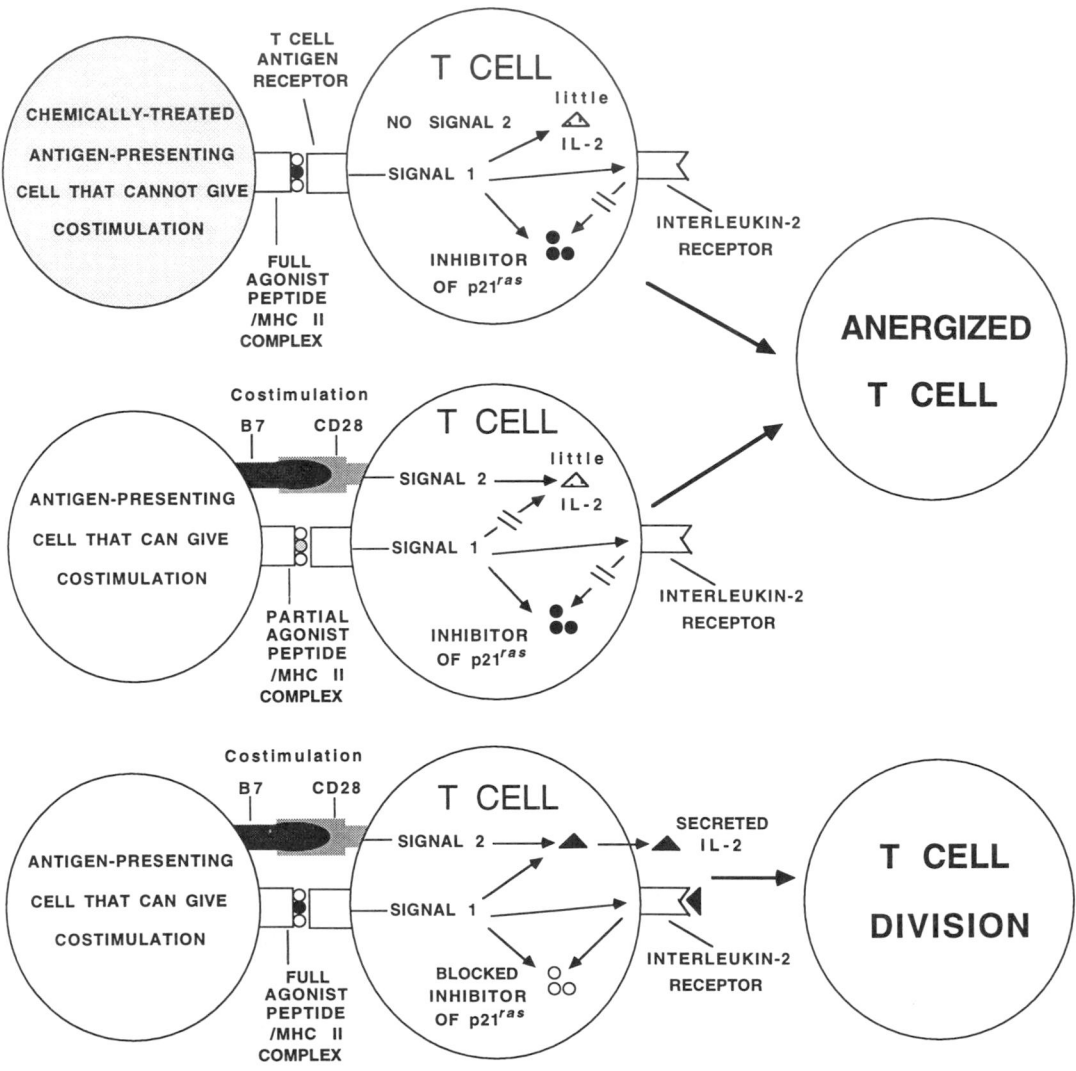

FIG. 8. T-cell anergy is induced in CD4[+] Th1 clones by either partial agonist peptides in the presence of costimulation or full agonist peptides in the absence of costimulation. Traditional anergy is induced using full agonist peptides and chemically fixed antigen-presenting cells and involves the generation of inhibitors of the Ras/MAP kinase pathway. Partial agonist peptides can achieve this same outcome even in the presence of full costimulation. The critical variable is induction of the inhibitors by TCR occupancy without blocking their formation or function through the production of IL-2, which occurs under normal activation conditions leading, to T-cell division.

blances to T-cell clonal models of anergy in tissue culture, where the T cells, on restimulation, fail to produce IL-2, and the unresponsive state is reversible (276).

There are several models for inducing T-cell anergy in nontransformed CD4$^+$ T clones. One, described earlier, is to stimulate the cell (either human or mouse) through its antigen-specific receptor in the absence of costimulation (230,276–278) (Fig. 8). This results in a signaling block in the Ras/MAP kinase pathway (279,280) following TCR stimulation, which disrupts formation and activation of the transcription factor AP-1 (281) via an increase in the GTP-bound form of Rap1 (282). This in turn prevents the cells from making IL-2. It also impedes the cell's ability to make IL-3 and TNF-β, but IFN-γ production is only slightly affected (283). In Th0 cells, IL-4 production is not inhibited, but, interestingly, the ability of the cell to respond to IL-4 is blocked (284). Hence, this state appears to represent a growth arrest of the lymphocyte rather than a complete shutdown of all responses.

Surprisingly, a similar state can be achieved if the T-cell clone is stimulated with peptide ligands of low affinity, even in the presence of full costimulation (285) (see Fig. 8). This appears to result from suboptimal TCR signal transduction, which is sufficient to induce the inhibitors of the Ras pathway, but not fully adequate to produce IL-2 (286–289). It is the IL-2 signaling and subsequent division that normally prevent the induction of the anergic state (289). A different model, also referred to as anergy, has been described in human clones stimulated with high concentrations of peptide antigen in the presence of costimulation (290,291). In contrast to the mouse models, however, this state appears to be a block in signaling through the calcium–calcineurin pathway, which prevents the cells from making all cytokines, including IL-4 (291–293). A similar block has been described for mouse clones; however, in this case, it is induced following stimulation with IL-2 and, it rapidly and spontaneously reverses in culture (294). By contrast, for all three anergy models (activation in the absence of costimulation, stimulation with low affinity ligands, and stimulation of human T cells with high concentrations of peptides), the unresponsive state induced is much more stable and can be reversed only by stimulating the cells to divide with IL-2 (283). It has been proposed that the two biochemical models of anergy be kept distinct by calling one ras-blocked anergy and the other calcium-blocked anergy (295).

Most of the *in vivo* models described as anergy have not been studied biochemically, and thus it is unclear what the underlying mechanism really is in each case. The one exception is in a model in which Mtv-7$^+$ spleen cells were injected into an Mtv-7$^-$ TCR transgenic mouse expressing Vβ8.1 on 90% of its T cells (296). The treated mice responded poorly in a proliferation assay to both anti-CD3 and Mtv-7 stimulation. The cells also showed a decreased response in the presence of additional IL-2, suggesting that there was a partial block in the upregulation of the IL-2 receptor or its signaling in addition to a block in IL-2 production. A biochemical analysis of early signal transduction events showed that certain defects in tyrosine phosphorylation resembled the pattern observed in stimulated anergic T-cell clones, suggesting the existence of this state *in vivo*. Not all investigators, however, have been able to demonstrate the induction of anergy in response to Mtv-7 (297). Furthermore, an analysis of some of the other *in vivo* anergy models has revealed suppression mechanisms mediated by cytokines such as IL-10 (298) or IFN-γ (299). Whatever the mechanisms, however, these *in vivo* manipulations can have important biologic consequences, such as impairment of an effective immune response to a viral infection (300).

A question has been raised as to whether anergy in T cells represents a prelude to cell death, as discussed in the section on B-cell anergy. For the T-cell clones, *in vitro* induction of anergy in the presence of anti-CD95 to block Fas signaling can lead to an increase in the number of anergic T cells (301); however, to date, no way has been found to inhibit anergy induction without also reducing apoptosis. Since ras-blocked anergy appears to be a growth arrest state without concomitant differentiation, my own opinion is that it represents an alternative outcome to TCR occupancy from that of proliferation, differentiation, or cell death.

Two-signal Models for the Activation of CD8$^+$ Cytotoxic T Cells

Naive CD8$^+$ T cells can be directly activated to proliferate by antigen and presenting cells (302). The amount of IL-2 they produce under optimal stimulation, however, is about tenfold less than CD4$^+$ T cells (303). At the low frequency of most antigen-specific cells and the less than optimal TCR occupancy in a typical immune response, the amount of IL-2 produced by CD8$^+$ cells is usually insufficient to sustain a response. Thus, most cytotoxic responses depend on concomitant priming of CD4$^+$ T cells to be effective. In a model system studied by Keene and Forman (304), the cytotoxic CD8$^+$ T-cell response to the class Ib MHC molecule Qa1 was shown to be dependent on the simultaneous CD4$^+$ T-cell response to the male-specific antigen H-Y, presumably because the frequency of Qa1-specific CD4$^+$ helpers is too low. The most effective help in this system was provided if the H-Y and Qa1 molecules were presented on the same APC. Thus, the optimal activation of this cytotoxic effector cell required a three-cell interaction.

Introduction of the Qa1 antigen on its own, in the form of either spleen cells (305) or a skin graft (306), failed to generate a cytotoxic response, because of the lack of help (Table 5). Interestingly, this prior exposure to antigen prevented a subsequent immune response to the Qa1 molecule in the presence of H-Y–specific help. The animals did not reject a skin graft, nor did their cells give a cytotoxic response *in vitro*. These results suggest that recognition of antigen by naive CD8$^+$ precytotoxic T cells in the absence of help can be a tolerogenic event. The data are compatible with the notion that a Bretscher and Cohn form of two-signal model operates during the activation of CD8$^+$ T cells (see Fig. 6). The antigen-specific signal 1 alone is tolerogenic, while this signal 1 plus the antigen-specific T-cell help as a second signal is activating. The molecular nature of the CD4$^+$ T-cell help has been postulated to be the production of IL-2 and other growth and differentiation cytokines in close proximity to the CD8$^+$ precytotoxic T cell on the same APC.

While these rules seem to apply to the generation of CTL against minor histocompatibility antigens such as Qa1, studies of viral infections have given a completely different picture. For both Sendai and influenza viruses, the generation of CD8$^+$ CTL was shown to take place in the complete absence of CD4$^+$ helpers (307,308). Although there were small quantitative differences in the level of cytotoxic activity obtained, the clear conclusion was reached that many of the CD8$^+$ T cells did not need an antigen-specific second signal. This is somewhat surprising because *in vitro* studies have clearly demonstrated that the activation of naive CD8$^+$ T cells from TCR transgenic mice absolutely requires non antigen-specific costimulation by either B7/CD28 or I-CAM/LFA-1 interactions and is optimal when both of these are present (258). One

TABLE 5. *Tolerance of CD8 T cells primed in the absence of CD4 help*

Qa-1b cell injection	H-Y specific CD4 helper cells	Qa-1b specific CD8 cytotoxic cells	Second in vivo injection	Killing of Qa1-b targets
Male cells	Yes	Yes	None	Yes
Female cells	No	Yes	None	No
Female cells	No	Yes	Male cells	No

A schematic summary of experiments from ref. 305.

way to reconcile this paradox has been proposed by Guerder and Matzinger (305). They postulated that the virus bypasses the need for T-cell help by infecting the APC and directly inducing the expression of non–antigen-specific costimulatory molecules. Such a potential bypass mechanism has been demonstrated by Wu and Liu (309), who showed that infection of mice with a CD4$^+$ helper–independent form of the influenza virus induced the expression of B7-2 on APCs, whereas a variant of the virus that largely depends on CD4$^+$ T-cell help for CTL generation did not. The induced B7-2 could thus provide enough direct costimulation for IL-2 production by the CD8$^+$ precytotoxic T cell, allowing this cell to proliferate and mature by itself. Therefore, in this case, a Dresser-type of two-signal model would apply (see Fig. 6).

Receptor Downmodulation

In addition to the question of whether CD8$^+$ T cells require costimulation for activation, several experiments have also raised the question of whether they are always inactivated by signal 1 alone. In the classical experiments of Lafferty and colleagues (310), on the acceptance of thyroid grafts that had been cultured *in vitro* to remove passenger leukocytes (presumably dendritic cells), the accepted grafts did not tolerize the recipients except in some cases after long periods of time. In this model, depletion of the dendritic cells removed the professional APC capable of delivering costimulation, but the remaining donor tissue cells expressing allogeneic MHC class I molecules did not inactivate the host T cells by delivering signal 1 alone. In more recent experiments, Ohashi et al. (311) and Oldstone et al. (312) created transgenic mice expressing the coat glycoprotein of the LCMV in the β cells of the pancreas, by engineering the gene to be under the control of the rat insulin promoter. These animals did not spontaneously react against the β cells, although these cells expressed the glycoprotein. Even crossing this mouse to a TCR transgenic expressing a receptor specific for the glycoprotein-derived peptide–MHC complex did not initiate autoimmunity (311). The CD8$^+$ T cells also were not deleted, and, in fact, the mice were not tolerant. Infection with the virus activated the T cells, which then caused diabetes by destroying the pancreatic β cells. Thus, the immune system in its resting state possessed T cells capable of recognizing the tissue-specific antigen, but the cells were neither activated nor inactivated by it. This situation has been called immunologic ignorance.

In contrast to these observations, a series of experiments performed by Schönrich et al. (313,314) showed that CD8$^+$ T cells from mice expressing an MHC class I molecule (K^b) expressed in three different peripheral tissues [liver, skin, or central nervous system (CNS)] were tolerant, as defined by their inability to reject skin grafts expressing K^b. The fate of the T cells was examined by crossing each transgenic mouse to a second TCR transgenic mouse whose receptor was specific for K^b. Expression of K^b in hepato-

cytes under the control of the albumin promoter led to peripheral T cells that had downmodulated their TCRs and their CD8 molecules. In the second model, expression of K^b in glial cells under the control of the fibrillary acidic protein promoter also resulted in receptor downmodulation; however, this was reversible in culture by stimulation with alloantigen. In the first model, the downmodulation was not reversible by alloantigen stimulation, but could be reversed by anti-CD2 stimulation. The molecular mechanisms responsible for the receptor downmodulation and reversal are not understood. In the third model, involving expression of K^b in epithelial cells under the control of the keratin IV promoter, both the receptor and CD8 levels on the T cells were normal. Reversal of the tolerant state in this case was achieved 2 weeks after transferring spleen cells into a nude mouse that did not express the antigen (315).

Several other experiments have suggested that expression of an antigen in a specific tissue outside of the thymus can lead to tolerance of the CD8$^+$ T-cell population, consistent with the observations of Schönrich et al., while others have not (316–318). Thus, the question of whether signal 1 alone is a negative signal for CD8$^+$ T cells is still being debated. One possible explanation for the differences is how much access the T cells have to the peripheral tissue (319). Small tissues like the β-cell islets in the pancreas may not be seen by many naive T cells, and thus these tissues would be ineffective at tolerizing all the T cells in a TCR transgenic mouse. In contrast, the liver is a bigger and hematologically more exposed organ. Thus, it is more likely to provide a large antigenic exposure to the immune system. Still, the most surprising result is that any peripheral tissue would be able to tolerize all of the T cells in a TCR transgenic mouse. This suggests that an encounter with antigen, when it occurs, delivers a signal to only a subset of T cells and that these cells are maintaining tolerance by some form of immunoregulation (see section on immunoregulation).

Veto Cells

Another mechanism for negatively signaling naive CD8$^+$ precytotoxic T cells has been described by Miller and colleagues (320,321). The initial observation was that cells from the spleen of a nude mouse were capable of suppressing a primary CTL response against allogeneic stimulators if the nude mouse expressed the same MHC molecules as the stimulator cells. Spleen cells from euthymic mice were not suppressive. Their model was that these unusual cells were recognized by the responding T cells in the culture and that the former inactivated the latter (Fig. 9); hence, the name veto cells (320).

Subsequent studies (322,323) showed that precultured T cells could acquire the ability to veto, and, eventually, cloned CD8$^+$ T-cell lines were developed that had this property (324–326). In mixed stimulator cultures, only CTLs specific for one stimulator

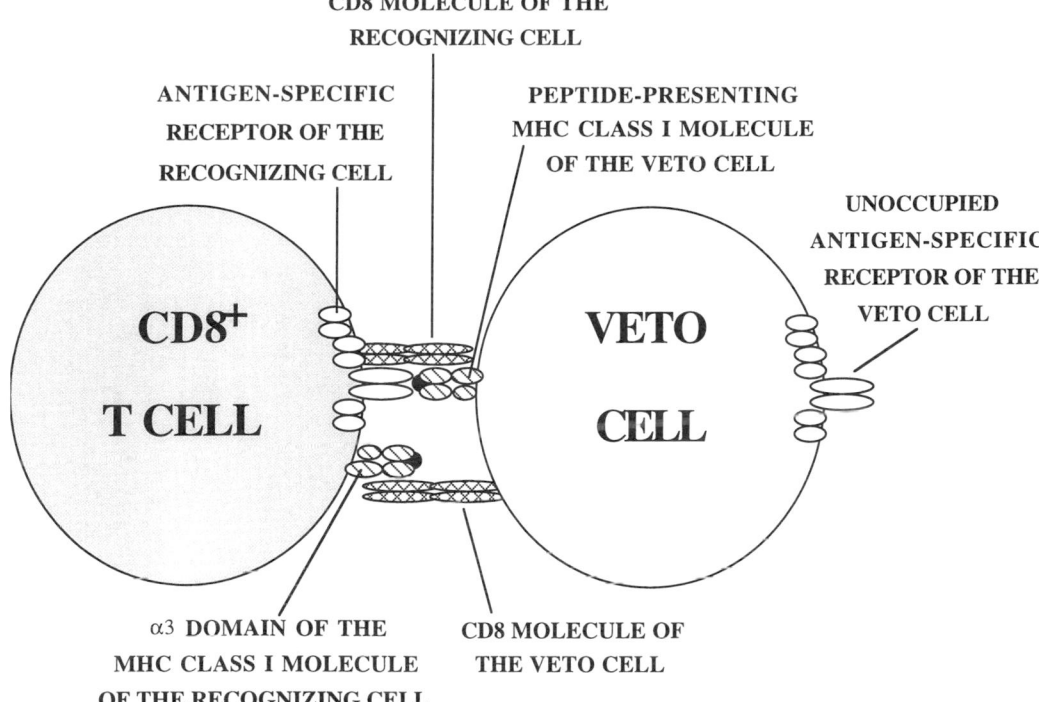

FIG. 9. The molecular mechanism of vetoing. The CD8+ T cell recognizes a peptide–MHC class I complex on the surface of a CD8+ veto cell using its antigen-specific receptor and its own CD8 molecule. Simultaneously, the CD8 molecules expressed by the veto cell engage the α3 domain of the MHC class I molecules on the recognizing cell. Signaling through the MHC molecule along with the TCR signaling leads to apoptosis. See refs. 330–332.

were inhibited, the one sharing MHC class I molecules with the veto cell. Veto cells acted late in culture (after 20 hours), mediated their effects by cell–cell interaction (not secreted products), and did not compete for lysis of target cells in the CTL assay (as they could be eliminated prior to the assay with anti-MHC antibodies and complement without reversing the effect). Primed responding T cells and T-cell clones were resistant to being vetoed. The phenomenon was not prevented by providing culture supernatants containing T-cell growth factors (such as IL-2) during the induction phase, and the vetoed population, when mixed with a normally induced CTL population, did not suppress the latter from killing. In the case of cloned CD8+ veto cells, it was clear that the TCR specificity of the veto cell did not matter and that engagement of its TCR was not required for its veto function. Instead, it was the recognition of cell surface MHC class I antigens on the veto cell by the responding T cell that led to the latter's inactivation (see Fig. 9).

Evidence that the veto phenomenon can operate *in vivo* came largely from the experiments of Rammensee, Fink, and Bevan (323,327,328). Injection of splenic T cells into mice differing at MHC class I loci resulted in inhibition of a subsequent *in vitro* CTL response against those class I molecules. Similarly, injection of parent A spleen cells, differing only in minor histocompatibility antigens, into an (A × B)F₁ host inhibited the subsequent CTL response to those minor antigens in the context of strain-A MHC class I molecules, but not strain-B class I molecules. These effects required the injection of live cells; irradiated cells primed the host when administered under the same experimental conditions. The most potent cell type capable of vetoing was a CD8+ T cell; however, Thy-1 negative spleen cells from nude mice were also capa

ble of inducing the effect. The latter cells were probably NK cells, which have been shown to manifest veto activity (329). The primary cell affected by the veto phenomenon is the precytotoxic T cell. Limiting dilution analysis in the presence of supernatants containing T-cell growth factors (to bypass any limitations in T-cell help) revealed a 200-fold decrease in functional CTL precursors. Again, the specificity of the veto cell did not matter, only that it expressed class I molecules and peptides recognized by the vetoed CTL. In fact, the vetoing cell could be completely tolerant of the host into which it was injected (328).

A molecular mechanism for vetoing has been described that involves signaling through MHC class I molecules following interaction with CD8 (see Fig. 9) (330,331). CD8-negative variants of clones capable of vetoing were found to lose their ability to veto. Furthermore, cell lines expressing the correct peptide–MHC complex, but which were not veto cells, became veto cells when transfected with a CD8 gene. Finally, a veto effect could be activated with peptide–MHC-positive, CD8-negative cells by adding a monoclonal antibody against the α3 domain of the MHC class I molecule (the molecular region for CD8 binding). Conversely, a CD8+ veto cell could be prevented from killing by a monoclonal antibody against CD8, which blocked its interaction with the MHC molecule. These results suggest that the veto signal is delivered by the interaction of CD8 on the veto cell with the α3 domain of an MHC class I molecule on the target cell, but only when the latter cell simultaneously becomes activated through its TCR via recognition of a peptide–MHC molecule on the veto cell (see Fig. 9). This is, in essence, a two-signal model in which both signals (TCR cross-linking and MHC class I molecule cross-linking) are required to tolerize the cell. NK cells could veto by a similar mechanism, since they can express low levels of CD8 when activated. The effect of this dual signaling by veto cells is to delete the responding T cells by apoptosis (332). The function of this mechanism in tolerance is not clear, but it may play a role in eliminating autoreactive CD8+ T cells specific for blast antigens expressed on activated CTLs.

IMMUNOREGULATION

In the past few years it has become clear that many states of unresponsiveness observed following the introduction of antigen to a mature immune system are actually the result of negative regulation of one type of immune response by another. This state is sometimes called "split" tolerance. In this section, I will summarize these various mechanisms, because tolerance in its broadest sense includes all nonharmful states of the immune system. The reader is referred to other chapters in the text for a more detailed discussion of help and suppression in the immune response.

Immune Deviation (Th1 Versus Th2 CD4+ Helpers)

The phenomenon of immune deviation was first described by Asherson and Stone (333). They injected guinea pigs with soluble or alum-precipitated antigens 2 weeks prior to challenge with the same antigen in CFA. The pretreatment prevented the usual DTH response measured as 24-hour skin reactions on rechallenge. In contrast, antibody production was normal, although the class of antibody was deviated from IgG2 toward IgG1. Parish and Liew (334) subsequently discovered a general reciprocal relationship between antibody production and DTH reactions as a function of antigen dose. When small doses of antigen were administered, the immune response was predominantly DTH. As the antigen dose was increased, an antibody response was observed, while the DTH response diminished. At very high doses of antigen, the antibody response also declined, and in some cases, the DTH response reemerged. These observations were interpreted by Bretscher (335) as reciprocal regulation between two interacting T-cell populations specific for the same antigen but with different effector functions. With the introduction of T-cell cloning technology, Mosmann and colleagues (336) discovered that fully differentiated mouse T-cell clones generally exhibit one of two discrete lymphokine production profiles. Th1 cells make IL-2, IFN-γ, and TNF-β, while Th2 cells make IL-4, IL-5, and IL-6 (337). This cellular dichotomy provided a potential explanation for immune deviation, because these two cell types can cross-regulate each other. Lymphokines produced by Th1 cells turned out to be primarily mediators for stimulating macrophage activation via induction of IFN-γ and complement fixing IgG2a antibodies, while those produced by Th2 cells were primarily mediators of helper T-cell function for B-cell IgG1, IgA, and IgE antibody production (338). The cross-regulation is also mediated by these lymphokines. Thus, IFN-γ inhibits the proliferation of Th2 cells (339) by blocking the costimulation of IL-1 (340), while IL-10 inhibits the stimulation of Th1 cells by blocking monocytic APC function (341) and by preventing production of IL-2 (342).

The forces that operate to determine the dominance of Th1 versus Th2 cells in any given immune response are not fully understood. The dose of antigen is critical, and the genetic constitution of the responding individual determines which particular doses are perceived as high and low. In the *Leishmania major* parasite model,

BALB/c mice make predominantly a nonprotective Th2 response, whereas C3H and C57BL/6 mice make predominantly a protective Th1 response (343). If, however, the BALB/c mice are inoculated with a minute number of parasites (<30), they become protected against a normal challenge dose due to deviation toward an IFN-γ response (344). The antigen specificity of the response is also a critical variable. A single immunodominant determinant of the *Leishmania* is recognized in the early response of the BALB/c mouse (345). If tolerance is induced to the protein containing this determinant, then the mouse mounts a protective Th1 immune response (346). Another critical parameter is the cytokine milieu. High concentrations of IL-4 deviate the response towards Th2 (347), while high concentrations of IL-12 deviate the response towards Th1 (348). Finally, the molecular form of the antigen is also influential, with particulate antigens favoring macrophage uptake and IL-12 production, which skews the response towards a Th1 phenotype (348,349).

Commitment to the Th1 or Th2 lineage begins with a naive CD4+ T cell capable of making only IL-2. Following antigen stimulation, the cell first passes through a Th0 stage, in which it is capable of making many of the different cytokines on restimulation (350). It then commits, to varying degrees, to the Th1 or Th2 lineage, if the antigen persists and the cytokine milieu is appropriate. The differentiation of CD4+ T cells to Th2 cells is often confused with the induction of clonal anergy, because IL-4 production can be turned on in both states (284,351). The two states can be distinguished, however, as anergy introduces a block in the proliferative response to IL-4. By contrast, Th2 cells remain responsive to IL-4, because they depend on it for their autocrine growth. Finally, CD8 subsets (Tc1 and Tc2) analogous to Th1 and Th2 CD4 cells have been described (352,353). The role of IL-4–producing CD8+ T cells is not yet clear, but they may serve an immunoregulatory function (see section on suppression). For CD4+ T cells, however, the involvement of IL-4–producing Th2 cells in certain "unresponsive" states has clearly been demonstrated (see sections on neonatal tolerance and the fetal–maternal relationship).

Oral Tolerance

The route of antigen introduction is a critical variable in determining the outcome of an immune response. Intravenous administration generally favors induction of tolerance (354,355), whereas subcutaneous administration favors immunity (356). Intravenous injection might allow antigen presentation by costimulatory molecule-deficient naive B cells in the spleen (357), whereas subcutaneous injection would favor uptake and presentation by Langerhans' cells, which, following activation, are very effective at initiating immune responses (358). Interestingly, ultraviolet light exposure transiently depletes the epidermis of Langerhans' cells and predisposes to tolerance induction when antigen is introduced into the treated area of skin (358,359).

Oral administration of antigen has also been reported to favor tolerance induction (360). From the earliest studies of Wells in 1911 (361), it was clear that this route of administration induces some form of immunoregulation. Orally immunized animals usually make an initial systemic antibody response, which subsequently diminishes (362). The tolerance state is often associated with large amounts of IgA production in the gut (363). In other cases (e.g., for myelin basic protein), in which the antigen is administered in a form (peptides) preferentially recognized by T cells rather than by B cells (364), the immunoregulation has been reported to be mediated either by T cells that secrete transforming growth factor β (TGF-β) on antigen stimulation (365) or by induction of clonal anergy and deletion (366,367). The mechanism observed depends on the antigen dose, with high doses inducing direct inactivation of the antigen-specific T cells and low doses eliciting TGF-β–mediated immunoregulation (368).

The T cells in the gut are unusual in that they can make substantial amounts of TGF-β following antigen stimulation (369). This cytokine acts as a critical switch factor for B cells, favoring the production of IgA (370). TGF-β is also an antiinflammatory cytokine, which blocks T-cell proliferation primarily at the G1 to S transition (371). Thus, when these activated gut T cells migrate to other sites in the body (e.g., the CNS in experimental allergic encephalomyelitis), they can act as suppressor cells if they recognize their peptide–MHC ligand at that site and release TGF-β (372). Clinical trials have suggested some success in treating autoimmune diseases by oral ingestion of tissue-specific antigens (372), although the results have not been overwhelming.

Suppression

Studies on suppressor T cells in immunoregulation and tolerance were a dominant theme in cellular immunology in the 1970s. Many model systems were established, but few were characterized at the molecular level. Looking back at those systems now, it is possible to classify some of them as forms of immune deviation. For example, in the classic suppression experiment of Okumura and Tada (373), the IgE response to DNP-Ascaris was inhibited by the injection of thymocytes from DNP-Ascaris but not DNP-BSA hyperimmunized rats. We now know that the IgE response is highly dependent on the production of IL-4 (374). Thus, one possible explanation for this early experiment is that the hyperimmunized thymocyte population contained recirculating mature Th1 cells that deviated the naive recipient T cells away from the Th2 response required for IgE production. In a typical immune deviation scheme, CD4+ Th1 cells would suppress Th2-cell proliferation by secreting IFN-γ (339). Another possibility is an interesting new CD4+ cell type that produces large amounts of IL-5, IL-10, and TGF β, and that suppresses naive T-cell proliferation (375). While cloned populations of CD4+ suppressor inducer cells have been described (376), the more typical T suppressor cell is CD8+ (377). Since CD8+ T cells are also particularly good at making IFN-γ (378), they should be capable of functioning as potent suppressors in immune deviation models. Experiments have demonstrated that Th2-like CD8+ T cells can also be generated under certain experimental conditions (352,353). These cells might have functioned in some of the suppression models in which CD4+ Th1 DTH responses were inhibited (379).

One new model of suppression that has received widespread attention, because of its relevance for organ transplantation, has been described by Qin et al. (380). They successfully induced tolerance to MHC class I and multiple minor transplantation antigens using injections of nondepleting anti-CD4 and anti-CD8 monoclonal antibodies (plus injection of donor bone marrow). Mice treated in this way accept donor skin grafts indefinitely. Injection of normal T cells into such an animal leads to rejection of a subsequent (second) skin graft, but only during a short period after T-cell transfer (381). By 2 weeks, the mice again accept donor skin grafts. This suppression of the normal T cells by the tolerant mice was shown with mixing experiments in an adoptive transfer assay to be mediated by a CD4+ suppressor T cell. When normal cells were injected into a tolerant transgenic mouse expressing human CD2 on its lymphocytes, elimination of the host T cells after 2 weeks with antihuman CD2 revealed that the injected normal cells themselves had become tolerant (381). Furthermore, they could suppress the response of a new cohort of normal T cells injected following anti-CD2 host-cell depletion. Thus, the phenomenon truly represents "infectious" tolerance, as originally defined by Gershon and Kondo (382). Part of the tolerance process involves a suppressive effect of IL-4, because anti–IL-4 antibody included in the adoptive transfer assay resulted in graft rejection (383). This is not the whole story, however, as the rejection time was still substantially delayed compared with a control group rejecting grafts in the absence of suppressor cells.

Overall, it now appears that regulatory cytokines will, in large part, provide a sufficient explanation for many of the previous models of suppression. Nonetheless, it still seems reasonable to refer to the cells that make such cytokines in a stable manner as suppressor T cells.

Neonatal Tolerance

The original experiments of Medawar and colleagues on neonatal tolerance, described at the beginning of the chapter, were carried out in an intellectual environment influenced by the observations of Owen (2) and the ideas of Burnet (8). In hindsight, it is clear that the success of those experiments hinged on the choice of particular experimental conditions. The mouse strain combination used by Billingham et al. (6) was A and CBA. This pair differs genetically only at the D end of the MHC complex as well as at multiple minor histocompatibility loci. Attempts to extend these observations to strain combinations involving MHC class II differences invariably failed, because the donor lymphoid tissue mounted a graft-versus-host response (136). To avoid this problem, all subsequent experiments were done by injecting (A × B)F1 adult spleen, or lymph node cells into strain-A neonates. In this version of the model, both the donor and the recipient were immunoincompetent; one from self-tolerance, the other from the small number of mature lymphocytes present in its immune system.

The success of the early experiments also depended heavily on the choice of antigen. Attempts by Burnet et al. (384) and subsequently Nossal (385) to use viruses or RBCs as the tolerogen in neonates were unsuccessful. The critical element of the spleen cell inoculum used by Medawar was that it contained hematopoietic stem cells, which, upon engraftment, set up a permanent state of chimerism. We know now that one can routinely detect donor cells that persist in tolerant hosts (386). Thus, as suggested by Billingham et al. (6), the model shows some analogy to the natural state of tolerance in dizygotic bovine twins.

The critical aspect of establishing a chimeric state is that it allows the antigen to persist. The importance of this parameter for maintaining tolerance was first demonstrated by Lubaroff and Silvers (386) (Fig. 10). CBA mice neonatally tolerized with (A × CBA)F1 spleen cells accepted strain-A skin grafts as adults. Injection with C3H lymphoid cells that were primed against strain-A MHC class I and minor antigens led to rejection of the chimeric F1 cells as well as the skin graft. This was subsequently followed by rejection of the C3H lymphoid cells by the CBA host, because CBA is not tolerant to C3H minor histocompatibility antigens. If the authors then administered a second A skin graft, it was rejected. They concluded that the CBA host had lost its tolerance for A antigens once the (A × CBA)F1 cells were eliminated.

T CELL POOL   MANIPULATION

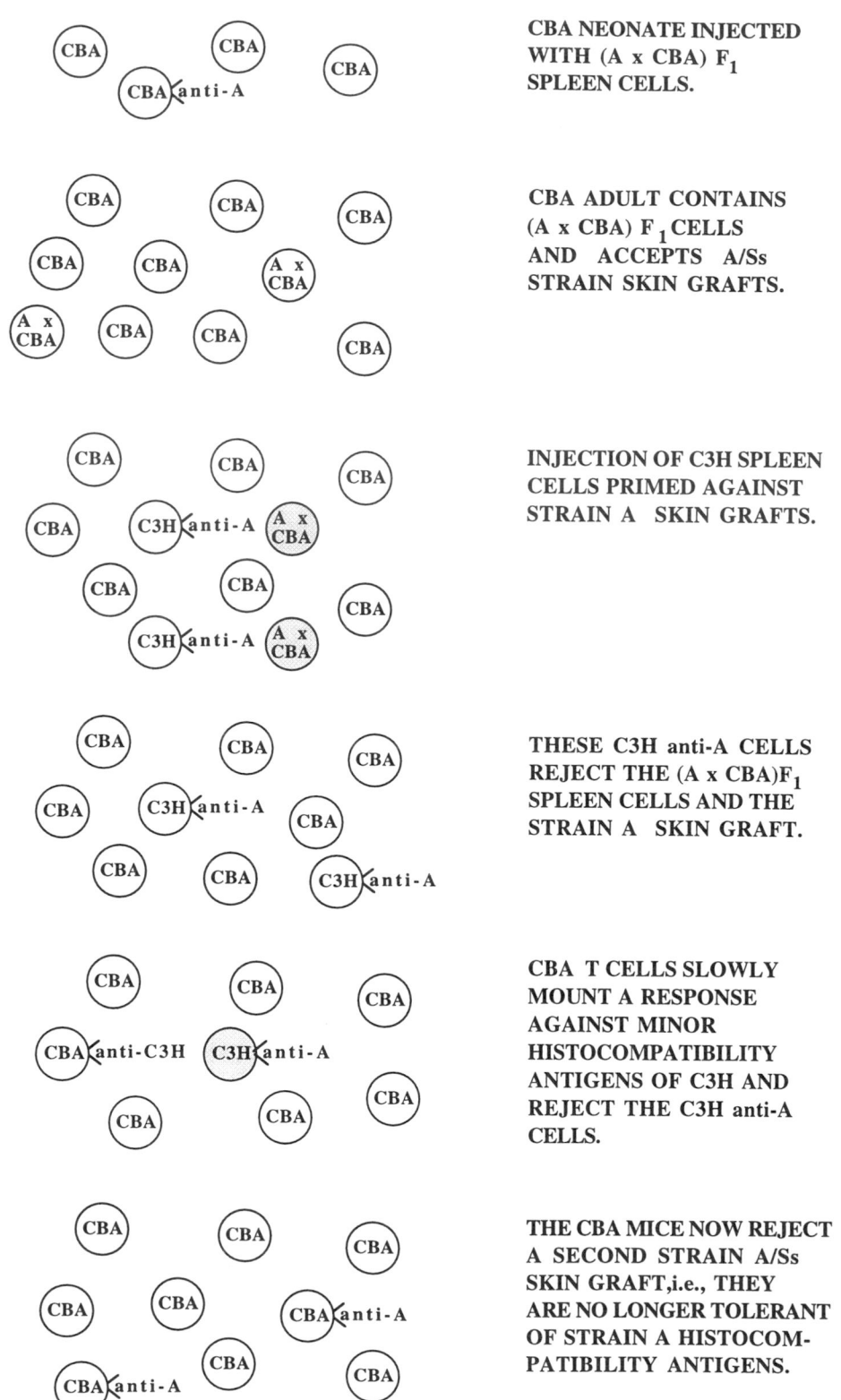

CBA NEONATE INJECTED
WITH (A x CBA) F₁
SPLEEN CELLS.

CBA ADULT CONTAINS
(A x CBA) F₁ CELLS
AND ACCEPTS A/Ss
STRAIN SKIN GRAFTS.

INJECTION OF C3H SPLEEN
CELLS PRIMED AGAINST
STRAIN A SKIN GRAFTS.

THESE C3H anti-A CELLS
REJECT THE (A x CBA)F₁
SPLEEN CELLS AND THE
STRAIN A SKIN GRAFT.

CBA T CELLS SLOWLY
MOUNT A RESPONSE
AGAINST MINOR
HISTOCOMPATIBILITY
ANTIGENS OF C3H AND
REJECT THE C3H anti-A
CELLS.

THE CBA MICE NOW REJECT
A SECOND STRAIN A/Ss
SKIN GRAFT,i.e., THEY
ARE NO LONGER TOLERANT
OF STRAIN A HISTOCOM-
PATIBILITY ANTIGENS.

FIG. 10. Antigen persistence is required for neonatal tolerance. Newborn mice have very few mature peripheral T cells. As a consequence they are easily tolerized by injection of F_1 spleen cells expressing foreign histocompatibility antigens. As adults, the tolerant mice accept skin grafts from the foreign donor parent. This tolerant state can be reversed, however, by injection of allogeneic T cells activated against the foreign parental histocompatibility antigens. These cells reject both the skin graft and the persisting F_1 spleen cells that are necessary to maintain the tolerant state. See ref. 386 for details.

To determine the mechanism by which the disrupted chimerism resulted in a loss of tolerance, Silvers (387) thymectomized the mice before injecting the primed C3H lymphoid cells. Under these circumstances, 60% of the mice failed to reject a second A skin graft. This suggested that tolerance induction in those animals involved an irreversible process such as clonal deletion and that the reversal of tolerance in nonthymectomized mice involved the generation of new T cells in the thymus. The other 40% of the mice, however, did reject a second A skin graft, suggesting that in those cases a peripheral regulatory mechanism was responsible for the tolerance, one that required persistence of the antigen to be maintained.

Neonatal tolerance induced across only an MHC class II barrier resulted in skin graft acceptance and loss of an allogeneic CTL response in the adult; but lymphoid cells from these mice still gave a mixed leuckocyte proliferative response (388). In contrast to a normal MLR, however, the response by cells from the tolerant mice was largely mediated by IL-4–producing cells (389). Furthermore, in a more traditional model involving a full MHC difference, (B6 × BALB/c)F$_1$ into BALB/c, the tolerant animals manifested a lupus-like autoimmune disease, including hypergammaglobulinemia, immune complex–mediated glomerulonephritis, and production of anti–single-stranded DNA antibodies of IgG1 isotype (390). The antibodies came from the chimeric F$_1$ B cells after interaction with host CD4$^+$ T cells (391). IL-4 plays a critical role in this process, as low doses of anti–IL-4 antibody administered 24 to 48 hours after injection of the tolerizing F$_1$ spleen cells prevented the autoimmune syndrome (392). Interestingly, higher doses of antibody prevented the tolerance induction as well. These results suggest that IL-4 producing Th2 cells are involved in initiating the tolerance process. Consistent with that notion, administration of IFN-γ at the time of neonatal priming blocked tolerance induction (393). Studies have also demonstrated the generation of Th2 cells in neonates when they are immunized with soluble protein antigens given in Freund's incomplete adjuvant (394). Thus, neonatal transplantation tolerance appears to result from a combination of (a) immune deviation and (b) clonal deletion following the establishment of donor-cell chimerism. The participation of other immunologic mechanisms, however, has not been ruled out (395).

Antibody-mediated Tolerance (Original Antigenic Sin)

Passive transfer of antibodies into a naive animal often prevents the priming of that animal with a subsequent injection of antigen (396). High-affinity antibodies are more effective than low-affinity ones (397). Some of this effect is due to formation and clearance of antigen–antibody complexes. The antibodies can also prevent the formation of particular peptides needed for T-cell recognition (398,399). The antigen–antibody complexes are also likely to be responsible for the phenomenon known as original antigenic sin (400), in which memory B cells, generated during a prior exposure to a cross-reacting antigen, prevent or downregulate the response to the unique new determinants on the antigen. This phenomenon was initially described in the immune response to influenza virus, where people infected with one strain of virus preferentially made an antibody response to that strain when subsequently infected with a second strain of the virus (401). Cross-reactivity in the memory B-cell response has been documented in the splenic focus assay for TNP and DNP (402). Primary B cells selectively respond to DNP or TNP, but secondary B cells can be stimulated to secrete

antibody by either hapten. It was proposed that memory B cells are more cross-reactive for their activation than are primary B cells because of increased affinity as a consequence of somatic hypermutation or because of class switching (402). By contrast, experiments from Linton et al. (201) have argued that the secondary B cells derive from a separate precursor population. Whatever the mechanism, memory B cells seem to have an advantage for rapid activation, and this early activation produces antibodies that feed back to inhibit the priming of new B cells possessing receptors that are specific for the second immunogen. This feedback mechanism is most likely mediated through antigen–antibody complexes, which interact with the Fcγ RIIb1 receptors on the naive B cells and inhibit signal transduction through their IgM receptors (403), possibly by bringing phosphatases into the receptor complex (404).

Antiidiotypic B-Cell Regulation

In 1974 Jerne proposed that antibody production could be regulated by other antibodies that recognized unique idiotypic determinants in the V regions of the first antibody (405). He postulated that an increase in the production of the first antibody could negatively regulate the production of antiidiotypic antibodies, and vice versa. Because of the interconnected pathways in such a network, perturbation of one segment would be dampened by the presence of other segments, and thus the original steady state would be buffered.

In recent years, studies have focused on the analysis of IgM hybridomas from nonimmunized neonatal mice (406) or IgM antibodies derived from human cord blood Epstein-Barr virus–transformed B cells (77,102,103,407). Interestingly, individual antibodies show the ability to react with several different self ligands, many of which are intracellular proteins, such as cytoskeletal proteins (74–76,103,408,409). In both species, their major source appears to be B1 (CD5$^+$) B cells (104,105). The interesting aspect with regard to immunologic networks is that these antibodies also interact with other members of the set (406,408). Administration of such antibodies to neonatal mice perturbs the B cell repertoire and affects the subsequent adult response to particular antigens (410). This effect is either positive or negative, depending on the timing and the antibody. Whether the natural dominance of B cells expressing certain idiotypes is related to such network interactions (411), or is due to early exposure to commensal bacteria (412) is still controversial. Support for the former idea comes from experiments in which bone marrow is transferred to syngeneic irradiated hosts; idiotypic dominance disappears unless small amounts of antiidiotypic antibodies are injected at the time of bone marrow transfer (413). Furthermore, clonally dominant idiotypes emerge in germ-free animals (414,415) and can be disrupted in their appearance by early antigen priming with heat-killed bacteria (416). Interestingly, the nonidiotype-positive antibodies elicited by this early priming proved *not* to be protective for subsequent challenge with virulent bacteria, suggesting that the network could play a crucial role in host defense (416,417).

Antiidiotypic T-Cell Regulation

Standard T-cell activation involves recognition of antigenic peptides bound to MHC molecules. The generation of regulatory T cells that could suppress an immune response by recognizing the receptor on responding T cells requires the recognition of unique peptides derived from that TCR. Evidence that this might occur comes from studies of experimental allergic encephalomyelitis (418,419). The CD4$^+$ T-cell response is dominated by cells expressing Vβ8 and Vα2 and 4. Animals immunized with a synthetic peptide corresponding to the CDR2 region of the TCR Vβ8 chain were protected against the demyelineating disease. Not all TCR peptides are effective, presumably because of the failure to bind to that animal's MHC molecules. The mechanism by which the regulatory process works is not clear. One possibility is that CD8$^+$ cytotoxic T cells are involved (420). Activation of the pathogenic CD4$^+$ T cell leads to clearing and cycling of its TCR. New receptor synthesis is initiated, which could give rise to endogenous peptides capable of binding to class I molecules. Such complexes could stimulate CD8$^+$ T cells if IL-2 produced by the CD4$^+$ T cell is a second signal for these cells. Once activated, the CD8 cells could then specifically lyse the CD4$^+$ cells. Sun et al. (421) have produced lines of CD8$^+$ T cells from Lewis rats that have some of these properties and that mediate resistance to disease induction *in vivo*.

IMMUNE PRIVILEGED SITES

Transplant surgeons have known for a long time that certain areas in the body are more favorable for grafting than others. In particular, the brain, the anterior chamber of the eye, and the testis seem to be privileged in their capacity to accept grafts readily (422). The idea thus emerged that antigens contained in these tissues could not be seen by the immune system because they were sequestered in some way, for example, by the blood–brain barrier. Subsequent studies, however, showed that lymphocytes do migrate into these tissues. Activated T cells acquire cell adhesion molecules (e.g., α4,β1 integrin) that allow the cells to cross the blood endothelium into the brain (423). The antigen specificity of the T cell does not matter. If, however, the cells recognize peptide antigens inside the brain, presented on microglia (bone marrow–derived APC), they can release lymphokines, resulting in tissue damage (424). On the other hand, the nervous system does have a number of mechanisms for preventing the initiation of an immune response. The tissue has few if any dendritic cells (cells expressing large amounts of MHC class II molecules), which are thought to be the primary initiating cells in most T-cell responses (425,426). It also has no lymphatic drainage, which is normally required to bring antigens to the lymph nodes for the priming of T cells (422). Finally, neurons do not express any MHC molecules, and, even in the presence of inflammatory lymphokines, they only express low levels of MHC class I molecules (426,427). Many other tissues (e.g., muscle) do not express MHC class II molecules and have only very low levels of MHC class I molecules, thus preventing the initiation of T-cell responses; but in the presence of an inflammatory reaction involving lymphokines such as IFN-γ, they increase their expression of MHC class I molecules to become more effective presenters of endogenous peptides (428,429).

Experiments have suggested an interesting mechanism by which a tissue may obtain privileged status, even if exposed to activated T cells: namely, by expression of Fas ligand on its cells. Although this would not impair freshly activated T cells from entering a tissue or a graft and initially having an effect, it would prevent sustained inflammatory responses by killing the T cells via a Fas–Fas ligand interaction. This would help reduce the immunopathology. The first nonlymphoid location where the presence of Fas Ligand was demonstrated is on the Sertoli cells of the testis (430). In a transplantation model, testis grafts from normal mice survived indefinitely under the kidney capsule of allogeneic recipients, while similar grafts from mice carrying a mutation in the Fas ligand (*gld*) gene were rejected. In a tissue destruction model, a viral infection of the anterior chamber of the eye of *gld* mice caused massive tissue damage, whereas the same infection in normal mice resulted in Fas/FasL-dependent killing of the inflammatory lymphoid cells (431). Fas ligand expression has been detected in corneal epithelial and endothelial cells (432). Interestingly, even some tumor cells have been shown to express Fas ligand, which might help them escape immune surveillance (433).

Another mechanism that has been described to participate in the immune privilege of the eye is called *anterior chamber–associated immune deviation* (ACAID) (434). Injection of exogenous antigens into the anterior chamber results in a systemic impairment of the production of complement-fixing antibodies and DTH to that antigen; that is, Th1 responses are blocked (435). The mechanism appears to be an effect of TGF-β secreted from the iris and ciliary body cells in the eye, which alters the presentation properties of the APCs such that class I–restricted CD8$^+$ regulatory T cells are induced in the spleen (436). How these cells suppress the DTH response has not yet been elucidated, but, interestingly, thymectomy and splenectomy experiments suggest that both the thymus and splenic B cells play a critical role in the process (437,438).

THE FETAL–MATERNAL RELATIONSHIP

A number of examples exist in the reproduction of vertebrates in which one organism successfully grafts itself onto another as a parabiont, completely circumventing rejection by the host's immune system (439). Perhaps the most interesting example of this natural tolerance induction is in viviparous mammals, in which the fetus successfully implants itself in the uterus (440). When any inbred mammalian strain-A female is mated to a strain-B male, the (A × B)F$_1$ fetus expresses histocompatibility antigens of the father to which the mother is not tolerant; yet the fetus is not rejected. This is also true for completely allogeneic fetuses that have been experimentally created by embryo transfer (441,442).

Witebski and Reich (443) were the first to suggest that this immune privilege might exist because the placenta does not express histocompatibility antigens. Evidence to support this idea is very good in primates. Syncytiotrophoblasts of the human fetus do not express polymorphic MHC class I or class II molecules (444,445). These cells are the closest in proximity to the maternal blood vessels in the villi of the placenta, and even when stimulated with IFN-γ, they do not express class I molecules (445). The remaining cells, cytotrophoblasts, express only the nonpolymorphic class Ib MHC molecule, HLA-G (446). Experiments have suggested that the major function of this molecule is to provide a ligand for the inhibitory receptor(s) on maternal NK cells, thus preventing them from killing the fetal cells (447). HLA-G is also expressed in thymic medullary epithelium, where it might ensure T-cell tolerance to this molecule (448). Finally, no cells expressing large amounts of class II molecules (dendritic cells) have been seen in the placenta. Possibly as a consequence of this limited MHC molecule expression, allogeneic fetuses do not prime for transplantation immunity, as measured by subsequent skin grafting (449). One puzzling fact, however, is that rodent placental cells do express classical polymorphic MHC class I molecules (450), yet these animals routinely produce live births. Hence other mechanisms must also play a role in fetal survival.

An effect of the fetus on the mother's immune system has been demonstrated in TCR transgenic female mice whose T cells are specific for a paternal MHC class I molecule (K^b) (451). During pregnancy, these cells were reduced in numbers and appeared to have downregulated their receptor levels. They were also functionally impaired, as the mother failed to reject K^b-bearing tumor grafts during this period. Following birth, the immune system returned to normal. Furthermore, these effects were antigen-specific, as they were not observed in syngeneic or non-K^b allogeneic pregnancies. Thus, pregnancy transiently results in a state of specific tolerance to paternal antigens.

Two mechanisms have been proposed for this transient tolerant state. One is expression of Fas ligand in the placenta, which, similar to its action in other privileged sites, would kill activated T cells entering the tissue (452). In the human placenta, Fas ligand is expressed early in cytotrophoblasts as well as at term in syncytiotrophoblasts (452,453). In the *gld* mouse, which lacks a functional Fas ligand, fetal resorption sites are common and litter sizes are small (453). A second mechanism is the production of cytokines and hormones by the placenta, which would inactivate the T cells or deviate these cells towards a Th2 response (454). Often after multiple pregnancies, the mother makes an antibody response to the father's histocompatibility antigens (455). Occasionally, the antibodies formed are harmful to the fetus, as in Rh incompatibility, causing erythrocyte destruction (456), but for the most part, the antibodies are not destructive. Several laboratories (457,458) have demonstrated that many of these antibodies do not fix complement. Furthermore, in some experiments on multiparous rodents, allogeneic paternal skin grafts on mothers that had been mated several times to males of that allogeneic strain were rejected more slowly than the same grafts placed on mothers that had been mated to syngeneic males (459,460). Thus, the fetus can induce noncytotoxic antipaternal MHC antibodies but does not prime or occasionally suppresses rejection of paternal skin grafts. This suggests that forces are at work in the placenta to deviate immune responses that the mother makes towards a Th2-like pattern.

In support of this idea, the cytokines usually associated with Th2 responses, such as IL-4, IL-5, and IL-10, have been detected in the placenta (454,461,462), as has an immunosuppressive cytokine related to TGF-β2 (463). Furthermore, progesterone, which is present in high concentrations in the placenta, has been shown to prolong allogeneic skin graft survival (464) and to favor the development of Th2 responses from antigen-specific T-cell lines and clones (465) A study of the effect of pregnancy on susceptibility to *Leishmania* infection in B6 mice, which normally resist the parasite with a vigorous Th1 response, showed an impaired clearance of the organism, resulting from a decreased IFN-γ response (466). Reciprocally, infection with *Leishmania* enhanced both spontaneous abortion and failed implantation rates, as well as decreased the production of IL-4 and IL-10 in the placenta (467). In humans, spontaneous abortions are also associated with an increased capability of producing IL-2 and IFN-γ and a decrease in IL-10 production (468). Finally, the excess fetal loss observed in the CBA and DBA/2 mouse mating combination is associated with decreased IL-4 and IL-10 production and can be reversed by administration of IL-10 or anti-IFN-γ antibody (469). Thus, the cytokine milieu of the placenta appears to play a critical role in the maternal acceptance of the fetus, and may provide another example of immune deviation leading to tolerance.

BREAKING OF TOLERANCE

Ehrlich's dogma (1) of *horror autotoxicus* went unchallenged for almost 40 years, until several groups began immunizing animals with CFA containing homogenates of proteins from peripheral tissues (470,471). This manipulation showed that the immune system was not fully tolerant to all self antigens and that immunopathology (autoimmunity) could result when the system was perturbed in certain ways. A detailed discussion of autoimmune diseases, both induced and spontaneous, is presented in Chapters 33 and 34. Here I will discuss only the general concepts of what must underlie this breakdown in tolerance when it occurs.

As presented earlier, not all demonstrable autoreactive B-cell clones are deleted during development. Thus, if a foreign protein that contains a self determinant or shares a determinant that closely mimics it, is introduced into an adult, tolerance can be broken at the B-cell level. The B cells bind and internalize the protein, and if any of the foreign peptides generated can bind to that individual's MHC molecules, the antigen will activate the T-cell help required for autoantibody production. In this way, tolerance at the T-cell level would be bypassed (78–81,113–115). Normally, such acute reactions that break tolerance are not a severe problem, because the antibody response helps clear the infectious agent and then disappears when the foreign antigen is cleared, because the T-cell help disappears. In some cases, however, an autoimmune disease can take place. For example, rheumatic carditis is thought to occur when antibodies elicited against determinants on the M-protein of Group A streptococci cross-react with cardiac myosin and cause acute damage and inflammation, which may lead to impairment of heart valve function (472,473).

At the T-cell level, the immune system appears to take extra precautions to ensure that autoreactive T-cell clones are deleted in the thymus. It does this by establishing a lower affinity threshold for negative selection than the threshold required for activation of T cells in the periphery (63–66). Nonetheless, low-affinity antiself T cells still emerge from the thymus. Furthermore, there will also be T cells that recognize tissue-specific peripheral antigens, which are unable to reach the thymus in large amounts. Cibotti et al. (474) studied a set of transgenic mice expressing different levels of hen eggwhite lysozyme, and showed that T cells specific for dominant determinants were always eliminated by clonal deletion, but that T cells specific for subdominant determinants were eliminated only when the circulating lysozyme concentration was high. Finally, even for peripheral antigens like myelin basic protein, which have been shown to be expressed at low levels in the thymus (475,476), low-affinity T cells have been clearly shown to survive thymic selection (477), presumably because not enough antigen is presented by thymic dendritic cells. It is such T cells that are activated by the antigen when it is administered in CFA (470) and that go on to initiate many autoimmune diseases.

What then is Freund's adjuvant doing, and how might this occur under "normal" environmental conditions to cause autoimmunity? Three basic models have been proposed. One suggests that inflammatory processes involving necrotic cell death, cytokine production, and the induction of costimulatory molecules in peripheral tissues lead to the activation of the low-affinity self-reactive T cells (478). The second suggests that these T cells are first activated by determinants from infectious agents to which the T cells have high affinity and that, once activated, a low-affinity cross-reaction on self peptides is sufficient to sustain them as a chronic immune response. This second model was referred to as molecular mimicry in its original formulation by Fujinami and Oldstone (479). The third model also invokes infectious agents, but postulates that it is a superantigen that they produce, which turns on the low-affinity antiself T cells (480–482).

TABLE 6. *Transgenic manipulations leading to autoimmune diabetes*

T cells	Costimulation	Inflammation	Diabetes
LCMV TCR transgenic	—	—	No
LCMV TCR transgenic	Islet B7	—	Yes
Normal	Islet B7	—	No
K^b TCR transgenic	Islet IL-2	—	Yes
Normal	Islet B7	Islet TNF-α	Yes
Normal	—	Islet TNF-α	No
Normal	—	Islet IFN-α	Yes
Normal	—	Islet IFN-γ	Yes

Data compiled from refs. 311, 487–491, and 499.

To test the inflammation hypothesis and to understand what Freund's complete adjuvant might be doing, a number of transgenic models have been created in which cytokine and costimulatory molecules have been expressed under the control of tissue-specific promoters (Table 6). To highlight some of the findings, we will focus on the induction of diabetes as an autoimmune disease, in which the immune system destroys the β cells of the pancreas (483) by a Fas-mediated mechanism (484). Although this destruction can be mediated by CD4⁺ T cells in TCR transgenic mice containing large numbers of T cells with receptors for an islet antigen (485), in NOD mice, which spontaneously get the disease, it is mediated by both CD8⁺ and CD4⁺ T cells (486).

In the model system of Ohashi et al. (311), described earlier, the LCMV glycoprotein was expressed in the β cells, but not recognized by an immune system containing large numbers of CD8⁺ T cells specific for a peptide from this protein, unless the T cells were activated by the virus. Interestingly, if these double transgenic mice were crossed to a third transgenic expressing the B7.1 costimulating molecule in the β cells, the triple transgenic spontaneously developed diabetes (487) (Table 6). None of the double transgenic permutations developed the disease. These results demonstrate that T cells are getting to the tissue even without viral activation, but that they are not sufficiently stimulated to cause disease. The failure of mice with a normal T-cell repertoire to get disease, even though they have B7.1 constitutively expressed in the islets, suggests that the frequency of T cells that get there, or that are stimulated there, is another critical variable in generating the disease process. In a different series of experiments, B7.1 expression in the islets was shown to result in spontaneous diabetes, if the proinflammatory cytokine TNF-α was also expressed (488). A mouse with only a TNF-α transgene in the islets did not get disease, although it did develop insulitis, in which T cells and macrophages were seen infiltrating the pancreas (489). Thus, under limiting conditions, when a few T cells with only low-affinity receptors for normal islet antigens are present, both an inflammatory signal to bring the T cells to the site and an aberrant costimulating signal to keep them activated there were necessary to induce islet destruction.

Two other studies have demonstrated that expression in the islets of IFN alone is sufficient to induce disease. Either IFN-γ or IFN-α resulted in diabetes (490,491). IFN-γ is known to upregulate MHC molecule expression on most cells, which could enhance presentation of islet antigens. Whether this could cause disease by synergizing with the inflammation that IFN-γ also induces via macrophage activation is unclear. IFN-γ and TNF-α together have been shown to cause MHC class II molecule expression on β cells

(492), which could facilitate local antigen presentation to CD4⁺ T cells specific for islet antigens. Whether this would help or hinder an immune response might depend on the presence of costimulation (493). The particular alleles of the MHC class II molecules expressed by an individual, either human (494) or mouse (495), play a critical role in predisposing to the onset of disease; however, whether this is important in antigen presentation in the islets (496) or tolerance induction in the thymus (497,498) is not clear. Finally, in another transgenic model (499), expression of IL-2 in the β cells facilitated diabetes induction, suggesting that prolonged local activation and survival of autoreactive T cells may be a major element in producing autoimmunity.

Overall, these experiments suggest that the critical variables for creating an autoimmune process involve stimulating a sufficient number of T cells by local production of inflammatory cytokines and upregulation of MHC and costimulatory molecules. CFA probably mimics this situation. The experimentalist, by providing the antigen together with CFA at the immunization site, can thus prime the low-affinity T cells in sufficient numbers to induce significant migration to tissues where the antigen is naturally expressed. Once in the tissue, the activated effector T cells initiate damage and inflammation at this location, allowing the native antigens to now be released and presented to the immune system in large enough amounts to sustain the immune response. Experimental support for such a process has come from the experiments of Lehmann et al. (500). Mice were immunized with the immunodominant peptide of myelin basic protein (MBP) in CFA. The initial T cells primed to the antigen were specific for this peptide. However, after 3 weeks, T cells specific for other, subdominant determinants on MBP were detected, even though these determinants were not present in the immunizing emulsion. The phenomenon, called determinant spreading, was not observed following immunization with a peptide from a nonself antigen, lysozyme. Their interpretation is that the initially primed T cells created an inflammatory process in the brain, which eventually allowed antigen presentation of the mouse's own MBP and activation of naive T cells specific for other determinants on the molecule.

Under nonexperimental conditions, this process is postulated to be initiated by an infectious agent. For example, coxsackie B3 virus is thought to initiate autoimmune disease in the heart by causing a local inflammatory process in the organ (478). This results in the presentation of cardiac myosin to the immune system, and the priming of T cells specific for this self antigen produces the autoimmune disease (501). Whether the initial T cells specific for cardiac myosin are actually primed by the virus is still not clear. Evidence for molecular mimicry between self proteins and foreign proteins is impressive (502,503); however, experimental data that show that immunization with a peptide from an infectious agent can elicit an autoimmune disease is sparse. In the original paper on molecular mimicry (479), immunization with a strong viral peptide mimic (six out of eight amino acids were the same as an immunodominant peptide from MBP) resulted in only very mild histologic evidence of immunopathology in a few of the rabbits. In fact, most experiments only show that viral or bacterial T-cell epitopes can stimulate T-cell clones isolated from patients or animals having the autoimmune disease (504).

The usual assumption in the molecular mimicry model is that the foreign determinant activates T-cells with TCRs that are cross-reactive for a peptide from a self protein. The possibility that a slightly different mechanism might operate has been suggested by the experiments of Lin et al. (505). Mice immunized with human cytochrome-c in CFA make a strong proliferative response when their T cells are restimulated with the antigen in culture. Immunization with mouse cytochrome-*c* in CFA does not result in a strong proliferative response. If, however, the mouse and human cytochromes are given together in CFA, a strong mouse-specific T cell–proliferative response is observed. Interestingly, this response did not result from the direct activation of T cells by the human cytochrome-*c* because this antigen could not stimulate mouse cytochrome-*c*–specific T-cell clones that were derived from the mixed culture. Rather, it appeared to involve a cross-reaction at the B-cell level, which allowed mouse cytochrome-*c* to be more effectively presented. Thus, B cells primed to human cytochrome-*c* made antibodies that cross-reacted with mouse cytochrome-*c*. Transfer of such B cells to a naive syngeneic mouse resulted in a T cell–proliferative response to mouse cytochrome-*c* when the animals were immunized with mouse cytochrome-*c* in CFA. Thus, molecular mimicry at the B-cell level could facilitate the priming or expansion of CD4$^+$ T cells specific for a self antigen, even if there is no cross-reactivity at the T-cell level.

Finally, there is a way in which a completely irrelevant protein might activate a T cell to become autoreactive. Because many T cells in the repertoire express more than one receptor, some cells with self-reactive receptors will escape clonal deletion in the thymus due to low expression of the self-reactive TCR. This was shown to be the case in a C5-specific TCR transgenic model expressing both C5 and the receptor. The T cells were all deleted on a Rag-1 knock-out backgound, which precludes endogenous receptor rearrangement. In contrast, many of the T cells escaped deletion if the mice were crossed to a second TCR transgenic mouse specific for another (nonself) antigen (506). These animals with two receptors appeared tolerant to the circulating C5 self antigen, presumably because of the low level of expression of the C5-specific receptor on the peripheral T cells. Interestingly, activation of these T cells with the antigen that was not present in the animal generated cells that were capable of killing targets that expressed the C5 antigen. These results suggest that autoreactivity can be generated from receptor downmodulated T cells upon stimulation with unrelated environmental antigens recognized by the second receptor on the cell.

The idea that a superantigen might initiate an autoimmune disease process has received some support from the isolation of a human endogenous retrovirus from diabetic patients (482). An enrichment of Vβ7-bearing T cells was observed in the pancreas of two diabetics (507), and this led to the identification of a superantigen at the N-terminus of the envelope glycoprotein of the mouse mammary tumor virus-related human retrovirus (482). The authors speculated that the endogenous retrovirus becomes activated to express the superantigen by environmental or hormonal stimulation and that this in turn activates T cells with low-affinity receptors for islet antigens, allowing them to migrate to the pancreas and initiate the autoimmunity. At this point, however, there is only a correlation between superantigen expression and disease, and further data will be required to establish cause and effect.

This discussion on the breaking of tolerance applies only to organ-specific autoimmune diseases. In contrast, systemic autoimmune diseases appear to result from dysregulations in the whole system. Either normal immune responses are unchecked by negative feedback regulation or the developing immune system is not adequately purged of autoreactive cells. These states can arise from genetic mutations such as the *lpr/lpr* mouse (508). In this case, the defect in Fas function allows lymphocytes to persist beyond their normal life span by interfering with the apoptotic cell death that they normally undergo following activation (509). When the *lpr*

gene is crossed into a mouse expressing a transgenic BCR specific for double-stranded DNA, the animals abnormally secrete large amounts of anti-DNA antibody (510), a characteristic of the autoimmune disease systemic lupus erythematosus. By contrast, B cells expressing this receptor on a non-*lpr* background are tolerized. Many other diseases of this type are discussed in Chapter 33, in which both genetic and environmental causes of immune system dysregulation are presented.

ACKNOWLEDGMENTS

I would like to thank Dr. Helen Quill for her scholarly review of the manuscript and for the many helpful suggestions she made, which improved it. The thoughtful comments of Dr. Colin Anderson are also gratefully acknowledged. This chapter is dedicated to A; may he live long and prosper.

REFERENCES

1. Ehrlich P, Morgenroth J. On haemolysins: third and fifth communications. In: *The Collected Papers on Paul Ehrlich*, vol 2. London: Pergamon, 1957:205–212, 246–255.
2. Owen RD. Immunogenetic consequences of vascular ananstomoses between bovine twins. *Science* 1945;102:400–401.
3. Lillie FR. The theory of the free-martin. *Science* 1916;43:611–613.
4. Burnet FM, Fenner F. In: *The production of antibodies*, 2nd ed. London: Macmillan, 1949:102–105.
5. Traub E. Factors influencing the persistence of choriomeningitis virus in the blood of mice after clinical recovery. *J Exp Med* 1938;68:229–250.
6. Billingham RE, Brent L, Medawar PB. Actively acquired tolerance of foreign cells. *Nature* 1953;172:603–606.
7. Hašek M. Parabiosis of birds during embryonic development. *Cesk Biol* 1953;2:265–270.
8. Burnet FM. A modification of Jerne's theory of antibody production using the concept of clonal selection. *Aust J Sci* 1957;20:67–69.
9. Triplett EL. On the mechanism of immunologic self recognition. *J Immunol* 1962;89:505–510.
10. Kappler JW, Roehm N, Marrack P. T cell tolerance by clonal elimination in the thymus. *Cell* 1987;49:273–280.
11. Blackman MA, Lund FE, Surman S, Corley RB, Woodland DL. Major histocompatibility complex-restricted recognition of retroviral superantigens by Vβ17$^+$ T cells. *J Exp Med* 1992;176:275–280.
12. Surh CD, Sprent J. T-cell apoptosis detected *in situ* during positive and negative selection in the thymus. *Nature* 1994;372:100–103.
13. MacDonald HR, Schneider R, Lees RK, et al. T-cell receptor V beta use predicts reactivity and tolerance to Mls^a-encoded antigens. *Nature* 1988;332:40–45.
14. Guidos CJ, Danska JS, Fathman CG, Weissman IL. T cell receptor-mediated negative selection of autorective T lymphocyte precursors occurs after commitment to the CD4 or CD8 lineages. *J Exp Med* 1990;172:835–845.
15. Hugo P, Boyd RL, Waanders GA, Petrie HT, Scollay R. Timing of deletion of autoreactive Vβ6$^+$ cells and down-modulation of either CD4 or CD8 on phenotypically distinct CD4$^+$8$^+$ subsets of thymocytes expressing intermediate or high levels of T cell receptor. *Int Immunol* 1990;3:265–272.
16. Kisielow P, Blüthmann H, Staerz UD, Steinmetz M, Von Boehmer H. Tolerance in T-cell receptor transgenic mice involves deletion of nonmature CD4$^+$8$^+$ thymocytes. *Nature* 1988;333:742–746.
17. Blüthmann H, Kisielow P, Uematsu Y, et al. T-cell-specific deletion of T-cell recptor transgenes allows functional rearrangement of endogenous alpha- and beta-genes. *Nature* 1988;334:156–159.
18. Sha WC, Nelson CA, Newberry RD, Kranz DM, Russell JH, Loh DY. Positive and negative selection of an antigen receptor on T cells in transgenic mice. *Nature* 1988;336:73–76.
19. Dent AL, Matis LA, Hooshmand F, Widacki SM, Bluestone JA, Hedrick SM. Self-reactive γδ T cells are eliminated in the thymus. *Nature* 1990;343:714–719.
20. Takahama Y, Kosugi A, Singer A. Phenotype, ontogeny, and repertoire of CD4$^-$CD8$^-$ T cell receptor αβ$^+$ thymocytes. *J Immunol* 1991;146:1134–1141.
21. Singer PA, Balderas RS, McEvilly RJ, Bobardt M, Theofilopoulos AN. Tolerance-related Vβ clonal deletions in normal CD4$^-$8$^-$, TCR-α/β$^+$ and abnormal lpr and gld cell populations. *J Exp Med* 1989;170:1869–1877
22. Bendelac A, Killeen N, Littman D, Schwartz RH. A subset of CD4$^+$ thymocytes selected by MHC class I molecules. *Science* 1994;263:1174–1178.
23. Poussier P, Edouard P, Lee C, Binnie M, Julius M. Thymus-independent development and negative selection of T cells expressing T cell receptor alpha/beta in the intestinal epithelium: evidence for distinct circulation patterns of gut- and thymus-derived T lymphocytes. *J Exp Med* 1992;176:187–199.

24. Takahama Y, Shores EW, Singer A. Negative selection of precursor thymocytes before their differentiation into CD4+CD8+ cells. *Science* 1992;258:653–656.

25. Pircher H, Bürki K, Lang R, Hengartner H, Zinkenagel RM. Tolerance induction in double specific T-cell receptor transgenic mice varies with antigen. *Nature* 1989;342:559–561.

26. MacDonald HR, Lees RK. Programmed death of autoreactive thymocytes. *Nature* 1990;343:642–644.

27. D'Adamio L, Awad KM, Reinherz EL. Thymic and peripheral apoptosis of antigen-specific T cells might cooperate in establishing self tolerance. *Eur J Immunol* 1993;23:747–753.

28. Kishimoto H, Sprent J. Negative selection in the thymus includes semimature T cells. *J Exp Med* 1997;185:263–271.

29. Sprent J, Lo D, Gao E-K, Ron Y. T cell selection in the thymus. *Immunol Rev* 1988;101:173–190.

30. Marrack P, Lo D, Brinster R, et al. The effects of thymus environment on T cell development and tolerance. *Cell* 1988;53:627–634.

31. Kyewski BA, Rouse RV, Kaplan HS. Thymocyte rosettes: multicellular complexes of lymphocytes and bone marrow-derived stromal cells in the mouse thymus. *Proc Natl Acad Sci USA* 1982;79:5646–5650.

32. Matzinger P, Guerder S. Does T-cell tolerance require a dedicated antigen-presenting cell. *Nature* 1989;338:74–76.

33. Swat W, Ignatowicz L, Von Boehmer H, Kisielow P. Clonal deletion of immature CD4+8+ thymocytes in suspension culture by extrathymic antigen-presenting cells. *Nature* 1991;351:150–153.

34. Sprent J, Von Boehmer H, Nabholz M. Association of immunity and tolerance to host H-2 determinants in irradiated F1 hybrid mice reconstituted with bone marrow cells from one parental strain. *J Exp Med* 1975;142:321–331.

35. Jenkinson EJ, Jhittay P, Kingston R, Owen JJT. Studies on the role of the thymic environment in the induction of tolerance to MHC antigens. *Transplantation* 1985;39:331–333.

36. Von Boehmer H, Schubiger K. Thymocytes appear to ignore class I major histocompatibility complex antigens expressed on thymus epithelial cells. *Eur J Immunol* 1984;14:1048–1056.

37. Gao E-K, Lo D, Sprent J. Strong T cell tolerance in parent → F1 bone marrow chimeras prepared with supralethal irradiation: evidence for clonal deletion and anergy. *J Exp Med* 1990;171:1101–1121.

38. Speiser DE, Pircher H, Ohashi PS, Kyburz D, Hengartner H, Zinkernagel RM. Clonal deletion induced by either radioresistant thymic host cells or lymphohemopoietic donor cells at different stages of class I-restricted T cell ontogeny. *J Exp Med* 1992;175:1277–1283.

39. Salaún J, Bandeira A, Khazaal I, et al. Thymic epithelium tolerizes for histocompatibility antigens. *Science* 1990;247:1471–1474.

40. Flajnik MF, Du Pasquier L, Cohen N. Immune responses of thymus/lymphocyte embryonic chimeras: studies on tolerance and major histocompatibility complex restriction in *Xenopus. Eur J Immunol* 1985;15:540–547.

41. Bonomo A, Matzinger P. Thymus epithelium induces tissue specific tolerance. *J Exp Med* 1993;177:1153–1164.

42. Jenkinson EJ, Anderson G, Owen JJT. Studies on T cell maturation on defined thymic stromal cell populations in vitro. *J Exp Med* 1992;176:845–853.

43. Berg LI, Fazekas de St Groth B, Pullen AM, Davis MM. Phenotype differences between αβ versus β T-cell receptor transgenic mice undergoing negative selection. *Nature* 1989;340:559–562.

44. Oehen S, Feng L, Xia Y, Surh CD, Hedrick SM. Antigen compartmentation and T helper cell tolerance induction. *J Exp Med* 1996;183: 2617–2626.

45. Schönrich G, Momburg F, Hämmerling GJ, Arnold B. Anergy induced by thymic medullary epithelium. *Eur J Immunol* 1992;22:1687–1691.

46. Hoffmann MW, Allison J, Miller JFAP. Tolerance induction by thymic medullary epithelium. *Proc Natl Acad Sci USA* 1992;89:2526–2530.

47. Van Ewijk W, Ron Y, Monaco J, et al. Compartmentalization of MHC class II gene expression in transgenic mice. *Cell* 1988;53:357–370.

48. Laufer TM, DeKoning J, Markowitz JS, Lo D, Glimcher LH. Unopposed positive selection and autoreactivity in mice expressing class II MHC only on thymic cortex. *Nature* 1996;383:81–85.

49. Shimonkevitz RP, Bevan MJ. Split tolerance induced by the intrathymic adoptive transfer of thymocyte stem cells. *J Exp Med* 1988;168:143–156.

50. Pircher H, Müller K-P, Kyewski BA, Hengartner H. Thymocytes can tolerize thymocytes by clonal deletion in vitro. *Int Immunol* 1992;4:1065–1069.

51. Pircher H, Brduscha K, Steinhoff U, et al. Tolerance induction by clonal deletion of CD4+8+ thymocytes in vitro does not require dedicated antigen-presenting cells. *Eur J Immunol* 1993;23:669–679.

52. Lederberg J. Genes and antibodies: do antigens bear instructions for antibody specificity or do they select cell lines that arise by mutation? *Science* 1959;129:1649–1653.

53. Scollay R, Shortman K. Cell traffic in the adult thymus: cell entry and exit, cell birth and death. In: Watson JD, Marbrook J, eds. *Recognition and regulation in cell-mediated immunity.* New York: Marcel Dekker Inc, 1985:3–30.

54. Page DM, Kane LP, Allison JP, Hedrick SM. Two signals are required for negative selection of CD4+8+ thymocytes. *J Immunol* 1993;151:1868–1880.

55. Punt JA, Osborne BA, Takahama Y, Sharrow SO, Singer A. Negative selection of CD4+8+ thymocytes by T cell receptor-induced apoptosis requires a costimulatory signal that can be provided by CD28. *J Exp Med* 1994;179:709–713.

56. Shahinian A, Pfeffer K, Lee KP, et al. Differential T cell costimulatory requirements in CD28-deficient mice. *Science* 1993;261:609–612.

57. Nelson AJ, Hosier S, Brady W, Linsley PS, Farr AG. Medullary thymic epithelium expresses a ligand for CTLA4 *in situ* and *in vitro. J Immunol* 1993;151: 2453–2461.

58. Van Parijs L, Ibraghimov A, Abbas AK. The roles of costimulation and Fas in T cell apoptosis and peripheral tolerance. *Immunity* 1996;4:321–328.

59. Douni E, Akassoglu K, Alexopoulou L, et al. Transgenic and knockout analyses of the role of TNF in immune regulation and disease pathogenesis. *J Inflamm* 1995;47:27–38.

60. Amakawa R, Hakem A, Kündig TM, et al. Impaired negative selection of T cells in Hodgkins disease antigen CD30-deficient mice. *Cell* 1996;84:551–562.

61. Bill J, Kanagawa O, Woodland D, Palmer E. The MHC molecule I-E is necessary but not sufficient for the clonal deletion of V(11 bearing T cells. *J Exp Med* 1989;169:1405–1419.

62. Gao E-K, Kanagawa O, Sprent J. Capacity of unprimed CD4+ and CD8+ T cells expressing Vβ11 receptors to respond to I-E alloantigens *in vivo. J Exp Med* 1989;170:1947–1957.

63. Yagi J, Janeway CA Jr. Ligand thresholds at different stages of T cell development. *Int Immunol* 1990;2:83–89.

64. Vasquez NJ, Kaye J, Hedrick SM. In vivo and in vitro clonal deletion of double-positive thymocytes. *J Exp Med* 1992;175:1307–1316.

65. Robertson K, Simon K, Schneider S, Timms E, Mitchison A. Tolerance of self induced in thymus organ culture. *Eur J Immunol* 1992;22:207–211.

66. Pircher H, Rohrer UH, Moskophidis D, Zinkernagel RM, Hengartner H. Lower receptor avidity required for thymic clonal deletion than for effector T-cell function. *Nature* 1991;351:482–485.

67. Robey EA, Ramsdell F, Gordon JW, et al. A self-reactive T cell population that is not subject to negative selection. *Int Immunol* 1992;4:969–974.

68. Auphan N, Jézo-Brémond A, Schönrich G, et al. Threshold tolerance in H-2Kb-specific TCR transgenic mice expressing mutant H-2Kb conversion of helper-independent to helper-dependent CTL. *Int Immunol* 1992;4:1419–1428.

69. Von Boehmer H. Developmental biology of T cells in T cell receptor transgenic mice. *Annu Rev Immunol* 1990;8:536–537.

70. Malissen M, Trucy J, Letourneur F, et al. A T cell clone expresses two T cell receptor alpha genes but uses one alpha beta heterodimer for allorecognition and self MHC-restricted antigen recognition. *Cell* 1988;55:49–59.

71. Padovan E, Casorati G, Dellabona P, Meyer S, Brockhaus M, Lanzavecchia A. Expression of two T cell receptor alpha chains: dual receptor T cells. *Science* 1993;262:422–424.

72. Bankhurst AD, Torrigiani G, Allison AC. Lymphocytes binding human thyroglobulin in healthy people and its relevance for autoantigens. *Lancet* 1973;1: 226–229.

73. Primi D, Smith CI, Hammarström L, Möller G. Sera from lipopolysaccharide (LPS)-injected mice exhibit complement-dependent cytotoxicity against syngeneic and autologous spleen cells. *Cell Immunol* 1977;32:252–262.

74. Dresser DW. Most IgM-producing cells in the mouse secrete auto-antibodies (rheumatoid factor). *Nature* 1978;274:480–483.

75. Steele EJ, Cunningham AJ. High proportion of Ig-producing cells making autoantibody in normal mice. *Nature* 1978;274:483–484.

76. Underwood JR, Pedersen JS, Chatmers PJ, Toh BH. Hybrids from normal, germ free, nude and neonatal mice produce monoclonal autoantibodies to eight different intracellular structures. *Clin Exp Immunol* 1985;60:417–426.

77. Prabhakar BS, Saegusa J, Onodera T, Notkins AL. Lymphocytes capable of making monoclonal antibodies that react with multiple organs are a common feature of the normal B cell repertoire. *J Immunol* 1984;133:2815–2817.

78. Iverson GM, Lindenmann J. The role of a carrier-determinant and T cells in the induction of liver-specific autoantibodies in the mouse. *Eur J Immunol* 1972;2: 195–197.

79. Lane DP, Silver DM. Isolation of a murine liver-specific alloantigen, F antigen, and examination of its immunogenic properties by radioimmunoassay. *Eur J Immunol* 1976;6:480–485.

80. Haba S, Nisonoff A. Induction of high titers of anti-IgE by immunization of inbred mice with syngeneic IgE. *Proc Natl Acad Sci USA* 1987;84:5009–5013.

81. Harris DE, Cairns L, Rosen FS, Borel Y. A natural model of immunologic tolerance. Tolerance to murine C5 is mediated by T cells, and antigen is required to maintain unresponsiveness. *J Exp Med* 1982;156:567–584.

82. Reichlin M. Localizing antigenic determinants in human haemoglobin with mutants: molecular correlations of immunological tolerance. *J Mol Biol* 1972; 64:485–496.

83. Urbanski GJ, Margoliash E. Topographic determinants on cytochrome c. 1. The complete antigenic structures of rabbit, mouse and guanaco cytochromes *c* in rabbits and mice. *J Immunol* 1977;118:1170–1180.

84. Pierres M, Devaux C, Dosseto M, Marchetto S. Clonal analysis of B- and T-cell responses to Ia antigens. 1. Topology of epitope regions on I-Ab and I-Eb molecules analyzed with 35 monoclonal alloantibodies. *Immunogenetics* 1981;14:481–495.

85. Stamatoyannopoulos G, Farquhar M, Lindsley D, Brice M, Papayannopoulou T, Nute PE. Monoclonal antibodies specific for globin chains. *Blood* 1983;61: 530–539.

86. Tsubata T, Nishikawa S, Katsura Y, Kumagai S, Imura H. B cell repertoire for anti-DNA antibody in normal and lupus mice: differential expression of precursor cells for high and low affinity anti-DNA antibodies. *Clin Exp Immunol* 1988; 71:50–55.

87. Nemazee DA, Bürki K. Clonal deletion of B lymphocytes in a transgenic mouse bearing anti-MHC class I antibody genes. *Nature* 1989;337:562–566.

88. Raff MC, Owen JJT, Cooper MD, Lawton AR, Megson M, Gathings WE. Differences in susceptibility of mature and immature mouse B lymphocytes to anti-immunoglobulin-induced immunoglobulin suppression *in vitro*: possible implications for B-cell tolerance to self. *J Exp Med* 1975;142:1052–1064.

89. Sidman CL, Unanue ER. Receptor-mediated inactivation of early B lymphocytes. *Nature* 1975;257:149–151.

90. Hartley SB, Cooke MP, Fulcher DA, et al. Elimination of self-reactive B lymphocytes proceeds in two stages: arrested development and cell death. *Cell* 1993; 72:325–335.

91. Hertz M, Nemazee D. BCR ligation induces receptor editing in IgM⁺ IgD⁻ bone marrow B cells *in vitro*. *Immunity* 1997;6:429–436.

92. Tiegs SL, Russell DM, Nemazee D. Receptor editing in self-reactive bone marrow B cells. *J Exp Med* 1993;177:1009–1020.

93. Gay D, Saunders T, Camper S, Weigert M. Receptor editing: an approach by autoreactive B cells to escape tolerance. *J Exp Med* 1993;177:999–1008.

94. Prak EL, Weigert M. Light chain replacement: a new model for antibody gene rearrangement. *J Exp Med* 1995;182:541–548.

95. Norvell A, Mandik L, Monroe JG. Engagement of the antigen-receptor on immature murine B lymphocytes results in death by apoptosis. *J Immunol* 1995;154: 4404–4413.

96. Kincade PW, Lawton AR, Bockman DE, Cooper MD. Suppression of immunoglobulin G synthesis as a result of antibody-mediated suppression of immunoglobulin M synthesis in chickens. *Proc Natl Acad Sci USA* 1970;67: 1918–1925.

97. Lawton AR, Asofsky R, Hylton MB, Cooper MD. Suppression of immunoglobulin class synthesis in mice, I. Effects of treatment with antibody to μ-chain. *J Exp Med* 1972;135:277–297.

98. Hartley SB, Crosbie J, Brink R, Kantor AB, Basten A, Goodnow CC. Elimination from peripheral lymphoid tissues of self-reactive B lymphocytes recognizing membrane-bound antigens. *Nature* 1991;353:765–769.

99. Osmond DG. Population dynamics of bone marrow B lymphocytes. *Immunol Rev* 1986;93:103–124.

100. Metcalf ES, Klinman NR. *In vitro* tolerance induction of neonatal murine B cells. *J Exp Med* 1976;143:1327–1340.

101. Nemazee D, Büerki K. Clonal deletion of autoreactive B lymphocytes in bone marrow chimeras. *Proc Natl Acad Sci USA* 1989;86:8039–8043.

102. Guilbert B, Dighiero G, Avrameas S. Naturally occurring antibodies against nine common antigens in normal humans. I. Detection, isolation and characterization. *J Immunol* 1982;128:2779–2787.

103. Dighiero G, Lymberi P, Holmberg D, Lundquist I, Coutinho A, Avrameas S. High frequency of natural autoantibodies in normal newborn mice. *J Immunol* 1985; 134:765–771.

104. Hayakawa K, Hardy RR, Honda M, Herzenberg LA, Steinberg AD, Herzenberg LA. Ly-1 B cells: functionally distinct lymphocytes that secrete IgM autoantibodies. *Proc Natl Acad Sci USA* 1984;81:2494–2498.

105. Lehuen A, Bartels J, Kearney JF. Characterization, specificity, and IgV gene usage of anti-lymphocyte monoclonal antibodies from perinatal mice. *Int Immunol* 1992;4:1073–1084.

106. Okamoto M, Murakami M, Shimizu A, et al. A transgenic model of autoimmune hemolytic anemia. *J Exp Med* 1992;175:71–79.

107. Erikson J, Radic MZ, Camper SA, Hardy RR, Carmack C, Weigert M. Expression of anti-DNA immunoglobulin transgenes in non-autoimmune mice. *Nature* 1991;349:331–334.

108. Radic MZ, Erikson J, Litwin S, Weigert M. B lymphocytes may escape tolerance by revising their antigen receptor. *J Exp Med* 1993;177:1165–1173.

109. Madaio MP, Hodder S, Schwartz RS, Stollar BD. Responsiveness of autoimmune and normal mice to nucleic acid antigens. *J Immunol* 1984;132:872–876.

110. Conger JD, Pike BL, Nossal GJV. Clonal analysis of the anti-DNA repertoire of murine B lymphocytes. *Proc Natl Acad Sci USA* 1987;84:2931–2935.

111. Gilkeson GS, Grudier JP, Karounos DG, Pisetsky DS. Induction of anti-double stranded DNA antibodies in normal mice by immunization with bacterial DNA. *J Immunol* 1989;142:1482–1486.

112. Rumore PM, Steinman CR. Endogenous circulating DNA in systemic lupus erythematosus. *J Clin Invest* 1990;86:69–74.

113. Adelstein S, Pritchard-Briscoe H, Anderson TA, et al. Induction of self-tolerance in T cells but not B cells of transgenic mice expressing little self antigen. *Science* 1991;251:1223–1225.

114. Chiller JM, Habicht GS, Weigle WO. Kinetic differences in unresponsiveness of thymus and bone marrow cells. *Science* 1971;171:813–815.

115. Basten A, Brink R, Peake P, et al. Self tolerance in the B-cell repertoire. *Immunol Rev* 1991;122:5–19.

116. Teale JM, Layton JE, Nossal GJV. *In vitro* model for natural tolerance to self antigens; inhibition of the development of surface-immunoglobulin-negative lymphocytes into T-dependent responsive B cells by antigen. *J Exp Med* 1979; 150:205–217.

117. Carman JA, Wechsler-Reya RJ, Monroe JG. Immature stage B cells enter but do not progress beyond the early G1 phase of the cell cycle in response to antigen receptor signaling. *J Immunol* 1996;156:4562–4569.

118. Bretscher P, Cohn M. A theory of self-nonself discrimination: paralysis and induction involve the recognition of one and two determinants on an antigen, respectively. *Science* 1970;169:1042–1049.

119. Ovary Z, Benacerraf B. Immunological specificity of the secondary response with dinitrophenylated proteins. *Proc Soc Exp Biol Med* 1963;114:72–76.

120. Mitchison NA. Induction of immunological paralysis in two zones of dosage. *Proc R Soc Lond [Biol]* 1964;161:275–292.

121. Cudkowicz G, Bennett M. Peculiar immunobiology of bone marrow allografts. I. Rejection of parental grafts by resistant F₁ hybrid mice. *J Exp Med* 1971;134: 1513–1528.

122. Herberman RB, Nunn ME, Lavrin DH. Natural cytotoxic reactivity of mouse lymphoid cells against syngeneic and allogeneic tumors. I. Distribution of reactivity and specificity. *Int J Cancer* 1975;16:216–223.

123. Kiessling R, Klein E, Wigzell H. "Natural" killer cells in the mouse. I. Cytotoxic cells with specificity for mouse Moloney leukemia cell. Specificity and distribution according to genotype. *Eur J Immunol* 1975;5:112–117.

124. NK cells, MHC class I antigens and missing self. *Immunol Rev* 1997;155: 11–221.

125. Öhlén C, Kling G, Höglund P, et al. Prevention of allogeneic bone marrow graft rejection by H-2 transgene in donor mice. *Science* 1989;246:666–668.

126. Kärre K, Ljunggren HG, Piontek G, Kiessling R. Selective rejection of H-2 deficient lymphoma variants suggests alternative immune defense strategy. *Nature* 1986;319:675–678.

127. Bix M, Liao NS, Zijlstra M, Lorring J, Jaenisch R, Raulet D. Rejection of class I MHC-deficient haemopoietic cells by irradiated MHC-matched mice. *Nature* 1991;349:329–331.

128. Sykes M, Harty MW, Karlhofer FM, Pearson DA, Szot G, Yokoyama W. Hematopoietic cells and radioresistant host elements influence natural killer cell differentiation. *J Exp Med* 1993;178:223–229.

129. Olsson MY, Kärre K, Sentman CL. Altered phenotype and function of natural killer cells expressing the major histocompatibility complex receptor Ly-49 in mice transgenic for its ligand. *Proc Natl Acad Sci USA* 1995;92:1649–1653.

130. Held W, Dorfman JR, Wu MF, Raulet DH. Major histocompatibility complex class I dependent skewing of the natural killer cell Ly 49 receptor repertoire. *Eur J Immunol* 1996;26:2286–2290.

131. Salcedo M, Diehl AD, Olsson-Alheim MY, et al. Altered expression of Ly 49 inhibitory receptors on natural killer cells from MHC class I-deficient mice. *J Immunol* 1997;158:3174–3180.

132. Held W, Cado D, Raulet DH. Transgenic expression of the Ly 49A natural killer cell receptor confers class I major histocompatibility complex (MHC)–specific inhibition and prevents bone marrow allograft rejection. *J Exp Med* 1996;184: 2037–2041.

133. Johansson MH, Bicberich C, Jay G, Kärre K, Höglund P. Natural killer cell tolerance in mice with mosaic expression of major histocompatibility complex class I transgene. *J Exp Med* 1997;186:353–364.

134. Anderson D, Billingham RE, Lampkin GH, Medawar PB. The use of skin grafting to distinguish between monozygotic and dizygotic twins in cattle. *Heredity* 1951;5:379–397.

268. Billingham RE, Brent L. Quantitative studies on tissue transplantation immunity. IV. Induction of tolerance in newborn mice and studies on the phenomenon of runt disease. *Proc R Soc Lond [Biol]* 1959;242:439–477.

136. Boyse EA, Lance EM, Carswell EA, Cooper S, Old LJ. Rejection of skin allografts by radiation chimeras: selective gene action in the specification of cell surface structure. *Nature* 1970;227:901–903.

137. Boyse EA, Carswell EA, Scheid MP, Old LJ. Tolerance of Sk-incompatible skin grafts. *Nature* 1973;244:441–442.

138. Wachtel SS, Thaler HT, Boyse EA. A second system of alloantigens expressed selectively on epidermal cells of the mouse. *Immunogenetics* 1977;5:17–23.

139. Steinmuller D, Lofgreen JS. The "sk" (skin-specific) rejection phenomenon as evidence of the natural role of acquired tolerance. *Transplant Proc* 1977;9: 1385–1391.

140. Emery D, McCullagh P. Immunological reactivity between chimeric cattle twins. I. Homograft reaction. *Transplantation* 1980;29:4–9.

141. Chen H-D, Silvers WK. Influence of Langerhans cells on the survival of H-Y incompatible skin grafts in rats. *J Invest Dermatol* 1983;81:20–23.

142. Rollins-Smith LA, Cohen N. Self-pituitary grafts are not rejected by frogs deprived of their pituitary anlagen as embryos. *Nature* 1982;229:820–821.

143. McCallagh P. Interception of the development of self tolerance in fetal lambs. *Eur J Immunol* 1989;19:1387–1392.

144. Mathisen PM, Pease S, Garvey J, Hood L, Readhead C. Identification of an embryonic isoform of myelin basic protein that is expressed widely in the mouse embryo. *Proc Natl Acad Sci USA* 1993;90:10,125–10,129.

145. Kraal G, Breel M, Janse M, Bruin G. Langerhans' cells, veiled cells, and interdigitating cells in the mouse recognized by a monoclonal antibody. *J Exp Med* 1986;163:981–997.

146. Kyewski BA, Fathman CG, Kaplan HS. Intrathymic presentation of circulating non-major histocompatibility complex antigens. *Nature* 1984;308:196–199.

147. Lo D, Burkly LC, Widera G, et al. Diabetes and tolerance in transgenic mice expressing class I MHC molecules in pancreatic beta cells. *Cell* 1988;53: 159–168.

148. Lo D, Burkly LC, Flavell RA, Palmiter RD, Brinster RL. Tolerance in transgenic mice expressing class II major histocompatibility complex on pancreatic acinar cells. *J Exp Med* 1989;170:87–104.

149. Burkly LC, Lo D, Kanagawa O, Brinster RL, Flavell RA. T-cell tolerance by clonal anergy in transgenic mice with nonlymphoid expression of MHC class II I-E. *Nature* 1989;342:564–566.

150. Böhme J, Haskins K, Stecha P, et al. Transgenic mice with I-A on islet cells are normoglycemic but immunologically intolerant. *Science* 1989;244:1179–1183.

151. Miller J, Daitch L, Rath S. Selsing E. Tissue-specific expression of allogeneic class II MHC molecules induces neither tissue rejection nor clonal inactivation of alloreactive T cells. *J Immunol* 1990;144:334–341.

152. Murphy KM, Weaver CT, Elish M, Allen PM, Loh DY. Peripheral tolerance to allogeneic class II histocompatibility antigens expressed in transgenic mice: evidence against a clonal-deletion mechanism. *Proc Natl Acad Sci USA* 1989;86: 10034–10038.

153. Morahan G, Brennan FE, Bhathal PS, Allison J, Cox KO, Miller JFAP. Expression in transgenic mice of class I histocompatibility antigens controlled by the metallothionein promoter. *Proc Natl Acad Sci USA* 1989;86:3782–3786.

154. Jones-Youngblood SL, Wieties K, Forman J, Hammer RE. Effect of the expression of a hepatocyte-specific MHC molecule in transgenic mice on T cell tolerance. *J Immunol* 1990;144:1187–1195.

155. Wieties K, Hammer RE, Jones-Youngblood S, Forman J. Peripheral tolerance in mice expressing a liver-specific class I molecule: inactivation/deletion of a T cell subpopulation. *Proc Natl Acad Sci USA* 1990;87:6604–6608.

156. Russell DM, Dembic Z, Morahan G, Miller JFAP, Nemazee D. Peripheral deletion of self reactive B cells. *Nature* 1991;354:308–311.

157. Felton LD. Significance of antigen in animal tissues. *J Immunol* 1949;6: 107–117.

158. Dixon FJ, Maurer PH. Immunological unresponsiveness induced by protein antigens. *J Exp Med* 1955;101:245–257.

159. Dresser DW. Specific inhibition of antibody production. II. Paralysis in adult mice by small quantities of protein antigen. *Immunology* 1962;5:378–388.

160. Frei PC, Benacerraf B, Thorbecke GJ. Phagocytosis of the antigen, a crucial step in the induction of the primary response. *Proc Natl Acad Sci USA* 1965;53:20–23.

161. Havas HF. The effect of the carner protein on the immune response and on the induction of tolerance in mice to the 2,4-dinitrophenyl determinant. *Immunology* 1969;17:819–829.

162. Golan DT, Borel Y. Nonantigenicity and immunologic tolerance: the role of the carner in the induction of tolerance to the hapten. *J Exp Med* 1971;134: 1046–1061.

163. Katz DH, Hamaoka T, Benacerraf B. Induction of immunological tolerance in bone marrow derived lymphocytes of the IgE antibody class. *Proc Natl Acad Sci USA* 1973;70:2776–2780.

164. Nossal GJV, Pike BL, Katz DH. Induction of B cell tolerance *in vitro* to 2,4-dinitrophenyl coupled to a copolymer of D-glutamic acid and D-lysine (DNP-D-GL). *J Exp Med* 1973;138:312–317.

165. Katz DH, Davie JM, Paul WE, Benacerraf B. Carrier function in anti-hapten antibody responses. IV. Experimental conditions for the induction of hapten-specific tolerance or for the stimulation of anti-hapten anamnestic responses by "nonimmunogenic" hapten-polypeptide conjugates. *J Exp Med* 1971;134:201–233.

166. Diener E, Paetkau VH. Antigen recognition: early surface-receptor phenomena induced by binding of a tritium-labeled antigen. *Proc Natl Acad Sci USA* 1972; 69:2364–2368.

167. Aldo-Benson M, Borel Y. Hapten-bearing cell in carrier-determined tolerance. *Eur J Immunol* 1977;7:175–179.

168. Aldo-Benson M, Borel Y. Loss of carrier-determined tolerance *in vitro* with loss of receptor blockade. *J Immunol* 1976;116:223–226.

169. Howard JG, Mitchison NA. Immunological tolerance. *Progr Allergy* 1975;18: 68–72.

170. Parish CR, Ada GL. Tolerance inducing properties in rats of bacterial flagellin cleaved at the methionine residues. *Immunology* 1969;17:153–164.

171. Andersson B. Induction of immunity and immunologic paralysis in mice against polyvinyl pyrrolidone. *J Immunol* 1969;102:1309–1313.

172. Miranda JJ, Zola H, Howard JG. Studies on immunological paralysis. X. Cellular characteristics of the induction and loss of tolerance to levan (polyfructose). *Immunology* 1973;23:843–855.

173. Feldmann M. Induction of immunity and tolerance to the dinitrophenyl determinant *in vitro*. *Nature New Biol* 1971;231:21–23.

174. Dintzis HM, Dintzis RZ, Vogelstein B. Molecular determinants of immunogenicity: the immunon model of immune response. *Proc Natl Acad Sci USA* 1976;73:3671–3675.

175. Dintzis RZ, Okajima M, Middleton MH, Greene G, Dintzis HM. The immunogenicity of soluble haptenated polymers is determined by molecular mass and hapten valence. *J Immunol* 1989;143:1239–1244.

176. Waldschmidt TJ, Borel Y, Vitetta ES. The use of haptenated immunoglobulins to induce B cell tolerance in vitro. The roles of hapten density and the Fc portion of the immunoglobulin carrier. *J Immunol* 1983;131:2204–2209.

177. Sinclair, NRStC, Chan PL. Regulation of the immune response. IV. The role of the Fc-fragment in feedback inhibition by antibody. *Adv Exp Med Biol* 1971;12: 609–615.

178. Daëron M. Fc receptor biology. *Annu Rev Immunol* 1997;15:203–234.

179. Katz DH, Hamaoka T, Benacerraf B. Immunological tolerance in bone marrow-derived lymphocytes. I. Evidence for an intracellular mechanism of inactivation of hapten-specific precursors of antibody-forming cells. *J Exp Med* 1972;136: 1404–1429.

180. Hamaoka T, Katz DH. Immunological tolerance in bone marrow-derived lymphocytes. II. Effects of allogeneic cell interactions and enzymatic digestion with trypsin on inactivated hapten-specific precursors of antibody-forming cells. *J Exp Med* 1974;139:1446–1463.

181. Klinman NR, Schrater AF, Katz DH. Immature B cells as the target for *in vivo* tolerance induction. *J Immunol* 1981;126:1970–1973.

182. Möller G, Gronowicz E, Persson U, et al. Spleen cells from animals tolerant to a thymus-dependent antigen can be activated by lipopolysaccharide to synthesize antibodies against the tolerogen. *J Exp Med* 1976;143:1429–1438.

183. Pike BL, Abrams J, Nossal GJV. Clonal anergy: inhibition of antigen-driven proliferation among single B lymphocytes from tolerant animals, and partial breakage of anergy by mitogens. *Eur J Immunol* 1983;13:214–220.

184. Nossal GJV, Pike BL. Clonal anergy: persistence in tolerant mice of antigen-binding B lymphocytes incapable of responding to antigen or mitogen. *Proc Natl Acad Sci USA* 1980;77:1602–1606.

185. Goodnow CC, Crosbie J, Adelstein S, et al. Altered immunoglobulin expression and functional silencing of self-reactive B lymphocytes in transgenic mice. *Nature* 1988;334:676–682.

186. Bell SE, Goodnow CC. A selective defect in IgM antigen receptor synthesis and transport causes loss of cell surface IgM expression on tolerant B lymphocytes. *EMBO J* 1994;13:816–826.

187. Goodnow CC, Crosbie J, Jorgensen H, Brink RA, Basten A. Induction of self tolerance in mature peripheral B lymphocytes. *Nature* 1989;342:385–391.

188. Eris JM, Basten A, Brink RA, Doherty K, Kehry MR, Hodgkin PD. Anergic B-reactive B cells present self antigen and respond normally to CD40-dependent T cell signals but are defective in antigen-receptor mediated functions. *Proc Natl Acad Sci USA* 1994;91:4392–4396.

189. Goodnow CC, Brink R, Adams E. Breakdown of self-tolerance in anergic B lymphocytes. *Nature* 1991;352:532–536.

190. Lenschow DJ, Sperling AI, Cooke MP, et al. Differential up-regulation of the B7-1 and B7-2 costimulatory molecules after Ig receptor engagement by antigen. *J Immunol* 1994;153:1990–1997.

191. Cooke MP, Heath AW, Shokat KM, et al. Immunoglobulin signal transduction guides the specificity of B cell-T cell interactions and is blocked in tolerant self-reactive B cells. *J Exp Med* 1994;179:425–438.

192. Healy JI, Dolmetsch RE, Timmerman LA, et al. Different nuclear signals are activated by the B cell receptor during positive versus negative signaling. *Immunity* 1997;6:419–428.

193. Fulcher DA, Basten A. Reduced life span of anergic self-reactive B cells in a double-transgenic model. *J Exp Med* 1994;179:125–134.

194. Cyster JG, Hartley SB, Goodnow CC. Competition for follicular niches excludes self-reactive cells from the recirculating B-cell repertoire. *Nature* 1994;371: 389–395.

195. Rathmell JC, Cook MP, Ho WY, et al. CD95 (Fas)-dependent elimination of self-reactive B cells upon interaction with CD4+ T cells. *Nature* 1995;376:181–184.

196. Rathmell JC, Townsend SE, Xu JC, Flavell RA, Goodnow CC. Expansion or elimination of B cells *in vivo*: dual roles for CD40- and Fas (CD95)-ligands modulated by the B cell antigen receptor. *Cell* 1996;87:319–329.

197. Tarlington DM, Smith KG. Apoptosis and the B cell response to antigen. *Int Rev Immunol* 1997;15:53–71.

198. Matiba B, Mariani SM, Krammer PH. The CD95 system and the death of a lymphocyte. *Semin Immunol* 1997;9:59–68.

199. Mountz JD, Zhou T, Su X, et al. Autoimmune disease results from multiple interactive defects in apoptosis induction molecules and signaling pathways. *Behring Inst Mitt* 1996;97:200–219.

200. Nunez G, Hockenbery D, McDonnell TJ, Sorensen CM, Korsmeyer SJ. Bcl-2 maintains B cell memory. *Nature* 1991;353:71–73.

201. McDonnell TJ, Korsmeyer SJ. Progression from lymphoid hyperplasia to high-grade malignant lymphoma in mice transgenic for the t(14;18). *Nature* 1991; 349:254–256.

202. Strasser A, Whittingham S, Vaux DL, et al. Enforced BCL2 expression in B-lymphoid cells prolongs antibody responses and elicits autoimmune disease. *Proc Natl Acad Sci USA* 1991;88:8661–8665.

203. Jacob J, Kelsoe G. *In situ* studies of the primary immune response to (4-hydroxy-3-nitrophenyl) acetyl. II. A common clonal origin for periarteriolar lymphoid sheath-associated foci and germinal centers. *J Exp Med* 1992;176: 679–687.

204. Linton PJL, Decker DJ, Klinman DR. Primary antibody-forming cells and secondary B cells are generated from separate precursor cell subpopulations. *Cell* 1989;59:1049–1059.

205. MacLennan IC. Germinal centers. *Annu Rev Immunol* 1994;12:117–139.

206. Tew JG, Wu J, Qin D, Helm S, Burton GF, Szakal AK. Follicular dendritic cells and presentation of antigen and costimulatory signals to B cells. *Immunol Rev* 1997;156:39–52.

207. Kearney ER, Pape KA, Loh DY, Jenkins MK. Visualization of peptide-specific T cell immunity and peripheral tolerance induction *in vivo*. *Immunity* 1994;1: 327–339.

208. Shokat KM, Goodnow CC. Antigen-induced B-cell death and elimination during germinal-centre immune responses. *Nature* 1995;375:334–338.

209. Pulendran B, Kannourakis G, Nouri S, Smith KG, Nossal GJ. Soluble antigen can cause enhanced apoptosis of germinal-centre B cells. *Nature* 375:331–334.

210. Coutinho A, Möller G. Thymus-independent B-cell induction and paralysis. *Adv Immunol* 1975;21:114–236.

211. Coutinho A, Gronowicz E, Möller G. Mechanisms of B-cell activation and paralysis by thymus-independent antigens. Additive effects between NNP-LPS and LPS in the specific response to the hapten. *Scand J Immunol* 1975;4:89–94.

212. Mond JJ, Lees A, Snapper CM. T cell-independent antigens type 2. *Annu Rev Immunol* 1995;13:655–692.

213. Feldmann M, Basten A. The relationship between antigenic structure and the

requirement for thymus-derived cells in the immune response. *J Exp Med* 1971; 134:103–119.

214. Pryjma J, Humphrey JH, Klaus GGB. C3 activation and T-independent B cell stimulation. *Nature* 1974;252:505–506.

215. Mosier DE, Mond JJ, Goldings EA. The ontogeny of thymic-independent antibody responses *in vitro* in normal mice and mice with an X-linked B lymphocyte defect. *J Immunol* 1977;119:1874–1878.

216. Schreier MH, Andersson J, Lernhardt W, Melchers F. Antigen-specific T-helper cells stimulate H-2 compatible and H-2-incompatible B cell blasts polyclonally. *J Exp Med* 1980;151:194–203.

217. Pecanha LMT, Snapper CM, Finkelman FD, Mond JJ. Dextran-conjugated anti-Ig antibodies as a model for T cell-independent type 2 antigen-mediated stimulation of Ig secretion *in vitro*. I. Lymphokine dependence. *J Immunol* 1991;146:833–839.

218. Ales-Martinez JE, Cuende E, Gaur A, Scott DW. Prevention of B cell clonal deletion and anergy by activated T cells and their lymphokines. *Semin Immunol* 1992;4:195–202.

219. Carter H, Spycher MO, Ng YC, Hoffman R, Fearon DT. Synergistic interaction between complement receptor type 2 and membrane IgM on B lymphocytes. *J Immunol* 1988;141:457–463.

220. Boussiotis VA, Nadler LM, Strominger JL, Goldfield AE. Tumor necrosis factor α is an autocrine growth factor for normal human B cells. *Proc Natl Acad Sci USA* 1994;91:7007–7011.

221. Snapper CM, Yamaguchi H, Moorman MA, Sneed R, Smoot D, Mond JJ. Natural killer cells induce activated murine B cells to secrete Ig. *J Immunol* 1993; 151:5251–5260.

222. Bachmann MF, Hengartner H, Zinkernagel RM. T helper cell-independent neutralizing B cell response against vesicular stomatitis virus: role of antigen patterns in B cell induction? *Eur J Immunol* 1995;25:3445–3451.

223. Fehr T, Bachmann MF, Bluethmann H, Kikutani H, Hengartner H, Zinkernagel RM. T-independent activation of B cells by vesicular stomatitis virus: no evidence for the need of a second signal. *Cell Immunol* 1996;168:184–192.

224. Lane PJL, Gray D, Oldfield S, MacLennan ICM. Differences in the recruitment of virgin B cells into antibody responses to thymus-dependent and thymus-independent type-2 antigens. *Eur J Immunol* 1986;16:1569–1575.

225. Hayakawa K, Hady RR. Normal autoimmune and malignant CD5 B cells: the Ly-1 B lineage. *Annu Rev Immunol* 1988;6:197–218.

226. Liou L-B, Warner GL, Scott DW. Can peritoneal B cells be rendered unresponsive? *Int Immunol* 1992;4:15–21.

227. Rajewsky K, Förster I, Cumano A. Evolutionary and somatic selection of the antibody repertoire in the mouse. *Science* 1987;238:1088–1094.

228. Ying-Zi C, Rabin E, Wortis HH. Treatment of murine CD5⁻ B cells with anti-Ig but not LPS induces surface CD5: two B cell activation pathways. *Int Immunol* 1991;3:467–476.

229. Zinkernagel RM. Immunology taught by viruses. *Science* 1996;271:173–178.

230. Schwartz RH, Mueller DL, Jenkins MK, Quill H. T-cell clonal anergy. *Cold Spring Harb Symp Quant Biol* 1989;54:605–610.

231. Jenkins MK, Schwartz RH. Antigen presentation by chemically modified splenocytes induces antigen-specific T cell unresponsiveness *in vitro* and *in vivo*. *J Exp Med* 1987;165:302–319.

232. Quill H, Schwartz RH. Stimulation of normal inducer T cell clones with antigen presented by purified Ia molecules in planar lipid membranes: specific induction of a long-lived state of proliferation nonresponsiveness. *J Immunol* 1987;138: 3704–3712.

233. Jenkins, MK, Ashwell JD, Schwartz RH. Allogeneic non-T spleen cells restore the responsiveness of normal T cell clones stimulated with antigen and chemically modified antigen presenting cells. *J Immunol* 1988;140:3324–3330.

234. Mueller DI, Jenkins MK, Schwartz RH. An accessory cell-derived costimulatory signal acts independently of protein kinase C activation to allow T cell proliferation and prevent induction of unresponsiveness. *J Immunol* 1989;142: 2617–2628.

235. Jenkins MK, Taylor PS, Norton SD, Urdahl KB. CD28 delivers a costimulatory signal involved in antigen-specific IL-2 production by human T cells. *J Immunol* 1991;147:2461–2466.

236. Linsley PS, Brady W, Grosmaire L, Aruffo A, Damle NK, Ledbetter JA. Binding of the B cell activation antigen B7 to CD28 costimulates T cell proliferation and interleukin 2 mRNA accumulation. *J Exp Med* 1991;173:721–730.

237. Freeman GJ, Gray GS, Gimmi CD, et al. Structure, expression and T cell costimulation activity of the murine homologue of the B lymphocyte activation antigen. B7. *J Exp Med* 1991;174:625–631.

238. Nabavi N, Freeman GJ, Gault A, Godfrey D, Nadler LM, Glimcher LH. Signalling through the MHC class II cytoplasmic domain is required for antigen presentation and induces B7 expression. *Nature* 1992;360:266–268.

239. Lafferty KJ, Cunningham AJ. A new analysis of allogeneic interactions. *Aust J Exp Biol Med Sci* 1975;53:27–42.

240. Janeway CA Jr. Approaching the asymptote? Evolution and revolution in immunology. *Cold Spring Harb Symp Quant Biol* 1989;54 Pt 1:1–13.

241. Janeway CA Jr. The immune system evolved to discriminate infectious nonself from noninfectious self. *Immunol Today* 1992;13:11–16.

242. Matzinger P. Tolerance, danger and the extended family. *Annu Rev Immunol* 1994;12:991–1045.

243. Ryser JE, MacDonald HG. Limiting dilution analysis of alloantigen-reactive T lymphocytes. I. Comparison of precursor frequencies for proliferative and cytolytic responses. *J Immunol* 1979;12:1691–1696.

244. Wilson D, Blyth J, Nowell P. Quantitative studies on the mixed lymphocyte interaction in rats. V. Tempo and specificity of the proliferative response and the number of reactive cells from immunized donors. *J Exp Med* 1971;133: 442–453.

245. Sprent J. Fate of H-2 activated T lymphocytes in syngeneic hosts. I. Fate in lymphoid tissues traced with ³H-thymidine, ¹²⁵I-deoxyuridine and ⁵¹chromium. *Cell Immunol* 1976;21:278–302.

246. Sprent J, Miller JFAP. Fate of H-2-activated T lymphocytes in syngeneic hosts. III. Differentiation into long-lived recirculating memory cells. *Cell Immunol* 1976;21:314–326.

247. Webb S, Morris C, Sprent J. Extrathymic tolerance of mature T cells: clonal elimination as a consequence of immunity. *Cell* 1990;63:1249–1256.

248. Kawabe Y, Ochi A. Programmed cell death and extrathymic reduction of Vβ8⁺ CD4⁺ T cells in mice tolerant to *Staphylococcus aureus* enterotoxin B. *Nature* 1991;349:245–248.

249. Rocha B, Von Boehmer H. Peripheral selection of the T cell repertoire. *Science* 1991;251:1225–1228.

250. Russell JH, Rush B, Weaver C, Wang R. Mature T cells of autoimmune lpr/lpr mice have a defect in antigen stimulated suicide. *Proc Natl Acad Sci USA* 1993; 90:4409–4413.

251. Zheng L, Fisher G, Miller RE, Peschon J, Lynch DH, Lenardo MJ. Induction of apoptosis in mature T cells by tumour necrosis factor. *Nature* 1995;377: 348–351.

252. Dhein J, Walczak H, Baumler C, Debatin KM, Krammer PH. Autocrine T-cell suicide mediated by APO-1 *Nature* 1995;373:438–441.

253. Boise LH, Minn AJ, Noel PJ, et al. CD28 costimulation can promote T cell survival by enhancing the expression of Bcl-X_L. *Immunity* 1995;3:87–98.

254. Duke RC, Cohen JJ. IL-addiction: withdrawal of growth factor activates a suicide program in dependent T cells. *Lymphokine Res* 1986;5:289–299.

255. Lenardo M. Interleukin-2 programs mouse αβ T lymphocytes for apoptosis. *Nature* 1991;353:858–861.

256. Lindsten T, June CH, Ledbetter JA, Stella G, Thompson CB. Regulation of lymphokine messenger RNA stability by a surface-mediated T cell activation pathway. *Science* 1989;244:339–343.

257. Fraser JD, Irving BA, Crabtree GR, Weiss A. Regulation of interleukin-2 gene enhancer activity by the T cell accessory molecule CD28. *Science* 1991;251: 313–316.

258. Cai Z, Brunmark A, Jackson MR, Loh D, Peterson PA, Sprent J. Transfected Drosophila cells as a probe for defining the minimal requirements for stimulating unprimed CD8⁺ T cells. *Proc Natl Acad Sci USA* 1996;93:14736–14741.

259. Boehme SA, Zheng L, Lenardo MJ. Analysis of the CD4 coreceptor and activation-induced costimulatory molecules in antigen-mediated mature T lymphocyte death. *J Immunol* 1995;155:1703–1712.

260. Vella AT, McCormack JE, Linsley PS, Kappler JW, Marrack P. Lipopolysaccharide interferes with the induction of peripheral T cell death. *Immunity* 1995;2: 261–270.

261. Nakata Y, Matusda K, Uzawa A, Nomura M, Akash M, Suzuki G. Administration of recombinant human IL-1 by Staphylococcus enterotoxin B prevents tolerance induction *in vivo*. *J Immunol* 1995;155:4231–4235.

262. Jiang H, Ware R, Stall A, Flaherty L, Chess L, Pernis B. Murine CD8⁺ T cells that specifically delete autologous CD4⁺ T cells expressing V beta 8 TCR: a role of the Qa-1 molecule. *Immunity* 1995;2:185–194.

263. Miller RA, Stutman O. T cell repopulation from functionally restricted splenic progenitors. 10,000-fold expansion documented by limiting dilution analysis. *J Immunol* 1984;133:2925–2932.

264. Rocha BB. Population kinetics of precursors of IL-2 producing peripheral T lymphocytes: evidence for short life expectancy, continuous renewal and postthymic expansion. *J Immunol* 1987;139:365–372.

265. Rocha B, Penit C, Baron C, Vasseur F, Dautigny N, Freitas AA. Accumulation of bromodeoxyuridine-labeled cells in central and peripheral lymphoid organs: minimal estimates of production and turnover rates of mature lymphocytes. *Eur J Immunol* 1990;20:1697–1708.

266. Tanchot C, Rocha B. The peripheral T cell repertoire: independent homeostatic regulation of virgin and activated CD8⁺ T cells pools. *Eur J Immunol* 1995;25: 2127–2136.

267. Tanchot C, Lemonnier FA, Perarnau B, Freitas AA, Rocha B. Differential requirements for survival and proliferation of CD8 naive or memory T cells. *Science* 1997;276:2057–2062.

268. Ahmed R, Gray D. Immunological memory and protective immunity, understanding their relation. *Science* 1996;272:54–60.

269. Moskophidis D, Laine E, Zinkernagel RM. Peripheral clonal deletion of antiviral memory CD8⁺ T cells. *Eur J Immunol* 1993;23:3306–3311.

270. Moskophidis D, Lechner F, Pircher H, Zinkernagel RM. Virus persistence in acutely infected immunocompetent mice by exhaustion of antiviral cytotoxic effector T cells. *Nature* 1993;362:758–761.

271. Kawabe Y, Ochi A. Selective anergy of Vβ8⁺ CD4⁺ T cells in staphylococcus enterotoxin B. *J Exp Med* 1990;172:1065–1070.

272. Rellahan BL, Jones LA, Kruisbeek AM, Fry AM, Matis LA. *In vivo* induction of anergy in peripheral Vβ8⁺ T cells by staphylococcal enterotoxin B. *J Exp Med* 1991;172:1091–1100.

273. Rocha B, Grandien A, Freitas AA. Anergy and exhaustion are independent mechanisms of peripheral T cell tolerance. *J Exp Med* 1995;181:993–1003.

274. Rocha B, Tanchot C, Von Boehmer H. Clonal anergy blocks *in vivo* growth of

mature T cells and can be reversed in the absence of antigen. *J Exp Med* 1993; 177:1517–1521.

275. Lanoue A, Bona C, Von Boehmer H, Sarukhan A. Conditions that induce tolerance in mature CD4+ T cells. *J Exp Med* 1997;185:405–414.

276. Schwartz RH. A cell culture model for T lymphocyte clonal anergy. *Science* 1990;248:1349–1356.

277. Boussiotis VA, Freeman GJ, Gray G, Gribben J, Nadler LM. B7 but not intercellular adhesion molecule-1 costimulation prevents the induction of human alloantigen-specific tolerance. *J Exp Med* 1993;178:1753–1763.

278. Boussiotis VA, Barber DL, Nakarai T, et al. Prevention of T cell anergy by signaling through the gamma c chain of the IL-2 receptor. *Science* 1994;266: 1039–1042.

279. Li W, Whaley CD, Mondino A, Mueller DL. Blocked signal transduction to the ERK and JNK protein kinases in anergic CD4+ T cells. *Science* 1996;271: 1272–1276.

280. Fields PE, Gajewski, TF, Fitch FW. Blocked ras activation in anergic CD4+ T cells. *Science* 1996;271:1276–1278.

281. Kang S-M, Beverly B, Tran A-C, Brorson R, Schwartz RH, Lenardo MJ. Transactivation by AP-1 is a molecular target of T cell clonal anergy. *Science* 1992; 257:1134–1138.

282. Boussiotis VA, Freeman GJ, Berezovskaya A, Barber DL, Nadler LM. Maintenance of human T cell anergy: blocking of IL-2 gene transcription by activated Rap1. *Science* 1997;278:124–128.

283. Beverly B, Kang S-M, Lenardo MJ, Schwartz RH. Reversal of *in vitro* T cell clonal anergy by IL-2 stimulation. *Int Immunol* 1992;4:661–671.

284. Mueller DL, Chiodetti L, Bacon PA, Schwartz RH. Clonal anergy blocks the response to IL-4, as well as the production of IL-2, in dual-producing helper T cell clones. *J Immunol* 1991;147:4118–4125.

285. Sloan-Lancaster J, Evavold BD, Allen PM. Induction of T cell anergy by altered T-cell receptor ligand on live antigen-presenting cells. *Nature* 1993;363:156–159.

286. Sloan-Lancaster J, Shaw AS, Rothbard JB, Allen PM. Partial T cell signaling: altered phospho-zeta and lack of Zap70 recruitment in APL-induced T cell anergy. *Cell* 1994;79:913–922.

287. Madrenas J, Wange RL, Wang JL, Isakov N, Samelson LE, Germain RN. Zeta phosphorylation without ZAP-70 activation induced by TCR antagonists or partial agonists. *Science* 1995;267:515–518.

288. Sloan-Lancaster J, Steinberg TH, Allen PM. Selective activation of the calcium signaling pathway by altered peptide ligands. *J Exp Med* 1996;184:1525–1530.

289. Madrenas J, Schwartz RH, Germain RN. Interleukin 2 production, not the pattern of early T-cell antigen receptor-dependent tyrosine phosphorylation, controls anergy induction by both agonists and partial agonists. *Proc Natl Acad Sci USA* 1996;93:9736–9741.

290. Lamb JR, Skidmore BJ, Green N, Chiller JM, Feldmann M. Induction of tolerance in influenza virus-immune T lymphocyte clones with synthetic peptides of influenza hemagglutinin. *J Exp Med* 1983;157:1434–1447.

291. O'Hehir RE, Yssel H, Verma S, de Vries JE, Spits H, Lamb JR. Clonal analysis of differential lymphokine production in peptide and superantigen induced T cell anergy. *Int Immunol* 1991;3:819–826.

292. LaSalle JM, Hafler DA. T cell anergy. *FASEB J* 1994;8:601–608.

293. Wotton D, Higgins JA, O'Hehir RE, Lamb JR, Lake RA. Differential induction of the NF-AT complex during restimulation and the induction of T-cell anergy. *Hum Immunol* 1995;42:95–102.

294. Otten G, Herold KC, Fitch FW. Interleukin 2 inhibits antigen stimulated lymphokine synthesis in helper T cells by inhibiting calcium-dependent signaling. *J Immunol* 1987;139:1348–1353.

295. Schwartz RH. Models of T cell anergy: is there a common molecular mechanism? *J Exp Med* 1996;184:1–8.

296. Bhandoola A, Cho EA, Yui K, Saragoui HU, Greene MI, Quill H. Reduced CD3-mediated protein tyrosine phosphorylation in anergic CD4+ and CD8+ T cells. *J Immunol* 1993;151:2355–2367.

297. Hayden LA, Tough DF, Webb SR. *In vivo* response of mature T cells to Mls antigens. Long-term progeny of dividing cells include cells with a naive phenotype. *J Immunol* 1996;156:48–55.

298. Sundstedt A, Hoiden I, Rosendahl A, Kalland T, van Rooijen N, Dohlsten M. Immunoregulatory role of IL-10 during superantigen-induced hyporesponsiveness *in vivo*. *J Immunol* 1997;158:180–186.

299. Cauley LS, Cauley KA, Shub F, Huston G, Swain SL. Transferable anergy: superantigen treatment induces CD4+ T cell tolerance that is reversible and requires CD4− CD8− cells and interferon gamma. *J Exp Med* 1997;186:71–81.

300. Kündig TM, Shahinian A, Kawai K, et al. Duration of TCR stimulation determines costimulatory requirement of T cells. *Immunity* 1996;5:41–52.

301. Hargreaves RG, Borthwick NJ, Montani MS, et al. Dissociation of T cell anergy from apoptosis by blockade of Fas/Apo-1 (CD95) signaling. *J Immunol* 1997; 158:3099–3107.

302. Singer A, Munitz TI, Golding H, Rosenberg AS, Mizuochi T. Recognition requirements for the activation, differentiation and function of T-helper cells specific for class I MHC alloantigens. *Immunol Rev* 1987;98:143–170.

303. Pfizenmaier K, Schcurich P, Däubener W, Krönke M, Röllinghoff M, Wagner H. Quantitative representation of all T cells committed to develop into cytotoxic effector cells and/or interleukin 2 activity-producing helper cells within murine T lymphocyte subsets. *Eur J Immunol* 1984;14:33–39.

304. Keene J, Forman J. Helper activity is required for the *in vivo* generation of cytotoxic T lymphocytes. *J Exp Med* 1982;155:768–782.

305. Guerder S, Matzinger P. Activation versus tolerance: a decision made by T helper cells. *Cold Spring Harb Symp Quant Biol* 1989;54:799–805.

306. Rees MA, Rosenberg AS, Munitz TI, Singer A. *In vivo* induction of antigen-specific transplantation tolerance to Qa1 by exposure to alloantigen in the absence of T-cell help. *Proc Natl Acad Sci USA* 1990;87:2765–2769.

307. Hou S, Mo XY, Hyland L, Doherty PC. Host response to Sendri virus in mice lacking class II major histocompatibility complex glycoproteins. *J Virol* 1995;69: 1429–1434.

308. Tripp RA, Sarawar SR, Doherty PC. Characteristics of the influenza virus-specific CD8+ T cell response in mice homozygous for disruption of the H-2I-Ab gene. *J Immunol* 1995;155:2955–2959.

309. Wu Y, Liu Y. Viral induction of co-stimulatory activity on antigen-presenting cells bypasses the need for CD4+ T-cell help in CD8+ T-cell responses. *Curr Biol* 1994;4:499–505.

310. Lafferty KJ, Prowse SJ, Simeonovic CJ, Warren HS. Immunobiology of tissue transplantation: a return to the passenger leukocyte concept. *Annu Rev Immunol* 1983;1:143–173.

311. Ohashi PS, Oehen S, Buerki K, et al. Ablation of "tolerance" and induction of diabetes by virus infection in viral antigen transgenic mice. *Cell* 1991;65:305–317.

312. Oldstone MBA, Nerenberg M, Southern P, Price J, Lewicki H. Virus infection triggers insulin-dependent diabetes mellitus in a transgenic model: role of anti-self (virus) immune response. *Cell* 1991;65:319–331.

313. Schönrich G, Kalinke U, Momburg F, et al. Downregulation of T cell receptors on self-reactive T cells as a novel mechanism for extrathymic tolerance induction. *Cell* 1991;65:293–304.

314. Schönrich G, Momburg F, Malissen M, et al. Distinct mechanisms of extrathymic T cell tolerance due to differential expression of self antigen. *Int Immunol* 1992;4:581–590.

315. Alferink J, Schittek B, Schönrich PG, Hämmerling GJ, Arnold B. Long life span of tolerant T cells and the role of antigen in maintenance of peripheral tolerance. *Int Immunol* 1995;7:331–336.

316. Hanahan D, Jolicouer C, Alpert S, Skowronski J. Alternative self or nonself recognition of an antigen expressed in a rare cell type in transgenic mice: implications for self-tolerance and autoimmunity. *Cold Spring Harb Symp Quant Biol* 1989;54:821–835.

317. Lo D, Freedman J, Hesse S, Palmiter RD, Brinster RL, Sherman LA. Peripheral tolerance to an islet cell-specific hemagglutinin transgene affects both CD4+ and CD8+ T cells. *Eur J Immunol* 1992;22:1013–1022.

318. Kündig TM, Bachmann MF, DiPaolo C, et al. Fibroblasts as efficient antigen presenting cells in lymphoid organs. *Science* 1995;268:1343–1347.

319. Mackay CR, Marston WL, Dudler L. Naive and memory T cells show distinct pathways of lymphocyte recirculation. *J Exp Med* 1990;171:801–817.

320. Miller RG. The veto phenomenon and T cell regulation. *Immunol Today* 1986;7: 112–114.

321. Miller RG, Derry H. A cell population in *nu/nu* spleen can prevent generation of cytotoxic lymphocytes by normal spleen cells against self antigens of the *nu/nu* spleen. *J Immunol* 1979;122:1502–1509.

322. Muraoka S, Ehman DL, Miller RG. Irreversible inactivation of activated cytotoxic T lymphocyte precursor cells by "anti-self" suppressor cells present in murine bone marrow T cell colonies. *Eur J Immunol* 1984;14:1010–1016.

323. Rammensee HG, Nagy ZA, Klein J. Suppression of cell-mediated lymphocytotoxicty against minor histocompatibility antigens mediated by Lyt1+ Lyt2+ T cells of stimulator strain origin. *Eur J Immunol* 1982; 12:930–934.

324. Fink PJ, Rammensee HG, Bevan MJ. Cloned cytolytic T cells can suppress primary cytotoxic responses directed against them. *J Immunol* 1984;133:1775–1781.

325. Claesson MH, Miller RG. Functional heterogeneity in allospecific cytotoxic T lymphocyte clones I. CTL clones express strong anti-self suppressive activity. *J Exp Med* 1984;160:1702–1716.

326. Fink PJ, Rammensee HG, Benedetto JD, Staerz UD, Lefrancois L, Bevan MJ. Studies on the mechanisms of suppression of primary cytotoxic responses by cloned cytotoxic T lymphocytes. *J Immunol* 1984;133:1769–1774.

327. Rammensee HG, Fink PJ, Bevan MJ. Functional clonal deletion of class I-specific cytotoxic T lymphocytes by veto cells that express antigen. *J Immunol* 1984;133:2390–2396.

328. Fink PJ, Weissman IL, Bevan MJ. Haplotype specific suppression of cytotoxic T cell induction by antigen inappropriately presented on T cells. *J Exp Med* 1983; 157:141–154.

329. Cassell DJ, Forman J. Regulation of the cytotoxic T lymphocyte response against Qa-1 alloantigens. *J Immunol* 1990;144:4075–4081.

330. Hambor JE, Kaplan DR, Tykocinski ML. CD8 functions as an inhibitory ligand in mediating the immunoregulatory activity of CD8+ cells. *J Immunol* 1990;145: 1646–1652.

331. Sambhara SR, Miller RG. Programmed cell death of T cells signaled by the T cell receptor and the domain of class I MHC. *Science* 1991;252:1424–1427.

332. Zhang L, Martin DR, Fung-Leung W-P, Teh H-S, Miller RG. Peripheral deletion of mature CD8+ antigen-specific T cells after *in vivo* exposure to male antigen. *J Immunol* 1992;148:3740–3745.

333. Asherson GL, Stone SH. Selective and specific inhibition of 24 hour skin reactions in the guinea pig. I. Immune deviation: description of the phenomenon and the effect of splenectomy. *Immunology* 1965;9:205–217.

334. Parish CR, Liew FY. Immune response to chemically modified flagellin. III. Enhanced cell-mediated immunity during high and low zone antibody tolerance to flagellin. *J Exp Med* 1972;135:298–311.

335. Bretscher P. Hypothesis. On the control between cell-mediated, IgM and IgG immunity. Cell Immunol 1974;13:171–195.

336. Mosmann TR, Cherwinski H, Bond MW, Giedlin MA, Coffman RL. Two types of murine helper T cell clone: I. Definition according to profiles of lymphokine activities and secreted proteins. J Immunol 1986;136:2348–2357.

337. Mosmann TR, Coffman RL. Th1 and Th2 cells: different patterns of lymphokine secretion lead to different functional properties. Annu Rev Immunol 1989;7:145–173.

338. Abbas AK, Murphy KM, Sher A. Functional diversity of helper T lymphocytes. Nature 1996;383:787–793.

339. Gajewski TF, Fitch FW. Anti-proliferative effect of IFN-gamma in immune regulation. I. IFN-gamma inhibits the proliferation of Th2 but not Th1 murine helper T lymphocyte clones. J Immunol 1988;140:4245–4252.

340. Oriss TB, McCarthy SB, Morel BF, Campana MA, Morel PA. Crossregulation between T helper cell (Th)1 and Th2: inhibition of Th2 proliferation by IFN-gamma involves interference with IL-1. J Immunol 1997;158:3666–3672.

341. Fiorentino DF, Bond MW, Mosmann TR. Two types of mouse T helper cell. IV. Th2 clones secrete a factor that inhibits cytokine production by Th1 clones. J Exp Med 1989;170:2081–2095.

342. de Waal Malefyt R, Yssel H, de Vries JE. Direct effects of IL-10 on subsets of human CD4+ T cell clones and resting T cells. Specific inhibition of IL-2 production and proliferation. J Immunol 1993;150:4754–4765.

343. Locksley RM, Scott P. Helper T-cell subsets in mouse leishmaniasis induction, expansion and effector function. Immunol Today 1991;12:A58–A61.

344. Bretscher PA, Wei G, Menon JN, Bielefeldt-Ohmann H. Establishment of stable, cell-mediated immunity that makes "susceptible" mice resistant to Leishmania major. Science 1992;257:539–542.

345. Mougneau E, Altare F, Wakil AE, et al. Expression cloning of a protective Leishmania antigen. Science 1995;268:563–566.

346. Julia V, Rassoulzadegan M, Glaichenhaus N. Resistance to Leishmania major induced by tolerance to a single antigen. Science 1996;274:421–423.

347. Seder RA, Paul WE, Davis MM, de St Groth BF. The presence of interleukin 4 during in vitro priming determines the lymphokine-producing potential of CD4+ T cells from T cell receptor transgenic mice. J Exp Med 1992;176:1091–1098.

348. Hsieh CS, Macatonia SE, Tripp CS, Wolf SF, O'Garra A, Murphy KM. Development of Th1 CD4+ T cells through IL-12 produced by Listeria-induced macrophages. Science 1993;260:547–549.

349. Gieni RS, Yang X, Kelso A, Hayglass KT. Limiting dilution analysis of CD4 T-cell cytokine production in mice administered native versus polymerized ovalbumin: directed induction of T-helper type-1-like activation. Immunology 1996;87:119–126.

350. Kamogana Y, Minasi LA, Carding SR, Bottomly K, Flavell RA. The relationship of IL-4- and IFN gamma-producing T cells studied by lineage ablation of IL-4-producing cells. Cell 1993;75:985–995.

351. Seder RA, Paul WE. Acquisition of lymphokine-producing phenotype by CD4+ T cells. Annu Rev Immunol 1994;12:635–673.

352. Bloom BR, Salgame P, Diamond B. Revisiting and revising suppressor T cells. Immunol Today 1992;13:131–136.

353. Seder RA, Boulay JL, Finkelman F, et al. CD8+ T cells can be primed in vitro to produce IL-4. J Immunol 1992;148:1652–1656.

354. Cremer MA, Hernandez AD, Townes AS, Stuart JM, Kang AH. Collagen-induced arthritis in rats: antigen-specific suppression of arthritis and immunity by intravenously injected native type II collagen. J Immunol 1983;131.2995–3000.

355. Scherer MT, Chan DMC, Ria F, Smith JA, Perkins DL, Gefter ML. Control of cellular and humoral immune responses by peptides containing T-cell epitopes. Cold Spring Harb Symp Quant Biol 1989;54:497–504.

356. Ptak W, Rozycka D, Askenase PW, Gershon RK. Role of antigen-presenting cells in the development and persistence of contact hypersensitivity. J Exp Med 1980;151:362–375.

357. Eynon EE, Parker DC. Small B cells as antigen-presenting cells in the induction of tolerance to soluble protein antigens. J Exp Med 1992;175:131–138.

358. Streilein JW, Toews GT, Gilliam JN, Bergstresser PR. Tolerance or hypersensitivity to 2,4-dinitro-1-fluorobenzene: the role of Langerhans cell density within epidermis. J Invest Dermatol 1980,74:319–322.

359. Alcalay J, Craig JN, Kripe ML. Alterations in Langerhans cells and Thy1+ dendritic epidermal cells in murine epidermis during the evolution of ultraviolet radiation-induced skin cancers. Cancer Res 1989;49:4591–4596.

360. Chase M. Inhibition of experimental drug allergy by prior feeding of the sensitizing agent. Proc Soc Exp Biol 1946;61:257–259.

361. Wells HG. Studies on the chemistry of anaphylaxis (III). Experiments with isolated proteins, especially those of the hen's egg. J Infect Dis 1911,9.147–171.

362. Asherson GL, Zembala M, Perera MACC, Mayhew B, Thomas WR. Production of immunity and unresponsiveness in the mouse by feeding contact sensitizing agents and the role of suppressor cells in the Peyer's patches, mesenteric lymph nodes and other lymphoid tissues. Cell Immunol 1977;33:144–155.

363. André C, Heremans JF, Vaerman JP, Cambiaso CL. A mechanism for the induction of immunological tolerance by antigen feeding: antigen-antibody complexes. J Exp Med 1975;142:1509–1519.

364. Higgins PJ, Weiner HL. Suppression of experimental autoimmune encephalomyelitis by oral administration of myelin basic protein and its fragments. J Immunol 1988;140:440–445.

365. Miller A, Lider O, Roberts AB, Sporn MB, Weiner HL. Suppressor T cells generated by oral tolerization to myelin basic protein suppress both in vitro and in vivo immune responses by the release of transforming growth factor β after antigen-specific triggering. Proc Natl Acad Sci USA 1992;89:421–425.

366. Whitacre CC, Gienapp IE, Orosz CG, Bitar DM. Oral tolerance in experimental autoimmune encephalomyelitis. III. Evidence for clonal anergy. J Immunol 1991;147:2155–2163.

367. Chen Y, Inobe J, Marks R, Gonnella P, Kuchroo VK, Weiner HL. Peripheral deletion of antigen-reactive T cells in oral tolerance. Nature 1995;376:177–180.

368. Friedman A, Weiner HL. Induction of anergy or active suppression following oral tolerance is determined by antigen dosage. Proc Natl Acad Sci USA 1994;91:6688–6692.

369. Chen Y, Kuchroo VK, Inobe J, Hafler DA, Weiner HL. Regulatory T cell clones induced by oral tolerance: suppression of autoimmune encephalomyelitis. Science 1994;265:1237–1240.

370. Coffman RL, Lebman DA, Shrader B. Transforming growth factor beta specifically enhances IgA production by lipopolysaccharide-stimulated murine B lymphocytes. J Exp Med 1989;170:1039–1044.

371. Bright JJ, Kerr LD, Sriram S. TGF-beta inhibits IL-2-induced tyrosine phosphorylation and activation of Jak-1 and Stat 5 in T lymphocytes. J Immunol 1997;159:175–183.

372. Weiner HL, Friedman A, Miller A, et al. Oral tolerance: immunologic mechanisms and treatment of animal and human organ-specific autoimmune diseases by oral administration of autoantigens. Annu Rev Immunol 1994;12:809–837.

373. Okumura K, Tada T. Regulation of homocytotropic antibody response in the rat. VI. Inhibitory effect of thymocytes on the homocytotropic antibody response. J Immunol 1971;107:1682–1689.

374. Finkelman FD, Katona IM, Urban JF Jr, Snapper CM, Ohara J, Paul WE. Suppression of in vivo polyclonal IgE responses by monoclonal antibody to the lymphokine BSF-1. Proc Natl Acad Sci USA 1986;83:9675–9678.

375. Groux H, O'Garra A, Bigler M, et al. A CD4+ T-cell subset inhibits antigen-specific T-cell responses and prevents colitis. Nature 1997;389:737–742.

376. Asano Y, Hodes RJ. T cell regulation of B cell activation. Cloned Lyt-1+2− suppressor cells inhibit the major histocompatibility complex-restricted interaction of T helper cells with B cells and/or accessory cells. J Exp Med 1983;158:1178–1190.

377. Cantor H, Shen FW, Boyse EA. Separation of helper T cells from suppressor T cells expressing different Ly components. II. Activation by antigen: after immunization, antigen-specific suppressor and helper activities are mediated by distinct T-cell subclasses. J Exp Med 1976;143:1391–1401.

378. Sandrig S, Laskay T, Anderson J, De Ley M, Andersson U. Gamma-interferon is produced by CD3+ and CD3− lymphocytes. Immunol Rev 1987;97:51–65.

379. Bach BA, Sherman L, Benacerraf B, Greene MI. Mechanisms of regulation of cell-mediated immunity. II. Induction and suppression of delayed-type hypersensitivity to azobenzenearsonate-coupled syngeneic cells. J Immunol 1978;121:1460–1468.

380. Qin S, Cobbold S, Benjamin R, Waldmann H. Induction of classical transplantation tolerance in the adult. J Exp Med 1989;169:779–794.

381. Qin S, Cobbold SP, Pope H, et al. "Infectious" transplantation tolerance. Science 1993;259:974–977.

382. Gershon RK, Kondo K. Infectious immunological tolerance. Immunology 1971;21:903–914.

383. Davies JD, Martin G, Phillips J, Marshall SE, Cobbold SP, Waldmann H. T cell regulation in adult transplantation tolerance. J Immunol 1996;157:529–533.

384. Burnet FM, Stone JD, Edney M. The failure of antibody production in the chick embryo. Aust J Exp Biol Med Sci 1950;28.291–297.

385. Nossal GJV. The immunological response of foetal mice to influenza virus. Aust J Exp Biol Med Sci 1957;35:549–558.

386. Lubaroff DM, Silvers WK. Importance of chimerism in maintaining tolerance of skin allografts in mice. J Immunol 1973;111:65–71.

387. Silvers W. Is the presence and persistence of antigen required? In: The tolerance workshop, 1986, vol 1. Basel: Editiones Roche, 1987:122–126.

388. Mohler KM, Streilein JW. Tolerance to class II major histocompatibility complex molecules is maintained in the presence of endogenous, interleukin-2-producing, tolerogen-specific T lymphocytes. J Immunol 1987;139:2211–2219.

389. Powell TJ, Streilein JW. Neonatal tolerance induction by class II alloantigens activates IL-4-secreting, tolerogen-responsive T cells. J Immunol 1990;144:854–859.

390. Goldman M, Feng H, Engers H, Hochman A, Louis J, Lambert PH. Autoimmunity and immune complex disease after neonatal induction of transplantation tolerance in mice. J Immunol 1983;131:251–258.

391. Merino J, Schurmans S, Duchosal M, Izui S, Lambert PH. Autoimmune syndrome after induction of neonatal tolerance to alloantigens: CD4+ T cells from the tolerant host activate autoreactive F1 B cells. J Immunol 1989;143:2202–2208.

392. Schurmans S, Heusser CH, Qin H-Y, Merino J, Brighouse G, Lambert P-H. In vivo effects of anti-IL-4 monoclonal antibody on neonatal induction of tolerance and on an associated autoimmune syndrome. J Immunol 1990;145:2465–2473.

393. Chen N, Gao Q, Field EH. Prevention of Th1 response is critical for tolerance. Transplantation 1996;61:1076–1083.

394. Forsthuber T, Yip HC, Lehmann PV. Induction of TH1 and TH2 immunity in neonatal mice. Science 1996;271:1728–1730.

395. Coutinho A, Salaun J, Corbel C, Bandeira A, Le Douarin N. The role of thymic epithelium in the establishment of transplantation tolerance. Immunol Rev 1993;133:225–240.

396. Uhr JW, Möller G. Regulatory effect of antibody on the immune response. *Adv Immunol* 1968;8:81–127.

397. Siskind GW, Dunn P, Walker JG. Studies on the control of antibody synthesis. II. Effect of antigen dose and of suppression by passive antibody on the affinity of antibody synthesized. *J Exp Med* 1968;127:55–66.

398. Ozaki S, Berzofsky JA. Antibody conjugates mimic specific B cell presentation of antigen: relationship between T and B cell specificity. *J Immunol* 1987;138: 4133–4142.

399. Manca F, Fenoglio D, Kunkl A, Cambiaggi C, Sasso M, Celada F. Differential activation of T cell clones stimulated by macrophages exposed to antigen complexed with monoclonal antibodies. A possible influence of paratope specificity on the mode of antigen processing. *J Immunol* 1988;140:2893–2898.

400. Fazekas de St Groth B, Webster RG. Disquisitions on original antigenic sin. I. Evidence in man. *J Exp Med* 1966;124:331–345.

401. Davenport FM, Hennessy AV, Francis T. Epidemiologic and immunologic significance of age distribution of antibody to antigenic variants of influenza virus. *J Exp Med* 1953;98:641–656.

402. Klinman NR, Press JL, Segal GP. Overlap stimulation of primary and secondary B cells by cross-reacting determinants. *J Exp Med* 1973;138:1276–1281.

403. Amigorena S, Bonnerot C, Drake JR, et al. Cytoplasmic domain heterogeneity and functions of IgG Fc receptors in B lymphocytes. *Science* 1992;256:1808–1812.

404. D'Ambrosio D, Hippen KL, Minskoff SA, et al. Recruitment and activation of PTP1C in negative regulation of antigen receptor signaling by Fc gamma RII B1. *Science* 1995;268:293–297.

405. Jerne N. Toward a network theory of the immune system. *Ann Immunol (Paris)* 1974;125C:373–389.

406. Holmberg D, Forsgren S, Forni L, Ivars F, Coutinho A. Reactions among IgM antibodies derived from normal neonatal mice. *Eur J Immunol* 1984;14: 435–441.

407. Logtenberg T, Kroon A, Gemlig-Meyling FHJ, Ballieux RE. Analysis of the human tonsil B cell repertoire by somatic hybridization: occurrence of both "monospecific" and "multispecific" (auto) antibody-secreting cells. *Eur J Immunol* 1987;17:855–859.

408. Vakil M, Kearney JF. Functional characterization of monoclonal auto-anti-idiotype antibodies isolated from the early B cell repertoire of BALB/c mice. *Eur J Immunol* 1986:16:1151–1158.

409. Souroujon M. White-Scharff ME, André-Schwartz J, Gefter ML, Schwartz RS. Preferential autoantibody reactivity of the preimmune B cell repertoire in normal mice. *J Immunol* 1988;140:4173–4179.

410. Lundkvist I, Coutinho A, Varela F, Holmberg D. Evidence for a functional idiotypic network among natural antibodies in normal mice. *Proc Natl Acad Sci USA* 1989;86:5074–5078.

411. Pollok BA, Kearney JF. Identification and characterization of an apparent germline set of auto-anti-idiotypic regulatory B lymphocytes. *J Immunol* 1984; 132:114–121.

412. Marion TN, Dzierzak EA, Lee HS, Adams RL, Janeway CA Jr. Non-dinitrophenyl-binding immunoglobulin that bears a dominant idiotype (Id460) associated with antidinitrophenyl antibody is specific for an antigen on *Pasteurella pneumotropica*. *J Exp Med* 1984;159:221–233.

413. Augustin AA, Julius MH, Cosenza H. Changes in the idiotypic pattern of an immune response following syngeneic haemopoietic reconstitution of lethally irradiated mice. In: Sercarz E, Herzenberg LA, Fox C, eds. *ICN-UCLA symposia on molecular and cellular biology. Immune system: genetics and regulation*, vol VI. New York: Academic Press, 1977:195–199.

414. Sigal NH, Pickard AR, Metcalf ES, Gearhart PJ, Klinman NR. Expression of phosphorylcholine-specific B cells during murine development. *J Exp Med* 1977;146:933–948.

415. Etlinger HM, Heusser CH. T15 dominance in BALB/c mice is not controlled by environmental factors. *J Immunol* 1986;136:1988–1991.

416. Vakil M, Briles DE, Kearney JF. Antigen-independent selection of T15 idiotype during B-cell ontogeny in mice. *Dev Immunol* 1991;1:203–212.

417. Briles DE, Nahm M, Schroer K, et al. Antiphosphocholine antibodies found in normal mouse serum are protective against intravenous infection with type 3 *Streptococcus pneumoniae*. *J Exp Med* 1981;153:694–705.

418. Vandenbark A, Hashim G, Offner H. Immunization with a synthetic T-cell receptor V-region peptide protects against EAE. *Nature* 1989;341:541–544.

419. Howell MD, Winters ST, Olee T, Powell HC, Carlo DJ, Brostoff SW. Vaccination against experimental allergic encephalomyelitis with T cell receptor peptides. *Science* 1989;246:668–670.

420. Gaur A, Haspel R, Mayer PJ, Fathman CG. Requirement for CD8+ cells in T-cell receptor peptide-induced clonal unresponsiveness. *Science* 1993;259:91–94.

421. Sun D, Qin Y, Chluba J, Epplen JT, Wekerle H. Suppression of experimentally induced autoimmune encephalomyelitis by cytolytic T-T cell interactions. *Nature* 1988;332:843–845.

422. Barker CF, Billingham RE. Immunologically privileged sites. *Adv Immunol* 1977;25:1–54.

423. Yednock TA, Cannon C, Fritz LC, Sanchez-Madrid F, Steinman L, Karin N. Prevention of experimental autoimmune encephalomyelitis by antibodies against alpha 4 beta 1 integrin. *Nature* 1992;356:63–66.

424. Zamvil SS, Steinman L. The T lymphocyte in experimental allergic encephalomyelitis. *Annu Rev Immunol* 1990;8:579–621.

425. Hart DNJ, Fabre JW. Demonstration and characterization of Ia-positive dendritic cells in the interstitial connective tissues of rat heart and other tissues, but not brain. *J Exp Med* 1981;154:347–361.

426. Wong GHW, Barlett PF, Clark-Lewis I, Battye F, Schrader JW. Inducible expression of H-2 and Ia antigens on brain cells. *Nature* 1984;310:688–691.

427. Daar AS, Fuggle SV, Fabre JW, Ting A, Morris JP. The detailed distribution of HLA-A, B, C antigens in normal human organs. *Transplantation* 1984;38: 287–292.

428. Mantegazza R, Gebbia M, Mora M, et al. Major histocompatibility complex class II molecule expression on muscle cells is regulated by differentiation: implications for the immunopathogenesis of muscle autoimmune diseases. *J Neuroimmunol* 1996;46:53–60.

429. Ohba Y, Fujikura Y, Sawada T, Tokuda N, Morimatsu M, Fukumoto T. Major histocompatibility complex expression in muscle of rats with graft-versus-host disease. *Histol Histopathol* 1996;11:97–102.

430. Bellgrau D, Gold D, Selawry H, Moore J, Franzusoff A, Duke RC. A role for CD95 ligand in preventing graft rejection. *Nature* 1995;377:630–632.

431. Griffith TS, Brunner T, Fletcher SM, Green DR, Ferguson TA. Fas ligand-induced apoptosis as a mechanism of immune privilege. *Science* 1995;270: 1189–1192.

432. Wilson SE, Li Q, Weng J, et al. The Fas-Fas ligand system and other modulators of apoptosis in the cornea. *Invest Ophthalmol Vis Sci* 1996;37:1582–1592.

433. Niehans GA, Brunner T, Frizelle SP, et al. Human lung carcinomas express Fas ligand. *Cancer Res* 1997;57:1007–1012.

434. Streilein JW. Immunological non-responsiveness and acquisition of tolerance in relation to immune privilege in the eye. *Eye* 1995;9:236–240.

435. Kosiewicz MM, Streilein JW. Intraocular injection of class II-restricted peptide induces an unexpected population of CD8 regulatory cells. *J Immunol* 1996;157: 1905–1912.

436. Okamoto S, Hara Y, Streilein JW. Induction of anterior chamber-associated immune deviation with lymphoreticular allogeneic cells. *Transplantation* 1995; 59:377–381.

437. Niederkorn JY, Mayhew E. Role of splenic B cells in the immune privilege of the anterior chamber of the eye. *Eur J Immunol* 1995;25:2783–2787.

438. Wang Y, Goldschneider I, Foss D, Wu DY, O'Rourke J, Cone RE. Direct thymic involvement in anterior chamber-associated immune deviation: evidence for a nondeletional mechanism of centrally induced tolerance to extrathymic antigens in adult mice. *J Immunol* 1997;158:2150–2155.

439. Beer AE, Billingham RE. Transplantation in nature. *Perspect Biol Med* 1979;22: 155–169.

440. Medawar PB. Some immunological and endocrinological problems raised by the evolution of viviparity in vertebrates. *Symp Soc Exp Biol* 1953;7:320–338.

441. Heape W. Preliminary note on the transplantation and growth of mammalian ova within a uterine foster mother. *Proc R Soc Lond [Biol]* 1891;48:457–458.

442. Mintz B. Gene control of mammalian pigmentary differentiation. I. Clonal origin of melanocytes. *Proc Natl Acad Sci USA* 1967;58:344–351.

443. Witebsky E, Reich H. Zur gruppenspezifischen differenzierung der placentarorgane. *Klin Wochenschr* 1932;11:1960–1961.

444. Faulk WP, Temple A. Distribution of beta-2-microglobulin and HLA in chorionic villi of human placentae. *Nature* 1976;262:799–802.

445. Hunt JS, Yelavarthi KK, Yang Y, Fishback JL. Class I major histocompatibility genes in trophoblast cells: studies on expression, regulation and function. In: Chaouat G, Mowbray J, eds. *Cellular and molecular biology of the materno-fetal relationship*. Colloque Inserem, vol 212. London: John Libbey, Eurotex Ltd, 1991:51–59.

446. Wei X, Orr HT. Differential expression of HLA-E, HLA-F, and HLA-G transcripts in human tissue. *Hum Immunol* 1990;29:131–142.

447. Pazmany L, Mandelboim O, Vales-Gomez M, Davis DM, Reyburn HT, Strominger JL. Protection from natural killer cell-mediated lysis by HLA-G expression on target cells. *Science* 1996;274:792–795.

448. Crisa L, McMaster MT, Ishii KJ, Fisher SJ, Salomon DR. Identification of a thymic epithelial cell subset sharing expression of the class Ib HLA-G molecule with fetal trophoblasts. *J Exp Med* 1997;186:289–298.

449. Billingham RE. Immunobiology of the maternal-fetal relationship. In: *Reproductive immunology*. New York: Alan R. Liss, 1981:63–75.

450. Hedley ML, Drake BL, Head JR, Tucker PW, Forman J. Differential expression of the class I MHC genes in the embryo and placenta during midgestational development in the mouse. *J Immunol* 1989;142:4046–4053.

451. Tafuri A, Alferink J, Moller P, Hämmerling GJ, Arnold B. T cell awareness of paternal alloantigens during pregnancy. *Science* 1995;270:630–633.

452. Runic R, Lockwood CJ, Ma Y, Dipasquale B, Guller S. Expression of Fas ligand by human cytotrophoblasts: implications in placentation and fetal survival. *J Clin Endocrinol Metab* 1996;81:3119–3122.

453. Hunt JS, Vassmer D, Ferguson TA, Miller L. Fas ligand is positioned in mouse uterus and placenta to prevent trafficking of activated leukocytes between the mother and the conceptus. *J Immunol* 1997;158:4122–4128.

454. Lin H, Mosmann TR, Guilbert L, Tuntipopipat S, Wegmann TG. Synthesis of T helper 2-type cytokines at the maternal-fetal interface. *J Immunol* 1993;151: 4562–4573.

455. Doughty RW, Gelsthorpe K. An initial investigation of lymphocyte antibody activity through pregnancy and in eluates prepared from placental material. *Tissue Antigens* 1974;4:291–298.

456. Levine P, Burnham L, Katzin EM, Vogel P. The role of isoimmunization in the pathogenesis of erythroblastosis fetalis. *Am J Obstet Gynecol* 1941;49:925–937.

457. Voisin GA, Chaouat GJ. Demonstration, nature and properties of maternal antibodies fixed on placenta and directed against paternal antigens. *J Reprod Fertil* 1974;21[Suppl]:89–103.

458. Rocklin RE, Kitzmiller JL, Kaye MD. Immunobiology of the maternal-fetal relationship. *Annu Rev Med* 1979;30:375–404.

459. Breyere EJ, Barrett MK. Prolonged survival of skin homografts in parous female mice. *J Natl Cancer Inst* 1960;25:1405–1410.

460. Beer AE, Head JR, Smith WG, Billingham RE. Some immunoregulatory aspects of pregnancy in rats. *Transplant Proc* 1976;8:267–273.

461. Delassus S, Coutinho GC, Saucier C, Darche S, Kourilsky P. Differential cytokine expression in maternal blood and placenta during murine gestation. *J Immunol* 1994;152:2411–2420.

462. Marzi M, Vigano A, Trabattoni D, et al. Characterization of type 1 and type 2 cytokine production profile in physiologic and pathologic human pregnancy. *Clin Exp Immunol* 1996;106:127–133.

463. Clark DA, Flanders KC, Banwatt D, et al. Murine pregnancy decidua produces a unique immunosuppressive molecule related to transforming growth factor β-2. *J Immunol* 1990;144:3008–3014.

464. Clemens LE, Siiteri PK, Stites DP. Mechanism of immunosuppression on maternal lymphocyte activation during pregnancy. *J Immunol* 1979;122:1978–1985.

465. Piccinni MP, Giudizi MG, Biagiotti R, et al. Progesterone favors the development of human T helper cells producing Th2-type cytokines and promotes both IL-4 production and membrane CD30 expression in established Th1 cell clones. *J Immunol* 1995;155:128–133.

466. Krishnan L, Guilbert LJ, Russell AS, Wegmann TG, Mosmann TR, Belosevic M. Pregnancy impairs resistance of C57BL/6 mice to Leishmania major infection and causes decreased antigen-specific IFN-gamma response and increased production of T helper 2 cytokines. *J Immunol* 1996;156:644–652.

467. Krishnan L, Guilbert LJ, Wegmann TG, Belosevic M, Mosmann TR. T helper 1 response against Leishmania major in pregnant C57BL/6 mice increases implantation failure and fetal resorptions. Correlation with increased IFN-gamma and TNF and reduced IL-10 production by placental cells. *J Immunol* 1996;156:653–662.

468. Hill JA, Polgar K, Anderson DJ. T-helper 1-type immunity to trophoblast in women with recurrent spontaneous abortion. *JAMA* 1995;273:1933–1936.

469. Chaouat G, Assal-Meliani A, Martal J, et al. IL-10 prevents naturally occurring fetal loss in the CBA and DBA/2 mating combination and local defect in IL-10 production in this abortion-prone combination is corrected by *in vivo* injection of IFN-tau. *J Immunol* 1995;154:4261–4268.

470. Kabat EA, Wolf A, Bezer AE. The rapid production of acute disseminated encephalomyelitis in rhesus monkeys by injection of heterologous and homologous brain tissue with adjuvants. *J Exp Med* 1947;85:117–130.

471. Rose NR, Witebsky E. Studies on organ specificity: V. Changes in the thyroid glands of rabbits following acute immunization with rabbit thyroid extracts. *J Immunol* 1956;76:417–427.

472. Dale JB, Beachey EH. Sequence of myosin-cross-reactive epitopes of streptococcal M proteins. *J Exp Med* 1986;164:1785–1790.

473. Kaplan MH, Bolande R, Rakita L, Blair J. Presence of bound immunoglobulins and complement in the myocardium in acute rheumatic fever. *N Engl J Med* 1964;271:637–645.

474. Cibotti R, Kanellopoulos JM, Cabaniols J-P, et al. Tolerance to a self-protein involves its immunodominant but does not involve its subdominant determinants. *Proc Natl Acad Sci USA* 1992;89:416–420.

475. Pribyl TM, Campagnoni C, Kampf K, Handley VW, Campagnoni AT. The major myelin protein genes are expressed in the human thymus. *J Neurosci* 1996;45:812–819.

476. Fritz RB, Zhao ML. Thymic expression of myelin basic protein (MBP). Activation of MBP-specific T cells by thymic cells in the absence of exogenous MBP. *J Immunol* 1996;157:5249–5253.

477. Zamvil SS, Steinman L. The T lymphocyte in experimental allergic encephalomyelitis. *Annu Rev Immunol* 1990;8:579–621.

478. Rose NR, Herskowitz A, Neumann DA, Neu N. Autoimmune myocarditis: a paradigm of post-infection autoimmune disease. *Immunol Today* 1988;9:117–119.

479. Fujinami RS, Oldstone MB. Amino acid homology between the encephalitogenic site of myelin basic protein and virus: mechanism for autoimmunity. *Science* 1985;230:1043–1045.

480. Cole BC, Griffiths MM. Triggering and exacerbation of autoimmune arthritis bt the Mycoplasma arthritidis superantigen MAM. *Arthritis Rheum* 1993;36:994–1002.

481. Brocke S, Gaur A, Piercy C, et al. Induction of relapsing paralysis in experimental autoimmune encephalomyelitis by bacterial superantigen. *Nature* 1993;365:642–644.

482. Conrad B, Weissmahr RN, Böni J, Arcari R, Schüpbach J, Mach B. A human endogenous retroviral superantigen as candidate autoimmune gene in type I diabetes. *Cell* 1997;90:303–313.

483. Castano L, Eisenbarth GS. Type 1 diabetes: a chronic autoimmune disease of human, mouse, and rat. *Annu Rev Immunol* 1990;8:647–679.

484. Chervonsky AV, Wang Y, Wong FS, et al. The role of Fas in autoimmune diabetes. *Cell* 1997;89:17–24.

485. Katz JD, Wang B, Haskins K, Benoist C, Mathis D. Following a diabetogenic T cell from genesis through pathogenesis. *Cell* 1993;74:1089–1100.

486. Bendelac A, Carnaud C, Boitard C, Bach JF. Syngeneic transfer of autoimmune diabetes from diabetic NOD mice to healthy neonates. Requirement for both L3T4+ and Lyt2+ T cells. *J Exp Med* 1987;166:823–832.

487. Harlan DM, Hengartner H, Huang ML, et al. Mice expressing both B7-1 and viral glycoprotein on pancreatic beta cells along with glycoprotein-specific transgenic T cells develop diabetes due to a breakdown of T-lymphocyte unresponsiveness. *Proc Natl Acad Sci USA* 1994;91:3137–3141.

488. Guerder S, Picarella DE, Linsley PS, Flavell RA. Costimulator B7-1 confers antigen-presenting-cell function to parenchymal tissue and in conjunction with tumor necrosis factor α leads to autoimmunity in transgenic mice. *Proc Natl Acad Sci USA* 1994;91:5138–5142.

489. Picarella DE, Kratz A, Li CB, Ruddle NH, Flavell RA. Transgenic tumor necrosis factor (TNF)-alpha production in pancreatic islets leads to insulitis, not diabetes. Distinct patterns of inflammation in TNF-alpha and TNF-beta transgenic mice. *J Immunol* 1993;150:4136–4150.

490. Sarvetnick N, Shizuru J, Liggitt D, et al. Loss of pancreatic islet tolerance induced by beta-cell expression of interferon-gamma. *Nature* 1990;346:844–847.

491. Stewart TA, Hultgren B, Huang X, Pitts-Meek S, Hully J, MacLachlan NJ. Induction of type I diabetes by interferon-alpha in transgenic mice. *Science* 1993;260:1942–1946.

492. Pujol-Borrell R, Todd I, Doshi M, et al. HLA class II induction in human islet cells by interferon-gamma plus tumor necrosis factor or lymphotoxin. *Nature* 1987;326:304–306.

493. Campbell IL, Oxbrow L, Harrison LC. Reduction in insulitis following administration of IFN-gamma and TNF-alpha in the NOD mouse. *J Autoimmun* 1991;4:249–262.

494. Todd JA. Genetic control of autoimmunity in type-1 diabetes. *Immunol Today* 1990;11:122–129.

495. Acha-Orbea H, McDevitt HO. The first external domain of the nonobese diabetic mouse class II I-Aβ chain is unique. *Proc Natl Acad Sci USA* 1987;84:2435–2439.

496. Ridgway WM, Fasso M, Lanctot A, Garvey C, Fathman CG. Breaking self-tolerance in nonobese diabetic mice. *J Exp Med* 1996;183:1657–1662.

497. Reich EP, Sherwin RS, Kanagawa O, Janeway Jr CA. An explanation for the protective effect of the MHC class II I-E molecule in murine diabetes. *Nature* 1989;341:326–328.

498. Schmidt D, Verdaguer J, Averill N, Santamaria P. A mechanism for the major histocompatibility complex-linked resistance to autoimmunity. *J Exp Med* 1997;186:1059–1075.

499. Heath WR, Allison J, Hoffmann MW, et al. Autoimmune diabetes as a consequence of locally produced interleukin-2. *Nature* 1992;359:547–549.

500. Lehmann PV, Forsthuber T, Miller A, Sercarz EE. Spreading of T-cell autoimmunity to cryptic determinants of an autoantigen. *Nature* 1992;358:155–157.

501. Smith SC, Allen PM. Myosin-induced acute myocarditis is a T cell-mediated disease. *J Immunol* 1991;147:2141–2147.

502. Baum H, Davies H, Peakman M. Molecular mimicry in the MHC: hidden clues to autoimmunity? *Immunol Today* 1996;17:64–70.

503. Roudier C, Auger I, Roudier J. Molecular mimicry reflected through database screening: serendipity or survival strategy? *Immunol Today* 1996;17:357–358.

504. Wucherpfennig KW, Strominger JL. Molecular mimicry in T cell-mediated autoimmunity: viral peptides activate human T cell clones specific for myelin basic protein. *Cell* 1995;80:695–705.

505. Lin R-H, Mamula MJ, Hardin JA, Janeway CA Jr. Induction of autoreactive B cells allows priming of autoreactive T cells. *J Exp Med* 1991;173:1433–1439.

506. Zal T, Weiss S, Mellor A, Stockinger B. Expression of a second receptor rescues self-specific T cells from thymic deletion and allows activation of autoreactive effector function. *Proc Natl Acad Sci USA* 1996;93:9102–9109.

507. Conrad B, Weidmann E, Trucco G, et al. Evidence for superantigen involvement in insulin-dependent diabetes mellitus aetiology. *Nature* 1994;371:351–355.

508. Murphy ED, Roths JB. Autoimmunity and lymphoproliferation: induction by mutant gene lpr and acceleration by a male-associated factor in strain BXSB mice. In: Rose NR, Bigazzi PE, Warner NL, eds. *Genetic control of autoimmune disease*. Amsterdam: Elsevier Science, 1979:207–220.

509. Itoh N, Yonehara S, Ishii A, et al. The polypeptide encoded by the cDNA for human cell surface antigen Fas can mediate apoptosis. *Cell* 1991;66:233–243.

510. Roark JH, Kuntz CL, Nguyen KA, Canton AJ, Erikson J. Breakdown of B cell tolerance in a mouse model of systemic lupus erythematosus. *J Exp Med* 1995;181:1157–1167.

Fundamental Immunology, Fourth Edition,
edited by William E. Paul
Published by Lippincott–Raven Publishers, Philadelphia 1999.

CHAPTER 21

Type I Cytokines and Interferons and Their Receptors

Warren J. Leonard

Overview and Issues of Nomenclature
Type I Cytokines and Receptors
Type I Cytokine Receptor Families and Their Relatives
Cytokine Pleiotropy, Cytokine Redundancy, Cytokine Receptor Pleiotropy, and Cytokine Receptor Redundancy
Soluble Receptors
Interferons (Type II Cytokines) and Their Receptors
Species Specificity of Cytokines
Signaling Through Interferon and Cytokine Receptors
Overview of Jaks and STATs
Activation of Jaks and the Jak–STAT Paradigm
Are There Other Jaks?
STAT Proteins Are Substrates for Jaks that at Least in Part Help Determine Specificity
Other Latent Transcription Factors as Examples of Cytoplasmic to Nuclear Signaling (NF-κB and NF-AT)
Other Substrates for JAKs
Other Signaling Molecules Important for Cytokines
Downmodulation of Cytokine Signals
The CIS Family of Inhibitory Adapter Proteins
Th1/Th2 Cells: The T-Helper Paradigm
Diseases of Cytokine Receptors and Related Molecules
Concluding Comments
References

W. J. Leonard: Laboratory of Molecular Immunology, National Heart, Lung, and Blood Institute, National Institutes of Health, Bethesda, Maryland 20892-1674.
This chapter was written by Dr. Warren J. Leonard in his private capacity. No official support or endorsement by the NHLBI or NIH is intended and none should be inferred.

OVERVIEW AND ISSUES OF NOMENCLATURE

Cytokines are proteins that are secreted by cells and exert actions on either the cytokine-producing cell (autocrine actions) or on other target cells (paracrine actions). Cytokines exert these effects by interacting with and transducing signals through specific cell surface receptors. Based on this operational type of definition, it is clear that the distinction between cytokines, growth factors, and hormones often may be imprecise. As a generalization, cytokines and growth factors can be thought of quite similarly, except that molecules involved in host defense that act on white blood cells (leukocytes) are generally called cytokines, whereas those that act on other somatic cell types are more typically described as growth factors. However, there is a major difference between cytokines and hormones. Cytokines generally act locally. For example, in the interaction between a T cell and an antigen-presenting cell, cytokines are produced and usually exert potent actions only locally, and have rather limited half-lives in the circulation. In contrast, after their release, hormones are generally disseminated by the bloodstream throughout the body, acting on a wide range of distal target organs.

In the immune system, terms such as "lymphokines" and "monokines" originally were used to identify the cellular source for the cytokine (1). Thus, interleukin-1 (IL-1), which was first recognized to be made by monocytes, was a monokine, whereas IL-2, which was first described as a T-cell growth factor, was a lymphokine. A major limitation of this nomenclature became evident when it was recognized that many of these lymphokines and monokines were in fact produced by a wide spectrum of cell types, resulting in the adoption of the term "cytokine," first coined by Stanley Cohen in 1974 (2,3). The term, in effect, refers to a factor made by a cell ("cyto") that acts on target cells. The range of actions of cytokines are diverse, including the abilities to induce growth, differentiation, cytolytic activity, apoptosis, and chemotaxis. The term "interleukin" refers to cytokines that are produced by one leukocyte and act on another leukocyte (4). In many cases, however, some interleukins (e.g., IL-1 and IL-6) are additionally produced by other cell types and can act on other cell types, and IL-7 is produced by stromal cells rather than by typical leukocytes.

Among the many different cytokines, the type I cytokines share a similar four α-helical structure, as detailed below, and correspondingly, their receptors also share characteristic features that have led to their description as the cytokine receptor superfamily, or type I cytokine receptors (5–8). Although many of the interleukins are type I cytokines, not all are. For example, of the proinflammatory cytokines IL-1, tumor necrosis factor (TNF)-α, and IL-6, IL-6 is a type I cytokine, whereas IL-1 and TNF-α are not (IL-1 and TNF-α are discussed in Chapter 22). One interleukin, IL-8, is a chemokine (see Chapter 22). Thus, the term "interleukin" refers to a relationship to leukocytes; in contrast, the characterization of a cytokine as a type I cytokine not only has implications regarding its three-dimensional structure, but also has implications related to the structure of its receptor and mechanisms of signal transduction.

In addition to molecules that primarily are of immunologic interest, other extremely important proteins, including growth hormone, prolactin, erythropoietin, thrombopoietin, and leptin, are also type I cytokines and their receptors are members of the same superfamily. As detailed below, these nonimmunologic cytokines share important signal transduction pathways with the type I cytokines of immunologic interest. Thus, the grouping in this chapter emphasizes evolution and signaling pathways, rather than common functions. Hence, although IL-6 exerts many overlapping actions with IL-1 and TNF-α, these latter molecules will be discussed elsewhere because the signaling pathways they use are very different from those common to type I cytokines and their receptors. This raises the important concept, however, that different end functions can be mediated via more than one type of signaling pathway.

The field of interferon (IFN) research has developed in parallel to the cytokine field. IFNs were first recognized as antiviral agents, and as such have been the source of great excitement both for basic science and for potential clinical uses. Over time, it has become clear that the type I cytokines and IFNs share a number of features that now for the first time result in their being addressed together in one chapter in this text. Correspondingly, it is noteworthy that the International Interferon Society changed its name to the International Society of Interferon and Cytokine Research and that the International Cytokine Society focuses on the IFNs, as well as cytokines, together emphasizing the importance of the common themes of IFNs and cytokines that will be the subject of part of this chapter.

TYPE I CYTOKINES AND RECEPTORS

Type I Cytokines: Structural Considerations

Despite the existence of extremely limited amino acid sequence similarities between different type I cytokines, it is striking that all type I cytokines whose three-dimensional structures have been solved (by nuclear magnetic resonance or x-ray crystallographic methods) have similar structures (5–8). Moreover, type I cytokines whose structures have not yet been solved also appear (based on modeling and comparison with the solved structures) to achieve similar three-dimensional structures (5–8). These cytokines are appropriately described as four α-helical bundle cytokines because their three-dimensional structures contain four α-helices (Fig. 1). The first two and last two of these α-helices are each connected by long-overhand loops. This results in an "up-up-down-down" topologic structure because the first two helices (A and B) can be oriented in an up orientation and the last two helices (C and D) can be oriented in a down orientation, as viewed from the NH₂- to COOH-terminal direction. As shown in Fig. 1, the N and C termini of the cytokines are positioned on the same part of the molecule.

Type I cytokines can be grouped as either short-chain or long-chain four α-helical bundle cytokines, based on their size (8). The

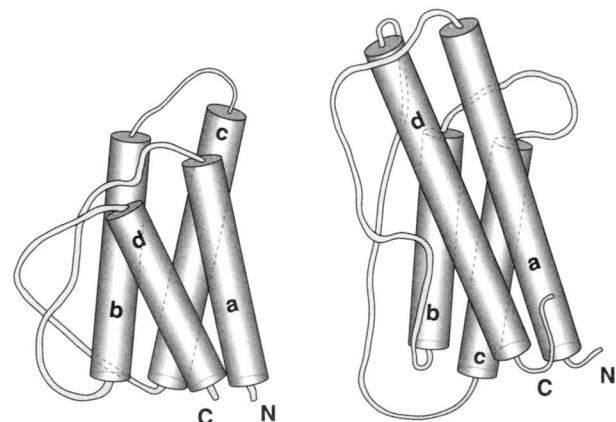

FIG. 1. Four α-helical bundle cytokines. Schematic drawing showing typical short-chain and long-chain four-helical bundle cytokines. Although these both exhibit an "up-up-down-down" topology to their four α helices, note that in the short-chain cytokines, the AB loop is behind the CD loop, whereas in the long-chain cytokines, the situation is reversed. Figure courtesy of Dr. Alex Wlodawer, National Cancer Institute.

short-chain cytokines include IL-2, IL-3, IL-4, IL-5, granulocyte-macrophage colony-stimulating factor (GM-CSF), IL-7, IL-9, IL-13, IL-15, monocyte-CSF (M-CSF), and stem cell factor (SCF), whereas the long-chain cytokines include growth hormone, pro-lactin, erythropoietin, thrombopoietin, leptin, IL-6, IL-11, leukemia inhibitory factor (LIF), oncostatin M (OSM), ciliary neu-rotrophic factor (CNTF), cardiotrophin-1 (CT-1), and G-CSF (Table 1) (8,9). In addition to a difference in the length of the helices, which typically are approximately 15 amino acids long for the short-chain helical cytokines and 25 amino acids long for the long-chain helical cytokines, there are differences in the angles between the pairs of helices, and the AB loop is "under" the CD loop in the short cytokines, but "over" the CD loop in the long cytokines (Fig. 1) (7,8,10). Short-chain, but not long-chain, cytokines have β sheet structures in the AB and CD loops. The groupings according to short-chain and long-chain cytokines have evolutionary considerations and also correlate with grouping of receptor chains for these two subfamilies of type I cytokines. An analysis of short-chain cytokines has shown that 61 residues com-prise the family framework, including most of the 31 residues that contribute to the buried inner core. The similarities and differences in the structures of IL-2, IL-4, and GM-CSF have been carefully analyzed (6). Among these cytokines, there is considerable varia-tion in the intrachain disulfide bonds that stabilize the structures. For example, IL-4 has three intrachain disulfide bonds, GM-CSF has two, and IL-2 has only one. In IL-4, the first disulfide bond (connecting residues 24 and 65) connects loop AB to BC, the sec-ond (connecting residues 46 and 99) connects helix B and loop CD, and the third (connecting residues 3 and 127) connects the residue preceding helix B with helix D. In GM-CSF, the N terminus of helix B and the N terminus of β strand CD are connected by one disulfide bond, whereas the other connects the C terminus of helix C and a strand following helix D. In IL-2, a single essential disul-fide bond connects residues 58 and 105 to connect helix B to strand CD. Thus, each cytokine has evolved distinct disulfide bonds to stabilize its structure, although it is typical that helix B is con-nected to the loop between helices C and D. The structures formed by helices A and D are more rigorously conserved than those formed by helices B and C, primarily due to the interhelical angles; helix D and the connecting region are the most highly conserved elements among the three cytokines (6). This is of particular inter-est because the regions of type I cytokines that are most important for cytokine–cytokine receptor interactions (based on analogy to the growth hormone receptor structure) include helices A and D and residues in the AB and CD loops, whereas helices B and C do not form direct contacts (6).

Certain variations on these typical structures can occur. For example, IL-5 is unusual in that it is a dimer, positioned in such a fashion so that the ends containing the N and C termini are juxta-posed (11). Helix D is "exchanged" between the two covalently attached molecules so that helix D of each molecule actually forms part of the four-helix bundle of the other monomer (11). M-CSF is also a helical cytokine dimer, but no exchange of helix D occurs (10). The IFNs achieve related albeit somewhat different structures and also are known as type II cytokines (8). IFN-β has an extra helix that is positioned in place of the CD strand (12). IFN-γ is a dimer, each of which consists of six helices (13), as can be seen in Fig. 2. Two of these helices are interchanged, including one from each four-helix bundle (10,13). IL-10, which is closely related to IFN-γ, has a similar structure (14). It is interesting that the major-ity of helical cytokines have four exons, with helix A in exon 1,

TABLE 1. *Four helical-bundle cytokines*

Short-chain cytokines	Long-chain cytokines
IL-2	IL-6
IL-4	IL-11
IL-7	Oncostatin M
IL-9	Leukemia inhibitory factor
IL-13	CNTF
IL-15	Cardiotropin-1
IL-3	Growth hormone
IL-5[a]	Prolactin
GM-CSF	Erythropoietin (EPO)
	Thrombopoietin (TPO)
M-CSF[a,b]	Leptin
SCF[b]	G-CSF

[a]Dimers.

[b]Different from the other four helical bundle cytokines in the M-CSF and SCF receptors (CSF-1R and c-kit, respectively) have intrin-sic tyrosine kinase activity and are not type I cytokine receptors.

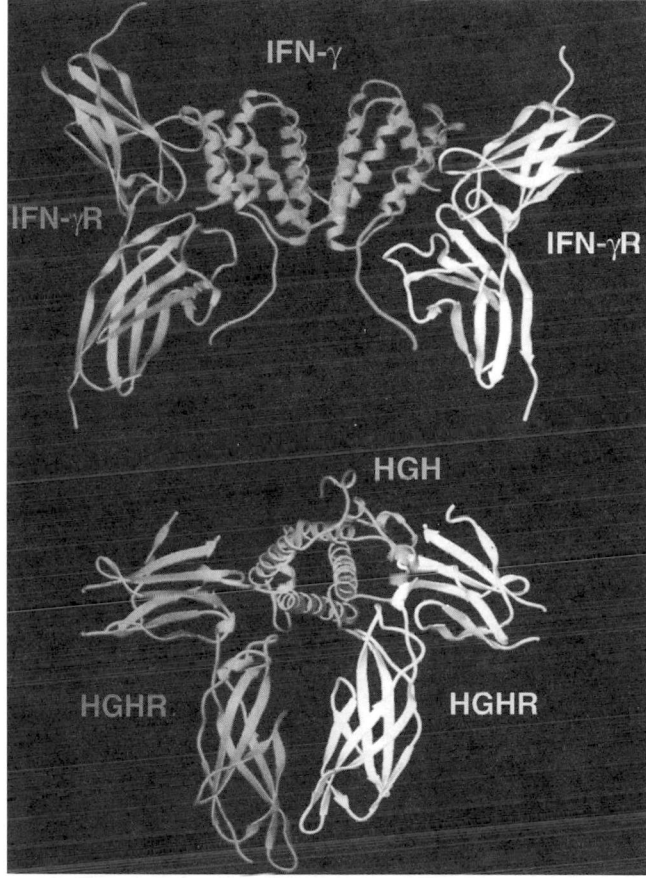

FIG. 2. Structure of the growth hormone and IFN-γ receptors. Shown are ribbon diagrams of the structures of the IFN-γ receptor (*above*) and growth hormone receptor (*below*) as examples of type II and type I cytokine receptors. In the IFN-γ receptor, only IFNGR-1 complexed to the IFN-γ dimer is shown because the full structure with IFNGR-2 is not available. For growth hormone, both growth hor-mone receptor monomers are shown. The coordinates for the growth hormone–growth hormone receptor structure are from ref. 21 and those for the IFN-γ–IFNGR-1 structure are from ref. 221. Figure cour-tesy of Dr. Alex Wlodawer, National Cancer Institute.

helices B and C in exon 3, and helix D in exon 4 (7). A related organization is found for IFN-γ, as well as the long-chain helical cytokines growth hormone and G-CSF. However, there are a number exceptions: for example, IL-15 is divided into five exons and IFN-β has only one exon, being devoid of introns (7).

Receptors for Type I Cytokines

The first published report suggesting that type I cytokine receptors had shared features came from a comparison of the sequences of the erythropoietin receptor and the IL-2 receptor β chain (15), but an analysis of a larger number of type I cytokine receptors provided a much clearer view of this new superfamily (16). Type I cytokine receptors are generally type I membrane–spanning glycoproteins (N-terminal extracellular, C-terminal intracellular), the only exceptions being proteins like the CNTF receptor α chain, which lacks a cytoplasmic domain and instead has a glycosylphosphoinositol (GPI) anchor; however, the orientation of this protein is otherwise similar to that of a type I membrane protein. In their extracellular domains, a number of conserved similarities have been noted (Table 2). These include four conserved cysteine residues that were predicted to be involved in intrachain disulfide bonding, and a tryptophan residue, located two amino acids C-terminal from the second conserved cysteine. In addition, a membrane proximal region WSXWS (trp-ser-X-trp-ser) motif was found to be generally conserved, although one exception to this relatively rigorous conservation is found in the growth hormone receptor, in which the motif is a substantially different YGEFS (tyr-gly-glu-phe-ser) sequence.

Interestingly, analysis of a number of the receptors showed that the two sets of cysteines are typically encoded in two adjacent exons, and the exon containing the WSXWS motif is typically just 5′ from the exon encoding the transmembrane domain. Although serines can be encoded by six different codons (i.e., six-fold degeneracy in codon usage), the codons used to encode the serines in WSXWS motif are far more limited, with two of the six possible codons (AGC and AGT) dominating. These data are consistent with a common ancestral precursor. Although many of the known cytokine receptors have been cloned based on expression cloning using a defined ligand, the limited degeneracy of the WSXWS motif has facilitated the complementary DNA (cDNA) cloning of new type I cytokine receptor members (via polymerase chain reaction [PCR]), leading to the first identification of IL-11R (17,18), IL-13Rα (19), and an oncostatin M receptor (20). Another shared feature of type I cytokine receptors is the presence of fibronectin type III domains. In some cases, such as the common cytokine receptor β chain (βc), which is shared by the IL-3, IL-5, and GM-CSF receptors, the extracellular domain is extended, containing

duplications of the domains comprising the four conserved cysteines and the WSXWS motif.

Overall, the different receptor molecules, analogous to the cytokines, have extremely limited sequence identity. Nevertheless, they appear to form similar structures, based on the known structures for the growth hormone prolactin and erythropoietin receptors (21–23), as well as the modeling of other cytokine receptor molecules based on the known structures. Thus, the available data indicate closely related three-dimensional structures for the different type I cytokines and closely related structures for type I cytokine receptors, despite the widely divergent sequences. It is important to note, however, that the only type I cytokine receptors whose structures have been solved correspond to long-chain type I cytokines. The cytokines and their receptors have presumably coevolved, with the differences in amino acid sequences between different cytokines allowing for their distinctive interactions with their cognate receptor chains. At times, however, as illustrated below, despite amino acid differences, a number of sets of cytokines are capable of interacting with shared receptor chains, allowing a number of the different cytokines and their receptors to be grouped into subfamilies (8).

In addition to the above noted similarities in the extracellular domains, there are sequence similarities that are conserved in the cytoplasmic domain of cytokine receptors. In particular, a membrane-proximal region known as the Box 1/Box 2 region is conserved (Table 2), with a proline-rich Box 1 region being the most conserved (24). This will be discussed in greater detail below.

Type I Cytokine Receptors Are Homodimers, Heterodimers, or Higher Order Receptor Oligomers

The first cytokine receptor structure to be solved was that for growth hormone (Fig. 2) (21). Before the x-ray crystallographic analysis, it was believed that growth hormone bound to its receptor with a stoichiometry of 1:1. Remarkably, however, the x-ray crystal structure solution provided the first evidence that a single growth hormone molecule interacted with a dimer of the growth hormone receptor, in which each receptor monomer contributes a total of seven β strands. Perhaps the most striking finding was that totally different parts of the growth hormone molecule interacted with the same general region of each growth hormone receptor monomer. The three-dimensional x-ray crystal structure for growth hormone and its receptor is shown in Fig. 2. Solving the structure also clarified the basis for growth hormone receptor assembly (21). Kinetically, growth hormone is believed to interact first with one receptor monomer via a relatively large and high-affinity interaction surface (site I), spanning approximately 1,230 Å^2. A second receptor monomer then interacts with the growth hormone–growth hormone receptor complex via two contact points—one on growth hormone (spanning approximately 900 Å^2)(site II), and the other on the first receptor monomer (spanning approximately 500 Å^2) (site III), located much more proximal to the cell membrane. Thus, a total of three extracellular interactions are responsible for the formation of the growth hormone–growth hormone receptor complex. Logically, mutations in site I might prevent receptor binding, whereas mutations in site II would potentially prevent dimerization and signal transduction, providing a rational method for the design of antagonists.

The growth hormone receptor structure showed that the growth hormone receptor extracellular domain is composed of two

---

TABLE 2. *Features common to type I cytokine receptors*

Extracellular domain
  Four conserved cysteine residues, involved in intrachain
    disulfide bonds
  WSXWS motif
  Fibronectin type III modules
Cytoplasmic domain
  Box 1/Box 2 regions—the Box 1 region is a proline-rich region
    that is involved in the interaction of Janus family tyrosine
    kinases

fibronectin type III modules, each of which is approximately 100 amino acids in length and contains seven β strands, yielding an immunoglobulinlike structure. The contact surface between ligand and receptor occurs in the hinge region that separates these two fibronectin type III modules. Analysis of a growth hormone–prolactin receptor complex showed the anticipated similar structure for the prolactin receptor (22).

The growth hormone–growth hormone receptor structure was obviously of great importance for researchers in the growth hormone field. In addition, however, the structure has been of perhaps even greater importance by serving as a model for the structures of all type I cytokine receptors. Because the growth hormone receptor forms a homodimer, it immediately served as a paradigm for other homodimers, such as the EPO receptor, whose structure also now has been solved (23). Interestingly, the structure of the EPO receptor complex was solved using a small protein (a peptide 20 amino acids long) mimetic of EPO that was identified using random phage display peptide libraries and affinity-selective methods (25). These studies on EPO provided direct evidence that a small molecule not only mimicked EPO action, but correspondingly, that it also induced dimerization of the EPO receptor, thereby forming a structure similar to that of the growth hormone receptor. The greatest difference, however, is that the site III stem region interaction surface in the EPO receptor is much smaller than that in the growth hormone receptor and comprises only 75 Å^2 (23).

In addition to the similarities between the structures for the growth hormone (21) and erythropoietin (23) receptors and presumably with other homodimeric receptors, it is immediately evident that the same type of structure can be achieved by heterodimeric receptors, as demonstrated by the growth hormone—growth hormone receptor/prolactin receptor structure (22), in which one of the growth hormone receptor monomers is replaced by the prolactin receptor. Thus, the growth hormone–growth hormone receptor system can be viewed as a specialized system in which two parts of growth hormone interact with the same receptor chain. It is reasonable to assume that cytokine receptor systems with a homodimeric receptor evolutionarily might be older than those with heterodimeric receptors, whereas the coordination of two different receptor chains might reflect an added level of specialization. Because the type I cytokines and their receptors are members of a superfamily, if one assumes that there was a single original primordial type I cytokine receptor molecule from which all the others have been derived, it is reasonable to hypothesize that the original type I cytokine receptor system might have involved a receptor that formed homodimers. It is therefore interesting that growth hormone and erythropoietin, whose actions are vital for growth and erythropoiesis, bind to receptors that are both homodimers, whereas the heterodimeric structures that typify the immune system are perhaps more specialized functions that have arisen later.

Interestingly, all helical cytokines known to interact with homodimers (growth hormone, prolactin, erythropoietin, and G-CSF) are long-chain helical cytokines, although other long-chain helical cytokines (e.g., the cytokines whose receptors contain glycoprotein [gp]130) interact with heterodimeric or heteromultimeric receptors. The short-chain cytokines that signal through homodimers are SCF and M-CSF, but in these cases the receptors (c-kit and CSF-1R, respectively) are different from type I cytokine receptors in that they contain intrinsic tyrosine kinase domains. Thus, SCF and M-CSF are not typical type I cytokines.

By analogy to the structure of the growth hormone receptor, for cytokines whose receptors are heterodimers, it is easy to envision

that heterodimeric receptors would occur with cytokines in which site II on the cytokine had evolved to a point wherein it now interacted with a different receptor molecule than site I, resulting in formation of a heterodimer rather than a homodimer. This latter situation is the case for many cytokines, including all short-chain type I cytokines except for SCF and M-CSF. Remarkably, there are a number of distinct groups of cytokines, with each group sharing at least one common receptor component. This phenomenon is true for certain sets of both short-chain and long-chain helical bundle cytokines, and the shared chain can interact either with site I or site II.

TYPE I CYTOKINE RECEPTOR FAMILIES AND THEIR RELATIVES

Cytokines that Share the Common Cytokine Receptor γ Chain

The receptors for five different immunologically important cytokines, IL-2, IL-4, IL-7, IL-9, and IL-15, share the common cytokine receptor γ chain, γ$_c$ (CD132) (26–37). These cytokines are all short-chain four-helical bundle cytokines; basic features of these cytokines are summarized in Table 3. The properties of these cytokines and their unique receptor chains will be summarized, followed by a discussion of the discovery that they share a common receptor component and the implications thereof.

Mature IL-2 is a peptide 133 amino acids long that is produced solely by activated T lymphocytes and is the major T-cell growth factor, in keeping with its original discovery as a T-cell growth factor (TCGF) (38). IL-2 has other important actions as well, however, including its ability to exert effects on a number of other lineages; most notably it can increase immunoglobulin synthesis and J-chain transcription in B cells (39–41), potently augment the cytolytic activity of natural killer (NK) cells (42–45), and induce the cytolytic activity of lymphokine-activated killer (LAK) cells (Table 3).

IL-2 is particularly important historically because it is the first type I cytokine that was cloned (46) and the first type I cytokine for which a receptor component was cloned (47,48). Many general principles were derived from this cytokine, including its being the first cytokine that was demonstrated to act in a growth factor-like fashion through specific high-affinity receptors, analogous to the growth factors being studied by endocrinologists and biochemists (49).

Although not produced by resting T cells, production of IL-2 is rapidly and potently induced after antigen presentation to resting T cells. As a result, transcription and synthesis of IL-2 are often used as key indicators of successful T-cell receptor activation. Although the antigen determines the specificity of the T-cell immune response, it is the interaction of IL-2 with high-affinity IL-2 receptors that regulates the magnitude and duration of the response, based on the amount of IL-2 produced, the levels of high-affinity receptors expressed, and the duration of IL-2 production and receptor expression (49). IL-2 can act in either an autocrine or paracrine fashion, depending on whether the producing cell is also the responding cell or whether the responding cell is a nonproducing cell. The gene encoding IL-2 is located on chromosome 4 (50), and like many other helical cytokines, its gene consists of four exons (7).

IL-2 binds to three different classes of receptors. These are formed by different combinations of three different chains. IL-2Rα

TABLE 3. *Features of cytokines whose receptors share γ_c*

Cytokine	Major source	Size[a]	Action	Chromosome location (h/m)[a]	Genomic org

IL-2	Activated T cells (Th1 cells)	h153 aa/20aa
		m169aa/20aa
		
		15.5 kDa
			T-cell growth factor
			B-cell growth, Ig production,
			  J chain expression
			Induce LAK activity
			Induce tumor infiltrating
			  lymphocyte activity
			Augment NK activity
			Stimulate
			  macrophage/monocytes
			Anti-tumor effects
				4q26–27/3	4 exons

IL-4	Activated T cells (Th2 cells) CD4⁺NK1.1⁺ Natural T cells	h153/24 aa m140 aa/20 aa 18 kDa	B-cell proliferation IgG1, IgE Augment MHC II, Fcε RII IL-4Rα and IL-2Rβ expression Th2 cell differentiation Anti-tumor effects	5q31.1/11	4 exons
IL-7	Stromal cells	h177 aa/25aa m154aa/25aa 17–25 kDa	Thymocyte growth T-cell growth Pre–B cell growth in mice but not humans	8q12–13/3	6 exons
IL-9	Activated helper T cells	 h144aa/18aa m144a/18aa 14 kDa	Th helper clones Erythroid progenitors B cells Mast cells Fetal thymocytes	5q31.1/13	5 exons
IL-15	Monocytes and many cells outside the immune system	h162aa/48aa m162aa/48aa 14–15 kDa	Mast cell growth NK cell development and activity T-cell proliferation	4q31/8	5 exons

[a]h and m refer to human and murine, respectively. The number of amino acids refers to the length of the open reading frame/length of signal peptide. The number of amino acids in the mature protein is therefore the difference between these numbers. Note that for IL-15, residues 1–29 have been identified as a signal peptide and 30–48 as a propeptide.

[b]More IL-15 mRNA is produced in skeletal muscle, kidney, placenta, and lung than in the thymus or spleen. It is important to note, however, that IL-15 mRNA is widely expressed without concomitant production of IL-15 protein, so that not all cells that express IL-15 mRNA necessarily produce biologically meaningful quantities of IL-15.

(47,48,51), IL-2Rβ (52–55), and a protein initially called IL-2Rγ (26) but now known as the common cytokine receptor γ chain (g$_c$) (28,34–37). The different classes of IL-2 receptors are discussed below.

IL-4, like IL-2, is produced principally by activated CD4⁺ T cells (56). It is also produced by the class of CD4⁺NK1.1⁺ natural T cells (57), and by mast cells and basophils (56). IL-4 is the major B-cell growth factor and is vital for immunoglobulin class switch, enhancing the production and secretion of IgG1 and IgE (56–60). IL-4 induces expression of class II *major histocompatibility complex* (MHC) molecules on B cells and increases cell surface expression of FcεRII (CD23) on B cells. However, IL-4 also can act as a T-cell growth factor, inducing proliferation in both human and murine T cells. Importantly, IL-4 can inhibit certain responses of cells to IL-2 (61). Moreover, IL-4 can exert actions on macrophages, hematopoietic precursor cells, stromal cells, and fibroblasts (56). Human IL-4 is 129 amino acids long, and its gene is located on human chromosome 5 (5q23.3-31.2) and mouse chromosome 11 (56,62), in the same region as IL-3, IL-5, and GM-CSF. Its receptor on T-cells and other hematopoietic cells consists of the 140-kDa IL-4Rα protein (63–65) and γ$_c$ (27,29). This form of receptor is known as the type I IL-4 receptor. Expression of IL-4Rα tends to be quite low, and cells that potently respond to IL-4 often express only a few hundred receptors per cell. As discussed below, in addition to the type I IL-4 receptor, an alternate form of the receptor, comprising IL-4Rα and IL-13Rα (now denoted IL-13Rα1) although not expressed on T-cells, is expressed on a number of other cell types and can transduce IL-4 signals into these cells.

IL-7 is not a lymphokine but instead is produced by stromal cells (66,67). Its major role is to enhance thymocyte growth, survival, and differentiation (68–71), but it also has some activity for the growth of mature T cells (69,72,73). It also is vital for the growth of murine pre-B cells (66,70,71,74), but based on humans with defective IL-7 signaling (patients with X-linked severe combined immunodeficiency), it is now clear that B cells can develop in the absence of IL-7 responsiveness, thereby indicating that IL-7 is not as vital for the growth of human pre-B cells as for thymocytes (75). Human IL-7 is 152 amino acids long (67), and its gene is located on chromosome 8 (76). The functional IL-7 receptor contains the 75-kDa IL-7Rα (77) and γ$_c$ (28,30). Based on chemical cross-linking experiments and Scatchard analyses, there is a suggestion, however, that the receptor may contain a third component as well (28).

IL-9 was originally described as a murine T-cell growth factor (78). Human and murine IL-9 are 126 amino acids long (78,79).

IL-9 is produced by activated T-cells and supports the growth of T-helper (Th) clones but not cytolytic clones (80,81). In contrast to IL-2, its production is much more delayed, suggesting its involvement in later, perhaps secondary signals. In the mouse, IL-9 also has been reported to exert effects on erythroid progenitors, B cells, mast cells, and fetal thymocytes. Regarding mast cells, IL-9 has been shown to be identical to mast cell growth-enhancing activity, a factor present in conditioned medium derived from splenocytes (82). IL-9 also can synergize with IL-3 for maximal proliferation (80). The action of IL-9 on thymocytes *in vitro* is interesting in view of the development of thymomas in IL-9 transgenic mice coupled to the observation that IL-9 is a major anti-apoptotic factor for thymic lymphomas (83). Although murine IL-9 is active on human cells, human IL-9 is not biologically active on murine cells (the opposite situation from that for IL-2). Human IL-9 is located on chromosome 5 in the 5q31-35 region (84) that is also the location for the genes encoding IL-3, IL-4, IL-13, and GM-CSF. In contrast, murine IL-9 is isolated on chromosome 13 (80), whereas IL-3, IL-4, IL-13, and GM-CSF are clustered on chromosome 11. IL-9 binds to the 64-kDa IL-9Rα binding protein, which is similar in size to γ_c (85), and the functional IL-9 receptor, which binds IL-9 with a K_d of 100 pM, consists of IL-9Rα plus γ_c (31,32).

IL-15 is the most recently identified of these cytokines (86,87). Although IL-15 *messenger RNA* (mRNA) is produced by a range of nonlymphocytic cell types, it is quite difficult to detect IL-15 protein production (88). Thus, a clear understanding of its physiologic cellular sources requires further investigation. IL-15 receptors are widely expressed, and it is becoming more clear that IL-15 plays a major role related to NK cell development and cytolytic activity (89-92). Interestingly, the receptor for IL-15 on T-cells contains IL-2Rβ (33,93), γ_c (33) and one unique protein, IL-15Rα. IL-15Rα shares a number of structural similarities with IL-2Rα (94), including close linkage of the IL2RA and IL15RA genes (95). An alternate form of receptor for IL-15, denoted IL-15RX has been detected on mast cells (96), with apparently distinctive signaling features, but cDNAs have not yet been reported. The existence of more than one type of IL-15 receptor raises the possibility that distinct types of IL-15 signals may be induced in distinct cell lineages.

Thus, IL-2, IL-4, IL-7, IL-9, and IL-15 collectively exhibit overlapping roles related to T cells, NK cells, B cells, and mast cells, and together would be expected to play vital roles in normal development or for the function of these cellular lineages. The fact that these five cytokines share γ_c is therefore of particular interest, and a historical review of the basis for the discovery that IL-2, IL-4, IL-7, IL-9, and IL-15 share a common chain is instructive.

X-Linked Severe Combined Immunodeficiency Disease Results from Mutations in γ_c

The γ chain was originally identified as a third component of the IL-2 receptor (26), after it became clear that IL-2 receptor α and β chains alone were not sufficient to transduce an IL-2 signal. The hypothesis that the γ chain was a shared component was motivated from a comparison of the clinical phenotypes in humans that result from defective expression of IL-2 versus γ_c. In 1993 it was reported that the γ chain was located on the X chromosome and that it was the gene that was mutated in X-linked severe combined immunodeficiency (XSCID; the disease is formally designated as SCIDX1) (97; see also Chapter 43) XSCID is characterized by profoundly

diminished numbers of T cells and NK cells (35,98–100) (Table 4). Although the B cells are normal in number, they are nonfunctional, apparently due to a lack of T-cell help as well as an intrinsic B-cell defect that is not corrected solely by the addition of T cells (35,98–100). In contrast to the profound decrease in the number of T cells in patients with XSCID, IL-2–deficient patients (101,102) and mice (103) were found to have normal numbers of T cells (the phenotypes of mice deficient in type I and type II cytokines and their receptor, Jak kinases, and STAT proteins are summarized in Table 15). This observation seemed to diminish the possibility that a component of the IL-2 receptor would be defective in XSCID, making the finding that the γ chain was mutated in XSCID all the more unexpected. Thus, the conundrum was why a defect in a component of a receptor would be more severe than a defect in the corresponding cytokine. This led to the hypothesis that the γ chain was part of other important cytokine receptors as well (97). In this model, the defects in XSCID are explained by the combination of defects resulting from simultaneous inactivation of multiple signaling pathways, rather than from a selective defect in IL-2 signaling (35,97,100,104). The initial two cytokines for which it was hypothesized that the γ chain might play a role were IL-4 and IL-7. The reasons for this were as follows (35,100):

1. IL-7 was known to be the major thymocyte growth factor, so that defective IL-7 signaling could potentially explain the basis for defective T-cell development.
2. Defective IL-4 and IL-7 signaling might explain the defects in B-cell function in XSCID. In XSCID, B-cell function was known to often not improve after successful bone marrow transplantation with T-cell engraftment, suggesting that there may be an intrinsic B-cell defect that persisted even when T-cell help was provided. Moreover, the γ chain appeared to be required for terminal B-cell differentiation, based on random X-inactivation patterns in immature surface IgM+ B cells of XSCID carrier females, but nonrandom X-inactivation patterns in their more mature surface IgM- B cells (i.e., only those B cells containing the active X with wild-type γ could mature) (98). Because IL-4 and IL-7 were both known to be important for B-cell function, defective IL-4 and IL-7 signaling could help to explain these defects.
3. At the time of the studies, only a single chain had been identified for both the IL-4 (63–65) and IL-7 (77) receptors, making it reasonable that a second type I cytokine receptor chain might form part of their receptors.
4. Like IL-2, both IL-4 and IL-7 could exert actions as T-cell growth factors; thus, it was possible that the sharing of a common chain might partially account for shared actions.

TABLE 4. *Features of XSCID*

1. Absent or profoundly diminished numbers of T cells and mitogen responses
2. Absence of NK cells
3. Normal numbers of B cells, but defective B cell responses
4. IgM can be normal, but immunoglobulins of other classes may be greatly diminished
5. XSCID carrier females exhibit nonrandom X-inactivation patterns in their T cells and NK cells. In B cells, the X-inactivation pattern is random in surface IgM-positive B cells, but nonrandom in more terminally differentiated B cells

5. In at least some situations, IL-2 and IL-4 were known to have opposing actions. If IL-2 and IL-4 competed for the recruitment of a shared receptor component present in limiting amounts, this could help to explain how they might have opposing actions (discussed below).

A series of experiments, including chemical cross-linking, Scatchard analyses on cells reconstituted with IL-4Rα γc or IL-7Rα γc, and functional analyses, led to the establishment that the γ chain was also an essential functional component of both the IL-4 and IL-7 receptors on T cells (27–30). In view of its multifactorial role, the γ chain was renamed as the common cytokine receptor γ chain, γc (28,29). IL-9, another T-cell growth factor, was subsequently shown to also use γc (31,32), whereas the receptor on T cells for IL-15, a cytokine quite similar to IL-2, shares both IL-2Rβ and γc (33) and differs only in that it has a different α chain. IL-15 appears even more dependent on IL-15Rα than is IL-2 on IL-2Rα for binding, because the IL-15–IL-2Rβ–γc complex appears to be less stable than the IL-2–IL-2Rβ–γc complex (105). Thus, at least five cytokines share γc (Fig. 3).

In view of the sharing of γc by five different cytokine receptors, XSCID is clearly a disease of defective cytokine signaling, and it is reasonable to try to explain the major deficiencies in XSCID in terms of the disrupted signaling pathways. Based on the dramatically diminished T-cell development in IL-7–deficient (71) or IL-7Rα–deficient mice (70), yet normal T-cell development in mice deficient in either IL-2 (103) or IL-4 (106,107) or both IL-2 and IL-4 (108), it seems likely that most if not all of the defect in T-cell development in patients with XSCID is due to defective IL-7 signaling. However, the analysis of mice deficient in IL-9 and IL-15, when they become available, will be of interest. Certainly, it is possible that IL-9 might partially contribute to thymic development, given the responsiveness of thymocytes to IL-9 and the development of thymomas in IL-9 transgenic mice, as noted above.

In addition to profoundly diminished numbers of T-cells, humans with XSCID lack NK cells. A question of considerable interest has been to clarify the γc-dependent cytokine(s) responsi-

ble for the lack of NK cell development in XSCID. Because IL-2–, IL-4–, and IL-7–deficient mice all have NK cells and significant actions of IL-9 on NK cells has not been described, it can be predicted that defective IL-15 signaling is responsible for the lack of NK-cell development, consistent with a variety of reports on the ability of IL-15 to drive NK-cell development (89–92).

In contrast to the greatly diminished number of T cells and absent NK cells in XSCID patients, the B-cell numbers are normal. This is in marked contrast to the greatly diminished numbers of B cells in γc–deficient mice (109–111) and mice deficient in either IL-7 or IL-7Rα, and strongly suggests that IL-7 is not required for pre-B cell development in humans. Although B cells develop, they are nonfunctional. This is due in part to a lack of T-cell help (given the near absence of T cells in XSCID), but a variety of data have suggested an intrinsic B-cell defect as well, including diminished activation of STAT (signal transducers and activators of transcription) proteins in XSCID B-cell lines in response to IL-4 (112). Indeed, defective γc-dependent signaling (and perhaps defective IL-4 signaling) may explain the transition from random to nonrandom X chromosome inactivation patterns in surface IgM⁺ versus IgM⁻ B cells from XSCID carrier females.

Rationale for the Sharing of γc

Why there should have been evolutionary pressure to maintaining the sharing of γc, given the obvious increased risk that sharing a receptor component has when mutations arise? There are at least two different types of models (35,104). First, given that IL-2, IL-4, IL-7, IL-9, and IL-15 can each act as T-cell growth factors, it was possible that γc would couple to signal transducing molecule(s) that would promote this function. The second type of model is diametrically different and suggests that the sharing of γc is a means by which each cytokine can modulate the signals of the other cytokines whose receptors contain γc. To understand this model, it is important to emphasize that cytokine receptor molecules individually are targeted to the cell surface and that the formation and/or stability of different receptor complexes is dependent on ligand. This was suggested above in the discussion of the growth hormone receptor, wherein the second receptor monomer recognizes the combined surface of growth hormone and the first growth hormone receptor monomer (21). Moreover, there are direct data for the IL-2 receptor, wherein γc was originally detected as a receptor component that could be coprecipitated with IL-2Rβ in the presence but not in the absence of IL-2 (113), and dimerization of IL-2Rβ and γc is known to be required for signaling (114,115). Thus, receptor heterodimerization at a minimum is stabilized by the cytokine and physiologically may be absolutely dependent on the presence of the cytokine. However, BIAcore optical biosensor experiments have indicated that under the proper experimental conditions, dimers between IL-2Rα and IL-2Rβ (only the latter of which is a type I cytokine receptor) can form in the absence of IL-2 (116,117). In the absence of stable preformed cytokine receptor complexes between γc and the other receptor chains, one can readily envision that γc could differentially associate with the different γc-dependent cytokine receptors depending on which cytokine was present. This provides for the possibility that γc is differentially recruited to different receptors based on the relative amount of a cytokine or its relative binding efficiency. In a situation where γc is limiting, a cytokine might then not only induce its own action but could also simultaneously inhibit the action of another cytokine that was less efficient at recruiting γc to its cognate receptor com-

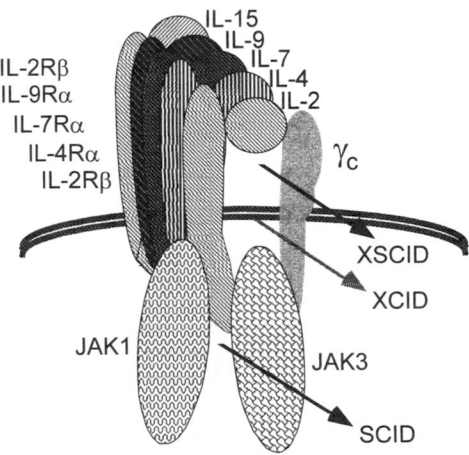

FIG. 3. Schematic of the receptors for IL-2, IL-4, IL-7, IL-9, and IL-15, showing interactions with Jak1 and Jak3. IL-2, IL-4, IL-7, IL-9, and IL-15 all share γc. IL-2Rα and IL-15Rα are not shown. Although the distinctive chains associate with Jak1, γc associates with Jak3. Mutations in γc cause XSCID or more moderate forms of X-linked immunodeficiency (XCID). Mutations in Jak3 cause an autosomal-recessive form of SCID.

plex. It is important to recognize that the two models as to why γ_c might be shared are not mutually exclusive.

An analysis of mice deficient in IL-2 (103), IL-2Rα (118), IL-2Rβ (119), and γ_c (109–111) provides the rather interesting observation that although the mice lacking γ_c have defective signaling in five different cytokine pathways, mice deficient in IL-2, IL-2Rα, and IL-2Rβ appear to be less healthy than the γ_c knock-out mice when maintained under *specific pathogen free* (SPF) conditions, although a direct comparison of all of the mice with the same genetic background in the same animal facility has not yet been performed. Although all of the mice have activated T cells, the development of autoimmunity is apparently less severe in γ_c-deficient mice. This suggests that the signals induced by IL-2 may normally be counterbalanced by signals from other γ_c-dependent cytokines. Thus, when γ_c itself is inactivated, there may be a normalization of the balance of signals due to the inactivation of both IL-2 and these other counterbalancing cytokines. These and other data suggest that γ_c plays a major role in regulating lymphoid homeostasis (120).

Cytokine Receptors that Share the Common β Chain β_c

The hematopoietic cytokines IL-3, IL-5, and GM-CSF (Table 5) are all synthesized by T cells and exert effects on cells of hematopoietic lineage (121–124). These cytokines are vital for proliferation as well as differentiation of myeloid precursor cells. IL-3 is the most pluripotent of these three cytokines (121,124) and historically was also called multi-CSF, reflecting the large number of lineages on which it can act. It can act to promote proliferation, survival, and development of multipotent hematopoietic progenitor cells and of cells that have become dedicated to a range of different lineages, including granulocyte, macrophage, eosinophil, mast cell, megakaryocyte, and erythroid lineages. IL-3 also can exert end-function effects, such as enhancing phagocytosis and cytotoxicity. GM-CSF is mainly restricted to the granulocyte and monocyte/macrophage lineages, but its actions are nevertheless still quite broad (122). It is both a growth and survival factor. In addition, it can expand the number of antigen-presenting cells, such as dendritic cells, and thereby may greatly expand the ability of the host to respond to antigen. Although IL-3 and GM-CSF can act on eosinophils, they act at much earlier stages than IL-5, presumably expanding the number of eosinophil-committed precursor cells, whereas IL-5 acts primarily to stimulate the eosinophilic lineage and eosinophil release from the bone marrow (123) and can enhance the killing activity of eosinophils against larvae from

Schistosoma mansoni. IL-5 also can induce immunoglobulin production in B cells activated by contact with activated Th cells in murine systems, but it has no role in stimulating human B-cell growth.

On cells that express receptors for more than one of these cytokines, such as eosinophilic progenitors that express receptors for IL-3, IL-5, and GM-CSF, or on murine pre-B cells, which express receptors for IL-3 and IL-5, the signals induced are indistinguishable (124). Thus, we can conclude that the differential lineage specificities of these cytokines are determined by the cellular distribution of their receptors rather than by fundamental differences in the signals that are induced by each cytokine. These observations are explained by studies demonstrating that each of these three cytokines has its own unique 60- to 80-kDa α chain (i.e., IL-3Rα, IL-5Rα, and GM-CSFRα) (125–130), but that they share a common 120- to 130-kDa β chain, β_c (131–133). The α chains have the principal binding activity for the cytokines, whereas the shared β_c can augment binding affinity but does not exhibit binding activity in the absence of the proper α chain. The α chains have relatively short cytoplasmic domains (approximately 55 amino acids each for IL-3Rα, IL-5Rα, and GM-CSFRα) and are not viewed as playing major roles in signaling function; thus, the signals of IL-3, IL-5, and GM-CSF are similar on cells that can respond to more than one of these cytokines because β_c, with its cytoplasmic domain of 432 amino acids, is the primary determinant of the signal. As a result, there is a relative compartmentalization of binding and signaling function for these cytokines, although the cytoplasmic domains of the GM-CSFRα and IL-5Rα chains (and by analogy, perhaps the IL-3Rα chains) appear to be capable of at least modulating the growth signals in transfected cells (134–136). The situation for the β_c family of cytokines is therefore quite different from the receptors for IL-2, IL-4, IL-7, IL-9, and IL-15, wherein the chains with the largest cytoplasmic domains (IL-2Rβ, IL-4Rα, IL-7Rα, and IL-9Rα) not only contribute most to signaling specificity, but also are the proteins principally involved in binding the ligands (note that in the case of IL-2 and IL-15, the IL-2Rα or IL-15Rα chains importantly cooperate with IL-2Rβ for this function). The shared chain, γ_c, serves a vital accessory function that when disrupted causes XSCID, but it plays little role in cytokine binding and does not provide an obvious basis for signaling specificity.

One of the surprising features of the hematopoietic cytokines is that despite their potent *in vitro* effects as well as some *in vivo* effects, there appears to be considerable redundancy of function, so that knockout mice that are lacking GM-CSF, IL-3, and IL-5 actions still exhibit relatively normal hematopoiesis. These observations do not minimize the potency of these particular cytokines,

TABLE 5. *Features of cytokines whose receptors share β_c*

Cytokine	Major Source	Size	Cellular targets	Chromosome location (h/m)	Exons
IL-3	T cells	h152/19aa m166/26aa 22–34 kDa	Multiple lineages	5q31.1/11	5
IL-5	T cells	h139/22aa m133/21aa 45 kDa dimer	eosinophils ? B cells	5q31.1/11	4
GM-CSF	T cells	h144/17aa m141/17aa 23 kDa	Granulocytes Macrophages	5q31.1/11	4

but instead underscore a substantial redundancy for a particularly important set of functions (124,137,138). It is noteworthy that these mice do exhibit defective host responses to some infectious challenges, suggesting that these hematopoietic cytokines play a vital role in promoting immune function.

Cytokine Receptors that Share gp130

There are now six cytokines that are known to utilize gp130 as a signal transducing molecule (17,139–143). Some of the properties of these cytokines are summarized in Table 6. This family is sometimes referred to as the IL-6 family of cytokines and includes IL-6, IL-11, OSM, LIF, CNTF, and CT-1. This group of cytokines comprises molecules with a diverse range of actions, ranging beyond the hematopoietic and immune systems to also include the central nervous system and cardiovascular systems, making them even more multifunctional than the γ_c and β_c families of cytokines, which appear to exert actions largely restricted to the lymphoid and hematopoietic systems.

IL-6 was the first member of this family to be recognized. It was originally identified and then cloned as a B-cell differentiation factor that stimulated terminal differentiation/maturation of B cells into antibody-producing plasma cells (144). However, IL-6 also can exert effects for T-cell growth and differentiation (and thus is a thymocyte comitogen), induce myeloid differentiation into macrophages, induce acute-phase protein synthesis of hepatocytes, and exert actions on keratinocytes, mesangial cells, hematopoietic stem cells, the development of osteoclasts, and neural differentiation of PC12 cells (145–147). IL-6 binds to an 80-kDa IL-6 binding protein, denoted IL-6Rα, which has a comparatively short 82–amino acid long cytoplasmic domain (148). This IL-6–IL-6Rα complex then interacts with and recruits the 130-kDa signal-transducing molecule gp130, which together with IL-6Rα can form a functional IL-6 receptor (139,149). gp130 is the molecule that is the common component of the receptors for the family of cytokines being discussed in this section. Interestingly, from a structural perspective, gp130 contains a total of six fibronectin type III modules, with the four conserved cysteine residues and the WSXWS motif being located in the second and third of these modules, starting from the N terminus (139). As such, these regions are topologically

positioned a greater distance external to the cell membrane than is the case for the other type I cytokine receptors discussed above.

Remarkably, the IL-6 system illustrates a novel twist on the properties of their principal binding proteins: the cytoplasmic domain of IL-6Rα is superfluous for signaling; a soluble form of the IL-6Rα extracellular domain is sufficient for ligand binding and coordination with gp130. Thus, in the presence of soluble IL-6Rα and IL-6, many cell types that express gp130 but not IL-6Rα are capable of signaling. It was observed that IL-6 signaling requires the dimerization of gp130 (150,151). In fact, subsequent data showed that IL-6 signals through a complex containing two molecules each of IL-6, IL-6Rα, and gp130 (a dimer of a trimer) (152), providing a possible paradigm for the stoichiometry of subunits for other members of the IL-6 family of cytokines.

IL-11 was originally identified as a factor produced by a stromal cell line in response to stimulation with IL-1 (153,154). It was noted to exert a number of effects on hematopoiesis, particularly in combination with IL-3 and stem cell factor. Because IL-11 exhibited IL-6–like activities, a cDNA was isolated based on the presence of IL-6–like activity in the presence of antibodies to IL-6 (155). Other actions of IL-11 include the ability to stimulate the proliferation of lymphoid and hematopoietic progenitor cells, stimulate megakaryocytic progenitors and megakaryocyte maturation, and stimulate erythroid progenitors (an action not shared by IL-6). Like IL-6, IL-11 can induce acute phase proteins and augment antigen-specific B-cell responses, but it does not stimulate human myeloma cells (153–156). Subsequently, adipogenesis inhibitory factor was cloned and found to be identical to IL-11 (157), revealing another action of IL-11. IL-11 signals through a receptor complex containing both IL-11Rα and gp130 (17). Interestingly, IL-11Rα mRNA can be alternatively spliced to yield a form lacking the cytoplasmic domain, and like IL-6Rα, a soluble form of IL-11Rα can coordinate with IL-11 to signal in cells expressing gp130 (158). Studies on the stoichiometry of the IL-11 receptor complex failed to reveal dimerization of gp130. Thus, assuming that it forms a hexameric receptor complex, only five of the members are known: two molecules of IL-11 and IL-11Rα, and one of gp130, suggesting that another component may still be found (159). IL-11 is located at 19q13.3–13.4.

Leukemia inhibitory factor is another multifunctional cytokine originally cloned based on the activity associated with its name

TABLE 6. *Cytokines whose receptors share gp130*

Cytokine	Chromosome location (h/m)
IL-6	7p21/5
IL-11	19q13.3–13.4/7
LIF	22q12.1–12.2/11
OSM	22q12.1–12.2/11
CNTF	11q12.2/19
CT1	16p11.1–11.2/?

Major action	IL-6	IL-11	LIF	OSM	CNTF	CT-1
Growth of myeloma cells	+	–	+	+	+	?
Maintenance of ES cell pluripotency	–	–	+	+	+	+
Induction of hepatic acute phase proteins	+	+	+	+	+	+
Induction of cardiac hypertrophy	–	+	+	+	+/–	+
Induction of osteoclast formation	–	+	+	+	?	?
Enhanced neuronal survival/differentiation	+	+	+	+	+	+
Inhibit adipogenesis	?	+	+	?	?	?

Most of the data in this table are derived from Taga and Kishimoto (147).

(160). LIF can suppress the differentiation of pluripotent embryonic stem cells, inhibit adipogenesis, and induce monocyte differentiation of the M1 murine leukemia cell line, thus mimicking a number of the actions of IL-6 (161). In addition, it exerts a number of actions in the central nervous system, and LIF was shown to be identical to cholinergic neural differentiation factor (162), a factor that can induce acetylcholine synthesis while simultaneously suppressing catecholamine production, thereby inducing cholinergic function while suppressing noradrenergic function (162). LIF was found to bind to a receptor (LIFRβ) that is structurally related to gp130 (163), but the functional LIF receptor requires the heterodimerization of LIFRβ and gp130 as well (140).

Ciliary neurotrophic factor was discovered based on its ability to promote neuronal survival (164,165). CNTF signals through a receptor comprising LIFRβ and gp130, but also requires a specific binding protein (166,167), now denoted CNTFRα. Interestingly, the CNTFRα chain lacks transmembrane and cytoplasmic domains and instead is a GPI-linked receptor molecule. Its sole function appears to be to provide a receptor-cytokine surface with which gp130 and LIFRβ can interact. Thus, CNTF is like IL-6 in that each requires initial binding to a receptor component (CNTFRα or IL-6Rα) which does not require its own cytoplasmic domain for signaling. Whereas IL-6 signaling involves homodimerization of gp130, CNTF (like LIF) signaling involves the heterodimerization of LIFRβ and gp130. In fact, the functional CNTF receptor appears to be a hexameric structure containing two molecules of CNTF, two of CNTFRα, and one each of gp130 and LIFRβ (168). The receptor is expressed largely within the nervous system and in skeletal muscle, accounting for largely restricted actions of CNTF (166).

Oncostatin M was originally identified based on its ability to inhibit the growth of A375 human melanoma cells (169), and cloning confirmed its actions as a growth regulator (170). Human OSM is a potent growth factor for Kaposi's sarcoma in patients with acquired immunodeficiency syndrome (AIDS) (171,172). Human OSM can bind directly to gp130 and signals through a receptor combination of gp130 and LIFRβ (140), but also has an alternative receptor comprising a specific OSM receptor subunit (OSMRβ) and gp130 (20). Interestingly, murine OSM can only act through the second type of receptor (172a).

Cardiotrophin 1 was initially isolated based on its actions on cardiac muscle cells (173). However, it is now clear that it is a multifunctional cytokine with hematopoietic, neuronal, and developmental effects, in additional to its effects on cardiac development and hypertrophy (174). The basis for these multifunctional actions became clear when it was found that like OSM and LIF, CT-1 can also signal through a heterodimer of LIFRβ and gp130 (143). Interestingly, more recent studies suggest that the CT-1 receptor on motor neurons involves a third receptor component, possibly GPI-linked (175,176).

Thus, six cytokines (IL-6, IL-11, LIF, CNTF, OSM, and CT-1) all have receptors that are dependent on gp130. These can be divided into two sets of cytokines: those known to not require LIFRβ, namely IL-6 and IL-11, and those that use both gp130 and LIFRβ (LIF, CT-1, and CNTF) (Table 7) with human OSM having two receptor forms. Within these two groups, each of the cytokines can be predicted to exert identical actions on cells that can respond to them. It is clear that the presence of IL-6Rα, IL-11Rα, and CNTFRα (either on the cell surface or as a soluble receptor form, discussed below) determines whether a cell can respond to IL-6, IL-11, and CNTF. This raises the interesting question as to whether functional homologs of IL-6Rα, IL-11Rα, and CNTFRα also will

TABLE 7. *Composition of receptors for the IL-6 family of cytokines*

Cytokines whose receptors do not contain LIFRβ

IL-6	IL-6Rα + gp130
IL-11	IL-11Rα + gp130
OSM	OSMRβ + gp130*

Cytokines whose receptors contain LIFRβ

LIF	LIFRβ + gp130
OSM	LIFRβ + gp130**
CNTF	CNTFRα + LIFRβ + gp130
CT1	LIFRβ + gp130 + ?CT1Rα

Note that there is evidence for CT1Rα but it has not been cloned. It is conceivable but unproven that OSMRα and LIFRα proteins also might exist.
*Human or mouse OSM.
**Human OSM.

exist for LIF, OSM, and CT-1. As noted above, this may well be the case for CT-1. There is added complexity, at least for human OSM, in that it also can signal through the OSMRβ/gp130 heterodimer in a fashion apparently independent of LIFRβ.

Significance of the Sharing of Receptor Chains

The common chains discussed above, γc, βc, and gp130, all contribute to signaling, but none of them has primary binding activity for cytokines. Instead, they each increase binding affinity in the context of the primary binding protein for each cytokine. Consequently, the capacity of a cell to respond to a given cytokine is determined by the unique binding chain, but signaling pathways can be shared.

Other Receptors with Similarities to gp130

As noted above, LIFRβ, and OSMRβ bear some similarities to gp130 (20). In addition, the G-CSFR, the leptin receptor (also denoted OB-R, for obesity receptor), and IL-12 receptor resemble gp130. The amino acid identity among these different receptors, compared pairwise, ranges from 18% to 32%, with LIFRβ and OSMRβ being the most similar.

Leptin

Leptin is the product of the obesity (ob) gene, an adipose tissue-derived signaling factor that plays a role in body weight homeostasis (177). The leptin receptor, OB-R, was cloned and was found to be most closely related to the gp130 signal transducer, G-CSFR, and LIFRβ (178). Interestingly, this receptor is encoded by the diabetes gene that is mutated in db/db mice (179). Chimeric constructs indicate that homooligomerization of the cytoplasmic domain is sufficient to transduce a signal (180), but it remains unclear whether additional receptor components also exist.

IL-12

IL-12 is also discussed in Chapters 17, 26, and 38. However, it is important to at least briefly mention this cytokine because its receptor chains are typical type I cytokine receptors. IL-12 is primarily produced by phagocytic cells in response to bacterial and intracellular parasites, such as *Toxoplasma gondii*, but it can be produced by other antigen-presenting cells, such as B cells, as well as by neutrophils (181). IL-12 potently induces the production of IFN-γ by NK cells and T cells and is also a growth factor for pre-activated NK and T cells, but not of resting T or NK cells, in keeping with its original discovery as *natural killer cell stimulatory factor* (NKSF) (182). IL-12 is a unique inducer of Th1 cell differentiation. IL-12 also can induce the production of IL-2, IL-3, GM-CSF, IL-9, TNF-α, and M-CSF, although inducing IFN-γ is probably its most important recognized action (181).

IL-12 can be thought of as having vital roles in both innate immunity and later adaptive immune responses. It is rapidly produced by NK cells and then T cells in response to antigens or foreign pathogens. This rapid response facilitates the activation of first-line defense against infections. In addition, however, IL-12 is also required for the subsequent differentiation of specialized T-cell populations, including the priming of Th1 cells for optimal production of IFN-γ and IL-2 (discussed below). IL-12 also has the ability to act synergistically with hematopoietic growth factors, such as IL-3 and stem cell factor, to support the proliferation and survival of hematopoietic stem cells (181). Structurally, IL-12 is a covalent dimer of 35- and 40-kDa peptides (181); thus, successful production of IL-12 requires that a cell can transcribe both the p35 and p40 genes (183). Interestingly, although p35 bears sequence similarity to IL-6 and G-CSF, p40 is homologous to the extracellular domains of IL-6Rα, CNTFRα, and G-CSFR and bears some of the features typical of type I receptors, including four conserved cysteines, a conserved tryptophan, and a WSEWAS motif, which has obvious similarity to the typical WSXWS motif (181). Moreover, because both IL-12 receptor (IL-12Rβ1 and IL-12Rβ2) chains bear some similarity to gp130 (184–186), one can think of p40 as a functional homolog of the soluble p80 IL-6Rα chain. Thus, for this cytokine, part of the receptor has become part of the cytokine. Interestingly, all the cells that produce IL-12 synthesize a much greater amount of p40 than p35, suggesting that the careful control of signaling is at the level of the primordial p35 cytokine part of IL-12. p40 is on human chromosome 5q31-33, whereas p35 is on 3p12-13.2 (181).

Other Examples of Shared Receptor Molecules

IL-7 and Thymic Stromal-Derived Lymphopoietin Share IL-7Rα

Although available data are still limited, in addition to IL-7, a second stromal factor, denoted *thymic stromal derived lymphopoietin* (TSLP) has been identified that shares at least some actions with IL-7, and shares the IL-7Rα chain (70). So far, TSLP has been identified only in the murine system.

Two Types of IL-4 Receptors, One of Which also Responds to IL-13

As detailed above, on T cells, IL-4 acts through a receptor comprising IL-4Rα and γ_c (now known as the type I IL-4 receptor) (27,29). However, it has been demonstrated that IL-4 also can signal through receptors on non-T cells (type II IL-4 receptors) that do not express γ_c (or Jak3, which is the Janus family tyrosine kinase that couples to γ_c, discussed below) (187). Other studies suggested that IL-13, another T cell–derived cytokine that shares actions with

IL-4 could induce identical signals to IL-4 on non-T cells that respond to IL-4, but had no effect in T cells because these cells do not bind IL-13 (188). The shared actions of IL-4 and IL-13 include the ability to (a) decrease expression of inflammatory cytokines, (b) induce MHC class II expression, (c) induce CD23 expression and IgE production by B cells, (d) inhibit IL-2–induced proliferation of chronic lymphocytic leukemia cells of B-cell origin, and (e) costimulate with anti-CD40 antibodies.

In addition to the shared biologic actions on non-T cells, other studies suggested that IL-4Rα was a component of both the IL-4 and IL-13 receptors (187–190), but that IL-4Rα could only bind IL-4. Specifically, antibodies to IL-4Rα inhibited both IL-4 and IL-13–induced proliferation, whereas soluble IL-4Rα could only inhibit IL-4–induced proliferation, consistent with its serving a major role for binding IL-4 but not IL-13. It was also shown that IL-13 as well as IL-4 could induce phosphorylation of IL-4Rα, again suggesting that it was a component of the IL-13 receptor. It was therefore hypothesized (187) and subsequently confirmed (19,191) that the type II IL-4 receptor consists of IL-4Rα plus IL-13Rα1, and that both IL-4 and IL-13 induce indistinguishable signals on cells expressing these receptors. Interestingly, IL-4 binds primarily to IL-4Rα, and IL-13 binds primarily to IL-13Rα1. This situation may be analogous to the situation for LIF, CT-1, and human OSM, which can all act through receptors containing LIFRβ and gp130, but differ in their abilities to directly interact with each of these receptor proteins. Recently, an additional IL-13 binding protein has been cloned, which has much higher binding affinity for IL-13 than does IL-13Rα1 (192). It is not yet clear if this protein (now denoted IL-13Rα2) is a component of a functional IL-13 receptor.

Using chimeric receptors, some investigators have artificially induced homodimerization of IL-4Rα and found that this can induce signals that are similar if not identical to those mediated by IL-4 on the same cells (193,194). However, it is important to recognize that this does not necessarily mean that IL-4 itself signals by homodimerizing IL-4Rα because IL-4 was shown to not be capable of dimerizing purified soluble IL-4Rα, even though it could form a heterotrimeric complex with IL-4Rα and γ_c (195). Moreover, IL-4 could not induce the tyrosine phosphorylation of insulin receptor substrate-1 (IRS-1) in murine fibroblasts expressing IL-4Rα alone (29). Instead, the chimeras might be able to function by artificially positioning a second Jak kinase close to the Jak1 that is physically associated with IL-4Rα, and this then is sufficient to mediate signaling function.

An Example of Multiple Affinities of Binding for a Single Cytokine: Three Classes of IL-2 Receptors

Although cytokines typically bind to a single class of high-affinity cell surface receptor, this is not always the case. One particularly well studied system in which there are three distinct classes of receptor is the IL-2 system. Above, we have discussed the high-affinity IL-2 receptor, which contains IL-2Rα, IL-2Rβ, and γ_c. The IL-2 system provides the very interesting illustration of a system with three classes of affinities of receptors (Table 8). In addition to the high-affinity receptor ($K_d = 10^{-11}$ M), there are both low-affinity (IL-2Rα alone, $K_d = 10^{-8}$ M) and intermediate-affinity (IL-2Rβ plus γ_c, $K_d = 10^{-9}$ M) receptors (34–37,196). Low- and high-affinity receptors are expressed on activated lymphocytes, whereas intermediate-affinity receptors are found on resting lymphocytes, particularly on NK cells.

TABLE 8. *Classes of IL-2 receptors*

Affinity	Kd	Where expressed	Composition	Functional
Low	10^{-8} M	Activated cells	IL-2Rα	No
Intermediate	10^{-9} M	Resting cells	IL-2Rβ and γc	Yes
High	10^{-11} M	Activated cells	IL-2Rα, IL-2Rβ, and γc	Yes

The intermediate- and high-affinity receptors can signal, thus suggesting that IL-2Rβ and γc are both necessary and sufficient for signaling, in keeping with the theme of dimerization indicated above. Given that the intermediate-affinity form is functional, why have an α chain, particularly in view of the fact that this non–type I cytokine receptor has an extremely short cytoplasmic domain that does not appear to play a role in signaling? The importance of the α chain has been clearly demonstrated by the severely abnormal phenotype of IL-2Rα–deficient mice, which exhibit autoimmunity, inflammatory bowel disease, and premature death (118), and more recently by the recognition that IL-2Rα mutations can cause SCID in humans (197). One of the clues to the importance of IL-2Rα comes from the kinetics of association of IL-2 with each chain. Although the α chain appears to lack a direct signaling function, it has a very fast "on" rate for IL-2 binding (49). Thus, the combination of this rapid on rate with the slow off rate from IL-2Rβ/γc dimers results in high-affinity binding that is vital for responding to the very low concentrations of IL-2 that are physiologically present *in vivo*. Moreover, because approximately 10-fold more low-affinity than high-affinity receptors are expressed on activated T cells, IL-2Rα may serve as an efficient means of recruitment and concentration of IL-2 on the cell surface, allowing more efficient formation of IL-2/IL-2Rβ/γc signaling complexes.

As mentioned above, IL-2Rα is not a type I cytokine receptor. In the mid-1980s, it was shown to have homology to the recognition domain of complement factor B (198). However, recently a second cytokine receptor has been identified that has a related structure, namely the IL-15 receptor α chain (94). This makes sense in view of the close relationship between IL-2 and IL-15 and the fact that the receptors for both IL-2 and IL-15 contain both IL-2Rβ and γc. It is important to recognize that as IL-2Rα cannot transduce a signal by itself, the detection of IL-2Rα on the cell surface does not necessarily reflect IL-2 responsiveness. Because IL-2Rα was the first chain identified, many early papers in the literature evaluated IL-2Rα expression without studying IL-2Rβ or γc. Thus, for example, the presence of IL-2Rα on a subpopulation of double negative thymocytes is a useful phenotypic marker corresponding to a stage of development, but it does not appear to reflect IL-2 responsiveness. Each of the components of the IL-2 receptor are located on different chromosomes: human IL-2Rα is located on chromosome 10p14-15 (199); IL-2Rβ is located at chromosome 22q (200,201); and γc is located at Xq13.1 (97).

Erythropoietin, Thrombopoietin, and Stem Cell Factor

Erythropoietin is vital for erythropoiesis and thrombopoietin for thrombopoiesis. These cytokines each bind to receptors that are homodimers (23,202–204). However, an extremely interesting finding related to erythropoietin is a report that erythropoietin signaling requires the functional cooperation of the erythropoietin receptor and c-kit (205), the receptor for stem cell factor (206). This latter receptor has intrinsic tyrosine kinase activity. This represents the only known example wherein a type I cytokine receptor appears to functionally require another receptor for its full function (205).

CYTOKINE PLEIOTROPY, CYTOKINE REDUNDANCY, CYTOKINE RECEPTOR PLEIOTROPY, AND CYTOKINE RECEPTOR REDUNDANCY

It is well recognized that many cytokines exhibit the phenomena of cytokine pleiotropy and redundancy (207). Cytokine pleiotropy refers to the ability of a cytokine to exert many different types of responses, often on different cell types, whereas cytokine redundancy refers to the fact that many different cytokines can induce similar signals. For example, cytokine pleiotropy is exhibited by a number of the cytokines whose receptors contain γc, which exert effects on a number of different lymphoid populations. Specifically, IL-2 can induce T-cell growth, B-cell immunoglobulin synthesis, and the activation of LAK and NK cells; IL-4 can induce B-cell growth and immunoglobulin class switch; and IL-7 plays a major role in thymocyte development, but also can stimulate mature T cells, and at least in the mouse, can act as a pre-B cell growth factor. IL-6 has even more diverse actions, ranging from that of a comitogen for thymocyte activation to that of a mediator of the acute phase response in liver. Regarding cytokine redundancy, it has already been highlighted that each of the cytokines whose receptors contain γc can act as T-cell growth factors and that IL-3 has actions that overlap with IL-5 and GM-CSF.

The recognition that cytokines share not only actions but also receptor components led to the concepts of cytokine receptor pleiotropy and cytokine receptor redundancy (34). The first of these terms can be defined by the ability of a single cytokine receptor subunit to function in more than one receptor. Thus, examples include the sharing of γc, βc, and gp130, as summarized above, as well as the sharing of IL-2Rβ by IL-2 and IL-15 receptors, and the sharing of IL-4Rα and IL-13Rα in type II IL-4 receptors and IL-13 receptors. Another way of viewing receptor pleiotropy is that certain receptor chains are useful modules. In other words, just as domains of proteins, such as SH2 and SH3, domains are used by many different proteins, one can think of shared receptor chains as an analogous situation in which an entire receptor chain is a module that functions in more than one context.

The final term, "cytokine receptor subunit redundancy," is the one with fewest examples. There is one well-documented example in mice, but not humans. IL-3 signals through IL-3Rα plus either βc or an alternative unique IL-3Rβ (208), which shares 91% amino acid identity with βc and is a completely functionally redundant protein for IL-3 signaling, but cannot substitute for βc in the context of IL-5 or GM-CSF signaling (133). Other potential examples exist. First, in type I and type II IL-4 receptors, as noted above, either γ_c or IL-13Rα can coordinate with IL-4Rα. Second, there is evidence for two types of human OSM receptors, both containing gp130, but one containing a specific OSMR and another containing LIFRβ. Third, IL-15 can apparently signal via what may be two completely different types of receptors depending on cell lineage. What remains unknown, however, is whether the signals mediated by these different types of receptors are the same so that there is redundancy, or whether there are distinctive features to the signals that IL-4, OSM, and IL-15 induce via the different receptors.

SOLUBLE RECEPTORS

Soluble forms of many cytokine receptors have been identified, including those for IL-1, IL-2, IL-4, IL-5, IL-6, IL-7, GM-CSF, type I and type II IFNs, and TNF (209,210). As is clear from this list of cytokines, soluble receptors are not restricted to receptors that are type I cytokine receptors, and in the case of IL-2, the principal soluble receptor protein is IL-2Rα, which is not a type I cytokine receptor. Soluble receptors can be created by alternative splicing that truncates the protein N-terminal to the transmembrane domain, resulting in a secreted protein rather than a membrane-anchored protein in the case of IL-4Rα, IL-5Rα, IL-6Rα, IL-7Rα, IFNαR β chain (IFNAR-2), and GM-CSFRα. Alternatively, they can be created by proteolytic cleavage of the membrane receptor, as is found for the receptors for IL-2Rα and TNFRI and TNFRII (210) (Table 9). Although it is theoretically possible that a soluble form of a receptor could be encoded by a distinct gene from the membrane-associated form of the receptor, no such examples have been reported. In the cases where proteolytic cleavage occurs, the identity of the proteases have not been identified. Three major questions relate to these soluble receptors:

1. Do they have physiologic or pathophysiologic functions?
2. How do their affinities compare with the corresponding cell surface receptor?
3. Do they have diagnostic, prognostic, and therapeutic applications?

Unfortunately, there is little information available on the *in vivo* role of soluble receptors. In general, in *in vitro* studies, soluble receptors can compete with their corresponding cell surface receptors, thereby serving a negative regulatory role. However, soluble IL-6Rα exerts an agonistic role because, as summarized above, IL-6 signaling occurs equally well via gp130 when the soluble rather than transmembrane form of IL-6Rα interacts with IL-6. Nevertheless, a mutated IL-6Rα that cannot interact with gp130 but still binds IL-6 can effectively inhibit (211). In the case of IL-2Rα, there is no reported physiologic function for soluble IL-2Rα

TABLE 10. *Soluble IL-2 receptors in human disease*

Malignancies
  Hematologic
    Adult T-cell leukemia
    Hairy cell leukemia
    Acute lymphocytic leukemia
    Chronic lymphocytic leukemia (B cell)
    Acute myelogenous leukemia
    Chronic myelogenous leukemia (especially in blast crisis)
    Malignant lymphomas
      Hodgkin's disease
      Non-Hodgkin's lymphomas
  Nonhematologic
    Adenocarcinoma of lung, breast, pancreas
    Small cell bronchogenic carcinoma
    Ovarian, cervical, and endometrial cancers
    Nasopharyngeal carcinoma
    Melanoma
Infections
  HIV
  Tuberculosis
  Rubeola
  Infectious mononucleosis
Other disease
  End-stage renal disease
  Rheumatoid arthritis
  Systemic lupus erythematosis
  Scleroderma
  Sarcoidosis
After transplantation
After IL-2 administration

In adults, the mean sIL-2Rα levels are 280 ± 161 u/ml (levels tend to be higher in pediatric populations). The situations here the levels exceed 5,000 u/ml are ATL, hairy cell leukemia, CML, and after IL-2 administration. The situations where levels are between 1,000 and 5,000 u/ml include AML, CLL, non-Hodgkin's lymphomas, AIDS associated with Kaposi's sarcoma, tuberculosis, rubeola, and end-stage renal disease. Data from Kurman et al. (209) and Fernandez-Betran et al. (210).

because the affinity of the released receptor is, as expected, similar to that of the low-affinity receptor ($K_d = 10^{-8}$ M), making it unlikely to effectively compete with the high-affinity cell surface receptor ($K_d = 10^{-11}$ M). However, this and other soluble receptors could serve as cytokine carrier proteins and potentially could increase stability of a cytokine by protecting it from proteolysis (210). There are potential diagnostic and prognostic uses for measuring these shed IL-2 receptors (Table 10).

INTERFERONS (TYPE II CYTOKINES) AND THEIR RECEPTORS

Interferons represent an evolutionarily conserved family (Table 11) of cytokines that, as noted above, are related to the type I cytokines. IFNs were originally discovered 40 years ago on the basis of their antiviral activity (212). Because of the existence of both type I and type II IFNs (213–216), the nomenclature of IFNs will be reviewed first. Type I IFNs include IFN-α (originally known as leukocyte IFN) and IFN-β (originally known as fibroblast IFN), and IFNω. IFN-ω is closely related to the IFN-αs and was formerly designated as an IFN-α. Unexpectedly, there are a very large number of IFN-αs, with at least 13 functional genes

TABLE 9. *Soluble cytokine receptors*

Generated by alternative splicing	Generated by proteolytic cleavage of mature receptor
sIL-4Rα	sIL-2Rα
sIL-5Rα	sTNFR
sIL-6Rα	
sIL-7Rα	
sGM-CSFRα	
sIFNAR-2	

TABLE 11. *Type II cytokines*

		Chromosomal location (h/m)
Type I interferons		
IFNα	13 genes[a]	9/4
IFNβ	single gene	9/4
IFNω	single gene[a]	9/4
IFNδ		
Type II interferon		
IFNτ	single gene	12/10
IL-10		
IL-10	single gene	1/1

[a]There are 12 known pseudogenes most closely related to the IFNα and IFNω genes.

(216). In contrast, the other type I IFNs, IFN-β and IFN-ω, are each encoded by single human and murine genes near the IFN-α cluster, and there are 12 pseudogenes most closely related to IFN-α and IFN-ω (216). The type I IFNs are clustered on human chromosome 9 and murine chromosome 4. Type II IFN is IFN-γ, which is encoded by a single gene on human chromosome 12 and murine chromosome 10 (213,215). In addition, another IFN, now denoted IFN-δ, has been reported (217,218).

The grouping of IFN-α and IFN-β together as type I IFNs is logical not only because of the similar amino acid sequences and structures of these IFNs, but also based on the fact that they share the same receptor and induce indistinguishable signals (219). These signals include antiproliferative and antiviral activities, as well as the ability to stimulate cytolytic activity in lymphocytes, NK cells, and macrophages. In contrast, IFN-γ has a distinct receptor. The type I and type II IFN receptors share a sufficient degree of similarity to each other so as to form a family (220). The structure of the IFN-γ receptor (221) is shown in Fig. 2. IFN receptors are referred to as type II cytokine receptors to reflect the substantial differences between these receptors and the type I cytokine receptors (8). Because both type I and type II IFNs bind to type II cytokine receptors, IFNs are occasionally referred to as type II cytokines, but more generally are referred to as IFNs. Based on the similarity of the IL-10 receptor to the IFN-γ receptors (8), IL-10 is considered to be a type II cytokine. Indeed, when its x-ray crystal structure was determined, IL-10 was found to be topologically related to IFN-γ (14). Among type II cytokines, IFN-γ has helices similar to those of the type I short-chain helical cytokines, but its short helices that occupy that AB and CD loop positions exhibit the AB over CD topology typical of long-chain type I cytokines. IL-10 and IFN-α/β have long chain structures (8).

Type I IFNs signal through a receptor containing a receptor known as the type I IFN receptor (222,223). The receptor consists of at least two chains (224–227). In contrast to the chains being denoted as α and β chains analogous to the nomenclature for type I cytokine receptors, the Interferon Nomenclature Committee has proposed that the chains be denoted as IFNAR-1 (previously also denoted IFN-αR1, IFNAR1, and IFN-Rα) and IFNAR-2 (previously also known as IFN-α/β receptor [IFN-α/βR], IFN-αR2, IFNAR2, and IFN-Rβ) (218). As such, this proposed nomenclature will be used in this chapter.

Interestingly, IFNAR-2 has both short and long forms as well as a soluble form (227). The long form has a much larger cytoplasmic domain and serves a more important role in signal transduction.

Whereas IFNAR-1 cannot bind IFNα, IFNAR-2 binds with low affinity, and the combination of both chains results in high-affinity binding (222) and function. As detailed below, IFNAR-1 binds the Janus family tyrosine kinase Tyk2, whereas IFNAR-2 binds Jak1. In addition to these cellular receptors, it is interesting that vaccinia virus and other orthopoxviruses encode a soluble form of type I IFN receptor that is related to the IL-1 receptors and that is capable of binding IFN-α, IFN-β, and IFN-ω (228,229). This form of IFN receptor is therefore not a member of the type II cytokine family but rather is a member of the immunoglobulin superfamily. Usually IFN-αs are species specific so that the human IFN-αs do not typically bind to the murine receptor. However, IFN-α8 is unusual in that it is one of the few or perhaps the only human type I IFNs that can bind to the mouse receptor. Thus, IFNAR-1 confers species specificity of binding (224).

IFN-γ was first recognized more than 30 years ago and was cloned in 1982 (213,230,231). IFN-γ is encoded by four exons on chromosome 12. IFN-γ forms a homodimer with an apparent molecular weight of 34 kDa. Little of the monomeric form can be detected, and it is not biologically active. As noted above, each IFN-γ monomer has six α helices, four of which resemble the short-chain helical cytokines, and there is no β sheet structure. The subunits interact in an antiparallel fashion. In contrast to the more ubiquitous production of IFN-α, IFN-γ is produced only by NK cells, CD8$^+$ T cells and the Th1 subclass of CD4$^+$ T cells (213). IFN-γ exerts its effects through specific receptors that are ubiquitously expressed, except on erythrocytes. Interestingly, even platelets express IFN-γ receptors, raising the possibility that they can serve a function in transporting IFN-γ in the circulation (213). The functional human receptor consists of two chains (232): IFNGR-1, also denoted IFNγR1 or IFNγRα (218,233), a 90-kDa protein whose gene is located on human chromosome 6q16-22 and murine chromosome 10 (231); and IFNGR-2, also denoted as IFN-γRβ (218,234,235), located on human chromosome 21q22.1 and murine chromosome 16 (231). IFNGR-1 is required for ligand binding, whereas IFNGR-2 plays a role in signaling. Jak1 associates with the Leu-Pro-Lys-Ser sequence in the membrane proximal region of the cytoplasmic domain of IFNGR-1 (236), whereas Jak2 binds to IFNGR-2 (237). Interestingly, as noted above, IFN-γ itself is a homodimer. Thus, binding of IFN-γ induces the homodimerization of IFNGR-1, which then allows the recruitment of IFNGR-2. Thus, the functional IFN-γ receptor is believed to contain two molecules each of IFNGR-1 and IFNGR-2.

In addition to the components of the IFN-α/β and IFN-γ receptors, there is an additional IFN receptor family member denoted CRF2-4 that is located on chromosome 21 within 35 kb of IFNGR-2 (238,239). This is now known to be a component of the IL-10 receptor (239a,b).

INTERLEUKIN-10, A TYPE II CYTOKINE

IL-10 is a cytokine that is produced by activated T cells, B cells, monocytes, and keratinocytes (240). The IL-10 gene is divided into five exons and is located on chromosome 1 in both mice and humans (240). IL-10 has an open reading frame of 178 amino acids, including the signal peptide, and the mature protein is 18 kDa. Human IL-10 receptor maps to 11q23.3 (241). It can inhibit the production of a number of cytokines, including IL-2, IL-3, IFN-γ, GM-CSF, and tumor necrosis factor and falls into the category of a Th2 cytokine (240). IL-10 inhibits monocyte-dependent

T-cell proliferation, in part by markedly decreasing synthesis of a variety of cytokines. Nevertheless, in addition to these indirect effects on T cells, IL-10 appears to exert direct stimulatory effects on thymocytes and T cells *in vitro*. Interestingly, the BCRF1 protein that is encoded by Epstein-Barr virus is very similar to IL-10 and shares many of its biologic properties as a macrophage deactivating factor and as a costimulator of proliferation of B cells (240,242). The EBV IL-10 homolog is a selective agonist, although its binding to the IL-10 receptor is somewhat impaired (242). IL-10 is a major inhibitor of Th1 functions (240). Although it may indirectly favor Th2 development by suppressing IL-12, it seems clear that IL-4 is the major differentiation factor for the development of Th2 cells.

As noted above, the IL-10 receptor is most closely related to IFN receptors, making it a type II, rather than type I cytokine receptor (243,244). This corresponds to the close structural relationship of IL-10 to IFN-γ, and as noted above CRF2-4 is also a component of the IL-10 receptor.

SPECIES SPECIFICITY OF CYTOKINES

There are no general rules for the species specificity of human and murine cytokines and how the cytokines and their receptor chains have coevolved. For example, human IL-2 can stimulate both human and murine cells, whereas murine IL-2 exhibits little action on human cells (40). Conversely, human IL-12 does not stimulate on murine cells, whereas murine IL-12 is biologically active on both murine and human cells (181). This selective property of IL-12 is dependent on the species origin of p35. Finally, IL-4 exhibits rather strict specificity so that human and murine IL-4 only induce responses on human and murine cells, respectively (56,62). Thus, virtually any combination of species specificities has been observed.

SIGNALING THROUGH INTERFERON AND CYTOKINE RECEPTORS

Our understanding of signaling through IFN and cytokine receptors has tremendously increased in the past few years. Multiple signaling pathways and molecules have been observed for various cytokines. Collectively, these include the Jak-STAT pathway, Src and Zap70 and related proteins, phosphatidylinositol 3-kinase (PI 3-kinase), IRS-1 and IRS-2, and phosphatases. Each of these pathways will be discussed in turn.

OVERVIEW OF JAKS AND STATS

The Jak-STAT pathway (230,245–254) is particularly exciting in that it serves as a rapid mechanism by which signals can be transduced from the membrane to the nucleus. Jak kinases are also known as Janus family tyrosine kinases and STAT proteins are signal transducers and activators of transcription that are substrates for Jak kinases. A tremendous amount of information is now available on Jaks and STATs that demonstrate their importance related to development, differentiation, proliferation, cellular transformation, and tumorigenesis.

Jaks

A schematic of Jak kinases is shown in Fig. 4. The Jak kinases are 116 to 140 kDa and comprise approximately 1,150 amino acids. The seven regions of conserved sequences in Jak kinases, denoted JH1 to JH7, are depicted. One of the hallmark features of the kinases is that in addition to the presence of a catalytic tyrosine kinase domain (JH1), there is also a pseudo-kinase region (JH2). The name "Janus kinase" reflects the two faces of the mythological Roman god, in this case one face representing the true kinase and the other the pseudo-kinase. Although the JH nomenclature has been used historically, the nomenclature has obvious limitations in that except for the JH1 catalytic domain and JH2 pseudokinase domain, it remains unclear whether or not the other JH regions correspond to discrete domains. Moreover, sequence analysis suggests that Jaks may have an SH2 domain, which approximately spans two of the JH domains.

There are four known Jak kinases, Jak1 (255), Jak2 (256), Jak3 (257,258), and Tyk2 (259). Interestingly, none of the Jak family kinases was cloned based on purification or function. Instead, the Jaks were all identified as parts of studies intended to identify new kinases (253). At least one Jak kinase has been found to be activated by every IFN and cytokine, and some cytokines activate two or three Jaks, but so far no cytokine has been found to activate all four Jaks (245–254). Table 12 lists a number of features of each Jak kinase, whereas Table 13 summarizes the Jak kinases that are activated by a variety of cytokines.

Given that the same cell generally expresses at least three of the Jak kinases (given the ubiquitous expression of Jak1, Jak2, and Tyk2), it is logical that the kinases that are activated are ones that can physically bind to the receptor chains. Jak kinases are known to bind to the membrane proximal Box 1/Box 2 regions of the cytoplasmic domains (260–263), and the N-terminal region of the Jaks

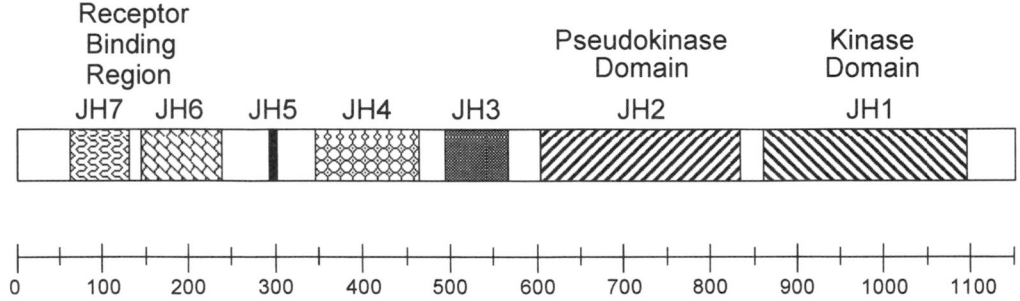

FIG. 4. Schematic of Jak kinases. Shown are the locations of the seven JH domains. JH1 is the catalytic domain. JH2 is the pseudo-kinase domain, the presence of which prompted the naming of this family as Janus family tyrosine kinases. As noted in the text, the JH nomenclature has limitations and in fact masks the presence of an SH2 domain that spans parts of the JH4 and JH3 domains. Also shown is the conserved tyrosine (Y1007 in Jak2) whose phosphorylation is required for maximal catalytic activity.

TABLE 12. *Features of Janus family kinases*

Kinase	Inducible vs. Constitutive	Size	Chromosome location (h/m)
Jak1	Constitutive	135 kDa	1p31.3/4
Jak2	Constitutive	130 kDa	9p24/19
Jak3	Inducible	116 kDa	19p13.1/8
Tyk2	Constitutive	140 kDa	19p13.2/?

is required for this function (264–266). The Box 1 region is proline rich (24,147), suggesting that Jak kinases may have SH3-like domains in their N-terminal regions to mediate these interactions. Because each receptor is a homodimer, heterodimer, or higher order oligomer, it is reasonable to assume that at least two Jak molecules (either two molecules of one Jak or one molecule each of two different Jaks) will be activated. Jak1, Jak2, and Tyk2 are ubiquitously expressed and are activated by a variety of different sets of cytokines (Tables 12 and 13). For example, Jak1 is activated not only by type I and II IFNs, but also by a number of interleukins (e.g., IL-2, IL-4, IL-7, IL-9, and IL-15), and Jak2 is activated not only by IFN-γ but also by growth hormone, erythropoietin, prolactin, and the hematopoietic cytokines IL-3, IL-5, and GM-CSF (245–250,253). Tyk2 is somewhat more restricted in that it is activated by IFN-α/β and IL-12. Interestingly, Jak1, Jak2, and Tyk2 are all recruited by all of the cytokines that share gp130 as a signal-transducing molecule, raising the question of whether in this context three Jak kinases are required or whether any one or two are sufficient. At least for IL-6, one study indicates that Jak1 is absolutely vital (267).

Jak3 is different from the other Jaks in that it is much more inducible. Furthermore, Jak3 is only activated by the cytokines whose receptors contain γ_c (35). It is interesting that each cytokine

TABLE 13. *Cytokines and the Jaks they activate*

Cytokine	Jak kinase(s) activated
IFN-α/β	Jak1, Tyk2
IFN-γ	Jak1, Jak2
Growth hormone	Jak2
Prolactin	Jak2
Erythropoietin	Jak2
Thrombopoietin	Jak2
IL-10	Jak1, Tyk2
IL-12	Jak2, Tyk2
G-CSF	Jak1, Jak2
γ_c family	
IL-2, IL-4[a], IL-7, IL-9, IL-15[b]	Jak1, Jak3
β_c family	
IL-3, IL-5, GM-CSF	Jak2, ?Jak1
gp130 family	
IL-6, IL-11, CNTF, LIF, OSM, CT-1	Jak1, Jak2, Tyk2

[a]Note that IL-4 activates Jak1 and Jak3 when it acts through the type I IL-4 receptor (IL-4Rα + γ_c, found, for example, on T cells). However, Jak3 is not activated when IL-4 signals through the type II IL-4 receptors (IL-4Rα + IL-13Rα1, a form of receptor that is expressed on a number of non-T cells, including fibroblasts).

[b]Note that IL-15 activates Jak1 and Jak3 when it acts through the type I IL-15 receptor (IL-15Rα + IL-2Rβ + γ, found, for example, on T cells). However, Jak2 is instead activated when IL-15 signals through the type II IL-15 receptor, denoted IL-15RX, found, for example, on mast cells.

whose receptor contains γ_c activates not only Jak3 but also Jak1. The basis for the activation of both Jak1 and Jak3 by IL-2, IL-4, IL-7, IL-9, and IL-15 is that Jak1 associates with each of the unique signaling chains (IL-2Rβ, IL-4Rα, IL-7Rα, and IL-9Rα) (31, 268–271), whereas Jak3 associates with γ_c (31,268,269). Although this could be coincidental, these observations raise the possibility that Jak1 is the Jak kinase that can most efficiently coordinate with Jak3. Given the wide range of cytokines that activate any particular Jak kinase and that in some cases multiple cytokines can activate the same set of Jaks, it is clear that the Jaks by themselves do not determine signaling specificity. For example, IL-2, IL-4, IL-7, IL-9, and IL-15 all activate Jak1 and Jak3, but induce a range of signals. Moreover, Jak2 is the only Jak activated by growth hormone and erythropoietin, cytokines with little in common in terms of function. Interestingly, Jak2 is the Jak that interacts with all cytokine receptors that form homodimers.

Importance of Jak Kinases in Signaling

In addition to the activation of Jak kinases by each of these cytokines, a variety of other data indicate their importance for signaling. Vital to the initial clarification of the importance of Jak kinases in IFN signaling were a group of mutant cell lines that were defective for IFN signaling, but wherein signaling could be rescued by genetic complementation (246). Defective IFN-α and IFN-β signaling was found in a mutant cell line lacking Tyk2 (U1 cells); defective IFN-α, IFN-β, and IFN-γ signaling was found in a mutant cell line lacking Jak1 (U4 cells); and defective IFN-γ signaling was found in cells lacking Jak2 (γ1 cells) (246). A variety of other data have indicated the importance of Jak kinases for other cytokine pathways. First, dominant negative Jak2 or Jak3 constructs inhibit signaling by erythropoietin, growth hormone, and IL-2 (272–274), and, as noted above, Jak1 is vital for IL-6 signaling (267). Second, humans (275,276) and mice (277–279) deficient in Jak3 exhibit developmental and signaling defects consistent with defective signaling. Third, in *Drosophila*, the *hopscotch* gene encodes a Jak kinase wherein loss of function alleles result in lethality and decreased proliferation, whereas a gain-of-function allele, *hopscotch*[Tumorous-lethal], results in melanotic tumors and hypertrophy of the hematopoietic organs (280,281). Fourth, in zebrafish, Jak1 is vital for normal cell migration and anterior specification (282). Fifth, as discussed below, Jak kinases are constitutively activated in many cell lines infected with a number of viruses, including HTLV-I, v-Abl, spleen focus forming virus, and v-src (283–286). Sixth, a Jak-2 inhibitor inhibited the growth of acute lymphoblastic leukemia cells *in vitro* (287). These data together demonstrate the vital role of Jaks in cytokine signaling. Depending on the function of the particular cytokine (e.g., development, differentiation, or proliferation), the particular Jak kinases may therefore be involved in a variety of processes, and when dysregulated, in at least certain settings appear to contribute to cellular transformation.

Jak3 Mutations Result in an Autosomal-Recessive Form of Severe Combined Immunodeficiency that Is Indistinguishable from XSCID

As mentioned above, mutations in γ_c result in XSCID in humans. At least 96 different mutations have been observed in XSCID (these are summarized on the World Wide Web; see http://www.nhgri.nih.gov/DIR/LGT/SCID/IL2RGbase.html). As might be expected, in cases where it has been examined, amino acid substitutions in the extracellular domain result in defective cytokine binding (35). In contrast, mutations or truncations in the γ_c cytoplasmic result in defective signaling. Analysis of an interesting family in which a number of males exhibit a moderate form of X-linked combined immunodeficiency (XCID) revealed that this disease also resulted from a mutation in γ_c (31). The mutation (Leu 271 → Gln) was found to result in a decrease, but not total loss of Jak3 association, in contrast to the loss of Jak3 interaction seen with cytoplasmic mutations that cause XSCID. Thus, the severity of the immunodeficiency appeared to inversely correlate with the degree of Jak3 activation. Thus, XSCID is truly a disease of defective cytokine signaling (35). Moreover, it was predicted that Jak3 was required for T-cell and NK-cell development and that mutations in Jak3 might result in a clinical phenotype indistinguishable from that in XSCID (31). Indeed, this is the case in humans (275,276). As one would hypothesize, a number of distinct mutations in Jak3 were found. Presumably, any mutation that interferes with its interaction with γ_c, with its catalytic activity, or with recruitment of substrates could result in clinical disease.

Analogous to the similarity of XSCID and SCID associated with Jak3 deficiency, mice deficient in either γ_c or Jak3 also have very similar phenotypes (109–111,277–279). These *in vivo* data underscored the vital role of Jak3 in mediating γ_c-dependent functions and suggested that Jak3 would be essential for most if not all γ_c-functions. Some *in vitro* data indicate that γ_c may do more than to recruit Jak3 (274,288), but the recruitment of Jak3 is clearly essential and the defects in T-cell and NK-cell development associated with γ_c or Jak3 deficiency are indistinguishable. Theoretically, it is possible that Jak3 might interact with other important cytokine receptor chain(s) that have not yet been identified. However, because Jak3 deficiency is not clinically or phenotypically worse than γ_c-deficiency, these *in vivo* data also demonstrate that Jak3 is likely to be associated only with γ_c. One report has suggested that Jak3 is associated with CD40 (289), raising the possibility of a role for Jak3 in a system distinct from cytokine receptors, although a functional role for Jak3 in CD40 signaling has not yet been established.

ACTIVATION OF JAKS AND THE JAK–STAT PARADIGM

Although the importance of Jak kinases should now be clear, it is equally important to understand how Jak kinases are activated, how they are regulated, and how they phosphorylate substrates. The paradigm of Jak–STAT activation is shown in Fig. 5, where IL-2 signaling is highlighted. After IFN or cytokine engagement, dimerization or higher order oligomerization of receptor complexes is induced. This in turn allows the juxtapositioning of Jak kinases, allowing their potential transphosphorylation and activation. In receptors with only two chains, the direct transphosphorylation of one Jak by the other makes sense. In more complex receptors, additional subtleties may exist. For example, for the IFN-γ system, because the receptor is a heterotetramer with two α (IFNGR-1) chains (each of which binds Jak1) and two β (IFNGR-2) chains (each of which binds Jak2), it was not clear if Jak1 and Jak2 transactivate each other or if one of them plays a dominant role. The available data now suggest that Jak2 may play the dominant role and that it is responsible for phosphorylating both itself and Jak1, thereby increasing the catalytic activities of both kinases (290). Jak1 in turn phosphorylates IFNGR-1, allowing the recruitment of

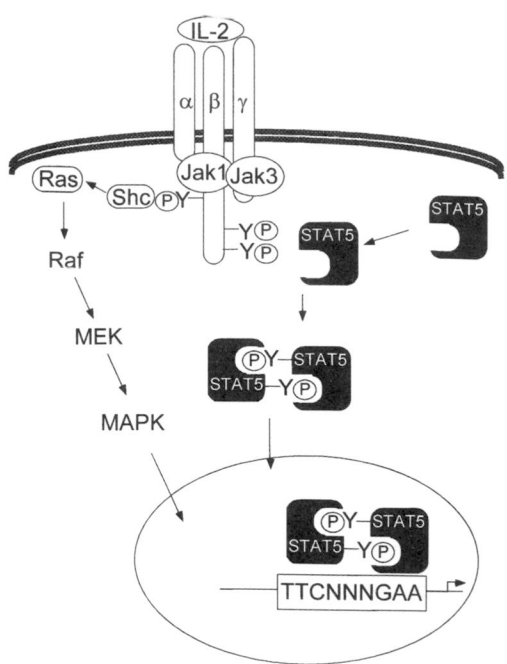

FIG. 5. Schematic of Jak-STAT paradigm in the context of IL-2 signaling. Shown is the association of two different Jak family kinases with different chains of the receptor. In this case, Jak1 associates with IL-2Rβ and Jak3 with γ_c. Activation of Jak kinases results in tyrosine phosphorylation of IL-2Rβ. This allows the docking of Stat5a or Stat5b via its SH2 domain. the STATs themselves are tyrosine phosphorylated, dimerize, and translocate to the nucleus, where they modulate expression of target genes. The schematic also indicates that another phosphotyrosine mediates recruitment of Shc, which then can couple to the Ras/Raf/MEK/MAP kinase pathway. These and other pathways are activated by many type I cytokines.

Stat1. In this model, it is additionally suggested that Jak2 phosphorylates Stat1 (290). Interestingly, a kinase dead mutant of Jak1 was able to mediate the induction of certain IFN-γ–induced genes, indicating a potential structural role for Jak1, but catalytically active Jak1 was essential for the establishment of the antiviral state (290), emphasizing the essential role of both Jak1 and Jak2 catalytic activities for normal IFN-γ function.

The above discussion assumes that cross-phosphorylation of Jak kinases is a mechanism for the amplification of catalytic activity. Unless other kinases are involved, however, implicit to this idea is that the Jak kinases themselves exhibit some basal activity that is amplified to a higher level by auto- or transphosphorylation. Consistent with Jak kinases being activated by phosphorylation, mutagenesis of a critical tyrosine in Tyk2 (291) or Jak2 (292) (e.g., tyrosine 1007 in the case of Jak2) in the activation loop of the kinase domain inhibits activity. It is conceivable that phosphorylation of other tyrosines on the Jaks may create appropriate motifs for the recruitment of additional signaling molecules, but at least so far, mutation of other tyrosines has not had obviously deleterious functional effects (293).

The function of the pseudo-kinase (JH2) domain remains unclear. No other metazoan protein tyrosine kinases contain such domains. The JH2 region is not a functional kinase for several reasons. First, it lacks the third glycine in the Gly-X-Gly-X-X-Gly motif; second, it is missing an aspartic acid that serves as the proton acceptor and is typically conserved in the catalytic loop of both tyrosine and serine kinases; and third, it lacks the conserved Phe in the Asp-Phe-Glu motif that binds ATP (253). The absence of the critical amino acids presumably explains the lack of catalytic function of the JH2 domain (255). Despite the lack of catalytic activity of the JH2 domain, there are increasing data in support of vital functions for this region. Although the kinase domain alone can act as an active kinase, it is interesting that a mutation in the Jak kinase JH2 domain can hyperactivate the *Drosophila* (*hop^{Tum-l}*/D-stat) Jak-STAT pathway and that the corresponding Glu695 to Lys mutation in murine Jak2 also resulted in increased autophosphorylation of Jak2 and phosphorylation of Stat5 in transfected cells (294). Moreover, the JH2 domain may play an important role in mediating the interaction of Jaks with STAT proteins (295).

Because Jaks are associated with cytokine receptors, it makes sense that Jak kinases might play important roles related to a variety of cytokine signals. These include roles in development (as demonstrated by the phenotype associated with Jak3 deficiency, a defect at least partially due to defective IL-7 signaling), roles in signaling in response to cytokines that are mitogenic growth factors (e.g., IL-2, IL-3, etc.), and roles in the antiviral response (IFNs). The analysis of the role of Jak1 in zebrafish was interesting not only in that it showed a role for Jak1 in early vertebrate development, but also because it was demonstrated that during early development Jak1 kinase was exclusively of maternal origin (282). These developmental roles for Jak1 in zebrafish are consistent with the importance of a Jak kinase in early *Drosophila* development as well (296).

ARE THERE OTHER JAKS?

Naturally, until and if additional Jaks are found, no one could possibly predict that they exist. So far, no obvious strong homologies are indicated in current data bases, suggesting that if other Jaks exist they might either be more divergent or might be encoded by relatively rare or lineage-restricted transcripts. Interestingly, splice variants have been found for at least Jak3 (297), a Jak that was originally detected as a gene expressed in breast carcinoma cells (298).

STAT PROTEINS ARE SUBSTRATES FOR JAKS THAT AT LEAST IN PART HELP DETERMINE SPECIFICITY

Given that the Janus family kinases cannot by themselves determine specificity (as demonstrated by the facts that different cytokines with different actions activate the same Jaks), a reasonable hypothesis was that the same Jaks might have different substrates, depending on the receptor. The best characterized substrates for Jaks are STATs (246–254). Among the mutant cell lines with defects in IFN signaling, in addition to the ones with defects in Jaks that are noted above, others were defective in STAT proteins. These data were among the first to prove a vital role for STAT proteins.

STAT proteins are latent transcription factors that initially exist in the cytosol and then are translocated to the nucleus. STATs were first discovered based on the identification of factors that were capable of binding to the promoters of IFN-inducible genes (254). There are now seven different STAT proteins that have been identified: Stat1 (299), Stat2 (300), Stat3 (301,302), Stat4 (303,304), Stat5a (305–309), Stat5b (307–310), and Stat6 (311). Table 14

TABLE 14. *Cytokines and the STATs they activate*

Cytokine	STAT activated
IFN-α/β	Stat1, Stat2
IFN-γ	Stat1
Growth hormone	Stat5a, Stat5b
Prolactin	Stat5a, Stat5b
Erythropoietin	Stat5a, Stat5b
Thrombopoietin	Stat5a, Stat5b
IL-10	Stat3
IL-12	Stat4, Stat3
G-CSF	Stat3
γc family	
IL-2, IL-7, IL-9, IL-15	Stat5a, Stat5b, Stat3
IL-4	Stat6
IL-13*	Stat6
βc family	
IL-3, IL-5, GM-CSF	Stat5a, Stat5b
gp130 family	
IL-6, IL-11, CNTF, LIF, OSM, CT-1	Stat3
Leptin	Stat3

*IL-13 is closely related to IL-14, but its receptor does not contain γc.

summarizes the cytokines that activate each of the STATs. Although the STATs conserve a reasonable level of homology, Stat5a and Stat5b are unusually closely related, with human Stat5a and Stat5b being 91% identical at the amino acid level (307–310). Although one might think that these proteins might have redundant functions, it is interesting that murine and human Stat5a are more related than are human Stat5a and human Stat5b or murine Stat5a and murine Stat5b. The same is true for murine and human Stat5b. Together, these data suggest that there has been evolutionary pressure to maintain the difference between Stat5a and Stat5b and that these two proteins will have important distinctive actions and may selectively activate different target genes. Because active STAT proteins exist as dimers, the ability of at least some STATs to form heterodimers [e.g., Stat1 with Stat2 or Stat3 (254) and Stat5a with Stat5b (307)] increases the number of different complexes that can form. Additional complexity can be generated by the ability of at least some of the STATs to exist in alternatively spliced forms (310,312). Some of these forms are inactive, and if alternative splicing of these forms were regulated, it would allow for negative regulation.

A schematic of STAT proteins is shown in Fig. 6. The STATs can be divided into two basic groups: those that are longer (Stat2 and Stat6, approximately 850 amino acids) and those that are shorter (Stat1, Stat3, Stat4, Stat5a, and Stat5b, between 750 and 800 amino acids). Interestingly, the chromosomal locations of the STATs suggests three different clusters. Murine Stat2 and Stat6 are both located on chromosome 10, Stat1 and Stat4 are located on chromosome 1, and Stat3, Stat5a, and Stat5b are located on chromosome 11 (313). Correspondingly, human Stat5a and Stat5b are closely positioned on chromosome 17q (310).

In order for STATs to be activated and to be able to function as transcriptional activators, a number of cellular events must occur. They must be able to bind to phosphorylated tyrosines, to be able to themselves be tyrosine phosphorylated, to dimerize, to translocate from the cytosol to the nucleus, to bind to target DNA sequences, and to activate gene expression. A number of conserved

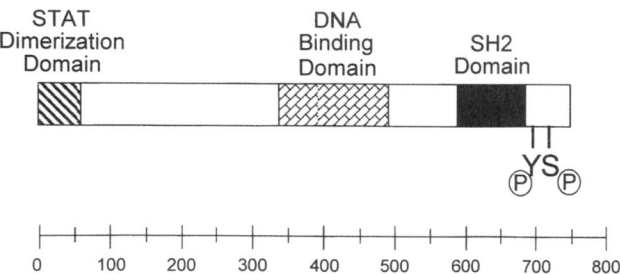

FIG. 6. Architecture of a typical STAT protein. Shown are the locations of the following important regions: (1) The N-terminal region has been shown to mediate the interaction of STAT dimers bound to adjacent GAS sites (known to be important for Stat1, but presumably true for all STATs); (2) the DNA-binding domain; (3) the SH2 domain that mediates STAT docking on receptors and STAT homodimerization/heterodimerization after tyrosine phosphorylation; and (4) the location of the conserved tyrosine whose phosphorylation allows the SH2-mediated dimerization. In Stat1 and Stat3, serine 727, which is C-terminal to the conserved tyrosine, is an important site for phosphorylation. In the case of Stat1, p48 interacts downstream from the STAT dimerization domain. CBP/p300 interacts with two sites, at both the N terminus and C terminus. Although it has been suggested that the region between the DNA-binding domains and the SH2 domain is an SH3 domain, this remains unproven and no interactions with proline-rich regions have been reported; as a result, I have omitted the labeling of this region as an SH3 domain. Note that this structure is typical of that for Stat1, Stat3, Stat4, Stat5a, and Stat5b. The main features are conserved in Stat2 and Stat6, but these are approximately 50 to 100 amino acids longer.

structural features common to all STATs help to explain these functions. These include an SH2 domain, a conserved tyrosine residue, a DNA binding domain, and a C-terminal transactivation domain, and an N-terminal STAT tetramerization region. Other regions as well contribute important functions. These special features of STATs are discussed below.

Docking of STATs on Receptors or Other Molecules, Tyrosine Phosphorylation of STATs, and STAT Dimerization

Each STAT protein has an SH2 domain that plays two important roles: (a) for receptor docking, for example, as has been shown for Stat1 docking on IFNGR-1 (314), Stat2 docking on IFNAR-1 (315), Stat3 docking on gp130 (316), Stat5 docking on IL-2Rβ and IL-7Rα (187,317), and Stat6 docking on IL-4Rα (318), and (b) for STAT dimerization. In the case of the IFN-α receptor, no Stat1 docking site on IFNAR-1 or IFNAR-2 has been identified, and it is believed that Stat1 may interact with Stat2 after Stat2 is itself tyrosine phosphorylated (290). It is also possible that STATs can dock on Jaks, given the ability to directly coprecipitate Jaks and STATs (283,295). After docking has occurred, a conserved tyrosine (tyrosine 701 in Stat1, tyrosine 694 in Stat5a, etc.) can be phosphorylated. This phosphorylation is required for the SH2 domain–mediated dimerization of STATs, and likely occurs while the STAT is docked on the receptor. After STAT phosphorylation, the STAT dissociates, and its dimerization with itself or another STAT is then favored over its reassociation with the receptor chain. One reason for this is that STAT dimerization involves two phosphotyrosine–SH2 interactions (a bivalent interaction), whereas docking on a receptor involves only one (monovalent interaction). Thus, efficient activation of STATs requires the presence in STATs of a conserved SH2 domain and a key tyrosine.

It is interesting that although IFNGR-1 (314) and IL-7Rα (187) each has only a single STAT docking site (for Stat1 and Stat5), respectively, a number of receptor molecules, including IL-2Rβ (187,317), IL-4Rα (318), gp130 (316), the erythropoietin receptor (319), and IL-10Rα (320), have more than one docking site for their respective STATs. The presence of more than one site provides functional redundancy, but also potentially could allow the simultaneous activation of two STATs, providing a high local concentration of phosphorylated STATs and thereby facilitating their dimerization.

STAT Nuclear Translocation and DNA Binding

After dimerization, the STATs translocate into the nucleus. The basis for the nuclear translocation is unknown. It is unclear whether dimerization reveals a nuclear localization domain, whether monomeric STATs are actively retained in the cytosol by a tethering protein, or whether STAT dimers associate with a chaperonin molecule to facilitate their nuclear translocation.

Whereas the majority of STAT dimers directly bind DNA, in the case of IFN-α/β, Stat1–Stat2 heterodimers are formed, and these bind DNA in conjunction with a 48-kDa DNA binding protein (254). In the case of other STAT dimers, accessory proteins are not required for DNA binding. The motif recognized by Stat1–Stat2–p48 complexes has an AGTTTNCNTTTCC motif (known as an ISRE for IFN-stimulated response element), whereas the other STAT complexes tend to bind more semipalindromic TTCN$_m$GAA motifs, where m = 3 or 4, with some variation being allowed even in these sequences.

DNA binding is determined by a region that has been defined as the DNA binding domain (318). A series of chimeric constructs formed by exchanging domains of different STATs was used to delineate a region of approximately 180 amino acids, with two conserved subdomains, as conferring DNA binding specificity. Although many of the STATs can bind to the same motifs, their relative efficiencies can vary considerably, indicating the fine specificities conferred by the different DNA binding domains. For example, although Stat1 homodimers favor a TTCN$_3$GAA motif, Stat6 prefers a TTCN$_4$GAA motif (318). These differences between the different STATs in terms of their DNA binding specificity provide part of the basis to explain why different STATs modulate the expression of nonidentical sets of target genes.

N-terminal regions can mediate cooperative DNA binding of STAT proteins when multiple STAT binding sites occur in proximity (321,322). Such situations have been shown for the IFN-γ gene, where multiple STAT binding sites occur, and likely also occurs for the IL-2 receptor α chain gene, where two gamma interferon activated sequence (GAS) motifs are closely juxtaposed and are known to functionally cooperate for IL-2–induced IL-2Rα transcription (323–325).

Historically, STAT proteins were the first tyrosine-phosphorylated transcription factors to be recognized. Previously, tyrosine phosphorylation was primarily associated with membrane-proximal events. A key feature of STATs was that the tyrosine phosphorylation in fact was associated with a membrane-proximal event, but this phosphorylation then allowed the dimerization that was a prerequisite for nuclear localization and DNA binding. STATs can interact directly with Jak kinases, as was first shown for Stat5 and Jak3 (283), providing added support for the idea that STATs are indeed phosphorylated by Jaks and also suggesting that STATs may at times dock on Jaks rather than on receptors.

Transcriptional Activation by STATs

An area of considerable interest is how STAT proteins trigger the initiation of transcription. In addition to tyrosine phosphorylation, some STATs can be phosphorylated on serine. For example, for Stat1 and Stat3, it has been shown that serine phosphorylation is required for full activity (326,327), whereas Stat2 is not serine phosphorylated (254). The phosphorylation site in these STATs (Ser 727) is located in the C-terminal region of the protein, within the C-terminal transactivation domain (328,329). Interestingly, the region of Ser 727 resembles a MAP kinase recognition site, and one study has indicated that MAP kinase activity is required for IFN-α/β–induced gene expression (330).

In addition to this regulated modification of the STAT proteins, considerable interest has focused on the ability of STATs to interact with other factors. As noted above, Stat1–Stat2 heterodimers bind

DNA only in the context of a DNA binding protein; the Stat1–Stat2–p48 complex is known as ISGF3 (247,254), and it is now clear that the region between amino acids 150 and 250 of Stat1 is required for the interaction with p48 (254). Stat1 has been reported to interact with and synergize with Sp1 for transcriptional activation in the ICAM-1 gene (331). An alternatively spliced shorter form of Stat3, denoted Stat3β, was found to associate with c-Jun in a yeast two-hybrid analysis and that this interaction enhanced transcriptional activity of a reporter construct (332). Moreover, both Stat1 and Stat2 have been shown to interact with the potent transcriptional activators CREB binding protein (CBP) and p300 (333–335). In the case of Stat1, this appears to be mediated by interactions involving both the N-terminal and C-terminal regions of Stat1 and the cyclic AMP response element binding protein (CREB) and E1A binding regions of CBP, respectively (334). Stat5a has been shown to associate with the glucocorticoid receptor (336). Additionally, the well-defined IL-2 response element in the IL-2Rα gene requires not only Stat5 binding but also the binding of Elf-1, an Ets family transcription factor, to a nearby site (324). Thus, active STAT complexes appear to involve the coordination of STAT proteins with other factors.

Specificity of STATs

In the analysis of STAT protein activation in response to different cytokines, it was observed that, analogous to the Jaks, the same STATs were induced by multiple cytokines. The degree of specificity conferred by the different STATs was therefore unclear. There are now published reports on at least the partial phenotypes of mice lacking expression of six of the seven STATs (Stat1, Stat3, Stat4, Stat5a, Stat5b, and Stat6) (see Table 15). Stat1 knock-out

---

TABLE 15. *Phenotypes of mice deficient in type I and type II cytokines, their receptors, Jaks, and STATs*

Type I cytokines and their receptors

γc family

IL-2 (103,431,432)	Normal thymic and peripheral T-cell development. Decreased polyclonal T-cell responses in vitro, but more normal *in vivo* responses to pathogenic challenges. Autoimmunity with marked changes in levels of serum immunoglobulin isotypes. Ulcerative colitis–like inflammatory bowel disease.
IL-4 (106,107)	Defective Th2 cytokine responses and class switch; defective IgG1 and IgE production.
IL-2/IL-4 (108)	Some features of both IL-2 and IL-4 knock-out mice. No gross abnormalities of T-cell development.
IL-7 (71)	Greatly diminished thymic and peripheral T-cell development and B-lymphopoiesis, resulting in profound lymphopenia.
IL-2Rα (118)	Normal initial lymphoid development, but massive enlargement of peripheral lymphoid organs, polyclonal T- and B-cell expansions, and activated T cells, with impaired activation-induced cell death. Autoimmunity with increasing age, including hemolytic anemia and inflammatory bowel disease.
IL-2Rβ (119)	Severe autoimmunity including autoimmune hemolytic anemia. Death within approximately 3 months. Deregulated T-cell activation. Dysregulated B-cell differentiation and altered immunoglobulin profile.
γc (109–111,120)	Greatly diminished thymic development, but double-negative, double-positive, and single-positive thymocytes are all represented. Age-dependent accumulation of peripheral CD4+ T cells with an activated memory phenotype. Greatly diminished numbers of conventional B cells, although B1 cells are present. No NK cells or γδ cells. Absent gut-associated lymphoid tissue, including Peyer's patches.
IL-7Rα (70)	Greatly diminished thymic and peripheral T-cell development and B-lymphopoiesis, resulting in profound lymphopenia.

βc family

IL-5 (433)	Decreased basal level of eosinophils and defective induction of eosinophils after infectious challenge. Developmental defect in CD5+ B1 cells. Normal antibody and cytotoxic T-cell responses.
GM-CSF (434,435)	Normal basal hematopoiesis. Unexpected abnormalities of the lung; abnormal pulmonary homeostasis.
IL-3Rβ (436)	No defects (due to redundant function of βc).

Table continues.

TABLE 15. *(Continued.)* *Phenotypes of mice deficient in type I and type II cytokines, their receptors, Jaks, and STATs*

β_c (137,436)	Defective responses to IL-5 and GM-CSF, but normal responses to IL-3 (due to redundant function of IL-3Rβ). Diminished eosinophils (both basal levels and in responses to infectious challenge). Unexpected abnormalities of the lung. In other words, the defects are a combination of those found in the IL-5 and GM-CSF–deficient mice.
gp130 family	
IL-6 (437)	Impaired acute phase responses after infection or tissue damage. Decreased numbers of hematopoietic progenitor cells.
gp130 (438,439)	Embryonic lethal. Extreme hypoplastic development of the myocardium; although the ventricular wall was very thin, trabeculation within the ventricle chamber was normal. Hematologic abnormalities characterized by greatly reduced CFU-S and somewhat reduced CFU-Gm and BFU-E. Markedly diminished size of thymus and numbers of thymocytes. Reduced primordial germ cells in embryonic gonads. Diminished size of placenta.
LIF (440–442)	Decreased hematopoietic progenitor cells. Normal sympathetic neurons but deficient neurotransmitter switch in vitro. Defective blastocyst implantation.
LIFRβ (443,444)	Postnatal lethality. Normal hematopoietic and germ cell compartments, but multiple neurologic, skeletal, placental, and metabolic defects. The greater severity than found in LIF deficient mice reflects that LIFRβ is shared by several cytokines, including CNTF, LIF, and CT1.
CNTF (445)	Progressive atrophy and loss of motor neurons.
CNTFRα (446)	Severe motor neuron deficiency resulting in perinatal mortality. The more severe phenotype than in CNTF-deficient mice was unexpected and suggests that another cytokine may use CNTFRα.
IL-12	
IL-12 p40 (447)	Impaired but not completely lacking in their ability to produce IFN-γ and to mount a Th1 response in vivo. Elevated secretion of IL-4, normal production of IL-2 and IL-10. Substantially decreased CTL responses.
IL-12Rβ1 (448)	Defective IL-12 signaling. IL-2 but not IL-12 could augment NK activity. Defective IFN-γ production in response to ConA or anti-CD3.
EPO, TPO, G-CSF, and M-CSF	
EPO (449)	Embryonic lethal. Complete block of fetal liver erythropoiesis, resulting in severe anemia, yet normal development of BFU-E and CFU-E progenitor cells.
EPOR (449,450)	Same as EPO-deficient mice.
TPOR (451)	Decreased megakaryocytes and platelets, but other hematopoietic cells are present in normal numbers.
G-CSF (452)	Neutropenia and impaired neutrophil mobility. Diminished granulocytes, and macrophage precursors.
M-CSF (138,453)	Osteopetrosis, absence of teeth. Females are infertile, suggesting an unexpected role for M-CSF.
M-CSF + GM-CSF (138)	A combination of defects of both M-CSF and GM-CSF, with osteopetrosis and alveolar proteinosis. Early death from pneumonia.
Type II cytokines and their receptors	
IFNAR-1 (454–456)	Normal development. Defective immune defense against most viral infections tested, including lymphocytic choriomeningitis virus, Semliki forest virus, Theiler's virus, vesicular stomatitis virus. Normal resistance to *Listeria monocytogenes, Leishmania major, Mycobacterium bovis,* and *M. avium.*
IFNγ (457,458)	Normal lymphoid development. Impaired resistance to *Listeria monocytogenes, Toxoplasma gondii, Leishmania major, Mycobacterium bovis,* and *M. avium.* Can mount curative responses to a number of viruses. CD4⁺ effector cells default to the Th2 pathway after infection with *Leishmania.*
IFNGR-1 (455,456,459)	Normal lymphoid development. Impaired resistance to *Listeria monocytogenes, Leishmania major, Mycobacterium bovis,* and *M. avium.* Can mount curative responses to a number of viruses.
IL-10 (460)	Normal lymphocyte development and antibody responses. Chronic enterocolitis, anemia, and growth retardation. Enhanced susceptibility in septic shock.
STATs and Jaks	
Stat1 (337,338)	Defective responses to both type I and type II IFNs.
Stat3 (339)	Embryonic lethal. Embryos implant but cannot grow. The fact that this phenotype is even more severe than that seen with gp130 suggests a role for Stat3 via a gp130-independent cytokine.
Stat4 (340,341)	Defect Th1 development, essentially the same phenotype as in IL-12–deficient mice.
Stat5a (345,346a)	Defective lobuloalveolar development in the mammary gland, a syndrome resulting from defective prolactin signaling. Defective IL-2 induced IL-2 Rα expression. Defective superantigen-induced expansion of Vβδ⁺ T cells.
Stat5b (346)	Defective growth analogous to Laron dwarfism, a disease of defective growth hormone signaling.
Stat6 (342–344)	Defective Th2 development, essentially the same phenotype as IL-4–deficient mice
Jak1 (461)	Perinatal lethality. Defective signaling by IFNs, γ_c-dependent cytokines, and gp130-dependent cytokines.
Jak2 (462,463)	Embryonic lethality. Lack of responsiveness to EPO, TPO, β_c-dependent cytokines, and IFNγ.

mice exhibit defects that are very selective for the actions of type I and type II IFNs, suggesting that Stat1 is only vital for the actions of IFNs, even though a variety of other cytokines have been reported to activate Stat1 (337,338). Although it is possible that Stat1 plays an important but redundant function for at least some of these other cytokines, the phenotype of Stat1-deficient mice indicates a need for caution in the interpretation of *in vitro* experiments that use very high concentrations of cytokines and cell lines expressing very large numbers of receptors because it is possible that these experiments may not always yield physiologically relevant patterns of STAT activation. Stat3-deficient mice are not born, and lethality is evident early in embryogenesis (339). Interestingly, the embryos implant, but there is defective development and growth. Stat4-deficient mice exhibit a phenotype indistinguishable from that of IL-12–deficient mice (i.e., defective Th1 development), a finding consistent with the observation that Stat4 is only activated by IL-12 (340,341). Analogously, Stat6-deficient mice exhibit a phenotype indistinguishable from that of IL-4–deficient mice (i.e., defective Th2 development) (342–344), in keeping with the observation that Stat6 is only activated by IL-4 and the closely related cytokine IL-13. Interestingly, mice lacking Stat5a exhibit a defect in prolactin-mediated effects, including defective lobuloalveloar proliferation (345), whereas mice lacking Stat5b have defective growth similar to that found in Laron dwarfism (346). Thus, although Stat5a and Stat5b appear to always be coordinately induced, it is clear that selective deletion of these similar STATs results in selective defects.

STATs Belong to an Ancient Phylogenetic Family

Just as *Drosophila* has a Jak kinase, there is a *Drosophila* STAT, denoted as either D3TAT or STAT92E (347,348). The existence of Jak kinases and STAT proteins in lower organisms suggest that the system is evolutionarily old, and these other systems may help to elucidate some of the subtleties of this system. Recently, a STAT has been identified in *Dictyostelium* that recognizes the sequence TTGA (349). This STAT has highest sequence similarity to Stat5b and can bind mammalian ISREs (349). Interestingly, *Saccharomyces cerevisiae* does not appear to have STATs because no SH2 domains have been identified in the entire *S. cerevisiae* genome.

What is the Function of STATs?

Given that STAT proteins translocate to the nucleus and bind DNA, it is self-evident that they can bind to the regulatory regions of the target genes and influence transcription. So far, STATs have only been shown to act as activators (and not repressors) of gene expression. STAT proteins were originally discovered based on the study of IFN-inducible genes as part of studies intended to understand the cellular differentiation events that lead to development of the antiviral state. However, there has been considerable discussion as to whether STAT proteins were solely differentiation factors or whether they would also play roles in mitogenic and proliferative responses that typify hematopoietic and immunologic cytokines, such as IL-3, IL-5, GM-CSF, IL-2, IL-4, and IL-7. Indeed, a variety of observations suggest possible roles in proliferation (252). First, a number of *in vitro* systems have demonstrated that viruses or viral oncogenes are associated with activated Jak-STAT pathways, suggesting a role for STATs in cellular transformation (283–286). Second, there is diminished pro-

liferation in a number of the STAT knock-out mice that have been analyzed. For example, Stat4-deficient mice exhibit diminished proliferation to IL-12 (340,341), whereas Stat6-deficient mice exhibit diminished proliferation to IL-4 (342–344). Third, a dominant-negative Stat5 construct can diminish IL-3–induced proliferation (350). Fourth, mutagenesis of tyrosines in the IL-2 receptor β chain that mediate STAT activation results in diminished proliferation (317,351). However, other data are not in agreement. First, one report indicates that mutation of tyrosines in the erythropoietin receptor that are required for STAT activation do not decrease proliferation (352), although another report came to the opposite conclusion (353), so the role of STATs in erythropoietin-induced proliferation remains unresolved. Second, Stat6-deficient mice exhibit decreased IL-4Rα expression, suggesting that the effect on proliferation may be indirect (344). Similarly, mutations of the key tyrosines in IL-2Rβ also result in a decrease in IL-2Rα expression (354). Thus, although there are strong data suggesting a role for a number of STATs in proliferation, in at least some cases the effect may be indirect, resulting from regulating the level of receptor components. Finally, it is interesting that Stat1 has been linked to cell growth arrest and induction of the cdk inhibitor p21$^{WAF1/CIP1}$ (355), and that activation of Stat1 occurs in thanatrophoric dysplasia type II dwarfism as the result of a mutant *fibroblast growth factor receptor* (FGFR3) (356). In this chondrodysplasia, the mutant FGFR3 induces nuclear translocation of Stat1, expression of p21$^{WAF1/CIP1}$, and growth arrest, suggesting a possible relationship to the disease. Thus, different STATs may potentially mediate either growth expansion or growth arrest. Moreover, STATs may potentially play other types of roles, as well. For example, Stat3 has been reported to serve as an adapter to couple phosphatidylinositol (PI) 3-kinase to the IFNAR-1 component of type I IFN receptors (357).

Are There Other STATs? Do Other Proteins Bind to GAS Motifs?

Efforts to identify STATs by low-stringency hybridization have not generally been successful, except for the cloning of Stat4 and Stat5b (the latter was in fact found by hybridization at high stringency). As a result, if other, somewhat more divergent STATs exist, they may need to be cloned by purification. Because each STAT identified so far appears to have relatively specific functions, it is reasonable that other specific functions might be identified that are subserved by specific STATs. Moreover, one non-STAT protein has now been discovered that binds to GAS motifs. The BCL-6 gene is frequently found to be mutated or to have undergone translocations in diffuse large-cell (B-cell) lymphomas. Interestingly, BCL-6 binds to GAS motifs capable of binding Stat6 and specifically can inhibit IL-4 action (358). These data suggest that dysregulated IL-4/IL-13 signaling may contributed to these lymphomas. Furthermore, mice lacking expression of BCL-6 exhibit defective germinal center formation, suggesting that formation of germinal centers is dependent on BCL-6 regulated (presumably negative) control of certain STAT-responsive genes (358).

OTHER LATENT TRANSCRIPTION FACTORS AS EXAMPLES OF CYTOPLASMIC TO NUCLEAR SIGNALING (NF-κB AND NF-AT)

One of the exciting features of STAT proteins is that they exist in an inactive form in the cytosol and then are rapidly translocated to the nucleus. The rapid transmission (within minutes) of signals from the cell membrane to nuclear DNA binding makes the STAT acronym seem very appropriate, in view of the urgency associated with "STAT" emergency physician orders in clinical medicine. The rapid activation of STAT proteins is somewhat analogous to NF-κB family proteins. However, in the case of NF-κB, the rapid nuclear translocation requires a completely different mechanism. In contrast to STAT proteins where the tyrosine phosphorylation of the STATs is an initiator of nuclear translocation, for NF-κB it is the serine phosphorylation or ubiquitination of IκB that results in its dissociation or destruction, allowing the release and translocation of NF-κB (359,360). A third example of cytosolic to nuclear translocation occurs with NF-AT (nuclear factor of activated T-cell) family proteins, which are vital for regulating transcription of a number of cytokines, including IL-2, IL-4, and GM-CSF (361,362). In this case, NF-AT is translocated to the nucleus, where it associates with AP-1 family proteins to form a functional complex. It is the activation of calcineurin and dephosphorylation of NF-AT that allows its nuclear translocation (361,362). Thus, three different types of mechanisms, each involving phosphorylation or dephosphorylation, have evolved to allow cytoplasmic to nuclear translocation of latent transcription factors.

OTHER SUBSTRATES FOR JAKS

Because Jaks are potent cytosolic tyrosine kinases, it is immediately evident that the activation of STATs may not be the sole function of Jaks. A variety of data indicate that Jaks have the ability to phosphorylate tyrosine on receptors where STAT proteins dock, as well as the ability to phosphorylate STATs. There are also *in vitro* data that indicate that Jak kinases can phosphorylate tyrosines on receptor chains other than those that are docking sites for STATs. For example, in overexpression experiments in COS cells, Jak1 appears to phosphorylate IL-2Rβ not only on tyrosines 392 and 510, which are needed for docking STAT proteins, but also on tyrosine 338, which is the docking site for Shc (317). Interestingly, in a reporter system, simultaneous mutation of all three of these tyrosines abrogates proliferation, suggesting that the molecules that dock on these tyrosines couple to vital pathways (317). Thus, Jak kinases may facilitate the recruitment of additional substrates to the receptors; in addition, it is well known that Jak kinases can autophosphorylate themselves or transphosphorylate other Jaks. Because Jak kinases contain a number of conserved tyrosine residues, it is possible that some of these are phosphorylated and serve as docking sites for important signaling molecules. One molecule that has recently been reported to be a substrate for Jaks is the STAM adapter molecule (363), which may play a role for cytokine-mediated proliferation. It seems likely that other additional substrates will be found. This is still an early area in need of further investigation.

OTHER SIGNALING MOLECULES IMPORTANT FOR CYTOKINES

Other Tyrosine Kinases Besides Jaks

In addition to their activation of Jak kinases, a number of cytokines can activate Src family kinases. For example, IL-2 can activate p56lck (364,365) in T cells and p59fyn and p53/p56lyn in B-cell lines (366,367). The activation of some of these kinases has been reported to be mediated by association with the A region of IL-2Rβ. Another tyrosine kinase, Syk, has been reported to associate with the S region of IL-2Rβ (368). However, the significance of these interactions is less clear than for Jak kinases. First, cells lacking Lck can vigorously proliferate in response to IL-2 (369,370). Second, when the A region is deleted, proliferation still occurs, albeit at a lower level than seen with wild-type IL-2Rβ (371). Although tyrosines 355 and 358 (Y355 and Y358) of IL-2Rβ have been reported to be the substrates for Lck (196), simultaneous mutation of these tyrosines did not affect proliferation in a reporter cell system (317). Instead, mutation of Y338, which is required for the recruitment of Shc via its PTB domain (317,372), but which is also in the A region, diminished proliferation (196). Thus, it is possible that the decrease in proliferation associated with deletion of the A region relates to the loss of Y338 than it does to the loss of association of Lck. Clearly, additional investigation is required to clarify the role of activation of Src family kinases by IL-2. The significance of the Syk interaction also remains unclear. Because Syk and Jak1 both associate with the S region of IL-2Rβ, mutations that delete the S region simultaneously prevent both associations, making it impossible if the effect is due solely to a loss of one of these elements. The fact that Syk-deficient mice exhibit normal IL-2 proliferation (373) further suggests that Syk may not play an important role in IL-2–induced proliferation. Analogously, the G-CSF receptor forms a complex with Lyn and Syk (374), but again Syk-deficient mice do not exhibit a defect in G-CSF signaling (373). Regarding other kinases, βc has been reported to interact with Src family kinases (375). gp130 has been reported to associate with a number of other kinases, including Btk, Tec, and Fes (376–378), and IL-4Rα has been shown to interact with Fes (379). Overall, relatively little is known about the significance of tyrosine kinases, other than Jak kinases, in cytokine signaling. It is possible that they play important roles that have been difficult to evaluate, perhaps in part due to the existence of redundant pathways.

IRS-1 and IRS-2

IRS-1 was originally noted to be a tyrosine phosphorylated substrate of the insulin receptor (380). Interestingly, both insulin and IL-4 induced tyrosine phosphorylation of an IRS-1–like molecule in hematopoietic cells (381). Moreover, 32D myeloid progenitor cells lack IRS-1 and could only signal in response to insulin or IL-4 when they were transfected with IRS-1 (382). In fact, another closely related molecule, IRS-2, also can mediate these functions (380), and it remains unclear to what extent these exhibit distinctive versus redundant functions. Both the insulin receptor and IL-4Rα proteins contain NPXY sequences that are important for IRS-1 or IRS-2 binding; in IL-4Rα, this is contained within a sequence denoted as the I4R motif (383).

Other cytokines have subsequently been shown to activate IRS-1 or IRS-2. For example growth hormone can induce phosphorylation of IRS-1 (384) and IRS-2 (385), IFN-γ and LIF induce phosphorylation of IRS-2 (385), and the γc-dependent cytokines, IL-2, IL-7, and IL-15, can induce tyrosine phosphorylation of IRS-1 and IRS-2 in T cells (386). The significance of these findings remains unclear, as 32D cells (which constitutively express γc) can proliferative vigorously in response to IL-2 when they are transfected with only IL-2Rβ (369), whereas, as noted above, in these same cells IL-4 responsiveness requires coexpression of both IL-4Rα and IRS-1. Thus, IL-2 proliferation is not strictly dependent on IRS-1, and the exact role of IRS-1 and IRS-2 in IL-2 signaling remains unclear.

Because IRS-1 and IRS-2 have a large number of phosphotyrosine docking sites, particularly for the p85 subunit of PI 3-kinase, they presumably serve to recruit important accessory molecules, and perhaps these differ in importance for mediating proliferation in response to different cytokines.

Phosphatidylinositol 3-Kinase

PI 3-kinase is a lipid kinase that consists of an 85-kDa regulatory subunit and a 110-kDa catalytic subunit (387). PI 3-kinase phosphorylation and activation can be induced by a number of cytokines (388–391), and the use of inhibitors, such as wortmannin or LY294002, has demonstrated its importance in cytokine signaling (391). IRS-1 has multiple docking sites for PI 3-kinase (YXXM motifs) and thus for some cytokines, such as IL-4, the association of IRS-1 might be the mechanism by which PI 3-kinase can be recruited.

DOWNMODULATION OF CYTOKINE SIGNALS

Much of the above discussion has centered on the induction of signals. Equally important are the mechanisms by which cytokine signals can be terminated. The potential levels at which this can occur include (a) a balance between the production (transcriptional and translational control) of the cytokine, its receptor, or downstream signaling molecules and the degradation of these same molecules; and (b) regulation of the activation state of the receptor and downstream signaling molecules.

Transcriptional control of cytokine production is a widely used mechanism. Many T cell–derived cytokines such as IL-2, IL-3, and IL-4 are only produced by activated T cells, and their production is lost with the loss of activation. This same is true for the IL-2 receptor α chain, but the transcriptional/translational control of most cytokine receptors is poorly studied. Given the constitutive expression of many of these proteins, additional control mechanisms besides transcriptional regulation are likely to be important.

Because phosphorylation events are vital for the creation of phosphotyrosine docking sites, dephosphorylation is an obvious mechanism of control. Indeed, two tyrosine phosphatases, Shp-1 (formerly also known as SHP, HCP, SH-PTP1, and PTP1C) and Shp-2 (formerly also known as Syp and PTP1D) have been shown to play roles related to cytokine signaling (392,393). The most well-studied example is Shp-1, mutations of which cause the motheaten (me) and viable motheaten (me^v) phenotypes in mice (394,395). The viable motheaten mouse had a less severe phenotype that is associated with increased numbers of erythroid progenitor cells and hyperresponsiveness to EPO (396), suggesting that Shp-1 might normally diminish responsiveness to EPO. Indeed, it was demonstrated that Shp-1 binds directly to the EPOR when Y429 is phosphorylated (397). This tyrosine is located in a negative regulatory region of the EPOR, and when mutated, EPO-responsive cells can grow in lower concentrations of EPO. After Shp-1 binding to Y429, dephosphorylation and inactivation of Jak2 are facilitated (397). Thus, the negative regulation of EPO signaling appears to be at the level of a receptor-dependent inactivation of a Jak kinase. Shp-1 also has been shown to interact with β$_c$ and to mediate diminished IL-3–induced signaling (398), and to be able to associate with both Tyk-2 (399) and Jak2 (400).

Shp-2 has generally been thought to be more of an activating phosphatase; it is therefore interesting that it has now been shown

that it can also interact with Jak1, Jak2, and Tyk2 (401). In addition to the presumed dephosphorylation of Jak kinases by phosphatases, STAT proteins also appear to be regulated at the level of tyrosine dephosphorylation (402). Finally, evolving data indicate the importance of another type of phosphatase, namely a lipid phosphatase known as SHIP, as a negative regulator of cytokine signals (403,404).

In addition to their dephosphorylation, another mode of negative regulation is by degradation. This degradation can occur at the level of receptor or other signaling molecules. Recently it was observed that Stat1 was regulated by the ubiquitin-proteasome pathway (405). Moreover, γ$_c$ can be cleaved by calpain, a calcium-activated neural protease, after T-cell receptor stimulation (405a). Finally, it is possible that regulation also can occur at the level of alternative splicing; in this regard, alternatively spliced versions of some of the STATs, including Stat1 and Stat5 (254,310,312), have been reported.

THE CIS FAMILY OF INHIBITORY ADAPTER PROTEINS

A new class of proteins has recently been identified that modulate the actions of cytokines. The prototype molecule was named CIS, for cytokine-inducible SH2 containing protein (406,407). CIS was observed to be rapidly induced by a variety of cytokines, including IL-2, IL-3, GM-CSF, and erythropoietin, to physically associate with both the β$_c$ and erythropoietin receptors, and to be a negative regulator of cytokine action (406,407). Recently, a related protein, variably denoted SOCS-1 (suppressor of cytokine signal-1), JAB (Jak-binding protein), and SSI-1 (STAT-induced STAT inhibitor-1), has been identified that appears to be capable of modulating activity of other cytokines, including IL-6 (408–410). Interestingly, this protein can associate with Jak family kinases, whereas this function has not been reported for CIS. Many other members of this family have now been cloned (408,410a,b) and their functions are being investigated.

TH1/TH2 CELLS: THE T-HELPER PARADIGM

Th1 and Th2 cells were originally described based on the patterns of cytokine production by murine T cells (411), but the paradigm has been extended to human cells as well (412–414)(discussed in detail in Chapter 26). Th1 cells secrete IL-2, IFN-γ, and lymphotoxin, whereas Th2 cells produce IL-4, IL-5, IL-6, IL-9, IL-10, and IL-13. The cytokines produced by Th1 and Th2 cells are sometimes referred to as type 1 and type 2 cytokines (for Th1 and Th2 cytokines); unfortunately, this results in potential confusion because IL-4 is a type I (four-helical bundle) cytokine that is functionally a type 2 cytokine (in that it is produced by Th2 cells).

In humans the Th1 and Th2 patterns are similar, but not all the cytokines are as tightly restricted (412–414). IFN-γ is the cytokine most reliably produced by Th1 cells, although IL-4, IL-5, and IL-9 are produced by Th2 cells. In both species, a number of cytokines, such as IL-3 and GM-CSF, are produced by both cells. The Th1/Th2 division of Th cells has proved useful in correlating the function of Th1 cells with cell-mediated immunity (inflammatory responses, delayed-type hypersensitivity, and cytotoxicity) and Th2 cells with humoral immunity. Of the Th2 cytokines, IL-4 is particularly important in driving IgE responses. Because the division of

Th1 and Th2 cells is not always perfect, when cells produce both Th1 and Th2 cytokines, they are called Th0 cells, whereas Th3 cells refer to cells that produce high levels of transforming growth factor-β.

The Th division of cells is useful because a number of murine and human physiologic and disease states correspond to Th1 or Th2 responses and patterns (412–414). In general, among infectious diseases, resistance to intracellular bacteria, fungi, and protozoa is linked to mounting a successful Th1 response. Th1 responses also can be linked to pathology, such as arthritis, colitis, and other inflammatory states. Effective protection against extracellular pathogens, such as helminths, requires a Th2 response, and the enhanced humoral immunity may result in successful neutralization of pathogens by the production of specific antibodies (412–414). In humans, Th1 and Th2 cytokines are each dominant in the different types of lesions found in leprosy, with Th1 cytokines dominating in tuberculoid lesions and Th2 cytokines dominating in lepromatous lesions. In human immunodeficiency virus (HIV), a simple Th1/Th2 pattern does not exist. The situation has been complicated by the fact that IL-4 expression is relatively transient, whereas IL-10 expression is more sustained (414). This has led to the current belief that IL-10 and IL-12 may be the most important cytokines controlling disease progression in AIDS (414). Interestingly, Th0 and Th2 cells seem to be more susceptible to HIV than Th1 cells, potentially explaining why the virus can persist even in the absence of Th1 cells (415).

It is believed that Th1 and Th2 cells are derived from a common precursor (Thp cells), and that IL-12 and a more recently recognized factor denoted IFN-γ inducing factor (IGIF) are the major driving force to induce Th1 differentiation (416), whereas IL-4 induces Th2 differentiation. IGIF is also called IL-1γ given structural considerations that it is processed by IL-1β converting enzyme (caspase-1) (417,418). Corresponding to these findings, as discussed earlier in this chapter, Stat4-deficient mice are defective in IL-12 signaling and exhibit a defect in Th1 development, whereas Stat6-deficient mice are defective in IL-4 signaling and exhibit a defect in Th2 development.

One major difference between Th1 and Th2 cells is in their differential ability to transcribe the genes for IL-2 and IL-4. A clear understanding of the regulation of the IL-2 and IL-4 genes is therefore important to understanding the differences between these cell types. Interestingly, both of the genes are regulated by one or more NF-AT family members, so it is clear that a single NF-AT member is not solely responsible for controlling expression of both genes. Although no specific factor for Th1 cells and IL-2 transcription has been found, the c-maf protooncogene product appears to be absolutely specific for Th2 cells and to be essential for IL-4 transcription (419). This product, together with NF-AT and another NF-AT interaction protein denoted NIP-45, appears to be vital for regulating IL-4 production (420). An understanding of the factor(s) regulating these genes will provide more insights into the regulation of the Th2 response. So far, no analogous cooperating proteins have been discovered that are vital for regulating IL-2 production.

In addition to the major differences between Th1 and Th2 cells in the production of IFN-γ, it was observed that Th subsets differed markedly in their abilities to respond to IFN-γ, with the proliferation of Th2 clones being inhibited and that of Th1 clones not being inhibited (421). Although Thp cells respond to IFN-γ, IFNGR-2 expression decreases after exposure to IFN-γ. This occurs to some degree on Th2 cells but is more dramatic on Th1 cells, consistent with the IFN-γ produced during the generation of Th1 cells and the resulting lack of responsiveness of Th1 cells to IFN-γ (422,423).

Thus, Th1 cells produce IFN-γ and can thereby inhibit the proliferation of Th2 cells. As noted above, IL-12 is the major inducer of Th1 cells. Many Th2 cells do not respond to IL-12; this extinction of IL-12 signaling appears to result from IL-4–mediated loss of expression of the IL-12Rβ2 subunit of the IL-12 receptor (424). This is not a stable differentiation, however, because treatment with IFN-γ for as little as 4 hours can restore IL-12 responsiveness (425). The abilities of mice to survive infections can be critically linked to the Th patterns of cytokines. For example, the ability to survive infection with *Toxoplasma gondii* is strictly dependent on IFN-γ/IL-12 production (a Th1 pattern) (412–414).

DISEASES OF CYTOKINE RECEPTORS AND RELATED MOLECULES

Range of Cytokine-Related Causes of SCID

As detailed above, mutation of the common cytokine receptor γ chain, γc, causes a profound immunodeficiency known as XSCID. One of the striking features of the discovery was that it demonstrated that XSCID was a disease of defective cytokine signaling, which allowed the hypothesis that defects in molecules in the downstream signaling pathways might also result in clinical disease. Indeed, it was directly confirmed that Jak3 mutations also resulted in SCID. Given that Stat5a and Stat5b are signaling molecules downstream of the Jaks, it remains an open question as to whether mutations in these STAT proteins cause human disease. Although it might have been assumed that mutations in either Stat5a or Stat5b alone might cause no phenotype due to similarity and potential redundancy, as noted above, these proteins have major distinctive actions. For example, Stat5a-deficient female mice exhibit a prolactin-related deficiency (345), whereas Stat5b-deficient mice have defective growth and a syndrome not dissimilar to that found in Laron dwarfism (346). It is not yet clear whether an immunodeficiency is associated with Stat5a or Stat5b deficiency.

It can be predicted that human immunodeficiencies might also result from mutations in some of the cytokines whose receptors contain γc, or from mutations in other components of the receptors for these cytokines. Indeed, as noted above, patients with IL-2 deficiency exhibit a SCID-like syndrome, due to inadequate function of their T cells, and recently an unusual immunodeficiency has been found to result from a mutation in IL-2Rα (197). Mutations in IL-2Rβ have not yet been described in humans, but an IL-2Rβ–deficient mouse has a phenotype (119) that suggests that some cases of human SCID may result from mutations in IL-2Rβ. Correspondingly, mutations in IL-7 (71) and IL-7Rα (70) seem like excellent candidates for causing human immunodeficiency syndromes. It is reasonable to predict that IL-7- or IL-7Rα–deficient patients might exhibit defective T-cell development analogous to that found in XSCID or Jak3 deficiency, but in contrast, they might not exhibit a defect in NK-cell development, given that IL-15 signaling would not be compromised. Conversely, mutations in IL-15 might cause a phenotype with a rather selective defect in NK cells (89–92). The analysis of IL-15 and IL-15Rα–deficient mice, when they are available, will therefore be important. It is also possible that defects in IL-9 will cause immunologic defects, given that IL-9 transgenic mice develop thymomas (81). At least for the moment, mutations in IL-2, IL-2Rα, γc, and Jak3 are the only cytokine-related mutations that have been found to cause SCID. More time will be required to determine whether mutations in other cytokines, cytokine receptors, Jaks, or STATs also can cause SCID.

Other Diseases Associated with Cytokine Receptors

A number of other diseases have been reported that are related to cytokine receptors (426). First, mutations in the growth hormone receptor have been found in a form of dwarfism (Laron dwarfism) in which target cells cannot respond to growth hormone (427). Second, a single patient with a form of congenital neutropenia (Kostmann's syndrome) has been found to have a mutation in one of his G-CSF receptor alleles (428). Third, a kindred of patients with familial erythrocytosis has truncation in the erythropoietin receptor, resulting in hypersensitivity to erythropoietin (429). Finally, it is interesting that the thrombopoietin receptor (c-mpl) was first identified as an orphan cytokine receptor when a viral oncogene, v-mpl, was originally identified as the oncogene of the *myeloprolif-erative leukemia virus* (MPLV) (430).

CONCLUDING COMMENTS

Type I cytokines and IFNs are involved in the regulation of an enormous number of immunologic and nonimmunologic processes. In the past several years, a new vision of these molecules has evolved: there has been a progressive transition from viewing these as discrete molecules with special actions to sets of molecules that can be grouped according to shared receptor components and common signaling pathways. Signaling is one area where our understanding has greatly expanded, but in truth, the pathways that are activated are similar for many cytokines, even when the biologic functions they induce are dramatically different. Although some of the differences can be explained by compartmentalization according to which cells produce the cytokine and which cells express receptors that allow them to respond to the cytokine, a tremendous amount still needs to be learned about how distinctive signals are triggered, as well as regarding the sets of genes that are induced by each cytokine. These will provide vital information important to the quest to understand the mechanisms by which type I cytokines and IFNs effect their actions.

REFERENCES

1. Dumonde DC, Wolstencroft RA, Panayi GS, Matthew M, Morley J, Howson WT. Lymphokines: non-antibody mediators of cellular immunity generated by lymphocyte action. *Nature* 1969;224:38.
2. Cohen S, Bigazzi PE, Yoshida T. Commentary. Similarities of T cell function in cell-mediated immunity and antibody production. *Cell Immunol* 1974;12:150.
3. Waksman BH, Oppenheim JJ. The contribution of the cytokine concept to immunology, In: Gallagher RB, Gilder J, Nossal FJV, Salvatore G, eds. *Immunology, the making of a modern science.* San Diego: Academic Press, 1995:33.
4. Oppenheim JJ, Gery I. From lymphodrek to interleukin 1 (IL-1). *Immunol Today* 1993;14,232.
5. Bazan JF. Neurotropic cytokines in the hematopoietic fold. *Neuron* 1991;7:1.
6. Wlodawer A, Pavlovsky A, Gustchina A. Hematopoietic cytokines: similarities and differences in the structures, with implications for receptor binding. *Protein Sci* 1993;2:1373.
7. Rozwarski DA, Gronenborn AM, Clore GM, et al. Structural comparisons among the short-chain helical cytokines. *Structure* 1994;2:159.
8. Sprang SR, Bazan JF. Cytokine structural taxonomy and mechanisms of receptor engagement. *Curr Opin Struc Biol* 1993;3:815.
9. Zhang F, Basinski MB, Beals JM, et al. Crystal structure of the obese protein leptin E100. *Nature* 1997,387:206.
10. Davies DR, Wlodawer A. Cytokines and their receptor complexes. *FASEB J* 1995;9:50.
11. Milburn MV, Hassell AM, Lambert MH, et al. A novel dimer configuration revealed by the crystal structure at 2.4 resolution of human interleukin-5. *Nature* 1993;363.172.
12. Senda T, Shimazu T, Matsuda S, et al. Three-dimensional crystal structure of recombinant murine interferon-β. *EMBO J* 1992;11:3193.
13. Ealick SE, Cook WJ, Vijay-Kumar S, et al. Three-dimensional structure of recombinant human interferon-γ. *Science* 1991;252:698–702.
14. Zdanov A, Schalk-Hihi C, Gustchina A, Tsang M, Weatherbee J, Wlodawer A. Crystal structure of interleukin-10 reveals the functional dimer with an unexpected topological similarity to interferon γ. *Structure* 1995;3:591.
15. D'Andrea AD, Fasman GD, Lodish HF. Erythropoietin receptor and interleukin-2 chain β: a new receptor family. *Cell* 1989;58:1023.
16. Bazan JF. Structural design and molecular evolution of a cytokine receptor superfamily. *Proc Natl Acad Sci USA* 1990;87:6934.
17. Hilton DJ, Hilton AA, Raicevic A, et al. Cloning of a murine IL-11 receptor α-chain: requirement for gp130 for high affinity binding and signal transduction. *EMBO J* 1994;13:4765.
18. Cherel M, Sorel M, Lebeau B, et al. Molecular cloning of two isoforms of a receptor for the human hematopoietic cytokine interleukin-11. *Blood* 1995;86:2534.
19. Hilton DJ, Zhang J-G, Metcalf D, Alexander WS, Nicola NA, Wilson TA. Cloning and characterization of a binding subunit of the interleukin 13 receptor that is also a component of the interleukin 4 receptor. *Proc Natl Acad Sci USA* 1996;93:497.
20. Mosley B, De Imus C, Friend D, Boiani N, Thoma B, Park LS, Cosman D. Dual oncostatin M (OSM) receptors: cloning and characterization of an alternative signaling subunit conferring OSM-specific receptor activation. *J Biol Chem* 1996;271:32635.
21. de Vos AM, Ultsch M, Kossiakoff AA. Human growth hormone and extracellular domain of its receptor: crystal structure of the complex. *Science* 1992;255:306.
22. Somers W, Ultsch M, De Vos AM, Kossiakoff AA. The X-ray structure of a growth hormone-prolactin receptor complex. *Nature* 1994;372:478.
23. Livnah O, Stura EA, Johnson DL, et al. Functional mimicry of a protein hormone by a peptide agonist: the EPO receptor complex at 2.8 Å. *Science* 1996;273:464.
24. Murakami M, Narazali M, Hibi M, et al. Critical cytoplasmic region of the interleukin 6 signal transducer gp130 is conserved in the cytokine receptor family. *Proc Natl Acad Sci USA* 1991;88:11349.
25. Wrighton NC, Farrell FX, Chang R, et al. Small peptides as potent mimetics of the protein hormone erythropoietin. *Science* 1996;273:458.
26. Takeshita T, Asao H, Ohtani K, et al. Cloning of the γ chain of the human IL-2 receptor. *Science* 1992;257:379.
27. Kondo M, Takeshita T, Ishii N, et al. Sharing of the interleukin-2 (IL-2) γ chain between receptors for IL-2 and IL-4. *Science* 1993;262:1874.
28. Noguchi M, Nakamura Y, Russell SM, et al. Interleukin-2 receptor γ chain; a functional component of the interleukin-7 receptor. *Science* 1993;262:1877.
29. Russell SM, Keegan AD, Harada N, et al. Interleukin-2 receptor γ chain: a functional component of the interleukin-4 receptor. *Science* 1993;262:1880.
30. Kondo M, Takeshita T, Higuchi M, et al. Functional participation of the IL-2 receptor γ chain in IL-7 receptor complexes. *Science* 1994;263:1453.
31. Russell SM, Johnston JA, Noguchi M, et al. Interaction of IL-2Rβ and γc chains with Jak1 and Jak3: implications for XSCID and XCID. *Science* 1994;266:1042.
32. Kimura M, Ishii N, Nakamura M, Van Snick J, Sugamura K. Sharing of the IL-2 receptor γ chain with the functional IL-9 receptor complex. *Int Immunol* 1995; 7:115.
33. Giri JG, Ahdieh M, Eisenman J, et al. Utilization of the β and γ chains of the IL-2 receptor by the novel cytokine IL-15. *EMBO J* 1994;13:2822.
34. Leonard WJ, Shores EW, Love PE. Role of the common cytokine receptor γ chain in cytokine signaling and lymphoid development. *Immunol Rev* 1995; 148:97.
35. Leonard WJ. The Molecular basis of X-linked combined immunodeficiency: defective cytokine receptor signaling. *Annu Rev Med* 1996;47:229.
36. Sugamura K, Asao H, Kondo M, et al. The interleukin-2 receptor γ chain: its role in the multiple cytokine receptor complexes and T cell development in XSCID. *Annu Rev Immunol* 1996;14:179.
37. Sugamura K, Asao H, Kondo M, et al. The common γ-chain for multiple cytokine receptors. *Adv Immunol* 1995;59:225.
38. Morgan DA, Ruscetti FW, Gallo R. Selective in vitro growth of T lymphocytes from normal human bone marrows. *Science* 1976;193:1007.
39. Mingari MC, Gerosa F, Carra G, et al. Human interleukin-2 promotes proliferation of activated B cells via surface receptors similar to those of activated T cells. *Nature* 1984;312:641.
40. Waldmann TA. The multi-subunit interleukin-2 receptor. *Annu Rev Biochem* 1989;58:875.
41. Blackman MA, Tigges MA, Minie ME, Koshland ME. A model system for peptide hormone action in differentiation: interleukin 2 induces a B lymphoma to transcribe the A chain gene. *Cell* 1986;47:609.
42. Siegel JP, Sharon M, Smith PL, Leonard WJ. The IL-2 receptor β chain (p70): role in mediating signals for LAK, NK, and proliferative activities. *Science* 1987;238:75.
43. Leonard WJ, Siegel JP. The interleukin-2 receptor complex and its role in the induction of a nonspecific cytotoxicity. In: Lotzova E, Herberman RB, eds. *Interleukin-2 and killer cells in cancer.* Boca Raton, FL: CRC Press, 1990:305.
44. Lanier LL, Phillips JH. Natural killer cells. *Curr Opin Immunol* 1992;4:38.
45. Janssen RAJ, Mulder NH, The TH, de Leij L, The immunobiological effects of interleukin-2 in vivo. *Cancer Immunol Immunother* 1994;39:207.
46. Taniguchi T, Matsui H, Fujita T, et al. Structure and expression of a cloned cDNA for human interleukin-2. *Nature* 1983;302:305.

47. Leonard WJ, Depper JM, Crabtree GR, et al. Molecular cloning and expression of cDNAs for the human interleukin-2 receptor. *Nature* 1984;311:625.

48. Nikaido T, Shimizu A, Ishida N, et al. Molecular cloning of cDNA encoding human interleukin-2 receptor. *Nature* 1984;311:631.

49. Smith KA. The interleukin 2 receptor. *Ann Rev Cell Biol* 1989;5:397.

50. Siegel LJ, Harper ME, Wong-Staal F, Gallo RC, Nash WG, O'Brien SJ. Gene for T-cell growth factor: location on human chromosome 4q and feline chromosome B1. *Science* 1984;223:175.

51. Leonard WJ, Depper JM, Uchiyama T, Smith KA, Waldmann TA, Greene WC. A monoclonal antibody that appears to recognize the receptor for human T-cell growth factor: partial characterization of the receptor. *Nature* 1982;300:267.

52. Sharon M, Klausner RD, Cullen BR, Chizzonite R, Leonard WJ. Novel interleukin-2 receptor subunit detected by cross-linking under high affinity conditions. *Science* 1986;234:859.

53. Tsudo M, Kozak RW, Goldman CK, Waldmann TA. Demonstration of a non-Tac peptide that binds interleukin-2: a potential participant in a multichain interleukin-2 receptor complex. *Proc Natl Acad Sci USA* 1986;83:9694.

54. Teshigawara K, Wang HM, Kata K, Smith KA. Interleukin-2 high affinity receptor expression requires two distinct binding proteins. *J Exp Med* 1987;165:223.

55. Hatakeyama M, Tsudo M, Minamoto S, et al. Interleukin-2 receptor β chain gene: generation of three receptor forms by cloned human α and β cDNAs. *Science* 1989;244:551.

56. Paul WE. Interleukin-4: a prototypic immunoregulatory lymphokine. *Blood* 1991;77:1859.

57. Yoshimoto T, Bendelac A, Watson C, Hu-Li J, Paul WE. Role of NK1.1+ T cells in a TH2 response and in immunoglobulin E production. *Science* 1995;270:1845.

58. Lee F, Yokota T, Otsuka T, et al. Isolation and characterization of a mouse interleukin cDNA clone that expresses B-cell stimulatory factor-1 activities and T cell and mast cell stimulating activities. *Proc Natl Acad Sci USA* 1986;83:2061.

59. Noma Y, Sideras P, Naito T, et al. Cloning of cDNA encoding the murine IgG1 induction factor by a novel strategy using ST6 promoter. *Nature* 1986;319:640.

60. Yokota T, Otsuka T, Mosmann T, et al. Isolation and characterization of a human interleukin cDNA clone, homologous to mouse B-cell stimulatory factor-1, that expresses B-cell and T cell stimulating activities. *Proc Natl Acad Sci USA* 1986;83:5894.

61. Paul WE. The role of IL-4 in the regulation of B cell development, growth, and differentiation. In: Spits H, ed. *IL-4: structure and function.* Boca Raton, FL: CRC Press, 1992:57.

62. Boulay J-L, Paul WE. Hematopoietin sub-family classification based on size, gene organization and sequence homology *Curr Biol* 1993;3:573.

63. Mosley B, Beckmann MP, March CJ, et al. The murine interleukin-4 receptor: molecular cloning and characterization of secreted and membrane bound forms. *Cell* 1989;59:335.

64. Idzerda RL, March CJ, Mosley B, et al. Human interleukin 4 receptor confers biological responsiveness and defines a novel receptor superfamily. *J Exp Med* 1990;171:861.

65. Galizzi J-P, Zuber CE, Harada N, et al. Molecular cloning of a cDNA encoding the human interleukin 4 receptor. *Int Immunol* 1990;2:669.

66. Namen AE, Lupton S, Hjerrild K, et al. Stimulation of B-cell progenitors by cloned murine interleukin-7. *Nature* 1988;333:571.

67. Goodwin RG, Lupton S, Schmierer A, et al. Human interleukin-7: molecular cloning and growth factor activity on human and murine B-lineage cells. *Cell* 1990;60:940.

68. Watson JD, Morrissey PJ, Namen AE, Conlon PJ, Widmer MB. Effect of IL-7 on the growth of fetal thymocytes in culture. *J Immunol* 1989;143:1215.

69. Murray R, Suda T, Wrighton N, Lee F, Zlotnik A. IL-7 is a growth and maintenance factor for mature and immature thymocyte subsets. *Int Immunol* 1989;1:526.

70. Peschon J, Morrissey PJ, Grabstein KH, et al. Early lymphocyte expansion is severely impaired in interleukin 7 receptor-deficient mice. *J Exp Med* 1994;180:1955–1960.

71. von Freeden-Jeffry U, Vieira P, Lucian LA, McNeil T, Burdach SE, Murray R. Lymphopenia in interleukin (IL)-7 gene-deleted mice identifies IL-7 as a nonredundant cytokine. *J Exp Med* 1995;181:1519–1526.

72. Chazen GD, Pereira GMB, LeGros S, Shevach EM. Interleukin 7 is a T-cell growth factor. *Proc Natl Acad Sci USA* 1989;86:5923.

73. Morrissey PJ, Goodwin RG, Nordan RP, et al. Recombinant interleukin 7, pre-B cell growth factor, has costimulatory activity on purified mature T cells. *J Exp Med* 1989;169:707.

74. Namen AE, Schmierer AE, March CJ, et al. B cell precursor growth-promoting activity: purification and characterization of a growth factor active on lymphocyte precursors. *J Exp Med* 1988;167:988.

75. Leonard WJ. The defective gene in X-linked severe combined immunodeficiency encodes a shared interleukin receptor subunit: implications for cytokine pleiotropy and redundancy. *Curr Opin Immunol* 1994;6:631–635.

76. Brunton LL, Lupton SD. An STS in the human IL7 gene located at 8p12-13. *Nucleic Acids Res* 1990;18:1315.

77. Goodwin RG, Friend D, Ziegler SF, et al. Cloning of the human and murine interleukin-7 receptors: demonstration of a soluble form and homology to a new receptor superfamily. *Cell* 1990;60:940.

78. Van Snick J, Goethals A, Renauld J-C, et al. Cloning and characterization of a cDNA for a new mouse T cell growth factor, (P40). *J Exp Med* 1989;169:363.

79. Yang Y, Ricciardi S, Ciarletta A, Kelleher K, Clark SC. Expression cloning of a

80. Renauld J-C, Kermouni A, Vink A, Louahed J, Van Snick J. Interleukin-9 and its receptor: involvement in mast cell differentiation and T cell oncogenesis. *J Leukoc Biol* 1995;57:353.

81. Renauld J-C, Houssiau F, Uyttenhove C, Vink A, Van Snick J. Interleukin-9: a T-cell growth factor with a potential oncogenic activity. *Cancer Invest* 1993;11:635.

82. Hultner L, Moeller J, Schmitt E, et al. Thiol-sensitive mast cell lines derived from mouse bone marrow respond to a mast cell growth-enhancing activity different from both IL-3 and IL-4. *J Immunol* 1989;142:3440.

83. Renauld J-C, Vink A, Louahed J, Van Snick J. Interleukin-9 is a major anti-apoptotic factor for thymic lymphomas. *Blood* 1995;85:1300.

84. Modi WS, Pollock DD, Mock BA, Banner C, Renauld J-C, Van Snick J. Regional localization of the human glutaminase (GLS) and interleukin-9 (IL9) genes by in situ hybridization. *Cytogenet Cell Genet* 1991;57:114.

85. Renauld J-C, Druez C, Kermouni A, et al. Expression cloning of the murine and human interleukin 9 receptor cDNAs. *Proc Natl Acad Sci USA* 1992;89:5690.

86. Grabstein KH, Eisenman J, Shanebeck K, et al. Cloning of a T cell growth factor that interacts with the β chain of the interleukin-2 receptor. *Science* 1994;264:965.

87. Burton JD, Famford RN, Peters C, et al. A lymphokine, provisionally designated interleukin T and produced by a human adult T-cell leukemia line, stimulates T-cell proliferation and the induction of lymphokine-activated killer cells. *Proc Natl Acad Sci USA* 1994;91:4935.

88. Tagaya Y, Bamford RN, DeFllippis AP, Waldmann TA. IL-15: a pleiotropic cytokine with diverse receptor signaling pathways whose expression is controlled at multiple levels. *Immunity* 1996;4:329.

89. Carson WE, Giri JG, Lindemann MJ, et al. Interleukin (IL) 15 is a novel cytokine that activates human natural killer cells via components of the IL-2 receptor. *J Exp Med* 1994;180:1395.

90. Cavazzana-Calvo M, Hacein-Bey S, de Saint Basile G, et al. Role of interleukin-2 (IL-2), IL-7, and IL-15 in natural killer cell differentiation from cord blood hematopoietic progenitor cells and from γc transduced severe combined immunodeficiency X1 bone marrow cells. *Blood* 1996;88:3901.

91. Leclercq G, Debacker V, de Smedt M, Plum J. Differential effects of interleukin-15 and interleukin-2 on the differentiation of bipotential T/natural killer progenitor cells. *J Exp Med* 1996;184:325.

92. Puzanov IJ, Bennett M, Kumar V. IL-15 can substitute for the marrow microenvironment in the differentiation of natural killer cells. *J Immunol* 1996;157:4282.

93. Bamford RN, Grant AJ, Burton JD, et al. The interleukin (IL) 2 receptor β chain is shared by IL-2, and a cytokine, provisionally designated IL-T, that stimulates T-cell proliferation and the induction of lymphokine-activated killer cells. *Proc Natl Acad Sci USA* 1994;91:4940.

94. Giri JG, Kumaki S, Ahdieh M, et al. Identification and cloning of a novel IL-15 binding protein that is structurally related to the α chain of the IL-2 receptor. *EMBO J* 1995;14:3654.

95. Anderson DM, Kumaki S, Ahdieh M, et al. Functional characterization of the human interleukin-15 receptor α chain and close linkage of IL15RA and IL2RA genes. *J Biol Chem* 1995;270:29862.

96. Tagaya T, Burton JD, Miyamoto Y, Waldmann TA. Identification of a novel receptor signal transduction pathway for IL-15/T in mast cells. *EMBO J* 1995;15:4928.

97. Noguchi M, Yi H, Rosenblatt HM, et al. Interleukin-2 receptor γ chain mutation results in X-linked severe combined immunodeficiency in humans. *Cell* 1993;73:147.

98. Conley ME. Molecular approaches to analysis of X-linked immunodeficiencies. *Annu Rev Immunol* 1992;10:215.

99. Fischer A, Cavazzana-Calvo M, de Saint Basile G, et al. Naturally occurring primary deficiencies of the immune system. *Annu Rev Immunol* 1997;15:93.

100. Leonard WJ, Noguchi M, Russell SM, McBride OW. The molecular basis of X-linked severe combined immunodeficiency: the role of the interleukin-2 receptor γ chain as a common γ chain, γc. *Immunol Rev* 1994;138:61.

101. Weinberg K, Parkman R. Severe combined immunodeficiency due to a specific defect in the production of interleukin-2. *N Engl J Med* 1990;322:1718.

102. Chatila T, Castigli E, Pahwa R, et al. Primary combined immunodeficiency resulting from defective transcription of multiple T-cell lymphokine genes. *Proc Natl Acad Sci USA* 1990;87:10033.

103. Schorle H, Holtschke T, Hunig T, Schimpl A, Horak I. Development and function of T cells in mice rendered interleukin-2 deficient by gene targeting. *Nature* 1991;352:621.

104. Leonard WJ. Dysfunctional cytokine receptor signaling in severe combined immunodeficiency. *J Invest Med* 1996;44:303.

105. de Jong JL, Farner NL, Widmer MB, Giri JG, Sondel PM. Interaction of IL-15 with the shared IL-2 receptor β and γc subunits. The IL-15/β/γc receptor-ligand complex is less stable than the IL-2/β/γc receptor-ligand complex. *J Immunol* 1996;156:1339.

106. Kuhn R, Rajewsky K, Muller W. Generation and analysis of interleukin-4 deficient mice. *Science* 1991;254:707.

107. Kopf M, Le Gros G, Bachmann M, Lamers MC, Bluethmann H, Kohler G. Disruption of the murine IL-4 gene blocks Th2 cytokine responses. *Nature* 1993;362:245.

108. Sadlack B, Kuhn R, Schorle H, Rajewsky K, Muller W, Horak I. Development

and proliferation of lymphocytes in mice deficient for both interleukins-2 and -4. *Eur J Immunol* 1994;24:281.

109. DiSanto JP, Muller W, Guy-Grand D, Fischer A, Rajewsky K. Lymphoid development in mice with a targeted deletion of the interleukin 2 receptor γ chain. *Proc Natl Acad Sci USA* 1995;92:377–381.

110. Cao X, Shores EW, Hu-Li J, et al. Defective lymphoid development in mice lacking expression of the common cytokine receptor γ chain. *Immunity* 1995;2:223.

111. Ohbo K, Suda T, Hashiyama M, et al. Modulation of hematopoiesis in mice with a truncated mutant of the interleukin-2 receptor γ chain. *Blood* 1996;87:956.

112. Izuhara K, Heike T, Otsuka T, et al. Signal transduction pathway of interleukin-4 and interleukin-13 in human B cells derived from X-linked severe combined immunodeficiency patients. *J Biol Chem* 1996;271.619.

113. Takeshita T, Asao H, Suzuki J, Sugamura K. An associated molecule, p64, with high-affinity interleukin 2 receptor. *Int Immunol* 1990;2:477.

114. Nakamura Y, Russell SM, Mess SA, et al. Heterodimerization of the interleukin-2 receptor β and γ cytoplasmic domains is required for signaling. *Nature* 1994;369:330.

115. Nelson B, Lord JD, Greenberg PD. Cytoplasmic domains of the interleukin-2 receptor β and γ chains mediate the signal for T-cell proliferation. *Nature* 1994;369:333.

116. Balasubramanian S, Chernov-Rogan T, Davis AM, et al. Ligand binding kinetics of IL-2 and IL-15 to heteromers formed by extracellular domains of the three IL-2 receptor subunits. *Int Immunol* 1995;7:1839.

117. Myszka DG, Arulanantham PR, Sana T, Wu Z, Morton TA, Ciardelli TL. Kinetic analysis of ligand binding to interleukin-2 receptor complexes created on an optical biosensor surface. *Protein Sci* 1996;5:2468.

118. Willerford DM, Chen J, Ferry JA, Davidson L, Ma A, Alt FW. Interleukin-2 receptor α chain regulates the size and content of the peripheral lymphoid compartment. *Immunity* 1995;3:521.

119. Suzuki H, Kundig TM, Furlonger C, et al. Deregulated T cell activation and autoimmunity in mice lacking interleukin-2 receptor β. *Science* 1995;268:1472.

120. Nakajima H, Shores EW, Noguchi M, Leonard WJ. The common cytokine receptor γ chain plays an essential role in regulating lymphoid homeostasis. *J Exp Med* 1997;185:189–196.

121. Ihle JN. Interleukin-3 and hematopoiesis. In: Kishimoto T, ed. *Interleukins: molecular biology and immunology.* Basel, Switzerland: Karger, 1992:65.

122. Metcalf D. *The hematopoietic colony stimulating factors.* Amsterdam: Elsevier, 1984.

123. Takatsu K, Tominaga A, Harada N, et al. T-cell replacing factor (TRF)/interleukin 5 (IL-5): molecular and functional properties. *Immunol Rev* 1988;102:107.

124. Hara T, Miyajima A. Functional and signal transduction mediated by the interleukin 3 receptor system in hematopoiesis. *Stem Cells* 1996;14.605.

125. Kitamura T, Sato N, Arai K, Miyajima A. Expression cloning of the human IL-3 receptor cDNA reveals a shared β subunit for the human IL-3 and GM-CSF receptors. *Cell* 1991;66:1165.

126. Hara T, Miyajima T. Two distinct functional high affinity receptors for mouse IL-3. *EMBO J* 1992;10:1875.

127. Takaki S, Tominaga A, HitoshY, Mita S, Sonoda E, Yamaguchi N, Takatsu K. Molecular cloning and expression of the murine interleukin-5 receptor. *EMBO J* 1990;9:4367.

128. Tavernier J, Devos R, Cornelis S, et al. A human high affinity interleukin-5 receptor (IL-5R) is composed of an IL-5-specific α chain and a β chain shared with the receptor for GM-CSF. *Cell* 1991;66:1174.

129. Gearing DP, King JA, Gough NM, Nicola NA. Expression cloning of a receptor for human granulocyte-macrophage colony stimulating factor. *EMBO J* 1989;8:3667.

130. Park LS, Martin U, Sorensen R, et al. Cloning of the low-affinity murine granulocyte-macrophage colony stimulating factor receptor and reconstitution of a high-affinity receptor complex. *Proc Natl Acad Sci USA* 1992;89:4295.

131. Gorman DM, Itoh N, Kitamura T, et al. Cloning and expression of a gene encoding an interleukin 3 receptor-like protein: identification of another member of the cytokine receptor gene family. *Proc Natl Acad Sci USA* 1990;87:5459.

132. Hayashida K, Kitamura T, Gorman DM, Arai K-I, Yokota T, Miyajima A. Molecular cloning of a second subunit of the receptor for human granulocyte-macrophage colony-stimulating factor (GM-CSF): reconstitution of a high affinity GM-CSF receptor. *Proc Natl Acad Sci USA* 1990;87:9655..

133. Miyajima A, Kitamura T, Harada N, Yokota T, Arai K. Cytokine receptors and signal transduction. *Annu Rev Immunol* 1992;10:295.

134. Sakamaki K, Miyajima I, Kitamura T, Miyajima A. Critical cytoplasmic domains of the common β subunit of the human GM-CSF, IL-3 and IL-5 receptors for growth signal transduction and tyrosine phosphorylation. *EMBO J* 1992;11:3541.

135. Cornelis S, Fache I, Van der Heyden J, et al. Characterization of critical residues in the cytoplasmic domain of the human interleukin-5 receptor α chain required for growth signal transduction. *Eur J Immunol* 1995;25:1857.

136. Kouro T, Kikuchi Y, Kanazawa H, et al. Critical proline residues of the cytoplasmic domain of the IL-5 receptor α chain and its function in IL-5–mediated activation of Jak kinase and Stat5. *Int Immunol* 1996;8:237.

137. Nishinakamura R, Miyajima A, Mee PJ, Tybulewicz VL, Murray R. Hematopoiesis in mice lacking the entire granulocyte-macrophage colony stimulating factor/interleukin-3/interleukin-5 functions. *Blood* 1996;88:2458.

138. Metcalf D. The granulocyte-macrophage regulators: reappraisal by gene inactivation. *Exp Hematol* 1995;23:569.

139. Hibi M, Murakami M, Saito M, Hirano T, Taga T, Kishimoto T. Molecular cloning and expression of an IL-6 signal transducer, gp130. *Cell* 1990;63:1149.

140. Gearing DP, Comeau MR, Friend DJ, et al. The IL-6 signal transducer, gp130; an oncostatin M receptor and affinity converter for the LIF receptor. *Science* 1992;255:1434.

141. Taga T, Narazaki M, Yasukawa K, et al. Functional inhibition of hematopoietic and neurotrophic cytokines by blocking the interleukin 6 signal transducer gp130. *Proc Natl Acad Sci USA* 1992;89:10998.

142. Yin T, Taga T, Tsang ML, Yasukawa K, Kishimoto T, Yang YC. Involvement of IL-6 signal transducer gp130 in IL-11–mediated signal transduction. *J Immunol* 1993;151:2555.

143. Pennica D, Shaw KJ, Swanson TA, et al. Cardiotrophin-1. Biological activities and binding to the leukemia inhibitory factor receptor/gp130 signaling complex. *J Biol Chem* 1995;270:10915.

144. Hirano T, Yasukawa K, Harada H, et al. Complementary DNA for a novel human interleukin (BSF-2) that induces B lymphocytes to produce immunoglobulin. *Nature* 1986;324:73.

145. Kishimoto T, Akira S, Narazaki M, Taga T. Interleukin-6 family of cytokines and gp130. *Blood* 1995;86:1243.

146. Hibi M, Nakajima K, Hirano T. IL-6 cytokine family and signal transduction: a model of the cytokine system. *J Mol Med* 1996;74:1.

147. Taga T, Kishimoto T. Gp130 and the interleukin-6 family of cytokines. *Annu Rev Immunol* 1997;15:797.

148. Yamasaki K, Taga T, Hirata Y, et al. Cloning and expression of the human interleukin-6 (BSF-2/IFNβ2) receptor. *Science* 1988;241:825.

149. Taga T, Hibi M, Hirata Y, et al. Interleukin-6 triggers the association of its receptor with a possible signal transducer, gp130. *Cell* 1989;58:573.

150. Murakami M, Hibib M, Nakagawa N, et al. IL-6-induced homodimerization of gp130 and associated activation of a tyrosine kinase. *Science* 1993;260:1808.

151. Panonessa G, Graziani R, Serio AD, et al. Two distinct and independent sites on IL-6 trigger gp130 dimer formation and signalling. *EMBO J* 1995;14:1942.

152. Ward LD, Howlett GJ, Discolo G, et al. High affinity interleukin-6 receptor is a hexameric complex consisting of two molecules each of interleukin-6, interleukin-6 receptor, and gp-130. *J Biol Chem* 1994;269:23286.

153. Du XX, Williams DA. Interleukin-11: a multifunctional growth factor derived from the hematopoietic microenvironment. *Blood* 1994;83:2023

154. Goldman SJ. Preclinical biology of interleukin 11: a multifunctional hematopoietic cytokine with potent thrombopoietic activity. *Stem Cells* 1995;13:462.

155. Paul SR, Bennett F, Calvetti JA, et al. Molecular cloning of a cDNA encoding interleukin 11, a stromal derived lymphopoietic and hematopoietic cytokine. *Proc Natl Acad Sci USA* 1990;87:7512

156. Kobayashi S, Teramura M, Oshi K, Mizoguchi H. Interleukin-11. *Leuk Lymph* 1994;15:45.

157. Kawashima I, Ohsumi J, Mita-Honjo K, et al. Molecular cloning of cDNA encoding adipogenesis inhibitory factor and identity with interleukin-11. *FEBS Lett* 1991;283:199.

158. Baumann H, Wang Y, Morella KK, et al. Complex of the soluble IL-11 receptor and IL-11 acts as IL-6-type cytokine in hepatic and nonhepatic cells. *J Immunol* 1996;157:284.

159. Neddermann P, Graziani R, Ciliberto G, Paonessa G. Functional expression of soluble human interleukin-11 (IL-11) receptor α and stoichiometry of in vitro IL-11 receptor complexes with gp130. *J Biol Chem* 1996;271:30986.

160. Gearing DP, Gough NM, King JA, et al. Molecular cloning and expression of cDNA encoding a murine myeloid leukaemia inhibitory factor (LIF). *EMBO J* 1987;6:3995.

161. Hilton DJ, Gough NM. Leukemia inhibitor factor: a biological perspective. *J Cell Biochem* 1991;46:21.

162. Yamamori T, Kukada K, Abersold R, Korsching S, Fann MJ, Patterson PH. The cholinergic neuronal differentiation factor from heart cells is identical to leukemia inhibitory factor. *Science* 1989;246:1412.

163. Gearing DP, Thut CJ, VandenBos T, et al. Leukemia inhibitory factor receptor is structurally related to the IL-6 signal transducer, gp130. *EMBO J* 1991;10:2839.

164. Lin L-FH, Mismer D, Lile JD, et al. Purification, cloning, and expression of ciliary neurotrophic factor (CNTF). *Science* 1989;246:1023.

165. Stockli KA, Lottspeich F, Sendtner M, et al. Molecular cloning, expression and regional distribution of rat ciliary neurotrophic factor. *Nature* 1989;342:920.

166. Davis S, Aldrich TH, Valenzuela DM, et al. The receptor for ciliary neurotrophic factor. *Science* 1991;253:59.

167. Davis S, Aldrich TH, Stahl N, et al. LIFRβ and gp130 as heterodimerizing signal transducers of the tripartite CNTF receptor. *Science* 1993;260:1805.

168. De Serio A, Graziani R, Laufer R, Ciliberto G, Paonessa G. In vitro binding of ciliary neurotrophic factor to its receptors: evidence for the formation of an IL-6-type hexameric complex. *J Mol Biol* 1995;254:795.

169. Zarling JM, Shoyab M, Marquardt H, Hanson MB, Lioubin MN, Todaro GJ. Oncostatin M: a growth regulator produced by differentiated histiocytic lymphoma cells. *Proc Natl Acad Sci USA* 1986;83:9739.

170. Malik N, Kalestad JC, Gunderson NL, et al. Molecular cloning, sequence analysis, and functional expression of a novel growth regulator, oncostatin M. *Mol Cell Biol* 1989;9:2847.

171. Nair BC, DeVico AL, Nakamura S, et al. Identification of a major growth factor for AIDS-Kaposi's sarcoma cells as oncostatin M. *Science* 1992;255:1430.

172. Miles SA, Martinez-Maza O, Rezai A, et al. Oncostatin M as a potent mitogen for AIDS–Kaposi's sarcoma derived cells. *Science* 1992;255:1432.

172a. Ichihara M, Hara T, Kim H, Morate T, Miyajima A. Oncostatin M and leukemia inhibitory factor do not use the same functional receptor in mice. *Blood* 1997;90:165.

173. Pennica D, King KL, Shaw KL, et al. Expression cloning of cardiotrophin-1, a cytokine that induces cardiac myocyte hypertrophy. *Proc Natl Acad Sci USA* 1995;92:1142.

174. Pennica D, Wood WI, Chien KR. Cardiotrophin-1: a multifunctional cytokine that signals via LIF receptor-gp130 dependent pathways. *Cytokine Growth Factor Rev* 1996;1:81.

175. Pennica D, Arce V, Swanson TA, et al. Cardiotrophin-1, a cytokine present in embryonic muscle, supports long-term survival of spinal motoneurons. *Neuron* 1996;17:63.

176. Robledo O, Fourcin M, Chevalier S, et al. Signaling of the cardiotrophin-1 receptor. Evidence for a third receptor component. *J Biol Chem* 1997;272:4855.

177. Zhang Y, Proenca R, Maffei M, Barone M, Leopold L, Friedman JM. Positional cloning of the mouse obese gene and its human homologue. *Nature* 1994;372: 425 [erratum *Nature* 1995;374:479].

178. Tartaglia LA, Dembski M, Weng X, et al. Identification and expression cloning of a leptin receptor, OB-R. *Cell* 1995;83:1263.

179. Chen H, Charlat O, Tartaglia LA, et al. Evidence that the diabetes gene encodes the leptin receptor: identification of a mutation in the leptin receptor gene in db/db mice. *Cell* 1996;84:491.

180. White DW, Kuropatwinski KK, Devos R, Baumann H, Tartaglia LA. Leptin receptor (OB-R) signaling. Cytoplasmic domain mutational analysis and evidence for receptor homo-oligomerization. *J Biol Chem* 1997;272:4065.

181. Trinchieri G. Interleukin-12: a proinflammatory cytokine with immunoregulatory functions that bridge innate resistance and antigen-specific adaptive immunity. *Annu Rev Immunol* 1995;13:251.

182. Kobayash M, Fitz L, Ryan M, et al. Identification and purification of natural killer cell stimulatory factor (NKSF), a cytokine with multiple biologic effect on human lymphocytes. *J Exp Med* 1989;170:827.

183. Gubler U, Chua AO, Schoenhaut DS, et al. Coexpression of two distinct genes is required to generate secreted bioactive cytotoxic lymphocyte maturation factor. *Proc Natl Acad Sci USA* 1991;88:4143.

184. Chua AO, Wilkinson VL, Presky DH, Gubler U. Cloning and characterization of a mouse IL-12 receptor-β component. *J Immunol* 1995;155:4286.

185. Presky DH, Yang H, Minetti LJ, et al. A functional interleukin 12 receptor complex is composed of two β-type cytokine receptor subunits. *Proc Natl Acad Sci USA* 1996;93:14002.

186. Gubler U, Presky DH. Molecular biology of interleukin-12 receptors. *Ann N Y Acad Sci* 1996;795:36.

187. Lin J-X, Migone T-S, Tsang M, et al. The role of shared receptor motifs and common Stat proteins in the generation of cytokine pleiotropy and redundancy by IL-2, IL-4, IL-7, IL-13, and IL-15. *Immunity* 1995;2:331.

188. Zurawski G, de Vries JE. Interleukin 13, an interleukin 4–like cytokine that acts on monocytes and B cells, but not on T cells. *Immunol Today* 1994;15:19.

189. Smerz-Bertling C, Duschl A. Both interleukin 4 and interleukin 13 induce tyrosine phosphorylation of the 140-kDa subunit of the interleukin 4 receptor. *J Biol Chem* 1994;270:966.

190. Zurawski SM, Chomarat P, Djossou O, et al. The primary binding subunit of the human interleukin-4 receptor is also a component of the interleukin-13 receptor. *J Biol Chem* 1995;270:13869.

191. Aman MF, Tayebi N, Obiri NI, Puri RK, Modi WS, Leonard WJ. cDNA cloning and characterization of the human interleukin-13 receptor α chain. *J Biol Chem* 1996;271:29265.

192. Caput D, Laurent P, Kaghad M, Lelias J-M, Lefort S, Vita N, Ferrara P. Cloning and characterization of α specific interleukin (IL)-13 binding protein structurally related to the IL-5 receptor α chain. *J Biol Chem* 1996;271:16921.

193. Kammer W, Lischke A, Moriggl R, et al. Homodimerization of interleukin-4 receptor alpha chain can induce intracellular signaling. *J Biol Chem* 1996;271:23634.

194. Lai SY, Molden J, Liu KD, Puck JM, White MD, Goldsmith MA. Interleukin-4–specific signal transduction events are driven by homotypic interactions of the interleukin-4 receptor α subunit. *EMBO J* 1996;15:4506.

195. Hoffman RC, Castner BJ, Gerhart M, et al. Direct evidence of a heterotrimeric complex of human interleukin-4 with its receptors. *Protein Sci* 1995;4:382.

196. Taniguchi T. Cytokine signaling through nonreceptor protein tyrosine kinases. *Science* 1995;268:251.

197. Sharfe N, Dadi HK, Shahar M, Roifman CM. Human immune disorder arising from mutation of the α chain of the interleukin-2 receptor. *Proc Natl Acad Sci USA* 1997;94:3168.

198. Leonard WJ, Depper JM, Kanehisa M, et al. Structure of the human interleukin-2 receptor gene. *Science* 1985;230:633.

199. Leonard WJ, Donlon TA, Lebo RV, Greene WC. The gene encoding the human interleukin-2 receptor is located on chromosome 10. *Science* 1985;228:1547.

200. Gnarra JR, Otani H, Wang MG, McBride OW, Sharon M, Leonard WJ. Human interleukin 2 receptor β chain gene: chromosomal localization and identification of 5′ regulatory sequences. *Proc Natl Acad Sci USA* 1990;87:3440.

201. Shibuya H, Yoneyama M, Nakamura Y, et al. The human interleukin-2 receptor β chain gene: genomic organization, promoter analysis and chromosomal assignment. *Nucleic Acids Res* 1990;18:3697.

202. Watowich SS, Yoshimura A, Longmore GD, Hilton DJ, Yoshimira Y, Lodish HF. Homodimerization and constitutive activation of the erythropoietin receptor. *Proc Natl Acad Sci USA* 1992;89:2140.

203. Lodish HF, Hilton DJ, Klingmuller U, Watowich SS, Wu H. The erythropoietin receptor: biogenesis, dimerization, and intracellular signal transduction. *Cold Spring Harb Symp Quant Biol* 1995;60:93.

204. Watowich SS, Wu H, Socolovsky M, Klingmuller U, Constantinescu SN, Lodish HF. Cytokine receptor signal transduction and the control of hematopoietic cell development. *Ann Rev Cell Dev Biol* 1996;12:91.

205. Wu H, Klingmuller U, Besmer P, Lodish HF. Interaction of the erythropoietin and stem-cell-factor receptors. *Nature* 1995;377:242.

206. Lev S, Blechman JM, Givol D, Yarden Y. Steel factor and c-kit protooncogene: genetic lessons in signal transduction. *Crit Rev Oncol* 1994;5:141.

207. Paul WE. Pleiotropy and redundancy: T cell-derived lymphokines in the immune response. *Cell* 1989;57:521.

208. Itoh N, Yonehara S, Schreurs J, et al. Cloning of an interleukin-3 receptor gene: a member of a distinct receptor gene family. *Science* 1990;247:324.

209. Kurman CC, Rubin LA, Nelson DL. Soluble products of immune activation: soluble interleukin-2R (sIL-2R, Tac protein). In: Rose NR, deMacario EC, Fahey JL, Friedman H, Penn GM, eds. *Manual of clinical laboratory immunology.* Washington, DC: American Society for Microbiology, 1992:256.

210. Fernandez-Botran R, Chilton PM, Ma Y. Soluble cytokine receptors: their roles in immunoregulation, disease, and therapy. *Adv Immunol* 1996;63:269.

211. Salvati AL, Lahm A, Paonessa G, Ciliberto G, Toniatti C. Interleukin-6 (IL-6) antagonism by soluble IL-6 receptor α mutated in the predicted gp130-binding interface. *J Biol Chem* 1995;270:12242.

212. Isaacs A, Lindemann J. Virus interference. I. The interferon. *Proc R Soc Lond [Biol]* 1957;147:258.

213. Farrar MA, Schreiber RD. The molecular cell biology of interferon-γ and its receptor. *Annu Rev Immunol* 1993;11:571.

214. Diaz MO, Testa D. Type I interferon genes and proteins. *Biotherapy* 1996;8:157.

215. van den Broek MF, Muller U, Huang S. Zinkernagel RM, Aguet M. Immune defence in mice lacking type I and/or type II interferon receptors. *Immunol Rev* 1995;148:5.

216. Hayes MP, Zoon KC. Production and action of interferons: new insights into molecular mechanisms of gene regulation and expression. *Prog Drug Res* 1994; 43:239.

217. Lefevre F, Boulay V. A novel and atypical type I interferon gene expressed by trophoblast during early pregnancy. *J Biol Chem* 1993;268:19760.

218. International Society for Interferon and Cytokine Research Newsletter. Nomenclature for Interferon Receptors and interferon δ. 1997;4:1.

219. Langer J, Garotta G, Pestka S. Interferon receptors. *Biotherapy* 1996;8:163.

220. Bazan JF. Shared architecture of hormone binding domains in type I and type II interferon receptors. *Cell* 1990;61:753.

221. Walter MR, Windsor WT, Nagabhushan TL, et al. Crystal structure of a complex between interferon-γ and its soluble high-affinity receptor. *Nature* 1995;376: 230–235.

222. Domanski P, Colamonici OS. The type-1 interferon receptor: the long and short of it. *Cytol Growth Fact Rev* 1996;7:143.

223. Uze G, Lutfalla G, Mogensen KE. α and β interferons and their receptor and their friends and relations. *J Interfer Cyt Res* 1995;15:3.

224. Uze G, Lutfalla G, Gresser I. Genetic transfer of a functional human interferon receptor into mouse cells: cloning and expression of its cDNA. *Cell* 1990;60: 225.

225. Novick D, Cohen B, Rubinstein M. The human interferon α/β receptor: characterization and molecular cloning. *Cell* 1994;77:391.

226. Domanski P, Witte M, Kellum M, et al. Cloning and expression of a long form of the β subunit of the interferon α receptor that is required for interferon signaling. *J Biol Chem* 1995;270:21606.

227. Lutfalla G, Holland SJ, Cinato E, et al. Mutant U5A cells are complemented by an interferon αβ receptor subunit generated by alternative processing of a new member of a cytokine receptor gene cluster. *EMBO J* 1995;14:5100.

228. Symons JA, Alcami A, Smith GL. Vaccinia virus encodes a soluble type I interferon receptor of novel structure and broad species-specificity. *Cell* 1995;81: 551.

229. Spriggs MK. Poxvirus-encoded soluble cytokine receptors. *Virus Res* 1994;33:1.

230. Gray PW, Leung DW, Pennica D, et al. Expression of human immune interferon cDNA in *E. coli* and monkey cells. *Nature* 1982;295:503.

231. Bach EA, Aguet M, Schreiber RD. The IFNγ receptor: a paradigm for cytokine receptor signaling. *Annu Rev Immunol* 1997;15:563.

232. Marsters SA, Pennica D, Bach E, Schreiber RD, Ashkenazi A. Interferon γ signals via a high-affinity multisubunit receptor complex that contains two types of polypeptide chain. *Proc Natl Acad Sci USA* 1995;92:5401.

233. Aguet M, Dembic Z, Merlin G. Molecular cloning and expression of the human interferon-γ receptor. *Cell* 1988;55:273.

234. Soh J, Donnelly RJ, Kotenko S, et al. Identification and sequence of an accessory factor required for activation of the human interferon γ receptor. *Cell* 1994; 76:793.

235. Hemmi S, Bohni R, Stark G, Di Marco F, Aguet M. A novel member of the interferon receptor family complements functionality of the murine interferon γ receptor in human cells. *Cell* 1994;76:803.

236. Kaplan DH, Greenlund AC, Tanner JW, Shaw AS, Schreiber RD. Identification of an interferon-γ receptor α chain sequence required for JAK-1 binding. *J Biol Chem* 1996;271:9.

237. Sakatsume M, Igarashi K, Winestock KD, Garotta G, Larner AC, Finbloom DS. The Jak kinases differentially associate with the α and β (accessory factor) chains of the interferon γ receptor to form a functional receptor unit capable of activating STAT transcription factors. *J Biol Chem* 1995;270:17528.

238. Lutfalla G, Gardiner K, Uze G. A new member of the cytokine receptor gene family maps on chromosome 21 at less than 35 kb from IFNAR. *Genomics* 1993;16:366.

239. Fibbs VC, Pennica D. CRF2-4: isolation of cDNA clones encoding the human and mouse proteins. *Gene* 1997;186:97.

239a.Kotenko SV, Krause CD, Izotova LS, et al. Identification and functional characterization of a second chain of the interleukin-10 receptor complex. *EMBO J* 1997;16:5894–5903.

329b.Spencer SD, Di Marco F, Hooley J, et al. The orphan receptor CRF2-4 is an essential subunit of the interleukin-10 receptor. *J Exp Med* 1998;187:571–581.

240. Moore KW, O'Garra A, de Waal Malefyt R, Vieira P, Mosmann TR. Interleukin-10. *Annu Rev Immunol* 1993;11:165.

241. Taniyama T, Takai S, Miyazaki E, et al. The human interleukin-10 receptor gene maps to chromosome 11q23.3. *Hum Genet* 1995;95:99.

242. Ying L, de Waal Malefyt R, Briere F, et al. The EBV IL-10 homologue is a selective agonist with impaired binding to the IL-10 receptor. *J Immunol* 1997;158:604.

243. Ho AS, Liu Y, Khan TA, Hsu DH, Bazan JF, Moore KW. A receptor for interleukin 10 is related to interferon receptors. *Proc Natl Acad Sci USA* 1993;90:11267.

244. Liu Y, Wei SH, Ho AS, de Waal Malefyt R, Moore KW. Expression cloning and characterization of a human IL-10 receptor. *J Immunol* 1994;152:1821.

245. Ziemiecki A, Harpur AG, Wilks AF. Jak protein tyrosine kinases: their role in cytokine signaling. *Trends Cell Biol* 1994;4:207.

246. Darnell JE Jr, Kerr IM, Stark GR. Jak-STAT pathways and transcriptional activation in response to IFNs and other extracellular signaling proteins. *Science* 1994;264:1415.

247. Schinder C, Darnell JE Jr. Transcriptional responses to polypeptide ligands: the Jak-STAT pathway. *Annu Rev Biochem* 1995;64:621.

248. Ihle JN, Witthuhn BA, Quelle FW, Yamamoto K, Silvennoinen O. Signaling through the hematopoietic cytokine receptors. *Annu Rev Immunol* 1995;13:369.

249. Wilks AF, Oates AC. The JAK/STAT pathway. *Cancer Surv* 1996;27:139.

250. Darnell JE Jr. The JAK-STAT pathway: summary of initial studies and recent advances. *Recent Prog Horm Res* 1996;51:391.

251. Ihle JN. STATs: signal transducers and activators of transcription. *Cell* 1996;84:331.

252. Leonard WJ. Stats and cytokine specificity. *Nature Med* 1996;2:968.

253. Leonard WJ, OShea JJ. Jaks and STATS: biological implications. *Annu Rev Immunol* 1998;16:293–322.

254. Horvath CM, Darnell JE. The state of the STATs: recent developments in the study of signal transduction to the nucleus. *Curr Opin Cell Biol* 1997;9:233.

255. Wilks AF, Harpur AG, Kurban RR, Ralph SJ, Zurcher G, Ziemiecki A. Two novel protein-tyrosine kinases, each with a second phosphotransferase-related catalytic domain, define a new class of protein kinase. *Mol Cell Biol* 1991;11:2057.

256. Harpur AG, Andres AC, Ziemiecki A, Aston RR, Wilks AF. JAK2, a third member of the JAK family of protein tyrosine kinases. *Oncogene* 1992;7:1347.

257. Johnston JA, Kawamura M, Kirken RA, et al. Phosphorylation and activation of the Jak-3 Janus kinase in response to interleukin-2. *Nature* 1994;370:151.

258. Witthuhn BA, Silvennoinen O, Miura O, et al. Involvement of the Jak-3 Janus kinase in signalling by interleukins 2 and 4 in lymphoid and myeloid cells. *Nature* 1994;370:153.

259. Krolewski JJ, Lec R, Eddy R, Shows TB, Dalla-Favera R. Identification and chromosomal mapping of new human tyrosine kinase genes. *Oncogene* 1990;5:277.

260. Witthuhn BA, Quelle FW, Silvennoinen O, et al. JAK2 associates with the erythropoietin receptor and is tyrosine phosphorylated and activated following stimulation with erythropoietin. *Cell* 1993;74:227.

261. DaSilva L, Howard OMZ, Rui H, Kirken RA, Farrar WL. Growth signaling and Jak2 association mediated by membrane-proximal cytoplasmic regions of the prolactin receptor. *J Biol Chem* 1994;269:18267.

262. Gurney AL, Wong SC, Henzel WJ, de Sauvage FJ. Distinct regions of c-mpl cytoplasmic domain are coupled to the JAK-STAT signal transduction pathway and Shc phosphorylation. *Proc Natl Acad Sci USA* 1995;92:5292.

263. Tanner JW, Chen W, Young RL, Longmore GD, Shaw AS. The conserved box 1 motif of cytokine receptors is required for association with Jak kinases. *J Biol Chem* 1995;270:6523.

264. Zhao, Y, Wagner F, Frank SJ, Kraft AS. The amino-terminal portion of the Jak2 protein kinase is necessary for binding and phosphorylation of the granulocyte-macrophage colony-stimulating factor receptor β_c. *J Biol Chem* 1995;270:13814.

265. Kohlhuber F, Rogers NC, Watling D, et al. A JAK1/JAK2 chimera can sustain alpha and γ interferon responses. *Mol Cell Biol* 1997;17:695.

266. Chen M, Cheng A, Chen Y-Q, et al. The amino terminus of JAK3 is necessary and sufficient for binding to the common γ chain and confers the ability to transmit interleukin 2–mediated signals. *Proc Natl Acad Sci USA* 1997;94:6910–6915.

267. Guschin D, Rogers N, Briscoe J, et al. A major role for the protein tyrosine kinase JAK1 in the JAK/STAT signal transduction pathway in response to interleukin-6. *EMBO J* 1995;14:1421.

268. Boussiotis VA, Barber DL, Nakarai T, et al. Prevention of T cell anergy by signaling through the γ_c chain of the IL-2 receptor. *Science* 1994;266:1039.

269. Miyazaki T, Kawahara A, Fujii H, et al. Functional activation of Jak1 and Jak3 by selective association with IL-2 receptor subunits. *Science* 1994;266:1045.

270. Yin T, Tsang ML, Yang YC. JAK1 kinase forms complexes with interleukin-4 receptor and 4PS/insulin receptor substrate-1–like protein and is activated by interleukin-4 and interleukin-9 in T lymphocytes. *J Biol Chem* 1994;269:26614.

271. Demoulin J-P, Uyttenhove C, van Roost E, et al. A single tyrosine of the interleukin-9 (IL-9) receptor is required for STAT activation, antiapoptoic activity, and growth regulation by IL-9. *Mol Cell Biol* 1996;16:4710.

272. Zhuang H, Patil SV, He T-C, Sonsteby SK, Niu Z, Wojchowski DM. Inhibition of erythropoietin-induced mitogenesis by a kinase-deficient form of Jak2. *J Biol Chem* 1994;269:21411.

273. Frank SJ, Yi W, Zhao Y, et al. Regions of the JAK2 tyrosine kinase required for coupling to the growth hormone receptor. *J Biol Chem* 1995;270:14776.

274. Kawahara A, Minami Y, Ihle JN, Taniguchi T. Critical role of the interleukin 2 (IL-2) receptor γ-chain-associated Jak3 in the IL-2 induced c-fos and c-myc but not bcl-2 induction. *Proc Natl Acad Sci USA* 1995;92:8724.

275. Macchi P, Villa A, Gillani S, et al. Mutations of Jak-3 gene in patients with autosomal severe combined immune deficiency (SCID). *Nature* 1995;377:65.

276. Russell SM, Tayebi N, Nakajima H, et al. Mutation of Jak3 in a patient with SCID: essential role of Jak3 in lymphoid development. *Science* 1995;270:797.

277. Thomis DC, Gurniak CB, Tivol E, Sharpe AH, Berg LJ. Defects in B lymphocyte maturation and T lymphocyte activation in mice lacking Jak3. *Science* 1995;270:794–797.

278. Nosaka T, van Deursen JMA, Tripp RA, et al. Defective lymphoid development in mice lacking Jak3. *Science* 1995;270:800–802.

279. Park SY, Saijo K, Takahash T, et al. Developmental defects of lymphoid cells in Jak3 kinase-deficient mice. *Immunity* 1995;3:771–82.

280. Luo H, Hanratty WP, Dearolf CR. An amino acid substitution in the Drosophila hop^Tum-l Jak kinase causes leukemia-like hematopoietic defects. *EMBO J* 1995;14:1412.

281. Harrison DA, Binari R, Nahreini TS, Gilman M, Perrimon N. Activation of a Drosophila Janus kinase (JAK) causes hematopoietic neoplasia and developmental defects. *EMBO J* 1995;14:2857.

282. Conway G, Margoliath A, Wong-Madden S, Roberts RJ, Gilbert W. Jak1 kinase is required for cell migrations and anterior specification in zebrafish embryos. *Proc Natl Acad Sci USA* 1997;94:3082.

283. Migone T-S, Lin J-X, Cereseto A, et al. Constitutively activated Jak-STAT pathway in T cells transformed with HTLV-I. *Science* 1995;269:79.

284. Danial NN, Pernis A, Rothman PB. Jak-STAT signaling induced by the v-abl oncogene. *Science* 1995;269:1875.

285. Ohashi T, Masuda M, Ruscetti SK. Induction of sequence-specific DNA-binding factors by erythropoietin and the spleen focus-forming virus. *Blood* 1995;84:1454–1462.

286. Yu CL, Meyer DJ, Campbell GS, et al. Enhanced DNA-binding activity of a Stat3-related protein in cells transformed by the Src oncoprotein. *Science* 1995;269:81.

287. Meydan N, Grunberger T, Dadi H, et al. Inhibition of acute lymphoblastic leukaemia by a Jak-2 inhibitor. *Nature* 1996;379:645.

288. Nelson BH, McIntosh BC, Rosencrans LL, Greenberg PD. Requirement for an intial signal from the membrane-proximal region of the interleukin 2 receptor γ_c chain for Janus kinase activation leading to T cell proliferation. *Proc Natl Acad Sci USA* 1997;94:1878.

289. Hanissian SH, Geha RS. Jak3 is associated with CD40 and is critical for CD40 induction of gene expression in B cells. *Immunity* 1997;6:379.

290. Briscoe J, Rogers NC, Witthuhn BA, et al. Kinase-negative mutants of JAK1 can sustain interferon-γ inducible gene expression but not an antiviral state. *EMBO J* 1996;15:799.

291. Gauzzi MC, Velazaquez L, McKendry R, Mogensen KE, Fellous M, Pellegrini S. Interferon-α–dependent activation of Tyk2 requires phosphorylation of positive regulatory tyrosines by another kinase. *J Biol Chem* 1996;271:20494.

292. Feng J, Witthuhn BA, Matsuda T, Kohlhuber F, Kerr IM, Ihle JN. Activation of Jak2 catalytic activity requires phosphorylation of Y1007 in the kinase activation loop. *Mol Cell Biol* 1997;17:2497.

293. Kohlhuber F, Rogers NC, Watling D, et al. A JAK1/JAK2 chimera can sustain alpha and γ interferon responses. *Mol Cell Biol* 1997;17:695.

294. Luo H, Rose P, Barber D, et al. Mutation in the Jak kinase JH2 domain hyperactivates Drosophila and mammalian Jak-Stat pathways. *Mol Cell Biol* 1997;17:1562.

295. Fujitani Y, Hibi M, Fukada T, et al. An alternative pathway for STAT activation that is mediated by the direct interaction between JAK and STAT. *Oncogene* 1997;14:751–761.

296. Binari R, Perrimon N. Stripe-specific regulation of pair-rule genes by hopscotch, a putative Jak family tyrosine kinase in Drosophila. *Genes Dev* 1994;8:300.

297. Lai KS, Jin Y, Graham DK, Witthuhn BA, Ihle JN, Liu ET. A kinase-deficient splice variant of the human JAK3 is expressed in hematopoietic and epithelial cancer cells. *J Biol Chem* 1995;270:25028.

298. Cance WG, Craven RJ, Weiner TM, Liu ET. Novel protein kinases expressed in human breast cancer. *Int J Cancer* 1993;54:571.

299. Fu XY. A transcription factor with SH2 and SH3 domains is directly activated by an interferon alpha-induced cytoplasmic protein tyrosine kinase(s). *Cell* 1992;70:323.

300. Fu XY, Schindler C, Improta T, Aebersold R, Darnell JE. The proteins of ISGF-3, the interferon alpha-induced transcriptional activator, define a gene family involved in signal transduction. *Proc Natl Acad Sci USA* 1992;89:7840.

301. Zhong Z, Wen Z, Darnell JE Jr. Stat3: a STAT family member activated by tyrosine phosphorylation in response to epidermal growth factor and interleukin-6. *Science* 1994;264:95.

302. Akira S, Nishio Y, Inoue M, et al. Molecular cloning of APRF, a novel IFN-stimulated gene factor 3 p91-related transcription factor involved in the gp130-mediated signaling pathway. *Cell* 1994;77:63.

303. Zhong Z, Wen Z, Darnell JE, Jr. Stat3 and Stat4: members of the family of signal transducers and activators of transcription. *Proc Natl Acad Sci USA* 1994;91:4806.

304. Yamamoto K, Quelle FW, Thierfelder WE, et al. Stat4, a novel γ interferon activation site-binding protein expressed in early myeloid differentiation. *Mol Cell Biol* 1994;14:4342.

305. Wakao H, Gouilleux F, Groner B. Mammary gland factor (MGF) is a novel member of the cytokine regulated transcription factor gene family and confers the prolactin response. *EMBO J* 1994;13:2182.

306. Hou J, Schindler U, Henzel WJ, Wong SC, McKnight SL. Identification and purification of human Stat proteins activated in response to interleukin-2. *Immunity* 1995;2:321.

307. Mui AL, Wakao H, O'Farrell A, Harada N, Miyajima A. Interleukin-3, granulocytes-macrophage colony stimulating factor and interleukin-5 signal through two STAT5 homologs. *EMBO J* 1995;14:1166.

308. Azam M, Erdjument-Bromage H, Kreider BL, et al. Interleukin-3 signals through multiple isoforms of Stat5. *EMBO J* 1995;14:1402.

309. Liu X, Robinston GW, Gouilleux F, Groner B, Hennighausen L. Cloning and expression of Stat5 and an additional homolgue (Stat5b) involved in prolactin signal transduction in mouse mammary tissue. *Proc Natl Acad Sci USA* 1995;92:8831.

310. Lin J-X, Mietz J, Modi WS, John S, Leonard WJ. Cloning of human Stat5B: reconstitution of interleukin-2–induced Stat5A and Stat5B DNA binding activity in COS-7 cells. *J Biol Chem* 1996;271:10738.

311. Hou J, Schindler U, Henzel WJ, Ho TC, Brasseur M, McKnight SL. An interleukin-4 induced transcription factor: IL-4 Stat. *Science* 1994;265:1701.

312. Wang D, Stravopodis D, Teglund S, Kitazawa J, Ihle JN. Naturally occurring dominant negative variants of Stat5. *Mol Cell Biol* 1996;16:6141–6148.

313. Copeland NG, Gilbert DJ, Schindler C, et al. Distribution of the mammalian Stat gene family in mouse chromosomes. *Genomics* 1995;29:225.

314. Greenlund AC, Farrar MA, Viviano BL, Schreiber RD. Ligand induced IFNγ receptor phosphorylation couples the receptor to its signal transduction system (p91). *EMBO J* 1994;13:1591.

315. Yan H, Krishnan K, Greenlund AC, et al. Phosphorylated interferon-alpha receptor 1 subunit (IFNαR1) acts as a docking site for the latent form of the 113 kDa STAT2 protein. *EMBO J* 1996;15:1064.

316. Stahl N, Farruggella TJ, Boulton TG, Zhong Z, Darnell JE Jr, Yancopoulos GD. Choice of STATs and other substrates specified by modular tyrosine-based motifs in cytokine receptors. *Science* 1995;267:1349.

317. Friedmann MC, Migone T-S, Russell SM, Leonard WJ. Different interleukin 2 receptor β-chain tyrosines couple to at least two signaling pathways and synergistically mediate interleukin 2–induced proliferation. *Proc Natl Acad Sci USA* 1996;93:2077.

318. Schindler U, Wu P, Rother M, Brasseur M, McKnight SL. Components of a Stat recognition code: evidence for two layers of molecular selectivity. *Immunity* 1995;2:686.

319. Klingmuller U, Bergelson S, Hsiao JG, Lodish HF. Multiple tyrosine residues in the cytosolic domain of the erythropoietin receptor promote activation of STAT5. *Proc Natl Acad Sci USA* 1996;93:8324.

320. Weber-Nordt RM, Riley JK, Greenlund AC, Moore KW, Darnell JE, Schreiber RD. Stat3 recruitment by two distinct ligand-induced, tyrosine-phosphorylated docking sites in the interleukin-10 receptor intracellular domain. *J Biol Chem* 1996;271:27954.

321. Xu X, Sun Y-L, Hoey T. Cooperative DNA binding and sequence-selective recognition conferred by the STAT amino-terminal domain. *Science* 1996;273:794.

322. Vinkemeier U, Cohen SL, Moarefi I, Chait BT, Kuriyan J, Darnell JE Jr. DNA binding of in vitro activated Stat1 alpha, Stat1 beta and truncated Stat1: interaction between NH2-terminal domains stabilizes binding of two dimers to tandem DNA sites. *EMBO J* 1996;15:5616.

323. Sperisen P, Wang SM, Soldaini E, et al. Mouse interleukin-2 receptor α gene expression. Interleukin-1 and interleukin-2 control transcription via distinct cis-acting elements. *J Biol Chem* 1995;270:10743.

324. John S, Robbins CM, Leonard WJ. An IL-2 response element in the human IL-2 receptor α chain promoter is a composite element that binds Stat5, Elf-1, HMG-I(Y), and a GATA family protein. *EMBO J* 1996;15:5627.

325. Lecine P, Algarte M, Rameil P, et al. Elf-1 and Stat5 bind to a critical element in a new enhancer of the human interleukin-2 receptor α gene. *Mol Cell Biol* 1996;16:6829.

326. Zhang, X, Blenis, Li HC, Schindler C, Chen-Kiang S. Requirement of serine phosphorylation for formation of STAT-promoter complexes. *Science* 1995;267:1990.

327. Wen Z, Zhong Z, Darnell JE Jr. Maximal activation of transcription by Stat1 and Stat3 requires both tyrosine and serine phosphorylation. *Cell* 1995;82:241.

328. Horvath CM, Darnell JE Jr. The antiviral state induced by alpha interferon and γ interferon requires transcriptionally active Stat1 protein. *J Virol* 1996;70:647.

329. Morrigl R, Berchtold S, Friedrich K, et al. Comparison of the transactivation domains of Stat5 and Stat6 in lymphoid cells and mammary epithelial cells. *Mol Cell Biol* 1997;17:3663.

330. David M, Petricon E III, Benjamin C, Pine R, Weber MJ, Larner AC. Requirement for MAP kinase (ERK2) activity in interferon alpha and interferon beta stimulated gene expression through Stat proteins. *Science* 1995;269:1721.

331. Look DC, Pelletier MR, Tidwell RM, Roswit WT, Holtzman MJ. Stat1 depends on transcriptional synergy with Sp1. *J Biol Chem* 1995;270:30264.

332. Schaefer TS, Sanders LK, Nathans D. Cooperative transcriptional activity of Jun and Stat3 beta, a short form of Stat3. *Proc Natl Acad Sci USA* 1995;92:9097.

333. Bhattacharya S, Eckner R, Grossman S, et al. Cooperation of Stat2 and p300/CBP in signalling induced by interferon-α. *Nature* 1996;383:344.

334. Zhang JJ, Vinkemeier U, Gu W, Chakravarti D, Horvath CM, Darnell JE Jr. Two contact regions between Stat1 and CBP/p300 in interferon γ signaling. *Proc Natl Acad Sci USA* 1996;93:15092.

335. Horvai AE, Xu L, Korzus E, et al. Nuclear integration of JAK/STAT and Ras/AP-1 signaling by CBP and p300. *Proc Natl Acad Sci USA* 1997;94:1074.

336. Stocklin E, Wissler M, Gouilleux F, Groner B. Functional interactions between Stat5 and the glucocorticoid receptor. *Nature* 1996;383:726–728.

337. Meraz MA, White JM, Sheehan KC, et al. Targeted disruption of the Stat1 gene in mice reveals unexpected physiologic specificity in the JAK-STAT signaling pathway. *Cell* 1996;84:431.

338. Durbin JE, Hackenmiller R, Simon MC, Levy DE. Targeted disruption of the mouse Stat1 gene results in compromised immunity to viral disease. *Cell* 1996;84:443.

339. Takeda K, Noguchi K, Shi W, et al. Targeted disruption of the mouse Stat3 gene leads to early embryonic lethality. *Proc Natl Acad Sci USA* 1997;94:3801.

340. Thierfelder WE, van Deursen J, Yamamoto K, et al. Requirement for Stat4 in interleukin-12–mediated responses of natural killer cells. *Nature* 1996;382:171.

341. Kaplan MH, Sun Y-L, Hoey T, Grusby MJ. Impaired IL-12 responses and enhanced development of Th2 cells in Stat4-deficient mice. *Nature* 1996;382:174.

342. Kaplan MH, Schindler U, Smiley ST, Grusby MJ. Stat6 is required for mediating responses to IL-4 and for the development of Th2 cells. *Immunity* 1996;4:313.

343. Takeda K, Tanaka T, Shi W, et al. Essential role of Stat6 in IL-4 signalling. *Nature* 1996;380:627.

344. Shimoda K, van Deursen J, Sangster MY, et al. Lack of IL-4–induced Th2 response and IgE class switching in mice with disrupted Stat6 gene. *Nature* 1996;380:630.

345. Liu X, Robinson GW, Wagner K-U, Garrett L, Wynshaw-Boris A, Hennighausen L. Stat5a is mandatory for adult mammary gland development and lactogenesis. *Genes Dev* 1997;11:179.

346. Udy GB, Towers RP, Snell RG, et al. Requirement of STAT5b for sexual dimorphism of body growth rates and liver gene expression. *Proc Natl Acad Sci USA* 1997;94:7239–7244.

346a.Nakajima H, Liu X-W, Wynshaw-Boris A, et al. An indirect effect of STAT5A in IL-2-induced proliferation: A critical role for STAT5a in IL-2-mediated IL-2 receptor α chain induction. *Immunity* 1997;7:691–701.

347. Hou XS, Melnick MB, Perrimon N. Marelle acts downstream of the Drosophila HOP/JAK kinase and encodes a protein similar to the mammalian STATs. *Cell* 1996;84:411.

348. Yan R, Small S, Desplan C, Dearolf R, Darnell JE Jr. Identification of a Stat gene that functions in Drosophila development. *Cell* 1996;84:421.

349. Kawata T, Shevchenko A, Fukuzawa M, et al. SH2 signaling in a lower eukaryote: a STAT protein that regulates stalk cell differentiation in Dictyostelium. *Cell* 1997;89:909.

350. Mui A, Wakao H, Kinosha T, Kitamura T, Miyajima A. Suppression of interleukin-3–induced gene expression by a C-terminal truncated Stat5: role of Stat5 in proliferation. *EMBO J* 1995;15:2425.

351. Goldsmith MA, Lai SY, Xu W, et al. Growth signal transduction by the human interleukin-2 receptor requires cytoplasmic tyrosines of the β chain and non-tyrosine residues of the γc chain. *J Biol Chem* 1995;270:21729.

352. Quelle FW, Wang D, Nosaka T, et al. Erythropoietin induces activation of Stat5 through association with specific tyrosines on the receptor that are not required for a mitogenic response. *Mol Cell Biol* 1996;16:1622.

353. Damen JE, Wakao H, Miyajima A, et al. Tyrosine 343 in the erythropoietin receptor positively regulates erythropoietin-induced cell proliferation and Stat5 activation. *EMBO J* 1995;14:5557–5568.

354. Ascherman DP, Migone T-S, Friedmann M, Leonard WJ. Interleukin-2 (IL-2)–mediated induction of the IL-2 receptor α chain gene: critical role of two functionally redundant tyrosine residues in the IL-2 receptor β chain cytoplasmic domain and suggestion that these residues mediate more than Stat5 activation. *J Biol Chem* 1997;272:8704.

355. Chin YE, Kitagawa M, Su WC, You ZH, Iwamoto Y, Fu XY. Cell growth arrest and induction of cyclin-dependent kinase inhibitor p21 WAF1/CIP1 mediated by STAT1. *Science* 1996;272:719.

356. Su W-C S, Kitagawa M, Xue N, et al. Activation of Stat1 by mutant fibroblast growth-factor receptor in thanatrophoric dysplasia type II dwarfism. *Nature* 1997;386:288.

357. Pfeffer LM, Mullersman JE, Pfeffer SR, Murti A, Shi W, Yang CH. STAT3 as an adapter to couple phosphatidylinositol 3-kinase to the IFNAR1 chain of the type I interferon receptor. *Science* 1997;276:1418.

358. Dent AL, Shaffer AL, Yu X, Allman D, Staudt LM. Control of inflammation, cytokine expression and germinal center formation by BCL-6. *Science* 1997;276:589.

359. Baldwin AS Jr. The NF-κB and IκB proteins: new discoveries and insights. *Annu Rev Immunol* 1996;14:649.

360. Lee FS, Hagler J, Chen ZJ, Maniatis T. Activation of the IkappaB alpha kinase complex by MEKK1, a kinase of the JNK pathway. *Cell* 1997;88:213.

361. Rao A, Luo C, Hogan PG. Transcription factors of the NFAT family. *Annu Rev Immunol* 1997;15:707.

362. Crabtree GR, Clipstone NA. Signal transmission betwen the plasma membrane and nucleus of T-lymphocytes. *Annu Rev Biochem* 1994;63:1045.

363. Takeshita T, Arita T, Higuchi M, et al. STAM, signal transducing adaptor molecule, is associated with Janus kinases and involved in signaling for cell growth and c-myc induction. *Immunity* 1997;6:449.

364. Horak ID, Gress RE, Lucas PJ, Horak EM, Waldmann TA, Bolen JB. T-lymphocyte interleukin 2-dependent tyrosine protein kinase signal transduction involves the activation of p56^lck. *Proc Natl Acad Sci USA* 1991;88:1996.

365. Hatakeyama M, Kono T, Kobayash N, et al. Interaction of the IL-2 receptor with the src-family kinase p56^lck: identification of novel intermolecular association. *Science* 1991;252:1523.

366. Torigo T, Saragovi HU, Reed JC. Interleukin-2 regulates the activity of the lyn protein tyrosine kinase in a B-cell line. *Proc Natl Acad Sci USA* 1992;89:2674.

367. Kobayashi N, Kono T, Hatakeyama M, et al. Functional coupling of the src-family protein tyrosine kinases p59fyn and p53/56lyn with the interleukin 2 receptor: implications for redundancy and pleiotropism in cytokine signal transduction. *Proc Natl Acad Sci USA* 1993;90:4201.

368. Minami Y, Nakagawa Y, Kawahara A, et al. Protein tyrosine kinase Syk is associated with and activated by the IL-2 receptor: possible link with the c-myc induction pathway. *Immunity* 1995;2.89.

369. Otani H, Siegel JP, Erdos M, et al. Interleukin (IL)-2 and IL-3 induce distinct but overlapping responses in murine IL-3 dependent 32D cells transduced with human IL-2 receptor β chain: involvement of tyrosine kinases other than p56^lck. *Proc Natl Acad Sci USA* 1992;89;2789.

370. Karnitz L, Sutor SL, Torigoe T, et al. Effects of p56lck deficiency on the growth and cytolytic effector function of an interleukin-2-dependent cytotoxic T-cell line. *Mol Cell Biol* 1992;12:4521.

371. Hatakeyama M, Mori H, Doi T, Taniguchi T. A restricted cytoplasmic region of IL-2 receptor β chain is essential for growth signal transduction but not for ligand binding and internalization. *Cell* 1989;59:837.

372. Ravichandran KS, Igras V, Shoelson SE, Fesik SW, Burakoff SJ. Evidence for a role for the phosphotyrosine-binding domain of Shc in interleukin 2 signaling. *Proc Natl Acad Sci USA* 1996;93:5275.

373. Turner M, Mee PJ, Costello PS, et al. Perinatal lethality and blocked B-cell development in mice lacking the tyrosine kinase Syk. *Nature* 1995;378:298.

374. Corey SJ, Burkhardt AL, Bolen JB, Geahlem RL, Tkatch LS, Tweardy DJ. Granulocyte colony-stimulating factor receptor signaling involves the formation of a three-component complex with lyn and syk protein tyrosine kinases. *Proc Natl Acad Sci USA* 1994;91:4683.

375. Rao P, Mufson RA. A membrane proximal domain of the human interleukin-3 receptor β_c subunit that signals DNA synthesis in NIH 3T3 cells specifically binds a complex of src and Janus family tyrosine kinases and phosphatidylinositol 3-kinase. *J Biol Chem* 1995;270:6886.

376. Ernst M, Gearing DP, Dunn AR. Functional and biochemical association of Hck with the LIF/IL-6 receptor signal transducing subunit gp130 in embryonic stem cells. *EMBO J* 1994;13:1574.

377. Matsuda T, Fukada T, Takahashi-Tezuka M, et al. Activation of Fes tyrosine kinase by gp130, an interleukin-6 family cytokine signal transducer, and their association. *J Biol Chem* 1995;270:11037.

378. Matsuda T, Takahashi-Tezuka M, Fukada T, et al. Association and activation of Btk and Tec tyrosine kinases by gp130, a signal transducer of the interleukin-6 family of cytokines. *Blood* 1995;85:627.

379. Izuhara K, Feldman RA, Greer P, Harada N. Interaction of the c-fes proto-oncogene product with the interleukin-4 receptor. *J Biol Chem* 1994;269:18623.

380. Myers MG Jr, White MF. Insulin signal transduction and the IRS proteins. *Annu Rev Pharmacol Toxicol* 1996;36:615.

381. Wang L-M, Keegan AD, Li W, et al. Common elements in interleukin 4 and insulin signaling pathways in factor-dependent hematopoietic cells. *Proc Natl Acad Sci USA* 1993;90.4032.

382. Wang L-M, Myers MG Jr, Sun S-J, Aaronson SA, White M, Pierce JH. IRS-1: essential for insulin- and IL-4-stimulated mitogenesis in hematopoietic cells. *Science* 1993;261:1591.

383. Keegan AD, Nelms K, White M, Wang L-M, Pierce JH, Paul WE. An IL-4 receptor region containing an insulin receptor motif is important for IL-4 mediated IRS-1 phosphorylation and cell growth. *Cell* 1994;76:811.

384. Ridderstrale M, Degerman E, Tornqvist H. Growth hormone stimulates the tyrosine phosphorylation of the insulin receptor substrate-1 and its association with phosphatidylinositol 3-kinase in primary adipocytes. *J Biol Chem* 1995;270:3471.

385. Argetsinger LS, Norstedt G, Billestrup N, White MF, Carter-Su C. Growth hormone, interferon-γ, and leukemia inhibitory factor utilize insulin receptor substrate-2 in intracellular signaling. *J Biol Chem* 1996;271:29415.

386. Johnston JA, Wang LM, Hanson EP, et al. Interleukins 2, 4, 7, and 15 stimulate tyrosine phosphorylation of insulin receptor substrates 1 and 2 in T cells. Potential role of JAK kinases. *J Biol Chem* 1995;270:28527.

387. Kapeller R, Cantley LC. Phosphatidylinositol 3-kinase. *Bioessays* 1994;16:565.

388. Truitt KE, Mills GB, Turck CW, Imboden JB. SH2-dependent association of phosphatidylinositol 3'-kinase 85-kDa regulatory subunit with the interleukin-2 receptor β chain. *J Biol Chem* 1994;269:5937.

389. Damen JE, Cutler RL, Jiao H, Yi T, Krystal G. Phosphorylation of tyrosine 503 in the erythropoietin receptor (EpR) is essential for binding of the p85 subunit of phosphatidylinositol (PI) 3-kinase and for EpR-associated PI 3-kinase activity. *J Biol Chem* 1995;270:23402.

390. Jucker M, Feldman RA. Identification of a new adapter protein that may link the common β subunit of the receptor for granulocyte/macrophage colong stimulating factor, interleukin-3 (IL-3), and IL-5 to phosphatidylinositol 3-kinase. *J Biol Chem* 1995;270:27817.

391. Karnitz LM, Burns LA, Sutor SL, Blenis J, Abraham RT. Interleukin-2 triggers a novel phosphatidylinositol 3-kinase-dependent MEK activation pathway. *Mol Cell Biol* 1995;15:3049.

392. Neel BG, Tonks NK. Protein tyrosine phosphatases in signal transduction. *Curr Opin Cell Biol* 1997;9:193.

393. Denu JE, Stuckey JA, Saper MA, Dixon JE. Form and function of protein dephosphorylation. *Cell* 1996;87:361.

394. Tsui HW, Siminovitch KA, de Souza L, Tsui FW. Motheaten and viable motheaten mice have mutations in the haematopoietic cell phosphatase gene. *Nat Genet* 1993;4:124.

395. Shultz LD, Schweitzer PA, Rajan TV, et al. Mutations at the murine motheaten locus are within the hematopoietic cell protein-tyrosine phosphatase (Hcph) gene. *Cell* 1993;73:1445.

396. van Zant G, Schultz L. Hematologic abnormalities of the immunodeficient mouse mutant, viable motheaten (mcV). *Exp Hematol* 1989;17;81.

397. Klingmuller U, Lorenz U, Cantley LC, Neel BG, Lodish HF. Specific recruitment of SH-PTP1 to the erythropoietin receptor causes inactivation of JAK2 and termination of proliferative signals. *Cell* 1995;80:729.

398. Yi T, Mui AL, Krystal G, Ihle JN. Hematopoietic cell phosphatase associates with the interleukin-3 (IL-3) receptor β chain and down-regulates IL-3 induced tyrosine phosphorylation and mitogenesis. *Mol Cell Biol* 1993;13:7577.

399. Yetter A, Uddin S, Krolewski JJ, Jiao H, Yi T, Platanias LC. Association of the interferon-dependent tyrosine kinase Tyk-2 with the hematopoietic cell phosphatase. *J Biol Chem* 1995;270:18179.

400. Jiao H, Berrada K, Yang W, Tabrizi M, Platanias LC, Yi T. Direct association with and dephosphorylation of Jak2 kinase by the SH2-domain-containing protein tyrosine phosphatase SHP-1. *Mol Cell Biol* 1996;16.6985.

401. Yin T, Shen R, Feng GS, Yang YC. Molecular characterization of specific interactions between SHP 2 phosphatase and JAK tyrosine kinases. *J Biol Chem* 1997;272:1032–1037.

402. Haspel RL, Salditt-Georgieff M, Darnell JE Jr. The rapid inactivation of nuclear tyrosine phosphorylated Stat1 depends upon a protein tyrosine phosphatase. *EMBO J* 1996;15:6262.

403. Damen JE, Liu L, Rosten P, Humphries RK, Jefferson AB, Majerus PW, Krystal G. The 145-kDa protein induced to associate with Shc by multiple cytokines is an inositol tetraphosphate and phosphatidylinositol 3,4,5,-trisphosphate 5-phosphatase. *Proc Natl Acad Sci USA* 1996;93:1689.

404. Ware MD, Rosten P, Damen JE, Liu L, Humphries RK, Krystal G. Cloning and characterization of human SHIP, the 145-kD inositol 5-phosphatase that associates with SHC after cytokine stimulation. *Blood* 1996;88:2833.

405. Kim TK, Maniatis T. Regulation of interferon γ activated STAT1 by the ubiquitin-proteasome pathway. *Science* 1996;273:1717.

405a. Noguchi M, Sarin A, Aman MJ, et al. Functional cleavage of the common cytokine receptor γ chain (γ_c) by calpain. *Proc Natl Acad Sci USA* 1997;94:11534–11539.

406. Yoshimura A, Ohkubo T, Kiguchi T, et al. A novel cytokine-inducible gene CIS encodes an SH2-containing protein that binds to tyrosine-phosphorylated interleukin 3 and erythropoietin receptors. *EMBO J* 1995;14:2816.

407. Matsumoto A, Masuhara M, Mitsui K, et al. CIS, a cytokine inducible SH2 protein, is a target of the JAK-STAT5 pathway and modulates STAT5 activation. *Blood* 1997;89:3148.

408. Starr R, Willson TA, Viney EM, et al. A family of cytokine-inducible inhibitors of signalling. *Nature* 1997;387:917–921.

409. Endo TA, Masuhara M, Yokouchi M, et al. A new protein containing an SH2 domain that inhibits JAK kinases. *Nature* 1997;387:921–924.

410. Naka T, Narazaki M, Hirata M, et al. Structure and function of a new STAT-induced STAT inhibitor. *Nature* 1997;387:924–929.

410a. Aman MJ, Leonard WJ. Cytokine signaling: Cytokine inducible signaling inhibitors. *Curr Biol* 1997;12:R784.

410b. Hilton DJ, Richardson RT, Alexander WS, et al. Twenty proteins containing a C-terminal SOCS box from five structural classes. *Proc Natl Acad Sci USA* 1998; 95:114-119.

411. Mossmann TR, Cherwinski H, Bond MW, Giedlin MA, Coffman RL. Two types of murine helper T cell clones. 1. Definition according to profiles of lymphokine activities and secreted proteins. *J Immunol* 1986;136:2348.

412. Mosmann TR, Sad S. The expanding universe of T-cell subsets: Th1, Th2 and more. *Immunol Today* 1996;17:138.

413. Abbas AK, Murphy KM, Sher A. Functional diversity of helper T lymphocytes. *Nature* 1996;383:787.

414. Lucey DR, Clerici M, Shearer GM. Type 1 and type 2 cytokine dysregulation in human infectious, neoplastic, and inflammatory diseases. *Clin Microbiol Rev* 1996;9:532.

415. Maggi E, Mazzetti M, Ravina A, et al. Ability of HIV to promote a Th1 to Th0 shift and to replicate preferentially in Th2 and Th0 cells. *Science* 1994;265:244.

416. Okamura H, Tsutsi H, Komatsu T, et al. Cloning of a new cytokine that induces IFN-γ production by T cells. *Nature* 1995;378:88–91.

417. Gu Y, Kuida K, Tsutsui H, et al. Activation of interferon-γ inducing factor mediated by interleukin-1 β converting enzyme. *Science* 1997;;275:206–209.

418. Ghayur T, Banerjee S, Hugunin M, et al. Caspase-1 processes IFN-γ–inducing factor and regulates LPS-induced IFN-γ production. *Nature* 1997;386:619-23.

419. Ho IC, Hodge MR, Rooney JW, Glimcher LH. The proto-oncogene c-maf is responsible for tissue-specific expression of interleukin-4. *Cell* 1996;85:973.

420. Hodge MR, Chun HJ, Rengarajan J, Alt A, Lieberson R, Glimcher LH. NF-AT-driven interleukin-4 transcription potentiated by NIP45. *Science* 1996;274:1903.

421. Gajewski TF, Fitch FW. Anti-proliferative effect of IFN-γ in immune regulation. I IFN-γ inhibits the proliferation of Th2 but not Th1 murine helper T lymphocyte clones. *J Immunol* 1988;140:4245.

422. Pernis A, Gupta S, Gollob KJ, et al. Lack of interferon γ receptor β chain and the prevention of interferon γ signaling in TH1 cells. *Science* 1995;269:245.

423. Bach EA, Szabo SJ, Dighe AS, et al. Ligand-induced regulation of IFN-γ receptor β chain expression in T helper cell subsets. *Science* 1995;270:1215.

424. Szabo SJ, Dighe AS, Gubler U, Murphy KM. Regulation of the interleukin (IL)-12Rβ2 subunit expression in developing T helper 1 (Th1) and Th2 cells. *J Exp Med* 1997;185:817.

425. Hu-Li J, Huang H, Ryan J, Paul WE. In differentiated CD4⁺ T cells, interleukin 4 production is cytokine-autonomous, whereas interferon γ production is cytokine-dependent. *Proc Natl Acad Sci USA* 1997;94:3189–3194.

426. d'Andrea AD. Cytokine receptors in congenital hematopoietic disease. *N Engl J Med* 1994;330:839.

427. Amselem S, Duquesnoy P, Attree O, et al. Laron dwarfism and mutations of the growth hormone receptor gene. *N Engl J Med* 1989;321:989.

428. Dong F, Hoefsloot LH, Schelen AM, et al. Identification of a nonsense mutation in the granulocyte-colony-stimulating factor receptor in severe congenital neutropenia. *Proc Natl Acad Sci USA* 1994;91:4480.

429. de la Chapelle A, Traskelin AL, Juvonen E. Truncated erythropoietin receptor causes dominantly inherited benign human erythrocytosis. *Proc Natl Acad Sci USA* 1993;90:4495.

430. Souyri M, Vigon I, Penciolelli J-F, Heard J-M, Tambourin P, Wendling F. A putative truncated cytokine receptor gene transduced by the myeloproliferative leukemia virus immortalizes hematopoietic progenitors. *Cell* 1990;63:1137.

431. Kundig TM, Schorle H, Bachmann MF, Hengartner H, Zinkernagel RM, Horak I. Immune responses in interleukin-2–deficient mice. *Science* 1993;262:1059–1061.

432. Sadlack B, Merz H, Schorle H, Schimpl A, Feller AC, Horak I. Ulcerative colitis-like disease in mice with a disrupted interleukin-2 gene. *Cell* 1993;75:253–261.

433. Kopf M, Brombacher F, Hodgkin PD, et al. IL-5–deficient mice have a developmental defect in CD5⁺ B-1 cells and lack eosinophilia but have normal antibody and cytotoxic T cell responses. *Immunity* 1996;4:15–24.

434. Dranoff G, Crawford AD, Sadelain M, et al. Involvement of granulocyte-macrophage colony-stimulating factor in pulmonary homeostasis. *Science* 1994;264:713–716.

435. Stanley E, Lieschke GJ, Grail D, et al. Granulocyte/macrophage colony-stimulating factor–deficient mice show no major perturbation of hematopoiesis but develop a characteristic pulmonary pathology. *Proc Natl Acad Sci USA* 1994;91:5592–5596.

436. Nishinakamura R, Nakayama N, Hirabayashi Y, et al. Mice deficient for the IL-3/GM-CSF/IL-5 βc receptor exhibit lung pathology and impaired immune response while βIL-3 receptor-deficient mice are normal. *Immunity* 1995;2:211–222.

437. Kopf M, Baumann H, Freer G, et al. Impaired immune and actue-phase responses in interleukin-6–deficient mice. *Nature* 1994;368:339–342.

438. Yoshida K, Taga T, Saito M, et al. Targeted disruption of gp130, a common signal transducer for the interleukin 6 family of cytokines, leads to myocardial and hematological disorders. *Proc Natl Acad Sci USA* 1996;93:407–411.

439. Akira S, Yosha K, Tanaka T, Taga T, Kishimoto T. Targeted disruption of the IL-6 related genes: gp130 and NF-IL6. *Immunol Rev* 1995;148:221–253.

440. Stewart CL, Kaspar P, Brunet LJ, et al. Blastocyst implantation depends on maternal expression of leukaemia inhibitory factor. *Nature* 1992;359:76–79.

441. Escary JL, Perreau J, Dum'enil D, Eziune S, Brulet P. Leukaemia inhibitory factor is necessary for maintenance of hematopoietic stem cells and thymocyte stimulation. *Nature* 1993;363:361–364.

442. Rao MS, Sun Y, Escary JL, Perreau J, Tresser S. Leukaemia inhibitory factor mediates an injury response but not a target-directed developmental transmitter switch in sympathetic neurons. *Neuron* 1993;11:1175–1185.

443. Ware CB, Horowitz MC, Renshaw BR, Hunt JS, Liggitt D. Target disruption of the low-affinity leukaemia inhibitory factor receptor gene causes placental, skeletal, neural and metabolic defects and results in perinatal death. *Development* 1995;121:1283–1299.

444. Li M, Sendtner M, Smith A. Essential function of LIF receptor in motor neurons. *Nature* 1995;378:724–727.

445. Masu Y, Wolf E, Holtmann B, Sendtner M, Brem G, Thoenen H. Disruption of the CNTG gene results in motor neuron degeneration. *Nature* 1993;365:27–32.

446. DeChiara TM, Bejsada R, Poueymirou WT, et al. Mice lacking the CNTF receptor, unlike mice lacking CNTF, exhibit profound motor neuron deficits at birth. *Cell* 1995;83:313–322.

447. Magram J, Connaughton SE, Warrier RR, et al. IL-12–deficient mice are defective in interferon-γ production and type 1 cytokine responses. *Immunity* 1996;4:471–481.

448. Wu C, Ferrante J, Gateley MK, Magram J. Characterization of IL-12 receptor β1 chain (IL-12Rβ1)-deficient mice. *J Immunol* 1997;159:1658–1665.

449. Wu H, Liu X, Jaenisch R, Lodish HF. Generation of committed erythroid BFU-E and CFU-E progenitors does not require erythropoietin or the erythropoietin receptor. *Cell* 1995;83:59–67.

450. Lin CS, Lim SK, D'Agati V, Costantini F. Differential effects of an erythropoietin receptor gene disruption on primitive and definitive erythropoiesis. *Genes Dev* 1996;10:154–164.

451. Gurney AL, Carver-Moore K, de Sauvage FJ, Moore MW. Thrombocytopenia in c-mpl deficient mice. *Science* 1994;265:1445–1447.

452. Lieschke GJ, Grail D, Hodgson G, et al. Mice lacking granulocyte colony-stimulating factor have chronic neutropenia, granulocyte and macrophage progenitor cell deficiency, and impaired neutrophil mobilization. *Blood* 1994;84:1737–1746.

453. Yoshida H, YayashS-I, Kunisada T, et al. The murine mutation osteopetrosis is in the coding region of the macrophage colony stimulating factor gene. *Nature* 1990;345:442.

454. Muller U, Steinhoff U, Reis LF, et al. Functional role of type I and type II interferons in antiviral defense. *Science* 1994;264:1918–1921.

455. van den Broek MF, Muller U, Huang S, Zinkernagel RM, Aguet M. Immune defence in mice lacking type I and/or type II interferon receptors. *Immunol Rev* 1995;148:5–18.

456. van den Broek MF, Muller U, Huang S, Aguet M, Zinkernagel RM. Antiviral defense in mice lacking both alpha/beta and γ interferon receptors. *J Virol* 1995;69:4792–4796.

457. Dalton DK, Pitts-Meek S, Keshav S, Figari IS, Bradley A, Stewart TA. Multiple defects of immune cell function in mice with disrupted interferon-γ genes. *Science* 1993;259:1739–1742.

458. Wang ZE, Reiner SL, Zheng S, Dalton DK, Locksley RM. CD4⁺ effector cells default to the Th2 pathway in interferon γ–deficient mice infected with Leishmania major. *J Exp Med* 1994;179:1367–1371.

459. Huang S, Hendriks W, Althage A, et al. Immune response in mice that lack the interferon γ receptor. *Science* 1993;259:1742–1745.

460. Kuhn R, Lohler J, Rennick D, Rajewsky K, Muller W. Interleukin-10–deficient mice develop chronic enterocolitis. *Cell* 1993;75:263–274.

461. Rodig SJ, Meraz MA, White JM, et al. Disruption of the Jak1 gene demonstrates obligatory and nonredundant roles of the Jaks in cytokine-induced biologic responses. *Cell* 1998;93:373–383.

462. Parganas E, Wang D, Stravopodis D, et al. Jak2 is essential for signaling through a variety of cytokine receptors. *Cell* 1998;93:385–395.

463. Neubauer H, Cumano A, Muller M, et al. Jak2 deficiency defines an essential developmental checkpoint in definitive hematopoiesis. *Cell* 1998;93:397–409.

Fundamental Immunology, Fourth Edition,
edited by William E. Paul
Published by Lippincott–Raven Publishers, Philadelphia 1999.

CHAPTER 22

Proinflammatory Cytokines

TNF and IL-1 Families, Chemokines, TGF-β, and Others

Teresa Krakauer, Jan Vilcek, and Joost J. Oppenheim

This chapter focuses on those intercellular mediators whose major activity is to promote innate and subsequent immunologically regulated inflammatory responses. These so-called proinflammatory cytokines therefore play vital roles in host defense, but, when present in excess or in the course of inappropriate autoimmune responses, can have self-destructive effects. Ever-increasing numbers of cytokines are being identified as contributors to host defense. Consequently, this chapter has had to be totally revised and covers the tumor necrosis factor and interleukin-1 family members, chemokines, transforming growth factor β (TGF-β), and the more recently discovered interleukins 16 and 17. This chapter emphasizes cytokine–receptor interactions, signal transduction, and the effects of gene targeting and relies on reviews and the previous edition for coverage of older literature concerning the myriad biologic effects of these intercellular signals.

T. Krakauer: Department of Immunology and Molecular Biology, USAMRIID, Fort Detrick, Frederick, Maryland 21702.

J. Vilcek: Department of Microbiology, New York University Medical Center, New York, New York 10016.

J. J. Oppenheim: Laboratory of Molecular Immunoregulation, National Cancer Institute, FDRDC, Frederick, Maryland 21702-1201.

TUMOR NECROSIS FACTOR FAMILY

Tumor necrosis factor (TNF) was originally described as a factor responsible for lipopolysaccharide (LPS)-induced hemorrhagic necrosis of tumors in animals (1) and was later independently identified as "cachectin," a factor responsible for wasting of animals during parasitic infections (2). Cloning of the TNF cDNA and purification of the TNF protein (3,4) revealed that TNF is structurally related to lymphotoxin (5,6), a product of activated T cells that is now termed LT-α. (Until recently, lymphotoxin was also termed TNF-β, and the "original" TNF was, and still is, sometimes referred to as TNF-α. Throughout this chapter, we will use the designations "TNF" and "LT-α.") Although TNF and LT-α are produced by different cells in response to different stimuli, they utilize the same receptors and thus can produce similar biologic activities (Table 1, Fig. 1). However, as will be discussed, LT-α also forms a heterocomplex with LT-β, and the latter complex utilizes a different receptor (LT-β receptor) and thus performs biologic functions different from those of LT-α alone. TNF and LT-α are the first-identified members of what has now become a large (and still growing) family of ligands and receptors (7) that also includes LT-β (8), the Fas/Apo1 receptor and its ligand (9–11), TRAIL/Apo2L

TABLE 1. *Tumor necrosis factor family: receptors, their ligands and major functions*

Receptors	Ligands	Functions
TNF-RI (p55)	TNF and LT-α	Host defense, inflammation, cell death
TNF-RII (p75)	TNF and LT-α	Host defense, inflammation
LT-βR	LT-α/β complex	Lymph node development, cell death
CD40	CD40L	Ig class switching and costimulation of T cells
CD27	CD27L	Costimulation of T cells
CD30	CD30L	Costimulation of T and B cells
OX40	OX40L	Costimulation of T cells
4-1BB	4-1BBL	Costimulation of T cells
Fas/Apo-1	FasL/Apo-1L	Cell death, NF-κB activation, elimination of autoreactive T cells
DR4	TRAIL/Apo-2L	Cell death
Apo3/DR3/Wsl-1/TRAMP	Apo3L	Cell death, NF-κB activation
TRAMP	?	NF-κB activation, cell death
CAR1	?	Receptor for avian leukosis-sarcoma virus
HVEM	LIGHT and LT-α	Coreceptor for herpes simplex virus
GITR	?	Protection from T cell receptor–mediated cell death
Osteoprotegerin (OPG)	Osteoclast + differentiation factor	Regulation of bone mass
p75 NGF-R	NGF, neurotrophins[a]	Neuronal differentiation, cell death

[a]Whereas the p75 NGF receptor (low-affinity NGF receptor) is structurally related to other members of the TNF receptor family, NGF and neurotrophins are not related to members of the TNF family ligands.
Adapted from ref. 15.

and its receptor (12,13), CD40 (14), and many others (see Table 1). CD40, CD40 ligand, and some other members of the TNF receptor and ligand family that affect primarily T- or B-cell functions are more extensively discussed in other chapters of this volume.

With the exception of LT-α, the ligands of this family are synthesized as type II membrane proteins, consisting of a C-terminal extracellular domain and transmembrane and intracellular domains. Homology among the ligand family members is most pronounced in the extracellular domains. Most of the ligands exist as integral transmembrane proteins, and only some, notably LT-α, TNF and FasL, are functional in a soluble form (15–17).

All members of the TNF family of receptors are type I membrane proteins. They show partial structural homology to one another in the extracellular ligand-binding domains, which contain varying numbers of characteristic repeating cysteine-rich domains (see Fig. 1). In addition to the homology in the extracellular domains, some of the receptors of this family also share some 80 amino acid–long "death-domain" regions within their intracellular domains. Death domains, important for the generation of the apoptotic signal, are present in the cytoplasmic regions of TNF-RI, Fas/Apo1, DR3/WSL-1, DR4, CAR1, TRAMP, and p75 NGF-R (17–21). Ligands for several more recently identified members of the TNF family of receptors (22–26) have not yet been identified (see Table 1).

Genes

The human TNF gene is located within the class III region of the major histocompatibility complex (MHC) on chromosome 6 (8,27,28). On its sides the TNF gene is flanked by the genes encoding LT-α and LT-β, respectively. (The LT-β gene is in reverse orientation.) Although the expression of these three genes is independently regulated, they closely resemble each other in genomic organization, with each of the three genes consisting of four exons arranged over approximately 3 kb of DNA. The similarly arranged murine TNF/LT genes are located on chromosome 17 within the murine MHC gene cluster (29,30). These structural features

strongly suggest that the TNF, LT-α, and LT-β genes arose from a single ancestral gene by duplication. Despite these similarities, distinct differences exist in the regulation of gene expression, tissue specificity of expression, and even in the biologic functions of the three proteins.

Analysis of the transcriptional regulatory elements within the 5′-flanking region of the TNF gene has led to the identification of several elements that, along with other elements, are important in the regulation of TNF gene expression (31,32). In addition to the regulation at the level of transcription, there is evidence that the rate of TNF synthesis is also controlled at the level of mRNA elongation, mRNA processing, and at the level of translation (33). Another regulatory site is at the level of proteolytic cleavage of the transmembrane TNF protein that results in the release of soluble TNF (see below). The location of the TNF gene within the MHC gene cluster has raised the possibility that polymorphisms within this locus may play a role as genetic determinants of susceptibility to autoimmune and infectious diseases that are known to be MHC-linked. A specific polymorphism within the TNF promoter has been shown to be associated with autoimmunity and increased TNF production (34).

The FasL gene is located on human and mouse chromosome 1 in the vicinity of the gene encoding the OX40 ligand gene (35). The FasL gene contains five exons, with its organization somewhat resembling that of TNF.

Proteins

Human TNF is synthesized as a 233 amino acid–long, 26-kDa transmembrane protein (Table 2). There is ample evidence that this transmembrane form of TNF is biologically active; that is, it can cross-link TNF receptors, either TNF-RI or TNF-RII (see Fig. 1). It appears, however, that the transmembrane form of TNF preferentially activates TNF-RII, rather than TNF-RI, suggesting that the transmembrane and soluble forms perform somewhat different functions (36). The soluble form of TNF, consisting of 157 amino acids, is derived from the transmembrane precursor by proteolytic

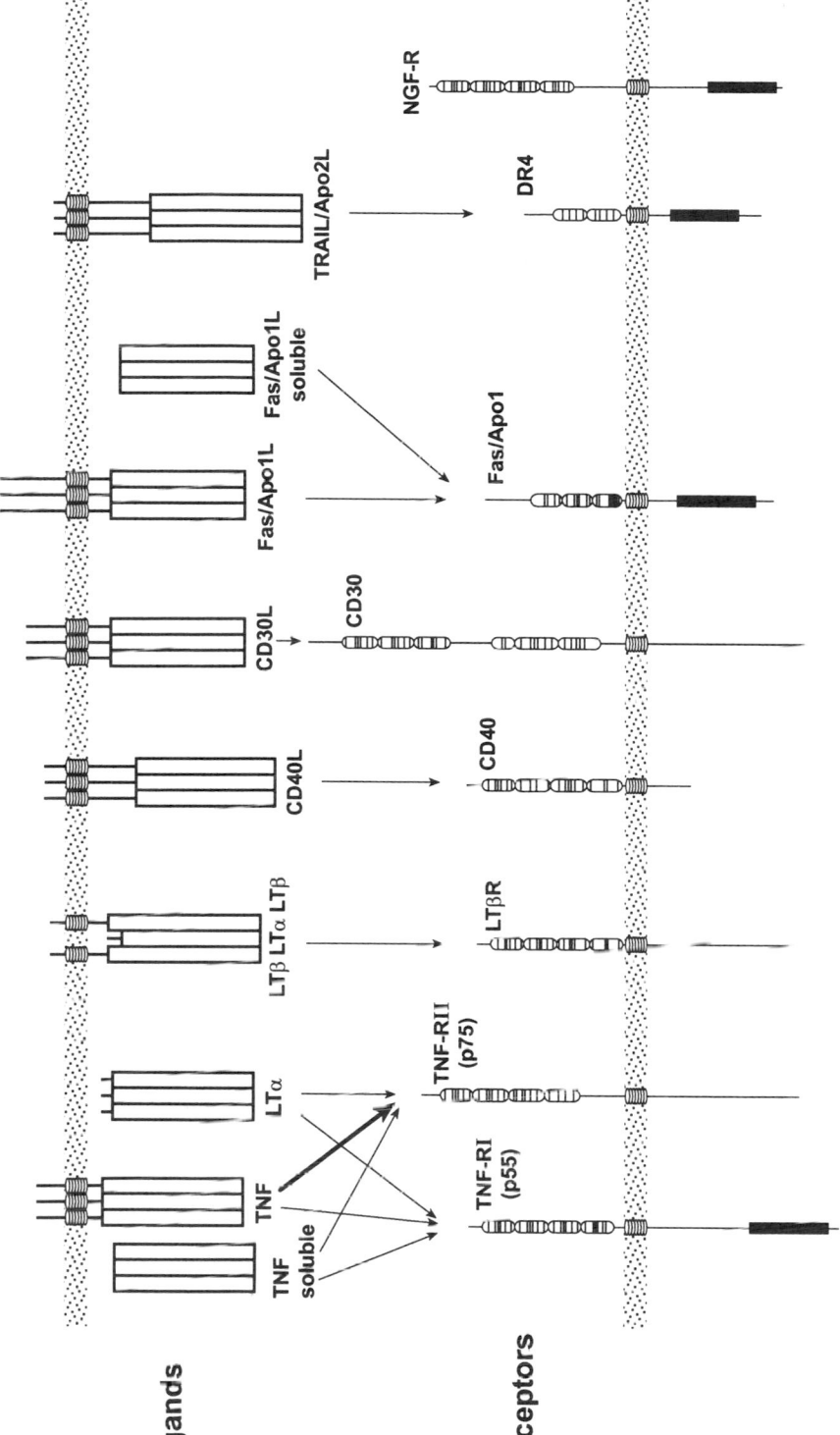

FIG. 1. Ligands and receptors of the TNF family (adapted from ref. 141). Of the ligands, only lymphotoxin-α (LT-α) is a secreted protein. All other ligands are synthesized as type II membrane proteins. TNF and Fas/Apo1 also exist in soluble form, derived from the membrane forms after cleavage by specific metalloproteinases. It is believed that the active forms of most TNF family ligands are homotrimers, LT-α and LT-β form heterotrimers. A hallmark of the TNF family receptors is the presence of three to six repeating cysteine-rich domains in the extracellular regions. In addition, some TNF family receptor's feature an approximately 80 amino acid–long death-domain region within their cytosolic portions (indicated by *solid rectangle*). For a more complete list of ligands and receptors of the TNF family, see Table 1.

TABLE 2. *Comparison of human and murine TNF and lymphotoxin-α*

Feature	TNF	LT-α
Cellular sources	Monocytes–macrophage, T cells, B cells, NK cells, vascular endothelial cells, keratinocytes, smooth muscle cells, mast cells, neutrophils, astrocytes, microglia cells	T cells (T_h1 and T_c), B cells
Chromosomal location	Chr. 6 (human) Chr. 17 (murine)	Chr. 6 (human) Chr. 17 (murine)
Gene organization	3 introns	3 introns
Size of precursor protein (amino acids)	233 (human) 235 (mouse)	205 (human) 202 (murine)
Release from cells	By cleavage of membrane protein by specific metalloproteinase (TACE)	Via secretory pathway
Size of released protein (amino acids)	157 (human) 156 (murine)	171 (human) 169 (murine)
Cysteine residues[a]	2 (human) 2 (murine)	None (human) 1 (murine)
Methionine residues[a]	None	3
N-glycosylation	No (human) Yes (murine)	Yes (human) Yes (murine)
Quaternary structure	Trimer	Trimer
Other features		Forms either homotrimer or heterotrimer with LT-β

[a]In released protein.

cleavage. The specific metalloproteinase responsible for this process (TNF converting enzyme or TACE) is an 824-amino acid transmembrane protein whose catalytic portion is part of the extracellular domain (37,38). TACE belongs to a family of membrane-anchored metalloproteinase disintegrins dubbed "protein ectodomain sheddases" (39). TACE cleaves the extracellular portion of the TNF precursor between Ala76 and Val77, leaving the transmembrane and intracytoplasmic domains intact. The resulting 157 amino acid–long soluble TNF peptide forms a homotrimer, a feature that is important in the cross-linking of TNF receptors (40). As the transmembrane form of TNF can bind and activate TNF receptors, it is likely that it, too, exists as a trimer, but formal proof of this is not available. The soluble form of human TNF was crystallized and found to form an elongated, antiparallel β-pleated sheet sandwich with a "jelly-roll" topology (41,42). The monomers associate intimately about a threefold axis of symmetry to form compact bell-shaped trimers. Available evidence indicates that LT-α and other members of the TNF ligand family also bind to the receptors as trimers and that the site of interaction with receptors is at the base of the trimers (43).

LT-α is unique among the TNF family ligands in that it is synthesized as a conventional secretory protein containing a cleavable signal peptide sequence (44). In contrast, LT-β, as well as other members of the TNF ligand family, are synthesized as type II membrane proteins. Secreted LT-α protein forms a homotrimer, which recognizes the same two cell surface receptors as TNF (see Table 1, Fig. 1). However, LT-α also forms a heterotrimer with LT-β (8,15). LT-β is a type II membrane protein that is not secreted. Thus, LT-β serves to anchor LT-α at the cell surface in the LT-α/β heterotrimer. It is believed that LT-α is released from cells only when it is produced in excess; that is, as long as LT-β is available at the cell surface, newly synthesized LT-α preferentially forms the LT-α/β heterotrimer. The more common form of the heterotrimer consists of one LT-α molecule complexed with two LT-β subunits (45). Significantly, the cell surface–bound LT-α/β heterotrimer binds to a receptor called LT-β R (46), distinct from the receptors recognized by LT-α (see Table 1, Fig. 1). Since LT-α and LT-α/β recognize different receptors, it is not surprising that they perform different biologic functions (see below).

The FasL protein is similar to TNF in that it is synthesized as a type II transmembrane protein, which may be released from the cell surface as a result of cleavage by specific metalloproteinases (47). Thus, like TNF, FasL exists in two forms, a 40-kDa transmembrane form and a 26-kDa soluble form (35,47).

Producers and Inducers

Mononuclear phagocytes are the major cellular source of TNF, but many other nucleated cells are capable of producing it (see Table 2). Among the cells that were shown to produce TNF upon appropriate stimulation are T cells (Th1 and Tc cells), B cells, natural killer (NK) cells, vascular endothelial cells, keratinocytes, smooth muscle cells, mast cells, neutrophils, astrocytes, and glial cells (48). Agents that stimulate the production of TNF often lead to the induction of interleukin (IL-1) as well (48). Among the most widely employed stimuli are various bacterial products, especially LPS, but also zymosan, phorbol esters, ultraviolet light, virus infection, allogenic B cells (in T cells), protozoa, and other microorganisms. The production of TNF can also be upregulated by a variety of cytokines and other endogenous mediators, including TNF itself, IL-1, interferon-γ (IFN-γ), IFN-α, granulocyte-macrophage colony-stimulating factor (GM-CSF), IL-2, transforming growth factor β (TGF-β, substance P, and platelet activating factor (48). Other endogenous substances were shown to inhibit TNF synthesis at the level of transcription or translation, including prostaglandins, corticordosteroids, IL-4, IL-6, and TGF-β (48). The fact that so many exogenous and endogenous agents can affect TNF production points to the complexity of events that regulate the production of this cytokine in the intact organism. Although TNF generation is initially triggered by an exogenous agent (e.g., infection), the process is fine-tuned by complex regulatory circuits controlled by cytokines.

Expression of LT-α is restricted to activated B cells, T cells, and possibly NK cells (49,50). LT-β is also expressed in lymphocytes, but its expression may not be as highly regulated as that of LT-α (51). It appears that the level of LT-α/β heterotrimer expression on the surface of lymphocytes is regulated mainly by the level of LT-α synthesis. LT-α synthesis, in turn, is regulated mainly at the level of transcription, but the transcription factors and enhancer elements important in the regulation of the LT-α gene expression have not been fully identified (49). Posttranscriptional regulatory mechanisms are also thought to affect the level of LT-α synthesis. LT-α (as well as TNF) is produced more readily by the Th₁ subset of the CD4⁺ cells and is thought to contribute to macrophage activation during the inflammatory response (52).

FasL is produced mainly by activated T cells, whereas B cells, macrophages, endothelial, and many other types of cells were not found to produce FasL mRNA or protein (35). However, FasL expression was found in tissues of the testis and the eye, suggesting a role for FasL in making the eyes and testes immunologically privileged sites, presumably by the induction of apoptosis in Fas-expressing activated lymphocytes that enter these sites (17,53,54).

Receptors

As noted earlier, two separate receptors, TNF-RI and TNF-RII, can bind both TNF and LT-α homotrimers (see Table 1, Fig. 1). [However, there is uncertainty about the ability of soluble murine LT-α to activate TNF-RI or TNF-RII (55).] Although the presence of repeating cysteine-rich regions in their extracellular domains characterizes TNF-RI and TNF-RII as members of the same receptor family, no structural homology is found in their intracellular domains, indicating that they signal by distinct mechanisms (56–59). TNF-RI contains a characteristic death domain region within its cytosolic portion (18). TNF receptors are widely distributed among different tissues, and many cells express both TNF receptors, but TNF-RI is more commonly expressed, especially in cells of nonhematopoietic lineage (15,58,59).

A number of agents were shown to regulate the level of TNF receptor expression. IFN-γ produced an upregulation of TNF receptor expression on many cell types, which may be partly responsible for the widely documented synergy between TNF and IFN-γ (60,61). Resting T cells do not express TNF receptors, but their expression can be induced by treatment with IL-2 (62). Among the agents that downregulate TNF receptors are phorbol esters, IL-1, IL-6, TGF-β, retinoids, and TNF itself (reviewed in refs. 63, 64). Most of the latter agents were also shown to induce the shedding of TNF-RI and/or TNF-RII from the cell surface. The enzymes responsible for the TNF receptor ectodomain cleavage that leads to shedding have not been identified. The shed, soluble TNF receptors retain the ability to bind TNF, thereby neutralizing the biologic activity of TNF. Soluble TNF receptors (both TNF-RI and TNF-RII) are found in the urine and plasma of healthy humans (65), and their levels become elevated in patients with various infections, immune disorders, and cancer (64). It has been suggested that levels of soluble TNF receptors in the serum can serve as markers of disease activity in autoimmune diseases, human immunodeficiency virus (HIV) infection and cancer (64). By binding TNF, soluble TNF receptors in body fluids can neutralize TNF activity. However, since the binding is reversible and the complexes of TNF with soluble receptors are less readily cleared than free TNF, soluble TNF receptors can also prolong the retention of TNF in the body (66).

Signaling from cell surface TNF receptors is triggered by their aggregation, resulting from the cross-linking of two or three receptor chains (either TNF-RI or TNF-RII) by the TNF or LT-α trimers. That homoaggregation of TNF receptors is sufficient for the initiation of signaling was first demonstrated by the fact that bivalent antibodies to the extracellular domains of the TNF receptors could mimic TNF action (67,68). It should be noted that the modus operandi of TNF receptors differs significantly from that of other cytokine receptors, most of which are heterodimers or heterotrimers. In common with most other cytokine receptors, both TNF receptors lack catalytic domains. Signaling is initiated by ligand-induced receptor clustering and the resulting recruitment of a variety of intracellular signaling proteins to the receptor complex. TNF-RI is the main signaling receptor, and many actions of TNF, including cytotoxicity, fibroblast proliferation, activation of NF-kB, and activation of many genes, can be elicited in the absence of TNF-RII engagement (69–71). Whereas TNF-RII can transmit some signals on its own (68), it is also thought to serve an auxiliary function by first binding TNF molecules and then passing them on to TNF-RI ("ligand passing" function) (72,73). Ligand passing may be facilitated by a faster on–off rate of TNF-RII compared to TNF-RI. In addition, evidence indicates that there is "cross-talk" between the intracellular domains of TNF-RI and TNF-RII, mediated by cytosolic adapter proteins (see below).

While the soluble LT-α homotrimer binds TNF-RI and TNF-RII, the LT-α₁β₂ heterotrimer binds to a separate receptor, termed LT-β R (see Table 1, Fig. 1) (46). FasL recognizes a receptor termed Fas, another important (and one of the earliest recognized) member of the TNF receptor family, whose major function is the triggering of apoptosis (9–11). Whereas FasL expression is largely restricted to lymphoid cells, Fas is expressed in a wide variety of different tissues, including tumor cells (17,35). Expression of Fas in some cells is increased after treatment with IFN-γ or TNF (35). Fas comprises a death domain region partially homologous to similar regions found in TNF-RI, DR3/WSL-1, DR4, CAR1, TRAMP, and p75 NGF-R (see Table 1) (17,74). The role of this region in signaling is discussed below.

Intracellular Signaling

Receptors of the TNF family contain no catalytic domains, and, with the exception of the death domain regions present in TNF-RI, Fas, p75 NGF-R, and some other members of this family (see above), no significant sequence homologies in the intracellular regions of these receptors have been reported. As is also true for most other cytokine receptors, activation of signal transduction pathways by TNF family receptors is initiated by the recruitment of various intracellular adapter proteins–signal transducers to the intracellular domains of the activated receptors. However, the number of intracellular proteins that participate in the transduction of signals generated by the TNF family of receptors is much greater than the number of intracellular proteins involved in the transduction of signals from other cytokine receptors (e.g., the interferon receptors) in which the JAK-Stat pathway provides the major mechanism of signaling. The much greater variety and complexity of signals produced by the TNF receptors matches the enormous diversity of biologic actions generated by these receptors. We shall review primarily signaling pathways that affect gene expression and differentiation, whereas the pathways activated by the TNF family of receptors (mainly TNF-RI and Fas) that trigger apoptosis are addressed in greater detail elsewhere in this volume.

TNF Receptor-associated Factors

The earliest isolated intracellular signaling proteins involved in TNF actions are TNF receptor–associated factors 1 and 2 (TRAF1 and TRAF2) (75). TRAF2 is a ubiquitously expressed 56-kDa protein that binds constitutively to the C-terminal region of TNF-RII. TRAF1, a approximately 45-kDa protein, whose expression is restricted mainly to spleen and lung tissue, is recruited to TNF-RII indirectly by virtue of its binding to TRAF2. Of the four other distinct TRAF proteins that have been identified (reviewed in refs. 16, 76), TRAF3 interacts with CD40 and the Epstein-Barr–transforming protein LMP1, TRAF5 associates with CD40 and the LT-β receptor, and TRAF6 plays a key role in IL-1 signaling (see below). A hallmark of all of these proteins is the presence of a characteristic approximately 230 amino acid–long TRAF domain that is important in homo- and heterooligomerization of the TRAF proteins, their binding to specific sequences in the intracellular regions of receptors, and the interaction with downstream targets (77). Most TRAF proteins also contain a RING finger motif and zinc finger sequences (75). TRAF2 appears to play a role in TNF-induced activation of the NF-kB transcription factor by both TNF-RI and TNF-RII (see below).

Death-domain Proteins

Another important family of signal transducers comprises proteins that share sequence homology with the death domains present in TNF-RI, Fas, and some other receptors of the TNF family (reviewed in refs. 16, 76). TRADD, an ubiquitously expressed 34-kDa protein, was identified as a protein interacting with the death domain of TNF-RI (78). FADD/MORT (79,80) and RIP (81) were originally isolated on the basis of their ability to associate with the intracellular domain of Fas (Fig. 2). A fourth member of this family is RAIDD (82). In addition to the self-associating death domains, some of these proteins contain other sequences that promote their associations with the ICE-like proteases MACH/FLICE (Caspase 8) and ICH-1 (Caspase 2), thus triggering the cell death pathway (reviewed in ref. 83). Remarkably, some of the death-domain proteins, specifically TRADD and RIP, can also associate with the TRAF domain of TRAF2 and thereby promote NF-kB activation (see below) (84). Thus, the death-domain proteins not only trigger cell death, but also lead to the activation of the NF-kB transcription factor, which, by inducing the synthesis of protective proteins, prevents cell death by apoptosis (85,86).

Pathways of NF-kB Activation

Although cell death triggered by TNF or Fas receptors occurs in the absence of protein synthesis, other important actions by members of the TNF family are attributed to the activation of gene expression and the resulting increased synthesis of the encoded proteins. A very large number of cellular genes are known to be inducible by TNF, including genes encoding various cytokines, growth factors, receptors, cell adhesion molecules, acute phase proteins, and transcription factors (reviewed in ref. 87). Induction of many of these genes can be attributed to the activation of cellular transcription factors, such as AP-1 and,

especially, NF-kB. The intracellular signaling cascade leading to NF-kB activation by TNF has been largely elucidated. It has been known for some time that triggering of either TNF-RI or TNF-RII can lead to NF-kB activation. It was also shown that overexpression of TRAF2, or overexpression of the death-domain proteins TRADD, FADD/MORT, or RIP, leads to NF-kB activation (83). In fact, RIP was found to be essential for TNF-induced NF-κB activation in the Jurkat T-cell line (84). It appears that the ability of the death-domain proteins to directly or indirectly associate with TRAF2 and the resulting TRAF2 activation is central to this pathway (see Fig. 2). TRAF2, in turn, associates with, and thereby activates, a serine–threonine kinase termed *NF-kB–activating kinase* (NIK) (88). NIK shows significant sequence homology to upstream activators of mitogen-activated protein (MAP) kinases, the so-called MAP kinase kinases (MEKKs) (88). NIK does not activate NF-kB directly, but acts as the upstream activator of yet another serine–threonine kinase, the long-elusive IkB-α kinase (89,90). In most vertebrate cells, NF-kB proteins are present in a latent form, sequestered in the cytoplasm by members of the IkB family of inhibitory proteins (91). The IkB-α kinase is responsible for phosphorylating serines 32 and 36 on IkB-α (the major inhibitory subunit of NF-kB), thereby targeting IkB-α for ubiquination and degradation by the proteasome pathway (89,90). The same kinase may also be responsible for phosphorylating IkB-β, another inhibitory subunit of NF-kB. IkB phosphorylation and resulting degradation then lead to the release of activated NF-kB proteins and their translocation to the nucleus.

Although the main function of Fas is the activation of the cell death pathway, the work of Malinin et al. (88) suggests that Fas triggering can also lead to NF-kB activation through TRAF2 and NIK, presumably mediated by FADD/MORT, TRADD, and/or RIP (see Fig. 2). The isolation of NIK also helped to explain the pathway of NF-kB activation by IL-1 (88). Available evidence suggests that NIK is at the point of convergence of TNF- and IL-1– signaling pathways (see Fig. 2). As explained in another part of this chapter (see Fig. 3), IL-1 leads to the activation of the kinase IRAK and of another member of the TRAF protein family, termed TRAF6. Like TRAF2 in TNF-treated cells, TRAF6 is likely to function as the immediate upstream activator of NIK in IL-1– stimulated cells. Thus, it is now possible to explain in molecular terms why TNF and IL-1, cytokines that are structurally unrelated and bind to completely distinct receptors, activate so many identical target genes and produce so many identical biologic actions. However, it is not yet known whether IkB kinase is the only target of NIK, or whether there perhaps are other NIK substrates that might mediate actions of TNF (and IL-1) independent of NF-kB activation.

Other Intracellular Adapter Proteins

In addition to the TRAFs and death-domain proteins, a large number of other intracellular proteins have been implicated in TNF signaling (reviewed in ref. 76). Most of these proteins have been isolated by the yeast two-hybrid screening method, based on their interaction with the intracellular domains of the TNF receptors or with other intracellular proteins implicated in TNF signaling (Table 3). With some of these proteins, overexpression of the complete protein or of dominant negative constructs produced detectable effects, which suggested their possible cellular functions. However, the physiologic roles of most of these proteins in the signaling cascades activated by TNF or other members of the

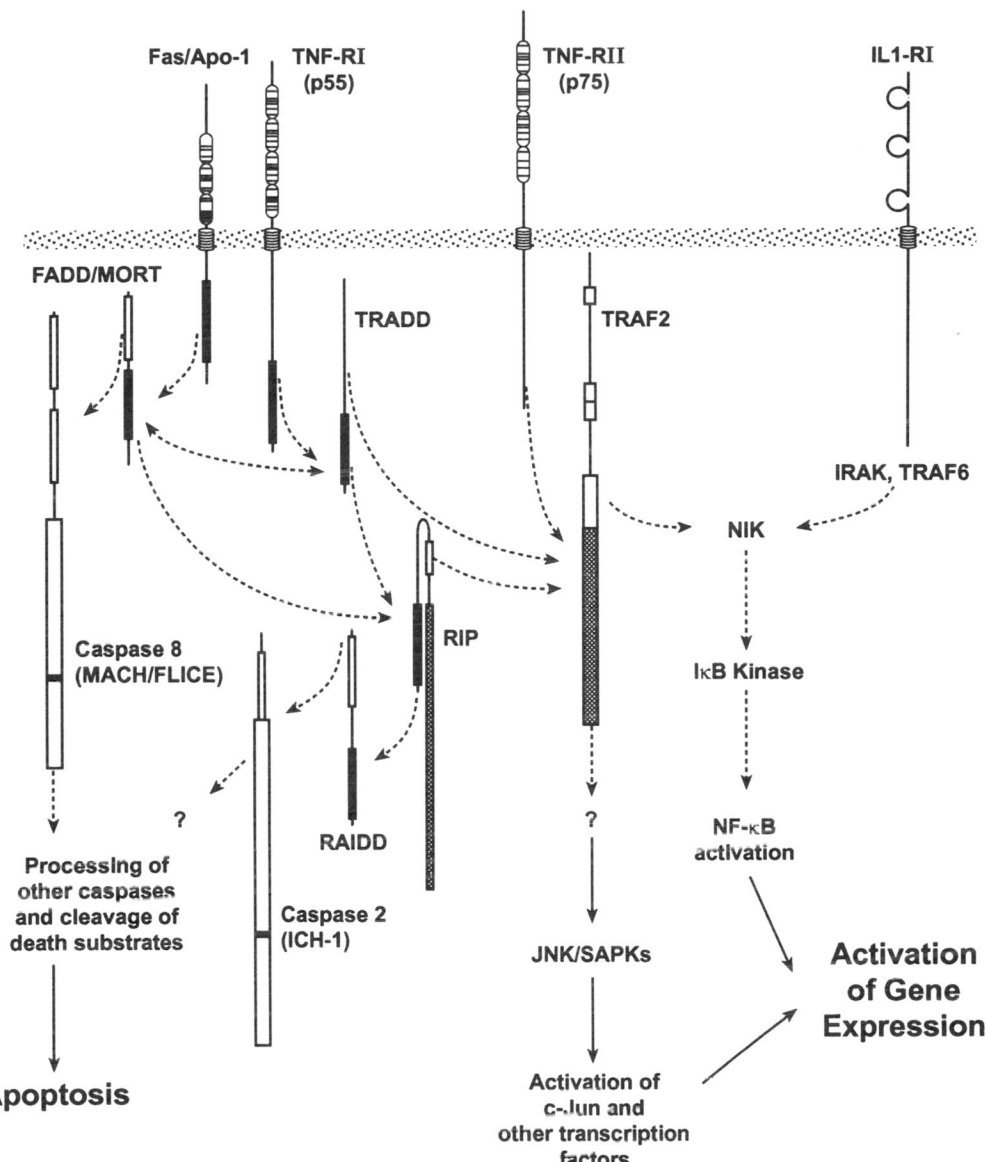

FIG. 2. Diagrammatic representation of some important signaling pathways activated by the TNF receptors and Fas/Apo1 (adapted from ref. 83). Although the intracellular domains of TNF receptors I (p55 receptor) and II (p75 receptor) share no sequence homology, they can signal cooperatively as a result of interactions among intracellular adapter proteins. The death domain–containing proteins (primarily TRADD) bind to the death domain of TNF-RI. However, TRADD also interacts with other death domain–containing proteins (FADD/MORT1 and RIP) as well as with TRAF2. TRAF2, in turn, binds directly to TNF-RII and serves as the downstream activator of a pathway leading to their activation of the JNK/SAPK subfamily of MAP kinases. TRAF2 can also directly bind and thereby activate NIK (a kinase), which then phosphorylates the IkB kinase, leading to IkB-α and IkB-β phosphorylation and resulting NF-kB activation. In addition, recruitment of the death-domain proteins leads to the activation caspases that in some cells will trigger cell death by apoptosis. The intracellular domain of Fas/Apo1 comprises a death domain similar to that found in TNF-RI. Consequently, Fas/Apo1 activates similar intracellular signaling pathways as TNF-RI, but it is generally more efficient in triggering apoptosis than in activating gene expression. Also shown in the diagram is that signaling from the IL-1 receptor, through the involvement of the kinase IRAK and of TRAF6, leads to NIK activation and subsequent NF-kB activation, similar to that produced by the TNF receptors. The IL-1 receptor also signals JNK/SAPK activation (not shown) through a still unknown pathway. The pathways of p38 MAP kinase activation by the TNF and IL-1 receptors are also not known and not shown in the diagram.

TNF family are not yet well understood. It is interesting that two of the proteins listed in Table 3 (A20 and I-TRAF/TANK) were shown to affect NF-kB activation by both TNF and IL 1, but the targets of their action within the IL-1 activated signaling cascade have not yet been elucidated.

Mitogen-activated Protein Kinases

MAP kinases play prominent roles in transcytoplasmic signalling to the nucleus by activating gene expression through the phosphorylation of transcription factors (92). MAP kinases become acti-

TABLE 3. *Intracellular proteins implicated in TNF signaling whose physiologic roles have not yet been firmly established*

Protein	Interacting partner(s)	Provisional function	Ref.
FAN	TNF-RI (a.a. 309–319)	Activation of neutral sphingomyelinase	105
Sentrin	TNF-RI (death domain)	Inhibits apoptosis	142
TRAP1	TNF-RI (N-terminus)	?	143
55.11	TNF-RI (N-terminus)	?	144
cIAP1 and 2	TRAF2 and TRAF1	? (related to inhibitors of apoptosis in insects)	145
A20	TRAF2 and TRAF1	Inhibits NF-κB activation by TNF and IL-1	146, 147
I-TRAF/TANK	TRAFs	Inhibits (or potentiates?) NF-κB activation by TNF, IL-1, and CD40	148, 149
TRIP	TRAFs	Inhibits NF-κB activation by TNF and CD30	150
Casper/FLIP	Caspases, FADD/MORT1, TRAF1 and 2	Inhibits (or potentiates?) apoptosis	151, 152

vated as a result of threonine–tyrosine phosphorylation by dual specificity MAPK kinases or MKKs, which in turn are activated as a result of serine phosphorylation by MAPKK kinases or MEKKs. Three major subfamilies of structurally related MAP kinases have been identified in mammalian cells: the extracellular signal-regulated kinases (ERKs), the c-Jun N-terminal kinases–stress-activated protein kinases (JNK/SAPKs), and the p38 kinases. Whereas ERKs are characteristically associated with cell proliferation and protection from apoptosis, JNKs and p38s can promote apoptosis. ERK-1 (p42) and ERK-2 (p44) were the first members of the MAP kinase family shown to be activated by TNF (and IL-1) in some types of cells (93,94). The exact pathway whereby TNF activates ERKs remains unclear. In addition, little is known about the functional significance of the ERKs in TNF actions. Compared with growth factors, such as EGF, ERK activation by TNF in many cells is relatively weak and short-lasting, leading to the notion that ERKs are not central to TNF actions (95). However, TNF (and IL-1) act as strong activators of the JNK/SAPKs and the p38 kinases (96,97). TNF-induced JNK activation is dependent on TRAF2: Not only does overexpression of TRAF2 (and not TRAF1 or TRAF3) lead to JNK activation, but dominant-negative TRAF2 blocks TNF-induced (and not IL-1–induced) JNK activation (86,98). The exact pathway that leads from TRAF2 to JNK activation (i.e., how TRAF2 produces activation of the upstream kinases required for JNK activation) is not known. Whether TNF-induced p38 activation also requires TRAF2 function (a likely possibility) has not been reported. Selective inhibitors of p38 MAP kinase activity were shown to suppress TNF and IL-1 production by activated macrophages, but the mechanism of this inhibition has not been fully elucidated (99). The roles of JNKs and p38s in TNF actions are only beginning to be analyzed. Since MAP kinases produce PLA$_2$ activation (100), they are thought to be important in TNF-induced arachidonic acid production by PLA$_2$ and the resulting generation of proinflammatory metabolites. It is likely that JNK and p38 are important for the TNF-induced activation of genes that requires the AP-1 transcription factor, because JNK phosphorylates and thereby activates c-Jun, and both JNK and p38 phosphorylate and activate ATF-2 (101). There is also preliminary evidence for a role of p38 kinase in NF-kB-mediated activation of the IL-6 gene by TNF (102).

Ceramide

Many studies have been devoted to the analysis of the role the lipid mediator ceramide as a potential second messenger in TNF (and IL-1) actions (reviewed in ref. 103). Treatment of many cells with TNF leads to the rapid activation of two types of cellular sphingomyelinases that cause sphingomyelin breakdown and the generation of ceramide: a membrane-bound neutral sphingomyelinase (104) and an acidic sphingomyelinase (105). Although both sphingomyelinases are activated via TNF-RI, their activation is by distinct pathways. Activation of the neutral sphingomyelinase involves the adapter protein FAN, which binds to a membrane-proximal site in the intracellular domain of TNF-RI above the death domain (105), whereas the acidic sphingomyelinase becomes activated through the action of DAG generated by a phosphatidylcholine-specific phospholipase C (PLC) (106). It has been postulated that ceramide generated by the latter pathway contributes to TNF-induced IkB degradation and resulting NF-kB activation, whereas ceramide generated by the acidic sphingomyelinase promotes apoptosis in response to TNF or Fas and initiates a protein kinase cascade that ultimately results in the activation of JNKs (107). A ceramide-activated protein kinase that phosphorylates Raf-1 has been described (108). Another consequence of ceramide generation is the activation of protein kinase Cζ (PKCζ) (109). Several reports have questioned the role of ceramide in TNF-induced NF-kB activation (110,111), and although it is clear that treatment of cells with cell-permeable C2-ceramide can lead to JNK activation and/or apoptosis in many types of cells, no consensus has yet emerged on the significance of ceramide as a second messenger in the actions of TNF and other members of the TNF family.

Biologic Functions

Of all cytokines, TNF and IL-1 display the broadest spectrum of pleiotropic activities. The literature describing the myriad demonstrated TNF actions in cell cultures, isolated tissues, and experimental animals and humans is so vast that any effort to review it fairly is doomed to failure. As TNF receptors are expressed ubiquitously and their triggering sets in motion an array of parallel signaling pathways, it is not surprising that the exposure of cells and tissues to TNF results in a multitude of biologic actions. It has been difficult to determine which of the many reported activities are physiologically or pathophysiologically relevant and which of them belong to the realm of interesting artifacts of experimentation. The generation of mice with targeted deletions of genes encoding various TNF family ligands and receptors (reviewed in ref. 112) has been extremely helpful in the identification of the "real" biologic functions of the major TNF family members and has led to the discovery of some previously unknown functions (Table 4). Thus, studies in gene knock-out mice have revealed a role for TNF in hematopoiesis (113), in obesity-induced insulin resistance (114),

TABLE 4. *Phenotypes of mice with TNF family gene deficiences*

Targeted gene	Major phenotypic abnormalities
TNF	Lower LPS lethality post D-galactosamine. Lack of germinal centers and abnormal IgG synthesis. Reduced resistance to intracellular microorganisms.
TNF-RI (p55)	Lower LPS lethality post D-galactosamine and reduced IL-6 production. Lack germinal centers and abnormal IgG synthesis. Reduced resistance to intracellular organisms.
TNF-RII (p75)	Lower LPS lethality without D-galactosamine.
LTα (TNF-β)	Failure of lymph node development, absent Peyer's patches and splenic hypoplasia. Defective isotype switching.
LTβ	Failure of lymph node development (except mesenteric and cervical), absent Peyer's patches and splenic hypoplasia.
CD40 ligand	No immunoglobulin response to T-dependent antigen. Hyper IgM syndrome with neutropenia and infections.
Fas ligand	Failure of T cell and CTL target-cell apoptosis. *gld* gene mouse defect results in autoimmune state.
Fas / Apo1	Failure to delete lymphocytes yields hyperplasia. *lpr/lpn* mice and human autoimmune lymphoproliferative syndrome have autoimmune diseases.

and in the development of germinal centers and IgG response to immunization (115–117). Even more surprising was the demonstration of the essential role for LT-α/β and of a somewhat distinct role for LT-α in normal lymph node development (118–121). Additional valuable information has been gained from clinical studies with monoclonal antibodies to TNF or soluble TNF receptor constructs.

Host Resistance to Infections

A wealth of evidence demonstrates the important role of TNF in the early stages of host resistance to infection with *Listeria monocytogenes* (reviewed in refs. 112, 122). Mice lacking TNF-RI or the structural gene for TNF succumbed to inoculation with very small doses of bacteria, whereas wild-type mice survived such infection. Bacteria multiplied to much higher titers in the mutant mice, and the mutant animals died with signs of a widespread infection of internal organs. A similar defect in resistance to *L. monocytogenes* was seen in mice with a targeted disruption of the IFN-γ receptor. Mice that lack either TNF-RI or the IFN-γ receptor are also much more susceptible to infection with mycobacteria and with *Toxoplasma gondii*. Together, these data indicate that both TNF and IFN-γ are essential for the development of resistance to intracellular pathogens, and that these two pathways are not redundant. Resistance to intracellular pathogens is known to involve the initial activation of macrophages and neutrophils, which secrete TNF and IL-12. These two cytokines stimulate NK cells to produce IFN-γ, and the latter cytokine together with TNF is then largely responsible for the activation of macrophages necessary for their microbicidal action, (e.g., through the efficient generation of NO). This brief (and undoubtedly oversimplified) scenario explains the requirement for both TNF and IFN-γ in host resistance to these organisms. Although TNF was demonstrated to inhibit the replication of some viruses in tissue culture (reviewed in ref. 123), there is no direct evidence for a protective role of TNF in virus infections in the intact organism. However, such a role is suggested by the fact that some poxviruses acquired genes encoding homologues of soluble TNF receptors, and the presence of this gene in myxoma virus contributes to virus virulence (124).

Along with the protective effect, the production of TNF in the course of infections can produce toxic manifestations and aggravate the course of disease. A case in point is the contribution of TNF to the pathogenesis of septic shock (see below). Another well-documented example is the role of TNF as an essential mediator of murine cerebral malaria and circumstantial evidence that TNF pro-

duction correlates with the severity of falciparum malaria in humans (125).

Lipopolysaccharide Toxicity and Septic Shock

The beneficial effects of TNF in resistance to infections are thought to be the result of modest amounts of TNF production at local sites of infection. In contrast, the production of larger amounts of TNF, which leads to a systemic distribution or the production of TNF in organs that are highly susceptible to its toxicity (e.g., the brain), leads to adverse effects and even death. The key role of TNF in the pathogenesis of septic shock is supported by several lines of evidence: (a) Antibodies to TNF were shown to protect animals from septic shock produced by lethal bacteremia (126), (b) administration of high doses of TNF to experimental animals or humans produces symptoms similar to septic shock, (c) TNF is produced in animals and in humans during experimental and clinical septic shock, and (d) clear evidence for the role of TNF in some forms of LPS-induced toxicity has been obtained in gene knock-out animals.

Normal mice are highly resistant to the toxicity of LPS, as they can survive injections with doses of 500 μg or more. However, LPS toxicity can be increased dramatically by concurrent administration of the hepatotoxic agent D-galactosamine. The role of TNF in the lethal action of LPS in D-galactosamine–treated mice was clearly demonstrated by several groups of investigators, who showed that mice with a targeted deletion of TNF-RI can survive injections with 100-fold higher doses of LPS than can wild-type mice (reviewed in ref. 122). Interestingly, toxicity produced by very high doses of LPS in the absence of D-galactosamine was not significantly affected by the deletion of TNF-RI, while being modestly reduced in mice that lacked TNF-RII (127). Thus, in the absence of D-galactosamine treatment, the lethal effect of LPS does not appear to be mediated primarily by TNF. Attempts to treat septic shock in humans with monoclonal antibodies to TNF or with soluble receptor constructs that neutralize TNF have so far failed to provide clear evidence of therapeutic benefit. At least two factors may be responsible for this failure. First, unlike in experimental animals, treatment in patients can be initiated only after the onset of disease symptoms. Second, as is also clear from animal studies, septic shock syndrome is not a single pathogenetic entity, and the relative contribution of TNF may vary from one form to another. Therapy with TNF antibodies or soluble TNF receptor constructs might have a better chance of success if tests were available that could differentiate between the forms of sepsis that are TNF-mediated and those that are not.

Lymphoid Organogenesis, Germinal Center Development, and Immunoglobulin-G Class Switching

Analysis of the phenotype of mice with a targeted deletion of the LT-α gene unexpectedly revealed that these mice are born without lymph nodes or Peyer's patches, and that they show gross abnormalities in splenic architecture (119). These findings led to the correct prediction that lymphoid development is regulated by the LT-α/β heterotrimer and mediated by the LT-β receptor, the binding site for LT-α/β . Another unexpected finding was that mice devoid of TNF-RI or the structural gene for TNF, although not showing defects in splenic architecture, fail to develop splenic germinal centers and follicular dendritic cell networks upon immunization, and they show a reduced IgG antibody response with impaired isotype switching 112,115,128–130). A summary of the various lymphoid organ abnormalities seen in mice with targeted deletions of LT-α, LT-β, TNF, TNF-RI, or TNF-RII is shown in Table 5.

Autoimmune Diseases

Evidence strongly implicates TNF as a pathogenetic factor in autoimmune diseases, especially rheumatoid arthritis and Crohn's disease. In some lines of transgenic mice, in which high levels of human TNF are produced in the synovial tissue, a large proportion of mice develop arthritis within 2 months after birth (131). Administration of monoclonal antibodies to human TNF alleviated disease activity in the transgenic animals. [Interestingly, treatment of these transgenic mice with antibody to the type I IL-1 receptor also suppressed the development of arthritis, indicating the close interdependence of TNF and IL-1 in pathogenesis (132).] These and other studies in which interactions among cytokines in rheumatoid arthritis tissues were analyzed, served as the impetus for the use of monoclonal antibodies to TNF in patients with severe forms of rheumatoid arthritis. A marked improvement in the clinical condition and laboratory parameters was seen in a large proportion of patients with rheumatoid arthritis treated with antibodies to TNF (133). There is also evidence for the pathogenetic role of TNF in experimental colitis in mice (134), and antibodies to TNF given to patients with severe Crohn's disease induced remissions in a significant proportion of

patients (135). In NOD mice, TNF treatment during the first 3 weeks of age was shown to promote the development of autoimmune diabetes (136). On the other hand, repeated administration of TNF to adult mice delayed the onset of diabetes in NOD mice and also suppressed the development of the lupus-like disease in NZB/W mice (137). The difference between the effects of TNF in young and adult mice was attributed to the possible role of TNF as a growth factor for T cells during development, as opposed to the suppression of T-cell function resulting from the chronic TNF exposure in adult mice (137).

Neoplasia

Despite its original description as "tumor necrosis factor," evidence for the role of TNF in host resistance to cancer is still largely indirect. TNF is directly cytotoxic for some tumor cells, and TNF production by monocytes contributes to the killing of TNF-sensitive tumor-cell lines *in vitro*. However, in some experimental malignancies, TNF appears to promote tumor progression (138). A better understanding of the role of TNF in the pathogenesis of malignancies is likely to emerge from studies on mice with targeted deletions of the genes for TNF or its receptors. Attempts to use TNF as an antitumor agent in patients have been largely abandoned because of severe systemic toxicity. Some therapeutic success has been achieved in patients with advanced soft-tissue sarcomas of the extremities, who were treated with high doses of TNF given by "isolated limb perfusion" (139).

In summary, studies in genetically altered mice support the view that the major function of TNF is as a key regulator of inflammation, and that its actions are especially important in host responses to infectious agents and in autoimmunity. The most surprising information derived from more recent studies in knock-out mice is the demonstration of the roles of TNF, LT-α and LT-α/β in lymphoid organ development. The proinflammatory actions and the effects on lymphoid tissue development may be related because, as pointed out (112,140), chronic local overexpression of TNF or LT-α can lead to lymphoid neogenesis, resulting in the appearance of lymph node-like structures at local inflammatory sites. However, rather than acting merely as a mediator of inflammation, in some situations TNF may actually limit the inflammatory response and promote the repair process (129).

TABLE 5. *Development and organization of secondary lymphoid organs in mice with targeted deletions of TNF family genes*

Analyzed feature	Knockout mice examined				
	LT-α–/–	LT-β–/–	TNF–/–	TNF-RI–/–	TNF-RII–/–
Peripheral lymph node development	–	–	+	+	+
Peyer's patch development	–	–	+(?)	–(?)	+
Cervical and mesenteric lymph node development	–	+	+	+	+
Splenic primary B cell follicles	–	–	–	–	+
Splenic follicular dendritic cell networks	–	–	–	–	+
Splenic germinal centers	–	–	–	–	+
MAdCAM-1 expression in splenic marginal zone	–	–	?	–	+
MOMA-1 expression in splenic marginal zone	–	–	?	+	+

+, present; –, absent.
MAdCAM-1 is an adhesion molecule and MOMA-1 staining is characteristic for metallophilic macrophages.
Adapted from ref. 111.

INTERLEUKIN-1 FAMILY

Interleukin 1 (IL-1) was originally described by Gery and Waksman as a macrophage-derived, lymphocyte-activating factor (LAF) with comitogenic effects on thymocytes and T cells (153). IL-1 is now known to have multiple biologic activities and is a regulator of the host response to infection and injury (154–156). The IL-1 family consists of three distinct but structurally related molecules: IL-1α and IL-1β, which elicit biologic responses, and a specific antagonist, termed IL-1 receptor antagonist (IL-1ra) (Table 6). IL-1ra was initially detected as an IL-1 inhibitor found in the urine of patients with fever or myelomonocytic leukemia (157). IL-1ra is the only known naturally occurring cytokine antagonist that acts as a competitive inhibitor of IL-1α and IL-1β by binding to IL-1 receptors without transducing a signal.

Genes

Molecular cloning and subsequent studies identified the three members of the IL-1 family as products of different genes located close to one another on human chromosome 2. The genomic organizations of both IL-1α and IL-1β consist of seven exons spanning 11 kb and 7.5 kb, respectively, whereas IL-1ra has four exons (158–161). The homology between human IL-1α and IL-1β is 45% at the nucleotide level, and the interspecies homologies (human verus mouse) is 62% for IL-1α and 67% for IL-1β. Analysis of gene sequences and mutational rates for IL-1α, IL-1β, and IL-1ra suggests that all three molecules arose from a common ancestral gene through the process of gene duplication about 350 million years ago.

The regulatory sequences in IL-1α, IL-1β, and IL-1ra genes differ, suggesting differential regulation. The typical transcriptional promotor motifs, TATA box and CAAT box, are found immediately upstream from the transcription initiation site in IL-1β, but are absent in IL-1α. AP-1 sites, a NF-IL-6 site, a CRE, and a novel LPS-inducible site have been identified in the IL-1β promotor (162). Glucocorticoid regulatory elements are present in both IL-1α and IL-1β genes. A lipophosphoglycan-responsive promotor sequence, located downstream from AP-1 sites of IL-1β, which acts as a "gene silencer," has been identified (163). This sequence is responsible for downregulating LPS-induced IL-1β mRNA. The promoter regions of the two forms of IL-1ra differ; intracellular IL-1ra (icIL-1ra) lacks a TATA box, whereas secretory IL-1ra (sIL-1ra) has a TATA box with consensus sequences for possible NF-kB,

NF-IL-1βA, AP-1, and CRE binding sites (164). The intracellular variants are generated by alternative splicing of 5' exons.

Transcription results in a 2.1-kb, 1.6-kb, and 1.8-kb mRNA for IL-1α, IL-1β, and IL-1ra respectively. The 3' untranslated region (UTR) of IL-1ra mRNA lacks the AU-rich sequence associated with mRNA instability of other cytokines, but this sequence is present in both IL-1α and IL-1β. In addition, the 3' UTR of IL-1β mRNA contains an LPS response element and augments IL-1β production (165). The genes for IL-1α, IL-1β, as well as IL-1ra are rapidly transcribed upon stimulation. The production of IL-1 and IL-1ra are differentially regulated at both the transcriptional and posttranscriptional levels, depending on the particular cell types and stimulants used for their induction.

Proteins

Both IL-1α and IL-1β are synthesized as 31-kDa precursors (271 amino acids for IL-1α and 269 amino acids for IL-1β), which are then proteolytically cleaved to generate the mature, 17-kDa proteins (159 amino acids for IL-1α and 153 amino acids for IL-1β) (see Table 6). Both lack the conventional, hydrophobic signal sequence of secretory proteins and are not secreted via the classical secretory pathway. IL-1 is found in the cytoplasm but not in the endoplasmic reticulum or Golgi. Most IL-1α is stored as intracellular pro-IL-1α, while the rest is either phosphorylated or myristoylated and becomes membrane-bound by a lectin interaction involving mannose residues on IL-1α (166,167). Both pro-IL-1α and membrane-IL-1α are biologically active, but pro-IL-1β has no biologic activity. Serine proteases, elastase, plasmin, chymotrypsin, cathepsin G, or a specific intracellular cysteine protease, named *IL-1β–converting enzyme* (ICE), which cleaves pro-IL-1β specifically between asparagine 116 and alanine 117, are required to generate the 17-kDa mature IL-1β (168,169). ICE is a 45.2 kDa proenzyme found in most cells and itself requires two proteolytic cleavages for activation. It is likely that pro-IL-1β is proteolytically processed during transport across the plasma membrane (170). Both LPS and IFN-γ upregulate the expression of ICE. ICE does not cleave pro-IL-1α, but mice lacking the ICE gene fail to secrete both IL-1β and IL-1α, presumably because IL-1β induces IL-1α (171). Pro-IL-1α is cleaved by calpain and other extracellular nonspecific proteases (172). Depending on the cell type and the stimulant used, the release or processing of IL-1 may not occur, and pro-IL-1 may accumulate intracellularly. IL-1 release *in vitro* may also occur as a consequence of cell injury and cell death.

TABLE 6. *IL-1 family*

	IL-1α	IL-1β	IL-1ra
Precursor protein	271 amino acids	269 amino acids	177 amino acids
Mature protein	159 amino acids	153 amino acids	152 amino acids
Signal sequence	None	None	25 amino acids
Biologically active forms	Intracellular (Pro-IL-1α)		Intracellular (ic IL-1ra)
	Extracellular	Extracellular	Extracellular
	Membrane IL-1α		
Cell source: nucleated cell types	Some released	Released	Especially keratinocytes
	Mostly as cell-associated form		Tissue macrophages
			Epithelial cells
Receptors	IL-1RI>IL-1RII	IL-1RII>IL-1RI	IL-1RI>1RII
Signal-transducing unit	IL-1RI+II -1R AcP	IL-1RI+IL-1R-AcP	Binding but no signal transduction

IL-1ra is synthesized as a nonglycosylated precursor peptide of 177 amino acids with a 25-amino acid signal sequence (155,173) IL-1ra is secreted extracellularly through the endoplasmic reticulum and Golgi of adherent IgG-stimulated monocytes as three structural variants of 18 to 22 kDa (152 amino acids), differing in the extent of glycosylation. These forms of secretory IL-1ra exhibit identical receptor binding, indicating that the N-linked sugar is not essential for the inhibitory activity. The intracellular variant of IL-1ra (icIL-1ra) has no signal sequence and is released only by the process of cell disruption (death) (174,175).

Crystallographic studies indicated that IL-1β is a globular protein and resembles a tetrahedron structure, with the triangular faces formed by 12 antiparallel β strands connected by highly hydrophilic loops well exposed on the surface (176). Both N- and C-termini are exposed, and receptor-binding sites are located in a number of discontinued regions along the primary sequence, held together in a certain conformation. The hydrophilicity plot of IL-1ra is similar to that of IL-1β, suggesting similarities in tertiary structure. However, IL-1ra shows only 26% sequence similarity to IL-1β and less to IL-1α.

Deletion mutation studies suggested that the minimum polypeptide size for retaining biologic activities for IL-1α is 140 amino acids, representing amino acids 128 through 267. The minimum size for IL-1β is 147 amino acids, extending from 120 through 266. Most attempts to identify smaller fragments of IL-1 failed, but a fragment of nine residues of human IL-1β (fragment 163–171), when fused to an antigen, has been reported to have significant immunoadjuvant activity (177). This fragment, which constitutes a crucial binding site for IL-1β to IL-1 receptor, is absent in IL-1ra. Another loop (amino acids 202–214), identified through binding and functional analysis of mutants, is also an important site for binding to the signaling IL-1 receptor (178). There are substantial differences between IL-1β and IL-1ra in the amino acid sequences of this region.

Producers and Inducers

Mononuclear phagocytes are the major cell source of IL-1, but all other nucleated cells are capable of producing IL-1. Normal cells must be stimulated to produce IL-1. Infections, immunologic and inflammatory processes, endogenous mediators, and cell and tissue injury can trigger IL-1 production (156,179). Thus IL-1 production by macrophages can be triggered by a wide variety of stimuli, including bacterial cell wall products, LPS, microbial superantigens, zymosan, phorbol esters, muramyl dipeptide, antigens, mitogens, endogenous cytokines, leukotrienes, activated complement components (C5a), immune complexes, ultraviolet irradiation, silica particles, viruses, parasites, and other microorganisms. Agents that activate lymphocytes can stimulate macrophages to produce IL-1 either by direct cell contact, which is genetically controlled by MHC class II, or by producing cytokines, such as TNF-α, GM-CSF, or IL-1 itself, which can stimulate macrophages and other cells to produce more IL-1. The nature of the stimulant determines whether IL-1 accumulates intracellularly or is secreted. Latex particles, LPS, and zymosan stimulate increases in both intracellular and extracellular IL-1, whereas silica particles and phorbol myristate acetate (PMA) induce mainly extracellular IL-1.

IL-1ra is also produced by many cell types; tissue macrophages and keratinocytes are good producers (180). The production of IL-1β and IL-1ra in human monocytes is reciprocally regulated. *In vitro* studies showed that LPS stimulates equivalent amounts of IL-1β and IL-1ra in human monocytes, but adherent IgG selectively induces high levels of IL-1ra due to enhanced transcription and prolonged mRNA stability. The mechanism of this differential regulation of IL-1 and IL-1ra may involve cross-linking of different carbohydrate groups on the cell surface, resulting in different signaling events. Production of IL-1β and IL-1ra are also differentially regulated by cytokines. For example, IL-4, IL-10, and TGF-β increase synthesis of IL-1ra, but they can concommitantly decrease production of IL-1β in monocytes. Corticosteroids suppress the production of IL-1α and IL-1β but have no effect on IL-1ra. Studies of the kinetics of IL-1 production reveal that IL-1β production usually precedes IL-1α, and IL-1ra is made last. In addition, patients treated with IL-1β develop elevated plasma IL-1ra levels, indicating that IL-1 is an excellent inducer of IL-1ra production (181).

Many cell types express all three IL-1 genes, but levels of IL-1α, IL-1β, and IL-1ra vary widely. Keratinocytes express mostly IL-1α and icIL-1ra. Human monocytes produce predominantly IL-1β, while mouse macrophages produce mostly IL-1α. During differentiation of monocytes into macrophages, production of IL-1ra is enhanced, while that of IL-1β is decreased. Thus, IL-1ra is a major product of tissue macrophages, particularly during disease. The ratio of IL-1/IL-1ra production might change with certain viral infections. For example, more IL-1ra than IL-1 is induced *in vitro* by monocytes stimulated by HIV and neutrophils stimulated by Epstein-Barr virus (EBV) (182,183). Most of the IL-1 activity detected in the circulation is IL-1β, whereas IL-1α is more often found associated with the cell membrane. Plasma concentrations of IL-1β in normal subjects are usually undetectable (less than 40 pg per ml), except in women after ovulation and in subjects after strenuous exercise (184). Circulating levels of IL-1ra in normal human subjects are in the range of 200 to 300 pg per ml. There is no consistent correlation of increases of serum levels of IL-1 during various infectious diseases. However, peak levels of 150 to 200 pg per ml of IL-1β can be observed at 3 to 4 hours during experimental endotoxemia (185). Peak levels of IL-1ra are usually higher, about 6,000 to 8,000 pg per ml at 4 hours and remain high for another 8 hours (186).

Receptors

Two distinct IL-1 receptors, IL-1 receptor types I and II (IL-1RI and IL-1RII), have been cloned and characterized (187–190). In addition, a receptor accessory protein (IL-1R-AcP), which is the putative signal-transducing subunit of the IL-1 receptor complex has been identified (191). Both type I and type II receptors are members of the immunoglobulin superfamily. The human type I receptor is an 80-kDa transmembrane protein with 552 amino acids. It has a single 22-amino acid transmembrane region and a long cytoplasmic tail of 212 amino acids, which participates in signal transduction. Its extracellular ligand-binding region consists of three immunoglobulin-like domains. The type II receptor is a 60-kDa protein and is similar to the type I receptor in its extracellular and transmembrane regions. However, the type II receptor has a short cytoplasmic tail of 29 amino acids and is incapable of signaling. The type II receptor actually competitively inhibits IL-1 activity by acting as a "decoy" receptor for IL-1 and downregulates the level of extracellular IL-1. IL-1 receptor accessory protein is a

66-kDa transmembrane protein of 570 amino acids. Although the extracellular portion of IL-1R-AcP also consists of three immunoglobulin-like domains and shares homology with IL-1RI, it does not bind IL-1 or IL-1ra directly.

IL-1 binds to IL-1 receptors on target cells with high affinity (KD of 10–10 M). Type I receptors are found on most cells, including T cells, endothelial cells, hepatocytes, fibroblasts, and keratinocytes. Type II receptors have a more restricted distribution and are the predominant receptor on B cells, monocytes, and neutrophils. IL-1a, IL-1b, and IL-1ra each can bind to both types of IL-1 receptors but with different affinities. IL-1α binds preferentially with higher affinity to type I receptor ($K_D = 2 \times 10_{-10}$ M) and IL-1b binds preferentially to type II receptor ($K_D = 10_{-10}$ M). IL-1α binds type I receptor with considerably higher affinity ($K_D = 10_{-10}$ M) than it binds type II decoy receptor ($K_D = 10_{-8}$ M), and it can block the binding to type I receptor and the biologic responses of both IL-1α and IL-1β. However, a ten- to 500-fold excess of IL-1ra is necessary to achieve a 50% inhibition of the biologic effects of IL-1 in vitro. Both pro and mature forms of IL-1α bind to receptor with equal affinity, and their biologic activities appear to be similar. Pro-IL-1β does not bind or signal through type I receptor, but the mature IL-1β cleavage product does. IL-1 receptor accessory protein forms a complex with IL-1R1 after it is bound by either IL-1α or IL-1β, but not IL-1ra. Despite the low number of type I receptors (200 per cell), all biologic responses of IL-1 are mediated by type I receptors complexed with IL-1R-AcP. A receptor occupancy of less than 5% per cell is sufficient for cell activation. These data suggest that a major amplification of IL-1 signal must occur after IL-1 binding to an IL-1R1/IL-1R-AcP heterodimeric complex.

Expression of both type I and type II IL-1 receptors is tightly regulated to control inflammatory and immune responses. Transgenic mice transfected to overexpress IL-1RI on epidermal keratinocytes exhibited an exaggerated inflammatory response when challenged with known inducers of IL-1, suggesting that type I IL-1 receptors mediate the response to IL-1 (192). The extracellular domain of both type I and type II receptors is shed by activated neutrophils and monocytes, and the solubilized shed receptor binds and inhibits IL-1β functions (193–195). It was shown that vaccinia and cowpox viruses express genes that encode for a protein with 30% sequence homology to the soluble type II IL-1 receptor (196,197). This so-called virokine protein counteracts the host inflammatory response to these viruses, because viruses genetically engineered to inactivate these genes become less pathogenic. This and reports of the acquisition of inhibitors of ICE by certain viruses again underscore the importance of IL-1 in host defense (198).

Signal Transduction by IL-1

The functional signal-transducing IL-1 receptor consists of IL-1RI and IL-1R-AcP as a two-subunit receptor complex that binds both IL-1α and IL-1β with higher affinity but IL-1ra less well (191,199). IL-1, like other proinflammatory cytokines, activates two transcription factors, NF-kB and AP-1, which translocate to the nucleus and activate many of the cytokine-inducible genes (200–202). In most cells, NF-kB is normally retained in the cytoplasm by inhibitory proteins, designated IkB. In response to IL-1 and a variety of other extracellular stimuli, such as TNF α, mitogens, oxidative stress, and LPS, IkB is degraded, releasing NF-kB to enter the nucleus, where it binds DNA and activates transcription (Fig. 3).

Although IL1-R1 does not possess intrinsic kinase activity, IL-1 binding leads to rapid phosphorylation of serine and threonine residues in a number of proteins (203). An IL-1 receptor–associated kinase activity (IRAK) that coimmunoprecipitates with human IL-1R1 has been identified and cloned (204,205). IRAK is a 100-kDa protein with a highly conserved protein kinase domain and bears homology to the *Drosophila* Pelle protein, a serine–threonine kinase that is essential for the activation of an NF-kB homologue in *Drosophila*. IRAK rapidly associates with the IL-1R1 complex upon IL-1 binding and becomes autophosphorylated (see Fig. 3). Another protein, TRAF6, a member of the TNF receptor–associated protein family, was also identified as a signal transducer for IL-1 (206). It is likely that upon IL-1 binding to the heterodimeric IL-1R1/IL-1R-AcP, IRAK becomes phosphorylated and associates with TRAF6. This phosphorylated IRAK/TRAF6 complex subsequently binds to the cytoplasmic tail of the IL-1R1 and IL-1R-AcP heterodimer, leading to NF-kB activation and induction of proinflammatory genes.

Numerous secondary messengers and signaling cascades have been proposed to be initiated by IL-1 (207,208). One potential pathway involves the activation of a neutral sphingomyelinase with subsequent hydrolysis of sphingomyelin to ceramide (209,210). Ceramide then stimulates a ceramide-activated protein kinase that phosphorylates a specific set of cellular proteins, thereby altering their function. A cloned protein kinase, NIK, participates in an NF-KB–inducing signaling cascade common to IL-1R1 and to receptors of the TNF/NGF family (88). The isolation of NIK helps to explain the pathway of NF-kB activation by IL-1. Available evidence suggests that NIK is at the point of convergence of TNF and IL-1 signaling pathways (see Fig. 3). As mentioned earlier in this chapter, IL-1 leads to the activation of the kinase IRAK and of another member of the TRAF protein family, termed TRAF6. Like TRAF2 in TNF-treated cells, TRAF6 is the immediate upstream activator of NIK in IL-1–stimulated cells. Thus, it is now possible to explain in molecular terms why TNF and IL-1, cytokines that are structurally unrelated and bind to completely distinct receptors, activate so many identical target genes and produce so many identical biologic actions. In addition, other kinases, including p38 MAPK, JNK/SAPK (c-Jun N-terminal kinase/stress-activated protein kinase or p54 MAPK), IkB kinase, and β-casein kinase, are also activated by IL-1 (211). These kinases are all implicated in the downstream phosphorylation of various nuclear binding proteins, through multiple phosphorylation steps and interactions, which then activate new gene expression. The precise order of these signaling cascades has not been determined. Different types of responding cells may utilize diverse signal transduction pathways for IL-1, resulting in cellular specificity. For example, IL-1 activates JNK, which phosphorylates ATF-2 and c-Jun, thereby increasing the transactivating potency of these factors in endothelial cells (212).

Translocation of transcription factors to the nucleus resulting from the various pathways activated after IL-1 receptor interactions induces many genes. AP-1 and NF-kB–binding sites are found in the promoter regions of certain IL-1–inducible genes, including those of IL-6, IL-8, IL-2 receptor, and endothelial cell adhesion molecule. IL-1 also activates two other transcription factors, Jun-1 and Jun-2, that bind to the promoter of *c-Jun*, leading to increased gene transcription (213). *c-Fos* is also activated, and the Jun and Fos proteins join to form AP-1 (214). Many of the biologic activities of IL-1 are mediated through the binding of these factors to the AP-1 and NF-kB sites of IL-1–inducible genes.

Inflammatory and Immunologic Effects

Biologic activities of IL-1 are mostly the indirect result of induction of a cascade of other mediators. Its biologic activities largely overlap with those of TNF-α and IL-6 (154,156). IL-1 is a pleiotropic mediator of the host response to infections and injurious insults, and it coordinates the activities of other cells and cytokines. Many of the effects of IL-1 are mediated through its capacity to increase the production of other cytokines, such as granulocyte colony-stimulating factor (G-CSF), GM-CSF, TNF-α, IL-6, IL-8, and homologous members of the chemokine family, platelet-derived growth factor (PDGF), and IL-11. Further amplification of the biologic effects of IL-1 is achieved by the ability of IL-1 to upregulate receptor expression for itself, for the IL-2 receptor α chain, and for the receptors for IFN-γ, IL-3, and GM-CSF, and the consequent synergistic action of some of these cytokines with IL-1.

IL-1 is active over low concentrations of 10^{-9} to 10^{-15} M. When produced locally by stimulated cells, IL-1 acts as an autocrine or paracrine costimulant of early innate inflammatory and later specific immune responses. When released in larger quantities into the circulation, IL-1 acts systemically to exert endocrine effects, such as activation of the fever center, the hypothalamus–pituitary–adrenal (HPA) axis, and in inducing acute-phase proteins.

IL-1 stimulates a variety of cells that function as effectors of immune and inflammatory responses. IL-1 is a comitogen for T cells by upregulating IL-2 production and the expression of IL-2 receptors on T cells (215). IL-1 acts preferentially as a costimulator for Th_2 cells activated through the T-cell antigen receptor, resulting in increased proliferation and IL-9 production (216). IL-1 augments antigen-induced T cell–proliferative and functional responses partly because IL-1 coinduces MHC class II expression on antigen-presenting cells (217). IL-1 also induces the production IL-6 and TNF-α. One study showed that IL-1 production within the thymic microenvironment induces expression of IL-2 receptor α chain on early immature thymocytes (218). Thus, IL-1 can contribute to thymocyte maturation and $CD4^+CD8^+$ differentiation. Despite this, thymic development in knock-out mice that lack the IL-1 type I receptor is normal, presumably based on redundancy of cytokine activities and compensatory pathways.

IL-1 can also promote B-cell maturation and differentiation, as evidenced by the induction of κ light chain synthesis by pre-B cells (219). IL-1 augments B-cell proliferation, surface IgM expression, and antibody production. However, knock-out mice that lack the IL-1 type I receptor have normal serum immunoglobulin levels and a normal immune response. IL-1 acts on monocytes and neutrophils, inducing secretion of several cytokines, including IL-8 and IL-1 itself (154,220). IL-1 is reported to prolong the survival of neutrophils *in vitro*. IL-1 augments the antigen-presenting capacity of dendritic cells (221).

IL-1 participates in the recruitment of leukocytes to inflammatory sites by inducing the expression of adhesion molecules (ICAM, ELAM, and VCAM) on vascular endothelium and a number of chemokines that attract neutrophils, eosinophils, macrophages, and lymphocytes to sites of injury (220,222–224). Other mediators, such as IL-1, IL-6, prostanoids, platelet-activating factor (PAF), and procoagulant factor (tissue factor), are also produced by endothelial cells in response to IL-1.

Other Biologic Functions

IL-1 is an important regulator of hematopoiesis (225), although the phenotype of IL-1β–deficient mice is remarkably normal (226). IL-1 induces the production of GM-CSF, G-CSF by bone marrow stromal cells and receptors for GM-CSF. Thus IL-1 synergizes with GM-CSF to stimulate growth of early hematopoietic bone marrow progenitor cells and can counteract the myelosuppressive effects of radiotherapy and chemotherapy (227,228). The latter effect is mediated partly through the induction of mitochondrial manganese superoxide dismutase activity that scavenges potentially toxic superoxide radicals.

IL-1, an endogenous pyrogen (229), has been shown to induce fever, induce the duration of slow-wave sleep, and decrease appetite, perhaps by inducing the production of leptins (230). Brain and endocrine organs have type I receptors. Neurons and glial cells can synthesize IL-1, suggesting that IL-1 may modulate interneuronal interactions (231). The synthesis of IL-1 in the central nervous system (CNS) is increased during development and in response to injury. IL-1, by itself or in combination with IFN-γ or TNF-α, stimulates astrocytes, but not microglia, to express the inducible form of nitric oxide synthase (232). IL-1 also stimulates the hypothalamus to produce corticotropin-releasing hormone (CRH), resulting in the expression of the proopiomelanocortin (POMC) gene by the pituitary gland, with production of endorphins, α-melanocyte-stimulating hormone (α-MSH), and adrenocorticotropic hormone (ACTH), all of which have antiinflammatory effects. This activation of the HPA axis culminates in induction of the production of glucocorticoids by the adrenals. Glucocorticoids also act as endogenous negative-feedback downregulators of the production of IL-1 and as upregulators of both type I and type II IL-1 receptors (233). The pivotal role of glucocorticoids in moderating the effects of IL-1 is shown by the fact that adrenalectomized animals become much more sensitive to the inflammatory and toxic effects of IL-1, indicating that normal adrenal activity buffers IL-1 activity (234). IL-1 also inhibits the release of gonadotropin-releasing hormones, thus suppressing reproductive function in face of immune challenge. IL-1 inhibits the release of luteinizing hormone (LH), as well as thyroid-stimulating hormone (TSH), and decreases plasma thyroid hormone.

FIG. 3. IL-1–induced signaling pathways. IL-1 binding to IL-1RI leads to interaction with IL-1R-AcP, and this complex transduces a signal. Binding of IL-1 to IL-1RII, which has a short cytoplasmic tail, does not transmit signals. IL-1ra, which lacks a second binding site, cannot interact properly with IL-1RI, and does not bind IL-1R-AcP, also produces no signal upon binding to IL-1RI. An intracellular kinase, IL-1 receptor–associated kinase (IRAK) rapidly associates with the IL-1RI and IL-1-AcP heterodimeric complex upon IL-1 binding. Binding of a TNF receptor–associated protein (TRAF6) to autophosphorylated IRAK leads to downstream activation of multiple kinases. Early membrane-associated events also may result in the release of ceramide from membrane sphingomyelin, which leads to activation of the kinase cascade. Activation of JNKK and other mitogen-activated protein (MAP) kinases lead to phosphorylation of p54 MAPK, p38 MAPK, and hsp27. Another pathway that contributes to singaling is the activation of a NFkB-inducing kinase (NIK), leading to NFkB activation. Translocation to the nucleus and binding of nuclear factors (NFkB and the heterodimer of jun and fos) to DNA initiate gene expression induced by IL-1.

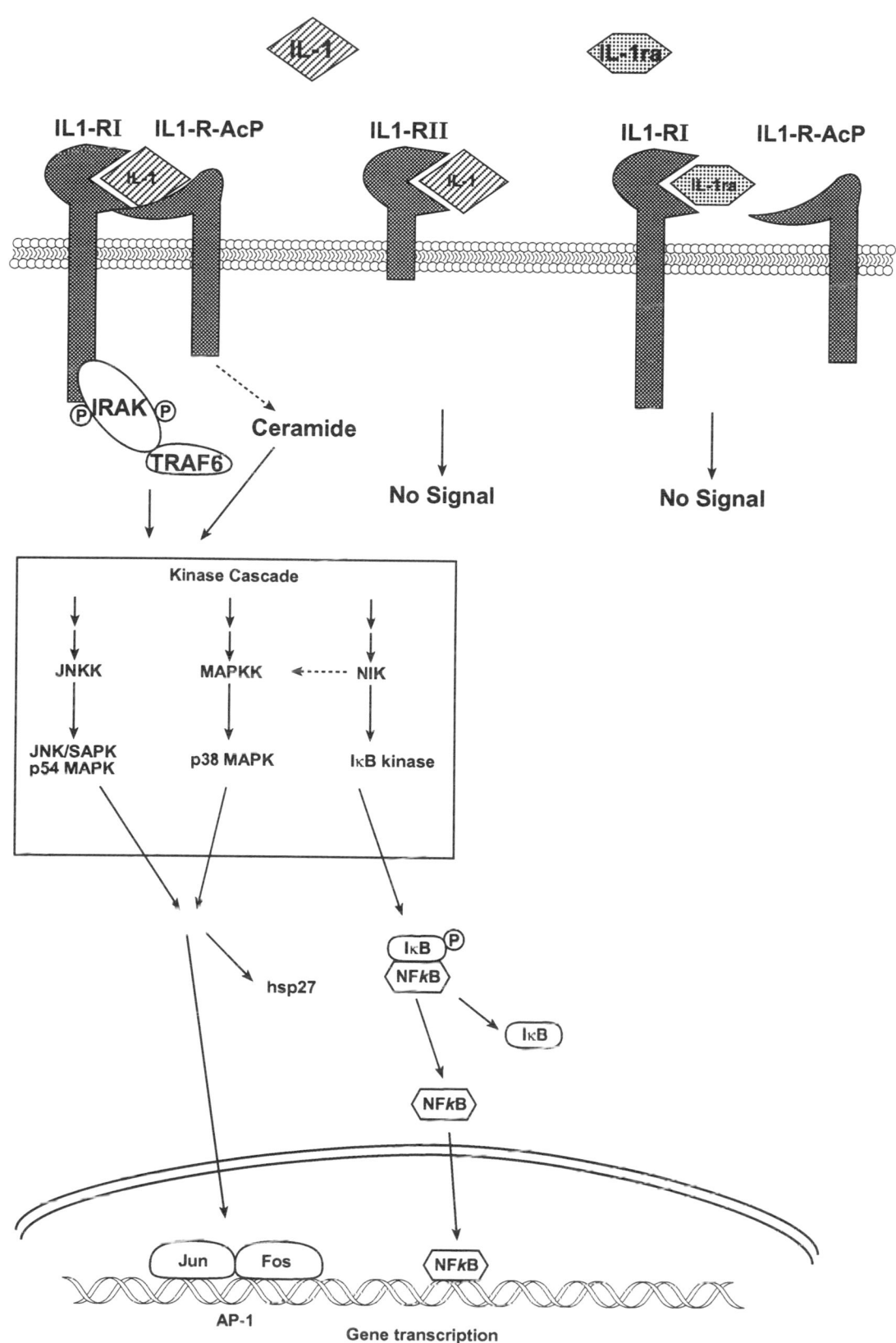

IL-1 is postulated to play a major role in destructive joint disease, such as rheumatoid arthritis (235). IL-1 stimulates bone resorption by inducing metalloprotease secretion by chondrocytes, resulting in cartilage breakdown and proteoglycan release. IL-1 induces tissue-type macrophages to secrete gelatinase and participates in extracellular matrix destruction (236). IL-1 stimulates fibroblast proliferation and secretion of collagenase, IL-6, IL-8, and G-CSF. IL-1 also induces cyclooxygenase synthesis and hence prostaglandin release from fibroblasts, but it suppresses expression of mRNA for matrix proteins. Adjuvant-induced arthritis in animal models can be markedly suppressed by the administration of IL-1ra or neutralizing antibodies to IL-1 (237,238).

IL-1 can have antitumor as well as tumor growth–promoting effects (239–241). IL-1 acts both as an cytostatic and a cytocidal agent for a number of tumor cell lines *in vitro*. This activity is asociated with inhibition of ornithine decarboxylase activity by IL-1. IL-1 increases the innate antitumor activity of NK cells as well as T cell–dependent tumor immunity *in vivo*. Fibrosarcoma tumor-cell lines transfected to overexpress IL-1α are more readily rejected and induce the development of immune resistance upon rechallenge. However, systemic administration of IL-1 has been reported to promote the development of tumor metastases in some animal models. Thus, under some circumstances, IL-1 can promote tumorogenesis.

IL-1 is also implicated in the induction of insulin secretion and stimulation of apoptosis of β cells of the pancreatic islet, presumably through induction of nitric oxide (242). Thus, the production of IL-1 by local inflammatory cells initiated by an unknown autoimmune process in insulin-dependent diabetes mellitus may contribute to the destruction of β cells.

One report suggested that intracellular IL-β acts as an endogenous inhibitor of Fas-mediated apoptosis, and this could prolong the release of IL-1β by inhibiting apoptosis of macrophages (243). An antisense oligodeoxynucleotide of IL-1α was shown to prolong the life span of cultured human endothelial cells (244). Thus, intracellular IL-1 may regulate senescence and plays a role in normal cell survival as well. However, once again, these activities are not defective in knock-out mice.

The intracellular functions of icIL-1ra, if any, are even less clear than those of IL-1α and IL-1β. IL-1ra is concentrated intracellularly in the stratum granulosum of normal skin, consistent with the observation from *in vitro* studies of enhanced production by differentiated keratinocytes. IcIL-1ra attenuates and destabilizes IL-1–induced GRO mRNA in ovarian cancer cells and limits IL-1 responsiveness at a point downstream of the cytokine–receptor interaction (245).

Inhibitors and Antagonists

Because of the potent proinflammatory effects of IL-1, its production, secretion, and biologic activities are tightly regulated (Table 7). The biologic effects of IL-1 are modulated by IL-1ra and also by the shed soluble forms of the IL-1 receptors (sIL-1R) (246–250). The findings of high plasma and tissue levels of IL-1ra in patients suffering from various inflammatory diseases indicate that endogenously produced IL-1ra may be a normal homeostatic response to limit the proinflammatory, pathogenic effects of IL-1. A markedly significant decrease in the intestinal mucosal IL-1ra/IL-1 ratio is associated with inflammatory bowel diseases (251). A similiar imbalance of IL-1ra/IL-1β production is also observed in cells from rheumatoid synovium (252).

Because of the differential affinities of IL-1 for receptors, sIL-1R1 inhibits preferentially IL-1α, and soluble IL-1RII present in normal plasma, serum, and synovial inflammatory exudate functions as a specific inhibitor of IL-1β. The affinity of sIL-1RII remains the same for IL-1α and IL-1β, but it decreases by a factor of 2,000 for IL-1ra when compared with cell surface IL-1RII (194). In addition, sIL-1RII also blocks the processing of pro-IL-1β by binding the propeptide with higher affinity. IL-1ra and sIL-1RII, in combination, have an additive effect in inhibiting the binding of IL-1β to IL-1RI. In contrast, IL-1ra and sIL-1RI potentially counteract each other's inhibitory effect (see Table 7).

A number of other naturally occurring inhibitors of IL-1 are present in serum. α-MSH inhibits the synthesis and activities of IL-1. PGE$_2$ suppresses the synthesis and release of IL-1, but enhances the expression of both IL-1 receptors. CRH inhibits IL-1–induced anorexia, sleep, and prostaglandin synthesis. Corticosteroids suppress expression of IL-1 mRNA, but increase the expression of both IL-1 receptors and sIL-1RII. TGF-β downregulates the production of IL-1 and IL-1R1, but induces IL-1ra synthesis. IL-4, IL-10, and IL-13 inhibit IL-1 production, but upregulate IL-1ra production. In addition, IL-4 and IL-13 also increase the expression of both receptors as well as the shedding of IL-1RII. Chemotactic agents, including IL-8, FMLP, C5a, leukotriene B$_4$, and PAF, induce rapid shedding of IL-1RII from human polymorphonuclear leukocytes (253). The ability of these cytokines and hormones to inhibit IL-1 production and to induce the expression and shedding of the decoy receptor may account for the antiinflammatory efects of these agents.

Despite the fact that knock-out mice with deficient IL-1 functions show only mild phenotypic defects, IL-1 is the only cytokine that is regulated by a natural competitive homologue, IL-1ra. Studies with IL-1ra–deficient mice suggest that IL-1ra is involved with normal development, as IL-1ra deficient mice have decreased body mass compared with wild-type controls (254). IL-1ra can block IL-1–induced T-cell proliferation and LPS-induced IL-8 production in mononuclear cells. IL-1ra also decreases IL-2 receptors and secretion of IL-1α, IL-1β, IL-2, and TNF in these cells *in vitro*. Several studies have shown that inhibition of IL-1ra by neutralizing antibodies results in considerable excerbation of inflammatory diseases. For example, administration of neutralizing antibodies to IL-1ra

TABLE 7. *Effects of IL-1 inhibitors on IL-1, IL-1ra, and IL-1R*

Inhibitors	IL-1	IL-1ra[a]	IL-1RII	sIL-1RII[a]	IL-1RI
Glucocorticoids	↓	↑	↑	↑	↑
IL-4 and IL-13	↓	↑	↑	↑	↑
IL-10	↓	↑	ND	ND	ND
TGF-β	↓	↑	ND	ND	↓
PGE$_2$	↓	ND	↑	ND	↑

[a]IL-1ra and sIL-1RII are also IL-1 inhibitors. The upregulatory or downregulatory effects of these inhibitors are shown with arrows.
ND, not determined.

markedly exacerbates colitis induced in an animal model (255). Thus, IL-1ra plays a role in downregulating *in vivo* inflammatory reactions. In animal models, IL-1–induced hypotension can be inhibited by pretreating the animals with large doses of IL-1ra. However, the large amounts of IL-1ra (10,000-fold molar excess, 2.5 g per day estimated for human use) required to counteract IL-1–mediated effects limit the clinical usefulness of IL-1ra. Thus, IL-1ra as yet has no significant therapeutic potential in human phase III clinical trials for sepsis. Improved delivery systems of providing a local source of IL-1ra may make IL-1ra more effective (256,257).

Other therapeutic approaches to block IL-1–mediated responses include the use of anti-IL-1 antibodies, anti-IL-1 receptor antibodies, soluble IL-1 receptors, and inhibitors of ICE to inhibit IL-1β processing. In another study, by comparing the receptor–binding affinities and antagonistic activities of different IL-1ra mutants, a better antagonist than IL-1ra, with increased binding to IL-1RI but decreased binding to IL-1RII, had been identified (249).

Gene Deletions

Despite the plethora of IL-1 activities, knock-out mice defective in the production of IL-1α or IL-1β or in the expression of IL-1 type I receptor are viable and show only relatively limited phenotypic deficiencies (258–260 (Table 8). IL-1β–deficient mice are resistant to fever induction and have an impaired acute-phase response to a local injection of turpentine, although systemic administration of LPS gave a normal inflammatory response in these mice. This normal response to LPS is based on redundancy in the activities of IL-1α, IL-1β, TNF-α, LT-α, and IL-6.

IL-1ra–deficient mice are more susceptible than controls to lethal endotoxemia but are less susceptible to infection with *L. monocytogenes*. Conversely, transgenic IL-1ra overproducers are protected from the lethal effects of endotoxin but are more susceptible to listeriosis. Serum levels of IL-1 after endotoxin challenge are decreased in IL-1ra–deficient mice and increased in IL-1ra overproducers. Thus, IL-1ra acts as a positive regulator of IL-1 levels to balance the potentially beneficial effects of IL-1 against the excessive production during infection.

In summary, IL-1 plays a central role in regulating immune responses, often by inducing other mediators and cytokines. IL-1 is the only cytokine for which a natural endogenous inhibitor with specificity exists, IL-1ra, to counteract its biologic effects. Thus, multiple mechanisms, such as the shedding of IL-1 receptors, corticosteroids, and IL-1ra, regulate the levels and activities of IL-1. Although mice with homologous deletions of IL-1α, IL-1β, or IL-1R1 show surprisingly few deficiencies, the best evidence that IL-1 plays an important role in host defense comes from observations

that a number of viruses produce IL-1 receptor homologues that subvert the host defense mechanisms and, if deleted, reduce the pathogenicity of these viruses.

CHEMOKINES

The burgeoning family of *chemo*attractant cyto*kines*, now known as chemokines, comprises the most diverse and largest subset of cytokines identified to date. Chemokines are characterized by their capacity to induce the directional migration and activation of leukocytes, as well as other somatic cell types, and thus play major roles in acute and chronic inflammation. Chemokines also promote humoral and cell-mediated immune reactions; regulate cell adhesion, angiogenesis, leukocyte trafficking, and homing; and contribute to lymphopoiesis and hematopoiesis (as reviewed in refs. 261–265). Chemokines are produced by a wide variety of leukocytes and other cell types in response to irritants, polyclonal stimulants, antigens, and endogenous cytokines. A variety of chemokines has been detected at local inflammatory sites in a great number of disease states (265). Studies of the *in vivo* effects of neutralizing antibodies and homologous deletion of chemokine genes reveal that chemokines play a central role in host defense against infectious organisms, including HIV-1 (266). Furthermore, chemokines participate in the pathogenesis of diverse conditions such as reperfusion injuries, including strokes, acute respiratory distress syndrome (ARDS), immune complex -induced glomerulonephritis, atherosclerosis, and autoimmune reactions (265,267). However, in contrast to other proinflammatory cytokines, such as IL-1 and TNF, circulating chemokines generally do not induce other cytokines, acute-phase responses, or fever, but induce other effector molecules, such as histamine, enzymes, and defensins. At higher concentrations, circulating chemokines have desensitizing effects and can suppress local inflammation. Because identification and studies of human chemokines are more advanced, our chapter will relate to human chemokines, unless otherwise specified.

Subfamilies

Four chemokine subfamilies have been identified, based on their structures. They include the CXC (α), CC (β), C (γ), and CX₃C subfamilies (261). The chemokine genes in each subset are usually clustered closely on the same chromosomes, indicating that they arose by repeated gene duplication. Nine of the members of the CXC chemokine α subset are clustered on human chromosome 4 (q12–21), whereas the SDF-1 gene is on chromosome 10. They all have one amino acid (x) separating the first two of their four conserved cysteine residues. Eleven of the CC chemokine β subset are located on human chromosome 17 (q11–21), but four newly characterized members are found on chromosomes 2, 9, and 16 (268). They have no intervening amino acid separating the first two of their four, or in the case of I-309, six cysteine residues. In both subfamilies, the first cysteine forms a disulfide bond with the third, and the second with the fourth, resulting in a stable tertiary structure ranging from 7 to 9 kDa in MW. Lymphotactin (Lptn), the only member of the chemokine γ group, is located on human chromosome 11, is 16 kDa in MW, and has only one pair of cysteines near its N-terminus (269). Lptn is produced by NK cells and acts on NK as well as T cells (270). The newest CX₃C chemokine, known as fractalkine or neurotactin, has three amino acids between the amino terminal cysteines and is on human chromosome 16 (271,272). It is larger than the other chemokines, with a MW of about 38 kDa. Fractalkine has an 18-amino acid hydrophobic sequence near the carboxyl end, which

TABLE 8. *Phenotypes of mice with IL-1 family gene knockouts*

Targeted gene	Major phenotypic abnormalities
IL-1β	Reduced production of IL-6 and acute-phase responses to turpentine
IL-1R type 1	Absence of fever and anorexic response to turpentine. Absence of IL-1–mediated signaling. Greater susceptibility to *Listeria monocytogenes*.
IL-1RA	Decreased body mass. Higher LPS lethality. Reduced susceptibility to *Listeria monocytogenes*.
ICE	Lower LPS lethality. Defect in both IL-1α and IL-1β release.

appears to act as an endothelial cell membrane-anchoring motif. The chemokine components, consisting of about 80 amino acids, may be cleaved off its 240-amino acid mucin-like stalk, but fractalkine may function largely in a cell-bound manner.

Chemokines are produced as inactive precursors, enzymatically cleaved intracellularly and secreted by the classical pathway. The carboxyl ends of the basic chemokine molecules all exhibit low-affinity (kDa 10^{-5} M) heparin-binding properties and bind to glycosaminoglycan (GAG) molecules and other negatively charged sugar molecules on cell surfaces and tissue matrix glycoproteins (273). This enables chemokines to adsorb onto endothelial cells (ECs) lining the blood vessels, connective tissue, and extracellular matrices. Consequently, chemokines also have the capacity to induce directional "haptotactic" migration of cells along GAG-coated surfaces.

Receptors and Signal Transduction

Chemokines exhibit high-affinity (kDa 10^{-8} to 10^{-9} M) interactions with a growing subfamily of homologous seven-transmembrane G protein–coupled receptors (7TMR) (262,263). Other proinflammatory chemoattractants, such as PAF, LTB4, C5a, and fMLP, also use a 7TMR with lower homology to the chemokine receptors. Hydropathy analysis revealed that the chemokine receptors consist of an extracellular N-terminus, seven hydrophobic transmembrane domains, resulting in three extracellular and three intracellular loops, and an intracellular carboxyl terminus that contains a number of serine and threonine residues. These residues are subject to phosphorylation and participate in signaling and desensitization. Chemokine ligands usually interact with both the N-terminal end and a second site located on one of the extracellular loops of the receptor. The heterotrimeric G protein is usually coupled to one of the intracellular loops of the receptor (274). The "DRY" motif (Asp-Arg-Tyr), which is generally located in the second intracellular loop, also has been implicated in signal transduction (275). To date, four receptors have been cloned and identified as CXCR1–4 for the CXC subfamily, and eight (CCR1–8) for the CC chemokines. The chemokines exhibit considerable redundancy in their receptor utilization, and leukocytes express multiple receptors (Fig. 4). Thus, chemokines, like the other cytokines, are pleiotropic in their activities.

Microbial organisms and viruses have also adapted chemokine receptors to their own advantage (262,275). The Duffy antigen, also known as DARC, has been identified as a 7TMR that binds many CXC and CC chemokines and provides a binding site on red blood cells for the invasion of *Plasmodium vivax* malaria parasites (276). Although DARC also has been detected on postcapillary venules, Purkinje cells, and activated T cells, ligation of this receptor does not transduce signals, and it is thought to transport and facilitate the clearance of circulating chemokines (Table 9). Furthermore, several herpes viruses have genes that encode for chemokine-binding molecules. Cytomegaloviruses (CMVs) cause infected lymphocytes to express a functional binding site for MCP-1, MIP-1α, MIP-1β, and RANTES. This CMV-encoded chemokine receptor, US28, has been shown to permit HIV-1 infection of CD4+ cells, possibly accounting for the exacerbated disease status of acquired immunodeficiency syndrome (AIDS) patients who are superinfected with CMV (277). Herpes virus saimiri (HVS)–infected lymphocytes express CXCR2-like binding sites (see Table 9). A gene from the human herpes virus 8 (HHV8), which was recovered from Kaposi sarcoma of AIDS patients, encodes an IL-8 like receptor (278). This receptor constitutively transduces signals and, thus (like IL-8) may promote tumor angiogenesis and account for the excessive vascularization of this tumor type.

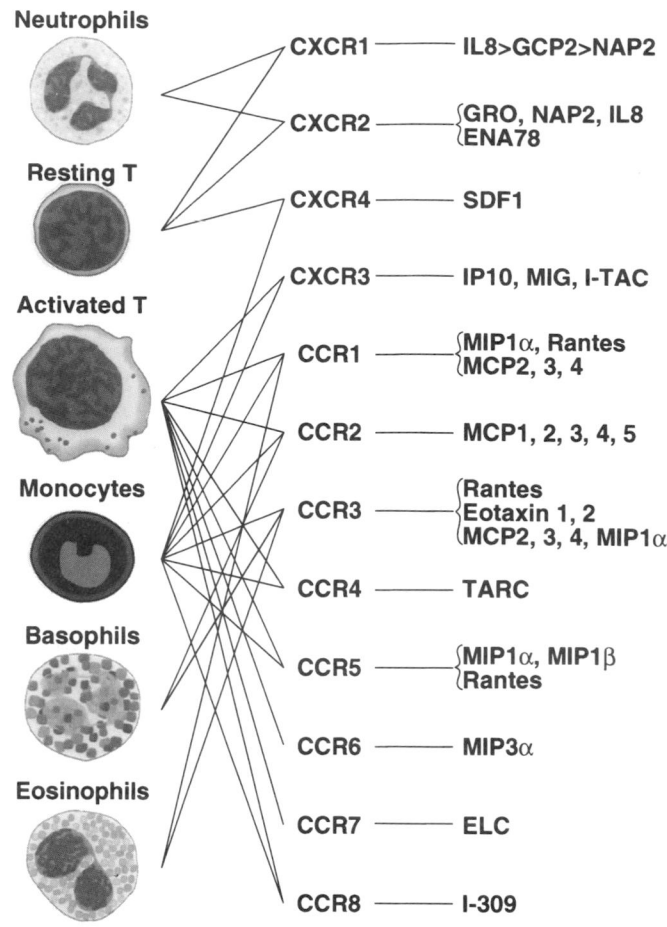

FIG. 4. Human leukocyte receptors for chemokines. Human leukocytes express multiple seven-transmembrane receptors that interact with one or more of the chemokines. (Adapted from drawings and data provided by Drs. Charles Mackay, Barrett Rollins, and Andrew Luster.)

The expression of chemokine receptors is closely regulated by exogenous and endogenous stimuli. With some exceptions, activated leukocytes express a greater number of receptors than do unstimulated resting leukocytes. For example, the transcription and expression of CXCR2 on human T-lymphocytes decrease with *in vitro* incubation at 37°C and are restored by incubation in the presence of monocytes or IFN-γ (279). Activated T-lymphocytes express more CCR1 through CCR7, whereas resting T cells express more CXCR1, 2, and 4 (280). It has also been shown that memory (CD45RO+) T cells cultured for four or more days with IL-2 express more CCR1, 2, and 5 and are more readily chemoattracted by CC chemokines, but not IL-8 (281). *In vitro* incubation of neutrophils with G-CSF enhances, whereas LPS inhibits, the expression of CXCR2 mRNA, IL-8 binding, and neutrophil chemotactic responses to IL-8 (282). LPS and other microbial agents also rapidly reduce the expression by mononuclear phagocytes of CCR2, and to a lesser extent, of CCR1 and CCR5, mRNA, with a concomitant reduction in their binding and chemotactic responses to MCP-1 (283). In contrast, IL-2 can augment CCR2 expression.

Signal transduction by chemokine receptors requires an initial coupling with G proteins, which initiates a cascade of cellular signals and eventual biologic responses (Fig. 5). The G proteins con-

TABLE 9. *Interactions of microbial pathogens and chemokines*

Pathogen-derived signal	Receptor	Chemokine ligands
Monotropic HIV-1 gp120	CCR5 > CCR3 and CCR2, STRL33	MIP-1β, α, RANTES, Eotaxin, MCP-2
Lymphotrophic HIV-1 gp120	CXCR4 and STRL33	SDF-1α
Plasmodium vivax	DARC	IL-8, GROα, Eotaxin, MCP-1, 2, 3, 4, MIP-1α, RANTES
Herpes CMV US28 genes	US28 (CCR-like receptor)	MCP-1, MIP-1α, RANTES
Herpes saimiri virus—ECRF3 genes	ECRF3 (CXCR-like receptor)	GROα, NAP-2, IL-8
Herpes virus 8: codes for MIP1α and IL-6 homologues	IL8R-like constitutively activated receptor CCR1, 3 and 5.	IL-8(?)
Myxoma (pox) virus	Virally derived inhibitors with GAG-binding sites	Carboxyl-terminal tail of many CC and CXC chemokines

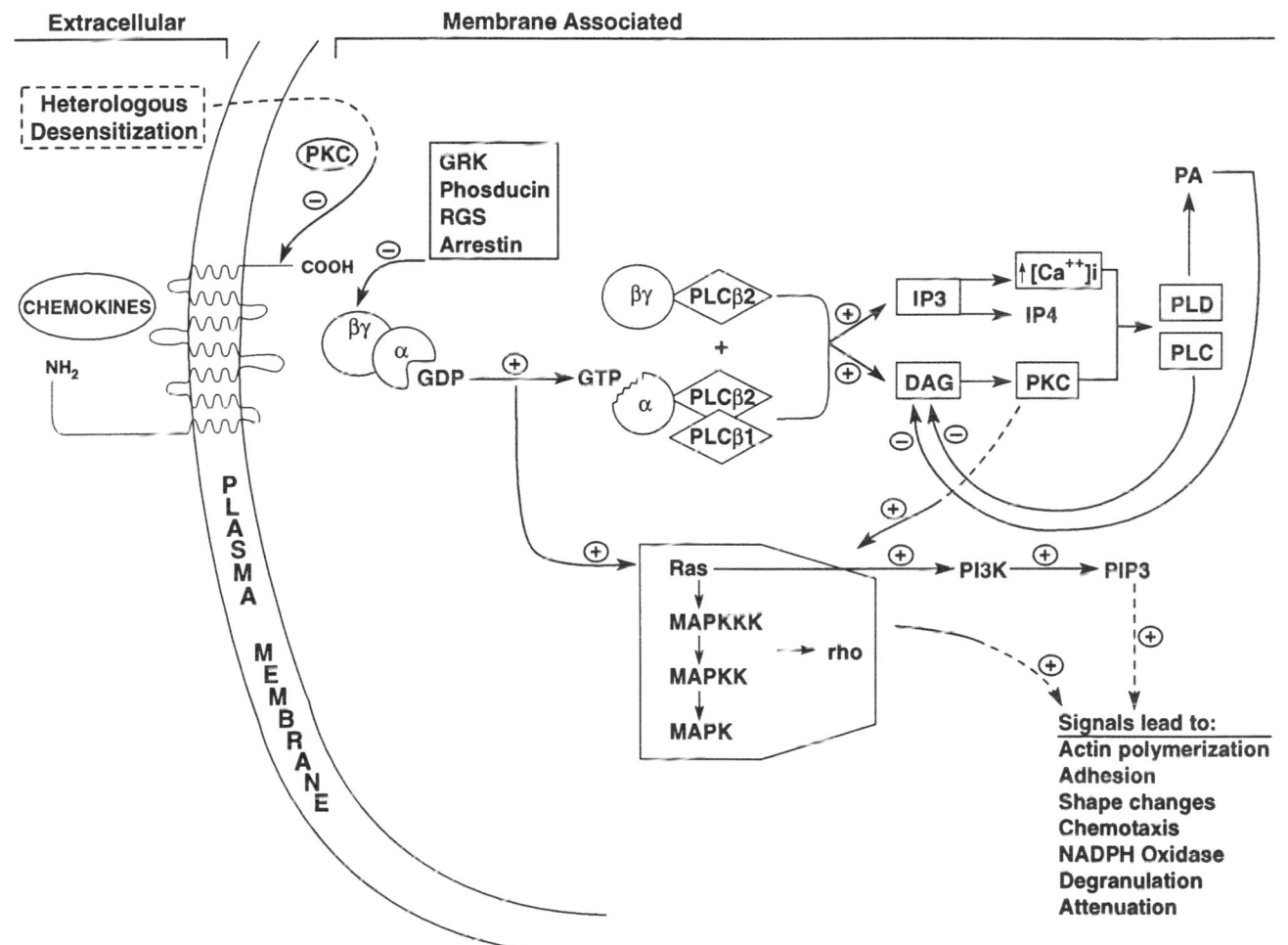

FIG. 5. Signal transduction by chemokines. Receptor coupling results in an exchange of the G protein from a GDP- to GTP-bound state. This can be prevented by uncoupling of G protein due to heterologous desensitization, signaling via PKC or a number of other downregulatory molecules. Otherwise, the α and βγ subunits of G protein activate PLCβ1 and PLCβ2, generating IP3 and DAG. IP$_3$ mobilizes calcium, whereas DAG stimulates PKC to phosphorylate downstream effectors such as MAP kinases, which culminates in cell mobilization, adhesion, degranulation, enzyme activation, and other cellular functions. PLC, phospholipase C; RGS, regulator of G-protein signal; PIP$_2$, phosphatidylinositol 4,5-bisphosphate; IP$_3$, inositol 1,4,5-trisphosphate; DAG, diacylglycerol; PLD, phospholipase D; PA, phosphatidic acid; PKC, protein kinase C; MAPK, mitogen-activated protein kinase; MAPKK, MAPK kinase; MAP-KKK, MAPKK kinase.

sist of a large gene family coding for at least 16 α, four β, and multiple γ subunits. The chemokine receptor signal is often inhibited by pertussis toxin (PT), which uncouples certain G proteins (Gαi 2 and 3) from chemokine receptors (284). Receptor coupling typically results in an exchange in the α subunit of the G protein from a GDP- to GTP-bound state, resulting in dissociation of the α from the β and γ subunits. These subunits then activate PLCβ1 and PLCβ2, followed by hydrolysis of phosphatidylinositol 4,5-biphosphonate (PIP$_2$) yielding inositol triphosphate (IP$_3$) and diacylglycerol (DAG). IP$_3$ mobilizes Ca^{2+} from intracellular stores, which accounts for the capacity of chemokines to induce a calcium flux in many cell types (261–263). The DAG stimulates PKC, which phosphorylates and activates a number of effectors, such as MAP kinases. MCP-1 is an exception, and does not induce CCR2 to signal PIP$_2$ turnover and IP$_3$ production (285). MCP-1 and 3 depend on external Ca^{2+} to induce a Ca2+ flux, whereas MCP-2 and MIP-1β are weak inducers of Ca^{2+} fluxes in monocytes. The chemokines also frequently induce tyrosine phosphorylation, which participates in the downstream MAP kinase cascade. G protein–dependent signals lead to actin polymerization, reconfiguration of adhesion proteins, and other cellular responses contributing to cell migration. This pathway can be dissociated from Ca^{2+} flux and PKC-dependent responses, whereas tyrosine phosphorylation and DAG/PLD interaction promote superoxide production.

CXC Chemokine Subsets

Those CXC chemokines with an ELR sequence (glu-leu-arg) at positions 4, 5, and 6 near the N-terminus, all interact with CXCR2 with equally high affinity (see Fig. 4). This receptor is highly expressed on neutrophils and accounts for the acute inflammatory effects of IL-8, GRO, NAP-2, ENA78, and GCP-2 (286). The ELR$^+$ CXC chemokines chemoattract neutrophils and promote their adherence to EC, their subsequent transmigration through blood vessel walls, tissue invasion, and migration along chemokine gradients on matrix proteins and cell surfaces to local inflammatory sites (Table 10). At higher concentrations, chemokines activate neutrophils to produce oxygen radicals and degranulate with consequent release of their granule contents, which can further amplify ongoing inflammatory and immunologic reactions (264. Modification of the ELR sequence inactivates these chemokines by abrogating their ability to interact with CXCR2 (261). The angiogenic effects of CXC chemokines are presumed to be based on their capacity to induce the proliferation and directional migration of ECs, thus leading to the formation of new vasculature (287). Although there are reports that some ECs can express CXCR1 (288), and at sites of wound healing, CXCR2 (289); others consider the effects of chemokines on ECs to be indirect (290). Many tumors have been shown to constitutively secrete IL-8, GRO, or ENA78, and neutralization of these chemokines by interfering with tumor vascularization reduces both tumor growth and metastatic spread (291). By contrast, CXC chemokines that do not possess N-proximal ELR sequences (e.g., IP-10 and MIG) have no effect on neutrophils, but are chemotactic for monocytes and T-lymphocytes as well as being potent angiostatic factors (292) (Table 11). PF4 is an exception in that it is chemotactic for fibroblasts as well as angiostatic. PF4 has actually been evaluated clinically for its angiostatic antitumor activity, but lacked potency when administered alone (293).

Gene Regulation

The genes for CXC chemokines consist of four exons and three intervening introns. The open reading frames of CXC chemokine

TABLE 10. *Properties of human CXC-ELR+ chemokine α subfamily*

Chemokine	Cell sources	Stimulants	Chemoattracted target cells	Major *in vitro* effects	Major *in vivo* effects
IL-8	M N F EC K NK T SMC	LPS Mitogens Particulates Viruses Bacteria IL-1 TNF IL-3	N Fresh T MC EC NK BS	Activate neutrophil adhesion, shape changes, degranulation, enzyme release, and respiratory burst EC proliferation, inhibits IL-4–mediated IgE production	Mobilize BM neutrophils Antibacterial Acute and chronic inflammation Angiogenesis
GRO (α, β, γ)/MGSA	M F EC MC	LPS IL-1 TNF	N MC EC F Fresh T	Neutrophil activation Melanoma cell proliferation EC proliferation Fibroblast proliferation Activates T cells	Acute inflammation Fibroplasia Angiogenesis
NAP-2	Plt M	Platelet activation	N EC	Neutrophil activation	Acute inflammation Clot resorbtion
ENA-78	K F M EC SMC	LPS IL-1 TNF-α	N EC	EC proliferation Neutrophil activation	Acute inflammation Angiogenesis Mobilize BM neutrophils
GCP-2	Osteosarcoma cells		N EC	Neutrophil gellatinase-β release	Acute inflammation

Abbreviations: M, monocytes-macrophages; N, neutrophil; F, fibroblasts; EC, endothelial cells; K, keratinocytes; NK, natural killer cells; T, T cells; SMC, smooth muscle cells; P, platelets; BS, basophils; MC, melanoma cells; BM, bone marrow.

TABLE 11. *Properties of human CXC (ELR⁻) C+CX₃C chemokine subfamilies*

Chemokine	Cell sources	Stimulants	Major *in vitro* effects	Major *in vivo* effects
PF-4 (CXC)	Plt	Plt aggregation	Inhibits EC proliferation Attracts fibroblasts	Angiostatic
IP-10 (CXC)	M T F EC K	IFN-α, β, γ TNF-α LPS	Inhibits EC Attracts resting > activated T cells, NK cells, and monocytes	Immunostimulant Angiostatic Antitumor immunity
MIG (CXC)	M Hepatic cells	IFN-γ	Inhibits EC Attracts T cells (resting > activated)	Angiostatic Host resistance to bacterial infection
I-TAC (CXC)	Astrocytes M T	IFN-β	Attracts T cells	
SDF-1 (CXC)	BM stroma	Constitutive	Attracts naive more than memory T cells	Competes with T tropic HIV-1 B-cell development Lymphocyte trafficking
Lymphotactin (LPTN) (C)	CD8 > CD4 T Cells NK 1.1 CD4⁺T cells		Attracts thymocytes, DC, T, and NK Cells	Lymphocyte trafficking
Fractalkine (neurotactin) (CX₃C)	EC Microglial cells M	TNF-α IL-1	Transmigration of EC by mononuclear cells Attracts T, M, and N	Brain inflammation Adhesion to EC

genes encode precursor proteins, which are shortened by removal of a signal sequence and by further cell type–dependent proteolysis of the NH2 terminus. In the case of IL-8, two major natural forms are produced: a 77-amino acid form generated by tissue cells, such as ECs and fibroblasts, and a more active 72-amino acid form produced by leukocytes (294). As is the case with many proinflammatory cytokines, the mRNA for CXC chemokines such as IL-8 contains a 3′ AU-rich sequence that causes the mRNA to be highly unstable and to be degraded, with a half-life of less than 1 hour (295).

Numerous exogenous agents and endogenous proinflammatory stimulants, such as endotoxin, lectins, hypoxia, viruses, bacteria, and cytokines, stimulate CXC chemokine production in a wide variety of cell types by stabilization of their mRNA as well as by activation of gene transcription (263). It is notable that proinflammatory IL-1 and TNF are major endogenous stimulants of ELR⁺ CXC chemokines, whereas IFNs, which also have angiostatic effects, rather than proinflammatory cytokines, are the major endogenous inducers of the non-ELR⁺ CXC chemokines. Furthermore, IFNs actively suppress the production of angiogenic chemokines such as IL-8 (296). IFN downregulation of TNF-α–induced ELR⁺ CXC chemokine gene expression acts at the transcriptional level via the NF-KB and NF-IL-6 sites (297). In the case of IL-8, the genomic sequence contains putative binding sites for several transcription regulatory elements in the 5′ flanking region preceding the first exon, including sites for NF-KB, NF-IL-6-C/EBP, AP-1, glucocorticoid receptor, hepatocyte nuclear factor-1, IFN regulatory factor-1, and an octamer-binding motif (298,299). Glucocorticoids, such as dexamethasone, are potent antiinflammatory hormones that have a marked inhibitory effect on gene transcription of numerous proinflammatory cytokines, including IL-8 and other chemokines. A glucocorticoid-responsive promotor element in a number of genotypes might contribute to inhibition of chemokine expression observed with dexamethasone. However, dexamethasone also suppresses IL-1–induced IL-8 production by inhibiting NF-KB activity (298).

Interleukin-8

Despite the redundancy in chemokines, IL-8 has been implicated as a major contributing factor in a variety of acute as well as more chronic inflammatory states. IL-8 has been detected in virtually every acute inflammatory response using immunohistologic and *in situ* hybridization assays (300). Conversely, neutralization of IL-8 by anti-IL-8 antibodies blocks the inflammatory response to IL-8 (267) and even reduces the delayed hypersensitivity response in rabbits to purified protein derivative of mycobacterium tuberculosis (PPD) (301). These results have provided clear evidence of the central role of IL-8 in a number of acute inflammatory states, including hypoxia-induced reperfusion injuries, ARDS, endotoxin-induced local inflammatory reactions, immune complex–induced glomerulonephritis, and others (267). In contrast with the proinflammatory cytokines, which by inducing one another are interdependent and act in synergy, the chemokines do not induce one another and are weak inducers of proinflammatory cytokines. This suggests that IL-8 and other chemokines have a direct causal role in galvanizing inflammatory reactions.

Although IL-8 can bind with equal affinity to CXCR1 and CXCR2, and different regions of IL-8 bind selectively to either CXCR1 or CXCR2 (302), there are conflicting reports that IL-8 preferentially utilizes CXCR1 or CXCR2. It has been suggested that higher doses of IL-8 are more effective on CXCR1-expressing cells, and lower doses are more effective on CXCR2-expressing cells. Consequently, CXCR2 is proposed to act over greater distances from an inflammatory site than CXCR1 (303). Mice lack a clear-cut homologue for IL-8, but they have functional murine homologues for human GRO α, β, γ (KC and MIP-2α and β), ENA78, mu LIX, GCP-2, and NAP-2. Mice express only one receptor for ELR⁺ CXC chemokines with homology to both human CXCR1 and CXCR2. This murine receptor has been deleted by homologous recombination (Table 12), and consequently, ELR⁺ murine chemokines are no longer chemotactic for "IL-8 receptor homologue" deficient murine neutrophils (304). These knock-out mice exhibit splenomegaly, bone

TABLE 12. *Phenotypes of murine chemokine, ligand, and receptor knockouts*

Targeted gene	Phenotypic abnormalities
IL-8R homologue	Defective chemotactic response to MIP2
	Increased bone marrow myelopoiesis with splenomegaly, lymphadenopathy, and plasmacytopoiesis only in conventional germ-laden environment.
CCR1	Defective granulomatous response to *S. mansoni* and neutrophil antifungal rresponse.
CCR5	Mice have reduced resistance to challenge with *Listeria monocytogenes,* although humans with defect are apparently normal.
SDF-1α	Mice die shortly after birth with immunodeficiency due to lack of B- and T-lymphocytes and cardiac ventricular septal defect.
MIP-1α	Reduced pulmonary mononuclear infiltrate to challenge with influenza virus, resulting in higher titers of influenza virus. Less severe autoimmune myocarditis after *Coxsackie* viral infection.
Eotaxin	Diminished number of circulating eosinophils and 60% reduction in tissue eosinophils in response to an allergen challenge.

marrow myeloid hyperplasia, and lymph node B-cell hyperplasia and plasmacytosis secondary to a compensatory overproduction of these lineages in response to conventional microbial challenges. These phenotypic abnormalities do not develop in knock-out mice kept in a germ-free environment (305). Consequently, the overactive myelopoiesis becomes apparent in receptor-deficient mice only when they are stressed by environmental pathogens. The normal microbial flora induce a large expansion of myeloid progenitors, suggesting that the IL-8 receptor homologue normally downregulates myeloid and B-cell generation (306).

Subcutaneous injections of human IL-8 into mice or rats within 3 to 4 hours results in local neutrophil infiltration with little or no edema or erythema. This is followed at 48 and 72 hours by a considerable T-lymphocyte infiltration. Although this may in part be attributable to the T-cell chemotactic effects of IL-8, the neutrophil degranulation by IL-8 results in the release of defensins, CAP37/azurocidin, and cathepsin G, which can recruit T cells, monocytes, and additional neutrophils to the injection site (307,308). In addition, defensins and cathepsin G are comitogenic and mitogenic for T cells, respectively; enhance the production of IFN-γ and IL-4; and promote the *in vivo* production of antibodies in response to an antigenic stimulus. Thus, chemokines, such as IL-8 by degranulating neutrophils, can initiate an immunostimulating cascade that helps to convert an innate into an immunologically specific host response.

Other CXC Chemokines

There are three variants of GRO (α, β, and γ) that are about 95% similar in amino acid sequence and interact equally well with CXCR2. The mouse homologues of GROα, β, and γ are known as KC, MIP-2α, and MIP-2β, which chemoattract human as well as murine neutrophils. In addition MIP-2 costimulates hematopoietic colony formation with CSF-1 and GM-CSF. *GROα,* or melanoma growth stimulatory activity (MGSA), was first discovered as a product of oncogene transfected cell lines and concomitantly as an autocrine growth factor for melanoma cell lines (309,310). GROα also indirectly promotes melanoma tumor growth based on its angiogenic activity. GRO also induces fibroblast proliferation, but the fibroblast receptor for GRO is not as yet identified (311), and GROα as well as IL-8 have been isolated from psoriatic tissues (265).

Neutrophil-activating peptide-2 (NAP-2) is a cleavage product of platelet alpha granule–derived platelet basic protein (PBP),

which is exocytosed and subsequently cleaved again, losing nine more amino acids to yield CTAPIII (263). Cleavage of another four amino acids at the N-terminus yields β thromboglobulin (βTG), while loss of another 11 amino acids forms the 70-amino acid neutrophil chemoattractant, NAP-2. Although NAP-2 has only about one-twentieth of the affinity of IL-8 for CXCR1, it has equal affinity for CXCR2 (312). NAP-2 is released by aggregation of platelets and contributes to attracting neutrophils to sites of injury, hemorrhage, and thrombosis, including atherosclerotic plaques (265).

Although epithelial cell–derived neutrophil-activating peptide-78 (ENA78) has only 22% homology with IL-8, it is equal in potency to GRO and NAP-2 in its activating effects on neutrophils and ECs (313). ENA78 is produced by monocytes subsequent to IL-8 in response to LPS, IL-1, and TNF-α and is detected in many inflammatory disease states. It is also an autocrine growth factor for a variety of tumors, based on its potent angiogenic activity. Granulocyte chemoattractant protein-2 (GCP-2) has 71% homology to ENA78. GCP-2 not only exhibits high-affinity interaction with CXCR2, but also interacts with CXCR1 with about one-tenth of the affinity of IL-8 (314). However, both GCP-2 and ENA78 proteins are produced in lower concentrations than is IL-8. Murine LPS–induced CXC chemokine (LIX) is the most recently described ELR+ CXC chemokine (315). It is most closely related to ENA78 and GCP-2, but has a longer carboxyl terminus. As yet, no clear-cut human homologue has been identified for LIX.

IP-10 was originally identified as an IFN-γ–inducible protein of 10 kDa from the human U937 monocytic leukemia cell line (316). IP-10 exerts antitumor activity based on its angiostatic effects, and in addition, administration of tumor cells transfected to express IP-10 results in T cell–dependent antitumor immunity (317). IFN-γ induces expression of IP-10 through an interferon stimulated response element present in the region flanking the transcription start site, and enhanced IP-10 transcription by TNFα acts via NF-KB (318). IL-4 can inhibit IFN-γ and subsequent IP-10 induction by activation of a negative regulator that competes for the ISRE site. LPS also stimulates IP-10 expression via the ISRE through the intermediate expression of endogenous IFN-α/β and through two NF-KB sites. As for the IL-8 gene, optimal expression of IP-10 by either IFN-γ or LPS requires cooperation between at least two upstream sites.

The monokine induced by IFN-γ (MIG) is a CXC chemokine that was discovered by differential screening of a cDNA library prepared from lymphokine-activated macrophages (319). MIG is chemotactic for activated T cells and NK cells, but not resting T cells, B cells, monocytes, or neutrophils. MIG is expressed maximally by hepatocytes and, unlike IP-10, is absolutely IFN-γ dependent (320). Monocytes also can be induced to produce IP-10, but not MIG in response to IFN-α/β and LPS. Hu MIG and IP-10 exhibit 37% identity in their amino acid sequences and use the same receptor: CXCR3 (321). Despite this, these CXC chemokines appear to act in a nonredundant manner *in vivo,* with MIG having greater systemic distribution, whereas IP-10 is expressed together with IFN-γ and may be more active at local tissue sites. I-TAC was the most recent non-ELR CXC chemokine to be identified by differential display in an IL-2–activated astrocyte cDNA library (322). IP-10, MIG, and I-TAC cross-desensitize one another, indicating that they all share CXCR3.

Stromal cell–derived factor 1 (SDF-1) was originally cloned from bone marrow stromal cells but has since been found to be expressed in a broad range of tissues (323). Because SDF-1 shows equidistant homology to CXC and CC chemokines and is strongly evolutionarily conserved, it may be considered a primordial chemokine. SDF-1 is constitutively produced and present at detectable levels in the plasma. SDF-1 is a potent chemoattractant of lymphocytes and monocytes and may play a greater role in mononuclear cell homing and development than in inflammation. SDF-1 is also chemotactic for CD34$^+$ hematopoietic progenitor cells and mobilizes them from the bone marrow to the peripheral blood (324). Mice with targeted disruption of the SDF-1 gene die perinatally, with severely reduced numbers of B-cell progenitors, T-cell deficiencies, reduced bone marrow myelopoiesis, and a ventricular septal defect (see Table 12) (325). SDF-1 utilizes the fusin orphan receptor (CXCR4), which also acts as coreceptor for T-lymphocyte and neuronal cell invasion by lymphotropic HIV-1 (326). CXCR4 is expressed during embryogenesis and by many organs and T cells of adult mice.

CC Chemokine Proteins and Genes

More than 25 human and murine CC chemokines have been identified and cloned. The genes for the CC chemokines consist of three exons and two intervening introns. Following stimulation, the genes are rapidly transcribed, and this peaks at 3 to 4 hours. The genes encode 92 to 99 amino acid precursors, with initial 20 to 25 amino acid leader sequences, which are cleaved off to yield mature proteins that exhibit 28% to 73% homology (261).

Nuclear magnetic resonance studies revealed that the tertiary structure of CC chemokine monomers is similar to those of the CXC chemokines (327). However, the quartenary structure of the homodimers is distinct. On the other hand, exchanging the amino acids in positions 28 and 30 of MCP-1 for those in IL-8 generated a mutein that selectively attracted neutrophils rather than monocytes, presumably by enabling it to bind to receptors for IL-8 (328). This suggests that the receptor-binding domains of MCP-1 and IL-8 are rather similar.

Studies of gene regulation of some of the CC chemokines have revealed potential binding sites for NF-KB, NF-IL-6, AP-1, and AP-2 in the 5′ flanking region of the mouse MCP-1 (JE) gene (329). NF-IL-6 (C/EPB), NF-KB, and c-Ets sites have been identified in the promoter region for MIP-1α (330). Subsequently it was shown that LPS and IFN-γ rapidly upregulate MIP-1α mRNA expression in macrophages. Much remains to be discovered about the activation elements regulating CC chemokine expression.

CC chemokines show the usual pattern of cytokine responses, with an increase in mRNA expression on cell activation, whereas constitutive expression is often seen with transformed cell lines. Although the CC chemokines are produced by a wide variety of cell types, it is notable that a number of them are T cell–derived (Table 13). Activation of T cells by polyclonal stimulants or antigens induces the production of RANTES, MIP-1α, MIP-1β, and I-309, suggesting that they contribute to immunologically regulated as well as innate host responses.

Receptors

Eight receptors that react to one or more of the CC chemokines, called CCR1–8, have been cloned and expressed (see Fig. 4). In addition, CMV-infected T-lymphocytes express the US28 gene product, which is a 7TMR that binds MIP-1α, MIP-1β, RANTES, and MCP-1 (262). Expression of this receptor by infected T cells presumably is advantageous to the virus. US28 also can serve as a coreceptor for HIV-1 entry, thus making CMV infection a potentially lethal accomplice in AIDS (331).

Functions

With few exceptions, CC chemokines chemoattract T cells and monocytes, but not neutrophils (see Fig. 4). A subgroup of the CC chemokines can be identified on the basis of their chemotactic effects on leukocytes participating in allergic reactions. Eotaxin 1, 2, MCP-4, and to a lesser extent, RANTES, MCP-2, 3, and MIP-1α are chemotactic for eosinophils, whereas eotaxin 1, 2, RANTES, and MCP-1, 2, 3, and 4, all chemoattract basophils and by inducing degranulation, cause rapid histamine release (332). MCP-1, 2, 3, RANTES, and MIP-1α are also chemotactic for murine mast cells, but they have not been reported to induce them to release histamine (265).

The chemokines also contribute to hematopoiesis. Based on inhibition of *in vitro* GM-CSF– and SCF-induced colony-forming assays, MIP-1α, IP-10, PF4, IL-8, MCP-1, eotaxin 2 (Mu MPIF-2), LARC (also known as MIP-3α or Exodus), MRP-1 and 2, and Mu MPIF-1 have all been reported to downregulate hematopoiesis (333–335), whereas eotaxin 1, Mu MIP-2, and IL-8 apparently enhance early hematopoietic progenitor cell growth (336). However, because mice with homologous deletion of MIP-1α, MCP-1, CCR1, and CCR5 genes normally do not exhibit any defects in hematopoiesis, chemokines appear to act in a redundant fashion. However, when CCR1$^{-/-}$ mice are stressed by an endotoxin challenge, they show diminished numbers of myeloid progenitor cells in the spleen and circulation, perhaps due to decreased mobilization of progenitor cells from the bone marrow (337).

Inflammatory and Immunologic Activities

As would be predicted from their chemoattractive effects for mononuclear cells, many of the CC chemokines have been detected by immunohistologic studies and *in situ* hybridization at sites of chronic inflammation due to persistent infections, autoimmune conditions, transplant rejection, and so on (264,265,300). Injections of CC chemokines such as MCP-1, 2, 3, RANTES, and MIP-1α result in mononuclear cell infiltration, beginning at 4 hours at local sites (338). However, mice transfected to overexpress MCP-1 in their skin fail to develop any cutaneous inflammation unless

TABLE 13. *Characteristics, cell sources, and activities of human (C-C) chemokines*

C-C subfamily	Chromosome	Cell sources	Property	Major activites
MCP-1	17(q11–q21)	Most nonlymphocytes		Chronic inflammation, activates macrophages, promotes TH_2 immunity, basophil histamine release
MCP-2	17(q11–q21)	Monocytes	62% homology with MCP-1	Like MCP-1, but also reduces HIV-1 uptake also by CCR5
MCP-3	17(q11–q21)	Monocytes	73% homology with MCP-1	Like MCP-1, but also attracts eosinophils
MCP-4	17(q11–q21)	Monocytes and epithelium	56%–61% homology with MCP1–3 70% homology to Eotaxin	Activates monocytes, basophils, and eosinophils
MCP-5	17(q11–q21)	Monocytes and SMC	60% homology to Eotaxin	Like MCP-1
MIP-1α	17(q11–q21)	T cells, monocytes, mast cells, and fibroblasts		Antiviral host defense, promotes TH_1 CMI
MIP-1β	17(q11–q21)	T cell, monocytes, and fibroblasts	72% homology with MIP-1α	Reduces HIV-1 uptake
LARC/MIP-3α/ exodus	2	Liver and lung, monocytes, DC		Chronic inflammation
MIP-3β/ELC	9	Monocytes, thymus, LN, spleen		
RANTES	17(q11–q21)	T cells, EC, and platelets		Early T-cell product that promotes mononuclear infiltrating
Eotaxin	17(q11–q21)	EC, M, epithelium, lung, LN	70% homology to MCPI–4	Present in tracheobronchial tissues in pulmonary allergies
I-309	17(q11–q21)	T cells, mast cells	Contains six cysteines	Attracts T cells and induces tumor immunity Antiapoptotic for T lymphoma cells
PARC	17(q11–q21)	Lung, thymus, LN, monocytes	61% homology to MIP-1α	Mononuclear inflammation
SLC	9	Spleen, LN, intestine		Mononuclear inflammation
TARC (TECK)	16	DC and EC, lung, colon and thymic DC	Homology to MIP-1γ	Mononuclear inflammation

exposed to a contact sensitizer or irritant (339). It therefore appears as if chemokines are necessary, but not sufficient, to induce inflammation. It has been proposed that a second signal by proinflammatory cytokines such as IL-1 and TNF is needed to activate ECs, which can then interact effectively with chemokine-activated leukocytes.

Some of the CC chemokines at micromolar concentrations, such as RANTES, MIP-1α, MIP-1β, MCP-1, and MCP-3, have a costimulatory role in T-cell activation. They enhance T-cell proliferation, IL-2 production, and IL-2Rα expression by anti-TCR and antigen-activated T-lymphocytes (340). This costimulatory effect can be detected only by using suboptimal concentrations of antigens or mitogens. Addition of CC chemokines to optimally antigen-stimulated T-cell clones actually had a suppressive effect. On the other hand, addition of neutralizing anti-RANTES antibodies partially inhibited the polyclonal response of T cells, suggesting that normally produced RANTES contributes to this response. These costimulating effects of the CC chemokines may be based in part on enhancing the capabilities of antigen presentation by APC. This is supported by data showing that the CC chemokines augment the expression of B7 costimulatory molecules on APC (340). A human CC chemokine that was abundantly expressed by dendritic cells was cloned and identified as DC-CK1 (341). This chemokine is present in dendritic cells located in germinal centers and T-cell areas of secondary lymphoid organs. DC-CK1 preferentially attracts naive CD45RA$^+$ T cells and may contribute to the induction of immune responses.

Chemokines promote the release of granule proteins by neutrophils and monocytes, which can promote tumor-cell cytolysis. Although chemokines do not promote LAK cell or antibody-dependent cytolytic responses, a number of the CC chemokines (e.g., MCP-1, 3, RANTES, and MIP-1α and MIP-1β) enhance CTL and NK cell–mediated killing of trans-target cells (C82). Chemokine-mediated augmentation of CTL- and NK-cell killing was dependent on the expression of β$_2$ integrin, which presumably promoted killer–target cell interactions. Chemokines also induce degranulation of lymphocytes, with subsequent release of serine esterases (340). This process is also blocked by PT and impaired in MIP-1α knock-out mice (343). Thus, degranulation of killer cells may serve to deliver lethal molecules to target cells.

Numerous studies have been aimed at linking chemokines to Th$_1$-dependent cellular immune responses or Th$_2$-dependent humoral immune responses. MCP-1 has been shown to enhance the production of IL-4 by Th$_2$-lymphocytes and diminishes the production of IL-12 and consequently IFN-γ by Th$_1$ lymphocytes (344). MCP-1 participates in Th$_2$-based chronic secondary inflammatory reactions to *Schistosoma mansoni* eggs, whereas MIP-1α plays a greater role in Th$_1$-dependent granulomatous response due to *M. tuberculosis* (345). In fact, costimulation of antigen-stimulated Th$_0$-cell clones with MIP-1α results in their differentiation into a Th$_1$ (IFN-γ–producing) phenotype, whereas exposure to MCP-1 drives them to differentiate into IL-4–producing Th$_2$ cells (346). The pivotal role of MIP-1α in Th$_1$-dependent cellular immunity is further supported by the observation that mice with homologous deletion of the CCR1 receptor for MIP-1α show markedly reduced Th₁-type granulomatous reactions together with decreased IFN-γ and increased IL-4 production by their lymph node cells (377).

Unique Properties

RANTES is a pleiotropic CC chemokine that is produced by immune as well as nonimmune cells and is detected at sites of acute allergic as well as chronic inflammatory reactions. RANTES was shown to be constitutively produced by unstimulated T cells, and its mRNA and protein expression is increased following T-cell activation. The regulation of RANTES expression is therefore unique and suggests a distinct physiologic role for this chemokine (347). RANTES is rapidly produced before the other CC chemokines and can activate cells expressing multiple receptors (CCR1, 3, and 5). At higher micromolar concentrations, RANTES is apparently mitogenic for T cells; it induces lymphokine production and IL-2Rα expression (348). This T-cell response is herbimycin A- rather than PT-sensitive, suggesting that it is mediated by tyrosine kinases. MIP-1α acts through the same receptors, but it is functionally distinct from RANTES, suggesting that each of them may use as yet unidentified receptors. Although MIP-1α and MIP-1β exhibit 78% sequence homology, MIP-1β is a much less potent chemoattractant of mononuclear cells and is known to interact mostly with CCR5. Mice with homozygous defective MIP-1α genes, when challenged by an influenza infection, have a reduced pulmonary mononuclear inflammatory response and develop higher titers of influenza virus (343). They also have a less severe autoimmune myocarditis following coxsackie viral infections (see Table 12). Thus, despite the redundancy in MIP-1α functions and receptor utilization, it plays a vital role in promulgating antiviral host defenses.

I-309 and its murine homologue TCA3 have three pairs of cysteines and are produced by activated T cells, but the gene is also expressed in monocytes (349). TCA3-transfected tumor cells become immunogenic, indicating that this T-cell chemoattractant has immunostimulating capabilities (350). I-309 is also unique in that it is the only chemokine that has been demonstrated to have antiapoptotic effects and can protect lymphocytes from dexamethasone-induced lysis (351). None of the other chemokines have been shown to influence in vitro cell survival.

The MCPs and eotaxins constitute a functional CC chemokine subfamily. MCP-1 was initially discovered as an IL-1–induced product of adherent mononuclear cells (332), while eotaxin was purified from bronchoalveolar fluids of guinea pigs undergoing an allergic response (352). MCP-1, 2, 3, and 4 share about 65% homology with each other and eotaxin 1, but only 35% with eotaxin 2. Murine MCP-5 is most homologous to human MCP-1. The intron–exon structures of the MCP-1 through 5 and eotaxin genes are similar, and they all cluster on human chromosome 17 and murine chromosome 11. All of the MCPs utilize CCR2 on T cells and macrophages, while MCP-2, 3, and 4 also utilize CCR1 and share CCR3, which is expressed by eosinophils and basophils with the eotaxins (see Fig. 4). Studies of the in vivo effects of eotaxin have revealed that it cooperates with IL-5 in promoting tissue eosinophilia (332,352). IL-5 induces bone marrow release and primes eosinophils, which are then attracted more readily by eotaxins to local sites. Mice with targeted disruption of eotaxin genes have diminished peripheral blood eosinophils, and after allergen challenge, eosinophilic infiltration of tissues is reduced by about 60% (353). This indicates that eotaxin plays an important, but not exclusive role in attracting eosinophils. Although MCP-4 is also a potent attractant for eosinophils, the MCPs have more potent effects on basophils than the do the eotaxins.

A novel CC chemokine, murine MIP-1γ, was discovered as a product of murine I-A⁺ Langerhans' cells as well as splenic and bone marrow–derived dendritic cells (354). MIP-1γ shows most homology to murine C10, but less so to MIP-1α and MIP-1β, and utilizes the CCR1 receptors (as does MIP-1α) present on murine neutrophils. MIP-1γ is uniquely produced constitutively by dendritic cells in relatively large amounts, and its production is not increased by IL-1β, TNFα, or IL-6. Consequently, mouse serum normally contains detectable levels of MIP-1γ. It must be noted that dendritic cells also produce TARC, Mu C10, and MCP-1, but only in response to inflammatory stimuli. MIP-1γ attracted both activated and unactivated CD4⁺ and CD8⁺ T cells (354).

Two novel murine CC chemokines were discovered to be inhibitors of two distinct classes of hematopoietic progenitors (335). MPIF-1 (CKβ8) is expressed predominantly by macrophages and ECs in lung, liver, bone marrow, and placenta. It is most similar to Mu MIP-1α in sequence, and they share receptors. MPIF-1 attracts resting T cells, monocytes, and also neutrophils, to a limited extent. MPIF-1 inhibits (low proliferative potential) LPP-CFC and CFU-GM of human and murine origin. MPIF-1 is a more potent inhibitor of hematopoietic progenitors than is MIP-1α and acts on T cells at a different stage of activation. MPIF-1 is also homologous to human MRP-2, and they share more functional similarities. Mu MPIF-2 is now also known as eotaxin 2 and is functionally similar to eotaxin 1 because they share CCR3. It also shows homology to MCP-3 and MIP-1α. MPIF-2 chemoattracts resting T cells and eosinophils. Eotaxin 2, as opposed to eotaxin 1, inhibits murine HPP-CFC multipotent hematopoietic precursors. The in vivo relevance of these hematopoietic effects of CC chemokines remains to be established.

Five additional CC chemokines have been identified, cloned, and expressed. They are TARC (TECK), LARC/MIP-3α, ELC/MIP-3β, SLC, and PARC (268). They are constitutively expressed by lymphoid tissues, but in the case of TARC, are particularly highly expressed in the thymus; LARC by the liver and lymphoid tissues and PARC by pulmonary tissues. MIP-3α and MIP-3β expression are readily downregulated by IL-10 (355). With the exception of TARC, which is specific for T-lymphocytes, these chemokines are selectively chemotactic only for T and B cells. They each appear to largely interact with a single receptor, which has been identified as CCR4 for TARC, CCR6 for LARC, and CCR7 for ELC (see Fig. 4). With the exception of PARC, which is located on chromosome 17 near all the other CC chemokines, the other four genes are located on other chromosomes. The specialized features of these CC chemokines suggest that they may be more involved in homeostatic regulation and homing of lymphocyte subsets to lymphoid tissues (268). This is certainly the role in development of the BCA-1 ligand for a chemokine receptor named BLR1 (356). To establish the function of this ligand, gene-targeted mice lacking BRL1 were prepared; they no longer expressed this receptor on their B cells and a memory subset of T cells. Such mice lacked inguinal lymph nodes and had only a few phenotypically abnormal Peyer's patches. Their primary lymphoid follicles were deficient in B cells, and their spleen lacked germinal centers, all of which indicated that this receptor is necessary for B-cell homing and localization. In contrast, SLC appears to be the pivotal regulator of T-cell homing.

Role of Chemokines in Acquired Immunodeficiency Syndrome

Throughout this chapter there are numerous references to the pivotal role of various chemokines in mobilizing inflammatory cells in response to infectious challenges. Chemokines also contribute to host resistance to HIV-1, and SDF-1α inhibits the invasion of T-lymphocytes by lymphotropic HIV-1 strains, whereas RANTES, MIP-1α, and MIP-1β prevent HIV-1 infection of a monocytic cell line (357). CXCR4, CCR5, and to a lesser extent, CCR3 and CCR2b are essential coreceptors for invasion of human CD4+ lymphocytes, monocytes, and eosinophils by lymphocytotropic, monocytotropic, and dual-tropic HIV-1 strains (358). A novel chemokine receptor, STRL33, has been identified as a fusion cofactor for both monocytotropic and lymphocytotropic HIV-1 strains on T cells (359). The strongest evidence of a role for chemokines in resistance to HIV-1 infection is that although 1% of Caucasians with defective CCR5 are apparently phenotypically normal, they are, with a few exceptions, totally resistant upon repeated exposure to transmission of HIV-1 infection (360). Mice lacking CCR5 have reduced resistance to challenge with *Listeria monocytogenes* (361). Consequently, these chemokine receptors, especially CCR5, have become relevant targets for the design of antagonistic therapeutic agents with anti-HIV-1 activity.

Suppression of Chemokine Responses

Some of the best evidence documenting the unique and vital roles of various chemokines has been generated by homologous recombinations resulting in gene deletions or inactivation (see Table 12). As is the case for cytokines, chemokines can also behave as two-edged swords: they are essential for host defense, but they can also contribute to self-destructive inflammatory responses in autoimmune diseases, traumatic injury, and hypoxic states. As has been mentioned, neutralizing antibodies to IL-8 by suppressing acute inflammation can ameliorate reperfusion injury and ARDS (267), while anti-MIP-1α can reduce the severity of EAE (346). On the other hand, anti-MIP-2 (GRO) can exacerbate *Klebsiella pneumoniae* infections in mice (362). The production of chemokines is downregulated by a number of endogenous antiinflammatory mediators, including corticosteroids, IL-10, and TGF-β (261). Chemokine-receptor interactions can also be competitively blocked by a variety of mutated chemokine ligands (363). Finally, studies of myxoma viruses has identified a more effective means of blocking chemokine effects, by expressing gene products that bind and neutralize the activities of a number of the chemokines (364,365). Deletion of these myxoma genes restores the host defense of rabbits against the myxoma viruses. These poxvirus-derived inhibitors apparently bind to the lower affinity GAG-binding domains of various CXC and CC chemokines (see Table 9).

There are also several downregulatory pathways resulting in desensitization of chemokine reactions, which result in blocking of signal transduction due to uncoupling of G proteins. Homologous desensitization or "attenuation" of the response occurs in response to ligands interacting with a given receptor. This process occurs at higher concentrations of ligands, involves receptor phosphorylation with or without internalization, and is reversed by receptor dephosphorylation and recycling of the receptor onto the cell surface (366). This is best illustrated by the report that transgenic mice transfected to overexpress mu JE(MCP-1) and that have 5- to 20-ng per ml plasma levels of mu JE (MCP-1) actually have deactivated macrophages and defective host reactions to infectious challenges (367). Macrophages from these mice are chronically desensitized in their response to MCP-1, and, in addition, the elevated chemokine levels in their circulatory compartments interfere with the formation of a peripheral MCP-1 gradient. In contrast, heterologous desensitization occurs in response to physiologic doses of other chemoattractant ligands interacting with distinct G protein–coupled receptors, resulting in cross-phosphorylation and deactivation of unrelated receptors. For example, prior interactions of opiates, for more than 1 hour, with μ and δ opioid receptors can inhibit chemokine receptor–dependent chemotaxis in response to IL-8 or RANTES (368). This is not associated with internalization of the chemokine receptors, but is associated with phosphorylation by the chemokine receptors in response to the opiates. Furthermore, preincubation of monocytes with gp120 also suppresses their chemotactic response to a variety of chemokines and fMLP (369). Consequently, more prolonged exposure to heterologous ligands may depress the capacity of cells to mobilize in response to host chemoattractants. These data illustrate the potential effectiveness of chemokine antagonists that can competitively interfere with chemokine-receptor interactions or desensitizers of receptor-dependent signal transduction. Development of such inhibitors of chemokine activities may yield potent antiinflammatory agents without numerous undesirable side effects.

TRANSFORMING GROWTH FACTOR β

TGF-β is a multifunctional cytokine that regulates the growth and differentiation of many cell types, and it has proinflammatory as well as immunosuppressive activities (Tables 14 and 15). TGF-β was first described as an activity produced by a murine sarcoma virus–transformed cell line that stimulated normal rat kidney fibroblasts to grow in an anchorage-independent manner, although it did not actually transform the cells (370). Many normal cells and tissues express TGF-β constitutively and produce more when stimulated. These include platelets, macrophages, B- and T-lymphocytes, fibroblasts, ECs, osteoblasts and osteoclasts, astrocytes, and microglial cells.

TABLE 14. *TGF-β*

Proteins

Pro-TGF-β	2 polypeptides of 390–412 amino acids with signal sequence
TGF-β1, -β2, or -β3	110–140 amino acids, 25-kD homodimer, biologically active
TGF-β1, -β2	25-kD heterodimer
Latent TGF-β	Noncovalent complex of LAP + TGF-β dimer

Producers

T and B cells, macrophages, thymus and bone marrow, fibroblasts, platelets, placenta, and bone

Receptors

Type I (53 kD) "signalling chain"
Type II (70–80 kD) "binding chain"
Type III (200–300 kD), betaglycans "presenting site"
200–2,000 type I and II receptors/cell, $K_D = 3$–30 pM, β1=β3 > β2
<20,000 type III sites/cell, $K_D = 50$–500 pM, β1=β2=β3
Signal-transducing unit = type I + type II heterodimer

TABLE 15. *Activities of TGF-β*

Mitogen for fibroblasts
Antiproliferative for most other cell types
Suppresses hematopoiesis and lymphopoiesis
Suppresses polyclonal antibody production
Suppresses CTL, NK, and LAK activity
Deactivates macrophages
Promotes oral tolerance
Induces IL-1ra and downregulates IL-1RI
Suppresses *in vivo* inflammation
Promotes wound healing and angiogenesis
Stimulates chemotaxis of fibroblasts, PMN, monocytes, mast cells, and T cells
Induces local inflammation and fibrosis
Stimulates extracelluular matrix deposition
Promotes switch to IgA

Five isoforms of TGF-β have been identified, but only the first three isoforms—TGF-β1, -β2, -β3—with 70% to 76% sequence homology are expressed in mammals. Each isoform is highly conserved among different species (95% to 99%), as exemplified by a single amino acid change in human TGF-β1 and the murine peptide. *In vitro* biologic activities of these isoforms are nearly identical (371,372). However, immunohistochemical and *in situ* hybridization techiques revealed a differential pattern of expression for the TGF-β isoforms during murine embryogenesis (373,374), suggesting functional differences between the isoforms, which have been confirmed by the phenotype difference in the TGF-β knock-out mice (375–377). Thus, TGF-β2 and TGF-β3 are important regulators of cellular differentiation and affect development and embryogenesis, whereas the effects of TGF-β1 are mostly immunologic.

Genes

The gene for each of the mammalian isoforms is located on a different chromosome, but they have the same genomic organization, with seven exons at homologous positions. Phylogenic analysis suggests that the TGF-β isoforms arose by the process of gene duplication and sequence divergence. Sequence analysis of the promoter regions of the genes for the three TGF-β isoforms revealed little homology and suggests differential regulation of their expression (378). The TGF-β2 and TGF-β3 promoters contain classic TATA box and CRE/ATF elements, whereas the TGF-β1 promoter contains AP-1, NF-1, and Sp1 binding sites and GC-rich regions, but lack a TATA consensus sequence (379,380). These AP-1 sites, which mediate autoinduction of TGF-β1 (381), may account for the increases in TGF-β1 transcription observed in pathologic conditions. The differential activation of the TGF-β2 promoter is most likely due to distinct cell type–dependent interactions of activating transcription factors with CRE sites adjacent to the TATA box. A feature common to all three isoforms is the presence of very long 5′ UTRs, which allow further transcriptional and translational regulation. Computer analysis of 5′ UTRs of TGF-β1 identified stable stem-loop structures that may serve as binding sites for cell type–specific cytoplasmic factors and affect translation. Overall, expression of TGF-β is regulated differentially at both transcriptional and posttranscriptional levels, which accounts for the cell–tissue and developmental expression of specific TGF-β isoforms in response to a variety of external stimuli.

Proteins

The biologically active forms of TGF-β are disulfide-linked dimers of 25 kDa containing highly conserved subunits of 110 to 140 amino acids (372,382). The subunits are synthesized as the C-terminal portion of larger precursors (of 390 to 412 amino acids) with N-terminal signal sequences of 20 to 23 amino acids and a prodomain. The prodomain is also well conserved and may assist in folding, dimerization, and secretion of TGF-β. The precursor is cleaved by a peptidase in the secretory pathway at a dibasic or RXXR site to release a mature carboxy-terminal sequence of 110 to 140 amino acids. The dimerized prodomain, also called *latency-associated protein* (LAP), remains noncovalently associated with the C-terminal fragment to produce a latent complex of high molecular weight, which includes another glycoprotein of 125 kDa, called *latent TGF-β–binding protein* (LTBP). Latent TGF-β is localized on the cell surface and in the extracellular matrix via binding to mannose-6-phosphate–insulin-like growth factor type II receptors or other glycosylated binding proteins (383). It is converted to active TGF-β at these sites by unknown, but presumably highly regulated, mechanisms. Because the secreted form of TGF-β is biologically inactive, the activation of latent TGF-β is a critical step in the regulation of TGF-β activity. Latent TGF-β can be converted to active TGF-β *in vitro* by plasmin, cathepsin D, or thrombospondin, or by disrupting noncovalent interactions through treatment with heat or acid pH, and chaotropic agents. In some cells, latent TGF-β activation requires the cascade action of other molecules, including tissue type II transglutaminase, LTBP, plasmin, and urokinase-type plasminogen activator (384). In addition, latent TGF-β can also be activated by interactions between cells. For example, coculture of bovine endothelial and smooth muscle cells generates active TGF-β through a plasmin-dependent mechanism. Only the dimeric form of mature TGF-β can interact with cell surface TGF-β receptors and generate signal transduction.

TGF-β cytokines share a similar three-dimensional structure, and the spacing of seven cysteines within the mature region is nearly invariant in members of the TGF-β family.

Receptors and Signal Transduction

TGF-β receptors are widely distributed and expressed by most cell types, including lymphoid and hematopoietic cells. Three types of TGF-β receptors were initially identified, based on their high-affinity binding to radiolabeled TGF-β. These are termed type I, type II, and type III receptors, based on their approximate sizes of 53, 70 to 80, and 200 to 300 kDa, respectively (372,385,386). Type I and type II receptors are transmembrane proteins with a relatively short, cysteine-rich extracellular region, a hydrophobic transmembrane helix, and a cytoplasmic domain with serine–threonine kinase activity. Antibodies to either type I or type II receptors coimmunoprecipitate both receptors after cross-linking in the presence of ligand. Studies with mutagenized cell lines indicated that type II receptor binds ligand efficiently, but that type I receptor can bind ligand only in the presence of type II receptor (387). The use of chimeric receptors showed that homodimers of either type I or type II receptors are incapable of generating biologic responses (388). Consequently, ligand binding to type II receptor induces a conformational change, which facilitates the recruitment of type I receptor to form a heteromeric receptor complex (389–391). Type II receptor, which is a constitutively active kinase, phosphorylates and activates the type I receptor, which then propagates the signal to intracellular substrates.

In addition to the signaling receptors, many cells express type III receptors, also known as betaglycans, and a set of isoform-specific TGF-β–binding proteins. Betaglycan is a proteoglycan with a large extracellular domain, a single transmembrane domain, and a short cytoplasmic tail with no known signaling motifs. It can interact with the extracellular matrix (ECM) via its extracellular glycosaminoglycan chains. Betaglycan binds all three TGF-β isoforms with the same affinity (K_D = 50 to 500 pM). There are many type III receptors on cells (fewer than 20,000 per cell), and their function is to present TGF-β to the signaling receptors. Thus, the affinity of TGF-β2 for the signaling receptors is increased 20-fold by its association with betaglycan. In contrast, although cells express fewer type I and type II receptors (200 to 2,000 per cell), the binding affinity of TGF-β1 and TGF-β3 is higher for these receptors (K_D = 3 to 30 pM).

Other TGF-β–binding proteins include endoglin, decorin, α2-macroglobulin, and thrombospondin. These proteins modulate ligand access to the signaling receptor complex. Endoglin, a membrane-anchored proteoglycan, is closely related in structure to betaglycan, is highly expressed in endothelial and mesangial cells, and binds only TGF-β1 and TGF-β3, but not TGF-β2. Thrombospondin can activate latent TGF-β, and the reduction in production of thrombospondin caused by a mutation of p53 in human tumors may contribute to tumorogenesis (392).

TGF-β receptors are rapidly internalized upon binding of dimeric ligand. The signaling pathways are not completely defined, but two signal transducers, Smad2 and DPC4, have been identified (393). Smads are a group of evolutionarily conserved proteins that have been implicated as key mediators for receptors of bone morphogenetic protein (BMP) and activin, members of the TGF-β superfamily. A related protein, DPC4, a tumor-suppressor gene product, also mediates TGF-β actions, as shown by a cotransfection experiment in a human breast carcinoma cell line (MDA-MB468). Within 10 minutes after addition of TGF-β, Smad2 is phosphorylated, and then forms a complex with DPC4. Nuclear translocation of this heterodimeric complex of Smad2 and DPC4 leads to specific TGF-β responses. The deletion of DPC4 in some cancer cells disables this signaling pathway for TGF-β. In immature B-cell lymphomas, TGF-β1 can induce IkBα, thereby inhibiting NF-kB/Rel activity. This downmodulation of NF-*K*B/Rel reduces c-myc expression, leading to apoptosis of these B cells in response to TGF-β (394).

Immunologic Activities

TGF-β elicits many opposing cellular effects, depending on cell type, maturation–differentiation status of the responding cell, and the local physiologic cellular environment. Thus, it suppresses the immune system at the systemic level, but stimulates the immune and inflammatory responses at the local level (395,396).

The immunosuppressive effects of systemic TGF-β are clearly illustrated in TGF-β1–deficient mice obtained through targeted gene disruption (375,376). These mice develop a multifocal inflammatory response with massive leukocyte infiltration in numerous organs, accompanied by increased expression of TNF-α, IFN-γ, MIP-1α, and class I and II MHC antigens, resulting in death at 3 to 5 weeks. TGF-β1–deficient mice also exhibit high levels of circulating autoantibodies, similar to that exhibited by autoimmune MRP/lpr mice, and have IgG deposits in their renal glomeruli. Thus, TGF-β1 normally acts as an active suppressor of inflammation.

TGF-β can suppress the proliferation and differentiation of both T- and B-lymphocytes and monocytes–macrophages (372,397). It suppresses immunoglobulin secretion of mature B cells but promotes a switch to IgA production (398). The generation of cytotoxic T cells, NK-cell activity, and LAK activity are all inhibited by TGF-β (399). TGF-β inhibits mitogen-induced synthesis of IFN-γ, IL-2, IL-3, GM-CSF, and TNF-α. TGF-β suppresses hematopoiesis by inhibiting bone marrow stem-cell proliferation and downregulating the expression of receptors for SCF (400), IL-3, and GM-CSF on hematopoietic cells. TGF-β can deactivate macrophages by reducing their capacity to release superoxide and nitric oxide, suppressing their cytotoxic activity, downregulating their expression of MHC class II, inhibiting the production of TNF-α and IL-1, and antagonizing the effects of these cytokines (401). These regulatory T cells can suppress ongoing inflammatory reactions in an antigen-nonspecific manner. TGF-β also suppresses inflammation by downregulating E-selectin and IL-8 on endothelial cells, thereby inhibiting the adhesion and transmigration of neutrophils and lymphocytes through cytokine-activated endothelial cells (402).

TGF-β also promotes oral tolerance (403). Oral administration of antigens (myelin basic protein) to multiple sclerosis patients generates antigen-specific TGF-β1–secreting Th3 cells (404). One of the primary mechanisms of oral tolerance is active suppression of immune responses through the induction of regulatory T cells in the gut-associated lymphoid tissue. These Th3 cells secrete TGF-β, IL-4, and IL-10, which downregulate Th1 and other immune cells.

At the site of inflammation and tissue injury, TGF-β induces the chemotaxis of neutrophils, monocytes, lymphocytes, mast cells, and fibroblasts (405,406); activates these cells to produce inflammatory cytokines (IL-1, TNF, and IL-6); and enhances leukocyte adhesion to the vessel wall and ECM (407).

Other Activities

TGF-β as a stimulant of connective tissue cells is also a potent regulator of tissue repair and a promoter of wound healing due to its unique effect in stimulating the deposition of ECM based on increased synthesis of matrix proteins and decreased matrix degradation, achieved both by decreasing protease synthesis and enhancing synthesis of protease inhibitors. TGF-β also increases the synthesis of integrin receptors, thereby enhancing interaction between cell and ECM. Because of the regulatory effects of TGF-β on ECM and the immune system, TGF-β has been proposed as a contributing factor in many chronic inflammatory diseases, which include rheumatoid arthritis, glomerulonephritis, pulmonary fibrosis, systemic sclerosis, and chronic hepatitis (408). TGF-β1 circulates in the plasma complexed with IgG in autoimmune MPR/lpr mice, and in some patients with SLE, IgG-bound active TGF-β1 is 500-fold more potent than uncomplexed active TGF-β1 in the suppression of neutrophil function *in vitro* and host defense against *Staphylococcus aureus* infection *in vivo* (409).

The critical regulatory functions of TGF-β in embryogenesis and development are demonstrated in the abnormal lung development and cleft palate seen in TGF-β3–deficient mice (377,410). Thus, TGF-β3 controls mesenchymal–epithelial cell interactions and regulates cellular differentiation and proliferation. It promotes growth of mesenchymal cells, but acts as a potent growth inhibitor for most other cell types, including epithelial cells, endothelial cells, lymphocytes, and hematopoietic progenitor cells. Studies have shown that TGF-β1 promotes the development of dendritic cells from hemopoietic progenitor cells *in vitro* by protecting precursor cells from apoptosis (411), and that endogenous TGF-β1 is essential for normal murine Langerhans' cell development and epidermal localization (412).

Due to its potent antiproliferative effects, TGF-β normally functions as a tumor suppressor in human malignancies (413). However, cancer cells develop resistance to TGF-β late in tumor progression by using multiple mechanisms, including TGF-β–receptor mutations, cell-signaling defects, and altered interactions between cell and ECM. TGF-β1 is present normally at nanogram-per-milliliter levels (0.1 to 6.3 ng per ml) in plasma but is elevated in plasma of patients with renal-cell carcinoma and invasive prostate cancer (414) and depressed in advanced atherosclerosis (415).

The importance of TGF-β in growth, development, and maintenance of immunologic homoeostasis is well substantiated by studies of TGF-β1– and TGF-β3–deficient mice. It is a key suppressor of inflammation, as autoimmunity results in its absence, and it serves to downregulate immune activation in immunologically privileged sites, such as the eye. It also inhibits tumor growth, whereas mutational inactivation of TGF-β type II receptors contributes to tumor growth and progression.

INTERLEUKIN-16

IL-16 was detected in 1982 as a peripheral blood mononuclear cell–derived T-lymphocyte chemoattractant factor (LCF) of the CD4+ subset (416). It is structurally distinct from chemokines and in its active form is a homotetramer composed of four 16.3-kDa chains. Its mRNA is constitutively expressed in both CD4+ and CD8+ T cells, but the tetramer is present only in CD8+ T cells. IL-16 is also produced by CD4+ T cells, mast cells, and eosinophils. It is secreted in response to serotonin, histamine, and mitogenic activation of lymphocytes. An intracellular 90-kDa precursor form has been detected that is cleaved at the carboxyl end to yield the unique monomer. IL-16 does not have a leader sequence. The IL-16 gene is located on human chromosome 15q26.1 and is highly conserved in primate and rodent species. Since synthetic peptide analogues of the 15 hydrophillic C-terminal region and antisera against this C-terminal region both inhibit IL-16 functions, the C-terminus may contribute to IL-16 receptor interactions.

There are a number of lines of evidence that CD4 may be a receptor for IL-16. Monomeric Fab of anti-CD4 inhibits IL-16 functions. The chemotactic activity of murine and rat IL-16 for human CD4+ T cells is blocked by soluble CD4, and, conversely, transfection of a mouse T-cell hybridoma with human CD4 enables the cells to migrate in response to IL-16. Studies of IL-16–induced signal transduction suggest a key role for p56 lck (417). Wortmannin, a selective PI3 kinase inhibitor, blocks IL-16–induced chemotaxis, as do selective inhibitors of PKC. However, CD4 may not be the sole receptor for IL-16, because IL-16 activities are also PT-sensitive, implicating the participation of Gi-protein signals.

IL-16 is chemotactic for resting as well as activated T cells, eosinophils, and monocytes. IL-16 promotes CD4+ T-cell adhesion, expression of IL 2Rα (CD25), and HLA-DR, as well as cytokine synthesis (e.g., IL-3, GM-CSF, and IFN-γ). IL-16 suppresses antigen- and alloantigen (MLR)-induced lymphocyte proliferation

(418) and represses the transcription of HIV and simian immunodeficiency virus (419). However, unlike the CC chemokines, IL-16 does not competitively inhibit the binding of HIV gp120. IL-16 acts as a potent survival factor and counters apoptotic effects of growth-inducing cytokines such as IL-2 (416). IL-16 has been detected in bronchial airway epithelial cells and fluid of asthmatics, and because it is induced by histamine, IL-16 may exacerbate allergic reactions. Immunohistologic assays have detected high levels of IL-16 in granulomas in patients with sarcoidosis and mycobacterium tuberculosis. These observations suggest that IL-16 is yet another proinflammatory and immunomodulatory cytokine.

INTERLEUKIN-17

Murine IL-17 was initially cloned by subtractive hybridization from an activated T-cell hybridoma and was termed *murine CTL–associated antigen-8* (mCTLA-8) (420). The 150 amino acid–long CTLA-8 was renamed IL-17 because it displayed characteristics of a cytokine, such as a hydrophobic N-terminus resembling a signal peptide and AU-rich repeats in the 3' UTR associated with mRNA instability. The expression of human and rodent CTLA-8 is tightly restricted to memory CD4+ lymphocytes, and it induces epithelial, endothelial, and fibroblastic cells to activate NFKB and to produce IL-6, IL-8, G-CSF, and PGE$_2$, but not IL-1 or TNF (421,422). A homologous "virokine" with 57% amino acid and functional similarity to IL-17 has been identified as ORF13 of herpes virus saimiri. IL-17 is located on murine chromosome 1A and human chromosome 2q31. The murine receptor for IL-17 has also been cloned and is more widely expressed than the ligand on a variety of stromal cells (423). IL-17 induces fibroblasts to better support the growth and differentiation of CD34+ progenitor cells. Thus, IL-17 can be considered an inducer of stromal cell proinflammatory and hematopoietic cytokines.

MIGRATION INHIBITORY FACTOR

It is fitting that we end this chapter with a review of the status of migratory inhibitor factor (MIF), one of the first lymphocyte-derived cytokine activities, discovered more than 30 years ago as an inhibitor of macrophage migration (424,425). This activity was ascribed to IFN-γ and IL-4 until the cloning and sequencing of a novel MIF molecule in 1989 by John David and colleagues, which, in the presence of PHA, also inhibited monocyte migration (426). However, this newly cloned, active MIF has been found to have some very surprising, unique properties of its own (427). MIF was codiscovered as an LPS-induced 12.5-kDa secreted product of a murine pituitary cell line (AtT-20). MIF is stored in considerable quantity in the granules of anterior pituitary cells and, like ACTH, is released by CRF. Initiation of a stress response by administration of LPS to rodents results in the release of pituitary granule contents and raises the normal plasma level of 10 to 15 ng per ml MIF to 50 ng per ml. The release is blocked by hypophysectomy, however, leaving MIF stored in peripheral monocytes and T cells as the other source of MIF.

In vitro and *in vivo* studies have revealed MIF to be a proinflammatory cytokine. MIF induces TNF α production by macrophages, and TNF-α, in turn, induces secretion of MIF. Furthermore, MIF potentiated IFN-γ–induced production of NO by murine macrophages. Coinjection into mice of MIF with LPS exacerbates lethal endotoxemia, whereas neutralizing anti-MIF antibodies protect mice from lethal doses of LPS. Anti-MIF antibody reduces LPS-induced circulating TNF-α levels by 35%. MIF mRNA and protein are also prominently expressed at sites of delayed hypersensitivity (DTH) reactions, and anti-MIF antibodies reduce the development of DTH in mice. Unexpectedly, glucocorticoids (GCs) were shown to directly induce the release of MIF from mononuclear cells. Thus, MIF is a proinflammatory cytokine that is uniquely released rather than suppressed by GCs and may function as a counterregulator of GCs. In fact, MIF overrides, in a dose-dependent manner, the GC-induced inhibition of TNF-α, IL-1β, IL-6, and IL-8 production by monocytes cultured with LPS. Conversely, anti-MIF antibodies markedly potentiate the inhibitory effects of GCs on LPS-induced TNF-α production. MIF also overrides the antiproliferative effect of GCs on antigen and polyclonaly stimulated T cells. MIF blocks the protective effect of GCs on LPS lethality in mice.

The mechanistic basis of these activities of MIF are not clearly defined. The gene contains enhancer–promoter motifs that bind to transcription factors such as NFKB, Ck-1, nGRE, and CREB. MIF appears to have enzymatic activity and catalyzes an isomerization reaction. The three-dimensional crystal structure of human MIF revealed it to be unique and to consist of a trimer with identical subunits. There is no information concerning a receptor for MIF. Although the preceding observations do not provide a clear identification of the prehistoric MIF activity, they have led to the identification of an another fascinating regulator of host-defense responses.

CONCLUSION

In conclusion, it is challenging to generalize about this diverse group of proinflammatory cytokines. However, we must emphasize that although we have reviewed the properties of each of the cytokines individually, they act in concert in the presence of many other mediators and hormones *in vivo*. Consequently, it is at times very difficult to predict the *in vivo* role of cytokines based on their *in vitro* activities. The cytokines are subject to multiple interactions, which drastically modify their net effects. The interactions of IL-1, TNF, and IL-6 represent a classical example of cytokines that not only induce one another, but also synergize, resulting in dramatic amplification of their impact in pathophysiologic reactions. Furthermore, the phenotypes of cytokine knock-out mice have usually had less than the predicted deficits because of the corrective effect of redundant cytokines, and at other times they have revealed totally unexpected cytokine activities, as for LTα. *In vivo veritas* remains trite but true, and *in vivo* experiments provide data concerning the essential cytokine functions and also provide the critical models for the development of therapeutic cytokine inhibitors and antagonists.

ACKNOWLEDGMENTS

We express our great appreciation for the constructive criticisms of Drs. Adit Ben-Baruch, Michael Grimm, O.M. Zach Howard, Dennis Taub, Sergei Nedospasov, Scott Durum, and Ji Ming Wang, and for the superb secretarial assistance of Cheryl Fogle and Ilene Totillo.

REFERENCES

Selected TNF Family

1. Carswell EA, Old LJ, Kassel RL, Green S, Fiore N, Williamson B. An endotoxin-induced serum factor that causes necrosis of tumors. *Proc Natl Acad Sci USA* 1975;72:3666–3670.
2. Beutler B, Mahoney J, LeTrang N, Pekala P, Cerami A. Purification of cachectin, a lipoprotein lipase-suppressing hormone secreted by endotoxin-induced RAW 264.7 cells. *J Exp Med* 1985;161:984–995.
3. Pennica D, Nedwin GE, Hayflick JS, et al. Human tumour necrosis factor: precursor structure, expression and homology to lymphotoxin. *Nature* 1984;312:724–729.
4. Aggarwal BB, Kohr WJ, Hass PE, et al. Human tumor necrosis factor. Production, purification, and characterization. *J Biol Chem* 1985;260:2345–2354.
5. Ruddle NH, Waksman BH. Cytotoxicity mediated by soluble antigen and lymphocytes in delayed hypersensitivity. 3. Analysis of mechanism. *J Exp Med* 1968;128:1267–1279.
6. Granger GA, Williams TW. Lymphocyte cytotoxicity in vitro: activation and release of a cytotoxic factor. *Nature* 1968;218:1253–1254.
7. Bazzoni F, Beutler B. The tumor necrosis factor ligand and receptor families. *N Engl J Med* 1996;334:1717–1725.
8. Browning JL, Ngam-ek A, Lawton P, et al. Lymphotoxin β, a novel member of the TNF family that forms a heteromeric complex with lymphotoxin on the cell surface. *Cell* 1993;72:847–856.
9. Yonehara S, Ishii A, Yonehara M. A cell-killing monoclonal antibody (anti-Fas) to a cell surface antigen co-downregulated with the receptor of tumor necrosis factor. *J Exp Med* 1989;169:1747–1756.
10. Trauth BC, Klas C, Peters AM, et al. Monoclonal antibody-mediated tumor regression by induction of apoptosis. *Science* 1989;245:301–305.
11. Itoh N, Yonehara S, Ishii A, et al. The polypeptide encoded by the cDNA for human cell surface antigen Fas can mediate apoptosis. *Cell* 1991;66:233–243.
12. Wiley SR, Schooley K, Smolak PJ, et al. Identification and characterization of a new member of the TNF family that induces apoptosis. *Immunity* 1995;3:673–682.
13. Pan G, O'Rourke K, Chinnaiyan AM, et al. The receptor for the cytotoxic ligand TRAIL. *Science* 1997;276:111–113.
14. Banchereau J, Bazan F, Blanchard D, et al. The CD40 antigen and its ligand. *Annu Rev Immunol* 1994;12:881–922.
15. Ware CF, VanArsdale S, VanArsdale TL. Apoptosis mediated by the TNF-related cytokine and receptor families. *J Cell Biochem* 1996;60:47–55.
16. Baker SJ, Reddy EP. Transducers of life and death: TNF receptor superfamily and associated proteins. *Oncogene* 1996;12:1–9.
17. Nagata S. Apoptosis by death factor. *Cell* 1997;88:355–365.
18. Tartaglia LA, Ayres TM, Wong GHW, Goeddel DV. A novel domain within the 55 kd TNF receptor signals cell death. *Cell* 1993;74:845–853.
19. Casaccia-Bonnefil P, Carter BD, Dobrowsky RT, Chao MV. Death of oligodendrocytes mediated by the interaction of nerve growth factor with its receptor p75. *Nature* 1996;383:716–719.
20. Chinnaiyan AM, O'Rourke K, Yu GL, et al. Signal transduction by DR3, a death domain-containing receptor related to TNFR-1 and CD95. *Science* 1996;274:990–992.
21. Kitson J, Raven T, Jiang Y-P, et al. A death-domain-containing receptor that mediates apoptosis. *Nature* 1996;384:372–375.
22. Brojatsch J, Naughton J, Rolls MM, Zingler K, Young JAT. CAR1, a TNFR-related protein, is a cellular receptor for cytopathic avian leukosis-sarcoma viruses and mediates apoptosis. *Cell* 1996;87:845–855.
23. Montgomery RI, Warner MS, Lum BJ, Spear PG. Herpes simplex virus-1 entry into cells mediated by a novel member of the TNF/NGF receptor family. *Cell* 1996;87:427–436.
24. Nocentini G, Giunchi L, Ronchetti S, et al. A new member of the tumor necrosis factor/nerve growth factor receptor family inhibits T cell receptor-induced apoptosis. *Proc Natl Acad Sci USA* 1997;94:6216–6221.
25. Bodmer J-L, Burns K, Schneider P, et al. TRAMP, a novel apoptosis-mediating receptor with sequence homology to tumor necrosis factor receptor 1 and Fas(Apo-1/CD95). *Immunity* 1997;6:79–88.
26. Simonet WS, Lacey DL, Dunstan CR, et al. Osteoprotegerin: a novel secreted protein involved in the regulation of bone density. *Cell* 1997;89:309–319.
27. Nedwin GE, Naylor SL, Sakaguchi AY, et al. Human lymphotoxin and tumor necrosis factor genes: structure, homology and chromosomal localization. *Nucleic Acids Res* 1985;13:6361–6373.
28. Spies T, Morton CC, Nedospasov SA, Fiers W, Pious D, Strominger JL. Genes for the tumor necrosis factors alpha and beta are linked to the human major histocompatibility complex. *Proc Natl Acad Sci USA* 1986;83:8699–8702.
29. Nedospasov SA, Hirt B, Shakhov AN, et al. The genes for tumor necrosis factor (TNF-alpha) and lymphotoxin (TNF-beta) are tandemly arranged on chromosome 17 of the mouse. *Nucleic Acids Res* 1986;14:7713–7725.
30. Muller U, Jongeneel CV, Nedospasov SA, Lindahl KF, Steinmetz M. Tumour necrosis factor and lymphotoxin genes map close to H-2D in the mouse major histocompatibility complex. *Nature* 1987;325:265–267.
31. Shakhov AN, Collart MA, Vassalli P, Nedospasov SA, Jongeneel CV. kB-type enhancers are involved in lipopolysaccharide-mediated transcriptional activation

of the tumor necrosis factor α gene in primary macrophages. *J Exp Med* 1990;171:35–47.

32. Kuprash DV, Udalova IA, Turetskaya RL, Rice NR, Nedospasov SA. Conserved kB element located downstream of the tumor necrosis factor α gene: distinct NF-kB binding pattern and enhancer activity in LPS activated murine macrophages. *Oncogene* 1995;11:97–106.

33. Han J, Thompson P, Beutler B. Dexamethasone and pentoxifylline inhibit endo-toxin-induced cachectin/tumor necrosis factor synthesis at separate points in the signaling pathway. *J Exp Med* 1990;172:391–394.

34. Wilson AG, Symons JA, McDowell TL, McDevitt HO, Duff GW. Effects of a polymorphism in the human tumor necrosis factor alpha promoter on transcrip-tional activation. *Proc Natl Acad Sci USA* 1997;94:3195–3199.

35. Nagata S, Golstein P. The Fas death factor. *Science* 1995;267:1449–1456.

36. Grell M, Douni E, Wajant H, et al. The transmembrane form of tumor necrosis factor is the prime activating ligand of the 80 kDa tumor necrosis factor recep-tor. *Cell* 1995;83:793–802.

37. Moss ML, Jin S-L, Milla ME, et al. Cloning of a disintegrin metalloproteinase that processes precursor tumour-necrosis factor-α. *Nature* 1997;385:733–736.

38. Black RA, Rauch CT, Kozlosky CJ, et al. A metalloproteinase disintegrin that releases tumour-necrosis factor-α from cells. *Nature* 1997;385:729–733.

39. Blobel CP. Metalloprotease-disintegrins: links to cell adhesion and cleavage of TNFα and notch. *Cell* 1997;90:589–592.

40. Smith RA, Baglioni C. The active form of tumor necrosis factor is a trimer. *J Biol Chem* 1987;262:6951–6954.

41. Jones EY, Stuart DI, Walker NP. Structure of tumour necrosis factor. *Nature* 1989;338:225–228.

42. Eck MJ, Sprang SR. The structure of tumor necrosis factor-α at 2.6 A resolution. Implications for receptor binding. *J Biol Chem* 1989;264:17595–17605.

43. Banner DW, D Arcy A, Janes W, et al. Crystal structure of the soluble human 55 kd TNF receptor-human TNF β complex: implications for TNF receptor activa-tion. *Cell* 1993;73:431–445.

44. Gray PW, Aggarwal BB, Benton CV, et al. Cloning and expression of cDNA for human lymphotoxin, a lymphokine with tumour necrosis activity. *Nature* 1984; 312:721–724.

45. Androlewicz MJ, Browning JL, Ware CF. Lymphotoxin is expressed as a het-eromeric complex with a distinct 33-kDa glycoprotein on the surface of an acti-vated human T cell hybridoma. *J Biol Chem* 1992;267:2542–2547.

46. Crowe PD, VanArsdale TL, Walter BN, et al. A lymphotoxin-β-specific receptor. *Science* 1994;264:707–710.

47. Tanaka M, Suda T, Haze K, et al. Fas ligand in human serum. *Nat Med* 1996;2: 317–322.

48. Neta R, Sayers TJ, Oppenheim JJ. Relationship of TNF to interleukins. In: Aggarwal BB, Vilcek J, eds. *Tumor necrosis factors: structure, function, and mechanism of action.* New York: Marcel Dekker Inc, 1992:499–566.

49. Turetskaya RL, Fashena SJ, Paul NL, Ruddle NH. Genomic structure, induction, and production of TNF-β. In: Aggarwal BB, Vilcek J, eds. *Tumor necrosis fac-tors: structure, function, and mechanism of action,* vol 56.New York: Marcel Dekker Inc, 1992:35–60.

50. Ware CF, Crowe PD, Grayson MH, Androlewicz MJ, Browning JL. Expression of surface lymphotoxin and tumor necrosis factor on activated T, B, and natural killer cells. *J Immunol* 1992;149:3881–3888.

51. Millet I, Ruddle NH. Differential regulation of lymphotoxin (LT), lymphotoxin-β (LT-β), and TNF-α in murine T cell clones activated through the TCR. *J Immunol* 1994;152:4336–4346.

52. Mosmann TR, Cherwinski H, Bond MW, Giedlin MA, Coffman RL. Two types of murine helper T cell clone. I. Definition according to profiles of lymphokine activities and secreted proteins. *J Immunol* 1986;136:2348–2357.

53. Griffith TS, Brunner T, Fletcher SM, Green DR, Ferguson TA. Fas ligand-induced apoptosis as a mechanism of immune privilege. *Science* 1995;270: 1189–1192.

54. Bellgrau D, Gold D, Selawry H, Moore J, Franzusoff A, Duke RC. A role for CD95 ligand in preventing graft rejection. *Nature* 1995;377:630–632.

55. MacKay F, Bourdon PR, Griffiths DA, et al. Cytotoxic activities of recombinant soluble murine lymphotoxin-α and lymphotoxin-α/β complexes. *J Immunol* 1997;159:3299–3310.

56. Loetscher H, Pan Y-CE, Lahm H-W, et al. Molecular cloning and expression of the human 55 kd tumor necrosis factor receptor. *Cell* 1990;61:351–359.

57. Schall TJ, Lewis M, Koller KJ, et al. Molecular cloning and expression of a receptor for human tumor necrosis factor. *Cell* 1990;61:361–370.

58. Smith CA, Davis T, Anderson D, et al. A receptor for tumor necrosis factor defines an unusual family of cellular and viral proteins. *Science* 1990;248: 1019–1023.

59. Dembic Z, Loetscher H, Gubler U, et al. Two human TNF receptors have similar extracellular, but distinct intracellular, domain sequences. *Cytokine* 1990;2: 231–237.

60. Aggarwal BB, Eessalu TE, Hass PE. Characterization of receptors for human tumour necrosis factor and their regulation by γ-interferon. *Nature* 1985;318: 665–667.

61. Tsujimoto M, Yip YK, Vilcek J. Interferon-γ enhances expression of cellular receptors for tumor necrosis factor. *J Immunol* 1986;136:2441–2444.

62. Owen-Schaub LB, Crump Wd, Morin GI, Grimm EA. Regulation of lymphocyte tumor necrosis factor receptors by IL-2. *J Immunol* 1989;143:2236–2241.

63. Tsujimoto M, Oku N. Regulation of TNF receptors. In: Aggarwal BB, Vilcek J,

64. Aderka D. The potential biological and clinical significance of the soluble tumor necrosis factor receptors. *Cytokine Growth Factor Rev* 1996;7:231–240.

65. Engelmann H, Aderka D, Rubinstein M, Rotman D, Wallach D. A tumor necro-sis factor-binding protein purified to homogeneity from human urine protects cells from tumor necrosis factor toxicity. *J Biol Chem* 1989;264:11974–11980.

66. Aderka D, Engelmann H, Maor Y, Brakebusch C, Wallach D. Stabilization of the bioactivity of tumor necrosis factor by its soluble receptors. *J Exp Med* 1992; 175:323–329.

67. Engelmann H, Holtmann H, Brakebusch C, et al. Antibodies to a soluble form of a tumor necrosis factor (TNF) receptor have TNF-like activity. *J Biol Chem* 1990;265:14497–14504.

68. Tartaglia LA, Goeddel DV, Reynolds C, et al. Stimulation of human T-cell pro-liferation by specific activation of the 75-kDa tumor necrosis factor receptor. *J Immunol* 1993;151:4637–4641.

69. Smith DM, Tran HM, Soo VW, et al. Enhanced synthesis of tumor necrosis fac-tor-inducible proteins, plasminogen activator inhibitor-2, manganese superoxide dismutase, and protein 28/5.6, is selectively triggered by the 55-kDa tumor necrosis factor receptor in human melanoma cells. *J Biol Chem* 1994;269: 9898–9905.

70. Tartaglia LA, Rothe M, Hu YF, Goeddel DV. Tumor necrosis factor's cytotoxic activity is signaled by the p55 TNF receptor. *Cell* 1993;73:213–216.

71. van der Poll T, Jansen PM, Van Zee KJ, et al. Tumor necrosis factor-α induces activation of coagulation and fibrinolysis in baboons through an exclusive effect on the p55 receptor. *Blood* 1996;88:922–927.

72. Tartaglia LA, Goeddel DV. Two TNF receptors. *Immunol Today* 1992;13: 151–153.

73. Tartaglia LA, Pennica D, Goeddel DV. Ligand passing: the 75-kDa tumor necro-sis factor (TNF) receptor recruits TNF for signaling by the 55-kDa TNF recep-tor. *J Biol Chem* 1993;268:18542–18548.

74. Itoh N, Nagata S. A novel protein domain required for apoptosis. Mutational analysis of human Fas antigen. *J Biol Chem* 1993;268:10932–10937.

75. Rothe M, Wong SC, Henzel WJ, Goeddel DV. A novel family of putative signal transducers associated with the cytoplasmic domain of the 75 kDa tumor necro-sis factor receptor. *Cell* 1994;78:681–692.

76. Darnay BG, Aggarwal BB. Early events in TNF signaling: a story of associations and dissociations. *J Leukoc Biol* 1997;61:559–566.

77. Takeuchi M, Rothe M, Goeddel DV. Anatomy of TRAF2. Distinct domains for nuclear factor-kB activation and association with tumor necrosis factor signaling proteins. *J Biol Chem* 1996;271:19935–19942.

78. Hsu H, Xiong J, Goeddel DV. The TNF receptor 1-associated protein TRADD signals cell death and NF-kB activation. *Cell* 1995;81:495–504.

79. Chinnaiyan AM, O'Rourke K, Tewari M, Dixit VM. FADD, a novel death domain-containing protein, interacts with the death domain of Fas and initiates apoptosis. *Cell* 1995;81:505–512.

80. Boldin MP, Varfolomeev EE, Pancer Z, Mett IL, Camonis JH, Wallach D. A novel protein that interacts with the death domain of Fas/APO1 contains a sequence motif related to the death domain. *J Biol Chem* 1995;270:7795–7798.

81. Stanger BZ, Leder P, Lee TH, Kim E, Seed B. RIP: a novel protein containing a death domain that interacts with Fas/APO-1 (CD95) in yeast and causes cell death. *Cell* 1995;81:513–523.

82. Duan H, Dixit VM. RAIDD is a new 'death' adaptor molecule. *Nature* 1997;385: 86–89.

83. Wallach D. Cell death induction by TNF: a matter of self control. *TIBS* 1997;22: 107–110.

84. Ting AT, Pimentel-Muinos FX, Seed B. RIP mediates tumor necrosis factor receptor 1 activation of NF-κB but not Fas/APO-1-initiated apoptosis. *EMBO J* 1996;15:;6189–6196.

85. Beg AA, Baltimore D. An essential role for NK-kB in preventing TNF-α-induced cell death. *Science* 1996;274:782–784.

86. Liu Z-G, Hsu H, Goeddel DV, Karin M. Dissection of TNF receptor 1 effector functions: JNK activation is not linked to apoptosis while NF-kB activation pre-vents cell death. *Cell* 1996;87:565–576.

87. Vilcek J, Lee TH. Tumor necrosis factor. New insights into the molecular mech-anisms of its multiple actions. *J Biol Chem* 1991;266:7313–7316.

88. Malinin NL, Boldin MP, Kovalenko AV, Wallach D. MAP3K-related kinase involved in NF-kB induction by TNF, CD95 and IL-1. *Nature* 1997;385: 540–544.

89. Regnier CH, Song HY, Gao X, Goeddel DV, Cao Z, Rothe M. Identification and characterization of an IkB kinase. *Cell* 1997;90:373–383.

90. DiDonato JA, Hayakawa M, Rothwarf DM, Zandi E, Karin M. A cytokine-responsive IkB kinase that activates the transcription factor NF-kB. *Nature* 1997;388:548–554.

91. Baldwin AS Jr. The NF-kB and I kB proteins: new discoveries and insights. *Annu Rev Immunol* 1996;14:649–683.

92. Cano E, Mahadevan LC. Parallel signal processing among mammalian MAPKs. *Trends Biochem Sci* 1995;20:117–122.

93. Victor I, Schwenger P, Li W, Schlessinger J, Vilcek J. Tumor necrosis factor-induced activation and increased tyrosine phosphorylation of mitogen-activated protein (MAP) kinase in human fibroblasts. *J Biol Chem* 1993;268: 18994–18999.

94. Van Lint J, Agostinis P, Vandevoorde V, et al. Tumor necrosis factor stimulates

multiple serine/threonine protein kinases in Swiss 3T3 and L929 cells. Implication of casein kinase-2 and extracellular signal-regulated kinases in the tumor necrosis factor signal transduction pathway. *J Biol Chem* 1992;267:25916–25921.

95. Minden A, Lin A, Smeal T, et al. c-Jun N-terminal phosphorylation correlates with activation of the JNK subgroup but not the ERK subgroup of mitogen-activated protein kinases. *Mol Cell Biol* 1994;14:6683–6688.

96. Kyriakis JM, Banerjee P, Nikolakaki E, et al. The stress-activated protein kinase subfamily of c-Jun kinases. *Nature* 1994;369:156–160.

97. Raingeaud J, Gupta S, Rogers JS, et al. Pro-inflammatory cytokines and environmental stress cause p38 mitogen-activated protein kinase activation by dual phosphorylation on tyrosine and threonine. *J Biol Chem* 1995;270:7420–7426.

98. Natoli G, Costanzo A, Ianni A, et al. Activation of SAPK/JNK by TNF receptor 1 through a noncytotoxic TRAF2-dependent pathway. *Science* 1997;275:200–203.

99. Lee JC, Laydon JT, McDonnell PC, et al. A protein kinase involved in the regulation of inflammatory cytokine biosynthesis. *Nature* 1994;372:739–746.

100. Lin L-L, Wartmann M, Lin AY, Knopf JL, Seth A, Davis RJ. cPLA₂ is phosphorylated and activated by MAP kinase. *Cell* 1993;72:269–278.

101. Read MA, Whitley MZ, Gupta S, et al. Tumor necrosis factor α-induced E-selectin expression is activated by the nuclear factor-kB and c-JUN N-terminal kinase/p38 mitogen-activated protein kinase pathways. *J Biol Chem* 1997;272:2753–2761.

102. Beyaert R, Cuenda A, Vanden Berghe W, et al. The p38/RK mitogen-activated protein kinase pathway regulates interleukin-6 synthesis in response to tumour necrosis factor. *EMBO J* 1996;15:1914–1923.

103. Kolesnick R, Golde DW. The sphingomyelin pathway in tumor necrosis factor and interleukin-1 signaling. *Cell* 1994;77:325–328.

104. Kim MY, Linardic C, Obeid L, Hannun Y. Identification of sphingomyelin turnover as an effector mechanism for the action of tumor necrosis factor alpha and gamma-interferon. Specific role in cell differentiation. *J Biol Chem* 1991;266:484–489.

105. Adam-Klages S, Adam D, Wiegmann K, et al. FAN, a novel WD-repeat protein, couples the p55 TNF-receptor to neutral sphingomyelinase. *Cell* 1996;86:937–947.

106. Heller RA, Krönke M. Tumor necrosis factor receptor-mediated signaling pathways. *J Cell Biol* 1994;126:5–9.

107. Verheij M, Bose R, Lin XH, et al. Requirement for ceramide-initiated SAPK/JNK signalling in stress-induced apoptosis. *Nature* 1996;380:75–79.

108. Yao B, Zhang Y, Delikat S, Mathias S, Basu S, Kolesnick R. Phosphorylation of Raf by ceramide-activated protein kinase. *Nature* 1995;378:307–310.

109. Muller G, Ayoub M, Storz P, Rennecke J, Fabbro D, Pfizenmaier K. PKC ζ is a molecular switch in signal transduction of TNF-α, bifunctionally regulated by ceramide and arachidonic acid. *EMBO J* 1995;14:1961–1969.

110. Gamard CJ, Dbaibo GS, Liu B, Obeid LM, Hannun YA. Selective involvement of ceramide in cytokine-induced apoptosis. Ceramide inhibits phorbol ester activation of nuclear factor kB. *J Biol Chem* 1997;272:16474–16481.

111. Zumbansen M, Stoffel W. Tumor necrosis factor α activates NF-kB in acid sphingo-myelinase-deficient mouse embryonic fibroblasts. *J Biol Chem* 1997;272:10904–10909.

112. Pasparakis M, Alexopoulou L, Douni E, Kollias G. Tumour necrosis factors in immune regulation: everything that's interesting is...new. *Cytokine Growth Factor Rev* 1996;7:223–229.

113. Zhang Y, Harada A, Bluethmann H, et al. Tumor necrosis factor (TNF) is a physiologic regulator of hematopoietic progenitor cells: increase of early hematopoietic progenitor cells in TNF receptor p55-deficient mice in vivo and potent inhibition of progenitor cell proliferation by TNF alpha in vitro. *Blood* 1995;86:2930–2937.

114. Uysal KT, Wiesbrock SM, Marino MW, Hotamisligil GS. Protection from obesity-induced insulin resistance in mice lacking TNF-α function. *Nature* 1997;389:610–614.

115. Le Hir M, Bluethmann H, Kosco-Vilbois MH, et al. Differentiation of follicular dendritic cells and full antibody responses require tumor necrosis factor receptor-1 signaling. *J Exp Med* 1996;183:2367–2372.

116. Pasparakis M, Alexopoulou L, Episkopou V, Kollias G. Immune and inflammatory responses in TNF alpha-deficient mice: a critical requirement for TNF α in the formation of primary B cell follicles, follicular dendritic cell networks and germinal centers, and in the maturation of the humoral immune response. *J Exp Med* 1996;184:1397–1411.

117. Matsumoto M, Mariathasan S, Nahm MH, Baranyay F, Peschon JJ, Chaplin DD. Role of lymphotoxin and the type I TNF receptor in the formation of germinal centers. *Science* 1996;271:1289–1291.

118. Banks TA, Rouse BT, Kerley MK, et al. Lymphotoxin-α-deficient mice. Effects on secondary lymphoid organ development and humoral immune responsiveness. *J Immunol* 1995;155:1685–1693.

119. De Togni P, Goellner J, Ruddle NH, et al. Abnormal development of peripheral lymphoid organs in mice deficient in lymphotoxin. *Science* 1994;264:703–707.

120. Koni PA, Sacca R, Lawton P, Browning JL, Ruddle NH, Flavell RA. Distinct roles in lymphoid organogenesis for lymphotoxins α and β revealed in lymphotoxin β-deficient mice. *Immunity* 1997;6:491–500.

121. Alimzhanov MB, Kuprash DV, Kosco-Vilbois MH, et al. Abnormal development of secondary lymphoid tissues in lymphotoxin β-deficient mice. *Proc Natl Acad Sci USA* 1997;94:9302–9307.

122. Bluethmann H. Physiological, immunological and pathological functions of TNF revealed by TNF deficient mice. In: Durum SK, Muegge K, eds. *Contemporary immunology: cytokine knockouts.* Totowa, NJ: Humana Press, 1998:69–88.

123. Rubin BY. TNF and viruses: multiple interrelationships. In: Aggarwal BB, Vilcek J, eds. *Tumor necrosis factors: structure, function, and mechanism of action.* New York: Marcel Dekker Inc, 1992:331–340.

124. Upton C, Macen JL, Schreiber M, McFadden G. Myxoma virus expresses a secreted protein with homology to the tumor necrosis factor receptor gene family that contributes to viral virulence. *Virology* 1991;184:370–382.

125. Grau GE, Taylor TE, Molyneux ME, et al. Tumor necrosis factor and disease severity in children with falciparum malaria. *N Engl J Med* 1989;320:1586–1591.

126. Tracey KJ, Fong Y, Hesse DG, et al. Anti-cachectin/TNF monoclonal antibodies prevent septic shock during lethal bacteraemia. *Nature* 1987;330:662–664.

127. Erickson SL, de Sauvage FJ, Kikly K, et al. Decreased sensitivity to tumour-necrosis factor but normal T-cell development in TNF receptor-2-deficient mice. *Nature* 1994;372:560–563.

128. Matsumoto M, Fu YX, Molina H, Chaplin DD. Lymphotoxin-α-deficient and TNF receptor-I-deficient mice define developmental and functional characteristics of germinal centers. *Immunol Rev* 1997;156:137–144.

129. Marino MW, Dunn A, Grail D, et al. Characterization of tumor necrosis factor-deficient mice. *Proc Natl Acad Sci USA* 1997;94:8093–8098.

130. Pasparakis M, Alexopoulou L, Grell M, Pfizenmaier K, Bluethmann H, Kollias G. Peyer's patch organogenesis is intact yet formation of B lymphocyte follicles is defective in peripheral lymphoid organs of mice deficient for tumor necrosis factor and its 55-kDa receptor. *Proc Natl Acad Sci USA* 1997;94:6319–6323.

131. Keffer J, Probert L, Cazlaris H, et al. Transgenic mice expressing human tumour necrosis factor: a predictive genetic model of arthritis. *EMBO J* 1991;10:4025–4031.

132. Probert L, Plows D, Kontogeorgos G, Kollias G. The type I interleukin-1 receptor acts in series with tumor necrosis factor (TNF) to induce arthritis in TNF-transgenic mice. *Eur J Immunol* 1995;25:1794–1797.

133. Feldmann M, Brennan FM, Maini RN. Role of cytokines in rheumatoid arthritis. *Annu Rev Immunol* 1996;14:397–440.

134. Neurath MF, Fuss I, Pasparakis M, et al. Predominant pathogenic role of tumor necrosis factor in experimental colitis in mice. *Eur J Immunol* 1997;27:1743–1750.

135. van Deventer SJ, Camoglio L. Monoclonal antibody therapy of inflammatory bowel disease. *Pharm World Sci* 1997;19:55–59.

136. Yang XD, Tisch R, Singer SM, et al. Effect of tumor necrosis factor alpha on insulin-dependent diabetes mellitus in NOD mice. I. The early development of autoimmunity and the diabetogenic process. *J Exp Med* 1994;180:995–1004.

137. Cope AP, Liblau RS, Yang XD, et al. Chronic tumor necrosis factor alters T cell responses by attenuating T cell receptor signaling. *J Exp Med* 1997;185:1573–1584.

138. Naylor MS, Stamp GW, Foulkes WD, Eccles D, Balkwill FR. Tumor necrosis factor and its receptors in human ovarian cancer. Potential role in disease progression. *J Clin Invest* 1993;91:2194–2206.

139. Eggermont AM, Schraffordt Koops H, Klausner JM, et al. Isolated limb perfusion with tumor necrosis factor and melphalan for limb salvage in 186 patients with locally advanced soft tissue extremity sarcomas. The cumulative multicenter European experience. *Ann Surg* 1996;224:756–764.

140. Kratz A, Campos-Neto A, Hanson MS, Ruddle NH. Chronic inflammation caused by lymphotoxin is lymphoid neogenesis. *J Exp Med* 1996;183:1461–1472.

141. Wallach D. Suicide by order: some open questions about the cell-killing activities of the TNF ligand and receptor families. *Cytokine Growth Factor Rev* 1996;7:211–221.

142. Okura T, Gong L, Kamitani T, et al. Protection against Fas/APO-1- and tumor necrosis factor-mediated cell death by a novel protein, sentrin. *J Immunol* 1996;157:4277–4281.

143. Song HY, Dunbar JD, Zhang YX, Guo D, Donner DB. Identification of a protein with homology to hsp90 that binds the type 1 tumor necrosis factor receptor. *J Biol Chem* 1995;270:3574–3581.

144. Boldin MP, Mett IL, Wallach D. A protein related to a proteasomal subunit binds to the intracellular domain of the p55 TNF receptor upstream to its 'death domain'. *FEBS Lett* 1995;367:39–44.

145. Rothe M, Sarma V, Dixit VM, Goeddel DV. TRAF2-mediated activation of NF-kappa B by TNF receptor 2 and CD40. *Science* 1995;269:1424–1427.

146. Opipari AW Jr, Boguski MS, Dixit VM. The A20 cDNA induced by tumor necrosis factor alpha encodes a novel type of zinc finger protein. *J Biol Chem* 1990;265:14705–14708.

147. Song HY, Rothe M, Goeddel DV. The tumor necrosis factor-inducible zinc finger protein A20 interacts with TRAF1/TRAF2 and inhibits NF-kB activation. *Proc Natl Acad Sci USA* 1996;93:6721–6725.

148. Rothe M, Xiong J, Shu HB, Williamson K, Goddard A, Goeddel DV. I-TRAF is a novel TRAF-interacting protein that regulates TRAF-mediated signal transduction. *Proc Natl Acad Sci USA* 1996;93:8241–8246.

149. Cheng G, Baltimore D. TANK, a co-inducer with TRAF2 of TNF- and CD 40L-mediated NF-kB activation. *Genes Dev* 1996;10:963–973.

150. Lee SY, Lee SY, Choi Y. TRAF-interacting protein (TRIP): a novel component of the tumor necrosis factor receptor (TNFR)- and CD30-TRAF signaling complexes that inhibits TRAF2-mediated NF-kB activation. *J Exp Med* 1997;185:1275–1285.

151. Irmler M, Thome M, Hahne M, et al. Inhibition of death receptor signals by cellular FLIP. *Nature* 1997;388:190–195.
152. Shu H-B, Halpin DR, Goeddel DV. Casper is a FADD- and caspase-related inducer of apoptosis. *Immunity* 1997;6:751–763.

Selected IL-1 Family

153. Gery I, Gershon RK, Waksman BH. Potentiation of the T lymphocyte response to mitogens. I. The responding cell. *J Exp Med* 1972;136:128–138.
154. Dinarello CA. Biologic basis for Interleukin-1 in disease. *Blood* 1996;87:2095–2147.
155. Arend WP. Interleukin-1 receptor antagonist. *Adv Immunol* 1993;54:167–227.
156. Durum SK, Schmidt JA, Oppenheim JJ. Interleukin 1: an immunological perspective. *Annu Rev Immunol* 1986;3:263–287.
157. Seckinger P, Lowenthal JW, Williamson K, Dayer JM, MacDonald JR. A urine inhibitor of interleukin 1 activity that blocks ligand binding. *J Immunol* 1987;139:1546–1552.
158. Auron PE, Webb AC, Rosenwasser LJ, et al. Nucleotide sequence of human monocyte interleukin 1 precursor cDNA. *Proc Natl Acad Sci USA* 1984;81:7907–7911.
159. LoMedico PT, Gubler U, Hellmann CP, et al. Cloning and expression of murine interleukin 1 cDNA in Escherichia coli. *Nature* 1984;312:458–462.
160. Eisenberg SP, Evans RJ, Arend WP, et al. Primary structure and functional expression from complementary DNA of a human interleukin-1 receptor antagonist. *Nature* 1990;343:341–343.
161. Carter DB, Deibel MR, Dunn CJ, et al. Purification, cloning, expression and biological characterization of an interleukin-1 receptor antagonist protein. *Nature* 1990;344:633.
162. Tsukada J, Saito K, Waterman WR, Webb AR, Auron PE. Transcription factors NF-IL6 and CREB recognize a common essential site in the human prointerleukin 1 β gene. *Mol Cell Biol* 1994;14:7285–7291.
163. Hatzigeorgiou DF, Geng J, Zhu B et al. Lipophosphoglycan from leishmania suppresses agonist-induced IL-1β gene expression in human monocytes via a unique promoter sequence. *Proc Natl Acad Sci USA* 1996;93:14708–14713.
164. Smith MF, Eidlen D, Brewer MT, Eisenberg SP, Arend WP, Gutierrez-Hartmann, A. Human IL-1 receptor antagonist promoter: cell type-specfic activity and identification of regulatory regions. *J Immunol* 1992;149:2000–2006.
165. Kern JA, Warnock LJ, McCafferty JD. The 3′ untranslated region of IL-1β regulates protein production. *J Immunol* 1997;58:1187–1193.
166. Koyabashi Y, Appella E, Yamada M, Copeland TD, Oppenheim JJ, Matsushima K. Phosphorylation of intracellular precursors of human IL-1. *J Immunol* 1988;140:2279–2284.
167. Brody DT, Durum SK. Membrane IL1: IL-1 alpha precursor binds to the plasma membrane via a lectin like interaction. *J Immunol* 1989;143:1183–1188.
168. Kostura MJ, Tocci MJ, Limjuco G, et al. Identification of a monocyte specific preinterleukin 1 beta convertase activity. *Proc Natl Acad Sci USA* 1989;86:5227–5231.
169. Thornberry NA, Bull HG, Calaycay JR, et al. A novel heterodimeric cystein protease is required for interleukin-1beta processing in monocytes. *Nature* 1992, 356:768–774.
170. Singer II, Scott S, Chin J et al. The IL-1β-converting enzyme (ICE) is localized on the exernal cell surface membranes and in the cytoplasmic ground substance of human monocytes by immuno-electron microscopy. *J Exp Med* 1995;182:1447–1459.
171. Kuida K, Lipke JA, Ku G, et al. Altered cytokine export and apoptosis in mice deficient in interleukin-1β converting enzyme. *Science* 1995;267:2000–2002.
172. Kobayashi Y, Yamamoto K, Saido T, Kawasaki H, Oppenheim JJ, Matsushima K. Identification of calcium-activated neutral protease as a processing enzyme of human interleukin 1 alpha. *Proc Natl Acad Sci USA* 1990;97:5548–5552.
173. Hannum CH, Wilcox CJ, Arend WP, et al. Interleukin-1 receptor antagonist activity of a human interleukin-1 inhibitor. *Nature* 1990;343:336–339
174. Haskill S, Martin M, Van Le L, et al. cDNA cloning of an intracellular form of the human interleukin 1 receptor antagonist associated with epithelium. *Proc Natl Acad Sci USA* 1991;88:3681–3685.
175. Muzio M, Polentarutti N, Sironi M, et al. Cloning and characterization of a new isoform of the IL-1 receptor antagonist. *J Exp Med* 1995;182:623–628.
176. Priestley JP, Schar HP, Grutter MG. Crystallographic refinement of interleukin-1 at 2.0 A resolution. *Proc Natl Acad Sci USA* 1989;86:9667–9671.
177. Hakim I, Levy S, Levy R. A nine-amino acid peptide from IL-1β augments antitumor immune responses induced by protein and DNA vaccines. *J Immunol* 1996;157:5503–5511.
178. Boraschi D, Bossu P, Ruggiero P, et al. Mapping of receptor binding sites on IL-1β by reconstruction of IL-1ra-like domains. *J Immunol* 1995,155:4719–4725.
179. Dinarello CA. The interleukin-1 family. 10 years of discovery. *FASEB J* 1994;8:1314–1325.
180. Arend WP. Interleukin 1 receptor antagonist. A new member of the interleukin 1 family. *J Clin Invest* 1991;88:1445–1451.
181. Kopp WC, Urba WJ, Rager HC, et al. Induction of interleukin-1 receptor antagonist after interleukin 1 therapy in patients with cancer. *Clin Cancer Res* 1996;2:501–506.
182. Roberge CJ, Poubelle PE, Beaulieu AD, Heitz D, Gosselin J. The IL-1 and IL-1 receptor antagonist (IL-1Ra) response of human neutrophils to EBV stimulation. *J Immunol* 1996;156:4884–4891.
183. Zavala F, Rimaniol AC, Boussin F, Dormont D, Bach JF, Deschamps-Latscha B. HIV predominantly induces IL-1 receptor antagonist over IL-1 synthesis in human primary monocytes. *J Immunol* 1995;155:2784–2790.
184. Cannon JG, Dinarello CA. Increased plasma interleukin-1 activity in women after ovulation. *Science* 1985;227:1247–1250.
185. Cannon JG, Tompkins RG, Gelfand JA, et al. Circulating interleukin-1 and tumor necrosis factor in septic shock experimental endotoxin fever. *J Infect Dis* 1990;161:79–84.
186. Granowitz EV, Santos A, Poutsiaka DD, et al. Circulating interleukin-1 receptor antagonist levels during experimental endotoxemia in humans. *Lancet* 1991;338:1423–1424.
187. Sims JE, March CJ, Cosman D, et al. Expression cloning of the IL-1 receptor, a member of the immunoglobulin superfamily. *Science* 1988;241:585–588.
188. McMahan CJ, Slack JL, Moslwy B, et al. A novel IL1 receptor, cloned from B cells by mammalian expression, is expressed in many cell types. *EMBO J* 1991;10:2821–2826.
189. Sims JE, Giri JG, Dower SK. The two interleukin-1 receptors play different roles in IL-1 actions. *Clin Immunol Immunopathol* 1994;72:9–14.
190. Colotta F, Dower SK, Sims JE, Mantovani A. The type II "decoy" receptor: a novel regulatory pathway for interleukin 1. *Immunol Today* 1994;15:562–566.
191. Greenfeder SA, Nunes P, Kwee L, Labow M, Chizzonite RA, Ju G. Molecular cloning and characterization of a second subunit of the interleukin-1 receptor complex. *J Biol Chem* 1995;270:13757–13765.
192. Groves RW, Rauschmayr T, Nakamura K, Sarkar S, Williams IR, Kupper TS. Inflammatory and hyperproliferative skin disease in mice that express elevated levels of the IL-1 receptor (type I) on epidermal keratinocytes. *J Clin Invest* 1996;98:336–344.
193. Symons JA, Eastgate JA, Duff GW. Purification and characterization of a novel soluble receptor for interleukin 1. *J Exp Med* 1991;174:1251–1258.
194. Symons JA, Young PR, Duff GW. Soluble type II IL-1 receptor binds and blocks processing of IL-1β precursor and loses affinity for IL-1 receptor antagonist. *Proc Natl Acad Sci USA* 1995;92:1714–1718.
195. Giri JG, Wells J, Dower SK, et al. Elevated levels of shed type II IL-1 receptor in sepsis. *J Immunol* 1994;153:5802–5807.
196. Spriggs MK, Hruby DE, Maliszewski CR, et al. Vaccinia and cowpox viruses encode a novel secreted interleukin-1 binding protein. *Cell* 1992;71:145–152.
197. Alcami A, Smith GL. A soluble receptor for interleukin-1β encoded by vaccinia virus: a novel mechanism of virus modulation of the host response to infection. *Cell* 992;71:153–160.
198. Ray CA, Black RA, Kronheim SR, et al. Viral inhibition of inflammation: cowpox virus encodes an inhibitor of the interleukin-1β converting enzyme. *Cell* 1992;69:597–604.
199. Sims JE, Gayle MA, Slack JL, et al. Interleukin-1 signalling occurs exclusively via the type I receptor. *Proc Natl Acad Sci USA* 1993;90:6155–6160.
200. Lenardo MJ, Baltimore D. NFKB: a pleiotropic mediator of inducible and tissue-specific gene control. *Cell* 1988;58:227–229.
201. Barnes PJ, Karin M. Nuclear factor-KB a pivotal transcription factor in chronic inflammatory diseases. *N Engl J Med* 1997;336:1066–1071.
202. Chiu R, Boyle WJ, Meek J, Smeal T, Hunter T, Karin M. The c-fos protein interacts with c-jun/AP-1 to stimulate transcription of AP-1 responsive genes. *Cell* 1988;54:541–549.
203. Guy GR, Chua SP, Wong NS, et al. Interleukin 1 and tumor necrosis factor activate common multiple protein kinases in human fibroblasts. *J Biol Chem* 1991;266:14343–14352.
204. Cao Z, Henzel WJ, Gao X. IRAK: a kinase associated with the interleukin 1 receptor. *Science* 1996;271:1128–1131.
205. Croston GE, Cao Z, Goeddel DV. NF-kB activation by IL-1 requires an IL-1 receptor-associated protein kinase activity. *J Biol Chem* 1995;270:16514–16517.
206. Cao Z, Xiong J, Takeuchi M, Kurama T, Goeddel DV. TRAF6 is a signal transducer for interleukin 1. *Nature* 1996;383:443–446
207. Saklatvala J, Davis W, Guesdon F. Interleukin 1 and tumor necrosis factor signal transduction. *Philos Trans R Soc Lond Biol Sci* 1996;351:151–157.
208. Kuno K, Matsushima K. The IL-1receptor signaling pathway. *J Leukoc Biol* 1994;56:542–547.
209. Kolesnick R, Golde DW. The sphingomyelin pathway in tumor necrosis factor and interleukin-1 signalling. *Cell* 1994;77:325–331.
210. Mathias S, Younes A, Kan CC, Orlow I, Joseph C, Kolesnick RN. Activation of the sphingomyelin signaling pathway in intact EL4 cells and in a cell-free system by IL-1β. *Science* 1993;259:519–522.
211. Ridley SH, Sarfield SJ, Lee JC, et al. Actions of IL-1 are selectively controlled by p38 mitogen-activated protein kinase. *J Immunol* 1997;158:3165–3173.
212. Karmann K, Min W, Fanslow WC, Pober JS. Activation and hologous desensitization of human endothelial cells by CD40 ligand, tumor necrosis factor and interleukin 1. *J Exp Med* 1996;184:173–182.
213. Muegge K, Vila M, Gusella GL, et al. IL-1 induction of the c-jun promoter. *Proc Natl Acad Sci USA* 1993;90:7054–7057.
214. Muegge K, Williams TM, Kant J, et al. Interleukin 1 costimulatory activity on the interleukin 2 promoter via AP-1. *Science* 1989;246:249–252.
215. Rothenberg EV, Diamond RA, Pepper KA, Yang JA. IL-2 gene inducibility in T cells before T cell receptor expression. Changes in signaling pathways and gene expression requirements during intrathymic maturation. *J Immunol* 1990;144:1614–1619.

216. Schmitt E, Beuscher HU, Huels C, et al. IL1 serves as a secondary signal for IL9 expression. *J Immunol* 1991;147:3848–3853.
217. Krakauer T, Oppenheim JJ. IL-1 and TNFα each up-regulate both the expression of IFNγ receptors and enhance IFNγ induced HLA-DR expression on human monocytes and a human monocytic cell line (THP-1). *J Immunol* 1993;150: 1205–1211.
218. Zuniga-Pflucker JC, Jiang D, Lenardo MJ. Requirement for TNF-α and IL-1α in fetal thymocyte commitment and differentiation. *Science* 1995;268:1906–1909.
219. Giri JG, Kincade PW, Mizel SB. Interleukin 1-mediated induction of kappa-light chain synthesis and surface immuno-globulin expression on pre-B cells. *J Immunol* 1984;132:223–227.
220. Oppenheim JJ, Zachariae COC, Mukaida N, Matsushima K. Properties of the novel proinflammatory supergene "intercrine" cytokine family. *Annu Rev Immunol* 1991;9:617–648.
221. Koide SL, Inaba K, Steinman RM. Interleukin 1 enhances T-dependent immune responses by amplifying the function of dendritic cells. *J Exp Med* 1987;165: 515–519.
222. Bevilacqua MP. Endothelial-leukocyte adhesion molecules. *Annu Rev Immunol* 1993;11:767–804.
223. Dustin ML, Rothlein R, Bhan AK, Dinarello CA, Springer TA. Induction by IL1 and interferon-gamma: tissue distribution, biochemistry, and function of a natural adherence molecule (ICAM-1). *J Immunol* 1986;137:245.
224. Sanz MJ, Weg VB, Bolanowski MA, Nourshargh S. IL-1 is a potent inducer of eosinophil accumulation in rat skin. *J Immunol* 1995;154:1364–1373.
225. Bagby GC. Interleukin 1 and hematopoiesis. *Blood Rev* 1989;3:152–159.
226. Fantuzzi G, Dinarello CA. The inflammatory response in interleukin-1β-deficient mice: comparison with other cytokine-related knock-out mice. *J Leukoc Biol* 1996;59:489–493.
227. Laver J, Abboude M, Gasparetto C, et al. Effects of IL-1 on hematopoietic progenitors after myelosuppressive chemoradiotherapy. *Biotherapy* 1989;1:293–300.
228. Neta R, Douches S, Oppenheim JJ. Interleukin-1 is a radioprotector. *J Immunol* 1986;136:2483–2488.
229. Duff GW, Durum SK. The pyrogenic and mitogenic actions of interleukin-1 are related. *Nature* 1983;304:449–452.
230. Grunfeld C, Zhao C, Fuller J, et al. Endotoxin and cytokines induce expression of leptin, the ob gene product, in hamsters. A role for leptin in the anorexia of infection. *J Clin Invest* 1996;97:1–6.
231. Besedovsky HO, Del Rey A. Immune-neuro-endocrine interactions: facts and hypotheses. *Endocr Rev* 1996;17:64–76.
232. Liu J, Zhao ML, Brosnan CF, Lee SC. Expression of type II nitric oxide synthase in primary human astrocytes and microglia. *J Immunol* 1996;157:3569–3576.
233. Fantuzzi G, Ghezzi P. Glucocorticoids as cytokine inhibitors: role in neuroendocrine therapy of inflammatory diseases. *Mediator Inflamm* 1993;2:263–268.
234. Bertini R, Bianchi M, Ghezzi P. Adrenalectomy sensitizes mice to the lethal effects of interleukin-1 and tumor necrosis factor. *J Exp Med* 1988;167: 1708–1714.
235. Dinarello CA, Wolff SM. The role of interleukin-1 in disease. *N Engl J Med* 1993;328:106–113.
236. Saren P, Welgus HG, Kovanen PT. TNFα and IL-1β selectively induce expression of 92-kDa gelatinase by human macrophages. *J Immunol* 1996;157: 4159–4165.
237. Wooley PH, Whalen JD, Chapman DL, et al. The effect of an IL-1 receptor antagonist protein on type II collagen-induced arthritis in mice. *Arthritis Rheum* 1993;36:1305–1310.
238. van den Berg WB, Joosten LA, Helsen M, van de Loo FA. Amelioration of established murine collagen-induced arthritis with anti-IL-1 treatment. *Clin Exp Immunol* 1994;95:237–242.
239. Onozaki K, Matsushima K, Aggarwal BB, Oppenheim JJ. Human interleukin-1 is a cytocidal factor for several tumor cell lines. *J Immunol* 1985;135: 3962–3968.
240. North RJ, Neubauer RH, Huang JJH, Newton RC, Loveless SE. Interleukin 1-induced, T cell-mediated regression immunogenic murine tumor. *J Exp Med* 1988;168:2031–2043.
241. Mori N, Shirakawa F, Murakami S, Oda S, Eto S. IL-1α as an autocrine growth factor for acute lymphoblastic leukaemia cells. *Br J Haematol* 1994;86:386–391.
242. Mandrup-Poulsen T, Zumsteg U, Reimers J, et al. Involvement of IL-1 and IL-1 antagonist in pancreatic β-cell destruction in insulin-dependent diaetes mellitus. *Cytokine* 1993;5:185–191.
243. Tatsuta T, Cheng J, Mountz JD. Intracellular IL-1β is an inhibitor of FAS-mediated apoptosis. *J Immunol* 1996;157:3949–3957.
244. Maier JA, Voulalas P, Roeder D, Maciag T. Extension of the life-span of human endothelial cells by an interleukin-1 alpha antisense oligomer. *Science* 1990;249: 570–574.
245. Watson JM, Lofquist AK, Rinehart CA, et al. The intracellular IL-1 receptor antagonist alters IL-1-inducible gene expression without blocking exogenous signaling by IL-1β. *J Immunol* 1995;155:4467–4475.
246. Arend WP, Malyak M, Smith MF, et al. Binding of IL-1α, IL-1β, and IL-1 receptor antagonist by soluble IL-1 receptors and levels of soluble IL-1 receptors in synovial fluids. *J Immunol* 1994;153:4766–4774.
247. Dinarello CA, Thompson RC. Blocking IL-1: interleukin 1 receptor antagonist in vivo and in vitro. *Immunol Today* 1994;12:404–410.
248. Van Zee KJ, Coyle SM, Calvano SE, et al. Influence of IL-1 receptor blockade on the human response to endotoxemia. *J Immunol* 1995;154:1499–1507.
249. Ruggiero P, Bossu P, Macchia G. et al. Inhibitory activity of IL-1 receptor antagonist depends on the balance between binding capacity for IL-1 receptor type 1 and IL-1 receptor type II. *J Immunol* 1997;158:3881–3887.
250. Burger D, Chicheportiche R, Giri JG, Dayer JM. The inhibitory activity of human IL-1 receptor antagonist is enhanced by type II IL-1 soluble receptor and hindered by type I IL-1 soluble receptor. *J Clin Invest* 1995;96:38–41.
251. Casini-Raggi V, Kam L, Chong YJT, Fiocchi C, Pizarro TT, Cominelli F. Mucosal imbalance of IL-1 and IL-1 receptor antagonist in inflammatory bowel disease. *J Immunol* 1995;154:2434–2440.
252. Chomarat P, Vannier E, Dechanet J, et al. Balance of IL-1 receptor antagonist/IL-1β in rheumatoid synovium and its regulation by IL-4 and IL-10. *J Immunol* 1995;154:1432–1439.
253. Colotta F, Orlando S, Fadlon EJ, Sozzani S, Matteucci C, Mantovani A. Chemoattractants induce rapid release of the IL-1 type II decoy receptor in human polymorphonuclear cells. *J Exp Med* 1995;181:2181–2188.
254. Hirsch E, Irikura VM, Paul SM, Hirsh D. Functions of interleukin 1 receptor antagonist in gene knockout and overproducing mice. *Proc Natl Acad Sci USA* 1996;93:11008–11013.
255. Ferretti M, Casini-Raggi V, Pizarro TT, Eisenberg SP, Nast CC, Cominelli F. Neutralization of endogenous IL-1 receptor antagonist exacerbates and prolongs inflammation in rabbit immune colitis. *J Clin Invest* 1994;94:449–453.
256. Muller-Ladner U, Roberts CR, Franklin BN, et al. Human IL-1ra gene transfer into human synovial fibroblasts is chondroprotective. *J Immunol* 1997;158: 3492–3498.
257. Caron JP, Fernandes JC, Martel-Pelletier J, et al. Chondroprotective effect of intraarticular injections of IL-1 receptor antagonist in experimental osteoarthritis suppression of collagenase-1 expression. *Arthritis Rheum* 1996;39: 1535–1541.
258. Zheng H, Fletcher D, Kozak W, et al. Resistance to fever induction and impaired acute-phase response in interleukin-β-deficient mice. *Immunity* 1995;3:9–19.
259. Li P, Allen H, Banerjee S, et al. Mice deficient in IL-1β-converting enzyme are defective in production of mature IL-1β and resistant to endotoxic shock. *Cell* 1995;80:401–411.
260. Fantuzzi G, Ku G, Harding MW, et al. Response to local inflammation of IL-1β-converting enzyme-deficient mice. *J Immunol* 1997;158:1818–1828. Selected Chemokine Reviews and References
261. Baggiolini M, Dewald B, Moser B. Human chemokines: an update. *Annu Rev Immunol* 1997;15:675–705.
262. Murphy PM. Chemokine receptors: structure, function and role in microbial pathogenesis. *Cytokine Growth Factor Rev* 1996;7:47–64.
263. Ben-Baruch A, Michiel DF, Oppenheim JJ. Signals and receptors involved in recruitment of inflammatory cells. *J Biol Chem* 1995;270:11703–11706.
264. Taub DD. Chemokine-leukocyte interactions. *Cytokine Growth Factor Rev* 1996;7:355–376.
265. Oppenheim JJ, Wang JM, Chertov O, Taub DD, Ben-Baruch, A. The role of chemokines in transplantation biology. In: Tilney NL, Strom TB, Paul LC, eds. *Cellular and molecular aspects.* Philadelphia: Lippincott-Raven Publishers, 1996:187–200.
266. Moore JP, Trkola A, Dragic T. Co-receptors for HIV entry. *Curr Opin Immunol* 1997;9:557–562.
267. Harada A, Sekido N, Akahoshi T, Wada T, Mukaida N, Matsushima K. Essential involvement of interleukin-8 (IL-8) in acute inflammation. *J Leukoc Biol* 1994;56:559–564.
268. Yoshie O, Irnai T, Nomiyama H, et al. Novel lymphocyte-specific CC chemokines and their receptors. *J Leukoc Biol* 1997;62:634–644.
269. Kelner GS, Kennedy J, Bacon KB, et al. Lymphotactin: a cytokine that represents a new class of chemokine. *Science* 1994;266:1395–1399.
270. Hedrick JA, Saylor V, Figueroa D, et al. Lymphotactin is produced by NK cells and attracts both NK cells and T cells in vitro. *J Immunol* 1997;158:1533–1540.
271. Bazan JF, Bacon KB, Hardiman G, et al. A new class of membrane-bound chemokine with a CX3C motif. *Nature* 1997;385:640–644.
272. Pan Y, Lloyd C, Zhou H, et al. Neurotactin, a novel membrane-anchored chemokine that is upregulated in brain inflammation. *Nature* 1997;387:611–617.
273. Witt DP, Lander AD. Differential binding of chemokines to glycosaminoglycan subpopulations. *Curr Biol* 1994;4:392–400.
274. Damaj BB, McColl SR, Neote K, et al. Identification of G-protein binding sites of the human interleukin-8 receptors by functional mapping of the intracellular loops. *FASEB J* 1996;10:1426–1434.
275. Horuk R. The interleukin-8 receptor family: from chemokines to malaria. *Immunol Today* 1994;15:169–174.
276. Chitnis CE, Chaudhuri A, Horuk R, Pogo AO, Miller LH. The domain on the Duffy blood group antigen for binding Plasmodium vivax and P. Knowlesi malarial parasites to erythrocytes. *J Exp Med* 1996;184:1531–1536.
277. Pleskoff O, Treboue C, Brelot A, Heveker N, Seman M, Alizon M. Identification of a chemokine receptor encoded by human cytomegalovirus as a cofactor for HIV-1 entry. *Science* 1997;276:1874–1878.
278. Guo HG, Browning P, Nicholas J, et al. Characterization of a chemokine receptor-related gene in human herpesvirus 8 and its expression in Kaposi's sarcoma. *Virology* 1997;228:371–378.
279. Tani K, Utsunomiya I, Xu L, Oppenheim JJ, Wang JM. Interferon-gamma maintains the binding and functional capacity of receptors for IL-8 on cultured human T cells. *Eur J Immunol* 1998;28:502–507.
280. Bleul CC, Wu L, Hoxie JA, Springer TA, Mackay C. The HIV coreceptors

CXCR4 and CCR5 are differentially expressed and regulated on human T lymphocytes. *Proc Natl Acad Sci USA* 1997;94:1925–1930.

281. Loetscher P, Seitz M, Baggiolini M, Moser B. Interleukin-2 regulates CC chemokine receptor expression and chemotactic responsiveness in T lymphocytes. *J Exp Med* 1996;184:569–577.

282. Lloyd AR, Oppenheim JJ, Kelvin DJ, Taub DD. Chemokines regulate T cell adhesion to endothelium and extracellular matrix proteins. *J Immunol* 1996; 156:932–938.

283. Sica A, Saccani A, Borsatti A, et al. Bacterial lipopolysaccharide rapidly inhibits expression of C-C chemokine receptors in human monocytes. *J Exp Med* 1997;185:969–974.

284. Al-Aoukaty A, Schall T, Maghazaci A. Differential coupling of CC chemokine receptors to multiple heterotrimeric G proteins in human interleukin-2 activated natural killer cells. *Blood* 1996;87:4255–4260.

285. Charo IF, Myers SJ, Hemman A, Franci G, Connoly AJ, Coughlin SK. Molecular cloning and functional expression of two monocyte chemoattractant protein 1 receptors reveals alternative splicing of the carboxyl-terminal tails. *Proc Natl Acad Sci USA* 1994;91:2752–2756.

286. Ahuja SK, Murphy PM. The CXC chemokines growth-regulated oncogene (GRO)α, GROβ, GROγ, neutrophil-activating peptide-2, and epithelial cell-derived neutrophil-activating peptide-78 are potent agonists for the type B, but not the type A, human interleukin-8 receptor. *J Biol Chem* 1996;271: 20545–20550.

287. Strieter RM, Polverini PJ, Kunkel SL, et al. The functional role of the ELR motif in CXC chemokine-mediated angiogenesis. *J Biol Chem* 1995;270:27348–27357.

288. Schonbeck S, Brandt E, Petersen F, Flad HD, Loppnow H. IL-8 specifically binds to endothelial but not smooth muscle cells. *J Immunol* 1995;154:2375–2383.

289. Nanney LB, Mueller SG, Bueno R, Peiper SC, Richmond A. Distributions of melanoma growth stimulatory activity of growth-regulated gene and the interleukin-8 receptor B in human wound repair. *Am J Pathol* 1995;147:1248–1260.

290. Petzelbauer P, Watson CA, Pfan SE, Pober JS. Il-8 and angiogenesis: evidence that human endothelial cells lack receptors and do not respond to IL-8 in vitro. *Cytokine* 1995;7;267–272.

291. Arenberg DA, Kunkel SL, Polverini PJ, Glass MC, Burdick M, Strieter RM. Inhibition of interleukin-8 reduces tumorigenesis of human non-small cell lung cancer in SCID mice. *J Clin Invest* 1996;97:2792–2802.

292. Angiolillo AL, Sgadari C, Taub DD, et al. Human interferon-inducible protein 10 is a potent inhibitor of angiogenesis in vivo. *J Exp Med* 1995;182:155–162.

293. Kolber DL, Knisely TL, Maione TE. Inhibition of development of murine melanoma lung metastases by systemic administration of recombinant platelet factor 4. *J Natl Cancer Inst* 1995;87:304 309.

294. Nourshargh S, Perkins JA, Showell HJ, Matsushima K, Williams TJ, Collins PD. A comparative study of the neutrophil stimulatory activity in vitro and proinflammatory properties in vivo of 72 amino acid and 77 amino acid IL-8. *J Immunol* 1992;148:106–111.

295. Abruzzo LV, Thornton AJ, Liebert M, et al. Cytokine-induced gene expression of interleukin-8 in human transitional cell carcinomas and renal cell carcinomas. *Am J Pathol* 1992;140:365–373.

296. Gusella GL, Musso T, Bosco MC, Espinoza-Delgado I, Matsushima K, Varesio L. IL-2 upregulates, but IFN-γ suppresses IL-8 expression in human monocytes. *J Immunol* 1993;151:2725–2732.

297. Olivera IC, Mukaida N, Matsushima K, Vilcek J. Transcriptional inhibition of the IL-8 gene by interferon is mediated by the NF-kB site. *Mol Cell Biol* 1994;14: 5300–5308.

298. Mukaida N, Morita M, Ishikawa Y, et al. Novel mechanism of glucocorticoid-mediated gene repression: nuclear factor kB is a target for glucocorticoid mediated IL-8 gene repression. *J Biol Chem* 1994;269:13289–13295.

299. Stein B, Baldwin AS Jr. Distinct mechanisms for regulation of the interleukin-8 gene involves synergism and cooperativity between C/EBP and NF-kappa B. *Mol Cell Biol* 1993;13:7191–7198.

300. Taub DD, Oppenheim JJ. Chemokines, inflammation and the immune system. *Ther Immunol* 1994;1:29–246.

301. Larsen CG, Thomsen MK, Gesser B, et al. The delayed-type hypersensitivity reaction is dependent on IL-8. *J Immunol* 1995;155:2151–2157.

302. Schraufstatter IU, Barritt DS, Ma M, Oades ZG, Cochrane CG. Multiple sites on IL-8 responsible for binding to α and β IL-8 receptors. *J Immunol* 1993;151: 6418–6428.

303. Chuntharapai A, Kim KJ. Regulation of the expression of IL-8 receptor A/B by IL-8: possible function of each receptor. *J Immunol* 1993;155:2587–2594.

304. Cacalano G, Lee J, Kikly K, et al. Neutrophil and B cell expansion in mice that lack the murine IL-8 receptor homolog. *Science* 1994;265:682–684.

305. Shuster DE, Kehrli ME Jr, Ackerman MR. Neutrophilia in mice that lack the murine IL-8 receptor homolog. *Science* 1995;269:1590–1591.

306. Broxmeyer HE, Cooper S, Cacalano G, Hague NL, Bailish E, Moore MW. Involvement of IL-8 receptor in negative regulation of myeloid progenitor cells in vivo: evidence from mice lacking the murine IL-8 receptor homologue. *J Exp Med* 1996;184:1825–1832.

307. Chertov O, Michiel DF, Xu L, et al. Identification of defensin-1, defensin-2 and CAP37/Azurocidin as selective T-cell chemoattractant proteins released from IL-8-stimulated neutrophils. *J Biol Chem* 1996;271:2935–2940.

308. Chertov O, Ueda H, Xu LL, et al. Identification of human neutrophil derived cathepsin G and azurocidin/CAP37 as chemoattractants for mononuclear cells and neutrophils. *J Exp Med* 1997;186:739 748.

309. Richmond A, Balentein E, Thomas HG, et al. Molecular characterization and chromosomal mapping of melanoma growth stimulatory activity, a growth factor structurally related to β-thromboglobulin. *EMBO J* 1988;7:2025–2033.

310. Haskill S, Peace A, Morris J, et al. Identification of three related human GRO genes encoding cytokine functions. *Proc Natl Acad Sci USA* 1990;87: 7732–7736.

311. Unemori EN, Amento EP, Bauer EA, Horuk R. Melanoma growth-stimulatory activity/GRO decreases collagen expression by human fibroblasts. Regulation by C-X-C but not C-C cytokines. *J Biol Chem* 1993;268:1338–1342.

312. Ben-Baruch A, Bengali K, Tani K, Xu L, Oppenheim JJ, Wang J. IL-8 and NAP2 differ in their capacities to bind and chemoattract 293 cells transfected with either IL-8 receptor A or B. *Cytokine* 19977;9:37–45.

313. Walz A, Schmutz P, Mueller C, Schnyder-Candrian L. Regulation and function of the CXC chemokine ENA-78 in monocytes and its role in disease. *J Leukoc Biol* 1997;62:604–611.

314. Van Damme J, Wuyts A, Froyen G, et al. Granulocyte chemotactic protein-2 and related CXC chemokines: from gene regulation to receptor usage. *J Leukoc Biol* 1997;62:563–569.

315. Smith JB, Rovai RE, Herschman HR. Sequence similarities of a subgroup of CXC chemokines related to murine LIX: implications for the interpretations of evolutionary relationships among chemokines. *J Leukoc Biol* 1997;62:598–603.

316. Luster AD, Ravetch JV. Genomic characterization of a gamma-interferon-inducible gene (IP-10) and identification of an interferon-inducible hypersensitive site. *Mol Cell Biol* 1987;7:3723–3731.

317. Luster AD, Leder P. IP-10, a C-X-C chemokine, elicits a potent thymus-dependent antitumor response in vitro. *J Exp Med* 1993;178:1057–1065.

318. Ohmori Y, Hamilton T. The interferon-stimulated response element and a kB site mediate synergistic induction of murine IP-10 gene transcription by IFN-gamma and TNF-α. *J Immunol* 1995;154:5235–5244.

319. Farber JM. A macrophage mRNA selectively induced by interferon encodes a member of the platelet factor 4 family of cytokines. *Proc Natl Acad Sci USA* 1990;87:5238–5242.

320. Liao F, Rabin RL, Yannelli JR, Koniares LG, Vanguri P, Farber JM. Human MIG chemokine: biochemical and functional characterization. *J Exp Med* 1995;182:1301–1314.

321. Loetscher M, Gerber B, Loetscher P, et al. Chemokine receptor specific for IP10 and MIG: structure, function, and expression in activated T-lymphocytes. *J Exp Med* 1996;184:963–969.

322. Cole KE, Strick CA, Paradis TJ, et al. Interferon inducible T cell alpha chemoattractant (I-TAC): A novel non-ELR CXC chemokine with potent activity on activated T cells through high affinity binding to CXC-R3. *J Exp Med* 1998;187:1–13.

323. Bleul CC, Fuhlbrigge RC, Casasnovas JM, Aiuti A, Springer TA. A highly efficacious lymphocyte chemoattractant, SDF-1. *J Exp Med* 1996;184:1101–1109.

324. Aiuti A, Webb I J, Bleul C, Springer T, Gutierree-Ramos JC. The chemokine SDF-1 is a chemoattractant for human CD34+ hematopoietic progenitor cells and provides a new in mechanism to explain the mobilization of CD34+ progenitors to peripheral blood. *J Exp Med* 1997;185:111–120.

325. Nagasawa T, Hirota S, Tachibana K, et al. Defects of B cell lymphopoiesis and bone marrow myelopoiesis in mice lacking the CXC chemokine PBSF/SDF-1. *Nature* 1996;382:635–638.

326. Nagasawa T, Nakajuma T, Tachibana K, et al. Molecular cloning and characterization of murine pre-B cell growth stimulating factor/pre-B cell-derived factor 1 entry coreceptor fusin. *Proc Natl Acad Sci USA* 1996;93:14726–14729.

327. Gronenborn AM, Clore CM. Modeling the three-dimensional structure of the monocyte chemo-attractant and activating protein MCAF/MCP-1 on the basis of the solution structure of interleukin-8. *Protein Eng* 1991;4:263–269.

328. Beall CJ, Mahajan S, Kolattukudy PE. Conversion of monocyte chemo-attractant protein-1 into a neutrophil attractant by substitution of two amino acids. *J Biol Chem* 1992;267:3455–3459.

329. Ueda A, Okuda K, Ohno S, et al. NF kB and Sp1 regulate transcription of the human monocyte chemoattractant protein 1 gene. *J Immunol* 1994;153: 2052 2063.

330. Grove M, Plumb M. C/EBP, NF-kB and C-Est family members and transcriptional regulation of the cell specific and inducible macrophage inflammatory protein 1α immediate early gene. *Mol Cell Biol* 1993;13:5276–5289.

331. Pleskoff O, Treboute C, Brelot A, Hereker N, Seman M, Alizon M. Identification of a chemokine receptor encoded by human cytomegalovirus as a cofactor for HIV-1 entry. *Science* 1997;276:1874–1878.

332. Luster A, Rothenberg M. Role of chemokines in allergy. *J Leukoc Biol* 1997;62:620–633.

333. Broxmeyer HE, Sherry B, Cooper S, et al. Comparative analysis of the human macrophage inflammatory protein family of cytokines (chemokines) on proliferation of human myeloid progenitor. *J Immunol* 1993;150:3448 3458.

334. Youn B-S, Jang I-K, Broxmeyer HE, et al. A novel chemokine MRP-2 inhibits colony formation of bone marrow myeloid progenitors. *J Immunol* 1995;155: 2661–2667.

335. Patel VP, Kreider BL, Li Y, et al. Molecular and functional characterization of two distinct classes of myeloid progenitors. *J Exp Med* 1997;185:1163–1172.

336. Keller JR, Bartelmer SH, Situoha E, et al. Distinct and overlapping direct effects of MIP 1α and TGFβ on hematopoietic progenitor cell growth. *Blood* 1994;84: 21275–21281.

337. Gao JL, Wynn TA Chang Y, et al. Impaired host defense, hematopoiesis granu-

lomatous inflammation and type 1–type 2 cytokine balance in mice lacking CCR1. *J Exp Med* 1997;185:1959–1968.

338. Taub DD, Oppenheim JJ, Anver M, Kelvin DJ, Longo DL, Murphy W. T lymphocyte recruitment by interleukin 8 (IL-8): IL-8 induced degranulation of neutrophils releases potent chemoattractants for human T lymphocytes both in vitro and in vivo. *J Clin Invest* 1996;97:1931–1941.

339. Nakamura K, Williams IR, Kupper TS. Keratinocyte-derived monocyte chemoattractant protein 1 (MCP-1): analysis in a transgenic model demonstrates MCP-1 can recruit dendritic and Langerhans cells to skin. *J Invest Dermatol* 1995;105:635–643.

340. Taub DD, Ortaldo JR, Turcovki-Corrales SM, Key ML, Longo Dl., Murphy WJ. Beta chemokines costimulate lymphocyte cytolysis, proliferation and lymphokine production. *J Leukoc Biol* 1996;59:81–89.

341. Gosse JA, Hartgers F, Verstraten R, et al. A dendritic-cell-derived C-C chemokine that preferentially attracts naive T cells. *Nature* 1997;387:713–717.

342. Taub DD, Sayers T, Carber C, Ortaldo J. Alpha and β chemokines induce NK cell migration and enhance NK cell cytolytic activity via cellular degranulation. *J Immunol* 1995;155:3877–3888.

343. Cook DN, Beck MA, Coffman TM. Requirement of MIP-1α for an inflammatory response to viral infection. *Science* 1995;269:1583–1585.

344. Chensue SW, Warmington KS, Ruth JH, Sanghi PS, Lincoln P, Kunkel SL. Role of monocyte chemoattractant protein-1 (MCP-1) in TH1 (mycobacterial) and TH2 (Schistosomal) antigen-induced granuloma formation. *J Immunol* 1996;157:4602–4608.

345. Lukacs NW, Kunkel SL, Strieter RM, Warmington K, Chensue SW. The role of MIP-1α in Schistosoma mansoni egg induced granulomatous inflammation. *J Exp Med* 1993;177:1551–1559.

346. Karpus WJ, Kennedy KJ. MIP-1α and MCP-1 differentially regulate acute and relapsing autoimmune encephalomyelitis as well as TH1/TH2 lymphocyte differentiation. *J Leukoc Biol* 1997;62:681–687.

347. Schall TJ. Biology of the RANTES/sis cytokine family. *Cytokine* 1991;3:165–183.

348. Bacon KB, Premack BA, Gardner B, Schall TJ. Activation of dual T cell signaling pathways by the chemokine RANTES. *Science* 1995;269:1727–1730.

349. Selvan RS, Zhou LJ, Krangel MS. Regulation of I-309 gene expression in human monocytes by endogenous interleukin-1. *Eur J Immunol* 1997;27:687–694.

350. Laning J, Kawasaki H, Tanaka E, Luo Y, Dorf ME. Inhibition of in vivo tumor growth by the beta chemokine, TCA3. *J Immunol* 1994;153:4625–4635.

351. Van Snick J, Houssiau F, Proost P, Van Damme J, Renauld JC. I-309/T cell activation gene-3 chemokine protects murine T cell lymphomas against dexamethasone-induced apoptosis. *J Immunol* 1996;157:2570–2576.

352. Jose PJ, Griffith-Johnson DA, Collins PD, et al. Eotaxin, a potent eosinophil chemoattractant cytokine detected in a guinea pig model of allergic airways inflammation. *J Exp Med* 1994;179:881–887.

353. Rothenberg ME, MacLean JA, Pearlman E, Luster AD, Leder P. Targeted disruption of the chemokine eotaxin partially reduces antigen-induced tissue eosinophilia. *J Exp Med* 1997;185:785–790.

354. Mohamadzadek M, Poltorak AN, Bergstresser PR, Beutler B, Takashima A. Dendritic cells produce MIP-1γ, a new member of the CC chemokine family. *J Immunol* 1996;156:3102–3106.

355. Rossi DL, Vicari AP, Franz-Bacon K, McClanahan TK, Zlotnik A. Identification through bio informatics of two new macrophage proinflammatory human chemokines: MIP-3α and MIP-3β. *J Immunol* 1997;158:1033–1036.

356. Forster R, Mattis AE, Kremmer E, Wolf E, Brem G, Lipp M. A putative chemokine receptor, BRL1, directs B cell migration to defined lymphoid organs and specific anatomic compartments of the spleen. *Cell* 1996;87:1037–1047.

357. Cocchi F, DeVico AL, Garzino-Demo A, Arya SK, Gallo RC, Lusso P. Identification of RANTES, MIP-1α, and MIP-1β as the major HIV-suppressive factors produced by CD8⁺ T cells. *Science* 1995;270:1811–1815.

358. Moore J, Trkola A. HIV type-1 coreceptors, neutralization, serotypes and vaccine development. *AIDS Res Hum Retroviruses* 1997;13:733–736.

359. Liao F, Alkhatib G, Peden KWC, Sharma S, Berger EA, Farber JM. STRL33, a novel chemokine receptor-like protein, functions as a fusion cofactor for both macrophage-tropic and T cell line tropic HIV-1. *J Exp Med* 1997;

360. Samson M, Libert F, Doranz BJ, et al. Resistance to HIV-1 infection in caucasian individuals bearing mutant alleles of the CCR-5 chemokine receptor gene. *Nature* 1996;382:722–725.

361. Zhou Y, Kurihara T, Ryseck R-P, et al. Impaired macrophage function and enhanced T-cell dependent immune response in mice lacking CCR5, the mouse homologue of the major HIV-1 coreceptor. *J Immunol* 1998;160:4018–4025.

362. Greenberger MJ, Strieter RM, Kunkel SL, et al. Neutralization of macrophage inflammatory protein-2 attenuates neutrophil recruitment and bacterial clearance in murine Klebsiella pneumonia. *J Infect Dis* 1996;173:159–165.

363. Howard OMZ, Ben-Baruch A, Oppenheim, JJ. Chemokines progress in identifying molecular targets for therapeutic agents. *Trends Biotechnol* 1996;46–51.

364. McFadden G, Kelvin D. New strategies for chemokine inhibition and modulation. *Biochem Pharmacol* 1997;53:1271–1280.

365. Lalani AS, McFadden G. Secreted poxvirus chemokine binding proteins. *J Leukoc Biol* 1997;62:570–576.

366. Ben-Baruch A, Bengali K, Xu L, Oppenheim JJ, Wang JM. IL8 and NAP 2 differ in their capacities to bind and chemo-attract 293 cells transfected with either IL8 receptor type A or type B. *Cytokine* 1997;9:37–45.

367. Rutledge BJ, Rayburn H, Rosenberg R, et al. High level MCP-1 expression in

transgenic mice increases their susceptibility to intracellular pathogens. *J Immunol* 1995;155:4838–4843.

368. Grimm MC, Ben-Baruch A, Taub DD, et al. Opiate inhibition of chemokine induced chemotaxis is based on δ and μ opiate receptor mediated heterologous desensitization. *J Exp Med* 1998 *(in press)*.

369. Wang JM, Ueda H, Chertov O, et al. The inhibitory effect of HIV-1 envelope gp120 on monocyte chemoattractant receptors involves activation of CD4. *J Immunol* 1998 *(in press)*.

Selected TGF and Other Cytokines

370. DeLarco J, Todaro G. Growth factors from sarcoma virus-transformed cells. *Proc Natl Acad Sci USA* 1978;75:4001–4005.

371. Roberts AB, Sporn MB. The transforming growth factor-βs. *Handbook Exp Pharm* 1990;95:419–475.

372. Massague J. The transforming growth factor-β family. *Annu Rev Cell Biol* 1990;6:597–674.

373. Heine U, Munoz EF, Flanders KC, et al. Role of transforming growth factor-beta in the development of the mouse embryo. *J Cell Biol* 1987;105:2861–2876.

374. Millan FA, Denhez F, Kondaiah P, Akhurst RJ. Embryonic gene expression patterns of TGF-β1, β2, and β3 suggest different development functions in vivo. *Development* 1991;111:131–143.

375. Shull MM, Ormbbsby I, Kier AB, et al. Targeted disruption of mouse TGF-β1 gene results in multifocal inflammatory disease. *Nature* 1990;359:693–696.

376. Letterio JJ, Roberts AB. Transforming growth factor-β1-deficient mice: identification of isoform-specific activities in vivo. *J Leukoc Biol* 1996;59:769–774.

377. Proetzel G, Pawlowski SA, Wiles MV, et al. Transforming growth factor-β3 is required for secondary palate fusion. *Nature* 1995;11:409–414.

378. Roberts AB, Sporn MB. Differential expression of the TGF-β isoforms in embryogenesis suggests specific roles in developing and adult tissues. *Mol Reprod Dev* 1992;32:92–97.

379. O'Reilly MA, Geiser AG, Kim SJ, et al. Identification of an activating transcription factor (ATF) binding site in the transforming growth factor-β2 promotor. *J Biol Chem* 1992;267:19938–19943.

380. Kim SJ, Park K, Koeller D, et al. Post-transcriptional regulation of the human transforming growth factor-β1 gene. *J Biol Chem* 1992;267:13702–13707.

381. Kim SJ, Jeang KT, Glick A Sporn MB, Roberts AB. Promoter sequences of the human transforming growth factor-β1 gene responsive to transforming growth factor-β1 autoinduction. *J Biol Chem* 1989;264:7041–7045.

382. Kingsley DM. The TGF-β superfamily: new members, new receptors, and new genetic tests of function in different organisms. *Genes Dev* 1994;8:133–146.

383. Dennis PA, Rifkin DB. Cellular activation of latent transforming growth factor-β requires binding to the cation-independent mannose 6-phosphate/insulin-like growth factor type II receptor. *Proc Natl Acad Sci USA* 1991;88:580–584.

384. Nunes I, Shapiro RL, Rifkin DB. Characterization of latent TGF-β activation by murine peritoneal macrophages. *J Immunol* 1995;155:1450–1459.

385. Lin HY, Lodish HF. Receptors for the TGF-β superfamily. *Trends Cell Biol* 1993;3:14–19.

386. Attisano L, Wrana JL, Lopez-casillas F, Massague J. TGF-β receptors and actions. *Biochim Biophys Acta* 1994;1222:71–80.

387. Laiho M, Weis FMB, Boyd FT, Ignotz RA, Massague J. Responsiveness of TGF-β restored by complementation between cells defective in TGF-β receptors I and II. *J Biol Chem* 1991;266:9108–9112.

388. Vivien D, Attisano L, Ventura F, Wrana JL, Massague J. Signalling activity of homologous and heterogous TGF-β receptor kinase complexes. *J Biol Chem* 1995;270:7134–7141.

389. Wrana JL, Attisano L, Wieser R, Ventura F, Massague J. Mechanism of activation of the TGF-β receptor. *Nature* 1994;370:341–347.

390. Chen RH, Moses HL, Maruoka EM, Derynck R, Kawabata M. Phosphorylation-dependent interaction of the cytoplasmic domains of the type I and type II TGF-β receptors. *J Biol Chem* 1995;270:12235–12241.

391. Attisano L, Wrana JL. Signal transduction by members of the transforming growth factor-β superfamily. *Cytokine Growth Factor Rev* 1996;7:327–339.

392. Markowitz SD, Roberts AB. Tumor suppressor activity of the TGF-β pathway in human cancers. *Cytokine Growth Factor Rev* 1996;7:93–102.

393. Lagna G, Hata A, Hemmati-Brivanlou A, Massague J. Partnership between DPC4 and SMAD proteins in TGF-β signalling pathways. *Nature* 1996;383:832–836.

394. Arsura M, Wu M, Sonenshein GE. TGF-β1 inhibits NF-kB/Rel activity inducing apotosis of B cells: transcriptional activation of IkBα. *Immunity* 1996;5:31–40.

395. McCartney-Francis NL, Wahl SM. Transforming growth factor: a matter of life and death. *J Leukoc Biol* 1994;55:401–409.

396. Sporn MB, Roberts AB. TGF-β: problems and prospects. *Cell Reg* 1990;1:875–882.

397. Kerl JH, Taylor A, Kim SJ, Fauci AS. Transforming growth factor β is a potent negative regulator of human lymphocytes. *Ann NY Acad Sci* 1991;628:345–353.

398. Kerl JH, Thenvenin C, Rieckmann P, Fauci AS. Transforming growth factor β suppresses human B lymphocyte Ig production by inhibiting synthesis and the switch from the membrane form to the secreted form of Ig mRNA. *J Immunol* 1991;146:4016–4023.

399. Ruscetti F, Varesio L, Ochoa A, Ortaldo J. Peiotropic effects of transforming growth factor-β on cells of the immune system. *Ann NY Acad Sci* 1993;685:488–500.

400. Dubois C, Ruscetti F, Stankova J, Keller J. Transforming growth factor β regulates c-kit message stability and cell-surface expression in hematopoietic progenitors. *Blood* 1994;83:3138–3145.

401. Tsunawaki S, Sporn M, Ding A, Nathan C. Deactivation of macrophages by transforming growth factor-β. *Nature* 1988;334:260–262.

402. Smith WB, Noack L, Khew–Goodall Y, Isenmann S, Vadas MA, Gamble JR. Transforming growth factor-β1 inhibits the production of IL-8 and the transmigration of neutrophils through activated endothelium. *J Immunol* 1996;157:360–368.

403. Weiner HL. Oral tolerance. *Proc Natl Acad Sci USA* 1994;91:10762–10765.

404. Fukaura H, Kent SC, Pietrusewicz MJ, Khoury SJ, Weiner HL, Hafler DA. Induction of circulating myelin basic protein and proteolipid protein-specific TGF-β1-secreting Th3 T cells by oral administration of myelin in multiple sclerosis patients. *J Clin Invest* 1996;98:70–77.

405. Wahl SM, Hines KL, Christ M, et al. Adhesion, recruitment, and activation of mononuclear phagocytes in inflammation. *J Leukoc Biol* 1993;54:74–81.

406. Reibman J, Meixler S, Lee TC, Gold, et al. Transforming growth factor β1, a potent chemoattractant for human neutrophils, bypasses classic signal-transduction pathways. *Proc Natl Acad Sci USA* 1991;88:6805–6809.

407. Wahl SM. Transforming growth factor β in inflammation: a cause and a cure. *J Clin Immunol* 1992;12:61–74.

408. Border WA, Noble NA. Transforming growth factor β in tissue fibrosis. *N Engl J Med* 1994;331:1286–1292.

409. Caver TE, O'Sullivan FX, Gold LI, Gresham HD. Intracellular demonstration of active TGF-β1 in B cells and plasma cells of autoimmune mice. *J Clin Invest* 1996;98:2496–2506.

410. Kaartinen V, Voncken JW, Shuler C, Warburton DB, Heisterkamp N, Groffen J. Abnormal lung development and cleft palate in mice lacking TGF-β3 indicates defects of epithelial-mesenchymal interaction. *Nat Genet* 1995;11:415–421.

411. Strobl H, Reidl E, Scheinecker C. TGF-β1 promotes in vitro development of dendritic cells from CD34+ hemopoietic progenitors. *J Immunol* 1996;157:1499–1507.

412. Borkowski TA, Letterio JJ, Farr AG, Udey MC. A role for endogenous TGF-β1 in Langerhans cell biology: the skin of TGF-β1 null mice is devoid of epidermal Langerhans cells. *J Exp Med* 1996;184:2417–2422.

413. Alexandrow MG, Moses HL. Transforming growth factor and cell cycle regulation. *Cancer Res* 1995;55:1452–1457.

414. Ivanovic V, Melman A, Davis-Joseph B, Valcic M, Geliebter J. Elevated plasma levels of TGF-β1 in patients with invasive prostrate cancer. *Nat Med* 1995;1:282–283.

415. Grainger DJ, Kemp PR, Metcalfe JC, et al. The serum concentration of active TGF-β is severely depressed in advanced atherosclerosis. *Nat Med* 1995;1:74–79.

416. Center DM, Kornfeld H, Cruikshank WW. Interleukin-16 and its function as a CD4 ligand. *Immunol Today* 1996;17:476–481.

417. T Ryan, WW Cruikshank, DM Center. Activation of CD4 associated p56 lck by the lymphocyte chemoattractant factor. Dissociation of kinase enzymatic activity with chemotactic response. *J Biol Chem* 1995;270:17081–17086.

418. Theodore AC, Center DM, Nicoll J, Fine G, Kornfeld H, Cruikshank WW. The CD4 ligand, IL-16, inhibits the MLR. *J Immunol* 1996;157:1958–1964.

419. Maciaszek JW, Parada NA, Cruikshank WW, Center DM, Kornfeld H, Vigliantis GA. Interleukin-16 represses HIV-1 promoter activity. *J Immunol* 1997;158:5–8.

420. Rouvier E, Luciani M-F, Mattei MG, Denizot F, Golstein P. CTLA-8 cloned from an activated T cell, bearing AU-rich mRNA instability sequences and homologs to a herpesvirus saimiri gene. *J Immunol* 1993;150:5445–5456.

421. Yao Z, Painter SL, Fanslow WC, et al. Human IL-17: a novel cytokine derived from T cells. *J Immunol* 1995;155:5483–5486.

422. Fossiez F, Djossou O, Chomarat P, et al. T cell interleukin-17 induces stromal cells to produce proinflammatory and hematopoietic cytokines. *J Exp Med* 1996;183:2593–2603.

423. Yao Z, Fanslow WC, Seldin MF, et al. Herpesvirus saimiri encodes a new cytokine IL-17, which binds to a novel cytokine receptor. *Immunity* 1995;3:811–821.

424. Bloom BR, Bennett B. Mechanism of a reaction in vitro associated with delayed-type hypersensitivity. *Science* 1966;153:8–82.

425. David J. Delayed hypersensitivity in vitro: its mediation by cell-free substances formed by lymphoid cell-antigen interaction. *Proc Natl Acad Sci USA* 1966;56:72–77.

426. Weiser WY, Temple PA, Witeek-Giannotti JS, Remold HG, Clark SC, David JR. Molecular cloning of a cDNA encoding a human macrophage migration inhibitory factor. *Proc Natl Acad Sci USA* 1989;86:7522–7526.

427. Bucala R. MIF re-discovered: pituitary hormone and glucocorticoid-induced regulator of cytokine production. *Cytokine Growth Factor Rev* 1996;7:19–24.

Fundamental Immunology, Fourth Edition,
edited by William E. Paul
Lippincott–Raven Publishers, Philadelphia © 1999.

CHAPTER 23

Apoptosis

Craig B. Thompson

In most cases an immune reaction is initiated in response to cell damage. The most catastrophic cell injury is cell death, and a number of intracellular contents are proinflammatory to the innate immune system. Thus, the release of intracellular contents from dying cells can serve as an early warning sign to the immune system that an organism is in danger. However, not all forms of cell death result in a proinflammatory signal. In most tissues, cells are constantly turning over. The cell death that occurs during normal tissue homeostasis was first reported to have unique histologic features by Kerr and colleagues (1). These investigators noted that even in normal tissues, a small percentage of cells died each day and that this cell death could be recognized by its distinctive morphology and the failure to initiate an inflammatory response. This physiologic form of cell death was termed apoptosis. Subsequent studies have demonstrated that apoptosis represents a form of cellular suicide in which the dying cell initiates its own death through the activation of an internally encoded and evolutionarily conserved death program (2–4).

MORPHOLOGIC AND BIOCHEMICAL FEATURES OF APOPTOSIS

Apoptotic cell death can be triggered by a variety of extrinsic and intrinsic signals (5). The physiologic control of apoptosis provides a mechanism for the elimination of cells that have been produced in excess, developed improperly, or sustained genetic damage. The hallmark of apoptosis is controlled autodigestion of the dying cell (Fig. 1). Cell death appears to be carried out through the activation of endogenous proteases (6–9). As a result of activation of these proteases, the integrity of the cytoskeleton is disrupted and the cell rounds up and begins to shrink in volume. In response to the contraction in cytoplasmic volume, the membrane begins to bleb and there is loss of the normal asymmetry of plasma membrane lipids. In healthy cells, phosphatidylserine is primarily distributed to the inner leaflet of the plasma membrane. During apoptosis, phosphatidylserine becomes exposed on the outer leaflet of the plasma membrane (10). Apoptosis also involves characteristic changes within the nucleus. Endonucleases are activated and begin to degrade nuclear DNA. In some cell types, DNA is degraded into fragments the size of oligonucleosomes, whereas in others larger DNA fragments are produced. Nuclear lamins also undergo degradation. As a result of these events, the nucleus becomes shrunken and pyknotic. The function of other organelles is also disrupted.

C.B. Thompson: Howard Hughes Medical Institute, Department of Medicine, The University of Chicago, Chicago, Illinois 60637-5420.

A)

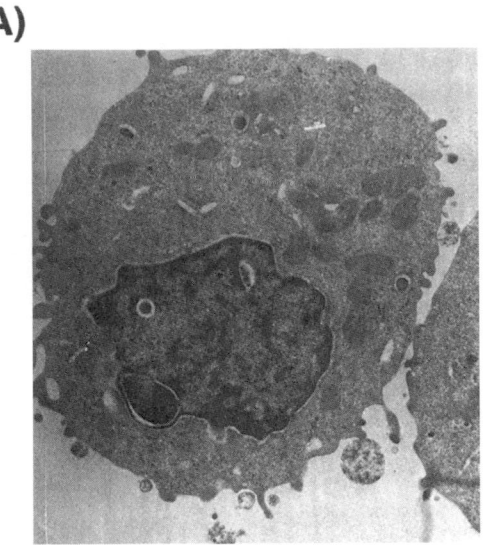

B)

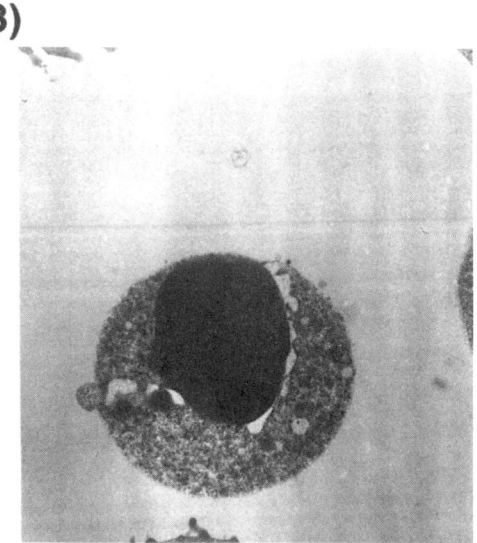

FIG. 1. Apoptotic cells have a distinct morphology. **A)** An electron micrograph of a WEHI 231 B lymphocyte grown in tissue culture. **B)** The appearance of a WEHI 231 cell 12 hours after crosslinking of its surface immunoglobulin receptor. This cell displays the classic morphologic characteristics of an apoptotic cell (see text for details, photomicrographs kindly provided by Alex Gottschalk and Jose Quintans).

Current evidence suggests that the decision to undergo apoptosis occurs within the cytoplasm. Cytoplasts devoid of nuclei can respond to apoptotic stimuli by shrinking in volume, losing plasma membrane asymmetry, and initiating the degradation of intracellular organelles (11). The loss of mitochondrial function has been suggested to be an early irreversible event that occurs during apoptotic cell death (12). Both the redistribution of cytochrome c from the mitochondrial intermembrane space and the loss of mitochondrial membrane potential have been observed during the initial stages of apoptotic cell death (13–15). The addition of cytochrome c to cytoplasmic extracts induces the activation of enzymes capable of carrying out the apoptotic destruction of exogenously added nuclei (16,17).

A key feature of apoptosis is that the plasma membrane remains intact. The alterations of the plasma membrane, including the exposure of phosphatidylserine, signal neighboring phagocytic cells to engulf the apoptotic cell and complete the degradation process (18). Interestingly, the phagocytosis of apoptotic cells is not associated with the upregulation of activation markers or cytokines by the phagocyte. Apoptotic cells that are not immediately phagocytized remain intact, breaking down to smaller membrane-bound fragments called apoptotic bodies. By maintaining plasma membrane integrity, apoptotic death promotes the elimination of the dying cell without the induction of an inflammatory response.

In contrast to apoptotic cell death, both necrotic cell death and traumatic cell death are pathologic forms of cell death resulting from acute cellular injury (19). Both are typified by rapid cell swelling and lysis, which results in leakage of cytoplasmic contents and the induction of an inflammatory response. The dying cell does not appear to play an active role in either necrotic or traumatic cell death. Therefore, the ability of a cell to respond to injury may play a critical role in whether its death is accompanied by inflammation. If the cellular damage overwhelms the cell, the cell will die by necrosis, resulting in the activation of an immune response. In con-

trast, if the dying cell is capable of a physiologic response to cell damage and is able to carry out its own orderly demise, the resulting apoptotic death may serve to terminate an organism's response to the initial insult. Viewed in this manner, the ability to carry out programmed cell death provides an important mechanism to regulate the extent of an immune response to tissue injury.

APOPTOTIC CELL DEATH IS GENETICALLY REGULATED

Many of the recent advances in the understanding of cell death have come from the discovery and characterization of genes that control apoptosis (2). These discoveries have demonstrated that the cell death that occurs during embryogenesis (often referred to as programmed cell death) and apoptosis are under common genetic regulation (Fig. 2). A number of genes that regulate this common cell death pathway are conserved in both invertebrates and vertebrates. Early experiments to identify genes that regulated cell death during the development of the nematode *Caenorhabditis elegans* led to the discovery of three genes that played a central role in regulating the fate of all cells genetically programmed to die during embryogenesis. A gain-of-function mutation in one of these genes,

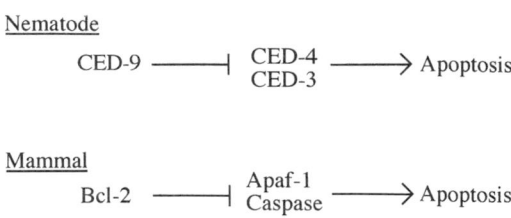

FIG. 2. The central genes involved in the regulation of apoptosis have been evolutionarily conserved.

CED-9, prevented programmed cell death in developing embryos (20). In contrast, the other two genes CED-3 and CED-4 were found to be required for the ability of cells to effect their own death during development (21,22). Mammalian homologs for all three genes have been identified (Fig. 2). When CED-9 was cloned, it was found to be related to the mammalian oncogene bcl-2 (23). The bcl-2 gene was originally identified because of its involvement in a human chromosomal translocation involving chromosomes 14 and 18 (24). This translocation is present in over 70% of lymphomas. The 14:18 translocation results in the juxtaposition of the bcl-2 gene on chromosome 18 to the immunoglobulin heavy chain enhancer on chromosome 14, resulting in increased expression of Bcl-2. Subsequent studies have shown that overexpression of Bcl-2 leads to a dramatic increase in the resistance of a cell to undergo programmed cell death in response to a wide range of apoptotic initiators. The conservation of function between Bcl-2 and CED-9 was confirmed by the demonstration that a Bcl-2 transgene could partially rescue cell death in CED-9–deficient worm (25).

The worm CED-3 protein was found to have sequence similarity to interleukin (IL)-1–converting enzyme, a cysteine protease now also referred to as caspase 1 (26). This observation led to the demonstration that overexpression of the active form of either protein was capable of inducing cell death that had all the morphologic features of apoptosis. Both enzymes carry out similar proteolytic cleavage reactions, cleaving their substrates after aspartic acid residues. A number of additional caspases have now been identified in mammals (27).

Recently a mammalian homolog for CED-4 has been identified and given the name *apoptotic protease activating factor* 1 (Apaf-1) (28). Apaf-1 was isolated as a cytoplasmic protein that is required for the ability of cytochrome c to induce apoptotic activity in cytosolic extracts. Similarly, CED-4 has been reported to be able to activate CED-3 (29). These data suggest that CED-4 and related proteins are likely to play a role in regulating the initial conversion of caspases from their inactive to active forms, thus facilitating protease activation and subsequent apoptosis. In view of the fact that both Bcl-2 and caspase 1 are members of multigene families in vertebrates, it is likely that additional mammalian CED-4 homologs will be identified. Such proteins might link caspase activation to stimuli in addition to mitochondrial release of cytochrome c.

APOPTOSIS MUST BE ACTIVELY SUPPRESSED IF A CELL IS TO MAINTAIN VIABILITY

In all multicellular organisms examined to date, individual cells will undergo apoptosis if cultured in the absence of exogenous survival factors or if treated with the serine kinase inhibitor staurosporine (30). In each of these instances, death occurs in the absence of new protein synthesis, suggesting that the proteins required to elicit apoptosis are constitutively expressed in all cells. Cell survival *in vivo* appears to be dependent on the constant supply of survival signals provided by neighboring cells, the extracellular matrix, or growth factors. This suggests that all cells within multicellular organisms are programmed to commit suicide if survival signals are not received from their environment either constantly or at regular intervals. Such a control system for cell survival could play a critical role in regulating the physiologic position or number of cells of a given cell lineage. For example, dependence on environmental signals for survival would prevent a liver cell from sur-

viving within the lung. In addition, because cell survival is dependent on extrinsic signals, cells such as hepatocytes are prevented from accumulating beyond the number that can be supported by stromal cell contacts or humoral survival factors.

CELLS CAN BE INSTRUCTED TO INITIATE APOPTOSIS

Apoptosis also can be initiated through an instructive mechanism. Specific cell surface receptors have been identified that can transduce signals that result in apoptosis in response to ligand binding (31). The best characterized cell death receptors are members of the tumor necrosis factor (TNF) receptor family such as Fas. Unlike cell death that occurs after limitations in survival signals, instructive cell death pathways do not appear to be constitutively expressed in all cells. In some instances instructive cell death involves the induction of apoptosis through mechanisms that require new protein synthesis. Initially the expression of cell death receptors was thought to be limited to cells that underwent cyclic expansions and contractions as a result of their normal physiologic roles such as lymphocytes or the cells of reproductive organs. More recently it has become apparent that most cells can be induced to express cell death receptors or their ligands as a result of the activation of various stress response pathways.

APOPTOSIS INITIATION

In addition to the extrinsic regulation of cell survival by growth factors and cell death receptors, intrinsic cellular events also can initiate apoptosis (Fig. 3). DNA damage has been shown to induce apoptosis. A major pathway through which DNA damage initiates apoptosis is mediated by p53 (32). Because resistance to programmed cell death can contribute to carcinogenesis, this may account for why the p53 gene is found mutated in so many human cancers. Virtually any cellular metabolic or cell cycle perturbation that persists also can induce apoptosis (5). These observations suggest that apoptosis may not be regulated by a single signaling pathway. Instead, the predisposition to undergoing programmed cell death may be regulated by the coordinated interactions of various signaling pathways. Although the specific points of integration of these metabolic or cell cycle disruptions in the regulation of programmed cell death have not yet been identified, several intracellular perturbations have been implicated in the regulation of cell survival. In a wide variety of cellular systems, elevations in intracellular calcium, decreases in cellular pH, and alterations in cellular redox potential have been shown to increase the propensity of the cell to undergo programmed cell death (33–41). How these perturbations contribute to the activation of the proteins that effect programmed cell death has not been elucidated.

Although all mammalian cells appear to be dependent on constant signaling for survival, how a loss of signaling initiates cell death also remains undefined. This form of apoptosis has been widely studied using growth factor–dependent cell lines that promptly initiate programmed cell death after growth factor withdrawal. A surprising feature of this form of cell death is that such cell lines all seem to respond in a similar manner to growth factor withdrawal despite being dependent on growth factors that use distinct signal transduction pathways. Growth factor withdrawal commonly results in an acute perturbation in cellular metabolism and the induction of cell cycle arrest. As noted above, such changes

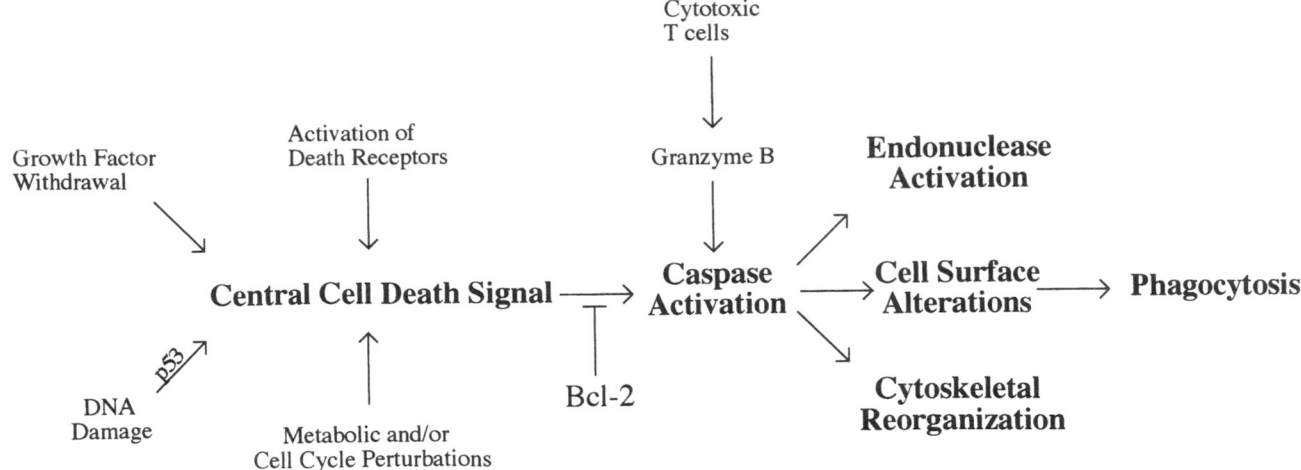

FIG. 3. Schematic representation of the central features of apoptotic cell death (see text for details).

have been reported to result in the activation of an apoptotic response. However, the mechanism(s) by which such changes result in cell death are at present unknown. Alternatively, growth factor withdrawal may result in the induction of a stress response that results in sensitization to signal transduction through cell death receptors.

In contrast to other apoptotic pathways, the signaling pathways through which cell surface receptors initiate apoptosis are beginning to be defined. For example, the signaling pathways initiated by TNF-related receptors appear to be integrated at a common step involving protease activation (42). The best characterized of the proteases capable of carrying out apoptosis in response to death receptor signal transduction are members of the caspase family.

CASPASES

Caspases are intracellular cysteine proteases that have the novel ability to carry out protein cleavage after aspartic acid residues, thus the name caspase (27). To date, 10 mammalian caspases have been identified (Fig. 4). All cell lines that have been carefully studied express one or more of such caspases constitutively. In viable cells, caspases are expressed as proenzymes that only become activated upon proteolytic cleavage (3,7). Proteolytic activation results in the removal of the amino-terminal prodomain and the processing of the remaining polypeptide into the two subunits of the active protease. The active enzyme appears to be a heterotetramer composed of two copies each of the active protein subunits. In the cases that have been reported, proteolytic activation occurs through cleavage at aspartic acid residues, suggesting that the major mechanism for the activation of caspases is either by autocatalysis or through processing by other family members. Once activated, most caspases have the ability to catalyze the activation of multiple other members of the caspase family, resulting in a positively amplifying cascade of proteolysis. If physiologically unchecked in a cell, caspase activation has been shown to be sufficient to initiate all the morphologic changes associated with apoptosis (26).

A number of caspase substrates that undergo proteolytic cleavage during apoptosis have been identified. These substrates include proteins involved in cell repair, such as poly-ADP ribose polymerase (PARP), DNA-dependent protein kinase, and MDM2; pro-

teins involved in cell cycle control, such as the retinoblastoma protein, cyclin dependent kinase, and the tyrosine kinase c-Abl; proteins involved in signal transduction, such as PAK2; and proteins involved in the structural integrity of the cell, such as nuclear lamins, fodrin, gelsolin, and actin (42–46). In most cases caspase

A)

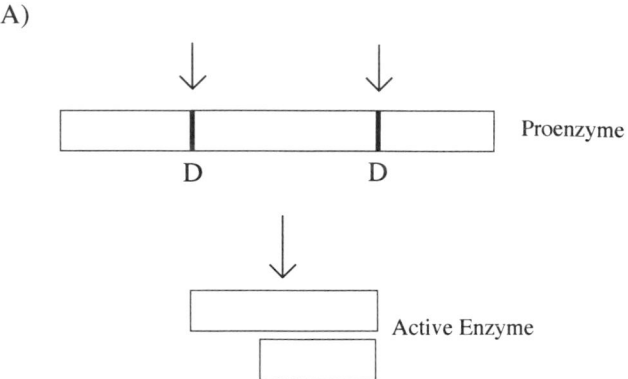

B) **Human Caspases**

Current Names	Original Names
Caspase 1	ICE
Caspase 2	ICH-1
Caspase 3	CPP32, Yama, apopain
Caspase 4	ICH-2, TX, ICE $_{rel}$ $^{-II}$
Caspase 5	ICE $_{rel}$ $^{-III}$, TY
Caspase 6	Mch2
Caspase 7	Mch3, ICE-LAP3, CMH-1
Caspase 8	FLICE, MACH, Mch5
Caspase 9	ICE-LAP6, Mch6
Caspase 10	Mch4

FIG. 4. The caspase gene family. **A)** A typical caspase is expressed as a proenzyme. The aminoterminal domain represents a prodomain which is involved in mediating protein/protein interactions and activation of the caspase. (D) Represents an aspartic acid residue that serves as a cleavage site. Conversion of the proenzyme to an active enzyme involves cleavage of the prodomain and processing of the remaining protein into the two subunits that form a catalytically active enzyme. **B)** Current nomenclature for human caspases.

cleavage results in the inactivation of the substrate. However, in some cases caspase cleavage has been shown to result in constitutive activation of the substrate. For example, caspase cleavage of PAK2 results in a constitutively active kinase (47). Whether any or all of these proteins represent the caspase targets that result in irreversible cell death remains to be determined. Caspases also are required to perform proteolytic activation of two cytokines, IL-1β and IL-18 (48). Whether the activation of these cytokines plays a role in regulating the response of a phagocyte to an apoptotic cell has not been determined.

Cell death initiated by activation of a death receptor such as Fas has been shown to be completely inhibited by caspase inhibitors (49). Thus, the physiologic proteases involved in receptor-mediated apoptosis are the caspases. However, in other forms of apoptosis, the central role of caspases as death effectors has not been firmly established (50). For example, although caspase inhibitors can prevent the morphologic changes associated with apoptosis that occur after growth factor withdrawal, most such caspase-protected cells fail to recover after growth factor readdition (51). Although caspase activity may be essential for the morphologic features of apoptosis, caspase activation may occur subsequent to irreversible cellular damage.

Caspases are not the only proteases that can initiate an apoptotic response. A wide variety of proteases when microinjected into a cell can induce apoptotic cell death (6). This suggests that although caspases may be the major physiologic effectors of programmed cell death, other proteases can function as initiators of apoptotic death. Alternatively, other proteases may induce apoptosis through the proteolytic activation of the caspases.

BCL-2 PROTEINS

The rate at which apoptotic signaling events initiate or amplify caspase activity can be regulated by proteins of the Bcl-2 family (24). Current evidence suggests that Bcl-2 does not work to inhibit a specific step in programmed cell death but rather alters the so-called apoptotic threshold of a cell (5). Bcl-2 overexpressing cells can still carry out programmed cell death in response to a wide variety of apoptotic initiators. However, the dose of the initiator necessary to induce programmed cell death in the presence of Bcl-2 is significantly greater than in the absence of Bcl-2.

A number of Bcl-2–related proteins have been identified (Fig. 5) (24,52,53). Paradoxically, some of these family members have

Anti-apoptotic Proteins	Pro-apoptotic Proteins	Proteins with Only BH3 Homology
Bcl-2	Bax	Bad
Bcl-x$_L$	Bak	Bid
Bcl-w	Bcl-x$_S$	Bik
Mcl-1		Hrk
NR-13		

FIG. 5. Bcl-2 related proteins. The Bcl-2 related proteins can be divided into three subfamilies based on overall sequence similarity. Although both anti-apoptotic and pro-apoptotic proteins display considerable sequence similarity throughout their entire length, the third class of Bcl-2-related proteins display only limited sequence similarity to other family members. The sequence similarity in these proteins is confined to a single a-helical domain known as the BH3 homology region.

been shown to promote cell survival, whereas others have been shown to enhance the sensitivity of a cell to programmed cell death. Five homologs of Bcl-2 have been identified that have antiapoptotic properties, including Bcl-x$_L$, Bcl-w, Mcl-1, NR-13, and A-1. In contrast, two proapoptotic members of the Bcl-2 family, Bax and Bak, have been reported (54–56). These proteins are capable of antagonizing the survival-promoting activity of either Bcl-2 or Bcl-x$_L$. A common feature of Bcl-2–related proteins is the ability to form either homo- or heterodimers with other family members. For example, Bcl-2 and Bcl-x$_L$ can form heterodimers with Bax. The ratio of Bcl-2 to Bax in transfected cells correlates with the apoptotic threshold (57). An excess of Bcl-2 promotes cell survival, whereas an excess of Bax promotes cell death. Although Bcl-2 family members have been traditionally subgrouped by their ability to promote or inhibit apoptosis, recent evidence suggests that depending on the cellular circumstances, an individual family member can be either pro- or antiapoptotic (58). Based on the extensive primary amino acid sequence similarities of these proteins, this suggests that the Bcl-2–related proteins may function along a biochemical continuum. One common feature of all Bcl-2-related proteins is that each of these proteins contains a carboxy-terminal hydrophobic domain that is both necessary and sufficient for insertion into the endoplasmic reticular membrane, the outer mitochondrial membrane, and the outer nuclear membrane (53,58). This pattern of intracellular distribution is unusual for a protein involved in signal transduction and suggests that Bcl-2–related proteins may have a novel biochemical function.

The three-dimensional structure of the Bcl-2–related protein Bcl-x$_L$ has been solved. This allowed the identification of two additional functional domains. The first consists of a large flexible loop that is dispensable for the antiapoptotic function of the protein. This loop domain comprises approximately one fourth of the protein and appears to be an important region for posttranslational regulation of protein function (59). The remaining portion of the protein is composed of seven α-helices and two central hydrophobic helices surrounded by five amphipathic helices (60). The top of this α-helical bundle is a hydrophobic cleft similar to the ligand binding sites present in cell surface receptors (61). This hydrophobic cleft has been shown to be necessary and sufficient for the ability of Bcl-x$_L$ to bind to a 16–amino acid α-helix present in the proapoptotic proteins Bak and Bax. This α-helical region in Bak and Bax has been termed the Bcl-2 homology domain 3 (BH3). BH3 domains have now been reported in a number of additional molecules capable of forming heterodimers with Bcl-x$_L$, including Bad, Bik, Hrk, and Bid (57,62–64). This subgroup of proteins can promote apoptosis by inactivating the antiapoptotic function of Bcl-x$_L$. Interestingly, mutations within the hydrophobic cleft of Bcl-x$_L$ have been reported that inhibit the ability of Bcl-x$_L$ to form heterodimers with BH3-containing proteins (65). These Bcl-x$_L$ mutants retain potent antiapoptotic properties.

Recently, several laboratories have suggested that Bcl-2 and Bcl-x$_L$ promote cell survival by forming inactivating heterodimers with proteins that are involved in caspase activation. One such protein is the proapoptotic worm protein CED-4. Bcl-2, Bcl-x$_L$, and the worm Bcl-2 homolog CED-9 have all been shown to bind CED-4 in transfected mammalian cells (66–68). Furthermore, Bax binding prevents Bcl-x$_L$ from binding to CED-4 (66). This suggests a model in which Bcl-x$_L$ and Bcl-2 prevent apoptosis by sequestering mammalian CED-4 homologs, thus preventing these proteins from activating caspases. In this model, Bax would be proapoptotic because it binds to Bcl-2, freeing CED-4 to activate caspases.

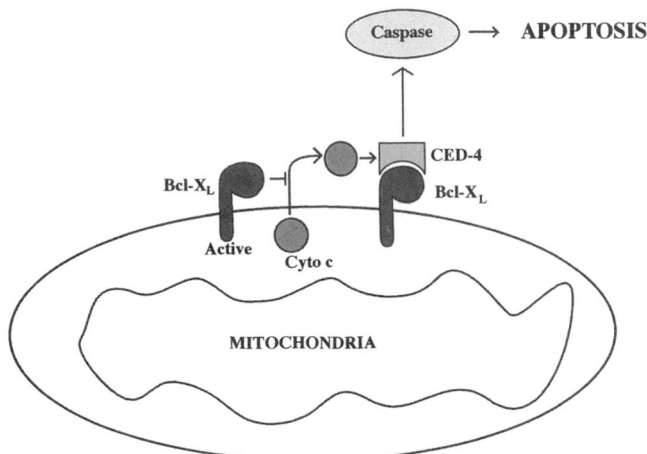

FIG. 6. Theoretical model of the potential mechanisms by which Bcl-x_L can regulate cytosolic caspase activation. Bcl-x_L has been reported to prevent cytochrome c redistribution from mitochondria by maintaining mitochondrial outer membrane integrity. In addition, Bcl-x_L has been shown to bind the pro-apoptotic protein CED-4. The mammalian CED-4 homolog, Apaf-1, is a direct caspase activator in the presence of cytochrome c. Thus, Bcl-x_L might prevent apoptosis by binding CED-4 and preventing its interaction with cytochrome c thus preventing the activation of caspases. Alternatively, CED-4 may bind and inactivate Bcl-x_L thus promoting cytochrome c redistribution and the induction of apoptosis.

However, it remains equally possible that CED-4 binding to Bcl-2–related proteins serves to inhibit the antiapoptotic function of the Bcl-2 homolog.

The three-dimensional structure of the antiapoptotic domain of Bcl-x_L has significant homology to the pore-forming domains of bacterial colicins (60). In colicins this pore-forming domain has the ability to insert and form a transmembrane pore in biologically active membranes. The localization of Bcl-2–related proteins to intracellular membranes–including the endoplasmic reticulum, outer mitochondrial membrane, and outer nuclear membrane— suggests that Bcl-x_L may have an analogous function in eukaryotic cells. Consistent with this possibility, Bcl-x_L can form an ion-conducting pore in synthetic lipid bilayers (69). Bcl-2 and Bax also have been shown to form ion-conducting pores in synthetic membranes (70–72). Perhaps one mechanism through which Bcl-2 proteins maintain homeostasis is through the regulation of the permeability of the membranes to which they distribute. Depending on its properties, such a pore might promote cell death by dissipating essential electrochemical gradients within the cell or promote cell survival by maintaining ion or protein homeostasis between intracellular compartments.

Consistent with the hypothesis that Bcl-2 proteins can serve to regulate membrane permeability, Bcl-2 expression promotes mitochondrial integrity (51). Cytochrome c has been reported to induce apoptosis when injected into the cytosol of viable cells (73). Normally cytochrome c is localized to the intermembrane space of mitochondria. Early in the apoptotic response, cytochrome c redistributes into the cytosol (13,14,51). In the presence of adenosine triphosphate and the mammalian CED-4-homolog Apaf-1, cytosolic cytochrome c is a potent caspase activator (16,28). Both high levels of endogenous Bcl-2 or exogenously added Bcl-2 can prevent cytochrome c release from mitochondria in response to a wide

variety of apoptotic stimuli. Mixing experiments involving Bcl-2–containing and Bcl-2–deficient mitochondria have demonstrated that only mitochondria that have Bcl-2 on their surface are prevented from releasing cytochrome c (14). These experiments seem to favor the hypothesis that Bcl-2 maintains cell survival by directly or indirectly promoting membrane integrity. However, one group has recently suggested that Bcl-2 prevents cytochrome c release from mitochondria because cytochrome c is a Bcl-x_L ligand (74). Therefore, it remains an open question whether the ligand-binding ability or pore-forming ability of Bcl-2–related proteins plays the more critical role in the ability of these proteins to regulate programmed cell death (Fig. 6).

VIRAL PATHOGENS ENCODE PROTEINS THAT INHIBIT HOST CELL APOPTOSIS

For viruses to sustain themselves, the host cell must survive until the virus has completed its life cycle. The ability of infected cells to undergo apoptosis in response to internal metabolic perturbations provides a multicellular organism with a first line of defense to limit viral spread. Apoptotic death, because it involves the ordered destruction of intracellular contents, undoubtedly results in the destruction of the viral genome and nascent viral particles. Viruses have incorporated into their genomes a variety of genes whose products can inhibit host cell apoptosis (Fig. 7). Some of these gene products work through the modulation of signaling pathways. Some of these viral proteins appear to function as autocrine survival factors for infected cells. Other viral proteins can suppress the function of death receptors. For example, several poxviruses encode secreted forms of the TNF receptor (74). Virally infected cells secrete this protein, which competes for TNF binding, thus preventing TNF from inducing the apoptosis of infected cells. Herpes viruses also encode proteins that regulate apoptotic pathways. Several herpes viruses encode proteins that inhibit Fas and TNF signal transduction (75,76). In addition, herpes viruses and adenoviruses can encode Bcl-2 homologs (77,78). These Bcl-2–related proteins when overproduced by transfection have been found to be antiapoptotic.

The most common viral intracellular apoptosis targets are the caspases. Poxviruses encode crmA, a potent inhibitor of caspase 1 (79). By inhibiting caspase 1, crmA not only partially blocks apoptosis but also prevents host cell conversion of pro–IL-1 to active IL-1, thus limiting the immune response. Insect baculoviruses encode two distinct caspase inhibitors. p35 is a broadly active caspase inhibitor that

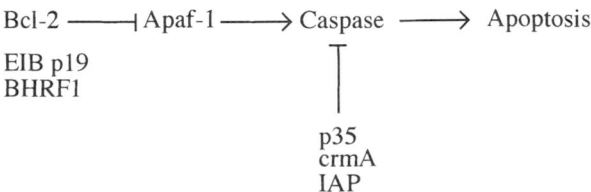

FIG. 7. Viral genes that regulate the central cell death pathway. Viral Bcl-2 homologs have been found in both the herpes virus (BHRF1) and adenovirus (E1B p19) families. Caspase inhibitors have been found in the genomes of baculoviruses (p35, IAP) and Pox viruses (crmA)

functions by being a caspase substrate that, once cleaved, remains bound to the active enzyme (80). In contrast, baculoviral inhibitors of apoptosis proteins (IAPs) appear to be nonsubstrate inhibitors of caspases 3 and 7, which are thought to be the major effector caspases in many forms of programmed cell death (81,82). Recently several mammalian homologs of IAP that inhibit apoptosis have been identified (83–85). These proteins when overproduced also prevent programmed cell death through the inhibition of caspases. In addition, IAP proteins appear to be involved in signal transduction pathways involving TNF-related receptors, although the role IAP proteins play in these pathways has not been defined (86).

The above observations support the hypothesis that viruses have coopted cellular proteins that regulate programmed cell death in order to promote host cell survival and viral replication. The genomes of additional viruses are currently being screened for genes that encode proteins that interfere with apoptosis. The identification and characterization of these genes is likely to define additional key regulatory steps in the apoptotic response.

APOPTOTIC CELL DEATH AS AN EFFECTOR COMPONENT OF THE IMMUNE SYSTEM

The constitutive expression of proteins that can carry out apoptosis and the existence of signaling pathways that can initiate apoptotic cell death have important implications for the immune system. One mechanism by which cytotoxic T cells can initiate the death of a target cell is through the intracellular introduction of proteins that can initiate an apoptotic response in the target cell (87). For example, cytotoxic T cells can induce apoptosis in target cells through the combined actions of perforin and granzyme B, two proteins stored in cytotoxic granules and released in response to target cell recognition. Perforin facilitates the entry of granzyme B into the target cell, where granzyme B can activate caspases (88–92). Granzyme B is the only known protease other than the caspases that cleaves after an aspartic acid residue. The fact that all cells within vertebrates endogenously express the proteases necessary to carry out apoptosis provides a mechanism that cytotoxic T cells can use to initiate the death of any target cell. Cytotoxic T cells also can engage cell death receptors to specifically induce signal transduction pathways that result in the activation of these proteases (87). Because cellular stress can induce the expression of cell death receptors in stromal cells, the use of a receptor-based cell death pathway may play an important role in the ability of cytotoxic T cells to selectively kill damaged cells within the complex environment of an inflammatory response. The ability of the cytotoxic T cell to initiate apoptosis in both damaged and infected target cells may provide an important mechanism through which cytotoxic cells can eradicate an infection while limiting tissue injury.

Unfortunately, the ability of immune cells to coopt a constitutively present, internally encoded system to eradicate infected or potentially damaged cells can have negative consequences for the host. In many cell lineages, the maintenance of lineage function is regulated by a balance of cell proliferation and cell death. However, some cell types, such as neural cells, have a limited capacity for self-renewal. Most neurons survive for the life of the organism. Mechanisms by which immune cell-mediated death is limited in such tissues are just beginning to be identified. Although such protective mechanisms may prevent the deletion of irreplaceable cells,

resistance to immune-induced apoptosis also may contribute to instances in which the immune system fails to eradicate either infected or abnormal cells.

REGULATION OF LYMPHOCYTE SURVIVAL

As with other cell types, lymphocyte accumulation is regulated not only by cell proliferation but also by apoptosis. The mechanisms that regulate cell survival in the immune system are just beginning to be understood. Apoptosis is essential for the regulation of lymphocyte development and homeostasis. Due to the imprecise nature of V(D)J recombination, the vast majority of cells that initiate differentiation into either the B- or T-cell lineage develop improperly. In order to prevent the accumulation of dysfunctional cells, such cells must be eliminated. Lymphocytes that fail to produce either an effective T-cell receptor (TCR) or a surface immunoglobulin receptor complex undergo apoptosis. In addition, potentially autoreactive B or T cells can be deleted during development by negative selection. During negative selection cells die by undergoing apoptosis (93,94). Thus, the factors that regulate the survival of developing lymphocytes play a critical role in shaping the immune response.

Once a vertebrate reaches adulthood, the number of lymphocytes that the animal maintains over its lifetime are relatively constant. Nevertheless, lymphocytes undergo cyclic expansions and contractions as a result of participating in host defense. In order to provide an effective immune response, antigen-specific lymphocytes must be capable of large clonal expansion to be able to rid the host of a pathogen. However, after successful eradication of a pathogen, lymphocytes must undergo a comparable reduction in cell number in order to maintain lineage cell number over time. The role of apoptosis in regulating lymphocyte development and survival are considered in the following sections.

THE ROLE OF APOPTOSIS IN REGULATING LYMPHOCYTE DEVELOPMENT

Due to imprecision in V(D)J recombination, the majority of developing lymphocytes fail to produce an expressible antigen receptor. Even the successful recombination of antigen receptor genes that leads to cell surface expression of an immunoglobulin receptor or TCR is not sufficient to guarantee that a lymphocyte will complete development. It is estimated that in the thymus over 95% of thymocytes create a TCR that can be neither positively nor negatively selected through interactions with self-encoded major histocompatibility complex (MHC) molecules (93). TCR-positive thymocytes that fail to undergo selection die with a half-life of approximately 4 days. Bcl-2 proteins can regulate the survival of these neglected thymocytes. Gene elimination studies suggest that bcl-x_L plays a critical role in maintaining the half-life of such cells because bcl-x_L null thymocytes die by neglect with a half-life of approximately 1 day (95). Increased constitutive expression of either Bcl-2 or Bcl-x_L leads to the enhanced accumulation of double-positive thymocytes. Similar observations have been made in studies of developing B cells (96). Bcl-x_L elimination decreases the survival of pre-B cells, whereas enhanced Bcl-x_L expression can lead to the accumulation of immature cells.

Overexpression of Bcl-2 family members does not appear to significantly affect the outcome of thymic selection (96a). The cell death that occurs in response to negative selection is either not related to apoptosis, involves a Bcl-2–independent form of apoptosis, or involves inactivation of Bcl-2 function. The first possibility is unlikely because the morphology of thymocyte death during negative selection has all the features of programmed cell death (93,94). A recent demonstration that Bcl-2 proteins can be posttranslationally inactivated suggest that inactivation of Bcl-2 proteins during negative selection remains a possibility that will need further examination (59). Alternatively, negative selection may provide such a persistent or strong signal that it overcomes the apoptotic threshold imposed by Bcl-2 proteins no matter how high the level of Bcl-2 expression. This is consistent with the hypothesis that negative selection results from a high-avidity signal through the TCR. A strong or persistent TCR signal in an immature thymocyte may set up a conflict in cell cycle progression or cellular metabolism that overwhelms the apoptotic threshold set by a Bcl-2 protein. This would be consistent with the hypothesis that cell survival results from the integration of the strength and persistence of signals from a variety of pro- and antiapoptotic signaling pathways. Cell death of thymocytes in response to TCR engagement involves new protein synthesis, suggesting that gene products involved in promoting cell death are induced in response to TCR signal transduction. Several transcriptionally induced genes, including Nur 77 and related steroid receptors, have been implicated in thymocyte apoptosis (97,98).

REGULATION OF PERIPHERAL LYMPHOCYTE HOMEOSTASIS

The vast majority of peripheral B and T cells that circulate within the primary lymphoid organs and the peripheral blood are in a quiescent or resting state. Although naive cells may have a shorter life span than memory cells, the life span of naive cells can still be measured in weeks or months. The survival of these quiescent cells is critical for the maintenance of an anticipatory immune system. This is particularly true after puberty, when the thymus involutes and the rate of new T-cell production is severely reduced. Like other cells, the survival of a resting lymphocyte is dependent on survival signals the cell receives from its environment. Removal of quiescent lymphocytes from a lymph node or the spleen results in the rapid induction of apoptosis that can be prevented by caspase inhibitors (99).

Two types of extracellular signals have been identified that support the survival of quiescent lymphocytes. The first is survival information the cell receives from its stromal environment. The failure of cells to migrate to appropriate environments within lymph nodes and spleen is associated with decreased survival (100). Survival information for a resting lymphocyte appears to be received in part through the antigen receptor. B cells lacking an antigen receptor rapidly undergo apoptosis in peripheral lymphoid organs (101). T cells transferred into MHC-deficient animals have shortened survivals (102). In addition, the survival of quiescent lymphocytes recruited to an inflammatory site is promoted by inflammatory cytokines. The cytokines produced in inflammatory lesions can promote lymphocyte survival in the absence of antigen receptor activation (103,104). This prevents the deletion of cells in the proapoptotic environment of an inflammatory lesion, preventing the inappropriate deletion of cells that may contribute to the protective immune repertoire.

In addition to extracellular survival signals, both resting B and T cells are also dependent on the intrinsic expression of Bcl-2 (105,106). Bcl-2 appears to be constitutively expressed by resting lymphocytes. Animals deficient in the bcl-2 gene rapidly become immunodeficient as a result of the progressive loss of resting lymphocytes. Thus, Bcl-2 is critical for the long-term survival of quiescent lymphocytes.

Antigen receptor engagement of a quiescent lymphocyte will induce the cell to enter the cell cycle (Fig. 8). However, this signaling alone does not appear to be sufficient to sustain cell survival. In the absence of additional growth factors or costimulatory receptors, antigen-activated cells become susceptible to undergoing apoptosis. The mechanism by which antigen receptor activation results in increased susceptibility of programmed cell death remains controversial. Signal transduction through costimulatory receptors such as the CD28 receptor on T cells or the CD40 receptor on B cells during antigen-dependent activation promotes not only cell proliferation but also cell survival (107–112). The clonal amplification of activated cells is regulated by the availability of progression growth factors, including IL-2, IL-4, IL-6, IL-7, IL-9, and IL-15. Such growth factors both promote cell survival as well as progression through the cell cycle (103,113–116). The clonal expansion of activated cells is limited by these factors, and cells deprived of these growth factors during the expansion phase of an immune response die by apoptosis.

Once antigen or costimulatory ligands becomes limiting at the end of an immune response, the expanded clonal cells become susceptible to deletion through cell death receptors, including Fas and the type 1 and type 2 TNF receptors (TNF-R1 and TNF-R2) (43,117–125). Fas-deficient animals fail to delete cells properly after a productive immune response. This leads to progressive accumulation of resting lymphocytes. Such animals also have an increased propensity to develop autoimmune disease (124,125). The phenotype of Fas-deficient animals can be made significantly worse by a concomitant deficiency of TNF-R1 (123). This suggests that these two receptors have partially redundant roles in promoting the deletion of excess of immune cells at the end of an inflammatory response. The factors that determine which cells produced during an inflammatory response survive and which cells go on to become memory cells have not been elucidated. Survival could potentially be on a stochastic basis. For example, only a limited number of cells may reach sites within a lymphoid follicle that will support the long-term persistence of the cell and prevent deletion by Fas ligand–bearing cells.

The above data suggest a model in which the survival of an active lymphocyte is determined by the integration of three distinct signaling pathways (126). After antigen receptor activation, survival and clonal expansion is controlled by cytokine receptors, whereas cell deletion is controlled by cell death receptors that include Fas and TNF-R1. Costimulatory receptors can play a potent role in preventing cell death in response to growth factor limitation or death receptor signal transduction. However, none of these signaling pathways is dominant in an all-or-none sense. It appears that the *in vivo* response of a cell is based on the integration of the net signaling information provided through these distinct signaling pathways.

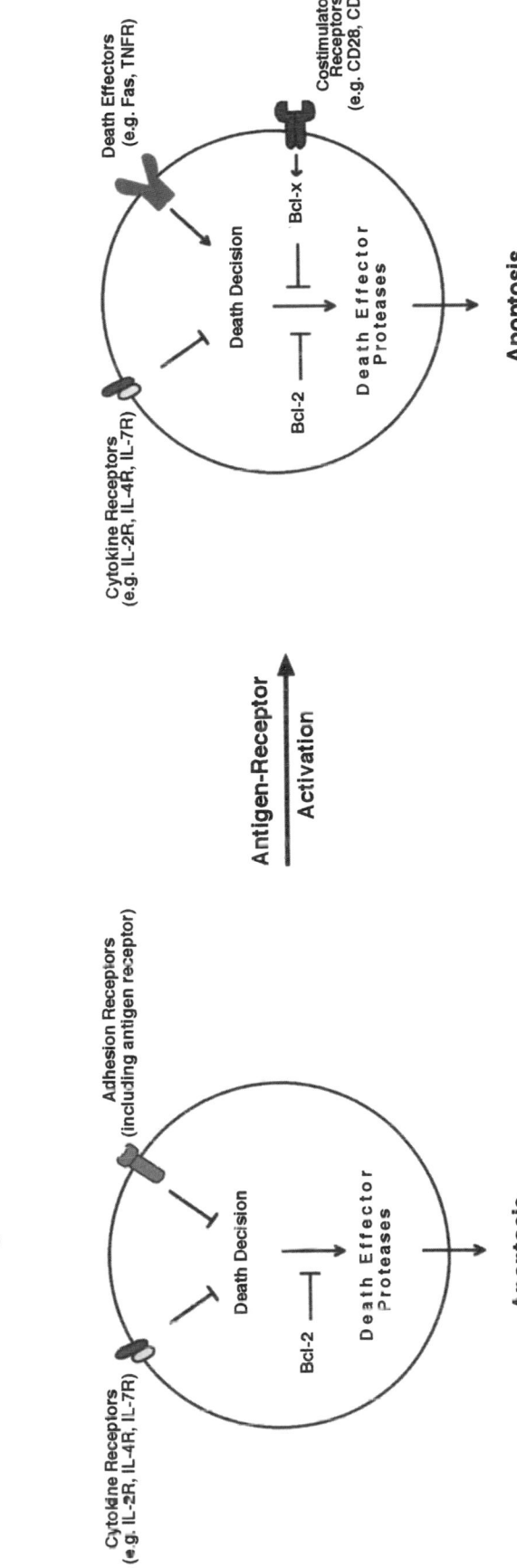

FIG. 8. Schematic representation of the factors that regulate the susceptibility of resting and activated lymphocytes to undergo apoptosis (see text for details).

COSTIMULATORY RECEPTORS ENHANCE THE EXPRESSION OF BCL-X$_L$

One common mechanism by which CD28 and CD40 promote cell survival is through the specific and transient upregulation of the Bcl-2–related protein Bcl-x$_L$ (107,108,111,112). Bcl-x$_L$ expression has been reported to prevent cell death in response to growth factor limitation or Fas signal transduction (107,127). Signal transduction through CD28 or CD40 induces Bcl-x$_L$ expression only in antigen-activated cells. In the absence of antigen receptor engagement, CD40 engagement appears to promote cell death (128,129). The induction of Bcl-x$_L$ by either CD28 or CD40 is transient, lasting 3 to 4 days (107,111). Protection of cells from cell death persists only for the period of time Bcl-x$_L$ is expressed.

CYTOKINE-INDUCED CELL SURVIVAL

Relatively little is known about the mechanisms by which growth factors promote the survival of activated lymphocytes.

Recently, one example of how growth factors promote cell survival has been elucidated (Fig. 9). IL-3 receptor signal transduction activates kinases that result in the phosphorylation of the Bcl-x$_L$ inhibitor Bad (130). One growth factor–dependent kinase that can phosphorylate Bad is Akt (131,132). Because Akt activation is phosphatidylinositol 3-kinase dependent, one mechanism by which both of these kinases can support cell survival is through the phosphorylation of Bad (133–137). Phosphorylated Bad is incapable of binding to Bcl-x$_L$. This releases Bcl-x$_L$ to promote cell survival either by binding other cell death effector molecules or by regulating membrane permeability as an ion-forming channel. When IL-3 signal transduction is withdrawn, Bad rapidly becomes dephosphorylated. Dephosphorylated Bad can then bind to Bcl-x$_L$, thereby potentially displacing bound death activators or inhibiting Bcl-x$_L$ from undergoing the conformational change that would be required for membrane insertion. Thus, Bad appears to regulate Bcl-x$_L$ function in a growth factor–dependent manner. Whether other Bcl-x$_L$ inhibitors such as Bik and Bid are similarly regulated has not been explored.

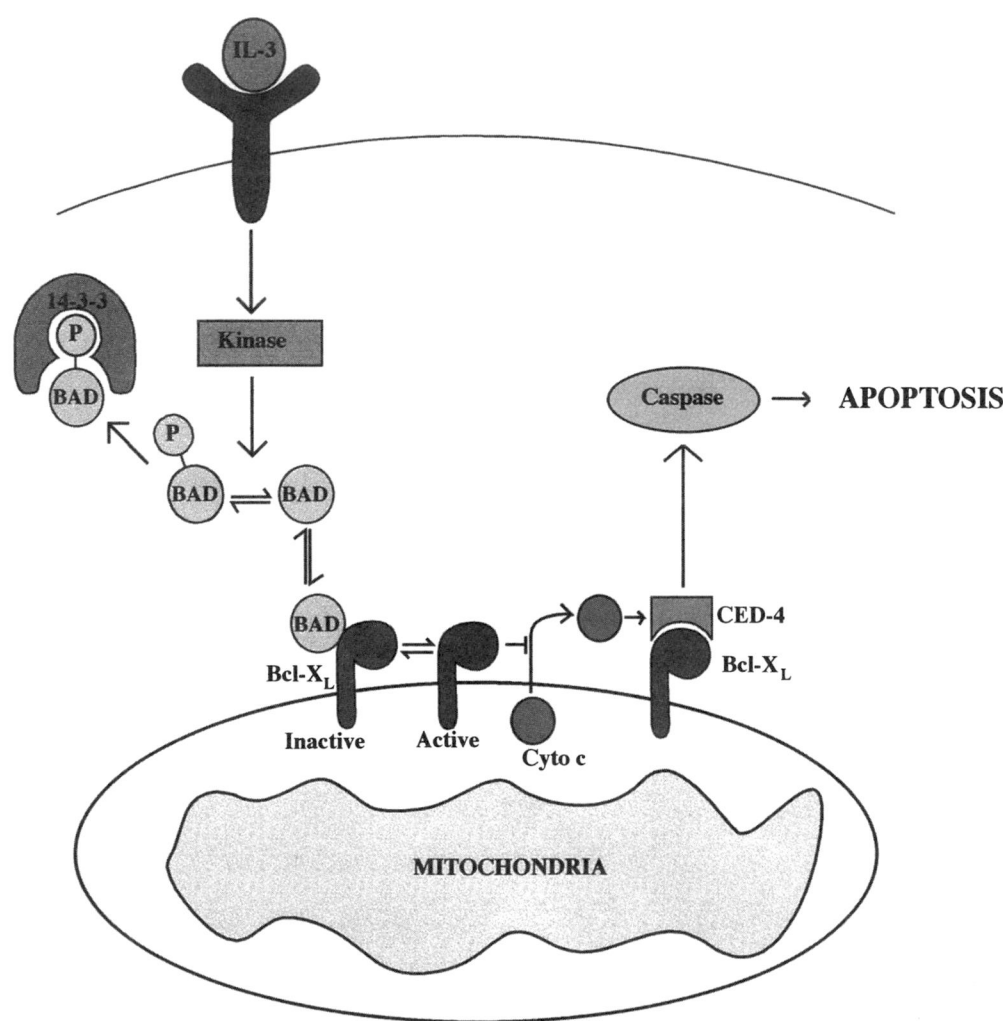

FIG. 9. Schematic representation of the molecular mechanism by which growth factors such as IL-3 promote cell survival by inactivating the Bcl-2 inhibitor Bad. Recent evidence suggest that one kinase which can lead to the phosphorylation of Bad is Akt. Phosphorylated Bad is sequestered in the cytosol through its interaction with the 14-3-3 proteins. Both phosphorylation and sequestration prevent Bad interaction with Bcl-x$_L$ leaving Bcl-x$_L$ in an active conformation that can regulate programmed cell death.

SIGNAL TRANSDUCTION THROUGH TNF RECEPTORS

One source of the controversy concerning the regulation of cell death involves the ability of Bcl-2 proteins to prevent cell death initiated through the TNF receptor–related protein Fas (138–142). Like other members of the TNF receptor family, Fas is believed to undergo ligand-induced trimerization (Fig. 10). Such trimerization results in the recruitment of an adaptor, the Fas-associated death domain–containing protein (FADD, also called MORT1) (143,144). FADD, in turn, contains a protein–protein interaction domain termed a death effector domain, which promotes dimerization with other proteins that contain a death effector domain. Recently one such protein has been identified and termed FLICE/MACH1/Mch5 (caspase 8) (145,146). Caspase 8 is a member of the caspase family, which contains two independent death effector domains in its amino terminus. Caspase 8 recruitment to the Fas signal transduction complex by FADD results in the autocatalyic cleavage of caspase 8, releasing the active protease subunits. Once activated, caspase 8 functions to activate additional caspases as well as degrade intracellular substrates.

Thus, the Fas signal transduction pathway involves a single adaptor molecule for the recruitment and activation of a caspase. This makes it difficult to understand how proteins of the Bcl-2 family can prevent Fas-induced cell death. Nevertheless, in several cellular systems, overexpression of Bcl-2 or Bcl-xL can prevent Fas-mediated cell death (140,142,147,148). Two distinct hypotheses for the ability of Bcl-2 to prevent Fas-induced cell death have been proposed. Recent biochemical evidence has suggested that the protein Bcl-xL can directly or indirectly bind and sequester cas-

pase 8 (66). By sequestering caspase 8 to intracellular organelles, Bcl-xL could prevent the recruitment of caspase 8 to the Fas receptor complex. However, other investigators have found relatively normal Fas-dependent activation of caspase 8 in Bcl-2–expressing cells (148,149). Instead, their data suggest that Bcl-xL prevents Fas-induced signal transduction downstream from Caspase 8 activation either by limiting caspase amplification or protecting intracellular organelles such as the mitochondria from the effects of caspase-mediated proteolysis. These two molecular mechanisms are not mutually exclusive, and both are consistent with the reported ability of Bcl-2 proteins to bind proapoptotic proteins and to regulate membrane permeability.

One curious aspect of the TNF receptor family is that although some members such as Fas, TNF-R1, DR3, DR4, and DR5 contain death domains that allow these receptors to recruit and activate caspases (150–156), other TNF-related receptors seem to be potent inducers of cell survival (157). The TNF-related protein CD40 is the major costimulatory receptor of B cells (Fig. 11). CD40 signal transduction provides a potent stimulus for B-cell survival, proliferation, and differentiation (158). In response to ligand-induced trimerization, CD40 recruits a set of adaptor molecules known as TNF receptor–associated factors (TRAFs). There are currently six TRAF proteins that share a common C-terminal TRAF domain, which is necessary and sufficient for receptor recruitment (159–163). Interaction with the TRAF domain also results in the recruitment of inhibitors of apoptosis proteins (IAPs) to receptor-associated complexes. The three known IAPs—cIAP1, cIAP2, and ILP (x-IAP)—are all potent inhibitors of apoptosis (83–85). In addition, the N terminus of TRAF proteins appears to be important in the activation of NF-κB and Jun C-terminal kinase activity as a

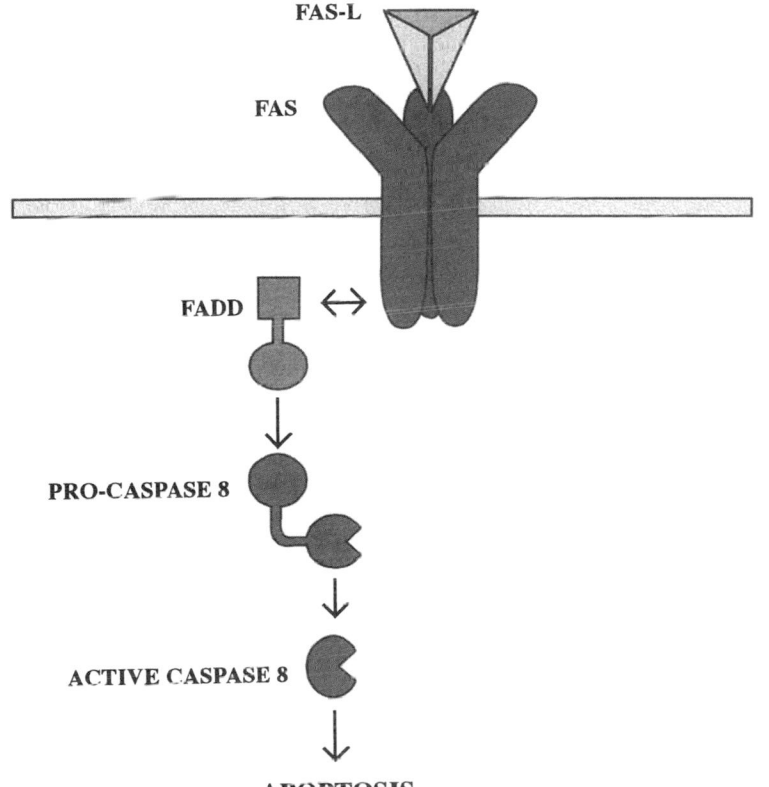

FIG. 10. Schematic representation of the cell death pathway activated through the Fas receptor (see text for details).

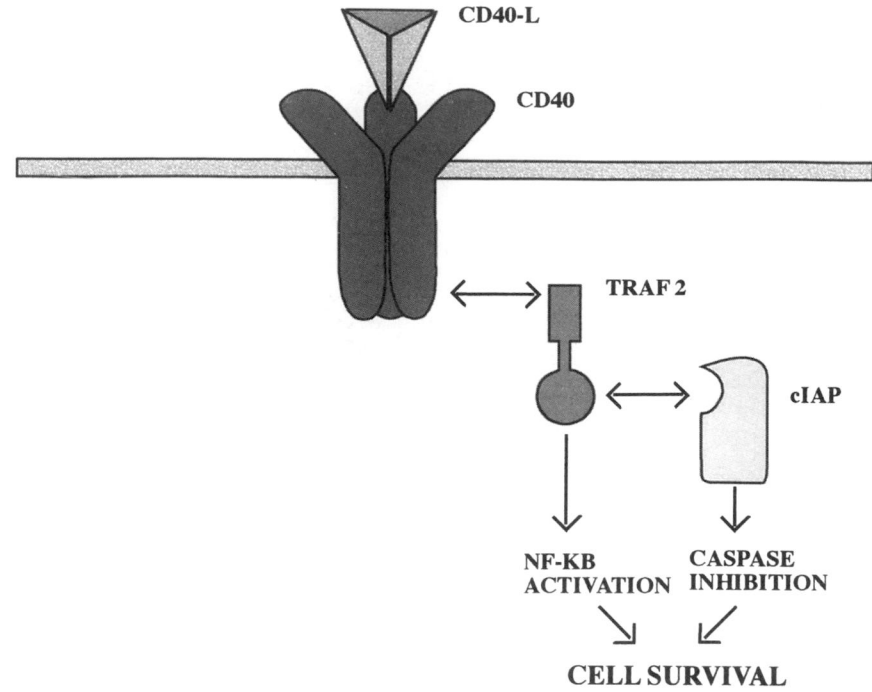

FIG. 11. Schematic representation of the CD40 signal transduction pathway that leads to the induction of cell survival (see text for details).

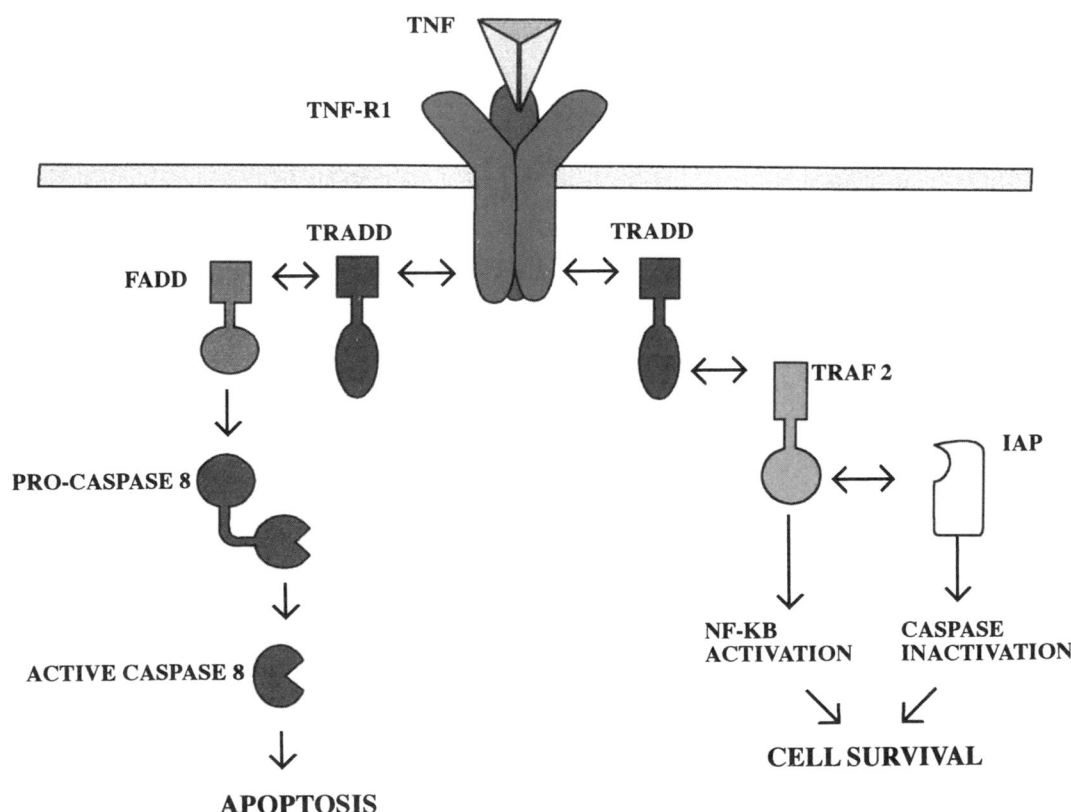

FIG. 12. Potential alternative forms of signal transduction initiated through the TNF-R1 receptor (see text for details).

result of receptor–ligand interaction (164,165). In addition to CD40, three TNF receptors associated with T-cell costimulation—CD30, OX-40, and 4-1BB—have been shown to be coupled to NF-κB activation through the TRAF family of adaptor proteins (166,167). One interesting consequence of CD40 and CD30 signal transduction is that although the primary effects of these intracellular receptors is to promote lymphocyte survival, a secondary effect is to induce increased sensitivity to the cell death–inducing members of the TNF receptor family, including Fas and TNF-R1 (128,129,168,169). This suggests that signal transduction through CD40 and CD30, although initially promoting cell survival, also serves to establish mechanisms that will facilitate the deletion of cells at the end of an immune response.

The receptor-mediated activation of NF-κB induces the transcription of genes that promote cellular survival (170–172). The potential importance of NF-κB in sustaining lymphocyte survival is supported by the observation that the other major costimulatory receptor, CD28, leads to the potent and prolonged inhibition of IκB activity, resulting in substantial NF-κB activation (173). In contrast, glucocorticoids, which promote the death of peripheral lymphocytes, can potently inhibit NF-κB activation by two distinct mechanisms: the upregulation of IκB transcription and the inhibition of NF-κB DNA binding activity (174,175). Cells deficient in the NF-κB subunit p65 display decreased survival (176).

Signal transduction through the TNF-R1 receptor is even more complex than through Fas or CD40 (177) (Fig. 12). The adaptor molecule recruited to the death domain of TNF-R1 is TRADD. TRADD has the ability to signal either through TRAF 2, which results in NF-κB activation or through the recruitment of FADD, which in turn activates FLICE. Which molecular mechanism is chosen depends on a complex set of variables that have not yet been completely defined. Thus, the ability of some members of the TNF receptor family to promote either lymphocyte survival or death will be dependent on the state of cellular activation and the levels of the available intracellular adaptors. Recently both cellular TNF receptor decoys and FADD decoys have been reported. These molecules appear to compete for either ligand or receptor binding and inhibit apoptosis signal transduction (155,156,178,179).

CELL SURVIVAL PATHWAYS MUST BE DOMINANT TO CELL DEATH PATHWAYS DURING A PRODUCTIVE IMMUNE RESPONSE

Based on the timing and relative levels of signal transduction, the effects of either costimulatory or cytokine receptors or cell death receptors can predominate. For example, activated CD4 cells are sensitive to Fas-induced cell death. Nevertheless, CD4 cells can be exponentially expanded *in vitro* by repetitive antigen receptor engagement in the presence of continuous CD28 costimulation (180). Such cells constitutively express Fas and are induced to express Fas ligand in response to TCR engagement. However the cells fail to undergo apoptosis when cultured in the presence of CD28 costimulation. The transient nature of Fas ligand expression after T-cell activation may account for the failure of Fas ligand to induce the death of cells actively receiving survival signals through costimulatory and cytokine receptors. In contrast, constitutive expression of Fas ligand can lead to the deletion of activated T cells *in vivo*. Constitutive expression of Fas ligand by cells in a tissue graft has been shown to prevent immune rejection by inducing the death of lymphocytes activated in response to the graft (181).

Although the above experiments define the range of effects that can be mediated through optimal stimulation through either costimulatory or cell death receptors, current evidence suggests that the signal transduction that induces cell death is subordinate to cell survival signals under conditions that mimic the amplification phase of the immune response. However, the loss of antigen or costimulatory receptors at any time during the proliferative response appears to leave an activated cell sensitive to the induction of cell death by either Fas or TNF-R1. If anything, prior costimulatory signals or cytokine treatment serves to enhance the sensitivity of T cells to deletion after a proliferative response. Additional receptors are likely to play a role in promoting the deletion of activated lymphocytes. For example, the antiproliferative effects of transforming growth factor-β and CTLA-4 appear to sensitize T cells to subsequent deletion (182,183). This suggests that the termination of cell proliferation may promote lymphocyte deletion during an immune response. Antiproliferative receptors and cell death receptors may function synergistically to downregulate an immune response.

IMMUNE PRIVILEGE

The ability of cells expressing Fas ligand to cause deletion of activated lymphocytes has provided a potential explanation for the phenomenon of immune privilege (184,185). The eye has been found to be a site where foreign tissues can be introduced without an immune response. The molecular mechanism(s) that allow this site to tolerate the introduction of foreign antigens has been controversial. It has recently been shown that the epithelial cells in the eye constitutively express Fas ligand. The constitutive expression of Fas ligand by the epithelium appears to promote deletion of T cells activated within the eye (186). Animals with a deficiency in either Fas ligand or the Fas receptor fail to display significant immune privilege. The epithelial cells for the eye are not the only cells where Fas ligand appears to be constitutively expressed. The Sertoli cells of the testes also express Fas ligand (187). The expression of Fas ligand by the stromal cells of the testes and the cornea may explain why these tissues are readily accepted as allografts. Similar mechanisms have been suggested to explain fetal tolerance during pregnancy (188) and some forms of tumor immune escape (189).

One group of investigators has found that immune privilege in the eye can be established in animals lacking the Fas ligand if antigen is introduced into the anterior chamber of the eye together with apoptotic T cells (190). This suggests that immune privilege results not only from the lack of an inflammatory response but also from subsequent immune consequences of the accumulation of apoptotic immune cells within a tissue. Thus, immune cell apoptosis may be a signal for the termination of an inflammatory response. The accumulation of apoptotic cells during an evolving immune response could trigger the development of cells that function to downmodulate or suppress further immune activation.

APOPTOSIS AND AUTOIMMUNITY

Apoptotic cell death is associated with the activation of caspases, which have a unique proteolytic cleavage pattern when compared with other intracellular proteases. Thus, caspase activation has the potential to produce peptide fragments distinct from those produced during normal proteasome-dependent protein turnover. Such novel fragments could be produced in levels that initiate an immune response. However, because apoptotic cell death is an ongoing process beginning early in development and persisting in many tissues throughout the life of the animal, it would be expected that T cells reactive to peptides unique to apoptotic cells would be deleted or anergized. Surprisingly, many of the autoantigens identified in human autoimmune diseases are substrates of caspase cleavage during apoptotic cell death. Such antigens include poly-ADP ribose polymerase (PARP), Rho, U1-70, nuclear mitotic activator protein (NuMA), DNA-dependent protein kinase, and fodrin (191). These observations have led to the hypothesis that some forms of autoimmune disease may result from an abnormal response to apoptotic cell death. Although how such an abnormal response might occur has not been determined, these observations reinforce the hypothesis that apoptosis may play an active role in regulating the immune response. As stated at the start of this chapter, it was initially believed that apoptotic cell death was immunologically silent. However, recent evidence that apoptosis may play a role in establishing immune privilege and in the pathogenesis of autoimmune disease suggests that apoptotic cell death may play an active role in regulating an immune response.

REFERENCES

1. Kerr JFR, Wyllie AH, Currie AR. Apoptosis: A basic biological phenomenon with wide-ranging implications in tissue culture. *J Cancer* 1972;26:239–257
2. Ellis RE, Yuan J, Horvitz HR. Mechanisms and functions of cell death. *Annu Rev Cell Biol* 1991;7:663–698.
3. Chinnaiyan AM, Dixit VM. The cell-death machine. *Curr Biol* 1996;6:555–562.
4. Golstein P. Controlling cell death. *Science* 1997;275:1081–1082.
5. Thompson CB. Apoptosis in the pathogenesis and treatment of disease. *Science* 1995;267:1456–1462.
6. Williams MS, Henkart PA. Apoptotic cell death induced by intracellular proteolysis. *J Immunol* 1994;153:4247–4255.
7. Kumar S. ICE-like proteases in apoptosis. *TIBS* 1995;20:198–202.
8. Deiss LP, Galinka H, Berissi H, Cohen O, Kimchi A. Cathepsin D protease mediates programmed cell death induced by interferon-γ, Fas/APO-1 and TNF-α. *EMBO J* 1996;15:3861–3870.
9. Vaux DL, Wilhelm S, Häcker G. Requirements for proteolysis during apoptosis. *Mol Cell Biol* 1997;17:6502–6507.
10. Castedo M, Hirsch T, Susin SA, et al. Sequential acquisition of mitochondrial and plasma membrane alterations during early lymphocyte apoptosis. *J Immunol* 1996;157:512–521.
11. Jacobson MD, Burne JF, Raff MC. Programmed cell death and Bcl-2 protection in the absence of a nucleus. *EMBO J* 1994;13:1899–1910.
12. Zamzami N, Susin SA, Marchetti P, et al. Mitochondrial control of nuclear apoptosis. *J Exp Med* 1996;183:1533–1544.
13. Yang J, Liu X, Bhalla K, et al. Prevention of apoptosis by Bcl-2: release of cytochrome c from mitochondria blocked. *Science* 1997;275:1129–1132.
14. Kluck RM, Bossy-Wetzel E, Green DR, Newmeyer DD. The release of cytochrome c from mitochondria: a primary site for Bcl-2 regulation of apoptosis. *Science* 1997;275:1132–1136.
15. Susin SA, Zamzami N, Castedo M, et al. The central executioner of apoptosis: multiple connections between protease activation and mitochondria in Fas/APO-1/CD95– and ceramide-induced apoptosis. *J Exp Med* 1997;186:25–37.
16. Liu X, Kim CN, Yang J, Jemmerson R, Wang X. Induction of apoptotic program in cell-free extracts: requirement for dATP and cytochrome C. *Cell* 1996;86:147–157.
17. Kluck RM, Martin SJ, Hoffman BM, Zhou JS, Green DR, Newmeyer DD. Cytochrome c activation of CPP32-like proteolysis plays a critical role in a *Xenopus* cell-free apoptosis system. *EMBO J* 1997;16:4639–4649.
18. Ren Y, Silverstein RL, Allen J, Savill J. CD36 gene transfer confers capacity for phagocytosis of cells undergoing apoptosis. *J Exp Med* 1995;181:1857–1862.
19. Wyllie AH, Kerr JFR, Currie AR. Cell death: the significance of apoptosis. *Int Rev Cytol* 1980;68:251–306.
20. Hengartner MO, Ellis RE, Horvitz HR. *Caenorhabditis elegans* gene ced-9 protects cells from programmed cell death. *Nature* 1992;356:494–499.
21. Yuan J, Horvitz HR. The *Caenorhabditis elegans* genes ced-3 and ced-4 act cell autonomously to cause programmed cell death. *Dev Biol* 1990;138:33–41.
22. Yuan J, Horvitz HR. The *Caenorhabditis elegans* cell death gene ced-4 encodes a novel protein and is expressed during the period of extensive programmed cell death. *Development* 1992;116:309–320.
23. Hengartner MO, Horvitz HR. C. Elegans cell survival gene ced-9 encodes a functional homolog of the mammalian proto-oncogene bcl-2. *Cell* 1994;76:665–676.

24. Yang E, Korsmeyer SJ. Molecular thanatopsis: a discourse on the BCL2 family and cell death. *Blood* 1996;88:386–401.
25. Vaux DL, Weissman IL, Kim SK. Prevention of programmed cell death in *Caenorhabditis elegans* by human bcl-2. *Science* 1992;258:1955–1957.
26. Yuan J, Shaham S, Ledoux S, Ellis HM, Horvitz HR. The *C. elegans* cell death gene ced-3 encodes a protein similar to mammalian interleukin-1β–converting enzyme. *Cell* 1993;75:641–652.
27. Alnemri ES, Livingston DJ, Nicholson DW, et al. Human ICE/CED-3 protease nomenclature. *Cell* 1996;87:171.
28. Zou H, Henzel WJ, Liu X, Lutschg A, Wang X. Apaf-1, a human protein homologous to *C. elegans* CED-4, participates in cytochrome c–dependent activation of caspase-3. *Cell* 1997;90:405–413.
29. Seshagiri S, Miller LK. *Caenorhabditis elegans* CED-4 stimulates CED-3 processing and CED-3–induced apoptosis. *Curr Biol* 1997;7:455–460.
30. Raff MC. Social controls on cell survival and cell death. *Nature* 1992;356:397–400.
31. Nagata S. Apoptosis: telling cells their time is up. *Curr Biol* 1996;6:1241–1243.
32. Oren M. Relationship of p53 to the control of apoptotic cell death. *Semin Cancer Biol* 1994;5:221–227.
33. Buttke TM, Sandstrom PA. Oxidative stress as a mediator of apoptosis. *Immunol Today* 1994;15:7–10.
34. Meisenholder GW, Martin SJ, Green DR, Nordberg J, Babior BM, Gottlieb RA. Events in apoptosis. *J Biol Chem* 1996;271:16260–16262.
35. Lemasters JJ, DiGuiseppi J, Nieminen A-L., Herman B. Blebbing, free Ca^{2+} and mitochondrial membrane potential preceding cell death in hepatocytes. *Nature* 1987;325:78–81.
36. Briehl MM, Cotgreave IA, Powis G. Downregulation of the antioxidant defence during glucocorticoid-mediated apoptosis. *Cell Death Differ* 1995;2:41–46.
37. Déas O, Dumont C, Mollereau B, et al. Thiol-mediated inhibition of FAS and CD2 apoptotic signaling in activated human peripheral T cells. *Int Immunol* 1997;9:117–125.
38. Wright SC, Wei QS, Kinder DH, Larrick JW. Biochemical pathways of apoptosis: nicotinamide adenine dinucleotide–deficient cells are resistant to tumor necrosis factor or ultraviolet light activation of the 24-kD apoptotic protease and DNA fragmentation. *J Exp Med* 1996;183:463–471.
39. Hockenbery DM, Oltvai ZN, Yin X-M, Milliman CL, Korsmeyer SJ. Bcl-2 functions in an antioxidant pathway to prevent apoptosis. *Cell* 1993;75:241–251.
40. Hyde H, Borthwick NJ, Janossy G, Salmon M, Akbar AN. Upregulation of intracellular glutathione by fibroblast-derived factor(s): enhanced survival of activated T cells in the presence of low Bcl-2. *Blood* 1997;89:2453–2460.
41. Polyak K, Xia Y, Zweier JL, Kinzler KW, Vogelstein B. A model for p53-induced apoptosis. *Nature* 1997;389:300–304.
42. Fraser A, Evan G. A license to kill. *Cell* 1996;85:781–784.
43. Nagata S. Apoptosis by death factor. *Cell* 1997;88:355–365.
44. Casciola-Rosen L, Nicholson DW, Chong T, et al. Apopain/CPP32 cleaves proteins that are essential for cellular repair: a fundamental principle of apoptotic death. *J Exp Med* 1996;183:1957–1964.
45. Jänicke RU, Walker PA, Lin XY, Porter AG. Specific cleavage of the retinoblastoma protein by an ICE-like protease in apoptosis. *EMBO J* 1996;15:6969–6978.
46. Kothakota S, Azuma T, Reinhard C, et al. Caspase-3–generated fragment of gelsolin: effector of morphological change in apoptosis. *Science* 1997;278:294–305.
47. Rudel T, Bokoch GM. Membrane and morphological changes in apoptotic cells regulated by caspase-mediated activation of PAK2. *Science* 1997;276:1571–1574.
48. Ghayur T, Banerjee S, Hugunin M, et al. Caspase-1 processes IFN-γ–inducing factor and regulates LPS-induced IFN-γ production. *Nature* 1997;386:619–623.
49. Longthorne VL, Williams GT. Caspase activity is required for commitment to Fas-mediated apoptosis. *EMBO J* 1997;16:3805–3812.
50. McCarthy N, Whyte M, Gilbert C, Evan G. Inhibition of Ced-3/ICE–related proteases does not prevent cell death induced by oncogenes, DNA damage, or the Bcl-2 homologue Bak. *J Cell Biol* 1997;136:215–227.
51. Vander Heiden MG, Chandel NS, WIlliamson EK, Schumacker PT, Thompson CB. Bcl-x$_L$ regulates the membrane potential and volume homeostasis of mitochondria. *Cell* 1997;91:627–637.
52. White E. Life, death, and the pursuit of apoptosis. *Genes Dev* 1996;10:1–15.
52a. Cory S. Regulation of lymphocyte survival by the BCL-2 gene family. *Annu Rev Immunol* 1995;13:513–543.
53. Reed JC. Double identity for proteins of the Bcl-2 family. *Nature* 1997;387:773–776.
54. Chittenden T, Flemington C, Houghton AB, et al. A conserved domain in Bak, distinct from BH1 and BH2, mediates cell death and protein binding functions. *EMBO J* 1995;14:5589–5596.
55. Brady HJM, Gil-Gómez G, Kirberg J, Berns AJM. Baxa perturbs T cell development and affects cell cycle entry of T cells. *EMBO J* 1996;15:6991–7001.
56. Xiang J, Chao DT, Korsmeyer SJ. BAX-induced cell death may not require interleukin 1β-cinvertin enzyme-like proteases. *Proc Natl Acad Sci U S A* 1996;93:14559–14563.
57. Yang E, Zha J, Jockel J, Boise LH, Thompson CB, Korsmeyer SJ. Bad, a heterodimeric partner for Bcl-x$_L$ and Bcl-2, displaces Bax and promotes cell death. *Cell* 1995;80:285–291.
58. Gajewski TF, Thompson CB. Apoptosis meets signal transduction: elimination of a BAD influence. *Cell* 1996;87:589–592.

59. Chang BS, Minn AJ, Muchmore SW, Fesik SW, Thompson CB. Identification of a novel regulatory domain in Bcl-x$_L$ and Bcl-2. *EMBO J* 1997;16:968–977.

60. Muchmore SW, Sattler M, Liang H, et al. X-ray and NMR structure of human Bcl-x$_L$, an inhibitor of programmed cell death. *Nature* 1996;381:335–341.

61. Sattler M, Liang H, Nettesheim D, et al. Structure of Bcl-x$_L$–Bak peptide complex: recognition between regulators of apoptosis. *Science* 1997;275:983–986.

62. Boyd JM, Gallo GJ, Elangovan B, et al. Bik, a novel death-inducing protein shares a distinct sequence motif with Bcl-2 family proteins and interacts with viral and cellular survival-promoting proteins. *Oncogene* 1995;11:1921–1928.

63. Wang K, Yin X-M, Chao DT, Milliman CL, Korsmeyer SJ. BID: a novel BH3 domain-only death agonist. *Genes Dev* 1996;10:2859–2869.

64. Inohara N, Ding L, Chen S, Núñez. Harakiri, a novel regulator of cell death, encodes a protein that activates apoptosis and interacts selectively with survival-promoting proteins Bcl-2 and Bcl-x$_L$. *EMBO J* 1997;16:1686–1694.

65. Kelekar A, Chang BS, Harlan JE, Fesik SW, Thompson CB. Bad is a BH3 domain–containing protein that forms an inactivating dimer with Bcl-x$_L$. *Mol Cell Biol* 1997;17:7040–7046.

66. Chinnaiyan AM, O'Rourke K, Lane BR, Dixit VM. Interaction of CED-4 with CED-3 and CED-9: a molecular framework for cell death. *Science* 1997;275:1122–1126.

67. Wu D, Wallen HD, Nuñez G. Interaction and regulation of subcellular localization of CED-4 by CED-9. *Science* 1997;275:1126–1129.

68. James C, Gschmeissner S, Fraser A, Evan GI. CED-4 induces chromatin condensation in *Schizosaccharomyces pombe* and is inhibited by direct physical association with CED-9. *Curr Biol* 1997;7:246–252.

69. Minn AJ, Vélez P, Schendel SL, et al. Bcl-x$_L$ forms an ion channel in synthetic lipid membranes. *Nature* 1997;385:353–357.

70. Antonsson B, Conti F, Ciavatta AM, et al. Inhibition of Bax channel-forming activity by Bcl-2. *Science* 1997;277:370–372.

71. Schendel SL, et al. Channel formation by antiapoptotic protein Bcl-2. *Proc Natl Acad Sci U S A* 1997;94:5113–5118.

72. Schlesinger PH, Gross A, Yin X-M, et al. Comparison of the ion channel characteristics of proapoptotic BAX and antiapoptotic BCL-2. *Proc Natl Acad Sci U S A* 1997;94:11357–11362.

73. Duckett CS, Wang J, Li F, Tomaselli KJ, Thompson CB, Armstrong RC. Human IAP-like protein is a downstream regulator of programmed cell death. *Mol Cell Biol* 1998;18:608–615.

73a. Kharbanda S, Pandey P, Schofield L, et al. Role for Bcl-x$_L$ as an inhibitor of cytosolic cytochrome C accumulation in DNA damage-induced apoptosis. *Proc Natl Acad Sci USA* 1997;94:6939–6942.

74. Smith CA, Farrah T, Goodwin RG. The TNF receptor superfamily of cellular and viral proteins: activation, costimulation, and death. *Cell* 1994;76:959–962.

75. Thome M, Schneider P, Hofmann K, et al. Viral FLICE-inhibitory proteins (FLIPs) prevent apoptosis induced by death receptors. *Nature* 1997;386:517–520.

76. Bertin J, Armstrong RC, Ottilie S, et al. Death effector domain–containing herpesvirus and poxvirus proteins inhibit Fas- and TNFR1-induced apoptosis. *Proc Natl Acad Sci U S A* 1997;94:1172–1176.

77. Lee M-A, Yates JL. BHRF1 of Epstein-Barr virus, which is homologous to human proto-oncogene bcl2, is not essential for transformation of B cells or for virus replication in vitro. *J Virol* 1992;66:1899–1906.

77a. Cheng EH-Y, Nicholas J, Bellows DS, et al. A Bcl-2 homolog encoded by Kaposi sarcoma–associated virus, human herpesvirus 8, inhibits apoptosis but does not heterodimerize with Bax or Bak. *Proc Natl Acad Sci U S A* 1997;94:690–694.

78. Han J, Sabbatini P, Perez D, Rao L, Modha D, White E. The E1B 19K protein blocks apoptosis by interacting with and inhibiting the p53-inducible and death-promoting Bax protein. *Genes Dev* 1995;10:461–477.

79. Ray CA, Black RA, Kronheim SR, et al. Viral inhibition of inflammation: cowpox virus encodes an inhibitor of the interleukin-1β converting enzyme. *Cell* 1992;69:597–604.

80. Clem RJ, Fechheimer M, Miller LK. Prevention of apoptosis by a baculovirus gene during infection of insect cells. *Science* 1991;254:1388–1390.

81. Crook NE, Clem RJ, Miller LK. An apoptosis-inhibiting baculovirus gene with a zinc finger-like motif. *J Virol* 1993;67:2168–2174.

82. Deveraux QL, Takahashi R, Salvesen GS, Reed JC. X-linked IAP is a direct inhibitor of cell-death proteases. *Nature* 1997;388:300–304.

83. Duckett CS, Nave VE, Gedrich RW, et al. A conserved family of cellular genes related to the baculovirus iap gene and encoding apoptosis inhibitors. *EMBO J* 1996;15:2685–2694.

84. Uren AG, Pakusch M, Hawkins CJ, Puls KL, Vaux DL. Cloning and expression of apoptosis inhibitory protein homologs that function to inhibit apoptosis and/or bind tumor necrosis factor receptor associated factors. *Proc Natl Acad Sci U S A* 1996;93:4974–4978.

85. Liston P, Roy N, Tamai K, et al. Suppression of apoptosis in mammalian cells by NAIP and a related family of IAP genes. *Nature* 1996;379:349–353.

86. Rothe M, Pan M-G, Henzel WJ, Ayres TM, Goeddel DV. The TNFR2-TRAF signaling complex contains two novel proteins related to baculoviral inhibitor of apoptosis proteins. *Cell* 1995;83:1243–1252.

87. Henkart PA. Lymphocyte-mediated cytotoxicity two pathways and multiple effector molecules. *Immunity* 1994;1:343–346.

88. Kägi D, Ledermann B, Bürki K, et al. Cytotoxicity mediated by T cells and natural killer cells is greatly impaired in perforin-deficient mice. *Nature* 1994;369:31–37.

89. Sarin A, Williams MS, Alexander-Miller MA, Berzofsky JA, Zacharchuk CM, Henkart PA. Target cell lysis by CTL granule exocytosis is independent of ICE/Ced-3 family proteases. *Immunity* 1997;6:209–215.

90. Darmon AJ, Nicholson DW, Bleackley RC. Activation of the apoptotic protease CPP32 by cytotoxic T cell–derived granzyme B. *Nature* 1995;377:446–448.

91. Quan LT, Tewari M, O'Rourke K, et al. Proteolytic activation of the cell death protease Yama/CPP32 by granzyme B. *Proc Natl Acad Sci U S A* 1996;93:1972–1976.

92. Shresta S, MacIvor DM, Heusel DM, Russell JH, Ley TJ. Natural killer and lymphokine-activated killer cells require granzyme B for the rapid induction of apoptosis in susceptible target cells. *Proc Natl Acad Sci U S A* 1995;92:5679–5683.

93. Surh CD, Sprent J. T-cell apoptosis detected in situ during positive and negative selection in the thymus. *Nature* 1994;372:100–103.

94. Clayton LK, Ghendler Y, Mizoguchi E, et al. T-cell receptor ligation by peptide/MHC induces activation of a caspase in immature thymocytes: the molecular basis of negative selection. *EMBO J* 1997;16:2282–2293.

95. Ma A, Pena JC, Chang B, et al. Bcl-x regulates the survival of double positive thymocytes. *Proc Natl Acad Sci U S A* 1995;92:4763–4767.

96. Motoyama N, Wang F, Roth KA, et al. Massive cell death of immature hematopoietic cells and neurons in Bcl-x–deficient mice. *Science* 1995;267:1506–1510.

96a. Chao D, Linette GP, Boise LH, White LS, Thompson CB, Korsmeyer SJ. Bcl-x$_L$ and Bcl-2 repress a common pathway of cell death. *J Exp Med* 1995;182:821–828.

97. Woronicz JD, Calnan B, Ngo V, Winoto A. Requirement for the orphan steroid receptor Nur77 in apoptosis of T-cell hybridomas. *Nature* 1994;367:277–281.

97a. Cheng LE-C, Chan FK-M, Cado D, Winoto A. Functional redundancy of the Nur77 and Nor-1 orphan steroid receptors in T-cell apoptosis. *EMBO J* 1997;16:1865–1875.

98. Liu Z-G, Smith SW, McLaughlin KA, Schwartz LM, Osborne BA. Apoptotic signals delivered through the T-cell receptor of a T-cell hybrid require the immediate-early gene nur77. *Nature* 1994;367:281–284.

99. Noel PJ, Boise LH, Green JM, Thompson CB. CD28 costimulation prevents cell death during primary T cell activation. *J Immunol* 1996;157:636–642.

100. Cyster JG, Hartley SB, Goodnow CC. Competition for follicular niches excludes self-reactive cells from the recirculating B-cell repertoire. *Nature* 1994;371:389–395.

101. Lam K-P, Kühn R, Rajewsky K. In vivo ablation of surface immunoglobulin on mature B cells by inducible gene targeting results in rapid cell death. *Cell* 1997;90:1073–1083.

102. Tanchot C, Lemonnier FA, Pérarnau B, Freitas AA, Rocha B. Differential requirements for survival and proliferation of CD8 naïve or memory T cells. *Science* 1997;276:2057–2062.

103. Boise LH, Minn AJ, June CH, Lindsten T, Thompson CB. Growth factors can enhance lymphocyte survival without committing the cell to undergo cell division. *Proc Natl Acad Sci U S A* 1995;92:5491–5495.

104. Vella AT, McCormack JE, Linsley PS, Kappler JW, Marrack P. Lipopolysaccharide interferes with the induction of peripheral T cell death. *Immunity* 1995;2:261–270.

105. Veis DJ, Sorenson CM, Shutter JR, Korsmeyer SJ. Bcl-2-deficient mice demonstrate fulminant lymphoid apoptosis, polycystic kidneys, and hypopigmented hair. *Cell* 1993;75:229–240.

106. Nakayama K-i, Nakayama K, Negishi I, et al. Disappearance of the lymphoid system in Bcl-2 homozygous mutant chimeric mice. *Science* 1993;261:1584–1588.

107. Boise LH, Minn AJ, Noel PJ, et al. CD28 costimulation can promote T cell survival by enhancing the expression of Bcl-x$_L$. *Immunity* 1995;3:87–98.

108. Radvanyi LG, Shi Y, Vaziri H, et al. CD28 costimulation inhibits TCR-induced apoptosis during primary T cell response. *J Immunol* 1996;156:1788–1798.

109. Vella AT, Mitchell T, Groth B, et al. CD28 engagement and proinflammatory cytokines contribute to T cell expansion and long-term survival in vivo. *J Immunol* 1997;158:4714–4720.

110. Tsubata T, Wu J, Honjo T. B-cell apoptosis induced by antigen receptor crosslinking is blocked by a T-cell signal through CD40. *Nature* 1993;364:645–648.

111. Choi MSK, Boise LH, Gottschalk AR, Quintans J, Thompson CB, Klaus GGB. The role of bcl x$_L$ in CD40-mediated rescue from anti-µ–induced apoptosis in WEHI-231 B lymphoma cells. *Eur J Immunol* 1995;25:1352–1357.

112. Ishida T, Kobayashi N, Tojo T, Ishida S, Yamamoto T, Inoue J-I. CD40 signaling-mediated induction of Bcl-x$_L$, Cdk4, and Cdk6. *J Immunol* 1995;155:5527–5535.

113. Illera VA, Perandones CE, Stunz LL, Mower DA Jr, Ashman RF. Apoptosis in splenic B lymphocytes. *J Immunol* 1993;151:2965–2973.

114. Renauld J-C, Vink A, Louahed J, Van Snick J. Interleukin-9 is a major anti-apoptotic factor for thymic lymphomas. *Blood* 1995;85:1300–1305.

115. Chauhan D, Kharbanda S, Ogata A, et al. Interleukin-6 inhibits Fas-induced apoptosis and stress-activated protein kinase activation in multiple myeloma cells. *Blood* 1997;89:227–234.

116. Kuroda K, Yagi J, Imanishi K, et al. Implantation of IL-2–containing osmotic pump prolongs the survival of superantigen-reactive T cells expanded in mice injected with bacterial superantigen. *J Immunol* 1996;157:1422–1431.

117. Lenardo MJ. Fas and the art of lymphocyte maintenance. *J Exp Med* 1996;183:721–724.

117a.Crispe IN. Fatal interactions: Fas-induced apoptosis of mature T cells. *Immunity* 1994;1:347–349.

118. Dhein J, Walczak H, Bäumler C, Debatin K-M, Krammer PH. Autocrine T-cell suicide mediated by APO-1/(Fas/CD95). *Nature* 1995;373:438–440.

119. Brunner T, Mogil RJ, LaFace D, et al. Cell-autonomous Fas (CD95)/Fas-ligand interaction mediates activation-induced apoptosis in T-cell hybridomas. *Nature* 1995;373:441–443.

120. Ju S-T, Panka DJ, Cui H, et al. Fas(CD95)/FasL interactions required for programmed cell death after T-cell activation. *Nature* 1995;373:444–448.

121. Singer GG, Abbas AK. The Fas antigen is involved in peripheral but not thymic deletion of T lymphocytes in T cell receptor transgenic mice. *Immunity* 1994;1: 365–371.

122. Zheng L, Fisher G, Miller RE, Peschon J, Lynch DH, Lenardo MJ. Induction of apoptosis in mature T cells by tumor necrosis factor. *Nature* 1995;377:348–351.

123. Zhou T, Edwards CK III, Yang P, Wang Z, Bluethmann H, Mountz JD. Greatly accelerated lymphadenopathy and autoimmune disease in lpr mice lacking tumor necrosis factor receptor. *J Immunol* 1996;156:2661–2665.

124. Watanabe-Fukunaga R, Brannan CI, Copeland NG, Jenkins NA, Nagata S. Lymphoproliferation disorder in mice explained by defects in Fas antigen that mediates apoptosis. *Nature* 1992;356:314–317.

125. Rieux-Laucat F, Le Deist F, Hivroz C, et al. Mutations in Fas associated with human lymphoproliferative syndrome and autoimmunity. *Science* 1995;268: 1347–1349.

126. Boise LH, Thompson CB. Hierarchical control of lymphocyte survival. *Science* 1996;274:67–68.

127. Lagresle C, Mondière P, Bella C, Krammer PH, Defrance T. Concurrent engagement of CD40 and the antigen receptor protects naive and memory human B cells from APO-1/Fas–mediated apoptosis. *J Exp Med* 1996;183:1377–1388.

128. Garrone P, Neidhardt E-M, Garcia E, Galibert L, van Kooten C, Banchereau J. Fas ligation induces apoptosis of CD40-activated human B lymphocytes. *J Exp Med* 1995;182:1265–1273.

128a. Rathmell JC, Townsend SE, Xu JC, Flavell RA, Goodnow CC. Expansion or elimination of B cells in vivo: dual roles for CD40- and Fas (CD95)-ligand modulated by the B cell antigen receptor. *Cell* 1996;87:319–329.

129. Schattner EJ, Elkon KB, Yoo D-H, et al. CD40 ligation induces Apo-1/Fas expression on human B lymphocytes and facilitates apoptosis through the Apo-1/Fas Pathway. *J Exp Med* 1995;182:1557–1565.

130. Zha J, Harada H, Yang E, Jockel J, Korsmeyer SJ. Serine phosphorylation of death agonist BAD in response to survival factor results in binding to 14-3-3 not BCL-X(L). *Cell* 1996;87:589–592.

131. del Peso L, González-García M, Page C, Herrera R, Nuñez G. Interleukin-3–induced phosphorylation of BAD through the protein kinase Akt. *Science* 1997;278:687–689.

132. Datta SR, Dudek H, Tao X, et al. Akt phosphorylation of BAD couples survival signals to the cell-intrinsic death machinery. *Cell* 1997;91:231–241.

133. Kauffmann-Zeh A, Rodriguez-Viciana P, Ulrich E, et al. Suppression of c-Myc–induced apoptosis by Ras signalling through PI(3)K and PKB. *Nature* 1997;385:544–548.

134. Kulik G, Klippel A, Weber MJ. Antiapoptotic signalling by the insulin-like growth factor I receptor, phosphatidylinositol 3-kinase, and Akt. *Mol Cell Biol* 1997;17:1595–1606.

135. Dudek H, Datta SR, Franke TF, et al. Regulation of neuronal survival by the serine-threonine protein kinase Akt. *Science* 1997;275:661–664.

136. Franke TF, Kaplan DR, Cantley LC. PI3K: downstream AKTion blocks apoptosis. *Cell* 1997;88:435–437.

137. Kennedy SG, Wagner AJ, Conzen SD, et al. The PI 3-kinase/Akt signaling pathway delivers an anti-apoptotic signal. *Genes Dev* 1997;11:701–713.

138. Strasser A, Harris AW, Huang DCS, Krammer PH, Cory S. Bcl-2 and Fas/APO-1 regulated distinct pathways to lymphocyte apoptosis. *EMBO J* 1995;14:6136–6147.

139. Memon SA, Moreno MB, Petrak D, Zacharchuk CM. Bcl-2 blocks glucocorticoid- but not Fas- or activation-induced apoptosis in a T cell hybridoma. *J Immunol* 1995;155:4644–4652.

140. Galle PR, Hofmann WJ, Walczak H, et al. Involvement of the CD95 (APO-1/Fas) receptor and ligand in liver damage. *J Exp Med* 1995;182:1223–1230.

141. Van Parijs L, Ibraghimov A, Abbas AK. The roles of costimulation and Fas in T cell apoptosis and peripheral tolerance. *Immunity* 1996;4:321–328.

142. Rodriguez I, Matsuura K, Khatib K, Reed JC, Nagata S, Vassalli P. A bcl-2 transgene expressed in hepatocytes protects mice from fulminant liver destruction but not from rapid death induced by anti-Fas antibody injection. *J Exp Med* 1996;183:1031–1036.

143. Boldin MP, Varfolomeev EE, Pancer Z, Mett IL, Camonis JH, Wallach D. A novel protein that interacts with the death domain of Fas/APO-1 contains a sequence motif related to the death domain. *J Biol Chem* 1995;270:7795–7798.

144. Chinnaiyan AM, Tepper CG, Seldin MF, et al. FADD/MORT1 is a common mediator of CD95 (Fas/APO-1) and tumor necrosis factor receptor–induced apoptosis. *J Biol Chem* 1996;271:4961–4965.

145. Boldin MP, Goncharov TM, Goltsev YV, Wallach D. Involvement of MACH, a novel MORT1/FADD–interacting protease, in Fas/APO-1–and TNF receptor–induced cell death. *Cell* 1996;85:803–815.

146. Muzio M, Chinnaiyan AM, Kischkel FC, et al. FLICE, a novel FADD-homologous ICE/CED-3–like protease, is recruited to the CD95 (Fas/APO-1) death-inducing signaling complex. *Cell* 1996;85:817–827.

147. Zhang X, Li L, Choe J, et al. Up-regulation of Bcl-x_L expression protects CD40-activated human B cells from Fas-mediated apoptosis. *Cell Immunol* 1996;173: 149–154.

148. Boise LH, Thompson CB. Bcl-x_L can inhibit apoptosis in cells that have undergone Fas-induced protease activation. *Proc Natl Acad Sci U S A* 1997;94: 3759–3764.

149. Peter ME, Medema JP, Krammer PH. Does the *Caenorhabditis elegans* protein CED-4 contain a region of homology to the mammalian death effector domain? *Cell Death Differ* 1997;4:523–525.

150. Tartaglia LA, Ayres TM, Wong GHW, Goeddel DV. A novel domain within the 55 kd TNF receptor signals cell death. *Cell* 1993;74:845–853.

151. Walczak H, Degli-Esposti MA, Johnson RS, et al. TRAIL-R2: a novel apoptosis-mediating receptor for TRAIL. *EMBO J* 1997;16:5386–5397.

152. Pan G, O'Rourke K, Chinnaiyan AM, et al. The receptor for the cytotoxic ligand TRAIL. *Science* 1997;276:111–113.

153. Marsters SA, Sheridan JP, Donahue CJ, et al. Apo-3, a new member of the tumor necrosis factor receptor family, contains a death domain and activates apoptosis and NF-κB. *Curr Biol* 1996;6:1669–1676.

154. Kitson J, Raven T, Jiang Y-P, et al. A death-domain–containing receptor that mediates apoptosis. *Nature* 1996;384:372–375.

155. Pan G, Ni J, Wei Y-F, Yu G-L, Gentz R, Dixit VM. An antagonist decoy receptor and a death domain-containing receptor for TRAIL. *Science* 1997;277:815–818.

156. Sheridan JP, Marsters SA, Pitti RM, et al. Control of TRAIL-induced apoptosis by a family of signaling and decoy receptors. *Science* 1997;277:818–821.

157. Bazzoni F, Beutler B. The tumor necrosis factor ligand and receptor families. *Semin Med Beth Israel Hosp* 1996;334:1717–1725.

158. Kehry MR. CD40-mediated signaling in B cells balancing cell survival, growth, and death. *J Immunol* 1996;156:2345–2348.

159. Rothe M, Wong SC, Henzel WJ, Goeddel DV. A novel family of putative signal transducers associated with the cytoplasmic domain of the 75 kDa tumor necrosis factor receptor. *Cell* 1994;78:681–692.

160. Cheng G, Cleary AM, Ye Z-S, Hong DI, Lederman S, Baltimore D. Involvement of CRAF1, a relative of TRAF, in CD40 signaling. *Science* 1995;267:1494–1498.

161. Régnier CH, Tomasetto C, Moog-Lutz C, et al. Presence of a new conserved domain in CART1, a novel member of the tumor necrosis factor receptor–associated protein family, which is expressed in breast carcinoma. *J Biol Chem* 1995;270:25715–25721.

162. Nakano H, Oshima H, Chung W, et al. TRAF5, an activator of NF-κB and putative signal transducer for the lymphotoxin-β receptor. *J Biol Chem* 1996;271: 14661–14664.

163. Ishida T, Mizushima S-i, Azuma S, et al. Identification of TRAF6, a novel tumor necrosis factor receptor–associated factor protein that mediates signaling from an amino-terminal domain of the CD40 cytoplasmic region. *J Biol Chem* 1996; 271:28745–28748.

164. Rothe M, Sarma V, Dixit VM, Goeddel DV. TRAF2-mediated activation of NF-κB by TNF receptor 2 and CD40. *Science* 1995;269:1424–1427.

165. Song HY, Régnier CH, Kirschning CJ, Goeddel DV, Rothe M. Tumor necrosis factor (TNF)–mediated kinase cascades: bifurcation of nuclear factor-κB and c-jun N-terminal kinase (JNK/SAPK) pathways at TNF receptor–associated factor 2. *Proc Natl Acad Sci U S A* 1997;94:9792–9796.

166. Duckett CS, Gedrich RW, Gilfillan MC, Thompson CB. Induction of nuclear factor kB by the CD30 receptor is mediated by TRAF1 and TRAF2. *Mol Cell Biol* 1997;17:1535–1542.

167. Arch RH, Thompson CB. 4-1BB and Ox40 are members of a TNF/NGF receptor subfamily that bind TRAF proteins and activate nuclear factor κB. *Mol Cell Biol* 1998;18:558–565.

168. Lee SY, Park CG, Choi Y. T cell receptor–dependent cell death of T cell hybridomas mediated by the CD30 cytoplasmic domain in association with tumor necrosis factor receptor–associated factors. *J Exp Med* 1996;183:669–674.

169. Duckett CS, Thompson CB. CD30-dependent degradation of TRAF2: implications for negative regulation of TRAF signaling and the control of cell survival. *Genes Dev* 1997;11:2810–2821.

170. Wang C-Y, Mayo MW, Baldwin Jr AS. TNF- and cancer therapy–induced apoptosis: potentiation by inhibition of NF-κB. *Science* 1996;274:784–787.

171. Liu Z-g, Hsu H, Goeddel DV, Karin M. Dissection of TNF receptor 1 effector functions: JNK activation is not linked to apoptosis while NF-κB activation prevents cell death. *Cell* 1996;87:555–576.

172. Wu M, Lee H, Bellas RE, et al. Inhibition of NF-κB/Rel induces apoptosis of murine B cells. *EMBO J* 1996;15:4682–4690.

173. Lai J-H, Tan T-H. CD28 signaling causes a sustained down-regulation of IkBa which can be prevented by the immunosuppressant rapamycin. *J Biol Chem* 1994;269:3077–30080.

174. Scheinman RI, Cogswell PC, Lofquist AK, Baldwin AS Jr. Role of transcriptional activation of IκBα in mediation of immunosuppression by glucocorticoids. *Science* 1995;270:283–286.

175. Auphan N, DiDonato JA, Rosette C, Helmberg A, Karin M. Immunosuppression by glucocorticoids: inhibition of NF-κB activity through induction of IkB synthesis. *Science* 1995;270:286–290.

176. Beg AA, Baltimore D. An essential role for NF-kappaB in preventing TNF-alpha induced cell death. *Science* 1996;274:782–784.

177. Hsu H, Shu H-B, Pan M-G, Goeddel DV. TRADD-TRAF2 and TRADD-FADD interactions define two distinct TNF receptor 1 signal transduction pathways. *Cell* 1996;84:299–308.

178. Irmler M, Thome M, Hahne M, et al. Inhibition of death receptor signals by cellular FLIP. *Nature* 1997;388:190–195.

178a. Inohara N, Koseki T, Hu Y, Chen S, Núñez G. CLARP, a death effector domain–containing protein interacts with caspase-8 and regulates apoptosis. *Proc Natl Acad Sci U S A* 1997;94:10717–10722.

179. Shu H-B, Halpin DR, Goeddel DV. Casper is a FADD- and caspase-related inducer of apoptosis. *Immunity* 1997;6:751–763.

180. Levine BL, Bernstein WB, Connors M, et al. Effects of CD28 costimulation on long-term proliferation of CD4+ T cells in the absence of exogenous feeder cells. *J Immunol* 1997;159:5921–5930.

181. Lau HT, Yu M, Fontana A, Stoeckert CJ Jr. Prevention of islet allograft rejection with engineered myoblasts expressing FasL in mice. *Science* 1996;273:109–112.

182. Waterhouse P, Penninger JM, Timms E, et al. Lymphoproliferative disorders with early lethality in mice deficient in Ctla-4. *Science* 1995;270:985–988.

183. Shull MM, Ormsby I, Kier AB, et al. Targeted disruption of the mouse transforming growth factor-beta 1 gene results in multifocal inflammatory disease. *Nature* 1992;359:693–699.

184. Green DR, Ware CF. Fas-ligand: privilege and peril. *Proc Natl Acad Sci U S A* 1997;94:5986–5990.

185. Streilein JW, Ksander BR, Taylor AW. Immune deviation in relation to ocular immune privilege. *J Immunol* 1997;158:3557–3560.

186. Griffith TS, Brunner T, Fletcher SM, Green DR, Ferguson TA. Fas ligand–induced apoptosis as a mechanism of immune privilege. *Science* 1995;270:1189–1192.

187. Bellgrau D, Gold D, Selawry H, Moore J, Franzusoff A, Duke RC. A role for CD95 ligand in preventing graft rejection. *Nature* 1995;377:630–632.

188. Hunt JS, Vassmer D, Ferguson TA, Miller L. Fas ligand is positioned in mouse uterus and placenta to prevent trafficking of activated leukocytes between the mother and the conceptus. *J Immunol* 1997;158:4122–4128.

189. Hahne M, Rimoldi D, Schröter M, et al. Melanoma cell expression of Fas(Apo-1/CD95) ligand: implications for tumor immune escape. *Science* 1996;274:1363–1366.

190. Griffith TS, Yu X, Herndon JM, Green DR, Ferguson TA. CD95-induced apoptosis of lymphocytes in an immune privileged site induces immunological tolerance. *Immunity* 1996;5:7–16.

191. Casciola-Rosen LA, Anhalt G, Rosen A. Autoantigens targeted in systemic lupus erythematosus are clustered in two populations of surface structures on apoptotic keratinocytes. *J Exp Med* 1994;179:1317–1330.

Fundamental Immunology, Fourth Edition,
edited by William E. Paul
Published by Lippincott–Raven Publishers, Philadelphia 1999.

CHAPTER 24

Immunoglobulin Class Switching

Clifford M. Snapper and Fred D. Finkelman

Antibodies bind to specific targets and damage these by inducing different effector mechanisms. Antibody specificity and affinity are determined primarily by amino acid sequences of light-chain and heavy-chain variable regions, although immunoglobulin heavy-chain constant regions can, in some circumstances, influence antibody affinity (1). The avidity with which an antibody molecule binds a multivalent antigen increases both with increases in antibody affinity and with the number of antigen-binding sites per antibody molecule. The specific effector mechanisms that can be elicited by an antibody, on the other hand, are determined primarily by the class (isotype) of heavy chain expressed by the antibody molecule. This chapter considers the different immunoglobulin isotypes and discusses, sequentially, differences in function between different immunoglobulin isotypes, the cytokines, and other stimuli that control immunoglobulin isotype expression, and the molecular mechanisms through which these stimuli function.

IMMUNOGLOBULIN ISOTYPE FUNCTION

Classification of Immunoglobulin Isotypes in Mouse, Rat, and Human

In the three mammalian species in which immunoglobulin isotypes have been most thoroughly studied—mouse, rat, and human—five main classes of immunoglobulin heavy chains have been

demonstrated: IgM, IgD, IgG, IgA, and IgE. In addition, in all three species, four subclasses of IgG are produced (IgG1, IgG2a, IgG2b, and IgG3 in the mouse; IgG1, IgG2a, IgG2b, and IgG2c in the rat; IgG1, IgG2, IgG3, and IgG4 in the human). In the human, there are also two classes of IgA (IgA1 and IgA2). In addition to differences in size and valency, differences in the structures of the heavy chains of the different isotypes result in differences in *in vivo* half-life, binding to cellular receptors, complement fixation, sensitivity to digestion by proteolytic enzymes, and the tendency to form aggregates.

IgM

Initial antibody responses are primarily of the IgM isotype (2,3). Inasmuch as IgM antibodies generally express germline-determined variable regions that have not yet been modified by somatic mutation, they tend to bind antigens with low affinity (4,5). The low affinity of most IgM antibodies is compensated by their ten antigen-binding sites, which allow even a low-affinity antibody to bind with high avidity to an antigen that has multiple representations of the same epitope (6,7). In addition to their ability to bind avidly to multimeric antigens, IgM antibodies can destroy or opsonize targets through their very efficient fixation of complement (8). These same characteristics, however, create a potential danger, in that even low-affinity antibodies to self antigens that express multiple copies of the same epitope, such as erythrocytes, can produce substantial damage. A second limitation that results from the pentameric structure of IgM is its limited ability to diffuse rapidly from sites of local production to distant sites (9). For this reason, and because of its short *in vivo* half-life relative to IgG (10,11), IgM antibodies are probably less well adapted than IgG antibodies to protect against second infections by a pathogen.

C. M. Snapper: Department of Pathology, Uniformed Services University of the Health Sciences, Bethesda, Maryland 20814.
F. D. Finkelman: Division of Immunology, University of Cincinnati Medical Center, Cincinnati, Ohio 45267-0563.

IgM Versus Non-IgM Antibodies

Antibodies of the IgG, IgA, and IgE isotypes are made later than IgM antibodies during a primary immune response, but they account for most of the antibody that is produced during a memory response. Although isotype-switching and affinity maturation are independent processes, they usually occur simultaneously (12), so that the affinity of bivalent antibodies of isotypes other than IgM is great enough to allow for high-avidity binding of antigen. IgG antibodies are the predominant isotype in plasma and extravascular lymph (13), while IgA antibodies predominate in respiratory, digestive, and urogenital secretions (14).

IgG Subclasses

Functional Properties of IgG Subclasses

The different IgG subclasses share a long half-life, which facilitates the maintenance of high serum IgG levels. In mouse, rat, and human, the different IgG subclasses differ in effector function. Complement is fixed most effectively by IgG2a and IgG2b in the mouse (15,16), IgG2b in the rat (17), and IgG1 and IgG3 in human (18,19). Mouse IgG3 and possibly IgG1; rat IgG1, IgG2a, and IgG2c; and human IgG2 antibodies also have some ability to fix complement (17). Rodent and human IgG subclasses also differ in their abilities to bind to Fcγ receptors. FcγRI, which is expressed on rodent monocytes and macrophages, binds mouse IgG2a and rat IgG2b with high affinity (20–22). Mouse FcγRII (on macrophages, monocytes, B-lymphocytes, mast cells, and some T-lymphocytes) and FcγRIII [on macrophages, neutrophils, mast cells, and natural killer (NK) cells] bind mouse IgG2b > IgG2a > IgG1; all with low affinity (21,23). None of these receptors binds mouse IgG3 effectively. Human FcγRI (on monocytes, macrophages, and neutrophils) binds IgG1 and IgG3 most avidly and IgG2 to a lesser degree (21,23–25). Human FcγRII (on macrophages, monocytes, neutrophils, and B cells) and FcγRIII (on monocytes, macrophages, NK cells, neutrophils, and some T cells) selectively bind, with low affinity, IgG1 and IgG3 (21,23). In addition, some IgG isotypes (IgG1 in the mouse, IgG2a in the rat) bind to mast-cell receptors and can mediate mast-cell degranulation (26,27). IgG isotypes also bind to placental Fc receptors, which facilitate transport of maternal IgG (but not other isotypes) into the fetal circulation (28) and to FcRn, a major histocompatibility complex (MHC) class I–related receptor that promotes intestinal absorption of maternal IgG in young animals and extends the *in vivo* life span of IgG by returning pinocytosed IgG back to the extracellular space (29,30).

Different Antigenic Stimuli Induce the Production of Different IgG Subclasses

Soluble protein antigens stimulate predominantly IgG1 responses in the mouse (31,32), while carbohydrate antigens induce substantial IgG3 responses in the mouse (31,33), IgG2c responses in the rat (34), and IgG2 responses in the human (35–37). Viruses induce mostly IgG2a responses in the mouse (38) and IgG1 and IgG3 responses in the human (39). Gram-negative bacteria induce IgG2a and, to some extent, IgG3 responses in the mouse (40–42). Nematode parasites induce predominantly IgG1 responses in most mouse strains (43) and are associated with IgG4

responses in the human (44,45). Repeated immunization, especially with allergens that also induce IgE, also tends to induce humans to produce IgG4 antibodies (46).

Physiologic Role of IgG Subclasses

To some extent, the functional properties of particular IgG subclasses appear to make them particularly well suited to the binding or destroying of particular types of antigen or parasite. The ability of mouse IgG2a to effectively fix complement, to bind to the macrophage high-affinity receptor for IgG, and to interact with NK-cell Fcγ receptors would seem to make it particularly well suited to the control of viral and gram-negative bacterial infections. The ability of mouse IgG3 to self-aggregate *after* binding to an antigen that expresses repeated carbohydrate epitopes (47) allows it, unlike IgM, to diffuse easily into sites of bacterial invasion and, like IgM, to form high-avidity interactions with bacterial cell wall carbohydrate antigens, even though carbohydrate antigens tend to induce low-affinity antibody responses. However, human IgG2 antibodies, despite their association with carbohydrate antigens, have not been found to have this autoaggregating feature (47). The ability of mouse IgG1 antibodies to mediate mast-cell degranulation may confer increased resistance to nematode parasites, which typically induce mucosal mast-cell responses.

Role of IgG Subclasses in Disease

Functional properties that might be expected to enhance the ability of an immunoglobulin isotype to destroy a pathogen may also, however, contribute to its potential to damage the host. The autoaggregating properties of mouse IgG3 antibodies appear to make them more likely than other isotypes to be cryoglobulins that cause vascular damage and glomerulonephritis (48). The ability of human IgG1 and IgG3 antibodies to bind to Fcγ receptors makes them, rather than IgG2 and IgG4 antibodies, mediators of erythrocyte destruction in patients with hemolytic disease of the newborn (49). The ability of mouse IgG1 to mediate mast-cell degranulation may contribute to its ability to induce anaphylaxis (50).

Redundancy in the Functions of IgG Subclasses

The correlation, however, between functional properties of individual immunoglobulin isotypes and their expression in response to different antigens or pathogens should not be taken as evidence that individual IgG subclasses are essential for protection against different pathogens. Rabbits, for example, produce only a single IgG isotype (51), yet appear to be immunologically competent. It is possible, however, that the multiple IgA isotypes produced by rabbits substitute for the diversity of IgG isotypes that are present in mouse and human (51). Passive transfer studies, in which the protective effects of injecting rodents with antibodies of different IgG isotype against subsequent challenge with infectious agents have not consistently shown the expected preference for a particular IgG subclass in providing protection. Mouse IgG1, IgG2b, and IgG3 monoclonal antibodies, which bound to phosphocholine epitopes on pneumococcal polysaccharide and shared similar or identical variable regions, provided equivalent protection against infection with *Streptococcus pneumoniae* (52). Normal serum antibodies of the IgG1 or IgG2 isotype were equally efficacious at enabling passively immunized mice to clear *Trypanosoma cruzi*

(53). Monoclonal rat IgG1, IgG2a, IgG2b, and IgG2c anti-*E.coli* lipopolysaccharide (LPS) antibodies that have identical variable regions (isotype-switch variants) each effectively promoted hepatic clearance and killing of injected *E. coli* cells, while IgM, IgA, and IgE switch variants did not (54). A separate study, on the other hand, demonstrated that IgM monoclonal antibodies against *E. coli* LPS were more efficient at protecting mice against peritoneal challenge with *E. coli* than was an unrelated IgG2a antibody against the same determinant, and that the IgG2a antibody provided protection at a lower dose than did unrelated IgG1, IgG2b, or IgG3 monoclonal antibodies specific for that determinant (55). However, experiments performed by the same laboratory with isotype-switch variants of a monoclonal anti-*E. coli* LPS antibody have failed to confirm that different IgG isotypes differ in the efficiency with which they protect hosts against bacterial infection (M. Pollack, personal communication).

Evidence for Functional Specialization of IgG Subclasses

A few passive immunization studies do suggest some influence of IgG subclass on host protection against microbial pathogens. Only IgG2a antibodies from the serum of mice hyperimmunized with *Plasmodium yoelii* altered the course of a challenge infection in passively immunized mice (56); however, it is not clear whether this resulted from qualitative differences in the different isotypes or from differences in their concentrations. IgG2a and IgG2b switch variants of a monoclonal antibody to *Cryptococcus neoformans* provided better clearance of this pathogen from the lungs and spleen of mice infected with this pathogen than did an IgG1 switch variant of the same antibody; however, none of these antibodies influenced *C. neoformans* infection of brain or survival of infected mice (57). In another study, it was observed that an IgG3 monoclonal antibody to *C. neoformans* capsular polysaccharide inhibited the host-protective ability of an IgG1 monoclonal antibody that bound to the same epitope (58); this suggested that different properties of IgG1 and IgG3 antibodies allowed the former isotype to contribute more to host protection than the latter. In view of the strong association between viral infections and IgG2a antibody production in the mouse, it will be of interest to determine if this isotype is particularly effective at protecting against viral infection; however, no studies have been reported of the relative efficiencies of isotype-switch variants of an antivirus monoclonal antibody at protecting against infection.

IgG Subclasses and Human Disease

Studies of humans with deficiencies in the production of specific immunoglobulin isotypes provide data complementary to the mouse passive transfer studies in that they suggest that individual isotypes are not required for protection against infection. Although people with isolated IgG2 deficiency are more likely than people with normal IgG2 serum levels to have infections with encapsulated bacteria, most people with isolated IgG2 deficiency are clinically normal. Furthermore, it is not clear whether the association between low IgG2 level and infection represents a specific lack of IgG2 antibodies to carbohydrate epitopes on bacterial capsules or a lack of antibody specific for these epitopes, regardless of isotype (59). For similar reasons, it is difficult to interpret whether the association between low IgG1 and IgG3 levels and chronic lung

disease represents a requirement for these complement-fixing, Fcγ receptor–binding isotypes for host defense against certain pulmonary pathogens (60).

IgA

As with the IgG subclasses, it is easier to point out properties of IgA antibodies that should make them particularly well suited to protect against infection than to demonstrate that these properties are essential to protect the host. The association of one to two IgA dimers with a molecule of secretory component facilitates transport of this isotype into the gut lumen (61,62). The oligomeric nature of IgA enhances its ability to interact with high avidity with viruses and bacteria that are present in secretions (63), while the lack of barriers to diffusion in secretions removes the liability that would be associated with an antibody's high molecular weight in tissues. Although IgA lacks the ability to fix complement by the classical pathway, it is the most effective isotype at fixing complement by the alternative pathway (64). IgA antibodies, like IgG antibodies, bind well to Fc receptors on neutrophils (65). The high resistance of IgA antibodies to digestion by proteolytic enzymes (61,66) makes this isotype particularly well adapted to function in environments, such as the digestive tract, where host and bacterial proteases are present in high concentration. The affinity of IgA antibodies for *mucus* may reinforce the *mucus* barrier to pathogen penetration of the gut mucosa (67), and terminal mannose-containing oligosaccharides on the α chain of IgA antibodies inhibit interactions between fimbriae on enteric bacteria and oligosaccharides on mucosal epithelial cell plasma membranes that would otherwise promote bacterial adherence to these cells (68). Despite these apparent advantages, mice that have a selective inability to produce IgA have been reported to be no more susceptible than normal mice to infection with the mucosal pathogen, influenza virus (69). Furthermore, the frequency of isolated IgA deficiency in humans is approximately 0.1% (70,71), and most IgA-deficient individuals have no obvious deficiency in immune function (72). However, a minority of IgA-deficient individuals experiences respiratory infections, malabsorption, and autoimmune disorders at increased frequency (73). In most IgA-deficient individuals, IgM antibodies associate with secretory component and replace IgA antibodies as the predominant secretory isotype (74). In at least some of the IgA-deficient patients who have frequent infections, this substitution in secretions of IgM for IgA fails to occur, leading to a more global immune defect (74,75).

IgE

IgE antibodies have the unique ability to bind with high affinity to IgE receptors (FcεRI) on mast cells and basophils, and induce degranulation and cytokine production by these cells when they are crosslinked by antigen (76–79). In addition to its central role in the pathogenesis of atopic disorders, it has been speculated that IgE-mediated mast-cell degranulation, by its release of mediators that increase vascular permeability, has an important role in the initiation of immune responses in general (80–82). IgE may also have a role in the expulsion of gut and respiratory tract multicellular parasites (83). This role may be mediated indirectly through mast-cell degranulation-induced smooth muscle contraction and increased vascular permeability, and through promotion of eosinophil killing of parasites by IgE-mediated antibody-dependent cell-mediated cytotoxicity (ADCC) in rats and humans (82,84,85). However, neutralization of IgE antibodies *in vivo* has had little effect on the expulsion of such parasites in the mouse (I.M. Katona, J.F. Urban, Jr., and F.D. Finkelman, unpublished data), and, while IgE antibodies have been shown in transfer studies to have protective effects against infection with some parasites in rats, these effects were no greater than those that could be achieved by transfer of IgG antibodies (86). In addition to their ability to stimulate mast-cell degranulation and cytokine production, IgE antibodies have been shown to facilitate presentation of soluble antigens through a mechanism that involves binding to FcεRII (87). However, this effect is also not unique, as IgG antibodies can enhance antigen presentation by forming complexes with antigens that can then be bound by FcγR-expressing cells (88,89).

IgD

Even less is known about the function of secreted IgD antibodies. Antibodies of this isotype are present on most rodent and primate B-lymphocytes, where they are expressed with IgM but are secreted to only a very limited extent in mice and to a greater, but quite variable extent, in humans (90,91). Although IgD immune complexes appear to induce the expression of T-cell receptors that enhance helper T-cell function (92), the lack of an obvious defect in mice that have been treated from birth with anti-IgD antibody (93,94) or have had the gene for δ chain deleted by homologous recombination (R. Kühn, personal communication) makes it unlikely that secreted IgD antibodies have a unique role that dramatically affects host immunity.

Summary

These observations, in sum, indicate that (a) different antigenic stimuli tend to induce secretion of different immunoglobulin isotypes, with the exception that IgM secretion always precedes the secretion of other isotypes in a primary response; and (b) different isotypes have functional and structural features that probably make them particularly well suited to defend against different types of pathogen; but (c) the advantages conferred by production of a particular isotype may be both subtle and redundant, and have been difficult to demonstrate in *in vivo* studies.

CONTROL OF IMMUNOGLOBULIN ISOTYPE SWITCHING AT THE CELLULAR LEVEL

Associations between the antigens that are used for immunization and the immunoglobulin isotypes that are secreted during the course of the subsequent immune response suggested that switches from the secretion of IgM to the secretion of other isotypes were controlled, rather than chance events. The demonstration that the addition of culture supernatant produced by an activated, transformed mouse T-cell line to LPS-activated mouse B cells suppressed IgG3 secretion and stimulated IgG1 secretion (95,96) indicated that humoral factors could participate in the control of isotype switching. This observation also provided a starting point for efforts to identify and purify such factors, which culminated in the demonstration that interleukin-4 (IL-4) was responsible for both activities (97,98). Subsequent studies have identified stimuli that control switching to all isotypes other than IgD in mice, and to IgE, IgA, and at least three IgG subclasses in humans. To a more limited

extent, control of murine immunoglobulin isotype switching *in vivo* has also been investigated. At the cellular level, these studies have identified two different kinds of stimuli that are important for the induction of isotype switching: (a) Stimuli that are predominantly responsible for the specificity of the isotype-switch event: These include IL-4, interferon-γ (IFN-γ), transforming growth factor-β (TGF-β), and IL-10. They are all characterized by the ability to induce the transcription of an immature (germline) form of RNA for the heavy-chain isotype to which switching will be induced, as will be described in the final section of this chapter. These cytokines are often referred to as "switch factors." Stimuli that induce switching to one isotype often also stimulate switching to an additional isotype and inhibit switching to other isotypes. (b) Stimuli, or combinations of stimuli, that act in concert with switch factors, in a relatively nonspecific way, to induce DNA synthesis, immunoglobulin secretion, and immunoglobulin class switching: These stimuli may permit switching to occur to any of a number of different isotypes, depending on which of the specific stimuli are present, although some of these stimuli appear to block switching to some isotypes. These B-cell stimuli include LPS, cross-linking of mIg or CD40, IL-4, and IL-5 (for mouse B cells), and infection with Epstein-Barr virus (EBV), cross-linking of mIg; cross-linking of CD40, and cross-linking of the tumor necrosis factor-α (TNF-α) receptor (for human B cells). At the molecular level, *three* processes, under the collective influence of the above stimuli, are needed to induce immunoglobulin class switching: (a) DNA synthesis, (b) germline C_H transcription, and (c) additional factors that may lead to the production or activation of a switch recombinase or allow it to interact with its substrate. These will be discussed in detail later on.

These general principles are best illustrated by discussion of the specific factors that control switching to the different immunoglobulin isotypes (summarized in Table 1).

Control of Switching to IgG isotypes

Mouse IgG1

Interleukin-4 Stimulates Switching to IgG1

IL-4 primes mouse B-lymphocytes for switching to IgG1, as demonstrated by its ability to induce transcription of a germline form of the γ1 gene (99–102). Actual switching, as detected by the expression of mature γ1 mRNA and membrane and/or secreted IgG1, requires additional stimuli. Among the additional stimuli that can induce naive mouse B cells to switch to IgG1 in the presence of IL-4 are (a) LPS (95,103), (b) IL-5 plus a dextran (104) or Sepharose conjugate (105) of antiimmunoglobulin antibody, (c) ligation and cross-linking of CD40 (106–112), and (d) ligation and cross-linking of CD30 (113). IL-4 stimulates both large increases in the percentage of B-cell clones that secrete IgG1 and small increases in clone size in some of these systems (114). B cells do not necessarily need to be exposed to IL-4 at the same time that they are being activated by additional stimuli to be induced to switch to IgG1; this will still occur if they are first pulsed with IL-4 and then washed prior to stimulation with LPS (103).

Interleukin-4–independent Induction of IgG1

Although IL-4 stimulates switching to IgG1, it is not required to induce an IgG1 response. B cells cultured with Th1 cells, which secrete IL-2 and IFN-γ, but not IL-4 (115), secrete some IgG1, par-

TABLE 1. *In vitro cellular systems for murine Ig class switching*

Ig isotype	Effector	Effect	Mechanism	Other Stimuli present
IgG3	LPS	+	A	None
	IFN-γ	+	A	Anti-Ig-dex+IL-5
	IL-10	+	R	LPS
	IFN-γ	-	R	LPS
	IL-4	-	A	LPS, anti-Ig-dex+IL-5
IgG1	IL-4	+	A	LPS, CD40L, angi-Ig-dex+IL-5
	IFN-γ, TGF-β	-	A	(LPS, CD40L, ant-Ig-dex+IL-5)+IL-4
	Anti-Ig-dex	-	R	LPS+IL-4
IgG2b	LPS	+	A	None
	TGF-β	+	A	LPS
	IL-4, IFN-γ	-	A	LPS
IgG2a	IFN-γ	+	A	LPS, anti-Ig-dex+IL-5
	IL-4	-	A	(LPS, anti-Ig-dex+IL-5)+IFN-γ
IgE	IL-4	+	A	LPS, CD40L
	IFN-γ	-	A	(LPS, CD40L)+IL-4
	Anti-Ig-dex	-	A	LPS+IL-4
IgA	TGF-β	+	A	(LPS, CD40L)+IL-4+IL-5+anti-Ig-dex
	IL-4	+	R	(LPS, CD40L)+IL-5+anti-Ig-dex+TGF-β
	IL-5	+	R	(LPS, CD40L)+IL-4+anti-Ig-dex+TGF-β
	IL-10	-	R	(LPS, CD40L)+IL-4+IL-5+anti-Ig-dex+TGF-β

(+), induction; (-), suppression of Ig class switching; A, change in switching associated with corresponding change in germline C_H RNA expression (i.e., [A]ccessibility effect); R, change in switching *not* corresponding with change in germline C_H RNA expression (i.e., [R]ecombination effect).

ticularly if IFN-γ is neutralized and the cultures are supplemented with additional IL-2 (116). B cells will also secrete significant quantities of IgG1 if simulated with dextran-conjugated anti-IgD antibody plus culture supernatants of activated Th1 cells (104). *In vivo* studies demonstrate that IL-4 antagonists (anti–IL-4 or anti–IL-4 receptor monoclonal antibodies) considerably inhibit IgG1 responses to some chronic stimuli (graft-versus-host disease, mercuric chloride) (117,118), but have relatively little effect on at least some acute IgG1 responses (those induced by injection of anti-IgD antibody or inoculation with a nematode parasite) (119,120). Acute IgG1 responses still occur in mice that have had a functional IL-4 gene deleted by homologous recombination (121); however, serum IgG1 levels in these mice are very low prior to immunization, and IgG1 levels following immunization are only 10% to 50% of those observed in normal mice. It is not known whether the differences between the results observed in mice treated with IL-4 antagonists and in the IL-4 "gene knock-out" mice reflect incomplete inhibition of IL-4 activity in the former animals or a chronic effect of IL-4 absence in the genetically deprived mice that leads to increased production of cytokines that inhibit IgG1 responses. Regardless of the cause for this discrepancy, all data demonstrate that IL-4 promotes switching to IgG1 and can contribute importantly to the development of physiologic IgG1 responses, but that alternative mechanisms exist for stimulating switching to IgG1. The ability of resting B cells stimulated by cell membranes from an activated Th1 clone (122), with CD40 ligand (123), or with dextran-anti-Ig antibody (124) to express germline γ1 mRNA transcripts in the absence of IL-4 suggests mechanisms for IL-4–independent switching to IgG1.

Inhibition of Switching to IgG1

Switching to IgG1 is inhibited by IFN γ. This has been demonstrated in *in vitro* experiments in which IFN-γ decreases IgG1 secretion when added to cultures of B cells plus LPS and IL-4

(125,126), as well as in experiments in which anti–IFN-γ antibody enhances IgG1 secretion when added to cultures of B cells plus IFN-γ-secreting T cells (116). Similar results have been demonstrated *in vivo* (127). Recombinant IFN-γ inhibits IgG1 secretion in mice injected with anti-IgD antibody, while anti–IFN-γ antibody enhances IgG1 secretion in mice injected with anti-IgD antibody or with killed *Brucella abortus*. In addition, anti–IFN-γ antibody fully reverses the ability of killed *Brucella abortus* to inhibit IgG1 secretion in anti-IgD antibody-injected mice, suggesting that endogenous IFN-γ production is particularly important at downregulating IgG1 secretion. IFN-γ–deficient mice produce increased influenza-specific IgG1 in response to immunization with influenza virus (128). TGF-β also inhibits IgG1 secretion (129,130) and the generation of mIgG1+ cells (C.M. Snapper, unpublished data) in B cells cultured with LPS plus IL-4. The effects of TGF-β on immunoglobulin isotype expression *in vivo* are not known. IFN-α also inhibits secretion of IgG1 by B cells cultured with LPS plus IL-4; however, the ability of IFN-α to directly inhibit IgG1 secretion *in vivo* may depend on induction of increased IFN-γ production and/or decreased IL-4 production (131).

Mouse IgG2a

Interferon γ Stimulates Switching to IgG2a

The regulation of switching to IgG2a and the production of this isotype is, to a large extent, the reciprocal of regulation of IgG1 switching and secretion: IgG2a responses are induced by IFN-γ and suppressed by IL-4 (126). IFN-γ substantially enhances IgG2a production by LPS-activated mouse B cells, while it inhibits secretion of IgG1, IgG2b, and IgG3 by these cells (126,132). IFN-γ also induces IgG2a secretion by B cells stimulated with dextran-conjugated anti-IgD antibody (42), as well as by T cell–activated B cells (133). In addition, IFN-γ production by NK cells enhances *in vitro* and *in vivo*

IgG2a responses (134–136). Pulsing of resting mIgM⁺ B cells with IFN-γ enhances IgG2a production when the cells are subsequently washed and cultured with LPS (132), just as pulsing with IL-4 enhances LPS-induced IgG1 production (103). Promotion of isotype switching to IgG2a by IFN-γ is suggested by its ability to increase germline γ2a RNA levels (101,137) and to increase the precursor frequency of IgG2a-secreting cells in soft agar cultures (132).

Inhibition of Switching to IgG2a and Interferon-γ–independent Induction of IgG2a

Addition of IL-4 to B cells cultured with LPS and IFN-γ suppresses IgG2a responses (126). This reciprocal relationship between IL-4 and IFN-γ is also seen *in vivo*; IL-4 antagonists (120) and IFN-γ (40) enhance IgG2a responses in anti-IgD antibody–injected mice, and IgG2a antibody responses are elevated in mice that lack a functional IL-4 gene (121), while anti–IFN-γ antibody inhibits IgG2a responses in normal mice injected with anti-IgD antibody or killed *Brucella abortus* (127). However, inhibition of IgG2a production in these systems by anti–IFN-γ antibody is never complete, suggesting that both IFN-γ–dependent and IFN-γ–independent mechanisms exist for the induction of IgG2a responses. This partial dependence of switching to IgG2a on IFN-γ has been more conclusively shown by studies with IFN-γ receptor– and IFN-γ–deficient mice that demonstrate decreased baseline IgG2a levels and reduced IgG2a and/or increased IgG1 responses to several protein and microbial antigens in these mice (128,138,139).

Role of Interleukin-12 in IgG2a Induction

IL-12 stimulates switching to IgG2a by LPS-activated murine B cells *in vitro* through induction of IFN-γ by NK cells (140). IL-12 also stimulates the production of IgG2a *in vivo*, perhaps through induction of IFN-γ from T cells and NK cells. Administration of IL-12 to mice immunized with T-cell dependent (TD) antigens stimulates higher specific IgG2a responses relative to mice immunized with TD antigen alone (140,141). Similarly, injection of neutralizing anti–IL-12 antibody during a TD response can reduce specific serum IgG2a responses (141). Administration of IL-12 to unimmunized mice increases IFN-γ mRNA and protein expression and enhances serum concentrations of IgG2a (142). Other effects of IL-12 *in vivo* are more complex and dependent on the time, duration, and extent of IL-12 treatment and the quantity of IFN-γ that is produced in response to IL-12. These effects include selective enhancement of IgG2a and IgG3 responses and suppression of IgG1 and IgE production (all IFN-γ–dependent), suppression of all IgG production (IFN-γ–dependent and seen with high-dose,long-duration IL-12 treatment) (142), and enhanced maturation to immunoglobulin secretion, with increased IgG secretion in an isotype-nonspecific manner, through a direct effect on postswitched cells (IFN-γ–independent) after a transient early suppression that is IFN-γ–dependent (140).

Mouse IgG3

Interferon-γ Can Either Stimulate or Inhibit Switching to IgG3, Depending On the Nature of the B-Cell Activator

Switching to IgG3 resembles switching to IgG2a, in that both are inhibited by IL-4 and both are stimulated, in some circumstances,

by IFN-γ. IFN-γ stimulation of switching to IgG3 is suggested by its ability to substantially increase IgG3 secretion, the percentage of mIgG3⁺ cells, and germline Cγ3 RNA in resting, naive B cells cultured with dextran-conjugated anti-IgD antibody plus IL-5 (42). In addition, IFN-γ–producing, antigen-specific T-cell clones selectively induce IgG3 as well as IgG2a responses if they are transferred into mice that are injected with the antigen for which the T cell is specific (143). Mice immunized with live bacteria that induce considerable endogenous IFN-γ production generate large IgG3 as well as IgG2a antibody responses (144–146), and virus-infected IFN-γR⁻ᐟ⁻ mice make decreased IgG3 relative to IgG1 and IgG2b, as compared to wild-type mice (139). However, while IFN-γ enhances IgG2a production by B cells cultured with LPS, it inhibits the substantial IgG3 response that is induced by LPS in the absence of IFN-γ (126). There is also no evidence that anti–IFN-γ antibodies inhibit the LPS-induced IgG3 responses *in vitro,* or polysaccharide-induced IgG3 responses *in vivo* (C.M. Snapper, J.J. Mond, unpublished data). Thus, it seems likely that IFN-γ contributes to the induction of IgG3 responses in some, but not all, circumstances.

Interleukin-4 Inhibits Switching to IgG3

The ability of IL-4 to inhibit IgG3 responses, originally demonstrated by addition of this cytokine to B cells cultured with LPS (95), has also been observed *in vivo* in studies in which IL-4 antagonists increased serum IgG3 levels in mice immunized with anti-IgD antibody (A.D. Levine, personal communication) and in studies in which antigen-specific and total serum IgG3 levels were shown to be elevated in mice that lack a functional IL-4 gene (121).

Mouse IgG2b

Transforming Growth Factor-β Stimulates Switching to IgG2b

Addition of TGF-β to naive B cells cultured with LPS selectively enhances IgG2b secretion as well as the number of IgG2b-secreting cells (147–149). This effect of TGF-β is associated with an increase in the steady-state levels of germline γ2b RNA (147). However, TGF-β has no stimulatory effect on IgG2b secretion by B cells cultured with IL-5 plus dextran–anti-IgD (147), suggesting that TGF-β can only induce switching to IgG2b in the presence of the proper costimuli. No studies have yet demonstrated that TGF-β has a role in the induction of *in vivo* IgG2b responses. A soluble activity, which has only partially been characterized biochemically but is distinct from TGF-β and present in joint fluids from patients with rheumatoid arthritis, also selectively enhances IgG2b secretion by LPS-activated murine B cells *in vitro* (150–153). IL-4 has a direct or indirect suppressive effect on *in vivo* IgG2b production, as IgG2b responses are increased in mice that lack a functional IL-4 gene (121). IFN-γ has been shown to suppress IgG2b production in some *in vitro* systems (126), but there are no reports of *in vivo* studies that indicate that IFN-γ has a role in limiting IgG2b production.

Human IgG Isotypes

IL-4 stimulates IgG4 secretion by human B cells cultured with anti-CD40 antibody (154) or with the murine thymoma line, EL-4

(155), plus phorbol myristate acetate (PMA). Human IgG4 is similar to the mouse IgG isotype that is induced by IL-4, IgG1, in that neither antibody fixes complement well (18,19); however, these immunoglobulins differ in that IgG1 is the major mouse isotype produced in response to soluble proteins, while human IgG4 is usually present in small amounts in human serum (28,59).

IL-10 stimulates switching to IgG1 and IgG3, as demonstrated by (a) increased secretion of these isotypes by CD40-activated, naive mIgD$^+$ human B cells (156); (b) a selective increase in germline Cγ1 and Cγ3 RNA expression by IL-10–treated B cells (157); and (c) the production of the appropriate circular DNA switch excision products in IL-10–treated, CD40-activated human IgD$^+$ B cells (158).

Although IFN-γ stimulates switching to IgG2a in the mouse, the only evidence that this cytokine might induce switching to any human immunoglobulin isotype is its selective enhancement of germline γ2 RNA expression by resting mIgM$^+$mIgG B cells; it is not known whether this correlates with increased switching to IgG2 (159). Although IFN-γ enhances and anti–IFN-γ antibody inhibits spontaneous IgG2 secretion by human peripheral blood mononuclear cells (PBMCs) in vitro, this effect is abrogated by depletion of mIgG2$^+$ cells, suggesting that IFN-γ acts selectively on B cells that had already switched to this immunoglobulin isotype and is therefore not operating as a switch factor (160). In contrast, a still unidentified factor produced by human Th1 but not Th2 cells that is not IFN-γ or any other known cytokine appears to have the ability to switch activated human B cells to IgG2 expression in vitro (161).

Control of Switching to IgE

Interleukin-4 Stimulates Switching to IgE

IL-4 is an important stimulus of switching to IgE in both mouse and human. This cytokine stimulates IgE responses by purified mouse B cells cultured with either LPS (125,126,162,163), activated T cells (106,116,133), or CD40 ligand (111,164,165) or by purified human B cells cultured with EBV (166–171), anti-CD40 antibody (154,172) or CD40 ligand (173,174), cortisol (175–177), mouse EL-4 cells plus PMA (155), or activated T cells (154,178–188). Anti–IL-4 antibody blocks IgE production by mouse B cells cultured with rabbit antimouse IgM antibody plus IL-4–secreting T cells that are specific for rabbit IgG (106). In the same culture system, the presence of added IL-4 instead of anti–IL-4 antibody stimulates the majority of immunoglobulin-secreting B-cell clones to generate an IgE response, which suggests that IL-4 is inducing mIgM$^+$ B cells in this system to switch to IgE expression (106). IL-4 stimulation of a large increase in steady-state germline ε RNA expression (99–101,154,166,168,178,189,190) also provides evidence for IL-4 promotion of switching to IgE.

Regulation of In Vivo IgE Production

Early in vivo studies in mice supported the view that IgE production was absolutely dependent on IL-4. Primary and secondary polyclonal and antigen-specific IgE responses, induced by injection of anti-IgD antibody, immunization with antigen on alum, or inoculation with nematode helminths, are all blocked by anti–IL-4 or anti–IL-4 receptor antibodies by more than 99% (119,120,191,192). Mice that lack a functional IL-4 gene also fail

to develop a detectable IgE response to infection with Nippostrongylus brasiliensis (121,193). An in vivo IgE response that is not inhibitable by IL-4 antagonists can be stimulated in mice by injecting them with goat antimouse IgE antibody (192). This response is produced by B-lymphocytes that had switched to expression of mIgE prior to immunization; the resulting lack of a requirement for switching during the course of the response explains the lack of a requirement for IL-4 (194). Studies in mice, however, have provided evidence for IL-4–independent switching to IgE (195–198). IL-4–deficient and control mice have comparably elevated serum IgE levels during the course of a retrovirus-induced immunodeficiency disease (MAIDS) (195). Further, injection of IL-4–deficient mice with polyclonal goat antimouse IgD antibody stimulates a large increase in germline ε RNA levels, some Sμ-Sε recombination, and an increase in serum IgE levels that is detectable but less than 1% as large as that seen in similarly treated controls (195). IL-4–independent switching to IgE is down-regulated by IFN-γ, similar to the IL-4–dependent pathway (195). IgE production, at substantially reduced levels relative to controls, is observed in IL-4–deficient mice infected with Plasmodium chabaudi (197) or Leishmania major (198), but not in Brugia malayi– or N. brasiliensis–infected mice (195,199). Finally, injection of an agonistic anti-CD40 antibody into IL-4–deficient mice induces IgE secretion (196). Collectively, these studies demonstrate that IL-4–independent switching to IgE can occur in vivo and may depend on the nature of the activating signals, but that the vast amount of IgE produced by mice is IL-4–dependent.

Interleukin-13 Stimulates Switching to IgE in Human B Cells

IL-13 mimics many of the functions of IL-4 in human B cells, including induction of switching to IgE (200–203). IL-13 can bind to and signal through a receptor that contains the IL-4 receptor α chain and additional polypeptide chains (204). It is unlikely, however, that switching to IgE in IL-4 deficient mice is IL-13–dependent. Mouse B cells lack detectable IL-13 receptor and fail to respond to IL-13, and anti–IL-4 receptor α antibody fails to block the IgE response in IL-4–deficient mice immunized with anti-IgD antibody (195). The relative importance of IL-4 and IL-13 in human IgE responses is uncertain.

Sequential Switching from IgM to IgG to IgE

Although IL-4 stimulates switching by mouse B cells to both IgE and IgG1 and by human B cells to both IgE and IgG4, differences exist in the kinetics of switching to the different isotypes, in the concentrations of IL-4 that are required to induce switching and in the requirements for costimuli. There is a 12- to 16-hour delay in the generation of most of the IgE response, as compared with the IgG1 response, by mouse B cells cultured with LPS plus IL-4 (205). Similarly, human B cells stimulated with IL-4 plus anti-CD40 antibody secrete detectable IgG4 approximately 2 days earlier than they secrete detectable IgE (154) Both observations are consistent with the interpretation that the switch from IgM to IgE typically involves an initial switch to an IgG isotype, and then a second switch to IgE, as is discussed in the last section of this chapter.

Switching to IgE Depends on the Nature of the B-Cell Activator

Switching to IgE, at least in the mouse, depends not only on IL-4, but also on the method of B-cell activation. Thus, B cells activated with dextran–anti-IgD antibodies or anti-IgD antibodies bound to cell-associated FcγRI (206) fail to express germline Cε RNA or switch to IgE in the presence of IL-4 plus IL-5, despite making a substantial IgG1 response (104). The failure of these agents, which activate B cells by stringent cross-linking of their mIg, to induce IgE secretion, even in the presence of a high concentration of IL-4, may protect the host by inhibiting the generation of IgE responses to bacteria, inasmuch as such responses could lead to the extensive cross-linking of mast cells by multivalent bacteria, which could cause systemic anaphylaxis. Protein A–bearing *Staphylococcus aureus,* which activate human B cells by cross-linking mIg and induce these cells to secrete immunoglobulin isotypes other than IgE in the presence of the appropriate cytokines, also fail to induce an IgE response in the presence of IL-4 (207). However, mIg cross-linking does not always block the induction of IgE secretion, since an IgE response can be induced by culturing mouse B-lymphocytes with IL-4 plus anti-IgD antibody that has been conjugated to an insoluble matrix, such as agarose (104).

Cytokines Augment Interleukin-4–induced IgE Production

A number of cytokines act in concert with IL-4 to stimulate IgE synthesis. These include IL-2, IL-5, IL-6, and TNF-α. IL-2 acts synergistically with IL-4 to stimulate IgE secretion by human B cells cultured with PMA and mouse EL-4 thymoma cells (155). IL-5 enhances IgE secretion by mouse B cells cultured with LPS plus IL-4 (208), and by human PBMCs cultured with suboptimal concentrations of IL-4 (182). Endogenously produced IL-6 is critical for the generation of the IgE responses made by human PBMCs cultured with IL-4 (182) and by human B cells cultured with cortisol plus IL-4 (175) or with IL-4 plus anti-CD40 antibody (172), since, in each case, anti–IL-6 antibody abrogates the response. These cytokines have been implicated, however, in stimulating the differentiation of B cells into antibody-secreting cells, and it is unlikely that they are specifically involved in stimulating B cells to switch to IgE expression. By contrast, the increased IgE synthesis observed in the presence of TNF-α is associated with an increase in IL-4–dependent induction of germline Cε RNA as well as with a growth-promoting effect of TNF-α (209). Although *in vitro* data suggest a stimulatory role for these cytokines in IL-4–dependent IgE synthesis, neutralizing or blocking antibodies to IL-2, IL-2 receptor, IL-5, IL-6, and IL-6 receptor have failed to interfere with the *in vivo* IgE responses that are induced by injecting mice with anti-IgD antibody or inoculating mice with nematode parasites (F.D. Finkelman, J.F. Urban, Jr., unpublished data).

The Role of CD23 in IgE Synthesis

Another factor that may play a role in the induction of IgE responses is CD23, the low-affinity IgE receptor, which is upregulated on B cells by IL-4 (210–213). Some monoclonal antibodies to this receptor inhibit the IgE responses made by human PBMCs cultured with IL-4 (180,214) and by human B cells cultured with IL-4 plus cortisol (177). Soluble CD23 has been reported to upregulate IgE secretion in some systems (215,216). However, there is no evi-

dence that CD23 regulates switching to IgE, *per se,* and anti-CD23 antibodies do not inhibit the IgE responses made by B cells stimulated with IL-4 plus EBV (G.T. Thyphronitis, unpublished data) or IL-4 plus anti-CD40 antibody (154). Furthermore, an antibody that blocks IgE binding to mouse CD23 and modulates nearly all CD23 from mouse B cells when injected *in vivo* has no effect on IgE responses generated *in vitro* by stimulation with IL-4 plus LPS (217) or a Th2 clone (218), or *in vivo* by immunization with antigen on alum, anti-IgD antibody, or anti-IgE antibody, or by inoculation with nematode helminths (I.M. Katona, J.F. Urban, Jr., D. Conrad, F.D. Finkelman, unpublished data). Further, CD23-deficient mice make normal *in vivo* polyclonal IgG1 and IgE synthesis in response to infection with the nematode parasite *N. brasiliensis* (219).

Agents That Inhibit IgE Synthesis

While a single cytokine, IL-4, is required for nearly all IgE production in the mouse, a number of different compounds specifically inhibit IgE responses. The inhibitory effects of these compounds vary, however, depending on the costimulus that is employed to induce the IgE response. IFN-γ inhibits germline ε mRNA expression (220) and IgE secretion by mouse B cells cultured with IL-4 plus LPS (125,126), and specifically inhibits IgE secretion by human PBMCs cultured with IL-4 (178,180), and human B cells cultured with IL-4 plus EBV (169,221), or with IL-4 plus cell membranes of activated T cells (222). IFN-γ has no effect, however, on IgE secretion by human B cells cultured with IL-4 plus anti-CD40 antibody (154). IFN-α also inhibits IgE secretion by human PBMCs cultured with IL-4 (178,180) and by human B cells cultured with IL-4 plus EBV (169,221). Contrary to the observations made with mouse B cells, however, neither IFN-α nor IFN-γ inhibits IL-4 induction of increased steady-state levels of germline ε mRNA in human B cells (178). Another cytokine, IL-12, suppresses IgE secretion by human B cells stimulated with IL-4 plus cortisol (223). This cytokine suppresses IgE indirectly, by inducing IFN-γ production, as well as through a direct effect on B cells. IL-12 also suppresses *in vivo* IgE production in the mouse through effects that are predominantly indirect (inhibition of IL-4 secretion and stimulation of IFN-γ secretion) (184). Prostaglandins can inhibit IgE production in at least some systems (human PBMCs cultured with IL-4) (180), but they can enhance IgE production and steady-state germline ε mRNA levels in other systems (mouse B cells cultured with IL-4 plus LPS) (224,225). IFNγ (127), IFN-α (131), and a prostaglandin E2 analogue (226) have all been found to selectively inhibit *in vivo* mouse IgE responses to injection of anti-IgD antibody; however, the extent to which this inhibition is a direct effect on the B cell, rather than an effect of decreased IL-4 production, has not been determined. All of these observations can be summed up by the statement that IL-4 (or, in the human, IL-13) is a critical requirement for the induction of switching to IgE, but that different, although not all, costimuli can substitute for each other in allowing this response. The inhibitory effects of other agents on IgE responses appear to depend on the costimulus that is involved.

Control of Switching to IgA

Stimulation of IgA Secretion by Type II Cytokines

Initial studies demonstrated that a population of T cells, derived from the Peyer's patch, selectively induces mIgM⁺ B cells to undergo IgA class switching (227–229). Although the mechanism for this action was not determined, it has been subsequently shown that certain cytokines, especially the type II–derived cytokines (e.g., IL-4, IL-5, IL-6), released, in part, by T cells can stimulate IgA secretion. Indeed, a predominantly type II cytokine profile has been demonstrated in mucosal tissue, the major site of IgA production, both before and after purposeful immunization with soluble protein antigens (230–233). Initially, it was reported that IL-5 selectively enhanced IgA secretion by LPS-activated B cells *in vitro*, and that this could be further augmented by IL-4 (234–236). Subsequent studies demonstrated that IL-5 acts on mIgA$^+$, but not mIgA$^-$ B cells to stimulate IgA synthesis (237–239), indicating that it promotes maturation of mIgA$^+$ cells to IgA secretion, but does not induce IgA class switching. Administration of IL-5 to mice enhances mucosal IgA responses *in vivo* (240,241). However, local induction of virus-specific IgA in IL-5–deficient mice after intranasal inoculation with Influenza virus is similar to that observed in control mice, indicating that, at least in this system, IL-5 is not critical for induction of IgA *in vivo* (242). In IL-4–deficient mice, mucosal and systemic IgA responses to soluble proteins after oral immunization with soluble protein antigen plus cholera toxin are markedly reduced relative to controls (243). This is thought to result from a failure to induce specific T and B cells in the Peyer's patches, and not to defective differentiation of mIgA$^+$ B cells. In contrast, IL-4–deficient mice have intact mucosal and systemic IgA anticholera toxin production, indicating that IL-4 is not critical for all IgA responses. Experiments with IL-6–deficient mice have suggested that IL-6 has a major role in stimulating mucosal antibody responses, particularly IgA responses, that follow mucosal challenge with either ovalbumin in CFA or vaccinia virus (211), but not those made to KLH or OVA plus cholera toxin or infection with *H. felis* (244). The two cited reports differ about the importance of IL-6 for mucosal IgA production in unimmunized mice. The basis for the differences between these two studies is not known, although differences in microbial flora in the investigators' mouse colonies or the use of different antigens and adjuvants in their experiments may have played a role.

Transforming Growth Factor-β Stimulates Switching to IgA

TGF-β stimulates LPS-activated B cells to undergo IgA class switching (129,130,245–247). TGF-β selectively enhances IgA secretion by mIgA$^-$, but not mIgA$^+$, LPS-activated B cells and inhibits the LPS-induced synthesis of IgM, IgG3, and IgG1 (129,169,246). IL-2 and IL-5 strongly enhance IgA secretion induced by LPS plus TGF-β (129,245). IL-2 appears to act post-transcriptionally to enhance IgA production by B cells cultured with LPS plus TGF-β, since it fails to increase the number of IgA-secreting cells, steady-state α mRNA levels, or the ratio of membrane to secretory α mRNA (130).

In addition to its ability to induce IgA class switching by mouse B cells activated by LPS, TGF-β also stimulates a class switch to IgA by murine B cells activated by T cells (248), CD40-ligand (249) or by dextran-conjugated anti-IgD antibody (104,248). In addition, TGF-β selectively stimulates IgA class switching by human B cells in at least two systems (250–253). In one system, TGF-β, in the presence of pokeweed mitogen (PWM) and activated CD4$^+$ T cells, stimulates highly purified human mIgA$^-$, but not mIgA$^+$, B cells to secrete increased amounts of IgA, but not IgM or IgG (252). Induc-

tion of this IgA response requires both the presence of TGF-β during the initial culture period and the removal of this cytokine during the later stages of culture. In a second system, TGF-β plus anti-CD40 antibody induce mIgD$^+$, but not mIgD$^-$, B cells to secrete IgA. IL-10 is required to stimulate isotype-switched cells to mature into IgA-secreting cells in this (253) and other systems (254a). Of interest, PBMCs from patients with IgA deficiency (IgA-D) secrete IgM and IgG, but not IgA, on activation with anti-CD40 antibody plus *S. aureus* Cowan strain I (SAC), whereas control B cells make all three isotypes under these conditions (156). However, the combination of IL-10, anti-CD40 antibody, and SAC induces substantial IgA secretion *by IgA-deficient* PBMCs and further enhances IgA synthesis in controls. In another study, it was demonstrated that unstimulated PBMCs from IgA-D patients had lower levels of germline Cα RNA and Sμ-Sα recombination events relative to control patients (254b). However, stimulation of IgA-D PBMCs with PMA plus TGF-β *in vitro* led to an apparent restoration of germline Cα RNA levels relative to control donors. These two studies suggest that B cells from IgA-D patients are competent to switch to IgA but do not receive the appropriate stimuli *in vivo*. In contrast to the action of IL-10 on human B cells, IL-10 strongly inhibits the generation of mIgA$^+$ cells and Sμ-Sα recombination events in LPS-activated, but not CD40 ligand–activated, murine B cells stimulated with dextran–anti-IgD plus IL-4, IL-5 and TGF-β (255). Dendritic cells (DCs) may also augment switching to IgA (256). Thus, DCs alone induced the expression of mIgA on ~10% of CD40-activated naive human mIgD$^+$ B cells *in vitro* and, with the addition of IL-10 and TGF-β, increased the percentage of mIgA$^+$ cells from 5% to 40% to 50%.

Limiting dilution analysis indicates that TGF-β increases the frequency of LPS-activated IgA-secreting B-cell clones by 20- to 25-fold, but does not increase the size of IgA-secreting clones (245,257). In contrast to TGF-β, neither IL-2 nor IL-5 increases the frequency of IgA-secreting clones. Support for TGF-β induction of IgA class switching at the clonal level also comes from studies in which this cytokine induces the neoplastic B-cell lines, CH12.LX (258) and I.29, to switch from IgM to IgA secretion (259). Enthusiasm for TGF-β as the major physiologic inducer of switching to IgA was initially tempered, however, by the observation that this cytokine induces only a relatively small increase in the percentage of mIgA$^+$ cells (from 0.1% to 0.3% in the absence of TGF-β to 1.6% to 2.2% in the presence of TGF-β), a much lower percentage of mIgA$^+$ cells than that normally found in Peyer's patches (248). More recently, a murine *in vitro* system that induces much higher percentages of mIgA$^+$ cells has been demonstrated (249). B-cell cultures, initially mIgM$^+$mIgA$^-$, contain 10% to 20% mIgA$^+$ cells after activation for 4 days with either LPS or CD40 ligand in the presence of IL-4, IL-5, dextran–anti-IgD and TGF-β.

In light of the ability of TGF-β to strongly inhibit B-cell proliferation, it is of interest that the cell-cycle inhibitors, thymidine and hydroxyurea, also selectively increase the numbers of IgA-secreting cells induced by LPS (245). This suggests the possibilities that (a) inhibition of B cell proliferation may play a role in TGF-β induction of IgA switching, and (b) many physiologic inhibitors of B-cell proliferation may promote switching to IgA *in vivo*.

Vasoactive Intestinal Peptide Stimulates Switching to IgA

Vasoactive intestinal peptide (VIP) also induces switching to IgA in human adult and fetal B cells and in human pre-B cells derived from bone marrow (260). Thus, VIP stimulates both IgA1 and IgA2 production by small, resting mIgA1⁻ and mIgA2⁻ adult human B cells, respectively (260); mIgM⁺ fetal B cells; or mIgM⁻ CD19⁺ pre-B cells (261) that have been activated with anti-CD40 antibody, but it does not induce any other isotype. Two other neuropeptides, somatostatin and substance P, have no effect on switching to IgA.

Summary

The effects of cytokines on murine and human immunoglobulin class switching is summarized in Table 1. Several general conclusions can be drawn: (a) Cytokines typically induce switching to more than one immunoglobulin isotype within a population of B cells; this may occur in certain instances through a sequential process within an individual clone of B cells. (b) Cytokines that induce one set of immunoglobulin isotypes often inhibit other immunoglobulin isotypes. (c) The effect of a particular cytokine on immunoglobulin class switching often depends on the nature of the B-cell activator.

MOLECULAR BIOLOGY OF ISOTYPE SWITCHING

Immunoglobulin Class Switching Is Associated with C_H Gene Deletion

Observations that a single cell could switch from the production of an IgM antibody to an IgG antibody that had specificity for the same antigen (2,262) suggested that a process existed that could switch the same immunoglobulin V_H region from $C\mu$ to $C\gamma$. The finding that the great majority of plasmacytomas and hybridomas secrete a single immunoglobulin isotype suggested that the mechanism that accomplishes isotype switching might eliminate the ability to express the original isotype. In contrast, the demonstration that most mouse and human mature B-lymphocytes simultaneously express both mIgM and mIgD molecules, which, on individual cells, have identical antigen-binding specificities and idiotypic determinants, supported the view that single V_H regions could combine with different C_H regions, but suggested that these alternative combinations could occur simultaneously in the same cell. Identification and sequencing of the immunoglobulin heavy-chain gene complex demonstrated that immunoglobulin isotypes are encoded by constant heavy (C_H) genes, which are aligned, in tandem, in the same transcriptional orientation, 3′ to the V_HDJ_H gene, which encodes specificity for antigen. In the mouse, the C_H genes are located on chromosome 12 within a 200-kb region in the order 5′-μ, δ, γ3, γ1, γ2b, γ2a, ε, and α-3′ (263). In the human, C_H genes are positioned on chromosome 14 within a 300-kb region and aligned 5′-μ, δ, γ3, γ1, Ψε, α1, Ψγ, γ2, γ4, ε, and α2-3′ (264) (Fig. 1). Mature, resting B cells that coexpress mIgM and mIgD produce mature μ mRNA predominantly by termination of transcription immediately 3′ to the $C\mu$ membrane or secretory exon, while mature δ mRNA is produced by transcription of a long RNA transcript that contains V_HDJ_H, $C\mu$, and $C\delta$, followed by the splicing out of $C\mu$ (265–268). In contrast, studies of myelomas and hybridomas, and, later, of normal B cells, activated both *in vitro* and *in vivo*, demonstrated that an immunoglobulin isotype switch is associated with deletion of all C_H genes 5′ to the one being expressed, with juxtaposition of the V_HDJ_H gene, with its 5′ promoter and 3′ intronic enhancer, 5′ to the expressed C_H gene (269–273). This is true even for myelomas and hybridomas that secrete IgD (274–280). It is also true for normal B cells that express a membrane isotype other than IgM or IgD, but do not secrete Ig (281). Both the nonexpressed, as well as the expressed, Igh loci can undergo class switching, with V_H genes in both chromosomes in a given cell often switching to genes that encode the same C_H isotype (269,282–284). Deletional isotype switching is, in fact, independent of membrane expression of productively rearranged immunoglobulin heavy and light chains, as it can occur in pre-B-cell lines in addition to B cells (285–288).

Immunoglobulin Class Switch Recombination Is Mediated through Switch Regions

In addition to determining the sequence of C_H genes within the immunoglobulin heavy-chain gene complex, DNA sequencing studies demonstrated the presence of switch (S) regions, that are located 5′ to each C_H gene, except $C\delta$ (289–298). All S regions contain repeats of the nucleotides GAGCT and TGGGG (290,292,299,300), which suggests that these sequences play a pivotal role in the class-switch process. In addition, S regions preferentially contain the sequence (C or T)AGGTTG, which is typically located 5′ to switch recombination sites and has been suggested to be important, in combination with the GAGCT and TGGGG tandem repeats, in mediating class switching (301). The S regions for different C_H genes are not, however, identical. Distinct differences are observed in their size (2 to 10 kb in length) and composition. Sequence homology with $S\mu$ is in the following order, from greatest to least homology: $S\epsilon$, $S\alpha$, $S\gamma3$, and ($S\gamma1$, $S\gamma2b$, $S\gamma2a$), with $S\gamma1$, $S\gamma2b$, and $S\gamma2a$ having strong homology to each other, but little homology, outside of the pentamer repeats, with $S\mu$ (299). Some S regions also contain sequences that are unique (292,295,299,302), but what role, if any, these unique sequences play in the regulation of switching to specific isotypes is presently unclear. The presence of multiple, short recognition sequences within S regions may promote an increased efficiency of switching by increasing the chance for switch recombination to occur.

Looping Out and Deletion of C_H Genes by Nonhomologous Recombination Is the Major Mechanism for Immunoglobulin Class Switching

In theory, isotype switching that is accompanied by deletion of C_H genes 5′ to the expressed C_H gene could occur by homologous recombination (recombination between identical or nearly identical gene segments) or nonhomologous recombination (recombination between gene segments with different nucleotide sequences). Switching could occur by (a) recombination between two sites on the same segment of DNA, with looping out of the excised DNA segment (Fig. 2A); (b) recombination between two sites on sister chromatids, with one chromatid and the cell into which it segregated acquiring the "extra" C_H genes that were lost by its sister (Fig. 2B); or (c) recombination between two sites on homologous chromosomes, with one chromosome acquiring the C_H genes that were deleted from its homologue (Fig. 2C). Recombination could be directed toward specific sites within the S regions or could occur at multiple sites within the S regions. Experimental observations provide evidence that nonhomologous recombination

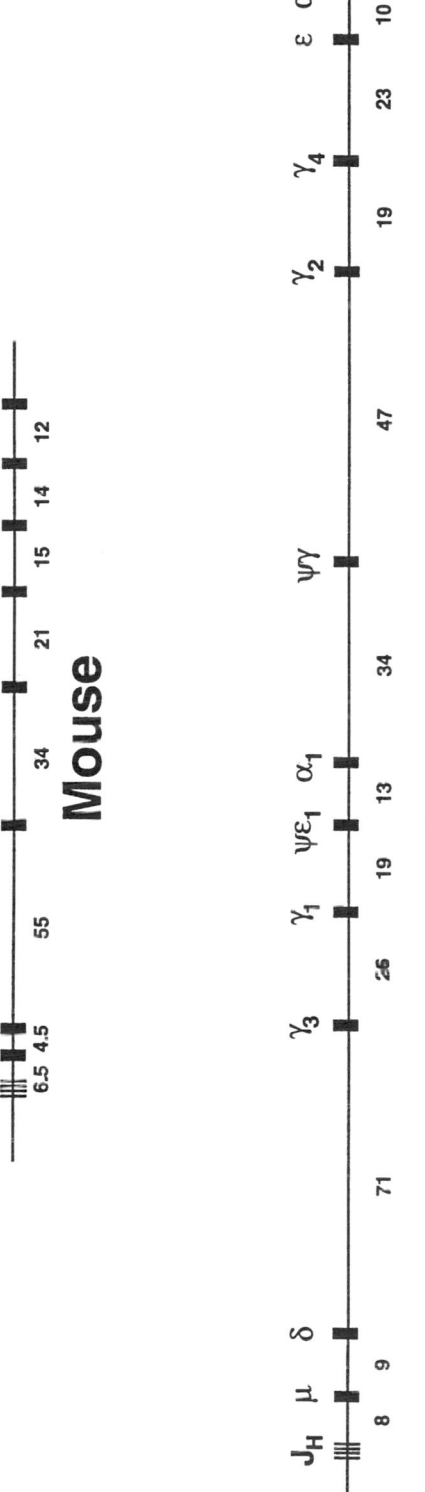

FIG. 1. Mouse and human IgH genes. The relative locations of J_H genes, C_H genes, and pseudogenes are shown. The approximate distances between genes (in kilobases) are indicated (263,264).

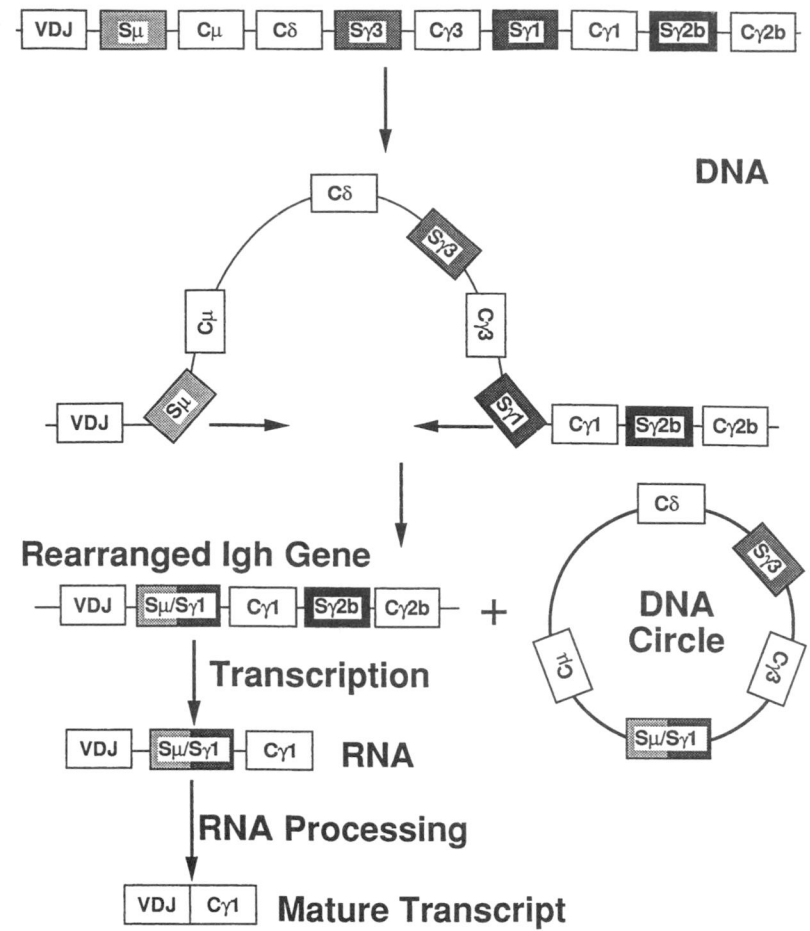

FIG. 2. Proposed mechanisms of Ig isotype switching. Five different possible mechanisms that would permit the synthesis of IgG1 by a mouse B cell that was originally expressing IgM are illustrated. **A:** Looping out: DNA recombination occurs between a site on Sμ and a site on Sγ1, with the production of a rearranged IgH gene that includes VDJ and Sγ1, separated by a recombined Sμ/Sγ1 intron. DNA 3′ to the Sμ recombination site, and 5′ to the Sγ1 recombination site, including Cμ, Cδ, and Cγ3, form a "looped out" DNA circle. RNA produced by transcription of the rearranged gene is processed to delete the recombined switch region, placing VDJ directly 5′ to Cγ1. I regions are not shown in this illustration, but are located 5′ to each S region.

FIG. 2. *(Continued).* **B:** Unequal crossing over between sister chromatids: Recombination is shown to occur between sister chromatids on one of two copies of mouse chromosome 12. The illustrated cross–over creates one chromatid in which Cμ, Cδ, and Cγ3 are deleted, so that VDJ and Cγ1 have become proximate, and a sister chromatid that has duplicated Cμ, Cδ, and Cγ3. Cell division segregates the rearranged sister chromatids, producing one daughter cell that is triploid for Cμ, Cδ, and Cγ3 and one daughter that is haploid for these exons. The cell that contains the rearranged C_H gene in which VDJ and Cγ1 are proximate could produce a γ1 mRNA transcript, as in Fig. 2A. (Continued on next page).

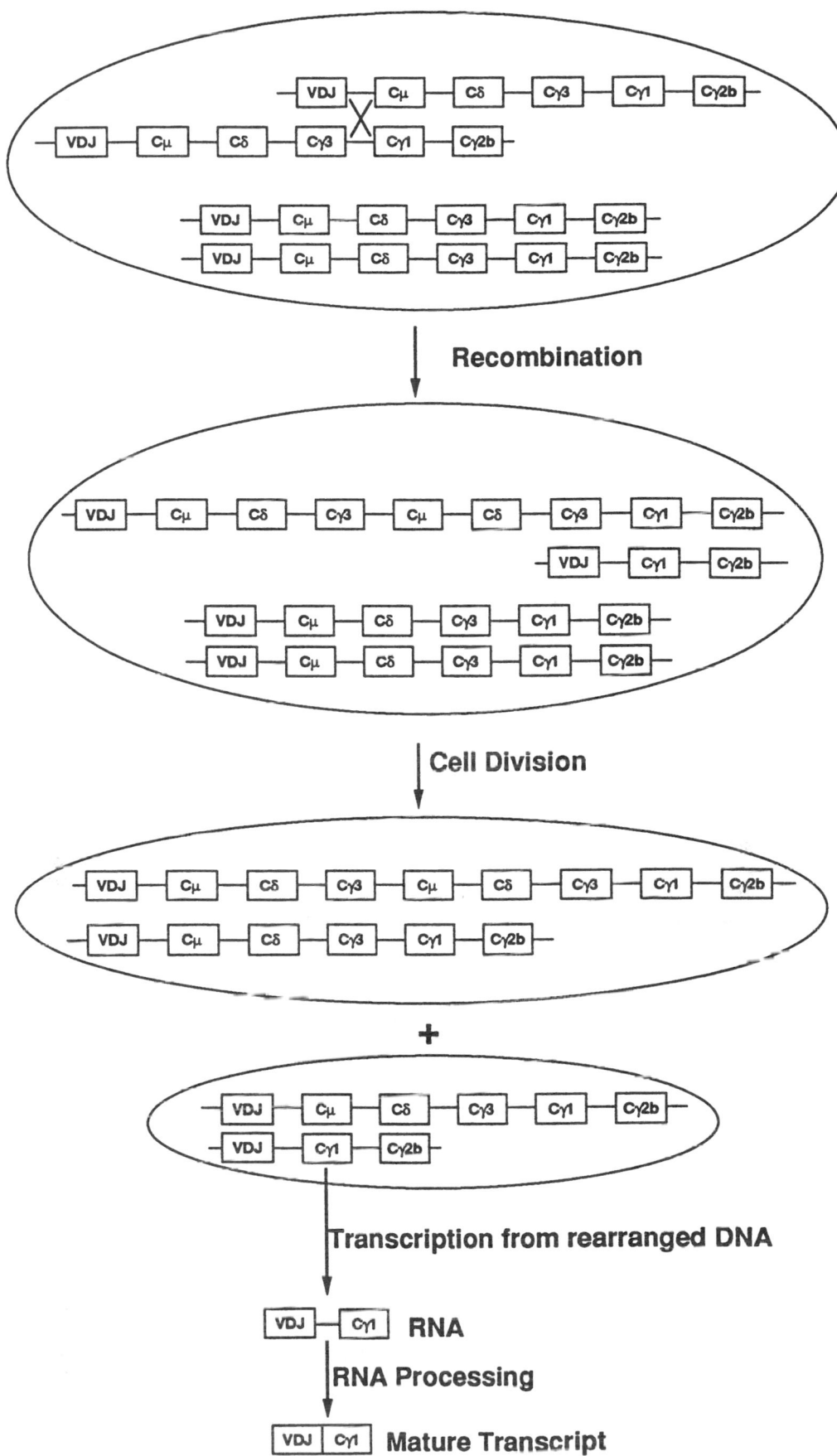

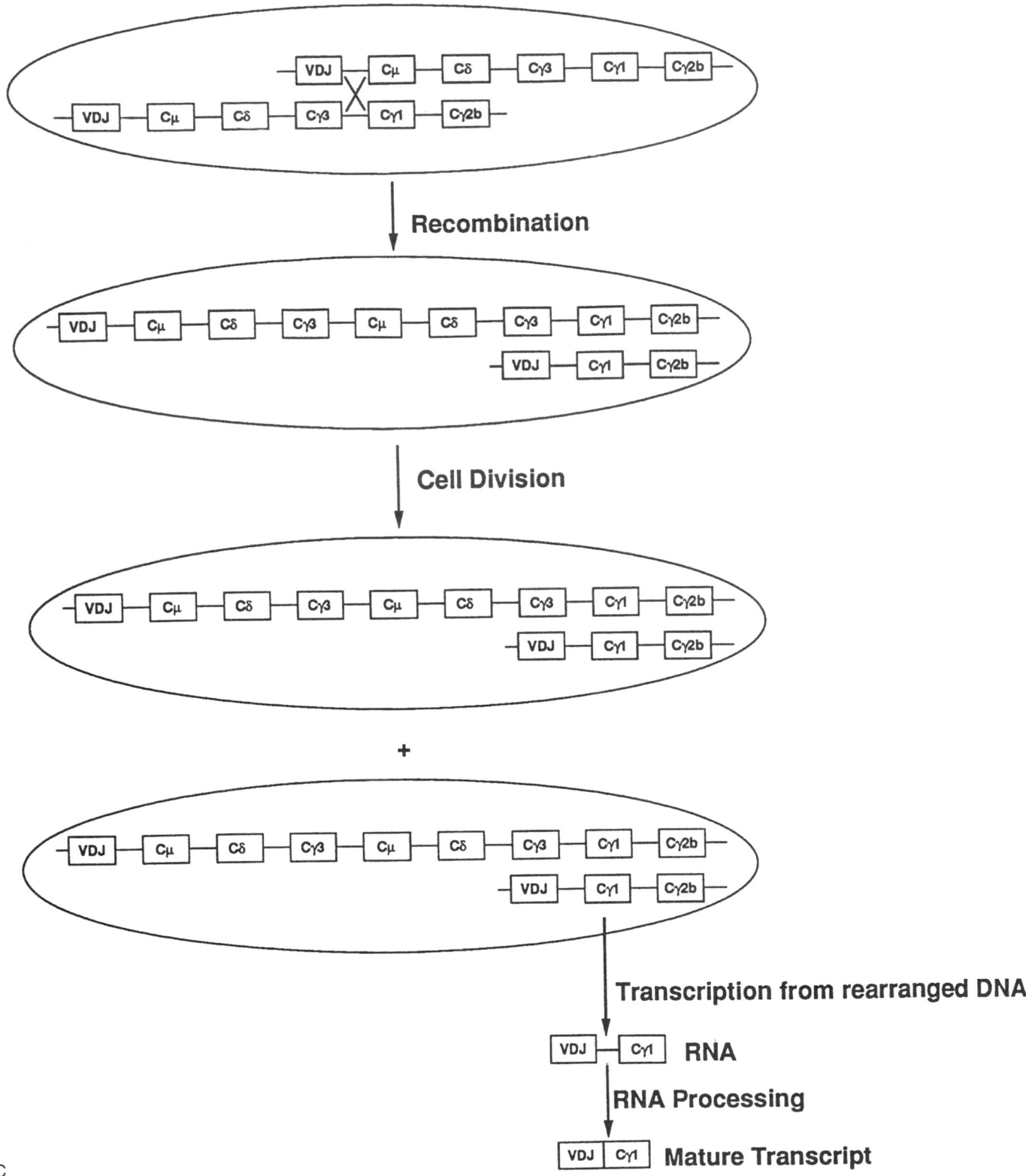

FIG. 2. *(Continued).* **C:** Unequal crossing over between homologous chromosomes: A cross-over between two copies of mouse chromosome 12 creates one IgH gene in which VDJ is proximate to Cγ1, and one in which these exons are separated by a duplication of the sequence Cμ–Cδ–Cγ3. The progeny of division of this cell contain copies of both rearranged chromosomes 12, and thus are diploid for all C$_H$ genes. A γ1 mRNA transcript could be produced from the deletion-containing IgH gene, as in Fig. 2A.

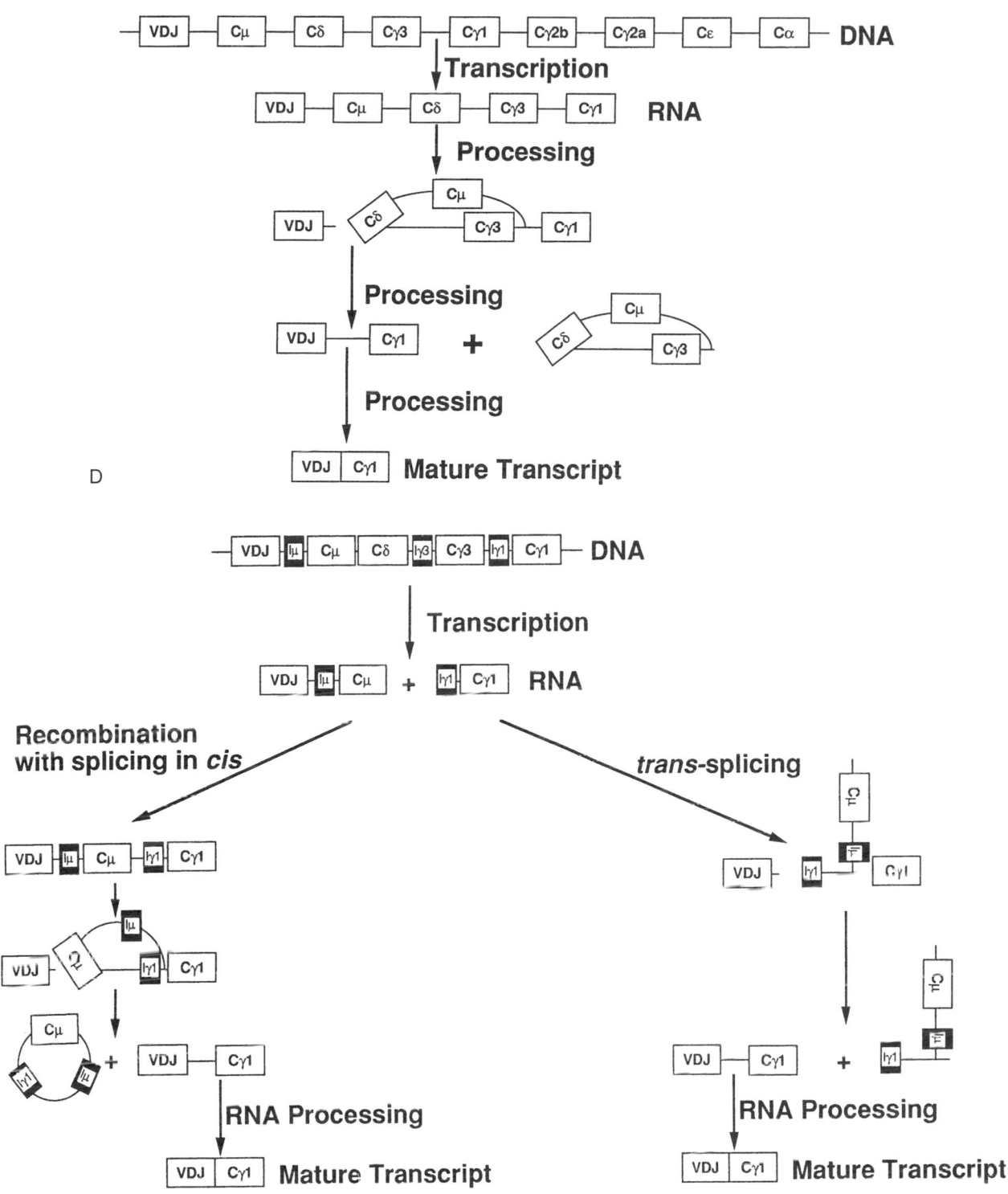

FIG. 2. *(Continued).* **D:** Processing of a long transcript: RNA that contains VDJ, Cμ, Cδ, Cγ3, and Cγ1, as well as all introns 3′ to VDJ and 5′ to Cγ1, is transcribed from an unrearranged IgH gene. Processing of this long transcript first splices out Cμ, Cδ, and Cγ3 (shown to occur by generation of a "lariat"), then splices out introns located between VDJ and Cγ1, to create mature γ1 mRNA. **E:** Discontinuous transcription and recombination: Productive μ mRNA and germline γ1 mRNA are both transcribed from an unrearranged IgH gene. These two transcripts are spliced to yield mature γ1 mRNA by one of two mechanisms. Splicing in *cis* (shown on the **left side** of this illustration) ligates the 3′ end of the VDJCμ transcript directly to the 5′ end of the Iγ1Cγ1 transcript. Cμ, the I exons, and the S introns (which are not shown) are subsequently spliced out by formation of a lariat. The generation of VDJCγ1 from the same RNA precursors by *trans*-splicing (shown on the **right side** of this illustration) involves, instead, steps in which (a) the 5′ end of IμCμ first ligates to Iγ1Cγ1 near the border between the Iγ1 and Cγ1 exons, creating a "Y branched intermediate" and freeing VDJ; and (b) subsequent splicing out of the Y-branched intermediate allows VDJ to ligate to Cγ1.

between two sites on the same DNA segment, with looping out of the deleted DNA, is the usual mechanism of deletional isotype switching, and that this recombination may occur at preferred sites within the S region. Analysis of circular DNA excision products, which are produced during isotype switching of normal B cells and which contain the deleted 5′ C_H genes, provides direct evidence that deletion occurs through formation and excision of a DNA loop (247,303–307). A similar process has been described for $V_L J_L$ recombination in B cells and for T-cell receptor α and β genes (308–310). The occasional occurrence of switch inversions, instead of deletions, in the genome of B-cell tumor lines (285,306,311,312) is consistent with the formation of a DNA loop.

Neither recombination between sister chromatids nor recombination between homologous chromosomes appears to be a typical mechanism of immunoglobulin isotype switching. Southern blot analysis of cells that have switched to an isotype other than IgM has revealed that the DNA for C_H genes 5′ to the expressed C_H gene is either totally absent or present only in haploid quantity (269–280), an observation that would be inconsistent with unequal crossing over between homologous chromosomes. However, as mentioned below, interchromosomal recombination between VDJ and the C_H gene cluster has been described for switching to IgA in the rabbit and may account for 3% to 7% of the switching to this isotype in this species (313a,313b). If unequal sister chromatid exchange were the mechanism of isotype switching, normal cells should be produced that express triploid quantities of $C\mu$ DNA; no such cells have been found (290,300,314,315). However, switching by sister chromatid exchange appears to occasionally occur (300).

Regions of homology exist between the S regions 5′ to the different C_H genes. However, sequencing of the recombined S regions located between $V_H DJ_H$ and the gene for the expressed C_H isotype in a clone that expresses an isotype other than IgM has indicated that S-region recombination typically occurs between DNA sequences that have either limited base pair homology or no homology at all (317). In addition, sequencing of DNA recombination sites from different clones that have switched isotype has demonstrated that recombination can occur at multiple sites within S regions (292,300,301,316). In fact, approximately 40% of sequenced chromosomal breakpoints in transformed B cells demonstrate recombination of a site within the S region 5′ to the expressed C_H gene to a sequence outside of $S\mu$ (275,317). It is not known whether the apparent lack of involvement of $S\mu$ in the chromosomal breakpoints reflects recombination that actually occurs outside of $S\mu$, or whether secondary deletional events in the long-term cultured cells used for these studies have obscured original recombination sites in which $S\mu$ was involved. The presence of $S\mu$ at the splice sites in the DNA circles that are looped out during isotype switching suggests that the latter possibility is more likely (247,303–307). However, even within these DNA circles, the recombined 5′ and 3′ S regions never have homologous sequences longer than 5 bp, and some recombination sites are found at DNA sequences that are entirely nonhomologous.

Analysis of DNA sequences from mouse hybridomas and plasmacytomas that secrete IgD has also provided evidence about the importance of S regions in isotype switching. These IgD-secreting cells, unlike mature B cells that express mIgM and mIgD, have deleted the $C\mu$ gene (274–280). Inasmuch as no S region is found between $C\mu$ and $C\delta$ in the mouse, this finding shows that a 3′ S region is not an absolute requirement for switching. The low frequency of switching to IgD in the mouse may, thus, reflect the absence of DNA sequences that facilitate, but are not required for

nonhomologous recombination. In addition, the frequent recombination of VDJ with an intron 3′ of the $C\delta 1$ exon in IgD-secreting cells, with the deletion of part of the gene that encodes the δ chain (274,275), suggests that 3′ S regions have an important function in directing switching to promote the production of intact C_H genes. Based on these observations, it has been proposed that the tandem repeats within S regions may be binding or assembly sites for proteins that control or facilitate the isotype-switching process, rather than sites at which recombination must occur. The importance for recombination of the limited DNA homology that is most frequently seen at recombination sites in DNA circles is still debated, as is the question of whether switching to IgD in the mouse utilizes similar recombinational mechanisms as does switching to other isotypes.

The one well-defined example of isotype switching that can involve classic homologous recombination is that which promotes switching from IgM to IgD in the human. Studies of human IgD–secreting myelomas as well as normal human B cells have shown that human $C\delta$ recombination occurs between two nearly identical 442- to 443-bp repeats 5′ and 3′ of the $C\mu$ gene, with joining at homologous sites of the 5′ and 3′ repeats (277, 318). However, analysis of two well-established IgD-secreting cell lines has indicated that human IgM to IgD switching can also occur outside of these repeats (318).

Molecular Parameters of the Switch Recombination Event

Recombination may require the alignment of specific regions of DNA into highly ordered structures through the binding of multiple proteins (319). Two DNA-binding protein complexes have been identified in the mouse that specifically interact with motifs within the $S\gamma$ tandem repeats (320–322). One protein complex, initially termed SNIP, is indistinguishable from NF-κB p50 homodimer, whereas the second protein complex, termed SNAP, is most likely a heterooligimer containing the product of the E2A gene, E47, a helix–loop–helix transcription factor. The breakpoints involved in switch recombination appear to cluster within the SNIP and SNAP binding regions (326). Similar SNIP and SNAP switch-binding regions have also been described in humans (323). Indeed, the SNIP site used most frequently in switching to human IgG3 was found to be mutated in patients with low serum IgG3 concentrations in association with the G3 m(g) allotype (323).

Because isotype switching requires the formation of breaks in both strands of DNA at switch sites, mechanisms that stimulate formation of double-strand breaks (DSBs) during switching have been investigated (328). B cells activated with LPS or dextran–anti-IgD plus IL-5, although not with dextran–anti-IgD alone, demonstrated DSBs within $S\gamma 3$, beginning 4 hours after activation and continuing for up to 44 hours. These DSBs were found to be (a) B cell–specific; (b) sequence-specific, occurring within a consensus sequence—5′-GRGNAGCT-3′—as read from the coding strand, and present at the boundaries of the SNAP binding site; (c) locus-specific; and (d) inducible, in that they were not present in resting B cells but appeared after activation. Although DSBs appear concomitantly with germline C_H RNA expression, it is not known whether transcription is required for the generation of DSBs. Sequences surrounding the DSBs contain short inverted repeats, which could facilitate the formation of stem-loop structures. It has been suggested that these secondary structures could play a role in recombinase targeting.

In addition to p50/NF-κB and E47, additional potential switch-binding proteins have been described (329,330). S regions are notable for their abundance of G-rich tandem repeats. Such repeats may form parallel four-stranded complexes, termed G4 (quadruplex) DNA, that could facilitate recombination between different sites on the same DNA strand. A protein, termed QUAD, has been described that binds specifically to this G4 conformation and could play a role in stabilizing this G-rich quadruplex DNA (329).

Switch and V$_H$DJ$_H$ Recombination Exhibit Both Distinct and Similar Molecular Features

The mechanism of switch recombination is distinct in certain fundamental ways from that which mediates V$_H$DJ$_H$ recombination. V$_H$DJ$_H$ recombination, unlike class switching, utilizes heptamer (CACTGTG) and nonamer (GGTTTTTGT) signal sequences of constant spacing (12 or 23 bp) (331,332), instead of the S-region tandem repeats of more variable alignment, and leads to precise joining of the V$_H$, D, and J$_H$ genes. This latter feature reflects the requirement for the recombined V$_H$DJ$_H$ to encode a translation product in which specificity for antigen is maintained, whereas S regions are spliced out of the mature C$_H$ mRNA. On this basis, it is likely that different enzyme systems are utilized to mediate these two processes, although the two processes will also likely share enzymes. Thus, although the RAG-1 (333) and RAG-2 (334) gene products have been implicated in recombination of V$_H$, D, and J$_H$ genes, these genes do not appear to be critical for switch recombination (335). However, as discussed below, the Ku protein complex appears to be critical for both switch (335) and V$_H$DJ$_H$ recombination, as well as for repair of damaged DNA (336–340).

Sequential Switching

Switching to a given C$_H$ gene by looping out and deletion does not always occur directly from Cμ but may occur through sequential deletional events. This was first suggested by the demonstration that S regions from some B-cell tumors that had undergone isotype switching contained a portion of Sμ that was ligated directly to S-region segments from two other non-IgM, non-IgD isotypes (292,297–299,341). Additional support for the existence of sequential switching came from studies in which circular DNA, which was obtained from actively switching normal B cells and represented the reciprocal deletion products from class-switch events, was shown to contain S-region sequences of Sμ ligated to two different Sγ sequences, Sμ ligated sequentially to an Sγ sequence and to Sε, and Sμ ligated sequentially to an Sγ sequence and to Sα (247,311,314). Restriction analysis of total, unselected circular DNA from LPS plus IL-4–stimulated cells indicated that the majority of Cγl-containing circles, generated by an IgE class switch, had rearranged Cγl DNA (205). In addition, DNA circles cloned from B cells stimulated to secrete IgE *in vivo* by infection with a nematode parasite that induces IL-4 production demonstrated sequences derived from Sγl as well as from Sμ and Sε (303). Both of these observations suggest that IgE switching may typically occur by a sequential IgM to IgG1 to IgE switch. Furthermore, Southern blot analysis of S regions present in chromosomal DNA that had been prepared from hybridomas made by fusion of *in vivo*-generated IgE-expressing B cells demonstrated that four of 12 Igh genes that had recombined VDJ to Cε had undergone an Sμ to Sγl to Sε switch recombination (311). This represented a minimal estimate of sequential switching, since recombination of Sμ/Sγl to Sε could have occurred so that the 5′ breakpoint was within Sμ, in which case Sγl would have been deleted.

At the cellular level, the occurrence of sequential switching is supported by the fact that (a) the majority of B cells induced to express mIgE by culture with LPS plus IL-4 coexpress mIgG1 (342); (b) anti-IgG1 antibody inhibits IgE secretion induced by LPS plus IL-4 by approximately 70% to 80% (205,311); and (c) approximately 5% of B cells that express cytoplasmic (c) [secretory] IgE after LPS plus IL-4 stimulation coexpress cIgG1 (205,311). Furthermore, the delay in approximately 80% of the LPS plus IL-4–induced IgE response, relative to the IgG1 response (205), suggests that most, but not all, IgE-secreting cells are generated in this system from cells that first switch to IgG1. Sequencing of S regions from human IgE-secreting cells has also provided evidence for the occurrence of sequential IgM/IgG/IgE switching (171,190,343). More recently, mono and double sequential switching from Sμ to Sε via Sγl, Sγ2, or Sγ4 has been demonstrated in patients infected with *Schistosoma mansoni* or with atopic dermatitis (344).

These observations are compatible with the possibilities that (a) sequential switching in the generation of an IgE response simply reflects the greater likelihood of B cells that are activated by some stimuli, such as LPS plus IL-4, to switch to IgG1 than IgE, so that most B cells that switch to IgE have already been induced to switch to IgG1; and (b) switching to IgE from IgG1 is more easily accomplished than is switching to IgE from IgM. Studies with human B cells favor the first hypothesis by providing evidence that some stimuli appear to favor a direct switch to IgE from IgM, while other stimuli appear to favor sequential switching to IgE through IgG. For example, human B cells induced to switch to IgE by culture with EBV plus IL-4 can switch to IgE via IgG (171), while human B cells cultured with IL-2, IL-4, and PMA-activated mouse EL-4 thymoma cells (345) or with anti-CD40 antibody plus IL-4 (189) appear to switch directly to IgE. The first hypothesis is also favored by data obtained from mice made genetically deficient in the 5′ flanking sequences of Sγl, which include the promoter elements and splice donor site of the γ1 germline RNA transcript, and which are unable to switch to IgG1 (346). B cells from such mice switched at normal frequencies to IgE in response to LPS plus IL-4 *in vitro* and to *N. brasiliensis* infection or NP-OVA immunization *in vivo* (347).

Molecular Requirements for Isotype-switching

At least three different processes appear to be necessary for the induction of most immunoglobulin isotype-switch events: (a) expression of a germline form of RNA for the C$_H$ gene to which switching will occur, (b) cell division, and (C) an additional, as yet undefined process.

Germline C$_H$ RNA and the Accessibility Model of Immunoglobulin Class Switching

Initial studies, which explored the mechanism through which directed switching might occur, utilized either an mIgM$^+$ murine B-cell lymphoma, I.29 (I.29μ), which spontaneously, or upon LPS treatment, switches *in vitro* to the expression of IgA, IgE, or IgG2a, but not IgG1 (348), or Abelson-transformed pre-B-cell lines (A-MuLV pre-B) that spontaneously switch from μ to γ2b production

(285). The studies with I.29μ suggested that the C_H genes that encoded the specific immunoglobulin isotypes to which this cell line would switch were transcriptionally active. Thus, I.29μ, which has the potential to switch to IgA but not IgG1, constitutively expresses steady-state levels of $C\alpha$ RNA, but no detectable RNA for $C\gamma 1$ prior to class switching. Similarly, the A-MuLV pre-B-cell lines that switch to $\gamma 2b$ constitutively express steady-state levels of $\gamma 2b$ RNA. Neither the $C\alpha$ gene in the 1.29μ line nor the $C\gamma 2b$ gene in the A-MuLV pre-B line is rearranged; thus they are transcribed in their germline configurations. Germline C_H RNA differs from mRNA encoded by a rearranged C_H gene in that it lacks an exon that encodes $V_H D J_H$. These germline C_H RNA transcripts thus fail to encode intact immunoglobulin heavy chains and are alternatively referred to as "sterile" RNA transcripts. Since it was known, in other contexts, that transcriptional activation serves to target genes for recombination (349–351), perhaps due to its association with an "open" chromatin configuration and accessibility to regulatory DNA binding proteins, a model was advanced (accessibility model) that proposed that C_H gene accessibility also targeted the C_H gene for switch recombination (285,348).

Cytokines Can Control Switching through Regulation of Germline C_H Gene Transcription

The accessibility model of immunoglobulin isotype switching established a basis for understanding the mechanism by which certain cytokines induce the expression of selective immunoglobulin classes by activated normal B cells. Thus, IL-4, which stimulates IgG1 secretion by LPS-activated murine B cells, induces an increase in the steady-state levels of germline $\gamma 1$ RNA within 24 to 48 hours after exposure to IL-4 (99–102). The IL-4 induction of germline $\gamma 1$ RNA precedes the onset of IgG1 class switching. In a similar fashion, it was observed that IL-4 selectively induces an early increase in the steady-state levels of germline ϵ RNA (99–101), IFN-γ stimulates increased germline $\gamma 2a$ (101) and $\gamma 3$ RNA (42) levels, and TGF-β enhances the levels of germline $\gamma 2b$ (147) and α (130,259,352) RNA in appropriately activated murine B cells. Likewise, IL-4 and TGF-β induce increased steady-state levels of germline ϵ (154,166,168,178,189,190) and α (250,251) RNA, respectively, in human B cells. Thus, in every instance studied, switching to a given immunoglobulin isotype is preceded by an induction or increase in steady-state levels of germline RNA specific for the targeted C_H gene. As discussed below, more recent data indicate that, whereas germline C_H gene activation is necessary for induction of switch rearrangement, it is not sufficient. The accessibility model predicts that an increase in steady-state levels of germline C_H RNA results from an increase in transcriptional rate of the C_H gene. However, an alternate possibility, which would be inconsistent with the accessibility model, is that increased steady-state C_H germline RNA solely reflects selective increases in RNA stability. To address this, more recent studies have employed nuclear run-on analysis of C_H transcription in B-cell tumors that were stimulated with either IL-4 or TGF-β. These studies demonstrated that IL-4 and TGF-β increase *de novo* transcription of germline ϵ (353) and α RNA (259), respectively, as predicted by the accessibility model.

Agents Other Than Cytokines Can Regulate Germline C_H Gene Expression

Agents other than cytokines may also regulate immunoglobulin isotype switching at the level of C_H gene accessibility. For exam-

ple, the bacterial mitogen, LPS, which predominantly stimulates immunoglobulin class switching to IgG3, induces increased steady-state levels of germline $\gamma 3$ RNA (101). Further, although LPS, alone, fails to induce germline ϵ RNA and stimulates only low levels of germline $\gamma 1$ RNA, it acts synergistically with IL-4 to enhance the expression of these transcripts (101,220,354). Resting B cells stimulated with cell membranes derived from a concavalin A- activated CD4$^+$ $T_H 1$ clone in the absence of IL-4, expressed increased steady-state levels of germline $\gamma 1$ RNA relative to freshly isolated B cells (122). Induction of germline $\gamma 1$ RNA was specific in that germline $\gamma 3$, $\gamma 2b$, ϵ, and α RNA levels were not increased. The induction of germline C_H RNA by activated T-cell membranes appears to be mediated, at least in part, by the CD40 ligand that is expressed on the the cell membranes of activated T cells. Membrane-bound CD40 ligand induces resting murine B cells to express germline $\gamma 1$ and ϵ RNA in the absence of exogenous cytokines, even in the presence of neutralizing anti–IL-4 antibody (123). Further, CD40 ligand and IL-4 synergistically induce germline $\gamma 1$ and ϵ RNA. Human B cells stimulated with anti–CD40 antibody, in the absence of exogenous cytokines, in contrast, express germline transcripts of all isotypes except for $\gamma 4$ and ϵ (355). However, a different study of human B cells failed to detect γ-subclass germline transcripts in response to activation with anti–CD40 antibody alone (356). The basis for the differing results of these two studies is unclear. The multivalent cross-linking of mIg on resting murine B cells by dextran–anti-Ig antibodies, like exposure to LPS or ligation of CD40, has been found to affect germline C_H transcription. Multivalent immunoglobulin cross-linking (a) induces the production of germline $\gamma 3$, $\gamma 1$, and $\gamma 2b$ RNA in the absence of other exogenous stimuli (124); (b) augments germline $\gamma 1$ RNA in LPS plus IL-4–activated B cells (124); (c) augments germline α RNA in B cells activated with LPS or CD40 ligand plus IL-4, IL-5, and TGF-β (P. Zelazowski, C.M. Snapper, unpublished); (d) inhibits germline ϵ RNA in B cells activated with LPS plus IL-4; (e) inhibits germline $\gamma 3$ and $\gamma 2b$ in B cells activated with LPS; and (f) inhibits germline $\gamma 2a$ RNA in B cells induced with LPS plus IFN-γ (124). In this regard, it has been demonstrated that either (Fab')$_2$ anti-IgM or PMA induces germline $\gamma 1$ promoter activity in B-cell lines and that IL-4 synergizes with these two agents for induction of the $\gamma 1$ promoter (386).

The Structure of the Germline C_H Transcript

Understanding of the mechanisms by which cytokines selectively induce transcriptional activation of C_H genes has been promoted by structural studies of germline C_H transcripts. cDNAs that encode germline transcripts have been isolated or identified for all murine immunoglobulin isotypes except IgD (288,352,354,357–361) and for human IgM (362), IgE (178), and IgA (251). All germline transcripts are composed of a complete C_H RNA that is spliced to an exon transcribed from DNA located 5' to the S region for that C_H gene. This latter structure is called the "I" region. Such $I_H C_H$ germline RNA results from transcription that initiates immediately 5' to the I region and proceeds contiguously through the S region and C_H genes, terminating near the same poly(A) sites that terminate mRNA that encodes mature immunoglobulin heavy chains. Subsequent splicing out of the S region creates the $I_H C_H$ transcript. Transcription initiation occurs at a promoter that, unlike classic promoters, lacks a TATA box and a CCAAT motif. This may explain why transcription of germline C_H RNA initiates at multiple sites

(220,358). Transcripts that initiate from the I region associated with one C_H isotype may, in some cases, transplice to the germline transcript for a different C_H isotype, to create chimeric germline C_H transcripts (IµCε, IεCµ, IµCγ4, IγCµ, IγCε, IεCγ, and Iγ4Cα1. These have been found, for example, in IgD⁺ (unswitched) human B cells after IL-4 stimulation (363). Spliced hybrid IµCγ transcripts also form subsequent to switch recombination, through processing of a single RNA transcript containing the juxtaposed Iµ and Cγ regions, and are coexpressed with the mature Cγ RNA (364).

What Is the Function, If Any, of Germline C_H RNA?

The structural similarities in the germline transcripts for different isotypes suggest that germline RNA may play a role in the switching process, although the functional significance of germline transcription of C_H genes as a prelude to immunoglobulin class switching remains to be determined. Several possibilities have been entertained: (a) Germline transcripts may have no function, and merely reflect transcriptional activation and accessibility of the C_H gene for the action of a recombinase. (b) Germline transcripts may actively participate in the switching process, perhaps by forming triplex structures with C_H DNA that stabilize the open DNA configuration (365); by forming strand-specific RNA:DNA hybrids (366) that might enhance the recombinagenic activity of S regions by facilitating formation of nuclease-sensitive, short stem-loop structures (367); or by some direct enzymatic activity that participates in recombination. (c) Germline transcripts might encode a regulatory protein. This latter possibility has been suggested by the finding of open reading frames, potentially encoding 43 and 48 amino acid proteins, respectively, in the germline transcripts for IgA (357) and IgG1 (359), with Met initiation codons that are positioned to allow for efficient translation. Furthermore, germline α transcripts comigrate with polyribosomes in sucrose gradients (357). One group has shown that a germline C_H transcript has the potential to encode a truncated Cµ protein in vitro (368). The observation that other germline transcripts with small open reading frames have Met initiation codons in poor contexts for translation, however, argues against this latter function as being critical for the class-switch process in general. (d) Germline C_H RNA could, in theory, participate in class switching by splicing to a VDJ-Cµ RNA, which would then allow for nondeletional expression of a new immunoglobulin class (369–372), as is discussed below.

The Switch Recombinase: Studies Using Switch Recombination Substrates

The identity and characterization of the switch recombinase, the putative enzyme or enzymes that mediate isotype switching, are not known. However, analyses of switch-recombinase substrates have provided insights into the mechanism of isotype switching. A number of studies demonstrate that substrates must be transcriptionally active to undergo switch rearrangement (373–375,377,378) and thus support the accessibility model of isotype switching. Several studies with switch-recombinase substrates also demonstrate that only the DNA strand that is being transcribed is subject to deletional rearrangement (365,366,378). Differences in the properties of switch-recombinase activity have been observed, however, between studies that used chromosomally integrated switch-recombinase substrates as opposed to episomal substrates. Extrachromosomal switch substrates (327,373,374,377,379) undergo recombination in inap-

propriate cell types and can produce non–S sequence recombination products (375,376,378). In contrast, recombinase activity appears to be B cell– and S sequence–specific in studies that use chromosomally integrated switch-recombinase substrates (373,374,377–379). Work with single-copy, chromosomally integrated retroviral substrates indicates that recombinase activity is not only B cell–specific but B cell stage–specific (restricted to cell lines representing late-stage pre-B and mature B cells) (379). In this study, the recombinase activity was found to act in a stochastic fashion upon transcribed S-region targets; that is, switch recombinations were found to be chance events that occur with similar probability from one cell generation to the next (379).

Regulation of Germline C_H Promoter Activity

The association of germline C_H transcripts with the isotype-switching process has focused attention on the mechanisms that regulate the initiation of C_H germline transcription at the I-region promoter. The observation that IL-4 induces the early appearance of a DNAse I hypersensitivity site in the region 5′ to Sγ1 (380,381), where Iγ1 is encoded, suggested that this cytokine might regulate Cγ1 promoter activity. DNAse I hypersensitivity sites are typically associated with regions of DNA that bind regulatory proteins that are important in transcriptional regulation (382). This notion was further supported by the demonstration that stimulation with LPS and IL-4, but not LPS alone, induces demethylation within 48 hours at an Msp I site 5′ of the Sγ1 region of B-cell DNA (383). Hypomethylated regions of C_H DNA are associated with transcriptional activation and may play a role in maintaining the activated state (384). More recently, regulation of C_H germline transcription has been studied by employing cloned I exon promoters as substrates for the binding of potential regulatory proteins. In these studies, constructs are produced in which the I exon promoters are ligated to reporter genes, such as chloramphenicol acetyl transferase (CAT) or luciferase, and then transfected into B-cell tumor lines, where the activity of the reporter gene is studied after various stimulations. Studies with such reporter gene constructs that contain γ1, ε, or α I exon promoters indicate that transcription driven by these promoters can be regulated by the same cytokines that control germline C_H RNA expression and direct switching to the corresponding isotypes in normal B cells (353,385–390a,b).

Regulation of the Cα Promoter

To study regulation of the Cα promoter, fusion genes were constructed in which different lengths of the region 5′ to Sα were covalently linked to luciferase (385). These plasmids were transfected into several B lymphoma–cell lines. Constitutive promoter activity was contained within a 106-bp segment located 5′ to the first transcription initiation site. The promoter activity of this DNA segment depended on the presence of an ATF/CRE consensus element, which is a previously characterized DNA sequence (cyclic AMP response element) that is a ligand for a DNA-binding protein (activation transcription factor) (391). Analysis of nuclear extracts from a variety of cell types by an electrophoretic mobility shift assay demonstrated specific binding of a putative transcription factor to the ATF/CRE motif. Any member of the ATF/CREB family of transcription factors may potentially bind to this site, although the ones involved in Iα promoter regulation are unknown. In addition to this constitutive activity, the germline Cα promoter was also inducible with TGF-β. Inducible activity depended on a region, located 105 to 127 bp 5′ to the transcription initiation site (and for this reason, numbered -127/-105), which contained two imperfect tandem repeats: 5′ CACAG(G)CCAGAC 3′. These repeats were not important for constitutive germline α expression. The -127/-105 tandem repeats functioned synergistically to activate transcription. These repeats bind a transcription factor(s), in a sequence-specific manner, from nuclear extracts of the TGF-β–inducible I.29μ lymphoma, but the binding itself appeared to be unaffected by prior TGF-β treatment. An additional TGF-β–inducible element was also located more than 826 bp 5′ to the initiation site (385). A similar CRE site has been demonstrated within a 327-bp segment in the human Iα1 and Iα2 promoters that is important for conferring responsiveness to PMA plus TGF-β (387). This segment also contains putative sites for Ets family members and Sp1, transcription factors that are important for basal promoter activity. Upstream distal elements are also observed that could negatively regulate Iα1 and Iα2 activity and might make germline a RNA expression B cell–specific.

Regulation of the Cγ1 and Cε Promoters

The γ1 and ε promoters are both positively regulated by IL-4 (123,261,386,388–390a,b,392–394). Further, IL-4 acts synergistically with LPS or CD40 ligation to induce germline γ1 and ε transcripts. CD40 ligation alone, but not LPS, can also induce IL-4–independent germline γ1 and ε RNA expression. In this regard, the γ1 and ε promoters appear to share common binding sites for transcription factors such as Stat6 (NF-IL-4), NF-κB/Rel proteins, and members of the C/EBP family. The binding of IL-4 or IL-13 to their receptors activates Stat6. Mutation of the Stat6-binding site in the ε or γ1 promoter ablates IL-4, but not CD40-ligand promoter activity in reporter gene assays (390,392,393,395). A study of B cells from Stat6-deficient mice suggests that Stat6 is required for IL-4–mediated stimulation of germline γ1 and ε RNA in CD40 ligand–activated B cells, although not for induction of γ1 and ε RNA by CD40 ligand alone (396). Little detectable switching to IgG1 and IgE has been observed in Stat6-deficient B cells in response to CD40 ligand plus IL-4. Other observations, however, suggest that IL-4 may promote switching to IgG1, but not IgE, by a Stat6-independent mechanism. IgG1 responses to gastrointestinal nematode parasites are considerably reduced in IL-4–deficient and IL-4 receptor α chain–deficient mice, but they are actually increased in Stat6-deficient mice (F. Finkelman, S. Morris, N. Noben-Trauth, J. Urban, unpublished data). In contrast, IgE responses to most stimuli are strongly and similarly suppressed in both IL-4–deficient and Stat6-deficient mice. These latter observations, if substantiated, would suggest that switching to IgG1 is stimulated by IL-4 through at least two mechanisms, and they could help to explain why switching to IgE requires stronger and more prolonged IL-4 stimulation than does switching to IgG1.

The ability of CD40 ligand to synergize with IL-4 for induction of germline γ1 and ε RNA, may lie, at least in part, on the induction by CD40 ligation of NF-κB/Rel proteins that bind to the γ1 and ε promoters (390a,390b,397). The CD40 response region (CD40RR) in the γ1 promoter contains three binding sites for NF-κB/Rel proteins, which are each required for optimal CD40 ligand–mediated promoter activity (397). CD40 ligand induces p50, p65, c-Rel, and RelB binding to the CD40RR. Experiments that used NF-κB/Rel expression vectors in a B-cell line demonstrated that p50 plus RelB

or p50 plus p65, but not p50 plus c-Rel, could transactivate the γ1 promoter. The ability of CD40 ligand, but not LPS, to induce germline γ1 RNA may be accounted for by the induction of different NF-κB/Rel proteins by these two stimuli and/or other regulatory factors that coregulate γ1 promoter activity. CD40 ligand induces the binding of NF-κB/Rel proteins to two tandem κB sites located 3′ to the IL-4–responsive region of the mouse germline ε promoter (390b). Mutation of the two κB sites abolishes the induction of promoter activity by CD40 ligand or by IL-4. The synergistic effects of CD40 ligand and IL-4 for induction of ε promoter activity may thus lie in the respective binding and interaction of NF-κB/Rel proteins and Stat6 at this site (390a,309b).

One or more members of the C/EBP family of transcription factors are also implicated in mediating γ1 and ε promoter activity (390,392). In reporter gene assays, mutation of the C/EBP binding site in the ε promoter reduced IL-4 induction of ε promoter activity (390). A similar role for C/EBP family members (i.e., C/EBPβ and C/EBPγ) in stimulating γ1 promoter activity has been suggested (392). C/EBPβ is induced by LPS in mature B cells and could account, at least in part, for the synergistic induction of γ1 and ε promoter activity by LPS and IL-4.

Several studies that used reporter gene constructs have suggested that B cell–specific activator protein (BSAP or Pax-5) plays a positive role in induction of the mouse germline ε promoter by LPS plus IL-4 (353,398). Although BSAP also binds to the human ε promoter, mutational analysis of reporter gene constructs concluded that BSAP played no key role in regulating its activity (399). However, a study that used both reporter constructs that contain the human ε promoter and mutational analysis in two EBV-negative B-cell lines has suggested that BSAP is essential for both IL-4 and anti-CD40 stimulation of ε germline transcription (400). The basis for these differing results is not clear.

Studies have also suggested that the murine germline ε promoter is repressed in the resting B cell (401,402). This repression appears to be mediated by two distinct binding sites: one for HMG-I(Y) and the other for Stat6. The authors suggest that at least one mechanism for IL-4 induction of germline Cε RNA expression is derepression of these sites. Of interest, these sites that mediate germline ε promoter repression also appear to be required for IL-4 inducibility of germline Cε gene transcription.

Studies using B cells that contain Cγ1 transgenes observed that a 17-kb transgene that includes Iγ1, Sγ1, and Cγ1 is regulated for induction of germline Cγ1 RNA expression in response to LPS, CD40 ligand, IL-4 and/or IFN-γ, similarly to the corresponding endogenous gene, without a requirement for additional elements (403,404). Surprisingly, regulatory elements located outside of Iγ1 were also important for germline Cγ1 RNA expression of the transgene (404). These elements may lie within a 900-bp region just 5′ to the main set of Sγ1 49-bp repeats or within a 600-bp fragment that includes the CH3 exon.

I Regions Target Isotype Switching in Addition to Inducing Transcription

In addition to inducing transcription, I regions target isotype switching to specific S regions (405,406). Lorenz et al. propose that spliced I$_H$C$_H$ RNA may also be required for switching (406). Bottaro et al. (405) show that when the LPS/IL-4–inducible Iε promoter and exon are replaced by an LPS-inducible Eμ enhancer–V$_H$ promoter, switching to IgE is inhibited, in cis, by ten- to 100-fold, in spite of substantial transcription through the targeted allele's Sε region (405). Lorenz et al. (406) report that the Iγ1 exon sequences encompassing the splice donor signal are necessary and sufficient for normal levels of switching to IgG1, implying that the spliced germline transcript or the spliceosome complex is in some way required for subsequent switch recombination. However, in this latter study, the mutant γ1 locus, which retained the I exon splice donor, possessed much higher transcriptional activity than the switching-defective, mutant γ1 locus, which lacked the same splice donor signal. Because the higher transcriptional activity might have promoted switching, a more direct role for the processed germline transcript or its splicing intermediate in subsequent switch recombination remains uncertain.

DNA Synthesis

In addition to germline C_H gene expression, DNA synthesis appears to be necessary to allow B cells to undergo isotype switching (96,407,408). DNA synthesis inhibitors, such as thymidine, hydroxyurea, and bromodeoxyuridine, selectively inhibit IgG, as opposed to IgM production by mitogen-stimulated B cells (96). Aphidicolin treatment of B cells stimulated with LPS plus IL-4 blocks both DNA synthesis and switching from IgM to IgG1; both are reversed when aphidicolin is washed out (409). Further, LPS activation of B cells in the presence of cytochalasin B, which inhibits cell division but not nuclear division, leads to the accumulation of polynucleated cells that express both IgM and IgG. This suggests that switching to IgG might involve an asymmetric cell division, in which one of the daughter cells secretes IgG, while the other secretes IgM (408). Computer modeling based on cell-cycle kinetics of LPS-activated B cells suggests that rearrangement at Sμ occurs during the first S phase after LPS induction (407). Compelling evidence for a direct association between DNA replication and immunoglobulin class switching also comes from studies with the B-cell lymphoma, I.29, which undergoes IgM to IgA class switching (410,411). Analysis of five clones that had recombined Sμ and Sα at identical sites with identical nucleotide sequences, and were, thus, descended from the same parent cell that had undergone an IgM to IgA switch (292,300,301,316), revealed that these clones segregated into two sets that differed from each other by several point mutations, small deletions, and duplications in the Sμ-Sα S region (324). These mutations, which could only occur during a period of DNA synthesis, arose on only one strand of DNA, which was passed during the subsequent cell division to half of the progeny of the cell that had switched to IgA (325). This pattern of B cells with identical Sμ–Sα S regions, which segregate into two groups that differ by several point, duplication, and deletion mutations, could not have been observed if the class switch preceded or followed the mutations by one or more cell divisions, or if cell divisions subsequent to the class switch were also accompanied by a high mutation rate in the S region. Collectively, the data strongly suggest that immunoglobulin class switching occurs during DNA replication, and that DNA synthesis that occurs during this time, but not subsequent to the switch, is error-prone within the S regions.

Additional Requirements for Isotype Switching

Germline C_H gene expression plus B-cell DNA synthesis appear to be required, but are not sufficient, for the induction of isotype switching. Thus, significant changes in isotype switching in response to cytokines, B-cell activators, or a pharmacologic agent, or under the influence of transcription factors have been documented in the absence of corresponding changes in germline C_H RNA expression (for review, see ref. 410). These data, summarized below, suggest that, in addition to changes in germline C_H gene accessibility, regulated processes that affect the switch recombinase and/or its targeting factors are also involved in control of isotype switching.

Interleukin-4

IL-4 promotes switching to IgA, in both transformed and normal murine B cells, without effecting a corresponding change in germline α RNA expression. Addition of anti–IL-4 mAb to cultures of mIgM⁺ I.29μ lymphoma cells inhibits the generation of mIgA⁺ cells in response to LPS or LPS plus TGF-β, but it does not alter the levels of germline α RNA (259). Addition of IL-4 alone induces up to 12% mIgA⁺ cells in cultures of mIgM⁺ CH12.LX lymphoma cells without altering germline α RNA expression (411). IL-4 also promotes switching to IgA by normal B cells activated with either LPS or CD40 ligand in the presence of TGF-β plus IL-5 and dextran–anti-IgD (249). IL-4 induction of mIgA⁺ cells and Sμ-Sα recombination events in this system is also not associated with corresponding changes in germline α RNA (P. Zelazowski, C.M. Snapper, unpublished).

Interleukin-5

IL-5 induces mIgG1⁺ cells and Sμ-Sγ1 recombination events in murine B cells activated with dextran–anti-IgD plus IL-4 without altering germline γ1 RNA expression (412). IL-5 also promotes switching to IgE, as well as IgG1, without altering the corresponding levels of germline ε and γ1 RNA, in Sepharose–anti-Ig–activated normal murine B-lymphoblasts cultured in the presence of LPS (105). Finally, IL-5 stimulates the development of mIgA⁺ cells and Sμ-Sα recombination events in murine B cells activated with either LPS or CD40 ligand in the presence of TGF-β plus IL-4 and dextran–anti-IgD (249) without altering the levels of germline α RNA (P. Zelazowski, C.M. Snapper, unpublished).

Interleukin-10

IL-10 augments the percentages of mIgG3⁺ cells and Sμ-Sγ3 recombination events in LPS-activated murine B cells without affecting the levels of germline γ3 RNA. Likewise, IL-10 inhibits mIgA⁺ cells and Sμ-Sα recombination events in B cells activated with LPS plus IL-4, IL-5, TGF-β, and dextran–anti-IgD without decreasing germline α RNA levels (255). As mentioned earlier, IL-10 also induces IgG1 and IgG3 secretion in mIgD⁺ human B cells activated with anti–CD40 antibody (156,158), but in contrast to the response of mouse B cells to IL-10, human B cells modulate germline C_H RNA in response to IL-10, which, thus, appears to regulate switching (157).

Interferon-γ

IFN-γ inhibits LPS-induced IgG3 secretion and the generation of murine mIgG3⁺ cells without altering expression of germline γ3

RNA (101,124,126). IFN-γ also inhibits IgE secretion by human B cells activated by T cells in the presence of IL-4, but it does not decrease germline ε RNA (168).

Membrane Immunoglobulin Cross-linking

Dextran–anti-IgD inhibits both IgG1 and IgE secretion and the generation of mIgG1$^+$ and mIgE$^+$ cells in cultures of murine B cells activated with LPS plus IL-4 (109). Whereas dextran–anti-IgD suppresses the levels of germline ε RNA in these cultures, consistent with the accessibility model, it induces a ~seven-fold *increase* in germline γ1 RNA (124).

CD40 Activation

Human B cells can be induced to switch to IgE if they are simultaneously infected with EBV and exposed to IL-4 (166–171). However, culture of cycling EBV-transformed B cells with IL-4 induces a large increase in germline ε RNA level, but it fails to stimulate switching to IgE or expression of mature ε mRNA, unless activated helper T cells are added to the culture (168). The T-cell help responsible for switching to IgE was not identified in this study, but it could have been CD40 ligand (154,172,189). One study demonstrated the ability of CD40 ligand to augment switching to IgA in cultures of mIgM$^+$ CH12.LX lymphoma cells that contained TGF-β without further increasing germline α RNA levels (411).

NF-κB/Rel Proteins (p50 and c-Rel)

Purified resting B cells from p50/NF-κB–deficient mice have a substantial defect in switching to IgA, although they express normal levels of germline α RNA (413). Although p50-binding sites have been identified near sites of recombination within Sγ3, Sγ1, and Sγ2b (320–322), which suggests a role for this factor in isotype switching, p50-deficient B cells switch at near-normal levels to IgG1. This indicates that p50 is not essential for switching to this isotype. Further, B cells from mice made genetically deficient in the transactivation domain of c-rel fail to switch to IgE, despite expressing normal levels of germline ε RNA relative to controls (414). In contrast, RelB-deficient (415) or p52-deficient (416) B cells demonstrate no obvious defects in isotype switching.

Disodium Cromoglycate

Disodium cromoglycate (DSCG), a drug commonly used in the prophylactic treatment of allergic disease, inhibits IgE secretion and Sμ-Sε rearrangement events in human B cells activated *in vitro* with anti–CD40 antibody plus IL-4 (417). These effects are not associated with a corresponding decrease in germline ε RNA.

A Role for Ku in Switch Recombination

The factors that mediate the switch recombination process are unknown, but they might include a variety of regulatory proteins that participate in DNA replication, repair, and/or recombination, and whose expression could, in theory, be regulated. Ku may represent one such protein complex. Ku plays a role in DNA strand-break repair and VDJ recombination (336–340). This complex consists of a Ku70/Ku86 heterodimer that recognizes and binds to double-stranded DNA ends, nicked DNA, or duplex DNA *that ends* in stem-loop structures. Once bound to DNA, the Ku70/Ku86 heterodimer binds and activates a DNA-dependent protein kinase (DNA-PK), which then can phosphorylate additional proteins with regulatory functions. In this regard, the ability of B-cell precursors from RAG-2–deficient and SCID mice to undergo Sμ-Sε recombination in response to anti–CD40 mAb plus IL-4 were compared (335). The RAG genes (RAG-1 and RAG-2) are key mediators of VDJ recombination (333,334). SCID mice lack the Ku70/Ku86-associated DNA-dependent serine–threonine protein kinase (DNA-PK; p350), which has also been implicated in VDJ recombination (418). B-cell precursors from both the RAG-2 and SCID mice expressed germline ε RNA in the presence of anti–CD40 mAb plus IL-4 (335). However, RAG-2–deficient, but not SCID, B-cell precursors undergo Sμ-Sε recombination under these conditions. This suggests that DNA-PK, although not RAG-2, is a key mediator of switch rearrangement.

The nuclear expression of Ku in normal murine B cells can be upregulated by stimuli that promote switch recombination (431). Resting B cells express relatively little nuclear Ku. Membrane immunoglobulin cross-linking using dextran–anti-IgD strongly stimulates nuclear Ku expression in resting B cells, and this may be further enhanced by IL-5. Likewise, the combination of IL-4 and CD40 ligand, but not either stimulant alone, strongly induces Ku expression. In contrast, IL-4 does not enhance Ku expression in dextran–anti-IgD–activated B cells (431).

In summary, although the nature of the switch recombination machinery and its targeting factors remain to be elucidated, the data cited above suggest that at least some of these parameters can be regulated by a number of cytokines, activators, drugs, and transcription factors. These model systems should help to elucidate the nature of these factors.

Nondeletional Switching

This chapter has focused on gene deletion and recombination as a mechanism for isotype switching. This emphasis was chosen both because the majority of studies favor this mechanism as the most important means of switching isotypes and because it is intuitively more likely that gene deletion and recombination would yield a stable isotype switch than would a mechanism that relied on transcriptional or posttranscriptional control. However, the precedent that IgM and IgD can simultaneously be expressed on the plasma membranes of mature B cells, and that the production of both isotypes by the same B cell is controlled at a transcriptional level (265,267), provided reason to believe that expression of other immunoglobulin isotypes might also be achieved without Cμ or Cδ gene deletion. Indeed, several studies suggest alternative means of expression of non-IgM/IgD isotypes. Cells that had been stimulated *in vitro* to express a C$_H$ gene 3′ of Cδ were reported to yield a long mRNA transcript that could be differentially spliced (see Fig. 2D) to encode μ chain or α chain (419); however, the methods used to perform this study were technically very difficult, and this result has not been confirmed. Another study reported that B cells could be stimulated *in vivo* to simultaneously express membrane IgM, IgD, and IgE without having undergone Cμ deletion (420); however, it is likely that the IgE expressed by these cells was cytophilic (i.e., produced by other cells and bound by an Fcε receptor on these cells) (421). Human B cells cultured with EBV plus helper T cells have been reported to secrete IgM, IgD and IgE without deleting Cμ or Cδ (422,423); however, analysis of these cells by other laboratories demonstrated only IgM secretion (G. Thyphronitis, F. Finkelman, unpublished data), and cloned EBV-transformed human B cells that secrete IgE have deleted the C_H genes 5' to Cε (170). This does not, of course, rule out the possibility that nonstable secretion of isotypes other than IgM might be accomplished by nondeletional mechanisms.

The best documented example of nondeletional isotype switching is a switch variant of the mouse B-cell lymphoma BCL_1, termed $BCL_1.B_2$, which coexpresses mIgM and mIgG1 and secretes both isotypes, which share identical idiotypic determinants. $BCL_1.B_2$ contains mRNA for both membrane and secreted forms of both μ and γ1 (424,425). These observations strongly suggest that the same VDJ is being used to encode both IgM and IgG1 (424). $BCL_1.B_2$ has two copies of chromosome 12, both of which have translocated to chromosome 16. One copy of chromosome 12 has deleted all C_H genes (425). The other copy of chromosome 12 contains a complete set of C_H genes, which display no rearrangement by Southern blot analysis (425). Dual μ/γ1 synthesis in this BCL_1 subclone occurs by a discontinuous transcription mechanism (372). Despite the observation that μ and γ1 are linked within the same nuclear pre-RNA, initiation of γ1 RNA synthesis occurs just upstream of Cγ1. Instead of a long, continuous pre-RNA of 150 kb, the length of the primary transcription unit for γ1 mRNA is similar (approximately 15 kb) to that for μ mRNA. This suggests that double-isotype expression can occur through the ligation of discontinuously produced RNA transcripts, rather than through differential splicing of a long RNA transcript (372). Mature γ1 mRNA could be produced in $BCL_1.B_2$ either through *trans*-splicing of the VDJCμ transcript with the Cγ1-containing transcript, or through ligation of these two RNAs followed by splicing in *cis* (see Fig. 2E). These two processes differ by the mechanism through which parts of two, discontinuously transcribed RNA molecules are joined. In *cis* splicing, joining is initiated by ligation of the 3' end of one transcript (e.g., VDJIμSμCμ) directly to the 5' end of the second transcript (e.g., Iγ1Sγ1Cγ1), with subsequent splicing out of the RNA that will not be part of the final, productive VDJCγ1 transcript. The generation of VDJCγ1 from the same RNA precursors by *trans*-splicing would involve, instead, steps in which (a) the 5' end of IμSμCμ first joined to Iγ1Sγ1Cγ1 near the border between the Sγ1 and Cγ1 exons, creating a "Y-branched intermediate" and freeing VDJ; and (b) subsequent splicing out of the Y-branched intermediate, allowing VDJ to ligate to Cγ1. *Trans*-splicing has been described in lower eukaryotes (299,300) and plant chloroplasts (426).

Additional evidence for discontinuous RNA transcription, by either mechanism, as a means for the simultaneous expression of two immunoglobulin isotypes, comes from studies of mice in which a human μ transgene was integrated into the mouse genome outside the IgH locus (369,370). In these experiments, LPS plus IL-4 activation of transgenic spleen cells *in vitro* resulted in a small percentage of cells that expressed immunoglobulin that contained hybrid heavy chains composed of human VDJ linked to mouse Cγ1 (369). These cells contained mRNA, in which the transgenic variable region was ligated to endogenous Cγ1. This RNA could not have arisen from intrachromosomal recombination, since the transgene was not physically located within the endogenous Igh locus on chromosome 12. Analysis of a purified population of cells that coexpressed the μ transgene and the endogenous mouse γ gene after LPS plus IL-4 stimulation (370) demonstrated expression of this hybrid RNA, but no detectable DNA rearrangement. This

argues against the possibility of interchromosomal recombination between S regions (S-S recombination) as an explanation for these findings. However, since cloned B cells that express the hybrid mRNA but have not rearranged DNA are not available, the possibility that the hybrid mRNA is derived from a small cell population that has undergone DNA rearrangement cannot be excluded.

By contrast, experiments with a system, in which an ARS-specific μ transgene was introduced into the mouse genome and found to associate with endogenous Cγ on immunization *in vivo*, provided evidence that this occurred by interchromosomal recombination (427,428). Sequence analysis of the recombined S region suggested that this interchromosomal recombination utilized the same enzymatic machinery that operates to mediate classic intrachromosomal switch recombination, rather than homologous recombination. The ARS and the human transgene systems differ in that the former system is antigen-driven, while the latter uses a mitogen and cytokines to induce polyclonal stimulation of B-cell proliferation and differentiation. It has been suggested (370) that the enormous clonal expansion that is characteristic of an *in vivo* response to antigenic stimulation might have greatly increased the number of descendents of B cells that were produced by a rare interchromosomal recombinant event. In contrast, such rare events would be less likely to be observed in a mitogen plus cytokine–driven system, in which less clonal expansion occurs.

That interchromosomal class switching can occur under more physiologic conditions is suggested by the finding that 3% to 7% of serum IgA from nonimmunized rabbits results from interchromosomal class switching *in vivo* (313a,313b). However, the mechanism for this is unknown. Interchromosomal class switching has also been reported in mouse hybridomas (429) and could explain the occasionally observed switching of a myeloma or hybridoma to the secretion of an isotype encoded by a C_H gene 5' to the one that was expressed earlier (430). Regardless of the mechanism, it remains unclear to what extent nondeletional class switching is important physiologically. It could, in theory, represent an intermediate stage in the class-switch process that allows for expression of new immunoglobulin isotypes and the potential for immunoglobulin isotype–specific B-cell regulation prior to looping out and deletion. In any event, the two mechanisms need not be mutually exclusive.

ACKNOWLEDGMENTS

We thank Ken Marcu, Michael Berton, Amy Kenter, Janet Stavnezer, and Fred Alt for helpful discussions; Janet Stavnezer, Barbara Birshtein, and Amy Kenter for critical review of this chapter; and multiple investigators for sharing their unpublished data.

REFERENCES

1. Pritsch O, Hudry-Clergeon G, Buckle M, et al. Can immunoglobulin C(H)1 constant region domain modulate antigen binding affinity of antibodies. *J Clin Invest* 1996;98:2235–2243.
2. Nossal GJV, Szenberg A, Ada GL, Austin GM. Single cell studies on 19S antibody production. *J Exp Med* 1964;119:485–502.
3. Wall R, Kuehl M. Biosynthesis and regulation of immunoglobulins. *Annu Rev Immunol* 1983;1:393–422.
4. Gearhart P, Johnson ND, Douglas R, Hood L. IgG antibodies to phosphorylcholine exhibit more diversity than their IgM counterparts. *Nature* 1981;291:29–34.
5. Wysocki L, Manser T, Gefter ML. Somatic evolution of variable region structures during an immune response. *Proc Natl Acad Sci USA* 1986;83:1847–1851.
6. Crothers DM, Metzger H. The influence of polyvalency on the binding properties of antibodies. *Immunochemistry* 1972;9:341–357.

7. Hornick CL, Karush F. Antibody affinity—III. The role of multivalence. *Immunochemistry* 1972;9:325–340.
8. Borsos T, Rapp HJ. Complement fixation on cell surfaces by 19S and 7S antibodies. *Science* 1965;150:505–506.
9. Solomon A, Fahey JL. Plasmapheresis therapy in macroglobulinemia. *Ann Intern Med* 1963;58:789–800.
10. Waldmann TA, Strober W. Metabolism of immunoglobulins. *Prog Allergy* 1969;13:1–110.
11. Vieira P, Rajewsky K. The half-lives of serum immunoglobulins in adult mice. *Eur J Immunol* 1988;18:313–316.
12. Fish S, Zenowich E, Fleming M, Manser T. Molecular analysis of original antigenic sin. I. Clonal selection, somatic mutation, and isotype switching during a memory B cell response. *J Exp Med* 1989;170:1191–1209.
13. Cohen S, Milstein C. Structure and biological properties of immunoglobulins. *Adv Immunol* 1967;7:1–89.
14. Tomasi TB, Bienenstock J. Secretory immunoglobulins. *Adv Immunol* 1968;9: 1–96.
15. Neuberger MS, Rajewsky K. Activation of mouse complement by monoclonal mouse antibodies. *Eur J Immunol* 1981;11:1012–1016.
16. Ey PL, Russel-Jones GJ, Jenkins CR. Isotypes of mouse IgG-I. Evidence for "non-complement-fixing" IgG1 antibodies and characterization of their capacity to interfere with IgG2 sensitization of target red blood cells for lysis by complement. *Mol Immunol* 1980;17:699–710.
17. Waldmann H. Manipulation of T-cell responses with monoclonal antibodies. *Ann Rev Immunol* 1989;7:407–444.
18. Bruggemann MG, Williams GT, Bindon CI, et al. Comparison of the effector functions of human immunoglobulins using a matched set of chimeric antibodies. *J Exp Med* 1987;166:1351–1361.
19. Dangl JL, Wensel TG, Morrison SL, Stryer L, Herzenberg LA, Oi VT. Segmental flexibility and complement fixation of genetically engineered chimeric human, rabbit and mouse antibodies. *EMBO J* 1988;7:1989–1994.
20. Unkeless JC, Eisen HN. The presence of two Fc receptors on mouse macrophages: evidence from a variant cell line and differential trypsin sensitivity. *J Exp Med* 1977;145:931–947.
21. Unkeless JC, Scigliano E, Freedman VH. Structure and function of human and murine receptors for IgG. *Annu Rev Immunol* 1988;6:251–281.
22. Denham S, Barfoot R, Jackson E. A receptor for monomeric IgG2b on rat macrophages. *Immunology* 1987;62:69–74.
23. Ravetch JV, Kinet J-P. Fc Receptors. *Annu Rev Immunol* 1991;9:457–492.
24. Looney RJ, Abraham GN, Anderson CL. Human monocytes and U937 cells bear two distinct Fc receptors for IgG. *J Immunol* 1986;136:1641–1647.
25. Guyre PM, Morganelli PM, Miller R. Recombinant immune interferon increases immunoglobulin G Fc receptors on cultured human mononuclear phagocytes. *J Clin Invest* 1983;72:393–397.
26. Bach MK, Bloch KH, Austen KF. IgE and IgG2a antibody-mediated release of histamine from rat peritoneal cells. II. Interaction of IgG2a and IgE at the target cell. *J Exp Med* 1971;133:772–784.
27. Conrad DH, Wingard JR, Ishizaka T. The interaction of human and rodent IgE with the human basophil IgE receptor. *J Immunol* 1983;130:327–333.
28. Jefferis, R. Structure-function relationships of IgG subclasses. In: Shakib F, ed. *The human IgG subclasses: molecular analysis of structure, function and regulation.* Oxford: Pergamon Press, 1990:93–108.
29. Ghetie V, Hubbard JG, Kim J-K, Tsen M-F, Lee Y, Ward ES. Abnormally short serum half-lives of IgG in β2-microglobulin-deficient mice. *Eur J Immunol* 1996;26:690–696.
30. Junghans RP, Anderson CL. The protection receptor for IgG catabolism is the β2-microglobulin-containing neonatal intestinal transport receptor. *Proc Natl Acad Sci USA* 1996;93:5512–5516.
31. Slack JH, Der-Balian G, Nahm MH, Davie JM. Subclass restriction of murine antibodies. II. The IgG plaque-forming response to thymus-independent type 1 and type 2 antigen in normal mice and mice expressing an X-linked immunodeficiency. *J Exp Med* 1980;151:853–862.
32. Scott MG, Fleischman JB. Preferential idiotype-isotype association in antibodies to dinitrophenyl antigens. *J Immunol* 1982;128:2622–2628.
33. Perlmutter R, Hansburg D, Briles DE, Nicolotti R, Davie JM. Subclass restriction of murine anti-carbohydrate antibodies. *J Immunol* 1978;121:566–572.
34. Der Balian GP, Slack J, Clevinger BL, Bazin H, Davie JM. Subclass restriction of murine antibodies. III. Antigens that stimulate IgG3 in mice stimulate IgG2c in rats. *J Exp Med* 1980;152:209–218.
35. Riesen WF, Skvaril F, Braun DG. Natural infection of man with group A streptococci. Levels; restriction in class, subclass, and type; and clonal appearance of polysaccharide group-specific antibodies. *Scand J Immunol* 1976;5:383–390.
36. Yount WJ, Dorner MM, Kunkel HG, Kabat EA. Studies on human antibodies. VI. Selected variations in subgroup composition and genetic markers. *J Exp Med* 1968;127:633–646.
37. Barrett DJ, Ayoub EM. IgG2 subclass restriction of antibody to pneumococcal polysaccharides. *Clin Exp Immunol* 1986;63:127–134.
38. Coutelier JP, Vanderlogt TTM, Heesen FWA, Vink A, Van Snick J. Virally induced modulation of murine IgG antibody subclasses. *J Exp Med* 1988;168: 2373–2378.
39. Skvaril F, Schilt U. Characterization of the subclass and light chain types of IgG antibodies to rubella. *Clin Exp Immunol* 1984;55:671–676.
40. Finkelman FD, Katona IM, Mosmann TR, Coffman RL. Interferon-γ regulates the isotypes of immunoglobulin secreted during in vivo humoral immune responses. *J Immunol* 1988;140:1022–1027.
41. Thyphronitis G, Kinoshita T, Inoue K, et al. Modulation of mouse complement receptors 1 and 2 suppresses antibody responses in vivo. *J Immunol* 1991;147: 224–230.
42. Snapper CM, McIntyre TM, Mandler R, et al. Induction of IgG3 secretion by interferon-γ: a model for T cell-independent class switching in response to T cell-independent type 2 antigens. *J Exp Med* 1992;175:1367–1371.
43. Zakroff SGH, Beck L, Spiegelberg HL. The IgE and IgG subclass responses of mice to four helminth parasites. *Cell Immunol* 1989;199:193–198.
44. Evengard B, Hammarstrom L, Smith CIE, Johansson SGO, Linder E. Subclass distribution and IgE responses after treatment in human schistosomiasis. *Clin Exp Immunol* 1989;73:383–388.
45. Otteson EA, Skvaril F, Tripathy SP, Poindexter RW, Hussain R. Prominence of IgG4 in the IgG antibody response to human filariasis. *J Immunol* 1985;134: 2707–2712.
46. Aalberse RC, van der Gaag R, Leewen J. Serologic aspects of IgG4 antibodies. I. Prolonged immunization results in an IgG4-restricted response. *J Immunol* 1983;130:722–726.
47. Greenspan NS, Cooper LJN. Intermolecular cooperativity: a clue to why mice have IgG3? *Immunol Today* 1992;13:164–168.
48. Berney T, Shibata T, Izui S. Murine cryoglobulinemia: pathogenic and protective IgG3 self-associating antibodies. *J Immunol* 1991;147:3331–3335.
49. Weiner E. The ability of IgG subclasses to cause the elimination of targets in vivo and to mediate their destruction by phagocytosis/cytolysis in vitro. In: Shakib F, ed. *The human IgG subclasses: molecular analysis of structure, function and regulation.* Oxford: Pergamon Press, 1990:135–160.
50. Lee HK, Lee HH, Park YM, Ha TY. Induction of active systemic anaphylaxis by IgG antibodies. *FASEB J* 1992;6:A1609.
51. Knight KL, Becker RS. Isolation of genes encoding bovine IgM, IgG, IgA, and IgE chains. *Vet Immunol Immunopathol* 1987;17:17–24.
52. Briles DE, Forman C, Hudak S, Claflin JL. The effects of subclass on the ability of anti-phosphocholine antibodies to protect mice from fatal infection with Streptococcus pneumoniae. *J Mol Cell Immunol* 1984;1:305–309.
53. Brodskyn CI, Silva AM, Takehara HA, Mota I. IgG subclasses responsible for immune clearance in mice infected with *Trypanosoma cruzi*. *Immunol Cell Biol* 1989;67:343–348.
54. Pelkonen S, Pluschke G. Use of hybridoma immunoglobulin switch variants in the analysis of the protective properties of anti-lipopolysaccharide antibodies in *Escherichia coli* K1 infection. *Immunology* 1989;68:260–264.
55. Oishi K, Koles NL, Guelde G, Pollack M. Antibacterial and protective properties of monoclonal antibodies reactive with *Escherichia coli* O111:B4 lipopolysaccharide: relation to antibody isotype and complement-fixing activity. *J Infect Dis* 1992;165:34–56.
56. White WI, Evans CB, Taylor DW. Antimalarial antibodies of the immunoglobulin IgG2a isotype modulate parasitemias in mice infected with *Plasmodium yoelii*. *Infect Immun* 1991;59:3547–3554.
57. Sanford JE, Lupan DM, Schlageter AM, Kozel TR. Passive immunization against Cryptococcus neoformans with an isotype-switch family of monoclonal antibodies reactive with cryptococcal polysaccharide. *Infect Immun* 1990;58: 1919–1923.
58. Nussbaum G, Yuan R, Casadevall A, Scharff MD. Immunoglobulin G3 blocking antibodies to the fungal pathogen *Cryptococcus neoformans*. *J Exp Med* 1996; 183:1905–1909.
59. Scott MG, Briles DE, Nahm MH. Selective IgG subclass expression: biologic, clinical and functional aspects. In: Shakib F, ed. *The human IgG subclasses: molecular analysis of structure, function and regulation.* Oxford: Pergamon Press, 1990:161–183.
60. Nilssen DE, Soderstrom R, Brandtzaeg P, et al. Isotype distribution of mucosal IgG-producing cells in patients with various IgG subclass deficiencies. *Clin Exp Immunol* 1991;83:17–24.
61. Mestecky J, McGhee JR. Immunoglobulin A (IgA): molecular and cellular interactions involved in IgA biosynthesis and immune response. *Adv Immunol* 1987;40:153–245.
62. Kühn LC, Kraehenbuhl J-P. The membrane receptor for polymeric immunoglobulin is structurally related to secretory component. *J Biol Chem* 1981;256: 12490–12495.
63. Taylor HP, Dimmock NJ. Mechanism of neutralization of influenza-virus by secretory IgA is different from that of monomeric IgA or IgG. *J Exp Med* 1985; 161:198–209.
64. Lucisano Valim YM, Lachmann PJ. The effect of antibody isotype and antigenic epitope density on the chimeric anti-PIP antibodies with human Fc regions. *Clin Exp Immunol* 1991;84:1–8.
65. Henson PM, Johnson HB, Spiegelberg HL. The release of granule enzymes from human neutrophils stimulated by aggregated immunoglobulins of different classes and subclasses. *J Immunol* 1972;109:1182–1192.
66. Killian M, Mestecky J, Russell MW. Defense mechanisms involving Fc-dependent functions of immunoglobulin A and their subversion by bacterial immunoglobulin proteases. *Microbiol Rev* 1988;52:296–303.
67. Magnusson K-E, Stjernström I. Mucosal barrier mechanisms. Interplay between secretory IgA (SIgA), IgG and mucins on the surface properties and association of salmonellae with intestine and granulocytes. *Immunology* 1982;45:239–248.
68. Wold AE, Mestecky J, Tomana M, et al. Secretory immunoglobulin A carries

oligosaccharide receptors for *Escherichia coli* type 1 fimbrial lectin. *Infect Immun* 1990;58:3073–3077.

69. Mbawuike IN, Pacheco S, Acuna CL, Walz KC, Harriman GR. IgA$^{-/-}$ knockout mice are not more susceptible to influenza virus infection. American Association of Immunologists Late Breaking Abstracts. LB28), 1997.

70. Bachman R. Studies on the serum gamma A-globulin level. III. The frequency of a-gamma A-globulinemia. *Scand J Clin Lab Invest* 1965;17:316–320.

71. Ropars C, Muller A, Paint N, Beige D, Avenard G. Large scale detection of IgA deficient blood donors. *J Immunol Methods* 1982;54:183–189.

72. Burks AW Jr, Steele RW. Selective IgA deficiency. *Ann Allergy* 1986;57:3–10.

73. Ammann AJ, Hong R. Selective IgA deficiency: presentation of 30 cases and a review of the literature. *Medicine (Baltimore)* 1971;50:223–236.

74. Bkrandtzaeg P, Fjellanger I, Gjeruldsen ST. Immunoglobulin M: local synthesis and selective secretion in patients with immunoglobulin A deficiency. *Science* 1968;160:789–791.

75. Mellander L, Bjorkander J, Carlsson B, Hanson LA. Secretory antibodies in IgA deficient and immunosuppressed individuals. *J Clin Immunol* 1986;6:284–291.

76. Ishizaka T, Tomioka H, Ishizaka K. Degranulation of human basophil leukocytes by anti-IgD antibody. *J Immunol* 1971;106:705–710.

77. Kulczycki A Jr, Metzger H. The interaction of IgE with rat basophilic leukemia cells. II. Quantitative aspects of the binding reaction. *J Exp Med* 1974;140:1676–1695.

78. Conrad DH, Bazin H, Sehan AH, Froese A. Binding parameters of the interactions between rat IgE and rat mast cell receptors. *J Immunol* 1975;114:1688–1691.

79. Ishizaka T, Ishizaka K. Triggering of histamine release from rat mast cells by divalent antibodies against IgE receptors. *J Immunol* 1978;120:800–805.

80. Wasserman SI. The mast cell and synovial inflammation: or, what's a nice cell like you doing in a joint like this? *Arthritis Rheum* 1984;27:841–844.

81. Bridges AJ, Malone DG, Jicinsky J, et al. Human synovial mast cell involvement in rheumatoid arthritis and osteoarthritis. Relation to disease type, clinical activity, and antirheumatic therapy. *Arthritis Rheum* 1991;34:1116–1124.

82. Peters SP, Schleimer RP, Naclerio RM, et al. The pathophysiology of human mast cells. *Am Rev Respir Dis* 1987;135:1196–1200.

83. Askenase PW. Immunopathology of parasitic disease: involvement of basophils and mast cells. *Springer Semin Immunopathol* 1980;2:417–442.

84. Capron M, Bazin H, Joseph M, Capron A. Evidence for IgE-dependent cytotoxicity by rat eosinophils. *J Immunol* 1981;126:1764–1768.

85. Kojima S, Yamamoto N, Kanazawa T, Ovary Z. Monoclonal IgE-dependent eosinophil cytotoxicity to haptenated schistosomula of *Schistosoma japonicum:* enhancement of the cytotoxicity and expression of Fc receptor for IgE by Nippostrongylus brasiliensis infection *J Immunol* 1985;134:2719–2722.

86. Ahmad A, Wang CH, Bell RG. A role for IgE in intestinal immunity: expression of rapid expulsion of *Trichinella spiralis* in rats transfused with IgE and thoracic duct lymphocytes. *J Immunol* 1991;146:3563–3570.

87. Kehry MR, Yamashita LC. Low-affinity IgE receptor (CD23) function on mouse B cells: role in IgE-dependent antigen focusing. *Proc Natl Acad Sci USA* 1989;86:7556–7560.

88. Cohen BE, Rosenthal AS, Paul WE. Antigen-macrophage interaction. II. Relative roles of cytophilic antibodies and other membrane sites. *J Immunol* 1973;111:820–828.

89. Celis E, Chang TW. Antibodies to hepatitis B surface antigen potentiate the response of human T lymphocyte clones to the same antigen. *Science* 1984;224:297–299.

90. Rowe DS, Fahey JL. A new class of human immunoglobulins. II. Normal serum IgD. *J Exp Med* 1965;121:185–199.

91. Finkelman FD, Woods VL, Berning A, Scher I. Demonstration of mouse serum IgD. *J Immunol* 1979;123:1253–1259.

92. Coico RF, Siskind GW, Thorbecke GJ. Role of IgD and T delta cells in the regulation of the humoral immune response. *Immunol Rev* 1988;105:45–67.

93. Finkelman FD, Mond JJ, Metcalf ES. Effects of neonatal anti-δ treatment on the murine immune system. I. Suppression of development of surface IgD$^+$ B cells and expansion of a surface IgM$^+$ IgD$^-$ B lymphocyte population. *J Immunol* 1983;131:593–605.

94. Metcalf ES, Mond JJ, Finkelman FD. Effects of neonatal anti-δ treatment on the murine immune system. II. Functional capacity of a stable sIgM$^+$sIa$^+$sIgD$^-$ B cell population. *J Immunol* 1983;131:601–605.

95. Isakson PC, Pure E, Vitetta ES, Krammer PH. T cell-derived B cell differentiation factor(s). Effect on the isotype switch of murine B cells. *J Exp Med* 1982;155:734–748.

96. Severinson E, Bergstedt-Lindqvist S, van der Loo W, Fernandez C. Characterization of the IgG response induced by polyclonal B cell activators. *Immunol Rev* 1982;67:73–85.

97. Vitetta ES, Ohara J, Myers CD, Layton JE, Krammer PH, Paul WE. Serological, biochemical, and functional identity of B cell-stimulatory factor 1 and B cell differentiation factor for IgG1. *J Exp Med* 1985;162:1726–1731.

98. Sideras P, Bergstedt-Lindqvist S, Severinson E. Partial biochemical characterization of IgG1-inducing factor *Eur J Immunol* 1985;15:593–598.

99. Stavnezer J, Radcliffe G, Lin Y-C, et al. Immunoglobulin heavy-chain switching may be directed by prior induction of transcripts from constant-region genes. *Proc Natl Acad Sci USA* 1988;85:7704–7708.

100. Rothman P, Lutzker S, Cook W, Coffman R, Alt FW. Mitogen plus interleukin 4 induction of Cε transcripts in B lymphoid cells. *J Exp Med* 1988;168:2385–2389.

101. Severinson E, Fernandez C, Stavnezer J. Induction of germ-line immunoglobulin heavy chain transcripts by mitogens and interleukins prior to switch recombination. *Eur J Immunol* 1990;20:1079–1084.

102. Esser C, Radbruch A. Rapid induction of transcription of unrearranged Sg1 switch regions in activated murine B cells by interleukin 4. *EMBO J* 1989;8:483–488.

103. Snapper CM, Paul WE. B cell stimulatory factor-1 (interleukin 4) prepares resting murine B cells to secrete IgG1 upon subsequent stimulation with bacterial lipopolysaccharide. *J Immunol* 1987;139:10–17.

104. Snapper CM, Peçanha LMT, Levine AD, Mond JJ. IgE class switching is critically dependent upon the nature of the B cell activator, in addition to the presence of IL-4. *J Immunol* 1991;147:1163–1170.

105. Purkerson JM, Isakson PC. Interleukin 5 (IL-5) provides a signal that is required in addition to IL-4 for isotype switching to immunoglobulin (Ig) G1 and IgE. *J Exp Med* 1992;175:973–982.

106. Lebman D, Coffman RL. Interleukin 4 causes isotype switching to IgE in T cell-stimulated clonal B cell cultures. *J Exp Med* 1988;168:853–862.

107. Hodgkin PD, Yamashita LC, Coffman RL Kehry MR. Separation of events mediating B cell proliferation and Ig production by using T cell membranes and lymphokines. *J Immunol* 1990;145:2025–2034.

108. Hodgkin PD, Yamashita LC, Seymour B, Coffman RL, Kehry MR. Membranes from both Th1 and Th2 T cell clones stimulate B cell proliferation and prepare B cells for lymphokine-induced differentiation to secrete Ig. *J Immunol* 1991;147:3696–3702.

109. Peçanha LMT, Yamaguchi H, Lees A, Noelle RJ, Mond JJ Snapper CM. Dextran-conjugated anti-IgD antibodies inhibit T cell-mediated IgE production but augment the synthesis of IgM and IgG. *J Immunol* 1993;150:2160–2168.

110. Hodgkin PD, Castle BE, Kehry MR. B cell differentiation induced by helper T cell membranes: evidence for sequential isotype switching and a requirement for lymphokines during proliferation. *Eur J Immunol* 1994;24:239–246.

111. Snapper CM, Kehry MR, Castle BE, Mond JJ. Multivalent, but not divalent, antigen receptor cross-linkers synergize with CD40 ligand for induction of Ig synthesis and class switching in normal murine B cells. *J Immunol* 1995;154:1177–1187.

112. Nakanishi K, Kiyoshi M, Kashiwamura S I, et al. IL-4 and anti-CD40 protect against Fas-mediated B cell apoptosis and induce B cell growth and differentiation. *Int Immunol* 1996;8:791–798.

113. Shanebeck KD, Maliszewski CR, Kennedy MK, et al. Regulation of murine B cell growth and differentiation by CD30 ligand. *Eur J Immunol* 1995;25:2147–2153.

114. Layton JE, Vitetta ES, Uhr JW, Krammer PH. Clonal analysis of B cells induced to secrete IgG by T cell-derived lymphokine(s). *J Exp Med* 1984;160:1850–1863.

115. Mosmann TR, Cherwinski H, Bond MW, Giedlin MA, Coffman RL. Two types of murine helper T cell clone. I. Definition according to profiles of lymphokine activities and secreted proteins. *J Immunol* 1986;136:2348–2357.

116. Coffman RL, Seymour BWP, Lebman DA, et al. The role of helper T cell products in mouse B cell differentiation and isotype regulation. *Immunol Rev* 1988;102:5–28.

117. Schurmans S, Heusser CH, Qin H-Y, Merino J, Brighouse, G Lambert P-H. In vivo effects of anti-IL-4 monoclonal antibody on neonatal induction of tolerance and on an associated autoimmune syndrome. *J Immunol* 1990;145:2465–2473.

118. Ochel M, Vohn H-W, Pfeiffer C, Gleichmann E. IL-4 is required for the IgE and IgG1 increase and IgG1 autoantibody formation in mice treated with mercuric chloride. *J Immunol* 1991;146:3006–3011.

119. Finkelman FD, Katona IM, Urban JFJ, Snapper CM, Ohara J, Paul WE. Suppression of in vivo polyclonal IgE responses by monoclonal antibody to the lymphokine B-cell stimulatory factor 1. *Proc Natl Acad Sci USA* 1986;83:9675–9678.

120. Finkelman FD, Urban JFJ, Beckmann MP, Schooley KA, Holmes JM, Katona IM. Regulation of murine in vivo IgG and IgE responses by a monoclonal anti-IL-4 receptor antibody. *Int Immunol* 1991;3:599–607.

121. Kühn R, Rajewsky K, Muller W. Generation and analysis of interleukin-4 deficient mice. *Science* 1991;254:707–710.

122. Schultz CL, Rothman P, Kuhn R, et al. T helper cell membranes promote IL-4-independent expression of germ-line Cγ1 transcripts in B cells. *J Immunol* 1992;149:60–64.

123. Warren WD, Berton MT. Induction of germ-line γ1 and ε Ig gene expression in murine B cells. *J Immunol* 1995;155:5637–5646.

124. Zelazowski P, Collins JT, Dunnick W, Snapper CM. Antigen receptor cross-linking differentially regulates germ-line C$_H$ ribonucleic acid expression in murine B cells. *J Immunol* 1995;154:1223–1231.

125. Coffman RL, Carty J. A T cell activity that enhances polyclonal IgE production and its inhibition by interferon-γ. *J Immunol* 1986;136:949–954.

126. Snapper CM, Paul WE. Interferon-γ and B cell stimulatory factor-1 reciprocally regulate Ig isotype production. *Science* 1987;236:944–947.

127. Finkelman FD, Katona IM, Mosmann T, Coffman RL. IFN-γ regulates the isotypes of Ig secreted during in vivo humoral immune responses. *J Immunol* 1988;140:1022–1027.

128. Graham MB, Dalton DK, Giltinan D, Braciale VL, Stewart TA Braciale TJ. Response to influenza infection in mice with a targeted disruption in the interferon γ gene. *J Exp Med* 1993;178:1725–1732.

129. Coffman RL, Lebman DA, Shrader B. Transforming growth factor β specifically

enhances IgA production by lipopolysaccharide-stimulated murine B lymphocytes. *J Exp Med* 1989;170:1039–1044.

130. Lebman DA, Lee FD, Coffman RL. Mechanism for transforming growth factor β and IL-2 enhancement of IgA expression in lipopolysaccharide-stimulated B cell cultures. *J Immunol* 1990;144:952–959.

131. Finkelman FD, Svetic A, Gresser I, et al. Regulation by interferon α of immunoglobulin isotype selection and lymphokine production in mice. *J Exp Med* 1991;174:1179–1188.

132. Snapper CM, Peschel C, Paul WE. IFN-γ stimulates IgG2a secretion by murine B cells stimulated with bacterial lipopolysaccharide. *J Immunol* 1988;140: 2121–2127.

133. Stevens TL, Bossie A, Sanders VM, et al. Regulation of antibody isotype secretion by subsets of antigen-specific helper T cells. *Nature* 1988;334:255–258.

134. Amigorena S, Bonnerot C, Fridman WH, Teillaud J-L. Recombinant interleukin 2-activated natural killer cells regulate IgG2a production. *Eur J Immunol* 1990; 20:1781–1787.

135. Michael A, Shao A, Yuan D. Productive interactions between B and natural killer cells. *Nat Immun Cell Growth Regul* 1991;10:71–82.

136. Wilder JA, Koh CY Yuan D. The role of NK cells during in vivo antigen-specific antibody responses. *J Immunol* 1996;156:146–152.

137. Collins JT Dunnick WA. Germline transcripts of the murine immunoglobulin γ2a gene: structure and induction by IFN-γ. *Int Immunol* 1993;5:885–891.

138. Huang S, Hendriks W, Althage A, et al. Immune response in mice that lack interferon-γ receptor. *Science* 1993;259:1742–1745.

139. Schijns VECJ, Haagmans BL, Rijke EO, Huang S, Aguet M Horzinek M. IFN-γ receptor-deficient mice generate antiviral Th1-characteristic cytokine profiles but altered antibody responses. *J Immunol* 1994;153:2029–2037.

140. Metzger DW, Buchanan JM, Collins JT, et al. Enhancement of humoral immunity by interleukin-12. *Ann NY Acad Sci* 1996;795:100–115.

141. McKnight AJ, Zimmer GJ, Fogelman I, Wolf SF, Abbas AK. Effects of IL-12 on helper T cell-dependent immune responses in vivo. *J Immunol* 1994;152: 2172–2179.

142. Morris SC, Madden KB, Adamovicz JJ, et al. Effects of IL-12 on in vivo cytokine gene expression and Ig isotype selection. *J Immunol* 1994;152:1047–1056.

143. Rizzo LV, DeKruyff RH, Umetsu DT. Generation of B cell memory and affinity maturation. Induction with Th1 and Th2 T cell clones. *J Immunol* 1992;148: 3733–3739.

144. Elzer PH, Jacobson RH, Nielsen KH, Douglas JT, Winter AJ. BALB/c mice infected with *Brucella abortus* express protracted polyclonal responses of both IgG2a and IgG3 isotypes. *Immunol Lett* 1994;42:145–150.

145. de Bagues MPJ, Elzer PH, Blasco JM, et al. Protective immunity to *Brucella ovis* in BALB/c mice following recovery from primary infections or immunization with subcellular vaccines. *Infect Immun* 1994;62:632–638.

146. Thatte J, Rath S, Bal V. Immunization with live versus killed *Salmonella typhimurium* leads to the generation of an IFN-γ-dominant versus an IL-4-dominant immune response. *Int Immunol* 1993;5:1431–1436.

147. McIntyre TM, Klinman DR, Rothman P, et al. Transforming growth factor-β selectively stimulates IgG2b secretion by LPS-activated murine B cells. *J Exp Med* 1993;177:1031–1037.

148. Sonoda E, Hitoshi Y, Yamaguchi N, et al. Differential regulation of IgA production by TGF-β and IL-5: TGF-β induces surface IgA-positive cells bearing IL-5 receptor, whereas IL-5 promotes their survival and maturation into IgA-secreting cells. *Cell Immunol* 1992;140:158–172.

149. Garcia B, Rodriguez R, Angulo I, Heath AW, Howard MC, Subiza LL. Differential effects of transforming growth factor-β1 on IgA vs. IgG2b production by lipopolysaccharide-stimulated lymph node B cells: a comparative study with spleen B cells. *Eur J Immunol* 1996;26:2364–2370.

150. Moller E, Strom H. Biological characterization of T cell-replacing factor in synovial fluid of rheumatoid arthritis patients. *Scand J Immunol* 1988;27:717–724.

151. Abedi-Valugerdi M, Ridderstad A, Strom H, Moller E. Relationship between IgG2b-inducing activity in rheumatoid arthritis synovial fluid and other well-known cytokines and inflammatory mediators. *Arthritis Rheum* 1991;34: 1461–1465.

152. Abedi-Valugerdi M, Ridderstad A, Strom H, Moller G, Moller E. Partial biochemical characterization and purification of IgG2b inducing factor as a new cytokine from synovial fluid of patients with rheumtoid arthritis. *Scand J Immunol* 1993;37:430–436.

153. Ridderstad A, Lettesjo H, Abedi-Valugerdi M, Moller E. Differential sensitivity to transforming growth factor (TGF)-β of CBA and of CBA/N B cells demonstrates that the IgG2b inducing factor in synovial fluid from rheumatiod arthritis patients is not identical to TGF-β. *Int Immunol* 1995;7:459–469.

154. Gascan H, Gauchat J-F, Aversa G, Van Vlasselaer P, De Vries JE. Anti-CD40 monoclonal antibodies or CD4+ T cell clones and IL-4 induce IgG4 and IgE switching in purified human B cells via different signaling pathways. *J Immunol* 1991;147:8–13.

155. Lundgren M, Persson U, Larsson P, et al. Interleukin 4 induces synthesis of IgE and IgG4 in human B cells. *Eur J Immunol* 1989;19:1311–1315.

156. Briere F, Servet-Delprat C, Bridon J-M, Saint-Remy J-M, Bancherau J. Human interleukin 10 induces naive surface immunoglobulin D+ (sIgD+) B cells to secrete IgG1 and IgG3. *J Exp Med* 1994;179:757–762.

157. Fujieda S, Saxon A, Zhang Ke. Direct evidence that gamma 1 and gamma 3 switching in human B cells is interleukin-10 dependent. *Mol Immunol* 1996;33: 1335–1343.

158. Malisan F, Briere F, Bridon J-M, et al. Interleukin-10 induces immunoglobulin G isotype switch recombination in human CD40-activated naive B lymphocytes. *J Exp Med* 1996;183:937–947.

159. Kitani A Strober W. Regulation of Cγ subclass germ-line transcripts in human peripheral blood B cells. *J Immunol* 1993;151:3478–3488.

160. Kawano Y, Noma T Yata J. Regulation of human IgG subclass production by cytokines. *J Immunol* 1994;153:4948–4958.

161. Servet-Delprat C, Bridon J-M, Djossou O, Yahia SA, Bancherau J, Briere F. Delayed IgG2 humoral response in infants is not due to intrinsic T or B cell defects. *Int Immunol* 1996;8:1495–1502.

162. Snapper CM, Finkelman FD, Paul WE. Differential regulation of IgG1 and IgE synthesis by interleukin 4. *J Exp Med* 1988;167:183–196.

163. Coffman RL, Ohara J, Bond MW, Carty J, Zlotnik A, Paul WE. B cell stimulatory factor-1 enhances the IgE response of lipopolysaccharide-activated B cells. *J Immunol* 1986;136:4538–4541.

164. Armitage RJ, Fanslow WC, Strockbine L, et al. Molecular and biological characterization of a murine ligand for CD40. *Nature* 1992;357:80–82.

165. Maliszewski CR, Grabstein K, Fanslow WC, Armitage R, Spriggs MK, Sato TA. Recombinant CD40 ligand stimulation of murine B cell growth and differentiation: cooperative effects of cytokines. *Eur J Immunol* 1993;23: 1044–1049.

166. Jabara HH, Schneider LC, Shapira SK, et al. Induction of germ-line and mature Cε transcripts in human B cells stimulated with rIL-4 and EBV. *J Immunol* 1990; 145:3468–3473.

167. Shapira SK, Jabara HH, Thienes CP, et al. Deletional switch recombination occurs in interleukin-4-induced isotype switching to IgE expression by human B cells. *Proc Natl Acad Sci USA* 1991;88:7528–7532.

168. Gauchat J-F, Gascan H, de Waal Malefyt R, de Vries JE. Regulation of germ-line ε transcription and induction of ε switching in cloned EBV-transformed and malignant human B cell lines by cytokines and CD4+ T cells. *J Immunol* 1992;148:2291–2299.

169. Thyphronitis G, Tsokos GC, June CH, Levine AD, Finkelman FD. IgE secretion by Epstein-Barr virus-infected purified human B lymphocytes is stimulated by interleukin 4 and suppressed by interferon-γ. *Proc Natl Acad Sci USA* 1989;86: 5580–5584.

170. Thyphronitis G, Max EE, Finkelman FD. Generation and cloning of stable human IgE-secreting cells that have rearranged the Cε gene. *J Immunol* 1991; 146:1496–1502.

171. Mills FC, Thyphronitis G, Finkelman FD, Max EE. Immunoglobulin μ-ε isotype switch in IL-4 treated human B lymphoblastoid cells; evidence for a sequential switch. *J Immunol* 1992;149:1075–1085.

172. Jabara HH, Fu SM, Geha RS, Vercelli D. CD40 and IgE: Synergism between anti-CD40 monoclonal antibody and interleukin 4 in the induction of IgE synthesis by highly purified human B cells. *J Exp Med* 1990;172:1861–1864.

173. Armitage RJ, Macduff BM, Spriggs MK, Fanslow WC. Human B cell proliferation and Ig secretion induced by recombinant CD40 lignad are modulated by soluble cytokines. *J Immunol* 1993;150:3671–3680.

174. Lederman S, Yellin MJ, Cleary AM, et al. T-BAM/CD40-L on helper T lymphocytes augments lymphokine-induced B cell Ig isotype switch recombination and rescues B cells from programmed cell death. *J Immunol* 1994;152:2163–2171.

175. Jabara HH, Ahern DJ, Vercelli D, Geha RS. Hydrocortisone and IL-4 induce IgE isotype switching in human B cells. *J Immunol* 1991;147:1557–1560.

176. Sarfati M, Luo H, Delespesse G. IgE synthesis by chronic lymphocytic leukemia cells. *J Exp Med* 1989;170:1775–1780.

177. Wu CY, Sarfati M, Heusser C, et al. Glucocorticoids increase the synthesis of immunoglobulin E by interleukin 4-stimulated human lymphocytes. *J Clin Invest* 1991;87:870–877.

178. Gauchat J-F, Lebman DA, Coffman RL, Gascan H, de Vries JE. Structure and expression of germline ε transcripts in human B cells induced by interleukin 4 to switch to IgE production. *J Exp Med* 1990;172:463–473.

179. Gascan H, Gauchat J-F, Roncarolo M-G, Yssel H, Spits H, de Vries JE. Human B cell clones can be induced to proliferate and to switch to IgE and IgG4 synthesis by interleukin 4 and a signal provided by activated CD4+ T cell clones. *J Exp Med* 1991;173:747–750.

180. Pene J, Rousset F, Briere F, et al. IgE production by normal human lymphocytes is induced by interleukin 4 and suppressed by interferons γ and α and prostaglandin E2. *Proc Natl Acad Sci USA* 1988;85:6880–6884.

181. Parronchi P, Tiri A, Macchia D, et al. Noncognate contact-dependent B cell activation can promote IL-4-dependent in vitro human IgE synthesis. *J Immunol* 1990;144:2102–2108.

182. Vercelli D, Jabara HH, Arai K-I, Yokota T, Geha RS. Endogenous interleukin 6 plays an obligatory role in interleukin 4-dependent human IgE synthesis. *Eur J Immunol* 1989;19:1419–1424.

183. DeKruyff RH, Turner T, Abrams JS, Palladino MA Jr, Umetsu DT. Induction of human IgE synthesis by CD4+ T cell clones. Requirement for interleukin 4 and low molecular weight B cell growth factor. *J Exp Med* 1989;170:1477–1493.

184. Del Prete G, Maggi E, Parronchi P, et al. IL-4 is an essential factor for the IgE synthesis induced in vitro by human T cell clones and their supernatants. *J Immunol* 1988;140:4193–4198.

185. Pene J, Rousset F, Briere F, et al. IgE production by normal human B cells induced by alloreactive T cell clones is mediated by IL-4 and suppressed by IFN-γ. *J Immunol* 1988;141:1218–1224.

186. Vercelli D, Jabara HH, Arai K, Geha RS. Induction of human IgE synthesis

requires interleukin 4 and T/B cell interactions involving the T cell receptor/CD3 complex and MHC class II antigens. *J Exp Med* 1989;169:1295–1307.

187. Gascan H, Aversa GG, Gauchat J-F, et al. Membranes of activated CD4+ T cells expressing T cell receptor (TcR) αβ or TcR γδ induce IgE synthesis by human B cells in the presence of interleukin-4. *Eur J Immunol* 1992;22:1133–1141.

188. Maggi E, Del Prete G, Macchia C, et al. Profiles of lymphokine activities and helper function for IgE in human T cell clones. *Eur J Immunol* 1988;18:1045–1050.

189. Shapira SK, Vercelli D, Jabara HH, Fu SM, Geha RS. Molecular analysis of the induction of immunoglobulin E synthesis in human B cells by interleukin 4 and engagement of CD40 antigen. *J Exp Med* 1992;175:289–292.

190. Jabara HH, Loh R, Ramesh N, Vercelli D, Geha RS. Sequential switching from μ to ε via γ4 in human B cells stimulated with IL-4 and hydrocortisone. *J Immunol* 1993;151:4528–4533.

191. Finkelman FD, Katona IM, Urban JF Jr, et al. IL-4 is required to generate and sustain in vivo IgE responses. *J Immunol* 1988;141:2335–2341.

192. Katona IM, Urban JFJ, Kang SS, Paul WE, Finkelman FD. IL-4 requirements for the generation of in vivo IgE responses. *J Immunol* 1991;146:4215–4221.

193. Kopf M, Gros GL, Bachmann M, Lamers MC, Bluethmann H, Koehler G. Disruption of the murine IL-4 gene blocks Th2 cytokine responses. *Nature* 1993;362:245–248.

194. Thyphronitis G, Katona IM, Gause WC, Finkelman FD. Germline and productive Cε gene expression during in vivo IgE responses. *J Immunol* 1993;151:4128–4136.

195. Morawetz RA, Gabriele L, Rizzo LV, et al. Interleukin (IL)-4-independent immunoglobulin class switch to immunoglobulin (Ig)E in the mouse. *J Exp Med* 1996;184:1651–1661.

196. Ferlin WG, Severinson E, Strom L, et al. CD40 signaling induces interleukin-4-independent IgE switching in vivo. *Eur J Immunol* 1996;26:2911–2915.

197. Von Der Weid T, Kopf M, Kohler G, Langhorne J. The immune response to *Plasmodium chabaudi* malaria in interleukin-4-deficient mice. *Eur J Immunol* 1994;24:2285–2293.

198. Noben-Trauth N, Kropf P, Muller I. Susceptibility to *Leishmania major* infection in interleukin-4-deficient mice. *Science* 1996;271:987–990.

199. Lawrence RA, Allen JE, Gregory WF, Kopf M, Maizels RM. Infection of IL-4-deficient mice with the parasitic nematode *Brugia malayi* demonstrates that the host resistance is not dependent on a T helper 2-dominated immune response. *J Immunol* 1995;154:5995–6001.

200. Punnonen J, Aversa G, Cocks BG, et al. Interleukin 13 induces interleukin 4-independent IgG4 and IgE synthesis and CD23 expression by human B cells. *Proc Natl Acad Sci USA* 1993;90:3730–3734.

201. Zurawski G, de Vries JE. Interleukin-13, an interleukin-4-like cytokine that acts on monocytes and B cells, but not on T cells. *Immunol Today* 1993;15:19–26.

202. Cocks BG, Malefyt RW, Galizzi J-P, de Vries JE Aversa G. IL-13 induces proliferation and differentiation of human B cells activated by the CD40 ligand. *Int Immunol* 1993;5:657–663.

203. Defrance T, Carayon P, Billian G, et al. Interleukin 13 is a B cell stimulating factor. *J Exp Med* 1994;179:135–143.

204. Hilton DJ, Zhang JG, Metcalf D, Alexander WS, Nicola NA, Willson TA. Cloning and characterization of a binding subunit of the interleukin 13 receptor that is also a component of the interleukin 4 receptor. *Proc Natl Acad Sci USA* 1996;93:497–501.

205. Mandler R, Finkelman FD, Levine AD, Snapper CM. Interleukin-4 induction of IgE class switching by LPS-activated murine B cells occurs predominantly through sequential switching. *J Immunol* 1993;150:407–418.

206. Cho S-W, Conrad DH. A new multivalent B cell activation model-anti-IgD bound to FcγRI. properties and comparison with CD40L-mediated activation. *Int Immunol* 1997;9:239–248.

207. Yokota T, Arai N, De Vries J, et al. Molecular biology of interleukin 4 and interleukin 5 genes and biology of their products that stimulate B cells, T cells, and hemopoietic cells. *Immunol Rev* 1988;102:137–187.

208. McHeyzer-Williams MG. Combinations of interleukins 2, 4, and 5, regulate the secretion of murine immunoglobulin isotypes. *Eur J Immunol* 1989;19:2025–2030.

209. Gauchat JF, Aversio G, Gascan H, de Vries, JE. Modulation of IL-4 induced germline ε RNA synthesis in human B cells by tumor necrosis factor-α, anti-CD40 monoclonal antibodies or transforming growth factor-β correlates with levels of IgE production. *Int Immunol* 1992;4:397–406.

210. Kikutani H, Suemura M, Owaki H, et al. Fcε receptor, a specific differentiation marker transiently expressed on mature B cells prior to isotype switching. *J Exp Med* 1986;164:1455–1469.

211. Defrance T, Aubry JP, Rousset F, et al. Human recombinant interleukin 4 induces Fcε receptors (CD23) on normal human B lymphocytes. *J Exp Med* 1987;165:1459–1467.

212. Hudak SA, Gollnick SO, Conrad DH, Kehry MR. Murine B cell stimulatory factor-1 (interleukin 4) increases expression of the Fc receptor for IgE on mouse B cells. *Proc Natl Acad Sci USA* 1987;84:4606–4610.

213. Conrad DH, Waldschmidt TJ, Lee WT, et al. Effect of B cell stimulatory factor-1 (interleukin 4) on Fcε and Fcγ receptor expression on murine B lymphocytes and B cell lines. *J Immunol* 1987;139:2290–2296.

214. Chretien I, Pene J, Briere F, de Waal Malefijt R, Rousset F, de Vries JE. Regulation of human IgE synthesis. I. Human IgE synthesis in vitro is determined by the reciprocal antagonistic effects of interleukin 4 and interferon γ. *Eur J Immunol* 1990;20:243–251.

215. Pene J, Chretien I, Rousset F, Briere F, Bonnefoy JY, De Vries J. Modulation of IL-4-induced human IgE production in vitro by IFN-γ and IL-5: the role of soluble CD23 (sCD23). *J Cell Biochem* 1989;39:253–264.

216. Delespesse G, Sarfati M, Hofstetter H. Human IgE-binding factors. *Immunol Today* 1989;10:159–164.

217. Conrad DH, Keegan AD, Kali KR, Van Dusen R, Rao M, Levine AD. Superinduction of low affinity IgE receptors on murine B lymphocytes by LPS and interleukin-4. *J Immunol* 1988;141:1091–1097

218. Keegan AD, Snapper CM, Van Dusen R, Paul WE, Conrad DH. Superinduction of the murine B cell FcεRII by T helper cell clones. Role of IL-4. *J Immunol* 1989;142:3868–3874.

219. Stief A, Texido G, Sansig G, Eibel H, Le Gros G, van der Putten H. Mice deficient in CD23 reveal its modulatory role in IgE production but no role in T and B cell development. *J Immunol* 1994;152:3378–3390.

220. Berton MT, Uhr JW, Vitetta ES. Synthesis of germ-line γ1 immunoglobulin heavy-chain transcripts in resting B cells: induction by interleukin 4 and inhibition by interferon γ. *Proc Natl Acad Sci USA* 1989;86:2829–2833.

221. Thyphronitis G, Banchereau J, Heusser C, Tsokos GC, Levine AD, Finkelman FD. Kinetics of interleukin-4 induction and inteferon-γ inhibition of IgE secretion by Epstein-Barr virus-infected human peripheral blood B cells. *Cell Immunol* 1991;133:408–419.

222. Aversa GG, Punnonen J, Gauchat JF, de Vries JE. The CD4+ T cell costimulatory signal required for IL-4 induced IgE switching is mediated by the 26 kD membrane form of TNF-α. *Eighth International Congress of Immunology Abstracts.* Budapest: Springer-Verlag, 1992:34.

223. Kiniwa M, Gately M, Guller V, Chizzonite R, Fargeas C, Delespesse G. Recombinant interleukin-12 suppresses the synthesis of immunoglobulin E by interleukin-4 stimulated human lymphocytes. *J Clin Invest* 1992;90:262–266.

224. Roper RL, Conrad DH, Brown DM, Warner GL, Phipps RP. Prostaglandin E₂ promotes IL-4-induced IgE and IgG1 synthesis. *J Immunol* 1990;145:2644–2651.

225. Roper RL, Phipps RP. Prostaglandin E enhances class switching to IgE and IgG1. *Eighth International Congress of Immunology Abstracts.* Budapest: Springer-Verlag, 1992:37.

226. Manning JA, Finkelman FD, Collins PW, Levine AD. Complete and selective inhibition of polyclonal IgE synthesis in vivo by a PGE₂ analogue (*submitted*).

227. Kiyono H, McGhee JR, Mosteller LM, et al. Murine Peyer's patch T cell clones. Characterization of antigen-specific helper T cells for immunoglobulin A responses. *J Exp Med* 1982;156:1115–1130.

228. Kawanishi H, Saltzman LE, Strober W. Mechanisms regulating IgA class-specific immunoglobulin production in murine gut-associated lymphoid tissues. I. T cell derived from Peyer's patches that switch sIgM B cells to sIgA B cells in vitro. *J Exp Med* 1983;157:433–450.

229. Kawanishi H, Saltzman LE, Strober W. Characteristics and regulatory function of murine Con-A-induced, clone T cells obtained from Peyer's patch and spleen: mechanisms regulating isotype-specific immunoglobulin production by Peyer's patch B cells. *J Immunol* 1982;129:475–479.

230. Xu-Amano J, Aicher WK, Taguchi T, Kiyono H, McGhee JR. Selective induction of Th2 cells in murine Peyer's patches by oral immunization. *Int Immunol* 1992;4:433–440.

231. Xu-Amano J, Kiyono H, Jackson RJ, et al. Helper T cell subsets for immunoglobulin A responses: oral immunization with tetanus toxoid and cholera toxin as adjuvant selectively induces Th2 cells in mucosa associated tissues. *J Exp Med* 1993;178:1309–1320.

232. Taguchi T, McGhee JR, Coffman RL, et al. Analysis of Th1 and Th2 cells in murine gut-associated tissues. Frequencies of CD4+ and CD8+ T cells that secrete IFN-γ and IL-5. *J Immunol* 1990;145:68–77.

233. Mega J, McGhee JR, Kiyono H. Cytokine and Ig-producing cells in mucosal effector tissues: analysis of IL-5 and IFN-γ-producing T cells, T cell receptor expression, and IgA plasma cells from mouse salivary gland-associated tissues. *J Immunol* 1992;148:2030–2039.

234. Coffman RL, Shrader B, Carty J, Mosmann TR, Bond MW. A mouse T cell product that preferentially enhances IgA production. I. Biologic characterization. *J Immunol* 1987;139:3685–3690.

235. Bond MW, Shrader B, Mosmann TR, Coffman RL. A mouse T cell product that preferentially enhances IgA production. II. Physicochemical characterization. *J Immunol* 1987;139:3691–3696.

236. Murray PD, McKenzie DT, Swain SL, Kagnoff MF. Interleukin 5 and interleukin 4 produced by Peyer's patch T cells selectively enhance immunoglobulin A expression. *J Immunol* 1987;139:2669–2674.

237. Harriman GR, Kunimoto DY, Elliott JF, Paetkau V, Strober W. The role of IL-5 in IgA B cell differentiation. *J Immunol* 1988;140:3033–3039.

238. Schoenbeck S, McKenzie DT, Kagnoff MF. Interleukin 5 is a differentiation factor for IgA B cells. *Eur J Immunol* 1989;19:965–969.

239. Sonoda E, Matsumoto R, Hitoshi Y, et al. Transforming growth factor β induces IgA production and acts additively with interleukin 5 for IgA production. *J Exp Med* 1989;170:1415–1420.

240. Pockley AG, Montgomery PC. In vivo adjuvant effect of interleukins 5 and 6 on rat tear IgA antibody responses. *Immunology* 1991;73:19–23.

241. Ramsay AJ, Kohonen Corish M. Interleukin-5 expressed by a recombinant virus vector enhances specific mucosal IgA responses in vivo. *Eur J Immunol* 1993;23:3141–3145.

242. Kopf M, Brombacher F, Hodgkin PD, et al. IL-5-deficient mice have a develop-

mental defect in CD5+ B-1 cells and lack eosinophilia but have normal antibody and cytotoxic T cell responses. *Immunity* 1996;4:15–24.

243. Vajdy M, Kosco-Vilbois MH, Kopf M, Kohler G, Lycke N. Impaired mucosal immune responses in interleukin 4-targeted mice. *J Exp Med* 1995;181:41–53.

244. Bromander AK, Ekman L, Kopf M, Nedrud JG, Lycke NY. IL-6-deficient mice exhibit normal mucosal IgA responses to local immunizations and *Helicobacter felis* infection. *J Immunol* 1996;156:4290–4297.

245. Kim P-H, Kagnoff MF. Transforming growth factor-β1 is a costimulator for IgA production. *J Immunol* 1990;144:3411–3416.

246. Sonoda E, Matsumoto R, Hitoshi Y, et al. Transforming growth factor β induces IgA production and acts additively with interleukin 5 for IgA production. *J Exp Med* 1989;170:1415–1420.

247. Matsuoka M, Yoshida K, Maeda T, Usuda S, Sakano H. Switch circular DNA formed in cytokine-treated mouse splenocytes: evidence for intramolecular DNA deletion in immunoglobulin class switching. *Cell* 1990;62:135–142.

248. Ehrhardt RO, Strober W, Harriman GR. Effect of transforming growth factor (TGF)-β1 on IgA isotype expression. TGF-β1 induces a small increase in sIgA+ B cells regardless of the method of B cell activation. *J Immunol* 1992;148:3830–3836.

249. McIntyre TM, Kehry MR, Snapper CM. Novel *in vitro* model for high-rate IgA class switching. *J Immunol* 1995;154:3156–3161.

250. Islam KB, Nilsson L, Sideras P, Hammarstrom L, Smith CIE. TGF-β1 induces germ-line transcripts of both IgA subclasses in human B lymphocytes. *Int Immunol* 1991;3:1099–1106.

251. Nilsson L, Islam KB, Olafsson O, et al. Structure of TGF-β1-induced human immunoglobulin Cα1 and Cα2 germ-line transcripts. *Int Immunol* 1991;3:1107–1115.

252. van Vlasselaer P, Punnonen J, de Vries JE. Transforming growth factor-β directs IgA switching in human B cells. *J Immunol* 1992;148:2062–2067.

253. Defrance T, Vanbervliet B, Briere F, Durand I, Rousset F, Banchereau J. Interleukin 10 and transforming growth factor β cooperate to induce anti-CD40-activated naive human B cells to secrete immunoglobulin A. *J Exp Med* 1992;175:671–682.

254a. Kitani A, Strober W. Differential regulation of Cα1 and Cα2 germ-line and mature mRNA transcripts in human peripheral blood B cells. *J Immunol*. 1994;153:1466–1477.

254b. Islam KB, Baskin B, Nilsson L, Hammarstrom L, Sideras P, Smith CIE. Molecular analysis of IgA deficiency: evidence for impaired switching to IgA. *J Immunol* 1994;152:1442–1452.

255. Shparago N, Zelazowski P, Jin L, et al. IL-10 selectively regulates murine Ig isotype switching. *Int Immunol* 1996;8:781–790.

256. Fayette J, Dubois B, Vandenabeele S, et al. Human dendritic cells skew isotype switching of CD40-activated naive B cells towards IgA1 and IgA2. *J Exp Med* 1997;185:1909–1918.

257. Kagnoff MF, Kim PH. Effects of transforming growth factor beta-1 and interleukin-5 on IgA isotype switching at the clonal level. *Immunol Res* 1991;10:396–399.

258. Whitmore AC, Prowse DM, Haughton G, Arnold LW. Ig isotype switching in B lymphocytes. The effect of T cell-derived interleukins, cytokines, cholera toxin, and antigen on isotype switch frequency of a cloned B cell lymphoma. *Int Immunol* 1991;3:95–103.

259. Shockett P, Stavnezer J. Effect of cytokines on switching to IgA and α germline transcripts in the B lymphoma I.29μ. *J Immunol* 1991;147:4374–4383.

260. Kimata H, Fujimoto M. Vasoactive intestinal peptide specifically induces human IgA1 and IgA2. *Eur J Immunol* 1994;24:2262–2265.

261. Kimata H, Fujimoto M. Induction of IgA1 and IgA2 production in immature human fetal B cells and pre-B cells by vasoactive intestinal peptide. *Blood* 1995;85:2098–2104.

262. Wabl MR, Forni L, Loor F. Switch in immunoglobulin class production observed in single clones of committed lymphocytes. *Science* 1978;199:1078–1080.

263. Shimizu A, Takahashi N, Yaoita Y, Honjo T. Organization of the constant-region gene family of the mouse immunoglobulin heavy chain. *Cell* 1982;28:499–506.

264. Hofker MH, Walter MA, Cox DW. Complete physical map of the human immunoglobulin heavy chain constant region gene complex. *Proc Natl Acad Sci USA* 1989;86:5567–5571.

265. Maki R, Roeder W, Traunecker A, et al. The role of DNA rearrangement and alternative RNA processing in the expression of immunoglobulin delta genes. *Cell* 1981;24:353–365.

266. Moore KW, Rogers J, Hunkapiller T, et al. Expression of IgD may use both DNA rearrangement and RNA splicing mechanisms. *Proc Natl Acad Sci USA* 1981;78:1800–1804.

267. Knapp MR, Liu C-P, Newell N, et al. Simultaneous expression of immunoglobulin μ and δ heavy chains by a cloned B-cell lymphoma: a single copy of the VH gene is shared by two adjacent CH genes. *Proc Natl Acad Sci USA* 1982;79:2996–3000.

268. Yuan D, Tucker PW. Transcriptional regulation of the μ-δ gene in normal murine B lymphocytes. *J Exp Med* 1984;160:564–583.

269. Coleclough C, Cooper D, Perry RP. Rearrangement of immunoglobulin heavy chain genes during B-lymphocyte development as revealed by studies of mouse plasmacytoma cells. *Proc Natl Acad Sci USA* 1980;77:1422–1426.

270. Rabbitts TH, Forster A, Dunnick W, Bentley DL. The role of gene deletion in the immunoglobulin heavy chain switch. *Nature* 1980;283:351–356.

271. Cory S, Adams JM. Deletions are associated with somatic rearrangement of immunoglobulin heavy chain genes. *Cell* 1980;19:37–51.

272. Honjo T, Kataoka T. Organization of immunglobulin heavy chain genes and allelic deletion model. *Proc Natl Acad Sci USA* 1978;75:2140–2144.

273. Snapper CM, Finkelman FD. Rapid loss of IgM expression by normal murine B cells undergoing IgG1 and IgE class switching after in vivo immunization. *J Immunol* 1990;145:3654–3660.

274. Mountz JD, Mushinski JF, Owens JD, Finkelman FD. The in vivo generation of murine IgD-secreting cells is accompanied by deletion of the Cμ gene and occasional deletion of the gene for the Cδ1 domain. *J Immunol* 1990;145:1583–1591.

275. Owens JD Jr, Finkelman FD, Mountz JD, Mushinski JF. Nonhomologous recombination at sites within the mouse JH-Cδ locus accompanies Cμ deletion and switch to immunoglobulin D secretion. *Mol Cell Biol* 1991;11:5660–5670.

276. Word CJ, White MB, Kuziel WA, Shen AL, Blattner FR, Tucker PW. The human immunoglobulin Cμ-Cδ locus: complete nucleotide and structural analysis. *Int Immunol* 1990;1:296–309.

277. Yasui H, Akahori Y, Hirano M, Yamada K, Kurosawa Y. Class switch from mu to delta is mediated by homologous recombination between σm and Σm sequences in human immunoglobulin gene loci. *Eur J Immunol* 1989;19:1399–1403.

278. Gilliam AC, Shen A, Richards JE, Blattner FR, Mushinski JF, Tucker PW. Illegitimate recombination generates a class switch from Cμ to Cδ in an IgD-secreting plasmacytoma. *Proc Natl Acad Sci USA* 1984;81:4161–4168.

279. Klein S, Sablitzky F, Radbruch A. Deletion of the IgH enhancer does not reduce immunoglobulin heavy chain production of a hybridoma IgD class switch variant. *EMBO J* 1984;3:2473–2476.

280. Sablitzky F, Radbruch A, Rajewsky K. Spontaneous immunoglobulin class switching in myeloma and hybridoma cell lines differs from physiological class switching. *Immunol Rev* 1982;67:59–72.

281. Irsch J, Burrows P, Cooper M, et al. Class switch recombination in human B lymphocytes. *Eighth International Congress of Immunology Abstracts.* Budapest: Springer-Verlag, 1992:35.

282. DePinho R, Kruger K, Andrews N, Lutzker S, Baltimore D, Alt FW. Molecular basis of heavy-chain class switching and switch region deletion in an Abelson virus-transformed cell line. *Mol Cell Biol* 1984;4:2905–2910.

283. Lang RB, Stanton LW, Marcu KB. On immunoglobulin heavy chain gene switching: two gamma-2b genes are rearranged via switch sequences in MPC11 cells but only one is expressed. *Nucleic Acids Res* 1982;10:611.

284. Radbruch A, Muller W, Rajewsky K. Class switch recombination is IgG1 specific on active and inactive IgH loci of IgG1-secreting B-cell blasts. *Proc Natl Acad Sci USA* 1986;83:3954–3957.

285. Yancopoulos GD, DePinho RA, Zimmerman KA, Lutzker SG, Rosenberg N, Alt FW. Secondary genomic rearrangement events in pre-B cells: VHDJH replacement by a LINE-1 sequence and directed class switching. *EMBO J* 1986;5:3259–3266.

286. Burrows PD, Beck-Engeser GB, Wabl MR. Immunoglobulin heavy-chain class switching in a pre-B cell line is accompanied by DNA rearrangement. *Nature* 1983;306:243–246.

287. Vogler LB, Crist WM, Bockman DE, Pearl ER, Lawton AR, Cooper MD. Pre-B-cell leukemia. A new phenotype of childhood lymphoblastic leukemia. *N Engl J Med* 1978;298:872–878.

288. Rothman P, Chen Y-Y, Lutzker S, et al. Structure and expression of germ line immunoglobulin heavy-chain ε transcripts: interleukin-4 plus lipopolysaccharide-directed switching to Cε. *Mol Cell Biol* 1990;10:1672–1679.

289. Davis MM, Calame K, Early PW, et al. An immunoglobulin heavy chain gene is formed by at least two recombinational events. *Nature* 1980;283:773–739.

290. Sakano H, Maki R, Kurosawa Y, Roeder W, Tonegawa S. Two types of somatic recombination are necessary for the generation of complete immunoglobulin heavy-chain genes. *Nature* 1980;286:676–683.

291. Dunnick W, Rabbitts TH, Milstein C. An immunoglobulin deletion mutant with implications for the heavy-chain switch and RNA splicing. *Nature* 1980;286:669–675.

292. Davis MM, Kim SK, Hood LE. DNA sequences mediating class switching in α-immunoglobulins. *Science* 1980;209:1360–1365.

293. Kataoka T, Miyata T, Honjo T. Repetitive sequences in class-switch recombination regions of immunoglobulin heavy chain genes. *Cell* 1981;23:357–368.

294. Stanton LW, Marcu K. Nucleotide sequence and properties of the murine γ3 immunoglobulin heavy chain gene switch region: implications for successive Cγ gene switching. *Nucleic Acids Res* 1982;10:5993–6006.

295. Mowatt MR, Dunnick WA. DNA sequence of the murine γ1 switch segment reveals novel structural elements. *J Immunol* 1986;136:2674–2683.

296. Szurek P, Petrini J, Dunnick W. Complete nucleotide sequence of the murine γ3 switch region and analysis of switch rebombination sites in two γ3-expressing hybridomas. *J Immunol* 1985;135:620–626.

297. Schultz C, Petrini J, Collins J, et al. Patterns and extent of isotype-specificity in the murine H chain switch DNA rearrangement. *J Immunol* 1990;144:363–370.

298. Hummel M, Berry JK, Dunnick W. Switch region content of hybridomas: the two spleen cell Igh loci tend to rearrange to the same isotype. *J Immunol* 1987;138:3539–3548.

299. Nikaido T, Yamawaki-Kataoka Y, Honjo T. Nucleotide sequences of switch regions of immunoglobulin Cε and Cγ genes and their comparison. *J Biol Chem* 1982;257:7322–7329.

300. Obata M, Kataoka T, Nakai S, et al. Structure of a rearranged γ1 chain gene and its implication to immunoglobulin class-switch mechanism. *Proc Natl Acad Sci USA* 1981;78:2437–2441.

301. Marcu KB, Lang RB, Stanton LW, Harris LJ. A model for the molecular requirements of immunoglobulin heavy chain switching. *Nature* 1982;298:87–89.

302. Wu TT, Reid-Miller M, Perry HM, Kabat EA. Long identical repeats in the mouse γ2b switch region and their implications for the mechanism of class switching. *EMBO J* 1984;3:2033–2040.

303. Yoshida K, Matsuoka M, Usuda S, Mori A, Ishizaka K, Sakano H. Immunoglobulin switch circular DNA in the mouse infected with Nippostrongylus brasiliensis: evidence for successive class switching from μ to ε via γ1. *Proc Natl Acad Sci USA* 1990;87:7829–7833.

304. Schwedler U, Jack H-M, Wabl M. Circular DNA is a product of the immunoglobulin class switch rearrangement. *Nature* 1990;345:452–455.

305. Iwasato T, Shimizu A, Honjo T, Yamagishi H. Circular DNA is excised by immunoglobulin class switch recombination. *Cell* 1990;62:143–149.

306. Jack H-M, McDowell M, Steinberg CM, Wabl M. Looping out and deletion mechanism for the immunoglobulin heavy-chain class switch. *Proc Natl Acad Sci USA* 1988;85:1581–1585.

307. Iwasato T, Arakawa H, Shimizu A, Honjo T, Yamagishi H. Biased distribution of recombination sites within S regions upon immunoglobulin class switch recombination induced by transforming growth factor β and lipopolysaccharide. *J Exp Med* 1992;175:1539–1546.

308. Davis DD, Yoshida K, Kingsbury L, Sakano H. Circular DNA resulting from recombination between V-(D)-J joining signals and switch repetitive sequences in mouse thymocytes. *J Exp Med* 1991;173:743–746.

309. Okazaki K, Davis DD, Sakano H. T cell receptor β gene sequences in the circular DNA of thymocyte nuclei: direct evidence for intramolecular DNA deletion in V-D-J joining. *Cell* 1987;49:477–485.

310. Fujimoto S, Yamagishi H. Isolation of an excision product of T-cell receptor α-chain gene rearrangements. *Nature* 1987;327:242–243.

311. Siebenkotten G, Esser C, Wabl M, Radbruch A. The murine IgG1/IgE class switch program. *Eur J Immunol* 1992;22:1827–1834.

312. Wabl M, Meyer J, Beck-Engeser G, Tenkhoff M, Burrows PD. Critical test of a sister chromatid exchange model for the immunoglobulin heavy chain class switch. *Nature* 1985;313:687–689

313a. Knight KL, Malek TR, Hanly WC. Recombinant rabbit secretory immunoglobulin molecules: alpha chains with maternal (paternal) variable-region allotypes and paternal (maternal) constant region allotypes. *Proc Natl Acad Sci USA* 1974;71:1169–1173.

313b. Knight, KL, Kingzette M, Crane MA, Zhai S-K. Transchromosomally derived Ig heavy chains. *J Immunol* 1995;155:684–691.

314. DePinho R, Kruger K, Andrews N, Lutzker S, Baltimore D, Alt FW. Molecular basis of heavy-chain class switching and switch region deletion in an Abelson virus-transformed cell line. *Mol Cell Biol* 1984;4:2905.

315. Tilley SA, Birshtein BK. Unequal sister chromatid exchange. A mechanism affecting immunoglobulin gene arrangement and expression. *J Exp Med* 1985;162:675.

316. Kim S, Davis M, Sinn E, Patten P, Hood L. Antibody diversity: somatic hypermutation of rearranged VH genes. *Cell* 1981;27:573–581.

317. Dunnick WA, Hertz GZ, Scappino LA, Gritzmacher CA. DNA sequences at immunoglobulin switch region recombination sites. *Nucleic Acids Res* 1993;21:365–372.

318. White MB, Word CJ, Humphries CG, Blattner FR, Tucker PW. Immunoglobulin D switching can occur through homologous recombination in human B cells. *Mol Cell Biol* 1990;10:3690–3699.

319. Matthews K. DNA looping. *Microbiol Rev* 1992;56:123–136.

320. Wuerffel R, Jamieson CE, Morgan L, Merkulov GV, Sen R, Kenter AL. Switch recombination breakpoints are strictly correlated with DNA recognition motifs for immunoglobulin Sγ3 DNA-binding proteins. *J Exp Med* 1992;176:339–349.

321. Kenter AL, Wuerffel R, Sen R, Jamieson CE, Merkulov GV. Switch recombination breakpoints occur at nonrandom postions in the Sγ tandem repeat. *J Immunol* 1993;151:4718–4731.

322. Ma L, Hu B, Kenter AL. Immunoglobulin Sγ specific DNA binding protein SNAP is related to the HLH transcription factor E47. *Int Immunol* 1997;9:1021–1029.

323. Pan Q, Rabbani H, Mills FC, Severinson E, Hammarstrom L. Allotype-associated variation in the human γ3 switch region as a basis for differences in IgG3 production. *J Immunol* 1997;158:5849–5859.

324. Dunnick W, Wilson M, Stavnezer J. Mutations, duplication, and deletion of recombined switch regions suggest a role for DNA replication in the immunoglobulin heavy-chain switch. *Mol Cell Biol* 1989;9:1850–1856.

325. Dunnick W, Stavnezer J. Copy choice mechanism of immunoglobulin heavy-chain switch recombination. *Mol Cell Biol* 1990;10:397–400.

326. Du J, Zhu Y, Shanmugam A, Kenter AL. Analysis of immunoglobulin Sγ3 recombination breakpoints by PCR: implication for the mechanism of isotype switching. *Nucleic Acids Res* 1997;25:3066–3073.

327. Li J, Daniels GA, Lieber MR. Asymmetric mutation around the recombination break point of immunoglobulin class switch sequences on extrachromosomal substrates. *Nucleic Acids Res* 1996;24:2104–2111.

328. Wuerffel RA, Du J, Thompson RJ, Kenter AL. Immunoglobulin Sγ3 DNA specific double strand breaks are induced in mitogen activated B cells and are implicated in switch recombination. *J Immunol* 1997;159:4139–4144.

329. Weisman-Shomer P, Fry M. QUAD, a protein from hepatocyte chromatin that binds selectively to guanine-rich quadruplex DNA. *J Biol Chem* 1993;268:3306–3312.

330. Muraiso T, Nomoto S, Yamazaki H, Mishima Y, Kominami R. A single stranded DNA binding protein from mouse tumor cells specifically recognizes the C-rich strand of the (AGG:CCT)n repeats that can alter DNA conformation. *Nucl Acids Res* 1992;20:6631–6635.

331. Sakano H, Huppi K, Heinrich G, Tonegawa S. Sequences at the somatic recombination sites of immunoglobulin light-chain genes. *Nature* 1979;280:288–294.

332. Max EE, Seidman JG, Leder P. Sequences of five potential recombination sites encoded close to an immunoglobulin kappa constant region gene. *Proc Natl Acad Sci USA* 1979;76:3450–3454.

333. Mombaerts P, Iacomini J, Johnson RS, Herrup K, Tonegawa S, Papaioannou VE. RAG-1 deficient mice have no mature B and T lymphocytes. *Cell* 1992;68:869–877.

334. Shinkai Y, Rathbun G, Lam K-P, et al. RAG-2-deficient mice lack mature lymphocytes owing to inability to initiate V(D)J rearrangement. *Cell* 1992;68:855–867.

335. Rolink A, Melchers F, Andersson J. The SCID but not the RAG-2 gene product is required for Sμ-Sε heavy chain class switching. *Immunity* 1996;5:319–330.

336. Rathmell WK, Chu G. A DNA end-binding factor involved in double-strand break repair and V(D)J recombination. *Mol Cell Biol* 1994;14:4741–4748.

337. Rathmell WK, Chu G. Involvement of the Ku autoantigen in the cellular response to DNA double strand breaks. *Proc Natl Acad Sci* 1994;91:7623–7627.

338. Taccioli GE, Gottlieb TM, Blunt T, et al. Ku80: product of the XRCC5 gene and its role in DNA repair and V(D)J recombination. *Science* 1994;265:1442–1445.

339. Smider V, Rathmell WK, Lieber MR, Chu G. Restoration of X-ray resistance and V(D)J recombination in mutant cells by Ku cDNA. *Science* 1994;266:288–291.

340. Boubnov NV, Hall KT, Wills Z, et al. Complementation of the ionizing radiation sensitivity, DNA end binding, and V(D)J recombination defects of double-strand break repair mutants by the p86 Ku autoantigen. *Proc Natl Acad Sci USA* 1995;92:890–894.

341. Kataoka T, Kawakami T, Takahashi N, Honjo T. Rearrangement of immunoglobulin γ1-chain gene and mechanism for heavy-chain class switch. *Proc Natl Acad Sci USA* 1980;77:919–923.

342. Snapper CM, Finkelman FD, Stefany D, Conrad DH, Paul WE. IL-4 induces co-expression of intrinsic membrane IgG1 and IgE by murine B cells stimulated with lipopolysaccharide. *J Immunol* 1988;141:489–498.

343. Zhang K, Mills FC, Saxon A. Switch circles from IL-4-directed ε class switching from human B lymphocytes. *J Immunol* 1994;152:3427–3435.

344. Baskin B, Islam KB, Evengard B, Emtestam L, Smith CIE. Direct and sequential switching from μ to ε in patients with Schistosoma mansoni infection and atopic dermatitis. *Eur J Immunol* 1997;27:130–135.

345. Brinkmann V, Müller S, Heusser CH. T cell dependent differentiation of human B cells: direct switch from IgM to IgE and sequential switch from IgM via IgG to IgA production. *Mol Immunol* 1997 (in press).

346. Jung S, Rajewsky K, Radbruch A. Shutdown of class switch recombination by deletion of a switch region control element. *Science* 1993;259:984–987.

347. Jung S, Siebenkotten G, Radbruch A. Frequency of immunoglobulin E class switching is autonomously determined and independent of prior switching to other classes. *J Exp Med* 1994;179:2023–2026.

348. Stavnezer-Nordgren J, Sirlin S. Specificity of immunoglobulin heavy chain switch correlates with activity of germline heavy chain genes prior to switching. *EMBO J* 1986;5:95–102.

349. Ikeda H, Matsumoto T. Transcription promotes rec A-independent recombination mediated by DNA-dependent RNA polymerase in *Escherichia coli. Proc Natl Acad Sci USA* 1979;76:4571–4575.

350. Voelkel-Meiman K, Keil RL, Roeder GS. Recombination-stimulating sequences in yeast ribosomal DNA correspond to sequences regulating transcription by RNA polymerase I. *Cell* 1987;48:1071–1079.

351. Blackwell KT, Moore MW, Yancopoulos GD, Suh H, Selsing E, Alt FW. Recombination between immunoglobulin variable region gene segments is enhanced by transcription. *Nature* 1986;324:585–589.

352. Lebman DA, Nomura DY, Coffman RL, Lee FD. Molecular characterization of germ-line immunoglobulin A transcripts produced during transforming growth factor type β-induced isotype switching *Proc Natl Acad Sci USA* 1990;87:3962–3966.

353. Rothman P, Li SC, Gorham D, Glimcher L, Alt F, Boothby M. Identification of a conserved lipopolysaccharide-plus-interleukin-4-responsive element located at the promoter of germ line ε transcripts. *Mol Cell Biol* 1991;11:5551–5561.

354. Gerondakis S. Structure and expression of murine germ-line immunoglobulin ε heavy chain transcripts induced by interleukin 4. *Proc Natl Acad Sci USA* 1990;87:1581–1585.

355. Jumper MD, Splawski JB, Lipsky PE, Meek K. Ligation of CD40 induces sterile transcripts of multiple Ig H chain isotypes in human B cells. *J Immunol* 1994;152:438–445.

356. Fujieda S, Zhang K, Saxon A. IL-4 plus CD40 monoclonal antibody induces human B cells γ subclass-specific isotype switch: switching to γ1, γ3, and γ4, but not γ2. *J Immunol* 1995;155:2318–2328.

357. Radcliffe G, Lin Y-C, Julius M, Marcu KB, Stavnezer J. Structure of germ line immunoglobulin α heavy-chain RNA and its location on polysomes. *Mol Cell Biol* 1990;10:382–386.

358. Lutzker S, Alt FW. Structure and expression of germ line immunoglobulin g2b transcripts. *Mol Cell Biol.* 1988;8:1849–1852.

359. Xu M, Stavnezer J. Structure of germline immunoglobulin heavy-chain γ1 transcripts in interleukin 4 treated mouse spleen cells. *Dev Immunol* 1990;1:11–17.

360. Lennon GG, Perry RP. Cμ-containing transcripts initiate heterogeneously within

the IgH enhancer region and contain a novel 5′-nontranslatable exon. *Nature* 1985;318:475–478.

361. Collins J, Dunnick W. Production and regulation of germline transcripts of the γ2a gene prior to switch recombination. *Eighth International Congress of Immunology Abstracts.* Budapest: Springer-Verlag, 1992:35.

362. Neale GA, Kitchingman GR. mRNA transcripts initiating within the human immunoglobulin mu heavy chain enhancer region contain a non-translatable exon and are extremely heterogeneous at the 5′ end. *Nucleic Acids Res* 1991; 19:2427–2433.

363. Fujieda S, Lin YQ, Saxon A, Zhang K. Multiple types of chimeric germ-line Ig heavy chain transcripts in human B cells: evidence for *trans*-splicing of human Ig RNA. *J Immunol* 1996;157:3450–3459.

364. Li SC, Rothman PB, Zhang J, Chan C, Hirsh D, Alt FW. Expression of Im-Cg hybrid germline transcripts subsequent to immunoglobulin heavy chain class switching. *Int Immunol* 1994;6:491–497.

365. Reaban ME, Griffin JA. Induction of RNA-stabilized DNA conformers by transcription of an immunoglobulin switch region. *Nature* 1990;348:342–344.

366. Daniels GA, Lieber MR. Strand specificity in the transcriptional targeting of recombination at immunoglobulin switch sequences. *Proc Natl Acad Sci USA* 1995;92:5625–5629.

367. Baar JN, Pennell M, Shulman MJ. Analysis of a hot spot for DNA insertion suggests a mechanism for Ig switch recombination. *J Immunol* 1996;157: 3430–3435.

368. Bachl JC, Truck W, Wabl M. Translatable immunoglobulin germ-line transcript. *Eur J Immunol* 1996;26:870–874.

369. Shimizu A, Nussenzweig MC, Mizuta T-R, Leder P, Honjo T. Immunoglobulin double-isotype expression by trans-mRNA in a human immunoglobulin transgenic mouse. *Proc Natl Acad Sci USA* 1989;86:8020–8023.

370. Shimizu A, Nussenzweig MC, Han J, Sanchez M, Honjo T. Trans-splicing as a possible mechanism for the multiple isotype expression of the immunoglobulin gene. *J Exp Med* 1991;173:1385–1393.

371. Han H, Okamoto M, Honjo T, Shimizu A. Regulated expression of immunogloulin trans-mRNA consisting of the variable region of a transgenic μ chain and constant regions of endogenous isotypes. *Int Immunol* 1991;3: 1197–1206.

372. Nolan-Willard M, Berton MT, Tucker P. Coexpression of μ and γ1 heavy chains can occur by a discontinuous transcription mechanism from the same unrearranged chromosome. *Proc Natl Acad Sci USA* 1992;89:1234–1238.

373. Ott DE, Alt FW, Marcu KB. Immunoglobulin heavy chain switch region recombination within a retroviral vector in murine pre-B cells. *EMBO J* 1987;6: 577–584.

374. Ott DE, Marcu KB. Molecular requirements for immunoglobulin heavy chain constant region gene switch-recombination revealed with switch-substrate retroviruses. *Int Immunol* 1989;1:582–591.

375. Leung H, Maizels N. Transcriptional regulatory elements stimulate recombination in extrachromosomal substrates carrying immunoglobulin switch-region sequences. *Proc Natl Acad Sci USA* 1992;89:4154–4158.

376. Leung H, Maizels N. Regulation and targeting of recombination in extrachromosomal substrates carrying immunoglobulin switch region sequences. *Mol Cell Biol* 1994;14:1450–1458.

377. Ballantyne J, Ozsvath L, Bondarchuk K, Marcu KB. Chromosomally integrated retroviral substrates are sensitive indicators of an antibody class switch recombinase-like activity. *Curr Top Microbiol Immunol* 1995;194:439–448.

378. Daniels GA, Lieber MR. RNA:DNA complex formation upon transcription of immunoglobulin switch regions: implications for the mechanism and regulation of class switch recombination. *Nucleic Acids Res* 1995a;23:5006–5011.

379. Ballantyne J, Henry DL, Marcu KB. Antibody class switch recombinase activity is B cell-stage specific and functions stochastically in the absence of targeted accessibility control. *Int Immunol* 1997;9:963–974.

380. Schmitz J, Radbruch A. An interleukin-4-induced DNase I hypersensitive site indicates opening of the γ1 switch region prior to switch recombination. *Int Immunol* 1989;1:570–575.

381. Berton MT, Vitetta ES. Interleukin 4 induces changes in the chromatin structure of γ1 switch region in resting B cells before switch recombination. *J Exp Med* 1990;172:375–378.

382. Elgin SCR. DNAaseI-hypersensitive sites of chromatin. *Cell* 1981;27:413–415.

383. Burger C, Radbruch A. Protective methylation of immunoglobulin and T cell receptor (TcR) gene loci prior to induction of class switch and TcR recombination. *Eur J Immunol* 1990;20:2285–2291.

384. Kolata G. Fitting methylation into development. *Science* 1985;228:1183–1184.

385. Lin Y-CA Stavnezer J. Regulation of transcription of the germ-line Igα constant region gene by an ATF element and by novel transforming growth factor-β1-responsive elements. *J Immunol* 1992;149:2914–2925.

386. Xu M, Stavnezer J. Regulation of transcription of immunoglobulin germ-line γ1 RNA: analysis of the promoter/enhancer. *EMBO J* 1992;11:145–155.

387. Nilsson L, Paschalis S. The human Iα1 and Iα2 germline promoter elements: proximal positive and distal negative elements may regulate the tissue specific expression of Cα1 and Cα2 germline transcripts. *Int Immunol* 1993;5:271–282.

388. Ichiki T, Takahashi W, Watanabe T. Regulation of the expression of human Cε germline transcript. *J Immunol* 1993;150:5408–5417.

389. Albrecht B, Peiritsch S, Woisetschlager M. A bifunctional control element in the human IgE germline promoter involved in repression and IL-4 activation. *Int Immunol* 1994;6:1143–1151.

390a. Delphin S, Stavnezer J. Characterization of an interleukin 4 (IL-4) responsive region in the immunoglobulin heavy chain germline ε promoter: regulation by NF-IL-4, a C/EBP family member and NF-κB/p50. *J Exp Med* 1995;181:181–192.

390b. Iciek LA, Delphin SA, Stavnezer J. CD40 cross-linking induces Igε germline transcripts in B cells via activation of NF-κ B. *J Immunol* 1997;158:4769–4779.

391. Lin YS, Green MR. Interaction of a common cellular transcription factor, ATF, with regulatory elements in both E1A- and cyclic AMP-inducible promoters. *Proc Natl Acad Sci USA* 1988;85:3396–3400.

392. Lundgren M, Larsson C, Femino A, Xu M, Stavnezer J, Severinson E. Activation of the Ig germ-line γ1 promoter. *J Immunol* 1994;153:2983–2995.

393. Berton MT, Linehan LA. IL-4 activates a latent DNA-binding factor that binds a shared IFN-γ and IL-4 response element present in the germ-line γ1 Ig promoter. *J Immunol* 1995;154:4513–4525.

394. Fujita K, Jumper MD, Meek K, Lipsky PE. Evidence for a CD40 response element, distinct from the IL-4 response element, in the germline ε promoter. *Int Immunol* 1995;7:1529–1533.

395. Hou J, Schindler W, Henzel WJ, Ho TC, Brasseur M, McKnight SL. An interleukin-4-induced transcription factor: IL-4 Stat. *Science* 1994;265:1701–1706.

396. Berton MT, Warren WD, Linehan LA, Grusby MJ. The role of Stat6 in IL-4- and CD40-mediated germline Ig gene transcription and switch recombination in murine B cells. *J Allergy Clin Immunol* 1997;99:S259.

397. Lin S-C, Stavnezer J. Activation of NF-κB/Rel by CD40 engagement induces the mouse germ line immunoglobulin Cγ1 promoter. *Mol Cell Biol* 1996;16: 4591–4603.

398. Liao F, Birshtein BK, Busslinger M, Rothman P. The transcription factor BSAP (NF-HB) is essential for immunoglobulin germ-line ε transcription. *J Immunol* 1994;152:2904–2911.

399. Albrecht B, Peiritsch S, Messner B, Woisetschlager M. The transcription factor B cell-specific activator protein is not involved in the IL-4-induced activation of the human IgE germline promoter. *J Immunol* 1996;157:1538–1543.

400. Thienes CP, De Monte L, Monticelli S, Busslinger M, Gould HJ, Vercelli D. The transcription factor B cell-specific activator protein (BSAP) enhances both IL-4- and CD40-mediated activation of the human ε germline promoter. *J Immunol* 1997;158:5874–5882.

401. Kim J, Reeves R, Rothman P, Boothby M. The non-histone chromosomal protein HMG-I(Y) contributes to repression of the immunoglobulin heavy chain germline ε RNA promoter. *Eur J Immunol* 1995;25:798–808.

402. Wang DZ, Cherrington A, Famakin-Mosuro B, Boothby M. Independent pathways for de-repression of the mouse Ig heavy chain germline ε promoter: an IL-4 NAF/NF-IL-4 site as a context-dependent negative element. *Int Immunol* 1996;8:977–989.

403. Elenich LA, Ford CS, and Dunnick WA. The γ1 heavy chain gene includes all of the cis-acting elements necessary for expression of properly regulated germ-line transcripts. *J Immunol* 1996;157:176–182.

404. Elenich LA, Ford CS, Collins JT, Dunnick WA. γ1 heavy chain transgenes are responsive to interferon-γ repression and CD40 ligation. *J Immunol* 1997;158: 4564–4573.

405. Bottaro A, Lansford R, Xu L, Zhang J, Rothman P, Alt FW. S region transcription per se promotes basal IgE class switch recombination but additional factors regulate the efficiency of the process. *EMBO J* 1994;13:665–674.

406. Lorenz M, Jung S, Radbruch A. Switch transcripts in immunoglobulin class switching. *Science* 1995;267:1825–1828.

407. Kenter AL, Watson JV. Cell cycle kinetics model of LPS-stimulated spleen cells correlates switch region rearrangements with S phase. *J Immunol Methods* 1987; 97:111–117.

408. van der Loo W, Severinson-Gronowicz E, Strober S, Herzenberg LA. Cell differentiation in the presence of cytochalasin B: studies on the "switch" to IgG secretion after polyclonal B cell activation. *J Immunol* 1979;122:1203–1208.

409. Chu CC, Paul WE, Max EE. Analysis of DNA synthesis requirement for deletional switching in normal B cells, *Eighth International Congress of Immunology Abstracts.* Bucapest: Springer-Verlag, 1992:34.

410. Snapper CM, Marcu KB, Zelazowski P. The Ig class switch: beyond "accessibility". *Immunity* 1997;6:217–223.

411. Nakamura M, Kondo S, Sugai M, Nazarea M, Imamura S, Honjo T. High frequency class switching of IgM⁺ B lymphoma clone CH12F3 to IgA⁺ cells. *Int Immunol* 1996;8:193–201.

412. Mandler R, Chu CC, Paul WE, Max EE, Paul WE, Snapper CM. Interleukin 5 induces Sμ-Sγ1 DNA rearrangement in B cells activated with dextran-anti-IgD antibodies and interleukin 4: a three component model for Ig class switching. *J Exp Med* 1993;178:1577–1586.

413. Snapper CM, Zelazowski P, Rosas FR, et al. B cells from p50/NF-κB konckout mice have selective defects in proliferation, differentiation, germ-line C_H transcription, and Ig class switching. *J Immunol* 1996;156:183–191.

414. Zelazowski P, Carrasco D, Rosas FR, Moorman MA, Bravo R, Snapper CM. B cells genetically deficient in the c-Rel transactivation domain have selective defects in germline C_H transcription and Ig class switching. *J Immunol* 1997;159:3133–3139.

415. Snapper CM, Rosas FR, Zelazowski P, et al. B cells lacking RelB are defective in proliferative responses but undergo normal B cell maturation to Ig secretion and Ig class switching. *J Exp Med* 1996;184:1537–1541.

416. Caamano JH, Rizzo C, Durham SK, et al. Nuclear factor (NF)-KB2 (p100/p52) is required for normal splenic microarchitecture and B cell-mediated immune responses. *J Exp Med* 1998;185–196.

417. Loh RKS, Jabara HH, Geha RS. Disodium cromoglycate inhibits Sµ-Sε deletional switch recombination and IgE synthesis in human B cells. *J Exp Med* 1994;180:663–671.

418. Blunt T, Finnie NJ, Taccioli GE, et al. Defective DNA-dependent protein kinase activity is linked to V(D)J recombination and DNA repair defects associated with the murine scid mutation. *Cell* 1995;80:813–823.

419. Perlmutter AP, Gilbert W. Antibodies of the secondary response can be expressed without switch recombination in normal mouse B cells. *Proc Natl Acad Sci USA* 1984;81:7189–7193.

420. Yaoita Y, Kumagai Y, Okumura K, Honjo T. Expression of lymphocyte surface IgE does not require switch recombination. *Nature* 1982;297:697–699.

421. Katona IM, Urban JF Jr, Finkelman FD. B cells that simultaneously express surface IgM and IgE in *Nippostrongylus brasiliensis*-infected SJA/9 mice do not provide evidence for isotype switching without gene deletion. *Proc Natl Acad Sci USA* 1985;82:511–515.

422. MacKenzie T, Dosch H-M. Clonal and molecular characteristics of the human IgE-committed B cell subset. *J Exp Med* 1989;169:407–430.

423. Chan MA, Benedict SH, Dosch HM, Hui MF, Stein LD. Expression of IgE from a nonrearranged epsilon locus in cloned B-lymphoblastoid cells that also express IgM. *J Immunol* 1990;144:3363–3368.

424. Chen Y-W, Word CJ, Jones S, Uhr JW, Tucker PW, Vitetta ES. Double isotype production by a neoplastic B cell line. I. Cellular and biochemical characteriza-

tion of a variant of BCL1 that expresses and secretes both IgM and IgG1. *J Exp Med* 1986;164:548–561.

425. Chen Y-W, Word C, Dev V, Uhr JW, Vitetta ES, Tucker PW. Double isotype production by a neoplastic B cell line. II. Allelically excluded production of µ and γ1 heavy chains without CH gene rearrangement. *J Exp Med* 1986;164:562–579.

426. Koller B, Fromm H, Galun E, Edelman M. Evidence for *in vivo* trans splicing of pre-mRNAs in tobacco chloroplasts. *Cell* 1987;48:111–119.

427. Durdik J, Gerstein RM, Rath S, Robbins PF, Nisonoff A, Selsing E. Isotype switching by a microinjected µ immunoglobulin heavy chain gene in transgenic mice. *Proc Natl Acad Sci USA* 1989;86:2346–2350.

428. Gerstein RM, Frankel WN, Hsieh C-L, et al. Isotype switching of an immunoglobulin heavy chain transgene occurs by DNA recombination between different chromosomes. *Cell* 1990;63:537–548.

429. Kipps TJ, Herzenberg LA. Homologous chromosome recombination generating immunoglobulin allotype and isotype switch variants. *EMBO J* 1986;5:263–268.

430. Radbruch A, Liseegand B, Rajewsky K. Isolation of variants of mouse myeloma X63 that express changed immunoglobulin class. *Proc Natl Acad Sci USA* 1980;77:2909–2913.

431. Zelazowski P, Max EE, Snapper CM. Induction of Ku in normal murine B cells by cytokines that promote switch recombination. *J Immunol* 1997;159:2559–2562.

Fundamental Immunology, Fourth Edition,
edited by William E. Paul
Lippincott–Raven Publishers, Philadelphia © 1999.

CHAPTER **25**

Affinity Maturation

Claudia Berek

Introduction
  One Cell–One Antibody Molecule · The Antibody
The Immune Response
  Introduction · Selection of the Initial Repertoire · Hypermutation and Selection · Accumulation of Somatic Mutations with Time · A Shift in the Repertoire
Germinal Centers
  Structure of the Germinal Center · Factors Required for the Development of a Germinal Center Reaction · Kinetics of Germinal Center Development · Affinity Maturation in Germinal Centers · Ectopic Germinal Centers
Somatic Hypermutation
  Definition of Hypermutation · The Analysis of Somatic Mutations · Control of the Hypermutation Mechanism · Mechanism of Hypermutation
Conclusions
References

INTRODUCTION

It has been known for many years that when a humoral immune response is induced, the affinity of the antigen-specific antibodies found in the serum often increases with time. This phenomenon of progressive increase in antibody affinity (or avidity) is termed maturation of the immune response (1). For a long time the mechanisms leading to the change in antibody affinity were quite unclear. These days we are able to describe the process in molecular terms, and some of the interactions at the cellular level that allow the maturation process to take place are understood in detail. Even today, however, the mechanisms are not fully understood. Before discussing details, I will give some background information to make the process of affinity maturation more understandable.

One Cell–One Antibody Molecule

According to the clonal selection theory of Burnet (2), one B cell produces one single type of antibody molecule. During B-cell development, the variable region of the heavy chain (V_H) is generated by the rearrangement of a specific V_H, D, or J_H gene element, the variable region of the light chain (V_L) through rearrangement of a specific V_L and J_L gene segment (3). These V(D)J elements and the unique rearrangement patterns produced during their joining can be regarded as the clonal marker of a particular B-cell clone. Thus, if before exposure to antigen the B cell is committed to the synthesis of a specific immunoglobulin (Ig) molecule of defined affinity and specificity, how is affinity maturation possible?

C. Berek: Deutsches Rheuma ForschungsZentrum, Berlin, D-10117 Berlin, Germany.

There are basically two ways to improve the quality of the immune response. The most obvious option would be to switch the population of B cells that are activated by antigen. In the 1960s, Nussenzweig and Benacerraf (4) noticed that after immunization there is a shift in the repertoire of specific antibodies in guinea pigs with time: the early response is dominated by low-affinity λ-bearing antibodies, and the late response is dominated by high-affinity-κ bearing molecules.

The second option is to use the same B-cell population but to alter their receptors. The work of Weigert et al. (1970) suggested that in B cells a hypermutation mechanism can be activated that leads to the diversification of the V-region genes (5). Sequencing 10 λ L chains derived from different myeloma proteins showed that six were identical, whereas the other four sequences differed by one to three amino acids (Fig. 1). Weigert concluded that all of these sequences are derived from a single V_λ germline gene and that the four variable sequences are diversified somatically by a hypermutation mechanism. This far-sighted suggestion set the stage for the experimental analysis of affinity maturation. However, it took a further 8 years before Weigert's conclusions were confirmed by the analysis of the mouse genomic DNA (6).

It is now known that from one B cell clone that expresses one antibody molecule [as defined by its V(D)J rearrangement] variants may be generated; some of the variants may by chance have a higher affinity for the antigen. In order for the generation of mutants to lead to affinity maturation, these high-affinity variants have to be preferentially selected to differentiate into antibody-secreting plasma cells. In this way the structure of the antibody molecule will change, although the same V(D)J rearrangement is retained.

Most recently it was found that antigen-activated B cells may reexpress enzymes such as Rag1 and Rag2, which are otherwise

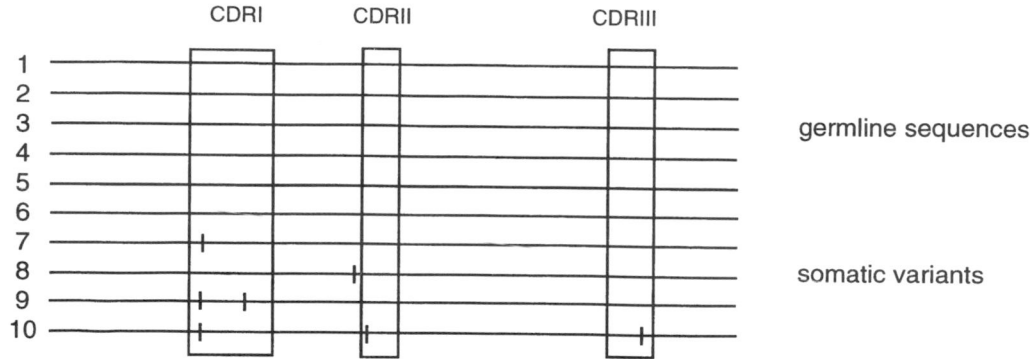

FIG. 1. Diagrammatic comparison of mouse Vλ protein sequences. A vertical bar indicates an amino acid difference. Complementarity determining regions (CDR) are indicated. Data from Weigert et al. (5).

seen only in premature B cells found in the bone marrow (7). These enzymes are required for V(D)J rearrangements to take place. Thus, one can no longer exclude the possibility that secondary rearrangements may occur in the mature IgD⁺/IgM⁺ B cells. These secondary rearrangements would then produce B cells with altered receptors.

The Antibody

A comparison across different V regions shows that diversity is concentrated in certain parts of the sequence (8). The variability plot of Kabat and Wu (see Chapter 3, Fig. 4) shows that some residues, those that are nescessary for the overall structure of the antibody molecule, are conserved, whereas other parts of the V region are highly variable. From the three-dimensional structure, it is clear that these hypervariable regions of the V_L and the V_H gene are brought together during protein folding to form the binding site of the antibody molecule. For this reason, these parts of the V region are referred to as the *complementarity determining regions* (CDR). The more conserved part of the V regions form the framework (FR).

Each of the V regions is composed of four framework regions (FR1, FR2, FR3, and FR4) interspersed by the three complementarity determining regions (CDR1, CDR2, and CDR3) (Fig. 1).

THE IMMUNE RESPONSE

Introduction

Given the number of available germline genes, their random combination, and the diversity generated during the joining of the various gene elements, a repertoire on the order of 10^{10} different B-cell receptors can in principle be generated in the mouse (9). From this enormous B-cell repertoire, many of the receptors will be able to bind to a protein antigen, like the hen egg lysozyme (Fig. 2), which has a complex surface structure. It is therefore not surprising that such a protein induces a heterogeneous immune response.

The crystal structure of three different antibodies with specificity for hen egg lysozyme complexed with lysozyme are shown in Fig. 2 (10). Each of these antibodies has a distinct target site on

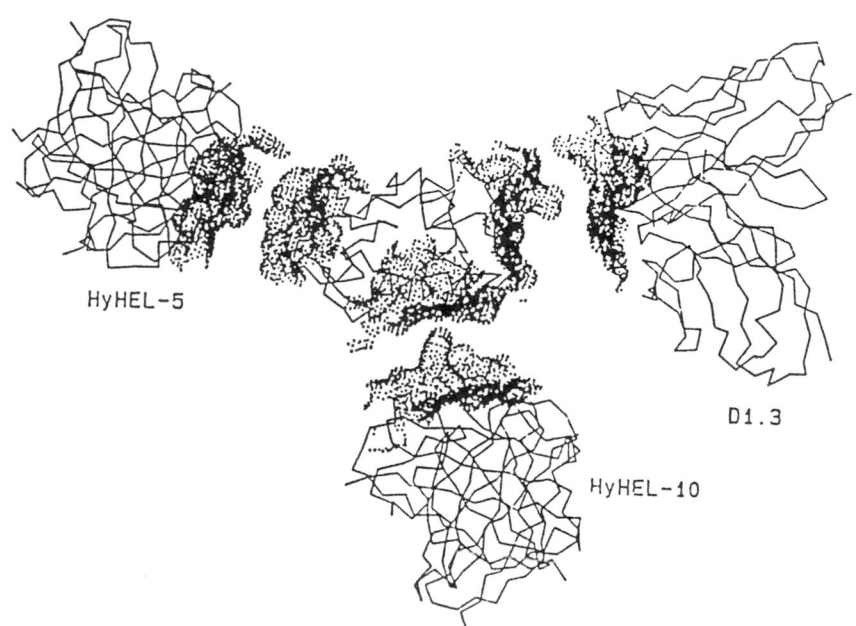

FIG. 2. View of lysozyme and three anti-lysozyme antibodies. Van der Waal's interactions between lysozyme and the CDR of three different antibodies, HyHEL-5, HyHEL-10 and D1.3, are shown (10).

the lysozyme surface. A tight interaction between the binding site of the antibody molecule and the protein surface is established through chemical forces such as hydrogen bonding or electrostatic and Van der Waals interactions. It follows that the degree of complementarity correlates with the binding affinity. After immunization with an antigen it is likely that the most frequent B cells available for activation will have a moderate degree of complementarity and hence a moderate affinity. On the other hand, the relatively rare B cells with a high-affinity receptor will have a higher chance of being activated by antigen. In this way, both frequency and affinity will determine the repertoire of the primary immune response.

In order to study the maturation of the response, one needs an antigen that will induce a rather restricted immune response. Small chemical compounds such as (4-hydroxy-3-nitrophenyl)-acetyl (NP), 2-phenyl-5-oxazolone (phOx), phosphorycholine (PC), or p-azophenylarsonate (Ars) are ideal. However, they will not by themselves induce an immune response. These small compounds, haptens, become immunogenic only when they are coupled to large carrier proteins. As an example, the immune response to the hapten phOx will be described in detail. Comparable results have been observed in immune reponses to the haptens NP (11–13), Ars (14,15), or PC (16–18), to protein antigens (19), and when mice were infected with a virus (20,21).

In addition to a restricted response, one needs techniques that allow a rapid analysis of the V_H and V_L genes expressed in the antigen-activated B cells. With the development of one important technology and the application of another, Milstein and his collaborators made it possible to study affinity maturation in molecular terms; the establishment of the hybridoma technology permitted the immortalization of antigen-activated B cells at different stages of the immune response (22), and the application of dideoxy sequencing to RNA permitted the direct analysis of V-region messenger RNA (mRNA) (23).

Selection of the Initial Repertoire

In order to look at the development of an immune response, BALB/c mice were injected with the hapten phOx coupled to the carrier protein chicken serum albumin (phOxCSA), and at various time points thereafter the immune response was analyzed (24). Spleen cells were fused with a nonsecreting fusion line, and hybridomas secreting phOx-specific antibodies were selected. The nucleotide sequences of the H- and L-chain V regions were determined by directly sequencing the mRNA. Figure 3 (upper part) shows the results of an experiment in which spleen cells were fused 7 days after immunization (25). This early response to phOx is surprisingly homogeneous. The majority of hybridoma lines use one particular V_L gene, referred to as VκOx1, and one particular V_H gene, referred to as V_HOx1 (25). There is little diversity, even in the CDRIIIs of the H-chain and the L-chain sequences. In the V_HOx1 sequences, the V-gene segment is joined to the D- and the J_H-gene segment in such a way that the overall length of the CDRIII is four amino acids. In all cases the first residue of the CDRIII is an aspartic acid and the third residue a glycine. Only the middle residue is variable (not shown in Fig. 3). Similarly, the majority of hybridoma lines express the same type of L chain. The VκOx1-gene segment is joined to Jκ5, resulting in the amino acid leucine at position 96. In the few cases where the VκOx1 gene is joined to Jκ4, leucine is generated again (not shown in Fig. 3) These hybridoma lines expressing the VκOx1–V_HOx1 combination

secrete antibodies with a relatively high affinity for the antigen phOx. B cells expressing low-affinity receptors for the antigen phOx are not seen in this experiment (9). These data suggest that from a diverse available repertoire only a few B cells emerge from a stringent selection process to participate in the affinity maturation.

Hypermutation and Selection

A comparison of the V regions showed that 7 days after induction of the immune response, sequences are unmutated. V_H and V_L regions derived from independent hybridoma lines are identical to germline sequences. The results looked very different when spleen cells were fused 2 weeks after immunization with antigen (26). Each of the V_H and Vκ sequences isolated showed multiple nucleotide exchanges when compared with the germline genes (Fig. 3, lower part). A somatic hypermutation mechanism has now diversified the germline-encoded receptors of the antigen-activated B cells.

Although the somatic mutations are rather randomly distributed in the V_H regions, the situation is different in the Vκ sequences (Fig. 3, lower part). Here the nucleotide exchanges accumulate at the border between CDRI and FR2. In all of the sequences, the histidine at position 34 in CDRI of the V region has been substituted by glutamine or asparagine. Furthermore, in many sequences, residue 36 (FR2), tyrosine, has changed into a phenylalanine. The triplet encoding histidine is CAC; seven different amino acids could be generated through a single nucleotide exchange. In the absence of selection, one would expect to see all of these exchanges occur with the same frequency. However, an amino acid substitution to proline, tyrosine, leucine, aspartic acid, or arginine is not observed in any of these sequences. The only two exchanges that are seen in the sequences derived from phOx-specific hybridoma lines are the changes to glutamine or to the very similar amino acid asparagine.

It has been shown that the single amino acid exchange from histidine to glutamine or asparagine results in an affinity increase of around 10-fold. Thus, 14 days after immunization, the repertoire of the B cells has been diversified by hypermutation, and a strong selection for high-affinity variants has occurred.

Accumulation of Somatic Mutations with Time

When the memory response was analyzed in the same way, nearly all hybridoma lines expressing the VκOx1 L chain carried the histidine to glutamine or asparagine replacement mutation at position 34 of the the CDRI (26,27). Thus, only high-affinity B cells differentiate into memory cells and become reactivated in the secondary and tertiary immune response. Furthermore, these sequences carried even more somatic mutations than the sequences isolated 14 days after immunization. From the early primary (□), to the late primary response (■), to the secondary (●), and finally the tertiary response (▲), the number of somatic mutations increases in the Vκ Ox1–V_HOx1 antibodies (Fig. 4) (25–27). One sees a stepwise accumulation of somatic mutations and at the same time an increase in affinity for the antigen phOx (Fig. 4). Thus, when memory cells become reactivated by antigen, the hypermutation mechanism is reinitiated (24). New variants are generated, and again those with the highest affinity will be selected to differentiate into plasma and further memory cells.

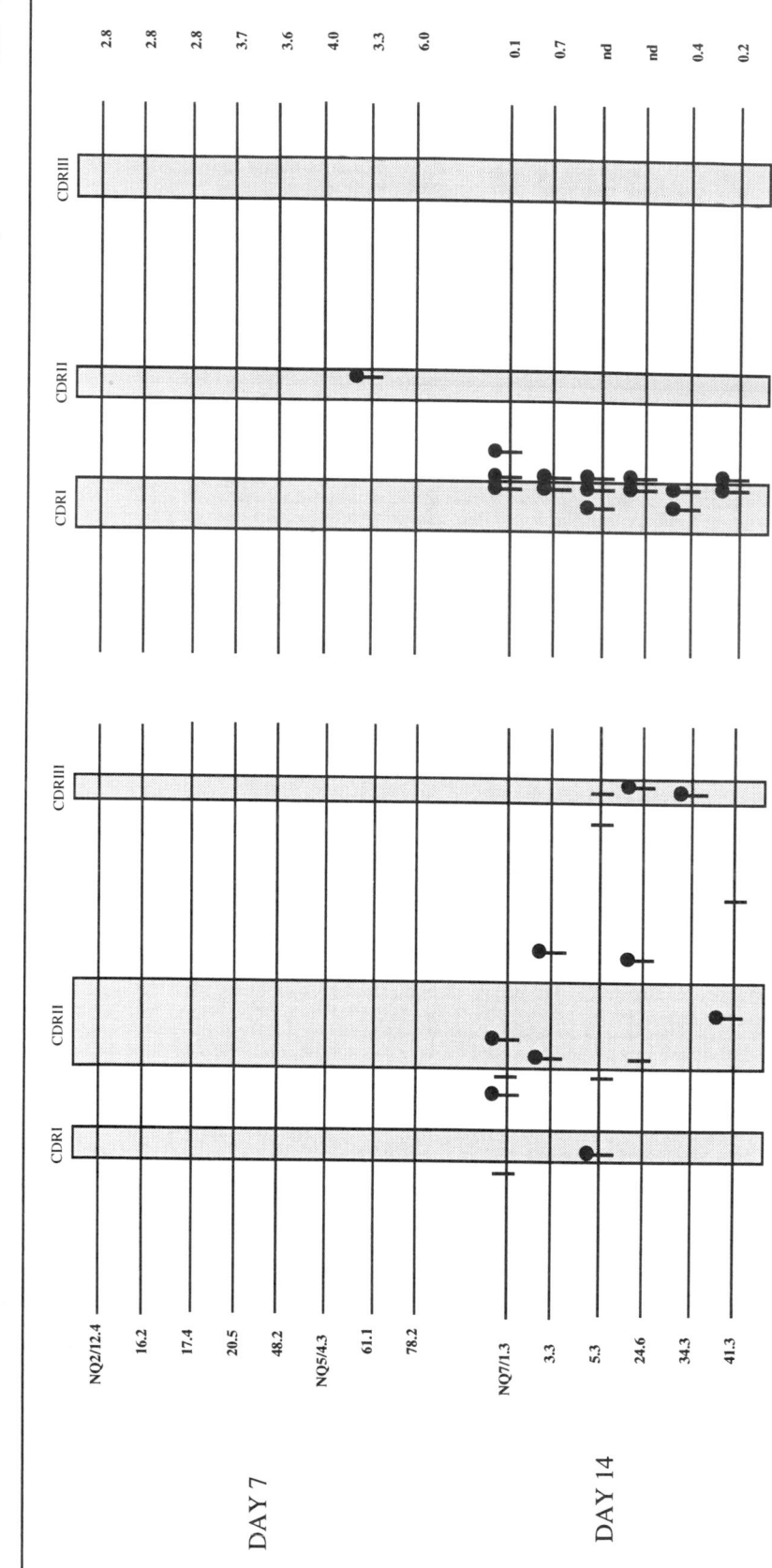

FIG. 3. The primary immune response to phOx. The somatic diversity seen in V_HOx1 and $V\kappa Ox1$ mRNA sequences is shown. Results from days 7 and 14 are compared. A vertical line indicates a silent mutation, and a circle above a line shows a replacement mutation. The affinity of the $V_HOx1-V\kappa Ox1$ antibodies is given on the right. Data from Kaartinen et al. (25) and Griffiths et al. (26).

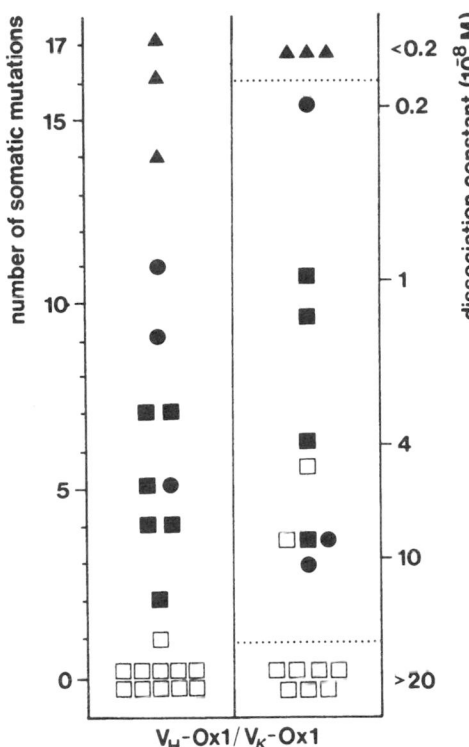

FIG. 4. The affinity increase in $V_H Ox1$–$V\kappa Ox1$ antibodies as a result of somatic mutations. The panel at left shows the number of somatic mutations seen in antibodies from the early primary (□), the late primary (■), the secondary (◆), and the tertiary (▲) immune response. The dissociation constants of these antibodies are shown on the right. Data from Kaartinen et al. (25), Griffiths et al. (26), and Berek et al. (27).

Data from other experimental systems have suggested that some memory cells may stop mutating. When memory cells were transferred into irradiated mice and reactivated by antigen, these cells were clonally expanded, although no further somatic mutations accumulated (28,29). In mice with autoimmune disease the long-term chronically activated memory cells still proliferate, but hypermutation is inactivated (30).

A Shift in the Repertoire

The generation of improved antibody binding sites through somatic mutation and selection is only part of affinity maturation. In addition, a shift in the repertoire is observed. Although the majority of the primary response hybridoma lines expressed the $V\kappa Ox1$-$V_H Ox1$ combination, there is a shift in the memory response toward antibodies where the $V\kappa Ox1$ L chain is seen in combination with other V_H regions (31). Comparing the CDRs in these V_H regions shows that CDRIII, which is generated through the joining of the V, D, and J elements, always has the canonical amino acid sequence seen in $V_H Ox1$ H chains (9). This striking finding supports the notion that in phOx-specific antibodies with a $V\kappa Ox1$ L chain, the highly conserved CDRIII of the H chain is essential for high-affinity binding. Additionally, in the memory response, hybridoma lines were isolated that expressed an H-chain–L-chain combination not seen in the early primary response (31). Comparable results were obtained in other hapten responses.

For example, in the immune response to NP there was a shift toward V_H regions in which the CDRIII of the $V_H 186.2$ gene, which encodes the H chain of most of the NP-specific antibodies in C57/Bl6 mice, showed a higher degree of N-region diversity in the 3′ half of the D segment (13). In other reponses a shift toward V_H and V_L combinations rarely seen in the primary response was found (17,20,21). Hence, it seems to be a general phenomenon that the repertoire of memory responses is more diverse than that of the primary. Although somatic hypermutation is a major factor in the diversification of the antigen-specific response, there is, in addition, a shift toward alternative V(D)J rearrangements. Both mechanisms may be of equal importance for the improvement of the antibody affinity.

The shift may be explained on kinetic grounds. In the memory response those V_H–$V\kappa$ combinations that have a faster "on-rate" constant than the canonical antibodies encoded by $V\kappa Ox1$ and $V_H Ox1$ are favored. The crystallographic structure of the phOx binding site revealed a deep and narrow binding pocket (32). Thus, binding to the hapten means overcoming a high-activation energy barrier. The affinity of the Ox1 antibodies is increased by point mutations that decrease k_{off} and hence prolong the lifetime of the hapten–antibody complex. B cells expressing a different V_H- and $V\kappa$-gene combination are kinetically superior in that they bind the antigen phOx more rapidly. Selection of B cells expressing such V_H and $V\kappa$ combinations into the memory response points to the biologic significance of the on-rate constant in the maturation of the immune response.

Various other mechanisms have been proposed to explain the shift in the repertoire observed between the primary and the memory responses, such as senescence of B-cell clones or regulation through the idiotypic network (9). But none of these has given an entirely satisfactory explanation. Just what drives the repertoire shift remains unclear.

GERMINAL CENTERS

The analysis of the V_H and V_L sequences expressed in hybridoma lines showed that within 14 days after activation by antigen, rapid changes take place in the antigen-specific B-cell population. First, the repertoire becomes diversified by the hypermutation mechanism; second, high-affinity B-cell clones are selected (Fig. 3). Where do these processes take place? In the first days after immunization, antigen-activated B cells migrate into the primary follicles of the peripheral lymphoid tissues, where rapid clonal expansion of the antigen-specific B cells leads to the formation of germinal centers (GCs) (33–36). The analysis of single GCs isolated directly from frozen tissue sections has demonstrated that B cells proliferating within the microenvironment of the GC undergo a process of somatic mutation so that a single initial B cell can give rise to variant progeny (37,38). The rare mutants that have improved affinity for the antigen are selected and differentiate into memory cells or into plasma cells (38–42).

Structure of the Germinal Center

Human tonsil tissue provides a source of classical GC (43). These GCs are composed of two zones, a dark zone and a light zone (Fig. 5). B cells in the dark zone are referred to as centroblasts, and it is in this part of the GC that proliferation takes place. B cells in the light zone are referred to as centrocytes and are in

GERMINAL CENTER

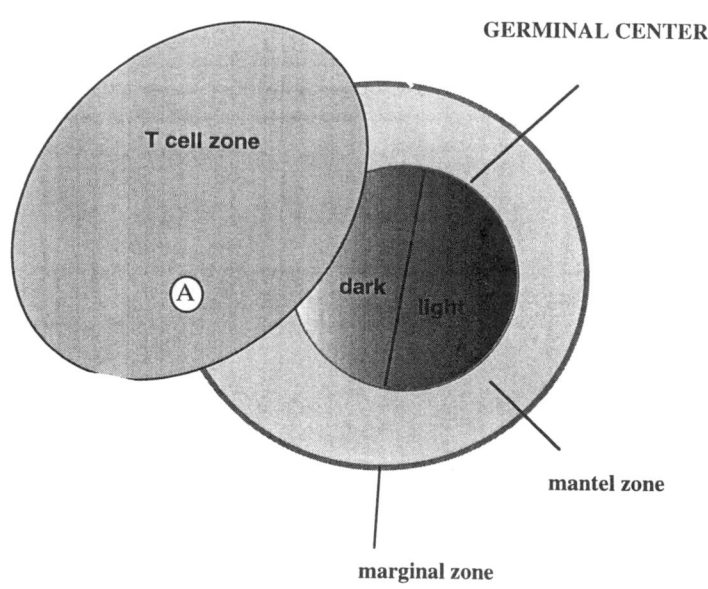

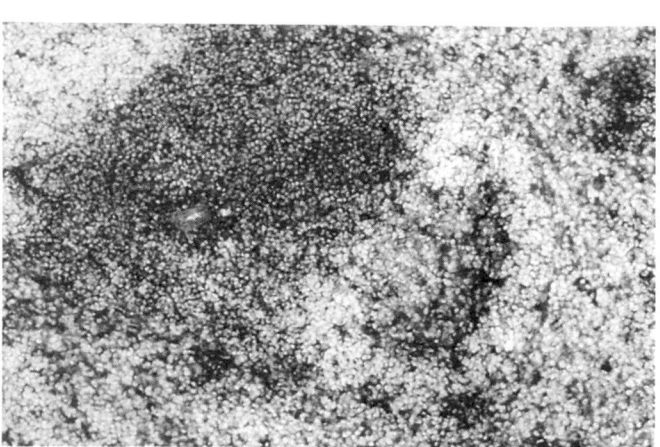

A

B

FIG. 5. The GC architecture. Diagrammatic representation **(A)** of a splenic tissue section **(B)**. Splenic tissue sections were prepared 10 days after immunization with phOx. Staining with an anti-CD3 antibody shows T cells mainly in the periarteriolar lymphocyte sheath. The dark zone of the GC is stained for proliferating cells (light shading), the light zone is stained with an antibody specific for FDC (dark shading) (62). In all cases the dark zone of the GC is adjacent to the T-cell zone, and the light zone is more distal. Kindly provided by S.A. Camacho.

close association with follicular dendritic cells (FDCs) (44–47), whose long branching cytoplasmic processes form a dense network that entangles the GC B cells. In contrast to dendritic cells, which present processed antigen in the form of peptides bound to the major histocompatibility complex (MHC) class II, FDC binds intact antigen complexed with antibody. These antigen–antibody complexes are bound to the surface of the FDC via the complement or the Fc receptor (46). It is thought that competition for the antigen presented on the surface of these FDCs positively selects high-affinity variants, allowing them to differentiate into memory cells and plasma cells. GC T cells, which are largely restricted to the light zone, are mainly CD4$^+$ cells of the helper type, which play a crucial role in the differentiation process (48). Those B cells that are not selected by antigen die through apoptosis (49), and the cell debris can be detected in the tingible body macrophages that are seen mainly at the border of the dark and the light zones.

Factors Required for the Development of a Germinal Center Reaction

The development of a GC is a complex process that is as yet only partly understood. However, a number of important aspects have so far been identified. For example, the generation of the appropriate tissue microarchitecture; activation of B cells; migration of B cells; T-/B-cell interactions, and the availability of the network of FDCs.

Tissue Microarchitecture

The molecular and cellular interactions necessary for the production of an intact functional lymphoid organ microarchitecture are largely unknown. However, experiments with knock-out mice have defined some of the essential elements. Correct lymphoid organogenesis is abberrant in animals in which the genes for any

of the cytokines tumor necrosis factor (TNF)-α, lymphotoxin (LT), LTα, and LTβ or any of their receptors, TNFRI and TNFR-RP (TNFRβ) are disrupted (50–53). In mice where either LTα or LTβ have been knocked out, the T-cell and B-cell zones (primary follicles) in the white pulp of the spleen (Fig. 6) are disorganized; hence, no GCs will develop (50,53). On the other hand, if TNF-α or the TNFR1 is knocked out, the microarchitecture of the spleen seems to develop normally (51); however, distinct primary follicles are missing (52). The migration of B cells via the marginal zone sinuses into the periarteriolar lymphocyte sheath (PALS) seems to be hindered. Instead, B cells appear to accumulate in the marginal zone (the border of the white and the red pulp of the spleen) (Fig. 6). A change in adhesion molecules expressed on endothelial cells of the marginal zone sinuses may block B-cell migration and hence prevent primary follicle formation. Furthermore, in mice deficient in TNF-α or the TNFRI, no FDC network develops. However, this effect may be secondary in that the development of a functional FDC network is dependent on the presence of mature B cells. In mice depleted of B cells or in SCID mice, the network of FDC is missing (54,55).

Activation of B Cells

Activation of naive B cells to a stage enabling GC formation requires more than signaling through the antigen receptor. Additional signals through the CD21–CD19 complex are required. In mice in which CD21 (the complement receptor CR2) has been disrupted, both the number and the size of the GC is reduced. This effect is reversed when syngeneic CD21$^+$ B cells are transferred into the CD21-deficient animals, indicating that coligation of the antigen receptor and the complement receptor by an antigen–complement complex enhances in the activated B cells the ability to initiate GC formation (56).

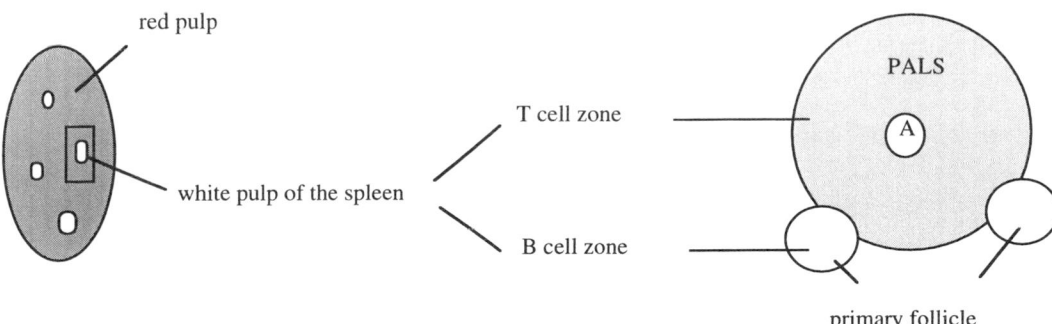

Antigen activation

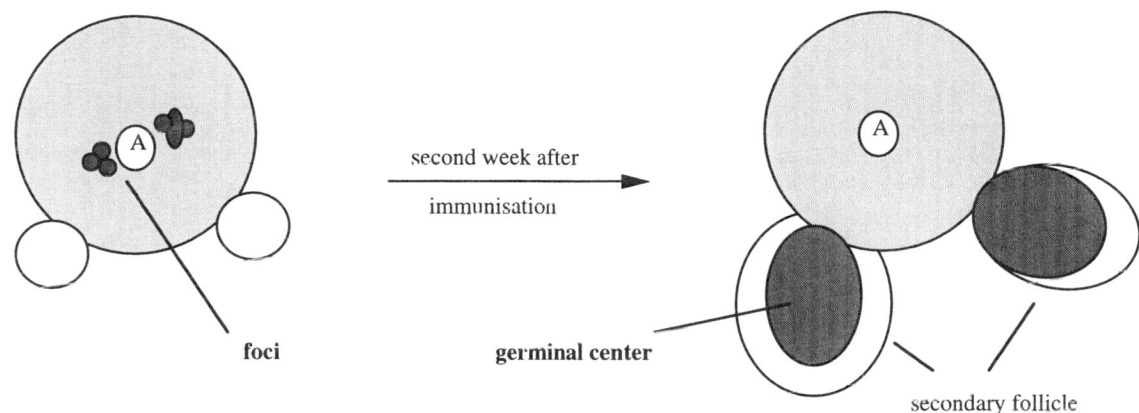

FIG. 6. The microanatomy of the spleen. In the white pulp of the spleen, a T- and a B-cell zone can be distinguished. T cells are in the PALS, whereas naïve IgD⁺/IgM⁺ B cells localize to form the primary follicle. After immunization, foci of antigen-activated B cells appear around the arteriole. These B cells are the precursors of short-lived plasma cells. By the second week, after immunization with a T cell–dependent antigen, GCs have fully developed; the primary follicle has changed into a secondary follicle.

Migration of B Cells

A characteristic of the mouse GC B cells is that they bind peanut agglutinin (PNA) strongly; hence, they are referred to as PNA^hi cells (57). This provides a convenient means of identification and isolation of GC B cells. An interesting observation was made in the spleen of mice deficient for the putative chemokine receptor BLR1. When these mice were immunized with a T cell–dependent antigen, PNA^hi B cells developed, although no GC formed in the spleen. PNA^hi cells accumulated in the T-cell zone, suggesting that in these mice the migration of B cells out of the PALS is impaired (58).

T-Cell/B-Cell Interaction

GCs are seen only in T cell–dependent immune responses, and the interaction between accessory molecules on T and B cells is crucial for normal GC development. Patients with hyper-IgM syndrome carry a mutation in the gene coding for CD40 ligand, which is expressed on T cells and is required for the interaction of T and B cells (59). In these patients, GCs are not formed and there is no diversification of the V-gene repertoire by hypermutation. In addition, B cells expressing IgM do not switch to IgG production, suggesting that class switching too may take place in the GC. CD40 and CD40 ligand are not the only molecules involved in T-/B-cell

interactions that are required to inititate GC formation. An interaction between B7 on B cells and CD28/CTL-4 on T cells also seems to be crucial (60). Mice deficient in both B7-1 and B7-2 fail to develop GCs when immunized with a T-dependent antigen. In transgenic mice that produce large amounts of soluble CTL-4, the T-/B-cell interaction is inhibited. These mice also lack the ability to form GCs and show a poor affinity maturation of their immune responses (61).

The Network of FDCs

The network of FDCs is essential both for the establishment of GCs and for the affinity maturation of the immune response. The first interaction between B cells and FDCs appears to be antigen independent and is mediated through adhesion molecules such as ICAM-1 and VCAM on the FDC surface (46). This interaction may initiate the GC formation by promoting the proliferation of antigen-activated B cells in the primary follicle. In addition, *in vitro* cultures have shown that B cells undergo phenotypic changes when interacting with FDCs (62). The expression of MHC class II is upregulated, and the B cells appear more blastlike. Furthermore, B cells proliferating in the network of FDC downregulate IgD and are, in contrast to B cells proliferating in PALS, positive only for IgM. However, the most important known function of the FDC network is the presentation of antigen–antibody complexes to the B cell (63,64). It is this function that drives the process by which high-affinity somatic mutants are selected to survive because competition for the antigen determines which B cells are selected to differentiate into memory or plasma cells.

Finally, the network of FDC functions as a store for antigen. Even months after the GC reaction has subsided, antigen–antibody complexes can be detected in association with FDC (44). It is thought that this antigen plays a crucial role for the maintenance of memory cells (65).

Kinetics of Germinal Center Development

The current general opinion is that in a T cell–dependent immune response B cells become activated in the PALS. Shortly after immunization, foci of proliferating B cells become apparent adjacent to the ateriole (66) (Fig. 6). Some of these cells will differentiate into plasma cells secreting IgM antibodies, whereas others may migrate into the primary follicle and become the precursors of the GC reaction. This viewpoint is supported by the finding of identical V(D)J rearrangements in B cells isolated from the PALS and adjacent GC structures (67). An alternative view is that the primary antibody-forming cells and the secondary memory cells are derived from different precursors. Peripheral B cells can be separated into two different subsets depending on the expression of the heat-stable antigen (J11d). Although J11d^{lo} cells are the precursors of the GC recation and give rise to memory cells, J11d^{hi} cells are the precursors of the primary antibody-forming cells (68).

Three to 4 days after immunization the first small clusters of proliferating PNA^{hi} B cells become apparent in the network of FDCs. At this early stage, GCs do not show the classical structure of a dark and a light zone. Practically all PNA^{hi}-binding B cells seem to be within the network of FDCs, although they express the Ki67 nuclear antigen characteristic for proliferating cells (62).

GC B cells rapidly proliferate with a cell cycle as short as 6 to 8 hours (69–71). Within a mere 3 days, a single cell may have developed into a clone of 1,000 cells, and by day 8 the FDC network has filled with centroblasts. The IgD$^+$/IgM$^+$ naive B cells of the primary follicle have been pushed out and form what is now called the mantel zone (Fig. 5). A primary follicle has developed into a secondary follicle. Over the next days, a classical GC structure with a dark and a light zone develops; fewer centroblasts are seen in the network of FDCs, and the dark zone seems to involute. By day 15, what remains of the GC is the FDC network filled with centrocytes, although even at this late stage of the GC reaction there are still groups of proliferating B cells detectable in the network of FDC.

Using PNA as a marker for GC B cells, it can be shown that the number of PNA^{hi} cells increases up to about 10 days postimmunization (72). By this time point, approximately 10% of splenic B cells are PNA^{hi} (Fig. 7). Thereafter, the number of PNA^{hi} cells decreases quickly, the majority dying through apoptosis. By 3 to 4 weeks after immunization, only residual GCs are seen in the splenic tissue. The GC reaction has subsided.

Affinity Maturation in Germinal Centers

Selection on the Repertoire

Although fully developed GCs are oligoclonal (73), a GC reaction may start from a heterogenous population of antigen-activated B cells. In order to study the diversity of GC B cells, techniques

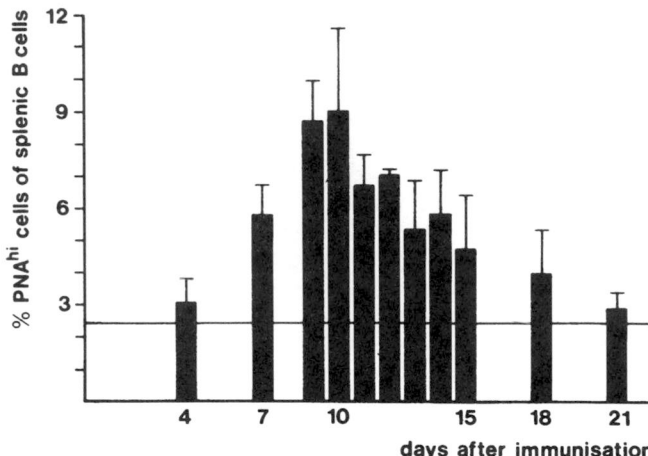

FIG. 7. The kinetics of the GC reaction. Mice were immunized with phOx, and spleen cells were prepared on various days. The percentage of PNA^{hi} cells as a fraction of all splenic B cells was determined by fluorescence activated cell sorting. Data from Apel and Berek (72), with permission.

were developed in the group of Rajewsky, which allow the analysis of single cells directly isolated from frozen tissue sections (74). The dark and the light zone of human tonsillar GCs were stained with specific antibodies. Single cells were picked, DNA was prepared, and the rearranged V-region genes amplified, cloned, and sequenced (74). A higher degree of clonal diversity was seen in the dark zone, supporting the notion that GCs become oligoclonal with time.

Similarly, a kinetic analysis of GC development in C57/Bl6 immunized with the antigen NP showed that a diverse population of NP-specific B cells participates in the early GC reaction (75). However, by day 8 the majority of B-cell clones express the V$_H$186.2/DFL16.1 characteristic of the high-affinity antibodies with specificity for NP. Interestingly, only these sequences accumulated somatic mutations.

Together these data suggest that B cells activated by antigen migrate into the primary follicles even when they are of low affinity. It seems that only those B cells with the highest affinity for the antigen succeed in establishing clonal descendents in the GC reaction. The other cells may die through apoptosis. In this way a rather polyclonal start is quickly reduced to an oligoclonal GC development.

Diversification of the B-Cell Repertoire in Germinal Centers

In 1991 a single GC was isolated by micromanipulation from a frozen tissue section, and the V-gene repertoire was determined (37). DNA was extracted from these NP-specific B cells, and the rearranged V$_H$186.2 gene was specifically amplified by PCR. Multiple sequences were isolated that had an identical V(D)J rearrangement and thus must have been derived from one single B-cell clone. However, these sequences differed by up to nine nucleotides from each other. Some somatic mutations were common to all sequences, whereas other mutations were only seen in single sequences. From the pattern of somatic mutations it is possible to draw a genealogic tree showing the stepwise intraclonal diversification of this B-cell clone (Fig. 8). These experiments

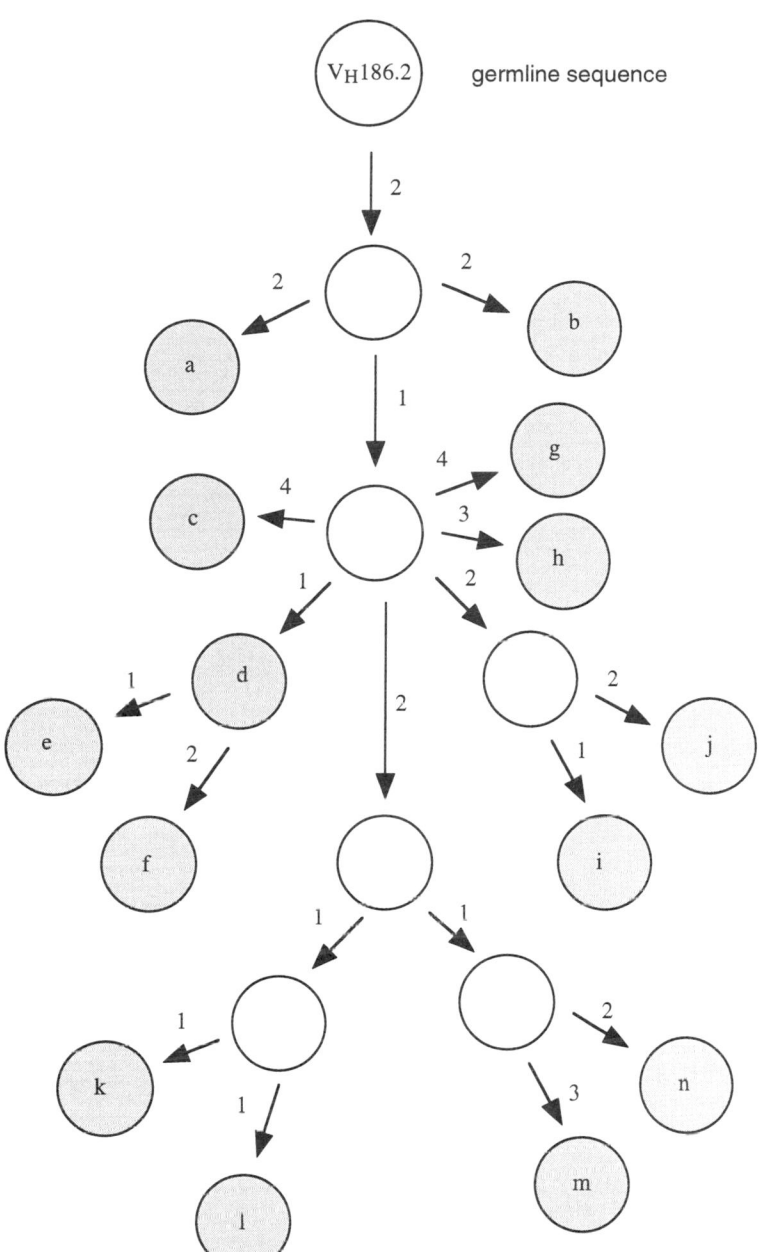

FIG. 8. Intraclonal diversification of V-gene sequences in GC B cells. The stepwise accumulation of somatic mutations is shown. Shaded circles indicate isolated sequences, open circles represent hypothetical intermediates. Numbers beside the arrows indicate the number of additional somatic mutations. Data from Jacob et al. (37), with permission.

demonstrate that during proliferation of B cells in the GC, nucleotide exchanges are introduced by a hypermutation mechanism and that the mutations accumulate in the V regions in a stepwise fashion.

Proof that the diversification of B cells takes place in the GC has been obtained also by separating different tonsillar B-cell populations by fluorescence-activated cell sorting (76). Using a panel of monoclonal antibodies binding to various B cell–specific surface antigens (CD antigens → clusters of differentiation), five different subsets of B cells could be distinguished (Table 1). The analysis of the V-region genes expressed in these populations showed that somatic mutations are seen only in GC (subsets Bm3 and Bm4) and memory B cells (subset Bm5). Thus, the hypermutation mechanism is switched on after the transition from the naive IgD+ (subsets Bm1 and Bm2) to the IgD− GC B cell (subsets Bm3 and Bm4) (76).

TABLE 1. *Tonsillar B-cell subsets*

	IgD	CD38	CD77	Somatic mutations	Differentiation stage
Bm1, Bm2	+	−		Germline	Naive B cells
Bm3	−	+	+	Mutated	Centroblasts
Bm4	−	+	−	Mutated	Centrocytes
Bm5	−	−		Mutated	Memory B cells

In fluorescence-activated cell sorting, CD38 is used as a marker for human GC cells, and CD77 distinguishes between centroblasts and centrocytes. Expression of IgD is used as a marker for naive B cells. Data are taken from ref. 76.

Affinity Selection in Germinal Centers

An amino acid exchange introduced into the sequence of the antibody molecule may be without effect, or it may lead to a change in the antibody's affinity for the antigen. From an evaluation of the V-region diversity and an analysis of the mutational pattern, Weigert (77) concluded that the majority of replacement mutations is disadvantageous for the antibody's affinity. Mutations that alter the protein's ability to fold correctly will lead to structurally nonfunctional antibodies. In addition, nonsense mutations or insertions or deletions may prevent expression of the protein. Replacement mutations in the CDR may reduce the affinity for the antigen or lead to antibodies with a specificity different from the parental cell line. Those replacement mutations in the CDR, or even in the FR, that improve the affinity for the antigen will be rather rare. Thus, without rigorous selection, an affinity maturation of the immune response based on somatic mutation would not be possible.

The analysis of single GCs isolated from the splenic tissue of mice immunized with the antigen phOx yielded an interesting result (38). In many GCs, all VκOx1 sequences found carried the key mutation in CDRI, which is an exchange from histidine to asparagine that increases the affinity by a factor of 10. These data suggest that those B cells that pick up a somatic mutation improving the affinity for the antigen gain a proliferative advantage over the other cells. Thus, B-cell clones in the GC develop by rapid expansion from the rare cells in which the affinity of the antigen receptor has been improved through somatic mutation.

One way to explain this efficient affinity selection is that cells in the GC cycle between phases in which the hypermutation mechanism is on or off (78). During proliferation, variants of various affinity are generated that then come into contact with antigen presented on the surface of FDCs where selection will take place. Whereas the majority of GC cells die by apoptosis, the few high-affinity mutants are selected to differentiate either into memory or plasma cells. Alternatively, selected cells may reenter a cycle of proliferation, diversification, and renewed selection. Like aiming for a peak while hiking through a rugged landscape, a high-affinity receptor is attained through multiple small steps (79).

The chance that a particular mutation is introduced at a particular position of the V region is low. Assuming a random mechanism for hypermutation, the chance to obtain the histidine-to-asparagine mutation at position 34 in the CDRI of the VκOx1 L chain is one in 900. Knowing that hypermutation becomes activated only in the second week postimmunization (39,40,75), GC B-cell clones may have reached a size that makes it likely that one of the cells picks up a mutation that improves the affinity. These are the cells that are selected to take over the GC and to differentiate into memory cells and plasma cells.

Little is known about the selection mechanism. Shortly after immunization, a high concentration of antigen will be present and will activate both B cells with low- and high-affinity receptors. It was initially thought that at lower concentrations antigen could be captured only by those B cells with high-affinity receptors (1). This was thought to lead to intense competition between the different mutant receptors for antigen. With the finding that complexed antigen bound to the surface of FDCs rather than free antigen directs the affinity maturation, this concept has to be modified. It may be that competition is indeed merely for access to the antigen in the immune complexes. On the other hand, B cells may actually physically remove antigen from these complexes, internalize and process it, and

express on their surface in association with MHC class II. These B cells could then monopolize the available T-cell help.

Development of Plasma Cells Secreting High-Affinity Antibodies

A successful B-cell response to an antigen involves the development from the naive B cell into two highly differentiated cell types. These are the plasma cells that synthesize and secrete antibody and the memory cells that provide the means of mounting a secondary response. In this section we will look at the ways in which plasma cells are selected.

As we have seen, antigen-activated B cells migrate into the T-cell zone of the spleen in the first days after immunization. Foci of proliferating B cells are seen in association with PALS (Fig. 6) (66). Many of these B cells will differentiate into plasma cells, which secrete antibodies of the IgM class that are unmutated and are in general of relatively low affinity. Nevertheless, these early antibodies may be essential for the survival of the organism. They are a first antigen-specific line of defense, which gives time for the T cell–dependent immune response to be established. During the second week of the response, when the primary follicles have developed into GCs containing secondary follicles, these foci involute (66,67).

Plasma cells secreting high-affinity antibodies develop in the GC. The affinity maturation of the serum antibody occurs during the primary response by the early selective differentiation of high-affinity variants into antibody-secreting cells. By day 14 after immunization, high-affinity plasma cells appear in the bone marrow (42). They seem to be responsible for the long-term production of high-affinity antibodies in the primary immune reponse.

V-region sequences isolated from bone marrow plasma cells (42) and from hybridoma lines derived from splenic tissue 2 weeks after immunization (26) carried only a few somatic mutations. However, the affinity-enhancing mutations were present in practically all sequences. In contrast, sequences derived from PNA^{hi} cells at the same time point showed (a) a higher frequency of somatic mutations and (b) that only some of them carried the affinity-enhancing mutation (39). These data indicate that early in the response, when the first B cells with high-affinity receptors are generated in the GC, some of them may be selected to differentiate into plasma cells. The high-affinity interaction with the antigen appears to switch off the hypermutation mechanism. Instead, these cells are pushed into a pathway of differentiation. In this way the system ensures that in the shortest possible time plasma cells secreting high-affinity antibodies are generated.

During infection with a cytopathic virus, such as the vesicular stomatitis virus, neutralizing antibodies are already seen within the first week after infection. These early antibodies have a surprisingly high affinity (21). They showed a binding avidity on the order of 10^{-9}. Even more surprising, V regions of the H and the L chains were devoid of somatic mutations. It seems that during evolution, a V-gene repertoire is selected that allows the rapid formation of high-affinity antibodies. IgG sequences isolated at later stages of the immune response accumulate somatic mutations in their V genes. The neutralizing capacity was about two orders of magnitude higher than that of the early primary response antibodies.

Ectopic Germinal Centers

GCs may develop not only in the spleen, tonsils, Peyer's patches, and other peripheral lymphoid organs, but, under certain cicumstances, also in nonlymphoid tissues. In a number of autoimmune diseases, GC-like structures have been found in the affected tissues: the thyroid gland of patients with Hashimoto's disease (80), the thymus in patients with myasthenia gravis (81), and the salivary gland in patients with Sjögren's syndrome (82). A GC reaction has also been demonstrated in the synovial tissue of patients with rheumatic diseases by directly isolating GC-like structures and analyzing the rearranged V-region genes. A sequence analysis showed a stepwise accumulation of somatic mutations in clonally related B cells, indicating that B cells proliferate and undergo hypermutation in the GC-like structures of the synovial tissue (83).

In these GC-like structures, a typical dark and light zone is not apparent and the network of FDCs is in the center. As expected, there are B cells in the network of FDCs, but the CD4+ T cells, normally found in a light zone, are missing.

An excessive production of proinflammatory cytokines in the chronically inflamed tissues may provide the milieu in which an ectopic GC-like structure can develop. The finding that a local overexpression of LTα induces the development of GC is in line with this interpretation (84).

SOMATIC HYPERMUTATION

Definition of Hypermutation

How are the mutations introduced into the rearranged V-region genes? One possibility would be by gene conversion (85), a mechanism that is used to generate the primary V-gene repertoire in chickens (86,87). Here, only one functional V gene exists, although many pseudogenes are available. The repertoire is generated by gene conversion, which copies short segments of the pseudogene sequences into the functional V gene. A rather similar system is used to generate the primary repertoire in rabbits (88). However, it is unlikely that gene conversion is the mechanism behind somatic hypermutation. All evidence speaks in favor of a somatic hypermutation mechanism that introduces single nucleotide exchanges stepwise into the rearranged V-region gene. Although in human sequences there is a slight tendency of mutations to cluster (89), single nucleotide substitutions generally are the most frequently observed changes. Furthermore, intensive searches for gene sequences that might function as donor sequences during the somatic diversification process have all failed.

Hypermutation is a tightly regulated process. In general, it is turned on only after antigenic activation of B cells (90), although in sheep the nucleotide substitutions are introduced into the V region of the H and the L chains during B-cell development to generate a diverse primary repertoire (91). Activation of B cells with a mitogen such as lipopolysaccharide (92) or with a T cell–independent antigen, such as a bacterial polysaccharide, will result in proliferation and differentiation but not in the accumulation of somatic mutations, and there is no affinity maturation (93). Thus, B-cell proliferation alone is not sufficient to induce hypermutation. Simultaneous stimulation through the B cell's own antigen receptor and through CD21, the complement receptor is necessary (56), as well as T-cell help (48) and interaction with the network of FDC (46). Only then will the microenvironment of the GC be built up, which is essential for affinity maturation.

Hypermutation introduces nucleotide exchanges into the rearranged V-region genes at a rate that is thought to be about a million times greater than the background rate of spontaneous

mutation. The actual rate of hypermutation is difficult to calculate. There are many variables such as the cell division time, the activation period of hypermutation or the frequency with which selectable mutations are generated. In addition, it is unclear whether the mutation rate is constant or whether cells oscillate between stages of high- and low-hypermutation rates. Interestingly, although rather different ways have been used for the calculation (11,24,94), it is generally agreed that the average rate of hypermutation has to be on the order of 10^{-3}/base pair/cell generation. Because the length of the V region is approximately 300 nucleotides, this means that with every third division one nucleotide exchange is introduced into the V region of the H chain and one into the V region of the L chain.

Hypermutation is a highly specific mechanism. Substitutions are seen only in rearranged V regions (95–97) and in their 3′ and 5′ flanking sequences (97–100). The target sequence is an array of approximately 1,500 nucleotides, referred to as the mutation domain (Fig. 9) (101). Figure 9 shows that the frequency of somatic mutations is highest over the rearranged V-region gene and falls off over the neighboring flanking sequences. The 5′ boundary of somatic mutations is within the leader intron, and mutations are only rarely seen upstream from the transcriptional start site (99). There are usually no somatic mutations in the constant region gene. An exception is the Cλ1 gene of the mouse, in which low numbers of somatic mutations have been described (100). This constant-region gene is unusually close to the J-region segments so that somatic mutations may simply spill over, resulting in substitutions both in the V and C regions.

No specific structural feature of the V gene sequence is required to make it a target for somatic hypermutation. The V-gene sequences have been replaced with a C-region domain, or with a completely unrelated DNA sequence, such as the human β-globin gene, drosophila intron DNA, bacterial neo or gpt, or even artificial sequences (102–105). In all these cases mutations are introduced at a similar rate as into the original V-region sequence.

The Analysis of Somatic Mutations

Does each base within a rearranged V gene have an equal probability of mutating? Because the pattern of somatic mutations seen in V- regions recovered from high-affinity B cells is strongly selected, these sequences cannot give us an accurate picture of the specificity of the mutator. In order to understand the mechanism, the pattern of somatic mutations in sequences that have not been exposed to selective pressure have to be analyzed. Examples are flanking region sequences (97–100), nonselected passenger transgenes, which pick up somatic mutations as a bystander effect (106,107), and nonfunctional rearranged V regions (108). Table 2 shows the distribution of nonselected somatic mutations seen in a passenger transgene (106). It is clear that transitions (A ↔ G and C ↔ T substitutions) are more frequent than transversions (A → C or T, G → C or T, T → A or G, and C → A or G). Furthermore, as assessed on the coding strand, G bases are more frequently substituted than C bases, and A bases more than T bases. This bias against exchanges of pyrimidines is not attributable to uneven base composition of the V genes. It is observed in V-gene sequences derived from both antigen-unselected (106) and -selected B cells (12,15,26,27,76). This suggests that the hypermutation machinery can discriminate between the two strands; one speaks of a strand bias in the hypermutation mechanism. Strand bias was observed

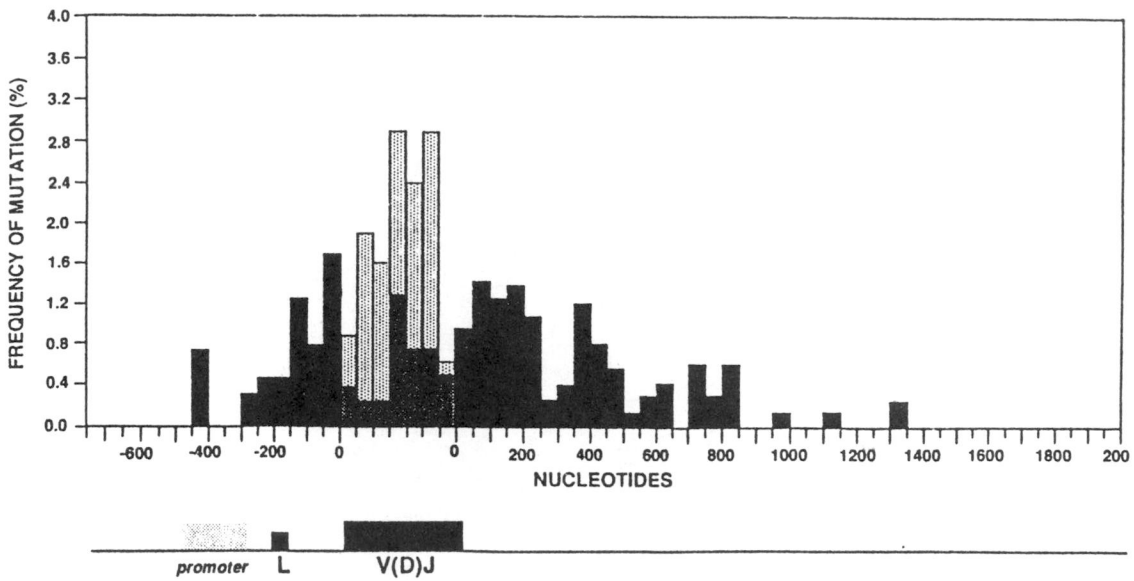

FIG. 9. The hypermutation domain. The data from 17 V$_H$ and V$_K$ segments rearranged to different J-gene segments are compiled (98). The drawing at bottom shows the position of the promotor, leader, and V(D)J gene. The abscissa of the graph is numbered as follows: negative numbers correspond to 5' flanking nucleotides; the coding region is not numbered but represents 350 bp; and positive numbers correspond to 3' flanking nucleotides. The ordinate designates the frequency of mutation per base pair averaged over 50-nucleotide increments. Black bars represent the frequency of flanking region mutations, light stippled bars are replacement mutations, and dark stippled bars are silent substitutions.

not only for Ig genes. It was also seen when a *neo* gene was inserted in place for a V gene, which means that the effect is not sequence specific (103).

As we have seen, the precise DNA sequence is not decisive for the definition of the 1,500–base pair mutational domain. There is nothing specific to the V-region sequence. However, when one looks closely at the mutational pattern, it becomes clear that the primary sequence does have an effect on the distribution of the somatic mutations within this domain. A comparison of the mutability of each of the possible triplets showed that some triplets are more likely to be targeted (hot spots for somatic mutations) than others (cold spots) (101,109). One of the favored targets for hypermutation is the consensus sequence RGYW (R = A or G; Y = C or T; W = A or T). It covers one of the first hot spots described, the AGY codon for serine 31 in the first CDR of many V-region genes. In both selected and unselected sequences the second residue, G, is frequently changed to either A or C (AGY → ACY or AAY). This hot spot is defined, at least in part, by the DNA sequence. Replacement of the AGC triplet by TCA, which also encodes serine, changes this site into a cold spot (110).

The CDRs are often hot spots for somatic hypermutation (91,106). For example, when one looks at the distribution of AGY and TCN serine codons in V-region genes, one finds that there is a preponderance of AGY over TCN serines in the CDRs (111). It looks as if CDRs have evolved in such a way that the somatic mutation mechanism preferentially targets mutations into this part of the V-region gene.

For each of the triplets, one can calculate an expected ratio of replacement (R) to silent (S) mutations. For example, the triplets encoding glycine are GGx. Six of the nine possible nucleotide substitutions result in an amino acid replacement mutation giving an R/S value of 2 (6/3). On the other hand, in the case of histidine (CAC) where eight out of nine possible substitutions lead to an amino acid exchange, the ratio is 8 (8/1). The analysis of V-region sequences has shown that evolution has selected for CDRs where the codon usage leads to a high ratio of R/S mutations. In this way it is more likely that amino acid exchanges are introduced into those positions of the V region that encode the binding site.

The ratio of replacement to silent mutations (R/S value) in the FR and the CDR of the V region is frequently used as an indirect marker for affinity maturation. Hot spots aside, somatic mutations are by and large introduced randomly. Any deviation from a random distribution can be taken as an indication that the selection mechanism is operative. However, one has to be careful with the interpretation of such data. In principle, one expects a low ratio of replacement mutations in the FR in order to preserve the three-dimensional structure. However, in the CDR either a high or a low value may be indicative of positive antigenic selection. At positions

TABLE 2. *Substitutions in a passenger transgene*

| From | To | | | | % of observed mutations |
	A	G	C	T	
A	—	46	29	25	33 (33)
G	68	—	24	8	35 (38)
C	20	0	—	80	21 (18)
T	14	14	72	—	10 (11)

Somatic mutations in the coding strand of a passenger transgene have been analyzed. For each of the four bases, the number of base substitutions as a percentage of the total is given. The values in parentheses give the corrected value, taking into account that in the V-region gene analyzed the four bases occur with different frequency. Data taken from ref. 106.

where an amino acid exchange is disadvantagous, one would expect a negative selection for replacement mutations and a positive selection for silent mutations. In such a case, silent mutations will accumulate even in a CDR (24).

Control of the Hypermutation Mechanism

Transgenic mice expressing an additional V gene in their germline have been used to analyze the cis-acting sequence elements necessary to target the hypermutation mechanism to the V-region gene (Fig. 10). Using various constructs of an Ig kappa transgene, it was found that two elements are essential for effective hypermutation: (a) the promotor (112) and (b) the transcription enhancer sequences, which are the 3′ enhancer (E3′) and the intron-enhancer (Ei)/matrix attachment region (MAR) (113). A deletion of the E3′ will lead only to a reduction in the number of somatic mutations. Sequences are still mutated. In contrast, when the Ei/MAR region is deleted, no somatic mutations are detectable (113).

The promotor itself does not seem to contain any special sequences necessary for the activation of the hypermutation mechanism. Constructs where the V-gene promotor was replaced with a β-globin minimal promotor continued to mutate. However, an inactive Ig promotor is inefficient in driving mutations, which suggests that an active promotor is required for hypermutation (105). The importance of the promotor and the Ei/MAR region for the targeting of the hypermutation mechanism was underlined when these sequence elements were inserted 5′ and 3′ from the C-region sequence, respectively. By inserting a new transcription initiation site upstream from the C region, high numbers of somatic mutations accumulated in the C region (112).

Because a region 5′ from the V-region sequence defines the start of the hypermutation domain, it seems likely that a process initiated here carries a mutator factor into the gene. Such a sequence has been described for the intronic region, separating the leader and the Vκ germline gene (114). However, an equivalent sequence in the intronic region of V_H germline genes could not be detected.

Mechanism of Hypermutation

The hypermutation mechanism is activated in proliferating cells. Thus, it was initially thought that the mechanism might be linked to DNA replication. Brenner and Milstein (115) originally suggested that hypermutation may result from error-prone DNA synthesis. A DNA polymerase was postulated that lacks a proofreading 3′ to 5′ exonuclease activity and therefore was more likely to lead to the incorporation of mismatches. To explain the strand bias of somatic mutations, a mechanism has been proposed that targets hypermutation either to the lagging or the leading strand in replicating DNA. However, attempts to link either hypermutation to the activity of particular DNA polymerases have been unsuccessful.

A number of observations imply that hypermutation is a form of error-prone DNA repair mechanism that is activated during transcription: (a) hypermutation is dependent on an active promotor (105,112), (b) the hypermutation domain starts downstream of the promotor region (97–99), (c) the transcription enhancer sequences are required for hypermutation (113), and (d) there is strand bias (101). Although transcription can give rise to errors in the mRNA, one does not usually think of it as being mutagenic for the DNA. Thus, the question arises, how are somatic mutations introduced specifically into the rearranged V-region gene and its flanking sequences during transcription? One idea is that sequences in the intron enhancer/MAR region may initiate regional single-strand nicking. In order for transcription to proceed, these lesions must be repaired. An error-prone DNA polymerase may be recruited to do

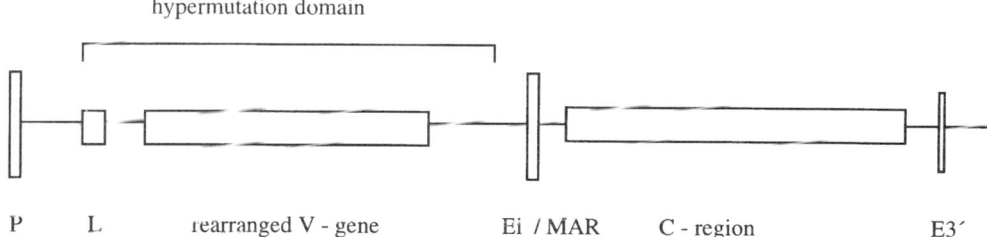

changes introduced	somatic mutations
replacement of the promotor	+
replacement of the V-region sequence	+
deletion of the Ei / MAR	−
deletion of the E3′	↓

FIG. 10. The effect of cis-acting elements on hypermutation in κ transgenes. For the activation of hypermutation an active promotor (P) and the presence of the Ei/MAR are necessary (101). The number of somatic mutations decreases (↓) when E3′ is deleted.

this job, and single nucleotide mismatches might be introduced during repair into the transcribed DNA strand (101). Another possibility that has been discussed is that a mutator factor associates with the transcription initiation complex (112). It is assumed that the mutator factor interferes with the RNA polymerase II, inducing pausing in the absence of DNA damage. A gratuitous transcription-coupled repair (112) may introduce mutations into the transcribed DNA strand. Only after cell division do mismatches introduced into the DNA become fixed as somatic mutations in the daughter cells. The size of the mutation domain would predict that no pausing of the RNA polymerase occurs later than approximately 2,000 nucleotides downstream from the transcription initiation site.

Despite intensive efforts, the mechanism of somatic hypermutation is still not understood. What has been missing is an *in vitro* system to study the mechanism. Recently, however, it has become possible to initiate the hypermutation mechanism *in vitro* by activating a Burkitt's lymphoma cell line through cross-linking the Ig receptors. By coculturing with an activated T-cell line, B cells will proliferate and accumulate somatic mutations (116). Such *in vitro* systems may help to identify the long sought after mechanisms of hypermutation.

CONCLUSIONS

It is just over 100 years since Flemming (117) first noted areas of massive proliferation in the follicles of lymphatic tissue. Because he thought that the white blood cells were generated here, he called these areas germinal centers. We now know that this interpretation was only partly correct because the primary B-cell repertoire in the adult is generated in the bone marrow rather than in the peripheral lymphatic tissue. However, the GC is indeed the site where the repertoire of mature high-affinity B cells is generated.

The term "affinity maturation" was first introduced in the 1960s to describe the phenomenon whereby the affinity of a humoral immune response typically increases with time. Since then we have learned a great deal about the molecular and cellular processes that lead to the generation of high-affinity B cells. However, as this brief review shows, there are still many open questions. The molecular basis of the hypermutation mechanism and the nature of the cellular interactions required to permit affinity maturation are currently not well understood. Progress has been made in defining the requirements for generating the special microenvironment of the GC and in delineating the intercellular contacts and signals that are necessary for the activation of B cells, their migration into the primary follicle, and finally the selective differentiation into high-affinity effector or long-term memory cells. Still, much remains to be done before any of these fundamental processes is fully understood. GCs and the processes that take place within them will remain fascinating fields of research for many years to come.

REFERENCES

1. Siskind GW, Benacerraf B. Cell selection by antigen in the immune response. *Adv Immunol* 1969;10:1–50.
2. Burnet FM. *The clonal selection theory of immunity.* London: Cambridge University Press, 1959.
3. Tonegawa S. Somatic generation of antibody diversity. *Nature* 1983;302:575–581.
4. Nussenzweig V, Benacerraf B. Quantitative variations in the L chain types in guinea pig antihapten antibodies. *J Exp Med* 1966;124:805–818.
5. Weigert MG, Cesari IM, Yonkovitch SJ, Cohn M. Variability in the lambda light chain sequences of mouse antibody. *Nature* 1970;228:1045–1047.
6. Bernard O, Hozumi N, Tonegawa S. Sequences of mouse immunoglobulin light chain genes before and after somatic changes. *Cell* 1978;15:1133–1144.
7. Han S, Zheng B, Schatz DG, Spanapoulou E, Kelsoe G. Neoteny in lymphocytes: Rag1 and Rag2 expression in germinal center B cells. *Science* 1996;274:2094–2097.
8. Kabat EA, Wu TT, Perry HM, Gottesman KS, Foeller C. Sequences of proteins of immunological interest. Bethesda, MD: NIH Publication, 1991.
9. Berek C, Milstein C. The dynamic nature of the antibody repertoire. *Immunol Rev* 1988;105:5–26.
10. Davies DR, Sheriff S, Padlan EA, Silverton EW, Cohen GH, Smith-Gill SJ. Three dimensional structures of two Fab complexes with lysozyme. In: Smith-Gill SJ, Sercarz EE, eds. *The immune response to structurally defined proteins: the lysozyme model.* Schenectady, NY: Adenine Press, 1989.
11. Allen D, Cumano A, Dildrop R, et al. Timing, genetic requirements and functional consequences of somatic hypermutation during B-cell development. *Immunol Rev* 1987;96:5–22.
12. Weiss U, Zoebelein R, Rajewsky K. Accumulation of somatic mutants in the B cell compartment after primary immunization with a T cell-dependent antigen. *Eur J Immunol* 1992;22:511–517.
13. Weiss U, Rajewsky K. The repertoire of somatic antibody mutants accumulating in the memory compartment after primary immunization is restricted through affinity maturation and mirrors that expressed in the secondary response. *J Exp Med* 1990;172:1681–1689.
14. Wysocki L, Manser T, Gefter ML. Somatic evolution of variable region structures during an immune response. *Proc Natl Acad Sci U S A* 1986;83:1847–1851.
15. Manser T, Wysocki LJ, Margolies MN, Gefter ML. Evolution of antibody variable region structure during the immune response. *Immunol Rev* 1987;96:141–162.
16. Gearhart PJ, Johnson ND, Douglas R, Hood L. IgG antibodies to phosphorylcholine exhibit more diversity than their IgM counterparts. *Nature* 1981;291:29–34.
17. Stenzel-Poore MP, Rittenberg MB. Clonal diversity, somatic mutation, amd immune memory to phosphorylcholine-keyhole limpet hemocyanin. *J Immunol* 1989;143:4123–4133.
18. Chien NC, Pollock RR, Desaymard C, Scharff MD. Point mutations cause the somatic diversification of IgM and IgG2a anti phosphorylcholine antibodies. *J Exp Med* 1988;167:945–973.
19. Kocks C, Rajewsky K. Stepwise intraclonal maturation of antibody affinity through somatic hypermutation. *Proc Natl Acad Sci U S A* 1988;85:8206–8210.
20. Clarke SH, Staudt LM, Kavaler J, Schwartz D, Gerhard WU, Weigert MG. V region gene usage and somatic mutation in the primary and secondary reponses to influenza virus hemagglutinin. *J Immunol* 1990;144:2795–2801.
21. Kalinke U, Bucher EM, Ernst B, et al. The role of somatic mutation in the generation of the protective humoral immune response against vesicular stomatitis virus. *Immunity* 1996;5:639–652.
22. Köhler G, Milstein C. Continuous cultures of fused cells secreting antibody of predefined specificity. *Nature* 1975;256:495–497.
23. Hamlyn PH, Browniee GG, Cheng CC, Gait MJ, Milstein C. Complete sequence of constant and 3′ noncoding regions of an immunoglobulin mRNA using the dideoxynucleotide method of RNA sequencing. *Cell* 1978;15:1067–1075.
24. Berek C, Milstein C. Mutation drift and repertoire shift in the maturation of the immune response. *Immunol Rev* 1987;96:23–41.
25. Kaartinen M, Griffiths GM, Markham AF, Milstein C. mRNA sequences define an unusually restricted IgG response to 2-phenyloxazolone and its early diversification. *Nature* 1983;304:320–324.
26. Griffiths GM, Berek C, Kaartinen M, Milstein C. Somatic mutation and the maturation of the immmune response to 2-phenyloxazolone. *Nature* 1984;312:271–275.
27. Berek C, Jarvis JM, Milstein C. Activation of memory and virgin B cell clones in hyperimmune animals. *Eur J Immunol* 1987;17:1121–1129.
28. Siekevitz M, Kocks C, Rajewsky K, Dildrop R. Analysis of somatic mutation and class switching in naive and memory B cells generating adoptive primary and secondary responses. *Cell* 1987;48:757–770.
29. Dell CL, Lu YX, Claflin JI. Molecular analysis of clonal stability and longevity in B cell memory. *J Immunol* 1989;143:3364–3370.
30. Shlomchik MJ, Marshak-Rothstein A, Wolfowicz CB, Rothstein TL, Weigert MG. The role of clonal selection and somatic mutation in autoimmunity. *Nature* 1987;328:805–811.
31. Berek C, Griffiths GM, Milstein C. Molecular events during maturation of the immune response to oxazolone. *Nature* 1985;316:412–418.
32. Foote J, Milstein C. Kinetic maturation of the immune response. *Nature* 1991;352:530–532.
33. Coico RF, Bhogal BS, Thorbecke GJ. Relationship of germinal centers in lymphoid tissue to immunologic memory. VI. Transfer of B cell memory with lymph node cells fractionated according to their receptors for peanut agglutinin. *J Immunol* 1983;131:2254–2257.
34. Rouse RV, Reichert RA, Gallatin WM, Weissman IL, Butcher EC. Localization of lymphocyte subpopulations in peripheral lymphoid organs: directed lymphocyte migration and segregation into specific microenvironments. *Am J Anat* 1984;170:391–405.
35. Nieuwenhuis P, Opstelten D. Functional anatomy of germinal centers. *Am J Anat* 1984;170:421–435.

36. MacLennan IC, Gray D. Antigen-driven selection of virgin and memory B cells. *Immunol Rev* 1986;91:61–85.

37. Jacob J, Kelsoe G, Rajewsky K, Weiss U. Intraclonal generation of antibody mutants in germinal centres. *Nature* 1991;354:389–392.

38. Ziegner M, Steinhauser G, Berek C. Development of antibody diversity in single germinal centers: selective expansion of high-affinity variants. *Eur J Immunol* 1994;24:2393–2400.

39. Berek C, Berger A, Apel M. Maturation of the immune response in germinal centers. *Cell* 1991;67:1121–1129.

40. McHeyzer-Williams MG, McLean MJ, Lalor PA, Nossal GJ. Antigen-driven B cell differentiation in vivo. *J Exp Med* 1993;178:295–307.

41. Liu AH, Jena PK, Wysocki LJ. Tracing the development of single memory-lineage B cells in a highly defined immune response. *J Exp Med* 1996;183:2053–2063.

42. Smith KGC, Light A, Nossal GJV, Tarlington DM. The extent of affinity maturation differs between memory and antibody-forming cell compartments in the primary immune response. *EMBO J* 1997;16:2996–3006.

43. Liu Y-J, Johnson GD, Gordon J, MacLennan IC. Germinal centres in T-cell–dependent antibody responses. *Immunol Today* 1992;13:17–21.

44. Nossal GJV, Ada GL. *Antigens, lymphoid cells and the immune response*. New York: Academic Press, 1971.

45. Mandel TE, Phipps RP, Abbot A, Tew JG. The follicular dendritic cell: long term antigen retention during immunity. *Immunol Rev* 1980;53:29–59.

46. Schriever F, Nadler LM. The central role of follicular dendritic cells in lymphoid tissues. *Adv Immunol* 1992;51:243–284.

47. Rademakers LHPM. Dark and light zones of germinal centres of the human tonsil: an ultrastructural study with emphasis on heterogeneity of follicular dendritic cells. *Cell Tissue Res* 1994;269:359–368.

48. MacLennan ICM. Germinal centers. *Ann Rev Immunol* 1994;12:117–139.

49. Liu Y-J, Joshua DE, Williams GT, Smith CA, Gordon J, MacLennan IC. Mechanism of antigen-driven selection in germinal centres. *Nature* 1989;342:929–931.

50. De Togni P, Goeller J, Ruddle NH, et al. Abnormal development of peripheral lymphoid organs in mice deficient in lymphotoxin. *Science* 1994;264:703–707.

51. Matsumoto M, Mariathasan S, Baranyay F, Peschon JJ, Chaplin DD. Role of lymphotoxin and the type I TNF receptor in the formation of germinal center. *Science* 1996;271:1289–1291.

52. Pasparakis M, Alexopoulou L, Episkopou V, Kollias G. Immune and inflammatory responses in TNFα-deficient mice: a critical requirement for TNFα in the formation of primary B cell follicle, follicular dendritic cell networks and germinal centres, and in the maturation of the humoral immune response. *J Exp Med* 1996;184:1397–1411.

53. Koni PA, Sacca R, Lawton P, Browning JL, Ruddle NH, Flavell RA. Distinct roles in lymphoid organogenesis for lymphotoxins α and β revealed in lymphotoxin b–deficient mice. *Immunity* 1997;6:491–500.

54. Cerny A, Zinkernagel RM, Groscurth P. Development of follicular dendritic cells in lymph nodes of B-cell–depleted mice. *Cell Tissue Res* 1988;254:449–454.

55. Yoshida K, van den Berg TK, Dijkstra CD. The functional state of follicular dendritic cells in severe combined immunodeficient (SCID) mice: role of lymphocytes. *Eur J Immunol* 1994;24:464–468.

56. Ahearn JM, Fischer MB, Croix D, et al. Disruption of the Cr2 locus results in a reduction in B-1a cells and in an impaired B cell response to T-dependent antigen. *Immunity* 1996;4:251–262.

57. Rose ML, Birbeck MC, Wallis VJ, Forrester JA, Davies AJS. Peanut lectin binding properties of germinal centres of mouse lymphoid tissue. *Nature* 1980;284:364–366.

58. Förster R, Mattis AE, Kremmer E, Wolf E, Brem G, Lipp M. A putative chemokine receptor, BLR1, directs B cell migration to defined lymphoid organs and specific anatomic compartments of the spleen. *Cell* 1996;87:1037–1047.

59. Facchetti F, Appiani C, Salvi L, Levy J, Notarangelo LD. Immunologic analysis of ineffective CD40–CD40 ligand interaction in lymphoid tissues from patients with X-linked immunodeficiency with hyper-IgM. Abortive germinal center cell reaction and severe depletion of follicular dendritic cells. *J Immunol* 1995;154:6624–6633.

60. Borriello F, Sethna MP, Boyd SD, et al. B7-1 and B7-2 have overlapping, critical roles in immunoglobulin class switching and germinal center formation. *Immunity* 1997;6:303–313.

61. Lane P, Burdet C, Hubele S, et al. B cell function in mice transgenic for mCTLA4-H gamma 1: lack of germinal centers correlated with poor affinity maturation and class switching despite normal priming of CD4+ T cells. *J Exp Med* 1994;179:819–830.

62. Kosco-Vilbois MH, Zentgraf H, Gerdes J, Bonnefoy J-Y. To B or not to B a germinal center? *Immunol Today* 1997;18:225–230.

63. Klaus GG, Humphrey JH, Kunkl A, Dongworth DW. The follicular dendritic cell: its role in antigen presentation in the generation of immunological memory. *Immunol Rev* 1980;53:3–28.

64. Szakal AK, Kosco MH, Tew JG. Microanatomy of lymphoid tissue during humoral immune responses: structure functions relationships. *Ann Rev Immunol* 1989;7:91–109.

65. Gray D, Skarvall H. B-cell memory is short-lived in the absence of antigen. *Nature* 1988;336:70–73.

66. Jacob J, Kassir R, Kelsoe G. In situ studies of the primary immune response to (4-hydroxy-3-nitrophenyl)acetyl. I. The architecture and dynamics of responding cell populations. *J Exp Med* 1991;173:1165–1175.

67. Jacob J, Kelsoe G. In situ studies of the primary immune response to (4-hydroxy-3-nitrophenyl)acetyl. II A common clonal origin for periarteriolar lymphoid sheath-associated foci and germinal centers. *J Exp Med* 1992;176:679–687.

68. Linton PJ, Decker DJ, Klinman NR. Primary antibody-forming cells and secondary B cells are generated from separate precursor cell subpopulations. *Cell* 1989;59:1049–1059.

69. Fliedner TM, Kesse M, Crokite EP, Robertson JS. Cell proliferation in germinal centers of the rat spleen. *Ann N Y Acad Sci* 1964;113:578–594.

70. Zaitoun AM. Cell population kinetics of the germinal centres of lymph nodes of BALB/c mice. *J Anat* 1980;130:131–137.

71. MacLennan IC, Johnson GD, Liu YJ, Gordon J. The heterogeneity of follicular reactions. *Res Immunol* 1991;142:253–257.

72. Apel M, Berek C. Differentiation of B cells in germinal centers. In: Imhof BA, Berrih-Aknin S, Ezine S, eds. *Lymphatic tissues and in vivo immune responses.* New York: Marcel Dekker, 1991:355–359.

73. Kroese FGM, Timens W, Nieuwenhuis P. Germinal center reaction and B lymphocytes: morphology and function. *Curr Top Pathol* 1990;84:103–100.

74. Küppers R, Zhao M, Hansmann M-L, Rajewsky K. Tracing B cell development in human germinal centers by molecular analysis of single cells picked from histological sections. *EMBO J* 1993;12:4955–4967.

75. Jacob J, Przylepa J, Miller C, Kelsoe G. In situ studies of the primary immune response to (4-hydroxy-3-nitrophenyl)acetyl. III. The kinetics of V region mutation and selection in germinal centers. *J Exp Med* 1993;178:1293–1307.

76. Pascual V, Liu YJ, Magalski A, de Bouteiller O, Banchereau J, Capra JD. Analysis of somatic mutation in five B cell subsets of human tonsil. *J Exp Med* 1994;180:329–339.

77. Weigert M. The influence of somatic mutation on the immune response. *Prog Immunol* 1986;VI:138–142.

78. Kepler TB, Perelson AS. Cyclic re-entry of germinal center B cells and the efficiency of affinity maturation. *Immunol Today* 1993;14:412–415.

79. Kauffman SA, Weinberger ED, Perelson AS. Maturation of the immune response via adaptive walks on affinity landscapes. In: Perelson AS, ed. *Theoretical immunology.* Part one: SFI studies in the sciences of complexity. Reading, MA: Addison-Wesley, 1988:349–382.

80. Bigazzi PE. Hashimoto's disease. In: Bona AC, Siminovitch KA, Zanetti M, Theophilopoulos AN, eds. *The molecular pathology of autoimmune diseases.* Chur: Harwood Academic Publishers, 1993:493–510.

81. Guigou V, Emilie D, Berrih-Aknin S, Fumoux F, Fougerau M, Schiff C. Individual germinal centres of myasthenia gravis human thymuses contain polyclonal activated B cells that express all the VH and Vκ families. *Clin Exp Immunol* 1991;83:267–266.

82. Friemark BR, Fantozzi R, Bone R, Bordin G, Fox R. Detection of clonally expanded salivary gland lymphocytes in Sjögren's syndrome. *Arthritis Rheum* 1989;32:859–869.

83. Schröder AE, Greiner A, Seyfert C, Berek C. Differentiation of B cells in the nonlymphoid tissue of the synovial membrane of patients with rheumatoid arthritis. *Proc Natl Acad Sci U S A* 1996;93:221–225.

84. Kratz A, Campos-Neto A, Hanson MS, Ruddle NH. Chronic inflammation caused by lymphotoxin is lymphoid neogenesis. *J Exp Med* 1996;183:1461–1472.

85. Maizels N. Somatic hypermutation: how many mechanisms diversify V region sequences? *Cell* 1995;83:9–12.

86. Reynaud C-A, Anquez V, Grimal H, Weill J-C. A hyperconversion mechanism generates the chicken light chain preimmune repertoire. *Cell* 1987;48:379–388.

87. McCormack WT, Thompson CB. Chicken IgL variable region gene conversions display pseudogene donor preference and 5 to 3 polarity. *Genes Dev* 1990;4:548–558.

88. Becker RS, Knight KL. Somatic diversification of immunoglobulin heavy chain VDJ genes: evidence for somatic gene conversion in rabbits. *Cell* 1990;63:987–997.

89. Klein R, Jaenichen R, Zachau HG. Expressed human immunoglobulin k genes and their hypermutation. *Eur J Immunol* 1993;23:3248–3271.

90. Manser T, Gefter ML. The molecular evolution of the immune response: idiotope-specific suppression indicates that B cells express germ-line–encoded V genes prior to antigenic stimulation. *Eur J Immunol* 1986;16:1439–1444.

91. Reynaud CA, Garcia C, Hein WR, Weill J-C. Hypermutation generating the sheep immunoglobulin repertoire is an antigen-independent process. *Cell* 1995;80:115–125.

92. Manser T. Mitogen-driven B cell proliferation and differntiationare not accompanied by hypermtation of immunoglobulin variable region genes. *J Immunol* 1987;139:234–238.

93. Maizels N, Bothwell A. The T cell independent immune response to the hapten NP uses a large repertoire of heavy chain genes. *Cell* 1985;43:715–720.

94. McKean D, Huppi K, Bell M, Staudt L, Gerhard W, Weigert M. Generation of antibody diversity in the immune response of BALB/c mice to influenza virus hemagglutinin. *Proc Natl Acad Sci U S A* 1984;81:3180–3184.

95. Gorski J, Rollini P, Mach B. Somatic mutations of immunoglobulin variable genes are restricted to the rearranged V gene. *Science* 1983;220:1179–1181.

96. Roes J, Huppi K, Rajewsky K, Sablitzky F. V gene rearrangement is required to

fully activate the hypermutation mechanism in B cells. *J Immunol* 1989;142: 1022–1026.

97. Weber JS, Berry J, Litwin S, Claflin JL. Somatic hypermutation of the JC intron is makedly reduced in unrearranged kappa and H alleles and is unevenly distributed in rearranged alleles. *J Immunol* 1991;146:3218–3226.

98. Lebecque SG, Gearhart PJ. Boundaries of somatic mutation in rearranged immunoglobulin genes: 5′ boundary is near the promotor, and 3 boundary is about 1 kb from V(D)J gene. *J Exp Med* 1990;172:1717–1727.

99. Rothenfluh HS, Taylor L, Bothwell ALM, Both GW, Steele EJ. Somatic hypermutation in 5′ flanking regions of heavy chain antibody variable regions. *Eur J Immunol* 1993;23:2152–2159.

100. Motoyama N, Miwa T, Suzuki Y, Okada H, Azuma T. Comparison of somatic mutation frequency among immunoglobulin genes. *J Exp Med* 1994;179: 395–403.

101. Wagner SD, Neuberger MS. Somatic hypermutation of immunoglobulin genes. *Ann Rev Immunol* 1996;14:441–457.

102. Azuma T, Motoyama N, Fields LE, Loh DY. Mutations of the chloramphenicol acetyl transferase transgene driven by the immunoglobulin promotor and intron enhancer. *Int Immunol* 1993;5:121–130.

103. Yelamos J, Klix N, Goyenechea B, et al. Targeting of non-Ig sequences in place of the V segment by somatic hypermutation. *Nature* 1995;376:225–229.

104. Storb U, Peters A, Klotz E, et al. *Sem Immunol* 1997;8:131–140.

105. Tumas-Brundage K, Manser T. The transcriptional promotor regulates hypermutation of the antibody heavy chain locus. *J Exp Med* 1997;185:239–250.

106. Betz AG, Rada C, Pannell R, Milstein C, Neuberger MS. Passenger transgenes reveal intrinsic specificity of the antibody hypermutation mechanism: clustering, polarity, and specific hot spots. *Proc Natl Acad Sci U S A* 1993;90: 2385–2388.

107. Hackett J Jr, Rogerson BJ, O'Brien RL, Storb U. Analysis of somatic mutations in kappa transgenes. *J Exp Med* 1990;172:131–137.

108. Dörner T, Brezinschek RI, Foster SJ, Domiati R, Lipsky PE. Analyis of the frequency and pattern of somatic mutations within nonproductively rearranged human variable heavy chain genes. *J Immunol* 1997;158:2779–2789.

109. Smith DS, Creadon G, Jena PK, Portanova JP, Kotzin BL, Wysocki LJ. Di- and trinucleotide target preferences of somatic mutagenesis in normal and autoreactive B cells. *J Immunol* 1996;156:2642–2652.

110. Goyenechea B, Milstein C. Modifying the sequence of an immunoglobulin V-gene alters the resulting pattern of hypermutation. *Proc Natl Acad Sci U S A* 1996;93:13979–13984.

111. Wagner SD, Milstein C, Neuberger MS. Codon bias targets mutation. *Nature* 1995;376:732.

112. Peters A, Storb U. Somatic hypermutation of immunoglobulin genes is linked to transcription initiation. *Immunity* 1996;4:57–65.

113. Betz AG, Milstein C, González-Fernández A, Pannel R, Larson T, Neuberger MS. Elements regulating somatic hypermutation of an immunoglobulin kappa gene: critical role for the intron enhancer/matrix attachment site. *Cell* 1994; 77:239–148.

114. Rada C, González-Fernández A, Jarvis JM, Milstein C. The 5′ boundary of somatic hypermutation in a Vκ gene is in the leader intron. *Eur J Immunol* 1994; 1453–1457.

115. Brenner S, Milstein C. Origin of antibody variation. *Nature* 1966;211:242–243.

116. Denepoux S, Razanajaona D, Blanchard D, Meffe G, Capra JD, Banchereau J. Induction of somatic mutation in a human B cell line in vitro. *Immunity* 1997; 6:35–46.

117. Flemming W. Schlussbemerkungen über die Zellvermehrung in den lymphoiden Drüsen. *Arch Mikrosk Anat* 1997;24:355.

Fundamental Immunology, Fourth Edition,
edited by William E. Paul
Published by Lippincott–Raven Publishers, Philadelphia 1999.

CHAPTER 26

Differentiation of Effector Phenotypes of CD4⁺ and CD8⁺ T Cells

Differentiation of Effector Phenotypes of CD4$^+$ and CD8$^+$ T Cells

Robert A. Seder and Timothy M. Mosmann

Role of Apoptosis in Selectively Regulating T Helper 1 and T Helper 2 Effector Cells
Differentiation of CD8 T-Cell Subsets
   Evidence for CD8 Cytokine Subsets · Cytokine Regulation of Differentiation into Tc1 or Tc2 Cells · Other Influences on CD8 Differentiation · Effector Functions of CD8 T-Cell Subsets · Further Differentiation of Tc1 CD8 T Cells
Conclusion
References

The immune system employs a highly complex mechanism designed to generate responses to protect us against a variety of foreign pathogens while at the same time preventing responses against self antigens. In addition to deciding whether to respond (antigen specificity), the immune system must also choose appropriate effector functions to deal with each pathogen (effector specificity). A cell critical in mediating and regulating these effector functions is the CD4$^+$ T cell. Furthermore, it is the elaboration of specific cytokines from CD4$^+$ T cells that appears to be the major mechanism by which they mediate their functions. Thus, characterizing the types of cytokines made by CD4$^+$ T cells as well as how their secretion is controlled is extremely important in understanding how the immune response is regulated.

The characterization of cytokine production from long-term mouse CD4$^+$ T cell clones was first published more than 10 years ago (1). In these studies, it was shown that CD4$^+$ T cells produced two distinct patterns of cytokine production, which were designated T helper 1 (Th1) and T helper 2 (Th2). Th1 cells were found to exclusively produce interleukin-2 (IL-2), interferon-γ (IFN-γ) and lymphotoxin (LT), while Th2 clones exclusively produced IL-4, IL-5, IL-6, and IL-13 (2). Somewhat later, additional cytokines, IL-9 and IL-10, were isolated from Th2 clones (3,4). Finally, additional cytokines, such as IL-3, granulocyte-macrophage colony-stimulating factor (GM-CSF), and tumor necrosis factor-α (TNF-α) were found to be secreted by both Th1 and Th2 cells (Table 1).

The observation that CD4$^+$ T cells could be segregated into distinct subsets based on the types of cytokines they produced was of great interest, because Th1 cytokines (i.e., IL-2, IFN-γ) were associated with cellular immune functions such as delayed-type hypersensitivity (5–8), while Th2 cytokines (i.e., IL-4, IL-5, IL-6, IL-10, IL-13) enhance antibody production from B cells and induce several aspects of the allergic response (6). In addition, it was soon appreciated that these specific cytokines produced from Th1 and Th2 cells (IFN-γ and IL-4, respectively) were also potent cross-inhibitors of the two cell types (9). Thus, these differences in cytokine profiles allowed for different effector functions as well as the ability to cross-regulate each other's function. In the following section, the evidence supporting the existence of Th1 and Th2 cells is discussed and a working definition that will be used as the conceptual basis for the remainder of the chapter is provided.

R. A. Seder: Clinical Immunology Section, Laboratory of Clinical Investigation, National Institute of Allergy and Infectious Diseases, National Institutes of Health, Bethesda, Maryland 20892.

T. M. Mosmann: Written in part during the tenure as Fogarty Scholar-in-Residence at the National Institutes of Health.

TABLE 1. *Expression of cytokines by CD4 T-cell subsets*

Cytokine	Th1	Th2	Th0	Thp
FN-γ	+	−	+	−
Lymphotoxin	+	−		−
IL-2	+(−)	−	+	+
IL-3	+	+	+	−
GM-CSF	+	+	+	
Tumor necrosis factor-α	+	+		
MIP-1α	+	+		
MIP-1β	+	+		
TCA-3 (I-309)	+	+		
IL-4	−	+	+	−
IL-5	−	+	+	−
IL-6	−(+)	+		
IL-9	−	+		
IL-10	−(+)	+		−
IL-13	−(+)	+		

All cytokines shown are expressed by the corresponding T-cell subset only after activation, normally through the T-cell antigen receptor.
Gaps indicate that synthesis is unknown.
Results in parenthesis indicate alternative possibilities, particularly in human cells. The synthesis of IL-6, IL-10 and IL-13 by human cells is not restricted to the Th2 subset, although Th2 cells normally synthesize higher amounts of these cytokines.

DEFINING T HELPER 1 AND T HELPER 2 PHENOTYPES

Evidence for Heterogeneity in Cytokine-producing CD4$^+$ T Cells: Are There Differences between Mouse and Human Cells?

The initial characterization of Th1 and Th2 cells from mouse CD4$^+$ T-cell clones ignited significant interest in determining whether these phenotypes extended to human cells as well as to *in vivo* immune responses. Although initial studies suggested that many human T-cell clones produced both Th1 and Th2 cytokines (10–12), it was subsequently established that human T-cell clones specific for allergens mostly showed a Th2 pattern, whereas clones specific for mycobacterial antigens secreted Th1 cytokines (13–15).

While these studies showed the existence of polarized mouse and human Th1 and Th2 cells, it is also evident that some mouse (16,17) and especially some human clones are capable of producing both IL-4 and IFN-γ. These cells have been designated Th0 cells and may be intermediates in the differentiation of Th1 or Th2 cells or end-stage cells that have their own characteristic effector functions. In addition, studies examining cytokine mRNA expression and protein production using short-term T-cell lines and clones showed that substantial heterogeneity existed with regard to cytokine production (17–19). These data have led some to speculate that at the single-cell level, there is a broad spectrum and/or continuum of cytokine profiles rather than the existence of distinct Th1 and Th2 cells (20). This is further supported by data showing that cytokine coexpression patterns are random in some panels of clones (20). However, in other sets of clones, even those made without exogenous cytokine influences during differentiation, recognizable and nonrandom Th1- and Th2-like patterns can be discerned (21). Overall, there appears little doubt that the extreme Th1 and Th2 cytokine patterns represent stable differentiated states, but it is not yet clear whether other cytokine-secretion phenotypes represent a continuum or additional discrete subsets.

Evidence for the Existence of T Helper 1 and T Helper 2 Cells at the Clonal and Population Levels

As we have highlighted above, while classification of T cells into distinct Th1 and Th2 cells may represent an oversimplification of a complex and dynamic process, it is important to note that, based on experimental *in vitro* models and *in vivo* models of infectious and autoimmune disease, substantial evidence exists supporting the fact that Th1 and Th2 cells do exist in a physiologic context at both the single-cell and population level. As there is clear-cut polarization of cytokine synthesis patterns to either Th1 or Th2 patterns during many major immune responses, it is important to describe the functions and interregulation of these major T-cell phenotypes. Other phenotypes undoubtedly exist and contribute to many responses, but their functions are not yet understood as clearly.

In Vitro Evidence that Interferon-γ and Interleukin-4–producing Cells Exist at the Population and Single-cell Levels

Once the Th1 and Th2 paradigm was established from mouse CD4+ T-cell clones, it became of great interest to develop experimental models to study the factors that regulated the differentiation of Th1 and Th2 cells. To this end, *in vitro* models of T-cell priming were developed in which naive CD4+ T cells were stimulated with polyclonal mitogen or specific antigen in short-term cultures for several days under various defined conditions and then assessed for IL-4 and IFN-γ production from supernatants following restimulation (22–25). In these studies, while it was clear that IL-4 and IFN-γ production could be segregated at the population level, there was little to no understanding of the frequency of cells producing IL-4 or IFN-γ at the single-cell level. This question was initially addressed by performing single-cell analysis of cytokine gene expression during CD4+ T-cell differentiation (26). While relatively low frequencies of IL-4– and IFN-γ–producing cells were induced following secondary stimulation, the expression of IL-4 and IFN-γ was indeed segregated, providing evidence for a dichotomous response at the single-cell level. More recently, cytokine expression was assessed using immunofluorescence to detect intracellular production of IL-4 and IFN-γ protein at the single-cell level, and IL-4 and IFN-γ were found to be expressed in separate cells (27) Following short-term stimulation of mouse T-cell receptor (TCR)/Tγ CD4+ T cells in conditions favoring IFN-γ induction, approximately 85% of the cells stained for IFN-γ, but none for IL-4 (28). By contrast, cells cultured in conditions favoring IL-4 induction had approximately 51% of the cells staining for IL-4 and none for IFN-γ. In similar types of *in vitro* priming studies, human neonatal CD4+ T cells that were repetitively stimulated with polyclonal mitogens in conditions favoring the differentiation of Th1 or

Th2 cells were found to have 32% of the cells expressing IFN-γ and 12% producing IL-4, respectively (29). Thus, these studies showed that stimulating human or mouse T cells under well-defined conditions favoring Th1 or Th2 differentiation resulted in cells producing either IFN-γ or IL-4, respectively, at both the population and single-cell levels.

In Vivo Evidence for the Existence of T Helper 1 and T Helper 2 Cells

The concept that T cells could be segregated into distinct cytokine-producing subsets that could provide different functionalities remained an interesting *in vitro* observation until it was demonstrated that Th1 and Th2 patterns of cytokine expression or production existed in defined experimental *in vivo* mouse models of infectious or autoimmune disease, or from cells of humans with various diseases. The first and perhaps best example of Th1 and Th2 cells existing *in vivo* was in an experimental model of *Leishmania major* infection. Disease susceptibility and resistance correlated with a Th2 or Th1 response, respectively (30,31). Furthermore, the striking finding that susceptible mice could be made resistant by converting the Th2 to a Th1 response further established the Th1/Th2 paradigm as being important *in vivo*. In addition to *L. major,* several other infectious pathogens elicit either a predominant Th1 or Th2 response *in vivo* (see Chapter 38). Human CD4+ T-cell clones from patients with allergic disease showed a strong bias toward Th2 cytokine production (13,14). Additional studies examining cytokine production from patients with a variety of allergic, infectious, and autoimmune diseases also showed that the cytokine profiles from many of these diseases were strongly biased toward Th1 or Th2 cytokine production (32,33). More recently, it has become appreciated that in several mouse experimental models of autoimmune diseases, Th1 responses correlate with disease severity, while Th2 responses are protective (34) (see Chapter 34). Although Th2 effector mechanisms can also cause autoimmune pathology [e.g., in experimental allergic encephalomyelitis (EAE) in the absence of Th1 cells] (35,36), most organ-specific autoimmune models studied so far appear to the Th1-mediated. However, Th2 responses may be involved in some systemic autoimmune responses (37), such as mercury-induced autoimmunity (38,39), as well as human systemic lupus erythematosus (SLE) (40) and the NZB/W (41), but not the MRL (42) mouse model of SLE.

To conclude, it seems clear from both *in vitro* and *in vivo* studies that there can exist a strong bias toward Th1 and Th2 cytokine production at the population level. Furthermore, the appearance of Th1-type and Th2-type responses is best demonstrated in well-defined *in vitro* and *in vivo* experimental conditions in which there is repetitive stimulation with a particular specific antigen or polyclonal mitogen. Thus, while there may be heterogeneity with respect to the types of cytokines produced at the single-cell level within a cell population, the net biologic outcome is often predicated on there being a predominance of either a Th1 or a Th2 response. Therefore, Th1 and Th2 refer to CD4 T cells secreting IFN-γ plus LT or IL-4 plus IL-5, respectively, whereas the terms *type 1* or *type 2 responses* (43) refer to responses that include a preponderance of Th1 or Th2 cytokines, respectively, without necessarily implying that these cytokines are produced by CD4 T cells. Thus, a type 1 response may include IFN-γ produced by CD8 cells or natural killer (NK) cells, as well as IL-12 produced by macrophages. Similarly, a type 2 response may include IL-4 produced by basophils or mast cells, or IL-10 produced by keratinocytes or macrophages.

Although IL-10 has often been used as a marker for a Th2 response, it is important to note that an additional, and perhaps the major, physiologic source for IL-10 is macrophages (44). Moreover, IL-10 and IL-4 expressions do not always correlate, as IL-10 may also be expressed during an antiinflammatory as well as a Th2 response. Finally, the fact that B cells can also produce IL-10 (45), and some CD4$^+$ T cells and clones produce both IFN-γ and IL-10, makes IL-10 a relatively nonspecific marker for Th2 responses (46–48).

Variability of Cytokine Expression Patterns according to Stimulus

Although the cytokine secretion patterns of fully differentiated Th1 or Th2 cells are relatively stable, there are conditions that can alter these patterns. Stimulation with calcium ionophore plus phorbol myristate acetate (PMA) can induce the synthesis of cytokines in addition to those secreted in response to antigen or lectin (49,50), and the cytokine pattern can be altered by antigen concentration or by cytokine signals (discussed below). Thus, caution must be used in extrapolating from the cytokine patterns induced by strong activation *in vitro* to the cytokines that may be expressed during the actual response *in vivo*.

Additional T Helper Phenotypes

In addition to defining discrete phenotypes based on Th1 and Th2 cytokine patterns, there have been many well-characterized populations of CD4$^+$ T cells producing additional cytokine patterns. In addition to the Th0 cells, described above, that account for a substantial proportion of human T-cell clones specific for certain antigens, there is a population of T cells producing IFN-γ and IL-10 but not IL-4 (27,51). Because IL-10 is a potent inhibitor of many immune functions, including IFN-γ production, this type of cell may serve to autoregulate a Th1 response. Another cell population described from CD4$^+$ T-cell lines or clones, which produces only transforming growth factor-β (TGF-β) but not IL-4 or IFN-γ, has been termed a *Th3 cell*. This type of cell has been suggested to be important in mediating immune suppression in autoimmune disease (52,53).

Cell Surface Markers Potentially Distinguishing T Helper 1 and T Helper 2 Cells

There has been intense interest in determining whether there are cell surface markers that can distinguish between differentiated Th1 and Th2 cells. Many of the early studies focused on whether differences in expression of CD45, a cell surface molecule that is altered following T-cell activation, may be such a marker (54,55). Furthermore, more recent studies have suggested that other cell surface markers, such as CD27 (56,57), CD30 (58–61), and CD31 (62), are preferentially expressed on cells producing IFN-γ or IL-4. While in some in some studies, there was a bias toward production of Th1 and Th2 type cytokines from cells expressing these surface molecules, other studies found that these markers are not specific for distinguishing Th1 and Th2 cells but rather are markers for T-cell activation or responses to cytokines. For example, CD30 expression is induced by IL-4 and inhibited by IFN-γ (63), so that

Th2, but not Th1 clones, may express CD30, whereas in a mixed population, the expression of CD30 on both cell types may depend on the cytokine balance. In addition to the aforementioned activation markers, a cell surface glycoprotein expressed on activated human CD4$^+$ T cells was cloned and given the designation of SLAM (64). While expression of SLAM does not distinguish cells producing IL-4 versus IFN-γ, engagement of SLAM enhanced the production of IFN-γ, but not IL-4 or IL-5, from CD4$^+$ T cells, even from Th2 cells. Thus, SLAM induces a selective Th1 cytokine profile upon activation.

Can Differential Expression of Cytokine or Chemokine Receptors Be Used to Distinguish between T Helper 1– and T Helper 2–type Cells?

In studies examining whether committed IL-4–producing Th2 cells were reversible (could be induced to produce IFN-γ by IL-12), it became clear that short-term *in vitro*-generated Th2 cells were resistant to the effects of IL-12 due to the failure of these cells to express a functional IL-12 Rβ2 subunit (65,66). Based on these findings, it was suggested that the IL-12 Rβ2 subunit could be used as a marker for differentiating Th1 and Th2 cells. Several reports also suggest that Th1- and Th2-type cells can be distinguished on the basis of differential expression of the IFN-γRβ chain subunit. Both mouse (67,68) and human (69) *in vitro* models demonstrated a striking decrease in the expression of IFN-γRβ chain on Th1-type cells. In contrast, Th2-type cells retained expression of this receptor subunit. Based on these studies, it was suggested that IFN-γRβ chain could be used as a marker for Th2-type cells, and that the selective expression of the IFN-γRβ chain on Th2 cells could allow IFN-γ to alter the effector function of these cells (see section on cross-regulation below). It is important to note, however, that exposure of Th2 cells to IFN-γ results in a decrease in the expression of the IFN-γRβ chain (70), and anti–IFN-γ antibodies induced IFN-γRβ expression on Th1 cells (70). These data suggest that autocrine production of IFN-γ from Th1 cells is responsible for downregulation of its own receptor and explains why there would diminished expression on Th1 but not Th2 clones. Thus, in a mixed population of cells *in vivo*, local production of IFN-γ would result in downregulation of IFN-γ receptor on all T cells, not just Th1 cells. Similarly, IL-12 Rβ2 may be expressed on more than just the Th1 cells in a mixed population, as IFN-γ induced expression of IL-12 Rβ2 on Th2 cells (65) and IFN-γ was required for IL-12 responsiveness of Th1 cells (71). Also, the presence or absence of these receptor chains may not unequivocally identify Th1 or Th2 cells, as either of them may also be expressed on other cell types, such as Th0 cells. Taken together, while these *in vitro* studies are provocative, further analysis of expression of the IL-12 Rβ2 and IFN-γRβ subunits on CD4$^+$ T cells from individuals with various diseases will be required to determine whether these are useful physiologic markers distinguishing between fully differentiated Th1 and Th2 cells taken *ex vivo*. Current information about the expression of cytokine receptor chains is summarized in Fig. 1.

The chemokine receptor CCR3, which binds the CC chemokine Eotaxin, is expressed preferentially on Th2 cells (72). Although CCR3$^+$ cells, even in a Th1-biased population, preferentially synthesized IL-4, both CCR3$^+$ and CCR3$^-$ populations could also contain some cells with a Th0 phenotype (72). Thus, as with some of the other markers described above, the Eotaxin receptor may not be an absolute marker for Th2 cells.

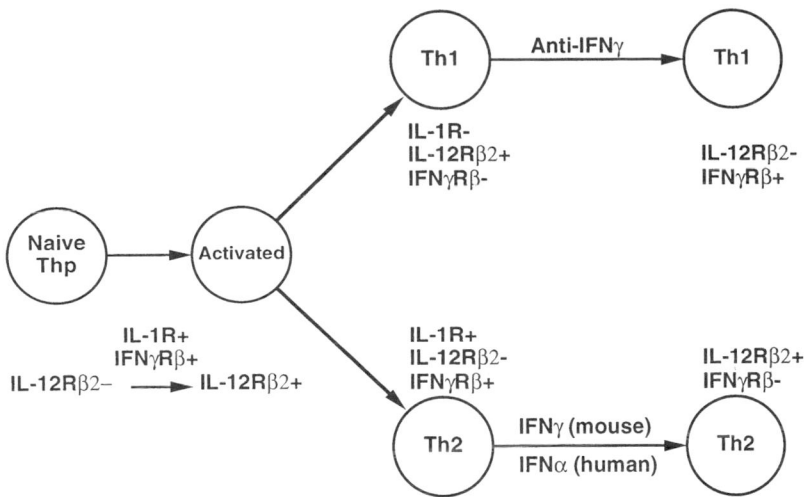

FIG. 1. Modulation of cytokine receptor expression on effector T cells before and after Th1/Th2 differentiation.

DIFFERENTIATION OF T HELPER 1 AND T HELPER 2 CELLS FROM NAIVE CD4⁺ T CELLS *IN VITRO*

T Helper 1 and T Helper 2 Cells Derive from a Common Interleukin–producing Precursor

To define the factors that regulate the differentiation of Th1 and Th2 cells, it is important to start with a homogeneous population of cells that must undergo activation to develop into cells capable of producing differentiated cytokines such as IFN-γ and IL-4 upon restimulation. To this end, small, dense lymphocytes expressing a surface phenotype of CD44^{lo}, CD62L^{hi}, CD45RB^{hi} (mouse) and CD45RA^{+} (human) that produce IL-2 but not IFN-γ or IL-4 following primary stimulation have been used in both mouse and human *in vitro* studies to study Th1 and Th2 differentiation. The TCR specificity does not appear to influence differentiation, as T cells in transgenic mice expressing a single TCR can differentiate into either Th1 or Th2 cells (25,73,74). This is confirmed by the ability of single IL-2–secreting CD4^{+} T cells, which have been referred to as precursor T helper cells (Thp), to develop into either IL-2– or IL-4–producing cells (75) or into Th1 or Th2 cells (76), depending on the conditions in which they were stimulated. These results provide strong evidence that Th1 and Th2 cells develop from a common precursor. The precursor cell may be a naive, small, resting T cell that is CD45RB^{hi}, CD62L^{hi}, CD44^{lo}, or an activated, proliferating T-cell precursor (Thpp) that is CD45RB^{lo}, CD62L^{lo}, CD44^{hi}, but for both cell types, subsequent differentiation into Th1 or Th2 subsets is regulated by similar cytokine effects (76).

Do Precursor CD4⁺ T Cells Go through an Intermediate Step in Their Differentiation toward T Helper 1 and T Helper 2 Cells?

An important but as yet unresolved question is whether IL-2–secreting precursor CD4^{+} T cells proceed by a stochastic process in their differentiation toward Th1 or Th2 cells or, alternatively, by an orderly transition through a defined intermediate cytokine-producing state. In addressing this question, studies were done using CD4^{+} T cells from transgenic mice in which a herpes virus thymidine kinase gene (HSV-TK) was placed under control of the IL-4 promotor. Activation of these CD4^{+} T cells in the presence of gancylovir (modified to a toxic product by HSV-TK) prevented the development of both IL-4– and IFN-γ–producing cells, demonstrating that effector cells producing IFN-γ or IL-4 proceed through a common pathway in which IL-4 mRNA is expressed (77). However, in a separate study using *in situ* hybridization to assess cytokine gene expression during T-cell development, it was noted that there were very few cells producing IL-4 during initial stimulation. Furthermore, these studies did not report significant numbers of cells producing both IL-4 and IFN-γ (26). Although these apparently conflicting results may be due to technical considerations, they leave open the question of whether intermediate steps in the differentiation of Th1 or Th2 cells exist.

Effector CD4⁺ T Helper Cells

Following short-term *in vitro* or *in vivo* stimulation, naive (precursor) CD4^{+} T cells develop into cells capable of producing IFN-γ or IL-4 upon restimulation. The ability of these activated CD4^{+} T cells to rapidly produce large amounts of the aforementioned cytokines is likely to have important physiologic consequences, and in this regard, these cells have been referred to as *effector* T helper cells. In contrast to naive *precursor* CD4^{+} T cells, effector cells generated following short-term *in vitro* stimulation are large, but return to a small, resting state that can be activated immediately to produce large amounts of cytokines, with a surface phenotype that is CD44^{hi}, CD62L^{lo}, CD45RB^{lo} (mouse), and CD45RO^{+} (human).

In this chapter we have predominantly used IL-4 rather than IL-5 as the cytokine representative of Th2 cells, based on the fact there has been more work done in examining the cellular, biochemical, and molecular factors regulating IL-4 production than IL-5 production. Also, IL-4 is significant in two ways for Th2 responses: It is responsible for some of the characteristic Th2 effector functions, and it is the major inducer of further differentiation of precursors into Th2 cells. Alternatively, with regard to Th1 cells, IL-2 and IFN-γ have both been used as markers for Th1 responses. However, because uncommitted precursor CD4^{+} Thp and Thpp cells, as well as differentiated Th1 cells, all produce IL-2, while some mature Th1 cells only produce IFN-γ and not IL-2, we have used IFN-γ as the specific cytokine for Th1 cells. As with IL-4, IFN-γ also enhances differentiation of cells producing more of the same cytokine. Although lymphotoxin is Th1-specific in both mice and humans, this cytokine is technically difficult to assay, as it shares bioactivities with TNF-α, and currently available ELISA reagents are not as effective as those for other cytokines. In the following section, several factors involved in the differentiation of naive CD4⁺ T cells into IFN-γ– and IL-4–producing effector cells are discussed.

CYTOKINES EFFECTING T HELPER 1 DIFFERENTIATION

At the outset of this section, while we highlight many factors involved in regulating the induction of Th1 and Th2 cells *in vitro*, it is clear that the single most important factors influencing this process are the types and amounts of cytokines present in the culture. The influences of cytokines and other soluble factors in stimulating preferential Th1 or Th2 differentiation are shown in Figs. 2 and 3.

Role of Interleukin-12 in Priming for Interferon-γ

Interleukin 12 is a heterodimeric cytokine first described as a stimulatory factor for cytotoxic lymphocyte (CTL) or NK responses (78,79). Importantly, it is a potent inducer of IFN-γ production by both NK cells (80) and T cells (81–83). Based on its ability to stimulate IFN-γ production, several investigators studied its role in the differentiation of Th1 type cells *in vitro*. In a series of mouse *in vitro* studies, the ability of both endogenous and exogenous IL-12 to direct Th1 differentiation was examined. In a seminal paper examining how endogenous production of IL-12 by antigen-presenting cells (APCs) could influence the Th1 response, it was shown that macrophages exposed to heat-killed *L. monocytogenes* (HKLM) induced Th1 development (81) and inhibited the generation of IL-4–producing cells. Furthermore, anti–IL-12 inhibited the ability of macrophages exposed to HKLM to induce IFN-γ, providing definitive proof that APCs, through their production of cytokines (IL-12), could influence the type of T helper response generated (see below). In additional studies using a similar *in vitro* priming model, it was shown that the presence of exogenous IL-12 could directly induce IFN-γ by purified CD4⁺ T cells in an accessory cell–independent manner (82,84). These studies established IL-12 as a major inducer of IFN-γ–producing Th1 cells.

In parallel studies using human CD4⁺ T cells, it was shown that the presence of IL-12 in lymphocyte bulk cultures stimulated with the allergen *Dermatophagoides pteronyssinus* group I (an antigen used to generate Th2-type cell lines) caused the outgrowth of cell lines that produced less IL-4 and more IFN-γ. In contrast, bulk cells cultured in PPD (an antigen used to generate Th1-type cell lines) in the presence of anti–IL-12 led to outgrowth of PPD-specific T-cell lines showing increased ability to produce IL-4 and clones showing a Th0 instead of a Th1 phenotype (83). In a subse-

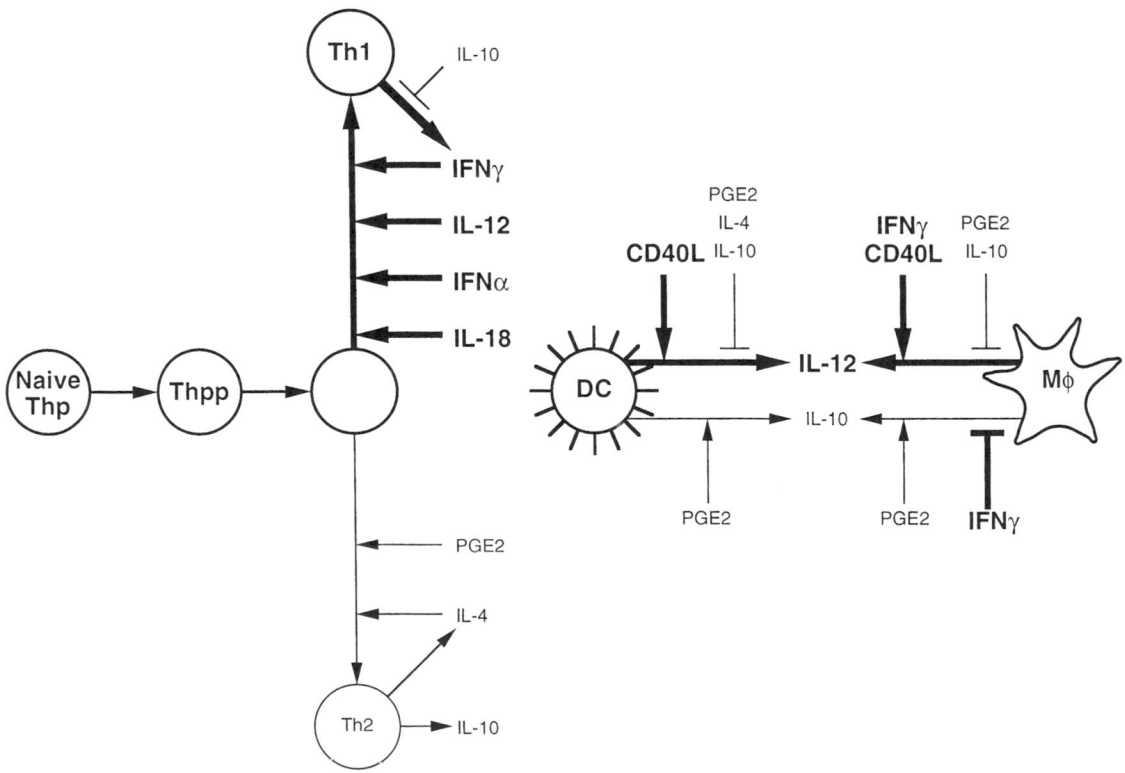

FIG. 2. Soluble factors enhancing the differentiation of Th1 cells. *Heavy arrows* represent stimulatory effects, whereas *bars* represent inhibitory or blocking effects. Several of the major known cytokine influences are shown, and the regulation of cytokine synthesis by macrophages and dendritic cells is also depicted. Although there are other APC (e.g., B cells) or cytokine sources that may influence this choice, less is known about their regulation.

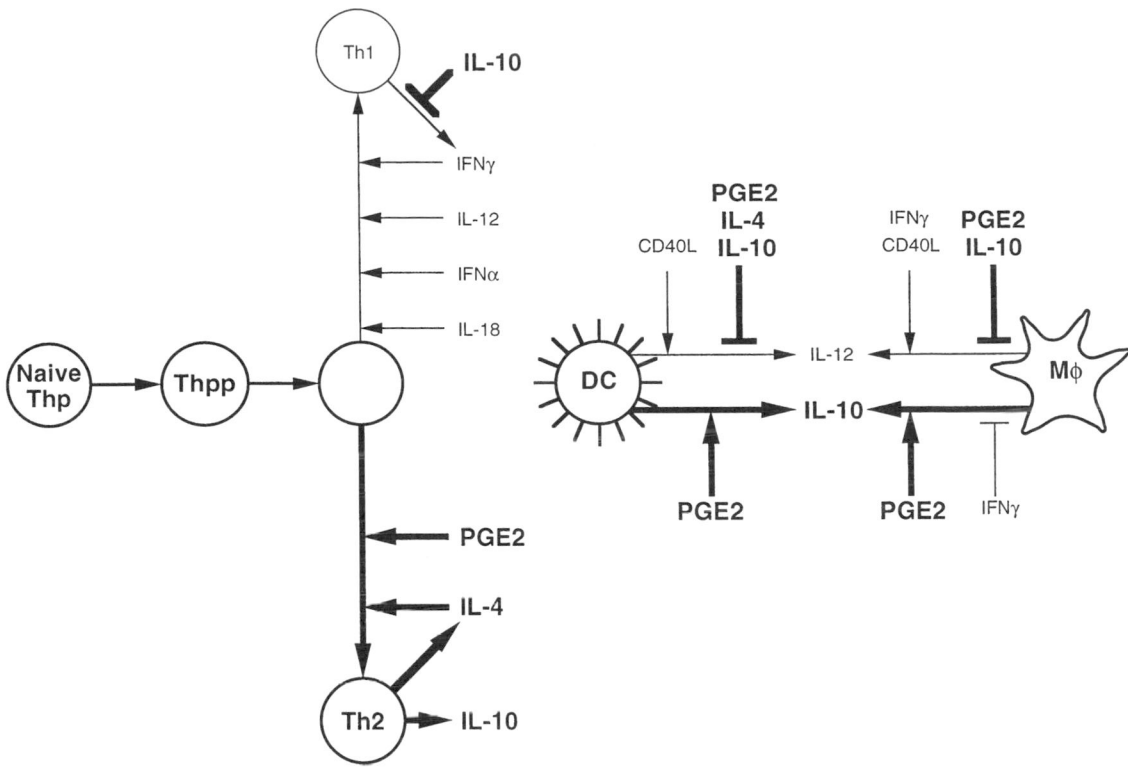

FIG. 3. Soluble factors enhancing the differentiation of Th2 cells.

quent study, IL-12 primed the clonal progenitors to differentiate into high IFN-γ–producing clones, although it did not cause suppression of IL-4–producing cells (85). Thus, similar to the effects seen in the mouse *in vitro* priming model above, the presence of IL-12 has a striking influence on the magnitude of IFN-γ production from cells stimulated with specific antigen or by polyclonal stimuli. However, the presence of IL-12 in the human priming cultures does not appear to have the clear-cut effect of generating only IFN-γ–producing Th1 cells and inhibiting IL-4–producing Th2 cells, as is seen in the mouse *in vitro* priming model (see section on reversibility of phenotypes). This point further suggests that human T cells are less easily polarized into Th1 or Th2 phenotypes than are mouse cells.

Finally, the most convincing evidence for IL-12 having a role in regulating IFN-γ responses was shown in studies using IL-12–deficient mice (86). Following *in vitro* and *in vivo* stimulation, there was a substantial (80% to 85%) but not absolute impairment in IFN-γ production. In addition, there was also a striking impairment in IFN-γ production in mice deficient in STAT4 (a protein that mediates IL-12 signaling) (87,88). Taken together, these data suggest that while IL-12 may not be absolutely essential for the development of a Th1 response, it is likely required to generate a functional Th1 response in the initiation phase of the immune response. Moreover, in some instances (i.e., autoimmune disease), IL-12 may be required to maintain a Th1 response (89,90). To conclude, the evidence to date suggests that IL-12 is the single most important physiologic factor in regulating the differentiation and magnitude of the Th1 response; however, this should not preclude the possibility that, in certain immune responses, additional factors may be found to have a compensatory role in regulating IFN-γ in the absence of IL-12.

Role of Interferon-γ in Regulating the Differentiation of T Helper 1 Cells

One of the most interesting and often confusing facets of studying the differentiation of Th1 and Th2 cells is that the factors that influence differentiation toward a specific T helper phenotype are also the factors used to define the phenotype. Thus, with regard to Th1 differentiation, the role that IFN-γ itself has on priming for IFN-γ production has been extensively studied. Initial work in both mouse and human *in vitro* models showed that the presence of IFN-γ in priming cultures resulted in the outgrowth of Th1 but not Th2 clones (91–93). It was postulated at that time that IFN-γ was differentially suppressing the proliferation of Th2 but not Th1 cells. In subsequent *in vitro* studies, the role of both endogenous and exogenous IFN-γ has been carefully examined with respect to its effect on IFN-γ induction. It seems clear from a majority of these studies that addition of exogenous IFN-γ to priming cultures does not cause a significant enhancement in IFN-γ induction following restimulation. By contrast, CD4+ T cells stimulated in an APC-independent manner (i.e., immobilized anti-CD3) in the presence of neutralizing anti-IFN-γ antibody had a striking reduction in IFN-γ following restimulation, suggesting that under these stimulatory conditions, there was a direct role for IFN-γ in regulating induction of IFN-γ (82,94,95). It should be noted, however, that under more physiologic conditions in which CD4+ T cells were stimulated with APCs and specific antigen, inhibiting endogenous IFN-γ led to a more modest (less than twofold) decrease in IFN-γ production following restimulation, compared with the APC-independent priming. Furthermore, and perhaps more importantly, the presence of anti–IFN-γ in priming cultures partially diminished (less than twofold) the ability of IL-12 to augment IFN-γ production

(94,96,97). This latter finding was consistent with evidence showing that IFN-γ leads to upregulation of the IL-12 Rβ chain subunit on mouse CD4⁺ T cells (65). Finally, it is important to note that the role of IFN-γ in regulating induction of IFN-γ appears to be restricted to naive CD4⁺ T cells defined by surface expression of CD62L (97).

To conclude, the ability of IFN-γ to augment IL-12 production from monocytes (98,99) and enhance responsivity to IL-12 by increasing the expression of the high-affinity IL-12 Rβ2 chain on mouse CD4⁺ T cells provides conclusive evidence as to its important role in regulating the magnitude of the Th1 response (94,97) *in vitro*. However, evidence from experimental models of infection in mice deficient for the IFN-γ receptor suggests that IFN-γ is not essential for the induction of a type 1 response under physiologic conditions *in vivo*. The receptor-deficient mice allow one to evaluate IFN-γ production in the absence of IFN-γ signaling through its receptor. In these experiments, IFN-γR⁻/⁻ infected with *L. major* (100), pseudorabies virus (101), or *L. monocytogenes* (102) produced similar if not greater amounts of IFN-γ than the did the wild-type controls. Thus, these results provide strong evidence that IFN-γ signaling through its own receptor was not required for IFN-γ production. Furthermore, IL-12 p40 was readily detected from spleen cells from IFN-γR⁻/⁻ mice infected with *L. monocytogenes* (102), suggesting that IL-12 was responsible for the IFN-γ induced. Taken together, these results would suggest that IFN-γ is not required for IFN-γ production *in vivo* in response to the aforementioned intracellular pathogens and that IL-12 is the major regulator of its induction.

Role of Interferon-α in Priming for Interferon-γ

IFN-α, a type I interferon, also influences IFN-γ production in a variety of experimental models. In studies in which antigen-specific T-cell clones were derived from human peripheral blood mononuclear cells (PBMCs), the presence of IFN-α in bulk cultures before cloning inhibited the development of Th2 cells and favored the development of antigen-specific Th1 clones (103,104). In additional human *in vitro* studies, addition of polyinosinic acid–polycytidylic acid (poly I:C), an inducer of IFN-α, to bulk cultures of lymphocytes stimulated with the allergen from *D. pteronyssinus* resulted in reduced ability to produce IL-4 and IL-5 and enhanced outgrowth of Th1 clones. Furthermore, the ability of poly I:C to enhance Th1-cell outgrowth was limited by the addition of antibodies against IFN-α and IL-12 to the cultures, providing additional evidence for IFN-α in the development of Th1 clones (105). In more recent studies, the presence of IFN-α in cultures led to a striking enhancement in IFN-γ production following restimulation. Interestingly, this occurred even in the presence of neutralizing antibodies to IL-12, suggesting that IFN-α directly induces IFN-γ from CD4⁺ T cells (66). In addition, it was shown in the same study that IFN-α also increased expression of the IL-12Rβ chain, leading to enhanced IL-12 responsiveness and production of IFN-γ.

The role of IFN-α and its interactions with IFN-γ and IL-12 have also been studied in a mouse *in vitro* model of Th1 development (97). In contrast to the results seen above, the addition of IFN-α *in vitro* had little effect on augmenting IFN-γ production, although there was a modest decrease in IL-4 production. Furthermore, IFN-α inhibited the production of IL-12 and IFN-γ *in vitro* and *in vivo* during viral infections in mice (106), suggesting a negative role for IFN-α in Th1 induction. However, mice injected with IFN-α or

poly I:C had a decrease in IL-4 mRNA and an increase in IFN-γ mRNA (107). These results suggest that, in mice, IFN-α may have either a positive or a negative role in Th1 differentiation. Overall, these data seem to support a more definitive role for IFN-α in regulating IFN-γ from human CD4⁺ T cells than from mouse T cells.

Role of Transforming Growth Factor-β in Priming for Interferon-γ

TGF-β can enhance the generation of Th1 cells *in vitro*. However, this cytokine has complex regulatory effects on many cell types, and it now appears that TGF-β can have both enhancing and inhibitory effects on Th1 responses. This is discussed in more detail below in the section on cross-regulation of responses.

Role of Interleukin-18 in Priming for Interferon-γ

A novel cytokine (IL-18), originally designated IFN-γ–inducing factor (IGIF), was isolated based on its ability to augment NK activity from spleen cells. In subsequent studies, IL-18 stimulated human T cells to secrete large amounts of IFN-γ (108). The effect of IL-18 may depend on IL-12, as IL-12 induces expression of the IL-18 receptor on T cells (109). This may explain the striking synergy seen in terms of IFN-γ production from cells stimulated in the presence of IL-12 and IL-18. Thus, additional studies will be needed to clarify whether IL-18 has an IL-12-independent role in regulating immune responses *in vivo*.

CYTOKINES EFFECTING T HELPER 2 DIFFERENTIATION

Role of Interleukin-4 in Priming for Mouse Interleukin-4 Production

The role of IL-4 in directing the differentiation of IL-4–producing cells from naive CD4⁺ T cells was first elucidated from mouse *in vitro* experiments in which cells were stimulated with polyclonal mitogens for several days under various conditions and then restimulated to evaluate the types of cytokines produced. In these studies, it was clearly shown that the development of Th2 cells from naive precursors is regulated by the presence of IL-4 in the priming cultures (22,24,110,111). Several additional points were noted. First, substantial amounts of IL-4 were required for the induction of IL-4–producing cells. Second, IL-4 could lead to the differentiation of IL-4–producing cells in an APC–independent manner, providing evidence for a direct effect of IL-4 on CD4⁺ T cells (24). Cells cultured in the presence of IL-4 for as little as 2 days produced IL-4 upon restimulation, suggesting that the differentiation of IL-4–producing cells can occur relatively soon after antigen stimulation. Finally, similar studies were done, using CD4⁺ T cells from TCR/transgenic mice specific for a particular antigen, such as cytochrome C or ovalbumin. These systems provided a more physiologic model than did the priming experiments highlighted above, in which polyclonal mitogens were used to stimulate T cells. In addition, it allowed one to vary the type of APC and the amount of antigen to see if they also had an effect on the differentiation of IL-4–producing cells (see below). Similar to the findings discussed above, the presence of IL-4 in priming cultures directed the development of IL-4–producing cells regardless of the type of APC used in the priming culture (23,25).

The most definitive evidence for IL-4 having a role in regulating IL-4 production was shown using IL-4, STAT 6-, or IL-4Rα–deficient mice. Experiments in IL-4–deficient mice showed that IgG1 and IgE production were markedly diminished following infection with *N. brasiliensis,* a nematode shown to cause IL-4–dependent elevations in IgE production from wild-type mice (112). Levels of the Th2 cytokines IL-5 and IL-9 were also reduced (113). In addition, mice deficient in IL-4Rα or STAT6 (a protein that is critical for IL-4 signaling) showed a striking impairment in IL-4 production in response to *N. brasiliensis* (114–117). Thus, these *in vivo* findings substantiated the *in vitro* results discussed above in establishing IL-4 as the major regulator of IL-4 production from naive CD4+ T cells. Furthermore, the finding that the inducer (IL-4) for IL-4 differentiation is the same molecule as the ultimate effector cytokine raises the question as to the initial source of IL-4 that drives the response. This is discussed in a separate section below

Role of Interleukin-4 in Priming for Human Interleukin-4 Production

The ability of IL-4 to influence the differentiation of human CD4+ T cells has also been extensively studied. In the initial studies examining the role of IL-4 in Th2 differentiation, bulk PBMCs were first stimulated *in vitro* with antigens that were likely to bias toward a Th1 or Th2 cytokine profile and then restimulated with polyclonal mitogens to elicit IL-4 or IFN-γ production. In these studies, bulk PBMCS stimulated with a Th1-inducing antigen such as PPD developed into PPD-specific T-cell lines and clones producing IFN-γ but little IL-4; however, bulk cultures stimulated with PPD in the presence of IL-4 resulted in the development of PPD-specific T-cell lines and clones producing not only IFN-γ, but also IL-4 and IL-5. On the other hand, bulk PBMCS stimulated with IL-4 and a Th2-inducing antigen such as the allergen Der P 1 developed into Der p 1–specific T-cell lines and clones producing IL-4 and IL-5 but little IFN-γ. The presence of anti–IL-4 in priming cultures markedly inhibited the development of Der p I-specific T cells into IL-4–producing T-cell lines (93). In follow-up studies evaluating the *in vitro* maturation of human neonatal CD4+ T cells, the presence of IL-4 in cultures stimulated with immobilized anti-CD3 resulted in enhanced production of IL-4 and IL-5 and a decrease in IFN-γ following restimulation. These results were consistent with the previous report showing that IL-4 can induce T cells in bulk culture toward a relative but not absolute Th2 phenotype (118).

Thus, while these results support a major role for IL-4 in regulating the differentiation of human Th2 cells, as noted in the introductory section, the ability of cytokines to influence the differentiation (frequency) of human CD4+ T cells into Th2-type cells appears less polarized as compared with short-term mouse Th1 and Th2 lines.

Role of Interleukin-2 in Priming for Interleukin-4 Production

In addition to the prominent role that IL-4 plays on the differentiation of Th2-producing cells *in vitro*, IL-2 is also required in the *in vitro* cultures (24,119). IL-2 was not simply required to maintain cell viability and cell proliferation in these cultures, because the presence of IL-4 in priming cultures was able to maintain cell viability even if endogenous IL-2 were neutralized. Additional *in vivo*

evidence supporting a role for IL-2 in IL-4 priming was shown in an experimental model of mouse leishmaniasis, in which a susceptible strain of animals that normally produce IL-4 in response to infection was made resistant if they were treated with anti–IL-2 at the time of infection (120). This correlated with a decrease in IL-4 production.

While IL-2 appears to be important in Th2 differentiation *in vitro*, there is also strong evidence to suggest that IL-2 is not absolutely essential for *in vivo* production of IL-4. This is supported by the finding that both IL-2−/− and IL-2 Rβ-chain−/− mice had higher serum levels of IgG1 and IgE, suggesting that IL-4 was produced. It is interesting to note, however, that these mice develop a severe colitis if kept in a non–germ-free environment, which has been correlated with enhanced production of IFN-γ at the site of disease (121,122), suggesting that both Th1 and Th2 responses may be increased and that the IL-2−/− mouse represents lack of regulation rather than a bias in either the Th1 or Th2 direction. Moreover, thymocytes from IL-2−/− mice produce substantially less IL-4 in response to *in vivo* immunization with TNP-KLH compared with similarly stimulated cells from IL-2−/− wild-type mice (123). These results are all consistent with a model in which IL-2 amplifies T-cell responses in general, and IL-4 production can be augmented or suppressed, depending on whether a Th1 or a Th2 response is dominant.

Role of Interleukin-6 in Priming for Intreleukin-4 Production

It has been reported that the presence of IL-6 in priming cultures supported the induction of IL-4–producing cells in a mouse *in vitro* culture system (124). Importantly, the ability of IL-6 to enhance the differentiation of IL-4–producing cells was inhibited if neutralizing antibodies against IL-4 were added into the priming cultures. These results suggest that IL-6 can rapidly induce enough endogenous IL-4 to lead to Th2 differentiation and further underscores the importance of IL-4 in regulating this process. Finally, since IL-6 is produced from various APCs, it provides a potential mechanism for APCs to control the differentiation of Th2 cells. Further studies examining the role of IL-6 in mediating *in vivo* Th2 responses should provide insight into whether this molecule has a physiologic role in IL-4 induction.

Role of Interleukin-1 in Priming for Interleukin-4 Production

IL-1 was initially shown to be important in maintaining the proliferative capacity of established mouse Th2 but not Th1 clones (91,125,126). This observation raised the issue of whether IL-1 was involved in regulating the differentiation of IL-4-producing cells, but addition of exogenous IL-1 or inhibition of endogenous IL-1 did not alter priming for IL-4 production in an *in vitro* mouse model (25,127).

In contrast, IL-1 does appear to have a role in regulating IL-4 induction from naive human CD4+ T cells. This was first shown in experiments in which the presence of an IL-1 inhibitor in bulk cultures stimulated with an allergen (Der.p.I) led to antigen-specific CD4+ T-cell clones showing a Th0/Th1-like phenotype rather than a Th0/Th2 phenotype (128). In a separate study, evaluating the requirements for IL-4 induction from naive human CD4+ T cells *in vitro*, cells stimulated with immobilized anti-CD3 in the presence of exogenous IL-1β and anti-CD28 showed enhanced production of IL-4 following secondary stimulation. This result was particularly striking, in that the induction of IL-4 in secondary cultures was not inhibited by the presence of anti–IL-4 in the primary cultures. Thus, these results suggest that in an APC-independent priming system, IL-1b and anti-CD28 in priming cultures can lead to an enhancement of IL-4–producing cells in an IL-4–independent manner (129). One caveat to these studies is that the regulation of IL-4 might be different using immobilized anti-CD3 as a stimulus rather than activation occurring through antigen presented by an APC.

COSTIMULATORY MOLECULES

In addition to cytokines, another influence on T helper cell differentiation is the interaction of costimulatory molecules on the surface of APCs with their cognate receptors on T cells. The most well-studied costimulatory interactions mediating T-cell activation and differentiation are the B7/CD28 and CD40/CD40L costimulatory pathways. Although the role of CD40/CD40L interactions in regulating Th1 responses is fairly clear, the role of B7/CD28 costimulation in regulating Th1 and Th2 differentiation is complex and not fully resolved. In this section, the mechanisms by which these costimulatory pathways affect T helper cell differentiation are reviewed.

Role of B7/CD28 Costimulation in Regulating T Helper 1 and T Helper 2 Responses

The B7/CD28 costimulatory pathway plays an integral part in the initial activation of naive T cells, preventing cells from becoming nonresponsive or anergic (130). Due to the importance of this interaction in T-cell activation, the role of B7/CD28 costimulation in regulating T helper cell differentiation has been an area of intense investigation. The studies examining how B7/CD28 costimulation affected T helper cell development were somewhat complicated by the fact that there existed at least two different B7 molecules (B7-1 and B-2) on APC that were each capable of interacting with two counterreceptors on T cells: CD28, which is constitutively expressed and delivers an activating signal; and CTLA4, which is expressed on activation and delivers an inhibitory signal (131). Furthermore, expression of B7-1 and B7-2 can vary greatly, depending on the type and state of activation of the particular APC (132,133). Thus, these data presented the possibility that these distinct costimulatory molecules (B7-1, B7-2) have a role in qualitatively and/or quantitatively altering specific cytokine production from CD4$^+$ T cells. The following sections discuss potential mechanisms by which the B7/CD28 costimulatory pathway may affect CD4$^+$ T helper cell differentiation.

Direct Effects of B7-1 and B7-2 in Differentially Regulating T Helper 1 and T Helper 2 Differentiation

The first evidence that B7-1 and B7-2 can differentially affect the types of cytokines produced from CD4$^+$ T cells was shown in an experimental mouse model of EAE. In this study, it was suggested that B7-1 and B7-2 costimulation enhanced the production of IFN-γ and IL-4, respectively (134). The idea that B7-2 may have a more selective role in IL-4 induction was further substantiated by

in vitro studies using human CD4$^+$ T cells, showing that stimulation with B7-2 but not B7-1 transfected fibroblasts led to induction of IL-4 (135,136). However, additional mouse (137) and human (138) in vitro studies showed that both B7-1 and B7-2 transfectants were able to stimulate IFN-γ and IL-4 from previously activated CD4$^+$ T cells, while neither B7-1 nor B7-2 transfectants could elicit IL-4 production from highly purified naive CD4$^+$ T cells. In more recent mouse in vitro (139) and in vivo studies (140), it was noted that neither B7-1 nor B7-2 had an obligatory or selective role in eliciting production of IL-4 or IFN-γ. Thus, since at present there is no clear biochemical evidence showing that B7-1 and B7-2 deliver qualitatively different signals to CD4$^+$ T cells, causing them to differentiate preferentially toward a Th1 or Th2 phenotype evidence (141), it is possible that the effects of B7-1 and B7-2 in differentially regulating IFN-γ and IL-4 production are related to the timing of costimulation.

Temporal Expression of B7-1 and B7-2 May Play a Role in Regulating Cytokine Production from CD4$^+$ T Cells

The timing with which B7-1 and B7-2 appear on APCs in the course of an immune response may play an important role in regulating IFN-γ and IL-4 induction, both at the initiation of a response and after a response is established. At the initiation of a response, B7-2 is expressed at higher levels than B7-1 on certain APCs, such as dendritic cells (133). Consistent with the idea that CD28 stimulation may be more important in inducing IL-4 than IFN-γ, blocking B7-2 at the initiation of a response diminishes IL-4 induction (134,142), and inhibiting both B7.1 and B7.2 using CTLA-4Ig reduced Th2 cytokine induction but maintained the Th1 response (143–145). These data all substantiate the importance of activation as a mechanism for controlling Th2 cytokine production at the initiation of a response. It is important to note that once CD4$^+$ T cells are activated, the requirements for CD28/B7 costimulation in regulating IL-4 and IFN-γ production may be different. Both in vitro (146,147) and in vivo (148) differentiated mouse Th1 cells continued to require B7 for activation, whereas Th2 cells were able to respond in the absence of B7. Thus anti–B7-2 may block Th2 responses because early B7-2 expression matches the early costimulation requirement of Th2 differentiation, whereas anti–B7-1 may inhibit Th1 responses because the later expression of B7-1 matches the continued requirement of differentiated Th1 cells for costimulation. These possibilities are diagrammed in Fig. 4.

Strength of Costimulation

Regardless of possible differential effects of B7-1 or B7-2, the B7/CD28 costimulatory pathway may regulate the differentiation of Th1 and Th2 cells by affecting the intensity of CD4$^+$ T-cell activation (149,150). For example, under relatively low T cell–stimulatory conditions, IFN-γ production can be induced, and at higher levels of stimulation, IL-4 is induced. This concept is supported by both mouse (137) and human (151–153) in vitro studies showing that repetitive stimulation of CD4$^+$ T cells with B7-transfected cells or through direct CD28 stimulation was required to induce or increase production of IL-4 (154). Additional direct evidence that CD28 stimulation has a role in IL-4 production was suggested by the finding that CD28-deficient mice bred onto NOD mice were relatively deficient in their in vitro production of IL-4 (155). It

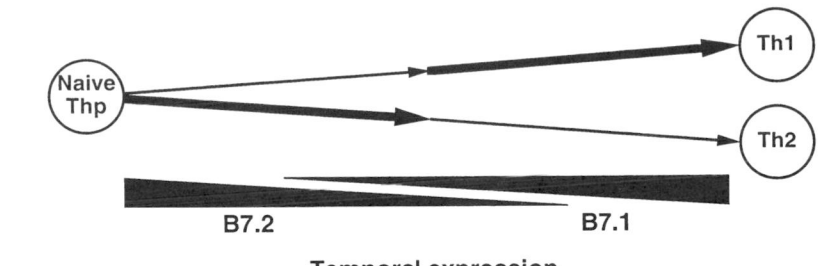

Temporal expression

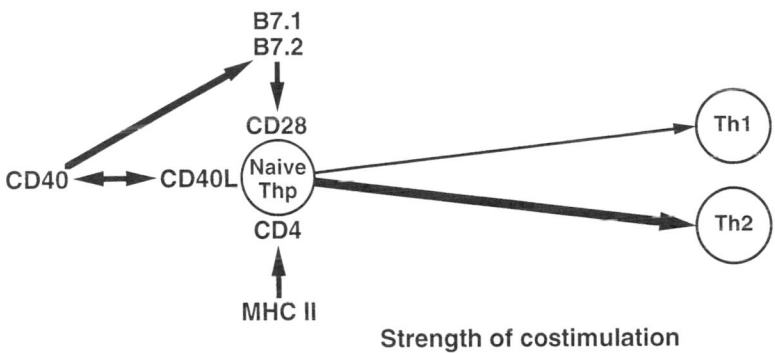

Strength of costimulation

FIG. 4. Possible effects of costimulation on Th1 and Th2 differentiation. Two potential effects of different costimulators on the Th1/Th2 choice are shown. First, the earlier and later expression of B7.2 and B7.1, respectively, may coincide with the earlier and later requirements for CD28 costimulation during Th2 and Th1 differentiation. Second, Th2 differentiation may be enhanced by the overall strength of costimulation through CD40L, CD28, and CD4.

should be noted, however, that there are also data showing that B7/CD28 costimulation may not be essential for IL-4 production. This is supported by *in vitro* studies showing that IL-4 production is readily induced from CD4$^+$ T cells in the absence of B7/CD28 costimulation, provided IL-2 is present (119,156). Moreover, the demonstration that CD28-deficient mice infected with *H. polygyrus* maintained their Th2 profile (157), coupled with the fact that these mice, bred on resistant and susceptible genetic backgrounds, maintained their respective IFN-γ- and IL-4-producing phenotypes In response to infection with *L. major*, demonstrates that both IFN-γ and IL-4 production can be achieved *in vivo* in the absence of CD28 costimulation (158). Taken together, these data suggest that the CD28/B7 dependence of Th2 cytokine induction is not absolute and can vary depending on the type of immune stimulation. Thus, for rapidly dividing infectious pathogens (i.e., *H. polygyrus, L. major*), there may be sufficient stimulation to obviate the need for CD28 stimulation in eliciting IL-4 production. Alternatively, for protein or autoantigens (i.e., NOD), CD28 stimulation may be required to provide a threshold of activation to elicit IL-4 production. These latter examples support the concept that the level of stimulation achieved through the CD28 costimulatory pathway may be able to influence the type of response generated and that IL-4 production may be more dependent on there being a greater degree of T-cell activation.

The association of stronger costimulation with IL-4 responses contrasts with the ability of higher concentrations of antigen to mostly induce Th1 responses, whereas lower doses induce Th2 responses (see below). This suggests that Th1 or Th2 differentiation may be influenced quite differently by the strength of signals through the CD3/TCR complex versus signals delivered through costimulators and their associated enzymes.

To summarize, the ability of B7-1 and B7-2 to regulate T helper responses is most likely due to the strength and/or timing of costimulation imposed by B7-1 and/or B7-2 on the CD4$^+$ T cells. Additional factors, such as the cytokine milieu, the influence of additional costimulatory interactions (CD40L/CD40; see below), and the nature of the antigenic stimulus (i.e., infectious versus autoantigen) at the time of initial T-cell activation, may also contribute to the ability of B7 costimulation to regulate Th1 or Th2 responses.

Role of CD40L/CD40 in Regulating T Helper 1 and T Helper 2 Responses

The CD40-ligand (CD40L)/CD40 costimulatory pathway is also a central regulator of the immune response. Initial work showed CD40L/CD40 stimulation to be important in B-cell activation and isotype switching (159,160). More recently, it has become evident that this pathway is also critical in regulating CD4$^+$ T cell–proliferative and cytokine responses (e.g., IL-4 and IFN-γ) (161–163). The mechanism by which CD40L/CD40 costimulation regulates the aforementioned responses has been shown to be through its ability to enhance expression of various costimulatory ligands, such as B7 (164,165). In addition, *in vitro* studies showing that CD40L/CD40 interaction induced a striking increase in the production of IL-12 from both monocytes and dendritic cells suggested that this interaction would have an important influence on Th1 differentiation (166–168). This latter mechanism was supported by *in vivo* studies showing that when CD40L$^{-/-}$ mice of a normally resistant strain were infected with *L. major*, they were markedly deficient in production of both IFN-γ and IL-12 (169,170). Thus the CD40L/CD40 costimulatory pathway appears to have an important indirect role in regulating CD4+ T cell–dependent Th1 responses, through B7/CD28 costimulation and/or IL-12 induction.

Role of Signaling through CD4 in Regulating T Helper 1 and T Helper 2 Responses

CD4 is thought to have two roles in T-cell activation: First, CD4 binds to the TCR–major histocompatibility (MHC) class II complex and increases the strength of binding; and second, the cytoplasmic tail of CD4 is associated with the protein kinase p56lck, resulting in signaling through CD4 (171,172). These functions of CD4 appear to be more important for Th2 differentiation, as blocking the CD4/MHC class II interaction with an MHC peptide induced a bias towards IFN-γ responses in vitro (173), and CD4-deficient mice were able to mount Th1 but not Th2 responses against protein or parasite antigens (174,175). A tailless CD4 mutant restored some but not all Th2 responses (175), suggesting that both adhesion and signaling properties of CD4 might contribute to the Th2 differentiation pathway.

ANTIGEN DOSE

The amount of antigen can strongly influence the type of effector functions induced during an immune response. Early work on immunization of rats with flagellin indicated that low doses gave better priming for subsequent delayed-type hypersensitivity (DTH) reactions, whereas high antigen doses primed for antibody production, and very high doses again primed for DTH (176). As the DTH and antibody responses are often due to polarization of cytokine production into Th1 or Th2 patterns, respectively, there have been a number of studies testing the effects of antigen dose on the polarization of cytokine responses.

Antigen Dose Effects during Polyclonal Responses to Proteins or Peptides

In vivo and in vitro mouse responses against human collagen type II show a clear dichotomy, depending on the MHC of the responding mouse: H2s mice mount a Th1-like DTH response, whereas H2b mice produce antibodies and Th2 cytokines (177). This correlates with the ability of I-As to bind the dominant collagen peptide with higher affinity, in contrast to the weaker binding of this peptide to I-Ab. High-affinity binding correlates with increased numbers of peptide–MHC complexes on the APC (178). Thus, high ligand density may preferentially induce Th1 responses, and this was supported by the induction of Th1 responses in H2b cells by higher peptide doses in vitro. Similar results were obtained using variants of the collagen peptide: One that bound more weakly to I-As induced Th2 responses, whereas one that bound more tightly to I-Ab induced a Th1 response (179). Also, in another peptide antigen system (180), immunization with a high-affinity peptide in vivo induced a Th1 response, whereas a low-affinity peptide induced a Th2 response at lower doses and a Th1 response at higher doses.

Antigen Dose Effects with Defined T-Cell Receptors

TCR-transgenic mice, recognizing a defined peptide antigen, have provided further evidence for the role of antigen dose in the choice between Th1 and Th2 differentiation. High doses of antigen peptide induced in vitro Th1 differentiation of naive T cells recognizing a moth cytochrome-c peptide, whereas low doses induced a Th2 response (181). However, in a similar study, which used a TCR transgene recognizing an ovalbumin peptide, very low, moderate, and very high doses of antigen induced Th2, Th1, and Th2 responses, respectively (182). Although it is difficult to compare concentrations of different TCRs and peptides because of the different affinities of the peptides for MHC and the TCRs, it is possible to reconcile these results if it is assumed that the very low and moderate doses in one study (182) correspond to the low and high doses in the other study (181). However, these results show that the effects of antigen dose may be more complex than a single dose-dependent switch.

It is also possible that some of the effects of different peptides may be due to qualitatively, rather than quantitatively different signals induced by different peptides. A wild-type peptide of moth cytochrome-c primed only for Th1 differentiation, whereas a peptide with reduced binding to the TCR but normal affinity for MHC primed differentiation of both IL-4 and IFN-γ–producing T cells at all doses tested (183). The altered peptide may actually have primed only Th2 differentiation at all doses, as some uncommitted precursor cells would be expected to have persisted after the 4-day primary culture, and the wild-type peptide may have induced these to differentiate into Th1 cells during the secondary stimulation (183). The low-affinity peptide may have functioned as a partial agonist, which could not induce high levels of signaling, even at saturating concentrations, and hence induced only Th2 differentiation (184).

The alteration of these differentiation pathways by antigen dose can be overcome by cytokine manipulation (182,183), suggesting that cytokine effects are dominant or that antigen dose effects are mediated via altered cytokine production.

In Vivo Effects of Pathogen Dose

The effects of pathogen dose in vivo are difficult to reconcile with the results obtained with soluble antigens or peptides, either in vitro or in vivo. BALB/c mice are normally susceptible to L. major infection because they mount a strong Th2 response. A healing, Th1 response can be induced by manipulating cytokine levels (30) or by reducing the number of parasites in the inoculum (185). In another infectious disease model, with opposite cytokine requirements, Trichuris infection in Balb/K mice is normally resolved by a strong Th2 response, but inoculation of low numbers of Trichuris eggs results in a Th1-biased response and parasite persistence (186). Thus, in both of these infectious models, high and low antigen levels induce Th2 and Th1 responses, respectively.

Although the in vivo results may be explained by assuming that low and high doses of infecting organisms in vivo correspond to moderate and very high doses in vitro (182), altering the dose of an infectious agent would be expected to have a very different effect from altering the dose of a peptide or soluble protein antigen (Fig. 5). Low numbers of infecting organisms would reduce the number of foci of infection, but each APC, particularly in the case of Leishmania-infected macrophages, might still present large amounts of antigen peptides. Thus at low infective doses, T cells would be stimulated by rare APCs with high antigen levels, which may give very different results from the stimulation that would occur in low-dose peptide experiments (i.e., frequent APCs with low peptide levels). The influence of a low infective dose may be analogous to the effect of depleting CD4 T cells during Leishmania infection in

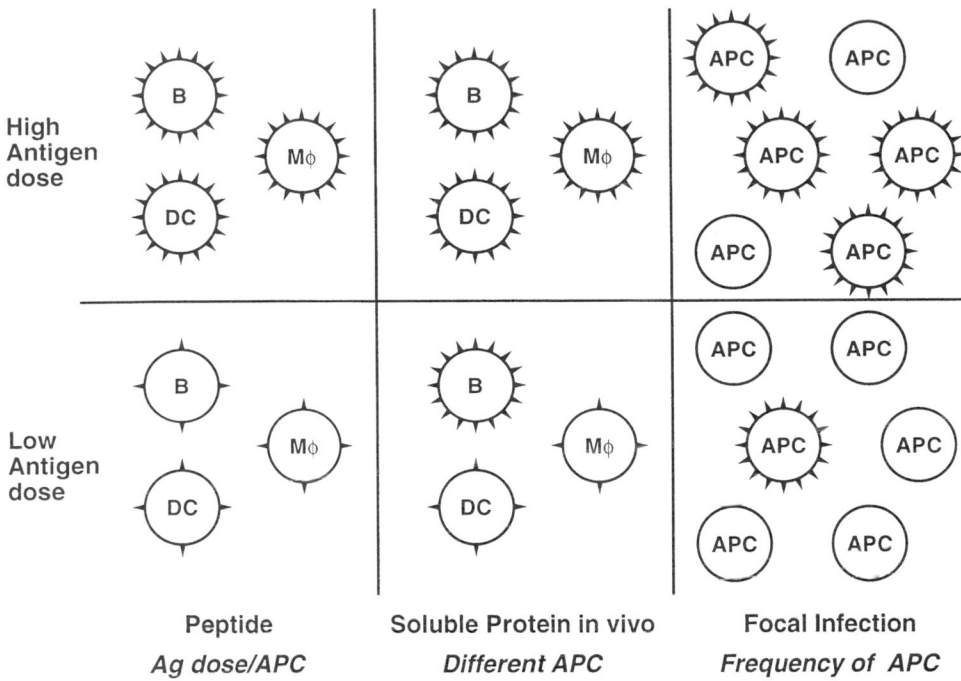

FIG. 5. Three ways in which high or low antigen doses may be presented to T cells. Peptides *in vivo* and *in vitro* may bind uniformly to APCs, so the main difference between high or low doses will be the peptide amount per APC. Soluble proteins may be captured preferentially by antigen-specific B cells at low antigen concentrations, but by all APCs at higher concentrations. During infection, particularly by intracellular parasites, APCs may be less frequent and/or localized to particular locations, but each APC may still present high amounts of antigen.

susceptible BALB/c mice (187). This manipulation decreases the number of responding T cells and results in a switch to a Th1 response and disease resistance.

An additional caution is that similar results *in vitro* and *in vivo* may not be due to the same mechanisms. *In vitro* results, in simple systems with nonreplicating APCs, may be due to the effect of ligand density, whereas *in vivo*, different antigen doses may be presented by different APCs (see Fig. 5). For example, low amounts of protein may be preferentially captured, processed, and presented by antigen-specific B cells, which will proliferate during the early stages of the response. Although B cells can support Th1 differentiation at high ligand densities (188), they can preferentially induce Th2 responses *in vitro* and *in vivo* (see below). Thus, the induction of Th2 responses at low protein or peptide doses *in vivo* could be due either to preferential presentation by B cells or to ligand density effects as observed *in vitro*.

A further possibility to explain the effects of antigen dose *in vivo* is that APCs such as dendritic cells or macrophages may express different cytokines or accessory molecules, depending on the intensity of the infection. The inherent ability of APCs to produce cytokines can drastically affect the nature of the response, and the balance of IL-12 and IL-10 produced by APCs could conceivably be affected by different levels of infection.

Effects of Antigen Dose on Effector T Cells

Different antigen doses also affect the functions of fully differentiated effector T cells. Although Th2 cells can be fully activated by a wide range of antigen concentrations, Th1 cells are activated by intermediate concentrations, but not by high concentrations (189). Similarly, transfer of Th1 or Th2 clones showed that high antigen doses favored expression of Th2 helper functions, whereas low antigen doses were more effective at inducing Th1 helper functions (190). Even the cytokines produced by the T cells can vary according to the dose of antigen: Allergen-specific human T-cell clones produced IL4 at low antigen concentrations, but both IL4 and IFN-γ at higher antigen concentrations (191). In a similar study, allergen-specific peripheral blood cells produced more IL-4 when stimulated by low doses of antigen, particularly on B cells, and less IL-4 when stimulated by high doses, particularly on monocytes (192).

Overall, the antigen dose clearly can have strong effects on the type of response obtained. Depending on the experimental system, these effects can be in opposite directions, suggesting that more than one mechanism is involved. As discussed above for costimulators such as B7, the effects of antigen dose may be related to other effects, such as the identity of initial APC, the duration of antigen persistence, and the potential expansion of the antigen-specific B-cell population.

T-CELL REPERTOIRE

Different antigens often induce characteristic Th1 or Th2 responses; for example, allergens normally induce Th2 responses, and mycobacterial antigens induce Th1 responses. There has been considerable interest in the relationship between the TCR specificity and the cytokine phenotype of T cells. In general, it appears that these two properties are not directly related, although unusual

T-cell populations with restricted TCR specificities have been identified as an early source of IL-4 in some systems (discussed below).

In several antigen systems, the same epitope of an antigen can induce either Th1 or Th2 responses (193–198). Mouse Th1 and Th2 cells recognizing *L. major* can recognize the same epitope and use very similar TCR α and β genes (74). Further evidence, suggesting that TCR specificity is unlinked to cytokine-secretion phenotype, is provided by the ability of TCR-transgenic T cells, expressing a single TCR, to differentiate into either Th1 or Th2 cells, depending on their cytokine environment during differentiation (23,25). Finally, individual naive CD4 precursor cells can differentiate into either Th1 or Th2 phenotypes (75,76). Thus, an individual naive T cell, already committed to TCR expression and hence antigen specificity, is still uncommitted with regard to cytokine-secretion phenotype.

However, there is also evidence for the preferential induction of either Th1 or Th2 responses by particular antigens or epitopes (199–201). This is unlikely to be due to a direct linkage between TCR specificity and cytokine patterns, but may be due to one or more of the following: The physical nature of the antigen (even a peptide) may direct antigen processing to a particular location or APC type; certain antigens may have adjuvant properties that nonspecifically stimulate particular APCs; the antigens may have different half-lives, resulting in different kinetics of stimulation; or the antigen or peptide may cross-react with an antigen that previously induced a polarized response, resulting in reactivation of a particular cytokine pattern that can influence the new response.

Overall, the data are consistent with a model in which naive T cells are bipotential or multipotential; that is, the specificity of the TCR does not directly determine subsequent differentiation into Th1, Th2, or other phenotypes.

ROLE OF ANTIGEN-PRESENTING CELLS IN THE DIFFERENTIATION OF T HELPER 1 AND T HELPER 2 CELLS

APCs, by their ability to present antigen in the context of MHC class II, have a major influence in the generation of antigen-specific CD4+ T-cell responses. It is widely appreciated that there is a hierarchy in the ability of different APCs to stimulate primary immune responses. In this regard, there is a general consensus that dendritic cells are the most potent APC on a per-cell basis for stimulating primary T-cell activation, although macrophages and activated B cells may also be sufficient for primary T-cell activation (202). While many of the different effects that APCs exert are through the expression of various costimulatory molecules, it is now clear that APCs are also potent producers of immunoregulatory cytokines that can influence the type of T helper response generated. This section will focus on how differential production of cytokines and expression of costimulatory molecules from APCs can influence the generation of Th1- and Th2-type cells.

Dendritic Cells

In experimental models of mouse *in vitro* priming, it was initially shown that dendritic cells elicited substantial production of either IFN-γ or IL-4 from naive CD4+ T cells, depending on the absence or presence of IL-4 in the priming culture, respectively (25). Subsequent work showing that IL-12 could be produced by dendritic cells (203,204) in response to CD40L/CD0 costimulation

(166–168,205) provided a mechanism by which dendritic cells themselves could lead to enhanced priming for IFN-γ specifically. While these latter data would suggest that antigen presentation by dendritic cells would bias toward Th1 responses, it has been shown *in vivo* that dendritic cells may also induce Th2-type responses (206). The ability of dendritic cells to enhance IL-4 production may be due to the cytokine milieu that might be present at the time a dendritic cell may interact with a naive CD4+ T cell. As noted above, if sufficient IL-4 is present at the time of initial stimulation, then dendritic cells induce substantial production of IL-4. Moreover, since IL-10 has been shown to inhibit dendritic cell stimulation of IFN-γ production by Th1 cells (207), probably by inhibiting production of IL-12 (208), it is possible that the presence of IL-10 at the time of initial stimulation would bias the response. Similarly, evidence has shown that other signals [e.g., prostaglandin E2 (PGE2)] can induce differentiation of potent APCs with dendritic morphology, which produce low IL-12 and high IL-10 levels and preferentially induce Th2 differentiation (209). Finally, since dendritic cells express relatively high levels of MHC class II and constitutively express costimulatory molecules such as B7-2, they could induce a relatively high level of T-cell activation, leading to the production of IL-4 by mechanisms outlined above. Thus, as perhaps the major APC-initiating immune responses, dendritic cells can guide either a Th1 or Th2 response, depending on the conditions present at the time of stimulation.

Monocytes and Macrophages

Some of the early mouse *in vitro* studies, examining the role of APCs in influencing Th1 and Th2 cells, suggested that using macrophages rather than B cells as APCs induced the production of IFN-γ from naive T cells (210). In subsequent *in vitro* studies, it was demonstrated that IL-12 was induced from phagocytic cells in response to bacterial products (211), providing a mechanism by which macrophages could selectively induce production of IFN-γ. The ability of macrophages to direct induction of IFN-γ was definitively shown in experiments in which macrophages infected with *L. monocytogenes* enhanced the differentiation of Th1 cells through an IL-12–dependent pathway (81,96). These *in vitro* studies and additional *in vivo* studies, demonstrating that many other intracellular infections (212–214) known to target macrophages are potent inducers of Th1 responses through their production of IL-12, provide clear evidence that macrophages can direct Th1 cytokine production. Th1 responses may also be enhanced by the direct production of IFN-γ by F4/80+ peritoneal macrophages stimulated by IL-12 (215). Alternatively, it should be noted that macrophages are also capable of producing IL-10, a potent counterregulatory cytokine to IL-12, in response to many of these same stimuli. Another macrophage cytokine, IL-6, may also enhance Th2 differentiation under some circumstances (124). Thus, macrophages could have a dual role in T helper cell differentiation, depending on the predominance of IL-12 or IL-10 production.

B Cells

B cells have also been suggested to be important in directing T helper responses. Similar to macrophages and dendritic cells, B cells are also capable of secreting cytokines that could influence the generation of Th1- or Th2-type cells. Since IL-12 was originally cloned from a lymphoblastoid B-cell line, it could theoretically serve to influence a Th1 response, although the physiologic relevance of IL-12 production from normal B cells *in vitro* and *in vivo* remains to be established. In addition, CD5[+] (B1) B cells are a source of IL-10 (216), which could lead to downregulation of Th1, as noted above (207), and indirectly enhance the development of IL-4–producing cells. This type of regulation is suggested from *in vivo* studies in which mice depleted of B cells showed impaired priming of T-cell responses to protein but not peptide antigens (217) or had decreased IL-4 and IL-10 production with enhanced production of IFN-γ in response to infection with *Plasmodium chabaudi chabaudi* (218). Further *in vivo* evidence was obtained using a transgenic TCR model in which the T cells recognized complement C5a. In these mice, B-cell antigen presentation biased towards Th2-like responses (219). Additional support for a role of B cells inducing Th2 responses comes from studies in which mice injected with anti-IgD antibody (which induces polyclonal B-cell activation) leads to potent IL-4 induction (220). Moreover, the ability of anti-IgD to enhance IL-4 production is abrogated in CD28[-/-] mice, suggesting that T-cell activation through the B7/CD28 pathway plays an important role in IL-4 induction, as described above (221). B cells may have a role in regulating IL-4 production, especially at low antigen concentrations, by their ability to more efficiently bind antigen through their surface receptor, resulting in a high density of antigen–MHC complexes (192,222–224). Although high ligand density, even on B cells, can cause Th1 differentiation (188), the selective focusing of low amounts of antigen on B cells may enhance Th2 responses, because the B cells are inherently more likely to induce Th2 differentiation, either by expression of Th2-inducing cytokines or costimulators, or because of a lack of Th1-inducing signals, such as IL-12. Finally, despite the considerable evidence that B cells can selectively enhance Th2 responses, there are *in vivo* data showing that IL-4 is induced in the absence of B cells (206), demonstrating that other APCs (i.e., dendritic cells) are sufficient to induce Th2 differentiation.

In summary, there appear to be two major mechanisms by which APCs can influence the type of T helper response induced. First, APCs, through their production of cytokines such as IL-12, would directly enhance Th1 responses, while production of IL-10 would diminish Th1 responses and indirectly increase Th2 cytokine production. Second, APCs, through differences in their relative expression of MHC class II and/or costimulatory molecules (e.g., B7, CD40) or in their ability to present antigen, would influence the type of T helper response generated by providing different degrees of activation to the CD4[+] T cells. It is important to reiterate that the cytokine milieu present at the time a T cell encounters the APC may be the most dominant factor in regulating Th1 and Th2 differentiation. This is supported by *in vitro* studies alluded to in the previous section, showing that addition of exogenous IL-4 or IL-12 to priming cultures leads to the induction of IL-4– or IFN-γ–producing cells irrespective of the type of APC used for stimulation (25). Furthermore, additional immunoregulatory cytokines such as IL-10 and TGF-β, which can influence the types of cytokines and costimulatory molecules expressed by APCs, are also likely to have an important effect in directing the type of T helper response that is generated.

GENETIC REGULATION OF T HELPER 1 AND T HELPER 2 DIFFERENTIATION

In studying the *in vitro* differentiation of Th1 and Th2 cells, it was noted that naive CD4[+] T cells derived from BALB/c mice stim-

ulated under neutral conditions (in the absence of exogenous IL-4 or IL-12) produced more IL-4 upon restimulation than did similarly stimulated CD4[+] T cells derived from B10.D2 mice (225). These data were consistent with the fact that BALB/c mice, through enhanced production of IL-4, are susceptible to infection with *L. major*, while B10.D2 mice, which are resistant to infection, have diminished IL-4 and enhanced IFN-γ production (31). Taken together, these results suggested an inherent bias of T cells from BALB/c mice to produce more IL-4 in response to antigenic stimulation. The importance of this early production of IL-4 in influencing the development and stability of a Th2 response has been shown to be due to its ability to downregulate the expression of the IL-12 Rβ2 subunit and subsequently IL-12 responsiveness (68). Thus, current work is focused on defining a genetic basis for enhanced IL-4 production in BALB/c mice, which may have important applications in regard to whether Th2 responses are preferentially generated and maintained in allergic and parasitic diseases. The potential complexity of this regulation is illustrated by the identification of at least six genes involved in resistance to *Leishmania* infection (226).

MOLECULAR BASIS FOR T HELPER 1 AND T HELPER 2 CELL DIFFERENTIATION

Intracellular Signaling in T-Cell Subsets Is Mediated by STAT Proteins

Because IL-12 and IL-4 are major determinants in controlling the differentiation of Th1 and Th2 cells, respectively, there has been substantial interest in defining the molecular mechanisms by which these cytokines regulate IFN-γ and IL-4 production. Over the past several years, the identification of a class of proteins involved in cytokine-induced signal transduction and activation of transcription (STAT) has led to a better understanding of how cytokines can specifically regulate the differentiation of CD4[+] T cells into Th1 and Th2 cells. In response to specific cytokine-receptor interaction, these STAT proteins, which exist in latent form in the cytoplasm, become phosphorylated by members of the Janus kinase (JAK) family of tyrosine kinases, dimerize, and are then translocated to the nucleus, where they bind to specific DNA sequences to regulate gene transcription (227,228). The fact that certain STAT proteins (see below) were specifically activated by IL-4 and IL-12 provided a molecular mechanism by which IL-4 and IL-12 could regulate the differentiation of Th2 and Th1 cells, respectively.

With regard to the role of IL-4 in Th2 differentiation, several groups have shown that IL-4, upon coupling to its specific receptor, induced phosphorylation of a transcription factor, which was called STAT 6 or IL-4 STAT (229,230). Phosphorylated STAT6 bound to a site on the IL-4 promotor, which was capable of directing transcription of a reporter gene in response to IL-4, providing a direct correlation of IL-4–mediated STAT6 activation and Th2 differentiation (230). Furthermore, definitive evidence for a role for STAT6 in regulating Th2 responses was shown by several groups using STAT6-deficient mice (114–116). In these studies, it was demonstrated that T cells were markedly deficient in their ability to differentiate into IL-4–producing cells in response to *in vitro* or *in vivo* stimulation. Thus, these data were consistent with the findings, discussed above, that IL-4 is critical for induction of IL-4–producing cells and clearly links the effects of IL-4 to the STAT6-signaling pathway (230).

With regard to the role of IL-12 in Th1 development, it was shown that IL-12 induced selective activation of STAT4, providing a specific mechanism to control IFN-γ production (231). Again, definitive evidence for a role of IL-12, and subsequently STAT4, in regulating Th1 differentiation was shown in studies using mice deficient in STAT4. In these studies, IFN-γ production in response to *in vitro* or *in vivo* stimulation with IL-12 was markedly impaired, demonstrating the critical role of STAT4 in mediating responses to IL-12 and regulating the differentiation of Th1 cells (87,88).

Role of Biochemical Intermediates and Transcription Factors in T Helper Cell Differentiation

Several investigators have focused on the role that certain biochemical intermediates have in regulating cytokine production from T helper clones. Based on these studies, it appears that both Th1 and Th2 clones increase free intracellular Ca^{2+} in response to stimulation (232,233); however, in these studies, it appears that Th2 clones use a signaling pathway for IL-4 production that is independent of protein tyrosine kinase, PIP2 breakdown, and protein kinase C, while Th1 production of IL-2 is more dependent on these pathways (232–234). One caveat is that most of these studies used established Th1 and Th2 clones stimulated with immobilized anti-CD3 or other pharmacologic agents. Thus, the ability to extrapolate these findings to primary $CD4^+$ T cells stimulated in a more physiologic context remains to be determined.

Another intense area of investigation has been to understand the molecular basis of regulating subset-specific expression of IL-4 and/or IFN-γ from T cells. Work by several groups, analyzing regions of the IL-4 promotor, initially identified NF-AT and AP-1 proteins as potentially important in regulating IL-4 transcription (235–239). More recently, additional transcriptional regulatory proteins, such as NF-IL-6 (240), IκB and NFκB (241), c-maf (242), NIP45 (243), and GATA3 (244), have been shown to be involved in IL-4 transcription. It should be noted, however, that while c-maf, NF-AT p, and NIP45 were relatively specific for selected Th2 clones and enhanced IL-4 production from Th1 clones and B cells following transfection (237,242–246), the tissue-specific expression of these factors with regard to IL-4–producing cells in the course of a physiologic *in vivo* immune response remains to be determined. Thus, as noted above, the clearest molecular mechanism by which IL-4 and IL-12 regulate Th2 and Th1 differentiation occurs initially through their ability to rapidly induce phosphorylation of specific STAT proteins, which then directly or indirectly leads to regulation of transcription.

SOURCES OF CYTOKINES INFLUENCING THE T HELPER 1–T HELPER 2 CHOICE

As described above, the major influences on T-cell precursor differentiation are cytokines, particularly IL-4, IFN-γ, and IL-12. Although IL-4 and IFN-γ are produced by T cells, the number of effector cells producing these cytokines may be very low at the beginning of an immune response. Thus, there has been considerable interest in defining other sources of these cytokines that may play an important role early in immune responses. There are a wide variety of cell types that can secrete cytokines that are important in Th1/Th2 regulation, and it is likely that the balance of these cytokines and cell types is often responsible for the direction of T-cell differentiation.

Keratinocytes

Keratinocytes are abundant cells that are among the first cells to be exposed to infections that enter through skin. In response to damage, both human and mouse keratinocytes can produce cytokines, such as the IL-10 that is secreted in response to UVB irradiation and during Th2 responses (247–249). This IL-10 is responsible for suppression of DTH responses (249). However, keratinocytes can also produce IL-12 (250–253) and IL-18 (254), which would bias immunity towards a Th1 response. Thus, the immune response bias induced by keratinocytes may depend on the balance between the production of IL-10 and IL-12, and this in turn may depend on other local factors.

Conventional T Cells

Although naive conventional CD4 or CD8 T cells do not make significant amounts of IFN-γ or IL4 following acute stimulation (17,255–257), there are two ways in which T cells with unrestricted, very diverse TCR specificities may nevertheless provide a strong differentiative signal during primary responses. First, there may be memory or effector cells that have been induced to differentiate in response to a previous antigen, and that cross-react with the new antigen during a primary exposure to an infection. Depending on the Th1 or Th2 bias of these memory cells, this may provide cytokines that influence the direction of the differentiation of concomitantly activated naive T cells. Second, there may be an ongoing immune response against a different pathogen, and this response may provide a cytokine milieu that strongly influences *de novo* T-cell differentiation. Examples of this include immune responses against antigens or other pathogens during helminth infections, which show enhanced production of IgE specific for ovalbumin (258), or reduced Th1 responses against a viral infection (259). Both of these mechanisms apply to CD4, CD8, and γδ T cells, as all three of these cell types can synthesize either Th1- or Th2-like cytokine patterns (6,43,257,260).

T-Cell Subpopulations Expressing Restricted T-Cell Receptors

A T-cell subpopulation with restricted TCR expression has been identified during the response to *L. major* infection. Vβ4, Vα8 TCRs were expressed by either protective Th1 or exacerbating Th2 clones specific for LACK antigen (74), and cells expressing this restricted TCR were responsible for a rapid burst of IL-4 expression (peaking at 16 hours) in susceptible mice (261). Vβ4-deficient BALB/c mice lacked this early IL-4 response and mounted Th1 responses against *Leishmania*. It is not yet clear if these Vβ4, Vα8 T cells are derived by a separate pathway, as are the NK T (NKT) cells (see below), or whether they represent a population of conventional T cells that has been expanded in response to a cross-reactive environmental antigen.

Natural Killer T Cells

A subpopulation of T cells, bearing the NK1.1 marker in appropriate mouse strains, produces cytokines rapidly on stimulation (262). These NKT cells can be $CD4^+$ $CD8^-$ or $CD4^-$ $CD8^+$, and they can express a very restricted pattern of TCRs, normally Vβ8 and Vα14 (263). These cells are restricted to the nonclassical MHC class I protein CD1 (264), rather than to MHC class II, and so these cells are absent in mice lacking expression of CD1 or MHC class I (e.g., β2-microglobulin (β2m)- or CD1-deficient mice (265–267). CD1 may bind glycolipid antigens such as those obtained from mycobacteria (268), and so the restricted repertoire of NKT cells may recognize common bacterial lipids. NKT cells produce large amounts of IL-4 within a few hours of activation by polyclonal activators such as anti-CD3 antibody. The ability of these cells to secrete large amounts of IL-4 without apparent priming prompted speculation that NKT cells could be an important source of early IL-4 that might bias the immune response. This was supported by the apparent requirement for NK1.1[+] cells for the IL-4 and IgE response to anti-IgD antibodies (269) and the increased expression of IL-4 and IgE in mice transgenic for the Vα14 TCR (270).

However, NKT cells do not appear to be important for several Th2 responses. Although polyclonal activation by anti-CD3 *in vivo* induces IL-4 production by NKT cells and a subsequent Th2 response, other T-cell responses are not dependent on NKT cells. In contrast to the results mentioned above, CD1-deficient mice mount Th2 responses after anti-IgD immunization (267). Normal Th2 responses also occur during *Leishmania* infection in β2m-deficient or anti-NK1.1–depleted BALB/c mice (271,272), and Th2 responses induced by protein antigens, *Schistosome* egg antigen or *Nippostrongylus* infection all occur normally in β2m-deficient mice (271). Thus, a role for these cells in Th2 responses against infection has not yet been shown. However, because of their rapid and high-level production of IL-4, NKT cells remain strong candidates for initiating Th2 responses under some circumstances, particularly in such tissues as the liver, where they are abundant.

Natural Killer Cells

NK cells, expressing the NK1.1 marker (in appropriate strains) but not the TCR, synthesize IFN-γ on stimulation through Fc receptors or by IL-12 (79,273). As NK cells are more abundant than T cells during the early stages of an immune response, IFN-γ production by NK cells can provide an early Th1 push to the immune system. During *Leishmania* infection in C3H/HeN mice, depletion of NK cells results in a more Th2-biased response and increased susceptibility (274). Although other cytokines may be produced by NK cells under some conditions (275), the major cytokine bias contributed by NK cells appears to be toward Th1 differentiation.

Macrophages

Macrophages are a major source of cytokines early in immune responses, and they can be stimulated by a variety of microbial products, other cytokines, and cell signals. Macrophages can be strong stimulators of Th1 responses, as IL-12 production is induced by heat-killed *L. monocytogenes,* CD40L, or IFN-γ (81,99,205, 276,277). However, macrophages can also produce IL-6 and IL-10, and depending on the balance of IL-10 and IL-12, the relative strength of Th1 induction can vary. IL-10 synthesis can be enhanced by PGE2 (278) and inhibited by IFN-γ (279). Although IL-10 does not directly enhance Th2 differentiation, its ability to inhibit IFN-γ and IL-12 secretion may decrease Th1 responses, which in turn may allow increased Th2 development.

Dendritic Cells

Cytokine synthesis by dendritic cells shows some parallels to that of macrophages. Stimulation by CD40L induces production of IL-12 (166,168), and IL-12 mRNA can be detected in purified Langerhans' cells by polymerase chain reaction (PCR) (280,281). However, culture of bone marrow cells in the presence of PGE2 results in the differentiation of cells with dendritic morphology that synthesize lower amounts of IL-12, but increased IL-10, which induce Th2 differentiation (282). Furthermore, IL-10 inhibits IL-12 production by dendritic cells (208). As dendritic cells are thought to be the major initiating APCs for activation of naive T cells, it is obviously important that dendritic cells should have the ability to induce either Th1 or Th2 differentiation, depending on the type of antigen and the surrounding cytokine milieu.

Mast Cells, Basophils, and Eosinophils

Both mouse and human mast cells can produce IL-4 on stimulation of the cells by IgE cross-linking (283,284). Thus, allergen may induce higher IL-4 levels, serving to amplify the allergic response. As helminth infections are often accompanied by extensive mucosal mast-cell infiltration, the release of IL-4 by mast cells potentially contributes to the Th2-biased responses against many helminths. However, not all mast cells may be Th2-biased. Differentiation of bone marrow precursors in the presence of IL-3 induces the formation of mucosa-like mast cells that produce IL-4, whereas stem-cell factor induces the differentiation of connective tissue–like mast cells that produce IL-12 (285). Cytokine production is discussed in more detail in Chapter 35.

Human basophils also produce IL-4, and both IL-4 and IL-13 have been reported to be preformed in granules (286–288). IL-4 is released on stimulation by complement C5a, IL-3, or IgE cross-linking (289,290). Although mouse basophils are difficult to recognize by histochemistry, the mouse basophil equivalent may be represented by a cell type that is a non-B, non-T, non-NK, non-mast cell and that releases substantial amounts of IL-4 on cross-linking of surface IgE receptors (291).

Eosinophils also synthesize IL-4, which is stored in granules and released on triggering by serum-coated beads (292). As with several other cell types, eosinophils may also have the ability to synthesize cytokines that induce either Th1 or Th2 responses, as eosinophils containing either IL-4 or IFN-γ have been described (293).

In summary, there are several cell types that can synthesize Th1- or Th2-directing cytokines. In any one response, a particular cytokine source may be crucial, but overall it is likely that all of these sources can play a role in T-cell differentiation in one system or another. Another general point that should be made is that many of the cell types secreting these polarizing cytokines can exist in at least two forms, inducing either Th1 or Th2 differentiation. This means not only that the decision between Th1 and Th2 differentiation is regulated by the activation of different cell types in the vicinity, but also that each of these cell types, in turn, responds to other signals in the environment.

NONPROTEIN INFLUENCES ON T-CELL DIFFERENTIATION

In addition to the effects of cytokines, antigen dose, costimulators, and other protein mediators on the regulation of T-cell subsets, there are also a number of other mediators that affect this choice. These include several stress and reproductive steroids, eicosanoids, several drugs that interfere with cyclic adenosine monophosphate (cAMP), β-adrenergic receptors, and histamine receptors. In many cases, these signals may allow other systems to influence the immune system's choice of cytokine pattern.

Sex Steroid Hormones

During pregnancy, type 1 responses are often suppressed (294), and at least part of this inhibition may be due to direct effects of progesterone and estradiol. Progesterone induces preferential differentiation of human T cells *in vitro* towards the Th2 phenotype, and it also induces transient IL-4 expression from established Th1 clones (295).

Coxsackie virus B3 induces a type 1 inflammatory response in male mice, but a type 2 response in females (296). Treatment of female mice with testosterone, or male mice with estradiol, reverses these phenotypes and also alters the cytokine subset balance, suggesting that these hormones also have effects on T-cell differentiation. Testosterone in female mice decreases the frequency of IL-4– and IL-5–producing clones, while estradiol in male mice increases the frequency of IL-4– and IL-5–producing clones and decreases the frequency of IL-2– and IFN-γ–producing clones. However, dihydrotestosterone (DHT, a metabolic product of testosterone) treatment *in vivo* prevented diabetes in the NOD mouse, and this was accompanied by an increase in IL-4 production (297). Finally, testosterone or DHT could inhibit both IL-4 and IFN-γ production *in vitro* (298). Thus, androgens and estrogens can clearly influence the choice between Th1 and Th2 responses, but it is not yet possible to easily classify the effects in one direction or the other.

Stress Steroid Hormones

Different types of stress can inhibit IFN-γ production by T cells. Inescapable tail shock reduced the ability of rat cells to produce IFN-γ and IgG2a antibody in response to KLH, but IgG1 antibody was not affected (299). The corticosteroid antagonist RU-486 blocked this effect, suggesting the involvement of corticosteroids. In mice, restraint stress increased circulating levels of corticosterone during viral infection and reduced synthesis of IL-2, IL-10, and IFN-γ (300). Again, RU-486 blocked these effects. In humans, surgical stress was also associated with reduced IFN-γ responses to mitogen stimulation *in vitro*, whereas IL-4 levels were enhanced (301). During sarcoidosis, a Th1-like cytokine pattern prevails in lung lavage fluid. Corticosteroid treatment reduced IFN-γ levels and elevated IL-4 levels (302).

In vitro treatment with corticosteroids provides similar results. Although high-dose hydrocortisone treatment suppressed the synthesis of both IFN-γ and IL-4 by human T cells, lower doses enhanced IL-4 production (303). Naive cells were very sensitive to corticosteroid inhibition, and low concentrations present during differentiation inhibited subsequent production of both IFN-γ and IL-4, but enhanced IL-10 production (304). After differentiation, the T cells were less sensitive to corticosteroids, and synthesis of IFN-γ was inhibited, whereas effects on IL-4 depended on the origin of the effector cells. Dexamethasone treatment during differentiation of rat CD4 T cells inhibited subsequent production of IFN-γ, but enhanced IL-4, IL-10, and IL-13 synthesis (305). Overall, corticosteroids appear to consistently inhibit Th1-like responses,

whereas the effects on Th2 cytokines are often stimulatory, but sometimes inhibitory.

Corticosteroids also affect the class of immune response at the level of the APC. Corticosteroid treatment during stimulation of whole human blood with lipopolysaccharide reduced IL-12 but not IL-10 production (306), and exposure of monocytes to corticosteroids reduced IL-12 production and enhanced the differentiation of T cells producing IL-4 (307). Thus, at the level of the APC, T-cell differentiation, and T-cell activation, corticosteroids appear to bias the immune response toward Th2 reactions, consistent with the effects of stress and corticosteroid treatment *in vivo*.

Other Steroid Hormones

Dehydroepiandrosterone (DHEA) and its sulfated product (DHEAS) are intermediates in sex hormone synthesis, but they also stimulate mouse T cells *in vivo* and *in vitro* and human cells *in vitro* to synthesize increased amounts of IL-2 but not IL-4 (308, 309). DHEA also reversed the inhibition of IL-2 synthesis and enhancement of IL-4 synthesis induced by glucocorticoids (308). In mice tolerized for DTH responses, DHEA restored the DTH response, increased IFN-γ production, and decreased IL-4 and IL-6 synthesis (310). In a mouse model of retroviral infection with suppressed Th1 and enhanced Th2 functions, DHEAS also increased IL-2 and IFN-γ production while reducing IL-6 and IL-10 production (311). DHEA therefore selectively enhances Th1 response, particularly in systems in which the Th1 response has been suppressed. Enhancement by DHEA of IL-2 synthesis by fresh CD4 T cells also suggests that DHEA may enhance cytokine production by uncommitted precursor cells.

Prostaglandin E2

PGE2 is produced by macrophages during inflammatory reactions and can regulate the choice between Th1 and Th2 differentiation at three levels: (a) PGE2 inhibits production of IL-12 and enhances IL-10 production by human monocytes (312). This effect appears to be mediated by induction of cAMP, as other cAMP inducers had similar effects. The inhibitory effects of PGE2 on IL-12 production were not mediated via IL-10. (b) PGE2 also biased the differentiation of naive T-cell precursors from cord blood by inhibiting the development of cells that could secrete IL-2 and IFN-γ, while allowing differentiation of Th2 cells (313). Again, other cAMP inducers had a similar effect. (c) Effector Th1 and Th2 cells are also differentially sensitive to PGE2. Synthesis of IL-2 and IFN-γ is inhibited, whereas IL-4 or IL-5 synthesis is unchanged or even enhanced (314,315). Continued synthesis of IL-4 and IL-5 is dependent on IL-2, as PGE2 inhibits the synthesis of all cytokines in the absence of IL-2 (316).

As all of these effects would selectively inhibit Th1 responses, PGE2 appears to be a potent mechanism for switching responses towards Th2. This is supported by the correlation of PGE2 production and type 2 responses in leprosy (317), *Leishmania* (318), atopic dermatitis (319), and high antibody responses (320).

Adrenergic Receptor Agonists

The β2-adrenergic receptor is expressed on Th1 but not Th2 clones (321), and agonists for this receptor selectively suppress IFN-γ synthesis *in vitro* (321); increase IL-4, IL-5, and IL-10 synthesis in spleen cells from treated mice; and increase IgE levels *in vivo* (322). Also, epinephrine and norepinephrine inhibit IL-12 production, but they enhance IL-10 production (306). Thus, stimulation of the β2-adrenergic receptor appears to bias immunity towards Th2 responses.

Vitamins A and D

Vitamin A deficiency in rats and mice caused increased IFN-γ responses, suggesting that vitamin A directly or indirectly inhibits Th1 responses (323,324). *In vivo,* vitamin A deficiency converted the normal Th2 response against *Trichinella* into a Th1 response (325). These alterations could be reversed by retinoic acid both *in vivo* and *in vitro* (324–326), and retinoic acid treatment suppressed disease and the accompanying type 1 immune response in EAE (327). The effect of vitamin A may not be quite as simple as inhibition of Th1 responses, however, as vitamin A deficiency also reduced DTH responses (323).

Calcitriol (1,25 dihydroxy vitamin D3, the active metabolite of vitamin D) also selectively inhibited IL-2 and IFN-γ synthesis by human peripheral blood T cells stimulated by several methods (328–330). Inhibition of IFN-γ synthesis also occurred with T-cell clones derived from psoriatic lesions (331), which may account for at least part of the beneficial effect of vitamin D analogues in the treatment of psoriasis. Interestingly, IFN-γ enhanced the synthesis of calcitriol by alveolar and bone marrow macrophages (332,333) and keratinocytes (334), suggesting the existence of a negative regulatory loop.

REVERSIBILITY OF T HELPER PHENOTYPES

Stability of T Helper 1 and T Helper 2 Cells

Because the production of IFN-γ and IL-4 can play an important role in normal immune regulation and dysregulation in a variety of diseases states, a question of biologic and potential clinical importance is whether established T helper phenotypes are irreversibly committed or can be altered through various immune mechanisms. The concept of reversibility refers to the induction of IL-4 or IFN-γ from a previously committed Th1 (IFN-γ-producing) or Th2 (IL-4-producing) cell, respectively. As will be discussed below, cytokine patterns can be altered transiently, but true reversibility would mean the stable, long-term acquisition of a new cytokine secretion pattern. Moreover, it is important to note that in studying the differentiation of Th1 and Th2 type cells *in vitro*, although the starting population of naive CD4- T cells is homogeneous and the culture conditions are maximized so that all cells should theoretically respond, the number of cells that differentiate toward production of IFN-γ or IL-4 can vary greatly. In fact, there often exists a relatively large population of activated cells that are not producing IL-4 or IFN-γ. This latter population may be uncommitted precursors, which can replicate extensively without differentiating (76). Thus, in studying reversibility, it is important to determine whether IL-4 or IFN-γ is produced from a population of the opposite phenotype by differentiation of previously uncommitted Thpp precursor cells, by induction of double-producing Th0 cells, or by reversal of committed Th1 or Th2 cells.

The reversibility of Th1 and Th2 populations has been extensively studied in both mouse and human *in vitro* models of T-cell priming. Initial mouse *in vitro* studies showed that at the population level, Th2 cells generated after 1 week of stimulation were irre-

versibly committed to IL-4 production, while Th1 populations could be induced to secrete IL-4 (29,335,336), suggesting a difference in the stability between Th1 and Th2 populations, or that complete differentiation occurs more rapidly in Th2 differentiation conditions. The second possibility is very likely, because in at least one of these studies, the secretion of IL-4 was subsequently shown to be derived from persisting uncommitted precursors in the population, rather than from actual redifferentiation of Th1 cells (337). In additional studies, using intracellular cytokine staining to determine the frequency of IL-4– and IFN-γ–producing cells following *in vitro* priming, it was shown that repetitive stimulation of cells over the course of 3 weeks resulted in populations of IFN-γ– or IL-4–producing cells that were irreversibly committed (338).

More recently, in a similar *in vitro* mouse model, using TCR-transgenic mice derived on a different background, it was shown that fully differentiated Th1 cells were irreversibly committed, while Th2 populations could be induced to secrete IFN-γ under certain conditions (see below) (339). Moreover, similar results were noted in studying the frequency of IL-4– and IFN-γ–producing cells derived from naive human CD4+ T cells (29). In these studies, IL-4–producing populations, induced after 1 or 3 weeks of stimulation, were not stable and were induced to produce IFN-γ in response to IL-12. By contrast, differentiated IFN-γ–producing cells could not be induced to produce IL-4 by further stimulation in the presence of IL-4. Although these population data are subject to the reservations noted above—that production of the opposite cytokine could be due to differentiation of uncommitted precursors—the production of IFN-γ from fully differentiated Th2 cells has been demonstrated by showing that IL-12 could temporarily induce small amounts of IFN-γ from established human Th0 and Th2 clones (61,85,340,341). However, this is a transient effect and does not appear to represent redifferentiation of Th2 cells into Th0 or Th1 cells.

Molecular Basis for Conditional Production of Interferon-γ by T Helper 2 Cells

From the results discussed above, it appears that Th2 cells can be induced by IL-12 to secrete IFN-γ in some systems but not in others. A molecular basis for these apparently discrepant results was elucidated by the finding that the presence of IL-4 in early priming cultures (which is required for IL-4 priming) inhibited the expression of the IL-12Rβ2 subunit, which is required for functional IL-12 signaling through STAT4 (65,68). Importantly, the addition of exogenous IFN-γ to priming cultures of early developing Th2 cells could induce IL-12 Rβ2 expression, allowing for the maintenance of IL-12–induced IFN-γ production, which was consistent with an earlier study, which showed that IFN-γ and IL-12 could induce the production of IFN-γ from *L. major*-specific Th2 cells (336). In parallel *in vitro* studies using human T cells, IL-12 Rβ2 expression was also selectively found on differentiating Th1 but not Th2 cells. In contrast to the mouse data, IFN-α but not IFN-γ induced IL-12 Rβ2 expression and was able to maintain IL-12 responsiveness, suggesting that type I (IFN-α) and type II (IFN-γ) have differential effects in maintaining IL-12 responsiveness in human and mouse CD4+ T cells, respectively.

To conclude, many factors determine the stability and reversibility of Th1 and Th2 cells. Perhaps the most important determinant for the development of stable Th1 and Th2 cells would be the cytokine milieu present at the time of initial priming, as well as during the course of a recall response. Thus, for mouse CD4+ T

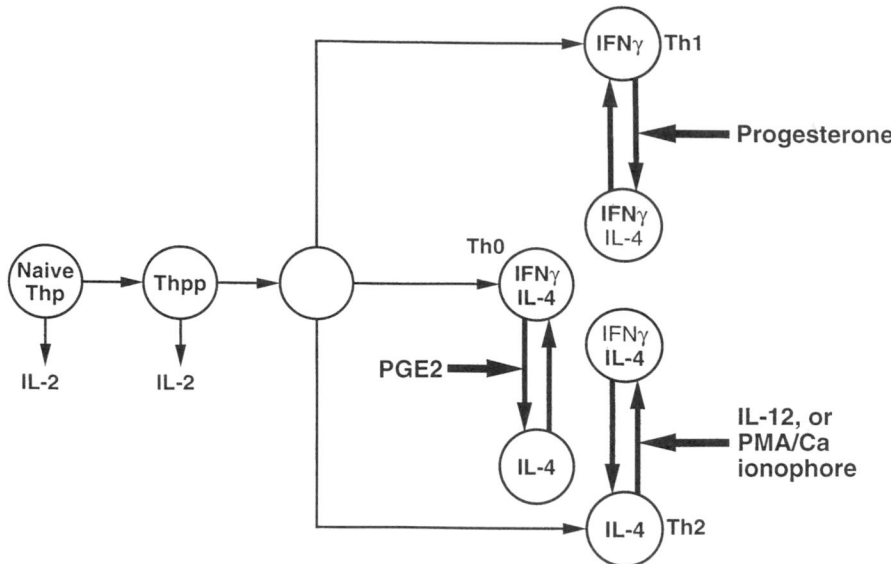

FIG. 6. Transient alterations in cytokine synthesis of differentiated T cells. After differentiation into Th1, Th2, or Th0 cells, further modifications in cytokine synthesis can occur. For example, IL-12 treatment of Th2 cells induces the temporary ability to synthesize IFN-γ. As these effects are transient, they do not represent reversability of the phenotypes.

cells, the presence of IL-4 and absence of IFN-γ and IL-12 would predispose a cell toward a stable Th2-type cell; however, the presence of IFN-γ and IL-12 may subsequently render even Th2 cells responsive to IL-12 through the upregulation of the IL-12 Rβ2 subunit, allowing for induction of IFN-γ. For human CD4+ T cells, the presence of IFN-α rather than IFN-γ would be important in regulating responsiveness to IL-12. Thus, in both mouse and human systems, it appears that transient IFN-γ synthesis can be induced from IL-4–producing cells. By contrast, fully differentiated Th1 cells appear relatively stable, with little capacity to produce IL-4, even in the presence of IL-4, although progesterone may be able to induce transient IL-4 synthesis by Th1 clones (295). Although these transient alterations in cytokine synthesis can be induced in both Th1 and Th2 cells (Fig. 6), it has not yet been possible to switch a fully differentiated Th1 cell into a stable Th2 cell, or vice versa.

INFLUENCE OF CYTOKINES IN CROSS-REGULATING T HELPER 1 AND T HELPER 2 CELLS AT BOTH THE DIFFERENTIATION AND EFFECTOR PHASES OF THE RESPONSE

As noted in the previous sections, cytokines such as IL-12 and IL-4 have direct effects on influencing the differentiation of IFN-γ (Th1-type) and IL-4 (Th2-type) producing cells, respectively. In addition IL-12, IL-4 and several additional cytokines can also negatively regulate or cross-regulate the differentiation of Th2 and Th1 cells, respectively. Moreover, cytokines can exert potent cross-regulatory influences on fully differentiated effector cells as well. In this section, the effects that cytokines have in counterregulating Th1 and Th2 responses at both the differentiation and effector stages are discussed.

Interferon-γ Versus Interleukin-4

During T helper cell differentiation, IL-4 has a direct effect on the induction of IL-4–producing cells (24). In addition, IL-4 appears to inhibit the induction of IFN-γ production cells *in vitro*

and *in vivo* (23–25). One mechanism in the mouse system by which IL-4 would prevent the development of IFN-γ–producing Th1 cells would be its ability to inhibit the expression of the IL-12 Rβ-chain subunit, making cells unresponsive to IL-12 stimulation (65,342). Thus, IL-4 would cross-regulate IFN-γ production indirectly through inhibiting IL-12 responsiveness.

The ability of IFN-γ to cross-regulate the induction of IL-4–producing cells was first suggested by studies showing that IFN-γ selectively inhibited the proliferation of Th2 clones (91,92) and caused the preferential outgrowth of Th1 clones (343). This differential sensitivity of Th2 clones to the growth inhibitory effects of IFN-γ may be due to maintenance of the IFN-γ receptor β chain (67–70). Thus, IFN-γ may have a counterregulatory role at both the differentiation and effector phases of the response. Finally, since IFN-γ can enhance both IL-12 production and responsiveness, it is likely that many of the effects of IFN-γ are mediated indirectly through IL-12 (see below).

Interleukin-12 Versus Interleukin-4

In the course of T helper cell differentiation, there is clear evidence that IL-12 can suppress IL-4 mRNA induction, both directly (344) and indirectly, through induction of IFN-γ (345–347). In addition, it should be noted that in the absence of IFN-γ, IL-12 has been shown to actually enhance Th2 responses (348). Thus, the ability of IL-12 to cross-regulate IL-4 production may be different at the differentiation and effector phases of the response, depending on the presence of IFN-γ.

The ability of IL-4 to cross-regulate IL-12 is complex. IL-4 has been shown to inhibit IL-12 production from both mouse dendritic cells (166) and human PBMCs (349). By contrast, human *in vitro* studies have also shown that pretreatment of cells with IL-4 before stimulation actually enhanced IL-12 production (349). While this latter finding is of interest, it remains to be determined whether this type of regulation occurs *in vivo*. Finally, evidence that IL-4 decreases IL-12 responsiveness through downregulation of the IL-12 Rβ2 chain (65) provides an additional mechanism by which IL-4 can cross-regulate the effects of IL-12 at both the differentiation and effector phases of the response.

Interferon-α Versus Interleukin-4

In addition to the role of type II interferon (IFN-γ) in cross-regulating IL-4 production, there is also evidence that type I interferons contribute to downregulation of Th2 responses. This was initially shown by treatment of mice with IFN-α or an inducer of IFN-α, which led to a decrease in production of IL-4 (107). More recent mouse *in vitro* studies have also shown that IFN-α could downregulate IL-4 production, but only when IL-12 was also present in the cultures (97). In human cultures, IFN-α causes preferential induction of IFN-γ and inhibition of antigen- or allergen-specific IL-4–producing cells (103–105,350). Moreover, a report that the inhibitory effect of IFN-α on IL-4 induction is independent of IL-12 provides additional evidence that IFN-α plays an important role in regulating the induction of IL-4–producing cells (66). As IFN-α also caused an increase in IFN-γ, additional work will be needed to determine whether the ability of IFN-α to downregulate IL-4 is a direct effect or indirect, through its enhancement of IFN-γ.

Interleukin-10 Versus Interferon-γ

IL-10 is a potent counterregulatory cytokine capable of inhibiting production of IFN-γ from established effector Th1 cells or clones (4). The principal mechanism by which IL-10 inhibits IFN-γ production was shown to be indirect, through its ability to inhibit IL-12 production from APCs (166,351). Reduction of IFN-γ synthesis will in turn reduce further Th1 differentiation, and thus, IL-10 exerts a potent but indirect cross-regulatory influence at both the differentiation and effector phases of the response.

Because IL-10 has such potent effects on inhibiting a developing Th1 response, it would be important to develop mechanism(s) to downregulate production of IL-10 in order to generate a functional Th1 response. This would especially apply to the development of primary immunity to a variety of infectious pathogens. In this regard, IFN-γ has been shown to be a potent inhibitor of IL-10 production from monocytes (352,353), providing a favorable environment for the development of a Th1 response.

Interleukin-12 Versus Interleukin-10

While there is clear antagonism between IL-10 and IL-12 in regulating IFN-γ production, there are several reports from human studies that IL-12 actually induces IL-10 in addition to IFN-γ from T cells *in vitro* (46–48). This ability of IL-12 to enhance IL-10 production from T cells may be a mechanism by which a developing or established Th1 response is mitigated. Additional studies examining the role of IL-10 from T cells in controlling ongoing responses should be helpful in determining whether this is an operative regulatory mechanism.

As noted in the previous section, IL-10 has been shown in many models to be a potent inhibitor of IL-12 from APCs, providing an indirect mechanism to inhibit IFN-γ production. Alteration of the ratio between IL-10 and IL-12 expression by APCs is probably a major regulatory point in the Th1/Th2 differentiation pathways.

Transforming Growth Factor-β as a Regulator of T Helper 1 and T Helper 2 Responses

TGF-β is a pleiotropic cytokine that is thought to be important in downregulating excessive proinflammatory responses in a variety of experimental mouse and human autoimmune diseases (354).

The role of TGF-β in the development of Th1 and Th2 cells is still not entirely clear. Initial mouse *in vitro* priming studies showed that TGF-β can induce (76,355) or inhibit (356) the induction of IFN-γ–producing cells, depending on the mouse strain used and the amount of IL-2 present in the priming culture (357). TGF-β also inhibited the differentiation of both IFN-γ– and IL-4–producing human T cells (72). *In vivo*, there is also evidence for multiple effects of TGF-β. In two experimental models of intracellular infection, TGF-β administration clearly inhibited the generation of Th1 responses (358,359). In one of these studies, it was also shown that TGF-β inhibited IL-12 production, further supporting a cross-regulatory role for TGF-β in the generation of Th1 cells (359). Induction of TGF-β–producing cells has also been shown to be important in suppressing inappropriate host responses that mediate autoimmune disease (360,361). Some of these inhibitory effects on Th1 responses may be due to inhibition of the effector stage, as TGF-β can inhibit both immediate and delayed hypersensitivity responses (362). However, endogenous TGF-β appeared to inhibit IL-4 production and enhance the protective Th1 response during *Candida albicans* infection (363). Thus, in these *in vivo* models, the presence of TGF-β mostly inhibits but can sometimes enhance Th1 responses. Overall, TGF-β has complex effects: It can inhibit Th2 differentiation and effector function, inhibit Th1 effector function, and either inhibit or enhance Th1 differentiation. TGF-β may thus be a general dampener of immune responses, consistent with its role in enhancing wound repair (364).

ROLE OF APOPTOSIS IN SELECTIVELY REGULATING T HELPER 1 AND T HELPER 2 EFFECTOR CELLS

The immune response must not only initiate a response against a potential pathogen, but also find a way to mitigate this response once it has completed its effector function. The ability to regulate T helper responses would be especially important with regard to Th1 cytokine production, since it has been shown in many *in vivo* models of both infectious and autoimmune disease that excessive and sustained Th1 cytokine production may provoke deleterious proinflammatory responses. One mechanism to regulate excessive cell activation that is central to all biology is the process of apoptosis. With regard to T cells, it has been shown that activation-induced apoptosis is mediated by interaction of Fas ligand (FasL) with its cognate receptor Fas. Th1 clones expressed high levels of FasL, while Th2 cells expressed only low levels (365), and Th1 cultures showed higher levels of activation-induced apoptosis, although Th2 cells could be killed in the presence of activated Th1 cells. Thus, the expression of FasL on Th1 cells may be an important mechanism in preventing continued expansion of a proinflammatory Th1 response.

DIFFERENTIATION OF CD8 T-CELL SUBSETS

Evidence for CD8 Cytokine Subsets

Human CD8 T cells producing low levels of IL-4 were found among a panel of T-cell clones (10), and higher levels of IL-4 were expressed by antigen-specific CD8 T cells from patients with lepromatous leprosy, the form associated with type 2 cytokine expression (43). CD8 clones with a full Th2-like cytokine pattern were isolated by mitogen stimulation from HIV-infected patients with Job's-like syndrome, which includes high levels of IgE (366).

Although many mouse CD8 T cells produced IFN-γ (367), and a set of mouse allospecific clones produced the Th1 set of cytokines (368), IL-4 can also be produced by mouse CD8 T cells. IL-4 production could be induced by treatment of mouse CD8 T cells with IL-4 (369), and PMA–ionomycin treatment of mouse CD8 T cells converted them into a noncytotoxic, CD8⁻ population that secreted IL-4 (370). Mouse CD8 cells secreting IL-4 and IL-5 were induced by stimulation of naive CD8 T cells in the presence of IL-4 (371), and clones of CD8 T cells expressing cytokine patterns similar to those of Th1 or Th2 cells were isolated after alloantigen stimulation of naive CD8 cells (257). In this chapter, the names *Tc1* and *Tc2* will be used for these two CD8 T-cell subsets. T1 and T2, or type 1 and type 2, CD8 T cells have also been used. Rat CD8 T cells can also be induced to differentiate into IL-4– and IL-5–secreting cells (372). Thus, in all three species, CD8 cells can produce either Th1-like or Th2-like patterns of cytokines, although CD8 cells are normally more likely to become Tc1 cells.

In addition to the identification of IL-4–secreting cells during AIDS and lepromatous leprosy, the existence of Tc2 cells has been confirmed in additional situations. Antipeptide CD8 T cells in the lung were induced to secrete IL-5 by the induction of a strong bystander CD4 Th2 response against a different antigen (373). Although Tc2-like cells clearly occur in these situations, spleen and lymph node CD8 cells display the Tc1 phenotype during most responses. In contrast, CD8 cells isolated from the normal human peritoneum show a substantial proportion of Tc2 cells, and CD8 T cells purified from mouse Peyer's Patches contained mRNA for Th1 as well as Th2 cytokines, raising the possibility that different subpopulations of CD8 cells may be found in different locations (374,375). Although the existence of IL-4–secreting CD8 T cells

has therefore been substantiated *in vivo* in several different systems, the functions of these cells *in vivo* are not yet understood.

Cytokine Regulation of Differentiation into Tc1 or Tc2 Cells

There are many similarities between CD4 and CD8 T-cell differentiation (257,371,376) (Figs. 7 and 8), although much less is known about the detailed requirements for CD8 T-cell differentiation. Naive CD8 T cells in the periphery are precursor cells that do not synthesize either Th1 or Th2 cytokine patterns when first activated (255,368). After antigen activation, the cells proliferate and differentiate within a few days, normally into the Tc1 phenotype. In contrast to CD4 cells, there appears to be a strong inherent bias for CD8 T cells to differentiate along the Tc1 pathway. IFN-γ or IL-12 enhances this preference (257,371). Differentiation into Tc2 cells requires the presence of IL-4, and normally also requires a strong Th2 environment or blockade of the effects of IFN-γ (Figs. 7 and 8). Thus, Tc2 cells may normally arise only during strongly biased type 2 responses *in vivo*, consistent with their identification mainly in such situations (43,366,373).

Other Influences on CD8 Differentiation

Many of the noncytokine influences on CD4 differentiation, such as antigen amount, costimulatory molecules, and different APC, have not yet been investigated thoroughly for CD8 T-cell differentiation. *In vitro*, spleen cells, dendritic cells, B-cell blasts, or a B-cell tumour, M12, can provide all necessary signals for cytokine-

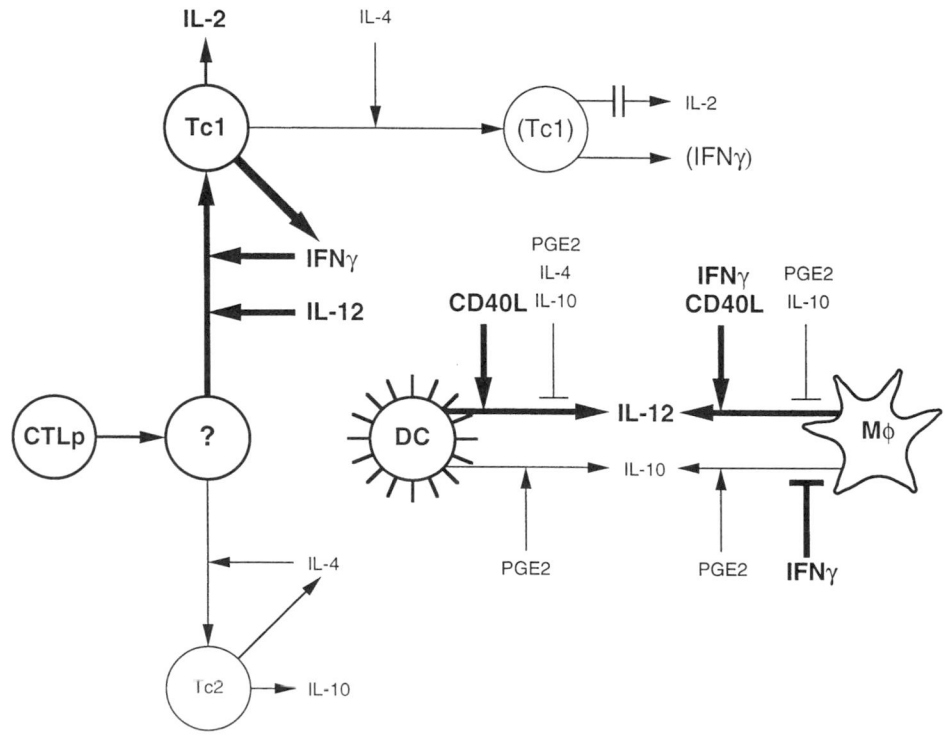

FIG. 7. Soluble factors enhancing the differentiation of CD8 Tc1 cells. *Heavy arrows* represent stimulatory effects, whereas *bars* represent inhibitory or blocking effects.

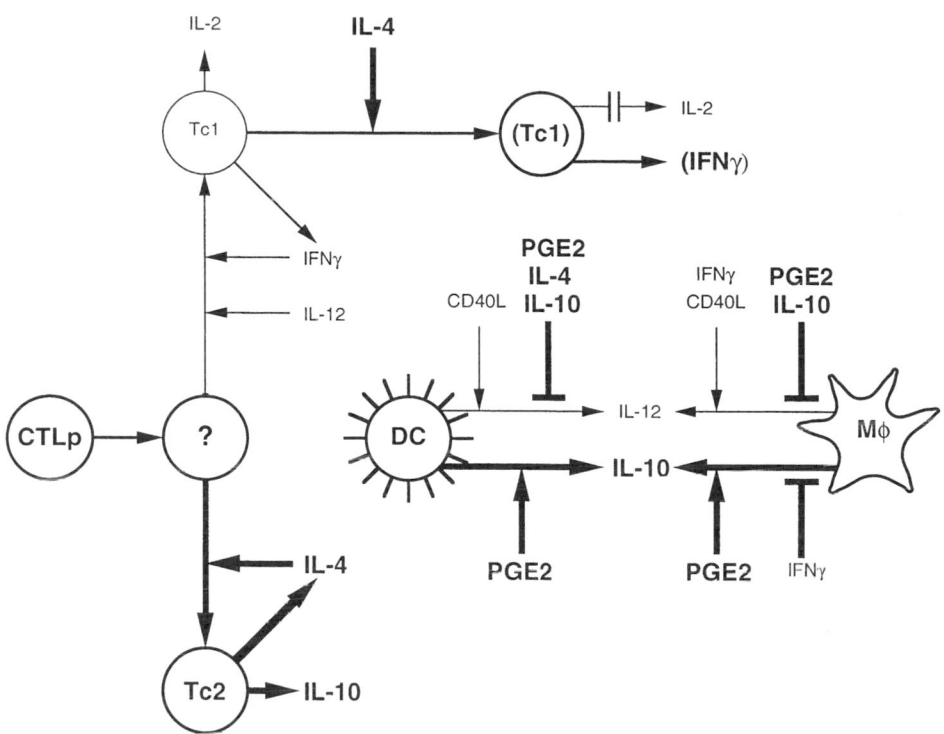

FIG. 8. Soluble factors enhancing the differentiation of CD8 Th2 cells.

driven differentiation of CD8 T cells into either Tc1 or Tc2 phenotypes (257,371).

Effector Functions of CD8 T-Cell Subsets

Both Tc1 and Tc2 cells are cytotoxic, and both use the perforin–granzyme killing pathway, as shown by the sensitivity of killing to a calcium chelating agent and the reduced cytotoxicity of Tc1 or Tc2 cells from perforin-deficient mice (377,378). Killing by Tc2 cells is less than that by Tc1 cells in some studies (366,374,377), although the cytotoxic ability of Tc1 and Tc2 cells depends on the growth conditions of the cells, and it is difficult to compare the two cell types directly. Although it is clear that the Tc1 subset also kills effectively by the FasL-mediated pathway, this pathway has been reported to be absent (377) or present (379) in Tc2 cells. Both Tc1 and Tc2 cells effectively kill activated B cells in the absence of perforin (379).

Tc2 cells can enhance B-cell antibody synthesis when stimulated by anti-CD3 antibodies (257,366,371,376). This probably represents bystander help for the B cells, as both Tc1 and Tc2 cells kill antigen-bearing targets, including B cells (379). In an allohelper system, Tc2 cells killed and did not help B cells, whereas the inclusion of anti-CD3 resulted in increased antibody synthesis and decreased killing. The cytokine pattern of Tc2 cells includes a number of B cell–stimulating cytokines, and after antigen activation, Tc2 cells express low levels of CD40L (376,379). Thus, Tc2 cells may contribute to an ongoing antibody response, but only by bystander activation, as cognate interaction would result in death of the B cell. This is consistent with the known antigen-processing pathways of B cells: Antigen captured by the B-cell surface antibody is processed and presented on MHC class II for presentation to CD4 cells, particularly Th2s, whereas antigen presented on class

I MHC to CD8 cells is normally derived from intracellular proteins, implying infection. Although a pathway for associating peptides from external antigens with MHC class I has been described (380), this may operate chiefly in phagocytes and has not yet been described in normal B cells.

Among CD4 T-cell subsets, Th1 cells induce DTH (5) and Th1 cytokines are associated with sites of DTH reactions (8,43). However, both Tc1 and Tc2 cells induced inflammatory reactions when allospecific CD8 cells were injected into mouse footpads (381). These reactions were similar in the kinetics of swelling, the numbers and types of infiltrating cells, and the extent of edema. However, cytokine expression *in vivo* during the reaction was quite distinct: IFN-γ was expressed only in Tc1 reactions, whereas IL-4 and IL-5 were present only in Tc2 reactions. The DTH reaction induced by Tc2 cells did not appear to be secondary to the killing of target cells, as Tc1 and Tc2 cells from perforin-deficient mice were also able to induce inflammation (381). Thus the Th2/Tc2 cytokine pattern can be associated with inflammatory reactions, as shown also by the injection of preactivated Th2 clones (382) and the stimulatory role of Th2 cytokines in granulomas induced by schistosome egg antigens (383).

Further Differentiation of Tc1 CD8 T Cells

After differentiation of naive precursor CD8 T cells into Tc1 effector cells producing IFN-γ, further differentiation is possible. Activation under conditions of low costimulation, or treatment with IL-4, converts Tc1 cells into a phenotype that is still cytotoxic but no longer synthesizes IL-2 (384–386). IL-4 induces the IL-2-deficient state in the presence or absence of antigen stimulation or APC. These IL-2-deficient Tc1 cells retain their ability to kill antigen-bearing targets by either the perforin or Fas pathways, but they are no longer capable of sustaining proliferation by autocrine production of IL-2. The synthesis of other cytokines in the aforementioned studies was also impaired, although the loss in IL-2 production was the most severe. Although the deficiency in cytokine synthesis was also expressed *in vivo,* both normal and IL-4–treated Tc1 cells induced similar inflammatory reactions. This phenotype of Tc1 cells appeared to be irreversible and may represent another way in which Th1/Tc1 responses are cross-regulated by Th2/Tc2 responses. Exposure of Tc1 cells to IL-4 would be expected to prevent future independent proliferation but allow continued short-term effector functions, and even proliferation, in the presence of an ongoing immune response that would supply growth factors.

CONCLUSION

Overall, the regulation of T-cell differentiation is very complex, including many positive and negative signals, with different accessory cell types playing opposite roles, depending on their environment. It is surprising that so many positive-feedback loops have been identified, either enhancing like responses or inhibiting opposite responses. This is consistent with the strong polarization seen in some chronic infections, but additional negative-feedback or homeostatic mechanisms may await discovery, these may help to explain many immune responses that comprise a more mixed cytokine pattern.

REFERENCES

1. Mosmann TR, Cherwinski H, Bond MW, Giedlin MA, Coffman RL. Two types of murine helper T-cell clone. I. Definition according to profiles of lymphokine activities and secreted proteins. *J Immunol* 1986;136:2348–2357.
2. Cherwinski HM, Schumacher JH, Brown KD, Mosmann TR. Two types of mouse helper T cell clone. III. Further differences in lymphokine synthesis between Th1 and Th2 clones revealed by RNA hybridization, functionally monospecific bioassays, and monoclonal antibodies. *J Exp Med* 1987;166:1229–1244.
3. van Snick J, Goethals A, Renauld J-C, et al. Cloning and characterization of a cDNA for a new mouse T cell growth factor (P40). *J Exp Med* 1989;169:363–368.
4. Fiorentino DF, Bond MW, Mosmann TR. Two types of mouse T helper cell. IV. Th2 clones secrete a factor that inhibits cytokine production by Th1 clones. *J Exp Med* 1989;170:2081–2095.
5. Cher DJ, Mosmann TR. Two types of murine helper T cell clone. II. Delayed-type hypersensitivity is mediated by TH1 clones. *J Immunol* 1987;138:3688–3694.
6. Mosmann TR, Coffman RL. TH1 and TH2 cells: different patterns of lymphokine secretion lead to different functional properties. *Ann Rev Immunol* 1989;7:145–173.
7. Yamamura M, Uyemura K, Deans RJ, et al. Defining protective responses to pathogens: cytokine profiles in leprosy lesions. *Science* 1991;254:277–279.
8. Tsicopoulos A, Hamid Q, Varney V, et al. Preferential messenger RNA expression of Th1-type cells (IFN-gamma+, IL-2+) in classical delayed-type (tuberculin) hypersensitivity reactions in human skin. *J Immunol* 1992;148:2058–2061.
9. Seder RA, Paul WE. Acquisition of lymphokine-producing phenotype by CD4+ T cells. *Annu Rev Immunol* 1994;12:635–673.
10. Paliard X, de Waal Malefijt R, Yssel H, et al. Simultaneous production of IL-2, IL-4, and IFN-gamma by activated human CD4+ and CD8+ T cell clones. *J Immunol* 1988;141:849–855.
11. Maggi E, Del Prete G, Macchia D, et al. Profiles of lymphokine activities and helper function for IgE in human T cell clones. *Eur J Immunol* 1988;18:1045–1050.
12. Umetsu DT, Jabara HH, DeKruyff RH, Abbas AK, Abrams JS, Geha RS. Functional heterogeneity among human inducer T cell clones. *J Immunol* 1988;140:4211–4216.
13. Wierenga EA, Snoek M, de Groot C, et al. Evidence for compartmentalization of functional subsets of CD2+ T lymphocytes in atopic patients. *J Immunol* 1990;144:4651–4656.
14. Del Prete GF, De Carli M, Mastromauro C, et al. Purified protein derivative of Mycobacterium tuberculosis and excretory-secretory antigen(s) of Toxocara canis expand in vitro human T cells with stable and opposite (type 1 T helper or type 2 T helper) profile of cytokine production. *J Clin Invest* 1991;88:346–350.
15. Haanen JB, de Waal Malefijt R, Res PC, et al. Selection of a human T helper type 1-like T cell subset by mycobacteria. *J Exp Med* 1991;174:583–592.
16. Firestein GS, Roeder WD, Laxer JA, et al. A new murine CD4+ T cell subset with an unrestricted cytokine profile. *J Immunol* 1989;143:518–525.
17. Street NE, Schumacher JH, Fong TA, et al. Heterogeneity of mouse helper T cells: evidence from bulk cultures and limiting dilution cloning for precursors of Th1 and Th2 cells. *J Immunol* 1990;144:1629–1639.
18. Bucy RP, Panoskaltsis-Mortari A, Huang GQ, et al. Heterogeneity of single cell cytokine gene expression in clonal T cell populations. *J Exp Med* 1994;180:1251–1262.
19. Kelso A, Groves P, Troutt AB, Francis K. Evidence for the stochastic acquisition of cytokine profile by CD4+ T cells activated in a T helper type 2-like response in vivo. *Eur J Immunol* 1995;25:1168–1175.
20. Kelso A. Th1 and Th2 subsets: paradigms lost?. *Immunol Today* 1995;16:374–379.
21. Mosmann TR, Sad S. The expanding universe of T cell subsets- Th1, Th2 and more. *Immunol Today* 1996;17:138–146.
22. Swain SL, Weinberg AD, English M, Huston G. IL-4 Directs the development of Th2-like helper effectors. *J Immunol* 1990;145:3796–3806.
23. Hsieh C-S, Heimberger AB, Gold JS, O'Garra A, Murphy KM. Differential regulation of T helper phenotype development by interleukins 4 and 10 in an alpha beta T-cell-receptor transgenic system. *Proc Natl Acad Sci USA* 1992;89:6065–6069.
24. Le Gros G, Ben Sasson SZ, Seder R, Finkelman FD, Paul WE. Generation of interleukin-4 (IL-4)-producing cells in vivo and in vitro—IL-2 and IL-4 are required for in vitro generation of IL-4-producing cells. *J Exp Med* 1990;172:921–929.
25. Seder RA, Paul WE, Davis MM, Fazekas de St Groth B. The presence of interleukin 4 during in vitro priming determines the lymphokine-producing potential of CD4+ T cells from T cell receptor transgenic mice. *J Exp Med* 1992;176:1091–1098.
26. Bucy RP, Karr L, Huang GQ, et al. Single cell analysis of cytokine gene coexpression during CD4+ T-cell phenotype development. *Proc Natl Acad Sci USA* 1995;92:7565–7569.
27. Assenmacher M, Schmitz J, Radbruch A. Flow cytometric determination of cytokines in activated murine T helper lymphocytes: expression of interleukin-10 in interferon-gamma and in interleukin-4-expressing cells. *Eur J Immunol* 1994;24:1097–1101.
28. Openshaw P, Murphy EE, Hosken NA, et al. Heterogeneity of intracellular cytokine synthesis at the single-cell level in polarized T helper 1 and T helper 2 populations. *J Exp Med* 1995;182:1357–1367.
29. Sornasse T, Larenas PV, Davis KA, de Vries JE, Yssel H. Differentiation and stability of T helper 1 and 2 cells derived from naive human neonatal CD4+ T cells, analyzed at the single-cell level. *J Exp Med* 1996;184:473–483.
30. Scott P, Pearce E, Cheever AW, Coffman RL, Sher A. Role of cytokines and CD4+ T-cell subsets in the regulation of parasite immunity and disease. *Immunol Rev* 1989;112:161–182.
31. Reiner SL, Locksley RM. The regulation of immunity to Leishmania major. *Annu Rev Immunol* 1995;13:151–177.
32. Parronchi P, Macchia D, Piccinni MP, et al. Allergen- and bacterial antigen-specific T-cell clones established from atopic donors show a different profile of cytokine production. *Proc Natl Acad Sci USA* 1991;88:4538–4542.
33. Romagnani S. Lymphokine production by human T cells in disease states. *Annu Rev Immunol* 1994;12:227–257.
34. Liblau RS, Singer SM, McDevitt HO. Th1 and Th2 CD4+ T cells in the pathogenesis of organ-specific autoimmune diseases. *Immunol Today* 1995;16:34–38.
35. Lafaille JJ, Van de Keere F, Hsu AL, et al. Myelin basic protein specific T helper 2 (Th2) cells cause experimental autoimmune encephalomyelitis in immunodeficient hosts rather than protect them from the disease. *J Exp Med* 1997;186:307–312.
36. Pakala SV, Kurrer MO, Katz JD. T helper 2 (Th2) T cells induce acute pancreatitis and diabetes in immune-compromised nonobese diabetic (NOD) mice. *J Exp Med* 1997;186:299–306.
37. Kroemer G, Hirsch F, Gonzalez-Garcia A, Martinez C. Differential involvement of Th1 and Th2 cytokines in autoimmune diseases. *Autoimmunity* 1996;24:25–33.
38. Goldman M, Druet P, Gleichmann E. TH2 cells in systemic autoimmunity: insights from allogeneic diseases and chemically-induced autoimmunity. *Immunol Today* 1991;12:223–227.
39. Gillespie KM, Saoudi A, Kuhn J, et al. Th1/Th2 cytokine gene expression after mercuric chloride in susceptible and resistant rat strains. *Eur J Immunol* 1996;26:2388–2392.
40. Richaud-Patin Y, Alcocer-Varela J, Llorente L. High levels of TH2 cytokine gene expression in systemic lupus erythematosus. *Rev Invest Clin* 1995;47:267–272.
41. Nakajima A, Hirose S, Yagita H, Okumura K. Roles of IL-4 and IL-12 in the development of lupus in NZB/W F1 mice. *J Immunol* 1997;158:1466–1472.
42. Takahashi S, Fossati L, Iwamoto M, et al. Imbalance towards Th1 predominance is associated with acceleration of lupus-like autoimmune syndrome in MRL mice. *J Clin Invest* 1996;97:1597–1604.
43. Salgame P, Abrams JS, Clayberger C, et al. Differing lymphokine profiles of functional subsets of human CD4 and CD8 T cell clones. *Science* 1991;254:279–282.
44. de Waal Malefyt R, Abrams J, Bennett B, Figdor CG, de Vries JE. Interleukin 10 (IL-10) inhibits cytokine synthesis by human monocytes: an autoregulatory role of IL-10 produced by monocytes. *J Exp Med* 1991;174:1209–1220.

45. O'Garra A, Stapleton G, Dhar V, et al. Production of cytokines by mouse B cells: B lymphomas and normal B cells produce interleukin 10. *Int Immunol* 1990;2: 821–832.

46. Gerosa F, Paganin C, Peritt D, et al. Interleukin-12 primes human CD4 and CD8 T cell clones for high production of both interferon-gamma and interleukin-10. *J Exp Med* 1996;183:2559–2569.

47. Jeannin P, Delneste Y, Seveso M, Life P, Bonnefoy JY. IL-12 synergizes with IL-2 and other stimuli in inducing IL-10 production by human T cells. *J Immunol* 1996;156:3159–3165.

48. Windhagen A, Anderson DE, Carrizosa A, Williams RE, Hafler DA. IL-12 induces human T cells secreting IL-10 with IFN-gamma. *J Immunol* 1996;157: 1127–1131.

49. Yssel H, Johnson KE, Schneider PV, et al. T cell activation-inducing epitopes of the house dust mite allergen Der p I. Proliferation and lymphokine production patterns by Der p I-specific CD4+ T cell clones. *J Immunol* 1992;148:738–745.

50. Li Y, Richards D, Noble A, Kemeny DM. Cytokine production by highly purified human CD8+ T cells. *Int Arch Allergy Immunol* 1995;107:354–355.

51. Svetic A, Jian YC, Lu P, Finkelman FD, Gause WC. Brucella abortus induces a novel cytokine gene expression pattern characterized by elevated IL-10 and IFN-gamma in CD4+ T cells. *Int Immunol* 1993;5:877–883.

52. Chen Y, Kuchroo VK, Inobe J, Hafler DA, Weiner HL. Regulatory T cell clones induced by oral tolerance: suppression of autoimmune encephalomyelitis. *Science* 1994;265:1237–1240.

53. Fukaura H, Kent SC, Pietrusewicz MJ, Khoury SJ, Weiner HL, Hafler DA. Induction of circulating myelin basic protein and proteolipid protein-specific transforming growth factor-beta1-secreting Th3 T cells by oral administration of myelin in multiple sclerosis patients. *J Clin Invest* 1996;98:70–77.

54. Luqman M, Johnson P, Trowbridge I, Bottomly K. Differential expression of the alternatively spliced exons of murine CD45 in Th1 and Th2 cell clones. *Eur J Immunol* 1991;21:17–22.

55. Lee WT, Yin XM, Vitetta ES. Functional and ontogenetic analysis of murine CD45Rhi and CD45Rlo CD4+ T cells. *J Immunol* 1990;144:3288–3295.

56. Elson LH, Shaw S, Van Lier RA, Nutman TB. T cell subpopulation phenotypes in filarial infections: CD27 negativity defines a population greatly enriched for Th2 cells. *Int Immunol* 1994;6:1003–1009.

57. Elson LH, Nutman TB, Metcalfe DD, Prussin C. Flow cytometric analysis for cytokine production identifies T helper 1, T helper 2, and T helper 0 cells within the human CD4+CD27- lymphocyte subpopulation. *J Immunol* 1995;154: 4294–4301.

58. Chilosi M, Facchetti F, Notarangelo LD, et al. CD30 cell expression and abnormal soluble CD30 serum accumulation in Omenn's syndrome: evidence for a T helper 2-mediated condition. *Eur J Immunol* 1996;26:329–334.

59. Bengtsson A, Johansson C, Linder MT, Hallden G, van der Ploeg I, Scheynius A. Not only Th2 cells but also Th1 and Th0 cells express CD30 after activation. *J Leukoc Biol* 1995;58:683–689.

60. Del Prete G, De Carli M, D'Elios MM, et al. CD30-mediated signaling promotes the development of human T helper type 2-like T cells. *J Exp Med* 1995;182: 1655–1661.

61. Hamann D, Hilkens CM, Grogan JL, et al. CD30 expression does not discriminate between human Th1- and Th2-type T cells. *J Immunol* 1996;156: 1387–1391.

62. Demeure CE, Byun DG, Yang LP, Vezzio N, Delespesse G. CD31 (PECAM-1) is a differentiation antigen lost during human CD4 T-cell maturation into Th1 or Th2 effector cells. *Immunology* 1996;88:110–115.

63. Nakamura T, Lee RK, Nam SY, et al. Reciprocal regulation of CD30 expression on CD4+ T cells by IL-4 and IFN-gamma. *J Immunol* 1997;158:2090–2098.

64. Cocks BG, Chang CC, Carballido JM, Yssel H, de Vries JE, Aversa G. A novel receptor involved in T-cell activation. *Nature* 1995;376:260–263.

65. Szabo SJ, Dighe AS, Gubler U, Murphy KM. Regulation of the interleukin (IL)-12R beta 2 subunit expression in developing T helper 1 (Th1) and Th2 cells. *J Exp Med* 1997;185:817–824.

66. Rogge L, Barberis-Maino L, Biffi M, et al. Selective expression of an interleukin-12 receptor component by human T helper 1 cells. *J Exp Med* 1997;185: 825–831.

67. Pernis A, Gupta S, Gollob KJ, et al. Lack of interferon gamma receptor beta chain and the prevention of interferon gamma signaling in TH1 cells. *Science* 1995;269:245–247.

68. Szabo SJ, Jacobson NG, Dighe AS, Gubler U, Murphy KM. Developmental commitment to the Th2 lineage by extinction of IL-12 signaling. *Immunity* 1995;2: 665–675.

69. Groux H, Sornasse T, Cottrez F, et al. Induction of human T helper cell type 1 differentiation results in loss of IFN-gamma receptor beta-chain expression. *J Immunol* 1997;158:5627–5631.

70. Bach EA, Szabo SJ, Dighe AS, et al. Ligand-induced autoregulation of IFN-gamma receptor beta chain expression in T helper cell subsets. *Science* 1995; 270:1215–1218.

71. Guler ML, Jacobson NG, Gubler U, Murphy KM. T cell genetic background determines maintenance of IL-12 signaling: effects on BALB/c and B10.D2 T helper cell type 1 phenotype development. *J Immunol* 1997;159:1767–1774.

72. Sallusto F, Mackay CR, Lanzavecchia A. Selective expression of the Eotaxin receptor CCR3 by human T helper 2 cells. *Science* 1997;277:2005–2007.

73. Hsieh CS, Heimberger AB, Gold JS, O'Garra A, Murphy KM. Differential regulation of T helper phenotype development by interleukins 4 and 10 in an alpha

74. Reiner SL, Wang Z-E, Hatam F, Scott P, Locksley RM. T$_{H}$1 and T$_{H}$2 cell antigen receptors in experimental leishmaniasis. *Science* 1993;259:1457–1460.

75. Rocken M, Saurat JH, Hauser C. A common precursor for CD4+ T cells producing IL-2 or IL-4. *J Immunol* 1992;148:1031–1036.

76. Sad S, Mosmann TR. Single IL-2-secreting precursor CD4 T cell can develop into either Th1 or Th2 cytokine secretion phenotype. *J Immunol* 1994;153: 3514–3522.

77. Kamogawa Y, Minasi LA, Carding SR, Bottomly K, Flavell RA. The relationship of IL-4- and IFN gamma-producing T cells studied by lineage ablation of IL-4-producing cells. *Cell* 1993;75:985–995.

78. Kobayashi M, Fitz L, Ryan M, et al. Identification and purification of natural killer cell stimulatory factor (NKSF), a cytokine with multiple biologic effects on human lymphocytes. *J Exp Med* 1989;170:827–845.

79. Wolf SF, Temple PA, Kobayashi M, et al. Cloning of cDNA for natural killer cell stimulatory factor, a heterodimeric cytokine with multiple biologic effects on T and natural killer cells. *J Immunol* 1991;146:3074–3081.

80. Chan SH, Perussia B, Gupta JW, et al. Induction of interferon gamma production by natural killer cell stimulatory factor: characterization of the responder cells and synergy with other inducers. *J Exp Med* 1991;173:869–879.

81. Hsieh CS, Macatonia SE, Tripp CS, Wolf SF, O'Garra A, Murphy KM. Development of TH1 CD4+ T cells through IL-12 produced by Listeria-induced macrophages. *Science* 1993;260:547–549.

82. Seder RA, Gazzinelli R, Sher A, Paul WE. Interleukin 12 acts directly on CD4+ T cells to enhance priming for interferon gamma production and diminishes interleukin 4 inhibition of such priming. *Proc Natl Acad Sci USA* 1993;90: 10188–10192.

83. Manetti R, Parronchi P, Giudizi MG, et al. Natural killer cell stimulatory factor (interleukin 12 [IL-12]) induces T helper type 1 (Th1)-specific immune responses and inhibits the development of IL-4-producing Th cells. *J Exp Med* 1993;177:1199–1204.

84. Schmitt E, Hoehn P, Germann T, Rude E. Differential effects of interleukin-12 on the development of naive mouse CD4+ T cells. *Eur J Immunol* 1994;24: 343–347.

85. Manetti R, Gerosa F, Giudizi MG, et al. Interleukin 12 induces stable priming for interferon gamma (IFN-gamma) production during differentiation of human T helper (Th) cells and transient IFN-gamma production in established Th2 cell clones. *J Exp Med* 1994;179:1273–1283.

86. Magram J, Connaughton SE, Warrier RR, et al. IL-12-deficient mice are defective in IFN gamma production and type 1 cytokine responses. *Immunity* 1996;4: 471–481.

87. Kaplan MH, Sun YL, Hoey T, Grusby MJ. Impaired IL-12 responses and enhanced development of Th2 cells in Stat4-deficient mice. *Nature* 1996;382: 174–177.

88. Thierfelder WE, van Deursen JM, Yamamoto K, et al. Requirement for Stat4 in interleukin-12-mediated responses of natural killer and T cells. *Nature* 1996;382: 171–174.

89. Reiner SL, Seder RA. T helper cell differentiation in immune response. *Curr Opin Immunol* 1995;7:360–366.

90. Seder RA, Kelsall BL, Jankovic D. Differential roles for IL-12 in the maintenance of immune responses in infectious versus autoimmune disease. *J Immunol* 1996;157:2745–2748.

91. Fernandez-Botran R, Sanders VM, Mosmann TR, Vitetta ES. Lymphokine-mediated regulation of the proliferative response of clones of T helper 1 and T helper 2 cells. *J Exp Med* 1988;168:543–558.

92. Gajewski TF, Fitch FW. Anti-proliferative effect of IFN-gamma in immune regulation. I. IFN-gamma inhibits the proliferation of Th2 but not Th1 murine helper T lymphocyte clones. *J Immunol* 1988;140:4245–4252.

93. Maggi E, Parronchi P, Manetti R, et al. Reciprocal regulatory effects of IFN-gamma and IL4 on the in vitro development of human TH1 and TH2 clones. *J Immunol* 1992;148:2142–2147.

94. Bradley LM, Dalton DK, Croft M. A direct role for IFN-gamma in regulation of Th1 cell development. *J Immunol* 1996;157:1350–1358.

95. Hsieh CS, Macatonia SE, O'Garra A, Murphy KM. Pathogen-induced Th1 phenotype development in CD4+ alpha beta-TCR transgenic T cells is macrophage dependent. *Int Immunol* 1993;5:371–382.

96. Macatonia SE, Hsieh C-S, Murphy KM, O'Garra A. Dendritic cells and macrophages are required for Th1 development of CD4+ T cells from αβ transgenic mice: IL12 substitution for macrophages to stimulate IFNγ production is IFNγ-dependent. *Int Immunol* 1993;5:1119–1128.

97. Wenner CA, Guler ML, Macatonia SE, O'Garra A, Murphy KM. Roles of IFN-gamma and IFN-alpha in IL-12-induced T helper cell-1 development. *J Immunol* 1996;156:1442–1447.

98. Ma X, Chow JM, Gri G, et al. The interleukin 12 p40 gene promoter is primed by interferon gamma in monocytic cells. *J Exp Med* 1996;183:147–157.

99. Hayes MP, Wang J, Norcross MA. Regulation of interleukin-12 expression in human monocytes: selective priming by interferon-gamma of lipopolysaccharide-inducible p35 and p40 genes. *Blood* 1995;86:646–650.

100. Swihart K, Fruth U, Messmer N, et al. Mice from a genetically resistant background lacking the interferon gamma receptor are susceptible to infection with Leishmania major but mount a polarized T helper cell 1-type CD4+ T cell response. *J Exp Med* 1995;181:961–971.

101. Schijns VE, Haagmans BL, Rijke EO, Huang S, Aguet M, Horzinek MC. IFN-gamma receptor-deficient mice generate antiviral Th1-characteristic cytokine profiles but altered antibody responses. *J Immunol* 1994;153:2029–2037.

102. Szalay G, Ladel CH, Blum C, Kaufmann SH. IL-4 neutralization or TNF-alpha treatment ameliorate disease by an intracellular pathogen in IFN-gamma receptor-deficient mice. *J Immunol* 1996;157:4746–4750.

103. Parronchi P, De Carli M, Manetti R, et al. IL-4 and IFN (alpha and gamma) exert opposite regulatory effects on the development of cytolytic potential by Th1 or Th2 human T cell clones. *J Immunol* 1992;149:2977–2983.

104. Brinkmann V, Geiger T, Alkan S, Heusser CH. Interferon alpha increases the frequency of interferon gamma-producing human CD4+ T cells. *J Exp Med* 1993;178:1655–1663.

105. Manetti R, Annunziato F, Tomasevic L, et al. Polyinosinic acid: polycytidylic acid promotes T helper type 1-specific immune responses by stimulating macrophage production of interferon-alpha and interleukin-12. *Eur J Immunol* 1995;25:2656–2660.

106. Cousens LP, Orange JS, Su HC, Biron CA. Interferon-alpha/beta inhibition of interleukin 12 and interferon-gamma production in vitro and endogenously during viral infection. *Proc Natl Acad Sci USA* 1997;94:634–639.

107. Finkelman FD, Svetic A, Gresser I, et al. Regulation by interferon alpha of immunoglobulin isotype selection and lymphokine production in mice. *J Exp Med* 1991;174:1179–1188.

108. Okamura H, Tsutsi H, Komatsu T, et al. Cloning of a new cytokine that induces IFN-gamma production by T cells. *Nature* 1995;378:88–91.

109. Ahn HJ, Maruo S, Tomura M, et al. A mechanism underlying synergy between IL-12 and IFN-gamma-inducing factor in enhanced production of IFN-gamma. *J Immunol* 1997;159:2125–2131.

110. Swain SL, McKenzie DT, Weinberg AD, Hancock W. Characterization of T helper 1 and 2 cell subsets in normal mice. Helper T cells responsible for IL-4 and IL-5 production are present as precursors that require priming before they develop into lymphokine-secreting cells. *J Immunol* 1988;141:3445–3455.

111. Betz M, Fox BS. Regulation and development of cytochrome C-specific Il-4-producing T-cells. *J Immunol* 1990;145:1046–1052.

112. Kuhn R, Rajewsky K, Muller W. Generation and analysis of interleukin-4 deficient mice. *Science* 1991;254:707–710.

113. Kopf M, Le Gros G, Bachmann M, Lamers MC, Bluethmann H, Köhler G. Disruption of the murine IL-4 gene blocks Th2 cytokine responses. *Nature* 1993;362:245–248.

114. Kaplan MH, Schindler U, Smiley ST, Grusby MJ. Stat6 is required for mediating responses to IL-4 and for development of Th2 cells. *Immunity* 1996;4:313–319.

115. Takeda K, Tanaka T, Shi W, et al. Essential role of Stat6 in IL-4 signalling. *Nature* 1996;380:627–630.

116. Shimoda K, van Deursen J, Sangster MY, et al. Lack of IL-4-induced Th2 response and IgE class switching in mice with disrupted Stat6 gene. *Nature* 1996;380:630–633.

117. Noben-Trauth N, Shultz LD, Brombacher F, Urban JF Jr, Paul WE. An Interleukin 4 (IL-4)-independent pathway for CD4+ T cell IL-4 production is revealed in IL-4 receptor-deficient mice. *Proc Natl Acad Sci USA* 1997;94:10838–10843.

118. Demeure CE, Wu CY, Shu U, et al. In vitro maturation of human neonatal CD4 T lymphocytes. II. Cytokines present at priming modulate the development of lymphokine production. *J Immunol* 1994;152:4775–4782.

119. Seder RA, Germain RN, Linsley PS, Paul WE. CD28-mediated costimulation of interleukin 2 (IL-2) production plays a critical role in T cell priming for IL-4 and interferon gamma production. *J Exp Med* 1994;179:299–304.

120. Heinzel FP, Rerko RM, Hatam F, Locksley RM. IL-2 is necessary for the progression of leishmaniasis in susceptible murine hosts. *J Immunol* 1993;150:3924–3931.

121. Kundig TM, Schorle H, Bachmann MF, Hengartner H, Zinkernagel RM, Horak I. Immune responses in interleukin-2-deficient mice. *Science* 1993;262:1059–1061.

122. Suzuki H, Kundig TM, Furlonger C, et al. Deregulated T cell activation and autoimmunity in mice lacking interleukin-2 receptor beta. *Science* 1995;268:1472–1476.

123. Ehrhardt RO, Ludviksson BR, Gray B, Neurath M, Strober W. Induction and prevention of colonic inflammation in IL-2-deficient mice. *J Immunol* 1997;158:566–573.

124. Rincon M, Anguita J, Nakamura T, Fikrig E, Flavell RA. Interleukin (IL)-6 directs the differentiation of IL-4-producing CD4+ T cells. *J Exp Med* 1997;185:461–469.

125. Kurt-Jones EA, Hamberg S, Ohara J, Paul WE, Abbas AK. Heterogeneity of helper/inducer T lymphocytes. I. Lymphokine production and lymphokine responsiveness. *J Exp Med* 1987;166:1774–1787.

126. Greenbaum LA, Horowitz JB, Woods A, Pasqualini T, Reich EP, Bottomly K. Autocrine growth of CD4+ T cells. Differential effects of IL-1 on helper and inflammatory T cells. *J Immunol* 1988;140:1555–1560.

127. Abbas AK, Williams ME, Burstein HJ, Chang TL, Bossu P, Lichtman AH. Activation and functions of CD4+ T-cell subsets. *Immunol Rev* 1991;123:5–22.

128. Manetti R, Barak V, Piccinni MP, et al. Interleukin-1 favours the in vitro development of type 2 T helper (Th2) human T-cell clones. *Res Immunol* 1994;145:93–100.

129. Kalinski P, Hilkens CM, Wierenga EA, et al. Functional maturation of human naive T helper cells in the absence of accessory cells. Generation of IL-4-producing T helper cells does not require exogenous IL-4. *J Immunol* 1995;154:3753–3760.

130. Linsley PS, Ledbetter JA. The role of the CD28 receptor during T cell responses to antigen. *Annu Rev Immunol* 1993;11:191–212.

131. Chambers CA, Krummel MF, Boitel B, et al. The role of CTLA-4 in the regulation and initiation of T-cell responses. *Immunol Rev* 1996;153:27–46.

132. Hathcock KS, Laszlo G, Pucillo C, Linsley P, Hodes RJ. Comparative analysis of B7-1 and B7-2 costimulatory ligands: expression and function. *J Exp Med* 1994;180:631–640.

133. Inaba K, Witmer-Pack M, Inaba M, et al. The tissue distribution of the B7-2 costimulator in mice: abundant expression on dendritic cells in situ and during maturation in vitro. *J Exp Med* 1994;180:1849–1860.

134. Kuchroo VK, Das MP, Brown JA, et al. B7-1 and B7-2 costimulatory molecules activate differentially the Th1/Th2 developmental pathways: application to autoimmune disease therapy. *Cell* 1995;80:707–718.

135. Freeman GJ, Boussiotis VA, Anumanthan A, et al. B7-1 and B7-2 do not deliver identical costimulatory signals, since B7-2 but not B7-1 preferentially costimulates the initial production of IL-4. *Immunity* 1995;2:523–532.

136. Lanier LL, O'Fallon S, Somoza C, et al. CD80 (B7) and CD86 (B70) provide similar costimulatory signals for T cell proliferation, cytokine production, and generation of CTL. *J Immunol* 1995;154:97–105.

137. Natesan M, Razi-Wolf Z, Reiser H. Costimulation of IL-4 production by murine B7-1 and B7-2 molecules. *J Immunol* 1996;156:2783–2791.

138. Levine BL, Ueda Y, Craighead N, Huang ML, June CH. CD28 ligands CD80 (B7-1) and CD86 (B7-2) induce long-term autocrine growth of CD4+ T cells and induce similar patterns of cytokine secretion in vitro. *Int Immunol* 1995;7:891–904.

139. Schweitzer AN, Borriello F, Wong RC, Abbas AK, Sharpe AH. Role of costimulators in T cell differentiation: studies using antigen-presenting cells lacking expression of CD80 or CD86. *J Immunol* 1997;158:2713–2722.

140. Greenwald RJ, Lu P, Halvorson MJ, et al. Effects of blocking B7-1 and B7-2 interactions during a type 2 in vivo immune response. *J Immunol* 1997;158:4088–4096.

141. Ghiotto-Ragueneau M, Battifora M, Truneh A, Waterfield MD, Olive D. Comparison of CD28-B7.1 and B7.2 functional interaction in resting human T cells: phosphatidylinositol 3-kinase association to CD28 and cytokine production. *Eur J Immunol* 1996;26:34–41.

142. Subramanian G, Kazura JW, Pearlman E, Jia X, Malhotra I, King CL. B7-2 requirement for helminth-induced granuloma formation and CD4 type 2 T helper cell cytokine expression. *J Immunol* 1997;158:5914–5920.

143. Lu P, Zhou X, Chen SJ, et al. CTLA-4 ligands are required to induce an in vivo interleukin 4 response to a gastrointestinal nematode parasite. *J Exp Med* 1994;180:693–698.

144. Corry DB, Reiner SL, Linsley PS, Locksley RM. Differential effects of blockade of CD28-B7 on the development of Th1 or Th2 effector cells in experimental leishmaniasis. *J Immunol* 1994;153:4142–4148.

145. Lu P, Zhou XD, Chen SJ, et al. Requirement of CTLA-4 counter receptors for IL-4 but not IL-10 elevations during a primary systemic in vivo immune response. *J Immunol* 1995;154:1078–1087.

146. McKnight AJ, Perez VL, Shea CM, Gray GS, Abbas AK. Costimulator dependence of lymphokine secretion by naive and activated CD4+ T lymphocytes from TCR transgenic mice. *J Immunol* 1994;152:5220–5225.

147. Murphy EE, Terres G, Macatonia SE, et al. B7 and interleukin 12 cooperate for proliferation and interferon gamma production by mouse T helper clones that are unresponsive to B7 costimulation. *J Exp Med* 1994;180:223–231.

148. Sayegh MH, Akalin E, Hancock WW, et al. CD28-B7 blockade after alloantigenic challenge in vivo inhibits Th1 cytokines but spares Th2. *J Exp Med* 1995;181:1869–1874.

149. Thompson CB. Distinct roles for the costimulatory ligands B7-1 and B7-2 in T helper cell differentiation? *Cell* 1995;81:979–982.

150. Lenschow DJ, Walunas TL, Bluestone JA. CD28/B7 system of T cell costimulation. *Annu Rev Immunol* 1996;14:233–258.

151. Brinkmann V, Kinzel B, Kristofic C. TCR-independent activation of human CD4+ 45RO- T cells by anti-CD28 plus IL-2: induction of clonal expansion and priming for a Th2 phenotype. *J Immunol* 1996;156:4100–4106.

152. King CL, Stupi RJ, Craighead N, June CH, Thyphronitis G. CD28 activation promotes Th2 subset differentiation by human CD4+ cells. *Eur J Immunol* 1995;25:587–595.

153. Yang LP, Demeure CE, Byun DG, Vezzio N, Delespesse G. Maturation of neonatal human CD4 T cells: III. Role of B7 co-stimulation at priming. *Int Immunol* 1995;7:1987–1993.

154. Rulifson IC, Sperling AI, Fields PE, Fitch FW, Bluestone JA. CD28 costimulation promotes the production of Th2 cytokines. *J Immunol* 1997;158:658–665.

155. Lenschow DJ, Herold KC, Rhee L, et al. CD28/B7 regulation of Th1 and Th2 subsets in the development of autoimmune diabetes. *Immunity* 1996;5:285–293.

156. Kuiper HM, De Jong R, Brouwer M, Lammers K, Wijdenes J, Van Lier RA. Influence of CD28 co-stimulation on cytokine production is mainly regulated via interleukin-2. *Immunology* 1994;83:38–44.

157. Harada Y, Watanabe S, Yssel H, Arai K. Factors affecting the cytokine production of human T cells stimulated by different modes of activation. *J Allergy Clin Immunol* 1996;98:S161–S173.

158. Brown DR, Green JM, Moskowitz NH, Davis M, Thompson CB, Reiner SL. Limited role of CD28-mediated signals in T helper subset differentiation. *J Exp Med* 1996;184:803–810.

159. Callard RE, Armitage RJ, Fanslow WC, Spriggs MK. CD40 ligand and its role in X-linked hyper-IgM syndrome. *Immunol Today* 1993;14:559–564.

160. Bancherau J, Bazan F, Blanchard D, et al. The CD40 antigen and its ligand. *Annu Rev Immunol* 1994;12:881–922.

161. Roy M, Aruffo A, Ledbetter J, Linsley P, Kehry M, Noelle R. Studies on the interdependence of gp39 and B7 expression and function during antigen-specific immune responses. *Eur J Immunol* 1995;25:596–603.

162. Grewal IS, Xu J, Flavell RA. Impairment of antigen-specific T-cell priming in mice lacking CD40 ligand. *Nature* 1995;378:617–620.

163. van Essen D, Kikutani H, Gray D. CD40 ligand-transduced co-stimulation of T cells in the development of helper function. *Nature* 1995;378:620–623.

164. Grewal IS, Foellmer HG, Grewal KD, et al. Requirement for CD40 ligand in costimulation induction, T cell activation, and experimental allergic encephalomyelitis. *Science* 1996;273:1864–1867.

165. Yang Y, Wilson JM. CD40 ligand-dependent T cell activation: requirement of B7-CD28 signaling through CD40. *Science* 1996;273:1862–1864.

166. Koch F, Stanzl U, Jennewein P, et al. High level IL-12 production by murine dendritic cells: upregulation via MHC class II and CD40 molecules and downregulation by IL-4 and IL-10. *J Exp Med* 1996;184:741–746.

167. Shu U, Kiniwa M, Wu CY, et al. Activated T cells induce interleukin-12 production by monocytes via CD40-CD40 ligand interaction. *Eur J Immunol* 1995;25:1125–1128.

168. Cella M, Scheidegger D, Palmer-Lehmann K, Lane P, Lanzavecchia A, Alber G. Ligation of CD40 on dendritic cells triggers production of high levels of interleukin-12 and enhances T cell stimulatory capacity: T-T help via APC activation. *J Exp Med* 1996;184:747–752.

169. Campbell KA, Ovendale PJ, Kennedy MK, Fanslow WC, Reed SG, Maliszewski CR. CD40 ligand is required for protective cell-mediated immunity to Leishmania major. *Immunity* 1996;4:283–289.

170. Kamanaka M, Yu P, Yasui T, et al. Protective role of CD40 in Leishmania major infection at two distinct phases of cell-mediated immunity. *Immunity* 1996;4:275–281.

171. Veillette A, Bookman MA, Horak EM, Samelson LE, Bolen JB. Signal transduction through the CD4 receptor involves the activation of the internal membrane tyrosine-protein kinase p56lck. *Nature* 1989;338:257–259.

172. Doyle C, Strominger JL. Interaction between CD4 and class II MHC molecules mediates cell adhesion. *Nature* 1987;330:256–259.

173. Shen X, Hu B, McPhie P, et al. Peptides corresponding to CD4-interacting regions of murine MHC class II molecules modulate immune responses of CD4+ T lymphocytes in vitro and in vivo. *J Immunol* 1996;157:87–100.

174. Fowell DJ, Magram J, Turck CW, Killeen N, Locksley RM. Impaired Th2 subset development in the absence of CD4. *Immunity* 1997;6:559–569.

175. Brown DR, Moskowitz NH, Killeen N, Reiner SL. A role for CD4 in peripheral T cell differentiation. *J Exp Med* 1997;186:101–107.

176. Parish CR. The relationship between humoral and cell mediated immunity. *Transplant Rev* 1972;13:35–66.

177. Murray JS, Pfeiffer C, Madri J, Bottomly K. Major histocompatibility complex (MHC) control of CD4 T cell subset activation. II. A single peptide induces either humoral or cell-mediated responses in mice of distinct MHC genotype. *Eur J Immunol* 1992;22:559–565.

178. Schountz T, Kasselman JP, Martinson FA, Brown L, Murray JS. MHC genotype controls the capacity of ligand density to switch T helper (Th)-1/Th-2 priming in vivo. *J Immunol* 1996;157:3893–3901.

179. Pfeiffer C, Stein J, Southwood S, Ketelaar H, Sette A, Bottomly K. Altered peptide ligands can control CD4 T lymphocyte differentiation in vivo. *J Exp Med* 1995;181:1569–1574.

180. Chaturvedi P, Yu Q, Southwood S, Sette A, Singh D. Peptide analogs with different affinities for MHC alter the cytokine profile of T helper cells. *Int Immunol* 1996;8:745–755.

181. Constant S, Pfeiffer C, Woodard A, Pasqualini T, Bottomly K. Extent of T cell receptor ligation can determine the functional differentiation of naive CD4(+) T cells. *J Exp Med* 1995;182:1591–1596.

182. Hosken NA, Shibuya K, Heath AW, Murphy KM, O'Garra A. The effect of antigen dose on CD4+ T helper cell phenotype development in a T cell receptor-alpha beta-transgenic model. *J Exp Med* 1995;182:1579–1584.

183. Tao X, Grant C, Constant S, Bottomly K. Induction of IL-4-producing CD4+ T cells by antigenic peptides altered for TCR binding. *J Immunol* 1997;158:4237–4244.

184. Constant SL, Bottomly K. Induction of Th1 and Th2 CD4+ T cell responses: the alternative approaches. *Annu Rev Immunol* 1997;15:297–322.

185. Bretscher PA, Wei G, Menon JN, Bielefeldt Ohmann H. Establishment of stable, cell-mediated immunity that makes "susceptible" mice resistant to Leishmania major. *Science* 1992;257:539–542.

186. Bancroft AJ, Else KJ, Grencis RK. Low-level infection with Trichuris muris significantly affects the polarization of the CD4 response. *Eur J Immunol* 1994;24:3113–3118.

187. Sadick MD, Heinzel FP, Shigekane VM, Fisher WL, Locksley RM. Cellular and humoral immunity to Leishmania major in genetically susceptible mice after in vivo depletion of L3T4+ T cells. *J Immunol* 1987;139:1303–1309.

188. Murray JS, Kasselman JP, Schountz T. High-density presentation of an immunodominant minimal peptide on B cells is MHC-linked to Th1-like immunity. *Cell Immunol* 1995;166:9–15.

189. Fitch FW, McKisic MD, Lancki DW, Gajewski TF. Differential regulation of murine T lymphocyte subsets. *Annu Rev Immunol* 1993;11:29–48.

190. Rizzo LV, DeKruyff RH, Umetsu DT, Caspi RR. Regulation of the interaction between Th1 and Th2 T cell clones to provide help for antibody production in vivo. *Eur J Immunol* 1995;25:708–716.

191. Carballido JM, Faith A, Carballido-Perrig N, Blaser K. The intensity of T cell receptor engagement determines the cytokine pattern of human allergen-specific T helper cells. *Eur J Immunol* 1997;27:515–521.

192. Secrist H, DeKruyff RH, Umetsu DT. Interleukin 4 production by CD4+ T cells from allergic individuals is modulated by antigen concentration and antigen-presenting cell type. *J Exp Med* 1995;181:1081–1089.

193. Evavold BD, Williams SG, Hsu BL, Buus S, Allen PM. Complete dissection of the Hb(64-76) determinant using T helper 1, T helper 2 clones, and T cell hybridomas. *J Immunol* 1992;148:347–353.

194. van der Veen RC, Chen PJ, McMillan M. Myelin proteolipid protein-induced Th1 and Th2 clones express TCR with similar fine specificity for peptide and CDR3 homology despite diverse V beta usage. *Cell Immunol* 1995;166:291–295.

195. Ogawa T, Uchida H, Yasuda K. Mapping of murine Th1 and Th2 helper T-cell epitopes on fimbriae from Porphyromonas gingivalis. *J Med Microbiol* 1995;42:165–170.

196. Robinson JH, Case MC, Kehoe MA. Characterization of a conserved helper-T-cell epitope from group A Streptococcal M proteins. *Infect Immun* 1993;61:1062–1068.

197. Spiegelberg HL, Beck L, Stevenson DD, Ishioka GY. Recognition of T cell epitopes and lymphokine secretion by rye grass allergen Lolium perenne I-specific human T cell clones. *J Immunol* 1994;152:4706–4711.

198. van Neerven RJ, van de Pol MM, Wierenga EA, Aalberse RC, Jansen HM, Kapsenberg ML. Peptide specificity and HLA restriction do not dictate lymphokine production by allergen-specific T-lymphocyte clones. *Immunology* 1994;82:351–356.

199. Kurup VP, Hari V, Guo J, et al. Aspergillus fumigatus peptides differentially express Th1 and Th2 cytokines. *Peptides* 1996;17:183–190.

200. Milich DR, Peterson DL, Schodel F, Jones JE, Hughes JL. Preferential recognition of hepatitis B nucleocapsid antigens by Th1 or Th2 cells is epitope and major histocompatibility complex dependent. *J Virol* 1995;69:2776–2785.

201. Ashbridge KR, Backstrom BT, Liu HX, et al. Mapping of T helper cell epitopes by using peptides spanning the 19-kDa protein of Mycobacterium tuberculosis. Evidence for unique and shared epitopes in the stimulation of antibody and delayed-type hypersensitivity responses. *J Immunol* 1992;148:2248–2255.

202. Metlay JP, Pure E, Steinman RM. Distinct features of dendritic cells and anti-Ig activated B cells as stimulators of the primary mixed leukocyte reaction. *J Exp Med* 1989;169:239–254.

203. Heufler C, Koch F, Stanzl U, et al. Interleukin-12 is produced by dendritic cells and mediates T helper 1 development as well as interferon-gamma production by T helper 1 cells. *Eur J Immunol* 1996;26:659–668.

204. Macatonia SE, Hosken NA, Litton M, et al. Dendritic cells produce IL-12 and direct the development of Th1 cells from naive CD4+ T cells. *J Immunol* 1995;154:5071–5079.

205. Kennedy MK, Picha KS, Fanslow WC, et al. CD40/CD40 ligand interactions are required for T cell-dependent production of interleukin-12 by mouse macrophages. *Eur J Immunol* 1996;26:370–378.

206. Ronchese F, Hausmann B, Le Gros G. Interferon-gamma- and interleukin-4-producing T cells can be primed on dendritic cells in vivo and do not require the presence of B cells. *Eur J Immunol* 1994;24:1148–1154.

207. Macatonia SE, Doherty TM, Knight SC, O'Garra A. Differential effect of IL-10 on dendritic cell-induced T cell proliferation and IFN-gamma production. *J Immunol* 1993;150:3755–3765.

208. De Smedt T, Van Mechelen M, De Becker G, Urbain J, Leo O, Moser M. Effect of interleukin-10 on dendritic cell maturation and function. *Eur J Immunol* 1997;27:1229–1235.

209. Kapsenberg M. PGE2 on DC, to Th2. *J Immunol* 1997;28–35.

210. Schmitz J, Assenmacher M, Radbruch A. Regulation of T helper cell cytokine expression: functional dichotomy of antigen-presenting cells. *Eur J Immunol* 1993;23:191–199.

211. D'Andrea A, Rengaraju M, Valiante NM, et al. Production of natural killer cell stimulatory factor (interleukin 12) by peripheral blood mononuclear cells. *J Exp Med* 1992;176:1387–1398.

212. Gazzinelli RT, Hieny S, Wynn TA, Wolf S, Sher A. Interleukin 12 is required for the T-lymphocyte-independent induction of interferon gamma by an intracellular parasite and induces resistance in T-cell-deficient hosts. *Proc Natl Acad Sci USA* 1993;90:6115–6119.

213. Zhou P, Sieve MC, Bennett J, et al. IL-12 prevents mortality in mice infected with Histoplasma capsulatum through induction of IFN-gamma. *J Immunol* 1995;155:785–795.

214. Cooper AM, Roberts AD, Rhoades ER, Callahan JE, Getzy DM, Orme IM. The role of interleukin-12 in acquired immunity to Mycobacterium tuberculosis infection. *Immunology* 1995;84:423–432.

215. Puddu P, Fantuzzi L, Borghi P, et al. IL-12 induces IFN-gamma expression and secretion in mouse peritoneal macrophages. *J Immunol* 1997;159:3490–3497.

216. O'Garra A, Chang R, Go N, Hastings R, Haughton G, Howard M. Ly-1 B (B-1) cells are the main source of B cell-derived interleukin 10. *Eur J Immunol* 1992;22:711–717.

217. Constant S, Schweitzer N, West J, Ranney P, Bottomly K. B lymphocytes can be competent APCs for priming CD4(+) T cells to protein antigens in vivo. *J Immunol* 1995;155:3734–3741.

218. Taylor-Robinson AW, Phillips RS. B cells are required for the switch from Th1- to Th2-regulated immune responses to Plasmodium chabaudi infection. *Infect Immun* 1994;62:2490–2498.

219. Stockinger B, Zal T, Zal A, Gray D. B cells solicit their own help from T cells. *J Exp Med* 1996;183:891–899.

220. Finkelman FD, Snapper CM, Mountz JD, Katona IM. Polyclonal activation of the murine immune system by a goat antibody to mouse IgD. IX. Induction of a polyclonal IgE response. *J Immunol* 1987;138:2826–2830.

221. Gause WC, Chen SJ, Greenwald RJ, et al. CD28 dependence of T cell differentiation to IL-4 production varies with the particular type 2 immune response. *J Immunol* 1997;158:4082–4087.

222. Malynn BA, Romeo DT, Wortis HH. Antigen-specific B cells efficiently present low doses of antigen for induction of T cell proliferation. *J Immunol* 1985;135:980–988.

223. Lanzavecchia A. Antigen-specific interaction between T and B cells. *Nature* 1985;314:537–539.

224. Abbas AK, Haber S, Rock KL. Antigen presentation by hapten-specific B lymphocytes. II. Specificity and properties of antigen-presenting B lymphocytes, and function of immunoglobulin receptors. *J Immunol* 1985;135:1661–1667.

225. Hsieh CS, Macatonia SE, O'Garra A, Murphy KM. T cell genetic background determines default T helper phenotype development in vitro. *J Exp Med* 1995;181:713–721.

226. Beebe AM, Mauze S, Schork NJ, Coffman RL. Serial backcross mapping of multiple loci associated with resistance to Leishmania major in mice. *Immunity* 1997;6:551–557.

227. Ihle JN. Cytokine receptor signalling. *Nature* 1995;377:591–594.

228. Schindler C, Darnell JE Jr. Transcriptional responses to polypeptide ligands: the JAK-STAT pathway. *Annu Rev Biochem* 1995;64:621–651.

229. Hou J, Schindler U, Henzel WJ, Ho TC, Brasseur M, McKnight SL. An interleukin-4-induced transcription factor: IL-4 Stat. *Science* 1994;265:1701–1706.

230. Lederer JA, Perez VL, DesRoches L, Kim SM, Abbas AK, Lichtman AH. Cytokine transcriptional events during helper T cell subset differentiation. *J Exp Med* 1996;184:397–406.

231. Jacobson NG, Szabo SJ, Weber-Nordt RM, et al. Interleukin 12 signaling in T helper type 1 (Th1) cells involves tyrosine phosphorylation of signal transducer and activator of transcription (Stat)3 and Stat4. *J Exp Med* 1995;181:1755–1762.

232. Tamura T, Nakano H, Nagase H, et al. Early activation signal transduction pathways of Th1 and Th2 cell clones stimulated with anti-CD3. Roles of protein tyrosine kinases in the signal for IL-2 and IL-4 production. *J Immunol* 1995;155:4692–4701.

233. Tamura T, Yanagida T, Nariuchi H. Difference in signal transduction pathway for IL-2 and IL-4 production in T helper 1 and T helper 2 cell clones in response to anti-CD3. *J Immunol* 1993;151:6051–6061.

234. Kawakami K, Parker DC. Differences between T helper cell type I (Th1) and Th2 cell lines in signalling pathways for induction of contact-dependent T cell help. *Eur J Immunol* 1992;22:85–93.

235. Bruhn KW, Nelms K, Boulay J-L, Paul WE, Lenardo MJ. Molecular dissection of the mouse interleukin-4 promoter. *Proc Natl Acad Sci USA* 1993;90:9707–9711.

236. Szabo SJ, Gold JS, Murphy TL, Murphy KM. Identification of cis-acting regulatory elements controlling interleukin-4 gene expression in T cells: roles for NF-Y and NF-ATc. *Mol Cell Biol* 1993;13:4793–4805.

237. Rooney JW, Hoey T, Glimcher LH. Coordinate and cooperative roles for NF-AT and AP-1 in the regulation of the murine IL-4 gene. *Immunity* 1995;2:473–483.

238. Hodge MR, Rooney JW, Glimcher LH. The proximal promoter of the IL-4 gene is composed of multiple essential regulatory sites that bind at least two distinct factors. *J Immunol* 1995;154:6397–6405.

239. Song Z, Casolaro V, Chen R, Georas SN, Monos D, Ono SJ. Polymorphic nucleotides within the human IL-4 promoter that mediate overexpression of the gene. *J Immunol* 1996;156:424–429.

240. Davydov IV, Krammer PH, Li-Weber M. Nuclear factor-IL6 activates the human IL-4 promoter in T cells. *J Immunol* 1995;155:5273–5279.

241. Lederer JA, Liou JS, Kim S, Rice N, Lichtman AH. Regulation of NF-kappa B activation in T helper 1 and T helper 2 cells. *J Immunol* 1996;156:56–63.

242. Ho IC, Hodge MR, Rooney JW, Glimcher LH. The proto-oncogene c-maf is responsible for tissue-specific expression of interleukin-4. *Cell* 1996;85:973–983.

243. Hodge MR, Chun HJ, Rengarajan J, Alt A, Lieberson R, Glimcher LH. NF-AT-driven interleukin-4 transcription potentiated by NIP45. *Science* 1996;274:1903–1905.

244. Zheng W, Flavell RA. The transcription factor GATA-3 is necessary and sufficient for Th2 cytokine gene expression in CD4 T cells. *Cell* 1997;89:587–596.

245. Hodge MR, Ranger AM, Charles de la Brousse F, Hoey T, Grusby MJ, Glimcher LH. Hyperproliferation and dysregulation of IL-4 expression in NF-ATp-deficient mice. *Immunity* 1996;4:397–405.

246. Rooney JW, Hodge MR, McCaffrey PG, Rao A, Glimcher LH. A common factor regulates both Th1- and Th2-specific cytokine gene expression. *EMBO J* 1994;13:625–633.

247. Enk CD, Sredni D, Blauvelt A, Katz SI. Induction of IL-10 gene expression in human keratinocytes by UVB exposure in vivo and in vitro. *J Immunol* 1995;154:4851–4856.

248. Nickoloff BJ, Fivenson DP, Kunkel SL, Strieter RM, Turka LA. Keratinocyte interleukin-10 expression is upregulated in tape-stripped skin, poison ivy dermatitis, and Sezary syndrome, but not in psoriatic plaques. *Clin Immunol Immunopathol* 1994;73:63–68.

249. Ullrich SE. Mechanism involved in the systemic suppression of antigen-presenting cell function by UV irradiation. Keratinocyte-derived IL-10 modulates antigen-presenting cell function of splenic adherent cells. *J Immunol* 1994;152:3410–3416.

250. Enk CD, Mahanty S, Blauvelt A, Katz SI. UVB induces IL-12 transcription in human keratinocytes in vivo and in vitro. *Photochem Photobiol* 1996;63:854–859.

251. Aragane Y, Riemann H, Bhardwaj RS, et al. IL-12 is expressed and released by human keratinocytes and epidermoid carcinoma cell lines. *J Immunol* 1994;153:5366–5372.

252. Muller G, Saloga J, Germann T, et al. Identification and induction of human keratinocyte-derived IL-12. *J Clin Invest* 1994;94:1799–1805.

253. Yawalkar N, Limat A, Brand CU, Braathen LR. Constitutive expression of both subunits of interleukin-12 in human keratinocytes. *J Invest Dermatol* 1996;106:80–83.

254. Stoll S, Muller G, Kurimoto M, et al. Production of IL-18 (IFN-gamma-inducing factor) messenger RNA and functional protein by murine keratinocytes. *J Immunol* 1997;159:298–302.

255. Budd RC, Cerottini JC, MacDonald HR. Selectively increased production of interferon-gamma by subsets of Lyt-2+ and L3T4+ T cells identified by expression of Pgp-1. *J Immunol* 1987;138:3583–3586.

256. Swain SL, Weinberg AD, English M. CD4+ T cell subsets: lymphokine secretion of memory cells and of effector cells which develop from precursors in vitro. *J Immunol* 1990;144:1788–1799.

257. Sad S, Marcotte R, Mosmann TR. Cytokine-induced differentiation of precursor mouse CD8+ T cells into cytotoxic CD8+ cells secreting Th1 or Th2 cytokines. *Immunity* 1995;2:271–279.

258. Kojima S, Ovary Z. Effect of Nippostrongylus brasiliensis infection on anti-hapten IgE antibody response in the mouse. II. Mechanism of potentiation of the IgE antibody response to a heterologous hapten-carrier conjugate. *Cell Immunol* 1975;17:383–391.

259. Actor JK, Marshall MA, Eltoum IA, Buller RM, Berzofsky JA, Sher A. Increased susceptibility of mice infected with Schistosoma mansoni to recombinant vaccinia virus: association of viral persistence with egg granuloma formation. *Eur J Immunol* 1994;24:3050–3056.

260. Ferrick DA, Schrenzel MD, Mulvania T, Hsieh B, Ferlin WG, Lepper H. Differential production of interferon-gamma and interleukin-4 in response to Th1- and Th2-stimulating pathogens by gamma delta T cells in vivo. *Nature* 1995;373:255–257.

261. Launois P, Maillard I, Pingel S, et al. IL-4 rapidly produced by V beta 4 V alpha 8 CD4+ T cells instructs Th2 development and susceptibility to Leishmania major in BALB/c mice. *Immunity* 1997;6:541–549.

262. Yoshimoto T, Paul WE. CD4pos, NK1.1pos T cells promptly produce interleukin 4 in response to in vivo challenge with anti-CD3. *J Exp Med* 1994;179:1285–1295.

263. Lantz O, Bendelac A. An invariant T cell receptor alpha chain is used by a unique subset of major histocompatibility complex class I-specific CD4+ and CD4-8- T cells in mice and humans. *J Exp Med* 1994;180:1097–1106.

264. Bendelac A. Positive selection of mouse NK1+ T cells by CD1-expressing cortical thymocytes. *J Exp Med* 1995;182:2091–2096.

265. Bendelac A, Killeen N, Littman DR, Schwartz RH. A subset of CD4+ thymocytes selected by MHC class I molecules. *Science* 1994;263:1774–1778.

266. Chen YH, Chiu NM, Mandal M, Wang N, Wang CR. Impaired NK1+ T cell development and early IL-4 production in CD1-deficient mice. *Immunity* 1997;6:459–467.

267. Smiley ST, Kaplan MH, Grusby MJ. Immunoglobulin E production in the absence of interleukin-4-secreting CD1-dependent cells. *Science* 1997;275:977–979.

268. Prigozy TI, Sieling PA, Clemens D, et al. The mannose receptor delivers lipoglycan antigens to endosomes for presentation to T cells by CD1b molecules. *Immunity* 1997;6:187–197.

269. Yoshimoto T, Bendelac A, Watson C, Hu-Li J, Paul WE. Role of NK1.1+ T cells in a Th2 response and in immunoglobulin E production. *Science* 1995;270:1845–1847.

270. Bendelac A, Hunziker RD, Lantz O. Increased interleukin 4 and immunoglobulin E production in transgenic mice overexpressing NK1 T cells. *J Exp Med* 1996;184:1285–1293.

271. Brown DR, Fowell DJ, Corry DB, et al. Beta 2-microglobulin-dependent NK1.1+ T cells are not essential for T helper cell 2 immune responses. *J Exp Med* 1996;184:1295–1304.

272. von der Weid T, Beebe AM, Roopenian DC, Coffman RL. Early production of IL-4 and induction of Th2 responses in the lymph node originate from an MHC class I-independent CD4+NK1.1- T cell population. *J Immunol* 1996;157:4421–4427.

273. Trinchieri G. Biology of natural killer cells. *Adv Immunol* 1989;47:187–216.

274. Scharton TM, Scott P. Natural killer cells are a source of interferon gamma that drives differentiation of CD4+ T cell subsets and induces early resistance to Leishmania major in mice. *J Exp Med* 1993;178:567–577.

275. Warren HS, Kinnear BF, Phillips JH, Lanier LL. Production of IL-5 by human NK cells and regulation of IL-5 secretion by IL-4, IL-10, and IL-12. *J Immunol* 1995;154:5144–5152.

276. Yoshida A, Koide Y, Uchijima M, Yoshida TO. IFN-gamma induces IL-12 mRNA expression by a murine macrophage cell line, J774. *Biochem Biophys Res Commun* 1994;198:857–861.

277. Kato T, Hakamada R, Yamane H, Nariuchi H. Induction of IL-12 p40 messenger RNA expression and IL-12 production of macrophages via CD40-CD40 ligand interaction. *J Immunol* 1996;156:3932–3938.

278. Berger S, Ballo H, Stutte HJ. Immune complex-induced interleukin-6, interleukin-10 and prostaglandin secretion by human monocytes: a network of pro- and anti-inflammatory cytokines dependent on the antigen:antibody ratio. *Eur J Immunol* 1996;26:1297–1301.

279. Donnelly RP, Freeman SL, Hayes MP. Inhibition of IL-10 expression by IFN-gamma up-regulates transcription of TNF-alpha in human monocytes. *J Immunol* 1995;155:1420–1427.

280. Kang K, Kubin M, Cooper KD, Lessin SR, Trinchieri G, Rook AH. IL-12 synthesis by human Langerhans cells. *J Immunol* 1996;156:1402–1407.

281. Yawalkar N, Brand CU, Braathen LR. IL-12 gene expression in human skin-derived CD1a+ dendritic lymph cells. *Arch Dermatol Res* 1996;288:79–84.

282. Kalinski P, Hilkens CM, Snijders A, Snijdewint FG, Kapsenberg ML. IL-12-deficient dendritic cells, generated in the presence of prostaglandin E2, promote type 2 cytokine production in maturing human naive T helper cells. *J Immunol* 1997;159:28–35.

283. Plaut M, Pierce JH, Watson CJ, Hanley-Hyde J, Nordan RP, Paul WE. Mast cell lines produce lymphokines in response to cross-linkage of Fc RI or to calcium ionophores. *Nature* 1989;339:64–67.

284. Bradding P, Feather IH, Howarth PH, et al. Interleukin 4 is localized to and released by human mast cells. *J Exp Med* 1992;176:1381–1386.

285. Smith TJ, Ducharme LA, Weis JH. Preferential expression of interleukin-12 or interleukin-4 by murine bone marrow mast cells derived in mast cell growth factor or interleukin-3. *Eur J Immunol* 1994;24:822–826.

286. Gibbs BF, Haas H, Falcone FH, et al. Purified human peripheral blood basophils release interleukin-13 and preformed interleukin-4 following immunological activation. *Eur J Immunol* 1996;26:2493–2498.

287. Li H, Sim TC, Alam R. IL-13 released by and localized in human basophils. *J Immunol* 1996;156:4833–4838.

288. Mueller R, Heusser CH, Rihs S, Brunner T, Bullock GR, Dahinden CA. Immunolocalization of intracellular interleukin-4 in normal human peripheral blood basophils. *Eur J Immunol* 1994;24:2935–2940.

289. Ochensberger B, Rihs S, Brunner T, Dahinden CA. IgE-independent interleukin-4 expression and induction of a late phase of leukotriene C4 formation in human blood basophils. *Blood* 1995;86:4039–4049.

290. Kasaian MT, Clay MJ, Happ MP, Garman RD, Hirani S, Luqman M. IL-4 production by allergen-stimulated primary cultures: identification of basophils as the major IL-4-producing cell type. *Int Immunol* 1996;8:1287–1297.

291. Ben-Sasson SZ, Le Gros G, Conrad DH, Finkelman FD, Paul WE. Cross-linking Fc receptors stimulate splenic non-B, non-T cells to secrete interleukin 4 and other lymphokines. *Proc Natl Acad Sci USA* 1990;87:1421–1425.

292. Moqbel R, Ying S, Barkans J, et al. Identification of messenger RNA for IL-4 in human eosinophils with granule localization and release of the translated product. *J Immunol* 1995;155:4939–4947.

293. Lamkhioued B, Aldebert D, Gounni AS, et al. Synthesis of cytokines by eosinophils and their regulation. *Int Arch Allergy Immunol* 1995;107:122–123.

294. Wegmann TG, Lin H, Guilbert LJ, Mosmann TR. Bidirectional cytokine interactions in the maternal-fetal relationship: is successful pregnancy a Th2 phenomenon? *Immunol Today* 1993;14:353–356.

295. Piccinni MP, Giudizi MG, Biagiotti R, et al. Progesterone favors the development of human T helper cells producing Th2-type cytokines and promotes both IL-4 production and membrane CD30 expression in established Th1 cell clones. *J Immunol* 1995;155:128–133.

296. Huber SA, Pfaeffle B. Differential Th1 and Th2 cell responses in male and female BALB/c mice infected with coxsackievirus group B type 3. *J Virol* 1994;68:5126–5132.

297. Toyoda H, Takei S, Formby B. Effect of 5-alpha dihydrotestosterone on T-cell proliferation of the female nonobese diabetic mouse. *Proc Soc Exp Biol Med* 1996;213:287–293.

298. Araneo BA, Dowell T, Diegel M, Daynes RA. Dihydrotestosterone exerts a depressive influence on the production of interleukin-4 (IL-4), IL-5, and gamma-interferon, but not IL-2 by activated murine T cells. *Blood* 1991;78:688–699.

299. Fleshner M, Brennan FX, Nguyen K, Watkins LR, Maier SF. RU-486 blocks differentially suppressive effect of stress on in vivo anti-KLH immunoglobulin. *Am J Physiol* 1996;271:R1344–R1352.

300. Dobbs CM, Feng N, Beck FM, Sheridan JF. Neuroendocrine regulation of cytokine production during experimental influenza viral infection: effects of restraint stress-induced elevation in endogenous corticosterone. *J Immunol* 1996;157:1870–1877.

301. Decker D, Schondorf M, Bidlingmaier F, Hirner A, von Ruecker AA. Surgical stress induces a shift in the type-1/type-2 T-helper cell balance, suggesting down-regulation of cell-mediated and up-regulation of antibody-mediated immunity commensurate to the trauma. *Surgery* 1996;119:316–325.

302. Milburn HJ, Poulter LW, Dilmec A, Cochrane GM, Kemeny DM. Corticosteroids restore the balance between locally produced Th1 and Th2 cytokines and immunoglobulin isotypes to normal in sarcoid lung. *Clin Exp Immunol* 1997;108:105–113.

303. Snijdewint FG, Kapsenberg ML, Wauben-Penris PJ, Bos JD. Corticosteroids class-dependently inhibit in vitro Th1- and Th2-type cytokine production. *Immunopharmacology* 1995;29:93–101.

304. Brinkmann V, Kristofic C. Regulation by corticosteroids of Th1 and Th2 cytokine production in human CD4+ effector T cells generated from CD45RO− and CD45RO+ subsets. *J Immunol* 1995;155:3322–3328.

305. Ramirez F, Fowell DJ, Puklavec M, Simmonds S, Mason D. Glucocorticoids pro-

306. mote a TH2 cytokine response by CD4+ T cells in vitro. *J Immunol* 1996;156:2406–2412.

306. Elenkov IJ, Papanicolaou DA, Wilder RL, Chrousos GP. Modulatory effects of glucocorticoids and catecholamines on human interleukin-12 and interleukin-10 production: clinical implications. *Proc Assoc Am Physicians* 1996;108:374–381.

307. Blotta MH, DeKruyff RH, Umetsu DT. Corticosteroids inhibit IL-12 production in human monocytes and enhance their capacity to induce IL-4 synthesis in CD4+ lymphocytes. *J Immunol* 1997;158:5589–5595.

308. Daynes RA, Dudley DJ, Araneo BA. Regulation of murine lymphokine production in vivo. II. Dehydroepiandrosterone is a natural enhancer of interleukin 2 synthesis by helper T cells. *Eur J Immunol* 1990;20:793–802.

309. Suzuki T, Suzuki N, Daynes RA, Engleman EG. Dehydroepiandrosterone enhances IL2 production and cytotoxic effector function of human T cells. *Clin Immunol Immunopathol* 1991;61:202–211.

310. Kim HR, Ryu SY, Kim HS, et al. Administration of dehydroepiandrosterone reverses the immune suppression induced by high dose antigen in mice. *Immunol Invest* 1995;24:583–593.

311. Araghi-Niknam M, Liang B, Zhang Z, Ardestani SK, Watson RR. Modulation of immune dysfunction during murine leukaemia retrovirus infection of old mice by dehydroepiandrosterone sulphate (DHEAS). *Immunology* 1997;90:344–349.

312. van der Pouw Kraan TC, Boeije LC, Smeenk RJ, Wijdenes J, Aarden LA. Prostaglandin-E2 is a potent inhibitor of human interleukin 12 production. *J Exp Med* 1995;181:775–779.

313. Katamura K, Shintaku N, Yamauchi Y, et al. Prostaglandin E2 at priming of naive CD4+ T cells inhibits acquisition of ability to produce IFN-gamma and IL-2, but not IL-4 and IL-5. *J Immunol* 1995;155:4604–4612.

314. Betz M, Fox BS. Prostaglandin E2 inhibits production of Th1 lymphokines but not of Th2 lymphokines. *J Immunol* 1991;146:108–113.

315. Snijdewint FG, Kalinski P, Wierenga EA, Bos JD, Kapsenberg ML. Prostaglandin E2 differentially modulates cytokine secretion profiles of human T helper lymphocytes. *J Immunol* 1993;150:5321–5329.

316. Hilkens CM, Vermeulen H, van Neerven RJ, Snijdewint FG, Wierenga EA, Kapsenberg ML. Differential modulation of T helper type 1 (Th1) and T helper type 2 (Th2) cytokine secretion by prostaglandin E2 critically depends on interleukin-2. *Eur J Immunol* 1995;25:59–63.

317. Misra N, Selvakumar M, Singh S, et al. Monocyte derived IL-10 and PGE2 are associated with the absence of Th 1 cells and in vitro T cell suppression in lepromatous leprosy. *Immunol Lett* 1995;48:123–128.

318. Milano S, Arceleo F, Dieli M, et al. Ex vivo evidence for PGE2 and LTB4 involvement in cutaneous leishmaniasis: relation with infection status and cytokine production. *Parasitology* 1996;112:13–19.

319. Chan S, Henderson WR Jr, Li SH, Hanifin JM. Prostaglandin E2 control of T cell cytokine production is functionally related to the reduced lymphocyte proliferation in atopic dermatitis. *J Allergy Clin Immunol* 1996;97:85–94.

320. Phillips C. Prostaglandin E2 production is enhanced in mice genetically selected to produce high affinity antibody responses. *Cell Immunol* 1989;119:382–392.

321. Sanders VM, Baker RA, Ramer-Quinn DS, Kasprowicz DJ, Fuchs BA, Street NE. Differential expression of the beta2-adrenergic receptor by Th1 and Th2 clones: implications for cytokine production and B cell help. *J Immunol* 1997;158:4200–4210.

322. Coqueret O, Petit-Frere C, Lagente V, Moumen M, Mencia-Huerta JM, Braquet P. Modulation of IgE production in the mouse by beta 2-adrenoceptor agonist. *Int Arch Allergy Immunol* 1994;105:171–176.

323. Wiedermann U, Hanson LA, Kahu H, Dahlgren UI. Aberrant T-cell function in vitro and impaired T-cell dependent antibody response in vivo in vitamin A-deficient rats. *Immunology* 1993;80:581–586.

324. Cantorna MT, Nashold FE, Hayes CE. Vitamin A deficiency results in a priming environment conducive for Th1 cell development. *Eur J Immunol* 1995;25:1673–1679.

325. Cantorna MT, Nashold FE, Hayes CE. In vitamin A deficiency multiple mechanisms establish a regulatory T helper cell imbalance with excess Th1 and insufficient Th2 function. *J Immunol* 1994;152:1515–1522.

326. Cantorna MT, Nashold FE, Chun TY, Hayes CE. Vitamin A down-regulation of IFN-gamma synthesis in cloned mouse Th1 lymphocytes depends on the CD28 costimulatory pathway. *J Immunol* 1996;156:2674–2679.

327. Racke MK, Burnett D, Pak SH, et al. Retinoid treatment of experimental allergic encephalomyelitis. IL-4 production correlates with improved disease course. *J Immunol* 1995;154:450–458.

328. Matsui T, Takahashi R, Nakao Y, et al. 1,25-Dihydroxyvitamin D3-regulated expression of genes involved in human T-lymphocyte proliferation and differentiation. *Cancer Res* 1986;46:5827–5831.

329. Rigby WF, Denome S, Fanger MW. Regulation of lymphokine production and human T lymphocyte activation by 1,25-dihydroxyvitamin D3. Specific inhibition at the level of messenger RNA. *J Clin Invest* 1987;79:1659–1664.

330. Reichel H, Koeffler HP, Tobler A, Norman AW. 1 alpha,25-Dihydroxyvitamin D3 inhibits gamma-interferon synthesis by normal human peripheral blood lymphocytes. *Proc Natl Acad Sci USA* 1987;84:3385–3389.

331. Barna M, Bos JD, Kapsenberg ML, Snijdewint FG. Effect of calcitriol on the production of T-cell-derived cytokines in psoriasis. *Br J Dermatol* 1997;136:536–541.

332. Koeffler HP, Reichel H, Bishop JE, Norman AW. gamma-Interferon stimulates production of 1,25-dihydroxyvitamin D3 by normal human macrophages. *Biochem Biophys Res Commun* 1985;127:596–603.

333. Reichel H, Koeffler HP, Norman AW. Synthesis in vitro of 1,25-dihydroxyvitamin D3 and 24,25-dihydroxyvitamin D3 by interferon-gamma-stimulated normal human bone marrow and alveolar macrophages. *J Biol Chem* 1987;262: 10931–10937.

334. Bikle DD, Pillai S, Gee E, Hincenbergs M. Regulation of 1,25-dihydroxyvitamin D production in human keratinocytes by interferon-gamma. *Endocrinology* 1989;124:655–660.

335. Perez VL, Lederer JA, Lichtman AH, Abbas AK. Stability of Th1 and Th2 populations. *Int Immunol* 1995;7:869–875.

336. Mocci S, Coffman RL. Induction of a Th2 population from a polarized Leishmania-specific Th1 population by in vitro culture with IL-4. *J Immunol* 1995; 154:3779–3787.

337. Mocci S, Coffman RL. The mechanism of in vitro T helper cell type 1 to T helper cell type 2 switching in highly polarized Leishmania major-specific T cell populations. *J Immunol* 1997;158:1559–1564.

338. Murphy E, Shibuya K, Hosken N, et al. Reversibility of T helper 1 and 2 populations is lost after long-term stimulation. *J Exp Med* 1996;183:901–913.

339. Hu-Li J, Huang H, Ryan J, Paul WE. In differentiated CD4+ T cells, interleukin 4 production is cytokine-autonomous, whereas interferon gamma production is cytokine-dependent. *Proc Natl Acad Sci USA* 1997;94:3189–3194.

340. Yssel H, Fasler S, de Vries JE, de Waal Malefyt R. IL-12 transiently induces IFN-gamma transcription and protein synthesis in human CD4+ allergen-specific Th2 cell clones. *Int Immunol* 1994;6:1091–1096.

341. Jeannin P, Delneste Y, Life P, Gauchat JF, Kaiserlian D, Bonnefoy JY. Interleukin-12 increases interleukin-4 production by established human Th0 and Th2-like T cell clones. *Eur J Immunol* 1995;25:2247–2252.

342. Launois P, Swihart KG, Milon G, Louis JA. Early production of IL-4 in susceptible mice infected with Leishmania major rapidly induces IL-12 unresponsiveness. *J Immunol* 1997;158:3317–3324.

343. Gajewski TF, Joyce J, Fitch FW. Antiproliferative effect of IFN-gamma in immune regulation. III. Differential selection of Th1 and Th2 murine helper T lymphocyte clones using recombinant IL-2 and recombinant IFN-gamma. *J Immunol* 1989;143:15–22.

344. Wang ZE, Zheng S, Corry DB, et al. Interferon gamma-independent effects of interleukin 12 administered during acute or established infection due to Leishmania major. *Proc Natl Acad Sci USA* 1994;91:12932–12936.

345. Via CS, Rus V, Gately MK, Finkelman FD. IL-12 stimulates the development of acute graft-versus-host disease in mice that normally would develop chronic, autoimmune graft-versus-host disease. *J Immunol* 1994;153:4040–4047.

346. Finkelman FD, Madden KB, Cheever AW, et al. Effects of interleukin 12 on immune responses and host protection in mice infected with intestinal nematode parasites. *J Exp Med* 1994;179:1563–1572.

347. Morris SC, Madden KB, Adamovicz JJ, et al. Effects of IL-12 on in vivo cytokine gene expression and Ig isotype selection. *J Immunol* 1994;152:1047–1056.

348. Germann T, Rude E, Schmitt E. The influence of IL12 on the development of Th1 and Th2 cells and its adjuvant effect for humoral immune responses. *Res Immunol* 1995;146:481–486.

349. D'Andrea A, Ma X, Aste-Amezaga M, Paganin C, Trinchieri G. Stimulatory and inhibitory effects of interleukin (IL)-4 and IL-13 on the production of cytokines by human peripheral blood mononuclear cells: priming for IL-12 and tumor necrosis factor alpha production. *J Exp Med* 1995;181:537–546.

350. Parronchi P, Mohapatra S, Sampognaro S, et al. Effects of interferon-alpha on cytokine profile, T cell receptor repertoire and peptide reactivity of human allergen-specific T cells. *Eur J Immunol* 1996;26:697–703.

351. D'Andrea A, Aste-Amezaga M, Valiante NM, Ma X, Kubin M, Trinchieri G. Interleukin 10 (IL-10) inhibits human lymphocyte interferon gamma-production by suppressing natural killer cell stimulatory factor/IL-12 synthesis in accessory cells. *J Exp Med* 1993;178:1041–1048.

352. Chomarat P, Rissoan M-C, Banchereau J, Miossec P. Interferon gamma inhibits interleukin 10 production by monocytes. *J Exp Med* 1993;177:523–527.

353. Libraty DH, Airan LE, Uyemura K, et al. Interferon-gamma differentially regulates interleukin-12 and interleukin-10 production in leprosy. *J Clin Invest* 1997; 99:336–341.

354. Weiner HL. Oral tolerance: immune mechanisms and treatment of autoimmune diseases. *Immunol Today* 1997;18:335–343.

355. Swain SL, Huston G, Tonkonogy S, Weinberg A. Transforming growth factor-beta and IL-4 cause helper T cell precursors to develop into distinct effector helper cells that differ in lymphokine secretion pattern and cell surface phenotype. *J Immunol* 1991;147:2991–3000.

356. Schmitt E, Hoehn P, Huels C, et al. T helper type 1 development of naive CD4+ T cells requires the coordinate action of interleukin-12 and interferon-gamma and is inhibited by transforming growth factor-beta. *Eur J Immunol* 1994;24: 793–798.

357. Hoehn P, Goedert S, Germann T, et al. Opposing effects of TGF-beta 2 on the Th1 cell development of naive CD4+ T cells isolated from different mouse strains. *J Immunol* 1995;155:3788–3793.

358. Barral Netto M, Barral A, Brownell CE, et al. Transforming growth factor-beta in leishmanial infection: a parasite escape mechanism. *Science* 1992;257:545–548.

359. Hunter CA, Bermudez L, Beernink H, Waegell W, Remington JS. Transforming growth factor-beta inhibits interleukin-12-induced production of interferon-gamma by natural killer cells: a role for transforming growth factor-beta in the regulation of T cell-independent resistance to Toxoplasma gondii. *Eur J Immunol* 1995;25:994–1000.

360. Weiner HL, Friedman A, Miller A, et al. Oral tolerance: immunologic mechanisms and treatment of animal and human organ-specific autoimmune diseases by oral administration of autoantigens. *Annu Rev Immunol* 1994;12:809–837.

361. Powrie F, Carlino J, Leach MW, Mauze S, Coffman RL. A critical role for transforming growth factor-beta but not interleukin 4 in the suppression of T helper type 1-mediated colitis by CD45RB(low) CD4+ T cells. *J Exp Med* 1996;183: 2669–2674.

362. Meade R, Askenase PW, Geba GP, Neddermann K, Jacoby RO, Pasternak RD. Transforming growth factor β1 inhibits murine immediate and delayed type hypersensitivity. *J Immunol* 1992;149:521–528.

363. Spaccapelo R, Romani L, Tonnetti L, et al. TGF-beta is important in determining the in vivo patterns of susceptibility or resistance in mice infected with Candida albicans. *J Immunol* 1995;155:1349–1360.

364. Roberts AB, Sporn MB. Physiological actions and clinical applications of transforming growth factor-β (TGF-β). *Growth Factors* 1993;8:1–9.

365. Ramsdell F, Seaman MS, Miller RE, Picha KS, Kennedy MK, Lynch DH. Differential ability of Th1 and Th2 T cells to express Fas ligand and to undergo activation-induced cell death. *Int Immunol* 1994;6:1545–1553.

366. Maggi E, Giudizi MG, Biagiotti R, et al. Th2-like CD8+ T cells showing B cell helper function and reduced cytolytic activity in human immunodeficiency virus type 1 infection. *J Exp Med* 1994;180:489–495.

367. Kelso A, Glasebrook AL. Secretion of interleukin 2, macrophage-activating factor, interferon, and colony-stimulating factor by alloreactive T lymphocyte clones. *J Immunol* 1984;132:2924–2931.

368. Fong TA, Mosmann TR. Alloreactive murine CD8+ T cell clones secrete the Th1 pattern of cytokines. *J Immunol* 1990;144:1744–1752.

369. Seder RA, Boulay JL, Finkelman F, et al. CD8+ T cells can be primed in vitro to produce IL-4. *J Immunol* 1992;148:1652–1656.

370. Erard F, Wild MT, Garcia Sanz JA, Le Gros G. Switch of CD8 T cells to noncytolytic CD8-CD4- cells that make Th2 cytokines and help B cells. *Science* 1993; 260:1802–1805.

371. Croft M, Carter L, Swain SL, Dutton RW. Generation of polarized antigen-specific CD8 effector populations: reciprocal action of interleukin (IL)-4 and IL-12 in promoting type 2 versus type 1 cytokine profiles. *J Exp Med* 1994;180: 1715–1728.

372. Noble A, Kemeny DM. Interleukin-4 and interferon-gamma regulate differentiation of CD8+ T cells into populations with divergent cytokine profiles. *Int Arch Allergy Immunol* 1995;107:186–188.

373. Coyle AJ, Erard F, Bertrand C, Walti S, Pircher H, Le Gros G. Virus-specific CD8+ cells can switch to interleukin 5 production and induce airway eosinophilia. *J Exp Med* 1995;181:1229–1233.

374. Birkhofer A, Rehbock J, Fricke H. T lymphocytes from the normal human peritoneum contain high frequencies of Th2-type CD8+ T cells. *Eur J Immunol* 1996;26:957–960.

375. Lagoo AS, Eldridge JH, Lagoo-Deenadalayan S, et al. Peyer's patch CD8+ memory T cells secrete T helper type 1 and type 2 cytokines and provide help for immunoglobulin secretion. *Eur J Immunol* 1994;24:3087–3092.

376. Cronin DC, Stack R, Fitch FW. IL-4-producing CD8+ T cell clones can provide B cell help. *J Immunol* 1995;154:3118–3127.

377. Carter LL, Dutton RW. Relative Perforin- and Fas-mediated lysis in T1 and T2 CD8 effector populations. *J Immunol* 1995;155:1028–1031.

378. Sad S, Kagi D, Mosmann TR. Perforin and Fas killing by CD8+ T cells limits their cytokine synthesis and proliferation. *J Exp Med* 1996;184:1543–1548.

379. Sad S, Krishnan L, Bleackley RC, Kagi D, Hengartner H, Mosmann TR. Cytotoxicity and weak CD40 ligand expression of CD8+ type 2 cytotoxic T cells restricts their potential B cell helper activity. *Eur J Immunol* 1997;27:914–922.

380. Rock KL. A new foreign policy: MHC class I molecules monitor the outside world. *Immunol Today* 1996;17:131–137.

381. Li L, Sad S, Kagi D, Hengartner H, Mosmann TR. CD8 Tc1 and Tc2 cells secrete distinct cytokine patterns in vitro and in vivo, but induce similar inflammatory reactions. *J Immunol* 1997;158:4152–4161.

382. Müller KM, Jaunin F, Masouyé I, Saurat J-H, Hauser C. Th2 cells mediate IL-4-dependent local tissue inflammation. *J Immunol* 1993;150:5576–5584.

383. Chensue SW, Warmington KS, Ruth JH, Lincoln P, Kunkel SL. Cytokine function during mycobacterial and schistosomal antigen-induced pulmonary granuloma formation. Local and regional participation of IFN-gamma, IL-10, and TNF. *J Immunol* 1995;154:5969–5976.

384. Otten GR, Germain RN. Split anergy in a CD8+ T cell: receptor-dependent cytolysis in the absence of interleukin-2 production. *Science* 1991;251: 1228–1231.

385. Sad S, Mosmann TR. IL-4, in the absence of antigen stimulation, induces an anergy-like state in differentiated CD8+ Tc1 cells: loss of IL-2 synthesis and autonomous proliferation but retention of cytotoxicity and synthesis of other cytokines. *J Exp Med* 1995;182:1505–1515.

386. Sad S, Li L, Mosmann TR. Cytokine-deficient CD8+ Tc1 cells induced by IL-4: retention of inflammation and perforin- and Fas-cytotoxicity but compromised long-term killing of tumor cells. *J Immunol* 1997;159:606–613.

Fundamental Immunology, Fourth Edition,
edited by William E. Paul
Lippincott–Raven Publishers, Philadelphia © 1999.

CHAPTER 27

The Mucosal Immune System

Jerry R. McGhee and Hiroshi Kiyono

Organization of the Mucosal Immune System
Mucosal Inductive Sites · Mucosal Effector Tissues
Regulation of Mucosal Immune Responses
Regulatory T Cells and Cytokines in the Mucosal Immune System · Relevance of Coreceptors in Lymphocyte Activation for Mucosal Immunity · Induction and Regulation of Mucosal CTLs
Mucosal IgA and Its Transport
Mucosal IgA1 and IgA2 Synthesis · Polymeric IgA and IgM Transport
The Mucosal Epithelium as a Unique Immune Compartment
Accessory Roles for Epithelial Cells · Cytokines, Receptors, and APC Functions for Epithelial Cells · Intraepithelial T Lymphocytes: A Major Cellular Component of the Epithelium
Mucosal Homing and the Common Mucosal Immune System
Lymphocyte Homing in the Gastrointestinal Tract · Lymphocyte Homing as a Basis for the CMIS · Homing of CD4$^+$ Regulatory T Cells · Role of αEβ7 for Adhesion of Intraepithelial T Lymphocytes to Epithelial Cells
Mucosal Immunity to Vaccines
Specialized Roles for S-IgA Antibodies in Mucosal Immunity · Mucosal Adjuvants · Oral Versus Intranasal Vaccination Strategies
Mucosally Induced Tolerance
The Concept of Mucosally Induced Tolerance · Mechanisms of Mucosally Induced Tolerance: Roles for Both $\alpha\beta$ and $\gamma\delta$ T Cells · Clinical Applications for Mucosally Induced Tolerance
Mucosal Inflammation
Murine Models of Inflammatory Bowel Disease
IgA Deficiency
Summary
Acknowledgments
References

That a highly integrated and finely regulated mucosal immune system exists alongside and separate from the peripheral system might at first seem redundant and puzzling. Why should such a separate and sophisticated system be necessary when the peripheral system already seems to ensure immunity for the host? There can be no doubt about the sophistication and elegance of the mucosal immune system. It presents a well-tuned, two-part defense, one more structured and localized, one more diffuse (1). In the first, foreign antigens are encountered and selectively taken up into highly structured sites for the initiation of immune responses. In the second, diffuse collections of effector cells, such as B- and T-lymphocytes, differentiated plasma cells, macrophages, and other antigen-presenting cells (APCs), as well as eosinophils,

basophils, and especially mast cells. Together, the two either produce mucosal and serum antibody responses and T cell–mediated immunity (CMI) or systemic anergy, commonly termed mucosally induced tolerance. Such a separate and sophisticated system may well have evolved as a major defense mechanism against mucosally encountered infectious agents. However, such protection of mucosal surfaces makes certain unique demands. In the human adult, the mucosal surface is enormous (e.g., the gastrointestinal [GI] tract alone is larger than 300 m^2) and so requires a significant expenditure of lymphoid cells and effector molecules for immunity. Effector elements include T-lymphocytes, of both CD4$^+$ and CD8$^+$ phenotypes, and APCs, together accounting for more than 60% of the entire cell population, as well as immunoglobulin A (IgA)-producing plasma cells. IgA is the major antibody isotope, representing more than twice the amount (approximately 70 mg/kg) of other isotypes, including IgG subclasses. This chapter will highlight the multiple roles for lymphoreticular cells and effector molecules, including IgA, in mucosal immunity, tolerance, and inflammation.

J. R. McGhee: Department of Microbiology, The University of Alabama at Birmingham, Birmingham, Alabama 35294-2170.

H. Kiyono: Department of Mucosal Immunology, Research Institute for Microbial Diseases, Osaka University, Osaka 565, Japan.

ORGANIZATION OF THE MUCOSAL IMMUNE SYSTEM

The mammalian host has evolved organized secondary lymphoid tissues in the upper respiratory and GI tract regions that facilitate antigen uptake, processing, and presentation for induction of mucosal immune responses. Collectively, these tissues are known as *inductive sites*. Although the gut-associated lymphoreticular tissues (GALT), e.g., Peyer's patches, are major inductive sites in all of the most common experimental mammalian systems, the degree of bronchus-associated lymphoreticular tissue (BALT) developed at airway branches for defense against intranasal/inhaled antigens differs considerably among species. In rabbits, rats, and guinea pigs, such BALT development is significant, whereas in humans and mice it is negligible (2,3) unless chronic inflammation, such as panbron-cholitis or rheumatoid arthritis, occurs (4,5). Instead, the major inductive tissues for intranasal/inhaled antigens in humans and mice apear to be the palatine tonsils and adenoids

(nasopharyngeal tonsils), which together form a physical barrier of lymphoid tissues termed the Waldeyer's ring, now more frequently referred to as a nasopharyngeal-associated lymphoreticular tissue (NALT) (6,7). To summarize, then, NALT and GALT in humans and mice and NALT, BALT, and GALT in other experimental mammalian systems comprise a mucosa-associated lymphoreticular tissue (MALT) network (8,9) whose integration is only partly understood.

Two major features distinguish MALT from the other systemic lymphoid tissues. First, the epithelium, which separates the tissue from the lumen, contains a specialized cell type termed M cells that are closely associated with lymphoreticular cells. Together this epithelial cell network is called the *follicle-associated epithelium* (FAE). Second, MALT contains organized regions that include a subepithelial area (dome), B-cell zones with germinal centers containing IgA-committed B cells (surface [s]IgA+ B cells) and adjacent T-cell regions with APCs and high endothelial venules (HEVs). Naive, recirculating B and T lymphocytes enter MALT

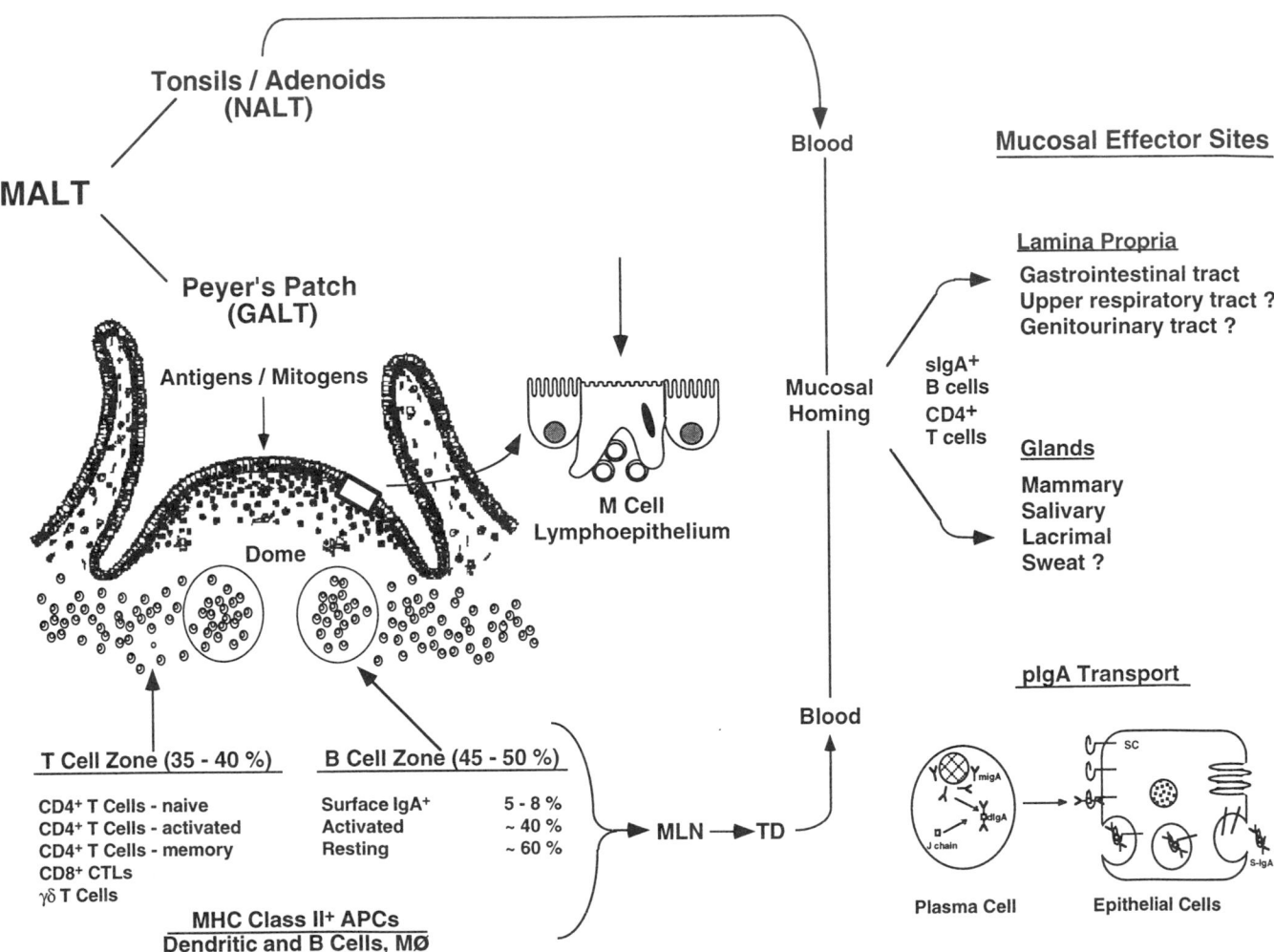

FIG. 1. The role of inductive and effector sites for mucosal IgA responses. Antigen uptake by M cells occurs in MALT (GALT, BALT, and NALT) and results in the initial induction of the immune response. Antigen-sensitized, precursor sIgA+ B cells, CD4+ Th cells, and CD8+ CTLs in GALT leave via efferent lymphatics and migrate to MLNs and then into the thoracic duct (TD) to reach the bloodstream. These migrating cells enter the IgA effector sites, where terminal differentiation, synthesis, and transport of S-IgA occurs. This induction in MALT and exodus of cells to effector sites is termed the common mucosal immune system (CMIS).

through HEVs. Antigen-activated and memory B- and T-cell populations then emigrate from the inductive environment via lymphatic drainage, circulate through the blood stream, and home to mucosal effector sites (Fig. 1). These effector sites include more diffuse tissues, where antigen-specific T and B lymphocytes ultimately reside and perform their respective functions (i.e., CMI, cytotoxic T lymphocyte [CTL], and regulatory functions or antibody synthesis, respectively) to protect mucosal surfaces.

Mucosal Inductive Sites

Mucosal inductive sites of the GI tract include Peyer's patches, the appendix, and solitary lymphoid nodules, which collectively comprise the GALT (8,9), whereas the tonsils and adenoids, or NALT, likely serve as the mucosal inductive sites for the upper respiratory tract and the nasal/oral cavity (6,7). The most extensively studied mucosal inductive tissues are the Peyer's patches of the murine GI tract, although in recent years several groups also have characterized NALT, albeit to a lesser extent than GALT, and salient characteristics of both are presented below.

Gut-Associated Lymphoreticular Tissue

Murine Peyer's patches contain a dome, underlying follicles (B-cell zones with germinal centers), and parafollicular regions enriched with T cells (Fig. 1). The surface of the dome region is covered by the specialized FAE, 10% to 20% of which is composed of M cells that exhibit thin extensions around lymphoreticular cells (10–15). These extensions, which almost surround B and T lymphocytes and occasional macrophages, form an apparent pocket (10,14,15). The M cells, which have short microvilli, small cytoplasmic vesicles, and few lysosomes, are adept at uptake and transport of lumenal antigens, including proteins and particulates such as viruses, bacteria, small parasites, and microspheres (13–16). Investigators in this field disagree on whether M cells are able to process and present antigen. Some believe that antigen uptake by M cells and transcellular passage results in delivery of intact antigen into the underlying lymphoid tissue (13,15). Others, however, contend that findings such as M-cell expression of major histocompatibility complex (MHC) class II molecules and acidic endosomal–lysosomal compartments suggest that M cells also may be involved in antigen processing and presentation (17). It is possible that the nature of endocytosed antigen influences M cell activation and their potential to express MHC class II molecules. Until M cells can be isolated or cultured in vitro, the ability of this unique cell type to process and present antigen will remain controversial.

In addition to serving as a means of transport for lumenal antigens, the M cells also provide an entry way for pathogens. Invasive strains of Salmonella typhimurium initiate murine infection by invading the M cells of the Peyer's patches (18). Although M cells are able to transport lumenal antigen, noninvasive strains of S. typhimurium cannot penetrate M cells and thus are avirulent. Reoviruses also initiate infection of the mouse through the M cell (19), an ability that has been associated with the reovirus sigma protein (20). Identification of bacterial and viral virulence factors associated with invasion or infection of M cells may provide tools to construct more efficient attenuated bacterial or viral vectors or to target mucosal vaccines to the inductive environment of MALT. Furthermore, it is possible that M cells are also involved in the induction of mucosally induced tolerance (e.g., oral tolerance). If antigen deposi-

tion via MALT is essential for induction of systemic unresponsiveness, it is likely that optimization of antigen delivery vehicles (including live vectors) that target M cells may improve immunization schema for development of mucosally induced tolerance.

The underlying dome region of the Peyer's patch consists of sparse plasma cells, as well as B and T lymphocytes (9,15), and this suggests that immediate antigen presentation may occur in the dome area after antigen uptake. It is also possible that T- and B-cell interactions in the dome area provide necessary protection for the Peyer's patch. The presence of macrophages (21), including the tingible body type, suggests that significant apoptosis occurs, but this is yet to be proven. A recent immunohistologic study has called into question whether dome macrophages are indeed a major cell type (22). This important study has described a major APC population in the dome with characteristics of dendritic cells (DCs) (22). Interestingly, the dome DCs were N418$^+$ (anti-CD11c) and could be differentiated from more classical DCs present in the interfollicular area (T-cell zone), demonstrating that two DC subsets occur in key antigen sampling areas of the Peyer's patch (22). This study also suggested that fewer numbers of B220$^+$ B cells occur in the dome area of mouse GALT. Recent studies of the lymphocyte populations associated with human M-cell pockets, the area where lumenal antigen may first be recognized by T and B lymphocytes, have provided evidence for a characteristic T-cell distribution. For example, M-cell pockets in human Peyer's patches contain approximately equal numbers of CD3$^+$ T-lymphocytes and CD19$^+$/CD20$^+$ B-lymphocytes with fewer CD68$^+$ macrophages (10). Of the T cells in this location, approximately 75% exhibited a T-helper (Th) cell phenotype.

Distinct follicles (B-cell zones) are located beneath the dome area of the Peyer's patches and contain germinal centers where significant B-cell division is seen. These germinal centers, which contain the majority of sIgA$^+$ B cells (23–27), are considered to be sites where frequent B-cell switches to IgA and affinity maturation occur. However, unlike immune lymph nodes and the spleen in the systemic compartment, plasma cell development does not occur.

All major T-cell subsets are found in the T cell–dependent areas adjacent to follicles (Table 1). The parafollicular T cells are mature, and more than 97% of these T cells use the αβ heterodimer form of the T-cell receptor (TCR). Approximately two-thirds of Peyer's patch αβ TCR$^+$ T cells are CD4$^+$, CD8$^-$ and exhibit properties of Th cells, including support for IgA responses (28). Approximately one third of the αβ T cells in GALT are CD4$^-$, CD8$^+$; this cell subset contains precursors of CTLs (29,30), whereas other CD8$^+$ T-cell subsets appear to contribute to mucosally induced tolerance.

Nasopharyngeal-Associated Lymphoreticular Tissue

Although the mouse has been the major model used to study Peyer's patches, the human tonsils are the most accessible secondary lymphoid tissue for study of NALT, and as such, a great deal is known about the component cells. Although the palatine and nasopharyngeal tonsils (adenoids) are largely covered by a squamous epithelium and are often not appreciated as mucosal tissues, the palatine tonsils usually contain 10 to 20 crypts, which increases their surface area (Fig. 2). The deeper regions of these crypts appear to contain M cells that may take up encountered antigens (Fig. 2) (15,31). Although it is not universally accepted that palatine tonsillar crypts have M cells, it has been shown that dyes and proteins penetrate tonsils in this region in rabbits and pigs (32,33)

TABLE 1. *Major mouse lymphocyte subpopulations associated with the mucosal immune system*

Mucosal sites	Example	Lymphocyte subsets	Distribution (%)	Possible functions
Inductive tissues	**Peyer's patches**	CD3$^+$ T cells	35–40	
		CD4$^+$, CD8$^-$	65	Major T-helper cells for mucosal immunity
		CD4$^-$, CD8$^+$	30	CTL precursors; regulatory/anergy
		CD4$^-$, CD8$^-$	2–4	Express $\gamma\delta$ TCRs
		Naive	30–40	Circulate within the mucosal system
		Effector (activated)	30–35	Stimulated through M-cell pathways
		Memory	30–40	Homing to effector sites
		B220$^+$ B cells	45–47	Include germinal center where >60% are sIgA$^+$B cells
		sIgA$^+$	~8–10	Committed to IgA
	Lamina propria lymphocytes	CD3$^+$ T cells	40–50	
		CD4$^+$ CD8$^-$	~60–65	Difficult to activate via TCR
		CD4$^-$, CD8$^+$	~30–35	Mature CTLs; other subset functions?
		CD4$^-$, CD8$^-$	~2–5	Express $\gamma\delta$ TCRs
		Memory	>90	
		sIgA$^+$ B cells	30–50	
		IgA plasma cells	10–15	Highest numbers of plasma cells in the mammalian immune system
Effector tissues	**Intraepithelial lymphocytes**	CD3$^+$ T cells	85–95	
		CD4$^+$, CD8$^-$	~5–8	All express $\alpha\beta$ TCRs
		CD4$^-$, CD8$^+$	~75–80	2/3 are CD8 $\alpha\alpha$; 80% $\gamma\delta^+$; 50% $\alpha\beta^+$
		CD4$^+$, CD8$^+$	~7–10	All express of $\alpha\beta$ TCRs
		CD4$^-$, CD8$^-$	~5–8	All express $\gamma\delta$ TCRs
		No B cells/plasma cells		

and the M-like cells express vimentin and cathepsin E, which are also associated with GALT M cells (34,35). Although there is evidence for antigen presentation by class II–positive (HLA-DR$^+$) epithelial cells, their precise role has not yet been documented. The tonsils contain all major classes of APCs, including dendritic and Langerhans' cells, macrophages, class II–positive B cells, and antigen-retaining follicular dendritic cells in B-cell germinal centers (Fig. 2). Tonsillar APCs can induce T-cell proliferative and cytokine responses after *in vitro* restimulation with appropriate vaccines such as tetanus and diphtheria toxoid and purified protein derivative (PPD) of *Mycobacterium.*

Approximately one half of tonsillar cells are B-lymphocytes and mainly occur in follicles containing germinal centers. Most human tonsillar B cells are actually sIgG$^+$; however, significant numbers of sIgM$^+$ and sIgA$^+$ B cells are also present. Furthermore, *in situ* staining of B cell blasts/plasma cells indicates a predominance of IgG blasts in germinal centers and of plasma cells in the parafollicular area. The overall ratio of Ig$^+$ cells was 65:30 for IgG versus IgA (36). It is not accurate to suggest that the tonsils are only a mucosal IgA inductive site, due to the presence of B cells committed to other isotypes, especially for IgG subclasses. Approximately 40% of tonsillar cells are T cells, and more than 98% express the $\alpha\beta$ TCR. Furthermore, somewhat higher CD4:CD8 ratios are found in tonsils (3:1) when compared with peripheral blood or murine GALT. In summary, the tonsils clearly exhibit not only features of mucosal inductive sites, but also characteristics of effector sites with high numbers of plasma cells. The role of the tonsils in host mucosal immunity after intranasal immunization is not yet fully established.

In order to understand the precise contribution of NALT to the induction of IgA responses to inhaled antigens, recent attempts were made to isolate and characterize lymphoid cells from NALT of mice and rats (6,37–39). In these species, NALT consists of bilateral strips of nonencapsulated lymphoid tissue underlying the epithelium on the ventral aspect of the posterior nasal tract and exhibits a bell-like shape in cross sections (40). Although dense aggregates of lymphocytes have been observed in the NALT of normal mice, germinal centers are absent but could be induced by nasal application of antigen (39). Thus, uncommitted B cells (sIgM$^+$) have been found in high proportions (80% to 85%), whereas low numbers of sIgA$^+$ and sIgG$^+$ B cells (3% to 4% and 0% to 1%, respectively) have been noted in mononuclear cells isolated from NALT (38). In contrast to GALT, where a high frequency (10% to 15%) of sIgA$^+$ B cells occur, NALT was found to contain fewer IgA-committed B cells. Characterization of isolated NALT mononuclear cells showed that approximately 30% to 40% of these cells are CD3$^+$ T cells, with a CD4:CD8 ratio of approximately 3.0 (38,39). The majority of NALT CD3$^+$ T cells coexpress CD45RB, suggestive of naive, resting T cells (38,39). Because transcriptional single cell analysis showed the expression of messenger RNA (mRNA) for both Th1 and Th2 cytokines, the majority of CD4$^+$ T cells are considered Th0 types (39). Furthermore, stimulation via the TCR–CD3 complex resulted in differentiation of both Th1- and Th2-type cells. These results support the notion that NALT exhibits characteristics of mucosal inductive sites.

Mucosal Effector Tissues

After initial exposure to antigen in MALT, mucosal lymphocytes leave the inductive site and home to mucosal effector tissues. This pathway, which results in immunity at several mucous membrane

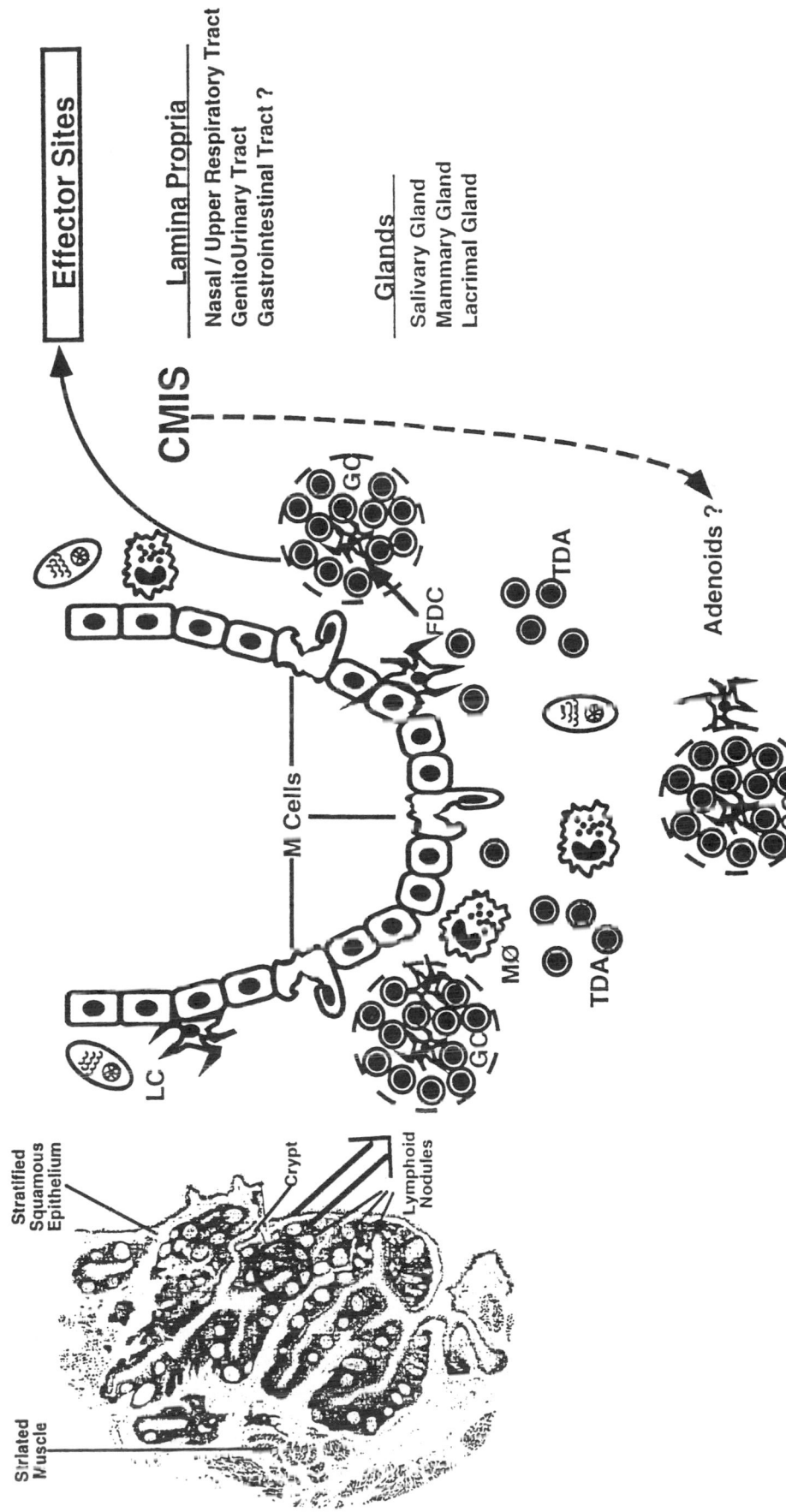

FIG. 2. The potential role of NALT as an inductive site for development of mucosal immunity. A palatine tonsil with deep crypts illustrates the microanatomy. The drawn portion shows the major APCs (LC, Langerhans' cells; MØ, macrophages), B-cell germinal centers, and parafollicular T cell–dependent areas (TDA). Effector/memory lymphocyte homing occurs via the CMIS.

sites, is referred to as the *Common Mucosal Immune System* (CMIS) (Fig. 1). Effector sites for mucosal immune responses include the lymphoid cells in the lamina propria (LP) regions of the GI, the upper respiratory and reproductive tracts, as well as secretory glandular tissues such as mammary, salivary, and lacrimal glands (9). In addition, most evidence suggests that the lymphocytes that reside in the epithelium (i.e., the intraepithelial lymphocytes [IELs]) also serve as effector cells; however, it has been difficult to precisely define IEL functions (41). Antigen-specific mucosal effector cells include IgA-producing plasma cells as well as B and T lymphocytes. IgA is the primary Ig involved in protecting mucosal surfaces and is locally produced in effector tissues (9). Again, the presence of antigen-specific secretory (S)-IgA antibodies at mucosal surfaces other than the inductive site where antigen uptake initially occurred is definitive evidence of the CMIS. Thus, it would suggest that immunization of either NALT or GALT could induce mucosal immune responses in all mucosal effector tissues.

Effector mechanisms used to protect mucosal surfaces include CTLs, as well as effector CD4[+] Th cells for CMI (Th1) and for S-IgA antibody (Th2) responses (42–44). Indeed, both CTL and S-IgA responses have been associated with protection against infection at mucosal surfaces, and both may be important for resistance to, or more importantly, prevention of mucosal infection with viruses, including human immunodeficiency virus (HIV) (45). Although little information regarding protective CD4[+] Th1-CMI responses is available, mucosal CMI appears to be important in tolerance and in control of infections by intracellular pathogens.

However, it must be remembered that effector sites, which must serve as a barrier against numerous environmental foreign antigens and mucosal pathogens with which the inductive sites need not contend, will offer mechanisms of protection significantly different from those at the inductive sites. The high concentration of IgA plasma cells [estimated at more than 10^{10} IgA plasma cells per meter of human small intestine (40)] has traditionally been viewed as the most distinctive trait of the immunity offered at these effector sites. However, as important, if not more so, are the large numbers of B and T lymphocytes (e.g., lamina propria lymphocytes [LPLs]), more than 60% of which are T cells.

When presented with an environmental antigen, epithelial cells endocytose it and in some cases themselves express class II MHC molecules, processing antigens with subsequent association of immunogenic peptides with MHC class II (49). It also has been shown that Langerhans-like cells occur on the lumenal side of the intestine at epithelial junctions between epithelial cells that could also provide accessory functions (50). When confronted with microorganisms and even with soluble proteins that can transverse the tight junctions between epithelial cells, the APCs at the effector sites may process them and so induce B- and T-cell responses. Some investigators have suggested that MHC class II–positive sIgA[+] B cells may bind antigen through endocytic pathways, and process and present peptides to CD4[+] Th cells. Macrophages in LP regions also could function in this manner for more complex antigens. Freshly isolated mouse intestinal LP CD4[+] T cells contain high numbers of interleukin (IL)-5–secreting Th2-type cells in addition to interferon (IFN)-γ–secreting Th1-type cells, suggesting that the effector regions of the mucosal immune system are somewhat biased toward a Th2 phenotype (51). Furthermore, recent findings obtained by a single cell reverse-transcriptase polymerase chain reaction analysis of CD4[+] T cells from murine nasal passages showed a high frequency of CD4[+] T cells expressing Th2 cytokine-specific mRNA (39). In summary, mucosal effector tissues contain

all the necessary cellular components, including epithelial cells, Th1/Th2-type CD4[+] T cells, CTLs, and IgA-producing cells for a multilayer barrier against the numerous environmental foreign antigens and mucosal pathogens.

REGULATION OF MUCOSAL IMMUNE RESPONSES

The development of mucosal immunity, inflammation, or tolerance to protein-based vaccines, viral and bacterial pathogens, allergens, and autoantigens requires T cells, including CD4[+] Th cell subsets, CD8[+] CTLs, and T-cell subsets for induction of mucosal tolerance. Of course, B-cell commitment (μ → α switching) and B-/T-cell interactions that result in the induction of plasma cells producing polymeric IgA (pIgA) are of central importance to mucosal immunity. Cytokines produced by CD4[+] and CD8[+] T cell subsets and by classical APCs (e.g., dendritic cells, MØ and B cells) as well as by nonclassical APCs (e.g., epithelial cells) contribute to all aspects of normal mucosal immunity, tolerance, and inflammation in the immune response.

Regulatory T Cells And Cytokines in the Mucosal Immune System

Regulatory T cells, which normally exhibit either a CD4[+] or CD8[+] phenotype, can be classified as (a) naive, or those which have not yet encountered antigen, (b) activated (effector), or (c) memory, where both effector and memory T cells have engaged in the immune response. CD8[+] T cells also occur in the same categories and will be discussed below. The mucosal migration patterns of these three subsets, along with the homing of B lymphocytes, form the cellular basis of the CMIS. Naive CD4[+] precursors of Th cells (pTh) normally recognize foreign peptide in association with MHC class II on APCs and express an αβ TCR[+], CD3[+], CD4[+], CD8[−] phenotype. On the other hand, precursor CTLs (pCTLs) express αβ TCRs which usually recognize foreign peptide in the context of MHC class I on target cells and normally exhibit a phenotype of CD3[+], CD4[−], CD8[+]. Thus, encounter with foreign antigen (peptides) will result in development of effector T cells that are either helper (Th) types for cell-mediated or antibody responses, or that lyse infected target cells (CTLs). Thus, the MALT can be considered as significant reservoirs of pTh cells and pCTLs such that encounter with bacterial or viral pathogens can result in the induction of CD4[+] Th cell and CD8[+] CTL responses.

Mucosal CD4[+] T-Helper Cells

Th1 And Th2 Subsets

As CD4[+] Th cells mature in response to foreign antigens, they assume unique characteristics such as production of distinct cytokine arrays. The pTh cells first produce IL-2 in response to stimuli and develop into T cells, producing multiple cytokines (including both IFN-γ and IL-4), a stage often termed Th0 (53,54). The environment and cytokine milieu greatly influences the further differentiation of these Th0 cells (Fig. 3). For example, stimulation by certain pathogens such as intracellular bacteria leads to the differentiation of Th1 cells producing IFN-γ, IL-2, and tumor necrosis factor-beta (TNF-β). These cells often develop after production of IL-12 by macrophages (55,56), activated by the ingestion of

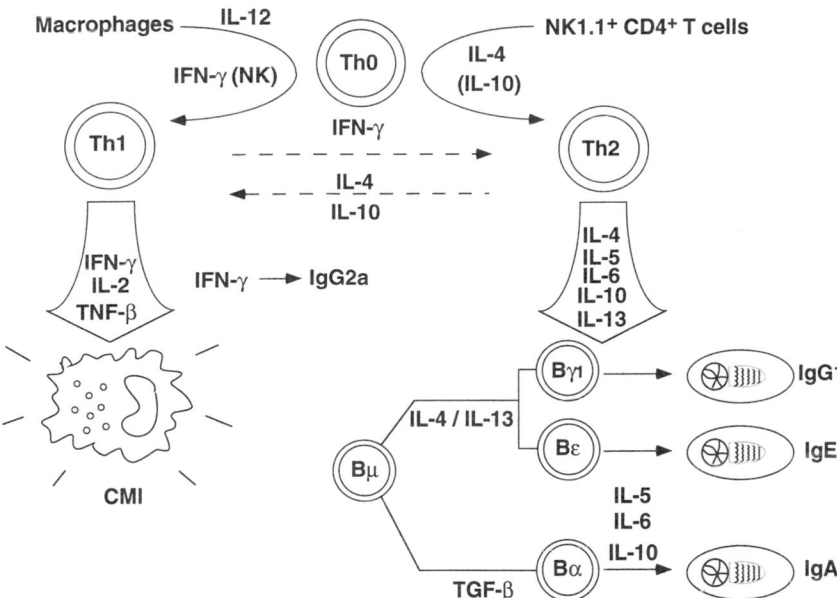

FIG. 3. The concept of functional subsets of helper T cells for the mucosal immune system. pTh cells (naive T cells) respond to vaccine with the production of IL-2, which supports autocrine growth. Antigen encounter can result in Th cells producing multiple cytokines, e.g., IFN-γ and IL-4 (Th0 cells). The environment in which the vaccine/microbe is present can determine the outcome, e.g., uptake of intracellular microbes by macrophages with production of IL-12 can induce Th cells capable of effective CMI responses (Th1 cells) via production of IFN-γ, TNF-β, and IL-2. Other vaccine/APC pathways induce Th2-type responses, and their cytokine array can determine the nature of B-cell help, e.g., IL-4 for IgG1 and IgE responses, and IL-5, IL-6, and IL-10 for mucosal IgA responses. The solid line indicates upregulation; the dotted line represents a negative signal.

intracellular pathogens (Fig. 3). There is compelling evidence that secreted IL-12 induces natural killer (NK) cells to produce IFN-γ (57,58), which, together with IL-12, triggers Th0 cells to differentiate along the Th1 pathway (Fig. 3). Furthermore, murine Th1-type responses are associated with development of CMI as manifested by delayed-type hypersensitivity (DTH) as well as by B-cell responses with characteristic patterns. For example, IFN-γ induces μ → γ2a switches (59) and production of complement-fixing IgG2a antibodies.

On the other hand, exogenous antigen in mucosal environments can trigger CD4+, NK1.1+ T cells (60–62) as well as other precursor cells that produce IL-4 for initiation of Th2-type responses (from Th0 cells). CD4+ Th2-type cells also produce IL-4 for expansion of this subset, as well as IL-5, IL-6, IL-9, IL-10, and IL-13 (63–65) (Fig. 3). This Th2 cell array may include production of IL-4 with other Th2 cytokines; however, individual cytokines are regulated through different signal transduction pathways so that all Th1 or Th2 cells do not produce the entire array. The production of IL-4 by Th2 cells is supportive of B-cell switches from sIgM expression to IgG1 and to IgE (66–68). Furthermore, the Th2 cell subset is considered to be the major helper phenotype for supporting IgA isotype in addition to IgG1, IgG2b, and IgE responses in the mouse system (44).

Mucosal Th Cell Clones

Clones of antigen-specific Peyer's patch Th cells were shown to support proliferation and differentiation of sIgA+ B cells into IgA-producing plasma cells (69,70). These Th-cell clones were derived from Peyer's patches of mice fed sheep erythrocytes (SRBCs), and SRBC-specific Th-cell clones were categorized based on the antibody response induced. The first category supported IgM, IgG1, and high IgA anti-SRBC responses, and although these studies preceded discovery of Th1 and Th2 subsets, in retrospect these clones would have properties of Th2-type cells. A second group of clones that supported only IgA anti-SRBC responses (70) may be considered as level 2 Th2-type cells. In this regard, it was recently suggested that

CD4+ Th cells preferentially producing IgA-enhancing cytokines (e.g., IL-6 and IL-10) were induced in a Th1-type dominant environment after oral immunization with recombinant *Salmonella typhimurium* (71). This subset of Th2 cells was termed level 2 Th2-type cells, in contrast to level 1 CD4+ T cells producing a full array of Th2 cytokines (IL-4, IL-5, IL-6, and IL-10). Furthermore, several studies have shown that Peyer's patch CD4+ T cells produce IL-5, IL-6, and IFN-γ (52,72), and this cytokine array also may support induction of sIgA+ B cells to differentiate into IgA-secreting plasma cells. More recent studies have formally shown that most Peyer's patch CD4+ Th clones induced in mice by oral immunization with SRBC indeed exhibit a Th2 phenotype (73).

Cytokine Regulation Of IgA Production

Earlier studies showed that addition of culture supernatants from dendritic cell (DC)–T cell clusters, T-cell clones, or T-cell hybridomas to cultures of Peyer's patch or splenic B cells resulted in enhanced secretion of IgA (74–77). One factor responsible for this activity was subsequently shown to be IL-5 (78–84). Removal of sIgA+ B cells from Peyer's patch B-cell cultures abrogated IgA synthesis, demonstrating that this cytokine affected postswitched IgA-committed B cells (82). No *in vitro* stimulus was required for Peyer's patch B cells, and IL-4 did not further enhance the effect of IL-5 (78). If splenic B cells were used, these cells required stimulation with LPS before increased IgA secretion occurred. Using LPS-stimulated splenic B cells, the IgA-enhancing effect of IL-5 could be further increased by addition of IL-2 or IL-4. Taken together, these results suggest that IL-5 induces sIgA+ B cells, which are in cell cycle (blasts) to differentiate into IgA-producing cells. Interestingly, another B-cell population, the peritoneal cavity B-1 cells, has been shown to contain precursors of LP IgA plasma cells (85). This population also contains cells that can be induced by IL-5 to secrete IgA (86). Human IL-5 is thought to act mainly as an eosinophil differentiation factor and thus may have little effect on B-cell isotype switching and differentiation. It has been reported, however, that human B cells, when stimulated with the bacterium *Branhamella catarrhalis*, could be induced by IL-5 to secrete IgA and to possibly undergo isotype switching to IgA (87). This effect could not be demonstrated using other more conventional B-cell mitogens, a finding that demonstrates the importance of the primary *in vitro* activation signal for B-cell switching.

Interleukin-6, when added to Peyer's patch B cells in the absence of any *in vitro* stimulus, causes a marked increase in IgA secretion with little effect on either IgM or IgG synthesis (88). In these studies, IL-6 induced two- to threefold more IgA secretion than IL-5 (88). The removal of sIgA$^+$ B cells abolished the effect of IL-6, demonstrating that like IL-5, this cytokine also acted on postswitched B cells. In mice where the IL-6 gene had been inactivated (IL-6 gene knock-outs; IL-6$^{-/-}$), the numbers of IgA$^+$ B cells in the LP were markedly reduced and antibody responses after mucosal challenge with ovalbumin or vaccinia virus were greatly diminished. Although the findings from these studies demonstrate the *in vivo* importance of IL-6 for mucosal IgA responses (89), others have shown that IL-6$^{-/-}$ mice exhibit normal LP distributions of IgA plasma cells and respond to oral protein when cholera toxin (CT) is used as mucosal adjuvant (90). These discrepant results are difficult to explain; however, it is possible that compensatory pathways may become activated in IL-6$^{-/-}$ mice for support of IgA responses. Of relevance to this discussion was the finding that human appendix sIgA$^+$ B cells express IL-6 receptors, whereas other B-cell subsets present do not. Furthermore, appendix B cells are induced by IL-6 to secrete both IgA1 and IgA2 in the absence of any *in vitro* activation (91). This effect was also shown in IgA-committed B cells, again demonstrating the importance of IL-6 for inducing the terminal differentiation of sIgA$^+$ B cells into IgA plasma cells.

An additional Th2 cytokine, IL-10, also has been shown to play an important role in the induction of IgA synthesis in humans (92–94). Stimulation of human B cells with anti-CD40 and *Staphylococcus aureus* Cowan (SAC) resulted in B-cell differentiation for IgM and IgG synthesis in patients with IgA deficiency. The addition of IL-10 to the anti–CD40- and SAC-stimulated B-cell cultures induced IgA production (92). Cultured B cells from common variable immunodeficiency patients also produce IgA in addition to IgM and IgG in the presence of anti-CD40 and IL-10 (93). Furthermore, naive sIgD$^+$ B cells could be induced to produce IgA after coculture with IL-10 in the presence of transforming growth factor (TGF)-β and anti-CD40 (94). Taken together, these findings demonstrate that Th2 cytokines such as IL-5, IL-6, and IL-10 all play major roles in the induction of IgA responses.

Because IL-2 produced by pTh or Th1-type cells has been shown to enhance IgA synthesis in LPS-stimulated B-cell cultures, it would be too simplistic to conclude that Th2-type cells and their derived cytokines are the only cytokines important in the generation of IgA responses (79). IL-2 also synergistically augmented IgA synthesis in B-cell cultures in the presence of LPS and TGF-β (95). Although IFN-γ is not directly involved in the enhancement of IgA B-cell responses, this cytokine has been shown to enhance the expression of polymeric Ig receptor (pIgR) or secretory component (SC), an essential molecule for the transport of S-IgA (96). B cells activated via surface Ig in the presence of IFN-γ became potent APCs for T cells (97). In addition, IFN-γ enhances the expression of B7-2, which may be a key costimulatory molecule for the induction of Th2-type cells (98). In summary, an optimal relationship between Th1- and Th2-derived cytokines is essential for the induction, regulation, and maintenance of appropriate IgA responses in mucosa-associated tissues.

Regulation of Mucosal Immunity by Th Cell Subsets

As discussed above, clear evidence has been presented that CD4$^+$ Th cells and derived clones from mucosal inductive sites can support the IgA response (69,70,94–101). However, it still remains to be shown that immune responses to mucosally presented antigens will fall into distinct classes of Th1- and Th2-type responses. Nevertheless, it is clear that Th1 and Th2 cells are sensitive to cross-regulation by the opposite cell type. For example, IFN-γ produced by Th1 cells inhibits proliferation of Th2 cells, is responsible for an isotype switch from IgM to IgG2a (102), and inhibits isotype switching induced by IL-4 (103,104). Th2 cells regulate the effects of Th1 cells by secreting IL-10, which inhibits cytokine secretion by Th1 cells (e.g., inhibition of IFN-γ secretion), in turn decreasing IFN-γ–mediated inhibition of Th2 cells. Therefore, it is important to determine the antigen-specific cytokine secretion profile as well as the antigen-specific IgG subclasses and IgE and IgA responses to fully characterize immune responses induced by mucosal antigens.

Recent studies have shown that oral immunization with a combined vaccine containing protein antigens (e.g., tetanus toxoid [TT]) together with the mucosal adjuvant cholera toxin (CT) resulted in protein-specific CD4$^+$ T cells in GALT and spleen that preferentially produce IL-4 and IL-5, but not IFN-γ or IL-2 (105). This immunization protocol also induces serum IgG responses characterized by high IgG1 titers with low or undetectable IgG2a antibodies (106), as well as increased antigen-specific IgE responses (106). Coadministration of other antigens such as ovalbumin (OVA) or hen egg white lysozyme (HEL) with CT using the same mucosal immunization schedule produced similar findings. It would appear then that oral immunization with soluble proteins with CT as adjuvant results in the induction of Th2-type responses. Others also have found that oral immunization of C3H/He, SWR/J, and DBA/1 mice with two doses of 200 μg of the soluble protein HEL and 5 to 10 mg CT separated by 3 weeks induces antigen-specific IgG (predominantly IgG1), IgA, and IgE responses (107). Additionally, systemic challenge of orally immunized mice with HEL led to a fatal anaphylactic reaction due to the high levels of antigen-specific IgE (107). Oral immunization of C57BL/6 mice with keyhole limpet hemocyanin (KLH) and CT (0.5 μg) and B subunit of CT (CT-B) (10 μg) on three occasions at 10-day intervals resulted in both Peyer's patch and LPL populations that produced low levels of IL-2, IFN-γ, and higher levels of IL-4 and IL-5 (108). The results from this study support the conclusion that oral immunization with soluble protein antigen and CT as an adjuvant induces Th2-type immune responses.

In addition to CT, heat-labile toxin (LT) from enterotoxigenic *Escherichia coli* is an effective immunogen and adjuvant for the induction and regulation of antigen-specific IgA responses (109,110). Oral immunization with LT resulted in the induction of antigen-specific serum IgG as well as mucosal IgA responses (111), and assessment of LT-specific IgG subclass responses showed high IgG1, IgG2a, and IgG2b, which contrasted with IgG subclass responses induced by CT (e.g., dominant IgG1 without IgG2a). Furthermore, lower IgE responses were observed after oral immunization with LT than with CT (111). With regard to the profile of isotype and subclass of antigen-specific responses induced by orally administered LT or CT, both bacterial enterotoxins supported mucosal IgA responses, although LT and CT behaved differently for the induction of serum IgG subclass and IgE responses. Large amounts of IFN-γ and IL-5 but little IL-4 were detected in

LT-specific CD4+ T cells from Peyer's patches and spleens of mucosally immunized mice. In marked contrast to CT, LT induced both Th1 and Th2-type responses. The production of IFN-γ by mucosally induced LT-specific Th1-type cells may lead to the induction of level 2 Th2-type cells, where the IgA enhancing cytokine, IL-5, is produced without IL-4. In this regard, LT could be used as a mucosal adjuvant for induction of both Th1 and Th2 type responses after mucosal immunization, whereas CT could be considered as a selective Th2 inducer in the murine system. These findings suggest that one can manipulate the outcome of Th1- or Th2-type responses after mucosal immunization using enterotoxins such as CT and LT.

T Cells and Cytokines for IgA Isotype Switching

CD4+ T cells and select cytokines are essential for the generation of IgA-producing cells. For example, depletion of CD4+ T cell subsets *in vivo* with monoclonal antibodies (mAbs) or by knock-out of the CD4 coreceptor gene markedly affects mucosal immune responses (99–101). Loss of CD4+ T cells is associated with diminished levels of IgA plasma cells (100) and with deficient Th cell–regulated IgA responses (99). B-cell isotype switching and gene rearrangements are discussed elsewhere in this book (see Chapters 5 and 6). This chapter focuses on the role of T cells and specific cytokines involved in switches to IgA. It is known that cytokines exert profound influences on B-cell switching from sIgM and sIgD expression to downstream isotypes, including IgG subclasses IgE and IgA. For B-cell terminal differentiation, IL-6, possibly in combination with other cytokines, appears essential for the continued presence of plasma cells undergoing high-rate secretion of IgA antibodies (86,88). Although many presume that isotype switching to IgA (i.e., μ → α) occurs in mucosal inductive sites such as GALT and that terminal differentiation into plasma cells producing IgA is a major event in effector sites, only indirect evidence is at hand to support these assumptions. In this regard, most studies of μ → α switching have been performed with nonmucosal lymphoid cells, e.g., splenic B cells, whereas *in vitro* studies of B-cell differentiation to IgA synthesis normally use Peyer's patch B cells (a mucosal inductive site) to support the idea that this also occurs in effector mucosal sites such as LP and exocrine glands. Moreover, cytokine knock-out mice have been used to determine the relevance of particular cytokines for mucosal immunity, an approach discussed below.

T Cells for μ → α Switching

Clear evidence was presented that clones of T cells from murine GALT, when mixed with noncommitted sIgM+ B cells, induced isotype switching to B cells expressing sIgA (112,113). The initial studies with murine T switch (Tsw) cells used T-cell clones derived by mitogen stimulation and IL-2–supported outgrowth, and when Tsw cells were added to sIgM+, sIgA- B-cell cultures resulted in marked increases in sIgA+ cells (112). Peyer's patch Tsw cells did not induce IgA synthesis, even when incubated with sIgA+ B cell–enriched cultures; however, addition of B-cell growth and differentiation factors readily induced IgA secretion (113). Additional experiments showed that Tsw cells were autoreactive and suggested that continued uptake of gut lumenal antigens in Peyer's

patches resulted in a unique microenvironment for T-/B-cell interactions and subsequent IgA responses (114). This result suggests that cognate interactions between Tsw and B cells are required for induction of the IgA class switch.

More recent studies have shown that T-/B-cell interactions support B-cell switches and have postulated a major role for the CD40 receptor on germinal center B cells with CD40L on activated T cells (115–117). In the presence of antigen, the B cells may alter the affinity and functions of the antibody receptor through somatic mutation of variable region genes, with cytokines such as IL-4 (for IgG1 and IgE) and TGF-β (for IgA) directing heavy-chain (isotype) switching. Furthermore, the environment of the B cell may play a role in switching (118). Germane to this discussion are studies with an effective APC, the DC, which resides in the dome region as well as T-cell zones of the Peyer's patches, and influences switching to IgA. For example, coculture of activated T cells and DC from Peyer's patches with purified sIgM+, sIgA- B cells resulted in the synthesis of large amounts of IgA, whereas the DC–T cell mixture isolated from spleen were less effective (74). Additional studies showed that the DC–T cell mixture from Peyer's patches also induced isotype switching to IgA in a pre-B cell line, whereas DC–T cell mixtures from spleen were without effect (119). Although these studies purported to show that the DC was the major cell type promoting B-cell switches to IgA, it remains possible that the Peyer's patch DC–T cell mixtures harbored contaminating B cells producing IgA, and thus more definitive proof that the DC is directly involved in B-cell switches to IgA is required.

Evidence for Tsw cells in human IgA responses has stemmed from an earlier study with malignant T cells from a patient RAC (T$_{RAC}$ cells) who suffered from a mycosis fungoides/Sezary-like syndrome. The T$_{RAC}$ cells induced tonsillar sIgM+ B cells to switch and secrete IgG and IgA (120). Furthermore, T$_{RAC}$ cells, when added to B-cell cultures obtained from patients with hyper-IgM immunodeficiency, induced eight of nine cultures to secrete IgG and three of nine to produce IgA (75). T-cell clones also have been obtained from human appendix, and these clones and their derived culture supernatants exhibited preferential help for IgA synthesis (76). Direct evidence also was provided that CD3+, CD4+, CD8 T-cell clones induced μ → α B-cell switches as well as terminal differentiation of sIgA+ B cells into IgA-producing plasma cells (76).

Cytokines that Induce Switches to IgA

Isotype switching involves the recombination between tandem repetitive DNA sequences (switch or S regions) located 5' from the respective C$_H$ genes (see Chapter 6). Switching is an irreversible DNA deletional event in which recombination between upstream and downstream S regions forms a DNA circle containing the deleted intervening C$_H$ genes. In addition to the IgA isotype switching induced by Tsw cells, isotype switching also can be induced by cytokines in combination with activation signals provided by mitogens such as LPS or through the more physiologic T cell–CD40L and B cell–CD40 interactions discussed above. The two best studied switch cytokines are IL-4, which induces switching to IgG1 and IgE in cultures of LPS-stimulated mouse splenic B cells (121,122), and TGF-β, which induces μ → α switches discussed in detail below. Several tangible events including demethylation of 5' flanking region DNA, DNAse hypersensitivity and transcription of unrearranged H chain genes precede cytokine-induced switching. The germline transcripts correspond to the immunoglobulin isotype to which the B cell will switch, where IL-4 will induce $C_{\gamma1}$ and C_ϵ germline transcripts before the expression of either IgG1 or IgE in LPS-stimulated splenic B cells. IFN-γ also has been shown to induce germline Cγ2a transcription and isotype switching to IgG2a in mouse splenic B-cell cultures (102). The germline transcription initiates 5' from the targeted C_H gene upstream from so-called I region exons that contain stop codons in all translational reading frames; thus, the resulting transcripts are sterile. I exons have been identified for all isotypes and subclasses, and their deletion, for example, in I exon knock-out mice, generally results in impaired switching to that isotype or subclass (123–126). An apparent exception has been observed for IgA switching, where replacement of the Iα exon with an irrelevant human gene construct in the gene transcriptional orientation did not impair B-cell switching to IgA (127). These studies rule out a direct role for the I exon in controlling switch recombination. However, transcription of the Cα locus was found to be constitutive in the Iα-targeted mice, in contrast to other I region knock-out mice (123–126). It seems likely that cytokine-induced transcription of the germline transcripts themselves direct cytokine-regulated isotype switching (128).

The most definitive studies to date suggest that TGF-β is the major cytokine for B-cell switching to IgA (129–134). The first studies showed that addition of TGF-β to LPS-triggered mouse splenic B-cell cultures resulted in switching to IgA, and IgA synthesis was markedly enhanced by IL-2 (129) or IL-5 (84). The effect of TGF-β on sIgM$^+$, sIgA$^-$ B cells was not due to selective induction of terminal B-cell differentiation. It was shown that TGF-β induced sterile Cα germline transcripts (130,131), an event that clearly precedes actual switching to IgA. Interestingly, deficient Ia mice apparently lose their requirement for TGF-β–induced switching, presumably because the Cα locus is constitutively activated and LPS alone is sufficient for induction of $\mu \rightarrow \alpha$ B-cell switches (127). Subsequent studies showed that TGF-β induced human B cells to switch to either IgA1 or IgA2, an event clearly shown to be preceded by formation of Cα1 and Cα2 germline transcripts (132,133). It can be presumed that TGF-β induces $\mu \rightarrow \alpha$ switches in normal physiologic circumstances because sIgM$^+$, sIgD$^+$ B cells triggered through CD40 were induced to switch to IgA by TGF-β and to secrete IgA in the presence of IL-10 (94,135).

It should be emphasized that all studies to date with TGF-β–induced switches have been performed in B-cell cultures stimulated with mitogens or via coreceptor signaling (129–135). These studies show that only 2% to 5% of B cells actually switch to IgA, making it difficult to explain the high rate of switching that normally occurs in Peyer's patch germinal centers (more than 60%). This point was recently addressed in a system where B cells were triggered with anti-CD40 and anti-dextran, both of which mimic T-dependent and T-independent stimuli, respectively. It was shown that TGF-β together with IL-4 and IL-5 induced sIgA$^+$ B-cell populations of up to 15% to 20% (136). Although one would predict that deletion of the TGF-β gene would lead to a negative influence on the IgA immune system, the TGF-β gene knock-out mouse unfortunately dies from a generalized lymphoproliferative disease 3 to 5 weeks after birth, making it difficult to use this model to investigate the role of TGF-β in IgA regulation *in vivo*. The recent finding that pulmonary disease and death in TGF-β knock-out mice are prevented by treatment with rapamycin may now allow analysis of B-cell switching in this unique mouse strain (137).

Relevance of Coreceptors in Lymphocyte Activation for Mucosal Immunity

Specificity of the immune response is determined by the antigen receptors on B and T cells. The B-cell antigen receptor is membrane Ig, which is cross-linked after binding to an antigen epitope, and which internalizes the antigen. The signal can result in activation, anergy, or death (by apoptosis). It is now recognized that the sIg (antibody) receptor is associated with a protein complex consisting of Igα and Igβ proteins. These proteins contain cytoplasmic domains involved in binding to kinases, leading to signal transduction (138). Likewise, T-lymphocytes express heterodimeric receptors for either $\alpha\beta$ or $\gamma\delta$ chains in association with the CD3 protein complex. For $\alpha\beta$ T cells, specific interactions with foreign peptide associated with MHC class II or class I and CD4$^+$ or CD8$^+$ T cells, respectively, result in signal transduction pathways mediated in part by cytoplasmic domains of CD3-associated peptides (139,140). In both cases, interaction of B-cell Ig receptors or T-cell $\alpha\beta$ TCR is insufficient for cell activation, division (proliferation), or terminal differentiation. The delivery of the first signal (antigen-specific) alone results in T- or B-cell anergy, whereas the second signal provided by costimulatory molecules and other corresponding ligands leads to the activation of cells. Thus, a two-signal model of B- and T-lymphocyte activation indicates that the antigen-specific and costimulatory signals are both required (141).

Costimulation of T Lymphocytes

The most widely studied coactivation signal for T-cell growth is delivered by CD28 (142–145), a costimulatory receptor expressed on naive T cells. This receptor recognizes on APCs one of two similar coligands, B7-1 (CD80) or B7-2 (CD86) (146–151). Stimulation and signal transduction through the CD28 receptor synergize with $\alpha\beta$ TCR–CD3 signaling and result in IL-2 production by pTh cells with subsequent cell division. A related costimulatory molecule, CTLA-4, also binds to B7-1 and was originally thought to be specific for activated CD8$^+$ CTLs. Though CTLA-4 has a higher affinity for B7-1 than does CD28, it is expressed at much lower levels than CD28 (152). For example, unlike CD28, CTLA-4 is not expressed on naive CD4$^+$ Th cells and occurs at only 2% to 3% of the level of CD28 on activated T cells (152). Evidence is now available that expression of CTLA-4 is associated with attenuation, and this molecule may be important in the downregulation of T-cell responses (153).

Dendritic cells in T-cell parafollicular areas of systemic and mucosal inductive sites are now considered to be the initial APCs responsible for inducing naive T cells to become antigen-responsive effectors or memory T cells (154,155). Although the DC expresses B7-1 constitutively with less B7-2, cytokines such as granulocyte-macrophage colony-stimulating factor (GM-CSF) maximize expression of both receptors (156). In humans whose monocytes express B7-2, activation by IFN-γ results in upregulation of expression of B7-1 (147,157), whereas in the mouse IFN-γ increases B7-2 and decreases B7-1 expression (158). Finally, B cells are also effective APCs, and IL-4 treatment markedly upregulates both B7-1 and B7-2 expression on B cells (159), whereas IFN-γ enhances expression of B7-2 on B cells stimulated via the Ig receptor (97).

Several studies have tested the hypothesis that T-cell differentiation into Th1 and Th2 subsets may be caused by differences in the second signal received from APCs expressing either B7-1 or B7-2 coreceptors and that different APC types may selectively trigger either Th1 or Th2 responses (160–164). However, other studies have shown that the same APC can function equally well for both responses (165). It is clear that CD28 is involved in activation of T cells for both IL-2 and IL-4 expression (166,167), although anti-CD28 suppresses production of IL-2 and IFN-γ (Th1) but is without effect on IL-4 (Th2) production (168). Recent studies also have presented evidence that B7-1 and B7-2 can play distinct roles in the differentiation of Th1- or Th2-type cells (98). One study, which used the murine experimental autoimmune encephalitis (EAE) model induced with a proteolipid protein showed that pretreatment with anti–B7-1 induced Th2-type cells that were associated with protection from EAE. On the other hand, pretreatment with anti–B7-2 induced Th1-type cells, increasing the severity of the EAE autoimmunity (98). Thus, it would be premature to conclude that B7-1 and B7-2 function equally for costimulation of Th1- and Th2-type subsets. It will be important to directly determine if differences in APC expression of B7-1 and B7-2 in mucosal inductive sites regulate Th1- and Th2-type responses to mucosal antigens.

Studies also have directly assessed the role of B7-1 and B7-2 expression on transfected APCs to determine possible effects on T-cell activation and cytokine production (169). Interestingly, both B7-1 and B7-2 provided second signals for CD4$^+$ Th1- and Th2-type responses, as well as for cytokine production by CD8$^+$ T cells (169). Evidence that both B7-1 and B7-2 can trigger T-cell activation via CD28 was shown in B7-1–deficient mice, which exhibited normal immune functions, presumably mediated through CD28–B7-2 interactions (148,149).

When this information is applied to the mucosal immune system, one may visualize dynamic, intricately regulated mucosal cell interactions via cytokines and corresponding receptors, as well as costimulatory molecules and their ligands. Both IFN-γ–producing Th1-type and IL-5– and IL-6–secreting Th2-type CD4$^+$ T cells reside in mucosa-associated tissues; however, the latter T-cell subset is directly involved in the induction of IgA B-cell responses. IFN-γ produced by Th1-type cells could be an essential cytokine for the activation of APCs on mucosal DCs, M cells, and sIgA$^+$ B cells, inducing the expression of B7-1 or B7-2 and other costimulatory molecules. If CD28–B7-2 interactions lead to preferential Th2-type responses (98), it is possible that IFN-γ production by mucosal Th1 cells is also involved. For example, IFN-γ could induce APC B7-2 expression, which in turn could lead to a series of signal transduction pathways for Th2-type responses. Thus, signal transduction initiated by the cognate interactions between mucosal CD4$^+$ T cells and APCs via the TCR–CD3 complex and peptide antigen with MHC class II together with CD28 and B7-1–B7-2 signaling may lead to the induction of IgA enhancing Th2 cytokines such as IL-5, IL-6, and IL-10. This scenario would lead to the preferential generation of IgA-producing cells in mucosal effector tissues.

Recent studies have begun to address the issue of APC–T cell costimulation in mucosal immune responses. For example, it was shown that a mutant of CTLA4-Ig, which selectively bound to B7-1, could alter the outcome of airway eosinophilia induced by intranasal delivery of ovalbumin (OVA) (170). Blockade of B7-1–CD28 with the mutant CTLA-4 markedly reduced airway inflammation, presumably by preventing inflammatory Th1-type responses, but did not affect systemic eosinophilia and IgE responses, which are regulated by IL-4 and IL-5 (Th2 cells) (170). Perhaps the level of expression of B7-1–B7-2 and CD28 determines the outcome of the response (171–173). Thus, lower signal

expression may selectively promote Th1-type inflammatory responses, whereas "strong" signal expression, for example, as may be provided by CT, preferentially induces Th2-type responses (171–173). It is reasonable to suggest that mucosally administered CT and LT may provide stimulation signals for the enhanced expression of B7-1 or B7-2 on APCs, leading to the generation of selective Th1 or Th2 cytokine expression by mucosal CD4$^+$ Th cells as discussed above.

Costimulation of B Lymphocytes

An important second receptor of B-cell activation is CD40, a 277–amino acid glycoprotein member of the TNF receptor superfamily (174). The receptor for CD40 is CD40 ligand (CD40L), a 261–amino acid glycoprotein that is expressed on activated T cells (and other cell types) and is considered a major determinant in direct T-/B-cell interactions (174). Most interestingly, cross-linking of CD40 via cells that express CD40L or bind anti-CD40 antibody via Fc receptors induced B cells to divide and, in the presence of additional cytokines such as IL-4, resulted in generation of long-term B-cell clones (175–178). This model has been useful in analysis of continuous B-cell clonal growth because the only previously available human B-cell lines had been either tumors or Epstein-Barr virus–transformed cells (175). This recent advance has prompted investigation of the events that occur in response to antigen, events that presumably lead to the formation of germinal centers (175). For example, resting B cells activated through CD40 are induced to enter cell cycle and to express CD23, class II MHC, and B7-1 (175). Addition of IL-4 to this system results in the generation of B cells with a memory phenotype as well as in sustained B-cell division (175). This novel system for clonal B-cell growth has naturally led to studies of B-cell isotype switching, including switches to IgA, as discussed above. Although it is still not known whether Tsw cells are a family of Th1- or Th2-type cells, the exchange of two signals between mucosal T cells and sIgM$^+$ B cells via the CD40L and CD40 as well as via cytokines including TGF-β (and IL-10?) appears essential to the induction of IgA isotype switching.

Induction and Regulation of Mucosal CTLs

In the mucosal setting, natural infection of the epithelium by enteric (rotavirus or reovirus) or by respiratory (influenza, respiratory syncytial virus [RSV]) viral pathogens leads to endogenous viral peptide processing, which induces pCTLs to become effector (activated) and memory CTLs. Most virus-specific CTLs are CD8$^+$, $\alpha\beta$ TCR$^+$, and recognition of viral peptides is associated with MHC class I presentation by infected cells (179,180). In this regard, high numbers of CD8$^+$ T cells reside in the mucosal epithelium as a subpopulation of IELs (41,181). These CD8$^+$ IELs are thought to represent an important cytotoxic effector population that can eliminate virus-infected epithelial cells. When freshly isolated IELs were examined using a redirected cytotoxicity assay, these T lymphocytes were found to constitutively possess lytic activity (182–184).

Significant progress is being made in areas related to the roles of APCs for induction of pCTLs and for mechanisms of perforin-mediated (185,186) or Fas-Fas ligand associated killing of target cells (187). Remaining issues include the importance of MHC class II–restricted CD4$^+$ Th1-type (and Th2-type) cells for regulation of pCTL differentiation into effector and memory CTLs (180). This section briefly reviews the significant progress in the area of mucosal CTL induction and regulation as it pertains to viral infections. It should be noted that the same processes occur during host responses to intracellular bacteria, to tumor-associated antigens, and in certain mucosal parasite infections. Although this focus is on CD8⁺ CTLs, cell-mediated and antibody-mediated cytotoxicity and NK cell activity are major responses associated with IELs (181,188–193).

An obvious question is how a CTL immune response is initiated given that mucosal inductive sites, which harbor pCTLs, are separate from effector sites, such as infected epithelial cells, where activated CD8⁺ CTLs function. A partial answer is that the M cell has specific receptors for mucosal viruses, best exemplified by reovirus. Through production of sigma protein (194) the reovirus enters the M cell in both NALT and GALT (196,197). It is likely, though less well documented, that other enteric viruses, such as rotavirus and respiratory pathogens, such as influenza and RSV, also enter the mucosal inductive pathway via M cells (194,195). Furthermore, it has been established that administration of virus into the GI tract results in the induction of increased pCTL frequencies in Peyer's patches (198,199). For example, reoviruses localize to T-cell regions and are clearly associated with both increased CD8⁺ pCTLs and memory B-cell responses (200). Oral administration of vaccinia virus to rats results in the induction of virus-specific CTLs in Peyer's patches and mesenteric lymph nodes (MLNs) (201). These findings suggest that, after enteric infection or immunization, antigen-stimulated CTLs are disseminated from Peyer's patches into mesenteric lymph nodes via lymphatic drainage (201). Furthermore, virus-specific CTLs are also generated in mucosa-associated tissues by oral immunization with reovirus and rotavirus (198,199). A high frequency of virus-specific CTLs was seen in Peyer's patches as early as 6 days after oral immunization. Furthermore, virus-specific CTLs also were found among LPLs, IELs, and spleen cells of mice mucosally immunized with reovirus or rotavirus (198,199,202). Although mucosal effector tissues such as intestinal epithelium contain high numbers of γδ T cells in addition to αβ T cells, virus-specific CTLs in IELs were associated with the latter T-cell subset (203). These studies suggest that oral immunization with live virus can induce antigen-specific CTLs in both mucosal inductive and effector tissues and in systemic lymphoid tissues. The murine system has been invaluable for discerning the pathways used by mucosal viruses and the importance of effector CTLs in immunity to infection. It should be borne in mind that CTLs do not function alone, and mucosal antibody responses are also of central importance in immunity. However, the focus here will be on the induction and functions of mucosal CTLs.

Enteric Viruses And Mucosal CTLs

The pCTLs induced by reovirus in GALT have been shown in kinetic studies to migrate to the systemic compartment (204,205). Such homing occurs to specialized effector compartments, including the epithelium of the small intestine. Thus, reovirus-specific CD8⁺ CTLs are present among IELs and are associated with the αβ T-cell population (205). Clear evidence also has been presented that oral delivery of rotavirus induces increased pCTLs in GALT, which are then disseminated throughout the murine lymphoid system within 3 weeks (199). Furthermore, effector CTLs were shown to protect against gastritis in the suckling mouse model (206). In a

series of elegant studies whose purpose was to define the host determinants of rotavirus immunity, it was shown that CD8⁺ T cells mediated clearance of rotavirus infection of SCID mice (207–209). It was further established that both S-IgA antibodies and CD8⁺ CTLs are of central importance in rotavirus immunity (210). Evidence also was presented that intracellular neutralization within epithelial cells by pIgA was a major contributor to immunity (210), a function for pIgA discussed below (210).

Respiratory Viruses and Mucosal CTLs

Detailed studies of immune responses after intranasal infection with influenza virus have revealed that immune pathways are involved in virus clearance. In this model, use of CD4–coreceptor knock-outs or depletion of this subset did not affect induction of pCTLs or significantly alter the clearance of infection (211). It also has been shown that using mice lacking CD8⁺ T cells (β2 microglobulin [β2m] knock-out mice) or treating with anti-CD8 mAbs did not alter clearance of influenza. These results support the presence of multiple pathways for immunity and suggest that CD4⁺ Th cell pathways are important for mucosal antibody responses and CD8⁺ CTLs for respiratory tract immunity (212). In this model, as clearance occurs, γδ T cells with several Vδ specificities increase in the infected site, suggesting an associated regulatory role for γδ T cells in antiviral immunity (213).

Several studies have established that effector CTLs protect mice from RSV infection. In one, the RSV F determinant, a 22-kDa glycoprotein was shown to induce protective CTLs (214,215). In a separate line of investigation, the murine RSV model was used to determine the relative importance of CD4⁺ T cells, including Th1 and Th2 subsets, which resulted in inflammation versus immunity. These ongoing studies clearly suggest that CD4⁺ IFN-γ–producing Th1 cells as well as CD8⁺ T cells are associated with recovery, whereas CD4⁺ Th2-type pathways are not (216,217). Interestingly, priming with inactivated RSV or F glycoprotein induced CD4⁺ Th2 cells, whereas live RSV elicited the Th1-type pathway (216,217). When one considers mucosal vaccine development for virus infections, these findings suggest that the outcome of Th1-type (including induction of CTLs) and Th2-type immune responses could be regulated by the nature and form of viral antigen used for immunization.

A Mucosal AIDS Model for CTL Responses

It is now clear that more than 80% of new HIV-1 infections result from sexual transmission, and significant efforts are now focused on development of mucosal immunity in the genitourinary tract. The vaginal infection model of rhesus macaques with simian immunodeficiency virus (SIV) has been useful in studies of immunity to SIV in the female reproductive tract (218–220). Recent studies in this model have provided direct evidence that pCTLs occur in female macaque reproductive tissues and that infection with SIV induced CTL responses (221). This important finding was recently extended to vaginal infection with an SIV/HIV-1 chimeric virus (SHIV) containing the HIV-1 89.6 env gene (222). Interestingly, all macaques infected with this reovirus pathogenic SHIV resisted two challenges with virulent SIV, and functional, gag-specific CTLs were found in the peripheral blood (222). Although it should be emphasized that vaginal antibodies were also induced, these results clearly indicate the importance of mucosal CTL responses in immunity to HIV infection. A discussion concerning the use of peptides to induce antiviral CTL responses is beyond the scope of this chapter; however, recent work has shown that intranasal immunization with SIV/HIV components induce antibody responses in vaginal secretions (223). Interestingly, intranasal immunization of mice with HIV-1 T-cell epitopes and the mucosal adjuvant CT has been shown to induce functional CTLs in spleen and cervical lymph node (224). Such evidence suggests that mucosal delivery of SIV/HIV components can induce mucosal CTLs, which will contribute to both systemic and mucosal immunity.

Other Mucosal CTL Systems

Recent studies have shown that not only viral infections but also recombinant *Salmonella* (225) or *Toxoplasma gondii* (226,227) can induce CD8[+] T cells, including CTL responses to expressed proteins. Significant questions remain regarding the mechanisms by which naive CD8[+] T cells are induced to expand into pCTLs and the rules for expression of effector CTLs and memory in the actual mucosal compartment that manifests the infection. It is tempting to suggest that pCTLs arising in mucosal inductive sites, although programmed to respond, do not do so until encounter occurs with infected mucosal epithelial cells. If this is the case, APC–CD4[+] T-cell regulation of pCTL induction would be a separate event from the generation of mucosal effector CD8[+] T cells. In this regard, it has been shown that pCTLs accumulate in immunologic privileged sites but do not develop cytotoxic function until encounter occurs with infected, MHC class I–presenting target cells (228). Perhaps this mechanism protects the Common mucosal immune system from undesirable cytotoxic inflammatory events.

MUCOSAL IgA AND ITS TRANSPORT

Mucosal IgA1 and IgA2 Synthesis

Human IgA occurs as two subclasses, IgA1 and IgA2, and differences occur in their distribution in serum and in various external secretions (9,42,44,46). For example, 90% to 95% of serum IgA is of the IgA1 subclass, and most is monomeric in nature. On the other hand, various glandular secretions contain 50 to 70% IgA1 and 30% to 50% IgA2, and the latter subclass is found in higher proportions in external secretions. The α1 and α2 H chains are both approximately 60 kDa in size and exhibit one V_H and three C_H domains; however, significant functional differences are noted (see Chapter 3). For example, a deletion of 13 amino acids is seen in the hinge region of α2, whereas only a 20–amino acid difference occurs between α1 and α2 over the entire 360–amino acid sequence. Interestingly, the unusual structure of the hinge in IgA2 confers the molecule a high degree of resistance to proteolytic enzymes (9,42). On the other hand, a number of bacterial pathogens produce proteases that selectively cleave IgA1 into Fab and Fc fragments (9,42). Generally, IgA1 proteases cleave the proline-threonine or the proline-serine peptide bonds in the IgA1 hinge region, and the potential significance of IgA1 proteases has been reviewed in detail elsewhere (9,42).

A characteristic array of IgA1 and IgA2 plasma cells occurs in mucosal effector sites. For example, the respiratory tract–associated tissues are rich in IgA1-producing cells, e.g., the nasal tract mucosa contains 90% to 95% IgA1, whereas the lacrimal glands

consist of 80% IgA1 and 20% IgA2 plasma cells (46). In contrast, higher numbers of IgA2 plasma cells occur in the LP of the GI tract, and the large intestine consists of more than 60% IgA2-producing cells (46).

If one assumes that tonsils are representative of NALT and that the human appendix is somewhat typical of GALT, then the pattern that emerges is that the inductive tissue harbors IgA1 or IgA2 precursors for predominant IgA1 or IgA2 responses. For example, more than 95% of IgA produced by tonsillar B cells is IgA1 subclass, supporting the notion that tonsils are a possible site for precursor IgA1[+] B cells in the nasopharynx (91). Likewise, although the human appendix, which may be representative of GALT, contains both IgA1[+] and IgA2[+] B cells, IL-6 induces much higher IgA2 responses in appendix B-cell cultures (91). This would suggest that GALT is a major source of IgA precursor B cells that populate the effector regions of the small and large intestine with some preference for the IgA2 subclass.

The epithelium that covers the upper respiratory and gastrointestinal tracts largely consist of columnar epithelial cells that are continuously renewed from less differentiated crypt cells. Epithelial cells not only provide a physical barrier but also produce a variety of glycoproteins, peptides, and receptors important to mucosal immunity (229–231). Together with IELs, mast cells, and other cell types, they form an intranet to protect the mucosa. Adjacent goblet cells contribute to innate mucosal immunity and produce different mucin forms that cover the epithelium (130,224,229,230). An important exception is in the lymphoepithelium that covers MALT, where the sparse numbers of goblet cells and the lack of mucin production are thought to facilitate antigen uptake by M cells (231).

Polymeric IgA and IgM Transport

A major function of epithelial cells in mucosal immune responses is the active transport of polymeric IgA (pIgA) produced in the mucosal and glandular tissues to the mucosal surface. The molecule responsible for transport of pIgA into mucosal secretions is the polymeric Ig receptor (pIgR) (232–234). A major hallmark of the mucosal immune response is the presence of Ag-specific S-IgA antibodies in external secretions. As discussed above, S-IgA in humans occurs as S-IgA1 and S-IgA2 subclasses, with a preponderance of the former in the upper respiratory and upper GI tracts, and the latter in the lower ileum and large intestine (9,235). Plasma cells in LP and acinar regions of exocrine glands produce pIgA associated with the 15.6-kDa peptide J chain (9,236). Initially it was thought that J chain was involved in polymerization of intracellular mIgA or mIgM (237); however, recent studies indicate that aberrant polymers of IgM occur in the absence of J chain (238). Furthermore, J-chain knockout mice exhibit IgA in external secretions; however, only monomeric IgA (mIgA) is transported in this mouse (239,240). Taken together, this suggests that J chain is required in the formation of pIgA and the correct pentameric form of IgM (236–240).

As indicated above, epithelial cells in glands and in basolateral crypts of the gastrointestinal (GI) and upper respiratory tract (URT) produce the full-length 100-kDa pIgR, which associates with the nonserosal surface of epithelial cells (241). The binding of pIgA/pIgM is followed by endocytosis and transcytosis across the epithelial cell (241). During transcytosis, disulfide bonds form between pIgR and pIgA, and secretion of S-IgA follows cleavage of a 20-kDa component of pIgR and exocytosis, the entire process requiring less than an hour (9,241) (Fig. 1). The disulfide-bonded portion of the pIgR termed secretory component (SC) stabilizes S-IgA and renders the molecule more resistant to proteolytic digestion (9,241). This transport process is highly efficient, and a normal adult produces 2.8 to 3.0 g of S-IgA per day in the GI tract alone.

THE MUCOSAL EPITHELIUM AS A UNIQUE IMMUNE COMPARTMENT

Accessory Roles for Epithelial Cells

In addition to their role in transport of pIgA from the mucosal effector tissues to mucosal secretions, mucosal epithelial cells also play an active role in the induction of mucosal immune responses and systemic unresponsiveness (mucosally induced tolerance). A number of studies have provided evidence that intestinal epithelial cell lines produce cytokines and express cytokine receptors and adhesion molecules that may affect the induction of mucosal immune responses (242–256). The rat intestinal epithelial cell line IEC-6 has been shown to produce IL-6, an important cytokine for the generation of IgA plasma cells from sIgA$^+$ B cells. Treatment of IEC-6 cells with TGF-β enhanced IL-6 production (88,91,242), whereas TGF-β acted synergistically with IL-1β to enhance IL-6 secretion (243). The mucosal adjuvant CT also increased IL-6 production and acted synergistically with TGF-β, IL-1β, and TNF-α (244). Others have shown that addition of CT to IEC-17 intestinal epithelial cells stimulates the production of inflammatory cytokines IL-1 and IL-6 (245). Taken together, these results suggest that intestinal epithelial cells have the ability to produce cytokines that could play a role in the induction and maintenance of both mucosal immune responses and intestinal inflammation.

Epithelial cell lines also have been useful in delineating the mechanisms that lead to inflammatory cytokine and chemokine responses after mucosal infection with pathogenic bacteria. Responding to stimuli such as live Escherichia coli and Salmonella, epithelial cells produce IL-6 (246–248) and IL-8 (249,250). IL-8 production is also elicited by other Gram-negative bacteria and by Helicobacter pylori infection of gastric epithelium and cell lines (251,252). In addition to inducing IL-6 and IL-8 production, Salmonella have been shown to cause epithelial cells to produce a characteristic array of inflammatory cytokines shortly after infection/stimulation (253). A similar cytokine array was produced after infection with Chlamydia, but its production was delayed and dependent on infection of cultured cells (254). Taken together, these studies suggest that epithelial cells are major players in both the inflammatory process and in immunity, where they produce antiinflammatory and immunoregulatory cytokine pathways.

Cytokines, Receptors, and APC Functions for Epithelial Cells

Human intestinal epithelial cells have been examined for their ability to produce cytokines. Both cell lines and freshly isolated human intestinal epithelial cells have been shown to produce IL-8 (255,256), the former also expressing mRNA for IL-1α, IL-1β, IL-10, and TNF-α, but not mRNA for IL-2, IL-4, IL-5, IL-6, or IFN-γ (255). Others have shown that the adhesion of Salmonella typhimurium to T84 human colonic epithelial cell lines induces the production of IL-8 (257) and is associated with an increased transepithelial migration of neutrophils, although this process appears not to be regulated by IL-8 (257).

In addition to the production of cytokines, intestinal epithelial cell lines have been shown to express adhesion molecules necessary for APCs to interact with lymphocytes. Both intracellular adhesion molecule (ICAM)-1 and lymphocyte-function associated antigen (LFA)-3 were constitutively expressed at low levels by human intestinal epithelial cell lines, and expression of ICAM-1 was enhanced by exposure to the inflammatory cytokines IFN-γ, TNF-α, IL-1β, and IL-6 (258). This observation provides support for the finding that rat intestinal epithelial cells are able to present processed antigen to antigen-specific CD4$^+$ T cells (259). Taken together, the findings that intestinal epithelial cells produce cytokines such as IL-1, IL-6, and IL-8, express the adhesion molecules ICAM-1 and LFA-3, and are able to present antigen to sensitized T-lymphocytes suggest that intestinal epithelial cells may play an important role in the maintenance of mucosal immune responses in mucosal effector sites. In addition, it is also likely that epithelial cells exhibit APC functions responsible for some forms of T-cell anergy in mucosally induced tolerance.

Intraepithelial T lymphocytes: A Major Cellular Component of the Epithelium

In addition to epithelial cells, the mucosal epithelium, an important interface between the host and its environment, contains a large number of IELs (41,181,260). As the name IEL indicates, these lymphocytes reside at the basolateral surface of epithelial cells that cover the GI, nasal, and reproductive tracts. It has been estimated that one IEL can be found for every four to six epithelial cells (261,262). Thus, tremendous numbers of lymphocytes, most of them T cells (more than 90%) of both αβ and γδ types, are situated in the mucosal epithelium, where they are continuously exposed to mucosally encountered antigens. As discussed above, a subset of IELs (i.e., CD4$^-$, CD8$^+$ T cells) possesses cytotoxic functions that may be an important cell-mediated immune defense against viral and intracellular bacterial infections. Furthermore, intraepithelial T lymphocytes serve as regulatory T cells (e.g., with Th1/Th2 cytokine production) for humoral immune responses, including IgA production (52,263,264). More recent evidence suggests that intraepithelial T cells communicate with epithelial cells via cytokine and corresponding receptor signaling pathways to ensure reciprocal regulation and to maintain an appropriate immunologic homeostasis (265,266). These findings strongly suggest that IELs are important for the induction and regulation of the mucosal immune response.

Origin and Development of IELs

The heterogeneity in subpopulations of intraepithelial T lymphocytes and the nature of their developmental processes mirror those of T cells in the thymus. The epithelia of the thymus shares the same embryonic endodermal origin as that of the GI tract, and both are important cellular components in T-cell selection. In contrast to T cells residing in the secondary lymphoid tissues (e.g., spleen and peripheral lymph nodes), IELs contain four subsets based on their expression of CD4 and CD8 and include CD4$^+$, CD8$^-$ and CD4$^-$, CD8$^+$ single-positive T cells; CD4$^+$, CD8$^+$ double-positive (DP) T cells; and CD4$^-$, CD8$^-$, double-negative (DN) T cells (52,267,268). Another parallel between IEL T cells and those of the thymus is suggested by the fact that both homodimeric (αα) and heterodimeric (αβ) chains of CD8 develop among CD8$^+$ T-lymphocytes in both. Such findings have led some to speculate that $\alpha\alpha$ CD8$^+$ and $\alpha\beta$ CD8$^+$ T cells represent extra- versus intrathymic IEL T-cell development, respectively (270). Moreover, the role played by the thymus in IEL production remains controversial. Although studies have suggested that some IEL T cells develop locally without thymic influence, others have provided evidence that intraepithelial $\alpha\beta$ T cells, including $\alpha\alpha$ CD8$^+$ T cells, arise from thymus (272,273). In the former, the bone marrow of both thymectomized and nonthymectomized RAG-2 deficient mice was reconstituted with that from MHC-matched nude mouse donors. Euthymic recipients produced normal numbers of IELs that were phenotypically similar to those observed in conventional mice (271), whereas athymic mice showed reduced numbers of IELs. Furthermore, CD4$^+$ and $\alpha\beta$ CD8$^+$ T cells were absent in the IEL compartment of athymic mice, whereas $\alpha\alpha$ CD8$^+$ T cells were present (271). In the studies that seemed to support a thymic origin for intraepithelial $\alpha\beta$ T cells, including $\alpha\alpha$ CD8$^+$ T cells in addition to CD8$^+$ T cells, athymic chimeric mice possessed similar numbers of $\alpha\alpha$ CD8$^+$ and $\alpha\beta$ CD8$^+$ T cells, as did euthymic mice (273). In addition, it was shown that all $\alpha\beta$ T-cell subsets were produced in normal numbers in these athymic radiation chimeras (274,275) and that $\alpha\alpha$ CD8$^+$ T cells could be derived from intrathymic precursors after activation with mitogen or T cell-derived cytokines (276,277). Although these discrepant results regarding a thymic role in IEL production are difficult to reconcile, some suggest that intraepithelial $\gamma\delta$ T cells may develop *in situ* (269,272). These $\gamma\delta$ T cells are found in both congenitally athymic nude mice and athymic radiation chimeras (269,272). It is important to point out that high numbers of $\gamma\delta$ T cells (40% to 50%) are found in the epithelium (41,278,279), whereas only small numbers occur in the underlying LP regions.

Unique Features of Intraepithelial T Lymphocytes

Naive and resting T cells are first stimulated to develop into effector (e.g., Th1 and Th2) or memory T cells when they encounter antigen in the natural milieu of mucosal tissues. T cells in the natural environment of the mucosal immune system are continuously exposed to a large array of antigens encountered by inhalation or ingestion via the epithelium, whereas systemic T cells in lymphoid tissues are anatomically isolated from direct and continuous burdens of environmental antigens. This constant antigen exposure could help explain the development of several immunologically unique types of intraepithelial T cells. For example, intraepithelial and splenic T cells behave differently in response to activation signals provided by T-cell mitogens as well as anti-TCR and anti-CD3 antibodies (280,281). As one might expect, elevated DNA replication (proliferation) was noted in splenic T-cell cultures in response to these stimuli, whereas IELs were unresponsive. However, highly purified $\alpha\beta$ and $\gamma\delta$ T cells from murine intestinal epithelium were capable of responding to stimulation signals via the TCR-CD3 complex (282). It has been suggested that neighboring epithelial cells may provide downregulatory signals for intraepithelial T cells *in situ* in order to avoid development of T-cell hyperreactive regions in the mucosal epithelium. Cell cycle analysis supported this view by revealing that the majority of intraepithelial $\gamma\delta$ and $\alpha\beta$ T cells were found in the G$_0$ and G$_1$ phases (283). These findings indicate that most IELs are in a resting stage despite continuous exposure to mucosally encountered antigens. However, when levels of RNA including Th1- and Th2-specific mRNA were examined, a subset of $\alpha\beta$ and $\gamma\delta$ T cells expressed higher levels of

mRNA than did splenic T cells (283,284). Furthermore, a higher frequency of Th1 and Th2 cytokine-producing T cells was noted in IELs than in spleen (52,283).

The unique properties of intraepithelial T cells could be explained by the formation of the TCR–CD3 complex. When ζ chain gene-deficient mice were examined, several interesting differences were observed between intraepithelial and systemic T-cell compartments (285–288). Because the expression of the ζ chain is required for appropriate intracellular assembly, trafficking, and membrane expression of the TCR–CD3 complex, the removal of this gene results in sharp reductions in the TCR–CD3 complex and diminution of the peripheral T-cell pool (10% of wild-type, control mice) (285,288). In marked contrast, the levels of TCR-CD3 complex expression on intraepithelial $\alpha\beta$ T cells were not nearly as affected by the absence of the ζ chain as were T cells in spleen (285,288). The extensive biochemical characterization of the TCR–CD3 complex on intraepithelial and peripheral T cells showed that the former subset expresses the TCR–CD3 complex associated with FcϵR γ homodimers in the absence of the ζ chain, whereas the TCR–CD3 complex–expressed cells were reduced in the latter T cells (285,287,289). Furthermore, it was shown that intraepithelial cells, especially $\gamma\delta$ T cells, preferentially use the FcR γ chain as part of their CD3 complex (289). These findings suggest that intraepithelial T cells differ from peripheral T cells with regard to assembly of the TCR–CD3 complex, and these differences may influence their ability to respond to activation signals.

Functions of Intraepithelial T Lymphocytes

IELs may be assumed to be a primary source of effector T cells in the natural environment of the mucosal epithelium. Such effector cells form a first line of defense against translocation of the mucosal microflora and against invading microbial pathogens. To this end, it has been shown that intraepithelial CD8$^+$ T cells possess cytolytic activity, a prerequisite for the generation of MHC class I–restricted virus-specific CTLs. In addition to the antiviral activity of IELs, some subsets of intestinal intraepithelial T cells have been shown to contribute to a regional host defense against intestinal infection with bacterial pathogens (290–292). During *Listeria monocytogenes* infection, IFN-γ production and target cell lysis by CD8$^+$, $\alpha\beta$ T cells are crucial for clearance of the pathogen (293). It was also shown that both CD4$^+$ $\alpha\beta$ and $\gamma\delta$ T cells can contribute to optimum protection after systemic challenge with *L. monocytogenes* (293). After oral inoculation with this intracellular bacterium, intestinal listeriosis induced IFN-γ–producing $\gamma\delta$ T cells in the epithelium (290). A separate study showed that IFN-γ–producing T cells could be induced regardless of the presence of β2m, an essential gene for the expression of MHC class Ia chains as well as MHC class I–like molecules, including CD1 and TL (291). In this study, mice deficient in β2m that were orally infected with *L. monocytogenes* exhibited IFN-γ–producing T cells. This finding further suggested that in addition to classical $\alpha\beta$ CD8 T cells, biologically functional $\alpha\alpha$ CD8$^+$ T cells, including both $\alpha\beta$ and $\gamma\delta$ T cells, are involved in immune defense against this bacterium. These T cells develop independently of β2m (291), because $\alpha\alpha$ CD8$^+$ but not $\alpha\beta$ CD8$^+$ T cells are present in β2m$^{-/-}$ mice (294). Taken together, these findings demonstrate that intraepithelial T cells can serve as effector cells against mucosal infection by bacteria and viruses.

Subsets of intraepithelial T lymphocytes have been shown to function as regulatory cells for the induction and regulation of mucosal immune responses. Thus, $\alpha\beta$ and $\gamma\delta$ T cells from intestinal IELs are capable of producing Th1 and Th2 cytokines (52,264,283,295). In addition to IFN-γ, both CD4$^+$, CD8$^-$ and CD4$^+$, CD8$^+$ (DP) T cell subsets of $\alpha\beta$ T cells were shown to actively produce Th2-type, IgA-enhancing cytokines that provide helper functions for B-cell responses (264,295). Such helper cytokines have been shown to be spontaneously produced by T cells contained in these two subsets of IELs. Purified cells from both IEL subsets induced Ig-producing cells, including those of the IgA isotype, when cocultured with Peyer's patch B cells (295). When CD4$^+$, CD8$^-$ and DP T cells from IELs of mice orally immunized with T-cell dependent antigen (e.g., sheep erythrocytes) were incubated with B cells and accessory cells, both T-cell subsets supported antigen-specific IgM, IgG, and IgA antibody responses (264). These findings demonstrate that subsets of intraepithelial $\alpha\beta$ T cells, especially CD4$^+$ T cells are capable of providing helper function for mucosal immune responses.

IELs are unique in that they consist not only of $\alpha\beta$ T cells but also of a large number of $\gamma\delta$ T cells that appear to be important regulatory T cells for the induction and regulation of IgA responses in the mucosal compartment (284,296). In the presence of mucosally induced tolerance (e.g., oral tolerance), these mucosal $\gamma\delta$ T cells are major regulatory T cells that maintain Th2 cytokine-dependent, antigen-specific IgA responses in mucosal effector sites and block systemic responsiveness (296). Furthermore, analysis of TCR$\delta^{-/-}$ mice lacking $\gamma\delta$ T cells has shown that the numbers of IgA-producing cells are significantly more reduced in mucosa-associated tissues than in background control mice (TCR$\delta^{+/+}$ mice) (297). When both TCR$\delta^{-/-}$ and TCR$\delta^{+/+}$ mice were orally immunized with a combined mucosal vaccine of TT and CT as adjuvant, the levels of antigen-specific IgA responses were lower in the $\gamma\delta$ T cell–deficient mice in comparison with the control group.

In addition to such upregulatory functions, $\gamma\delta$ T cells have been shown to provide downregulatory signals in mucosally induced immune responses. Thus, $\gamma\delta$ T cells reduced antigen-specific IgE responses in mice and rats, which were given OVA by repetitive respiratory aerosols (298,299). Furthermore, hapten-specific $\gamma\delta$ T cells also inhibited IFN-γ–producing CD4$^+$ $\alpha\beta$ T cells from effecting the development of contact hypersensitivity (300). Taken together, these intriguing results provide new insights into the dual regulatory functions of mucosal $\gamma\delta$ T cells that can provide both stimulatory and inhibitory signals for CD4$^+$ $\alpha\beta$ T cells dependent on the isotype of the antigen-specific immune response.

A Mucosal Intranet: Epithelial Cell–T Cell Interactions for Mucosal Immunity

Epithelial cells and intraepithelial T cells in mucosal tissues form a cellular and molecular network of cross-talk in order to induce and maintain an appropriate immunologic barrier against inhaled and ingested antigens, including allergens, food products, and microorganisms. T cell–derived cytokines, including IFN-γ, IL-4, and TNF-α have been shown to influence epithelial cell functions such as the production of the pIgR (301,302). These cytokines were produced by both $\alpha\beta$ and $\gamma\delta$ T cells in the mucosal epithelium (263,264,295). Intraepithelial $\gamma\delta$ T cells have been shown to support the growth of epithelial cells by the production of keratinocyte growth factor (303). Studies with $\gamma\delta$ T cell–deficient mice, whose TCRδ gene had been deleted, have demonstrated the important role played by intraepithelial T cells in epithelial growth. In $\gamma\delta$ T cell–deficient mice, the turnover of epithelial cells in intestinal villi

of TCR$\delta^{-/-}$ mice and the levels of MHC class II expression were both lower than in background (control) mice (304). These findings suggest that intraepithelial $\gamma\delta$ T cells provide essential cytokines for the growth and function of epithelial cells.

Regulation is bidirectional because epithelial cells can also influence $\gamma\delta$ T-cell development and function. When mice deficient in stem cell factor (SCF) or its receptor c-kit (S1/S1^d and w/w^v, respectively) were assessed, peripheral T cells appeared normal in both mutants; however, the IELs were markedly affected (305). For example, the numbers of intraepithelial $\gamma\delta$ T cells were greatly reduced in S1/S1^d and w/w^v mice. Because SCF and c-kit are the products of epithelial cells and IELs, respectively, this cytokine signaling pathway from epithelial cells to intestinal $\gamma\delta$ T cells is essential for the growth of mucosal $\gamma\delta$ T cells. The SCF and c-kit network has also been shown to be important for intestinal fluid secretion induced by Vibrio cholerae (306). Using a ligated intestinal loop model, it was shown that both S1/S1^d and w/w^v mice produced significantly less intestinal fluid in response to CT challenge than did their control littermates. The interaction of SCF with its receptor was further shown to be important in Salmonella infections (307). Both human and murine intestinal epithelial cell lines have been shown to express high levels of SCF mRNA after exposure to Salmonella, and when c-kit mutant and control background mice were challenged with oral S. typhimurium, w/w^v mice had an enhanced susceptibility to infection in comparison with littermate controls. These findings provide important information that interactions between SCF and c-kit play an essential role as a first line of defense at the mucosal epithelium.

In addition to the SCF–c-kit cascade, cytokine signaling interaction between IL-7 and its receptor (IL-7R) also contributes to development and activation of intraepithelial $\gamma\delta$ T cells. It was shown that both human and murine intestinal epithelial cells express specific mRNA for IL-7 (266,308). The analysis of intestinal $\gamma\delta$ T cells shows that the corresponding receptor is expressed on a subset of $\gamma\delta$ T cells (266). Thus, cocultivation of intestinal $\gamma\delta$ T cells and recombinant IL-7 results in the activation of T cells for proliferative responses (266). Stimulatory signals provided via IL-7 as well as those provided via the IL-7R pathway (between epithelial cells and $\gamma\delta$ T cells), also induce IL-2R expression on the latter cell fraction. Furthermore, IL-2 provides a synergistic activation signal for further activation of $\gamma\delta$ T cells. IL-7 and IL-7R gene deleted mice (IL-7$^{-/-}$ and IL-7R$^{-/-}$) provide a unique opportunity to directly demonstrate the importance of this pathway for intestinal $\gamma\delta$ T-cell development. The deletion of the IL-7 gene resulted in reduction of intestinal $\gamma\delta$ T cells (309–311), whereas depletion of IL-7R completely depletes them (309,311). These findings support the idea that epithelial cell–derived IL-7 is an essential cytokine for the development and activation of neighboring IL-7R$^+$ $\gamma\delta$ T cells. Thus, epithelial cells and intraepithelial T cells are major players in the formation of a mucosal internet and can reciprocally regulate each other via select cytokines and corresponding receptor interactions.

MUCOSAL HOMING AND THE COMMON MUCOSAL IMMUNE SYSTEM

Interest in lymphocyte migration was sparked by early efforts to understand the cellular basis for the CMIS (8,315,316). It has since blossomed into the field of lymphocyte homing. The early studies showed a predisposition of B lymphocytes to migrate from Peyer's patches and draining mesenteric lymph nodes and ultimately into the LP regions of the gastrointestinal tract (312–314). These difficult but elegant studies clearly showed that GALT B cells had a propensity to migrate to mucosal effector sites, including not only the LP of the GI tract but also the mammary, salivary, and lacrimal glands (8,315–319). This section briefly summarizes the significant progress that has been made in understanding the GALT portion of the CMIS and outlines what is known of the as yet poorly understood but important NALT lymphocyte migration to mucosal effector tissues. Lymphocyte homing can be divided into several steps: lymphocyte adhesion (rolling) to HEVs, secondary adhesion (arrest), cell migration to HEV endothelial cell junctions, transmigration across the HEV, and chemotaxis into the appropriate lymphoid tissue compartment. These steps involve expression of receptors and ligands that mediate these events, and the details are beyond this discussion (320–324). For the purpose of this chapter, it will be sufficient to discuss only the unique expressional array of mucosal lymphocyte homing receptors and their ligand targets displayed on HEVs and HEV-like structures in mucosal inductive and effector sites, especially in the GI tract.

Lymphocyte Homing in the Gastrointestinal Tract

The mucosal immune system, like its peripheral system counterpart, has evolved the ability to respond to its environment, one of those responses being defense against pathogens. This response primarily depends on functioning lymphocytes that continuously traffic into organized lymphoid tissues (e.g., GALT and NALT) and, after antigen encounter, from inductive into effector sites. It is important that a full repertoire of naive lymphocytes stand poised to respond to mucosal antigens and that activated (effector) as well as memory cells migrate into effector regions where antigen exposure/pathogen damage has occurred. As a means to properly perform these important functions, lymphocytes express an array of homing receptors, and HEV endothelial cells express reciprocal ligands termed addressins (320–324). Adhesion molecules are major components of both lymphocyte homing receptors as well as endothelial cell addressins. The particular array of adhesion molecules/homing receptors or of adhesion molecules/addressin expression determines the immune compartment in which they function. For the purpose of this section, emphasis will be placed on the mucosal immune compartment in the GI tract and on how it contrasts with the peripheral immune compartment. Studies in this area have tended to discuss lymphocyte homing in the GI tract as if it were synonymous with mucosal homing, when in fact it is clear that it is only one component of the mucosal immune system.

Addressins selectively expressed on the endothelial cells include the P- and L-selectins (CD62P and CD62L, respectively), as well as glycolipid ligands, simply termed peripheral lymph node and mucosal vascular addressins, or peanut aggulinin addressin (PNAd) and mucosal addressin cell adhesion molecule-1 (MAdCAM-1), respectively (325–329) (Fig. 4B). In addition, ICAM-1 and ICAM-2 addressins function by interacting with LFA on lymphocytes that are also homing receptors (Fig. 4B). Although lymphocytes express an array of homing receptors, certain of these receptors, including selectins and β1 and β7 integrins, differentiate between mucosal and peripheral lymphocytes. For example, although L-selectin is a major homing receptor for PNAd and thus for peripheral lymph node (PLN) homing (Fig. 4B), it also plays a role in mucosal homing (325,326).

The integrins represent a large class of molecules characterized by a heterodimeric structure of α and β chains. Both chains are essential determinants for mucosal lymphocyte homing; for example, the α4 chain may pair with either β1 or β7 (324,330). The ligand for α4β1 is VCAM-1 (and fibronectin) and is associated with expression in inflamed sites (331,332). Pairing of α4 with β7 represents the major integrin form present for lymphocyte homing to MAdCAM-1 expressed on HEVs in Peyer's patches and GI tract LP (333). A number of studies have now established α4β7 MAdCAM-1 as the major mucosal homing receptor ligand. For example, monoclonal anti-α4 prevents lymphocyte binding to Peyer's patch HEV in vitro (333) and in vivo in rats (334) and mice (335). Furthermore, in vivo binding was also inhibited to a similar degree by mAbs to β7 and an α4β7 combined epitope but not with mAb to β1 (335). Such results clearly establishe α4β7 as a major mucosal homing receptor and MAdCAM-1 on Peyer's patch and LP HEV as their addressin (ligand).

Lymphocyte Homing as a Basis for the CMIS

Studies in humans have shown that parenteral vaccination results in a transient increase in peripheral blood B cells that produce antibodies to the vaccine and that oral immunization induces a similarly transient increase in antigen-specific antibody-forming cells (AFCs) (337,338). It is assumed that peripheral blood B cells are homing to systemic lymphoid tissue for plasma cell development (336), but a recent study offers strong evidence that they are also destined for mucosal effector sites in the GI tract. In this study, an oral cholera vaccine elicited transient IgA AFC in blood and subsequent IgA anticholera toxin AFC in duodenal tissues (339). Other studies have directly assessed the actual expression of mucosal (α4β7) and peripheral (α4β1) homing receptor expression on normal human peripheral blood T- and B-cell subpopulations (340). Interestingly, αEβ7+ T cells express high amounts of α4β7 and bind MAdCAM-1 well, clearly demonstrating their presence in peripheral blood mononuclear cells. Furthermore, B cells are separable into α4β7 and α4β1 subsets, with binding affinity for MAdCAM-1 and PNAd, respectively, suggesting that both B and T subsets are present in the blood circulation and are migrating to mucosal inductive or effector sites (340).

In a recent study, the avirulent live vaccine Salmonella typhi Ty21A was administered by both parenteral and oral immunization, and the resulting levels of AFCs in circulating B cells were compared (341). Peripheral blood cells were separated into α4β7+/α4β7−, or L-selectin+/L-selectin− subsets and assessed for anti-Ty21A AFCs. Interestingly, α4β7 was expressed on 99% of AFCs of subjects orally immunized, but only on 58% of those given parenteral Ty21A vaccine. On the other hand, more than 80% of AFCs from parenterally immunized subjects were L-selectin+, whereas only about 40% L-selectin+ AFCs were seen in subjects given oral Ty21A (341). Taken together, these results indeed suggest that mucosal immunization triggers α4β7+ B cells, which then migrate into the bloodstream. It is assumed that these cells are trafficking to the GI tract and enter MAdCAM-1+ HEVs for subsequent IgA plasma cell responses. In summary, homing receptors and addressins are major determinants for the CMIS, and this homing pathway is becoming reasonably well characterized for the GI tract in experimental models and in humans.

Homing of CD4+ Regulatory T Cells

Regulatory T cells in the CD4+ subset can be separated into naive, activated (effector) and memory cells, and, as discussed above,

A. Mucosal Homing For A CMIS

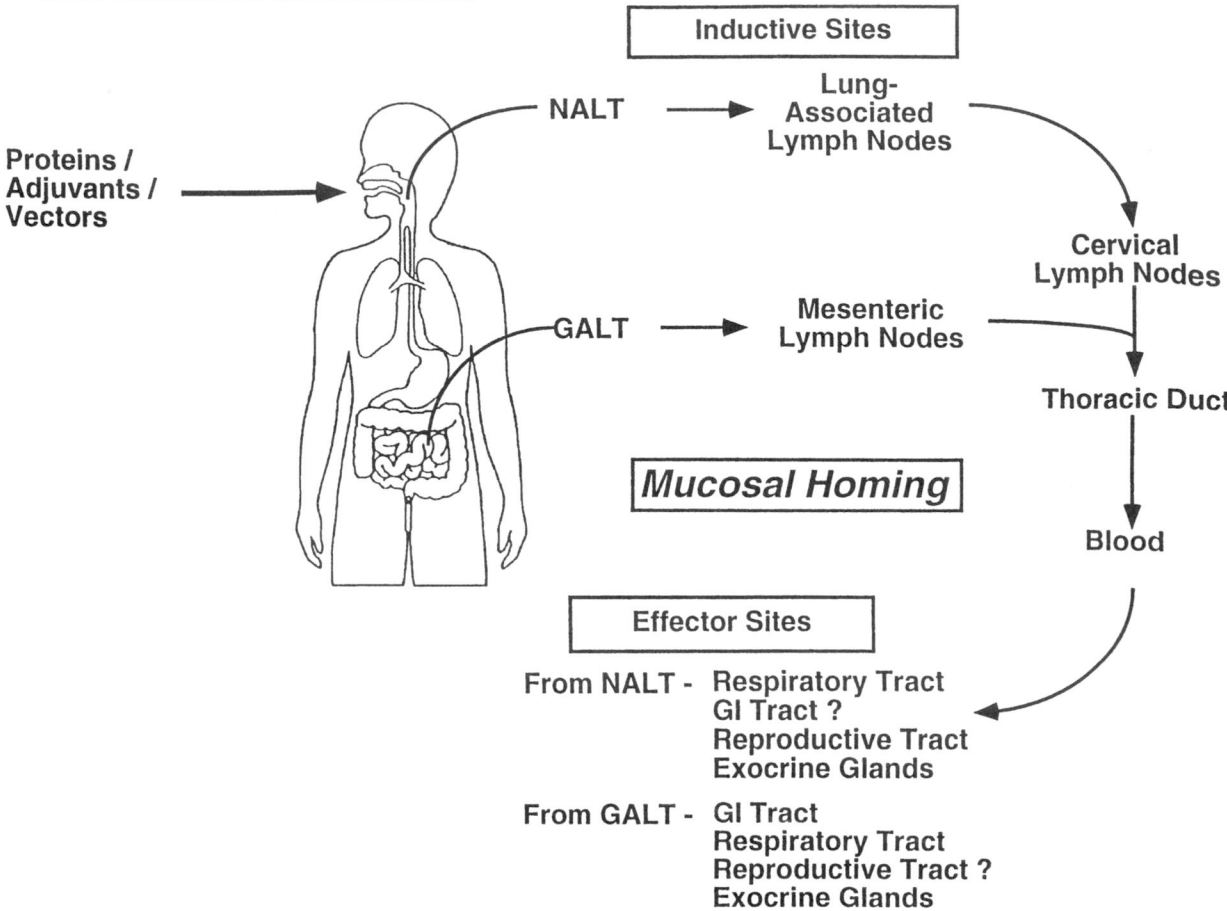

FIG. 4. Lymphocyte homing pathways for the CMIS (**A**), which is composed of IgA inductive and effector tissues. Antigen uptake and presentation in NALT and GALT results in the priming of Th1 or Th2 cells and sIgA⁺ B cells. These antigen-stimulated lymphocytes leave the inductive tissues and migrate to distant effector sites via the mucosal homing pathway (or CMIS). *Continued on next page.*

these T-cell subsets also express homing receptors (Fig. 4B). For example, CD4⁺ T cells with a naive phenotype (CD44^{lo}, CD45RB^{hi}, IL-2R⁻) represent approximately 65% of the entire population in mouse Peyer's patches. These cells presumably recirculate within the peripheral and mucosal immune systems (Fig. 4B) and display homing receptors for addressins expressed either by PLN or MLN. It remains possible that a subset of naive T cells in GALT develop mucosal homing receptors, such as α4β7 and then possibly recirculate to other mucosal inductive tissues. Approximately one fourth to one third of the GALT CD4⁺ T-cell subsets are activated (i.e., in cell cycle), most likely as a result of recent antigen exposure. These cells express α4β7 and recirculate within the mucosal immune system, at least within the portion associated with the GI tract. Memory CD4⁺ T cells (CD44^{hi}, CD45RB^{lo}, IL-2R⁻) also occur in GALT. Although estimates of their frequency vary, it is likely that more than 30% are present. Furthermore, these T cells also express mucosal homing receptors and are involved in population of effector sites in the GI tract (Fig. 4B). In this regard, more than 90% of CD4⁺ T cells isolated from either mouse (342) or human (343,344) LP regions exhibit characteristics of memory T cells. The precise relationship between repopulation of LP by activated (effector, CD44^{hi}, CD45RB^{lo}, IL-2R⁺) versus memory CD4⁺ T cells is not yet

resolved. Furthermore, it is not known if recently migrated effector cells function immediately for regulation of a local immune response. A major unresolved question regards the requirements for activation of memory T cells in effector sites, but the studies necessary to resolve this question are difficult to perform because LP T cells are notoriously unresponsive. Nevertheless, evidence suggests that LP T cells do not recirculate and that they undoubtedly play a major role in regulation of both Th1- and Th2-type responses that occur in this effector site.

Role of αEβ7 for Adhesion of Intraepithelial T Lymphocytes to Epithelial Cells

A family of integrins, αEβ7 (now CD103), was originally defined by the HML-1 and M290 monoclonal antibodies in humans and mice, respectively (345,346). It was shown that these monoclonal antibodies strongly react with IELs in mucosal epithelium and with *in vitro* activated CD8⁺ T cells from peripheral blood (345–347). Furthermore, the αEβ7 molecule was also strongly expressed by rat and chicken T cells (348,349). Recent evidence has demonstrated that αEβ7 mediates adhesion of intraepithelial T

B. Mucosal Homing - Regulatory T Cells

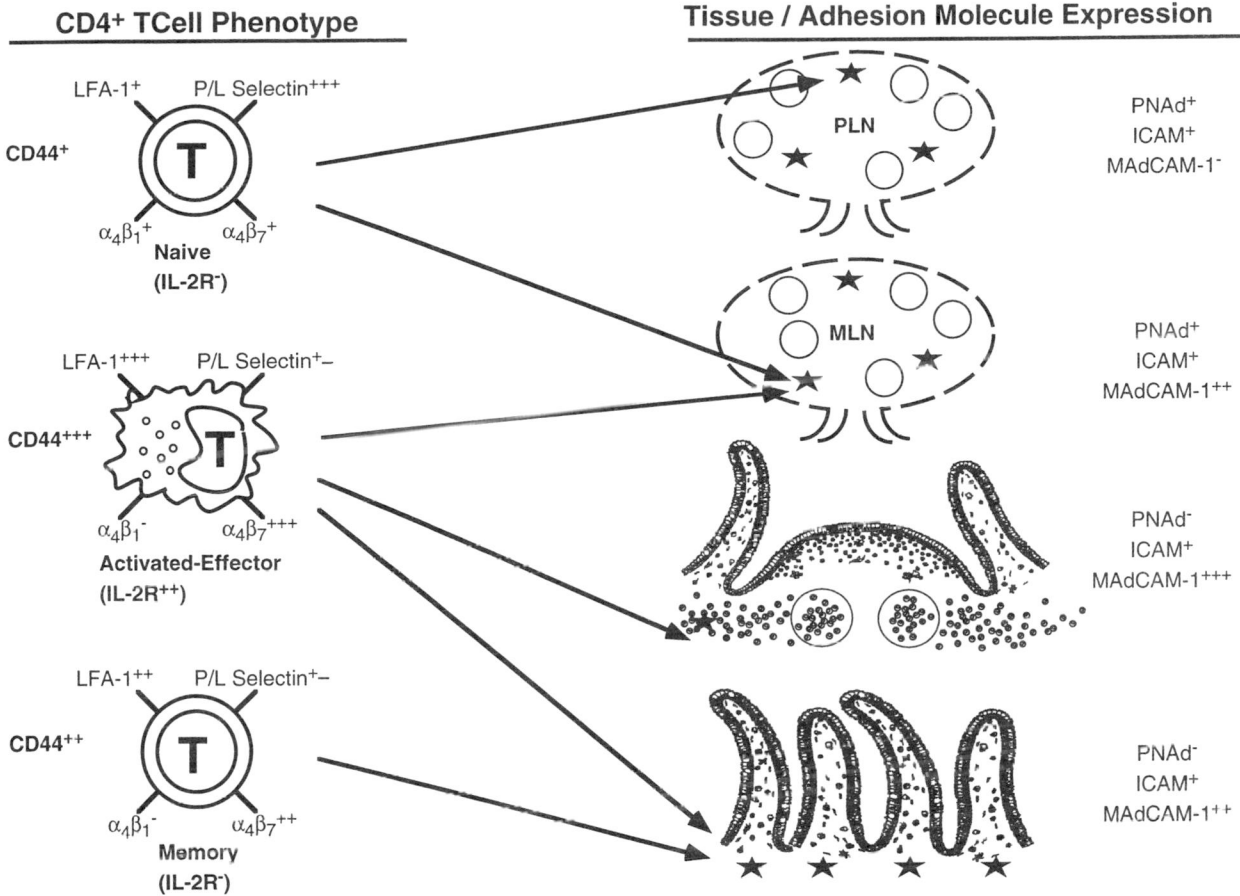

FIG. 4. *(Continued).* **(B)** After antigen stimulation, mucosal lymphocytes express distinct homing molecules for migration to GALT/NALT and to effector tissues.

lymphocytes to epithelial cells (350–352). For example, cultured intestinal IEL appears to bind to epithelial cells obtained from human intestine and breast tissues via αEβ7 because the binding is blocked by a monoclonal antibody specific for CD103 (350). Furthermore, because TGF-β can induce expression of αEβ7 instead of α4β7 (350,353,354), this cytokine downregulates α4 expression and induces the αE chain that associates with β7 to form αEβ7. Because epithelial cells can produce TGF-β (355), α4β7-expressing T-cell subsets that have recently arrived from mucosal inductive tissues may become αEβ7+ T cells under the influence of epithelial cell–derived TGF-β, thus allowing them to adhere T cells to epithelial cells. Other studies have elucidated the mechanism for recruitment of T cells into the epithelium. It has been shown that epithelial cells are capable of producing chemokines such as IL-8, MIP1α, and MIPβ (356,357). The epithelial cell ligand for CD103 has been identified as E-cadherin, which was previously termed epithelial cell membrane protein because of its function in homophilic interactions between epithelial cells, formation of adherent junctions, and epithelial cell morphogenesis (358). Thus, an interaction between αEβ7 and E-cadherin or between intraepithelial T cells and epithelial cells is important in cell-to-cell interactions in the mucosal epithelium. Although it remains to be shown directly, this molecular interaction likely mediates lymphocyte

homing into the epithelial cell layer and may be involved in the exchange of regulatory signals between intraepithelial T cells and epithelial cells. These hypotheses are supported by the fact that incubation of IELs with monoclonal anti-CD103 results in the activation of intraepithelial T cells (359). In addition, E-cadherin has been shown to be involved in the growth of epithelial cells (360).

MUCOSAL IMMUNITY TO VACCINES

Jenner introduced vaccination 200 years ago with the use of *Vaccinia* virus to prevent smallpox. However, since this auspicious beginning, fewer than 50 vaccines have been approved for human use, and in some instances these vaccines are merely improved versions of earlier forms. All but three of the current vaccines are administered parenterally and as such do not induce significant mucosal immunity. Nevertheless, almost all viral and bacterial pathogens to which vaccines would be desirable invade mucosal tissues where cell-mediated and antibody-mediated immunity would be most effective. Perhaps the most important example of the importance of the mucosal immune system in vaccine development is the realization that more than 80% of current HIV infections occur through sexual transmission. Hardly less striking are the strides that would be made against respiratory infections ranging from influenza (requiring yearly vaccination) to bacterial pneumonia and the enteric infections ranging from diarrhea- inducing bacterial enteropathies (cholera, *Shigella,* and *E. coli*) to infant rotavirus infections, should research into mucosal immunity become a research priority worldwide. Furthermore, an advantage of mucosal vaccination is that this mode can induce both mucosal and systemic immune responses, which result in two layers of host protection against infectious diseases.

In mucosal vaccine development, it is crucial to select an appropriate immunization route, and most current mucosal vaccine delivery is intended to mimic the natural encounter of mucosal inductive sites with environmental antigens and pathogens. Mucosal vaccination is usually performed by either oral (enteric) or intranasal (respiratory tract) application. In fact, many new vaccines are being tested by both routes to determine which induces immune responses via the CMIS most effectively. In many cases, intranasal immunization is more effective and in general requires smaller vaccine doses with less adjuvant. The occasional inefficiency of oral immunization is due in part to degradation of vaccine by the acidic gastric pH and proteolytic enzymes as well as by the potential for induction of mucosally induced tolerance.

Numerous studies over the past 25 years have shown that induction of precursor IgA B cells and Th cells in MALT results in the dissemination of B and Th cells to remote effector sites, including the LP regions of the GI, upper respiratory and genitourinary tracts, and exocrine glands (Fig. 1) for subsequent S-IgA antibody responses. In this regard, IgA precursor B cells from NALT, BALT, or GALT populate remote secretory sites, including the mammary, salivary, lacrimal, and uterine cervical glands. Using various oral vaccines, it was further shown that orally administered antigens resulted in the appearance of S-IgA antibodies in secretions from these remote sites, suggesting that antigen-specific IgA precursors originating in GALT follow a homing cycle to ultimately reach effector sites (361). Adoptive transfer of antigen-specific cells from mesenteric lymph nodes (presumably derived from Peyer's patches) repopulated the LP of the GI tract and mammary tissue of the host into which they were introduced to become antigen-specific plasma cells (317). It was also shown that S-IgA responses were identical in individual animals, clearly suggesting a clonal origin in MALT (362). Peyer's patches were first considered major IgA inductive sites after the observation that immunization of isolated intestinal segments containing a Peyer's patch could induce S-IgA antibodies even in adjacent nonimmunized segments, whereas immunized segments not containing a Peyer's patch did not (363). The MALT, especially the Peyer's patches, and NALT are major IgA inductive sites, which lead to S-IgA responses in remote external secretions via a CMIS (315).

Specialized Roles for S-IgA Antibodies in Mucosal Immunity

Efforts are underway to elucidate the potential use of the pIgR (SC) transport system to develop novel strategies to provide S-IgA antibodies in appropriate effector tissues. Although the mouse model has been useful (see below), we still do not understand how monomeric antibodies of IgG or IgA isotype appear in external secretions. Nevertheless, varying levels can occur and the potential that additional transport mechanisms are operative in mammals still exists. The importance of S-IgA transport across epithelial surfaces and into external secretions should be considered when vac-

cines are designed to prevent infections that occur at mucosal surfaces. Passive transfer studies in mice using antigen-specific monoclonal IgA have provided evidence that IgA antibodies alone are able to protect against intranasal infection with influenza (364), intestinal infection with *Vibrio cholerae* (365,366) or *S. typhimurium* (367), and gastric infection with *Helicobacter felis* (368). Specific S-IgA antibodies presumably bind with the colonizing pathogen and thereby inhibit its interaction with host epithelial cells. Furthermore, passive transfer of IgA anti–*S. typhimurium* antibodies provides protection against oral challenge with virulent *S. typhimurium.* However, it is unable to prevent infection when the organisms are injected intraperitoneally, suggesting that mechanisms for protection at a mucosal surface do not correlate with protection from systemic challenge (367). This model also has been used to show that passive transfer of IgA leads to high titers of serum IgA, which are indicative of high levels of IgA at mucosal surfaces. Furthermore, mice with high titers of serum IgA are protected from infection by *S. typhimurium,* whereas all mice with low serum IgA titers become infected (367). Therefore, specific S-IgA antibody responses may provide a means to completely prevent bacterial or viral infections or at least greatly reduce the size of the infectious inoculum at the mucosal sites where initial contact with most infectious agents occurs.

A series of elegant *in vitro* studies with polymeric IgA (pIgA) and pIgR$^+$ epithelial cells have now suggested that pIgA can actually mediate intracellular virus neutralization as well as transport of immune complexes across epithelial cells (369–372). These additional functions would be beneficial in preventing or inhibiting infection at mucosal surfaces. Virus-specific pIgA has been shown to neutralize Sendai virus intracellularly in pIgR$^+$ cells (371); such neutralization requires the expression of pIgR by infected cells (for intracellular transport of IgA) as well as antigen-specific pIgA. Because IgG is not transported by the pIgR, this isotype is unable to neutralize virus intracellularly (371). Another potential function mediated by pIgA in pIgR$^+$ epithelial cells involves transcytosis of noxious antigens as immune complexes and their release into the external secretions (369,370,372). In one study, immune complexes formed with antigen and pIgA were transported across pIgR$^+$ epithelial cells and released in the same manner as polymeric IgA transported across pIgR$^+$ epithelial cells (369). In additional studies, it was shown that immune complexes containing antigen, antigen-specific monomeric IgA, or IgG also could be transported across epithelial cells in a pIgR-dependent fashion as long as the immune complex contained polymeric IgA (370). Direct evidence for the *in vivo* relevance of this intracellular neutralization model for S-IgA function has recently been published (373). In this study, the tumor backpack model was used to allow production of monoclonal IgA antibody to rotavirus VP4 and VP6. Interestingly, two mAbs to VP6, which is an inner capsid protein not amenable to neutralization, were protective when delivered via backpack, but were not when presented at the mucosal surfaces of the GI tract (373). Additional studies should provide more details regarding the intracellular compartments involved in virus assembly versus transcellular transport of pIgA by the pIgR.

Mucosal Adjuvants

The introduction of proteins including vaccines into mucosal inductive sites is an effective way to induce systemic unresponsiveness (mucosally induced tolerance). Although mucosally induced tolerance is considered a useful approach to prevent autoimmune diseases, this modality could result in loss of the host's ability to respond to infection. Thus, mucosal adjuvants are required not only to boost mucosal and systemic immunity, but also to prevent the induction of mucosally induced tolerance. The major enterotoxins produced by *Vibrio cholerae* and *Escherichia coli,* termed, respectively, cholera toxin (CT) and heat-labile toxin (LT), are macromolecules composed of two structurally, functionally, and immunologically separate A and B subunits (374–376). The B subunits of both toxins consist of five identical 11.6 kDa peptides but differ from each other in that the B subunit of CT (CT-B) only binds to GM1 ganglioside (377), whereas the B subunit of LT (LT-B) is more promiscuous and binds GM1 as well as asialo GM1 and GM2 (378). After binding of the B subunit to epithelial cell GM1 or GM2 receptors, the A subunit reaches the cytosol and, after activation, binds to NAD and catalyzes ADP-ribosylation of Gsα (379). This GTP-binding protein activates adenyl cyclase with subsequent elevation of cyclic adenosine monophosphate, resulting in epithelial cells in secretion of water and chloride ions into the small intestine (380).

Mucosal exposure of CT and LT, which are both immunogenic, results in S-IgA and serum antibodies, which are almost entirely restricted to CT-B or LT-B (381). More importantly, both toxins are potent mucosal adjuvants for coadministered, unrelated proteins when given by oral, intranasal, or even parenteral routes (105,381,382). Recent studies have shown that induction of maximal mucosal S-IgA and serum IgG antibody response correlates directly to the presence of antigen-specific CD4+ Th cells secreting IL-4 and IL-5 in mice orally immunized with protein antigen and CT as adjuvant (105). Further detailed analysis has shown that CT elicits adjuvant responses by inducing antigen-specific CD4+ Th2-type cells, which in turn produce high levels of IL-4, IL-5, IL-6, and IL-10. These support subsequent development of systemic IgG1 and IgG2b subclass, IgE and mucosal S-IgA antibody responses (106). On the other hand, oral immunization with LT results in IgM, IgG1, IgG2a, IgG2b, and S-IgA antibody responses, which are associated with a mixed CD4+ Th1- and Th2-type response with IFN-γ, IL-5, IL-6, and IL-10 production (111). Furthermore, when IL-4 levels produced by CD4+ T cells are compared, antigen-specific IL-4 production was significantly lower when LT as adjuvant was used as opposed to CT (106,111).

It is now well known that both CT and LT cause severe diarrhea in humans and account for the clinical manifestations of cholera and enterotoxigenic *E. coli* enteritis; thus, neither is suitable for use as a mucosal adjuvant in humans. Earlier studies have attempted to dissociate the diarrhoeagenicity and adjuvanticity of these two molecules; however, it has been shown that a mutant of LT, termed E112K (383), which contains a single amino acid substitution in the ADP-ribosyltransferase active center (384), is nontoxic and also lacks adjuvanticity (385). More recently, it was reported that single amino acid substitution mutants of LT, R7K (386), and R192G (387), which are outside of the adenosine diphosphate (ADP)–ribosyltransferase cleft, are nontoxic but retain adjuvant properties when coadministered with protein by the intranasal or oral route, respectively (386,387). In addition, another LT mutant, designated S63K, was shown to be without toxicity (388). This mutant exhibited relatively low mucosal adjuvant properties when administered intranasally (389). On the other hand, two mutants of CT (mCTs), designated S61F and E112K, which harbor single amino acid substitutions in the ADP–ribosyltranferase active center, completely lack ADP–ribosyltransferase activity and diar-

rhoeagenicity (390). Both mCTs are effective adjuvants and are comparable with native CT (nCT) when given parenterally (390) or nasally (391).

The questions of adjuvanticity of CT-B also have been addressed by the creation of fusion proteins from hybrid genes. The advantages of using fusion proteins rather than chemically coupled ones are that they are free of contaminating holotoxin and are uniform in structure. It has been shown that fusion of a portion of glucosyl transferase (GftB) to alkaline phosphatase (PhoA) or to CT-B does not affect the functional activity of either PhoA or CT-B as determined by enzyme activity or GM1 binding, respectively (392,393). The CT-B conjugates induce serum IgG and IgA anti–CT-B antibodies, whereas antibodies to GftB are only detectable when a high dose of the GftB–CT-B conjugate is used for immunization. Furthermore, the IgG titers are low and no IgA anti–Gtf-B is detected. Others have created fusions between protein and CT-B–CT-A2 mutants, which lack the toxic A1 subunit (394). Interestingly, oral administration of this chimeric vaccine induces serum IgG antibodies; however, maximum mucosal IgA responses require an additional adjuvant. Thus, it appears that CT-B is an excellent carrier molecule due to its ability to bind to GM1 but at best exhibits low adjuvant properties. Full adjuvanticity requires both the A and B subunits of the holotoxin.

Oral Versus Intranasal Vaccination Strategies

A full discussion of recent studies with either oral or intranasal vaccines is beyond the scope of this chapter and more detail is provided elsewhere (395–397). However, it is now realized that the nature of the delivery system as well as the route of immunization influence the nature of Th-cell subsets induced and markedly affect the outcome of systemic and mucosal immunity. For example, use of native CT or mutant CTs with vaccines given orally tend to induce CD4+ Th2-type cells with characteristic serum IgG1, IgG2b, IgE, and IgA as well as mucosal S-IgA responses (105,106). On the other hand, oral immunization with recombinant bacteria, e.g., *Salmonella*-expressing proteins, tends to induce not only CD4+ Th1-type cells and CMI but characteristics of level CD4+ Th2-type cells as well. These CD4+ Th cells produce cytokines such as IL-6 and IL-10 that appear to support mucosal S-IgA responses (71,398). In this section, we have selected studies that illustrate the development of oral and intranasal immunization strategies using either mucosal adjuvants or live vectors, and in the following section we have outlined the plethora of vector strategies currently under investigation for mucosal vaccine development.

Oral Vaccines

We have purposely selected a small subset of studies to illustrate the nature of murine immune responses that result from oral immunization with microbial vaccines (Table 2). It is important to emphasize that immune responses vary depending on the nature of antigen used as well as mouse strains selected for study. However, proteins such as TT or HEL with CT as mucosal adjuvant induce predominantly serum IgG1 and IgE antibodies (106,107). Furthermore, in one study it was shown that systemic challenge of mice orally immunized with HEL and CT led to a fatal anaphylactic response (107). Thus, all studies that use CT or its derivatives should consider untoward reactions that may occur due to induction of IgE antibody responses.

TABLE 2. *General characteristics of murine immune responses after oral immunization with protein-based combined vaccines*

| Vaccine delivery system | Pattern of antigen specific antibody responses | | | | Profile of Th1 and Th2 responses | | Comments |
| | Serum | | | Secretions | | | |
	IgG1	IgG2a	IgE	S-IgA	Th1	Th2	
Protein antigen + CT	+++	+	+	++	+	+++	In general, CT supports a dominant Th2-regulated immune response. However, in some cases (e.g., parasite antigen can support Th1 induction).
Protein antigen + LT	++	++	±	++	++	++	LT activates both Th1 and Th2 pathways.
rSalmonella	+	+++	-	++	+++	+	rSalmonella induces dominant Th1 responses in the presence of level two Th2 cells producing selective cytokines for IgA.

**[a]Antigen plus mucosal adjuvant or recombinant bacterial vectors.

Oral immunization of mice with KLH or TT and CT as adjuvant have been shown to induce Ag-specific CD4⁺ Th cells with a characteristic Th2 phenotype (105,106,108). For example, both Peyer's patch and LP lymphocytes, when restimulated with KLH, produced significant quantities of IL-4 and IL-5, with minimal levels of IFN-γ and IL-2 (Table 2) (108). Thus, several studies now support the notion that oral immunization with soluble proteins and CT as adjuvant induce Th2-type responses that provide help for characteristic serum IgG1 and IgE as well as mucosal S-IgA antibodies (Table 2).

There is evidence that orally coadministered CT also can induce antigen-specific CD4⁺ Th1-type responses. For example, mice given a soluble preparation of *Toxoplasma gondii* on three occasions at 10-day intervals harbored splenic *T. gondii*–specific T cells (399). Further *in vitro* restimulation resulted in increased levels of both IFN-γ and IL-2, whereas IL-4 and IL-5 levels were similar to those seen in mice orally immunized with *T. gondii* only (399). A more revealing study used the mouse parasite *Trichuris muris* in a soluble form with CT and assessed IFN-γ and IL-5 levels as markers for Th1 or Th2-type responses, respectively (400). Interestingly, oral *T. muris* plus CT induced T cells that produced IL-5 before parasite challenge, but which switched to IFN-γ production after *T. muris* infection. This shift suggests that the infection itself results in CD4⁺ Th1-type responses, even in the presence of a predominant Th2-type response. One study has shown that oral immunization with parasite antigen and CT elicits both serum IgG and mucosal IgA responses (401). This study, which also assessed antiparasite antibodies in bile (where IgA was the predominant isotype), showed that oral immunization normally induces serum IgA, and in experimental species such as mice, rats, and rabbits, in which the serum IgA is predominantly polymeric, the pIgA is transported into the GI tract. Thus, all studies that assess intestinal IgA responses should ensure that the response actually occurs locally and should therefore perform assays to detect IgA producing plasma cells in LP regions of the GI tract.

Attenuated avirulent *Salmonella* strains have received considerable attention as mucosal vaccine delivery vectors for recombinant proteins associated with virulence (402–405). After oral administration, *Salmonella* replicates directly in the mucosa-associated tissues (e.g., Peyer's patches) and thereafter disseminates via the MALT to systemic sites (e.g., spleen). This characteristic dissemination pattern of growth in both mucosal and systemic sites allows *Salmonella* to induce broad-based immune responses, including cell-mediated as well as serum IgG and mucosal S-IgA antibody responses. Although a large number of genes from bacteria,

viruses, parasites, and mammalian species have been expressed in attenuated *Salmonella* (402,403), few studies have fully characterized both T- and B-cell responses to the expressed protein antigen. In particular, the balance between antigen-specific CD4⁺ Th1 and Th2 cells and their subsequent influence on subclass-specific IgG and mucosal IgA responses have received little attention in these systems. Such clarity is paramount to the development of delivery protocols that will provide the appropriate immune response to a given pathogen.

A pioneering study in this area showed that mice given an oral attenuated *S. typhimurium*–expressing *Leishmania* surface protein (gp63) elicited CD4⁺ T cells that produced IFN-γ and IL-2, but not IL-4 (406). The results at first might appear puzzling. Because it appears that mucosal S-IgA responses are dependent on Th2 cells and cytokines such as IL-5, IL-6, and IL-10, by what mechanisms do these attenuated recombinant Salmonella (rSalmonella)- expressing foreign protein antigens induce S-IgA responses? Recent studies have addressed this issue by use of rSalmonella expressing the Tox C gene of TT. Oral administration of rSalmonella Tox C resulted in predominant serum IgG2a and IgG2b anti-TT as well as mucosal S-IgA anti-TT antibody responses (71). Splenic and Peyer's patch CD4⁺ T cells selectively produced IFN-γ and IL-2 as well as the Th2 cytokine IL-10 (71). Furthermore, macrophages from these mice produced heightened levels of IL-6 (71). Clear verification that IL-4 is not involved was shown by oral immunization of IL-4 knock-out (IL-4⁻/⁻) mice, which produced serum IgG2a and mucosal S-IgA antibodies. Interestingly, CD4⁺ T cells in these mice exhibited two cytokine patterns: a Th1 phenotype as well as T cells that produced IL-6 and IL-10, but not IL-5 (398). The latter subset of Th2 cells, which produce only IgA enhancing cytokines, has been termed level 2 Th2-type cells in contrast to so-called level 1 Th2-type cells producing an array of IL-4, IL-5, IL-6, and IL-10.

Intranasal Vaccines

Intranasal immunization has emerged as perhaps the most effective route for induction of both peripheral and mucosal immune responses. Again, most studies can be divided into those that use soluble vaccine components with mucosal adjuvants such as CT (as well as protein–CT-B conjugates) versus studies with attenuated vectors. A series of extensive studies using the influenza (flu) model demonstrated that intranasal immunization with flu vaccine provides more effective protective immunity than oral immunization (397,407). Intranasal immunization with trivalent vaccines in the presence of CT-B containing a trace amount of A subunit provides cross-protection against a broad range of viruses (408). It was also shown that intranasal immunization with flu vaccine together with LT-B (containing a trace amount of LT) induces antigen-specific immune responses in humans (409). These findings show that an appropriate intranasal vaccine can provide effective immunity against infection.

With regard to vectors, most studies have been limited to respiratory tract viral pathogens, which have been subjected to attenuating mutations or genomic deletions. It is interesting that recombinant adenoviruses (r-Ad), currently used for gene therapy, are also candidates for mucosal delivery of vaccine proteins. In most current protocols, vaccine is instilled into each nostril (usually 10 mg per nostril) and inhaled, resulting in effective delivery of vaccine presumably into NALT. Larger aliquots are subsequently swallowed, producing oral immunization. For this reason, any intranasal protocol cannot avoid some oral delivery, whereas most studies of oral immunization use gastric intubation to avoid potential nasal immunization. It also should be noted that two routes of pulmonary immunization have been used: intratracheal and intranasal delivery. In general, it appears that intratracheal immunization tends to induce responses in the lower lungs and associated lymph nodes, including BALT, whereas intranasal immunization sensitizes NALT and associated cervical lymph nodes.

Several studies can be used to illustrate principles associated with intranasal immunization. In one, intranasal administration of inactivated respiratory syncytial virus (RSV) with CT resulted in nasal IgA and serum IgG anti-RSV responses (410). Analysis of IgG subclasses suggest that both IgG1 and IgG2a are induced (410). Interestingly, infection with RSV and subsequent Th1-type responses are characterized by a favorable outcome, whereas Th2-type responses are associated with significant pathology (216,411). Intranasal immunization with the C fragment of tetanus toxoid (fragment C) and CT as adjuvant resulted in serum antibody responses characterized by comparable IgG1, IgG2a, and IgG2b anti–fragment C titers, suggesting that the use of CT as an adjuvant with fragment C induces a response characterized by both Th1- and Th2-type responses (412). However, when fragment C is administered intranasally with pertussis toxin (PT) or a mutated form of PT known as PT-9K/129G as mucosal adjuvants, anti-fragment C IgG1 predominates, suggesting that an immune response biased toward the Th2 type has been induced. Direct comparisons between CT and PT or PT-9K/129 in this study are difficult because the use of CT is associated with much more potent anti–Frg C IgG responses. Further investigation will be needed to determine the role that adjuvants, the vaccine antigen, and the route of immunization play in induction of CD4+ Th1 and Th2 responses.

Recombinant adenoviruses have proven to be rather successful delivery agents of foreign genes to mucosal tissues for therapy of genetic disorders such as cystic fibrosis, as well as good vehicles for vaccination with expressed genes for certain infectious diseases. It is interesting that in these two instances host immune responses develop both to r-Ad and to the transgene. In gene therapy, the expression is transient, whereas in vaccination the immune response to r-Ad precludes boosting of foreign gene–specific immunity. Thus, in both instances the host immune response renders the use of r-Ad suboptimal. Despite these drawbacks, the use of r-Ad remains a promising approach in both arenas. Most studies to date have been performed with r-Ad from which the E1 and E3 genes have been deleted, rendering virus replication defi-

cient. However, the virion retained full competence for infection of mucosal epithelial cells in the respiratory tract (413). In recent studies, r-Ad expressing herpes simplex virus glycoprotein B was shown to be a most effective vaccine when given by the intranasal route to mice (414). This regimen induced serum IgG as well as pulmonary IgA anti–glycoprotein B responses, which correlated with protection from challenge. Furthermore, this vaccine induced an effective CTL response (414). This mucosal route of immunization also appears to be safe and effective because intranasal delivery of rAd-expressing HIV envelope and gag proteins to chimpanzees resulted in significant serum antibody responses (415). These antibody responses were broad based, and boosting with a gp160 subunit vaccine elicited serum-neutralizing antibodies (415). A major advantage of the current generation of r-Ad vectors is their capacity to accommodate large amounts of exogenous complementary DNA (7 to 8 kilobases). Of course, this feature has been used to express virulence genes from a number of viral pathogens. For example, human r-Ad vectors were used to express vesicular stomatitis virus and were effective for induction of systemic antibody responses after oral delivery (416). r-Ad also has been used as vector for rabies virus in order to orally vaccinate foxes (417). In addition, r-Ad expressing respiratory syncytial virus and hepatitis B proteins have been given orally to dogs and chimpanzees with successful induction of circulating antibody responses (418,419).

A major goal in developing an AIDS vaccine is to elicit mucosal immunity to HIV. In this regard, it is important to consider mucosal delivery for induction of effective immunity in the genitourinary tract. The infection of rhesus macaques with SIV via the genitourinary tract has served as a useful model to study mucosal immunity to HIV (218,420). In an important study, groups of macaques were immunized with SIV in biodegradable microspheres by oral, intratracheal, or intramuscular routes (220). It was shown that intratracheal priming was more effective than oral dosing for induction of serum IgA responses. Although all three routes of immunization resulted in vaginal anti-SIV antibodies, only the intratracheal route induced a long-lasting response. When immunized macaques were challenged with two vaginal ID$_{50}$ (50% infectious dose) of SIV$_{mac251}$, three of four naive macaques and all macaques immunized solely by the oral route were infected. Of the animals primed by the intramuscular route, only two of three intratracheally boosted and one of three orally boosted monkeys were infected. Although CMI responses were not examined in this study, and further investigation is needed to determine the role of vaginal anti-SIV antibodies in protection, the model provides evidence that protection against SIV (and possibly HIV) at mucosal surfaces may be an attainable goal (220). This view has (50% infectious dose) also has been supported by recent evidence that intranasal immunization of rhesus macaque with SIV p55 and CT induced antigen-specific IgG and IgA antibodies in serum and mucosal secretions, respectively (421). In addition, oral immunization with the combined vaccine (p55 and CT) resulted in the Th1/Th2-type response as well as antigen-specific IgG and IgA antibody production (422).

A recent murine study used an HIV peptide containing T-helper, CTL, and B-cell epitopes in the V3 loop with CT as mucosal adjuvant. This study showed that intranasal immunization induced serum-neutralizing IgG antibodies that are predominantly of the IgG1 subclass (423). Significant vaginal anti-HIV IgA responses were induced, and these antibodies were associated with the secretory component, suggesting a mucosal origin (423). This study also showed that strong CMI or DTH responses are elicited with this regimen. A second study evaluated the efficacy of CT to induce CTL responses. Intranasal immunization with HIV-1 peptide and CT resulted in peptide-specific CTLs in both cervical lymph nodes and spleen (424). Thus, it would appear that mucosal adjuvants such as CT and its mutant derivatives possessing HIV peptides offer the possibility of a vaccine that can generate both antibody-mediated and CTL responses.

MUCOSALLY INDUCED TOLERANCE

In addition to the beneficial induction of antigen-specific S-IgA and serum IgG responses by mucosal immunization, this route of immunization also can induce an opposite type of immune response, namely the induction of systemic unresponsiveness (e.g., oral tolerance). Thus, mucosal immunization can up- or downregulate systemic immune responses. As discussed above, for the purpose of mucosal vaccine development against infectious diseases, the goal would be induction of both mucosal and systemic immunity in order to provide two layers of protection. In contrast, inhibition of antigen-specific immune responses in systemic compartments by mucosal immunization is important for the prevention of allergic responses to food proteins and allergens. Furthermore, this system can be applied to the prevention and treatment of autoimmune diseases by feeding self antigens.

Oral administration of a single high dose or repeated oral delivery of low doses of proteins have been shown to induce systemic unresponsiveness in the presence of mucosal IgA responses (425–427). These immunologically distinct responses in mucosa-associated versus systemic-associated lymphoid tissues were originally termed oral tolerance (425). More recent studies have shown that intranasal administration of proteins also induces systemic unresponsiveness (428–433) and has led to the more general term "mucosally induced tolerance." Nevertheless, even though antigen-specific systemic unresponsiveness can be induced by oral or nasal antigen administration, the bulk of studies in this area have been performed by antigen feeding. Thus, most available information applies to oral tolerance with the assumption that the same principles may apply to nasally induced tolerance.

The Concept of Mucosally Induced Tolerance

Mucosal administration of antigen is a long-recognized method of inducing peripheral unresponsiveness or tolerance (434). The effect is often referred to as oral tolerance because it was initially documented by the effect of oral administration of antigen for the induction of reduced immune responses in the systemic immune compartment. This is a unique immune reaction and is characterized by the fact that experimental animals fed large quantities of protein antigen become refractory or have a diminished capability to develop an immune response when reexposed to that same antigen introduced by the systemic route (e.g., by injection) (425,435). This unique response is an important natural physiologic mechanism whereby the host avoids development of DTH reactions to many ingested food proteins and other antigens (426). Furthermore, the development of mucosally induced tolerance against pollen and dust antigens could also be essential for the inhibition of allergic reactions, including IgE-mediated hypersensitivity. Although several possible mechanisms for the induction of mucos-

ally induced tolerance have been proposed, the primary ones appear to be mediated by T cells involved in the generation of active suppression or clonal anergy or deletion (436). For example, high doses of antigen given by the oral route induced clonal deletion or anergy (437–439), characterized by the absence of T-cell proliferation and diminished IL-2 production as well as IL-2R expression. However, frequently administered low doses of antigen induced active suppression by CD4$^+$ or CD8$^+$ T cells that secreted cytokines such as TGF-β, IL-4, and IL-10 (440,441). It is interesting to note that the latter scenario involves cytokines that are also known to upregulate IgA production (442) and is thus compatible with the observation that secretory immune responses and systemic tolerance may develop concomitantly (425,443). Because tolerance can be transferred by both serum and cells from tolerized animals, it is possible that humoral antibodies (IgG and IgA? anti-idiotype antibody? immune complexes?), circulating undegraded antigens, or tolerogenic antigen fragments and cytokines may act synergistically to confer T-cell unresponsiveness (435). Because oral tolerance is specific for the antigen initially ingested or inhaled and thus does not influence the development of systemic immune responses against other antigens, its manipulation has become an increasingly attractive strategy for preventing and possibly treating illnesses associated with or resulting from the development of untoward immunologic reactions against specific antigens encountered or expressed (autoantigens) in nonmucosal tissues.

Mechanisms of Mucosally Induced Tolerance: Roles for Both αβ and γδ T Cells

In the late 1970s and early 1980s, mucosal immunologists had already made attempts to investigate the possible mechanisms of oral tolerance at a time when the immune system was not characterized at the cellular and molecular levels. Although several possible mechanisms (e.g., B-cell tolerance, antiidiotypic antibody, intestinal antigen-processing events for tolerogen and APCs) have been shown to be involved in the induction of oral tolerance (435), the most compelling evidence to date suggests that T cells are the major cell type involved in the induction of mucosally induced tolerance. In earlier work, it was shown that systemic unresponsiveness was induced by adoptive transfer of T cells from rats orally fed bovine serum albumin (444). Subsequently, a large number of studies demonstrated that oral immunization of protein antigen induces CD4$^+$ Th cells in mucosa-associated tissues that support IgA responses, whereas suppressor T cells were induced in systemic compartments such as spleen and downregulate antigen-specific IgM, IgG, and IgE responses (445–451). For example, oral feeding of OVA to mice led to the generation of Th cells supporting IgA responses and suppressor T cells for IgG and IgE responses in GALT (448,450,451). Furthermore, the former T cells for IgA responses remained in Peyer's patches, whereas the suppressor T cells migrated into the systemic compartment (e.g., spleen). These observations were considered to be logical explanations for cellular mechanisms of oral tolerance where Peyer's patch–derived CD4$^+$ Th cells supported IgA responses, while splenic T-suppressor cells induced systemic unresponsiveness. It is now generally agreed that a functional suppressor mechanism exists for the downregulation of systemic immune responses; however, the nature and properties of these suppressor T cells are disputed.

αβ T Cells in Mucosally Induced Tolerance

Considering the past and recent studies concerning cellular and molecular mechanisms of oral tolerance, αβ T cells appear to be involved in the downregulation of systemic immune responses to orally administered antigens (Table 3). It is also currently assumed that the status of oral tolerance can be explained by clonal anergy or deletion of T cells, as well as by active suppression by T cells via the secretion of inhibitory cytokines (436,437,439,452–456). Low doses of oral antigen favor the latter form of inhibition, whereas higher doses of feeding induce clonal anergy of immunocompetent T cells (436,452–454). These two forms of oral tolerance are not mutually exclusive and may occur simultaneously after oral administration of antigens.

T-Cell Anergy

A condition of anergy is defined as a state of T-cell unresponsiveness characterized by the lack of proliferation and of IL-2 synthesis, as well as diminished IL-2R expression (457). This state can be reversed by preculturing T cells with IL-2 (458). Anergy recently was demonstrated under one condition of oral tolerance in which a large dose of protein antigen induced anergy in OVA-specific T cells (439). Furthermore, oral administration of myelin basic protein (MBP) diminished IL-2 and IFN-γ synthesis (437). These findings suggest that Th1 type T cells may be susceptible to the induction of anergy after oral feeding. To this end, it has been shown that Th1 type cells appear to be more sensitive to the induction of tolerance in vitro than Th2 type cells (459). In vivo evidence has demonstrated that Th1 cells are likely to be anergized in oral tolerance (455). In order to identify which lymphocyte compartment (e.g., CD4+ versus CD8+ T cells) preferentially mediates the induction of oral tolerance, cell transfer experiments were recently performed using SCID and nu/nu mice (454). Adoptive transfer of splenic lymphocytes from mice orally tolerized with bovine α-

casein resulted in the induction of tolerance in these immunocompromised mice. It was shown that oral tolerance was induced by anergized CD4+ but not CD8+ T cells. Taken together, a form of oral tolerance can be achieved by the induction of anergic CD4+ T cells in the systemic compartment.

An Imbalanced Th1/Th2 Cytokine Network

It has been suggested that the induction of tolerance can also be explained by dysregulation of homeostasis between Th1- and Th2-type cells. For example, preferential activation of Th2 cells may lead to downregulation of Th1-CMI responses by Th2 cytokines such as IL-4 and IL-10 (460). In addition, and as described above, Th1-type cells are much more sensitive to anergy induction after oral administration of protein antigens (Table 3). These findings suggest the possibility that oral tolerance is associated with selective downregulation of Th1 cells by Th2 cells via their respective cytokines in the systemic immune compartment. This possibility is consistent with the fact that oral tolerance has more profound effects on Th1-regulated CMI responses than on Th2-mediated antibody responses. However, recent studies have shown that feeding high doses of OVA inhibited production of both Th1 (IL-2 and IFN-γ) and Th2 (IL-4, IL-5, and IL-10) cytokines and resulted in the reduction of IFN-γ– and IL-4–dependent antigen-specific IgG2a and IgG1 antibody responses, respectively (452). These findings indicate that both subsets of Th cells are equally involved in the induction of oral tolerance (Table 3).

A recent study has suggested that oral administration of a high dose of protein antigen can induce brisk IFN-γ production, which may contribute to inhibition of IgG-enhancing cytokines such as IL-4 by Th2 cells, leading to reduced B-cell responses (461). Thus, mucosally induced tolerance was not induced in IFN-γ gene-disrupted mice. The role of IFN-γ for the induction of mucosally induced tolerance is further supported by recent studies in which spleen cells taken from mice given OVA by the oral route showed Ag-specific IFN-γ production when restimulated in vitro (462). Another recent study demonstrated that repeated oral administration of high doses of OVA to OVA-specific TCR mice results in IFN-γ–dominated immune responses in the Peyer's patches (463). The regulatory mechanisms for the induction and maintenance of mucosally induced tolerance by IFN-γ are not yet known; however, it is well established that IFN-γ contributes to inhibition of IL-4–producing Th2-type cells, which favor production of IgG B-cell responses (63–66). Taken together, the immunologic consequences of systemic B-cell tolerance induced by a high dose of oral antigen could be due to IFN-γ–mediated immune regulation, with significant suppression of Th2-type cells.

Role of Active Suppression in Mucosally Induced Tolerance

As summarized above, numerous past studies have demonstrated that a form of suppression is an important element of oral tolerance. Recent reports have provided evidence that CD8+ T cells producing inhibitory cytokines are induced in oral tolerance (427). Oral administration of MBP induces CD8+ T cells to produce TGF-β (456,464) (Table 3), which inhibits antigen-specific immune responses both in vivo and in vitro. These TGF-β–producing CD8+ T cells were found in Peyer's patches 24 to 48 hours after oral

TABLE 3. Mechanisms of mucosally-induced tolerance and potential clinical applications

Concept
Inhibition of antigen-specific immune responses in the systemic compartment in the presence of mucosal immune response after oral or intranasal administration of protein antigens.
Possible mechanisms
Downregulation of systemic immune responses
1. T-cell anergy
2. T-cell clonal deletion
3. Imbalance in cross-regulation of Th1 and Th2 cells
4. Suppression by TGF-β producing Th3 cells or CD8+ T cells
Maintenance of mucosal immune responses
1. Regulation by mucosal γδ T cells
2. GALT-derived Th2 cells
Possible clinical applications
Prevention and treatment of autoimmune diseases
1. Multiple sclerosis (bovine myelin)
2. Rheumatoid arthritis (chicken type II collagen)
3. Uveoretinitis (bovine S antigen)
4. Type I diabetes (human insulin)
Prevention of allergy
1. Food allergy (milk protein)
2. Pollen allergy (craj)

administration of MBP, indicating that they were initially induced in GALT (427). It is possible that these GALT-derived T cells migrate to systemic sites and mediate active bystander suppression. Thus, T cells from MBP-fed animals suppressed OVA responses when stimulated with fed antigen (465). In a similar fashion, T cells from OVA-fed animals inhibited MBP responses upon restimulation with the fed antigen. Induction of active suppression has been shown to be dependent on antigen dosage and frequency of feeding (e.g., low-dose oral tolerance) (436). Recent results that were obtained by the characterization of MBP-specific T cell lines from patients with multiple sclerosis who have been orally treated with MBP daily for 2 years provided evidence for the induction of a high frequency of antigen-specific TGF-β–producing T cells (461). When coproduction of an array of Th1 (IFN-γ) and Th2 (IL-4) cytokines was examined, the majority of antigen-specific TGF-β–producing T cells did not produce IFN-γ or IL-4 (466). Thus, it was suggested that oral administration of MBP induced TGF-β–secreting Th3 cells responsible for the generation of oral tolerance.

Regulatory Mucosal γδ T Cells Support IgA Responses in Mucosally Induced Tolerance

Most investigators agree that a subset of regulatory T cells in mucosa-associated tissue plays an important role in maintaining an antigen-specific mucosal IgA response in the presence of systemic unresponsiveness (Table 3). It is well established that mucosal immune compartments such as the intestinal epithelium contain large numbers of γδ T cells in addition to αβ T cells (41), as does the endothelium and LP regions of the small intestine (467). Because γδ T cells are localized in mucosa-associated tissues, it may be hypothesized that mucosal γδ T cells are involved in the maintenance of antigen-specific IgA responses in the presence of systemic unresponsiveness after oral administration of antigens.

As discussed above, IEL T cells from mice orally immunized with SRBCs were separated into γδ and αβ T cells. When purified γδ and αβ T cells were adoptively transferred to mice orally tolerized with SRBC, a conversion of systemic unresponsiveness to IgM, IgG, and IgA anti-SRBC responses was achieved in mice that received γδ but not αβ T cells (296). A more recent study also has demonstrated that γδ T cells isolated from mucosa-associated tissues of mice orally immunized with protein vaccine (LT-B) exhibit a similar activity. That is, IEL γδ T cells from LT-B–fed mice (which were tolerized) abrogate systemic unresponsiveness after adoptive transfer to syngeneic mice orally tolerized with LT-B (468). Mucosal γδ T cells thus appear to be important in the maintenance of appropriate immunologic homeostasis between local IgA responses and systemic unresponsiveness in oral tolerance.

Clinical Applications for Mucosally Induced Tolerance

Mucosally induced tolerance was earlier proposed as a strategy to reduce or suppress immune responses against self antigens (469–473) (Table 3). Mucosal deposition of autoantigens onto the intestinal (by feeding) or respiratory (by aerosolization or intranasal instillation) mucosa has made it possible to delay the onset or to decrease the severity of experimentally induced autoimmune diseases in a variety of animal systems. Pilot clinical trials of oral tolerance have recently been conducted in patients with

autoimmune diseases, and promising clinical benefits have been reported (427). Despite encouraging results that have been reported regarding oral delivery of autoantigens for the prevention and treatment of autoimmune diseases, the most recent results provide an unfortunate alternative possibility. Oral feeding of autoantigen in mice resulted in the generation of antigen-specific CD8+ CTL responses, which could lead to the aggravation of autoimmune disease (474). Furthermore, it was shown that the feeding of insulin to nonobese diabetic mice induced CD8+ T cells that enhanced the disease after adoptive transfer (475). Thus, one must also keep in mind that oral administration of autoantigen may induce undesirable CD8+ CTLs, which may worsen the disease instead of preventing the development of autoimmune diseases.

Oral administration of antigens had earlier been proposed to prevent or treat allergic reactions to common allergens such as house dust components or substances present in grass pollen (476,477). Although the above examples indicate that oral tolerance offers promise for inducing antigen-specific immunologic tolerance, its therapeutic potential remains limited by practical problems. Indeed, large quantities of orally administered antigens (e.g., milligrams to kilograms) are required to induce systemic unresponsiveness in experimental animals and humans.

MUCOSAL INFLAMMATION

This chapter has emphasized that numerous clinical disorders including inflammatory diseases can affect mucosal surfaces. Of course, most allergens are inhaled, and the primary lesions affect the respiratory tract. A full discourse on mucosal inflammation is beyond the scope of this chapter; however, the recent development of murine models for human inflammatory bowel diseases (IBD) serve as an excellent example of current attempts to determine how aberrant immune responses lead to mucosal inflammation.

Murine Models of Inflammatory Bowel Disease

Human IBDs are characterized by episodes of diarrhea, bloody stools, weight loss, and intestinal inflammation. It is generally agreed that human IBDs are multifactorial, with immunologic, environmental, and genetic contributions making systematic studies difficult. To obviate these difficulties, mice have been treated with chemical haptens or modified immunologically to induce colonic inflammation. In all models, some mouse strains exhibit greater susceptibility, suggesting significant genetic control in the development of IBD. One of these models is based on local exposure of colonic mucosa to the contact-sensitizing agent trinitrobenzene sulfonic acid (TNBS), first established in rats (478) and more recently in mice (479,480). The colonic administration of a single dose of TNBS in 50% ethanol induces chronic distal colitis in rats that could persist for 2 months or more (478), and a similar, single dose also induces colitis in mice (479,480). Contact-sensitizing agents such as TNBS are covalently reactive compounds that attach to autologous proteins and stimulate a DTH response to hapten (TNP)-modified self antigens, a reaction that is regulated by complex interactions among various functional subsets of CD4+ T cells (481,482). This model was used to contrast the potential roles for Th1-inducing cytokines in stimulating development of IBD or in ameliorating the disease. It was first shown that T cells from mice with TNBS colitis produced both IL-2 and IFN-γ (Th1 type), and *in situ* analysis of IBD lesions showed increased IFN-γ production

(479). Treatment of mice with anti–IL-12 markedly decreased the severity of TNBS-induced colitis (479).

Chronic enteric inflammation is also induced in mice by manipulating T cells or cytokines by gene targeting. TCR α-chain knock-out mice develop a chronic colitis accompanied by enhanced production of IFN-γ by gut-associated cells (483,484). Chronic intestinal inflammation also has been shown to develop in IL-2 knock-out mice, which exhibited abnormal B-cell responses, including colon autoantibodies (485). IL-10 knock-out mice develop severe focal inflammation in both small and large intestines and have an elevated production of the Th1 cytokine IFN-γ (486). Another well-characterized model involves adoptive transfer of CD45RB^{Hi} (naive) T cells to SCID mouse recipients, which subsequently develop a colitis characterized by expansion of CD4$^+$ T cells producing IFN-γ (487). It is interesting that TGF-β is corrective in the CD45RB^{Hi} transfer system as well as in the TNBS colitis model (488,489), suggesting that TGF-β downregulates mucosal inflammation and induces tolerance. Yet another model involves the adoptive transfer of T cell–depleted bone marrow from normal mice into TCR-defective CD3$_\varepsilon$ transgenic mice (490). Additional studies have now shown that both CD4$^+$ αβ$^+$ as well as γδ$^+$ T cells producing IFN-γ and TNF-α characterize the colonic inflammatory lesion of these CD3$_\varepsilon$ transgenic mice (491). Thus, compelling evidence is at hand to suggest that dysregulated T-cell responses are associated with murine IBD and that exaggerated Th1-type cells producing IFN-γ are the major effector population. These effector T cells respond to autoantigens and intestinal flora, to which they are normally tolerant (492). Abrogation of tolerance is an important aspect in Th1-type dysregulation in the various IBD models.

A genetic, heritable model of colitis also has been established in the C3H/HeJBir substrain of C3H/HeJ mice (493). These mice were noted to spontaneously develop a predominantly right-sided colitis early in life with resolution (493). These mice developed high-titered IgG antibodies to enteric bacterial antigens, and the response pattern was highly restricted. Furthermore, CD4$^+$ T cells from C3H/HeJBiR mice responded to enteric bacterial proteins with cytokine arrays of a Th1 type. Adoptive transfer of bacterial protein–activated T cells from C3H/HeJBir mice into SCID recipients induces colitis, whereas transfer of similarly treated CD4$^+$ T cells from C3H/HeJ mice does not. Studies are currently underway to identify the genes responsible by quantitative trait locus mapping. Although the susceptibility to IBD is most likely multigenic, this approach should reveal the genes that contribute to disease. Such information, when combined with data from T-cell studies suggesting hyper Th1-type responses, could be used to develop therapeutic intervention strategies to treat the human forms of IBD.

IgA DEFICIENCY

After AIDS, human IgA deficiency is the most common immune defect, occurring in 1.67 individuals per 1,000 of European descent. A complete discussion of human immunodeficiency diseases is presented in Chapter 42. However, we have summarized salient features and currently available models to study this condition. IgA deficiency is clinically diagnosed based on less than 5 mg% (50 mg/ml) of IgA in human serum; however, almost all IgA-deficient subjects exhibit loss of both S-IgA1 and S-IgA2 in their external secretions. Thus, IgA deficiency affects both the mucosal and systemic immune compartments, and only rare individuals

exhibit a deficiency solely in either IgA1 or IgA2 subclasses. However, approximately one fourth of IgA-deficient individuals exhibit other immune abnormalities, including T-cell defects and associated IgG-subclass deficiencies (495).

About half of IgA-deficient subjects exhibit clinical manifestations that include infections in both mucosal sites and systemic tissues. Mucosal infections include sinusitis, otitis media, bronchitis, and pneumonias of viral or bacterial origin (494,495), as well as acute diarrhea, again caused by viruses, bacteria, or *Giardia lamblia* parasites. A high incidence of autoimmunity also can occur in IgA deficiency and is accompanied by production of autoantibodies (494,495). Other respiratory problems seen in IgA deficiency include allergies, sinusitis, asthma, and eczema (495), and it is tempting to suggest that loss of normally protective S-IgA antibodies facilitates the development of IgE-type responses. A higher occurrence of serum antibodies to milk antigens in IgA deficiency (340) also suggests that normal S-IgA responses protect the host from continued bombardment with environmental antigens.

Although two views on potential mechanisms to account for IgA deficiency will be given, it should be stressed that the underlying cause of this disease remains unknown. From a simplistic standpoint, one could consider loss of IgA at the B-cell level, at the T-cell level, or from the standpoint of aberrant immunoregulation (e.g., by T cells or cytokines) (Fig. 5). For example, loss of Cα1/Cα2 genes, failure to switch to IgA, or lack of IgA B-cell terminal differentiation could all lead to IgA deficiency (Fig. 5). At the gene level, loss of both Cα1 and Cα2 would at a minimum be accompanied by loss of Cγ2, Cγ3, and Cε, and no examples of this tandem deficiency have been found (496). On the other hand, rare occurrences of gene deletion of Cα1 or Cα2 genes have been described (495), but this cannot account for this disease.

Earlier studies had suggested that T cells regulate IgA class switching (Tsw), but more recently it was shown that CD40L or CD40 interactions between T and B cells, respectively, precede signals to initiate isotype switching in germinal centers. Certainly, loss of CD40L or CD40 through gene deletion results in impaired T-/B-cell interactions, and these mice exhibit an antigen-specific IgA deficiency (Fig. 5). TGF-β is a major switch factor for IgA; however, it has been difficult to assess this cytokine's role *in vivo*, especially in TGF-β$^{-/-}$ mice because they die at 3 to 5 weeks of age from a wasting syndrome together with an inflammatory lung disorder. The next major B-cell stage susceptible to external influence involves terminal differentiation into plasma cells (Fig. 5). Obviously, Th cells and cytokines are of central importance for this response, and the important Th subsets and cytokines is shown in Fig. 5.

The alternative view to explain IgA deficiency does not encompass a loss of Cα genes, lack of μ → α switching, or a failure of IgA-committed B cells to terminally differentiate. Instead, it suggests that large numbers of regulatory cell pathways are involved in normal mucosal IgA responses, and interruption at multiple points could all lead to IgA deficiency. The availability of gene knock-out mice has allowed a rather systemic analysis of the presence/absence of a functioning mucosal IgA system. The pattern emerging is that a number of genes and products are important for mucosal IgA responses, and their loss also results in an IgA deficiency. In Fig. 5, we have presented a total of 12 knock-out situations that can lead to various forms of IgA deficiency. These range from switch factors to T cell deficiencies, including T-/B-cell coreceptors. Furthermore, both switch and Th2-type cytokines exhibit marked influences on IgA responses. The specific nature

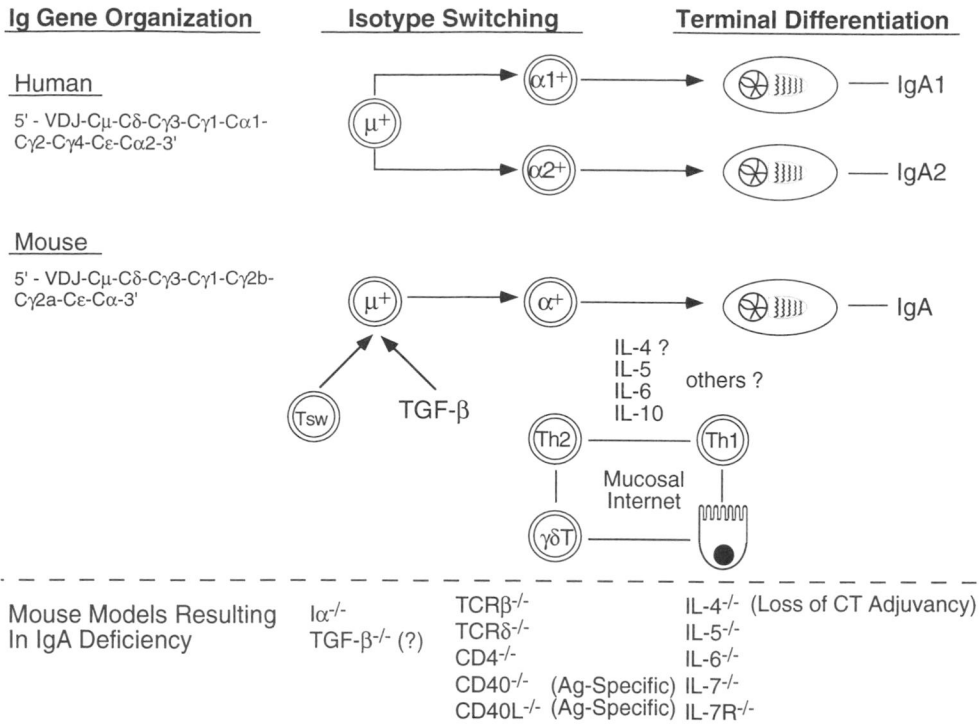

FIG. 5. The gene organization, switching to IgA and IgA plasma cell formation, is illustrated for both humans and mice. Production of IgA is regulated at several steps, including Tsw cells, switch cytokines (TGF-β), and Th cell subsets and cytokines, which promote IgA synthesis. In the lower panel, various mouse knock-outs are shown that either impair or block mucosal IgA responses. Individual knock-out mouse studies are described in more detail in the text.

of the mucosal IgA defect has been described in original papers; however, the underlying general principle is that the mucosal IgA system is so intricately regulated that a disruption of multiple pathways can lead to IgA deficiency.

SUMMARY

The mucosal immune system in higher mammals, and a related form in other vertebrates, consists of an integrated network of lymphoid tissues and mucous membrane–associated cells and effector molecules that work together to achieve host protection. Major effector molecules include antibodies, largely of IgA isotype, as well as cytokines, chemokines, and their receptors, which function in synergy with innate host factors such as defensins. The goal of this system is protective immunity; however, like the systemic immune system, it is susceptible to immunologic diseases, including IgA deficiency, allergy, hypersensitivity, and inflammation. Furthermore, immunologic unresponsiveness (tolerance) is a key feature of the mucosal immune system, and deliberate or natural immunization can effectively elicit mucosally induced tolerance. The mucosal immune system is unique in that it can provide both positive and negative signals for the induction and regulation of immune responses in both mucosal and systemic compartments after mucosal antigen exposure. Intertissue communication is important for mucosal immunity, and homing of lymphocytes via adhesion molecules, which recognize mucosal addressins expressed on high endothelial venule cells, is the major pathway by which the mucosal immune system connects the diverse compartments located in the gastrointestinal, pulmonary, and genitourinary tracts,

and exocrine glands. Such unique properties distinguish the mucosal from the systemic immune system. As we have emphasized in this chapter, the induction of peripheral immune responses by parenteral antigen does not result in significant mucosal immunity. However, mucosal immunization, e.g., oral or nasal administration of antigen, can induce antigen-specific S-IgA and CTL responses in distant mucosa-associated tissues. Moreover, induction of mucosal immune responses often results in both cell-mediated and humoral responses in the systemic lymphoid compartment.

ACKNOWLEDGMENTS

We thank Drs. Peter Burrows, Taeko Dohi, James Lillard, Mariarosaria Marinaro, Ichiro Takahashi, Shingo Yamamoto, and John VanCott for critical comments and advice. We also thank Wendy Jackson for preparing the figures and editing the manuscript. Special thanks are extended to Kim McGhee for editorial advice and help. Studies from the authors laboratories are supported by U.S. Public Health Service Grants AI 18958, DE 09837, AI 35344, AI 35544, DE 08228, and DK 44240; DMID-NIAID contracts AI 65298 and AI 65299; and grants from the Ministry of Education, Science, Sports and Culture and Ministry of Health and Welfare in Japan.

REFERENCES

1. Conley ME, Delacroix DL, Intravascular and mucosal immunoglobulin A: two separate systems of mucosal defense? *Ann Intern Med* 1987;106:892–899.
2. Pabst R. Is BALT a major component of the human lung immune system? *Immunol Today* 1992;13:119–122.

3. Kolopp-Sarda MN, Bene MC, Massin N, Moulin JJ, Faure GC. Immunohisto-logical analysis of macrophages, B-cells and T-cells in the mouse lung. *Anat Rec* 1994;239:150–157.

4. Sato A, Chida K, Iwata M, Hayakawa H. Study of bronchus-associated lymphoid tissues in patients with diffuse panbronchiolitis. *Am Rev Res Dis* 1992;146: 473–478.

5. Sato A, Hayakawa H, Uchiyama H, Chida K. Cellular distribution of bronchus-associated lymphoid tissue in rheumatoid arthritis. *Am J Respir Crit Care Med* 1996;154:1903–1907.

6. Kuper CF, Koornstra PJ, Hameleers, DM, et al. The role of nasopharyngeal lymphoid tissue. *Immunol Today* 1992;13:219–224

7. Bernstein JM. Mucosal immunology of the upper respiratory tract. *Respiration* 1992;59(suppl 3):3–13.

8. Bienenstock J, McDermott M, Befus D, O'Neill M. A common mucosal immunologic system involving the bronchus, breast and bowel. *Adv Exp Med Biol* 1978;107:53–59.

9. Mestecky J, McGhee JR. Immunoglobulin A (IgA): molecular and cellular interactions involved in IgA biosynthesis and immune response. *Adv Immunol* 1987;40:153–245.

10. Farstad IN, Halstensen TS, Fausa O, Brandtzaeg P. Heterogeneity of M-cell–associated B and T cells in human Peyer's patches. *Immunology* 1994;83:457–464.

11. Bockman DE, Cooper MD. Pinocytosis by epithelium associated with lymphoid follicles in the bursa of Fabricius, appendix and Peyer's patches. An electron microscopic study. *Am J Anat* 1973;136:455–477.

12. Owen RL, Jones AL. Epithelial cell specialization within human Peyer's patches: an ultrastructural study of intestinal lymphoid follicles. *Gastroenterology* 1974;66:189–203.

13. Wolf, JL, Bye WA. The membranous epithelial (M) cell and the mucosal immune system. *Annu Rev Med* 1984;35:95–112.

14. Neutra MR, Frey A, Kraehenbuhl J-P. Epithelial M cells: gateways for mucosal infection and immunization. *Cell* 1996;86:345–348.

15. Gebert A, Rothkötter H-J, Pabst R. M cells in Peyer's patches of the intestine. *Intern Rev Cytol* 1996;167:91–159.

16. Ermak TH, Dougherty EP, Bhagat HR, Kabok Z, Pappo J. Uptake and transport of copolymer biodegradable microspheres by rabbit Peyer's patch M cells. *Cell Tissue Res* 1995;279:433–436.

17. Allan CH, Mendrick DL, Trier JS. Rat intestinal M cells contain acidic endosomal-lysosomal compartments and express class II major histocompatibility complex determinants. *Gastroenterology* 1993;104:698–708.

18. Jones BD, Ghori N, Falkow S. Salmonella typhimurium initiates murine infection by penetrating and destroying the specialized epithelial M cells of the Peyer's patches. *J Exp Med* 1994;180:15–23.

19. Wolf JL, Rubin, DH, Finberg R, et al. Intestinal M cells: a pathway for entry of reovirus into the host. *Science* 1981;212:471–472.

20. Nibert ML, Furlong DB, Fields BN. Mechanisms of viral pathogenesis. Distinct forms of reoviruses and their roles during replication in cells and host. *J Clin Invest* 1991;88:727–734.

21. Sminia T, van der Ende MB. Macrophage subsets in the rat gut: an immunohistochemical and enzyme-histochemical study. *Acta Histochem* 1991;90:43–50.

22. Kelsall BL, Strober W. Distinct populations of dendritic cells are present in the subepithelial dome and T cell regions of the murine Peyer's patch. *J Exp Med* 1996;183:237–247.

23. Lebman DA, Griffin PM, Cebra JJ. Relationship between expression of IgA by Peyer's patch cells and functional IgA memory cells. *J Exp Med* 1987;166: 1405–1418.

24. Butcher EC, Rouse RV, Coffman RL, Nottenburg CN, Hardy RR, Weissman IL. Surface phenotype of Peyer's patches germinal center cells: implications for the role of germinal centers in B-cell differentiation. *J Immunol* 1982;129:2698–2707.

25. George A, Cebra, JJ. Responses of single germinal-center B cells in T-cell-dependent microculture. *Proc Natl Acad Sci U S A* 1991;88:11–15.

26. Weinstein PD, Cebra JJ. The preference for switching to IgA expression by Peyer's patch germinal center B cells is likely due to the intrinsic influence of their microenvironment. *J Immunol* 1991;147:4126–4135.

27. Weinstein PD, Schweitzer PA, Cebra-Thomas JA, Cebra JJ. Molecular genetic features reflecting the preference for isotype switching to IgA expression by Peyer's patch germinal center B cells. *Intern Immunol* 1991;3:1253–1263.

28. Kiyono H, McGhee JR, Wannemuehler MJ, et al. *In vitro* immune responses to a T cell-dependent antigen by cultures of disassociated murine Peyer's patch. *Proc Natl Acad Sci U S A* 1982;79:596–600.

29. London SD, Rubin DH, Cebra JJ. Gut mucosal immunization with reovirus serotype 1/L stimulates specific cytotoxic T-cell precursors as well as IgA memory cells in Peyer's patches. *J Exp Med* 1987;165:830–844.

30. London SD, Cebra-Thomas JA, Rubin DH, Cebra JJ. CD8 lymphocyte subpopulations in Peyer's patches induced by reovirus serotype 1 infection. *J Immunol* 1990;144:3187–3194.

31. Owen RL, Nemanic P. Antigen processing structures of the mammalian tract: an SEM study of lymphoepithelial organs. *Scanning Electron Microscopy* 1978;2: 367–378.

32. Oláh I, Surján L, Toro I. Electronmicroscopic observations on the antigen reception in the tonsillar tissue. *Acta Biol Acad Sci Hun* 1972;23:61–93.

33. Williams DM, Rowland AC. The palatine tonsil of the pig—an afferent route to the lymphoid tissue. *J Anat* 1972;113:131–137.

34. Finzi G, Cornaggia M, Capella C, et al. Cathepsin E in follicle associated epithelium of intestine and tonsils: localization to M cells and possible role in antigen processing. *Histochemistry* 1993;99:201–211.

35. Gebert A, Identification of M-cells in the rabbit tonsil by vimentin immunohistochemistry and *in vivo* protein transport. *Histochem Cell Biol* 1995;104:211–220.

36. Brandtzaeg P, Surjan L Jr, Berdal P. Immunoglobulin systems of human tonsils. I. Control subjects of various ages: quantification of Ig-producing cells, tonsillar morphometry and serum Ig concentrations. *Clin Exp Immunol* 1978;31:367–381.

37. Asanuma H, Inaba Y, Aizawa C, Kurata T, Tamura S. Characterization of mouse nasal lymphocytes isolated by enzymatic extraction with collagenase. *J Immunol Methods* 1995;187:41–51.

38. Wu HY, Nikolova EB, Beagley KW, Russell MW. Induction of antibody-secreting cells and T-helper and memory cells in murine nasal lymphoid tissue. *Immunology* 1996;88:493–500.

39. Hiroi T, Iwatani K, Iijima H, Kodama S, Yanagita M, Kiyono H. Nasal immune system: Distinctive Th0 and Th1/Th2-type environments in murine nasal-associated lymphoid tissues (NALT) and nasal passages, 1998 (*submitted for publication*).

40. Mair TS, Batten EH, Stokes CR, Bourne FJ. The histological features of the immune system of the equine respiratory tract. *J Comp Pathol* 1987;97:575–586.

41. Kiyono H, McGhee JR, eds. Mucosal immunology: intraepithelial lymphocytes. *Adv Host Defense Mechanisms* 1994;9:1–204.

42. Kilian M, Russell MW, Function of mucosal immunoglobulins. In: Ogra PL, et al., eds. *Handbook of mucosal immunology.* San Diego: Academic Press, 1994: 127–137.

43. London SD, Cytotoxic lymphocytes in mucosal effector sites. In: Ogra PL, et al., eds. *Handbook of mucosal immunology.* San Diego: Academic Press, 1994: 325–332.

44. McGhee JR, Mestecky J, Elson CO, Kiyono H, Regulation of IgA synthesis and immune response by T cells and interleukins. *J Clin Immunol* 1989;9:175–199.

45. Staats HF, Jackson RJ, Marinaro M, Takahashi I, Kiyono H, McGhee JR. Mucosal immunity to infection with implications for vaccine development. *Curr Opin Immunol* 1994;6:572–583.

46. Brandtzaeg P, Distribution and characterization of mucosal immunoglobulin-producing cells. In: Ogra PL, Mestecky J, Lamm M, et al., eds. *Handbook of mucosal immunology.* San Diego: Academic Press, 1994:251–262.

47. James SP, Fiocchi C, Graeff AS, Strober W, Phenotypic analysis of lamina propria lymphocytes. Predominance of helper-inducer and cytolytic T-cell phenotypes and deficiency of suppressor-inducer phenotypes in Crohn's disease and control patients. *Gastroenterology* 1986;91:1483–1489.

48. Abreu-Martin, MT, Targan SR. Lamina propria lymphocytes: a unique population of mucosal lymphocytes. In: Kagnoff MF, Kiyono H, eds. *Essentials of mucosal immunology.* San Diego: Academic Press, 1996:227–245.

49. Mayer L, Shlien R, Evidence for function of Ia molecules on gut epithelial cells in man. *J Exp Med* 1987;166:1471–1483.

50. Miller CJ, McChesney JM, Moore PF. Langerhans cells, macrophages and lymphocyte subsets in the cervix and vagina of rhesus macaques. *Lab Invest* 1992;67: 628–634.

51. Edwards JNT, Morris HB. Langerhans cells and lymphocyte subsets in the female genital tract. *Br J Obstet Gynecol* 1985;92:974–980.

52. Taguchi T, McGhee JR, Coffman RL, et al. Analysis of Th1 and Th2 cells in murine gut-associated tissues. Frequencies of CD4+ and CD8+ T cells that secrete IFN-γ and IL-5. *J Immunol* 1990;145.68–77.

53. Weinberg AD, English M, Swain SL. Distinct regulation of lymphokine production is found in fresh versus *in vitro* primed murine helper T cells. *J Immunol* 1990;144:1800–1807.

54. Powers GD, Abbas AK, Miller RA. Frequencies of IL 2 and IL-4–secreting T cells in naive and antigen-stimulated lymphocyte populations. *J Immunol* 1988; 140:3352–3357.

55. Hsieh CS, Macatonia SE, Tripp CS, Wolf SF, O'Garra A, Murphy KM. Development of Th1 CD4+ T cells through IL-12 produced by *Listeria*-induced macrophages. *Science* 1993;260:547–549.

56. Trinchieri G. Interleukin-12: a proinflammatory cytokine with immunoregulatory functions that bridge innate resistance and antigen-specific adaptive immunity. *Annu Rev Immunol* 1995;13:251–276.

57. Kobayashi M, Fitz L, Ryan M, et al. Identification and purification of natural killer cell stimulatory factor (NKSF), a cytokine with multiple biologic effects on human lymphocytes. *J Exp Med* 1989;170:827–845.

58. Chan SH, Perussia B, Gupta JW, et al. Induction of interferon gamma production by natural killer cell stimulatory factor: characterization of the responder cells and synergy with other inducers. *J Exp Med* 1991;173:869–879.

59. Snapper CM, Paul WE. Interferon-gamma and B cell stimulatory factor-1 reciprocally regulate Ig isotype production. *Science* 1987;236:944–947.

60. Yoshimoto T, Paul WE, CD4Pos NK1.1Pos T cells promptly produce interleukin-4 in response to *in vivo* challenge with anti-CD3. *J Exp Med* 1994;179.1285–1295.

61. Yoshimoto T, Bendelac A, Watson C, Hu-Li J, Paul WE. Role of NK1.1+ T cells in a Th2 response and in immunoglobulin E production. *Science* 1995;270: 1845–1847.

62. Arase H, Arase N, Nagawa K, Good RA, Onoe K, NK1.1+ CD4+ CD8+ thymocytes with specific lymphokine secretion. *Eur J Immunol* 1993;23:307–310.

63. Seder RA, Acquisition of lymphokine-producing phenotype by CD4+ T cells. *J Allergy Clin Immunol* 1994;94;1195–1202.

64. Mosmann TR, Coffman RL. Th1 and Th2 cells: different patterns of lymphokine secretion lead to different functional properties. *Annu Rev Immunol* 1989;7: 145–173.

65. Coffman RL, Varkila K, Scott P, Chatelain R, Role of cytokines in the differentiation of CD4⁺ T-cell subsets *in vivo*. *Immunol Rev* 1991;123:189–207.

66. Coffman RL, Seymour BW, Lebman DA, et al. The role of helper T cell products in mouse B cell differentiation and isotype regulation. *Immunol Rev* 1988;102:5–28.

67. Esser C, Radbruch A. Immunoglobulin class switching: molecular and cellular analysis. *Annu Rev Immunol* 1990;8:717–735.

68. Finkelman FD, Holmes J, Katona IM, et al. Lymphokine control of *in vivo* immunoglobulin isotype selection. *Annu Rev Immunol* 1990;8:303–333.

69. Kiyono H, McGhee JR, Mosteller LM, et al. Murine Peyer's patch T-cell clones: characterization of antigen-specific helper T cells for immunoglobulin A responses. *J Exp Med* 1982;156:1115–1130.

70. Kiyono H, Cooper MD, Kearney JF, et al. Isotype-specificity of helper T cell clones: Peyer's patch Th cells preferentially collaborate with mature IgA B cells for IgA responses. *J Exp Med* 1984;159:798–811.

71. VanCott JL, Staats HF, Pascual PW, et al. Regulation of mucosal and systemic antibody responses by T helper cell subsets, macrophages and derived cytokines following oral immunization with live recombinant *Salmonella*. *J Immunol* 1996;156:1504–1514.

72. Tonkonogy SL, Swain SL. Distinct lymphokine production by CD4⁺ T cells isolated from mucosal and systemic lymphoid organs. *Immunology* 1993;80:574–580.

73. Xu-Amano J, Aicher WK, Taguchi T, Kiyono H, McGhee JR. Selective induction of Th2 cells in murine Peyer's patches by oral immunization. *Intern Immunol* 1992;4:433–445.

74. Spalding DM, Williamson SI, Koopman WJ, McGhee JR. Preferential induction of polyclonal IgA secretion by murine Peyer's patch dendritic cell–T cell mixtures. *J Exp Med* 1984;160:941–946.

75. Mayer L, Kwan SP, Thompson C, et al. Evidence for a defect in "switch" T cell in patients with immunodeficiency and hyperimmunoglobulinemia, M. *N Engl J Med* 1986;314:409–413.

76. Benson EB, Strober W. Regulation of IgA secretion by T cell clones derived from the human gastrointestinal tract. *J Immunol* 1988;140:1874–1882.

77. Kiyono H, Mosteller-Barnum LM, Pitts AM, Williamson SI, Michalek SM, McGhee JR. Isotype-specific immunoregulation: IgA-binding factors produced by Fcα receptor⁺ T cell hybridomas regulate IgA responses. *J Exp Med* 1985;161:731–747.

78. Beagley KW, Eldridge JH, Kiyono H, McGhee JR. The identification of murine Peyer's patch T cell-derived factors which enhance IgA isotype-specific responses. *Adv Exp Med Biol* 1988;237:641–647.

79. Coffman RL, Shrader B, Carty J, Mosmann TR, Bond MW. A mouse T cell product that preferentially enhances IgA production. I. Biologic characterization. *J Immunol* 1987;139:3685–3690.

80. Harriman GR, Kunimoto DY, Elliot JF, Paetkau V, Strober W. The role of IL-5 in IgA B cell differentiation. *J Immunol* 1988;140:3033–3039.

81. Beagley KW, Eldridge JH, Kiyono H, et al. Recombinant murine IL-5 induces high rate IgA synthesis in cycling IgA-positive Peyer's patch B cells. *J Immunol* 1988;141:2035–2042.

82. Murray PD, McKenzie DT, Swain SL, Kagnoff MF. Interleukin 5 and interleukin 4 produced by Peyer's patch T cells selectively enhance immunoglobulin A expression. *J Immunol* 1987;139:2669–2674.

83. Lebman DA, Coffman RL. The effects of IL-4 and IL-5 on the IgA response by murine Peyer's patch B cell subpopulations. *J Immunol* 1988;141:2050–2056.

84. Sonoda E, Matsumoto R, Hitoshi Y, et al. Transforming growth factor β induces IgA production and acts additively with interleukin 5 for IgA production. *J Exp Med* 1989;170:1415–1420.

85. Kroese FG, Butcher EC, Stall AM, Lalor PA, Adams S, Herzenberg LA. Many of the IgA producing plasma cells in murine gut are derived from self-replenishing precursors in the peritoneal cavity. *Intern Immunol* 1989;1:75–84.

86. Beagley KW, Black CA, Dunkley ML, McGhee JR. Regulation of mucosal immunity. In: Snapper CM, ed. *Cytokine regulation of humoral immunity: basic and clinical aspects.* New York: John Wiley and Sons, 1996:391–408.

87. Benson EM, Bertolini JN, Brodtmann ME. T cell regulation of immunoglobulin isotypes in health and disease. *J Pediatr Infect Dis* 1990;9:525.

88. Beagley KW, Eldridge JH, Lee F, et al. Interleukins and IgA synthesis. Human and murine IL-6 induce high rate IgA secretion in IgA-committed B cells. *J Exp Med* 1989;169:2133–2148.

89. Ramsay AJ, Husband AJ, Ramshaw IA, et al. The role of interleukin-6 in mucosal IgA antibody responses *in vivo*. *Science* 1994;264:561–563.

90. Bromander AK, Ekman L, Kopf M, Nedrud JG, Lycke NY. IL-6–deficient mice exhibit normal mucosal IgA responses to local immunizations and *Helicobacter felis* infection. *J Immunol* 1996;156:4290–4297.

91. Fujihashi K, McGhee JR, Lue C, et al. Human appendix B cells naturally express receptors for and respond to interleukin 6 with selective IgA1 and IgA2 synthesis. *J Clin Invest* 1991;88:248–252.

92. Briere F, Bridon JM, Chevet D, et al., Interleukin 10 induces B lymphocytes from IgA-deficient patients to secrete IgA. *J Clin Invest* 1994;94:97–104.

93. Nonoyama S, Farrington M, Ishida H, Howard M, Ochs HD. Activated B cells from patients with common variable immunodeficiency proliferate and synthesize immunoglobulin. *J Clin Invest* 1993;92:1282–1287.

94. DeFrance T, Vanbervliet B, Briere F, Durand I, Rousset F, Banchereau J. Interleukin 10 and transforming growth factor beta cooperate to induce anti-CD40-activated naive human B cells to secrete immunoglobulin A. *J Exp Med* 1992;175:671–682.

95. Lebman DA, Lee FD, Coffman RL. Mechanism for transforming growth factor β and IL-2 enhancement of IgA expression in lipopolysaccharide-stimulated B cell cultures. *J Immunol* 1990;144:952–959.

96. Youngman KR, Fiocchi C, Kaetzel CS. Inhibition of IFN-γ activity in supernatants from stimulated human intestinal mononuclear cells prevents up-regulation of the polymeric Ig receptor in an intestinal epithelial cell line. *J Immunol* 1994;153:675–681.

97. Morokata T, Kato Y, Igarashi O, Nariuchi H, Mechanism of enhanced antigen presentation by B cells activated with anti-μ plus interferon-γ: role of B7-2 in the activation of naive and memory CD4⁺ T cells. *Eur J Immunol* 1995;25:1992–1998.

98. Kuchroo VK, Das MP, Brown JA, et al. B7-1 and B7-2 costimulatory molecules activated differentially the Th1/Th2 developmental pathways: application to autoimmune disease therapy. *Cell* 1995;80:707–718.

99. Hörnqvist E, Goldschmidt TJ, Holmdahl R, Lycke N. Host defense against cholera toxin is strongly CD4⁺ T cell dependent. *Infect Immun* 1991;59:3630–3638.

100. Mega J, Bruce MG, Beagley KW, et al. Regulation of mucosal responses by CD4⁺ T lymphocytes: effects of anti-L3T4 treatment on the gastrointestinal immune system. *Intern Immunol* 1991;3:793–805.

101. Hörnquist CE, Ekman L, Grdic KD, Schön K, Lycke NY. Paradoxical IgA immunity in CD4-deficient mice. Lack of cholera toxin-specific protective immunity despite normal gut mucosal IgA differentiation. *J Immunol* 1995;155:2877–2887.

102. Snapper CM, Paul WE. Interferon-gamma and B cell stimulatory factor-1 reciprocally regulate Ig isotype production. *Science* 1987;236:944–947.

103. Gajewski TF, Fitch FW. Anti-proliferative effect of IFN-γ in immune regulation. I. IFN-γ inhibits the proliferation of Th2 but not Th1 murine helper T lymphocyte clones. *J Immunol* 1988;140:4245–4252.

104. Golding B. Cytokine regulation of humoral immune responses. *Top Vaccine Adjuvant Res* 1991;25:37.

105. Xu-Amano J, Kiyono H, Jackson RJ, et al. Helper T cell subsets for immunoglobulin A responses: oral immunization with tetanus toxoid and cholera toxin as adjuvant selectively induces Th2 cells in mucosa associated tissues. *J Exp Med* 1993;178:1309–1320.

106. Marinaro M, Staats HF, Hiroi T, et al. Mucosal adjuvant effect of cholera toxin in mice results from induction of T helper 2 (Th2) cells and IL-4. *J Immunol* 1995;155:4621–4629.

107. Snider DP, Marshall JS, Perdue MH, Liang H. Production of IgE antibody and allergic sensitization of intestinal and peripheral tissues after oral immunization with protein Ag and cholera toxin. *J Immunol* 1994;153:647–657.

108. Wilson AD. Bailey M, Williams NA, Stokes CR. The *in vitro* production of cytokines by mucosal lymphocytes immunized by oral administration of keyhole limpet hemocyanin using cholera toxin as an adjuvant. *Eur J Immunol* 1991;21:2333–2339.

109. Walker RI, Clements JD. Use of heat-labile toxin of enterotoxigenic *Escherichia coli* to facilitate mucosal immunization. *Vaccine Res* 1993;2:1.

110. Spangler BD. Structure and function of cholera toxin and related *Escherichia coli* heat-labile enterotoxin. *Microbiol Rev* 1992;56:622–647.

111. Takahashi I, Marinaro M, Kiyono H, et al. Mechanisms for mucosal immunogenicity and adjuvant of *Escherichia coli* labile enterotoxin. *J Infect Dis* 1996:173:627–635.

112. Kawanishi H, Saltzman L, Strober W. Mechanisms regulating IgA class-specific immunoglobulin production in murine gut-associated lymphoid tissues. I. T cells derived from Peyer's patches that switch sIgM B cells to SIgA B cells *in vitro*. *J Exp Med* 1983;157:433–450.

113. Kawanishi H, Saltzman L, Strober W. Mechanisms regulating IgA class-specific immunoglobulin production in murine gut-associated lymphoid tissues. II. Terminal differentiation of postswitch sIgA-bearing Peyer's patch B cells. *J Exp Med* 1983;158:649–669.

114. Kawanishi H, Ozato K, Strober W. The profilerative response of cloned Peyer's patch switch T cells to syngeneic and allogenic stimuli. *J Immunol* 1985;134:3586–3591.

115. Fuleihan R, Ramesh N, Geha RS. Role of CD40-CD40-ligand interaction in Ig-isotype switching. *Curr Opin Immunol* 1993;5:963–967.

116. Banchereau J, Bazan F, Blanchard D, et al. The CD40 antigen and its ligand. *Annu Rev Immunol* 1994;12:881–922.

117. MacLennan IC. Germinal centers. *Annu Rev Immunol* 1994;12:117–139.

118. Weinstein PD, Cebra JJ. The preference for switching to IgA expression by Peyer's patch germinal center B cells is likely due to the intrinsic influence of their microenvironment. *J Immunol* 1991;147:4126–4135.

119. Spalding DM, Griffin JA. Different pathways of differentiation of pre-B cell lines are induced by dendritic cells and T cells from different lymphoid tissues. *Cell* 1986;44:507–519.

120. Mayer L, Posnett DN, Kunkel HG. Human-malignant T cells capable of inducing an immunoglobulin class switch. *J Exp Med* 1985;161:134–144.

121. Isakson PC, Pure E, Vitetta ES, Krammer PH. T cell-derived B cell differentiation factor(s). Effect on the isotype switch of murine B cells. *J Exp Med* 1982;155:734–748.

122. Coffman RL, Seymour BW, Lebman DA, et al. The role of helper T cell products in mouse B cell differentiation and isotype regulation. *Immunol Rev* 1988;102:5–28.

123. Jung S, Rajewsky K, Radbruch A. Shutdown of class switch recombinant by deletion of a switch region control element. *Science* 1993;259:984–989.

124. Xu L, Groham B, Li SC, Bottaro A, Alt FW, Rothman P. Replacement of germ-

line E promoter by gene targeting alters control of immunoglobulin heavy chain class switching. *Proc Natl Acad Sci U S A* 1993;90:3705–3709.

125. Zhang J, Bottaro A, Li S, Stewart V, Alt FW. A selective defect in IgG2b switching as a result of targeted mutation of the I gamma 2b promoter and exon. *EMBO J* 1993;12:3529–3537.

126. Bottaro A, Lansford R, Xu L, Zhang J, Rothman P, Alt FW. S region transcription per se promotes basal IgE class switch recombination but additional factors regulate the efficiency of the process. *EMBO J* 1994;13:665–674.

127. Harriman GR, Bradley A, Das S, Rogers-Fani P, Davis AC. IgA class switch in Ia exon-deficient mice. Role of germline transcription in class switch recombination. *J Clin Invest* 1996;97:477–485.

128. Snapper CM, McIntyre TM, Mandler R, et al. Induction of IgG3 secretion of interferon g: A model for T cell-independent class switching in response to T cell-independent type 2 antigens. *J Exp Med* 1992;175:1367–1371.

129. Coffman RL, Lebman DA, Schrader B. Transforming growth factor β specifically enhances IgA production by lipopolysaccharide-stimulated murine B lymphocytes. *J Exp Med* 1989;170:1039–1044.

130. Lebman DA, Nomura DY, Coffman RL, Lee FD. Molecular characterization of germ-line immunoglobulin A transcripts produced during transforming growth factor type β-induced isotype switching. *Proc Natl Acad Sci U S A* 1990;87:3962–3966.

131. Lebman DA, Lee FD, Coffman RL. Mechanism for transforming growth factor β and IL-2 enhancement of IgA expression in lipopolysaccharide-stimulated B cell cultures. *J Immunol* 1990;144:952–959.

132. Islam KB, Nilsson L, Sideras P, Hammarstrom L, Smith CI. TGF-β1 induces germ-line transcripts of both IgA subclasses in human B lymphocytes. *Intern Immunol* 1991;3:1099–1106.

133. Nilsson L, Islam KB, Olafsson O, et al. Structure of TGF-β1-induced human immunoglobulin Cα1 and Cα2 germ-line transcripts. *Intern Immunol* 1991;3:1107–1115.

134. Stavnezer J. Regulation of antibody production and class switching by TGF-β. *J Immunol* 1995;155:1647–1651.

135. Rousset F, Garcia E, Banchereau J. Cytokine-induced proliferation and immunoglobulin production of human B lymphocytes triggered through their CD40 antigen. *J Exp Med* 1991;173:705–710.

136. McIntyre TM, Kehry MR, Snapper CM. Novel *in vitro* model for high-rate IgA class switching. *J Immunol* 1995;154:3156–3161.

137. Borkowski TA, Letterio JJ, Farr AG, Udey MC. A role for endogenous transforming growth factor β1 in Langerhans cell biology: the skin of transforming growth factor β1 null mice is devoid of epidermal Langerhans cells. *J Exp Med* 1996;184:2417–2422.

138. Cambier JC, Pleiman CM, Clark MR. Signal transduction by the B cell antigen receptor and its coreceptors. *Annu Rev Immunol* 1994;12:457–486.

139. Chan AC, Desai DM, Weiss A. The role of protein tyrosine kinases and protein tyrosine phosphatases in T cell antigen receptor signal transduction. *Annu Rev Immunol* 1994;12:555–592.

140. Cantrell D. T cell antigen receptor signal transduction pathways. *Annu Rev Immunol* 1996;14:259–274.

141. Langman RE, Cohn M. Terra firma: a retreat from "danger." *J Immunol* 1996;157:4273–4276.

142. June CH, Bluestone JA, Nadler LM, Thompson CB. The B7 and CD28 receptor families. *Immunol Today* 1994;15:321–331.

143. Linsley PS, Ledbetter JA. The role of the CD28 receptor during T cell responses to antigen. *Annu Rev Immunol* 1993;11:191–212.

144. Schwartz RH. Costimulation of T lymphocytes: the role of CD28, CTLA-4, and B7/BB1 in interleukin-2 production and immunotherapy. *Cell* 1992;71:1065–1068.

145. Allison JP. CD28-B7 interaction in T-cell activation. *Curr Opin Immunol* 1994;6:414–419.

146. Freeman GJ, Freedman AS, Segil JM, Lee G, Whitman JF, Nadler LM. B7, a new member of the Ig superfamily with unique expression on activated and neoplastic B cells. *J Immunol* 1989;143:2714–2722.

147. Azuma M, Ito D, Yagita H, et al. B70 antigen is a second ligand for CTLA-4 and CD28. *Nature* 1993;366:76–79.

148. Freeman GJ, Borriello F, Hodes RJ, et al. Uncovering of functional alternative CTLA-4 counter-receptor in B7-deficient mice. *Science* 1993;262:907–909.

149. Freeman GJ, Gribben JG, Boussiotis VA, et al. Cloning of B7-2: a CTLA-4 counter-receptor that costimulates human T cell proliferation. *Science* 1993;262:909–911.

150. Reiser H, Freeman GJ, Razi-Wolf Z, Gimmi CD, Benacerraf B, Nadler LM. Murine B7 antigen provides an efficient costimulatory signal for activation of murine T lymphocytes via the T-cell receptor/CD3 complex. *Proc Natl Acad Sci U S A* 1992;89.271–275.

151. Boussiotis VA, Freeman GJ, Gribben JG, Daley J, Gray G, Nadler LM. Activated human B lymphocytes express three CTLA-4 counterreceptors that costimulate T-cell activation. *Proc Natl Acad Sci U S A* 1993;90:11059–11063.

152. Linsley PS, Greene JL, Tan P, et al. Coexpression and functional cooperation of CTLA-4 and CD28 on activated T lymphocytes. *J Exp Med* 1992;176:1595–1604.

153. Lenschow DJ, Walunas TL, Bluestone JA. CD28/B7 system of T cell costimulation. *Annu Rev Immunol* 1996;14:233–258.

154. Metlay JP, Pure E, Steinman RM. Distinct features of dendritic cells and anti-Ig activated B cells as stimulators of the primary mixed leukocyte reaction. *J Exp Med* 1989;169:239–254.

155. Lassila O, Vainio O, Matzinger P. Can B cells turn on virgin T cells? *Nature* 1988;334:253–255.

156. Larsen CP, Ritchie SC, Hendrix R, et al. Regulation of immunostimulatory function and costimulatory molecule (B7-1 and B7-2) expression on murine dendritic cells. *J Immunol* 1994;152:5208–5219.

157. Freedman AS, Freeman GJ, Rhynhart K, Nadler LM. Selective induction of B7/BB-1 on interferon-gamma stimulated monocytes: a potential mechanism for amplification of T cell activation through the CD28 pathway. *Cell Immunol* 1991;137:429–437.

158. Hathcock KS, Laszlo G, Pucillo C, Linsley P, Hodes RJ. Comparative analysis of B7-1 and B7-2 costimulatory ligands: expression and function. *J Exp Med* 1994;180:631–640.

159. Stack RM, Lenschow DJ, Gray GS, Bluestone JA, Fitch FW. IL-4 treatment of small splenic B cells induces costimulatory molecules B7-1 and B7-2. *J Immunol* 1994;152:5723–5733.

160. Weaver CT, Hawrylowicz CM, Unanue ER. T helper subsets require the expression of distinct costimulatory signals by antigen-presenting cells. *Proc Natl Acad Sci U S A* 1988;85:8181–8185.

161. Magilavy DB, Fitch FW, Gajewski TF. Murine hepatic accessory cells support the proliferation of Th1 but not Th2 helper T lymphocyte clones. *J Exp Med* 1989;170:985–990.

162. Fabry Z, Sandor M, Gajewski TF, et al. Different activation of Th1 and Th2 CD4+ cells by murine brain microvessel endothelial cells and smooth muscle/pericytes. *J Immunol* 1993;151:38–47.

163. Fox BS. Antigen presenting cell-derived co-stimulatory signals can selectively regulate IL-2 and IL-4 production from a Th0 cell hybridoma. *Int Immunol* 1993;5:323–330.

164. Goodman RE, Nestle F, Naidu YM, et al. Keratinocyte-derived T cell costimulation induces preferential production of IL-2 and IL-4 but not IFN-gamma. *J Immunol* 1994;152:5189–5198.

165. Abbas AK, Murphy KM, Sher A. Functional diversity of helper T lymphocytes. *Nature* 1996;383:787–793.

166. Seder RA, Germain RN, Linsley PS, Paul WE. CD28-mediated costimulation of interleukin 2 (IL-2) production plays a critical role in T cell priming for IL-4 and interleukin gamma production. *J Exp Med* 1994;179:299–304.

167. McKnight AJ, Perez VL, Shea CM, Gray GS, Abbas AK. Costimulator dependence of lymphokine secretion by naive and activated CD4+ lymphocytes from TCR transgenic mice. *J Immunol* 1994;152:5220–5225.

168. Tan P, Anasetti C, Hansen JA, et al. Induction of alloantigen-specific hyporesponsiveness in human T lymphocytes by blocking interaction of CD28 with its natural ligand B7/BB1. *J Exp Med* 1993;177:165–173.

169. Levine BL, Ueda Y, Craighead N, Huang ML, June CH. CD28 ligands CD80 (B7-1) and CD86 (B7-2) induce long-term autocrine growth of CD4+ T cells and induce similar patterns of cytokine secretion *in vitro. Int Immunol* 1995;7:891–904.

170. Harris N, Peach R, Naemura J, Linsley PS, LeGros G, Ronchese F. CD80 costimulation is essential for the induction of airway eosinophilia. *J Exp Med* 1997;185:177–182.

171. Corry DB, Reiner SL, Linsley PS, Locksley RM. Differential effects of blockade of CD28-B7 on the development of Th1 or Th2 effector cells in experimental leishmaniasis. *J Immunol* 1994;153:4142–4148.

172. Lu P, Zhou X, Chen SJ, et al. CTLA-4 ligands are required to induce an *in vivo* interleukin 4 response to a gastrointestinal nematode parasite. *J Exp Med* 1994;180:693–698.

173. Rulifson IC, Sperling AI, Fields PE, Fitch FW, Bluestone JA. CD28 costimulation promotes the production of Th2 cytokines. *J Immunol* 1997;158.658–665.

174. Banchereau J, Bazan F, Blanchard D, et al. The CD40 antigen and its ligand. *Annu Rev Immunol* 1994;12:881–922.

175. Kansas GS, Tedder TF. Transmembrane signals generated through MHC Class II, CD19, CD20, CD39, and CD40 antigens induce LFA 1-dependent and independent adhesion in human B cells through a tyrosine kinase-dependent pathway. *J Immunol* 1991;147:4094–4102.

176. Gordon J, Millsum MJ, Guy GR, Ledbetter JA. Synergistic interaction between interleukin 4 and anti-Bp50 (CDw40) revealed in a novel B cell restimulation assay. *Eur J Immunol* 1987;17:1535–1538.

177. Gordon J, Millsum MJ, Guy GR, Ledbetter JA. Resting B lymphocytes can be triggered directly through the CDw40 (Bp50) antigen. A comparison with IL-4 mediated signaling. *J Immunol* 1988;140:1425–1430.

178. Rousset F, Garcia E, Banchereau J. Cytokine-induced proliferation and immunoglobulin production of human B lymphocytes triggered through their CD40 antigen. *J Exp Med* 1991;173:705–710.

179. Marrack P, Kappler J. The T cell receptor. *Science* 1987;238:1073–1079.

180. Kägi D, Ledermann B, Bürki K, Zinkernagel RM, Hengartner H. Molecular mechanisms of lymphocyte-mediated cytotoxicity and their role in immunological protection and pathogenesis *in vivo. Annu Rev Immunol* 1996;14:207–232.

181. Ernst PB, Befus AD, Bienenstock J. Leukocytes in the intestinal epithelium: An unusual immunologic compartment. *Immunol Today* 1985;6:50.

182. Lefrancois L, Goodman T. *in vivo* modulation of cytolytic activity and Thy-1 expression in TCR-γδ+ intraepithelial lymphocytes. *Science* 1989;243:1716–1718.

183. Guy-Grand D, Malassis-Seris M, Briottet C, Vassalli P. Cytotoxic differentiation of mouse gut thymodependent and independent intraepithelial T lymphocytes is induced locally. Correlation between functional assays, presence of perforin and granzyme transcripts and cytoplasmic granules. *J Exp Med* 1991;173:1549–1552.

184. Viney JL, Kilshaw PL, MacDonald TT. Cytotoxic αβ+ and γδ+ T cells in murine intestinal epithelium. *Eur J Immunol* 1990;20:1623–1626.

185. Kägi D, Ledermann B, Bürki K, et al. Cytotoxicity mediated by T cells and natural killer cells is greatly impaired in perforin-deficient mice. *Nature* 1994;369: 31–37.

186. Walsh CM, Matloubian M, Liu C-C, Ueda R, Kurahara CG, Clark WR. Immune functions in mice lacking the perforin gene. *Proc Natl Acad Sci U S A* 1994;91: 10854–10858.

187. Tartaglia LA, Ayres TM, Wong GH, Goeddel DV. A novel domain within the 55 kd TNF receptor signals cell death. *Cell* 1993;74:845–853.

188. Croitoru K, Ernst PB. Intraepithelial lymphocyte lineage and function. The interactions between the intestinal epithelium and the intraepithelial lymphocyte. In: Kigono H, McGhee JR, eds. *Advances in host defense mechanisms* 1997;9: 79–88.

189. Davies MD, Parrott DM. Cytotoxic T cells in small intestine epithelial, lamina propria and lung lymphocytes. *Immunology* 1981;44:367–371.

190. Guy-Grand D, Griscelli C, Vassalli P. The mouse gut T lymphocyte, a novel type of T cell: nature, origin, and traffic in mice in normal and graft-versus-host conditions. *J Exp Med* 1978;148:1661–1677.

191. MacDermott RP, Franklin GO, Jenkins KM, Kodner IJ, Nash GS, Weinrieb IJ. Human intestinal mononuclear cells. 1. Investigation of antibody-dependent, lectin-induced and spontaneous cell-mediated cytotoxic capabilities. *Gastroenterology* 1980;78:47–56.

192. Nauss KM, Pavlina TM, Kumar V, Newberne PM. Functional characteristics of lymphocytes isolated from the rat large intestine. Responses to T-cell mitogen and natural killer cell activity. *Gastroenterology* 1984;86:468–475.

193. Tagliabue A, Luini W, Soldateschi D, Boraschi D. Natural killer activity of gut mucosal lymphoid cells in mice. *Eur J Immunol* 1981;11:919–922.

194. Neutra MR, Kraehenbuhl J-P. Cellular and molecular basis for antigen transportation in the intestinal epithelium. In: Ogra PL, Mestecky J, Lamm M, et al., eds. *Handbook of mucosal immunology.* San Diego: Academic Press, 1994;27–39.

195. Nibert ML, Furlong DB, Fields BN. Mechanisms for viral pathogenesis. Distant forms of reoviruses and their roles during replication in cells and host. *J Clin Invest* 1991;88:727–734.

196. Wolf JL, Rubin DH, Finberg R, et al. Intestinal M cells: a pathway for entry of reovirus into the host. *Science* 1981;212:471–472.

197. Morin MJ, Warner A, Fields BN, A pathway for entry of reoviruses into the host through M cells of the respiratory tract. *J Exp Med* 1994;180:1523–1527.

198. London SD, Rubin DH, Cebra JJ. Gut mucosal immunization with reovirus serotype 1/L stimulates virus-specific cytotoxic T cell precursors as well as IgA memory cells in Peyer's patches. *J Exp Med* 1987;165:830–847.

199. Offit PA, Cunningham SL, Dudzik KI. Memory and distribution of virus-specific cytotoxic T lymphocytes (CTLs) and CTL precursors after rotavirus infection. *J Virol* 1991;65:1318–1324.

200. London SD, Cebra-Thomas JA, Rubin DH, Cebra JJ. CD8 lymphocyte subpopulations in Peyer's patches induced by reovirus serotype 1 infection. *J Immunol* 1990;144:3187–3194.

201. Issekutz TB. The response of gut-associated T lymphocytes to intestinal viral immunization. *J Immunol* 1984;133:2955–2960.

202. Offit PA, Dudzik KI. Rotavirus-specific cytotoxic T lymphocytes appear at the intestinal mucosal surface after rotavirus infection. *J Virol* 1989;63:3507–3512.

203. Cebra JJ, Cuff CF, Rubin DH. Relationship between alpha/beta T cell receptor/CD8 precursors for cytotoxic T lymphocytes in the murine Peyer's patches and the intraepithelial compartment probed by oral infection with reovirus. *Immunol Res* 1991;10:321–323.

204. George A, Kost SI, Witzleben CL, Cebra JJ, Rubin DH. Reovirus-induced liver disease in severe combined immunodeficient (SCID) mice. A model for the study of viral infection, pathogenesis, and clearance. *J Exp Med* 1990;171:929–934.

205. Cuff CF, Cebra CK, Rubin DH, Cebra JJ, Developmental relationship between cytotoxic α/β T cell receptor-positive intraepithelial lymphocytes and Peyer's patch lymphocytes. *Eur J Immunol* 1993;23:1333–1339.

206. Offit PA, Dudzik KI, Rotavirus-specific cytotoxic T lymphocytes passively protect against gastroenteritis in suckling mice. *J Virol* 1990;64:6325–6328.

207. Dharakul T, Labbe M, Cohen J, et al. Immunization with baculovirus-expressed recombinant rotavirus proteins VP1, VP4, VP6 and VP7 induces CD8+ T lymphocytes that mediate clearance of chronic rotavirus infection in SCID mice. *J Virol* 1991;65:5928–5932.

208. Franco MA, Greenberg HB. Role of B cells and cytotoxic T lymphocytes in clearance of and immunity to rotavirus infection in mice. *J Virol* 1995;69: 7800–7806.

209. Franco MA, Tin C, Rott LS, VanCott JL, McGhee JR, Greenberg HB. Evidence for CD8+ T cell immunity to murine rotavirus in the absence of perofrin, fas and gamma interferon. *J Virol* 1997;71:479–486.

210. Burns JW, Siadat-Pajouh M, Krishnaney AA, Greenberg HB. Protective effect of rotavirus VP6-specific IgA monoclonal antibodies that lack neutralizing activity. *Science* 1996;272:104–107.

211. Allan W, Tabi Z, Cleary A, Doherty PC. Cellular events in the lymph node and lung of mice with influenza. Consequences of depleting CD4+ T cell. *J Immunol* 1990;144:3980–3986.

212. Eichelberger M, Allan W, Zijlstra M, Jaenisch R, Doherty PC. Clearance of influenza virus respiratory infection in mice lacking class I major histocompatibility complex-restricted CD8+ T cells. *J Exp Med* 1991;174:875–880.

213. Carding SR, Allan W, Kyes S, Hayday A, Bottomly K, Doherty PC. Late dominance of the inflammatory process in murine influenza by γ/δ+ T cells. *J Exp Med* 1990;172:1225–1231.

214. Muñoz JL, McCarthy CA, Clark ME, Hall CB, Respiratory syncytial virus infection in C57BL/6 mice: clearance of virus from the lungs with virus-specific cytotoxic T cells. *J Virol* 1991;65:4494–4497.

215. Nicholas JA, Rubino KL, Levely ME, Meyer AL, Collins PL. Cytotoxic T cell activity against the 22-kDa protein of human respiratory syncytial virus (RSV) is associated with a significant reduction in pulmonary RSV replication. *Virology* 1991;182:664–672.

216. Graham BS, Bunton LA, Wright PF, Karzon DT. Role of T lymphocyte subsets in the pathogenesis of primary infection and rechallenge with respiratory syncytial virus in mice. *J Clin Invest* 1991;88:1026–1033.

217. Graham BS, Henderson GS, Tang Y-W, Lu X, Neuzil KM, Colley DG. Priming immunization determines T helper cytokine mRNA expression patterns in lungs of mice challenged with respiratory syncytial virus. *J Immunol* 1993;151: 2032–2040.

218. Miller CJ, Alexander NJ, Sutjipto S, et al. Genital mucosal transmission of simian immunodeficiency virus: animal model for heterosexual transmission of human immunodeficiency virus. *J Virol* 1989;63:4277–4284.

219. Miller CJ, Alexander NJ, Sutjipto S, et al. Effect of virus dose and nonoxynol-9 on the genital transmission of SIV in rhesus macaques. *J Med Primatol* 1990;19: 401–409.

220. Marx PA, Compans RW, Gettie A, et al. Protection against vaginal SIV transmission with microencapsulated vaccine. *Science* 1993;260:1323–1327.

221. Lohman BL, Miller CJ, McChesney MB. Antiviral cytotoxic T lymphocytes in the vaginal mucosa of simian immunodeficiency virus-infected rhesus macaques. *J Immunol* 1995;155:5855–5860.

222. Miller CJ, McChesney MB, Lü X, et al. Rhesus macaques previously infected with simian/human immunodeficiency virus are protected from vaginal challenge with pathogenic SIVmac239. *J Virol* 1997;71:1911–1921.

223. Miller CJ. Mucosal transmission of SIV. *Curr Top Microbiol Immunol* 1994; 188:107–122.

224. Porgador A, Staats HF, Faiola B, Gilboa E, Palker TJ. Intranasal immunization with CTL epitope peptides from HIV-1 or ovalbumin and the mucosal adjuvant cholera toxin induces peptide-specific CTLs and protection against tumor development *in vivo. J Immunol* 1997;158:834–841.

225. Aggarwal A, Kumar S, Jaffe R, Hone D, Gross M, Sadoff J. Oral *Salmonella*: circumsporozoite recombinants induce specific CD8+ cytotoxic T cells. *J Exp Med* 1990;172:1083–1090.

226. Khan IA, Ely KH, Kasper LH. A purified parasite antigen (p30) mediates CD8+ T cell immunity against fatal *Toxoplasma gondii* infection in mice. *J Immunol* 1991;147:3501–3506.

227. Hakim FT, Gazzinelli RT, Denkers E, Hieny S, Shearer GM, Sher A. CD8+ T cells from mice vaccinated against *Toxoplasma gondii* are cytotoxic for parasite-infected or antigen-pulsed host cells. *J Immunol* 1991;147:2310–2316.

228. Ksander BR, Streilein JW. Failure of infiltrating precursor cytotoxic T cells to acquire direct cytotoxic function in immunologically privileged sites. *J Immunol* 1990;145:2057–2063.

229. Podolsky DK. Oligosaccharide structure of isolated human colonic mucin species. *J Biol Chem* 1985;260:15510–15515.

230. Sanderson IR, Walker WA. Mucosal barrier. In: Ogra PL, Mestecky J, Lamm M, et al., eds. *Handbook of mucosal immunology.* San Diego: Academic Press, 1994:41–55.

231. Kato T, Owen RL, Structure and function of intestinal mucosal epithelium. In: Ogra PL, Mestecky J, Lamm M, et al., eds. *Handbook of mucosal immunology.* San Diego: Academic Press, 1994:11–26.

232. Mostov KE, Kraehenbuhl JP, Blobel G. Receptor-mediated transcellular transport of immunoglobulin: synthesis of secretory component as multiple and larger transmembrane forms. *Proc Natl Acad Sci U S A* 1980;77:7257–7261.

233. Mostov KE, Friedlander M, Blobel G. The receptor for transepithelial transport of IgA and IgM contains multiple immunoglobulin-like domains. *Nature* 1984; 308:37–43.

234. Krajci P, Kvale D, Taskén K, Brandtzaeg P. Molecular cloning and exon-intron mapping of the gene encoding human transmembrane secretory component (the poly-Ig receptor). *Eur J Immunol* 1992;22:2309–2315.

235. Brandtzaeg P. Distribution and characteristics of mucosal immunoglobulin-producing cells. In: Ogra PL, Mestecky J, Lamm M, et al., eds. *Handbook of mucosal immunology.* San Diego: Academic Press, 1994:251–262.

236. Brandtzaeg P. Presence of J chain in human immunocytes containing various immunoglobulin classes. *Nature* 1974;252:418–420.

237. Brandtzaeg P, Prydz H. Direct evidence for an integrated function of J chain and secretory component in epithelial transport of immunoglobulins. *Nature* 1984; 311:71–73.

238. Niles MJ, Matsuuchi L, Koshland ME. Polymeric IgM assembly and secretion in lymphoid and nonlymphoid cell lines: evidence that J chain is required for pentamer IgM synthesis. *Proc Natl Acad Sci U S A* 1995;92:2884–2888.

239. Hendrickson BA, Conner DA, Ladd DJ, et al. Altered hepatic transport of immunoglobulin A in mice lacking J chain. *J Exp Med* 1995;182:1905–1911.

240. Hendrickson BA, Rindisbacher L, Corthesy B, et al. Lack of association of secretory component with IgA in J chain-deficient mice. *J Immunol* 1996;157:750–754.

241. Mostov KE. Transepithelial transport of immunoglobulins. *Annu Rev Immunol* 1994;12:63–84.

242. McGee DW, Beagley KW, Aicher WK, McGhee JR. Transforming growth fac-

tor-β enhances interleukin-6 secretion by intestinal epithelial cells. *Immunology* 1992;77:7–12.

243. McGee DW, Beagley KW, Aicher WK, McGhee JR. Transforming growth factor-β and IL-1β act in synergy to increase IL-6 secretion by the intestinal epithelial cell line, IEC-6. *J Immunol* 1993;151:970–978.

244. McGee DW, Elson CO, McGhee JR. Enhancing effect of cholera toxin on interleukin-6 secretion by IEC-6 intestinal epithelial cells: mode of action and augmenting effect of inflammatory cytokines. *Infect Immun* 1993;61:4637–4644.

245. Bromander AK, Kjerrulf M, Holmgren J, Lycke N. Cholera toxin enhances alloantigen presentation by cultured intestinal epithelial cells. *Scand J Immunol* 1993;37:452–458.

246. Hedges S, Agace W, Svanborg C. Epithelial cytokine responses and mucosal cytokine networks. *Trends Microbiol* 1995;3:266–270.

247. Hedges S, Svensson M, Svanborg C. Interleukin-6 response of epithelial cell lines to bacterial stimulation in vitro. *Infect Immun* 1992;60:1295–1301.

248. Agace U, Andersson J, Ceska M, Svanborg C. Selective cytokine production by epithelial cells following exposure to Escherichia coli. *Infect Immun* 1993;61: 602–609.

249. Agace WW, Hedges SR, Ceska M, Svanborg C. Interleukin-8 and the neutrophil response to mucosal gram-negative infection. *J Clin Invest* 1993;92:780–785.

250. Eckmann L, Kagnoff MF, Fierer J. Epithelial cells secrete the chemokine interleukin-8 in response to bacterial entry. *Infect Immun* 1993;61:4569–4574.

251. Crowe SE, Alvarez L, Dytoc M, et al. Expression of interleukin 8 and CD54 by human gastric epithelium after *Helicobacter pylori* infection in vitro. *Gastroenterology* 1995;108:65–74.

252. Sharma SA, Tummuru MK, Miller GG, Blaser MJ. Interleukin-8 response of gastric epithelial cell lines to *Helicobacter pylori* stimulation in vitro. *Infect Immun* 1995;63:1681–1687.

253. Jung HC, Eckmann L, Yang SK, et al. A distinct array of proinflammatory cytokines is expressed in human colon epithelial cells in response to bacteria invasion. *J Clin Invest* 1995;95:55–65.

254. Rasmussen SJ, Eckmann L, Quayle AJ, et al. Secretion of proinflammatory cytokines by epithelial cells in response to *Chlamydia* infection suggests a central role for epithelial cells in chlamydial pathogenesis. *J Clin Invest* 1997;99: 77–87.

255. Eckmann L, Jung HC, Schürer-Maly C, Panja A, Morzycka-Wroblewska E, Kagnoff MF. Differential cytokine expression by human intestinal epithelial cell lines: regulated expression of interleukin 8. *Gastroenterology* 1993;105: 1689–1697.

256. Schürer-Maly C-C, Eckmann L, Kagnoff MF, Falco MT, Maly F-E. Colonic epithelial cell lines as a source of interleukin-8: stimulation by inflammatory cytokines and bacterial lipopolysaccharide. *Immunology* 1994;81.85–91.

257. McCormick BA, Colgan SP, Delp-Archer C, Miller SI, Madara JL. *Salmonella typhimurium* attachment to human intestinal epithelial monolayers: transcellular signalling to subepithelial neutrophils. *J Cell Biol* 1993;123:895–907.

258. Kvale D, Krajci P, Brandtzaeg P. Expression and regulation of adhesion molecules ICAM-1 (CD54) and LFA-3 (CD58) in human intestinal epithelial cell lines. *Scand J Immunol* 1992;35:669–676.

259. Brandeis JM, Sayegh MH, Gallon L, Blumberg RS, Carpenter CB. Rat intestinal epithelial cells present major histocompatibility complex allopeptides to primed T cells. *Gastroenterology* 1994;107:1537–1542.

260. LeFrancois L. Intraepithelial lymphocytes of the intestinal mucosa: Curiouser and couriouser. *Semin Immunol* 1991;3:99–108.

261. Ferguson A, Parrott DM, The effect of antigen deprivation on thymus-dependent and thymus-independent lymphocytes in the small intestine of mouse. *Clin Exp Immunol* 1972;12:477–488.

262. Crowe PT, Marsh MN. Morphometric analysis of intestinal mucosa. VI. Principals in enumerating intra-epithelial lymphocytes. *Virchows Arch* 1994;424:301–306.

263. Barrett TA, Gajewski TF, Danielpour D, Chang EB, Beagley KW, Bluestone JA. Differential function of intestinal intraepithelial lymphocyte subsets. *J Immunol* 1992;149:1124–1130.

264. Fujihashi K, Yamamoto M, McGhee JR, Kiyono H. αβ TCR+ IELs with CD4+, CD8- and CD4+, CD8+ phenotypes from orally-immunized mice provide Th2-like function for B cell responses. *J Immunol* 1993;151:6681–6691.

265. Komano H, Fujiura Y, Kawaguchi M, et al. Homeostatic regulation of intestinal epithelia by intraepithelial γδ T cells. *Proc Natl Acad Sci U S A* 1995;92:6147–6151.

266. Fujihashi K, Kawabata S, Hiroi T, et al. Interleukin 2 (IL-2) and interleukin 7 (IL-7) reciprocally induce IL-7 and IL-2 receptors on γδ T cell receptor-positive intraepithelial lymphocytes. *Proc Natl Acad Sci U S A* 1996;93:3613–3618.

267. Lefrancois L, Phenotypic complexity of intraepithelial lymphocytes of the small intestine. *J Immunol* 1991;147:1746–1751.

268. Mosley, RL, Styre D, Klein JR, CD4+, CD8+ murine intestinal intraepithelial lymphocytes. *Int Immunol* 1990;2:361–365.

269. Guy-Grand D, Cerf-Bensussan N, Malissen B, Malassis-Seris M, Briottet C, Vassalli P. Two gut intraepithelial CD8+ lymphocyte populations with different T cell receptors: a role for the gut epithelium in T cell differentiation. *J Exp Med* 1991; 173:471–481.

270. Rocha B, Vassalli P, Guy-Grand D. The extrathymic T-cell development pathway. *Immunol Today* 1992;13:449–454.

271. Rocha B, Vassali P, Guy-Grand D. Thymic and extrathymic origins of gut intraepithelial lymphocyte population in mice. *J Exp Med* 1994;180:681–686.

272. Poussier P, Julius M. Intestinal intraepithelial lymphocytes: The plot thickens. *J Exp Med* 1994;180:1185–1189.

273. Klein JR, Mosley RL. Phenotypic and cytotoxic characteristics of intraepithelial lymphocytes. *Adv Host Def Mech* 1993;9:33.

274. Poussier P, Edouard P, Lee C, Binnie M, Julius M. Thymus-independent development and negative selection of T cells expressing T cell receptor αβ in the intestinal epithelium: evidence for distinct circulation patterns of gut and thymus-derived T lymphocytes. *J Exp Med* 1992;176:187–199.

275. Mosley RL, Styre D, Klein JR. Differentiation and functional maturation of bone marrow derived intestinal epithelial T cells expressing membrane T cell receptor in athymic radiation chimeras. *J Immunol* 1990;145:1369–1375.

276. Hori T, Paliard X, de Waal, Malefijit R, Ranes M, Spits H, Comparative analysis of CD8-expressed on mature CD4+, CD8+ T cell clones cultured with IL-4 and that on CD8+ T cell clones: implication for functional significance of CD8b. *Int Immunol* 1991;3:737–741.

277. MacDonald HR, Schreyer M, Howe RC, Bron C. Selective expression of CD8a (Ly-2) subunit on activated thymic γδ cells. *Eur J Immunol* 1990;20:927–930.

278. Goodman T, Lefrancois L. Expression of the γδ T cell-receptor on intestinal CD8+ intraepithelial lymphocytes. *Nature* 1988;333:855–858.

279. Bonneville M, Janeway CA Jr, Ito K, et al. Intestinal intraepithelial lymphocytes are a distinct set of γδ T cells. *Nature* 1988;336:479–481.

280. Mosley RL, Whetsell M, Klein JR. Proliferative properties of murine intestinal intraepithelial lymphocytes (IEL): IEL expressing TCR αβ or TCR tau delta are largely unresponsive to proliferative mediated signals via conventional stimulation of the CD3-TCR complex. *Int Immunol* 1991;3:563–569.

281. Mowat AM, MacKenzie S, Baca ME, Felstein MV, Parrott DM. Functional characteristics of intraepithelial lymphocytes from mouse small intestine. II. in vivo and in vitro responses of intraepithelial lymphocytes to mitogenic and allogenic stimuli. *Immunology* 1986;58:627–634.

282. Yamamoto M, Fujihashi K, Amano M, McGhee JR, Beagley KW, Kiyono K. Cytokine synthesis and apoptosis by intestinal intraepithelial lymphocytes: signaling of high density αβ TCR+ and γδ TCR+ T cells via TCR-CD3 complex result in IFN-γ and IL-5 production, while low density T cells undergo DNA fragmentation. *Eur J Immunol* 1994;24:1301–1306.

283. Yamamoto M, Fujihashi K, Beagley KW, McGhee JR, Kiyono H. Cytokine synthesis by intestinal intraepithelial lymphocytes. Both γδ TCR+ and αβ TCR+ T cells in the G1 phase of cell cycle produce IFN-γ and IL-5. *J Immunol* 1993;150: 106–114.

284. Fujihashi H, Yamamoto Y, McGhee JR, Kiyono H. Intraepithelial lymphocytes. Immunoregulatory function and cytokine production by αβ TCR+ and γδ TCR+ T cells for mucosal immune responses. *Adv Host Def Mech* 1993;9:89.

285. Liu, CP, Ueda R, She J, et al. Abnormal T cell development in CD3-zeta-/- mutant mice and identification of a novel T cell population in the intestine. *EMBO J* 1993;12:4863–4875.

286. Love PE, Shores EW, Johnson MD, et al. T cell development in mice that lack the zeta chain of the T cell antigen receptor complex. *Science* 1993;261: 918–921.

287. Malissen M, Gillet A, Rocha B, et al. T cell development in mice lacking the CD3-5 In gene. *EMBO J* 1993;12:4347–4355.

288. Ohno H, Aoe T, Taki S, et al. Developmental and functional impairment of T cells in mice lacking CD3 zeta chains. *EMBO J* 1993;12:4357–4366.

289. Ohno H, Ono S, Hirayama N, Shimada S, Saito T. Preferential usage of the Fc receptor δ chain in the T cell antigen receptor complex by γδ T cells localized in epithelia. *J Exp Med* 1994;179:365–369.

290. Yamamoto S, Russ F, Teixeira HC, Conradt P, Kaufmann SH. *Listeria monocytogenes*-induced gamma interferon secretion by intestinal intraepithelial γ/δ T lymphocytes. *Infect Immun* 1993;61:2154–2161.

291. Emoto M, Neuhaus O, Emoto Y, Kaufmann SH. Influence of β2-microglobulin expression on gamma interferon secretion and target cell lysis by intraepithelial lymphocytes during intestinal *Listeria monocytogenes* infection. *Infect Immun* 1996;64:569–575.

292. Roberts SJ, Smith AL, West AB, et al. T cell αβ (+) and γδ (+) deficient mice display abnormal but distinct phenotypes towards a natural, widespread infection of the intestinal epithelium. *Proc Natl Acad Sci U S A* 1996;93:11774–11779.

293. Kaufmann SH, Immunity to intracellular bacteria. *Annu Rev Immunol* 1993;11: 129–163.

294. Zijlstra M, Bix M, Simister NE, Loring JM, Raulet DH, Jaenisch R. β2-microglobulin deficient mice lack CD4-8+ cytolytic T cells. *Nature* 1990;344: 742–746.

295. Fujihashi K, Yamamoto M, McGhee JR, Beagley KW, Kiyono H. Function of αβ TCR+ intestinal intraepithelial lymphocytes: Th1- and Th2-type cytokine production by CD4+ CD8- and CD4+ CD8+ T cell for helper activity. *Int Immunol* 1993;5:1473–1481.

296. Fujihashi K, Taguchi T, Aicher WK, et al. Immunoregulatory functions for murine intraepithelial lymphocytes: γ/δ T cell receptor-positive (TCR+) T cells abrogate oral tolerance, while α/β TCR+ T cells provide B cell help. *J Exp Med* 1992;175:695–707.

297. Fujihashi K, McGhee JR, Kweon M-N, et al. γ/δ T cell-deficient mice have impaired mucosal immunoglobulin A responses. *J Exp Med* 1996;183:1929–1935.

298. McMenamin C, Pimm C, McKersey M, Holt PG. Regulation of IgE responses to inhaled antigen in mice by antigen specific γδ T cells. *Science* 1994;265: 1869–1871.

299. McMenamin C, McKersey M, Kuhnlein P, Hunig T, Holt PG, γδ T cells down regulate primary IgE responses in rats to inhaled soluble protein antigens. *J Immunol* 1995;154:4390–4394.

300. Szczepanik M, Anderson LR, Ushio H, et al. γδ T cells from tolerized αβ T cell receptor (TCR)-deficient mice inhibit contact sensitivity-effector T cells in vivo, and their interferon-γ production in vitro. J Exp Med 1996;184:2129–2139.

301. Kvale D, Lovhaug D, Sollid LM, Brandtzaeg P. Tumor necrosis factor-α up-regulates expression of secretory component, the epithelial receptor for polymeric Ig. J Immunol 1988;140:3086–3089.

302. Phillips JO, Everson MP, Moldoveanu Z, Lue C, Mestecky J. Synergistic effect of IL-4 and IFN-γ on the expression of polymeric Ig receptor (secretory component) and IgA binding by human epithelial cells. J Immunol 1990;145:1740–1744.

303. Boismenu R, Havran WL. Modulation of epithelial cell growth by intraepithelial γδ T cells. Science 1994;266:1253–1255.

304. Komano H, Fujiura Y, Kawaguchi M, et al. Homeostatic regulation of intestinal epithelia by intraepithelial γδ T cells. Proc Natl Acad Sci U S A 1995;92:6147–6151.

305. Puddington L, Olson S, Lefrancois L. Interactions between stem cell factor and c-kit are required for intestinal immune system homeostasis. Immunity 1994;1:733–739.

306. Klimpel GR, Chopra AK, Langley KE, et al. A role for stem cell factor and c-kit in the murine intestinal tract secretory response to cholera toxin. J Exp Med 1995;182:1931–1942.

307. Klimpel GR, Langley AK, Wypych J, et al. A role for stem cell factor: c-kit interaction(s) in the intestinal tract response to Salmonella typhimurium infection. J Exp Med 1996;184:271–276.

308. Watanabe M, Veno Y, Yajima T, et al. Interleukin 7 is produced by human intestinal epithelial cells and regulates the proliferation of intestinal mucosal lymphocytes. J Clin Invest 1995;95:2945–2953.

309. Maki K, Sunaga S, Komagata Y, et al. Interleukin 7 receptor-deficient mice lack γδ T cells. Proc Natl Acad Sci U S A 1996;93:7172–7177.

310. Moore TA, von Freeden-Jeffry U, Murray R, Zlotnik A. Inhibition of γδ T cell development and early thymocyte maturation in IL-7-/- mice. J Immunol 1996;157:2366–2373.

311. Fujihashi K, McGhee JR, Yamamoto M, et al. An interleukin-7 internet for intestinal intraepithelial T cell development: knockout of ligand or receptor reveal differences in the immunodeficient state. Eur J Immunol 1997;27:2133–2138.

312. Gowans JL, Knight EJ. The route of recirculation of lymphocytes in the rat. Proc R Soc Lond [Biol] 1964;159:257–282.

313. Craig SW, Cebra JJ. Peyer's patches: an enriched source of precursors for IgA-producing immunocytes in the rabbit. J Exp Med 1971;134:188–200.

314. Craig SW, Cebra JJ. Rabbit Peyer's patches, appendix and popliteal lymph node B lymphocytes: a comparative analysis of their membrane immunoglobulin components and plasma cell precursor potential. J Immunol 1975;114:492–502.

315. McDermott MR, Bienenstock J. Evidence for a common mucosal immunologic system. I. Migration of B immunoblasts into intestinal, respiratory and genital tissues. J Immunol 1979;122:1892–1898.

316. McWilliams M, Phillips-Quagliata JM, Lamm ME. Characteristics of mesenteric lymph node cells homing to gut-associated lymphoid tissue in syngeneic mice. J Immunol 1975;115:54–58.

317. McWilliams M, Phillips-Quagliata JM, Lamm ME. Mestenteric lymph node B lymphoblasts which home to the small intestine are precommitted to IgA synthesis. J Exp Med 1977;145:866–875.

318. Husband A-J, Gowans JL. The origin and antigen-dependent distribution of IgA-containing cells in the intestine. J Exp Med 1978;148:1146–1160.

319. Roux ME, McWilliams M, Phillips-Quagliata JM, Lamm ME, Origin of IgA-secreting plasma cells in the mammary gland. J Exp Med 1977;146:1311–1322.

320. Butcher EC, Picker LJ. Lymphocyte homing and homeostasis. Science 1996;272:60–66.

321. Picker LJ. Control of lymphocyte homing. Curr Opin Immunol 1994;6:394–406.

322. Bradley LM, Watson SR, Lymphocyte migration into tissue: the paradigm derived from CD4 subsets. Curr Opin Immunol 1996;8:312–320.

323. Butcher EC. Leukocyte-endothelial cell recognition: three (or more) steps to specificity and diversity. Cell 1991;67:1033–1036.

324. Springer TA. Traffic signals for lymphocyte recirculation and leukocyte emigration: the multistep paradigm. Cell 1994;76:301–314.

325. Streeter PR, Rouse BT, Butcher EC. Immunohistologic and functional characterization of a vascular addressin involved in lymphocyte homing into peripheral lymph nodes. J Cell Biol 1988;107:1853–1862.

326. Berg EL, Robinson MK, Warnock RA, Butcher EC. The human peripheral lymph node vascular addressin is a ligand for LECAM-1, the peripheral lymph node homing receptor. J Cell Biol 1991;114:343–349.

327. Berlin C, Berg EL, Briskin MJ, et al. α4/β7 integrin mediates lymphocyte binding to the mucosal vascular addressin MadCAM-1. Cell 1993;74:185.

328. Briskin MJ, McEvoy LM, Butcher EC. MAdCAM-1 has homology to immunoglobulin and mucin-like adhesion receptors and to IgA1. Nature 1993;363:461–464.

329. Streeter PR, Berg EL, Rouse BT, Bargatze RF, Butcher EC. A tissue-specific endothelial cell molecule involved in lymphocyte homing. Nature 1988;331:41–46.

330. Altevogt P, Hubbe M, Ruppert M, et al. The α integrin chain is a ligand for α4β7 and α4β1. J Exp Med 1995;182:345–355.

331. Bevilacqua MP. Endothelial-leukocyte adhesion molecules. Annu Rev Immunol 1993;11:767–804.

332. Osborn L. Leukocyte adhesion to endothelium in inflammation. Cell 1990;62:3–6.

333. Holzmann B, McIntyre BW, Weisman IL. Identification of a murine Peyer's patch-specific lymphocyte homing receptor as an integrin molecule with an α chain homologous to human VLA-4a. Cell 1989;56:37–46.

334. Bell RG, Issekutz T. Expression of a protective intestinal immune response can be inhibited at three distinct sites by treatment with anti-α4 integrin. J Immunol 1993;151:4790–4802.

335. Hamann A, Andrew DP, Jablonski-Westrich D, Holzmann B, Butcher EC. Role of α4-integrins in lymphocyte homing to mucosal tissues in vivo. J Immunol 1994;152:3282–3293.

336. Rott LS, Briskin MJ, Andrew DP, Berg EL, Butcher EC. A fundamental subdivision of circulating lymphocytes defined by adhesion to mucosal addressin cell adhesion molecule-1. Comparison with vascular cell adhesion molecule-1 and correlation with β7 integrins and memory differentiation. J Immunol 1996;156:3727–3736.

337. Kantele A, Arvilommi H, Jokinen I. Specific immunoglobulin-secreting human blood cells after peroral vaccination against Salmonella typhi. J Infect Dis 1986;153:1126–1131.

338. Czerkinsky C, Prince SJ, Michalek SM, et al. IgA antibody-producing cells in peripheral blood after antigen ingesiton: evidence for a common mucosal immune system in humans. Proc Natl Acad Sci U S A 1987;84:2449–2453.

339. Quiding M, Nordstrom I, Kilander A, et al. Intestinal immune responses in humans. Oral cholera vaccination induces strong intestinal antibody responses and interferon-γ production and evokes local immunological memory. J Clin Invest 1991;88:143–148.

340. Buckley RH, Dees SC. Correlation of milk precipitins with IgA deficiency. N Engl J Med 1969;281:465–469.

341. Kantele A, Kantele JM, Savilahti E, et al. Homing potential of circulating lymphocytes in humans depend on the site of activation: oral, but nor parenteral, typhoid vaccination induces circulating antibody-secreting cells that all bear homing receptors directing them to the gut. J Immunol 1997;158:574–579.

342. Schieferdecker HL, Ullrich R, Weiss-Breckwoldt AN, et al. The HML-1 antigen of intestinal lymphocytes is an activation antigen. J Immunol 1990;144:2541–2549.

343. Schieferdecker HL, Ullrich R, Zeitz M, Phenotype of HML-1-positive T cells in the human intestinal lamina propria. Immunol Res 1991;10:207–210.

344. James SP, Zeitz M, Human gastrointestinal mucosal T cells. In: Ogra PL, Mestecky J, Lamm M, et al., eds. Handbook of mucosal immunology. San Diego: Academic Press, 1994:275–285.

345. Cerf-Bensussan N, Jarry A, Brousse N, et al. A monoclonal antibody (HML-1) defining a novel membrane molecule present on human intestinal lymphocytes. Eur J Immunol 1987;17:1279–1285.

346. Kilshaw PJ, Murant SJ. A new surface antigen on intraepithelial lymphocytes in the intestine. Eur J Immunol 1990;20:2201–2207.

347. Schieferdecker HL, Ullrich R, Weiss-Breckwoldt AN, et al. The HML-1 antigen of intestinal lymphocytes is an activation antigen. J Immunol 1990;144:2541–2549.

348. Cerf-Bensussan N, Guy-Grand D, Lisowska-Grospierre B, et al. A monoclonal antibody specific for rat intestinal lymphocytes. J Immunol 1986;136:76–82.

349. Haury M, Kasahara Y, Schaal S, Bucy RP, Cooper MD. Intestinal lymphocytes in the chicken express an integrin-like antigen. Eur J Immunol 1993;23:313–319.

350. Cepek KL, Parker CM, Madara JL, Brenner MB. Integrin αEβ7 mediates adhesion of T lymphocytes to epithelial cells. J Immunol. 1993;150:3459–3470.

351. Benmerah A, Badrichani A, Ngohou K, et al. Homotypic aggregation of CD103 (αEβ7)+ lymphocytes by an anti-CD103 antibody, HML-4. Eur J Immunol 1994;24:2249–2249.

352. Roberts K, Kilshaw DJ, The mucosal T cell integrin αM290β7 recognizes a ligand on mucosal epithelial cell lines. Eur J Immunol 1993;23:1630–1635.

353. Kilshaw DJ, Murant SJ. Expression and regulation of β7 (βP) integrins on mouse lymphocytes: Relevance to the mucosal immune system. Eur J Immunol 1991;21:2591–2597.

354. Parker CM, Cepek KL, Russell GJ, et al. A family of β7 integrins on human mucosal lymphocytes. Proc Natl Acad Sci U S A 1992;89:1924–1928.

355. Barnard JA, Warwick GJ, Gold LI. Localization of transforming growth factor β isoforms in the normal murine small intestine and colon. Gastroenterology 1993;105:67–73.

356. Tanaka Y, Adams DH, Shaw S. Proteoglycans on endothelial cells present adhesion-inducing cytokines to leukocytes. Immunol Today 1993;14:111–115.

357. Yang SK, Eckmann L, Kagnoff M. Colon epithelial cells express a broad array of chemokines. Clin Immunol Immunopathol 1995;76:520.

358. Cepek KL, Shaw SK, Parker CM, et al. Adhesion between epithelial cells and T lymphocytes mediated by E-cadherin and the αEβ7 integrin. Nature 1994;372:190–193.

359. Sarnacki S, Begue B, Buc H, et al. Enhancement of CD3-induced activation of human intestinal intraepithelial lymphocytes by stimulation of the β7-containing integrin defined by HML-1 antibody. Eur J Immunol 1992;22:2887–2892.

360. Peifer M, Cancer, catenins and cuticle pattern: a complex connection. Science 1993;262:1667–1668.

361. Mestecky J. The common mucosal immune system and current strategies for induction of immune responses in external secretions. J Clin Immunol 1987;7:265–276.

362. McWilliams M, Phillips-Quagliata JM, Lamm ME. Mestentric lymph node lymphoblasts which home to the small intestine are precommitted to IgA synthesis. J Exp Med 1977;145:866–875.

363. Montgomery PC, Ayyildiz A, Lemaitre-Coelho IM, Vaerman J-P, Rockey JH. Induction and expression of antibodies in secretions: the ocular immune system. Ann NY Acad Sci 1983;409:428–440.

364. Robertson SM, Cebra JJ. A model for local immunity. *Ric Clin Lab* 1976;6(suppl 3):105.

365. Winner L III, Mack J, Weltzin R, Mekalanos JJ, Kraehenbuhl JP, Neutra MR. New model for analysis of mucosal immunity: intestinal secretion of specific monoclonal immunoglobulin A from hybridoma tumors protects against *Vibrio cholerae* infection. *Infect Immun* 1991;59:977–982.

366. Lee CK, Weltzin R, Soman G, Georgakopoulos KM, Houle DM, Monath TP. Oral administration of polymeric immunoglobulin A prevents colonization with *Vibrio cholerae* in neonatal mice. *Infect Immun* 1994;62:887–891.

367. Michetti P, Mahan MJ, Slauch JM, Mekalanos JJ, Neutra MR. Monoclonal secretory immunoglobulin A protects mice against oral challenge with the invasive pathogen *Salmonella typhimurium*. *Infect Immun* 1992;60:1786–1792.

368. Czinn SJ, Cai A, Nedrud JG. Protection of germ-free mice from infection by *Helicobacter felis* after active oral or passive IgA immunization. *Vaccine* 1993; 11:637–642.

369. Kaetzel CS, Robinson JK, Chintalacharuvu KR, Vaerman JP, Lamm ME. The polymeric immunoglobulin receptor (secretory component) mediates transport of immune complexes across epithelial cells: a local defense function for IgA. *Proc Natl Acad Sci U S A* 1991;88:8796–8800.

370. Kaetzel CS, Robinson JK, Lamm ME. Epithelial transcytosis of monomeric IgA and IgG cross-linked through antigen to polymeric IgA. A role for monomeric antibodies in the mucosal immune system. *J Immunol* 1994;152:72–76.

371. Mazanec MB, Kaetzel CS, Lamm ME, Fletcher D, Nedrud JG. Intracellular neutralization of virus by immunoglobulin A antibodies. *Proc Natl Acad Sci U S A* 1992;89:6901–6905.

372. Mazanec MB, Nedrud JG, Kaetzel CS, Lamm ME. A three-tiered view of the role of IgA in mucosal defense. *Immunol Today* 1993;14:430–435.

373. Burns JW, Siadat-Pajouh M, Krishnaney AA, Greenberg HB. Protective effect of rotavirus VP6-specific IgA monoclonal antibodies that lack neutralizing activity. *Science* 1996;272:104–107.

374. Spangler BD. Structure and function of cholera toxin and the related *Escherichia coli* heat-labile enterotoxin. *Microbiol Rev* 1992;56:622–647.

375. Gill DM. The arrangement of subunits in cholera toxin. *Biochemistry* 1976;15: 1242–1248.

376. Gill DM, Clements JD, Robertson DC, Finkelstein RA. Subunit number and arrangement in *Escherichia coli* heat-labile enterotoxin. *Infect Immun* 1981;33: 677–682.

377. van Heyningen S. Cholera toxin: interaction of subunits with ganglioside GM1. *Science* 1974;183:656.

378. Fukuta S, Magnani JL, Twiddy EM, Holmes RK, Ginsburg V. Comparison of the carbohydrate-binding specificities of cholera toxin and *Escherichia coli* heat-labile enterotoxins LTh-I, LT-IIa, and LT-IIb. *Infect Immun* 1988;56: 1748–1753.

379. Gill DM, King CA. The mechanisms of action of cholera toxin in pigeon erythrocyte lysates. *J Biol Chem* 1975;250:6424–6432.

380. Field M, Rao MC, Chang EB. Intestinal electrolyte transport and diarrheal disease I. *N Engl J Med* 1989;321:800–806.

381. Elson CO, Ealding W. Generalized systemic and mucosal immunity in mice after mucosal stimulation with cholera toxin. *J Immunol* 1984;132:2736–2741.

382. Clements JD, Hartzog NM, Lyon FL. Adjuvant activity of *Escherichia coli* heat-labile enterotoxin and effect on the induction of oral tolerance in mice to unrelated protein antigens. *Vaccine* 1988;6:269–277.

383. Tsuji T, Inoue T, Miyama A, Okamoto K, Honda T, Miwatani T. A single amino acid substitution in the A subunit of *Escherichia coli* enterotoxin results in a loss of its toxic activity. *J Biol Chem* 1990;265:22520–22525.

384. Sixma TK, Pronk SE, Kalk KH, van Zanten BA, Berghuis AM, Hol WG. Lactose binding to heat-labile enterotoxin revealed by X-ray crystallography. *Nature* 1992;355:561–564.

385. Lycke N, Tsuji T, Holmgren J. The adjuvant effect of *Vibrio cholerae* and *Escherichia coli* heat-labile enterotoxins is linked to their ADP-ribosyltransferase activity. *Eur J Immunol* 1992;22:2277–2281.

386. Douce G, Turcotte C, Cropley I, et al. Mutants of *Escherichia coli* heat-labile toxin lacking ADP-ribosyltransferase activity act as nontoxic, mucosal adjuvants. *Proc Natl Acad Sci U S A* 1995;92:1644–1648.

387. Dickinson BL, Clements JD. Dissociation of *Escherichia coli* heat-labile enterotoxin adjuvanticity from ADP-ribosyltransferase activity. *Infect Immun* 1995;63: 1617–1623.

388. Pizza M, Domenighini M, Hol W, et al. Probing the structure-activity relationship of *Escherichia coli* LT-A by site-directed mutagenesis. *Mol Microbiol* 1994; 14:51–60.

389. Di Tommaso A, Saletti G, Pizza M, et al. Induction of antigen-specific antibodies in vaginal secretions by using a nontoxic mutant of heat-labile enterotoxin as a mucosal adjuvant. *Infect Immun* 1996;64:974–979.

390. Yamamoto S, Takeda Y, Yamamoto M, et al. Mutants in the ADP-ribosyltransferase cleft of cholera toxin lack diarrhoeagenicity but retain adjuvanticity. *J Exp Med* 1997;185:1203–1210.

391. Yamamoto S, Kiyono H, Yamamoto M, et al. A nontoxic mutant of cholera toxin elicits Th2-type responses for enhanced mucosal immunity. *Proc Natl Acad Sci U S A* 1997;94:5267–5272.

392. Dertzbaugh MT, Elson CO. Comparative effectiveness of the cholera toxin B subunit and alkaline phosphatase as carriers for oral vaccines. *Infect Immun* 1993;61:48–55.

393. Dertzbaugh MT, Peterson DL, Macrina FL. Cholera toxin B-subunit gene fusion: structural and functional analysis of the chimeric protein. *Infect Immun* 1990;58: 70–79.

394. Hajishengallis G, Hollingshead SK, Koga T, Russell MW. Mucosal immunization with a bacterial protein antigen genetically coupled to cholera toxin A2/B subunits. *J Immunol* 1995;154:4322–4332.

395. Holmgren J, Czerkinsky C, Lycke N, Svennerholm A-M. Mucosal immunity: implications for vaccine development. *Immunobiology* 1992;184:157–179.

396. Holmgren J, Czerkinsky C, Lycke N, Svennerholm A-M. Strategies for the induction of immune responses at mucosal surfaces making use of cholera toxin B subunit as immunogen, carrier and adjuvant. *Am J Trop Med Hyg* 1994; 50:42–54.

397. Tamura S-I, Kurata T. Intranasal immunization with influenza vaccine. In: Kiyono H, Ogra PL, McGhee JR, eds. *Mucosal vaccines*. San Diego: Academic Press, 1996:425–436.

398. Okahashi N, Yamamoto M, VanCott JL, et al. Oral immunization of interleukin-4 (IL-4) knockout mice with a recombinant *Salmonella* strain or cholera toxin reveals that CD4$^+$ Th2 cells producing IL-6 and IL-10 are associated with mucosal immunoglobulin A responses. *Infect Immun* 1996;64:1516–1525.

399. Bourguin I, Chardes T, Bout D. Oral immunization with *Toxoplasma gondii* antigens in association with cholera toxin induces enhanced protective and cell-mediated immunity in C57BL/6 mice. *Infect Immun* 1993;61:2082–2088.

400. Robinson K, Bellaby T, Wakelin D. Efficacy of oral vaccination against the murine intestinal parasite *Trichuris muris* is dependent upon host genetics. *Infect Immun* 1995;63:1762–1766.

401. Zhang T, Li E, Stanley SL Jr. Oral immunization with the dodecapeptide repeat of the serine-rich *Entamoeba histolytica* protein (SREHP) fused to the cholera toxin B subunit induces a mucosal and systemic anti-SREHP antibody response. *Infect Immun* 1995;63:1349–1355.

402. Curtiss R III, Kelley SM, Hassan JO. Live oral avirulent *Salmonella* vaccines. *Vet Microbiol* 1993;37:397–405.

403. Roberts M, Chatfield SN, Dougan G. Salmonella as carriers of heterologous antigens. In: O'Hagan DT, eds. Novel delivery systems for oral vaccines. Boca Raton, FL: CRC Press, 1994:27–35.

404. Chatfield S, Roberts M, Londono P, Cropley I, Douce G, Dougan G. The development of oral vaccines based on live attenuated *Salmonella* strains. *FEMS Immunol Med Microbiol* 1993;7:1–7.

405. Doggett TA, Brown PK. Attenuated *Salmonella* as vectors for oral immunization. In: Kiyono H, et al. Mucosal vaccines. San Diego: Academic Press, 1996: 105–108.

406. Yang DM, Fairweather N, Button LL, McMaster WR, Kahl LP, Liew FY. Oral *Salmonella typhimurium* (AroA$^-$) vaccine expressing a major leishmanial surface protein (gp 63) preferentially induces T helper 1 cells and protective immunity against leishmaniasis. *J Immunol* 1990;145:2281–2285.

407. Hirabayashi Y, Kurata H, Funato H, et al. Comparison of intranasal inoculation of influenza HA vaccine combined with cholera toxin B subunit with oral or parenteral vaccination. *Vaccine* 1990;8:243–248.

408. Tamura S, Ito Y, Asanuma H, et al. Cross-protection against influenza virus infection afforded by trivalent inactivated vaccines inoculated intranasally with cholera toxin B subunit. *J Immunol* 1992;149:981–988.

409. Hashigucci K, Ogawa H, Ishidate T, et al. Antibody responses in volunteers induced by nasal influenza vaccine combined with *Escherichia coli* heat-labile enterotoxin B subunit containing a trace amount of the holotoxin. *Vaccine* 1996;14:113–119.

410. Freihorst PD, Keely SP, Schiff GM. Similar subclass antibody responses after intranasal immunization with UV-inactivated RSV mixed with cholera toxin or live RSV. *J Med Virol* 1991;35:192–197.

411. Graham BS, Bunton LA, Rowland J, Wright PF, Karzon DT. Respiratory syncytial virus infection in anti-μ treated mice. *J Virol* 1991;65:4936–4942.

412. Roberts M, Bacon A, Rappuoli R, et al. A mutant pertussis toxin molecule that lacks ADP-ribosyltransferase activity, PT-9K/129G, is an effective mucosal adjuvant for intranasally delivered proteins. *Infect Immun* 1995;63:2100–2108.

413. Graham FL, Smiley J, Russell WC, Nairn R. Characterization of a human cell line transformed by DNA from human adenovirus type 5. *J Gen Virol* 1977;36: 59–74.

414. Gallichan WS, Johnson DC, Graham FL, Rosenthal KL. Mucosal immunity and protection after intranasal immunization with recombinant adenovirus expressing herpes simplex glycoprotein B. *J Infect Dis* 1993;168:622–629.

415. Lubeck MD, Natuk RJ, Chengalvala M, et al. Immunogenicity of recombinant adenovirus-human immunodeficiency virus vaccines in chimpanzees following intranasal administration. *AIDS Res Hum Retrovir* 1994;10:1443–1449.

416. Prevec K, Schneider M, Rosenthal KL, Belbeck LW, Derbyshire JB, Graham FL. Use of human adenovirus-based vectors for antigen expression in animals. *J Gen Virol* 1989;70:429–434.

417. Prevec L, Campbell JB, Christie BS, Belbeck L, Graham FL. A recombinant human adenovirus vaccine against rabies. *J Infect Dis* 1990;161:27–30.

418. Hsu KH, Lubeck MD, Davis AR, et al. Immunogenicity of recombinant adenovirus-respiratory syncytial virus vaccines with adenovirus types 4, 5 and 7 vectors in dogs and a chimpanzee. *J Infect Dis* 1992;166:769–775.

419. Lubeck MD, Davis AR, Chengalvala M, et al. Immunogenicity and efficacy testing in chimpanzees of an oral hepatitis B vaccine based on live recombinant adenovirus. *Proc Natl Acad Sci U S A* 1989;86:6763–6767.

420. Miller CJ, Vogel P, Alexander NJ, Sutjipto S, Hendrickx AG, Marx PA. Localization of SIV in the genital tract of chronically infected female rhesus macaques. *Am J Pathol* 1992;141:655–660.

421. Imaoka, K, Miller C, Someya K, et al. Nasal immunization of non-human primates with simian immunodeficiency virus (SIV) p55 gag and cholera toxin (CT) adjuvants induces Th1/Th2 help for anti-viral immunity. (*Submitted for publication.*)

422. Kubota M, Miller C, Imaoka, K, et al. Oral immunization with simian immunodeficiency virus (SIV) p55 gag and cholera toxin elicits both mucosal IgA and systemic IgG1 immune responses in non-human primates. *J Immunol* 1997;158: 5321–5329.

423. Staats HF, Nichols WG, Palker TJ. Mucosal immunity to HIV-1: Systemic and vaginal antibody responses after intranasal immunization with the HIV-1 C4/V3 peptide T1SP10 MN(A). *J Immunol* 1996;157:462–472.

424. Porgador A, Staats HF, Faiola B, Gilboa T, Palker TJ. Intranasal immunization with CTL epitope peptides from HIV-1 or ovalbumin and the mucosal adjuvant cholera toxin induces peptide-specific CTLs and protection against tumor development *in vivo*. *J Immunol* 1997;158:834–841.

425. Tomasi TB Jr. Oral tolerance. *Transplantation* 1980;29:353–356.

426. Mowat AM, The regulation of immune responses to dietary protein antigens. *Immunol Today* 1987;8:93.

427. Weiner HL, Friedman A, Miller A, et al. Oral tolerance: immunologic mechanisms and treatment of animal and human organ-specific autoimmune diseases by oral administration of autoantigens. *Annu Rev Immunol* 1994;12:809–837.

428. McMenamin C, Holt PG. The natural immune response to inhaled soluble protein antigens involves major histocompatibility complex (MHC) class I-restricted CD8+ T cell-mediated but MHC class II-restricted CD4+ T cell-dependent immune deviation resulting in selective suppression of immunoglobulin E production. *J Exp Med* 1993;178:889–899.

429. Hoyne GF, O'Hehir RE, Wraith DC, Thomas WR, Lamb JR. Inhibition of T cell and antibody responses to house dust mite allergens by inhalation of the dominant T cell epitope in naive and sensitized mice. *J Exp Med* 1993;178: 1783–1788.

430. Dick, AD, Cheng YF, McKinnon A, Liversidge J, Forrester JV. Nasal administration of retinal antigens suppresses the inflammatory response in experimental allergic uveoretinitis. A preliminary report of intranasal induction of tolerance with retinal antigens. *Br J Ophthalmol* 1993;77:171–175.

431. Metzler B, Wraith DC. Inhibition of experimental autoimmune encephalomyelitis by inhalation but not oral administration of the encephalitogenic peptide: influence of MHC binding affinity. *Int Immunol* 1993;5:1159–1165.

432. Ma CG, Zhang GX, Xiao BG, Link J, Olsson T, Link H. Suppression of experimental autoimmune myasthenia gravis by nasal administration of acetylcholine receptor. *J Neuroimmunol* 1995;58:51–60.

433. Tian J, Atkinson MA, Clare-Salzler M, et al. Nasal administration of glutamate decarboxylase (GAD65) peptides induces Th2 responses and prevents murine insulin-dependent diabetes. *J Exp Med* 1996;183:1561–1567.

434. Wells H, Studies on the chemistry of anaphylaxis III. Experiments with isolated proteins, especially those of hen's egg. *J Infect Dis* 1911;9:147.

435. Mowat AM. Oral tolerance and regulation of immunity to dietary antigens. In: Ogra PL, Mestecky J, Lamm M, et al., eds. *Handbook of mucosal immunology*. San Diego: Academic Press, 1994:185:201.

436. Friedman A Weiner HL. Induction of anergy or active suppression following oral tolerance is determined by antigen dosage. *Proc Natl Acad Sci U S A* 1994;91: 6688–6692.

437. Whitacre CC, Gienapp, IE, Orosz CG, Bitar DM. Oral tolerance in experimental autoimmune encephalomyelitis. III. Evidence for clonal anergy. *J Immunol* 1991;147:2155–2163.

438. Chen Y, Inobe J, Marks R, Gonnella P, Kuchroo VK, Weiner HL. Peripheral deletion of antigen-reactive T cells in oral tolerance. *Nature* 1995;376:177–180.

439. Melamed D, Friedman A. Direct evidence for anergy in T lymphocytes tolerized by oral administration of ovalbumin. *Eur J Immunol* 1993;23:935–942.

440. Chen Y, Inobe J, Weiner HL. Induction of oral tolerance to myelin basic protein in CD8-depletion mice: both CD4+ and CD8+ cells mediate active suppression. *J Immunol* 1995;155:910–916.

441. Khoury SJ, Hancock WW, Weiner HL. Oral tolerance to myelin basic protein and natural recover from experimental autoimmune encephalomyelitis are associated with downregulation of inflammatory cytokines and differential upregulation of transforming growth factor β, interleukin 4, and prostagladin E expression in the brain. *J Exp Med* 1992;176:1355–1364.

442. Czerkinsky C, Holmgren J. The mucosal immune system and prospects for anti-infectious and anti-inflammatory vaccines. *Immunologists* 1995;3:97.

443. Challacombe SJ, Tomasi TB Jr. Systemic tolerance and secretory immunity after oral immunization. *J Exp Med* 1980;152:1459–1472.

444. Thomas HC, Parrott MV. The induction of tolerance to a soluble protein antigen by oral administration. *Immunology* 1974;27:631–639.

445. Kagnoff MF. Effects of antigen-feeding on intestinal and systemic immune responses. IV. Similarity between the suppressor factor in mice after erythrocyte-lysate injection and erythrocyte feeding. *Gastroenterology* 1980;79:54–61.

446. Kiyono H, Babb JL, Michalek SM, McGhee JR. Cellular basis for elevated IgA responses in C3H/HeJ mice. *J Immunol* 1980;125:732–737.

447. Kiyono H, McGhee JR, Wannemuehler MJ, Michalek SM. Lack of oral tolerance in C3H/HeJ mice. *J Exp Med* 1982;155:605–610.

448. Mattingly JA Waksman BH. Immunologic suppression after oral administration of antigen. I. Specific suppressor cells formed in rat Peyer's patches after oral administration of sheep erythrocytes and their systemic migration. *J Immunol* 1978;121:1878–1883.

449. Mowat AM, Lamont AG, Parrott DM. Suppressor T cells, antigen-presenting cells and the role of I-J restriction in oral tolerance to ovalbumin. *Immunology* 1988;64:141–145.

450. Richman LK, Graeff AS, Yarchoan R, Strober W. Simultaneous induction of antigen-specific IgA helper T cells and IgG suppressor T cells in the murine Peyer's patch after protein feeding. *J Immunol* 1981;126:2079–2083.

451. Ngan J, Kind LS, Suppressor T cells for IgE and IgG in Peyer's patches of mice made tolerant by the oral administration of ovalbumin. *J Immunol* 1978;120: 861–865.

452. Garside P, Steel M, Worthey EA, et al. T helper 2 cells are subject to high dose oral tolerance and are not essential for its induction. *J Immunol* 1995;154: 5649–5655.

453. Gregerson DS, Obritsch WF, Donoso LA. Oral tolerance in experimental autoimmune uveoretinitis. Distinct mechanisms of resistance are induced by low dose vs. high dose feeding protocols. *J Immunol* 1993;151:5751–5761.

454. Hirahara K, Hisatsune T, Nishijima K, Kato H, Shiho O, Kaminogawa S. CD4+ T cells anergized by high dose feeding establish oral tolerance to antibody responses when transferred in SCID and nude mice. *J Immunol* 1995;154: 6238–6245.

455. Melamed D Friedman A. *In vivo* tolerization of Th1 lymphocyte following a single feeding with ovalbumin: anergy in the absence of suppression. *Eur J Immunol* 1994;24:1974–1981.

456. Miller A, Lider O, Roberts AB, Sporn MB, Weiner HL. Suppressor T cells generated by oral tolerization to myelin basic protein suppress both *in vitro* and *in vivo* immune responses by the release of transforming growth factor β after antigen-specific triggering. *Proc Natl Acad Sci U S A* 1992;89:421–425.

457. Schwartz RH. A cell culture model for T lymphocyte clonal anergy. *Science* 1990;248:1349–1356.

458. DeSilva DR, Urdahl KB, Jenkins MK. Clonal anergy is induced *in vitro* by T cell receptor occupancy in the absence of proliferation. *J Immunol* 1991;147: 3261–3267.

459. Williams ME, Lichtman AH, Abbas AK. Anti-CD3 antibody induces unresponsiveness to IL-2 in Th1 clones but not in Th2 clones. *J Immunol* 1990;144: 1208–1214.

460. Burstein HJ, Abbas AK. *In vivo* role of interleukin 4 in T cell tolerance induced by aqueous protein antigen. *J Exp Med* 1993;177:457–463.

461. Kweon M-N, Fujihashi K, VanCott JL, et al. Lack of orally-induced systemic unresponsiveness in interferon-gamma knockout mice. *J Immunol* 1998;160: 1687–1693.

462. Mowat AM, Steel M, Worthey EA, Kewin PJ, Garside P. Inactivation of Th1 and Th2 cells by feeding ovalbumin. In: Weiner HL, Mayer LF, eds. *Oral tolerance: mechanisms and applications*. New York: New York Academy of Science, 1996: 122–132.

463. Marth T, Strober W, Kelsall BL. High dose oral tolerance in ovalbumin TCR-transgenic mice: systemic neutralization of IL-12 augments TGF-β secretion and T cell apoptosis. *J Immunol* 1996;157:2348–2357.

464. Lider O, Santos LM, Lee CS, Higgins PJ, Weiner HL. Suppression of experimental autoimmune encephalomyelitis by oral administration of myelin basic protein II. Suppression of disease and *in vitro* immune responses is mediated by antigen-specific CD8+ T lymphocytes. *J Immunol* 1989;142:748–752.

465. Miller A, Lider O, Weiner HL. Antigen-driven bystander suppression after oral administration of antigens. *J Exp Med* 1991;174:791–798.

466. Fukaura H, Kent SC, Pietrusewicz MJ, et al. Induction of circulating myelin basic protein and proteolipid protein-specific transforming growth factor-β1-secreting Th3 T cells by oral administration of myelin in multiple sclerosis patients. *J Clin Invest* 1996;98:70–77.

467. Aicher WK, Fujihashi K, Yamamoto M, Kiyono H, Pitts AM, McGhee JR. Effects of the lpr/lpr mutation on T and B cell populations in the lamina propria of the small intestine, a mucosal effector site. *Intern Immunol* 1992;4:959–968.

468. Takahashi I, Nakagawa I, Kiyono H, McGhee JR, Clements JD, Hamada S. Mucosal T cells induce systemic anergy for oral tolerance. *Biochem Biophys Res Commun* 1995;206:414–420.

469. Chase MW. Inhibition of experimental drug allergy by prior feeding of the sensitizing agent. *Proc Soc Exp Biol* 1946;61:257.

470. Bitar DM, Whitacre CC. Suppression of experimental autoimmune encephalomyelitis by the oral administration of myelin basic protein. *Cell Immunol* 1988;112:364–370.

471. Higgins PJ, Weiner HL. Suppression of experimental autoimmune encephalomyelitis by oral administration of myelin basic protein and its fragments. *J Immunol* 1988;140:440–445.

472. Thompson HS, Staines NA. Gastric administration of type II collagen delays the onset and severity of collagen-induced arthritis in rats. *Clin Exp Immunol* 1986;64:581–586.

473. Nagler-Anderson C, Bober LA, Robinson ME, Siskind GW, Thorbecke GJ. Suppression of type II collagen-induced arthritis by intragastric administration of soluble type II collagen. *Proc Natl Acad Sci U S A* 1986;83:7443–7446.

474. Blanas E, Carbone FR, Allison J, Miller JF, Heath WR. Induction of autoimmune diabetes by oral administration of autoantigen. *Science* 1996;274:1707–1709.

475. Bergerot I, Fabien N, Maguer V, et al. Oral administration of human insulin to NOD mice generates CD4+ T cells that suppress adoptive transfer of diabetes. *Autoimmunity* 1994;7:65.

476. Wortmann F. Oral hyposensitization of children with pollinosis or house-dust asthma. *Allergol Immunopathol* 1977;5:15–26.

477. Rebien W, Puttonen E, Maasch HJ, Stix E, Wahn U. Clinical and immunological response to oral and subcutaneous immunotherapy with grass pollen extracts. A prospective study. *Eur J Pediatry* 1982;138:341–344.

478. Morris GP, Beck PL, Herridge MS, Depew WT, Szewczuk MR, Wallace JL. Hapten-induced model of chronic inflammation and ulceration in the rat colon. *Gastroenterology* 1989;96:795–803.

479. Neurath MF, Fuss I, Kelsall BL, Stuber E, Strober W. Antibodies to interleukin 12 abrogate established experimental colitis in mice. *J Exp Med* 1995;182:1281–1290.

480. Elson CO, Beagley KW, Sharmanov AT, et al. Hapten-induced model of murine inflammatory bowel disease. Mucosa immune responses and protection by tolerance. *J Immunol* 1996;157:2174–2185.

481. Miller SD, Butler LD. T cell responses induced by the parenteral injection of antigen-modified syngeneic cells. I. Induction, characterization, and regulation of antigen-specific T helper cells involved in delayed-type hypersensitivity responses. *J Immunol* 1983;131:77–85.

482. Greene MI, Ginsburg CH, Benacerraf B. The regulation of hapten-specific granuloma formation. *Clin Immunol Immunopathol* 1982;23:275–285.

483. Mombaerts P, Mizoguchi E, Grusby MJ, Glimcher LH, Bhan AK, Tonegawa S. Spontaneous development of inflammatory bowel disease in T cell receptor mutant mice. *Cell* 1993;75:274–282.

484. Mizoguchi A, Mizoguchi E, Chiba C, et al. Cytokine imbalance and autoantibody production in T cell receptor-α mutant mice with inflammatory bowel disease. *J Exp Med* 1996;183:847–856.

485. Sadlack B, Merz H, Schorle A, Schimpl A, Feller A, Horak I. Ulcerative colitis-like disease in mice with disrupted interleukin-2 gene. *Cell* 1993;75:253–261.

486. Kuhn R, Lohler J, Rennick D, Rajewsky K, Muller W. Interleukin-10–deficient mice develop chronic enterocolitis. *Cell* 1993;75:263–274.

487. Powrie F, Leach MW, Mauze S, Menon S, Caddle LB, Coffman RL. Inhibition of Th1 responses prevents inflammatory bowel disease in SCID mice reconstituted with CD45RB^{hi} CD4$^+$ T cells. *Immunity* 1994;1:553–562.

488. Powrie F, Carlino J, Leach MW, Mauze S, Coffman RL. A critical role for transforming growth factor-b but not interleukin 4 in the suppression of T helper type 1-mediated colitis by CD45RB^{low} CD4$^+$ T cells. *J Exp Med* 1996;183:2669–2674.

489. Neurath MF, Fuss I, Kelsall BL, Presky DH, Waegell W, Stober W. Experimental granulomatous colitis in mice is abrogated by induction of TGF-β-mediated oral tolerance. *J Exp Med* 1996;183:2605–2616.

490. Hollander GA, Simpson SJ, Mizoguchi E, et al. Severe colitis in mice with aberrant thymic selection. *Immunity* 1995;3:27–38.

491. Simpson SJ, Hollander GA, Mizoguchi E, et al. Expression of pro-inflammatory cytokines by TCR αβ$^+$ and TCR γδ$^+$ T cells in an experimental model of colitis. *Eur J Immunol* 1997;27:17–25.

492. Duchmann, R, Schmitt E, Knolle P, Meyer Zum Buschenfelde KH, Neurath M. Tolerance towards resident intestinal flora in mice is abrogated in experimental colitis and restored by treatment with interleukin-10 or antibodies in interleukin-12. *Eur J Immunol* 1996;26:934–938.

493. Sundberg JP, Elson CO, Bedegian H, Birkenmeier EH. Spontaneous heritable colitis in a new substrain of C3H/HeJ mice. *Gastroenterology* 1994;107:1726–1735.

494. Koskinen S, Long-term follow-up of health in blood donors with primary selective IgA deficiency. *J Clin Immunol* 1996;16:165–170.

495. Burrows PD, Cooper MD. IgA deficiency. *Adv Immunol* 1997;65:245–276.

496. Hammarström L, Carlsson B, Smith CI, Wallin J, Wieslander L. Detection of IgA heavy chain constant region genes in IgA deficient donors: evidence against gene deletions. *Clin Exp Immunol* 1985;60:661–664.

Fundamental Immunology, Fourth Edition,
edited by William E. Paul
Lippincott–Raven Publishers, Philadelphia © 1999.

CHAPTER 28

Aging and Immune Function

Richard A. Miller

Evolutionary forces weaken as individual animals age (1). Selective pressures may sculpt the immune system of 10-year-olds to meet an unremitting onslaught of infectious threats, because immunocompetent adolescents are far more likely to reproduce than their immunodeficient siblings. But the selective pressure on the immune system of 100-year-old people is minimal: As the chances of surviving to a specific age drop (and drop they would, even if biologic aging were not a factor), so will the force of natural selection subside in parallel. Indeed, genetic variants that promote survival of youngsters do very well in a population, even if as a side effect they lead to unfortunate decrepitude at advanced ages (i.e., at ages beyond those at which most reproducing takes place). The genetic mechanisms still at play in the elderly are a collection of leftovers and compromises; the successes of the elderly immune system are attributable to inertia and lucky accident.

Gerontologists interested in the immune system are a fortunate bunch, because as the juggernaut of modern molecular and cellular immunology proceeds to lay bare the inner workings of this complex, multicellular, vital set of defenses, it leaves in its wake highly detailed models and tools for understanding the way in which immune cells and their products protect (and sometimes fail to protect) young mice and young people. The challenge to the immunogerontologist is then to capitalize on this rich inheritance of ideas and reagents to identify the modes of failure that convert teenagers nearly invulnerable to all but the most exotic of infectious and neoplastic agents into their grandparents, ridden with shingles, cancers, and potentially fatal bouts of influenza or tuberculosis that might have gone unnoticed, or occasioned, at worst, a few lost workdays, six decades earlier.

Complex, homeostatic systems are just the sort whose gradual failure typifies the pathobiology of aging, but many such systems present formidable obstacles to reductionist analysis. Dissociated brains, kidneys, and limbs do not think, excrete, or walk in tissue culture, but dissociated immune systems can perform a fairly credible imitation of an immune response *in vitro*, in part because so much of physiologic immunity requires interactions among mobile cellular elements. Much of the work done to delineate the effects of aging on immunity has exploited the leverage provided by *in vitro* technology, although the discipline of cross-checking key conclusions in intact animals has been slower to emerge, and unexplained inconsistencies among results obtained with slightly different culture systems frequently plague the field.

The interested reader may wish to consult other review articles for detailed discussions of T-cell subsets and cytokine production

R. A. Miller: Department of Pathology, University of Michigan, Ann Arbor, Michigan 48109-0946.

(2), B-lymphocyte aging (3), or suppressor T-cell function (4), and can turn to other general essays on immune senescence for surveys of the earlier literature and thoughtful discussions from alternate perspectives (5–8).

EXPERIMENTAL GERONTOLOGY FOR IMMUNOLOGISTS: A PRIMER

Before embarking on a description of what aging does to immune responses, it might be helpful to outline a few useful facts and main ideas in modern experimental aging research for those who rarely encounter a mouse older than 10 weeks.

The question, "How old is an old mouse?" does not, of course, have a simple answer, but median survival times for many of the common laboratory inbred strains, in a well-run specific pathogen–free (SPF) colony, typically range between 22 and 26 months, while F1 hybrid strains typically survive a few months longer. The life span of laboratory rats is roughly equal to, or slightly greater than, that of mice. Thus, a group of unselected mice or rats aged 30 months is almost certain to contain many animals that are near death, and even at 24 months of age, a random sample is likely to include many individuals with some form of degenerative or neoplastic disease.

Studies that deal only with young individuals—for example, one comparing 2-month-old to 6-month-old mice (i.e., a study in which the oldest subjects are still well below the age at which mortality risks become easily perceptible)—may yield important insights into developmental biology but provide little information about the effects of aging per se. Although it is tempting to assume that aging is just like development, but later, such an assumption would be rash and poorly justified. The principles that govern the assembly of a complex structure, such as the construction of a car, say, from glass, metal, latex, and blueprints, are altogether different from those that convert new vehicles to junkers. Evolutionary pressures exert fine-grained control over the assembly of young adults, but they affect the process of senescent decay only indirectly, in the same way that the pace of automobile senescence depends on the thickness of the rustproofing and the materials used for the brake pads. The aging process results from the failure of evolutionary pressures to affect fitness at advanced ages, and it is not surprising that new principles and new modes of failure become apparent only in older animals.

Too many studies of aging select subjects from only two age groups, typically very young adults and very old adults. Designs of this sort are tempting; the hope is that large age differences will lead to large effects on outcome and thus improved statistical power, but can lead to serious errors. First, such a survey may fail to note changes at intermediate ages that can be at least as informative as those at the very end of life. Figure 1 gives some hypothetical examples of this sort. Second, very old animals or human subjects are much more likely to be ill, and the range of illness may include syndromes not detectable even by a careful necropsy or careful physical examination. A change that occurs progressively across a wide range of late-life ages is more likely to represent a robust effect of aging than one that occurs only in the very oldest age ranges. Conversely, diffcrences between populations of very aged and young subjects may represent selection artifacts, that is, the survival into old age of an atypical subset of individuals that were unusually resistant to disease, perhaps because of unusually

strong immune responses. The use of very young individuals (e.g., 6-week-old mice or teen-aged humans) as controls is also a common mistake, and may make it difficult to distinguish aging effects from the effects of maturation.

Economic considerations also mitigate against the use of very old animals. Because the risk of mortality rises exponentially over time, the production cost of laboratory rodents also increases exponentially, rather than linearly, as a function of age. A *per diem* cost of $0.15 per mouse per day translates to about $50 for a 1-year-old mouse. To produce a 3-year-old mouse, however, would cost not $150, but well over $1,500, adjusting for the cost of the 90% to 95% of the mice that would die before reaching 3 years of age. A sensible decision to use only disease-free animals would increase the cost of the oldest mice still further.

Studies of the effects of aging on human immunity often make use of more-or-less stringent exclusionary criteria, and interpretation of the data from these reports is tightly tied to these details. Some groups, for example, use a set of criteria recommended by a European research consortium, the so-called Senieur screen (9), which excludes up to 90% of the individuals at the oldest ages. It is by no means clear whether the immune status of the healthiest 10% of the population should be accepted as usefully representative of the effects of aging on the population more generally. On the other hand, studies of elderly people that include subjects afflicted with chronic or acute neoplastic or inflammatory diseases, or individuals who are receiving drugs likely to alter immune status, are also of only limited value. An intermediate procedure, which excludes only those with obviously confounding conditions (such as acute infection, chemotherapy, steroid treatment) and treats other factors as recorded covariates, is likely to be more informative than either of the two extreme approaches, but requires more effort in both the data-gathering and the analysis stages.

Unfortunately, studies of aging rodents are less often able to incorporate explicit exclusion criteria, except perhaps for tumor incidence, skin lesions, or splenomegaly. Experimental rodents are not screened for disease as thoroughly as are human volunteers and are not able to communicate information about their symptoms. Because a detailed necropsy can add $50 or more, per animal, to the cost of a study, most laboratories content themselves with a casual inspection, if indeed they carry out any postmortem analysis at all. Protocols that require pooling of tissues from several mice or rats are particularly at risk of artifact, because pooling increases the likelihood that some of the cells studied have come from diseased subjects. The traditional use of inbred or F1 hybrid animals, in which all subjects are genetically identical and thus likely to exhibit similar pathologic changes and physiologic idiosyncrasies, poses problems of its own and makes it harder to extrapolate key findings. Studies using conventionally housed rodents (i.e., those not known to be free of specific infectious pathogens) are still all too frequent. Variations in endemic flora can lead to unsuspected discrepancies between studies in different laboratories, or even between studies carried out in the same laboratory at different times. The practice of obtaining animals from an SPF supplier and then housing them in a conventional colony for a few weeks before experimental study is particularly bad, because it greatly increases the chance that the animals are studied during a period of acute infectious illness. Such complications can be especially troublesome in studies of elderly rodents, which are particularly prone to infection.

A

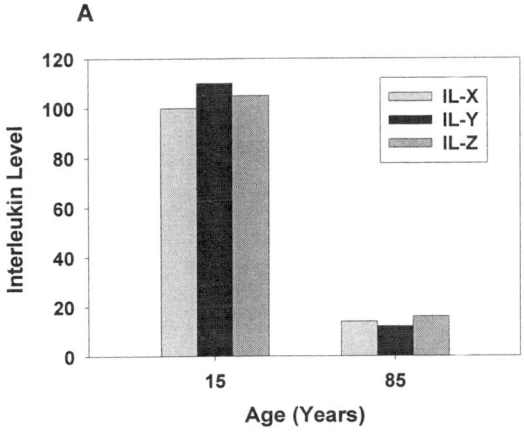

B

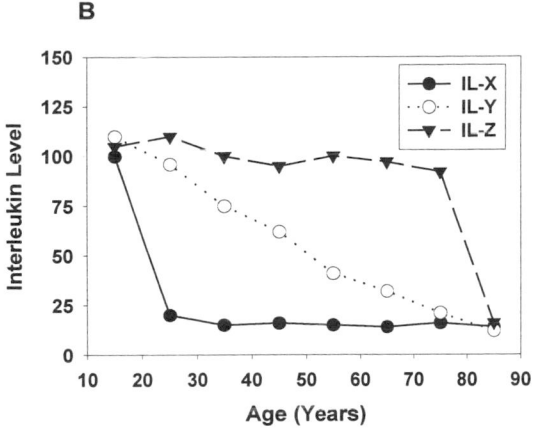

C

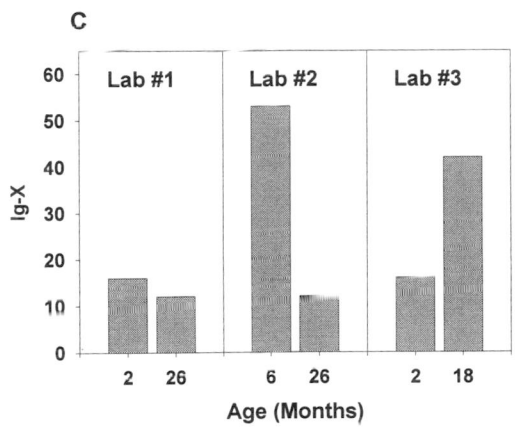

D

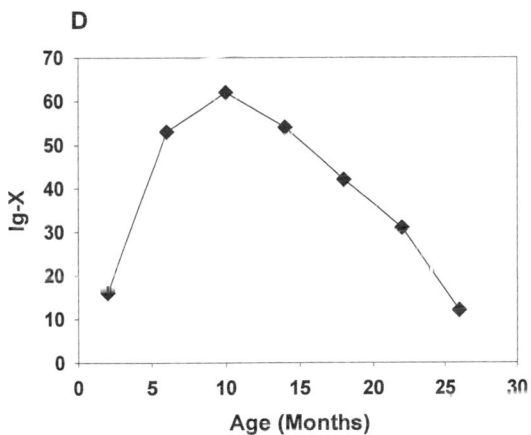

FIG. 1. Experimental design in immunogerontology: appropriate selection of age groups. **Panel A:** A hypothetical report on age-related changes in interleukins X, Y, and Z in two groups of women, aged, respectively, 15 and 85 years. All three cytokines appear to fall with age. **Panel B:** The same hypothetical data set in more detail, this time with adequate sampling of intermediate age groups. Interleukin-X falls rapidly between ages 15 and 25, but changes little thereafter; this decline may reflect maturation rather than an effect of aging per se. Interleukin-Z declines only in very old people; this decline could reflect an effect of disease or perhaps a selection effect (low IL-Z levels protecting against early death.) **Panel C:** Hypothetical results from three different laboratories concerning age effects on production of mouse Ig-X. Each laboratory reaches different conclusions. **Panel D:** The same Ig-X dataset, but with more appropriate sampling of age groups; also shown is that Ig-X increases in early adult life and declines thereafter, a pattern missed by each of the three laboratories shown in **Panel C**.

AGE-DEPENDENT CHANGES IN T-LYMPHOCYTE SUBSETS

In the 1960s and 1970s, a small number of laboratories began to examine the effects of aging on immune responses, using *in vivo* tests, such as delayed-type hypersensitivity, graft-versus-host reactions, and antibody production, and *in vitro* culture methods based on mitogen-induced proliferation and immunoglobulin secretion. With rare exceptions, these investigations demonstrated a decline with age in both cell-mediated and humoral responses to soluble, particulate, and alloantigens, both in humans and in rodents. Table 1 lists some of the most reproducible and dramatic of the age-associated changes in immune responsiveness, together with representative citations. Effects that are equally dramatic, but less reproducible or more controversial, are excluded from Table 1

and are discussed in detail later in this chapter. More comprehensive and detailed summaries of the phenomenology can be found in a number of review articles (5–8).

The task of analyzing the cellular and molecular basis for the decline in protective immune responses was greatly facilitated by two developments in basic immunology: the realization that surface antigenic markers could discriminate functionally distinct subsets of T and B cells, and the discovery that T cells produced an antigen-nonspecific factor, interleukin-2 (IL-2), that promoted clonal expansion of other lymphocytes in the context of antigen-driven reactions.

Early work on what later came to be called CD4 and CD8 antigens emphasized their ability to distinguish T cells with differing functional capabilities, and prompted a spate of reports on age-related changes in CD4 and CD8 cell numbers that continues

TABLE 1. *Age-related changes in immune function: selected examples*

Immune response	Effect of age	Ref.
Proliferative response to T-cell mitogen PHA *in vitro*	Twenty-fold decline, 6- to 30-mo mice	288
Proliferative response to T-cell mitogens Con A and PHA *in vitro*	Fourfold decline, 20- to 80-year-old humans	289
IgG plaque-forming cells after DNP-BGG immunization	Seven-fold decline, 2- to 25-mo mice	290
Production of antierythrocyte antibodies *in vivo*	Nine-fold decline, 2- to 19-mo mice	291
In vitro generation of cytolytic T cells after allogeneic immunization	>16-fold decline, 2- to 19-month mice	292
Spleen-cell NK activity	>fourfold decline, 3- to 22-mo mice	223
Skin graft rejection times (MHC-incompatible)	Threefold increase, 2- to 28-mo rats	293
Primary skin sensitization to dinitrochlorobenzene	Twenty-three percent nonresponders at 20 to 40 yr: 77% Nonresponders at >65 yr (humans)	294

unabated to the present generation. A list of 24 such reports is tabulated in ref. 10. Approximately half of the papers find no change in the relative or absolute numbers of CD4 and CD8 cells in human peripheral blood (PBL) or mouse or rat spleen, and those that do report age-dependent alterations are evenly divided between small increases in CD4/CD8 ratios and small decreases in the same ratio. Age does seem to lead fairly consistently to a decline in CD4 cells (as a proportion of total T cells) in mouse blood (11–13), but neither human PBL nor mouse spleen and lymph node tissues show a similar degree of consistency (10). The safest conclusion is that although specific inbred strains or specific populations may sometimes show progressive changes in CD4 or CD8 subset proportions in late life, the changes are inconsistent and too small to provide a plausible explanation for the large changes in T-cell responsiveness.

Aging does, however, lead to a consistent change in the distribution of other T-cell subsets, specifically a shift from naive- to memory-cell phenotypes within both the CD4 and CD8 pools. The proportion of mouse T cells expressing the memory-cell marker CD44 increases with age in the blood, spleen, and peripheral lymph nodes of both the CD4 and CD8 pools (12,14,15). The proportion of CD45RB^hi (i.e., naive) T cells in the CD4 pool declines in aging mice (15,16), consistent with the data on CD44 expression. Expression of another marker of CD4 naive cells, 3G11, also declines with age in mice (15,17), as does CD62L (Mel-14), a marker of naive cells in both the CD4 and CD8 lineages (18). Studies of T-cell subsets in aging humans have also documented an increase in the proportion of cells expressing the memory markers CD45R0 and CD29, and a decline in the naive population marked by CD45RA (19–23). Because some authorities argue that loss of CD45RA (or CD45RB in mice) and acquisition of CD45R0 should be considered a sign of T-cell activation rather than of memory cell status, it is worth noting that aging does not lead to an increase in the proportion of T cells expressing the IL-2 receptor chain CD25 or class II major histocompatibility complex (MHC) molecules (22,24).

Studies of aging mice have also documented an increase in the proportion of T cells that express P-glycoprotein (25), better known for its role in endowing neoplastic cells with multiple drug resistance. T cells expressing P-glycoprotein increase with age in the naive and memory pools of both CD4 and CD8 lineages of aging CB6F1 mice (25); genetically heterogeneous mice (13) and TCR-transgenic mice (26) also exhibit an age-dependent increase in P-glycoprotein expression, as monitored by the ability to extrude the fluorochrome R123. The proportion of T cells expressing P-glycoprotein also increases with age in humans (27), although much of the change seems to be accomplished in early adulthood.

The extent to which the decline in naive cells and parallel increase in memory cells, or the accumulation of cells expressing

P-glycoprotein, might have implications for T-cell function, and the extent to which these shifts might be explained by thymic or post-thymic changes, will both be considered later in this chapter.

T-CELL FUNCTION

Interleukin-2

The first report of an age-related decline in IL-2 production (28) appeared only 3 years after the initial development of a reproducible bioassay for this T-cell growth factor, and it has since been followed by many other reports of diminished IL-2 production by T cells from aged mice and humans (see refs. 10, 29 for lists of citations) in responses initiated by mitogenic lectins or antibodies to components of the T-cell receptor (TCR)/CD3 complex. There are a few apparent exceptions to the general rule. (a) Immobilized anti-CD3 antibody induces high-level IL-2 production in T cells from both young and old mice (30), perhaps by providing an unusually strong stimulus that overcomes barriers to activation of aged T cells. Interestingly, the strong response of T cells from old mice to immobilized anti-CD3 can be inhibited by antibodies to IL-4, suggesting that IL-4–dependent activation of IL-2 production may be particularly potent in cultures of old T cells (31). (b) Young and old rats show equivalent IL-2 production in some (32,33), but not all (34–36) studies. The age-dependent decline in IL-2 secretion is accompanied by a parallel decline in IL-2 mRNA production (37–39). Both limiting dilution and *in situ* hybridization methods show a decline with age in the proportion of T cells that can respond to plant lectins (40,41) or superantigens (16) by IL-2 production.

Production of IL-2 *in vitro* by T cells from older humans is notoriously variable (42), with some subjects producing levels of IL-2 that are well within the normal range for young controls, and there is poor agreement even between samples obtained from the same individual at different times (43). Poor production of IL-2 *in vitro* in responses to plant lectins are associated, in T cells from elderly people, with high levels of serum IL-2 and with poor responsiveness to influenza vaccination, while vaccination itself induces a transient (i.e., 2-week) decline in the ability to produce IL-2 in culture (44). These data suggest a model in which *in vitro* immune responses are dampened by inhibitory factors secondary to infections—perhaps subclinical—that may be more common among the elderly.

The observation that IL-2 production declined with age prompted a flurry of interest in the idea of IL-2 supplementation as a potential antidote to age-related immunodeficiency. Although large doses of exogenous IL-2 added to *in vitro* cultures can indeed improve the responses of T cells from old donors (45,46), reports of age-related declines in mitogen-induced activation of the IL-2 receptor (47–49) showed that T-cell deficits in old age were not attributable to a single biochemical lesion, and indeed most groups find that exogenous IL-2 is largely ineffective in restoring function of T cells from old donors *in vitro* (see ref. 10 for citations). Aging leads to changes in the proportion of stimulated cells that express the high-affinity IL-2–binding complex (50,51), and a decline in the proportion of mitogen-exposed T cells that can proliferate in IL-2 containing limiting dilution cultures (41). In addition, there is an age-dependent decline in responsiveness to IL-2, even among those cells that do express the IL-2 receptor (48,50,52); the molecular basis for this defect is not known.

Thus the poor *in vitro* proliferation of T cells exposed to polyclonal stimuli seems to reflect a constellation of defects: low IL-2 production, low expression of IL-2 receptors, and poor response to IL-2 by receptor-positive blasts. Can these changes be explained by intrinsic differences between naive T cells, which are common in young individuals, and memory T cells, which predominate in old age? Consistent with this idea, limiting-dilution experiments suggest that naive mouse T cells are much more likely than memory T cells to produce IL-2 in cultures stimulated by concanavalin A (Con A) or by the superantigen SEB (16,41), and more likely to proliferate in response to IL-2 after activation by mitogens or alloantigens (41,53). Indeed, the nonlinear titration curves seen in limiting-dilution experiments using T cells from old mice can be reproduced by mixing naive and memory cells from young mice at ratios similar to those naturally seen in older animals (54). On the other hand, analysis of naive-cell function using transgenic mice, most of whose T cells express a receptor specific for pigeon cytochrome C, has suggested that aging may also impair the ability of naive T cells to respond to cognate antigen (26). There are also instances (discussed below) in which T cells from old donors produce lower levels of cytokines typically secreted only by memory cells, and in which alterations in signal transduction pathways seem to affect both naive and memory cells equally. In transgenic mice in which most of the naive CD4 T cells express a TCR specific for a fragment of pigeon cytochrome C, aging leads to a decline in the ability of the transgene-positive naive cells to produce IL-2 (26). Although this change cannot be ascribed to an antigen-dependent transition from the naive to the memory subset, it is noteworthy that expression of P-glycoprotein by these transgene-positive cells does increase with age, and the idea that the P-glycoprotein–positive cells are themselves hypofunctional deserves to be tested. Aging also diminishes the mitogen responsiveness of purified human naive and memory T cells, as well as the proliferative responses of memory cells to a recall antigen, the A/Taiwan strain of influenza virus (55). The shift from naive to memory predominance thus seems to contribute to the decline in production of and response to IL-2, but cannot by itself provide a complete explanation for age-related declines in cellular immune responsiveness.

Interleukin-4, Interleukin-5, and Interleukin-10

Because IL-4 is principally a product of memory T cells, an increase with age in memory T-cell number might be expected to lead to an increase in IL-4 production. Aging also leads, however, to declines in T-cell activation pathways (see below), including those needed for the activation of memory cells. Thus, data on IL-4 production by old T cells could be expected to shed light on the relative importance of these two contrary trends. Unfortunately, the

published data are somewhat inconsistent. For mouse cells, most of the data suggest an age-related increase in IL-4 production (15,56–58) in short-term *in vitro* cultures. In contrast, though, aging seems to have no effect on IL-4 production by mouse T cells when anti-CD28 is included as a costimulus together with anti-CD3 (59), and leads to a decrease in IL-4 secretion in cultures where the anti-CD3 signal is accompanied by IL-2 (60). Production of IL-4 by human T cells also seems to decline with age (61,62), as does production of IgE, whose secretion is largely IL-4–dependent. Limiting-dilution assays of virus-responsive human T cells show no decline with age in the proportion of IL-4–producing cells (63), while flow cytometric analyses of IL-4–containing T cells after mitogen activation *in vitro* show a large decline with age in mice (64).

The data on production of IL-5 and IL-10 are more limited, but similarly inconsistent. IL-5 production by mouse T cells in short-term serum-free cultures is reported to increase with age (57), as does accumulation of IL-5 and IL-5 mRNA by mouse cells stimulated with immobilized anti-CD3 (30). Cultures in which anti-CD3 stimulation is accompanied by any of several costimuli [anti-CD28, phorbol myristate acetate (PMA), or IL-4], however, show a decline with age in IL-5 production (65). IL-10 production by T cells from old mice has been reported to increase (66,67) when anti-CD3 is used as stimulus, but to decrease when costimuli, including IL-2 and/or IL-4, are added (65). IL-10 production by purified memory T cells is reported to increase with age in anti-CD3–stimulated cultures (66), but antigen-induced IL-10 production by memory CD4 cells from KLH-primed mice declines with age (N Bining and RA Miller, submitted); the latter defect reflects the accumulation of a subset of CD4 memory cells expressing P-glycoprotein, which make much less IL-10 than the P-glycoprotein–negative cells that predominate in old mice.

It is thus unclear at this point whether the accumulation of memory T cells, balanced against age-related declines in memory-cell function, necessarily leads to increased production of IL-4, IL-5, and IL-10 in old age, because the effect of aging on production of these cytokines seems to depend on details of the species, stimulus, and culture conditions chosen.

Interferon-γ

Most reports of interferon-γ (IFN-γ) production by human T cells show a decline with age, including experiments using Con A (62,68), phytohemagglutinin (PHA) (69), and anti-CD3 (70). Results from protocols using antigen-specific stimulation are also consistent: Exposure of human T cells to influenza virus *in vitro* induces threefold more IFN-γ–producing cells from young than from old donors (71), and limiting-dilution cultures show a decline with age in the frequency of human T cells able to secrete IFN-γ when challenged with varicella zoster virus (63).

The data on polyclonal stimulation of IFN-γ production by mouse T cells are internally consistent but at odds with the data on human T-cell responses: Nearly all laboratories report an increase with age in IFN-γ and IFN-γ mRNA production after stimulation by Con A or anti-CD3 antibodies (59) (and see ref. 10 for six other citations). IFN-γ mRNA induction by IL-12 in the context of an alloantigen response is also unimpaired by aging (72). Interestingly, the P-glycoprotein–positive subset of CD4 memory cells in old mice, which are unable to generate IL-4, IL-5, or IL-10, do retain the ability to secrete IFN-γ in response to anti-CD3 and IL-

12, and indeed produce more IFN-γ than the corresponding subset from young mice (65); this specialization for IFN-γ production may contribute to the preservation of IFN-γ production in old age. IFN-γ production by CD8 memory T cells is also unimpaired by aging in mice, and the accumulation of memory CD8 cells thus contributes to age-related increases in mouse IFN-γ production (18).

Studies of mouse T cells using antigen-specific stimuli, however, are consistent with the human results and are thus inconsistent with most murine studies with polyclonal stimuli: IFN-γ production by T cells from influenza-primed mice declines with age (73), as does IFN-γ secretion in *Legionella*-stimulated mouse T-cell cultures (74). The basis for the discrepancy between mitogen-stimulated and antigen-stimulated cultures deserves further investigation, and provides a warning against overinterpretation of studies that utilize potent polyclonal stimuli alone.

In summary, then, the questions of whether the age-related increase in the memory T-cell pool leads to corresponding increases in production of the memory-cell products IFN-γ, IL-4, IL-5, and IL-10, and whether there is, with age, a shift in the balance between Th1- and Th2-related cytokines cannot be answered in a simple way. Some experiments, such as those involving polyclonal activation of mouse T cells in short-term cultures, typically show an increase, with age, in both IFN-γ and IL-4 production, but studies using costimuli or antigen-dependent activation reveal a more complex picture, and analyses of mouse responses do not in all cases predict the outcome of similar studies using human peripheral blood cells.

Responses to Interferon-γ and Interleukin-4

Macrophage activation by IFN-γ seems to decline with age. Peritoneal macrophages, for example, tested after activation by IFN-γ plus lipopolysaccharide (LPS), are less potent in antitumor cytotoxic tests when they are derived from aged mice (75). Macrophage production of hydrogen peroxide and nitric oxide after IFN-γ activation also declines with age in mice (76). The decline in antitumor cytotoxicity by LPS-stimulated human monocytes is accompanied by increased cyclic adenosine monophosphate (cAMP) and diminished translocation of protein kinase C (PKC) (77), but whether this is attributable specifically to altered IFN-γ responsiveness has not been determined.

Some, but not all, assays of responsiveness to IL-4 also show age-dependent defects. Three tests for mouse B-cell response to IL-4 expression of class II antigens, anti-IgM costimulated proliferation, and IgE expression in LPS-stimulated cultures all decline with age (78), but T-cell proliferation to PMA plus IL-4 is unaffected. IL-4–mediated suppression of human *in vitro* antibody responses to tetanus toxoid is also diminished by age (61). In contrast, IgE production in IL-4–stimulated cultures of peripheral blood lymphocytes is unimpaired by aging in humans (62).

T-Cell Cytotoxic Function

The decline with age in the production of cytotoxic T cells *in vitro* is at least partially due to the parallel decline in the ability of helper T cells to produce IL-2 (79–81), but defects in the ability of resting CD8 cells to generate clones of cytotoxic effectors when exposed to activating agents plus IL-2 also contribute to this deficit (41,53,79,82). The question of whether cytotoxic effectors, once generated, show an age-dependent decline in lytic function is controversial, with data on both sides of the issue (83,84). Rejection of skin grafts bearing class II alloantigens, which depends principally on CD4 cells, is more severely impaired by aging than the rejection of class I alloantigen-bearing skin (85). The poor protective responses of aged mice to influenza virus are correlated with lower cytotoxic T-cell generation, and heterotypic (i.e., cross-reactive) immunity is particularly weak, but the available data do not rule out an important effect of virus-specific helper function in this system (86,87). A discussion of the role of T cells in promotion of antibody production is postponed until after the section on aging and B-cell function.

T-LYMPHOCYTE ACTIVATION

The process by which antigen (or, in many experimental systems, polyclonal activators) converts resting T cells to proliferating blasts involves a cascade of changes in calcium ion flux, protein kinase–mediated phosphorylations, and new gene transcription. Although the details of this process are under intensive investigation in many laboratories, much less is so far known about the effects of aging on the activation process. Progress on this front is impeded in part by the heterogeneity of natural T-cell populations, in that differences between T cells from young and older donors might reflect either an effect of age on intracellular processes or merely a difference between the naive cells that predominate in young donors and the memory cells that predominate in older subjects, or a combination of both effects. The high cost of producing sufficient quantities of purified T cells for typical assays of enzyme activity poses another serious obstacle: While the cost of materials to produce, say, 10^9 Jurkat cells is approximately $50, production of 10^9 CD8 memory T cells from 2-year-old mice would cost about $1,500 to $6,000 for mouse purchase alone, and would yield much lower amounts of cellular protein. Despite these difficulties, information has gradually begun to accumulate on three aspects of early T-cell activation: calcium signal generation, protein kinase function, and induction of DNA-binding proteins that regulate gene expression. These data taken together indicate that abnormalities of T-cell activation can be demonstrated within the first few minutes after encounter with mitogenic stimuli.

Calcium Signals

Mitogenic lectins and antibodies to the CD3/TCR complex induce a rapid change in free calcium ion concentration ($[Ca]_I$) from a resting level near 100 nM to activated levels between 300 nM and 1 μM within 20 to 60 seconds; $[Ca]_I$ then subsides to a plateau level that remains elevated above baseline for hours. Although this process is highly dependent on IP3 activity in lymphoma cells traditionally used for exploration of calcium signal development, release of IP3-triggered internal Ca^{2+} stores is quantitatively much less important for normal lymphocytes (88), which depend heavily on a calcium gradient across the plasma membrane, particularly after the first 30 to 60 seconds of the response. The mechanisms that control $[Ca]_I$ immediately after T-cell activation are not well understood, but presumably reflect a balance among calcium influx (through poorly characterized plasma membrane channels), calcium efflux mediated by the adenosine triphosphate (ATP)-dependent extrusion pump, and transport to and from intracellular stores.

Aging leads to a decline in the ability of T cells from humans (62,89–91), mice (92–94), and monkeys (95) to increase [Ca]ᵢ after stimulation by a polyclonal activator. Both CD4 and CD8 cells are affected in spleen and blood of a variety of mouse strains (12,92,96). The decline in the average level of [Ca]ᵢ produced by T cells from old mice reflects a decline in the proportion of cells able to generate a signal, and this in turn reflects the replacement of naive by memory cells, since memory T cells are more resistant to calcium signal production, whether this is induced by Con A, anti-CD3, or ionomycin (96–98). The accumulation of cells that do not generate a calcium signal after exposure to a polyclonal activator largely accounts for the decline, with age, in the proportion of T cells that can make IL-2 or proliferate in response to Con A plus IL-2, in that isolation of the calcium-nonresponsive cells, from mice of any age, enriches cells that fail to respond in these functional assays (99,100). Whether the cells that resist calcium signal development might be specialized for other functions, such as IL-4 or IFN-γ production, is still an open question.

The molecular basis for the resistance of T cells from older donors, and memory T cells from mice of any age, to the development of calcium signals is still uncertain. The rate of influx of calcium ions across the plasma membrane is stimulated to a small extent by Con A, and this stimulation declines with the age of the T-cell donor (101), but the stimulation for influx is very transient (102) and cannot fully explain the much longer lasting mitogen-induced change in calcium ion concentration, which represents a balance reflecting rates of influx, efflux, and sequestration. Age-related declines in IP3 production have been reported by some groups (93,103), while others find no effect on production by T cells of IP3 or IP4 (91,101). Although the contribution of IP3-releasable intracellular calcium stores is very small in normal lymphocytes, the possibility of an age-dependent change in response to IP3 or in restocking of an IP3-releasable pool from extracellular sources cannot be ruled out. Exposure of T cells to very small doses of ionomycin induces a change in [Ca]ᵢ to a plateau level, above the resting level, that is likely to represent a changed balance between (ionomycin-facilitated) calcium influx and the ability of the ATP-dependent plasma membrane calcium pump to remove calcium ions from the cytoplasm. T cells from old mice are more resistant than cells from young mice to ionomycin-mediated increases in [Ca]ᵢ, and this resistance cannot be attributed to diminished penetration of the ionomycin–calcium complex into the cells, suggesting that aging may lead to an increase in the activity or calcium-sensitivity of the membrane calcium pump (104–106). In mice, ionomycin-resistant T cells are predominantly in the memory T-cell subset, are found in both the CD4 and CD8 subpopulations, and are hyporesponsive in limiting dilution tests for IL-2 production and IL-2 responsiveness (96,99,100). Studies of the functional properties of human T cells separated on the basis of differential calcium signal development have not been reported, but indirect evidence suggests that poor proliferation of CD8 T cells from aged humans is not linked to abnormalities of calcium signal generation (89).

Protein Kinase Function

Early studies used antiphosphotyrosine immunoblotting methods or electrophoretic separation of ³²P-labeled phosphoproteins to document age-related defects in protein phosphorylation within 1 to 10 minutes after exposure to Con A or anti-CD3 antibodies

(107,108). Although these studies provided no information about the role of specific kinases or defined protein substrates in the alterations, they did demonstrate (a) that aging altered the pattern of protein phosphorylation, decreasing phosphorylation of most substrates while increasing phosphorylation of a small number of others; (b) that both CD4 and CD8 cells were affected; (c) that small changes could be seen in mice as young as 11 months of age, which increased progressively through the rest of the life span; and (d) that many of the defects were seen even when PMA (an activator of PKC) and/or ionomycin were used to bypass ligand-dependent steps in the activation cascade. Some of the changes in tyrosine-specific phosphorylation could be attributed to differences between naive and memory T cells—the latter more frequent in old age and less responsive at any age—while the changes detected using ³²P, presumably involving phosphorylation on serine and threonine residues, affected both naive and memory CD4 cells equally.

More recent work has focused on kinases and substrates whose role in T-cell activation is better defined, although data relevant to age effects are still fragmentary. Activation of the MEK/ERK sequence in the MAP kinase pathway has been shown to decline with age in CD3-stimulated human (109) and mouse (110) T cells. Translocation of PKC from cytosol to plasma membrane declines with age in Con A–stimulated mouse T cells (93,103), and PMA-mediated phosphorylation of most, but not all substrates, also declines with age in mice (107). In this context, it is of interest to note major changes, with age, in PKC isoenzyme distribution in both resting and activated human T cells (111). PKCα and PKCε are both almost entirely cytoplasmic in resting T cells from young individuals, but they are often found membrane-associated in T cells from older people. Anti-CD3 stimulation induces translocation, to the membrane, of several PKC isoenzymes (α, β, δ, and ε) in T cells from young donors, but induces only PKCβ translocation in T cells from old donors (Fig. 2). It is possible that differences among these isoforms in substrate preference or sensitivity to various intracellular activators might contribute to changes with age in responses to PKC-dependent signals. A separate group, however, found no age-dependent change in PKCα or PKCβ activation or translocation in human T cells (112); this discrepancy will require clarification by additional experimentation.

A study of tyrosine-specific phosphorylation of the ζ chain of the mouse CD3 complex has revealed age-dependent changes in both resting and activated cells. Normal resting T cells, in contrast to lymphoma cells frequently used for exploration of activation pathways, have a substantial fraction of their ζ chains in a tyrosine-phosphorylated state. The level of ζ-chain phosphorylation in resting T cells declines about threefold in aged mice (113). At least four isoforms of ζζ dimers can be discriminated by electrophoresis in nonreducing gels, and three of these isoforms are phosphorylated in mouse CD4 cells in response to anti-CD3 cross-linked to anti-CD4; the level of inducible phosphorylation of these three isoforms also declines about threefold in old mice. Information on the implications of altered TCR/CD3 signaling on downstream events is still sparse. Tyrosine phosphorylation of phospholipase-Cγ1 after stimulation of mouse T cells with anti-CD3 declines with age, as does phosphorylation of a 35- to 36-kDa protein that associates with this enzyme, and two phosphoproteins that associate with the SH2 domains of a ras-GTPase–activating protein (114). Phosphorylation of Shc, which is thought to couple TCR signals to the ras activating protein mSOS, also declines with age in CD3-stimulated mouse T cells (115). Interestingly, anti-CD4 stimulation leads to a threefold age-associated

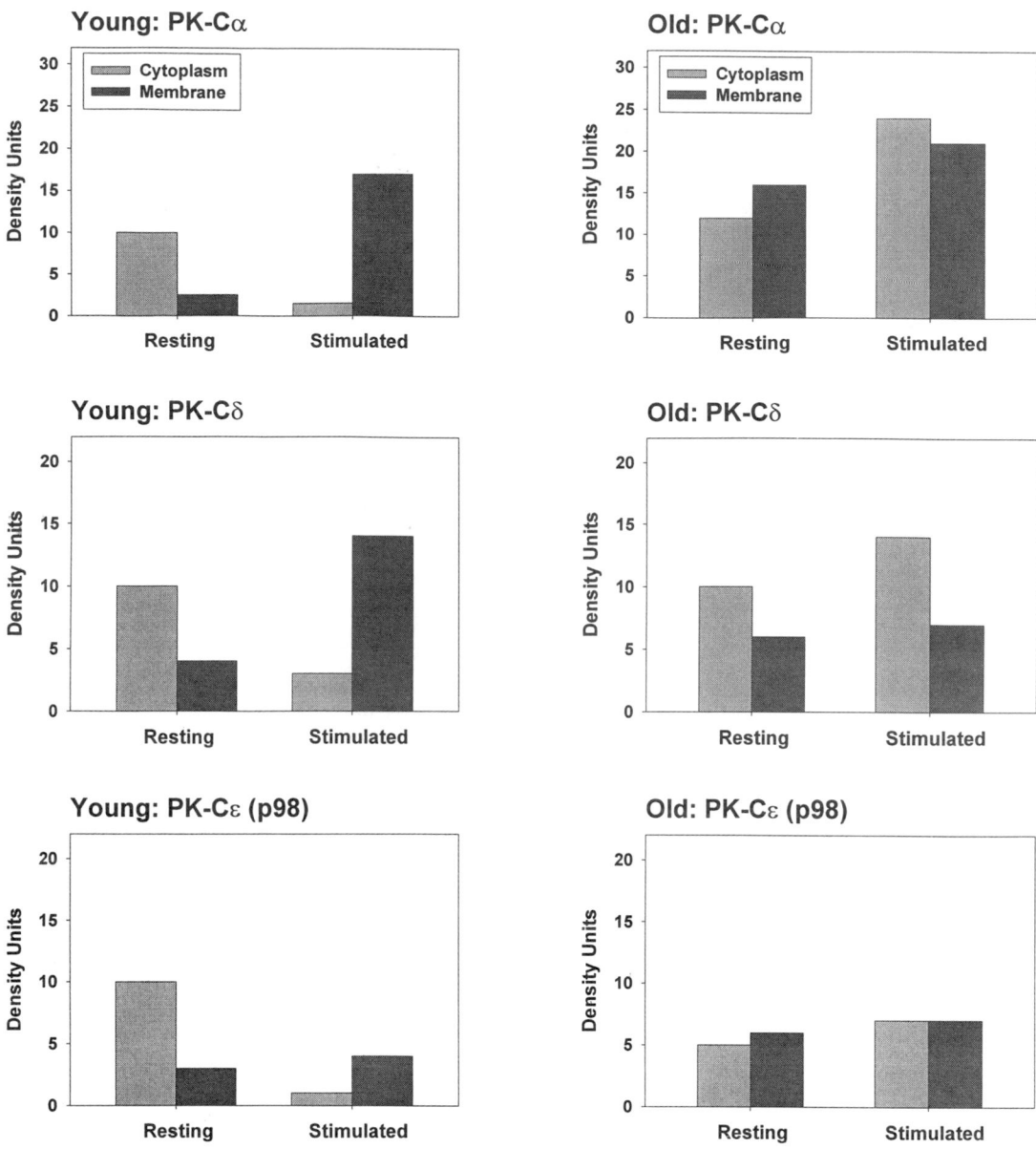

FIG. 2. Effects of age on PKC distribution in resting or stimulated peripheral blood T cells from young or old humans. Panels (**top to bottom**) show three distinct isoenzymes: PKCα, PKCβ, and the p98 form of PKCε; values represent means quantitated by densitometry of Western blots, with the value of 10 arbitrary units assigned to the PKC found in the cytoplasmic fraction of resting young cells for each isoenzyme. Activation was achieved by exposure to mouse anti-CD3 for 10 minutes, followed by sheep anti-mouse IgG for 5 minutes. (From ref. 111)

increase in Shc phosphorylation, consistent with the idea that complexes between CD4 and the src-family tyrosine protein kinase p56[lck] may be distributed differently in T cells from old and young mice. Studies of age-related alterations in other components of the T-cell activation process are badly needed, and may reveal qualitative as well as quantitative alterations in coupling mechanisms.

Gene Activation by DNA-binding Factors

Work in this area is also still fragmentary, and a satisfactory synopsis of the differences in mitogen-dependent gene activation between T cells from young and old individuals cannot yet be provided. There are reports of age-related declines in expression of several genes whose products are expressed early after activation, including c-myc, c-myb, c-fos, c-jun, and the formation of the AP-1 DNA-binding protein that includes the fos/jun complex (116–120). The picture that emerges from these reports is not fully consistent: Not all older individuals are clearly different from young controls, and the effect of age is seen for some mitogens but not for others. In some cases (such as in the studies of c-myc expression), it is not clear whether the alterations represent alterations in gene transcription or in translation (116,117). Systematic descriptive work is still needed to decide whether these changes in early gene expression are consistent and important influences on the commitment to later steps in the mitogenic process, to determine to what extent the age effects reflect changes in the proportions of different T-cell subsets in old and young individuals, and to link the changes in gene transcription to the parallel alterations in protein kinase and calcium-mediated upstream signals.

T-CELL DEVELOPMENT

The dramatic decline in thymic size and emigration rate in childhood, referred to as thymic involution, has long been considered the most reasonable cause of the age-associated decline in T-cell function, while the possible role of postthymic changes as a cause of functional immunosenescence has been badly neglected. The loss in thymic mass and cellularity, and the replacement of parenchymal tissue by fat and connective tissue (121), are accompanied by a loss in the developmentally active CD4(+), CD8(+) (double-positive) subset (122,123) and at least a 90% decline, by 6 months of age in mice, in the daily output of thymic emigrants (124). Tests of the ability of transplanted thymic tissue to support the maturation of bone marrow–derived prothymocytes into mature T cells have also shown a dramatic decline in function within the first 3 months of life in mice (125), although the extent and pace of this change have been called into question by further results from the same laboratory (126). The combination of irradiation, bone marrow transplantation, and implantation of a syngeneic infant thymus gland can restore excellent T-cell function to an old mouse, and indeed repeated applications of this procedure can maintain immunocompetence throughout the life span of mice (127).

Can these age-related changes in thymic function be explained by alterations in the function of prothymocytes that initiate T-cell development upon arrival in the thymus gland? In reconstitution protocols, the age of the bone marrow donor seems to have little effect on functional restoration of the adoptive host, at least when the recipients are tested within a few months of construction (128,129), although there is some evidence that T-cell regeneration from bone marrow cells of old mice is not as long lasting as regeneration from younger marrow donors (130,131). The number of prothymocytes in the marrow does not change with age (132), but prothymocytes from old donors are at a slight disadvantage when compared with cells from younger mice in a competitive repopulation assay using thymic rudiment organ cultures (133). The ability of growth hormone to increase thymic size in old mice has suggested the possibility that this or other changes in hormonal milieu may contribute to thymic involution, but it should be noted that this increase in thymic mass is not accompanied by more than marginal improvements in peripheral T-cell function in treated animals (134,135), and that dw/dw mutant mice have two- to threefold higher responses to T-cell mitogens, at 15 months of age, than their littermate controls (136), despite a virtual absence of circulating growth hormone in the dw/dw animals.

Two studies have shown a shift, with age, in the proportions of subsets within the pool of thymocytes, marked by absence of CD4 and CD8, that give rise to all subsequent classes in the differentiation sequence. The earliest subset within this double-negative pool, which expresses CD44 but not CD25, is reported to remain unaltered by aging, while its immediate progeny (CD44$^+$/CD25$^+$, CD44$^-$/CD25$^+$, and CD44$^-$/CD25$^-$ cells) do decline with age (137,138). These data suggest that thymic maturation in old age may be blocked at a very early stage, just prior to the rearrangement of the Vβ gene from its germline constituents. Whether this block is intrinsic to the T-cell lineage or represents an age-associated failure to provide a needed environmental signal requires further investigation.

Two animal models in which thymic involution is absent or delayed—a strain of Buffalo rat that exhibits thymic hyperplasia (139) and a transgenic mouse line in which Fas expression in T cells is driven by the CD2 promoter (67)—show a retardation of the age-associated decline of T-cell function. The molecular basis for hyperplasia in the rat model is unclear, as is the pathway by which overexpression of the apoptosis-inducing Fas protein delays thymic involution in the transgenic mouse strain. Transgenic mice that express fully rearranged Vα and Vβ chains driven by the CD2 promoter also fail to show thymic involution in old age (137), although the effects of aging on peripheral T-cell function have not yet been tested in this model. Investigation of these and other strains in which thymic degeneration is altered may shed additional light on this process and its implications for T-cell functional decline.

Although it is tempting to attribute T-cell dysfunction in old age simply to thymic involution, to do so would be a serious oversimplification, and much more work is needed on the role of peripheral renewal of T-cell populations in aging. The number of cells exported daily by the thymus of a young adult mouse is only a few percent of the number that would be needed to account for cell turnover (140,141), and peripheral T cells can expand by a factor of 10^4 or more, in a thymic-independent fashion, when called on to repopulate a depleted immune system (142,143). T-cell immunity in adult thymectomized mice is also easily distinguished from that seen in old mice (144–146). The balance between naive and memory cells is maintained not by a simple process of thymic replenishment, but rather by a subtle balance between cell expansion and cell death in antigen-driven (147) and perhaps also antigen-independent processes.

The effects of aging on these postthymic processes are, at present, almost entirely mysterious, but there is growing evidence for age-related shifts in T-cell repertoire. Aged mice (148) and aged humans (149) show imbalances in the relative proportions of CD8 cells expressing specific TCR Vβ chains; these are idiosyncratic in the sense that the Vβ distribution patterns are typically different for each individual mouse or person. In the mouse, these abnormalities seem to be less common in SPF animals, and the generality of the finding in humans has been called into question (150), in part because the original report (149) used cord blood as controls, rather than samples from young adult subjects. In the human subjects (149), these accumulations appear to represent the products of clonal expansion, and the expanded clones are found predominantly in the CD28-negative subset of CD8 cells. This CD28-negative subset increases with age in humans and has short average telomere lengths, consistent with an extended proliferative history (151). The fact that each aged mouse has its own pattern of TCR Vβ abnormalities implies that there is no change in the average distribution of Vβ chains with age, and thus explains the negative findings of a study of Vβ mRNA in which RNA samples were pooled across mice before analysis (122). Spectratyping methods that display the distribution of sizes in the TCR-Vβ complementarity-determining region 3 (CDR3) from individual mice reveal individually specific distortions of the CDR3 distribution in both the CD4 and CD8 cells of every mouse tested above 15 months of age (RL Mosley, MM Koker, and RA Miller, unpublished data, Fig. 3). These abnormalities are likely to represent the expansion of rare T-cell clones that

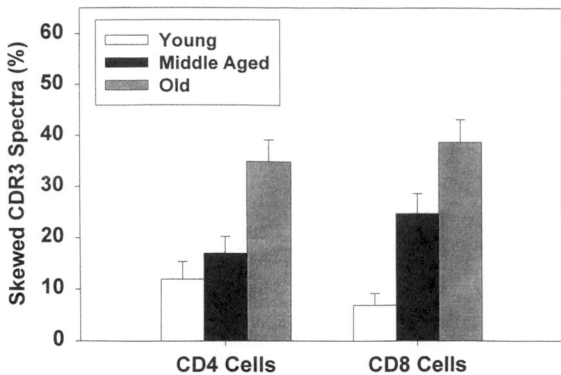

FIG. 3. Proportions of skewed TCR-Vβ CDR3 (complementarity determining region 3) size distributions in young (8-month), middle-aged (16-month), and old (24-month) SPF CB6F1 mice. *Bars* show proportions and standard errors for N = 93 to 132 spectratypes derived from six mice of each age group. The age trend is significant by linear regression for both CD4 and CD8 cell types. (From RL Mosley, MM Koker, and RA Miller, unpublished data.)

have lost the ability to cease proliferation or undergo clonal deletion at the end of a period of antigen-stimulated growth. Similar methods have also revealed an increase in clonally expanded T cells in both the CD4 and CD8 lineages in human subjects (152). The functional implications, if any, of these changes in T-cell repertoire are unclear. Although one group has reported a decline, with age, in Fas expression and susceptibility to apoptosis (67), three other studies have shown an age-related increase in apoptosis and/or Fas expression after activation in mouse (153) and human (154,155) T cells, and both the molecular basis for these changes and their implications for protective immunity are still open questions.

AGE-RELATED CHANGES IN B LYMPHOCYTES

Intrinsic Alterations in B-Cell Function

The difficulty in devising tests for age-related changes in B-cell function, typically measured as proliferation or antibody secretion, lies in assuring that the changes seen do not merely reflect alterations in the activity of accompanying T cells. Studies in which strong B-cell mitogens are used or in which T-cell help is provided in excess show an age-related decline in the magnitude of B-cell response about half the time, and they find no difference between young and old donors in the other half of the cases (see ref. 10 for list of citations). The frequency of B cells that can respond to synthetic haptens in T cell–containing splenic fragment cultures typically declines about twofold with age (156), with responses to phosphorylcholine (PC) a notable exception that will be discussed in more detail below (157). Studies of B cell–responder frequencies in limiting-dilution cultures are in conflict, with one report showing a 20-fold decline in the frequency of LPS-reactive B cells in mice (158), another finding no change in this index of B-cell function (159), and third, using a filter-paper colony assay, reporting a two- to threefold decline with age (160). Work on signal transduction defects in B cells is in its infancy, with some data indicating changes in PKC (161), and perhaps also MAP kinase activation (162) in some but not all elderly humans.

Evidence of possible changes, with age, in functionally distinct subsets of mature B cells is still sketchy. Using surface IgM and IgD levels as indices of B-cell diversity, one group has noted that individual aged mice frequently have levels of different B-cell subsets that are either higher or lower than those seen in young controls, but found no change, with age, in the average subset distribution (163). Increases in the proportion of B cells expressing the CD5 marker have been reported in female mice of some strains (164), but these changes are not seen in male mice (165,166) and are thus unlikely to be responsible for most changes in B-cell function, which are not limited to female animals. The numbers and functional properties of B cells expressing high levels of a heat-stable antigen, said to mark precursors of memory B cells, are also not altered by aging (167).

Antibody Levels, Repertoire, and Autoreactivity

There is a surprising lack of agreement among various reports on possible age-related changes in the concentrations of immunoglobulin isotypes in serum. Two groups, studying several strains of inbred mice, have reported very large (i.e., up to fivefold) increases with age in the serum concentrations of IgM, IgA, and all four IgG subclasses (168,169). A third group (170), however, found no age-associated changes, except in IgG2b (twofold) and IgG1 (threefold), and a fourth found no evidence for changes, except for a small increase in IgG2a (171). The results in humans are also in conflict, with some studies reporting no change in immunoglobulin isotypes (172,173) and others finding fourfold increases in IgA levels and smaller increases in other isotypes (174).

Three studies of the effects of age on utilization of immunoglobulin V_H and V_L gene families have similarly left a lack of consensus. One group found no change, in aged BALB/c mice, in use of the J558, S107, and 7183 V_H genes among mitogen-stimulated B-cell colonies (175). A second laboratory found no effects of age on use of eight V_H and eight V_L families in BALB/c or C57BL/6 mice, except for an increase in V_H-S107 use by old BALB/c mice (160). A third report, however, noted increased use of J558 genes in older C57BL/6 mice and overexpression of different V_H gene families—not including S107—in each of three aged BALB/c mice (176). It is difficult to judge whether these results, which included a clonal expansion step to produce a sufficient number of cells for study, are representative of the larger number of B cells that do not proliferate vigorously to generate large colonies *in vitro*. Information about differential usage of D and J segments in the aged is limited to an analysis of hybridoma cells produced from a single 15-month-old BALB/c mouse (177). Compared with a panel of sequences derived from a single young mouse, the sequences from the old donor showed differences in the frequency of utilization of specific D and J fragments, and an increase in the average amount of D-derived sequence used in the mature mRNA. Duplicate sequences were much more common in the old mouse than in the young control; this overrepresentation of certain sequences is reminiscent of the TCR data presented earlier. More work will be needed—using more mice, of different strains, and in humans—to test the robustness of these conclusions and their functional implications.

Studies of the idiotypically restricted response of BALB/c mice to the PC hapten, which plays a critical role in the protective response to pneumococcal infection, have led to a number of provocative observations. Although the response of young mice to

PC is almost entirely derived from B cells expressing V_H-S107 and a defined combination of D and J segments, aged BALB/c mice show a dramatic shift toward the use of other V genes for their anti-PC response (178,179). The preferential use of V_K22 by young mice is also lost with age in several strains of mice (180). Although the molecular basis for these changes in gene selection is unknown, the reliance on noncanonical V_H sequences by the older mice does lead to production of low-affinity antibody pools that are less protective against pneumococcal infection in passive immunization protocols (181). The possible role of T cells in modulation of the B-cell repertoire is discussed below.

Aging leads to increases in the serum concentrations of antibodies reactive with self antigens in humans (182) and in mice (183) (and see refs. 10, 29 for additional citations). Because these antibodies are of low affinity and are found in as many as 80% of elderly persons and animals, they seem unlikely to have great pathologic significance. The classical autoimmune syndromes seen in young and middle-aged adults can, however, be retarded by the caloric restriction protocols that also retard most age-dependent changes in immune function (184), and it is possible that alterations in the relative amounts of different cytokines, or idiosyncratic expansions of T- or B-cell clones in the elderly, could contribute both to autoimmune diseases and to nonpathologic autoantibody formation. Animal models of cell-mediated autoimmunity have found evidence for increased (185), decreased (186), or unaltered (187) susceptibility in old animals, and it is clear that details of strain (or genotype), antigen, and route of immunization must interact in complex ways with the effects of aging on autoimmune responses.

B-Cell Development: Intrinsic and T Cell–dependent Changes

Analysis of pre-B and pro-B cells, detectable in bone marrow by flow cytometry, have documented an age-dependent decline in the

number of B-cell precursors in mice (188,189); in addition, the ability of these cells to generate mature B cells in a number of *in vitro* culture models declines with age (189). B-cell repopulation by bone marrow cells transferred into depleted host mice is also impaired by aging (190). These data support the idea that aging may lead to defects in the B-cell production pathway, but they do not provide insights into the importance, if any, of such a defect.

There is some evidence that T cells from old mice can influence the B-cell developmental process and mold a B-cell pool that has the properties typically seen in aged animals. Adoptive transfer protocols, in which B cells mature from marrow progenitors in the presence of T cells from old donors, reproduce the decline in the frequency of reactive B cells (191), the production of autoantibodies specific for B-cell immunoglobulin idiotypes (192), and other age-specific aspects of the expressed B-cell antibody repertoire (193).

Interactions between T and B Cells in Humoral Immunity

The age-related decline in humoral immune responses to thymic-dependent antigens reflects changes in both T- and B-cell function (194,195). A part of this decline could be attributable to changes in production of cytokines by T-cells and/or B-cell response to these cytokines. As discussed above, some studies suggest that aging may lead to increases in production of IL-4 and IL-5 *in vitro*. If, in fact, production of these cytokines in the course of an *in vivo* humoral response does increase with age, then the decline in antibody production might be more plausibly tied to changes in IL-2 production and/or defects in contact-dependent events. The ability of mouse CD4 T cells to promote production, by young B cells, of IgM, IgA, and four IgG subclasses is diminished at least two- to fourfold by aging in cultures containing optimal doses of IL-2, IL-4, and IL-5 (196); these results are consistent

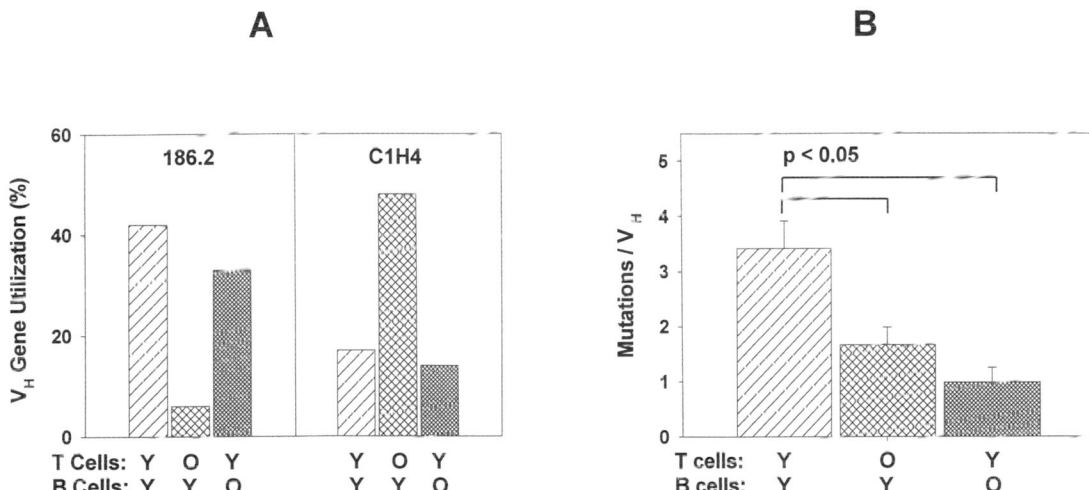

A   **B**

FIG. 4. Collaboration between T and B cells in the anti-NP response. SCID/SCID mice were reconstituted with CD4+ T cells and B cells from mice of the indicated ages [Y, young (2 to 3 months); O, old (21 to 25 months)], and then immunized with NP-KLH. Rearranged V_H genes from genomic DNA of germinal center B cells were amplified by polymerase chain reaction and sequenced. **Panel A:** The effect of donor age on usage of two V_H genes, 186.2 and C1H4, from the J558 family. Use of the 186.2 gene required T cells from young donors, but did not require young B cells. **Panel B:** The mean number of somatic mutations per V_H chain (means and standard errors for N = six or seven germinal centers). Use of either old T cells or old B cells diminishes the number of somatic mutations per gene. (From ref. 201.)

with the idea that contact-dependent signals from T cells to B cells may be impaired by aging. This decline in B-cell activation by T cells was accompanied by, and may perhaps be attributable to, a fivefold decline in the proportion of T cells able to express CD40 ligand after activation by anti-CD3 antibodies (196). Changes in expression of B-cell surface receptors may also be relevant in this context. Aging leads, for example, to a decline in germinal center B-cell expression of the B7-2 molecule, which is involved in reciprocal signaling interactions with T-cell CD28 (197), and monoclonal antibodies to CD40 fail to correct the proliferative defects in B cells from aged human donors (198). Aging also leads to a decline in the ability of T cells to respond to activation by expression of a receptor for B-cell surface IgD (199). This T-cell Fc receptor may play a role in activation of IgD-positive B cells, and it is interesting to note the strong correlation between poor expression of T-cell IgD receptor and poor responses to influenza vaccination among elderly subjects (200).

A study using adoptive transfer of T- and B-cell mixtures into severe combined immunodeficiency (SCID) mice has provided important insights into the role of T cells in molding B-cell repertoire (201). Adoptive hosts that received both CD4 T and B cells from young donors prior to immunization with the NP hapten produced antibodies that utilized the canonical V_H gene V186.2 and had high rates of somatic hypermutation. Anti-NP responses in mice that had received both T and B cells from old mice generated much lower rates of somatic mutation, and used a different V_H gene, C1H4. Construction of mice that had received either T or B cells from aged donors showed that the use of the V186.2 gene required the presence of young CD4 T cells, and that the development of high rates of somatic mutation required both T and B cells from young donors. Figure 4 illustrates the key findings in this system. Affinity maturation does occur in the germinal centers of old mice, but in the absence of somatic mutation, this is limited by the available (i.e., unmutated) repertoire and is less able to give rise to new, higher affinity B-cell clones (202).

ACCESSORY-CELL FUNCTION

Two aspects of the function of macrophages, dendritic cells, and their cognates in the initiation and support of antigen-specific immune responses have been examined from a gerontologic perspective: (a) support for T-cell activation and (b) production of cytokines and other nonspecific effector molecules.

There are many studies in which antigen-presenting cells (APCs) from aged donors have been tested for their ability to support T-cell activation; the majority show no effect of aging on this aspect of APC function (10,29). None of these studies did a systematic analysis of antigen uptake, processing, or presentation, and few took the trouble to distinguish among the various cell types that could contribute in different ways to T-cell activation; more work, with modern methods and reagents, is clearly called for. Analysis of APC function in vivo has been more productive. Early work (203) showed that although old mice are able to convey immune complexes into both spleen and lymph nodes after injection of radioactive antigen into passively immunized hosts, transport of the complexes into the lymph node follicles was impaired in older mice. The follicular dendritic cells (FDCs), which in the lymph nodes of young mice process immune complexes into highly immunogenic vesicles, are much less active in older animals (204). Indeed, the secondary immune response in old mice after reconsti-

tution with primed T and B cells from young donors is weak, but it can be restored by adding immune complexes on vesicles produced artificially by sonication of FDCs from old donors (205). In the skin, there is a small decline with age in the number of Langerhans' dendritic cells, which seems not to contribute to declines in cutaneous immune responses (206,207). Splenic dendritic cells from aged rats are relatively ineffective at presenting conalbumin to primed T cells in vitro; this defect does not reflect any change in ICAM-1 or class II MHC antigen expression on a per-cell basis (208).

The effects of aging on production of IL-1 and tumor necrosis factor-α (TNF-α) by macrophages are very inconsistent. The earliest studies (see ref. 29 for citations) relied on bioassays that are now known not to discriminate among a variety of proinflammatory agents, and did not pay sufficient attention to the interactions of stimulus, timing, and assay methodology with aging. More comprehensive studies, however, show these experimental details to be very influential. Thus IL-1 production by peritoneal macrophages collected from mice after injection of complete Freund's adjuvant (CFA) is increased by age when Candida cells are used as eliciting stimulus, but is decreased in cultures stimulated by staphylococci and exhibit no age effect using E. coli cells as stimulus (209); these data are illustrated in Fig. 5. The age effects on production of TNF-α were parallel to those on IL-1 production, except that some doses of E. coli led to an age-dependent increase in this monokine. A related report (210) noted that aging led to an increase in IL-1, TNF, and IL-6 production in vitro by thioglycolate-elicited mouse macrophages, but to a decline in monokine production by resident macrophages taken without stimulation from the peritoneum, or by CFA-stimulated cells. Reports of age-related increases in plasma levels of IL-6 or in spontaneous production of IL-6 in primary cell cultures (168,211) are disputed by reports of declines (212) or the absence of age effects (213). Production of IL-6 and TNF-α production after LPS injection in vivo increases with age in rats (214), as does TNF-α production in LPS-injected mice (215). Further progress in this area will depend on more explicit consideration of

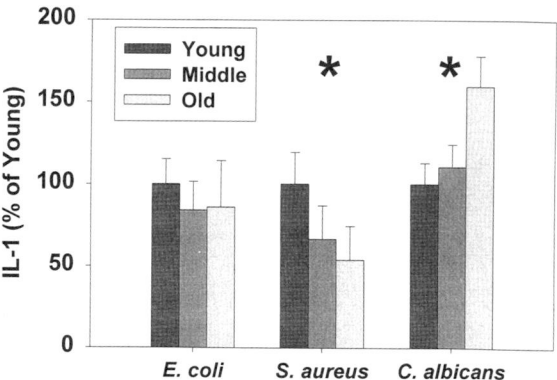

FIG. 5. Age effect on production of IL-1 by mouse peritoneal cells varies with stimulus. IL-1 bioactivity measured in supernatants obtained after 24-hour culture with either *E. coli, Staphylococcus aureus,* or *Candida albicans* at ratios of 4:1, 20:1, or 10:1 (microbe:cell), respectively. *Bars* show means ± standard errors for N = eight to 12 experiments, relative to the mean level of IL-1 produced by young mice in response to the same stimulus. The *asterisks* indicate significant increase or decline with age (p < 0.01) by Bonferroni-adjusted Student's *t* test. (Data from ref. 209.)

cellular heterogencity and interactions, together with better consideration of stimulus, dose, and timing. Nearly all of the published work on monokine production has, for experimental convenience, relied on cells activated *in vivo* by exposure to potent inflammatory agents, and thus the question of age-related changes in monokine production during the course of specific immune responses to antigenic stimuli has not been addressed. Because addition of IL-1 does not restore youthful levels of function to T-cell cultures from older donors (48,216), it seems unlikely that deficient production of IL-1 is itself a major contributor to age-related defects in T-cell function.

Several lines of evidence suggest that prostaglandin production by macrophages may contribute to poor immune responsiveness in old age. Prostaglandin synthesis inhibitors have been reported to improve both antibody production and proliferative responses to T-cell mitogens in cultures derived from old donors (217,218), although this effect has been disputed (219). Vitamin E–containing diets, which diminish macrophage prostaglandin synthesis, can also improve mouse T-cell responses (220), and *in vitro* production of prostaglandin-E2 increases with age in Con A–stimulated mouse splenocytes (221). The extent to which these changes undermine the natural immune response *in vivo* is uncertain, and it is noteworthy that macrophage-free cultures, in which costimulation is provided by anti-CD28 antibody, still exhibit an age-dependent decline in proliferative response (89).

NATURAL KILLER CELLS

Nearly all reports of natural killer (NK) cell function in humans find no effect, or at most a small decline (see ref. 222 and five other reports cited in ref. 29). These data are, however, derived from studies of peripheral blood; mouse data, derived principally from studies of splenic or lymph node NK cells, typically reveal a dramatic decline in NK function in middle-aged or older animals (for example, in refs. 68 and 223 and other papers cited in ref. 29). The discrepancy between these two series of studies probably reflects a difference between blood and internal lymphoid tissues, rather than between humans and mice, because NK function in the blood of mice, like that in humans, shows no effect of age (224). Data on NK function in spleen and lymph node tissues of elderly humans would therefore be of great interest. If it were found that aging humans, like aging mice, do show a severe decline in internal NK function, this might provide an opportunity for pharmacologic intervention to prevent or treat viral and neoplastic disease in the elderly, because in mice, at least, the ability to increase NK function by exposure to IL-2 and IFN-γ seems to be preserved in old age (223,225,226).

RESTORATION OF IMMUNE FUNCTION IN THE ELDERLY

A major goal of immunogerontology is to help develop strategies for improving immune function in middle-aged and older people, toward the goal of preventing or perhaps treating infectious or neoplastic illness among elderly people. Because our understanding of the fundamental cell and molecular bases for immune failure in old age is still highly imperfect, most of the intervention strategies tried have rested on empirical or quasispeculative foundations. The list of agents examined include dehydroepiandros-

terone (DHEA), melatonin, growth hormone, and substances alleged to be thymic hormones, as well as a number of vitamins and micronutrients.

DHEA and DHEA-S

DHEA, produced by the adrenal cortex, is, in its sulfated form DHEA-S, the most abundant adrenal steroid in human blood. (The term *DHEA(S)* will be used in this chapter to refer to both substances together). Interest in DHEA(S) as an immunomodulator was stimulated by evidence that its level falls dramatically with age in adult humans (227), and that low plasma DHEA(S) concentrations in middle-aged adults are associated with increased risks of heart disease (228) and breast cancer (229). Later work, however, failed to confirm the original impression of protective effects on cardiovascular disease (230), and demonstrated (231) that breast cancer incidence was actually higher in premenopausal women with above-average levels of DHEA(S). Furthermore, DHEA(S), though produced at high levels in some primates, is virtually absent in most other mammals, including mice and rats; levels of DHEA(S) in adult rat serum are at least 300-fold lower than in human serum (232), and there is no evidence for any effect of age on rodent DHEA(S) concentrations. Nonetheless, administration of DHEA or DHEA(S) to aged mice has been reported to generate a dramatic restoration of immune function. Thus, for example, a single injection of DHEA just prior to antigen administration is said to fully restore the ability of aged mice to produce antibodies to a foreign protein antigen (57) and to lead to strong secondary antibody responses in mice primed in the presence of DHEA. Dramatic improvement (i.e., a tenfold increase in antibody titer) was also reported in old mice vaccinated by hepatitis B antigen (233). This group has also reported that a single DHEA injection reverses a sixfold age-associated increase in mouse IL-6 levels and a threefold increase in serum amyloid P, and that 2 months of treatment with oral DHEA-S reverses age-related increases in autoantibody production and serum immunoglobulin levels (168). None of these impressive results has been replicated in another laboratory, however, and reports of DHEA-S effects on IL-2 production in culture (234) have been contradicted by two other groups (235,236). DHEA administered to elderly humans for a 6- to 12-month period apparently does not improve response to influenza or tetanus vaccination (237), and 20-week treatment with oral DHEA did not alter spontaneous IL-6 production by cultured lymphocytes (238). In this latter study, small changes in induced production of IL-6 and IL-2 were seen at occasional time points in a long series of measurements, and they almost certainly represent a multiple-comparisons artifact. Interest in DHEA as a candidate immunostimulator is likely to fade unless this agent can be shown to have strong reproducible effects in several laboratories.

Melatonin

Melatonin, the principal hormonal product of the pineal, has also been touted as a potential stimulator of immunity in old age, but the evidence for such an effect is very weak. Melatonin, like DHEA, is not produced by any of the commonly used strains of laboratory mice (239), and it is thus clear that alterations in melatonin levels cannot contribute to the decline in immune function seen in laboratory mice as they age. Melatonin seems to have no effects on *in vitro* mitogen responses or on syngeneic or allogeneic mixed-lymphocyte reactivity (240), and no effect *in vivo* on contact sensitivity to oxazalone (241). There is some evidence that melatonin may improve the response of old mice to sheep erythrocytes (242), although this effect seems to be small and limited to a very small dose range (243); there is no evidence for a melatonin effect on responses to other, more representative, antigens.

Growth Hormone

Interest in growth hormone (GH) as a potential inducer of immune rejuvenation stems in part from the observation (135) that a GH-secreting pituitary cell line could increase thymic size in aged rats. Peripheral immune function, however, was not improved dramatically either in the original study (135) or in follow-up studies using purified hormone (134) or pituitary transplantation (244). The one report of a positive effect of GH administration on immune responsiveness (245) is complicated by the death of 61% of the control animals during the 13-week treatment period; indeed, all of the control mice died prior to 21 months of age, of unexplained causes. The original suggestion that GH treatment could prevent thymic involution in GH-deficient dw/dw mice (246) has since been shown to be an artifact related to the timing of weaning (247). Indeed GH-deficient mutant mice are unusually long-lived (248) and lose T-cell mitogen responses more slowly than hormonally normal controls (136). Surgical removal of the pituitary also improves immune function in aged mice (249). Thus, on balance, there is little reason to suspect that GH deficiency is a key cause of immune senescence or to regard GH therapy as a promising avenue of immune restoration.

Thymic Hormones

The idea that thymic involution is a key element in immune aging has stimulated a good deal of research into the thymus as a potential source of soluble immunoregulators, the so-called thymic hormones, despite serious reservations about the strength of the evidence for such hormonal influences (250) and growing evidence that many products suspected to be thymic hormones were indeed produced by a variety of tissues (251). The literature contains a number of credible reports that synthetic peptides, with sequences derived from those of thymic products, can lead to improvements in immune response when administered to aged mice, monkeys, or humans (56,252–254). Reports of replication of these initial studies, however, are rare, and a comprehensive and systematic survey of both short- and long-term effects of several such thymic products (255,256) failed to produce strong evidence for immunoenhancing effects at any of the several dose regimens used. Current models for T-cell maturation in the thymus emphasize contact-dependent events involving T-lineage cells and thymic stromal cells, and the observation that implanted thymic epithelial cells can restore T-cell immune function to aged mice (257) justifies additional attention to the potential role of the nonlymphoid thymic cells, or their nonsecreted products, in immunotherapeutic strategies.

Nutritional Interventions

There are several hints that administration of vitamins or trace minerals may improve immunity in old mice or people, whether by correction of physiologic deficiencies or by pharmacologic means. Thus, a daily dose of tablets containing a number of trace elements and vitamins at levels at or only slightly above recommended minimal requirements was found to improve IL-2 production, NK function, and *in vitro* antibody production, and also lower the rate of serious infectious illness, in a 1-year placebo-controlled trial in healthy elderly persons (258). Vitamin E also has positive effects on immunity in aged mice (220) and humans (259), perhaps through effects on prostaglandin secretion, discussed above. Effects of zinc supplementation have been noted in some (260), though not other (261), studies. Detailed work on possible immune restoration by manipulation of micronutrients is just beginning.

The one nutritional approach that has a large and reproducible effect on immunity in aging rodents is the caloric restriction regime, which retards age-dependent changes in so many physiologic systems (262,263), including various aspects of T cell–mediated immunity (264–266). It is not yet clear if a similar approach will work in primates, and, indeed, preliminary evidence on immune function in calorically restricted monkeys is not encouraging in this respect (267). The restriction model makes it clear, however, that it is possible to retard immune decline in mammals by environmental manipulation, and further insights into the mechanism of the food restriction effect could well suggest new strategies for prevention of immune decline in humans.

IMMUNITY AND LATE-LIFE DISEASE

There are several approaches that have begun to yield information about the possible contribution of immune senescence to late-life illness. Analyses of immune responses to infectious agents or neoplastic cells give insights into mechanisms that could connect altered immunity to disease, but they often say little about the relative importance of immune factors and other influences on pathogenesis. Correlation analyses can provide clues about the amount of risk attributable to immune factors, but they provide little information about the basis for the associations seen, and they can be complicated by confounding factors that might influence both disease and immunity in parallel.

Studies in mice show that aging is accompanied by a decline in resistance to infection by a wide range of organisms, and that in most well-studied cases, changes in T-cell function are probably to blame. Adoptive transfer studies, in which T cells from young or old mice are transplanted into a set of young hosts and then tested for ability to inhibit infection, have shown that young T cells convey superior protection in responses to polio virus (268), tuberculosis (269), and *Listeria* (270). Declines in T-cell immunity also contribute to poor resistance of aged mice to influenza virus infection (86,87) and to trypanosomes (271).

The effects of aging on responses to influenza virus and to vaccination against influenza have been particularly well studied, with a view toward overcoming the increased risk of lethal influenza infection in elderly persons. Aging is not associated, in people, with an increased risk of infection during influenza epidemics, but it is associated with increased severity of illness and higher mortality. The ability to generate cytotoxic T cells after influenza infection declines with age in infected mice (86) and vaccinated humans (272), and the decline in heterotypic immunity (i.e., protection conferred by exposure to a cross-reacting strain of virus) is particularly associated with a loss in ability to control viral spread from nasal tissues to lungs (87). The possible role of alterations in helper

T cell function in the host response to influenza has been less well explored, but there are hints that helper memory cells produced in older people may be less long-lived than those produced in younger individuals (273). Mice primed to influenza at 8 weeks of age retain strong helper and cytotoxic responses for at least 2 years (274), although an age-related decline in memory-cell function contributes to recrudescence of active tuberculosis in mice infected when young (275).

Generation of specific cytotoxic T-cell immunity to syngeneic tumors also declines with age (276,277), although it is unclear whether studies of responses to transplantable tumors are germane to the issue of immune protection against early stages in tumor development. The question of whether immune deficits in old age contribute to increased cancer incidence in the elderly is controversial (278,279), with little strong evidence on either side. Mice selected, from genetically heterogeneous stock, for high levels of early-life humoral immunity do exhibit a diminished risk of spontaneous neoplasia (280), and high levels of CD4 memory T cells—characteristic of old mice—predict early development of neoplasia when seen in young adult mice (281). Among apparently healthy, elderly humans, anergic skin test responses to common recall antigens are associated with about a twofold increased risk of cancer mortality during a 9-year follow-up period, but the effect was not statistically significant in a sample of 229 subjects, and there was no association between anergy and cancer incidence (282). Large (e.g., 400-fold) age-dependent increases in susceptibility to transplanted tumors can be associated with much smaller (e.g., twofold) changes in the outcome of *in vitro* tests for generation of antitumor effectors (283), and it is possible that modest defects in complementary arms of the immune system—perhaps including the changes in NK-cell function discussed above—act in concert to generate a more serious impairment of host antitumor defense.

There are reports that immunologic tests have useful prognostic value for predictions of all-cause mortality, but these are, in general, not very satisfactory. Some of the early studies, showing associations between poor immunity and low survival in elderly people (284,285), failed to adjust statistically for potential confounding variables (such as age and sex), and studies that focus on extremely old subjects (e.g., mean ages in the 80s) and include comparatively short-term follow-up periods (typically 2 years) are plagued by the possibility that preexisting illness may alter the outcome of immunologic tests while also hastening death. An analysis of all-cause mortality in a younger group of elderly subjects, and with a longer follow-up period, found a twofold increase in mortality risk among anergic subjects, which just failed to meet conventional criteria for statistical significance ($p = 0.06$) after adjustment for subject age. Anergy was also shown to predict infection, particularly pneumonia, as well as all-cause mortality, among a group of 225 elderly nursing home residents (286). Strategies that pool information from a number of immune assays, including lymphocyte subset distributions and *in vitro* mitogen responses, also show some promise as predictors of mortality rates in humans (287).

Analogous studies in mice have the potential to compare prognostic tests with pathologic outcomes over a much larger percentage of the total life span, but they are, in general, hampered by the difficulty of obtaining adequate sample sizes without harm to the animal. An early report (11) showed an association between high proportions of peripheral blood CD8 cells and poor survival in CBA mice, but this particular colony exhibited large age-association changes in CD8-cell proportions that are not usually seen in other laboratories. High proportions of CD4 memory T cells in the peripheral blood predict short life span, regardless of the specific cause of death, in a population of 20-month-old genetically heterogeneous mice, in which most deaths were attributable to a variety of forms of neoplasia (R.A. Miller et al., submitted), consistent with models in which prematurely aged immune systems predispose to spontaneous cancer and early death. The basis for this correlation, and its possible extension to human disease, clearly require additional work.

SUMMARY AND PROSPECTUS

Knowledge of the normal (i.e., young) immune system is now sufficiently well advanced as to provide great opportunities for gerontologic research, and the gerontological community is just starting to return the favor by revealing immunologically interesting phenomena that were inapparent in studies of younger subjects. Exploitation of immune models is providing important clues to the effects of aging on cell activation, gene expression, and intercellular communication, and on the connections between physiologic aging and late-life diseases. Studies of the balance between naive and memory T cells, of alterations in immunoglobulin gene selection and T-cell repertoire, and of heterogeneity among memory cells with different functional capabilities are likely to be of continuing interest both to experimental gerontologists and to the larger community of immunologic researchers.

REFERENCES

1. Rose MR. *Evolutionary biology of aging.* New York: Oxford University Press, 1991.
2. Hobbs MH, Ernst DN. T cell differentiation and cytokine expression in late life. *Dev Comp Immunol* 1997;21:461–470.
3. Klinman NR. The basis for decreased B cell responsiveness with aging: the legacy and the challenge. *Ageing: Immunol Infect Dis* 1994;5:203–210.
4. Gottesman SRS, Thorbecke GJ, Walford RL. Specific and nonspecific suppressor cells in aged animals. In: Goidl E, ed. *Aging and the immune response.* New York: Marcel Dekker Inc, 1986:243–270.
5. Makinodan T, Kay MMB. Age influence on the immune system. *Adv Immunol* 1980;29:287–330.
6. Murasko DM, Goonewardene IM. T-cell function in aging: mechanisms of decline. *Annu Rev Gerontol Geriatr* 1990;10:71–96.
7. Hausman PB, Weksler ME. Changes in the immune response with age. In: Finch CF, Schneider EL, eds. *Handbook of the biology of aging.* New York: Van Nostrand Reinhold, 1985:414–432.
8. Thoman ML, Weigle WO. The cellular and subcellular bases of immunosenescence. *Adv Immunol* 1989;46:221–261.
9. Ligthart GJ, Corberand JX, Geertzen HG, Meinders AE, Knook DL, Hijmans W. Necessity of the assessment of health status in human immunogerontological studies: evaluation of the SENIEUR protocol. *Mech Ageing Dev* 1990;55:89–105.
10. Miller RA. Immune system. In: Masoro E, ed. *Handbook of physiology. Section 11: physiology of aging.* New York: Oxford University Press, 1995:555–590.
11. Boersma WJA, Steinmeier FA, Haaijman JJ. Age-related changes in the relative numbers of Thy-1 and Lyt-2-bearing peripheral blood lymphocytes in mice: a longitudinal approach. *Cell Immunol* 1985;93:417–430.
12. Grossmann A, Maggio Price L, Jinneman JC, Rabinovitch PS. Influence of aging on intracellular free calcium and proliferation of mouse T-cell subsets from various lymphoid organs. *Cell Immunol* 1991;135:118–131.
13. Miller RA. Age-related changes in T cell surface markers: a longitudinal analysis in genetically heterogeneous mice. *Mech Ageing Dev* 1997;96:181–196.
14. Lerner A, Yamada T, Miller RA. PGP-1hi T lymphocytes accumulate with age in mice and respond poorly to Concanavalin A. *Eur J Immunol* 1989;19:977–982.
15. Ernst DN, Hobbs MV, Torbett BE, et al. Differences in the expression profiles of CD45RB, Pgp-1, and 3G11 membrane antigens and in the patterns of lymphokine secretion by splenic CD4+ T cells from young and aged mice. *J Immunol* 1990;145:1295–1302.
16. Flurkey K, Stadecker M, Miller RA. Memory T lymphocyte hyporesponsiveness to non-cognate stimuli: a key factor in age-related immunodeficiency. *Eur J Immunol* 1992;22:931–935.
17. Hayakawa K, Hardy RR. Phenotypic and functional alteration of CD4+ T cells after antigenic stimulation. Resolution of two populations of memory T cells that both secrete Interleukin 4. *J Exp Med* 1989;169:2245–2250.

18. Ernst DN, Weigle WO, Noonan DJ, McQuitty DN, Hobbs MV. The age-associated increase in IFN-γ synthesis by mouse CD8+ T cells correlates with shifts in the frequencies of cell subsets defined by membrane CD44, CD45RB, 3G11, and MEL-14 expression. *J Immunol* 1993;151:575–587.

19. De Paoli P, Battistin S, Santini GF. Age-related changes in human lymphocyte subsets: progressive reduction of the CD4 CD45R (suppressor inducer) population. *Clin Immunol Immunopathol* 1988;48:290–296.

20. Pilarski LM, Yacyshyn BR, Jensen GS, Pruski E, Pabst HF. β1 integrin (CD29) expression on human postnatal T cell subsets defined by selective CD45 isoform expression. *J Immunol* 1991;147:830–837.

21. Serra HM, Krowka JF, Ledbetter JA, Pilarski LM. Loss of CD45R (Lp220) represents a post-thymic T cell differentiation event. *J Immunol* 1988;140:1435–1441.

22. Utsuyama M, Hirokawa K, Kurashima C, et al. Differential age-change in the numbers of CD4+CD45RA+ and CD4+CD29+ T cell subsets in human peripheral blood. *Mech Ageing Dev* 1992;63:57–68.

23. Walker D, Gauchat JF, De Weck AL, Stadler BM. Analysis of leukocyte markers in elderly individuals. *Aging: Immunol Infect Dis* 1990;2:31–43.

24. Kendig NE, Chrest FJ, Nagel JE, Chaisson RE, Saah AJ, Adler WH. Age-related changes in the immune function of HIV-1 seropositive adults. *Aging: Immunol Infect Dis* 1991;3:67–80.

25. Witkowski JM, Miller RA. Increased function of P-glycoprotein in T lymphocytes of aging mice. *J Immunol* 1993;150:1296–1306.

26. Linton PJ, Haynes L, Klinman NR, Swain SL. Antigen-independent changes in naive CD4 T cells with aging. *J Exp Med* 1996;184:1891–1900.

27. Pilarski LM, Paine D, McElhaney JE, Cass CE, Belch AR. Multidrug transporter P-glycoprotein 170 as a differentiation antigen on normal human lymphocytes and thymocytes: modulation with differentiation stage and during aging. *Am J Hematol* 1995;49:323–335.

28. Gillis S, Kozak R, Durante M, Weksler ME. Immunological studies of aging. Decreased production of and response to T cell growth factor by lymphocytes from aged humans. *J Clin Invest* 1981;67:937–942.

29. Miller RA. Aging and the immune response. In: Schneider EL, Rowe JW, eds. *Handbook of the biology of aging.* San Diego: Academic Press, 1996:355–392.

30. Hobbs MV, Weigle WO, Noonan DJ, et al. Patterns of cytokine gene expression by CD4+ T cells from young and old mice. *J Immunol* 1993;150:3602–3614.

31. Dobber R, Tielemans M, de Weerd H, Nagelkerken L. Mel14+ CD4+ T cells from aged mice display functional and phenotypic characteristics of memory cells. *Int Immunol* 1994;6:1227–1234.

32. Goya RG, Brooks K, Meites J. A comparison between hormone levels and T lymphocyte function in young and old rats. *Mech Ageing Dev* 1991;61:275–285.

33. Holbrook NJ, Chopra RK, McCoy MT, et al. Expression of interleukin 2 and the interleukin 2 receptor in aging rats. *Cell Immunol* 1989;120:1–9.

34. Davila DR, Kelley KW. Sex differences in lectin-induced interleukin-2 synthesis in aging rats. *Mech Ageing Dev* 1988;44:231–240.

35. Odio M, Brodish A, Ricardo MJ Jr. Effects on immune responses by chronic stress are modulated by aging. *Brain Behav Immun* 1987;1:204–215.

36. Wrabatz LG, Antel JP, Oger JJF, Arnason BGW, Goust JM, Hopper JE. Age-related changes in in vivo immunoglobulin secretion: comparison of responses to T-dependent and T-independent polyclonal activators. *Cell Immunol* 1982;74:398–403.

37. Thoman ML, Weigle WO. Partial restoration of Con A-induced proliferation, IL-2 receptor expression, and IL-2 synthesis in aged murine lymphocytes by phorbol myristate acetate and ionomycin. *Cell Immunol* 1988;114:1–11.

38. Nagel JE, Chopra RK, Chrest FJ, et al. Decreased proliferation, interleukin 2 synthesis, and interleukin 2 receptor expression are accompanied by decreased mRNA expression in phytohemagglutinin-stimulated cells from elderly donors. *J Clin Invest* 1988;81:1096–1102.

39. Wu WT, Pahlavani M, Cheung HT, Richardson A. The effect of aging on the expression of interleukin 2 messenger ribonucleic acid. *Cell Immunol* 1986;100:224–231.

40. Fong TC, Makinodan T. In situ hybridization analysis of the age-associated decline in IL-2 mRNA expressing murine T cells. *Cell Immunol* 1989;118:199–207.

41. Miller RA. Age-associated decline in precursor frequency for different T cell-mediated reactions, with preservation of helper or cytotoxic effect per precursor cell. *J Immunol* 1984;132:63–68.

42. Hessen MT, Kaye D, Murasko DM. Heterogeneous effects of exogenous lymphokines on lymphoproliferation of elderly subjects. *Mech Ageing Dev* 1991;58:61–73.

43. Brill S, Kukulansky T, Tal E, et al. Individual changes in T lymphocyte parameters of old human subjects. *Mech Ageing Dev* 1987;40:71–79.

44. Huang Y-P, Pechere J-C, Michel M, et al. In vivo T cell activation, in vitro defective IL-2 secretion, and response to influenza vaccination in elderly women. *J Immunol* 1992;148:715–722.

45. Thoman ML, Weigle WO. Reconstitution of in vivo cell-mediated lympholysis responses in aged mice with Interleukin 2. *J Immunol* 1985;134:949–952.

46. Beckman I, Dimopoulos K, Xu XN, Bradley J, Henschke P, Ahern M. T cell activation in the elderly: evidence for specific deficiencies in T cell/accessory cell interactions. *Mech Ageing Dev* 1990;51:265–276.

47. Ernst DN, Weigle WO, McQuitty DN, Rothermel AL, Hobbs MH. Stimulation of murine T cell subsets with anti-CD3 antibody. Age-related defects in the expression of early activation molecules. *J Immunol* 1989;142:1413–1421.

48. Negoro S, Hara H, Miyata S, et al. Mechanisms of age-related decline in antigen-specific T cell proliferative response: IL-2 receptor expression and recombinant IL-2 induced proliferative response of purified TAC-positive T cells. *Mech Ageing Dev* 1986;36:223–241.

49. Vie H, Miller RA. Decline, with age, in the proportion of mouse T cells that express IL-2 receptors after mitogen stimulation. *Mech Ageing Dev* 1986;33:313–322.

50. Nagel JE, Chopra RK, Powers DC, Adler WH. Effect of age on the human high affinity interleukin 2 receptor of phytohaemagglutinin stimulated peripheral blood lymphocytes. *Clin Exp Immunol* 1989;75:286–291.

51. Schwab R, Pfeffer LM, Szabo P, Gamble D, Schnurr CM, Weksler ME. Defective expression of high affinity IL-2 receptors on activated T cells from aged humans. *Int Immunol* 1990;2:239–246.

52. Thoman ML. Impaired responsiveness of IL-2 receptor-expressing T lymphocytes from aged mice. *Cell Immunol* 1991;135:410–417.

53. Nordin AA, Collins GD. Limiting dilution analysis of alloreactive cytotoxic precursor cells in aging mice. *J Immunol* 1983;131:2215–2218.

54. Dozmorov IM, Kalinichenko VV, Sidorov IA, Miller RA. Antagonistic interactions among T cell subsets of old mice revealed by limiting dilution analysis. *J Immunol* 1995;154:4283–4293.

55. Hallgren HM, Ambroziak J, O'Leary JJ, Degelau JJ. Changes with age in CD4+ memory and naive T lymphocyte proliferative responses to both mitogen and recall antigens in healthy humans. *Aging: Immunol Infect Dis* 1994;5:109–119.

56. Cillari E, Milano S, Dieli M, et al. Thymopentin reduces the susceptibility of aged mice to cutaneous leishmaniasis by modulating CD4 T cell subsets. *Immunology* 1992;76:362–366.

57. Daynes RA, Araneo BA. Prevention and reversal of some age-associated changes in immunologic responses by supplemental dehydroepiandrosterone sulfate therapy. *Aging: Immunol Infect Dis* 1992;3:135–154.

58. Nagelkerken L, Hertogh-Huijbregts A, Dobber R, Drager A. Age-related changes in lymphokine production related to a decreased number of CD45RBhi CD4+ T cells. *Eur J Immunol* 1991;21:273–281.

59. Engwerda CR, Fox BS, Handwerger BS. Cytokine production by T lymphocytes from young and aged mice. *J Immunol* 1996;156:3621–3630.

60. Li SP, Miller RA. Age-associated decline in IL-4 production by murine T lymphocytes in extended culture. *Cell Immunol* 1993;151:187–195.

61. Burns EA, L'Hommedieu GD, Cunning JL, Goodwin JS. Effects of interleukin-4 on antigen-specific antibody synthesis by lymphocytes from old and young adults. *Lymphokine Cytokine Res* 1994;13:227–231.

62. al-Rayes H, Pachas W, Mirza N, Ahern DJ, Geha RS, Vercelli D. IgE regulation and lymphokine patterns in aging humans. *J Allergy Clin Immunol* 1992;90:630–636.

63. Zhang Y, Cosyns M, Levin MJ, Hayward AR. Cytokine production in varicella zoster virus-stimulated limiting dilution lymphocyte cultures. *Clin Exp Immunol* 1994;98:128–133.

64. Green-Johnson JM, Haq JA, Szewczuk MR. Effects of aging on the production of cytoplasmic interleukin-4 and 5, and interferon-γ by mucosal and systemic lymphocytes after activation with phytohemagglutinin. *Aging: Immunol Infect Dis* 1991;3:43–57.

65. Bining N, Miller RA. Cytokine production by subsets of CD4 memory T cells differing in P-glycoprotein expression: effects of aging. *J Gerontol A Biol Sci Med Sci* 1997;52:B137–B145.

66. Hobbs MV, Weigle WO, Ernst DN. Interleukin-10 production by splenic CD4+ cells and cell subsets from young and old mice. *Cell Immunol* 1994;154:264–272.

67. Zhou T, Edwards CK, Mountz JD. Prevention of age-related T cell apoptosis defect in CD2-fas-transgenic mice. *J Exp Med* 1995;182:129–137.

68. Albright JW, Albright JF. Age-associated impairment of murine natural killer activity. *Proc Natl Acad Sci USA* 1983;80:6371–6375.

69. Abb J, Abb H, Deinhardt F. Age-related decline of human interferon alpha and interferon gamma production. *Blut* 1984;48:285–289.

70. Gauchat JF, DeWeck AL, Stadler BM. Decreased cytokine mRNA levels in the elderly. *Aging: Immunol Infect Dis* 1988;1:191–204.

71. Salkind AR. Influence of age on the production of Fos and Jun by influenza virus-exposed T cells. *J Leukoc Biol* 1994;56:817–820.

72. Bloom ET, Thompson WC, Horvath-Arcidiacono JA, Burd PR. Differential effects of interleukin-12 treatment on gene expression by allostimulated T cells from young and aged mice. *Mech Ageing Dev* 1995;85:109–124.

73. Mbawuike IN, Acuna C, Caballero O, et al. Reversal of age-related deficient influenza virus-specific CTL responses and IFN-gamma production by monophosphoryl lipid A. *Cell Immunol* 1996;173:64–78.

74. Fujio H, Kawamura I, Miyamoto H, Mitsuyama M, Yoshida S. Decreased capacity of aged mice to produce interferon-gamma in Legionella pneumophila infection. *Mech Ageing Dev* 1995;81:97–106.

75. Wallace PK, Eisenstein TK, Meissler JJ Jr, Morahan PS. Decreases in macrophage mediated antitumor activity with aging. *Mech Ageing Dev* 1995;77:169–184.

76. Ding A, Hwang S, Schwab R. Effect of aging on murine macrophages. Diminished response to IFN-gamma for enhanced oxidative metabolism. *J Immunol* 1994;153:2146–2152.

77. McLachlan JA, Serkin CD, Morrey KM, Bakouche O. Antitumoral properties of aged human monocytes. *J Immunol* 1995;154:832–843.

78. Thoman ML, Keogh EA, Weigle WO. Response of aged T and B lymphocytes to IL-4. *Aging: Immunol Infect Dis* 1988;1:245–253.

79. Gottesman SRS, Walford RL, Thorbecke GJ. Proliferative and cytotoxic immune functions in aging mice. III. Exogenous interleukin-2 rich supernatant only partially restores alloreactivity in vitro. *Mech Ageing Dev* 1985;31:103–113.

80. Askonas BA, Mullbacher A, Ashman RB. Cytotoxic T-memory cells in virus infection and the specificity of helper T cells. *Immunology* 1982;45:79–84.

81. Miller RA, Stutman O. Decline, in aging mice, of the anti-TNP cytotoxic T cell response attributable to loss of Lyt-2⁻, IL-2 producing helper cell function. *Eur J Immunol* 1981;11:751–756.

82. Saxena RK, Saxena QB, Adler WH. Lectin-induced cytotoxic activity in spleen cells from young and old mice. Age-related changes in types of effector cells, lymphokine production and response. *Immunology* 1988;64:457–461.

83. Gottesman SRS, Edington J. Proliferative and cytotoxic immune functions in aging mice: V. Deficiency in generation of cytotoxic cells with normal lytic function per cell as demonstrated by the single cell conjugation assay. *Aging: Immunol Infect Dis* 1990;2:19–29.

84. Bloom ET, Kubota LF, Kawakami K. Age-related decline in the lethal hit but not the binding stage of cytotoxic T-cell activity in mice. *Cell Immunol* 1988;114: 440–446.

85. Rosenberg AS, Sechler JM, Horvath JA, Maniero TG, Bloom ET. Assessment of alloreactive T cell subpopulations of aged mice in vivo. CD4+ but not CD8+ T cell-mediated rejection response declines with advanced age [published erratum appears in *Eur J Immunol* 1994 Oct;24(10):2571]. *Eur J Immunol* 1994;24: 1312–1316.

86. Bender BS, Johnson MP, Small PA. Influenza in senescent mice: impaired cytotoxic T-lymphocyte activity is correlated with prolonged infection. *Immunology* 1991;72:514–519.

87. Bender BS, Small PA Jr. Heterotypic immune mice lose protection against influenza virus infection with senescence. *J Infect Dis* 1993;168:873–880.

88. Gelfand EW, Cheung RT, Mills GB, Grinstein S. Uptake of extracellular Ca²⁺ and not recruitment from internal stores is essential for T lymphocyte proliferation. *Eur J Immunol* 1988;18:917–922.

89. Grossmann A, Ledbetter JA, Rabinovitch PS. Reduced proliferation in T lymphocytes in aged humans is predominantly in the CD8+ subset, and is unrelated to defects in transmembrane signaling which are predominantly in the CD4+ subset. *Exp Cell Res* 1989;180:367–382.

90. Gupta S. Membrane signal transduction in T cells in aging humans. *Ann NY Acad Sci* 1989;568:277–282.

91. Whisler RL, Newhouse YG, Donnerberg RL, Tobin CM. Characterization of intracellular ionized calcium responsiveness and inositol phosphate production among resting and stimulated peripheral blood T cells from elderly humans. *Aging: Immunol Infect Dis* 1991;3:27–36.

92. Grossmann A, Ledbetter JA, Rabinovitch PS. Aging-related deficiency in intracellular calcium response to anti-CD3 or concanavalin A in murine T-cell subsets. *J Gerontol Biol Sci* 1990;45:B81–B86.

93. Proust JJ, Filburn CR, Harrison SA, Buchholz MA, Nordin AA. Age-related defect in signal transduction during lectin activation of murine T lymphocytes. *J Immunol* 1987;139:1472–1478.

94. Miller RA, Jacobson B, Weil G, Simons ER. Diminished calcium influx in lectin-stimulated T cells from old mice. *J Cell Physiol* 1987;132:337–342.

95. Grossmann A, Rabinovitch PS, Lane MA, et al. Influence of age, sex, and dietary restriction on intracellular free calcium responses of CD4+ lymphocytes in rhesus monkeys (*Macaca mulatta*). *J Cell Physiol* 1995;162:298–303.

96. Philosophe B, Miller RA. Diminished calcium signal generation in subsets of T lymphocytes that predominate in old mice. *J Gerontol Biol Sci* 1990;45:B87–B93.

97. Rajasekar R, Augustin A. Antigen-dependent selection of T cells that are able to efficiently regulate free cytoplasmic calcium levels. *J Immunol* 1994;153: 1037–1045.

98. Lohmiller JJ, Roellich KM, Toledano A, Rabinovitch PS, Wolf NS, Grossmann A. Aged murine T-lymphocytes are more resistant to oxidative damage due to the predominance of the cells possessing the memory phenotype. *J Gerontol A Biol Sci Med Sci* 1996;51:B132–B140.

99. Miller RA, Flurkey K, Molloy M, Luby T, Stadecker MJ. Differential sensitivity of virgin and memory T lymphocytes to calcium ionophores suggests a buoyant density separation method and a model for memory cell hyporesponsiveness to Con A. *J Immunol* 1991;147:3080–3086.

100. Philosophe B, Miller RA. T lymphocyte heterogeneity in old and young mice: functional defects in T cells selected for poor calcium signal generation. *Eur J Immunol* 1989;19:695–699.

101. Lerner A, Philosophe B, Miller RA. Defective calcium influx and preserved inositol phosphate generation in T cells from old mice. *Aging: Immunol Infect Dis* 1988;1:149–157.

102. Freedman MH, Raff MC, Gomperts B. Induction of increased calcium uptake in mouse T lymphocytes by concanavalin A and its modulation by cyclic nucleotides. *Nature* 1975;255:378–382.

103. Kawanishi H. Activation of calcium (Ca)-dependent protein kinase C in aged mesenteric lymph node T and B cells. *Immunol Lett* 1993;35:25–32.

104. Miller RA, Philosophe B, Ginis I, Weil G, Jacobson B. Defective control of cytoplasmic calcium concentration in T lymphocytes from old mice. *J Cell Physiol* 1989;138:175–182.

105. Negoro S, Hara H. The effect of taurine on the age-related decline of the immune response in mice: the restorative effect on the T cell proliferative response to costimulation with ionomycin and phorbol myristate acetate. *Adv Exp Med Biol* 1992;315:229–239.

106. Ran Q, Li D, Zhen Y. [Changes of proto-oncogene expression and cytosolic free calcium in activated T-lymphocytes of aged mice]. *Chung Hua I Hsueh Tsa Chih* 1995;75:466–9, 509–510.

107. Patel HR, Miller RA. Age-associated changes in mitogen-induced protein phosphorylation in murine T lymphocytes. *Eur J Immunol* 1992;22:253–260.

108. Shi J, Miller RA. Tyrosine-specific protein phosphorylation in response to anti-CD3 antibody is diminished in old mice. *J Gerontol Biol Sci* 1992;47: B147–B153.

109. Whisler RL, Newhouse YG, Bagenstose SE. Age-related reductions in the activation of mitogen-activated protein kinases p44^mapk/ERK1 and p42^mapk/ERK2 in human T cells stimulated via ligation of the T cell receptor complex. *Cell Immunol* 1996;168:201–210.

110. Gorgas G, Butch ER, Guan KL, Miller RA. Diminished activation of the MAP kinase pathway in CD3-stimulated T lymphocytes from old mice. *Mech Ageing Dev* 1997;94:71–83.

111. Fulop T Jr, Leblanc C, Lacombe G, Dupuis G. Cellular distribution of protein kinase C isozymes in CD3-mediated stimulation of human T lymphocytes with aging. *FEBS Lett* 1995;375:69–74.

112. Whisler RL, Newhouse YG, Grants IS, Hackshaw KV. Differential expression of the alpha- and beta-isoforms of protein kinase C in peripheral blood T and B cells from young and elderly adults. *Mech Ageing Dev* 1995;77:197–211.

113. Garcia GG, Miller RA. Differential tyrosine phosphorylation of zeta chain dimers in mouse CD4 T lymphocytes: effect of age. *Cell Immunol* 1997;175: 51–57.

114. Grossmann A, Rabinovitch PS, Kavanagh TJ, et al. Activation of murine T-cells via phospholipase-C gamma 1-associated protein tyrosine phosphorylation is reduced with aging. *J Gerontol A Biol Sci Med Sci* 1995;50:B205–B212.

115. Ghosh J, Miller RA. Rapid tyrosine phosphorylation of Grb2 and Shc in T cells exposed to anti-CD3, anti-CD4, and anti-CD45 stimuli: differential effects of aging. *Mech Ageing Dev* 1995;80:171–187.

116. Buckler A, Vie H, Sonenshein G, Miller RA. Defective T lymphocytes in old mice: diminished production of mature c-myc mRNA after mitogen exposure not attributable to alterations in transcription or RNA stability. *J Immunol* 1988;140: 2442–2446.

117. Gamble DA, Schwab R, Weksler ME, Szabo P. Decreased steady state c-myc mRNA in activated T cell cultures from old humans is caused by a smaller proportion of T cells that transcribe the c-myc gene. *J Immunol* 1990;144:3569–3573.

118. Pieri C, Recchioni R, Moroni F, Marcheselli F, Lipponi G. Phytohemagglutinin induced changes of membrane lipid packing, c-myc and c-myb encoded protein expression in human lymphocytes during aging. *Mech Ageing Dev* 1992;64: 177–187.

119. Song L, Stephens JM, Kittur S, et al. Expression of c-fos, c-jun and jun B in peripheral blood lymphocytes from young and elderly adults. *Mech Ageing Dev* 1992;65:149–156.

120. Whisler RL, Liu B, Wu LC, Chen M. Reduced activation of transcriptional factor AP-1 among peripheral blood T cells from elderly humans after PHA stimulation: restorative effect of phorbol diesters. *Cell Immunol* 1993;152:96–109.

121. Nakahama M, Mohri N, Mori S, Shindo G, Yokoi Y, Machinami R. Immunohistochemical and histometrical studies of the human thymus with special emphasis on age-related changes in medullary epithelial and dendritic cells. *Virchows Arch B Cell Pathol* 1990;58:245–251.

122. Gonzalez-Quintial R, Theofilopoulos AN. V beta gene repertoires in aging mice. *J Immunol* 1992;149:230–236.

123. el Demellawy M, el Ridi R. Age-associated decrease in proportion and antigen expression of CD8+/CD4+ thymocytes in BALB/c mice. *Mech Ageing Dev* 1992;62:307–318.

124. Scollay RG, Butcher EC, Weissman IL. Thymus cell migration. Quantitative aspects of cellular traffic from the thymus to the periphery in mice. *Eur J Immunol* 1980;10:210–218.

125. Hirokawa K, Makinodan T. Thymic involution: effect on T cell differentiation. *J Immunol* 1975;114:1659–1664.

126. Utsuyama M, Kasai M, Kurashima C, Hirokawa K. Age influence on the thymic capacity to promote differentiation of T cells: induction of different composition of T cell subsets by aging thymus. *Mech Ageing Dev* 1991;58:267–277.

127. Hirokawa K, Utsuyama M. The effect of sequential multiple grafting of syngeneic newborn thymus on the immune functions and life expectancy of aging mice. *Mech Ageing Dev* 1984;28:111–121.

128. Gozes Y, Umiel T, Trainin N. Selective decline in differentiating capacity of immunohemopoietic stem cells with aging. *Mech Ageing Dev* 1982;18:251–259.

129. Harrison DE, Astle CM, Delaittre JA. Loss of proliferative capacity in immunohemopoietic stem cells caused by serial transplantation rather than aging. *J Exp Med* 1978;147:1526–1531.

130. Averill LE, Wolf NS. The decline in murine splenic PHA and LPS responsiveness with age is primarily due to an intrinsic mechanism. *J Immunol* 1985;134: 3859–3863.

131. Hirokawa K, Kubo S, Utsuyama M, Kurashima C, Sado T. Age-related change in the potential of bone marrow cells to repopulate the thymus and splenic T cells in mice. *Cell Immunol* 1986;100:443–451.

132. Basch RS. Thymic repopulation after irradiation in aged mice. *Aging: Immunol Infect Dis* 1990;2:229–235.

133. Eren R, Zharhary D, Abel L, Globerson A. Age-related changes in the capacity of bone marrow cells to differentiate in thymic organ cultures. *Cell Immunol* 1988;112:449–455.

134. McCormick KR, Harr JL, Taubenberger JK, Krieg RJ. A murine model for regeneration of the senescent thymus using growth hormone therapy. *Aging: Immunol Infect Dis* 1991;3:19–26.

135. Kelley KW, Brief S, Westly HJ, et al. GH3 pituitary adenoma cells can reverse thymic aging in rats. *Proc Natl Acad Sci USA* 1986;83:5663–5667.

136. Flurkey K, Harrison DE. Use of genetic models to investigate the hypophyseal regulation of senescence. In: Harrison DE, ed. *Genetic effects on aging II*. Caldwell, NJ: The Telford Press, 1990:437–456.

137. Aspinall R. Age-associated thymic atrophy in the mouse is due to a deficiency affecting rearrangement of the TCR during intrathymic development. *J Immunol* 1997;158:3037–3045.

138. Thoman ML. The pattern of T lymphocyte differentiation is altered during thymic involution. *Mech Ageing Dev* 1995;82:155–170.

139. Paolini R, Jouvin M-H, Kinet J,-P. Phosphorylation and dephosphorylation of the high-affinity receptor for immunoglobulin E immediately after receptor engagement and disengagement. *Nature* 1991;353:855–858.

140. Rocha B, Penit C, Baron C, Vasseur F, Dautigny N, Freitas AA. Accumulation of bromodeoxyuridine-labeled cells in central and peripheral lymphoid organs: minimal estimates of production and turnover rates of mature lymphocytes. *Eur J Immunol* 1990;20:1697–1708.

141. Stutman O. Postthymic T cell development. *Immunol Rev* 1986;91:159–194.

142. Rocha B, Dautigny N, Pereira P. Peripheral T lymphocytes: expansion potential and homeostatic regulation of pool sizes and CD4/CD8 ratios in vivo. *Eur J Immunol* 1989;19:905–911.

143. Miller RA, Stutman O. T cell repopulation from functionally restricted splenic precursors: 10,000 fold expansion documented by using limiting dilution analyses. *J Immunol* 1984;133:2925–2932.

144. Kappler JW, Hunter PC, Jacobs D, Lord E. Functional heterogeneity among the T-derived lymphocytes of the mouse. I. Analysis by adult thymectomy. *J Immunol* 1974;113:27–38.

145. Metcalf D. Delayed effect of thymectomy in adult life on immunological competence. *Nature* 1965;208:1336.

146. Miller JFAP. Effect of thymectomy in adult mice on immunological responsiveness. *Nature* 1965;208:1337–1338.

147. Ahmed R, Gray D. Immunological memory and protective immunity: understanding their relation. *Science* 1996;272:54–60.

148. Callahan JE, Kappler JW, Marrack P. Unexpected expansions of CD8-bearing cells in old mice. *J Immunol* 1993;151:6657–6669.

149. Posnett DN, Sinha R, Kabak S, Russo C. Clonal populations of T cells in normal elderly humans: the T cell equivalent to "benign monoclonal gammapathy" [published erratum appears in *J Exp Med* 1994 Mar 1;179(3):1077]. *J Exp Med* 1994;179:609–618.

150. Ruiz M, Esparza B, Barranquero M, Sabino E, Merino F. T cell receptor V-segment frequencies in aged individuals. *Immunol Invest* 1996;25:111–114.

151. Effros RB. Insights on immunological aging derived from the T lymphocyte cellular senescence model. *Exp Gerontol* 1996;31:21–27.

152. Schwab R, Szabo P, Manavalan JS, et al. Expanded CD4+ and CD8+ T cell clones in elderly humans. *J Immunol* 1997;158:4493–4499.

153. Chrest FJ, Buchholz MA, Kim YH, Kwon TK, Nordin AA. Anti-CD3-induced apoptosis in T-cells from young and old mice. *Cytometry* 1995;20:33–42.

154. Phelouzat MA, Arbogast A, Laforge T, Quadri RA, Proust JJ. Excessive apoptosis of mature T lymphocytes is a characteristic feature of human immune senescence. *Mech Ageing Dev* 1996;88:25–38.

155. Lechner H, Amort M, Steger MM, Maczek C, Grubeck-Loebenstein B. Regulation of CD95 (APO-1) expression and the induction of apoptosis in human T cells: changes in old age. *Int Arch Allergy Immunol* 1996;110:238–243.

156. Zharhary D, Klinman NR. Antigen responsiveness of the mature and generative B cell populations of aged mice. *J Exp Med* 1983;157:1300–1308.

157. Zharhary D, Klinman NR. A selective increase in the generation of phosphorylcholine-specific B cells associated with aging. *J Immunol* 1986;136:368–370.

158. Andersson J, Coutinho A, Melchers F. Frequencies of mitogen-reactive B cells in the mouse. I. Distribution in different lymphoid organs from different inbred strains of mice at different ages. *J Exp Med* 1977;145:1511–1530.

159. Hooijkaas H, Preesman AA, Van Oudenaren A, Benner R, Haaijman JJ. Frequency analysis of functional immunoglobulin C and V gene expression in murine B cells at various ages. *J Immunol* 1983;131:1629–1633.

160. Schulze DH, Mancillas P, Kaushik A, Bona C, Kelsoe G. Mitogen-induced V_H and V_K expression is similar in young adult and aged mice. *Aging: Immunol Infect Dis* 1992;3:127–134.

161. Whisler RL, Grants IS. Age-related alterations in the activation and expression of phosphotyrosine kinases and protein kinase C (PKC) among human B cells. *Mech Ageing Dev* 1993;71:31–46.

162. Whisler RL, Beiqing L, Newhouse YG, Walters JD, Breckenridge MB, Grants IS. Signal transduction in human B cells during aging: alterations in stimulus-induced phosphorylations of tyrosine and serine-threonine substrates and in cytosolic calcium responsiveness. *Lymphokine Cytokine Res* 1991;10:463–473.

163. Subbarao B, Morris J, Kryscio RJ. Phenotypic and functional properties of B lymphocytes from aged mice. *Mech Ageing Dev* 1990;51:223–241.

164. Weksler ME, Schwab R, Huetz F, Kim YT, Coutinho A. Cellular basis for the age-associated increase in autoimmune reactions. *Int Immunol* 1990;2:329–335.

165. Linton P-J, Klinman NR. Functionality of B-cell subsets in aged mice. *Aging: Immunol Infect Dis* 1993;4:135–137.

166. Gottesman SRS, Edington J, Tsiagbe VK, Thorbecke GJ. Influence of cytokines and the effect of aging on colony formation by B-cell subsets. *Aging: Immunol Infect Dis* 1993;4:197–211.

167. Linton P-J. The status of progenitors of memory B cells in aged mice. *Aging: Immunol Infect Dis* 1993;4:35–46.

168. Daynes RA, Araneo BA, Ershler WB, Maloney C, Li G-Z, Ryu S-Y. Altered regulation of interleukin-6 production with normal aging: possible linkage to the age-associated decline in dehydroepiandrosterone (DHEA) and its sulfated derivative. *J Immunol* 1993;150:5219–5230.

169. Goidl EA, Stashak PW, McEvoy SJM, Hiernaux JR. Age-related changes in serum immunoglobulin isotypes and isotype sub-class levels among standard long-lived and autoimmune and immunodeficient strains of mice. *Aging: Immunol Infect Dis* 1988;1:227–236.

170. Haaijman JJ, van den Berg P, Brinkhof J. Immunoglobulin class and subclass levels in the serum of CBA mice throughout life. *Immunology* 1977;32:923–927.

171. Albright JW, Holmes KL, Albright JF. Fluctuations in subsets of splenocytes and isotypes of Ig in young adult and aged mice resulting from Trypanosoma musculi infections. *J Immunol* 1990;144:3970–3979.

172. Lyngbye J, Kroll J. Quantitative immunoelectrophoresis of proteins in serum from a normal population: season-, age-, and sex-related variations. *Clin Chem* 1971;17:495–500.

173. French MAH, Harrison G. Serum IgG subclass concentrations in healthy adults: a study using monoclonal antisera. *Clin Exp Immunol* 1984;56:473–475.

174. Paganelli R, Quinti I, Fagiolo U, et al. Changes in circulating B cells and immunoglobulin classes and subclasses in a healthy aged population. *Clin Exp Immunol* 1992;90:351–354.

175. Ravichandran KS, Osborne BA, Goldsby RA. Quantitative analysis of the B cell repertoire by limiting dilution analysis and fluorescent in situ hybridization. *Cell Immunol* 1994;154:309–327.

176. Viale AC, Chies JA, Huetz F, et al. VH-gene family dominance in ageing mice. *Scand J Immunol* 1994;39:184–188.

177. Bangs LA, Sanz IE, Sanz JM. Comparison of D, J_H, and junctional diversity in the fetal, adult, and aged B cell repertoires. *J Immunol* 1991;146:1996–2004.

178. Nicoletti C, Cerny J. The repertoire diversity and magnitude of antibody responses to bacterial antigens in aged mice: I. Age-associated changes in antibody responses differ according to the mouse strain. *Cell Immunol* 1991;133:72–83.

179. Riley SC, Froscher BG, Linton PJ, Zharhary D, Marcu K, Klinman NR. Altered V_h gene segment utilization in the response to phosphorylcholine of aged mice. *J Immunol* 1989;143:3798–3805.

180. Nicoletti C, Borghesi-Nicoletti C, Yang X, Schulze DH, Cerny J. Repertoire diversity of antibody response to bacterial antigens in aged mice. II. Phosphorylcholine-antibody in young and aged mice differ in both V_H/V_L gene repertoire and in specificity. *J Immunol* 1991;147:2750–2755.

181. Nicoletti C, Yang X, Cerny J. Repertoire diversity of antibody response to bacterial antigens in aged mice. III. Phosphorylcholine antibody from young and aged mice differ in structure and protective activity against infection with Streptococcus pneumoniae. *J Immunol* 1993;150:543–549.

182. Goodwin JS, Searles RP, Tung KSK. Immunological responses of a healthy elderly population. *Clin Exp Immunol* 1982;48:403–410.

183. Hayashi Y, Utsuyama M, Kurashima C, Hirokawa K. Spontaneous development of organ-specific autoimmune lesions in aged C57BL/6 mice. *Clin Exp Immunol* 1989;78:120–126.

184. Fernandes G, Friend P, Yunis EJ, Good RA. Influence of dietary restriction on immunologic function and renal disease in (NZB × NZW) F1 mice. *Proc Natl Acad Sci USA* 1978;75:1500–1504.

185. Ben-Nun A, Ron Y, Cohen IR. Spontaneous remission of autoimmune encephalomyelitis is inhibited by splenectomy, thymectomy or ageing. *Nature* 1980;288:389–390.

186. Tomer Y, Mendlovic S, Kukulansky T, Mozes E, Shoenfeld Y, Globerson A. Effects of aging on the induction of experimental systemic lupus erythematosus (SLE) in mice. *Mech Ageing Dev* 1991;58:233–244.

187. Romball CG, Weigle WO. The effect of aging on the induction of experimental autoimmune thyroiditis. *J Immunol* 1987;139:1490–1495.

188. Riley RL, Kruger MG, Elia J. B cell precursors are decreased in senescent BALB/c mice, but retain normal mitotic activity in vivo and in vitro. *Clin Immunol Immunopathol* 1991;59:301–313.

189. Zharhary D. Age-related changes in the capability of the bone marrow to generate B cells. *J Immunol* 1988;141:1863–1869.

190. Francus T, Chen YW, Staiano-Coico L, Hefton JM. Effect of age on the capacity of the bone marrow and the spleen cells to generate B lymphocytes. *J Immunol* 1986;137:2411–2417.

191. Zharhary D. T cell involvement in the decrease of antigen-responsive B cells in aged mice. *Eur J Immunol* 1986;16:1175–1178.

192. Kim YT, Goidl EA, Samarut C, Weksler ME, Thorbecke GJ, Siskind GW. Bone marrow function. I. Peripheral T cells are responsible for the increased auto-anti-idiotype response of older mice. *J Exp Med* 1985;161:1237–1242.

193. Weksler ME, Russo C, Siskind GW. Peripheral T cells select the B-cell repertoire in old mice. *Immunol Rev* 1989;110:173–185.

194. Callard RE, Basten A. Immune function in aged mice. IV. Loss of T cell and B cell function in thymus-dependent antibody responses. *Eur J Immunol* 1978;8:552–558.

195. Liu JJ, Segre M, Segre D. Changes in suppressor, helper, and B-cell functions in aging mice. *Cell Immunol* 1982;66:372–382.

196. Li SP, Verma S, Miller RA. Age-related defects in T cell expression of CD40 ligand and induction of in vitro B cell activation. *Aging: Immunol Infect Dis* 1995;6:79–93.

197. Miller C, Kelsoe G, Han S. Lack of B7-2 expression in the germinal centers of aged mice. *Aging: Immunol Infect Dis* 1994;5:249–257.

198. Whisler RL, Williams JW Jr, Newhouse YG. Human B cell proliferative responses during aging. Reduced RNA synthesis and DNA replication after signal transduction by surface immunoglobulins compared to B cell antigenic determinants CD20 and CD40. *Mech Ageing Dev* 1991;61:209–222.

199. Coico RF, Gottesman SRS, Thorbecke GJ. Physiology of IgD. VIII. Age-related decline in the capacity to generate T cells with receptors for IgD and partial reversal of the defect with IL-2. *J Immunology* 1987;138:2776–2781.

200. Wei C-F, Wali A, Cherniack EP, et al. Correlation between the ability of elderly individuals to respond to influenza vaccination and the capacity of their peripheral blood lymphocytes to express receptors for IgD. *Aging: Immunol Infect Dis* 1992;3:195–202.

201. Yang X, Stedra J, Cerny J. Relative contribution of T and B cells to hypermutation and selection of the antibody repertoire in germinal centers of aged mice. *J Exp Med* 1996;183:959–970.

202. Miller C, Kelsoe G. Ig VH hypermutation is absent in the germinal centers of aged mice. *J Immunol* 1995;155:3377–3384.

203. Holmes KL, Schnizlein CT, Perkins EH, Tew JG. The effect of age on antigen retention in lymphoid follicles and in collagenous tissue of mice. *Mech Ageing Dev* 1984;25:243–255.

204. Szakal AK, Taylor JK, Smith JP, Kosco MH, Burton GF, Tew JG. Morphometry and kinetics of antigen transport and developing antigen retaining reticulum of follicular dendritic cells in lymph nodes of aging mice. *Aging: Immunol Infect Dis* 1988;1:7–22.

205. Burton GF, Kosco MH, Szakal AK, Tew JG. Iccosomes and the secondary antibody response. *Immunology* 1991;73:271–276.

206. Choi KL, Sauder DN. Epidermal Langerhans cell density and contact sensitivity in young and aged BALB/c mice. *Mech Ageing Dev* 1987;39:69–79.

207. Belsito DV, Derarkissian RM, Thorbecke GJ, Baer RL. Reversal by lymphokines of the age-related hyporesponsiveness to contact sensitization and reduced Ia expression on Langerhans cells. *Arch Dermatol Res* 1987;279:S76–S80.

208. Yuan A, Baird MA. Changes in the frequency and function of rat spleen dendritic cells occur with age. *Aging: Immunol Infect Dis* 1994;5:121–132.

209. Chen Y, Ramsey MA, Bradley SF. Differential monokine production by macrophages from aged mice stimulated with various microorganisms. *Aging: Immunol Infect Dis* 1993;4:155–167.

210. Chen Y, Bradley SF. Aging and eliciting agents: effect on murine peritoneal macrophage monokine bioactivity. *Exp Gerontol* 1993;28:145–159.

211. Wei J, Xu H, Davies JL, Hemmings GP. Increase of plasma IL-6 concentration with age in healthy subjects. *Life Sci* 1992;51:1953–1956.

212. Effros RB, Svoboda K, Walford RL. Influence of age and caloric restriction on macrophage IL-6 and TNF production. *Lymphokine Cytokine Res* 1991;10:347–351.

213. Fagiolo U, Cossarizza A, Scala E, et al. Increased cytokine production in mononuclear cells of healthy elderly people. *Eur J Immunol* 1993;23:2375–2378.

214. Foster KD, Conn CA, Kluger MJ. Fever, tumor necrosis factor, and interleukin-6 in young, mature, and aged Fischer 344 rats. *Am J Physiol* 1992;262:R211–R215.

215. Chorinchath BB, Kong LY, Mao L, McCallum RE. Age-associated differences in TNF-alpha and nitric oxide production in endotoxic mice. *J Immunol* 1996;156:1525–1530.

216. Bruley-Rosset M, Vergnon I. Interleukin 1 synthesis and activity in aged mice. *Mech Ageing Dev* 1984;24:247–264.

217. Delfraissy JF, Galanaud P, Wallon C, Balavoine JF, Dormont J. Abolished in vitro antibody response in elderly: exclusive involvement of prostaglandin-induced T suppressor cells. *Clin Immunol Immunopathol* 1982;24:377–385.

218. Goodwin JS, Messner RP. Sensitivity of lymphocytes to prostaglandin E2 increases in subjects over age 70. *J Clin Invest* 1979;64:434–439.

219. Sohnle PG, Larson SE, Collins-Lech C, Guansing AR. Failure of lymphokine-producing lymphocytes from aged humans to undergo activation by recall antigens. *J Immunol* 1980;124:2169–2174.

220. Meydani SN, Meydani M, Verdon CP, Shapiro AA, Blumberg JB, Hayes KC. Vitamin E supplementation suppresses prostaglandin E2 synthesis and enhances the immune response of aged mice. *Mech Ageing Dev* 1986;34:191–201.

221. Hayek MG, Meydani SN, Meydani M, Blumberg JB. Age differences in eicosanoid production of mouse splenocytes: effects on mitogen-induced T-cell proliferation. *J Gerontol* 1994;49:B197–207.

222. Pross HF, Baines MG. Studies of human natural killer cells. I. In vivo parameters affecting normal cytotoxic function. *Int J Cancer* 1982;29:383–390.

223. Weindruch R, Devens BH, Raff HV, Walford RL. Influence of dietary restriction and aging on natural killer cell activity in mice. *J Immunol* 1983;130:993–996.

224. Lanza E, Djeu JY. Age-independent natural killer cell activity in murine peripheral blood. In: Herberman RB, ed. *NK cells and other natural effectors*. New York: Academic Press, 1982:335–340.

225. Kawakami K, Bloom ET. Lymphokine-activated killer cells and aging in mice: significance for defining the precursor cell. *Mech Ageing Dev* 1987;41:229–240.

226. Ho SP, Kramer KE, Ershler WB. Effect of host age upon interleukin-2-mediated anti-tumor responses in a murine fibrosarcoma model. *Cancer Immunol Immunother* 1990;31:146–150.

227. Orentreich N, Brind JL, Rizer RL, Vogelman JH. Age changes and sex differences in serum dehydroepiandrosterone sulfate concentrations throughout adulthood. *J Clin Endocrinol Metab* 1984;59:551–555.

228. Barrett-Conner E, Khaw K-T, Yen SSC. A prospective study of dehydroepiandrosterone sulfate, mortality, and cardiovascular disease. *N Engl J Med* 1986;315:1519–1524.

229. Bulbrook RD, Hayward JL, Spicer CC. Relation between urinary androgen and corticoid secretion and subsequent breast cancer. *Lancet* 1971;2:395–398.

230. Barrett-Connor E, Goodman-Gruen D. Dehydroepiandrosterone sulfate does not predict cardiovascular death in postmenopausal women. The Rancho Bernardo Study. *Circulation* 1995;91:1757–1760.

231. Gordon GB, Bush TL, Helzlsouer KJ, Miller SR, Comstock GW. Relationship of serum levels of dehydroepiandrosterone and dehydroepiandrosterone sulfate to the risk of developing postmenopausal breast cancer. *Cancer Res* 1990;50:3859–3862.

232. Wichmann U, Wichmann G, Krause W. Serum levels of testosterone precursors, testosterone and estradiol in 10 animal species. *Exp Clin Endocrinol* 1984;83:283–290.

233. Araneo BA, Woods ML, Daynes RA. Reversal of the immunosenescent phenotype by dehyrdoepiandrosterone: hormone treatment provides an adjuvant effect on the immunization of aged mice with recombinant hepatitis B surface antigen. *J Infect Dis* 1993;167:830–840.

234. Araneo BA, Dowell T, Diegel M, Daynes RA. Dihydrotestosterone exerts a depressive influence on the production of interleukin-4 (IL-4), IL-5, and γ-interferon, but not IL-2 by activated murine T cells. *Blood* 1991;78:688–699.

235. Padgett DA, Loria RM. In vitro potentiation of lymphocyte activation by dehydroepiandrosterone, androstenediol, and androstenetriol. *J Immunol* 1994;153:1544–1552.

236. Pahlavani MA, Harris MD. Effect of dehydroepiandrosterone on mitogen-induced lymphocyte proliferation and cytokine production in young and old F344 rats. *Immunol Lett* 1995;47:9–14.

237. Araneo B, Dowell T, Woods ML, Daynes R, Judd M, Evans T. DHEAS as an effective vaccine adjuvant in elderly humans. Proof-of-principle studies. *Ann NY Acad Sci* 1995;774:232–248.

238. Yen SS, Morales AJ, Khorram O. Replacement of DHEA in aging men and women. Potential remedial effects. *Ann NY Acad Sci* 1995;774:128–142.

239. Ebihara S, Marks T, Hudson DJ, Menaker M. Genetic control of melatonin synthesis in the pineal gland of the mouse. *Science* 1986;231:491–493.

240. Maestroni GJ, Conti A, Pierpaoli W. The pineal gland and the circadian, opiatergic, immunoregulatory role of melatonin. *Ann NY Acad Sci* 1987;496:67–77.

241. Pierpaoli W, Regelson W. Pineal control of aging: effect of melatonin and pineal grafting on aging mice. *Proc Natl Acad Sci USA* 1994;91:787–791.

242. Caroleo MC, Doria G, Nistico G. Melatonin restores immunodepression in aged and cyclophosphamide-treated mice. *Ann NY Acad Sci* 1994;719:343–352.

243. Maestroni GJ, Conti A, Pierpaoli W. Role of the pineal gland in immunity: II. Melatonin enhances the antibody response via an opiatergic mechanism. *Clin Exp Immunol* 1987;68:384–391.

244. Cross RJ, Campbell JL, Markesbery WR, Roszman TL. Transplantation of pituitary grafts fail to restore immune function and to reconstitute the thymus glands of aged mice. *Mech Ageing Dev* 1990;56:11–22.

245. Khansari DN, Gustad T. Effects of long-term, low-dose growth hormone therapy on immune function and life expectancy of mice. *Mech Ageing Dev* 1991;57:87–100.

246. Fabris N, Pierpaoli W, Sorkin E. Lymphocytes, hormones and ageing. *Nature* 1972;240:557–559.

247. Cross RJ, Bryson JS, Roszman TL. Immunologic disparity in the hypopituitary dwarf mouse. *J Immunol* 1992;148:1347–1352.

248. Brown-Borg HM, Borg KE, Meliska CJ, Bartke A. Dwarf mice and the ageing process. *Nature* 1996;384:33.

249. Harrison DE, Archer JR, Astle CM. The effect of hypophysectomy on thymic aging in mice. *J Immunol* 1982;129:2673–2677.

250. Stutman O. Role of thymic hormones in T cell differentiation. *Clin Immunol Allergy* 1983;3:9–81.

251. Clinton M, Frangou-Lazaridis M, Panneerselvam C, Horecker BL. Prothymosin alpha and parathymosin: mRNA and polypeptide levels in rodent tissues. *Arch Biochem Biophys* 1989;269:256–263.

252. Ershler WB, Coe CL, Laughlin N, et al. Aging and immunity in non-human primates. II. Lymphocyte response in thymosin treated middle-aged monkeys. *J Gerontol* 1988;43:B142–B146.

253. Meroni PL, Barcellini W, Frasca D, et al. In vivo immunopotentiating activity of thymopentin in aging humans: increase of IL-2 production. *Clin Immunol Immunopathol* 1987;42:151–159.

254. Goso C, Frasca D, Doria G. Effect of synthetic thymic humoral factor (THF-gamma 2) on T cell activities in immunodeficient ageing mice. *Clin Exp Immunol* 1992;87:346–351.

255. Hiramoto RN, Ghanta VK, Soong SJ. Effect of thymic hormones on immunity and lifespan. In: Goidl E, ed. *Aging and the immune response*. New York: Marcel Dekker Inc, 1986:177–198.

256. Ghanta VK, Hiramoto NS, Soong SJ, Hiramoto RN. Survey of thymic hormone effects on physical and immunological parameters in C57Bl/6NNia mice of different ages. *Ann NY Acad Sci* 1991;621:239–255.

257. Haar JL, Taubenberger JK, Doane L, Kenyon N. Enhanced in vitro bone marrow cell migration and T-lymphocyte responses in aged mice given subcutaneous thymic epithelial cell grafts. *Mech Ageing Dev* 1989;47:207–219.

258. Chandra RK. Effect of vitamin and trace-element supplementation on immune responses and infection in elderly subjects. *Lancet* 1992;340:1124–1127.

259. Meydani SN, Barklund MP, Liu S, et al. Vitamin E supplementation enhances cell-mediated immunity in healthy elderly subjects [see comments]. *Am J Clin Nutr* 1990;52:557–563.

260. Mocchegiani E, Santarelli L, Muzzioli M, Fabris N. Reversibility of the thymic involution and of age-related peripheral immune dysfunctions by zinc supplementation in old mice. *Int J Immunopharmacol* 1995;17:703–718.

261. Remarque EJ, Witkamp L, Masurel N, Ligthart GJ. Zinc supplementation does not enhance antibody formation to influenza virus vaccine in the elderly. *Aging: Immunol Infect Dis* 1993;4:17–23.

262. Weindruch R, Walford RL. *The retardation of aging and disease by dietary restriction.* Charles C. Thomas Publisher, Springfield, IL: 1988.

263. Yu BP. Putative interventions. In: Masoro EJ, ed. *Handbook of physiology. Section 11: Aging.* New York: Oxford University Press, 1995:613–631.

264. Miller RA. Caloric restriction and immune function: developmental mechanisms. *Aging: Clin Exp Res* 1991;3:395–398.

265. Effros RB, Walford RL, Weindruch R, Mitcheltree C. Influences of dietary restriction on immunity to influenza in aged mice. *J Gerontol Biol Sci* 1991;46:B142–B147.

266. Grossmann A, Maggio-Price L, Jinneman JC, Wolf NS, Rabinovitch PS. The effect of long-term caloric restriction on function of T-cell subsets in old mice. *Cell Immunol* 1990;131:191–204.

267. Roecker EB, Kemnitz JW, Ershler WB, Weindruch R. Reduced immune responses in rhesus monkeys subjected to dietary restriction. *J Gerontol [A]* 1996;51A:B276–B279.

268. Bentley DM, Morris RE. T cell subsets required for protection against age-dependent polioencephalomyelitis of C58 mice. *J Immunol* 1982;128:530–534.

269. Orme IM, Griffin JP, Roberts AD, Ernst DN. Evidence for a defective accumulation of protective T cells in old mice infected with Mycobacterium tuberculosis. *Cell Immunol* 1993;147:222–229.

270. Patel PJ. Aging and antimicrobial immunity. Impaired production of mediator T cells as a basis for the decreased resistance of senescent mice to Listeriosis. *J Exp Med* 1981;154:821–831.

271. Utsuyama M, Albright JW, Holmes KL, Hirokawa K, Albright JF. Changes in the subsets of CD4+ T cells in Trypanosoma musculi infection: delay of immunological cure in young mice and the weak ability of aged mice to control the infection. *Int Immunol* 1994;6:1107–1115.

272. Powers DC. Influenza A virus-specific cytotoxic T lymphocyte activity declines with advancing age. *J Am Geriatr Soc* 1993;41:1–5.

273. McElhaney JE, Meneilly GS, Beattie BL, et al. The effect of influenza vaccination on IL2 production in healthy elderly: implications for current vaccination practices. *J Gerontol Med Sci* 1992;47:M3–M8.

274. Ashman RB. Persistence of cell-mediated immunity to influenza A virus in mice. *Immunology* 1982;47:165–168.

275. Orme IM. A mouse model of the recrudescence of latent tuberculosis in the elderly. *Am Rev Respir Dis* 1988;137:716–718.

276. Urban JL, Schreiber H. Rescue of the tumor-specific immune response of aged mice in vitro. *J Immunol* 1984;133:527–534.

277. Flood PM, Urban JL, Kripke ML, Schreiber H. Loss of tumor-specific and idiotype-specific immunity with age. *J Exp Med* 1981;154:275–290.

278. Ershler WB. The influence of an aging immune system on cancer incidence and progression. *J Gerontol Biol Sci* 1993;48:B3–B7.

279. Miller RA. Aging and cancer—another perspective. *J Gerontol Biol Sci* 1993;48:B8–B9.

280. Covelli V, Mouton D, Di Majo V, et al. Inheritance of immune responsiveness, life span, and disease incidence in interline crosses of mice selected for high or low multispecific antibody production. *J Immunol* 1989;142:1224–1234.

281. Miller RA, Turke P, Chrisp C, et al. Age-sensitive T cell phenotypes covary in genetically heterogeneous mice and predict early death from lymphoma. *J Gerontol* 1994;49:B255–B262.

282. Wayne SJ, Rhyne RL, Garry PJ, Goodwin JS. Cell-mediated immunity as a predictor of morbidity and mortality in subjects over 60. *J Gerontol Med Sci* 1990;45:M45–M48.

283. Goodman SA, Makinodan T. Effect of age on cell-mediated immunity in long-lived mice. *Clin Exp Immunol* 1972;19:533–542.

284. Murasko DM, Weiner P, Kaye D. Association of lack of mitogen-induced lymphocyte proliferation with increased mortality in the elderly. *Aging: Immunol Infect Dis* 1988;1:1–6.

285. Roberts-Thomson IC, Whittingham S, Youngchaiyud U, Mackay IR. Ageing, immune response, and mortality. *Lancet* 1974;2:368–370.

286. Mulvihill M, Cohen C, Martemucci W, et al. Anergy in the frail elderly is associated with an increased rate of infection and mortality. *Aging: Immunol Infect Dis* 1995;6:1–13.

287. Ferguson FG, Wikby A, Maxson P, Olsson J, Johansson B. Immune parameters in a longitudinal study of a very old population of Swedish people: a comparison between survivors and nonsurvivors. *J Gerontol A Biol Sci Med Sci* 1995;50:B378–B382.

288. Hori Y, Perkins EH, Halsall MK. Decline in phytohemagglutinin responsiveness of spleen cells from aging mice. *Proc Soc Exp Biol Med* 1973;144:48–53.

289. Murasko DM, Weiner P, Kaye D. Decline in mitogen induced proliferation of lymphocytes with increasing age. *Clin Exp Immunol* 1987;70:440–448.

290. Goidl EA, Innes JB, Weksler ME. Immunological studies of aging. II. Loss of IgG and high avidity plaque-forming cells and increased suppressor cell activity in aging mice. *J Exp Med* 1976;144:1037–1048.

291. Kishimoto S, Tsuyuguchi I, Yamamura Y. Immune responses in aged mice. *Clin Exp Immunol* 1969;5:525–530.

292. Bach MA. Lymphocyte-mediated cytotoxicity: effects of ageing, adult thymectomy and thymic factor. *J Immunol* 1977;119:641–647.

293. Tielen FJ, van Vliet AC, de Geus B, Nagelkerken L, Rozing J. Age-related changes in CD4+ T-cell subsets associated with prolonged skin graft survival in aging rats. *Transplant Proc* 1993;25:2872–2874.

294. Girard JP, Paychere M, Cuevas M, Fernandes B. Cell-mediated immunity in an ageing population. *Clin Exp Immunol* 1977;27:85–91.

Fundamental Immunology, Fourth Edition,
edited by William E. Paul
Lippincott–Raven Publishers, Philadelphia © 1999.

CHAPTER 29

Complement

Wolfgang M. Prodinger, Reinhard Würzner, Anna Erdei, and Manfred P. Dierich

A LOOK BACK IN HISTORY

W. M. Prodinger, R. Würzner, and M.P. Dierich: Institut für Hygiene, University of Innsbruck, Innsbruck, A 6020, Austria.

A. Erdei: Department of Immunology, Eötvös Lorand University, Göd, H-2131, Hungary.

In the beginning, i.e., in the second half of the 19th century, research on complement was intertwined with the investigation of humoral immunity and proceeded in parallel with the discovery of important bacterial pathogens (1). Nuttall, Buchner, and others contributed to the first major conceptual advance that a heat-labile fraction in normal serum (i.e., complement) and a heat-stable component of immune serum (i.e., antibody) were necessary for killing bacteria. Buchner named the labile fraction alexin (Greek for "without a name") and postulated an enzymatic mode of action for alexin. Bordet demonstrated a similar mode of action using lysis of erythrocytes by immune serum as a system that was fundamental for his development of the complement fixation test.

The term "complement" itself was coined by Paul Ehrlich in 1899, when he applied his *Seitenkettentheorie* (side-chain theory), which he had developed to explain immune bacteriolysis, to the understanding of hemolysis by sera of sensitized animals (2). "Complement" thus replaced "alexin." Ehrlich thought of complement as a group of factors that would not strictly rely on each other, whereas others (e.g., Bordet) considered complement a uniform substance. The chemical nature of complement was initially considered to be detergentlike or otherwise lipid destroying; the protein nature of complement components became clear much later. From this initial concept of complement (solely) as an effector mechanism of antibody, the entities of C1, C2, and C4 were the first to be differentiated by early biochemical methods until the 1920s. The proteins C3, C5, C6, C7, C8, and C9, however, were still thought of as one factor, as "classical C3."

A major step forward in the understanding of neglected aspects of complement was made by Louis Pillemer in the 1940s and 1950s. He extended previous findings with yeast cells and substances such as cobra venom, which activated complement in the absence of antibody. Pillemer demonstrated that classical C3 was consumed by zymosan, a yeast cell wall mannoprotein, without consumption of C1, C2, and C4 (3). In 1954, he postulated the existence of a serum factor he called properdin (Latin for "destruction-bringing") and understood the properdin system as a second, antibody-independent mode of complement activation (4). Pillemer's hypothesis was heavily criticized initially, and the controversy was ended for some time by his death. However, as the factors of the properdin system were isolated and characterized later on, this concept (now called the alternative pathway of complement activation) became accepted.

The role of C3 as the pivotal factor in both the classical and the alternative pathway and of C5 through C9 forming the terminal complex common to both became clear when classical C3 was biochemically dissected into the individual proteins during the 1960s. Hans Müller-Eberhard and his collaborators identified the C3 protein (according to the current nomenclature) as a major constituent of human plasma and also purified the components C5 to C9 (5). Robert Nelson's and Paul Klein's groups achieved the same for guinea pig C3 (6–8).

The concept of complement-mediated lysis was advanced by Manfred Mayer, who hypothesized that one complex containing all complement components is sufficient to lyse one red cell (9). His "doughnut hypothesis" later summarized results from several groups and postulated that C5b through C9 together formed a channel-like structure in the membrane (the membrane attack complex) (10). Since then, there has been a constant debate whether destruction of a nucleated cell is brought about by the pore character of the membrane attack complex (i.e., by osmotic swelling of the cell) or accomplished through destabilization of membrane integrity. This dispute is still unresolved because there is experimental evidence to support both contentions.

More recently, a second antibody-independent way of complement-activation, the mannan-binding lectin (MBL) pathway (named MBLectin pathway), has been established. MBL recognizes pathogens via their carbohydrate-rich exterior. MASP-2, a serine-esterase associated with MBL and cloned in 1997, is the youngest member in the family of complement proteins to date (11).

Besides research on the complement activation mechanism, there has been early recognition of its proinflammatory effects, such as opsonization and anaphylaxis. At the beginning of the 20th century it was noted that treatment with nonheated serum not only promoted lysis of bacteria, but also their clearance by phagocytosis. This nondestructive effect of serum causing improved uptake of bacteria by phagocytic cells was called opsonization (Greek for "preparation for ingestion"). Due to their heat-labile nature, the underlying serum factors were postulated to be related to complement early on, but proven to be mainly C3 fragments decades later. The existence of receptors for deposited complement components on cells was first postulated in 1953 by Nelson. He demonstrated that bacteria treated with immune serum gain the ability to bind to erythrocytes and called this phenomenon immune adherence. Complement receptors were subsequently identified on phagocytic cells and lymphocytes as well and shown to be specific for fragments of C3.

Heat lability also characterized anaphylaxis, a phenomenon observed after administration of immune complex–treated serum. Like opsonization, anaphylaxis was thus proposed to relate to complement. The generation of a complement-derived anaphylatoxin and another, chemotactic factor was proven by Boyden in the 1960s. These were finally characterized as C3a and C5a.

With the advent of molecular cloning in the early 1980s, the deduced amino-acid sequences were unraveled for all of the known human complement proteins, and the chromosomal locations of their genes have been clarified. The recognition of structural motifs conserved between the individual mosaic proteins allowed the definition of functional groups of components as well as a look back in evolution. Animals genetically deficient for a component as well as transgenic mice have been established and are a field of intense investigation.

Although there have been many contributions on involvement of complement in clinical disorders, it appears that only now, after 100 years of complement research including detailed biochemistry and molecular genetics, the role of complement in a broad spectrum of diseases becomes the focus of research. It concerns, among others, atherosclerosis, Alzheimer's disease, cancer, and, of course, infection and transplantation. It remains an unachieved goal to find ways to interfere with unwanted or excessive complement activation. Clinical use of recombinant proteins such as soluble CR1 or of humanized monoclonal antibodies has started, but to date there are no chemical substances at the disposal of clinical medicine that can selectively and effectively block individual components.

GENERAL OVERVIEW

As suggested by its name, complement serves as an auxiliary system in immunity, both on its own and by interaction with humoral immunity. On its own, it represents a primitive surveillance for microbes, independent from antibodies or T cells. During evolution, it became intertwined with the humoral immune system at multiple levels and now represents a major effector system for antibodies.

The complement system comprises more than 30 plasma or membrane proteins (Tables 1 and 2). Its activation as a whole relies initially on a cascade of proteolytic steps performed by serine pro-

TABLE 1. *Complement components: the plasma proteins involved in activation*

Component	Molecular weight in kDa of the intact protein (of subunits)	Concentration in plasma (μg/mL)
Common to all activation pathways		
C3	185 (α,110; β,75)	1,200–1,300
Alternative pathway		
Factor B	93	200
Factor D	24	2
Properdin (predominant oligomers)	110, 165, 200 (monomer: 55)	25
Classical pathway		
C1q	460 (six subunits with three chains each: A,26; B,26, C,24)	150
C1r	85	50
C1s	85	50
C4	205 (α,97; β,75; γ,33)	300–600
C2	102	20
MBLectin pathway		
MBL (predominant forms)	200, 300, 400 (two to four subunits with three chains of 32 kDa each)	1 (0.01–20)
MASP-1	100	1.5–12
MASP-2	76	nd
Terminal complement pathway		
C5	190 (α,115; β,75)	80
C6	110	45
C7	100	90
C8	150 (α,64; β,64; γ,22)	55
C9	70	60

MBL, mannan binding lectin; MASP, MBL-associated serine protease; nd, not determined.

TABLE 2. *Complement control proteins*

Component	Molecular weight in kDa of the intact protein (of subunits)	Concentration in plasma (μg/mL)
In plasma		
Factor I	88 (50 + 38)	35
Factor H	150	300–450
C1-INH	105	240
C4bp	550 (7 × 70, 1 × 45)	250
S protein (Vitronectin)	84	500
Clusterin (SP-40,40)	70 (35 + 35)	50
Carboxypeptidase N (anaphylatoxin inactivator)	280 (2 × 90, 2 × 50)	35
Related molecules with unclear function		
FHL-1	42	5–20
FHR-1, FHR-2	39/42, 24/29	40–60
FHR-3	55	nd
FHR-4	86	nd

Component (CD number)	Molecular weight (kDa) of the intact protein	Tissue distribution
On cell membranes		
CR1 (CD35)	190 (most common allotype)	(see Table 4)
DAF (CD55)	70	Very wide: peripheral blood cells (except NK cells), erythrocytes, epithelial and secretory cells, endothelial and mesenchymal cells
MCP (CD46)	45–70 (due to glycosylation)	Same as DAF (but not on erythrocytes)
CD59 antigen	18–20	Same as DAF

C1-INH, C1 Inhibitor; FHL, factor H–like protein; FHR, factor H–related protein; nd, not determined; CR, complement receptor; DAF, decay-accelerating factor; MCP, membrane cofactor protein.

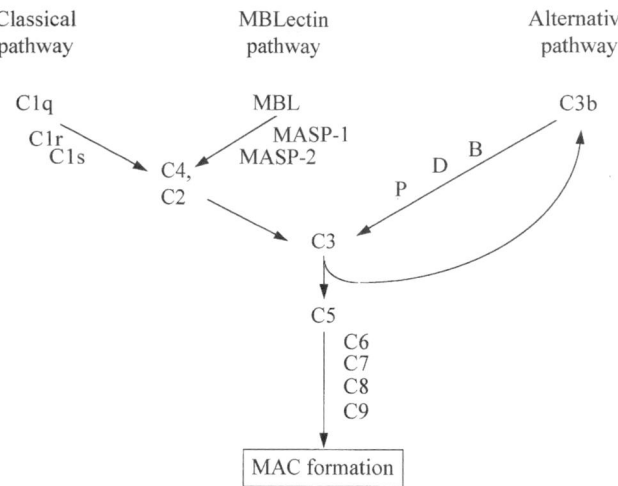

FIG. 1. Overview: the pathways of complement activation.

tease domains in the components involved. Three different pathways of activation have been recognized (Fig. 1), triggered by either target-bound antibody (the classical pathway), by polysaccharide structures of microbes (the MBLectin pathway) or by recognition of "foreign" surface structures by complement itself (the alternative pathway). All three merge into the pivotal activation of C3 and, subsequently, of C5. In the common terminal pathway, further complement components are activated in a nonproteolytic manner and assembled into the membrane attack complex (MAC), which can directly bring about lysis of a microbe.

Such a powerful machinery needs safe, redundant control mechanisms. Therefore, about half of the complement components serve for controlling the critical steps in activation, especially those dealing with C3b generation. In addition to direct killing of microbes by the MAC, complement recruits other branches of the host's defense system (Fig. 2). Opsonization, the coating of microbes with C3 fragments, leads to their uptake into phagocytic cells via complement receptors. The solubility of immune complexes and the immunogenicity of antigens are improved by attachment to C3 fragments. On the other hand, cells of the unspecific defense system (like neutrophils, macrophages, or mast cells) become stimulated by the anaphylatoxins, small peptides generated in the course of proteolytic complement activation.

COMPLEMENT

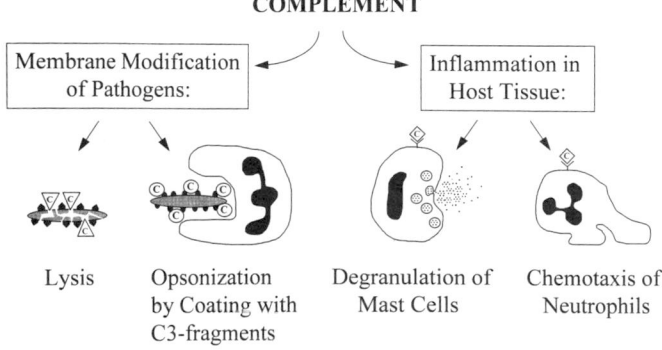

FIG. 2. Overview: the contributions of complement activation to infection control.

COMPLEMENT NOMENCLATURE

Due to historical reasons the components of the classical and terminal pathways are numbered from C1 to C9, with the biochemical reaction sequence being C1-C4-C2-C3-C5-C6-C7-C8-C9. Additional proteins operating in the alternative pathway are called factors and distinguished by letters (factors B, D, H, I, P). Up to C5, activation involves a proteolytic cleavage step, liberating smaller fragments from C2 through C5, which in part exert biologic effects. The larger fragments remain bound in a complex required for the next activation step. By convention, the smaller fragments are denoted by the letter a (e.g., C3a, C5a), the larger by b (e.g., C3b), with the notable exception being C2 (C2a is the larger, active fragment). For C3 and C4, inactivation of C3b or C4b yields smaller fragments (not participating further in complement activation), denoted C3c, C3d, etc. The activation products must not be confused with the terms denoting the protein chains in molecules consisting of disulfide-linked chains, such as C3, C4, and C5, which are indicated by Greek letters (e.g., C3α). Still different is the classification of the two allelic forms of the C4 gene, C4A and C4B. The encoded isotypic proteins C4A and C4B differ in characteristic amino acid residues, which determine the preference of the thioester bond to react with either amino groups (C4A) or hydroxyl groups (C4B) on acceptor molecules. The nomenclature of C3 convertases used here is according to Müller-Eberhard (12). The membrane proteins in the complement system are named under several points of view: either by the function they exert (e.g., decay accelerating factor [DAF]) or by using the cluster of differentiation (CD) system (e.g., CD55 for DAF). The four complement receptors are also simply numbered consecutively (CR1 to CR4).

BIOSYNTHESIS OF COMPLEMENT: LOCATION AND REGULATION

The liver is the major site of production for complement proteins. About 90% of the plasma complement components are synthesized in the liver (13). Only few components have their origin predominantly outside of the liver: C1 in the intestinal epithelium and monocytes/macrophages, and factor D in adipose tissue. C7 of hepatic origin was found to contribute less than 60% to plasma C7 (14,15). Bone marrow–derived cells, particularly granulocytes, apparently represent a major source of plasma C7 (15,16). The main source for plasma properdin has not yet been identified (13).

In addition to the liver, complement component biosynthesis has been detected in many other organs and cell types, such as monocytes/macrophages, endothelial cells, lymphocytes, glial cells, renal epithelium, reproductive organs and many others. Notably, production of virtually all components has been observed in monocytes/macrophages and, interestingly, in astrocytes (17). The contribution of extrahepatic complement production has not been clearly defined: as for astrocytes or other glial cells, they are the only source for complement beyond an intact blood–brain barrier. Hence, the role of complement in the brain is an emerging field of interest in several, primarily noninfectious diseases. Macrophages, by their presence in an activated state at sites of infection, may add to the locally effective levels of complement.

Complement production is augmented in the acute-phase response that follows tissue injury. This pertains to most components, although the extent of induction varies substantially (from about three- to 50-fold). The main common transcriptional inducer of complement genes is interferon (IFN)-γ, with other important acute-phase mediators being interleukin (IL)-1– and IL-6–type cytokines (IL-1α, IL-1β, tumor necrosis factor [TNF]-α, IL-6, IL-11, and others) (18).

Membrane-anchored complement regulators are expressed on a variety of tissues (13). Even complement receptors are widely distributed, although expression may be weak and noticed only upon cell activation.

GENETIC FAMILIES AND STRUCTURAL MOTIFS AMONG COMPLEMENT COMPONENTS

Proteins Endowed with an Internal Thioester

C3, C4, and C5 are proteins considered to be evolutionarily derived from one ancestral protein. Upon proteolytic cleavage at a conserved site during complement activation, they undergo a gross conformational change associated with the exposition of several new epitopes and (in C3 and C4) the ability to covalently bind to other molecules. This capability is linked with the formation of an internal thioester in the native molecule between a glutamyl residue and a cysteine two residues apart (Fig. 3) (19). This thioester is present in C3, C4, and the related α2 macroglobulin, but has been lost in C5 during evolution. Hidden in the native proteins, the thioester is exposed upon activation to react with the NH_2 or OH residues of surrounding molecules. The two isotypic forms of C4, C4A and C4B, differ by the presence and absence, respectively, of a histidine 115 amino acids downstream, which acts as the catalyst for the formation of ester bonds. Hence, C4B and C3, which behaves similar to C4B, preferentially form ester bonds with OH residues, whereas C4A forms amide bonds with NH_2-groups (19). It has been suggested that formation during biosynthesis needs the presence of chaperone molecules that may be different for the individual thioester proteins (19).

Proteins with Short Consensus Repeats

The regulator of complement activation (RCA) gene cluster comprises the genes for factor H and related proteins of the factor H family, for C4bp (several loci), and for DAF, CR2, CR1, and MCP (20). The RCA proteins consist of four to 34 short consensus repeats (SCRs) (Fig. 4), eventually in addition to short transmem-

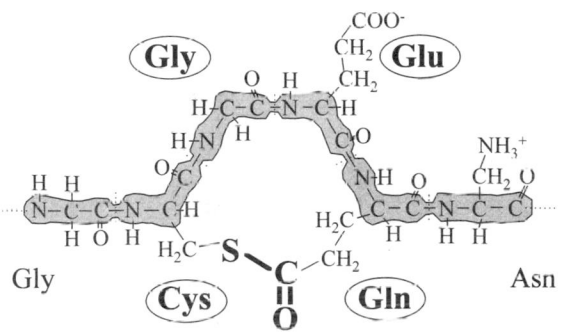

FIG. 3. The thioester region of human C3: the backbone of peptide bonds (*shaded*) and the four amino acids forming the thiolactone ring (*oncircled*). The thioester bond is shown in bold print.

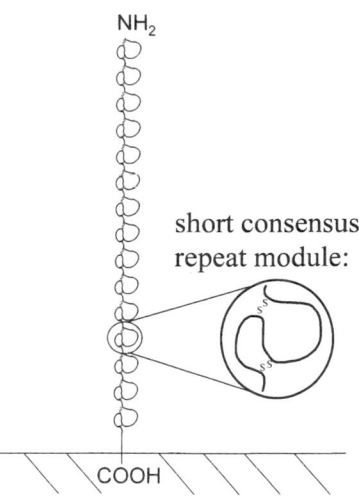

FIG. 4. The structure of the SCR and of SCR-based complement regulators (e.g., for CR2).

brane and intracytoplasmic parts (CR1, CR2, MCP) or glycosylphosphatidylinositol (GPI) anchors, as in the case of DAF (21). The consensus SCR is a globular domain of about 60 amino acids, with distinct conserved residues, e.g., tryptophane, prolines, or, most importantly, four cysteines that form two disulfide bonds (Cys_1 to Cys_3 and Cys_2 to Cys_4) (22). The RCA proteins are elongated in shape, with CR1 and CR2 extending 90 and 28 nm, respectively, from the cell membrane (Fig. 4). Electron microscopy has shown the plasma protein factor H to have an elongated, hairpinlike structure.

The RCA gene cluster is thought to have evolved from one ancestral prototypic SCR by duplication and gene conversion events as a family of genes for proteins controlling C3 and C4 activation (23). Interestingly, though, binding of activated C3/C4 can be attributed only to a few distinct SCRs in each RCA member (24). Few SCRs are present in mosaic proteins such as factor B, C2, C1r, C1s, MASP-1, MASP-2, C6, and C7, all of which interact with C3/C4/C5. SCRs are also found in noncomplement proteins as factor XIIIB of the clotting system, IL-2 receptor α chain (CD25) and selectins. Because each SCR is usually encoded by a separate exon, these combinations of domains can be seen as the result of exon shuffling.

Modified Serine Proteases

Serine proteases are crucially involved in the early, amplifying steps of complement activation. Serine protease domains are present in C1r, C1s, MASP-1, MASP-2, C2, factor B, factor I, factor D, and many other noncomplement enzymes (e.g., trypsin).

Thrombospondinlike Repeats Containing Proteins

A 30–amino acid module also found in the extracellular matrix protein thrombospondin is present in constituents of the terminal pathway and in properdin (25). C6 has three thrombospondinlike repeats (TSRs), C7, C8α, and C8β all have two TSRs; and C9 possesses a single TSR module. Six tandem TSRs are found in properdin. These proteins have amphiphilic character, allowing them to act in plasma and on lipid membranes, which is the important feature for MAC formation.

Members of Other Structural Families

Serpins comprise proteins acting as serine protease inhibitors. Among the many serine proteases active in the complement system, only C1s and C1r are inhibited by a serpin, namely C1 inhibitor (C1-INH).

MBL is a collectin, a lectin with structural resemblance to collagen in the stalk parts of its subunits. Although C1q does not bind to carbohydrates, it is structurally related to the collectins, primarily MBL. Both form collagenous and globular domains and share the feature of assembly from several identical subunits.

C9, apart from including a TSR, is homologous to perforin, the pore-forming protein of cytotoxic T cells and natural killer cells. The terminal pathway components also comprise one low density lipoprotein-receptor domain and one epidermal growth factor (EGF) module.

CR3 and CR4 belong to the large integrin family of heterodimeric proteins. Their β chain is of the β2-integrin type, which is also present in leukocyte function antigen-1. Integrins are mainly involved in cell–cell and cell–matrix interactions. CR3 and CR4 have similar properties as well.

The receptors for the anaphylatoxins C3a and C5a belong to the G-protein–linked receptors (seven-pass transmembrane receptors), which cross the cell membrane seven times with α-helical stretches and are coupled to (intracellular) G proteins.

COMPLEMENT ACTIVATION: THE PIVOTAL ROLE OF C3 ACTIVATION

Activation of C3 by cleavage to C3b is the pivotal reaction in the activation cascade (Fig. 5). This reaction is common to all three activating pathways and catalyzed by two different C3 convertases. Although some other proteases (like plasmin) or toxins (e.g., cobra venom factor) can activate C3, the C3 convertases are the only physiologically relevant effectors. Of all complement components, C3 is present in the highest concentration (1 to 1.4 mg/ml plasma) and is one of the most abundant plasma proteins. Due to the presence of an intramolecular thioester, C3, together with its closest relative C4, is the only component able to form covalent bonds with various targets.

It appears that the complement system has evolved around the capability of this protein (or its ancestor) to covalently bind to other molecules. An ancestral C3 protein might have resembled the thioester-containing protease inhibitor α2 macroglobulin, which binds covalently to various proteases if they cleave α2 macroglobulin and hence induce its active conformation.

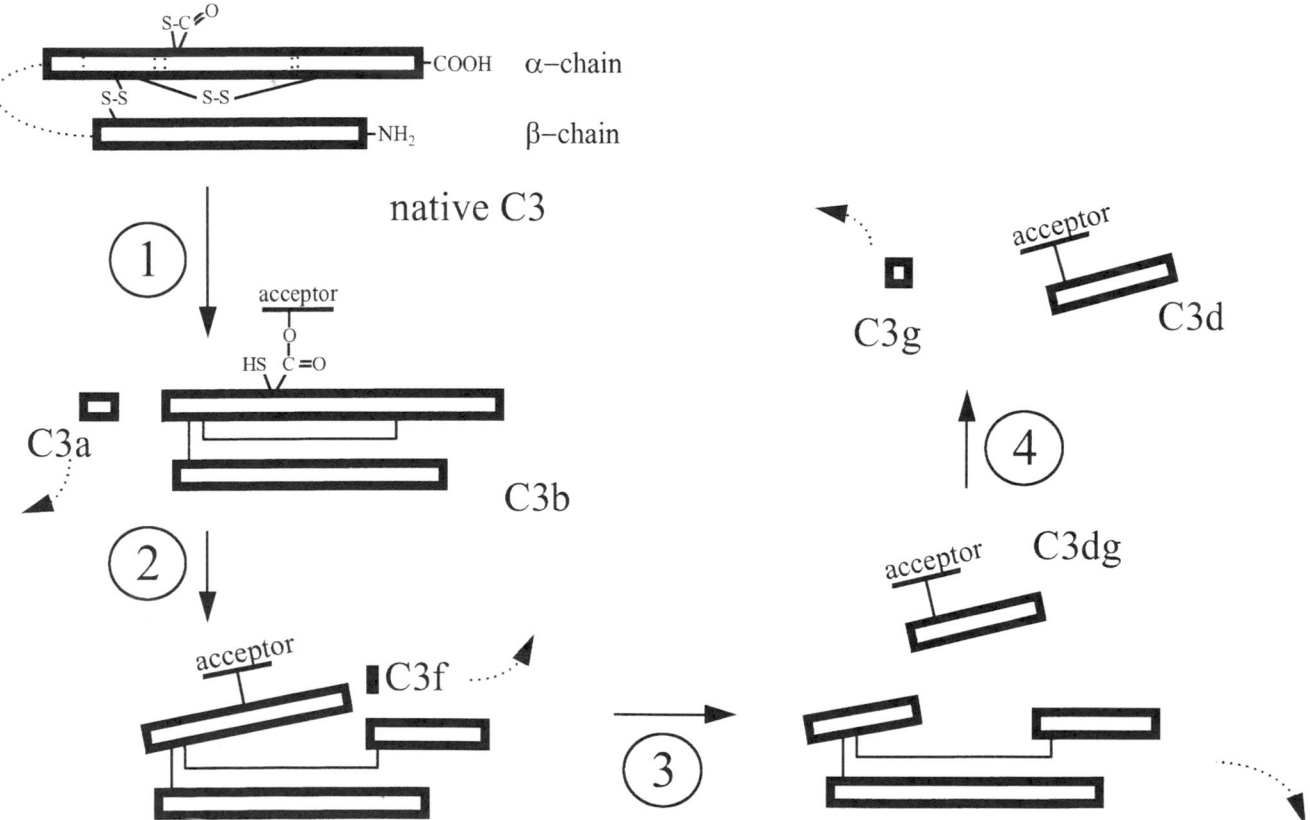

FIG. 5. Activation, inactivation, and degradation of C3. (**1**) Activation of native C3 by C3 convertases yields C3b (bound to an acceptor molecule) and C3a. (**2**) C3b is inactivated to iC3b by factor I and a cofactor that cleaves off C3f. (**3**) iC3b is further degraded by factor I and CR1 to C3dg and C3c. (**4**) Acceptor-bound C3dg is trimmed by plasma proteases to C3d.

Four functional entities act on C3 and its derivatives:

1. The C3 convertases, two homologous enzymatic complexes (C3b,Bb and C4b,2a, respectively) that consist of an activated serine protease and C3b or C4b; they activate native C3 by cleaving it into C3a and C3b.
2. Factor I, a plasma serine protease specific for C3b (and C4b); it inactivates C3b (and C4b) by cleaving it into iC3b (and iC4b). Factor I requires a cofactor.
3. Proteins of the RCA family consisting of four to 34 SCRs; they negatively regulate C3 (and/or C4) activation by disintegrating the convertases and serving as cofactors for factor I.
4. The receptors for fragments of C3, comprising genetically unrelated proteins such as integrins, seven-pass transmembrane proteins, or RCA family members; they exploit the remnants of C3 activation for the activation or attraction of cells (e.g., in opsonophagocytosis).

Through the action of either C3 convertase, the native C3 molecule is cleaved at a specific arginine residue in the α chain into C3a and C3b. The peptide C3a (77 amino acids) is a potent anaphylatoxin and exerts its effects more distant from the site of C3 activation. The major part, nascent C3b, acts within its life span of 60 microseconds. Nascent C3b immediately changes its conformation and exposes the buried internal thioester bond. Via the now highly reactive thioester, nascent C3b is enabled to bind covalently to proper nucleophils, either OH or NH_2 groups of any surrounding molecule (termed acceptor molecule), including H_2O molecules.

THE ALTERNATIVE PATHWAY

Phylogenetically the oldest of the C3-activating pathways, the alternative pathway represents the first line in defense against invading microorganisms (Table 1 and Fig. 6). It can be activated

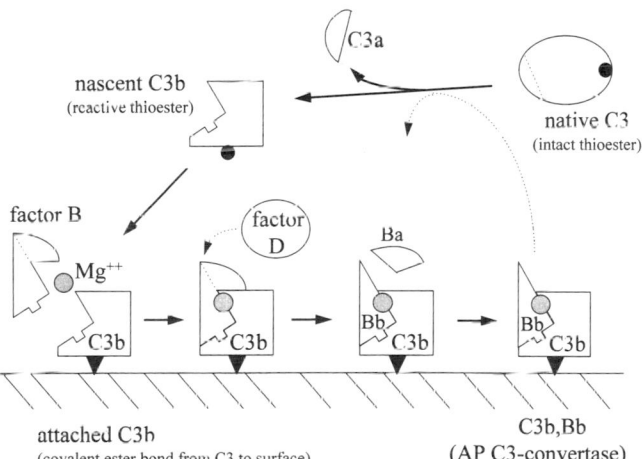

FIG. 6. C3b amplification by the alternative pathway (AP). By action of the alternative pathway, C3 convertase C3b,Bb native C3 is activated, changes its conformation, and exposes the reactive thioester (●). Some of the nascent C3b attaches covalently to an activator surface via the thioester (▼), where it associates with factor B in the presence of Mg^{2+}. Bound factor B is cleaved by factor D, Ba is released, and Bb remains bound to C3b, thus forming a new AP C3 convertase.

and amplified instantaneously in the presence of foreign (nonself) material. The alternative pathway defines "foreign" by other criteria, as do antibodies, and hence represents a primitive immune system on its own. An ancestral alternative pathway system was probably present about 500 million of years ago and is found in the most primitive vertebrates like lamprey and hagfish (23). Circumstantial evidence supports the existence of a primitive alternative pathway or a C3 analog in nonvertebrates like the horseshoe crab or even insects, possibly linked to an ancestral humoral immune system based on recognition of (foreign) carbohydrates.

After the evolution of the immunoglobulin system, it became as a new trigger to the old effectors through the classical pathway.

The proteins participating in the alternative pathway are C3 (and C3b) and the factors B and D. These proteins can establish a positive feedback loop of C3 activation (the C3b amplification loop). Properdin (factor P) favors the amplification loop by stabilizing the convertase C3b,Bb. Proteins controlling the alternative pathway are factor I (together with its cofactors factor H, CR1 and MCP) and DAF.

Initiation by iC3

A longstanding conceptual problem was to explain generation of the first C3b. From in vitro experience rather then from plasma level measurements, the concept of alternative pathway was formulated that relies on the initiation by inactive C3 (iC3 or C3b-like C3).

This concept is based on a continuous background turnover of native C3 into iC3 (termed "tickover of C3"). iC3 results from spontaneous reaction of the internal thioester bond with water [hence its former name $C3(H_2O)$]. Thus, iC3 represents uncleaved, but hemolytically inactive C3 with C3b-like conformation. iC3 forms in plasma at a constant low rate, and its actual presence in plasma has been proved years after being postulated and was shown to be 0.5% of the amount of native C3 (26).

iC3 can associate with factor B in a Mg^{2+}-dependent reaction. In this complex, the zymogen factor B is accessible to cleavage by factor D. The enzymatically active Bb fragment remains attached to iC3, thus forming iC3,Bb, the initial C3 convertase of the alternative pathway. It is thought that this initial convertase is constantly formed in the fluid phase but has a very short half-life. iC3,Bb is quickly disassembled by factor H, and iC3 is readily cleaved by factor I in analogy to C3b (Fig. 5). Nevertheless, this would still allow the generation of some nascent C3b molecules that could attach at random to nearby plasma or surface molecules.

The fate of such a surface-bound C3b molecule would be determined by the activator or nonactivator character of the surface. Whether a particle is an activator (evoking massive C3 activation and C3b deposition on its surface) or a nonactivator (effectively limiting this reaction) is determined by the relative affinities of bound C3b to factor H, the negative regulator, and factor B, the positive regulator of the alternative pathway. The ratio of factor H to factor B affinity is mainly influenced by the decreased affinity of factor H to activator surfaces (about tenfold less), whereas factor B affinity is similar to activator or nonactivator surfaces.

Amplification of C3b by the Alternative Pathway on Activator Surfaces

With a first C3b molecule randomly attached to an activator surface, however, amplification of C3b proceeds rapidly (Fig. 6).

First, factor B associates with C3b in the presence of Mg^{2+} and is activated by factor D, a serine protease present in plasma in minute amounts. Factor D is brought into its active conformation through recognition of its substrates, C3b,B or iC3,B (27). After generating C3b,Bb and releasing Ba, factor D returns to its inactive state. The surface-attached C3b,Bb activates further C3 molecules, and some of the new nascent C3b will attach again to the surface. C3b,Bb remains active as long as Bb remains bound to C3b, and properdin stabilizes the convertase against decay by binding to both Bb and C3b.

Inactivation of C3b on Nonactivator Surfaces

On nonactivator surfaces such as host cell membranes, the binding of factor H is promoted by its affinity to negatively charged residues like multiple sialic acid molecules. Their presence on the carbohydrate part of glycoproteins allows C3b bound to host cells to be quickly bound to factor H and subsequently cleaved by factor I. Factor H also can dissociate C3b,Bb enzymes, which have eventually formed on nonactivators or which are present in the fluid phase (see section on "Control of the Complement System" and Fig. 10).

THE CLASSICAL PATHWAY

Proteins of the Classical Pathway

The proteins forming the activation cascade of the classical pathway comprise C1, C4, C2, and C3, in that order (Table 1 and Figs. 1 and 7). C1 inhibitor (C1-INH), C4-binding protein (C4bp), CR1, factor I, DAF, and MCP function as control proteins.

C1 is a large molecule (MW = 750 kDa) consisting of one C1q molecule noncovalently associated with two C1r and two C1s molecules (Fig. 7). Calcium ions are required for formation of this stable complex, $C1q(C1r)_2(C1s)_2$. In plasma, about 70% of the C1 components are present in C1 complexes at a given time. The C1q protein is assembled from six identical subunits, each of which consists of three homologous chains (A, B, and C). The chains form a globular domain at one end, a neck portion, and a stalk part where the three α-helices are twisted around each other and, like in the collagen molecule, form a coil. The six subunits are held together in their collagen-like parts. This appearance of C1q is often likened to "a bouquet of six tulips." The globular domains of C1q bind to the Fc portion of immunoglobulins. A similar overall structure applies to MBL.

C1q interacts with C1r and C1s in its stalk part. The $C1r_2C1s_2$ tetramer has been shown by electron microscopy to form a linear chain of subcomponents (28). Each C1s and C1r possesses a serine protease domain (catalytic domain) and a contact domain. Before activation, all four catalytic domains are placed inside the cone-shaped stalk part of C1q (Fig. 7).

Complement Activation via the Classical Pathway

Physiologically most important, activation of C1 is initiated by its binding to antigen-bound IgG or IgM. Nevertheless, other triggers of C1 activation besides immunoglobulins have been found and include bacterial lipopolysaccharide (LPS), polyanionic compounds, myelin, the acute-phase reactant C-reactive protein, and some viruses (e.g., human immunodeficiency virus [HIV]-1). When binding to immunoglobulin, C1q recognizes the Fc region, which has undergone conformational alteration upon binding to

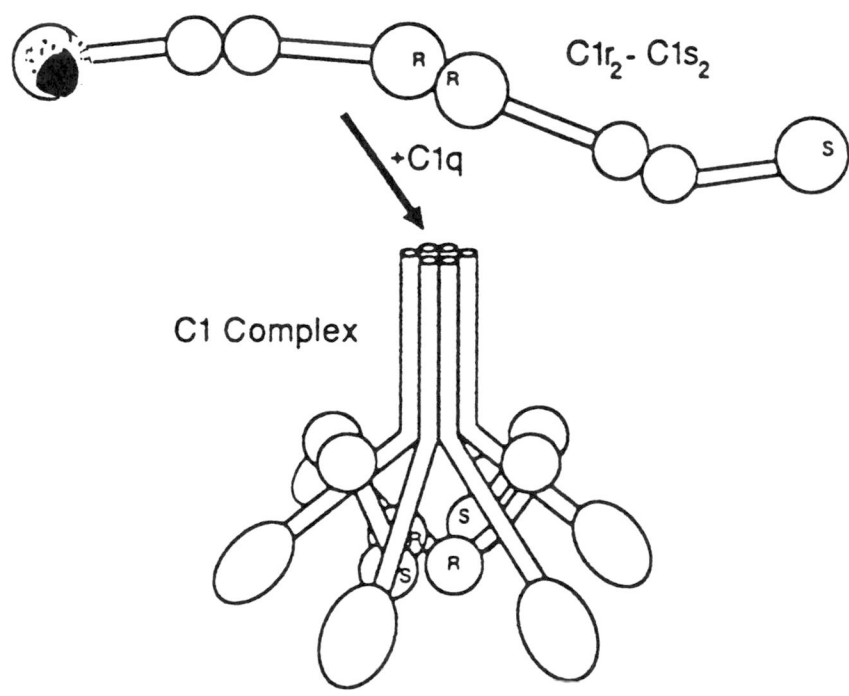

FIG. 7 The C1 complex. The model for the C1 complex proposes that the folding of the rodlike C1r2-C1s2 around the arms of C1q causes the catalytic domains of C1s to contact the catalytic domains of C1r.

antigen. C1q must at least bind with two of its six C-terminal globular domains, one IgM (having five Fc regions per molecule) or at least two IgG molecules are required to trigger complement activation, and they must be in sufficient proximity (not more than 40 nm apart). Therefore, with IgG the activation of C1 will only be effective on surfaces with a critical density of bound antibodies. Among human IgG subclasses, the potential for C1q binding increases in the order IgG4 < IgG2 < IgG1 < IgG3.*

The positions of the serine esterase domains of the two C1r relative to each other change due to conformational alteration of C1q after immunoglobulin binding. This allows for reciprocal cleavage of the C1r molecules. Activated C1r then cleaves (activates) C1s, which is the enzyme activating C4 and C2. Cleavage of C1r and C1s does not liberate proteolytic fragments.

C1s and C1r are tightly controlled by C1-INH in the unbound C1 molecule, which tends toward autoactivation. Activated C1r and C1s are rapidly inactivated by covalent binding of C1-INH to both in a stoichiometric relationship [yielding two C1rC1s(C1-INH)$_2$ molecules per C1]. Nevertheless, although the half-life of active C1 is thus very short, one active C1 molecule can cleave about 35 C4 molecules due to its low K_m value and the high plasma concentration of C4 (29). C4 is cleaved into the short C4a fragment, which exhibits low chemotactic activity, and the large C4b, which undergoes a gross change in conformation. As a result, the internal thioester region within C4b is exposed and forms covalent amide or ester bonds with surrounding molecules (proteins, carbohydrates, water). These reactions take place within microseconds (19). Most of the nascent C4b gets lost by reacting with water, but about 5% of C4b becomes covalently attached to the particle surface in the immediate vicinity of the focus of the activating immunoglobulin–C1 complex (30). In this way a cell or particle surface becomes covered with C4b clustered around central C1 molecules.

Due to its lower plasma concentration, activation of C2 proceeds less effectively than C4 activation (12). About four C2 molecules are activated during the life span of one active C1 molecule. C2 compensates for this by forming an Mg^{2+}-dependent complex with C4b. In this complex, C2 is accessible for cleavage by C1s into C2a (larger fragment remaining associated to C4b) and C2b (liberated smaller fragment exhibiting kinin activity). Free C2 is much less likely to be cleaved by C1s. C2a is the enzymatically active fragment in C4b,2a, the classical pathway C3 convertase. It is active only as long as it is associated with C4b, and once dissociated, it cannot bind to C4b again. The C3 convertase activates C3 and contributes to C5 activation, which then initiates the terminal pathway.

Role of the Classical Pathway

The classical pathway is the phylogenetically youngest among the three activation pathways. It developed after the emergence of the immunoglobulin system in the vertebrates as a potent effector mechanism for humoral immunity. The formation of specific antibodies requires several days, during which defense against infection has to rely on natural immunity: the alternative and MBLectin pathway, opsonization and phagocytosis, other plasma defense proteins (CRP, α2 macroglobulin), and NK cells. By triggering C3 activation via the C1-C4-C2 cascade, Ig combines the effective C3b amplification loop of the older alternative pathway and the formation of membrane attack complexes with a much more potent release mechanism.

THE MBLECTIN PATHWAY (OR LECTIN PATHWAY)

The concept of the MBLectin pathway of complement activation has emerged only recently (see Fig. 1). Its main constituent is the plasma protein mannan-binding lectin (also called mannose-binding lectin), MBL (31).†

MBL is a protein of the collectin family, meaning that it comprises collagenous structures (α-helical parts of three subunit chains twisted around each other to form a coiled-coil bundle) and also functions as lectin. This means it recognizes specific carbohydrate residues by the C-terminal globular part of each subunit chain. MBL is a C-type lectin that binds to its preferred sugars dependent on Ca^{2+}. Among other collectin family members are the lung surfactant proteins SP-D and SP-A and the bovine serum protein conglutinin. The overall structures of the individual collectins are quite different, with MBL resembling C1q in its "bouquet of tulips" appearance. Although C1q is not further included in the collectin family, C1q and the collectins share several features: the subunit structure with its collagenous part and its C-terminal globular domains and the assembly of several subunits by disulfide bonds into the final molecule.

MBL has originally been characterized in other species (33). Human MBL is present in plasma as a mixture of oligomers of its subunit with trimers/tetramers and pentamers/hexamers, constituting approximately 80% and 15% of the pool, respectively (34). MBL levels increase during an acute-phase response by about threefold, which is a less strong induction than seen with several other acute-phase proteins (35). Normal plasma levels also differ substantially between individuals (10 µg/ml to 20 µg/ml; see Table 1) and are genetically determined (36,37). Additionally, distinct allelic forms of MBL are known to be differently effective with respect to complement activation. It is thought that these quantitative and qualitative differences influence predisposition to infections. In fact, deficiency in MBL had been recognized as a functional defect of serum in some patients much earlier and termed defective yeast opsonization (38). The underlying molecule and mechanism, however, was unraveled only recently, when MBL was shown to activate the classical pathway (39).

MBL does so after binding with its globular heads (the carbohydrate recognition domain [CRD]) to sugar residues like N-acetylglucosamin or mannose. Because the ligand affinity of the individual CRD is low (K_d of approximately 10^{-3} M), MBL will only bind if several of its CRDs become attached to oligo- or polysaccharide residues. Such repetitive carbohydrate patterns are often encountered with LPS or other microbial surface structures. The distance between the individual CRDs is big enough not to allow binding of one MBL to a single mammalian glycoprotein (31). On the other

---

*Some mouse immunoglobulin subclasses can also activate human complement, which is exploited for selective killing of human cells by monoclonal antibodies and human serum (e.g., to achieve pure preparations of lymphocyte subsets). However, the isotype order is different from that of humans.

†Because MBL is the only lectin to activate complement, the term "MBLectin pathway" was suggested by C. Janeway as a substitute for "lectin pathway." The former terms for MBL, mannan-binding protein or mannose-binding protein (MBP), were proposed to be discontinued to avoid confusion with maltose-binding protein or myelin basic protein (32).

hand, several pathogens have been shown to bind MBL, e.g., *Salmonella, Listeria, Neisseria* species or *Candida albicans,* and *Cryptococcus neoformans,* whereas the presence of a bacterial capsule significantly impairs MBL binding (31). A conformational change accompanying ligand binding leads to activation of two MBL-associated serine proteases, MASP-1 and MASP-2 (11). MASP-1 and MASP-2 are both homologous to C1r and C1s, emphasizing the analogy between MBL and C1q. Active MASP-2, like C1s, activates C4 and leads to C1-independent formation of classical pathway C3 convertase C4b,2a. Control of the MBL pathway seems to be exerted through α2-macroglobulin and C1-INH, both of which can bind covalently to the activated MBLectin/ MASP complexes (40,41). In contrast to the C1 complex, very little is known about the sites involved in complex formation between MBL and MASP-1/MASP-2 to date.

Complement activation is not the only contribution of MBL to host defense. Bound MBL is recognized by the collectin receptor (42). Because the affinity of MBL to the collectin receptor is low, clustering of the receptor on the cell membrane and the presence of multiple ligands are required for a strong interaction. Whether this collectin receptor actually mediates the opsonic effect on phagocytes is still a controversial issue.

ACTIVATION OF C5

All three pathways of complement activation unite, as outlined, in the activation of C3 by two different C3 convertases (Fig. 8). These same molecular complexes are also used for the next activation step in the cascade, the cleavage of C5, but they need an additional C3b molecule covalently deposited immediately next to them. This C3b acts like an anvil for C5: it interacts with C5 and presents C5 in the correct conformation for cleavage by the C2a part or the Bb part of the respective C3 convertase. Hence C3b,Bb,C3b and C4b,2a,3b constitute the two different C5 convertase complexes. Both require Mg^{2+} ions. Cleavage of C5 in the α chain generates the 11-kDa C5a peptide and the larger fragment C5b. C5a is a very potent chemoattractant peptide that acts distantly from the site of complement activation. C5b is the starter molecule for the formation of the membrane attack complex.

THE TERMINAL COMPLEMENT PATHWAY

The terminal complement pathway is the same whether activation is initiated via the classical, alternative, or MBLectin pathway (see Figs. 1 and 8). After cleavage of C5 by either the classical or the alternative C5 convertase, the terminal complement components C6, C7, C8 and C9 are sequentially, but nonenzymatically, activated, resulting in the formation of the terminal complement complex (TCC) (43).

TCC can be generated on a biologic target membrane as potentially membranolytic MAC, or in extracellular fluids as nonlytic SC5b-9 in the presence of S protein (also called vitronectin). Both forms consist of C5b and the complement proteins C6, C7, C8, and C9. After cleavage of C5, C5b undergoes conformational changes and exposes a binding site for C6. The ability of C5b, staying near the C5 convertase on the target surface, to bind C6 decays rapidly, but once bound, C5b6 forms a stable bimolecular complex. C5b6 binds C7, resulting in the exposure of membrane binding sites and incorporation into target membranes. If C7 concentrations near the

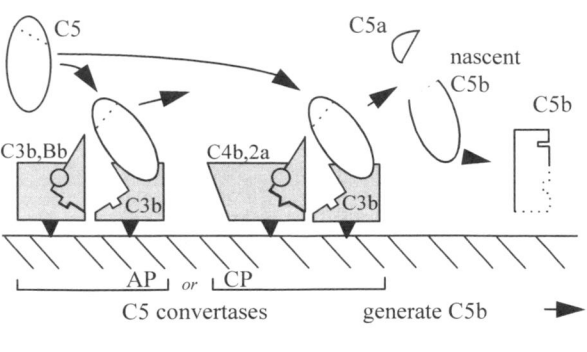

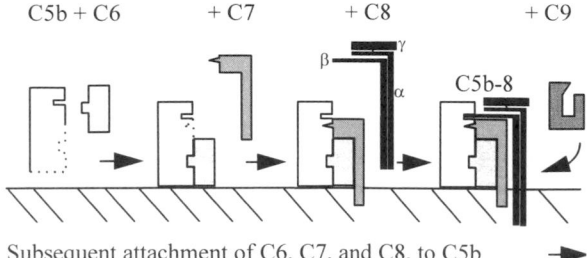

Subsequent attachment of C6, C7, and C8, to C5b

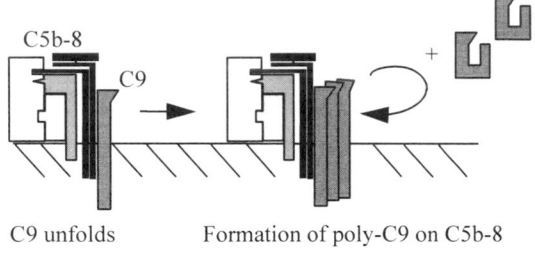

C9 unfolds   Formation of poly-C9 on C5b-8

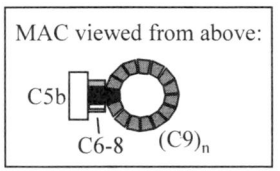

FIG. 8. Activation of C5 and terminal complement pathway. C5 is activated by C5 convertases of the classical or alternative pathway. Nascent C5b interacts sequentially with C6, C7, and C8 and attaches to lipid membranes. As a last step, C9 polymerization on C5b-8 completes the MAC.

site of complement activation are limiting, the stable bimolecular C5b6 complex dissociates from the C5 activating complex and accumulates in solution. In the presence of C7, fluid phase C5b-7 is formed that will not necessarily stay soluble because it has a transient ability to secondarily attach to membranes and initiate lysis, a process called reactive lysis (44). Both the membrane-bound C5b-7 complex as well as the fluid phase C5b-7 complex are capable of binding C8. C8 consists of three nonidentical polypeptide chains: the α and γ chains are covalently linked by a disulfide bond, and the β chain is attached by noncovalent forces. Nascent C5b-7 binds to C8 β via C5b. The C8 γ chain does not appear to have a function in complement lysis, probably because it does not lie adjacent to the membrane but faces the extracellular plasma (Fig. 8).

Although some lytic activity is expressed by the C5b-8 complex, efficient lysis is dependent on an interaction with C9, facilitated by the α-moiety of C8. C5b-8 acts as a polymerizing agent for C9. The first C9, after binding to C5b-8, undergoes major structural changes, enabling formation of an elongated molecule, and allows binding of further C9 molecules and insertion of C9 cylinders into the target membrane (Fig. 8). Whereas only one molecule of each terminal component C5b, C6, C7, and C8 is involved in TCC formation, the number of C9 molecules varies from one to three in the fluid phase and from one to 12 in the membrane-bound form, although polymers containing up to 15 C9 molecules are also possible, provided sufficient amounts of C9 are available. Due to the different number of C9 molecules involved, the tubular structure is not homogeneous. In solution, C9 is also capable of polymerizing with itself without binding to C5b 8, and this tendency toward polymerization can be increased by the presence of metal ions.

The precise mechanism of terminal complement-mediated cytotoxicity after insertion of C9, however, remains unresolved. Currently, two popular hypotheses that do not necessarily exclude each other have been proposed and vigorously defended. According to one model, the polar domains of inserted complement proteins, particularly C9, cause local distortion of the phospholipid bilayer, resulting in leaky patches (45). The other theory postulates that the terminal complement proteins form a hydrophilic channel (pore) through the membrane with consequent disruption of the cell (46).

Membrane perforation by complement is not a unique feature. Perforin, which is contained in the cytoplasmic granules of cytotoxic T-lymphocytes and natural killer cells, is capable of polymerizing on target membranes, thereby forming transmembrane channels. It shares a strong homology with C9. Thus, after antibodies or T cells have identified a target, unspecific destructive forces (i.e., C9 or perforin) take action.

Biological Properties of the Terminal Complement Complex

The TCC has been implicated in a large number of diseases because of its presence in diseased tissues or its elevated levels in the blood, although it is usually not clear whether the detected TCC has a significant pathogenic role. However, its lytic properties are important in host defense against bacterial and viral infections (Fig. 9).

On nucleated cells that are not unequivocally identified as nonself, complement activation is often sublytic (48). The term "sublytic" is of a quantitative, not qualitative, nature (i.e., the number but not the structure of TCC complexes is different. Sublytic attack offers some protection to the cell because it can withstand single (and erroneous) attacks, unlike erythrocytes, which are lysed by a single hit. Furthermore, previous sublytic effects exerted on nucleated cells even protect from further, otherwise lytic doses, favoring those cells that are constantly in contact with complement, as host cells (49). Sublytic attack not only protects host cells, but it also stimulates their protein neosynthesis and arachidonic acid metabolism and activates polymorphonuclear leukocytes. In particular, sublytic TCC on nucleated cells transiently increases intracellular Ca^{2+} and activates protein kinase C and guanine nucleotide binding regulatory proteins (G proteins) (50). It also has the potential to

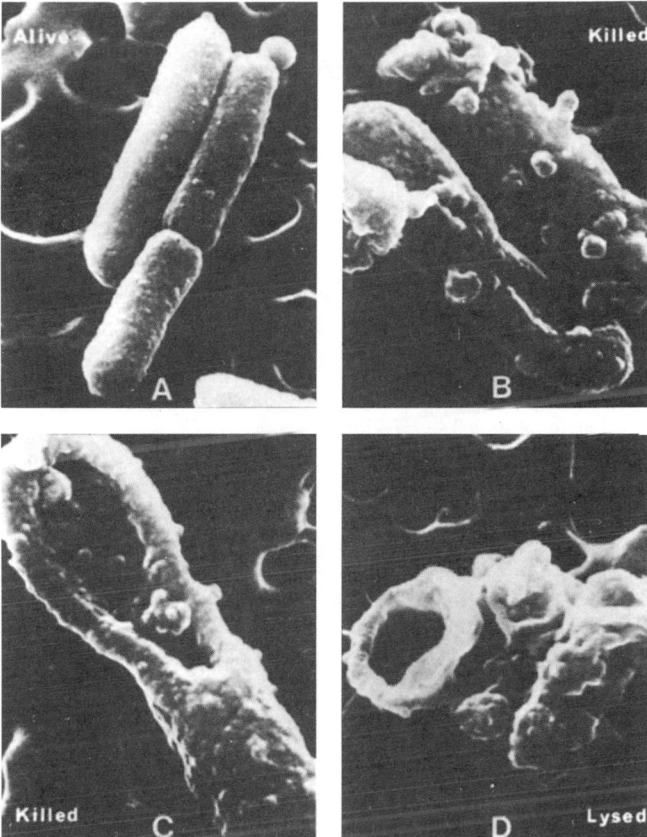

FIG. 9. The structure of *Escherichia coli* as seen in scanning electron micrographs before and after killing by complement. **A:** Intact bacteria. **B and C:** Bacteria killed by purified complement proteins. **D:** Bacteria killed by the combined action of complement and lysozyme (a circulating enzyme that helps degrade bacterial cell walls). Reprinted with permission (47).

induce procoagulant and proinflammatory activities (48,51). Likewise, the presence of TCC on the surface of viable immune cells suggests a modulating role in the physiology of cells to which it attaches (52). Thus, the main biologic functions of the terminal complement cascade as an important humoral effector arm of host defense thus extend far beyond those originally described. Whether SC5b-9 represents simply the inactivated form of the TCC or whether it plays a role in immune defense remains controversial.

CONTROL OF COMPLEMENT ACTIVATION

As a potentially self-damaging mechanism, complement activation has to be avoided or at least to be restricted on autologous cells (see Table 3 and Figs. 5 and 10). The control efforts are not evenly distributed throughout the activation cascade, but are rather focused on the key events of the pathways leading to C3 activation and on polymerization of C9 (generation of the MAC). There are proteins controlling activation in the fluid phase, i.e., plasma and other membrane-localized proteins that are only effective on the surfaces of autologous or allogeneic cells, but not on xenogeneic cells.

For the classical pathway, activated C1 is soon inactivated by covalent binding of C1-INH to active C1r and C1s. In this complex,

TABLE 3. *Mode of action of complement control proteins*

Control protein	Main site of action	Decay acceleration of convertases[a]		Cofactor activity[b]	
		C3b,Bb	C4b,2a	C3b	C4b
C4 activation					
C1-INH	Plasma	Binds covalently to active C1s and C1r			
C3 and C5 activation					
Factor H	Plasma and nonactivator membranes	+	−	+	−
C4bp	Plasma	−	+	−	+
CR1	Self[c] membranes (restricted tissue distribution)	+	+	+	+
MCP	Self[c] membranes (wide tissue distribution)	−	−	+	+
DAF	Self[c] membranes (wide tissue distribution)	+	+	−	−
Formation of the membrane attack complex					
S protein	Plasma	Binds to soluble C5b-7 and blocks its Integration into membranes			
Clusterin	Plasma	Binds to soluble C5b-7 and blocks its Integration into membranes			
CD59	Self[c] membranes (wide tissue distribution)	Inhibits binding of C9 and its polymerization			

[a]Decay acceleration is the ability to dissociate the C3 convertases C3b, Bb or C4b,2a.
[b]Cofactor activity for the cleavage of C3b or C4b by factor I.
[c]In this context, "self" stands for "within the same species." Control proteins are mostly inactive for complement of other species.

A:

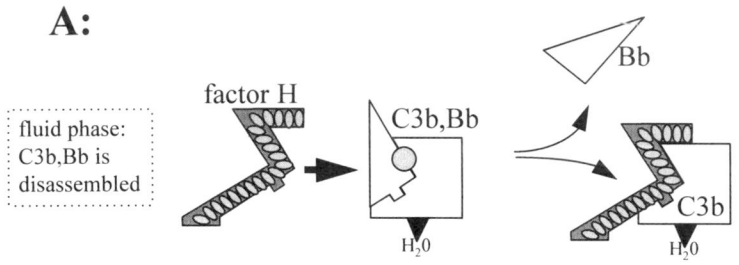

B:

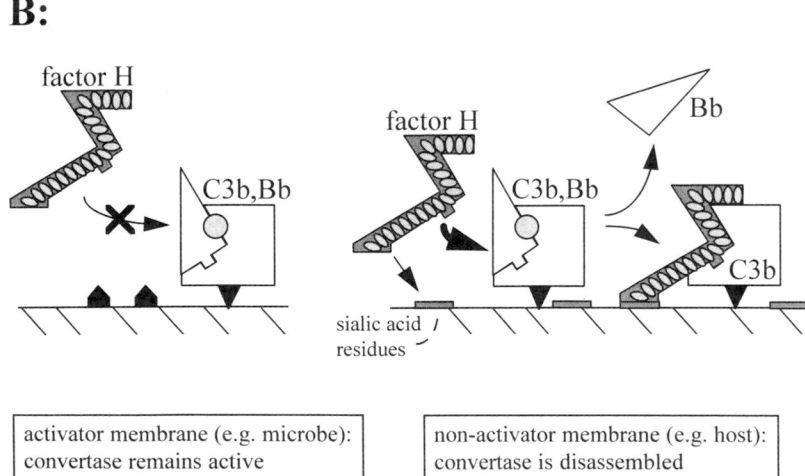

activator membrane (e.g. microbe): convertase remains active

non-activator membrane (e.g. host): convertase is disassembled

FIG. 10. Control of C3b amplification by factor H. **A:** Factor H destroys C3 convertases circulating in plasma by displacing Bb and rendering C3b accessible for cleavage by factor I. **B:** The same occurs on nonactivator membranes (*right part*) which facilitate factor H binding through sialic acid residues. On activator membranes (*left part*), factor H binding is not promoted and C3b,Bb remains active.

C1s has lost C4 cleaving potential. C1-INH is normally present in a relatively high plasma concentration, and deficiency of C1-INH has been recognized as the cause for hereditary angioedema. C1-INH is probably also involved in the control of MASP-1 and MASP-2.

The next step in control occurs through cleavage of C4b by factor I, which requires C4bp (in fluid phase) or CR1 or MCP (on membranes) as a cofactor. Additionally, the squidlike C4bp binds C4b not attached to a surface, thus preventing association of C4b with C2 in the fluid phase. Control is then exerted on the assembled C3 convertase C4b,2a: the complex is attacked by DAF or CR1 and dissociated into C4b and inactive C2a. This mechanism is equally effective for the C5 convertase of the classical pathway.

The tightest control is afforded for the alternative pathway C3b amplification loop. Convertases present on nonactivator surfaces (Fig. 10B) or in the fluid phase (Fig. 10A) are dissociated into C3b and Bb, which irreversibly deprives Bb of its enzymatic activity, and C3b is cleaved to iC3b, which prevents (re-) formation of a new convertase. First, decay of C3b,Bb is accelerated by the membrane-anchored molecules DAF or CR1 or by the plasma protein factor H. All three are able to displace Bb from C3b, and factor H and CR1 bind to C3b themselves, which is intrinsic for the subsequent cleavage by factor I. Factor H is the main control protein in plasma, but also contributes to dissociation of C3b,Bb on those parts of the cell membrane that are not accessible to DAF (12). Interestingly, DAF uses different SCRs for dissociating C4b,2a or C3b,Bb. It has to be pointed out that without decay accelerators the C3 convertases decay spontaneously, having only a short half-life of 2 minutes. This is important because they are very powerful enzymes and even on activator surfaces C3 activation must be limited.

The inactivation of C3b to iC3b relies on factor I and its cofactors factor H, CR1, or MCP. Due to the high plasma concentration of H, virtually all C3b present in plasma (i.e., nascent C3b that has reacted with water) quickly binds to H. The low value of the Michaelis constant (K_m) of factor I for C3b,H permits an efficient cleavage of C3b (and iC3) even at the low factor I levels in human plasma.

C3b degradation (see Fig. 5) serves two purposes: dangerous C3b is destroyed, but the C3b fragments iC3b and C3dg remain on the activating surface, tagging it for opsonophagocytosis. Factor I cleaves C3b three times: after cleavages 1 and 2, C3b is inactivated to iC3b. The third cleavage releases the larger, biologically inert C3c, whereas the smaller C3dg fragment remains bound to the target as it comprises the thioester region (see Fig. 5). C3dg may be further trimmed by several plasma proteases to C3d.

The physiologic role of the ever-growing family of factor H–like or factor H–related proteins in C3b control is currently not understood (53). Cofactor activity is present in FHL-1, but the low plasma concentration suggests that the protein may have additional characteristics that could be more important (54). FHR-1 and FHR-2 do not have cofactor activity, but share homology in the C terminus of factor H, a site contributing to binding of C3b.

The terminal pathway is controlled both before the integration of the assembling membrane attack complex into the membrane and at the stage of pore formation (association of C8 and polymerization of C9). A number of different membrane and plasma molecules are involved in modulating TCC assembly, of which C8 is probably the most important. It represents not only an essential component of the lytic complex but, paradoxically, also prevents membrane damage by binding to the nascent C5b-7 complex in the fluid phase, thereby precluding its firm insertion into the membrane.

Not only C8, but also the abundant S protein (55), clusterin (also called SP-40,40) (56), lipoproteins, antithrombin III, and proteoglycans such as heparin and protamine, the powerful antidote to heparin, are able to bind to nascent C5b-7 and to prevent its membrane insertion. In addition, numerous interactions have been observed among these inactivators, of which some occur preferably under acidic conditions as reviewed elsewhere (57).

The extent to which these complex interactions affect host defense *in vivo* is not fully understood. The final step of MAC assembly, subsequent to C5b-7 insertion, when the MAC becomes more firmly inserted into the lipid bilayer, is safeguarded by cell membrane proteins, termed homologous restriction factors because they show some degree of species restriction, i.e., they prevent lysis by autologous complement attack (58): (a) a 65- to 68-kDa molecule (C8bp, HRF, MIP), which remains less well characterized and which is supposed to predominantly bind to C8; and (b) an 18- to 20-kDa well-characterized glycolipid-anchored membrane molecule (CD59), which protects against complement-mediated lysis by interfering with the particular C9 interaction site on the C8 α chain that is needed for membrane insertion and subsequent polymerization of C9.

CD59 is found on nucleated cells, including those beyond an (intact) blood–brain barrier (17) and on erythrocytes, but also in serum, urine, seminal plasma, colostrum, and milk. Recently, pigs transgenic for human CD59 have been generated for the envisaged use of xenotransplants in humans, which may be of benefit regarding the shortage of compatible human donors. Such organs have been shown to be protected *in vitro* from hyperacute rejection by expressing human CD59.

COMPLEMENT RECEPTORS

Several biologic activities of complement are mediated by complement receptors that react with activation products generated in the course of one of the activation pathways (see Figs. 4, 11, and 12). Each red and white blood cell expresses cell membrane receptors for various complement fragments (Table 4). It is important to note that native, intact components do not bind to these receptors; the ligands are generated upon activation.

The best studied complement receptors are the cell membrane molecules binding C3 fragments bound covalently to activating surfaces. C3 undergoes degradation that results in cells or particles bearing C3b, iC3b, and C3dg/C3d fragments, forming the ligands for various receptors (Fig. 11). All the receptor binding sites are localized on the α chain of C3. The most important physiologic functions of complement mediated by C3 receptors are the uptake of opsonized particles and activation of various complement receptor–bearing cells.

Complement Receptor Type 1 (CR1, C3b Receptor, CD35)

This single-chain membrane protein binds C3b and C4b with high affinity, and besides serving as a cell membrane receptor, it is involved in the regulation of complement activation (59). CR1 occurs in four polymorphic forms containing up to 34 SCRs. Two of the codominantly expressed allelic forms have MWs of 220 and 250 kDa, and the two other less common forms have MWs of 190

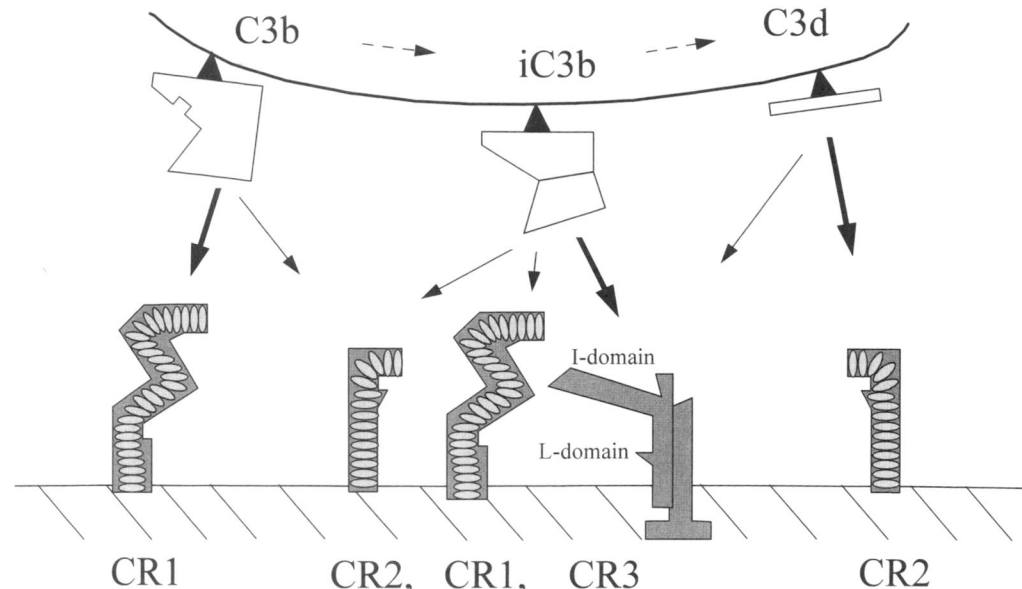

FIG. 11. Specificity of complement receptors for the various fragments of C3. CR1 and CR2 consist of SCRs (shown as ovals), whereas CR3 is a heterodimer (integrin). Higher affinity of a C3 fragment to a certain CR is shown by thicker arrows.

and 280 kDa. The extracellular part of the most common form of CR1 is composed of 30 tandemly arranged SCR domains. These are organized into four groups called long homologous repeats with seven repeated SCRs each (SCRs 1 to 7, 8 to 14, 15 to 21, and 22 to 28) plus two additional SCRs at the C terminus. The ligand binding sites are located on the second SCR in the first three LHRs, providing the basis for multivalent interaction with C3b- or C4b-coated cells and particles.

CR1 is present on erythrocytes, monocytes/macrophages, eosinophils, neutrophils, follicular dendritic cells, and T- and B-lymphocytes. The number of CR1 on erythrocytes is only about 500 per cell, in contrast to leukocytes, where up to 50,000 CR1 per cell can be found. Nevertheless, more than 85% of CR1 in blood is present on the red blood cells because of the vast number of erythrocytes.

The Functions of CR1

The phenomenon of immune adherence, i.e., the binding of opsonized microbes to primate erythrocytes, was the first recognized complement-mediated cellular reaction. This reaction is mediated by CR1 expressed on erythrocytes, a process important for the clearance of immune complexes from the circulation. Soluble antigen–antibody complexes such as toxin–antitoxin complexes are formed after most antibody reactions. These activate the complement system, and C3b that is generated binds covalently to the immune complexes. CR1-expressing erythrocytes adsorb these complexes and transport them to the phagocytic cells of the liver and the spleen for removal.

CR1 expressed on macrophages and polymorphonuclear cells serves as an opsonin receptor. Most probably one of the major defense mechanisms against systemic bacterial and fungal infections is C3b- and iC3b-dependent phagocytosis. On unactivated phagocytes, CR1 alone cannot mediate phagocytosis but efficiently cooperates with Fc receptors and CR3 to bind and ingest opsonized particles. The T cell–derived cytokine IFN-γ and the anaphylatoxic peptide C5a, however, are able to activate macrophages to ingest microbes coated with C3b/iC3b via CR1 only. Triggering of monocytes via their CR1 has been reported to lead to phosphorylation of the receptor and to induce the nuclear translocation of the NF-κB complex (60). As mentioned previously, CR1 also regulates complement activation by the inhibition of C3 convertase activity, thus protecting host cells from comple-

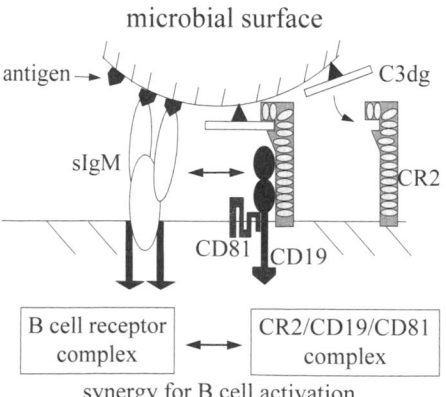

FIG. 12. Interaction of the B-cell receptor complex and the CR2–CD19–CD81 complex for B-cell activation. Antigens coated with C3d bind to the specific surface IgM and to CR2 and cross-link the two receptor complexes. The additional signal triggered via CR2 augments stimulation of the B cell about 100-fold, depending on the amount of C3d bound to the antigen.

TABLE 4. *Complement receptors*

Type	Ligand	Structure, MW	Distribution	Function
CR1 (CD35)	C3b>C4b>iC3b	Single chain, 160–250 kDa, glycoprotein, four allotypes, consists of 28–34 SCRs	Monocytes, macrophages, neutrophils, eosinophils, erythrocytes, B and T cells, FDC	Immune adherence, phagocytosis, immune complex clearance, immune complex localization to germinal centers, control of activation
CR2 (CD21)	C3db/C3d>iC3b EBV, CD23, IFNα	Single chain, 140–145 kDa, glycoprotein, two isoforms: CD2⁻ S (15 SCRs), CD21L (16 SCRs)	B cells, activated T cells, epithelial cells, FDC (CD21L)	B-cell activation, immune complex localization to germinal centers, rescue of germinal center cells from apoptosis
CR3 (CD11b/CD18)	iC3b, factor X, ICAM-1, fibrinogen, LPS, certain carbohydrates	Heterodimer of glycoproteins. α chain: 165 kDa β chain: 95 kDa	Monocytes, macrophages, neutrophils, NK cells, FDC, T cells, mast cells	Phagocytosis, cell adhesion, signal transduction, oxydative burst
CR4 (CD11c/CD18)	iC3b, fibrinogen	Heterodimer of glycoproteins. α chain: 150 kDa β chain: 95 kDa	Monocytes, macrophages, neutrophils, NK cells, T cells, mast cells	Phagocytosis, cell adhesion

ment-mediated damage. Additionally, the genetically engineered soluble form of CR1 also has been shown to inhibit both pathways of complement activation (24). CR1 expressed on follicular dendritic cells in the lymph nodes and spleen plays an important role in maintaining immunologic memory. These cells trap complement-coated immune complexes, enabling the antigen to persist longer in the germinal centers.

Complement Receptor Type 2 (CR2, C3d Receptor, CD21)

Two isoforms of this single-chain glycoprotein have been described: the well-characterized short form of CR2 (CD21S), which comprises 15 SCRs, and the recently reported long CR2 (CD21L), containing an additional exon (encoding an additional SCR 10a). The shorter isoform is expressed on B-lymphocytes, activated T cells, and epithelial cells, but not on monocytes, macrophages, granulocytes, or erythrocytes. The longer CR2 isoform appears to be selectively expressed on follicular dentritic cells (FDC). The ligand binding site of CR2 resides in the first two SCRs. It binds C3dg, C3d, and (weakly) iC3b and also interacts with CD23, the low-affinity Fcε-receptor on B cells. This interaction is thought to be important for isotype switching and survival of germinal center cells (61). However, the highest affinity for CR2 is seen with the envelope protein gp350/220 of Epstein-Barr virus (EBV). Human and mouse CR1 and CR2 proteins are homologous. However, although human CR1 and CR2 are encoded by two separate genes, mouse CR1 and CR2 arise from alternative splicing of a common gene encoding the C3b and C4b binding sites.

The Functions of CR2

Probably the most important physiologic function of CR2 is its recently recognized involvement in B-cell activation by the association with CD19 and TAPA-1 (CD81) in the B-cell membrane (62). Cross-linking of the trimolecular complex to the membrane Ig complex lowers the threshold for B-cell activation and, depending on the number of C3d fragments complexed to the antigen, may enhance Ig production 10- to 10,000-fold (Fig. 12).

Like CR1, CR2 on FDC has been shown to trap immune complexes in germinal centers, most probably playing a role in the development of B-cell memory. The recently described long isoform expressed exclusively on FDC may provide a clue for explaining the mechanism of this process. Pathogenetically very important, CR2 is also the port of entry for EBV, enabling the virus to enter B cells or other CR2-expressing cells. This is achieved without the involvement of complement.

Complement Receptor Type 3 (CR3, Mac-1, CD11b/CD18)

CR3 is a heterodimer containing the 165-kDa α chain (CD11b) and the 95-kDa β chain (CD18) (see Fig. 11). The latter polypeptide is identical with the β chains of LFA-1 and p150,95, the related leukocyte integrins (also named β2 integrins). It is the α chain of the receptor that possesses the binding site for iC3b (and, with lower affinity, for C3b and C3dg). Binding of the ligands to integrins is Ca^{2+} dependent.

The Functions of CR3

CR3 is expressed on mononuclear phagocytes, neutrophils, cytotoxic T cells, FDCs, NK cells, and mast cells. Its most important role is the mediation of binding and phagocytosis of particles and microorganisms opsonized by iC3b. Unlike the interaction between C3b and CR1, binding of iC3b to CR3 is sufficient on its own to initiate phagocytosis. In addition to binding iC3b (via the I-domain), CR3 has carbohydrate-binding capacity (via its lectin or L domain) and in this way interacts with other membrane constituents. Also, some yeasts, such as *Saccharomyces cerevisiae,* and some bacteria, including *Staphylococcus epidermidis,* bind to this receptor without the involvement of complement. Triggering of CR3 via its L domain results in oxidative burst in neutrophils and mononuclear phagocytes. By binding to ICAM-1, CR3 enhances the adhesion of monocytes and neutrophils to the endothelium in the absence of complement proteins and facilitates the accumulation of these cells at sites of tissue injury. Other ligands for CR3 include fibrinogen and clotting factor X. On certain cells, GPI-anchored membrane proteins use CR3 as an adapter for transducing signals across the plasma membrane. The physical and functional association of CR3 with the LPS receptor (CD14) after LPS binding, with the urokinase plasminogen activator receptor (uPAR; CD87) after binding uPA, and with the Fcγ receptor type III (CD16) was demonstrated (63).

Complement Receptor Type 4 (CR4, p150/95, CD11c/CD18)

CR4 is also a heterodimer, containing the 150-kDa α chain and the β chain, which is identical to that of CR3. Both the ligand specificity and the tissue distribution of this receptor is very similar to that of CR3.

RECEPTORS FOR THE ANAPHYLATOXIC PEPTIDES: C5aR (CD88) AND C3aR

In the course of complement activation, peptides of 74 to 77 amino acids are cleaved from the N termini of the α chains of components C4, C3, and C5 (Table 5 and Fig. 13). The cleavage occurs after an arginyl residue, resulting in C4a, C3a, and C5a peptides with C-terminal arginine residues. Receptor molecules for C5a and C3a have been cloned (64). Both C3aR and C5aR are members of the rhodopsin superfamily of receptors, which have seven hydrophobic transmembrane regions and are coupled to G proteins in the cytoplasma (Fig. 13). They are homologous to receptors mediating chemotactic signals, such as the fMLP receptor (which binds bacterial peptides), the receptor for IL-8, or the receptor for RANTES (i.e., chemokine receptor type 5). The deduced MW of C5aR is 43 kDa, whereas C3aR is larger (48 kDa; see Table 5) due to a longer second extracellular loop, most probably conferring ligand specificity.

Functions of C5aR and C3aR

Regarding several of the known biologic activities, C5a is the most potent of all the small activation products, followed by C3a and C4a. Binding of these peptides to their corresponding recep-

TABLE 5. *Receptors for anaphylatoxins and receptors for C1q or factor H*

Type	Ligand	Structure, MW	Distribution	Function
C3aR	C3a	Single chain 48 kDa, G-protein linked, contains seven transmembrane segments	Mast cells, basophils, smooth muscle cells, lymphocytes	Increases vascular permeability, triggers serosal type mast cells
C5aR (CD 88)	C5a, C5a desArg	43 kDa, single chain, G-protein linked, contains seven transmembrane segments	Mast cells, basophils, neutrophils, monocytes, macrophages, endothelial cells, smooth muscle cells, lymphocytes	Increases vascular permeability, triggers serosal type mast cells, promotes chemotaxis
cC1qR, "collectin-receptor"	Collagen region of C1q, "collectins": MBL, CL-43, SP-A, conglutinin	Single chain, 60 kDa, acidic glycoprotein; identical to endoplasmic reticulum protein calreticulin?	B cell, monocytes, macrophages, platelets, endothelial cells, fibroblasts	
gC1qR	Globular heads of C1q, thrombin, heparin binding form of S protein, Hageman factor, high molecular weight kininogen	33 kDa, acidic protein, tetramer under nondissociating conditions; probably not a surface receptor, but with mitochondrial protein	B cells, monocytes, macrophages platelets, endothelial cells, neutrophils	
C1qR$_p$	Collagenous regions of C1q, MBL, SP-A	Single chain 126 kDa membrane protein, highly glycosylated	Monocytes, macrophages, neutrophils, endothelial cells, microglia	Phagocytosis
fH-R	Factor H	Two species: 150 kDa with 50-kDa subunits 170 kDa, single chain	B cells and B-cell lines, monocytes, macrophages, neutrophils	Activation of B cells, stimulation of respiratory burst, release of factor I, prostaglandin E and thromboxane

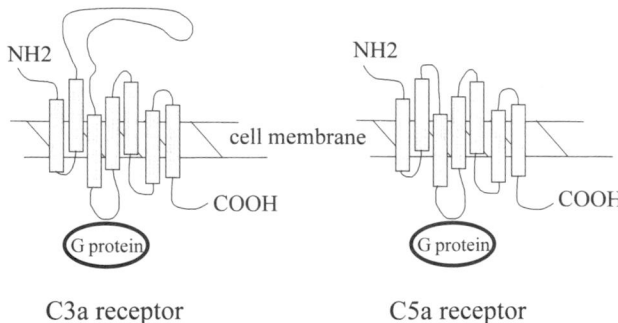

C3a receptor   C5a receptor

FIG. 13. Structure of the receptors for the anaphylatoxins C3a and C5a. Both belong to the family of seven-pass transmembrane receptors. They signal by interaction of their second cytoplasmic loop with intracellular guanosine triphosphate–binding proteins.

tors induces local inflammatory reactions; therefore, they are often referred to as anaphylatoxins. They induce the contraction of smooth muscle and increase vascular permeability. Consequently, antibodies, complement, and phagocytes are recruited to the site of infection, and a locally developing edema restricts the movement of phagocytes. All these processes contribute to the initiation of adaptive immune responses.

Both C3a and C5a trigger the degranulation of serosal type mast cells, resulting in the release of histamine and other vasoactive mediators from these cells. C3aR and C5aR are widely expressed on different lymphoid cells, and their messenger RNAs have been detected in various nonlymphoid organ tissues. Various cell types respond differently to the anaphylatoxic peptides. On neutrophils, C5a has a strong chemotactic activity and induces the expression of adhesion molecules. These cells are also triggered by the complement peptides to produce oxygen free radicals, prostaglandins, and eicosanoids.

C5a has a short half-life in circulation because the plasma enzyme carboxypeptidase N (also called anaphylatoxin inactivator) cleaves off its C-terminal arginine. C5a desArg generated this way is much less active in several biologic systems than is C5a. In analogy with C5a, serum carboxypeptidase N generates desArg peptides with greatly reduced biologic activity from C3a and C4a.

C1q RECEPTORS

A cell membrane protein named C1qR$_p$, reacting with the collagenlike stalks of C1q, has been cloned recently. This highly glycosylated 126-kDa protein is expressed on phagocytic cells, but not on T- or B-lymphoblastoid cells. It has a C-type carbohydrate recognition domain and five EGF-like domains.

There are two other types of surface proteins that bind to specific regions of the complement subcomponent C1q, although their location at the plasma membrane, and thus their potential to serve as receptors, has recently been questioned (65). The 60-kDa glycoprotein that binds the collagenlike portion of C1q is named cC1qR. This protein is also referred to as the collectin receptor because in addition to C1q, it binds to other members of the collectin family, such as MBL, conglutinin, SP-A and CL-43 (see Table 5). Several cell types, including monocytes, macrophages, B cells, granulo-

cytes, endothelial cells and platelets possess this receptor. Its peptide sequence shows almost complete identity to the complementary DNA–derived sequence of calreticulin, a Ca^{2+} binding protein resident in the endoplasmic reticulum. The relationship between cC1qR and calreticulin is not fully understood. The other acidic cellular protein reacts with the globular heads of C1q and hence has been named gC1qR (see Table 5). The distribution of this 33-kDa protein is very similar to that of cC1qR.

Functions of C1q Receptors

C1q receptors have been reported to mediate several responses of various cells, such as the augmentation of the uptake of bacteria opsonized with MBL and immune complexes having C1q, regulating phagocytosis, eliciting the production of oxygen radicals, and enhancing cell-mediated cytotoxicity.

FACTOR H RECEPTOR

A receptor for factor H has been detected on B-lymphoblastoid cells, monocytes, and neutrophils. Using factor H–sepharose for the isolation of the receptor, a protein complex was identified consisting of two disulfide-linked components of 50 kDa each with an additional 50-kDa chain attached noncovalently. Another cell membrane factor H–binding protein was also isolated from tonsil B cells and from B-lymphoblasts by affinity chromatography. This single-chain protein species was found to be 170 kDa in MW.

Functions of Factor H Receptor

Regarding the possible function of factor H receptor, it has been shown that factor H serves as a growth factor for B-cell lines. Moreover, it stimulates B-lymphocytes and lymphoblastoid cell lines to release endogenous factor I. Factor H also has been demonstrated to trigger the oxydative metabolism of monocytes.

THE ROLE OF COMPLEMENT IN LINKING INNATE IMMUNITY TO ADAPTIVE RESPONSES

Elements of the innate immunity such as the complement system, macrophages, NK cells, and granulocytes are the first-line defense in higher vertebrates. These cells and molecules are able to recognize foreign material and come into action within minutes (or hours) of infection. Several microbes trigger the complement cascade immediately after entering the body in the absence of antibodies by activating either the alternative or the MBL pathway. Complement and complement receptor–mediated processes link innate immunity to adaptive responses in several ways:

- Complement is involved in the initiation of adaptive immune responses because antibody-independent, complement-mediated opsonization of microbes facilitates uptake and presentation of antigens via complement receptor–bearing antigen-presenting cells.
- Antigen-bound C3d facilitates B-cell activation via cross-linking membrane IgM to the CR2/CD19/TAPA-1 complex.

- CR1 and CR2 expressed on follicular dendritic cells are essential for the formation of memory B cells by localizing immune complexes in the germinal centers.
- Complement activation generates anaphylatoxic peptides at sites of infection and, by recruiting inflammatory cells, contributes to the elimination of the antigen.
- Complement plays an important role in the processing of immune complexes by inhibiting the formation of large immune complexes and by solubilizing complexes that have already been precipitated.
- Complement activation resulting in lysis of cells and bacteria is essential for the elimination of several pathogens.

INTERSECTIONS OF THE COMPLEMENT SYSTEM WITH THE CLOTTING AND THE KININ SYSTEM

A biochemical relatedness exists between the complement system and the two other plasma protein systems. For one, the concept for activation in all three relies on consecutive proteolytic cleavages of multiple components, with modified serine protease domains being the effectors. On the other hand, some active components of one system exert effects in one of the others.

For example, C1-INH not only controls C1r and C1s, but also inhibits kallikrein, plasmin, and factors XII and XI of the clotting system (66). Although more potent means of inactivation exist for plasmin or factors XII and XI within the fibrinolytic and clotting system, this is a good example for the overlapping function of a serpin molecule. Plasmin, on its part, is capable of activating C3. Although this is not of importance under physiologic conditions, it is relevant in shock conditions such as disseminated intravascular coagulation or adult respiratory distress syndrome, where concomitant activation of all three systems occurs (67).

COMPLEMENT QUANTITATION

The traditional assay to measure serum complement activity is the total hemolytic complement assay (CH_{50}). In this assay, sheep red blood cells are incubated with an antierythrocyte antibody (amboceptor) and incubated with human serum at various dilutions. The reciprocal of the dilution at which serum lyses 50% of the erythrocytes is the CH_{50} value. This assay measures the functional capacity of only the classical and terminal pathways and is usually combined with immunochemical assays for measuring C3 and C4 protein. These immunochemical assays, which assess the presence and integrity of a protein but not their functional activities, comprise radial immunodiffusion (Mancini), electroimmunodiffusion (rocket electrophoresis, Laurell) and enzyme immunoassay (EIA).

Detecting a reduction in the level of the uncleaved component is less sensitive for assessing complement activation than detecting the increase in cleavage products (C4d, C3dg, C3a, C5a) or complexes containing that particular component (e.g., the TCC). This is readily understood: an increase of a particular concentration from 1% to 5% is much easier to detect (fivefold increase) than a decrease from 99% to 95% (which is within the error of the assay). For these reasons, assays based on activation-specific, so-called neoepitope-specific, and native-restricted monoclonal antibodies have been successfully used to specifically measure only the activated or the native molecule, respectively (68). For accurate assessments they are best run simultaneously because low amounts of native proteins in the first place cannot generate as much activation product as high concentrations. The application of activation-specific antibodies markedly improved both specificity and sensitivity of complement activation assessment in biologic fluids and is used to follow the course of a disease, to reveal exacerbations, and to evaluate the success of a treatment. In particular, these novel methods have been used to assess the biocompatibility of extracorporeal membranes or to distinguish complete from subtotal complement deficiencies. For the latter, the TCC EIA, based on a neoepitope-specific anti-C9 monoclonal antibody, has an additional advantage because it can serve as a functional assay: TCC can only be generated when all preceding proteins, including the one present in limited amounts, are functionally active. However, even these sophisticated assays do not allow, although widely practiced, the assumption that approximately half normal concentrations indicate heterozygous deficiency; even heterozygous subjects may present with almost normal concentrations of the component in question.

COMPLEMENT GENETICS

The study on genetics of complement proteins was originally initiated by the discovery of complement deficiencies in animals and humans. It has been used to detect both homozygous deficient individuals and heterozygous carriers in family studies and to compile further evidence for disease associations with certain complement alleles. However, complement genetics also has been a valuable tool to investigate plasma protein genetics in general and their evolution. The chromosomal assignment of the genes coding for complement proteins (Fig. 14) shows interesting linkage groups of structurally homologous components, confirming previous assumptions, based on homology studies on the protein level, that the majority of complement proteins has evolved by duplication from only a small number of precursor genes (69).

Because complement receptors and certain regulatory proteins are expressed on erythrocytes, they have the potential to represent blood group antigens: the Knops, McCoy, Swain-Langley, and York antigens are known to be on CR1. Variations in the DAF antigen are responsible for the Cromer blood group system, with the rare Inab phenotype lacking DAF altogether. Chido and Rogers blood group antigens are associated with C4 (69). In this respect, complement genetics has been widely applied to anthropologic investigations and forensic medicine.

Recently, progress on the molecular level has facilitated the characterization of complement allotypes on the molecular level. Both phenotypical assessments of protein variants (phenotyping) and characterization of genomic DNA (genotyping) are currently used (70). Phenotyping is traditionally performed using methods analyzing the mobility or isoelectric point of proteins in agarose or polyacrylamide gel electrophoresis. In addition, monoclonal antibodies have been described that distinguish between certain complement allotypes. Genotyping is performed by studying restriction fragment length polymorphisms or by polymerase chain reaction using specific primers followed by enzymatic digestion or sequencing. Phenotyping has the advantage that the product and, depending on

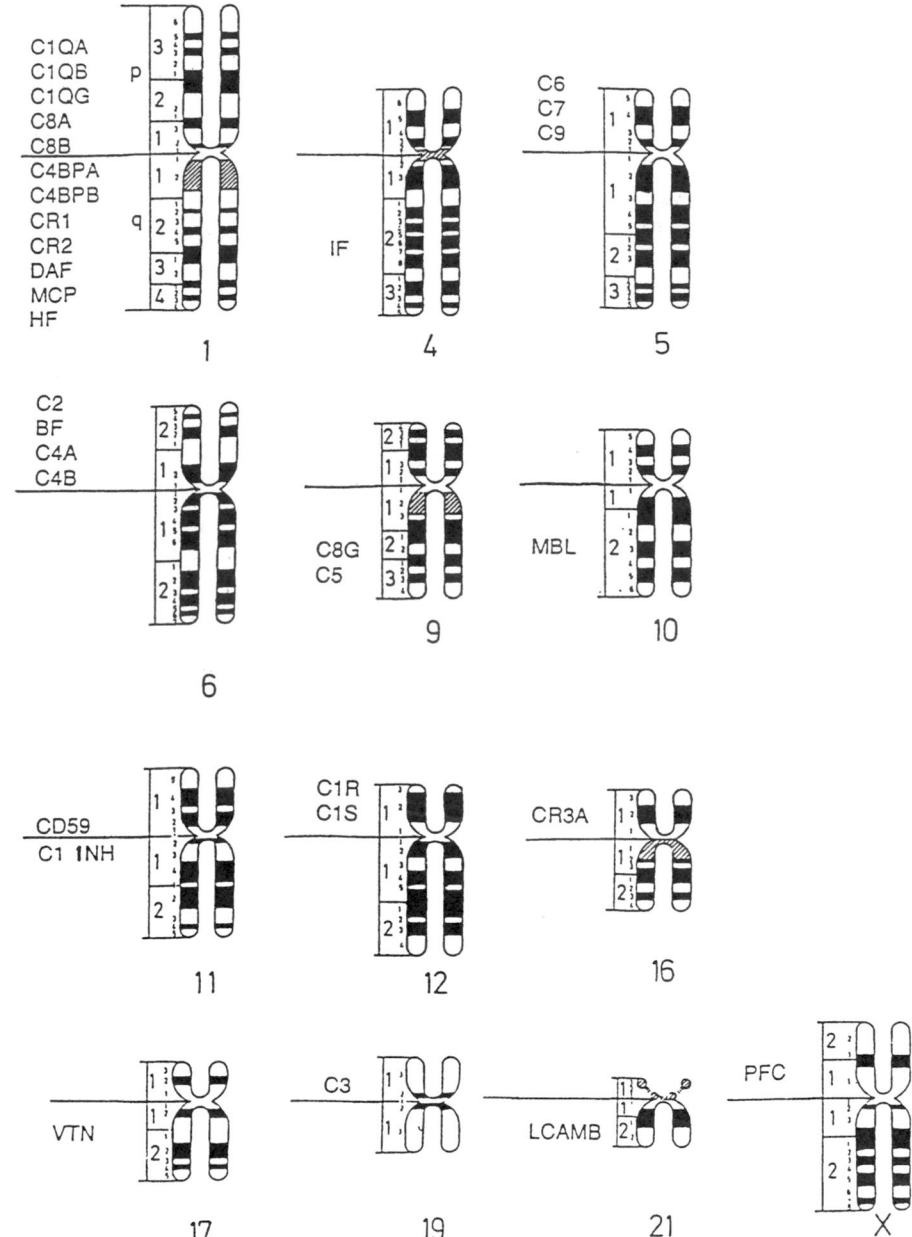

FIG. 14. Schematic diagram of the location of structural genes of complement or related proteins within the human chromosome set, indicated on the left (according to the Paris Nomenclature, Paris Conference, 1971). Only chromosomes carrying complement genes are shown. C1QA, C1q α chain; C1QB, C1q β chain; C1QG, C1q γ chain, all at 1p34-36; C8A, C8 α chain; C8B, C8 β chain, both at 1p22; C4BPA, C4 binding protein α chain; C4BPB, C4 binding protein β chain; CR1, CR2, DAF, MCP, and HF, factor H, all at 1q32 (RCA gene cluster); IF, factor I at 4q25; C6, C7, and C9 at 5p14-p12 (MAC gene cluster); BF, factor B at 6p21 within the MHC III cluster together with C2, C4A, and C4B; C8G, C8 γ chain at 9q22-32 with C5 at 9q33; MBL at 10q22; CD59 at 11p13; C1-INH at 11q12-13; C1R and C1S at 12p13; CR3A, CR3 α chain (CD11b) at 16p13-11; VTN, vitronectin at 17q11; C3 at 19p13; LCAMB, leucocyte adhesion molecule β chain (CD18), common for all β2 integrins, including CR3 at 21q22; PFC, properdin at Xp11.

the method applied, even the functional activity of a protein coded by the allele can be ascertained. Genotyping does not allow identification of silent or null alleles as such; however, once a mutation is known, a defective gene may be traced in family studies, providing a basis for genetic counseling for the afflicted family.

COMPLEMENT AS PATHOGENIC FACTOR IN DISEASE

The complement system contributes to inflammation and tissue damage in neurodegenerative and autoimmune diseases, especially at renal and dermatologic manifestations but also in ischemic and reperfusion injury or shock situations. Evidence has included the detection of complement activation products in biologic fluids or tissues and information from animal models of disease where complement can be efficiently inhibited. Table 6 presents an incomplete summary of these many conditions. In almost all of these, complement is not the cause but is one of several factors involved in pathogenesis [71]. In particular, complement is critical to proper immune complex processing. When excessive quantities of complexes are deposited in tissue, ongoing complement activation will also affect and destroy surrounding tissue, such as vascular endothelial cells, leading to vasculitis.

There are probably two ways in which complement fixation influences the fate of immune complexes [72]. First, the fixation of C4 and C3 into the antigen–antibody lattice alters the size of the immune complex, giving rise to a large number of small complexes as opposed to a small number of large ones. The latter may precipitate locally and cause Arthus reactions or immune complex disease. Thus, complement helps to solubilize initial immune complexes (detergentlike effect of complement). Second, and probably more important, the presence of C4b and C3b on the immune complex facilitates transport predominantly via the CR1 on red cells in circulation. Under physiologic conditions, erythrocyte-bound immune complexes are sequestered in the liver, where antigenic material can be removed by reticulohistiocytic cells (Fig. 15). If adequate complement fixation on these complexes fails, they can be taken up by endothelial cells and sequestered at peripheral sites, giving rise to further inflammation and immune complex formation.

TABLE 6. *Complement in disease*

System/Disease	Assay[a]	Histology[b]	Model[c]
Biocompatibility/shock			
Postbypass syndrome	Yes	Yes	Yes
Catheter reactions	Yes	Yes	No
ARDS	Yes	Yes	Yes
Anaphylaxis	Yes	No	No
Transplant rejection	Yes	Yes	Yes
Preeclampsia	Yes	Yes	No
Dermatological			
Pemphigus/pemphigoid	No	Yes	No
Phototoxic reactions	Yes	Yes	Yes
Vasculitis	Yes	Yes	No
Neurological			
Myasthenia gravis	Yes	Yes	Yes
Multiple sclerosis	Yes	Yes	Yes
Cerebral lupus	Yes	No	No
Guillain-Barré syndrome	Yes	Yes	Yes
Alzheimer's disease	No	Yes	No
Renal			
Lupus nephritis	Yes	Yes	Yes
Membranproliferative GN	Yes	Yes	Yes
Membranous nephritis	Yes	Yes	Yes
Rheumatological			
Rheumatoid arthritis	Yes	Yes	Yes
SLE	Yes	Yes	Yes
Behcet's syndrome	Yes	Yes	No
Juvenile rheumatoid	Yes	No	No
Sjogren's syndrome	Yes	No	No
Other			
Atheroma	Yes	Yes	No
Bowel inflammation	Yes	Yes	No
Thyroiditis	Yes	Yes	Yes
Infertility	Yes	Yes	No

[a]Measurement of complement activation products in biological fluids.
[b]Detection of complement products in diseased tissue.
[c]Animal models of disease. Modified [71] with permission.

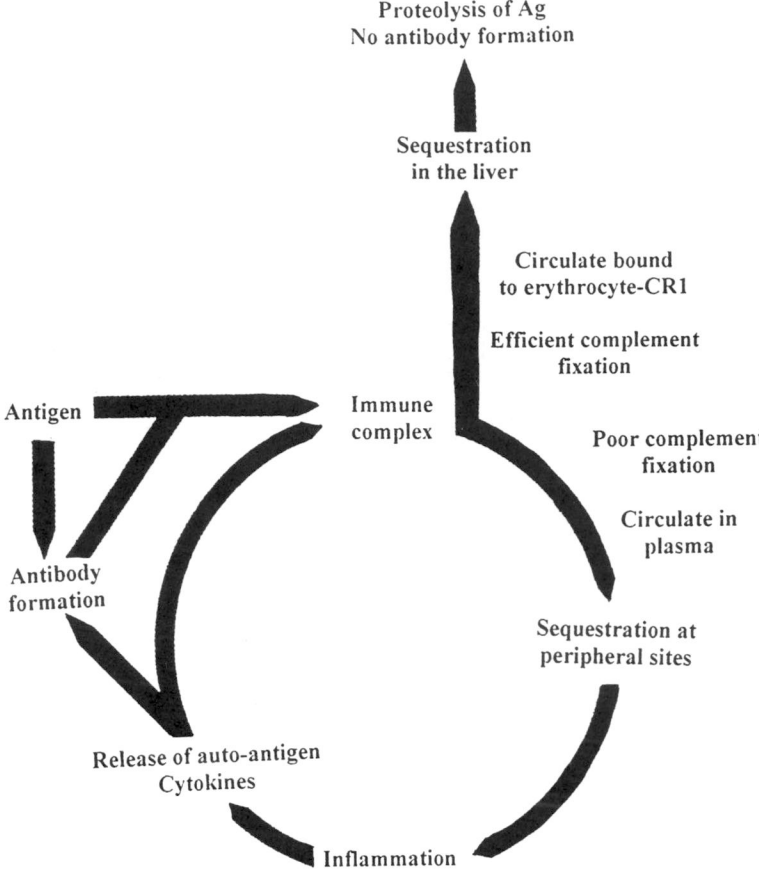

Proteolysis of Ag
No antibody formation

Sequestration
in the liver

Circulate bound
to erythrocyte-CR1

Efficient complement
fixation

Antigen

Immune
complex

Poor complement
fixation

Antibody
formation

Circulate in
plasma

Sequestration at
peripheral sites

Release of auto-antigen
Cytokines

Inflammation

FIG. 15. Schema to show the role of complement in immune complex handling and of defective complement function in giving rise to autoimmune immune complex disease. Reprinted with permission from Oxford University Press (72).

COMPLEMENT DEFICIENCIES

Inherited deficiencies have been described for most complement components and regulatory proteins (Table 7). These abnormalities are relatively rare and usually inherited in an autosomal-recessive manner because only homozygous subjects are readily detected and susceptible to disease. An important exception is hereditary angioedema, which is inherited as an autosomal-dominant trait and also presents in the heterozygote. Complement deficiencies may be considered as important *in vivo* experiments of nature, defining the role of the particular components in the immune system, giving insights into their normal function. Two mutated alleles of the particular gene are usually responsible for the deficiency.

A particular deficiency is paroxysmal nocturnal hemoglobinuria (PNH), which is primarily not a complement deficiency. Mutations in the PIG-A gene affect the synthesis of a competent GPI anchor, which leads to failure of expression of all molecules attached to the membrane via this anchor, including CD55 and CD59. The lack of these two complement control proteins is responsible for the extreme susceptibility of PNH erythrocytes to lysis by complement, activated either by the alternative pathway or via acidic generation of C5-C6 complexes, especially at the physiologically lower blood pH in the night.

The by far most acute, and if untreated potentially lethal, complement deficiency is hereditary angioedema (HAE) due to dysfunctional or missing C1-INH. This disease is intermittently recurring when the patient experiences trauma or infection that forms a trigger for complement activation. Because there is no back-up for C1-INH, activation of C1 will indifferently proceed with generation of C4 and C2 and activation of kinins. The latter are primarily responsible for the classical symptoms of HAE: abdominal colics and suffocation due to larynx edema.

The incidence of complement deficiency states has been difficult to ascertain. A large and representative number of individuals need to be screened, and data available now suggest that the incidence varies considerably depending on the ethnic and geographic background for each component. Study of the relatives of complement-deficient patients and population screening also have led to the identification of a relatively large number (up to 10% to 20%, depending on the component) of healthy deficient individuals.

However, usually complement-deficient subjects are detected because of their increased propensity to infection or in association with immune complex diseases, such as systemic lupus erythematosus (SLE) (Table 7). Particularly striking is the association between SLE and deficiencies of the early classical pathway components. Because only C4 and C2 are coded on the same chromosome (on chromosome 6 within the MHC III gene locus), the possibility that these deficiencies are all linked to a disease susceptibility gene has to be excluded, and there is no reason to question that the increased incidence of these (auto)immune complex diseases is a direct consequence of complement deficiency. Thus, early classical pathway deficiency can be regarded as one of the very few, if not the only, examples where a single defect is sufficient (however, not necessary) for the development of an autoimmune disease (72).

TABLE 7. *Complement deficiency states*

Component	No. of reported patients	Functional defect	Disease associations[a]
C1	50–100	Impaired immune complex handling	SLE, bacterial infections
C4	20–50	Impaired immune complex handling	SLE, bacterial infections
C2	>100	Impaired immune complex handling	SLE, bacterial infections
C3	20–50	Impaired opsonization	Bacterial infections
C1-INH	>>100	Excessive C2 and kinin activation	HAE
B	None		Incompatible with life?
D	3	Impaired alternative pathway activation	Bacterial infections?
P	50–100	Impaired alternative pathway activation	Meningococcal infections
H	<20	Excessive alternative pathway activation	Meningococcal infections, glomerulonephritis
H	20–50	Excessive alternative pathway activation	Bacterial infections
C5	20–50	Impaired chemotaxis, absent lytic activity	Meningococcal infections
C6	>100	Absent lytic activity	Meningococcal infections
C7	>100	Absent lytic activity	Meningococcal infections
C8	>100	Absent lytic activity	Meningococcal infections
C9	>100	Impaired lytic activity	Meningococcal infections

Only strong and established associations are listed, i.e., more than 50% of the diseased subjects have this disease. Note, however, that healthy complement deficient subjects have been found by family studies.

In individuals with homozygous C3 deficiency, pyogenic infections with encapsulated bacteria are severe, recurrent, and life threatening, usually in early childhood. Deficiencies of either factor I or factor H are associated with the inability to degrade C3b, leading to uncontrolled amplification of cleavage of C3 by an unregulated C3b,Bb C3 convertase and result in a state of acquired, severe C3 deficiency (73). Interestingly, the disease associations are not uniform because factor H deficiency, in contrast to C3 or factor I deficiency, predisposes also to glomerulonephritis, which is supported by studies on pig factor H deficiency (74). Deficiency in the factor H–related protein FHR-1 is commonly encountered but has not been linked to any disease (75).

Hereditary deficiency of a terminal complement component leads to an inability to generate a functional terminal complement complex with consecutive absence of hemolysis and bactericidal activity. The particularly frequent occurrence of terminal complement deficiencies in patients with meningococcal infections suggests that the cytolytic activity of the complement system is important in resistance to *Neisseria meningitidis* (76). The data available suggest that either recurrent infection or infection with uncommon serogroups should alert the clinician in Western countries, whereas recurrent disease is the important indicator in endemic areas (77). In addition, it is a quite striking feature that, although *Neisseriae* or Gram-negative bacteria in general have been accused to cause disease in terminal complement deficient subjects, the incidence of gonococcal infections is not increased in deficient subjects, possibly because infections by gonococci are initially restricted to the local mucous membrane and are usually not as fulminantly penetrating into circulation and brain as menongococci. Association of terminal complement deficiencies with susceptibility to autoimmune diseases or nonneisserial infections has been previously mentioned. It was proposed that deficiency might slow down the clearance of these organisms, allowing them to persist for long enough to evoke an abnormal immune response and hence disease (73). Nevertheless, a close examination of the cases available suggests that these associations are very unlikely and probably the result of ascertainment artefacts (77). For example, SLE is found among homozygous terminal complement–deficient subjects, but the frequency is very low and not significantly higher than that found for complement-competent patients.

Several features of terminal complement deficiency have been accumulated in recent years:

1. Low amounts (subtotal deficiency) of functionally active terminal complement proteins may be sufficient for preventing meningococcal disease, suggesting that there is a wide safety margin.

2. Although the incidence of meningococcal infection is much higher, the case fatality rate and the percentage of fulminant cases appears to be lower in terminal complement–deficient subjects when compared with normal subjects. A failure to generate the membrane attack complex with the consequent inability to lyse foreign and autologous cells may lead to a milder form of disease with lower endotoxin concentrations and less host cell injury. In addition, fewer organisms are required for systemic infection. However, in many families of patients investigated, there are often unaccounted deaths of siblings in early childhood, and the possibility of ascertainment artefacts cannot be excluded.

3. The mean age of the first meningococcal attack in complement-deficient individuals tends to be higher than in complement sufficient patients, and the percentage of deficient subjects among meningococcal patients is highest in areas where *N. meningitidis* infections are rare. This reveals that terminal complement deficiency is less likely to be detected in situations where meningococcal infection is common (in early childhood and in meningitis belt countries such as the Sahel zone) and shows that TCC is only one of the means to successfully tackle meningococci.

COMPLEMENT DEFENSE AGAINST INFECTION

Evasion Strategies and Escape of Microorganisms

Microorganisms invading the human body are usually classified by the immune system as nonself. Nonself structures are attacked first by alternative and MBLectin pathways (triggered by the surface composition of the invader) and second by the classical pathway (triggered by specific antibodies targeted toward the intruder, or directly as in the case of several viruses). Chemotaxis of phagocytic cells, opsonization, and lysis of the microbe then mostly lead to limitation of the attack and control of the infection. This sort of host defense is executed on a number of bacteria, viruses, or fungi, and here typically plays a crucial role.

However, evolution of both host and microorganisms has also created a commensual relationship between humans and several microbes so that in many cases potentially infectious microorganisms are not attacked and live in symbiosis with the host. Most of them only cause disease when the host defense is considerably weakened.

The third type of relationship is medically very important and scientifically the most interesting: microorganisms that are highly pathogenic but nevertheless either evade appropriate recognition or constrain suitable attack and destruction (78). To achieve these goals, a range of strategies has been developed by microorganisms during evolution, including both biochemical and biophysical measures to resist C3b deposition, opsonophagocytosis, or complement-mediated cytolytic damage (Table 8) or the remarkable mimicking of complementlike structures or functions (Table 9). A number of microorganisms even use complement receptors to initiate infection in two ways. More commonly, the microorganisms have refined complement-activating properties, which lead to nonopsonic attachment of C3 fragments on their surface, resulting in an inappropriate recognition by polymorphonuclear cells (PMNs) (disguise) (Table 8). On the surface

TABLE 8. *Resistance to complement-mediated damage by interfering with or using complement, excluding molecular mimicry*

Interference with complement activation via poorly activating molecules on the surface of the pathogen	
Lipopolysaccharide	*Salmonella spp., Klebsiella pneumoniae*
Sialic acids	*Schistosoma mansoni*
Trypsin/sialidase sensitive molecules	*Trypanosoma cruzi*
Serum-resistant promastigotes	*Leishmania spp.*
Interference with complement activation via C1q/C1s binding proteins on the surface of the pathogen	
Inhibiting[a]	*Salmonella minnesota* porin, 39 kDa
Inhibiting	*Schistosoma mansoni* paramyosin
Inhibiting	*Taenia solium* paramyosin
Enhancing[a]	HIV-gp41
Interference with C3 convertases	
Blocking of assembly	*Streptococcus spp., Campylobacter spp.*
Prevention of access of phagocytes to cell surface C3 fragments	
Development of capsules	Several encapsulated bacteria
Adsorption of C3 fragments on the pathogen to gain entry into a target cell (usually monocyte/macrophage)	
Utilization of Cr1, target cell: erythrocyte	*Babesia rodhaini, Plasmodium spp.* merozoites
Utilization of CR1 and CR3	*Legionella pneumophila, Mycobacterium leprae*
	Mycobacterium tuberculosis, Leishmania major
Utilization of CR2	HIV-1
Utilization of CR3	HIV-1
	West Nile virus
Interference with complement activation after C3 generation	
No deposition of C6 or C9 on membrane	*Borrelia burgdorferi*
Inhibition or inactivation of C5b6	*Escherichia coli* (traT)
C3b binding far from membrane, no MAC assembly	*Klebsiella pneumoniae*
Interference with C5b-9 insertion into the cytoplasmic membrane	
Insertion distant from membrane due to	
Hydrophobic outer membrane constituents	*Salmonella spp.* (rck), *Trypanosoma cruzi*
Restriction of bactericidal process[a]	*Neisseria gonorrhoeae* (porin PI)
?	*Yersinia enterocolitica* (YadA)
?	*Moraxella catarrhalis*
Incorporation into soluble C5b-9, clusterin binding	*Streptococcus pyogenes* A (SIC)
Adsorption, incorporation or expression of complement regulatory proteins	
Attachment of factor H	*Streptococcus* A (M-protein)
Adsorption of DAF	HIV-1
Incorporation of DAF	Cytomegalovirus
Expression of DAF	*Schistosoma mansoni*
Expression of MCP	Cytomegalovirus
Incorporation of CD59	HIV-1
Proteolytic cleavage of complement components	
Cleavage of C1q and C3	*Pseudomonas deruginosa*, elastase and alkaline protease
Cleavage of C1-INH	*Serratia marcescens*, protease, 56 kDa
Cleavage of C3	*Porphyromonas gingivalis*, trypsin-like protease, 80 kDa
	Entamoeba histolytica, cystein protease, 56 kDa
	Leishmania major, acid protease, gp63
Cleavage of C3 and C9	*Schistosoma mansoni*, serine protease, 28 kDa
Cleavage of C4, C3, C5–C9	*Serratia liquefaciens*, metalloprotease, 53 kDa

[a]assumed/proposed.
? not known.

TABLE 9. *Resistance to complement-mediated damage by mimicking complement proteins*

	Ligand	Functional mimicry	Structural similarity	Antigenic cross-reactivity	Sequence homology
Mimicry of C3 Convertase controlling proteins (DAF, C4bp)					
Blocking assembly of CP C3 convertase					
Trypanosoma cruzi gp60	C3b				DAF
Blocking assembly of AP C3 convertase					
Trypanosoma cruzi gp160		CR1, DAF			
Trypanosoma cruzi gp58/68		CR1			C4bp,DAF,MCP
Blocking assembly of CP and AP and accelerating decay of CP C3 convertase					
Vaccinia virus VCP, gp35	C4b, C3b		C4bp		C4bp
Accelerating decay of AP C3 convertase					
Herpes simplex virus-1/2 gC 1/2	C3b;iC3b	CR1		CR1*	CR1
Epstein-Barr virus	C3b;iC3b,C4	CR1			
Herpes virus Saimiri CCPH (ORF-4)	C4bp	DAF		C4bp,DAF,MCP	
Accelerating decay of CP and AP C3 convertase					
Trypanosoma cruzi gp87–93	C3, C4	CR1, DAF		DAF	
Schistosoma mansoni		CR1			
Unknown mode					
HIV-1 gp120	iC3,C3b,C4b	C4bp		C4bp	C4bp
Mimicry of C3 and C4 facilitating receptor binding					
Epstein-Barr virus gp350/220	CR2	C3d/C3dg		C3d/C3dg	C3d/C3dg
HIV-1 gp41	CR3	C3			C3
Mycobacterium tuberculosis	CR3	iC3b			
Leishmania major/donovani gp63	CR3, CR4	iC3b			
Histoplasma capsulatum	CR3, CR4	iC3b			
Measles virus	MCP				
Streptococcus pyogenes A M-protein	MCP				
Enteroviruses (ECHO, Coxsackie)	DAF				
HIV-1 gp41	P,H	C3			
Streptococcus pyogenes A	C4bp	C4bp			C3
Mimicry of thrombospondin repeat containing proteins					
HIV-1 gp120	C3b,H	P			
Plasmodium falciparum TRAP and CSP	CR1^a			P	P
Trypanosoma cruzi hemolysin, 75 kDa	C9		P,C6-C9	C9	
Mimicry of complement receptors facilitating adhesion					
HIV-1 gp120	C3b	CR3			
Candida albicans, CR3-like, 188 kDa	iC3b	CR3	CR3 (CD11b)	CR3 (CD11b)	CR3 (CD11b)
Candida albicans, CR2-like	C3b	CR2		CR2	CR3 (CD11b)
Mimicry of CD59 limiting membrane attack					
Herpes virus Saimiri ORF-15 (ORF-LS)	C9^a	CD59	CD59	CD59	
Entamobea histolytica adhesin, 260 kDa	C8, C9	CD59		CD59	
Schistosoma mansoni, SCIP-1	C8, C9	CD59			CD59

^a assumed/proposed.
AP alternative pathway; CP, classical pathway

of some microorganisms, however, proteins antigenically or functionally mimicking C3 are present that can bind to complement receptors, mediating uptake in a complement-independent manner, i.e., the uptake does not rely on prior opsonization of the invader (Table 9). By both means, disguise and mimicry, the pathogen avoids destruction by complement and antibody and can harness the cellular machinery for its own reproduction. However, it should be stressed that complement resistance may depend on molecules other than proteins.

An interesting additional feature is the proteolytic degradation of complement proteins by microorganisms protecting them from opsonization or lysis (Table 8). Cleavage of C1-INH by proteases leads to constant consumption of C1 and cleavage of C3, leading to proinflammatory responses and reactive lysis of bystander cells. These microbes must have a highly sophisticated regulation to ensure that enough but not too much detrimental activation occurs. This is also true for pathogens, using a particular receptor for their entry into the host cells. Cleavage has to be very accurate so that most of the surface-deposited C3 is present in the optimum form (C3b or iC3b) for receptor binding.

Another mechanism is the use of complement proteins provided by the host. When HIV-1 is leaving an infected cell (budding process), it is encoated by a lipid bilayer obtained from the host cell membrane and as a consequence carries, in addition to viral, also host cell membrane proteins. Of the latter, DAF and CD59 are of particular importance because they protect HIV-1 from complement lysis (79). Attachment of factor H to C3b on the virus and to several sites on the external portion of gp41 and to one site on gp120 additionally protects against efficient destruction (80,81).

Mimicry of Complement Structures by Microorganisms

During millions of years of coevolution alongside their obligate hosts, several pathogenic microorganisms have evolved functional properties identical to those used by normal mammalian cells to prevent their own destruction by complement. In particular, a number of distinct microbial proteins have been identified that share structural or genetic similarities (antigenic cross-reactivity, sequence homology) with complement proteins or receptors. Such molecular mimicry not only enables the pathogens to avoid destruction by complement, but also facilitates complement-mediated infection via complement receptors (82). Under certain circumstances, mimicry can even lead to development of autoimmunity.

Furthermore, in some instances only a certain principle is adopted. Several microorganisms attack human cells by drilling holes into the lipid bilayer using polymerization and cylinder formation of their specific cytolysins: streptococcal streptolysin-O, *E. coli* hemolysin, or staphylococcal α-toxin (83). The presence of these pore-forming proteins is strongly associated with the virulence of their carriers. However, although using a similar biologic principle as C9, these microbial toxins do not exhibit structural homology on the amino acid sequence level to each other or to C9 or perforin. A number of these molecules bringing about lysis have been identified (84). Some of the microbial proteins mimicking complement proteins are listed in Table 9, comprising mostly those that have yet been defined on the molecular level. For some of these, however, data are insufficient to support their postulated involvement *in vivo* in immune evasion, and many more are awaited to fill this list.

The question is how these molecules have evolved. Teleologically, some of the complementlike molecules are expressed as a consequence of selection on the basis of facilitation of attachment, penetration into host cells, or escape from lysis (84). In the case of vaccinia virus, the DNA encoding VCP, a functionally CR1-like and structurally C4bp-like complement control protein, was presumably originally acquired from the host. Over an evolutionary period, the captured gene was constantly manipulated to retain only the most essential domains because any further manipulation of the small viral protein results in loss of function, indicating that the gene has achieved a maximum efficiency to encode a protein with the minimum number of amino acids (85). In other pathogens, molecular mimicry may represent the conservation of important ancestral molecular recognition motifs. Some of the molecules listed in Table 9 are discussed here in more detail. Many are related to mammalian CR1, DAF, MCP, or C4bp, confirming the importance of C3- and C4-binding molecules.

The overall homology of HIV envelope proteins gp41 and gp120 with complement proteins is very low; in certain short stretches, however, remarkable similitaries were discovered. The respective sites appear to be involved in complement binding and may facilitate virus uptake via complement receptors or play a role in the noncovalent association between gp41 and gp120 (80).

The trematode *Schistosoma mansoni* appears to have the most elaborate anticomplement arsenal: first, it can modify its surface sialic acids, thus modulating activation; second, it can acquire DAF to accelerate decay of surface-bound C3; third, it can bind and cleave C4 and C3 mimicking CR1; fourth, it can cleave C9, preventing MAC assembly; and fifth, but probably not last, it encodes a protein mimicking CD59, inhibiting membrane attack.

The yeast *Candida albicans* possesses an integrin/CR3-like molecule on its surface that is involved in morphology changes representing a virulence factor (86). Furthermore, it appears to facilitate cellular adherence like all members of the human integrin gene family. Interestingly, this molecule is not only functionally (87) but also antigenically and structurally related to human CR3. There is strong evidence that HIV-1 is able to bind to *Candida* directly, possibly via C3-like regions on gp41 and CR3-like regions on *Candida* (88). This interaction enhances candidial proteinase release and suppresses phagocytosis by PMNs (89). Thus, the concerted mimicry of both pathogens may contribute to the virulence of both *Candida* and HIV (88).

It has been proposed that sites of molecular mimicry may represent useful sites for vaccine development (90). However, considering the multiple as yet unrevealed interactions, a detrimental effect of such a vaccine cannot be excluded.

COMPLEMENT DISORDERS AND CLINICAL THERAPY

Effector functions arising from activated complement proteins are potentially harmful with the consequence of inflammatory tissue destruction. This is manifested clinically in various diseases, including sepsis and multiple organ failure. In animals, complement depletion or the use of hereditary deficient species has been effective in reducing tissue injury and ameliorating disease.

Therapeutic interventions to prevent complement activation, to control complement-mediated inflammation, and to minimize host cell lysis are promising and offer tremendous clinical potential for treating a wide variety of acute and chronic diseases. Attempts to efficiently inhibit complement include the following:

1. The application of endogenous purified complement inhibitors (C1-inhibitor)
2. The use of recombinant soluble complement inhibitors (recombinant soluble CR1)
3. The administration of antibodies blocking key steps in the cascade reaction, such as the formation of TCC assembly or C5a generation (anti-C5)
4. The treatment with neutralizing antibodies that inhibit anaphylatoxin effects on host tissue (inflammation, anti-C5a, anti-C5aR)
5. The use of antibodies interfering with adhesion of inflammatory cells to the vascular endothelium (anti-CR3)
6. The incorporation of membrane-bound complement regulators into organs of transgenic animals (pigs) as xenograft sources (CD55, CD46, and CD59) (91)

SUMMARY AND CONCLUSIONS

When immunologists started to dissect the functional entities of the humoral immune response in the second half of the last century, one of the fundamental observations was the discrimination between heat-stable and heat-labile factors. The heat-stable, antigen-specific component was termed the antibody, whereas the heat-labile factor was thought to assist antibodies of diverse specificities in their destructive work and hence given the name "complement" by Paul Ehrlich. However, the role of an executor in the course of the humoral immune response characterizes only one (i.e., the classical pathway) of three pathways leading to the pivotal step of complement activation, i.e., generation of C3b from C3 and its covalent deposition on the activating surface. Likewise, the common endpiece of all complement activation pathways, the terminal pathway, finally leads to assembly of the pore-forming, lytic membrane-attack complex.

Phylogenetically older than the classical pathway, the alternative pathway forms a primitive immune system on its own. It recognizes microbial surfaces in a way distinct from antibody and directs deposition of C3b to these particles. Host tissue is protected by a powerful, redundant control mechanism from self-destructive alternative pathway activation.

The more recently discovered MBLectin pathway has most of the biochemical steps in common with the classical pathway, but is triggered by binding of MBL to polysaccharides present on the surface of many microbes. The importance of all three pathways for innate and acquired immunity is reflected by genetically caused deficiencies that either relate to increased susceptibility to infection or to immune-complex disease.

The molecular core of complement is formed by two main protein families. First, the thioester proteins C3 and C4 possess the unique ability to attach covalently to surfaces upon activation, which causes a profound conformational change. Second, several plasma and membrane proteins interact with the thioester proteins via SCR modules. The SCR is a structural unit that comprises about 60 amino acids (10 to 16 highly conserved). On the one hand, SCRs are found in complement proteins that advance complement activation (e.g., C1r and C1s, C2, factor B). Additionally, these proteins possess serine protease domains to perform the initial proteolytic steps on C3 and C4 required for the amplification of the activation cascade. On the other hand, SCRs are abundantly present in complement receptors (CR1, CR2) or in complement regulatory proteins (e.g., factor H, DAF), which restrict complement activation by binding to activated forms of C3 or C4 and bringing about their inactivation. The genes of these proteins constitute the RCA gene cluster.

The complement system has been present throughout the evolution of the vertebrates, and primitive forms of it are found among nonvertebrates. Ever since, pathogens have tried to overcome this major obstacle or to use it to their advantage. Molecular mimicry is documented among all sorts of pathogens, from nematodes and protozoa to bacteria and viruses. For example, *Trypanosoma cruzi* disposes of proteins that resemble complement regulators present on the host cell and thus help the parasite to evade complement attack. Other pathogens like *Leishmania* or the Epstein-Barr virus use the host cell's complement receptors as their port of entry.

Although designed to combat microbes, complement activation may become harmful to the host himself under certain circumstances. Excessive complement activation contributes to the pathology of immune-complex diseases or autoimmune syndromes. To interfere with such unwanted complement activation has been a longstanding goal of complement research. Recent achievements like recombinantly produced forms of complement regulator proteins (soluble CR1) or humanized monoclonal antibodies against C5 have met the first expectations for a use in several clinical settings. On the other hand, the range of pathologic disorders, where the role of complement is being scrutinized, is broadening. Besides infectious or rheumatic diseases, it now also encompasses atherosclerosis, Alzheimer's disease, and cancer. Consequently, renewed clinical interest will lead the way into the second century of complement research.

ACKNOWLEDGMENT

The authors are supported in their research by the Austrian Fonds zur Förderung der wissenschaftlichen Forschung (FWF).

REFERENCES

1. Ross GD. Introduction and history of complement research. In: Ross GD, ed. *Immunobiology of the complement system.* New York: Academic Press, 1986:1–19.
2. Ehrlich P, Morgenroth J. Über Hämolysine. Zweite Mittheilung. *Berl Klin Wochenschr* 1899;36:481–486.
3. Pillemer L, Lepow IH, Blum L. The requirement for a hydrazine-sensitive serum factor and heat-labile serum factors in the inactivation of human C'3 by zymosan. *J Immunol* 1953;71:339–345.
4. Pillemer L, Blum L, Lepow IH. The properdin system and immunity. I. Demonstration and isolation of a new serum protein, properdin, and its role in immune phenomena. *Science* 1954;120:279–285.
5. Müller-Eberhard HJ, Nilsson UR. Relation of a β1-glycoprotein of human serum to the complement system. *J Exp Med* 1960;111:217–234.
6. Klein PG, Wellensieck HJ. Multiple nature of the third component of guinea-pig complement. I. Separation and characterization of three factors a, b, and c, essential for haemolysis. *Immunology* 1965;8:590–603.
7. Wellensieck HJ, Klein PG. Multiple nature of the third component of guinea-pig complement. II. Separation and description of two additional factors beta and d: preparation and characterization of four intermediate products. *Immunology* 1965; 8:590–603.
8. Nelson RAJ, Jensen J, Gigli I, Tamura N. Methods for the separation, purification and measurement of nine components of hemolytic complement in guinea-pig serum. *Immunochemistry* 1966;3:111–135.
9. Mayer MM. Development of a one-hit theory of immune hemolysis. In: Heidelberger M, Plescia DJ, eds. *Immunochemical approaches to problems in microbiology.* New Brunswick: Rutgers, 1961:268–279.
10. Mayer MM. Mechanism of cytolysis by complement. *Proc Natl Acad Sci U S A* 1972;69:2954–2958.
11. Thiel S, Vorup-Jensen T, Stover CM, et al. A second serine protease associated with mannan-binding lectin that activates complement. *Nature* 1997;386:506–510.
12. Muller-Eberhard HJ. Molecular organization and function of the complement system. *Annu Rev Biochem* 1988;57:321–347.

13. Morgan BP, Gasque P. Extrahepatic complement biosynthesis: where, when and why? *Clin Exp Immunol* 1997;107:1–7.

14. Würzner R, Joysey VC, Lachmann PJ. Complement component C7. Assessment of in vitro synthesis after liver transplantation reveals that hepatocytes do not synthesize the majority of the C7. *J Immunol* 1994;152:4624–4629.

15. Naughton MA, Walport MJ, Würzner R, Carter MJ, Alexander GJ. Organ-specific contribution to circulating C7 levels by the bone. *Eur J Immunol* 1996;26: 2108–2112.

16. Hogasen AK, Würzner R, Abrahamsen TG, Dierich MP. Human polymorphonuclear leukocytes store large amounts of. *J Immunol* 1995;154:4734–4740.

17. Morgan BP, Gasque P. Expression of complement in the brain: role in health and disease. *Immunol Today* 1996;17:461–466.

18. Volanakis JE. Transcriptional regulation of complement genes. *Annu Rev Immunol* 1995;13:277–305.

19. Law SKA, Dodds AW. The internal thioester and the covalent binding properties of the complement proteins C3 and C4. *Protein Sci* 1997;6:263–274.

20. Heine-Suner D, Diaz-Guillen MA, Pardo F, et al. A high resolution map of the regulator of the complement activation gene cluster on 1q32 that integrates new genes and markers. *Immunogenetics* 1997;45:422–427.

21. Nicholson Weller A. Decay accelerating factor (CD55). *Curr Top Microbiol Immunol* 1992;178:7–30.

22. Janatova J, Reid KB, Willis AC. Disulfide bonds are localized within the short consensus repeat units of complement regulator proteins: C4b-binding protein. *Biochemistry* 1989;28:4754–4761.

23. Farries TC, Atkinson JP. Evolution of the complement system. *Immunol Today* 1991;12:295–300.

24. Kalli KR, Hsu P, Fearon DT. Therapeutic uses of recombinant complement protein inhibitors. *Springer Semin Immunopathol* 1994;15:417–431.

25. Reid KB, Day AJ. Structure-function relationships of the complement components. *Immunol Today* 1989;10:177–180.

26. Hack CE, Paardekooper J, Van Milligen F. Demonstration in human plasma of a form of C3 that has the conformation of "C3b-like C3." *J Immunol* 1990; 144:4249–4255.

27. Volanakis JE, Narayana SV. Complement factor D, a novel serine protease. *Protein Sci* 1996;5:553–564.

28. Tschopp J, Villiger W, Fuchs H, Kilchherr E, Engel J. Assembly of subcomponents C1r and C1s of the first component of complement: electron microscopic and ultracentrifugal studies. *Proc Natl Acad Sci U S A* 1980;77:7014–7018.

29. Ziccardi R. Activation of the early components of the classical complement pathway under physiologic conditions. *J Immunol* 1981;126:1769–1773.

30. Morgan BP. *Complement*. London: Academic Press, 1990.

31. Turner MW. Mannose-binding lectin: the pluripotent molecule of the innate. *Immunol Today* 1996;17:532–540.

32. Kolble K, Lu J, Mole SE, Kaluz S, Reid KB. Assignment of the human pulmonary surfactant protein D gene (SFTP4) to 10q22-q23 close to the surfactant protein A gene cluster. *Genomics* 1993;17:294–298.

33. Kawasaki T, Etoh R, Yamashina I. Isolation and characterization of a mannanbinding protein from rabbit liver. *Biochem Biophys Res Commun* 1978;81: 1018–1024.

34. Lu JH, Thiel S, Wiedemann H, Timpl R, Reid KB. Binding of the pentamer/hexamer forms of mannan-binding protein to zymosan activates the proenzyme forms of the C1r2C1s2 complex, of the classical pathway of complement, without involvement of C1q. *J Immunol* 1990;144:2287–2294.

35. Thiel S, Holmskov U, Hviid L, Laursen SB, Jensenius JC. The concentration of the C-type lectin, mannan-binding protein, in human plasma increases during an acute phase response. *Clin Exp Immunol* 1992;90:31–35.

36. Lipscombe RJ, Lau YL, Levinsky RJ, Sumiya M, Summerfield JA, Turner MW. Identical point mutation leading to low levels of mannose binding protein and poor C3b mediated opsonisation in Chinese and Caucasian populations. *Immunol Lett* 1992;32:253–257.

37. Ryley NG, Heryet AR, Lu J, Reid KB, Fleming KA. Comparison between liver and serum concentrations of mannan binding protein. *J Clin Pathol* 1993;46: 259–263.

38. Super M, Thiel S, Lu J, Levinsky RJ, Turner MW. Association of low levels of mannan-binding protein with a common defect of opsonisation. *Lancet* 1989;2:1236–1239.

39. Ikeda K, Sannoh T, Kawasaki N, Kawasaki T, Yamashina I. Serum lectin with known structure activates complement through the classical pathway. *J Biol Chem* 1987;262:7451–7454.

40. Storgaard P, Nielsen EH, Andersen O, et al. Isolation and characterization of porcine mannan-binding proteins of different size and ultrastructure. *Scand J Immunol* 1996;43:289–296.

41. Terai I, Kobayashi K, Matsushita M, Fujita T, Matsuno K. Alpha 2-macroglobulin binds to and inhibits mannose-binding protein-associated serine protease. *Int Immunol* 1995;7:1579–1584.

42. Malhotra R, Willis AC, Jensenius JC, Jackson J, Sim RB. Structure and homology of human C1q receptor (collectin receptor). *Immunology* 1993;78:341–348.

43. Müller-Eberhard HJ. The membrane attack complex of complement. *Annu Rev Immunol* 1986;4:503–528.

44. Thompson RA, Lachmann PJ. Reactive lysis: the complement-mediated lysis of unsensitized cells. I. The characterization of the indicator factor and its identification as C7. *J Exp Med* 1970;131:629–641.

45. Esser AF. Big MAC attack: complement proteins cause leaky patches. *Immunol Today* 1991;12:316–318.

46. Bhakdi S, Tranum Jensen J. Complement lysis: a hole is a hole. *Immunol Today* 1991;12:318–320.

47. Schreiber RD, Morrison DC, Podack ER, Müller-Eberhard HJ. Bactericidal activity of the alternative complement pathway generated from 11 isolated plasma proteins. *J Exp Med* 1979;149:870–882.

48. Morgan BP. Complement membrane attack on nucleated cells: resistance, recovery and non-lethal effects. *Biochem J* 1989;264:1–14.

49. Reiter Y, Ciobotariu A, Fishelson Z. Sublytic complement attack protects tumor cells from lytic doses of antibody and complement. *Eur J Immunol* 1992;22:1207–1213.

50. Niculescu F, Rus H, Shin ML. Receptor-independent activation of guanine nucleotide-binding regulatory proteins by terminal complement complexes. *J Biol Chem* 1994;269:4417–4423.

51. Sims PJ, Wiedmer T. Induction of cellular procoagulant activity by the membrane attack complex of complement. *Semin Cell Biol* 1995;6:275–282.

52. Würzner R, Xu H, Franzke A, Schulze M, Peters JH, Götze O. Blood dendritic cells carry terminal complement complexes on their cell surface as detected by newly developed neoepitope-specific monoclonal antibodies. *Immunology* 1991; 74:132–138.

53. Zipfel PF, Skerka C. Complement factor H and related proteins: an expanding family of. *Immunol Today* 1994;15:121–126.

54. Misasi R, Huemer HP, Schwaeble W, Sölder E, Larcher C, Dierich M. Human complement factor H: an additional gene product of 43 kDa isolated from human plasma shows cofactor activity for the cleavage of the third component of complement. *Eur J Immunol* 1989;19:1765–1768.

55. Preissner KT. Structure and biological role of vitronectin. *Annu Rev Cell Biol* 1991;7:275–310.

56. Jenne DE, Tschopp J. Clusterin: the intriguing guises of a widely expressed glycoprotein. *TIBS* 1992;17:154–159.

57. Würzner R, Schuff Werner P, Franzke A, et al. Complement activation and depletion during LDL-apheresis by heparin-induced extracorporeal LDL-precipitation (HELP). *Eur J Clin Invest* 1991;21:288–294.

58. Lachmann PJ. The control of homologous lysis. *Immunol Today* 1991;12:312–315.

59. Ahearn JM, Fearon DT. Structure and function of the complement receptors, CR1 (CD35) and CR2 (CD21). *Adv Immunol* 1989;46:183–219.

60. Thieblemont N, Haeffner Cavaillon N, Haeffner A, Cholley B, Weiss L, Kazatchkine MD. Triggering of complement receptors CR1 (CD35) and CR3 (CD11b/CD18) induces nuclear translocation of NF-kappa B (p50/p65) in human monocytes and enhances viral replication in HIV-infected monocytic cells. *J Immunol* 1995;155:4861–4867.

61. Bonnefoy JY, Gauchat JF, Life P, Graber P, Aubry JP, Lecoanet Henchoz S. Regulation of IgE synthesis by CD23/CD21 interaction. *Int Arch Allergy Immunol* 1995;107:40–42.

62. Fearon DT, Carter RH. The CD19/CR2/TAPA-1 complex of B lymphocytes: linking natural to acquired immunity. *Annu Rev Immunol* 1995;13:127–149.

63. Stockinger H. Interaction of GPI-anchored cell surface proteins and complement receptor type 3. *Exp Clin Immunogenet* 1997;14:5–10.

64. Wetsel RA. Structure, function and cellular expression of complement. *Curr Opin Immunol* 1995;7:48–53.

65. Reid KBM, Colomb MG, Loos M. Complement component C1 and the collectins: Parallels between routes of acquired and innate immunity. *Immunol Today* 1998;19:56–59.

66. Büscher KH, Opferkuch W. Control mechanisms: C1 inhibitor. In: Rother K, Till GO, eds. *The complement system*. Berlin: Springer, 1988:168–175.

67. Rother U. Shock and shock fragments. In: Rother K, Till GO, eds. *The complement system*. Berlin: Springer, 1988:504–510.

68. Würzner R, Mollnes TE, Morgan BP. Immunochemical assays for complement components. In: Johnstone AP, Turner MW, eds. *Immunochemistry 2: a practical approach*. Oxford, England: Oxford University Press, 1997:197–223.

69. Schneider PM, Rittner C. Complement genetics. In: Dodds A, Sim RB, eds. *Complement—a practical approach*. Oxford, England: Oxford University Press, 1997: 165–198.

70. Mauff G, Würzner R. Complement genetics. In: Herzenberg LA, Weir DM, Blackwell C, eds. *Weir's handbook of experimental immunology*. Malden, MA: Blackwell Science, 1997:77.1–77.11.

71. Morgan BP. Clinical complementology: recent progress and future trends. *Eur J Clin Invest* 1994;24:219–228.

72. Lachmann PJ. Complement. In: McGee JOD, Isaacson PG, Wright NA, eds. *Oxford textbook of pathology*. Oxford, England: Oxford University Press, 1992: 259–266.

73. Morgan BP, Walport MJ. Complement deficiency and disease. *Immunol Today* 1991;12:301–306.

74. Hogasen K, Jansen JH, Mollnes TE, Hovdenes J, Harboe M. Hereditary porcine membranoproliferative glomerulonephritis type II is caused by factor H deficiency. *J Clin Invest* 1995;95:1054–1061.

75. Feifel E, Prodinger WM, Mölgg M, et al. Polymorphism and deficiency of human factor H-related proteins p39 and p37. *Immunogenetics* 1992;36:104–109.

76. Figueroa JE, Densen P. Infectious diseases associated with complement deficiencies. *Clin Microbiol Rev* 1991;4:359–395.

77. Würzner R, Orren A, Lachmann PJ. Inherited deficiencies of the terminal components of human complement. *Immunodefic Rev* 1992;3:123–147.

78. Joiner KA. Complement evasion by bacteria and parasites. *Annu Rev Microbiol* 1988;42:201–230.

79. Marschang P, Sodroski J, Würzner R, Dierich MP. Decay-accelerating factor (CD55) protects human immunodeficiency virus type I from inactivation by human complement. *Eur J Immunol* 1995;25:285–290.

80. Stoiber H, Schneider R, Janatova J, Dierich MP. Human complement proteins C3b, C4b, factor H and properdin react with specific sites in gp120 and gp41, the envelope protein of HIV-1. *Immunobiology* 1995;193:98–113.

81. Stoiber H, Pinter C, Siccardi AG, Clivio A, Dierich MP. Efficient destruction of human immunodeficiency virus in human serum by inhibiting the protective action of complement factor II. *J Exp Med* 1996;183:307–310.

82. Cooper NR. Complement evasion strategies of microorganisms. *Immunol Today* 1991;12:327–331.

83. Bhakdi S, Tranum Jensen J. Damage to cell membranes by pore-forming bacterial cytolysins. *Prog Allergy* 1988;40:1–43.

84. Fishelson Z. Complement-related proteins in pathogenic organisms. *Springer Semin Immunopathol* 1994;15:345–368.

85. Kotwal GJ. The great escape: immune evasion by pathogens. *Immunologist* 1997;4:157–164.

86. Gale C, Finkel D, Tao N, et al. Cloning and expression of a gene encoding an integrin-like protein in *Candida albicans. Proc Natl Acad Sci U S A* 1996;93:357–361.

87. Heidenreich F, Dierich MP. *Candida albicans* and *Candida stellatoidea,* in contrast to other *Candida* species, bind iC3b and C3d but not C3b. *Infect Immun* 1985;50:598–600.

88. Würzner R, Gruber A, Stoiber H, et al. Human immunodeficiency virus type I gp41 binds to Candida albicans via complement C3-like regions. *J Infect Dis* 1997 176:492–498.

89. Gruber A, Lukasser-Vogl E, Borg-von Zepelin M, Dierich MP, Würzner R. Human immunodeficiency virus type 1 gp160/gp41 binding to *Candida albicans* enhances candidal virulence in vitro. *J Infect Dis* 1998;177:1057–1063.

90. Fishelson Z. Complement evasion by parasites: search for "Achilles' heel." *Clin Exp Immunol* 1991;86(suppl 1):47–52.

91. Kirschfink M. Controlling the complement system in inflammation. *Immunopharmacology* 1997;38:57–62.

Fundamental Immunology, Fourth Edition,
edited by William E. Paul
Lippincott–Raven Publishers, Philadelphia © 1999.

CHAPTER 30

Phagocytosis

Samuel L. Jones, Frederik P. Lindberg, and Eric J. Brown

PHAGOCYTOSIS AND INFLAMMATION

A major requirement for the survival of multicellular organisms is protection from potential threats in the environment, including traumatic injury, injury due to noxious conditions such as anoxia or exposure to chemical toxins, and destruction by potential pathogens. The mechanisms by which multicellular organisms protect themselves from infection by bacteria, viruses, and unicellular eukaryotes such as fungi and protozoa are collectively referred to as host defense. Many of the cellular and molecular mechanisms of host defense against these invaders are used in recognition and repair of tissue injury by other mechanisms as well. The vertebrate host defense system is best viewed as a set of highly integrated layers of response to any of these threats. Evolutionarily early "primitive" systems, such as lysis via the complement cascade, are very rapid but not very discriminatory on their own and are relatively easily evaded by potential pathogens. Phagocytosis and killing of invading organisms by polymorphonuclear and mononuclear leukocytes is a marked improvement in both the range of effector mechanisms and the detection of noxious agents. The antigen-specific mechanisms of T cells and B cells are the most advanced, precise mechanism of host defense. Yet none of these facets of host defense successfully protects the host independent of the others. Since the host defense function of phagocytes has evolved in the presence of the com-

plement system, the cells are highly dependent on the complement cascade for activating and discriminating signals. Adaptive immunity has evolved in the presence of both of these systems, and thus is highly dependent on complement and phagocytes for antigen recognition as well as effector functions. Moreover, antibodies produced by the specific immune system are used to augment the function of underlying defense systems, such as in antibody-mediated complement activation and antibody-dependent phagocytosis.

Although it is often convenient to examine the contribution of individual cells and systems in isolation, the components of host defense, tissue repair, and homeostasis systems are highly integrated. For example, a simple laceration leads to exposure of blood to tissue phospholipids, which in turn causes activation of the clotting cascade and complement, as well as platelet activation and aggregation. Platelet activation leads to the release of factors such as thrombin, histamine, adenosine diphosphate (ADP) and adenosine triphosphate (ATP), and platelet-activating factor (PAF), which dilate the microvasculature and activate the surrounding endothelium to express new adhesion molecules for circulating leukocytes. Activation of the coagulation and complement cascades aids the recruitment of neutrophils, which also can be activated directly by thrombin, PAF, ATP, cytokines, and other inflammatory factors. Tissue-resident macrophages and mast cells are activated as well and release more chemoattractants for neutrophils, monocytes, and lymphocytes. Neutrophils also release chemoattractants, which augment neutrophil influx. Biochemical transcellular cooperation among neutrophils, platelets, and endothelial cells occurs in the synthesis of leukotrienes such as LTB4. These effects are directed toward limiting the extent of trauma and preventing infection by

---

S.L. Jones, Department of Molecular Biology and F.P. Lindberg, and E.J. Brown: Department of Internal Medicine, Division of Infectious Diseases, Washington University School of Medicine, St. Louis, Missouri 63110.

potential pathogens. The repair process is initiated by these same cooperative events. Platelet-released platelet-derived growth factor (PDGF) leads to contraction and proliferation of the smooth muscle cells in the blood vessels. PDGF and neutrophil- and macrophage-released growth factors and chemokines lead to invasion by fibroblasts, wound contraction, and scar formation. Phagocytosis, the process by which cells internalize other cells, cell fragments, protein aggregates, and foreign bodies, has an essential role in this complex pattern of events, which occurs in response to purturbation of homeostasis. This chapter will review the cell biology and biochemistry of phagocytosis, in the context of the current understanding of the role of phagocytic cells in host defense.

While targets for engulfment by the process of phagocytosis may be any size, the term *phagocytosis* is generally reserved for those particles that are more than 1 μ in diameter, because at this size the mechanisms for internalization clearly differ from those used for endocytosis of soluble material (1). Phagocytosis was first described by Elie Metchnikoff who observed that there were cells in starfish larvae capable of ingesting and destroying foreign substances or invaders (2,3). This led him to propose the hypothesis that phagocytosis by these cells and their equivalents in other multicellular organisms was an essential aspect of host defense. Although controversial at that time, this hypothesis has been proven over the ensuing decades. Indeed, phagocytosis is a component of many different physiologic processes. For example, amoebae phagocytose bacteria and other organisms as a food source, and certain plant roots harbor bacteria in compartments resembling phagocytic vacuoles to benefit from their nitrogen-fixing capacity. In metazoans, the most prominent roles for phagocytosis include removal of tissue debris after injury, removal of apoptotic cells during development, and destruction of invading pathogens.

TYPES AND DERIVATION OF PHAGOCYTES

As an essential element of host defense, phagocytosis is a part of the mechanism by which most potential pathogens are ultimately destroyed. The host defense aspects of phagocytosis require recognition of potential pathogens and are a function primarily of specialized leukocytes, the myeloid cells known as *polymorphonuclear neutrophils* (PMNs) and monocytes or macrophages, collectively referred to as "professional phagocytes". PMNs and monocytes migrate through blood and tissues, surveying for disruptions of homeostasis, which require repair. All phagocytes are bone marrow–derived. PMNs mature from committed precursors for 6 days in the marrow and then are released into the vasculature to circulate for only 6 to 12 hours (4), following which they enter various tissues, where they ultimately apoptose and are efficiently removed by resident macrophages. During infection, PMNs are released from the bone marrow in greater numbers and sometimes prior to full maturation. The existence of increased numbers and/or immature PMNs in the blood has been used clinically for many years as a sign of infection. Nonetheless, the signals and mechanisms leading to PMN release during either homeostasis or infection are not well understood.

Myeloid granulocytes are divided based on the staining properties of their granules into neutrophils, eosinophils, and basophils. PMNs are the most abundant, constituting about 95% of the total granulocytes. Mature PMNs contain at least three different classes of granules, termed *primary, secondary,* and *tertiary,* which differ in their contents. In general, the granules contain lysosomal enzymes and/or bacteriostatic or bacteriocidal molecules and act as a repository for membrane molecules, which can be rapidly mobilized to the cell surface for use in host defense. The regulated secretion of granule contents is a critical component of host defense, as demonstrated by the markedly increased susceptibility of patients lacking one or more classes of neutrophil granules (5–8). Eosinophils represent 2% to 4% of circulating granulocytes, with granules that contain proteolytic and glycolytic enzymes, basic proteins, and peroxidase. They are especially important in host defense against parasitic infections, and their numbers increase during allergic reactions. Basophils and the tissue-resident, long-lived mast cells have acidic granules that contain heparin and histamine. Basophils and mast cells have surface IgE receptors, which when cross-linked by antigen, cause degranulation with secretion of histamine and other vasoactive mediators. Mast cells have an important role in the inital events of host defense against invading bacteria (9,10). This is probably because mast-cell degranulation is required for the generation of inflammation and influx of phagocytic cells, rather than because of a direct toxic effect of the mast-cell granule contents on the invading bacteria.

Mononuclear phagocytes are released from the bone marrow as monocytes, which migrate into different tissues, where they further differentiate into mature macrophages. The phenotype of these cells is highly dependent on the tissue in which they are found. Much of the role of these cells is to remove dead and damaged cells and particulate matter from the tissues. As Kupffer cells in liver and spleen sinusoids, they remove senescent erythrocytes from the bloodstream. Kupffer cells also remove other debris, such as fibrin degradation products and immune complexes, from the circulation. As alveolar macrophages, they ingest and remove inhaled particles that are small enough to reach the terminal airways. As microglia in the central nervous system, they ingest degenerated myelin. They also are found in the submucosa of the gastrointestinal and urogenital tracts, in the skin, and in the synovial membranes lining the joint cavities. At these sites, as well as in the peritoneal and pleural cavities, they remove the small numbers of bacteria that frequently leak into these tissues from the bowel or the lung.

Monocytes circulate with a half-time of 16 to 20 hours prior to migration into tissue to become tissue macrophages (11). Whether migration into tissue in the absence of inflammation is stochastic or if, alternatively, there are subpopulations of monocytes predestined for certain tissues is unknown. Fully differentiated resident macrophages have a lifetime of 4 to 15 days in their home tissues. During inflammation, monocyte accumulation at the perturbed site is greatly increased. This is due primarily to increased influx from circulating monocytes and only minimally to proliferation of resident macrophages. These inflammatory macrophages have a different phenotype than the resident tissue cells, including expression of myeloperoxidase, increased phagocytic capacity, and enhanced ability to generate toxic oxygen and nitrogen metabolites.

Phagocyte Recruitment to Sites of Host Defense

Leukocyte Rolling

The initial steps in successful host defense require that the professional phagocytes recognize and migrate to sites of pathogen invasion. Since all of the PMNs and the vast majority of the macrophages present at such sites come from the blood, migration to the site of perturbation requires recognition of endothelium overlying the inflammatory site, movement through the blood vessel wall, and then movement through the extracellular matrix. This process of migration to a site of infection requires specific receptors by which the phagocyte recognizes the inflammatory site, adheres to and migrates through the endothelium and other elements of the vascular wall, and then moves to and destroys the inciting stimulus. The current model is that this is a multistep process involving sequential adhesion events (Fig. 1). The most acute response of small venular endothelium overlying a site of inflammation to thrombin, PAF, interleukin-1 (IL1), histamine, and other mediators released by clotting, platelet activation, or mast-cell activation is expression of an adhesion molecule, P-selectin, on the lumenal plasma membrane (12–14). P-selectin is stored in a regulated secretory compartment of the endothelial cell known as Weibel-Palade bodies and can be mobilized to the cell surface within seconds after exposure to the appropriate inflammatory stimulus. P-selectin is one of three known Ca^{2+}-dependent carbohydrate-binding proteins involved in interaction between leukocytes and endothelium: P-selectin, L-selectin, and E-selectin, also known as CD62P, CD62L, and CD62E (14,15). PMNs express a P-selectin ligand and a second member of the selectin family, L-selectin, which recognizes a ligand on the endothelial cells (15,16). Together, P- and L-selectin interactions with their ligands lead to transient binding of leukocytes to endothelium, which markedly slows the rate at which PMNs transit through the blood vessels at the site of inflammation (17–19). This is the first step in specific recognition of an inflammatory site by leukocytes, but selectin-mediated interaction is not sufficient to cause transendothelial migration of leukocytes, or even to firm adhesion between the PMNs and the endothelial cells. Rather, these interactions lead to the phenomenon of leukocyte rolling along blood vessels overlying sites of inflammation.

The phagocyte-rolling process serves to bring these cells into close contact with the endothelium, and to slow their passage in regions of tissue damage and inflammation. Captured by the endothelial surface glycocalyx are numerous mediators synthesized by activated endothelial cells or the underlying tissue. Ligation of phagocyte receptors by these mediators is the next step in leukocyte recruitment (20). PMNs have on their surfaces high-affinity (nM) receptors for a number of chemoattractants or chemokines, notably the complement fragment C5a, IL-8, PAF, LTB4, Gro-alpha, and N-formylated peptides [e.g., formylmethionylleucylphenylalanine (fMLP)] present in bacterial but not eukaryotic proteins (21,22). Monocytes have receptors for an overlapping but distinct set of molecules found at sites of inflammation (23,24).

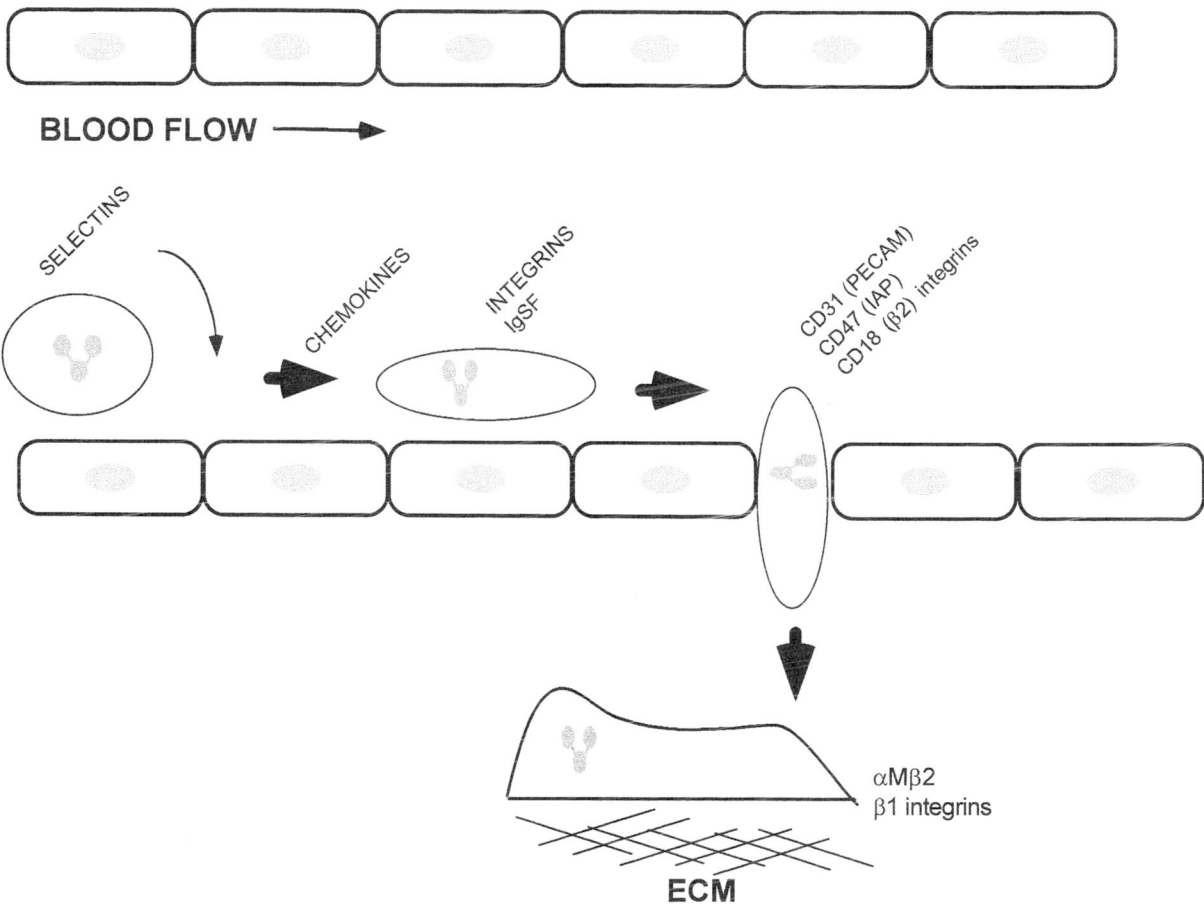

FIG. 1. Leukocyte emigration to sites of inflammation. On recognition of endothelium overlying sites of inflammation, leukocytes initially roll on the endothelial apical membrane, then develop more stable, firm adhesion in response to chemokines, histamine, thrombin, or other mediators of inflammation. Leukocytes leave the vasculature at interendothelial junctions and then migrate through the extravascular spaces by chemotaxis on extracellular matrix proteins.

Response to chemokines is likely to provide much of the specificity in leukocyte recruitment to particular sites of inflammation. For example, monocytes and macrophages have receptors for a number of chemokines, such as MIP-1α and MCP-1, that are not recognized by PMNs (25). On the other hand and in contrast to PMNs, macrophages do not respond to IL-8 (26,27). Among granulocytes, eosinophils are unique in that they respond to the complement fragment C3a as a chemoattractant (28). RANTES, MIP-1α, MCP-3, and eotaxin also are chemotactic for eosinophils, but not for neutrophils (29–31). All of these chemoattractant receptors are members of the seven-transmembrane family of G protein–coupled receptors (32).

Firm Adhesion to Endothelium

As leukocytes have been slowed down by selectin-mediated interactions and exposed to locally produced chemokines, they become activated within a few cell diameters from the site of original contact. Firm adhesion at this stage is a prerequisite for subsequent transendothelial migration. Leukocyte integrins (CD18 or β2 integrins) binding endothelial immunoglobulin family members are the major mediators of this event (see Fig. 1).

Integrins are heterodimeric cell surface receptors, composed of polypeptide chains from two gene families, known as α and β. There are 14 polypeptides in the α-chain family, and eight in the β, which can make 22 distinct combinations that express overlapping ligand specificities (33). Both chains are type I membrane proteins with a large extracellular amino terminal portion (around 160 kDa for α and 90 kDa for β), a transmembrane segment, and a short (20 to 50 amino acids) cytoplasmic tail. The integrin family is ubiquitously expressed, and all integrin receptors are involved in adhesion events. Integrins may mediate cell attachment to extracellular matrix (ECM) or to other cells. Leukocytes express integrins of the β1, β2, β3, β5, and β7 subfamilies. While many of these are expressed on other cells as well, β2 and β7 integrins are expressed exclusively on leukocytes and are especially important in the regulated adhesive events that occur as lymphocytes circulate through lymph nodes or phagocytes migrate to sites of inflammation. Leukocyte integrins can exist in at least two different states (active and inactive), marked primarily by a large difference in ability to mediate adhesion (34–39). As leukocytes circulate in the blood, their integrins are inactive and poorly adhesive. Exposure of slowly rolling leukocytes to chemokines on the endothelial surface activates integrins to a much more adhesive state. These activated integrins mediate rapid, firm leukocyte adhesion to the endothelial cells.

Transendothelial Migration and Chemotaxis to Extravascular Sites

The migration of phagocytes through the vascular wall is less well understood than these initial events leading to firm adhesion. β2 integrins and the immunoglobulin superfamily members PECAM-1 (CD31) and integrin-associated protein (IAP) (CD47) all appear to have a role, as may an additional integrin, αvβ3 (40–45). Endothelial cell-produced IL-8 also is believed to have a critical role in this process (46). Once through the endothelium, the phagocytes may adhere to other cells during migration to the site of inflammation, for example, smooth muscle cells of the vascular wall or fibroblasts in the connective tissue. These interactions also are dependent on the leukocyte-specific β2 integrins αMβ2 and αXβ2 (47,48). Migration through the ECM to a site of trauma or infection also is integrin-mediated. In these interactions, cell surface β1, β3, and β5 integrins recognize specific protein ligands in the ECM (49). These integrin-mediated interactions, like interactions with the endothelial cells, require integrin activation to a high-avidity state by chemoattractants produced at the site of inflammation. The chemoattractants also have a critical role in determination of the direction of phagocyte migration, because the cells will move toward higher concentrations of many different chemoattractants, a process called chemotaxis. In this way, the PMNs and inflammatory macrophages arrive at the site of highest chemoattractant concentration, which is the focus of infection or inflammation. Cell migration through ECM also depends on protease activity associated with the phagocytes, presumably to degrade ECM to allow easier migration (50,51). Once at these sites, the effector functions latent in the phagocytes are activated. These include generation of toxic oxygen and nitrogen metabolites, release of proteases and other destructive enzymes, and synthesis of cytokines and chemoattractants, which amplify the host defense response, as well as phagocytosis.

CELL BIOLOGY OF PHAGOCYTOSIS

Phagocytosis can be thought of as occuring in four basic steps (Fig. 2). The initial event is recognition of the target by the phagocytic cell. Recognition of a phagocytic target can be either direct, through phagocyte receptor interaction with specific aspects of the target that the phagocyte recognizes as "foreign," or through the process of opsonization. Opsonization occurs when host proteins interact with invading pathogens, apoptotic cells, or cellular debris. In the next step of the engulfment process, receptor–ligand interaction causes specific cellular responses through signal transduction pathways. These responses are required for membrane and cytoplasmic changes that lead to engulfment and also are accompanied by other aspects of inflammation, such as enzyme secretion, adhesion, degranulation, and respiratory burst. The third step is the actual process of internalization, which requires one or more membrane fusion events by the phagocytic cell to bring the phagocytic target from the extracellular milieu to the intracellular vesicular network. Finally, the ingested particle enters the lysosomal system in the phagocyte, where it is degraded. The study of the response to many infectious organisms, and the mechanisms by which virulent organisms evade ingestion and killing, have helped elucidate many steps in the process.

Recognition of the Phagocytic Target

Nonopsonic Recognition

The initial event of phagocytosis is recognition of the particle to be ingested by the phagocytic cell. In "professional phagocytes," this occurs because of expression on the phagocytic cell of a set of receptors that have evolved to recognize invading organisms and devitalized cells or tissues. A number of these receptors recognize specific features that differentiate the target from normal cells or tissue. For example, there are phagocyte receptors for bacterial lipopolysaccharide, a component of the gram-negative bacterial cell wall, for peptidoglycan of gram-positive organisms, for certain carbohydrates, for denatured proteins, and for phosphatidylserine (a surface-exposed component of apoptotic cells) (52–58). Nonopsonic phagocytic receptors are enumerated in Table I. These receptors fail to attain very broad recognition of potential pathogens,

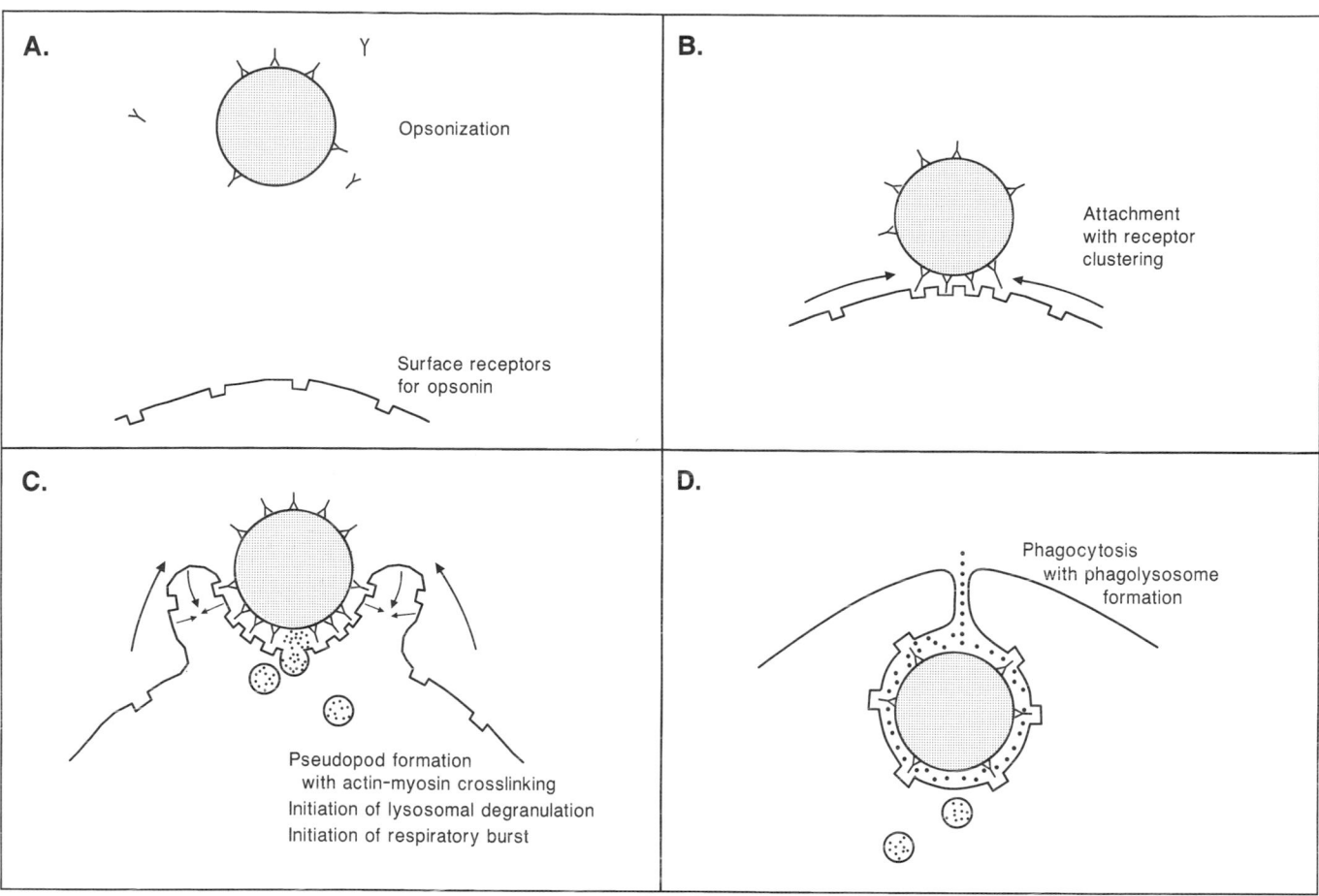

FIG. 2. The four steps of phagocytosis. Initial recognition of a phagocytic target can be either direct; through phagocyte receptors for bacteria, apoptotic cells, or cellular debris; or through the process of opsonization, as depicted in **panel A**. Initial interaction leads to a coordinated series of changes in phagocyte membrane and cytoskeleton, which lead to pseudopod extension around the target (**panel B**). Initiation of engulfment is accompanied by a series of changes in the composition of the plasma membrane and fluid milieu at the site of ingestion, resulting from degranulation and regulated secretion (**panel C**). Finally, the phagocyte plasma membrane fuses, causing the internalization of the phagocytic target with phagocyte membrane in a phagosome (**panel D**).

however, because many virulent bacteria and parasites have evolved mechanisms to evade this rather small cohort of receptors. Teleologically, these receptors represent the first line of host protection, and as bacterial strategies for evasion have evolved, the host has had to evolve correspondingly more sophisticated mechanisms for recognition of the wide variety of potential pathogens.

One of the major classes of nonopsonic phagocytic receptors are the scavenger receptors (57,59). These receptors recognize a wide variety of ligands, including modified proteins, polyanions (including nucleic acids), and acidic phospholipids, including lipopolysaccharide of gram-negative bacteria and the lipoteichoic acid of gram-positive bacteria. This array of ligands makes it seem likely that these receptors are involved in removal of damaged tissue and debris, as well as in host defense against a wide variety of potential pathogens. The ability of members of the family to recognize both low- and high-density lipoproteins suggest they may have a role in the pathologic process of atherosclerosis as well (60,61). Structurally, the family of scavenger receptors is large and diverse (57). The unifying feature of these receptors is the presence of one or more cysteine-rich domains, known as *scavenger receptor cysteine-rich* (SRCR) (57). Further sequence homologies define three subgroups of SRCR domains; the structural distinctions among the subgroups of scavenger receptors are reflected in different ligand-binding properties. Scavenger receptors also can mediate macrophage adhesion (62,63).

Another class of nonopsonic receptors for phagocytosis are the C-type lectins (64). The major macrophage phagocytic C-type lectin is the mannose receptor. The mannose receptor is a 175-kDa type I membrane protein present on macrophages with eight C-type lectin domains, although not all are active in mannose binding (65). Mannose receptors transfected into Chinese hamster ovary cells mediate phagocytosis (66), in contrast to at least one class of IgG Fc receptors (see below). Mannose receptor expression is decreased by IFN-γ, lipoposlysaccharide, and immune complexes (64). The phagocytic function of other lectin receptors reported on phagocytic cells, including the β-glucan receptor, fucose receptor, advanced glycosylation end-products receptor, and galactose receptor, has not been studied.

Opsonin Receptors

Successful homeostasis has required the evolution of other mechanisms for recognition and destruction of invaders or dam-

TABLE 1. *Direct recognition of ingestion targets by phagocyte receptors*

Ligand on phagocytic target	Phagocyte receptors	Receptor family	Involvement in phagocytosis	Refs.
Lipopolysaccharide	CD14	GPI-linked	Possibly	54
	CD11b/Cd18	Integrin	Yes	287
Phosphatidylserine	?Croque mort	Scavenger receptor	Apoptotic cells	150
	Other	Not known	Apoptotic cells	58
Peptidoglycan	Scavenger receptor type I		Yes	55
Carbohydrate	Mannose receptor	C-type lectin	Yes	64

aged tissue. The host response to this challenge has been to evolve a series of soluble proteins that recognize invaders and in turn are recognized by specific receptors on phagocytic cells (Table 2). These plasma proteins increase the range of microbes recognized as possible pathogens, or extracellular debris recognized as damaged or defective, and they engage potentially more efficient mechanisms for signaling the removal and destruction of the targets to which they attach than do the nonopsonic receptors discussed above. The plasma proteins are called opsonins, from the Greek *opson*, "to prepare to eat." The major opsonins of plasma are immunoglobulin and complement, for which there are a variety of receptors on phagocytes, which, when engaged, mediate the effector mechanisms of host defense, including phagocytosis.

Fc Receptors

Fc receptors bind to the Fc portion (immunoglobulin domains C2-C3 of the heavy chain) of IgG, IgA, and IgE molecules (67,68). IgE receptors are not expressed on phagocytes, but IgG receptors (FcγR) and IgA receptors (FcαR) are (69,70). FcγR and FcαR are immunoglobulin family members with three (FcγRIA) or two (other Fc receptors) extracellular immunoglobulin domains, a transmembrane segment and a relatively short cytoplasmic tail, except for human FcγRIIIB, which is anchored to the membrane through a glycan phosphoinositol (GPI) linkage and thus lacks transmembrane and intracellular domains (71). Phagocyte Fc receptors are listed in Table 3. All Fcγ receptor genes are located within a small region of chromosome 1 in both human and mouse. Most likely, the different genes evolved from a single ancestral FcγR by a series of duplications. While FcγRI can bind monomeric IgG with nM affinity, FcγRII and FcγRIII are mainly receptors for polyvalent IgG, such as occurs in immune complexes or on antibody-coated bacteria, viruses, or cellular debris (72). The affinity

of the different Fcγ receptors differs considerably for immune complexes made with different IgG subclasses (73).

FcγRI

FcγRI, with its three immunoglobulin domains, is a high-affinity (1 to 10 nM) receptor for IgG. There are three FcγRI genes, FcγRIA through FcγRC. FcγRIA is normally expressed on macrophages and monocytes (see Table 3); expression of the protein products of the other two genes is not certain. FcγRI is not normally expressed on PMNs but can be induced by IFN-γ or granulocyte colony-stimulating factor (G-CSF) (74). Like the FcεRI, FcγRIA is associated with an additional membrane molecule, the γ-chain dimer (75). γ chain, named because of its association with the α and β chains of the high-affinity IgE receptor of basophils, is a relative of the ζ chain of the T-cell antigen receptor, and, like it, mediates receptor signaling via immune-tyrosine activation motifs (ITAMs) and binding of syk-family kinases. In contrast to FcεRI and the T-cell antigen receptor, FcγRIA surface expression is not dependent on expression of this signaling chain. FcγRI is the only FcγR that has sufficient affinity for ligand to bind monomeric IgG well. While it is capable of mediating phagocytosis of IgG opsonized targets, FcγRI is saturated with monomeric IgG on circulating monocytes. Thus, it may addition-

TABLE 2. *Some opsonins for phagocyte recognition of invading pathogens or apoptotic cells*

Opsonin	Phagocyte receptors	Refs.
Antibody	IgG Fc	288, 289
Complement		
C3 fragments	CR1, CR3, CR4	125, 290
C1q	C1qR	291, 292
Lectins		
Mannose binding protein	?C1qR	131, 293
C-reactive protein	?	136
Fibrinogen	several integrins	294, 295
Fibronectin	several integrins	296, 297
Thrombospondin	αVβ3, CD36, CD47	298

TABLE 3. *Phagocyte receptors for immunoglobulin Fc region*

Receptor	CD	Mr (kD)	Cell distribution
FcγRI[a]	64	75	Monocytes
			Macrophages
			IFN-γ treated PMN
FcγRIIA[b]	32	40	PMN
			Monocytes
			Macrophages
			Platelets
FcγRIIB[b]	32	40	Monocytes
			Macrophages
			B-lymphocytes
			Mast cells
FcγRIIIA[c]	16	50–65	Macrophages
			NK cells
			Mast cells
FcγRIIIB[c]	16	50	Primate PMN
FcαR	89	55–75	Granulocytes
			Monocytes
			Macrophages

[a]There are three genetic loci encoding FcγRI proteins.
[b]Antibodies do not distinguish the extracellular domains of FcγRIIA and FcγRIIB.
[c]The extracellular domains of FcγRIIIA and FcγRIIIB are identical.

ally function as a cytophilic antibody similar to the high-affinity IgE receptor on basophils, requiring only dimeric antigen to induce cell activation.

FcγRII

FcγRII is a medium-affinity Fcγ-receptor. Like FcγRI, there are three gene loci that encode FcγRII proteins (FcγRIIA, FcγRIIB, and FcγRIIC). PMNs express only FcγRIIA. Monocytes and macrophages express some FcγRIIB, but FcγRIIA predominates. FcγRIIC has not been detected at the protein level. A polymorphism in the membrane-proximal immunoglobulin domain (H131R) of human FcγRIIA leads to an isoform with substantially reduced IgG$_2$ affinity. This may affect host defense, as homozygousity for the high-affinity 131H allele is associated with a lower incidence of infections with encapsulated bacteria (76,77).

There are significant differences in function between FcγRIIA and FcγRIIB because of differences in sequence in the cytoplasmic tails of the two receptors. FcγRIIA and FcγRIIB differ in their ability to support phagocytosis. While attachment via FcγRIIA leads to particle engulfment, attachment via FcγRIIB does not (78,79). This may result from failure of FcγRIIB to activate the leukocyte-specific tyrosine kinase syk, as well as its constitutive association with actin microfilaments, which may exclude it from membrane domains active in phagocytosis (78,80). FcγRIIA activates phagocytes through a tyrosine kinase cascade requiring syk. While FcγRIIA may, like other phagocyte Fc receptors, associate with the transmembrane ITAM-containing γ chain (81), its signaling activity critically depends on two of the three tyrosines in its cytoplasmic tail (82,83). These two tyosines are in YXXL motifs, like the tyrosines of ITAMs, but the spacing between the two YXXL sequences is 12 amino acids rather than the six to eight of the typical ITAM. Nonetheless, syk appears to bind directly to FcγRIIA and to be activated when these tyrosines are phosphorylated (83–86), suggesting that the FcγRIIA cytoplasmic tail does express a functional ITAM. In contrast, FcγRIIB does not have an ITAM sequence; instead, its phosphorylated tyrosine is within a sequence that binds the inhibitory SH2 domain containing inositol phosphatase SHIP (87–90). Thus, while ligation of FcγRIIA activates phagocytes, ligation of FcγRIIB diminishes cell activation.

FcγRIII

FcγRIII is encoded by two nearly identical genes, FcγRIIIA and FcγRIIIB. FcγRIIIA is a transmembrane protein with two immunoglobulin domains. There are nine nucleotide differences between the genes encoding FcγRIIIA and FcγRIIIB. A single nucleotide change leads to substitution of Phe at amino acid 185 in FcγRIIIA with Ser in FcγRIIIB, a difference that creates a signal for addition of a GPI anchor rather than a transmembrane domain in FcγRIIIB. FcγRIIIA has intermediate affinity for IgG (30 nM), whereas FcγRIIIB binds monomeric IgG very poorly, suggesting that the γ chain association of FcγRIIIA may affect ligand affinity (91). Macrophages, some monocytes, natural killer (NK) cells, and some T-lymphocytes express FcγRIIIA. Only neutrophils constitutively express FcγRIIIB, which is expressed on eosinophils after exposure to IFN-γ (74). FcγRIIIA has a sequence in its transmembrane segment that leads to retention in the endoplasmic reticulum, unless it is associated with the γ chain. Thus, not only its signaling but also its surface expression is dependent on association with a γ

chain. In this way, it differs from both FcγRI and FcγRII, which associate with the γ-chain dimer for signaling, but do not require this association for plasma membrane expression. Loss of FcγRIIIB expression through a chromosomal deletion of FcγRIIIB (and part of FcγRIIC) does not cause an obvious increased susceptibility to bacterial infections (92).

Soluble Fcγ Receptors

Several FcγRs can be secreted after synthesis from alternatively spliced mRNAs or released from the cell surface by proteolytic cleavage (93). These soluble products are increased in inflammatory diseases and in situations in which phagocyte numbers or turnover are increased. While these proteins in vitro can inhibit immune complex–mediated phagocyte activation by blocking immune complex interaction with cellular Fc receptors, the in vivo significance of these receptor fragments is unclear.

FcαR

FcαR is expressed on monocytes and PMNs (70). The receptor has nM affinity for IgA and associates with the γ-chain dimer, like Fcγ receptors (94). Like FcγRI and FcγRIIA, FcαR expression is not dependent on γ-chain association. Because of its relatively high affinity for IgA and its γ-chain association, FcαR may have functions similar to those of FcγRI. Although FcαR-mediated phagocytosis has been reported, its phagocytic capacity has not been studied extensively. IgA antibody to some bacteria and viruses actually increases susceptibility to systemic infection and blocks opsonization and phagocytosis in vitro, suggesting that IgA does not have a potent opsonic effect (95–98). The polymeric immunoglobulin receptor, which transports IgA across mucosal barriers (99), is essential for normal host defense, but is not expressed on phagocytes.

Complement Receptors

The complement component C3 is the second major opsonin of serum. During complement activation, C3 is cleaved to C3b and then further to iC3b, both of which are covalently attached to the complement-activating surface. Phagocytes express receptors for both of these C3 fragments, and these complement receptors are involved in phagocytosis. Complement receptors are not competent for ingestion in unactivated cells, while they phagocytose C3-opsonized targets efficiently after cell activation in vivo or in vitro (100,101). Thus, the capacity of these receptor for ingestion is not constitutive but depends on many other cellular events. The molecular nature of the events governing the ability of complement receptors to phagocytose is only partially understood. Because the primary role of phagocytosis in host defense is at sites of infection and inflammation, where activating stimuli abound, it is likely that at these sites complement receptors make an important contribution to the phagocytic potential of the responding cells.

CR1

CR1 is a single-chain type I transmembrane protein that is expressed on erythrocytes and glomerular podocytes as well as phagocytes and some lymphocytes (102). The molecule is made up of multiple loose repeats of an approximately 60-amino acid highly disulfide-bonded domain, known as the short consensus repeat. There are allellic polymorphisms in the number of SCRs expressed by CR1, which have been associated with differences in immune complex clearance and with autoimmunity (103), but these are not known to affect the phagocytic function of CR1. Opsonization by C3b alone and ligation and cross-linking of CR1 does not lead to phagocytosis by unactivated phagocytes. On the other hand, when protein kinase C (PKC) is activated exogenously, for example, by phorbol esters, C3b-opsonized particles are phagocytosed by both PMNs and monocytes (100,104). This suggests that CR1 ligation fails to activate a PKC required for engulfment, but much less is known about signal transduction from CR1 ligation than about Fc receptors.

Integrin Complement Receptors

Two phagocyte-specific integrins of the β2 family act as receptors for the iC3b fragment of C3 (105,106). These two are αMβ2 (also known as complement receptor 3/CR3, Mac1, and CD11b/CD18) and αXβ2 (also known as CR4, p150, 95, or CD11c/CD18). These same two receptors have roles in transendothelial migration and chemotaxis through ECM, as discussed above. As with other integrins on leukocytes, these two phagocyte iC3b receptors require activation for high-affinity ligand binding (37). Thus, these receptors, like CR1, are not competent to mediate phagocytosis in resting unactivated phagocytes, but are activated after phagocyte exposure to cytokines and chemoattractants.

CR3 (αMβ2) has a very special and central role in many PMN adhesion-dependent functions, such as phagocytosis, because its expression is required for multiple other receptors to interact appropriately with the phagocyte cytoskeleton for adhesion and ingestion. The central role of this integrin on PMNs is best appreciated by the phenotype of humans, cows, or dogs with leukocyte adhesion deficiency (LAD), type I, a complete or almost complete absence of expression of the β2-integrin chain (107,108). PMNs from these patients are unable to migrate into sites of inflammation, leading to uncontrolled tissue infection and delays in clearance of debris and

wound healing (109). A characteristic feature of these patients is failure to resorb the umbilical stump. This defect results from failure of leukocytes to adhere to endothelium and/or to migrate through ECM, a recognized role for all three β2 integrins (20,110). LAD PMNs also fail to activate appropriately in response to inflammatory signals, as manifest by their failure to phagocytose IgG- or C3b-opsonized targets appropriately (111,112), to make a normal amount of LTB4 after immune complex binding (113), to generate a normal increase in intracytoplasmic Ca^{2+} in response to Fcγ receptor ligation (114), to make a respiratory burst in response to tumor necrosis factor-α (TNF-α) (115), and to phosphorylate the cytoskeleton protein paxillin after multiple activating stimuli (116,117). Failure to activate is due to absence of αMβ2 specifically, as is the failure of LAD PMNs to adhere to or migrate on a variety of different surfaces *in vitro* (118). Because integrins are known to bind indirectly to the actin cytoskeleton through their cytoplasmic tails, these various effects of αMβ2 deficiency suggest that PMN activation is intimately linked to integrin-dependent effects on cytoskeleton. However, the requirement for Mac-1, even when there is no obvious ligand for this integrin, is surprising, and suggests that one function of Mac-1 may be to mediate lateral interactions with other receptors on the phagocyte plasma membrane (119). There is significant evidence for these lateral interactions, which have been studied most intensively between αMβ2 and Fcγ receptors or the urokinase receptor, uPAR (120). αMβ2 cocaps with both FcγRIIIB and uPAR in PMNs. When FcγRIIIB is transfected into fibroblasts, it is not competent to mediate phagocytosis of IgG-opsonized particles, but when αMβ2 is cotransfected, IgG-mediated ingestion occurs (121). The demonstration of resonance energy transfer between FcγRIIIB and αMβ2 also suggests a close lateral association, as does the demonstration that contransfection of αMβ2 slows the diffusion in the cell membrane of the GPI-linked FcγRIIIB (122). Other data support a functional and physical association of FcγRIIA with αMβ2 in PMNs (113,123,124). Together these data support the hypothesis that the role of αMβ2 in phagocyte effector mechanisms extends beyond its function as a complement receptor and that it may be an essential component of the adhesive and phagocytic functions of diverse phagocyte plasma membrane receptors (Fig. 3).

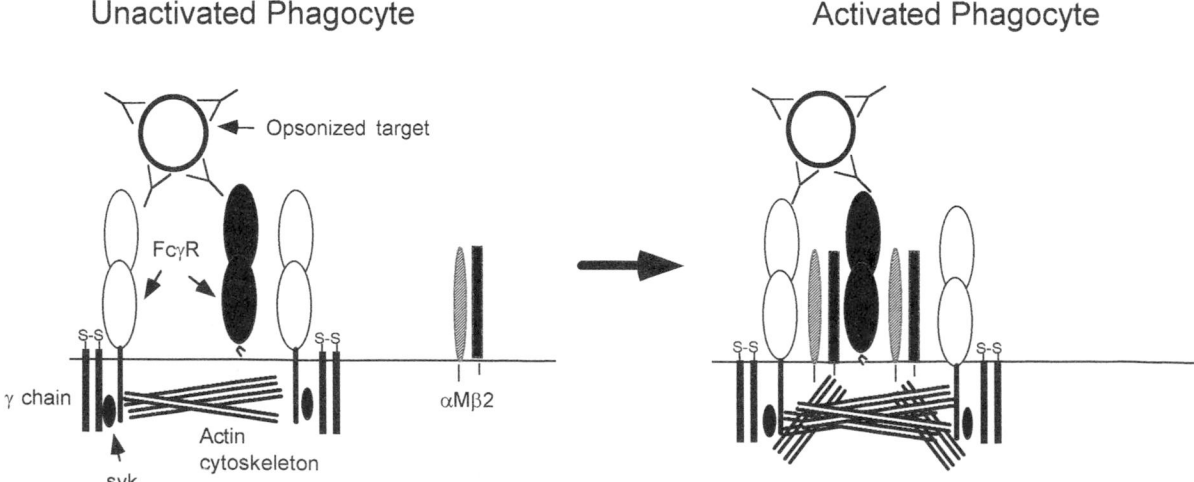

FIG. 3. Role of αMβ2 in phagocytosis. αMβ2 has a role in phagocytosis beyond its function as a complement receptor. Although not proven, the most likely role for this phagocyte-specific integrin is in effecting more efficient interactions between the actin cytoskeleton and the phagosome plasma membrane.

Another remarkable feature of αMβ2 is the large number of ligands thought to bind to it, including ICAM-1, fibrinogen, factor X, particulate lipopolysaccharides, heparan sulfates, and lipopeptidoglycan of *Leishmania*, in addition to iC3b (125). While iC3b, ICAM-1, fibrinogen, and factor X have been shown to bind directly, many of the other putative ligands have been defined by antibody inhibition of adhesion to ligand-coated particles and surfaces. Because of the apparently fundamental role of Mac-1 in PMN adhesion to any surface, studies of ligand binding using these techniques must be interpreted with caution.

αXβ2 (complement receptor 4 [CR4], CD11c/CD18) is less abundant than αMβ2 on PMNs and monocytes, but increases in expression as monocytes differentiate into macrophages *in vitro* and in tissues. In mice, αXβ2 expression seems to be confined to dendritic cells (126). Like αMβ2, αXβ2 binds iC3b and fibrinogen, although there is no evidence that it binds any other of the wide spectrum of ligands thought to interact with αMβ2. The sites on fibrinogen recognized by the two integrins differ (127,128). While both integrins can mediate phagocyte adhesion, there appear to be differences in function. For example, adhesion via αXβ2 but not αMβ2 activates the respiratory burst in PMNs (129), and αXβ2 seems to have a more important role in transendothelial migration of monocytes than does αMβ2 (130). Because αMβ2 and αXβ2 have identical β chains, differences in function are assumed to be encoded in the distinct α chains. However, no detailed analysis of the molecular basis for the differences in function of the two closely related integrins has been made.

Other Opsonin Receptors

There are a variety of other opsonins that can bind to bacteria and to phagocytic cells, leading to phagocytosis. A major class of opsonic molecules are the collectins, soluble molecules expressing an amino-terminal collagen domain, a neck region, and a globular carboxy-terminal C-type lectin domain (131). A characteristic of all collectins is that they form high order oligomers. For example, mannose-binding protein (MBP), a 32-kDa monomer, circulates as oligomers of nine to 18 polypeptide chains. Binding of the multimer to mannose-rich surfaces, as occurs on many bacteria, allows the MBP to activate both the classical and the alternative pathways of complement (132–134). Nonsense mutations in MBPs have been reported to lead to an immunodeficiency characterized by frequent bacterial infections (135). C-reactive protein (CRP), another collectin, can activate both the classical and the alternative complement pathways after binding its ligand, the C carbohydrate of *Streptococcus pneumoniae* (136). In addition, CRP may have its own cellular receptor (137). While mice express only trace amounts of CRP, transgenic overexpression of CRP is protective in *S. pneumoniae* bacteremia and several other experimental inflammatory diseases (138–140).

Plasma proteins, which incorporate into blood clots or ECM, can sometimes bind to invading pathogens. For example, fibrinogen and fibronectin can bind to various streptococci, fibronectin can bind to *Staphyococcus aureus* and many mycobacteria, and vitronectin can bind to *Pneumocystis carinii* (141). Although these interactions with bacteria are often regarded as enhancing pathogenicity, because they allow retention in tissue, they clearly can mediate binding to phagocytes as well. Indeed, one of the original descriptions of fibronectin was as a serum opsonin mediating the clearance of denatured collagen (142,143).

Phagocytosis of Apoptotic Cells

Apoptosis is a characteristic feature of normal embryogenesis and of T-lymphocyte development and can be a mechanism for prevention of development of malignancy. In addition, apoptosis is a normal component of the resolution of inflammation, because neutrophils present at an inflammatory site rapidly undergo apoptosis. One role for macrophages is phagocytosis of apoptotic cells, both during the resolution of inflammation (144) and during embryogenesis (145). Macrophage phagocytosis of apoptotoic cells occurs both through receptors for direct recognition and through opsonization (Fig. 4). The platelet-derived protein thrombospondin, often a component of the ECM at inflammatory sites, can opsonize apoptotic PMNs, with subsequent recognition of the thrombospondin-opsonized PMNs by macrophage CD36 and the αvβ3/CD47 complex (146,147). CD36 is a member of the scavenger receptor superfamily (61,148). In addition, direct, nonopsonic macrophage recognition of phosphatidylserine, which appears in the outer leaflet of the plasma membrane of apoptotic cells, has been implicated in macrophage phagocytosis of apoptotic PMNs and thymocytes (149). However, the macrophage receptor responsible for recognition of phosphatidylserine has not been identified. A *Drosophila* macrophage receptor that binds apoptotic cells has been identified. Termed *croquemort* ("catcher of death"), it is structurally related to CD36 but appears to interact directly with the apoptotic target rather than with thrombospondin (150). CD36 also has been implicated in phagocytosis of rod outer segments by retinal pigment epithelial cells (151). It is possible that the CD36 family is one of primordial phagocytic receptors, and that the original function of phagocytosis was actually in removal of apoptotic cells and cellular debris during development. Phagocytosis as a major mechanism of host defense may be a later evolutionary adaptation. There may be differences in the mechanism of phagocytosis of apoptotic cells and of invading pathogens. For example, an anion transporter implicated in phagocytosis of apoptotic cells apparently has no role in phagocytosis of yeast (152,153).

Signal Transduction during Phagocytosis

More than 20 years ago, Silverstein et al. proposed a model for phagocytosis that has guided much of the research in the field. This model, called the zipper hypothesis, states that phagocytosis requires repeated interactions between ligands on the target particle and receptors on the phagocytic cell, and that interruption of formation of new interactions at any point prevents ingestion of the particle (154,155). In this model, the phagocytic cell moves over the target like a zipper (Fig. 5). Interaction between the plasma membrane and the phagocytic target is close at the leading edge of the zipper, but more distant at the base of the phagocytic cup. Actin microfilaments polymerize and organize at the leading edge of the zipper as well, while the actin at the base of the phagocytic cup is less organized. The evidence in favor of this model includes electron microscopic observations of phagocytes in the process of ingestion of IgG-coated particles, use of antireceptor antibodies, and removal of opsonin from a portion of the phagocytic target by capping (155) (Fig. 6). Another important feature of the model is that the membrane events that lead to engulfment are very localized. When unactivated macrophages (which have nonphagocytic complement receptors) bound complement-opsonized erythrocytes and IgG-opsonized pneumo-

Apoptotic Cell

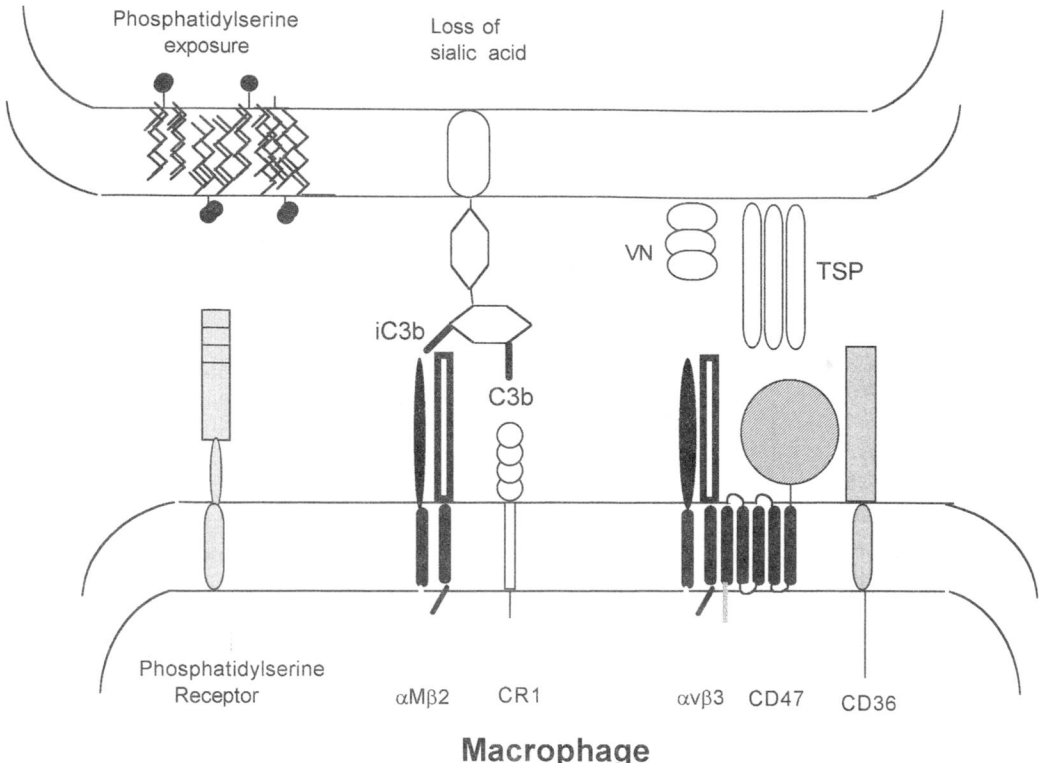

FIG. 4. Phagocytosis of apoptotic cells. Some interactions important in the phagocytosis of apoptotic cells by macrophages include recognition of phosphatidylserine (58), vitronectin (146), thrombospondin (147), and C3 fragments deposited because of loss of cell surface sialic acid (310).

cocci, only the IgG-opsonized bacteria were ingested, even though the red cells and pneumococci adhered to contiguous regions of the plasma membrane (156). These basic aspects of the model are largely accepted to this day, although many details have been modified and expanded. The implications of this model are, first, that there is continuous communication between phagocytic receptors engaged by ligand and the underlying cytoplasm and cytoskeleton, and, second, that the communication is spatially and kinetically lim-

ited. Thus, the signal for phagocytosis is not propagated through the plasma membrane. The third implication of this model is that because signaling is limited in time and space, the signal transduction pathways involved in a phagocytic signal may be quite distinct from the signaling designed to transfer information from the plasma membrane to the nucleus, such as after engagement of hormone or growth factor receptors. For these receptors, the final outcome of signal transduction initiated at the plasma membrane may not occur

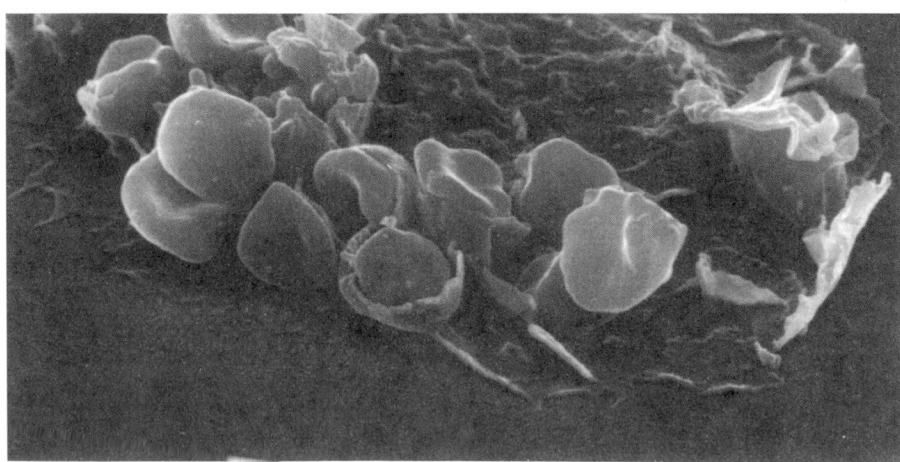

FIG. 5. Scanning electron micrograph of macrophage phagocytosis of IgG-opsonized sheep erythrocytes. Thirty minutes after adding IgG-opsonized targets to macrophages, phagocytosis is proceeding in accord with the zipper hypothesis. Note the close apposition of the phagocyte membrane associated with erythrocytes and the projection of macrophage membrane into pseudopods, which surround the target. (From ref. 244, with permission.) (Photo kindly provided by N. Araki.)

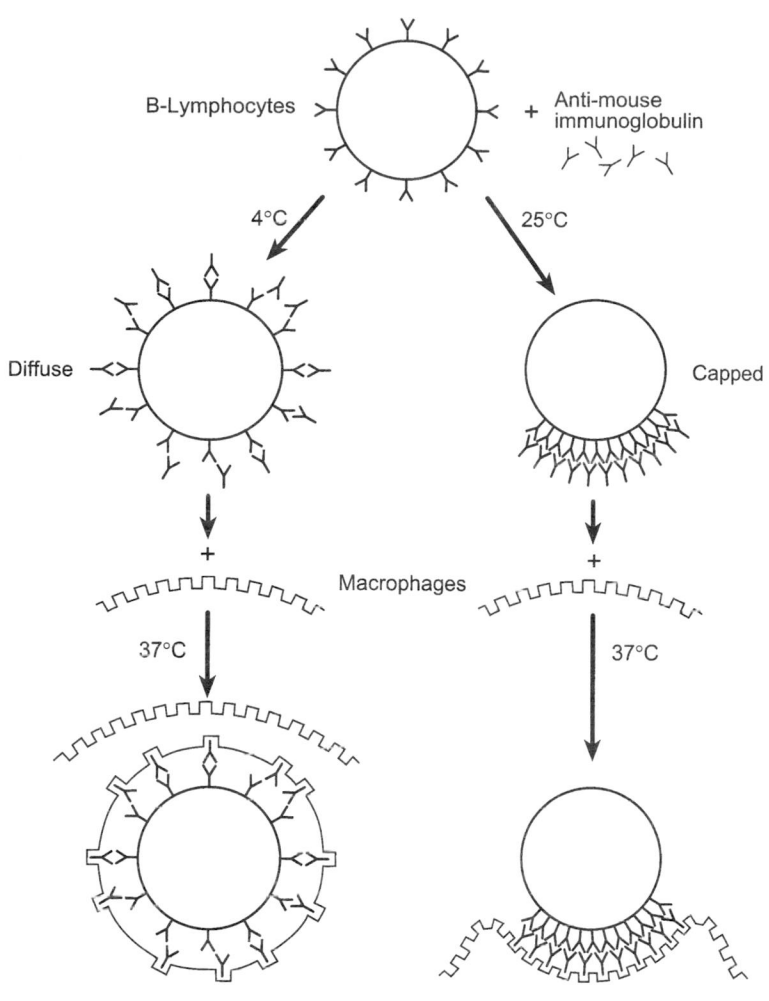

Fig. 6. Zippering phagocytosis requires sequential interactions between phagocyte and target. A schematic representation of the classic experiment of Griffin and Silverstein (154). When the lymphocyte target of ingestion was circumferentially opsonized, phagocytosis proceeded; when the target had capped opsonin, it was recognized and bound by the macrophage but could not be ingested.

for hours; the cytoskeletal and membrane rearrangements that occur during phagocytosis are completed within minutes.

Whether the zipper hypothesis explains all phagocytosis is still debated. Early studies that compared IgG-mediated phagocytosis and complement-mediated phagocytosis suggested that they were ultrastructurally distinct (157). Pseudopod extension, an important component of zippering, was not apparent in complement-mediated phagocytosis or in phagocytosis of damaged erythrocytes (158). Moreover, differential sensitivity to cytochalasin D and colchicine suggested that IgG-mediated ingestion was more dependent on actin microfilaments than complement-mediated internalization, and complement-mediated phagocytosis was more sensitive to the microtubule inhibitor. These studies were performed prior to the elucidation of the diversity of Fcγ and complement receptors. More recent studies have confirmed and extended these by demonstrating that αMβ2 is the important complement receptor in this ingestion and that the distribution of cytoskeletal and signaling molecules on phagosomes differs in αMβ2- and FcγR-mediated ingestion (159). The significance of these differences for the cell biology of phagocytosis is not yet resolved.

It is clear that not all cell surface molecules on phagocytes are competent to mediate ingestion. Although this may be expected, because phagocytic receptors must communicate cytoskeletal elements and signaling components which modulate cytoskeletal assembly, comparison of the cytoplasmic domains of receptors capable of mediating phagocytosis has not revealed common amino acid motifs clearly relevant to particle ingestion.

Tyrosine Kinase Signaling in Phagocytosis

FcγR-mediated ingestion has been the primary paradigm for understanding signal transduction in phagocytosis. The family of FcγRs includes ligand-binding transmembrane proteins with highly homologous extracytoplasmic domains but often quite distinct intracytoplasmic sequences. The family members, which have been shown to mediate ingestion (FcγRI, FcγRIIA, and FcγRIIIA) share the ability to propagate a tyrosine kinase cascade, at least in part through their association with the γ-chain dimer. γ chain can activate the tyrosine kinase syk after phosphorylation; the ITAM-like sequence in the FcγRIIA cytoplasmic tail may do the same (80). Syk activation is required for phagocytosis (86), and direct activation of syk by clustering induces ingestion and actin polymerization (160), suggesting that this is the critical step for initiating FcγR-mediated phagocytosis. The downstream effectors of syk in phagocytosis and actin polymerization are not known. There is evidence for involvement of phosphatidylinositol (PI) 3-kinase in

FcγR-mediated ingestion (161), and PI3-kinase can be activated by tyrosine kinase signaling. Because PI3-kinase can regulate cell shape and spreading through effects on integrins and actin polymerization (162,163), it is likely to be an important intermediary in the signaling cascade that induces phagocytosis.

Phospholipase Cγ (PLCγ) also is activated by FcγR ligation as a downstream effect of syk activation (84). This leads to generation of both IP3, with the consequent release of intracellular Ca^{2+} stores into the cytoplasm, and diacylglycerol, which activates several isoforms of PKC. PKC activity is required for phagocytosis (164–166). PKC-α rapidly associates with the nascent phagosome and remains associated throughout its maturation (166). The major PKC substrates in macrophages, myristoylated alanine-rich C-kinase substitute (MARCKS) and MacMARCKS, likely are involved in regulation of actin assembly during formation of the phagosome (167). Because phorbol myristate acetate, a pharmacologic activator of PKC, can induce the phagocytic competence of αMβ2 in unactivated cells, it is likely that the difference between active and inactive αMβ2 is the ability to recruit PKC to the nascent phagosome.

The importance of the other consequence of PLCγ activation, increased [Ca^{2+}]$_i$, in phagocytosis is more controversial. Although some studies report normal phagocytosis in cells buffered at very low [Ca^{2+}]$_i$, others report inhibition under the same conditions (83,168,169). A likely resolution of these differences is whether the phagocytosis involves recruitment of αMβ2 (170). When FcγR alone is involved in the phagocytic event, an increase in [Ca^{2+}]$_i$ is unimportant. However, FcγR-mediated phagocytosis requires αMβ2 when phagocytes are stimulated to their maximal phagocytic potential at sites of inflammation (111), and an increase in [Ca^{2+}]$_i$ likely is necessary for this maximally stimulated ingestion. The reason for the differential requirement for [Ca^{2+}]$_i$ in different mechanisms of ingestion is unknown. Ca^{2+} can regulate PKC activation, interaction of actin with various binding proteins, and calmodulin-dependent processes, including interaction with myosin I (171), any of which might be differentially required for basal and stimulated ingestion. When an increase in [Ca^{2+}]$_i$ is involved in ingestion, as in IgG-mediated ingestion stimulated by PAF or formylated bacterial peptides, the stimulus for release of Ca^{2+} from intracellular stores must be generated at the nascent phagosome, and signals for release of intracellular Ca^{2+} stores generated at a distance from the phagocytic target cannot substitute (170). Moreover, intracellular Ca^{2+} stores redistribute in phagocytosing cells to concentrate around the forming phagosome (172). These facts emphasize the local nature of the signaling and the spatial and temporal organization of the signals required for phagocytosis.

Phospholipases other than PLCγ play important roles in the phagocytic process. Phospholipase D (PLD) cleaves phospholipids, especially phosphatidylcholine, to phosphatidic acid and choline. PLD activity correlates closely with complement receptor–mediated ingestion and appears to be required for it (165,173,174). Tyrosine kinase cascades and seven-transmembrane receptors can synergize to enhance PLD activity, suggesting a mechanism by which multiple signals at inflammatory sites, including adhesion, chemokines, complement, and bacterial peptides, regulate the phenotype of phagocytes that migrate to these sites. How the products of PLD activation influence phagocytosis is unknown. It is possible that the phosphatidic acid generated by PLD could provide an alternative source of diacylglycerol for PKC activation.

Phospholipases A2 (PLA2) cleave fatty acids from the R2 position of various phospholipids. Pharmacologic experiments have suggested that a specific PLA2 isoform has an important role in phagocytosis (175). This PLA2 is distinct from the PLA2 primarily responsible for providing arachidonate to the cyclooxygenase and leukotriene pathways. The phagocytic PLA2 is Ca^{2+}-independent, prefers phosphatidylserine as substrate, and is activated by PKC (176,177). This PLA2 apparently is involved in endosome–endosome fusion (178) and thus is a candidate for mediating the final membrane fusion that allows the forming phagosome to bud from the plasma membrane (see Fig. 2) and may well play a role in vessicle fusion with the nascent phagosome as well (178).

The extent to which these signaling pathways elucidated for FcγR-mediated ingestion are relevant to complement-mediated phagocytosis is unclear. Unike the FcγRs, complement receptors are not tyrosine phosphorylated and thus not obviously involved in initiation or propagation of tyrosine kinase cascades. However, αMβ2 may associate with a tyrosine kinase called pyk2, cakb, or raftk in phagocytes (179,180). The significance of this interaction for phagocytosis is unknown. Complement-mediated ingestion does require PKC activation (181).

Cytoskeleton in Phagocytosis

Actin Cytoskeleton in Phagocytosis

The immediate target of signal transduction during phagocytosis is the actin cytoskeleton. An important feature of leukocytes, critical for phagocytosis, is the ability to rapidly change shape in response to activation. The actin cytoskeleton is critical for membrane remodeling that must occur for a cell to adhere, migrate, and phagocytose particles. The role of the actin cytoskeleton in effector functions that require membrane remodeling is twofold. First, the actin cytoskeleton provides a mechanical framework to accomplish shape changes. While the force that drives extension and contraction of the membrane when pseudopodia, lamellae, filopodia, or phagosomes form is not elucidated completely, there is evidence that suggests that actin–myosin complexes provide a motor to drive such formations (182). Second, the actin cytoskeleton regulates signal transduction events that are important for the development of the effector phenotype. The cytoskeleton acts as a platform to bring surface receptors, activatable enzymes, and their substrates into close proximity. This dual role of the cytoskeleton is illustrated by the finding that depolymerizing agents such as cytochalasin D not only inhibit shape changes, such as those associated with the process of phagocytosis (183), but also inhibit signals initiated by receptor ligation, such as the rise in intracellular calcium concentration induced by FcγR ligation with immune complexes (184).

While it is clear that actin filament assembly and disassembly underlie the process of phagocytosis, little is certain about the molecular details of assembly and regulation of the actin cytoskeleton during phagocytosis. However, information from other leukocyte processes and other cells is probably highly relevant to the process of ingestion, and in the years since the zipper model of phagocytosis was first proposed, a model for regulation of the cytoskeleton during phagocytosis has begun to emerge. During fibroblast integrin–mediated adhesion to ECM, structures called focal adhesions form that are sites of interaction between the cytoskeleton and the plasma membrane (185). Focal adhesions are the points of closest apposition of the fibroblast to the substrate on which it adheres. These sites may be analogous to the points of close apposition of phagocyte membrane and phagocytic target during the zippering process, where actin polymerization also occurs. On the cytoplasmic face of focal contacts, integrin receptors interact with actin filaments via several proteins, including vinculin, talin, α-actinin, and filamin (185).

Focal adhesions are also sites of concentration of signaling molecules, such as tyrosine and serine–threonine kinase and phosphatases, lipid kinases, and small guanosine triphosphatases (GTPases) (185,186). It is likely, but not certain, that equivalent structures form in leukocytes. Adherent phagocytes have multiple points of close contact with the substrate, called podosomes. Podosomes are characterized by punctate accumulations of F-actin, and contain clusters of integrins as well as many of the actin-binding proteins found in focal contacts (187,188). However, the morphologic organization of podosomes is quite distinct from focal contacts. For example, leukocytes rarely make stress fibers, the F-actin bundles that terminate in focal contacts in fibroblasts. Whether substrate adhesion and phagocytosis are equivalent processes is not known. Adhesion to target particles is a critical step in phagocytosis, and there are morphologic and molecular similarities between the cytoskeletal structures that form in adherent phagocytes and in phagocytic cups (159). Many cytoskeletal molecules have been identified in phagocytic cups and phagosomes, which are found in focal adhesions and podosomes, such as α-actinin, L-plastin (LPL), talin, vinculin, and paxillin (see Table 4 for a more comprehensive list). These morphologic studies have helped determine the cytoskeletal components that are potentially involved in phagocytosis. Although detailed studies of cytoskeletal regulation during phagocytosis are lacking, a five-step model can be proposed based on the work in other systems.

1. *F-actin nucleation and actin polymerization* When the target particle initially contacts the phagosome membrane, one of the first events is rapid actin polymerization. Consistent with the zipper hypothesis, active actin polymerization occurs in the tip of the pseudopod as it advances around the target. Although it has been known for years that actin polymerization is required for phagocytosis, the regulation of actin polymerization in phagocytes remains unclear. The importance of the small GTPases rac, rho, and cdc42 in regulation of phagocyte function has been recognized only during the past decade (189). These guanosine triphosphate (GTP) hydrolases coordinate cell adhesion and actin filament polymerization in a number of cells, including phagocytes (190–192). Cdc42, rac, and rho are activated in a hierarchical fashion in response to growth factor stimulation (193). Expression of constitutively active cdc42 and rac results in filopodia extension and membrane ruffling, respectively. In cells expressing constitutively active cdc42 and rac, small punctate actin aggregates form that are distinct from focal adhesions and resemble podosomes found in adherent phagocytes (193,194). Rho activation induces stress fibers and classical focal adhesions to form (195). Because phagocytosis has many features in common with adhesion, it is likely that these structures and the GTPases that regulate them are highly relevant to the process of phagocytosis. However, no experimental analysis of this hypothesis has yet been published. The small GTPases have been shown to activate serine–threonine kinases called p21-activated kinases, or paks (196,197). Whether paks control organization of actin cytoskeleton or are more important in rac-mediated activation of stress protein kinases such as p38 and jun kinase is uncertain (198,199). Expression of the constitutively active form of pak1, a rac/cdc42-activated serine–threonine kinase, results in membrane ruffling and actin accumulation in lamellipodia and formation of large focal adhesion–like complexes in fibroblasts (200). Although a role for these molecules has not been established in phagocytosis, FcγR ligation induces pak1 activation with kinetics similar to

TABLE 4. *Cytoskeletal and signaling proteins associated with phagosomes*

Cytoskeletal protein	Phagocytic target	Refs.
F-actin	COZ[a], IgG-LB[b], LB[c], *Shigella*[d]	159, 299, 300
Vinculin	COZ, IgG-LB, *Shigella*	159, 300
Paxillin	COZ, IgG-LB, IgG-E[a] *Shigella*	159, 236, 300
α-actinin	COZ, IgG-LB, LB, *Shigella*	159, 299, 300
Talin	COZ, IgG-LB, IgG-E, *Shigella*	159, 300, 301
MARCKS, MacMARCKS	COZ, IgG-LB	159, 221
Moesin	LB	299
L-plastin	LB	299
T-plastin	*Shigella*	302
α-tubulin	LB	299
β-tubulin	LB	299
Cortactin	*Shigella*	303
Myosin I	COZ	166
PKCα	COZ	166
Calreticulin	LB	299
Calnexin	LB	299
Rab5, rab7	LB	299
Rap1	LB	299
$G_{\beta 1}$, $G_{\beta 2}$	LB	299
BiP	LB	299
annexin II, VI	LB	299

[a]Complement-opsonized zymosan
[b]IgG-opsonized latex beads
[c]Unopsonized latex beads. Many as yet unidentified proteins also associate with latex bead–induced phagosomes (299).
[d]*Shigella* invasion is mediated by the integrin α5β1.
[e]IgG-opsonized sheep erythrocytes

the kinetics of phagocytosis in PMNs, and pak1 activation correlates with the activation of αMβ2-mediated adhesion (200a).

The mechanism by which the small GTPases regulate the formation of various actin cytoskeletal structures is as yet unknown. However, studies using a permeabilized platelet model have shown that active Rac induces uncapping of the barbed end of actin filaments through the synthesis of D3 and D4 phosphoinositides (201). D4 phosphoinositides bind capping protein and gelsolin to inhibit their capping activity, exposing actin filament barbed ends, which can act as nucleation sites (202,203). A similar pathway, involving GTP-binding proteins, also leads to filament uncapping and actin polymerization in PMN (192,204). Gelsolin severs actin filaments in a calcium-dependent manner, creating additional free barbed ends. PIP$_2$ regulates ADF/cofilin- and profilin-G actin association (205,206), and agonist-induced increases in PIP$_2$ promote actin polymerization (201). Additionally, talin, which specifically binds PIP$_2$ and localizes to phagosomal membranes, nucleates actin and anchors actin filaments to the membrane (207). Thus, an early event in phagocytosis likely is the activation of small GTPases rac and cdc42, and PI3-kinase, which in turn activate actin polymerization. It should be emphasized that while this model presents a hypothesis concerning the mechanism of regulating actin filament polymerization in response to external stimuli, its relevance to phagocytosis has not been experimentally verified.

2. *Association of F-actin with the phagosome membrane.* The newly assembled F-actin must interact with the plasma membrane to exert the force required for engulfment of target particles. At least two mechanisms anchor actin microfilaments to the membrane of phagosomes. The first is via MARCKS or MacMARCKS, described in detail below. The second is via association of actin-binding proteins such as α-actinin, filamin, and talin–vinculin complexes with integrin β-chain cytoplasmic tails (185). This mechanism may account in part for the importance of αMβ2 in FcγR-mediated phagocytosis (111).

3. *Regulation of F-actin organization.* The dynamic regulation of the three-dimensional structure of the cytoskeletal complexes that associate with phagosomes is complex. Actin filaments within pseudopods of phagocytic cups are arranged in parallel arrays that are cross-linked by several actin-cross-linking proteins, such as LPL, ABP-120, and α-actinin (208,209). At the base of the phagocytic cup, the actin filaments are less ordered. Actin-binding proteins found in phagosome cytoskeletal structures such as LPL, vinculin, cortactin, ABP-120, α-actinin, MARCKS, moesin, and ezrin, regulate the stability of the filaments and membrane association with F-actin. The cytoskeletal architecture of phagosomes forming around complement- and IgG-opsonized particles differ (159), suggesting that actin filament organization is regulated differently in response to complement receptor and FcγR ligation. Coopsonization of particles with IgG and complement leads to markedly enhanced phagocytosis, as compared with IgG or complement alone (210), establishing that signals from both IgG and complement receptors are required for optimal phagocytic function. It may be that their cooperativity occurs in part through synergy in regulation of the phagosome cytoskeleton.

4. *Localization of signaling proteins to the phagosome.* It is likely that the cytoskeletal structures that form at the phagosome membrane are similar to focal adhesions, in that they form a scaffold for recruitment of signaling molecules such protein kinases and phosphatases, lipid-modifying enzymes, and many adapter and regulatory proteins, which are important for coordination of the events of phagocytosis. This function of the cytoskeleton provides a mechanism to bring phagocytic receptors, activatable enzymes, and their substrates into close proximity at the site of the forming phagosome. Because multiple and sequential receptor ligation events must occur during phagocytosis (see Fig. 5), the signals generated by a single receptor ligation event are not sufficient to trigger the process. Therefore, the molecular events of phagocytosis must be regulated locally, and the signals generated by each receptor ligation are confined to the vicinity of the receptor. Thus, the cytoskeletal structures analagous to podosomes that form during the process of phagocytosis allow localization of molecules that enable further formation of the phagosome.

5. *Generation of the forces necessary for engulfment.* Three models exist that may explain the generation of the forces required to extend pseudopodia and engulf particles during phagocytosis (211). The first model predicts that the force generated by actin polymerization is sufficient to result in pseudopodia and lamellipodia extension. This model is supported by the fact that active actin polymerization occurs at the advancing tip of the pseudopod. However, this model does not account for the contractile forces required for internalization of the phagosome. The second predicts that the osmotic forces generated during actin polymerization in the phagocytic cup expand the membrane into protrusions. However, very little evidence exists to support this model. The third model predicts that actin–myosin complexes generate a motor force that drives phagocytosis. Genetic evidence from *Dictyostelium* demonstrates a very important role for myosin I in this process (182), but other nonclassical myosins may participate as well. These models are not mutually exclusive, and aspects of both the first and the third models be important to explain the generation of the forces necessary for phagocytosis.

Based on this model for the role of the cytoskeleton in phagocytosis, some actin-binding and -signaling molecules are likely to play a key role in ingestion. These proteins are described in more detail below.

L-plastin

LPL is a 65-kDa actin-bundling protein, also called fimbrin, that is expressed in leukocytes, embryonic endoderm, and transformed cells (212,213). Two closely related isoforms, I- and T-plastin, are expressed in epithelia and solid tissues, respectively (212,214). The sequences of plastins are highly conserved among yeast, mouse, rat, human, and chicken, suggesting a function conserved through evolution. LPL localizes to phagocytic cups, phagosomes, and podosomes in phagocytes, but it is not clear what role LPL plays in these processes. Most of the undertanding of the function of LPL is inferred from the phenotype of the yeast fimbrin-null mutant (215). Internalization of α-factor is impaired in fimbrin-null cells, suggesting that it is critical for yeast actin-dependent receptor-mediated endocytosis, a process similar to phagocytosis. Actin filaments are unstable in fimbrin-null yeast or yeast with mutations in actin that inhibit fimbrin binding (216).

LPL is unique among fimbrins because it is phosphorylated within the N-terminal regulatory region in response to cellular activation by a variety of agonists, especially stimuli that cause shape changes, migration, adhesion, and/or phagocytosis (217–220), during which the ability to rapidly regulate the actin cytoskeleton is critical. It is tempting to speculate that LPL phosphorylation allows an additional mechanism of regulation of LPL function, but direct evidence supporting this hypothesis is lacking. The kinetics of phosphorylation of LPL are correlated with phagocytosis of IgG-opsonized beads and adhesion to immune-complex coated surfaces in PMNs as well as activation of the integrin αMβ2 (217). Thus, LPL is likely important in the formation and stabilization of F-actin filaments during phagocytosis.

MARCKS

MARCKS and related family member MacMARCKS have been implicated in macrophage activation and phagocytosis (166,221). Both MARCKS and MacMARCKS have been found to associate with forming phagosomes in macrophages and cycle between the plasma membrane and lysosomes in fibroblasts (159,166,222). J774 macrophages transfected with a dominant negative Mac-MARCKS do not phagocytose zymosan, but receptor-mediated endocytosis continues at normal levels (222). Expression of the dominant-negative mutant also inhibits integrin-mediated adhesion to culture dishes and to surfaces coated with immune complexes, two processes that require the integrin αMβ2 (221). MARCKS cross-links actin filaments (223) and associates with the plasma membrane via the myristoylation site and a highly basic region called the effector domain (224), providing a mechanism for anchoring actin filaments to the plasma membrane in a regulated manner. MARCKS and MacMARCKS are specific substrates for PKC. Activation of PKC causes phosphorylation of serine residues in the effector domain and inhibits both membrane association and actin cross-linking activity of MARCKS, releasing the MARCKS and actin filaments from the membrane (225). Regulation of membrane–actin linkage by phosphorylation of MARCKS may explain the finding that PKC inhibitors block phagocytosis (166). Calmodulin binding to the effector domain in the presence of calcium also inhibits actin cross-linking, but not membrane association (223). A model has been proposed (226) in which MARCKS mediates actin filament cross-linking and association with the membrane in unactivated cells, anchoring the filaments in a rigid state. On activation of PKC, MARCKS is phosphorylated and the filaments are released from the membrane. Dephosphorylation of MARCKS allows it to reassociate with the membrane, but calcium transients induced by activation of the cell induce calmodulin binding. Under these conditions, MARCKS binds to, but will not cross-link, actin filaments and potentially provides a less rigid anchor of actin filaments to the membrane. Thus, MARCKS and MacMARCKS may have important roles in regulating actin filament association with the plasma membrane.

Myosins

Much attention has focused on the role of myosin as a molecular motor-regulating cell movement and phagocytosis because of the importance of actin in these processes. Myosin has long been known to localize to phagocytic cups in macrophages and PMNs (227,228). However, the diversity of the myosin family has made the study of specific myosin functions difficult. Myosins comprise a very large family of proteins, with at least 11 subfamilies (229). The filamentous myosin II, or muscle myosin, is present in non-muscle cells including leukocytes, but it is not present in the phagocytic cup or in extending pseudopods during locomotion (230). Mutant Dictyostelium lacking myosin II or expressing truncated protein is perfectly capable of chemotaxis and phagocytosis (231,232). In contrast, non-muscle myosins are likely candidates for regulating membrane remodeling during phagocytosis. Myosins I have been the most studied of the unconventional non-muscle myosins. Several genes encode distinct myosins I, and more than one may be expressed in a single tissue (233). Myosins I are characterized by a single globular headpiece that is highly conserved, but they have unrelated tails that each contain an actin-binding site and a basic region that binds acidic phospholipid and may regulate actin myosin association with plasma membrane during migration and phagocytosis (233,234).

Myosin I isoforms have been found in the mouse macrophage cell line J774, mouse bone marrow–derived macrophages, and human peripheral blood leukocytes (229). Immunolocalization studies in nonleukocytes have shown that myosin I localizes mainly to motile extension of cells, such as filopodia, lamellipodia, and growth cones (235). Myosin I localizes to the phagocytic cup, particularly in the distal regions of pseudopodia, but not phagosomes, in peritoneal macrophages, and to lamellipodia during migration and phagocytic cups during ingestion in Dictyostelium (230). These data suggest that the role of myosin I is in extension of membrane structures. Genetic analysis of myosin I function in Dictyostelium has shown that two isoforms of myosin I, myoB and myoC, have an important role in phagocytosis (182). While deletion of either gene caused marked defects in phagocytosis, deletion of both genes does not further inhibit phagocytosis, suggesting that the role for each gene product is distinct and that the two myosins I act sequentially. By analogy, myosin I is thought to have a role in vertebrate phagocytosis, but no data are available to indicate which isoforms of myosin I are involved in phagocytosis in vertebrates.

Paxillin

Paxillin is a broadly expressed 68-kDa protein that localizes to the actin cytoskeleton during membrane remodeling events and is tyrosine and serine phosphorylated during integrin-mediated adhesion and phagocytosis (236–238). Paxillin associates with several important signaling molecules in focal adhesions, including focal adhesion kinase (FAK), crk, and src, but lacks any enzyme activity itself, suggesting that it is an adaptor molecule that regulates signal transduction events in cytoskeletal structures (185,239). Recruitment of paxillin to the actin cytoskeleton probably occurs by binding to vinculin and to FAK (185,239).

Paxillin localizes to podosomes in adherent macrophages and PMNs and to phagocytic cups in macrophages (159,236). Tyrosine phosphorylation and localization to the actin cytoskeleton occurs as a result of integrin ligation in adherent cells (240–243). While paxillin is found in phagocytic cups and becomes tyrosine phosphorylated during FcγR-induced phagocytosis of IgG-opsonized particles, tyrosine phosphorylation of paxillin requires β2 integrins, even if no apparent β2 ligand is present (116,117). In the absence of β2 integrins, neither adhesion to immune complexes nor phagocytosis of IgG-coated particles induces paxillin tyrosine phosphorylation, perhaps explaining the requirement of β2 integrins for FcγR-mediated phagocytosis and adhesion, events that require actin-based membrane remodeling.

Phagosome Formation and Fusion

After the phagocytic target has attached to the phagocyte membrane, it is rapidly internalized. Internalization requires the actin cytoskeleton, and the models for its initiation, propagation, and regulation are discussed above. The final event in phagosome formation requires membrane fusion, both by the phagosome and at the plasma membrane (see Fig. 2). While this fusion event is very poorly understood, there is evidence that it requires both an intracellular calcium-independent PLA2 (176) and PI3-kinase (244). Indeed, during phagocytosis, the surface area of the plasma membrane of the cell changes little, implying an increased rate of delivery of intracellular membrane to the cell surface during the ingestion process. There is evidence for increased lipid synthesis during phagocytosis, consistent with cell repletion of membrane during engulfment (245).

During phagosome formation, a complex series of fusions with intracellular vesicles also occurs. The models for this process owe much to the detailed understanding of the cytoskeleton-independent process of fluid endocytosis (246,247). However, unlike the orderly process of endosome maturation, in which endosome–lysosome fusion does not occur for about 20 minutes after ligand internalization, phagosomes fuse with lysosomes extremely rapidly. Indeed, lysosomes begin to fuse with phagosomes even prior to budding of the phagosome from the plasma membrane (248). At the same time, endosomes of various states of maturation fuse with phagosomes. While endosome–phagosome fusion is independent of the increase in $[Ca^{2+}]_i$ that often accompanies ingestion, controversy exists about the calcium dependence of phagosome–lysosome fusion (249,250). Many of the molecular requirements for phagosome–endosome fusion are identical to those defined for endosome–endosome fusion (247).

As would be predicted, the phagosome rapidly becomes an acidic compartment enriched in proteases found in vesicles throughout the endocytic pathway. In addition, the NADPH oxidase and nitric oxide synthase, which are important for pathogen destruction, become associated with phagosomes (251). Thus, the phagosome is a cell compartment specialized for the destruction of engulfed material. To counter this killing machinery, a variety of intracellular pathogens have developed the ability to inhibit phagosome maturation, as will be discussed in detail below. After engulfment, phagosomes migrate from the cell periphery, where they are formed, to a perinuclear region. The significance of this intracellular migration is unknown.

Regulation of Phagocytosis

Like many fundamental immunologic processes, phagocytosis is a highly regulated function in phagocytes. Because ingestion often is accompanied by tissue-destructive phenomena, such as release of lysosomal enzymes, and the generation of high-energy oxygen and nitrogen metabolites, it is reasonable that it is a process largely confined to sites of infection or inflammation. Thus, resting, circulating phagocytes are capable only of minimal ingestion, and they develop their full phagocytic potential after exposure to additional signals, such as bacterial peptides, fragments of complement or clotting proteins, arachidonate metabolites, cytokines, and other molecules found predominantly at sites of inflammation.

Cytokine and Extracellular Matrix Regulation of Ingestion

As discussed above, stimulation of phagocytosis at sites of inflammation depends on the phagocyte-specific integrin $\alpha M\beta 2$.

In unactivated cells, $\alpha M\beta 2$ is in a basal state that is not adherent. With cell stimulation from any of a variety of signals, $\alpha M\beta 2$ achieves its activated state, in which it is highly adherent to a large variety of ligand-coated surfaces (252). Activation of $\alpha M\beta 2$ thus at least enhances adhesion of the phagocyte to its ingestion target and likely has additional signaling effects as well. In the absence of $\alpha M\beta 2$, circulating phagocytes cannot activate their full phagocytic potential, and some receptors, such as CR1 (CD35), cannot induce phagocytosis at all, despite optimal stimulation. Thus, the abilities of cytokines to stimulate phagocytosis very closely parallels their activation of $\alpha M\beta 2$-mediated adhesion. Cytokines that induce phagocyte adhesion will stimulate phagocytosis; these include G-CSF, granulocyte-macrophage colony-stimulating factor (GM-CSF), and TNF-α (253). The molecular mechanisms involved in $\alpha M\beta 2$ activation remain poorly understood, but they may include tyrosine kinase cascades and PI3-kinase (254).

A major mechanism to enhance the rate and extent of phagocytosis by PMNs and monocytes is adhesion to ECM proteins. Teleologically, this is a way for the normally circulating phagocytes to understand that they are out of the bloodstream, at a site of infection or injury, where their full phagocytic potential is required. The signal for enhanced phagocytosis from many ECM proteins appears to be mediated by a short peptide sequence, Arg-Gly-Asp, present in many of these proteins. While Arg-Gly-Asp–containing proteins may interact with multiple integrins, the $\alpha v\beta 3$ integrin is critical for the phagocyte activation response to these proteins. Both PMNs and macrophages express the $\alpha v\beta 3$ integrin on their surfaces. The mechanism of signal transduction for PMN activation by $\alpha v\beta 3$ has been studied in depth (255). $\alpha v\beta 3$-mediated signaling for PMN activation requires at least one more plasma membrane protein, the immunoglobulin superfamily member, integrin-associated protein (IAP, CD47) (256). IAP and $\alpha v\beta 3$ physically interact to create a signaling complex that leads ultimately to $\alpha M\beta 2$ activation (257,258). Certain microorganisms have taken advantage of this integrin crosstalk between $\alpha v\beta 3$ and $\alpha M\beta 2$ to invade monocytes. This has been elegantly shown for *Bordetella pertussis* (259). Its filamentous hemagglutinin expresses both an RGD for binding $\alpha v\beta 3$/IAP and a less well defined site for binding $\alpha M\beta 2$. Bacterial attachment to monocytes proceeds via interaction with $\alpha v\beta 3$/IAP and consequent activation of the $\alpha M\beta 2$ high-affinity state, which then enables firm attachment of the bacteria to the monocyte, and phagocytosis of the attached organisms. A similar mechanism of attachment and engulfment by macrophages has been found for nonpathogenic strains of the rickettsial agent of Q fever, *Coxiella burnetii*.

Several ECM proteins activate phagocytes via a mechanism distinct from $\alpha v\beta 3$/IAP. Entactin (260) and laminin (261) can stimulate phagocytosis through mechanisms independent of Arg-Gly-Asp sequences in the ligands. This effect is mediated by the $\alpha 3\beta 1$ integrin. Collagen gels stimulate macrophage phagocytosis, apparently through $\alpha 2\beta 1$ (262). These data suggest that $\beta 1$-integrin ligation can activate $\alpha M\beta 2$, but this possibility has not been tested directly.

Signaling Interactions between Fc Receptors and Other Receptors

Cooperation between plasma membrane receptors is a fundamental aspect of the regulation of phagocytosis. This was first recognized in the early 1970s as a synergistic effect of complement and IgG opsonization of phagocytic targets on subsequent engulfment by PMNs and monocytes (210). At the time, this was interpreted as complement receptor–mediated adhesion increasing the efficiency of presentation of IgG to its receptor on the phagocytes. However, subsequent studies have demonstrated that the interaction is more complex. In the absence of $\alpha M\beta 2$, Fc receptor–mediated ingestion is defective, although not absent. Furthermore, although normal PMNs demonstrate strong, sustained adhesion to immune complexes (a process known as "frustrated phagocytosis"), $\alpha M\beta 2$-deficient PMNs adhere only transiently and never polarize (113). Thus, critical elements of the communication between Fc receptors and the cell cytoskeleton depend on $\alpha M\beta 2$. The signaling effects of the two receptors are synergistic, because $\alpha M\beta 2$ activation requires the tyrosine kinase cascade induced by aggregation of FcγRIIA by immune complexes, through a PI3-kinase–dependent mechanism. Subsequently, activated $\alpha M\beta 2$ amplifies the signaling, adhesion, degranulation, and phagocytosis initiated by FcγR ligation. As discussed above, the molecular mechanism for this synergy may involve direct interaction between the extracellular domains of Mac-1 and PMN FcγR.

Cooperative signaling also occurs between the two FcγRs of PMNs. Coligation of the two receptors, as would occur when PMNs recognize immune complexes, leads to a synergisitic stimulation of degranulation, respiratory burst, and increased $[Ca^{2+}]_i$ (263,264). FcγRIIIB can associate with the src family tyrosine kinase hck. FcγRIIIB-associated hck can phosphorylate the FcγRIIA cytoplasmic tail (264). Because phosphorylation of FcγRIIA is sufficient to activate syk and its downstream effector cascades, hck-induced phosphorylation may be the mechanism for FcγRIIIB synergy with FcγRIIA. However, additional mechanisms, such as sustained opening of a plasma membrane Ca^{2+} channel (265), may contribute importantly to synergy as well.

MICROBES AND PHAGOCYTOSIS

Phagocytosis is a major defense mechanism against invading pathogens such as bacteria and protozoa. It is therefore not surprising that pathogenic microbes have evolved mechanisms to subvert the process of phagocytosis to enhance their ability to survive within a host. In fact, a group of microbes, termed *intracellular pathogens,* have used phagocytosis to their advantage as a mechanism of invasion, as well as a strategy to avoid the hostile extracellular environment of the host by taking refuge within host cells. The strategies used by various pathogens to induce phagocytosis by host cells, both professional and nonprofessional phagocytes, are

quite diverse. There has been an explosion of information over the past decade that has begun to unravel the strategies used by several model pathogens to control phagocytosis, as well as the fate of the microbe, once phagocytosis has occurred. This information not only has increased our understanding of how microbes infect and survive within their host, but also has been valuable for understanding the fundamental host processes of phagocytosis, cytoskeletal regulation, and vesicular trafficking.

Ingestion by Nonprofessional Phagocytes

Fibroblasts and epithelial cells are capable of ingestion. Although phagocytosis by these cells is considerably slower than for the professional phagocytes, it is morphologically similar. Fibroblasts and epithelial cells are clearly devoid of receptors for IgG or complement opsonins; hence the standard recognition mechanisms of professional phagocytes are unavailable for phagocytosis by these cells. Instead, microorganisms interact with other cell surface proteins that mediate adhesion. These cells will ingest not only through endogenous receptors, such as integrins or cadherins (266,267), but also by using transfected Fcγ or mannose receptors. The ability of these cells, which do not express syk, to phagocytose via Fcγ receptors suggests that syk likely augments the rate and extent of ingestion via this receptor in professional phagocytes, rather than being absolutely required. Moreover, the specialized bacterial killing mechanisms of professional phagocytes, such as nitric oxide synthase and NADPH oxidase, are absent from these cells. Therefore, many potential pathogens have exploited the phagocytic potential of these cells to cross anatomic barriers in invasion of the host. In these cases, phagocytosis turns from a mechanism of host defense to a mechanism of pathogenesis by the invading microorganism, such as integrins.

Pathogenic organisms must invade the external defenses, including the cellular barriers or epithelia, to infect a host. Perhaps the best-understood pathogen invasion techniques have come from enteric organisms such as *Salmonella, Yersinia, Listeria,* and *Shigella.* These organisms use unique strategies to invade the host gastrointestinal epithelium through specialized cells, called M cells, overlying Peyer's patches (268). M cells are derived from normal mucosal epithelium by contact with lymphocytes (269). Specific bacterial proteins bind cellular receptors to induced uptake into the cell (Table 5). The mechanism of uptake induced by these pathogens falls into two general categories, zippering, which resembles conventional phagocytosis, and triggering, which resembles macropinocytosis.

TABLE 5. *Microbe–host cell interactions*

Microbe	Ligand	Receptor	Cell	Refs.
Yersinia	Invasin	β_1 integrins	M cells–epithelia	270
Legionella	C3bi	$\alpha M\beta 2$(CR3, Mac-1)	Macrophages	286
Rhodococcus equi	C3bi	$\alpha M\beta 2$	Macrophages	279
Listeria	C3bi	$\alpha M\beta 2$	Macrophages	304
	Internalin	E cadherin	Epithelia	305
Mycobacteria	C3b	$\alpha M\beta 2$, CR1	Macrophages	306, 307
	FAP/Fn	$\alpha 5\beta 1$	M cells–epithelia	308
Shigella	IpaA/B/C	$\alpha 5\beta 1$	M cells–epithelia	309
Leishmania	C3bi	$\alpha M\beta 2$	Macrophages	270
	LPG	$\alpha M\beta 2$	Macrophages	312
Histoplasma	C3bi	$\alpha M\beta 2$	Macrophages	270

An example of uptake by the zippering mechanism is *Yersinia pseudotuberculosis. Y. pseudotuberculosis* expresses a virulence gene, called invasin, which is a protein that binds to integrins of the β1 family present on the apical membranes of M cells and the basolateral membrane of other epithelial cells (270). On binding to the integrin, phagocytosis is induced, which is associated with the accumulation of actin and actin-binding proteins similar to focal adhesions, leading to tyrosine phosphorylation of FAK and cas (271,272). Once they have invaded the host tissue, *Yersinia* species live within Peyer's patches and lymph nodes as extracellular pathogens (273). As extracellular organisms, they secrete essential virulence factors called Yops which, on contact with host phagocytes, are translocated into the cytosol and inhibit phagocytosis (274). One such Yop, YopH, is a tyrosine phosphatase that dephosphorylates several host proteins, including cas and FAK in HeLa cells (271,272); YopH expression is required for *Yersinia*'s inhibition of phagocytosis (275). A second Yop, YopE, is a cytotoxin that depolymerizes actin filaments by an unknown mechanism (276). Evidently, *Yersinia* can induce phagocytosis by nonprofessional phagocytes, such as epithelial cells, for invasion, but can then avoid phagocytosis by professional phagocytes, to survive extracellularly within the host.

The classic example of microbial invasion induced by a triggering mechanism rather than conventional zippering phagocytosis is provided by *Salmonella* (277). On contact with the host fibroblasts or macrophages, *Salmonella* induces membrane ruffling that leads to bacterial engulfment in a process resembling macropinocytosis (Fig. 7). The key feature of this mechanism is that while only virulent *Salmonella* can induce membrane ruffling, the process of uptake does not discriminate between pathogenic or nonpathogenic *Salmonella* (278). Thus, this mechanism of ingestion fails to exhibit the exquisite specificity that characterizes zippering phagocytosis. The membrane ruffling is similar to that induced by growth factor receptors. In fact, ligation of the epidermal growth factor receptor can induce uptake of nonpathogenic *Salmonella* (278).

Ingestion by Professional Phagocytes

Many intracellular pathogens seek refuge within macrophages, presumably because within the macrophage the organisms avoid recognition and destruction by PMNs, complement, and other elements of host defense. The ability to survive within the seemingly hostile macrophage is a common feature of such pathogens, but the strategies used to subvert the microbicidal activities of the phagocyte are quite diverse (Fig. 8). These intracellular pathogens often invade macrophages by inducing phagocytosis. Many pathogens, including *Listeria, Leishmania, Rhodococcus,* and *Mycobacterium,* are opsonized by the complement fragment C3bi, which induces phagocytosis by ligating the macrophage integrin complement receptors αMβ2 and αXβ2 (270,279,280). In contrast to FcγR-mediated phagocytosis, phagocytosis mediated by the complement receptors does not induce respiratory burst activity (281). This mechanism provides a relatively safe way to invade phagocytes, but some pathogens are able to further suppress activation of the cell by directly inhibiting signaling pathways such as PKC-dependent activation of the respiratory burst (282).

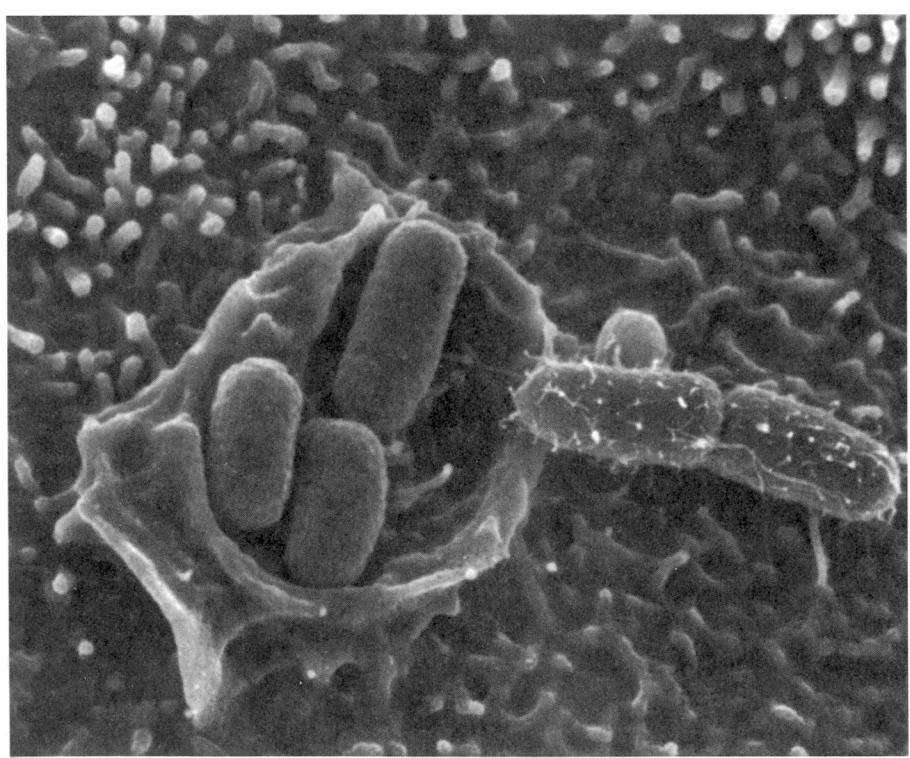

FIG. 7. Phagocytosis without zippering. High-resolution scanning electron microscopy of cultured Madin-Darby canine kidney cells infected with wild-type *Salmonella typhimurium*. Within 30 minutes after infection, bacteria associated with host cell membrane ruffles are readily apparent, but there is no pseudopod extension around adherent bacteria (compare Fig. 5). (From ref. 311, with permission.) (Photo kindly provided by J. Galán.)

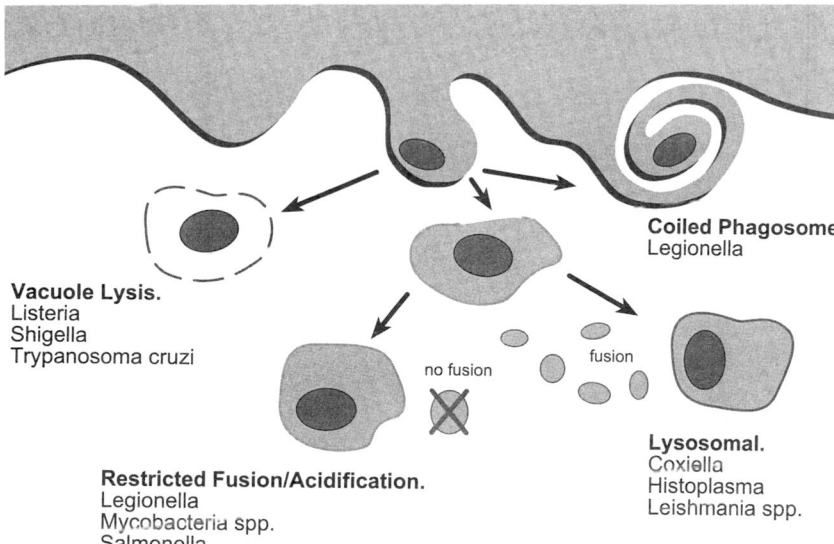

Coiled Phagosome.
Legionella

Vacuole Lysis.
Listeria
Shigella
Trypanosoma cruzi

no fusion   fusion

Restricted Fusion/Acidification.
Legionella
Mycobacteria spp.
Salmonella
Toxoplasma gondii

Lysosomal.
Coxiella
Histoplasma
Leishmania spp.

FIG. 8. Macrophage invasion and survival strategies of intracellular pathogens. Intracellular pathogens in macrophages can protect themselves from normal host defense by many mechanisms, including altering the mode of phagocytosis (coiling phagocytosis), escape from the phagosome, inhibition of phagosome acidification, and/or fusion with other effector vacuoles. Other organisms are able to survive within phagolysosomes.

Once inside a phagosome, pathogens use a variety of methods to modify the environment to allow them to survive and proliferate. Some, like *Listeria* and *Shigella*, express hemolysins, which lyse the phagosome, allowing the bacteria to escape into the cytosol, where they can grow effectively (283). Both *Listeria* and *Shigella* induce the formation of cytoskeletal structures called comets, because these actin-rich structures resemble comet tails (283). These comets are required for cell-to-cell spread of infection, because the bacteria use the polymerizing actin of the infected host cell to propel themselves through the cytosol and to induce protrusions containing the bacteria to extend from the cell surface and be ingested by neighboring phagocytes. Some pathogens can tolerate the acid pH and acid hydrolase of the phagolysosome, while still others alter the maturation of the phagosome or prevent fusion with lysosomes (284). *Mycobacterium* prevents acidification of the vesicular compartment by secreting NH_3 and by preventing phagosome acquisition of the Na/H adenosine triphosphatase (285). The high pH inhibits activation of many lysosomal hydrolases, which act optimally only at the normally low pH of the lysosome. *Legionella* species induce their own ingestion through a process known as coiling phagocytosis (286). The organism wraps itself in macrophage plasma membrane, which is then internalized by the macrophage. These internalized layers of membrane become associated with a complex of organelles containing rough endoplasmic reticulum, which is thought to be important for providing nutrients for the bacteria (286). While elegant studies over the past decade have provided insight as to how pathogens modify vesicular trafficking (284), the understanding of the mechanisms used by many pathogens to modify the intracellular environment is still rudimentary.

CONCLUSIONS

Phagocytosis is an evolutionarily ancient adaptation of cell adhesion mechanisms to specific requirements in host defense, wound repair, and development. While specialized receptors and signaling mechanisms have developed that increase the efficiency and responsiveness of the ingestion process in professional phagocytes,

the basic cell biology of phagocytosis still shares many features with regulated cell adhesion. In metazoan host defense, these processes are highly interactive. Professional phagocytes must be able to migrate rapidly into solid tissues to meet a potential pathogen and to interact effectively with that pathogen to assure its elimination. Phagocyte adhesion and engulfment can be dangerous to the host as well, and diseases as diverse as autoimmunity and atherosclerosis may result in part from abnormalities of adhesion and phagocytosis. The future holds the hope that further understanding of the molecular mechanisms underlying these related processes will allow clinically relevant pharmacologic regulation of inflammation and host defense.

REFERENCES

1. Brown EJ, Steinberg TH. Phagocytosis. In: Lee AG, ed. *Endocytosis and exocytosis.* Greenwich, CT: JAI Press Inc, 1996:33–64.
2. Metchnikoff E. Uber eine Sprosspilzkankheit der Daphnei: Beitrag zur libre uber den Kampf der phagocyten gegen Darmkrankheitserreger. *Virchows Arch* 1884; 96:177.
3. Metchnikoff E. Sur la lutte des cellules de l'organisme contre l'invasion des microbes. *Ann Inst Pasteur* 1887;1:321.
4. Bainton DF. Developmental biology of neutrophils and eosinophils. In: Gallin JI, Goldstein IM, Snyderman R, eds. *Inflammation: basic principles and clinical correlates.* New York: Raven Press, 1992:303–324.
5. Gallin JI. Neutrophil specific granule deficiency. *Annu Rev Med* 1985;36: 263–274.
6. Davis WC, Douglas SD. Defective granule formation and function in the Chediak-Higashi syndrome in man and animals. *Semin Hematol* 1972;9:431–450.
7. Root RK. Host defenses against infection: importance of phagocytic mechanisms from the study of genetic disorders of leukocyte function [review, 75 refs]. *Bull NY Acad Med* 1982;58:669–680.
8. Baehner RL. Neutrophil dysfunction associated with states of chronic and recurrent infection. *Pediatr Clin North Am* 1980;27:377–401.
9. Malaviya R, Ikeda T, Ross E, Abraham SN. Mast cell modulation of neutrophil influx and bacterial clearance at sites of infection through TNF-alpha. *Nature* 1996;381:77–80.
10. Echtenacher B, Mannel DN, Hultner L. Critical protective role of mast cells in a model of acute septic peritonitis. *Nature* 1996;381:75–77.
11. Van Furth R. Development and distribution of mononuclear phagocytes. In: Gallin JI, Goldstein IM, Snyderman R, eds. *Inflammation: basic principles and clinical correlates.* 2nd ed. New York: Raven Press, 1992:325–339.
12. McEver RP. Selectins: novel receptors that mediate leukocyte adhesion during inflammation. *Thromb Haemost* 1991;65:223–228.
13. Albelda SM, Smith CW, Ward PA. Adhesion molecules and inflammatory injury. *FASEB J* 1994;8:504–512.
14. McEver RP. Selectins. *Curr Opin Immunol* 1994;6:75–84.

15. Kansas GS. Selectins and their ligands—current concepts and controversies. *Blood* 1996;88:3259–3287.

16. Spertini O, Luscinskas FW, Kansas GS, et al. Leukocyte adhesion molecule-1 (LAM-1, L-selectin) interacts with an inducible endothelial cell ligand to support leukocyte adhesion. *J Immunol* 1991;147:2565–2573.

17. Lawrence MB, Springer TA. Leukocytes roll on a selectin at physiologic flow rates: distinction from and prerequisite for adhesion through integrins. *Cell* 1991;65:859–873.

18. Von Andrian UH, Chambers JD, McEvoy LM, Bargatze RF, Arfors K-E, Butcher EC. Two-step model of leukocyte-endothelial cell interaction in inflammation: distinct roles for LECAM-1 and the leukocyte β_2 integrins in vivo. *Proc Natl Acad Sci USA* 1991;88:7538–7542.

19. Ley K, Bullard DC, Arbones ML, et al. Sequential contribution of L- and P-selectin to leukocyte rolling in vivo. *J Exp Med* 1995;181:669–675.

20. Springer TA. Traffic signals for lymphocyte recirculation and leukocyte emigration: the multistep paradigm. *Cell* 1994;76:301–314.

21. Wilkinson PC. Chemotactic factors: an overview. *Methods Enzymol* 1988;162:127–132.

22. Zwahlen R, Walz A, Rot A. In vitro and in vivo activity and pathophysiology of human interleukin-8 and related peptides [review, 48 refs]. *Int Rev Exp Pathol* 1993;34:27–42.

23. Premack BA, Schall TJ. Chemokine receptors: gateways to inflammation and infection. *Nat Med* 1996;2:1174–1178.

24. Graves DT, Jiang Y. Chemokines, a family of chemotactic cytokines. *Crit Rev Oral Biol Med* 1995;6:109–118.

25. Leonard EJ, Yoshimura T. Human monocyte chemoattractant protein-1 (MCP-1). *Immunol Today* 1990;11:97–101.

26. Leonard EJ, Yoshimura T, Tanaka S, Raffeld M. Neutrophil recruitment by intradermally injected neutrophil attractant/activation protein-1. *J Invest Dermatol* 1991;96:690–694.

27. Yoshimura T, Matsushima K, Tanaka S, et al. Purification of a human monocyte-derived neutrophil chemotactic factor that has peptide sequence similarity to other host defense cytokines. *Proc Natl Acad Sci USA* 1987;84:9233–9237.

28. Daffern PJ, Pfeifer PH, Ember JA, Hugli TE. C3a is a chemotaxin for human eosinophils but not for neutrophils. I. C3a stimulation of neutrophils is secondary to eosinophil activation. *J Exp Med* 1995;181:2119–2127.

29. Lukacs NW, Strieter RM, Warmington K, Lincoln P, Chensue SW, Kunkel SL. Differential recruitment of leukocyte populations and alteration of airway hyperreactivity by C-C family chemokines in allergic airway inflammation. *J Immunol* 1997;158:4398–4404.

30. Kitaura M, Nakajima T, Imai T, et al. Molecular cloning of human eotaxin, an eosinophil-selective CC chemokine, and identification of a specific eosinophil eotaxin receptor, CC chemokine receptor 3. *J Biol Chem* 1996;271:7725–7730.

31. Rot A, Krieger M, Brunner T, Bischoff SC, Schall TJ, Dahinden CA. RANTES and macrophage inflammatory protein 1 alpha induce the migration and activation of normal human eosinophil granulocytes. *J Exp Med* 1992;176:1489–1495.

32. Birnbaumer L. Transduction of receptor signal into modulation of effector activity by G proteins: the first 20 years or so. *FASEB J* 1990;4:3068–3078.

33. Hynes RO. Integrins: versatility, modulation, and signaling in cell adhesion. *Cell* 1992;69:11–25.

34. Ginsberg MH, Loftus JC, D'Souza S, Plow EF. Ligand binding to integrins: common and ligand specific recognition mechanisms. *Cell Differ Dev* 1990;32:203–214.

35. O'Toole TE, Katagiri Y, Faull RJ, et al. Integrin cytoplasmic domains mediate inside-out signal transduction. *J Cell Biol* 1994;124:1047–1059.

36. Faull RJ, Kovach NL, Harlan JM, Ginsberg MH. Stimulation of integrin-mediated adhesion of T lymphocytes and monocytes: two mechanisms with divergent biological consequences. *J Exp Med* 1994;179:1307–1316.

37. Wright SD, Meyer BC. Phorbol esters cause sequential activation and deactivation of complement receptors on polymorphonuclear leukocytes. *J Immunol* 1986;136:1758–1764.

38. Hogg N, Harvey J, Cabanas C, Landis RC. Control of leukocyte integrin activation. *Am Rev Respir Dis* 1993;148:S55–S59.

39. Brown E, Hogg N. Where the outside meets the inside: integrins as activators and targets of signal transduction cascades. *Immunol Lett* 1996;54:189–193.

40. Cheng Y-F, Clyman RI, Enenstein J, Waleh N, Pytela R, Kramer RH. The integrin complex $\alpha_v\beta_3$ participates in the adhesion of microvascular endothelial cells to fibronectin. *Exp Cell Res* 1991;194:69–77.

41. Piali L, Hammel P, Uherek C, et al. CD31/PECAM-1 is a ligand for alpha v beta 3 integrin involved in adhesion of leukocytes to endothelium. *J Cell Biol* 1995;130:451–460.

42. Luscinskas FW, Lawler J. Integrins as dynamic regulators of vascular function. *FASEB J* 1994;8:929–938.

43. Albelda SM, Muller WA, Buck CA, Newman PJ. Molecular and cellular properties of PECAM-1 (endoCAM/CD31): A novel vascular cell-cell adhesion molecule. *J Cell Biol* 1991;114:1059–1068.

44. Muller WA, Weigl SA, Deng X, Phillips DM. PECAM-1 is required for transendothelial migration of leukocytes. *J Exp Med* 1993;178:449–460.

45. Cooper D, Lindberg FP, Gamble JR, Brown EJ, Vadas MA. The transendothelial migration of neutrophils involves integrin associated protein (CD47). *Proc Natl Acad Sci USA* 1995;92:3978–3982.

46. Rot A. Endothelial cell binding of NAP-1/IL-8: role in neutrophil emigration [review, 47 refs]. *Immunol Today* 1992;13:291–294.

47. Gao JX, Issekutz AC. Mac-1 (CD11b/CD18) is the predominant beta 2 (CD18) integrin mediating human neutrophil migration through synovial and dermal fibroblast barriers. *Immunology* 1996;88:463–470.

48. Burns AR, Simon SI, Kukielka GL, et al. Chemotactic factors stimulate CD18-dependent canine neutrophil adherence and motility on lung fibroblasts. *J Immunol* 1996;156:3389–3401.

49. Brown EJ, Lindberg FP. Matrix receptors of myeloid cells. In: Horton MA, ed. *Blood cell biochemistry.* Vol 5: *Macrophages and related cells.* New York: Plenum Press, 1993:279–306.

50. Mandeville JT, Lawson MA, Maxfield FR. Dynamic imaging of neutrophil migration in three dimensions: mechanical interactions between cells and matrix. *J Leukoc Biol* 1997;61:188–200.

51. Owen CA, Campbell MA, Sannes PL, Boukedes SS, Campbell EJ. Cell surface-bound elastase and cathepsin G on human neutrophils: a novel, non-oxidative mechanism by which neutrophils focus and preserve catalytic activity of serine proteinases. *J Cell Biol* 1995;131:775–789.

52. Chow CW, Grinstein S, Rotstein OD. Signaling events in monocytes and macrophages. *New Horiz* 1995;3:342–351.

53. Morrison DC, Lei MG, Kirikae T, Chen TY. Endotoxin receptors on mammalian cells. *Immunobiology* 1993;187:212–226.

54. Ziegler-Heitbrock HW, Ulevitch RJ. CD14: cell surface receptor and differentiation marker. *Immunol Today* 1993;14:121–125.

55. Dunne DW, Resnick D, Greenberg J, Krieger M, Joiner KA. The type I macrophage scavenger receptor binds to gram-positive bacteria and recognizes lipoteichoic acid. *Proc Natl Acad Sci USA* 1994;91:1863–1867.

56. Stahl PD. The mannose receptor: current status. *Am J Respir Cell Mol Biol* 1990;2:317–318.

57. Resnick D, Pearson A, Krieger M. The SRCR superfamily: a family reminiscent of the Ig superfamily. *Trends Biochem Sci* 1994;19:5–8.

58. Fadok VA, Savill JS, Haslett C, et al. Different populations of macrophages use either the vitronectin receptor or the phosphatidylserine receptor to recognize and remove apoptotic cells. *J Immunol* 1992;149:4029–4035.

59. Krieger M, Herz J. Structures and functions of multiligand lipoprotein receptors: macrophage scavenger receptors and LDL receptor-related protein (LRP). *Annu Rev Biochem* 1994;63:601–637.

60. Acton S, Rigotti A, Landschulz KT, Xu S, Hobbs HH, Krieger M. Identification of scavenger receptor SR-BI as a high density lipoprotein receptor [see comments]. *Science* 1996;271:518–520.

61. Rigotti A, Acton SL, Krieger M. The class B scavenger receptors SR-BI and CD36 are receptors for anionic phospholipids. *J Biol Chem* 1995;270:16221–16224.

62. Hughes DA, Fraser IP, Gordon S. Murine macrophage scavenger receptor: in vivo expression and function as receptor for macrophage adhesion in lymphoid and non-lymphoid organs. *Eur J Immunol* 1995;25:466–473.

63. Hughes DA, Fraser IP, Gordon S. Murine M phi scavenger receptor: adhesion function and expression. *Immunol Lett* 1994;43:7–14.

64. Stahl PD. The mannose receptor and other macrophage lectins. *Curr Opin Immunol* 1992;4:49–52.

65. Taylor ME. Recognition of complex carbohydrates by the macrophage mannose receptor. *Biochem Soc Trans* 1993;21:468–473.

66. Ezekowitz RA, Sastry K, Bailly P, Warner A. Molecular characterization of the human macrophage mannose receptor: demonstration of multiple carbohydrate recognition-like domains and phagocytosis of yeasts in Cos-1 cells. *J Exp Med* 1990;172:1785–1794.

67. Gergely J, Sarmay G. The two binding-site models of human IgG binding Fc-gamma receptors. *FASEB J* 1990;4:3275–3283.

68. Powell MS, Hulett MD, Brinkworth RI, Hogarth PM. Human FcgR:Ligand interactions. In: van de Winkel JGJ, Capel PJA, eds. *Human IgG Fc receptors.* Austin, TX: R.G. Landes Company, 1996:5–24.

69. Erbe DV, Collins JE, Shen L, Graziano RF, Fanger MW. The effect of cytokines on the expression and function of Fc receptors for IgG on human myeloid cells. *Mol Immunol* 1990;27:57–67.

70. Shen L. Receptors for IgA on phagocytic cells [review, 40 refs]. *Immunol Res* 1992;11:273–282.

71. Salmon JE, Edberg JC, Kimberly RP. FcgR on Neutrophils. In: van de Winkel JGJ, Capel PJA, eds. *Human IgG Fc receptors.* Austin, TX: R.G. Landes Company, 1996:79–106.

72. Kurlander RJ, Batker J. The binding of human immunoglobulin G1 monomer and small, covalently cross-linked polymers of immunoglobulin G1 to human peripheral blood monocytes and polymorphonuclear leukocytes. *J Clin Invest* 1982;69:1–8.

73. Van de Winkel JGJ, Capel PJA. Human IgG Fc receptor yellow pages. In: van de Winkel JGJ, Capel PJA, eds. *Human IgG Fc receptors.* Austin, TX: R.G. Landes Company, 1997:227–237.

74. Fanger NA, Yeaman GR, Guyre PM. Regulation of FcgR expression and function by cytokines and hormones. In: van de Winkel JGJ, Capel PJA, eds. *Human IgG Fc receptors.* Austin, TX: R.G. Landes Company, 1996:123–148.

75. Ernst LK, Duchemin AM, Anderson CL. Association of the high-affinity receptor for IgG (Fc gamma RI) with the gamma subunit of the IgE receptor. *Proc Natl Acad Sci USA* 1993;90:6023–6027.

76. Sanders LA, van de Winkel JG, Rijkers GT, et al. Fc gamma receptor IIa (CD32) heterogeneity in patients with recurrent bacterial respiratory tract infections. *J Infect Dis* 1994;170:854–861.

77. Bredius RG, Derkx BH, Fijen CA, et al. Fc gamma receptor IIa (CD32) polymorphism in fulminant meningococcal septic shock in children. *J Infect Dis* 1994;170:848–853.

78. Miettinen HM, Matter K, Hunziker W, Rose JK, Mellman I. Fc receptor endocytosis is controlled by a cytoplasmic domain determinant that actively prevents coated pit localization. *J Cell Biol* 1992;116:875–888.

79. Indik Z, Kelly C, Chien P, Levinson AI, Schreiber AD. Human Fc$_{gamma}$RII, in the absence of other Fc$_{gamma}$ receptors, mediates a phagocytic signal. *J Clin Invest* 1991;88:1766–1771.

80. Indik ZK, Park JG, Hunter S, Schreiber AD. The molecular dissection of Fcgamma receptor mediated phagocytosis. *Blood* 1995;86:4389–4399.

81. Masuda M, Roos D. Association of all three types of Fc gamma R (CD64, CD32, and CD16) with a gamma-chain homodimer in cultured human monocytes. *J Immunol* 1993;151:7188–7195.

82. Mitchell MA, Huang M-M, Chien P, Indik ZK, Pan XQ, Schreiber AD. Substitutions and deletions in the cytoplasmic domain of the phagocytic receptor FcgammaRIIA: effect on receptor tyrosine phosphorylation and phagocytosis. *Blood* 1994;84:1753–1759.

83. Edberg JC, Lin CT, Lau D, Unkeless JC, Kimberly RP. The Ca^{2+} dependence of human Fcgamma receptor-initiated phagocytosis. *J Biol Chem* 1995;270:22301–22307.

84. Shen Z, Lin CT, Unkeless JC. Correlations among tyrosine phosphorylation of Shc, p72syk, PLC-gamma 1, and [Ca2+]i flux in Fc gamma RIIA signaling. *J Immunol* 1994;152:3017–3023.

85. Hunter S, Kamoun M, Schreiber AD. Transfection of an Fc[gamma] receptor cDNA induces T cells to become phagocytic. *Proc Natl Acad Sci USA* 1994;91:10232–10236.

86. Matsuda M, Park JG, Wang DC, Hunter S, Chien P, Schreiber AD. Abrogation of the Fc gamma receptor IIA-mediated phagocytic signal by stem-loop Syk antisense oligonucleotides. *Mol Biol Cell* 1996;7:1095–1106.

87. Ono M, Bolland S, Tempst P, Ravetch JV. Role of the inositol phosphatase ship in negative regulation of immune function by mast cell Fc receptors. *Nature* 1996;383:263–266.

88. Takai T, Ono M, Hikida M, Ohmori H, Ravetch JV. Augmented humoral and anaphylactic responses in Fc gamma RII-deficient mice. *Nature* 1996;379:346–349.

89. Muta T, Kurosaki T, Misulovin Z, Sanchez M, Nussenzweig MC, Ravetch JV. A 13-amino-acid motif in the cytoplasmic domain of Fc gamma RIIB modulates B-cell receptor signalling. *Nature* 1994;369:340

90. Ono M, Okada H, Bolland S, Yanagi S, Kurosaki T, Ravetch JV. Deletion of SHIP or SHP-1 reveals two distinct pathways for inhibitory signaling. *Cell* 1997;90:293–302.

91. Miller KL, Duchemin AM, Anderson CL. A novel role for the Fc receptor gamma subunit: enhancement of Fc gamma R ligand affinity. *J Exp Med* 1996;183:2227–2233.

92. De Haas M, Kleijer M, Van Zwieten R, Roos D, Von dem Borne AEGK, von dem Borne AE. Neutrophil FcgammaRIIIb deficiency, nature, and clinical consequences: a study of 21 individuals from 14 families. *Blood* 1995;86:2403–2413.

93. Koene HR, De Haas M, Roos D, Von dem Borne AEGK. Soluble FcgRIII: biology and clinical implications. In: van de Winkel JGJ, Capel PJA, eds. *Human IgG Fc receptors.* Austin, TX: R.G. Landes Company, 1996:181–194.

94. Morton HC, van den Herik-Oudijk IE, Vossebeld P, et al. Functional association between the human myeloid immunoglobulin A Fc receptor (CD89) and FcR gamma chain. Molecular basis for CD89/FcR gamma chain association. *J Biol Chem* 1995;270:29781–29787.

95. Scott CB, Ratcliffe DR, Cramer EB. Human monocytes are unable to bind to or phagocytize IgA and IgG immune complexes formed with influenza virus in vitro. *J Immunol* 1996;157:351–359.

96. Nikolova EB, Russell MW. Dual function of human IgA antibodies: inhibition of phagocytosis in circulating neutrophils and enhancement of responses in IL-8-stimulated cells. *J Leukoc Biol* 1995;57:875–882.

97. Saito K, Kato C, Katsuragi H, Komatsuzaki A. IgA-mediated inhibition of human leucocyte function by interference with Fc gamma and C3b receptors. *Immunology* 1991;74:99–106.

98. Griffiss JM. Biologic function of the serum IgA system: modulation of complement-mediated effector mechanisms and conservation of antigenic mass. *Ann NY Acad Sci* 1983;409:697–707.

99. Mostov KE. Transepithelial transport of immunoglobulins. *Annu Rev Immunol* 1994;12:63–84.

100. Wright SD, Silverstein SC. Tumor-promoting phorbol esters stimulate C3b and C3b′ receptor-mediated phagocytosis in cultured human monocytes. *J Exp Med* 1982;156:1149–1164.

101. Bianco C, Griffin FM Jr, Silverstein SC. Studies of the macrophage complement receptor. Alteration of receptor function upon macrophage activation. *J Exp Med* 1975;141:1278–1291.

102. Holers VM. Complement receptors. *Year Immunol* 1989;4:231–240.

103. Liszewski MK, Atkinson JP. The role of complement in autoimmunity. *Immunol Ser* 1991;54:13–37.

104. Roubey RAS, Ross GD, Merrill JT, et al. Staurosporine inhibits neutrophil phagocytosis but not iC3b binding mediated by CR3 (CD11b/CD18). *J Immunol* 1991;146:3557–3562.

105. Wright SD, Rao PE, Wesley C, et al. Identification of the C3bi receptor of human monocytes and macrophages by using monoclonal antibodies. *Proc Natl Acad Sci USA* 1983;80:5699–5703.

106. Myones BL, Dalzell JG, Hogg N, Ross GD. Neutrophil and monocyte cell surface p150,95 has iC3b receptor (CR4) activity. *J Clin Invest* 1988;82:640–651.

107. Todd RF, Freyer DR. The CD11/CD18 leukocyte glycoprotein deficiency. *Hematol Oncol Clin North Am* 1988;2:13–31.

108. Etzioni A. Adhesion molecule deficiencies and their clinical significance. *Cell Adhes Commun* 1994;2:257–260.

109. Anderson DC, Schmalsteig FC, Finegold MJ, et al. The severe and moderate phenotypes of heritable Mac-1, LFA-1 deficiency: their quantitative definition and relation to leukocyte dysfunction and clinical features. *J Infect Dis* 1985;152:668–689.

110. Butcher EC. Leukocyte-endothelial cell recognition: three (or more) steps to specificity and diversity. *Cell* 1991;67:1033–1036.

111. Gresham HD, Graham IL, Anderson DC, Brown EJ. Leukocyte adhesion deficient (LAD) neutrophils fail to amplify phagocytic function in response to stimulation: evidence for CD11b/CD18-dependent and -independent mechanisms of phagocytosis. *J Clin Invest* 1991;88:588–597.

112. Arnaout MA, Todd RF III, Dana N, Melamed J, Schlossman SF, Colten HR. Inhibition of phagocytosis of complement C3- or immunoglobulin G-coated particles and of C3bi binding by monoclonal antibodies to a monocyte granulocyte membrane glycoprotein (Mo1). *J Clin Invest* 1983;72:171–179.

113. Graham IL, Lefkowith JB, Anderson DC, Brown EJ. Immune complex-stimulated neutrophil LTB4 production is dependent on beta2 integrins. *J Cell Biol* 1993;120:1509–1517.

114. Sehgal G, Zhang K, Todd RF, Boxer LA, Petty HR. Lectin-like inhibition of immune-complex receptor-mediated stimulation of neutrophils—effects on cytosolic calcium release and superoxide production. *J Immunol* 1993;150:4571–4580.

115. Nathan C, Srimal S, Farber C, et al. Cytokine-induced respiratory burst of human neutrophils: dependence on extracellular matrix proteins and CD11/CD18 integrins. *J Cell Biol* 1989;109:1341–1349.

116. Fuortes M, Jin W, Nathan C. β2 integrin-dependent tyrosine phosphorylation of paxillin in human neutrophils treated with tumor necrosis factor. *J Cell Biol* 1994;127:1477–1483.

117. Graham IL, Anderson DC, Holers VM, Brown EJ. Complement receptor 3 (CR3, Mac-1, Integrin alpha-M beta-2, CD11b/CD18) is required for tyrosine phosporylation of paxillin in adherent and nonadherent neutrophils. *J Cell Biol* 1994;127:1139–1147.

118. Coxon A, Rieu P, Barkalow FJ, et al. A novel role for the beta-2 integrin CD11b/CD18 in neutrophil apoptosis—a homeostatic mechanism in inflammation. *Immunity* 1996;5:653–666.

119. Petty HR, Todd RF. Integrins as promiscuous signal transduction devices. *Immunol Today* 1996;17:209–212.

120. Sitrin RG, Todd RF, Petty HR, et al. The urokinase receptor (cd87) facilitates cd11b/cd18-mediated adhesion of human monocytes. *J Clin Invest* 1996;97:1942–1951.

121. Krauss JC, Poo H, Xue W, Mayo-Bond L, Todd RF, Petty HR. Reconstitution of antibody-dependent phagocytosis in fibroblasts expressing Fc gamma receptor IIIB and the complement receptor type 3. *J Immunol* 1994;153:1769–1777.

122. Poo H, Krauss JC, Mayobond L, Todd RF, Petty HR. Interaction of Fc-gamma receptor type IIIB with complement receptor type 3 in fibroblast transfectants—evidence from lateral diffusion and resonance energy transfer studies. *J Mol Biol* 1995;247:597–603.

123. Zhou M-J, Brown EJ. CR3 (Mac-1, α$_M$β$_2$, CD11b/CD18) and Fc(gamma)RIII cooperate in generation of a neutrophil respiratory burst: requirement for Fc(gamma)RII and tyrosine phosphorylation. *J Cell Biol* 1994;125:1407–1416.

124. Brown EJ, Bohnsack JF, Gresham HD. Mechanism of inhibition of immunoglobulin G-mediated phagocytosis by monoclonal antibodies that recognize the Mac-1 antigen. *J Clin Invest* 1988;81:365–375.

125. Brown EJ. Complement receptors and phagocytosis. *Curr Opin Immunol* 1991;3:76–82.

126. Metlay JP, Witmer Pack MD, Agger R, Crowley MT, Lawless D, Steinman RM. The distinct leukocyte integrins of mouse spleen dendritic cells as identified with new hamster monoclonal antibodies. *J Exp Med* 1990;171:1753–1771.

127. Wright SD, Weitz JI, Huang AJ, Levin SM, Silverstein SC, Loike JD. Complement receptor type three (CD11b/CD18) of human polymorphonuclear leukocytes recognizes fibrinogen. *Proc Natl Acad Sci USA* 1988;85:7734–7738.

128. Loike JD, Sodeik B, Cao L, et al. CD11c/CD18 on neutrophils recognizes a domain at the N terminus of the Aα chain of fibrinogen. *Proc Natl Acad Sci USA* 1991;88:1044–1048.

129. Berton G, Laudanna C, Sorio C, Rossi F. Generation of signals activating neutrophil functions by leukocyte integrins: LFA-1 and gp150/95, but not CR3, are able to stimulate the respiratory burst of human neutrophils. *J Cell Biol* 1992;116:1007–1017.

130. Keizer GD, te Velde AA, Schwarting R, Figdor CG, de Vries JE. Role of p,150,95 in adhesion, migration, chemotaxis, and phagocytosis of human monocytes. *Eur J Immunol* 1987;17:1317.

131. Epstein J, Eichinger Q, Sheriff S, Ezekowitz RA. The collectins in innate immunity. *Curr Opin Immunol* 1996;8:29–35.

132. Schweinle JE, Ezekowitz RA, Tenner AJ, Kuhlman M, Joiner KA. Human mannose-binding protein activates the alternative complement pathway and enhances serum bactericidal activity on a mannose-rich isolate of Salmonella. *J Clin Invest* 1989;84:1821–1829.

133. Matsushita M, Fujita T. Activation of the classical complement pathway by man-

nose-binding protein in association with a novel C1s-like serine protease. *J Exp Med* 1992;176:1497–1502.

134. Matsushita M, Fujita T. Cleavage of the third component of complement (C3) by mannose-binding protein-associated serine protease (MASP) with subsequent complement activation. *Immunobiology* 1995;194:443–448.

135. Summerfield JA. The role of mannose-binding protein in host defence. *Biochem Soc Trans* 1993;21:473–477.

136. Mold C, Du Clos TW, Nakayama S, Edwards KM, Gewurz H. C-reactive protein reactivity with complement and effects on phagocytosis. *Ann NY Acad Sci* 1982;389:251–262.

137. Crowell RE, Du Clos TW, Montoya G, Heaphy E, Mold C. C-reactive protein receptors on the human monocytic cell line U-937. Evidence for additional binding to Fc gamma RI. *J Immunol* 1991;147:3445–3451.

138. Xia D, Samols D. Transgenic mice expressing rabbit C-reactive protein are resistant to endotoxemia. *Proc Natl Acad Sci USA* 1997;94:2575–2580.

139. Ahmed N, Thorley R, Xia D, Samols D, Webster RO. Transgenic mice expressing rabbit C-reactive protein exhibit diminished chemotactic factor-induced alveolitis. *Am J Respir Crit Care Med* 1996;153:1141–1147.

140. Szalai AJ, Briles DE, Volanakis JE. Human C-reactive protein is protective against fatal Streptococcus pneumoniae infection in transgenic mice. *J Immunol* 1995;155:2557–2563.

141. Hook M, McGavin MJ, Switalski LM, et al. Interactions of bacteria with extracellular matrix proteins. *Cell Differ Dev* 1990;32:433–438.

142. Saba TM, Blumenstock FA, Weber P, Kaplan JE. Physiologic role of cold-insoluble globulin in systemic host defense: implications of its characterization as the opsonic alpha 2-surface-binding glycoprotein. *Ann NY Acad Sci* 1978;312:43–55.

143. Saba TM. Fibronectin: relevance to phagocytic host response to injury. *Circ Shock* 1989;29:257–278.

144. Savill J. Apoptosis in resolution of inflammation. *J Leukoc Biol* 1997;61:375–380.

145. Morris L, Graham CF, Gordon S. Macrophages in haemopoietic and other tissues of the developing mouse detected by the monoclonal antibody F4/80. *Development* 1991;112:517–526.

146. Savill J, Dransfield I, Hogg N, Haslett C. Vitronectin receptor-mediated phagocytosis of cells undergoing apoptosis. *Nature* 1990;343:170–173.

147. Savill J, Hogg N, Ren Y, Haslett C. Thrombospondin cooperates with CD36 and the vitronectin receptor in macrophage recognition of neutrophils undergoing apoptosis. *J Clin Invest* 1992;90:1513–1522.

148. Ryeom SW, Silverstein RL, Scotto A, Sparrow JR. Binding of anionic phospholipids to retinal pigment epithelium may be mediated by the scavenger receptor CD36. *J Biol Chem* 1996;271:20536–20539.

149. Hart SP, Haslett C, Dransfield I. Recognition of apoptotic cells by phagocytes. *Experientia* 1996;52:950–956.

150. Franc NC, Dimarcq JL, Lagueux M, Hoffmann J, Ezekowitz RA. Croquemort, a novel Drosophila hemocyte/macrophage receptor that recognizes apoptotic cells. *Immunity* 1996;4:431–443.

151. Ryeom SW, Sparrow JR, Silverstein RL. CD36 participates in the phagocytosis of rod outer segments by retinal pigment epithelium. *J Cell Sci* 1996;109:387–395.

152. Luciani M-F, Chimini G. The ATP binding cassette transporter ABC1 is required for the engulfment of corpses generated by apoptotic cell death. *EMBO J* 1996;15:226–235.

153. Polte T, Newman W, Raghunathan G, Venkat Gopal T. Structural and functional studies of full-length vascular cell adhesion molecule-1: internal duplication and homology to several adhesion proteins. *DNA Cell Biol* 1991;10:349–357.

154. Griffin FM Jr, Griffin JA, Silverstein SC. Studies on the mechanism of phagocytosis: II. The interaction of macrophages with anti-immunoglobulin IgG-coated bone marrow-derived-lymphocytes. *J Exp Med* 1976;144:788–809.

155. Griffin FM Jr, Griffin JA, Leider JE, Silverstein SC. Studies on the mechanism of phagocytosis: I. Requirements for circumferential attachment of particle-bound ligands to specific receptors on the macrophage plasma membrane. *J Exp Med* 1975;142:1263–1282.

156. Griffin FM Jr, Silverstein SC. Segmental response of the macrophage plasma membrane to a phagocytic stimulus. *J Exp Med* 1974;139:323–336.

157. Kaplan G. Differences in the mode of phagocytosis with Fc and C3 receptors in macrophages. *Scand J Immunol* 1977;6:797–807.

158. Kaplan G, Bertheussen K. The morphology of echinoid phagocytes and mouse peritoneal macrophages during phagocytosis in vitro. *Scand J Immunol* 1977;6:1289–1296.

159. Allen LAH, Aderem A. Molecular definition of distinct cytoskeletal structures involved in complement- and Fc receptor-mediated phagocytosis in macrophages. *J Exp Med* 1996;184:627–637.

160. Greenberg S, Chang P, Wang DC, Xavier R, Seed B. Clustered syk tyrosine kinase domains trigger phagocytosis. *Proc Natl Acad Sci USA* 1996;93:1103–1107.

161. Ninomiya N, Hazeki K, Fukui Y, et al. Involvement of phosphatidylinositol 3-kinase in Fc gamma receptor signaling. *J Biol Chem* 1994;269:22732–22737.

162. Shimizu Y, Mobley JL, Finkelstein LD, Chan ASH. Role for phosphatidylinositol 3-kinase in the regulation of β1 integrin activity by the CD2 antigen. *J Cell Biol* 1995;131:1867–1880.

163. Hotchin NA, Hall A. Regulation of the actin cytoskeleton, integrins and cell growth by the Rho family of small GTPases. *Cancer Surv* 1996;27:311–322.

164. Zheleznyak A, Brown EJ. IgG-mediated phagocytosis by human monocytes requires protein kinase C activation: evidence for protein kinase C translocation to phagosomes. *J Biol Chem* 1992;267:12042–12048.

165. Fällman M, Gullberg M, Hellberg C, Andersson T. Complement receptor-mediated phagocytosis is associated with accumulation of phosphatidylcholine-derived diglyceride in human neutrophils. Involvement of phospholipase D and direct evidence for a positive feedback signal of protein kinase C. *J Biol Chem* 1992;267:2656–2663.

166. Allen LH, Aderem A. A role for MARCKS, the alpha isozyme of protein kinase C and myosin I in zymosan phagocytosis by macrophages. *J Exp Med* 1995;182:829–840.

167. Aderem A. The MARCKS family of protein kinase-C substrates. *Biochem Soc Trans* 1995;23:587–591.

168. Lew DP, Andersson T, Hed J, Di Virgilio F, Pozzan T, Stendahl O. Ca2+-dependent and Ca2+-independent phagocytosis in human neutrophils. *Nature* 1985;315:509–511.

169. DiVirgilio F, Meyer BC, Greenberg S, Silverstein SC. Fc receptor-mediated phagocytosis occurs in macrophages at exceedingly low cytosolic Ca^{2+} levels. *J Cell Biol* 1988;106:657–666.

170. Rosales C, Brown EJ. Two mechanisms for IgG Fc-receptor-mediated phagocytosis by human neutrophils. *J Immunol* 1991;146:3937–3944.

171. Collins K, Sellers JR, Matsudaira P. Calmodulin dissociation regulates brush border myosin I (110-kD-calmodulin) mechanochemical activity in vitro. *J Cell Biol* 1990;110:1137–1147.

172. Stendahl O, Krause K-H, Krischer J, et al. Redistribution of intracellular Ca^{2+} stores during phagocytosis in human neutrophils. *Science* 1994;265:1439–1441.

173. Serrander L, Fallman M, Stendahl O. Activation of phospholipase D is an early event in integrin-mediated signalling leading to phagocytosis in human neutrophils. *Inflammation* 1996;20:439–450.

174. Kusner DJ, Hall CF, Schlesinger LS. Activation of phospholipase D is tightly coupled to the phagocytosis of *Mycobacterium tuberculosis* or opsonized zymosan by human macrophages. *J Exp Med* 1996;184:585–595.

175. Lennartz MR, Brown EJ. Arachidonic acid is essential for Fc-receptor-mediated phagocytosis by human monocytes. *J Immunol* 1991;147:621–626.

176. Lennartz MR, Lefkowith JB, Bromley FA, Brown EJ. Immunoglobulin G-mediated phagocytosis activates a calcium-independent, phosphatidylethanolamine-specific phospholipase. *J Leukoc Biol* 1993;54:389–398.

177. Karimi K, Lennartz MR. Protein kinase C activation precedes arachidonic acid release during IgG-mediated phagocytosis. *J Immunol* 1995;155:5786–5794.

178. Mayorga LS, Colombo MI, Lennartz M, et al. Inhibition of endosome fusion by phospholipase-a(2) (PLA2) inhibitors points to a role for PLA2 in endocytosis. *Proc Natl Acad Sci USA* 1993;90:10255–10259.

179. Manie SN, Beck AR, Astier A, et al. Involvement of p130(Cas) and p105(HEF1), a novel Cas-like docking protein, in a cytoskeleton-dependent signaling pathway initiated by ligation of integrin or antigen receptor on human B cells. *J Biol Chem* 1997;272:4230–4236.

180. Salgia R, Avraham S, Pisick E, et al. The related adhesion focal tyrosine kinase forms a complex with paxillin in hematopoietic cells. *J Biol Chem* 1996;271:31222–31226.

181. Allen LAH, Aderem A. Mechanisms of phagocytosis. *Curr Opin Immunol* 1996;8:36–40.

182. Jung G, Wu XF, Hammer JA. Dictyostelium mutants lacking multiple classic myosin I isoforms reveal combinations of shared and distinct functions. *J Cell Biol* 1996;133:305–323.

183. Zigmond SH, Hirsch JG. Effects of cytochalasin B on polymorphonuclear leucocyte locomotion, phagocytosis and glycolysis. *Exp Cell Res* 1972;73:383–393.

184. Rosales C, Jones SL, McCourt D, Brown EJ. Bromophenacyl bromide binding to the actin bundling protein l-plastin inhibits IP$_3$-independent [Ca^{+2}]$_i$ rise in human neutrophils. *Proc Natl Acad Sci USA* 1994;91:3534–3538.

185. Burridge K, Chrzanowska-Wodnicka M. Focal adhesions, contractility, and signaling. *Ann Rev Cell Dev Biol* 1996;12:463–518.

186. Yamada KM, Geiger B. Molecular interactions in cell adhesion complexes. *Curr Opin Cell Biol* 1997;9:76–85.

187. Gaidano G, Bergui L, Schena M, et al. Integrin distribution and cytoskeleton organization in normal and malignant monocytes. *Leukemia* 1990;4:682–687.

188. Marchisio PC, Bergui L, Corbascio GC, et al. Vinculin, talin, and integrins are localized at specific adhesion sites of malignant B lymphocytes. *Blood* 1988;72:830–833.

189. Bokoch GM, Knaus UG. The role of small GTP-binding proteins in leukocyte function. *Curr Opin Immunol* 1994;6:98–105.

190. Tapon N, Hall A. Rho, rac and cdc42 gtpases regulate the organization of the actin cytoskeleton. *Curr Opin Cell Biol* 1997;9:86–92.

191. Allen WE, Jones GE, Pollard JW, Ridley AJ. Rho, Rac, and Cdc42 regulate actin organization and cell adhesion in macrophages. *J Cell Sci* 1997;110:707–720.

192. Zigmond SH, Joyce MP, Borleis J, Bokoch GM, Devreotes PN. Regulation of actin polymerization in cell-free systems by GTPgammaS and Cdc42. *J Cell Biol* 1997;138:363–374.

193. Nobes CD, Hall A. Rho, rac, and cdc42 GTPases regulate the assembly of multimolecular focal complexes associated with actin stress fibers, lamellipodia, and filopodia. *Cell* 1995;81:53–62.

194. Hotchin NA, Hall A. The assembly of integrin adhesion complexes requires both extracellular matrix and intracellular rho/rac GTPases. *J Cell Biol* 1995;131:1857–1865.

195. Ridley AJ, Hall A. The small GTP-binding protein rho regulates the assembly of focal adhesions and actin stress fibers in response to growth factors. *Cell* 1992;70.389–399.

196. Manser E, Leung T, Salihuddin H, Zhao ZS, Lim L. A brain serine/threonine protein kinase activated by Cdc42 and Rac1. *Nature* 1994;367:40–46.

197. Knaus UG, Morris S, Dong HJ, Chernoff J, Bokoch GM. Regulation of human leukocyte p21-activated kinases through G protein–coupled receptors. *Science* 1995;269:221–223.

198. Lamarche N, Tapon N, Stowers L, et al. Rac and Cdc42 induce actin polymerization and G1 cell cycle progression independently of p65PAK and the JNK/SAPK MAP kinase cascade. *Cell* 1996;87:519–529.

199. Joneson T, McDonough M, Bar-Sagi D, Van Aelst L. RAC regulation of actin polymerization and proliferation by a pathway distinct from Jun kinase. *Science* 1996;274:1374–1376.

200. Sells M, Knaus U, Bagrodia S, Ambrose D, Bokoch G, Chernoff J. Human p21-activated kinase (Pak1) regulates actin organization in mammalian cells. *Curr Biol* 1997;7:202–210.

200a.Jones SL, Knaus UG, Bokoch GM, Brown EJ. Two signalling mechanisms for activation of αMβ2 avidity in polymorphonuclear leukocytes. *J Biol Chem.* 1998;273:10556–10566.

201. Hartwig JH, Bokoch GM, Carpenter CL, et al. Thrombin receptor ligation and activated Rac uncap actin filament barbed ends through phosphoinositide synthesis in permeabilized human platelets. *Cell* 1995;82:643–653.

202. Schafer DA, Jennings PB, Cooper JA. Dynamics of capping protein and actin assembly in vitro: uncapping barbed ends by polyphosphoinositides. *J Cell Biol* 1996;135:169–179.

203. Barkalow K, Witke W, Kwiatkowski DJ, Hartwig JH. Coordinated regulation of platelet actin filament barbed ends by gelsolin and capping protein. *J Cell Biol* 1996;134:389–399.

204. Tardif M, Huang S, Redmond T, Safer D, Pring M, Zigmond SH. Actin polymerization induced by GTP gamma S in permeabilized neutrophils is induced and maintained by free barbed ends. *J Biol Chem* 1995;270:28075–28083.

205. Lassing I, Lindberg U. Specific interaction between phosphatidylinositol 4,5-bisphosphate and profilactin. *Nature* 1985;314:472–474.

206. Theriot JA. Accelerating on a treadmill: ADF/cofilin promotes rapid actin filament turnover in the dynamic cytoskeleton. *J Cell Biol* 1997;136:1165–1168.

207. Kaufmann S, Kas J, Goldmann WH, Sackmann E, Isenberg G. Talin anchors and nucleates actin filaments at lipid membranes. A direct demonstration. *FEBS Lett* 1992;314:203–205.

208. Dubreuil RR. Structure and evolution of the actin crosslinking proteins. *Bioessays* 1991;13:219–226.

209. Matsudaira P. Modular organization of actin crosslinking proteins [review, 26 refs]. *Trends Biochem Sci* 1991;16:87–92.

210. Ehlenberger AG, Nussenzweig V. The role of membrane receptors for C3b and C3d in phagocytosis *J Exp Med* 1977;145:357–371.

211. Mitchison TJ, Cramer LP. Actin-based cell motility and cell locomotion [review, 76 refs]. *Cell* 1996;84:371–379.

212. Lin CS, Park T, Chen ZP, Leavitt J. Human plastin genes: comparative gene structure, chromosome location, and differential expression in normal and neoplastic cells. *J Biol Chem* 1993;268:2781–2792.

213. Chafel MM, Shen W, Matsudaira P. Sequential expression and differential localization of I-, L-, and T-fimbrin during differentiation of the mouse intestine and yolk sac. *Dev Dyn* 1995;203:141–151.

214. Lin CS, Shen W, Chen ZP, Tu YH, Matsudaira P. Identification of I-plastin, a human fimbrin isoform expressed in intestine and kidney *Mol Cell Biol* 1994;14:2457–2467.

215. Kubler E, Riezman H. Actin and fimbrin are required for the internalization step of endocytosis in yeast. *EMBO J* 1993;12:2855–2862.

216. Karpova TS, Tatchell K, Cooper JA. Actin filaments in yeast are unstable in the absence of capping protein or fimbrin. *J Cell Biol* 1995;131:1483–1493.

217. Jones SL, Brown EJ. FcgammaRII-mediated adhesion and phagocytosis induce L-plastin phosphorylation in human neutrophils. *J Biol Chem* 1996;271:14623–14630.

218. Messier JM, Shaw LM, Chafel M, Matsudaira P, Mercurio AM. Fimbrin localized to an insoluble cytoskeletal fraction is constitutively phosphorylated on its headpiece domain in adherent macrophages. *Cell Motil Cytoskeleton* 1993;25:223–233.

219. Shinomiya H, Hagi A, Fukuzumi M, Mizobuchi M, Hirata H, Utsumi S. Complete primary structure and phosphorylation site of the 65-kDa macrophage protein phosphorylated by stimulation with bacterial lipopolysaccharide. *J Immunol* 1995;154:3471–3478.

220. Shibata M, Ohoka T, Mizuno S, Suzuki K. Characterization of a 64-kd protein phosphorylated during chemotactic activation with IL-8 and fMLP of human polymorphonuclear leukocytes. I. Phosphorylation of a 64-kd protein and other proteins. *J Leukoc Biol* 1993;54:1–9.

221. Li J, Aderem A. MacMARCKS, a novel member of the MARCKS family of protein kinase C substrates. *Cell* 1992;70:791–801.

222. Zhu Z, Bao Z, Li J. MacMARCKS mutation blocks macrophage phagocytosis of zymosan. *J Biol Chem* 1995;270:17652–17655.

223. Hartwig JH, Thelen M, Rosen A, Janmey PA, Nairn AC, Aderem A. MARCKS is an actin filament crosslinking protein regulated by protein kinase C and calcium-calmodulin. *Nature* 1992;356:618–622.

224. Seykora JT, Myat MM, Allen LAH, Ravetch JV, Aderem A. Molecular determinants of the myristoyl-electrostatic switch of MARCKS. *J Biol Chem* 1996;271:18797–18802.

225. Thelen M, Rosen A, Nairn AC, Aderem AA. Regulation by phosphorylation of reversible association of a myristoylated protein kinase C substrate with the plasma membrane. *Nature* 1991;351:320–322.

226. Aderem A. The MARCKS brothers: A family of protein kinase C substrates. *Cell* 1992;71:713–716.

227. Stendahl OI, Hartwig JH, Brotschi EA, Stossel TP. Distribution of actin-binding protein and myosin in macrophages during spreading and phagocytosis. *J Cell Biol* 1980;84:215–224.

228. Valerius NH, Stendahl OI, Hartwig JH, Stossel TP. Distribution of actin-binding protein and myosin in neutrophils during chemotaxis and phagocytosis. *Adv Exp Med Biol* 1982;141:19–28.

229. Bement WM, Hasson T, Wirth JA, Cheney RE, Mooseker MS. Identification and overlapping expression of multiple unconventional myosin genes in vertebrate cell types [published erratum appears in *Proc Natl Acad Sci USA* 1994 Nov 22;91(24):11767]. *Proc Natl Acad Sci USA* 1994;91:6549–6553.

230. Fukui Y, Lynch TJ, Brzeska H, Korn ED. Myosin I is located at the leading edges of locomoting Dictyostelium amoebae. *Nature* 1989;341:328–331.

231. Manstein DJ, Titus MA, De Lozanne A, Spudich JA. Gene replacement in Dictyostelium: generation of myosin null mutants. *EMBO J* 1989;8:923–932.

232. Knecht DA, Loomis WF. Antisense RNA inactivation of myosin heavy chain gene expression in Dictyostelium discoideum. *Science* 1987;236:1081–1086.

233. Ostap EM, Pollard TD. Overlapping functions of myosin-I isoforms? [comment] [review, 40 refs]. *J Cell Biol* 1996;133:221–224.

234. Hasson T, Mooseker MS. Molecular motors, membrane movements and physiology—emerging roles for myosins. *Curr Opin Cell Biol* 1995;7:587–594.

235. Wagner MC, Barylko B, Albanesi JP. Tissue distribution and subcellular localization of mammalian myosin I. *J Cell Biol* 1992;119:163–170.

236. Greenberg S, Chang P, Silverstein SC. Tyrosine phosphorylation of the gamma subunit of Fcgamma receptors, p72syk, and paxillin during Fc receptor-mediated phagocytosis in macrophages. *J Biol Chem* 1994;269:3897–3902.

237. Turner CE, Glenney JR Jr, Burridge K. Paxillin: a new vinculin-binding protein present in focal adhesions. *J Cell Biol* 1990;111:1059–1068.

238. De Nichilo MO, Yamada KM. Integrin alpha v beta 5-dependent serine phosphorylation of paxillin in cultured human macrophages adherent to vitronectin. *J Biol Chem* 1996;271:11016–11022.

239. Clark EA, Brugge JS. Integrins and signal transduction pathways: the road taken [review]. *Science* 1995;268:233–239.

240. Burridge K, Nuckolls G, Otey C, Pavalko F, Simon K, Turner C. Actin-membrane interaction in focal adhesions. *Cell Differ Dev* 1990;32:337–342.

241. Burridge K, Turner CE, Romer LH. Tyrosine phosphorylation of paxillin and pp125FAK accompanies cell adhesion to extracellular matrix: a role i cytoskeletal assembly. *J Cell Biol* 1992;119:893–903.

242. Turner CE, Miller JT. Primary sequence of paxillin contains putative SH2 and SH3 domain binding motifs and multiple LIM domains: identification of a vinculin and pp125FAK binding region. *J Cell Sci* 1994;107:1583–1591.

243. Schaller MD, Otey CA, Hildebrand JD, Parsons JT. Focal adhesion kinase and paxillin bind to peptides mimicking β integrin cytoplasmic domains. *J Cell Biol* 1995;130:1181–1187.

244. Araki N, Johnson MT, Swanson JA. A role for phosphoinositide 3-kinase in the completion of macropinocytosis and phagocytosis by macrophages. *J Cell Biol* 1996;135:1249–1260.

245. Sbarra AJ, Karnovsky ML. The biochemical basis of phagocytosis: II. Incorporation of C14-labeled building blocks into lipid, protein, and glycogen of leukocytes during phagocytosis. *J Biol Chem* 1960;235:2224–2229.

246. Mayorga LS, Bertini F, Stahl PD. Fusion of newly formed phagosomes with endosomes in intact cells and in a cell-free system. *J Biol Chem* 1991;266:6511–6517.

247. Funato K, Beron W, Yang CZ, Mukhopadhyay A, Stahl PD. Reconstitution of phagosome-lysosome fusion in streptolysin o-permeabilized cells. *J Biol Chem* 1997;272:16147–16151.

248. Joiner KA, Ganz T, Alabert A, Rotrosen D. The opsonizing ligand on Salmonella typhimurium influences incorporation of specific, but not azurophil, granule constituents into neutrophil phagosomes. *J Cell Biol* 1989;109:2771–2782.

249. Lew PD, Monod A, Waldvogel FA, Dewald B, Baggiolini M, Pozzan T. Quantitative analysis of the cytosolic free calcium dependency of exocytosis from three subcellular compartments in intact human neutrophils. *J Cell Biol* 1986;102:2197–2204.

250. Zimmerli S, Majeed M, Gustavsson M, Stendahl O, Sanan DA, Ernst JD. Phagosome-lysosome fusion is a calcium independent event in macrophages. *J Cell Biol* 1996;132:49–61.

251. Rotrosen D. The respiratory burst oxidase. In: Gallin JI, Goldstein IM, Snyderman R, eds. *Inflammation: basic principles and clinical correlates.* 2nd ed. New York: Raven Press, 1992:589–601.

252. Brown EJ. Adhesive interactions in the immune system. *Trends Cell Biol* 1997;7:289–295.

253. Rosales C, Brown EJ. Neutrophil receptors and modulation of the immune response. In: Abramson JS, Wheeler JG, eds. *The neutrophil.* Oxford: IRL Press, 1993:23–62.

254. Shimizu Y, Hunt SW III. Regulating integrin-mediated adhesion: one more function for PI 3-kinase? *Immunol Today* 1996;17:565–573.

255. Brown EJ. Signal transduction from leukocyte integrins. In: Hemler ME, Mihich E, eds. *Cell adhesion molecules.* New York: Plenum Press, 1993:105–126.

256. Brown EJ, Lindberg FP. Leucocyte adhesion molecules in host defence against infection. *Ann Med* 1996;28:201–208.

257. Van Strijp JAG, Russell DG, Tuomanen E, Brown EJ, Wright SD. Ligand specificity of purified complement receptor type 3 (CD11b/CD18, Mac-1, alphaM beta2): indirect effects of an Arg-Gly-Asp sequence. *J Immunol* 1993;151: 3324–3336.

258. Zhou M-J, Brown EJ. Leukocyte response integrin and integrin associated protein act as a signal transduction unit in generation of a phagocyte respiratory burst. *J Exp Med* 1993;178:1165–1174.

259. Ishibashi Y, Claus S, Relman DA. *Bordetella pertussis* filamentous hemagglutinin interacts with a leukocyte signal transduction complex and stimulates bacterial adherence to monocyte CR3 (CD11b/CD18). *J Exp Med* 1994;180:1225–1233.

260. Gresham HD, Graham IL, Griffin GL, et al. Domain-specific interactions between entactin and neutrophil integrins—g2 domain ligation of integrin alpha(3)beta(1) and e domain ligation of the leukocyte response integrin signal for different responses. *J Biol Chem* 1996;271:30587–30594.

261. Gresham HD, Goodwin JL, Anderson DC, Brown EJ. A novel member of the integrin receptor family mediates Arg-Gly-Asp-stimulated neutrophil phagocytosis. *J Cell Biol* 1989;108:1935–1943.

262. Newman SL, Tucci MA. Regulation of human monocyte/macrophage function by extracellular matrix. Adherence of monocytes to collagen matrices enhances phagocytosis of opsonized bacteria by activation of complement receptors and enhancement of Fc receptor function. *J Clin Invest* 1990;86:703–714.

263. Vossebeld PJM, Kessler J, Von dem Borne AEGK, Roos D, Verhoeven AJ. Heterotypic FcgammaR clusters evoke a synergistic Ca²⁺ response in human neutrophils. *J Biol Chem* 1995;270:10671–10679.

264. Zhou M-J, Lublin DM, Link DC, Brown EJ. Distinct tyrosine kinase activation and Triton X-100 insolubility upon FcgammaRII or FcgammaRIIIB ligation in human polymorphonuclear leukocytes: implications for immune complex activation of the respiratory burst. *J Biol Chem* 1995;270:13553–13560.

265. Watson F, Gasmi L, Edwards SW. Stimulation of intracellular Ca²⁺ levels in human neutrophils by soluble immune complexes: functional activation of Fc[gamma]RIIIb during priming. *J Biol Chem* 1997;272:17944–17951.

266. Mengaud J, Ohayon H, Gounon P, Mege R, Cossart P. E-cadherin is the receptor for internalin, a surface protein required for entry of L. monocytogenes into epithelial cells. *Cell* 1996;84:923–932.

267. Isberg RR. Uptake of enteropathogenic Yersinia by mammalian cells. *Curr Top Microbiol Immunol* 1996;209:1–24.

268. Neutra MR, Frey A, Kraehenbuhl JP. Epithelial M cells: gateways for mucosal infection and immunization [review, 19 refs]. *Cell* 1996;86:345–348.

269. Kerneis S, Bodganova A, Kraehenbuhl JP, Pringault E. Conversion by Peyer's patch lymphocytes of human enterocytes into M cells that transport bacteria. *Science* 1997;277:949–952.

270. Isberg R, Tran Van Nhieu G. Binding and internalization of microorganisms by integrin receptors. *Trends Microbiol* 1994;2:10–14.

271. Persson C, Carballeira N, Wolfwatz H, Fallman M. The PTPase YopH inhibits uptake of Yersinia, tyrosine phosphorylation of P130(CAS) and FAK, and the associated accumulation of these proteins in peripheral focal adhesions. *EMBO J* 1997;16:2307–2318.

272. Black DS, Bliska JB. Identification of P130(CAS) as a substrate of Yersinia YopH (Yop51), a bacterial protein tyrosine phosphatase that translocates into mammalian cells and targets focal adhesions. *EMBO J* 1997;16:2730–2744.

273. Fallman M, Persson C, Wolf-Watz H. Yersinia proteins that target host cell signaling pathways [Review, 35 refs]. *J Clin Invest* 1997;99:1153–1157.

274. Pettersson J, Nordfelth R, Dubinina E, et al. Modulation of virulence factor expression by pathogen target cell contact [see comments]. *Science* 1996;273: 1231–1233.

275. Bliska JB, Guan KL, Dixon JE, Falkow S. Tyrosine phosphate hydrolysis of host proteins by an essential Yersinia virulence determinant. *Proc Natl Acad Sci USA* 1991;88:1187–1191.

276. Rosqvist R, Magnusson KE, Wolf-Watz H. Target cell contact triggers expression and polarized transfer of Yersinia YopE cytotoxin into mammalian cells. *EMBO J* 1994;13:964–972.

277. Pace J, Hayman MJ, Galan JE. Signal transduction and invasion of epithelial cells by S. typhimurium. *Cell* 1993;72:505–514.

278. Francis CL, Ryan TA, Jones BD, Smith SJ, Falkow S. Ruffles induced by Salmonella and other stimuli direct macropinocytosis of bacteria. *Nature* 1993;364: 639–642.

279. Hondalus MK, Diamond MS, Rosenthal LA, Springer TA, Mosser DM. The intracellular bacterium Rhodococcus equi requires Mac-1 to bind to mammalian cells. *Infect Immun* 1993;61:2919–2929.

280. Marra A, Isberg RR. Common entry mechanisms. Bacterial pathogenesis [review, 14 refs]. *Curr Biol* 1996;6:1084–1086.

281. Wright SD, Silverstein SC. Receptors for C3b and C3bi promote phagocytosis but not the release of toxic oxygen from human phagocytes. *J Exp Med* 1983; 158:2016–2023.

282. Reiner NE. Altered cell signaling and mononuclear phagocyte deactivation during intracellular infection [review, 70 refs]. *Immunol Today* 1994;15:374–381.

283. Theriot JA. The cell biology of infection by intracellular bacterial pathogens [review, 106 refs]. *Ann Rev Cell Dev Biol* 1995;11.213–239.

284. Garcia-del Portillo F, Finlay B. The varied lifestyles of intracellular pathogens within eukaryotic vacuolar compartments. *Trends Microbiol* 1995;3:373–380.

285. Sturgill-Koszycki S, Schlesinger PH, Chakraborty P, et al. Lack of acidification in *Mycobacterium phagosomes* produced by exclusion of the vesicular proton-ATPase. *Science* 1994;263:678–681.

286. Horwitz MA. Interactions between macrophages and Legionella pneumophila [review, 102 refs]. *Curr Top Microbiol Immunol* 1992;181:265–282.

287. Wright SD, Levin SM, Jong MTC, Chad Z, Kabbash LG, Jong MT. CR3 (CD11b/CD18) expresses one binding site for Arg-Gly-Asp-containing peptides and a second site for bacterial lipopolysaccharide. *J Exp Med* 1989;169:175–183.

288. Schreiber AD, Rossman MD, Levinson AI. The immunobiology of human Fcgamma receptors on hematopoietic cells and tissue macrophages. *Clin Immunol Immunopathol* 1992;62:S66–S72.

289. Edwards SW. Cell signalling: by integrins and immunoglobulin receptors in primed neutrophils. *Trends Biochem Sci* 1995;20:362–367.

290. Brown EJ, Joiner KA, Frank MM. Complement. In: Paul WE, ed. *Fundamental immunology*. New York: Raven Press, 1984:645–668.

291. Guan E, Robinson SL, Goodman EB, Tenner AJ. Cell-surface protein identified on phagocytic cells modulates the C1q-mediated enhancement of phagocytosis. *J Immunol* 1994;152:4005–4016.

292. Alvarez-Dominguez C, Carrasco-Marin E, Leyva-Cobian F. Role of complement component C1q in phagocytosis of Listeria monocytogenes by murine macrophage-like cell lines. *Infect Immun* 1993;61:3664–3672.

293. Tenner AJ, Robinson SL, Ezekowitz RA. Mannose binding protein (MBP) enhances mononuclear phagocyte function via a receptor that contains the 126,000 M(r) component of the C1q receptor. *Immunity* 1995;3:485–493.

294. Francois P, Vaudaux P, Foster TJ, Lew DP. Host-bacteria interactions in foreign body infections. *Infect Control Hosp Epidemiol* 1996;17:514–520.

295. Shen W, Steinruck H, Ljungh A. Expression of binding of plasminogen, thrombospondin, vitronectin, and fibrinogen, and adhesive properties by Escherichia coli strains isolated from patients with colonic diseases. *Gut* 1995;36:401–406.

296. Hasty DL, Courtney HS. Group A streptococcal adhesion. All of the theories are correct. *Adv Exp Med Biol* 1996;408:81–94.

297. Westerlund B, Van Die I, Hoekstra W, Virkola R, Korhonen TK. P fimbriae of uropathogenic Escherichia coli as multifunctional adherence organelles. *Zentralbl Bakteriol* 1993;278:229–237.

298. Zareba TW, Pascu C, Hryniewicz W, Wadstrom T. Binding of extracellular matrix proteins by enterococci. *Curr Microbiol* 1997;34:6–11.

299. Desjardins M, Celis JE, van Meer G, et al. Molecular characterization of phagosomes. *J Biol Chem* 1994;269:32194–32200.

300. Galan JE, Bliska JB. Cross-talk between bacterial pathogens and their host cells [review, 172 refs]. *Ann Rev Cell Dev Biol* 1996;12:221–255.

301. Greenberg S, Burridge K, Silverstein SC. Colocalization of F-actin and talin during Fc receptor-mediated phagocytosis in mouse macrophages. *J Exp Med* 1990;172:1853–1856.

302. Adam T, Arpin M, Prévost M-C, Gounon P, Sansonetti PJ. Cytoskeletal rearrangements and the functional role of T-plastin during entry of *Shigella flexneri* into HeLa cells. *J Cell Biol* 1995;129:367–381.

303. Dehio C, Prevost MC, Sansonetti PJ. Invasion of epithelial cells by Shigella flexneri induces tyrosine phosphorylation of cortactin by a pp60c-src-mediated signalling pathway. *EMBO J* 1995;14:2471–2482.

304. Drevets DA, Campbell PA. Roles of complement and complement receptor type 3 in phagocytosis of *Listeria monocytogenes* by inflammatory mouse peritoneal macrophages. *Infect Immun* 1991;59:2645–2652.

305. Mengaud J, Ohayon H, Gounon P, Mege R-M, Cossart P. E-cadherin is the receptor for internalin, a surface protein required for entry of L. monocytogenes into epithelial cells. *Cell* 1996;84:923–932.

306. Schlesinger LS, Horwitz MA. Phagocytosis of *Mycobacterium leprae* by human monocyte-derived macrophages is mediated by complement receptors CR1 (CD35), CR3 (CD11b/CD18), and CR4 (CD11c/CD18) and IFN-gamma activation inhibits complement receptor function and phagocytosis of this bacterium. *J Immunol* 1991;147:1983–1994.

307. Schlesinger LS, Horwitz MA. Phagocytosis of leprosy bacilli is mediated by complement receptors CR1 and CR3 on human monocytes and complement component C3 in serum. *J Clin Invest* 1990;85:1304–1314.

308. Schorey JS, Li Q, McCourt DW, et al. A *Mycobacterium leprae* gene encoding a fibronectin binding protein is used for efficient invasion of epithelial cells and Schwann cells. *Infect Immun* 1995;63:2652–2657.

309. Watarai M, Funato S, Sasakawa C. Interaction of ipa proteins of shigella flexneri with alpha(5)beta(1) integrin promotes entry of the bacteria into mammalian cells. *J Exp Med* 1996;183:991–999.

310. Brown EJ, Joiner KA, Frank MM. Interactions of desialated guinea pig erythrocytes with the classical and alternative pathways of guinea pig complement in vivo and in vitro. *J Clin Invest* 1983;71:1710–1719.

311. Ginocchio CC, Olmsted SB, Wells CL, Galan JE. Contact with epithelial cells induces the formation of surface appendages on Salmonella typhimurium. *Cell* 1994;76:717–724.

312. Talamas-Rohana P, Wright SD, Lennartz MR, Russsell DG. Lipophosphoglycan from Leishmania mexicana promastigotes binds to members of the CR3, p150.95 and LFA-1 family of leukocyte integrins. *J Immunol* 1990;144:4817–4824.

Fundamental Immunology, Fourth Edition,
edited by William E. Paul
Published by Lippincott–Raven Publishers, Philadelphia 1999.

CHAPTER 31

Cytotoxic T Lymphocytes

Pierre A. Henkart

Lymphocytes share with macrophages the unusual cellular property of being able to destroy other cells. Not surprisingly, this activity must be tightly controlled in order to prevent harm to the host, and this chapter will summarize our current understanding of the cytotoxic functions of lymphocytes. I will emphasize cytotoxic T-lymphocytes (CTLs) because more study has been devoted to their properties, but the description of the post-triggering events of the granule exocytosis pathway applies to natural killer (NK) cells as well. For more detailed descriptions of NK cell properties, the reader is referred to Chapter 16. In some cases basic advances in our knowledge of the cytotoxic mechanism was made in NK cells first.

Because cytotoxic lymphocytes that acquire cytotoxic activity are also important producers of cytokines, confusion may sometimes arise in trying to implicate the easily demonstrable *in vitro* cytotoxic activity of these cells in various *in vivo* phenomena. This chapter does not attempt to describe the cytokine secretion activities of cytotoxic lymphocytes because these do not seem uniquely different from such secretion by noncytotoxic lymphocytes. It

rather focuses on the unique activity of cytotoxic lymphocytes related to their ability to destroy other cells.

CYTOTOXIC LYMPHOCYTES ARE DEFINED BY THEIR *IN VITRO* FUNCTIONAL ACTIVITY

Cytotoxicity assays are conveniently performed via short-term (4- to 18-hour) microculture in which cytotoxic effector cells are mixed with target cells at varying ratios, followed by assessment of target cell death. Such a functional definition raises questions of *in vivo* relevance, but the simplicity and quantitative nature of *in vitro* cytotoxicity assays has allowed molecular definitions of this lymphocyte effector function. This, in turn, has allowed the design of definitive experiments to address *in vivo* relevance, as discussed below.

In vitro target cell death can be assessed by measurement of two distinct but related classes of target cell properties. The most commonly used property is plasma membrane integrity, and lymphocyte cytotoxic activity was initially discovered by microscopic observations of target cell lysis, or loss of such integrity. Satisfactory quantitation of this death was achieved with the development of the chromium release assay (1), which for many years has been the stan-

P. A. Henkart: Experimental Immunology Branch, National Cancer Institute, National Institutes of Health, Bethesda, Maryland 20892-1360.

dard technique in this field. This cytotoxicity assay uses target cells loaded with the isotope ^{51}Cr by preincubation with tracer levels of the oxidant $^{51}Cr_2O_7^{-2}$. Target cell death is measured by the lytic release into incubation supernatants of the isotope, which is reduced intracellularly to $^{51}Cr^{+3}$ and complexed with intracellular polyanions (2). Such complexes are not taken up by living cells and can be readily quantitated by sampling the supernatant. Recently, comparably sensitive nonradioactive techniques for quantitating target lysis have been developed, including some that measure release of preloaded impermeant soluble fluorescent dyes (3), or of chelators detectable by time-resolved fluorescence of rare earth complexes (4). The lytic release of cytoplasmic enzymes unique to particular target cells or of cytoplasmically expressed viral proteins provides another alternative approach that is potentially applicable *in vivo* (5,6).

A second target cell property reflecting death that is conveniently measured is based on measurement of DNA fragmentation. As discussed below, this is part of the characteristic pattern of apoptotic nuclear damage associated with cell death by many agents, including cytotoxic lymphocytes. Fragmented DNA is released from nuclei, allowing its release into detergent lysates (7) or using automated cell harvesters (8). Lysis and DNA fragmentation readouts typically correlate well (9), although DNA fragmentation represents a commitment to target cell death that can sometimes be measured earlier than lysis (10,11). However, some target cells or experimental conditions may dissociate these two death measurements. Fibroblasts, particularly when not dividing, show minimal DNA release during CTL-induced lysis (12,13). Thus, the term "cell death" can potentially be misleading unless it is precisely and experimentally defined.

Measurements of target cell death by the above approaches are not suitable for direct comparisons of the cytotoxic potency of different cell populations because target cell death is not linearly related to the input of cytotoxic cells. Furthermore, within the assay culture, some cytotoxic lymphocytes may be more efficient than others in mediating cytotoxicity. A practical means of comparing the cytotoxic capacity of different populations is to compare the number of effector cells required to achieve a given level of target lysis in a given assay system. The results are expressed in lytic units, which are inversely related to the effector cell number required (14).

BASIC PROPERTIES OF LYMPHOCYTE-MEDIATED CYTOTOXICTY

Many elegant studies of cytotoxic lymphocyte mechanisms were conducted before the recognition of several different molecular pathways of target cell damage, and the results of such older studies must be interpreted cautiously. Nevertheless, such studies clearly established that cytotoxic lymphocytes have the ability to kill target cells quickly, sequentially, and selectively. Bystander cells lacking antigen intimately mixed with lysed target cells are generally spared destruction (15), although low levels of CTL bystander lysis can be detected in some systems (16–18). In time-lapse cinematography studies of the cytotoxic process, CTLs have been observed to bind target cells and inflict visible injury within a few minutes, with target death in some cases following within another few minutes (19,20). Such studies show that single CTLs can kill multiple target cells within a few hours, as also seen by examination of CTL–target clusters (21). The rapid CTL-induced death process was not blocked by inhibitors of protein synthesis (22), suggesting preformed lytic mediators. One of the most striking aspects of CTL-induced cytotoxicity has been its generally

strict T-cell receptor (TCR)-defined specificity, and the phenomenon of major histocompatibility complex (MHC) restriction was first defined using cytotoxicity as a rapid and convenient readout of TCR recognition (23). Use of IL-2 and other cytokines has allowed the culture of cloned CTL lines exhibiting a potent cytotoxicity that can mediate the complete destruction of target cells within a few hours when mixed at less than a 1:1 ratio (24).

During the 1970s, studies of the CTL killing mechanism defined three distinct phases of the process (25,26). The first is CTL–target adhesion, defined as formation of a firm attachment that cannot be disrupted by mild shearing forces. This adhesion step requires several minutes at 37°C, occurs in the absence of calcium if magnesium is provided, and is blocked by cold temperatures and a range of drugs. This is followed by a second step called lethal hit or programming for lysis, which also requires several minutes. Its hallmark property is a requirement for calcium in the medium; like adhesion, it is blockable by cold temperatures and a range of drugs. The final target cell disintegration stage of CTL cytotoxicity ends with lysis and is the most prolonged, with a mean half-life of 1.7 hours. This stage involves only the target cell because it is unaffected if CTLs are eliminated, e.g., by complement treatment. It is characterized by its independence of divalent cations, and no drugs have been found that effectively block lysis of the lethally injured target cell.

DISTINGUISHING THE TWO MAJOR MECHANISMS OF LYMPHOCYTE CYTOTOXICITY

As schematically shown in Fig. 1 and described in detail below, CTLs use two distinct cytolytic pathways in 4- to 6-hour assays *in vitro*: the perforin-dependent granule exocytosis pathway and the FasL/Fas pathway. Because distinct effector molecules are required

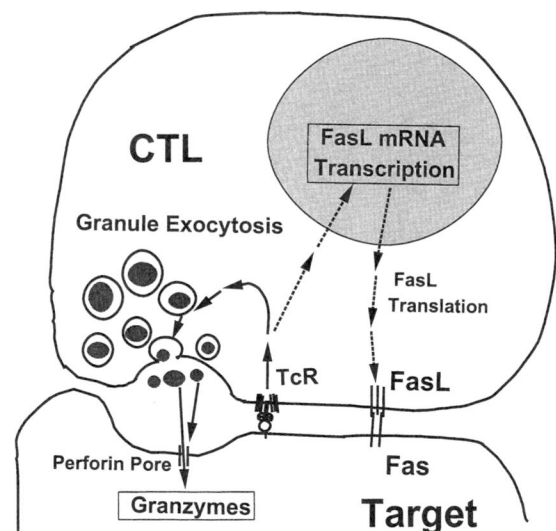

FIG. 1. The two cytotoxicity pathways used by CTLs *in vitro*. Both pathways are initiated via TCR cross-linking by target cell antigen, which is made possible by adhesive interactions between the cells. In the CTL, common initial signaling steps are shared by both pathways, which then diverge. The granule exocytosis pathway on the left side is a typical receptor controlled secretion process resulting in the release of perforin and granzymes from the granule cores into the synapselike junctional region between the CTL and its target. The FasL/Fas pathway on the right requires *de novo* transcription of Fas ligand mRNA and its subsequent surface expression on the CTL, where it cross-links target cell Fas.

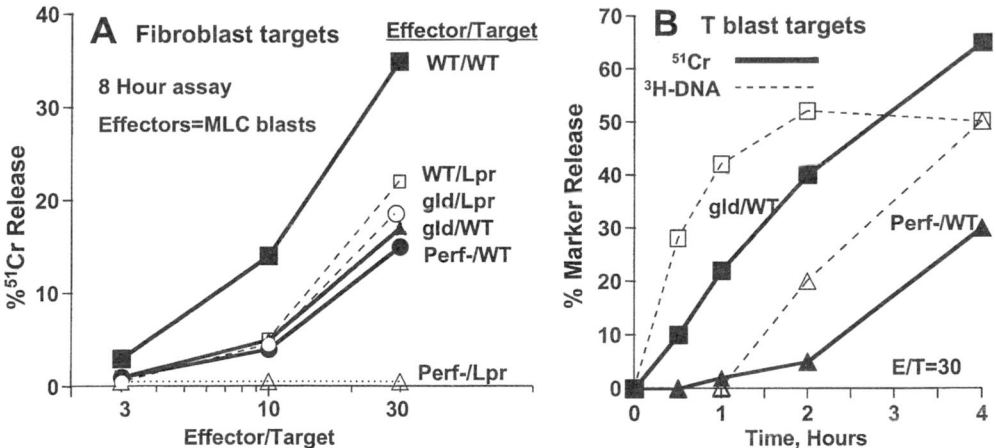

FIG. 2. Cytotoxicity by the two CTL pathways. **A:** A comparison of fibroblast lysis after 8 hours by *in vitro* CTL derived from MLC blasts from mice defective in one or both cytotoxicity pathways. The CTL effector/fibroblast target combinations are: ■, wild-type/wild-type; □, wild-type/Lpr (Fas defective); ○, gld (FasL defective)/Lpr; ▲, gld/wild-type; ●, perforin defective/wild type; Δ, perforin defective/Lpr. Data from Lowin et al. (29). **B:** A comparison of the kinetics of lysis (filled symbols and solid lines) and DNA fragmentation (open symbols and dashed lines) by the two pathways. DNA fragmentation was measured by the release of thymidine label from prepulsed targets into the supernatant. Effector and target combinations as in A except that the target cells were ConA-stimulated T cell blasts. Data from Lowin et al. (27).

for the function of each pathway, it has recently become possible to block each pathway selectively and thus assess their relative importance to particular CTL–target combinations. As shown in Fig. 2, the FasL/Fas pathway can be selectively blocked by several approaches: (a) use of CTL effectors from gld mutant mice lacking functional FasL; (b) use of Fas negative targets, particularly those derived from lpr mutant mice; and (c) use of non-cross-linking anti-Fas antibody or soluble Fas constructs to block FasL-Fas binding. Inhibitors of transcription and translation provide another possible approach (27), but in addition to problems with side effects of such drugs, some CTLs may bear preexisting FasL. The perforin-dependent granule exocytosis pathway can be blocked most cleanly by using effector cells from perforin knock-out mice (28,29). Potentially useful pharmacologic approaches to blocking the granule exocytosis pathway include treatment of effector cells with concanamycin A (30) or pretreating with Sr^{+2} to trigger degranulation (31). With target cells bearing fully functional Fas, the FasL/Fas pathway can contribute as much as half the cytotoxicity in a 4- to 6-hour assay. However, for most CTL–target cell combinations, such short-term assays are dominated by the granule exocytosis pathway (28,29). As shown in Fig. 2, when both pathways are blocked, CTLs lose all detectable cytotoxicity in short-term assays. For assays of 12 to 20 hours' duration, the Fas/FasL mechanism can be more prominent in some Fas-bearing target cells (27). For such longer term assays, a third mechanism using tumor necrosis factor (TNF) produced by CTLs also can contribute to cytotoxicity of TNF-sensitive target cells (32).

CYTOTOXIC LYMPHOCYTE SECRETORY GRANULES

"Regulated" Versus "Constitutive" Protein Secretory Pathways

Cellular secretion occurs via a membrane fusion process, termed exocytosis, in which an intracellular vesicle or granule membrane fuses with the plasma membrane, thus releasing the material enclosed within the granule to the extracellular space. Such secretion

has been categorized as either regulated, if the exocytosis occurs in preformed granules in response to a membrane signal, or constitutive, if vesicles containing newly synthesized proteins exocytose without delay (33). Most lymphocyte protein secretion (antibodies, cytokines) is constitutive because it occurs without detectable intracellular storage of newly secreted proteins. This secretion is greatly stimulated in response to lymphocyte activation and differentiation, especially as B-lymphocytes mature into plasma cells, and in this sense the constitutive secretory pathway is highly regulated in lymphocytes. The regulated secretory pathway is prominent in many nonlymphoid cell types and is characterized by an initial vesicular transport of newly synthesized proteins to larger secretory granules, where they are stored for indefinite periods. Degranulation is typically triggered by a plasma membrane receptor.

CTLs use both regulated and constitutive secretory pathways. Cytokines such as interferon-γ appear to be secreted by CTL via the consitutive pathway (34). Even cytotoxic mediators principally secreted by the regulated pathway are secreted by the constitutive pathway immediately after antigen triggering of cloned CTLs (35), and such constitutive secretion may mediate some bystander killing. Chapter 25 describes the control of cytokine secretion by CD8+ T cells.

The presence of secretory granules in lymphocytes is not always obvious because they are few in number compared with granulocytes or mast cells. Sensitive immunostaining for granule components shows that resting naive TCR-α T cells have few if any granules, whereas most resting TCR-δ T cells and NK cells have detectable granules (36). Antigen-triggered activation results in granule formation in CD8+ and to some extent in CD4+ T cells, and granules are detectable in most resting blood CD45RO+ memory phenotype CD8+ T cells.

Granule Morphology

Figure 3A shows images of CTL granules as seen in electron micrographs (EMs) of *in vitro* grown cloned CTLs. Such granules are typically 0.5 to 1 μm in diameter and have a heterogeneous structure, consisting of two components. Granule cores are densely

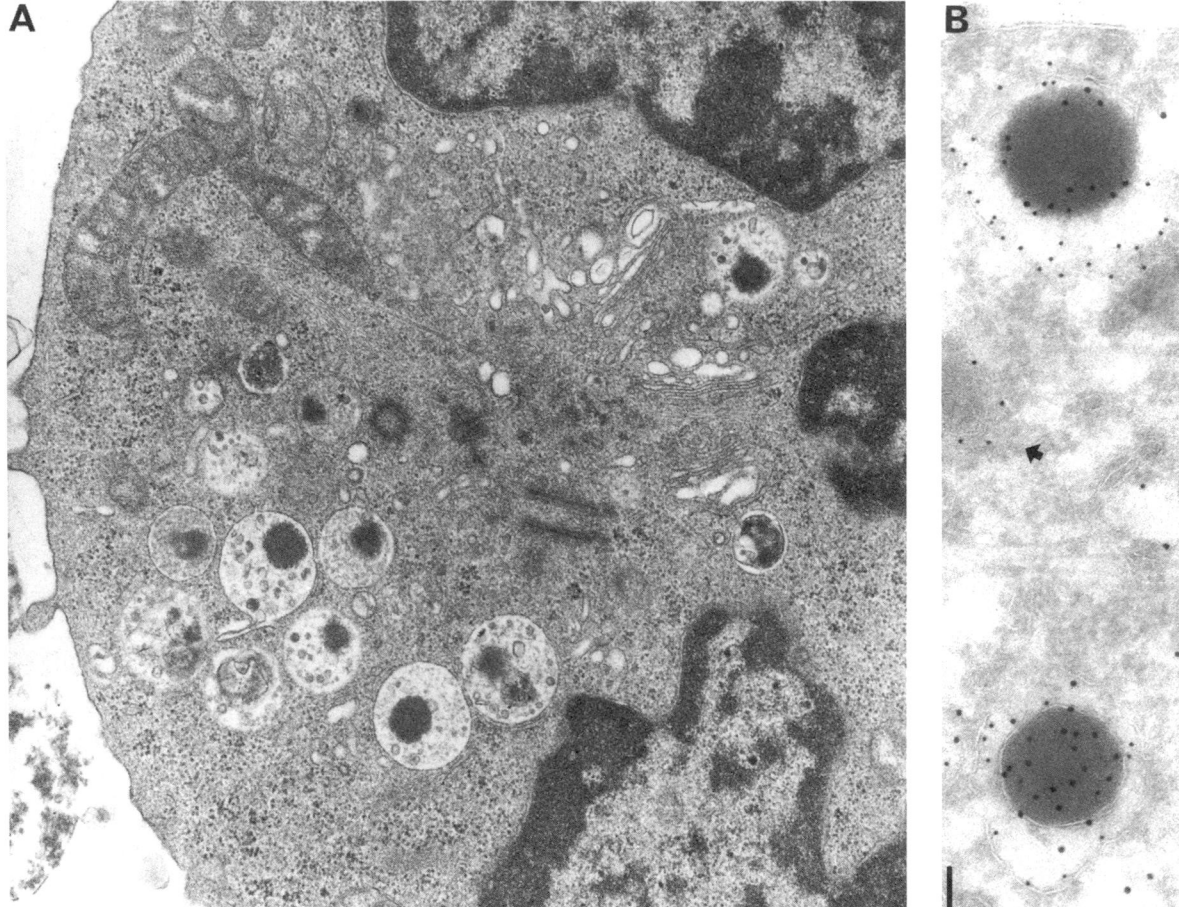

FIG. 3. CTL granules as seen by electron microscopy. **A:** Human CTL clone showing major cytoplasmic organelles including granules. This section shows cores in most granules, which are of the intermediate type because they also contain a prominent multivesicular region. The cytoplasm also contains mitochondria (with christae), endoplasmic reticulum (smaller empty vesicles), Golgi, and centrioles. **B:** Immunogold-labeled granules of a human CTL clone showing localization of granzyme B (large particles) in the cores and the lysosomal membrane marker LAMP1 (small particles) in the surrounding membrane. The size bar is 100 nm (37). Images provided by Dr. Peter Peters, University of Utrecht.

staining homogeneous regions that show some similarity to cores of granules of mast cells. In some granules, the cores are surrounded by a double membrane, whereas in other cases the cores are not bound by membranes (Fig. 3B) (37). The other granule component is multivesicular, composed of numerous membrane vesicles ranging from 30 to 150 nm in diameter. Granules have been classified on the basis of the dominance of these components, with type I granules defined as those dominated by cores, with only a small cortical rim of the multivesicular component. In contrast, type II granules contain only the multivesicular component with no cores. These appear similar to late endosomes or prelysosomes in other cells. Intermediate granules contain both components, with smaller cores than type I granules.

Electron micrograph studies using immunogold staining (Fig. 3B) have shown that the granule cores contain perforin, granzymes, and proteoglycan, whereas the multivesicular regions contain lysosomal enzymes and lysosomal membrane markers (37). Evidence that the vesicles are derived from the plasma membrane by endocytosis comes from EM studies using immunogold, showing the presence of TCR, CD8, and class I MHC molecules. These proteins are oriented with the normally extracellular domains facing the lumen of the granules, as expected from an endocytic origin.

In conjunction with microscopy, weak base pH probes show that CTL granules have an acidic interior, with an estimated internal pH of 5.4 (38). Similar estimates have been obtained for secretory granules in other cell types, but this pH is not as low as that found in mature lysosomes.

Components of Cytotoxic Lymphocyte Granules

Cytotoxic lymphocyte granules have been purified from homogenates of cloned lymphocytes grown *in vitro*. When analyzed biochemically, such granules show a limited number of prominent protein bands. The most abundant proteins are perforin and the granzymes, components that have been studied for their functional role in target cell death. The biochemical properties of these components are discussed in this section, and their functional roles in cytotoxicity are discussed in the next section.

Perforin (Cytolysin, PFP)

Perforin appears to be uniquely expressed in cytotoxic lymphocyte granules and is required for the function of the granule exocytosis pathway of cytotoxicity. It is a 555–amino acid glycoprotein of 65 to 75 kDa that in the presence of calcium has the ability to insert into lipid bilayer membranes, polymerize, and form structural and functional pores that can lead to cell lysis (39). Although perforin is a water-soluble protein after careful isolation from granules, exposure to calcium concentrations normally found extracellularly appears to trigger a conformational change that exposes hydrophobic groups and renders it amphipathic. In the presence of calcium, perforin inserts into pure lipid membranes and self-associates into stable polymeric forms, which appear by EM to be porelike structures with striking homology to those formed by complement (Fig. 4). The internal diameter of these structures is larger for perforin than for complement, but the overall shape is similar. Such porelike structures can be detected on the surface of target cells killed by large granular lymphocytes or CTLs (40–42), providing evidence that effector cell degranulation accompanies target cell death.

As shown in Fig. 4, cloning and sequence analysis of perforin from three species has shown two regions of sequence homology of probable functional importance: (a) a complement homology domain related to proteins of the complement membrane attack complex (C6, C7, C8a, C8b, and C9), which associate to form lytic pores (43–46) and (b) a C2 domain related to those in other calcium-binding, lipid-interacting proteins (47). These are connected by a short cysteine-rich region. The amino-terminal third of the molecule does not show significant homology to data base proteins. The COOH terminal peptide has been found to be removed by proteolytic processing of the newly synthesized perforin molecule between the Golgi and granules, activating the C2 domain for phospholipid binding (48).

It has been difficult to relate the functional pore-forming properties of perforin to its structure. Typical membrane-spanning motifs of about 20 hydrophobic amino acids characteristic of α-helical transmembrane domains are absent. Analysis of the sequence for periodic occurrence of hydrophobic amino acids that would make amphipathic helices reveals candidate sequences that could interact with membranes in this manner, the most prominent being at the amino-terminal end of the complement homology domain (49). Because hydrophobic probes react with membrane-

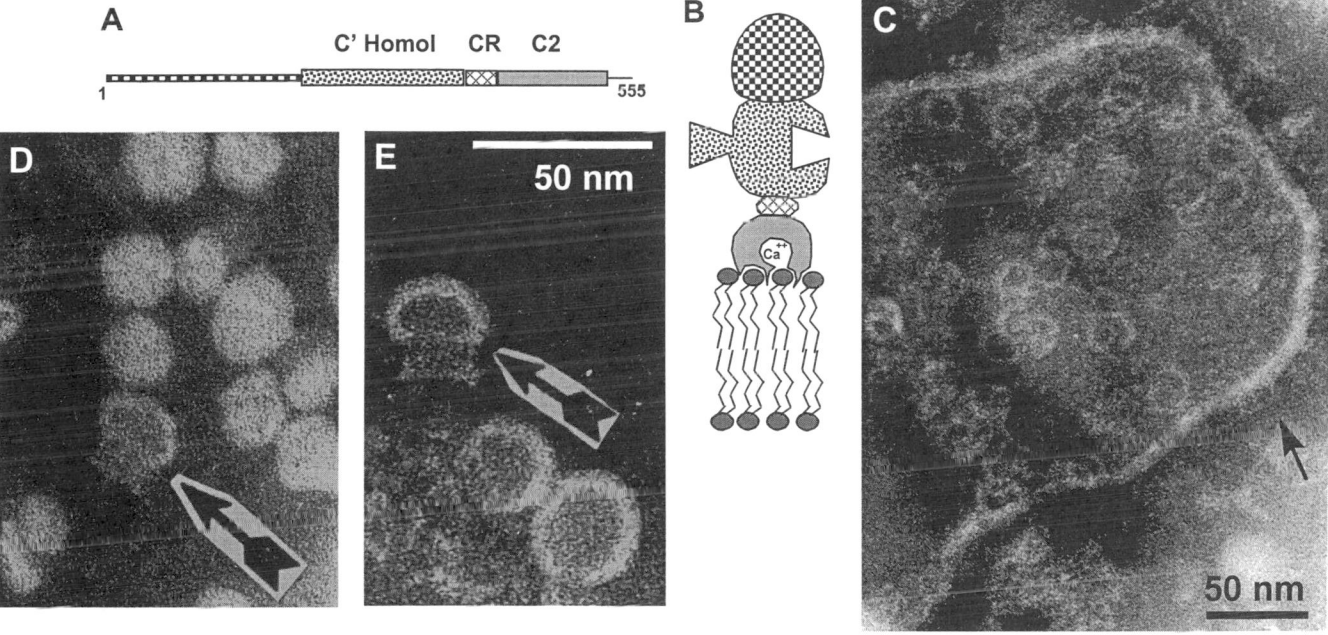

FIG. 4. Perforin sequence and porelike structures. **A:** Schematic view of perforin protein sequence. The amino-terminal portion of the molecule shows no homology to data base proteins. The stippled central region (C Homol) shows significant but distant homology to complement components C6, C7, C8a, and C9 and contains a putative amphipathic helix at its left end. This is followed by a short cysteine-rich (CR) region of unknown significance, and then by the C2 homology domain implicated in calcium-dependent phospholipid interactions, and finally by the COOH peptide, which is removed by processing before granule storage. **B:** A speculative schematic depiction of the perforin domains in the monomer bound to membrane before its polymerization and membrane insertion. The C2 domain is shown binding calcium and phospholipid headgroups. The C homology domain is shown with motifs that allow self-aggregation because C9 forms polymers and the other complement proteins bind other homologous proteins in forming the membrane attack complex. The regions of membrane interaction after aggregation and insertion remain unknown. **C:** Electron micrographic images of negative stained perforin porelike structures on the surface of resealed red cell ghosts attacked by human large granular lymphocytes in antibody-dependent cell-mediated cytotoxicity (ADCC) (40). Similar but slightly smaller structures had been previously described from red cells lysed by complement (315). Arrow points to edge view of the porelike structure, suggesting they are short cylinders embedded in the membrane. In this ADCC system, previous functional experiments with this system had indicated a porelike sieving behavior of released marker proteins (64). Micrograph courtesy of Robert Dourmashkin. **D:** Small unilamellar liposomes treated with low concentration of purified perforin in the presence of calcium. Under these conditions, soluble markers were released from these liposomes. Arrow shows one liposome with the perforin porelike structure inserted in its membrane. This liposome has become permeable to the dark negative stain. **E:** Liposomes treated with a higher concentration of purified perforin releasing a high percentage of trapped marker. Arrow shows porelike structure inserted into lipid bilayer. D and E reprinted with permission (60).

associated C9 within a 150–amino acid span, which includes the region homologous to perforin, a highly speculative model in which this region is part of a membrane pore has been proposed (50). There is no clear experimental evidence implicating any region of perforin in membrane interactions. Functional studies of synthetic peptides from the N terminus have shown lytic activity and pore-forming activity in artificial membranes (51), but the physiologic relevance of these findings remains unclear. Recombinant perforin expressed in baculovirus has calcium-dependent lytic activity, and constructs lacking the amino-terminal region show a generally similar but less calcium-dependent activity (52,53).

Although both the amino-terminal and carboxy-terminal portions of the complement homology region of perforin show significant homology to the complement proteins C6, C7, C8α, and C9, the functional implications are open to question. These complement proteins all associate with membranes by poorly understood interactions (54), but only C9 forms large functional pores and porelike structures homologous to perforin. The molecular basis for C9 polymerization and pore formation remains an unsolved problem (54) and offers limited insights for perforin.

Although calcium is critical to its function, perforin sequences show no typical EF hand calcium-binding motifs such as found in calmodulin domains. However, recently a homology was recognized with the C2 domain family originally described in several phospholipase C isoforms (55). These domains are found in other proteins showing a calcium-dependent interaction with lipids, including protein kinase C isoforms, v-SNARE proteins, and ras-GTPase activating proteins (47). The domain is composed of a sandwiched pair of four-stranded antiparallel β sheets, with the connecting loops forming a pocket binding one to two Ca^{+2} ions at one end. Significantly, the five aspartic acid residues ligating the Ca^{2+} ions are present in all three perforin sequences along with the most of the consensus amino acids forming the strands. In other proteins where it is present, C2 domains seem to be responsible for calcium-dependent binding to phospholipid head groups in membranes.

Perforin has been shown to form calcium-dependent reversible complexes with cellular membranes at low temperatures or low ionic strength (56–59), and it seems plausible that this interaction involves the C2 domain. A phosphosphoryl choline head group interaction has been proposed on the basis of inhibition of perforin-mediated lysis by soluble and membrane-associated phosphorylcholine (59), but perforin forms pores in liposomes containing no phosphorylcholine head groups (60). The head group specificity of C2 domain membrane binding appears to be variable (47). Binding of calcium and lipid by C2 domains has been postulated to trigger conformational changes in neighboring protein domains, suggesting a model for perforin function in which such a change accompanies exposure of hydrophobic protein groups, membane insertion, and polymerization. Polymerization implies two different surfaces of intermolecular interaction, as shown in Fig. 4. Although these may be in the complement homology domain by analogy to C9, it is possible that the C2 domain also may be involved (61).

The porelike structure of aggregated perforin on membranes immediately suggests a central hydrophilic core surrounded by protein molecules lining the membrane (Fig. 4). However, such fully aggregated porelike structures may not be necessary to form smaller pores capable of allowing passage of ions and small molecules. Electrical studies of planar lipid bilayers show that perforin pores induce large ion-permeable channels that are heterogeneous in size (39,62,63). Studies examining the ability of labeled macromolecules to cross perforin-treated cell membranes show it forms functional pores capable of allowing passage of proteins and dextrans with diameters of up to 10 to 14 nm, i.e., globular proteins of over 100 kDa (64,65). These estimates are thus in reasonable agreement with the 14-nm inner diameter of the pore structure seen in the EM.

In the presence of calcium, perforin is an extremely potent lytic agent when assayed for red blood cell lysis or for its ability to permeabilize liposomes. Studies of perforin's lytic activity on nucleated cells show that 10 to 100 times more perforin is required to achieve lysis compared with red cells (66,67), as is found for other pore-forming agents (68). As discussed below, this is presumably due to repair mechanisms present in nucleated cells. CTL-delivered perforin pores appear not to lyse nucleated target cells directly, but rather to function by permeablizing target cells to granzymes. Although complement and perforin lyse red cell targets by a colloid osmotic mechanism, this does not explain their action on nucleated target cells (69), and it may be that such pores kill cells by directly allowing passage of vital intracellular molecules.

Several properties of perforin help explain its function in cytotoxic lymphocytes. Its lytic activity drops off rapidly as the pH diminishes below 7 (66), so that it would not be expected to make pores in the acidic granule membranes. Its functional activity is efficiently inhibited by hydrophobic substances, including lipoproteins and membranes. Thus, the postsecretion amphipathic form arising after exposure to calcium and neutral pH rapidly inserts into any hydrophobic surface nearby. The presence of lipoproteins and neighboring membranes assures that bystander lysis is minimized after secretion. This also raises the issue of CTL self-protection discussed below.

The mechanism by which newly synthesized perforin is sorted to granules after passage through the Golgi is unknown. This protein does not have covalently attached mannose-6-phosphate groups as is the case with granzymes and lysosomal proteins. However, lysosomal proteins appear to also use an uncharacterized second system for sorting, and it is possible that perforin shares this. It is also not clear what perforin properties are important to its ability to form the granule core complexes with proteoglycan and granzymes, although cationic regions of the sequence can be identified.

Granzymes

Granzymes are serine proteases present in the granules of cytotoxic lymphocytes and show minimal expression in other sites or in the granules of other tissues (70). Their protein sequence shows a clear homology to serine proteases including conservation of the amino acids of the classical serine protease catalytic triad (71). Based on sequence homology, granzymes form a monophyletic subfamily of serine proteases, along with granule proteases of mast cells, macrophages, and neutrophils (72). This subfamily is characterized by a conserved PYMPHSRA motif near the amino terminus of the mature enzyme. The term "granzyme" has been used only to describe the members of this subfamily expressed in lymphocytes.

Although the physiologic substrates of granzymes remain a matter of speculation, synthetic peptide substrates have been found for some of these proteases, allowing biochemical studies (73). Table 1 summarizes properties of the known granzymes. Mouse granzymes A and B are the only ones detectable in the highly lytic CTLs found in the peritoneal cavity after alloimmunization and are expressed within a few days of activation of CD8+ CTLs *in vitro* (74). It is interesting that these two proteases have enzymatic speci-

TABLE 1. *Lymphocyte granzymes*

Granzyme	P1 aa at Cleavage	Expressed in	Species	Other features
A	Lys/Arg	CD8$^+$ CTL, NK, $\gamma\delta$	M,H,R	SS dimer
B	Asp	CD8$^+$ CTL, NK, $\gamma\delta$	M,H,R	Glycosylation variable
C	?	CD8$^+$ CTL clones	M,R	Not glycosylated
D	Lys/Arg	CD8$^+$ CTL clones	M	Highly glycosylated
E	?	CD8$^+$ CTL clones	M	Highly glycosylated
F	?	CD8$^+$ CTL clones	M	Highly glycosylated
G	?	CD8$^+$ CTL clones	M	
H	?	CD8$^+$ CTL, NK	H	
Tryp-2	Lys/Arg	CD8$^+$ CTL, NK	R,H	
Met-1	Met/Leu	NK	M,H,R	

ficities that are distinctly different from each other, as well as from most of the remaining granzymes. Granzyme B has a substrate recognition unique among mammalian serine proteases in that it requires aspartic acid as the P1 amino acid (i.e., cleavage occurs, leaving a carboxy-terminal aspartic acid). It has been widely speculated that this specificity allows it to activate target cell apoptosis, as discussed below. Granzyme A is highly active against the lysine thioester benzoyl lysine thioester (BLT), and the presence of this activity in lymphocyte homogenates appears limited to cytotoxic lymphocytes. However, related tryptases are found in mast cell granules.

After longer periods of *in vitro* culture, CD8$^+$ CTLs increasingly express the other mouse granzymes (C-G). Limited biochemical studies of these granzymes have been conducted, and their proteolytic specificities remain undefined. For all granzymes studied, enzymatic activity is maximal at neutral pHs rather than at the acidic pH of the granules. Therefore, it has been considered unlikely that the granzyme functional substrates are intragranular because they appear designed to operate in the neutral pH environment after exocytosis.

Like many other proteases, granzymes are synthesized as inactive proenzymes and must be proteolytically processed in order to become enzymatically active. All known granzymes contain an activation dipeptide after the signal sequence before the consensus amino terminal sequence IIGG of the mature enzyme. The activation dipeptide is removed in the granule by dipeptidyl peptidase I. It has been proposed that the granzyme PHSRPYM motif interacts with granule proteoglycan to maintain the proper conformation for activation processing performed by dipeptidyl peptidase.

Granzymes are highly positively charged proteins at neutral pH. Although these charges are clearly important to the formation of ionic complexes with granule proteoglycans, they also may mediate binding to extracellular polyanionic components after secretion. Unlike some other serine proteases, granzymes do not contain extra protein domains beyond the catalytic domain.

Dipeptidyl Peptidase I (Cathepsin C)

The lysosomal enzyme dipeptidyl peptidase I (DPPI) cleaves an amino terminal dipeptide from pregranzymes to produce the mature and enzymatically active proteases. Functional and sequence studies show this enzyme to be part of the cysteine protease family, related to the lysosomal cathepsins, and it shares with them a requirement for proteolytic processing for its own activity. Coexpression of both DPPI and granzymes in nonhematopoietic cells allows expression of enzymatically active granzymes A (75)

and B (76), whereas expression of the granzyme alone results in the inactive prograzyme.

DPPI expression confers sensitivity to cytolysis by esters of hydrophobic amino acids and dipeptides, particularly leucine-leucine methyl ester (LLOMe). Such membrane-permeant weak bases accumulate in secretory granules because of their low pH, and DPPI catalyzes a peptide synthesis reaction that results in the formation of longer chain hydrophobic peptides that are lysolytic detergents (77). Thus, LLOMe can be used to deplete lymphoid populations of macrophages, NK cells, and CTL precursors while sparing most other cells (78). Nevertheless, DPPI is widely expressed at lower levels in lysosomes of other tissues including liver (79).

Proteoglycan

Proteoglycans are found in secretory granules of many hematopoietic cells (80) and are known to play an important role in binding other granule components to form an insoluble complex visualized as the granule core. CTLs and NK granule proteoglycans are heterogeneous molecules composed of a serglycin protein backbone with a variable number of covalently attached glycosaminoglycan chains. The serglycin protein backbone is a 17- to 20-kDa protein containing an unusual interior domain with the repeat sequence (ser-gly)$_n$, where n = 9 to 24, depending on the species. These serines are substituted with 50- to 85-kDa chondroitin sulfate chains to form high molecular weight proteoglycans. The sulfate groups of chondroitin sulfate maintain their negative charge even at the low intragranular pH, thus allowing the formation of an ionic complex with the cationic granzymes as well as binding perforin by less defined forces (81). Evidence for such an ionic complex between proteoglycans, granzymes, and perforin comes from the isolation of an insoluble complex from granules in low salt and its dissociation at physiological pH and salt. Parallel ionic complexes between proteoglycans and granule proteases (as well as small cationic mediators) can be found in mast cell granules (82).

Other Lysosomal Enzymes

A variety of normal lysosomal enzymes are detectable in granules of cytotoxic lymphocytes by histochemical and biochemical techniques. This has led to their characterization as secretory lysosomes, which also describes mast cell granules, azurophilic granules of neutrophils, and platelet granules, as well as a subpopulation of lysosomes in fibroblasts and endothelial cells (83). Lysosomes with a classical appearance are rare in CTLs, and it appears that their normal internal digestive functions are largely taking place in the secretory granules. Because lysosomal enzymes have a low pH optimum or are unstable at neutral pH, they are generally considered unlikely to participate in target cell damage after exocytosis, and no evidence for this has been produced. However, early EM studies of CTL–target interactions showed their exocytosis and suggested such a possibility (84). It remains unclear why the secretory and lysosomal compartments are not separated in cells such as CTLs because they are in nonhematopoietic lineages. The protease cathepsin D has been localized to the cortical region of CTL granules between the membrane vesicles, where it is found with endocytosed bovine serum albumin (85).

Granule Membrane Proteins

Granule membrane proteins can be divided into several categories. The lysosomal membrane proteins LAMP1, LAMP2 (CD107a and b), CD63 (granulophysin), and the cation-independent mannose-6-phosphate receptor are found on both the vesicles and the internal surface of the outer granule membrane (37). LAMP1 and LAMP2 become exposed on the cell surface after exocytosis but are rapidly removed by endocytosis (86). This category of granule membrane proteins is presumed to be largely involved with lysosomal functions of these granules, but their surface exposure after exocytosis could be important in CTL self-protection.

The second category of membrane proteins in granules is composed of normal surface proteins that are present on the cortical vesicles of CTL granules. They include the TCR, CD8, and MHC class 1 (85). These appear to arise as a result of the budding processes of compound endocytosis, which may be part of the lysosomal functions of these granules. Because the cortical granule vesicles are secreted in the vicinity of target cells and they can presumably attach specifically to target cells via their TCRs, it has been suggested that they contribute to target cell damage (87). However, their interior is topologically cytoplasmic rather than intragranular, so that their fusion with target cell membranes cannot readily be envisioned as a means of delivering secreted material, and there is presently no clear experimental evidence in favor of a functional role for these vesicles.

The low intragranular pH is maintained by a membrane proton pump termed the vacuolar-type adenosine triphosphatase (V-ATPase) (88). This pump is selectively inhibited by the macrolide antibiotic concanamycin A, which neutralizes CTL granules and triggers a degradation of intragranular perforin but not granzymes, with concomitant loss of cytotoxic activity (89). Because the Fas pathway does not involve granules, concanamycin A provides a useful experimental tool for distinguishing the granule exocytosis and Fas pathways of lymphocyte cytotoxicity (30).

TIA-1 is a protein component unique to CTL granules that is localized in the outer granule membranes with the protein domain exposed to the cytoplasm (90). TIA-1 also can be localized to the interior of some of the intragranular vesicles derived from these membranes by budding. The protein is expressed as two isoforms—a 15-kDa form and a 40-kDa form—with the former comprising the carboxy-terminal third of the latter protein. The dominant isoform in CTL granules is the 15-kDa species. Although the 40-kDa protein binds RNA and is homologous to other RNA-binding proteins described in various species, the 15-kDa protein lacks this activity. A functional role for TIA-1 in cytotoxicity has been proposed but remains speculative (91).

Granulysin (NK-lysin/519)

A small protein termed granulysin has recently been described in CTL granules (92) and is homologous to NK-lysin in porcine T- and NK-cell granules (93). Granulolysin was originally recognized as a T cell–specific messenger RNA (mRNA) that was upregulated several days after activation. Granulysin protein occurs in two forms: a 15-kDa form present only in immature granules and a further processed 9-kDa form that is secreted in response to TCR cross-linking as well as present in both mature and immature granules. Granulysin has lytic activity against tumor targets in 4-hour assays and is also lytic to bacteria. The 9-kDa protein sequence shows homology to the amoebapore family of lytic proteins from *Entamoeba histolytica,* the previously described lytic protein NK lysin, and two lipid hydrolyases. Although the importance of granulysins to the lytic function of CTLs is still unclear, it is reasonable to speculate that these proteins could interact with perforin to foster its insertion into lipid membranes.

Calreticulin

Calreticulin is an acidic 46-kDa protein known as a calcium-binding protein and molecular chaperone expressed in the endoplasmic reticulum (ER) of most cells. It was identified as a CTL granule component based on its copurification with perforin in granule extracts (94). It appears likely that calreticulin binds to perforin at least in part due to its lectinlike function in binding carbohydrates that have not been terminally processed by ER glycosidases (95). Immunolocalization studies show that calreticulin resides in CTL granules as well as in the ER, and it is secreted in response to TCR stimulation. Calreticulin's calcium-binding abilities may play a functional role, but because most of the calcium-binding capacity of calreticulin is low affinity it is not clear whether such binding is relevant to granules in the cell. After exocytosis, calreticulin could play a role as a local calcium chelator.

FUNCTIONAL STEPS IN THE GRANULE EXOCYTOSIS CYTOTOXIC MECHANISM

Figure 5 illustrates the basic properties of the granule exocytosis mechanism for lymphocyte cytotoxicity. It consists of discrete steps that have been defined in varying levels of detail as discussed below. The process is viewed as cyclical, reflecting microscopic observations that cytotoxic lymphocytes can kill up to a dozen target cells in the course of several hours without themselves suffering noticeable damage (19). The essential feature of this mechanism is the exocytosis step in which preformed mediators in secretory granules are released locally from the polarized CTLs into a synapselike region formed between the CTL and its bound target cell. A number of important molecular details of this cytotoxic pathway remain to be elucidated, including the terminal steps leading to target lysis. Although all short-term *in vitro* target cell cytotoxicity via this pathway is perforin dependent, it is quite possible that important noncytotoxic mediators may be secreted by the granule exocytosis pathway, which has the advantage of being more rapid than other cytotoxicity pathways requiring protein synthesis.

Adhesion

Time-lapse cinematography observations of CTLs interacting with target cells show CTLs moving on the substrate in apparently

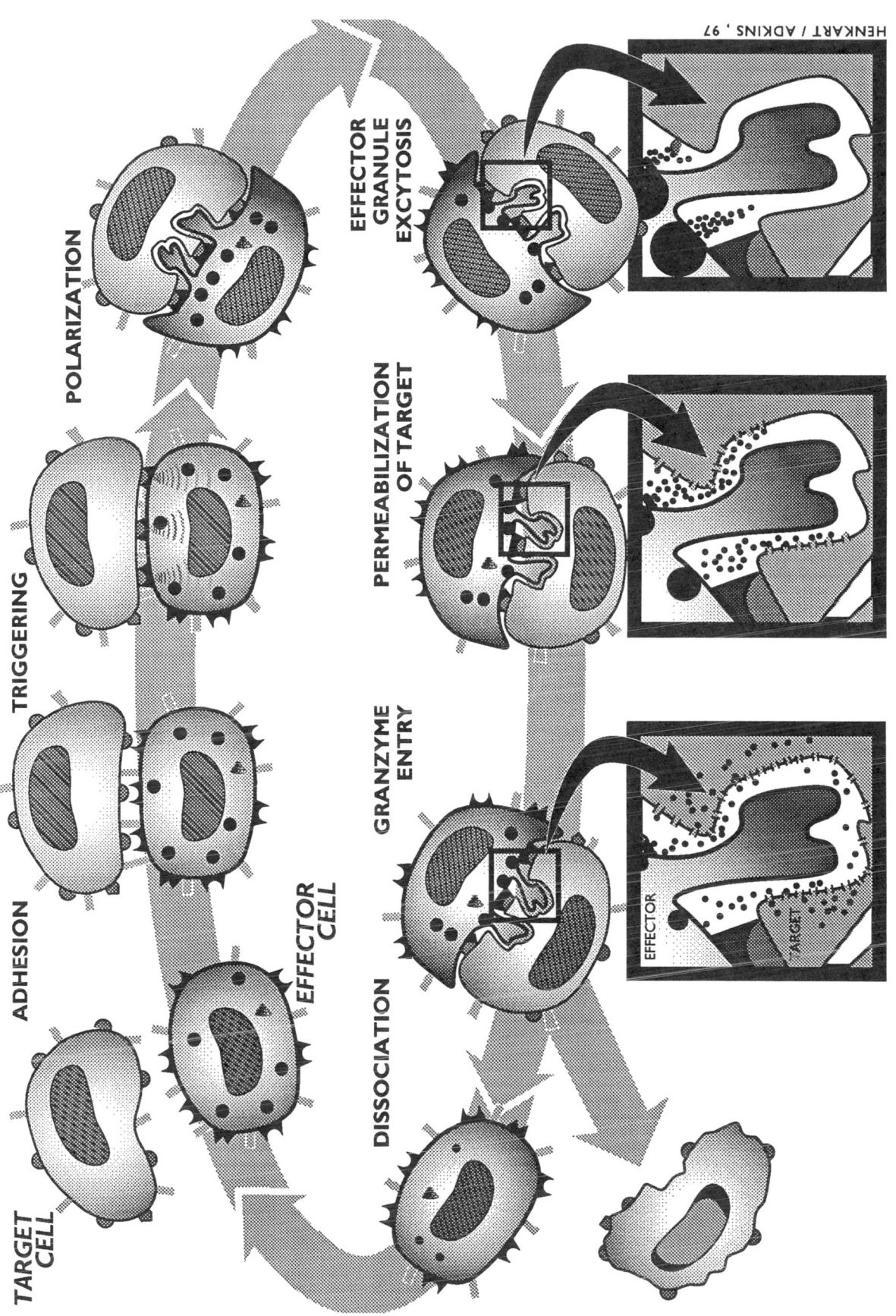

FIG. 5. The granule exocytosis cytotoxic mechanism, depicting the sequential stages of the process described in detail in the text.

random motion before encountering other cells (19,20,96,97). When contact is made via fine membrane processes, a firmer adhesion involving membrane–membrane contact appears to follow rapidly, with the CTLs moving along the surface of the typically larger cells (Fig. 6). In some cases the CTL soon detaches and resumes its random motion, even with target cells of appropriate specificity. In other cases, the adhesion is maintained for minutes to hours until signs of target cell damage can be observed. EMs of CTLs bound to target cells show considerable areas of close membrane–membrane contact with some gaps in the center of this contact area (Fig. 7).

CTL–target adhesion has been studied by isolation of conjugates, which are CTL–target clusters observed after CTLs have been centrifuged into contact with nonadherent tumor target cells and gently resuspended (98). By varying the ratio of CTLs and targets, clusters containing more than one target or CTL can be observed. Study of isolated 1:1 conjugates between allogeneic tumor target cells and potent *in vivo* CTLs showed that target cells were killed with 2 hours of further incubation (21). Classically conjugates have been enumerated by microscopic counting, with target cells identified by use of a prelabeled fluorescent marker, but two-color flow cytometry has recently been used for such studies (99). When potent *in vivo*–derived CTLs from the peritoneal exudate after rejection of allogeneic tumors are used, the specificity of conjugate formation generally reflects TCR recognition, with a variable background of nonspecific conjugates that are not lysed. However, when cloned CTLs grown in long-term *in vitro* cultures are used, this nonspecific conjugate formation may dominate (100),

apparently due to the stronger expression of adhesion molecules such as LFA-1 and CD2 on such CTLs.

Specific CTL–target conjugate formation requires a few minutes of incubation at 37°C after CTL–target contact to achieve the stability necessary to survive the isolation-induced shear forces. This adhesion does not take place in the cold, is blockable by inhibitors of intracellular energy generation, and requires magnesium in the medium (101). The latter appears to be due to the interaction of the CTL adhesion molecule LFA-1 with its target cell ligands intracellular adhesion molecule (ICAM)-1 or ICAM-2, which also requires magnesium. A temperature-sensitive strengthening of the adhesion of specific CTL–target pairs can be measured by varying the shear forces required to disrupt binding (102).

Specific CTL–target conjugate formation (as well as cytotoxicity) can be blocked by antibodies against adhesion molecules, and this approach led to the identification of the two pairs of nonspecific adhesion molecules. LFA-1 on the CTL surface interacts with ICAMs on target cells, and CD2 on the CTL surface interacts with LFA-3 on target cells (103). The dependence of such nonspecific adhesive interactions for successful CTL–target interactions appears to vary with the CTL (104).

Adhesion Strengthening

The most simple view of adhesion molecules is that they provide additional adhesive forces between interacting cell membranes and hence allow a more efficient interaction of the specific receptor–ligand interactions. However, there is now considerable evidence

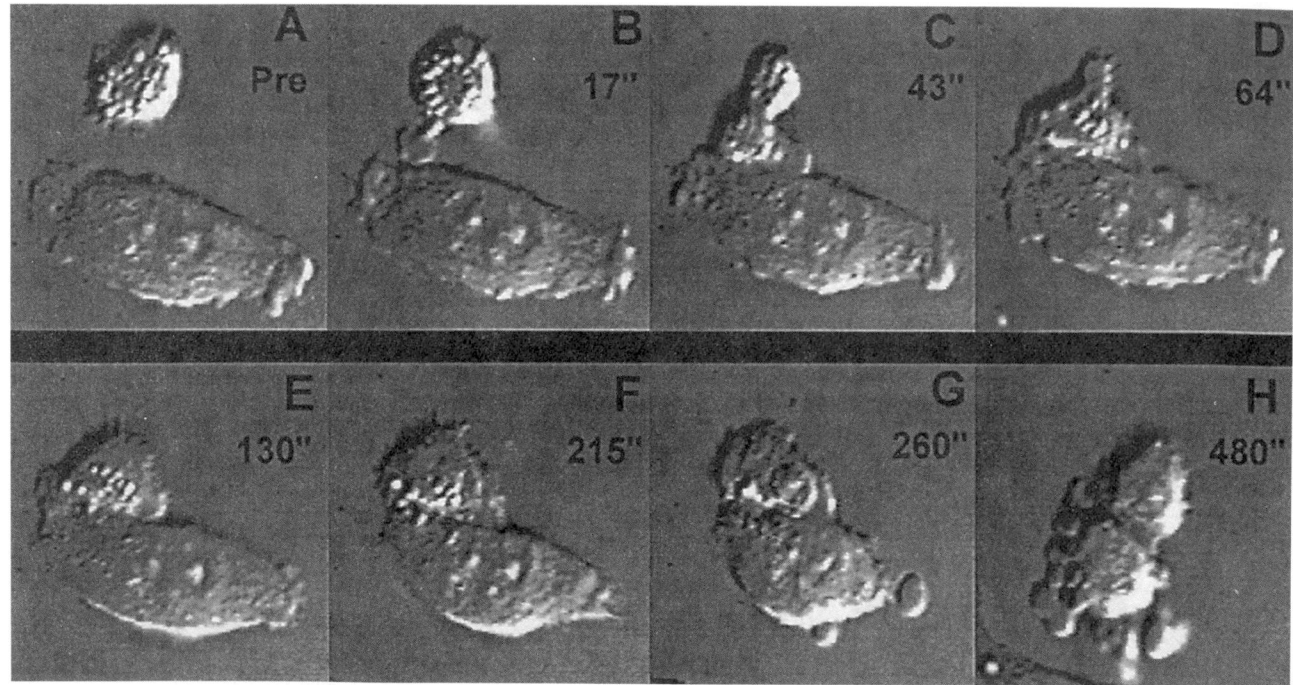

FIG. 6. Time-lapse frames of cytotoxicity by a cloned MHC class I–allospecific CD8+ CTL on a fibroblast target cell as seen with differential interference contrast microscopy. **A:** The CTL approaching the target cell before contact, with random ruffling and extension of small lamellae. **B** to **H:** Sequential images after contact, with the time in seconds after contact indicated. A single large lamella connects the CTL and target (**B**), followed by the extension of membrane-membrane contact along the target surface (**C** and **D**). Granule movement from the initially dispersed array toward the bound target cell (**D–G**), followed by granule disappearance (**F–H**). Membrane blebbing, a sign of target injury, is first seen in **G**, and becomes more dramatic in **H**. Images provided by Dr. Klaus Hahn, Scripps Clinic and Research Foundation (124) with permission.

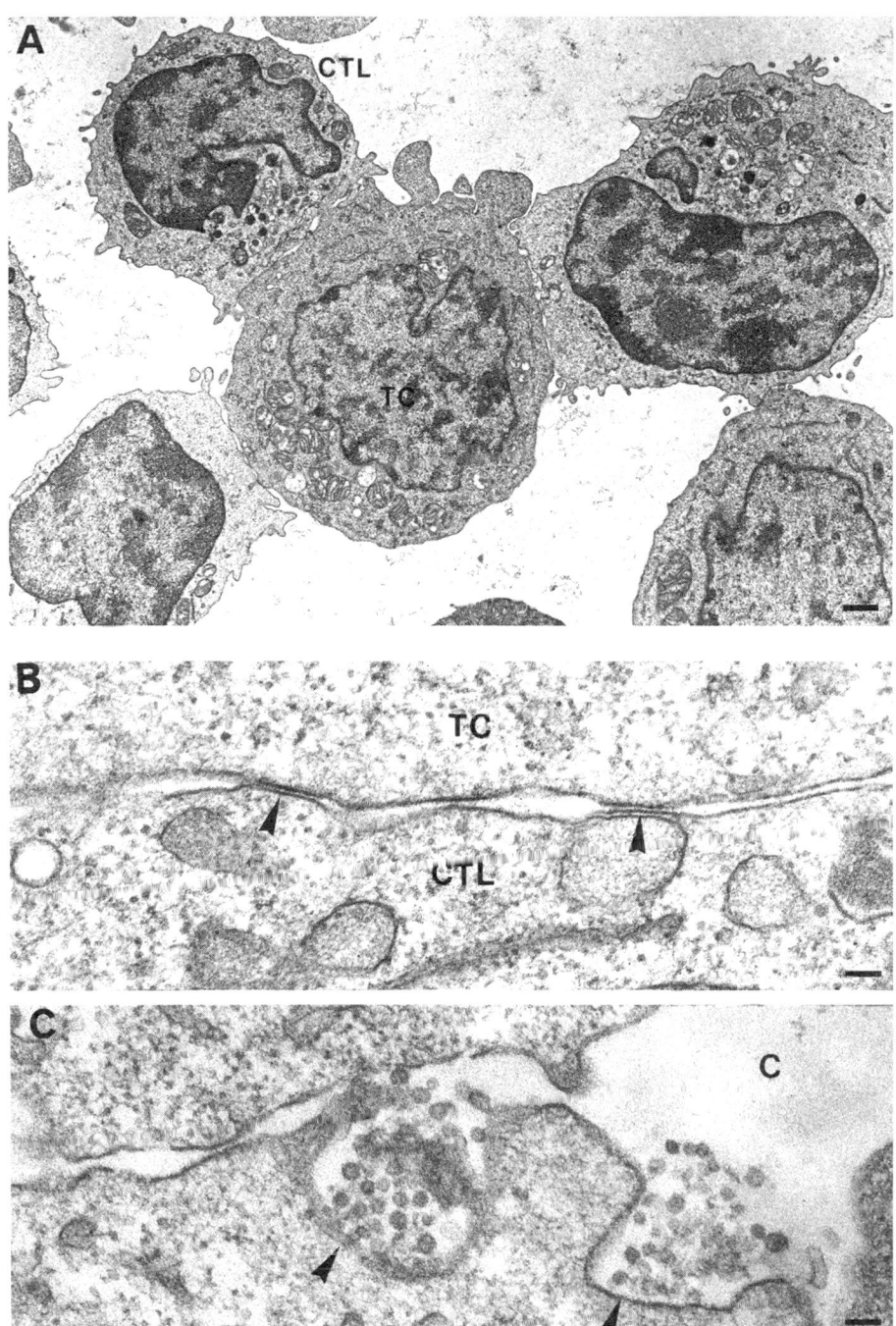

FIG. 7. Rapid polarization and exocytosis induced by target cells in a human CTL clone. **A:** Three CTLs adherent to one target cell (TC) fixed 1 minute after mixing the two cell types. Polarization is seen only in the CTL in the upper left (CTL label). Size bar, 1 µm. **B:** CTL–target interface fixed at 1 minute after mixing at higher power showing two sites of close apposition of CTL and target cell plasma membranes (*arrowheads*). Size bar, 0.1 µm. **C:** CTL–target interface fixed 10 minutes after mixing showing exocytosis of granules containing membrane vesicles. Granule cores are not seen in this section. Size bar, 0.1 µm. Courtesy of Dr. Peter Peters, University of Utrecht (85) with permission.

for a more complex set of interactions between the TCR–MHC peptide interaction, CD8–MHC interaction, and the engagement of CTL adhesion molecules with their target ligands. It has become clear that the adhesion molecules and CD8 are capable of generating signals within the CTL, and that TCR engagement leads to a strengthening of the avidity of the LFA-1–ICAM interaction (105)

as well as the CD8–MHC interaction (106). Thus, the initial weak interactions between CTL adhesion molecules and target ligands promote interaction between TCR and target MHC peptide. This in turn induces a further strengthening of LFA-1–ICAM and CD8–MHC interaction, which gives strong adhesion. The cytoskeleton may play a role in these interactions because cytochalasins block adhesions that lead to conjugate formation. It is clear that although adhesion molecules can generate intracellular signals, these alone do not account for the LFA-1 requirement because its augmentation of CTL function requires its colocalization with the TCR cross-linking agent (107).

Studies of CTL triggering by surface-immobilized purified class I MHC antigens have shown the importance of the CTL CD8 coreceptor (106). In this system, soluble anti-CD3 triggers the binding of CTL to irrelevant class I molecules via CD8, which indicates that the TCR signaling induces an enhancement in CD8–MHC binding by an unknown mechanism. Because CTL–target conjugates form stable adhesion in the absence of extracellular calcium, a functionally useful definition of the adhesion and adhesion strengthening phase of the CTL lytic process is that this is the calcium-independent, magnesium-dependent step.

Triggering the Lethal Hit

The positively reinforcing adhesion–receptor–coreceptor interactions induce a functional triggering of further steps in the CTL lytic mechanism. The second messengers include an increase in intracellular calcium, which accompanies many examples of T-cell activation (108). Using single-cell imaging with intracellular calcium-sensitive fluorescent dyes, CTLs were shown to undergo a rapid cytoplasmic calcium increase after engagement of specific target cells (109,110). Resting CTL calcium levels of about 100 nM increased to a mean of approximately 500 nM within a few minutes before declining to baseline over the course of about 20 minutes. Multiple cycles of Ca_i increase were sometimes seen (111). The antigen-induced Ca_i increase was blunted and transient if extracellular calcium was removed, suggesting an influx of external calcium through the plasma membrane as the major source. However, the calcium channel blocker verapamil does not inhibit this increase, which occurs via a potential sensitive calcium channel activated in response to depletion of intracellular calcium stores (112,113). The target cell–induced calcium increase in CTLs is correlated with the calcium-requiring lethal hit phase of the CTL mechanism described from functional measurements earlier.

The strong stimulatory effect of the protein kinase C activator PMA on CTL degranulation in the presence of calcium ionophores (34) suggests an involvement of protein kinases in CTL intracellular signaling similar to that in other T cells. Anti-TCR antibody stimulation of CTLs induces tyrosine phosphorylation of a discrete set of substrates including p56[lck], with additional substrates phosphorylated upon CD8 binding to class I (114). These results show that CD8 engagement provides costimulation signals via protein kinases. However, TCR-induced protein kinase activation was found to be stronger in CD8-dependent CTLs than in CD8-independent CTLs (115). In this system, TCR engagement increased the association of p56[lck] with CD8 and recruited ZAP-70 to the TCR complex. These studies of protein kinases in CTLs activated by target recognition suggest similar TCR signaling pathways to those found in other T cells. However, it is not yet clear at what point signaling for cytoplasmic polarization and degranulation diverges from signaling for gene expression (e.g., Fas ligand and interferon-γ).

Effector Polarization

Microscopic studies of CTL–target conjugates show that a pronounced polarization exists in CTLs bound to specific target cells,

as can be seen in Figs. 6 and 7A. Under favorable circumstances polarization can be observed within 1 minute after CTL–target contact (Fig. 7). Lysosomal enzymes now known to be granule associated (116), the Golgi apparatus (117) and microtubule organizing centers (MTOCs) (118) are found to be preferentially localized toward the target cell, and it appears that the majority of the cytoplasmic organelles are coordinately moved in response to target recognition. Such polarization could arise from previously polarized CTL binding target cells via an asymmetrically displayed receptor, or could be induced in a previously nonpolarized CTL as a result of target binding. Two types of studies show that the latter model is correct.

Using fluorescence microscopy to assess the intracellular localization of microtubule organizing centers and the cytoskeletal protein talin, cytoplasmic polarization was observed only in cloned CTLs or NK cells bound to a target that was later lysed (119). When CTL–target conjugates were formed in the absence of calcium, the CTLs were not polarized, but subsequent addition of calcium induced asymmetry within a few minutes (120). Effector polarization was found to be blocked by microtubule-disrupting drugs (121). It was found that the CTL Golgi apparatus and MTOC oriented sequentially toward each bound target before its death (120), and similar findings were made in the unidirectional killing of CTL–CTL conjugates (122). Based on observations of conjugates in which one effector cell is bound to multiple target cells and of conjugates in which two mutually antagonistic CTL were mixed, target cell lysis was shown to be a highly polarized event (98). The observation of CTL cytoplasmic polarization provides a mechanistic correlate to these results, which together document a dramatic rapid triggered cytoplasmic reorganization of CTL in response to contact with specific target cells (123).

Time lapse cinematographic studies of CTL killing using Nomarski optics strongly support the induced polarization model (96,124). Studies of calcium signaling show that motile T cells have a higher antigen sensitivity along their leading edge, where they are likely to encounter antigen-presenting cells (APCs), than their trailing surface (125). On the other hand, CTL cytoplasmic granules are normally localized toward the rear of the cell (124). As shown in Fig. 6, at the time of CTL–target contact, the CTL granules generally are located away from the target cell, but within seconds a rapid coordinated movement of granules toward the target can be seen. Granule movement appears to be part of an overall polarization of the CTL and occurs at a step after the increased membrane contact between CTL and target, as shown in Fig. 6D to F. When the same CTL later came into contact with control cells not engaging the TCR, no similar granule reorientation was observed (124).

Exocytosis

Secretion is the result of a membrane fusion event between the granule membrane and plasma membrane, termed exocytosis, which results in a continuity between the granule interior and the extracellular space. Many examples of polarized secretion can be found in cell biology, but few if any follow a rapid induced polarization such as occur after target binding by cytotoxic lymphocytes. Basic molecular aspects of the critical exocytosis process are still poorly understood, although progress is being made (126). Images from high-resolution time-lapse cinematographic studies of CTL-induced cytotoxicity show what appear to be granule exocytosis after CTL–target contact (96,124). In these images, visible granules close to the CTL membrane disappear shortly after reorientation but before visible target injury. EM images (Fig. 7C) strongly suggest granule exocytosis in progress near the bound target cell, and similar images were seen with NK cell–target conjugates (127,128). Other EM studies of effector–target conjugates have shown transfer of the CTL lysosomal enzyme acid phosphatase into the space between CTL and target (84), as well as a similar transfer of the NK lysosomal enzyme aryl sulfatase (129).

CTL and NK-cell granule exocytosis can be measured by assessing the release of granule components into the medium. Because of its sensitivity, the BLT-esterase assay of granzyme A (and tryptase-2) activity is most convenient and widely used (130). Degranulation of cloned CTLs is observed within a few hours of culture in the presence of target cells, on immobilized antibodies against the TCR complex, or in response to stimulatory lectins such as concanavalin A (ConA). MHC-restricted granzyme A secretion from purified T splenocytes from LCMV-infected mice was shown to occur within 3 hours in response to viral antigen on target cells (131). NK-cell degranulation was first measured in cloned human NK cells by following release of ^{35}S-labeled granule proteoglycan into the medium in response to target cells (132,133).

In common with most other types of secretion via the regulated secretory pathway, CTL degranulation triggered by anti-TCR antibodies and antigen is blocked by removal of extracellular calcium (131,134). Granzyme A secretion is not blocked by inhibitors of RNA and protein synthesis, in striking contrast to that of interferon-γ by the same CTL (34). A combination of the calcium ionophore and the protein kinase C activator phorbol myristyl acetate can trigger degranulation in the absence of TCR cross-linking (34).

Like other secretory granules, CTL granules move through the cytoplasm toward the plasma membrane and exocytosis guided by microtubules. Isolated granules have been shown to undergo a kinesin-dependent translational motility along microtubules *in vitro* (135).

Target Permeabilization

EM observations of complementlike, porelike structures on target cells attacked by cytotoxic large granular lymphocytes and CTLs strongly suggested that analogous membrane damage was responsible for target cell death by both complement and cytotoxic lymphocytes (40–42). Subsequent studies have raised a number of

issues that have forced a significant revision of this paradigm without denying the importance of membrane damage. Both complement and isolated perforin cause the death of nucleated target cells within a few minutes at 37°C (66,67), but CTL–target cells lethally injured by CTLs require an average of 1.7 hours between inflicting the lethal damage and target lysis (25). It has been established that nucleated cells have a cytoplasmic system of protection against membrane injury. This has been characterized in studies with complement as due to a calcium-dependent shedding of vesicles containing pore structures into the medium (68), and in studies with physical wounding of cell membranes as due to a calcium-dependent exocytosis of internal membranes (136). Such repair mechanisms can explain the ability of cells to recover within minutes from the permeability increases induced by sublytic perforin concentrations (137,138), as well as the cross-protection from lysis observed among different channel-forming agents (139).

As described below, most target cells killed by CTL or NK cells acquire an apoptotic death phenotype as seen by microscopy or by DNA fragmentation (140,141). Because pore-forming agents including purified perforin induce a nonapoptotic death (142), the granule exocytosis model does not explain the apoptotic target death phenotype if perforin pores are the critical lethal target damage. As summarized in Fig. 8, studies with noncytolytic RBL mast cell tumors show that perforin expression confers a potent cytolytic activity against red cell targets but only a modest lytic activity against tumor targets, which was not accompanied by DNA fragmentation (143). These results argue that unlike mammalian erythrocytes, nucleated cells have defensive systems that can normally repair the membrane damage due to pore formation induced by high local concentrations of perforin after degranulation. However, it is clear from results with the perforin knock-out mice that perforin is absolutely required for rapid lethal damage of Fas-negative cells induced by CTL and NK cells (144). Given the evidence discussed above that perforin pores are capable of allowing passage of macromolecules, and the evidence discussed below for a role for granzymes in target cell damage, it appears that the primary role for perforin is to permeabilize the target membrane to granzymes, although other interpretations are viable (145).

Granzyme Entry and Internal Proteolysis

The strongest evidence for a role for granzymes in cytolysis comes from the experiments with transfected RBL mast cells sum-

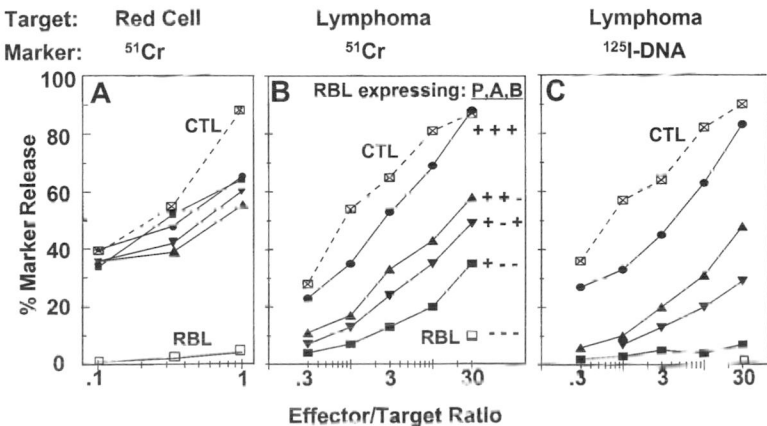

FIG. 8. Cytotoxic activity of RBL mast cells expressing perforin, granzyme A, and granzyme B. Data shown are means of transfectant clones of RBL mast cell tumors expressing perforin, granzyme A and granzyme B (●), perforin and granzyme A (▲), perforin and granzyme B (▼), perforin alone (■), untransfected parental RBL line (□), and CTL clone control (⊠). RBL IgE FcR triggering of TNP hapten-modified target cells was achieved with IgE anti-TNP, and CTLs were redirected by anti-CD3×anti-TNP heteroconjugated antibody. Data shows marker release from 4-hour incubations. **A:** Lysis of human red cells. **B:** Lysis of EL-4 lymphoma cells. **C:** DNA release from CL-4 lymphoma cells. Data replotted from Shiver and Henkart (143).

marized in Fig. 8. Unlike the case with red cell targets (Fig. 8A), in order to achieve an RBL cytolytic activity comparable with CTLs on tumor targets, expression of granzymes A and B are required along with perforin (Fig. 8B) (146,147). Analysis of transfectant clones showed that their cytolytic activity on tumor targets was quantitatively correlated with granzyme but not perforin expression levels (although perforin expression was required for activity) (147).

Another approach to granzyme function has been to examine the function of CTL and NK cells from knock-out mice. Granzyme B–deficient mice show normal CTL- and LAK-induced target lysis and a roughly twofold reduction in NK-induced lysis rate (148, 149). Target cell DNA fragmentation is significantly retarded compared with controls with all three cytotoxic effector cells lacking granzyme B, but significant nuclear damage remains. With granzyme A knock-out mice, neither CTL nor NK effectors showed any *in vitro* defects in target lysis or DNA fragmentation (150). Thus, the granzyme knock-out results show that neither granzyme A nor B are required for good *in vitro* target cell lysis, but do not address the possibility that other granule proteases may supplant the role of the one deleted in these mice.

Several possibilities can be envisioned to explain the ability of granzymes to potentiate target killing in the RBL transfectant studies. Granzymes could proteolytically process perforin either before or after exocytosis to produce a more active protein, and the effects of protease inhibitors on perforin hemolytic activity have been interpreted as favoring this model (151). However, no such perforin cleavage has been biochemically defined, and the cytotoxic activity of recombinant perforin (52) argues against this. Another possibility is that granzymes could act on target cell surface proteins to enhance perforin insertion or pore formation. However, there is no evidence for this, and perforin's potent ability to permeabilize liposomes and red cells suggests that it may not be necessary.

A more likely possibility is that granzymes enter the target cell and trigger a preexisting apoptotic death pathway. Although there is currently no direct evidence that granzymes enter target cells, the ability of the granzyme inhibitor aprotinin to block lysis and apoptotic nuclear damage by granzyme-expressing effector cells is highly suggestive. Aprotinin was found to block target lysis when loaded into the target cell cytoplasm (152) or coupled to the target membrane (153) but not in the medium, and blocking was not seen with RBL expressing perforin only (152).

Considerable evidence exists that granzymes can trigger apoptotic nuclear damage in target cells. Fig. 8C shows that without granzymes the limited target lysis by perforin-expressing RBL cells is not accompanied by DNA fragmentation. However, expression of either granzyme alone confers some nuclear damage, whereas both together give target DNA release approaching the levels of lysis, as seen with CTLs. It has been found that granzyme A causes DNA fragmentation in detergent-permeabilized cells (154) and that granzymes A, B, and tryptase-2 mediate this effect in cells treated with sublytic doses of perforin (the rat granzymes with this activity were termed fragmentins) (155). The mechanism for these effects has been pursued by several laboratories. Granzyme A has been shown to cleave the nuclear protein nucleolin (156). Granzyme B binds to the nucleus of permeabilized target cells, where it can be localized to the heterochromatin (157). In the presence of sublytic doses of perforin, granzymes A, B, and tryptase-2 trigger apoptotic nuclear damage in tumor cells, with granzyme B the most potent effector (155). Granzyme B was shown to act by triggering dephosphorylation and consequent activation of the cyclin-dependent protein kinase p34^{cdc2} (158), which

normally becomes activated just before mitosis during the cell cycle. Both granzyme B–induced apoptosis and the p34^{cdc2} kinase activation are blocked by overexpression of its negative regulator, wee1 kinase (159). Although the functional granzyme B substrate in this system has not been clearly identified, caspases are required in at least some cell types (160).

A recent series of experiments has addressed the possibility that granzyme B acts by proteolytically processing and hence activating caspases, a family of cytoplasmic cysteine proteases that are the mammalian analogs of the *C. elegans* death protease ced-3. Caspases share with granzyme B the unusual cleavage specificity requiring aspartic acid at the P1 amino acid, and such cleavages appear to be required for the death-associated activation of the precaspases normally present in cells. Thus, it has been shown that purified granzyme B can process and activate caspases 3, 7, 8, 9, and 10 but not caspases 1 or 2. Furthermore, CTLs have been shown to specifically induce the processing of caspase 3 in target cells (161), which does not occur with CTLs lacking granzyme B (162).

The role of caspases in CTL-induced cytotoxicity has been tested using caspase inhibitors, which block most apoptotic death in a variety of *in vitro* and *in vivo* systems (163). Both cell-permeant peptide-based caspase inhibitors and the protein inhibitor baculovirus p35 effectively block the lysis and apoptotic nuclear damage induced by the CTL FasL/Fas pathway in several different target cell types. Using the granule exocytosis pathway, CTL-induced lysis of these targets was unaffected by either of these types of caspase inhibitor. However, target nuclear damage measured by morphology or DNA fragmentation was completely blocked (164), compatible with the idea that granzyme B activates caspases that trigger nuclear damage but not lysis. These results are compatible with the scheme in Fig. 9, in which caspases play a central role in cell death via the FasL/Fas pathway but not the granule exocytosis pathway.

Does the CTL Granule Exocytosis Pathway Kill Target Cells by Triggering Apoptosis?

Observations of apoptotic morphology (140) and DNA fragmentation (141) in CTL targets led to the idea that CTLs trigger target cell apoptosis. Although this is clearly a useful way of thinking about the FasL/Fas pathway, the experiments with caspase inhibitors raise questions about whether this correctly describes target death induced by the granule exocytosis pathway. A major problem is the lack of a molecular definition of apoptosis, which is often functionally defined by nuclear damage accompanying death. For CTL-induced death, target cell double-stranded DNA cleavage is usually but not always found (12,165,166). The role of the nucleus in CTL-induced target cell death was addressed in experiments using enucleated cytoplasts. Such target cells were fully lysable by CTLs using both the granule exocytosis and Fas death pathways, and the 10-fold increase in effector potency due to granzyme expression in RBL effector cells was seen in such targets (167). These results are parallel to some other apoptotic death inducers, which also do not require target nuclei (168) and show that granzyme-triggered apoptotic nuclear damage is not required for CTL-induced target cell lysis.

Although target cell death via the granule exocytosis pathway does not require the nucleus or caspases, it may still be considered apoptotic if the downstream portion of its death pathway merges with the apoptotic pathway as shown in Fig. 9. Further experiments are needed to resolve this issue.

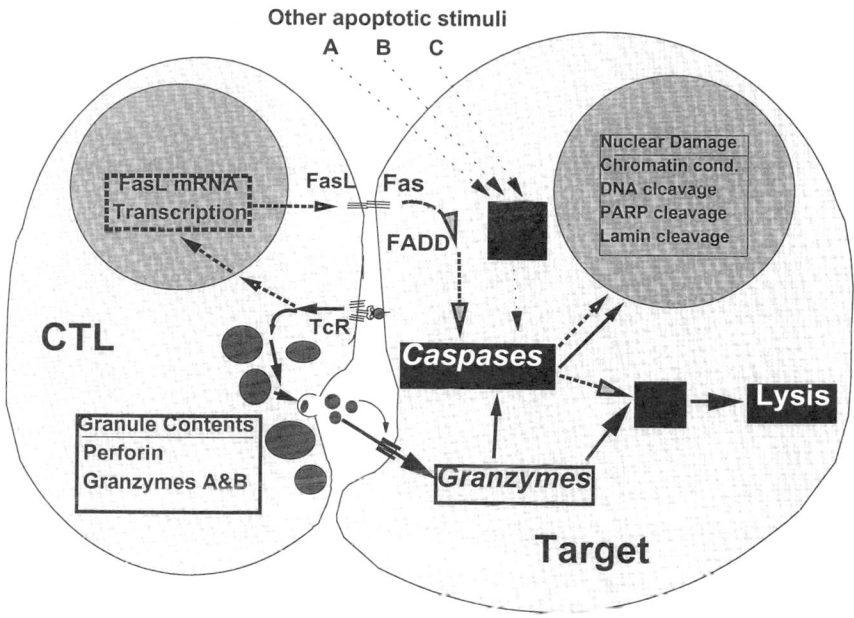

FIG. 9. Target cell death pathways induced by CTLs. The FasL/Fas pathway is depicted by dashed arrows, whereas the granule exocytosis pathway is depicted by solid arrows. This scheme assumes the two pathways converge downstream from caspases, which are part of the FasL/Fas death pathway but which participate only in nuclear damage by the granule exocytosis pathway.

The Bcl-2 family of intracellular proteins has been shown to have a major influence on apoptotic cell death by a number of input pathways. Most members of the Bcl-2 family, including Bcl-2 and Bcl-x, inhibit most apoptotic deaths in lymphoid and other cell lineages (169), but for CTL-induced death there is no consensus. Bcl-2 has been reported by different laboratories to inhibit or have no effect on the CTL FasL/Fas and granule exocytosis death pathways (170–172). Whether Bcl-2 functional effects on CTL killing depends on the target cell type or these conflicting reports are due to technical issues awaits further clarification.

Another intracellular regulator of apoptotic death is the protein kinase Bcr-abl, which has been shown to be overexpressed in cancer cells with the Philadelphia chromosome (173). Such cells are resistant to death induced by a variety of input pathways that induce an apoptotic death in other cells (174), and this effect of Bcr-abl expression may be accounted for by its Ras-mediated upregulation of Bcl-2 (175). CTL-induced death of two different transfected cell lines is not affected by Bcr-abl overexpression, which strongly protects against death by radiation (176). Furthermore, K562 cells have been derived from a patient with chronic myelogenous leukemia with the Philadelphia chromosome, and they are resistant to death by radiation and chemotherapeutic agents. However they are the classical target cells sensitive to human NK cells, which induce an apoptotic death (177). These experiments are compatible with the model shown in Fig. 9, if it is assumed that the granzyme-triggered death pathway bypasses the precaspase control points used by Bcr-abl and probably Bcl-2.

CTL Detachment

Time-lapse cinematography of CTL-induced cytotoxicity shows that CTLs detach from target cells, move away, and subsequently kill more neighboring target cells. The mechanism of this detachment is unclear, and it is hard to tell if the CTLs remain attached until target lysis or if an active decision is made before lysis but after the lethal injury has been delivered (178). A model for detachment based on a spreading wave of adhesion molecule off signals is appealing but needs further experimental verification (106).

Self-Protection of Cytotoxic Lymphocytes

A major question facing the granule exocytosis model has always been why the effector cells are not themselves lysed after degranulation releases lethal mediators at high local concentrations. Microscopic studies established that CTL can kill multiple target cells without suffering detectable damage themselves. Numerous subsequent investigations addressed the question of whether CTLs are themselves susceptible targets to attack by other CTLs. Early studies found that uncloned CTLs were inactivated by other CTLs, and it was assumed that they were killed. However, more recent studies indicate that such target CTLs are not necessarily killed when other CTLs inactivate them (179). Cloned CTLs have frequently found to be highly resistant to lysis after recognition by other CTLs (179–182). Thus, CTLs appear to express a permanent global resistance to their own lethal mediators. CTLs are resistant to perforin-induced lysis relative to other lymphoid cells (183–185). Such resistance is not absolute, and it is not clear that CTLs are uniquely resistant to perforin lysis because there is a wide range of resistance among non-CTL targets. Protective membrane proteins have been proposed to be responsible for this resistance, e.g., by binding perforin molecules before membrane insertion or before inserted molecules aggregate and form functional pores (186), but satisfactory molecular identification and functional experiments establishing their role in CTL self-protection have not been performed. Another explanation for CTL perforin resistance is that CTLs have a particularly active system of removing functional pores from their membranes as discussed above.

As suggested by experiments in which cytoplasmic loading of the granule inhibitor aprotinin protected against CTL-induced lysis (187), the cytoplasm is another potential level of CTL self-protection. A serpin inhibitor of granzyme B has been identified in CTLs and other cells (188), but critical experiments implicating such intracellular protease inhibitors in CTL self-protection remain to be conducted.

Despite the above evidence in favor of a global system of CTL self-protection, a variety of studies show that CTLs can kill other CTLs, implying that the above resistance can be overcome. Thus, enriched populations of *in vivo*–derived CTLs are lysed by other CTLs, hapten-specific cloned CTLs kill other hapten-specific cloned CTLs, and peptide-specific cloned CTLs kill each other in the presence of peptide (180,189,190). These findings continue to pose a challenge for the granule exocytosis model and suggest that other local or temporary protective systems exist in CTLs to prevent self-destruction after degranulation. Because granule membrane components become locally incorporated into the plasma membrane after exocytosis, they are one class of candidates. Another possibility is a transient global protection triggered by target recognition. These speculative possibilities have been difficult to test experimentally. Because the RBL mast cell tumors did not detectably self-destruct upon killing target cells after they had been transfected with perforin and granzyme A, the self-protection property appears not be unique to CTLs (146).

EXPRESSION OF GRANULE CYTOTOXIC MEDIATORS

A general survey of normal tissues for expression of perforin mRNA or protein shows it is expressed exclusively in lymphoid tissue, and closer examination shows that its expression is highly correlated with cytotoxic lymphocytes. For example, in normal human peripheral blood, perforin protein was detected in more than 95% of the $CD56^+$ NK cells and more than 97% of the $\gamma\delta$ T cells (36). Both of these populations show cytolytic activity using redirected lysis. Although blood $CD4^+$ T cells were negative for perforin expression and cytotoxicity, $CD8^+$ cells with memory phenotype showed substantial cytotoxic activity and perforin expression. Naive and cord blood $CD8^+$ T cells lack detectable perforin expression (191,192). After *in vitro* activation, $CD4^+$ T cells remained negative for perforin expression and cytotoxicity, whereas $CD8^+$ T cells increased their perforin expression and cytotoxicity (36).

Granzyme mRNA and protein expression is not detectable in resting peripheral T-lymphocytes, but is detected in resting NK cells (74,193). *In vitro* activation increases expression of all granzymes in both $CD4^+$ and $CD8^+$ T cells as well as in NK cells. Granzyme A and B mRNA expression is detectable in immature thymocytes, but declines at the $CD4^+8^+$ stage (194). In $CD4^-8^+$ thymocytes, granzyme A mRNA and enzymatic activity are detectable.

Peritoneal exudate lymphocytes induced by allostimulation have been a classical source of highly potent CTLs (98). These cells express perforin and granzymes, but at lower levels than do CTLs grown *in vitro* (195,196). After *in vitro* culture in IL-2, such CTLs acquire higher levels of these granule mediators (197).

The metrial gland develops near the placenta in pregnant rodents and contains a granulated cell whose function has been obscure. The granules in these cells contain perforin and granzyme A (198), and the isolated granulated cells have NK activity (199), although the significance of this for the physiology of pregnancy remains unknown.

THE FASL/FAS PATHWAY OF CYTOTOXICITY

The existence of additional pathways of lymphocyte-mediated cytotoxicity *in vitro* besides granule exocytosis was inferred by experiments indicating that some target cells were killed by CTLs under conditions of calcium chelation, preventing granule exocytosis and perforin lytic activity (200–202). Studies with a CTL hybridoma and peritoneal exudate CTL showed that expression of

Fas on the target cell is required for this calcium-independent cytotoxicity pathway (203), but as described below, under most conditions extracellular calcium is necessary for the full activity of this pathway. The description of Fas ligand and its upregulation on T-lymphocytes after activation (204,205) allowed a more complete description of this cytotoxicity pathway. As shown in Fig. 1, the use of cytotoxic cells lacking perforin and the effect of the gld and lpr mutations in FasL and Fas, respectively, have allowed studies of this pathway both *in vitro* and *in vivo*. Although this cytotoxicity pathway appears to play a role in some *in vivo* phenomena long thought to be attributable to cytotoxic lymphocytes, studies of lpr and gld mice suggest that the major role of Fas and FasL appears to be regulating immune responses (206,207).

One major difference between the granule exocytosis and FasL/Fas pathways is that a number of other cell types besides cytotoxic lymphocytes can express FasL and have been shown to function as effector cells capable of killing target cells *in vitro* (208). These include macrophages, dendritic cells, neutrophils, neurons, and a variety of tumor cells. The role of such FasL expression in immune regulation and tissue destruction *in vivo* is currently under investigation.

Molecular Mechanism of the FasL/Fas Cytotoxicity Pathway

Detailed studies of the initial stages of CTL–target interaction leading to death via the FasL/Fas pathway have not been performed. However, it is likely that these are identical to those described for the granule exocytosis pathway. As shown in Fig. 1, TCR triggering is required for triggering both CTL-mediated death pathways, and the magnesium-dependent adhesion steps needed to achieve this activation would appear identical for the two pathways. However, it is possible that the threshold levels of TCR engagement with antigen required to trigger the two pathways may differ.

Even after TCR triggering has led to FasL expression, the FasL/Fas pathway may require adhesion molecules for efficient cross-linking of target cell Fas by FasL on the CTL. Experimental evidence that FasL expression alone is inadequate was provided by findings that EGTA blocks Fas-dependent lytic function but not FasL upregulation in CTL clones in response to antigen (209).

Studies of CTLs derived from primary *in vitro* allosensitization cultures have shown that the FasL/Fas pathway can be dissected into two phases (210). The first is an activation phase of 1 to 3 hours that can be triggered by antigen, antibodies against the TCR complex, or PMA and ionomycin. This phase requires extracellular calcium and RNA and protein synthesis, which are required for FasL expression (27). This phase appears to account for the kinetic lag in target cytotoxicity shown in Fig. 2. The second phase of this cytotoxicity pathway is initiated by FasL-mediated cross-linking of target Fas, as described below. Other studies of such primary *in vitro*–derived allo-CTLs have compared the activities of (presumably $CD8^+$) CTLs from perforin-deficient and FasL-defective gld mice. Calcium chelation eliminated cytotoxic activity by both pathways, whereas inhibitors of protein and RNA synthesis blocked the FasL/Fas pathway but not the perforin-dependent pathway.

The FasL/Fas Pathway in T-Cell Clones

$CD4^+$ Th1 clones and hybridomas show cytotoxic activity via the FasL/Fas pathway when activated in cultures containing Fas-bearing target cells. Cytotoxicity is observed whether or not the target cells bear ligands recognized by the TCR, and such bystander cytotoxic activity was also found when such clones are preactivated (211). Similar to the primary allospecific CTLs, the activation phase of CD4$^+$ T cell–mediated cytotoxicity requires protein synthesis and extracellular calcium, but cytotoxicity by preactivated Th1 clones requires neither.

Cultured CD8$^+$ CTL lines use the FasL/Fas cytotoxicity pathway in addition to the granule exocytosis pathway, and studies on the mechanism of TCR-induced FasL upregulation have been performed in such cells. Inhibitor studies have implicated src-like protein tyrosine kinases, phosphatidylinositol-3 kinase, and the phosphatase calcineurin in such signaling (205,212). It is of interest to understand how TCR signaling mediates the distinct degranulation versus FasL mRNA upregulation responses, and how the latter is distinctly regulated from cytokine genes such as interferon-γ.

Although one possibility is that qualitatively identical signals trigger degranulation and FasL upregulation with potentially different thresholds, it is also possible that qualitatively different signaling is required. In support of the latter, several studies of CD8$^+$ CTL clones have shown that although the original peptide used for generating these CTLs induced both the granule exocytosis and FasL/Fas pathways of target lysis, the FasL/Fas pathway can be selectively triggered by altered peptide ligands (213–215). These results parallel findings with such variant peptides in differentially inducing responses in CD4$^+$ T cells (216). Further evidence for qualitatively different signaling for the two cytotoxicity pathways comes from studies of a granule-bearing CD8$^+$ influenza HA-specific CTL clone variant that lost its ability to kill by granule exocytosis and was found to retain the ability to kill via the FasL/Fas pathway and secrete interferon-γ (217). This variant clone had an unusually high resting intracellular calcium level but little or no TCR-induced calcium increase. Thus, distinct signaling requirements were inferred for the two cytotoxicity pathways.

Target Cell Death by Fas Cross-linking

The target cell events in the FasL/Fas cytotoxic pathway begins with cross-linking of target cell Fas by FasL on the effector cell. This phase of target cell death does not require macromolecular synthesis or extracellular calcium. Because FasL appears to be trimeric (218), it provides a potent ability to cross-link Fas and trigger the signals leading to a target cell apoptotic response. As described in detail in Chapter 22, Fas cross-linking leads to activation of intracellular caspases via FADD. Studies with caspase inhibitors show that CTL-induced target lysis and nuclear damage via the FasL/Fas pathway are caspase dependent (164). The postcaspase events in this death process are still undefined but are presumed to be common to other apoptotic death pathways.

Studies of lymphocyte death induced by Fas cross-linking make it clear that surface expression of Fas does not ensure target susceptibility to death by Fas cross-linking, and there appear to be unexplained susceptibility factors operating. Thus, T-lymphocytes are resistant to Fas-induced death for some time after activation despite adequate Fas expression (218,219), and cytokines can protect against apoptotic death of B-lymphocytes by Fas cross-linking (220). Because Bcl-2 blocks Fas-mediated death inefficiently (221), other susceptibility factors such as Bcl-x (222) may be responsible. Such factors may influence death in other target cells via the FasL/Fas pathway.

Bystander Lysis by the Fas/FasL Pathway

Depending on the polarity and kinetics of FasL surface expression and downregulation after TCR engagement, this cytotoxicity pathway may give rise to bystander lysis of Fas$^+$ target cells. Minimal bystander lysis is expected if (a) FasL surface expression is polarized so that it occurs only in the junctional region where the antigenic target cell is bound and (b) FasL expression is highly transient so that it is downregulated by the time the CTL detaches from the bound target. Using a long-term CTL line from perforin-deficient mice, one study reported minimal bystander lysis by the FasL/Fas pathway (223). However, another study detected considerable bystander lysis by this pathway (18), and given the above considerations, the occurrence of bystander lysis may be dependent on the particular effectors and bystanders.

PROPERTIES OF CYTOTOXIC LYMPHOCYTES

Classical CTLs Are CD8$^+$ T Cells Recognizing Target Cells via Their TCR

The major CTL responses to alloimmunization and viral infection are due to CD8$^+$ T cells in which cytotoxicity is triggered by the αβ TCR recognizing complexes of peptide antigen and MHC class I. The discovery that virus-specific CTL recognition of target cells is restricted by MHC class I historically provided the basis for the present concept of TCR recognition (23). Virtually all older studies on CTL mechanisms used such CD8$^+$ CTLs. The availability of monoclonal antibodies against CD8 allowed the demonstration that most CTL effector cells express this surface marker and that CD8$^+$ T cells are required in vivo for antiviral host defense (224).

Although normally they comprise only a minor component of CTL responses, γδ CTLs can play important functional roles in responses to particular antigens. Such CTLs may have unusual properties (225), but have been reported to use the granule exocytosis pathway (36).

CD4$^+$ CTLs

Despite abundant results indicating that CD8$^+$ T cells dominate the CTL response under most activation conditions, it is clear that CD4$^+$ T cells can become cytotoxic in some circumstances, particularly via the FasL/Fas pathway. However, they also have the potential to express the granule exocytosis pathway. When CD8$^+$ T cells are removed from the responding population of an in vitro mixed lymphocyte culture, CD4$^+$ T cells respond to allostimulation by becoming cytotoxic, and such cells predominantly use the granule exocytosis pathway (226). Similarly, if viral antigens are presented in vitro on class II but not class I MHC molecules, CD4$^+$ T cells can respond by becoming cytotoxic, e.g., in β2 microglobulin knock-out mice, which develop only minimal numbers of CD8$^+$ T cells. Such mice respond to LCMV and Sendai virus infection with CD4$^+$ CTLs instead of the CD8$^+$ CTLs characteristic of their normal counterparts (227). These results imply a negative regulatory influence of the CD8$^+$ T-cell response on the ability of CD4$^+$ T cells to differentiate into CTLs.

CD4$^+$ T cells can express Fas ligand transiently after TCR cross-linking, and most of the cytotoxic activity associated with this lymphocyte subpopulation is thought to be attributable to this pathway (228). Because of the great potential for such cytotoxic effects regulating immune responses, it is important to understand the details of FasL regulation in normal T-lymphocytes. CD4$^+$ T-cell clones responding to soluble antigens presented on class II antigens often have been found to be cytotoxic to target cells bearing the appropriate antigen, including APCs. Among clones with the Th1 cytokine profile (228,229), many have been found to use the FasL/Fas cytotoxic pathway.

CD4$^+$ CTLs may have the ability to regulate immune responses by killing APCs that are required for the activation of other lymphocytes. Cloned CD4$^+$ CTLs recognizing peptides from a soluble protein carrier have been shown to specifically reduce an *in vitro* antihapten antibody response based on that carrier (230). Thus, some suppressor T cells may actually be cytotoxic T cells that lyse antigen-presenting T cells. Similarly, CD4$^+$ CTL can potentially regulate antibody responses by killing B cells bearing antigenic peptide complexed to MHC class II. However, antigen binding by B-cell surface immunoglobulin M has been shown to protect B cells against the FasL/Fas cytotoxicity pathway, an effect not found when B cells were stimulated by CD40 ligand (231). These experiments demonstrate that CD4$^+$ CTLs have the potential to regulate immune responses *in vivo*.

CTLs Can Detect a Small Number of Peptide–MHC Complexes on Target Cells

With the molecular definition of the peptide-MHC complexes recognized by particular cloned CTLs, it has become possible to estimate the number of such complexes required for target recognition leading to lysis. A mass action law predicts the ability of cloned CTLs to lyse targets, such that for moderate TCR affinities the product of TCR affinity and epitope density (peptide–MHC complexes per cell) is constant (232,233). At high TCR affinities, a ceiling is reached and the epitope density required for half-maximal lysis was estimated at less than 10 peptide–MHC complexes per cell. Using a highly radioactive labeled peptide, binding studies were combined with target lysis measurements. At titrated peptide concentration where 50% of the target cells were lysed, most cells had an epitope density of fewer than five complexes per cell, leading to a suggestion that a single complex can trigger a cytolytic response (234).

Using a peptide titration approach, the CTL cytotoxic response appears to have a particularly low sensitivity threshold compared with other TCR-triggered responses. Thus, a CTL clone gave a half-maximal cytotoxic response at about 10^{-11} M peptide, whereas the half-maximal concentrations for the interferon-γ response, the CD3 downregulation response, and the Ca$_i$ increase were about 10^{-8} M peptide (235). Other studies estimated that the interferon-γ response threshold of CTL clones occurred at about three to five peptide–MHC complexes on the APC–target cell (236).

The above studies of cytotoxicity by peptide-specific CTLs did not distinguish between the granule exocytosis and FasL/Fas pathways, and the possibility must be considered that these two pathways may have different TCR signaling thresholds. Recent results with several different CD4$^+$ T-cell clones recognizing the same peptide suggest that there is a consistent hierarchy of TCR thresholds for different T-cell responses (237). For both the original and variant peptides recognized by the TCR, target cell killing via the granule exocytosis pathway is at the sensitive end of that hierarchy, requiring minimal concentrations of peptide for cytolysis, whereas cytolysis by the FasL/Fas pathway is at the least sensitive end of that hierarchy. The thresholds for secretion of several cytokines were intermediate between those of the two cytotoxicity pathways.

Thus, receptor-induced signaling for degranulation may have a lower threshold than other responses requiring transcriptional activation in the same cells.

Redirected Lysis by CTLs

A number of means have been developed to redirect the normal TCR-based recognition of target cells (238). The simplest approach is the use of TCR-binding lectins such as ConA or phytohemagglutinin, which agglutinate targets to CTL while crosslinking the TCR. A more selective approach is to use target cells bearing IgG Fc receptors (e.g., the classical CTL target P815 mastocytoma) and IgG monoclonal antibodies against the TCR complex on the CTL. Binding of such antibodies to the target FcR leaves it coated with anti-TCR antibodies that cross-link this receptor on CTLs. More elaborate approaches to redirected cytotoxicity include creation of bispecific antibodies that bind both TCR and target cell (239) by chemically cross-linking antireceptor and antitarget antibodies, producing hybrid hybridomas with one antibody V region recognizing the TCR and the other target antigen, or using recombinant technology to produce a single-chain bispecific antibody (240).

Redirected cytotoxicity can be used to show that CTLs are capable of lysing such simple target cells as nonnucleated red cells (241) or other cells bearing no appropriate MHC antigens. In addition to its use as a laboratory tool, approaches involving bifunctional antibodies with tumor specificity have been proposed for *in vivo* tumor therapy (242).

Some CTLs Recognize Target Cells by Receptors Other than the TCR

Although the TCR is generally the major means by which target cells are triggered for cytotoxicity, in some cases other receptors can play this role. For example, CD44 can redirect the lysis of some human CTLs (243), and a combination of B7.1 and ICAM overexpression on target cells triggers TCR-independent lysis (244). By culturing cloned CTLs with classical TCR-mediated, MHC-restricted target recognition in high levels of IL-2, the CTL lines become promiscuous, killing many tumor targets regardless of the original CTL specificity. This altered recognition appears similar to that shown by lymphokine-activated killer (LAK) cells, resulting from culture of NK cells with high levels of IL-2 (245).

Generation of CTLs

The description of CTLs in this chapter refers to T cells that have become differentiated *in vivo* or *in vitro* to become effector CTLs. This differentiation process normally takes place in response to antigen and represents a major difference between CTLs and NK cells, which are found in a differentiated state in naive lymphoid tissue. The differentiation process giving rise to effector T cells begins with naive CTL precursors (nCTLp) and involves a substantial development of secretory granules and their protein components as well as an enhancement of functional TCR-induced FasL expression. The CD8$^+$ population of T cells giving rise to CTLs shows parallels in this differentiation with the CD4$^+$ population, which has been studied principally with respect to cytokine secretion (246).

In Vivo

Early studies with mouse allografts showed that allospecific CTLs with *ex vivo* cytotoxic activity could be detected in lymphoid organs after graft rejection. A particularly enriched and highly active alloreactive CTL population was identified in peritoneal exudates after rejection of intraperitoneal allogeneic tumors (98). It has been estimated that such CTLs represent close to 50% of the lymphocytes in such populations. Testing lymphocytes in the exudate shows that this CTL response increases rapidly 5 to 10 days after tumor innoculation and decreases slowly starting at about 2 weeks, which correlates with the disappearance of the tumor. The differentiation of such CTLs has been difficult to study in this *in vivo* system. Other types of allografts also give rise to CTL generation *in vivo*, generally correlating with rejection. However, difficulties in purifying lymphocytes infiltrating most engrafted organs has hampered their study, and draining lymph nodes are often a more convenient source of active CTLs. One useful system for studying allogeneic or xenogeneic CTLs *in vivo* is the sponge matrix allograft in which plastic sponges coated with foreign fibroblasts are implanted into mice. The infiltrating lymphocytes including CTLs can be expelled from the sponge after removal from the animal and studied *in vitro* (247).

Murine virus-specific CTLs become detectable in the spleen after infection with some viruses (e.g., LCMV or ectromelia), and this response generally correlates well with the resolution of the infection (248). In humans, HIV-specific CTLs are detectable in the blood of infected individuals (249). However, in most cases of viral infection, CTLs are not detectable by assaying murine splenocytes or human peripheral blood lymphocytes directly *ex vivo*. They may be detectable at the site of infection or in the regional lymph nodes draining the site of infection (250). However, after resolution of the infection, an increased frequency of CTL precursors (CTLp) becomes detectable in the spleen or blood if CTL activity is measured after a secondary *in vitro* stimulation culture. These memory CTLs (mCTLs) are considered further below.

The decline in effector CTL detectable directly *ex vivo* after resolution of a viral infection appears to be due to the *in vivo* death of CTLs. Apoptotic CD8$^+$ T cells are detectable *in vivo*, and the number of such dying cells peaks during the decline of the CTL response (251). Evidence against the hypothesis that this occurs via the FasL/Fas pathway was obtained when lpr and gld mice were LCMV infected and found to show normal levels of CD8$^+$ T-cell apoptosis and decline in LCMV-specific CTLs (252).

Recently it has been shown that protein and peptide antigens recognized by CTLs can be used to induce pCTLs *in vivo*. Intravenous injection of antigenic MHC class I–binding peptides can specifically prime spleen T cells for subsequent *in vitro* induction of antipeptide CTLs (253). *In vitro* pulsing of dendritic cells with protein antigens followed by injection into mouse foot pads gives rise to primed CTLs in lymph nodes draining the site of injection (254). Similar peptide pulsing of dendritic cells is capable of priming spleen cells for subsequent *in vitro* CTL induction (255) or inducing CTLs that protect mice against tumors expressing the peptide (256).

Although vaccines have traditionally been designed to stimulate the formation of antibodies *in vivo*, interest recently has focused on vaccines to elicit CTLs as well. A number of promising approaches have been developed using various forms of antigen and adjuvants, which are discussed in Chapter 41.

In Vitro

The classic *in vitro* source of alloreactive CTLs is from short-term mixed lymphocyte cultures in which irradiated spleen stimulator cells are cocultured with spleen cells of a different MHC haplotype (257). In such cultures, CTL activity becomes detectable in 3 to 4 days and peaks at 5 to 6 days. The active CTLs are CD8$^+$ blasts. With further culture, activity declines slowly, with no obvious increase in cell death observable in the culture. After a rest, the cells can be restimulated to obtain a more enriched secondary effector cell population, and such cultures can be maintained in IL-2 with periodic restimulation. Using limiting dilutions, cloned cells can be obtained, expanded, and propagated for years.

In vitro generation of virus-specific CTL cultures has classically been initiated using T cells from mice that have been previously primed *in vivo* by a viral infection. Subsequent stimulation by viral antigen expressed in syngeneic infected or transfected cells *in vitro* gives rise to CTLs recognizing viral antigen. However, when dendritic cells are used to present antigen, primary *in vitro* CTL responses can be generated against viral antigens (258).

As discussed above, immunization of mice with peptides can specifically prime T cells to generate CTLs *in vitro*. CTLs also can be induced directly *in vitro* with MHC class I–binding peptides, particularly when dendritic cells are used as presenting cells (259, 260).

Cytokine Regulation of CTL Generation

When tested for their ability to enhance CTL generation when added to MLR cultures, several recombinant cytokines can be seen to significantly enhance CTL activity measured at the end of culture. These include IL-2 (261), IL-4 (262), IL-7 (263), IL-10 (264), IL-12 (265), and IL-15 (266). The extent of enhancement appears to depend on the particular antigen and responding cell populations used, but IL-2 is a particularly potent inducer of cytotoxicity in such experiments. The observed effects can be accounted for by a combination of a differentiation effect (inducing expression of relevant genes) and a more efficient growth of individual CTL clones responding to antigen. Other cytokines may negatively regulate the differentiation of lymphocyte cytotoxicity. For example, transforming growth factor-beta has the ability to block the IL-2–mediated enhancement of cytotoxicity and granule protein upregulation *in vitro* (267).

In order to determine which endogenously produced cytokines are important for CTL generation, the effect of adding anticytokine antibodies to such cultures has been examined, and lymphocytes from knock-out mice selectively lacking cytokines have been tested. These results point to IL-2 as the one critically important endogenous cytokine because cells from IL-2–deficient mice show compromised CTL production *in vitro* (268) and addition of anti–IL-2 (269) or anti–IL-2R (270) antibodies have been shown to block CTL generation.

Costimulation Requirement for CTL Generation from Naive Precursors

The simplest system for studying CTL generation is to start with a purified population of small resting naive CD8$^+$ T cells and determine what conditions are required to drive their differentiation into cytotoxic effectors (271). The starting population has no cytotoxic activity by redirected assay using anti-CD3, nor does it

TABLE 2. *CTL/CTLp accessory molecules*

T-cell receptor/target (APC) ligand	Adhesion molecule: CTL effector/target	Costimulatory molecule: CTLp/APC
CD28/B7-1,B7-2	No	Yes
LFA-1/ICAM	Yes	Yes
CD2/LFA-3	Yes	Yes
X/HSA	No	Yes (?CTL mem)
X/CD44	No	Yes
X/DNAM-1	Yes	?
CD8/MHC I	Yes	?

have detectable levels of the granule mediator proteins perforin or granzymes. When incubated with anti-CD3 coated target cells bearing B7-1, cytotoxicity could be detected starting at 6 hours. This slow-starting cytotoxicity has several properties that strongly contrast to normal CTL effectors: (a) it is dependent on target cell B7-1 expression; (b) it is blocked by anti-CD28 antibodies; and (c) it is inhibited by inhibitors of RNA and protein synthesis. Thus, in this system functional CTLs were generated within several hours in response to TCR stimulation and CD28 costimulation. The requirement for costimulation appears to be a clear distinction between nCTLp and differentiated CTL effectors, which show no similar requirement for target recognition. Such CD8$^+$ nCTLp are thus similar to naive CD4$^+$ T cells in their requirement for costimulation for some cytokine responses. However, IL-2 cannot overcome the costimulation requirement for CTLp differentiation (272). More complex *in vitro* and *in vivo* systems measuring CTL generation have confirmed the requirement for costimulation in order to generate CTLs from CTLp. The importance of CD28 in generating costimulation signals is demonstrated by the blocking of CTL generation by CTLA4Ig (273), which avidly binds CD28 and blocks its engagement with ligands on antigen-bearing cells. However, other receptor–ligand pairs also have the ability to costimulate CTLp with antigen to drive their differentiation to CTL in some experimental systems. As shown in Table 2, these include CD2/LFA-3 (274) and heat-stable antigen on macrophages (275).

Memory CTLs

Memory CTLs can be defined as those T cells present in immunized animals which give rise to progeny CTLs comprising the enhanced cytotoxic response after a subsequent challenge. They are thus an alternative form of CTLp to nCTLp, and in practical terms mCTLs are similar to nCTLp in that they are defined by their ability to give rise to cytolytically active effector CTLs after restimulation with antigen, typically *in vitro*. CTLp are typically assayed by limiting dilution assays in which T cells are diluted into wells containing APCs and cultured for 5 to 7 days, and the frequency of wells containing CTL activity is determined by adding target cells to wells. In most systems, unimmunized animals have a small or undetectable frequency of CTLp so that any increase in response to immunization becomes defined as the mCTL population. For example, for virus-specific CTLp, spleen cells from unimmunized animals typically contain nCTLp at a frequency of 10^{-6}, which increases to 10^{-3} to 10^{-2} during viral infection when

effector CTL are included, and then decreases back to 10^{-5} to 10^{-4} with time (276). The net 10- to 100-fold increase in CTLp frequency after the infection thus comprises mCTLs. This increase accounts for at least part of the overall enhanced immune memory response to viruses, allowing more rapid and stronger development of CTL responses after priming. The decline in CTLp frequency from its peak during the infection to the stable level maintained after infection is attributable to apoptotic death.

Because limiting dilution assays do not allow a direct means of analyzing CTLp, their characterization is largely limited to analysis of their surface phenotype by sorting or depleting cells reacting with antibodies before the restimulation culture. Virus-specific mCTLs are CD8$^+$, CD44^{hi}, and variable in their expression of L-selectin and CD25 (250,277). No distinctive surface marker identifying functionally defined mCTLs has been described because the above markers also may reside on previously activated T cells that cannot differentiate into CTLs. There is currently considerable debate about the requirement for antigen and the need for cell cycling for the maintenance of mCTLs *in vivo* (276,278). As is found for nCTLp, induction of CTLs from mCTLs *in vitro* requires B7-1 costimulation (279).

The pathways of differentiation of mCTLs from nCTLp have been investigated both *in vivo* and *in vitro*. However, the basic question of whether mCTLs are derived from CTLs or arise directly from an antigen-responsive CD8$^+$ progenitor is still the subject of debate (278,280). Because there are no specific surface markers distinguishing CTLs and mCTLs, the most direct experiments are not possible. Because CTLs and mCTLs share memory/activation markers such as CD44 and because the decline of CTL activity in MLR cultures *in vitro* is not accompanied by detectable cell death, it has been assumed that CTLs give rise to mCTLs (281). However, recent experiments examining the induction of memory and effector CTL responses to influenza in the absence of CD28-mediated costimulation indicate that mCTLs can be induced from nCTLp without detectable CTL intermediates when stimulated by antigen and the weaker HSA costimulator (279).

LYMPHOCYTE CYTOTOXICITY *IN VIVO*

Although cytotoxic lymphocytes are defined by their *in vitro* activity, their potential *in vivo* activities have provided the major motivation for the intense interest in their mechanism of action. However, *in vivo* studies of cell death have proven difficult. Histological studies often do not reveal dying cells in circumstances where a high rate of cell death is predicted from other studies. For example, most thymocytes die during the course of normal development, but until sensitive assays measuring apoptotic DNA fragmentation *in situ* were used (282), cell death was not apparent in sections of normal thymus tissue. An explanation for this has emerged from the recognition that an important feature of apoptotic death is the consequent recognition and phagocytosis of dying cells by tissue macrophages. Because both lymphocyte cytotoxicity pathways typically induce apoptotic features in their target cells, it is likely that lymphocyte cytotoxicity is difficult to observe by histology. Even when sensitive DNA fragmentation assays are applied under conditions where substantial CTL-induced death is expected, only a small number of apoptotic cells may be observable before phagocytosis destroys the evidence. Studies of liver destruction by adoptively transferred hepatitis B–specific cloned CTLs have shown that hepatocyte death is detectable by the release of liver enzymes into the circulation (283). In this case of acute CTL-mediated death, careful histologic examination shows some apoptotic hepatocytes associated with CTLs.

One approach to show *in vivo* function for lymphocytes generally is adoptive transfer to naive animals of *in vitro*–characterized lymphocyte populations and examination of the recipients for the *in vivo* response of interest. With respect to the cytotoxic function of CTLs and NK cells, this approach has the problem that the injected cytotoxic lymphocytes themselves secrete cytokines and potentially perform other functions as well as mediate cytotoxicity. A particular problem is that CTLs and NK cells are major sources of interferon-γ, which is known to stimulate macrophages to become cytotoxic. Thus, the adoptive transfer approach can identify lymphocyte phenotypes required for *in vivo* events but leaves open the nature of the effector cells and the mechanism of *in vivo* cell death.

The difficulties in measuring cell death *in vivo* can give rise to misleading conclusions in considering the effects of adoptively transferred CTLs. Thus, in the murine hepatitis B model system, *in vivo* injection of CTL results in detectable hepatocyte lysis and eliminates viral replication (284). However, viral replication in the liver was abolished by antibodies against interferon-γ and TNF, which did not influence hepatocyte lysis (284). Furthermore, perforin-deficient CTLs failed to kill the hepatocytes but did abolish viral replication. Thus, in this model, CTL-induced cytokine secretion but not cytotoxicity appears to play a major role in viral protection (285). Furthermore, in some cases of viral infection, CTL-induced cytotoxicity appears to play a major role in the pathogenic consequences of viral infection (286).

One immunologic approach to cancer therapy involves adoptive transfer of cytotoxic lymphocytes specific for the tumor into patients (287). With the increasing identification of tumor antigens that can be recognized by CTLs (see Chapter 36), the prospect of a vaccine designed to elicit tumor-specific CTLs becomes more appealing. The culture of tumor-infiltrating lymphocytes (TILs) has been accomplished from surgical specimens of tumor to allow the treatment of patients with more than 10^{11} cells resulting from *in vitro* expansion (288). Clinical tumor regression is most often seen with melanomas, and the probability of such a successful response was noted to correlate with the *in vitro* cytotoxic activity against autologous tumor cells (as well as cytokine secretion) (289).

Studies of Mice Lacking Cytotoxic Mediators

As discussed above, several laboratories have prepared perforin defective mice by targeted gene disruption of embryonic stem cells, and these have been the source of a number of important *in vivo* studies as well as providing a source of CTLs crippled in the granule exocytosis pathway. Similarly, the mutant mice defective in the FasL/Fas pathway can reveal *in vivo* functions of this cytotoxicity pathway, but in this case other alterations in the control of immune responses discussed below complicate interpretation of this line of experiments. In addition to the major biologic processes where *in vivo* CTL-induced death had been implicated, CTL-induced death of antigen-reactive T cells or of APCs has been proposed to regulate immune responses. Study of immune responses of mice defective in the perforin or FasL/Fas cytotoxicty pathways allows the most meaningful approach to assessment of CTL function *in vivo*.

Effects on Normal Physiology and Regulation of Immune Responses

Perforin-deficient mice appear to have normal fertility and life spans under laboratory conditions (144). Analysis of lymphocyte numbers and phenotypes as well as histology of various lymphoid organs indicate no detectable differences from normal immune systems, although perforin-defective mice may have more activated macrophages and higher cytokine production levels in the absence of experimental infection, perhaps as a result of subclinical bacterial infections attributable to immune defects (223). Activation of T cells by alloantigen or virus showed normal cell proliferation and expansion of the CD8+ T cell subset. Granzyme content and TCR-induced exocytosis also were found to be normal in perforin-deficient animals (223). These studies suggest that perforin does not play a significant role in overall normal physiology or general lymphocyte homeostasis. No enhanced immune responses attributable to negative regulatory activities have been reported in perforin-deficient mice *in vivo*, but in cultures where APCs are limiting, CD8+ but not CD4+ T cells from such mice have enhanced proliferative and cytokine secretion responses to antigen *in vitro* (290). This effect is attributable to killing of the APC by the granule exocytosis pathway.

A surprising result of studies examining perforin mRNA expression *in vivo* was that pregnant mice express perforin in the granular metrial gland, an organ not found in humans. The cells of this gland appear to be NK-like by phenotypic markers and have been proposed to use their cytotoxic activity during normal embryonic physiology. However, the normal fertility of perforin-deficient inbred mice argues against a vital physiologic role for such cytotoxicity activity, despite differences in the histology of the uterus and placenta compared with normal animals (226).

Mice defective in Fas (lpr) and FasL (gld) arose by spontaneous mutation and were studied for their lymphoproliferative phenotype before identification of the molecular basis of these defects (291). Several considerations suggest caution in interpreting results with these mice as due to defects in the FasL/Fas lymphocyte cytotoxicity pathway. FasL is expressed on cells other than cytotoxic lymphocytes, and such expression has been proposed to alter immune responses (208), and Fas has been proposed to have functions other than cytotoxicity (206). Both gld and lpr strains show similar phenotypes characterized by lymphadenopathy and splenomegaly increasing with age. The enlarged organs become populated by nonfunctional lymphocytes, which complicate experimental use of these mice. However, young lpr and gld mice have minimal lymphoproliferative disease, and these animals appear more suitable for experiments examining the role of the FasL/Fas death pathway. However, double-deficient mice in which perforin knock-out mice are crossed with gld mice show a more dramatic and lethal autoimmune disease, making their use in experiments very difficult (292).

Mice defective in either granzyme A or granzyme B by targeted gene disruption have been reported to have normal fertility, life span, and lymphoid cell development (148,150), as expected if these proteases function exclusively in cytotoxic lymphocyte granules.

In addition to the granule exocytosis and FasL/Fas-dependent pathways that are dominant in *in vitro* cytotoxicity, TNF-α and lymphotoxin (LT, TNF-β) must be considered as potential mediators of lymphocyte cytotoxicity *in vivo*. Although traditionally known for their selective *in vitro* cytotoxic activity on tumor cells, these cytokines are cytotoxic for activated T-lymphocytes (293, 294) and may well be cytotoxic to other normal cells *in vivo*. Effects of anti-TNF antibodies or the use TNF/TNFR-deficient mice cannot readily be interpreted as attributable to TNF from CTLs because macrophages are the major *in vivo* source of TNF. LT had been considered as a candidate CTL lethal mediator, but studies of LT-deficient mice show normal *in vitro* CTL function despite a gross defect in lymph node structure (295).

In Vivo Resistance to Infections and Infection-Induced Immunopathology

Because CTLs had long been shown to be capable of lysing cells infected with viruses and intracellular bacteria *in vitro*, the ability of perforin-deficient mice to resist infection has been tested with a number of viruses and bacteria. Intravenous injection of the non-cytopathic virus LCMV was previously found to be cleared by CD8$^+$ T cells, which also cause an immunopathogenic hepatitis (286). In perforin-deficient mice, intravenous LCMV doses that are cleared in normal mice cause a wasting disease and death, with no hepatitis. When perforin-deficient mice expressing high numbers of LCMV-recognizing CD8$^+$ T cells were constructed, there was no evidence that these cells were capable of protecting mice from LCMV infections, nor was priming with LCMV antigen effective in overcoming this functional defect (296). In normal mice, intracerebral LCMV injection causes a lethal choriomeningitis mediated chiefly by CD8$^+$ T cells, whereas in perforin-deficient mice such viral injections were accompanied by weight loss without lethality (144). Thus, a perforin-dependent process is required for this immunopathogenic response. In contrast to perforin-deficient mice, both lpr and gld mice had no detectable alterations in their responses to LCMV infection compared with controls, including both viral protection and immunopathology (296).

Cytopathic viruses that kill their host cells in the process of replication appear not to be controlled by lymphocyte cytotoxicity. Infection of perforin-deficient mice with the cytopathic viruses vaccinia, vesicular stomatitis virus, and Semliki forest virus showed normal levels of protection (297), and a similar result was obtained when gld mice were tested (297).

Of several mouse models for infection by intracellular bacteria, *Listeria monocytogenes* is known to be principally controlled by macrophages activated by interferon-γ. When perforin-defective mice were compared with controls for their ability to resist *Listeria* infection, at high doses of bacteria there was no difference in survival, whereas at low doses there was a modest delay in bacterial clearance from the spleen but not liver. However, when primed by a sublethal infection, perforin-defective mice showed a 10-fold and 100-fold defect in their ability to clear a secondary *Listeria* challenge from spleen and liver, respectively (298). Perforin-deficient as well as gld mice have been examined for their ability to resist infections by mycobacteria, a model for human tuberculosis. Using both the nonvirulent *Mycobacterium bovis* and the virulent *Mycobacterium tuberculosis*, it was found that neither perforin-defective nor gld mice had detectable differences in the numbers of bacteria in the lungs, liver, or spleen after intravenous injection of the mycobacteria (299). Thus lymphocyte-mediated cytotoxicity does not appear to play a required role in the normal resistance to these infections, although studies with β2 microglobulin–deficient mice has suggested that CD8$^+$ T cells confer protection (300).

Although granzyme A–deficient CTLs have no detectable defect in cytotoxic function (150), granzyme A–deficient mice were tested for their ability to resist infection with the cytopathic virus ectromelia (301), for which protection by CD8$^+$ T cells and NK cells had been previously shown. Although a normal virus-specific CTL response was elicited in spleen T cells by this infection in both normal and granzyme A–defective mice, virus growth was dramatically greater in the granzyme A–defective mice in both spleen and liver, with a lethality not seen in controls. These experiments suggest that a noncytotoxic function of granzyme A may be important to *in vivo* virus protection, although it is possible that the target cells used in the *in vitro* experiments were not representative of the cells critical to *in vitro* protection.

Allograft Rejection

Perforin- and FasL/Fas-deficient mice have been used as organ donors and recipients to assess whether these cytotoxicity pathways play a role in immune-based rejection phenomena. It was found that allogeneic grafts differing at MHC class I, MHC class II, fully allogeneic, and xenogeneic rat skin allografts were rejected normally by both perforin-deficient and gld mice (302). Skin grafts from allogeneic lpr mice were also rejected normally. Thus, it appears that the two major pathways of lymphocyte-mediated cytotoxicity are not required for such skin graft rejection.

Similar results were obtained with transplantation of pancreatic islet cells in mice. Perforin-deficient recipients rejected fully allogeneic pancreatic islet cell grafts identically to control recipients, whereas syngeneic grafts were accepted. Allogeneic lpr donor islet cells were also rejected normally by perforin-deficient recipients (303), indicating that neither of the two cytotoxicity pathways nor a combination is required for such rejection.

Vascularized fully allogeneic heart grafts were acutely rejected by perforin-deficient as well as normal mice within 6 days, and similar mononuclear infiltrates were found in the rejecting tissue in both cases (304). Allospecific CTLs were generated in response to such grafts in the normal but not perforin-deficient mice. However, when such heart grafts were performed with mice differing at only MHC class I, perforin-defective recipient mice showed prolonged graft survival compared with control mice (88 versus 31-day mean survival) (304). The role of the FasL/Fas pathway in this cardiac allograft model was tested using gld and lpr mice as donors and recipients (305). Cardiac myocytes from normal but not lpr mice were found to express functional Fas and gld recipients showed slower rejection of cardiac allografts. However, the role of the FasL/Fas pathway could not be inferred from these results because hearts from allogeneic lpr mice were quickly rejected as controls, and lpr recipients showed delayed rejection. These results suggest that the general immune disorder in these mutant mice may account for the observed differences in graft rejection rather than a specific defect in the FasL/Fas pathway of lymphocyte-mediated cytotoxicity. The perforin knock-out results with this model of the heart allograft system suggest that different tissues may have different rejection mechanisms.

Fas-negative, TNF-resistant allogeneic tumors were found to be rejected normally in perforin-defective mice, although CTLs were generated as expected from the normal controls (306). Thus, the data make it clear that perforin-dependent cytotoxicity is not the major mediator of rejection of allogeneic or xenogeneic tissue in most cases, although this pathway does appear to play a significant role in some models with clinical relevance such as heart transplants.

Graft-Versus-Host Disease

Graft-versus-host disease (GVHD), due to an immunologic attack by transplanted foreign lymphocytes on the host, has been studied using donor mice defective in both major cytotoxic pathways. Perforin-deficient T cells from fully allogeneic mice or MHC-matched mice differing at minor histocompatibility loci induced all symptoms of acute lethal GVHD but with delayed kinetics (292,307). In contrast, when similar graft of T cells from gld mice was given, cachexia and lethality were intact (although delayed), but no evidence of the characteristic skin pathology was observed (307). The profound lymphoid hyperplasia and B-cell functional defects associated with this GVHD model were fully present in perforin-defective mice but absent in gld mice (308). These results show that lymphocyte cytotoxicity plays a major role in GVHD pathology, and that both cytotoxicity pathways are used in these in vivo models.

The function of granzyme B in GVHD was tested using the murine model of lethal GVHD induced by allogeneic T cells (309). The lethal disease induced by CD8+ class I mismatched T cells was found to be significantly less potent with granzyme B–deficient cells compared with normals. However, a parallel GVHD induced by CD4+ T cells was normal. To test the role of granzyme B function in NK cells in vivo, a hybrid resistance model measuring engraftment of parental bone marrow into F2 hybrid hosts was used. Granzyme B deficient hosts showed full resistance to these grafts despite their compromised CTL-induced target DNA damage in vitro.

Autoimmune Disease

The role of cytotoxic lymphocytes in autoimmune diabetes has been tested using perforin-deficient mice in a transgenic model in which LCMV glycoprotein is expressed in pancreatic beta cells (310). In normal transgenic mice, such LCMV expression leads to a T-cell response resulting in the rapid development of diabetes, whereas in perforin-deficient transgenic mice, no diabetes arose despite demonstrable pancreatitis due to T-cell infiltration of the pancreas. Thus, cytotoxic T cells using the perforin pathway are required for the development of autoimmune diabetes in this model. Interestingly, using this same model system the role of interferon-γ was tested by using LCMV transgenic mice bearing a defective gene for this cytokine (311). No resulting diabetes was observed with these mice either, although anti-LCMV CTL activity was induced. In this case, T-cell infiltration into the pancreas was not observed, nor was the pancreatic MHC class I and II upregulation associated with this inflammation. Thus, it is clear that other aspects of inflammation are also required in order to eliminate functional islet cells.

Another murine diabetes model is available in the nonobese diabetic (NOD) mice strain, which shows a high rate of spontaneous diabetes. When NOD animals expressing the lpr defective form of Fas were prepared, they did not develop diabetes and they were resistant to the rapid diabetogenic effect of injected CD8+ T cells from diabetic mice (312). These data strongly implicate the FasL/Fas pathway in pancreatic β-cell destruction in this model and raise the possibility that different mouse models of diabetes use different effector pathways.

Tumor Immunity

Perforin-deficient mice were found to be highly prone to tumor development after injection of syngeneic fibrosarcoma cells rejected by normal mice in a CD8+ T cell–dependent process (144). Several other tumor lines gave similar results, with 10- to 100-fold more tumor cells required to produce tumors in normal mice than perforin-deficient mice. However, other examples were found in which tumor resistance was normal in perforin-deficient mice (313). Similarly perforin-deficient mice were defective in their ability to control growth of tumors lacking MHC class I expression, which in normal mice occurs via NK cells (314). When mice were first primed with irradiated tumor cells to give tumor immunity as shown by their increased resistance to tumor generation, perforin-deficient mice were clearly defective in this immunity with some tumors but not others (313).

A role for the FasL/Fas cytotoxic pathway in tumor protection in vivo was implicated by the finding that some Fas-transfected tumors were more efficiently rejected with and without priming than their Fas-negative parental tumor cells (313). However, findings that some tumors express FasL that might compromise immune responses by inducing death in Fas-bearing lymphocytes recognizing tumor antigens (208) indicate that the role of this pathway in tumor immunity may be complex.

Treatment of mice with chemical carcinogens or oncogenic viruses and after tumor development over the course of time provides a model of in vivo tumor surveillance. It was found that perforin-deficient mice were clearly more sensitive than control mice to tumors induced by the carcinogen methylcholanthrene, as seen by the occurrence of more tumors at low carcinogen doses and earlier appearance of tumors at all carcinogen doses (313). However, skin papillomas induced by the carcinogen DMBA and the cocarcinogen TPA were not different in perforin-deficient and normal mice, and tumors induced by Moloney sarcoma virus arose with similar kinetics in the two types of mice, whereas rejection was slower in the perforin-deficient case (313). Thus, cytotoxic lymphocytes using a perforin-dependent pathway are implicated in the prevention of tumor development in at least some animal models of immune surveillance.

These studies with perforin-deficient mice confirm that the cytotoxic activity of lymphocytes long studied in vitro is able to mediate the in vivo destruction of tumors, and they support the continued development of tumor therapy based on CTL cytotoxic activity. The role of the FasL/Fas pathway is clearly complex, and it may play a role in suppressing tumor immunity that mediates destruction of tumors. The current evidence does not argue against additional roles for cytokines, which may enhance cytotoxic activity in various ways.

SUMMARY AND CONCLUSIONS

Cytotoxic T and NK lymphocytes have a unique ability to specifically trigger the apoptotic death of target cells in vitro by two distinct processes, both of which are significantly more rapid than the apoptotic cell deaths produced by other agents. Both types of cytotoxic lymphocyte possess cytoplasmic secretory granules that are secreted in a polarized response to target binding in the granule exocytosis cytotoxicity pathway. Target cells bearing Fas also may be killed by the FasL/Fas pathway, which has been characterized chiefly in cytotoxic T-lymphocytes.

The granule exocytosis pathway is initiated when target cell binding induces a rapid polarization of CTL cytoplasm, allowing a secretion of granule mediators into the synapselike junctional region between the CTL and its bound target. Secreted perforin forms pores in target cell membranes, which directly or indirectly allow cosecreted granzymes to enter the target cell cytoplasm

Granzyme B processes and activates target caspases to trigger nuclear damage, but caspase inhibitors do not block target lysis. Thus, the terminal steps in molecular pathway of target cell death remain unknown.

The FasL/Fas cytotoxic pathway used by CTLs is also initiated by TCR cross-linking, which triggers the transcriptional upregulation of Fas ligand in the effector cells. Surface expression of Fas ligand allows efficient cross-linking of target cell Fas, which in turn engages FADD and activates caspase 8 in the target cell cytoplasm. Target cell lysis as well as apoptotic nuclear damage via this pathway is dependent on caspases. The requirement for *de novo* synthesis of Fas ligand means that target cell lysis via the FasL/Fas pathway exhibits a kinetic lag, but this pathway is also rapid compared with other apoptotic death processes.

Studies of mice lacking mediators of the cytotoxic pathways defined by their *in vitro* functional activity provide evidence that lymphocyte cytotoxicity is important to a number of *in vivo* immunologic processes. Perforin-deficient mice are clearly defective in a number of systems in which CTL effectors had been implicated by other studies. They have decreased resistance to infection to the noncytopathic virus LCMV, are resistant to vaccine-conferred protection against *Listeria* infection, are resistant to diabetes triggered by LCMV expressed in pancreatic islets, and are defective in resistance to some transplanted and chemically induced tumors. On the other hand, perforin-deficient mice show normal behavior in other parallel phenomena where CTLs had also been implicated. In particular, rejection of allogeneic transplants is generally normal in perforin-deficient mice. Thus, although perforin-dependent cytotoxicity comprises one element of *in vivo* effector mechanisms, destruction of foreign tissue can occur by other pathways as well.

In vivo studies of the FasL/Fas cytotoxicity pathway are complicated by the role of this pathway in immunoregulatory phenomena. Because mice specifically defective in this pathway have abnormal immune responses, it is difficult to assess the importance of the FasL/Fas pathway as an immune effector mechanism.

REFERENCES

1. Martz E. The 51Cr release assay for CTL-mediated target cell lysis. In: *Cytotoxic cells. Recognition, effector function, generation, and methods.* Boston: Birhauser, 1993:457–467.
2. Sanderson CJ. The uptake and retention of chromium by cells. *Transplantation* 1976;21:526–529.
3. Lichtenfels R, Biddison WE, Schulz H, Vogt AB, Martin R. CARE-LASS (calcein-release assay), an improved fluorescence-based test system to measure cytotoxic T lymphocyte cytotoxicity. *J Immunol Methods* 1994;172:227–239.
4. Blomberg K, Hautala R, Lovgren J, Mukkala VM, Lindqvist C, Akerman K. Time-resolved fluorometric assay for natural killer activity using target cells labelled with a fluorescence enhancing ligand. *J Immunol Methods* 1996;193:199–206.
5. Zinkernagel RM, Haenseler E, Leist T, Cerny A, Hengartner H, Althage A. T cell–mediated hepatitis in mice infected with lymphocytic choriomeningitis virus. Liver cell destruction by H-2 class I–restricted virus-specific cytotoxic T cells as a physiological correlate of the 51Cr-release assay. *J Exp Med* 1986;164:1075–1092.
6. Kyburz D, Speiser DE, Battegay M, Hengartner H, Zinkernagel RM. Lysis of infected cells *in vivo* by antiviral cytolytic T cells demonstrated by release of cell internal viral proteins. *Eur J Immunol* 1993;23:1540–1545.
7. Russell JH, Masakowski V, Rucinsky T, Phillips G. Mechanisms of immune lysis. III. Characterization of the nature and kinetics of the cytotoxic T lymphocyte–induced nuclear lesion in the target. *J Immunol* 1982;128:2087–2094.
8. Matzinger P. The JAM test. A simple assay for DNA fragmentation and cell death. *J Immunol Methods* 1991;145:185–192.
9. Russell JH, Masakowski VR, Dobos CR. Mechanisms of immune lysis. I. Physiological distinction between target cell death mediated by cytotoxic T lymphocytes and antibody plus complement. *J Immunol* 1980;124:1100–1105.
10. Russell JH, Dobos CR. Mechanisms of immune lysis. II. CTL-induced nuclear disintegration of the target begins within minutes of cell contact. *J Immunol* 1980;125:1256–1261.
11. Duke RC, Chervenak R, Cohen JJ. Endogenous endonuclease-induced DNA fragmentation: An early event in cell-mediated cytolysis. *Proc Natl Acad Sci U S A* 1983;80:6361–6365.
12. Sellins KS, Cohen JJ. Cytotoxic T lymphocytes induce different types of DNA damage in target cells of different origins. *J Immunol* 1991;147:795–803.
13. Nishioka WK, Welsh RM. Susceptibility to cytotoxic T lymphocyte–induced apoptosis is a function of the proliferative status of the target. *J Exp Med* 1994;179:769–774.
14. Bryant J, Day R, Whiteside TL, Herberman RB. Calculation of lytic units for the expression of cell-mediated cytotoxicity. *J Immunol Methods* 1992;146:91–103.
15. Cerottini JC, Nordin AA, Brunner KT. Specific *in vitro* cytotoxicity of thymus-derived lymphocytes sensitized to alloantigens. *Nature* 1970;228:1308–1309.
16. Fleischer B. Lysis of bystander target cells after triggering of human cytotoxic T lymphocytes. *Eur J Immunol* 1986;16:1021–1024.
17. Burrows SR, Fernan A, Argaet V, Suhrbier A. Bystander apoptosis induced by CD8+ cytotoxic T cell (CTL) clones: implications for CTL lytic mechanisms. *Int Immunol* 1993;5:1049–1058.
18. Kuwano K, Arai S. Involvement of two distinct killing mechanisms in bystander target cell lysis induced by a cytotoxic T lymphocyte clone. *Cell Immunol* 1996;169:288–293.
19. Rothstein TL, Mage M, Jones G, McHugh LL. Cytotoxic T lymphocyte sequential killing of immobilized allogeneic tumor target cells measured by time-lapse microcinematography. *J Immunol* 1978;121:1652–1656.
20. Sanderson CJ. The mechanism of T cell mediated cytotoxicity. II. Morphological studies of cell death by time-lapse microcinematography. *Proc R Soc Lond* 1976;192:241–255.
21. Zagury D, Bernard J, Thierness N, Feldman M, Berke G. Isolation and characterization of individual functionally reactive cytotoxic T lymphocytes: conjugation, killing and recycling at the single cell level. *Eur J Immunol* 1975;5:818–822.
22. Thorn RM, Henney CS. Studies on the mechanism of lymphocyte mediate cytolysis. VI. A reappraisal of the requirement for protein synthesis during T cell–mediated lysis. *J Immunol* 1976;116:146–149.
23. Zinkernagel RM, Doherty PC. The discovery of MHC restriction. *Immunol Today* 1997;18:14–17.
24. Gillis S, Smith KA. Long term culture of tumor specific cytotoxic T cells. *Nature* 1977;268:154–156.
25. Martz E. Mechanism of specific tumor cell lysis by alloimmune T lymphocytes: resolution and characterization of discrete steps in the cellular interaction. *Contemp Top Immunobiol* 1977;7:301–361.
26. Golstein P, Smith ET. Mechanism of T-cell–mediated cytolysis: the lethal hit stage. *Contemp Top Immunobiol* 1977;7:273–300.
27. Lowin B, Mattman C, Hahne M, Tschopp J. Comparison of Fas(Apo-1/CD95)– and perforin-mediated cytotoxicity in primary T lymphocytes. *Int Immunol* 1996;8:57–63.
28. Kagi D, Vignaux F, Ledermann B, et al. Fas and perforin pathways as major mechanisms of T cell–mediated cytotoxicity. *Science* 1994;265:528–530.
29. Lowin B, Hahne M, Mattmann C, Tschopp J. Cytolytic T-cell cytotoxicity is mediated through perforin and Fas lytic pathways. *Nature* 1994;370:650–652.
30. Kataoka T, Shinohara N, Takayama H, et al. Concanamycin A, a powerful tool for characterization and estimation of contributed perforin- and Fas-based lytic pathways in cell-mediated cytotoxicity. *J Immunol* 1996;156:3678–3686.
31. Stenger S, Mazzaccaro RJ, Uyemura K, et al. Differential effects of cytolytic T cell subsets on intracellular infection. *Science* 1997;276:1684–1687.
32. Ratner A, Clark WR. Role of TNF-α in CD8+ cytotoxic T lymphocyte–mediated lysis. *J Immunol* 1993;150:4303–4314.
33. Burgess TL, Kelly RB. Constitutive and regulated secretion of proteins. *Annu Rev Cell Biol* 1987;3:243–293.
34. Fortier AH, Nacy CA, Sitkovsky MV. Similar molecular requirements for antigen receptor–triggered secretion of interferon and granule enzymes by cytolytic T lymphocytes. *Cell Immunol* 1989;124:64–76.
35. Isaaz S, Baetz K, Olsen K, Podack E, Griffiths GM. Serial killing by cytotoxic T lymphocytes: T cell receptor triggers degranulation, re-filling of the lytic granules and secretion of lytic proteins via a non-granule pathway. *Eur J Immunol* 1995;25:1071–1079.
36. Nakata M, Kawasaki A, Azuma M, et al. Expression of perforin and cytolytic potential of human peripheral blood lymphocyte subpopulations. *Int Immunol* 1992;4:1049–1054.
37. Peters PJ, Borst J, Oorschot V, et al. Cytotoxic T lymphocyte granules are secretory lysosomes, containing both perforin and granzymes. *J Exp Med* 1991;173:1099–1109.
38. Burkhardt JK, Hester S, Lapham CK, Argon Y. The lytic granules of natural killer cells are dual-function organelles combining secretory and pre-lysosomal compartments. *J Cell Biol* 1990;111:2327–2340.
39. Young JD, Cohn ZA, Podack ER. The ninth component of complement and the pore-forming protein (perforin 1) from cytotoxic T cells: structural, immunological, and functional similarities. *Science* 1986;233:184–190.
40. Dourmashkin RR, Deteix P, Simone CB, Henkart PA. Electron microscopic demonstration of lesions on target cell membranes associated with antibody-dependent cytotoxicity. *Clin Exp Immunol* 1980;43:554–560.
41. Podack ER, Dennert G. Assembly of two types of tubules with putative cytolytic function by cloned natural killer cells. *Nature* 1983;302:442–445.
42. Dennert G, Podack ER. Cytolysis by H-2 specific T killer cells. Assembly of tubular complexes on target membranes. *J Exp Med* 1983;157:1483–1495.

43. Shinkai Y, Takio K, Okumura K. Homology of perforin to the ninth component of complement (C9). *Nature* 1988;334:525–527.

44. Lowrey DM, Aebischer T, Olsen K, et al. Cloning, analysis, and expression of murine perforin 1 cDNA, a component of cytolytic T-cell granules with homology to complement component C9. *Proc Natl Acad Sci U S A* 1989;86:247–251.

45. Ishikawa H, Shinkai YI, Yagita H, et al. Molecular cloning of rat cytolysin. *J Immunol* 1989;143:3069–3073.

46. Lichtenheld MG, Olsen KJ, Lu P, et al. Structure and function of human perforin. *Nature* 1988;335:448–451.

47. Nalefski EA, Falke JJ. The C2 domain calcium-binding motif: structural and functional diversity. *Protein Sci* 1996;5:2375–2390.

48. Uellner R, Jones J, Griffiths GM. Perforin is activated by proteolytic cleavage during biosynthesis which reveals a phospholipid binding domain. 1997 (*submitted for publication*).

49. Yagita H, Nakata M, Kawasaki A, Shinkai Y, Okumura K. Role of perforin in lymphocyte-mediated cytolysis. *Adv Immunol* 1992;51:215–242.

50. Peitsch MC, Amiguet P, Guy R, Brunner J, Maizel JV Jr, Tschopp J. Localization and molecular modelling of the membrane-inserted domain of the ninth component of human complement and perforin. *Mol Immunol* 1990;27:589–602.

51. Liu CC, Persechini PM, Young JD. Perforin and lymphocyte-mediated cytolysis. *Immunol Rev* 1995;146:145–175.

52. Liu CC, Persechini PM, Young JD. Characterization of recombinant mouse perforin expressed in insect cells using the baculovirus system. *Biochem Biophys Res Commun* 1994;201:318–325.

53. Liu CC, Persechini PM, Young JD. Expression and characterization of functionally active recombinant perforin produced in insect cells. *J Immunol* 1996;156: 3292–3300.

54. Esser AF. The membrane attack complex of complement. Assembly, structure and cytotoxic activity. *Toxicology* 1994;87:229–247.

55. Ponting CP, Parker PJ. Extending the C2 domain family: C2s in PKCs gamma, epsilon, eta, theta, phospholipases, GAPs, and perforin. *Protein Sci* 1996;5: 162–166.

56. Young JD, Damiano A, DiNome MA, Leong LG, Cohn ZA. Dissociation of membrane binding and lytic activities of the lymphocyte pore-forming protein (perforin). *J Exp Med* 1987;165:1371–1382.

57. Kuta AE, Reynolds CR, Henkart PA. Mechanism of lysis by large granular lymphocyte granule cytolysin: generation of a stable cytolysin-RBC intermediate. *J Immunol* 1989;142:4378–4384.

58. Kuta AE, Bashford CL, Pasternak CA, Reynolds CW, Henkart PA. Characterization of non-lytic cytolysin-membrane intermediates. *Mol Immunol* 1991;28: 1263–1270.

59. Tschopp J, Schäfer S, Masson D, Peitsch MC, Heusser C. Phosphorylcholine acts as a Ca²⁺-dependent receptor molecule for lymphocyte perforin. *Nature* 1989;337:272–274.

60. Blumenthal R, Millard PJ, Henkart MP, Reynolds CW, Henkart PA. Liposomes as targets for granule cytolysin from cytotoxic LGL tumors. *Proc Natl Acad Sci U S A* 1984;81:5551–5555.

61. Damer CK, Creutz CE. Calcium-dependent self-association of synaptotagmin I. *J Neurochem* 1996;67:1661–1668.

62. Henkart P, Blumenthal R. Interaction of lymphocytes with lipid bilayer membranes: a model for the lymphocyte-mediated lysis of target cells. *Proc Natl Acad Sci U S A* 1975;72:2789–2793.

63. Young JD, Nathan CF, Podack ER, Palladino MA, Cohn ZA. Functional channel formation associated with cytotoxic T-cell granules. *Proc Natl Acad Sci U S A* 1986;83:150–154.

64. Simone CB, Henkart P. Permeability changes induced in erythrocyte ghost targets by antibody-dependent cytotoxic effector cells: evidence for membrane pores. *J Immunol* 1980;124:954–963.

65. Sauer H, Pratsch L, Tschopp J, Bhakdi S, Peters R. Functional size of complement and perforin pores compared by confocal laser scanning microscopy and fluorescence microphotolysis. *Biochim Biophys Acta* 1991;1063:137–146.

66. Henkart PA, Millard PJ, Reynolds CW, Henkart MP. Cytotoxic activity of purified cytoplasmic granules from cytotoxic rat LGL tumors. *J Exp Med* 1984; 160:75–93.

67. Podack ER, Konigsberg PJ. Cytolytic T cell granules. Isolation, biochemical and functional characterization. *J Exp Med* 1984;160:695–710.

68. Morgan BP. Complement membrane attack on nucleated cells: resistance, recovery, and non-lethal effects. *Biochem J* 1989;264:1–14.

69. Kim SH, Carney DF, Papadimitriou JC, Shin ML. Effect of osmotic protection on nucleated cell killing by C5b-9: cell death is not affected by the prevention of cell swelling. *Mol Immunol* 1989;26:323–331.

70. Smyth MJ, O'Connor MD, Trapani JA. Granzymes: a variety of serine protease specificities encoded by genetically distinct subfamilies. *J Leukoc Biol* 1996;60: 555–562.

71. Jenne DE, Masson D, Zimmer M, Haefliger JA, Li WH, Tschopp J. Isolation and complete structure of the lymphocyte serine protease granzyme G, a novel member of the granzyme multigene family in murine cytolytic T lymphocytes. Evolutionary origin of lymphocyte proteases. *Biochemistry* 1989;28:7953–7961.

72. Lutzelschwab C, Pejler G, Aveskogh M, Hellman L. Secretory granule proteases is rat mast cells. Cloning of 10 different serine proteases and a carboxypeptidase A from various rat mast cell populations. *J Exp Med* 1997;184: 13–29.

73. Odake S, Kam C-M, Narasimhan L, et al. Human and murine cytotoxic T lymphocyte serine proteases: subsite mapping with peptide thioester substrates and inhibition of enzyme activity and cytolysis by isocoumarins. *Biochemistry* 1991; 30:2217–2227.

74. Garcia-Sanz JA, MacDonald HR, Jenne DE, Tschopp J, Nabholz M. Cell specificity of granzyme gene expression. *J Immunol* 1990;145:3111–3118.

75. Kummer JA, Kamp AM, Citarella F, Horrevoets AJG, Hack CE. Expression of human recombinant granzyme A zymogen and its activation by the cysteine proteinase cathepsin C. *J Biol Chem* 1996;271:9281–9286.

76. Smyth MJ, McGuire MJ, Thia KY. Expression of recombinant human granzyme B. A processing and activation role for dipeptidyl peptidase I. *J Immunol* 1995; 154:6299–6305.

77. Thiele DL, Lipsky PE. The action of leucyl-leucine methyl ester on cytotoxic lymphocytes requires uptake by a novel depeptide-specific facilitated transport system and dipeptidyl peptidase I–mediated conversion to membranolytic products. *J Exp Med* 1990;172:183–194.

78. Thiele DL, Lipsky PE. The immunosuppressive activity of L-leucyl-L-leucine methyl ester: selective ablation of cytotoxic lymphocytes and monocytes. *J Immunol* 1986;136:1038–1048.

79. Kominami E, Ishido K, Muno D, Sato N. The primary structure and tissue distribution of cathepsin C. *Biol Chem Hoppe Seyler* 1992;373:367–373.

80. Kolset SO, Gallagher JT. Proteoglycans in haemopoietic cells. *Biochim Biophys Acta* 1990;1032:191–211.

81. Masson D, Peters PJ, Geuze HJ, Borst J, Tschopp J. Interaction of chondroitin sulfate with perforin and granzymes of cytolytic T cells is dependent on pH. *Biochemistry* 1990;29:11229–11235.

82. Stevens RL, Kamada MM, Serafin WE. Structure and function of the family of protcoglycans that reside in the secretory granules of natural killer cells and other effector cells of the immune response. *Curr Top Microbiol Immunol* 1989; 140:93–108.

83. Rodriguez A, Webster P, Ortego J, Andrews NW. Lysosomes behave as Ca2⁺-regulated exocytic vesicles in fibroblasts and epithelial cells. *J Cell Biol* 1997; 93–104

84. David A, Bernard J, Thiernesse N, Nicolas G, Cerottini JC, Zagury D. Le processus d'exocytose lysosomale localisee est-il responsable de l'action cytolytique des lymphocytes T tuers? *C R Acad Sci* 1979;288:441–444.

85. Peters PJ, Geuze HJ, van der DH, et al. Molecules relevant for T cell–target cell interaction are present in cytolytic granules of human T lymphocytes. *Eur J Immunol* 1989;19:1469–1475.

86. Kannan K, Stewart RM, Bounds W, et al. Lysosome-associated membrane proteins h-LAMP1 (CD107a) and h-LAMP2 (CD107b) are activation-dependent cell surface glycoproteins in human peripheral blood mononuclear cells which mediate cell adhesion to vascular endothelium. *Cell Immunol* 1996;171:10–19.

87. Peters PJ, Geuze HJ, van der DH, Borst J. A new model for lethal hit delivery by cytotoxic T lymphocytes. *Immunol Today* 1990;11:28–32.

88. Mellman I, Fuchs R, Helenius A. Acidification of the endocytic and exocytic pathways. *Annu Rev Biochem* 1986;55:663–700.

89. Kataoka T, Takaku K, Magae J, et al. Acidification is essential for maintaining the structure and function of lytic granules of CTL: effect of concanamycin A, an inhibitor of vacuolar type H⁺-ATPase, on CTL-mediated cytotoxicity. *J Immunol* 1994;153:3938–3947.

90. Anderson P, Nagler-Anderson C, O'Brien C, et al. A monoclonal antibody reactive with a 15-kDa cytoplasmic granule-associated protein defines a subpopulation of CD8⁺ T cells. *J Immunol* 1990;144:574–582.

91. Anderson P. TIA-1: structural and functional studies on a new class of cytolytic effector molecule. *Curr Top Microbiol Immunol* 1995;198:131–143.

92. Pena SV, Hanson DA, Carr BA, Goralski TJ, Krensky AM. Processing, subcellular localization, and function of 519 (Granulysin), a human late T cell activation molecule with homology to small lytic granule proteins. *J Immunol* 1997;158: 2680–2688.

93. Andersson M, Gunne H, Agerberth B, et al. NK-lysin, a novel effector peptide of cytotoxic T and NK cells. Structure and cDNA cloning of the porcine form, induction by interleukin 2, antibacterialo and antitumor activity. *EMBO J* 1995;14:1615–1625.

94. Dupuis M, Schaerer E, Krause KH, Tschopp J. The calcium-binding protein calreticulin is a major constituent of lytic granules of cytolutic T lymphocytes. *J Exp Med* 1993;177:1–7.

95. Helenius A, Trombetta ES, Hebert DN, Simons JF. Calnexin, calreticulin and the folding of glycoproteins. *Trends Cell Biol* 1997;7:193–200.

96. Yannelli JR, Sullivan JA, Mandell GL, Engelhard VH. Reorientation and fusion of cytotoxic T lymphocyte granules after interaction with target cells as determined by high resolution cinemicrography. *J Immunol* 1986;136:377–382.

97. Waters JB, Oldstone MBA, Hahn KM. Changes in the cytoplasmic structure of CTLs during target cell recognition and killing. *J Immunol* 1996;157:3396–3403.

98. Berke G. Interaction of cytotoxic T lymphocytes and target cells. *Prog Allergy* 1980;27:69–133.

99. Perez P, Bluestone JA, Stephany DA, Segal DM. Quantitative measurements of the specificity and kinetics of conjugate formation between cloned cytotoxic T-lymphocytes and splenic target cells by dual parameter flow cytometry. *J Immunol* 1985;134:478–485.

100. Martz E. LFA-1 and other accessory molecules functioning in adhesions of T and B lymphocytes. *Hum Immunol* 1987;18:3–37.

101. Martz E. Immune T lymphocyte to tumor cell adhesion. Magnesium sufficient, calcium insufficient. *J Cell Biol* 1980;84:584–598.

102. Hubbard BB, Glacken MW, Rodgers JR, Rich RR. The role of physical forces on cytotoxic T cell–target cell conjugate stability. *J Immunol* 1990;144:4129–4138.

103. Martz E, Davignon D, Kurzinger K, Springer TA. The molecular basis of cytolytic T lymphocyte function: analysis with blocking monoclonal antibodies. *Adv Exp Med Biol* 1982;146:447–468.

104. Springer TA, Davignon D, Ho M-K, Kurzinger K, Martz E, Sanchez-Madrid F. LFA-1 and Lyt-2,3, molecules associated with T lymphocyte-mediated killing; and Mac-1, an LFA-1 homologue associated with complement receptor function. *Immunol Rev* 1982;68:171–195.

105. Griffiths GM, Namikawa R, Mueller C, et al. Granzyme A and perforin as markers for rejection in cardiac transplantation. *Eur J Immunol* 1991;21:687–692.

106. Mescher MF. Molecular intereactions in the activation of effector and precursor cytotoxic T lymphocytes. *Immunol Rev* 1995;146:177–210.

107. Berg NN, Ostergaard HL. Characterization of intercellular adhesion molecule-1 (ICAM-1)–augmented degranulation by cytotoxic T cells. ICAM-1 and anti-CD3 must be co-localized for optimal adhesion and stimulation. *J Immunol* 1995;155:1694–1702.

108. Gartner P. Calcium and T lymphocyte activation. *Cell* 1989;59:15–20.

109. Poenie M, Tsien RY, Schmidt-Verhulst AM. Sequential activation and lethal hit measured by [Ca²⁺] in individual cytolytic T cells and targets. *EMBO J* 1987;6: 2223–2232.

110. Gray LS, Gnarra JR, Engelhard VH. Demonstration of a calcium influx in cytolytic T lymphocytes in response to target cell binding. *J Immunol* 1987;138:63–69.

111. Gray LS, Gnarra JR, Sullivan JA, Mandell GL, Engelhard VH. Spatial and temporal characteristics of the increase in intracellular Ca²⁺ induced in cytotoxic T lymphocytes by cellular antigen. *J Immunol* 1988;141:2424–2430.

112. Gray LS, Gnarra JR, Russell JH, Engelhard VH. The role of K⁺ in the regulation of the increase in intracellular Ca²⁺ mediated by the T lymphocyte antigen receptor. *Cell* 1987;50:119–127.

113. Densmore JJ, Haverstick DM, Szabo G, Gray LS. A voltage-operable current is involved in Ca²⁺ entry in human lymphocytes whereas ICRAC has no apparent role. *Am J Physiol* 1996;271:C1494–C1503.

114. Anel A, O'Rourke AM, Kleinfeld AM, Mescher MF. T cell receptor and CD8-dependent tyrosine phosphorylation events in cytotoxic T lymphocytes: activation of p56lck by CD8 binding to class I protein. *Eur J Immunol* 1996;26: 2310–2319.

115. Anel A, Martinez-Lorenzo MJ, Schmitt-Verhulst AM, Boyer C. Influence on CD8 of TCR/CD3-generated signals in CTL clones and CTL precursor cells. *J Immunol* 1997;158:19–28.

116. Thiernesse N, David A, Bernard J, Jeanesson P, Zagury D. Activitie phosphatasique acide de la cellule T cytolytique au cours du processus de cytolyse. *C R Acad Sci* 1977;285:713–715.

117. Bykovskaja SN, Rytenko AN, Rauschenbach MO, Mykovsky AF. Ultrastructural alteration of cytolytic T lymphocytes following their interaction with target cells. I. Hypertrophy and change of orientation of the Golgi apparatus. *Cell Immunol* 1978;40:164–174.

118. Geiger B, Rosen D, Berke R. Spatial relationships of microtubule-organizing centers and the contact area of cytotoxic T lymphocytes and target cells. *J Cell Biol* 1982;95:137–130.

119. Kupfer A, Dennert G. Reorientation of the microtubule-organizing center and the Golgi apparatus in cloned cytotoxic lymphocytes triggered by binding to lysable target cells. *J Immunol* 1984;133:2762–2766.

120. Kupfer A, Dennert G, Singer SJ. The reorientation of the Golgi apparatus and the microtubule-organizing center in the cytotoxic effector cell is a prerequisite in the lysis of bound target cells. *J Mol Cell Immunol* 1985;2:37–49.

121. Kupfer A, Dennert G, Singer SJ. Polarization of the Golgi apparatus and the microtubule-organizing center within cloned natural killer cells bound to their targets. *Proc Natl Acad Sci U S A* 1983;80:7224–7228.

122. Kupfer A, Singer SJ, Dennert G. On the mechanism of unidirectional killing in mixtures of two cytotoxic T lymphocytes. Unidirectional polarization of cytoplasmic organelles and the membrane-associated cytoskeleton in the effector cell. *J Exp Med* 1986;163:489–498.

123. Kupfer A, Singer SJ. Cell biology of cytotoxic and helper T cell functions: immunofluorescence microscopic studies of single cells and cell couples. *Annu Rev Immunol* 1989;7:309–337.

124. Hahn K, DeBiasio R, Tishon A, et al. Antigen presentation and cytotoxic T lymphocyte killing studied in individual, living cells. *Virology* 1994;201:330–340.

125. Negulescu PA, Krasieva TB, Khan A, Kerschbaum HH, Cahalan MD. Polarity of T cell shape, motility, and sensitivity to antigen. *Immunity* 1996;4:421–430.

126. Schneider SW, Sritharan KC, Geibel JP, Oberleithner H, Jena BP. Surface dynamics in living acinar cells imaged by atomic force microscopy: identification of plasma membrane structures involved in exocytosis. *Proc Natl Acad Sci U S A* 1997;94:316–321.

127. Henkart MP, Henkart PA. Lymphocyte mediated cytolysis as a secretory process. *Adv Exp Med Biol* 1982;146:227–242.

128. Frey T, Petty HR, McConnell HM. Electron microscopic study of natural killer cell–tumor cell conjugates. *Proc Natl Acad Sci U S A* 1982;79:5317–5321.

129. Zucker-Franklin D, Grusky G, Yang JS. Arylsulfatase in natural killer cells: its possible role in cytotoxicity. *Proc Natl Acad Sci U S A* 1983;80:6977–6981.

130. Pasternack MS, Verret CR, Liu MA, Eisen HN. Serine esterase in cytolytic T lymphocytes. *Nature* 1986;322:740–743.

131. Welsh RM, Nishioka WK, Antia R, Dundon PL. Mechanism of killing by virus-induced cytotoxic T lymphocytes elicited *in vivo*. *J Virol* 1990;64:3726–3733.

132. Schmidt RE, MacDermott RP, Bartley G, et al. Specific release of proteoglycans from human natural killer cells during target lysis. *Nature* 1985;318:289–291.

133. MacDermott RP, Schmidt RE, Caulfield JP, et al. Proteoglycans in cell-mediated cytotoxicity. Identification, localization, and exocytosis of a chondroitin sulfate proteoglycan from human cloned natural killer cells during target cell lysis. *J Exp Med* 1985;162:1771–1787.

134. Takayama H, Trenn G, Sitkovsky MV. A novel cytotoxic T lymphocyte activation assay. Optimized conditions for antigen receptor triggered granule enzyme secretion. *J Immunol Methods* 1987;104:183–190.

135. Burkhardt JK, McIlvain JM, Sheetz MP, Argon Y. Lytic granules from cytotoxic T cells exhibit kinesin-dependent motility on microtubules *in vitro*. *J Cell Sci* 1993;104:151–162.

136. Miyake K, McNeil PL. Vesicle accumulation and exocytosis at sites of plasma membrane disruption. *J Cell Biol* 1995;131:1737–1745.

137. Bashford CL, Menestrina G, Henkart PA, Pasternak CA. Cell damage by cytolysin: spontaneous recovery and reversible inhibition by divalent cations. *J Immunol* 1988;141:3965–3974.

138. Allbritton NL, Verret CR, Wolley RC, Eisen HN. Calcium ion concentrations and DNA fragmentation in target cell destruction by murine cloned cytotoxic T lymphocytes. *J Exp Med* 1988;167:514–527.

139. Reiter Y, Ciobotariu A, Jones J, Morgan BP, Fishelson Z. Complement membrane attack complex, perforin, and bacterial exotoxins induce in K562 cells calcium-dependent cross-protection from lysis. *J Immunol* 1995;155:2203–2210.

140. Sanderson CJ, Glaueret AM. The mechanism of T cell mediated cytotoxicity. V. Morphological studies by electron microscopy. *Proc R Soc Lond* 1977;198: 315–323.

141. Russell JH. Internal disintegration model of cytotoxic lymphocyte-induced target damage. *Immunol Rev* 1983;72:97–118.

142. Duke RC, Persechini PM, Chang S, Liu CC, Cohen JJ, Young JD. Purified perforin induces target cell lysis but not DNA fragmentation. *J Exp Med* 1989; 170:1451–1456.

143. Shiver JW, Henkart PA. A noncytotoxic mast cell tumor line exhibits potent IgE-dependent cytotoxicity after transfection with the cytolysin/perforin gene. *Cell* 1991;62:1174–1181.

144. Kagi D, Ledermann B, Burki K, et al. Cytotoxicity mediated by T cells and natural killer cells is greatly impaired in perforin-deficient mice. *Nature* 1994;369:31–37.

145. Shi L, Mai S, Israels S, Browne K, Trapani JA, Greenberg AH. Granzyme B (GraB) autonomously crosses the cell membrane and perforin initiates apoptosis and GraB nuclear localization. *J Exp Med* 1997;185:855–866.

146. Shiver JW, Su L, Henkart PA. Cytotoxicity with target DNA breakdown by rat basophilic leukemia cells expressing both cytolysin and granzyme A. *Cell* 1992; 71:315–322.

147. Nakajima H, Park HL, Henkart PA. Synergistic roles of granzymes A and B in mediating target cell death by RBL mast cell tumors also expressing cytolysin/perforin. *J Exp Med* 1995;181:1037–1046.

148. Heusel JW, Wesselschmidt RL, Shresta S, Russell JH, Ley TJ. Cytotoxic lymphocytes require granzyme B for the rapid induction of DNA fragmentation and apoptosis in allogeneic target cells. *Cell* 1994;76:977–987.

149. Shresta S, MacIvor DM, Heusel JW, Russell JH, Ley TJ. Natural killer and lymphokine-activated killer cells require granzyme B for the rapid induction of apoptosis in susceptible target cells. *Proc Natl Acad Sci U S A* 1995;92: 5679–5683.

150. Ebnet K, Hausmann M, Lehmann-Grube F, Müllbacher A, Kopf M, Lamers M, Simon MM. Granzyme A–deficient mice retain potent cell-mediated cytotoxicity. *EMBO J* 1995;14:4230–4239.

151. Hudig D, Ewoldt GR, Woodard SL. Proteases and lymphocyte cytotoxic killing mechanisms. *Curr Opin Immunol* 1993;5:90–96.

152. Nakajima H, Henkart PA. Cytotoxic lymphocyte granzymes trigger a target cell internal disintegration pathway leading to cytolysis and DNA breakdown. *J Immunol* 1994;152:1057–1063.

153. Wagner L, Avery RK, Bensinger L, Hibberd PL, Pasternack MS. Inhibition of cytotoxic T-lymphocyte–triggered apoptosis by target cell surface–coupled aprotinin. *Mol Immunol* 1995;32:853–864.

154. Hayes MP, Berrebi GA, Henkart PA. Induction of target cell DNA release by the cytotoxic T lymphocyte granule protease granzyme A. *J Exp Med* 1989;170: 933–946.

155. Shi L, Kam CM, Powers JC, Aebersold R, Greenberg AH. Purification of three cytotoxic lymphocyte granule serine proteases that induce apoptosis through distinct substrate and target cell interactions. *J Exp Med* 1992;176:1521–1529.

156. Pasternack MS, Blier KJ, McInerney TN. Granzyme A binding to target cell proteins. Granzyme A binds to and cleaves nucleolin *in vitro*. *J Biol Chem* 1991; 266:14703–14708.

157. Pinkoski MJ, Winkler U, Hudig D, Bleackley RC. Binding of granzyme B in the nucleus of target cells-Recognition of an 80-kilodalton protein. *J Biol Chem* 1996;271:10225–10229.

158. Shi L, Nishioka WK, Th'ng J, Bradbury EM, Litchfield DW, Greenberg AH. Premature p34cdc2 activation required for apoptosis. *Science* 1994;263:1143–1145.

159. Chen G, Shi L, Litchfield DW, Greenberg AH. Rescue from granzyme B-induced apoptosis by Wee1 kinase. *J Exp Med* 1995;181:2295–2300.

160. Shi L, Chen G, MacDonald G, et al. Activation of an interleukin 1 converting enzyme-dependent apoptosis pathway by granzyme B. *Proc Natl Acad Sci U S A* 1996;93:11002–11007.

161. Darmon AJ, Nicholson DW, Bleackley RC. Activation of the apoptotic protease CPP32 by cytotoxic T cell–derived granzyme B. *Nature* 1995;377:446–448.

162. Darmon AJ, Ley TJ, Nicholson DW, Bleackley RC. Cleavage of CPP-32 by

granzyme B represents a critical role for granzyme B in the induction of target cell DNA fragmentation. *J Biol Chem* 1996;271:21709–21712.

163. Henkart PA. ICE family proteases: mediators of all apoptotic cell death? [Review]. *Immunity* 1996;4:195–201.

164. Sarin A, Williams MS, Alexander-Miller MA, Berzofsky JA, Zacharchuk CM, Henkart PA. Target cell lysis by CTL granule exocytosis is independent of ICE/Ced-3 family proteases. *Immunity* 1997;6:209–215.

165. Ucker DS, Obermiller PS, Eckhart W, Apgar JR, Berger NA, Meyers J. Genome digestion is a dispensable consequence of physiological cell death mediated by cytotoxic T lymphocytes. *Mol Cell Biol* 1992;12:3060–3069.

166. Nishioka WK, Welsh RM. Inhibition of cytotoxic T lymphocyte–induced target cell DNA fragmentation, but not lysis, by inhibitors of DNA topoisomerases I and II. *J Exp Med* 1992;175:23–27.

167. Nakajima H, Golstein P, Henkart PA. The target cell nucleus is not required for cell-mediated granzyme- or Fas-based cytotoxicity. *J Exp Med* 1995;181:1905–1909.

168. Jacobson MD, Burne JF, Raff MC. Programmed cell death and Bcl-2 protection in the absence of a nucleus. *EMBO J* 1994;13:1899–1910.

169. Yang E, Korsmeyer SJ. Molecular thanatopsis: a discourse on the Bcl2 family and cell death. *Blood* 1996;88:386–401.

170. Chiu VK, Walsh CM, Liu C-C, Reed JC, Clark WR. Bcl-2 blocks degranulation but not fas-based cell-mediated cytotoxicity. *J Immunol* 1995;154:2023–2032.

171. Lee RK, Spielman J, Podack ER. bcl-2 protects against fas-based but not perforin-based T cell–mediated cytolysis. *Int Immunol* 1996;8:991–1000.

172. Schroter M, Lowin B, Borner C, Tschopp J. Regulation of Fas(Apo-1/CD95)– and perforin-mediated lytic pathways of primary cytotoxic T lymphocytes by the protooncogene bcl-2. *Eur J Immunol* 1995;25:3509–3513.

173. Barton K, Westbrook CA. Chronic myelogenous leukemia: a model for the genetic and biochemical basis of neoplasia. In: *Biochemical and molecular aspects of selected cancers*. New York: Academic Press, 1994.1–17.

174. Cotter TG. BCR-ABL: an anti-apoptosis gene in chronic myelogenous leukemia. *Leuk Lymphoma* 1995;18:231–236.

175. Sanchez-Garcia I, Martin-Zanca D. Regulation of Bcl-2 gene expression by BCR-ABL is mediated by Ras. *J Mol Biol* 1997;267:225–228.

176. Fuchs EJ, Bedi A, Jones RJ, Hess AD. Cytotoxic T cells overcome BCR-ABL–mediated resistance to apoptosis. *Cancer Res* 1995;55:463–466.

177. Roger R, Issaad C, Pallardy M, et al. BCR-ABL does not prevent apoptotic death induced by human natural killer or lymphokine-activated killer cells. *Blood* 1996;87:1113–1122.

178. Martz E. Overview of CTL–target adhesion and other critical events in the cytotoxic mechanism. In: *Cytotoxic cells: Recognition, effector function, generation, and methods*. Boston: Birkhauser, 1993:9–45.

179. Gorman K, Liu CC, Blakely A, Young JD, Torbett BE, Clark WR. Cloned cytotoxic T lymphocytes as target cells. II. Polarity of lysis revisited. *J Immunol* 1988;141:2211–2215.

180. Luciani MF, Brunet JF, Suzan M, Denizot F, Golstein P. Self-sparing of long-term *in vitro*–cloned or uncloned cytotoxic T lymphocytes. *J Exp Med* 1986;164:962–967.

181. Bensussan A, Leca G, Corvaïa N, Boumsell L. Selective induction of autocytotoxic activity through the CD3 molecule. *Eur J Immunol* 1990;20:2615–2619.

182. Kranz DM, Eisen HN. Resistance of cytotoxic T lymphocytes to lysis by a clone of cytotoxic T lymphocytes. *Proc Natl Acad Sci U S A* 1987;84:3375–3379.

183. Verret CR, Firmenich AA, Kranz DM, Eisen HN. Resistance of cytotoxic T lymphocytes to the lytic effects of their toxic granules. *J Exp Med* 1987;166:1536–1547.

184. Shinkai Y, Ishikawa H, Hattori M, Okumura K. Resistance of mouse cytolytic cells to pore-forming protein–mediated cytolysis. *Eur J Immunol* 1988;18:29–33.

185. Persechini PM, Young JD, Almers W. Membrane channel formation by the lymphocyte pore-forming protein: comparison between susceptible and resistant target cells. *J Cell Biol* 1990;110:2109–2116.

186. Müller C, Tschopp J. Resistance of CTL to perforin-mediated lysis: Evidence for a lymphocyte membrane protein interacting with perforin. *J Immunol* 1994;153:2470–2478.

187. Williams MS, Henkart PA. Apoptotic cell death induced by intracellular proteolysis. *J Immunol* 1994;153:4247–4255.

188. Sun J, Bird CH, Sutton V, et al. A cytosolic granzyme B inhibitor related to the viral apoptotic regulator cytokine response modifier A is present in cytotoxic lymphocytes. *J Biol Chem* 1996;271:27802–27809.

189. Schick B, Berke G. The lysis of cytotoxic T lymphocytes and their blasts by cytotoxic T lymphocytes. *Immunology* 1990;71:428–433.

190. Su MW-C, Walden PR, Eisen HN. Cognate peptide-induced destruction of CD8+ cytotoxic T lymphocytes is due to fratricide. *J Immunol* 1993;151:658–667.

191. Berthou C, Legros-Maida S, Soulie A, et al. Cord blood T lymphocytes lack constitutive perforin expression in contrast to adult peripheral blood T lymphocytes. *Blood* 1995;85:1540–1546.

192. Azuma M, Cayabyab M, Phillips JH, Lanier LL. Requirements for CD28-dependent T cell–mediated cytotoxicity. *J Immunol* 1993;150:2091–2101.

193. Smyth MJ, Browne KA, Kinnear BF, Trapani JA, Warren HS. Distinct granzyme expression in human CD3- CD56+ large granular and CD3- CD56+ small high density lymphocytes displaying non–MHC-restricted cytolytic activity. *J Leukoc Biol* 1995;57:88–93.

194. Ebnet K, Levelt CN, Tran TT, Eichmann K, Simon MM. Transcription of granzyme A and B genes is differentially regulated during lymphoid ontogeny. *J Exp Med* 1995;181:755–763.

195. Nagler-Anderson C, Lichtenheld M, Eisen HN, Podack ER. Perforin mRNA in primary peritoneal exudate cytotoxic T lymphocytes. *J Immunol* 1989;143:3440–3443.

196. Munger WE, Berrebi G, Henkart PA. Granule exocytosis by cytotoxic T lymphocytes generated *in vivo*. *Ann Inst Pasteur Immunol* 1987;138:301–304.

197. Berke G, Rosen D. Highly lytic *in vivo* primed cytolytic T lymphocytes devoid of lytic granules and BLT-esterase activity acquire these constituents in the presence of T cell growth factors upon blast transformation *in vitro*. *J Immunol* 1988;141:1429–1436.

198. Zheng LM, Ojcius DM, Liu CC, Kramer MD, Simon MM, Parr EL, Young JD. Immunogold labeling of perforin and serine esterases in granulated metrial gland cells. *FASEB J* 1991;5:79–85.

199. Croy BA, Reed N, Malashenko B-A, Kim K, Kwon BS. Demonstration of YAC target cell lysis by murine granulated metrial gland cells. *Cell Immunol* 1991;133:116–126.

200. Tirosh R, Berke G. T-Lymphocyte–mediated cytolysis as an excitatory process of the target. I. Evidence that the target cell may be the site of Ca^{2+} action. *Cell Immunol* 1985;95:113–123.

201. Trenn G, Takayama H, Sitkovsky MV. Exocytosis of cytolytic granules may not be required for target cell lysis by cytotoxic T lymphocytes. *Nature* 1987;330:72–74.

202. Ostergaard HL, Kane KP, Mescher MF, Clark WR. Cytotoxic T lymphocyte mediated lysis without release of serine esterase. *Nature* 1987;330:71–72.

203. Rouvier E, Luciani MF, Golstein P. Fas involvement in Ca^{2+}independent T cell–mediated cytotoxicity. *J Exp Med* 1993;177:195–200.

204. Suda T, Takahashi T, Golstein P, Nagata S. Molecular cloning and expression of the Fas ligand, a novel member of the tumor necrosis factor family. *Cell* 1993;78:1169–1178.

205. Anel A, Buferne M, Boyer C, Schmitt-Verhulst A-M, Golstein P. T cell receptor–induced Fas ligand expression in cytotoxic T lymphocyte clones is blocked by protein tyrosine kinase inhibitors and cyclosporin A. *Eur J Immunol* 1994;24:2469–2476.

206. Lynch DH, Ramsdell F, Alderson MR. Fas and FasL in the homeostatic regulation of immune responses. *Immunol Today* 1995;16:569–574.

207. Abbas AK. Die and let live: Eliminating dangerous lymphocytes. *Cell* 1996;84:655–657.

208. Walker PR, Saas P, Dietrich PY. Role of Fas Ligand (CD95L) in immune escape: The tumor cell strikes back. *J Immunol* 1997;158:4521–4524.

209. Glass A, Walsh CM, Lynch DH, Clark WR. Regulation of the fas lytic pathway in cloned CTL. *J Immunol* 1996;156:3638–3644.

210. Vignaux F, Vivier E, Malissen B, Depraetere V, Nagata S, Golstein P. TCR/CD3 coupling to Fas-based cytotoxicity. *J Exp Med* 1995;181:781–786.

211. El-Khatib M, Stanger BZ, Dogan H, Cui H, Ju ST. The molecular mechanism of FasL-mediated cytotoxicity by CD4+ Th1 clones. *Cell Immunol* 1995;163:237–247.

212. Anel A, Simon AK, Auphan N, et al. Two signaling pathways can lead to Fas ligand expression in CD8+ cytotoxic T lymphocyte clones. *Eur J Immunol* 1995;25:3381–3387.

213. Cao W, Tykodi SS, Esser MT, Braciale VL, Braciale TJ. Partial activation of CD8+ T cells by a self-derived peptide. *Nature* 1995;378:295–298.

214. Brossart P, Bevan MJ. Selective activation of Fas/Fas ligand–mediated cytotoxicity by a self peptide. *J Exp Med* 1996;183:2449–2458.

215. Kessler BM, Bassanini P, Cerottini JC, Luescher IF. Effects of epitope modification on T cell receptor–ligand binding and antigen recognition by seven H-2kd–restricted cytotoxic T lymphocyte clones specific for a photoreactive peptide derivative. *J Exp Med* 1997;185:629–640.

216. Sloan-Lancaster J, Allen PM. Altered peptide ligand–induced partial T cell activation: Molecular mechanisms and role in T cell biology. *Annu Rev Immunol* 1996;14:1–27.

217. Esser MT, Krishnamurthy B, Braciale VL. Distinct T cell receptor signaling requirements for perforin- or FasL-mediated cytotoxicity. *J Exp Med* 1996;183:1697–1706.

218. Suda T, Tanaka M, Miwa K, Nagata S. Apoptosis of mouse naive T cells induced by recombinant soluble Fas ligand and activation-induced resistance to Fas ligand. *J Immunol* 1996;157:3918–3924.

219. Klas C, Debatin KM, Jonker RR, Krammer PH. Activation interferes with the APO-1 pathway in mature human T cells. *Int Immunol* 1993;5:625–630.

220. Rothstein TL. Signals and susceptibility to programmed death in b cells. *Curr Opin Immunol* 1996;8:362–371.

221. Memon SA, Moreno MB, Petrak D, Zacharchuk CM. Bcl-2 blocks glucocorticoid- but not Fas- or activation-induced apoptosis in a T cell hybridoma. *J Immunol* 1995;155:4644–4652.

222. Boise LH, Minn AJ, Noel PJ, et al. CD28 costimulation can promote T cell survival by enhancing the expression of Bcl-xL. *Immunity* 1995;3:87–98.

223. Kojima H, Shinohara N, Hanaoka S, et al. Two distinct pathways of specific killing revealed by perforin mutant cytotoxic T lymphocytes. *Immunity* 1994;1:357–364.

224. Leist TP, Cobbold SP, Waldmann H, Aguet M, Zinkernagel RM. Functional analysis of T lymphocyte subsets in antiviral host defense. *J Immunol* 1987;138:2278–2281.

225. Bluestone JA, Khattri R, Sciammas R, Sperling AI. TCRgammaδ cells: a spe-

cialized T-cell subset in the immune system. *Annu Rev Cell Biol* 1995;11: 307–353.

226. Williams NS, Engelhard VH. Identification of a population of CD4⁺ CTL that utilizes a perforin- rather than a Fas ligand–dependent cytotoxic mechanism. *J Immunol* 1996;156:153–159.

227. Muller D, Koller BH, Whitton JL, LaPan KE, Brigman KK, Frelinger JA. LCMV-specific, class II–restricted cytotoxic T cells in beta 2-microglobulin–deficient mice. *Science* 1992;255:1576–1578.

228. Hahn S, Gehri R, Erb P. Mechanism and biological significance of CD4-mediated cytotoxicity. *Immunol Rev* 1995;146:57–79.

229. Yagita H, Hanabuchi S, Asano Y, Tamura T, Nariuchi H, Okumura K. Fas-mediated cytotoxicity—a new immunoregulatory and pathogenic function of Th1 CD4- T cells. *Immunol Rev* 1995;146:223–239.

230. Shinohara N, Huang Y, Muroyama A. Specific suppression of antibody responses by soluble protein-specific, class II–restricted cytolytic T lymphocyte clones. *Eur J Immunol* 1991;21:23–27.

231. Rothstein TL, Wang JK, Panka DJ, et al. Protection against Fas-dependent Th1-mediated apoptosis by antigen receptor engagement in B cells. *Nature* 1995;374: 163–165.

232. Sykulev Y, Cohen RJ, Eisen HN. The law of mass action governs antigen-stimulated cytolytic activity of CD8⁺ cytotoxic T lymphocytes. *Proc Natl Acad Sci U S A* 1995;92:11990–11992.

233. Schodin BA, Tsomides TJ, Kranz DM. Correlation between the number of T cell receptors required for T cell activation and TCR–ligand affinity. *Immunity* 1996; 5:137–146.

234. Sykulev Y, Joo M, Vturina I, Tsomides TJ, Eisen HN. Evidence that a single peptide–MHC complex on a target cell can elicit a cytolytic T cell response. *Immunity* 1996;4:565–571.

235. Valitutti S, Müller S, Dessing M, Lanzavecchia A. Different responses are elicited in cytotoxic T lymphocytes by different levels of T cell receptor occupancy. *J Exp Med* 1996;183:1917–1921.

236. Brower RC, England R, Takeshita T, et al. Minimal requirements for peptide mediated activation of CD8⁺ CTL. *Mol Immunol* 1994;31:1285–1293.

237. Hemmer B, Stefanova I, Vergelli M, Germain RN, Martin R. The activating properties of TCR agonists and partial agonists reflect hierarchical effector response thresholds of the T-cell and the potency and signal induction quality of the ligand. 1997 (*submitted for publication*).

238. Segal DM, Jost CR, George AJT. Targeted cellular cytotoxicity. In: *Cytotoxic cells. Recognition, effector function, generation, and methods.* Boston: Birkhauser, 1993:96–110.

239. Fanger MW, Marganelli PM, Guyre PM. Bispecific antibodies. *Crit Rev Immunol* 1992;12:101–124.

240. Kurucz I, Titus JA, Jost CR, Jacobus CM, Segal DM. Retargeting of CTL by an efficiently refolded bispecific single-chain Fv dimer produced in bacteria. *J Immunol* 1995;154:4576–4582.

241. Lanzavecchia A, Staerz UD. Lysis of nonnucleated red blood cells by cytotoxic T lymphocytes. *Eur J Immunol* 1987;17:1073–1074.

242. Beun GDM, Van de Velde CJH, Fleuren GJ. T-cell based cancer immunotherapy: direct or redirected tumor-cell recognition. *Immunol Today* 1994;15:11–15.

243. Gagliardi MC, De Petrillo G, Salemi S, et al. Presentation of peptides by cultured monocytes or activated T cells allows specific priming of human cytotoxic T lymphocytes *in vitro. Int Immunol* 1995;7:1741–1752.

244. Nishio M, Spielman J, Lee RK, Nelson DL, Podack ER. CD80 (B7.1) and CD54 (intracellular adhesion molecule-1) induce target cell susceptibility to promiscuous cytotoxic T cell lysis. *J Immunol* 1996;157:4347–4353.

245. Brooks CG, Holscher M. Cell surface molecules involved in NK recognition by cloned cytotoxic lymphocytes. *J Immunol* 1987;138:1331–1337.

246. Swain SL, Croft M, Dubey C, Haynes L, Rogers P, Zhang X, Bradley LM. From naive to memory T cells. *Immunol Rev* 1997;150:143–167.

247. Ascher NL, Chen S, Hoffman RA, Simmons RL. Maturation of cytotoxic T cells within sponge matrix allografts. *J Immunol* 1983;131:617–621.

248. Zinkernagel RM, Doherty PC. MHC-restricted cytotoxic T cells: studies on the biological role of polymorphic major transplantation antigens determining T-cell restriction-specificity, function, and responsiveness. *Adv Immunol* 1979;27: 51–177.

249. Rosenberg ZF, Fauci AS. The immunopathogenesis of HIV infection. *Adv Immunol* 1989;47:377–431.

250. Doherty PC. Cytotoxic T cell effector and memory function in viral immunity. *Curr Top Microbiol Immunol* 1996;206:1–14.

251. Razvi ES, Jiang Z, Woda BA, Welsh RM. Lymphocyte apoptosis during the silencing of the immune response to acute viral infections in normal, lpr, and Bcl-2-transgenic mice. *Am J Pathol* 1995;147:79–91.

252. Lohman BL, Razvi ES, Welsh RM. T-lymphocyte downregulation after acute viral infection is not dependent on CD95 (Fas) receptor–ligand interactions. *J Virol* 1996;70:8199–8203.

253. Carbone FR, Bevan MJ. Induction of ovalbumin-specific cytotoxic T cells by *in vivo* peptide immunization. *J Exp Med* 1989;169:603–612.

254. Inaba K, Metlay JP, Crowley MT, Steinman RM. Dendritic cells pulsed with protein antigens *in vitro* can prime antigen-specific, MHC-restricted T cells *in situ. J Exp Med* 1990;172:631–640.

255. Porgador A, Gilboa E. Bone marrow–generated dendritic cells pulsed with a class I–restricted peptide are potent inducers of cytotoxic T lymphocytes. *J Exp Med* 1995;182:255–260.

256. Celluzzi CM, Mayordomo JI, Storkus WJ, Lotze MT, Falo LD Jr. Peptide-pulsed dendritic cells induce antigen-specific CTL-mediated protective tumor immunity. *J Exp Med* 1996;183:283–287.

257. Berke G, Sullivan KA, Amos DB. Tumor immunity *in vitro*: destruction of a mouse ascites tumor through a cycling pathway. *Science* 1972;177:433–434.

258. Macatonia SE, Taylor PM, Knight SC, Askonas BA. Primary stimulation by dendritic cells induces antiviral proliferative and cytotoxic T cell responses *in vitro. J Exp Med* 1989;169:1255–1264.

259. Carbone FR, Moore MW, Sheil JM, Bevan MJ. Induction of cytotoxic T lymphocytes by primary *in vitro* stimulation with peptides. *J Exp Med* 1988;167: 1767–1779.

260. De Bruijn ML, Nieland JD, Schumacher TN, Ploegh HL, Kast WM, Melief CJ. Mechanisms of induction of primary virus-specific cytotoxic T lymphocyte responses. *Eur J Immunol* 1992;22:3013–3020.

261. Hefeneider SH, Conlon PJ, Henney CS, Gillis S. *In vivo* interleukin 2 administration augments the generation of alloreactive cytolytic T lymphocytes and resident natural killer cells. *J Immunol* 1983;130:222–227.

262. Widmer MB, Acres RB, Sassenfeld HM, Grabstein KH. Regulation of cytolytic cell populations from human peripheral blood by B cell stimulatory factor 1 (interleukin 4). *J Exp Med* 1987;166:1447–1455.

263. Alderson MR, Sassenfeld HM, Widmer MB. Interleukin 7 enhances cytolytic T lymphocyte generation and induces lymphokine-activated killer cells from human peripheral blood. *J Exp Med* 1990;172:577–587.

264. Chen WF, Zlotnik A. IL-10: a novel cytotoxic T cell differentiation factor. *J Immunol* 1991;147:528–534.

265. Pardoux C, Asselin-Paturel C, Chehimi J, Gay F, Mami-Chouaib F, Chouaib S. Functional interaction between TGF-beta and IL-12 in human primary allogeneic cytotoxicity and proliferative response. *J Immunol* 1997;158:136–143.

266. Kanai T, Thomas EK, Yasutomi Y, Letvin NL. IL-15 stimulates the expansion of AIDS virus–specific CTL. *J Immunol* 1996;157:3681–3687.

267. Smyth MJ, Strobl SL, Young HA, Ortaldo JR, Ochoa AC. Regulation of lymphokine-activated killer activity and pore-forming protein gene expression in human peripheral blood CD8+ T lymphocytes: inhibition by transforming growth factor-β. *J Immunol* 1991;146:3289–3297.

268. Gately MK, Warrier RR, Honasoge S, et al. Administration of recombinant IL-12 to normal mice enhances cytolytic lymphocyte activity and induces production of IFN-gamma *in vivo. Int Immunol* 1994;6:157–167.

269. Gillis S, Gillis AE, Henney CS. Monoclonal antibody directed against interleukin 2. I. Inhibition of T lymphocyte mitogenesis and the *in vitro* differentiation of alloreactive cytolytic T cells. *J Exp Med* 1981;154:983–988.

270. Leist TP, Kohler M, Eppler M, Zinkernagel RM. Effects of treatment with IL-2 receptor specific monoclonal antibody in mice. Inhibition of cytotoxic T cell responses but not of T help. *J Immunol* 1989;143:628–632.

271. Azuma M, Lanier LL. The role of CD28 costimulation in the generation of cytotoxic T lymphocytes. *Curr Top Microbiol Immunol* 1995;198:59–74.

272. Guerder S, Carding SR, Flavell RA. B7 costimulation is necessary for the activation of the lytic function in cytotoxic T lymphocyte precursors. *J Immunol* 1995;155:5167–5174.

273. Harding FA, Allison JP. CD28-B7 interactions allow the induction of CD8+ cytotoxic T lymphocytes in the absence of exogenous help. *J Exp Med* 1993;177: 1791–1796.

274. Parra E, Wingren AG, Hedlund G, Kalland T, Dohlsten M. The role of B7-1 and LFA-3 in costimulation of CD8⁺ T cells. *J Immunol* 1997;158:637–642.

275. De Bruijn ML, Peterson PA, Jackson MR. Induction of heat-stable antigen expression by phagocytosis is involved in *in vitro* activation of unprimed CTL by macrophages. *J Immunol* 1996;156:2686–2692.

276. Zinkernagel RM, Bachmann MF, Kündig TM, Oehen S, Pirchet H, Hengartner H. On immunological memory. *Annu Rev Immunol* 1996;14:333–367.

277. Razvi ES, Welsh RM, McFarland HI. *In vivo* state of antiviral CTL precursors: Characterization of a cycling cell population containing CTL precursors in immune mice. *J Immunol* 1995;154:620–632.

278. Ahmed R, Gray D. Immunological memory and protective immunity: understanding their relation. *Science* 1996;272:54–60.

279. Liu Y, Wenger RH, Zhao M, Nielsen PJ. Distinct costimulatory molecules are required for the induction of effector and memory cytotoxic T lymphocytes. *J Exp Med* 1997;185:251–262.

280. Mullbacher A, Flynn K. Aspects of cytotoxic T cell memory. *Immunol Rev* 1996; 150:113–127.

281. Cerottini J-C, MacDonald HR. The cellular basis of T-cell memory. *Annu Rev Immunol* 1989;7:77–89.

282. Surh CD, Sprent J. T-cell apoptosis detected in situ during positive and negative selection in the thymus. *Nature* 1994;372:100–103.

283. Ando K, Guidotti LG, Wirth S, et al. Class I–restricted cytotoxic T lymphocytes are directly cytopathic for their target cells *in vivo. J Immunol* 1994;152: 3245–3253.

284. Guidotti LG, Ishikawa T, Hobbs MV, Matzke B, Schreiber R, Chisari FV. Intracellular inactivation of the hepatitis B virus by cytotoxic T lymphocytes. *Immunity* 1996;4:25–36.

285. Guidotti LG, Chisari FV. To kill or to cure: options in host defense against viral infection. *Curr Opin Immunol* 1996;8:478–483.

286. Kägi D, Ledermann B, Bürki K, Zinkernagel RM, Hengartner H. Molecular mechanisms of lymphocyte-mediated cytotoxicity and their role in immunological protection and pathogenesis *in vivo. Annu Rev Immunol* 1996;14:207–232.

287. Melief CJM. Tumor eradication by adoptive transfer of cytotoxic T lymphocytes. *Adv Cancer Res* 1992;58:143–176.

288. Yannelli JR, Hyatt C, McConnell S, et al. Growth of tumor-infiltrating lymphocytes from human solid cancers: summary of a 5-year experience. *Int J Cancer* 1996;65:413–421.

289. Schwartzentruber DJ, Hom SS, Dadmarz R, et al. *In vitro* predictors of therapeutic response in melanoma patients receiving tumor-infiltrating lymphocytes and interleukin-2. *J Clin Oncol* 1994;12:1475–1483.

290. Sad S, Kagi D, Mosmann TR. Perforin and Fas killing by CD8+ T cells limits their cytokine synthesis and proliferation. *J Exp Med* 1996;184:1543–1547.

291. Cohen PL, Eisenberg RA. Lpr and gld: single gene models of systemic autoimmunity and lymphoproliferative disease. *Ann Rev Immunol* 1991;9:243–269.

292. Braun MY, Lowin B, French L, Acha-Orbea H, Tschopp J. Cytotoxic T cells deficient in both functional fas ligand and perforin show residual cytolytic activity yet lose their capacity to induce lethal acute graft-versus-host disease. *J Exp Med* 1996;183:657–661.

293. Zheng L, Fisher G, Miller RE, Peschon J, Lynch DH, Lenardo MJ. Induction of apoptosis in mature T cells by tumour necrosis factor. *Nature* 1995;377:348–351.

294. Sarin A, Conan-Cibotti M, Henkart PA. Cytotoxic effect of tumor necrosis factor and lymphotoxin on T lymphoblasts. *J Immunol* 1995;155:3716–3718.

295. De Togni P, Goellner J, Ruddle NH, et al. Abnormal development of peripheral lymphoid organs in mice deficient in lymphotoxin. *Science* 1994;264:703–707.

296. Tanaka M, Suda T, Haze K, et al. Fas ligand in human serum. *Nature Med* 1996;2:317–322.

297. Kagi D, Seiler P, Pavlovic J, et al. The roles of perforin- and Fas-dependent cytotoxicity in protection against cytopathic and noncytopathic viruses. *Eur J Immunol* 1995;25:3256–3262.

298. Kagi D, Ledermann B, Burki K, Hengartner H, Zinkernagel RM. CD8+ T cell-mediated protection against an intracellular bacterium by perforin-dependent cytotoxicity. *Eur J Immunol* 1994;24:3068–3072.

299. Laochumroonvorapong P, Wang J, Liu CC, et al. Perforin, a cytotoxic molecule which mediates cell necrosis, is not required for the early control of mycobacterial infection in mice. *Infect Immun* 1997;65:127–132.

300. Flynn JL, Goldstein MM, Triebold KJ, Koller B, Bloom BR. Major histocompatibility complex class I–restricted T cells are required for resistance to *Mycobacterium tuberculosis* infection. *Proc Natl Acad Sci U S A* 1992;89:12013–12017.

301. Mullbacher A, Ebnet K, Blanden RV, et al. Granzyme A is critical for recovery of mice from infection with the natural cytopathic viral pathogen, ectromelia. *Proc Natl Acad Sci U S A* 1996;93:5783–5787.

302. Selvaggi G, Ricordi C, Podack ER, Inverardi L. The role of the perforin and Fas pathways of cytotoxicity in skin graft rejection. *Transplantation* 1996;62:1912–1915.

303. Ahmed KR, Guo TB, Gaal KK. Islet rejection in perforin-deficient mice: the role of perforin and Fas. *Transplantation* 1997;63:951–957.

304. Schulz M, Schuurman H-J, Joergensen J, et al. Acute rejection of vascular heart allografts by perforin-deficient mice. *Eur J Immunol* 1995;25:474–480.

305. Seino K, Kayagaki N, Bashuda H, Okumura K, Yagita H. Contribution of Fas ligand to cardiac allograft rejection. *Int Immunol* 1996;8:1347–1354.

306. Clark WR, Walsh CM, Glass AA, Huang MT, Ahmed R, Matloubian M. Cell-mediated cytotoxicity in perforin-less mice. *Int Rev Immunol* 1995;13:1–14.

307. Baker MB, Altman NH, Podack ER, Levy RB. The role of cell-mediated cytotoxicity in acute GVHD after MHC-matched allogeneic bone marrow transplantation in mice. *J Exp Med* 1996;183:2645–2656.

308. Baker MB, Riley RL, Podack ER, Levy RB. Graft-versus-host-disease–associated lymphoid hypoplasia and B cell dysfunction is dependent upon donor T cell-mediated Fas-ligand function, but not perforin function. *Proc Natl Acad Sci U S A* 1997;94:1366–1371.

309. Graubert TA, Russell JH, Ley TJ. The role of granzyme B in murine models of acute graft-versus-host disease and graft rejection. *Blood* 1996;87:1232–1237.

310. Kagi D, Odermatt B, Ohashi PS, Zinkernagel RM, Hengartner H. Development of insulitis in transgenic mice lacking perforin-dependent cytotoxicity. *J Exp Med* 1996;183:2143–2152.

311. van Herrath MG, Oldstone MB. Interferon-gamma is essential for destruction of beta cells and development of insulin-dependent diabetes mellitus. *J Exp Med* 1997;185:531–539.

312. Chervonsky AV, Wang Y, Wong FS, Visintin I, Janeway CA, Matis LA. The role of Fas in autoimmune disease. *Cell* 1997;89:17–24

313. van den Broek M, Kagi D, Ossendorp F, et al. Decreased tumor surveillance in perforin-deficient mice. *J Exp Med* 1996;184:1781–1790.

314. van den Broek MF, Kagi D, Zinkernagel RM, Hengartner H. Perforin dependence of natural killer cell-mediated tumor control *in vivo*. *Eur J Immunol* 1995;25:3514–3516.

315. Humphrey JH, Dourmashkin RR. The lesions in cell membranes caused by complement. *Adv Immunol* 1969;11:75–115.

Fundamental Immunology, Fourth Edition,
edited by William E. Paul
Published by Lippincott–Raven Publishers, Philadelphia 1999.

CHAPTER 32

Inflammation

Helene F. Rosenberg and John I. Gallin

HISTORICAL PERSPECTIVE AND OVERVIEW

Inflammation is the physiologic process by which vascularized tissues respond to injury. During the inflammatory process, soluble mediators and cellular components work together in a systematic fashion in the attempt to contain and eliminate the agents causing physical distress. While inflammation is clearly crucial to maintaining the health and integrity of an individual organism, when poorly controlled, the inflammatory process can result in massive tissue destruction. For this reason, the concept of inflammation as a double-edged sword has taken hold.

The first observations on the inflammatory process are credited to Cornelius Celsus, who described the cardinal clinical signs of inflammation during the first century of the Common Era. His signs—rubor (redness), dolor (pain), calor (heat), and tumor (swelling)—remain as focal points for study. Another early contributor to this field was John Hunter (1793), who was the first to appreciate inflammation as host defense, as opposed to a disease process (1). In the 1800s, Julius Cohnheim provided the first microscopic descriptions of the inflammatory process (2). Paul Ehrlich contributed to the overall understanding of the inflamma-

tory process with his observations on the role of antibodies, and Elie Metchnikoff, with his observations on phagocytosis; both were awarded the Nobel prize for their work in 1908. Other crucial discoveries included those of Wright, who described the plasma proteins (opsonins) that coat and tag foreign substances for phagocytic destruction, and Dale and Laidlaw, who demonstrated the vasoactive role of histamine (3). In recent history, many investigators have contributed observations on the soluble mediators known as cytokines (which include chemokines, interleukins, interferons, and colony-stimulating factors) and the role played by cytokines and their specific receptors in modulating nearly every event characteristic of the inflammatory response.

Inflammation has been traditionally divided into acute and chronic responses. Acute inflammation is the rapid, short-lived (minutes to days), relatively uniform response to acute injury, characterized by accumulations of fluid, plasma proteins, and neutrophilic leukocytes. In contrast, chronic inflammation is of longer duration and includes influx of lymphocytes and macrophages and fibroblast growth.

The highlights of the events characteristic of acute and chronic inflammation are as depicted in Fig. 1. For more detail on all topics covered in this chapter, the reader is referred to the textbook entitled, *Inflammation* (4).

An injuring agent evades or destroys primary barriers (epithelial or endothelial cells and their specialized structures), initiating

H. F. Rosenberg and J. I. Gallin: Laboratory of Host Defenses, National Institute of Allergy and Infectious Diseases, National Institutes of Health, Bethesda, Maryland 20892-1504.

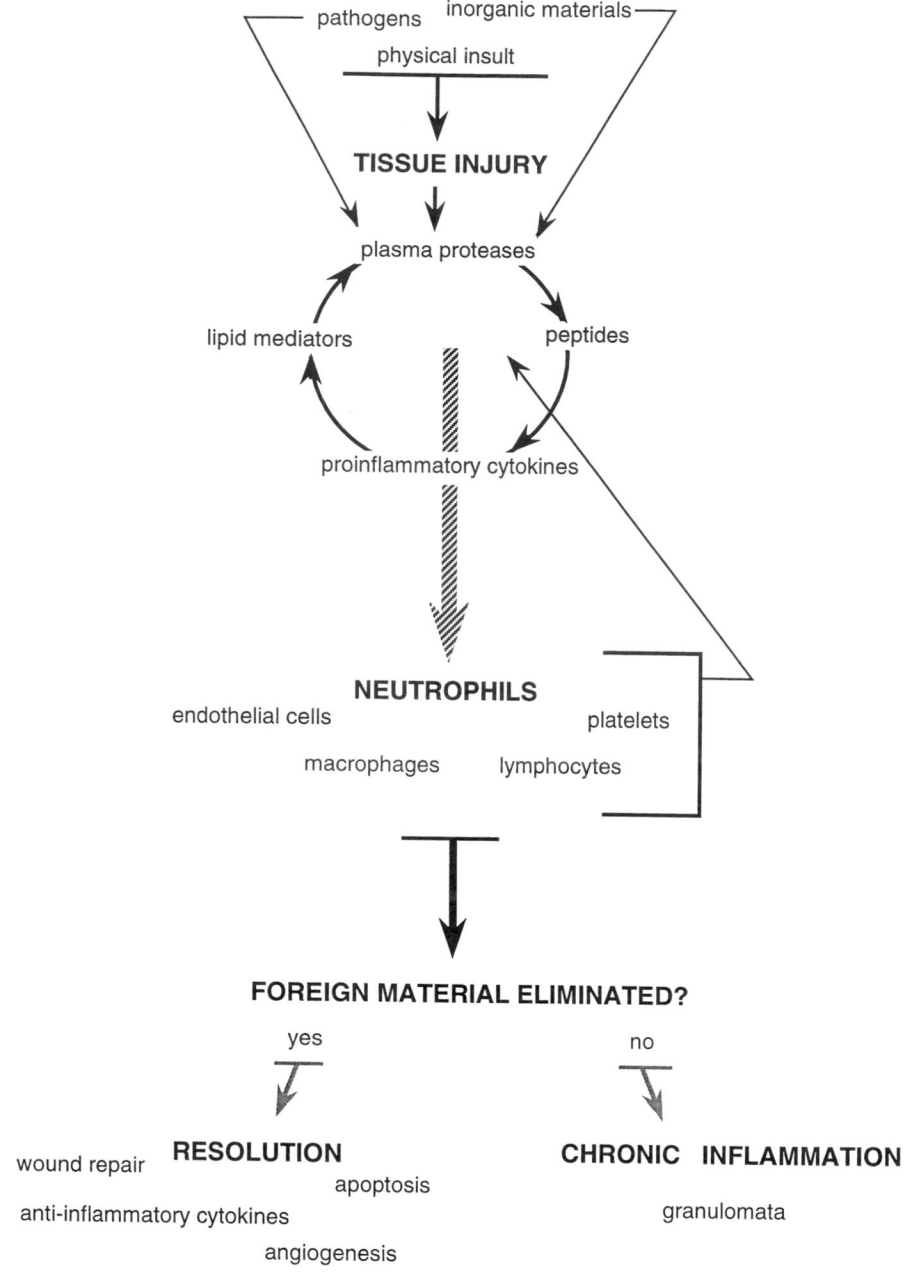

FIG. 1. Molecular and cellular events of the inflammatory response.

acute inflammation. Examples of injurious agents include pathogens (e.g., bacteria, viruses, parasites), foreign bodies from exogenous (e.g., asbestos) or endogenous (e.g., urate crystals, immune complexes) sources, as well as physical (e.g., burns) or chemical (e.g., caustics) agents.

Tissue damage initiates a series of molecular events, resulting in the production of soluble proinflammatory mediators that promote the hallmark physical signs of inflammation, including increased blood flow and vascular permeability, migration of leukocytes from the peripheral blood into the tissues, accumulation of these leukocytes at the inflammatory focus, and activation of the leukocytes to destroy and (if possible) eliminate the foreign substance. These soluble mediators include the plasma protease systems, lipid mediators, and proinflammatory peptides and cytokines. Addi-

tional mediators secreted by activated leukocytes can serve to prolong the inflammatory response by both direct and indirect means.

As the foreign threat is eliminated, antiinflammatory mediators permit the process to wind down, so as to avoid unnecessary and excessive damage to the tissues surrounding the inflammatory focus. If this acute process results in only incomplete destruction and/or elimination of the foreign substance, the inflammatory process persists and expands its repertoire of soluble mediators and cellular components, a process referred to as chronic inflammation.

This chapter describes in some detail the physical, cellular, and molecular events underlying acute and chronic inflammation. We describe several clinical disorders in which deficient or deranged inflammatory responses play a crucial role, and conclude with a discussion of novel therapeutic agents designed to combat the ravages of an excessive inflammatory response. References have been selected to include recent reviews and textbook chapters that cover the individual topics in greater detail.

INITIATION OF THE ACUTE INFLAMMATORY RESPONSE

The way in which the inflammatory process is initiated depends in part on the nature and portal of entry of the foreign substance and, to some degree, the nature and circumstances of a particular individual. Pathogens can initiate inflammation by a number of distinct and idiosyncratic mechanisms, including activation of the plasma protease systems by interaction with degradation products of the bacterial cell walls and by secretion of toxins that can activate the inflammatory response directly (5). Injured cells can release degradation products that initiate one or more of the plasma protease cascades, and can upregulate expression of proinflammatory cytokines that augment the inflammatory process.

PHYSICAL RESPONSES TO ACUTE INJURY

Regardless of the initiating agent, the physiologic changes accompanying acute inflammation encompass four main features.

Vasodilation

Vasodilation (often preceded by a brief period of vasoconstriction) is one of the earliest physical responses to acute tissue injury. The arterioles are the first to be involved, followed by the capillary beds, resulting in a net increase in blood flow. The increased blood flow results in the characteristic heat and redness (calor and rubor) associated with foci of acute inflammation.

Increased Vascular Permeability

Under normal conditions, the vascular endothelial cells function as a semipermeable membrane, restricting the plasma proteins to the intravascular space. In response to inflammatory stimuli, endothelial cells lining the venules contract, widening the intercellular junctions to produce gaps, permitting passage of plasma proteins (tumor) (see ref. 6 for a more complete discussion). More severe injury is associated with endothelial cell necrosis and increased leakage of plasma proteins and blood cells.

Neutrophil Recruitment and Activation

One of the initial and most crucial responses to acute inflammation is the recruitment of leukocytes (primarily neutrophils) from the bloodstream (and ultimately from the bone marrow) to the focus of inflammatory activity. The first step observed in this process is margination, as the neutrophils appear to roll slowly along the periphery of the blood vessel. This is followed by a more definitive sticking, or adherence stage. Neutrophils then migrate into the tissue, traveling through the enlarged endothelial cell junctions and the basement membrane. Under the influence of soluble chemotactic agents (see below), neutrophils are targeted to the site of inflammation, where they collect to form an inflammatory exudate known as pus. At this site, the neutrophils ingest pathogenic material by a process known as phagocytosis, and detoxify and digest this material by the actions of endogenous oxidants and proteolytic enzymes.

Fever

Fever remains the most poorly understood of the acute inflammatory responses. Agents producing fever, known as pyrogens, are released from leukocytes in response to specific stimuli, such as bacterial endotoxin. Pyrogens exert their actions via the temperature-regulating mechanism of the hypothalamus. A number of soluble proinflammatory mediators (discussed below and in Chapter 22) have been implicated in this process, including interleukin-1 (IL-1), tumor necrosis factor-α (TNF-α) and prostaglandins. The beneficial role of fever with respect to the acute inflammatory response remains a mystery.

MOLECULAR MEDIATORS OF THE ACUTE INFLAMMATORY RESPONSE

The physiologic features of the inflammatory process are initiated, regulated, and ultimately eliminated by the actions of numerous entities collectively termed *soluble inflammatory mediators*. Some of these mediators exist in inactive form and are activated by products of acute inflammation; others are synthesized and/or released from cellular sources, also in response to the products of acute inflammation, or by other soluble inflammatory mediators. Although presented as separate components, it is important to appreciate that these mediators perform their functions via intersecting, coordinately regulated, and mutually augmenting pathways.

The Plasma Proteases

Among the central components of the inflammatory response are the three interacting groups of plasma proteases. It is through the actions of plasma proteins as they convert one another from inactive to active forms that many of the major soluble mediators of inflammation are generated.

Complement

This group of plasma proteins was initially identified on the basis of their ability to complement the bactericidal activities of antibodies. At present, there are nine proteins known as participants in the complement cascade, described in detail in Chapter 29. By serial and sequential proteolytic cleavage, the complement proteins become activated and promote the inflammatory response by binding to foreign organisms and enhancing phagocytosis (components C3b and C4b), by functioning as agents increasing vascular permeability and as chemoattractants for inflammatory cells (C3a and C5a), and by creating lytic multiprotein complexes (C5b-9) (7–11). The classical pathway of complement is activated by antigen-bound antibodies of the IgM or IgG class. The first complement component, C1, undergoes autocatalytic cleavage to produce C1s, which in turn catalyzes a specific cleavage of C4 to C4b and C4a; C4b then binds to the target antigen, and C4a combines with C2a (product of the proteolytic cleavage of C2 by C1s) to create a protease specific for the component C3, and so on. The alternative pathway is utilized by other initiating agents (e.g., bacterial endotoxin) and converges with the classical pathway at the cleavage of C3; in addition, proteases from bacteria and damaged tissue, as well as plasmin generated by the fibrinolytic system (see below), can catalyze the cleavage of C3. From this point, the cleavage product C3b goes on to cleave C5, and serial proteolysis leads to activation of proteins C6 through C9.

Inherited deficiencies in individual components of the complement system can result in increased susceptibility to infection, rheumatic disorders, or angioedema. Individual deficiencies of various components have been identified (12,13); among the more common of these conditions is C2 deficiency. Individuals with C2 deficiency cannot utilize the classical pathway of complement activation; this autosomal recessive trait predisposes affected individuals to both pyogenic infections and rheumatic disorders. A defect in a complement regulatory protein, C1-inhibitor, results in the clinical disorder known as hereditary angioedema (14,15). A more complete discussion of identified deficiencies in complement components, and the disorders to which they relate, can be found in Chapter 29.

Kinins

The kinins are a group of serum proteases whose ultimate product is bradykinin, an agent known to induce smooth muscle contraction, vasoconstriction, and increased permeability of smaller blood vessels (16–20). The kinin cascade is initiated by a number of by-products of tissue damage—collagen, cartilage, basement membranes—as well as by endotoxin and inorganic materials, which serve to activate factor XII (or Hageman factor, better known as a participant in the clotting cascade, as described below). Factor XII mediates the cleavage of prekallikrein to kallikrein, which not only serves to activate more factor XII, but also cleaves the proenzyme kininogen to produce bradykinin. Factor XII represents a crucial intersection, as it can also be activated by plasmin, a product of proteolytic cleavage among the fibrinolytic proteins, and by kallikrein, another protein of the kinin group.

Clotting and Fibrinolytic Proteins

In addition to the roles played by these proteins in hemostasis, they contribute significantly to the amplification of the inflammatory response via the direct activation of factor XII, as described above. Proteolytic cleavages initiated by activated factor XII ultimately result in the cleavage of fibrinogen to fibrin and to smaller fibrinopeptides, which serve as inflammatory modulators. Activated factor XII similarly activates the fibrinolytic system by generating the protease plasmin. Similar to factor XII, plasmin represents an important intersecting locus for all three protease systems, as its activity proceeds in a number of directions. Plasmin activity can generate fibrin split products, also inflammatory mediators, but more importantly, plasmin activity augments the production of activated factor XII, and in direct activation of the complement pathway via proteolytic cleavage of factor C3 (21–26).

Lipid Mediators

Lipid mediators are a complex group of chemicals that also participate in augmenting the inflammatory response. This group includes the prostaglandins, leukotrienes, platelet-activating factor (PAF), and a novel group known as lipoxins (27).

Prostaglandins

Prostaglandins are oxidized derivatives of the fatty acid arachidonate that mediate a number of the cardinal signs of inflammation, including fever, pain, and vascular permeability (28–33). The major sources of prostaglandin in acute inflammation include mononuclear phagocytes, endothelial cells, and platelets. Prostaglandin synthesis is augmented during inflammation by a number of stimuli, including bacterial endotoxin, immune complexes, complement component C3a, bradykinin, and IL-1. During inflammation, the production of prostaglandins is upregulated by a variety of mechanisms, including increased availability of fatty acid substrates, increased phospholipase activity, and increases in the level of cyclooxygenase activity. Prostaglandins mediate their proinflammatory effects through specific receptors present on target cells, and are known to promote the pain, fever, and edema characteristic of the acute inflammatory response.

Leukotrienes

Leukotrienes are also oxidation products of arachidonate that are synthesized in and released from neutrophilic, and to a lesser extent, eosinophilic leukocytes. LTA4 and its synthetic products LTB4 and LTC4 are synthesized and exported from these cells; LTA4 can then be taken up by erythrocytes, platelets, and endothelial cells, where conversion to LTB4 and LTC4 can also take place. LTD4 and LTE4 are additional metabolic conversion products of LTC4. Although evidence suggesting the existence for specific receptors for individual leukotrienes exists, these receptors remain undefined. Together, leukotrienes mediate a large array of proinflammatory activities, including vasoconstriction, increased vascular permeability, and increased endothelial adhesiveness, as well as neutrophil chemotaxis and activation (34–37). Most recently, leukotrienes have received attention as contributors to the pathophysiology of asthma (38–42).

Platelet-activating Factor

PAF (43–47) is a substituted derivative of glycerol phosphate that exists in both circulating and cellular forms. In its cellular form in endothelial cells, PAF has been shown to enhance neutrophil–endothelial cell adhesion. Specific receptors for PAF have been identified on neutrophils (48), and numerous antagonists have been identified (49–53).

Peptides and Amines

Histamine and Serotonin

Histamine, a decarboxylated derivative of the amino acid histidine was among the earliest of the soluble inflammatory mediators to be discovered (54–57). Tissue mast cells and basophils synthesize and store histamine, which is released in response to variety of physical and chemical stimuli (55). Histamine diffuses rapidly through tissues and into the bloodstream, and promotes many of the sequelae of acute inflammation, including vasodilation, increased vascular permcability, and interactions with the peripheral nervous system. As is the case with most other inflammatory mediators, histamine is recognized by specific receptors, in this case three distinct receptors, H1, H2, and H3 (58–66). Serotonin, a derivative of tryptophan, is stored in platelets, mast cells, and enterochromaffin cells of the gastrointestinal tract and is released through degranulation. Similar to histamine, serotonin has receptor-mediated vasoactive properties, although its role in acute inflammation is not well defined (54,67).

Neuropeptides

Neuropeptides are among the many components connecting the nervous system and the inflammatory response. As a group, neuropeptides are inflammatory mediators released from neurons in response to local tissue damage. This group of mediators includes substance P, vasoactive intestinal peptide, somatostatin, and calcitonin gene-related peptide (68–73). While numerous immunomodulatory activities have attributed to these mediators, the determination of the true physiologic roles and overall effects produced by these proteins is currently under study. Also under consideration are the roles played by neuropeptide-degrading enzymes, such as neutral endopeptidase, shown to be expressed on the neutrophil cell surface (74–76).

Nitric Oxide

Although its activity as both a neurotransmitter and an agent maintaining hemodynamic stability has been established, the role of nitric oxide in human host defense has been quite controversial (77–82). In initial studies, stimulation of human macrophages with lipopolysaccharide, interferon-γ (IFN-γ), granulocyte-macrophage colony-stimulating factor (GM-CSF), TNF-α, or heat-killed bacteria failed to elicit production of nitric oxide (83), in contrast to results obtained with a murine system. In contrast, a more recent study (84) demonstrated the generation of nitrite in human macrophage cultures in response to TNF-α and GM-CSF together with avirulent mycobacterial strains. Other groups have also demonstrated high levels of nitric oxide synthesis in response to a select group of stimuli (85–87). The molecular basis for this selectivity is currently an area of intense investigation.

Proinflammatory Cytokines

The identification and characterization of these soluble mediators has been one of the most active fields in current inflammation research (88–90). New cytokines are being discovered, and new activities for known cytokines are still emerging. It is often difficult to discuss the physiologic actions of an individual cytokine, as the interactions among cytokines and their cellular targets are complex. Rather than an exhaustive list, this is a brief overview of those mediators with major roles in the inflammatory response, and a review of some recent research focusing on the interplay of these mediators. A more comprehensive discussion of individual proinflammatory cytokines can be found in Chapter 22 and within the references listed.

Interleukin-1

IL-1 is a major inflammatory mediator, produced primarily by monocytes and activated macrophages (91–99). IL-1 activity is produced by two polypeptides (IL-1α and IL-1β) encoded by two distinct genes on chromosome 2. High-affinity receptors for IL-1 are found on lymphocytes and fibroblasts. Numerous local and systemic proinflammatory activities have been attributed to IL-1, including increasing local blood flow, fever, production of other soluble mediators, and enhanced expression of adhesion molecules. An unusual feature of IL-1 is the presence of a naturally occurring antagonist, IL1RA, which is expressed in neutrophils and monocytes (100,101).

Interleukin-4

IL-4 has a number of activities related to allergic inflammation, including stimulating basophil development, eosinophil chemotaxis, and expression of IgE receptors on B cells (102–108). IL-4 also participates in cell fusion related to the formation of granulomas, and also has antiinflammatory properties.

Interleukin-6

IL-6 is produced by T-lymphocytes, endothelial cells, monocytes, and fibroblasts, and has wide-reaching effects on T- and B-lymphocytes and macrophages, including promoting monocyte differentiation, increased number of circulating platelets, and synthesis of acute phase reactant proteins (including fibrinogen) in the liver (102,109–113).

Interleukin-8

IL-8 is a chemokine whose synthesis can be induced in a variety of cell types (monocytes, lymphocytes, and neutrophils) stimulated with IL-1α, IL-1β, or TNF. The activities of IL-8, however, appear to be restricted to neutrophils, enhancing both the chemotactic and degranulation responses. At the molecular level, IL-8 induces a net increase in the expression of cell surface adhesion molecules and elicits activation of the neutrophil NADPH oxidase (114–121).

Tumor Necrosis Factor

TNF (122–128) is derived from activated macrophages; TNF-α and TNF-β are two distinct but related polypeptides. TNF is associated with the production of fever and, similar to IL-1, promotes the increased expression of most other proinflammatory mediators, and it is prominently associated with the induction of cellular apoptosis (129–131).

Interferon-γ

IFN-γ (132–137) is a product of T cells and natural killer (NK) cells. Although initially recognized as an antiviral agent, IFN-γ activities are wide-ranging; best characterized is its ability to increase generation of highly reactive oxygen species such as superoxide anion and hydrogen peroxide and to alter the cell surface antigens of macrophages, permitting them to eliminate invading pathogens. IFN-γ also mediates activities of endothelial cells and, to a somewhat lesser extent, neutrophils. IFN-γ has been shown to have utility in preventing infections in certain patients with compromised host defenses or infections with intracellular pathogens (135). Research on a family with enhanced susceptibility to mycobacterial infection has demonstrated a role for the IFN-γ receptor in the pathogenesis of this disease (138,139).

Interleukin-12

IL-12 is a heterodimeric product of macrophages and B-lymphocytes that enhances the synthesis of IFN-γ and stimulates proliferation of NK, T helper 1 (Th1) cells, and cytotoxic T-lymphocytes. The role of IL-12 in host defense against intracellular bacteria is discussed in Chapter 40.

MODEL SYSTEMS OF INFLAMMATION

Two model systems have provided insight into the temporal appearance and importance of mediators in the various processes of inflammation in humans. In one model, small amounts of the lipid-A derivative of endotoxin are administered intravenously to normal human subjects, and mediator accumulation in peripheral blood is monitored (140). In the other model, mediator accumulation is monitored locally in the skin following creation of skin blisters by suction (141,142).

Response to Intravenous Endotoxin

Following intravenous endotoxin, a characteristic change in body temperature and white blood count is observed. Body temperature begins to increase after about 1 hour and reaches a maximum at about 4 hours. The leukocyte count shows a characteristic decrease at about 30 minutes, due to neutrophil and monocyte adherence to endothelial cells in the lung and spleen. This is followed by a leukocytosis characterized by the presence of immature neutrophils at about 4 hours, which can persist throughout 24 hours, with gradual return to baseline by 48 hours. The leukocytosis is predominantly due to mobilization of immature neutrophils from the bone marrow. The critical components of the inflammatory response—fever, neutrophil margination in the circulatory vessels, and then mobilization from the bone marrow—are associated with readily detected changes in circulating levels of certain mediators of inflammation. For example, TNF-α peaks within 2 hours (143) and is likely the predominant pyrogen associated with the febrile response. Plasma levels of the chemoattractant IL-8 increase early and peak by 4 hours. Early increases in IL-8 may relate to the transient decrease in the neutrophil count at 30 minutes (margination), since administration of intravenous chemoattractants in experimental animals is associated with a rapid neutropenia, likely a result of increased neutrophil expression of adhesion receptors (CR3) (144). In this regard, it is of interest that significant increases in plasma C5a and LTB4 were not detected following administration of intravenous endotoxin to humans, reinforcing the probable critical role of IL-8 in the process of neutrophil margination. Plasma concentrations of IL-6 also increased 2 to 4 hours following intravenous endotoxin. In addition to not detecting increases in plasma C5a, LTB4, or IL-1, no increases in circulating IL-2, IL-3, IL-4, IFN-γ, transforming growth factor-β (TGF-β), or nitrate–nitrite were detected following intravenous endotoxin, emphasizing the specificity of the responses observed. Kuhns and colleagues (145) have described a patient with recurrent bacterial infections that displayed hyporesponsiveness to both endotoxin and IL-1, attributable to a defect in signal transduction. Although the precise molecular basis of endotoxin activity has not been determined, there is evidence to suggest that endotoxin interacts with the cell surface antigen CD14 on the surface of phagocytes (146,147) and modulates the expression of nuclear factor κB (NF-κB), a factor that promotes the transcription of numerous proinflammatory mediators (148).

Temporal Analysis of Soluble Mediators in Blister Fluid

Soluble mediator accumulation at local inflammatory processes can be detected in raised skin blisters induced in normal volunteers (141). Mediators detected in blister fluid within 3 to 5 hours of the inflammatory response included LTB4, C5a, IL-8, and IL-6. In contrast, IL-1β, GM-CSF, and TNF-α were not detected until after 8 hours in the blister. Although IFN-γ was reported by Kuhns and colleagues (141) to be an early mediator in skin blister fluid, these results have not been repeated in subsequent studies (D.B. Kuhns and J.I. Gallin, unpublished results). Small amounts of IL-4 accumulated into the skin blisters, but IL-2 and IL-1α were not detected. Thus, the endotoxin and skin blister models of inflammation demonstrate that there are clear differences in the mediators that can be detected systemically and locally.

CELLULAR MEDIATORS OF THE ACUTE INFLAMMATORY RESPONSE

There are many who would argue that the entire interconnecting network of proinflammatory responses are designed to facilitate the recruitment of neutrophils to the site of tissue injury. Neutrophils are among the cells known as "professional phagocytes"; they respond to the soluble inflammatory mediators by migrating to the site of tissue injury and by ingesting and destroying invading pathogens and damaged tissue, leading the way to resolution and, ultimately, tissue repair. The recruitment of leukocytes (neutrophils, monocytes, and eosinophils) to foci of inflammation can be monitored by a both blister fluid and Rebuck skin window techniques, as discussed above. Other participants in the acute response include platelets, lymphocytes, and endothelial cells.

Neutrophils

Neutrophilic leukocytes are crucial to both immunity and inflammation, and prolonged neutropenia leads to inevitable demise as a result of overwhelming infection (149–151). Neutrophils normally represent between 40% and 50% of the circulating leukocyte population, and they are easily recognized on a Wright's stained blood smear by their size, their characteristic multilobed nuclei, and the presence of fine stippling, representing granules throughout the cytoplasmic compartment (Fig. 2). Primary and secondary granules contain distinct sets of their own proinflammatory mediators, as described below.

Development in the Bone Marrow

Neutrophils develop from undifferentiated precursors present in the bone marrow (152). The myeloblast is the first morphologically identifiable precursor of the neutrophil lineage, followed by the promyelocyte, myelocyte, metamyelocyte, and band form, which directly precedes the mature neutrophil (Fig. 3). Several products of activated T-lymphocytes, including GM-CSF, IL-3, and granulocyte colony-stimulating factor (G-CSF), participate in the process of neutrophil maturation by direct interactions with their respective receptors, which have been identified on neutrophil precursor cells. When mature, neutrophils are released into the circulation, where they can respond to the soluble proinflammatory mediators described above. Neutropenia may be related to chemotherapeutic

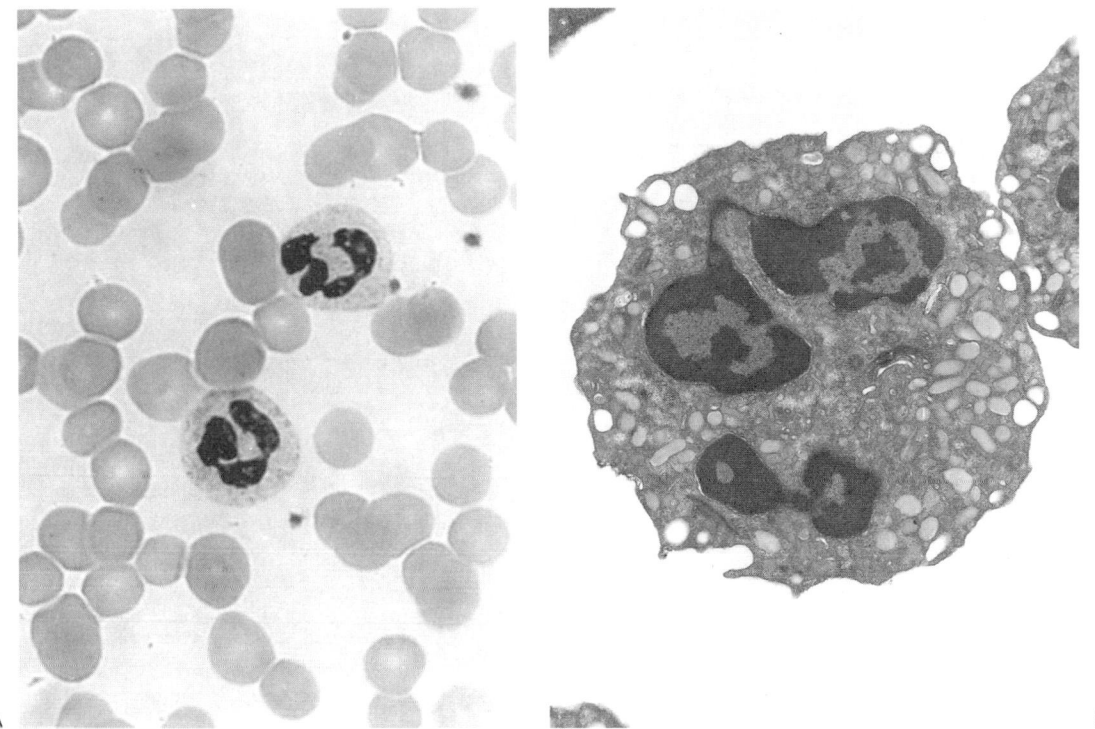

FIG. 2. A: Light and **(B)** electron microscopic views of a mature human peripheral blood neutrophil. (Illustrations courtesy of Dr. Douglas Kuhns.)

agents, autoantibodies, or infection. These conditions are often reversible; inherited disorders known as cyclic neutropenia and familial neutropenia have also been identified (153–157).

Activation and Priming

Neutrophils in the circulation are quiescent cells with only the potential to mediate a wide range of inflammatory activities. This potential is realized when neutrophils are activated (158,159). Neutrophils can be activated by a large (and increasing) number of specific agents (Table 1). As a group, these activating agents transmit signals to the neutrophils via interaction with specific cell surface receptors (149,158–164), many of which interact with intracellular components known as G proteins. G proteins catalyze the hydrolysis of guanosine triphosphate (GTP) to guanosine diphosphate (GDP) and inorganic phosphate, meanwhile initiating a series of events including activation of phospholipase C, initiation of calcium fluxes, and membrane depolarization. Once activated, neutrophils are able to adhere to endothelial cells, migrate through the endothelial barrier, and ingest and at least attempt to destroy

pathogens, foreign bodies, and remnants of tissue damage. An intriguing aspect of neutrophil activation is the phenomenon of priming. Neutrophils primed by brief exposure to activating agents (endotoxin, IL-1, f-Met-Leu-Phe, GM-CSF) exhibit an enhanced response to subsequent stimuli. Both short-term (including changes in cell shape, oxidative and phagocytic capacity) and long-term (prolonged cell viability) responses to priming agents have been observed. Overall, the phenomenon of priming suggests that neutrophil activation is a two-step process, requiring an initial switch from a nonreceptive to a receptive state. The molecular basis for this switch is currently under investigation.

Adherence

To participate effectively in the inflammatory process, neutrophils must ultimately leave the bloodstream and migrate into the tissues. The initial step in this process is adherence to the vascular endothelium. Neutrophil adherence is a two-step process, the first involving a class of cell surface molecules known as selectins (165–173). Selectins mediate the process in which neutrophils roll

myeloblast   promyelocyte   myelocyte   metamyelocyte   band   mature neutrophil

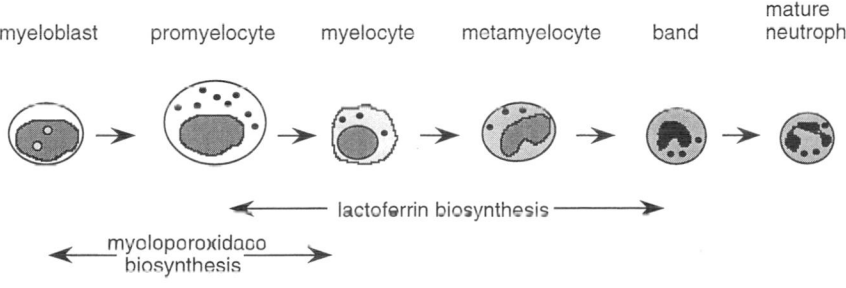

←—— lactoferrin biosynthesis ——→

←—— myeloperoxidase biosynthesis ——→

FIG. 3. Stages of neutrophil maturation in the bone marrow, from myeloblast to mature neutrophil. The *large black circles* represent the primary granules, and the *dark shading,* the secondary granules. The stages at which the proinflammatory mediators myeloperoxidase and lactoferrin are synthesized are as indicated by the *arrows.* (Adapted from ref. 300.)

TABLE 1. *Agents promoting neutrophil activation*

Agent	Function stimulated
LTB4	Chemoattractant; enhances adherence to endothelial cells; activates degranulation and NADPH oxidase activity
Complement fragment C5a	Chemoattractant; induces degranulation and adherence
PAF	Induces aggregation and adherence, chemoattractant degranulation
Histamine	Concentration-dependent changes in chemotaxis priming, and degranulation
IFN-γ	Increases antibody-dependent cytotoxicity, priming
G-CSF	Increases antibody-dependent cytotoxicity, priming; enhances phagocytosis; stimulates maturation within bone marrow
GM-CSF	Priming; stimulates maturation within bone marrow
TNF-α	Chemoattractant, priming; enhances phagocytosis and antibody-dependent cytotoxicity
IL-8	Chemoattractant; induces degranulation and NADPH oxidase activity
fMet-Leu-Phe	Chemoattractant; induces aggregation, degranulation, and NADPH oxidase activity

or slow down prior to their actual activation-dependent adherence to the endothelial cells. There are three classes of selectins that have been identified: L-selectins, which have been identified on all leukocytes; E-selectin, on the surface of activated endothelial cells; and P-selectin, found on endothelial cells and platelets. Selectins function by binding to carbohydrate ligands present on the adhering cell. The ligand for the endothelial E-selectin is sialylated Lewis-X antigen, found on the neutrophil, which, when absent, results in a marked immunodeficiency state.

The second part of the adherence process is the tight binding mediated by integrins (174–180). The leukocyte integrins are a subgroup of an extensive family of proteins that mediate a wide range of interactions between cells, and between cells and the extracellular environment. The leukocyte integrins—LFA-1 (CD11a/CD18), Mac-1 (CD11b/CD18), and p150,95 (CD11c/CD18)—are heterodimeric proteins with distinct α and shared β polypeptide chains. Mac-1 in particular has several well-characterized roles in the inflammatory process. Mac-1 is stored in the secondary granule compartment and is brought to the cell surface in conjunction with neutrophil activation. In addition to mediating specific adherence, Mac-1 participates in phagocytosis and chemotaxis, and in production of reactive oxygen species (see below). Intercellular cell adhesion molecule-1 (181), a cell surface protein found on endothelial cells, has been identified as a ligand for Mac-1.

Two forms of inherited defects of neutrophil adhesion have been identified: Leukocyte adhesion deficiency I (LAD I) involves a genetic defect in the biosynthesis of CD18, the shared β chain for all three leukocyte adhesion molecules (182–184). The defect is autosomal recessive and has been mapped to human chromosome 22q22.3. Individuals with this disorder have frequent and recurrent skin and soft-tissue infections, poor wound healing, and severe peridontal disease. In contrast, leukocyte adhesion deficiency II (LAD II) is a glycosylation defect that results in the inability to synthesize the sialyl-Lewis X carbohydrate ligand for E- and P-selectin (185,186). This condition results in a defect in neutrophil rolling that occurs prior to and facilitates neutrophil adherence to endothelial cells, and affected individuals likewise suffer from frequent severe bacterial infections.

Chemotaxis

As part of the activation process, neutrophils are capable of sensing and responding to concentration gradients of the activating agents that are highlighted in Table 1. By "crawling" across a surface, neutrophils can be seen to migrate toward a higher concentration of attractant. At the subcellular level, cell motility requires alterations in the neutrophil cytoskeleton, which is composed primarily of actin filaments. Although the precise mechanism by which signals are transmitted directly to the cytoskeleton is unclear, there is evidence to suggest that several actin-binding proteins (including profilin, cofilin, and gelsolin) participate in altering the actin filament structure, permitting net movement of the cell in response to a chemoattractant gradient (187–189).

Phagocytosis

Phagocytosis, or engulfment of foreign or damaged material, is the centerpiece of the inflammatory process and is discussed in detail in Chapter 30 (190,191). To engulf a particle, neutrophils extend pseudopodia, which encircle the offending material; the pseudopodia fuse, trapping the material inside the cell in a compartment known as a phagosome. Particles coated with immunoglobulins (or opsonized) are phagocytosed in a highly efficient fashion, as they are recognized by and bind directly to the Fc receptors present on the neutrophil cell surface. Particles opsonized by proteolytic products of complement (see above) are similarly phagocytosed in a specific, receptor-mediated fashion, involving CR1 and CR3.

Degranulation

The primary and secondary granules of neutrophils contain a number of distinct effector proteins, listed in Table 2. As part of the activation process, the cytoplasmic membrane-bound granules fuse with the phagosome, placing the effector proteins in direct contact with the ingested material. Among the highlights of the components of the primary (also known as azurophil) granules are lysozyme, which can digest the peptidoglycan component of most bacterial cell walls, and cathepsin G, defensins, and bacterial permeability-increasing protein (BPI), all with inherent antibacterial activity. Goldman and colleagues (192) have shown that human β-defensin-1 is inactivated in individuals with cystic fibrosis, and thus may be related to the pathogenesis of bacterial infections in affected individuals. Also among the more prominent components is myeloperoxidase, which converts hydrogen peroxide generated by the NADPH oxidase (see below) and hydrochloric acid to hypochlorous acid, another antimicrobial agent.

The secondary (or specific) granules contain several proteins whose role in the inflammatory response remains a bit mysterious.

TABLE 2. *Major components of neutrophil primary and secondary granules*

Primary granules	Secondary granules
Myeloperoxidase	Lactoferrin
Defensins	Gelatinase
BPI	Collagenase
Cathepsin G	Vitamin B 12–binding protein
Lysozyme	Lysozyme
Elastase	Cytochrome b558
Alkaline phosphatase	fMLP receptor
Proteinase 3	CD11b/CD18, CD11c/CD18 (integrins)
Beta glucuronidase	Complement receptor 3 (CR3)
Alpha fucosidase	Histaminase
Phospholipases A2, C, D	Plasminogen activator
Alpha mannosidase	

Among these proteins is lactoferrin, an iron-binding protein with some antibacterial activity (193). The secondary granules also contain stored sources of CR3 and other receptors for neutrophil activation agents, as well as stored membrane components of the NADPH oxidase.

Chediak-Higashi syndrome is a disorder in which neutrophils demonstrate abnormal morphology, abnormal chemotaxis, and failure to degranulate, and affected individuals are subjected to recurrent, severe bacterial and fungal infections. Three independent groups have reported the identification of the genetic defect in Chediak-Higashi syndrome, residing on human chromosome 1q42-43 (194–196). Disorders of neutrophils are specific granule deficiency, in which the secondary, or specific, granules are absent or, alternatively, are present, but without the granule protein components (197–199) and myeloperoxidase deficiency (200–202).

NADPH Oxidase

A crucial component of the neutrophil host defense mechanism is the enzyme complex known as the NADPH oxidase (Fig. 4) (203–210). This enzyme assembles on the phagosomal membrane from two integral membrane components (gp91-phox and p22-phox, for *pha*gocyte *ox*idase) and three cytosolic components (p47-phox, p67-phox, and rac) to catalyze the production of superoxide anion from molecular oxygen and free electrons; superoxide is then converted to the toxic metabolite hydrogen peroxide by the actions of superoxide dismutase, or to hypochlorous acid by the primary granule protein myeloperoxidase.

While the ability to generate toxic oxygen metabolites is crucial to host defense, these agents represent the sharpest part of the double-edged sword of inflammation. Superoxide anion is readily diffusible through membranes and can be converted to toxic metabolites outside the restricted locale of the phagosome. Products of oxygen radicals can create enlarged foci of tissue damage, thereby enhancing and augmenting the inflammatory process far beyond what was necessary to contain the initial insult. Similarly, oxidative injury has been implicated in the pathogenesis of cardiovascular, neoplastic, arthritic, and neurodegenerative disease. Chronic granulomatous disease is an inherited disorder in which neutrophils are rendered incapable of generating toxic oxygen metabolites (207,211–213). This results in an inability to mount an effective defense against bacteria (particularly catalase-positive strains) and fungi, and affected individuals often present with recurrent, life-threatening infections. Inherited defects in any one of the four oxidase proteins can disable the enzyme complex and result in disease. Therapy for this disorder includes prophylactic antibiotics and injections of the inflammatory modulating agent IFN-γ (214,215).

Protein Biosynthesis

Although neutrophils are generally perceived as "end-stage" cells, more recent work has shown that neutrophils are indeed capable of significant biosynthetic activity. The proteins expressed *de novo* in neutrophils include components of the NADPH oxidase and specific membrane receptors and antigens. Several proinflammatory mediators are released by activated neutrophils, including IL-1, TNF-α, IL-6, IL-8, GM-CSF, G-CSF, and plasminogen activator (149,211–215). Kuhns and Gallin (216) have shown that IL-8 is actively synthesized by exudate neutrophils. These mediators can "feed back" on the system and augment the overall inflammatory response.

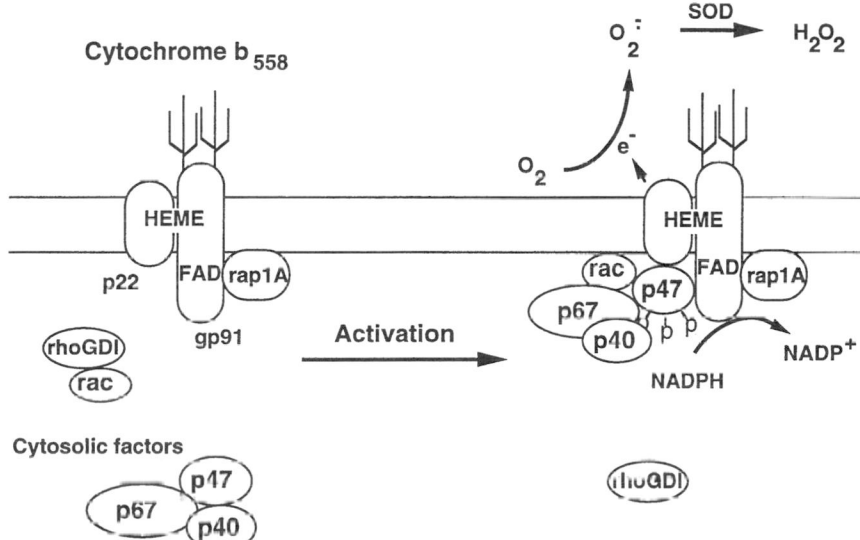

FIG. 4. Schematic of the protein components of the phagocyte NADPH oxidase. On activation, the cytoplasmic components rac, p67, p47, and p40 are translocated to the cell membrane to form the catalytic complex. Once formed, the complex can catalyze the conversion of molecular oxygen (O_2) to superoxide (O_2^-), which is then converted to the toxic oxygen metabolite, hydrogen peroxide (H_2O_2) by the actions of superoxide dismutase (*SOD*). The proteins associate via specific recognition sites, known as SH3 domains, as described in refs. 301–303 (Illustration courtesy of Dr. Thomas Leto.)

Monocytes and Macrophages

Monocytes, also within the "professional phagocyte" grouping, migrate into the tissues, as do the neutrophils (217–223). Activated macrophages, like neutrophils, are capable of phagocytosis and release antibacterial proteins and proinflammatory mediators. Macrophage functions complement those of neutrophils during the acute response, and they take on a more central role during chronic inflammation. The biology and physiology of macrophages are covered in detail in Chapter 15.

Eosinophils

Eosinophils are primarily tissue-dwelling granulocytes that are also recruited to sites of acute inflammation, seen most prominently in response to respiratory, gastrointestinal, and dermatologic allergens, and to generalized infection with helminthic parasites (224–228). Similar to neutrophils, eosinophils develop in the bone marrow, have receptor-mediated responses to specific activating agents (including RANTES, MIP-1α, and eotaxin), and contain cytoplasmic granules with oxidative and cationic proteins; in contrast to neutrophils, eosinophils are ineffective phagocytes and release the contents of their granules to the extracellular milieu. Interestingly, the detrimental features of eosinophils are among the best characterized, particularly their contributions to the pathogenesis of reactive airway disease (229–231), while the beneficial aspects of eosinophils in the inflammatory response remain poorly (if at all) understood.

Platelets and Lymphocytes

Platelets contribute to the inflammatory response by several different mechanisms (236–247). Platelets contain and can release numerous inflammatory mediators, including fibrinogen, plasminogen, and other components that participate in the plasma protease systems, lipids, and serotonin. Several of these mediators released from platelets are direct activating agents for neutrophils, and, conversely, mediators released by activated neutrophils (oxygen metabolites, granule proteins, lipids) serve to alter platelet function. Platelets interact with lymphocytes, providing the cell contact and reagents for prostaglandin synthesis. Platelets also interact with fibroblasts, stimulating collagen and fibronectin synthesis during resolution (see later discussion).

The complex biology of T- and B-lymphocytes and their role in specific immunity are discussed in detail in Chapters 6, 7, 10 and 11; the role of immunoglobulins in augmenting the inflammatory response and enhancing neutrophil phagocytosis has been discussed above. It is also important to emphasize that many of the soluble mediators discussed in the earlier sections (interleukins, IFN-γ) are produced by activated T-lymphocytes, as are a number of the antiinflammatory mediators to be discussed below.

Endothelial Cells

The role of endothelial cells in providing a base for neutrophil adherence has already been discussed. More recently appreciated is the fact that endothelial cells synthesize and release numerous proinflammatory mediators (236–247; see also references from selectins and integrins above).

ALLERGY AND INFLAMMATION

Allergy, also known as the immediate hypersensitivity response, is also a form of inflammation and is considered in detail in Chapter 35. The central components of this type of the allergic response are IgE, IgE receptors on basophils and mast cells, and histamine released from these cells upon IgE receptor–mediated interaction. The role of allergy in host defense remains controversial and is focused on the role of IgE and mucosal mast cells in the defense against gastrointestinal parasites (248–250); most of the literature on allergy focuses on its detrimental features.

RESOLUTION OF THE ACUTE INFLAMMATORY RESPONSE

Resolution, or the way in which the acute inflammatory response is downregulated, is currently an area of active research. The mediators promoting inflammatory resolution may ultimately be harnessed for use as therapeutic agents in limiting the injurious aspects of acute inflammation.

Cell Senescence or Apoptosis

A concept that has been appreciated only recently, apoptosis, or programmed cell death, is an active process in which cells, responding to specific stimuli, undergo a stereotypical pattern of morphologic changes (nuclear condensation, DNA "laddering") prior to their eventual demise. Granulocyte apoptosis as a means of inflammatory resolution is an intriguing avenue of current research (251–257). Several cytokines have been reported to modulate neutrophil apoptosis *in vitro,* including TNF-α, eicosanoids, IL-10, and antioxidants (258–262); the role of these mediators in the resolution of acute inflammation awaits future study (see also Chapter 23).

Antiinflammatory Mediators

The antiinflammatory effects of a number of soluble mediators have been characterized. There are most likely many others awaiting identification and characterization (see also Chapter 22).

Interleukin-4

In addition to the proinflammatory effects described previously, IL-4 downregulates IL-6 production and is involved in the downregulation of neutrophil superoxide production (263).

Transforming Growth Factor-β

TGF-β promotes several antiinflammatory effects, including suppression of hematopoiesis, reduction in production of proinflammatory cytokines, and inhibition of leukocyte adhesion (264–269). Perhaps most dramatic, TGF-β 1 knock-out mice develop severe inflammation in multiple tissues, suggesting the primary role of TFG-β as that of an antiinflammatory mediator (270,271). TGF-β is produced in many cell types, including platelets, macrophages, and T- and B-lymphocytes.

Interleukin-10 and Interleukin-13

IL-10 is produced by macrophages and CD8⁺ T-lymphocytes, and it has been shown to inhibit the activation of specific macrophage subsets, including inhibition of the production of proinflammatory cytokines and interference with the macrophage-mediated antigen presentation. IL-10 is also implicated in host response to both Epstein-Barr virus and human immunodeficiency virus infection (272–276). IL-13 has been observed to induce IL-4–independent IgE synthesis and to induce proliferation and differentiation of human B cells activated by the CD40 ligand (277–279).

Hypothalamo–Pituitary–Adrenocortical Axis

One of the more intriguing avenues of investigation is the connection between the central nervous system, the adrenal cortex, and the resolution of inflammation (280–284). An appreciation of this phenomenon relates to the observation that glucocorticoids, produced by the adrenal cortex, mediate immunosuppression, and thus may downregulate the acute inflammatory response. Numerous studies have suggested that IL-1, IL-6, and TNF-α promote marked increases in hypothalamic stimulation, leading to increases in serum ACTH and corticosterone in experimental animal systems; prostaglandins have also been implicated in this process.

Wound Repair and Angiogenesis

Several morphologic stages of wound repair have been described (264–268). Neutrophils and macrophages carry out the initial debridement, including removal of foreign material and cellular debris. Fibroblasts and epithelial and endothelial cells, responding to multiple inflammatory mediators, grow and divide to create new tissue and restore function. Angiogenesis is the process by which new tissue is revascularized. The formation of capillaries has been shown to proceed through several well-defined morphologic events, including vasodilation of the parent venule or capillary, removal of the preexisting basement membrane, migration and proliferation of endothelial cells, and formation of a new lumen. These events are promoted by numerous soluble mediators, including epidermal growth factor, keratinocyte growth factor, platelet-derived growth factor, fibroblast growth factors, TGF-α, TGF-β, and cellular mediators (macrophages, platelets, keratinocytes, endothelial cells, and mast cells) (285–289).

CHRONIC INFLAMMATION

When acute inflammation persists, either through incomplete clearance of the initial inflammatory focus or as a result of multiple acute events occurring in the same location, chronic inflammation takes over. In contrast to acute inflammation, which is characterized by a primarily neutrophil influx, the histologic findings in chronic inflammation include accumulation of macrophages and lymphocytes and growth of fibroblasts and vascular tissue. It is these latter two features that result in the tissue scarring that is typically seen at sites of prolonged or repeated inflammatory activity.

Among the most interesting sequelae of chronic inflammation is the formation of a tissue granuloma (290–296). A granuloma is a collection inflammatory cells—principally macrophages and lymphocytes, which are eventually surrounded by a fibrotic wall—that forms in tissues as part of the inflammatory response to a persistent irritant. Several unusual cell types are characteristic of granulomata, including epithelioid cells, which are macrophage derivatives, and multinuclear giant cells, which are fusions of epithelioid cells and

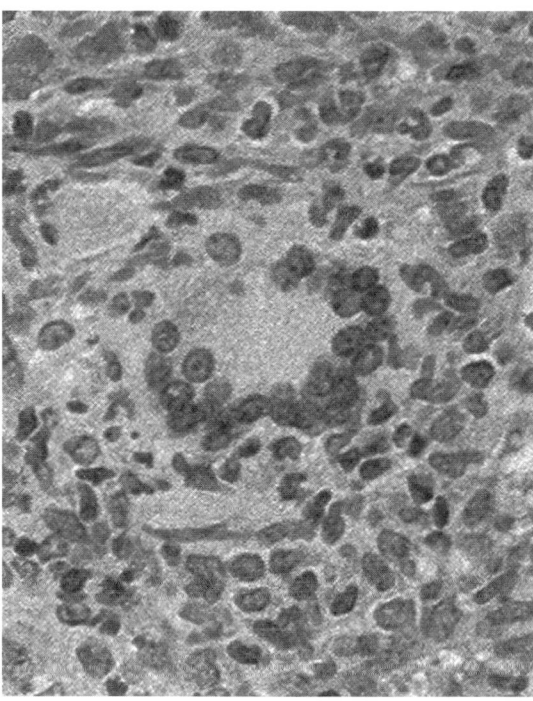

FIG. 5. Light microscopic image of a tissue granuloma from the murine CGD (p47 phox knock-out) model (304). Lymphocytes comprise the central core, which is surrounded by macrophages and fibroblasts.

macrophages (Fig. 5). Although the precise mechanism of granuloma formation and resolution is not yet clear, the actions of specifically sensitized T cells and their soluble mediators (including TNF-α and IFN-γ) participate in the formation and maintenance of granulomata in their active state. Several conditions predispose an individual to granuloma formation, most notably the presence of intracellular bacteria (e.g., tuberculosis; see Chapter 40) or inorganic antigens (e.g., berylliosis).

More recent work on the molecular mechanisms underlying chronic inflammation has focused on the role of NF-κB, a transcription factor originally identified as regulating the expression of the murine κ light chains. Since that time, NF-κB activation has been associated with endotoxin, cytokines, viruses, and oxidants, and NF-κB has been shown to regulate expression of adhesion molecules, E-selectin, and numerous chemotactic cytokines (297–299).

FUTURE DIRECTIONS: NOVEL ANTIINFLAMMATORY THERAPIES

The goal of antiinflammatory therapy is to eliminate the undesirable aspects of the double-edged sword—tissue destruction beyond what is absolutely necessary for containing and eliminating a pathogenic agent. At the same time, antiinflammatory therapy must be sufficiently short-lived and/or selective so as to avoid creating an immunocompromised host. To this end, several generalized antiinflammatory agents (e.g., glucocorticoids, nonsteroidal antiinflammatory agents) have been recognized for their broad scope of effectiveness. Specific agents on the horizon may be more effective at pinpointing specific aspects of the inflammatory response that might be more carefully controlled.

Immunophilin-binding Agents

Cyclosporine (CsA) and FK506 (tacrolimus) are the most current of this group of generalized antiinflammatory agents (305–310). CsA and FK506 are structurally unrelated agents that selectively inhibit T-lymphocyte activation by interfering with the transcription of several cytokine genes. In the most recently proposed molecular mechanism, CsA and FK506 interact with distinct intracellular-binding proteins, known as immunophilins, which have enzymatic activity that appears to be unrelated to their role in immunosuppression. The immunophilin-bound complexes formed interfere with calcineurin-mediated transcriptional activation, thus inhibiting transcription of the genes encoding the proinflammatory agents IL-2, IL-3, IL-4, GM-CSF, IL-8, and IFN-γ; the complexes also function by suppressing T-cell proliferation. Although used primarily as adjuvant therapy in organ transplantation, they have also been used in the treatment of rheumatoid arthritis and inflammatory bowel disease (311–314).

Experimental Antiinflammatory Agents

Several groups have experimented with agents that specifically inhibit individual proinflammatory mediators (315–332) or pathways (333–337), including specific cytokine and receptor antagonists. Other approaches take their lead from the actions of the immunophilin-binding proteins, and have considered ways to exert transcriptional control on one or more proinflammatory mediators (337,338). In the not too distant future, gene replacement therapy may emerge as an option, once the genetic bases of the complex inflammatory disorders have been identified and elucidated.

REFERENCES

1. Hunter J. *A treatise of the blood inflammation, and gunshot wounds.* vol I. London: J. Nicoll, 1794.
2. Cohnheim J. *Lectures in general pathology.* vol I. London: New Sydenham Society, 1889. McKee AD, translator, from the German edition.
3. Dale HH, Laidlaw PP. The physiologic action of b-imidazolyethylamine. *J Physiol* 1911;41:318–344.
4. Gallin JI, Goldstein IM, Snyderman R, eds. *Inflammation.* 2nd ed. New York: Raven Press, 1992.
5. Musher D, Cohen M, Baker C. Immune responses to extracellular bacteria. In: Rich RR, Fleisher TA, Schwartz, BD, Shearer WT, Strober W, eds. *Clinical immunology.* vol I. St. Louis: Mosby–Year Book, 1996:479–502.
6. Robbins SL, Cotran RS. Inflammation and repair. In: *Pathologic basis of disease.* 2nd ed. Philadelphia: WB Saunders, 1979:59–63.
7. Ward PA. Role of complement, chemokines, and regulatory cytokines in acute lung injury. *Ann NY Acad Sci* 1996;796:104–112.
8. Goldstein IM. Complement: biologically active products. In: Gallin JI, Goldstein IM, Snyderman R, eds. *Inflammation.* 2nd ed. New York: Raven Press, 1992:63–80.
9. Kozel TR. Activation of the complement system by pathogenic fungi. *Clin Microbiol Rev* 1996;9:34–46.
10. Muller-Eberhard HJ. Complement: chemistry and pathways. In: Gallin JI, Goldstein IM, Snyderman R, eds. *Inflammation.* 2nd ed. New York: Raven Press, 1992:33–62.
11. Holers VM. Complement. In: Rich RR, Fleisher TA, Schwartz BD Shearer WT, Strober W, eds. *Clinical immunology: principles and practice.* St. Louis: Mosby–Year Book, 1996:363–391.
12. Holers VM. Complement. In: Rich, RR, Fleisher TA, Schwartz BD, Shearer WT, Strober W, eds. *Clinical immunology: principles and practice.* St. Louis: Mosby–Year Book, 1996:363–391.
13. Ratnoff WD. Inherited deficiencies of complement in rheumatic diseases. *Rheum Dis Clin North* Am 1996;22:75–94.
14. Ono H, Kawaguchi H, Ishii N, Nakajima H. A point mutation in exon 7 of the C1-inhibitor gene causing type I hereditary angioedema. *Hum Genet* 1996;98:452–453.
15. Ernst SC, Circolo A, Davis AE, Gheesling-Mullis K, Fliesler M, Strunk RC. Impaired production of both normal and mutant C1 inhibitor proteins in type I hereditary angioedema with a duplication in exon 8. *J Immunol* 1996;157:405–410.
16. Busse R, Fleming I. Molecular responses of endothelial tissue to kinins. *Diabetes* 1996;45[Suppl 1]:S8–S13.
17. Gepetti P, Bertrand C, Ricciardolo FL, Nadel JA, Ricciardolo FL. New aspects on the role of kinins in neurogenic inflammation. *Can J Physiol Pharmacol* 1995;73:843–847.
18. Margolius HS. Kallikreins and kinins. Molecular characteristics and cellular and tissue responses. *Diabetes* 1996;45[Suppl 1]:S14–S19.
19. Margolius HS. Kallikreins and kinins. Some unanswered questions about system characteristics and roles in human disease. *Hypertension* 1995;26:221–229.
20. Mombouli JV, Vanhoutte PM. Kinins and endothelial control of vascular smooth muscle. *Annu Rev Pharmacol Toxicol* 1995;35:679–705.
21. Carmeliet P, Collen D. Gene targeting and gene transfer studies of the biological role of the plasminogen/plasmin system. *Thromb Haemost* 1995;74:429–436.
22. Altieri DC. Inflammatory cell participation in coagulation. *Semin Cell Biol* 1995;6:269–274.
23. Esmon CT, Fukudome K. Cellular regulation of the protein C pathway. *Semin Cell Biol* 1995;6:259–268.
24. Esmon CT. Inflammation and thrombosis: the impact of inflammation on the protein C anticoagulant pathway. *Haematology* 1995;80[Suppl 2]:49–56.
25. Salgado A, Boveda JL, Monasterio J, et al. Inflammatory mediators and their influence on haemostasis. *Haemostasis* 1994;24:132–138.
26. Benedict CR, Pakala R, Willerson JT. Endothelial-dependent procoagulant and anticoagulant mechanisms. Recent advances in understanding. *Tex Heart Inst J* 1994;21:86–90.
27. Brady HR, Serhan CN. Lipoxins: putative braking signals in host defense, inflammation and hypersensitivity. *Curr Opin Nephrol Hypertens* 1996;5:20–27.
28. Davies P, MacIntyre DE. Prostaglandins and inflammation. In: Gallin JI, Goldstein IM, Snyderman R, eds. *Inflammation.* 2nd ed. New York: Raven Press, 1992:123–138.
29. Wallace JL, Tigley AW. New insights into prostaglandins and mucosal defense. *Aliment Pharmacol Ther* 1995;9:227–35.
30. Vane JR, Botting RM. New insights into the mode of action of anti-inflammatory drugs. *Inflamm Res* 1995;44:1–10.
31. Goetzl EJ, An S, Smith WL. Specificity of expression and effects of eicosanoid mediators in normal physiology and human diseases. *FASEB J* 1995;9:1051–1058.
32. Seibert K, Masferrer J, Zhang Y, et al. Mediation of inflammation by cyclooxygenase-2. *Agents Actions Suppl* 1995;46:41–50.
33. Ashby B. Interactions among prostaglandin receptors. *Receptor* 1994;4:31–32
34. Lam BK, Austen KF. Leukotrienes: biosynthesis, release, and actions. In: Gallin JI, Goldstein IM, Snyderman R, eds. *Inflammation.* 2nd ed. New York: Raven Press, 1992:139–148.
35. Ford-Hutchinson AW. Regulation of leukotriene biosynthesis. *Cancer Metastasis Rev* 1994;13:257–267.
36. Henderson WR Jr. The role of leukotrienes in inflammation. *Ann Intern Med* 1994;121:684–697.
37. Obata T, Yamashita N, Nakagawa T. Leukotriene and thromboxane antagonists. *Clin Rev Allergy* 1994;12:79–93.
38. Busse WW. The role of leukotrienes in asthma and allergic rhinitis. *Clin Exp Allergy* 1996;26:868–879.
39. Spector SL. Leukotriene inhibitors and antagonists in asthma. *Ann Allergy Asthma Immunol* 1995;75:463–470.
40. Dahlen B, Dahlen SE. Leukotrienes as mediators of airway obstruction and inflammation in asthma. *Clin Exp Allergy* 1995;2:50–54.
41. Harris RR, Carter GW, Bell RL, Moore JL, Brooks DW. Clinical activity of leukotriene inhibitors. *Int J Immunopharmacol* 1995;17:147–156.
42. Israel E. Moderating the inflammation of asthma: inhibiting the production or action of products of the 5-lipoxygenase pathway. *Ann Allergy* 1994;72:279–284.
43. Kingsnorth AN. Platelet-activating factor. *Scand J Gastroenterol Suppl* 1996;219:28–31.
44. Bussolino F, Camussi G. Platelet-activating factor produced by endothelial cells. A molecule with autocrine and paracrine properties. *Eur J Biochem* 1995;229:327–337.
45. Pinckard RN, Woodard DS, Showell HJ, Conklyn MJ, Novak MJ, McManus LM. Structural and (patho)physiological diversity of PAF. *Clin Rev Allergy* 1994;12:329–359.
46. Snyder F. Metabolic processing of PAF. *Clin Rev Allergy* 1994;12:309–327.
47. Zimmerman, GA, Prescott SM, McIntyre TM. Platelet-activating factor: a fluid-phase and cell-associated mediator of inflammation. In: Gallin JI, Goldstein IM, Snyderman R, eds. *Inflammation.* New York: Raven Press, 1992:149–162.
48. Dent G, Ukena D, Chanez P, Sybrecht G, Barnes P. Characterization of PAF receptors on human neutrophils using the specific antagonist, WEB 2086. *FEBS Lett* 1989 244:365–368.
49. Hilger RA, Koller M, Konig W. Inhibition of leukotriene formation and IL-8 release by the PAF-receptor antagonist SM-12502. *Inflammation* 1996;20:57–70.
50. Catalan RE, Martinez AM, Aragones MD, Lombardia M, Garde E. PCA-4248, a PAF receptor antagonist, inhibits PAF-induced phosphoinositide turnover. *Eur J Pharmacol* 1995;290:183–188.
51. Canz MJ, Weg VG, Walsh DT, Williams TJ, Nourshargh S. Differential effects of the PAF receptor antagonist UK-74, 505 on neutrophil and eosinophil accumulation in guinea-pig skin. *Br J Pharmacol* 1994;113:513–521.
52. Yokota Y, Inamura N, Asano M, et al. Effect of FR128998, a novel PAF receptor antagonist on endotoxin-induced disseminated intravascular coagulation. *Eur J Pharmacol* 1994;258:239–246.

53. Underwood SL, Lewis SA, Raeburn D. RP 59227, a novel PAF receptor antagonist: effects in guinea pig models of airway hyperreactivity. *Eur J Pharmacol* 1992;210:97–102.
54. Atkinson TP, White MV, Kaliner MA. Histamine and serotonin. In: Gallin JI, Goldstein IM, Snyderman R, eds. *Inflammation.* 2nd ed. New York: Raven Press, 1992:193–210.
55. MacDonald SM. Histamine-releasing factors. *Curr Opin Immunol* 1996;8: 778–783.
56. Raud J, Thorlacius J, Xie X, Lindbom L, Hedqvist P. Interactions between histamine and leukotrienes in the microcirculation. Aspects of relevance to acute allergic inflammation. *Ann NY Acad Sci* 1994;744:191–198.
57. Greaves MW, Sabroe RA. Histamine: the quintessential mediator. *J Dermatol* 1996;23:735–740.
58. Gothert M, Garbarg M, Hey JA, Schlicker E, Schwartz JC, Levi R. New aspects of the role of histamine in cardiovascular function: identification, characterization and potential pathophysiological importance of H3 receptors. *Can J Physiol Pharmacol* 1995;73:558–564.
59. Du Buske LM. Clinical comparison of histamine H1-receptor antagonist drugs. *J Allergy Clin Immunol* 1996;98:S307–S318.
60. Roberts DJ. A preclinical overview of ebastine. Studies on the pharmacological properties of a novel histamine H1 receptor antagonist. *Drugs* 1996;S1:8–14.
61. Nielsen HJ. Histamine-2 receptor antagonists as immunomodulators: new therapeutic views? *Ann Med* 1996;28:107–113.
62. Leurs R, Vollinga RC, Timmerman H. The medicinal chemistry and therapeutic potentials of ligands of the histamine H3 receptor. *Prog Drug Res* 1995;45: 107–165.
63. Leurs R, Smit MJ, Timmerman H. Molecular pharmacological aspects of histamine receptors. *Pharmacol Ther* 1995;66:413–463.
64. Zingel V, Leschke C, Schunack W. Developments in histamine H1-receptor agonists. *Prog Drug Res* 1995;44:49–85.
65. Arrang JM, Drutel G, Garbarh M, Ruat M, Traffort E, Schwartz JC. Molecular and functional diversity of histamine receptor subtypes. *Ann NY Acad Sci* 31995; 757:314–323.
66. Arrang JM. Pharmacological properties of histamine receptor subtypes. *Cell Mol Biol* 1994;40:275–281.
67. Cazzola M, Matera MG, D Amato G, Rossi F. Effects of serotonin on airways: recent developments. *Allergy* 1995;50:1–10.
68. Chancellor-Freeland C, Zhu GF, Kage R, Beller DI, Leeman SE, Black PH. Substance P and stress-induced changes in macrophages. *Ann NY Acad Sci* 1995; 771:472–484.
69. Hanesch U. Neuropeptides in dural fine sensory nerve endings involvement in neurogenic inflammation? *Prog Brain Res* 1996;113:299–317.
70. Reubi JC, Laissue J, Waser B, Horisberger U, Schaer JC. Expression of somatostatin receptors in normal, inflamed and enoplastic human gastrointestinal tissues. *Ann NY Acad Sci* 1994;733:122–137.
71. Said SI. Vasoactive intestinal peptide and nitric oxide: divergent roles in relation to tissue injury. *Ann NY Acad Sci* 1996;805:379–387.
72. Weinstock JV. Vasoactive intestinal peptide regulation of granulomatous inflammation in murine Schistosomiasis mansoni. *Adv Neuroimmunol* 1996;6:95–105.
73. Reichlin S. Neuroendocrine-immune interactions. *N Engl J Med* 1993;329: 1246–1253.
74. Matsumura T, Kugiyama K, Sugiyama S, et al. Neutral endopeptidase 24.11 in neutrophils modulates protective effects of natriuretic peptides against neutrophil-induced endothelial cytotoxicity. *J Clin Invest* 1996;97:2192–2203.
75. Painter RG, Aiken ML. Regulation of N-formyl-methionyl-leucyl-phenylalanine receptor recycling by surface membrane neutral endopeptidease-mediated degradation of ligand. *J Leukoc Biol* 1995;58:468–476.
76. Fagny C, Marchant A, De Prez E, Goldman M, Deschodt-Lanckman M. Lipopolysaccharide induced upregulation of neutral endopeptidase 24.11 on human neutrophils: involvement of the CD14 receptor. *Clin Sci* 1995;89:83–89.
77. Denis M. Human monocytes/macrophages: NO or no NO? *J Leukoc Biol* 1994; 55:682–684.
78. Moncada S, Higgs A. The L-arginine-nitric oxide pathway. *N Engl J Med* 1993;329:2002–2012.
79. Schoedon G, Schneemann M, Walter R, Blau N, Hofer S, Schaffner A. Nitric oxide and infection: another view. *Clin Infect Dis* 1995;21[Suppl 2]:S152 S157.
80. Davies MG, Fulton GJ, Hagen PO. Clinical biology of nitric oxide. *Br J Surg* 1995;82:1598–1610.
81. Granger DL, Hibbs JB Jr. High-output nitric oxide: weapon against infection? *Trends Microbiol* 1996;4:46–47.
82. Lowenstein CJ, Dinerman JL, Snyder SH. Nitric oxide: a physiologic messenger. *Ann Intern Med* 1994;120:227–237.
83. Schneemann M, Schoedon G, Hofer S, Blau N, Guerrero L, Schaffner A. Nitric oxide synthase is not a constituent of the antimicrobial armature of human mononuclear phagocytes. *J Infect Dis* 1993;167:1358–1363.
84. Denis M. Tumor necrosis factor and granulocyte macrophage-colony stimulating factor stimulate human macrophages to restrict growth of virulent *Mycobacterium avium*: killing effector mechanism depends on the generation of reactive nitrogen intermediates. *J Leukoc Biol* 1991;49:380 382.
85. Hibbs JB, Westenfelder C, Taintor R, et al. Evidence for cytokine-inducible nitric oxide synthesis from L-arginine in patients receiving interleukin-2 therapy. *J Clin Invest* 1992;89:867–877.
86. Bukrinsky M, Schmidtmayerova H, Zybarth G, Dubrovsky L, Sherry B,

87. Enikolopov G. A critical role of nitric oxide in human immunodeficiency type 1-induced hyperresponsiveness of cultures monocytes. *Mol Med* 1996;2:460–468.
87. Zembala M, Siedlar M, Marcinkiewicz J, Pryjma J. Human monocytes are stimulated for nitric oxide release in vitro by some tumor cells but not by cytokines and lipopolysaccharide. *Eur J Immunol* 1994;24:435–439.
88. Howard OM, Ben-Baruch A, Oppenheim JJ. Chemokines: progress toward identifying molecular targets for therapeutic agents. *Trends Biotechnol* 1996;14:46–51.
89. Murphy PM. Chemokine receptors: structure, function and role in microbial pathogenesis. *Cytokine Growth Factor Rev* 1996;7:47–64.
90. Prieschl EE, Kulmburg PA, Baumruker T. The nomenclature of chemokines. *Int Arch Allergy Immunol* 1995;107:475–483.
91. Estrov Z, Kurzrock R, Talpaz M. Interleukin-1 and its inhibitors: implications for disease, biology and therapy. *Cancer Treat Res* 1995;80:51–82.
92. Dinarello CA. Interleukin-1 and interleukin-1 receptor antagonist. *Nutrition* 1995;11:492–494.
93. Dinarello CA. Biologic basis for interleukin-1 in disease. *Blood* 1996;87: 2095–2147.
94. Fantuzzi G, Dinarello CA. The inflammatory response in interleukin-1 beta deficient mice: comparison with other cytokine-related knock-out mice. *J Leukoc Biol* 1996;59:489–493.
95. Saklatvala J. Intracellular signalling mechanisms of interleukin 1 and tumour necrosis factor: possible targets for therapy. *Br Med Bull* 1995;51:402–418.
96. Kupper TS, Groves RW. The interleukin-1 axis and cutaneous inflammation. *J Invest Dermatol* 1995;105:62S–66S.
97. Burger D, Dayer JM. Inhibitory cytokines and cytokine inhibitors. *Neurology* 1995;45:S39–S43.
98. Dinarello CA. The biological properties of interleukin-1. *Eur Cytokine Netw* 1994;5:517–531.
99. van der Meer JW, Vogels MT, Kullberg BJ. Interleukin-1 and related proinflammatory cytokines in the treatment of bacterial infections in neutropenic and non-neutropenic animals. *Biotherapy* 1994;7:161–167.
100. Mantovani A, Muzio M, Ghezzi P, Colotta F, Introna M. Negative regulators of the interleukin-1 system: receptor antagonists and a decoy receptor. *Int J Clin Lab Res* 1996;26:7–14.
101. Lennard AC. Interleukin-1 receptor antagonist. *Crit Rev Immunol* 1995;15: 77–105.
102. Kopf M, Le Gros G, Coyle AJ, Kosco-Vilbois M, Brombacher F. Immune responses of IL-4, IL-5, IL-6 deficient mice. *Immunol Rev* 1995;148:45 69.
103. Puri RK. Structure and function of interleukin-4 and its receptor. *Cancer Treat Res* 1995;80:143–185.
104. Schroeder JT, Kagey-Sobotka A, MacGlashan DW, Lichtenstein LM. The interaction of cytokines with human basophils and mast cells. *Int Arch Allergy Immunol* 1995;107:79–81.
105. Tepper RI. The anti-tumor and proinflammatory actions of IL-4. *Res Immunol* 1993;144:633–637.
106. Ryan JJ, McReynolds LJ, Keegan A, et al. Growth and gene expression are predominantly controlled by distinct regions of the human IL-4 receptor. *Immunity* 1996;4:123–132.
107. Pernis A, Witthuhn B, Keegan AD, et al. Interleukin 4 signals through two related pathways. *Proc Natl Acad Sci USA* 1995;92:7971–7975.
108. Keegan AD, Johnston JA, Tortolani PJ, et al. Similarities and differences in signal transduction by interleukin 4 and interleukin 13: analysis of Janus kinase activation. *Proc Natl Acad Sci USA* 1995;92:7681–7685.
109. Sehgal PB. Interleukin-6-type cytokines in vivo: regulated bioavailability. *Proc Soc Exp Biol Med* 1996;213:238–247.
110. Biffl WL, Moore EE, Moore FA, Peterson VM. Interleukin-6 and the injured patient. Marker of injury or mediator of inflammation? *Ann Surg* 1996;224: 647–664.
111. Baatout S. Interleukin-6 and megakaryocytopoeisis: an update. *Ann Hematol* 1996;73:157–162.
112. Paquet P, Pierard GE. Interleukin-6 and the skin. *Int Arch Allergy Immunol* 1996; 109:308–317.
113. Luheshi G, Rothwell N. Cytokines and fever. *Int Arch Allergy Immunol* 1996; 109:301–307.
114. Harada A, Mukaida N, Matsushima K. Interleukin 8 as a novel target for intervention therapy in acute inflammatory diseases. *Mol Med Today* 1996;2: 482 489.
115. Hoch RC, Schraufstatter IU, Cochrane CG. In vivo, in vitro, and molecular aspects of interleukin-8 and the interleukin-8 receptors. *J Lab Clin Med* 1996; 128:134–145.
116. Kunkel SL, Lukacs N, Streiter RM. Chemokines and their role in human disease. *Agents Actions Suppl* 1995;46:11–22.
117. Baggiolini M, Loetscher P, Moser B. Interleukin-8 and the chemokine family. *Int J Immunopharmacol* 1995;17:103–108.
118. Ben-Baruch A, Michiel DF, Oppenheim JJ. Signals and receptors involved in recruitment of inflammatory cells. *J Biol Chem* 1995;270:11703–11706.
119. Harada A, Sekido N, Akahochi T, Wada T, Mukaida N, Matsushima K. Essential involvement of interleukin-8 (IL-8) in acute inflammation. *J Leukoc Biol* 1994;56:559–564.
120. Horuk R. The interleukin-8-receptor family: from chemokines to malaria. *Immunol Today* 1994;15:169–174.
121. Murphy PM, Tiffany HL. Cloning of a complementary DNA encoding a functional human interleukin-8 receptor. *Science* 1991;253:1280–1283.

122. Lynch DH. The role of FasL and TNF in the homeostatic regulation of immune responses. *Adv Exp Med Biol* 1996;406:135–138.

123. Barbara JA, van Ostade X, Lopez A. Tumour necrosis factor alpha (TNF-alpha): the good, the bad and the potentially very effective. *Immunol Cell Biol* 1996;74: 434–443.

124. Riches DW, Chan ED, Winston BW. TNF-alpha-induced regulation and signalling in macrophages. *Immunobiology* 1996;195:477–490.

125. Douni E, Akassoglou K, Alexopoulou L, et al. Transgenic and knockout analyses of the role of TNF in immune regulation and disease pathogenesis. *J Inflamm* 1995-6;47:27–38.

126. Gruss HJ, Duyster J, Hermann F. Structural and biological features of the TNF receptor and TNF ligand superfamilies. *Ann Oncol* 1996;4:19–26.

127. Cosman D. A family of ligands for the TNF receptor superfamily. *Stem Cells* 1994;12:440–455.

128. Beutler B. TNF, immunity and inflammatory disease: lessons of the past decade. *J Invest Med* 1995;43:227–235.

129. Cleveland JL, Ihle JN. Contenders in the FasL/TNF death signalling. *Cell* 1995; 81:479–482.

130. Ware CF, VanArsdale S, VanArsdale TL. Apoptosis mediated by the TNF-related cytokine and receptor families. *J Cell Biochem* 1996;60:47–55.

131. Baker SJ, Reddy EP. Transducers of life and death: TNF receptor superfamily and associated proteins. *Oncogene* 1996;12:1–9.

132. Young HA. Regulation of interferon-gamma gene expression. *J Interferon Cytokine Res* 1996;16:563–568.

133. Billiau A. Interferon-gamma: biology and role in pathogenesis. *Adv Immunol* 1996;62:61–130.

134. Young HA, Hardy KJ. Role of interferon-gamma in immune cell regulation. *J Leukoc Biol* 1995;58:373–381.

135. Gallin JI, Farber JM, Holland SM, Nutman TB. Interferon-gamma in the management of infectious diseases. *Ann Intern Med* 1995;123:216–224.

136. Appelberg R. Protective role of interferon gamma, tumor necrosis factor alpha and interleukin-6 in mycobacterium tuberculosis and M. avium infections. *Immunobiology* 1994;191:520–525.

137. Vilcek J, Oliveira IC. Recent progress in the elucidation of interferon-gamma actions: molecular biology and biological functions. *Int Arch Allergy Immunol* 1994;104:311–316.

138. Newport MJ, Huxley CM, Huston S, et al. A mutation in the interferon-gamma-receptor gene and susceptibility to mycobacterial infection. *N Engl J Med* 1996; 335:1941–1949.

139. Holland SM, Gerstberger SM, Pitha-Rowe IF, et al. Interferon gamma receptor deficiency in disseminated mycobacterium avium complex (DMAC) infection. *J Invest Med* 1997;45:199A.

140. Brown CC, Malech HL, Gallin JI. Intravenous endotoxin recruits distinct subset of human neutrophils, defined by monoclonal antibody 3108, from bone marrow to the peripheral circulation. *Cell Immunol* 1989;123:294–306.

141. Zimmerli W, Gallin JI. Monocytes accumulate on Rebuck skin window coverslips but not in skin chamber fluid. *J Immunol Methods* 1987;96:11–17.

142. Kuhns DB, DeCarlo E, Hawk DM, Gallin JI. Dynamics of the cellular and humoral components of the inflammatory response elicited in skin blisters in human. *J Clin Invest* 1992;89:1734–1740.

143. Martich GD, Danner RL, Ceska M, Suffredini AF. Detection of interleukin-8 and tumor necrosis factor in normal humans after intravenous endotoxin: the effects of anti-inflammatory agents. *J Exp Med* 1991;173:1021–1024.

144. Kishimoto TK, Anderson DC. The role of integrins in inflammation. In: Gallin JI, Goldstein IM, Snyderman R, eds. *Inflammation.* 2nd ed. New York: Raven Press, 1992:353–406.

145. Kuhns DB, Long Priel DA, Gallin JI. Endotoxin and IL-1 hyporesponsiveness in a patient with recurrent bacterial infections. *J Immunol* 1997;158:3959–3964.

146. Haziot A, Tsuberi BZ, Goyert SM. Neutrophil CD14: biochemical properties and role in the secretion of tumor necrosis factor alpha in response to lipopolysaccharide. *J Immunol* 1993;150:5556–5565.

147. Frey EA, Miller DS, Jahr TG, et al. Soluble CD14 participates in the response of cells to lipopolysaccharide. *J Exp Med* 1992;176;1665–1671.

148. Muller JM, Ziegler-Heitbrock HW, Bauerle PA. Nuclear factor kappa B, a mediator of lipopolysaccharide effects. *Immunobiology* 1993;187;233–256.

149. Smith JA. Neutrophils, host defense, and inflammation: a double-edged sword. *J Leukoc Biol* 1994;56:672–686.

150. Edwards SW. *Biochemistry and physiology of the neutrophil.* Cambridge: Cambridge University Press, 1994.

151. Domachowske JB, Malech HL. Phagocytes. In: Rich RR, Fleisher TA, Schwartz BD, Shearer WT, Strober W, eds. *Clinical immunology: principles and practice.* St. Louis: Mosby–Year Book, 1996:392–407.

152. Bainton DF. Developmental biology of neutrophils and eosinophils. In: Gallin JI, Goldstein IM, Snyderman R, eds. *Inflammation.* 2nd ed. New York: Raven Press, 1992:303–324.

153. Sievers EL, Dale DC. Non-malignant neutropenia. *Blood Rev* 1996;10:95–100.

154. Kim SK, Demetri GD. Chemotherapy and neutropenia. *Hematol Oncol Clin North Am* 196;10:377–395.

155. Bernini JC. Diagnosis and management of chronic neutropenia during childhood. *Pediatr Clin North Am* 1996;43:773–792.

156. Welte K, Dale D. Pathophysiology and treatment of severe chronic neutropenia. *Ann Hematol* 1996;72:158–165.

157. Souid AK. Congenital cyclic neutropenia. *Clin Pediatr* 1995;34:151–155.

158. Cohen MS. Molecular events in the activation of human neutrophils for microbial killing. *Clin Infect Dis* 1994;18[Suppl 2]:S170–S179.

159. Downey GP, Fukushima T, Fialkow L, Waddell TK. Intracellular signaling in neutrophil priming and activation. *Semin Cell Biol* 1995;6:345–356.

160. Sengelov H. Complement receptors in neutrophils. *Crit Rev Immunol* 1995;15: 107–131.

161. Edwards SW. Cell signalling by integrins and immunoglobulin receptors in primed neutrophils. *Trends Biochem Sci* 1995;20:362–367.

162. Murphy PM. The molecular biology of leukocyte chemoattractant receptors. *Annu Rev Immunol* 1994;12:593–633.

163. Wells TN, Lusti-Narsimhan M, Chung CW, et al. The molecular basis of selectivity between CC and CXC chemokines: the possibility of chemokine antagonists as anti-inflammatory agents. *Ann NY Acad Sci* 1996;796:245–256.

164. Hoch RC, Schraufstatter IU, Cochrane CG. In vivo, in vitro, and molecular aspects of interleukin-8 and the interleukin-8 receptors. *J Lab Clin Med* 1996; 128:134–145.

165. Symon FA, Wardlaw AJ. Selectins and their counter receptors: a bitter sweet attraction. *Thorax* 1996;51:1155–1157.

166. Crockett-Torabi E, Fantone JC. The selectins: insights into selectin-induced intracellular signalling in leukocytes. *Immunol Res* 1995;14:237–251.

167. Kansas GS. Selectins and their ligands: current concepts and controversies. *Blood* 1996;88:3259–3287.

168. Vestweber D. Ligand-specificity of the selectins. *J Cell Biochem* 1996;61: 585–591.

169. Tedder TF, Steeber DA, Chen A, Engel P. The selectins: vascular adhesion molecules. *FASEB J* 1995;9:866–873.

170. Rosen SD, Bertozzi CR. The selectins and their ligands. *Curr Opin Cell Biol* 1994;6:663–673.

171. McEver RP. Role of selectins in leukocyte adhesion to platelets and endothelium. *Ann NY Acad Sci* 1994;714:185–189.

172. McEver RP. Selectins. *Curr Opin Immunol* 1994;6:75–84.

173. Furie B, Furie BC. The molecular basis of platelet and endothelial cell interaction with neutrophils and monocytes: role of P-selectin and the P-selectin ligand PSGL-1. *Thromb Haemost* 1995;74:224–227.

174. Gille J, Swerlick RA. Integrins: role in cell adhesion and communication. *Ann NY Acad Sci* 1996;797:93–106.

175. Mazzone A, Ricevuti G. Leukocyte CD11/CD18 integrins: biological and clinical relevance. *Haematologica* 1995;80:161–175.

176. Edwards SW. Cell signalling by integrins and immunoglobulin receptors in primed neutrophils. *Trends Biochem Sci* 1995;20:362–367.

177. Luscinskas FW, Lawler J. Integrins as dynamic regulators of vascular function. *FASEB J* 1994;8:929–938.

178. Kishimoto TK, Rothlein R. Integrins, ICAMs and selectins: role and regulation of adhesion molecules in neutrophil recruitment to inflammatory sites. *Adv Pharmacol* 1994;25:117–169.

179. Patarroyo M. Adhesion molecules mediating recruitment of monocytes to inflamed tissue. *Immunobiology* 1994;191:474–477.

180. Carlos TM, Harlan JM. Leukocyte-endothelial adhesion molecules. *Blood* 1994; 84:2068–2101.

181. van de Stolpe A, van der Saag PT. Intercellular adhesion molecule-1. *J Mol Med* 1996;74:13–33.

182. Anderson DC, Schmalsteig FC, Finegold MJ, et al. The severe and moderate phenotypes of heritable Mac-1, LFA-1 deficiency: their quantitative definition and relation to leukocyte dysfunction and clinical features. *J Infect Dis* 1988; 152:668–689.

183. Anderson DC, Springer TA. Leukocyte adhesion deficiency and inherited defect in the Mac-1, LFA-1, and p150, 95 glycoproteins. *Ann Rev Med* 1987;175–194.

184. Kishimoto TK, Hollander N, Roberts TM, Anderson DC, Springer TA. Heterogeneous mutations in the beta subunit common to the LFA-1, Mac-1 and p150, 95 glycoproteins cause leukocyte adhesion deficiency. *Cell* 1987;50:193–202.

185. Etzioni A, Frydman M, Pollack S, et al. Brief report: recurrent severe infections caused by a novel leukocyte adhesion deficiency. *N Engl J Med* 1992;327: 1789–1792.

186. Etzioni A, Phillips LM, Paulson JC, Harlan JM. Leukocyte adhesion deficiency (LAD) II. *Ciba Found Symp* 1995;189:51–58.

187. Brown SS. Structure and function of profilin. *Cell Motil Cytoskeleton* 1990;17: 71–75.

188. Southwick FS, Stossel TP. Contractile proteins in leukocyte function. *Semin Hematol* 1984;30:305–310.

189. Stossel TP. The mechanical responses of white blood cells. In: Gallin JI, Goldstein IM, Snyderman R, eds. *Inflammation.* 2nd ed. New York: Raven Press, 1992:459–476.

190. Wright SD. Receptors for complement and the biology of phagocytosis. In: Gallin JI, Goldstein IM, Snyderman R, eds. *Inflammation.* 2nd ed. New York: Raven Press, 1992:477–496.

191. Allen LA, Aderem A. Mechanisms of phagocytosis. *Curr Opin Immunol* 1996; 8:36–40.

192. Goldman MJ, Anderson GM, Stolzenberg ED, Kari UP, Zasloff M, Wilson JM. Human beta-defensin-1 is a salt-sensitive antibiotic in lung that is inactivated in cystic fibrosis. *Cell* 1997;88:553–560.

193. Lonnerdal B, Iyer S. Lactoferrin: molecular structure and biological function. *Annu Rev Nutr* 1995;15:93–110.

194. Nagle DL, Karim MA, Woolf EA, et al. Identification and mutation analysis of the complete gene for Chediak-Higashi syndrome. *Nat Genet* 1996;14:307–311.

195. Barbosa MD, Nguyen QA, Tchernev VT, et al. Identification of the homologous beige and Chediak-Higashi syndrome genes. *Nature* 1996;382:262–265.

196. Barrat FJ, Auloge L, Pastural E, et al. Genetic and physical mapping of the Che-

diak-Higashi syndrome on chromosome 1q42-43. *Am J Hum Genet* 1996;59: 625–632.

197. Gallin JI. Neutrophil specific granule deficiency. *Annu Rev Med* 1985;36: 263–274.

198. Rosenberg HF, Gallin JI. Neutrophil specific granule deficiency includes eosinophils. *Blood* 1993;82:268–273.

199. Lomax KJ, Gallin JI, Rotrosen D, et al. Selective defect in myeloid cell lactoferrin gene expression in neutrophil specific granule deficiency. *J Clin Invest* 1989; 83:514–519.

200. Parry MF, Root RK, Metcalf JA, Delaney KK, Kaplow LS, Richar WJ. Myeloperoxidase deficiency: prevalence and clinical significance. *Ann Intern Med* 1981;95:293–301.

201. Nauseef WM, Brigham S, Cogley M. Hereditary myeloperoxidase deficiency due to a missense mutation of arginine 569 to tryptophan. *J Biol Chem* 1994;269: 1212–1216.

202. Nauseef WM, Cogley M, McCormack S. Effect of R569W missense mutation on the biosynthesis of myeloperoxidase. *J Biol Chem* 1996;271:9546–9549.

203. DeLeo FR, Quinn MT. Assembly of the phagocyte NADPH oxidase: molecular interaction of the oxidase proteins. *J Leukoc Biol* 1996;60:677–691.

204. Leusen JH, Verhoeven AJ, Roos D. Interactions between the components of the human NADPH oxidase: intrigues in the phox family. *J Lab Clin Med* 1996;128: 461–476.

205. Wientjes FB, Segal AW. NADPH oxidase and the respiratory burst. *Semin Cell Biol* 1995;6:357–365.

206. Henderson LM, Chappel JB. NADPH oxidase of neutrophils. *Biochim Biophys Acta* 1996;1273:87–107.

207. Segal AW. The NADPH oxidase and chronic granulomatous disease. *Mol Med Today* 1996;2:129–135.

208. Jones OT. The regulation of superoxide production by the NADPH oxidase of neutrophils and other mammalian cells. *Bioessays* 1994;16:919–923.

209. Bokoch GM. Regulation of the human neutrophil NADPH oxidase by the Rac GTP-binding proteins. *Curr Opin Cell Biol* 1994;6:212–218.

210. Mardiney MM, Jackson SH, Spratt SK, Li F, Holland SM, Malech HL. Enhanced host defense after gene transfer in the murine p47-phox-deficient model of chronic granulomatous disease. *Blood* 1997;89:2268–2275.

211. Lloyd AR, Oppenheim JJ. Poly's lament: the neglected role of the polymorphonuclear neutrophil in the afferent limb of the immune response. *Immunol Today* 1992;13:169–172.

212. Granelli-Piperno A, Vassalli JD, Reich E. Secretion of plasminogen activator by human polymorphonuclear leukocytes. *J Exp Med* 1977;149:284–289.

213. Shirafuji N, Matsuda S, Ogura H, et al. Granulocyte colony-stimulating factor stimulates human mature neutrophilic granulocytes to produce interferon-alpha. *Blood* 1990;75:17–19.

214. Tiku K, Tiku ML, Skosey JL. Interleukin 1 production by human polymorphonuclear neutrophils. *J Immunol* 1986;136:3677–3685.

215. Hughes V, Humphreys JM, Edwards SW. Protein synthesis is activated in primed neutrophils: a possible role in inflammation. *Biosci Rep* 1987;7:881–889.

216. Kuhns DB, Gallin JI. Increased cell-associated IL-8 in human exudative and A23187-treated peripheral blood neutrophils. *J Immunol* 1995;154:6556–6662.

217. van Furth R. Development and distribution of mononuclear phagocytes. In: Gallin JI, Goldstein IM, Snyderman R, eds. *Inflammation*. 2nd ed. New York: Raven Press, 1992.325–340.

218. Adams DO, Hamilton TA. Macrophages as destructive cells in host defense. In: Gallin JI, Goldstein IM, Snyderman R, eds. *Inflammation*. 2nd ed. New York: Raven Press, 1992:637–662.

219. Laskin DL, Pendino KJ. Macrophages and inflammatory mediators in tissue injury. *Annu Rev Pharmacol Toxicol* 1995;35:655–677.

220. Cavaillon JM. Cytokines and macrophages. *Biomed Pharmacother* 1994;48: 445–453.

221. Thepen T, Kraal G, Holt PG. The role of alveolar macrophages in regulation of lung inflammation. *Ann NY Acad Sci* 1994;725:200–206.

222. Seljelid R, Busund LT. The biology of macrophages: II. Inflammation and tumors. *Eur J Haematol* 1994;52:1–12.

223. Nielsen BW, Mukaida N, Matsushima K, Kasahara T. Macrophages as producers of chemotactic proinflammatory cytokines. *Immunol Ser* 1994;60:131–142.

224. Gleich GJ, Adolphson CR, Leiferman KM. Eosinophils. In: Gallin JI, Goldstein IM, Snyderman R, eds. *Inflammation*. 2nd ed. New York: Raven Press, 1992: 663–700.

225. Spry CJF. *Eosinophils: a comprehensive review and guide to the scientific and medical literature*. Oxford: Oxford University Press, 1988.

226. Martin LB, Kita H, Leiferman KM, Gleich GJ. Eosinophils in allergy: role in disease, degranulation and cytokines. *Int Arch Allergy Immunol* 1996;109: 207–215.

227. Makino S, Fukuda T. *Eosinophils: biological and clinical aspects*. Boca Raton, FL: CRC Press, 1993.

228. Wardlaw AJ. Eosinophils in the 1990s: new perspectives on their role in health and disease. *Postgrad Med J* 1994;70:536–552.

229. Makino S, Fukuda T. Eosinophils and allergy in asthma. *Allergy Proc* 1995;16: 13–21.

230. Seminario MC, Gleich GJ. The role of eosinophils in the pathogenesis of asthma. *Curr Opin Immunol* 1994;6:860–864.

231. Reed CE. The importance of eosinophils in the immunology of asthma and allergic disease. *Ann Allergy* 1994;72:376–380.

232. Weksler BB. Platelets. In: Gallin JI, Goldstein IM, Snyderman R, eds. *Inflammation*. 2nd ed. New York: Raven Press, 1992:727–746.

233. de Sousa JR, Palma-Carlos AG. Platelets and hypersensitivity. *J Investig Allergol Clin Immunol* 1995;5:12–17.

234. Herd CM, Page CP. Pulmonary immune cells in health and disease: platelets. *Eur Respir J* 1994;7:1145–1160.

235. Nash GB. Adhesion between neutrophils and platelets: a modulator of thrombotic and inflammatory events? *Thromb Res* 1994;74:S3–S11.

236. Tonnel AB, Gosset P, Molet S, Tillie-Leblond I, Jeannin P, Joseph M. Interactions between endothelial cells and effector cells in allergic inflammation. *Ann NY Acad Sci* 1996;796:9–20.

237. Kubes P, Granger DN. Leukocyte-endothelial cell interactions evoked by mast cells. *Cardiovasc Res* 1996;32:699–708.

238. Malik AB, Lo SK. Vascular endothelial adhesion molecules and tissue inflammation. *Pharmacol Rev* 1996;48:213–229.

239. Luscinskas FW, Gimbrone MA Jr. Endothelial-dependent mechanisms in chronic inflammatory leukocyte recruitment. *Annu Rev Med* 1996;47:413–421.

240. Garcia JG, Pavalko FM, Patterson CE. Vascular endothelial cell activation and permeability responses to thrombin. *Blood Coagul Fibrinolysis* 1995;6:609–626.

241. Chen CC, Manning AM. Transcriptional regulation of endothelial cell adhesion molecules: a dominant role for NF-kappa B. *Agents Actions Suppl* 1995;47: 135–141.

242. Bevilacqua MP, Nelson RM, Mannori G, Cecconi O. Endothelial-leukocyte adhesion molecules in human disease. *Annu Rev Med* 1994;45:361–378.

243. Vane JR, Botting RM. Mediators from the endothelial cell and their participation in inflammation. *Int J Tissue React* 1994;16:19–49.

244. Varani J, Ward PA. Mechanisms of neutrophil-dependent and neutrophil-independent endothelial cell injury. *Biol Signals* 1994;3:1–14.

245. Korthuis, RJ, Anderson DC, Granger DN. Role of neutrophil-endothelial cell adhesion in inflammatory disorders. *J Crit Care* 1994;9:47–71.

246. Granger DN, Kubes P. The microcirculation and inflammation. Modulation of leukocyte-endothelial cell adhesion. *J Leukoc Biol* 1994;55:662–675.

247. Benedict CR, Pakala R, Willerson JT. Endothelial-dependent procoagulant and anti-coagulant mechanisms. Recent advances in understanding. *Tex Heart Inst J* 1994;21:86–90.

248. Jarrett EEE, Bazin H. Elevation of total serum IgE in rats following helminth parasite infection. *Nature* 1974;251.541–543.

249. Jarrett E. Stimuli for the production and control of IgE in rats. *Immunol Rev* 1978;41:52–76.

250. Hussain R, Ottesen EA. IgE responses in human filiariasis. 3. Specificities of IgE and IgG antibodies compared by immunoblot analysis. *J Immunol* 1985;135: 1415–1420.

251. Anderson GP. Resolution of chronic inflammation by therapeutic induction of apoptosis. *Trends Pharmacol Sci* 1996;17:438–442.

252. Savill J, Haslett C. Granulocyte clearance as apoptosis in the resolution of inflammation. *Semin Cell Biol* 1995;6:385–393.

253. Bellamy CO, Malcomson RD, Harrsion DJ, Wyllie AH. Cell death in health and disease: the biology and regulation of apoptosis. *Semin Cancer Biol* 1995;6:3–16.

254. Savill J. Apoptosis in disease. *Eur J Clin Invest* 1994;24:715–723.

255. Haslett C, Savill JS, Whyte MK, Stern M, Dransfield I, Meagher LC. Granulocyte apoptosis and the control of inflammation. *Philos Trans R Soc London B Biol Sci* 1994;345:327–333.

256. Simon HU, Yousefi S, Blaser K. Tyrosine phosphorylation regulated activation and inhibition of apoptosis in human eosinophils and neutrophils. *Int Arch Allergy Immunol* 1995;107:338–339.

257. Liles WC, Klebanoff SJ. Regulation of apoptosis in neutrophils—Fas track to death? *J Immunol* 1995;155:3289–3291.

258. Cox G. IL-10 enhances resolution of pulmonary inflammation in vivo by promoting apoptosis of neutrophils. *Am J Physiol* 1996;27:L566–L571.

259. Gelrud AK, Carper HT, Mandell GL. Interaction of tumor necrosis factor-alpha and granulocyte colony-stimulating factor on neutrophil apoptosis, receptor expression, and bactericidal function. *Proc Assoc Am Physicians* 1996;108: 455–456.

260. Gon S, Gatanaga T, Sendo F. Involvement of two types of TNF receptor in TNF-alpha induced neutrophil apoptosis. *Microbiol Immunol* 1996;40:463–465.

261. Hebert MJ, Takano T, Holthofer H, Brady HR. Sequential morphologic events during apoptosis of human neutrophils. Modulation by lipoxygenase-derived eicosanoids. *J Immunol* 1996;157:3105–3115.

262. Oishi K, Machida K. Inhibition of neutrophil apoptosis by antioxidants in culture medium. *Scand J Immunol* 1997;45:21–27.

263. Abramson SL, Gallin JI. Interleukin-4 inhibits superoxide production by human mononuclear phagocytes. *J Immunol* 1990;144:625–630.

264. Lawrence DA. Transforming growth factor-beta: a general review. *Eur Cytokine Netw* 1996;7:363–374.

265. Kolodziejczyk SM, Hall BK. Signal transduction and TGF-beta superfamily receptors. *Biochem Cell Biol* 1996;74:299–314.

266. Markowitz SD, Roberts AB. Tumor suppressor activity of the TGF-beta pathway in human cancers. *Cytokine Growth Factor Rev* 1996;7:93–102.

267. Kingsley DM. The TGF-beta superfamily: new members, new receptors, and new genetic tests of function in different organisms. *Genes Dev* 1994;8:133–146.

268. Serra R, Moses HL. Tumor suppressor genes in the TGF-beta signaling pathway? *Nat Med* 1996;2:390–391.

269. Derynck R. TGF-beta-receptor-mediated signaling. *Trends Biochem Sci* 1994; 19:548–553.

270. Letterio JJ, Geiser AG, Kulkarni AB, et al. Autoimmunity associated with TGF-beta1-deficiency in mice is dependent on MHC class II antigen expression. *J Clin Invest* 1996;98:2109–2119.

271. Dang H, Geiser AG, Letterio JJ, et al. SLE-like autoantibodies and Sjogren's syndrome-like lymphoproliferation in TGF-beta knockout mice. *J Immunol* 1995; 155:3205–3212.

272. Moore KW, O Garra A, deWaal Malefyt R, Viera P, Mosmann TR. Interleukin-10. *Annu Rev Immunol* 1993;11:165–190.

273. Hoiden I, Moller G. CD8+ cells are the main producers of IL-10 and IFN gamma after superantigen stimulation. *Scand J Immunol* 1996;44:501–505.

274. Klein SC, Kube D, Abts H, Diehl V, Tesch H. Promotion of IL-8, IL-10, TNF-alpha and TNF-beta production by EBV infection. *Leuk Res* 1996;20:633–636.

275. Schuitemaker H. IL-4 and IL-10 as potent inhibitors of HIV-1 replication in macrophages in vitro. A role for cytokines in the in vivo virus host range? *Res Immunol* 1994;145:588–592.

276. Mosmann TR. Properties and functions of interleukin 10. *Adv Immunol* 1994;56: 1–26.

277. McKenzie AN, Culpepper JA, de Waal Malefyt R, et al. Interleukin 13, a T-cell-derived cytokine that regulated human monocyte and B-cell function. *Proc Natl Acad Sci USA* 1993;90:3735–3739.

278. de Vries JE, Punnonen J, Cocks BG, de Waal Malefyt R, Aversa G. Regulation of the human IgE response by IL-4 and IL-13. *Res Immunol* 1993;144:597–601.

279. Mossman T. Cytokines and immune regulation. In: Rich RR, Fleisher TA, Schwartz BD, Shearer WT, Strober W, eds. *Clinical immunology: principles and practice*. St. Louis: Mosby–Year Book, 1996:217–230.

280. Sternberg EM. Neuroendocrine factors in susceptibility to inflammatory disease: focus on the hypothalamic-pituitary-adrenal axis. *Horm Res* 1995;43: 159–161.

281. Buckingham JC, Loxley HD, Christian HC, Philip JG. Activation of the HPA axis by immune insults: roles and interactions of cytokines, eicosanoids and glucocorticoids. *Pharmacol Biochem Behav* 1996;54:285–298.

282. Derjik R, Sternberg EM. Corticosteroid action and neuroendocrine-immune interactions. *Ann NY Acad Sci* 1994;746:33–41.

283. Cunningham ET, de Souza EB. Interleukin-1 receptors in the brain and endocrine system. *Immunol Today* 1992;14:171–173.

284. Munck A, Guyre PM. Glucocorticoids and immune function. In: Ader R, Felton DL, Cohen N, eds. *Psychoneuroimmunology*. New York: Academic Press, 1991: 447–474.

285. Martin P. Wound healing—aiming for perfect skin regeneration. *Science* 1997; 276:75–81.

286. Davidson JM. Wound repair. In: Gallin JI, Goldstein IM, Snyderman R, eds. *Inflammation*. 2nd ed. New York: Raven Press, 1992:809–820.

287. Folkman J, Brem H. Angiogenesis and inflammation. In: Gallin JI, Goldstein IM, Snyderman R, eds. *Inflammation*. 2nd ed. New York: Raven Press, 1992: 821–840.

288. Strieter RM, Polverini PJ, Arenberg DA, Kunkel SL. The role of CXC chemokines as regulators of angiogenesis. *Shock* 1995;4:155–160.

289. Diaz-Flores L, Gutierrez R, Varela H. Angiogenesis: an update. *Histol Histopathol* 1994;9:807–843.

290. Boros DL. The role of cytokines in the formation of the schistosome egg granuloma. *Immunobiology* 1994;191:441–450.

291. Wynn TA, Cheever AW. Cytokine regulation of granuloma formation in schistosomiasis. *Curr Opin Immunol* 1995;7:505–511.

292. Stadecker M. The shrinking schistosomal egg granuloma: how accessory cells control T cell-mediated pathology. *Exp Parasitol* 1994;79:198–201.

293. Mornex JF, Leroux C, Greenland T, Ecochard D. From granuloma to fibrosis in interstitial lung diseases: molecular and cellular interactions. *Eur Respir J* 1994; 7:779–785.

294. Kunkel SL, Lukacs NW, Strieter RM, Chensue SW. Th1 and Th2 responses regulate experimental lung granuloma development. *Sarcoidosis Vasc Diffuse Lung Dis* 1996;13:120–128.

295. Hansch HC, Smith DA, Mielke ME, Hahn H, Bancroft GJ, Ehlers S. Mechanisms of granuloma formation in murine Mycobacterium avium infection: the contribution of CD4+ T cells. *Int Immunol* 1996;8:1299–1310.

296. Chensue SW, Warmington KS, Ruth JH, Lincoln P, Kunkel SL. Cytokine function during mycobacterial and schistosomal antigen-induced pulmonary granuloma formation. Local and regional participation of IFN-gamma, IL-10, and TNF. *J Immunol* 1995;154:5969–5976.

297. Barnes PJ, Karin M. Nuclear factor kappa-B—a pivotal transcription factor in chronic inflammatory diseases. *N Engl J Med* 1997;336:1066–1071.

298. Barnes PJ, Adcock I. Anti-inflammatory actions of steroids: molecular mechanisms. *Trends Pharmacol Sci* 1993;14:436–441.

299. Saatcioglu F, Claret FX, Karin M. Negative transcriptional regulation by nuclear receptors. *Semin Cancer Biol* 1994;5:347–359.

300. Rosenberg HF, Gallin JI. Neutrophils. In: Frank MM, Austen KF, Claman HN, Unanue ER, eds. *Samter's immunologic diseases*. 5th ed. Boston: Little, Brown and Company, 1995:247–250.

301. Leto TL, Adams AG, deMendez I. Assembly of the phagocyte NADPH oxidase: binding of Src homology 3 domains to proline-rich targets. *Proc Natl Acad Sci USA* 1994;91:10650–10654.

302. deMendez I, Garrett MC, Adams AG, Leto TL. The role of p67-phox SH3 domains in assembly of the NADPH oxidase system. *J Biol Chem* 1994;269: 16326–16332.

303. Sathyamoorthy M, deMendez I, Adams AG, Leto TL. P40 phox down-regulated NADPH oxidase activity through interactions with its SH3 domain. *J Biol Chem* 1997;272:9141–9146.

304. Jackson SH, Gallin JI, Holland SM. The p47 phox mouse knockout model of chronic granulomatous disease. *J Exp Med* 1995;182:751–758.

305. Marks AR. Cellular functions of immunophilins. *Physiol Rev* 1996;76:631–649.

306. Yocum DE. Cyclosporine, FK-506, rapamycin and other immunomodulators. *Rheum Dis Clin North Am* 1996;22:133–154.

307. Lee JI, Canafax DM. Cyclosporine pharmacology. *Transplant Proc* 1996;28: 2156–2158.

308. Khanna A, Li B, Sharma VK, Suthanthiran M. Immunoregulatory and fibrogenic activities of cyclosporine: a unifying hypothesis based on transforming growth factor-beta expression. *Transplant Proc* 1996;28:2015–2018.

309. Stiller CR. An overview of the first decade of cyclosporine. *Transplant Proc* 1996;28:2005–2012.

310. High KP. The anitmicrobial activities of cyclosporine, FK-506 and rapamycin. *Transplantation* 1994;57:1689–1700.

311. Emery P, van de Putte LB. New perspectives on controlling progression of severe rheumatoid arthritis—a summary of the potential role of cyclosporin. *Br J Rheumatol* 1996;35[Suppl 2]:1–3.

312. Yocum DE. Combination therapy with cyclosporin in rheumatoid arthritis. *Br J Rheumatol* 1996;35[Suppl 2]:19–23.

313. Forre O. Cyclosporin in rheumatoid arthritis: an overview. *Clin Rheumatol* 1995;14[Suppl 2]:33–36.

314. Yocum DE, Torley H. Cyclosporine in rheumatoid arthritis. *Rheum Dis Clin North Am* 1995;21:835–844.

316. Weckmann AL, Alcocer-Varela J. Cytokine inhbitors in autoimmune disease. *Semin Arthritis Rheum* 1996;26:539–557.

317. Feldmann M, Brennan FM, Williams RO, Elliott MJ, Maini RN. Cytokine expression and networks in rheumatoid arthritis: rationale for anti-TNF alpha therpay and its mechanism of action. *J Inflamm* 1995-6;47:90–96.

318. Sasayama S, Matsumori A. Vesnarinone: a potential cytokine inhbitor. *J Card Fail* 1996;2:251–258.

319. Maini RN. A perspective on anti-cytokine and anti-T cell-directed therapies in rheumatoid arthritis. *Clin Exp Rheumatol* 1995;13[Suppl 12]:S35–S40.

320. Bartalena L, Marcocci C, Pinchera A. cytokine antagonists: new ideas for the management of Graves' ophthalmopathy. *J Clin Endocrinol Metab* 1996;81: 446–448.

321. Ferrara JL. Cytokine inhibitors and graft-versus-host disease. *Ann NY Acad Sci* 1995;770:227–236.

322. Richardson CE, Emery P. Innovative treatment approaches for rheumatoid arthritis. New cyclo-oxygenase and cytokine inhibitors. *Baillieres Clin Rheumatol* 1995;9:731–758.

323. Elliott MJ, Maini RN. Anti-cytokine therapy in rheumatoid arthritis. *Baillieres Clin Rheumatol* 1995;9:633–652.

324. Schwiebert LA, Beck LA, Stellato C, Bickel CA, Bochner BS, Schleimer RP. Glucocorticosteroid inhibition of cytokine production: relevance to antiallergic actions. *J Allergy Clin Immunol* 1996;97:143–152.

325. Feldmann M, Brennan FM, Elliott MJ, Williams RO, Maini RN. TNF-alpha is an effective therapeutic target for rheumatoid arthritis. *Ann NY Acad Sci* 1995; 766:272–278.

326. Border WA, Noble NA, Ketteler M. TGF-beta: a cytokine mediator of glomerulosclerosis and a target for therapeutic intervention. *Kidney Int Suppl* 1995;49: S59–S61.

327. Devos R, Plaetinck G, Cornelis S, Guisez Y, van der Heyden J, Tavernier J. Interleukin-5 and its receptor: a drug target for eosinophilia associated with chronic allergic disease. *J Leukoc Biol* 1995;57:813–819.

328. Firestein GS. Cytokine networks in rheumatoid arthritis: implication for therapy. *Agents Actions Suppl* 1995;47:37–51.

329. Klein B, Brailly H. Cytokine-binding proteins: stimulating antagonists. *Immunol Today* 1995;16:216–220.

330. Tartour E, Lee RS, Fridman WH. Anti-cytokines: promising tools for diagnosis and immunotherapy. *Biomed Pharmacother* 1994;48:417–424.

331. Enayati P, Fong Y. Cytokine neutralizing strategies in experimental sepsis. *Prog Clin Biol Res* 1994;388:295–306.

332. Kinoshita T. Protection of host from its own complement by membrane-bound complement inhibitors: C3 convertase inhibitors vs. membrane attack complex inhibitors. *Res Immunol* 1996;147:100–103.

333. Mouthon L, Kaveri SV, Spalter SH, et al. Mechanisms of action of intravenous immune globulin in immune-mediated diseases. *Clin Exp Immunol* 1996; 104[Suppl 1]:3–9.

334. Ryan US. Complement inhibitory therapeutics and xenotransplantation. *Nat Med* 1995;1:967–968.

335. Smiley JD, Talbert MG. Southwestern Internal Medicine Conference: high-dose intravenous gamma globulin therapy: how does it work? *Am J Med Sci* 1995;309:295–303.

336. Corral LG, Muller GW, Moreira AL, et al. Selection of novel analogs of thalidomide with enhanced tumor necrosis factor alpha inhibitory activity. *Mol Med* 1996;2:506–515.

337. Wang P, Wu P, Siegel MI, Egan RW, Billah MM. Interleukin (IL)-10 inhibits nuclear factor kappa B (NF kappa B) activation in human monocytes: IL-10 and IL-4 suppress cytokine synthesis by different mechanisms. *J Biol Chem* 1995, 270:9558–9563.

338. Pahl HL, Krauss B, Schulze-Osthoff K, et al. The immunosuppressive fungal metabolite gliotoxin specifically inhibits transcription factor NF-kappa B. *J Exp Med* 1996;183:1829–1834.

Fundamental Immunology, Fourth Edition,
edited by William E. Paul
Lippincott–Raven Publishers, Philadelphia © 1999.

CHAPTER 33

Systemic Autoimmunity

Philip L. Cohen

The study of systemic autoimmune disease has held the interest of many immunologists for two important reasons. First, human systemic autoimmune diseases are an important cause of suffering and shortening of life. Second, the aberrations that lead to autoreactivity against multiple self antigens must hold the keys to understanding important aspects of the fundamental basis of self–nonself discrimination.

Systemic autoimmunity is mediated both by autoantibodies and by self-reactive T cells. The availability of human autoimmune sera and autoantigen-binding monoclonal antibodies has yielded considerable insight into the nature of autoantibodies and their binding to antigen. More recently, hybridoma technology has extended this knowledge to immunoglobulin genetics, mostly using autoantibodies derived from mice. The cellular basis for autoantibody formation, especially the participation of helper T-lymphocytes in these responses, has been much harder to study. In part, this reflects the difficulties of investigation in humans, the practical difficulties of studying cells versus serum, and the inadequacy of animal models. It seems likely that direct autoreactive T-cell injury is an important

part of many of the autoimmune diseases discussed below, but currently there is a poor understanding of the specificity and the regulation of T cells mediating systemic autoimmune disease.

A large number of potential etiologies have been put forth to explain systemic autoimmune disease. It seems unlikely that a single explanation is adequate to account for the diverse phenomena described in this chapter, yet there are common issues regarding self-reactive immune responses, regardless of the inciting causes. The comments regarding overall mechanisms of autoimmune disease may not apply to all diseases or models, but are intended to place systemic autoreactivity into the context of basic immunology and to focus future thought about mechanisms.

GENERAL CONSIDERATIONS

Systemic autoimmunity encompasses autoimmune conditions in which autoreactivity is not limited to a single organ or organ system. This definition would include systemic lupus erythematosus (SLE), systemic sclerosis (scleroderma), rheumatoid arthritis (RA), chronic graft-versus-host disease (GVHD), and the various forms of vasculitis. A truly satisfactory definition is elusive; the demonstration of autoimmunity as a cause of disease is difficult

P.L. Cohen. Departments of Medicine and Microbiology/Immunology, University of North Carolina, Chapel Hill, North Carolina 27599-7280.

and requires the replication of disease manifestation by transfer of antibody or T-lymphocytes. As these kinds of data are difficult to generate, the inference that a disease is autoimmune is made based on the presence of autoantibodies and the localization in diseased tissue of antibody, complement, and T-lymphocytes.

In addition to the human diseases, there are many animal models that are helpful in testing hypotheses about human illness and in gaining insights into fundamental mechanisms; however, some models may not be not representative of human diseases.

Certain features of systemic autoimmune disease stand out as clues to the possible etiology. The first is their variable course from person to person (or even from inbred mouse to inbred mouse) and their tendency to wax and wane in severity over time. In a single individual, disease activity can vary from life-threatening to asymptomatic, even without medical intervention. This suggests the operation of potent forces that can downregulate the autoimmune process.

A second characteristic of most systemic autoimmune conditions is the increased susceptibility of the female sex (1). Women are at least tenfold more likely to develop SLE, for instance (2). The female predominance is also true of most animal models of autoimmunity, with a few notable exceptions. Efforts to understand the female tendency to develop autoimmune disease have not been entirely successful, but hormonal influences play a major role, and endocrinologic abnormalities have been described (3,4).

A third feature of autoimmune disease is called overlap, the finding in individual patients of features of multiple systemic autoimmune disease (5). This leads to taxonomic confusion; for example, some patients have an autoimmune disease sometimes termed *mixed connective tissue disease,* which has features of SLE, scleroderma, and polymyositis (6).

It seems paradoxical that humans and animals with systemic autoimmune disease, despite their high immunoglobulin and autoantibody levels, respond poorly when immunized with exogenous antigens, as if their immune systems were preoccupied with responses to self antigens (7). Cell-mediated immunity is particularly impaired (8), possibly reflecting the lymphocytopenia characteristic of SLE but also seen in other disorders (9). This immunosuppression may be further exacerbated by medical efforts to suppress autoantibody formation; infection due to immunosuppression is a regrettably common feature in patients suffering from systemic autoimmune disease (10).

HISTORY

To early immunologists, the notion that autoantibodies or self-reactive cellular immunity could ever occur met with considerable resistance. It had been observed, for example, that immunization of animals with mixtures of self and foreign erythrocytes elicited antibody only against blood from other individuals. Ehrlich and others proposed that the consequences of the formation of self antibodies were so severe (*horror autotoxicus*) that the immune system stringently prohibited its occurrence (11). Although investigators as early as Donath observed clear evidence of anti-self agglutinins, acceptance of the concept that autoantibodies could cause immune injury came from the convincing experiments of Harrington in human idiopathic thrombocytopenic purpura (ITP) (12), in which the profoundly low platelet counts of the ITP patients were reproduced in the investigator and his colleagues by transfer of patient serum; and from the pioneering work of Rose and Witebsky in rabbit experimental thyroiditis (13). An important intellectual figure of the era was F.M. Burnet, who extended the clonal selection theory to postulate the elimination of self-reactive antibody-producing cells (14).

NONPATHOLOGIC SYSTEMIC AUTOIMMUNITY

Autoimmune disease must be distinguished from the many instances of nonpathologic self-recognition by the immune system. These include the ready isolation of self class II reactive T-lymphocytes (15) and the existence in normal individuals of low levels of autoantibodies to certain self proteins (16). The use of binding assays like ELISA further complicates the definition of autoantibodies, as low-titer, low-affinity autoantibodies can be readily detected in the sera of normal individuals using almost any assay system of sufficient sensitivity. Even when threshold values are set to exclude low-titer positives, antinuclear antibodies and rheumatoid factor (RF) are seen in small but significant numbers of normal humans (17) and become more prevalent among the aged and among hospitalized patients (18).

Autoantibodies to some self proteins may serve important physiologic functions. This has been best shown for RF, antibody against IgG. RF is mainly IgM, and a substantial fraction of IgM-bearing lymphocytes express this specificity (19). RF levels rise promptly after immunization with foreign antigens (20,21), and the antibody is commonly observed in the serum of patients with chronic infections (22). RF probably serves to eliminate immune complexes; its affinity for monomeric IgG is low, yet is much higher for the multimeric IgG that exists in complexes. The binding of RF to complexes very likely expedites their removal from the circulation via the mononuclear phagocyte system.

RF-bearing B cells may also serve an important function in presenting foreign antigens, by virtue of their binding of antigen–antibody complexes (23). Mice expressing a human RF transgene produce little circulating RF; their RF-producing B cells are found in primary B-cell follicles and the mantle zone of secondary splenic follicles (24). Spleen cells from these RF transgenic mice present human IgG antitetanus toxoid immune complexes with high efficiency. The resulting wave of T-cell help may serve to amplify the immune response, and its subsequent downregulation may be related to deletion of many of the RF-bearing cells (25).

As depicted in Fig. 1, low-affinity IgM antibodies against other self antigens have been observed in unimmunized animals (16,26–30). The function of these specificities is uncertain and may include shaping of the repertoire against exogenous antigens. The fetal repertoire is rich in such antibodies, which are derived from a limited set of VH and VL genes with limited somatic mutation (31).

The B1 subset of B-lymphocytes, which in rodents is concentrated in the peritoneal cavity, may have as its primary function the production of IgM autoantibodies such as RF (32). In mice, B1 cells may be responsible for production of antierythrocyte autoantibodies (33), but they are not the source of antichromatin antibodies or RF in the *lpr* model (34), nor do they produce such antibodies in GVHD (35). In SLE, both B1 and B2 cells secrete anti-DNA, but high-affinity autoantibody is derived from the B2 cells (36).

Autoantibodies to idiotypes are another form of nonpathogenic humoral autoimmunity. Antiidiotypes arise after immunization and have been shown to mediate both negative and positive feedback of humoral responses, in some systems, via regulatory T cells (37–39).

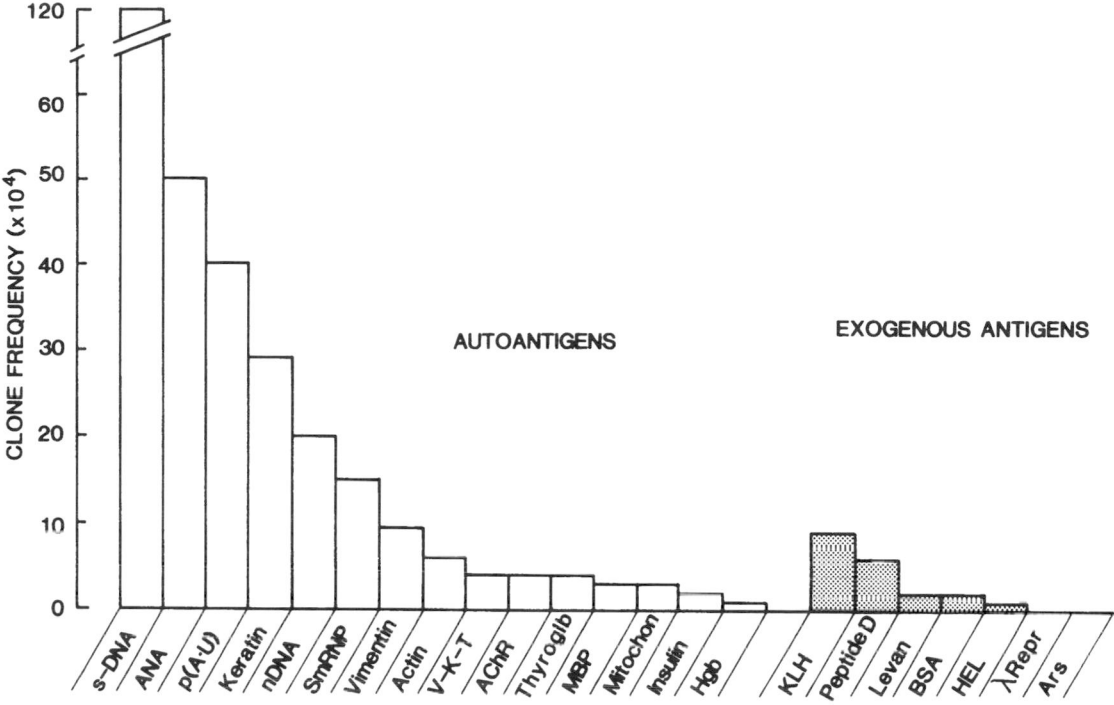

FIG. 1. The natural autoantibody repertoire in normal mice. Antibodies produced by 11,800 hybridomas prepared from splenic B cells of unimmunized 6-week-old A/J mice were screened for reactivity against a panel of autoantigens and foreign antigens. Note the high frequency of antibodies against nuclear and cytoskeletal antigens. (From Souroujon M, White-Scharff ME, Andre-Schwartz J, Gefter ML, Schwartz RS. Preferential autoantibody reactivity of the preimmune B cell repertoire in normal mice. *J Immunol* 1988;140:4173–4179, with permission.)

TOLERANCE AND AUTOIMMUNE DISEASE

The establishment and maintenance of immunologic tolerance is a key feature of the immune system, and is fully discussed elsewhere. The occurrence of autoimmunity may reflect the imperfect nature of the tolerance generated in the developing T- and B-cell repertoires. Very likely, peripheral tolerance mechanisms are required to prevent the emergence of autoimmunity in adult life. No autoimmune disorders have thus far been shown to involve deficits in intrathymic tolerance, and autoimmune diseases typically do not occur in the neonatal period.

Data show that intrathymic tolerance is of potential importance in establishing tolerance to nuclear antigens (40). B-cell tolerance to protein antigens may be abnormal in certain autoimmune disease models (41,42).

It is typical of systemic autoimmune disease, that, rather than a global loss of tolerance, there is a selective autoimmune response directed primarily against intracellular autoantigens, and especially against components of the nucleus (43).

Role of T cells in Systemic Autoimmune Disease

It is not difficult to find evidence in normals of T-cell autoreactivity to class II major histocompatibility complex (MHC) antigens (44). The degree to which this represents autoreactivity to self peptides, compared with reactivity to the class II MHC molecule itself, is difficult to determine. Perhaps contrary to expectation, self-Ia–reactive T cells are less abundant in human and murine systemic autoimmunity (45), and this defect may vary with disease activity. Cloned autoreactive T cells, on the other hand, are associated with induction of disease in some models. They elicit lesions typical of the inflammatory skin disease lichen planus (46) and are present among the hyperproliferative T cells found in mice expressing the *lpr* Fas mutant gene (47). Whether such self-reactive cells are involved in providing help for autoantibody production is unknown.

Besides any role as helpers, T cells may provoke cellular injury in systemic autoimmunity. In chronic GVHD, CD4- and CD8-bearing T cells cause inflammatory infiltrates in skin, intestine, and elsewhere (48). There is evidence that T cells in systemic lupus are spontaneously activated, as judged by increased expression of activation antigens (49,50). T-lymphocytes are found in inflammatory skin lesions (51) and may be responsible for some of the other nonrenal manifestations of the illness (52,53). For the most part, however, autoimmunity mediated directly by T cells seems to be more characteristic of organ-specific autoimmune disease such as experimental allergic encephalomyelitis (EAE) than it is of systemic autoimmune disease.

Systemic autoimmunity is thus usually mostly a problem of B-cell production of autoantibodies, yet the contribution of T cells to these autoantibody responses has been difficult to define. Thymectomy in SLE may lead to exacerbation or remission of disease (54). Human immunodeficiency virus (HIV) infection of SLE patients, with its depletion of CD4-bearing T cells, results in a remission in SLE activity (55,56), supporting a role for a continuing source of T-cell help for SLE autoantibodies.

Some properties of systemic autoimmune disease strongly suggest the involvement of helper T-lymphocytes. Autoantibody responses are high-affinity IgG responses (57), which appear to have undergone affinity maturation, a process that requires T cells. The protein antigens to which many antinuclear antigens are directed presumably require T-lymphocyte help, as they do not possess the repeating determinants characteristic of most T-independent antigens. Some of the treatments for SLE appear to act primarily at the T cell, e.g., cyclosporine A and cyclophosphamide.

Even in patients with high-titer autoantibodies, T-cell proliferation to nuclear autoantigens has been difficult to demonstrate. There are several well-documented examples, however: T cells from SLE patients respond to a recombinant form of the SLE-associated ribosomal protein P2 autoantigen. Under the same conditions, responses to tetanus toxoid are poor, suggesting that the autoantigen-specific response occurs despite generalized T-cell dysfunction (58). In another report, CD4$^+$ T cells against a recombinant snRNP protein were found in high frequency (1/4,000 → 1/25,000) but were not seen in normal subjects (59). In contrast, snRNP A protein-reactive T cells could be isolated both in normal individuals and in patients (60).

Some of the most extensive work on specificity of T helper cells in systemic autoimmunity comes from analysis of clones of SLE T cells which provide help for anti-DNA. These cells have charged motifs in the T-cell receptor (TCR) CDR3s, presumably promoting binding to peptides derived from charged DNA-binding nucleosomal proteins [high-mobility group (HMG) and histones]. Anti-DNA–specific B cells probably bind to the DNA, bringing along the attached proteins, and internalize and process them for presentation to CD4$^+$ T cells (61). It has been reported that at least some SLE T cells that provide help for antinuclear antibody production lack both CD4 and CD8 and express $\alpha\beta$ TCRs (62).

SLE mouse models have allowed *in vivo* experiments to define the role of T cells. Treatment of NZB/NZW mice with anti-Thy 1 or anti-CD4 prevents autoantibody production and renal disease (63). Thymectomy of this strain, on the other hand, exacerbates autoimmunity, reflecting complex T-cell interactions early in life. In the *lpr* model (64), thymectomy prevents disease if done within 72 hours of birth (65), and antibody depletion of T cells prevents both autoantibodies and lymphoid hyperplasia (66).

Even in these defined genetic models, the precise role of T cells and the amount of nonspecific versus specific help for autoantibodies has been elusive. The T-cell repertoire of NZB/NZW mice, despite its content of autoantigen-specific T cells, shows polyclonal and not oligoclonal T-cell activation (67). In MRL/*lpr* mice, disease fails to develop in animals in which a source of normal T cells is provided, but in which *lpr* T cells have been depleted, indicating that the T cells provide more than just a passive source of cytokines or nonspecific help and that they participate actively as helpers for autoantibody-producing B cells (68). The extreme restriction of the TCR repertoire imposed by expression of a TCR β transgene has been reported to result in lower autoantibody levels and increased survival in MRL/*lpr* mice (69), suggesting again that autoantigen-specific T-cell help is required for autoantibody production.

Because the transgenic studies could be confounded by the ability of mice to express endogenous α or β chains, MRL/*lpr* mice transgenic for both the α/β chains of a pigeon cytochrome C hybridoma have been constructed by breeding the TCR transgenes onto TCR α and β knock-out mice (70). These animals expressed only the transgenic TCR, yet hypergammaglobulinemia and autoantibodies to IgG, DNA, and snRNPs developed despite the lack of autoantigen-specific T-cell help. Lymphadenopathy, renal, salivary, and cutaneous disease were absent, suggesting that more specific T-cell help was required for these manifestations. These studies indicate that both antigen-specific and antigen-nonspecific T-cell help are required for full development of the MRL/*lpr* SLE syndrome. In this regard, chimera studies, in which *lpr* mice have been constructed using congenic donors in which T-B interactions could be analyzed, have shown that the T help required for autoantibody production is MHC-restricted; in other words, autoreactive T cells must share class II MHC determinants with autoreactive B cells in order for autoantibody production to occur (71).

The role of $\gamma\delta$ T cells has also been evaluated in MRL/*lpr* mice by comparing disease manifestations and autoimmunity in mice lacking $\gamma\delta$ T cells (72). In the absence of the latter, mice developed a more severe autoimmune syndrome, suggesting a regulatory role for $\gamma\delta$ T cells. In the converse situation, mice lacking $\alpha\beta$ T cells had only an attenuated SLE syndrome, implying that $\gamma\delta$ T cells were capable of providing significantly less help for autoantibody production than were $\alpha\beta$ T cells.

Autoantigen-reactive T cells have been studied in murine models. For MRL mice, which are prone to develop antibodies to the snRNP complex, snRNP-reactive T cells can be demonstrated in draining lymph nodes after immunization with purified snRNPs (73). While normal mice can generate T cells reactive to foreign snRNP, only MRL mice and mice expressing certain MHC alleles can recognize snRNP of murine origin (74). The ability of normal mice to recruit T cells reactive to self antigens after immunization with foreign nuclear antigen may reflect epitope spreading. This process entails the recruitment of T cells reactive to self peptides as a result of the presentation of self antigen by B cells cross-reactive with self proteins.

T cells reactive to overlapping core histone peptides have been described in SLE-prone SWR×NZB F1 mice (75). These antigenic determinants are apparently protected in intact chromatin, as responses to whole histone are not measurable. Interestingly, these T-cell antigenic regions of histones overlap with determinants recognized by antihistone autoantibodies. T-cell help for autoantibodies may also be mediated through T cells with specificity for the variable regions of autoantibody molecules.

NZB/NZW mice develop T cells that recognize peptides corresponding to the variable regions of anti-DNA antibodies (76). Presumably there is presentation to T cells of peptides derived from the processing of self immunoglobulin by B cells. The resulting helper T cells can provide autoantibody-specific help, and interference with their action has been reported to ameliorate autoimmune disease.

CD40 ligand (CD40L) may play a critical role in regulating autoantibody production in SLE. Expression of this T-cell activation-related molecule is increased in SLE patients, especially those with active disease, and also appears on some SLE B-lymphocytes (77). The latter observation may account for a relative T-independence of some SLE antibody formation. Treatment of NZB×SWR F1 mice with antibody to CD40L prevents autoimmune disease (78). MRL/*lpr* mice that are genetically deficient in CD40L, in contrast, develop autoantibodies to nuclear antigen, but these are skewed toward the IgM isotype, suggesting impairment of class switching (79). Renal disease appears to be diminished in such mice.

Role of Antigen

Unlike immune responses arising from deliberate immunization, it is not obvious that autoimmunity is initiated or perpetuated by self antigen. Other mechanisms can be conceived, and some have been seriously put forth. For instance, the diffuse activation of B cells by lipopolysaccharide (LPS) leads to limited systemic autoimmunity (chiefly IgM antibodies to DNA and RF) and may be a good model for the autoimmunity that accompanies certain infections [e.g., Epstein-Barr virus (EBV) and mycoplasma (80)]. It is also possible that aberrations in the web of idiotypes and antiidiotypes could result in autoimmunity without the need for autoantigen as immunogen. Yet considerable evidence supports the view that self antigens themselves act as immunogens for autoantibody responses

Autoimmunity against nuclear protein complexes such as the snRNP spliceosome is directed against multiple components of the autoantigen, as might be expected from an immune response to the intact particle (81). Analysis of the fine specificity of these responses has revealed a further complexity consistent with what might be expected from a high-affinity, antigen-driven response (82,83). Immunization with nuclear antigens, in some cases, may result in autoantibody formation and disease (84), although antigens need to be repeatedly administered in adjuvant, and the complexity of the resulting autoantibody response is usually much reduced.

Immunization of rabbits and mice with small peptide fragments of certain autoantigens has been reported to result in antigen not only to the immunogenic epitope, but also to other epitopes on the same antigen and even to autoantibodies to other nuclear antigens and clinical evidence of SLE (85). This may reflect epitope spreading (i.e., the recruitment of T cells reactive to additional epitopes on the autoantigen). As tolerance usually does not extend to all such "cryptic" epitopes, a mechanism that might be capable of enlisting progressively more autoreactive T cells might amplify any initial breakage of tolerance. The impetus for such responses might come from immunization with autoantigens from another species, which could elicit T-cell help against *bona fide* foreign determinants, along with the generation of antibody against the foreign antigen (86). B cells expressing antibody cross-reactive with self determinants could then selectively take up autoantigens, process them, and express autoantigenic peptides, including cryptic epitopes. The physical association of many autoantigens, such as Ro and La (87), or the many components of the snRNP complex, could lead to further diversification of an autoimmune response initiated by the breaking of tolerance to only a single autoantigen. For the La nuclear antigens, a hierarchy of immunogenic cryptic epitopes with differing potential for driving a full autoimmune response has been identified using peptide fragments of the intact antigen (88).

Immunization of animals with mammalian DNA generally does not lead to autoantibody unless the DNA is complexed to a cationic protein such as methylated bovine serum albumin (89). DNA that has been damaged by ultraviolet (UV) irradiation or by reactive oxygen species is much more immunogenic than unaltered DNA, which may be relevant to UV-induced SLE exacerbations (90). Much interest has focused on the potential of bacterial DNA to activate B cells and provoke autoimmune responses through CpG motifs not found in mammalian DNA (91). Exposure to bacterial DNA also accelerates genetically predetermined autoimmune disease in NZB/NZW mice (92). Although it is possible that microbial DNA is an immunogen in SLE, the bulk of the small amount of circulating DNA in SLE has been shown to be of human origin and mostly in the form of small complexes bound to histone (93,94).

If nuclear antigens serve as immunogens, how do they interact with the immune system? The most likely answer is that they are

released from senescent cells, or are presented on the surface of phagocytic cells that have ingested such debris. Cells undergoing apoptosis have been shown to express several important SLE nuclear antigens (95) and may serve as an important source of autoimmunogen. It seems doubtful that the apoptotic cell can serve as a competent antigen-presenting cell (APC) for these molecules; rather, it seems more likely that specialized APCs would serve to present these apoptosis-related nuclear antigens, perhaps the same cells that so avidly phagocytose apoptotic cells.

The elution of peptides from both class I and class II MHC molecules provides further reason to believe that nuclear autoantigens are presented to the immune system. Both in rodents and in humans, MHC molecules have been found to have peptides derived from such nuclear antigens as histone on their cell surfaces, presumably through the processing of nuclear debris (96). It is also possible that these peptides are derived from autoantigens processed from within normal antigen-processing cells using a class II pathway, although examples of such "inside out" class II processing are uncommon (97).

Regulatory T-Cell Abnormalities

Much evidence suggests that T cells can exert a controlling influence on the generation of autoantibodies and on the regulation of autoimmunity (98). Thymectomy of normal animals, in some systems, results in autoimmunity, both systemic and organ-specific (99). Nude mice develop autoantibodies and immune complex renal disease, and the process can be reversed by adoptive transfer of T cells (100,101). These studies imply that regulatory T cells may control antinuclear antibody production. In SLE, there are multiple reports of *in vitro* abnormalities of regulatory T-cell function both in animals and in humans (102). Much of the suppressor-cell literature of the 1970s is now better regarded in light of the current concepts of classification of both helper and cytotoxic cells into T helper 1 (Th1), Th2, TC1, and TC2 subsets based on their cytokine phenotype (103). It is likely that some of the observed phenomena represent the action of cytokines derived from these T-helper subsets, for example, interferon-γ (IFN-γ), interleukin-10 (IL-10), and IL-4, which have potent effects on the magnitude and character of humoral immune responses.

An important example of perturbation of regulatory T cells is the autoimmune and GVHD-like syndrome induced by cyclosporine treatment of irradiated rats reconstituted with autologous marrow (104). While animals become immunocompetent, the T-cell imbalance brought on by the protocol leads to autoimmune disease.

Cytokines in Systemic Autoimmune Disease

A multiplicity of cytokine abnormalities have been associated with systemic autoimmune diseases and models. Some occur late in illness and are probably not causal, while others may be actively involved in regulation and dysregulation of immune responses. In general, IL-2 levels and the expression of IL-2 receptors are diminished both in human and murine SLE (105) and in several related autoimmune disorders (105). Circulating IL-2 receptors may be increased, however, in parallel with other circulating receptors (106), although assays for these receptors are difficult. Efforts to characterize SLE as a Th2 or Th1 disease based on the phenotype of helper cells have met with difficulty, but IL-10 seems to be increased in human and murine SLE, along with IL-6. The ratio of

IL-10 to IFN-γ–secreting cells in SLE peripheral blood is increased, implying a predominance of Th2 cells in the circulation (107). Supporting the importance of Th2 cells in promoting systemic autoimmunity is the observation that some IL-4 transgenic mice develop SLE-like antinuclear antibodies, hemolytic anemia, and immune-mediated renal disease (108).

There have been several published surveys of cytokine production in murine SLE models. For chronic GVHD, a Th2 profile has been observed (109). For NZB/NZW and MRL/lpr, however, a complex pattern not fitting either Th1 or Th2 exists, with increases in IL-6, IL-4, and IL-10 (110). Tumor necrosis factor-α (TNF-α) may also be increased, and evidence has been published that allelic polymorphisms at this locus predispose to SLE (111,112).

APOPTOSIS ABNORMALITIES IN SYSTEMIC AUTOIMMUNE DISEASE

The realization that the autoimmune and lymphoproliferative syndrome of lpr and gld mice was due to mutations in the Fas apoptosis receptor and its ligand led to great interest in the possibility that impairment of apoptosis might be responsible for other autoimmune diseases. Because multiple pathways of apoptosis exist, many possibilities exist for potential lesions. In human SLE, spontaneous lymphocyte apoptosis appears increased (113). Expression of bcl-2 appears to be elevated (114), particularly in T cells (115). Fas expression is elevated (116), contrary to what might be expected from murine studies, and apoptosis through the Fas molecule is apparently intact (117). The status of Fas ligand (FasL) expression and function is not yet clear for SLE, and conflicting data have been presented. It is of great interest, however, that an SLE patient with a mutant FasL has been identified (118).

The Canale-Smith syndrome, also known as autoimmune and lymphoproliferative syndrome (ALPS), is a rare illness resulting in lymphoid enlargement and immune cytopenias (119,120). In a number of kindreds, the disorder results from a dominant nonfunctional Fas molecule. Like lpr and gld mice, children develop "double-negative" T cells and hypergammaglobulinemia. Unlike the murine mutations, however, affected patients rarely develop antinuclear antibodies or lupus-like renal pathology. It is significant that, in the few long-term observations of such patients, an increased susceptibility to malignancy has been noted.

The apoptosis resistance imparted by the mutant Fas molecule in lpr mice has been intensively studied. Thymic selection, as reflected by deletion of I-E and mammary tumor virus–reactive T cells, is normal in lpr mice. Nevertheless, there is evidence for abnormal thymic T-cell development in lpr mice, both in intact and in transgenic mice. The intense Fas expression on thymic T cells (121), however, makes it paradoxical that only subtle thymic selection defects are apparent in lpr and gld mice.

If thymic deletion is intact, how does the Fas apoptosis defect lead to autoimmunity? At least part of the answer is that peripheral T-cell tolerance is strongly dependent on the Fas/FasL system, as deduced from studies of tolerance in lpr mice transgenic for a pigeon cytochrome-C TCR (122). The imposition of the Fas defect on such transgenic mice leads to their inability to achieve tolerance in spleen and lymph nodes. Additional support for the idea that it is in the periphery that Fas/FasL contribute to tolerance comes from the observation that activation-induced cell death is abnormal in peripheral lpr T cells (123). The Fas/FasL interaction appears to

act as an important mechanism to eliminate errant autoreactive postthymic T cells. The delayed development of autoimmunity in lpr mice probably reflects the gradual appearance and clonal expansion of such autoreactive T cells.

Chimeric (124) and tetraparental (125) experiments in which lpr T or B cells coexist with cells of normal origin have shown that B cells must also express the Fas defect in order for autoimmunity to occur; there is direct evidence for defective B-cell apoptosis in lpr and gld mice (126). In vivo studies of tolerance using transgenic self-reactive antibodies have shown surprisingly little difference between lpr and normal mice. In the HEL-anti-HEL system, most B6/lpr mice maintain tolerance through early life. A significant minority, however, break through and generate autoantibodies at 5 months and beyond (42). These findings imply that other mechanisms can substitute effectively for the Fas/FasL system for maintenance of tolerance. Parallel results are reported for mice with an anti–H-2^k transgene: in a conventional facility, most mice maintain tolerance (127). When housed in a specific pathogen-free colony, however, tolerance is intact, suggesting an important role for microbial influences (see above).

Of potential importance regarding the relationship of apoptosis and autoantibody formation are data showing that SLE-related nuclear autoantigens such as Ro and La appear in blebs on the surface of apoptotic cells (95). These and other observations that SLE serum contains antibodies to proteins expressed in apoptotic cells (108) raise the possibility that the process of apoptosis may serve to expose autoantigens to the afferent limb of the immune system. Impairments of apoptosis, or of the process of rapid phagocytosis and disposition of apoptotic bodies, might serve to present autoantigens to the immune system and provoke T- and B-cell autoreactivity.

Among the other commonly used autoimmune mouse models, apoptosis resistance for NZB, NZB/NZW, and BXSB B cells has been reported and may contribute to the expression of disease in these models (128).

ENVIRONMENTAL INFLUENCES ON SYSTEMIC AUTOIMMUNITY

Systemic autoimmune disease may be provoked or exacerbated by a variety of environmental agents, including diet, drugs, infections, and toxins (129). UV-B radiation can provoke flares of SLE, and it is apparent that inflammatory skin lesions are usually limited to light-exposed areas.

The ingestion of certain drugs is clearly linked to development of an SLE-like syndrome (130,131). Unlike spontaneous SLE, renal and central nervous system involvement is rare, and the syndrome resolves after discontinuing the drug. Procainamide, used extensively for treatment of ventricular arrhythmias, is the best-studied agent provoking drug-induced SLE, but hydralazine, chlorpromazine, diphenylhydantoin, and many other drugs can also cause the SLE-like syndrome, characterized mainly by pleuropericarditis, arthritis, pulmonary infiltrates, and fever. Only about 10% of patients given procainamide develop clinically evident disease, but fluorescent antinuclear antibodies appear in the vast majority of patients taking the drug for prolonged periods. Antibodies are directed mostly against histones, and a distinct specificity and isotype pattern have been reported (132,133). No relationship to procainamide acetylator frequency governs SLE development. Efforts to reproduce the syndrome in animals have been largely unsuccessful. It has been proposed that procainamide exerts its action by hypomethylation of DNA, with consequent overexpression of LFA-1 on T-lymphocytes, leading to enhanced autoreactive T-cell help (134).

The contribution of infectious agents to systemic autoimmunity remains an active area of investigation. It is clear that systemic autoimmunity can arise as an immediate consequence of infection with EBV and mycoplasma, and probably other viral infections (135,136). Antinuclear antibodies arising after infectious mononucleosis are short-lived and probably are harmless. Systemic autoimmunity may also arise during the course of severe microbial infections, such as endocarditis and osteomyelitis. Occasionally, skin and kidney lesions are seen, probably representing deposits of immune complexes, possibly associated with RF(137).

Vasculitis, discussed in detail later, accompanies meningococcal, rickettsial, spirochetal, and many other bacterial infections. Systemic autoimmunity is also a sometime feature of HIV infection and may reflect imbalance of helper-cell subsets (138). Various bacterial superantigens have been implicated in autoimmune phenomena, including vasculitis, associated with infections (139). Kawasaki disease, caused by an unknown agent, causes a serious vasculitis and alterations in TCR V_β phenotype, suggesting the role of a superantigen (140).

The influence of infection on the development of SLE is unclear. NZB mice that are maintained germ-free still develop antierythrocyte autoantibodies (141); however, NZB mice in a germ-free environment developed lower levels of IgG and antinuclear antibodies and less renal disease. Immunization of NZB/NZW mice with bacterial DNA accelerates development of renal disease (92), and pristane-treated mice that are maintained in a conventional colony have a higher prevalence of autoantibodies and renal disease than do mice maintained in a pathogen-free environment. MRL/*lpr* mice, in contrast, develop similar levels of autoantibodies when raised in germ-free compared with conventional environments.

Certain toxins are capable of inducing systemic autoimmune disease. Mercuric chloride is the best-studied heavy metal associated with autoimmunity. Animals given $HgCl_2$ develop antinuclear antibodies and immune-complex nephritis. T cells are required, and background genes are important determinants of autoantibody specificity (117,142,143).

Systemic sclerosis and related fibrotic diseases believed to be of autoimmune origin may rarely be provoked by toxins. Workers exposed to polyvinyl chloride are at risk for a scleroderma-like syndrome (144), and an inflammatory and fibrotic scleroderma-like illness has been linked to the ingestion of rapeseed oil (145). An eosinophilic infiltrative disease is caused by a contaminant of L-tryptophan preparations (146). An area of great controversy has been the relationship between silicone breast implants and the development of scleroderma or other rheumatic diseases. Several studies have failed to find a true association (147,148), despite anecdotal reports.

GENETICS OF SYSTEMIC AUTOIMMUNE DISEASE

Susceptibility to SLE is strongly influenced by genetics. In studies of identical twins with SLE, the concordance rate has been reported to be between 28% and 57% (149,150). Multiple genes are involved in determining SLE susceptibility; even in inbred mouse models, the genetics is complex, with as many as 12 genes

contributing (151). Furthermore, genes that alone do not cause disease may interact with other genes to result in disease. For instance, neither the NZB nor the NZW parent strains develop renal disease or antinative DNA antibodies, yet the F1 hybrid resulting from their crossing develops severe SLE-like renal disease and antinative DNA. The most important NZW genetic contribution to murine SLE is linked to the MHC, probably MHC class II genes. NZB contributes a chromosome 4–linked gene that is most important for nephritis, but at least seven other genes have been reported to contribute. Surprisingly, the chromosome 4 gene determining nephritis susceptibility does not affect the levels of anti-DNA, antihistone, and antichromatin (152).

A study using microsatellite markers to analyze sib pairs with SLE defined a region of chromosome 1 linked to disease susceptibility (153). This region may be syntenic to the region of mouse chromosome 1 previously shown to encode renal disease and mortality in NZB mice. While the region encompassed by these studies is large and remains to be defined further, candidate genes include those for Fc receptor gamma 2 and 3; previous human epidemiologic studies have shown linkage in blacks of SLE nephritis to Fc receptor alleles (154)

Genetic deficiencies of complement result in increased risk of SLE (155). C2-deficient individuals are at greatly increased risk of developing SLE, as are those with inherited deficiencies of C8 and C5; the inheritance of a C4 null allele is also a risk factor (156). MHC influences on SLE susceptibility have been harder to define than for RA, insulin-dependent diabetes mellitus (IDDM), and other organ-specific autoimmune diseases (157). For North American blacks, one study found no overall DR association, both associations with subgroups divided according to clinical findings (158). For developing the disease-related autoantibodies anti-Ro and anti-La, susceptibility appears to be linked both to DR and to DQ genes (159).

NATURE OF THE AUTOANTIBODIES IN SYSTEMIC AUTOIMMUNE DISEASE

With some notable exceptions, the autoantibodies characteristic of systemic autoimmune disease are high-titer IgG antibodies (160). The genetic basis of autoantibodies has been best studied in mice, where hybridomas have been useful for sequence analysis (161). Several insights have emerged concerning antinuclear antibodies in NZB/NZW and MRL/*lpr* mice; within a single mouse, anti-DNA and other autoantibodies recovered from hybridomas tend to be clonally related (162). For anti-DNA and anti-Sm, there is evidence of extensive somatic mutation when sequences are compared to germline, and clonal lineages can be deduced (163). Many clones show dual reactivity, implying a common ancestry for at least part of these specificities (164). The binding site of antinuclear autoantibodies is dictated neither by the VH nor the VL hypervariable regions, but usually by a combination of both (165). Anti-DNA antibodies may arise from point mutations in the hypervariable regions of antibodies to exogenous antigens (166). For the S107 response to pneumococcal polysaccharide, a pathogenic anti-DNA antibody can arise from just such a mutation (167). It is not clear how widespread is this mechanism of diversion of normal immune responses to autoimmune responses.

Enough hybridoma autoantibodies from autoimmune mice have now been sequenced that generalizations can be made about VH and VL gene use. Although it appeared in early work that there was preferential use of 3′ VH genes, there are, at best, only modest degrees of bias, and it appears that the VH558 group is the most commonly used gene family, as is the case for antibodies to exogenous antigens (168).

Extensive epitope-mapping studies have been undertaken for many antinuclear antibodies. In most cases, it appears that the antibodies recognize multiple conformationally dependent, often discontinuous, epitopes of nuclear proteins (169,170). There is a predilection for binding to the active site of nuclear proteins; thus, the function of certain enzymes and other autoantigens may be inhibited by autoantibody-containing sera. Antibodies to RNA are often found together with antibodies to the protein components of the snRNP particle, as well in sera containing antibody to other RNA-binding proteins (171). Autoantibodies in systemic autoimmune disease usually bind with greater avidity to antigen derived from the same species, emphasizing their derivation through affinity maturation and their probable origin from immunization with self proteins.

Isotype switching from IgM to IgG has been observed for some but not all autoantibodies. Anti DNA antibodies in NZB/NZW mice undergo this process (172), as do certain serial samples of human sera. MRL/*lpr* anti-Sm sera, however, either switch too rapidly for the change to be measured, or are IgG at the outset (173). It is of interest that autoantibodies in human and murine SLE are mostly of the highly T-dependent IgG (human IgG1, mouse IgGa and IgG2a) subclasses, probably reflecting their T-cell dependence (174,175).

It is not understood why certain protein antigens are the targets of autoantibody formation in systemic autoimmune disease. Autoantigens are nearly always intracellular or cell surface proteins (RF is a prominent exception), and nuclear antigens account for most of the autoantigenic targets. Just why certain nuclear proteins are chosen is particularly obscure. It is not a question of abundance; for instance, the Ro and La proteins are far from the most abundant nuclear proteins, yet are characteristic SLE autoantigens (176).

Attention has been focused on certain aspects of nuclear autoantigens. Individuals with autoimmune diseases frequently have autoantibodies to multiple components of subcellular particles, such as ribosomal proteins, nucleoli, or snRNPs (177). This is suggestive of immunization by the particle itself. Autoantibodies also tend to be directed against nuclear antigens, which are present in greater amounts in cells undergoing proliferation. For instance, proliferating-cell nuclear antigen (PCNA), the centromeral proteins, and the nuclear mitotic apparatus protein NuMa are present in greatly increased concentrations during S and G2 phases of the cell cycle (178). Perhaps nuclear antigens are more available as immunogens at such times.

Antinuclear antibody levels can be quite high. In exceptional patients, 30% or more of the total antibody repertoire can be directed against a single specificity (179). Certain autoantibody levels fluctuate with disease activity (antinative DNA is the best known example), but in the more usual case, antibody levels are fairly constant over time.

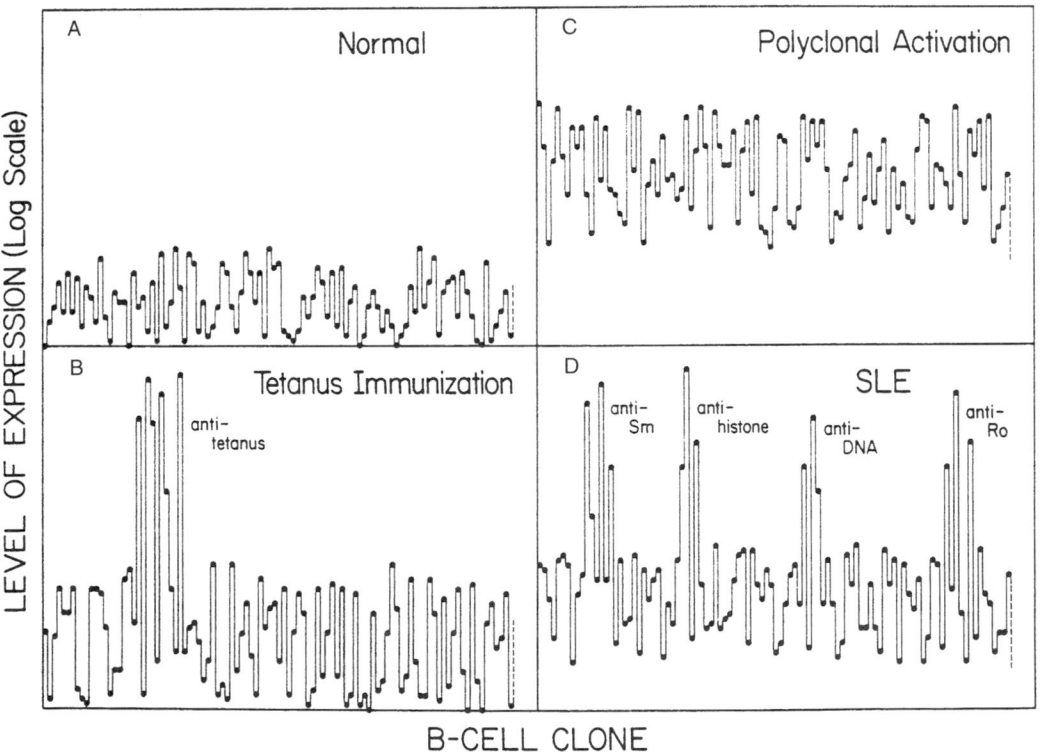

FIG. 2. Nature of autoantibody production in SLE. **Panel A:** Antibody arising from multiple B-cell clones in a normal individual. **Panel B:** Tetanus toxoid immunization is shown to provoke a group of tetanus-specific B-cell clones, along with a modest degree of polyclonal activation. **Panel C:** The effect of diffuse polyclonal activation resulting from exposure to bacterial lipopolysaccharide or other polyclonal B-cell activator. In contrast, **panel D** illustrates the usual situation in SLE and other systemic autoimmune diseases, namely, a background of polyclonal B-cell activation together with large amounts of autoantibody arising from a discrete number of clones of defined specificity. (Reprinted from Eisenberg RA, Cohen PL. Mechanisms of autoantibody production in systemic lupus erythematosus. Clin Asp Autoimmun 1988;2:11, with permission.)

TABLE 1. *Autoantibodies to nuclear proteins in systemic autoimmune disease*

Specificity	Antigen recognized	Disease association
Sm	U1,U2, U4–6 snRNPs	SLE
RNP	U1 snRNP	SLE, MCTD
Ro (SS-A)	60-KdtRNA-binding protein	SLE, Sjogren's syndrome
La (SS-B)	50-KdaRNA-binding protein	SLE, Sjögren's syndrome
Histone	H1, H2a, H2b, H3 (native)	SLE
Jo-1	Histidyl tRNA synthetase	Myositis
Scl-70	DNA topoisomerase I	Scleroderma
PCNA (cyclin)	DNA polymerase delta	SLE
Alu	Signal recogn. particle	SLE, myositis
PL-7	Threonyl tRNA synthetase	Myositis
tRNA-1	Alanyl tRNA synthetase	Myositis, SLE, JRA
RNA polymerase I		Scleroderma
DNA (native)	Double-stranded DNA	SLE
DNA (denatured)	Single-stranded DNA	SLE, RA, inflammation
Centromere	CENP A, B, C	Raynaud's syndrome, CREST

Autoantibodies in SLE and SLE models occur in the midst of diffuse polyclonal B-cell activation. Antibodies to haptens, such as DNP, and to viral antigens are increased on the order of five- to tenfold (180,181). In contrast, the levels of specific autoantibodies, such as antibodies to snRNP, or to Ro and La, are elevated far out of proportion to the polyclonal B-cell activation, and are not uncommonly thousands- or millions-fold greater than the weak binding that might be found in normal control serum (Fig. 2).

Certain SLE serologic specificities are seen in a variety of autoimmune and inflammatory diseases, and do not connote diagnostic specificity. Examples include antihistone and anti-DNA antibodies. Other autoantibodies, such as anti–double-stranded DNA, anti-Sm, and anti-Ro, are highly specific for the diagnosis of SLE and must in some way be linked to its pathogenesis (Table 1). Some marker autoantibodies serve as excellent diagnostic correlates of scleroderma [antitopoisomerase I, or Scl-70 (182)], of myositis [antihistidyl tRNA synthetase (183)], or of Sjögren's syndrome (anti-Ro and anti-La). Some of these autoantibodies are exquisitely specific for their autoantigens and are hard, if not impossible, to generate by deliberate immunization of rabbits or other experimental animals (87,184).

Individual patients with SLE tend to have distinctive profiles of autoantibodies that remain stable throughout the course of the illness. While the patient-to-patient variability in antibody spectrum is undoubtedly due in part to genetic diversity, it is surprising that even genetically homogeneous inbred mice show considerable differences in their autoantibody levels. Inbred mice maintained in the same colony under the same conditions have sharp differences in their autoantibody specificities. The anti-Sm response of MRL/*lpr* may give insight into the genesis of SLE autospecificities. Only about 25% of these mice develop anti-Sm, regardless of colony. Antibody levels show a true bimodal distribution; that is, anti-Sm–negative MRL/*lpr* mice have negligible amounts of anti-Sm, comparable to that of normal mice. When the lineage and microenvironment of anti-Sm–positive mice were traced, no genetic or environmental clustering could explain the appearance of autoantibody in certain mice but not others. The occurrence of the anti-Sm specificity in only a minority of mice was not due to the use of an uncommon V gene, nor to unusual gene rearrangements. These findings, which probably apply to antiribosomal P and anti-Su in MRL/*lpr* mice, have been interpreted as reflecting stochastic influences on the autoantibody repertoire of individuals. The individual

variability in the laboratory, and perhaps the clinical manifestations of SLE and other autoimmune diseases, may arise from analogous poorly understood stochastic influences (185).

Systemic Lupus Erythematosus

SLE is a multisystem disorder that most frequently affects young women. Arthritis, skin rash, central nervous system dysfunction, and renal disease are the most common clinical manifestations (186). The severity of illness has a remarkable tendency to fluctuate over time, confounding studies of drug treatment. Long-term survival is the rule, although there remain considerable morbidity and mortality, chiefly from renal disease (10).

Immunologic interest in SLE dates back to the 1940s, when elevated gamma-globulin levels were noted, and attention was called to marrow tart cells. The realization that the spontaneous neutrophil phagocytosis of nuclear material observed *in vivo* could also be seen in buffy coat preparations from patients, and could be induced in normal buffy coat cells by addition of patient serum, gave rise to the notion that antibodies to nuclear material were of key importance. This led to many investigations of SLE antinuclear factors, demonstrated to be IgG, and to the development of a universal highly sensitive test for SLE, the fluorescent antinuclear antibody test (FANA) (187). More than 95% of SLE patients have positive FANAs, and furthermore, that the pattern of fluorescence staining was related to the antinuclear antibodies present in individual SLE serum (188). Diffuse staining, for example, was shown to be due to antibodies to histones and other DNA-binding proteins, rim staining to be due to antinative DNA, and a speckled pattern to reflect antibodies to components of the splicing apparatus, such as snRNPs. Some antibodies, detected by more specific methods, such as double immunodiffusion or ELISA, are quite specific for SLE (anti-Sm, anti-Su, anti-Ro, anti-La, and antinative DNA, for example).

Although SLE is best known for its array of antinuclear antibodies, antibodies to many other self components are well described. With the exception of IgG, the antigens tend to be cell-bound (e.g., antibodies to lymphocytes, platelets, erythrocytes, neutrophils, and basement membranes). In the case of IgG and clotting factors, it is possible that the true autoantibody target is cell-bound, in the form of immune complexes or of activated clotting factors.

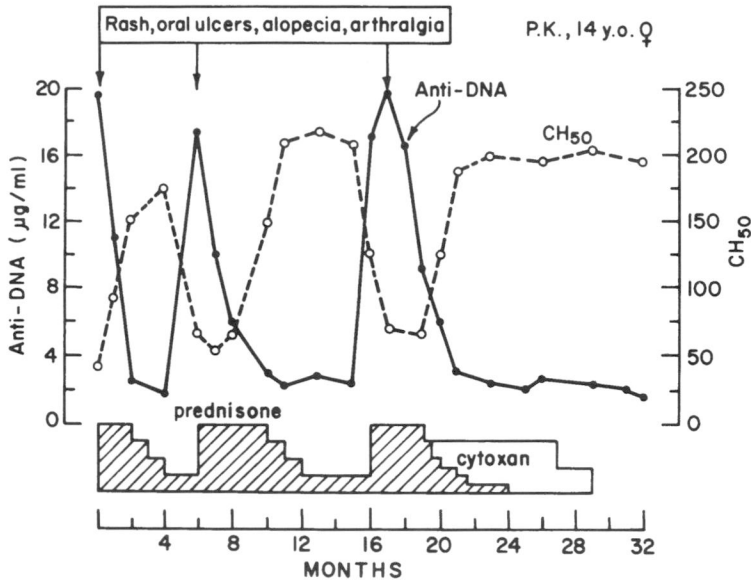

FIG. 3. Clinical course of a patient with systemic lupus erythematosus. Note the "mirror image" pattern of levels of anti-DNA antibodies and hemolytic complement (CH₅₀) in the serum. Exacerbations of the disease (*vertical arrows*) coincide with increased levels of anti-DNA antibodies.

Despite the wealth of information regarding SLE autoantibodies, it is useful to realize that only a few are implicated in disease pathogenesis. SLE renal disease has been attributed to DNA–anti-DNA complexes trapped in glomerular endothelium and epithelium, presumably triggering complement-mediated vascular injury and inflammation (189). This mechanism is supported by a correlation between anti-DNA levels and active renal disease when patients are followed serially, by an inverse correlation with circulating complement levels (Fig. 3) and by the finding of concentrated DNA–anti-DNA complexes in eluates from SLE glomeruli (190). Even for renal disease, however, studies supporting such immune-complex involvement for all histopathologic types are conflicting.

Although, presumably, nonrenal manifestations of SLE are autoantibody-mediated, few mechanistic data exist, except for the various cytopenias, for which an immune basis is well supported. Inflammatory skin disease (Fig. 4) appears to be T cell–mediated, although antibodies to Ro and La may be of importance (191). Infants born to SLE patients occasionally have thrombocytopenia and lesions typical of subacute cutaneous SLE, together with the Ro and La antibodies typical of this condition (192). Transplacental passage of IgG autoantibodies from mother to fetus explains the infant disease, as well as its spontaneous resolution, which is coincident with the disappearance of maternal antibody. Presumably, the heart block often seen in infants born to anti-Ro–positive mothers is also mediated by antibody that damages the developing cardiac conduction system.

Several other SLE manifestations have been difficult to relate to immune processes. Central nervous system involvement can lead to psychosis, seizures, and debilitating neurologic deficits (193). Nervous system tissue from affected patients is usually devoid of immunoglobulin deposition or evidence of cellular infiltration, the only usual finding being microvascular changes. Immunologic studies of arthritis and of pleural and pericardial inflammation are few, and an immune basis can be only presumed.

Rheumatoid Arthritis

RA is a common chronic inflammatory polyarthritis of worldwide distribution, with a female predominance of 3:1 and a peak onset in the fourth decade of life. Intense inflammation occurs in synovial joints, so that the normally delicate synovial membrane becomes infiltrated with mononuclear phagocytes, lymphocytes, and neutrophils (194). An inflammatory fluid is usually exuded by the inflamed synovium. In addition to pain and loss of mobility of joints, patients frequently develop systemic manifestations, namely anemia, subcutaneous nodules, pleurisy, pericarditis, interstitial lung disease, and manifestations of vasculitis such as nerve infarction, skin lesions, and inflammation of the ocular sclera. The course of RA is variable, but usually patients develop progressive loss of cartilage and bone around joints, with resulting diminished mobility.

Although the cause of RA remains unknown, a number of its features are suggestive of an autoimmune etiology. The pathology of arthritic joints suggests a T cell–mediated chronic inflammatory reaction (195,196). Susceptibility to RA is significantly greater in individuals with the DR4 haplotype, owing to the QKRAA motif in the hypervariable region, thereby suggesting a role for autoantigen presentation (197). Most patients (more than 80%) develop RF (19), mostly produced in the marrow, but with significant production by the inflamed synovium (198). The presence of intrasynovial immune complexes, together with diminished levels of complement components, implies an involvement of RF in some of the local pathology (199). In recent years, however, much interest has focused on the T cells and mononuclear phagocytes infiltrating the

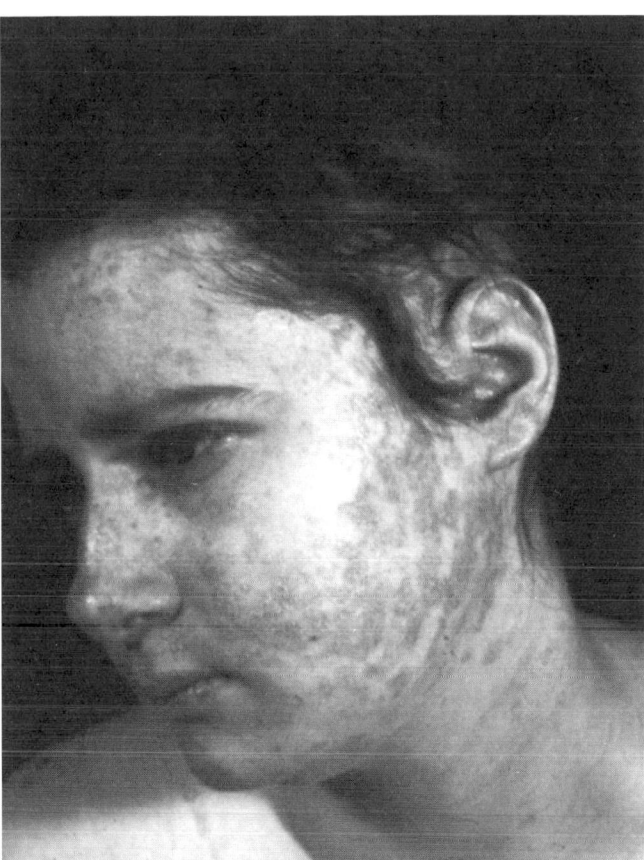

FIG. 4. Photosensitive rash in a patient with SLE. Note the erythematous and scaly quality of the rash, which crosses the bridge of the nose and gives rise to a "butterfly" pattern. No skin rash was noted in areas of the skin usually covered by clothing.

joint. T cells are probably polyclonal (187), although evidence for selective expansion of certain Vβ subsets exists and has led some investigators to propose a role for superantigens (200). Depletion of T cells by thoracic duct drainage (201) or by immunosuppressive drugs, such as cyclosporine, has resulted in improvement, implying an important role for T cells in the inflammatory process (202). Much work on intrasynovial cytokines, however, has pointed toward mononuclear phagocytes as the prime driving force of the inflammatory process (203).

The synovial fluid in RA contains primarily cytokines of mononuclear origin, namely, IL-1, IL-6, and TNF-α. IL-1 receptor antagonist can also be demonstrated in most fluids. In contrast, IL-2, IFN-γ, and other T-cell cytokines are usually present in only small quantities, with the possible exception of IL-17. Efforts to treat RA with T cell–depleting monoclonal antibodies have yielded disappointing results (204). In contrast, administration of monoclonal antibodies to TNF-α has resulted in marked reduction of inflammation (205). Modest improvement has also been reported for antibodies to IL-6 and with administration of IL-1 receptor antagonist.

Efforts to define the underlying etiology of RA have met with frustration. Numerous reports of isolation of viruses, mycoplasmas, and other infectious agents have not been confirmed. Because experimental anti-collagen immunity in rodents results in an RA like syndrome (206), it is possible that similar autoimmunity might be at work in RA. Although low levels of anti-collagen antibodies and reactive T cells have been reported in RA, there is little to support the involvement of anti-collagen immunity in this disorder (207).

The mechanism whereby joint inflammation results in cartilage and bone erosion in RA is incompletely understood (208). It seems unlikely that leakage into cartilage of neutrophil or mononuclear phagocyte-derived proteolytic enzymes is responsible. The diffusion through the cartilage matrix of cytokines, such as IL-1 and IL-6, probably stimulates breakdown of cartilage and bone through an action on chondrocytes and osteoclasts. The destruction of cartilage and bone is functionally much more devastating than the joint inflammation.

Reactive Arthritis and the Spondyarthritides

An important group of rheumatic diseases is characterized by inflammation mostly of large joints, with a predilection for the sacroiliac joints in chronic cases, often associated with infection by certain organisms, or with psoriasis or inflammatory bowel disease (209). These illnesses share a tendency for inflammation to heal with brisk fibroblastic proliferation, together with the formation of new bone. They are unlike RA in that periarticular cartilage loss and osteopenia are uncharacteristic. A remarkable feature of these illnesses is their association with the HLA-B27 class I MHC allele. For Reiter's disease, a form of reactive arthritis that often includes genitourinary, oral mucosal, uveal tract, and skin inflammation, approximately 90% of afflicted individuals have the B27 haplotype, compared with 7% of the normal population (210). Numerous outbreaks of Reiter's disease have been observed in HLA-B27–positive individuals following epidemic infections with diarrhea-causing bacteria (see below), as shown in Fig. 5.

Whether autoimmunity is operative in the pathogenesis of these forms of chronic arthritis is unclear (211). Autoantibodies to IgG are absent, as are antinuclear antibodies, and other autoantibodies are not described. There is some evidence that infection with inciting organisms (which include *Chlamydia, Yersinia, Salmonella,* and *Shigella*) may elicit antibodies or cell-mediated immunity that is cross-reactive with self antigen, but the pathogenesis of these illnesses is quite unclear (212). The class I association has given rise to the speculation that CD8 T cells are important in mediating self-reactivity, and this contention is supported by the occurrence of Reiter's disease, often severe, in HIV-infected individuals with severely depressed CD4 counts yet relative preservation of CD8+ T cells (213).

Rats expressing a human HLA-B27 transgene in high copy number develop arthritis, inflammatory bowel disease, and skin lesions (214). These are less severe in animals raised under germ-free conditions, implying a role for microbial flora. T cells are required for development of disease. Imposition of the HLA-B27 transgene in mice lacking class I MHC molecules also gives rise to a Reiter's-like arthritic and inflammatory syndrome (215).

Systemic Vasculitis

The susceptibility of the vascular system to injury from deposition within vessel walls of immune complexes or from intravascular cell-mediated lesions is the basis of a large group of disorders with multiple manifestations that depend on the severity of involvement and the nature of the affected blood vessel (216). Figure 6 shows typical involvement of a medium-sized artery. In

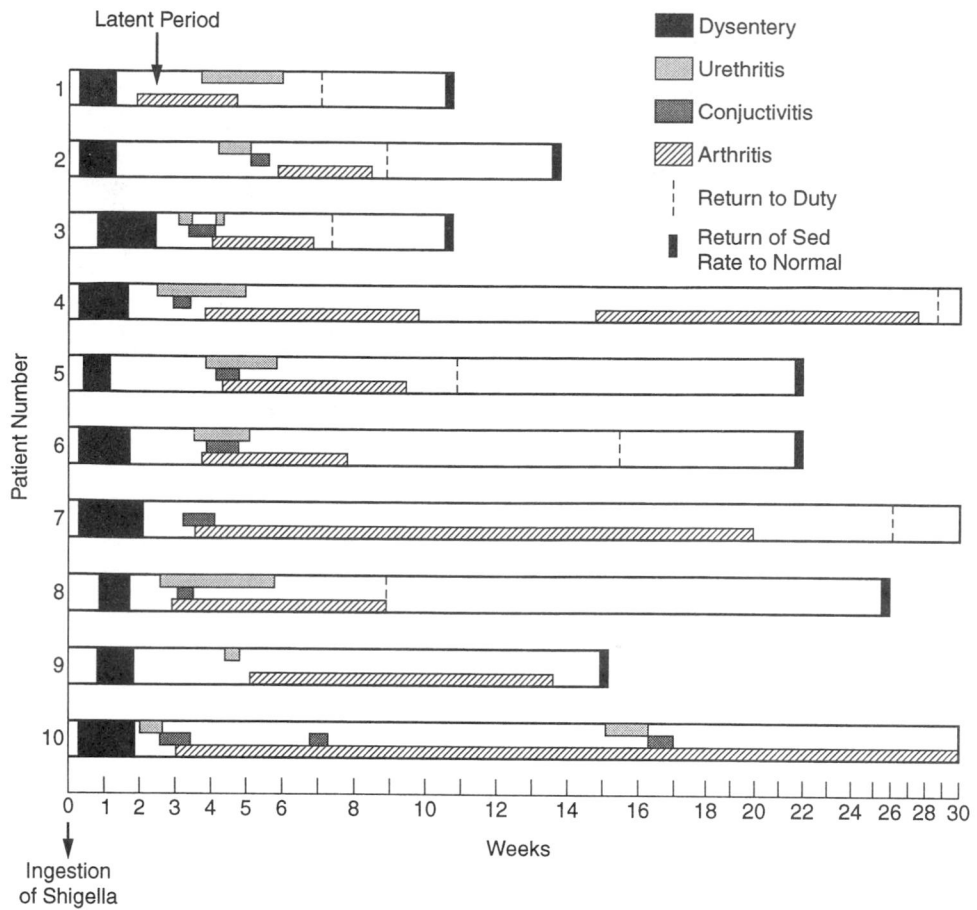

FIG. 5. The evolution of an outbreak of reactive arthritis among the crew of a naval vessel following an epidemic of *Shigella* dysentery is shown. Of over 600 crew members who developed diarrhea, only 11 developed features of Reiter's syndrome. Five of these sailors were traced 10 years later, and four were found to be HLA-B27–positive. (Reprinted from Noer HR. An "experimental" epidemic of Reiter's syndrome. *JAMA* 1966;198:693–698, with permission.)

some cases, the mechanism is immune complexes formed in response to exogenous antigens, such as viruses (especially hepatitis B and C) or drugs (217), while in other instances, autoantibodies or antibodies to as yet uncharacterized environmental agents are responsible.

Autoimmune vasculitis can be seen alone or together with SLE or other rheumatic diseases. Figure 7 demonstrates the deposition of C3 in the lumen of an inflamed small artery from an SLE patient with vasculitis. There is evidence for deposition of complexes of DNA–anti-DNA and IgG RF–IgG, with subsequent injury involving the complement system (218). On occasion, clinical disease correlates with cryoprecipitation of complexes in serum cooled below body temperature. A special example of vasculitis is that of mixed cryoglobulinemia (219), in which a monoclonal IgM (the product of a single aberrant B-cell clone) with autoantibody activity against IgG (i.e., RF activity) forms large circulating complexes that deposit in the walls of small and medium-sized arteries, causing ischemia and infarction of skin, nerves, and kidney.

Vasculitis manifestations can range from skin lesions alone (small vessel vasculitis) to ischemia of vital organs such as kidney, heart, brain, and liver. Attempts have been made to classify vasculitis based on known versus unknown etiology and

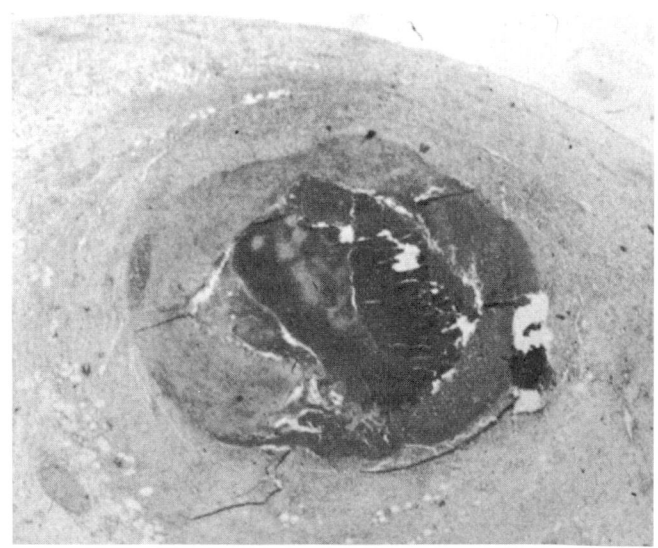

FIG. 6. Systemic necrotizing arteritis. Shown is a section of a subsegmental mesenteric artery of a 65-year-old man with severe abdominal pain and a bowel infarction. Note the disruption of the internal elastic lamina of the vessel, the intramural thrombus, and the leukocytic infiltrate. The patient had an excellent response to corticosteroids and cyclophosphamide.

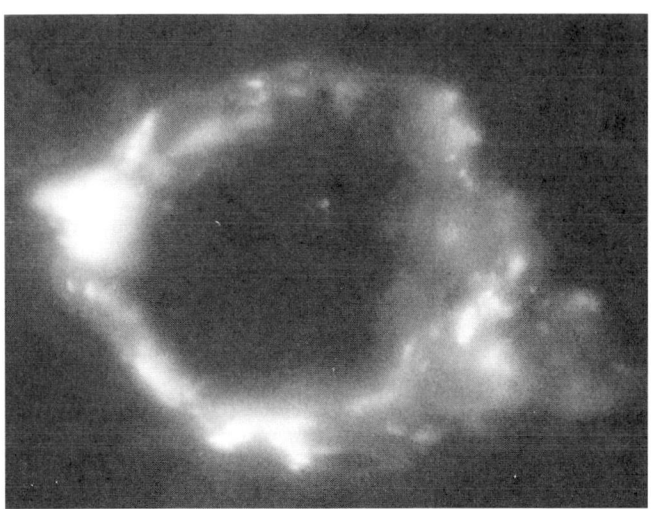

FIG. 7. Vasculitis in a patient with SLE. Note the presence of complement demonstrated using antihuman C3 in the wall of this artery.

rheumatic versus nonrheumatic. Figure 8 schematizes the type of involvement that results from inflammation of blood vessels of differing caliber.

Wegener's granulomatosis is a rare form of vasculitis featuring the formation of granulomas around blood vessels, with typical severe involvement of lung and kidney (220). The presence of antiproteinase 3 (c-ANCA) in most patients with this disorder has led to the hypothesis that ANCA-induced neutrophil activation is central to a chain of events leading to T-cell activation and a cellular immune response involving macrophage activation (221).

Sjögren's Syndrome

This lymphoproliferative and autoimmune disorder occurs in a primary form, not associated with a rheumatic disease, and as a complication of RA, SLE, or scleroderma. Patients develop infiltration of exocrine glands, mostly salivary and lacrimal glands, with activated polyclonal CD4+ T cells, together with hypergammaglobulinemia, autoantibodies, and, sometimes, vasculitis (222). Lymphocyte infiltration may extend beyond the exocrine glands to involve lungs, liver, and other viscera. Primary Sjögren's syndrome is associated with HLA-DR3 and with antibodies to Ro and La. There is an increased susceptibility to lymphoid malignancy, mostly B-cell lymphomas. An entity closely resembling Sjögren's syndrome has been described in HIV infection, with CD8- rather than CD4-bearing cells infiltrating exocrine glands (223).

Chronic Graft-Versus-Host Disease

In animals undergoing GVHD against class II determinants, a systemic autoimmune syndrome with SLE-like features produces antinuclear antibodies, immune-complex renal disease, and immune cytopenias (224). Clinical manifestations vary according to background genes and according to the genetic barrier between strains: I-E differences generate higher levels of antinuclear antibodies, yet I-A differences result in more renal disease. In murine chronic GVHD, induced across an MHC class II barrier, T and B cells interact in a cognate, MHC-restricted fashion, implying a specific form of T-cell help rather than the nonspecific effect on B cells of excessive cytokines (225).

"Homologous disease" occurs in rats subjected to chronic GVHD. Extensive sclerotic visceral lesions that are very like scleroderma occur (226). In human recipients of bone marrow, a chronic GVHD

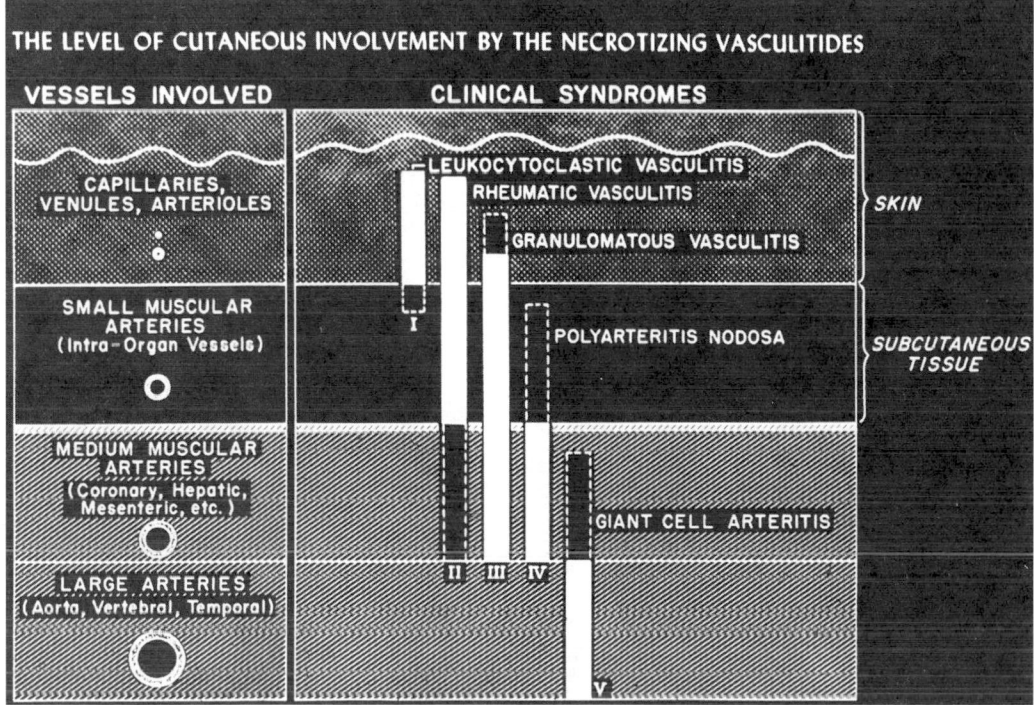

FIG. 8. The spectrum of vasculitis. The manifestations of vasculitis are dependent on the caliber of the involved vessel, which may in turn reflect the size, charge, or other physical properties of deposited immune complexes. Note that the resulting disease is dependent on the size of the inflamed vessel. (Courtesy of James A. Gilliam, M.D.)

syndrome is a major clinical problem, leading to fibrosis, skin pathology, and autoantibodies. The syndrome occurs even in recipients of autologous marrow, although in a milder form (227).

Scleroderma (Systemic Sclerosis)

This disease is marked by inflammation, followed by deposition in skin and viscera accompanied by certain antinuclear antibodies (228). Early lesions contain T-lymphocytes, and there is evidence of bias of the T-cell repertoire (229). Antibodies to topoisomerase I (Scl-70) correlate with visceral damage, and antibodies to centromere antigens connote a more benign course (230). Scleroderma is characterized by marked vascular abnormalities, the most dramatic of which is the episodic reduction in peripheral arterial perfusion (often provoked by cold temperatures), known as Raynaud's phenomenon. Impairment of circulation can lead to pain, infections, and ischemic amputation of the distal fingertips. Considerable disability can result from this and from the loss of hand mobility due to thickening of the overlying skin.

Patients with the severe form of scleroderma, known as progressive systemic sclerosis, develop serious injury to the skin, kidney, lung, and gastrointestinal tract. Therapy is usually ineffective. Despite the clear-cut evidence of serologic autoimmunity, the autoimmunity underlying the visceral and skin damage in the illness is only presumed, and nothing is known of the basic mechanism. A strain of chickens develops an illness with marked scleroderma-like features (231).

COMMONLY USED ANIMAL MODELS OF SYSTEMIC AUTOIMMUNE DISEASE

Several spontaneous murine models have been widely used to address SLE pathogenesis and treatment.

Lpr and gld Mice

The autosomal recessive *lpr* mutation of the Fas apoptosis gene causes progressive, spectacular lymphadenopathy (Fig. 9), multiple SLE-like autoantibodies, and hypergammaglobulinemia (232). As is also true for the other murine SLE models (*vide infra*),

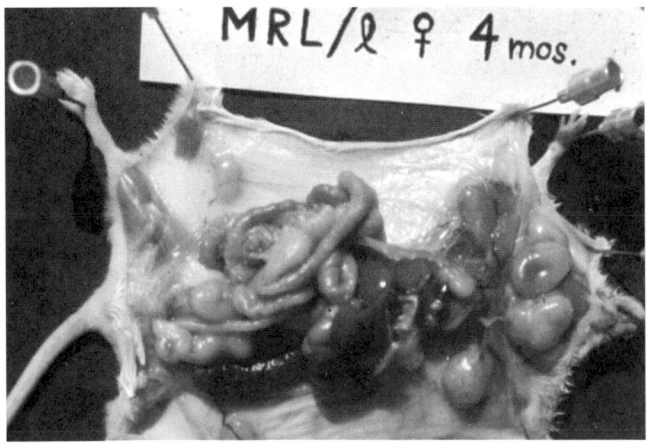

FIG. 9. MRL/*lpr* mouse (age 4 months). Note massive lymph node and spleen enlargement due to CD4⁻CD8⁻ T-cell infiltration. (Courtesy of Robert Eisenberg, M.D.)

expression of laboratory and clinical manifestations of disease is highly dependent on other, poorly understood background genes (233). Thus, MRL/*lpr* mice, which are the best-studied strain, develop severe glomerulonephritis and vasculitis and have a markedly foreshortened life span, while C57BL6/*lpr* (B6/*lpr*) mice manifest a milder syndrome, with nearly normal longevity. The *gld* gene leads to essentially identical syndromes on similar backgrounds.

The failure of the Fas/FasL system to delete autoreactive extrathymic T cells accounts for the accumulation of vast numbers of CD4⁻CD8⁻ anergic T cells, the unusual phenotype of which apparently represents a secondary mechanism for downregulating function, in the absence of deletion. The Fas mutation is also expressed in B cells, leading to a failure to delete autoantibody-forming cells but not to lymphoproliferation analogous to T cells (234).

T cells are required for development of both lymphadenopathy and autoantibodies. In *lpr* mice with deletion of MHC class II genes (235), or those lacking CD4 molecules (236), autoantibodies fail to develop, yet lymphadenopathy occurs; conversely, the absence of CD8 or β2-microglobulin (237) results in little change in autoantibody levels, but a marked decrease in lymphadenopathy. These and other studies support the idea that the abnormal double-negative T cells of *lpr* are descended primarily from CD8 precursors, which lose their CD8 as part of their evolution into anergic cells. The T cells that provide help for autoantibodies, on the other hand, are primarily CD4-bearing cells that recognize antigens (and presumably autoantigens) in the context of self class II MHC.

NZB and NZB/NZW F1 Mice

NZB mice develop autoimmune hemolytic anemia, antinuclear antibodies, and late-life lymphoreticular neoplasms (238). The F1 offspring of this strain and near-normal NZW mice suffer from a much more fulminant and SLE-like syndrome, leading to diffuse proliferative glomerulonephritis, high-titer antinuclear antibodies, and early death (especially in females). NZB×SWR F1 mice are another well-studied model that develops renal disease, offering the additional advantage that the SWR parents are free of endogenous retroviruses and without apparent additional immunopathology (239). The genetics of SLE in NZB crosses are complex and are discussed elsewhere. The SLE-like disease is characterized by both B- and T-cell defects, notably B-cell hyperactivity, even in fetal life, and a requirement for T cells for development of autoantibodies and disease (240).

BXSB Mice

These animals develop an age-dependent SLE-like syndrome that is much more severe in males because of a Y-chromosome gene (Yaa) (241). Unlike the *lpr* mutation, which provokes at least some degree of autoimmune disease regardless of genetic background, Yaa results in acceleration of autoimmunity only when bred onto the genomes of autoimmune mice. High-titer antinuclear antibodies and immune-complex nephritis lead to early mortality in males. Chimera studies using B6-Yaa mice have shown that it is largely the T-lymphocytes that are responsible for the autoimmune disease, as their elimination, but not the elimination of B cells, reduces disease in chimeras. It has been suggested that the basic defect in this strain involves enhanced T-B interaction, possibly through abnormal adherence. The presence of a functional I-E molecule reduces serologic and clinical disease, possibly through presentation of peptide fragments of I-E by the I-A element (242).

Induction of Systemic Lupus-like Syndrome in Mice through Injection of Pristane

Pristane, a branched alkane, is widely used to produce peritoneal inflammation, which primes mice for subsequent hybridoma implantation. It was fortuitously observed that mice receiving pristane alone developed a progressive autoimmune syndrome marked by development of SLE-like autoantibodies, including anti-Sm and other highly characteristic specificities (243). SLE-like glomerular changes are observed, together with deposition of immunoglobulin and complement. Serologic features of the syndrome are dependent on the genetic background of the mouse, with H-2 playing a prominent role. For instance, H-2^s mice develop antiribosomal protein autoantibodies, while autoantibodies appear only in low titer in H-2^b-expressing C57BL mice (244).

Systemic Autoimmunity Induced by Idiotype Infusion

A syndrome characterized by antinuclear antibodies, cytopenias, and immune-mediated renal disease occurs in mice given antibodies expressing the human 16/6 idiotype, which is found on certain human IgM monoclonal anti-DNA antibodies (245). Disease is preceded by antibodies to the 16/6 idiotype, and may represent precipitation of a cascade of aberrant idiotype–antiidiotype network interactions involving T cells, as SLE manifestations can also be induced by T-cell lines from idiotype-immunized mice (246). These mice have also been reported to have anticardiolipin antibodies and abnormalities of hemostasis.

The Viable Motheaten Mouse

Research has shown that the lethal motheaten (me) and viable motheaten (me^v) phenotypes, which result in a severe neonatal autoimmune syndrome with hypergammaglobulinemia and autoantibodies to DNA and erythrocytes, are due to a mutant tyrosine kinase expressed in hematopoietic cells (247). Virtually all of the mouse B cells are of the B1 subset, and death from an apparent autoimmune and inflammatory disease occurs by 3 weeks. The mechanism whereby the kinase deficiency results in autoreactivity is unclear, but it presumably reflects fundamental mechanisms controlling B-cell differentiation.

Severe Autoimmune Disease in Knock-out and Transgenic Strains

Mice homozygous for deletion of the transforming growth factor-β (TGF-β) gene suffer a severe and fulminant autoimmune disorder that is characterized by multiorgan inflammatory disease and death by 3 weeks. The disorder is mediated by T-lymphocytes and can be adoptively transferred to MHC-compatible normal mice (248). Apparently, the absence of the immunosuppressive and antiinflammatory effects of TGF-β permits unregulated spontaneous inflammatory disease. A parallel situation occurs in mice without functional CTLA4. The absence of negative regulation of T cells, which is normally mediated by this molecule, also leads to a severe neonatal autoimmune and inflammatory disease (249).

Striking autoimmune disease, especially involving the intestinal tract, but with hematologic and other systemic manifestations as well, occurs in mice with deleted IL-2 (250), IL-4 (251), and TCR genes (252). To some extent, the inflammatory disease is dependent on the microbiologic environment of the mice as well as the background strain, and has been attributed to the consequences of cytokine imbalances.

Mice transgenic for the bcl-2 oncogene expressed in B cells develop certain SLE-like autoantibodies (253). The combination of the bcl-2 apoptosis defect and the lpr Fas mutation results in mice with even further lymphoid hyperplasia, but no further increase in autoantibodies, suggesting that the apoptosis impairment resulting from the lpr mutation is maximal in terms of autoantibody production and cannot be further exacerbated (254).

The Tight-skin Mouse

The tsk mutation is a dominant mutation on chromosome 2, which is lethal in its homozygous form (255). The mice develop progressive skin tightening, together with pulmonary fibrosis and cardiomyopathy. Antibodies to topoisomerase I (256) and RNA polymerase I have been detected. Mice lacking CD4 cells fail to develop skin lesions, but develop visceral abnormalities; lack of CD8 cells has little influence on disease (257).

Models of Rheumatoid Arthritis

Several rodent models of RA have been widely used (258). A chronic polyarthritis results from the injection of peptidoglycan–polysaccharide in rats, with extensive joint destruction (259). It is dependent on the genetic background of the rat (Lewis is the prototype susceptible strain; Buffalo is resistant), partly due to MHC genes, and requires T-lymphocytes. Considerable evidence suggests that the inflammatory disease is due to the persistence of bacterial debris. A relapsing form of the disease can be induced by intraarticular bacterial LPS in animals that have had an earlier injection of peptidoglycan–polysaccharide (260).

A chronic inflammatory arthritis, also in general use, is induced by immunization with type II collagen in adjuvant (261). Collagen arthritis is mainly due to T-cell immunity to type II collagen, although antibody is also demonstrable and may provoke some of the injury. MHC influences and T-cell oligoclonality are important in this illness (262). A single injection of complete Freund's adjuvant alone causes a chronic arthritis in rats but not in mice. It has been used as a way of evaluating antiinflammatory drugs.

One of the most interesting more recent models of RA is the inflammatory arthritis in mice transgenic for human T-cell leukemia virus type I (HTLV-I) tax (263). Such animals develop chronic erosive arthritis with synovial proliferation and pathologic changes resembling RA. They produce anticollagen antibodies, RF, and anti–heat-shock proteins, and they also manifest T-cell immunity to collagen and heat-shock proteins. A Sjögren's-like autoimmune exocrinopathy has also been reported in these animals (264). These findings are of special interest because humans with HTLV infection may also develop inflammatory arthritis, alone or in the presence of myelopathy (265).

Mice transgenic for TNF-α also develop a spontaneous erosive arthritis, presumably due to the proinflammatory action of this cytokine (266). These studies support the proposed key role of TNF-α in RA.

IMMUNE INJURY IN SYSTEMIC AUTOIMMUNE DISEASE

The classification scheme of Gell and Coombs is still a useful way of subdividing injury mechanisms in systemic autoimmunity. Type I injury, mediated by IgE, is not important in these disorders. By contrast, tissue damage initiated by binding of autoantibody directly to target tissues is of importance, particularly in organ-specific autoimmune disease, but, to a great extent, also in systemic autoimmune disease, in which antibodies to cell and basement membranes, fibronectin, collagen, and other fixed components of tissue may exist. Binding of antibody to self tissue leads to inflammation through a complex series of events involving the complement and coagulation pathways, leading to chemotaxis of neutrophils and monocytes and to their phagocytosis and release of local inflammatory mediators. Platelet aggregation, dilatation of vascular smooth muscle, and activation of mast cells are all part of the series of events triggered by autoantibody binding to tissue in type II injury; these topics are discussed in detail elsewhere in this textbook. Examples of autoantibodies provoking these changes probably include anticollagen antibodies and antiglomerular basement antibodies. Figure 10 depicts the pathologic changes in Goodpasture's syndrome, a disorder that causes hemorrhagic lung and kidney lesions due to antibodies directed against the basement membrane proteins common to both organs.

Type III injury, mediated by immune complexes, is believed to account for much of the pathology of systemic autoimmune diseases, particularly SLE and vasculitis. In NZB/NZW mice, blocking of C5 using monoclonal antibody reduces nephritis and increases survival, supporting a role for classical pathway activation in the immune-complex disease of this strain (267). The protean nature of immune complexes, which can range from just a few molecules of antigen and antibody to huge complexes involving whole cells coated or cross-linked by antibody, accounts for the great variety of pathology encountered in type III injury. Much interest has focused on defining the offending antigens that are present in injurious immune complexes in SLE and related diseases, but with mixed success. SLE exacerbations are frequently preceded

or accompanied by a fall in hemolytic complement, together with a rise in levels of antibodies to native (double-stranded) DNA. These antibodies are concentrated in the glomeruli of patients with SLE renal disease (Fig. 11), consistent with the idea that DNA–anti-DNA complexes may deposit in SLE kidneys and provoke inflammation (268). Although it seems likely that DNA–anti-DNA is an important antibody system in SLE renal disease, it is very likely that other kinds of autoantibodies also contribute in important ways to glomerular injury (189). Antichromatin, for example, forms immune complexes that may localize on the glomerular basement membrane. Current studies focus on the charge, size, and antigenic characteristics of such antibodies in relation to their ability to bind and to injure glomeruli.

Type IV injury is due to T-lymphocytes, macrophages, and perhaps other cells that infiltrate tissues, sometimes causing granulomas. Some systemic autoimmune diseases are dominated by type IV injury, for example, Wegener's granulomatosis; yet it is more common for type IV mechanisms to coexist with types II and III. SLE, for example, is frequently accompanied by destructive and inflammatory skin lesions dominated by T-lymphocytes; similarly, the destructive inflammatory muscle lesions of polymyositis occur together with antisynthetase antibodies and other serologic autoimmunity. There may be some contribution of cell-mediated immunity to SLE renal disease, but expression of MHC class I or class II molecules is unnecessary for development of nephritis in MRL/*lpr* mice (269).

Autoantibodies may also exert damage through their effects on the coagulation system. The antiphospholipid syndrome is marked by arterial and venous thromboses, which may cause stroke, myocardial infarction, and thromboembolism. It is seen alone or as a feature of SLE and is due not to true antiphospholipid antibodies, but rather to antibodies to phospholipid-binding proteins, mainly β2-glycoprotein I (270). By an imperfectly understood mechanism, these antibodies enhance platelet aggregation and activation and promote thrombus formation while paradoxically prolonging the *in vitro* partial thromboplastin time, an indicator of coagulation. This *in vitro* phenomenon is termed the *lupus anticoagulant* and is present in a substantial minority of SLE patients as well as in many individuals with no other recognized illness. It is a major cause of

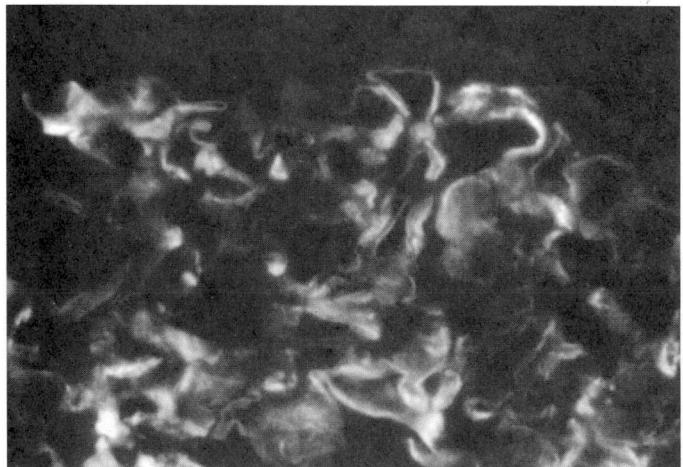 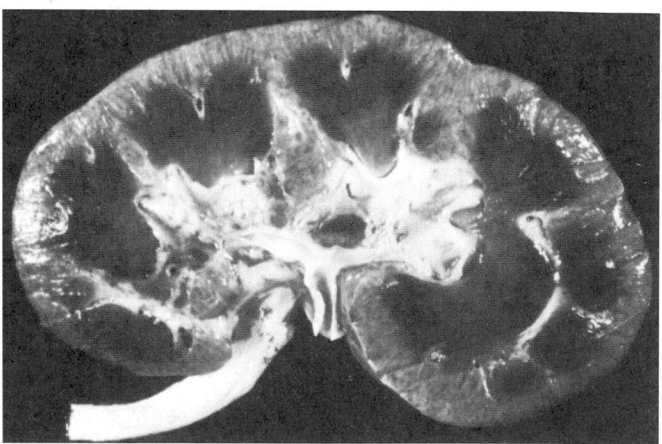

A   B

FIG. 10. Type II immune-mediated injury. **Panel A:** Linear deposition of IgG against antigens present on the glomerular basement membrane of a patient with Goodpasture's syndrome is illustrated using fluoresceinated antihuman IgG. Similar changes were seen in the lung. **Panel B:** Hemorrhagic changes are visible in the gross autopsy pathology specimen from this patient. (Courtesy of William J. Yount, M.D.)

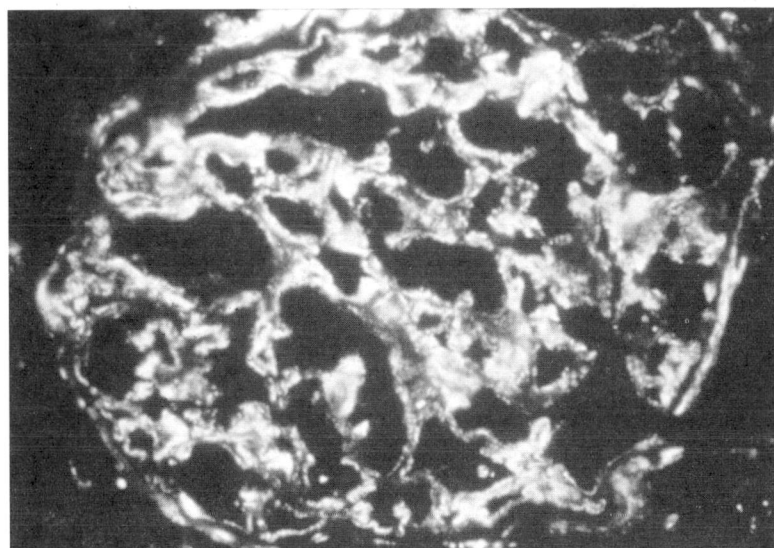

FIG. 11. Type III (immune-complex) injury in an SLE renal biopsy specimen. This patient had proteinuria and red blood cells in her urine. Note the granular (sometimes called "lumpy-bumpy") distribution of the immune deposits in this section stained with antibody to human C3.

early spontaneous abortion and may be an important cause of thrombotic disease in the general population.

Tissue damage may also be mediated through antibodies to neutrophil cytoplasmic antigens (ANCAs). These IgG antibodies, initially detected by immunofluorescence, have been divided by staining patterns into perinuclear (p-ANCA) and cytoplasmic (c-ANCA). p-ANCAs are directed against myeloperoxidase, while c-ANCAs are specific for proteinase 3 (221). These autoantibodies are useful markers for vasculitis, including Wegener's granulomatosis, pauciimmune necrotizing and crescentic pauciimmune glomerulonephritis, and polyarteritis nodosa, and their titers correlate with disease severity. The mechanism by which antibodies to these cytoplasmic antigens leads to blood vessel damage and inflammation is incompletely understood, but it may involve expression on activated neutrophils of proteinase 3 and myeloperoxidase, and possibly release of free proteinase 3. Antibodies to these molecules may provoke enhanced neutrophil chemotaxis and adhesion, together with triggering of the respiratory burst. This may lead to a series of events culminating in activation of T cells and macrophages and the formation of necrotizing granulomas.

APPROACHES TO THE TREATMENT OF SYSTEMIC AUTOIMMUNE DISEASE

In general, the management of human systemic autoimmune disease is empirical and unsatisfactory. For the most part, broadly immunosuppressive drugs, such as corticosteroids, are used in a wide variety of severe autoimmune and inflammatory disorders; in milder conditions, antiinflammatory agents acting on eicosenoid metabolism are often sufficient.

In addition to corticosteriods, other immunosuppressive agents are used in management of the systemic autoimmune diseases. Cyclophosphamide is an alkylating agent that causes profound depletion of both T- and B-lymphocytes and impairment of cell-mediated immunity. It is used in SLE nephritis and is particularly effective in granulomatous vasculitis and polyarteritis nodosa. Its use entails the risks of immunosuppression, along with an increased incidence of lymphoreticular malignancies. Azathioprine

and the closely related 6-mercaptopurine are used in parallel situations; these are somewhat less effective but are less toxic.

Cyclosporine, tacrolimus, and mycophenolate mofetil are natural products with specific properties of T-lymphocyte suppression, and they have been used with success in SLE, RA, and, to a limited extent, in vasculitis and myositis. They have significant renal toxicity in addition to their immunosuppressive effects.

Methotrexate is widely used as a "second-line" agent in RA, with the goal of reducing disease progression. It is also useful in polymyositis and other connective-tissue diseases. Its mechanism of action here is controversial and may relate to its action on adenosine receptors rather than to its more familiar role as an antimetabolite.

There is optimism that more specific treatment for autoimmune disorders can be devised when their mechanisms become better understood. Oral tolerance holds promise as a means of attracting immunosuppressive T-lymphocytes to sites of active autoimmune pathology and suppressing inflammation by a bystander effect, probably involving TGF-β (271). Other approaches under development are monoclonal antibodies that are intended to block the action of cytokines or to deplete lymphocytes (204). With the exception of anti–TNF-α in RA (205), these have been disappointing.

CONCLUSIONS

The mechanisms of systemic autoimmune disease are diverse and incompletely understood. Several points are worthy of emphasis. The rules and restrictions governing ordinary immune responses seem to apply to autoimmune responses: there is little that is extraordinary about the immunoglobulin or TCR genes used or in their means of rearrangement or diversification; antigen is required to initiate responses. Production of and response to cytokines and other mediators is similar to what is seen for responses to exogenous antigens, and T and B cells collaborate in an MHC-restricted fashion. The availability of transgenic and knock-out mice and continuing progress in the understanding of the genome seem likely to open novel and fruitful approaches to understanding disorders of systemic autoimmunity.

REFERENCES

1. Lahita RG. The connective tissue diseases and the overall influence of gender. *Int J Fertil Menopausal Stud* 1996;41:156–165.
2. Cervera R, Khamashta MA, Font J, et al. Systemic lupus erythematosus: clinical and immunologic patterns of disease expression in a cohort of 1,000 patients. *Medicine* 1993;72:113–124.
3. Lahita RG. Low plasma androgens in women with systemic lupus erythematosus. *Arthritis Rheum* 1987;30:241–248.
4. Ahmed SA, Penhale WJ, Talal N. Sex hormones, immune responses, and autoimmune diseases. Mechanisms of sex hormone action. *Am J Pathol* 1985;121:531–551.
5. Lorber M, Gershwin ME, Shoenfeld Y. The coexistence of SLE with other autoimune diseaes: the kaleidoscope of autoimmunity. *Semin Arthritis Rheum* 1994;24:105–113.
6. Sharp GC, Irvin WS, Tan EM, Gould RG, Holman HR. Mixed connective tissue disease—an apparently distinct rheumatic disease syndrome associated with a specific antibody to an extractable nuclear antigen (ENA). *Am J Med* 1972;52:148–159.
7. Gottlieb AB, Lahita RG, Chiorazzi N, Kunkel HG. Immune function in systemic lupus erythematosus: impairment of in vitro T-cell proliferation and in vivo antibody response to exogenous antigen. *J Clin Invest* 1979;63:885–892.
8. Hahn BH, Bagby MK, Osterland CK. Abnormalities of delayed hypersensitivity in systemic lupus erythematosus. *Am J Med* 1973;55:25–31.
9. Winfield JB, Winchester RJ, Kunkel HG. Association of cold-reactive anti-lymphocyte antibodies with lymphopenia in systemic lupus erythematosus. *Arthritis Rheum* 1975;18:587–594.
10. Estes D, Christian CL. The natural history of systemic lupus erythematosus by prospective analysis. *Medicine* 1971;50:85–95.
11. Ehrlich P, Morgenroth J. On haemolysis: third communication. In: *The collected papers of Paul Ehrlich*. F. Himmelweit, ed. vol 2. London: Pergamon, 1957:205–212.
12. Harrington WJ, Minnich V, Hollingsworth JW, Moore CV. Demonstration of a thrombocytopenic factor in the blood of patients with thrombocytopenic purpura. 1951. *J Lab Clin Med* 1990;115:636–645.
13. Rose NR, Witebsky E. Studies on organ specificity: V. Changes in the thyroid glands of rabbits following acute immunization with rabbit thyroid extracts. *J Immunol* 1956;76:417–423.
14. Burnet FM. A modification of Jerne's theory of antibody production using the concept of clonal selection. *Aust J Sci* 1957;20:67–69.
15. Kakkanaiah VN, Seth A, Nagarkatti M, Nagarkatti P. Autoreactive T cell clones isolated from normal and autoimmune-susceptible mice exhibit lymphokine secretory and functional properties of both Th1 and Th2 cells. *Clin Immunol Immunopathol* 1990;57:148–162.
16. Grabar P. Autoantibodies and the physiological role of immunoglobulins. *Immunol Today* 1983;4:337–339.
17. Hooper B, Whittingham S, Mathews JD, Mackay IR, Curnow DH. Autoimmunity in a rural community. *Clin Exp Immunol* 1972;12:79–87.
18. Hawkins BR, O'Connor KJ, Dawkins RL, Dawkins B, Rodger B. Autoantibodies in an Australian population. I. Prevalence and persistence. *J Clin Lab Immunol* 1979;2:211–215.
19. Chen PP, Fong S, Carson DA. Rheumatoid factor. *Rheum Dis Clin North Am* 1987;13:545–568.
20. Nemazee DA, Sato VL. Induction of rheumatoid antibodies in the mouse: regulated production of autoantibody in the secondary humoral response. *J Exp Med* 1983;158:529–545.
21. Welch MJ, Fong S, Vaughan J, Carson D. Increased frequency of rheumatoid factor precursor B lymphocytes after immunization of normal adults with tetanus toxoid. *Clin Exp Immunol* 1983;51:299–304.
22. Bonfa E, Llovet R, Scheinberg M, de Souza JM, Elkon KB. Comparison between autoantibodies in malaria and leprosy with lupus. *Clin Exp Immunol* 1987;70:529–537.
23. Roosnek E, Lanzavecchia A. Efficient and selective presentation of antigen-antibody complexes by rheumatoid factor B cells. *J Exp Med* 1991;173:487–489.
24. Tighe H, Heaphy P, Baird S, Weigle WO, Carson DA. Human immunoglobulin (IgG) induced deletion of IgM rheumatoid factor B cells in transgenic mice. *J Exp Med* 1995;181:599–606.
25. Tighe H, Chen PP, Tucker T, et al. Function of B cells expressing a human immunoglobulin M rheumatoid factor autoantibody in transgenic mice. *J Exp Med* 1993;177:109–118.
26. Chau V, Tobias JW, Bachmair A, et al. A multiubiquitin chain is confined to specific lysine in a targeted short-lived protein. *Science* 1989;243:1576–1583.
27. Klinman DM, Banks S, Hartman A, Steinberg AD. Natural murine autoantibodies and conventional antibodies exhibit similar degrees of antigenic cross-reactivity. *J Clin Invest* 1988;82:652–657.
28. Hartman AB, Mallett CP, Srinivasappa J, Prabhakar BS, Notkins AL, Smith-Gill SJ. Organ reactive autoantibodies from non-immunized adult BALB/c mice are polyreactive and express non-biased VH gene usage. *Mol Immunol* 1989;26:359–370.
29. Oldstone MBA. Molecular mimicry and autoimmune disease. *Cell* 1987;50:819–820.
30. Kieff E, Dambaugh T, Heller M, et al. The biology and chemistry of Epstein-Barr virus. *J Infect Dis* 1982;146:506–517.
31. Chen PP. From human autoantibodies to the fetal antibody repertoire to B cell malignancy: it's a small world after all. *Int Rev Immunol* 1990;5:239–251.
32. Casali P, Notkins AL. Probing the human B-cell repertoire with EBV: polyreactive antibodies and CD5+ B lymphocytes. *Annu Rev Immunol* 1989;7:513–535.
33. Murakami M, Tsubata T, Okamoto M, et al. Antigen-induced apoptotic death of Ly-1 B cells responsible for autoimmune disease in transgenic mice. *Nature* 1992;357:14–15.
34. Reap EA, Sobel ES, Cohen PL, Eisenberg RA. Conventional B cells, not B-1 cells, are responsible for producing autoantibodies in lpr mice. *J Exp Med* 1993;177:69–78.
35. Reap EA, Sobel ES, Jennette JC, Cohen PL, Eisenberg RA. Conventional B cells, not B1 cells, are the source of autoantibodies in chronic graft versus host disease. *J Immunol* 1993;151:7316–7323.
36. Casali P, Burastero SE, Balow JE, Notkins AL. High-affinity antibodies to ssDNA are produced by CD-B cells in systemic lupus erythematosus patients. *J Immunol* 1989;143:3476–3483.
37. Rajewsky K, Takemori T. Genetics, expression, and function of idiotypes. *Annu Rev Immunol* 1983;1:569–607.
38. Bona CA, Heber-Katz E, Paul WE. Idiotype-anti-idiotype regulation. I. Immunization with a levan-binding myeloma protein leads to the appearance of auto-anti-(anti-idiotype) antibodies and to the activation of silent clones. *J Exp Med* 1981;153:951–967.
39. Uner AH, Knupp CJ, Tatum AH, Gavalchin J. Treatment with antibody reactive with the nephritogenic idiotype, IdLNF1, suppresses its production and leads to prolonged survival of (NZB × SWR) F1 mice. *J Autoimmun* 1994;7:27–44.
40. Oukka M, Colucci-Guyon E, Tran PL, et al. CD4 T cell tolerance to nuclear proteins induced by medullary thymic epithelium. *Immunity* 1996;4:545–553.
41. Goldings EA. Defective B cell tolerance induction in New Zealand black mice I. Macrophage independence and comparison with other autoimmune strains. *J Immunol* 1983;131:2630–2634.
42. Rathmell JC, Goodnow CC. Effects of the lpr mutation on elimination and inactivation of self-reactive B cells. *J Immunol* 1994;153:2831–2842.
43. Staudt LM, Singh H, Sen R, Wirth T, Sharp PA, Baltimore D. A lymphoid-specific protein binding to the octamer motif of immunoglobulin genes. *Nature* 1986;323:640–643.
44. Nagarkatti PS, Snow EC, Kaplan AM. Characterization and function of autoreactive T-lymphocyte clones isolated from normal, unprimed mice. *Cell Immunol* 1985;94:32–48.
45. Sakane T, Steinberg AD, Arnett FC, Reinertsen JL, Green I. Studies of immune functions of patients with systemic lupus erythematosus. *Arthritis Rheum* 1979;22:770–776.
46. Saito K, Tamura A, Narimatsu H, Tadakuma T, Nagashima M. Cloned auto-Ia-reactive T cells elicit lichen planus-like lesion in the skin of syngeneic mice. *J Immunol* 1985;137:2485–2495.
47. Weston KM, Yeh ET, Sy MS. Autoreactivity accelerates the development of autoimmunity and lymphoproliferation in MRL/Mp-lpr/lpr mice. *J Immunol* 1987;139:734–742.
48. Deeg HJ. Graft-versus-host disease: host and donor views. *Semin Hematol* 1993;30:110–117.
49. Erkeller-Yusel F, Hulstaart F, Hannet I, Isenberg D, Lydyard P. Lymphocyte subsets in a large cohort of patients with systemic lupus erythematosus. *Lupus* 1993;2:227–231.
50. Wigfall DR, Sakai RS, Wallace DJ, Jordan SC. Interleukin-2 receptor expression in peripheral blood lymphocytes from systemic lupus erythematosus patients: relationship to clinical activity. *Clin Immunol Immunopathol* 1988;47:354–362.
51. Furukawa F, Tokura Y, Matsushita K, et al. Selective expansions of T cells expressing V beta 8 and V beta 13 in skin lesions of patients with chronic cutaneous lupus erythematosus. *J Dermatol* 1996;23:670–676.
52. Groen H, Aslander M, Bootsma H, van der Mark TW, Kallenberg CG, Postma DS. Bronchoalvelolar lavage cell analysis and lung function impairment in patients with systemic lupus erythematosus (SLE). *Clin Exp Immunol* 1993;94:127–133.
53. Alcocer-Varela J, Aleman-Hoey D, Alarcon-Segovia D. Interleukin-1 and interleukin-6 activities are increased in the cerebrospinal fluid of patients with CNS lupus erythematosus and correlate with local late T-cell activation markers. *Lupus* 1992;1:111–117.
54. Zandman-Goddard G, Lorber M, Shoenfeld Y. Systemic lupus erythematosus and thymoma—a double-edged sword. *Int Arch Allergy Immunol* 1995;108:99–102.
55. Molina JF, Citera G, Rosler D, et al. Coexistence of human immunodeficiency virus infection and systemic lupus erythematosus. *J Rheumatol* 1995;22:347–350.
56. Byrd VM, Sergent JS. Suppression of systemic lupus erythematosus by the human immunodeficiency virus. *J Rheumatol* 1996;23:1295–1296.
57. Eisenberg RA, Winfield JB, Cohen PL. Subclass restriction of anti-Sm antibodies in MRL mice. *J Immunol* 1982;129:2146–2149.
58. Crow MK, DelGiudice-Asch G, Zehetbauer JB, et al. Autoantigen-specific T cell proliferation induced by the ribosomal P2 protein in patients with systemic lupus erythematosus. *J Clin Invest* 1994;94:345–352.
59. Okubo M, Yamamoto K, Kato T, et al. Detection and epitope analysis of autoantigen-reactive T cells to the U1-small nuclear ribonucleoprotein A protein in autoimmune disease patients. *J Immunol* 1993;151:1108–1115.
60. Hoffman RW, Takeda Y, Sharp GC, et al. Human T cell clones reactive against

U-small nuclear ribonucleoprotein autoantigens from connective tissue disease patients and healthy individuals. *J Immunol* 1993;151:6460–6469.

61. Desai-Mehta A, Mao C, Rajagopalan S, Robinson T, Datta SK. Structure and specificity of T cell receptors expressed by potentially pathogenic anti-DNA autoantibody-inducing T cells in human lupus. *J Clin Invest* 1995;95:531–541.

62. Wen L, Pao W, Fong FS, et al. Germinal center formation, immunoglobulin class swiching, and autoantibody production driven by "non-alpha/beta" T cells. *J Exp Med* 1996;183:2271–2282.

63. Fujitsu T, Sakuma S, Seki N, Senoh H, Mori J, Kikuchi H. Effect of auranofin on autoimmune disease in a mouse model. *Int J Immunopharmacol* 1986;8:897–910.

64. Hang L, Theofilopoulos AN, Balderas RS, Francis SJ, Dixon FJ. The effect of thymectomy on lupus-prone mice. *J Immunol* 1984;132:1809–1813.

65. Steinberg AD, Roths JB, Murphy ED, Steinberg RT, Raveche ES. Effects of thymectomy or androgen administration upon the autoimmune disease of MRL/Mp-*lpr/lpr* mice. *J Immunol* 1980;125:871–873.

66. Wofsy D, Ledbetter JA, Roubinian JR, Seaman WE, Talal N. Thymic influences on autoimmunity in MRL-*lpr* mice. *Scand J Immunol* 1982;16:51–58.

67. Rozzo SJ, Drake CG, Chiang B-L, Gershwin ME, Kotzin BL. Evidence for polyclonal T cell activation in murine models of systemic lupus erythematosus. *J Immunol* 1994;153:1340–1351.

68. Sobel ES, Cohen PL, Eisenberg RA. *Lpr* T cells are necessary for autoantibody production in *lpr* mice. *J Immunol* 1993;158:4160–4167.

69. Mounty JD, Zhou T, Johnson L. Production of transgenic mice and application to immunology and autoimmunity. *Am J Med Sci* 1990;300:322–329.

70. Peng SL, Fatenejad S, Craft J. Induction of nonpathologic, humoral autoimmunity in lupus-prone mice by a class II-restricted, transgenic alpha beta T cell. Separation of autoantigen-specific and -nonspecific help. *J Immunol* 1996;157:5225–5230.

71. Sobel ES, Kakkanaiah VN, Kakkanaiah M, Cheek RL, Cohen PL, Eisenberg RA. T-B collaboration for autoantibody production in *lpr* mice is cognate and MHC-restricted. *J Immunol* 1994;152:6011–6016.

72. Peng SL, Madaio MP, Hughes DPM, et al. Murine lupus in the absence of alpha-beta T cells. *J Immunol* 1996;156:4041–4049.

73. Bernard NF, Eisenberg RA, Cohen PL. Response of MRL/Mp +/+ mice to mouse Sm: non-H-2-linked genes determine T cell recognition. *J Immunol* 1985;134:1422–1425.

74. Bernard NF, Eisenberg RA, Cohen PL. H-2 linked If gene control of the T cell recognition of the Sm nuclear autoantigen and the aberrant response of autoimmune MRL/Mp-+/+ mice. *J Immunol* 1985;134:3812–3818.

75. Mohan C, Adams S, Stanik V, Datta SK. Nucleosome: a major immunogen for pathogenic autoantibody-inducing T cells of lupus. *J Exp Med* 1993;177:1367–1381.

76. Ebling FM, Tsao BP, Singh RR, Sercarz E, Hahn BH. A peptide derived from an autoantibody can stimulate T cells in the (NZB × NZW)F1 mouse model of systemic lupus erythematosus. *Arthritis Rheum* 1993;36:355–364.

77. Desai-Mehta A, Lu L, Ramsey-Goldman R, Datta SK. Hyperexpression of CD40 ligand by B and T cells in human lupus and its role in pathogenic autoantibody formation. *J Clin Invest* 1996;97:2063–2073.

78. Mohan C, Shi Y, Laman JD, Datta SK. The interaction between CD40 and its ligand gp39 in the development of murine lupus nephritis. *J Immunol* 1995;154:1470–1480.

79. Ma J, Xu J, Madaio MP, et al. Autoimmune *lpr/lpr* mice deficient in CD40 ligand: spontaneous Ig class switching with dichotomy of autoantibody responses. *J Immunol* 1996;157:417–426.

80. Dziarski R. Preferential induction of autoantibody secretion in polyclonal activation by peptidoglycan and lipopolysaccharide: II. In vivo studies. *J Immunol* 1982;128:1026–1030.

81. Fisher DE, Reeves WH, Conner GE, Blobel G, Kunkel HG. Pulse labeling of small nuclear ribonucleoproteins in vivo reveals distinct patterns of antigen recognition by human autoimmune antibodies. *Proc Natl Acad Sci USA* 1984;81:3185–3189.

82. Rokeach LA, Jannatipour M, Haseloy JA, Hoch SO. Mapping of the immunoreactive domains of a small nuclear ribonucleoprotein-associated Sm-D autoantigen. *Clin Immunol Immunopathol* 1992;65:315–324.

83. Reeves WH, Pierani A, Chou CH, et al. Analysis of the assembly, DNA binding, and antigenicity of the Ku autoantigen using recombinant vaccinia viruses. *Mol Biol Rep* 1991;15:115.

84. Rosario MO, Fox OF, Koren E, Harley JB. Anti-Ro (SS-A) antibodies from Ro (SS-A)-immunized mice. *Arthritis Rheum* 1988;31:227–237.

85. James JA, Gross T, Scofield RH, Harley JB. Immunoglobulin epitope spreading and autoimmune disease after peptide immunization: Sm B/B′-derived PPPGMRPP and PPPGIRGP induce spliceosome autoimmunity. *J Exp Med* 1995;181:453–461.

86. Lin RH, Mamula MJ, Hardin JA, Janeway CA. Induction of autoreactive B cells allows priming of autoreactive T cells. *J Exp Med* 1991;173:1433–1439.

87. Slobbe RL, Pruijn GJM, van Venrooij WJ. Ro (SS-A) and La (SS-B) ribonucleoprotein complexes: structure, function and antigenicity. *Ann Med Interne* 1991;142:592–600.

88. Reynolds P, Gordon TP, Purcell AW, Jackson DC, McCluskey J. Hierarchical self-tolerance to T cell determinants within the ubiquitous nuclear self-antigen La (SS-B) permits induction of systemic autoimmunity in normal mice. *J Exp Med* 1996;184:1857–1870.

89. Fuchs S, Mozes E, Stollar BD. The nature of murine immune response to nucleic acids. *J Immunol* 1975;114:1287–1291.

90. Cooke MS, Mistry N, Wood C, Herbert KE, Lunec J. Immunogenicity of DNA damaged by reactive oxygen species—implications for anti-DNA antibodies in lupus. *Free Radic Biol Med* 1997;22:151–159.

91. Krieg AM, Yi AK, Matson S, et al. CpG motifs in bacterial DNA trigger direct B-cell activation. *Nature* 1995;374:546–549.

92. Gilkeson GS, Ruiz P, Pippen AM, Alexander AL, Lefkowith JB, Pisetsky DS. Modulation of renal disease in autoimmune NZB/NZW mice by immunization with bacterial DNA. *J Exp Med* 1996;183:1389–1397.

93. Rumore PM, Steinman CR. Endogenous circulating DNA in systemic lupus erythematosus. Occurrence as multimeric complexes bound to histone. *J Clin Invest* 1990;86:69–74.

94. Li JZ, Steinman CR. Plasma DNA in systemic lupus erythematosus. Characterization of cloned base sequences. *Arthritis Rheum* 1989;32:726–733.

95. Casciola-Rosen L, Rosen A, Petri M, Schliessel M. Surface blebs on apoptotic cells are sites of enhanced procoagulant activity: implications for coagulation events and antigenic spread in systemic lupus erythematosus. *Proc Natl Acad Sci USA* 1996;93:1624–1629.

96. Rudensky AY, Preston-Hurlburt P, Hong SC, Barlow A, Janeway CA. Sequence analysis of peptides bound to MHC class II molecules. *Nature* 1991;353:622–627.

97. Nygard NR, Bono C, Brown LR, et al. Antibody recognition of an immunogenic influenza hemagglutinin-human leukocyte antigen class II complex. *J Exp Med* 1991;174:243–251.

98. Asherson GL. Antigen-specific T-helper and -suppressor factors in the control of the immune response. *Immunol Suppl* 1988;1:53–56.

99. Bonomo A, Kehn PJ, Shevach EM. Post-thymectomy autoimmunity: abnormal T-cell homeostasis. *Immunol Today* 1995;16:61–67.

100. Monier JC, Costa O, Souweine G, Rigal D. Lupus-like syndrome in some strains of nude mice. *Thymus* 1980;1:241–255.

101. Morse III HC, Steinberg AD, Schur PH, Reed ND. Spontaneous "autoimmune disease" in nude mice. *J Immunol* 1974;113:688–696.

102. Sy MS, Benacerraf B. Suppressor T cells, immunoglobulin and Igh restriction. *Immunol Rev* 1988;101:133–148.

103. Moller G. Do suppressor T cells exist? *Scand J Immunol* 1988;27:247–250.

104. Urdahl KB, Pardoll DM, Jenkins MK. Cyclosporine A inhibits positive selection and delays negative selection in alpha beta TCR transgenic mice. *J Immunol* 1994;152:2853–2859.

105. Alcocer-Varela J, Alarcon-Segovia D. Longitudinal study on the production of and cellular response to interleukin-2 in patients with systemic lupus erythematosus. *Rheumatol Int* 1995;15:57–63.

106. Spronk PE, ter Borg EJ, Huitema MG, Limburg PC, Kallenberg CG. Changes in levels of soluble T-cell activation markers, sIL-2R, sCD4 and sCD8, in relation to disease exacerbations in patients with systemic lupus erythematosus: a prospective study. *Ann Rheum Dis* 1994;53:235–239.

107. Hagiwara E, Gourley MF, Lee S, Klinman DM. Disease severity in patients with systemic lupus erythematosus correlates with an increased ratio of interleukin-10-interferon gamma-secreting cells in the peripheral blood. *Arthritis Rheum* 1996;39:379–385.

108. Erb KJ, Rueger B, von Brevern M, Ryffel B, Schimpl A, Rivett K. Constitutive expression of interleukin (IL)-4 in vivo causes autoimmune-type disorders in mice. *J Exp Med* 1997;185:329–339.

109. Rus V, Svetic A, Nguyen P, Gause WC, Via CS. Kinetics of Th1 and Th2 cytokine production during the early course of acute and chronic murine graft-versus-host disease. Regulatory role of donor CD8+ T cells. *J Immunol* 1995;155:2396–2406.

110. Handwerger BS, Rus V, da Silva L, Via CS. The role of cytokines in the immunopathogenesis of lupus. *Springer Semin Immunopathol* 1994;16:153–180.

111. Jacob CO, Fronek Z, Lewis GD, Koo M, Hansen JA. Heritable major histocompatibility complex class II-associated differences in production of tumor necrosis factor alpha: relevance to genetic predisposition to systemic lupus erythematosus. *Proc Natl Acad Sci USA* 1990;87:1233–1237.

112. Jacob CO, Hwang F. Definition of microsatellite size variants for TNFa and Hsp70 in autoimmune and nonautoimmune mouse strains. *Immunogenetics* 1995;36:182–188.

113. Emlen W, Niebur J, Kadera R. Accelerated in vitro apoptosis of lymphocytes form patients with systemic lupus erythematosus. *J Immunol* 1994;152:3685–3692.

114. Gatenby PA, Irvine M. The bcl-2 proto-oncogene is overexpressed in systemic lupus erythematosus. *J Autoimmun* 1994;7:623–631.

115. Aringer M, Wintersberger W, Steiner CW, et al. High levels of bcl-2 protein in circulating T lymphocytes, but not B lymphocytes, of patients with systemic lupus erythematosus. *Arthritis Rheum* 1994;37:1423–1430.

116. Amasaki Y, Kobayashi S, Takeda T, et al. Up-regulated expression of Fas antigen (CD95) by peripheral naive and memory T cell subsets in patients with systemic lupus erythematosus (SLE): a possible mechanism for lymphopenia. *Clin Exp Immunol* 1995;99:245–250.

117. Jiang Y, Moller G. In vitro effects of HgCl2 on murine lymphocytes. I. Selective activation of T cells expressing certain V beta TCR. *Int Immunol* 1996;8:1729–1736.

118. Wu J, Wilson J, He J, Xiang L, Schur PH, Mountz JD. Fas ligand mutation in a patient with systemic lupus erythematosus and lymphoproliferative disease. *J Clin Invest* 1996;98:1107–1113.

119. Fisher GH, Rosenberg FJ, Straus SE, et al. Dominant interfering Fas gene mutations impair apoptosis in a human autoimmune lymphoproliferative syndrome. *Cell* 1994;81:935–946.

120. Drappa J, Vaishnaw AK, Sullivan KE, Chu JL, Elkon KB. Fas gene mutations in the Canale-Smith syndrome, an inherited lymphoproliferative disorder associated with autoimmunity. *N Engl J Med* 1996;335:1643–1649.

121. Drappa J, Brot N, Elkon KB. The Fas protein is expressed at high levels on CD4-CD8- thymocytes and activated mature lymphocytes in normal mice but not in the lupus-prone strain, MRL *lpr/lpr. Proc Natl Acad Sci USA* 1993;90:10340–10344.

122. Singer GG, Abbas AK. The Fas antigen is involved in peripheral but not thymic deletion of T lymphocytes in T cell receptor transgenic mice. *Immunity* 1994;1:365–371.

123. Russell JH, Wang R. Autoimmune *gld* mutation uncouples suicide and cytokine/proliferation pathways in activated, mature T cells. *Eur J Immunol* 1993;23:2379–2382.

124. Perkins DL, Glaser RM, Mahon CA, Michaelson J, Marshak-Rothstein A. Evidence for an intrinsic B cell defect in *lpr/lpr* mice apparent in neonatal chimeras. *J Immunol* 1990;145:549–555.

125. Katagiri T, Azuma S, Toyoda Y, et al. Tetraparental mice reveal complex cellular interactions of the mutant, autoimmunity-inducing *lpr* gene. *J Immunol* 1992;148:430–438.

126. Reap EA, Leslie D, Abrahams M, Eisenberg RA, Cohen PL. Apoptosis abnormalities of splenic lymphocytes in autoimmune *lpr* and *gld* mice. *J Immunol* 1995;154:936–943.

127. Rubio CF, Kench J, Russell DM, Yawger R, Nemazee D. Analysis of central B cell tolerance in autoimmune-prone MRL/*lpr* mice bearing autoantibody transgenes. *J Immunol* 1996;157:65–71.

128. Casiano CA, Tan EM. Recent developments in the understandng of antinuclear autoantibodies. *Int Arch Allergy Immunol* 1996;111:308–313.

129. Yoshida S, Gershwin ME. Autoimmunity and selected environmental factors of disease. *Semin Arthritis Rheum* 1993;22:399–419.

130. Yung RL, Richardson BL. Drug-induced lupus. *Rheum Dis Clin North Am* 1994;20:61–86.

131. Blomgren SE, Condemi JJ, Vaughan JH. Procainamide-induced lupus erythematosus. *Am J Med* 1972;52:338–348.

132. Rubin RL, Nusinow SR, Johnson AD, Rubenson DS, Curd JG, Tan EM. Serologic changes during induction of lupus-like disease by procainamide. *Am J Med* 1986;80:999–1002.

133. Rubin RL, McNally EM, Nusinow SR, Robinson CA, Tan EM. IgG antibodies to the histone complex H2A-H2B characterize procainamide-induced lupus. *Clin Immunol Immunopathol* 1985;36:49–59.

134. Yung RL, Johnson KJ, Richardson BC. New concepts in the pathogenesis of drug-induced lupus. *Lab Invest* 1995;73:746–759.

135. Sutton RNP, Emond RT, Thomas DB, Doniach D. The occurrence of autoantibodies in infectious mononucleosis. *Clin Exp Immunol* 1974;17:427–436.

136. Whittingham S, McNeilage J, Mackay IR. Primary Sjogren's syndrome after infectious mononucleosis. *Ann Intern Med* 1985;102:490–493.

137. Maisch B. Autoreactive mechanisms in infective endocarditis. *Springer Semin Immunopathol* 1989;11:439–456.

138. Itescu S. Rheumatic aspects of acquired immunodeficiency syndrome. *Curr Opin Rheumatol* 1996;8:346–353.

139. Johnson HM, Torres BA, Soos JM. Superantigens: structure and relevance to human disease. *Proc Soc Exp Biol Med* 1996;212:99–109.

140. de Inocencio J, Hirsch R. The role of T cells in Kawasaki disease. *Crit Rev Immunol* 1995;15:349–357.

141. East J, Prosser PR, Holborow EJ, Jaquet H. Autoimmune reactions and virus-like articles in germ-free NZB mice. *Lancet* 1967;i:755–757.

142. Hultman P, Eneström S, Pollard KM, Tan EM. Anti-fibrillarin autoantibodies in mercury-treated mice. *Clin Exp Immunol* 1989;78:470–477.

143. Pelletier L, Pasquier R, Rossert J, Vial MC, Mandet C, Druet P. Autoreactive T cells in mercury-induced autoimmunity. *J Immunol* 1988;140:750–754.

144. Black C, Pereira S, McWhirter A, Welsh K, Laurent R. Genetic susceptibility to scleroderma-like syndrome in symptomatic and asymptomatic workers exposed to vinyl chloride. *J Rheumatol* 1986;13:1059–1062.

145. Yoshida SH, German JB, Fletcher MP, Gershwin ME. The toxic oil syndrome: a perspective on immunotoxicological mechanisms. *Regul Toxicol Pharmacol* 1994;19:60–79.

146. Kaufman LD. The eosinophilia-myalgia syndrome: current concepts and future directions. *Clin Exp Rheumatol* 1992;10:87–91.

147. Hochberg MC, Perlmutter DL, Medsger TA Jr, et al. Lack of association between augmentation mammoplasty and systemic sclerosis. *Arthritis Rheum* 1996;39:1125–1131.

148. Wong O. A critical assessment of the relationship between silicone breast implants and connective tissue diseases. *Regul Toxicol Pharmacol* 1996;23:74–85.

149. Leslie RD, Hawa M. Twin studies in auto-immune disease. *Acta Genet Med Gemellol* 1994;43:71–81.

150. Block SR, Winfield JB, Lockshin MD, D'Angelo WA, Christian CL. Studies of twins with systemic lupus erythematosus. A review of the literature and presentation of 12 additional sets. *Am J Med* 1975;59:533–552.

151. Vyse TJ, Kotzin BL. Genetic basis of systemic lupus erythematosus. *Curr Opin Immunol* 1996;8:843–851.

152. Drake CG, Rozzo SJ, Vyse TJ, Palmer E, Kotzin BL. Genetic contributions to lupus-like disease in (NZB×NZW) F1 mice. *Immunol Rev* 1995;144:51–74.

153. Tsao BP, Cantor TM, Kalunian KC, et al. Evidence for linkage of a candidate chromosome 1 region to human systemic lupus erythematosus. *J Clin Invest* 1997;99:725–731.

154. Salmon JE, Millard S, Schacter LA, et al. Fc gamma RIIA alleles are heritable risk factors for lupus nephritis in African Americans. *J Clin Invest* 1996;97:1348–1354.

155. Ruddy S. Rheumatic diseases and inherited complement deficiencies. *Bull Rheum Dis* 1996;45:6–8.

156. Hauptmann G, Tappeiner G, Schifferli JA. Inherited deficiency of the fourth component of human complement. *Immunodef Rev* 1988;1:3–22.

157. Arnett FC, Bias WB, Reveille JD. Genetic studies in Sjogren's syndrome and systemic lupus erythematosus. *J Autoimmun* 1989;2:403–413.

158. Reveille JD, Schrohenloher RE, Acton RT, Barger BO. DNA analysis of HLA-DR and DQ genes in American blacks with systemic lupus erythematosus. *Arthritis Rheum* 1989;32:1243–1251.

159. Fujisaku A, Frank MB, Neas B, Reichlin M, Harley JB. HLA-DQ gene complementation and other histocompatibility relationships in man with anti-Ro/SSA autoantibody response of systemic lupus erythematosus. *J Clin Invest* 1990;86:606–611.

160. Rothfield NF, Stollar BD. The relation of immunoglobulin class, pattern of antinuclear antibody, and complement-fixing antibodies to DNA in sera from patients with systemic lupus erythematosus. *J Clin Invest* 1967;46:1785–1794.

161. Radic MZ, Weigert M. Origins of anti-DNA antibodies and their implications for B-cell tolerance. *Ann NY Acad Sci* 1995;764:384–396.

162. Shlomchik MJ, Aucoin AH, Pisetsky DS, Weigert MG. Structure and function of anti-DNA autoantibodies derived from a single autoimmune mouse. *Proc Natl Acad Sci USA* 1987;84:9150–9154.

163. Shlomchik M, Mascelli M, Shan H, et al. Anti-DNA antibodies from autoimmune mice arise by clonal expansion and somatic mutation. *J Exp Med* 1990;171:265–292.

164. Bloom DD, Davignon J-L, Cohen PL, Eisenberg RA, Clarke SH. Overlap of the anti-Sm and anti-DNA responses of MRL/Mp-*lpr/lpr* mice. *J Immunol* 1993;150:1579–1590.

165. Ibrahim SM, Weigert M, Basu C, Erikson J, Radic MZ. Light chain contribution to specificity in anti-DNA antibodies. *J Immunol* 1995;155:3223–3233.

166. Diamond B, Scharff MD. Somatic mutation of the T15 heavy chain gives rise to antibody with autoantibody specificity. *Proc Natl Acad Sci USA* 1984;81:5841–5844.

167. Behar SM, Scharff MD. Somatic diversification of the S107 (T15) Vh11 germline gene that encodes the heavy-chain variable region of antibodies to double-stranded DNA in (NZB × NZW) F1 mice. *Proc Natl Acad Sci USA* 1988;85:3970–3974.

168. Bloom DD, Davignon J-L, Retter MW, et al. V region gene analysis of anti-Sm hybridomas from MRL/Mp-*lpr/lpr* mice. *J Immunol* 1993;150:1591–1610.

169. Miller FW, Twitty SA, Biswas T, Plotz PH. Origin and regulation of a disease-specific autoantibody response. Antigenic epitopes, spectrotype stability, and isotype restriction of anti-Jo-1 autoantibodies. *J Clin Invest* 1990;85:468–475.

170. Huff JP, Roos G, Peebles CL, Houghten R, Sullivan KF, Tan EM. Insights into native epitopes of proliferating cell nuclear antigen using recombinant DNA protein products. *J Exp Med* 1990;172:419–429.

171. Patton JR, Habets W, van Venrooij WJ, Pederson T. U1 small nuclear ribonucleoprotein particle-specific proteins interact with the first and second stem-loops of U1 RNA, with the A protein binding directly to the RNA independently of the 70K and Sm proteins. *Mol Cell Biol* 1989;9:3360–3368.

172. Papoian R, Pillarisetty R, Talal N. Immunological regulation of spontaneous antibodies to DNA and RNA. II. Sequential switch from IgM to IgG in NZB/NZW F1 mice. *Immunology* 1977;32:75–79.

173. Eisenberg RA, Craven SY, Cohen PL. Isotype progression and clonality of anti-Sm autoantibodies in MRL/Mp-*lpr/lpr* mice. *J Immunol* 1987;139:728–733.

174. Rubin RL, Tang FL, Chan EK, Pollard KM, Tsay G, Tan EM. IgG subclasses of autoantibodies in systemic lupus erythematosus, Sjogren's syndrome, and drug-induced autoimmunity. *J Immunol* 1986;137:2528–2534.

175. Eisenberg RA, Winfield JB, Cohen PL. Subclass restriction of anti-Sm antibodies in MRL mice. *J Immunol* 1982;129:2146–2149.

176. Nakamura RM, Tan EM. Autoantibodies to nonhistone nuclear antigens and their clinical significance. *Hum Pathol* 1983;14:392–400.

177. Habets WJ, Hoet MH, De Jong BA, Van der Kemp A, van Venrooij WJ. Mapping of B cell epitopes on small nuclear ribonucleoproteins that react with human autoantibodies as well as with experimentally-induced mouse monoclonal antibodies. *J Immunol* 1989;143:2560–2566.

178. Kozono Y, Kotzin BL, Holers VM. Resting B cells from New Zealand Black mice demonstrate a defect in apoptosis induction following surface IgM ligation. *J Immunol* 1996;156:4498–4503.

179. Maddison PJ, Reichlin M. Quantitation of precipitating antibodies to certain soluble nuclear antigens in SLE. *Arthritis Rheum* 1977;20:819–824.

180. Budman DR, Merchant EB, Steinberg AD, et al. Increased spontaneous activity of antibody-forming cells in the peripheral blood of patients with active SLE. *Arthritis Rheum* 1977;20:829–833.

181. Hollinger FB, Sharp JT, Lidsky MD, Rawls WE. Antibodies to viral antigens in systemic lupus erythematosus. *Arthritis Rheum* 1971;14:1–10.

182. Maul GG, French BT, van Venrooij WJ, Jiminez SA. Topoisomerase I identified by scleroderma 70 antisera: enrichment of topoisomerase I at the centromere in mouse mitotic cells before anaphase. *Proc Natl Acad Sci USA* 1986;83:5145–5149.

183. Mathews MB, Bernstein RM. Myositis autoantibody inhibits histidyl-tRNA synthetase: a model for autoimmunity. *Nature* 1983;304:177–179.
184. Mamula MJ, Fox OF, Yamagata H, Harley JB. The Ro/SSA autoantigen as an immunogen. Some anti-Ro/SSA antibody binds IgG. *J Exp Med* 1986;164:1889–1901.
185. Eisenberg RA, Craven SY, Warren RW, Cohen PL. Stochastic control of anti-Sm autoantibodies in MRL/Mp-*lpr/lpr* mice. *J Clin Invest* 1987;80:691–697.
186. Hochberg MC, Boyd RE, Ahearn JM, et al. Systemic lupus erythematosus: a review of clinico-laboratory features and immunogenetic markers in 150 patients with emphasis on demographic subsets. *Medicine* 1985;64:285–295.
187. Friou GJ. Setting the scene: a historical and personal view of immunologic diseases, autoimmunity, and ANA. *Clin Exp Rheumatol* 1994;12[Suppl 11]:S23–S25.
188. Friou GJ. Antinuclear antibodies: diagnostic significance and methods. *Arthritis Rheum* 1967;10:151–159.
189. Lefkowith JB, Gilkeson GS. Nephritogenic autoantibodies in lupus. *Arthritis Rheum* 1996;39:894–903.
190. Koffler D, Agnello V, Carr RI, Kunkel HG. Anti-DNA antibodies and the renal lesions of patients with systemic lupus erythematosus. *Transplant Proc* 1969;1:933–938.
191. Lee LA, Gaither KK, Coulter SN, Norris DA, Harley JB. Pattern of cutaneous immunoglobulin G deposition in subacute cutaneous lupus erythematosus is reproduced by infusing purified anti-Ro (SSA) autoantibodies into human skin-grafted mice. *J Clin Invest* 1989;83:1556–1562.
192. Buyon JP, Ben-Chetrit E, Karp S, et al. Acquired congenital heart block: pattern of maternal antibody response to biochemically defined antigens of the SSA/Ro-SSB/La system in neonatal lupus. *J Clin Invest* 1989;84:627–634.
193. Elkon K, Weissbach H, Brot N. Central nervous system function in systemic lupus erythematosus. *Neurochem Res* 1990;15:401–406.
194. Palmer DG. The anatomy of the rheumatoid lesion. *Br Med Bull* 1995;51:286–295.
195. Salmon M, Gaston JS. The role of T-lymphocytes in rheumatoid arthritis. *Br Med Bull* 1995;51:332–345.
196. DeKeyser F, Elewaut D, Vermeesch J, DeWever N, Cuvelier C, Veys EM. The role of T cells in rheumatoid arthritis. *Clin Rheumatol* 1995;14[Suppl 2]:5–9.
197. Winchester RJ, Gregersen PK. The molecular basis of susceptibility to rheumatoid arthritis: the conformational equivalence hypothesis. *Springer Semin Immunopathol* 1988;10:119–139.
198. Smiley JD, Hoffman WL, Moore SE, Paradies LH. The humoral immune response of the rheumatoid synovium. *Semin Arthritis Rheum* 1985;14:151–162.
199. Winchester RJ, Agnello V, Kunkel HG. Gamma globulin complexes in synovial fluids of patients with rheumatoid arthritis. Partial characterization and relationship to lowered complement levels. *Clin Exp Immunol* 1970;6:689–706.
200. Paliard X, West SG, Lafferty JA, et al. Evidence for the effects of a superantigen in rheumatoid arthritis. *Science* 1991;253:325–329.
201. Vaughan JH, Fox RI, Abresch RJ, Tsoukas CD, Curd JG, Carson DA. Thoracic duct drainage in rheumatoid arthritis. *Clin Exp Immunol* 1984;58:645–653.
202. Sany J. Immunological treatment of rheumatoid arthritis. *Clin Exp Rheumatol* 1990;8[Suppl 5]:81–88.
203. Feldmann M, Brennan FM, Maini RN. Role of cytokines in rheumatoid arthritis. *Annu Rev Immunol* 1996;14:397–440.
204. Fox DA. Biological therapies: a novel approach to the treatment of autoimmune disease. *Am J Med* 1995;99:82–88.
205. Elliott MJ, Maini RN, Feldmann M, et al. Randomised double-blind comparison of chimeric monoclonal antibody to tumour necrosis factor alpha (cA2) versus placebo in rheumatoid arthritis. *Lancet* 4997;344:1105–1110.
206. Nabozny GH, David CS. The immunogenetic basis of collagen induced arthritis in mice: an experimental model for the rational design of immunomodulatory treatments of rheumatoid arthritis. *Adv Exp Med Biol* 1994;347:55–63.
207. Ronnelid J, Klareskog L. Local versus sytemic immunoreactivity to collagen and the collagen-like region of C1q in rheumatoid arthritis and SLE. *Scand J Rheumatol* 1995;101[Suppl]:57–61.
208. Zvaifler NJ, Firestein GS. Pannus and pannocytes. Alternative models of joint destruction in rheumatoid arthritis. *Arthritis Rheum* 1994;37:783–789.
209. Hughes RA, Keat AC. Reiter's syndrome and reactive arthritis: a current view. *Semin Arthritis Rheum* 1994;24:190–210.
210. Lopez-Larrea C, Gonzalez-Roces S, Alvarez V. HLA-B27 structure, function, and disease association. *Curr Opin Rheumatol* 1996;8:296–308.
211. Careless DJ, Inman RD. Etiopathogenesis of reactive arthritis and ankylosing spondylitis. *Curr Opin Rheumatol* 1995;7:290–294.
212. Geczy AF, Sullivan JS. Possible role of HLA-B27 associated cytotoxic T lymphocyte activity in the pathogenesis of the seronegative arthropathies. *Ann Rheum Dis* 1995;54:329–330.
213. Kaye BR. Rheumatologic manifestations of infection with human immunodeficiency virus (HIV). *Ann Intern Med* 1989;111:158–167.
214. Taurog JD, Hammer RE. Experimental spondyloarthropathy in HLA-B27 transgenic rats. *Clin Rheumatol* 1996;15[Suppl 1]:22–27.
215. Khare SD, Luthra HS, David CS. Spontaneous inflammatory arthritis in HLA-B27 transgenic mice lacking beta 2-microglobulin: a model of human spondyloarthropathies. *J Exp Med* 1995;182:1153–1158.
216. Bacon PA. Systemic vasculitis syndromes. *Curr Opin Rheumatol* 1993;5:5–10.
217. Mader R, Keystone EC. Infections that cause vasculitis. *Curr Opin Rheumatol* 1992;4:35–38.
218. Sunday JS, Haynes BF. Pathogenic mechanisms of vessel damage in vasculitis syndromes. *Rheum Dis Clin North Am* 1995;21:861–881.
219. Invernizzi F, Pietrogrande M, Sagramoso B. Classification of the cryoglobulinemic syndrome. *Clin Exp Rheumatol* 1995;13[Suppl]13:S123–S128.
220. Hoffman GS, Kerr GS, Leavitt RY. Wegener's granulomatosis: an analysis of 158 patients. *Ann Intern Med* 1992;116:488–498.
221. Gross WL, Schmitt WH, Csernok E. ANCA and associated diseases: immunodiagnostic and pathogenetic aspects. *Clin Exp Immunol* 1993;91:1–12.
222. Price EJ, Venables PJ. The etiopathogenesis of Sjogren's syndrome. *Semin Arthritis Rheum* 1995;25:117–133.
223. Bruze M, Krook G, Ljunggren B. Fatal connective tissue disease with antinuclear antibodies following PUVA therapy. *Acta Derm Venereol* 1984;64:157–160.
224. Van Rappard-Van der Veen FM, Kiesel U, Poels L, et al. Further evidence against random polyclonal antibody formation in mice with lupus-like graft-vs-host disease. *J Immunol* 1984;132:1814–1820.
225. Morris SC, Cheek RL, Cohen PL, Eisenberg RA. Autoantibodies in chronic graft versus host result from cognate T-B interactions. *J Exp Med* 1990;171:503–517.
226. Stastny P, Stembridge VA, Ziff M. Homologous disease in the adult rat, a model for autoimmune disease. I. General features and cutaneous lesions. *J Exp Med* 1963;118:635–648.
227. Kennedy MJ, Hess AD. Autologous graft-versus-host disease. *Med Oncol* 1995;12:149–156.
228. Smiley JD. The many faces of scleroderma. *Am J Med Sci* 1992;304:319–333.
229. White B. Immunologic aspects of scleroderma. *Curr Opin Rheumatol* 1995;7:541–545.
230. Weiner ES, Earnshaw WC, Senecal J-L, Bordwell B, Johnson P, Rothfield NF. Clinical associations of anticentromere antibodies and antibodies to topoisomerase I: a study of 355 patients. *Arthritis Rheum* 1988;31:378–385.
231. Gershwin ME, Abplanalp H, Castles JJ, et al. Characterization of a spontaneous disease of white leghorn chickens resembling progressive systemic sclerosis. *J Exp Med* 1981;153:1640–1659.
232. Cohen PL, Eisenberg RA. *Lpr* and *gld*: single gene models of systemic autoimmunity and lymphoproliferative disease. *Annu Rev Immunol* 1991;9:243–269.
233. Izui S, Kelley VE, Masuda K, Yoshida H, Roths JB, Murphy ED. Induction of various autoantibodies by mutant gene *lpr* in several strains of mice. *J Immunol* 1984;133:227–233.
234. Perkins DL, Glaser RM, Mohan CA, Michaelson J, Marshak-Rothstein A. Evidence for an intrinsic B cell defect in *lpr/lpr* mice apparent in neonatal chimerias. *J Immunol* 1990;145:549–555.
235. Jevnikar AM, Grusby JJ, Glimcher LH. Prevention of nephritis in major histocompatibility complex class II-deficient MRL-*lpr* mice. *J Exp Med* 1994;179:1137–1143.
236. Koh D-R, Ho A, Rahemtulla A, Fung-Leung WP, Griesser H, Mak T-W. Murine lupus in MRL/*lpr* mice lacking CD4 or CD8 T cells. *Eur J Immunol* 1995;25:2558–2562.
237. Maldonado MA, Eisenberg RA, Roper E, Cohen PL, Kotzin BL. Greatly reduced lymphoproliferation in *lpr* mice lacking major histocompatibility complex class I. *J Exp Med* 1995;181:641–648.
238. Theofilopoulos AN, Dixon FJ. Murine models of systemic lupus erythematosus. *Adv Immunol* 1985;37:269–390.
239. Datta SK. A search for the underlying mechanisms of systemic autoimmune disease in the NZB × SWR model. *Clin Immunol Immunopathol* 1989;51:141–156.
240. Reininger L, Winkler TH, Kalbere CP, Jourdan M, Melchers F, Rolink AG. Intrinsic B cell defects in NZB and NZW mice contribute to systemic lupus erythematosis in (NZB × NZW) F1 mice. *J Exp Med* 1996;184:853–861.
241. Izui S, Iwamoto M, Fossati L, Merino R, Takahashi S, Ibnou-Zekri N. The Yaa gene model of systemic lupus erythematosus. *Immunol Rev* 1995;144:137–156.
242. Merino R, Fossati L, Lacour M, Lemoine R, Higaki M, Izui S. H-2-linked control of the Yaa gene-induced acceleration of lupus-like autoimmune disease in BXSB mice. *Eur J Immunol* 1992;22:295–299.
243. Satoh M, Kumar A, Kanwar YS, Reeves WH. Anti-nuclear antibody production and immune-complex glomerulonephritis in BALB/c mice treated with pristane. *Proc Natl Acad Sci USA* 1995;92:10934–10938.
244. Satoh M, Hamilton KJ, Ajmani AK, et al. Autoantibodies to ribosomal P antigens with immune complex glomerulonephritis in SJL mice treated with pristane. *J Immunol* 1996;157:3200–3206.
245. Shoenfeld Y, Mozes E. Pathogenic idiotypes of autoantibodies in autoimmunity: lessons from new experimental models of SLE. *FASEB J* 1990;4:2646–2651.
246. Fricke H, Mendlovic S, Blank M, Shoenfeld Y, Ben-Bassat M, Mozes E. Idiotype specific T-cell lines inducing experimental systemic lupus erythematosus in mice. *Immunology* 1991;73:421–427.
247. Kozlowski M, Mlinaric-Rascan I, Feng GS, Shen R, Pawson T, Siminovitch KA. Expression and catalytic activity of the tyrosine phosphatase PTP1C is severely impaired in motheaten and viable motheaten mice. *J Exp Med* 1993;178:2157–2163.
248. Letterio JJ, Geiser AG, Kulkarni AB, et al. Autoimmunity associated with TGF-beta1-deficiency in mice is dependent on MHC class II antigen expression. *J Clin Invest* 1996;98:2109–2119.
249. Marengere LE, Waterhouse P, Duncan GS, Mittrucker HW, Feng GS, Mak TW. Regulation of T cell receptor signaling by tyrosine phosphatase SYP association with CTLA-4. *Science* 1996;272:1170–1173.
250. Sadlack B, Merz H, Schorle H, Schimpl A, Feller AC, Horak I. Ulcerative colitis-like disease in mice with a disrupted interleukin-2 gene. *Cell* 1993;75:203–205.

251. Kuhn R, Lohler J, Rennick D, Rajewsky K, Muller W. Interleukin-10-deficient mice develop chronic enterocolitis. *Cell* 1993;75:263–274.

252. Mombaerts P, Mizoguchi E, Grusby MJ, Glimcher LH, Bhan AK, Tonegawa S. Spontaneous development of inflammatory bowel disease in T cell receptor mutants. *Cell* 1993;75:203–205.

253. Strasser A, Whittingham S, Vaux DL, et al. Enforced BCL2 expression in B-lymphoid cells prolongs antibody responses and elicits autoimmune disease. *Proc Natl Acad Sci USA* 1991;88:8661–8665.

254. Reap EA, Felix NJ, Wolthusen PA, Kotzin BL, Eisenberg RA. bcl-2 transgenic *lpr* mice show profound enhancement of lymphadenopathy. *J Immunol* 1995;155:5455–5462.

255. Green MD, Sweet HO, Bunker LE. Tight-skin, a new mutation of the mouse causing excessive growth of connective tissue and skeleton. *Am J Pathol* 1976;892:493–512.

256. Hatakeyama A, Kasturi KN, Wolf I, Phelps RG, Bona CA. Correlation between the concentration onf serum anti-topoisomerase I autoantibodies and histological and biochemical alterations in the skin of tight skin mice. *Cell Immunol* 1996;167:135–140.

257. Wallace VA, Kondo S, Kono T, et al. A role for CD4+ T cells in the pathogenesis of skin fibrosis in tight skin mice. *Eur J Immunol* 1994;24:1463–1466.

258. Houri JM, O'Sullivan FX. Animal models in rheumatoid arthritis. *Curr Opin Rheumatol* 1995;7:201–205.

259. Cromartie WJ, Craddock JG, Schwab JH, Anderle SK, Yang CH. Arthritis in rats after systemic injection of streptococcal cells or cell walls. *J Exp Med* 1977;146:1585–1602.

260. Stimpson SA, Esser RE, Carter PB, Sartor RB, Cromartie WJ, Schwab JH. Lipopolysaccharide induces recurrence of arthritis in rat joints previously injured by peptidoglycan-polysaccharide. *J Exp Med* 1987;165:1688–1702.

261. Castro JE, Listman JA, Jacobson BA, et al. Fas modulation of apoptosis during negative selection of thymocytes. *Immunity* 1996;5:617–627.

262. Naboczny GH, David CS. Collagen arthritis in T cell receptor congenic mice. A unique approach to study the role of T cell receptor genotypes in autoimmune arthritis. *Adv Exp Med Biol* 1995;383:99–104.

263. Iwakura Y, Tosu M, Yoshida E, et al. Induction of inflammatory arthropathy resembling rheumatoid arthritis in mice transgenic for HTLV-1. *Science* 1991;253:1026–1028.

264. Green JE, Hinrich SH, Vogel J, Jay G. Endocrinopathy resembling Sjogren's syndrome in HTLV-1 tax transgenic mice. *Nature* 1989;341:72–74.

265. Nishioka K, Maruyama I, Sato K, Kitajima I, Nakajima T, Osame M. Chronic inflammatory arthopathy associated with HTLV-1. *Lancet* 1989;i:441–441.

266. Brennan FM. Transgenic models for arthritis: useful clues to be gained? *Ann Med* 1996;28:271–274.

267. Wang Y, Hu Q, Madri JA, Rollins SA, Chodra A, Matis LA. Amelioration of lupus-like autoimmune disease in NZB/W F1 mice after treatment with a blocking monoclonal antibody specific for complement component C5. *Proc Natl Acad Sci USA* 1996;93:8563–8568.

268. Koffler D, Schur PH, Kunkel HG. Immunological studies concerning the nephritis of systemic lupus erythematosus. *J Exp Med* 1967;126:607–624.

269. Mukherjee R, Zhang Z, Zhong R, Yin Z-Q, Roopenian DC, Jevnikar AM. Lupus nephritis in the absence of renal major histocompatibility complex class I and class II molecules. *J Am Soc Nephrol* 1996;7:2445–2452.

270. Roubey RAS. Immunology of the antiphospholipid antibody syndrome. *Arthritis Rheum* 1996;39:1444–1454.

271. Kagnoff MF. Oral tolerance: mechanisms and possible role in inflammatory joint diseases. *Baillieres Clin Rheumatol* 1996;10:41–54.

Fundamental Immunology, Fourth Edition,
edited by William E. Paul
Published by Lippincott–Raven Publishers, Philadelphia 1999.

CHAPTER 34

Organ-specific Autoimmunity

Ethan M. Shevach

The Major Organ-specific Autoimmune Diseases of Humans and Experimental Animals
Insulin-dependent Diabetes Mellitus · Multiple Sclerosis and Experimental Allergic Encephalomyelitis · Autoimmunity Secondary to a Deficiency of Regulatory T Cells · Inflammatory Bowel Disease · Transgenic Models of Organ-specific Autoimmune Disease
The Etiology and Pathogenesis of Organ-specific Autoimmunity
Molecular Mimicry · Determinant Spreading · The T Helper 1–T Helper 2 Balance · The Cytokine Milieu · The Role of Costimulation in the Activation and Inactivation of Autoreactive T Cells
Immunotherapeutic Approaches to Organ-specific Autoimmunity
Antigen-specific Therapy · T-Cell Receptor–based Immunoregulation · Oral Tolerance
Concluding Remarks
References

Autoimmune diseases have traditionally been divided into organ-specific (pancreas, brain, thyroid, gastrointestinal tract) or non–organ-specific (systemic lupus erythematosus, rheumatoid arthritis), depending on whether autoimmune responses are directed to an antigen confined to a particular organ or to an antigen that is widely distributed in the body. The characteristic feature of organ-specific autoimmunity is the selective targeting of a single organ or individual cell type; gross abnormalities of the immune system are absent. It should be pointed out, however, that this division may be quite artificial, as it remains possible that systemic and organ-specific autoimmune diseases share a common mechanism(s). In fact, in both humans and animals, one organ-specific disease is frequently associated with another (e.g., diabetes, gastritis, and thyroiditis) which raises the possibility that common immunologic, genetic, or environmental factors may play critical roles in the induction of pathology of both types of autoimmunity.

Organ-specific autoimmune disease is often considered to result from a deficiency in tolerance induction mechanisms, resulting in their failure to eliminate or deactivate self antigen–reactive lymphocytes. The role of autoantigens in events responsible for the breakdown of self-tolerance is poorly defined in most models of spontaneous autoimmune disease. For example, is the presence of the target autoantigen required for initiation and maintenance of the pathogenic immune responses which occur during the development of autoimmune diseases? Do antigen presentation and the initial activation of autoreactive lymphocytes take place exclusively at the target organ site, or could they occur at sites distant from the target organ? This chapter is divided into three sections. The first

describes the clinical and pathologic features of the major organ-specific autoimmune diseases of humans and their pertinent animals models. The second section analyzes common immunologic features of these diseases that have relevance to both etiology and pathogenesis. The third section is devoted to issues related to the immunotherapy of organ-specific autoimmune diseases.

THE MAJOR ORGAN-SPECIFIC AUTOIMMUNE DISEASES OF HUMANS AND EXPERIMENTAL ANIMALS

Insulin-dependent Diabetes Mellitus

Insulin-dependent diabetes mellitus (IDDM) is an autoimmune disease in which self-reactive lymphocytes mediate the complete destruction of pancreatic β cells. IDDM is a multifactorial autoimmune disease for which susceptibility is determined by environmental and genetic factors. Inheritance is polygenic, with the genotype of the major histocompatibility complex (MHC) being the strongest genetic determinant. The concordance rate in monozygotic twins is only 50%, and 90% of patients with newly diagnosed IDDM do not have an affected first-degree relative, which suggests that environmental factors play an important role. Numerous (approximately 19) other genetic regions may also play important roles in determining susceptibility. Susceptibility or resistance to IDDM is associated with different HLA-DR and DQ genotypes. Although only 45% of whites in the United States have HLA-DR3 or DR4, 95% of patients with diabetes have at least one of these HLA-DR antigens. The strong association that exists between specific MHC class II alleles and disease susceptibility implies that the diabetogenic response is antigen-driven. Extensive sequencing of the MHC class II alleles in humans, and the major animal model for IDDM, the NOD mouse,

E. M. Shevach: Laboratory of Immunology, National Institute of Allergy and Infectious Diseases, National Institutes of Health, Bethesda, Maryland 20892.

has revealed a complex interplay between alleles of the two major isotypes of the MHC class II molecules DQ and DR in humans and I-A and I-E in the mouse (1). The NOD mouse expresses an unusual MHC class II, I-A^{g7}, I-A allele (the mouse homologue of HLA-DQ), which carries a histidine residue at position 56 and a small amino acid residue (serine) at position 57, while all other strains have proline and aspartic acid at these positions. Susceptibility to IDDM is most strongly determined by DQ^β- and I-A^β-chain alleles that encode serine, alanine, or valine at position 57, while aspartic acid at this position mediates resistance to IDDM. Expression of I-E (β-chain position 57 aspartic acid–positive) in the NOD mouse, and of DRB1 chains expressing aspartic acid position 57, also mediates varying degrees of resistance to type I IDDM. Although DQB1 0602 (an IDDM-resistant allele)–positive siblings of diabetics rarely develop diabetes, they can produce high titers of autoantibodies to several islet-cell antigens. This indicates that resistant alleles do not cause resistance by inducing more self-tolerance to islet-cell antigens than do susceptible DQB1 allelles.

IDDM results from a chronic autoimmune process that usually exists for years in a preclinical phase (2,3). The most striking histologic feature of the pancreas of a patient with long-standing IDDM is the near total lack of insulin-secreting β cells. Cells secreting glucagon, somatostatin, or pancreatic polypeptide are preserved. At the time of onset of IDDM or shortly thereafter, most islets are deficient in β cells, and the remaining islets are involved by insulitis consisting of a chronic inflammatory infiltrate that is composed mostly of CD8$^+$ T cells plus variable numbers of CD4$^+$ T cells, B-lymphocytes, macrophages, and natural killer (NK) cells. The expression of HLA class I on β cells is increased, whereas class II molecules may be overexpressed on macrophages and endothelium. ICAM-1 on the vascular endothelium of the islets is also increased. The distribution of islets with insulitis in the pancreas of patients with newly diagnosed IDDM can be strikingly uneven, as the most metabolically active β cells are preferentially destroyed. Histologic studies suggest that an 80% reduction in volume of β cells is required to induce symptomatic IDDM.

Islet-cell cytoplasmic autoantibodies (ICAs) react with antigens located in the cytoplasm of all endocrine cells of the pancreatic islets and are detected by indirect fluorescence microscopy. The target antigens include insulin, carboxypeptidase H, peripherin, sulfatides, ICA512, and ICA89 (4). ICA512/IA-2 is a member of a multigene family of protein tyrosine phosphatases and is expressed predominantly in neuroendocrine cells, particularly in secretory granules. Two other antigens detected with the sera of diabetic subjects include antigens of MW 37 kDa and 40 kDa. The 40-kDa antigen has now been shown to be a prominant proteolytic fragment of the ICA512/IA-2 gene product, and the 37-kDa antigen is a proteolytic fragment of the product of a related but distinct gene that encodes the Phogrin molecule. Antibodies to these antigens are present in 0.5% of normals, 3% to 4% of nondiabetic relatives of patients with IDDM, and 70% to 80% of patients with newly diagnosed IDDM. Increased risk of developing diabetes is associated with younger age and higher autoantibody titers. Autoantibodies to insulin are present in about half of patients with newly diagnosed IDDM before any insulin is administered. The presence of antiinsulin autoantibodies together with with islet-cell cytoplasmic antibodies in a single person confers a much greater risk of the development of IDDM than does the presence of either autoantibody alone (4). The presence of antiinsulin antibodies in younger subjects may reflect a faster rate of islet-cell destruction and more rapid progression to IDDM. Glutamic acid decarboxylase (GAD) is considered to be one of the critical β-

cell autoantigens. GAD is an enzyme with two isoforms, GAD 65 and GAD 67, which catalyze the biosynthesis of the neurotransmitter γ-aminobutyric acid. The two GADs, GAD65 and GAD67, differ in molecular size and amino acid sequence (approximately 30% divergence of sequence), as well as in their intracellular distributions and interactions with the GAD cofactor, pyridoxal phosphate. The presence of anti-GAD antibodies in the sera of prediabetic individuals has proven to be a reliable predictive marker for progression to overt diabetes. The levels of anti-GAD autoantibodies decrease within a few years after diagnosis, and after 6 years, are indistinguishable from controls (5). The loss of these autoantibodies may be secondary to the destruction of GAD-containing β cells and a suppression of the antigen-driven immune response. A majority of diabetic patients with neuropathy continue to show high levels of anti-GAD, and this may reflect continued stimulation of the immune system by GAD in the peripheral nervous system. Patients with newly diagnosed IDDM may have antibodies to BSA and a 17-amino acid BSA peptide termed *ABBOS*. It has been hypothesized that ingestion of cow's milk in early life can initiate β-cell destruction through molecular mimicry between the ABBOS sequence common to both bovine serum albumin and a 69-kDa β-cell antigen. However, this concept remains quite controversial.

There is no evidence that suggests that autoantibodies play a role in the pathogenesis of IDDM, while considerable evidence indicates that islet β-cell damage and destruction is mediated by islet-cell antigen-specific T helper 1 (Th1) cells. Eight to ten islet β cell–expressed proteins have been identified as potential targets of the autoimmune process, and their biochemical identity has been determined over the past 5 to 8 years. Little is really known about the contribution of each antigen to the disease process and whether each one is actually pathogenic. Half of new-onset IDDM patients have T cell–proliferative responses to GAD, and some progress has been made in defining potential epitopes of GAD, which are presented by DR4 (6). The responsiveness of lymphocytes to GAD may be a better predictor of the development of IDDM than high titers of autoantibodies to GAD, but at the present time, peripheral T-cell reactivity cannot be considered a reliable indicator of individuals at risk for IDDM. Lymphocytes from patients with IDDM also proliferate on exposure to islet cells, a 38-kDa islet-cell antigen, and insulin. T cell–mediated pancreatic islet destruction may occur secondary to cytokines produced by Th1 cells themselves or induced in other inflammatory cells within the inflamed islets; alternatively, these cytokines may stimulate the production of nitric oxide by β cells, which can be lethal to these cells. Overall, it is still unclear which antigens play a primary role in initiating the autoimmune process, and it is still not possible to distinguish primary autoantigens from those autoantigens that elicit an autoimmune response as a secondary event due to inflammation.

The study of IDDM had been greatly facilitated by the availability of good animal models. The Biobreeding (BB) rat (7) and the NOD mouse develop a form of IDDM that is quite similar to the human disease (8,9). The NOD mouse has a reproducibly high frequency of disease (80% to 90% of females and 50% to 60% of males). Genetic analysis had shown that NOD diabetes is a polygenic disease. As discussed above, of the genes involved in diabetes (Idd), the MHC plays a key role. The strong parallel structure between the two susceptibility alleles of MHC class II in mouse and human has further supported the importance and relevance of the NOD model to human disease. Other recessive loci that predispose to IDDM have been identified, including genes on mouse chromosomes 3, 7, 11, and 14, which appear to play a cumulative role in increasing the frequency of IDDM. Idd-3 and Idd-10 on chromosome 3 predispose to insulitis and diabetes, whereas Idd-5 seems to predispose predominantly to insulitis. Insulitis and diabetes are not 100% correlated, as some strains of NOD mice show insulitis but little diabetes. Insulitis may be necessary but not sufficient for the induction of diabetes. Surprisingly, germ-free NOD mice have the highest incidence (nearly 100%) that has been seen in any NOD colony.

Insulitis in the NOD mouse appears spontaneously around 3 to 4 weeks of age and is well established by 10 weeks of age. Progression to overt diabetes occurs in 80% of female mice between 10 and 30 weeks of age. The role of T-lymphocytes in the pathogenesis of disease in NOD mice is clear. Immunohistologic analyses have revealed that the majority of cells in the insulitic lesion are T cells. Disease does not appear in NOD mice that are congenitally athymic or that have been neonatally thymectomized and is ameliorated or prevented by treatment with a number of anti–T cell reagents. Diabetes can be prematurely induced in irradiated young or unmanipulated newborn NOD mice by the transfer of T cells from sick animals, including cloned lines of T cells. A temporal analysis of β-cell reactivity in NOD mice suggests that only a few autoantigens are targeted in the early stages. As intrainsulitis progresses, additional β-cell destruction occurs, apparently resulting in the sensitization and recruitment of other β cell–specific T cells. The presence of β cells is required to maintain diabetogenic T cells in a functional state, because spleen cells from 6-month-old NOD mice whose β cells had been destroyed by treatment with the toxic agent alloxan did not transfer diabetes, while sialitis (another disease manifestation in NOD mice) did develop in the recipients (10). Furthermore, spleen cells from diabetic mice parked in the β cell–deficient mice also had a reduced capacity to transfer diabetes (Table 1).

The defined progression of disease in the NOD strain was confirmed by study of a T-cell receptor (TCR) transgenic mouse generated from a T-cell clone that recognized an islet-cell antigen (11). The BDC 2.5 clone was CD4+, diabetogenic, and proliferated when challenged with islet cells from any mouse strain and antigen-presenting cells (APCs) from NOD mice. Cells expressing the transgenic TCR were positively selected in the thymus of the transgenic mouse, migrated to the periphery, and did not appear to be in abnormal activation state. Insulitis set in abruptly at 3 weeks and very quickly became massive, involving all of the islets; even in the presence of overwhelming insulitis, diabetes only appeared much later and onset was widely spread over 10 to 25 weeks. These results in the BDC 2.5 transgenic mouse have led to the hypothesis that there are two critical time points in the evolution of disease in both the TCR transgenic mouse and in the conventional NOD mouse (12). Before 3 weeks of age, there is no insulitis, although large numbers of autoreactive T cells (in the transgenic) are circulating through the immune system, and checkpoint 1 marks the onset of insulitis. However, in spite of extensive insultis, intact β cells persist for long periods and no diabetes occurs. Eventually, this balance is lost and the insulitis becomes terminally aggressive. Checkpoint 2 marks the switch from insulitis to overt diabetes. While the BDC 2.5 transgenic has a preformed repertoire, the 3-week period before checkpoint 1 is needed in the NOD mouse to recruit and activate self-reactive cells. Checkpoint 1 may be related to weaning and the immunologic changes that take place at that time, including shifts in food intake and in intestinal flora. The broad stimulation that takes place at the time of weaning may modify the homing potential of T cells and endow them with the ability to migrate into pancreatic connective spaces or lead to changes in the pancreatic blood vessel endothelium, which facilitate the onset of insulitis. Splenocytes from TCR transgenic or NOD mice that have insulitis, but not diabetes, do not transfer diabetes to neonatal recipients, while those from overtly diabetic mice do. A number of factors may be involved in the control of checkpoint 2, including the cytokine producing capacity of the infiltrating T cells (Th1/Th2), an uncoupling of the signaling pathways that mediate negative control through cell surface molecules such as CTLA-4, or the the loss of inactivation of regulatory cell populations that would control insulitis by nonspecific interactions, such as the secretion of inhibitory cytokines (see discussion of the role of costimulation in the activation and inactivation of autoreactive T cells). Elimination of T cells displaying nontransgene-encoded specificities by crossing the transgenic mice to TCR α chain–deficient mice failed to prevent diabetes and actually accelerated its onset, suggesting that other cells (e.g., CD8+) were not required to break through checkpoint 2.

NOD mice also exhibit antibody reactivity to GAD and insulin at an age when minimal histologic signs of islet inflammation are observed and reactivity to other β-cell antigens, such as heat-shock protein (HSP) 60, peripherin, and carboxypeptidase H could not be detected (13). Anti-GAD reactivity may modulate initial events associated with intrainsulitis. NOD mice remain protected from diabetes when treated with GAD either at an age preceding islet inflammation or when exhibiting extensive intrainsulitis (14). Protection may be mediated by the induction of GAD-specific regulatory T cells that secrete lymphokines that nonspecifically suppress the diabetogenic response (see discussion of Th1/Th2 balance). Insulin is another β-cell autoantigen that appears to have a critical role in the diabetogenic response. Insulin-specific CD4+ T-cell clones can accelerate disease in young NOD mice or transfer disease to NOD–severe combined immunodeficiency (SCID) mice (15). Oral treatment of young NOD mice with insulin also protected animals from diabetes (see discussion of oral tolerance within the section on immunotherapeutic approaches). In contrast to young NOD mice treated with GAD, insulin-treated NOD mice continued to exhibit intrainsulitis, suggesting that antiinsulin reactivity may be necessary for more distal events in disease progression. Autoantibodies and T-cell reactivity specific for HSP 60 have also been detected in NOD mice. It is far from clear whether HSP 60 functions as a target in human diabetes. Treatment of NOD mice with HSP 60 also has been reported to protect animals from disease.

TABLE 1. *Islet cells are required for the induction and continued maintenance of diabetogenic T cells*

Donor	Disease Incidence (%)
A. Nondiabetic	89
B. Alloxan-treated	0
C. Diabetic → male	60
D. Diabetic → male/alloxan-treated	0

Spleen cells from 6-month-old nondiabetic NOD females (A) or from age-matched females that had been treated with alloxan at 3 weeks of age (B) were transferred to 8-week-old irradiated NOD male recipients. The incidence of diabetes was determined 12 weeks after transfer. Spleen cells from diabetic female mice were transferred into irradiated male mice (C) or irradiated male mice treated with alloxan (D). After a 28-day "parking," the cells from these recipients were assayed for the capacity to induce diabetes in irradiated male mice.
Adapted from ref. 10.

The NOD mouse model of IDDM has been widely used to dissect the pathogenic processes involved in destruction of pancreatic β cells. Most importantly, both CD4+ and CD8+ T-lymphocytes were seen to infiltrate the pancreatic islets of NOD mice, and the destruction of β cells following adoptive transfer of cells from newly diabetic NOD mice required both CD4+ and CD8+ T cells. These results were initially interpreted as indicating that CD4+ cells initiated the attack on the islets and then recruited the CD8+ cells, which were the effectors responsible for the final destruction of the β cells. It now appears more likely that CD8+ T cells play the major role in disease initiation, as NOD mice bred to MHC class I–deficient, β2-microglobulin (β2m) gene knock-out mice developed neither insulitis nor diabetes (16). The role of autoantigen-specific CD8+ T cells would be to initiate β-cell damage. As pancreatic β cells do not express MHC class II molecules, CD4+ T cells would then recognize processed soluble antigens from β cells in the context of MHC class II (I-Ag7) on NOD APCs. These findings are also consistent with the observation that when 6- to 8-week-old donors were used, there was an absolute dependence on both CD4+ and CD8+ T cells for transfer of disease, but when spleen cells from overtly diabetic donors were depleted of CD8+ T cells, only a decreased incidence of diabetes and delayed time to onset were seen.

The pathogenic role of CD8+ T cells in the NOD mouse was further supported by the isolation of islet-reactive CD8+ cytotoxic T-lymphocytes (CTL) clones from 7-week-old NOD mice, a time point at which the animals have insulitis but would not become diabetic for several weeks (17). These cells have been shown to be capable of destroying pancreatic β cells in vitro and rapidly (within 5 days) causing diabetes in the irradiated NOD mouse without cotransferred CD4+ cells. In addition, the CD8+ clones could transfer diabetes to SCID mice matched only for MHC class I antigens. In contrast to these results, other studies have demonstrated that CD8+ clones only induced disease when transferred with CD4+ clones. Injection of anti-CD8 monoclonal antibody (mAb) into young NOD mice at any time between 2 and 5 weeks of age inhibited the development of insulitis (18). It is unclear how the the absence of CD8+ T cells during the early weeks of life led to inhibition of insulitis for the life of the animal. It remains possible that during the first 2 to 5 weeks of life a critical autoantigen is expressed that primes CD8+ cells to make an anti–islet-cell response, and the resulting inflammation then triggers priming of an anti-islet response by CD4+ cells, leading ultimately to insulitis. The expression of this purported autoantigen could be turned on by the physiologic changes that take place at the time of weaning. The requirement for CD8+ T cells for disease is not absolute, as studies using cloned T cells have demonstrated that some CD4+ T-cell clones alone can cause diabetes in irradiated recipients and can accelerate diabetes in young NOD mice that have endogenous CD8+ cells. CD4+ T cells from diabetic NOD donors can also transfer disease into NOD/SCID mice that lack endogenous CD4+, CD8+, and β cells. Taken together, these data suggest that CD8+ T-lymphocytes are important in the initiation of diabetes in the NOD mouse, but once a CD4+ T-cell response develops, CD8+ T cells are not absolutely necessary. Diabetic spleen cells can adoptively transfer disease into the NOD-β2m–deficient mouse, but disease onset is delayed, suggesting that CD8+ cells may also play a direct effector role in causing diabetes. Although much less is known about the effector T cells responsible for the initiation of human IDDM, both CD4+ and CD8+ cells are found in the postmortem pancreatic sections

of patients who have died at the onset of disease and in pancreatic biopsy specimens from newly diagnosed patients (4).

A large number of CD4+ T-cell lines and clones have been generated that react with islet-cell antigens, but relatively few of these lines have been characterized with respect to pathologic activity (19). One problem with the analysis of the pathogenic potential of T-cells clones is that there is a very narrow window in which disease can be transferred to unirradiated NOD mice; the highest efficiency of transfer is seen in 8- to 14-day-old recipients. There appears to be a developmental event in the NOD mouse after 3 weeks of age that confers resistance to T-cell transfer of disease. While adoptive transfer of splenocytes from diabetic NOD mice to NOD/SCID mice reproducibly resulted in full-blown diabetes within a 3- to 4-week period, not all CD4+ clones induced diabetes following transfer to NOD/SCID animals; in many cases, only insulitis and not overt diabetes was seen. Many of the pathogenic T-cell clones recognized an antigenic fraction isolated from the β-granule membrane. Because insulin comprises approximately 80% of the β-cell protein, its role as an autoantigen is of great interest. Insulin is also the major secretory product of the β cell that does not require cell death for release of large amounts of antigen. Insulin-specific clones have been isolated from the islets of NOD mice and appear to preferentially respond to a peptide encompassing residues 9–23 of the insulin B chain. When other strains of mice are immunized with insulin, they respond to the insulin A chain or to a combinatorial A chain–B chain determinant. T cells specific for insulin 9–23 are present within islet lesions when NOD mice are first tested at 4 weeks of age. They are pathogenic and rapidly lead to insulitis and diabetes when injected into young NOD mice. When the α and β chains of TCRs of B 9–23 reactive clones were sequenced, no TCR β-chain restriction was found; however, a majority of the clones used Vα 13 coupled with one of two homologous Jα segments (20). Although it has been suggested that GAD may be the primary antigen that initiates disease in the NOD mouse, GAD-reactive T cells cannot be isolated from islets.

Epidemiologic evidence in IDDM is consistent with the view that unknown environmental factors may play a role in either precipitating the disease or dominantly shaping its course. Autoimmunity to β cells could be initiated by an immune response against a viral protein that shares an amino acid sequence with a β-cell protein (see discussion of molecule mimicry within the section on etiology and pathogenesis of organ-specific autoimmunity), or bacterial and/or viral superantigens (SAGs) may lead to activation of peripheral autoreactive T cells. The function of SAGs is restricted by the presence of MHC class II on the surface of APCs and the expression of one or more defined Vβ TCR chains on T cells. In two patients who died with IDDM, a dominant expression of one Vβ family, Vβ7, was observed in the pancreas (21). When normal T cells were stimulated with surface membrane preparations derived from the pancreatic inflammatory lesions, but not with membranes from healthy control islets, a similar enhanced expression of Vβ7 was observed. This result raised the possibility of the presence of a surface membrane SAG. Indeed, a SAG was identified (22) in these two patients and was found to be encoded by a human endogenous retrovirus, IDDMK1,222, which is related to the murine retrovirus, MMTV. In contrast to MMTV, the IDDM-associated SAG is encoded within the retroviral env gene rather than with the 3' LTR. Retroviral RNA sequences were also detectable in the plasma of IDDM patients at disease onset, but not in the plasma of age-matched healthy controls. It is possible that this endogenous retroviral SAG expressed in APCs induces a systemic activation of the Vβ T-cell subset. Some of these activated Vβ7-expressing T cells would then migrate to the pancreas, and subsequent pancreatic β-cell destruction would be mediated by the islet cell–reactive T cells within the subset of Vβ7 SAG-activated T-lymphocytes. The expression of the SAG could be modulated by physiologic stimuli such as steroid hormones, infectious agents, or ubiquitous pathogens. Although the identification of an IDDM-associated SAG is an exciting finding, it still remains possible that the activation of SAG function in these patients is the result of rather than the cause of the inflammation. The retrovirus could be a second stimulus for precipitation of β-cell destruction by cells that had invaded the pancreas in response to other stimuli.

Multiple Sclerosis and Experimental Allergic Encephalomyelitis

Multiple sclerosis (MS) is a relapsing neurologic disorder that most commonly affects young adults. The evidence supporting an immune-mediated mechanism in MS is circumstantial (23–25). The striking appearance of inflammatory cells in the brain, spinal cord, and cerebrospinal fluid (CSF) in MS supports the view that an immune attack directed against some component of central nervous system (CNS) myelin is central to the pathogenesis of MS. Histopathologic similarities between postvaccinial encephalitis (PVE) and MS support the hypothesis that the latter is immune-mediated. PVE is characterized pathologically by perivascular inflammation and demyelination. An early sign of lesion development in MS is breakdown of the blood–brain barrier (BBB), which can be visualized by magnetic resonance imaging (MRI) as leakage of paramagnetic substances into the parenchyma. The characteristic lesion in MS is the plaque, which refers to the macroscopic appearance of a demyelinating lesion. Plaques are found throughout the the brain and spinal cord and are of different ages. The histologic appearance of the plaques is different in different stages of the disease. In active lesions, the BBB is damaged, permitting extravasation of serum proteins into the extracellular space. Inflammatory cells are seen in perivascular cuffs and throughout the white matter and activated monocytes–macrophages predominate. CD4$^+$ TCRαβ$^+$ T cells expressing activation markers accumulate around postcapillary venules at the edge of the plaque and also are scattered in the white matter. CD8$^+$ cells are more prominent in long-standing lesions.

The factors responsible for triggering the influx of activated T cells and monocytes into the CNS are still poorly characterized. Upregulation of adhesion molecules and MHC antigens, as well as T-cell activation antigens, is seen. Macrophages are primarily involved in the intial steps of myelin destruction. Demyelination is seen throughout the plaque, and thinly myelinated axons at the margins of the plaque represent attempts at remyelination. In early lesions, oligodendrocytes are not destroyed, but in the chronic phase of the disease, oligodendrocytes are lost. T cells expressing the γδ TCR are also found in MS lesions and may be involved in selective destruction of oligodendrocytes. The nature of early MS lesions indicates that demyelination occurs in the presence of an active immune response. In chronic plaques, inflammatory infiltrates are less pronounced and there is reactive gliosis and abortive attempts at remyelination. The role of antimyelin antibodies in the pathogenesis of MS lesions is not clear, although they may mediate demyelination in chronic MS; β cells and plasma cells are commonly found in chronic plaques.

Increased amounts of immunoglobulin in the CSF have been consistently demonstrated, and this finding is frequently used a diagnostic criterion. This elevation is due to increased synthesis of IgG and some IgM and IgA. Separation of immunoglobulin by electrophoresis or isoelectric focusing shows a limited number of distinct bands. These so-called oligoclonal bands are observed in more than 90% of patients. Oligoclonal immunoglobulins in the CSF of MS patients can be specific for several different viruses.

As the autoantigen-specific T cells responsible for MS have not been isolated, it is very difficult to ascertain the role of cytokines in the pathogenesis of MS. Indeed, the contribution of cytokines to the disease process has largely been inferred from the success and/or failure of various treatment modalities. For example, a therapeutic trial of interferon-γ (IFN-γ) in MS resulted in the development of exacerbations in seven of the 18 treated patients, and the study had to be terminated (25). Conversely, treatment of MS patients with a recombinant human IFN-β (IFN-β-1b), in which one of the cysteine residues at position 17 of the molecule had been substituted with serine, resulted in a one-third reduction of all attacks of MS and a reduction by one-half of the frequency of severe attacks. Clinical improvement was paralleled by changes in the MRI. A highly significant reduction in disease activity, as measured by numbers of active scans and appearance of new lesions, was noted; a clear-cut beneficial effect on disability status was not demonstrated. The mechanism of action of IFN-β in MS is not known, but it may be related to its antiproliferative effects on T cells or its ability to inhibit the effects of IFN-γ in upregulating adhesion molecule expression on endothelial cells, MHC class II molecule expression on monocytes and astrocytes, or tumor necrosis factor (TNF) production. IFN-β may also augment transforming growth factor-β (TGF-β) production by activated T cells. IFN-β has been shown to have some therapeutic efficacy in relapsing–remitting MS, but it has not yet been tested in chronic progressive MS.

Concordance of MS has been demonstrated in 26% of monozygotic and 2.3% of dizygotic twins, and some of the clinically normal monozygotic twins had MRI studies showing lesions consistent with MS. Thus, genetic factors play a clear role in the development of MS, although, as in IDDM, concordance is far from 100% in monozygotic twins. Different HLA-DR specificities are associated with MS in different ethnic groups; strong association of MS with MHC class II genes DR2 and DQ6 is seen in Northern Europeans. Studies of the TCR germline repertoire suggest that genes within the TCR α- and β-chain complex may confer risks that are independent of HLA genes.

The geographic distribution of MS is not uniform and the prevalance is higher in regions with cooler climates of both hemispheres. Furthermore, individuals that migrate before the age of 15 acquire the risk of getting MS that is found in the geographic region to which they migrate. Individuals that migrate after age 15 carry the risk of developing the disease that is seen in the geographic region of origin. Epidemics of MS have occurred. The most extensively studied is the occurrence of MS on the Faroe islands, where there were no cases of MS prior to 1940. Subsequent to the occupation of the islands by the British troops during World War II, the disease appeared. The epidemiologic data indicated that MS was related to an infectious agent encountered between ages 13 and 26 years. Twelve different viruses, ranging from paramyxo- to retroviruses, have been implicated in the etiology of MS, but no single agent related to the disease has been identified. The association of HTLV-I with a chronic, inflammatory, demyelinating disease led to extensive studies to identify an HTLV-I–like retrovirus in MS patients, but the presence of an HTLV-I–like agent has not been confirmed. The role of viruses in the pathogenesis of MS has focused on two viral families, the paramyxoviridae and the herpesviridae. The key observation is a frequently increased antibody titer to measles virus in MS patients in CSF directed to measles virus fusion protein. In the herpes virus family, Epstein-Barr virus (EBV), herpes simplex virus type I, and human herpes virus 6 have been proposed as candidates (26). A purported MS-associated retrovirus (MSRV) has been isolated repeatedly from leptomeningeal, choroid plexus, and EBV-immortalized B cells of MS patients (27).

T cells reactive with myelin basic protein (MBP) can be demonstrated in the peripheral blood, and MBP-specific T-cell lines can be generated from the PBL of MS patients and healthy individuals. The significance of this finding with regard to MBP as a target antigen in MS is far from clear. Although limiting-dilution studies have shown that the number of MBP-specific T cells in the blood and CSF of MS patients is higher than that of healthy individuals, it is very difficult to exclude the possibility that the higher numbers of MBP-specific T cells in MS patients result from a secondary expansion of preexisting MBP-specific T cells following myelin release during the disease. MBP-specific T cells can also be activated during the course of infections in the blood after postinfectious encephalomyelitis, postmeasles, and in the CSF during Lyme disease and rubella. The presence of MBP-specific T cells in the blood of healthy controls shows that cells specific to CNS autoantigens belong to the normal T-cell repertoire and that these cells may be expanded during the course of viral infection. Alternatively, self-reactive T cells could be activated by the recognition of epitopes shared by virus and autoantigen. Most MBP-specific T-cell lines were CD4$^+$ and secreted substantial amounts of IFN-γ and TNF-α. The sequence defined by amino acids 87–106 of MBP is recognized in the context of the four HLA molecules previously associated with MS in different ethnic groups. The minimal-sequence epitope is located between amino acids 89 and 99. There is little agreement among the studies of TCR usage by MBP-specific T cells derived from the blood of MS patients, and dominant TCR usage has not been established.

The major animal model for the study of MS is experimental allergic encephalomyelitis (EAE) (28,29). Paradoxically, this animal model of human disease was actually derived from the analysis of the pathogenesis of the neurologic sequelae that were seen shortly after the introduction of attenuated rabies vaccine by Pasteur in 1885. Although it was initially assumed that PVE was secondary to the live rabies virus itself, neurologic complications persisted even after the introduction of the killed virus vaccine in 1919. Recipients of the vaccine developed antibodies that reacted with brain extracts; the neurologic complications were therefore due to sensitization by nervous system antigens associated with the virus preparation. In 1935, Rivers established this point experimentally by giving repeated injections of CNS extracts to monkeys and reproducing PVE (30). The vaccine was prepared by growing the virus in rabbit spinal cord, and control animals that were immunized with normal spinal cord also developed PVE. Neuropathologic examination of affected animals showed extensive areas of myelin destruction associated with perivenular infiltration of lymphocytes and monocytes. It was later shown that EAE could be induced by a single injection of CNS extract in adjuvant. Chemical characterization of the encephalitogen showed that the antigen resided in myelin. Although MBP was the major component in the CNS extract that caused the disease, other components of myelin, such as proteolipid protein (PLP) were later shown to be capable of inducing EAE. PLP is highly hydrophobic and difficult to work with, but some of the technical difficulties have been overcome by using synthetic peptides. There are many other proteins in the oligodendrocyte–myelin membrane that could function as target antigens in EAE. These include myelin-associated glycoprotein (MAG) and myelin oligodendrocyte glycoprotein (MOG). EAE can be monophasic, but relapsing–remitting models have also been developed. Pathologically, EAE consists of perivascular inflammatory cells, but the cellular composition and extent of demyelination vary in the different models. In the Lewis rat, in which immunization with MBP leads to monophasic disease, the major pathologic feature is perivascular inflammation with minimal demyelination, while in guinea pigs, there is much more demyelination.

EAE is mediated by antigen-specific CD4$^+$ T cells, and T-cell lines and clones that adoptively transfer the disease in SJL and PL/J mice have been described (31). Host factors, particularly the animal species chosen for study, are critically important. Although EAE has been induced in outbred rabbits, guinea pigs, rats, and primates, certain inbred strains of rats, guinea pigs, and mice are susceptible, while others are relatively resistant (32). Inbred Lewis rats are uniformly susceptible, while Brown Norway rats are relatively resistant and do not develop disease when immunized under the same conditions. Similarly, inbred strain 13 guinea pigs are relatively susceptible, while strain 2 animals are relatively resistant. The term *relatively resistant* is used because EAE may be induced in resistant strains by modification of the immunization procedure. Most inbred MHC congenic and mutant strains of mice that have been tested for susceptibility to MBP-induced EAE are resistant or weakly susceptible. The expression and intensity of disease can be related to the composition of the encephalitogenic inoculum. For example, certain strains of mice are resistant to MBP-induced EAE, but not to spinal cord homogenate-induced EAE. The source of the CNS tissue or MBP preparation is also important in some species. Guinea pig MBP is much more encephalitogenic in Lewis rats than is rat MBP. The composition and preparation of the emulsion, the site of injection, and the number of injections can influence the production of EAE. *Bordetella pertussis* is widely administered as a cofactor for the production of EAE in mice. It is believed that its mode of action is mediated by increasing vascular permeability.

MBP exists in several isoforms that vary in number and structure in different animal species. Five isoforms have been identified in the mouse. The isoforms vary in molecular weight from 14.0 to 21.5 kDa and are generated by alternative mRNA splicing mechanisms. The biologic function of each of the isoforms has not been elucidated. MBP is highly conserved among species. There is no single region of the molecule that serves as a general encephalitogen for all species. Different sequences are encephalitogenic for different species. For example, the sequence 70–90 of guinea pig MBP is highly encephalitogenic in Lewis rats but is not encephalitogenic in the mouse. In mice, different regions of the molecule are encephalitogenic for different inbred strains. Residues 1–9 are encephalitogenic for H-2^u mice, while at least two epitopes (91–102 and 95–108) are encephalitogenic for SJL (H-2^s) mice. It is likely that the finding of unique encephalitogenic determinants in each species or strain is secondary to differences in T-cell repertoires, antigen processing, exposure of epitopes in the CNS, or differences in binding of peptides to MHC class II molecules. I-A^s interacts with peptide 91–103 in SJL mice to form the dominant epitope, and the T-cell response would be predominantly against this region of the molecule, while peptide 1–9 would interact with I-A^u. This would not preclude other MBP peptides from interaction with I-A^s or I-A^u to form subdominant or suppressor epitopes. T cells taken from MBP or peptide-immune SJL mice proliferated vigorously when cultured with MBP or peptide 91–102 and can transfer disease adoptively to naive recipients. The same lymph node cells proliferated well to peptide 1–39, but did not transfer disease adoptively. Encephalitogenic and nonencephalitogenic T-cell clones may recognize the same peptide epitopes, and the factors that render an MBP-specific T-cell encephalitogenic have not fully been determined (33). Properties intrinsic to the T cell, in addition to specific reactivity with an encephalitogenic epitope, may play critical roles. Other biologic and biochemical properties of EAE effector cells may be important in the pathogenesis of EAE, including their ability to produce a particular set of lymphokines, to home to a particular region, or to interact with the target peptide antigen presented by specialized APCs (astrocytes, endothelial cells, microglia). Lymphoid cell infiltration in CNS in EAE is thought to depend on the adherence of peripheral blood cells to brain capillary endothelia, with resulting damage to endothelial cells and migration of lymphoid cells into perivascular space. The adhesion proteins implicated in these lymphocyte–endothelial cell interactions are VLA-4 (integrin $\alpha 4\beta 1$) and VCAM-1, and the encephalitogenicity of the T-cell clones correlated with their ability to express VLA-4. Furthermore, anti-VLA-4 prevented transfer of EAE by T-cell clones in rats and mice (34).

EAE is considered to be the prototypic Th1-mediated organ-specific autoimmune disease. The CD4$^+$ T-cell lines and clones that transfer EAE invariably produce IFN-γ and/or TNF-α/LTα on antigenic challenge in vitro (31). Interventions to block the activity of the Th1 cytokine, TNF-α, by the use of neutralizing antibodies, soluble TNF I receptors, or type I phosphodiesterase inhibitors led to reversal of EAE, while injection of TNF-α triggered relapses (35,36). Interleukin-12 (IL-12) plays a critical role in the development of EAE effector T cells (37). The adoptive transfer of T cells cultured in vitro with PLP and IL-12 resulted in a more prolonged and progessive disease than that induced when T cells were cultured with antigen alone. Similarly, mice treated with IL-12 after transfer of antigen-stimulated lymph node cells developed a more severe and prolonged course of the disease. Treatment of mice with an antibody to IL-12 after cell transfer completely prevented paralysis, with only 40% of the mice developing mild disease. No data are available on the use of anti–IL-12 therapeutically beginning after the onset of disease. IL-12 has been shown to be critical for the induction of EAE effectors in both wild-type and IFN-γ–deficient (-/-) mice (38).

Immunization with MBP in incomplete adjuvant leads to suppression of clinical EAE upon subsequent challenge with MBP in complete adjuvant (39). When synthetic peptides were tested in this model, the protective effect exactly paralleled their encephalitogenic activity when administered in complete adjuvant. Thus, only encephalitogenic peptides were effective for protection. The suppression seen when mice are preimmunized with MBP in incomplete adjuvant could be transferred with spleen cells. In rats, EAE is monophasic, and, following recovery from the acute episode, additional immunizations do not lead to disease (40). This resistance may be due to the induction of regulatory T cells (see discussion of Th1/Th2 balance within the section on etiology and pathogenesis). Treatment with antibody to MHC class II antigens

prevented EAE, presumably by altering presentation of encephalitogenic epitopes to CD4$^+$ T cells. Similarly, antibodies against CD4$^+$ T cells reversed EAE in rats and mice. In some susceptible strains, such as the B10.PL and PL, the T-cell population responding to MBP peptides exhibits a restricted repertoire. TCR Vβ8 is expressed on 16% to 25% of peripheral T cells from unimmunized PL mice. When LN cells from PL mice immunized with MBP 1 to 11 were sorted into Vβ8$^+$ and Vβ8$^-$ subsets and assessed for their capacity to proliferate in response to the MBP 1–11 peptide, the responding cells were found in the Vβ8$^+$ pool (41). Furthermore, administration of anti-Vβ8 mAb prevented the induction of EAE after immunization with MBP 1–11 in CFA. It is unlikely that such a TCR-targeted approach would be useful in other strains, where the T-cell repertoire of the anti-MBP responder population is much more heterogeneous.

The relatively homogeneous T-cell repertoire of the anti-MBP response of certain strains of mice has also facilitated the analysis of environmental factors that may play a role in susceptiblity to autoimmune disease. Infection has been proposed as a major inciting factor in the pathogenesis of clinical relapses that occur in most autoimmune diseases, including MS (42). The bacterial SAG staphylococcal entertotoxin B (SEB) activates Vβ8-expressing T cells. In those strains of mice whose T-lymphocytes use the Vβ8 TCR to recognize MBP, injection of SEB (Table 2) induced exacerbation or relapses of paralytic disease in mice that were in clinical remission following an initial episode of paralysis and triggered paralysis in mice with subclinical disease (43). Thus, the microbial SAG can influence the course of autoimmune disease through a direct action on pathogenic T cells once autoreactivity has been initiatied.

A second approach that has proven useful for exploring the role of environmental influences on autoimmune disease induction has been the construction of trangenic mice expressing genes encoding a rearranged T-cell receptor specific for MBP. MBP-specific T cells from such a transgenic animal were not clonally deleted, did not become anergic, proliferated in response to MBP, and secreted cytokines (44). TCR transgenic mice were also highly susceptible to induction of EAE following injection of antigen in adjuvant and pertussis toxin. Some transgenic animals developed disease following injection of pertussis toxin alone. MBP-specific autoantibodies were detected following injection of pertussis toxin alone, suggesting that endogenous MBP can be presented in a form that is recognized by the transgenic T cells. Relapsing disease did not occur after disease induction, which suggested that the induction of chronic relapsing EAE depended on other factors. When mice were maintained in a conventional facility or in a specific pathogen-free

TABLE 2. *Bacterial superantigens induce relapses of EAE*

Treatment	Increase in disease incidence (%)
PBS	14–20
SEB	67–86

EAE was induced by immunization with MBP Ac1-11 and pertussis toxin. Three to 4 weeks later, when the mice had recovered from the acute disease, they were challenged with PBS or SEB. Disease scores were measured over the next 2 weeks.
Adapted from ref. 43.

facility, marked differences in disease susceptibility were noted. Under clean conditions, spontaneous disease was not seen, and disease could not be induced with adjuvant alone, but required coadministration of pertussis toxin; in contrast, in the dirty facility, some mice developed EAE spontaneously, and some mice that received MBP in adjuvant alone developed disease.

Although these results strongly suggest that infection-related cofactors are required in addition to specific autoantigen to precipitate disease, very different results were obtained (45) with another anti-MBP TCR transgenic line. In these studies, the MBP TCR transgenic mice were crossed to RAG-1$^{-/-}$ mice to obtain transgenic mice that only have T cells that express the transgenic TCR. In Rag-1$^{-/-}$ mice, lymphocytes can mature only if they express rearranged antigen receptor transgenes. Only approximately 14% of the conventional TCR transgenic mice developed spontaneous EAE, while 100% of the TCR transgenic RAG-1$^{-/-}$ mice developed spontaneous EAE within 12 months. These results conclusively demonstrate that no other cell populations, including CD4$^+$ T cells, CD8$^+$ T cells, γδ T cells, or B cells, were required for the generation of EAE lesions and clinical symptoms. The data indicate that EAE can be mediated by a single population of lymphocytes that express a single TCR and that responses to other peptides derived from the same autoantigen or other antigens in the same tissues are not required for full-blown disease to be seen (see discussion of determinant spreading within the section on etiology and pathogenesis). On the other hand, these studies also indicate that complex interactions occur between disease-inducing and -protective cells. The mechanisms responsible for the protection afforded by the nontransgenic lymphocytes or by lymphocytes that express two TCRs (one for self antigen and one for foreign antigen) in the conventional TCR transgenics remain to be elucidated. It is possible that TCR specific for foreign peptides interfered with the inflammatory responses of the disease-initiating cells by secreting antiinflammatory cytokines, or that MBP peptide presentation by B cells induced the production of protective T cells. Collectively, these studies on anti-MBP TCR transgenics, which in some respect have reached opposing conclusions, reflect the subtle role environmental factors can play in the initiation and progression of autoimmune disease.

Autoimmunity Secondary to a Deficiency of Regulatory T Cells

The mechanisms that mediate self–nonself discrimination among T cells may be classified into two broad types (46). The first group of mechanisms are passive or recessive, because they depend on a functional absence of autoreactive cells or the presentation of self antigens in a nonimmunogenic form. The mechanisms of passive tolerance include clonal deletion for those self antigens expressed intrathymically, T-cell anergy, or T-cell indifference for those exclusively expressed extrathymically. These mechanisms are passive in the sense that they all depend either on the intrathymic death of autoreactive T cells or on processes that extrathymically induce intrinsic nonresponsiveness of cells that are not deleted. The second group of mechanisms are active, or dominant, because they prevent the activation of other T cells that have the potential to cause autoimmunity. The mechanisms of active tolerance involve the active control of autoreactive T cells by other regulatory T cells. A number of organ-specifc autoimmune diseases can be induced in rodent strains that do not normally develop autoimmunity, by procedures that interfere with normal T-cell maturation or by rendering the animals partially T cell–deficient. The ability of a defined subset of T cells from syngeneic healthy donors to prevent the development of autoimmunity on transfer to these lymphopenic animals indicates that an intact immune system contains T cells with the capacity to prevent the activation of autoreactive T cells.

The earliest experiments on the role of regulatory T cells in the prevention of organ-specific autoimmunity were derived from functional studies of rat CD4$^+$ T cells that could be divided into two subsets based on their differential expression of the CD45RC isoform of the leukocyte common antigen (47). In normal adult rats, one-third of the CD4$^+$ population are CD45RC^{low} cells and two-thirds are CD45RC^{high} cells. CD45RC^{low} cells secrete Th2-like cytokines and are functional in providing help for B cells in secondary antibody responses, while CD45RC^{high} T cells secrete Th1-like cytokines and mediate alloreactvity in graft-versus-host disease (GVHD). Surprisingly, athymic rats injected with the CD45RC^{high} subset developed a fatal systemic wasting disease with a mononuclear cell infiltrate in different organs, such as liver, stomach, pancreas, and thyroid. Rats injected with the CD45RC^{low} subset remained healthy and were more resistant to infection than were noninjected *nu/nu* rats. The coinjection of the RC^{low} subset with the RC^{high} subset prevented the wasting disease and the multiorgan mononuclear cell infiltration. Thus, regulatory T cells in the normal repertoire dominated over the pathogenic T cells.

Typical organ-specific autoimmunity has developed following the use of other approaches for the elimination of regulatory T-cell subsets (48). The PVG.RT1^u strain of rats does not spontaneously develop autoimmune disease, but when these rats were thymectomized (Tx) at 6 weeks of age and sublethally irradiated with 4 doses of 250 rads at 2-week intervals, IDDM developed. Eight to 10 weeks after the final dose of irradiation, all of the males and 70% of the females developed autoimmune diabetes with selective destruction of the β cells of the pancreas. The disease could be completely prevented by the intravenous injection of CD45RC^{low} T cells from syngeneic normal donors. The injection of a neutralizing antibody to IL-4 did not abrogate the protection mediated by the CD45RC^{low} cells. Penhale and coworkers originally demonstrated that thyroiditis developed in PVG.RT1^c rats treated by an identical regimen (49). Some of these animals also became diabetic, and the disease was transferable. In addition to these studies, which involve manipulation of T-cell subsets in normal animals, it should be emphasized that the BB strain of rats, which develops spontaneous IDDM, is genetically lymphopenic and lacks a subset of rat T cell that express the RT6 antigen; the spontaneous diabetes that develops in this rat strain can be prevented by transfer of RT6$^+$ T cells from a nondiabetic congenic line (50).

Although the mechanism by which the CD45RC^{low} T cells prevent disease is not known, some of the properties of this unique subpopulation have been characterized. CD45RC^{low} T cells from long-term Tx donors were at least as potent in preventing diabetes as similar cells from normal donors. Thus, the protective CD4$^+$ subset was long-lived in the periphery and its regulatory effect was not dependent on continued replenishment from the thymus. A striking feature of the prevention of diabetes by the injection of CD45RC^{low} CD4$^+$ T cells was the change in surface phenotype of T cells recovered from the thoracic duct lymph of Tx-irradiated rats. The percentage of CD4$^+$ T cells that expressed activation markers was reduced to about half of that found in prediabetic animals, and there was a marked increase in CD45RC^{high} cells. It appeared that injection of the CD45RC^{low} subset resulted in the development of a CD4$^+$ T-cell subset distribution that more closely approximates that of a normal rat. CD4$^+$8$^-$ thymocytes were actually more effective at preventing disease in this model than were RC^{low} peripheral T cells. This suggests that the protective effect mediated by the regulatory T cells in the periphery is unlikely to be secondary to their priming to environmental antigens in the periphery (51).

Autoimmunity induced by neonatal Tx exemplifies another experimental system, in which attenuation of the T-cell pool leads to autoimmune disease. Tx on day 3 of life of selected strains of mice resulted in the development of several organ-specific autoimmune diseases, such as thyroiditis, gastritis, oophoritis, or orchitis (52,53). Autoimmune disease in these models could be prevented by reconstituting the Tx animals with adult CD4$^+$ T cells from syngeneic normal animals within the first 14 days of life. These studies suggest that normal thymus begins to produce pathogenic self-reactive T cells shortly after birth; Tx on day 3 abrogates the peripheralization of mature T cells with autoimmune preventive activity, thereby producing a relative dominance of the self-reactive T cells that have peripheralized before the Tx. A similar spectrum of autoimmune disease could be produced by the CD4$^+$CD5^{low} subset of normal T cells following transfer to syngeneic nu/nu recipients. Disease could be prevented by coinjection of the CD4$^+$CD5^{high} subset of normal cells. Although the regulatory T cells in this model were originally shown to express high levels of the CD5 antigen, this marker is difficult to use, as all mouse CD4$^+$ cells are also CD5$^+$. CD25 expression has been shown to be more specific for CD4$^+$ cells with autoimmune preventive activity than CD5^{high} or CD45RB/RC^{low} expression, because depletion of CD25$^+$ cells eliminated only a fraction of CD4$^+$CD5^{high} or RB^{low} cells; autoimmune disease was elicited at an even higher incidence and in a wider spectrum of organs than depletion of CD5^{high} or CD45RB^{low} populations (54). Induction of autoimmunity could be prevented by cotransfer of the CD4$^+$CD25$^+$ population. CD25$^+$ T cells constitute approximately 10% of peripheral CD4$^+$ cells and less than 1% of CD8$^+$ cells in normal unimmunized mice. The majority of them do not express the IL-2R β chain (CD122). In addition to organ-specific autoimmune disease, transfer of CD25$^-$ cells to nu/nu recipients led to immune-complex glomerulonephritis, arthritis, and a GVHD-like wasting disease. In addition to antibodies directed to the involved organs, IgG isotype anti-dsDNA autoantibodies were also seen, as well as hypergammaglobulinemia and spontaneous antihapten antibodies. Disease could be transferred from the nu/nu recipients with cells that were CD25$^+$ and had differentiated from the transferred CD25$^-$ cells.

These experiments demonstrate that removal of a particular T-cell subpopulation suffices to activate self-reactive T cells and elicit autoimmune disease under conditions in which the self antigens are normally expressed in physiologic concentrations. Although it has been proposed (55) that any CD4$^+$ T cell that has become activated to express CD25 may be capable of suppressing autoreactive T cells, other data suggest that a distinct population of CD4$^+$CD25$^+$ that is specialized for autoimmune suppressive function is responsible for this activity (56). First, CD4$^+$CD25$^+$ cells are the only population capable of preventing the development of autoimmunity post d3Tx, as reconstitution of d3Tx animals with spleen-cell populations depleted of CD25$^+$ cells failed to prevent disease (Table 3). It thus appears that the regulatory cell population that prevents the normal CD4$^+$CD25$^-$ T cells from inducing autoimmunity upon transfer to nu/nu mice is identical to the one that controls the development of autoimmunity post-d3Tx. Second, when d3Tx animals were reconstituted with a homogeneous popu-

TABLE 3. *Inhibition of gastritis post-d3 Tx by CD25$^+$ T cells*

Reconstitution	Disease incidence (%)
No cells	59
Normal spleen	0
CD25-depleted spleen	59
TCR transgenic SCID	60
TCR transgenic SCID/immunization	55

BALB/c mice were thymectomized on day 3 of life. On day 10, they were reconstituted with the indicated cell populations. Some of the animals reconstituted with TCR transgenic SCID T cells were immediately immunized with the antigen recognized by the transgenic TCR to induce CD25 expression. Gastritis was assayed after 6 weeks.

Adapted from ref. 56.

lation of CD4$^+$ T cells from a TCR transgenic mouse on a SCID background, suppression of disease was not seen. Most importantly, even after activation of the transgenic T cells with antigen, which induced expression of CD25 on greater than 50% of the CD4$^+$ cells in the animal, prevention of disease was not observed. These results are most consistent with the concept that the active immunoregulatory population contained within the CD4$^+$CD25$^+$ population in normal mice represents a lineage of cells with unique immunoregulatory properties. In addition to suppressing the disease induced following d3Tx, CD4$^+$CD25$^+$ cells can also inhibit the disease induced by transfer of cloned autoantigen-specific cells into nu/nu mice. Thus, not only precursors, but also effectors of organ-specific autoimmunity can be inhibited by the CD4$^+$CD25$^+$ population. A number of important questions remain to be addressed about the CD4$^+$CD25$^+$ population, including the nature of the physiologic ligand recognized by their TCR, whether they must be activated via the TCR to exert their suppressive functions, and how they mediate their suppressive effects.

Immunoregulatory T cells have also been demonstrated to play a role in other organ-specific models of autoimmunity. Lewis rats have a monophasic course of EAE following immunization with MBP, and attempts to induce further episodes of disease by repeated immunization did not result in relapses (40). No evidence was found for destruction or induction of nonresponsiveness of encephalitogenic T cells, as splenocytes from animals that had recovered from EAE could be reactivated in culture with MBP and could transfer EAE to unimmunized recipients. An active process appeared to be taking place in rats that recovered from EAE; such animals become progressively more resistant to passive EAE induced by the transfer of encephalitogenic cells, and refractoriness was antigen-specific. As discussed in the previous section, the differential susceptibility of anti-MBP TCR transgenic mice on a conventional compared to a RAG$^{-/-}$ background is strongly suggestive of the presence of immunoregulatory cells in the former case, and these have been shown to be T cells that express the $\alpha\beta$ TCR (57)

The need for irradiation in order to render nondiabetic adult NOD mice susceptible to diabetes transfer appears around 5 weeks of age in females and around 3 weeks of age in males (58). Cyclophosphamide, a cytotoxic drug used to induce lymphopenia, has also been shown to accelerate the autoimmune diabetes that occurs spontaneously in NOD mice and to increase the incidence in males. The induction of early diabetes in young male and female NOD mice by injection of cyclosphophamide and the requirements for preirradiation to transfer disease suggest a role for suppressive autoimmune phenomena. Furthermore, lymphoid cells from NOD mice (before the onset of diabetes) can delay or suppress the transfer of diabetes induced by spleen cells from overtly diabetic mice into sublethally irradiated NOD recipients (58), but suppression of insulitis was not seen. The suppression was mediated by CD4$^+$ T cells, which were absent from female mice thymectomized at 3 weeks of age. Protective activity detected in spleen cells reached its highest level at 8 weeks of age in nondiabetic NOD mice. In neonates, the activity was undetectable in spleens, although it was present in thymocytes. Neonatal Tx abrogated both the suppressor and effector activities. Similarly, the ability of splenocytes from diabetic NOD donors to transfer disease to NOD/SCID recipients was inhibited (Table 4) by cotransfer of CD4$^+$, but not CD8$^+$, T cells from nondiabetic mice (59); the suppressor activity was localized to the CD45RB^{low} subset of CD4$^+$ cells.

Some attempts have been made to characterize the cells responsible for adoptive transfer of suppression in the NOD models. T-cell clones capable of suppressing IDDM have been isolated (60,61). These clones appear to exhibit properties that are quite different from one another, indicating a diversity in the population of regulatory T cells involved in modulating disease in NOD mice. At present, the repertoire of regulatory T cells capable of inhibiting IDDM, their requirements for activation, their cellular targets, TCR diversity, and their molecular basis for protection are poorly understood. In one study, an unusual group of clones were isolated that recognized both normal syngeneic B-cell blasts and antigens expressed on islets (62). These clones significantly inhibited adoptive transfer of IDDM. A poorly characterized factor was isolated from the clones that inhibited the mixed-lymphocyte reaction, and their protective capacity correlated with the production of this suppressor factor. The T-cell clones inhibited intra-islet, but not peri-islet, lymphocyte infiltration.

The conclusions to be drawn from these studies are that normal healthy animals possess T cells with the potential to cause organ-specific autoimmune diseases, but regulatory T cells play a dominant role in maintaining self-tolerance. The major question that remains to be addressed is the nature of the antigenic specificity of the regulatory T cells that are responsible for the dominant tolerance. It has been proposed that the T cells that mediate dominant tolerance do so by recognizing the tolerated antigen or antigenic peptides derived from it (51). A difficulty with this model is that the regulatory T cells would have to be generated in the thymus at the same time clonal deletion of T cells with high-affinity receptors for self antigens was taking place. Such a regulatory cell repertoire would also be limited to those self antigens that were expressed intrathymically, and it is difficult to understand how such a repertoire would control autoreactive T cells specific for antigens that were only expressed extrathymically. It is also possible that such

TABLE 4. *Inhibition of diabetes by regulatory CD4$^+$ T cells*

Effector cells	Regulatory cells	Disease incidence (%)
Diabetic NOD spleen	None	90
Diabetic NOD spleen	CD4$^+$ nondiabetic	20
Diabetic NOD spleen	CD8$^+$ nondiabetic	70

Splenocytes from a recently diabetic NOD mouse were transferred to NOD/SCID recipients together with splenic CD4$^+$ or CD8$^+$ T cells from young (7- to 12-week-old) nondiabetic NOD mice. Disease incidence was determined 8 weeks after cell transfer.
Adapted from ref. 59.

regulatory T cells mediate inhibition by TCR-based immunoregulation (see discussion of TCR-based immunoregulation within the section on immunotherapeutic approaches to organ-specific autoimmunity). Other targets for their inhibitory effects have been proposed (63), but any model selected must deal with the difficult problem of how the suppressor cells distinguish autoreactive T cells from T cells specific for determinants of foreign antigens, particularly pathogens. At present, no human autoimmune disease has been identified whose pathogenesis is secondary to a deficiency of regulatory T cells. On the other hand, it has been known for a number of years that there is an increased incidence of autoimmunity in patients with immunodeficiencies associated with lymphopenia (64).

Inflammatory Bowel Disease

Inflammatory bowel disease (IBD) in humans is a chronic, presumably noninfectious, inflammation of the bowel (65). Two distinct disease entities have been described. Ulcerative colitis (UC) is limited to the large bowel and pathologically is a relatively superficial, ulcerative inflammation. In contrast, Crohn's disease (CD) can occur anywhere along the gastrointestinal tract and is characterized as a transmural granulomatous inflammation. The etiology of CD and UC are unknown, but it is likely that they have an autoimmune basis. The immune system is exposed to an enormous number of antigens in the intestine, including those derived from food and bacteria, yet mucosal immune responses are characterized by a lack of cell-mediated immune responses to these antigens. There are regulatory mechanisms in place that actively prevent development of immune responses to antigens present in the gut, and oral exposure to antigens may lead to a state of immunologic tolerance (see discussion of oral tolerance within the section on immunotherapeutic approaches). Immune homeostasis in the mucosal immune system relies on a delicate balance between the ability to react to the presence of potential gut pathogens and the ability not to react with common, ubiquitous gut constituents. The large intestine contains the bulk of the bacterial flora, raising the possibility that colitis develops as a result of dysregulated cell-mediated immune responses against components of the enteric flora. Bacterial SAGs themselves may activate T cells, while bacterial products may activate the innate immune system to produce IL-12, which tips the balance to the development of a Th1 response. IBD results from an upset of this balance, but it is not clear whether inflammatory bowel disease is a classical autoimmune disease involving either a reaction against a self constituent or a gut constituent that cross-reacts with a self constituent. Ulcerative colitis does appear to be an organ-specific autoimmune disease in the sense that antibodies to self constituents have been described. The specificity of the antibodies ranges from bacterial components that cross-react with epithelial cell products to epithelial cell antigens, or neutrophil cytoplasmic antigens. It is not clear what role these autoantibodies play in disease pathogenesis. It is possible that they mediate damage by mediating antibody-dependent cytotoxicity.

All studies on animal and human models of IBD suggest hyperresponsiveness to normal gut constituents as a cause of the various forms of the disease. Distinct changes in the number of macrophages, B cells, and T cells, as well as elevated levels of cytokines, have been noted in colonic tissues from patients with IBD. Studies of patients with IBD have shown that inflammatory cytokines are produced with markedly increased levels of IL-1, IL-

6, and TNF-α, as one would expect in any inflammatory immune response (66). IL-2 production in one study, by both peripheral and intestinal lymphocytes, of patients with IBD was found to be lower, while other studies have shown that IL-2 mRNA levels and IL-2 secretion in the serum and mucosal lesions are increased. Evidence of reduced IL-2 secretion has come from studies of mitogen-stimulated T cells, whereas evidence of increased production has come from studies of spontaneous IL-2 secretion.

There are four broad groups of animal models that have proven to be useful for the study of IBD: (a) mice with alterations in T-cell subpopulations and T-cell selection, including TCR α chain– and β chain–deficient mice, MHC class II–deficient mice, SCID mice reconstituted with CD45RB^{high} T cells, HLA-B27 transgenic rats, and human CD3ϵ transgenic mice reconstituted with T cell–depleted F1 bone marrow cells; (b) mice with targeted disruptions of the IL-2 (67), IL-10, and TGF-β genes; (c) mice lacking signaling proteins—and Gα_{i2}-deficient mice; and (d) mice and rats that develop colitis subsequent to the intrarectal introduction of an inflammatory hapten such as trinitrobenzene sulfonic acid (TNBS). The inflammatory conditions that develop in these different mouse models may represent different diseases.

In contrast to animal models of IDDM and MS, in which it has been possible to clone and, in many instances, characterize the fine autoantigen specificity of effector cells, studies of animal models of IBD have yielded very few clues as to the nature of effector cells, but they have emphasized the role of regulatory T cells in the prevention of disease (68). Indeed, IBD may be the best example of an animal model of human autoimmune disease that is secondary to a deficiency of regulatory T cells (see previous discussion of autoimmunity secondary to a deficiency of regulatory T cells). Some studies suggest that T cells are mandatory for regulation of colitis, but are optional for its induction. Colitis developed in mice that lacked the majority of $\alpha\beta$ T cells or CD4$^+$ T cells, while $\gamma\delta$-deficient mice remained disease-free (69). These results suggest that a population of class II–restricted $\alpha\beta$ T cells is important for the prevention of colitis. Disease still developed in mice that lacked both $\alpha\beta$ and $\gamma\delta$ T cells, indicating that cells other than T cells, such as B cells or NK cells, may be involved in the disease process.

Rats that are transgenic for HLA-B27 spontaneously develop gastroduodenitis, colitis, arthritis, and spondylitis (70), and this model has proven to be the most instructive in implicating enteric bacteria as causative agents in the induction of IBD. Diarrhea is the earliest clinical manifestation and develops between 5 and 20 weeks of age. B27 transgenic rats raised under germ-free conditions do not develop colitis and arthritis, but continue to develop orchitis, alopecia, and dermatitis with an incidence and severity similar to that of conventionalized B27 transgenic rats. When the germ-free animals are conventionalized with pathogen-free enteric bacteria, they develop arthritis and gastrointestinal inflammation. Thus, it is likely that bacteria present in the normal flora are responsible for the pathogenesis of chronic intestinal inflammation, as pathogenic bacteria, viruses, and parasites were absent. When the transgenic rats were exposed to bacteria, increased expression of IFN-γ and the monokines IL-1α/β, IL-1RA, TNF-α, and IL-6 were observed in the inflamed colons.

In contrast to human IBD, of which little is known about the cytokines produced by the effector T cells, studies in several of the mouse models have yielded major insights into the potential involvement of pathogenic and protective cytokines. The best-studied disease model in this respect is that seen when CD45RB^{high} CD4$^+$ T cells are transferred to SCID mice (71,72). Curiously, these mice

exclusively develop a colitis with a high frequency of deep ulcers, resembling the colonic lesions that occur in CD; however, the lack of lesions in the small intestine and the high incidence of rectal involvement in this model are more characteristic of UC. In many respects, this animal most closely resembles the disease seen in 15% to 25% of patients with CD who have lesions restricted to the colon. Reactivity to intestinal flora plays some role in this model, as wasting disease in CD45RB^{high} to SCID recipients was prevented by antibiotic treatment. The transmural infiltrate in diseased mice is composed predominantly of macrophages and CD4$^+$ T cells.

Colitis in this model has the features of a pathogenic Th1 response, as the CD4$^+$ T cells from the lamina propria of mice with severe colitis produced very high levels of IFN-γ and lower levels of IL-4 and IL-10 upon polyclonal stimulation *in vitro*. IFN-γ has direct effects on epithelial cells, including enhanced polymorphonuclear transmigration and increased permeability of a colonic epithelial cell line. IFN-γ also activates macrophages, and in synergy with TNF-α, enhances adhesion molecule expression, and in synergy with lipopolysaccharide (LPS), increases the production of a number of inflammatory mediators, such as reactive oxygen and nitrogen intermediates, TNF-α, and IL-1. Furthermore, the disease was almost completely abrogated by treatment of the recipients with anti–IFN-γ or administration of IL-10 (Table 5). It is likely that the blocking effects anti–IFN-γ were secondary to changes in the development of pathogenic Th1 cells, as only two doses of the antibody, given 1 and 4 days after reconstitution, led to significant protection up to 10 weeks later, when neutralizing levels of the antibody were no longer present. Th2 cells were not induced following anti–IFN-γ therapy. Blocking of TNF-α and TNF-β (LTα) by weekly administration of anti-TNF led to protection from wasting disease and a significant reduction in the development of colitis. Anti–IFN-γ was much more effective at preventing colitis than was anti-TNF. Anti-TNF had no effect when given only during the first 2 weeks after T-cell reconstitution; disease occurred 4 weeks after ending treatment in mice that received the anti-TNF for 8 weeks. IL-10 may function by preventing the induction of Th1 cytokines, because administration of IL-10 suppressed levels of IFN-γ and TNF mRNA in the colon. Protection was dependent on the continued presence of IL-10, as disease developed when treatment was stopped, indicating that IL-10 prevented activation of the inflammatory subset of T cells rather than modulated the development or differentiation of Th1 cells. IL-4 treatment failed to prevent development of colitis in this model.

TABLE 5. *Role of cytokines in the pathogenesis and treatment of IBD induced by transfer of CD4$^+$CD45RB^{high} T cells of SCID recipients*

Treatment	Effect on disease
Anti-IFN-γ (days 1+4)	Substantial protection
Anti-TNF (days 1+4)	No protection
Anti-TNF (weekly)	Protection during treatment only
IL-10	Protection during treatment only
IL-4	No protection
CD4$^+$CD45RB^{low} T cells	Complete protection
CD4$^+$CD45RB^{low} + anti-IL-4	Complete protection
CD4$^+$CD45RB^{low} + anti-IL-10	Complete protection
CD4$^+$CD45RB^{low} + anti-TGFβ	No protection

SCID mice were injected with CD4$^+$CD45RB^{high} T cells to induce IBD. Reconstituted mice were treated as indicated. Disease was assayed 12 weeks after transfer.
Adapted from refs. 72–74.

One unique aspect of this model is that has also offered major insights into the mechanism of protection from disease by regulatory T cells (73,74). When CD45RB^low cells were cotransferred with CD45RB^high cells, neutralizing antibodies against IL-10 were unable to reverse the inhibition of colitis. In contrast, when mice were treated with anti–TGF-β mAb at the time of reconstitution, followed by weekly injections for 6 weeks and then killed at 7 weeks, inhibition of colitis by CD45RB^low cells was completely abolished (see Table 5). Protection could not be blocked by anti–IL-4, and CD4RB^low cells isolated from IL-4–deficient mice were able to protect from colitis as well as the same population isolated from wild-type mice. Thus, the TGF-β–dependent regulatory mechanism developed and functioned normally in the absence of IL-4. These studies provide direct evidence that TGF-β is an important mediator of the natural immune regulatory mechanisms involved in control of intestinal immune responses (68) and are consistent with the phenotype of TGF-β1–deficient mice, which developed a severe multiple-organ inflammatory disease that was lethal by 3 to 5 weeks of age, with the most severe lesions being present in the heart and lungs (75). The cellular infiltration in affected organs of these mice was associated with increases in the inflammatory cytokines IFN-γ and TNF-α, suggesting that TGF-β is important for the prevention of dysregulated inflammatory responses in many organs.

The dominant role of regulatory T cells in preventing IBD is also implicated in the disease observed in transgenic mice that overexpress the human CD3ε gene (76). These mice are characterized by a very early arrest in T-cell development and a highy abnormal thymic microenvironment; the mice lack both T cells and NK cells in the periphery. Transplantation of these mice with normal T cell–depleted F1 bone marrow led to severe colitis, which was prevented when the same mice were simultaneously transplanted with normal fetal thymus. Transfer of a small number of lymph node T cells from diseased mice caused severe colitis in RAG^−/− recipients. Colonic T cells from diseased mice had a phenotype of activated CD4^+ cells and also displayed greatly enhanced cytotoxic activity. Large numbers of CD4^+ and CD8^+ TCR αβ^+ T cells, which produced IFN-γ and TNF-α, were identified in sick animals (77). An involvement of γδ T cells was also seen in this model when bone marrow cells from TCR αβ^−/− donors were transplanted into the transgenic animals. Disease in these mice correlated with the development of peripheral and colonic TCR γδ^+ T cells capable of IFN-γ production. The dramatic skewing of TCR αβ^+ and γδ^+ T cells towards IFN-γ production is consistent with the other IBD models and could be secondary to polyclonal and/or nonspecific activation of T cells by products derived from luminal bacteria of the colon. This model suggests that T-cell development through the aberrant thymus resulted in a population of T cells that lacked the regulatory subpopulation and were thus able to induce a pathogenic response in the intestine. Regulatory T cells developed normally in the microenvironment of the grafted fetal thymus, and these cells prevented the induction of colitis by the pathogenic T cells, which differentiated in the abnormal thymus. It remains unclear why regulatory T cells fail to be selected in the aberrant thymus, whereas pathogenic T cells develop normally; it is also unclear why these mice only develop inflammatory disease exclusively in the colon.

The involvement of pathogenic CD4^+ Th1 T cells in IBD and the critical role of IL-12 in their generation were prominently seen when the hapten, 2,4,6-trinitrobenzene sulfonic acid (TNBS), was administered intrarectally to mice (78). TNBS haptenates autologous colonic proteins with TNP, which then induce an intense immune response and a massive transmural inflammation resembling the pathology of CD (diarrhea, rectal prolapse, weight loss, and granulomatous inflammation). The persistence of such inflammation, along with the fact that it can be transferred to naive recipients with CD4^+ T cells, suggested that the initial response to TNP-substituted protein was eventually superseded by respones to cross-reactive antigens in the mucosal lumen. The responding T cells in vitro produce greatly increased amounts of IFN-γ and IL-2 and reduced amounts of IL-4. Cells in the inflamed tissues produced increased amounts of IL-12 as well as IFN-γ. Anti–IL-12 antibodies or anti-IFN-γ antibodies prevented colitis when administered at the time of induction, and the disease could be abrogated by anti–IL-12 treatment well after colitis was established (79). CD4^+ T cells isolated from the lamina propria of anti–IL-12 treated mice failed to secrete IFN-γ on in vitro stimulation. This suggests that the presence of IL-12 is essential to maintain TNBS-induced colitis and a persistent local Th1 response of intestinal lamina propria T cells. Administration of TNBS did not induce disease in IFN-γ^−/− mice.

If Th1 cells play a prominent role in IBD, then one might assume that a dysregulated Th1 response would also result in induction of disease. Indeed, IL-10–deficient mice (80) developed a generalized enterocolitis under conventional housing conditions, but under pathogen-free conditions, intestinal inflammation was less severe and occurred only in the mucosa of the proximal colon. Disease began as small focal areas of inflammation and minimal epithelial hyperplasia in the cecum, ascending, and transverse colon. Early lesions contain increased numbers of T cells and epithelial cells aberrantly expressing MHC class II molecules. Pathologic changes occurred at weaning, when significant colonization of the gastrointestinal tract with normal flora takes place. The regions where the lesions take place in young IL-10^−/− mice are known to be colonized with the greatest number and types of bacteria. The disease is more severe in adult mice, with multifocal lesions in multiple segments of the colon and occasionally in the duodenum; ultimately, the disease is characterized by an increased number of focal ulcerations and transmural lesions.

It has been hypothesized that the intestinal disease in the IL-10^−/− mice is due to the absence of the general suppressive effects of IL-10 on cytokine production by macrophages and Th1 T cells. Intestinal tissue from diseased IL-10^−/− mice spontaneously produced elevated amounts of IL-1α, TNF, IL-6, and NO levels in vitro. Immunohistochemistry identified very high numbers of macrophages, and it is likely that uncontrolled cytokine production by macrophages was taking place. Abnormally high numbers of activated CD4^+ and CD8^+ T cells were also detected in the colonic lesions and produced large amounts of IFN-γ, but no IL-4 (81). The ability of IFN-γ to synergize with luminal bacterial products to enhance cytokine production by macrophages would further heighten the inflammatory response, particularly in the absence of negative regulation by IL-10. When IL-10^−/− mice were treated at weaning with anti–IFN-γ for 6 weeks, a smaller proportion (31%) developed colitis, as compared with weanlings treated with control antibody (93%). Established colitis in adult animals was not altered by anti–IFN-γ treatment, although the levels of MHC class II expression on epithelial cells were markedly diminished. Thus, IFN-γ may be required for initiation of the response, but not for its continuation. Two months of IL-10 therapy were very effective in modulating disease in young IL-10^−/− mice; IL-10 therapy failed to cure established disease in adults, but did reduce the incidence of adenocarcinoma and duodenitis associated with progressive disease.

G proteins are signal-transducing proteins that couple a large family of receptors to effectors, such as adenyl cyclase, phospholipase C, and ion channels. Mice deficient for the G protein subunit α_{i2} displayed growth retardation and developed a lethal diffuse colitis with clinical and histopathologic features closely resembling UC in humans, including the development of adenocarcinoma of the colon (82). These typical features of human UC are unique to this animal model. These mice also have profound alterations in thymocyte maturation and functions. Deficient mice have increased numbers of single-positive thymocytes with high-intensity CD3 staining; normal numbers of T cells are present in the spleen. Thymocytes and peripheral T cells from $\alpha_{i2}^{-/-}$ mice produced IL-2, IFN-γ, and TNF at levels that were 80-fold higher than controls, while IL-4 was only modestly enhanced. Although marked abnormalities of B-cell development or function were not seen, elevated levels of plasma IgG and IgA were detected in the deficient mice. Increased numbers of blood neutrophils were present in the deficient mice. Neutrophils may be unable to migrate out of blood vessels, as α_{i2} plays a role in coupling receptors for chemokines. In contrast to many of the other animal models of IBD, $G\alpha_{i2}$-deficient mice in a specific pathogen-free barrier facility developed disease with the wasting and histopathologic features of colitis and adenocarcinoma. The complex factors that link this interesting genetic defect, the abnormalities in immune function, and IBD remain to be explored.

Transgenic Models of Organ-specific Autoimmune Disease

Study of organ-specific autoimmunity has been limited in the past to the study of the few spontaneous disease models that develop in inbred animals or to those diseases that occur following the injection of autoantigens in adjuvant. Animal models are needed that can serve as tools to understand the pathogenetic processes involved in the initial phase of autoimmune reactions. The availability of transgenic technologies has allowed the development of animal models of human diseases, which should facilitate our understanding of the basic mechanisms of disease and the development of effective therapeutic approaches (83). Strains expressing molecules in a tissue-specific manner have proven to be particularly useful, for example, the expression of transgenes in the islets of Langerhans under control of the rat insulin promoter (RIP). The foreign (viral or microbial) gene is integrated into the host genome, passed on to progeny, and, in essence, becomes a self antigen. Experiments that address the issues of peripheral tolerance in autoimmunity have used animals that express such "foreign" antigens; studies directed to understanding pathogenesis have used animals that express cytokines or costimulatory molecules (see previous discussion of autoimmunity secondary to a deficiency of regulatory T cells). Several models have been established that use both of these systems, separately or together, which allow autoreactive immune responses to be precisely followed. Because there is ample evidence that autoreactive T cells exist in healthy individuals and animals (52,84), transgenic models have proven to be particularly useful in addressing the question of the fate of those autoreactive T cells that have the potential to respond to antigens not represented within the thymus, but unique to extrathymic tissues.

The question of whether tolerance can be induced to extrathymic self antigens was initially investigated by injecting the gene for the class I molecule, K^b, linked to the RIP into mice of non–H-2^b haplotype, to create transgenic mice expressing the K^b gene in the insulin-producing β cells of the islets of the pancreas (85). The RIP-K^b mice were then crossed to mice transgenic for genes encoding an anti-K^b–specific TCR so that a large proportion of the T cells of the double transgenic offspring were K^b-specific and of a single clonotype. Although these doubly transgenic mice developed neither diabetes nor insulitis, interpretation of these studies was complicated because the T cells with the highest density of expression of the transgenic TCR were deleted, presumably because expression of the transgene was leaky; K^b was not exclusively expressed in the pancreas, and a certain level of expression was present in the thymus. On the other hand, young transgenic mice did have CD8$^+$ T cells with a low density of the clonotypic receptor and were capable of rejecting K^b-expressing skin grafts. It appeared that the K^b molecule on the pancreatic β cells was ignored by antigen-specific T-cells. Even after skin grafting and rejection, there was no infiltration of the islets.

Similar results were also observed when single transgenic RIP-K^b mice were thymectomized, irradiated, and reconstituted with bone marrow from anti-K^b transgenic mice and thymus grafts from nontransgenic mice. Under these conditions, the thymus could not express K^b, and these mice showed no deletion of the T cells that expressed high levels of the anti-K^b TCR. Nevertheless, these animals did not develop diabetes and remained ignorant or indifferent to antigens expressed on the β cells, but rejected skin grafts as rapidly as did control mice. When these animals were primed with K^b-expressing cells, islet-cell infiltration by CD8$^+$ T cells was seen within 3 weeks of priming, but infiltration was not sustained and was not seen at later time points unless multiple primings were done. Taken together, these studies clearly demonstrate that most naive T cells do not usually circulate through nonlymphoid tissues, and unprimed autoreactive T cells do not inflict damage on target tissues. Furthermore, these results suggest that for the development of autoimmune disease, a single priming of autoreactive T cells by a cross-reacting infectious agent may not be sufficient to cause disease, and a more sustained priming, such as that seen during chronic infections, may be needed to maintain a pathogenic response.

The role of T-cell ignorance in maintaining tolerance of antigens that are only expressed in nonlymphatic organs and the contribution of an infectious insult in breaking the tolerant state are well illustrated in the model in which the glycoprotein (GP) of lymphocytic choriomeningitis virus (LCMV) was expressed in pancreatic β cells under the control of the RIP (86). Although potentially autoreactive, GP-specific CTL can be easily detected in the periphery of these mice following priming *in vitro*, they never develop diabetes spontaneously because the self antigen is ignored. Following infection with LCMV, β cells expressing GP are destroyed within 8 to 14 days in RIP/GP transgenic mice and within 4 days in double transgenics, expressing both RIP/GP and an anti-GP–specific transgenic TCR (87). T cells that infiltrated the islets were specific for the viral gene product (GP) and could lyse virus-infected target cells *in vitro*. The presence of CD8$^+$ lymphocytes was mandatory for generating immunopathology, and their depletion resulted in abrogation of IDDM. In contrast to the induction of disease following LCMV, infection of RIP/GP transgenic mice with a recombinant vaccinia virus expressing LCMV/GP (VAC/GP) failed to induce autoimmune diabetes, but did so by day 8 in the TCRXGP double transgenics. Thus, the induction of autoimmunity has a quantitative aspect, as infection of mice with LCMV generated 100 to 1,000 times higher CTL activity than infection with VAC/GP. VAC/GP infection still led to insulitis in

RIP-GP mice, but was not sufficient to induce overt diabetes. The increased frequency of CTL precursors in the double transgenics compensated for the weak antigenic stimulus, and mice developed diabetes after infection with the VAC/GP.

In addition to the numbers of precursors specific for an autoantigen, the affinity of their TCR may also determine whether autoimmune damage results following infection. This is best illustrated by the findings of Oldstone's group (83,88), who generated LCMV RIP/GP transgenic mice in manner very similar to those described above. Following infection with LCMV, these mice developed slowly progressive injury of β cells, leading to IDDM only 3 to 6 months after LCMV infection, while in the mice developed by Ohashi et al. (86), IDDM rapidly developed within 7 to 4 days after challenge. It was later found that the discrepancy between these two studies was secondary to expression of the transgene in both the thymus and pancreas in Oldstone's animals, while in those generated by Ohashi et al., the transgene was exclusively expressed in the pancreas. In the former case, only low-affinity anti-self CTLs were identified in islet infiltrates and CD4+ T cells were required to generate the CD8+ CTLs. In many respects, this model may better mimic the process that takes place in the induction of autoimmunity in normal mice and humans. As the process of negative selection and deletion in the thymus is never 100% efficient, it will be the low-affinity anti-self precursors that are seeded at relatively low frequency to the periphery. Activation and expansion of such low-affinity autoreactive cells by an infectious agent will require repeated stimulation, and a long lag time will be present from the initiation of an autoimmune response until the onset of disease.

Although the RIP/LCMV model has been extensively studied, one should be cautious about drawing too many conclusions from a single system. For example, when the influenza virus hemagglutinin (HA) was expressed under control of the RIP (89), mice that expressed a conventional T-cell repertoire did not develop diabetes, even after immunization with influenza virus. When these mice were mated to TCR transgenics expressing an anti-HA receptor, CD8+ T cells accumulated within the islets of the double transgenic mouse and neonates developed diabetes within 10 days after birth. All other models have required local expression of additional transgenes or immunization of the mice with an exogenous form of the transgenic autoantigen. It is possible that in this model the mechanisms of self-tolerance are overwhelmed by the large number of autoreactive T cells expressing a transgenic TCR, that the particular T-cell clone in these studies may have a low threshold for activation that does not require costimulatory signals, or that HA could be reprocessed and presented by professional APCs residing in the islets.

In summary, the major lesson to be drawn from these transgenic models is that T-cell tolerance is rarely established against organ-specific (nonlymphohematopoietic) self antigens located in sequestered sites or expressed below a critical level. Autoreactive T cells specific for such self antigens are neither physically deleted nor functionally inactivated. These self antigens are mostly ignored. The autoreactive T cells remain harmless as long as their status of ignorance is not broken by the presentation of self antigens by professional APCs in the lymphoid tissues. Even the induction of experimental autoimmunity is only feasible in the presence of strong adjuvants and/or pertussis toxin. During an acute viral infection, the virus-infected host eliminates the virus with only a minute destruction of tissue. Self antigens would be released only transiently, in small amounts that are not sufficient to activate self-reactive T-lymphocytes. Autoimmunity is unlikely to occur unless the virus and the infected host share antigenic determinants by the

process of molecular mimicry (see discussion of molecular mimicry in the following section). During the inflammatory response seen in chronic viral infections, large amounts of self antigens may be released and transported to APCs in lymphoid tissues. Under these latter conditions, tolerance will be broken and cells that recognize tissue-specific autoantigens will be activated. Even under these conditions, induction of autoimmune T cells is exacting with respect to quantity, duration of antigen exposure, requirements for cytokines, and MHC antigen upregulation. As the incidence of autoimmunity is low, even severe tissue destruction and release of large amounts of self antigen are normally not sufficient to induce significant signs of autoimmune disease in most hosts. It should be pointed out that all of the transgenic models described above involve autoantigen recognition by CD8+ T cells; several mice that express transgenic autoreactive TCR in the CD4+ lineage do spontaneously develop autoimmune disease (11) or remain disease-free because the pathogenic T cells are controlled by regulatory T-cell populations (57).

THE ETIOLOGY AND PATHOGENESIS OF ORGAN-SPECIFIC AUTOIMMUNITY

Molecular Mimicry

Many of the clinical and epidemiologic studies on human autoimmune diseases and their animal models described above have indicated that infections are important in the induction of autoimmunity. The consistent inability to detect the pathogen in the target tissue led to the concept of "molecular mimicry" as the mechanism by which reactivity to foreign pathogens could be extended to self (90). Many viruses share antigenic sites with normal host-cell components. The identification of mAbs that reacted with both host and virus constituents suggested that viruses have the potential to trigger autoimmune responses and resultant disease. In a study of 600 mAbs to 11 different viruses, it was found that more than 3% of such antibodies also reacted with normal tissues (91). Microbial agents share determinants with host protein, and an immune response mounted by the host against a determinant of an infecting agent may cross-react with the mimicked host sequence, potentially leading to inflammation, tissue destruction, and autoimmunity. The immunopathologic process could continue chronically after the triggering agent has been eliminated, or be reinitiated by multiple viral infections. Host genetic factors also play a role, as host genes control immune responses to various pathogens, play a role in the expression of cellular receptors, and can influence replication of the infectious agent. The major difficulty in establishing a correlation between triggering events such as a viral infection and the actual autoimmune disease is the usually long lag period that often precedes the onset of disease. To date, molecular mimicry has been suggested to play a role in the pathogenesis of several human diseases, including IDDM, ankylosing spondylitis, Guillain-Barre syndrome, primary biliary cirrhosis (PBC), and MS, but it has yet to be conclusively shown to be the initiating factor of these autoimmune diseases. The conceptual strength of the molecular mimicry hypothesis is that it offers a physiologic explanation for the breakdown of immunologic self-tolerance in autoimmunity, which leads to organ-specific immunopathology. The mimicked epitope of the microbial pathogen is sufficiently different from self to allow an immune response to develop to it, with presumably severe consequences for the microbe, while the similarity to

TABLE 6. *Molecular mimicry between MBP and HBVP*

	66	75
MBP	Thr-Thr-His-Tyr-Gly-Ser-Leu-Pro-Gln-Lys	
	589	598
HBVP	Ile-Gly-Cys-Tyr-Gly-Ser-Leu-Pro-Gln-Glu	

Adapted from ref. 92.

self allows the breakdown of self-tolerance and an autoimmune response ensues to the mimicked self-determinant.

One of the first clear examples of molecular mimicry was the demonstration by Fujinami and Oldstone (92) that a cross-reaction between an 8- to 10- amino acid sequence of MBP (the encephalitogenic site of rabbit MBP, amino acids 66–75) and a viral protein could generate an autoimmune response (Table 6). Rabbits inoculated with the hepatitis B viral polymerase made a humoral and cellular immune response that cross-reacted with both MBP and the MBP peptide; some of the animals developed lesions characteristic of EAE. It has been postulated that in patients with MS that express HLA-DR2, the expansion of a relatively few MBP (84 to 102) reactive T cells could be secondary to the recognition of viral peptides with sufficient structural similarity to the immunodominant MBP peptide. Similarly, in IDDM, GAD65 and GAD67 share an amino acid sequence with the P2-C protein of coxsackie virus (Table 7), raising the possibility that in IDDM, autoimmunity may arise by molecular mimicry as a consequence of infection by coxsackievirus. Coxsackie infection would initiate the autoimmune attack on the pancreatic β cells. The resultant destruction of the β cells would result in the release of GAD, which could then stimulate lymphocytes already primed to the coxsackievirus peptide. The anti-GAD response would remain long after the virus infection subsided (5). Another well-characterized example of molecular mimicry is the high homology between a motif in region II of malaria CS protein, which mediates binding of the sporozoite to the hepatocyte, to a cytoadhesive motif found on thrombospondin and some members of the complement system.

One of the most interesting examples of molecular mimicry is seen in PBC, an autoimmune chronic cholestatic liver disease, which affects mainly women and leads to destruction of the intrahepatic bile ducts and death from liver failure (93). Molecular mimicry has been postulated to be responsible for the generation of the antimitochondrial antibodies in PBC because of homology between the E2 subunits of mammalian mitochondrial enzymes and the E2 subunits of the *E. coli* pyruvate dehydrogenase complex. In addition, HLA-DR α chains, which are abnormally expressed on the surface of bile duct epithelial cells in PBC, also share homology with the E2 epitope. A complex cascade of events may be involved in the pathogenic process in this disease.

Autoimmunity should only occur when the microbial peptide and the host determinants cross-react, yet are different enough to break immunologic tolerance. Tissue injury can take place in the absence of the infectious virus that initiated the immune response;

TABLE 7. *GAD and coxsackievirus P2-C share common sequences*

257		267
	K-M-F-P-E-V-K-E-K-G-M	
35		46
	K-I-L-P-E-V-K-E-K-H-E	

Adapted from ref. 5.

viral replication is also not required. The autoimmune response itself leads to tissue injury that in turn leads to the release of more self antigen, and the cycle continues. Viruses that persist may continuously or cyclically express viral antigens. Even in the absence of replication, production of the determinant or immunodominant region in common with that of the host could continue. The resulting antigen, properly presented, might then evoke immune responsiveness to the cross-reacting tissue antigen, leading to chronic and progressive disease. Molecular mimicry may also have a selective advantage for the virus by mimicking sites or regions on host molecules that are suppressive or tolerance-inducing so that a virus might be regarded as self and not be eliminated by an immune response. Immunologic injury could occur after removal of the infectious agent, as elements of the immune response mounted against it would continue to assault the host, resulting in release of self antigens that would then continue to stimulate the immune response and provoke further injury. This might account for the viral encephalopathies occurring after measles, mumps, vaccinia, or herpes zoster infections.

Viruses that cause latent and/or persistent infections may permit chronic antigenic stimulation of autoreactive populations. Based on the structural requirements for both MHC class II binding and TCR recognition of an immunodominant MBP peptide, criteria for a data base search were developed in which the degeneracy of amino acid side chains required for MHC class II binding and the conservation of those required for T-cell activation were considered (94). This study demonstrated that some TCRs actually recognize not a single peptide, but rather a limited repertoire of structurally related peptides derived from different antigens. This recognition did not merely represent a minor degree of cross-reactivity, because these peptides efficiently activated MBP-specific clones. The stimulatory mimicry peptides identified had only limited primary sequence similarity and cross-reactivity would not have been predicted based on simple alignments between MBP and viral antigens (Table 8). The diverse nature of the viral peptides that stimulated MBP-specific T-cell clones makes it unlikely that a single virus is responsible for initiating autoimmunity in MS. It appears that a group of common viral pathogens, particularly the herpes family (EBV, herpes simplex, and cytomegalovirus), influenza viruses, and papillomaviruses, could be involved in initiating the autoimmune process. It was widely believed that TCR recognition was exquisitely specific, because even minor substitutions in a T-cell epitope diminished or abrogated T-cell activation, but these studies demonstrate that there is also a significant degree of cross-reactivity. One of the complications of the need of a very large T-cell repertoire to deal with the large number of constantly changing pathogen-derived epitopes is the necessity that a certain percentage of these TCRs will also have a degree of self-reactivity.

TABLE 8. *Activation of MBP-specific T cells by viral peptides*

Peptide	Sequence	T-cell proliferation
MBP (85–99)	ENPVVHFFKNIVTPPR	70,350
EBV, DNA polymerase	TGGVYHFVKKHVHES	96,613
Influenza A, hemagglutinin	YRNLVWFIKKNTRYP	45,094

An MBP-specific, DR2-restricted T-cell clone could be activated to the same degree by MBP 85–99 and the other two unrelated peptides.

Adapted from ref. 94.

Such self-reactive T cells would likely be of relatively low affinity and have escaped thymic negative selection as well as peripheral tolerance by clonal deletion or induction of anergy.

A transgenic mouse model that allows direct testing of the molecular mimicry hypothesis has been developed (95). Mice were generated that expressed a viral protein exclusively in oligodendrocytes. To determine whether a virus-induced immune response would result in an autoimmune attack against the viral transgene product, adult transgenic mice were infected with a virus that encoded the same gene, but did not infect the CNS, and was quickly cleared by the host immune response. Infection of immunocompetent mice with LCMV results in the infection of many tissues, but not cells of the CNS. It was thus possible to determine if a viral infection in the periphery could result in immune attack against CNS components. Although the LCMV infection was cleared following infection, a chronic CNS autoimmune disease subsequently developed, which was enhanced by a second infection with LCMV or unrelated viruses that stimulated LCMV- specific memory immune responses. The cross-activation of memory T cells specific for an oligodendrocyte protein by subsequent viral infections may explain why patients with an autoimmune disease such as MS often exhibit disease exacerbation after infections by different viruses. This model is quite compatible with a model of MS in which infection by a virus sharing epitopes with a myelin component such as MBP could result in activation of self-reactive T cells that would cross the BBB and recognize oligodendrocytes presenting self peptides.

Determinant Spreading

One of the major goals in understanding the pathogenesis of organ-specific autoimmune disease is to define the inciting autoantigen. As will be discussed in the section on immunotherapeutic approaches, it is hoped that such information will lead to the development of antigen-specific immunotherapy protocols. Most attempts to identify target autoantigens even very early in the course of evolution of a spontaneous autoimmune disease such as IDDM in the NOD mouse model have demonstrated that multiple autoantigens may be recognized by antigen-specific T cells. Studies of immune responses to foreign antigens have led to the definition of two classes of antigenic epitopes (96). *Dominant* epitopes are defined as those epitopes to which an animal initially responds when primed to a protein or an infectious agent. Responses to other epitopes on an antigen, which arise later on hyperimmunization, are termed *secondary* or *cryptic*. An immune response targeting one or two dominant epitopes on an infectious agent is frequently not sufficient, so the immune system has evolved a mechanism for increasing the number of epitopes targeted during an infection. This results in the appearance of a response against cryptic epitopes but, as pointed out above, increases the likelihood that some of the responses to these cryptic epitopes can also cross-react with autoantigens.

Cryptic determinants of self antigens are probably not generated at all, or are generated during normal antigen processing at very low levels. Because the induction of T-cell tolerance to self during the process of negative selection in the thymus requires a certain level of peptide antigen expression, T cells specific for these cryptic epitopes may escape deletion and be present in the normal T-cell repertoire. The fundamental questions that remain to be answered include how epitopes that are normally cryptic become visible to the immune system, how autoaggressive cells specific for these

epitopes become activated, and how cryptic epitopes elicit sustained pathogenic responses. Although the mechanisms responsible for the priming of T cells specific for cryptic epitopes have not been defined, it is widely accepted that T cells that recognize the initiating self epitope induce an inflammatory cascade in the target organ, resulting in tissue damage (97). Tissue debris is taken up by macrophages, dendritic cells, or B cells, and presented to naive tissue–specific T cells that, once activated, perpetuate the inflammatory response. Presentation might be facilitated because of the increase in MHC class II synthesis and the upregulation of adhesion–costimulatory molecules, which occurs during the course of an inflammatory response. Antigen-specific B cells, which are highly efficient APCs, may play a major role in diversification of the immune response (98). Antibody can increase the efficiency of antigen capture in antigen-specific B cells and in Fc receptor–bearing APCs. Antibodies can also modulate antigen processing so that the production of some epitopes can be increased, while others are decreased. Cytokine production during the course of an inflammatory response may lead to upregulation of certain enzymes involved in antigen processing, which could also result in the enhancement of production of minor epitopes.

The acquired recognition of new self-determinants during the course of an autoimmune disease has been termed *determinant spreading*. Chronic relapsing EAE is the best example of a chronic autoimmune disease in which determinant spreading plays a major pathologic role. Lehmann et al (99) showed that immunoreactivity to nondominant determinants (35–47,81–100,121–140) of MBP occurred during the development of chronic EAE in (SJLXB10.PL)F1 mice immunized exclusively with the immunodominant I-A^u peptide MBP Ac1-11 (Table 9). Determinant spreading during the development of autoimmune disease is an ordered physiologic process in which defined self determinants are recognized in a sequential predictable manner (100). Inflammatory cytokines and chemokine activity associated with relapse and chronicity of autoimmune demyelination are due in part to spreading of T-cell recognition to new myelin self determinants. The order in which determinants are recognized during spreading does not follow the traditional immunodominant prior to nondominant heirarchy, nor does it favor an intramolecular bias (101). CNS myelin damage is necessary for the initiation of epitope spreading. An invariant relationship exists between the development of relapse–progression and the spreading of recognition to new immunodominant encephalitogenic determinants. A predictable sequence of both intermolecular and intramolecular epitope spreading has been seen in (SWRXSJL)F1 mice following induction of relapsing EAE with PLP 139–151; during disease progression, responses to PLP 249–273 appeared first, followed by responses to MBP 87–99, and then to PLP 173–198 (Table 10). PLP 173–198-specific T cells are demonstrable in the CNS of mice

TABLE 9. *Intramolecular Epitope Spreading Following Immunization with MBP Ac1–11*

Ac1–11	35–47	81–100	121–140
5/5	1/5	3/5	5/5

EAE was induced by immunization with MBP Ac1–11 and pertussis toxin. Twenty-one days later, spleen cells, were assayed for proliferative responses to the indicated peptides. Results are expressed as the number of animals tested that demonstrated a positive response to each peptide.
Adapted from ref. 99.

TABLE 10. *Intramolecular and intermolecular determinant spreading following immunization with PLP 139–151*

Antigen	Days following immunization			
	7	28	56	84
PLP 139–151	+	+	+	+
PLP 249–273	–	+	+	+
MBP 87–89	–	–	+	+
PLP 173–193	–	–	–	+

(+), response; (–), no response.

Animals were immunized with PLP 139–151, and proliferative responses to the different peptides were tested on the indicated days.

Adapted from ref. 100.

that are in remission from PLP 139–151-induced EAE. After EAE onset, the induction of peptide-specific tolerance to spreading, but not to nonspreading, encephalitogenic determinants prevented subsequent progression of EAE. Thus, induction of tolerance to intact PLP or to the relapse-associated PLP173–198 epitope, but not to the disease-inducing PLP 139–151 epitope, protected mice that were in remission from acute PLP 139–151-induced disease from renewed disease. Similarly, in (SWRXSJL)F1 mice with PLP 139–151-induced EAE, disease progression was blocked by tolerance to MBP 87–99.

Epitope spreading has also been observed in IDDM in NOD mice. Induction of neonatal tolerance to GAD65 via intrathymic or intravenous peptide injections blocked the activation of responses to other β-cell epitopes and the subsequent development of diabetes and insulitis (14). These results have supported the view that islet-cell destruction in NOD mice is initiated by a T-cell response against the 65-kDa isoform of GAD, which arises within 4 weeks of age, and that T-cell reactivity subsequently spreads to other pancreatic β-cell antigens, such as carboxypeptidase H, insulin, and HSP65. Epitope spreading may play a role in the pathogenesis of chronic and relapsing–remitting organ-specific and systemic human autoimmune diseases, such as SLE, rheumatoid arthritis, and MS. In MS, as in EAE, determinant spreading may correlate with disease progression (102).

T Helper 1–T Helper 2 Balance

The Th1/Th2 model of Th-cell differentiation proposes that, on activation by cognate ligand, naive Th cells differentiate into distinct functional subgroups, which are characterized by their pattern of cytokine secretion (see Chapter 26). Th1 cells secrete IFN-γ, activate macrophages, and elicit delayed-type hypersensitivity (DTH). Th2 cells produce IL-4, -5, -10, and -13; are important for IgE production; and suppress cell-mediated immunity. Cytokines produced by one subset cross-regulate the other subset's development and function. The best-characterized factors affecting the development of Th subsets are the lymphokines themselves. Polarized phenotypes are likely to be most relevant in chronic diseases such as persistent infection and autoimmunity.

Because it is likely that the fundamental immunologic reactions that control immune responses to foreign antigens are also operative in the recognition of self antigens during the course of autoimmune diseases, Th1 and Th2 phenotypes should also characterize these conditions (103). One might predict that Th1 cells will promote the development of organ-specific autoimmune diseases,

while Th2 cells should promote antibody-mediated systemic autoimmune diseases such as SLE. The first evidence of a role for cytokine phenotype in the pathogenesis of autoimmune diseases was derived from studies of mercuric chloride–induced lupus and chronic GVHD, which are both characterized by elevated levels of IgE. Administration of anti-IL-4 early in the immune response inhibited not only IgE production, but also the associated pathology, including splenomegaly and the nephrotic syndrome (104). The major role of Th1 cells as effector populations in all of the organ-specific autoimmune diseases, including IDDM, EAE, and IBD, has already been reviewed. In general, only Th1, not Th2, populations can induce these diseases on passive transfer. A logical extension of the analysis of the role of cytokines in the pathogenesis of autoimmunity is whether this information can be used to design immunotherapy regimens for the treatment of autoimmune diseases. Because Th1 and Th2 populations cross-regulate each other, it may be feasible to convert an autoimmune disease mediated by inflammatory pathogenic Th1 cells to one in which protective Th2 populations predominate, or to convert a disease mediated by Th2 cells to one in which Th1 cells exert protection.

The regulation of cytokine production during the course of EAE has been studied extensively. The inflammation observed in EAE lesions resembles that of a DTH reaction. In most studies, there is a strong correlation between the development of EAE and the DTH response to myelin. Kennedy et al. (105) have shown that IFN-γ dominated intracerebral cytokine production during the exacerbation phase of EAE, but was followed by a dramatic rise in IL-10 mRNA expression during recovery, with a concomitant waning of Th1 cytokine expression. The level of IL-10 mRNA remained elevated throughout the recovery phase. The selective intracerebral upregulation of IL-4 and IL-10, which closely parallels spontaneous recovery, has also been seen in other studies (106) using immunohistologic methods. IL-2, TNF-α, IFN-γ, but not IL-4, were present in the CNS tissues at the height of disease. During recovery, IFN-γ levels were lower, and IL-4, IL-10, and TGF-β dominated. These studies suggested that the therapeutic administration of either IL-4 or IL-10 might be of benefit in the treatment of EAE.

The ability to prime CD4⁺ T cells *in vivo* for IL-4 production in an antigen-specific fashion raised the question as to whether an ongoing immune response dominated by Th1 cells could be deviated *in vivo* to one dominated by Th2 cells. When naive SJL mice were inoculated with highly pathogenic MBP-specific Th1 lines and the recipient mice were treated with exogenous IL-4, clinical signs of EAE were suppressed (107). IL-4 administration was required immediately following the cell transfer during the time period in which T cells began to invade the CNS and were activated by the autoantigen. Th2-like CD4⁺ T cells could be isolated from the spleens of the recipients, but were surprisingly not associated with a downregulation of Th1 cytokine production. Once Th2 cells were induced, the animals remained protected from the clinical signs of EAE for at least 1 month without further therapy.

In the rat model of EAE, the systemic administration (days 0, 3, and 6 after immunization) of IL-10 during the initiation phase of disease was effective in markedly suppressing the subsequent induction of EAE (108). This suppression of clinical disease coincided with a significant elevation of MBP-specific autoantibody production, sustained T cell–proliferative responses to MBP, and a diminution of CNS infiltration. The presence of autoantigen-specific Th2 cells was not evaluated in these animals; nevertheless, the beneficial effects of IL-10 appeared to be secondary to an enhancement of Th2-like responses and a simultaneous reduction of Th1 cytokine production. It remains possible that all of the therapeutic effects of IL-10 were mediated by inactivation of microglial cells and brain-invading macrophages. IL-13 has also been shown to be a potent inhibitor of macrophage function in the rat. When IL-13–secreting cells were injected at the same time rats were immunized with MBP, marked suppression of the development of EAE was seen (109). This suppression of disease was not accompanied by reductions in MBP-specific T-cell proliferation nor in alteration of MBP-specific autoantibody production. These data suggest that IL-13 may exert its beneficial effects on the development of EAE mainly by its capacity to suppress the production of proinflammatory immune mediators by macrophage–microglial cells. Macrophages–microglial cells play a crucial role in the final effector phase of EAE and are responsible for tissue destruction and the manifestations of clinical symptoms. The most convincing argument for the central role of macrophages in EAE is the observation that depletion of this cell population shortly before the onset of clinical symptoms protects against disease.

Because IL-4 plays its critical role in inducing the differentiation of Th2 cells at the time of cytokine priming, it was also of interest to determine whether immunization against foreign antigens could inhibit the development of EAE by modifying the cytokine environment in which autoreactive T-cell clones develop, so that their cytokine profile was shifted from an inflammatory Th1 toward a protective Th2 type (110). SJL mice were preimmunized with KLH in incomplete adjuvant to induce a population of KLH-specific Th2 cells. When EAE was induced in these animals with MBP and the animals were simultaneously boosted with KLH, the clinical signs of EAE were markedly reduced (Table 11). Furthermore, the cytokine profile of the MBP-specific T cells was shifted from an inflammatory Th1 toward a protective Th2 type. It was concluded from these studies that the presence of IL-4 secreted by the KLH-specific memory Th2 cells in the lymphoid microenvironment in which the autoreactive T cells were being primed with MBP was able to bias their cytokine profile towards a protective Th2 phenotype. The protective effect of immunization with KLH was abrogated by IL-12, which inhibited the production of IL-4 and biased the autoimmune response to a predominantly Th1 type.

Additonal data in favor of the protective effects of induction of Th2 cells in EAE was derived from studies in which rats were treated with the encephalitogenic peptide of MBP covalently coupled to monoclonal anti-IgD antibody to target the autoantigen to B cells (111). Animals immunized by this protocol were resistant to the induction of EAE on concomitant challenge with MBP in CFA,

and leukocyte infiltration into the CNS was not observed. Nonresponsiveness was not induced, as *in vitro* stimulation of lymphocytes from nodes draining the site of challenge with MBP showed that such cells from anti-IgD peptide–pretreated donors proliferated as well to MBP as those from control rats, and anti-MBP antibody titers were readily detectable. The most likely explanation for these results was that the presentation of the antigen by B-lymphocytes, which are unable to secrete IL-12, polarized the resultant immune response to the Th2 phenotype. EAE induction was also suppressed when the antibody peptide conjugate was injected intravenously 14 and 7 days before immunization with MBP in adjuvant. T cells from pretreated rats produced consistently less IFN-γ on activation *in vitro,* transferred EAE weakly to naive recipients, and had mRNA levels for IL-4 and IL-13 approximately five to ten times higher than those from controls. The ability of a neutralizing anti-rat IL-4 to attenuate the protective effect of the anti-IgD peptide pretreatment is also consistent with the induction of IL-4–producing Th2 cells by this pretreatment regimen.

Taken together, all of these studies support the view that induction of autoantigen-specific Th2 cells by administration of IL-4, perhaps together with macrophage-deactivating cytokines such as IL-10/IL-13, would be of therapeutic benefit in Th1-mediated autoimmune diseases. However, it should be emphasized that the conclusions drawn from the above studies were largely based on a correlation between positive therapeutic results and evidence for induction of Th2 cells. In a small number of studies, adoptive transfer of autoantigen-specific Th2 or TGF-β–producing cells lines has protected mice from the development of disease (112,113) induced by the transfer of Th1 lines or clones or induced by active immunization. On the other hand, it is somewhat disturbing that in the majority of cell transfer studies using highly polarized autoantigen-specific T-cell lines, therapeutic effects of Th2 populations have been absent. Thus, while highly polarized PLP-specific Th1 cells caused severe EAE on transfer into naive hosts and highly polarized Th2 cells did not transfer disease, no protective effects were seen in cotransfer studies, even at high ratios of Th2 to Th1 cells (114). It remains possible that Th2 cells are much more effective in inhibiting the generation of Th1 cells from naive cells, but they fail to counteract already activated Th1 cells.

Studies of the Th1/Th2 balance in IDDM have led to many of the same conclusions as those derived from the EAE experiments. Although little information is available from studies in humans, the presence of high titers of antibodies to GAD (potentially indicating the involvement of Th2 cytokines) is associated with protection from clinical diabetes in families with autoimmune diabetes, while individuals whose T cells show a strong proliferative response to GAD (potentially indicating Th1 cytokines) have a high risk for developing IDDM (115). Although it is likely that pathogenic Th1 cells play a role in IDDM, cytokine production *in situ* has proven difficult to analyze in NOD mice, and only TNF-α and granzyme A transcripts have been found in the islets using *in situ* hybridization. By reverse-transcriptase–polymerase chain reaction (RT-PCR), T cells producing IFN-γ have been detected just prior to islet graft destruction. T-cell clones that are able to accelerate the onset of diabetes in young NOD mice produce Th1 patterns of cytokines when challenged with islets and APCs *in vitro*. T cells from NOD mice specific for GAD produce large amounts of IFN-γ in response to this protein. Anti–IFN-γ antibodies can prevent the development of diabetes induced in NOD mice either by cyclophosphamide or by adoptive transfer of diabetogenic cells (116). Systemic administration of IL-4 prevented diabetes in NOD females; the develop-

TABLE 11. *The cytokine milieu regulates the priming of autoreactive T cells*

| First Immunization | Disease | | |
	Second Immunization	Incidence	Score
PBS	Myelin/CFA	80	1.5
KLH/IFA	Myelin/CFA	80	1.8
KLH/IFA	Myelin/KLH/CFA	20	0.1

Animals were primed with KLH in IFA or injected with PBS. After 4 weeks, two groups were primed with myelin in CFA, while the third group received KLH with the myelin injection. All animals received pertussis toxin. Disease was evaluated 14 to 16 days after the second immunization.

Adapted from ref. 110.

ment of T-cell subsets was not examined in this study, and the mechanism of IL-4 protection was not determined (117).

One of the best-studied examples of the protective role of Th2 cytokines in IDDM was seen in studies (118) of TCR transgenic mice in which the majority of the CD4$^+$ T cells express a TCR that recognizes a peptide from influenza HA. When these mice were crossed with transgenic mice expressing HA as a neoantigen on their islets cells, the double transgenic mice showed no evidence for clonal deletion or inactivation. Two very distinct phenotypes occurred in double transgenic mice, depending on the genetic background of the strain to which they were backcrossed. On a BALB/c background, double transgenic mice did not develop diabetes, either spontaneously or after immunization with the relevant HA peptide or virus. In contrast, double transgenic mice on a B10.D2 background developed early spontaneous diabetes following a third backcross. The islet infiltrates in these mice were extensive, primarily comprising CD4$^+$ and CD8$^+$ T cells with B cells and dendritic cells. Whereas T cells from the B10.D2 mice secreted high levels of IFN-γ, but low and transient levels of IL-4, BALB/c T cells produced high levels of IFN-γ together with elevated, sustained levels of IL-4. Because the Th2 promoting activities of IL-4 may be dominant over the Th1-promoting cytokines IL-12 and IFN-γ, these data are consistent with a dominant BALB/c genetic predisposition towards Th2 differentiation, which confers resistance to spontaneous IDDM.

Disease in this transgenic model did not require induction with specific antigen or the use of adjuvants. This system demonstrates a dependence on genetic factors present in common inbred mouse strains and not on genes present only in NOD mice. These results emphasize that a common feature of rodent and human disease is that both MHC and non-MHC genes are known to be critical to the development of disease. Furthermore, the genetic effect noted here bears a striking resemblance to the genetic influence over immune responses to infection by the *Leishmania* parasite, in which BALB/c mice develop a predominant Th2 response, while C57BL/6 mice generate a Th1 inflammatory response, resulting in cure of the infection. Thus, while the BALB/c Th2 response may be protective against autoimmunity, it is maladaptive in the case of parasite infection. A similar dependence on non-MHC background genes has been described in autoimmunity induced by neonatal thymectomy (52). Here, susceptibility to a variety of organ-specific autoimmune syndromes was dependent on non-MHC genes in a large number of common inbred mouse strains. The contribution of non-MHC genes to disease susceptibility also parallels the situation in humans; among individuals with permissive a MHC haplotype, a much higher incidence of disease is seen within certain families.

NOD mice fail to express I-E and have a unique I-A β-chain allele, I-A^{g7}. When NOD mice were made transgenic for a normal MHC class II I-A allele, they did not develop diabetes, despite the continued expression of I-A^{g7}, and purified T cells from NOD mice transgenic for I-A^d could prevent the adoptive transfer of diabetes to nontransgenic NOD recipients (119). NOD transgenic mice have been made that have an I-A^{g7} allele that has been mutated at positions 56 and 57 (His-Ser>Pro-Asp) and were found to be protected from insulitis and diabetes (120). T cells from these mice inhibited the adoptive transfer of diabetes. In addition, such T cells failed to proliferate or make IFN-γ in response to β-cell antigens *in vitro*, despite the fact that these mice do contain T cells specific for β-cell antigens. The anti-GAD antibodies from conventional NOD mice are predominantly of the IgG2a subclass, as would be predicted by their T-cell production of IFN-γ in response to GAD; in contrast,

the NOD mice that express the mutant I-A^{g7} allele produced anti-GAD antibodies of the IgG1 and IgE subclasses, which is consistent with the presence of IL-4–producing T cells. In an adoptive transfer system, the prevention of diabetes by T cells from this transgenic was shown to be partially due to T-cell production of IL-4/IL-10. Thus, in this model, it appears that the MHC itself regulates the Th1/Th2 balance to an autoantigen. The mechanism by which the MHC regulates the phenotype of the differentiating T cells is still not clear. In these transgenic NOD mice, the MHC class II transgenes may have acted both intrathymically and extrathymically by influencing the positive selection of regulatory cells and then influencing their expansion. Autoantigen-specific immunoregulatory cells may have low-affinity TCR, which will allow them to escape negative selection in the thymus. These cells in the periphery could then control autoreactive T cells by the mechanism of immune deviation.

Although these studies on the Th1/Th2 balance in IDDM strongly support the concept that Th2 cells are protective, as in EAE, it has been exceedingly difficult to directly demonstrate protection by β cell-specific Th2 cells in adoptive transfer studies. The most insightful experiments were performed by using cells from BDC 2.5 transgenic animals, which express a TCR specific for an unknown islet-cell antigen, and stimulating them in culture under conditions that promote differentiation to Th1 cells or Th2 cells (121). When the disease-inducing capacity of these two populations was tested by adoptive transfer to neonatal NOD mice, the Th1 cells rapidly precipitated diabetes in almost all recipients, while very few of the recipients of the Th2 cells developed diabetes. Both cell types were capable of migrating to the pancreas, as lymphocytic infiltrates were present immediately after transfer in both groups of recipients, but by day 11, all of the islets of the recipients of the Th1 cells exhibited overwhelming insulitis, while the infiltrate in the recipients of the Th2 cells did not progress. The IgG1/IgG2a phenotype of isotype-switched B cells in the islets correlated with the known influence of Th1 and Th2 cytokines on immunoglobulin switching. When cell-mixing experiments were performed, the recipients of a 1:1 mix developed diabetes at a rate identical to that of the recipients of Th1-like cells alone, but when the number of Th1 cells was reduced to a ratio of 1:10, only a slight reduction in the disease was seen. These results provide direct evidence for the role of Th1 subsets in precipitating disease, but they do not support the concept that Th2 cells can mediate protection from disease.

Although cell transfer studies into normal animals have not revealed any role of Th2 cells in inducing organ-specific inflammatory responses, it should be emphasized that the induction of Th2 type immune responses may result in nonprotective immunity against intracellular microorganisms and can promote allergic reactions, raising the possibility that suppression of a DTH type of response in favor of a humoral response may, under certain circumstances, lead to pathologic consequences. Indeed, in an extension of the studies with polarized populations of Th1 and Th2 cells from BDC 2.5 mice, Pakala et al. (122) reported that, in contrast to the results observed when neonatal NOD mice were used as recipients, both Th1- and Th2-polarized T cells could transfer disease to NOD/SCID mice and other immune-deficient recipients (Table 12). The Th2-mediated diabetes in NOD/SCID recipients exhibited a longer prediabetic phase and a lower overall incidence. The lesions produced by the Th2 cells resembled allergic inflammation and contained a large eosinophilic infiltrate, islet necrosis, and abscess, and a severe pancreatitis with a destruction of both exo- and endocrine tissue. In contrast, Th1 cells produced focally confined infiltration

TABLE 12. *Th2 cells induce diabetes in NOD/SCID mice*

Cells transferred	Recipient	Rx	Disease Incidence (%)
Th1	Neonate	—	100
Th2	Neonate	—	0
Th1	NOD/SCID	—	100
Th2	NOD/SCID	—	60
Th2	NOD/SCID	Anti-IL-4	100
Th2	NOD/SCID	Anti-IL-10	20

Naive T cells from BDC 2.5 TCR transgenic mice were stimulated with islet cells under Th1- or Th2-polarizing conditions. The cells were then transferred to neonatal NOD or adult NOD/SCID mice. Some recipients were treated with anti-IL-4 or anti-IL-10. Disease incidence was determined 28 days after transfer.

Adapted from ref. 122.

of the islets and β-cell apoptosis, which spared the exocrine tissue. Anticytokine antibody-blocking studies demonstrated that the Th2-mediated destruction of the islet cells was produced by local IL-10, but not by IL-4. This result parallels the studies using NOD transgenics, which express either IL-4 or IL-10 in the islets where IL-4 expression was protective and IL-10 promoted disease (see upcoming discussion of the cytokine milieu). The precise mechanism whereby IL-10 induces immunopathology is unknown, but it has been postulated that IL-10 may produce changes in the endothelium with migration of inflammatory cells, or it may induce vascular damage, resulting in hypoxia and abscess formation.

A very similar result was observed when the TCR transgenics, which express an anti-MBP Ac1-10 TCR, were induced to differentiate into Th1 and Th2 populations *in vitro* and then transferred to adoptive recipients (57). MBP-specific Th1 cells, but not Th2 cells, were capable of causing EAE upon transfer into normal mice. Th2 cells failed to protect against Th1 cell–mediated EAE, but induced EAE by themselves when transferred to immunocompromised RAG$^{-/-}$ recipients. The appearance of the first clinical signs of EAE was delayed by approximately 10 days in recipients of Th2, as compared with Th1 cells. Although the cytokine responsible for the inflammatory encephalitis in the RAG$^{-/-}$ recipients of Th2 cells was not defined in these studies, an unusually high percentage of polymorphonuclear cells and mast cells was present in the CNS, but this was not the case in RAG$^{-/-}$ mice that had received Th1 cells.

It should also be emphasized that, in some circumstances, organ-specific autoimmunity may normally be a manifestation of a mixed Th1/Th2 pathologic immune response. EAE in the common marmoset, following immunization with MOG, is an example of such mixed pathogenic T-cell and B-cell responses. Indeed, under certain circumstances, the Th2 (or B-cell) component of the disease may actually dominate. Tolerization of marmosets by administration of soluble MOG intraperitoneally (a protocol that can suppress Th1 cells) on days 7 through 18 after administration of antigen in adjuvant resulted in suppression of disease (123). Surprisingly, after cessation of treatment, a rapidly progressive lethal form of hyperacute EAE developed that was more severe than that seen in the immunized controls. Changes were seen in the CNS of the tolerized animals that were consistent with the possibility that the demyelination was humorally mediated. Antibody titers were higher in the tolerized group, and tolerized animals had increased synthesis of IL-10 and IL-6 mRNA in response to stimulation with MOG. The shift from a Th1 to a Th2 pattern of cytokine production in response to MOG was present by day 14 after immunization

in the tolerized animals. It was concluded from these studies that a Th2 response was preferentially magnified by the administration of soluble antigen intraperitoneally and exacerbated autoimmunity by enhancing production of pathogenic autoantibodies.

In summary, all of the studies on the role of the Th1/Th2 balance in organ-specific immunity have suggested that genetic factors that tip this balance toward the Th2 pole have resulted in a reduced incidence or severity of disease. Once a Th1-mediated autoimmune disease has been established, it has been proposed that the induction of immune deviation by administration of exogenous IL-4 (124), the administration of altered peptide antigens (APLs) (see discussion of antigen-specific therapy in the section on immunotherapeutic approaches), or the induction of oral tolerance (see discussion of oral tolerance in the section on immunotherapeutic approaches) may be of therapeutic potential. On the other hand, interest in this therapeutic approach must be tempered by the large number of studies that fail to demonstrate any therapeutic efficacy of potent Th2 cells in cotransfer studies. Furthermore, the studies described above clearly demonstrate that, under certain conditions, Th2 T cells may produce acute pathology and disease. One notable feature of these studies is that, in the intact animal, pathogenic Th2 cells are tightly controlled by immunoregulatory T cells that express the αβ TCR, as Th2 populations have not induced disease in immunologically competent hosts. The nature of this immunoregulatory interaction vis-à-vis Th2 function remains to be be determined, and how the presence of other T cells affect the *in vivo* function of Th2 cells remains to be seen. Caution should be used before the adoption of immune deviation as a therapeutic paradigm in organ-specific autoimmunity. In humans with MS, myelin-specific autoantibodies are also present, and antibody- and complement-mediated damage may occur. In MS, induction of a Th2 response to myelin antigens might promote humoral autoimmunity.

The Cytokine Milieu

As there is little doubt that cytokines can influence the development of Th1/Th2 T-cell populations that mediate and regulate organ-specific autoimmune diseases, attempts have been made using transgenic and knock-out technologies to analyze the contribution of expression of a given cytokine, either at the whole animal level or at the level of the target organ. Overexpression of IL-2 in the pancreas of C57BL/6 mice resulted in a massive inflammatory response directed at pancreatic β cells, as well as destruction of islets, resulting in diabetes; adoptive transfer and islet transplantation demonstrated that β-cell destruction in these IL-2 transgenic mice was not due to antigen-specific immunity, as IL-2 expression in *nu/nu* and SCID mice was also shown to induce an inflammatory response and diabetes (125). Thus, local production of IL-2 in the islets mediated the recruitment and activation of cells capable of destroying islets by a nonantigen-specific mechanism. Nevertheless, these studies raised the possibility that local expression of IL-2 might augment the activity of effector T cells that had been activated by some other means. For example, when triple transgenic mice were created that expressed K^b and an anti-K^b TCR, as well as IL-2 in the pancreatic β cells, all of the mice developed diabetes 1 week after birth (126). The expression of IL-2 by the pancreatic β cells induced a large lymphocytic infiltrate, and a large proportion of the infiltrating cells were clonotype-positive CD8$^+$ cells, which expressed the IL-2R. The anti-K^b–specific T cells that escaped thymus deletion in these animals were of low avidity and were not able to cause islet-cell damage after priming by skin grafting; nevertheless, the rapid onset of islet destruction and diabetes in the triple transgenic mouse indicated that these low-avidity cells could be stimulated to aggression, provided sufficient help was available in the form of IL-2. The occurrence and progression of autoimmunity may depend on the avidity of the self-reactive T cells and may be influenced by exogenous IL-2 that could be provided even in paracrine fashion during the course of a chronic infection. High-avidity cells can produce their own IL-2 and respond independently of CD4$^+$ T-cell help.

Both NOD mice and resistant strains of mice have been used to study the outcome of the local expression of a number of different cytokine genes on the development of diabetes. The prediction that the overexpression of proinflammatory cytokines locally in the pancreas would facilitate the development of autoimmune disease was confirmed, as IFN-γ islet transgenic mice (127) developed massive infiltration of inflammatory cells and total destruction of insulin-secreting cells. When mice were made doubly transgenic for a viral GP from LCMV and IFN-γ, IFN-γ expression in islets abrogated the tolerance and spontaneously induced the development of anti-LCMV CTL, which resulted in insulitis and diabetes (128). Thus, cytokines secreted within target tissues may play critical roles in determining the loss of tolerance to self antigens. Indeed, local expression of IFN γ in pancreatic islets abolished tolerance to islet-cell antigens in a specific manner, because the IFN-γ transgenic mice rejected histocompatible islet grafts, but not pituitary transplants.

These results support the concept that, following viral infection and local cytokine secretion, immune reactivity may undergo dysregulation in specific target tissues of genetically predisposed individuals. Regional factors in a given tissue may also be important. IFN-γ activated T cells, but not antibody responses, when it was expressed in islets; however, when expressed in the motor end plate, it led to development of antibodies to motor end plates and a disease clinically similar to myasthenia gravis (129). Tissue-specific factors may therefore determine the pathogenicity of a local immune response. The local factor could involve making the target cells more visible to the activated immune system. When mice were thymectomized on day 3 of life, they developed autoimmune gastritis, and the target antigen has been shown to be the enzyme H/K adenosine triphosphatase (ATPase), expressed in the gastric parietal cell. When this antigen was expressed in islets and the mice were subjected to thymectomy on day 3, the mice developed gastritis and periinsulitis, but not diabetes. Lack of diabetes in the presence of periinsulitis strongly suggests that the target antigen is presented differently by gastric parietal cells and pancreatic islets cells (130).

Studies on the role of TNF-α in IDDM models initially involved the systemic administration of the cytokine and suggested that the early and late events that occur during the progression to clinical disease in NOD mice are separable and subject to distinct regulatory mechanisms. When TNF-α was administered to adult NOD mice, complete inhibition of the development of IDDM was observed. Although the administration of TNF-α to neonates exacerbated IDDM, it was difficult to determine if TNF-α was acting locally on the disease process in the islets or systemically (131). The early disease-aggravating effects of TNF-α may have been due to the effects of this cytokine on the thymus, with resultant alterations in lymphoid development of the circulating lymphocyte pool. As no infiltration of the pancreas by leukocytes was seen in TNF-α treated adult mice, it is likely that the protective effects could be accounted for by altered homing properties brought about by changes in adhesion capabilities of circulating leukocytes. A

similar pattern was seen when NOD mice were treated with anti–TNF-α; when the antibody was administered for the first 4 weeks of life, the incidence of diabetes in NOD mice was reduced, while administration for 8 weeks increased the incidence of diabetes.

The actions of pro- and antiinflammatory cytokines have been quite unpredictable when expressed individually within tissues in transgenic mice. TNF-α is a potent inflammatory mediator that activates endothelial cells *in vitro* to express a number of leukocyte adhesion molecules, including, E-selectin, VCAM-1, and ICAM-1; it also upregulates MHC class I on islet cells. Expression of TNF-α or TNF-β (LTα) in the resistant C57BL/6 background resulted in massive insulitis, but these mice did not develop diabetes, even after more than 1 year of observation (132). The damage in these mice was restricted to the islets, and included lymphocytic insulitis, endothelial cell alteration, fibrotic reactions, and disorganization of the endocrine cells. The insulitis consisted of CD4$^+$ and CD8$^+$ T cells; no polymorphonuclear infiltration was seen. All of these alterations resemble what is observed in NOD mice. Thus, an inflammatory infiltrate was not sufficient to cause autoimmune disease, and the TNF-α transgenic mice lacked secondary events required to precipitate β-cell damage. Some of these events are likely to be controlled by genes uniquely present in the NOD, particularly the MHC. Overexpression of TNF-α in NOD mice also resulted in massive insulitis, but expression of TNF-α paradoxically protected NOD mice from diabetes (133). The composition of the cellular infiltrate appeared to be the same as in normal NOD mice. Furthermore, splenic cells from TNF-α transgenic animals could not transfer disease into NOD/SCID recipients, but diabetes could be induced in the transgenics when cloned diabetogenic cells or cells from diabetic NOD mice were transferred to these mice, indicating that there was no inhibition of effector-cell functions.

In TNF-α transgenic NOD mice, TNF-α is not expressed in the neonatal period and expression only begins at 7 weeks of age, when infiltration into the islets is first seen. Sensitized autoreactive lymphocytes with the potential to cause diabetes were absent in the transgenic mice. T-cell responses were markedly diminished to GAD and other autoantigens contained in islet-cell extracts, but responses to foreign antigens were normal. It thus appeared that the expression of TNF-α downregulated the response to autoantigens and prevented the development of islet-specific autoaggressive T cells. Although the mechanism by which TNF-α mediated its protective effect in this NOD trangenic model remains unknown, it is possible that the lymphocytes that were recruited to the islets by TNF-α played a protective role, because they encountered islet autoantigens expressed at enhanced levels secondary to the effects of TNF-α on MHC antigen expression. Stimulation of the autoreactive cells under these circumstances might have induced anergy or apoptosis. It is also possible that the protective effects of TNF-α were targeted to the CD8$^+$ cells that initiate this disease; if the CD8$^+$ cells became anergic, they would have been unable to perpetuate the cascade of events that result in recruitment of CD4$^+$ effector cells, which are responsible for mediating the majority of the β-cell destruction. Other effects of TNF-α, such as the local inhibition of antigen presentation or processing, have not been ruled out. Overexpression of IL-6 in islets led to insulitis, but it also protected NOD mice from developing diabetes (134). Increased proliferation of islets as well as ductal and fibroblast cells was also seen in IL-6 islet transgenics and was probably secondary to the role of IL-6 in tissue repair. The protective effects of

TNF-α were much more pronounced than those of IL-6, which were only two- to threefold.

Expression of the antiinflammatory Th2 cytokine, IL-4, in NOD islets cells completely protected the mice from developing either insulitis or overt diabetes (135). IL-4 transgenic NOD mice still developed sialitis in their submandibular glands, indicating that IL-4 induced a local immunosuppressive effect in the pancreas, but not a generalized immunosuppression. Evidence of functional tolerance induction was also seen, because, when islets from young NOD mice were grafted under the kidney capsule of 10- to 11-month-old NOD/IL-4 mice, the grafts remained completely free of infiltrating inflammatory cells. When 8- to 10-week-old sublethally irradiated NOD/IL-4 mice and their nontransgenic littermates were injected with splenocytes from acutely diabetic mice, the NOD/IL-4 mice developed only periinsulitis and not diabetes, while the controls had massive inflammatory infiltrates and severe diabetes. Thus, the diabetogenic spleen cells were able to home to the NOD/IL-4 islets, but they were unable to initiate a destructive autoimmune attack. When NOD/IL-4 islets were grafted into diabetic recipients, the grafted islets were destroyed. NOD/IL-4 mice remained at the periinsulitis stage for their entire lives. In contrast to the TNF-α transgenics, splenocytes from the IL-4 transgenic mice responded to islet antigens. IL-4 may have regulatory capability during both the initial and ongoing phases of the disease process, while TNF-α blocks disease initiation. Although these results suggest that Th2-type cytokines such as IL-4 can prevent the development of an autoreactive immune response and destruction of islets, no evidence of skewing CD4+ T cells to develop into inhibitory Th2 cells was seen and GAD-specific Th2 cells could not be detected in the NOD/IL-4 mice. T cells from NOD/IL-4 mice did not possess any regulatory activity on cotransfer with splenocytes from diabetic NOD mice into NOD/SCID recipients. Furthermore, when NOD/IL-4 mice were bred to transgenic BDC2.5 mice (which express a transgenic TCR recognizing an unknown islet-cell antigen), limitation of T-cell diversity abrogated the protection by IL-4 (136). Collectively, these studies suggest that the regulatory effect of pancreatic IL-4 was localized to T cells present in the pancreas, but was not manifest systemically. Perhaps, the pancreatic IL-4 acted on APCs such as macrophages, which are required for disease to be manifest. IL-4 exposure could have eliminated the amplification of autoreactive responses and the generation of islet antigen-specific memory effector cells. Such a mechanism would be overwhelmed by the monoclonality of the pathogenic T cells in the BDC2.5 transgenic, but capable of inhibiting the diverse T-cell population within the diabetogenic NOD spleen.

An entirely different result was observed when the other major antiinflammatory Th2 cytokine, IL-10, was expressed in islets (137). Transgenic mice expressing IL-10 in the islets of a nondiabetes-prone strain developed periinsulitis, which never progressed to insulitis and diabetes, while IL-10 transgenic NOD mice rapidly developed diabetes. The expression of IL-10 promoted a Th2-like cytokine pattern, as determined by the level of IL-10 production by the infiltrating cells. Although this study is consistent with the observation that the secretion of IL-10 by Th2 cells can mediate IDDM (122), other genetic factors may also play important roles; for example, transgenic expression of IL-10 in β cells from BALB/c mice leads to peri-islet inflammation that does not progress to insulitis or diabetes.

Although the studies on the transgenic expression of IL-10 suggested that it mediated proinflammatory effects rather than antiinflammatory effects in the pancreas, PLP-specific T-cell clones have been genetically modified so as to express antigen-inducible IL-10 (138). When transferred to normal recipients, such clones prevented the onset of EAE and also had some therapeutic effects in the treatment of EAE after onset of neurologic signs. Similarly, IL-4 has been delivered to the CNS by MBP-specific T-cell clones that had been retrovirally transfected. Animals treated with these clones had a delayed onset and reduced severity of EAE (139). Exogenous IL-4 has also been delivered intraperitoneally to rats with TNBS colitis via a recombinant human type 5 adenovirus vector, with significant improvement of tissue damage and a decrease in IFN-γ levels in the colon (140). It is likely that future studies will validate the therapeutic potential of cellular or viral delivery of suppressive cytokines to sites of autoimmune inflammation.

Studies of mice genetically deficient in one of the proinflammatory or antiinflammatory cytokines have also proven to be very instructive in the analysis of the immunopathogenesis of both IDDM and EAE. IFN-γ$^{-/-}$ NOD mice do develop diabetes, although there is an increase in the time it takes to develop diabetes and a slight reduction in the percentage of mice that become diabetic (141). There were no obvious differences in the appearance of the islet infiltrates in the islets of IFN-γ$^{-/-}$ and IFN-γ$^{+/+}$ mice. There was a small decrease in the expression of TNF-α in the -/- mice. Both IL-4 and IL-10 were present in the +/+ mice, but were markedly reduced in the -/- mice. IL-2 was not detectable in the -/- mice, but was present in the +/+. Splenocytes from both types of mice could transfer disease to young +/+ mice with the same efficiency. In contrast to the studies in NOD mice, IDDM did not occur in IFN-γ$^{-/-}$ RIP-LCMV transgenic mice following infection with LCMV (142). Antiviral CTL trafficked to the pancreas and were found around the islets, but neither infiltration into the islets nor upregulation of MHC class I or class II molecules occurred. IFN-γ also was not necessary for clearance of acute LCMV infection *in vivo*. The failure of these mice to develop IDDM was probably secondary to the lack of upregulation of class I molecules on β cells and class II molecules on APCs. As a consequence, there was a lack of antigen presentation, and functional CTLs were not retained in the islets.

Although mice have not yet been generated that express cytokines locally in the CNS, which would faciliate the execution of studies similar to those reported in experimental models of IDDM, alteration in the systemic expression of cytokines, believed to be important in the pathogenesis of EAE, has yielded paradoxical results with respect to clinical outcome (Table 13). For example, the injection of neutralizing antibodies to IFN-γ exacerbated disease in several studies, and administration of IFN-γ has repeatedly been found to have a protective effect (143,144). EAE can easily be induced in IFN-γ$^{-/-}$ and IFN-γ–receptor$^{-/-}$ mice and is frequently more severe in the deficient mice than in the wild-type

TABLE 13. *EAE in cytokine-deficient mice*

Deficient gene	Antigen	Disease susceptibility
IFN-γ	MBP	Increased
IL-10	MBP	Increased
IL-4	MBP	Unchanged
IL-12	MBP	Decreased
TNFα	MOG	Increased
TNFα/LTα	Spinal Cord	Unchanged
LTα	MOG	Decreased
LTβ	MOG	Unchanged

Adapted from refs. 38, 143–150.

animals (145,146). These results suggest that IFN-γ can actually act to suppress the development of EAE, probably during the evolution of encephalitogenic effector cells. Surprisingly, IL-12$^{-/-}$ mice were resistant to EAE, and treatment of both IFN-γ$^{-/-}$ and IFN-γ$^{+/+}$ mice with anti–IL-12 prevented EAE. Thus, IL-12 appears to be indispensable for the clinical manifestations of EAE (38).

The simple application of the Th1/Th2 paradigm to EAE is also brought into question by the successful induction of disease in mice doubly deficient of the two other Th1 cytokines, TNF-α and LTα (147), and by the failure to induce a more severe form of EAE in IL-4$^{-/-}$ mice in comparison to wild-type counterparts (148). IL-10$^{-/-}$ mice have been shown to have enhanced susceptibility. It thus appears that the absence of one or more of the proinflammatory cytokines can compensate for the absence of another in disease pathogenesis. In certain situations, this redundancy may not operate, as LTα$^{-/-}$ mice have been reported to be resistant to EAE following immunization with a peptide derived from MOG, while LTβ$^{-/-}$ mice were susceptible (149). Curiously, mice deficient in TNF-α have an enhanced susceptibiity to MOG-induced EAE, and treatment of both TNF-α$^{-/-}$ and TNFα$^{+/+}$ mice with TNF-α reduced the severity of disease (150). The paradoxical enhancement of EAE in the absence of IFN-γ or TNF-α strongly suggests that some of the pleotropic effects of these proinflammatory cytokines are actually antiinflammatory.

Although much effort hase been focused on the role of cytokines in the pathogenesis of organ-specific autoimmune disease, any effector mechanism has to account for the extreme specificity of the disease process that leads to injury and/or elimination of target cells (e.g., islet β cells), but spares other cell types present in the pancreatic islets. Studies of effector mechanisms have focused on perforin-mediated cell lysis and Fas/Fas ligand (FasL)–dependent killing. In the RIP/LCMV model, the disease process seen upon infection with LCMV is dependent on the release of perforin, because RIP/LCMV transgenic mice with a disrupted perforin gene were unable to develop IDDM after LCMV infection (151). It should be noted that in perforin-competent, but IFN-γ–deficient, RIP/LCMV transgenic mice, IDDM also does not occur (142), despite the generation of high-affinity autoreactive CTLs. It is likely that IFN-γ is needed to mediate the MHC upregulation required for CTL-mediated killing. Other mechanisms, such as cytokines or Fas-dependent cytotoxicity, were not efficient enough to fully compensate for the lack of perforin-dependent cytotoxicity. Perforin-dependent mechanisms were most important in the late effector phase of the disease process and not in the early induction phase, as insulitis was present in recipients of perforin-deficient spleen cells. A role for perforin in β-cell death is suggested by the marked rise in perforin expression in CD8$^+$ T cells immediately preceding hyperglycemia following adoptive transfer of spleen cells from diabetic to young nondiabetic NOD mice.

CD95 (Fas) and its ligand (CD95L) are members of the TNF–nerve growth factor receptor and TNF family of proteins. The role of these molecules in the regulation of systemic autoimmune disease in lpr and gld mice is discussed in Chapter 33. The results of the studies on the perforin-deficient mice strongly suggested that the destruction of pancreatic β cells by CD8$^+$ T cells was mediated by direct recognition of a target on the β cells, and this necessitated T cell–β cell contact; it is also possible that the mere proximity of activated T cells to β cells led to their death. CD4$^+$ T cells recognize antigens shed from β cells that have been damaged by CD8$^+$ cells. Activated CD4$^+$ T cells might then kill the bystander β cells through Fas/FasL-mediated cell death, through the production

of soluble cytotoxic mediators, or by the activation of cytocidal macrophages. Although the expression of FasL by β cells might lead to the destruction of activated autoreactive Fas-expressing T cells, and thus protect the islets, FasL transgenic animals showed higher rates of diabetes and were more sensitive to diabetogenic T cells than were their nontransgenic lettermates (152). Conversely, NOD$^{lpr/lpr}$ mice were found to be resistant to the development of diabetes at the end of a 25-week observation period, while Fas-sufficient animals showed greater than 75% incidence. Fas expression on β cells was found to be upregulated at 12 weeks of age, the check point for the development of diabetes in NOD mice. If such Fas-expressing islets also express FasL, β cells would be destroyed by suicide or fratricide. It is likely that IFN-γ produced by either CD4$^+$ or CD8$^+$ T cells may be involved in upregulation of Fas on β cells. Similar results were observed in EAE (153,154). As in the NOD mouse, it was originally assumed that CD95L expressed in the CNS might prevent autoreactive cells from mediating damage, and the lpr and gld mutations might lead to an exacerbation of disease. Exactly the opposite was observed, as either mutation dramatically ameliorated clinical signs of EAE without affecting the development of a Th1 response or inflammatory cell infiltration into the CNS. Apoptotic cell death in the CNS was also diminished. It was hypothesized from these studies that CD95L expressed in activated CD4$^+$ T cells mediated bystander lysis of oligodendrocytes expressing CD95. Although CD95 mRNA was not expressed in normal tissues, it may be induced by inflammatory cytokines such as TNF-α and IFN-γ. Alternatively, as in the IDDM model, death of CNS cells may result from the suicide of FasL-positive CNS cells following the induction of Fas. Taken together, these studies strongly support the view that the Fas/FasL interaction is critically important in the induction or progression of organ-specific injury in autoimmunity. It is also apparent from these studies that multiple overlapping pathways are operative during the initiation, progression, and final effector phases of organ-specific autoimmunity.

The Role of Costimulation in the Activation and Inactivation of Autoreactive T Cells

Studies on the requirements for activation of normal CD4$^+$ T cells have demonstrated a critical requirement for two signals: Signal 1 is delivered through the TCR; signal 2 results from the delivery of costimulation (see Chapter 20). In vitro studies have demonstrated that delivery of signal 1 in the absence of signal 2 results in T-cell nonresponsiveness or anergy. Because costimulation appears to be pivotal in determining whether recognition of antigen by T cells leads to T-cell activation or to anergy, a role for costimulation in the development of autoimmune responses has been hypothesized. Although the studies in transgenic mouse models have offered strong support to the concept of T-cell ignorance, an alternative hypothesis is that the recognition of autoantigens on resting tissue APCs in the absence of costimulatory molecules results in the induction and maintenannce of T-cell tolerance to self antigens. Conversely, the aberrant expression of costimulators on APCs could activate self-reactive T cells, resulting in autoimmunity (155).

Transgenic studies have provided a way to test the hyothesis that peripheral tolerance is due to antigen presentation in the absence of costimulation. To assess the importance of absence of costimulation in the induction of peripheral tolerance, transgenic mice (non–diabetes susceptible) that specifically expressed B7-1

(CD80) on the islets of Langerhans were generated (156). Following expression of B7-1, pancreatic β cells became immunogenic to T cells *in vivo* and *in vitro*, but the transgenic mice expressing B7-1 on islets rarely became diabetic. It remained possible that a major additional factor was required for induction of autoimmunity and that local inflammation was needed to enhance the recruitment of lymphocytes to nonlymphoid tissues. Although TNF-α trangenic mice developed a massive islet infiltration, they did not develop diabetes (157). Double transgenic mice that expressed both B7-1 and TNF-α on their islets (158) rapidly developed tissue destruction and diabetes. Thus, neither costimulation alone nor recruitment of T cells to the tissues alone was sufficient to lead to autoimmunity, but the recruitment of the T cells into a tissue that had the capacity to trigger the expansion and activation of the autoreactive T cells was sufficient to lead to autoimmunity. It seems reasonable to assume that the local expression of TNF-α substituted for a natural initiating event, such as viral infection, in generating local inflammation. These results are most compatible with the view that tolerance to peripheral antigens results from immunologic ignorance rather than specific unresponsiveness. Because naive autoreactive T cells have limited access to nonlymphoid tissues, it is very unlikely that they would be rendered anergic by their recognition of tissue-specific antigens in the absence of a costimulatory signal.

Studies in the transgenic model of IDDM have clearly shown that a critical number of actitvated autoreactive CTLs is needed to induce disease. One pathway for the expansion of a low number of precursors of autoreactive T cells would be to provide a costimulatory signal for T-cell proliferation at the site of antigen recognition. Viral transgenes alone or B7-1 expression alone in the islets did not result in IDDM. In the double transgenic mice that expressed both the costimulatory molecule, B7-1, and LCMV-GP in the β cells, anti-self CTLs were activated without viral infection, and spontaneous IDDM developed (159). Furthermore, double transgenic mice expressing RIP/GP and RIP/B7-1 developed insulitis and diabetes after infection with VAC/GP, which was not observed in the RIP/GP-alone mice following infection with VAC/GP. In this model, it was also possible to reverse the state of T-cell ignorance by enhancing the trafficking of autoreactive cells to the target organ following the induction of a local inflammatory response. RIP/TNF-α and RIP/TNF-αXRIP/GP mice developed severe insulitis, but not diabetes; when infected with VAC/GP, the TNF-αXRIP/GP mice developed diabetes. The local secretion of TNF-α may have enhanced lymphocyte traffic and increased levels of local MHC antigen expression. Thus, when the frequency of autoreactive T cells is low, IDDM does not develop unless other factors are provided in the local milieu of the target organ.

Although little support has been obtained for the concept that autoreactive T cells are rendered anergic secondary to recognition of autoantigen in the absence of costimulation, a radically different view of the role of costimulatory molecules in controlling autoreactivity has emerged from studies of the differential functions of the CD28 molecule and the CTLA4 molecule in promoting and inhibiting T-cell activation, respectively (160). Direct evidence for a critical physiologic role for CTLA4 in negtively regulating T-cell activation and autoreactivity has been derived from the phenotype of mice lacking CTLA4 (161). These mice rapidly developed a spontaneous lymphoproliferative disease with massive lymphocytic infiltrates and tissue destruction in many organs. Myocarditis was particularly severe, and mice died by 3 to 4 weeks of age. They exhibited splenomegaly, lymphadenopathy, and elevated serum immunoglobulin. The peripheral T cells from these mice were acti-

vated, proliferated spontaneously *in vitro,* and produced abundant cytokines. This phenotype of the CTLA4 knock-out mouse has provided the first formal proof that dysregulation of costimulation can lead to activated T cells that mediate lethal tissue injury. These studies suggest that costimulation plays an essential role in maintaining tolerance to self antigens, and that negative signaling via CTLA4 plays an active role in downregulating autoreactive T cells. Indeed, anergy to certain autoantigens may be induced by engagement of CTLA4 during the process of antigen recognition on certain APCs; a failure of delivery of this downregulatory signal might then result in autoimmunity (162,163).

Even though the role of costimulatory molecules in inducing and/or maintaining the T cell–tolerant state remains to be further defined, there is little doubt that, following activation, the expansion of antigen-specific T cells is highly dependent on the delivery of costimulatory signals. A number of studies in animal models have been focused on the inhibition of the delivery of costimulation as a therapeutic approach to organ-specific autoimmunity. The soluble form of CTLA4 as an immunoglobulin fusion protein reacts with both B7-1 and B7-2 (CD86) and can prevent the interaction of these costimulatory molecules with both CD28 and CTLA4. Repeated injection of CTLA4 immunoglobulin (CTLA4Ig) prevented the induction of EAE in the active model with pertussis (164). However, PLP-primed cells from animals treated with CTLA4Ig, when activated in culture with PLP peptide, transferred typical EAE when given to naive recipients. It thus appears that administration of CTLA4Ig does not inhibit priming, and that pathogenic memory T cells can still be expanded from these animals by *in vitro* culture. The adoptive transfer model of EAE affords the ability to distinguish mechanisms involved in the loss of T-cell tolerance to MBP from those involved in the effector stages that result in inflammatory demyelination. The presence of CTLA4Ig during both the immunization and *in vitro* activation stages was most effective in preventing clinical signs of disease (165). This diminution in clinical disease was paralleled by a decreased proliferative response, but not IFN-γ production, after antigenic stimulation of encephalitogenic T cells *in vitro*. In contrast, CTLA4Ig treatment of recipient animals after the transfer of MBP-activated T cells affected neither the disease course nor the severity. The effector stage may be relatively independent of costimulation, as memory cells are less dependent on costimulatory signals. In adoptively transferred EAE, the combined use of anti–B7-1 and anti–B7-2 suppressed disease transfer, while the use of the antibodies individually did not (166). On the other hand, multiple injections of CTLA4Ig resulted in enhanced disease in an active model. The frequent use of CTLA4Ig may result in the use of other costimulatory pathways, or the constant presence of CTLA4Ig may prevent the delivery of a negative signal by B7-1 and B7-2 via CTLA4.

Divergent results have also been observed in the use of CTLA4Ig to treat EAE in the Lewis rat model (167). Systemic administration of CTLA4Ig suppressed clinical disease and was even effective when delayed until day 10 postimmunization, a time when pathologic disease was evident. The protection was not reversed by systemic administration of high-dose IL-2. Immunohistologic studies showed a suppressed inflammatory infiltrate with inhibition of Th1 cytokines, but sparing of Th2 cytokines. It was concluded from this study that blockade by CTLA4Ig led to the failure to expand encephalitogenic Th1 cells, but allowed the emergence of regulatory Th2 cells, which entered the CNS and protected animals against EAE. When rats were hyperimmunized so that they developed fatal EAE with 100% mortality by day 17 postimmunization (168), CTLA4Ig given from days 2 to 18 markedly decreased the incidence and severity of EAE, but delayed treatment with CTLA4Ig, beginning on day 7, did not affect the development of EAE. The protective effect of CTLA4Ig could also be completely reversed by the daily administration of recombinant IL-2 from days 0 to 10. Although blockade of CD28/CTLA4-B7/1B7-2 interactions early in the course of EAE in several models inhibited the initiation phases of disease induction, it appears that costimulatory signals delivered by this pathway are relatively less important for the subsequent effector phases. It is also possible that the delayed injection of CTLA4Ig does not suppress encephalitogenic T cells that have already traversed the BBB.

Costimulation specifically delivered in the local site of inflammation in autoimmune disease may play a role in chronic relapsing disease. In normal mice, B7-2 is expressed primarily on splenic macrophages, B cells, and dendritic cells, while B7-1 expression is not detectable. During the acute and remission phases of EAE, the expression of B7-1 on splenic macrophages and B cells increased, and in the CNS, the expression of B7-1 was markedly upregulated, particularly on infiltrating mononuclear cells (169). Clinical relapses could be decreased if the animals were treated with Fab fragments of anti-B7-1, starting during the recovery phase of the acute episode. Anti–B7-2 antibody administered at the same time had no significant effect on the incidence or severity of clinical relapses when given during remission. Histologic examination of the CNS demonstrated that treatment of the mice with anti-B7-1 Fab fragments decreased both the inflammatory response and demyelination. These results are consistent with a model in which B7-1 may function as a dominant costimulatory molecule involved in the presentation of antigen to EAE effector cells locally in the CNS and in recruiting naive T cells specific for secondary myelin peptides that are exposed during the first clinical episode.

Kuchroo et al. (113) were the first to suggest that the B7-1 and B7-2 molecules might activate different T helper cell pathways and in this way modulate autoimmune disease. Treatment of animals with EAE with anti–B7-1 reduced the incidence of disease, while anti–B7-2 increased the severity of disease. Neither antibody affected the priming of the T cells, but they appeared to modify the patterns of cytokines induced. Prevention of the initial secretion of IL-4 abrogated the protective effect of anti–B7-1. These studies were interpreted as demonstrating that B7-1 preferentially acted as a selective costimulatory molecule for the generation of Th1 cells, while B7-2 costimulated and induced Th2 cells. Thus, blocking B7-1 will inhibit the generation of Th1 cells, while enhancing the generation of Th2 cells; blocking B7-2 will have the opposite effect. Very few data have been obtained from other autoimmune disease models or from the study of the activation of antigen-specific Th1/Th2 cells specific for foreign antigens to support this hypothesis. It is quite possible that the anti-B7 antibodies cross-linked their target antigens on the surface of T cells, macrophages, and dendritic cells, which resulted in the production of specific cytokines (e.g., IL-12), and these changes in the cytokine milieu in the microenvironment resulted in polarization of Th-cell responses. Alternatively, anti–B7-1 and anti–B7-2 may differentially inhibit the interactions of their target ligands with CD28 or CTLA4 and thereby affect the overall strength of the autoreactive response.

The role of CD28/CTLA4 has also been examined in NOD mice (170). Female NOD mice treated at the onset of insulitis (2 to 4 weeks of age) with CTLA4Ig or anti–B7-2 did not develop diabetes. Although these reagents blocked the development of diabetes, they had little effect on the development or severity of insuli-

tis, and neither of these treatments altered the disease process when administered late (more than 10 weeks). In contrast, treatment with anti–B7-1 significantly accelerated disease in female mice and induced diabetes in normally resistant male mice. Treatment with anti–B7-1 resulted in a more rapid and severe infiltrate, and T cells isolated from the pancreases of mice treated with anti–B7-1 exhibited a more activated phenotype than did T cells isolated from other treatment groups. The effect of anti–B7-1 was dominant, as treatment of the animals with a combination of anti–B7-1 and anti–B7-2 also resulted in an acceleration of disease onset. The role of CD28-B7-1/B7-2 interactions in the development of diabetes has also been addressed by breeding the NOD mouse to mice that express CTLA4Ig driven by a skin-specific promoter, resulting in the expression 10- to 30-μ per ml soluble CTLA4Ig in the serum (171). This mouse displayed a more rapid onset, higher penetrance, and severity of diabetes than did littermate controls.

The role of CTLA4 in preventing the activation of autoreactive T cells was directly studied by using an anti-CTLA4 mAb (172). In the active disease model of EAE, a single injection of anti-CTLA4 on day 2 postimmunization resulted in enhanced disease. When CTLA4 blockade was delayed until after the onset of clinical symptoms, disease was markedly exacerbated. CTLA4 blockade also increased the production of proinflammatory cytokines, and some of the recipient mice died. Treatment of mice with a single injection of anti–B7-1 on day 2 postimmunization also resulted in exacerbation of disease, presumably by preventing downregulation of the immune response through CTLA4. Results very similar to these were also observed by Karandikar et al. (173). Anti-CTLA4 mAbs or their Fab fragments enhanced in vitro proliferation and proinflammatory cytokine production by PLP-primed T cells. Addition of either reagent to in vitro activation cultures potentiated the ability of T cells to adoptively transfer disease to naive recipients. In vivo administration of anti-CTLA4 mAb to recipients of PLP-specific T cells resulted in an accelerated and exacerbated disease.

Taken together, these studies demonstrate that inhibition of the interaction of B7-1/B7-2 with their receptors CD28 and CTLA4 can have complex effects on the ultimate manifestations of autoimmune diseases. Prevention of clonal expansion of autoreactive effectors with resultant inhibition of the clinical signs of disease can occur under certain conditions, particularly during disease initiation. CTLA4 has emerged as the major negative regulator of autoimmune T-cell functions both in vivo and in vitro. Blockade of CTLA4 interactions with its ligands results in enhancement of every T cell–effector function studied, with the final effects being an enhanced ability to maintain ongoing autoimmune disease and a greater incidence and severity of relapses. CTLA4-mediated inhibitory functions may be important both during the initial activation of autoreactive T cells, when they express low levels of CTLA4, and following clonal expansion, when activated T cells express higher levels of CTLA4. The enhancement of diabetes in the NOD model by anti–B7-1 or by the continuous presence of CTLA4Ig blockade may reflect the role of B7-1 early in the disease process in engaging CTLA4. Use of CD28 antagonists as therapeutic agents to treat organ-specific autoimmune diseases should be approached with considerable caution. Inhibition of this costimulatory pathway may result in distinct outcomes, depending on the stage of disease, relative expression of CD28/CTLA4 and their ligands during a given response, and perhaps the genetic predisposition of a strain toward the development of Th1 and Th2 responses.

Although little direct information is available on the contribution of the CD28/CTLA4 antigens and their ligands to autoimmune disease in humans, the expression of the costimulatory molecules CD80 and CD86 has been studied in MS lesions by RT-PCR and immunocytochemistry (174). Increased expression of CD80 was observed in acute MS plaques, but not in inflammatory infarcts. CD80 staining was localized predominantly to the lymphocytes in perivenular inflammatory cuffs, but not the parenchyma. CD86 was expressed predominantly on macrophages, both in MS lesions of varied age and in inflammatory infarcts. CD86 expression was clearly not specific for MS plaques and was seen in nonautoimmune and viral-mediated inflammation. Even the upregulation of CD80 expression could also be a secondary event due to a CNS virus infection and need not be indicative of autoimmune pathogenesis.

IMMUNOTHERAPEUTIC APPROACHES TO ORGAN-SPECIFIC AUTOIMMUNITY

Antigen-specific Therapy

A major goal in the treatment of autoimmune disease is the establishment of therapeutic modalities that selectively target the pathogenic T cells, leaving the remainder of the immune system intact. Ideally, such therapy should be effective when it is initiated after the onset of the disease. Systemic administration of soluble protein antigens was shown in the 1950s and 1960s to inhibit the subsequent immune response to that antigen and has been shown to induce effective antigen-specific T-cell tolerance (175). Insulin administered prior to the onset of diabetes can delay or prevent disease in NOD mice (176), and it appears that this is secondary to the immunologic rather than the metabolic effects of the hormone (177). Clonal anergy is one mechanism associated with T-cell unresponsiveness induced by systemic injection of antigen; the refractory state exhibited by T cells may also be the consequence of reduced levels of TCR and CD4/CD8. T-cell hyporesponsiveness can be reversed *in vivo* in the absence of antigen, suggesting that the continuous presence of antigen is necessary to maintain a state of anergy. The induction of clonal anergy might be effective when the inciting autoantigen is known, and would prevent determinant spreading only if administered early during the course of the disease. A combination of antigens might be needed in most human diseases.

A second mechanism by which systemic administration of antigen can modulate autoimmune disease is by the induction of apoptosis, which may be mediated by both FAS/FAS-L and TNF-dependent pathways. In an adoptive transfer model of EAE, repeated high intravenous injections of large doses of MBP or the MBP peptide Ac1-11 prevented disease; the T cells activated prior to transfer appeared to undergo clonal deletion on encounter with antigen in the adoptive recipient (178). Application of this model to humans may prove difficult, as it may be necessary to maintain the duration of the tolerogenic effect for a long period. It is also possible that systemic administration of autoantigen could enhance autoreactive T-cell responses (see later discussion of oral tolerance) or could activate CD4$^+$ and CD8$^+$ T cells to produce proinflammatory cytokines.

Exposure to high concentrations of antigen may also result in immune deviation. The conditions that lead to anergy or deletion of Th1 cells tend to promote activation of Th2 cells (179). Treatment of young NOD mice at an age prior to islet inflammation with the β-cell antigens GAD-65, GAD-67, insulin, and HSP 60 can effectively prevent disease. For example, treatment of female NOD mice with soluble GAD-65 as late as 12 weeks of age, when they exhibited islet-cell infiltration and maximum T- and B-cell anti–β-cell

responses, led to protection from diabetes and suppression of the progression of islet infiltration; this effect was probably mediated by Th2 cells (13). Again, it should be emphasized that the induction of an autoantigen-specific Th2 response may have unwarrented side effects, particularly when some of the effector mechanisms in the disease process may involve autoantibodies (see later discussion of oral tolerance). It may be possible to circumvent B-cell responses by the use of specific peptides rather than intact antigens, but peptides have a short half-life, which would require the development of a continuous delivery system.

Studies over the past five to ten years have attempted to design rational therapeutic strategies for the systemic administration of antigen based on the specific interaction between the TCRs and peptides bound to MHC molecules. Blocking of the antigen-presenting function of MHC by peptides capable of high-affinity binding to this molecule has been proposed as a potential immunotherapeutic intervention in MHC-linked diseases. The first description of peptide-induced inhibition of EAE in PL/J mice used an inhibitor peptide identical in sequence to the encephalitogenic peptide, with the exception of an Ala-for-Lys substitution at position 4 of the MBP Ac1-11 peptide. This endowed the molecule with an enhancement in binding affinity to the MHC-restricting element I-A^u, which enabled it to effectively compete with the encephalitogen for binding and presumably prevented disease induction (180). When the minimal structural requirements of MBP peptide Ac1-11 for interaction with I-A^u and with TCRs were examined, substitution with alanines at all but five amino acids in the MBP peptide did not alter its ability to bind MHC class II, to stimulate specific T cells, or to induce EAE (181). Most other amino acid side chains were essentially irrelevant for T-cell stimulation and for disease induction. Binding to I-A^u occurred with a peptide that consisted mainly of alanines with only three of the original residues of Ac1-11. When used as a coimmunogen, this peptide inhibited EAE, presumably by inhibiting the binding of the wild-type peptide to I-A^u. These results suggested that very few amino acids need to interact with MHC class II molecules and with TCRs to initiate specific responses *in vivo* resulting in autoimmune disease. A peptide unrelated to the immunizing peptide can fulfill this requirement as long as the peptide contains the critical MHC and TCR contact residues. This finding also favors the concept of molecular mimicry, as a pathogen that expresses an epitope with limited homology to self at a few amino acid residues may trigger autoimmune disease.

Inhibition of MHC binding by peptides in these studies required a detailed knowledge of the autoantigen and used inhibitor peptides that bore a close structural relationship to the encephalitogenic peptide; the use of highly related peptides raised the possibility that disease inhibition may also be occurring through an antigen-specific rather than an MHC-specific regulatory mechanism. Antigen competition for MHC binding by a peptide unrelated to the autoantigen has been used as an approach for the treatment of EAE in the Lewis rat (182). Induction of EAE in Lewis rats was inhibited by coimmunization with whole MBP and ovalbumin. As both of these peptides may be immunogenic, it remains possible that the peptides may inhibit disease by other mechanisms, such as the induction of tolerance or clonal immunodominance. The ideal peptide should be nonimmunogenic and should have a high affinity for the MHC allele. Inhibition of *in vivo* responses under these conditions would support the argument that MHC class II binding by the inhibitor is critical for suppression of disease. The peptide OVA 323–339 bound to I-A^u, but failed to initiate T-cell responses *in vivo*. More importantly, it inhibited EAE in (PL/JXSJL)F1 mice when administered as a coimmunogen with Ac1-9. Thus, MHC class II binding alone can modulate the induction of EAE. Inhibition of T-cell activation *in vitro* has also been used to identify antagonist peptides from a large panel of unrelated peptides (183). Peptides were also selected because they were relatively resistant to the proteolytic enzymes present in serum. One such peptide was effective in reducing the induction of EAE when administered together with, or separately from, PLP 139–151. Disease inhibition in this model was transient, leaving the animals susceptible to disease arising from a subsequent injection of PLP 139–151.

A peptide capable of blocking presentation of antigen by the NOD class II molecule, I-A^{g7}, was also identified by inhibition of antigen presentation to a T-cell hybridoma derived from an NOD mouse (184). This peptide was used for chronic treatment of young prediabetic NOD mice, beginning at the the age of 3 to 4 weeks, prior to the development of insulitis, continuing five times per week for 3 weeks, and then twice per week until 22 to 23 weeks (Table 14). The onset of diabetes was delayed, and the frequency of diabetic animals did not exceed 16% for the entire period of treatment (control group 60% diabetic by 22 weeks of age). The data demonstrated that MHC blockade may not permanently suppress disease, because manifestations of disease returned after cessation of treatment. In humans, a continuous treatment protocol may be necessary, or treatment may have to be administered repeatedly during clinical relapses in diseases such as MS. An important observation in this study was that peptides, although not immunogenic when admininstered short-term in soluble form, did induce antibody production with serious side effects (symptoms of immediate hypersensitivity) in a fraction of animals under long-term treatment. The development of antibodies to the therapeutic peptides may represent a major difficulty with their long-term use in humans. Although nonimmunogenic peptides with high affinity for the disease-linked MHC molecules may still represent potential immunotherapeutic agents for human autoimmune disease, the pharmacologic application of this strategy will likely require the development of small nonpeptidic MHC-blocking molecules.

Another problem with the use of MHC-blocking peptides has been that it has proven difficult to directly demonstrate that the mechanism of their disease-inhibiting effects is actually secondary to MHC blockade. When an I-A^{g7}–binding peptide was administered intraperitonally in incomplete adjuvant at the time of transfer of diabetogenic T cells, it markedly inhibited the development of disease (185). When tolerance to the peptide was first induced by intravenous injection before administration of the same peptide in incomplete adjuvant, the induction of tolerance abolished the therapeutic effect on diabetes cell transfer seen in the nontolerant mice. It is likely that the blocking effects seen in initial experiments in the NOD mouse were not caused by blockade of MHC presenta-

tion, but by other unknown effects related to the immunogenicity of the blocking peptide.

Because of the practical and theoretical problems with the design of pure nonimmunogenic MHC-blocking peptides, more recent approaches have focused on modifications of the residues within an antigenic peptide involved in the interaction with the TCR (186). Such an approach can yield peptides that strongly and specifically inhibit T-cell function. These so-called TCR antagonist peptides have been proposed as specific therapies for inhibiting organ-specific autoimmune diseases. The feasibility of using TCR antagonists to treat PLP-induced EAE in SJL mice has been extensively studied (187). Residue W144 was shown to be critical for TCR binding, because substitutions at this residue led to complete loss of antigenicity for several T-cell clones. Nonantigenic peptides that still retained good I-A^s–binding capacity were tested for TCR antagonism. Most peptides were antagonistic for at least one T-cell clone, but no peptide could be identified that simultaneously inhibited all of the different T-cell clones. A pool of the most effective inhibitory peptides was therefore used for *in vivo* studies. This pool of TCR antagonist peptides was found to be one to three orders of magnitude more potent than antigen-unrelated MHC-blocking peptides in inhibiting disease, and the pool resulted in effective inhibition at approximately equimolar amounts with the encephalitogenic PLP 139–151 peptide. This finding underlines the extreme potency of antigen analogues as antigen-specific immunomodulators. TCR antagonist peptides were not capable of inhibiting ongoing responses and were only modestly effective when used to preimmunize mice before administration of the encephalitogenic peptide. In general, both antigen and antagonist had to be administered simultaneously and presumably must be presented on the surface of the same APC in order for TCR antagonism to occur. A similar approach was used in the Lewis rat model of EAE induced by MBP peptide 87–99 (188). A number of inhibitory peptide analogues were identified that antagonized the proliferative response of an encephalitogenic line. Moreover, one of these analogues [91K>A] could prevent and reverse EAE. Rats coimmunized with peptide 87 99 and 91K>A downregulated the production of IFN-γ and TNF-α. As the most powerful inhibitory analogue was the peptide with the lowest affinity for binding to the MHC, it was unlikely that inhibition of MHC binding played a major role in the inhibition of disease.

Detailed studies of the individual residues of MBP peptide Ac1-9 that interact with the MHC or TCR (189) demonstrated that residues 3 and 6 define TCR interaction sites, while residues 4 and 5 determine binding to I-A^u (Fig. 1). Delivery of soluble Ac1-9 via the intraperitoneal route was effective in inducing unresponsiveness in adult mice. Peptides with a higher affinity for the MHC had a more profound inhibitory effect on EAE when used to tolerize animals *in vivo* by adminstration in soluble form. The tolerizing protocol also resulted in inhibition of T-cell proliferation as well as IL-2, IL-4, and IFN-γ production. The different peptide analogues

TABLE 14. *Prevention of diabetes in NOD mice with an MHC-blocking peptide*

	Disease Incidence (%)	
Treatment	22 wk	28 wk
Control peptide	60	60
I-A^{g7}-blocking peptide	16	40

NOD mice were treated with a control peptide or an I-A^{g7}-blocking peptide beginning at 3 weeks of age and continuing until 22 weeks of age.
Adapted from ref. 184.

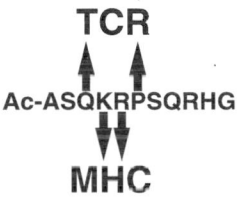

FIG. 1. MHC and TCR contact residues of peptide MBP Ac1-11.

were also shown to be effective in treatment of EAE when administered at the first sign of disease, but peptide treatment was less effective as the disease progressed. The affinity of self antigens for the MHC played an important role in dictating the fate of peripheral autoreactive cells. High-affinity peptides were more likely to induce tolerance, whereas low-affinity peptides allowed autoreactive cells to persist in healthy individuals. The mechanism of action of the high-affinity peptides is not known. It is unlikely that MHC blockade was operative, as a single dose of the highest MHC-binding peptide was even capable of inducing unresponsiveness in primed mice, while MHC blocking peptides primarily function when given at the time of immunization or administered continuously. Anergy and deletion are the most likely mechanisms in this model, as no evidence for immune deviation or induction of suppressor cells was noted.

The same group of high-affinity MHC-binding Ac1-11 peptides was also administered to TCR transgenic mice that express a TCR specific for Ac1-11 restricted to I-A^u (190). In contrast to the lack of an observable effect on T-cell activation when these peptides were injected into normal mice, in the transgenics, T-cell activation and apoptosis in the periphery were seen; the magnitude of the response was positively correlated with the affinity of the peptide for the MHC. A shift in the T helper phenotype of the surviving cells occurred such that the low-affinity peptides induced primarily a Th1 response, whereas the high-affinity peptides induced primarily a Th2 response. These observations raise the possibility that in addition to changing the interaction of the peptide with the MHC, the conformation of the peptide bound to the MHC may also be altered with a secondary change in the affinity of the TCR for the peptide MHC. Such an altered interaction could lead to a qualitatively different T-cell response, which in this case would be enhanced stimulatory capacity and enhanced ability to induce Th2 responses.

Most of the studies described above used peptides that differed in their MHC-binding properties. An alternative approach to define peptides that may alter the differentiation program of autoreactive T cells has been to identify peptides that do not differ in their MHC-binding properties, but only differ in TCR contact residues. The Q144 variant of PLP 139–151 fulfills this criterion. When mice were immunized with this peptide, they did not develop EAE, and coimmunization with the variant peptide and the native peptide reduced the incidence and mean severity of disease (191). Preimmunization with Q144 also resulted in inhibition of disease. T cells from animals immunized with native peptide (W144) proliferated and produced significant amounts of IL-2 and IFN-γ in vitro when stimulated with native peptide, but not Q144. LNC from animals immunized with Q144 proliferated to Q144 or W144 and produced IL-2, IFN-γ, and IL-10, but not IL-4. Short-term T-cell lines from animals immunized with Q144 were transferred to naive mice, which were then immunized with W144 to induce EAE. T-cell lines generated from mice immunized with Q144 and activated in vitro with Q144 conferred some protection from clinical disease, but the greatest protection was seen after transfer of the T-cell lines generated from mice immunized with Q144 and activated in vitro with W144. It appeared that the cells induced with Q144 were cross-reactive and needed to be activated by the W144 to mediate protection. Immunization with the altered peptide induced T cells of a mixed phenotype. In contrast to the other studies, which demonstrated that peptides inhibited disease by binding to the TCR as pharmacologic antagonists without triggering a response, Q144 in this model likely interacted with the TCR and induced changes in the responding cells without evoking a full repertoire of effector

functions. The T cells of mixed phenotype induced by Q144 were less autoaggressive than were the Th1 cells induced by the native peptide. When the Q144-specific T cells cross-reacted with the native peptide in the CNS, they secreted Th2 cytokines on activation. Although it is likely that Th2 cytokines were responsible for the amelioration of disease in this model, it should be emphasized that studies with neutralizing anticytokine antibodies were not performed.

In an attempt to understand the mechanism of inhibition by variant peptides, mice were coimmunized with PLP 139–151 and a variant peptide (L144/R147) with substitutions at TCR contact residues (192,193). The mice were protected from clinical disease, but still developed inflammatory foci within the CNS, which suggested that L144/R147 was not simply inhibiting the development of the PLP 139–151-specific T-cell response. Surprisingly, the L144/R147 peptide also protected animals from EAE induced by another encephalitogenic PLP peptide as well as by the unrelated MBP and MOG peptides. Protection was, therefore, not due to TCR antagonism in vivo. When T cells from animals immunized with L144/R147 were reactivated in vitro with L144/R147 and then transferred to animals that were then immunized with PLP 178–191 to induce disease, the mice that received cells from the L144/R147 animals were protected from disease. Immunization with L144/R147 induced regulatory T cells, which cross-reacted with the native PLP 139–151; transfer of these cross-reactive regulatory T-cell lines could protect against the development of EAE to other unrelated CNS antigens by a process of bystander suppression. T-cell lines and clones specific for L144/R147 frequently cross-reacted with PLP 139–151 and most commonly produced cytokines with a mixed Th1/Th2 phenotype. Engagement of the TCR of naive T cells with a lower avidity peptide may deliver a qualitatively different signal, which is sufficient to alter their differentiation to produce a mixture of Th1 and Th2 cytokines. Brocke et al. (194) successfully treated mice exhibiting paralysis and inflammatory infiltrates in the brain, induced by adoptive transfer of an encephalitogenic T-cell clone specific for MBP peptide 87–99, with a variant peptide (96P>A). Thus, a variant peptide could also be used to treat established EAE. In a second study, EAE was induced by transferring a T-cell line specific for MBP Ac1-11. The same mice were injected with the T-cell clone specific for MBP 87-99 six days later. When the variant peptide 96P>A was then injected, disease was ameliorated (Table 15). The transacting effect depended on the intralesional presence of the T-cell clone that recognized the 96P>A. Reversal of EAE by the variant peptide also depended on production of IL-4, because neutralizing antibodies against IL-4 blocked the therapeutic effect of the APL. As most autoimmune responses are of diverse antigen reactivity, which is further magnified by determinant spreading during the course of the inflammatory response, it is rather unlikely that a therapeutic approach directed to even a predominant T-cell population would prove useful. The demonstration that a peptide antagonist can induce regulatory T cells that are effective in ameliorating disease caused by a structurally unrelated myelin antigen underscores the therapeutic importance of this approach in many different autoimmune diseases.

Attempts have also been made to modulate cytokine secretion by human autoantigen reactive T-cell clones in vitro with variant peptides (195). Stimulation of human T-cell clones that recognize MBP 85–99 with variant peptides substituted at primary TCR contact residues failed to elicit any response, while stimulation with variant peptides substituted at secondary residues induced a switch in

TABLE 15. *Reversal of EAE with a variant peptide*

T cell transferred		Peptide Rx	Disease score	
Day 0	Day 6	Day 11	Day 10	Day 14
MBP Ac1–11	—	PBS	1.5	2.0
MBP Ac1–11	—	MBP 87–89 (96P→A)	1.5	2.0
MBP Ac1–11	MBP 87–89	PBS	2.0	2.5
Mbp Ac1–11	MBP 87–89	MBP 87–89 (96P→A)	2.0	1.2

All groups of mice were injected on day 0 with an anti-MBP Ac1–11 specific T-cell line. Some groups were injected on day 6 with an anti-MBP 87–89 specific T-cell clone. On day 11, following the first cell transfer, mice were treated with PBS or the variant peptide MBP 87–89 (96P→A).
Adapted from ref. 194.

the cytokine pattern from a mixed Th1/Th2 pattern to the TGF-β–secreting phenotype. The molecular mechanisms involved in the switch of cytokine secretion after stimulation of the T-cell clones with variant peptides are not known. Presumably, the qualitatively distinct signal delivered by the variant peptide during engagement of the the TCR leads to alterations in the final cytokine-secretion pattern. TGF-β is a potent downregulator of immune responses and ameliorates EAE (196,197).

T-Cell Receptor–based Immunoregulation

Ben-Nun et al. (198) were the first to demonstrate that T-cell clones that induced EAE in rodents may be used as a vaccine against the induction of EAE. This observation raised the possibility that the relevant antigen responsible for the protective effects of the cellular vaccine might be the TCR itself. The induction of EAE with either MBP or MBP peptides in B10.PL or PL/J mice often leads to a limited Vβ T-cell response, frequently limited to TCR Vβ8.2. In 1989, two groups demonstrated (199,200) that immunization with Vβ8.2 TCR peptides in the Lewis rat model of EAE completely protected the rats from subsequent active induction of EAE. It was later demonstrated that treatment of clinical EAE by vaccination with Vβ8.2 peptides not only prevented the induction of EAE, but also rapidly reversed disease symptoms (201). These studies led to the hypothesis that expansion of the original encephalitogenic T-cell response, mediated by T cells expressing TCR Vβ8.2, generated a counterregulatory immune response against Vβ8.2 T cells, and that this counterregulation could be boosted by Vβ8.2 TCR peptide vaccination to further downregulate the immune response and stop the disease. Indeed, T cells from MBP-immunized rats exhibiting clinical EAE proliferated vigorously to the protective TCR Vβ8.2 peptide, even though they had never been vaccinated with it. Although the response of SJL mice to MBP is characerized by a more heterogeneous TCR Vβ repertoire, including Vβ2, Vβ4, and Vβ17a, SJL mice treated with peptides from Vβ17a and Vβ4 also demonstrated decreased severity of disease and fewer relapses than did control mice.

Kumar and Sercarz (202) have further defined the nature of the immunoregulation induced by TCR-derived peptides in EAE. It is important to note at the outset that the clinical characteristics of the disease induced by MBP Ac1-10 peptide in B10.PL mice strongly suggest an active immunoregulatory process; the course of disease is acute but transitory, and a majority of mice recover permanently from EAE. B10.PL mice recovering from Ac1-9 induced EAE developed a population of T cells that recognized a defined peptide (B5, amino acids 76–101 from the framework region III) of Vβ8.2 in the absence of exogenous TCR peptide immunization (203).

When the anti-TCR Vβ8.2–reactive T cells were cloned and transferred to naive mice that were subsequently challenged with MBP in adjuvant, these mice demonstrated a decreased response to Ac 1-9 *in vitro* and were also protected against EAE *in vivo*. In addition, immunization of B10.PL mice with the Vβ8.2 76–101 peptide suppressed the immune response to Ac1-9 *in vitro* and protected the mice from EAE. The anti-Vβ8.2 T-cell clones predominantly expressed Vβ14 and could be stimulated by fresh spleen cells, suggesting that they recognized endogenously processed TCR peptide.

The Vβ14 T-cell clones specific for B5 were CD4+CD8− and MHC class II–restricted. It was hypothesized that the TCR peptide-reactive CD4+ T cells recognize TCR peptides in the context of MHC class II presented by APCs at the inflammatory sites. The mechanisms by which the regulatory T cells actually suppress disease is unknown. It is possible that they could secrete suppressor cytokines (TGF-β or IL-10), which would act locally on targets at the site of inflammation; alternatively, these cells could recruit CD8+ T cells that specifically recognize peptides from either the native α or β chains of the TCR presented in the context of class I on the surface of the MBP-reactive effector cells. The involvement of CD8+ T cells may explain why CD8-deficient mice have a delayed recovery from EAE (204). To directly demonstrate a role for TCR peptide–specific regulatory T cells in the maintenance of self-tolerance and prevention of disease, (SJLXB10.PL)F1 mice were treated with with mAbs to Vβ chains that are expressed on the regulatory CD4+ T cells. Such treatment resulted in a delayed recovery from acute EAE, and the mice developed chronic EAE. A similar role for regulatory anti-TCR peptide T cells has been demonstrated in collagen-induced arthritis (205). The pathogenic T cells that recognize collagen also express Vβ8.2, and the regulatory T cells also recognize the framework 3 region peptide B5, composed of amino acids 76–101 of the Vβ8.2 chain. Vaccination with TCR peptide B5, before or after immunization with collagen, protected mice from arthritis. The mechanism by which B5-specific T cells mediate protection from CIA is not yet clear, although B5 vaccination does not result in deletion of most Vβ8.2-expressing T cells.

Although these studies collectively suggest that the immune response to the autoantigen is largely regulated by a counterresponse to the predominant TCR, not all groups have been able to reproduce these findings, and significant technical differences exist when comparing all of these studies. It has also been demonstrated that TCR peptide immunization may induce a heterogeneous immune response, which may sometimes worsen disease (206). One of the major assumptions behind these experiments is that the immune response to autoantigens in organ-specific immunty is primarily composed of clonal or oligoclonal T-cell populations. The response of B10.PL mice to the Ac1-10 peptide of MBP clearly is one such an example of a restricted response, but in most other autoimmune diseases in experimental animals and in humans, it has proven difficult to identify a predominant T-cell clone, and in many studies, a clonal bias could not be detected (207).

Oral Tolerance

It has been known for more than 50 years that a state of antigen-specific hyporesponsiveness follows exposure to an orally delivered protein antigen. The gut-associated lymphoid tissue (GALT) has evolved not only to protect the host from ingested pathogens, but also to prevent the host from reacting to ingested proteins. Peyer's patches are interspersed among the villi and are one of the primary areas in the GALT where specific immune responses are generated. Although most dietary antigens are degraded by the time they reach the small intestine, some intact or partially degraded antigen is absorbed into the systemic circulation. Absorbed or processed antigen may be involved in inducing tolerance. Oral tolerance has been found to involve multiple mechanisms and is not a single immunologic event (208,209). The primary mechanisms by which oral tolerance is mediated include deletion, anergy, and active cellular suppression, and some studies suggest that the particular tolerogenic pathway chosen is determined by the dose of fed antigen. Low doses of antigen favor active suppression, and high doses favor deletion or anergy. In the Lewis rat, high doses of oral MBP resulted in clonal anergy, whereas lower doses induced transferable cellular suppression (210). Active suppression is mediated by the induction of regulatory T cells in the GALT, which then migrate to the systemic immune system. The primary mechanism of active cellular suppression is via secretion of suppressive cytokines, such as TGF-β, IL-4, and IL-10, following antigen-specific triggering (211). Priming to antigens in the GALT favors induction of Th2 cells, particularly T cells that secrete TGF-β. TGF-β also serves as a switch factor for IgA production in the mucosa of the gut and may be involved in the homing mechanisms of cells to high endothelial venules. TGF-β produced both by CD4$^+$ and CD8$^+$ GALT-derived T cells is an important mediator of the active suppression component of oral tolerance. Both CD4$^+$ and CD8$^+$ T cells can be generated during the induction or oral tolerance, but oral tolerance can be induced in CD8-deficient mice. In the CNS of low-dose fed animals, inflammatory cytokines such as TNF and IFN-γ are downregulated, while TGF-β is upregulated (106).

Bystander suppression results when regulatory T cells induced by oral antigen secrete cytokines after being triggered by the same antigen in the microenvironment where the antigen is localized. For a human organ-specific inflammatory disease, it is not necessary to know the specific antigen that is the target of an autoimmune response, but only to administer orally an antigen capable of inducing regulatory T cells, which then migrate to the target tissue. Even if MBP is not the target antigen in MS, oral exposure to MBP will trigger MBP-specific T-regulatory cells that will home to the CNS; they will be reactivated there by native MBP, secrete suppressor cytokines, and inhibit inflammatory responses mediated by T cells specific for any CNS autoantigen. Bystander suppression was demonstrated *in vitro* (Table 16) when it was shown that cells from animals fed MBP suppressed proliferation of an OVA-specific cell line across a transwell, but only when triggered by the fed antigen (212). *In vivo* studies (213) have demonstrated that feeding animals

TABLE 16. *Bystander suppression in vitro*

Upper	Lower	% suppression
	Ova line + OVA	0
MBP-Fed	Ova line + OVA	0
MBP-Fed + MBP	Ova line + OVA	51
PBS-Fed + MBP	Ova line + OVA	0
	MBP line + MBP	0
OVA-Fed	MBP line + MBP	6
OVA-Fed + OVA	MBP line + MBP	47
PBS-Fed + OVA	MBP line + MBP	5

MBP-specific or OVA-specific T cell lines were cultured in the lower chamber of a Transwell system in the presence of antigen. Cells from PBS-, OVA-, or MBP-fed donors were placed in the upper chamber and stimulated as indicated. T-cell proliferation was assayed after 72 hours.
Adapted from ref. 212.

MBP protected them from EAE induced by PLP (Table 17). Bystander suppression has been demonstrated in several other autoimmune disease models. In theory, bystander suppression could be used to target antiinflammatory cytokines to an organ where inflammation may play a role in disease pathogenesis, even if the disease is primarily not autoimmune in nature. Oral MBP decreased stroke size in a rat stroke model, presumably by decreasing inflammation associated with ischemic injury (214).

TGF-β has emerged over the past few years as the major downregulatory cytokine in normal immune reactions. The strongest evidence to support its critical role is the observation that animals homozygous for a mutated TGF-β gene succumb at 3 weeks of age to a wasting syndrome accompanied by a multifocal mixed inflammatory cell response and tissue necrosis (75). The potential role of TGF-β as the major mediator of oral tolerance is supported by studies on the use of this cytokine to treat autoimmune diseases. Exogenously administered TGF-β given on days 5 to 9 after immunization with spinal cord in complete Freund's adjuvant (CFA) protects against the development of acute EAE; such mice fail to develop disease, even up to day 48 (196,197). The proliferative responses of myelin-sensitized T cells taken from draining lymph nodes of control and TGF-β–treated mice were the same. This protection was not dependent on an inhibitory influence of exogenously administered TGF-β on the development of myelin protein–sensitized T cells, although cytokine secretion was not examined in these studies. Only a minor lymphoid cell infiltration in the CNS was seen in protected mice, suggesting that the sensitized cells failed to enter or to proliferate in the CNS. Treatment on days 1 to 5 during active sensitization was ineffective, while treatment on days 5 to 9 was most effective. At the time symptoms

TABLE 17. *Bystander suppression in vivo*

Fed Antigen	Clinical Score
Histone	4.0
MBP	1.8
PLP	2.2

Animals were fed histone (control), MBP, or PLP seven times over a 2-week period. All groups were then immunized with PLP to induce EAE. EAE induced by PLP was suppressed by feeding either PLP or MBP.
Adapted from ref. 213.

develop, no protection was afforded by treatment with TGF-β. TGF-β thus appears to inhibit the late induction–effector phase of the immune response rather than the early T cell–induction phase. In acute EAE, anti–TGF-β precipitated and enhanced disease symptoms when given on days 5 to 9 postimmunization, and neutralization later had no effect. Treatment with anti–TGF-β accelerated the appearance and increased the severity of relapses in relapsing EAE. It is not clear which cells are responsible for endogenous TGF-β production. The effect of anti-TNF on active and passive EAE is protective, as opposed to that of anti–TGF-β, and it is likely that endogenous production of TNF-α contributes to the severity of the disease by upregulating adhesion molecules or class II MHC antigens, or by promoting macrophage activation and the production of reactive oxygen and nitrogen intermediates. TGF-β may prevent entry of lymphoid cells to the CNS by antagonizing the effects of TNF-α on endothelial cells and may also inhibit the actions of TNF-α on macrophages.

Initial studies on the induction of regulatory T cells following feeding of antigens used bulk populations of T cells to adoptively transfer suppression. T-cell clones have been isolated from the mesenteric lymph nodes of SJL mice fed MBP (112). These clones were CD4+ and were structurally identical to Th1 encephalitogenic CD4+ clones in TCR usage, MHC restriction, and epitope recognition. Most of these clones produced TGF-β in addition to various amounts of one of the other Th2-type cytokines (IL-4 and IL-10). When SJL mice were immunized with MBP to induce EAE and were simultaneously injected with these mucosally derived clones, each of the clones suppressed EAE. These MBP-specific regulatory clones exerted bystander suppression as they suppressed PLP-induced disease. Treatment with antibodies to TGF-β reversed the bystander suppression induced by one of the clones. It has been proposed that TGF-β–secreting cells are a unique subset, termed *Th3 cells,* with both mucosal T helper function and downregulatory properties for Th1 cells.

Although regulatory populations of T cells have been reproducibly induced by mucosal exposure to antigen, both human and murine alloantigen- or antigen-specific CD4+ T cells with very similar cytokine profiles have been induced *in vitro* by chronic activation in the presence of IL-10 (215). These antigen-specific T-cell clones suppressed the proliferation of CD4+ T cells in response to antigen by secreting IL-10 and/or TGF-β and have been termed *T-regulatory cells* 1 (Tr1). Ovalbumin-specific Tr1 cells prevented the inflammatory bowel disease induced by transfer of CD4/CD45RB^high T cells to SCID mice, but only when the Tr1 cells were stimulated *in vivo* by feeding the mice ovalbumin. The relationship of Tr1 cells, which inhibit responses by an antigen-driven bystander suppression mechanism, to the Th2- or Th3-like cells, which have been seen after oral feeding of antigen, remains to be determined.

One of the problems in studying the regulatory mechanisms responsible for oral tolerance is the heterogenous effector-cell response of the host to the autoantigen, as well as the complex response to orally administered tolerogen. It would be desirable to dissect the initiating (triggering) antiself immune response from the immunosuppressive bystander effect induced by oral tolerization. The role of bystander suppression has been convincingly demonstrated in the transgenic model described in the discussion of transgenic models of organ-specific autoimmunity in the first section of this chapter, in which the viral nucleoprotein of LCMV is expressed in the β cells of the pancreas and in the thymus (216). A slow-onset IDDM developed in more than 95% of transgenic

animals, but not in controls, after challenge with LCMV. Oral treatment with 1 mg of insulin twice per week for 2 months, starting either 1 week before or 10 days after initiating LCMV infection, prevented the induction of IDDM by LCMV infection in more than 50% of the transgenic mice. In this slow-onset (1 to 6 months) IDDM model, high-affinity antiself CTLs are deleted, and CTLs found in the periphery are of low affinity. In the treated mice, the generation of the antiself CTL response was not inhibited. T-cell infiltration of islets occurred in protected mice, but the degree of infiltration was reduced and fewer β cells were destroyed. In the islets of the protected mice, the number of lymphocytes producing IL-4, IL-10, and TGF-β was increased, while in the unprotected mice, a higher proportion of T cells produced IFN-γ. MHC class I and II levels were also markedly reduced in transgenic mice receiving oral insulin and not developing IDDM. Oral insulin therapy was not effective in preventing the rapid-onset diabetes occurring in mice that only expressed the transgene in the pancreas. Presumably, the protective response induced by oral tolerance could not prevent a rapid autoimmune process that solely depends on high-affinity CTL. Nevertheless, this study convincingly demonstrated that oral administration of one self antigen is effective against an autoimmune disease induced to a different specific self antigen, even after the autoimmune process had been initiated and islet injury had begun.

Similar results were seen when animals that expressed a transgenic anti-MBP TCR were fed both high and low doses of antigen (217,218). Low-dose feeding induced cells producing significant amounts of IL-4, IL-10, and TGF-β. Administration of the higher concentrations of antigen did not lead to the production of these cytokines, nor did it result in a decrease in IFN-γ production. T cells from animals fed low-dose MBP markedly suppressed the development of EAE on adoptive transfer to syngeneic nontransgenic animals, which were then immunized with MBP. Furthermore, when transgenic animals were fed and then challenged with MBP in CFA, a marked reduction of clinical score was seen in the fed animals. Thus, cells bearing the same TCR and recognizing a defined epitope on MBP can differentiate either into effector cells when exposed to antigen in adjuvant or into regulatory T cells by exposure of antigen via the mucosal route.

Adoptive transfer and T-cell depletion studies (219) have shown that oral insulin suppressed insulitis and the development of diabetes in the NOD mouse by a T cell–dependent mechanism. Pancreatic tissues from NOD mice fed insulin showed less insulitis than did controls. The residual cellular infiltrate was composed mostly of CD4+ T cells expressing IL-4, IL-10, and TGF-β, but not IFN-γ and TNF-α (220), while islet mononuclear infiltration in the controls was composed of cells expressing Th1 cytokines such as IFN-γ and TNF-α. In addition to the oral delivery of insulin, intranasal administration of insulin and GAD65 (221) has also proven to be effective in suppressing disease. Intranasal administration of insulin B-chain peptide 9–23 given at 4 weeks of age and at 4-week intervals thereafter resulted in a dramatic delay in the time of onset of diabetes (222). The amount of peptide needed for protection by the intranasal route was much less than that required for oral tolerance–mediated protection. Although T cells from mice that received intranasal insulin had a lower proliferative response, cytokine-secretion profiles were not determined, and the mechanism by which intranasal administration of the insulin peptide conferred protection from diabetes is unknown.

A large number of other animal models of organ-specific autoimmune diseases have been successfully treated and/or prevented by the oral delivery of antigen. In the TNBS-induced model of IBD, disease can be prevented by induction of oral tolerance by feeding mice a mixture of colonic proteins that had been derivatized with the TNBS hapten (78). Mice fed TNBS proteins had T cells, which demonstrated a greatly increased capacity to secrete TGF-β, and a striking reduction of IL-12 heterodimer secretion was also observed. Oral adminsitration of type II collagen suppressed several models of arthritis, including collagen-induced, adjuvant-induced, pristane-induced, and antigen-induced arthritis (223). Type II collagen peptides given nasally also suppressed collagen-induced arthritis in mice. The oral administration of mycobacterial 65-kDa HSP suppressed the clinical severity of adjuvant arthritis as well as mycobacterial and HSP-specific responses (224). Suppression of adjuvant arthritis after oral administration of HSP can be adoptively transferred by spleen cells from tolerant animals. In this model, sensitization was necessary for expansion of regulatory T cells, because transfer of suppression was observed only when cells were obtained from animals that had been fed HSP and then immunized with CFA. Oral administration of retinal S antigen (S-Ag), which can induce experimental autoimmune uveitis, markedly diminished the clinical appearance of S-Ag–induced disease, as measured by ocular inflammation (225). Oral tolerization to adenoviral antigens permitted long-term gene expression using adenoviral vectors (226).

The use of an oral tolerance protocol for the treatment of autoimmune disease in humans represents an attractive therapeutic option. There are, however, a number of theoretical problems with the widespread adoption of oral tolerance in clinical trials. Although the induction of anergy or deletion of autoreactive T cells has been clearly demonstrated, particularly after oral delivery of high doses of antigen, it is unlikely that such a therapeutic approach would be applicable to humans because the target antigen in a given autoimmune disease would have to be well defined. Epitope spreading would predict that induction of oral tolerance with the initiating peptide epitope, after disease induction, would be an ineffective therapy. Progression of disease is likely to be mediated by T cells that recognize new epitopes on endogenous self antigens generated during the process of determinant spreading (see previous discussion of determinant spreading in the section on etiology and pathogenesis). The induction of regulatory T cells, which are capable of mediating bystander suppression, obviates the need for precisely knowing the target autoantigen, but the window of antigen dose in which such regulatory T cells can be induced may be extremely narrow, and it also may be difficult to readily extrapolate dosage from animal models. Although it has been relatively easy to prevent the induction of autoimmune diseases by oral feeding, it is still unclear whether feeding defined peptides can regulate an established autoimmune diseae such as EAE. Furthermore, even in some animal model studies it has been difficult to document the induction of regulatory T cells following "low or intermediate" doses of oral antigen. For example, a single oral dose of PLP 139–151 completely prevented acute and relapsing EAE induced by immunization with PLP 139–151. The oral tolerance regimen reduced T-cell proliferation as well as IL-2 and IFN-γ production and resulted in the significant elevation of IL-4, but not IL-10 or TGF-β, production; the increased IL-4 production was not directly responsible for inhibition of disease, because in vivo neutralization of IL-4 with antibody therapy had no effect on induction of oral tolerance or its ability to to prevent EAE (227). It appeared that feeding PLP 139–151 induced anergy, because in vitro culture of T cells from fed mice in IL-2 was able to reverse the nonresponsiveness.

Restoration of responsiveness by culture in IL-2 is one of the hallmarks of anergy and definitively demonstrates that not all of the PLP139–151-specific T cells were deleted. No evidence for the generation of suppressor cells or bystander suppression was obtained, and lower doses of antigen could not induce oral tolerance or prevent clinical symptoms.

In most studies, including those in humans, the oral administration of antigen has not resulted in harmful sequelae or progression of disease. On the other hand, the ability to induce cytotoxic T cells by feeding ovalbumin to animals has raised the possibility of whether the oral administration of antigen could induce autoreactive CTLs capable of causing autoimmune disease (228). When transgenic animals that expressed ovalbumin in pancreatic β cells were lethally irradiated and reconstituted with bone marrow from mice that expressed a transgenic TCR that recognized ovalbumin and was expressed in CD8+ CTL, the chimeras rarely became diabetic, but 50% of the animals had mild insulitis. When these mice were fed ovalbumin, about 40% became diabetic. It is difficult to generalize from this single study in a double transgene model, but these results do clearly suggest that oral exposure to autoantigens can stimulate CD8+ CTLs and emphasize that appropriate caution should be used in oral tolerance studies.

Only a limited number of studies of the induction of oral tolerance in humans have thus far been performed. The oral administration of keyhole limpit hemocyanin to human subjects has been reported to decrease subsequent cell-mediated immune responses, although antibody responses were not affected (229). Human trials of oral tolerance have been initiated in MS, rheumatoid arthritis, and uveitis (209,230). Trials of oral recombinant human insulin have also been initiated in new-onset diabetes and in subjects at risk. No evidence of systemic toxicity or exacerbation of disease was seen. One small preliminary trial of the oral administration of chicken collagen II to patients with rheumatoid arthritis showed that some patients had significantly less progression of disease, and 14 % of patients had complete resolution of disease; consistent clinical efficacy is yet to be demonstrated. In MS patients, MBP- and PLP-specific Th3-type cells have been observed in the peripheral blood of patients treated with oral bovine myelin preparations, but not in patients who were untreated (231). There was no increase in MBP- and PLP-specific IFN-γ–secreting cells in treated patients.

CONCLUDING REMARKS

Studies over the past 10 years, particularly those using transgenic mice, on the development and differentiation of T-lymphocytes during the process of positive and/or negative selection in the thymus have offered new insights to our understanding of the genesis of the T cells that mediate organ-specific autoimmunity. Although it would have been plausible that autoreactivity would have resulted from a failure or dysregulation of the process of negative selection in the thymus, or a failure to induce anergy or nonresponsiveness in the periphery, there are very few experimental data to support either of these pathways. Indeed, a large number of studies have clearly demonstrated that autoreactive T cells make up a significant percentage of the peripheral T-cell pool. Why, then, is the incidence of autoimmune disease so low? As has been described here in great detail, CD8+ autoreactive T cells exist in the periphery in a state of ignorance and/or indifference to autoantigens expressed on non-bone marrow–derived cells. The situation for CD4+ autoreactive cells is less clear, as fewer transgenic models are available for study. However, studies over the past 5 years have demonstrated the existence of suppressor or regulatory T-cell populations that control the potential pathogenicity of self-reactive CD4[+] cells. Regulatory T cells have been shown to play important roles in all of the animal models of human disease, including IDDM, EAE, and IBD. The mechanisms by which these regulatory cells exert their suppressive effects remain to be discovered.

Studies in the future will focus on those factors that tip the balance and lead to the activation of both autoreactive CD4[+] and CD8[+] T cells. Infectious agents appear to play a major role and may stimulate the production of powerful inducers of the activation of Th1 cells, such as IL-12. Perhaps, IL-12 inhibitors may be of clinical value in preventing the exacerbations of certain autoimmune diseases, such as MS, that are frequently seen following infections. The concept of molecular mimicry has influenced our thinking for many years, but newer studies on the activation of autoreactive T cells by mimicry peptides expressed by pathogens, which have only subtle homologies with native autoantigens, reemphasize the importance of infectious agents in inducing and perpetuating autoimmunity.

The explosion of new information on the role of cytokines in organ-specific autoimmunity has generated several new models for immunotherapy. The concept of the Th1/Th2 balance in organ-specific autoimmune disease has been repeatedly validated. Most organ-specific diseases in humans and animals are mediated by polarized populations of Th1 lymphocytes. It is still controversial whether autoantigen-specific Th2 cells are actually protective. Nevertheless, numerous attempts are being made to generate autoantigen-specific Th2 cells by the administration of Th2-polarizing cytokines, by injecting variant peptide antigens that preferentially activate a Th2-like program of cytokine production, or by stimulating mucosally derived Th2 or Th3 cells by the oral administration of antigen. Although some of these therapies are already being evaluated in controlled clinical trials in humans, more recent studies in mice that are genetically deficient in cytokines have raised concerns about the simplicity of the Th1/Th2 paradigm in autoimmunity. Several of the Th1 cytokines have been shown to exert protective effects in animal models of EAE (see Table 13). Furthermore, under certain conditions, autoantigen-specific Th2 populations have also been shown to induce organ-specific autoimmunity (57,122,123). Future studies will help to resolve these complex problems. Other therapeutic approaches, such as the enhancement of antigen-specific or antigen-nonspecific regulatory T-cells should also prove to be of interest. An ideal therapy for organ-specific autoimmune disease is one that does not involve the induction of generalized immunosuppression and that specifically targets the autoantigen-specific populations. This goal remains elusive.

REFERENCES

1. Tisch R, McDevitt H. Insulin-dependent diabetes mellitus. *Cell* 1996;85:291.
2. Bach J-F. Insulin-dependent diabetes mellitus as an autoimmune disease. *Endocr Rev* 1994;15:516.
3. Thomas JW, Powers AC. Immunology of diabetes. In: Rich R, ed. *Clinical immunology: principles and practice.* St. Louis: Mosby–Year Book, 1996: 1503–1522.
4. Atkinson MA, Maclaren NK. The pathogenesis of insulin-dependent diabetes mellitus. *N Engl J Med* 1994;331:1428.
5. Kaufman DL, Erlander MG, Clare-Salzler M, Atkinson MA, Maclaren NK, Tobin AJ. Autoimmunity to two forms of glutamate decarboxylase in insulin-dependent diabetes mellitus. *J Clin Invest* 1992;89:283.
6. Endl J, Otto H, Jung G, et al. Identification of naturally processed T cell epitopes from glutamic acid decarboxylase presented in the context of HLA-DR alleles by T lymphocytes of recent onset IDDM patients. *J Clin Invest* 1997;99:2405.
7. Crisa L, Mordes JP, Rossini AA. Autoimmune diabetes mellitus in the BB rat. *Diabetes Metab Rev* 1992;8:4.
8. Wicker LS, Todd JA, Peterson LB. Genetic control of autoimmune diabetes in the NOD mouse. *Annu Rev Immunol* 1995;13:179.
9. Delovitch TL, Singh B. The nonobese diabetic mouse as a model of autoimmune diabetes: immune dysregulation get the NOD. *Immunity* 1997;7:727.
10. Larger E, Becourt C, Bach JF, Boitard C. Pancreatic islet β cells drive T cell-immune responses in the non-obese diabetic mouse model. *J Exp Med* 1995;181: 1635.
11. Katz JD, Wang B, Haskins K, Benoist C, Mathis D. Following a diabetogenic T cell from genesis through pathogenesis. *Cell* 1993;74:1089.
12. Andre I, Gonzalez A, Wang B, Katz J, Benoist C, Mathis D. Checkpoints in the progression of autoimmune disease: lessons from diabetes models. *Proc Natl Acad Sci USA* 1996;93:2260.
13. Tisch R, Yang XD, Singer SM, Liblau RS, Fugger L, McDevitt HO. Immune response to glutamic acid decarboxylase correlates with insulitis in non-obese diabetic mice. *Nature* 1993;366:72.
14. Kaufman DL, Clare-Salzler M, Tian J, et al. Spontaneous loss of T-cell tolerance to glutamic acid decarboxylase in murine insulin-dependent diabetes. *Nature* 1993;366:69.
15. Daniel D, Gill RG, Schloot N, Wegmann D. Epitope specificity, cytokine production profile and diabetogenic activity of insulin-specific T cell clones isolated from NOD mice. *Eur J Immunol* 1995;25:1056.
16. Katz J, Benoist C, Mathis D. Major histocompatibility complex class I molecules are required for the development of insulitis in non-obese diabetic mice. *Eur J Immunol* 1993;23:3358.
17. Wong FS, Visintin I, Wen L, Flavell RA, Janeway CA Jr. CD8 T cell clones from young nonobese diabetic (NOD) islets can transfer rapid onset of diabetes in NOD mice in the absence of CD4 cells. *J Exp Med* 1996;183:67.
18. Wang B, Gonzalez A, Benoist C, Mathis D. The role of CD8[+] T cells in the initiation of insulin-dependent diabetes mellitus. *Eur J Immunol* 1996;26:1762.
19. Haskins K, Wegmann D. Diabetogenic t-cell clones. *Diabetes* 1996;45:1299.
20. Simone E, Daniel D, Schloot N, et al. T cell receptor restriction of diabetogenic autoimmune NOD T cells. *Proc Natl Acad Sci USA* 1997;94:2518.
21. Conrad B, Weissmahr RN, Boni J, Arcari R, Schupbach J, Mach B. A human endogenous retroviral superantigen as candidate autoimmune gene in type I diabetes. *Cell* 1997;90:303.
22. Conrad B, Weldmann E, Trucco G, et al. Evidence for superantigen involvement in insulin-dependent diabetes mellitus aetology. *Nature* 1994;371:351.
23. Noronha A, Arnason B. Demyelinating diseases. In: Rich R, ed. *Clinical immunology: principles and practice.* St. Louis: Mosby–Year Book, 1996: 1364–1376.
24. Hohlfeld R. Biotechnological agents for the immunotherapy of multiple sclerosis. Principles, problem, perspectives. *Brain* 1997;120:865.
25. Ruddick RA, Cohen JA, Weinstock-Guttman B, Kinkel RP, Ransohoff RM. Management of multiple sclerosis. *N Engl J Med* 1997;337:1604.
26. Soldan SS, Berti R, Salem N, et al. Association of human herpes virus 6 (HHV-6) with multiple sclerosis: increased IgM response to HHV-6 early antigen and detection of serum HHV-6 DNA. *Nat Med* 1997;3:1394.
27. Perron H, Garson JA, Bedin F, et al. Molecular identification of a novel retrovirus repeatedly isolated from patients with multiple sclerosis. *Proc Natl Acad Sci USA* 1997;94:7583.
28. Zamvil SS, Steinman L. The T lymphocyte in experimental allergic encephalomyelitis. *Annu Rev Immunol* 1990;8:579.
29. Martin R, McFarland HF, McFarlin DE. Immunological aspects of demyelinating diseases. *Annu Rev Immunol* 1992;10:153.
30. Rivers TM, Schwentker FF. Encephalomyelitis accompanied by myelin destruction experimentally produced in monkeys. *J Exp Med* 1935;61:689.
31. Powell MB, Mitchell D, Lederman J, et al. Lymphotoxin and tumor necrosis factor-alpha production by myelin basic protein-specific T cell clones correlates with encephalitogenicity. *Int Immunol* 1990;2:539.
32. Fritz RB, McFarlin DE. Encephalitogenic epitopes of myelin basic protein. In: Sercarz E, ed. *Antigenic determinants and immune regulation.* Basel: Karger. 1989;101-125.
33. Kuchroo VK, Martin CA, Greer JM, Ju ST, Sobel RA, Dorf ME. Cytokines and adhesion molecules contribute to the ability of myelin proteolipid protein-specific T cell clones to mediate experimental allergic encephalomyelitis. *J Immunol* 1993;151:4371.
34. Baron JL, Madri JA, Ruddle NH, Hashim G, Janeway CA. Surface expression of α4 integrin by CD4 T cells is required for their entry into brain parenchyma. *J Exp Med* 1993;177:57.
35. Ruddle NH, Bergman CM, McGrath KM, et al. An antibody to lymphotoxin and tumor necrosis factor prevents transfer of experimental allergic encephalomyelitis. *J Exp Med* 1990;172:1193.
36. Selmaj K, Paplerz W, Glabinski A, Kohno T. Prevention of chronic relapsing autoimmune encephalomyelitis by soluble tumor necrosis factor receptor. *J Neuroimmunol* 1995;56:135.
37. Leonard JP, Waldburger KE, Goldman SJ. Prevention of experimental autoimmune encephalomyelitis by antibodies against interleukin 12. *J Exp Med* 1995; 181:381.
38. Segal BM, Dwyer BK, Shevach EM. An interleukin (IL)-10/IL-12 immunoregulatory circuit controls susceptibility to autoimmune disease. *J Exp Med* 1998; 187:537.
39. Chou FCH, Chou CHJ, Fritz R, Kibler R. Prevention of experimental allergic

encephalomyelitis in Lewis rats with peptide 68-88 of guinea pig myelin basic protein. *Ann Neurol* 1980:7:336.

40. Swierkosz J, Swanborg R. Suppressor cell control of unresponsiveness to experimental allergic encephalomyelitis. *J Immunol* 1975;115:631.

41. Acha-Orbea H, Mitchell DJ, Timmerman L, et al. Limited heterogeneity of T cell receptors from lymphocyte mediating autoimmune encephalomyelitis allows specific immune intervention. *Cell* 1988;54:263.

42. Rocken M, Urban JF, Shevach EM. Infection breaks T-cell tolerance. *Nature* 1992;359:79.

43. Brocke S, Gaur A, Piercy C, et al. Induction of relapsing paralysis in experimental autoimmune encephalomyelitis by bacterial superantigen. *Nature* 1993; 365:642.

44. Goverman J, Woods A, Larson L, Weiner LP, Hood L, Zaller DM. Transgenic mice that express a myelin basic protein-specific T cell receptor develop spontaneous autoimmunity. *Cell* 1993;72:551.

45. Lafaille JJ, Nagashima K, Katsuki M, Tonegawa S. High incidence of spontaneous autoimmune encephalomyelitis in immunodeficient anti-myelin basic protein T cell receptor transgenic mice. *Cell* 1994:78:399.

46. Saoudi A, Seddon B, Heath V, Fowell D, Mason D. The physiological role of regulatory T cells in the prevention of autoimmunity: the function of the thymus in the generation of the regulatory T cell subset. *Immunol Rev* 1996149:195.

47. Fowell D, McKnight AJ, Powrie F, Dyke R, Mason D. Subsets of CD4+ T cells and their roles in the induction and prevention of autoimmunity. *Immunol Rev* 1991;123:37.

48. Fowell D, Mason D. Evidence that the T cell repertoire of normal rats contains cells with the potential to cause diabetes. Characterization of the CD4+ T cell subset that inhibits this autoimmune potential. *J Exp Med* 1993;177:627.

49. Penhale WJ, Farmer A, Irvine WJ. Thyroiditis in T cell-dpeleted rats. Influence of strain, radiation dose, adjuvants and antilymphocyte serum. *Clin Exp Immunol* 1975;21:362.

50. Greiner DL, Handler ES, Nakano K, Mordes JP, Rossini AA. Absence of the RT-6 T cell subset in diabetes-prone BB/W rats. *J Immunol* 1986;136:148.

51. Saoudi A, Seddon B, Fowell D, Mason D. The thymus contains a high frequency of cells that prevent autoimmune diabetes on transfer into prediabetic recipients. *J Exp Med* 1996;184:2393.

52. Sakaguchi S, Sakaguchi N. Thymus, T cells, and autoimmunity: various causes but a common mechanism of autoimmune disease. In: Coutinho A, Kazatchkine MD, eds. *Autoimmunity: physiology and disease.* New York: Wiley-Liss, 1994:203–227.

53. Gleeson PA, Toh B-H, van Driel IR. Organ-specific autoimmunity induced by lymphopenia. *Immunol Rev* 1996;149:97.

54. Sakaguchi S, Sakaguchi N, Asano M, Itoh M, Toda M. Immunologic self-tolerance maintained by activated T cells expressing IL-2 receptor α-chains (CD25): breakdown of a single mechanism of self-tolerance causes various autoimmune diseases. *J Immunol* 1995;155:1151.

55. Sakaguchi S, Toda M, Asano M, Itoh M, Morse SS, Sakaguchi N. T cell-mediated maintenance of natural self-tolerance: its breakdown as a possible cause of various autoimmune diseases. *J Autoimmun* 1996;9:211.

56. Suri-Payer E, Amar AZ, Thornton AM, Shevach EM. CD4+CD25+ T cells inhibit both the induction and effector function of autoreactive T cells and represent a unique lineage of immunoregulatory cells. *J Immunol* 1998;160:1212–1218.

57. Lafaille JJ, Van de Keere F, Hsu AL, et al. Myelin basic protein-specific T helper 2 (Th2) cells cause experimental autoimmune encephalomyelitis in immunodeficient hosts rather than protect them from the disease. *J Exp Med* 1997;186:307.

58. Boitard C, Yasunami R, Dardeene M, Bach JF. T cell-mediated inhibition of the transfer of autoimmune diabetes in nod mice. *J Exp Med* 1989;169:1669.

59. Shimada A, Charlton B, Rohane P, Taylor-Edwards C, Fathman CG. Immune regulation in type 1 diabetes. *J Autoimmun* 1996;9:263.

60. Pankewycz O, Strom TB, Rubin-Kelley VE. Islet-infiltrating T cell clones from non-obese diabetic mice that promote or prevent accelerated onset diabetes. *Eur J Immunol* 1991;21:873.

61. Diaz-Gallo C, Moscovitch-Lopatin M, Strom TB, Kelley VR. An anergic, islet-infiltrating T-cell clone that blocks interleukin 2/interleukin 4-dependent proliferation. *Proc Natl Acad Sci USA* 1992;89:8656.

62. Akhtar I, Gold JP, Pan L-Y, et al. CD4+ β islet cell-reactive T cell clones that suppress autoimmune diabetes in nonobese diabetic mice. *J Exp Med* 1995;182:87.

63. Shevach EM, Thornton A, Suri-Payer E. T lymphocyte mediated control of autoimmunity. *Ciba Found Symp* 1998;(in press).

64. Eisenstein EM, Sneller MC. Common variable immunodeficiency; diagnosis and managment. *Ann Allergy* 1994;73:285.

65. Strober W, Neurath MF. Immunologic diseases of the gastrointestinal tract. In: Rich R, ed. *Clinical immunology: principles and practice.* St. Louis: Mosby–Year Book, 1996:1401–1428.

66. Sartour RB, Cytokines in intestinal inflammation: pathophysiological and clinical considerations. *Gastroenterology* 1994:106:533.

67. Sadlack B, Merz H, Schorie H, Schimpl A, Feller AC, Horak I. Ulcerative colitis-like disease in mice with a disrupted interleukin-2 gene. *Cell* 1993;75:253.

68. Strober W, Kelsall B, Fuss I, et al. Reciprocal IFN-γ and TGF-β responses regulate the occurrence of mucosal inflammation. *Immunol Today* 1997;18:61.

69. Mombaerts P, Mizoguchi E, Grusby MJ, Glimcher LH, Bhan AK, Tonegawa S. Spontaneous development of inflammatory bowel disease in T cell receptor mutant mice. *Cell* 1993;75:275.

70. Rath HC, Herfarth HH, Ikeda JS, et al. Normal luminal bacteria, especially bacteroides species, mediate chronic colitis, gastritis, and arthritis in HLA-B27/human β2 microglobulin transgenic rats. *J Clin Invest* 1996;98:945.

71. Morrissey PJ, Charrier K, Braddy S, Liggitt D, Watson JD. CD4+ T cells that express high levels of CD45RB induce wasting disease when transferred into congenic severe combined immunodeficient mice. Disease development is prevented by cotransfer of purified CD4+ T cells. *J Exp Med* 1993;178:237.

72. Powrie F, Leach MW, Mauze S, Menon S, Caddle LB, Coffman RL. Inhibition of Th1 responses prevents inflammatory bowel disease in *scid* mice reconstituted with CD45RB[hi] CD4+ T cells. *Immunity* 1994;1:553.

73. Powrie F. T cells in inflammatory bowel disease: protective and pathogenic roles. *Immunity* 1995;3:171.

74. Powrie F, Carlino J, Leach MW, Mauze S, Coffman RL. A critical role for transforming growth factor-β but not interleukin 4 in the suppression of T helper type 1-mediated colitis by CD45RB[low] CD4+ T cells. *J Exp Med* 1996;183:2669.

75. Kulkarni AB, Huh C-G, Becker D, et al. Transforming growth factor β1 null mutation in mice causes excessive inflammatory response and early death. *Proc Natl Acad Sci USA* 1993;90:770.

76. Hollander GA, Simpson SJ, Mizoguchi E, et al. Severe colitis in mice with aberrant thymic selection. *Immunity* 1995;3:27.

77. Simpson SJ, Hollander GA, Mizoguchi E, et al. Expression of pro-inflammatory cytokines by TCRαβ+ and TCRγδ+ T cells in an experimental model of colitis. *Eur J Immunol* 1997;27:17.

78. Neurath MF, Fuss I, Kelsall BL, Presky DH, Waegell W, Strober W. Experimental granulomatous colitis in mice is abrogated by induction of TGF-β-mediated oral tolerance. *J Exp Med* 1996;183:2605.

79. Neurath MF, Fuss I, Kelsall BL, Stuber E, Strober W. Antibodies to interleukin 12 abrogaate established experimental colitis in mice. *J Exp Med* 1995;182: 1281.

80. Kuhn R, Lohler J, Rennick D, Rajewsky K, Muller W. Interleukin-10-deficient mice develop chronic enterocolitis. *Cell* 1993;75:263.

81. Berg DJ, Davidson N, Kuhn R, et al. Enterocolitis and colon cancer in interleukin-10-deficient mice are associated with aberrant cytokine production and CD4+ TH1-like responses. *J Clin Invest* 1996;98:1010.

82. Rudolph U, Finegold MJ, Rich SS, et al. Ulcerative colitis and adenocarcinoma of the colon in Gα12-deficient mice. *Nature* Genetics 1995;10:143.

83. von Herrath MG, Evans CF, Horwitz MS, Oldstone MBA. Using transgenic mouse models to dissect the pathogenesis of virus-induced autoimmune disorders of the islets of Langerhans and the central nervous system. *Immunol Rev* 1996;152:111.

84. Wekerle H, Bradl M, Linington C, Kaab G, Kojima K. The shaping of the brain-specific T lymphocyte repertoire in the thymus. *Immunol Rev* 1996;149:231.

85. Miller JFAP, Heath WR. Self-ignorance in the peripheral T-cell pool. *Immunol Rev* 1993:133:131.

86. Ohashi PS, Oehen S, Buerki K, et al. Ablation of "tolerance" and induction of diabetes by virus infection in viral antigen transgenic mice. *Cell* 1991;65:305.

87. Aichele P, Bachmann MF, Hengartner H, Zinkernagel RM. Immunopathology or organ-specific autoimmunity as a consequence of virus infection. *Immunol Rev* 1996;152:21.

88. Von Herrath MG, Dockter J, Oldstone MBA. How virus induces a rapid or slow onset insulin-dependent diabetes mellitus in a transgenic model. *Immunity* 1994; 1:231.

89. Morgan DJ, Liblau R, Scott B, et al. CD8+ T cell-mediated spontaneous diabetes in neonatal mice. *J Immunol* 1996;157:978.

90. Oldstone MBA. Molecular mimicry and autoimmune disease. *Cell* 1987;50:819.

91. Hall R. Molecular mimicry. *Adv Parasitol* 1994:34:81.

92. Fujinami RS, Oldstone MBA. Amino acid homology between the encephalitogenic site of myelin basic protein and virus: mechanism for autoimmunity. *Science* 1985;230:1043.

93. Burroughs AK, Butler P, Stemberg MJE, Baum H. Molecular mimicry in liver disease. *Nature* 1992;358:377.

94. Wucherpfennig KW, Strominger JL. Molecular mimicry in T cell-mediated autoimmunity: viral peptides activate human T cell clones specific for myelin basic protein. *Cell* 1995;80:695.

95. Evans CF, Horwitz MS, Hobbs MV, Oldstone MBA. Viral infection of transgenic mice expressing a viral protein in oligodendrocytes leads to chronic central nervous system autoimmune disease. *J Exp Med* 1996;184:2371.

96. Sercarz EE, Lehmann PV, Ametani A, Benichou G, Miller A, Moudagil K. Dominance and crypticity of T cell antigenic determinants. *Annu Rev Immunol* 1993; 11:729.

97. Lehmann PV, Sercarz EE, Forsthuber T, Dayan CM, Gammon G. Determinant spreading and the dynamics of the autoimmune T-cell repertoire. *Immunol Today* 1993;14:203.

98. Roth R, Gee RJ, Mamula M. B lymphocytes as autoantigen-presenting cells in the amplification of autoimmunity. *Ann NY Acad Sci* 1997;815:88.

99. Lehmann PV, Forsthuber T, Miller A, Sercarz EE. Spreading of T-cell autoimmunity to cryptic determinants of an autoantigen. *Nature* 1992;358:155.

100. Yu M, Johnson JM, Tuohy VK. A predictable sequential determinant spreading cascade invariably accompanies progression of experimental autoimmune encephalomyelitis: a basis for peptide-specific therapy after onset of clinical disease. *J Exp Med* 1996;183:1777.

101. McRae BL, Vanderlugt CL, Dal Canto MC, Miller SD. Functional evidence for epitope spreading in the relapsing pathology of experimental autoimmune encephalomyelitis. *J Exp Med* 1995;182:75.

102. Tuohy VK, Yu M, Weinstock-Guttman B, Kinkel RP. Diversity and plasticity of self recognition during the development of multiple sclerosis. *J Clin Invest* 1997; 99:1682.

103. Liblau RS, Singer SM, McDevitt HO. Th1 and Th2 CD4⁺ T cells in the pathogenesis of organ-specific autoimmune diseases. *Immunol Today* 1995;16:35.

104. Goldman M, Druet P, Gleichmann E. TH2 cells in systemic autoimmunity: insights from allogeneic diseases and chemically-induced autoimmunity. *Immunol Today* 1991;12:223.

105. Kennedy MK, Torrance DS, Picha KS, Mohler KM. Analysis of cytokine mRNA expression in the central nervous system of mice with experimental autoimmune encephalomyelitis reveals that IL-10 mRNA expression correlates with recovery. *J Immunol* 1992;149:2496.

106. Khoury SJ, Hancock WW, Weiner HL. Oral tolerance to myelin basic protein and natural recovery from experimental autoimmune encephalomyelitis are associated with downregulation of inflammatory cytokines and differential upregulation of transforming growth factor β, interleukin 4, and prostaglandin E expression in the brain. *J Exp Med* 1992;176:1355.

107. Racke MK, Bonomo A, Scott DE, et al. Cytokine-induced immune deviation as a therapy for inflammatory autoimmune disease. *J Exp Med* 1994;180:1961.

108. Rott O, Fleischer B, Cash E. Interleukin-10 prevents experimental allergic encephalomyelitis in rats. *Eur J Immunol* 1994;24:1434.

109. Cash E, Minty A, Ferrara P, Caput D, Fradelizi D, Rott O. Macrophage-inactivating IL-13 suppresses experimental autoimmune encephalomyelitis in rats. *J Immunol* 1994;153:4258.

110. Falcone M, Bloom BR. A T helper cell 2 (Th2) immune response against non-self antigens modifies the cytokine profile of autoimmune T cells and protects against experimental allergic encephalomyelitis. *J Exp Med* 1997;185:901.

111. Saoudi A, Simmonds S, Huitinga I, Mason D. Prevention of experimental allergic encephalomyelitis in rats by targeting autoantigen to B cells: evidence that the protective mechanism depends on changes in the cytokine response and migratory properties of the autoantigen-specific T cells. *J Exp Med* 1995;182:335.

112. Chen Y, Kuchroo VK, Inobe J-I, Hafler DA, Weiner HL. Regulatory T cell clones induced by oral tolerance: suppression of autoimmune encephalomyelitis. *Science* 1994;265:1237.

113. Kuchroo VK, Das MP, Brown JA, et al. B7-1 and B7-2 costimulatory molecules activate differentially the Th1/Th2 development pathways: application to autoimmune disease therapy. *Cell* 1995;80:707.

114. Khoruts A, Miller SD, Jenkins MK. Neuroantigen-specific Th2 cells are inefficient suppressors of experimental autoimmune encephalomyelitis induced by effector Th1 cells. *J Immunol* 1995;155:5011.

115. Harrison LC, Honeiman MC, DeAlpuzurua H, et al. Inverse relation between humoral and cellular immunity to glutamic acid decarboxylase in subjects at risk of insulin-dependent diabetes. *Lancet* 1993;341:1365.

116. Debray-Sachs M, Carnaud C, Boitard C, et al. Prevention of diabetes in NOD mice treated with antibody of IFNγ. *J Autoimmun* 1991;4:237.

117. Rapoport MJ, Jaramillo A, Zipris D, et al. Interleukin 4 reverses T cell proliferative unresponsiveness and prevents the onset of diabetes in nonobese diabetic mice. *J Exp Med* 1993;178:87.

118. Scott B, Liblau R, Degermann S, et al. A role for non-MHC genetic polymorphism in susceptibility to spontaneous autoimmunity. *Immunity* 1994;1:73.

119. Singer SM, Tisch R, Yang XD, McDevitt HO. An Abᵈ transgene prevents diabetes in nonobese diabetic mice by inducing regulatory T cells. *Proc Natl Acad Sci USA* 1993;90:9566.

120. Singer SM, Umetsu DT, McDevitt HO. High copy number I-Ab transgenes induce production of IgE throughan interleukin 4-dependent mechanism. *Proc Natl Acad Sci USA* 1996;93:2947.

121. Katz JD, Benoist C, Mathis D. T helper cell subsets in insulin-dependent diabetes. *Science* 1995;268:1185.

122. Pakala SV, Kurrer MO, Katz JD. T helper 2 (Th2) T cells induce acute pancreatitis and diabetes in immune compromised nonobese diabetic (NOD) mice. *J Exp Med* 1997;186:299.

123. Genain CP, Abel K, Belmar N, et al. Late complications of immune deviation therapy in a nonhuman primate. *Science* 1996;274:2054.

124. Rocken M, Shevach EM. Immune deviation—the third dimension of nondeletional T cell tolerance. *Immunol Rev* 1996;149:175.

125. Allison J, Malcom L, Chosich N, Miller JFAP. Inflammation but not autoimmunity occurs in transgenic mice expressing constitutive levels of interleukin-2 in islet beta-cells. *Eur J Immunol* 1992;22:1115.

126. Heath WR, Allison J, Hoffmann MW, et al. Autoimmune diabetes as a consequence of locally produced interleukin-2. *Nature* 1992;359:547.

127. Sarvetnick N, Liggitt D, Pitts SL, Hansen SE, Stewart TA. Insulin-dependent diabetes mellitus induced in transgenic mice by ectopic expression of class II MHC and interferon gamma. *Cell* 1988,52.773.

128. Lee MS, von Herrath MG, Reiser H, Oldstone MBA, Sarvetnick N. Sensitization to self (virus) antigen by in situ expression of murine interferon-γ. *J Clin Invest* 1995;95:486.

129. Gu D, Wogensen L, Calcutt NA, et al. Myasthenia gravis-like syndrome induced by expression of interferon γ in the neuromuscular junction. *J Exp Med* 1995;181:547.

130. Barrett SP, van Driel IR, Tan SS, Alderuccio F, Toh BH, Gleeson PA. Expression of a gastric autoantigen in pancreatic islets results in non destructive insulitis after neonatal thymectomy. *Eur J Immunol* 1995;25:2686.

131. Yang XD, Tisch R, Singer S, et al. Effect of tumor necrosis factor α on insulin-dependent diabetes mellitus in NOD mice. I. The early development of autoimmunity and the diabetogenic process. *J Exp Med* 1994;180:995.

132. Higuchi Y, Herrera P, Muniese P, et al. Expression of a tumor necrosis factor α

133. Grewal IS, Grewal KD, Wong FS, Picarella DE, Janeway CA Jr, Flavell RA. Local expression of transgene encoded TNFα in islets prevents autoimmune diabetes in nonobese diabetic (NOD) mice by preventing the development of autoreactive islet-specific T cells. *J Exp Med* 1996;184:1963.

134. Grewal IS, Flavell RA. New insights into insulin dependent diabetes mellitus from studies with transgenic mouse models. *Lab Invest* 1997;76:3.

135. Mueller R, Krahl T, Sarvetnick N. Pancreatic expression of interleukin-4 abrogates insulitis and autoimmune diabetes in nonobese diabetic (NOD) mice. *J Exp Med* 1996;184:1093.

136. Mueller R, Bradley LM, Krahl T, Sarvetnick N. Mechanism underlying counter-regulation of autoimmune diabetes by IL-4. *Immunity* 1997;7:411.

137. Wogensen L, Lee M-S, Sarvetnick N. Production of interleukin 10 by islet cells accelerates immune-mediated destruction of β cells in nonobese diabetic mice. *J Exp Med* 1994;179:1379.

138. Mathisen PM, Yu M, Johnson JM, Drazba JA, Tuohy VK. Treatment of experimental autoimmune encephalomyelitis with genetically modified memory T cells. *J Exp Med* 1997;186:159.

139. Shaw MK, Lorens JB, Dhawan A, et al. Local delivery of interleukin 4 by retrovirus-transduced T lymphocytes ameliorates experimental autoimmune encephalomyelitis. *J Exp Med* 1997;185:1711.

140. Hogaboam CM, Vallance BA, Kumar A, et al. Therapeutic effects of interleukin-4 gene transfer in experimental inflammatory bowel disease. *J Clin Invest* 1997;100:2766.

141. Hultgren B, Huang X, Dybdal N, Stewart TA. Genetic absence of γ-interferon delays but does not prevent diabetes in NOD mice. *Diabetes* 1996;45:812.

142. von Herrath MG, Oldstone MBA. Interferon-γ is essential for destruction of β cells and development of insulin-dependent diabetes mellitus. *J Exp Med* 1997;185:531.

143. Billiau A, Heremans H, Vandekerckhove F, et al. Enhancement of experimental allergic encephalomyelitis in mice by antibodies against IFNγ. *J Immunol* 1988;140:1506.

144. Krakowski M, Owens T. Interferon-γ confers resistance to experimental allergic encephalomyelitis. *Eur J Immunol* 1996;26:1641.

145. Ferber IA, Brocke S, Taylor-Edwards C, et al. Mice with a disrupted IFN-γ gene are susceptible to the induction of experimental autoimmune encephalomyelitis (EAE). *J Immunol* 1996;156:5.

146. Willenborg DO, Fordham S, Bernard CCA, Cowden WB, Ramshaw IA. IFN-γ plays a critical down-regulatory role in the induction and effector phase of myelin oligodendrocyte glycoprotein-induced autoimmune encephalomyelitis. *J Immunol* 1996;157:3223.

147. Frei K, Eugster H-P, Bopst M, Constantinescu CS, Lavi E, Fontana A. Tumor necrosis factor α and lymphotoxin α are not required for induction of acute experimental autoimmune encephalomyelitis. *J Exp Med* 1997;185:2177.

148. Steinman L. Some misconceptions about understanding autoimmunity through experiments with knockouts. *J Exp Med* 1997;185:2039.

149. Suen WE, Bergman CM, Hjelmstrom P, Ruddle NH. A critical role for lymphotoxin in experimental allergic encephalomyelitis. *J Exp Med* 1997;186:1233.

150. Liu J, Marino MW, Wong G, et al. TNF is a potent anti-inflammatory cytokine in autoimmune-mediated demyelination. *Nat Med* 1998;4:78.

151. Kagi D, Odermatt B, Ohashi PS, Zinkernagel RM, Hengartner H. Development of insulitis without diabetes in transgenic mice lacking perforin-dependent cytotoxicity. *J Exp Med* 1996;183:2143.

152. Chervonsky AV, Wang Y, Wong FS, et al. The role of Fas in autoimmune diabetes. *Cell* 1997;89:17.

153. Sabelko KA, Kelly KA, Nahm MH, Cross AH, Russell JH. Fas and Fas ligand enhance the pathogenesis of experimental allergic encephalomyelitis, but are not essential for immune privilege in the central nervous system. *J Immunol* 1997;159:3096.

154. Waldner H, Sobel RA, Howard E, Kuchroo VK. Fas- and FasL-deficient mice are resistant to induction of autoimmune encephalomyelitis. *J Immunol* 1997;159:3100.

155. Harlan DM, Abe R, Lee KP, June CH. Short analytical review. Potential roles of the B7 and CD28 receptor families in autoimmunity and immune evasion. *Clin Immunol Immunopathol* 1995;75:99.

156. Guerder S, Meyerhoff J, Flavell R. The role of the T cell costimulator B7-1 in autoimmunity and the induction and maintenance of tolerance to peripheral antigen. *Immunity* 1994;1:155.

157. Picarella DE, Kratz A, Li C-B, Ruddle NH, Flavell RA. Transgenic tumor necrosis factor (TNF)-α production in pancreatic islets leads to insulitis, not diabetes. *J Immunol* 1993;150:4136.

158. Guerder S, Picarella DE, Linsley PS, Flavell RA. Costimulator B7-1 confers antigen-presenting-cell function to parenchymal tissue and in conjunction with tumor necrosis factor α leads to autoimmunity in transgenic mice. *Proc Natl Acad Sci USA* 1994;91:5138.

159. von Herrath MG, Guerder S, Lewicki H, Flavell RA, Oldstone MBA. Coexpression of B7-1 and viral ("self") transgenes in pancreatic β cells can break peripheral ignorance and lead to spontaneous autoimmune diabetes. *Immunity* 1995;3:727.

160. Chambers CA, Krummel MF, Boitel B, et al. The role of CTLA-4 in the regulation and initiation of T-cell responses. *Immunol Rev* 1996;153:27.

161. Tivol EA, Borriello F, Schweitzer AN, Lynch WP, Bluestone JA, Sharpe AH. Loss of CTLA-4 leads to massive lymphoproliferation and fatal multiorgan tis-

sue destruction, revealing a critical negative regulatory role of CTLA-4. *Immunity* 1995;3:541.

162. Perez VL, Parijs LV, Biuckians A, Zheng XX, Strom TB, Abbas AK. Induction of peripheral T cell tolerance in vivo requires CTLA-4 engagement. *Immunity* 1997;6:411.

163. Van Parijs L, Perez VL, Biuckians A, Maki RG, London CA, Abbas AK. Role of interleukin 12 and costimulators in T cell anergy in vivo. *J Exp Med* 1997;186:1119.

164. Cross AH, Girard TJ, Giacoletto KS, et al. Long-term inhibition of murine experimental autoimmune encephalomyelitis using CTLA-4-Fc supports a key role for CD28 costimulation. *J Clin Invest* 1995;95:2783.

165. Perrin PJ, Scott D, Quigley L, et al. Role of B7: CD28/CTLA-4 in the induction of chronic relapsing experimental allergic encephalomyelitis. *J Immunol* 1995;154:1481.

166. Racke MK, Scott DE, Quigley L, et al. Distinct roles for B7-1 (CD-80) and B7-2 (CD-86) in the initiation of experimental allergic encephalomyelitis. *J Clin Invest* 1995;96:2195.

167. Khoury SJ, Akalin E, Chandraker A, et al. CD28-B7 costimulatory blockade by CTLA4Ig prevents actively induced experimental autoimmune encephalomyelitis and inhibits Th1 but spares the Th2 cytokines in the central nervous system. *J Immunol* 1995;155:4521.

168. Arima T, Rehman A, Hickey WF, Flye MW. Inhibition by CTLA4Ig of experimental allergic encephalomyelitis. *J Immunol* 1996;156:4916.

169. Miller SD, Vanderlugt CL, Lenschow DJ, et al. Blockade of CD28/B7-1 interaction prevents epitope spreading and clinical relapses of murine EAE. *Immunity* 1995;3:739.

170. Lenschow DJ, Ho SC, Sattar H, et al. Differential effects of anti-B7-1 and anti-B7-2 monoclonal antibody treatment on the development of diabetes in the nonobese diabetic mouse. *J Exp Med* 21995;181:1145.

171. Lenschow DJ, Herold KC, Rhee L, et al. CD28/B7 regulation of Th1 and Th2 subsets in the development of autoimmune diabetes. *Immunity* 1996;5:285.

172. Perrin PJ, Maldonado JH, Davis TA, June CH, Racke MK. CTLA-4 blockade enhances clinical disease and cytokine production during experimental allergic encephalomyelitis. *J Immunol* 1996;157:1333.

173. Karandikar NJ, Vanderlugt CL, Walunas TL, Miller SD, Bluestone JA. CTLA-4: a negative regulator of autoimmune disease. *J Exp Med* 1996;184:783.

174. Windhagen A, Newcombe J, Dangond F, et al. Expression of costimulatory molecules B7-1 (CD80), B7-2 (CD86), and interleukin 12 cytokine in multiple sclerosis lesions. *J Exp Med* 1995;182:1985.

175. Liblau R, Tisch R, Bercovici N, McDevitt HO. Systemic antigen in the treatment of T-cell-mediated autoimmune diseases. *Immunol Today* 1997;18:599.

176. Muir A, Peck A, Clare-Salzler M, et al. Insulin immunization of nonobese diabetic mice induces a protective insulitis characterized by diminished intraislet interferon-γ transcription. *J Clin Invest* 1995;95:628.

177. Karounos DG, Bryson JS, Cohen DA. Metabolically inactive insulin analog prevents type I diabetes in prediabetic NOD mice. *J Clin Invest* 1997;100:1344.

178. Critchfield JM, Racke MK, Zuniga-Pflucker JC, et al. T cell deletion in high antigen dose therapy of autoimmune encephalomyelitis. *Science* 1994;263:1139.

179. Burstein HJ, Abbas AK. *In vivo* role of interleukin 4 in T cell tolerance induced by aqueous protein antigen. *J Exp Med* 1993;177:457.

180. Wraith DC, Smilek DE, Mitchell DJ, Steinman L, McDevitt HO. Antigen recognition in autoimmune encephalomyelitis and the potential for peptide-mediated immunotherapy. *Cell* 1989;59:247.

181. Gautam AM, Pearson CI, Smilek DE, Steinman L, McDevitt HO. A polyalanine peptide with only five native myelin basic protein residues induces autoimmune encephalomyelitis. *J Exp Med* 1992;176:605.

182. Gautam AM, Pearson CI, Sinha AA, Smilek DE, Steinman L, McDevitt HO. Inhibition of experimental autoimmune encephalomyelitis by a nonimmunogenic non-self peptide that binds to I-A. *J Immunol* 1992;148:3049.

183. Lamont AG, Sette A, Fujinami R, Colon SM, Miles C, Grey HM. Inhibition of experimental allergic encephalomyelitis induction of SJL/J mice by using a peptide with high affinity for IA molecules. *J Immunol* 1990;145:1687.

184. Hurtenbach U, Lier E, Adorini L, Nagy ZA. Prevention of autoimmune diabetes in non-obese diabetic mice by treatment with a class II major histocompatibility complex-blocking peptide. *J Exp Med* 1993;177:1499.

185. Vaysburd M, Lock C, McDevitt H. Prevention of insulin-dependent diabetes mellitus in nonobese diabetic mice by immunogenic but not by tolerated peptides. *J Exp Med* 1995;182:897.

186. Kersh GJ, Allen PM. Essential flexibility in the T-cell recognition of antigen. *Nature* 1996;380:495.

187. Franco A, Southwood S, Arrhenius T, et al. T cell receptor antagonist peptides are highly effective inhibitors of experimental allergic encephalomyelitis. *Eur J Immunol* 1994;24:940.

188. Karin N, Mitchell DJ, Brocke S, Ling N, Steinman L. Reversal of experimental autoimmune encephalomyelitis by a soluble peptide variant of a myelin basic protein epitope: T cell receptor antagonism and reduction of interferon γ and tumor necrosis factor α production. *J Exp Med* 1994;180:2227.

189. Liu GY, Wraith DC. Affinity for class II MHC determines the extent to which soluble peptides tolerize autoreactive T cells in naive and primed adult mice implications for autoimmunity. *Int Immunol* 1995;7:1255.

190. Pearson CI, van Eqijk W, McDevitt HO. Induction of apoptosis and T helper 2 (Th2) responses correlates with peptide affinity for the major histocompatibility

191. complex in self-reactive T cell receptor transgenic mice. *J Exp Med* 1997;185:583.

191. Nicholson LB, Greer JM, Sobel RA, Lees MB, Kuchroo VK. An altered peptide ligand mediates immune deviation and prevents autoimmune encephalomyelitis. *Immunity* 1995;3:397.

192. Kuchroo VK, Greer JM, Kaul D, et al. A single TCR antagonist peptide inhibits experimental allergic encephalomyelitis mediated by a diverse T cell repertoire. *J Immunol* 1994;153:3326.

193. Nicholson LB, Murtaza A, Hafler BP, Sette A, Kuchroo VK. A T cell receptor antagonist peptide induces T cells that mediate bystander suppression and prevent autoimmune encephalomyelitis induced with multiple myelin antigens. *Proc Natl Acad Sci USA* 1997;94:9279.

194. Brocke S, Gijbels K, Allegretta M, et al. Treatment of experimental encephalomyelitis with a peptide analogue of myelin basic protein. *Nature* 1996;379:343.

195. Windhagen A, Scholz C, Hollsberg P, Fukaura H, Sette A, Hafler DA. Modulation of cytokine patterns of human autoreactive T cell clones by a single amino acid substitution of their peptide ligand. *Immunity* 1995;2:373.

196. Racke MK, Dhib-Jalbut S, Cannella B, Albert PS, Raine CS, McFarlin DE. Prevention and treatment of chronic relapsing experimental allergic encephalomyelitis by transforming growth factor-β₁. *J Immunol* 1991;146:3012.

197. Santambrogio L, Hochwald GM, Saxena B, et al. Studies on the mechanisms by which transforming growth factor-β (TGF-β) protects against allergic encephalomyelitis. *J Immunol* 1993;151:1116.

198. Ben-Nun, A, Wekerle H, Cohen IR. Vaccination against autoimmune encephalomyelitis using attenuated cells of a T lymphocyte line reactive against myelin basic protein. *Nature* 1981;292:60.

199. Howell MD, Winters ST, Olee T, Powell HC, Carlo DJ, Brostoff SW. Vaccination against experimental allergic encephalomyelitis with T cell receptor peptides. *Science* 1989;246:668.

200. Vandenbark AA, Hashim G, Offner H. Immunization with a synthetic T-cell receptor V-region peptide protects against experimental autoimmune encephalomyelitis. *Nature* 1989;341:541.

201. Offner H, Hashim G, Vandenbark A. T cell receptor peptide therapy triggers autoregulation of experimental encephalomyelitis. *Science* 1991;251:430.

202. Kumar V, Sercarz E. The involvement of T cell receptor peptide-specific regulatory CD4+ T cells in recovery from antigen-induced autoimmune disease. *J Exp Med* 1993;177:1609.

203. Kumar V, Stellrecht K, Sercarz E. Inactivation of T cell receptor peptide-specific CD4 regulatory T cells induces chronic experimental autoimmune encephalomyelitis (EAE). *J Exp Med* 1996;184:1609.

204. Jiang H, Zhang S, Pernis B. Role of CD8⁺ T cells in experimental allergic encephalomyelitis. *Science* 1992;256:1213.

205. Kumar V, Aziz F, Sercarz E, Miller A. Regulatory T cells specific for the same framework 3 region of the Vβ8.2 chain are involved in the control of collagen II-induced arthritis and experimental autoimmune encephalomyelitis. *J Exp Med* 1997;185:1725.

206. Desquenne-Clark L, Esch TR, Otvos L, Heber-Katz E. T-cell receptor peptide immunization leads to enhanced and chronic experimental allergic encephalomyelitis. *Proc Natl Acad Sci USA* 1991;88:7219.

207. Olive J. T cell receptor usage in autoimmune disease. *Immunol Cell Biol* 1995;73:297.

208. Weiner HL, Friedman A, Miller A, et al. Oral tolerance: immunologic mechanisms and treatment of animal and human organ-specific autoimmune diseases by oral administration of autoantigens. *Annu Rev Immunol* 1994;12:809.

209. Weiner HL. Oral tolerance: immune mechanisms and treatment of autoimmune diseases. *Immunol Today* 1997;18:335.

210. Friedman A, Weiner HL. Induction of anergy or active suppression following oral tolerance is determined by antigen dosage. *Proc Natl Acad Sci USA* 1994;91:6688.

211. Miller A, Lider O, Roberts AB, Sporn MB, Weiner HL. Suppressor T cells generated by oral tolerization to myelin basic protein suppress both *in vitro* and *in vivo* immune responses by the release of transforming growth factor β after antigen-specific triggering. *Proc Natl Acad Sci USA* 1992;89:421.

212. Miller A, Lider O, Weiner HL. Antigen-driven bystander suppression after oral administration of antigens. *J Exp Med* 1991;174:791.

213. Al-Sabbagh A, Miller A, Santos LMB, Weiner HL. Antigen-driven tissue-specific suppression following oral tolerance: orally administered myelin basic protein suppresses proteolipid protein-induced experimental autoimmune encephalomyelitis in the SJL mice. *Eur J Immunol* 1994;24:2104.

214. Becker KJ, McCarron RM, Ruetzler C, et al. Immunologic tolerance to myelin basic protein decreases stroke size after transient focal cerebral ischemia. *Proc Natl Acad Sci USA* 1997;94:10873.

215. Groux H, O'Garra A, Bigler M, et al. A CD4⁺ T-cell subset inhibits antigen-specific T-cell responses and prevents colitis. *Nature* 1997;389:737.

216. Von Herrath MG, Dyrberg T, Oldstone MBA. Oral insulin treatment suppresses virus-induced antigen-specific destruction of β cells and prevents autoimmune diabetes in transgenic mice. *J Clin Invest* 1996;98:1324.

217. Chen Y, Inobe J-I, Marks R, Gonnella P, Kuchroo VK, Weiner HL. Peripheral deletion of antigen-reactive T cells in oral tolerance. *Nature* 1995;376:177.

218. Chen Y, Inobe J-I, Kuchroo VK, Baron JL, Janeway CA, Weiner HL. Oral toler-

ance in myelin basic protein T-cell receptor transgenic mice: suppression of autoimmune encephalomyelitis and dose-dependent induction of regulatory cells. *Proc Natl Acad Sci USA* 1996;93:388.

219. Zhang ZJ, Davidson L, Eisenbarth G, Weiner HL. Suppression of diabetes in nonobese diabetic mice by oral administration of porcine insulin. *Proc Natl Acad Sci USA* 1991;88:10252.

220. Hancock WW, Polanski M, Zhang J, Blogg N, Weiner HL. Suppression of insulitis in non-obese diabetic (NOD) mice by oral insulin administration is associated with selective expression of interleukin-4 and-10, transforming growth factor-β, and prostaglandin-E. *Am J Pathol* 1995;147:1193.

221. Tian J, Atkinson MA, Clare-Salzler M, et al. Nasal administration of glutamate decarboxylase (GAD65) peptides induces Th2 responses and prevents murine insulin-dependent diabetes. *J Exp Med* 1996;183:1561.

222. Daniel D, Wegmann DR. Protection of nonobese diabetic mice from diabetes by intranasal or subcutaneous administration of insulin peptide B-(9-23). *Proc Natl Acad Sci USA* 1996;93:956.

223. Khare SD, Krco CJ, Griffiths MM, Luthra HS, David CS. Oral administration of an immunodominant human collagen peptide moldulates collagen-induced arthritis. *J Immunol* 1995;155:3653.

224. Haque MA, Yoshino S, Inada S, Nomaguchi H, Tokunaga O, Kohashi O. Suppression of adjuvant arthritis in rats by induction of oral tolerance to mycobacterial 65-kDa heat shock protein. *Eur J Immunol* 1996;26:2650.

225. Whitcup SM, Nussenblatt RB. Immunologic mechanisms of uveitis. New targets for immunomodulation. *Arch Ophthalmol* 1997;115:520.

226. Iian Y, Prakash R, Davidson A, et al. Oral tolerization to adenoviral antigens permits long-term gene expression using recombinant adenoviral vectors. *J Clin Invest* 1997;99:1098.

227. Karpus WJ, Kennedy KJ, Smith WS, Miller SD. Inhibition of relapsing experimental autoimmune encephalomyelitis in SJL mice by feeding the immunodominant PLP139-151 peptide. *J Neurosci Res* 1996;45:410.

228. Blanas E, Carbone FR, Allison J, Miller JFAP, Heath WR. Induction of autoimmune diabetes by oral administration of autoantigen. *Science* 1996;274:1707.

229. Husby S, Mestecky J, Moldoveanu Z, Holland S, Elson CO. Oral tolerance in humans. T but not B cell tolerance after antigen feeding. *J Immunol* 1994;152:4663.

230. Weiner HL, Mackin GA, Matsui M, et al. Double-blind pilot trial of oral tolerization with myelin antigens in multiple sclerosis. *Science* 1993;259:1321.

231. Fukaura H, Kent SC, Pietrusewicz MJ, Khoury SJ, Weiner HL, Hafler DA. Induction of circulating myelin basic protein and proteolipid protein-specific transforming growth factor-β1-secreting Th3 T cells by oral administration of myelin in multiple sclerosis patients. *J Clin Invest* 1996;98:70.

Fundamental Immunology, Fourth Edition,
edited by William E. Paul
Lippincott–Raven Publishers, Philadelphia © 1999.

CHAPTER 35

Allergy

Stephen J. Galli and Chris S. Lantz

Introduction and Historical Perspective

Features of IgE-associated Immune Responses, Including IgE-associated Clinical Allergies
Overview · Similarities and Differences between IgE-associated Reactions in Humans and in Experimental Animals

Allergens

Regulation of IgE Synthesis
Regulation of IgE Synthesis by Interleukin-4, Interleukin-13, and Other Cytokines · Regulation of IgE Synthesis by CD40 and CD40 Ligand · Regulation of IgE Synthesis by CD23 · Genetic Studies of IgE Production

Receptors for IgE
The High-affinity Receptor for IgE (FcεRI) · FcεRII/CD23

The Effector Cells and Mediators of IgE-associated Immune Responses
Overview · Development and Natural History of Mast Cells and Basophils · Mast-Cell Distribution and Heterogeneity · Mediators Derived from Mast Cells and Basophils · Mechanisms of Mast-Cell or Basophil Activation · Development and Natural History of Eosinophils · Mediators Derived from Eosinophils · Mechanisms of Activation and Recruitment · T Cells · Monocytes and Macrophages and Related Cells

Mechanisms of IgE-associated Acute and Late-phase Reactions and Chronic Allergic Inflammation
Overview · Acute Allergic Reactions · Late-phase Reactions · Chronic Allergic Inflammation · Mast Cell–Leukocyte Cytokine Cascades

Roles of IgE-associated Immune Responses in Host Defense

Features of IgE-associated Allergic Diseases
General Characteristics of Allergic Diseases · Examples of IgE-associated Allergic Diseases

Management Strategies for IgE-associated Allergic Disorders
Overview · Alter the Individual's Predisposition to Develop, or to Strongly and Persistently Express, Allergic Diseases · Reduce or Modify Exposure to Allergen · Inhibit or Modulate the IgE-associated Response Itself · Interfere with Effector-Cell Activation · Interfere with the Production of Mediators by Effector Cells · Block the Action of Mediators on Target Cells · Interrupt the Evolution of Inflammatory Responses by Targeting Adhesion Molecules · Counteract the End-organ Consequences of Allergic Responses

Concluding Remarks

Acknowledgments

References

The purpose of this chapter is to provide a broad overview of the topic of allergy and, in particular, to discuss the basic immunologic mechanisms that underlie the pathogenesis of IgE-associated allergic disorders. Many subjects relevant to the broad area of allergy, such as the biology of T cells, B cells, and antigen-presenting cells (APCs), or the clinical characteristics of specific allergic diseases, are considered in greater detail elsewhere in this volume or in other, more clinically oriented textbooks; such topics are addressed herein rather selectively, to illustrate general points regarding the development or expression of IgE-associated immunologic

responses. Other areas, which are central to our understanding of allergy but which are not treated extensively elsewhere in this volume, such as the biology of mast cells, basophils and eosinophils, the structure and function of the high-affinity receptor for IgE, and the biochemistry and function of the mediators of allergic reactions, are discussed in greater detail.

Because the term *allergy* is now most often used with a meaning that is quite different than the original definition of the term, we will begin by considering the origin of the concept of *allergy* and the subsequent changes in the usage of the word.

INTRODUCTION AND HISTORICAL PERSPECTIVE

The most general definition of *allergy* is altered reactivity to antigenic stimulation (1). Indeed, von Pirquet, who is credited with

S. J. Galli: Department of Pathology, Harvard Medical School, Division of Experimental Pathology, Beth Israel Deaconess Medical Center, Boston, Massachusetts 02215.

C. S. Lantz: Department of Pathology, Harvard Medical School and Beth Israel Deaconess Medical Center, Boston, Massachusetts 02215.

introducing the term *allergy,* intended that the term refer to *all* forms of changed reactivity to antigenic stimulation, whether this resulted in a response protective to the host (i.e., immunity) or to an adverse clinical reaction to the antigen (i.e., hypersensitivity) (1). Thus, when used in this original sense, *allergy* would encompass both beneficial and harmful manifestations of immune system function, whereas an *immune response* would refer to a protective response (1).

However, the term *immune response* is now often used to refer to any functional expression of the immune system, against either foreign or self antigens, and whether the consequences of these reactions are beneficial or harmful to the host. By contrast, the term *allergy* now is almost exclusively used, particularly in the clinical setting, to refer to a subset of potentially harmful immune responses. Moreover, common usage now primarily restricts the term *allergic reactions,* as encountered clinically, to responses to certain environmental antigens (by definition, these are referred to as *allergens,* see ref. 1), such as components of some foods, drugs, pollen, and so on. These *allergic reactions* both (a) reflect the expression of acquired immunologic responsiveness, involving preexisting specific antibodies and/or T cells, and (b) result in any of a number of symptoms, such as runny eyes and increased nasal secretions and sneezing (in hay fever), wheezing and coughing (in asthma), or redness and itching in the skin (in urticaria, i.e., hives, or in reactions to contact allergens, such as poison ivy). Thus, although laypersons may use a much broader definition of allergy (children have declared "allergies" to homework, for example), for the clinician, the *sine qua non* of the definition of allergic diseases is the establishment of an immunologic basis for the disorder.

One of the most enduring of the schemes to classify allergic disorders and other hypersensitivity reactions is that proposed by Coombs and Gell (2). In the initial formulation of this system, four major types of hypersensitivity reactions, or "allergic reactions that may be deleterious to the tissues and harmful to the host" (2), were identified: type I, now often referred to as immediate hypersensitivity, in which allergen or antigen reacts with tissue cells (e.g., mast cells) that have been passively sensitized with specific antibodies, resulting in the release of pharmacologically active mediators of inflammation; type II, now often called cytotoxic reactions, in which antibody reacts with a cell surface component or an antigen or hapten associated with the cell surface and in which complement activation is usually involved in effecting tissue damage; type III, Arthus reactions and other immune-complex reactions, in which toxicity is mediated by immune complexes that are formed by antibody reacting with excess antigen (it was originally proposed that the tissue damage in such reactions might also involve complement activation); and type IV, in which sensitized T cells react with antigen in the absence of any essential role for antibodies.

Coombs and Gell emphasized that their classification referred primarily to the *initiating mechanisms* of allergic reactions, and was not meant as an attempt to classify either the pathogenesis of the later stages in the disease process or the actual diseases themselves.

TABLE 1. *Modified Coombs/Gell classification of the four major types of initiating mechanisms of immunologically-mediated adverse (i.e., "hypersensitivity") reactions*

| Immunologic specificity | Type I: IgE antibody (+ IgG$_1$ in mouse) | Type II: IgG antibody | | Type III: IgG antibody | Type IV: T cells | | |
		a	b		a1 Th1 cells	a2 Th2 cells	b Cytolytic T cells
Antigen	Soluble antigen "allergen"	Cell- or matrix-associated antigen	Cell surface receptors	Soluble antigen	Soluble antigen	Soluble antigen	Cell-associated antigen
Effector mechanism	FcεRI or FcγRIII-dependent mast cell/basophil activation, with release of mediators/cytokines	Complement, FcγR+ professional phagocytes, NK cells	Antibody alters signaling	FcγR+ cells[a], complement	Th1-associated effectors (e.g., macrophages)	Th2-associated effectors (e.g., eosinophils, basophils)	Direct cytotoxicity
Initial consequences[b]	Rapidly developing (seconds to minutes) effects of mediators on target cells (usually not involving direct cytotoxicity)	Cell death and/or tissue injury	Pathology due to increased or diminished receptor-dependent cell function	Inflammation associated with recruitment and activation of neutrophils and other leukocytes	Chronic inflammation Reactions develop slowly (hours to days) and can persist for long periods	Chronic Inflammation	Death of target cells
Examples and notes	IgE- (or, in mouse, IgG$_1$-) dependent anaphylaxis (potentially fatal systemic reaction) or passive cutaneous anaphylaxis (a local reaction)	Certain drug reactions and reactions to incompatible blood transfusions	Graves disease (thyroid stimulating agonist antibody); myasthenia gravis (antagonist antibody to acetylcholine receptor)	(including mast cells in the mouse); Arthus reaction and other "immune complex"–mediated reactions	Contact dermatitis, tuberculin reaction	Chronic allergic inflammation (type I reactions may also contribute to chronic allergic inflammation)	Reactions to certain viral infected cells, certain forms of graft rejection

[a]This modification of the original scheme (refs 2) incorporates some of the features of the modifications presented elsewhere (3, 4).
[b]These are the major initial consequences; intense inflammatory responses (e.g., of types III or IVa1) can also sometimes lead to tissue injury and cell death at the site of the reactions, whereas extensive cell death by necrosis (e.g., in type IIa or IVb reactions) can induce the development of an inflammatory response.

Indeed, they felt that some individual immunologic diseases probably involved more than one of their "types" of allergic reactions (2). Nevertheless, subsequent modifications of the original scheme have not only proposed useful subdivisions of the original four types of allergic reactions, but have also attempted to classify various immunologic disorders as "examples" of such subtypes of the four major reaction patterns (3). In the scheme shown in Table 1, we have retained the modifications of the Coombs and Gell classification presented by Janeway and Travers (4) and, in slightly modified form, by Kay (3), but have included some additional comments on the classification and its relevance to specific allergic diseases.

It bears emphasis that certain clinical disorders may represent relatively "pure" manifestations of individual Coombs and Gell "types" of hypersensitivity reactions, whereas the pathogenesis of others may be much more complex. Anaphylaxis is a life-threatening systemic reaction that occurs in sensitized individuals within minutes of their exposure to the offending allergen; this reaction reflects largely, if not entirely, the effects of mediators released by the IgE antibody–dependent activation of specialized effector cells (see section on features of IgE-associated allergic diseases). Anaphylaxis is thought to represent a relatively pure form of a type I "immediate hypersensitivity" reaction. By contrast, allergic reactions to poison ivy, and other examples of cutaneous contact hypersensitivity responses, are thought to represent a relatively pure form of a type IV T cell–dependent "delayed hypersensitivity" reaction. But other clinical conditions resist such neat accommodation within the classical Coombs-Gell scheme.

Given the potential complexity of most allergic diseases (and many "models" of allergic diseases in experimental animals), we favor, whenever possible, avoiding the use of nomenclature or classification schemes that appear to imply a certainty about underlying mechanisms that, in fact, may not yet have been achieved. For example, the relative contributions of IgE antibodies, as opposed to T cells or other effector mechanisms, to the different individual pathologic features of human allergic asthma appear to vary, and some aspects of the disease may depend more on T cell–dependent (i.e., type IVa2) than IgE-dependent (i.e., type I) effector mechanisms (5,6). On the other hand, the notion that IgE antibodies importantly contribute to the pathogenesis of many allergic diseases in humans not only is firmly entrenched among most immunologists and allergists, but also is probably correct. Accordingly, in this chapter, we primarily will use the term *IgE-associated* (rather than either *type I, immediate hypersensitivity,* or *IgE-dependent*) to refer to examples of experimental or naturally occurring immune responses that include the development of a prominent IgE antibody response to the initiating allergens. By using this term, we mean to indicate that a robust antigen-specific IgE response is an important defining *phenotypic characteristic* of such immune responses, but we do not intend to imply that IgE-dependent reactions necessarily represent the only or even, in some cases, the most important pathogenetic mechanisms in the expression of these responses.

While all of the types of "allergic reactions" in the Coombs and Gell classification clearly can contribute to human diseases (some examples are given in Table 1), the majority of patients encountered in the clinical practice of allergy suffer from IgE-associated immune responses. For this reason, and because discussions of the mechanisms that underlie the expression of the other Coombs-Gell "types" of allergic reactions may be found elsewhere in this vol-

TABLE 2. *Definitions of key terms*

Allergy	*Original definition (von Pirquet):* Altered reactivity to antigenic stimulation, which may result in a protective response (i.e., immunity) or an adverse clinical reaction (i.e., hypersensitivity). *Current usage:* Clinically adverse reactions to environmental antigens (allergens, see below) which reflect the expression of acquired immunologic responsiveness involving allergen-specific antibodies and/or T cells. Often used to refer specifically to adverse immunologic responses that are associated with the production of allergen-specific IgE.
Allergens	Antigens that typically elicit a specific IgE response (in at least some individuals). Allergens ordinarily have little or no intrinsic toxicity (exceptions include components of *Hymenoptera* insect or other venoms), but induce pathology because of their ability to elicit an IgE-associated immune response, and, upon subsequent exposure, to elicit IgE- and/or T cell–dependent hypersensitivity reactions. Note: Antigens that can elicit contact hypersensitivity responses (a type IVa1 reaction in Table 1) are often called contact allergens, even though they may not also elicit an IgE response.
IgE-associated immune response	The group of immune responses (whether protective, e.g., against certain parasites, or clinically adverse, e.g., in allergic diseases) that are associated with the production of specific IgE to certain antigens (allergens) and in which IgE-mediated reactions (type I or immediate hypersensitivity reactions in the Coombs and Gell classification, see Table 1) are thought to have a role.
Immediate hypersensitivity reactions	These may also be called acute IgE-associated allergic reactions. The group of immunologically specific reactions, whether local or systemic, which typically occur within minutes of allergen exposure in sensitized individuals and which reflect the recognition of the allergen by IgE (and/or, in mice, IgG$_1$) antibodies bound to specific receptors on the surface of effector cells (primarily mast cells and basophils); this results in the aggregation of the receptors, leading to the activation of the effector cells to release mediators that produce the acute signs and symptoms of the reaction.
Allergic diseases	The group of clinical disorders (such as hay fever, allergic asthma, and atopic dermatitis) in which IgE-associated immune responses, typically directed against otherwise innocuous environmental allergens, are thought to have a pathogenetic role. Certain aspects of the pathology associated with these diseases, such as the chronic allergic inflammation that is characteristic of allergic asthma or atopic dermatitis, probably reflect significant "effector cell" contributions from T cells (especially Th2 cells), in addition to FcεRI+ effector cells.
Atopy	The propensity to develop immediate hypersensitivity reactions to common allergens. Note: Individuals who are "non-atopic," in that they lack skin test reactivity to common environmental allergens, may nonetheless exhibit life-threatening IgE-associated reactions to the venom of stinging insects.

ume, this chapter focuses largely on the IgE-associated immune responses. Definitions of some of the key terms that are used in this chapter are provided in Table 2.

FEATURES OF IgE-ASSOCIATED IMMUNE RESPONSES, INCLUDING IgE-ASSOCIATED CLINICAL ALLERGIES

Overview

The immune responses that are elicited in response to infections with many parasites, as well as in response to many otherwise innocuous environmental allergens that are not derived from parasites, are often associated with high levels of IgE production; such immune responses are now known to be promoted by antigen-specific T helper 2 (Th2) cells (7–10). These facts have supported the widely held view that unwanted IgE-associated immune responses (i.e., allergic diseases) are the unfortunate result of the immune system perceiving and responding to otherwise essentially harmless allergens as if they were derived from a parasite (Fig. 1).

In the context of either parasite infections or allergic diseases, allergen challenge of a sensitized host can result in a range of tissue responses, depending on such factors as the route and dose of allergen challenge, and whether the allergen challenge represents a single transient exposure, results in the persistence of the allergen, or occurs seasonally (as in hay fever) or in some other repetitive fashion; the tissue responses may also be affected importantly by the genetic background of the host and by diverse nongenetic factors (such as certain concurrent infections), which can modify the host's response to allergen.

Nevertheless, it is useful to think of the effector phases of IgE-associated immune responses as occurring in three temporal patterns: (a) *acute reactions,* which develop within seconds or minutes of allergen exposure; (b) *late-phase reactions,* which develop within hours of allergen exposure, often after at least some of the effects of the acute reaction have partially diminished; and (c) *chronic allergic inflammation,* which can persist for days to years (see Fig. 1). By selecting appropriate experimental model systems, it is possible to elicit examples of acute or late-phase reactions, or chronic allergic inflammation, for detailed analysis. However, the responses to allergen challenge in "naturally" sensitized subjects, whether the sensitization has occurred in the context of a parasite infection or an allergic disease, may represent very complex tissue responses, which reflect the overlapping or sequential expression of acute, late-phase, and chronic IgE-associated reactions. Important general features of IgE-associated immune responses are given in Table 3.

Similarities and Differences between IgE-associated Reactions in Humans and in Experimental Animals

The value of a number of mammalian species for studies of IgE-associated immune responses has been reviewed (11–17). While a detailed comparison of the features of IgE-associated immune responses in humans and the many other mammalian species in which such responses have been studied is beyond the scope of this chapter, some general points seem clear. Individual nonhuman species may have certain advantages (and disadvantages) for the analysis of particular aspects of IgE-associated immune responses (and individual investigators tend to be especially fond of the experimental species with which they work), yet most investigators would agree that the final proof of human relevance of findings initially made in other mammalian species requires the direct examination of the human system. On the other hand, there is no denying the experimental flexibility, and importance, of employing nonhuman mammalian species for studies of immune responses. The mouse (*Mus musculus*) is a particularly useful model, because it is possible to perform extensive genetic manipulation in this species, it is relatively inexpensive to maintain, it has a relatively short interval to reach reproductive age, and much is already known about its immune system. Accordingly, this chapter focuses primarily on results derived from studies performed in mice and in humans.

IgE-associated immune responses in mice and humans exhibit the general features presented in Table 3. However, the responses in the two species also exhibit some potentially significant differences, as listed in Table 4. Two of these need special emphasis.

First, there seems to be significantly more redundancy in mice than in humans with respect to the immunoglobulin isotypes that are both Th2 cell–driven and able to sensitize mast cells and other FcεRI$^+$ effector cells for release of mediators in response to challenge with specific allergen. In mice, IgG$_1$ is not only typically coordinately regulated with IgE, but it can also perform many of the same general functions as IgE (see section on regulation of IgE synthesis, below). By contrast, there is as yet no convincing evidence in humans to support the existence of a subclass of IgG that can substitute for IgE in the expression of "immediate-type" hypersensitivity responses. This fact has a number of important implications, not the least of which is that the phenotype of genetically IgE-deficient mice (which can still express multiple features of allergen-specific anaphylactic responses, including death; see ref. 18), probably does not accurately mimic the phenotype that might be expressed in humans who are rendered IgE-deficient.

Second, evidence indicates that, in humans, FcεRI (the high-affinity Fc receptor for IgE) can be expressed, at least under some

FIG. 1. Steps in the development (sensitization phase) and expression (effector phase) of IgE-associated immune responses, such as those elicited in response to allergens derived from parasites or from otherwise innocuous agents (e.g., pollen). *Dotted lines* in the diagram refer to potential interactions whose biologic importance is not yet clear. Note that dendritic cells, such as those in the respiratory mucosa and the Langerhans' cells in the skin, can occur within epithelia, placing them in position to interact with allergens at or near the epithelial surface. In the effector phase of IgE-associated responses, the extent to which mast cells versus Th2 cells contribute to the development of various features of late-phase reactions or chronic allergic inflammation in different settings may vary. It is not yet clear whether cells of monocytic lineage (e.g., macrophages, Langerhans' cells, or other dendritic cells), in addition to their function as APCs, also can represent important IgE-dependent sources of cytokines and other mediators. However, the APC function of such cells can be enhanced by the binding of allergen to IgE bound to the cells' surface.

DEVELOPMENT AND EXPRESSION OF IgE-ASSOCIATED IMMUNE RESPONSES

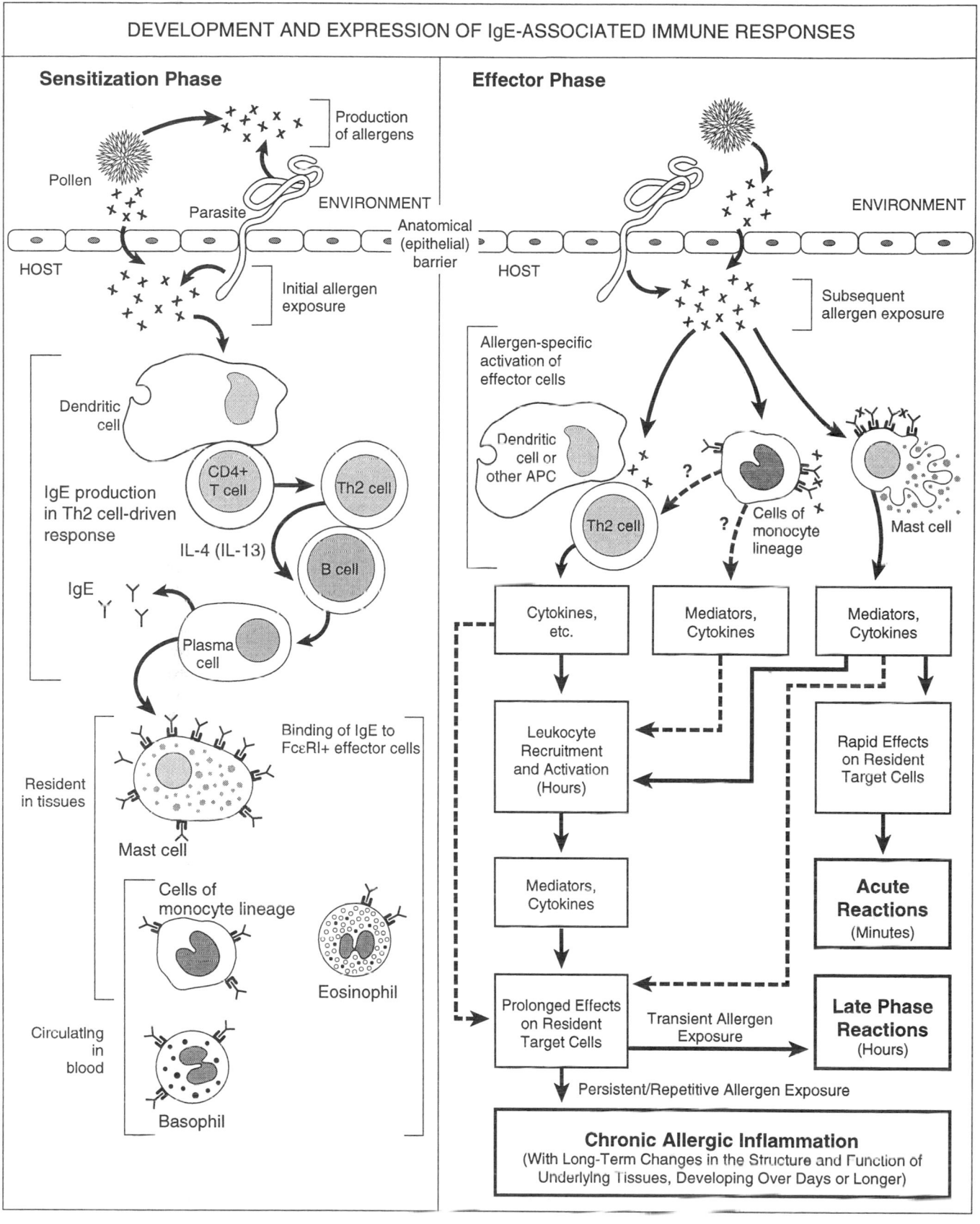

TABLE 3. *Major features of IgE-associated immune responses in humans and mice*

1. Responses are elicited by certain groups of antigens (i.e., allergens) derived from components of parasites or from diverse environmental substances (e.g., certain foods and drugs, and proteins derived from plant pollen, insects, or mammalian pets).
2. Depending on the circumstances, responses to allergen in sensitized subjects can result in acute reactions (which occur within seconds to minutes), late phase reactions (which occur hours after allergen challenge) and/or chronic allergic inflammation (which can persist for days to years).
3. Th2 cells and Th2 cell-associated cytokines are important in regulating various aspects of the responses. Th2 cells may also express effector functions in certain responses, particularly in certain late phase reactions and in chronic allergic inflammation.
4. Immunologic specificity of activation of FcR-bearing effector cells is conferred by IgE (and, in mice, IgG$_1$) antibodies.
5. Tissue mast cells and, in some cases, blood basophils, have an important effector role in acute reactions and may contribute to late-phase reactions and chronic allergic inflammation.
6. Binding to the FcεRI (the high-affinity receptor for IgE), which is expressed on mast cells and basophils in humans and mice, is the major mechanism by which IgE can express effector function in these responses. Note: In humans, but not in mice, FcεRI can be expressed on additional cells with potential effector or immunoregulatory roles in these reactions, including monocytes/macrophages, circulating dendritic cells, Langerhans' cells, and eosinophils.
7. Acute reactions reflect the actions of mediators derived from IgE/IgG$_1$-sensitized effector cells that are normally resident in the tissues (especially mast cells), whereas leukocytes recruited to the tissues make important contributions to late-phase reactions and chronic allergic inflammation.
8. Acute reactions typically do not result in permanent structural changes in the underlying tissues, whereas such changes typically do occur at sites of persistent chronic allergic inflammation.
9. These responses can be primarily harmful to the host, especially when they are elicited by otherwise essentially innocuous allergens, or may confer benefit in host defense, when they are elicited in response to infection with certain parasites.

circumstances, by many potential effector cells in addition to mast cells and basophils, including Langerhans' cells, blood monocytes and macrophages, circulating dendritic cells, and eosinophils (see section on receptors for IgE, below). Many of these cell types may exclusively express the αγ$_2$ form of the receptor, which in turn may mediate functional responses that are not identical to those mediated by the αβγ$_2$ form of the FcεRI that is expressed by mast cells and basophils (see section on receptors for IgE). Nevertheless, the presence of FcεRI on these cells certainly suggests that they may contribute to the expression of IgE-associated immune responses in humans. By contrast, normal mice appear to express FcεRI (of the αβγ$_2$ form) exclusively on mast cells and basophils (see section on receptors for IgE). However, mice express FcγRIII, which can bind IgG$_1$ and which utilizes the same β and γ chains as FcεRI, on monocytes and macrophages, neutrophils, and natural killer (NK) cells (19). Thus, in mice, the IgG$_1$ generated during a Th2 response may permit effectors other than mast cells and basophils to participate in the expression of IgE-associated immune responses, whereas, in humans, IgE itself appears to be able to sensitize multiple potential effector cells, in addition to mast cells and basophils, for the expression of allergen-specific function in IgE-associated immune responses.

ALLERGENS

Allergens are antigens that can elicit specific IgE responses that, in at least some individuals, are sufficiently robust to be associated with clinical evidence of IgE-associated hypersensitivity responses (20, 21). Both the ability of individual human or experimental animal subjects to develop specific IgE responses to particular potential allergens, and the overall strength of the IgE responses that can be expressed by individual subjects, are genetically determined (see section on regulation of IgE synthesis). As a result, a particular allergen will not be "allergenic" in all subjects. Nevertheless, individuals who are genetically predisposed to develop strong IgE responses (i.e., atopic humans) typically exhibit specific IgE responses to multiple distinct allergens.

Why do some foreign antigens represent potent allergens, whereas others do not? Unfortunately, even though there has been great progress in the cloning, sequencing, and physicochemical characterization of diverse allergens, the identification of a simple set of "general rules of allergenicity" has remained elusive. Perhaps this is not surprising, because the properties that would confer allergenicity on a substance that is experienced by the individual in minute quantities at mucosal surfaces (e.g., many allergens present in the air, or aeroallergens) may be quite different from

TABLE 4. *Important differences between IgE-associated immune responses in humans and mice*

1. In mice, either IgE or IgG$_1$-can function to sensitize mast cells for allergen-specific effector function, whereas there is no firm evidence for clinically important anaphylactogenic antibodies in humans other than those of the IgE isotype.
2. In normal mice, the FcεRI is apparently expressed only on mast cells and basophils, whereas, in humans, the αγ$_2$ form of FcεRI can be found on many other cell types, including monocytes/macrophages, circulating dendritic cells, Langerhans' cells, and eosinophils. Note: In IgE-associated immune responses in mice, it is likely that the participation of some of the effector cells which in humans express the αγ$_2$ form of FcεRI can be elicited via allergen-specific IgG antibodies and FcγR.
3. Some IgE-associated immune responses in mice are associated with striking hyperplasia of certain mast cell populations in the affected tissues (e.g., over 100-fold increases in intestinal mucosal mast cells in certain nematode infections); the changes in tissue mast cell numbers in corresponding settings in humans typically are much less impressive.
4. Basophils may represent a more important effector cell in these responses in humans than in mice (this cell type ordinarily is extremely infrequent in the blood of many strains of mice).

those of allergens that are presented to the immune system parenterally and in large doses (e.g., injected antibiotics). The first class would need to have properties that permit the substance to traverse various components of the mucosal barrier of the respiratory tract prior to presentation to the immune system, whereas, for the latter substances, the systemic distribution of the allergen is ensured by courtesy of the health care provider.

On the other hand, certain generalizations about the properties of allergens (almost all of which have exceptions) have emerged. Allergens typically are proteins (often, glycoproteins) or chemicals (haptens) that can become bound to proteins (21). These substances are named in accord with guidelines published in 1994 by the World Health Organization/International Union of Immunologic Sciences Allergen Nomenclature Sub-committee (22). The names incorporate the first three letters of the genus and the first (or first two, to avoid ambiguity) letter(s) of the species from which the allergen is derived, plus an Arabic numeral (which can be used to denote structurally homologous allergens from different species). For example, structurally similar allergens (antigen 5) from two species of *Vespula* wasps (*V. vulgaris* and *V. vidua*) are designated Ves v 5 and Ves vi 5, respectively. Four additional numbers can be used to identify specific isoallergens or variants. For example, four isoallergens derived from short ragweed (*Ambrosia artemisiifolia*), two of which are variants of the first, are designated Amb a 1.01, Amb a 1.0101 and Amb a 1.0102, and Amb a 1.02.

Efforts to identify, clone, and characterize allergens have been pursued to understand why certain substances are allergenic and for clinical purposes. Highly purified native allergen preparations and, increasingly, the corresponding recombinant proteins, can be used diagnostically, for example, to identify the presence of reactive (or cross-reactive) IgE (23), to perform clinical tests (e.g., skin tests or airway provocation studies), and to elicit specific IgE-associated allergic responses for experimental analyses. In some cases, such allergen preparations can also be used therapeutically, to elicit "desensitization" or in attempts to induce T-cell tolerance (see section on management strategies for IgE-associated allergic disorders, below).

Analyses of common allergens so far have not revealed why these substances induce a Th2 cell–driven, IgE-associated response. Antigenic fragments of allergens are presented to the T-cell receptor (TCR) via major histocompatibility complex (MHC) class II molecules on APCs, as for fragments of other antigens (24), and both DR-restricted and DP-restricted responses to allergens have been identified (25). Many allergens are enzymes, and it has been proposed that a widespread ability to express strong Th2-type responses to enzymes evolved because of selection pressure that favored the development of adequate immune responses to parasites (many of which depend on enzymes for successful invasion of, or migration through, host tissues), but that this response can also be elicited by otherwise "innocuous" enzymes, such as those allergenic enzymes produced by plants, insects, and companion animals (26–29). It is also possible that such enzymes, whether derived from pathogens such as parasites or comprising various innocuous allergens, may themselves be able to have certain effects (independent of their ability to function as antigens) that can initiate the development of Th2-type responses, for example, by directly inducing interleukin-4 (IL-4) or IL-13 production in mast cells, basophils, T cells, or other potential sources of these cytokines.

Both hypotheses are attractive, but the first (i.e., allergens represent substances that the immune system perceives as if they were components of parasites) may be difficult to confirm experimentally, whereas the second (i.e., allergens can themselves directly initiate Th2-type responses), while accessible to rigorous experimental verification, is yet to be firmly established. Allergenic enzymes might also have effects that promote allergenicity that are independent of their ability to induce cytokine production. For example, Der p 1, a proteolytically active house dust mite allergen, can release CD23 from the surface of human B cells (30). If soluble CD23 can significantly enhance IgE responses (31), or if the loss of CD23 from the B cell surface can diminish a negative feedback signal for IgE production (32) (and see section on receptors for IgE), then Der p 1 might promote the development of an IgE-associated immune response, at least in part, by altering the regulation of IgE production (30).

However, many allergens lack enzymatic activity (21). Also, many allergens are glycoproteins, and it is possible that the oligosaccharide side chains of some of these molecules may favor their binding to lectin receptors on APCs, and thus promote APC allergen uptake (21). Accordingly, perhaps the most reasonable working hypothesis is that different allergens may elicit Th2-type, IgE-associated responses by distinct mechanisms.

The clinical classification of allergens is based on specific aspects of their origin, or patterns of their distribution and/or dissemination within the environment. For example, *aeroallergens* refers to airborne allergens, typically associated with airborne particles (e.g., pollen grains, dust mite feces, animal danders). These are further subdivided into indoor or outdoor aeroallergens (e.g., the dust mite–, cockroach-derived, or household pet–derived allergens or the pollen-derived allergens, respectively) (21). Aeroallergens are typically relatively small proteins that are highly soluble in aqueous media (permitting them to disperse in mucus and other bodily fluids) and are associated with or derived from particles whose properties favor the survival or dispersal of the intact allergen (20,21). For example, dust mite–associated allergens, some of them derived from digestive enzymes (such as Der p 1, a 222-amino acid cysteine protease; see ref. 33), are incorporated into the fecal particles of dust mites (*Dermatophagoides pteronyssinus* and *D. farinae*). The survival and reproduction of these creatures, which subsist on the keratin disquamated from the surface of human skin, can be enhanced by a number of factors often associated with socioeconomic "progress," including the warm, relatively humid environment of well-insulated and heated homes and wall-to-wall carpets (which are difficult to clean adequately of the dust mite feces or keratin) (20). Moreover, Der p 1 and other mite allergens can remain intact in the dust mite fecal particles for long periods. The particles also represent a delivery system (for transporting the allergens to the skin surface or mucosa of the respiratory tract) and may also favor allergen presentation and/or processing by APCs (20).

Notably, the types of clinical problems associated with particular aeroallergens vary, although the extent to which this reflects the nature of the allergens, as opposed to the pattern of exposure to the allergens, is not clear. Thus, pollen-associated allergens typically are associated with allergic rhinitis (hay fever) to a greater extent than asthma, whereas the production of specific IgE to cockroach-, dust mite–, and cat-derived allergens represents a significant risk factor for the development of asthma, as well as allergic rhinitis (20,34).

Food allergens can be derived from a long list of food items, but allergens derived from peanuts and other legumes, tree nuts, fish and shellfish, crustacea and mollusks, cow's milk, hen's egg, and cereal grains account for a large fraction of clinically significant food allergies (21,35,36). The allergens are typically 10- to 70-kDa proteins that are relatively resistant to heat denaturation or acid hydrolysis, proteolysis, and digestion. However, there are important exceptions (e.g., many allergens in fresh fruit or vegetables are heat-labile). Allergic reactions to food allergens can be catastrophic, including fatal anaphylaxis (35–37).

Insect venoms contain allergens, many of them enzymes, that can induce IgE-associated responses in both atopic and nonatopic individuals (38,39), and the stings of *Hymenoptera* species (yellowjackets, bees, hornets, etc.) represent a common cause of anaphylaxis. This may reflect the fact that relatively large amounts of venom can be injected intradermally and/or subcutaneously during a single sting (approximately 50 μg; see ref. 38). Moreover, some *Hymenoptera*-associated allergens can be cross-reactive. Fortunately, allergen desensitization with *Hymenoptera* venom allergens can be performed in many sensitized subjects with a very high rate of success (38,39).

Most conventional pharmaceutical agents (drugs) are relatively low-molecular-weight compounds that become allergens only after their haptenization to endogenous proteins. Penicillin is associated with a relatively high incidence of allergic reactions (e.g., adverse reactions thought to be due to IgE were reported in approximately 3% of clinic patients receiving penicillin; see ref. 40), probably because both penicillin and its metabolic products are chemically highly reactive. Moreover, the drug is often administered parenterally, which greatly increases the probability that an adverse IgE-associated response will be fatal (41). Indeed, while the first recorded case of penicillin-induced anaphylaxis occurred in 1949, by 1972 this drug was thought to account for 75% of all recorded fatalities due to anaphylaxis (42). While protein-bound penicillin itself is the major allergen, some of its metabolic products (penicilloate and penilloate), although minor allergens, appear to induce a large fraction of the life-threatening reactions observed in patients treated with penicillin (40). However, many other drugs have also been associated with anaphylactic responses, including cephalosporin antibiotics (which are structurally similar to penicillin and which may be cross-reactive with IgE induced by penicillin), sulfonamide antibiotics, and quaternary ammonium compounds used as neuromuscular blocking agents (41).

It bears emphasis that the mechanisms that may produce adverse immunologic responses to drugs are not restricted to IgE-associated immediate hypersensitivity-type reactions, but can include all of the immunopathologic reactions in the Coombs and Gell classification (2,41) (see Table 1).

REGULATION OF IgE SYNTHESIS

In 1921, Prausnitz and Küstner (43) demonstrated that the passive transfer of a serum factor from a fish-allergic individual (in this case, Küstner himself) to an individual not allergic to fish (Prausnitz) permitted the nonallergic subject to exhibit sensitivity to a specific allergen. Decades later, this serum factor, also known as reagin, was conclusively shown to be a new immunoglobulin class (44), which was also recognized through analysis of the human myeloma protein IgND (45); this new immunoglobulin class was designated IgE. IgE not only has the shortest biologic half-life (2.5 days or less) of all classes of immunoglobulins (46,47), but also is present in serum at the lowest levels, usually less than 100 ng per ml in nonatopic individuals (48). While there is considerable overlap between IgE levels in normal and atopic adults, IgE concentrations in atopic or parasitized individuals can be 100- to more than 1,000-fold higher than those in nonatopic, nonparasitized adults (48,49). IgE is directly involved in mediating many allergic reactions as a result of its ability to bind to and, upon contact with multivalent allergen, to activate various effector cells, such as mast cells and basophils (see section on receptors for IgE and section on effector cells and mediators of IgE-associated immune responses).

The induction of IgE synthesis requires cytokines secreted by CD4$^+$ Th cells (Fig. 2). These cells can be subdivided into either Th1 or Th2 subsets based on their functional capabilities and the profile of cytokines that they produce (7–10). Th1 cells represent a major source of IL-2, interferon-γ (INF-γ), and tumor necrosis factor-β (TNF-β), cytokines important in the development of cell-mediated immune responses. Th2 cells secrete IL-4, IL-5, IL-6, IL-10, and IL-13, which are important in the development of humoral immune responses, including IgE-associated allergic responses. While not all immunologic diseases can be easily classified as being mediated predominantly by Th1 or Th2 cells, allergic diseases (as well as IgE-associated immune responses to many parasites) do appear to be predominantly dependent on Th2 cells (9,10).

Notably, the initial allergen-induced differentiation of naive Th cells to Th2 cells, while potentially influenced by many factors, appears to require the production of IL-4 early in the immune response (50) (see Fig. 2). The cellular source of this "early IL-4" (cells *X, Y,* and *Z* in Fig. 2) is not yet clear. While much attention had focused on NK1.1$^+$ CD4$^+$ T cells, which can rapidly produce large amounts of IL-4 upon suitable activation *in vivo,* these cells do not appear to be necessary for the induction of Th2 responses leading to IgE production (51–55). Other potential candidate sources of early IL-4 include naive CD4$^+$ T cells, mast cells, basophils, and eosinophils (56–58), and it is possible that different potential sources of the cytokine are responsible for producing early IL-4 in different examples of IgE-associated immune responses.

Whatever the source(s) of early IL-4, the induction of IgE synthesis also requires the binding of allergen by allergen-specific B cells via their membrane-bound immunoglobulin receptor (BCR) (see Fig. 2). The B cells then internalize and process the allergen, and present the processed allergen to Th2 cells as peptide fragments in association with MHC class II molecules (see Fig. 2). The peptide–MHC class II complex is then recognized by the TCR on Th2 cells. Once activated (e.g., by its interaction with allergen peptide–MHC class II complex on APCs or B cells), these T cells provide B cells with two signals that are crucial for IgE synthesis. First, activated Th2 cells begin to secrete the IgE-switching

FIG. 2. Major cellular interactions in the development of the sensitization phase of an IgE-associated immune response. Note that the cellular origin(s) of early IL-4 in this setting, as well as the factors that induce such cells to release this early IL-4, remain to be clarified. Also, it is likely that dendritic cells represent the most critical APCs in the primary response to allergen; these cells can acquire allergen at or near epithelial surfaces, then migrate to regional lymphoid tissue, where, as mature dendritic cells, they can present peptide–MHC complexes to naive T cells and deliver costimulatory signals for T-cell activation.

CELLULAR INTERACTIONS IN THE DEVELOPMENT OF AN IgE-ASSOCIATED IMMUNE RESPONSE

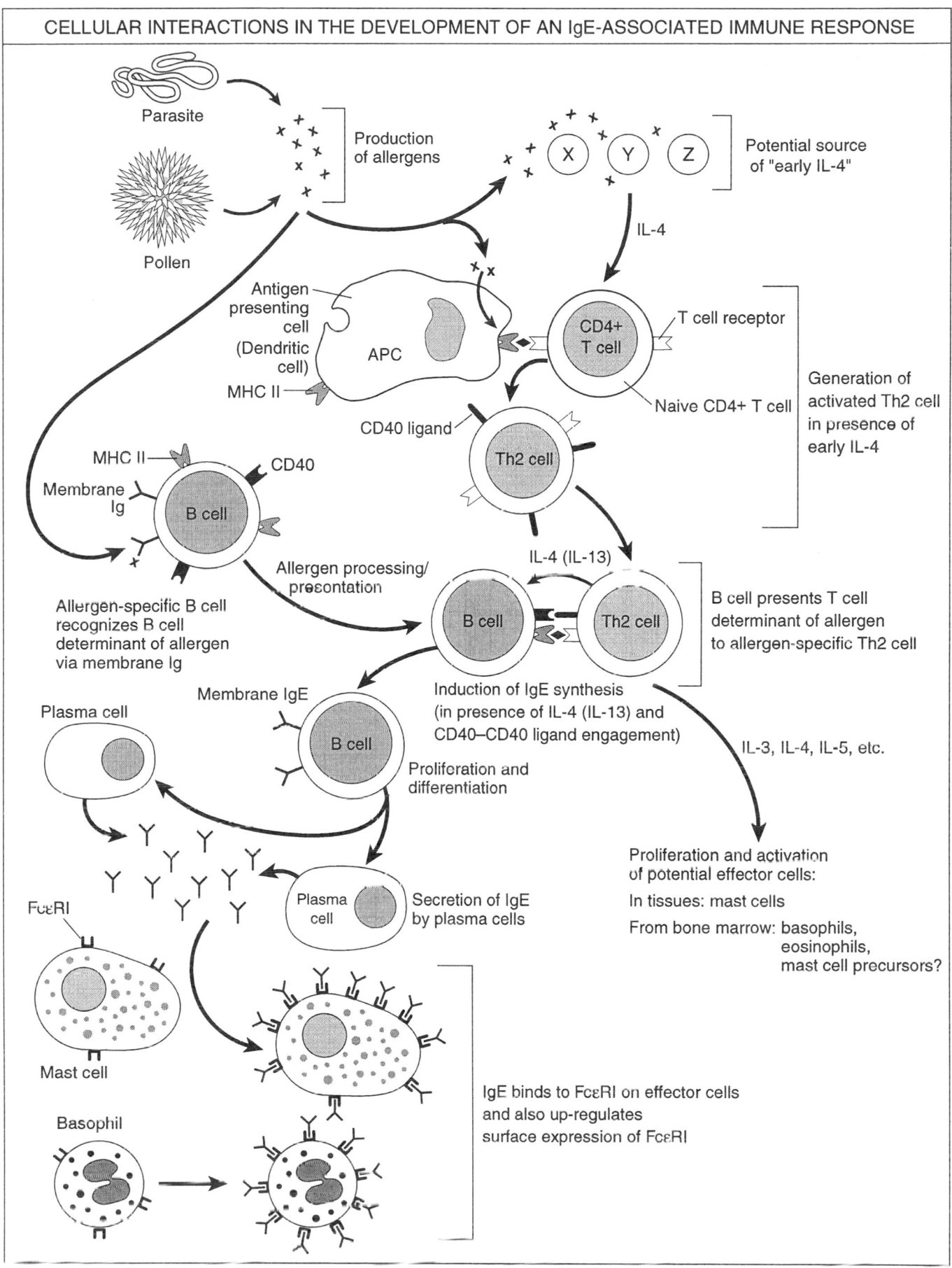

cytokines IL-4 and/or IL-13 (see below). In addition, cell-to-cell contact between B cells and T cells is required for IgE production, and this can be effected via binding of CD40 ligand (CD40L) expressed on the Th2 cell surface to CD40 expressed on B cells.

The switch from IgM to IgE by B cells appears to occur by sequential deletional events, such that mouse or human B cells initially switch to IgG_1 or IgG_4, respectively (see Chapter 24). The production of these particular IgG isotypes and IgE are subject to similar regulatory signals, and thus they are often coordinately expressed at high levels. The simplified two-signal model of IgE production described above is subject to fine positive and negative regulation by additional soluble and cell membrane–associated molecules (see Chapter 24). For example, a recent study indicates that interactions between either B7-1 or B7-2 on APCs and CD28 on T cells can provide the costimulatory signal needed for activation of T-cell IL-4 production during the evolution of the Th2-type response (59). The potential complexity of IgE production is further illustrated by the fact that, under some circumstances, IgE can be produced independently of T cells and/or IL-4, as discussed below.

It has been reported that several different variants of the IgE heavy chain can be produced as a result of alternative mRNA splicing (60). This observation raises the intriguing possibility (which, however, is yet to be confirmed) that these different isoforms of IgE may express different functional properties *in vivo* (60).

Regulation of IgE Synthesis by Interleukin-4, Interleukin-13, and Other Cytokines

IL-4 was initially described based on its ability to enhance B-cell growth and IgG_1 class switching (61,62). The central role of IL-4 in IgE induction was first described using LPS-stimulated mouse B cells and with human B cells cultured with activated T-cell clones or their supernatants (63–67). More recently, the role of IL-4 in IgE induction has been confirmed *in vivo* using mice that either overexpress IL-4 or are deficient in various steps in IL-4 signaling. Thus, IL-4 transgenic mice have very high levels of serum IgE and develop an allergic-like cutaneous disorder (68), whereas both polyclonal and antigen-specific IgE responses are severely impaired in mice treated with either anti–IL-4 or anti–IL-4 receptor antibodies (69,70). Similarly, IL-4 knock-out mice are unable to synthesize detectable amounts of IgE in response to infection with the nematode *Nippostrongylus brasiliensis* (71,72). While the vast majority of IgE synthesis in many contexts appears to require IL-4, IL-4–independent IgE class switching can occur in the mouse under certain circumstances. For instance, IL-4–deficient mice can make small amounts of IgE when infected with *Leishmania major*, *Plasmodium chabaudi*, or the retrovirus that causes mouse immunodeficiency disease (73–75).

Mouse and human IL-4 function in part by inducing transcription through the ε switch region, resulting in the synthesis of ε-germline transcripts. In the mouse, there are a number of highly conserved DNA sequences located 5′ to the major initiation sites for ε-germline RNA, which bind the transcription factors Stat6, NF-κB/Rel proteins, and members of the C/EMP family (76). Mutations of any of the binding sites for these transcription factors can severely impair the IL-4 inducibility of the ε promoter (76). In humans, it appears that the transcription factors Stat6 and the B cell lineage–specific activator protein (BSAP or Pax-5) activate the ε-germline promoter (77). Stat6 appears to be essential for IL-4–induced IgE synthesis, in that Stat6 knock-out mice exhibit little or no detectable levels of serum IgE either before or after immunization or infection with

nematodes (78–80). Notably, membrane expression of IgE is required for IgE secretion *in vivo*, because mice that lack the transmembrane and cytoplasmic domains of IgE exhibit profound (greater than 95%) reductions in serum IgE and give minimal specific responses to immunization with allergen (81).

IL-13 also can express IgE-switching activity in human B cells (82). IL-13 and IL-4 have many overlapping biologic properties, including the induction of B-cell activation, proliferation, and class switching to IgE and (in humans) IgG_4, and both cytokines are produced by activated T cells, mast cells, and basophils (82–95). However, mouse and human T cells and mouse B cells apparently lack detectable IL-13 receptors and do not respond to IL-13 (83). The similarity in function between IL-4 and IL-13 also extends to their receptors, in that the α chain of the IL-4R is a common component of both receptors (96). Both IL-13 and IL-4 activate Stat6, and T cells from Stat6 knock-out mice do not differentiate into Th2 cells in response to either cytokine (80). While IL-13 shares many functions with IL-4, more studies are needed to determine the relative contributions of IL-4 versus IL-13 to human IgE production *in vivo*.

A variety of other cytokines or factors have been shown to modulate IgE synthesis. Cytokines that have been shown to inhibit IgE synthesis, at least under some circumstances, include INF-γ, INF-α, TGF-β, IL-8, IL-10, and IL-12 (97), while enhancement has been observed with IL-5, IL-6, IL-9, TNF-α (97), and MIP-1α (98). These cytokines can either act by directly influencing B-cell IgE class switching or proliferation, or act indirectly through effects on T cells. Furthermore, the ability of some cytokines to modulate IL-4–induced IgE synthesis appears to differ depending on whether mouse or human B cells are employed, as well as on the conditions of culture (e.g., according to the type of costimulus that is used to induce the IgE response) (66,99,100). However, the specific mechanisms by which these cytokines modulate IgE synthesis are incompletely understood.

Regulation of IgE Synthesis by CD40 and CD40 Ligand

Although both IL-4 and IL-13 can induce ε-germline transcripts, the production of mature ε mRNA and IgE protein by B cells requires a physical interaction with T cells or other cell types. This event can be mediated by the interaction of CD40 present on B cells with its ligand (CD40L) that is expressed on activated, but not on resting, T cells and on certain other cells, including mast cells, basophils, and eosinophils (101,102). CD40 is a 50-kDa integral membrane glycoprotein that belongs to a family of transmembrane receptors that includes CD30, CD27, the *fas* antigen, and the receptors for TNF-α and nerve growth factor. CD40L is a 39-kDa type 2 membrane glycoprotein that is a member of a family that includes lymphotoxin, TNF-α, and the ligands for CD27 and CD30.

The importance of CD40 in IgE synthesis was first indicated in experiments using anti-CD40 antibodies, and later using CD40L protein (103,104), and was then confirmed by studies of CD40 and CD40L knock-out mice (105–108) and human patients with the hyper-IgM syndrome, which is caused by mutations in the CD40L or CD40 genes (101,102). In addition to T cells, mast cells, basophils, and eosinophils have also been shown to express CD40L, which appears to be able, at least under some circumstances, to induce B-cell IgE synthesis or proliferation *in vitro* (94,109,110). The *potential* influence of mast cells and/or basophils in regulating IgE production is further underscored by the fact that allergen-activated mast cells from patients with allergic rhinitis, or blood basophils from normal individuals, can promote B-cell IgE synthesis even in the absence of exogenous cytokines *in vitro* (94,110).

Given the evidence that they can express CD40L and produce IL-13 and/or IL-4, to what extent might mast cells, basophils, and/or eosinophils actually substitute for T cells in the development of IgE-associated immune responses *in vivo*? It is too early to tell. For one thing, current evidence indicates the mast cells may represent a relatively poor source of IL-4 relative to basophils (111–113), and there is yet to be a report proving that mast cells, basophils, or eosinophils actually promote IgE responses *in vivo*. However, it seems very unlikely that any one of these cells is essential for IgE production. For example, genetically mast cell–deficient mice appear to be able to generate apparently normal IgE responses (114,115). Perhaps mast cells, basophils, and eosinophils can influence the development of IgE responses in tissues in which these cells are relatively abundant, or can modulate the development of IgE responses that are driven primarily by the action of Th2 cells.

Regulation of IgE Synthesis by CD23

CD23, the low-affinity receptor for IgE (see section on receptors for IgE, below), has long been postulated to play a role in T cell–dependent IgE production (32,116,117). CD23 expression is upregulated by IL-4 and IL-13 (which also upregulate IgE production), and the expression of CD23 on lymphocytes and macrophages is often increased in patients with allergic diseases (118,119). CD23 is also expressed on many other cell types, including follicular dendritic cells, Langerhans' cells, monocytes, eosinophils, platelets, and some thymic epithelial cells (32). While many studies have suggested various roles for CD23 in the modulation of IgE production, its exact roles remain unclear. This is in part due to conflicting reports showing that CD23 can either enhance or inhibit B-cell IgE synthesis in humans or mice, respectively (120). These differences may reflect species differences in the structure and distribution of CD23 and its counterstructures (120). For example, studies with either CD23 knock-out or CD23 transgenic mice have suggested that CD23 can negatively regulate IgE production (121–123). However, IgE production was not affected in CD23 knock-out mice that had been infected with *N. brasiliensis* (*N.b.*) (123–125). By contrast, in one study (123) but not another (124), antigen-specific IgE was increased in CD23-deficient mice following immunization with DNP-OVA, a thymus-dependent antigen. In support of a suppressive role for CD23 in IgE production, mice that expressed a membrane CD23 transgene exhibited a decreased IgE response to infection with *N.b.* or immunization with anti-IgD, BPO-KLH, or DNP-KLH (121,122). However, such an effect was not seen in transgenic mice that overexpressed soluble CD23 (122), supporting previous findings that soluble CD23 has no effect on mouse IgE synthesis (126).

Unlike in some of the mouse systems described above, CD23 appears to promote IgE synthesis in rats and humans. IgE complexes, soluble CD23, and some antibodies to CD23 have been shown to inhibit IgE synthesis by human lymphocytes cultured *in vitro* (66,127–129), and administration to rats of a polyclonal antibody to CD23 strongly inhibited antigen-specific IgE synthesis *in vivo* (129). In addition to IgE, CD23 also binds CD21 (the Epstein-Barr virus receptor or complement receptor-2), and such an interaction has been demonstrated to increase human B-cell IgE synthesis in the presence of IL-4 (130). Therefore, in allergic patients

at least, it appears that the binding of CD23 on T cells to CD21 on B cells may promote T cell–B cell interactions, which in turn enhance B-cell IgE production (118).

Genetic Studies of IgE Production

Total serum IgE represents a composite of both antigen-specific and polyclonal fractions. High total serum IgE levels are strongly associated with the expression of allergic diseases, especially atopic allergic asthma (131), and studies with twins indicate that IgE concentrations are strongly influenced by genetic factors (132,133). Genetic linkage analyses using candidate gene approaches that have focused on limited regions of chromosomes near genes likely to be involved in allergic disease (e.g., IL-4) (134), as well as other types of genetic analyses, have shown that polyclonal IgE responses are strongly influenced by genes that map within the IL-4 cytokine–gene cluster on chromosome 5q31–33 (134–136). Genes located near 5q31–33 encode many cytokines that are known (or likely) to be important in the regulation of IgE responses and allergic diseases. These include IL-3, IL-4, IL-5, IL-9, IL-13, and granulocyte–macrophage colony-stimulating factor (GM-CSF), as well as other potential candidates, such as the transcription factor IRF1, whose gene product upregulates INF-γ. Given the role of IL-4 in Th2-cell differentiation and IgE class switching, these findings suggest that one or more functional polymorphisms in the IL-4 gene or its regulatory regions may account, at least in part, for genetic determination of total serum IgE levels (137).

By contrast, genes within the human leukocyte antigen D (HLA-D) region of chromosome 6p21.3 have been linked to antigen-specific IgE responses (138). Indeed, specific IgE responses to many clinically important allergens, including rye grass and dust mite allergens, are associated with HLA-linked immune response (Ir) genes (139). Given our current understanding of MHC-dependent restriction of Th-cell responses, it is not surprising that there is a strong Ir effect on IgE responses to many inhaled allergens. However, HLA class II haplotypes have not been shown to be clearly related to the likelihood of developing clinical disease.

Other studies of genetic factors in IgE production have implicated genes on additional chromosomes, including those in 11q13, in which polymorphisms for FcϵRIβ have been found (134,140–144) (and see next section), or chromosome 12q15-24.1, which contains several candidate genes, such as INF-γ and stem-cell factor (SCF) (145). Genome-wide searches for asthma susceptibility loci have confirmed the importance of many of these chromosomal regions in IgE production (146,147).

RECEPTORS FOR IgE

The High-affinity Receptor for IgE (FcϵRI)

The two major Fc receptors for IgE are distinguished by their structures and their relative affinities for IgE. The first, the high-affinity receptor for IgE (FcϵRI), binds monomeric IgE with an affinity (K_a) of about 10^{10} M^{-1}, while the second receptor for IgE, FcϵRII (CD23, see below), binds IgE with much lower affinity ($K_a = 10^8$ M^{-1}) (148).

FcϵRI was conclusively identified in 1970, shortly after the discovery of IgE, by studies that demonstrated that IgE preferentially bound to basophils and, subsequently, to mast cells (149). Although relatively high "constitutive" levels of expression of FcϵRI are restricted to mast cells and basophils, low levels of FcϵRI can be detected on human Langerhans' cells, peripheral blood dendritic cells, and monocytes, where it can function in IgE-mediated allergen presentation (150–155). In addition, FcεRI has been reported on human eosinophils, including those from atopic and nonatopic patients (156,157). However, most studies of FcεRI function have been conducted in rodent systems, primarily due to the availability of both IgE hybridomas of defined antigen specificity and useful cell lines, such as the rat basophilic leukemia cell line, RBL-2H3.

Many lines of evidence indicate that the activation of mast cells and basophils via FcεRI, resulting in the release of potent biologically active mediators, represents a primary (and in many cases, *the* primary) effector mechanism in allergic responses that are demonstrably IgE-dependent, such as those that can be transferred passively with antigen-specific IgE antibodies. The activation of mast cells or basophils by FcεRI aggregation initiates a coordinated sequence of biochemical and morphologic events that result in (a) exocytosis of secretory granules containing histamine and other preformed mediators; (b) synthesis and secretion of newly formed lipid mediators, such as prostaglandins and leukotrienes; and (c) synthesis and secretion of cytokines. Together, these mediators are responsible for the majority of the clinical symptoms associated with acute IgE-associated allergic reactions, and also contribute to the development of late-phase reactions and chronic allergic inflammation. The critical role of FcεRI in acute IgE-associated reactions has been demonstrated in mice by targeted gene disruption of the IgE-binding FcεRI α chain (158) or the intracellular γ chain common to FcεRI and FcγRII/III (159). When FcεRI α chain–deficient or FcR γ chain–deficient mice were injected intravenously with specific IgE followed by specific antigen, these mice did not show signs of systemic anaphylaxis, such as fluid extravasation, a drop in temperature, changes in pulmonary function, tachycardia, or death (158,160). Similar results were obtained when FcεRI α chain–deficient or FcR γ chain–deficient mice were challenged for IgE-dependent acute allergic reactions in a passive cutaneous anaphylaxis (PCA) model (158,161).

FcεRI Structure

In mast cells and basophils, FcεRI has a tetrameric structure composed of a single ligand-binding α chain, a single β chain, and two identical disulfide-linked γ chains (Fig. 3). In the mouse, the cDNA cloning of the α chain predicts an amino acid sequence containing 227 amino acid residues with six potential sites for N-linked glycosylation (162). The 181 N-terminal residues are located extracellularly and contain two immunoglobulin-like domains. The site of interaction of IgE with the α chain appears to involve both the Cε2 and Cε3 domains of the IgE heavy chain. The α chain has a single hydrophobic transmembrane domain of 21 amino acids and 25 C-terminal amino acid residues, which forms a short cytoplasmic tail. The β chain of mouse FcεRI is a 235-amino acid residue polypeptide whose structure is believed to transverse the membrane four times, with both the N-terminal and C-terminal segments exposed to the cytoplasm. The γ chain consists of only five extracellular amino acid residues, followed by one membrane-spanning segment and a cytoplasmic region of 36 residues. Sequence analysis of the γ chain indicates that it is highly homologous to the ζ chain of the TCR, and, in fact, human γ and ζ subunits are in some respects functionally interchangeable (163). As deduced from transfection experiments, all three subunits of rodent FcεRI must be present for efficient cell surface expression (162,164). In contrast, human FcεRI can be expressed efficiently when only the α chain and the γ chain are pre-

sent, and, in fact, this αγ2 FcεRI may be the only form of the receptor expressed on human APCs (see Fig. 3) (165).

FcεRI is member of the multichain immune recognition receptor family, which includes Fcγ receptors as well as the B- and T-cell antigen receptors (166). All contain extracellular ligand-binding protein(s) that are noncovalently associated with multiple protein subunits, which contain signaling motifs termed *immunoreceptor tyrosine-based activation motifs* (ITAMs) (167). This motif consists of six conserved amino acids spaced precisely over an approximately 26-amino acid sequence (D/EX$_7$D/EX$_2$YX$_2$LX$_7$YX$_2$L). Structurally, FcεRI shows the highest degree of homology with the low-affinity IgG receptor, FcγRIII, which is also expressed by mouse mast cells. Both receptors exhibit the same αβγ2 stoichiometry, share the same β and γ chains, and differ only slightly in the structure of their ligand-binding α chain (95% sequence homology). This high degree of homology is associated with similarities in function, in that aggregation of FcγRIII, like FcεRI, can lead to mast-cell activation and mediator release, both *in vitro* and *in vivo* (160,161,168). Moreover, in the mouse, the FcεRI and FcγRIII compete for limiting amounts of the β and γ chains, so that mice lacking FcεRIα exhibit enhanced expression of FcγRIII, and increased FcγRIII-dependent mast-cell activation, both *in vitro* and *in vivo* (160,161). Finally, FcγRIII can bind aggregates of IgE with low affinity (169).

FcεRI Signal Transduction

The aggregation or bridging of FcεRI that is occupied by IgE, as can occur in response to the recognition by this IgE of specific multivalent antigen, is sufficient for initiating downstream signal transduction events (170) (see Fig. 3). FcεRI activation also can be induced experimentally using antibodies to the FcεRI α chain, or by mitogens such as concanavalin A (which are thought to induce mediator release by binding to carbohydrates on the IgE molecules). It has been shown that the bridging of only a few hundred pairs of IgE molecules is sufficient to trigger human basophil histamine release (171). Because such a small fraction of the total surface FcεRI must be bridged to initiate the degranulation response (mast cells and basophils may express more than 1.0×10^5 FcεRI per cell, refs. 172, 173), basophils or mast cells may be sensitized simultaneously with IgE antibodies of many different specificities and therefore can react to stimulation by many different antigens.

Because FcεRI does not have any intrinsic enzymatic activity, it must interact with other membrane or cytoplasmic proteins in order to propagate a biochemical signal. The FcεRI γ chain is primarily responsible for transmitting cell-activation signals (168,174), while the β chain acts as an amplifier of signaling (175). The current model of the early events in FcεRI-mediated signaling is shown in Fig. 3. Immediately following FcεRI aggregation, the tyrosine kinase lyn, which appears to be constitutively associated, via its unique domain, with the C-terminal domain of the β chain (176), phosphorylates the ITAMs of both the β and γ chains. The tyrosine phosphorylation of the γ-chain ITAM induces its association with the syk tyrosine kinase, which then undergoes phosphorylation, permitting it to interact with and activate various downstream substrates.

A number of signaling pathways are either directly or indirectly activated by syk (Fig. 4). One substrate that can be directly tyrosine phosphorylated by syk is PLCγ1. PLCγ1 cleaves phosphatidylinositol 4,5-bisphosphate, generating diacylglycerol (DAG) and inositol 1,4,5-triphosphate (IP3). These second messengers then, respectively, activate protein kinase C (PKC) and stimulate the release of Ca^{2+} from the endoplasmic reticulum. FcεRI-dependent

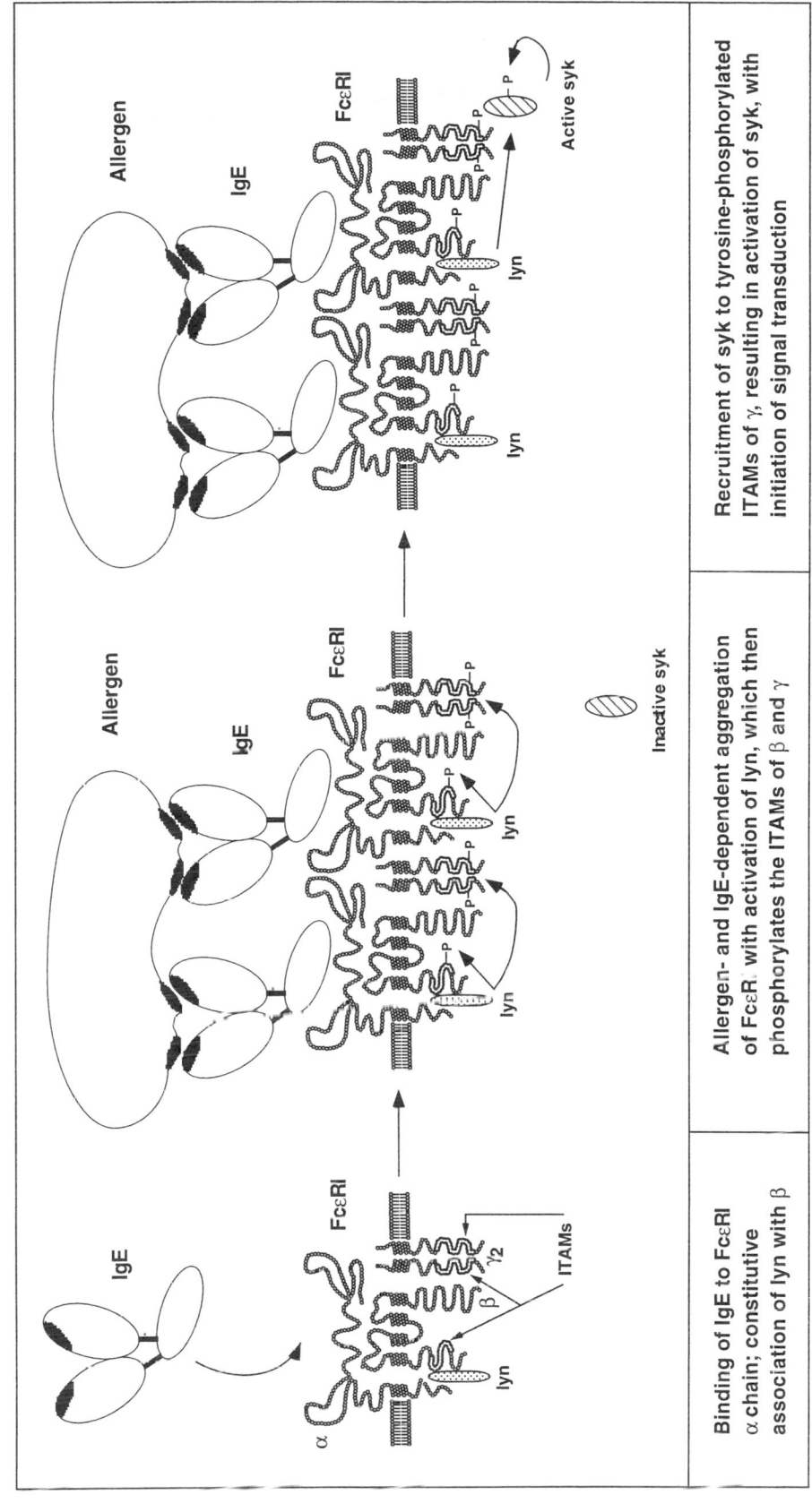

| Binding of IgE to FcεRI α chain; constitutive association of lyn with β | Allergen- and IgE-dependent aggregation of FcεRI, with activation of lyn, which then phosphorylates the ITAMs of β and γ | Recruitment of syk to tyrosine-phosphorylated ITAMs of γ, resulting in activation of syk, with initiation of signal transduction |

FIG. 3. Current model of the earliest steps in IgE- and antigen-dependent signal transduction through FcεRI. The illustration shows the αβγ2 form of the receptor that is expressed on mast cells and basophils. In humans, an αγ2 form of the receptor is expressed on cells in the monocytic lineage, including macrophages, Langerhans' cells, and dendritic cells (see text). Note that the illustration is greatly simplified. For example, it is not clear whether lyn is associated with the ITAM of the β chain; syk may undergo autophosphorylation, but it may also be phosphorylated by lyn and perhaps other mechanisms. (Modified after Figure 2 from Scharenberg AM, Kinet J-P. Early events in mast cell signal transduction. In: Marone G, ed. *Chem Immunol* vol 61. *Human basophils and mast cells: biological aspects.* Basel: Karger, 1995;72–87, with permission.)

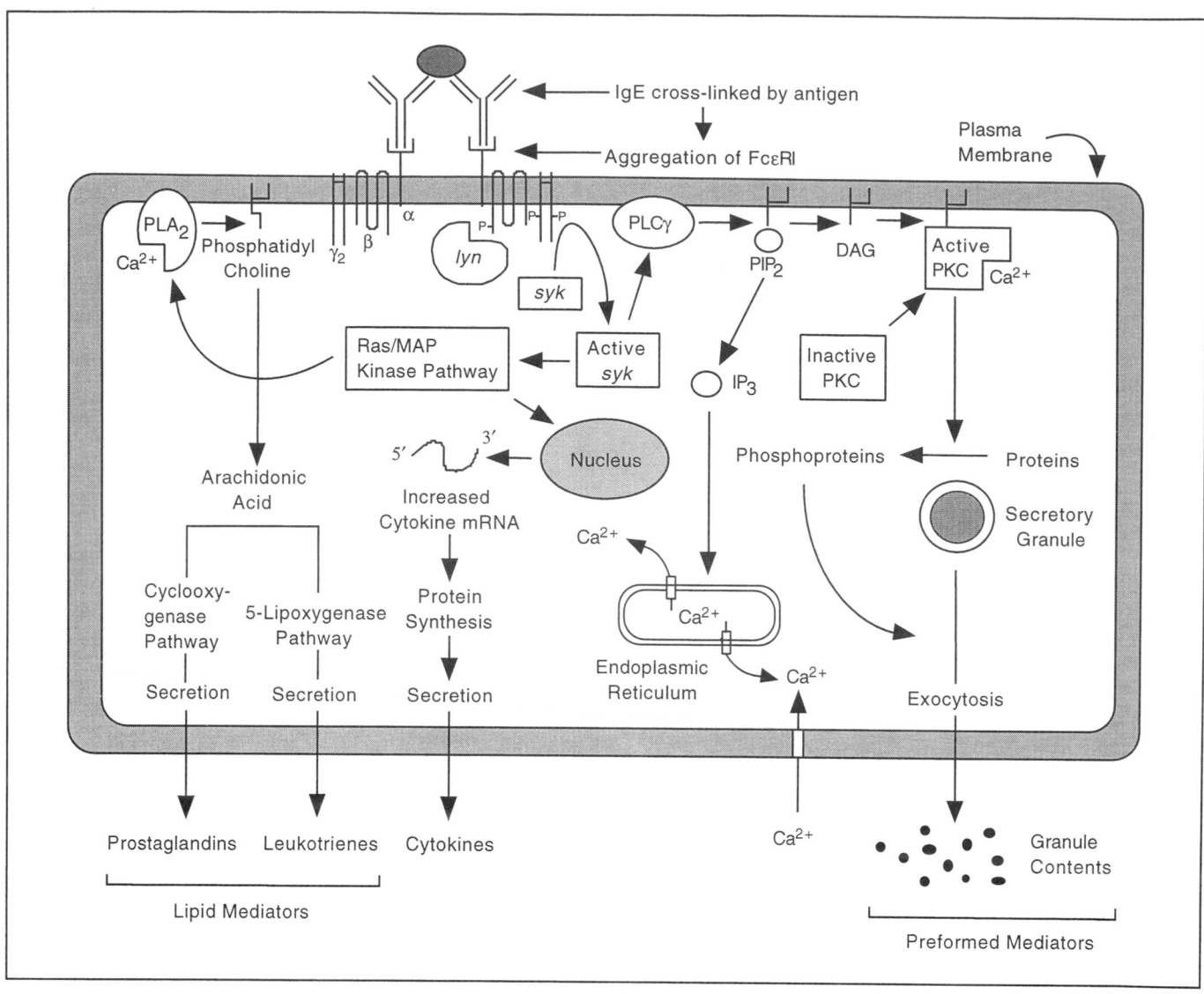

FIG. 4. Major biochemical events underlying the IgE- and FcεRI-dependent activation of mediator secretion by mast cells (see text for additional details). Note that at least some mast cells can release TNF-α and perhaps certain other cytokines from "preformed" pools, as well as from newly synthesized pools.

stimulation of mast cells also activates sphingosine kinase, triggering the release of sphingosine 1-phosphate, which may also contribute to calcium mobilization (177). Calcium mobilization is necessary for FcεRI-dependent exocytosis of granule-stored mediators and the release of lipid and cytokine mediators; accordingly, calcium ionophores such as ionomycin or A23187 are often used experimentally to induced mast-cell and basophil mediator release independently of the FcεRI. The Ras–mitogen-activated protein (MAP) kinase pathway is also activated following FcεRI aggregation (178–180) and has been shown to be syk-dependent (179). In addition to activating nuclear transcription factors, MAP kinase regulates the enzymatic activity of PLA2 and thus may play a role in the generation of prostaglandins and leukotrienes.

In addition, a variety of other proteins undergo tyrosine and/or serine–threonine phosphorylation following FcεRI aggregation (174,180–182). Some of the proteins that appear to be activated

include the following: (a) the tyrosine kinases Btk, Src, Yes, Fer, and Fak (183–186); (b) the Vav and Cbl protooncogenes (187,188); (c) the cytoskeletal protein, paxillin (189); (d) the tyrosine phosphatase, CD45 (190,191); and (e) Shc, Grb2, SOS, and other proteins linked to the activation of the Ras/MAP kinase pathway (192,193). Despite significant advances in identifying the potential involvement of these and other molecules in FcεRI-mediated secretion, the mechanisms and/or significance of their activation in this pathway are yet to be fully defined.

Negative Regulation of FcεRI Function by Immunoreceptor Tyrosine-based Inhibitory Motif–bearing and Other Cell Surface Receptors

Several cell surface receptors can function as negative regulators of ITAM-dependent signaling. These include type I transmembrane proteins that are members of the immunoglobulin superfamily, such as FcγRIIB on B cells, CTLA-4 on T cells, and killer cell–inhibitor receptors (KIRs) on NK cells (194). Each of these receptors possesses a conserved amino acid motif, originally described as a 13-amino acid sequence that was required for FcγRIIB-dependent inhibition of B-cell activation (195,196). This motif, termed an *immunoreceptor tyrosine-based inhibitory motif* (ITIM), has the general consensus sequence I/VxYxxL/V (197). ITIM-bearing receptors function while engaged in concert with an activating receptor [e.g., coaggregation of FcγRIIB with the B-cell antigen receptor (BCR) by cognate antigen and IgG]. In addition to FcεRI and FcγRIII, mouse mast cells and human basophils also express FcγRIIB. Coaggregation of FcγRIIB and FcεRI has been shown to diminish IgE-dependent activation *in vitro,* both in mouse mast cells and RBL cells, as well as in human basophils (198,199). Similarly, FcγRIIB knock-out mice show both increased FcγRIII-dependent mast-cell degranulation and increased IgG₁-induced PCA reactions (200). Rodent mast cells also express two other ITIM-bearing molecules, gp49b1 (201), a member of the immunoglobulin superfamily, and mast-cell function-associated antigen (MAFA), a type II transmembrane C-type lectin (202). Although the endogenous extracellular ligand(s) for either gp49 or MAFA have not yet been identified, aggregation of these receptors by specific antibodies can diminish IgE-dependent cell activation *in vitro* (201,202).

While studies of this type of inhibitory signaling are still limited, a few general themes have emerged. It appears that coclustering of antigen receptors with ITIM-bearing inhibitory receptors leads to the tyrosine phosphorylation of the ITIM and results in the recruitment of SH2-containing phosphatases (194). In B cells, phosphorylated FcγRIIB recruits the protein tyrosine phosphatase SHP-1 and the inositol-5-phosphatase, SHIP-1, while KIRs of NK cells appear to recruit only SHP-1. Notably, mast cells from motheaten mice, which lack SHP-1, are not inhibited by FcγRIIB (203). This suggests that, in mast cells, FcγRIIB may selectively recruit SHIP-1, which then inhibits downstream pathways that require elevations in inositol phosphates and/or intracellular calcium. However, the *in vivo* relevance of ITIM-bearing receptors in the regulation of IgE-dependent mast-cell or basophil activation remains to be determined.

The cell surface molecule CD81 has also been shown to inhibit FcεRI-mediated degranulation of RBL cells *in vitro,* and antibodies to CD81 can diminish the intensity of IgE- and mast cell-dependent PCA reactions *in vivo* (204). CD81 belongs to the transmembrane 4 superfamily (which includes CD9, CD53, CD63, and CD82); is broadly expressed on hematopoietic cells, including T and B cells, granulocytes, and monocytes; and lacks ITIM motifs (205). Notably, CD81 appears to regulate FcεRI activation without influencing aggregation-dependent tyrosine phosphorylation, calcium mobilization, or leukotriene synthesis (204).

IgE-dependent Upregulation of FcεRI Surface Expression

The expression of FcεRI on the surface of mouse mast cells appears to occur early in their differentiation and/or maturation *in vivo,* beginning around the time of granule formation *in vitro* (206,207). On the other hand, a small subpopulation of *in vitro*–derived mouse mast cells (which contain cytoplasmic granules) lacks detectable FcεRI expression (208). Moreover, the pro-

mastocytes present in the circulation of fetal mice also appear to express cytoplasmic granules, as well as mRNA for mouse mast cell-associated proteases, before they express mRNA for FcεRIα (209). Nevertheless, mRNA for FcεRIα is rapidly induced when promastocytes are cultured *in vitro* with IL-3 and SCF (209). And, as mast cells undergo further maturation in normal mice, the FcεRI is eventually expressed at levels that are in excess of 10^5 receptors per cell (172).

About 20 years ago, it was observed that there was a correlation between the serum concentration of IgE and the level of IgE receptor surface expression on circulating human basophils (173,210, 211). However, the basis for this association was not determined. Studies in both mice and humans have revealed that levels of FcεRI surface expression on mast cells and basophils can be regulated by levels of IgE (212–215). Moreover, genetically IgE-deficient mice exhibit a dramatic (greater than 80%) reduction in mast-cell and basophil FcεRI expression, which can be corrected by administration of monomeric IgE *in vivo* (212,213). Such IgE-dependent upregulation of FcεRI expression permits mouse or human mast cells to exhibit IgE-dependent mediator release at lower concentrations of specific antigen, and/or to secrete increased amounts of mediators at a given level of antigen or anti-IgE challenge, as well as to produce strikingly higher levels of certain cytokines (95,213, 216).

This work thus identifies a potentially important mechanism for enhancing the expression of effector-cell function in IgE-dependent allergic reactions or immunologic responses to parasites (Fig. 5). Because this process also can increase the ability of mast cells to produce IL-4 (213), IL-13 (95), and MIP-1α (216), all of which can promote IgE production (see section on regulation of IgE synthesis), IgE-dependent upregulation of FcεRI expression may also be part of a positive-feedback mechanism for inducing further production of IgE (see Fig. 5). While the mechanism(s) by which monomeric IgE regulates FcεRI expression are not yet clear, research in this area may suggest novel therapeutic approaches for the management of allergic disease.

The fact that mast cells and basophils from IgE −/− mice do express detectable, albeit greatly reduced, levels of FcεRI indicates that factors other than IgE must contribute to the regulation of FcεRI expression. Cytokines represent likely suspects. IL-4 has been reported to upregulate FcεRI expression on human umbilical cord blood–derived (217), nasal (94), or fetal liver–derived (218) mast cells *in vitro* (94,217), and studies of human fetal liver–derived (218) or umbilical cord blood–derived (95) mast cells show that IL-4 and IgE can act synergistically to enhance surface FcεRI expression *in vitro.* Furthermore, peritoneal mast cells and basophils of IL-4 −/− mice exhibit fewer FcεRI than do those of IL-4 +/+ mice (219). However, the reduction in FcεRI expression on mast cells and basophils of IL-4 −/− mice may reflect, at least in part, the low levels of IgE in these animals, because intravenous administration of IgE to these animals can increase FcεRI expression to wild-type levels (our unpublished results).

FcεRII/CD23

FcεRII (the B cell–differentiation antigen, CD23) is a type II integral membrane protein that belongs to the calcium-dependent animal lectin family (32,220). Thus, FcεRII/CD23 and FcεRI are structurally unrelated receptors, with the only similarity being the sharing of a common ligand. Compared with FcεRI, CD23 binds

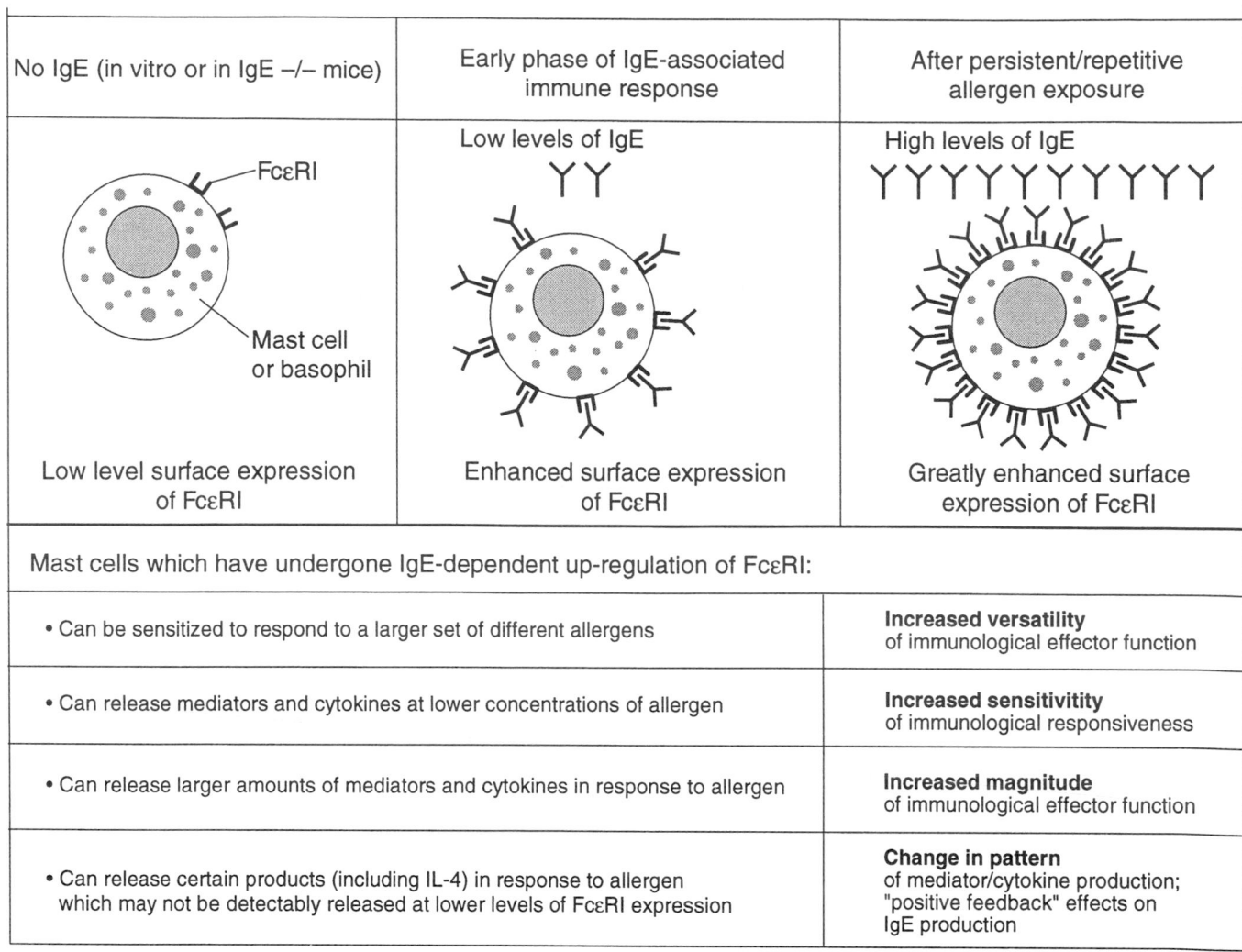

No IgE (in vitro or in IgE –/– mice)	Early phase of IgE-associated immune response	After persistent/repetitive allergen exposure
Low level surface expression of FcεRI	Enhanced surface expression of FcεRI	Greatly enhanced surface expression of FcεRI

Mast cells which have undergone IgE-dependent up-regulation of FcεRI:

• Can be sensitized to respond to a larger set of different allergens	**Increased versatility** of immunological effector function
• Can release mediators and cytokines at lower concentrations of allergen	**Increased sensitivity** of immunological responsiveness
• Can release larger amounts of mediators and cytokines in response to allergen	**Increased magnitude** of immunological effector function
• Can release certain products (including IL-4) in response to allergen which may not be detectably released at lower levels of FcεRI expression	**Change in pattern** of mediator/cytokine production; "positive feedback" effects on IgE production

FIG. 5. Potential consequences, on mast-cell and basophil effector and immunoregulatory functions, of IgE-dependent upregulation of surface expression of FcεRI.

IgE with a relatively low affinity ($Ka = 10^8$ M^{-1}). In addition to IgE, CD23 binds to CD21, the receptor for both the complement component, C3b, and the Epstein-Barr virus, as well as to the α chain of the β_2 integrins, CD11b and CD11c (130,221,222).

CD23 consists of an extracellular region composed of a C-terminal lectin domain and a single transmembrane segment and a short N-terminal cytoplasmic tail. Between the lectin domain and the transmembrane segment is a region consisting of a heptad repeat of hydrophobic residues, an element that is characteristic of proteins that exhibit an α-helical coiled-coil structure. Although CD23 is thought to be expressed on the cell membrane in a trimeric configuration, it can be cleaved by proteolysis into soluble fragments that retain IgE binding and other functional activities. Mouse and human CD23 are structurally related, but human CD23/FcεRII exists in two forms (CD23a/FcεRIIa, which is expressed primarily by B cells, and CD23b/FcεRIIb, which is expressed on B cells and other cell types), which differ by six amino acids in their intracellular amino terminus (118,223). In the mouse, CD23 is primarily expressed by B cells and follicular den-

dritic cells, while human CD23 can be expressed on additional cell types, including monocytes, eosinophils, platelets, T cells, Langerhans' cells, and some thymic epithelial cells (32).

A number of functions have been proposed for CD23, either as the intact cell-associated molecule or as a soluble fragment. In human (224,225) or mouse (226) B cells, CD23 can clearly mediate IgE-dependent antigen "focusing," with subsequent enhancement of antigen presentation to T cells *in vitro,* and the ability of passively transferred IgE to enhance IgG antibody responses is markedly impaired in CD23 –/– mice (124). Other proposed roles for CD23 include the regulation of IgE synthesis (see section on regulation of IgE synthesis), IgE-dependent phagocytosis, B-cell activation, B-cell homing in germinal centers, cellular adhesion, and, in the case of soluble CD23, various cytokine-like activities (32,118,220). However, partly because of the apparent differences in the biology of CD23 in mice and humans, and partly because of the apparently conflicting findings by different groups investigating CD23-deficient mice, there is, as yet, no consensus about the biologic importance or clinical relevance of many of these proposed functions of CD23.

THE EFFECTOR CELLS AND MEDIATORS OF IgE-ASSOCIATED IMMUNE RESPONSES

Overview

Mast cells, basophils, and eosinophils have long been regarded as important effector cells in IgE-associated allergic disorders, as well as in IgE-associated protective host responses to parasites. Indeed, it is thought that the cytoplasmic granule-associated and lipid mediators of mast cells (and, in systemic reactions, also of basophils) are primarily responsible for the signs and symptoms that are characteristic of acute IgE-associated allergic reactions. Mast cells, basophils, and eosinophils also probably contribute importantly to the development of late-phase reactions and chronic allergic inflammation. However, T cells, particularly Th2 cells, monocytes and macrophages, and neutrophils are also represented in the inflammatory cell infiltrates in both late-phase reactions and sites of chronic allergic inflammation; it is likely that these cells also contribute to the pathogenesis of such reactions.

Development and Natural History of Mast Cells and Basophils

While mast cells and basophils share several notable features, they are distinct cell types (Table 5). Both mast cells and basophils (a) contain prominent cytoplasmic granules, which exhibit metachromasia when stained with certain basic dyes; (b) are derived from bone marrow progenitor cells, (c) are major sources of histamine and other potent chemical mediators of inflammation; and (d) in all mammalian species yet analyzed, constitutively express FcεRI.

It once was thought that basophils might be circulating precursors of mast cells or that mast cells were "tissue basophils," but current evidence indicates that mature basophils are terminally differentiated circulating granulocytes that can infiltrate tissues or appear in exudates during a variety of inflammatory or immunologic processes. By contrast, morphologically identifiable mature mast cells do not normally circulate, but instead mature within the vascularized tissues in which they reside.

Routine methods of tissue fixation and processing are poorly suited for demonstration of mouse or human basophils and mast cells; optimal visualization is achieved in appropriately prepared 1-μm plastic sections or with ultrastructural approaches (227).

Ultrastructurally, human basophils typically exhibit a segmented nucleus with marked condensation of nuclear chromatin, and contain round or oval cytoplasmic granules (Fig. 6). By contrast, mast cells typically appear as either round or elongated cells with a nonsegmented or, occasionally, bi- or multilobed nucleus with moderate condensation of nuclear chromatin, and contain cytoplasmic granules that are usually smaller, more numerous, and generally more variable in appearance than those in basophils (see Fig. 6).

Like other granulocytes, basophils are derived from pluripotent CD34+ hematopoietic progenitor cells, ordinarily differentiate and mature in the bone marrow, and then circulate in the blood (228,229). IL-3 appears to be an important developmental factor for basophils, although other growth factors may also influence basophil development (228–230). The basophil is the least common blood granulocyte in humans, with a prevalence of approximately 0.5% of total leukocytes and approximately 0.3% of nucleated marrow cells (227). Basophils are also present in low numbers in the circulation or bone marrow of mice, with apparently significant variability among different strains (90,212,231,232). While human basophils appear to exhibit kinetics of production and peripheral circulation similar to those of eosinophils, unlike the eosinophil, the basophil ordinarily does not occur in peripheral tissues in significant numbers (227–229). Basophils can infiltrate sites of many immunologic or inflammatory processes, including IgE-associated late-phase reactions and sites of chronic allergic inflammation, often in association with eosinophils, and they also can participate in the inflammatory reactions to some tumors (233).

Mast cells are also derived from CD34+ hematopoietic progenitor cells (228,229,234). However, except for the small members of mast cells that are resident in the bone marrow, mast-cell maturation typically occurs in the peripheral tissues. Several lines of evidence indicate that interactions between the tyrosine kinase receptor c-kit, which is expressed on the surface of mast cells and their precursors, and the c-kit ligand, SCF, are essential for normal mast-cell development and survival (235). For example, mice with mutations that either result in markedly impaired c-kit function, or a marked reduction in the expression of membrane-associated SCF, virtually lack tissue mast cells (235,236), and subcutaneous administration of recombinant SCF (rSCF) can induce mast-cell hyperplasia in vivo in mice (230,237–239), rats (239), experimental primates (240), and humans (241). SCF is expressed on the plasma membrane of a vari-

TABLE 5. *Natural history of mast cells and basophils*

Characteristic	Mast cells	Basophils
Origin of precursor cells	CD34+ hematopoietic progenitor cells	CD34+ hematopoietic progenitor cells
Site of maturation	Connective tissue (a few in bone marrow)	Bone marrow
Mature cells in circulation	No	Yes (usually <1.0% of blood leukocytes)
Mature cells recruited into tissues from circulation	No	Yes
Mature cells normally residing in connective tissues	Yes (numbers can increase greatly at sites of certain IgE-associated immune responses or other types of chronic inflammation)	No
Proliferative ability of mature cells	Yes (under certain circumstances)	No
Life span	Weeks to months (according to studies in mice and rats)	Days
Major developmental factor	SCF	IL-3
Expression of FcεRI	Yes	Yes

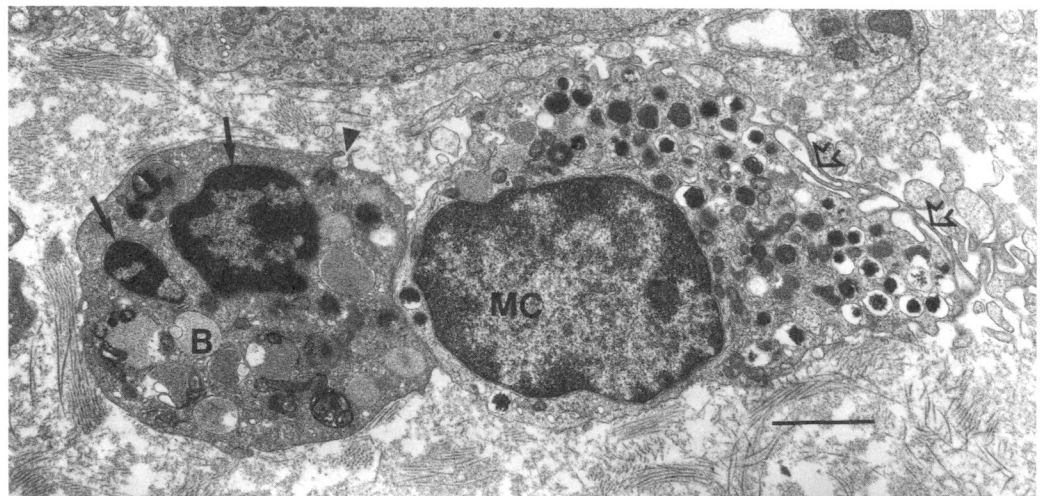

FIG. 6. A basophil (B) adjacent to a mast cell (MC) in the ileal submucosa of a patient with Crohn's disease. The basophil exhibits a bilobed nucleus (*solid arrows*), whose chromatin is strikingly condensed beneath the nuclear membrane. The basophil surface is relatively smooth, with a few blunt processes (*arrowhead*). The mast cell nucleus is larger and its chromatin less condensed than that of the basophil. The mast cell's granules are smaller, more numerous, and more variable in shape and content than those of the basophil. The mast-cell surface has numerous elongated, thin folds (*open arrows*). (Bar = 2 μm) (Modified from Dvorak AM, Monahan RA, Osage JE, Dickersin GR. Crohn's disease: transmission electron microscopic studies. II. Immunologic inflammatory response. Alterations of mast cells, basophils, eosinophils, and the microvasculature. *Hum Pathol* 1980;11:606–619, with permission.)

ety of cell types, including fibroblasts, bone marrow stromal cells, and vascular endothelial cells, and the extracellular domain of SCF can be released from these cells by proteolytic cleavage; both the membrane-associated and circulating soluble forms of SCF are biologically active (235). It is likely that local levels of SCF importantly regulate mast-cell numbers in normal tissues, and also contribute to the striking alterations in mast-cell numbers that have been noted in association with a variety of immunologic reactions, reparative responses, and disease processes (235,236,241–245).

However, it is also likely that the development and phenotypic characteristics of mouse or human mast-cell populations can be influenced by a complex interplay of cytokines and growth factors other than SCF (235,236,241–243). For example, in mice and rats, IgE-associated immune responses to nematodes are often associated with a striking hyperplasia of "mucosal mast cells" in the gastrointestinal tract (246,247). This process, long known to be T cell–dependent, probably primarily reflects the actions of IL-3 (230,248), IL-4 (249–251), and other cytokines (including IL-9; see ref. 252) that are produced by Th2 cells (and perhaps other cells) in response to parasite infection. Genetic approaches in mice have established that mucosal mast-cell hyperplasia in response to infection with the nematode *Strongyloides venezuelensis (S.v.)* requires both adequate SCF/c-kit function and IL-3 (230). Thus, genetically mast cell–deficient Kit^{W}/Kit^{W-v}, IL-3 +/+ mice exhibit a marked deficiency of mucosal mast-cell hyperplasia in response to *S.v.* infection (less than 3% of the levels in wild-type mice), but the response is diminished even further (virtually absent) in Kit^{W}/Kit^{W-v}, IL-3 −/− mice (230).

Mast-Cell Distribution and Heterogeneity

Mast cells are distributed throughout normal connective tissues, where they often lie adjacent to blood and lymphatic vessels, near or within nerves, beneath epithelial surfaces that are exposed to the external environment, such as those of the respiratory and gastrointestinal systems and the skin, and, in mice and rats, within

serosal cavities (235,236,242–245). Mast cells are also a normal, if numerically minor, component of the bone marrow and lymphoid tissues. However, unlike mature basophils, mature mast cells do not normally circulate in the blood.

In mice, humans, and many other mammalian species, mast-cell numbers in normal tissues exhibit considerable variation according to anatomic site, and these "baseline" numbers of mast cells can change in association with certain IgE-associated immune responses and other inflammatory or immunologic reactions (235, 236,242–245). For example, the numbers of mast cells at sites of chronic inflammation due to a variety of different causes, including that which develops in response to infections with some parasites, may well be many times higher than in the corresponding normal tissues (235,236,242–245).

The concept of "mast cell heterogeneity" is based on evidence derived from studies in humans and experimental animals, particularly the mouse, indicating that mast cells can vary in many aspects of phenotype, including morphology, histochemistry, mediator content, and response to drugs and stimuli of activation (235,236, 242–245). Although the regulation and functional significance of mast-cell heterogeneity remains to be fully defined, it is clear that many aspects of mast-cell phenotype can be regulated, particularly *in vitro*, by exposure to various cytokines (235,236,243). Moreover, it appears likely that phenotypically distinct mast-cell populations may express different functions in health and disease (235,236, 242–245). For example, mouse (253), rat (254,255), and human (256) mast cells exhibit subpopulations that vary in the types and amounts of trypsin-like or chymotrypsin-like proteases (i.e., tryptases and chymases) that are stored in their cytoplasmic granules, the patterns of lipid mediators that they produce in response to FcεRI-dependent activation (257,258), and, perhaps, the panels of cytokines that they can secrete (259).

In the mouse, many mast cells can be classified into T cell–dependent (or mucosal) and T cell–independent, or connective tissue (or serosal), subtypes (235,236,242,243). In humans, a major classification scheme is based on the presence or apparent absence of the granule-associated protease, chymase (256). The tryptase-positive, chymase-negative human mast-cell population is similar in some respects to mouse mucosal mast cells, whereas the tryptase-positive, chymase-positive human mast-cell population shares some features with mouse connective tissue-type mast cells (256). However, as discussed in detail elsewhere (235,242), such classifications should not be applied rigidly, because several lines of evidence indicate that the patterns of expression of many mast-cell phenotypic characteristics (a) can vary extensively, even within traditional murine mucosal or connective tissue–type populations; and (b) can exhibit reversible and bidirectional changes within clonal mast-cell populations. Moreover, some factors, including certain cytokines, may be able to alter the expression of some mast-cell phenotypic characteristics while having few or no effects on others (257,260). It appears that the mast-cell population, taken as a whole, can exhibit exquisitely fine regulation of important aspects of phenotype, and it may even be possible that, from the standpoint of the qualitative and quantitative aspects of all of its phenotypic characteristics, each individual mast cell may be unique.

Mediators Derived from Mast Cells and Basophils

Basophils and mast cells contain, or elaborate on appropriate stimulation, a diverse array of potent biologically active mediators (Table 6) (227–229,243,261–265). Some of these products are stored preformed in the cells' cytoplasmic granules (e.g., proteoglycans, proteases, histamine); others are synthesized upon activation of the cell by IgE and antigen or other stimuli [e.g., products of arachidonic acid oxidation through the cyclooxygenase or lipoxygenase pathways, and, in some cells, platelet activating factor (PAF)]. Cytokines are the most recently identified group of mast-cell and basophil mediators, at least one of which, TNF-α, can be released by activated mast cells from both preformed and newly synthesized pools (262,266–268).

Preformed Mediators

Mediators stored preformed in the cytoplasmic granules of mouse or human mast cells include histamine (mouse and rat, but not human, mast cells also contain serotonin), proteoglycans, serine proteases, carboxypeptidase A, and small amounts of sulfatases and exoglycosidases (227–229). Mast cells and basophils form histamine by the decarboxylation of histidine. Studies in genetically

mast cell–deficient and congenic normal mice indicate that mast cells account for nearly all of the histamine stored in normal tissues, with the exception of the glandular stomach and the central nervous system (CNS) (269). Basophils are the source of most of the histamine in normal human blood.

Mouse and human mast-cell populations contain variable mixtures of heparin (about 60 kDa) and chondroitin sulfate proteoglycans (228,243,261,263). Although the sulfated glycosaminoglycans of normal mouse or human blood basophils have not been characterized, chondroitin sulfates account for the majority of the proteoglycans in the basophils of patients with myelogenous leukemia. Mast-cell and basophil proteoglycans probably have several biologic functions both within and outside of the cells. By ionic interactions, they bind histamine, neutral proteases, and carboxypeptidases, and they may contribute to the packaging and storage of these molecules within the secretory granules. When the granule matrices are exposed to physiologic conditions of pH and ionic strength during degranulation, the various mediators associated with the proteoglycans dissociate at different rates—histamine very rapidly but tryptase and chymase much more slowly (228). In addition to regulating the kinetics of release of mediators from the granule matrices, proteoglycans can also regulate the activity of some of the associated mediators (see below).

Neutral proteases are the major protein component of mast-cell secretory granules. Both basophils and mast cells contain enzymes with TAME-esterase activity, which can be used as a marker of human mast-cell or basophil activation in vivo. By weight, tryptase is the major enzyme stored in the cytoplasmic granules of human mast cells, and this neutral protease occurs in most, if not all, human mast-cell populations (228). Human mast-cell tryptase is a serine endopeptidase that exists in the granule in active form as a tetramer of 134 kDa-containing subunits of 31 to 35 kDa, each of which contains an active site. Negligible amounts of tryptase have been identified in normal human basophils by immunoassay. Because this enzyme appears to be highly characteristic of, if not unique to, the human mast cell, measurements of mast-cell tryptase in biologic fluids such as plasma, serum, and inflammatory exudates have been used to assess mast-cell activation in these settings. Tryptase is stored in the cytoplasmic granules in the active tetrameric form as a complex that is stabilized by its association with heparin and perhaps other proteoglycans within the mast-cell granule. The function of mast-cell tryptase in vivo is unknown. Mast-cell chymase is also a serine protease that is stored in the active form, as a monomer with a molecular weight of 30 kDa, in

TABLE 6. *Products of human mast cells and basophils*

Mediators	Mast cells	Basophils
Major mediators stored performed in cytoplasmic granules	Histamine, heparin and/or chondroitin sulfates, neutral proteases (typically tryptase with or without chymase), many acid hydrolases, cathepsin G, carboxypeptidase	Histamine, chondroitin sulfates, neutral protease with bradykinin-generating activity, β-glucuronidase, elastase, cathepsin G-like enzyme, major basic protein, lysophospholipase (Charcot-Leyden crystal protein)
Major lipid mediators produced on appropriate activation	Prostaglandin D$_2$, leukotriene C$_4$, platelet-activating factor	Leukotriene C$_4$
Cytokines[a]	IL-4, IL-5, IL-6, IL-8, IL-13, TNF-α, MIP-1α, bFGF, VPF/VEGF	IL-4, IL-13

[a]In some cases, the listings are based on immunohistochemical evidence indicating that at least some mast cells contain immunoreactivity for the cytokine, rather than proof that the biologically active cytokine can be released from the cell.

the granules of some, but not all, human mast cells. Human basophils, like eosinophils, can form Charcot-Leyden crystals and contain Charcot-Leyden crystal protein (lysophospholipase) in quantities similar to that of eosinophils (228).

Newly Synthesized Lipid Mediators

The activation of mast cells or basophils with appropriate stimuli not only causes the secretion of preformed granule-associated mediators, but also can initiate the *de novo* synthesis of certain lipid-derived substances (Fig. 7). Of particular importance are the cyclooxygenase and lipoxygenase metabolites of arachidonic acid, which have potent inflammatory activities and which may also play a role in modulating the release process itself (263,265). The major cyclooxygenase product of mast cells is prostaglandin D_2 (PGD_2), and the major lipoxygenase products derived from mast cells and basophils are the sulfidopeptide leukotrienes (LTs): LTC_4 and its peptidolytic derivatives, LTD_4 and LTE_4. Human mast cells, but not

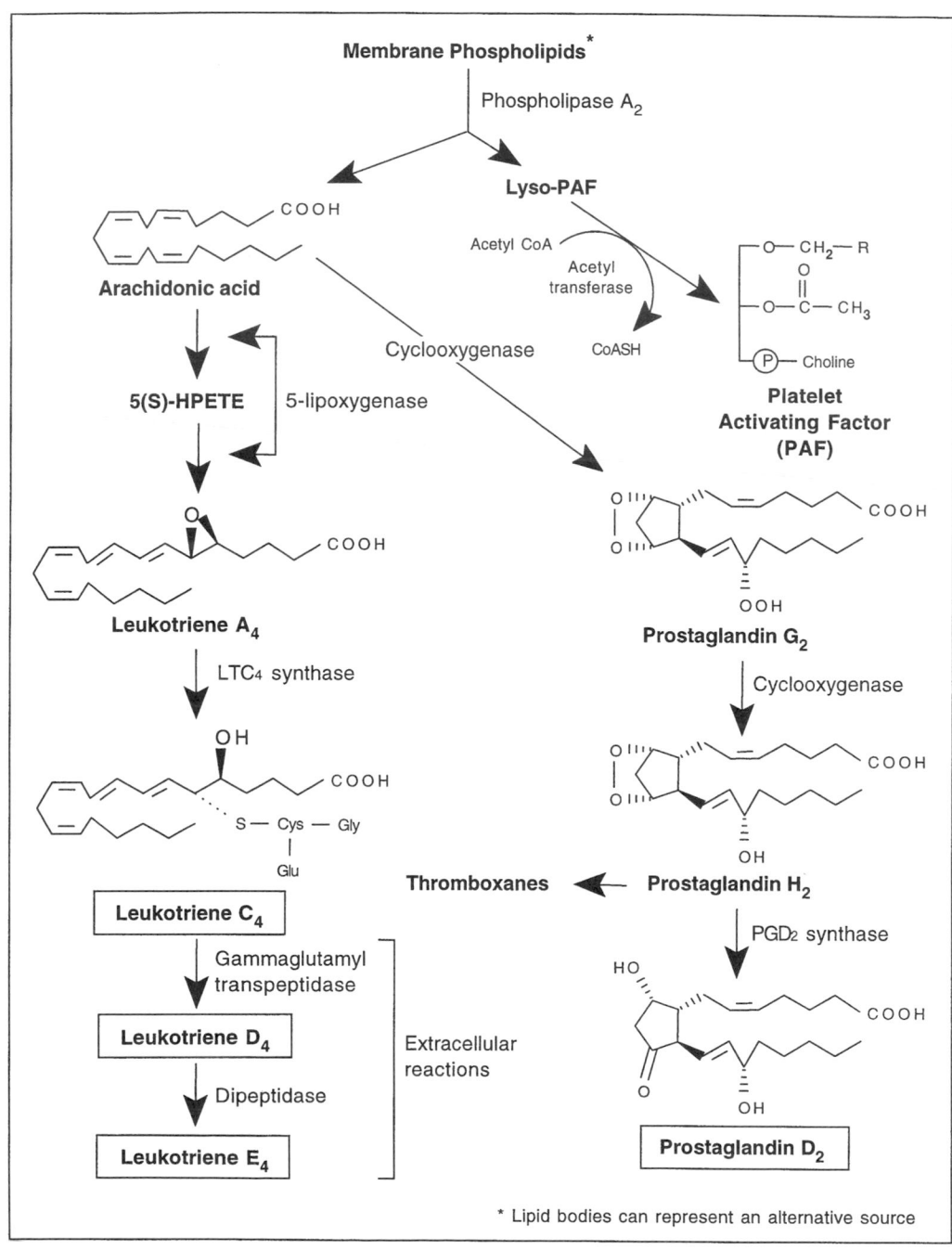

FIG. 7. Biosynthetic pathways of the major lipid mediators of mast cells. *Boxes* enclose the mediators that are thought to represent the most quantitatively and biologically important of the mast cell–derived products of arachidonic acid metabolism. In mast cells (and other cell types) that contain lipid bodies, these structures represent an alternative source of phospholipids for these pathways (see text).

human basophils, also can produce LTB$_4$, although in much smaller quantities than PGD$_2$ or LTC$_4$ (263,265).

There are at least three patterns of release of products of arachidonic acid metabolism by human mast cells and basophils: (a) Gut or lung mast cells produce similar amounts of LTC$_4$ and PGD$_2$, (b) skin mast cells produce largely PGD$_2$, and (c) basophils generate primarily LTC$_4$ and very little PGD$_2$. Studies of *in vitro*-derived mouse mast cells indicate that SCF and other cytokines can regulate the expression of phospholipase A$_2$ and other enzymes involved in arachidonic acid metabolism, which in turn influences the ability of the cells to release lipid mediators, including PGD$_2$ (257,270) and arachidonic acid itself (258).

Cytokines

Many cytokine-dependent processes are implicated in IgE-associated allergic inflammation, including the upregulation of the IgE response itself (e.g., IL-4, IL-13, and perhaps MIP-1α), the enhancement or induction of basophil recruitment (e.g., TNF-α, IL-4) or mediator production (e.g., IL-3, IL-4, MIP-1α), the promotion of eosinophil development and/or survival (e.g., IL-5, IL-3, GM-CSF) and recruitment (e.g., IL-3, IL-5, IL-16, GM-CSF, certain C-C chemokines), and the recruitment of monocytes and T cells (e.g., IL-16, certain C-C chemokines) (264). Much of the ability of certain cytokines, (i.e., IL-1 and TNF-α) to contribute to the development and perpetuation of allergic inflammation is thought to reflect the ability of these agents to enhance the recruitment of leukocytes, by inducing the increased expression of adhesion molecules, such as P- and E selectin, vascular cell adhesion molecule-1 (VCAM-1), and intercellular adhesion molecule-1 (ICAM-1), on vascular endothelial cells (264,271,272). However, cytokines may critically influence many other stages in the development of allergic inflammation, as well as regulate some of the local consequences of these responses.

The production of cytokines may represent one of the critical links between the IgE-dependent mast-cell activation that occurs immediately after allergen challenge in sensitized subjects, the inflammation that develops during the subsequent late-phase reactions to such provocation, and the persistent inflammation and associated tissue changes that are characteristic of chronic allergic disorders (262,273). For example, studies in mast cell–reconstituted genetically mast cell–deficient mice have demonstrated that mast cells are required for essentially all of the leukocyte infiltration observed in the skin or stomach wall after challenge with IgE and specific antigen (274,275). A similar approach was used to show that mast cells can importantly contribute to the eosinophil infiltration elicited in the lungs in certain protocols of aerosol allergen challenge in sensitized mice (276). In the skin, approximately 50% of such IgE- and mast cell–dependent leukocyte infiltration can be inhibited by using an antibody to recombinant mouse TNF-α (274).

Other cells present at sites of chronic allergic inflammation beside the mast cell also can produce TNF-α, such as macrophages, T cells, and B cells, but these cells apparently contain little or no preformed TNF-α bioactivity. By contrast, several lines of evidence indicate that certain mature, "resting" (nonactivated) mouse (266–268) or human (277,278) mast cells contain preformed stores of TNF-α available for immediate release upon appropriate stimulation of the cells (262,264). Thus, in IgE-dependent reactions, mast cells are likely to represent an important initial source of TNF-α.

Mast cells represent a potential source of many cytokines, in addition to TNF-α, that might influence IgE-associated allergic inflammation, and the synthesis and release of these products can be induced via IgE-dependent mechanisms. Thus, certain mouse mast cells activated via the FcεRI contain increased levels of mrnA for many cytokines [IL-1α, IL-3, IL-4, IL-5, IL-6, and GM-CSF and the chemokines MIP-1α, MIP-1β, MCAF (MCP-1), MARC, and I-309], and secrete substances with the corresponding bioactivities [IL-1, IL-3, IL-4, IL-6, IL-9, IL-13, GM-CSF and vascular permeability factor–vascular endothelial cell growth factor [VPF/VEGF]] (84,87,88,113,262,264,273,279). In part because of the difficulty of obtaining highly purified preparations of human mast cells, studies of human mast-cell cytokine production have been slow to emerge. However, *human* mast cells also appear to represent a potential source of many cytokines, including TNF-α, basic fibroblast growth factor (bFGF), IL-4, IL-5, IL-6, IL-8, IL-13, and VPF/VEGF (89,93–95,111–113,279,280).

Glucocorticoids can inhibit cytokine production in many cell types, as can cyclosporin A (CsA), and these effects have been proposed as one of the important mechanisms of action of these agents in patients with asthma (281). In mice, both glucocorticoids and CsA can diminish mast-cell cytokine production *in vitro* and can also suppress mast cell– and TNF-α–dependent allergic inflammation *in vivo* (282).

Although the ability of basophils to produce cytokines has been less extensively studied than mast-cell cytokine production, several reports have demonstrated that mature human basophils, isolated from peripheral blood, can release IL-4 and IL-13 in response to FcεRI-dependent activation, and that such release can be enhanced in basophils exposed to IL-3 but not to certain other cytokines (227–229). It is possible that IL-4, IL-13, and/or MIP-1α derived from mast cells or basophils at sites of allergic inflammation may play a role in enhancing IgE production or driving Th2-cell differentiation. Moreover, recent findings indicate that human basophils and mast cells also express CD40L and thus may be able to contribute to IgE production by promoting immunoglobulin class switching (94,110,227,264).

Mechanisms of Mast-Cell or Basophil Activation

The best-understood cellular event that underlies expression of basophil or mast-cell function is degranulation (or anaphylactic-type degranulation), a stereotyped constellation of stimulus-activated biochemical and morphologic events that result in the fusion of the cytoplasmic granule membranes with the plasma membrane (with external release of granule-associated mediators) (Fig. 8). Although a variety of agents can initiate basophil or mast-cell anaphylactic-type degranulation, the best-studied pathway of stimulation is transduced through FcεRI expressed on the basophil or mast-cell surface (see section on receptors for IgE). This process occurs without evidence of toxicity to the cell. Because mast cells are long-lived cells, they thus can potentially participate in multiple rounds of FcεRI-dependent activation. And, as noted in the aforementioned section, mast cells and basophils can be simultaneously sensitized with multiple IgE species of differing antigen specificities, permitting them to release mediators in response to challenge with numerous distinct allergens.

In addition to IgE and specific antigen, a variety of biologic substances, including products of complement activation and certain cytokines, chemical agents, and physical stimuli, can elicit release of basophil or mast-cell mediators (227,228,244,245,261,263,283).

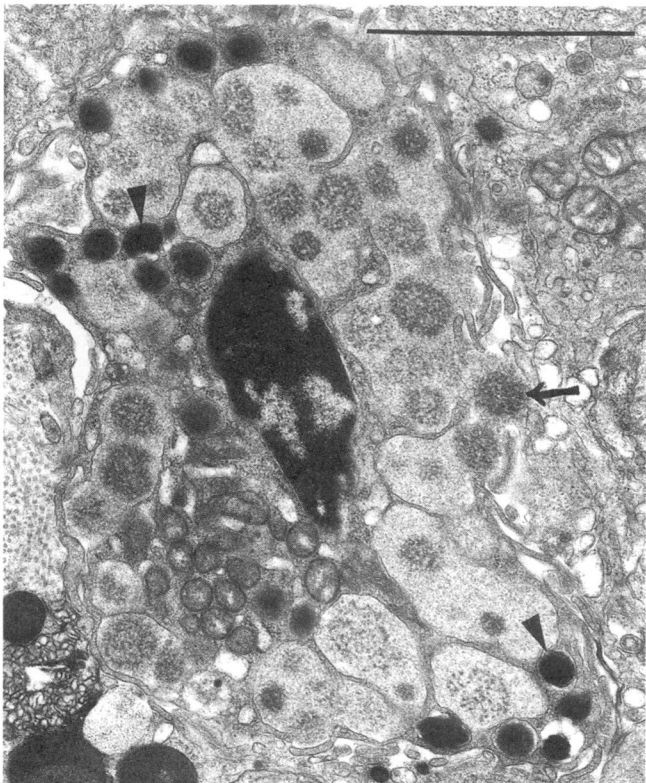

FIG. 8. "Anaphylactic-type" degranulation in a human mast cell in an ileostomy biopsy of a patient with Crohn's disease. Note intracytoplasmic degranulation channels formed by fusion of granule membranes that contain altered, swollen granule matrix material; one of these altered, membrane-free granules (*arrow*) has been extruded to the exterior through an opening in the plasma membrane. Some unaltered, dense granules (*arrowheads*) remain in the cytoplasm. (Bar = 5 µm) (Modified from Dvorak AM. Ultrastructure of human gastrointestinal system. Interactions among mast cells, eosinophils, nerves and muscle in human disease. In: Snape WJ Jr, Collins SM, eds. *Effects of immune cells and inflammation on smooth muscle and enteric nerves.* Boca Raton, FL: CRC Press, 1991:139–168, with permission.)

However, the responsiveness of human basophils and different populations of human mast cells to individual stimuli varies. For example, cutaneous mast cells appear to be much more sensitive to stimulation by neuropeptides or morphine than are pulmonary mast cells (244,245,261,263). Moreover, some of these stimuli can induce a pattern of mediator release different from that associated with FcεRI-dependent mast-cell activation. Similarly, certain cytokines can directly activate mast cells or basophils, and/or modulate the cells' ability to release mediators in response to IgE and antigen or other stimuli, but the effects of individual cytokines can be markedly different in various populations of mast cells or basophils (113,227–229). For example, SCF can induce degranulation and release of preformed and lipid mediators from some mast-cell populations (284–287), whereas basophils are relatively unresponsive (286). Moreover, some mast-cell populations release little or no preformed mediators in response to SCF, but they do secrete certain cytokines, such as IL-6 (288). Bacterial LPS can also induce the release of IL-6 to a greater extent than can preformed mediators in certain rat (289) or mouse (288) mast cells.

Taken together, these findings indicate that the participation of mast cells and basophils in inflammatory and immune responses can be recruited by complement activation and many other IgE-independent mechanisms, as well as by activation via FcεRI, and that the function of these effector cells in such settings can be modulated by cytokines. Moreover, because mast cells and basophils activated by such FcεRI-independent mechanisms can release many (if not all) of the same mediators that are produced by cells that have been activated via IgE and specific antigen, the signs and symptoms that develop in experimental animals or humans experiencing such IgE-independent activation of mast cells and basophils may be virtually indistinguishable from those observed with true IgE-associated reactions. Finally, morphologic evidence suggests that mast cells and basophils can release mediators by a secretory mechanism distinct from that of classical anaphylactic-type degranulation (233). This alternative mechanism, termed *piecemeal degranulation,* is most often noted in ultrastructural studies of basophils and mast cells in tissue specimens at sites of inflammation (233,290). Such studies, and related *in vitro* experiments, indicate that piece-meal degranulation may permit mast cells and basophils to release their mediators slowly and/or in relatively limited quantities, possibilities that, if confirmed, would have a number of interesting implications with respect to the function of these cell types (233).

Development and Natural History of Eosinophils

Eosinophils, like neutrophils and basophils, are a type of bone marrow-derived granulocyte (Table 7); eosinophils can be distinguished from other hematopoietic cells by the striking affinity of their cytoplasmic granules for acid aniline dyes such as eosin. While eosinophils contain several eosinophil-specific proteins in their cytoplasmic granules, no cell surface proteins unique to eosinophils have yet been recognized. Thus, the identification of eosinophils in blood and tissues is still based on the cells' staining properties and other morphologic features. However, under some circumstances, immunostaining for eosinophil granule proteins or eosinophil fluorescence after fluorescein isothiocyanate or Giemsa staining may be needed for optimal identification and quantitation of these cells. Eosinophilia, characterized by both heightened production of eosinophils in bone marrow and the accumulation of eosinophils in tissues and blood, is characteristically associated with a spectrum of immune responses or pathologic processes

TABLE 7. *Natural history of eosinophils*

Characteristic	
Origin of precursor cells	CD34+ hematopoietic progenitor cells
Site of maturation	Bone marrow
Mature cells in circulation	Yes
Mature cells recruited into tissues from circulation	Yes
Mature cells normally residing in certain connective tissues	Yes (especially near surfaces of gastrointestinal and respiratory tracts)
Proliferative ability of mature cells	No
Life span	Days to weeks
Major developmental factor	IL-5
Expression of FcεRI	Variable, low levels (compared with mast cells and basophils)

(291–293). These include IgE-associated allergic disorders and infections with helminth parasites, as well as a variety of other diseases with less-defined causes.

Eosinophils are similar in size to neutrophils but have bilobed nuclei and distinctive cytoplasmic granules (294). The abundant specific granules, with their structured packaging of cationic proteins, which render the cell eosinophilic, are the eosinophils' most characteristic morphologic feature (294). Ultrastructurally, these specific granules contain characteristic distinct, usually electron-dense, crystalloid cores (Fig. 9). Eosinophils also contain two other types of granules: primary granules, which lack a crystalloid core and develop early in eosinophil maturation, and smaller granules, which contain arylsulfatase and other enzymes. Prominent tubulovesicular structures are sometimes identified as a fourth population of "granules" (microgranules) (294). Eosinophils, also contain varying numbers of lipid bodies (295). Lipid bodies are non–membrane-bound, lipid-rich inclusions that are also found in macrophages and mast cells (296,297), and many other types of cells, and that can contribute to the formation of eicosanoid mediators (295).

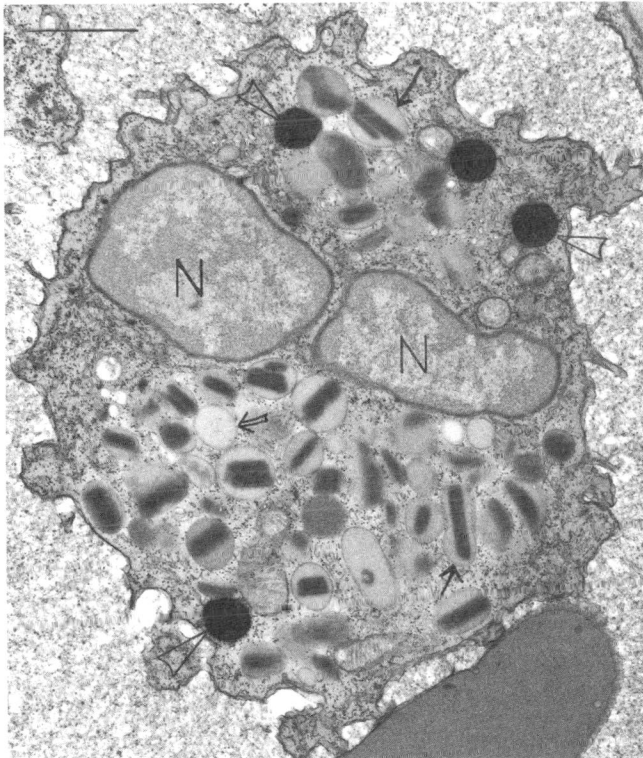

FIG. 9. Mature peripheral blood eosinophil from a patient with the idiopathic hypereosinophilic syndrome, showing the cell's bilobed nucleus (*N*); irregular, blunt surface processes; granules; and mitochondria. Dark cytoplasmic particles are monoparticulate glycogen. Four large, round, osmiophilic lipid bodies (*open arrowheads*) are present. Specific granules are elongated, membrane-bound structures with dense central crystal(s) and lightly dense matrix (*arrows*). Primary granules do not have central crystals (*open arrow*). The specimen was processed with the reduced osmium technique, osmium potassium ferrocyanide. (Bar = 1.4 µm) (Modified from Dvorak AM, Ackerman SJ, Weller PF, Subcellular morphology and biochemistry of eosinophils. In: Harris JR, ed. *Blood cell biochemistry.* vol 2. *Megakaryocytes, platelets, macrophages and eosinophils.* London: Plenum Publishing Corp., 1991:237–344, with permission.)

Eosinophils are terminally differentiated granulocytes that develop in the bone marrow but that, unlike basophils, normally reside in large numbers in the peripheral tissues (see Table 7). Eosinophils are most abundant in tissues with a mucosal epithelial interface with the environment, including the respiratory, gastrointestinal, and lower genitourinary tracts. Although their precise life span is not known, eosinophils live longer than neutrophils and may survive for weeks within tissues.

The development and differentiation of eosinophils are promoted by at least three cytokines. GM-CSF, IL-3, and IL-5 can each promote eosinophilopoiesis *in vivo*, but IL-5 has the most specific effects on eosinophil differentiation and production (298). IL-5 can also rapidly induce the release of developed eosinophils from the marrow into the circulation (299). While IL-5 is produced by Th2 cells and IL-3 and GM-CSF can be produced by both Th1 and Th2 cells, eosinophils (as well as mast cells) also can elaborate each of these cytokines (see below).

Mediators Derived from Eosinophils

Like mast cells and basophils, eosinophils can express function by the production and release of cytoplasmic granule-associated mediators, lipid mediators, and cytokines.

Intracellular Constituents

The specific granules of eosinophils contain lysosomal hydrolases, as well as the cationic proteins that are apparently unique to eosinophils and that can express toxicity to both parasites and host tissues (Table 8) (291). The crystalloid core of the granule is composed of major basic protein (MBP), and the noncore matrix contains eosinophil cationic protein (ECP), eosinophil-derived neurotoxin (EDN), and eosinophil peroxidase. Human eosinophil MBP has no recognized enzymatic activity, but it is toxic to helminthic parasites, tumor cells, and host cells (292). ECP is a markedly cationic polypeptide with toxicity to bacteria, helminths, and host cells (292). EDN is a protein that shares some sequence similarity with ECP (292). Its name is based on its ability (like ECP) to

TABLE 8. *Products of human eosinophils*

Mediators	
Major mediators stored preformed in cytoplasmic granules	Major basic protein (MBP), eosinophil cationic protein (ECP), eosinophil-derived neurotoxin (EDN), eosinophil peroxidase, lysosomal hydrolases, lysophospholipase (Charcot-Leyden crystals)
Major lipid mediators products on appropriate activation	Leukotriene C$_4$, lipoxins
Cytokines[a]	IL-1α, IL-2, IL-3, IL-4, IL-5, IL-6, IL-8, IL-10, IL-16, GM-CSF, TNF-α, RANTES, MIP-1α, eotaxin, TGF-α, TGF-β$_1$, VPF/VEGF

[a]In some cases, the listings are based on immunohistochemical evidence indicating that at least some eosinophils contain immunoreactivity for the cytokine, rather than proof that the biologically active cytokine can be released from the cell.

induce cerebrocerebellar dysfunction when injected intracerebrally into rabbits (292). Both EDN and ECP have partial sequence identity with pancreatic ribonuclease and have ribonuclease catalytic activity; however, EDN is about 100 times more potent as a ribonuclease than is ECP (292). Elevated concentrations of eosinophil-derived cationic proteins can be detected in the sputum of patients with asthma, in nasal and bronchoalveolar lavage fluids after the experimental inhalation of antigens, and within involved tissues (291–293). In allergic diseases, eosinophil granule proteins may cause damage and desquamation of airway epithelial cells, alter airway hyperreactivity and cilial function, and elicit local edema (291–293).

Eosinophil peroxidase, which is distinct from the myeloperoxidase of neutrophils and monocytes, consists of two polypeptides of about 15 and 55 kDa. It catalyzes the formation of hypohalous (e.g., hypochlorous or hypobromous) acid from hydrogen peroxide and halide ions (preferentially, bromide). Accordingly, in the presence of hydrogen peroxide and halide ions, eosinophil peroxidase is toxic to helminthic and protozoan parasites, bacteria, tumor cells, and host cells (292).

Human eosinophils represent a major source of the protein (also produced by human basophils) that forms Charcot-Leyden crystals; these bipyramidal crystals are often found in sputum, feces, and tissues in patients with allergic asthma and other eosinophil-related diseases characterized by significant eosinophilia. This 17-kDa hydrophobic protein with lysophospholipase activity composes approximately 5% of the eosinophil's total protein (293). It is found in the primary granules and is also associated with eosinophil cell membranes.

Lipid Mediators

Eosinophils can produce PAF and eicosanoid derivatives of arachidonic acid (300). Although eosinophils can synthesize prostanoids derived from the cyclooxygenase pathway, the principal eosinophil eicosanoids are products of arachidonate lipoxygenation via either the 5- or 15-lipoxygenase pathways. The predominant product of the 5-lipoxygenase pathway in human eosinophils is LTC_4 (300). The three sulfidopeptide leukotrienes, LTC_4 and its derivatives LTD_4 and LTE_4, are potent stimulants of vasoactivity, smooth muscle contraction, and mucous secretion. In addition, human eosinophils, unlike neutrophils, contain large quantities of 15-lipoxygenase (300). Lipoxins, products of double lipoxygenation, and certain peptide mediators, such as substance P, are also formed by eosinophils.

Cytokines

The recognition in recent years that eosinophils represent a potential source of many cytokines has suggested that these cells may influence IgE-associated immune responses, as well as other inflammatory reactions and biologic responses, through a broader spectrum of mechanisms than had previously been supposed (301–304). Immunohistochemical or immunocytochemical evidence has suggested that many of these eosinophil cytokines may be "stored" within specific granules. However, immunocytochemical approaches can be difficult in eosinophils (and mast cells), because of the occurrence of artifactual staining of the cells' granules; moreover, in many cases, it is not yet clear whether the detection of even valid immunoreactivity for cytokines in eosinophil or mast-cell granules necessarily reflects the presence of cytokine

bioactivity (304). Nevertheless, these findings suggest that eosinophils may contain potential "preformed" pools of cytokine that are available for release.

The cytokines elaborated by eosinophils may be grouped into four categories: (a) growth factors, including GM-CSF, IL-3, and IL-5, which may exert autocrine and parcrine effects on the survival and function of eosinophils and other cells; (b) chemokines, including RANTES, MIP-1α, and eotaxin; (c) cytokines involved in inflammation, fibrosis, and wound healing and repair, including TGF-α, TGF-β1, VEGF/VPF, TNF-α, IL-1α, IL-6, and IL-8; and (d) cytokines with potential activities in regulating immune responses, such as IL-2, IL-4, IL-10, and IL-16.

Mechanisms of Activation and Recruitment

IgE can bind to three structures on human eosinophils: the S-type lectin galectin-3, FcεRII/CD23, and FcεRI (305). Although both CD23 and FcεRI are detectable on eosinophils in sites of allergic reactions, including the airways (306), the extent to which eosinophil function in IgE-associated immune responses is dependent on expression of FcεRI versus CD23 largely remains to be determined. Human eosinophils also express receptors for IgG, typically FcγRI (CD64) and FcγRII (Cdw32) and IgA (FcαR) (305). The eosinophil receptor for IgA binds secretory IgA more strongly than other forms of IgA (307). Because eosinophils localize to mucosal surfaces of the respiratory, gastrointestinal, and genitourinary tracts, their IgA receptors could engage secretory IgA at these sites.

Eosinophils also express receptors for complement components [including those for C1q, C3b/C4b (CR1), iC3b (CR3), and C5a], for several cytokines (including those for IL-2, IL-3, IL-4, IL-5, IL-16, IFN-α, and GM-CSF), and for a number of ligands that are chemoattractants, many of which are likely to be generated at sites of allergic inflammation (including PAF, LTB_4, C5a, and several chemokines, such as eotaxin). These eosinophil chemoattractants can also stimulate eosinophil degranulation and the formation of superoxide anion and other oxidant derivatives. Eosinophils also have intracellular receptors for estrogens and glucocorticoids.

In addition to these receptors, eosinophils can express specific integrins, which not only may contribute to their preferential recruitment into sites of allergic diseases, but also may help to regulate their activation within extravascular tissues (308). Eosinophils (and lymphocytes), unlike neutrophils, can emigrate into sites of inflammation in patients with the leukocyte adhesion deficiency syndrome, indicating that eosinophils can migrate into tissues by mechanisms not dependent on CD18. Eosinophils express ligands for binding to both E-selectin and P-selectin (309). In addition, eosinophils express two α4 integrins, α4β1 and α4β7. The α4β1 integrin VLA-4 binds to VCAM and to domains within tissue fibronectin (310, 311). VLA-4/VCAM interactions may favor the preferential recruitment or activation of eosinophils (as well as basophils; see ref. 311) and mononuclear leukocytes to sites of allergic inflammation. The second α4 integrin of eosinophils, α4β7, can bind to the mucosal vascular addressin MAdCAM-1. The common expression of α4β7 by eosinophils and some lymphocyte populations, such as mucosal trophic CD4+ memory T-lymphocytes (312), may contribute to their colocalization within some lymphoid tissues. Treatment with certain mAbs to the α4 component of both α4β1 and α4β7 can prevent eosinophil influx into cutaneous or pulmonary sites of elicited IgE-associated allergic reactions (313,314). Moreover, blockade of α4 integrins can have beneficial effects on experimental IgE-associated allergic reactions, such as inhibiting pulmonary late-phase reactions, even without inhibiting eosinophil influx (315).

It needs to be emphasized that the functional properties (or state of "activation") of the eosinophils circulating in the blood of normal individuals may be quite different than those of eosinophils in tissues or exudates at sites of IgE-associated allergic inflammation, or in the blood of certain atopic or nonatopic subjects with markedly elevated levels of circulating eosinophils (i.e., eosinophilic subjects). For example, it has long been recognized that eosinophils from eosinophilic donors exhibit metabolic, morphologic, and functional changes, which are indicative of their being "activated" *in vivo* (291–293).

Moreover, many of the effector responses of eosinophils (e.g., degranulation, eicosanoid formation) can be enhanced by specific eosinophil-active cytokines, including GM-CSF, IL-3, and IL-5. Such cytokines may also influence the ability of eosinophils to express certain immunoregulatory functions. Thus, early eosinophil precursors that develop within the bone marrow ordinarily express class II MHC proteins, whereas blood eosinophils, from most normal and eosinophilic donors, lack expression of class II MHC proteins, even if these circulating eosinophils otherwise exhibit phenotypic evidence of *in vivo* activation. However, when mature, blood-derived human eosinophils are cultured *in vitro* with specific cytokines, including IL-3, GM-CSF, and IFN-γ, they are uniformly induced to synthesize and express HLA-DR (316). Eosinophils in the sputum of asthmatics have also been shown to express HLA-DR, as do airway, but not blood, eosinophils in allergic subjects challenged with antigen via segmental airways or by inhalation or in patients with chronic eosinophilic pneumonia.

While the eosinophil-active growth factor cytokines clearly may contribute to many aspects of eosinophil "activation" *in vivo*, these cytokines alone apparently cannot elicit all measures of eosinophil activation (317), such as enhanced expression of FcεRI (318) or CD40 (319) found on eosinophils from allergic subjects. Therefore, it is likely that other cytokines, and/or tissue- or extracellular matrix–derived activating stimuli, also contribute to the promotion of specific functional capabilities of eosinophils.

T Cells

In addition to their critical immunoregulatory role in the afferent phase of IgE-associated immunologic responses, a large body of evidence now indicates that T cells can also express effector-cell function in some examples of IgE-associated immune responses (5). T cells, particularly those that, according to *in situ* hybridization or immunohistochemical analyses, can produce Th2-type cytokines, are typically present in large numbers at sites of chronic allergic inflammation in the airways of patients with asthma (320) and can be recruited to late-phase reactions in the airways and other sites (5,320,321), and such T cells clearly may represent an important source of ongoing Th2-type cytokine production in these settings. The potential importance of T cells as a source of mediators that can account for features of chronic allergic inflammation is also supported by studies of models of IgE-associated immune responses in genetically mast cell–deficient Kit^W/Kit^{W-v} mice. Taken together, such work strongly supports the hypothesis that T cells can orchestrate the mast cell–independent recruitment of eosinophils to sites of allergen challenge (e.g., in the airways) (276, 322–325) and that this process can be associated with the develop-

ment of mast cell–independent airway hyperresponsiveness to methacholine (322).

Monocytes and Macrophages and Related Cells

Monocytes and macrophages are represented in the cellular infiltrates of late-phase reactions and chronic allergic inflammation, and these cells clearly represent a potential source of cytokines and other mediators in such settings (326,327). In these reactions, monocytes and macrophages may be activated independently of IgE, for example, by IgG (or complement components) that are generated in association with these immune responses. However, cells in the monocytic lineage, including dendritic cells such as Langerhans' cells, can express FcεRII/CD23 and, under some circumstances, FcεRI, in addition to other FcR (see section on receptors for IgE). There is *in vitro* evidence that both CD23 and FcεRI may permit at least some cells in the monocytic lineage to concentrate allergens recognized by cell surface–bound IgE, and then to present peptides derived from such allergens to T cells (see section on receptors for IgE). This work suggests that such cells may contribute to IgE-dependent mechanisms that can amplify and/or perpetuate the afferent components of Th2-type immune responses. The extent to which monocytes, macrophages, or dendritic cells can release mediators in response to signaling via IgE with FcεRI (of the αγ₂ type) largely remains to be determined.

MECHANISMS OF IgE-ASSOCIATED ACUTE AND LATE-PHASE REACTIONS AND CHRONIC ALLERGIC INFLAMMATION

Overview

Allergen challenge of sensitized individuals can elicit three types of responses: (a) acute allergic reactions, (b) late-phase reactions, and (c) chronic allergic inflammation. The major features of acute allergic reactions, which can be expressed seconds or minutes after exposure to allergen, primarily reflect the actions of mediators released from mast cells and other effector cells that are normally resident in the tissues at the site of allergen challenge. However, some of the mediators that are released in response to acute allergen challenge, in addition to having direct effects on cells resident in the affected tissues, such as vascular endothelial cells, secretory glands, sensory nerves, and vascular, respiratory, or gastrointestinal smooth muscle cells, also have effects that result in the recruitment of circulating leukocytes. Such recruited leukocytes can in turn influence the local characteristics of the evolving allergic responses, for example, by contributing to the reappearance or development of erythema (reflecting increased blood flow and stasis) and swelling (reflecting enhanced vascular permeability) in the skin or airway narrowing in the respiratory tract. These late-phase reactions characteristically do not develop until several hours after initial allergen challenge, in many cases after the signs and symptoms related to the acute allergic reaction have greatly diminished or even disappeared.

The third major pattern of allergic response, chronic allergic inflammation, typically occurs at anatomic sites that have been repeatedly challenged with allergen over prolonged periods. Sites of chronic allergic inflammation not only contain effector cells that have been recruited from the circulation, notably including increased numbers of eosinophils and T cells, many of them of the

Th2 phenotype, but also can be associated with striking, chronic (i.e., long-lasting) changes in the underlying tissues. For example, the chronic allergic inflammation that is characteristic of human allergic asthma, when persistent, can be associated with major structural changes in all layers of the affected airways, as well as with marked changes in the functional characteristics of the respiratory smooth muscle itself (see next section). Because repeated allergen challenge can also result in marked elevations of levels of total, as well as allergen-specific, IgE, which in turn may enhance the ability of mast cells and basophils to secrete IL-4, IL-13, and other mediators that can promote further IgE production, chronic allergic inflammation may also be associated with significant long-term enhancement of the individual's propensity to express Th2 cell–driven, IgE-associated immune responses.

In summary, acute allergic reactions, late-phase reactions, and chronic allergic inflammation differ in their time courses, their dependence on resident cells versus recruited leukocytes as sources of the mediators that determine their key characteristics, and the extent to which they can alter the structural and functional characteristics of the tissues in which they occur. Accordingly, these patterns of allergic reaction are thought to have distinct roles in adaptive immune responses involving IgE, and they certainly make distinct contributions to the clinical manifestations of allergic diseases.

Acute Allergic Reactions

PCA represents one of the simplest experimental models of an acute allergic reaction. In this model, IgE (and/or, in mice, IgG$_1$) antibodies of defined allergenic specificity are injected into the skin, and, at a suitable interval thereafter (for IgE-dependent PCA reactions, this is typically 24 to 48 hours), the specific allergen is administered intravenously (328,329). The ensuing FcεRI aggregation induced in cutaneous mast cells at the site where IgE was injected results in the secretion of all classes of mast cell-derived mediators (preformed, lipid, and cytokine). These products in turn produce multiple local effects, including enhanced local vascular permeability (leading to leakage of plasma proteins, including fibronogen, resulting in local deposition of cross-linked fibrin and tissue swelling), increased cutaneous blood flow, with intravascular trapping of red cells (due to arteriolar dilatation and increased loss of intravascular fluid from postcapillary venules, producing erythema), and other effects, such as itching, due to the stimulation of cutaneous sensory nerves by histamine (263,328,329) (Fig. 10).

Typically, such PCA reactions are detectable within a few minutes of allergen challenge (e.g., via measurements of changes in ear thickness, in reactions elicited at that site), reach a maximum, in features such as tissue swelling, in 30 to 60 minutes, and then rapidly wane. Many of the features of PCA reactions that have traditionally been measured, such as increased vascular permeability, tissue swelling, and, more recently, local fibrin deposition, diminish so rapidly after the reactions reach their peak that the responses may, at first glance, seem to have ceased entirely. Yet the consequences of strong PCA reactions, such as modest levels of tissue swelling or fibrin deposition, may still be detectable 24 hours or more after allergen challenge (274,330). For reasons that will be addressed below, the persistent swelling associated with IgE-dependent PCA reactions in the mouse probably represent part of the late-phase reaction at this site.

In normal mice, the FcεRI appears to be expressed only on mast cells and basophils. Moreover, genetically mast cell-deficient Kit^W/Kit^{W-v} mice, which essentially lack tissue mast cells but con-

tain basophils (230), are not able to express detectable PCA reactions (274,329,330). By contrast, IgE-dependent PCA reactions can be readily expressed in Kit^W/Kit^{W-v} mice at cutaneous sites that have been selectively repaired of their mast-cell deficiency by the adoptive transfer, several weeks before the experiment, of lineage-committed immature mast cells that had been derived in vitro from the bone marrow cells of the congenic wild-type mice (274,329). Similar approaches have been used to show that essentially all of the assessed acute consequences of IgE-dependent reactions elicited in the respiratory tract (331) or stomach (275) of mice are also mast cell–dependent. Based on this evidence, it appears very likely that mast cells are essential for the expression of at least the major features of IgE-dependent acute allergic reactions in mice.

It is clear that acute allergic reactions elicited in humans [e.g., in the skin at sites of allergen injection (332) or in the respiratory tract at sites of endobronchial challenge with allergens (333)] are also associated with extensive activation of mast cells, as judged by morphologic studies and by the detection of the release of mast cell—associated mediators (such as histamine and mast-cell tryptase) at the site of allergen challenge (228). However, in humans, the FcεRI can be expressed, at least under certain circumstances, on several cell types in addition to mast cells and basophils, including monocytes and macrophages, Langerhans' cells, circulating dendritic cells, and eosinophils (see section on receptors for IgE). As a result, it is possible that the expression of some acute allergic reactions in humans may include contributions from these cell types, as well as from mast cells and basophils.

Late-phase Reactions

The first description of what now might be called a *late-phase reaction* (LPRs) may have been that of Blackley, who noted in 1859 that the inhalation of an allergen can be associated with the occurrence of symptoms of asthma hours later (334). It is now clear that a large fraction of patients with allergic asthma (estimated at approximately 50% of adult asthmatics and 70% or more of children with asthma) express LPRs, or late responses, to inhaled allergens (335). The typical pattern of bronchial reactivity in subjects with allergic asthma is to develop an immediate or early asthmatic response, clinically detected by objective measurement of airflow obstruction, or bronchoconstriction, which occurs within approximately 10 minutes of allergen inhalation and which reaches a maximum by approximately 30 minutes and then completely, or nearly completely, resolves by 1 to 3 hours after challenge. The patients who develop LPRs then exhibit a second phase of bronchoconstriction, which usually is maximal at 6 to 12 hours and resolves by 24 hours.

Unlike acute allergic reactions, for which suitable animal models have been available for many years, models of LPRs in nonhuman subjects have been slower to develop and gain widespread acceptance. As a result, much of the data about the characteristics, and potential pathogenesis, of such responses have been derived from human studies. Several points about human LPRs appear to be well established: (a) The responses can be elicited by appropriate allergen challenge in the skin (see Fig. 10) and upper airways (nose), as well as in the lungs. (b) The reactions are almost always preceded by an acute allergic reaction, and at least some of the key pathologic features of these acute responses usually resolve before the onset of the LPR. (c) The signs (e.g., reddening and swelling of the skin, nasal discharge, airway narrowing) and symptoms (e.g., sneezing upon nasal challenge, wheezing and cough upon lower

Normal Skin

(in a host sensitized to express an IgE-associated immune response)

Epidermis

Arterioles

"Resting" mast cell with IgE on surface

Venule with single RBC in lumen

Dermis

Sensory nerve

Acute Allergic Reaction (minutes)

(1,2): Allergen and IgE-dependent mast cell activation; mast cell-derived mediators induce arteriolar dilatation (3), and increased venular permeability (4), leading to stasis of blood (5), resulting in erythema, and extravasation of plasma fluid and proteins (6), resulting in tissue swelling; histamine also stimulates sensory nerves (7), with antidromic stimulation of neuropeptide release, resulting in arteriolar dilatation (8) at periphery of site (peripheral "flare").

1 Allergen challenge

Late Phase Reaction (hours)

After partial or full resolution of many signs of the acute reaction, cytokines/mediators derived from mast cells (1) and, in some cases, Th2 cells (2) induce recruitment of circulating leukocytes (3), which, in turn, have multiple effects on resident cells, with reappearance of erythema and swelling.

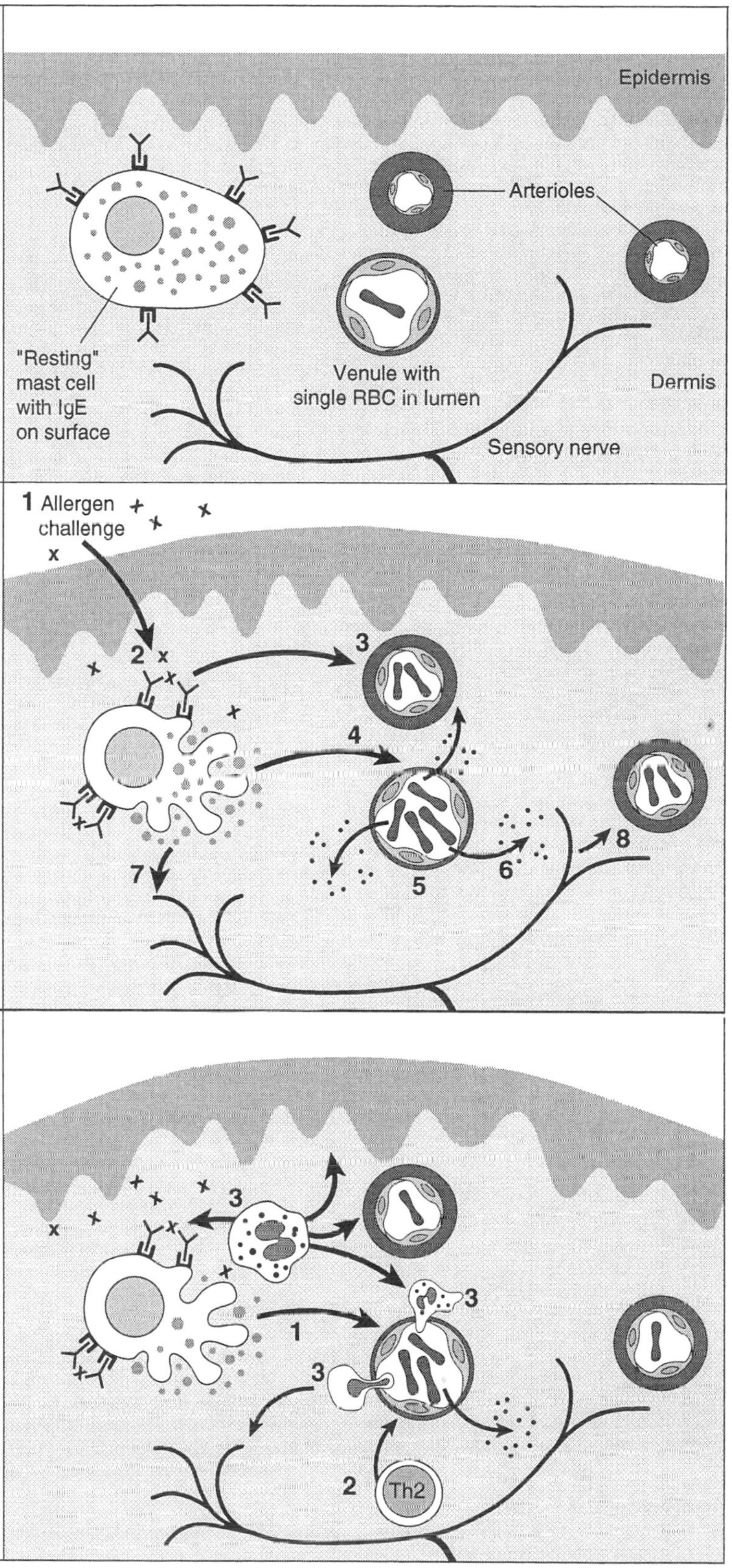

Th2

FIG. 10. Major cellular interactions and pathophysiologic events underlying the expression of IgE-associated acute and late-phase allergic reactions in the skin.

airway challenge) characteristic of LPRs are associated with the recruitment of circulating leukocytes to the sites of the reactions. (d) A variety of treatments, which are associated with a reduction in the leukocyte recruitment that is elicited at sites of LPRs, can also reduce the signs and symptoms that are characteristic of these responses (335–338).

It should also be noted that in humans, not all methods of mast-cell activation that yield an acute response will generate a subsequent LPR. For example, injection of codeine into the skin of normal individuals has been shown to produce an immediate cutaneous response that is clinically indistinguishable from that seen after allergen challenge, but it does not produce a subsequent "late" cellular response (339).

Given these findings, it is widely believed that many, and perhaps most, of the pathophysiologic changes that are associated with LPRs reflect, directly or indirectly, the function of the leukocytes that are recruited to the sites of these responses. In humans, the leukocytes recruited to sites of LPR include eosinophils, basophils, neutrophils, macrophages, and T cells; all of these cells may influence the reactions by providing additional proinflammatory mediators and cytokines. The recruitment and activation of basophils at LPR sites is supported by analyses of nasal lavage or bronchoalveolar lavage (BAL) fluids obtained several hours after antigen challenge, which demonstrate elevations in histamine, TAME-esterase activity, and LTC_4, but not PGD_2 or tryptase (227,228). Based on their representation in the infiltrates associated with LPRs, and their functional properties, Th2 cells may also contribute to the development of the pathology associated with certain LPRs (335).

Because of the great difficulties, in clinical studies in humans, in identifying the specific importance of individual elements in complex inflammatory responses, many basic questions about the pathogenesis of LPRs in humans remain unresolved. One of these is the relative importance of mast cells versus T cells in orchestrating the reactions. Rarely, clinical LPRs to allergen challenge can occur in subjects who appear to lack an antecedent acute allergic reaction (335). Moreover, allergen challenge of T-lymphocytes clearly can induce the cells to release cytokines, which might account for the recruitment and functional activation of eosinophils, basophils, and other circulating leukocytes, which are characteristic of LPRs (335). Finally, corticosteroids can markedly suppress the expression of LPRs; among their many activities, these agents can inhibit cytokine production by T cells but have little or no effect on the release of histamine and other preformed mediators by mast cells (281,340). These points have been used to support the hypothesis that LPRs are primarily dependent on Th2 cells, with lesser contributions from mast cells (335).

However, in mice that are sensitized solely by the passive transfer of IgE, IgE-dependent leukocyte recruitment in the skin (274) and stomach (275), and an IgE-dependent change in airway function, which is also observed in LPRs in humans (namely, increased airway responsiveness to the cholinergic agonist, methacholine) (331), are largely, if not entirely, mast cell-dependent. These findings support the view that certain important features of LPRs can be elicited at sites of allergen challenge, at least in mice, by IgE- and mast cell-dependent mechanisms. Moreover, a substantial amount of the IgE- and mast cell-dependent leukocyte recruitment that occurs in these murine reactions reflects the actions of TNF-α, and perhaps other cytokines, that can be derived from mast cells (274); corticosteroids and CsA, which can diminish cytokine production in mast cells (88,341,342) as well as in T cells (281,343), can markedly inhibit the development of IgE- and mast

cell-dependent cutaneous leukocyte recruitment in the mouse (282). Finally, it has been reported that late asthmatic responses can be elicited in some subjects by apparently allergen-independent mechanisms, including inhalation challenge with distilled water or by exercise (335). While the pathogenesis of such apparently IgE- and allergen-independent LPRs and their clinical significance remains to be fully elucidated, the occurrence of these phenomena support the hypothesis that there may be multiple pathogenetic routes to clinical LPRs, some of which almost certainly do not involve immune responses. However, it seems likely that *allergen-dependent* LPRs can be elicited by mechanisms that involve either IgE and mast cells (and/or other FcεRI-bearing cells) or T cells, and that, in many subjects, both types of mechanisms may contribute to the reactions.

Chronic Allergic Inflammation

In naturally occurring allergic diseases, such as allergic asthma, allergic rhinitis, and atopic dermatitis, patients typically experience repeated (perennial or seasonal) exposure to the offending allergens over a period of weeks to years. Although the specific features of the pathology of each of these diseases vary according to the anatomic site affected, certain general characteristics have been recognized: (a) The inflammatory infiltrates at such sites typically include eosinophils and T cells (particularly, Th2 cells), (b) the affected tissues exhibit persistent structural changes, and (c) the affected tissues exhibit significant alterations in their function.

It is widely believed that much, if not all, of the chronic tissue changes and alterations in organ function which develop at sites of chronic allergic inflammation are direct or indirect consequences of the inflammation itself (344,345). The evidence supporting this view is similar to that discussed above for the pathology associated with LPRs. Specifically, (a) the cells and mediators which are present at sites of chronic allergic inflammation have properties that might explain the structural and functional changes characteristic of tissues that are affected by these responses; and (b) treatments directed against the development of chronic allergic inflammatory responses (e.g., corticosteroids), cannot only reduce the extent of these inflammatory responses and their associated infiltrates of eosinophils and T cells, but can also eventually result in at least partial improvement in the structural and functional changes that are associated with these reactions (346–348).

Because the inflammatory cell infiltrates present at sites of human experimental LPRs and naturally occurring chronic allergic inflammation are similar in composition (prominent eosinophils and T cells, with smaller numbers of monocytes and macrophages and basophils), it is possible that the cellular infiltrates at sites of chronic allergic inflammation represent, largely, the result of multiple, overlapping LPRs elicited by persistent or repeated exposure to allergen. However, it has been shown that certain chronic inflammatory responses in mice can result in the cytokine-dependent local development of structures with features of lymphoid organs (349,350). Moreover, the persistence of large numbers of allergen-specific T cells at sites of chronic allergic inflammation clearly may result in enhanced local production of T cell-derived cytokines in these responses. Accordingly, the pathology associated with chronic allergic inflammation is typically qualitatively, as well as quantitatively, distinct from that observed at sites of experimentally induced LPRs.

Mast Cell–Leukocyte Cytokine Cascades

As described below (in section on features of IgE-associated allergic diseases), there has been much discussion of the relative importance of IgE and mast cells and other FcεRI⁺ effector cells, as opposed to T cells, in the pathogenesis of chronic allergic inflammation, particularly that associated with allergic asthma. While this remains an important area of active research, we feel that the key question is not whether IgE and mast cells, or T cells, are mainly responsible for the pathology associated with chronic allergic diseases (because both types of mechanisms are likely to be important), but to identify the extent to which particular clinically significant characteristics of these disorders reflect the specific contributions of distinct effector mechanisms.

Our group has formulated the hypothesis that a "mast cell–leukocyte cytokine cascade" critically contributes to the initiation and perpetuation of IgE-associated allergic inflammation in the airways and other sites (228,262,264,273). Specifically, it is proposed that the activation of mast cells through the FcεRI can initiate both the acute and late-phase components of the response, the latter in part through the release of TNF-α and other cytokines that can influence the recruitment and function of additional effector cells. These recruited cells then promote the further progression of the inflammatory response by providing additional sources of certain cytokines that may also be produced by mast cells stimulated by ongoing exposure to allergen, as well as new sources of cytokines and other mediators that may not be produced by mast cells. Certain mast-cell cytokines, such as TNF-α and TGF-β, may also contribute to chronic allergic inflammation through effects on fibroblasts and other cells resident at the sites of these reactions (351,352). Finally, mast-cell activation may directly or indirectly promote the release of cytokines from certain other cells resident in the tissues (e.g., in the respiratory tract, such cells would include alveolar macrophages, eosinophils, bronchial epithelial cells, vascular endothelial cells, fibroblasts, epithelial cells and nerves); together, the diverse cytokines that are released in these responses then contribute to the vascular and epithelial changes and to the tissue remodeling, angiogenesis, and fibrosis that can be so prominent in IgE-associated chronic allergic inflammation and many other disorders associated with mast-cell activation and leukocyte infiltration. At certain points in the natural history of these complex processes, cytokines and other mediators derived from mast cells, or from eosinophils or other recruited cells, may also contribute to the downregulation of the response.

In addition to their roles in allergic diseases, mast cell–leukocyte cytokine cascades may contribute to host defense, both in innate immunity to microbial infection, in which mast cells are activated independently of IgE (353–355), and in immune responses to parasites (see the following section) (356).

ROLES OF IgE-ASSOCIATED IMMUNE RESPONSES IN HOST DEFENSE

What selective advantage is (or, perhaps more to the point, was) conferred by IgE-associated immune responses? Circumstantial evidence has strongly suggested that this form of immune responsiveness developed as an important component of host defense against parasites, particularly helminths (worms) (246,247,357). Thus, infections from such parasites often induce strong primary and secondary IgE responses, and some of this IgE has specificity for antigens derived from the parasites. The responses to such infections frequently also exhibit other features characteristic of the Th2-type immune responses: (a) Circulating levels of eosinophils and basophils may be elevated during some phases of the infection; (b) tissues at sites of parasite infection (or parasite egg deposition) can exhibit inflammatory infiltrates which are similar in composition to those at sites of chronic allergic inflammation in human allergic diseases, with prominent representation of eosinophils, T cells, and basophils; (c) morphologic and biochemical analyses indicate that such infections can be associated with mast-cell degranulation and mediator release, and products derived from mast cells and basophils, including biogenic amines (which, in this context, may be derived predominantly from mast cells and basophils) and certain cytokines (which may be derived from mast cells and multiple other cell types present in the inflammatory infiltrates), can have direct or indirect effects which may promote parasite expulsion and/or diminish the organism's viability or fecundity; and (d) eosinophils, which typically are well represented in the inflammatory infiltrates at sites of parasite infection, can produce several proteins that can be directly toxic to the helminths.

Despite these general findings, it has been difficult to prove that individual components of IgE-associated immune responses to helminths, including IgE itself, are truly essential for the expression of protective host immunity to these parasites. Because of the intrinsic limitations of human studies, demonstrating the importance of IgE-associated immune responses in resistance to parasite infections in humans has been even more difficult. For example, there is a strong positive correlation between high levels of anti-schistosomal IgE and a reduced incidence of reinfection of human subjects with *Schistosoma haematobium* (358), but the basis for this correlation has not been established. Perhaps the difficulty in proving that IgE, mast cells, or eosinophils are critical for host defense against parasites should not be surprising, given the redundancy that apparently has been engineered into the expression of important immune responses. The maintenance of effective immune resistance to helminth parasites may simply be too critical to permit the response to be ablated by the loss of a single effector component, such as IgE, mast cells, or eosinophils. For example, the duration of experimental parasite infections with *Trichinella spiralis* and *Strongyloides ratti* was longer in genetically mast cell–deficient Kit^W/Kit^{W-v} mice than in the corresponding normal mice (359–362). However, it is not clear to what extent these defects reflected the mast cell deficiency of these mice, as opposed to c-kit–related abnormalities in other hematopoietic lineages (360–362). Moreover, the impairment of immunity to these parasites in mast cell-deficient mice was not as severe as in athymic nude mice, and in each instance the mast cell-deficient mice eventually were able to resolve the infection. Similarly, IgE −/− mice exhibit relatively modest abnormalities in their immune responses to *S. mansoni* (363).

Kit^W/Kit^{W-v} mast cell–deficient mice which are also genetically devoid of IL-3 exhibit a striking impairment in their ability to expel a primary infection with the nematode *Strongyloides venezuelensis* (*S.v.*); these mice also fail to develop an increase in bone marrow basophils in response to the infection, and they exhibit virtually no hyperplasia of mucosal mast cells in the intestines at sites of infection (230). However, IL-3 −/− mice also exhibit impaired cutaneous contact hypersensitivity responses, indicating a defect in certain T-cell functions (364). As a result, it is not yet possible to assess the extent to which the defect in immune response to *S.v.* infection in Kit^W/Kit^{W-v}, IL-3 −/− mice reflects their mast-cell and basophil deficiencies, as opposed to problems with T cells or other lineages that may be influenced by SCF/c-kit and/or IL-3.

The most compelling evidence for a critical role for mast cells or basophils in defense against parasites is in immune responses to ectoparasites such as ticks. However, the relative importance of basophils and mast cells in reactions to ticks appears to vary according to the species of host and the species of tick (227,365–367). Cutaneous mast cells and IgE appear to be essential for the local expression of acquired immune resistance to the feeding of larval *Haemaphysalis longicornis* ticks (365), whereas both mast cells and basophils may be involved in the cutaneous immune response to the larvae of a different species of ixodid tick, *Dermacentor variabilis* (366). Studies with antibasophil and antieosinophil antibodies suggest that, in guinea pigs, basophils and eosinophils are important effectors in acquired immune responses that impair the cutaneous feeding and promote the rejection of larval *Amblyomma americanum* ticks (367).

In certain settings, it appears that some elements of IgE-associated immune responses may have been co-opted by the parasite, and may contribute more to the pathology associated with these infections (or to the success of the parasite) than to effective immunity. For example, the preponderance of evidence from work in Kit^W/Kit^{W-v} mast cell-deficient mice indicates that mast cells are not critical for immune resistance to primary infections with the nematode *N. brasiliensis* (*N.b.*) (359). And in c-*kit* mutant *Ws/Ws* mast cell-deficient rats, the peak of egg output by *N.b.* (on day 8 of infection) was actually approximately 3.5-fold *lower* than in the corresponding +/+ (wild-type) rats (368). This was despite the much higher levels of mucosal mast-cell hyperplasia in the intestines of the +/+ than of the *Ws/Ws* rats. Similarly, in a different strain of normal rats, treatment with rrSCF *increased* levels of both mucosal mast-cell hyperplasia and egg production during primary infections with *N.b.* (369). By contrast, treatment of such rats with a neutralizing antibody to SCF markedly *decreased* the mucosal mast-cell hyperplasia response that was observed during *N.b.* infection and, in parallel, significantly *decreased* egg production by the parasite.

N.b. egg production in these models may have been affected by other SCF-responsive cell lineages besides the mast cell, including the cells responsible for electrical "pacemaker" activity in the intestines (interstitial cells of Cajal), which also express c-kit (370). Nevertheless, the findings are consistent with the possibility that mast cells may actually have some effects that favor parasite fecundity during *N.b.* infection. For example, perhaps the activation of mediator release from increased numbers of intestinal mucosal mast cells, and the resulting increased permeability of gut blood vessels and intestinal mucosa, promotes the nutrition of the parasites. This hypothesis is also consistent with the finding that suppression of IgE levels with an anti-IgE antibody can *decrease* both the worm burden and the parasite egg production associated with primary infection of *S. mansoni* in mice (371).

In other contexts, mast cells may have little or no detectable effect on parasite viability, but they may promote the tissue pathology that is associated with the immune response to that organism. For example, studies employing genetically mast cell-deficient Kit^W/Kit^{W-v} mice, which had been selectively repaired of their cutaneous mast-cell deficiency, showed that mast cells can significantly augment the intensity and maximal size of the cutaneous lesions at sites of experimental infection with the parasite *L. major* and, in some cases, substantially prolong the persistence of the reactions (372). However, the lesions ultimately resolved in both mast cell-deficient and congenic normal mice, and the presence or absence of mast cells had little or no effect on the numbers of viable parasites recovered from the cutaneous lesions (372).

It has long been thought that eosinophils represent important elements of host defense against helminthic parasites. However, more recent studies have questioned this role, because neutralizing anti–IL-5 antibody can abrogate the blood, bone marrow, and tissue eosinophilia associated with helminth infections, but *not* the severity of either the primary or the secondary infections (373,374). Thus, even though eosinophils clearly can function as helminthotoxic effector cells *in vitro,* the beneficial function of eosinophils in parasite host defense *in vivo* remains to be confirmed. On the other hand, eosinophils may contribute to the pathology associated with certain IgE-associated immune responses, because the eosinophil-derived cationic proteins which are toxic to helminths can also damage host tissues (see section on the effector cells and mediators of IgE-associated immune responses).

Finally, in rats, more than 99% of the IgE that is produced in the lamina propria of the intestines during infections with *Trichinella spiralis* does not enter the blood, but instead is transported into the intestinal lumen, where it is rapidly degraded; whether such intraintestinal IgE has a protective function in parasite immunity remains to be determined (357,375).

In summary, the emerging generalization appears to be that parasite-induced, IgE-associated immune responses can either protect or harm the host (or, in some cases, may have both types of effect), depending on the specific parasite, the genetically determined or acquired characteristics of the host's immunologic responsiveness, and, perhaps, many other factors.

IgE responses to certain viruses (376,377) or bacteria (378–380) have also been reported. While any protective functions of such responses remain to be confirmed, it has been proposed that IgE responses to respiratory viruses may contribute to the development of respiratory symptoms during infection (376,377) and that IgE antibodies to bacteria may contribute to exacerbations of bronchial asthma (378), atopic dermatitis (379), and chronic bronchitis (380). On the other hand, more recent work indicates that mast cells, and specifically mast cell-dependent leukocyte recruitment, can importantly contribute to host defense in innate immunity to bacterial infection (353–355). However, it appears that the release of mast-cell cytokines and other mast cell-derived mediators in these settings is elicited independently of IgE, for example, in response to products of complement activation (355) or derived from the bacteria themselves (354).

FEATURES OF IgE-ASSOCIATED ALLERGIC DISEASES

General Characteristics of Allergic Diseases

Allergic diseases are the group of hypersensitivity disorders that are (a) associated with the production of specific IgE to environmental allergens and (b) thought to involve, as part of their pathogenesis, IgE-mediated reactions. These disorders are prevalent. For example, allergic rhinitis (hay fever) affects 22% or more of the population in the United States (381,382), whereas allergic asthma is thought to affect at least 20 million residents of the United States (383,384). The economic impact of allergic diseases in the United States, including health care costs and lost productivity, were estimated at $6.4 billion in 1990 alone (385). Moreover, the incidence of these disorders, at least in populations for which reliable data are available, appears to be increasing (381–384).

A detailed description of the clinical features of allergic diseases, or a comprehensive consideration of the many factors that may contribute to the prevalence of these disorders, is beyond the scope for this chapter. However, we will present brief summaries of the characteristics of some of the major diseases, because this will help to illustrate how the various pathologic mechanisms which can result in the expression of IgE-associated hypersensitivity reactions, may contribute to specific clinical examples of such disorders.

Perhaps the best example of an acute allergic reaction is IgE-associated anaphylaxis, in which exposure of a sensitized individual to allergen (e.g., as the result of a bee sting or the ingestion of a certain food) induces, within minutes, a severe systemic reaction, which, if untreated, may rapidly result in death (see below). In this instance, IgE-dependent activation of mediator release by mast cells and basophils may account for virtually all of the pathology. By contrast, the pathology associated with atopic dermatitis may primarily reflect the consequences of chronic allergic inflammation, whereas the clinical manifestations of allergic rhinitis and asthma may reflect the contributions of all three patterns of IgE-associated hypersensitivity: acute, late-phase, and chronic.

The likelihood that a given individual will develop an allergic disease reflects a combination of genetic and environmental factors. Identical twins are significantly more likely than fraternal twins to demonstrate concordance for the occurrence of allergic diseases (386). However, the concordance of allergic diseases in identical twins, while high, is not 100% (386,387), nor will identical twins necessarily develop sensitivities to the same allergens (388). Similarly, individuals with two "atopic" parents are at greater risk of developing an allergic disease than those with only one atopic parent (approximately 47% versus approximately 24%; see ref. 389), but those individuals' specific allergic disease may be different than that of the parent(s) (387,389). Some of the genetic factors that may influence the development or expression of IgE-associated allergic diseases are discussed in the section on the regulation of IgE synthesis.

In addition to hereditary influences and the molecular features of specific allergens, it is likely that multiple environmental factors can importantly influence the development of allergic diseases, and that there may be complex interactions between many of these individual factors. Such factors can be considered to fall into three general categories: (a) the magnitude and pattern of allergen exposure, (b) the age at which exposure(s) occur, and (c) the presence of factors that can influence the nature of the individual's response to allergen exposure.

Magnitude and Pattern of Allergen Exposure

Induction of IgE responses to insect venoms can occur with a single or small number of exposures to the allergen, and these are typically "administered" intradermally and/or subcutaneously, at approximately 50 µg of the venom components per exposure (38). Moreover, individual subjects can develop potentially life-threatening hypersensitivity to insect venoms, even though they may exhibit no other manifestations of atopy, such as allergic rhinitis or asthma. The development of IgE responses to the dust mite allergen, Der p 1.0, has been reported to require exposure to at least 2 µg of allergen per gram of dust, and higher levels of exposure are

correlated with higher levels of development of allergic asthma in the affected populations (390,391). Moreover, allergens associated with atopic diseases (i.e., allergic rhinitis, allergic asthma, atopic dermatitis) are typically present in the environment of the patient for long periods (e.g., pollens, dust mite-, cockroach-, and companion animal-derived allergens, etc.). Clearly, many factors can influence the duration and magnitude of exposure to specific antigens: (a) geographic (species of plants and their pollens vary in their distribution); (b) economic [some individuals in lower socioeconomic groups may find it difficult to avoid exposure to cockroach-derived allergens, which are an important source of allergens in patients with asthma (34), whereas members of higher socioeconomic groups may have warmer and more humid houses, with low rates of indoor air turnover, which can favor the development of high levels of dust mite–related allergens (391,392)]; and (c) social (it has been suggested that relatively sedentary patterns of childhood activities may keep children indoors and thus prolong their exposure to indoor allergens [the TV theory of asthma (392)].

Age at Which Exposure Occurs

Several factors may contribute to the effect of age on the development of IgE responses (393). For example, the "barrier function" of the gastrointestinal epithelium—those properties that limit the ability of foreign substances to traverse the epithelium and thereby gain access to the interstitium—is not fully developed at birth (394). This probably contributes to the observation that genetically susceptible infants who are exposed to food allergens at an early age are at increased risk for the early development of IgE responses to such allergens (393). Exposure to such food allergens can occur as a result of either the diet of the infant or, if the infant is being breast fed, the diet of the mother (393,395,396). Such infants may also later exhibit an increased incidence of allergies to inhaled allergens, although the reason(s) for this correlation are not fully understood.

Age of exposure can also influence the development of allergies to inhaled allergens. For example, birch pollen–induced IgE responses and allergic rhinitis develop more frequently in Scandinavian children who were born in late winter or early spring than in those born in other seasons (397,398). The extent to which this increased susceptibility to IgE responses reflects factors related to the barrier function of the infants' respiratory epithelium, as opposed to factors related to the development of the immune system itself, remains to be determined. In any event, it is now clear that immune responses to allergens may develop very early in infancy or even, in some cases, in utero (393,399). Nevertheless, the majority of people who ultimately develop allergies in adulthood do not have a history of allergies in early childhood.

The Presence of Factors That Can Influence the Nature of the Individual's Response to Allergen Exposure

The elucidation of the critical role of cytokines in the initiation, and modulation, of immunologic allergic responses has suggested that factors that can influence cytokine production (or the effects of these molecules on their target cells) might also influence the ultimate expression of these responses. A number of candidate mechanisms have been put forward. Epidemiologic evidence has linked the striking increase in allergic rhinitis and asthma to Japanese cedar pollen in certain parts of Japan to a parallel sharp rise in those areas of the number of trucks that burn diesel fuel (400). At least three mechanisms have been proposed by which diesel particles might enhance the development of IgE responses: (a) the diesel particles adsorb pollen proteins, and help to deliver them to the lower airways [the pollen grains themselves, which are much larger than the diesel particles, are primarily deposited in the nasal turbinates (400)]; (b) the diesel particles function as a particulate adjuvant, which favors the development of IgE responses (400,401); and (c) the diesel particles contain certain aromatic hydrocarbons, which in turn can enhance IL-4 and CD40-dependent IgE synthesis by B cells *in vitro* (402). Exposure to second-hand tobacco smoke is also associated with an increased incidence of allergic diseases, although the responsible mechanisms are not yet fully understood (393,403). Finally, epidemiologic evidence has suggested that infections or immunizations that induce a Th1-type response early in life may reduce the subsequent risk of developing allergic diseases (404–406).

Examples of IgE-associated Allergic Diseases

Anaphylaxis

Anaphylaxis is an acute, systemic, hypersensitivity response to allergen, which typically involves multiple organ systems and which, if untreated, can lead rapidly to death (407,408). Because such reactions can be elicited by allergens derived from diverse agents that are otherwise relatively innocuous (Table 9), anaphylaxis represents the most grotesque imbalance between the costs and benefits of a response of the host's immune system to a foreign substance. When the term is used to refer to an example of an acute allergic reaction, anaphylaxis, by definition, refers to responses in which IgE antibodies (or, in mice, IgE and/or IgG$_1$ antibodies) have a critical pathogenic role. However, a clinical picture that may be indistinguishable from IgE-mediated anaphylaxis can occur by a number of other mechanisms that result in the systemic activation of mast cell–basophil mediator release. Such IgE-independent anaphylactoid reactions can be due to immune complexes (which may activate mast cells directly and/or via the activation of complement), complement activation by other mechanisms (including interaction with the surface of dialysis membranes or as a result of activation of the coagulation system), or agents that can directly activate mast cells or basophils (such as hyperosmolar solutions of 50% dextrose, mannitol, or certain radiocontrast materials) (407,408).

The great majority of anaphylactic or anaphylactoid reactions encountered clinically are due to IgE-dependent reactions to penicillin or other antibiotics, foods, or the venom of stinging insects, or they can reflect IgE-independent reactions to radiocontrast

TABLE 9. *Agents that have been shown to induce IgE-associated anaphylaxis or anaphylactoid (i.e., IgE-independent) reactions in humans, and the responsible mechanisms*

Mechanisms	Type of Inciting Agent	Examples
IgE-mediated reaction against proteins (native or transgenic) Note: Rarely, death can occur during allergen immunotherapy	Venoms[a]	Hymenoptera,[a] fire ant, snake
	Airborne allergens	Pollens, molds, "danders"
	Foods	Peanuts, milk, eggs, seafoods, grains
	Enzymes	Trypsin, chymopapain, streptokinase
	Heterologous serum	Tetanus antitoxin, antilymphocyte globulin
	Human proteins	Insulin, corticotropin, vasopressin, serum and seminal proteins
	Other	Latex, protamine
IgE-mediated reaction against protein–hapten conjugates	Antibiotics[b]	Penicillins, cephalosporins, sulfonamides
	Disinfectants	Ethylene oxide
Complement activation and generation of anaphylatoxins (which induce mast cell–basophil mediator release and have other effects)	Human proteins	Gamma globulins, other blood products
	Dialysis	Contact of blood with some dialysis membranes
Direct (IgE-independent) activation of mediator release from basophils and/or mast cells	Hypertonic solutions	Radiocontrast medium,[b] mannitol
	Drugs	Opiates, curare, *d*-tubocurarine, vancomycin
	Others	Dextran, fluorescein (for angiography)
Unknown	Nonsteroidal antiinflammatory drugs	Aspirin, indomethacin
	Anesthetics	Lidocaine, thiopental
	Preservatives	Metabisulfites, benzoates
	Steroids	Progesterone, hydrocortisone
	Exercise	
	Exercise and food	
	Idiopathic anaphylaxis	

[a]A common cause of serious anaphylaxis; as much as 25% of population may be at risk, tens of thousands of reactions (but <100 deaths) annually.

[b]Most common causes of serious anaphylactic or anaphylactoid reactions, about one reaction per 5,000 exposures (<10% are fatal, but these agents account for most deaths due to IgE-dependent or -independent anaphylaxis). Certain foods also account for many of the deaths due to IgE-dependent anaphylaxis.

Modified with permission from Bochner BS, Lichenstein LM. *N Engl J Med* 1991;324:1785.

material administered intravenously (407,408). Anaphylaxis to antibiotics or insect venom appears to occur regardless of atopic status, whereas life-threatening anaphylactic reactions to food allergens typically occur in subjects with other manifestations of atopic diseases (35–37).

The anaphylaxis that is induced in mice by the intravenous administration of relatively large amounts of allergen (e.g., 100 μg) can occur in genetically mast cell-deficient mice (114,115,409) or in mice that lack the IgE-binding α chain of the FcεRI (158,160). By contrast, both the mortality and most of the cardiopulmonary changes associated with this form of anaphylaxis do not occur in mice that lack the FcR γ chain that is common to both the FcεRI and FcγRIII (160,161). Mouse mast cells can be activated for mediator release by aggregation of either FcεRI or FcγRIII (19,168), and intravenous challenge of normal mice with an antibody (2.4G2) that binds to FcγRII/III induces a syndrome that resembles anaphylaxis (161). Both the physiologic changes and the mortality associated with 2.4G2-induced anaphylaxis are diminished but not completely absent in genetically mast cell–deficient mice (161). Taken together, this evidence indicates that, in the mouse, certain features of these models of anaphylaxis, including altered cardiopulmonary function and death, can occur independently of mast cells or of the FcεRI, but such FcεRI-independent effects are largely dependent on FcγRIII. Although the non–mast cell FcγRIII-bearing effector cell(s) responsible for the full expression of these models of anaphylaxis have not yet been defined, monocytes and macrophages represent attractive candidates (161).

These findings, together with the documentation of potentially fatal active anaphylaxis in genetically mast cell–deficient (114, 115) or IgE knock-out (18) mice, indicate that mast cells, FcεRI, and IgE are not required for the expression of anaphylaxis in mice, at least under certain experimental conditions. On the other hand, IgG$_1$- and FcγRIII-dependent murine anaphylaxis lacks some of the physiologic changes that can be associated with active anaphylaxis in the mouse, including the rapidly occurring and partially reversible airway narrowing that is associated with this response (160,161). Thus, even in the mouse, IgE and mast cells appear to be required for the full expression of the pathophysiologic changes that are associated with anaphylaxis to challenge with large amounts of allergen.

However, there may be important differences between the models of anaphylaxis that are typically studied in mice and naturally occurring anaphylaxis in humans. In humans, there is no evidence that antibodies other than IgE can induce FcR-dependent mast-cell activation in anaphylaxis. Moreover, life-threatening anaphylactic reactions can be induced in humans by exceedingly small amounts of allergen (407,408). When such reactions are induced by insect venoms (a well-studied example of anaphylaxis), they are associated with the appearance of high levels of mast-cell tryptase in the circulation, which is clear evidence of the extensive activation of this cell type (410). In anaphylaxis induced by food ingestion, serum levels of mast-cell tryptase may be normal or only slightly elevated (37); whether this reflects the types and anatomic location of the mast cells that are activated by ingestion of food allergens, a more prominent role for basophils than for mast cells in this example of anaphylaxis, or other factors, remains to be determined.

Nevertheless, it is widely believed that most, if not all, of the signs and symptoms of IgE-associated anaphylaxis in humans reflect (a) the systemic, FcεRI-dependent activation of mast cells and/or basophils and (b) the end-organ consequences of the release of mediators by these cells (407,408). Mild cases of acute systemic allergic reactions may primarily involve the skin, which exhibits widespread areas of increased vascular permeability, erythema, and itching, a condition termed *urticaria* or *hives*. Some authors consider such cases to represent mild cases of anaphylaxis, whereas others restrict the term *anaphylaxis* to acute systemic allergic reactions that include respiratory and/or cardiovascular manifestations. In more severe cases, greatly increased vascular permeability occurs in multiple organ systems, including the upper airways, leading to laryngeal edema and upper airway obstruction, as well as the rapid loss of intravascular fluid volume. The latter change, together with other consequences of mediator release in anaphylaxis, such as loss of tone in capacitance vessels and decreased contractility of the heart, leads to hypotension and shock. Breathing may also be impaired by marked narrowing of the lower airways, resulting in a severe case of acute asthma, and there may be pronounced gastrointestinal signs and symptoms (nausea, vomiting).

In some cases of severe anaphylaxis, initial stabilization of the patient's condition in response to appropriate management may be followed, several hours later, by a worsening of the condition. These systemic LPRs can occur even in patients who have been treated with glucocorticosteroids during the initial management of the anaphylactic episode, and it is not clear to what extent the pathogenesis of these responses resembles that of localized LPRs, such as those produced in the skin or airways of sensitized individuals by allergen challenge.

Allergic Rhinitis

Allergic rhinitis (hay fever) affects approximately 22% or more of the population of the United States, making it the most prevalent of the allergic diseases (381,382). Symptoms, which include sneezing, nasal congestion and itching, and rhinorrhea (increased production of nasal secretions), probably primarily reflect the IgE-dependent release of mediators by effector cells (primarily mast cells and basophils) in response to aeroallergens. Accordingly, symptoms may be seasonal (correlating with the presence of the offending grass, weed, or tree pollens, or mold spores) or year round (e.g., in subjects with dust mite or animal dander allergies). Some of the pathophysiology of allergic rhinitis clearly reflects the consequences of locally elicited, acute allergic reactions. Thus, symptoms typically develop rapidly upon natural or laboratory exposure to allergen, and the severity of some of the symptoms can be significantly diminished by H$_1$ antihistamines, although these agents typically provide only partial relief of the full symptom complex (337,411). However, the nasal tissues usually exhibit marked infiltration with eosinophils and other inflammatory cells, and laboratory studies have documented LPRs to experimental challenge with allergens, including the infiltration of eosinophils and basophils (337,412,413). Such LPRs can be largely blocked after local treatment with corticosteroids (413,414), which are also the most effective agents for the clinical management of the disorder (337,414). Accordingly, the pathophysiology of this disease appears to include elements of acute allergic reactions, LPRs, and chronic allergic inflammation.

Asthma

Asthma affects millions of people worldwide— more than 20 million in the United States alone—and its reported incidence is increasing dramatically in many developed nations; the human and economic costs of this disorder (in morbidity, health care expenses, lost productivity, and, most tragically, even mortality) are enormous (383,384). Rather than constituting a single "disease," it is now generally thought that asthma is a syndrome (i.e., potentially a group of different disorders, but with common clinical signs and symptoms), typically characterized by three major features: (a) intermittent and reversible airway obstruction, (b) airway "hyperresponsiveness" (i.e., a markedly increased sensitivity of the airways, as reflected in bronchoconstriction, to "immunologically nonspecific" stimuli such as histamine, cholinergic agonists, or cold air), and (c) airway inflammation. The syndrome of asthma may arise as a result of interactions between multiple genetic and environmental factors (383,384,415,416). Nevertheless, most cases of the disorder (the so-called atopic or allergic asthma) occur in subjects who also exhibit acute immediate hypersensitivity responses to defined environmental allergens, and challenge of the airways of such subjects with even very small amounts of these allergens can produce reversible airway obstruction (48,383,384,415,416). It is also known that the overall incidence of asthma in several different populations exhibits a strong positive correlation with serum concentrations of IgE (48,131,383,384,415). Moreover, it has also been demonstrated that IgE-sensitized mast cells, upon encounter with a specific antigen that is recognized by their FcεRI-bound IgE, secrete a broad panel of bioactive mediators that can promote reversible airway obstruction, bronchial hyperreactivity, and/or airway inflammation (263,264,384,415,416).

Although it once was thought that atopic or allergic asthma is a disease that primarily reflects the consequences of IgE- and allergen-dependent mast-cell activation (417), several findings have called into question the central role of mast cells in asthma. These include the demonstration that additional cell types, including eosinophils (293) and Th2 lymphocytes (418), both of which are well represented in the chronic inflammatory infiltrates in the airways of patients with asthma (384,415,416,419,420), also can produce cytokines or other mediators that may contribute to many of the features of the disease. Moreover, it has been shown that the high-affinity IgE receptor, FcεRI, which was once thought to be restricted to tissue mast cells and basophils, can also be expressed on the surface of monocytes (151), circulating dendritic cells (152), Langerhans' cells (154), and eosinophils (157), thus identifying these cells as additional potential sources of mediators in various IgE-dependent inflammatory responses.

As discussed in detail elsewhere (5,6,416), it may be very difficult, in settings as complex as allergic asthma, to assess the relative importance of individual effector mechanisms in the disorder. However, studies of mouse models of asthma support the following conclusions: (a) Airway hyperreactivity to cholinergic stimulation can occur by either mast cell-dependent mechanisms (which can be expressed even in the absence of leukocyte recruitment) or by CD4+ T cell-dependent mechanisms (which typically occur in a setting that also includes eosinophil infiltration of the airways); (b) mast cells are not necessary for the recruitment of Th2 cells or eosinophils to the airways after aerosol challenge with antigen, but they may contribute to their recruitment at "suboptimal" levels of antigen exposure; (c) the extent to which eosinophils are necessary for the expression of T cell-dependent changes in airway hyperreactivity in various murine models remains to be fully defined; and (d) in many experimental settings, particularly in various strains of normal mice, the expression of airway hyperresponsiveness (and other asthma-like features of these models) probably reflects the combined contributions of both mast cell- and T cell-dependent pathways.

In human allergic asthma, it seems very likely that IgE-dependent mast-cell activation importantly contributes to acute allergen-induced bronchoconstriction, and that mast cells can contribute to the airway inflammation associated with this disorder as well (263,264,273,383,415,416). However, a number of new findings indicate that IgE can influence the pathogenesis of asthma and other disorders associated with chronic allergic inflammation in additional, quite complex ways. For example, in humans, unlike in mice, the FcεRI can be expressed on several potential effector cells in addition to mast cells and basophils, including monocytes and macrophages (151) and eosinophils (157), and the form of the FcεRI expressed on monocytes and dendritic cells (which lacks the β chain) can function, via the binding of IgE, to enhance the processing and/or presentation of antigenic fragments of proteins, which are recognized by the cells' surface-bound IgE (150,152). IgE can also upregulate FcεRI expression on mast cells and basophils, and thereby prime them to release increased amounts of certain mediators, including IL-4, IL-13, MIP-1α, and other cytokines, under optimal conditions of antigen challenge (see section on receptors for IgE). Thus, in humans, IgE may not only serve to arm mast cells and other effectors of the efferent limb of acquired immune responses, but may also contribute, by enhancing IgE production, to the further development of such responses.

The clinical significance of these new findings largely remains to be established, but they point to previously unsuspected (or, at least, underappreciated) links between IgE- and mast cell-, or T cell-, dependent contributions to the pathogenesis of chronic allergic inflammation in asthma and other disorders. This emerging, more complex view of the pathogenesis of allergic asthma proposes that T cells and mast cells (and other FcεRIC+ cells) can have both effector cell and immunoregulatory roles in this disorder.

Atopic Dermatitis

This prevalent and troublesome chronic skin disease can be regarded as the cutaneous manifestation of atopy. The diagnosis is made based on a group of major and minor clinical and serologic features. To qualify, a patient must exhibit at least three of 24 minor features, one of which can be elevated serum IgE, as well as three of the four major features: (a) cutaneous itching, or pruritus; (b) involvement of the face and extensor surfaces in infants and children, and certain chronic changes in the skin of adults; (c) chronic or chronically relapsing inflammation of the skin, or dermatitis; and (d) personal or family history of atopy (i.e., asthma, allergic rhinitis, atopic dermatitis) (421,422). Although the reasons are not understood, the prevalence of this disorder has increased over the last few decades, with a study reporting a lifetime prevalence of atopic dermatitis of 20% in British children aged 3 to 11 years (423). The disease risk in monozygotic twins is 0.86 versus 0.21 (not different from that in non-twin siblings) for dizygotic twins (386).

While the pathogenesis of this disorder is not fully understood, 80% to 90% of patients have a family history of atopy and elevated serum IgE levels, and approximately 85% have positive immediate skin tests (i.e., an acute allergic reaction) to diverse food allergens or aeroallergens (421). However, much of the disease morbidity and pathology reflects chronic cutaneous inflammation, and the skin lesions typically include infiltrates of T cells, whose patterns of cytokine expression may be that of Th0, Th1, or Th2 cells, in part depending on the age of the lesions (424–426). Some of these

T cells include allergen-specific CD4$^+$ T cells, which exhibit a Th2 pattern of cytokine expression after cloning and expansion *in vitro* (427,428); such T cells, which also can express CLA, the marker of skin-homing T cells, are also recruited to the infiltrates that develop in the skin hours after the application of a patch containing a suitable allergen (429). The naturally occurring lesions of atopic dermatitis and the patch test–induced infiltrates in such patients also include eosinophils and their products, but the roles of eosinophils in this disorder are not yet clear (430,431).

How do allergens induce cutaneous inflammation in atopic dermatitis? Although more than one mechanism may be involved, most patients with the disease have IgE-bearing Langerhans' cells in the skin, which express the $\alpha\gamma_2$ form of FcεRI, as well as CD23 (154,155,432). Moreover, such Langerhans' cells can perform IgE-dependent antigen presentation to autologous T cells *in vitro* (433). *In vitro* studies with Epstein-Barr virus–transformed B cells which express CD23 indicate that the binding of antigen-specific IgE to B cell CD23 can enhance antigen presentation by these cells approximately 1,000-fold (434,435). Lines of evidence such as this suggest that the role of IgE in the pathogenesis of the chronic inflammation associated with atopic dermatitis may relate more to the enhancement of APC function by Langerhans' cells and perhaps other potential APCs than to the triggering of mediator and cytokine release by mast cells. On the other hand, it is well known that emotional stress can trigger itching and exacerbation of the lesions of atopic dermatitis (421). It has been suggested that a possible underlying mechanism for this finding is the induction of neuropeptide-dependent mast-cell activation of cutaneous mast cells (436).

MANAGEMENT STRATEGIES FOR IgE-ASSOCIATED ALLERGIC DISORDERS

Overview

One of the defining characteristics of acquired immune responses is the exhibition of long-term memory for the antigen that initially induced the response, and allergic diseases typically are experienced as long-lasting disorders. Indeed, the majority of patients with disorders such as allergic asthma, allergic rhinitis, and anaphylactic reactivity to allergens express these disorders for years and, in many cases, throughout their lifetimes. Allergic disorders, as a whole, are rarely fatal (some cases of anaphylaxis and, occasionally, allergic asthma representing unfortunate exceptions), but these conditions typically result in significant discomfort and reduced productivity. As a result, there has long been a need for effective approaches to prevent or diminish the occurrence of these disorders and to reduce the pathology and symptoms associated with these diseases in affected individuals. However, while efficacy (i.e., effectiveness in producing the desired clinical outcome) represents the *sine qua non* of a management approach for any disorder, other factors are also important. The first of these is safety, which is a particular concern in the design of treatments for allergic diseases. Ideally, the management approach must also be convenient (to promote patient compliance) and cost effective.

It cannot be emphasized too strongly that, while the design of therapeutic approaches must take into account both our understanding of the mechanism(s) of action of candidate drugs or biologicals and our concepts of the pathogenesis of the target disease, our knowledge in both of these areas may be quite incomplete. For example, sodium cromoglycate and nedocromil are useful and safe

for the treatment of some patients with asthma (437–439). While still widely regarded clinically as mast-cell stabilizers, which can prevent the release of mediators from mast cells, it is not clear whether this action represents the most important mechanism by which these drugs improve the pathology associated with allergic diseases [e.g., nedocromil has actions on other effector cells, such as eosinophils and, apparently, on nerves (439)]. Nor is it yet fully understood precisely how these drugs interfere with mast-cell activation, or why different patients with asthma either respond well to or are apparently unaffected by these agents (437–439). Given our current understanding that asthma does not "simply" reflect aberrant mast-cell activation (see below), it is likely that the actions of nedocromil on multiple potential effector cells may contribute to its usefulness in this disorder.

Table 10 presents the major management strategies currently employed for IgE-associated allergic diseases, as well as some selected newer approaches which are currently under investigation. Brief comments about these approaches are provided in the text.

Alter the Individual's Predisposition to Develop, or to Strongly and Persistently Express, Allergic Diseases

In the foreseeable future, it is difficult to envision a cost-effective and practical way to address this problem (e.g., via gene therapy). On the other hand, it has been proposed that early immunization to develop Th1-type immune responses may, through mechanisms that remain to be fully elucidated, decrease the incidence of Th2- and IgE-associated allergic diseases in the immunized population (404–406). If an effective and safe scheme of generic immunization could be developed to reduce significantly the occurrence or severity of IgE-associated diseases, this clearly would represent a practical and cost-effective component of the management strategy for these disorders. However, the ethical issues of performing such manipulations in infants or young children would have to be considered carefully.

Reduce or Modify Exposure to Allergen

Allergen avoidance, particularly in infancy (e.g., by eliminating common potential allergens from the infant's diet), may help to reduce the early onset of allergies to these allergens (36), but the long-term benefits of such approaches are not as clear (393). However, reduction in levels of key environmental allergens (e.g., by modifications in housekeeping to reduce house dust mites or cockroaches; by finding a new home for the cat; etc.) can reduce the severity of disease, days of hospitalization, and need for pharmacologic treatment of patients who have already developed allergies (391). Allergen avoidance is an extremely critical component of the management of patients who express anaphylaxis (35–39,407,408).

Unfortunately, there are a number of practical problems with such approaches. For optimal results, the patients (and/or their families) must be knowledgeable, highly motivated, and compliant (e.g., some cat-sensitive patients may want to keep their cat). In the case of anaphylaxis, it may be difficult to avoid the allergen (e.g., bee venom components in a beekeeper) or even to know when it might be present. For example, patients with life-threatening allergies to components of peanuts or other foods may consume products whose labeling (which may list several possible "alternative" ingredients) makes it virtually impossible for them to discern that

TABLE 10. *Management strategies for IgE-associated disorders*

Strategy	Examples	Status
Alter the individual's propensity to develop Th2-type responses	Early immunization to develop Th1-type responses	Theoretical
Reduce/modify exposure to allergens	Allergen avoidance by patients[a]	Key in prevention of anaphylaxis; important in asthma, allergic rhinitis; benefit in some patients with atopic dermatitis
	Reduce dietary exposure to allergens in infancy	May delay onset of, but may not prevent, sensitization
Inhibit/modify the IgE-associated response	Traditional immunotherapy with allergens[a]	Very useful in some settings (e.g., insect venom allergies)
	Induction of T-cell tolerance with peptides that are not recognized by IgE	In clinical testing (modest benefits so far)
	Immunotherapy with modified allergens that are not recognized by IgE	Preclinical studies
	Antibodies to IgE that do not cross-link IgE on FcεRI	In clinical testing
	IgE "vaccines" to ablate IgE	Preclinical studies
	Administer, modulate, and antagonize cytokines	Efficacy of IFN-γ in trials in atopic dermatitis
	Block binding of IgE to FcεRI	Preclinical studies
Interfere with activation of effector cells	Sodium cromoglycate, nedocromil sodium[a]	Benefit in some patients with asthma
	Enhance negative regulation of FcεRI-dependent effector cell activation by targeting cell surface structures	Preclinical studies
Interfere with mediator production by effector cells	5-lipoxygenase inhibitors[a]	Benefit in some patients with asthma, especially aspirin-sensitive asthma
	Corticosteroids[a]	Clinical efficacy probably reflects other actions also. See below.
	Cyclosporin A, FK506	Benefit in clinical trials in some patients with asthma and/or atopic dermatitis
Block actions of mediators on target cells	H_1 antihistamines[a]	Benefit in allergic rhinitis, ocular allergies, urticaria
	Leukotriene receptor antagonists	Benefit in some patients with asthma
Block cellular interactions with adhesion molecules	mAb to ICAM-1	Preclinical studies
Counteract end organ consequences of allergic responses	Epinephrine[a]	Essential in treatment of anaphylaxis
	β-adrenergic agonists[a]	Benefit in treating acute airway narrowing in asthma
	Costicosteroids[a]	Benefit in chronic allergic inflammation (asthma, allergic rhinitis, atopic dermatitis, etc.)

[a]Widely used in current management of IgE-associated disorders.

the offending allergen has been used in its preparation (440). The use of transgenic technology to alter foodstuffs will likely further complicate the utilization of allergen-avoidance approaches (441).

Inhibit or Modulate the IgE-associated Response Itself

In traditional immunotherapy or hypoimmunization therapy, the offending allergen is repeatedly (and carefully, to avoid eliciting anaphylaxis or other allergic reactions) administered to sensitive individuals in progressively increasing doses over a period of years. Both the effectiveness of the therapy and the levels of allergen-specific IgG (generally, IgG_4) antibodies obtained by treatment are allergen dose–dependent, and treatment eventually results in a

decline in levels of allergen-specific IgE and, in those with pollen allergies, a reduction in the postallergen season rise in IgE levels that are typically observed in untreated subjects (442,443). It once had been thought that the IgG antibodies induced by allergen injections "block" allergen-induced and IgE-dependent mast-cell and basophil activation, by binding allergen before it can be detected by IgE antibodies bound to FcεRI+ effector cells (442,443). An alternative possibility has been suggested: Allergen-specific IgG, by binding to FcγRIIB on the effector cell surface, can negatively regulate allergen- and IgE-dependent signaling via FcεRI (168).

However, it is not yet clear to what extent human mast cells express FcγRIIB that can function to downregulate FcεRI-dependent signaling. Nor is it even certain that the effectiveness of immunotherapy reflects its ability to influence levels of IgE or

IgG₄. For example, some patients exhibit clinical benefit from this approach before measurable changes in allergen-specific IgE levels can be detected and, in some cases, even before the onset of significant changes in levels of allergen-specific IgG isotypes (442–444). Moreover, there is evidence that immunotherapy can result in altered allergen-induced T-cell cytokine production, including decreased levels of IL-4 secretion, as well as reductions in levels of tissue mast cells and allergen-induced tissue infiltration by eosinophil and CD4⁺ T cells in the nasal mucosa (442,445,446). Despite the lack of a complete understanding of its mechanism of action, in certain settings, immunotherapy can be highly effective and safe. For example, in adult patients who have had anaphylactic reactions to insect venom components, the risk of developing another episode of anaphylaxis upon a subsequent sting is approximately 50% to 60% (447). However, after immunotherapy, the risk is less than 5% (38,39,447).

An extensive body of work in mouse models has indicated that the administration of certain antigenic peptides derived from allergens can induce T-cell tolerance and a marked reduction in levels of specific IgE and IgG (448–452). Clinical trials of peptides of this type are now underway, and some of the early results indicate that these approaches can reduce, albeit modestly, the signs and symptoms associated with allergic reactions to cat allergen in patients with allergic rhinitis or asthma (453–455). However, the clinical results do not yet indicate that such treatment protocols will be able to eliminate, or even markedly reduce, the pathology associated with allergic disease, or that such approaches are superior to or more cost effective than traditional immunotherapy. Whether this is because the treatment protocols have not yet been optimized, or because of intrinsic limitations of this approach, remains to be determined.

Attempts to improve conventional immunotherapy by chemically modifying allergens, in order to retain their ability to be recognized by T cells while reducing their ability to interact with IgE bound to mast cells or basophils, have shown promising results in certain animal models (456). Moreover, it has been reported that disruption of a disulfide bond that links the N- and C-terminal sequences of the major house dust mite allergen, Der f 2, virtually eliminated its ability to induce IgE-dependent histamine release from basophils in vitro, or skin test reactivity in vivo, while the altered allergen retained its ability to stimulate T-cell proliferation (457). This finding suggests that it may be possible to render certain common allergens safe (or, at least, safer) for use in standard allergen-based, rather than peptide-based, immunotherapy, by markedly reducing their ability to be recognized by IgE while retaining their expression of most T-cell epitopes (457). This approach, in theory, avoids one of the potential problems of peptide-based immunotherapy: the large number of different T-cell epitopes that can be recognized by the diversity of MHC and TCR structures expressed by different individuals.

Alternative approaches for manipulating Th2 cell- and IgE-associated allergic diseases have focused on the IgE response itself. To be therapeutically successful, such approaches clearly require that two assumptions be largely correct: (a) IgE is directly or indirectly responsible for a significant amount of the pathology associated with the disease that will be treated; and (b) in the treated patient population, the reductions in IgE necessary to reduce disease-related pathology will not result in significant negative consequences, such as increased susceptibility to infectious diseases. While several approaches for inhibiting the production or effective function of allergen-specific IgE have been developed and tested in

animal models, the method that has advanced furthest, and is now in clinical trials, is based on the subcutaneous administration of a humanized mAb that reacts with an epitope of human IgE that is masked when the IgE is bound to FcεRI (214). Accordingly, this mAb (214), like certain mAbs that are specific for IgE-producing B cells (458), has virtually no ability to cross-link IgE bound to FcεRI, and thus provoke "allergic" reactions. Furthermore, preclinical tests in animals have indicated that the extensive reductions in circulating levels of IgE that can be achieved with such approaches are not associated with increased pathology, even in animals infected with certain parasites that induce Th2 cell- and IgE-associated immune responses (371).

In human subjects, treatment with the mAb can reduce circulating levels of free IgE by up to 99% or more (214), which in turn results in reduced FcεRI expression by basophils and, probably, mast cells, and it can diminish significantly the ability of the blood basophils isolated from such subjects to release histamine in response to allergen challenge [particularly in subjects with multiple allergen sensitivities (214)]. This treatment also can significantly reduce (but not fully eliminate) the acute and late-phase bronchoconstriction responses to challenge with aerosolized allergen (459,460). Further studies are required to assess more fully the cost effectiveness and safety of this type of treatment approach and to define those clinical settings in which it may be useful.

Current evidence indicates that anti-IgE therapy based on mAb is reversible, in that IgE levels gradually return to pretreatment levels when therapy is discontinued (214). It has been proposed that long-term elimination of the IgE response could be achieved by linking toxins to anti-IgE (461) or by vaccinating subjects with certain peptides derived from IgE (462,463). The proposed mechanism in the first instance would be ablation of clones of IgE-producing B cells (461) and, in the second, the development of autoantibodies against IgE that do not cross-link IgE (and therefore do not induce activation of mast cells and basophils) (462–464). These approaches may have advantages, vis à vis mAb-based anti-IgE treatment, with respect to cost and convenience. However, the use of toxins in this setting, as well as the potential adverse consequences of achieving a long-term or even permanent elimination of IgE responses, have implications for the safety of these approaches which need to be carefully considered and evaluated.

Given the ability of cytokines to regulate IgE responses, there has been much consideration of the potential value of targeting the cytokines that promote IgE responses, the receptors for these cytokines, or the intracellular signaling pathways triggered by cytokines, for the management of allergic tissues. Major problems in this area are the complexity and redundancy in cytokine-dependent immunologic processes (465,466). For example, the finding that either IL-4 or IL-13 can promote IgE responses would suggest that elements that may be relatively specific to the IL-4/IL-13 signaling pathway, such as Stat 6 (467), may represent more attractive targets for efforts to reduce IgE responses than does either IL-4 or IL-13 itself, yet targeting intracellular molecules represents a challenge for drug-development efforts. An alternative approach to blocking pathways that upregulate Th2-cell responses is to attempt to downregulate such responses with cytokines, such as IFN-γ. This approach has exhibited safety and partial efficacy in clinical trials in patients with atopic dermatitis (468,469). However, such treatment is not regarded as effective as corticosteroid therapy, and subjects relapse shortly after discontinuation of IFN-γ injections (121). Furthermore, whether one attempts to reduce the production or action of positive regulators of the IgE response or to enhance the negative regulation of the response (e.g., by providing cytokines or cytokine mimics that have these effects), one must design and test such approaches with due consideration for the many potential consequences these manipulations might have on biologic processes other than IgE responses.

A final IgE-based approach for treating allergic diseases would be to interfere with binding of IgE to the α chain of the FcεRI (470). Given the high affinity of IgE for the FcεRI, the challenge here is to find an agent that can produce the desired biologic effect (i.e., substantially decreased IgE-dependent signaling in FcεRI+ effector cells) safely and at therapeutically achievable (and cost-effective) concentrations. However, this approach clearly has the potential advantage of rapid reversibility upon cessation of treatment with the agent.

Interfere with Effector-Cell Activation

Although their mechanisms of action are not fully understood, sodium cromoglycate and nedocromil sodium can diminish activation and mediator secretion from at least some mast-cell populations in vitro, and this effect of the drugs may, at least in part, explain their ability to diminish signs and symptoms of allergic disease in certain patients with allergic asthma, allergic rhinitis, or ocular allergic responses (439). However, in vitro studies indicate that nedocromil sodium also can inhibit eosinophil mediator release, chemotaxis, and survival, as well as diminish neuronally mediated contraction of airway tissue from experimental animals (439). Thus, the clinical efficacy of these compounds may reflect actions on multiple cell types.

β-adrenergic agonists, such as epinephrine, can also reduce mast cell–mediator production in response to FcεRI-dependent stimulation, presumably because of the ability of these agents to increase levels of cyclic adenosine monophosphate (cAMP) (471–473). However, the clinical efficacy of β-adrenergic agonists in asthma primarily reflects their ability to induce bronchodilatation (see below).

In theory, it may be possible to use approaches that are based on the engagement of receptors that negatively regulate FcεRI-dependent mediator secretion (i.e., FcγRIIB, gp49, CD81) in the management of allergic disorders. Such approaches have the advantage of targeting molecules that are expressed on the cell surface, and therefore are relatively accessible to potential therapeutic agents. Similarly, if the potential therapeutic agents could achieve effective intracellular concentrations, it may be possible to suppress effector-cell activation by targeting important components of the signaling pathways that link FcεRI aggregation with effector cell–mediator production. Signaling elements that are activated relatively proximal to FcεRI aggregation (such as syk), and therefore are critical for the production of all classes of mediators, represent particularly attractive targets.

In all approaches such as these, a key challenge is to achieve appropriate specificity of action. Thus, actions on cells other than mast cells and basophils can be desirable if these cells contribute to the pathology of allergic diseases, but they can also be undesirable if such cells have important roles in promoting health. On the other hand, the utilization of potential molecular targets, whether they are surface structures or intracellular signaling elements, by cells other than the effector cells of allergic diseases does not necessarily indicate that targeting such molecules carries unsurmountable risk. For example, approaches might be used that favor the delivery of the therapeutic agent to sites of pathology and/or to the target cells of interest (e.g., inhalation therapy in asthma); and it is possible that concentrations of the agent that are sufficient to produce a desired effect (i.e., diminished effector cell–mediator production) may not be sufficient to produce an untoward effect (e.g., diminished function of another cell type that utilizes the same targeted molecule).

Interfere with the Production of Mediators by Effector Cells

Clinical trials with inhibitors of 5-lipoxygenase (5-LO) indicate that this approach may be useful in settings where products of arachidonic acid metabolism via the 5-LO pathway importantly contribute to disease pathology. Such agents appear to be especially useful in patients with aspirin-sensitive asthma (474), and they also confer significant benefit in some subjects with allergic asthma (475,476).

Corticosteroids (also referred to as glucocorticosteroids or steroids) are currently the most effective class of drugs used for the treatment of asthma; they are also useful in other diseases associated with chronic allergic inflammation, such as atopic dermatitis and allergic rhinitis (281,414,421,477,478). Inhaled steroids are effective in all types of asthma, and are associated with fewer undesirable side effects than are systemic steroids. These agents are now used relatively early in the treatment of patients with asthma, reflecting the knowledge that airway inflammation is present in even mild cases of the disorder. However, despite intensive study, the mechanisms by which steroids confer their benefit are not fully understood. They certainly can diminish transcription of cytokine genes, and they have other effects that suppress cytokine production by multiple effector-cell types that can contribute to allergic diseases, including T cells, mast cells, basophils, eosinophils, and monocytes and macrophages (281,477). However, these agents have additional, diverse effects on these and many other cell types, and the extent to which the individual effects of these agents on particular cell types are responsible for their efficacy in allergic diseases is not yet known. For example, steroids decrease the transcription of genes for inducible phospholipase A_2, inducible cyclooxygenase, inducible nitric oxide synthetase, and adhesion molecules such as ICAM-1 or E-selectin (477). Steroids also can reduce the cytokine-dependent survival of eosinophils and other inflammatory cells (479), and they can diminish mast-cell survival (480), an effect that may, at least in part, reflect diminished production of SCF at sites of steroid treatment (481). Finally, steroids can have multiple direct and indirect affects on the resident tissue cells, such as epithelial cells, smooth muscle cells, fibroblasts, and vascular endothelial cells; some of these effects may also contribute to the clinical efficacy of steroids in diseases of chronic allergic inflammation (477).

Clinical studies indicate that the immunosuppressive agents CsA (482–484) and FK506 (485) may be effective in suppressing multiple aspects of allergic inflammation and its clinical consequences. While such studies provide proof-of-principle that immunosuppressive agents other than corticosteroids can have benefit in diseases associated with chronic allergic inflammation, the potential toxicity associated with such agents (at least, those that are currently available) may limit their utility in most patients with allergic diseases.

Block the Action of Mediators on Target Cells

The most widely used agents in this group are antihistamines, which block the binding of histamine to their receptors on target cells, such as vascular endothelial cells and vascular, respiratory, and gastrointestinal smooth muscle cells. Most of the pathologic effects of histamine in allergic diseases are thought to reflect the action of histamine on H_1 receptors, and agents that represent relatively specific antagonists of the binding of histamine to H_1 receptors are accordingly the most generally effective antihistamines for use in allergic diseases (486). Antihistamines are particularly helpful in settings in which alterations of vascular permeability and other consequences of the local actions of histamine (e.g., stimulation of nerve fibers responsible for itching) dominate the symptomatology: These include allergic rhinitis, ocular allergies, urticaria, and atopic dermatitis (486,487). However, they have been minimally beneficial in allergic asthma, probably because they both induce tachyphylaxis and have little ability to affect the expression of chronic allergic inflammation in the airways of these patients (487–491).

Drowsiness, due to the non-H_1 effects of the drugs (i.e., anticholinergic and antiserotonergic effects) in the CNS, has represented the most widespread and significant adverse effect of traditional antihistamines (486,487). This explains the great popularity of the more newly developed nonsedating antihistamines, which poorly cross the blood–brain barrier and have little or no anticholinergic or antiserotonergic effects in the CNS (486,487).

Several different leukotriene receptor antagonists are now in clinical trials, and these agents show promise in reducing the signs and symptoms of chronic allergic asthma, at least in some patients (491,492). Although these agents are clearly superior to antihistamines in this setting, they by no means completely eliminate clinical evidence of the disease. This probably reflects the fact that multiple mediators in addition to leukotrienes contribute to the pathology.

Because of the strong evidence implicating various cytokines in the pathogenesis of chronic allergic inflammation, there is interest in using agents that interfere with the actions of specific cytokines in this setting. IL-5 [because of its importance in regulating eosinophil production and function (493)], TNF-α [because of its role in recruiting leukocytes to sites of IgE-dependent mast-cell activation (274,494,495)], and eotaxin and other chemokines [because of their ability to promote the recruitment of eosinophils and other leukocytes to sites of allergic inflammation (496)] are considered to represent particularly attractive potential targets.

Based on *in vitro* studies and preclinical studies in animal models, PAF once was regarded as an attractive therapeutic target in asthma; however, several trials in asthma of agents that interfere with PAF production or antagonize its function have shown little or no benefit (497).

Interrupt the Evolution of Inflammatory Responses by Targeting Adhesion Molecules

The identification of the molecules that regulate the multiple steps whereby leukocytes are recruited to sites of inflammation has provided a number of potential therapeutic targets. Antibodies or other molecules that can block the binding of adhesion molecules (on vascular endothelial cells, epithelial cells, or other cells) to their counterreceptors on leukocytes have been of particular interest. For example, a mAb to ICAM-1 can inhibit the eosinophil infiltration and airway hyperresponsiveness observed shortly after allergen challenge in a primate model of allergic asthma (11,498). However, this treatment had little effect on chronic airway inflammation in experimental nonhuman primates (499), and it remains to be determined whether approaches that target cellular adhesion will be useful, safe, and cost effective in the treatment of allergic diseases in humans.

Counteract the End-organ Consequences of Allergic Responses

The pharmacologic modulation of the function of the target cells that are affected as a direct or indirect consequence of IgE-associated allergic reactions represents a major approach for the clinical management of these disorders. Notably, this approach represents the most essential component of the treatment of the most acute and catastrophic of the allergic disorders, anaphylaxis. The key drug used in this setting, which must be administered as soon as possible after the onset of symptoms, is epinephrine (407,408). Epinephrine, which is an endogenous agonist of α- and β-adrenergic receptors, has a number of important effects in this setting, including those dependent on α-adrenergic receptors (support of blood pressure and cardiac function) and β-adrenergic receptors (relaxation of respiratory smooth muscle cells, to open upper and lower airways and thereby to improve respiration); it may also, through β-adrenergic effects, diminish further mediator release by mast cells and basophils (407,408). Antihistamines and corticosteroids can also be useful in the management of anaphylaxis, but these agents should be used in addition to, rather than instead of, epinephrine (407,408).

β-adrenergic agonists also represent an important agent in the management of asthma, in which their main value is to promote relaxation of airway smooth muscle (500). However, careful attention must be given to the manner in which these agents are employed (501); indeed, it has been proposed that the inappropriate (i.e., excessive) use of these agents may actually increase the risk of death associated with asthma, perhaps in part by contributing to a delay in the institution of additional, more appropriate treatment modalities (500,502).

Among their many biologic activities, some of the beneficial effects of corticosteroids on chronic allergic inflammation are to alter the end-organ consequences of the responses (281,346,477). For example, these agents may suppress or, in part, reverse some of the chronic structural or functional consequences of allergic inflammation (347,348). However, chronic use of corticosteroids, particularly when the agents are administered systemically, may have a number of undesirable effects on multiple organs (477). Thus, the balance between the costs and benefits of such approaches can be quite delicate.

CONCLUDING REMARKS

Allergic disorders that are associated with IgE not only are widespread causes of significant morbidity and lost productivity, but also are increasing in incidence and in human and economic impact in many parts of the developed world. Since the publication of the last edition of this text, there has been substantial progress in our understanding of the genetic and environmental factors that influence these disorders, as well as the molecular mechanisms that underlie the expression of their associated pathology. And some of this progress has already been translated into new experimental approaches for the therapy of these diseases. Yet these encouraging signs of progress should not obscure how much remains to be done to understand more fully and manage more effectively these complex and troublesome disorders.

One of the most important developments (and one that we wish to encourage) is an abandonment of attempts to accommodate all of the IgE-associated allergic diseases within the Procrustean bed of the "type I" category of the original Coombs and Gell classification of the mechanisms that underlie disorders of immunologic hypersensitivity. Although acute allergic reactions, such as anaphylaxis, are still thought to represent a relatively pure example of a type I IgE- and mast cell– and basophil-mediated reaction, the most widespread of the allergic diseases, including asthma and atopic dermatitis, clearly are much more complex, with significant aspects of their pathology that probably reflect largely IgE- and mast cell–independent effector cell activities of T cells, particularly those with the Th2 phenotype.

On the other hand, the appreciation of the important contribution of chronic allergic inflammation, as well as the acute consequences of IgE-dependent mast-cell activation, to the pathogenesis of allergic diseases may have had an unintended consequence: diverting attention from the possibility that IgE and mast cells and other FcεRI⁺ effector cells may contribute to the chronic, as well as to the acute, manifestations of allergic diseases. The findings that mast cells (and basophils) represent potential sources of many cytokines, including those that can promote IgE production and/or leukocyte recruitment, and that mast cells can exhibit enhanced ability to generate such cytokines after IgE-dependent upregulation of their surface expression of FcεRI, immediately suggest mechanisms by which mast cells (and perhaps other FcεRI⁺ effector cells) may contribute to the amplification or persistence of Th2-type responses, as well as to local expressions of chronic allergic inflammation. Eosinophils also can produce multiple cytokines and express FcεRI and, like mast cells and basophils, can express certain properties that may permit them to function in antigen presentation to T cells and/or in the promotion of antibody production by B cells.

Taken together, these new insights into the functional capabilities of the traditional immunoregulatory cells (i.e., T cells) and effector cells (i.e., mast cells, basophils, and eosinophils) of allergic diseases suggest a more complex view of the pathogenesis of these disorders, in which T cells, mast cells, basophils, and eosinophils may have *both* effector and immunoregulatory roles. Indeed, one of the most critical current challenges of research in this area is to clarify to what extent the various *potential* effector and/or immunoregulatory cells of chronic allergic inflammation actually contribute to specific clinically important features of allergic diseases, and to define more precisely how such cellular functions are expressed and regulated. Addressing these issues is of considerable clinical importance, as the answers will carry clear implications for efforts to devise new approaches to prevent or treat IgE-associated allergic disorders.

ACKNOWLEDGMENTS

Our research work is supported by grants from the United States Public Health Service, National Institutes of Health. We thank John J. Costa and Andrew Scharenberg for helpful discussions and constructive criticism of the manuscript, and Ann M. Dvorak for the electron micrographs.

REFERENCES

1. von Pirquet C. Allergie. *Munch Med Wochenschr* (Translated from the German by Prausnitz C.). In: Gell PGH, Coombs RRA, eds. (1963) *Clinical aspects of immunology.* vol 30. Oxford: Blackwell Scientific Publications, 1906:1457.
2. Coombs RRA, Gell PGH. The classification of allergic reactions underlying disease. In: Gell PGH, Coombs RRA, eds. *Clinical aspects of immunology.* Oxford: Blackwell Scientific Publications, 1963:317–337.
3. Kay AB. Concepts of allergy and hypersensitivity. In: Kay AB, ed. *Allergy and allergic diseases.* vol 1. Oxford: Blackwell Science Ltd., 1997:23–35.
4. Janeway CA Jr, Travers P. *Immunobiology: the immune system in health and disease.* New York: Garland Publishing Inc., 1994;11:2.
5. Kay AB, Frew AJ, Corrigan CJ, Robinson DS. The T-cell hypothesis of chronic asthma. In: Kay AB, ed. *Allergy and allergic diseases.* vol 2. Oxford: Blackwell Science Ltd., 1997:1379–1394.
6. Galli SJ. Complexity and redundancy in the pathogenesis of asthma: reassessing the roles of mast cells and T cells. *J Exp Med* 1997;186:343–347.
7. Mosmann TR, Sad S. The expanding universe of T-cell subsets: Th1, Th2 and more. *Immunol Today* 1996;17:138–148.
8. Abbas AK, Murphy KM, Sher A. Functional diversity of helper T lymphocytes. *Nature* 1996;383:787–793.
9. Aebischer I, Stadler BM. Th1–Th2 cells in allergic responses: at the limits of a concept. *Adv Immunol* 1996;61:341–403.
10. Romagnani S. The Th1/Th2 paradigm. *Immunol Today* 1997;18:263–266.
11. Gundel RH. Primate models of allergic asthma. In: Kay AB, ed. *Allergy and allergic diseases.* vol 2. Oxford: Blackwell Science Ltd., 1997:1037–1044.
12. Abraham WM. Sheep models of allergic bronchoconstriction. In: Kay AB, ed. *Allergy and allergic diseases.* vol 2. Oxford: Blackwell Science Ltd., 1997: 1045–1055.
13. Geba GP, Askenase PW. Murine models of allergy, asthma and hyperresponsiveness. In: Kay AB, Coombs RRA, eds. *Allergy and allergic diseases.* vol 2. Oxford: Blackwell Science Ltd., 1997:1056–1067.
14. Chung KF. The allergic response in rats. In: Kay AB, ed. *Allergy and allergic diseases.* vol 2. Oxford: Blackwell Science Ltd., 1997:1068–1078.
15. Herd CM, Page CP. The rabbit as an animal model of allergy, asthma and airway hyperresponsiveness. In: Kay AB, ed. *Allergy and allergic diseases.* vol 2. Oxford: Blackwell Science Ltd., 1997:1079–1092.
16. Minshall E, Sanjar S. The sensitized guinea pigs as a model of allergic asthma. In: Kay AB, ed. *Allergy and allergic diseases.* vol 2. Oxford: Blackwell Science Ltd., 1997:1093–1102.
17. Emala C, Hirshman CA. Canine models of asthma and hyperresponsiveness. In: Kay AB, ed. *Allergy and allergic diseases.* vol 2. Oxford: Blackwell Science Ltd., 1997:1103–1110.
18. Oettgen HC, Martin TR, Wynshaw-Boris A, Deng C, Drazen JM, Leder P. Active anaphylaxis in IgE-deficient mice. *Nature* 1994;370:367–370.
19. Ravetch JV, Kinet J-P. Fc receptors. *Annu Rev Immunol* 1991;9:457–492.
20. Platts-Mills TAE, Solomon WR. Aerobiology and inhalant allergens. In: Middleton E Jr, Reed CE, Ellis EF, Adkinson NF Jr, Yunginger JW, Busse WW, eds. *Allergy: principles and practice.* vol I. St. Louis: Mosby–Year Book, 1993:469–528.
21. Cromwell O. Biochemistry of allergens. In: Kay AB, ed. *Allergy and allergic diseases.* vol 2. Oxford: Blackwell Science Ltd., 1997:797–810.
22. King TP, Hoffman D, Lowenstein H, Marsh DG, Platts-Mills TAE, Thomas W. Allergen nomenclature. *Clin Exp Allergy* 1995;25:27–37.
23. Thomas WR. Molecular cloning of allergens. In: Kay AB, ed. *Allergy and allergic diseases.* vol 2. Malden, MA: Blackwell Science, 1997:811–824.
24. O'Hehir RE, Garman RD, Greenstein JL, Lamb JR. The specificity and regulation of T-cell responsiveness to allergens. *Adv Immunol* 1991;9:67–95.
25. Higgins JA, Lamb JR, Marsh SGE, et al. Peptide-induced nonresponsiveness of HLA-DP restricted human T cells reactive with *Dermatophagoides* spp. (house dust mite). *J Allergy Clin Immunol* 1992;90:749–756.
26. McReynolds LA, Kennedy MW, Selkirk ME. The polyprotein allergens of nematodes. *Parasitol Today* 1993;9:403–406.
27. Stewart GA, Thompson PJ, McWilliam AS. Biochemical properties of aeroallergens: contributory factors in allergic sensitization? *Pediatr Allergy Immunol* 1993;4:163–172.
28. Smith AM, Dalton JP, Clough KA, et al. Adult *Schistosoma mansoni* express cathepsin L proteinase activity. *Mol Biochem Parasitol* 1994;57:11–19.
29. Brown A, Burleigh JM, Billett EE, Pritchard DI. An initial characterization of the proteolytic enzymes secreted by the adult stage of the human hookworm *Necator americanus. Parasitology* 1995;110:555–563.
30. Hewitt CRA, Brown AP, Hart BJ, Pritchard DI. A major house dust mite allergen disrupts the IgE network by selectively cleaving CD23. *J Exp Med* 1995;82: 1143–1145.
31. Pritchard DI, Kumar S, Edmonds P. Soluble CD23 levels in a parasitized population from Papua New Guinea. *Parasite Immunol* 1993;15:205–208.
32. Delespesse G, Sarfati M, Wu CY, Fournier S, Letellier M. The low-affinity receptor for IgE. *Immunol Rev* 1992;125:77–97.
33. Chua KY, Stewart GA, Thomas WR, et al. Sequence analysis of cDNA coding for a major house dust mite allergen, Der p 1. *J Exp Med* 1988;167:175–182.
34. Rosenstreich DL, Eggleston P, Kattan M, et al. The role of cockroach allergy and exposure to cockroach allergen in causing morbidity among inner-city children with asthma. *N Engl J Med* 1997;336:1356–1363.
35. Sampson HA. Adverse reactions to foods. In: Middleton E Jr, Reed CE, Ellis EF,

Adkinson NF Jr, Yunginger JW, Busse WW, eds. *Allergy: principles and practice.* vol II. St. Louis: Mosby–Year Book, 1993:1661–1686.

36. Sampson HA. Food allergy. In: Kay AB, ed. *Allergy and allergic diseases.* vol 2. Oxford: Blackwell Science Ltd., 1997:1517–1549.

37. Sampson HA, Mendelson L, Rosen JP. Fatal and near-fatal anaphylactic reactions to food in children and adolescents. *N Engl J Med* 1992;327:380–384.

38. Valentine MD. Anaphylaxis and stinging insect hypersensitivity. *JAMA* 1992; 268:2830–2832.

39. Yunginger JW. Insect allergy. In: Middleton E Jr, Reed CE, Ellis EF, Adkinson NF Jr, Yunginger JW, Busse WW, eds. *Allergy: principles and practice.* vol II. St. Louis: Mosby–Year Book, 1993:1511–1524.

40. Adkinson NF Jr. New developments in the assessment of sensitivity in beta lactam antibiotics. In: Postgraduate Education Course and Asthma Consultants Course Syllabus, 48th Annual Meeting, Orlando, Florida, 1992.

41. Pradal M, Vervloet D. Drug reactions. In: Kay AB, ed. *allergy and allergic diseases.* vol 2. Oxford: Blackwell Science Ltd., 1997:1671–1692.

42. Delage C, Irey NS. Anaphylactic deaths: a clinicopathologic study of 43 cases. *J Forensic Sci* 1972;17:215–218.

43. Prausnitz C, Küstner H. Studine uber die Ueberemfindlichkeil. *Zentralbl Bakteriol* 1921;86:160–169.

44. Ishizaka K, Ishizaka T, Hombrook MM. Physico-chemical properties of human reaginic antibody IV. Presence of a unique immunoglobulin as a carrier of reaginic activity. *J Immunol* 1966;97:75–85.

45. Johansson SGO, Bennich H. Immunochemical studies of an atypical (myeloma) immunoglobulin. *Immunology* 1967,13.381–394.

46. Waldmann TA. Disorders of immunoglobulin metabolism. *N Engl J Med* 1969; 281:1170–1177.

47. Tada T, Okumura K, Platteau B, Beckers A, Bazin H. Half lives of two types of rat homocytotropic antibodies in circulation and in the skin. *Int Arch Allergy Appl Immunol* 1975;48:116–131.

48. Ownby DR. Clinical significance of IgE. In: Middleton EJ, Reed CE, Ellis EF, Adkinson NF Jr, Yuninger JW, Busse WW, eds. *Allergy: principles and practice* vol I. St. Louis: Mosby–Year Book, 1993:1059–1076.

49. Merrett TG. Quantification of IgE both as total immunoglobulin and as allergenspecific antibody. In: Kay AB, ed. *Allergy and allergic diseases.* vol 2. Oxford: Blackwell Science Ltd., 1997:1012–1034.

50. Constant SL, Bottomly K. Induction of TH1 and TH2 CD4+ T cells: the alternative approaches. *Annu Rev Immunol* 1997;15:297–322.

51. Coffman RL, von der Weid T. Multiple pathways for the initiation of T helper 2 (Th2) responses. *J Exp Med* 1997;185:373–375.

52. Chen YH, Chiu NM, Mandal M, Wang N, Wang CR. Impaired Nk1(+) T cell development and early IL-4 production in CD1-deficient mice. *Immunity* 1997; 6:459–467.

53. Mendiratta SK, Martin WD, Hong S, Boesteanu A, Joyce S, Vankaer L. CD1d1 mutant mice are deficient in natural T cells that promptly produce IL-4. *Immunity* 1997;6:469–477.

54. Smiley ST, Kaplan MH, Grusby MJ. Immunoglobulin E production in the absence of interleukin-4-secreting CD1-dependent cells. *Science* 1997;275:977–979.

55. Brown DR, Fowell DJ, Corry DB, et al. Beta 2 microglobulin-dependent Nk1.1(+) T cells are not essential for T helper cell 2 immune responses. *J Exp Med* 1996;184:1295–1304.

56. Sabin EA, Kopf MA, Pearce EJ. Schistosoma mansoni egg-induced early IL-4 production is dependent upon IL-5 and eosinophils. *J Immunol* 1996;184:1871–1878.

57. Paul WE, Seder RA, Plaut M. Lymphokine and cytokine production by FcεRI+ cells. *Adv Immunol* 1993;53:1–29.

58. Rincon M, Anguita J, Nakamura T, Fikrig E, Flavell RA. Interleukin (IL)-6 directs the differentiation of IL-4-producing CD4+ T cells. *J Exp Med* 1997;185: 461–469.

59. Greenwald RJ, Lu P, Halvorson MJ, et al. Effects of blocking B7-1 and B7-2 interactions during a type 2 in vivo immune response. *J Immunol* 1997;158:4088–4096.

60. Saxon A, Diaz-Sanchez D, Zhang K. Regulation of the expression of distinct human secreted IgE proteins produced by alternative RNA splicing. *Biochem Soc Trans* 1997;25:383–387.

61. Coffman RL, Debman DA, Rothman P. Mechanism and regulation of immunoglobulin isotype switching. *Adv Immunol* 1993;54:229–270.

62. Paul WE. Interleukin-4: a prototypic immunoregulatory lymphokine. *Blood* 1991,77 1859–1870.

63. Snapper CM, Paul WE. Interferon-γ and B cell stimulatory factor-1 reciprocally regulate Ig isotype production. *Science* 1987;236:944–947.

64. Coffman RL, Carty JA. A T cell activity that enhances polyclonal IgE production and inhibition by interferon-γ. *J Immunol* 1986;136:949–954.

65. Coffman RL, Ohara J, Bond MW, Carty J, Jlotnik A, Paul WE. B cell stimulatory factor-1 enhances the IgE response of lipopolysaccharide-activated B cells. *J Immunol* 1986;136:4538–4541.

66. Pene J, Rousset F, Briere F, et al. IgE production by normal human lymphocytes is induced by interleukin 4 and suppressed by interferons γ and α and prostaglandin E2. *Proc Natl Acad Sci USA* 1988;85:6880–6884.

67. Del Prete G, Maggi E, Parronchi P, et al. IL-4 is an essential factor for the IgE synthesis induced in vitro by human T cell clones and their supernatants. *J Immunol* 1988;140:4193–4198.

68. Tepper RI, Levinson DA, Stanger BZ, Campos-Torres J, Abbas AK, Leder P. IL-4 induces allergic-like inflammatory disease and alters T cell development in transgenic mice. *Cell* 1990;62:457–467.

69. Finkelman FD, Urban JFJ, Beckmann MP, Schooley KA, Holmes JM, Katona IM. Regulation of murine in vivo IgG and IgE responses by a monoclonal anti-IL-4 receptor antibody. *Int Immunol* 1991;3:599–607.

70. Finkelman FD, Katona IM, Urban JFJ, Snapper CM, Ohara J, Paul WE. Suppression of in vivo polyclonal IgE responses by monoclonal antibody to the lymphokine B-cell stimulatory factor 1. *Proc Natl Acad Sci USA* 1986;83: 9675–9678.

71. Kopf M, Gros GL, Bachmann M, Lamers MC, Bluethmann H, Kohler G. Disruption of the murine IL-4 gene blocks Th2 cytokine responses. *Nature* 1993; 362:245–248.

72. Kuhn R, Rajewsky K, Muller W. Generation and analysis of interleukin-4 deficient mice. *Science* 1991;254:707–710.

73. Morawetz RA, Gabriele L, Rizzo LV, et al. Interleukin (IL)-4-independent immunoglobulin class switch to immunoglobulin (Ig)E in the mouse. *J Exp Med* 1996;184:1651–1661.

74. Noben-Trauth N, Kropf P, Muller I. Susceptibility to *Leishmania major* infection in interleukin-4-deficient mice. *Science* 1996;271:987–990.

75. von der Weid T, Kopf M, Kohler G, Langhorne J. The immune response to *Plasmodium chabaudi* malaria in interleukin-4-deficient mice. *Eur J Immunol* 1994; 24:2285–2293.

76. Delphin S, Stavnezer J. Characterization of an interleukin 4 (IL-4) responsive region in the immunoglobulin heavy chain germline ε promoter: regulation by NF-IL-4, a C/EBP family member and NF κB/p50. *J Exp Med* 1995,181: 181–192.

77. Thienes CP, De Monte L, Monticelli S, Busslinger M, Gould HJ, Vercelli D. The transcription factor B cell-specific activator protein (BSAP) enhances both IL-4- and CD40-mediated activation of the human ε germline promoter. *J Immunol* 1997;158:5874–5882.

78. Takeda K, Tanaka T, Shi W, et al. Essential role of Stat6 in IL-4 signalling. *Nature* 1996;380:627–630.

79. Shimoda K, van Deursen J, Sangster MY, et al. Lack of IL-4-induced Th2 response and IgE class switching in mice with disrupted Stat6 gene. *Nature* 1996;380:630–633.

80. Kaplan MH, Schindler U, Smiley ST, Grusby MJ. Stat6 is required for mediating responses to IL-4 and for the development of Th2 cells. *Immunity* 1996;4: 313–319.

81. Achatz G, Nitschke L, Lamers MC. Effect of transmembrane and cytoplasmic domains of IgE on the IgE response. *Science* 1997;276:409–411.

82. Punnonen J, Aversa G, Cocks BG, et al. Interleukin 13 induces interleukin 4-independent IgG4 and IgE synthesis and CD23 expression by human B cells. *Proc Natl Acad Sci USA* 1993;90:3730–3734.

83. de Vries JE. Molecular and biological characteristics of interleukin-13. *Chem Immunol* 1996;63:204–218.

84. Burd PR, Thompson WC, Max EE, Mills FC. Activated mast cells produce interleukin 13. *J Exp Med* 1995;181:1373–1380.

85. Gibbs BF, Haas H, Falcone FH, et al. Purified human peripheral blood basophils release interleukin-13 and preformed interleukin-4 following immunological activation. *Eur J Immunol* 1996;26:2493–2498.

86. Li HM, Sim TC, Alam R. IL-13 released and localized in human basophils. *J Immunol* 1996;156:4833–4838.

87. Plaut M, Pierce JH, Watson CJ, Hanley-Hyde J, Nordan RP, Paul WE. Mast cell lines produce lymphokines in response to cross-linkage of FcεRI or to calcium ionophores. *Nature* 1989;339:64–67.

88. Burd PR, Rogers HW, Gordon JR, et al. Interleukin 3-dependent and -independent mast cells stimulated with IgE and antigen express multiple cytokines. *J Exp Med* 1989;170:245–257.

89. Bradding P, Feather IH, Howarth PH, et al. Interleukin 4 is localized to and released by human mast cells. *J Exp Med* 1992;176:1381–1386.

90. Seder RA, Paul WE, Dvorak AM, et al. Mouse splenic and bone marrow cell populations that express high-affinity Fc epsilon receptors and produce interleukin 4 are highly enriched in basophils. *Proc Natl Acad Sci USA* 1991;88: 2835–2839.

91. Brunner T, Heusser CH, Dahinden CA. Human peripheral blood basophils primed by interleukin 3 (IL-3) produce IL-4 in response to immunoglobulin E receptor stimulation. *J Exp Med* 1993;177:605–611.

92. Arock M, Merle-Beral H, Dugas B, et al. IL-4 release by human leukemic and activated normal basophils. *J Immunol* 1993;151:1441–1447.

93. Jaffe JS, Raible DG, Post TJ, et al. Human lung mast cell activation leads to IL-13 mRNA expression and protein release. *Am J Respir Cell Mol Biol* 1996;15: 473–481.

94. Pawankar R, Okuda M, Yssel H, Okumura K, Ra C. Nasal mast cells in perennial allergic rhinitics exhibit increased expression of the FcεRI, CD40L, IL-4, and IL-13, and can induce IgE synthesis in B cells. *J Clin Invest* 1997;99: 1492–1499.

95. Yamaguchi M, Sayama K, Yano K, et al. IgE enhances FcεRI expression and IgE-dependent release of IL-13 from human umbilical cord blood-derived mast cells: synergistic effect of IL-4 and IgE on human mast cell FcεRI expression. 1997 (submitted).

96. Callard RE, Matthews DJ, Hibbert L. IL-4 and IL-13 receptors: are they one and the same? *Immunol Today* 1996;17:108–110.

97. Worm M, Henz BM. Molecular regulation of human IgE synthesis. *J Mol Med* 1997;75:440–447.

98. Kimata H, Yoshida A, Ishioka C, Fujimoto M, Lindley I, Furusho K. RANTES

and macrophage inflammatory protein 1 alpha selectively enhance immunoglobulin (IgE) and IgG4 production by human B cells. *J Exp Med* 1996;183: 2397–2402.

99. Thyphronitis G, Tsokos GC, June CH, Levine AD, Finkelman FD. IgE secretion by Epstein-Barr virus-infected purified human lymphocytes is stimulated by interleukin 4 and suppressed by interferon-γ. *Proc Natl Acad Sci USA* 1989;86: 5580–5584.

100. Gascan H, Gauchat JF, Aversa G, van Vlasselaer P, de Vries JE. Anti-CD40 monoclonal antibodies or CD4+ T cell clones and IL-4 induce IgG4 and IgE switching in purified human B cells via different signaling pathways. *J Immunol* 1991; 147:8–13.

101. Banchereau J, Bazan F, Blanchard D, et al. The CD40 antigen and its ligand. *Annu Rev Immunol* 1994;12:881–922.

102. Foy TM, Aruffo A, Bajorath J, Buhlmann JE, Noelle RJ. Immune regulation by CD40 and its ligand gp49. *Annu Rev Immunol* 1996;14:591–617.

103. Jabara HH, Fu SM, Geha RH, Vercelli D. CD40 and IgE: synergism between anti-CD40 monoclonal antibody and interleukin-4 in the induction of IgE synthesis by highly purified human B-cells. *J Exp Med* 1990;72:1861–1864.

104. Armitage RJ, Fanslow WC, Strockbine L, et al. Molecular and biological characterization of a murine ligand for CD40. *Nature* 1992;357:80–82.

105. Xu J, Foy TM, Laman JD, et al. Mice deficient for the CD40 ligand. *Immunity* 1994;1:423–431.

106. Renshaw BR, Fanslow WC, Armitage RJ, et al. Humoral immune responses in CD40 ligand-deficient mice. *J Exp Med* 1994;180:1889–1900.

107. Kawabe T, Naka T, Yoshida K, et al. The immune response in CD40 deficient mice: impaired immunoglobulin class switching and germinal center formation. *Immunity* 1994;1:167–78.

108. Castigli E, Alt FW, Davidson L, et al. CD40-deficient mice generated by recombination-activating gene-2-deficient blastocyst complementation. *Proc Natl Acad Sci USA* 1994;91:12135–12139.

109. Gauchat JF, Henchoz S, Fattah D, et al. CD40 ligand is functionally expressed on human eosinophils. *Eur J Immunol* 1995;25:863.

110. Gauchat JF, Henchoz S, Mazzei G, et al. Induction of human IgE synthesis in B cells by mast cells and basophils. *Nature* 1993;365:340–343.

111. Okayama Y, Petit-Frere C, Kassel O, et al. IgE-dependent expression of mRNA for IL-4 and IL-5 in human lung mast cells. *J Immunol* 1995;155:1796–1808.

112. Jaffe JS, Glaum MC, Raible DG, et al. Human lung mast cell IL-5 gene and protein expression: temporal analysis of upregulation following IgE-mediated activation. *Am J Respir Cell Mol Biol* 1995;13:665–675.

113. Costa JJ, Church MK, Galli SJ. Mast cell cytokines in allergic inflammation. In: Holgate ST, Busse W, eds. *Inflammatory mechanisms in asthma.* vol 199. New York: Marcel Dekker Inc, 1997:111–127.

114. Ha TY, Reed ND, Crowle PK. Immune response potential of mast cell-deficient W/W^v mice. *Int Arch Allergy Appl Immunol* 1986;80:85–94.

115. Takeishi T, Martin TR, Katona IM, Finkelman FD, Galli SJ. Differences in the expression of the cardiopulmonary alterations associated with anti-immunoglobulin E-induced or active anaphylaxis in mast cell-deficient and normal mice. Mast cells are not required for the cardiopulmonary changes associated with certain fatal anaphylactic responses. *J Clin Invest* 1991;88:598–608.

116. Sutton BJ, Gould HJ. IgE and IgE receptors. In: Kay AB, ed. *Allergy and allergic diseases.* vol 1. Oxford: Blackwell Science Ltd., 1997:81–95.

117. Sutton BJ, Gould HJ. The human IgE network. *Nature* 1993;366:421–428.

118. Bonnefoy J-Y, Lecoanet-Henchoz S, Aubry J-P, Gauchat J-F, Graber P. CD23 and B-cell activation. *Curr Opin Immunol* 1995;7:355–359.

119. Williams J, Johnson S, Mascali JJ, Smith H, Rosenwasser LJ, Borish L. Regulation of low affinity IgE receptor (CD23) expression on mononuclear phagocytes in normal and asthmatic subjects. *J Immunol* 1992;149:2823–2829.

120. Gordon J. B-cell signalling via the C-type lectins CD23 and CD72. *Immunol Today* 1994;15:411–417.

121. Cho SW, Kilmon MA, Studer EJ, Vanderputten H, Conrad DH. B cell activation and Ig, especially IgE, production is inhibited by high CD23 levels in vivo and in vitro. *Cell Immunol* 1997;180:36–46.

122. Texido G, Eibel H, Le Gros G, Van der Putten H. Transgene CD23 expression on lymphoid cells modulates IgE and IgG1 responses. *J Immunol* 1994;153: 3028–3042.

123. Yu P, Kosco-Vilbois M, Richards M, Kohler G, Lamers MC. Negative feedback regulation of IgE synthesis by murine CD23. *Nature* 1994;369:753–756.

124. Fujiwara H, Kikutani H, Suematsu S, et al. The absence of IgE antibody-mediated augmentation of immune responses in CD23-deficient mice. *Proc Natl Acad Sci USA* 1994;91:6835–6839.

125. Stief A, Texido G, Sansig G, Eibel H, Le Gros G, Van der Putten H. Mice deficient in CD23 reveal its modulatory role in IgE production but no role in T and B cell development. *J Immunol* 1994;152:3378–3390.

126. Bartlett WC, Conrad DH. Murine soluble FcεRII: a molecule in search of a function. *Res Immunol* 1992;143:431–436.

127. Sarfati M, Delespesse G. Possible role of human lymphocyte receptor for IgE (CD23) or its soluble fragments in the in vitro synthesis of human IgE. *J Immunol* 1988;141:2195–2199.

128. Sherr E, Macy E, Kimata H, Gilly M, Saxon A. Binding the low affinity FcεR on B cells suppresses ongoing human IgE synthesis. *J Immunol* 1989;142:481–489.

129. Flores-Romo L, Shields J, Humbert Y, et al. Inhibition of an in vivo antigen-specific IgE response by antibodies to CD23. *Science* 1993;261:1038–1041.

130. Aubry J-P, Pochon S, Graber P, Jansen KU, Bonnefoy J-Y. CD21 is a ligand for CD23 and regulates IgE production. *Nature* 1992;358:505–507.

131. Burrows B, Martinez ED, Halonen M, Barbee RA, Cline MG. Association of asthma with serum IgE levels and skin-test reactivity to allergens. *N Engl J Med* 1989;320:271–277.

132. Bazaral M, Orgel HA, Hamburger RN. Genetics of IgE and allergy: serum IgE levels in twins. *J Allergy Clin Immunol* 1974;54:288–304.

133. Blumenthal MN, Bonini S. Immunogenetics of specific immune responses to allergens in twins and families. In: Blumenthal MN, Marsh DG, eds. *Genetic and environmental factors in clinical allergy.* Minneapolis: University of Minnesota Press, 1990:20–31.

134. Ruffilli A, Bonini S. Susceptibility genes for allergy and asthma. *Allergy* 1997; 52:256–273.

135. Marsh DG, Neely JD, Breazeale DR, et al. Linkage analysis of IL-4 and other chromosome 5q31.1 markers and total serum immunoglobulin E concentrations. *Science* 1994;264:1152–1155.

136. Meyers DA, Postma DS, Panhuysen CIM, et al. Evidence for a locus regulating total serum IgE levels mapping to chromosome 5. *Genomics* 1994;23:464–470.

137. Rosenwasser LJ. Genetics of atopy and asthma–promoter-based candidate gene studies for IL-4. *Int Arch Allergy Immunol* 1997;113:61–64.

138. Marsh DG. Mapping the genes for IgE production and allergy. In: Sehon A, HayGlass KT, Kraft D, eds. *New horizons in allergy immunotherapy.* New York: Plenum Press, 1996:43–53.

139. Huang S, Marsh DG. Immunogenetics of allergic disease. In: Middleton E Jr, Reed CE, Ellis EF, Adkinson NF Jr, Yunginger JW, Busse WW, eds. *Allergy: principles and practice.* vol 1. St. Louis: Mosby–Year Book, 1993:60–72.

140. Cookson WOCM, Sharp PA, Faux JA, Hopkin JM. Linkage between immunoglobulin E responses underlying asthma and rhinitis and chromosome 11q. *Lancet* 1989;i:1292–1295.

141. Cookson WOCM, Young RP, Sandford AJ, et al. Maternal inheritance of atopic, IgE responsiveness on chromosome 11q. *Lancet* 1992;340:381–384.

142. Sandford AJ, Shirakawa T, Moffatt MF, et al. Localisation of atopy and β-subunit of high-affinity IgE receptor (FcεRI) on chromosome 11q. *Lancet* 1993;341: 332–334.

143. Shirakawa T, Li A, Dubowitz M, et al. Association between atopy and variants of the beta subunit of the high-affinity immunoglobulin E receptor. *Nat Genet* 1994;7:125–130.

144. Hopkin JM. Genetics of atopy. In: Kay AB, ed. *Allergy and allergic diseases.* vol 2. Oxford: Blackwell Science Ltd., 1997:1187–1195.

145. Barnes KC, Neely JD, Duffy DL, et al. Linkage of asthma and total serum IgE concentration to markers on chromosome 12q: evidence from afro-caribbean and caucasian populations. *Genomics* 1996;37:41–50.

146. Marsh DG, Maestri NE, Freidhoff LR, et al. A genome-wide search for asthma susceptibility loci in ethnically diverse populations. *Nat Genet* 1997;15: 389–392.

147. Daniels SE, Bhattacharyya S, James A, et al. A genome-wide search for quantitative trait loci underlying asthma. *Nature* 1996;383:247–250.

148. Kulczycki A, Metzger H. The interaction of IgE with rat basophilic leukemia cells. II. Quantitative aspects of the binding reaction. *J Exp Med* 1974;140:1676.

149. Ishizaka K, Tomioka H. Mechanisms of passive sensitization. I. Presence of IgE and IgG molecules on human leukocytes. *J Immunol* 1970;105:1459–1467.

150. Bieber T. FcεRI-expressing antigen-presenting cells: new players in the atopic game. *Immunol Today* 1997;18:311–313.

151. Maurer D, Fiebiger E, Reininger B, et al. Expression of functional high affinity immunoglobulin E receptors (FcεRI) on monocytes of atopic individuals. *J Exp Med* 1994;179:745–750.

152. Maurer D, Fiebiger E, Ebmer C, et al. Peripheral blood dendritic cells express FcεRI as a complex composed of FcεRIα- and FcεRIγ-chains, and can use this receptor for IgE-mediated allergen presentation. *J Immunol* 1996;157:607–616.

153. Wollenberg A, Kraft S, Hanau D, Bieber T. Immunomorphological and ultrastructural characterization of Langerhans cells and a novel, inflammatory dendritic epidermal cell (IDEC) population in lesional skin of atopic eczema. *J Invest Dermatol* 1996;106:446–453.

154. Wang B, Rieger A, Kilgus O, et al. Epidermal Langerhans cells from normal human skin bind monomeric IgE via FcεRI. *J Exp Med* 1992;175:1353–1365.

155. Bieber T, de la Salle H, Wollenberg A, et al. Human epidermal Langerhans cells express the high affinity receptor for immunoglobulin E (FcεRI). *J Exp Med* 1992;175:1285–1290.

156. Sihra BS, Kon OM, Grant JA, Kay AB. Expression of high-affinity IgE receptors (Fc epsilon RI) on peripheral blood basophils, monocytes, and eosinophils in atopic and nonatopic subjects: relationship to total serum IgE concentrations. *J Allergy Clin Immunol* 1997;99:699–706.

157. Gounni AS, Lamkhloued B, Ochiai K, et al. High-affinity IgE receptor on eosinophils is involved in defence against parasites. *Nature* 1994;367:183–473.

158. Dombrowicz D, Flamand V, Brigman KK, Koller BH, Kinet J-P. Abolition of anaphylaxis by targeted disruption of the high affinity immunoglobulin E receptor alpha chain gene. *Cell* 1993;75:969–976.

160. Miyajima I, Dombrowicz D, Martin TR, Ravetch JV, Kinet JP, Galli SJ. Systemic anaphylaxis in the mouse can be mediated largely through IgG1 and FcγRIII. Assessment of the cardiopulmonary changes, mast cell degranulation, and death associated with active or IgG1-dependent passive anaphylaxis. *J Clin Invest* 1997;99:901–914.

161. Dombrowicz D, Flamand V, Miyajima I, Ravetch JV, Galli SJ, Kinet JP. Absence of FcεRI α chain results in upregulation of FcγRIII-dependent mast cell degranulation and anaphylaxis. Evidence of competition between FcεRI and FcγRIII for limiting amounts of FcR β and γ chains. *J Clin Invest* 1997;99:915–925.

162. Ra C, Jouvin M-HE, Kinet J-P. Complete structure of the mouse mast cell receptor for IgE (FcεRI) and surface expression of chimeric receptors (rat-mouse-human) on transfected cells. *J Biol Chem* 1989;264:15323–15327.

163. Kinet J-P. The γ-ζ dimers of Fc receptors as connectors to signal transduction. *Curr Opin Immunol* 1992;4:43–48.

164. Blank U, Ra C, Miller L, White K, Metzger H, Kinet J-P. Complete structure and expression in transfected cells of the high affinity IgE receptor. *Nature* 1989; 337:187–189.

165. Miller L, Blank U, Metzger H, Kinet J-P. Expression of high-affinity binding of human immunoglobulin E by transfected cells. *Science* 1989;244:334–337.

166. Keegan AD, Paul WE. Multichain immune recognition receptors: similarities in structure and signaling pathways. *Immunol Today* 1992;13:63–68.

167. Cambier JC. Antigen and Fc receptor signaling: the awesome power of the immunoreceptor tyrosine-based activation motif (ITAM). *J Immunol* 1995;155: 3281–3285.

168. Daeron M. Fc receptor biology. *Annu Rev Immunol* 1997;15:203–234.

169. Takizawa F, Adamezewski M, Kinet J-P. Identification of the low affinity receptor for immunoglobulin E on mouse mast cells and macrophages, as Fc gamma RII and Fc gamma RIII. *J Exp Med* 1992;176:469–476.

170. Metzger H. Transmembrane signaling: the joy of aggregation. *J Immunol* 1992; 149:1477–1487.

171. Dembo M, Goldstein B, Sobotka AK, Lichtenstein LM. Degranulation of human basophils: quantitative analysis of histamine release and desensitization due to a bivalent penicilloyl hapten. *J Immunol* 1979;123:1864–1872.

172. Sterk AR, Ishizaka T. Binding properties of IgE receptors on normal mouse mast cells. *J Immunol* 1982;128:838–843.

173. Malveaux FJ, Conroy MC, Adkinson NF, Lichtenstein LM. IgE receptors on human basophils: relationship to serum IgE concentration. *J Clin Invest* 1978;62: 176–181.

174. Jouvin M-H, Numerof RP, Kinet J-P. Signal transduction through the conserved motifs of the high affinity IgE receptor FcεRI. *Semin Immunol* 1995;1:29–35.

175. Lin S, Cicaia C, Scharenberg AM, Kinet J-P. The FcεRIβ subunit functions as an amplifier of FcεRIγ-mediated cell activation signals. *Cell* 1996;85:985–995.

176. Vonakis BM, Chen H, Haleem-Smith H, Metzger H. The unique domain as the site on lyn kinase for its constitutive association with the high affinity receptor for IgE. *J Biol Chem* 1997;272:24072–24080.

177. Choi OH, Kim J-H, Kinet J-P. Calcium mobilization via sphingosine kinase in signalling by the FcεRI antigen receptor. *Nature* 1996;380:634–636.

178. Tsai M, Chen R-H, Tam S-Y, Blenis J, Galli SJ. Activation of MAP kinases, pp90rsk and pp70-S6 kinases in mouse mast cells by signaling through the c-kit receptor tyrosine kinase or FcεRI: rapamycin inhibits activation of pp70-S6 kinase and proliferation in mouse mast cells. *Eur J Immunol* 1993;23:3286–3291.

179. Hirasawa N, Scharenberg A, Yamamura H, Beaven MA, Kinet J-P. A requirement for Syk in the activation of the MAP kinase/phospholipase A₂ pathway by FcεRI is not shared by a G protein-coupled receptor. *J Biol Chem* 1995;270: 10960–10967.

180. Beaven MA, Baumgartner PA. Downstream signals initiated in mast cells by FcεRI and other receptors. *Curr Opin Immunol* 1996;8:766–772.

181. Bolen JB, Brugge JS. Leukocyte protein tyrosine kinases: potential targets for drug discovery. *Annu Rev Immunol* 1997,15:371–404.

182. Hamawy MM, Mergenhagen SE, Siraganian RP. Protein tyrosine phosphorylation as a mechanism of signalling in mast cells and basophils. *Cell Signal* 1995; 7:535–544.

183. Kawakami Y, Yao L, Miura T, Tsukada S, Witte ON, Kawakami T. Tyrosine phosphorylation and activation of bruton tyrosine kinase upon FcεRI cross-linking. *Mol Cell Biol* 1994;14:5108–5113.

184. Eiseman E, Bolen JB. Engagement of the high-affinity IgE receptor activates src protein-related tyrosine kinases. *Nature* 1992;355:78–80.

185. Penhallow RC, Class K, Sonoda H, Bolen JB, Rowley RB. Temporal activation of nontransmembrane protein-tyrosine kinases following mast cell Fc epsilon RI engagement. *J Biol Chem* 1995;270:23362–23365.

186. Hamawy MM, Mergenhagen SE, Siraganian RP. Tyrosine phosphorylation of pp125FAK by the aggregation of high affinity immunoglobulin E receptors requires cell adherence. *J Biol Chem* 1993;268:6851–6854.

187. Ota Y, Beitz LO, Scharenberg AM, Donovan JA, Kinet J-P, Samelson LE. Characterization of Cbl tyrosine phosphorylation and a Cbl-Syk complex in RBL-2H3 cells. *J Exp Med* 1996;184:1713–1723.

188. Ota Y, Samelson LE. The product of the proto-oncogene c-cbl: a negative regulator of the Syk tyrosine kinase. *Science* 1997;276:418–420.

189. Hamawy MM, Swaim WD, Minoguchi K, de Feijter AW, Mergenhagen SE, Siraganian RP. The aggregation of the high affinity IgE receptor induces tyrosine phosphorylation of paxillin, a focal adhesion protein. *J Immunol* 1994;153: 4655–4662.

190. Berger SA, Mak TW, Paige CJ. Leukocyte common antigen (CD45) is required for immunoglobulin E-mediated degranulation of mast cells. *J Exp Med* 1994;180:471–476.

191. Adamczewski M, Numerof RP, Koretzky GA, Kinet J-P. Regulation by CD45 of the tyrosine phosphorylation of high affinity IgE receptor beta- and gamma-chains. *J Immunol* 1995;154:3047–3055.

192. Jabril-Cuenod B, Zhang C, Scharenberg AM, et al. Syk-dependent phosphorylation of Shc. *J Biol Chem* 1996;271:16268–16272.

193. Turner H, Reif K, Rivera J, Cantrell DA. Regulation of the adapter molecule Grb2 by the Fc epsilon RI in the mast cell line RBL2H3. *J Biol Chem* 1995; 270:9500–9506.

194. Scharenberg AM, Kinet J-P. The emerging field of receptor-mediated inhibitory signaling: SHP or SHIP? *Cell* 1996;87:961–964.

195. Amigorena S, Salamero J, Davoust J, Fridman WH, Bonnerot C. Tyrosine-containing motif that transduces cell activation signals also determines internalization and antigen presentation via type III receptors for IgG. *Nature* 1992;358:337–341.

196. Muta T, Kurosaki T, Misulovin Z, Sanchez M, Nussenzweig MC, Ravetch JV. A 13-amino-acid motif in the cytoplasmic domain of the FcγRIIB modulates B-cell receptor signalling. *Nature* 1994;368:70–73.

197. Vivier E, Daeron M. Immunoreceptor tyrosine-based inhibition motifs. *Immunol Today* 1997;18:286–291.

198. Daeron M, Latour S, Malbec O, et al. The same tyrosine-based inhibition motif, in the intra-cytoplasmic domain of FcγRIIB, regulates negatively BCR-, TCR-, and FcR-dependent cell activation. *Immunity* 1995;3:635–646.

199. Daeron M, Malbec O, Latour S, Arock M, Fridman WH. Regulation of high-affinity IgE receptor-mediated mast cell activation by murine low-affinity IgG receptors. *J Clin Invest* 1995;95:577–585.

200. Takai T, Ono M, Hikida M, Ohmori H, Ravetch JV. Augmented humoral and anaphylactic responses in FcγRII-deficient mice. *Nature* 1996;379:346–349.

201. Katz HR, Austen KF. A newly recognized pathway for the negative regulation of mast cell-dependent hypersensitivity and inflammation mediated by an endogenous cell surface receptor of the gp49 family. *J Immunol* 1997;158:5065–5070.

202. Guthmann MD, Tal M, Pecht I. A new member of the C-type lectin family is a modulator of mast cell secretory response. *Int Arch Allergy Immunol* 1995; 107.82–86.

203. Ono M, Bolland S, Tempst P, Ravetch JV. Role of the inositol phosphatase SHIP in negative regulation of the immune system by the receptor FcγRIIB. *Nature* 1996;383:263–266.

204. Fleming TJ, Donnadieu E, Song CH, Van Laethem F, Galli SJ, Kinet J-P. Negative regulation of FcεRI-mediated degranulation by CD81. *J Exp Med* 1997;186: 1307–1314.

205. Wright MD, Tomlinson MG. The ins and outs of the transmembrane 4 superfamily. *Immunol Today* 1994;15:558–594.

206. Rottem M, Barbieri S, Kinet J-P, Metcalfe DD. Kinetics of the appearance of FcεRI-bearing cells in interleukin-3-dependent mouse bone marrow cultures: correlation with histamine content and mast cell maturation. *Blood* 1992;79:972–980.

207. Lantz CS, Huff TF. Murine KIT⁺ lineage⁻ bone marrow progenitors express FcγRII but do not express FcεRI until mast cell granule formation. *J Immunol* 1995;154:355–362.

208. Kinzer CA, Keegan AD, Paul WE. Identification of FcεRIneg mast cells in mouse bone marrow cultures. Use of a monoclonal anti-p161 antibody. *J Exp Med* 1995;182:575–579.

209. Rodewald H-R, Dessing M, Dvorak AM, Galli SJ. Identification of a committed precursor for the mast cell lineage. *Science* 1996;271:818–822.

210. Conroy MC, Adkinson NF, Lichtenstein LM. Measurement of IgE on human basophils: relation to serum IgE and anti-IgE-induced histamine release. *J Immunol* 1977;118:1317–1321.

211. Stallman PJ, Aalberse RC, Bruhl PC, Van Elven EH. Experiments on the passive sensitization of human basophils, using quantitative immunofluorescence microscopy. *Int Arch Allergy Appl Immunol* 1977;54.364–373.

212. Lantz CS, Yamaguchi M, Oettgen HC, et al. IgE regulates mouse basophil FcεRI expression in vivo. *J Immunol* 1997;158:2517–2521.

213. Yamaguchi M, Lantz CS, Oettgen HC, et al. IgE enhances mouse mast cell FcεRI expression in vitro and in vivo. Evidence for a novel amplification mechanism in IgE-dependent reactions. *J Exp Med* 1997;185:663–672.

214. MacGlashan DW Jr, Bochner BS, Adelman DC, et al. Down-regulation of FcεRI expression on human basophils during in vivo treatment of atopic patients with anti-IgE antibody. *J Immunol* 1997;158:1438–1445.

215. Shaikh N, Rivera J, Hewlett BR, Stead RH, Zhu F-G, Marshall JS. Mast cell FcεRI expression in the rat intestinal mucosa and tongue is enhanced during Nippostrongylus brasiliensis infection and can be up-regulated by in vivo administration of IgE. *J Immunol* 1997;158:3805–3812.

216. Yano K, Yamaguchi M, de Mora F, et al. Production of macrophage inflammatory protein-1α by human mast cells: increased anti-IgE-dependent secretion after IgE-dependent enhancement of mast cell IgE binding ability. *Lab Invest* 1997;77:185–193.

217. Toru H, Ra C, Nonoyama S, Suzuki K, Yata J, Nakahata T. Induction of the high-affinity IgE receptor (FcεRI) on human mast cells by IL-4. *Int Immunol* 1996;8: 1367–1373.

218. Xia H-Z, Du Z, Craig S, et al. Effect of recombinant human IL-4 on tryptase, chymase, and Fcε receptor type I expression in recombinant human stem cell factor-dependent fetal liver-derived human mast cells. *J Immunol* 1997;159: 2911–2921.

219. Banks EM, Coleman JW. A comparative study of peritoneal mast cells from mutant IL-4 deficient and normal mice: evidence that IL-4 is not essential for mast cell development but enhances secretion via control of IgE binding and passive sensitization. *Cytokine* 1996;8:190–196.

220. Conrad DH, Campbell KA, Bartlett WC, Squire CM, Dierks SE. Structure and function of the low affinity IgE receptor. *Adv Exp Med Biol* 1994;347:17–30.

221. Bonnefoy J-Y, Plater-Zyberk C, Lecoanet-Henchoz S, Gauchat J-F, Aubry J-P, Graber P. A new role for CD23 in inflammation. *Immunol Today* 1996;17: 418–420.

222. Lecoanet-Henchoz S, Gauchat J-P, Aubry J-P, et al. CD23 regulates monocyte activation through a novel interaction with the adhesion molecules CD11b-CD18 and CD11c-CD18. *Immunity* 1995;3:119–125.

223. Yokota A, Kikutani H, Tanaka T, et al. Two species of human Fcε receptor II (FcεRII/CD23): tissue-specific and IL-4-specific regulation of gene expression. *Cell* 1988;55:611–618.

224. Pirron U, Schlunck T, Prinz JC, Rieber EP. IgE-dependent antigen focusing by human B lymphocytes is mediated by the low-affinity receptor for IgE. *Eur J Immunol* 1990;20:1547–1551.

225. Mudde GC, Bheekha R, Bruijnzeel-Koomen CA. Consequences of IgE/CD23-mediated antigen presentation in allergy. *Immunol Today* 1995;16:380–383.

226. Kehry MR, Yamashita LC. Low-affinity IgE (CD23) function on mouse B cells: role in IgE dependent antigen focusing. *Proc Natl Acad Sci USA* 1989;86:7556–7560.

227. Costa JJ, Galli SJ. Mast cells and basophils. In: Rich R, Fleisher TA, Schwartz BD, Shearer WT, Strober W, eds. *Clinical immunology: principles and practice.* St. Louis: Mosby–Year Book, 1996:408–430.

228. Schwartz LB, Huff TF. Biology of mast cells and basophils. In: Middleton E, Reed CE, Ellis EF, Adkinson NF, Yunginger JW, Busse WW, eds. *Allergy: principles and practice.* vol I. St. Louis: Mosby–Year Book, 1993:135–168.

229. Valent P, Bettelheim P. The human basophil. *Crit Rev Oncol Hematol* 1990;10:327–352.

230. Lantz CS, Boesiger J, Song CH, et al. Role for interleukin-3 in mast cell and basophil development and in immunity to parasites. *Nature* 1998;392:90–93.

231. Urbina C, Ortiz C, Hurtado I. A new look at basophils in mice. *Int Arch Allergy Appl Immunol* 1981;66:158–160.

232. Dvorak AM, Nabel G, Pyne K, Cantor H, Dvorak HF, Galli SJ. Ultrastructural identification of the mouse basophil. *Blood* 1982;59:1279–1285.

233. Dvorak AM. Basophil and mast cell degranulation and recovery. In: Harris JR, ed. *Blood cell biochemistry.* vol 4. London: Plenum Press, 1991:1–415.

234. Kirshenbaum AS, Goff JP, Kessler SW, Mican JM, Zsebo KM, Metcalfe DD. Effect of IL-3 and stem cell factor on the appearance of human basophils and mast cells from CD34+ pluripotent progenitor cells. *J Immunol* 1992;148:772–777.

235. Galli SJ, Zsebo KM, Geissler EN. The kit ligand, stem cell factor. *Adv Immunol* 1994;55:1–96.

236. Kitamura Y. Heterogeneity of mast cells and phenotypic change between sub-populations. *Annu Rev Immunol* 1989;7:59–76.

237. Zsebo KM, Williams DA, Geissler EN, et al. Stem cell factor (SCF) is encoded at the *Sl* locus of the mouse and is the ligand for the c-*kit* tyrosine kinase receptor. *Cell* 1990;63:213–224.

238. Ando A, Martin TR, Galli SJ. Effects of chronic treatment with the c-*kit* ligand, stem cell factor, on immunoglobulin E-dependent anaphylaxis in mice: genetically mast cell-deficient *Sl/Sl^d* mice acquire anaphylactic responsiveness, but the congenic normal mice do not exhibit augmented responses. *J Clin Invest* 1993;92:1639–1649.

239. Tsai M, Shih L, Newlands GFJ, et al. The rat c-kit ligand, stem cell factor, induces the development of connective tissue-type and mucosal mast cells in vivo. Analysis by anatomical distribution, histochemistry, and protease phenotype. *J Exp Med* 1991;174:125–131.

240. Galli SJ, Iemura A, Garlick DS, Gamba-Vitalo C, Zsebo KM, Andrews RG. Reversible expansion of primate mast cell populations *in vivo* by stem cell factor. *J Clin Invest* 1993;91:148–152.

241. Costa JJ, Demetri GD, Harrist TJ, et al. Recombinant human stem cell factor (Kit ligand) promotes human mast cell and melanocyte hyperplasia and functional activation *in vivo.* *J Exp Med* 1996;183:2681–2686.

242. Galli SJ. New insights into "the riddle of the mast cell": microenvironmental regulation of mast cell development and phenotypic heterogeneity. *Lab Invest* 1990;62:5–33.

243. Stevens RL, Austen KF. Recent advances in the cellular and molecular biology of mast cells. *Immunol Today* 1989;10:381–386.

244. Church MK, Benyon RC, Rees PH, et al. Functional heterogeneity of human mast cells. In: Galli SJ, Austen KF, eds. *Mast cell and basophil differentiation and function in health and disease.* New York: Raven Press, 1989:161–170.

245. Bienenstock J, Befus AD, Denburg JA. Mast cell heterogeneity: basic questions and clinical implications. In: Befus AD, Bienenstock J, Denburg JA, eds. *Mast cell differentiation and heterogeneity.* New York: Raven Press, 1986:391–402.

246. Jarrett EEE, Miller HRP. Production and activities of IgE in helminth infection. *Prog Allergy* 1982;31:178–233.

247. Miller HRP, King SJ, Gibson S, Huntley JF, Newlands GFJ, Woodbury RG. Intestinal mucosal mast cells in normal and parasitized rats. In: Befus AD, Bienenstock J, Denburg JA, eds. *Mast cell differentiation and heterogeneity.* New York: Raven Press, 1986:239–255.

248. Ihle JN, Keller J, Orsozlan S, et al. Biological properties of homogeneous interleukin 3. I. Demonstration of WEHI-3 growth factor activity, mast cell growth factor activity, P cell stimulating factor activity and histamine producing factor activity. *J Immunol* 1983;131:282–287.

249. Lee F, Yokota T, Otsuka T, et al. Isolation and characterization of a mouse interleukin cDNA clone that expresses B cell stimulatory factor 1 activities and T cell and mast cell stimulating activities. *Proc Natl Acad Sci USA* 1986;83:2061–2065.

250. Hamaguchi Y, Kanakura Y, Fujita J, et al. Interleukin 4 as an essential factor for in vitro clonal growth of murine connective tissue-type mast cells. *J Exp Med* 1987;165:268–273.

251. Madden KB, Urban JF, Ziltener HJ, Schrader JW, Finkelman FD, Katona IM. Antibodies to IL-3 and IL-4 supress helminth-induced intestinal mastocytosis. *J Immunol* 1991;147:1387–1391.

252. Hültner L, Druez C, Moeller J, et al. Mast cell growth-enhancing activity (MEA) is structurally related and functionally identical to the novel mouse T cell growth factor P40/TCGFIII (interleukin 9). *Eur J Immunol* 1990;20:1413–1416.

253. Hunt JE, Stevens RL. Mouse mast cell proteases. In: Kitamura Y, Yamamoto S, Galli SJ, Greaves MW, eds. *Biological and molecular aspects of mast cell and basophil differentiation and function.* New York: Raven Press, 1995:149–160.

254. Lutzelschwab C, Pejler G, Aveskogh M, Hellman L. Secretory granule proteases in rat mast cells. Cloning of 10 different serine proteases and a carboxypeptidase A from various rat mast cell populations. *J Exp Med* 1997;185:13–29.

255. Miller HRP, Huntley JF, Newlands GFJ. Mast cell chymases in helminthosis and hypersensitivity. In: Caughey GH, ed. *Mast cell proteases in immunology and biology.* New York: Marcel Dekker Inc, 1995:203–235.

256. Schwartz LB. Heterogeneity of human mast cells. In: Kaliner MA, Metcalfe DD, eds. *The mast cell in health and disease.* New York: Marcel Dekker Inc, 1993:219–236.

257. Murakami M, Austen KF, Arm JP. Cytokine regulation of arachidonic acid metabolism in mast cells. In: Kitamura Y, Yamamoto S, Galli SJ, Greaves MW, eds. *Biological and molecular aspects of mast cell and basophil differentiation and function.* New York: Raven Press, Ltd., 1995:25.

258. Samet JM, Fonteh AN, Galli SJ, Tsai M, Fasano MB, Chilton FH. Alterations in arachidonic acid metabolism in mouse mast cells induced to undergo maturation in vitro in response to stem cell factor. *J Allergy Clin Immunol* 1996;97:1329–1341.

259. Bradding P, Okayama Y, Howarth PH, Church MK, Holgate ST. Heterogeneity of human mast cells based on cytokine content. *J Immunol* 1995;155:297–307.

260. Gurish MF, Ghildyal N, McNeil HP, Austen KF, Gillis S, Stevens RL. Differential expression of secretory granule proteases in mouse mast cells exposed to interleukin 3 and c-kit ligand. *J Exp Med* 1992;175:1003–1012.

261. Galli SJ, Lichtenstein LM. Biology of mast cells and basophils. In: Middleton E, Reed CE, Ellis EF, Adkinson JNF, Yunginger JW, eds. *Allergy: principles and practice.* St. Louis: Mosby–Year Book, 1988:106–134.

262. Gordon JR, Burd PR, Galli SJ. Mast cells as a source of multifunctional cytokines. *Immunol Today* 1990;11:458–464.

263. Holgate ST, Robinson C, Church MK. Mediators of immediate hypersensitivity. In: Middleton E, Reed CE, Ellis EF, Adkinson NF, Yunginger JW, Busse WW, eds. *Allergy: principles and practice.* St. Louis: Mosby–Year Book, 1993:267–301.

264. Galli SJ, Costa JJ. Mast cell-leukocyte cytokine cascades in allergic inflammation. *Allergy* 1995;50:851–862.

265. Valone FH, Boggs JM, Goetzl EJ. Lipid mediators of hypersensitivity and inflammation. In: Middleton E Jr, Reed CE, Ellis EF, Adkinson NF, Yunginger JW, Busse WW, eds. *Allergy: principles and practice.* St. Louis: Mosby–Year Book, 1993:302–319.

266. Young JD-E, Liu C, Butler G, Cohn ZA, Galli SJ. Identification, purification, and characterization of a mast cell-associated cytolytic factor related to tumor necrosis factor. *Proc Natl Acad Sci USA* 1987;84:9175–9179.

267. Gordon JR, Galli SJ. Mast cells as a source of both preformed and immunologically inducible TNF-alpha/cachectin. *Nature* 1990;346:274–276.

268. Gordon JR, Galli SJ. Release of both preformed and newly synthesized tumor necrosis factor alpha (TNF-alpha)/cachectin by mouse mast cells stimulated by the FcεRI. A mechanism for the sustained action of mast cell-derived TNF-alpha during IgE-dependent biological responses. *J Exp Med* 1991;174:103–107.

269. Yamatodani A, Maeyama K, Watanabe T, Wada H, Kitamura Y. Tissue distribution of histamine in a mutant mouse deficient in mast cells: clear evidence for the presence of non-mast-cell histamine. *Biochem Pharmacol* 1982;31:305–309.

270. Murakami M, Matsumoto R, Urade Y, Austen KF, Arm JP. c-Kit ligand mediates increased expression of cytosolic phospholipase A2, prostaglandin endoperoxide synthase-1, and hematopoietic prostaglandin D2 synthase and increased IgE-dependent prostaglandin D2 generation in immature mouse mast cells. *J Biol Chem* 1995;270:3239–3246.

271. Bochner BS, Schleimer RP. The role of adhesion molecules in human eosinophil and basophil recruitment. *J Allergy Clin Immunol* 1994;94:427–438.

272. Bevilacqua MP. Endothelial-leukocyte adhesion molecules. *Annu Rev Immunol* 1993;11:767–804.

273. Galli SJ. New concepts about the mast cell. *N Engl J Med* 1993;328:257–265.

274. Wershil BK, Wang Z, Gordon JR, Galli SJ. Recruitment of neutrophils during IgE-dependent cutaneous late phase responses in the mouse is mast cell dependent: partial inhibition of the reaction with antiserum against tumor necrosis factor-alpha. *J Clin Invest* 1991;87:446–453.

275. Wershil BK, Furuta GT, Wang Z-S, Galli SJ. Mast cell-dependent neutrophil and mononuclear cell recruitment in immunoglobulin E-induced gastric reactions in mice. *Gastroenterology* 1996;110:1482–1490.

276. Kung TT, Stelts D, Zurcher JA, et al. Mast cells modulate allergic pulmonary eosinophilia in mice. *Am J Respir Cell Mol Biol* 1995;12:404–409.

277. Klein LM, Lavker RM, Matis WL, Murphy GF. Degranulation of human mast cells induces an endothelial antigen central to leukocyte adhesion. *Proc Natl Acad Sci USA* 1989;86:8972–8976.

278. Walsh LJ, Trinchieri G, Waldorf HA, Whitaker D, Murphy GF. Human dermal mast cells contain and release tumor necrosis factor α, which induces endothelial leukocyte adhesion molecule 1. *Proc Natl Acad Sci USA* 1991;88:4220–4224.

279. Boesiger J, Tsai M, Maurer M, et al. Mast cells can secrete VPF/VEGF and exhibit enhanced release after IgE-dependent upregulation of FcεRI expression (submitted).

280. Robinson DS, Durham SR, Kay AB. Cytokines. III. Cytokines in asthma. *Thorax* 1993;148:401–406.

281. Schleimer RP. Glucocorticosteroids. Their mechanisms of action and use in allergic diseases. In: Middleton E Jr, Ellis EF, Adkinson NF Jr, Yunginger JW, Busse WW, eds. *Allergy: principles and practice.* St. Louis: Mosby–Year Book, 1993:893–925.

282. Wershil BK, Furuta GT, Lavigne JA, Choudhury AR, Wang Z-S, Galli SJ. Dexamethasone or cyclosporin A suppresses mast cell-leukocyte cytokine cascades. *J Immunol* 1995;154:1391–1398.

283. MacDonald SM, Rafnar T, Langdon J, Lichtenstein LM. Molecular identification of an IgE-dependent histamine-releasing factor. *Science* 1995;269:688–690.

284. Wershil BK, Tsai M, Geissler EN, Zsebo KM, Galli SJ. The rat c-*kit* ligand, stem cell factor, induces c-*kit* receptor-dependent mouse mast cell activation in vivo. Evidence that signaling through the c-*kit* receptor can induce expression of cellular function. *J Exp Med* 1992;175:245–255.

285. Nakajima K, Hirai K, Yamaguchi M, et al. Stem cell factor has histamine releasing activity in rat connective tissue-type mast cells. *Biochem Biophys Res Commun* 1992;183:1076–1083.

286. Columbo M, Horowitz EM, Botana LM, et al. The human recombinant *c-kit* receptor ligand, rhSCF, induces mediator release from human cutaneous mast cells and enhances IgE-dependent mediator release from both skin mast cells and peripheral blood basophils. *J Immunol* 1992;149:599–608.

287. Coleman JW, Holliday MR, Kimber I, Zsebo KM, Galli SJ. Regulation of mouse peritoneal mast cell secretory function by stem cell factor, IL-3 or IL-4. *J Immunol* 1993;150:556–562.

288. Gagari E, Tsai M, Lantz CS, Fox LG, Galli SJ. Differential release of mast cell interleukin-6 via c-kit. *Blood* 1997;89:2654–2663.

289. Leal-Berumen I, Conlon P, Marshall JS. IL-6 production by rat peritoneal mast cells is not necessarily preceded by histamine release and can be induced by bacterial lipopolysaccharide. *J Immunol* 1994;152:5468–5476.

290. Galli SJ, Dvorak AM, Dvorak HF. Basophils and mast cells: morphologic insights into their biology, secretory patterns, and function. *Prog Allergy* 1984; 34:1–141.

291. Gleich GJ, Adolphson CR. The eosinophilic leukocyte: structure and function. *Adv Immunol* 1986,39.177–253.

292. Gleich GJ, Adolphson CR, Leiferman KM. The biology of the eosinophilic leukocyte. *Annu Rev Med* 1993;44:85–101.

293. Weller PF. The immunobiology of eosinophils. *N Engl J Med* 1991;324: 1110–1118.

294. Weller PF, Dvorak AM. Human eosinophils development, maturation and functional morphology. In: Busse W, Holgate ST, eds. *Asthma and rhinitis.* Boston: Blackwell Scientific, 1994:225–274.

295. Bozza PT, Yu W, Penrose JF, Dvorak AM, Weller PF. Eosinophil lipid bodies: specific, inducible intracellular sites for enhanced eicosanoid formation. *J Exp Med* 1997;186:909–920.

296. Dvorak AM, Dvorak HF, Peters SP, et al. Lipid bodies: cytoplasmic organelles important to arachidonate metabolism in macrophages and mast cells. *J Immunol* 1983;131:2965–2976.

297. Hammel I, Dvorak AM, Peters SP, et al. Differences in the volume distributions of human lung mast cell granules and lipid bodies: evidence that the size of these organelles is regulated by distinct mechanisms. *J Cell Biol* 1985;100:1488–1492.

298. Sanderson CJ. Interleukin-5, eosinophils, and disease. *Blood* 1992;79: 3101–3109.

299. Collins PD, Marleau S, Griffiths-Johnson DA, Jose PJ, Williams TJ. Cooperation between interleukin-5 and the chemokine eotaxin to induce eosinophil accumulation in vivo. *J Exp Med* 1995;182:1169–1174.

300. Weller PF. Lipid, peptide and cytokine mediators elaborated by eosinophils. In: Smith H, Cook M, eds. *Immunopharmacology of eosinophils. The handbook of immunopharmacology.* London: Academic Press, 1993:25–42.

301. Galli SJ, Gordon JR, Wershil BK, et al. Mast cell and eosinophil cytokines in allergy and inflammation. In: Gleich GJ, Kay AB, eds. *Eosinophils: immunological and clinical aspects.* New York: Marcel Dekker Inc, 1994:255–280.

302. Moqbel R, Levi-Schaffer F, Kay AB. Cytokine generation by eosinophils. *J Allergy Clin Immunol* 1994;94:1183–1188.

303. Desreumaux P, Capron M. Eosinophils in allergic reactions. *Curr Opin Immunol* 1996;8:790–795.

304. Kita H. The eosinophil—a cytokine-producing cell. *J Allergy Clin Immunol* 1996;97:889–892.

305. Capron M, Soussi Gounni A, Morita M, et al. Eosinophils: from low- to high-affinity immunoglobulin E receptors. *Allergy* 1995;50:20–23.

306. Humbert M, Grant JA, Taborda-Barata L, et al. High-affinity IgE receptor (FcεRI)-bearing cells in bronchial biopsies from atopic and nonatopic asthma. *Am J Respir Crit Care Med* 1996;153:1931–1937.

307. Abu-Ghazaleh RI, Fujisawa T, Mestecky J, Kyle RA, Gleich GJ. IgA-induced eosinophil degranulation. *J Immunol* 1989;142:2393–2400.

308. Resnick MB, Weller PF. Mechanisms of eosinophil recruitment. *Am J Resp Cell Mol Biol* 1993;8:349–355.

309. Wein M, Sterbinsky SA, Bickel CA, Schleimer RP, Bochner BS. Comparison of human eosinophil and neutrophil ligands for P-selectin: ligands for P-selectin differ from those for E-selectin. *Am J Respir Cell Mol Biol* 1995;12:315–319.

310. Weller PF, Rand TH, Goelz SE, Chi-Rosso G, Lobb RR. Human eosinophil adherence to vascular endothelium mediated by binding to VCAM 1 and ELAM-1. *Proc Natl Acad Sci USA* 1991;88;7430–7433.

311. Bochner BS, Luscinskas FW, Gimbrone MA, et al. Adhesion of human basophils, eosinophils, and neutrophils to interleukin 1-activated human vascular endothelial cells: contributions of endothelial cell adhesion molecules. *J Exp Med* 1991;173:1553–1557.

312. Rott LS, Briskin MJ, Andrew DP, Berg EL, Butcher EC. A fundamental subdivision of circulating lymphocytes defined by adhesion to mucosal cell adhesion molecule-1. *J Immunol* 1996;156:3726–3727.

313. Weg VB, Williams TJ, Lobb RR, Nourshargh S. A monoclonal antibody recognizing very late activation antigen-4 inhibits eosinophil accumulation in vivo. *J Exp Med* 1993;177:561–566.

314. Pretolani M, Ruffie C, Lapa e Silva JR, Joseph D, Lobb RR, Vargaftig BB. Antibody to very late activation antigen 4 prevents antigen-induced bronchial hyperreactivity and cellular infiltration in the guinea pig airways. *J Exp Med* 1994; 180:795–805.

315. Abraham WM, Sielczak MW, Ahmed A, et al. Alpha 4-integrins mediate antigen-induced late bronchial responses and prolonged airway hyperresponsiveness in sheep. *J Clin Invest* 1994;93:776–787.

316. Weller PF, Rand TH, Barrett T, Elovic A, Wong DT, Finberg RW. Accessory cell function of human eosinophils. HLA-DR-dependent, MHC-restricted antigen-presentation and interleukin-α expression. *J Immunol* 1993;150:2554–2562.

317. Sedgwick JB, Quan SF, Calhoun WJ, Busse WW. Effect of interleukin-5 and granulocyte-macrophage colony stimulating factor on in vitro eosinophil function: comparison with airway eosinophils. *J Allergy Clin Immunol* 1995;96: 375–385.

318. Gounni AS, Lamkioued B, Delaporte E, et al. The high-affinity IgE receptor on eosinophils: from allergy to parasites or from parasites to allergy? *J Allergy Clin Immunol* 1994;94:1214–1216.

319. Ohkawara Y, Lim KG, Xing Z, et al. CD40 expression by human peripheral blood eosinophils. *J Clin Invest* 1996;97:1761–1766.

320. Robinson DS, Hamid Q, Bentley A, Ying S, Kay AB, Durham SR. Activation of CD4+ T cells, increased Th2-type cytokine mRNA expression, and eosinophil recruitment in bronchoalveolar lavage after allergen inhalation challenge in atopic asthmatics. *J Allergy Clin Immunol* 1993;92:313–324.

321. Bentley AM, Meng Q, Robinson DS, Hamid Q, Kay AB, Durham SR. Increases in activated T lymphocytes, eosinophils and cytokine messenger RNA for IL-5 and GM-CSF in bronchial biopsies after allergen inhalation challenge in atopic asthmatics. *Am J Respir Cell Mol Biol* 1993;8:35–42.

322. Takeda K, Hamelmann E, Joetham A, et al. Development of eosinophilic airway inflammation and airway hyperresponsiveness in mast cell-deficient mice. *J Exp Med* 1997;186:449–454.

323. Nogami M, Suko M, Okudaira H, et al. Experimental pulmonary eosinophilia in mice by *Ascaris suum* extract. *Am Rev Respir Dis* 1990;141:1289–1295.

324. Brusselle GG, Kips JC, Tavernier JH, et al. Attenuation of allergic airway inflammation in IL-4 deficient mice. *Clin Exp Allergy* 1994;24:73–80.

325. Coyle AJ, Wagner K, Betrand C, Tsuyuki S, Bews J, Heusser C. Central role of immunoglobulin (Ig) E in the induction of lung eosinophil infiltration and T helper 2 cell cytokine production: inhibition by a non-anaphylactogenic anti-IgE antibody. *J Exp Med* 1996;183:1303–1310.

326. Holt PG. Macrophages and dendritic cells in allergic reactions. In: Kay AB, ed. *Allergy and Allergic Diseases.* Vol. 1. Oxford: Blackwell Science Ltd., 1997: 228–243.

327. Rankin JA, Lee TH. Monocytes and macrophages. In: Middleton EJ, Reed CE, Ellis EF, Adkinson NFJ, Yunginger JW, Busse WW, eds. *Allergy. Principles and Practice.* Vol. 1. St. Louis: Mosby—Year Book, Inc., 1993:226–242.

328. Ovary Z. Quantitative studies in passive cutaneous anaphylaxis of the guinea pig. *Int Arch Allergy App Immunol* 1952;3:162–174.

329. Wershil BK, Mekori YA, Murakami T, Galli SJ. ¹²⁵I-fibrin deposition in IgE-dependent immediate hypersensitivity reactions in mouse skin. Demonstration of the role of mast cells using genetically mast cell-deficient mice locally reconstituted with cultured mast cells. *J Immunol* 1987;139:2605–2614.

330. Mekori YA, Galli SJ. [¹²⁵I]fibrin deposition occurs at both early and late intervals of IgE-dependent or contact sensitivity reactions elicited in mouse skin. *J Immunol* 1990;145:3719–3727.

331. Martin TR, Takeishi T, Katz HR, Austen KF, Drazen JM, Galli SJ. Mast cell activation enhances airway responsiveness to methacholine in the mouse. *J Clin Invest* 1993;91:1176–1182.

332. Alter SC, Schwartz LB. Tryptase: An indicator of mast cell-mediated allergic reactions. *Prov Chall Proc* 1989:167–183.

333. Wenzel SE, Fowler AAI, Schwartz LB. Activation of pulmonary mast cells by bronchoalveolar allergen challenge. *In vivo* release of histamine and tryptase in atopic subjects with and without asthma. *Am Rev Respir Dis* 1988;137:1002–1008.

334. Blackley CH. Experimental Researches on the Causes and Nature of Catarrhus Aestivus: Republished by Dawson's of Pall Mall (Balliere, Tindall and Cox, 1873), 1859:p.80.

335. Bentley AM, Kay AB, Durham SR. Human late asthmatic responses. In: Kay AB, ed. *Allergy and Allergic Diseases.* Vol. 2. Oxford: Blackwell Science Ltd., 1997. 1113–1130.

336. Frew AJ. Late-phase skin reactions. In: Kay AB, ed. *Allergy and Allergic Diseases.* Vol. 2. Oxford: Blackwell Science Ltd., 1997:1131–1138.

337. Peebles RS, Toglas A. Late-phase reactions in the nose. In: Kay AB, ed. *Allergy and Allergic Diseases.* Vol. 2. Oxford: Blackwell Science Ltd., 1997:1139–1160.

338. Lemanske RFJ, Kaliner MA. Late phase allergic reactions. In: Middleton EJ, Reed CE, Ellis EF, Adkinson NFJ, Yunginger JW, Busse WW, eds. *Allergy: Principles and Practice.* Vol. 1. St. Louis: Mosby—Year Book, Inc., 1993:320–361.

339. Dolovich J, Denberg J, Kwee YN, Belda T, Blajchman J, Hargreave FE. Does

non-immunologic mast cell mediator release/activation elicit a late cutaneous response? *Ann Allergy* 1983;50:241–244.

340. Schleimer RP. The effects of glucocortocoids on mast cells and basophils. In: Schleimer RP, Claman HN, Oronsky A, eds. *Anti-Inflammatory Steroid Action: Basic and Clinical Aspects.* San Diego: Academic Press, 1989:226.

341. Hatfield SM, Roehm NW. Cyclosporin and FK506 inhibition of murine mast cell cytokine production. *J Pharmacol Exp Ther* 1992;260:680–688.

342. Kaye RE, Fruman DA, Bierer BE, et al. Effects of cyclosporin A and FK506 on Fc epsilon receptor type I-initiated increases in cytokine mRNA in mouse bone marrow-derived progenitor mast cells: resistance to FK506 is associated with a deficiency in FK506-binding protein FKBP12. *Proc Natl Acad Sci USA* 1992; 89:8542–8546.

343. Sigal NH, Dumont FJ. Cyclosporin A, FK-506, and Rapamycin: pharmacologic probes of lymphocyte signal transduction. *Annu Rev Immunol* 1992;10:519–560.

344. Hogg JC. Post-mortem pathology in asthma. In: Kay AB, ed. *Allergy and Allergic Diseases.* Vol. 2. Oxford: Blackwell Science Ltd., 1997:1360–1365.

345. Holgate ST. Aetiology and pathogenesis of asthma. In: Kay AB, ed. *Allergy and Allergic Diseases.* Vol. 2. Oxford: Blackwell Science Ltd., 1997:1366–1378.

346. Barnes PJ. Inhaled glucocorticoids for asthma. *N Engl J Med* 1995;332:868–875.

347. Laitinen LA, Laitinen A, Haabtela T. A comparative study of the effects of an inhaled corticosteroid, budesonide, and of a β2-agonist, terbutaline, on airway inflammation in newly diagnosed asthma. *J Allergy Clin Immunol* 1992;90: 32–42.

348. Trigg CJ, Manolitsas ND, Wang J, et al. Placebo-controlled immunopathologic study of four months of inhaled corticosteroids in asthma. *Am J Respir Crit Care Med* 1994;150:17–22.

349. Kratz A, Campos-Neto A, Hanson MS, Ruddle NH. Chronic inflammation caused by lymphotoxin is lymphoid neogenesis. *J Exp Med* 1996;183: 1461–1472.

350. Koni PA, Sacca R, Lawton P, Browning JL, Ruddle NH, Flavell RA. Distinct roles in lymphoid organogenesis for lymphotoxins alpha and beta revealed in lymphotoxin beta-deficient mice. *Immunity* 1997;6:491–500.

351. Gordon JR, Galli SJ. Promotion of mouse fibroblast collagen gene expression by mast cells stimulated via the FcεRI. Role for mast cell-derived transforming growth factor β and tumor necrosis factor α. *J Exp Med* 1994;180:2027–2037.

352. Kendall JC, Li XH, Galli SJ, Gordon JR. Promotion of mouse fibroblast proliferation by IgE-dependent activation of mouse mast cells: Role for mast cell tumor necrosis factor-alpha and transforming growth factor-beta 1. *J Allergy Clin Immunol* 1997;99:113–123.

353. Echtenacher B, Männel DN, Hültner L. Critical protective role of mast cells in a model of acute septic peritonitis. *Nature* 1996;381:75–77.

354. Malaviya R, Ikeda T, Ross E, Abraham SN. Mast cell modulation of neutrophil influx and bacterial clearance at sites of infection through TNF-α. *Nature* 1996;381:77–80.

355. Prodeus AP, Zhou X, Maurer M, Galli SJ, Carroll MC. Impaired mast cell-dependent natural immunity in complement C3-deficient mice. *Nature* 1997;390: 172–175.

356. Galli SJ, Wershil BK. The two faces of the mast cell. *Nature* 1996;381:21–22.

357. Bell RG. IgE, allergies and helminth parasites: A new perspective on an old conundrum. *Immunol Cell Biol* 1996;74:337–345.

358. Woolhouse ME, Taylor P, Matanhire D, Chandiwana SK. Acquired immunity and epidemiology of *Schistosoma haematobium. Nature* 1991;351:757–759.

359. Reed ND. Function and regulation of mast cells in parasite infections. In: Galli SJ, Austen KF, eds. *Mast Cell and Basophil Differentiation and Function in Health and Disease.* New York: Raven Press, 1989:205–215.

360. Abe T, Nawa Y. Localization of mucosal mast cells in *W/W^v* mice after reconstitution with bone marrow cells or cultured mast cells, and its relation to the protective capacity to *Strongyloides ratti* infection. *Parasite Immunol* 1987;9: 477–485.

361. Abe T, Nawa Y. Reconstitution of mucosal mast cells in *W/W^v* mice by adoptive transfer of bone marrow-derived cultured mast cells and its effects on the protective capacity to *Strongyloides ratti*-infection. *Parasite Immunol* 1987;9:31–38.

362. Nawa Y, Kiyota M, Korenaga M, Kotani M. Defective protective capacity of *W/W^v* mice against *Strongyloides ratti* infection and its reconstitution with bone marrow cells. *Parasite Immunol* 1985;7:429–438.

363. King CL, Xianli J, Malhotra I, Liu S, Mahmoud AAF, Oettgen HC. Mice with a targeted deletion of the IgE gene have increased worm burdens and reduced granulomatous inflammation following primary infection with *Schistosoma mansoni. J Immunol* 1997;158:294–300.

364. Mach N, Lantz CS, Galli SJ, et al. Involvement of interleukin-3 in delayed-type hypersensitivity. *Blood* 1998;91:778–783.

365. Matsuda H, Watanabe N, Kiso Y, et al. Necessity of IgE antibodies and mast cells for manifestation of resistance against larval *Haemaphysalis longicornis* ticks in mice. *J Immunol* 1990;144:259–262.

366. Steeves EB, Allen JR. Basophils in skin reactions of mast cell-deficient mice infested with *Dermacentor variabilis. Int J Parasitol* 1990;20:655–667.

367. Brown SJ, Galli SJ, Gleich GJ, Askenase PW. Ablation of immunity to *Amblyomma americanum* by anti-basophil serum: cooperation between basophils and eosinophils in expression of immunity to ectoparasites (ticks) in guinea pigs. *J Immunol* 1982;129:790–796.

368. Arizono N, Kasugai T, Yamada M, et al. Infection of *Nippostrongylus brasiliensis* induces development of mucosal-type but not connective tissue-type mast cells in genetically mast cell-deficient Ws/Ws rats. *Blood* 1993;81:2572–2578.

369. Newlands GFJ, Miller HRP, MacKellar A, Galli SJ. Stem cell factor contributes to intestinal mucosal mast cell hyperplasia in rats infected with *Nippostrongylus brasiliensis* or *Trichinella spiralis,* but anti-stem cell factor treatment decreases parasite egg production during *N. brasiliensis* infection. *Blood* 1995;86: 1968–1976.

370. Maeda H, Yamagata A, Nishikawa S, et al. Requirement of c-kit for development of intestinal pacemaker system. *Development* 1992;116:369–375.

371. Amiri P, Haak-Frendscho M, Robbins K, McKerrow JH, Stewart T, Jardieu P. Anti-immunoglobulin E treatment decreases worm burden and egg production in *Schistosoma mansoni*-infected normal and interferon γ knockout mice. *J Exp Med* 1994;180:43–51.

372. Wershil BK, Theodos CM, Galli SJ, Titus RG. Mast cells augment lesion size and persistence during experimental *Leishmania major* infection in the mouse. *J Immunol* 1994;152:4563–4571.

373. Sher A, Coffman RL, Hieny S, Cheever AW. Ablation of eosinophil and IgE responses with anti-IL-5 or anti-IL-4 antibodies fails to affect immunity against *Schistosoma mansoni* in the mouse. *J Immunol* 1990;145:3911–3916.

374. Herndon FJ, Kayes SG. Depletion of eosinophils by anti-IL-5 monoclonal antibody treatment of mice infected with *Trichinella spiralis* does not alter parasite burden or immunologic resistance to reinfection. *J Immunol* 1992;149:3642–3647.

375. Negrão-Corrêa D, Adams LS, Bell RG. Intestinal transport and catabolism of IgE: a major blood-independent pathway of IgE dissemination during a *Trichinella spiralis* infection of rats. *J Immunol* 1996;157:4037–4044.

376. Welliver RC, Wong DT, Sun M, Middleton EJ, Vaughan RS, Ogra PL. The development of respiratory syncytial virus-specific IgE and the release of histamine in nasopharyngeal secretions after infection. *N Engl J Med* 1981;305:841–846.

377. Welliver RC, Wong DT, Middleton EJ, Sun M, McCarthy N, Ogra PL. Role of parainfluenza virus-specific IgE in pathogenesis of croup and wheezing subsequent to infection. *J Pediatr* 1982;101:889–896.

378. Pauwels R, Verschraegen G, van der Straeten M. IgE antibodies to bacteria in patients with bronchial asthma. *Allergy* 1980;35:665–669.

379. Abramson JS, Dahl MV, Walsh G, Blumenthal MN, Douglas SD, Quie PG. Anti-staphylococcal IgE in patients with atopic dermatitis. *J Am Acad Dermatol* 1982; 7:105–110.

380. Kjaergard LL, Larsen FO, Norn S, Clementsen P, Skov PS, Permin H. Basophil-bound IgE and serum IgE directed against Haemophilus influenzae and Streptococcus pneumoniae in patients with chronic bronchitis during acute exacerbation. *APMIS* 1996;104:61–67.

381. Turkeltaub PC, Gergen PJ. Prevalence of upper and lower respiratory conditions in the U.S. population by social and environmental factors: data from the second National Health and Nutrition Examination Survey, 1976 to 1980: NHANES II. *Ann Allergy* 1991;67:147–154.

382. Nathan RA, Meltzer EO, Selner JC, Storms W. Prevalence of allergic rhinitis in the United States. *J Allergy Clin Immunol* 1997;99:S808–S814.

383. Evans R. III. Epidemiology and natural history of asthma, allergic rhinitis, and atopic dermatitis. In: Middleton EJ, Reed CE, Ellis EF, Adkinson NFJ, Yuninger W, Busse WW, eds. *Allergy: principles and practice.* vol I. St. Louis: Mosby–Year Book, 1993:1109–1136.

384. Goldstein RA, Paul WE, Metcalfe DD, Busse WW, Reece ER. Asthma. *Ann Intern Med* 1994;121:698–708.

385. Sullivan SD, Weiss KB. Assessing cost-effectiveness in asthma care: building an economic model to study the impact of alternative intervention strategies. *Allergy* 1993;48:146–152.

386. Schultz LF. A genetic epidemiologic study in a population based twin sample. *J Am Acad Dermatol* 1986;15:487–494.

387. Sibbald B. Familial inheritance of asthma and allergy. In: Kay AB, ed. *Allergy and allergic diseases.* vol 2. Oxford: Blackwell Science Ltd., 1997:1177–1186.

388. Hanson B, McGue M, Roitman-Johnson B, Segal NL, Bouchard TJJ, Blumenthal MN. Atopic disease and immunoglobulin E in twins reared apart and together. *Am J Hum Genet* 1991;48:873–879.

389. Zeiger RS. Development and prevention of allergic disease in childhood. In: Middleton EJ, Reed CE, Ellis EF, Adkinson NFJ, Yunginger JW, Busse WW, eds. *Allergy: principles and practice.* vol II. St. Louis: Mosby–Year Book, 1993: 1137–1171.

390. Platts-Mills TAE, Hayden ML, Chapman MD, Wilkins SR. Seasonal variation in dust mite and grass-pollen allergens in dust from the houses of patients with asthma. *J Allergy Clin Immunol* 1987;79:781–791.

391. Platts-Mills TAE, Woodfolk JA. Dust mites and asthma. In: Kay AB, ed. *Allergy and allergic diseases.* vol 2. Oxford: Blackwell Science Ltd., 1997:888–899.

392. Platts-Mills TAE, Carter MC. Asthma and indoor exposure to allergens. *N Engl J Med* 1997;336:1382–1384.

393. Hide D, Warner JA. Prevention of allergy in the fetus and newborn. In: Kay AB, ed. *Allergy and allergic diseases.* vol 2. Oxford: Blackwell Science Ltd., 1997: 1715–1725.

394. Wershil BK, Walker WA. The mucosal barrier, IgE-mediated gastrointestinal events, and eosinophilic gastroenteritis. *Gastroenterol Clin North Am* 1992;21: 387–404.

395. Warner JO. Food allergy in fully breast-fed infants. *Clin Allergy* 1980;10: 133–136.

396. Stuart CA, Twiselton R, Nicholas MK, Hide DW. Passage of cows' milk protein in breast milk. *Clin Allergy* 1984;14:533–535.

397. Bjorksten F, Suoniemi I, Koski V. Neonatal birch-pollen contact and subsequent allergy to birch pollen. *Clin Allergy* 1980;10:585–591.

398. Bjorksten F, Suoniemi I. Time and intensity of first pollen contacts and risk of subsequent pollen allergies. *Acta Med Scand* 1981;209:299–303.

399. Jones AC, Miles EA, Warner JO, Colwell BM, Bryant TN, Warner A. Fetal peripheral blood mononuclear cell proliferative responses to mitogenic and allergenic stimuli during gestation. *Pediatr Allergy Immunol* 1996;7:109–116.

400. Takafuji S, Suzuki S, Muranaka M, Miyamoto T. Influence of environmental factors on IgE production. *Ciba Found Symp* 1989;147:188–204.

401. Takafuji S, Suzuki S, Koizumi K, et al. Enhancing effect of suspended particulate matter on the IgE antibody production in mice. *Int Arch Allergy Appl Immunol* 1989;90:1–7.

402. Takenaka H, Zhang K, Diaz-Sanchez D, Tsien A, Saxon A. Enhanced human IgE production results from exposure to the aromatic hydrocarbons from diesel exhaust: direct effects on B-cell IgE production. *J Allergy Clin Immunol* 1995; 95:103–115.

403. Arshad SH, Stevens M, Hide DW. The effect of genetic and environmental factors on the prevalence of allergic disorders at the age of two years. *Clin Exp Allergy* 1993;23:504–511.

404. Shirakawa T, Enomoto T, Shimazu S-i, Hopkin JM. The inverse association between tuberculin responses and atopic disorder. *Science* 1997;275:77–79.

405. Cookson WOCM, Moffatt MF. Asthma: an epidemic in the absence of infection? *Science* 1997;275:41–42.

406. Holt PG. A potential vaccine strategy for asthma and allied atopic diseases during early childhood. *Lancet* 1994;344:456–458.

407. Bochner BS, Lichtenstein LM. Anaphylaxis. *N Engl J Med* 1991;324:1785–1790.

408. Lane SJ, Lee TH. Anaphylaxis. In: Kay AB, ed. *Allergy and allergic diseases.* vol 2. Oxford: Blackwell Science Ltd., 1997:1550–1572.

409. Martin TR, Ando A, Takeishi T, Katona IM, Drazen JM, Galli SJ. Mast cells contribute to the changes in heart rate, but not hypotension or death, associated with active anaphylaxis in mice. *J Immunol* 1993;151:367–376.

410. Yunginger JW, Nelson DR, Squillace DL, et al. Laboratory investigation of deaths due to anaphylaxis. *J Forensic Sci* 1991;36:857–865.

411. Calderon-Zapata MA, Davies RJ. Treatment and management of allergic rhinitis. In: Kay AB, ed. *Allergy and allergic diseases.* vol 2. Oxford: Blackwell Science Ltd., 1997:1327–1343.

412. Naclerio RM, Proud D, Togias AG, et al. Inflammatory mediators in late antigen-induced rhinitis. *N Engl J Med* 1985;313:65–70.

413. Bascom R, Wachs M, Naclerio RM, Pipkorn U, Galli SJ, Lichtenstein LM. Basophil influx occurs after nasal antigen challenge: effects of topical corticosteroid pretreatment. *J Allergy Clin Immunol* 1988;81:580–589.

414. Naclerio RM. Allergic rhinitis. *N Engl J Med* 1991;325:860–869.

415. Pare PD, Bai TR. The consequences of chronic allergic inflammation. *Thorax* 1995;50:328–332.

416. Drazen JM, Arm JP, Austen KF. Sorting out the cytokines of asthma. *J Exp Med* 1996;183:1–5.

417. Austen KF. In: Kay AB, Austen KF, Lichtenstein LM, eds. *Asthma: physiology, immunopharmacology and treatment.* London: Academic Press, 1984:425.

418. Mosmann TR, Coffman RL. Heterogeneity of cytokine secretion patterns and functions of helper T cells. *Adv Immunol* 1989;46:111–147.

419. Bousquet J, Chanez P, Lacoste JY, et al. Eosinophilic inflammation in asthma. *N Engl J Med* 1990;323:1033–1039.

420. Robinson DS, Hamid Q, Ying S, et al. Predominant Th2-like bronchoalveolar T-lymphocyte population in atopic asthma. *N Engl J Med* 1992;326:298–304.

421. Bruijnzeel-Koomen CAFM, Mudde GC, Kapp A. Atopic dermatitis. In: Kay AB, ed. *Allergy and allergic diseases.* vol 2. Oxford: Blackwell Science, Ltd., 1997:1573–1585.

422. Hanifin J, Rajka G. Diagnostic features of atopic dermatitis. *Acta Dermatol Venereol* 1980;92:44–47.

423. Kay J, Gawkrodger DJ, Mortimer MJ, Jaron AG. The prevalence of childhood atopic eczema via general population. *J Am Acad Dermatol* 1994;30:35–39.

424. Grewe M, Gyufko K, Schopf E, Krutmann J. Lesional expression of interferon-gamma in atopic eczema. *Lancet* 1994;343:25–26.

425. Hamid Q, Boguniewicz M, Leung DYM. Differential *in situ* cytokine gene expression in acute versus chronic atopic dermatitis. *J Clin Invest* 1994;105:407–410.

426. Thepen T, Langeveld-Wildschut EG, Bihari IC, et al. Biphasic response against aeroallergen in atopic dermatitis showing a switch from an initial Th2 response to a Th1 response *in situ*: an immunocytochemical study. *J Allergy Clin Immunol* 1996;97:828–837.

427. Ramb-Lindhauer C, Feldmann A, Rotte M, Neumann C. Characterization of a grass pollen reactive T cell lines derived from lesional atopic skin. *Arch Dermatol Res* 1991;283:71–76.

428. van der Heyden FL, Wierenga EA, Bos JD, Kapsenberg MC. High frequency of IL-4 producing CD4+ allergen-specific T lymphocytes in atopic dermatitis lesional skin. *J Invest Dermatol* 1991;97:389–394.

429. van Reijsen FC, Bruijnzeel-Koomen CAFM, Kalthoff FS. Skin-derived aeroallergen-specific T cell clones of Th2 phenotype in patients with atopic dermatitis. *J Allergy Clin Immunol* 1992;90:184–193.

430. Kapp A. The role of eosinophils in the pathogenesis of atopic dermatitis eosinophil granule proteins as markers of disease activity. *Allergy* 1993;48:1–5.

431. Leiferman K, Ackerman S, Sampson H, Haugen H, Venencie P, Gleich G. Dermal deposition of eosinophil granule major basic protein in atopic dermatitis. *N Engl J Med* 1985;313:282–285.

432. Buckley C, Ivison C, Poulter LW, Rustin MH. CD23/FcɛRII expression in contact sensitivity reactions: a comparison between aeroallergen patch test reactions in atopic dermatitis and the nickel patch test reaction in non-atopic individuals. *Clin Exp Immunol* 1993;91:357–361.

433. Mudde GC, van Reijsen FC, Boland GJ, de Gast GC, Brunjzeel PLB, Brunjzeel-Koomen CAFM. Allergen presentation by epidermal Langerhans' cells from patients with atopic dermatitis is mediated by IgE. *Immunology* 1990;69:335–341.

434. Santamaria LF, Bheekha R, van Reijsen FC, et al. Antigen focusing by specific monomeric IgE bound to CD23 on EBV-transformed B cells. *Hum Immunol* 1993;37:23–30.

435. van der Heijden FL, van Neerven RJJ, van Katwijk M, Bos JD, Kapsenberg ML. Serum IgE-facilitated allergen presentation in atopic disease. *J Immunol* 1993; 150:3643–3650.

436. Tobin D, Nabarro G, Baart de la Faille H, van Vloten WV, van der Putte SCJ, Schuurman HJ. Increased immunoreactive fibers in atopic dermatitis. *J Allergy Clin Immunol* 1992;90:613–622.

437. Warner JO. Childhood asthma. In: Kay AB, ed. *Allergy and allergic diseases.* vol 2. Oxford: Blackwell Science Ltd., 1997:1451–1463.

438. Church MK, Warner JO. Sodium cromoglycate and related drugs. *Clin Allergy* 1985;15:311–320.

439. Eady RP, Norris AA. Nedocromil sodium and sodium cromoglycate: pharmacology and putative modes of action. In: Kay AB, ed. *Allergy and allergic diseases.* vol 1. Oxford: Blackwell Science Ltd., 1997:584–595.

440. Yunginger JW. Lethal food allergy in children. *N Engl J Med* 1992;327:421–422.

441. Nordlee JA, Taylor SL, Townsend JA, Thomas LA, Bush RK. Identification of a Brazil-nut allergen in transgenic soybeans. *N Engl J Med* 1996;334:726–728.

442. Durham SR, Varney VA. Allergen injection immunotherapy: mechanisms. In: Kay AB, ed. *Allergy and allergic diseases.* vol 2. Oxford: Blackwell Science Ltd., 1997:1227–1233.

443. Van Metre TEJ, Adkinson NFJ. Immunotherapy for aeroallergen disease. In: Middleton EJ, Reed CE, Ellis EF, Adkinson NFJ, Yunginger JW, Busse WW, eds. *Allergy: principles and practice.* vol II. St. Louis: Mosby–Year Book, 1993:1489–1509.

444. Hedlin G, Silber G, Naclerio R, Proud D, Eggleston P, Adkinson NFJ. Attenuation of allergen sensitivity early in the course of ragweed immunotherapy. *J Allergy Clin Immunol* 1989;84:390–399.

445. Otsuka H, Mezawa A, Ohnishi M, Okubo K, Seki H, Okuda M. Changes in nasal metachromatic cells during allergen immunotherapy. *Clin Exp Allergy* 1991;21:115–120.

446. Durham SR, Ying S, Varney VA, et al. Grass pollen immunotherapy inhibits allergen-induced infiltration of CD4+ T lymphocytes and eosinophils in the nasal mucosa and increases the number of cells expressing messenger RNA for interferon-gamma. *J Allergy Clin Immunol* 1996;97:1356–1365.

447. Hunt KJ, Valentine MD, Sobotka AK, Benton AW, Amodio FJ, Lichtenstein LM. A controlled trial of immunotherapy in insect hypersensitivity. *N Engl J Med* 1978;299:157–161.

448. Holt PG, Batty JE, Turner KJ. Inhibition of specific IgE responses in mice by pre-exposure to inhaled antigen. *Immunology* 1981;42:409–417.

449. Holt PG, McMenamin C. Defense against allergic sensitization in the healthy lung: the role of inhalation tolerance. *Clin Exp Allergy* 1989;19:255–262.

450. Hoyne GF, Hetzel C, Lamb JR. Immunological tolerance and T-cell anergy. In: Kay AB, ed. *Allergy and allergic diseases.* vol 1. Oxford: Blackwell Science Ltd., 1997:131–146.

451. Hoyne GF, Callow MG, Kuhlman J, Thomas WR. T-cell lymphokine response to orally administered antigens during priming and unresponsiveness. *Immunology* 1993;78:534–540.

452. Briner TJ, Kuo MC, Keating KM, Rogers BL, Greenstein JL. Peripheral T-cell tolerance induced in naive and primed mice by subcutaneous injection of peptides from the major cat allergen Fel d I. *Proc Natl Acad Sci USA* 1993;90:7608–7612.

453. Hoyne GF, Kristensen NM, Yssel H, Lamb JR. Peptide modulation of allergen-specific immune response. *Curr Opin Immunol* 1995;7:757–761.

454. Norman PS, Ohman JLJ, Long AA, et al. Treatment of cat allergy with T-cell reactive peptides. *Am J Respir Crit Care Med* 1996;154:1623–1628.

455. van Neerven RJJ, Ebner C, Yssel H, Kapsenberg ML, Lamb JR. T-cell responses to allergens: epitope specificity and clinical relevance. *Immunol Today* 1996;17:526–532.

456. Kudo K, Okudaira H, Miyamoto T, Nakagawa T, Horiuchi Y. IgE antibody response to mite antigen in the mouse. Suppression of an established IgE antibody response by chemically modified antigen. *J Allergy Clin Immunol* 1978;61:1–9.

457. Takai T, Yokota T, Yasue M, et al. Engineering of the major house dust mite allergen Der f 2 for allergen-specific immunotherapy. *Nat Biotechnol* 1997;15:754–758.

458. Chang TW, Davis FM, Sun NC, Sun CR, MacGlashan DW Jr, Hamilton RG. Monoclonal antibodies specific for human IgE-producing B cells: a potential therapeutic for IgE-mediated allergic diseases. *Biotechnology* 1990;8:122–126.

459. Boulet L P, Chapman KR, Cote J, et al. Inhibitory effects of an anti-IgE antibody E25 on allergen-induced early asthmatic response. *Am J Respir Crit Care Med* 1997;155:1835–1840.

460. Fahy JV, Fleming HE, Wong HH, et al. The effect of an anti-IgE monoclonal antibody on the early- and late-phase responses to allergen inhalation in asthmatic subjects. *Am J Respir Crit Care Med* 1997;155:1828–1834.

461. Lustgarten J, Waks T, Eshhar Z. Prolonged inhibition of IgE production in mice following treatment with an IgE-specific immunotoxin. *Mol Immunol* 1996;33: 245–251.

462. Hellman L. Profound reduction in allergen sensitivity following treatment with a novel allergy vaccine. *Eur J Immunol* 1994;24:415–420.

463. Stadler BM, Rudolf MP, Vogel M, Miescher S, Zurcher AW, Kricek F. Can active immunization redirect an anti-IgE immune response? *Int Arch Allergy Immunol* 1997;113:216–218.

464. Hellman L, Carlsson M. Allergy vaccines—a review of developments. *Clin Immunother* 1996;6:130–142.

465. Paul WE, Seder RA. Lymphocyte responses and cytokines. *Cell* 1994;76:241–251.

466. Paul WE. Pleiotropy and redundancy: T cell-derived lymphokines in the immune response. *Cell* 1989;50:328–332.

467. Takeda K, Kishimoto T, Akira S. STAT6: Its role in interleukin 4-mediated biological functions. *J Mol Med* 1997;75:317–326.

468. Boguniewicz M, Jaffe HS, Izu A, et al. Recombinant gamma interferon in treatment of patients with atopic dermatitis and elevated IgE levels. *Am J Med* 1990;88:365–369.

469. Hanifin JM, Schneider LC, Leung DYM, et al. Recombinant interferon gamma therapy for atopic dermatitis. *J Am Acad Dermatol* 1993;28:189–197.

470. Kinet J-P. The high-affinity receptor for IgE. *Curr Opin Immunol* 1990;2:499–505.

471. Church MK, Hiroi J. Inhibition of IgE-dependent histamine release from human dispersed lung mast cells by anti-allergic drugs and salbutamol. *Br J Pharmacol* 1987;90:421–429.

472. Peters SP, Schulman ES, Schleimer RP, MacGlashan DW Jr, Newball HH, Lichtenstein LM. Dispersed human lung mast cells. Pharmacologic aspects and comparison with human lung tissue fragments. *Am Rev Respir Dis* 1982;126:1034–1039.

473. Undem BJ, Peachell PT, Lichtenstein LM. Isoproterenol-induced inhibition of immunoglobulin E-mediated release of histamine and arachidonic acid metabolites from the human lung mast cell. *J Pharmacol Exp Ther* 1988;247:209–217.

474. Dahlen SE, Nizankowska E, Dahlen B. The Swedish-Polish treatment study with the 5-lipoxygenase inhibitor zileuton in aspirin-intolerant asthmatics. *Am J Respir Crit Care Med* 1995;151:A376(abst).

475. Israel E, Rubin P, Kemp JP, et al. The effect of inhibition of 5-lipoxygenase by zileuton in mild-to-moderate asthma. *Ann Intern Med* 1993;119:1059–1066.

476. Israel E, Cohn J, Dube L, Drazen JM. Effect of treatment with zileuton, a 5-lipoxygenase inhibitor, in patients with asthma—a randomized controlled trial. *JAMA* 1996;275:931–936.

477. Barnes PJ. Glucocorticosteroids. In: Kay AB, ed. *Allergy and allergic diseases.* vol 1. Oxford: Blackwell Science Ltd., 1997:619–641.

478. Barnes PJ. Treatment of chronic asthma in adults. In: Kay AB, ed. *Allergy and allergic diseases.* vol 2. Oxford: Blackwell Science Ltd., 1997:1429–1439.

479. Owens GP, Hahn WE, Cohen JJ. Identification of mRNAs associated with programmed cell death in immature thymocytes. *Mol Cell Biol* 1991;11:4177–4188.

480. Lavker RM, Schechter NM. Cutaneous mast cell depletion results from topical corticosteroid usage. *J Immunol* 1985;135:2368–2373.

481. Finotto S, Mekori YA, Metcalfe DD. Glucocorticoids decrease tissue mast cell number by reducing the production of the c-kit ligand, stem cell factor, by resident cells: in vitro and in vivo evidence in murine systems. *J Clin Invest* 1997;99:1721–1728.

482. Szczeklik A, Nezankowska E, Dworski R, Domagala B, Pinis G. Cyclosporin for steroid-dependent asthma. *Allergy* 1990;46:312.

483. Alexander AG, Barnes NC, Kay AB. Trial of cyclosporin in corticosteroid-dependent chronic severe asthma. *Lancet* 1992;339:324–328.

484. Granlund H, Erkko P, Sinisalo M, Reitamo S. Cyclosporin in atopic dermatitis: time to relapse and effect of intermittent therapy. *Br J Dermatol* 1995;132: 106–112.

485. Ruzicka T, Bieber T, Schopf E, et al. A short-term trial of tacrolimus ointment for atopic dermatitis. *N Engl J Med* 1997;337:816–821.

486. Du Buske LM. Clinical comparison of histamine H1-receptor antagonist drugs. *J Allergy Clin Immunol* 1996;98:S307–318.

487. Simons FER. Histamine and antihistamines. In: Kay AB, ed. *Allergy and allergic diseases.* vol 1. Oxford: Blackwell Science Ltd., 1997:421–438.

488. Taytard A, Beaumont D, Pujet JC, Sapene M, Lewis PJ. Treatment of bronchial asthma with terfenadine: a randomised controlled trial. *Br J Clin Pharmacol* 1987;24:743–746.

489. Gould CAL, Ollier S, Aurich R, Davies RJ. A study of the clinical efficacy of azelastine in patients with extrinsic asthma and its effect on airway responsiveness. *Br J Clin Pharmacol* 1988;26:515–525.

490. Ulbrich E, Nowak H. Long term, multicentre study with azelastine in patients with intrinsic asthma. *Arzneimittelforschung* 1990;40:1225–1230.

491. Kon OM, Barnes NC. New treatment drugs for asthma. In: Kay AB, ed. *Allergy and allergic diseases.* vol 2. Oxford: Blackwell Science Ltd., 1997:1726–1738.

492. Spector SL, Smith LJ, Glass M. Effects of 6 weeks of therapy with oral doses of ICI 204,219, a leukotriene D4 receptor antagonist, in subjects with bronchial asthma. *Am J Respir Crit Care Med* 1994;150:618–623.

493. Danzig M, Cuss F. Inhibition of interleukin-5 with a monoclonal antibody attenuates allergic inflammation. *Allergy* 1997;52:787–794.

494. Casale TB, Costa JJ, Galli SJ. TNF-alpha is important in human lung allergic reactions. *Am J Respir Cell Mol Biol* 1996;15:35–44.

495. Feldmann M, Brennan FM, Maini RN. Role of cytokines in rheumatoid arthritis. *Annu Rev Immunol* 1996;14:397–440.

496. Baggiolini M, Dewald B, Moser B. Human chemokines: an update. *Annu Rev Immunol* 1997;15:675–705.

497. Herd CM, Page CP. Platelets. In: Kay AB, ed. *Allergy and allergic diseases.* vol 1. Oxford: Blackwell Science Ltd., 1997:214–227.

498. Wegner CD, Gundel RH, Reilly P, Haynes N, Letts LG, Rothlein R. Intercellular adhesion molecule-1 (ICAM-1) in the pathogenesis of asthma. *Science* 1990; 247:456–459.

499. Gundel RH, Wegner CD, Rocellini CA, Letts LG. The role of intercellular adhesion molecule-1 in chronic airway inflammation. *Clin Exp Allergy* 1992;22: 569–575.

500. Bai TR. Adrenergic agonists and antagonists. In: Kay AB, ed. *Allergy and allergic diseases.* vol 1. Oxford: Blackwell Science Ltd., 1997:568–583.

501. Drazen JIM, Israel E, Boushey HA, et al. Comparison of regularly scheduled with as-needed use of albuterol in mild asthma. *N Engl J Med* 1996;335: 841–847.

502. Spitzer WO, Suissa S, Ernest P, et al. The use of beta-agonists and the risk of death and near death from asthma. *N Engl J Med* 1992;326:501–506.

Fundamental Immunology, Fourth Edition,
edited by William E. Paul
Lippincott–Raven Publishers, Philadelphia © 1999.

CHAPTER 36

Transplantation Immunology

Hugh Auchincloss, Jr., Megan Sykes, and David H. Sachs

Because the transplantation of tissues between members of a species does not occur in nature, a defense against transplantation provides no obvious advantage for the survival of the species. Thus, the allogeneic response (i.e., the immune response to the novel antigens of other members of the same species) probably did not evolve for the purpose of graft rejection, and issues of fundamental immunology cannot be explained on the basis of their importance to allogeneic immunity (1–3). Nevertheless, studies of transplantation biology have contributed significantly to our understanding of fundamental immunology by leading, for example, to the discovery of the major histocompatibility complex (MHC) antigens and by providing the mixed lymphocyte response (MLR) assay for the study of T-cell activation. Now, however, the emphasis has shifted. With the increasing importance of clinical transplantation, the goal is to apply our knowledge of fundamental immunology to the problem of graft rejection.

The common error in many summaries of transplantation immunology is to assume that the field can be understood simply by applying classical immunologic principles to describe the response to this particular set of foreign antigens. Allogeneic responses, however, differ from other immunologic responses in at least two fundamental ways. First, they exhibit extraordinary strength and, probably for that reason, they include unusual types of responses that cannot be detected in classical immunology. Second, they can be stimulated by two different sets of antigen-presenting cells (APCs): those of the donor and those of the recipient. In this chapter, we will emphasize these differences from classical immunology as we describe our current understanding of the several immune responses that cause graft rejection.

THE ORIGINS OF TRANSPLANTATION IMMUNOLOGY

Early History

The earliest known records of tissue transplantation are those of the Hindu surgeon Sushrutu who reported the use of a flap from a

H. Auchincloss, Jr.: Department of Surgery, Harvard Medical School and Massachusetts General Hospital, Boston, Massachusetts 02114-2696.
M. Sykes: Department of Surgery, Transplantation Biology Research Center, Harvard Medical School and Massachusetts General Hospital, Boston, Massachusetts 02129.
D. H. Sachs: Department of Surgery, Transplantation Biology Research Center, Harvard Medical School and Massachusetts General Hospital, Boston, Massachusetts 02129.

patient's forehead to repair an amputated nose (4). This procedure was probably practiced by Hindu surgeons as early as 700 B.C. In the 15th century, Italian surgeons began to practice rhinoplasty by means of flaps and extended the donor site to the patient's arm (5). In 1503, one such surgeon reported the first allograft: the grafting of skin from a slave for the reconstruction of the master's nose. A sizable legend grew out of such reports, although obviously unfounded in fact.

Skin grafting became an accepted practice in the late 1800s. Many surgeons, however, did not distinguish between autografts (donor and recipient the same individual) and allografts (donor and recipient of the same species) or even, sometimes, xenografts (donor and recipient of different species). The last of these formed the basis for an extensive practice known as zoografting, in which patients were subjected to grafts from animals ranging from pigs to frogs (6). Billingham points out that no one apparently cared whether the grafted skin "took" or merely promoted healing of the wound (7). The results of these efforts led to a period of confusion in transplantation. Without any clear understanding of the processes involved, surgeons embarked on all sorts of transplants, and a series of operations were reported that we know, from our present understanding of the laws of transplantation, could not possibly have been successful. Dr. Serge Voronoff, for example, attained considerable fame (and fortune) in Europe by developing an unusual grafting procedure in which testicles were transplanted from apes to man in order to restore men to youth and vitality (8).

The transplantation of internal organs awaited the development of techniques for vascular anastomosis. In 1908, Alexis Carrel, one of the pioneers of vascular surgery, reported the results of en bloc allotransplantation of both kidneys in a series of nine cats (9). He was able to obtain up to 25 days of urine output in some cats, but ultimately all of them died. Although other investigators repeated and modified Carrel's experiments, no major advances in prolonging the function of allografts or in understanding the cause for their failure were made for the following three decades.

During this same period, the closely related field of tumor transplantation gained momentum. In 1902, Jensen reported the transplantation of a mouse tumor through 19 successive generations of mice and was able to obtain tumor growth in some 50% of the mice he injected. Furthermore, he showed that mice in whom the tumor grew for a while and then regressed were resistant to subsequent challenge with the same tumor. He also was able to prevent successful tumor grafting by prior treatment with grafts of normal tissues (7).

Although it seems obvious to us now that these experiments provided much of the information essential to an understanding of transplantation immunology, this was not clear at the time. Many investigators still held to the Athrepsia Theory formulated by Paul Erlich in 1906 (10). According to this hypothesis, living tissues required a vital substance specific for each species and provided only by the intact organism. Thus, a transplanted tumor might grow for a while until it used up its supply of this substance. Other investigators who accepted a theory of immunity were nevertheless committed to the idea that they were studying an effect peculiar to tumor tissues. In his Harvey Lecture (11), Sir Peter Medawar summed up the confusion neatly by the statement, "Nearly everyone who supposed that he was using transplantation to study tumors was in fact using tumors to study transplantation."

In 1936, Voronoy, a Russian surgeon, reported the first clinical renal allograft (5). There was apparently a mismatch of blood types and the patient died having demonstrated only minimal renal func-

tion. The early postwar years saw reports of attempts at clinical renal homotransplantation from various world centers (12–15). In 1952 the first successful renal transplant was performed in Boston using the kidney of an identical twin (16–19).

One of the important contributions to the understanding of transplantation in this era was the work of Sir Peter Medawar. In 1943, Gibson and Medawar reported their experience with autologous and allogeneic skin grafts on a woman who had suffered extensive third-degree burns (20). The allografts in this case were taken from the patient's sibling, and for clinical reasons they were transplanted in two different stages about a week apart. The authors observed accelerated rejection of the second grafts. Appreciating the possible significance of these observations, Medawar followed them with a series of grafting experiments in rabbits and mice (21,22). By 1945, he was able to conclude that "resistance to homologous grafted skin therefore belongs to the general category of actively acquired immune reactions . . ." (23), thereby establishing the relationship of clinical transplantation to the field of immunology.

History, Principles, and Discoveries of Immunogenetics

Inbred Strains

Rodents have provided an invaluable model for the study of the genetic basis for graft rejection. One of the main features that has made them so valuable is the availability of a large number of inbred strains. Such strains consist of animals that have been produced by sequential pedigreed brother–sister matings for at least 20 generations and which are, therefore, essentially genetically identical. With the exception of the sex chromosomes, chromosomes in such strains are homozygous and therefore produce identical homozygous progeny.

The reason that sequential inbreeding leads to homozygosity is illustrated in Fig. 1. For the sake of simplicity, the first generation illustrated in this figure is indicated as a brother–sister mating in which for any given autosomal locus the alleles being bred will be of the form $AB \times AB$. The more general case of $AB \times CD$ also can be analyzed statistically by a similar, although slightly more complicated, mathematical treatment. The ratio of genotypes of the offspring from this breeding are given by the binomial formula ($AA:AB:BB = 1:2:1$). Thus, as illustrated at generation 2, when a single brother–sister pair is chosen, the chance that both animals will have the genotype AA at the locus in question is $1/16$. Similarly, the probability that the second generation mating will take the form $BB \times BB$ is also $1/16$. In either of these eventualities, all future generations will be fixed as homozygotes (either AA or BB); therefore, we speak of the locus as being fixed. Thus, the probability of fixation of a given autosomal locus at this generation is $1/8$.

For segregation of a large number of independent loci, it is mathematically equivalent to state that the probability of fixing a given locus is $1/8$, or that on the average $1/8$ of the segregating loci will be fixed. If the locus in question is not fixed during this random breeding, then the chances that it will be fixed at the next breeding are still approximately $1/8$ (actually a little larger). In other words, $1/8$ of the loci would be expected to fix at the second inbreeding generation, $1/8$ of the remaining unfixed loci would be expected to fix at the next generation, and so on. As indicated in Fig. 1, the probability of fixation (P_{fix}) is given by the following formula:

$$P_{fix} = 1 - (7/8)^{n-1}$$

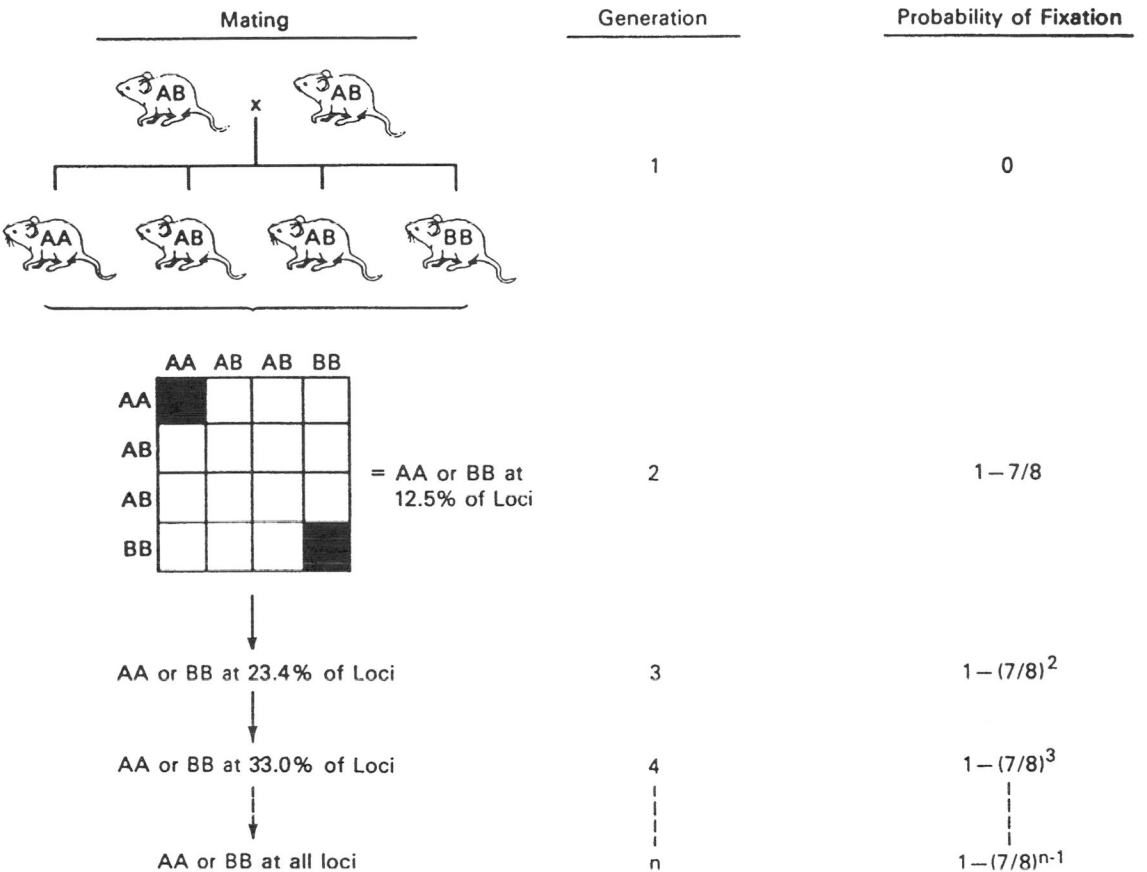

FIG. 1. Breeding scheme for inbred strains. A schematic representation of the inbreeding process. As indicated in the diagram, random selection of a single brother and sister at each generation provides a $\frac{1}{8}$ chance for fixation of any autosomal locus as either AA or BB. In other words, $\frac{1}{8}$ of the independently segregating loci will be expected to be fixed by each brother–sister mating.

This equation describes a curve that rises asymptotically toward a probability of 100% fixation (Fig. 2). Because genes travel at meiosis in groups rather than individually, there is a finite number of units of genetic information that segregate. Therefore, for practical purposes, one can consider a strain inbred after 20 such brother–sister matings, because at this point there is a very small chance that any locus will not have reached homozygosity. All loci will be of the genotype either AA or BB, and there will no longer be any loci of the heterozygous form AB. The strain so derived is defined as an inbred strain. Hundreds of such well-characterized inbred strains are now available.

During the procedure of sequential brother–sister matings to produce such inbred strains, there are, as expected, numerous cases in which lethal recessive genes become homozygous, leading to the loss of a particular line. However, because a very large number of sequential brother–sister pairs can be started and maintained from a single original breeding pair, it is generally possible to produce at least several inbred strains from the breeding of two outbred animals. If, for example, one sets up all possible brother–sister matings at the first two or three generations and then selects only a single brother–sister pair for all subsequent generations, one might easily obtain 10 successful inbred strains, even if 90% of the lines started were to succumb to lethal recessives. Because a large number of strains of mice can be housed in a small space, such a project is feasible in this species. Inbred

strains also have been produced in several other species, including rats, guinea pigs, and rabbits. However, both space requirements and other genetic features, such as gestation times, age of sexual maturity, and litter size, make production of inbred strains in larger species much more difficult.

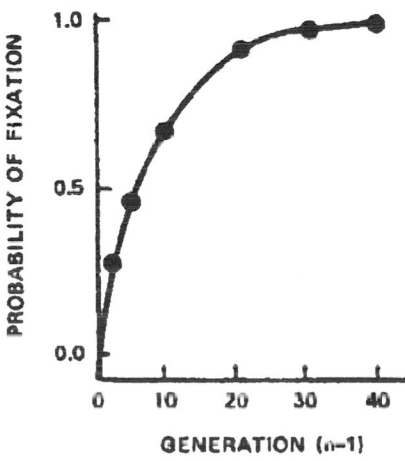

FIG. 2. Probability of fixation curve. The approach to fixation of all loci is asymptotic, given by the formula $P = 1 - (7/8)^{n-1}$ (see Fig. 1).

Several factors may mitigate against the generation of truly inbred animals. One such factor is known as forced heterozygosity. This situation arises when both possible alleles at a given locus are recessive lethals such that only heterozygotes are viable. In this case, the locus in question, as well as loci closely linked to this locus, will be maintained in a heterozygous state. This situation, although theoretically possible, has apparently been encountered only rarely during the production of inbred strains. A more common problem in obtaining true homozygosity is that of mutation, which is of course a continuously occurring phenomenon that cannot be avoided. The average mutation frequency for mammalian genes has been estimated to be approximately 10^{-6} per locus per meiosis. Because there are more than 10^6 genetic loci in mammalian organisms, one would expect at least one mutation to occur somewhere in the genome at every generation. Although one cannot avoid this source of reintroduction of heterozygosity, one can assure that such heterozygosity, once introduced, will not remain for very long by continuing to maintain a brother–sister pedigreed mating scheme for the reference line of any inbred strain. As indicated in Fig. 1, such a scheme will ensure that any mutation that occurs will either be lost or be fixed as a homozygous allele by this procedure. In order to assure that inbred lines stay inbred, therefore, pedigreed reference lines for each inbred strain must be maintained. A single brother–sister mating is chosen at each generation, and all other animals of the strain are bred from this pair or its progeny. Animals used for experiments in large numbers are bred in expansion and production colonies but should not be more than a few generations away from the reference pedigreed line.

If a particular inbred strain is maintained in two different colonies, the pedigreed reference lines will accumulate different mutations. The lines will therefore be said to drift from each other. If proper sequential brother–sister mating is performed in both colonies, each line will remain truly inbred, although eventually the two lines will be distinct at a number of genetic loci. Lines maintained separately are therefore called sublines and are designated by a series of letters following the strain designation, which indicate the origin and location of the pedigreed reference line. Thus, for example, the C3H/HeJ and C3H/HeN lines are two different sublines of the C3H strain. Both were originally maintained by Heston (He), one subline then being maintained at the Jackson Laboratory (C3H/HeJ) and the other at the National Institutes of Health (C3H/HeN). Although these strains are still quite similar for many properties, there are already several known differences between them, such as the responsiveness of their lymphocytes to lipopolysaccharide. Often differences between sublines are first detected when results from one laboratory are found difficult to reproduce in another.

Genetic Principles Governing Tissue Transplantation: The "Laws of Transplantation"

The earliest strains of inbred mice examined by geneticists had been produced for commercial rather than experimental purposes. Mouse fanciers in Europe and Japan had for many years attempted to maintain a variety of desirable characteristics in their mouse lines, such as coat color and behavioral patterns, and in selecting for such traits they had essentially inbred their mouse strains. In the early 1900s it was noted by tumor biologists that tumors arising in such animals could frequently be transplanted successfully to other animals of the same line, whereas this was usually impossible in outbred animals. Little and colleagues then studied this phenomenon systematically, in the process producing and characterizing a large number of inbred strains of mice (24).

In summarizing the results of these studies of tumor grafting in mice, Little described what have since been called the five laws of transplantation (Table 1). These are not really laws but rather a set of apparently confusing observations in which the capacity for graft rejection exists in the parental generation, is lost in the F1 generation, but is regained in the F2 generation in most cases. For those attempting to identify the genetic basis for tumor (graft) acceptance, this pattern did not appear in keeping with Mendelian genetics. Little's remarkable insight was to reconcile these observations with the classical Mendelian principles by suggesting the true fundamental principle of graft rejection and by identifying the genetic basis for the unusual outcomes (25,26). His fundamental principle was that recipients would reject grafts if the donor expressed a product of any histocompatibility (tissue compatibility) locus that was not expressed by the recipient (a principle that is now second nature to any student of transplantation immunology). His explanation for the unusual inheritance pattern was to suggest, first, that there must be codominant expression of the histocompatibility genes, and second, that there must be a relatively large number of histocompatibility loci. Under these conditions, members of the F1 generation would express both parental alleles at all histocompatiblity loci (and thus would fail to reject grafts from parental, F2, or subsequent generations), and members of the F2 generation would be unlikely to express all of the products of histocompatibility genes that are expressed by either parental generation (and thus would usually reject parental allografts).

Estimating the Number of Histocompatibility Genes

Given the availability of inbred strains and the genetic principles discussed above, one can experimentally determine the number of histocompatibility loci by which any two inbred strains differ. One breeds a large F2 population between these strains and then transplants tissues from one of the parental strains to all of the F2 offspring, measuring the fraction of grafts that survive. As illustrated in Fig. 3, if the two strains were to differ at only one histocompatibility locus, one would predict that $3/4$ of the grafts would survive. If, however, the two strains differed by two independently segregating histocompatibility loci, then one would predict that $(3/4)^2$ or $9/16$ of the grafts would survive because of the $3/4$ of animals accepting the graft due to histocompatibility at the first locus, only $3/4$ would be expected to be histocompatible for the second locus. Similarly, if there were n loci by which these two strains differed, one would expect $(3/4)^n$ to be the fraction of surviving grafts.

TABLE 1. *The laws of transplantation*

1. Transplants within inbred strains will succeed.
2. Transplants between inbred strains will fail.
3. Transplants from a member of an inbred parental strain to an F1 offspring will succeed, but those in the reverse direction will fail.
4. Transplants from F2 and all subsequent generations to F1 animals will succeed.
5. Transplants from inbred parental strains to the F2 generation will usually, but not always, fail.

Modified from ref. 774.

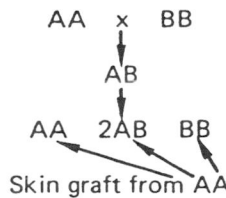

$$AA \quad \times \quad BB$$
$$\downarrow$$
$$AB$$
$$\downarrow$$
$$AA \quad 2AB \quad BB$$

Skin graft from AA

No. Loci	Expected Survivals
1	3/4
2	$(3/4)^2$
.	.
.	.
n	$(3/4)^n$

FIG. 3. Estimating the number of histocompatibility loci. Given two inbred strains, the number of independently segregating histocompatibility loci can be determined by skin grafting to the F2 generation.

When experiments designed to determine the number of histocompatibility loci were first performed, tumor grafts were used. The number of loci detected was between four and 10, depending on the particular parental strains chosen and the tumor used for transplantation. Subsequently these experiments were repeated using skin grafts as the challenging transplant. In this case, numbers for n as high as 30 to 50 have been reported (27 30). Because there are only 20 chromosome pairs in the mouse genome, these larger numbers imply that many chromosomes carry more than one histocompatibility locus.

Producing Congenic Strains: Identifying the MHC

There are thus a very large number of histocompatibility loci, each encoding a cell protein capable of contributing to rejection of a graft. However, in addition to Little's insight that there were multiple histocompatibility loci, the genetic principles he identified also suggested the process for breeding mice that would generate strains differing from one another genetically at only a single histocompatibility locus. This process, pursued especially by Snell at the Jackson Laboratories, involved the production of congenic strains (inbred strains that differ from one another at only one independently segregating genetic locus) using the rejection of parental skin grafts as the trait used to select successive matings (31). The resulting congenic strains were therefore called congenic-resistant strains because they resisted engraftment of tissues from one another. In the course of producing numerous congenic-resistant strains, it became apparent that one histocompatibility locus could be distinguished from all the others by the speed with which it caused skin graft rejection. This is now called the MHC. All of the other 30 to 50 histocompatibility loci have since been called minor histocompatibility loci. There are now a large number of H-2 congenic-resistant strains of mice available (Table 2), as well as some that isolate minor histocompatiblity loci, and some rat congenic-resistant strains.

One of the most useful breeding schemes to produce congenic-resistant lines is illustrated in Fig. 4. Starting with two inbred strains, labeled strain A and strain B, the objective is to obtain a strain that will share its entire genome with strain A except for the major histocompatibility locus H-2, which will be derived from strain B. The end product will be designated as strain A.B. Accord-

TABLE 2. *List of H-2 congenic resistant strains*

Strain	H-2 haplotype	Origin of background	MHC MHC
A	a	A	—
A.BY	b	A	Brackyury
A.CA	f	A	Caracal
A.SW	s	A	Swiss
BALB/c	d	BALB/c	BALB/c
BALB.B	b	BALB/c	C57BL/10
BALB.K	k	BALB/c	C3H
B6.AKR-H-2^k	k	C57BL/6	AKR
B6.SJL	s	C57BL/6	SJL
B10	b	C57BL/10	C57BL/10
B10.A	a	C57BL/10	A
B10.D2	d	C57BL/10	DBA/2
B10.M	f	C57BL/10	Outbred
B10.BR	k	C57BL/10	C57BR
B10.SM	v	C57BL/10	SM
B10.RIII	r	C57BL/10	RIII
B10.PL	u	C57BL/10	PL/J
C3H	k	C3H	C3H
C3H.SW	h	C3H	Swiss
C3H.JK	j	C3H	JK
C3H.NB	p	C3H	NB
D1.C	d	DBA/1	BALB/c
D1.LP	b	DDA/1	LP
LP.RIII	r	LP	RIII

ing to the cross-intercross scheme illustrated in Fig. 4, the two inbred strains are first crossed to produce an F1 generation. Because, as described above, both inbred strains can be presumed to be homozygous at all autosomal loci, all loci of the F1 generation will be heterozygous (ab). These F1 animals are then intercrossed to produce an F2 generation. The distribution of alleles at all autosomal loci in this generation follows the binomial expansion. At any locus, one fourth of the animals would be expected to be of genotype bb. A skin graft or tumor graft from strain A is next placed onto all of the F2 offspring. Animals that reject the graft must be of genotype bb for at least one histocompatibility locus. Obviously, because there are many histocompatibility loci, most animals at this generation will reject the graft. However, if only animals rejecting vigorously are chosen, and if numerous such animals are selected, then one can be reasonably certain to have selected bb homozygotes at the H-2 locus by this procedure.

The process is next repeated by mating rejectors back to strain A animals. For selected loci, therefore, the offspring once again are heterozygous. At all other, nonselected loci, offspring will have a 50% probability of being homozygous for aa alleles or of being heterozygous ab. Obviously, therefore, approximately half of the nonselected genetic information is caused by this process to revert to the inbred strain A type. Once again, these animals are intercrossed to produce the expected F2 distribution for selected loci. Another tissue graft from strain A is performed, and again rejecting animals are selected. The fraction of animals rejecting grafts vigorously at this generation will be smaller than it was at the previous generation. Once again, by selecting only vigorous rejectors, one will assure the selection of the bb homozygote at the H-2 locus. A cross to strain A is again performed, again producing the expected ab heterozygotes at the selected locus or loci. This time,

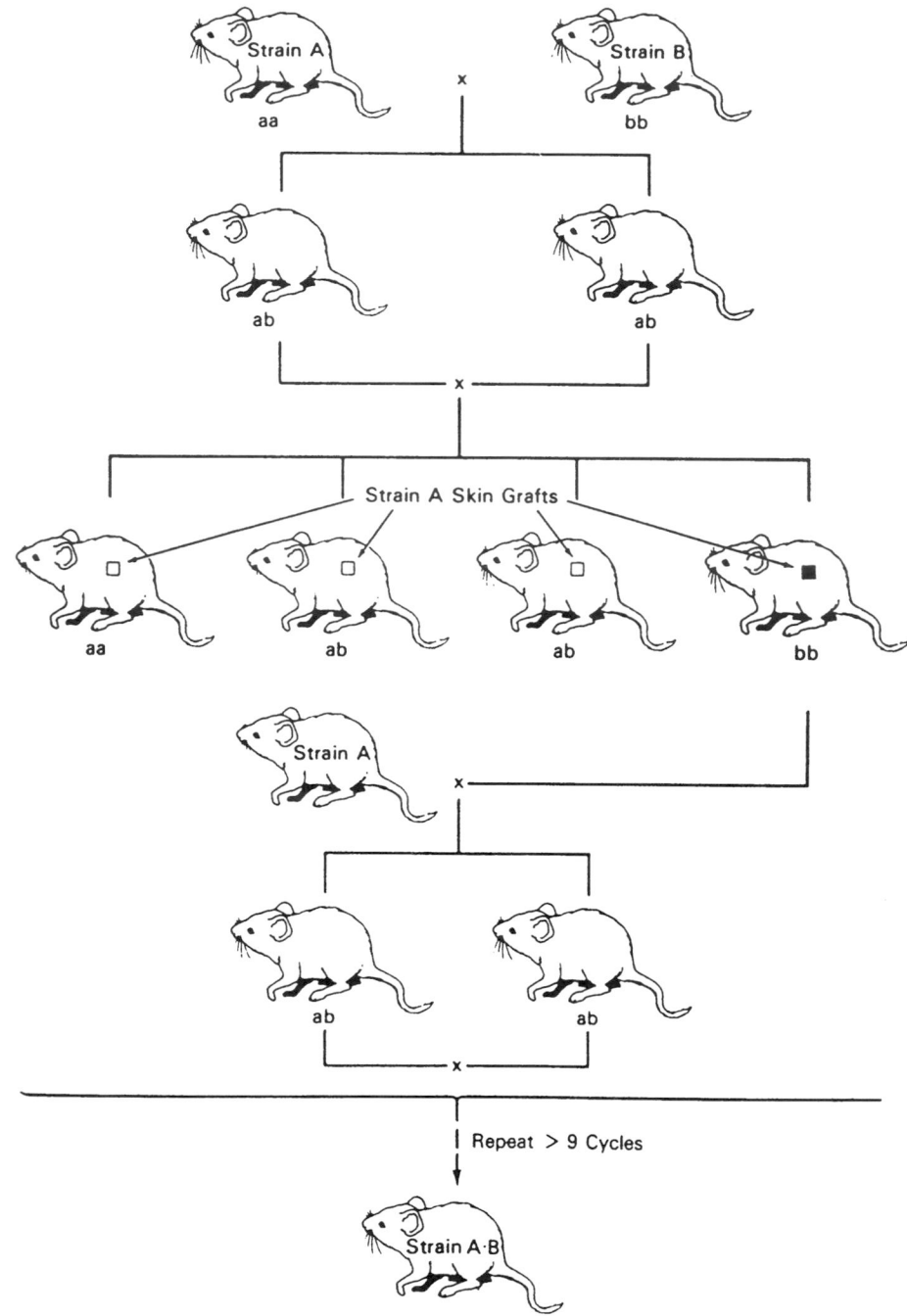

FIG. 4. Schematic representation for production of a congenic line (A.B). Illustrated is the intercross-backgross system, in which selection for histocompatibility genes is performed by skin grafting progeny of each intercross generation and selecting animals capable of rejecting grafts from the strain A parent.

however, the chances that any nonselected locus will still be heterozygous have decreased to 25%.

This process of crossing, intercrossing, and selecting by graft rejection is repeated sequentially. By the time nine cycles have been completed, one would expect there to be only one histocompatibility locus still segregating, so that only 25% of the intercross offspring should be capable of rejecting the graft. Assuming that vigorous rejection has been demanded throughout, one can be relatively certain that the selected locus will be H-2. In addition, the

chances that any other nonselected locus will still be heterozygous rather than having reverted to the homozygous aa genotype will have fallen to less than 0.2%. Stated another way, more than 99.8% of nonselected loci will be expected to be identical to their counterparts in strain A. A male and a female homozygote from the final intercross are selected and used to establish a pedigreed inbred congenic resistant line A.B.

Because mammalian genes are transferred as linked units in chromosomes, this process will always lead to the retention of a variable amount of bb genetic information at genes closely linked to the locus being selected. However, as described below, the occurrence of recombination during intercrossing generations also leads to fixation of the aa genotype at loci on the same chromosome as the MHC (chromosome 17 in mice), but at a variable distance from H-2. For practical purposes, animals that have been through at least nine cycles of such selected breeding are considered to be congenic.

As indicated in Table 2, there are now a large number of H-2 congenic mouse strains available on a variety of backgrounds. In general, the names of each of these strains follow the rule A.B, with Strain A being the background strain used in the production of the congenic, and strain B being the other parental strain from which the alternate allele at H-2 was selected. All of the early inbred mouse strains were assigned a small letter designation to represent the particular constellation of alleles that they possessed at genes in the MHC. This small letter designation is often called the haplotype designation, as indicated in Table 2. Thus, for example, strain C57BL/10 is assigned the haplotype designation H-2b and strain DBA/2 the haplotype designation H-2d. The shorthand designation for C57BL/10 is B10 and that for DBA/2 is D2. Thus, the congenic strain B10.D2 represents a congenic-resistant line in which the background is derived from the C57BL/10 and the MHC from DBA/2. It thus resembles in almost every way the C57BL/10 congenic partner, except that it differs from this partner for all properties controlled by MHC-linked genes. Similarly, the C3H.B10 strain was derived from an initial cross between C3H (H-2k) and C57BL/10 (H 2b).

The formal designation of a congenic-resistant line also includes, in parentheses after the letters, a designation such as (18M), distinguishing different congenic lines derived from the same cross. Because a large number of congenic-resistant lines have been developed in which histocompatibility loci other than H-2 have been transferred to the same background, these numbers are often included to distinguish different lines. However, for most purposes when one is describing an MHC congenic, one does not need to include its suffix. Thus, B10.D2 is a generally acceptable designation for the H-2 congenic between C57BL/10 and DBA/2.

Intra-MHC Recombinant Strains: Class I and II Antigens

As can be seen in Fig. 4, every alternate generation in this mating scheme involves the crossing of animals heterozygous at H-2. Whenever heterozygotes are bred, there is always a possibility of recombination between autosomal chromosomes at meiosis. During the production of congenic lines, such recombination will tend to decrease the amount of linked genetic information carried into the congenic from the H-2 source. Therefore, the more backcrosses a particular congenic line has been subjected to, the closer will be the boundaries on either side of H-2 at which the chromosome reverts to the background strain. Because it soon became apparent that the MHC was in fact made up of multiple loci, there was also the possibility for recombination within H-2 to occur during such crosses. Indeed, it was through the detection and characterization of such recombinants that the linkage map of H-2 was constructed. It is instructive to

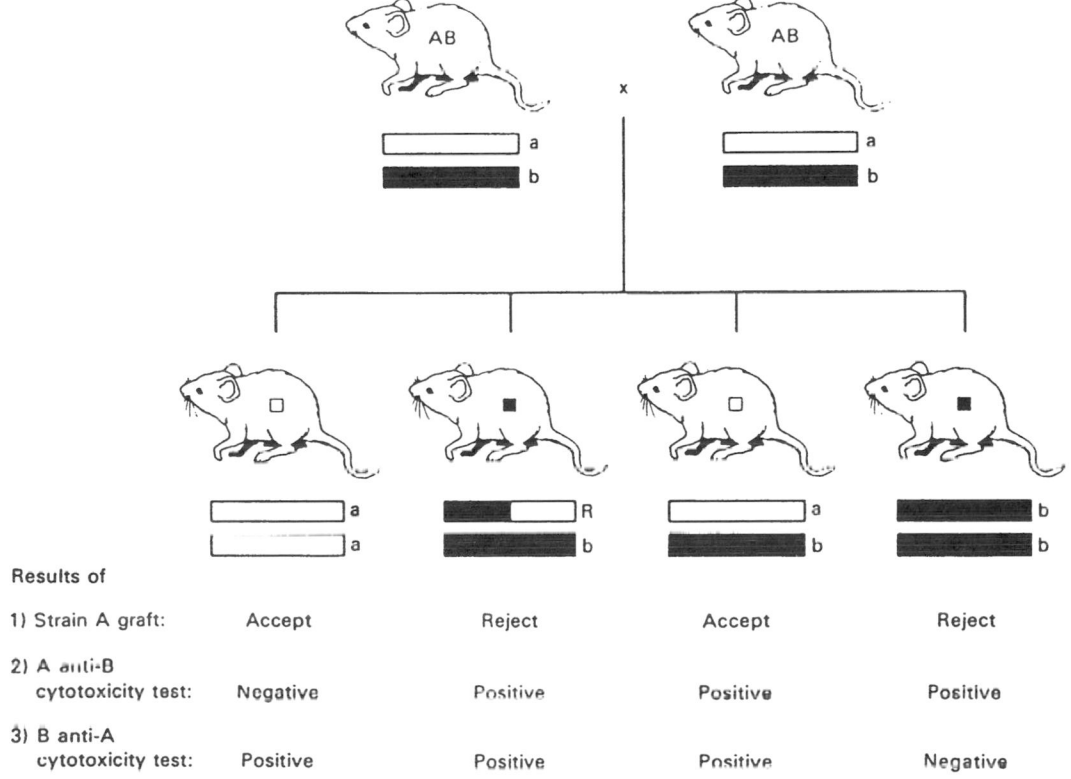

FIG. 5. Occurrence of intra-MHC recombination during the production of a congenic line. Illustrated is the occurrence of a recombination between H-2a and H-2b from one of the parents, leading to a new recombinant haplotype in one of the offspring.

examine how such recombinants would be detected and used in determining the genetic fine structure of the H-2 locus.

In order to detect a recombination event, one must examine the intercross or backcross progeny for more than one of the distinguishing features of the MHC described in the subsequent section of this chapter. This is because one can only detect the occurrence of a recombination event if the two properties examined do not behave comparably in the progeny. Thus, during the production of the hypothetical congenic resistant strain A.B, a recombination such as that illustrated in Fig. 5 might occur. In this case, let us assume that progeny are being examined both for ability to reject vigorously a strain A skin graft (i.e., genotype bb for a histocompatibility locus) and for presence of a or b gene products on lymphocyte surfaces as detected by a complement-mediated cytotoxic assay. The antisera used might be strain A anti-strain B (detecting products of bb) and strain B anti-strain A (detecting products of aa).

As seen in Fig. 5, an intra–H-2 recombinant event might lead to an animal that would type as bb by the skin graft analysis because it lacks a part of the H-2 complex that encodes products capable of causing skin graft rejection, but nevertheless type positively with both A anti-B and B anti-A antisera, suggesting an ab genotype. Such an animal would certainly not satisfy the requirement for an eventual A.B congenic line, so that other rejectors would be used for further crossing to produce the desired congenic. However, such an animal might be selected as a putative recombinant and backcrossed further to strain A to produce a congenic recombinant line designated A.B(1R). The next such putative recombinant found would be called A.B(2R), etc. In this way, a series of congenic lines might be obtained, each differing from the background strain A at the MHC, and from each other by different points of recombination within the MHC.

Fortunately, mouse geneticists were aware of this possibility and saved numerous recombinants during the production of H-2 congenic lines. Thus, for example, there are now a series of recombinants between strain C57BL/10(H-2b) and A/WySn(H-2a) which were isolated by Stimpfling during production of the B10.A CR line and which have provided a great deal of information on the genetic fine structure of the H-2 complex (32). Strains B10.A(2R) and B10.A(4R), for example, have been used to map a variety of immune response genes within the MHC. Table 3 lists many of the

most useful congenic recombinant strains now available and their known or presumed points of recombination. Among the most important contributions that came from the study of intra-MHC recombinant strains was the progressive understanding that the loci within the MHC encoded two general types of MHC antigens, now referred to as class I and class II MHC antigens.

DONOR ANTIGENS RESPONSIBLE FOR GRAFT REJECTION

Major Histocompatibility Antigens

As discussed above, the genetic analysis of graft rejection indicated that the antigens encoded within the MHC are of particular importance in graft rejection. Table 4 summarizes important aspects of the MHC antigens that are worth emphasizing in this chapter on transplantation. A much more detailed description of their structure and function can be found in Chapter 8.

Basic Features of MHC Antigens

Class I and Class II Antigens

Different loci within the complex encode two general types of MHC antigens, today called class I and class II antigens. Over the years the distinction between these two classes has been based on several different criteria; thus, the terminology applied to them has varied. Originally the class I antigens were identified most easily by serologic techniques, and they were therefore named *serologically defined* (SD) antigens. Class II antigens, however, were not originally detected by antibody responses but by proliferative responses of allogeneic lymphocytes. Class II antigens were therefore called *lymphocyte defined* (LD) antigens (33). Subsequently, serologic identification of class II antigens was accomplished and it was recognized that genes responsible for class II antigens were tightly linked to the I region of the mouse MHC (34). Thus, for a time, these antigens were called I region–associated (Ia) antigens. Among other differences, class I and class II MHC antigens evoke allogeneic responses that differ in both character and magnitude, as will be discussed below.

TABLE 3. *List of H-2 recombinant strains*

Recombinant interval haplotypes	Parental haplotypes	Haplotype designation	K A E S D	Presence of additional recombinant site	Strain bearing recombinant
K-A	b/m	bq1	b/k k k q	Yes	B10.MBR
	s/a1	t1	slk k k d	Yes	A.TL
A-E	a/b	h4	k k/b b b	No	B10.A(4R)
	b/a	i5	b b/k d d	Yes	B10.A(5R)
	b/a	i3	b b/k d d	Yes	B10.A(3R)
E-S	k/d	a	k k k/d d	No	A, B10.A
S-D	d/b	g	d d d d/b	No	HTG, B10.HTG
	d/k	o2	d d d d/k	No	C3H.OH
	a/b	h1,h2	k k k d/b	Yes	B10.A(2R)
	k/q	m	k k k k/q	No	AKR.M, B10.AKM
	q/a	y2	q q q q/d	No	B10.T(6R)
	s/a	t2	s s s s/d	No	A.TH

Congenic recombinant haplotypes available from The Jackson Laboratory.
Note that many of the recombinants involve at least one haplotype already containing a point of recombination. These are indicated by "Yes" and are listed only under the recombinant interval representing the most recent recombination in the haplotype's history.

TABLE 4. *Summary of the MHC*

Class I antigens	Single polymorphic chain Three domains: alpha 1,2,3 MW: 45,000 Associated with Beta 2 microglobulin A, B, and C loci in humans Expressed on all tissues and cells
Class II antigens	Two polymorphic chains: alpha and beta Each with two domains: alpha 1 and 2; Beta 1 and 2 MW: 33,000 and 28,000 DP, DQ, and DR loci in humans Expressed on macrophages, dendritic cells and B cells; vascular endothelium; activated human T cells

Polymorphism

The MHC antigens exhibit extraordinary polymorphism. This polymorphism presumably provides an advantage to members of the species by ensuring a broad capacity to present the peptides of, and thus respond to, a large number of foreign antigens. The high degree of polymorphism has important consequences for transplantation. The large number of alleles encoded by each locus combined with the presence of at least six individual loci in the MHC in humans make the likelihood of achieving identity for MHC antigens in two unrelated humans extremely small. Some have estimated this probability at one in a million, although the true probability varies enormously depending on an individual's genetic background.

Tissue Distribution

The tissue distribution of the two types of MHC antigens is not identical. Class I antigens are present on all nucleated cells of the body, but they may be sparsely represented on some types of cells, including certain APCs (35,36). Class II MHC antigens are more selective in their distribution (37). They are especially frequent on macrophages, dendritic cells, and B-lymphocytes. They may be present on other lymphoid cells under some circumstances, as well as on vascular endothelium. Their expression on some tissues of the body is not constant and varies according to several stimuli (38). Finally, the tissue distribution of class II MHC antigens is not the same in all species. One of the important distinctions between rodents and many larger species is the lack of expression of class II antigens on the vascular endothelium and other cell populations in rodents, whereas pigs, monkeys, and humans do express class II antigens on these tissues (39).

Physiologic Function of MHC Antigens

MHC antigens are called histocompatibility antigens because of their powerful role in causing graft rejection, yet they did not evolve in nature to prevent tissue grafting. Although the name serves to emphasize the historical importance of transplantation in the discovery of the MHC, the essential role of MHC antigens is now understood to involve the presentation of peptides of foreign antigens to responding T cells (see Chapter 9).

The Importance of MHC Antigens in Alloreactivity

Alloreactivity is the immune response to foreign antigens of other members of the same species. MHC antigens are exceptionally important in stimulating alloreactive responses, both *in vivo* and *in vitro*.

Vigorous Graft Rejection

Allogeneic MHC antigens are the most important antigens responsible for causing graft rejection. Their discovery depended largely on this feature because early experiments showed that mouse skin grafts differing only in their MHC antigens were typically rejected in 8 to 10 days, whereas grafts differing by only a single minor histocompatibility antigen were typically rejected in three or more weeks. Subsequent experiments have confirmed the importance of MHC antigens for other types of grafts. In pigs, primarily vascularized organs such as the kidney may survive indefinitely in some cases, even without immunosuppression, if all of their MHC antigens are matched, whereas MHC-mismatched kidneys are always rejected within 2 weeks (40).

However, the clear evidence for the importance of MHC antigens in causing graft rejection generally depends on there being disparities of both class I and II antigens together. Thus, there are examples in mice of skin grafts that have only class I or only class II MHC antigen disparities that are not rejected at all (41). Furthermore, the importance of MHC antigen matching becomes harder to detect, especially for skin graft survival, when comparing MHC–antigen mismatched grafts with grafts differing in multiple minor histocompatibility antigens.

Primary In Vitro MLR and CML

Allogeneic MHC antigens also stimulate an extraordinarily strong T-cell response *in vitro*. This strength is manifested partly by the ability to achieve primary *in vitro* cell-mediated responses to allogeneic MHC antigens, whereas *in vitro* responses to nominal antigens, such as ovalbumin, generally require *in vivo* priming. The greater strength also can be measured by the higher precursor frequency of alloreactive T cells compared with that for other foreign antigens presented in association with self MHC molecules. T cells reactive with an allogeneic MHC determinant may represent as many as 2% of the total T-cell population, whereas T cells reactive with an exogenous protein generally represent only approximately one in 10,000 of the same T-cell pool (42,43). This difference, representing at least two orders of magnitude, is not necessarily the result of a multiplicity of determinants on allo-MHC antigens because the same findings are obtained when precursor frequencies are measured for a mutant MHC antigen varying from the responder by only a single amino acid.

Explanations for the Strong Response to Allogeneic MHC Antigens

Originally, efforts to explain the strength of the immune response stimulated by allogeneic MHC antigens focused on possible physiologic benefits of a strong alloreactive response. For example, some considered the possibility that alloreactivity might be helpful in terminating pregnancy at parturition or that it might help prevent the spread of infectious diseases between individuals.

However, as the true physiologic function of MHC antigens has become better understood, most immunologists have concluded that the strong response to allogeneic MHC antigens is not physiologic, but rather an accidental occurrence that depends on two important features: first, that allogeneic MHC antigens are almost unique among foreign proteins in being able to stimulate an immune response without first being processed into peptides for presentation by self MHC molecules, and second, that because of this feature they can be recognized on allogeneic rather than just on self APCs.

Direct Recognition of Allogeneic MHC Antigens

All theoretical explanations for the extraordinary strength of alloreactivity are based on the unusual feature that T cells can recognize allogeneic MHC antigens without the usual requirement that peptides of these antigens be processed and presented by self MHC molecules. Transplantation immunologists refer to this special type of recognition as direct recognition of allogeneic MHC antigens. The capacity for direct recognition is believed to result from the similarity of the determinants formed by allo-MHC antigens with those created by the presentation of foreign peptides by self MHC antigens. In short-hand terminology, this has been referred to as "Allo = Self + X" (44,45). The evidence supporting this cross-reactive property comes from studies of T-cell clones that are specific for peptide antigens presented by self MHC molecules, but that also recognize allogeneic MHC antigens directly (44–46). Because the T-cell repertoire is selected in the thymus to recognize modified self MHC antigens preferentially (47), it therefore also includes large numbers of receptors capable of recognizing allo-MHC antigens directly.

Although it is widely agreed that direct recognition of allo-MHC antigens is an important component of the strength of alloreactivity, the mere presence of T cells that can respond directly to allo-MHC antigens does not explain why they should be present in higher frequency than the physiologically relevant T cells that respond to modified self MHC antigens. In the same short-hand terminology, the existence of T cells capable of recognizing allo-MHC antigens directly does not, in itself, predict "Allo >> Self + X."

The Strength of Direct Alloreactivity

Three different, but not mutually exclusive, hypotheses have been proposed to explain the high frequency of alloreactive T cells: (a) a genetic bias favoring T-cell receptor genes that are specific for MHC antigens, (b) a greater density of individual allogeneic MHC determinants on the surface of allogeneic APCs, and (c) a greater frequency of different allogeneic MHC determinants on the donor APCs.

Jerne was the first to propose that the genes that encode T-cell receptors might be maintained according to their ability to confer reactivity with the MHC antigens of the species (48). If so, then after the thymus removed self-reactive T cells, the mature T-cell repertoire would include a high frequency of cells reactive with all other MHC antigens. Jerne's hypothesis was proposed before immunologists had learned about associative recognition and positive thymic selection, but his theory became even more attractive in light of these considerations. Because the thymus only selects T cells with some degree of MHC reactivity, a T-cell receptor gene pool that encodes a broad range of specificities (as is the case for B cells) would produce many useless precursors. A narrower pool of T-cell receptor genes, however, as suggested by Jerne's hypothesis, would allow for more efficient thymic selection. There is some evidence to support Jerne's hypothesis (49–55), although the selection of mature T cells within the thymus appears nonetheless to be extremely inefficient (56).

The second explanation for strong alloreactivity, sometimes called the determinant density hypothesis, considers the difference in the expression of nominal antigens, presented as peptides by self MHC molecules on self APCs, and the expression of allogeneic MHC molecules on allogeneic APCs (57). As illustrated in Fig. 6A, the density of nominal antigen determinants expressed by a self APC would be quite low (because most MHC antigens present other peptides), whereas the density of an allogeneic MHC determinant on allogeneic APCs would be very high (because every MHC antigen would represent a foreign determinant). According to this hypothesis there might not really be a higher precursor frequency of alloreactive T cells, but they would appear to exist in larger numbers because the more powerful stimulus of an allogeneic APC would activate many T cells with relatively low affinities.

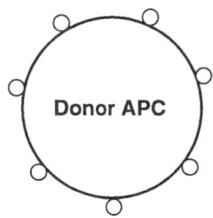 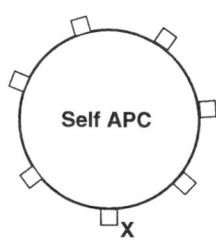 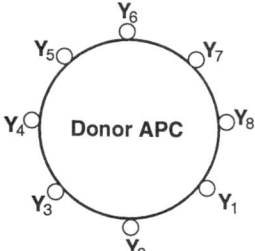 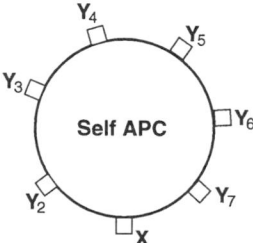

Donor APC with donor MHC antigens (○) all of which are foreign.

Self APC with self MHC molecules (□). The rare self MHC molecule presents a peptide (**X**) of an environmental pathogen.

Donor MHC antigens (○). Each presents different "self peptides" generating different foreign determinants.

Self MHC molecules (□) also present self peptides (Y₁...ₙ), but these are all self determinants.

A

B

FIG. 6. A: Determinant density hypothesis. Donor APC with donor MHC antigens (○), all of which are foreign (left). Self APC with self MHC molecules (□). The rate at which self MHC molecules present a peptide (x) of an environmental pathogen is very low (right). **B:** Determinant frequency hypothesis. Donor MHC antigens (○), each present different self peptides generating different foreign determinants (left). Self MHC molecules (□) also present self peptides ($Y^{1\cdots n}$), but these are all self determinants.

The third explanation for alloreactivity, sometimes referred to as the determinant frequency hypothesis, was developed on the basis of the idea that T cells specific for allogeneic MHC antigens might be influenced by the peptides presented by these MHC molecules (58). If the MHC molecules on self APCs often present peptides of self proteins (say $X_{1, 2, \ldots n}$), then allogeneic MHC antigens would also present peptides of allogeneic self proteins (e.g., Allo + X_1, Allo + X_2, . . Allo + X_n") (Fig. 6B). In some cases, the self peptides presented by self or allogeneic MHC molecules might be identical, but the peptides of self proteins presented by allogeneic MHC also might differ from those presented on a self APC. In either case, however, the set of determinants represented by "Self + $X_{1 \ldots n}$" would differ from that represented by "Allo + $X_{1 \ldots n}$." T cells responsive to self peptides on self APCs (Self + X_1, Self + X_2, etc.) are eliminated by the induction of self tolerance, leaving only the rare self MHC molecule, presenting a peptide of a nominal antigen, to stimulate an immune response. On the other hand, self tolerance would not affect the response to the many self peptides on allogeneic APCs (Allo + X_1, Allo + X_2, etc.). Thus, the determinant frequency hypothesis suggests that alloreactive T cells really are more frequent because each allogeneic MHC antigen generates a large number of different foreign determinants.

Choosing between the determinant density and frequency hypotheses depends on the degree to which alloreactive T cells are influenced by the peptides presented by allo-MHC molecules. Although there is some evidence that alloreactive T cells can recognize determinants that are not influenced by peptide presentation (59–61), most evidence suggests that they generally do see "Allo + X" (62–67). Thus, the available information tends to support the determinant frequency hypothesis, although no formal proof of this conclusion is available.

The finding that alloreactivity is so strong often generates confusion in light of the discussion of T-lymphocyte development in Chapter 11. There it was pointed out that the process of positive selection in the thymus generates a T-cell repertoire that is strongly biased toward recognition of peptides presented by self MHC molecules and against the recognition of peptides presented by allogeneic MHC molecules. This would seem to suggest that the response to allogeneic MHC antigens ought to be weak, not strong. However, this confusion occurs only if one forgets that the experiments demonstrating the principles of positive selection could only be performed after T-cell alloreactivity to a particular set of foreign MHC antigens was first eliminated. Under these circumstances, an individual "A" who was tolerant to self and tolerant to "B," whose T-cell repertoire developed in an "A" thymus, would develop T cells capable of recognizing "A + X" much more efficiently than "B + X." However, under ordinary circumstances, an individual "A" who was tolerant only to self, whose T-cell repertoire developed in an "A" thymus, would develop T cells capable of recognizing "A + X" and "B + X," but would also be capable of recognizing "B without X," even in the absence of *in vivo* priming. Thus, the recognition of "B + X" would be uninterpretable in these experiments. Therefore, the phenomenon of positive selection represents the enrichment of T-cell receptors capable of seeing modified MHC antigens after those receptors with strong affinity for the same MHC antigens plus self peptides have been removed. Alloreactivity can occur despite the influence of positive selection because negative selection never occurs for the vast majority of T cells recognizing allogeneic MHC antigens.

Minor Histocompatibility Antigens

The experimental process that initially defined the "major" histocompatibility complex similarly defined the "minor" loci by the slower rejection caused by their antigens. As understanding of MHC antigens increased, however, it became apparent that the separation between major and minor antigens could not depend on the speed of graft rejection alone. Class I or II MHC antigens alone, for example, do not necessarily cause rapid skin graft destruction in mice, whereas the combination of several minor histocompatibility discrepancies may bring about rejection as rapidly as a whole MHC difference (68,69). Thus, the identification of a major histocompatiblity antigen depends in part on the location of the genes encoding the molecule and in part on the well-characterized structure of both class I and class II antigens (see Chapter 8). For example, Qa and Tla antigens are generally considered class I–like products because of their structure, even though they are weak transplantation antigens in terms of rejection. Thus, minor histocompatibility antigens are those capable of causing cell-mediated graft rejection, but which lack the structural characteristics of MHC products (70). This definition of minor histocompatibility antigens does not include all non-MHC alloantigens, but rather focuses on those capable of eliciting a T-cell immune response. Other glycoproteins, such as blood group antigens, which can cause rejection through B-cell responses, are considered below.

For a long time investigators tended to assume that the minor histocompatibility antigens were other allelic cell surface proteins, similar in nature if not in strength to the MHC antigens. We now recognize that this is not the case. The minor histocompatibility antigens, defined on the basis of cell-mediated rejection, are peptides of donor proteins that are presented by MHC molecules (71–78). Thus, the minor histocompatiblity antigens are analogous to nominal foreign antigens, the peptide fragments of which are presented by MHC molecules to evoke a T-cell response. Of course, individuals are tolerant to the peptides derived from their own proteins and can only respond to the peptides of another individual's proteins that have allelic variation, i.e., polymorphism.

During the past several years, some of the peptides representing minor histocompatibility antigens have been isolated (76–78) and, in several cases, the proteins from which they are derived have been identified. As expected, these proteins are not surface glycoproteins, but are instead intracellular proteins such as nuclear transcription factors. Presumably any cellular protein with allelic variation could function as a minor histocompatibility antigen as long as it contains a peptide expressing that allelic variation that is capable of being presented by an MHC antigen in an immunogenic form.

The notion that the minor antigens are peptides recognized in association with MHC molecules has explained many of the features of these antigens that were known, but poorly understood, for a long time (79,80). First, it is difficult, if not impossible, to detect humoral responses to minor antigens. This is probably because most minor histocompatibility antigens come from intracellular proteins and, thus, even if an antibody response did occur, we would not know how to detect it without knowing the protein. Second, minor antigens do not stimulate a primary *in vitro* cell-mediated response, whereas MHC antigens evoke a powerful primary response in both MLR and CML assays. This is in keeping with the general difficulty in detecting *in vitro* T-cell responses to peptides of nominal antigens unless *in vivo* priming has occurred. Third, the recognition of minor antigens is MHC restricted, i.e., secondary responses require that the minor antigens be presented in association with the same MHC molecules as during the primary exposure (71–75). This would be expected for any antigen that evokes a T-cell response by the presentation of its peptides in the cleft of an MHC molecule. Fourth, when multiple minor antigen discrepancies exist, the immune response to one of these antigens often predominates in a phenomenon known as immunodominance (81–86). This is not due to weak recipient responsiveness to some of the minor antigens because slight changes in the donor–recipient combination sometimes produce strong responses to antigens that evoked weak or no responses before. This phenomenon may be due to competition between peptides of different minor antigens for presentation by MHC molecules.

Although this discussion of minor histocompatibility antigens has emphasized general conclusions, it is based on studies of the responses to individual minor antigens. Several studies have been reported using a variety of congenic-resistant strains that were generated on the basis of weak rejection in order to isolate minor histocompatibility loci (e.g.. H-1, H-3, H-41, or H-42) (87–90). In addition, one of the most thoroughly studied minor antigens has been the H-Y antigen, encoded on the Y chromosome, that is therefore expressed only by males of a given species (91–93). There is no reproducible antibody response to this antigen, primary *in vitro* cellular responses cannot be obtained, and secondary *in vitro* cell-mediated responses are MHC restricted. In addition, analysis of the anti–H-Y response has shown that (a) some strains can generate this response whereas others cannot, (b) the immune response genes determining responsiveness are encoded both within and outside the MHC, and (c) the rejection of grafts on the basis of the H-Y antigen alone requires that the antigen generate both helper determinants, recognized by CD4$^+$ cells in association with class II MHC antigens, and cytotoxic determinants, recognized by CD8$^+$ cells in association with class I antigens. This last feature suggests that to be identified as a minor histocompatibility antigen, a protein or perhaps a combination of proteins, probably has to generate at least two different peptide fragments that show allelic variation (94).

Other Antigens of Potential Importance

The minor histocompatibility antigens, defined by their ability to evoke cell-mediated rejection, do not account for all of the non-MHC antigens that can elicit transplantation rejection. Several other groups of antigens also should be considered.

Superantigens

Superantigens share the feature with MHC antigens that they can stimulate primary *in vitro* T-cell proliferative responses and activate an unusually high proportion of the T-cell repertoire. However, these antigens are not presented as peptides in the binding groove of MHC molecules, but instead bind to distinct regions of class II MHC molecules and engage nonvariable portions of Vβ components of the T-cell receptor, rather than the hypervariable regions that recognize peptides. Furthermore, it does not appear that endogenous superantigens can serve as transplantation antigens, perhaps because they are not expressed by endothelial cells or parenchymal cells of most tissues (95–99). Thus, superantigens cannot be classified as transplantation antigens of any type.

Tissue-Specific Antigens

There is evidence that some peptides presented by MHC molecules may be derived from proteins with limited tissue distribution (100–102). For example, T-cell clones specific for allogeneic cells of one type do not always recognize cells of a different type from the same individual (103).

The only well-described tissue-specific antigen that causes graft rejection is that for skin, referred to as the Sk antigen (100). Because it was identified on the basis of T cell–mediated responses, this antigen most likely represents a peptide, derived from a protein expressed only in skin, that is presented by an MHC molecule. This tissue-specific protein differs from the minor antigens, however, in that it need not necessarily show allelic variation because the determinant formed by "Allo + X_{sk}" (where X_{sk} is a peptide derived from the skin-specific protein) would be different from that formed by "Self + X_{sk}." Hence, T cells can be tolerant to the skin-specific antigen expressed on their own tissues, but responsive to this same antigen of a different individual. The tissue specificity of this antigen occurs because "Allo + X_{sk}" is expressed only by donor skin and not by other donor tissues.

The existence of tissue-specific antigens has importance in several ways. First, *in vitro* assays to measure T-cell responsiveness to donor antigens may be misleading when they use donor lymphohematopoietic cells as the stimulating population if the actual T-cell response is specific for donor tissue–specific antigens. Second, the need to develop self-tolerance to tissue-specific antigens emphasizes that the induction of tolerance might not be accomplished entirely in the thymus by a central process (104). Finally, the existence of tissue-specific antigens suggests that transplantation tolerance induced by one set of donor cells might not always induce complete tolerance to donor cells of a different sort.

Endothelial Glycoproteins

Blood Group Antigens

The blood group antigens do not evoke cell-mediated responses and hence are not classified as minor histocompatibility antigens. They are expressed on many types of cells and, importantly, are present on vascular endothelium where they may serve as the targets for an antibody-mediated attack on blood vessels.

Blood group antigens were identified because of their importance in transfusions (105). They represent the effects of glycosylation enzymes such that A and B individuals each express their respective antigen but O individuals have neither. The natural antibodies that develop against these antigens probably do so as a result of cross-reactions with common carbohydrate determinants of environmental microorganisms as long as the individual does not already express those determinants. Thus, O individuals will develop antibodies to the antigens of A and B donors, whereas A and B individuals will only develop antibodies reactive with antigens from each other, and AB individuals will develop responses to neither. Therefore, O recipients can only receive transfusions from O donors; A and B recipients can receive transfusions from O donors or from individuals sharing their blood type; and AB recipients can receive blood from donors of any blood type. The same rules apply to the transplantation of most primarily vascularized organs in humans because the vascular endothelium expresses ABO antigens (106,107). In addition to the ABO locus, there are other loci determining blood group antigens on erythrocytes, but these are irrelevant to organ transplantation because they are not expressed on vascular endothelium.

Other Allogeneic Endothelial Glycoproteins

In addition to the well-known blood group antigens, other glycoproteins expressed on the vascular endothelium may serve as targets for humoral responses. Rarely, preformed antibodies to these antigens may give rise to hyperacute rejection of primarily vascularized organs. In addition, antibody responses to endothelial glycoproteins can be detected after kidney transplantation between MHC identical, blood group matched individuals (108). However, these induced antibodies may not have any role in graft rejection.

Species-Specific Carbohydrate Determinants

Closely analogous to the blood group antigens are the carbohydrate determinants expressed on vascular endothelium that show species specificity. For example, pigs have a glycosyl-transferase enzyme that is not expressed by humans, that glycosylates N-acetyllactosamine to form a gal-α(1,3)α-gal determinant. In humans, a fucosyltransferase generates instead the H substance from the same substrate, leading to blood group O. Preformed or "natural" antibodies are present in human serum that react to the novel pig determinant. Similarly, natural antibodies are present between all but the most closely related species combinations. Like the blood group antibodies, these natural antibodies probably arise from cross-reactions with environmental microorganisms (109,110), and they also cause hyperacute rejection of most primarily vascularized xenogeneic transplants. They also may be recognized by other components of the innate immune system, such as macrophages and NK cells.

The Hh locus

In apparent violation of the laws of transplantation described above, a phenomenon has been described in mice whereby (A × B) F1 offspring can reject bone marrow from parental donors. This phenomenon, as well as the phenomenon of rapid rejection of fully allogeneic marrow, was shown in studies by Cudkowicz and colleagues to be mediated by natural killer (NK) cells (111). However, the identity of what appeared to be recessively inherited transplantation antigens responsible for this rejection could not be determined. Recently, it has become clear that the specificity of NK cell–mediated marrow rejection is due to the expression by NK cells of receptors that recognize specific class I MHC ligands on target cells, and that transmit an inhibitory signal to the NK cell upon such recognition. The absence of some self class I molecules on, for example, AA parental hematopoietic cells permits subsets of (A × B)F1 NK cells that recognize class I molecules from the B parent to destroy AA cells. The nature of NK-cell recognition of class I MHC is discussed in detail in Chapter 17.

COMPONENTS OF THE IMMUNE SYSTEM INVOLVED IN GRAFT REJECTION

Antigen Presenting Cells

Types of APCs

The role of specialized APCs in the process of immune activation is discussed elsewhere in this textbook (see Chapters 9,15, and

16). The critical role of APCs in graft rejection is best exemplified by the prolonged survival of some types of grafts when APCs of the donor have been eliminated (112–116).

Several types of cells have antigen-presenting capability, including dendritic cells, macrophages, and activated B cells (117–121). In addition, several organ-specific cell populations, such as Kuppfer cells in the liver and Langerhans' cells in the skin are probably subpopulations of dendritic cells. Not all APCs are equally effective, and those of the dendritic lineage are the most potent on a per-cell basis (122). All of the "professional" APCs are derived from bone marrow progenitors.

Antigen-presenting cells express MHC class II antigens constitutively, and the level of class II antigen expression can be further increased by various lymphokines, including interferon (IFN)-γ and tumor necrosis factor (TNF)-α (123–125). Some APCs may express relatively low levels of MHC class I antigens, which might serve to protect these crucial cells from destruction by the activated immune response before they can provide their full helper function (35).

An important feature of transplantation immunology is that the APCs responsible for T-cell activation may potentially originate from either the donor graft or from the recipient. The types of APCs in each case are unlikely to be the same because those from the donor will generally be the tissue-specific APCs (such as Langerhans' cells), whereas those from the recipient will generally be those associated with lymphoid tissues. Furthermore, the MHC antigens expressed by the two different sets of APCs often will be different and, thus, the specificities of the T cells stimulated by the two different sets of APCs will generally differ. Unless there is matching of MHC antigens between donor and recipient, only the determinants expressed on donor APCs will also be expressed by parenchymal cells of the graft.

Direct Versus Indirect Antigen Presentation

Because the distinction between the two potential sets of APCs is so important in describing and understanding the mechanisms of graft rejection, transplantation immunologists have developed a terminology to describe the two potential processes of T-cell sensitization. The direct pathway refers to antigen presentation by APCs derived from the donor graft, whereas the indirect pathway refers to donor antigen presentation by recipient APCs (75,126,127). Of course, indirect recognition corresponds to the form of presentation used in classical immunology; thus, the term "indirect" unfortunately seems to suggest that this is not the physiologic process for stimulating an immune response. Actually, direct recognition is the nonphysiologic pathway.

The use of the terms "direct presentation" and "indirect presentation" sometimes becomes confusing. The definition is based on which set of APCs (donor versus recipient) is involved in T-cell activation, not on the mechanisms of antigen presentation. Therefore, although indirect presentation must clearly involve peptide processing, direct presentation also may do so. For example, if peptides of donor MHC class I molecules are presented by donor class II antigens (or even other donor class I antigens), this would still represent direct presentation, even though it involves antigen processing and peptide presentation. In addition, the terms may be confusing in cases where the donor and recipient share some MHC antigens. Under these circumstances, the determinants formed by direct and indirect presentation may be identical. Nonetheless, the distinction between donor and recipient APC stimulation of T cells is still valid and may be important. Finally, the term "indirect" sensitization, which refers to the process of T-cell stimulation by an APC, can be confused with terms describing effector mechanisms. One frequently encounters discussions of possible indirect effector mechanisms of graft rejection, referring to cases in which T cells appear to recognize determinants expressed only on recipient APCs but not in the donor graft. If such effector mechanisms exist, they would be stimulated by the indirect pathway (afferent arm of the immune response) and they would also mediate graft destruction (efferent arm) indirectly because the graft would lack the target antigen. The two events are obviously related, but the word "indirect" applies to two different phases of the T-cell response.

Trafficking of APCs After Transplantation

Because APCs are the critical element in stimulating immune responses, an important issue in the regulation of transplant rejection and tolerance is which APCs are available and where they are located. Studies in mice show that changes in the location of both donor and recipient APCs take place almost immediately after transplantation. Donor APCs begin to migrate from the graft to the recipient lymphoid compartments, finding their way to both draining lymph nodes and the spleen of the recipient (122). Simultaneously, bone marrow–derived APCs from the recipient begin entering the graft and gradually replace the donor APCs. The time required for this change probably varies for different organs. In the case of murine skin grafts, the replacement of donor by recipient APCs seems to require many months, whereas the shift may occur over weeks in the case of pig kidney and human liver grafts (128–132).

Anatomic Sites of Sensitization

Although activation of T cells generally involves contact with APCs, and allogeneic APCs are especially powerful stimulators, it does not necessarily follow that cell sensitization occurs within the donor graft. Because donor APCs migrate to recipient lymphoid compartments, sensitization may occur primarily in these locations. Experiments by Barker and others have suggested that draining lymph nodes are the primary site of sensitization for skin graft rejection (133–136). They showed that skin grafts on vascular pedicles that had been deprived of lymphatic drainage failed to undergo rejection and failed to prime the recipient against donor antigens. These grafts, however, were susceptible to rejection if the recipient was sensitized by normal skin grafts placed concurrently.

The notion that allogeneic sensitization occurs primarily in draining lymph nodes is in keeping with the principles of fundamental immunology. Naive T cells generally traffic in the lymphoid circulation, waiting for foreign antigens to be concentrated there (137). Only T cells that have been previously activated are allowed to migrate into the nonlymphoid tissues, seeking the source of the antigen challenge (138,139). On the other hand, some memory T cells that were previously activated by "Self + X" determinants may cross-react with allogeneic determinants of a new graft. Thus, it is not surprising that there is also evidence suggesting that activation, or perhaps reactivation, of alloreactive T cells can occur within grafts, especially when they are primarily-vascularized and express donor endothelial cells (135,140,141).

B Cells and Antibodies
Preformed Antibodies

Anti-donor antibodies that are present before transplantation are extremely important in causing rejection of many types of primarily vascularized organ transplants. If they are present in sufficient quantity and recognize determinants expressed on vascular endothelium, preformed antibodies can cause hyperacute rejection. The preformed antibodies that do this are of two general types: natural antibodies and antibodies generated by previous exposure to transplantation antigens.

Natural Antibodies

Natural antibodies include those directed at blood group antigens and species-specific carbohydrate determinants. Their existence does not require previous exposure to transplanted tissues because they are probably generated in response to carbohydrate determinants on microorganisms. They tend to be of the immunoglobulin (Ig)M class, although IgG isotypes also may occur. Their presence is generally thought to be T cell independent, and their receptors are often in, or near, germline configuration.

Preformed Antibodies from Prior Sensitization

Recipients also may express antidonor antibodies if they have been previously exposed to cells expressing the donor antigens. This can occur by prior blood transfusion, as a result of pregnancy, or from previous organ transplantation. The antibodies formed in this way are usually IgG in isotype, are directed at protein rather than carbohydrate determinants (usually against MHC antigens), and have much higher binding affinities than the natural antibodies. Probably because of the density of MHC antigen expression and high affinity of the antibodies, lower titers of these antibodies cause organ damage more consistently than even higher titers of natural antibodies.

Induced Antibodies

After transplantation, new antibodies may be formed to the novel determinants expressed on donor tissue. Often this antibody response is directed at MHC antigens, although antibody responses to other molecules with allelic variation also may occur, especially if the recipient is repeatedly immunized. Induced antibody responses start with IgM antibody formation and then convert to IgG production in a T cell–dependent fashion.

In most cases induced antibodies are not responsible for acute graft rejection, either because they appear too late, after T-cell responses have already caused rejection, or because they appear so slowly, in the face of immunosuppression, that they fail to cause acute graft destruction. However, there are exceptions to this rule that are best demonstrated by primarily vascularized xenotransplants between closely-related species (142–144). In these cases, the induced antibody response occurs especially rapidly and causes an accelerated form of rejection targeted at the vascular endothelium. A similar form of rejection occurs only rarely in allogeneic combinations, when antidonor antibodies appear unusually early, probably reflecting prior sensitization. Induced antibodies after transplantation may play a role in chronic graft rejection. This process also involves injury primarily to the donor vessels, but occurs over a much longer period of time.

T Cells

Most allograft rejection involves T cell–mediated responses. The particular importance of T cells has been confirmed experimentally by the demonstration that athymic mice accept tissue grafts indefinitely from other members of the same species, and usually from members of other species (145). Furthermore, repopulation of these mice with purified T cells reconstitutes their ability to reject grafts (41,146,147). In humans, the use of reagents that specifically block T-cell responses, as well as the correlation of their effectiveness with their ability to eliminate T cells, supports the central role of T cells in graft rejection (148).

Because there is no phenotypic marker that correlates precisely with the function of particular T-cell subsets, it has been difficult to determine the exact role of the various subsets that participate in graft rejection. Nonetheless, a distinction between helper and effector functions can be made and is important in understanding the process. In the case of T-dependent B-cell responses, the role of T cells as helper cells for B cells that produce alloantibodies has been demonstrated well (149). There have also been *in vivo* experiments that have indicated a distinction between helper and effector T-cell functions for cell-mediated rejection. For example, there are particular cases of skin grafts that are not rejected unless simultaneous grafts that express both the antigenic determinants of the first graft and additional determinants are placed elsewhere on the same recipient (41,150). The rejection of both grafts under these circumstances indicates that a T-cell effector mechanism was potentially available for the rejection of the first graft, but that it required an additional T-cell helper function to allow the effector response to occur. These types of experiments have defined the distinction between helper and effector T-cell functions for graft rejection *in vivo,* and they have suggested the terms "helper determinants" and "effector determinants" based on which determinants were expressed on the first or second grafts. Because in these types of experiments the effector determinants have usually been presented by class I antigens, which are likely to stimulate CD8+ cells, whereas the helper determinants have usually been presented by class II antigens, which stimulate CD4+ cells, the results of these experiments have supported the idea that CD4+ T cells often provide help for CD8+ cells, at least in those cases where the two functions reside in separate cell populations.

Other Cells

Natural Killer Cells

Natural killer cells are large granular lymphocytes that lack T-cell receptors and have the ability to mediate cytolysis against certain tumor targets and hematopoietic cells. NK cells also produce a number of proinflammatory cytokines, including TNF-α and IFN-γ. NK cells can be activated and triggered to kill through a number of different cell surface receptors, some of which may still be undefined, and they represent a first line of defense against a variety of microorganisms. It has recently become clear that NK cells of both humans and mice express clonally distributed surface receptors that are capable of recognizing specific class I MHC molecules. These class I receptors, which are type II C lectin membrane proteins in the mouse (Ly49 family) and are either Ig supergene family members (p58/p70) or dimers of CD94 with NKG2 lectins in the human, are referred to as killer cell inhibitory receptors (KIRs). Recognition by a KIR of a class I molecule results in intracellular transmission of an inhibitory signal via an immune receptor tyrosine-based inhibitory motif (ITIM) that interacts with a tyrosine phosphatase and counteracts activating signals transmitted from other cell surface molecules. Recognition of self class I inhibitory ligands is believed to be important in preventing the NK cell from killing normal autologous cells (151,152).

Although the role of NK cells in mediating hybrid resistance and allogeneic marrow rejection is well-established in mice, the amount of resistance mediated by NK cells to allogeneic pluripotent hematopoietic stem cells is limited and can be readily overcome by increasing the dose of donor stem cells administered (153). Furthermore, despite the fact that human NK cells, like those of mice, have class I–dependent recognition mechanisms that inhibit lysis of targets expressing those class I molecules, a role for NK cells in resisting human allogeneic marrow engraftment has not been clearly demonstrated. However, studies in the mouse indicate a greater role for NK cells in resisting xenogeneic marrow (154) than allogeneic marrow engraftment (153,155).

Natural killer cells are also prominent in infiltrates found in rejecting allogeneic organs and sponge allografts. However, there is no clear evidence that NK cells contribute to solid organ allograft rejection. If they do, NK cells must be dependent on T cells because mice lacking T cells are unable to reject nonhematopoietic allografts. Furthermore, whereas bone marrow allografts from class I–deficient donors (β2 microglobulin [β2m] negative) are subject to potent NK-mediated rejection [because these cells cannot trigger inhibitory receptors on host NK cells (156)], β2m− skin grafts are not rejected by β2m+ recipients (157). These results are consistent with the likelihood that NK cells do not reject solid tissue allografts.

Inhibitory receptors on NK cells are quite broad in their class I specificity (158), and recognition of even fully allogeneic class I molecules can confer some protection from NK-mediated marrow destruction compared with that observed for cells deficient in class I expression (156,159). Because of the increased disparity of xenogeneic compared with allogeneic MHC molecules, a greater role might be expected for NK cells in rejecting xenografts than allografts. Indeed, NK cells appear to mount greater resistance to xenogeneic than to allogeneic marrow engraftment in mice (154,155).

Consistent with the hypothesis that NK cells are poorly inhibited by xenogeneic compared with allogeneic MHC molecules, NK cells also have been implicated in the accelerated rejection (160) that can destroy solid organ xenografts that have escaped hyperacute rejection. Because one mechanism by which NK cells mediate cytolysis is via antibody-dependent cell-mediated cytotoxicity (ADCC), it is possible that IgG natural antibodies play a significant role in initiating NK cell–mediated rejection. NK cells also release cytokines, such as IFN-γ and TNF-α, that activate macrophages and endothelial cells and induce inflammation (160). In addition to failing to receive inhibitory signals from xenogeneic MHC molecules, NK cells also may be activated by direct recognition of xenogeneic determinants. For example, it has recently been suggested that lectins on the surface of human NK cells can activate cytolysis when xenogeneic carbohydrate determinants such as α1,3 gal are recognized (161).

Recent studies in allogeneic bone marrow chimeras have suggested that bone marrow engraftment induces a state of tolerance among NK cells so that both donor and host class I MHC antigens are regarded as self by the NK cells. Similar to the T-cell repertoire, the development of a self-tolerant NK-cell repertoire is adaptively acquired (159,162–164) and is determined by the expression of particular members of the family of molecules (Ly-49 molecules in the murine system) that recognize class I antigens (162). This capacity of hematopoietic cells to tolerize host NK cells may prove to be an important advantage of the mixed chimerism approach for xenotransplantation.

T Cells that Express NK Cell–Associated Markers

In recent years, a subset of murine T cells that express NK cell–associated phenotypic surface markers has been defined. It appears that some of these cells are thymus-dependent (165) and others thymus-independent (166,167) and that they produce a variety of cytokines, including IFN-γ and interleukin (IL)-4 (168). These cells appear to recognize the nonclassical class I molecule CD1 (169) and have been suggested as a possible initial source of IL-4 that can drive T-helper type 2 responses in naive T cells. The cells can be either CD4+CD8- or CD4-CD8-. Humans appear to have a parallel subset of cells (170,171) that use a similar invariant α chain with restricted Vβ gene usage in their T-cell receptor (172,173). This T-cell subset has been reported to play a role in the phenomenon of hybrid resistance in mice (174).

Monocytes/Macrophages

A role in graft rejection for other nonspecific cellular effectors such as monocytes has been suggested (160), especially in xenograft rejection (175). It is likely that proinflammatory cytokines produced by activated monocytes and macrophages, such as IL-1 and TNF-α, play a role in endothelial cell activation. Chemoattractants produced by the inflammatory process may partially explain monocyte recruitment.

MECHANISMS OF GRAFT REJECTION

At least four distinct mechanisms that can cause graft rejection have been identified so far, and it is likely that additional mechanisms will be characterized in the future. It is convenient to describe these mechanisms according to the time frame in which

they tend to occur in clinical practice, especially because their names (hyperacute rejection, accelerated rejection, acute rejection, and chronic rejection) have a clear temporal distinction. However, it is increasingly possible to characterize these mechanisms according to the cell types and processes involved and, in some cases, they may occur at uncharacteristic times.

Rejection Caused by Preformed Antibodies (Hyperacute Rejection)

Hyperacute rejection is said to occur when a vascularized organ suffers from rejection within minutes to hours after transplantation. The phenomenon is visible and dramatic. Transplanted kidneys that have initially perfused well turn blue and mottled shortly after vascularization is established. Urine output ceases and recovery does not occur. Microscopically, organs show evidence of extensive vascular thrombosis and hemorrhage with little evidence of a mononuclear cell infiltrate (176).

There are several important components involved in the mechanism of hyperacute rejection. First, there are donor endothelial MHC antigens or carbohydrate determinants as described above. Second, there are preformed antibodies that can bind these antigens. Third, the complement and coagulation cascades are activated by the binding of preformed antibodies to the donor antigens. Finally, there are complement regulatory proteins that can modify complement activation, and anticoagulants that can modify the coagulation pathway. The target of the hyperacute rejection process is the donor vascular endothelium.

The interaction of these components leading to hyperacute rejection is diagrammed in Fig. 7. The crucial event in the process is the formation of the membrane attack complex (MAC), made up of C5–9 of the complement cascade (177,178). In allogeneic combinations, this is always initiated by antibody–antigen binding, which activates complement through the classical pathway. In a few xenogeneic combinations, complement activation also can occur through the alternative pathway and thus does not require antibody binding (179). Complement activation is controlled by several regulatory molecules, including complement receptor 1, decay accelerating factor (DAF, CD55), membrane cofactor protein (CD46), and CD59, which act at different stages along the cascade (see Chapter 29). Many of these molecules are produced by the vascular endothelial cells. Because these regulatory proteins prevent unwanted complement activation in the face of low levels of per-

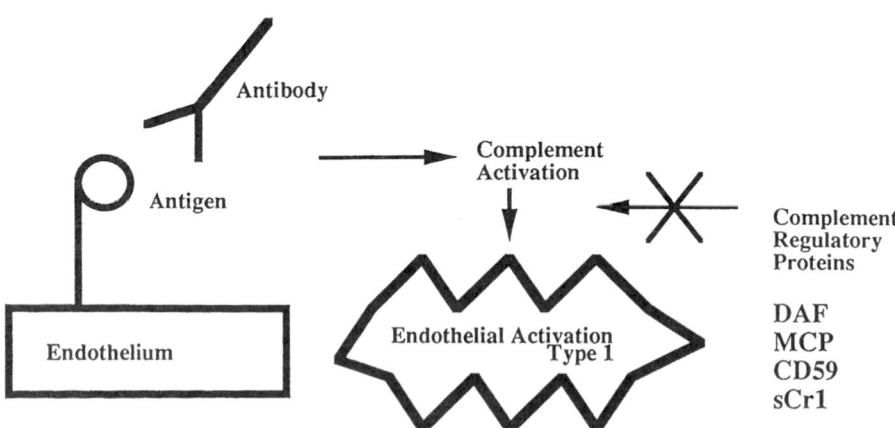

FIG. 7. Schematic representation of hyperacute rejection.

turbation to the system, the initial stimulus for activation must be strong enough to overcome these downregulating molecules. Thus, the titer and avidity of the preformed antibodies must be relatively high. Preformed antibodies directed at MHC antigens almost always accomplish this activation, whereas the lower affinity blood group antibodies lead to hyperacute rejection in only about 25% of cases. One of the reasons that hyperacute rejection is such an important feature in xenogeneic transplantation is that the complement regulatory proteins produced by the donor vascular endothelium of one species do not always function effectively with complement molecules derived from a different species (180). Because of this homologous restriction, lower levels of an initial triggering signal lead to explosive complement activation.

Although the MAC is often thought of as a lytic molecule, its effect on the donor vascular endothelium, even before cell lysis, is to cause endothelial activation (181). This occurs rapidly, before there is time for new gene transcription or protein synthesis, and has been referred to as type I endothelial activation. The two principal manifestations of this activation are cell retraction, leading to gaps between endothelial cells, and the loss of antithrombotic molecules from the endothelium (182). Thus, type I endothelial activation is responsible for the two principal pathologic findings in hyperacute rejection: (a) extravascular hemorrhage and edema and (b) intravascular thrombosis.

There are no known treatments that can stop the process of hyperacute rejection once it has started; thus, it is essential to avoid the circumstances that initiate it. Experimentally, this can be accomplished for relatively short periods of time by administration of cobra venom factor, which depletes complement (183). In clinical practice, this is accomplished by avoiding transplantation in the face of preformed antibodies, both by avoiding blood group antigen disparities and by testing recipients before transplantation to determine whether they have preformed anti-MHC antibodies that react with the donor's MHC antigens. This test is referred to as a cross-match and is usually performed by adding recipient serum to a suspension of donor lymphocytes and measuring cell lysis in the presence of an exogenous source of complement (184). In a small number of cases, allogeneic transplantation in the face of preformed antibodies has been attempted after first removing antidonor antibodies by plasmapheresis (185). This has been successful in some cases involving blood group disparities, but rarely in cases involving preformed anti-MHC antibodies. Discordant xenogeneic transplantation always involves preformed antibodies and thus cannot be accomplished without initial efforts to modify the process of hyperacute rejection.

Not all organs and tissues are equally susceptible to hyperacute rejection. Most primarily vascularized organs, such as kidneys and hearts, are susceptible, but the liver often can survive without hyperacute rejection despite preexisting antidonor antibodies (186–188). It is not clear whether this unusual feature of the liver reflects the large surface area of its vascular endothelium or an intrinsic property of liver endothelial cells. It is possible that because of its anatomic position in the portal circulation, the liver has more powerful mechanisms to prevent endothelial activation resulting from antigen–antibody complexes. Nonetheless, hyperacute rejection of the liver has occurred in some cases, especially involving xenogeneic transplantation, indicating that its resistance to hyperacute rejection is not absolute. The other types of transplants that are resistant to hyperacute rejection are those that do not immediately expose donor vascular endothelium to the recipient's circulation. For example, skin grafts do not suffer hyperacute rejec-

tion because their blood vessels are not in communication with those of the recipient until about a week after transplantation (189). After this, large doses of exogenously administered antidonor antibodies can destroy skin grafts through a complement-dependent mechanism (190). Nonetheless, long-term survival of xenogeneic skin grafts has been achieved despite the presence of natural antibodies, suggesting that the threshold for initiating this late antibody-mediated rejection is hard to achieve (191). Fresh pancreatic islets appear to behave like skin grafts, but cultured pancreatic islets (which lose their endothelial components in culture) are probably never susceptible to hyperacute rejection (192–194). Free cellular transplants, such as bone marrow cells or hepatocytes, do not have an endothelium and thus are not susceptible to the mechanisms of hyperacute rejection. However, in many cases these cell transplants do express some of the antigens recognized by preformed antibodies, and there is evidence indicating that the presence of these antibodies can lead to resistance to engraftment (195). Although this resistance can be overcome by transplanting larger numbers of cells, this finding suggests that preformed antibodies can cause cellular graft rejection by mechanisms that are distinct from hyperacute rejection.

Although hyperacute rejection is a dramatic and powerful mechanism of graft rejection, it is rarely encountered in clinical practice. The understanding of its causes, and the use of standard immunologic assays to detect preformed antidonor antibodies, has largely eliminated its occurrence. This is one of the best examples where an understanding of immunology has had an important impact on clinical transplantation.

Early Rejection Caused by Induced Antibodies (Accelerated Rejection)

A second mechanism of rejection, usually caused by antibodies, is almost as infrequent as hyperacute rejection. It occurs as a result of antibodies that are induced rapidly after a transplant is performed. This type of rejection has sometimes been called accelerated rejection because it typically occurs within the first 5 days, but there is no consensus regarding this name. The process is characterized by fibrinoid necrosis of donor arterioles with intravascular thrombosis (196).

Accelerated rejection is rare in allogeneic combinations because it requires that an antibody response occur before the T-cell response that is typically responsible for early rejection episodes. Indeed, in allogeneic combinations, accelerated rejection is sufficiently rare that some investigators have questioned its existence. Other investigators who have studied this mechanism of rejection in xenogeneic combinations have given it several different names, such as acute vascular rejection (197) or delayed xenograft rejection (198), thereby generating confusion about what may be a single process involving endothelial activation occurring later than the type I activation described above. In some xenogeneic cases, accelerated rejection may occur even without an antibody response and may result from endothelial activation by NK cells or other components of the innate immune system.

There are several causes for the difficulty in characterizing accelerated rejection. First, the clinical circumstances are rare in which induced antibodies appear before T cell–mediated rejection. Second, some patients develop antidonor alloantibodies weeks or months after their transplant, but without suffering an acute rejection episode. Finally, it is difficult experimentally to induce a B-cell response in the absence of T-cell immunity. Thus, it has been hard to prove that an induced B-cell response, rather than an especially vigorous T-cell response, is responsible for a unique rejection mechanism.

Given these difficulties, the best characterization of accelerated rejection has been achieved using primarily vascularized organ transplants from closely related xenogeneic species (142). In these cases, the levels of preformed antibodies are not sufficient to cause hyperacute rejection, but antidonor antibodies appear rapidly (within 3 to 4 days) in association with the onset of rejection (142–144). Vigorous anti-T cell immunosuppression has little effect on this early rejection, whereas immunosuppression with reagents that affect B-cell responses, such as cyclophosphamide, delays its onset until more typical T cell–mediated rejection occurs (142). The two types of immunosuppression together can lead to prolonged graft survival, unless release of the B-cell suppression allows the appearance of antidonor antibodies and the concurrent initiation of rejection (142). The pathology in these cases shows a paucity of lymphocytes infiltrating the donor graft, antibody binding to donor vascular endothelium, and fibrinoid necrosis of the donor vessels.

These studies of concordant xenograft rejection have indicated that the most important feature in accelerated rejection is the early appearance of antidonor antibodies. In fact, these antibodies appear so early, and despite the presence of anti-T cell immunosuppression, that they probably do not represent a primary response to the donor's antigens in most cases. For xenografts, they may represent a rapid increase in the levels of natural antibodies that were present before transplantation, but at undetectable levels. In the case of allografts, low levels of preformed antibodies also exist occasionally as a result of previous exposure to donor MHC antigens, but with the levels having fallen to a point where they are not detected in the standard cross-match. Thus, it is probably the unusual rapidity and perhaps the especially high levels of the antibody response that are critical in causing accelerated rejection.

As in hyperacute rejection, the process of accelerated rejection is usually initiated by antibody binding to antigens on the donor vascular endothelium. In this case, however, the subsequent endothelial changes occur more slowly, allowing time for gene transcription and new protein synthesis. This later form of activation has been called type II endothelial activation (198). Many of its features appear to be mediated by the transcription factor NF-κB, which generates many of the responses associated with inflammation, including the secretion of inflammatory cytokines such as IL-1 and IL-8 and the expression of adhesion molecules such as E-selectin and intercellular adhesion molecule (ICAM)-1 (199). In addition, type II endothelial activation causes the loss of thrombomodulin and other prothrombotic changes (200). Thus, the events following type II endothelial activation are associated with the pathologic changes that occur with accelerated rejection, including the tendency toward intravascular thrombosis and the inflammatory destruction of donor vessels that occurs in the absence of infiltrating lymphocytes.

Just as there are regulatory processes for complement activation, there are regulatory molecules that counter the tendency toward intravascular coagulation and the process of type II endothelial activation. For example, the expression of tissue factor protein inhibitor by vascular endothelium tends to inhibit factor Xa of the clotting cascade (201). In addition, the tendency toward type II endothelial activation is inhibited by the expression of a number of protective molecules, including, bcl-x$_L$, bcl-2, and A20 (198).

Although these are often thought of as antiapoptotic molecules, they also tend to inhibit activation mediated by NF-κB. Just as the regulatory molecules of complement may not function across species differences, so too some of the regulatory molecules involved in type II endothelial activation may show homologous restriction (201). Thus, in addition to the more rapid appearance of antidonor antibodies, loss of regulation also may be responsible for the finding that accelerated rejection is an important aspect of xenogeneic graft rejection (once hyperacute rejection is avoided), whereas it is rarely seen in allografts.

Although vigorous early antibody responses generate type II endothelial activation and accelerated rejection, later antibody responses usually fail to do so. The process that enables transplanted organs to survive in the face of circulating antibodies that can bind endothelial antigens has been called accommodation. In xenogeneic combinations, and some allogeneic combinations with preformed blood group antibodies, accommodation has been achieved by the removal of preformed antibodies for a period of 1 to 2 weeks and the allowance of their slow return after this time. Similarly, resistance to type II endothelial activation has been achieved *in vitro* by pretreatment with low levels of antiendothelial antibodies that are insufficient to trigger activation (202). The achievement of accommodation is associated with increased expression of the antiapoptotic genes described above and with changes in the isotype of the recipient's antibody responses (198).

Although both hyperacute rejection and accelerated rejection occur early after transplantation and depend on antidonor antibodies, there are a number of important differences between the two. One of these is that although hyperacute rejection is primarily mediated by complement activation, accelerated rejection can occur in the absence of complement. On the other hand, accelerated graft rejection may involve different secondary mediators, such as monocytes and macrophages. In xenogeneic combinations (where the inhibition of NK cells by class I molecules is lost), NK cells also may participate in accelerated rejection using antibodies to generate an ADCC response. Possibly NK cells alone can cause type II endothelial activation in xenogeneic combinations, even in the absence of antidonor antibodies, perhaps by triggering through activating lectin molecules that recognize xenogeneic carbohydrate moieties (161).

Another important difference between the two early forms of antibody-mediated rejection involves treatment. Once hyperacute rejection is initiated, there is no known therapy that can stop graft destruction, whereas accelerated rejection can sometimes be reversed by vigorous therapy. This has usually included plasmapheresis to remove antidonor antibodies and treatment with anti–B cell reagents such as cyclophosphamide (142–144). These reagents also may have a direct effect on the donor endothelium, blocking the process of type II endothelial activation. Although treatment of accelerated rejection is possible, it is not always successful. In current clinical practice, this form of humoral rejection may be responsible for many of the relatively few cases in which immunologically mediated graft loss occurs during the first several months after transplantation.

Rejection Caused by T Cells (Acute Rejection)

Although in clinical practice few allogeneic organs suffer either hyperacute or accelerated rejection after careful cross-matching, rejection episodes occurring toward the end of the first week after transplantation are not infrequent, despite the use of immunosuppression. These episodes are separable from the humoral rejection processes by the later timing of their occurrence, by the absence in many cases of antidonor antibodies in the recipient, and by the cellular infiltrate usually present in the biopsy. Called acute rejection episodes, most rejection treated by clinicians is of this type. Acute rejection may occur at any time after the first few days following transplantation, but with decreasing frequency after the first 3 months. However, rejection that appears to be similar in mechanisms may occur much later after transplantation, especially if immunosuppressive medication is withdrawn.

Acute rejection of organ allografts is T cell mediated. Therefore, treatment is usually with increased doses of standard immunosuppressive drugs or with antilymphocyte antibodies. These strategies are so likely to be successful that the diagnosis of acute rejection is doubtful if they are not (148).

Because T cell–mediated acute allograft rejection plays such an important role in clinical transplantation, there has been considerable study of the mechanisms involved. Nonetheless, the following discussion will indicate that many important issues regarding this rejection process remain to be resolved. On the other hand, most current clinical therapies to control cell-mediated rejection have been developed in the absence of a thorough understanding of the process but have still been extremely effective in controlling it. Whereas 30 years ago the majority of transplant recipients experienced one, or several, rejection episodes, and only about half of the recipients were able to keep their transplanted organ for a full year, the use of newer immunosuppressive drugs and monoclonal anti-T cell antibodies has changed these numbers considerably. Recent studies have shown that as many as 80% of kidney transplant recipients never experience an episode of acute rejection (203), and it is now rare to lose a transplanted organ to cell-mediated rejection during the first year after transplantation. These impressive results suggest that further analysis of cell-mediated rejection is unlikely to lead to better short-term survival of transplanted organs.

Nonetheless, the experimental study of cell-mediated rejection continues to receive considerable attention for several reasons. First, T cell–mediated responses may contribute to the process of chronic rejection. Second, a better understanding of the mechanisms of T cell–mediated rejection may help to identify assays that would accurately measure the state of a particular recipient's immune responsiveness to their transplanted organ, which therefore might help identify those individuals who needed more or less immunosuppression. More importantly, a better understanding of how T cells cause graft rejection may help in the design of strategies to eliminate this response altogether, by inducing tolerance to the donor antigens. Achievement of this goal would be the ultimate accomplishment of transplantation immunology.

The study of cell-mediated rejection in vivo has used four types of experiments. First, there have been the studies of clinical transplants, which are obviously highly relevant and provide frequent tissue for analysis, but which are always performed in the presence of immunosuppression and without the capacity to manipulate important variables. Second, there have been studies of skin grafts or islet transplants using rodents, which provide large amounts of controlled data, but which may not accurately reflect the processes of rejection for primarily vascularized organs. Third, there have been studies of heart transplants and occasionally other types of primarily vascularized organ transplants in rodents, although these types of transplants are too easily accepted compared with similar transplants in human beings. Finally, there have been studies of primarily vascularized organ transplants performed in large animals,

such as monkeys or pigs, which have obvious clinical relevance, but which are expensive and difficult to perform in large numbers. The conclusions suggested by these different approaches have not always been the same; thus, the description of the general mechanisms of T cell–mediated rejection is complicated by the need to identify exceptions and features that occur only in special cases.

The Simple, Classical Model of T Cell–Mediated Allograft Rejection

The description above of the donor antigens involved in rejection indicated that allogeneic MHC antigens play a special role in stimulating T-cell responses, especially by direct recognition of these antigens. In addition, the description of the components of the recipient's immune system involved in rejection indicated that APCs play an important role in sensitizing T cells and that sensitized helper T cells lead to the development of an effector mechanism for T cell–mediated graft rejection. Based on these considerations, the simplest model of a T-cell rejection mechanism is that shown in Fig. 8. This model emphasizes the importance of direct recognition of donor class II MHC antigens by recipient CD4+ T cells, which then serve as helper cells for recipient CD8+ cells, which are sensitized by direct recognition of donor class I MHC antigens. The CD8+ cells then provide the effector mechanism for graft rejection based on the direct recognition of parenchymal cells throughout the donor graft that express class I antigens.

A powerful feature of the model shown in Fig. 8 is that it emphasizes that T cell responses to allografts cannot be thought of strictly in terms of the classical mechanisms of T-cell activation described throughout this textbook on fundamental immunology. This is because alloreactivity has the unique feature that donor MHC antigens do not require processing and presentation of their peptides by recipient MHC molecules in order to stimulate a T-cell response. By concentrating on the direct recognition of donor MHC antigens, expressed on donor APCs, the model in Fig. 8 seems to capture the critical features that distinguish allograft rejection from other immune responses, determine its strength, and explain the particular importance of MHC compared with other donor antigens. Nonetheless, as will be described in detail below, the model in Fig. 8 fails to predict the outcome of transplantation experiments under a variety of different experimental conditions. For example, this simple model would predict that the elimination of either CD4+ or CD8+ T cells from the recipient would prevent graft rejection, whereas MHC-disparate skin grafts can be rejected by either subpopulation alone (149,204). This, and many other examples described below, make it clear that the simple model shown in Fig. 8 is inadequate to describe T cell–mediated graft rejection.

There are at least two basic weaknesses with the simple model in Fig. 8. On the one hand, it fails to emphasize sufficiently the importance of direct recognition and the strength of this response. As a result of the high precursor frequency of T cells that respond to allogeneic MHC antigens directly, populations of T cells that ordinarily have minimal significance become functionally important. For example, CD8+ T cells that recognize allogeneic class I antigens directly can generate their own IL-2 and function independently of CD4+ helper cells. On the other hand, the second weakness with the model in Fig. 8 is that this simple model may overemphasize the importance of direct recognition by ignoring the potential contribution of recipient APCs and their capacity to present peptides of donor antigens in the manner of a classical immune response.

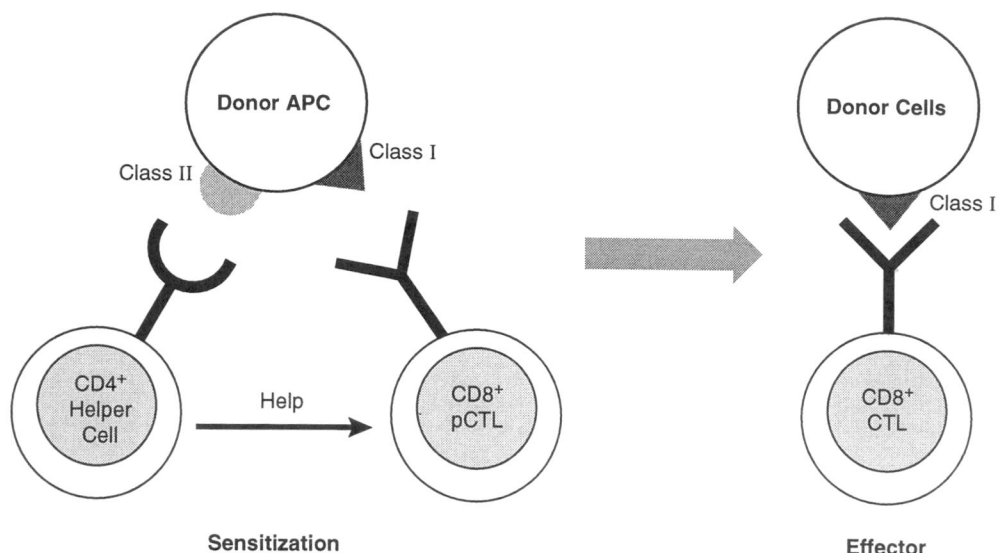

FIG. 8. Simple model of T cell–mediated rejection.

The primary finding from experimental studies of T cell–mediated rejection is that there are multiple ways in which T cells can be sensitized to donor antigens and probably several types of effector mechanisms of graft destruction. Thus, it has become common to talk about pathways of alloreactivity to describe the multiple processes that may be involved. For example, experimental systems have been developed to investigate graft rejection that depends on the indirect pathway alone or that depends on direct recognition by CD8+ cells in the absence of CD4+ cells. This reductionist approach to the analysis of T cell–mediated rejection has become possible because of the availability of antibodies that deplete selected T-cell subpopulations in the recipient, because of mutant and genetically engineered strains of donor mice that express isolated class I or class II antigen disparities, and because of genetically engineered strains of mice that lack the expression of class I or class II antigens. The results of the numerous experiments, both *in vitro* and *in vivo,* that have examined the pathways of alloreactivity are described below, leading to the generation of a more complex model of T cell–mediated graft rejection.

Pathways of Alloreactivity: Helper Responses

Alloreactive Helper Activation Measured In Vitro

The standard *in vitro* assay of helper function in cellular immunity is the MLR. This assay measures proliferation of T cells after allogeneic stimulation. More recently, investigators have found it useful to quantify and characterize the helper response more precisely by measuring the production of particular lymphokines such as IL-2 using biologic assays, enzyme-linked immunosorbent assays, and semiquantitative polymerase chain reaction (PCR). Extensive investigation of the pathways of alloreactive helper activation has been undertaken using these *in vitro* techniques (205–210). A summary of the experimental results is shown in Table 5, which indicates the magnitude of the helper response for each T-cell subpopulation in response to each type of antigenic

challenge. It should be noted that in some cases where the response is shown in Table 5 to be absent (based on bulk culture experiments), there have been T-cell clones derived (presumably exceptional cases) that demonstrate this specificity.

The results summarized suggest that there are three main pathways of alloreactive helper activation *in vitro*: CD4+ lymphocytes responding directly to allogeneic class II stimulation, CD4+ lymphocytes responding to peptides of alloantigens presented in association with responder-type class II MHC molecules, and CD8+ lymphocytes responding directly to class I alloantigens. The CD4+ direct response is easily measured. The ability to measure the CD4+ indirect response usually requires *in vivo* priming, although there is an unexpected, weak primary response to peptides of allogeneic MHC antigens presented by self MHC molecules. The ability to measure the CD8+ direct response is often enhanced if IL-2 production rather than just proliferation is measured, especially if an anti–IL-2 receptor antibody is used to prevent IL-2 consumption (207). In addition, detection of the CD8+ direct response requires depletion of the CD4+ population or stimulation with just a class I antigen disparity because helper responses generated by whole MHC differences are generally dominated by CD4+ cells (211). Although CD8+ helper cells can be activated directly by alloantigens *in vitro*, it has been much harder to demonstrate CD8+ helper cells in response to modified self class I antigens. They have not been found in response to TNP-modified self class I molecules (205), but have been detected after *in vivo* priming with virus followed by *in vitro* stimulation with virus-modified class I antigens

TABLE 5. In vitro *pathways of alloreactivity*

	Helper pathways				Cytotoxic pathways	
	Direct		Indirect			
	I	II	I	II	I	II
CD4+	–	++++	–	+++	–	++
CD8+	++	–	±	–	++++	++

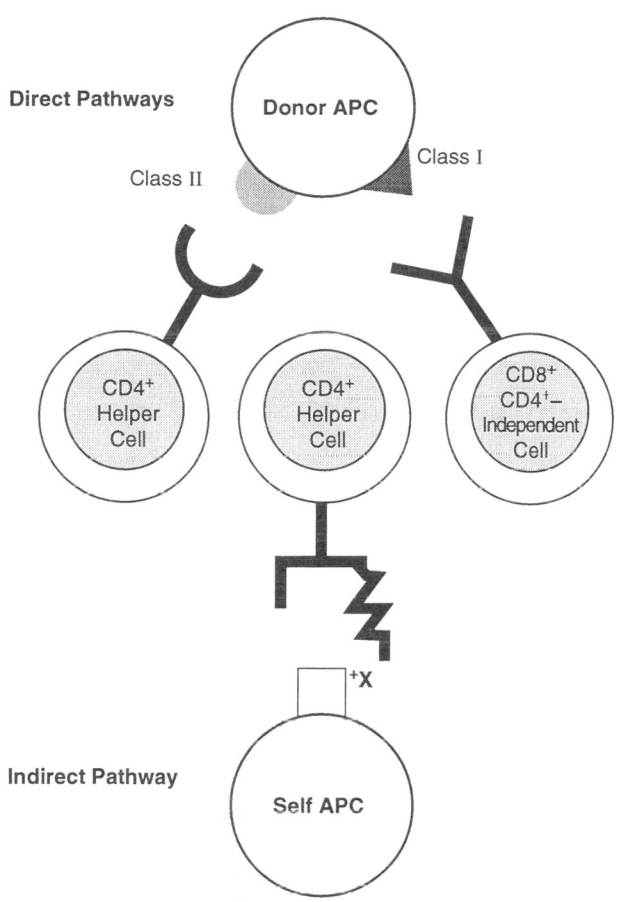

FIG. 9. Complex model of T-cell sensitization pathways.

The role of the direct pathway in stimulating CD4[+] cells has been demonstrated using genetically engineered class II knock-out mice as recipients after reconstitution of their CD4[+] T-cell population. These mice lack class II antigens on their own APCs and therefore cannot generate an indirect response. Thus, CD4-dependent rejection of grafts by these recipients must reflect direct sensitization of CD4[+] cells in vivo (227).

CD4[+] Indirect Activation In Vivo. lthough indirect CD4[+] activation has been easily demonstrated in vitro, it has been difficult to prove that the indirect pathway for CD4[+] activation actually contributes to graft rejection in vivo. This experimental difficulty stems from the powerful CD4[+] direct response that is almost always present, making it difficult to isolate the effect of indirect activation. Furthermore, some experiments looking for evidence of CD4[+] indirect helper activation using class II–matched, class I–mismatched murine skin grafts failed to demonstrate a role for the indirect pathway (41,146). However, accumulating evidence now suggests that indirect activation can contribute to graft rejection:

1. MHC-mismatched APC-depleted endocrine grafts are not rejected, whereas similarly depleted MHC-matched grafts sometimes are, suggesting that an indirect response to determinants expressed on the donor graft may be responsible for rejection (228,229).
2. Xenograft rejection in mice is very dependent on CD4[+] function, even though CD4[+] direct activation measured *in vitro* is very weak (230).
3. Antibody blocking of recipient class II antigens *in vivo* can sometimes prevent rejection (231).
4. Immunization of recipients with peptides of donor antigens before transplantation can speed subsequent graft rejection (232).
5. Rejection of some grafts lacking class II antigen expression has been shown to be dependent on CD4[+] T cells, which were therefore presumably stimulated by modified class II antigens of the recipient (233).
6. Some manipulations that alter the immune response to peptides of donor MHC antigens have been found to prevent rejection of grafts expressing the intact MHC antigens, suggesting that the indirect response to these antigens may be dominant over the direct response in causing graft rejection (234,235).

CD8[+] Direct Activation In Vivo. CD8[+] T cells alone can reject some types of grafts, including skin grafts that express an MHC class I antigen disparity (41,146,149,236). These results suggest that CD8[+] direct activation also can contribute to graft rejection.

Direct CD8[+] activation does not appear to be as powerful as direct CD4[+] activation because grafts expressing only class I antigen disparities are usually rejected more slowly than class II–disparate grafts, and responses dependent on CD8[+] helper responses are more easily suppressed by cyclosporine (237–239). Probably as a result of this weakness, rejection that depends on CD8[+] direct activation is influenced by several factors that do not seem to be as important for CD4[+] direct activation. First, CD8[+] direct activation is dependent on the relative number of donor APCs in a graft (149,233). This may explain why many primarily vascularized grafts that express a class I antigen disparity still require CD4[+] cells to initiate rejection. Second, CD8[+] helper cells recognize modified self class I antigens poorly (87,205). Therefore, CD8[+] direct activation fails to initiate rejection of grafts with only a small number of minor antigen disparities and provides only a weak helper response even when there are a large number of foreign minor antigens.

(212). The CD8[+] cells that have helper function in allogeneic responses have been found to have particularly high affinity for class I alloantigens (213).

Alloreactive Helper Activation Measured In Vivo

Two basic approaches have been used to study the pathways of alloreactive helper activation *in vivo*. First, selected T-cell subpopulations have been depleted *in vivo* (149,204,214–221), and second, selected T-cell subpopulations have been transferred into nude or severe combined immunodeficient (SCID) recipients, which themselves lack the T-cell components of graft rejection (41,146,147,217,222–224). In both cases, the approach has been modified by placing grafts with narrow antigenic disparities or by using different types of tissues for transplantation. The results of these studies suggest that all three alloreactive helper pathways detected *in vitro* also can be detected *in vivo*.

CD4[+] Direct Activation In Vivo. CD4[+] T cells alone can cause rejection of many types of grafts, including those with a class II antigen disparity and those with multiple minor antigen disparities (204,223,225). Thus, CD4[+] cells must provide the helper function in these cases. Furthermore, CD4[+] cells have been shown to contribute to rejection of almost every type of graft, the only exception being the rejection of some types of class I–only disparate murine skin grafts (41,146). Thus, CD4[+] helper function is an important component in vivo in most cases of graft rejection (226).

CD8[+] helper cells also differ from CD4[+] helper cells in being unable to provide help for other cell populations (240). Apparently the IL-2 produced by these cells is used by the cells themselves as they develop effector function. Therefore, CD8[+] helper cells cannot provide help for CD8[+] cells with a different specificity and cannot provide help for B-cell antibody responses.

A More Complex Model of the Sensitization Pathways of Alloreactivity

The results of the experiments described above indicate that the simple diagram of alloreactive pathways shown in Fig. 8 is not sufficient and that the more complex model shown in Fig. 9 more accurately depicts the possible routes of sensitization that can initiate graft rejection. Not all of these pathways are available in every case, however, and their availability may change over time, especially because donor APCs are replaced by recipient APCs. Determining the relative importance of the alloreactive pathways is one of the important issues in transplantation immunology at this time.

Which Pathways Are Important in Graft Rejection?

We cannot yet determine precisely the relative importance of the three alloreactive pathways of helper activation of naive T cells in graft rejection. Probably the particular helper activation pathway used depends on the type of graft involved, the antigenic disparity, the time after transplantation, and the previous history of the recipient. In general, the *in vitro* and *in vivo* data suggest that the CD4[+] direct pathway is more important than the CD8[+] direct pathway unless CD4[+] T cells are depleted or class I antigen disparities alone are present. In addition, *in vitro* studies suggest that it is more difficult to suppress either one of the direct pathways than the CD4[+] indirect pathway and that it is harder to suppress the CD4[+] direct pathway than the CD8[+] direct pathway (237,241). Of the various helper pathways, the CD8[+] direct response is probably the least important *in vivo* because most studies of rejection, except those using skin grafts, indicate that CD4[+] cells are essential for initiating rejection.

The Emerging Emphasis on Indirect Recognition

These results would seem to suggest that although there may be many pathways of alloreactivity, as shown in Fig. 9, the classical CD4[+] direct response shown in Fig. 8 is nonetheless the dominant response. However, an important event in transplantation immunology over the past several years has been an increasing tendency to stress the importance of indirect recognition (242–246). This trend has been supported by several different observations. First, it has long been recognized in clinical practice that the amount of immunosuppression needed to achieve prolonged graft survival does not make transplant recipients immunologically crippled. This observation is contrary to the prediction, inherent in Fig. 8, that because of the strength of direct recognition, the immune response leading to graft rejection should be much stronger than any ordinary immune response. Second, a number of investigators have sought to correlate rejection activity in clinical patients with *in vitro* measures of T-cell sensitization. In some cases, they have suggested that an increase in the precursor frequency of T cells responding through the indirect pathway provides the best correla-

tion with clinical events (247–254). Third, recent studies with the class II knock-out mice, in which graft rejection may be studied under conditions where either direct or indirect pathways are available in isolation, have indicated that rejection mediated through the indirect pathway is a powerful event, and that it is often as difficult to control as rejection depending on direct recognition. In some cases, helper responses mediated by indirect recognition even appear to be suppressed by sensitization through the direct pathway (227). Fourth, the recent studies using peptides of allogeneic MHC antigens to suppress the rejection of grafts expressing the intact MHC molecules suggest that manipulations that can only affect the indirect response can have a dominant effect on graft rejection (255–258). These results not only indicate that indirect responses participate in graft rejection, but they also suggest that indirect recognition may be more important than direct recognition. On the other hand, descriptions of graft rejection that emphasize the indirect pathway must deal with several new issues that emerge from this shift in orientation.

Special Problems Associated with Indirect Recognition

Explaining The Importance of MHC Antigen Matching. One of the most attractive features of the classical model shown in Fig. 8 is that it provides a clear basis for explaining the importance of allogeneic MHC antigens in causing graft rejection. As described above, direct recognition of intact allogeneic MHC antigens gives rise to an unusually powerful (if not physiologic) immune response, whereas peptides of donor antigens would not be expected to be any more powerful than those of other histocompatibility antigens. If the recent trend toward emphasizing the importance of indirect responses is correct, then new explanations will be required for why allogeneic MHC antigens are more important than other donor antigens in causing graft rejection.

Indirect Presentation and Donor-Specific Tolerance. The availability of indirect recognition also has implications regarding the potential effectiveness of some strategies to achieve donor-specific nonresponsiveness. Many of these strategies seek to present donor antigens to immunocompetent recipients in a manner that leads to T-cell downregulation rather than activation. If these strategies only involve manipulations of donor APCs, they may be ineffective in preventing indirect immune responses because these depend on recipient APCs (246).

Why Does Donor APC Depletion Prolong Graft Survival? Numerous studies have demonstrated that depletion of donor APCs can prolong graft survival (112–116,259). Although this result is in keeping with the central role ascribed to APCs in graft rejection, it is not obvious why donor APC depletion should be effective if the indirect pathway is available to initiate graft rejection. A possible explanation for this observation may be that the donor APCs transfer antigens from the graft to recipient APCs in the draining lymph nodes. Thus, donor APC depletion might prevent both direct and indirect activation at least until APCs of the recipient repopulated the donor graft. An alternative explanation might be that donor APCs are essential for the sensitization of the effector cells responsible for graft rejection, whereas indirect presentation is available for the sensitization of helper cells. Potential effector cells therefore might undergo anergy as a result of encountering donor antigens directly only on parenchymal cells of a graft. In this case, donor APCs also would be required despite the potential importance of the indirect pathway.

Communication Between Indirect Helper Cells and Direct Effector Cells. The possibility that helper cells might be sensitized by recipient APCs while effector cells might be sensitized by donor APCs highlights a special feature of alloreactivity compared with ordinary immunology: that in the case of graft rejection, two different populations of APCs, potentially expressing different MHC antigens, may be involved in the process. This special circumstance creates a unique problem in transplantation immunology: that sensitization of different subpopulations of T cells may occur without the physical linkage afforded by the expression of different determinants on a single APC. The absence of such physical linkage may be important in limiting the availability of help from one subpopulation during the sensitization of another subpopulation. This issue is discussed in more detail below, in the section on the regulation of graft rejection.

Presentation of Donor Antigens by Recipient Class I versus Class II Antigens. Another conceptual problem associated with indirect pathways stems from the general principle in fundamental immunology that peptides of exogenous antigens tend to be presented by MHC class II antigens while those of endogenous antigens are generally presented by MHC class I molecules (260,261). Strictly applied, this principle would imply that indirect recognition would only generate responses to donor peptides presented by self class II molecules, whereas sensitization to donor peptides in association with class I molecules would have to occur by direct presentation. However, numerous exceptions to this principle have been reported, and there is good evidence that peptides of exogenous allogeneic antigens can be presented by recipient class I molecules (262–264).

Bevan demonstrated that indirect sensitization of CD8+ cells can occur in vivo when he described the phenomenon of cross-priming (75). He showed that when minor antigen-disparate grafts with MHC antigens of type A were placed on MHC (A × B) F1 recipients, the CD8+ cells of these recipients became sensitized to the minor antigens presented by both A and B types of class I MHC molecules. Despite these findings, it is still far more common to talk about indirect responses in terms of CD4+ T cells than in terms of CD8+ sensitization by modified self class I molecules. As a mechanism for sensitization of helper cells, indirect CD8+ sensitization is unlikely to be important because the help generated by CD8+ cells has been found to be useful only for the CD8+ cells themselves. Because CD8+ effectors, sensitized indirectly, would not generally recognize determinants expressed in the graft, the CD8+ helper response, which might generate such CD8+ effectors, has generally been thought to be irrelevant for purposes of graft rejection. On the other hand, there is increasing interest in the possibility that indirect effector mechanisms may contribute to graft rejection. In addition, even if the effector mechanisms are unimportant, the cytokines produced by CD8+ cells sensitized indirectly may contribute to the overall regulation of the immune response (265). Thus, the question of how CD8+ indirect sensitization might affect graft rejection remains one of the open issues in transplantation immunology.

Indirect Effector Mechanisms. The classical model of rejection in Fig 8 suggested that the effector population was sensitized directly just as the helper population was. However, with recognition that helper sensitization could occur through the indirect pathway, it was natural to consider the possibility that effector populations also could be sensitized indirectly, or that inflammatory processes stimulated by indirect helper T cells might cause graft rejection without the participation of any effector T cells that rec-

ognize donor antigens directly. These types of rejection mechanisms have been referred to as indirect effector mechanisms and are considered more fully in the next section.

Pathways of Alloreactivity: Effector Mechanisms

Although there are many controversial aspects of helper T-cell function, there is even more uncertainty about the effector mechanisms of cell-mediated graft rejection. Originally, the delayed-type hypersensitivity (DTH) response was the only in vivo mechanism known for cell-mediated tissue destruction; thus, for many years transplantation immunologists assumed that it was responsible for graft rejection. Subsequently, the cytotoxic function of T cells was identified, with the attractive feature that a mechanism involving these cells could account for the precise selectivity of graft destruction. Therefore, many transplantation immunologists began to assume that cytotoxic T cells were the important effector cells, and this was the assumption incorporated in the model shown in Fig. 8. As with the helper pathways, recent evidence has suggested that the depiction of effector function in Fig. 8 is too simple. An especially troublesome issue is to determine whether cell-mediated effector mechanisms necessarily require T cells that are specific for antigens expressed by the donor tissue or whether an indirect effector mechanism initiated by T cells specific for modified self MHC antigens also might be sufficient. The following discussion reviews the important data available on these issues and suggests that the almost conflicting conclusions drawn from different types of experiments make it likely that more than one effector mechanism is available, depending on the circumstances.

In Vitro *Studies of Effector Mechanisms*

In vitro studies have been used to examine T cell effector functions in transplantation immunology just as they have for the analysis of helper function. A standard assay measuring an alloreactive effector function is the cytotoxic T-lymphocyte (CTL) or cell-mediated lympholysis (CML) assay measuring T cell–mediated cytotoxicity against allogeneic targets. Alloreactive CTLs can easily be generated from naive T cells after about 5 to 7 days of in vitro stimulation with MHC-disparate cells. Generation of CTLs to peptides of minor antigens presented by self MHC molecules, however, requires that the T cells first be primed in vivo. The amount of cytotoxicity measured in vitro is a function of both the helper activation and the number of precursor CTLs available at the start of the in vitro culture. Therefore, to focus on just the cytotoxic effector function, the assay is often performed with the addition of exogenous helper factors, such as IL-2, in order to provide an excess of help. The assay also can be quantified by measuring precursor frequencies of cytotoxic T cells using limiting dilution cultures.

Because alloreactive T cells to foreign MHC antigens can be measured even in naive animals, the standard CML assay is inadequate to determine whether CTLs have been primed in recipients that have rejected MHC-disparate grafts. Therefore, efforts have been made to modify the assay to measure the effect of in vivo events. For example, peritoneal T cells from mice that have recently rejected grafts can kill donor targets even without the period of in vitro sensitization. In addition, determination of the precursor frequency of alloreactive T cells, measured under modified conditions, can sometimes differentiate recently activated from naive cytotoxic T cells (266). In general, however, it has been difficult to measure reliably the effect of *in vivo* CTL priming to MHC alloantigens. On the other hand, generation of cytotoxic T cells to minor histocompatibility antigens does require *in vivo* priming and therefore reflects *in vivo* sensitization.

The *in vitro* CML assay has been used to determine the pathways of alloreactive T-cell cytotoxic function. The results of these assays are summarized in Table 5. CD8⁺ cytotoxic T cells reactive with donor class I antigens are the most frequent effectors *in vitro,* and CD8⁺ cytotoxic cells specific for self class I antigens modified by allogeneic peptides also can be detected after *in vivo* priming (267–269). In addition, CD8⁺ cytotoxic cells specific for allogeneic class II antigens can be detected, although they would not be predicted in classical immunology (206). CD4⁺ cytotoxic cells, specific for allogeneic class II antigens, also can be measured *in vitro* (211). Thus, as for helper cells, there are multiple pathways for generating alloreactive cytotoxic T cells *in vitro.*

In Vivo *Analysis of the Cellular Effector Mechanism*

The Selectivity of Allograft Rejection. A critical feature when considering in vivo effector mechanisms of graft rejection is the selectivity by which the process destroys foreign but not self tissues. Experiments illustrating this selectivity have been performed by placing syngeneic skin grafts adjacent to allogeneic grafts on a single bed. The inflammation of rejection shows a perfect demarcation at the division between the two grafts (270,271). An even more dramatic demonstration of this selectivity has been achieved using skin grafts from tetraparental (allophenic) donors, animals produced by fusing embryonic cells of two parental pairs. Grafts from these animals represent a mosaic of two kinds of cells, interspersed throughout the tissue, each cell bearing one of the two sets of parental MHC antigens. When these grafts are placed on animals that are syngeneic with one of the sets of MHC antigens, there is at first a generalized inflammatory process that appears to destroy the entire epithelium, but some syngeneic tissue remains after the rejection process subsides and all the allogeneic cells have been destroyed (272–274). Thus even when different cell types exist side-by-side, the process of graft rejection shows selectivity.

Experiments such as these often have been taken to imply that graft rejection must take place by the cell-by-cell destruction of allogeneic tissue. This is not the only interpretation, however, because the syngeneic elements that eventually survived from the tetraparental grafts might actually represent the product of epithelial seeding by a few syngeneic cells that remained as the tissue around them died. Furthermore, the experiments with the allophenic skin grafts did reveal a nonspecific inflammatory process early in the rejection process (274). Other types of experiments mixing donor and recipient cell types in a single skin graft also have been performed, using skin from bone marrow chimeras in which the APCs of the skin have been replaced by cells derived from the donor bone marrow (275). When transplanted to syngeneic recipients, skin grafts from these chimeras provide a graft in which only the APCs express alloantigens. The results of these experiments showed that entire skin grafts can be rejected when only the APCs are foreign, although this rejection is more apt to occur when there are large antigenic disparities and when the recipient has been previously sensitized to the foreign antigens. Thus, nonselective destruction of grafted tissue can occur, especially if the inflammatory response is sufficiently vigorous.

Analysis of the Cells Invading Allografts and the Immunopathology of Rejection. Another approach to study the effector mechanisms of graft rejection has been to identify the actual cells that invade a graft by immunohistochemical staining. Such studies, using sponge matrix allografts and rejecting allogeneic organs, have shown that many types of cells are present during graft rejection, including CD4⁺ and CD8⁺ T cells, NK cells, and macrophages (276–284). There are relatively few B cells, however, and some T-cell subpopulations (including L-selectin cells) are largely excluded from the graft (285,286). Therefore, some selectivity must exist in the process that recruits the invading cell populations.

The number of invading T cells in a graft is not necessarily related to the speed of the resulting rejection. Whole MHC and class II–disparate grafts generally elicit dense cellular infiltrates, whereas class I–disparate grafts are generally sparsely infiltrated. Indeed, the density of the cellular infiltrate in the case of a class I only difference is not significantly different from the density in a syngeneic graft (285), and the number of invading cells sometimes appears insufficient to mediate rejection by cell-to-cell contact with every allogeneic target. This finding has suggested that certain critical elements of the graft, such as its blood vessels, are the actual site of graft destruction and, indeed, endothelialitis is an important hallmark of clinically significant rejection activity (287). The number of cells within minor antigen–disparate grafts is generally far greater than the number invading grafts with class I only differences, even when the rejection of the class I grafts is faster (285). In addition to the implication that the degree of cellular infiltrate may not correlate with the strength of active rejection, these findings also suggest the possibility that only a small portion of the T cells within a graft may actually have specificity for the allogeneic antigens. The role, if any, of the other invading lymphocytes in rejection is unclear.

Further analysis of the invading cells within rejecting allografts has been undertaken by in vitro propagation of the T cells derived from rejecting organs (283,288–295). Most reports of such efforts have indicated that these T cells are polyclonal and that both cytotoxic and IL-2–producing lymphocytes of both CD4⁺ and CD8⁺ lineages can be obtained (296,297). A few reports have suggested that an oligoclonal T-cell response occurs during allograft rejection (298). Overall, however, because so many cell types with so many functions have been identified in rejecting allografts, this type of phenotypic and functional analysis of the invading cells has not been helpful in identifying the effector mechanisms of graft rejection.

In addition to phenotypic and functional analyses of invading T cells, interesting studies recently have been performed correlating the onset of graft rejection with the ability to detect immunologically active proteins in the invading lymphocytes (299–307). For example, PCR has revealed high levels of message for IL-5 in liver grafts showing clinical evidence of rejection, although the role of this cytokine in the rejection mechanism is not clear (308). In addition, graft rejection can be correlated with the presence of perforin, granzymes, and proteases associated with cell-mediated cytotoxicity (309–316).

Studies of Effector Mechanisms Using Knock-Out Mice. Genetically engineered mice lacking the expression of particular genes have been used to study the mechanisms of graft destruction in at least two ways. First, mice lacking the expression of some of their MHC antigens have been used as donors to determine whether grafts can be rejected when they fail to express the determinant recognized by the effector T cells. For example, skin grafts from class II knock-out mice have been placed on SCID or nude recipients reconstituted with CD4$^+$ but not CD8$^+$ T cells. These experiments have shown that the class II–deficient grafts can be rejected by CD4$^+$ cells alone, but much more slowly than when CD8$^+$ cells are also present (224). Thus, an indirect effector mechanism mediated by CD4$^+$ cells in this case appears to be much less effective than one involving direct recognition of donor antigens. The ultimate experiment to test the effectiveness of an indirect effector mechanism would be to use completely MHC-deficient donors (317). Experiments of this type have been performed using the mice generated by crossing class II and β2m knock-out animals (318). Unfortunately, the results of these experiments have indicated that there is sufficient residual class I antigen expression by the double knock-out mice that rejection of skin grafts can still be mediated by CD8$^+$ effector cells specific for the class I antigens, making the use of skin grafts from these donors ineffective for answering the experimental question (227,319). On the other hand, the rejection of other types of tissues, such as pancreatic islets, is diminished substantially by the reduced expression of donor MHC antigens unless the MHC-deficient islets are placed in xenogeneic recipients (320–324). Thus, these results again suggest that an indirect effector mechanism is a relatively ineffective way of destroying transplanted tissue, unless the inflammation generated by the indirect response is especially powerful.

The other way that genetically engineered mice have been used to examine rejection mechanisms has been to use mice lacking the expression of particular genes as recipients of transplants. A striking result of these types of experiments is that rejection of all types of organ transplants can occur in the absence of the key components of T-cell cytotoxicity such as perforin and Fas ligand (325,326). Thus, despite the strong correlation between expression of perforin and evidence of clinical rejection described above, these experiments strongly suggest that cytotoxicity is not essential for graft rejection. Cytotoxicity by T cells may represent one of several mechanisms for graft destruction, or the presence of cytotoxic T cells in rejecting allografts may simply be a marker for the sensitization of effector T cells that actually utilize a different mechanism. The use of other types of knock-out mice as recipients lacking various cytokines also has failed to reveal any single molecule that is essential for the mechanism of graft destruction (327–330).

Correlation Between In Vitro and In Vivo Results

Another approach to analyzing effector mechanisms has been to examine the correlation between graft rejection *in vivo* and the ability to measure *in vitro* cell-mediated cytotoxicity. A strong correlation would support a T cell–mediated cytotoxic mechanism, whereas a breakdown in this correlation would suggest alternative mechanisms.

One way to measure this correlation is to deplete selected T cells *in vivo* before placing grafts with limited antigenic disparities. For example, such studies have shown that CD4$^+$ cells alone but not CD8$^+$ cells alone can reject skin grafts with only class II antigen disparities (41,146,147,221). This result correlates with the *in vitro* experiments showing that both CD4$^+$ and CD8$^+$ cells contain precursors of cytotoxic cells specific for allogeneic class II antigens, but that only the CD4$^+$ population has a helper pathway to generate mature class II specific CTLs. The outcome of many other experiments of this sort correlate with the *in vitro* results for CTL generation.

The most controversial experiments of this type have involved studies of rejection of class I–only disparate grafts by recipients depleted of CD8$^+$ T cells (41,146,147,214,220,221,331). Graft rejection frequently has been demonstrated in this situation even though *in vitro* assays have generally failed to reveal cytotoxic CD4$^+$ cells specific for class I alloantigens. Thus, these results appear to violate the correlation between graft rejection and the ability to measure *in vitro* cytotoxicity. Rosenberg and Singer, however, demonstrated that mice depleted of CD8$^+$ T cells by antibody treatment still have a population of cytotoxic precursors (apparently of the CD8$^+$ lineage despite the absence of the CD8 antigen) that require *in vivo* priming and help from CD4$^+$ T cells for their activation. These investigators have demonstrated the presence of CD4$^+$, CD8$^+$, αβ$^+$ cytotoxic T cells after graft rejection in the mice that were treated with anti-CD8 antibodies (222,332). These results suggest that depletion of CD8$^+$ cells *in vivo* may not always eliminate all cytotoxic cells of this lineage and that the rejection of class I–disparate skin grafts apparently by CD4$^+$ cells alone is not actually a violation of the correlation between *in vitro* CTL activity and *in vivo* graft rejection. Other investigators have disputed Rosenberg and Singer's conclusions, suggesting that they apply only to the limited antigenic disparities generated by the comparison of the class I mutant H-2^{bm} mice with wild-type H-2b mice. These other investigators suggest that the larger number of foreign peptides generated by more disparate class I antigens are sufficient to generate an effector mechanism mediated by CD4$^+$ cells specific for class I peptides presented by class II molecules (333). These results do not distinguish a direct from an indirect effector mechanism because the class II molecules of the donor and recipient are identical in these experiments, but they do suggest a lack of correlation between *in vivo* rejection and *in vitro* cytotoxicity because CD4$^+$ cytotoxic T cells have not been detected after rejection in these experiments.

Another important challenge to the hypothesis that cytotoxic T cells cause graft rejection comes from examination of *in vitro* cytotoxicity after rejection of grafts that differ only in minor histocompatibility antigens. Because CTL activity to minor antigens can only be measured *in vitro* after *in vivo* priming, minor disparate graft rejection provides a good opportunity to test whether every case of rejection is associated with the development of CTL activity. A particularly good model to test this correlation is the rejection of murine skin grafts, which differ by only the H-Y antigen because some strains, but not others, can reject skin grafts with only this single minor antigen disparity. Experiments from Simpson's laboratory have indicated that the rejection of H-Y grafts is not always associated with measurable *in vitro* cytotoxicity, whereas in other cases the development of CTLs *in vitro* occurs despite the absence of graft rejection (334–336). Although these results obviously challenge the role of CTLs in graft rejection, they too are controversial.

Uncertainties Regarding the Effector Mechanisms of Graft Rejection

All of the approaches described above have failed to provide clear evidence demonstrating a single effector mechanism for graft destruction. Although the results do suggest that cytotoxic T cells are not the only effector cells involved, they do not demonstrate what other effector mechanisms are involved and they fail to answer the basic question of whether effector T cells must necessarily recognize donor MHC antigens directly in order to achieve the selectivity of graft destruction. As diagrammed in Fig. 10, the evidence is consistent with the complex view that multiple effector mechanisms exist, some involving cytotoxicity and some not, and some with specificity for donor antigens, and others involving an indirect effector process (221,281,337–346). The evidence at this point does suggest that indirect effector mechanisms are less efficient than ones involving direct recognition unless the stimulus to a nonspecific inflammatory response is especially powerful. All of these conclusions are tenuous at this time, however.

Potential Final Mediators of T Cell–Dependent Effector Mechanisms

Whether or not there are indirect effector mechanisms for graft destruction, the final mediators of cell-mediated rejection may not be T cells themselves, but rather other components of the immune system that depend on helper T cells. There are several candidates for such mediators of graft destruction. Classical DTH responses are thought to depend on the activation of macrophages by helper T cells through production of IFN-γ. In turn, the destruction of tissues by activated macrophages often may involve the production of toxic molecules such as nitric oxide (347). Although an effector mechanism involving macrophages would appear to lack selectivity, the process might still cause limited tissue destruction if the donor cells (such as pancreatic islets) are especially sensitive to these inflammatory mediators, or if donor blood vessels in the immediate vicinity of the activated cells are especially likely to be injured by the inflam-

matory response. Cytokines are clearly involved in the mechanisms of graft rejection. However, most of the obvious examples of their participation involve their role in the helper mechanisms of T-cell sensitization. It is likely, however, that some cytokines, such as TNF-α, may themselves be toxic to allogeneic tissues.

Chronic Rejection (B and/or T Cell-Mediated)

Most experimental studies of rejection are performed without immunosuppression. Therefore, graft destruction usually occurs within the first several weeks by one of the mechanisms described above. In clinical practice, however, the use of immunosuppression usually allows graft survival for much longer periods of time. Nonetheless, clinical survival statistics show that even when 1-year graft survival has been achieved, the loss of transplanted organs continues to occur at a rate of about 3% to 5% per year, and a significant portion of this loss appears to be due to immunologic mechanisms. The term "chronic rejection" has been used to describe this late process of graft destruction. Because immunosuppressive reagents have become more effective at controlling acute rejection, chronic rejection has emerged as one of the most important problems in clinical practice. Indeed, Fig. 11 shows that although there has been ongoing improvement over the past 30 years in the 1-year graft survival rates for kidney transplants, the half-life for organs that have survived for 1 year has not changed significantly over that entire period of time (348). As a result of this ongoing loss, only about 50% of transplants are still functioning 10 years later.

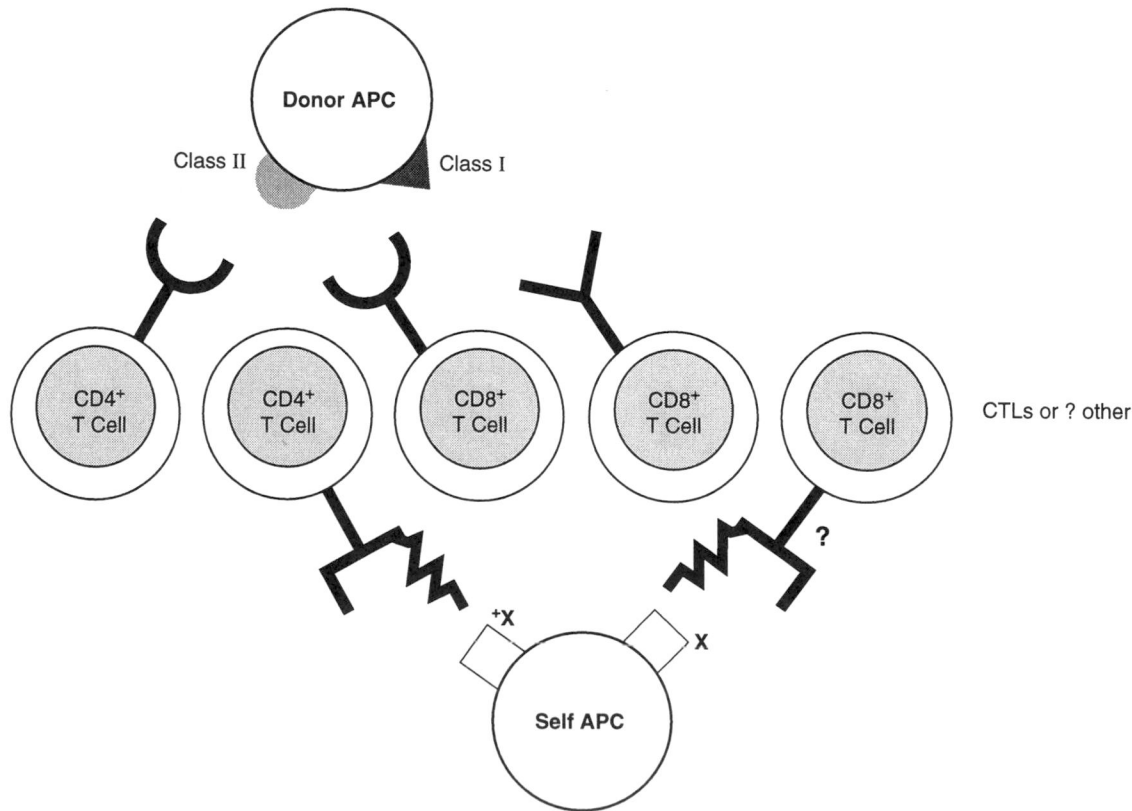

FIG. 10. Complex mode of T-cell effector pathways.

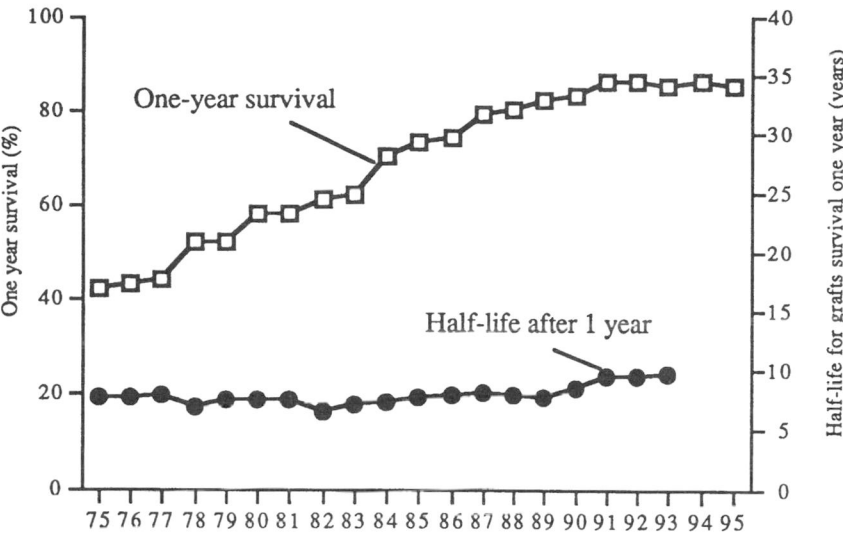

FIG. 11. One-year graft survival and chronic half-life over time for kidney transplants.

Although almost every type of organ transplant suffers from chronic rejection, the pathologic manifestations are different in each case. Kidney biopsies tend to show interstitial fibrosis along with arterial narrowing from hyalinization of the vessels. In the heart, the process is manifested principally as a diffuse myointimal hyperplasia proceeding to fibrosis of the coronary arteries that has often been referred to as accelerated atherosclerosis. Chronic rejection in lung transplants primarily affects the bronchioles with progressive narrowing of these structures and is referred to as bronchiolitis obliterans. The liver may be the one type of organ transplant that is relatively resistant to chronic rejection, but the progressive destruction of bile ducts referred to as the vanishing bile duct syndrome may be another manifestation of this process.

Some of the causes of chronic graft destruction may not be immunologic in origin (349,350). Potential factors that have been considered include the initial ischemic insult, the reduced mass of transplanted tissue (especially in the case of kidney transplants leading to hyperfiltration injury), the denervation of the transplanted organ, the hyperlipidemia and hypertension associated with immunosuppressive drugs, the immunosuppressive drugs themselves, and chronic viral injury. Nonetheless, although these factors undoubtedly contribute to the process, there is a marked difference in survival between syngeneic and allogeneic transplants in experimental models. In addition, native hearts in kidney transplant recipients do not show manifestations of chronic rejection and vice versa. Thus, there is almost certainly an important immunologic component in most cases of chronic rejection.

Several important observations regarding chronic rejection have emerged from clinical practice. First, the process is frequently associated with the presence of antidonor antibodies. This was first recognized in the case of kidney transplants when a high correlation was found between the presence of alloantibodies and the hyalinization of renal arteries on late biopsy specimens (351). The same correlation has been found for other organs as well (352). Second, the process of chronic rejection is usually refractory to increases in immunosuppressive therapy, in contrast to acute rejection episodes, which almost always respond to treatment. Third, there is a high correlation between the onset of chronic rejection and a history of early acute rejection episodes (353). Together these clinical observations have suggested to some that chronic rejection is the result of chronic B-cell alloantibody production. They have suggested to others that chronic rejection requires the early sensitization of the immune system to donor antigens. Both suggestions may be correct, but neither the logic nor the evidence fully supports these conclusions. In the first place, alloantibody production often reflects indirect T-cell sensitization; hence, it might equally well be a marker for other rejection mechanisms as opposed to a cause of chronic rejection. In addition, early rejection episodes probably reflect primarily the degree of antidonor immunoreactivity and may not themselves be required for chronic rejection. Therefore, even if sufficient immunosuppression were given to prevent acute rejection, chronic rejection still might occur when the suppression was reduced to levels tolerable over the long term, even if acute rejection had never occurred. Finally, experimental studies have suggested that the mechanisms of chronic rejection are not absolutely dependent on either antibody formation nor on the occurrence of acute rejection episodes (354,355).

The uncertainties that arise from the interpretation of the clinical data make it important to develop experimental models for studying the mechanisms of chronic rejection. However, it is difficult in the laboratory to mimic a process that may take 5 or 10 years to develop in patients treated with immunosuppressive drugs. Thus, the effort to study chronic rejection experimentally has depended on surrogate short-term pathologic markers that are thought to predict the long-term changes of chronic rejection. In particular, these studies have concentrated on the development of the myointimal proliferation that is thought to be the precursor of the chronic vascular changes typically observed in patients. Both in rodents and in pigs, this has often been done with heart transplants after an initial period of immunosuppression that prevents acute rejection (354). All of these experimental studies are subject to the caveat that the surrogate pathologic lesion occurs much earlier than the typical changes of chronic rejection in clinical patients. Thus, the process being studied experimentally may not be the same as the clinical process.

Pathologic Manifestations of Experimental Chronic Rejection

The typical pathologic features of the experimental lesion associated with chronic rejection are shown in Fig. 12 (356). The marked narrowing of the vascular lumen is caused by the substantial proliferation of endothelial and then smooth muscle cells. Associated with this proliferation is progressive destruction of the media. With further time, the cellular proliferation becomes less pronounced and is replaced by concentric fibrosis that narrows the vascular lumen. Immunohistologic staining indicates that there is increased expression of several adhesion molecules during the early manifestations of this process (354) and easily detectable levels of several cytokines and factors (357–361), including nitric oxide synthase (362), acidic fibroblast growth factor (363), insulin-like growth factor (364), and endothelin (365,366).

Immunologic Mechanisms of Chronic Rejection

With the availability of animal models, it has become possible to examine the immunologic mechanisms responsible for chronic rejection, using the same genetic modifications and manipulations of the recipient that have been useful in the studies of other rejection mechanisms. Studies in pigs have suggested that the vascular changes are more apt to develop when there are class I antigenic disparities than when there are only class II disparities and have suggested that the lesion depends especially on CD8$^+$ T cells (367). Mouse studies, however, have indicated that either CD4$^+$ or CD8$^+$ T cells can produce the lesion and that either class I or class II antigenic disparities are sufficient to stimulate chronic rejection (368). The finding that class II antigenic disparities are themselves sufficient is especially important because in mice these antigens are not expressed on the vascular endothelium, indicating that the lesion can develop even when a target antigen is not expressed on the cell type that shows the most striking proliferation (354). In keeping with the prediction of many clinical studies, adoptive transfer

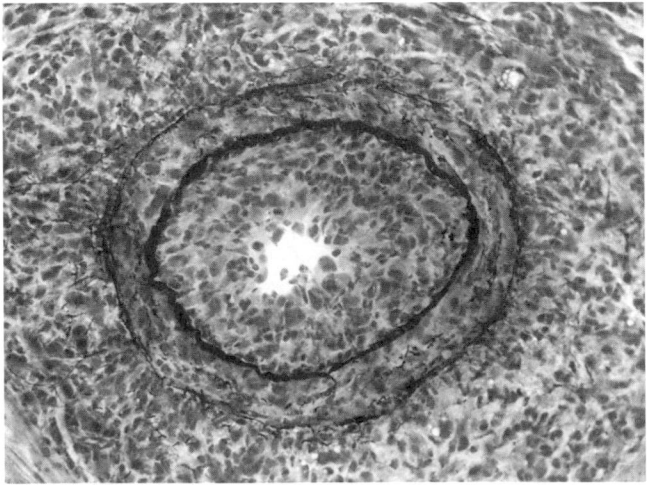

FIG. 12. Moderately advanced (stage 3) arterial lesion in an experimental form of chronic rejection, showing marked cellular expansion of the intima, luminal stenosis, and a prominent adventitial infiltrate that invades the media. B10.A to B10.BR mouse heart transplant on day 56, × 200, elastic tissue stain. Reprinted with permission (354).

experiments into SCID mice have shown that alloantibodies in the absence of T cells can induce the typical pathologic vascular changes (369). However, T cells without B cells also have been shown to cause the lesion, although there may be somewhat less tendency to progress to end-stage fibrosis (355). Several studies have indicated that the induction of donor-specific tolerance can prevent the development of the vascular changes of chronic rejection, although not all of the short-term manipulations that have been effective in preventing acute rejection have necessarily prevented the later onset of chronic rejection.

From these data, it is difficult to determine a single immunologic mechanism that is the cause of chronic rejection. Probably, the process represents the manifestation of chronic injury from many different types of ongoing immune response and that the particular manifestation of this injury depends on the organ involved. In most cases, the injury is reflected in the vascular changes described above, but in the case of the lung or the liver, chronic injury may cause changes most prominently in the bronchioles or the bile ducts. Because it is assumed that stimulation of direct immune responses is likely to diminish over time as donor APCs are replaced by recipient APCs, it is commonly assumed that the predominant immune response that causes chronic rejection occurs through the indirect pathway. However, there is no evidence at this time to support this assumption.

PHYSIOLOGIC INTERACTIONS REGULATING GRAFT REJECTION

The preceding sections have described the interactions between donor antigens and the recipient immune system that lead to graft rejection. This section addresses the regulatory elements that control this process. Because the regulation of complement and endothelial activation already have been described in the sections on humoral mechanisms of rejection, this discussion will concentrate on the regulation of T-cell responses. First, we consider the process of T-cell sensitization, then we consider the interactions required between sensitized helper and effector cells, and finally we consider the regulation of effector cell activity.

Regulation of Sensitization

Tissue Damage and Inflammatory Signals

Although it is possible for T-cell sensitization to occur in the presence of resting dendritic cells, many types of APCs require activation before they gain full APC function. For this reason, and also because of changes in adhesion molecule expression and cell trafficking, one of the important elements controlling T-cell sensitization is the release of inflammatory cytokines, such as IFN-γ, with its potent ability to activate macrophages (370). Tissue injury from any source is an important stimulus for releasing such cytokines; thus, the concept that a danger signal helps regulate graft rejection is important in transplantation immunology (371). All forms of transplantation involve ischemic and traumatic injury to the donor tissue, which may be one of the reasons that rejection episodes occur most frequently early after transplantation. In addition, later nonimmunologic inflammation, either occurring in the transplanted organ or perhaps elsewhere in the body, may trigger late rejection episodes. On the other hand, it would be wrong to picture the role of nonspecific danger signals as the dominant feature controlling graft rejection. For example, skin transplants placed on SCID recipients can be allowed to heal for long periods before immunologic reconstitution of the recipients, but rejection always occurs when this is done. Similarly, even achieving organ transplant survival for many years in clinical practice is rarely sufficient to allow the cessation of immunosuppression. Thus, it is better to picture the antigenic disparity and the recipient's immunoresponsiveness as the dominant features controlling graft rejection, while danger signals may influence the timing, intensity, or character of the immune response.

Costimulatory Signals Involved in T-Cell Activation

The special features of APCs involve not only their ability to present foreign antigens on their surface but also to provide additional signals for T-cell activation. This second component of T-cell activation is often referred to as the "second signal", although it more likely involves several different elements (372–375). The likely components of the second signal include the lymphokines secreted by APCs, including IL-1, and signals transmitted after binding of T-cell accessory molecules with their ligands on APCs. These include the interaction of CD4 or CD8 with monomorphic determinants on MHC antigens, LFA-1 with ICAM-1, 2, or 3, CD2 with LFA-3 (CD48), CD40 with CD40 ligand, CD28 with B7.1 and B7.2, and the function of 4-1BB. In addition, lymphokines secreted by T cells, such as IL-2, may further contribute to the second signal for both themselves and other cell populations (376–378).

An important feature of the second signal is that in the absence of some or all of its components, T cells stimulated through their antigen receptor may be anergized (as discussed below in the section on tolerance induction). Because many of the cells of a transplanted organ are not APCs, the induction of anergy would seem likely to be initiated after every organ transplant, a process that is in competition with the activation events stimulated by APCs. Early after transplantation, this competition probably favors APC activation because allograft rejection is almost universal, but the stimuli may be more evenly balanced months or years after transplantation when the donor APCs have mostly been replaced.

Downregulating Signals Following T-Cell Activation

It has become increasingly apparent in recent years that cell-mediated immune responses are controlled by downregulating interactions, such as by the ligation of CTLA-4 and by the interaction between Fas and Fas ligand (379–381). In transplantation, there is evidence that high levels of expression of Fas ligand on some or all of the cells of donor tissue may prevent rejection (382) and that Fas ligand may be partly responsible for lack of rejection when tissues are transplanted to some privileged sites, such as the testis or the anterior chamber of the eye (382). These findings suggest that a promising approach for preventing rejection might be to manipulate these molecular interactions (381). However, our understanding of these downregulating signals is not adequate at this time to generate effective strategies for this purpose. For example, overexpression of Fas ligand in pancreatic islets has tended to make them more susceptible to destruction rather than to provide them with protection from rejection, and CD28 knock-out mice have been found to reject allografts, despite unopposed signaling through CTLA-4 (383). It is likely, however, that a better understanding of the downregulating events controlling immune

responses will provide new approaches for preventing graft rejection in years to come.

Regulatory Cytokines

Many cytokines play a role in the regulation of graft rejection. However, because almost none of the cytokine or cytokine receptor knock-out mice have demonstrated a defective phenotype for graft rejection, it is impossible to describe more precisely which cytokines provide particular regulatory functions. It is usually assumed that IL-2 is important as a helper cytokine for effector T cells, but its role can apparently be performed by other molecules (377). IFN-γ is thought to play a role in activating other cells in the process of graft destruction and in upregulating the expression of antigens, especially on donor vascular endothelium (384). However, graft rejection also occurs rapidly on the IFN-γ knock-out mice (385,386). Several studies with antiinflammatory cytokines, such as IL-10 or transforming growth factor (TGF)-β, suggest that these may modify the process of graft destruction (387–389), whereas proinflammatory cytokines such as TNF-α are thought to enhance the process (361). On the other hand, IL-10 can enhance cytolytic mechanisms of islet graft rejection (390). Studies of tolerance induction have suggested that in some cases shifts in the balance of Th1 and Th2 cytokines may be important in determining graft rejection versus acceptance (391). However, the difference in outcome based on Th1 versus Th2 production is far from clear, as will be discussed further below (392–397). Thus, although cytokines are undoubtedly of enormous importance in causing and regulating the processes of graft rejection, our understanding of their role is poor at this time.

The Presence of the Transplanted Organ

Although early rejection episodes occur with most types of organ transplants, there are some exceptions to this rule. Kidney and liver transplants in mice can survive for long periods without immunosuppression even with MHC disparities (398–400), and there have been cases of prolonged liver transplant survival in pigs without immunosuppression (401). In addition, many types of rodent transplants, such as mouse heart transplants, require only a short course of immunosuppression to achieve prolonged survival (402,403). Furthermore, in the experimental animal studies, the long survival of these transplanted organs often diminishes, or even prevents, the subsequent rejection of antigenically identical skin grafts that would have been rejected rapidly by naive animals (398,404). Even in clinical transplantation it appears that the long survival of a transplanted organ may diminish the rejection response because much less immunosuppression is required late after transplantation than in the early period. Thus, there is substantial evidence that the mere survival of a transplanted organ generates a powerful regulating force that inhibits the specific anti-donor immune response.

As discussed below, the induction of anergy, as donor grafts lose their APCs, is one possible mechanism by which this might occur. However, it is also possible that downregulating signals from the allograft, even potentially from allogeneic APCs, or that changes in cytokine production contribute to the inhibition of graft rejection caused by the persistent survival of the organ.

There are two important features to emphasize regarding the capacity of transplanted organs to regulate their own survival. First, their capacity to do so often confuses the results of experimental studies designed to test tolerance-inducing strategies. For example, it is frequently reported that a particular form of immunosuppression induces tolerance when provided at the time of murine cardiac transplantation. Although the result may be accurate, the conclusion that the form of immunosuppression used leads to tolerance is not justified. The long survival of the transplanted heart, rather than the immunosuppression that achieved it, may be responsible for the tolerant condition. This issue can be tested by removing the transplanted organ to see if tolerance persists, or by testing the particular form of immunosuppression with other types of antigenic challenge from the donor. Second, it is important to understand that the processes that downregulate graft rejection as a result of long-term graft survival may be inhibited by the standard forms of immunosuppression that are used clinically to achieve excellent graft survival (405). This is probably because many of the standard immunosuppressive drugs inhibit T-cell signaling and therefore inhibit active processes of tolerance induction. In other words, if T cells never learn that they have encountered donor antigens, they may not generate donor-specific mechanisms that inhibit graft rejection.

Communication Between Helper and Effector Cells

APCs play a role in regulating immune responses by serving as the focus for the interaction between helper and effector cells.

A Three-Cell Model of Helper and Effector Cell Interactions

An important tenet of fundamental immunology is that the cell–cell interactions that generate an immune response generally require intimate contact between the individual cells involved. Mitchison demonstrated this principle in studies of the T–B collaborations leading to antibody production. He showed that T cells, B cells, and the APCs that stimulate them must join together in a three-cell cluster to achieve effective collaboration between the helper T cells and effector B cells (406). Findings such as these have led to the concept that the lymphokines involved in helper function tend to function like neurotransmitters, working only between two closely spaced cells, rather than as hormones acting over large distances (407–409).

In addition to Mitchison, others have performed experiments suggesting that the three-cell cluster model also applies to the interactions between helper T cells, effector T cells, and APCs involved in graft rejection (146,215,410,411). For example, tail skin grafts from class I mutant mice (bm7) placed on B6 recipients are not rejected, apparently because of a lack of helper stimulation. On the other hand, grafts from (bm12 × bm7) F1 mice, which express an additional class II antigen disparity, are rejected. A bm12 graft on one side of a B6 mouse, although itself rejected, does not induce the rejection of a bm7 graft on the other side of the same animal, whereas a (bm12 × bm7) F1 graft on one side of a recipient does induce rejection of a bm7 graft on the other side. These results suggest that the helper factors elicited during rejection of a bm12 graft cannot function elsewhere in the body to assist potential effector cells specific for the bm7 graft. On the other hand, when both the bm12 and bm7 antigens are expressed on the same graft, and therefore on the same APCs, effector cells are generated that can function elsewhere in the body. As diagrammed in Fig. 13, it appears that the helper cells, effector cells, and stimulat-

ing APCs must join together in a three-cell cluster to allow efficient helper function for graft rejection (150,412). An attractive feature of the three-cell model is that it provides a mechanism for regulating the availability of help. Responses occurring elsewhere in the body, perhaps stimulated by environmental pathogens, will not generally initiate an immune response to the donor graft.

T-Cell Help for B-Cell Alloantibody Production

T-cell help for B-cell alloantibody production is an example in which several cell populations need to interact to achieve an immune response. Although it is commonly assumed that the B-cell production of antibodies to protein (usually MHC) antigens involves first the production of IgM antibodies, in a T cell–independent process, and later the conversion to IgG antibodies, requiring T-cell help, studies of alloantibody production, at least after skin graft rejection, have actually suggested that even the initial IgM response also depends on CD4$^+$ T cells (149). However, there are two potential pathways by which CD4$^+$ T cells might provide help for alloreactive B cells (413). First, as diagrammed in Fig. 14 on page 1216, recipient CD4$^+$ helper cells might recognize donor class II antigens directly, whereas recipient B cells recognize donor class I MHC antigens. Alternatively, recipient CD4$^+$ cells might recognize donor peptides presented by recipient APCs through the indirect pathway and then provide help to recipient B cells that recognize donor antigens directly. In the first case, the T and B cells would be in close physical association, but in the second case the T cells would interact with the B cells even more intimately, through their recognition of the B cell's class II antigens presenting donor peptides. Experiments to examine these two possibilities have been performed using class II knock-out mice as either donors or recipients and then testing alloantibody production (414). The results have indicated that there are two levels of help that can be provided by CD4$^+$ T cells for B cells. First, the help provided by T cells brought into physical association with B cells through the direct pathway allows B-cell IgM production. Second, the help provided by T cells sensitized indirectly allows B cells to produce IgM antibodies and to convert from IgM to IgG production. In addition to indicating the importance of the indirect pathway in this form of T-cell helper sensitization, these results also suggest that the conversion to IgG alloantibody production can be used as a marker to demonstrate that indirect sensitization of CD4$^+$ T cells has occurred (415–417).

Can a Four-Cell Cluster Activate Effector T Cells?

It is easy to picture how donor APCs, stimulating T-cell responses through direct presentation, provide the focus for a three-cell interaction during T cell–mediated graft rejection because donor APCs can express both the helper determinants and the effector determinants necessary to bring the two T-cell populations together. On the other hand, when the indirect pathway for helper sensitization is considered, recipient APCs will not necessarily express donor MHC antigens and therefore will not generally express the same effector determinants that are present in the graft. Therefore, if an indirect helper response is to generate effector cells that recognize donor antigens directly, CD4$^+$ cells stimulated by recipient APCs would have to provide help for CD8$^+$ cells that would be sensitized by donor APCs. The three-cell model would not predict that productive helper–effector communication would occur under these circumstances. Nonetheless, although the evidence is clear that APCs from one graft and APCs from a second

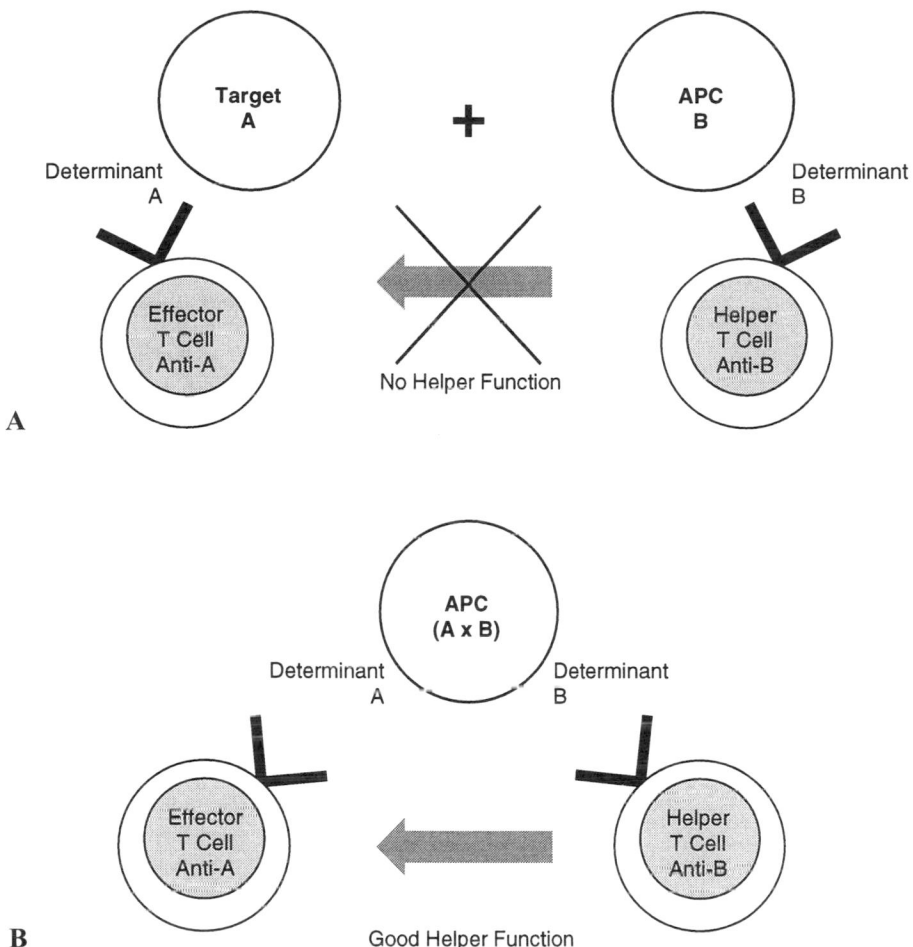

FIG. 13. The three-cell cluster model of sensitization. **A:** Two populations of APCs *in vivo* cannot stimulate help for each other's determinants. **B:** One population of APCs can stimulated help for the different determinants expressed by that population.

graft cannot work together, there is evidence that APCs from a graft and APCs from the recipient can join in a four-cell cluster with helper and effector cells to initiate graft rejection (227,418).

Effector Cell Regulation

The third level of regulatory interactions in graft rejection involves the effector cells after they have been sensitized by contact with donor antigens and been augmented by activated helper cells. Once activated, the effector cells appear capable of functioning anywhere in a recipient where they encounter donor antigens, in contrast to the limited range of helper function (112,419 422). Nonetheless, the function of effector T cells is controlled by regulation of the trafficking of the effector cells and by the accessory molecules involved in the interaction of effector cells with their target cells.

Adhesion Molecules Regulate Effector Cell Trafficking

The regulation of lymphoid cell trafficking by adhesion molecules is one of the expanding areas of fundamental immunology

(see Chapter 14). A key feature of this regulation is that naive T cells are kept within lymphatic tissues and that only activated or memory T cells are allowed to circulate into peripheral tissues. This pattern is controlled through the expression of L-selectin and other adhesion molecules expressed by naive T cells that keep them in the lymphatic circulation (423). Activated cells lose this expression and are free to circulate more widely (138).

In addition to allowing activated cells out of lymphatic tissue, adhesion molecules control the entry of cells into foreign tissues. Inflammation alters the trafficking patterns of lymphoid cells through the expression of ICAM-1, ELAM, VCAM-1, and perhaps other adhesion molecules expressed on vascular endothelium (424–427). These molecules bind lymphoid cells, polymorphonuclear lymphocytes, and macrophages to sites of inflammation by halting their passage within vessels and stimulating the transmigration of these cells across the vascular endothelium The expression of these adhesion molecules changes over time in response to various cytokines and other factors (308,424,425,428).

The cellular infiltrate associated with graft rejection is a special case of inflammation, and recent studies have investigated the unique features associated with allogeneic compared with syngeneic grafts (429). Both types of grafts show a cellular infiltrate during the first

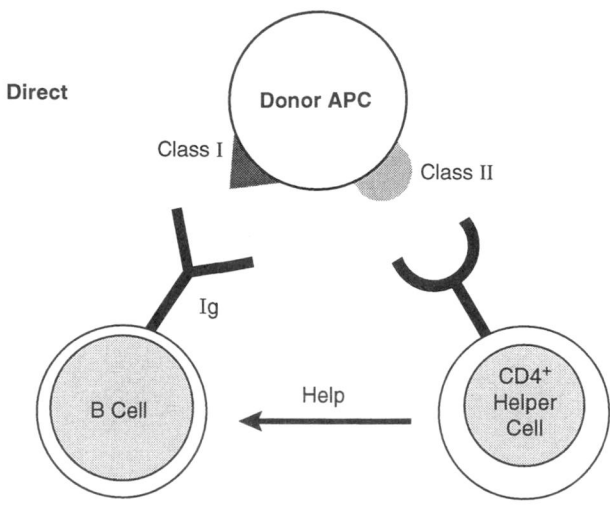

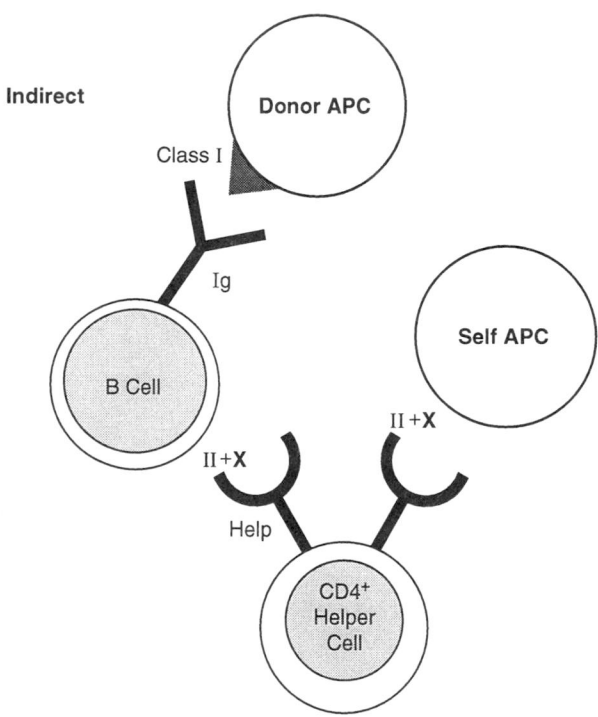

FIG. 14. T-cell help for B-cell alloantibody production.

several days following transplantation, and both types express ICAMs and ELAMs. By about the fourth day after transplantation, however, allografts can be distinguished from syngeneic grafts by the expression of VCAM-1 and by the appearance of IL-2, IL-4, and IFN-γ (430). Further studies of this type may help to elucidate the regulatory elements of effector cell function in graft rejection.

Target Cell Accessory Molecules and Effector Cell Function

In addition to altering cell trafficking, cell surface molecules are important in controlling the interaction of effector T cells with their targets. The T-cell antigen receptor and CD3 proteins are naturally critical in this interaction. The CD4 and CD8 coreceptors, which bind to monomorphic determinants on MHC antigens, also are important (431), as is the interaction of ICAM-1 with LFA-1 (432). Of course these same molecules are also involved in the early stages of T-cell sensitization, but their additional role at the effector stage suggests that interruption of these interactions may alter graft rejection even after T cells have been activated (433,434).

MANIPULATIONS TO PREVENT GRAFT REJECTION

The importance of transplantation immunology lies ultimately in the application of its principles to clinical transplantation. Thus, the critical issue is to determine how the components and regulatory interactions involved in graft rejection might be manipulated to allow graft acceptance. One level of immunosuppression involves nonspecific approaches, reducing the overall immunocompetence of the recipient to all foreign antigens, and the second level seeks to prevent responses only to the antigens of a particular donor. Ultimately the goal is to achieve tolerance, which is lasting donor-specific nonresponsiveness.

Nonspecific Techniques

Standard Drugs

It is beyond the scope of this chapter to review the pharmacology of the nonspecific immunosuppressive drugs commonly used in clinical transplantation. It is important to acknowledge, however, that the major advances in clinical transplantation have been made possible largely by such agents. Most recipients of allogeneic organs receive exogenous immunosuppression in the form of steroids, azathioprine, mycophenolate, cyclosporine, or FK-506. In general terms, both standard and experimental immunosuppressive drugs suppress immune responses by inhibiting lymphocyte gene transcription (e.g., cyclosporine, FK-506), cytokine signal transduction (rapamycin, leflunomide), nucleotide synthesis (e.g., azathioprine, mycophenolate mofetil), or differentiation (15-deoxyspergualin).

Corticosteroids have pleiotropic effects, including inhibition of T-cell proliferation and cytokine gene transcription (435). Azathioprine is an analog of 6-mercaptopurine that acts by inhibiting purine metabolism so as to block cell division. Mycophenolate mofetil is a prodrug of the active metabolite mycophenolic acid, which is related to azathioprine in its inhibition of purine synthesis. Its effect is limited, however, to the enzymatic pathways involved in lymphocyte proliferation, theoretically allowing normal development of other hematopoietic elements. However, significant side effects, including leukopenia, were observed in double-blind randomized trials comparing mycophenolate to azathioprine in renal allograft recipients. A significant reduction in rejection episodes, without any overall effect on early graft survival, was observed in the mycophenolate groups in these trials (436,437). Cyclosporine blocks the generation of IL-2 by T cells and thereby prevents sensitization (438–440). The discovery of cyclosporine played a major role in making cardiac and liver allo-transplantation feasible, and it has become a mainstay of many immunosuppressive regimens. The complex of cyclosporine and its cytoplasmic receptor cyclophilin binds to and blocks the phosphatase activity of calcineurin, which is an intracellular signaling protein that is essential for transcriptional activation of the IL-2 gene. FK-506 is a macrolide that binds to a member of the intracellular FK-506 binding protein (FKBP) family of intracellular receptors. The FK-506–FKBP12 complex binds to and inactivates calcineurin, and thus has effects quite similar to those of cyclosporine (441).

In addition to the standard drugs for clinical transplantation, several other drugs are sometimes used. Cyclophosphamide is roughly equivalent to azathioprine in its effects at the doses used in transplantation. It is sometimes substituted for azathioprine to avoid particular side effects or with the hope of controlling B-cell responses. Prostaglandin E1 has been found to be immunosuppressive in some experimental models, and it may reduce some of the toxicities associated with other agents. Actinomycin D inhibits bone marrow function and is used occasionally.

Experimental Drugs

The list of standard drugs will almost certainly be modified in the near future by the addition of drugs that are now considered experimental. Rapamycin is a macrocyclic triene antibiotic somewhat analogous to FK-506 (442). Despite binding to the same intracellular binding protein (FKBP12) as FK506, the FKBP12–rapamycin complex does not block calcineurin activity. Instead, rapamycin has a different ultimate target protein known as the mammalian target of rapamycin, and it inhibits T-cell proliferation by blocking signal transduction mediated by IL-2 and other cytokines, not by inhibiting IL-2 production (442). Rapamycin has proved to be a potent immunosuppressive agent in animal studies, although it is not without significant toxicity (442). It is currently being evaluated in clinical trials in combination with other immunosuppressive agents. 15-Deoxyspergualin is a distinctly different agent that has no effect on IL-2 production or utilization (443). It appears to prevent activated T and B cells from differentiating into mature effector cells. It is currently under clinical evaluation for rejection crises and for prophylaxis in highly sensitized patients. Leflunomide is an orally bioavailable prodrug that is converted to the active metabolite A77 1726, which has shown promise in treating acute and chronic rejection in animal models. It prevents lymphocyte proliferation both by inhibiting *de novo* pyrimidine synthesis and by inhibiting the activity of tyrosine kinases associated with cytokine receptors. Leflunomide also can prevent smooth muscle proliferation, and hence may be beneficial in preventing graft vasculopathy (435). Leflunomide has not only prolonged allo- and xenograft survival but also has prevented the production of antidonor antibodies in animal models (444,445).

Anti–T Cell Antibodies

Another form of nonspecific immunosuppressive therapy used both clinically and experimentally is that achieved with antibodies specific for T cells of the recipient. Originally anti–T cell antibodies were obtained from heterologous antisera prepared against lymphocytes or thymocytes of the recipient species (ATG or ALS) (446,447). These powerful immunosuppressants are still used in some induction regimens and for the treatment of rejection episodes. Their major side effects include serum sickness and infectious complications. More recently, monoclonal antibodies (mAbs) such as OKT3, a mouse antibody directed against the CD3

antigen of humans, has become widely used in clinical transplantation (148). Like polyclonal sera, OKT3 is highly efficacious in reversing rejection episodes and is also used in many centers in the first week or two posttransplant to prevent rejection episodes. Other pan–T cell antibodies have been used in clinical trials, including CAMPATH-1, T-12, CBL1, and BTI-322, but none has yet proven more effective than OKT3.

Numerous experimental studies and a few clinical trials have explored the use of monoclonal anti–T cell antibodies that are more selective for subpopulations of T cells (448–451). Subset-specific antibodies such as those recognizing CD4 or CD8 have helped define the pathways of alloreactivity in animal models, but it is unclear whether knowledge of these pathways could be used to predict accurately which antibodies will be effective clinically and under what circumstances. Monoclonal antibodies to the α chain of the IL-2 receptor (CD25) have been evaluated in an effort to achieve greater antigen specificity with anti–T cell antibodies (452–456). Because CD25 is only transiently expressed when T cells are activated, such therapy might selectively eliminate only those T cells activated at the time of allogeneic challenge. Although clinical results with rodent anti-CD25 antibodies were disappointing, more recent studies suggest that humanized versions of anti-CD25 antibodies are more efficacious (457).

Monoclonal antibodies also have been used to block the effector mechanism of graft rejection. Anti-ICAM antibodies are immunosuppressive in monkeys and may function at the effector stage (434), and anti-TNF antibodies also have been tested experimentally. Agents that suppress T-cell costimulation via CD28 or CD40 ligand and anti-CD2 mAbs have shown promise, particularly when given in combination in animal models (458–460), and they are likely to be clinically evaluated in the near future.

Although mAb therapy has been extremely effective (461,462), several problems still exist. First, the interaction of the mAb OKT3 with the CD3 antigen initially activates T cells, stimulating release of several lymphokines, before the target cells are depleted (463). Some of these lymphokines, including TNF-α, can cause significant clinical side effects, including fever, chills, and pulmonary edema. These side effects usually can be well controlled and are seldom life threatening. Second, OKT3 and many of the mAbs that have been evaluated in humans are mouse proteins. When these are injected, human recipients generally respond in time with antibody production against both constant region and idiotypic determinants of the mAb (462). These antibody responses may hinder both repeated courses of therapy with the original antibody and treatment with other mAbs of different specificity, although higher dose therapy can usually overcome a recipient's antibody response. Third, mAb therapy may not always eliminate the target T-cell population. For example, during OKT3 treatment, cells of T-cell lineage expressing CD4 and CD8 antigens, but without the CD3 antigen, usually return to the circulation. This phenomenon is referred to as modulation of the target antigen (461). In the case of OKT3, the absence of the CD3 surface structure renders T cells immunologically incompetent (464). The loss of other surface antigens, however, may not be as immunosuppressive. Finally, OKT3 provides broad, nonspecific immunosuppression that renders the recipient significantly immunoincompetent. Although OKT3 does not cause permanent nonresponsiveness to environmental antigens, unfortunately neither does it achieve permanent tolerance to the antigens of the graft.

Many of the difficulties associated with mAb therapy are associated with the constant region of the antibody. For example, T-cell activation does not occur when F(ab)'2 antibodies are used, and antiantibody responses by the recipient are much weaker in the absence of the constant region (465). Considerable effort has therefore been devoted to engineering ideal therapeutic antibodies. One approach has been to construct chimeric mouse antibodies with human Fc portions, or to graft the hypervariable (CDR3) component of a murine antibody to an otherwise human molecule. This latter process is known as humanizing an mAb from another species. Another promising approach has been to couple toxic elements, such as ricin or diphtheria toxin, to the antibody (466,467).

Donor-Specific Tolerance Induction

The Need for Tolerance-Inducing Regimens

Specific immunosuppression in transplantation immunology involves suppression of the immune response to donor allo- or xenoantigens but not to other antigens. The ultimate form of specific unresponsiveness is tolerance, in which the donor-specific nonresponsiveness is maintained permanently without further treatment. The achievement of transplantation tolerance has been the goal of transplantation immunology for over 40 years, for three major reasons. First, although improvements in immunosuppressive therapy have dramatically increased the success of clinical organ transplantation, these drugs are associated with life-long increased risks of infection and malignancy. Chronic drug treatment would not be required in tolerant recipients. Second, despite improved immunosuppression, chronic rejection is still a major problem and leads to constantly downsloping long-term survival curves for organ allografts. Chronic rejection would not occur in tolerant recipients. Third, a critical shortage of allogeneic organs has increased interest in the use of other species as xenogeneic donors. However, immune barriers to xenografts may be even greater than those to allografts (468), and the induction of both B-cell and T-cell tolerance may be essential to the ultimate success of xenotransplantation.

Central and Peripheral Tolerance

Other chapters in this book describe the mechanisms by which tolerance to self antigens is achieved (see Chapter 20). For developing T cells, these processes take place in the thymus, which is the central organ for T-cell development. Hence, induction of tolerance among developing thymocytes is referred to as "central," as distinguished from the peripheral tolerance that may develop among already mature T cells when they encounter antigen in the peripheral tissues.

B cells are also susceptible to tolerance induction by several mechanisms during development in the marrow. However, unlike T cells, the term "central tolerance" is not generally used in this context, largely because the marrow, the major organ for B-lymphopoiesis in mammals, is not dedicated exclusively to this activity.

Mechanisms of Transplantation Tolerance

The known mechanisms for inducing T- and B-cell tolerance can be grouped into the categories deletion, anergy, and suppression. In addition, a graft may simply be ignored by recipient lymphocytes. Each of these mechanisms will be described briefly below, and then particular strategies designed to capture these mechanisms to alter transplantation tolerance will be discussed.

Clonal Deletion

Recent studies have demonstrated that a major mechanism by which self tolerance normally develops among both B and T cells is deletion of developing lymphocyte with specificity for self antigens.

Studies using Ig receptor transgenic mice suggest that B cells are susceptible to deletion at particular stages of development upon recognition of membrane-bound antigen (469). Antigen expression on either radioresistant host cells or on a small population of hematopoietic cells appears to be sufficient to delete immature B cells specific for that antigen (470). Cells of the B1 subset, which are thought to be the major source of the natural antibodies responsible for xenograft hyperacute rejection, can be deleted by an apoptotic process in mice when their surface Ig is cross-linked by cell-bound antigen (471).

Deletion of self-reactive T cells is believed to occur when the avidity of an interaction between an immature thymocyte and an APC in the thymus is sufficiently high to induce apoptotic cell death (472,473). This high avidity is often due, at least in part, to a relatively high-affinity interaction between a rearranged TCR and a self peptide–MHC complex presented in the thymus. Several marrow-derived cell types, including dendritic cells (474), B cells (475), and thymocytes (476,477), as well as nonhematopoietic cells of the thymic stroma (371,478,479), have the capacity to induce intrathymic tolerance by both deletional and nondeletional mechanisms. Tolerance induced by intrathymic deletion should be reliable because the absence of lymphocytes with reactivity to the donor would ensure that a specific response to donor antigens could not be induced under any circumstances.

Peripheral deletion also has been described for mature T cells upon exposure to antigen in vivo (480–482). In addition, veto cells can delete alloreactive CTL precursors (CTLp).

Anergy

Anergy is another consequence that may result when T cells recognize peptide–MHC complexes, but without receiving adequate accessory or costimulatory signals. A lymphocyte is considered to be anergic if it cannot respond to APCs expressing the antigen for which it is specific. Frequently, in the case of T cells, the anergic state is associated with a lack of IL-2 production and can be overcome by providing exogenous IL-2 (373). Numerous methods of inducing T- and B-cell anergy have been described (469,483–486). In some cases anergy has been associated with TCR or Ig receptor downregulation (469,482,487–489). In the case of B-cell tolerance, the induction of anergy versus activation may be dependent on antigen concentration (469). T cells typically become anergic if they encounter antigen without costimulation, but they also may undergo anergy if they encounter peptide ligands for which they have low affinity (472,473). It appears that thymocytes (in addition to mature peripheral T cells) are also susceptible to anergy induction, particularly by antigens presented on thymic epithelium or dendritic cells (475). Anergy is generally reversible in vivo and can be overcome by infection (490) or by removal of antigen (491,492).

Suppression

A potential form of antibody-mediated suppression might be through the recognition of idiotypes of antidonor receptors. Idiotypes are unique antigenic determinants that characterize the binding sites of antibody or T-cell receptors and can therefore be detected by antiidiotypic antibodies (493,494). In the case of transplantation responses, such antiidiotypic reagents might have the potential to specifically modify responses to subsequent transplants. For this reason, the antiidiotype approach to specific immunosuppression has received considerable attention in the past. We now know, however, that the determinants recognized by B cells and the genes encoding B-cell receptors are different from those involved in T-cell responses. Thus, it is unlikely that cellular immunity can be modified by antiidiotypic reagents raised against B cells. It continues to be an intriguing question whether normal regulatory mechanisms for B-cell responses might include antiidiotypes, as suggested by Jerne. However, efforts to control transplantation using exogenous antiidiotypic antibodies to either T- or B-cell receptors have been disappointing (495).

Antibodies also can induce tolerance through a process known as enhancement. Enhancement is defined as prolongation of graft survival achieved by the presence of antigraft antibodies (496). This phenomenon was first described in experiments involving allogeneic tumor growth (497). Subsequently, Stuart et al. (498) and Batchelor (499) demonstrated that enhancing regimens using anti-MHC antibodies or soluble antigen could produce long-term tolerance for rodent allogeneic kidney transplants (500). The simple interpretation was that anti-MHC antibodies bind to the antigen and thereby block the immune response, but this explanation has not turned out to be sufficient. For example, tolerance after enhancement can be transferred by cells and not serum from enhanced recipients. Apparently, the administered antibody sets up a host reaction that leads to specific immunosuppression. An idiotype antiidiotype network would be an attractive explanation for this phenomenon. Unfortunately, the spectacular success obtained using enhancement for kidney graft survival in rats has not been observed for grafts in other species.

Another form of suppression promoting graft acceptance may be mediated by cell populations. Suppression of T-cell responses has been attributed to both T cells and non–T cells, and may show varying degrees of specificity. In some instances, nonspecific suppressive effector molecules may be secreted in response to a specific antigenic stimulus, thus conferring apparent specificity. In the ensuing discussion, we categorize mechanisms of suppression in terms of the degree of specificity of their ability to suppress transplant rejection.

Nonspecific Suppression. Nonspecific suppression can result from secretion by cells, in a non–antigen-specific manner, of soluble molecules that downmodulate immune function, such as cytokines (501,502), nitric oxide (503,504), and prostaglandins (505,506). Nonspecific suppressive cell populations such as natural suppressor (NS) cells may mediate suppression, at least in part, via soluble mediators (507–511). Obviously, nonspecific suppressive mechanisms would only be of interest for tolerance induction if they could be induced temporarily during a critical period when alloreactivity was present. In the absence of mechanisms for ensuring specific tolerance, nonspecific suppressive cells offer no advantage over other nonspecific immunosuppressive therapies. Facilitation of specific suppressor cell development by nonspecific, phenotypically null natural suppressor cells has been described (512–514).

Veto Activity. Veto activity, which is the ability to inactivate CTLp reacting against alloantigens expressed on the surface of the veto cell (515,516), confers suppression of CTL responses directed against any antigens shared by the veto cell. CTLs themselves (517), as well as activated NK cells (518) and poorly characterized cell types in hematopoietic tissues (515), have been found to have veto activity. Although the mechanism of vetoing is poorly understood, in some instances it may involve signaling through the MHC class I molecule of the CTLp upon ligation by CD8 expressed on the veto cells (519–521). However, not all veto cells express CD8, so this mechanism cannot explain all veto phenomena. Veto activity has been suggested to involve the immunosuppressive cytokine TGF-β (501).

Antigen-Specific Suppression. Although functional evidence for the existence of alloantigen-specific suppressor cells has been obtained in several transplantation models (450,522–529), such cells have been cloned in only a few instances (530), and suppressor cell–specific surface markers have not been identified. In addition, mechanisms of specific suppression of alloreactivity have not been well characterized. In several instances, antiidiotypic T-cell recognition by other T cells has been implicated in mediating specific suppression of graft rejection or graft-versus-host responses (523,526,529).

It is possible that some antigen-specific suppressive phenomena might be explained by the recently described dichotomy of T-helper cell function (531). A shift to the IL-4– and IL-10–producing T-helper type 2 (Th2) type of response from a proinflammatory Th1 (IL-2– and IFN-γ–producing) response has been associated with allograft acceptance (532–537). Because Th1 and Th2 responses mutually downregulate one another, these observations have led to the hypothesis that Th2 responses are tolerogenic. Th2 responses may influence APCs in a manner that prevents them from providing costimulation that could cause naive T cells to differentiate into Th1 cells. Thus, the APC might serve as an important intermediary for this and other infectious forms of tolerance. For practical purposes, an immune response that is nondestructive and inhibits the development of destructive responses could provide a powerful means of ensuring graft acceptance. However, most of the data merely demonstrate an association of Th2-dominant responses with graft acceptance, and only limited data exist to implicate an active role for Th2 cells in tolerance induction (538,539). It is clear that Th2 responses are not always benign because Th2 cells and Th2-associated cytokines can mediate or contribute to allograft rejection (540–543). It has recently been suggested that the xenograft reaction in at least one species combination is associated with a predominant Th2-type response (544). However, Th2-associated cytokines also have been detected in accepted xenografts in which accommodation had occurred (146). Furthermore, the Th1/Th2 dichotomy of cytokine production is not always clear-cut, and future studies are likely to better clarify the role of individual cytokines in inducing graft acceptance and rejection. Recently, a subset of murine and human CD4+ cells that produces IL-10 but not IL-4 has been reported to suppress *in vitro* responses as well as inflammatory bowel disease *in vivo* (545).

Lymphocytes Ignoring Graft Antigens (Ignorance)

Experimental situations have been described in which antigens are ignored by T cells (489,546,547) or B cells (469) that can recognize them. This may be due to the presentation of these antigens by nonprofessional APCs that are unable to activate T cells, or it may reflect a failure of recipient T cells to migrate to the graft tissue and encounter donor antigens. The level of peripheral antigen expression, how recently the responding T cell has emerged from the thymus (489,548), and the presence of proinflammatory cytokines (549,550) and upregulated costimulatory molecules within peripheral tissues (551) all may influence the decision of a T cell to ignore or respond to peripheral antigens. However, in contrast to a state of systemic tolerance, ignorance may be a more precarious state that can be upset by additional immunologic stimuli provoked by inflammation that may be induced, for example, by infections (547) or by presentation of antigen on professional APCs, as has been described for endocrine allografts that are depleted of APCs before transplantation (552).

Strategies for Inducing Transplantation Tolerance

Strategies to Achieve Central Tolerance

Mixed Chimerism. The pioneering work of Owen, Medawar, and others, beginning 50 years ago, led to the observation that hematopoietic chimerism can be associated with a state of donor-specific tolerance (553). The capacity of hematopoietic cells to induce tolerance results largely from their ability to induce intrathymic clonal deletion of thymocytes specific for antigens expressed by the hematopoietic cells. Thus, bone marrow engraftment can reliably induce tolerance to the most immunogenic allografts, such as fully MHC-mismatched skin grafts and small bowel grafts (155,554). In view of this powerful tolerance-inducing capacity, it may seem surprising that hematopoietic cell transplantation has not yet been applied to the induction of tolerance in humans. However, bone marrow transplantation (BMT) for tolerance induction has traditionally involved recipient treatment with lethal whole-body irradiation to eliminate mature recipient T cells and to make hematopoietic space for the marrow allograft. Removal of mature donor T cells before transplantation can prevent graft-versus-host disease (GVHD) (555–558). Under these circumstances, a new immune system can develop that is tolerant to both donor and recipient antigens. Although this approach has been successful in rodents, MHC-mismatched allogeneic BMT in larger animals, including humans, has proved to be less successful and more dangerous because of the unacceptable toxicity associated with myeloablative conditioning, and the inordinately high risks of GVHD and engraftment failure (559). Therefore, it will be useful to develop more specific and effective methods of overcoming the barriers to marrow engraftment. Achievement of this goal will require an understanding of the immunologic and physiologic obstacles to the engraftment and function of allogeneic and xenogeneic hematopoietic cells. It would be most desirable to achieve a state of mixed hematopoietic chimerism rather than full donor reconstitution in completely MHC-mismatched combinations. Improved immunocompetence has been observed in mixed chimeras, which contain host-type APCs in the peripheral tissues, presumably because these allow optimal antigen presentation to T cells that have developed in the host thymus, and which may therefore preferentially recognize peptide antigens presented by host-type MHC molecules (560,561).

Several approaches have been developed to permit the use of BMT to achieve mixed chimerism and specific tolerance. The use of total lymphoid irradiation (TLI) plus BMT has been studied extensively in rodents (562,563). The long bones are shielded during the radiation preparative regimen, so BMT results in mixed chimerism rather than full donor reconstitution. Mice treated in this way have been shown to be both resistant to GVHD and tolerant to

skin grafts from donor but not third-party animals. The mechanism by which TLI induces this tolerance is incompletely understood, and its success varies depending on the species involved. In rodent models, Th2-type responses appear to predominate when antigens are introduced after TLI, and this Th1 to Th2 shift may play a role in permitting graft acceptance (564,565). Natural suppressor cells that inhibit IL-2 production also have been implicated in tolerance induction after TLI (566). In clinical transplantation, TLI also has been used successfully, although it is cumbersome, especially in the case of cadaver donor transplantation (567,568). Donor-specific tolerance has been demonstrated in a small number of patients in whom immunosuppressive therapy was terminated after kidney transplantation under cover of TLI (569). Posttransplant TLI has been shown to have beneficial effects in conjunction with antithymocyte globulin in a primate model (570).

Mixed chimerism also can be achieved in rodents by administering a combination of T cell–depleted syngeneic and allogeneic bone marrow cells to lethally irradiated recipients. Mixed bone marrow chimeras are fully immunocompetent (560) and are specifically tolerant to subsequent skin grafts from the donor (571,572). More recently, mixed chimerism and donor-specific tolerance across MHC barriers has been achieved in mice without myeloablative conditioning (155). This model involves host treatment with depleting anti–T cell mAbs followed by a sublethal dose of whole-body irradiation to create hematopoietic space and a higher dose of local irradiation to the thymus to eliminate thymocytes that are not depleted by the mAbs. Several other regimens involving various combinations of anti–T cell antibodies, irradiation, and immunosuppressive drugs also have permitted the achievement of mixed chimerism in both large (573) and small (574–577) animals. The successful induction of tolerance in a primate model using the non-myeloablative approach to inducing mixed chimerism (573) has been used as the basis for a pilot clinical trial.

Mouse studies involving the use of mAbs to permit marrow engraftment have helped to elucidate the immune barriers to such grafts (155,578,579). As expected, CD4$^+$ cells resist engraftment of class II–mismatched marrow, and CD8 cells reject class I–disparate marrow grafts. However, CD8$^+$ cells also mount significant resistance to class II–mismatched marrow, and CD4$^+$ host cells pose a weak but detectable barrier to class I–mismatched marrow (578,579). Although NK cells resist allogeneic myeloid progenitor cell engraftment, as is described above, they actually present only a weak barrier to the engraftment of allogeneic long-term multilineage repopulating, pluripotent hematopoietic stem cells (PHSCs) (153,580). However, NK cells may play a more significant role in resisting the engraftment of xenogeneic marrow (154).

Gene Therapy of Autologous Marrow for the Induction of Tolerance. An alternative to using allogeneic hematopoietic engraftment to achieve tolerance is to reconstitute recipients with autologous bone marrow cells that have been transfected with genes encoding foreign transplantation antigens. This approach has permitted markedly prolonged survival of class I–disparate skin grafts bearing the class I gene that was introduced into the autologous marrow (581). If the genes selected encode particularly important antigens (such as those determining class II antigens), then tolerance to these antigens may have a significant effect on the rejection of subsequent grafts expressing these and other transplantation antigens and can lead to transplantation tolerance (582).

Extension of the Mixed Chimerism Approach to Xenotransplantation. Host treatment with mAbs to T cells and NK cells along with sublethal irradiation also has permitted rat marrow engraftment in mice, resulting in mixed xenogeneic chimerism and donor-specific tolerance (154). However, hematopoietic function depends on interactions between adhesion molecules and their ligands (583) and on a number of specific molecular interactions between the stroma and hematopoietic cells. It is probably the species specificity of some of these interactions (cytokines, adhesion molecules, other cell surface signaling molecules) that accounts for the competitive advantage enjoyed by recipient marrow over xenogeneic rat marrow that becomes increasingly evident as recovery of the host from low-dose whole-body irradiation occurs (584,585).

Achievement of xenogeneic hematopoietic repopulation has proved to be an even more formidable challenge in more disparate species combinations. Human and pig progenitor cells have been shown to be capable of repopulating murine recipients at low levels (586–588), but the species specificity of critical regulatory molecules may limit the level of donor repopulation. Administration of exogenous donor species-specific cytokines can partially overcome this barrier (587,589).

Xenogeneic Thymic Transplantation. Because of the difficulties encountered in inducing xenogeneic hematopoietic cells to migrate to a recipient thymus and induce central tolerance, an alternative approach might involve replacement of the recipient thymus with a xenogeneic donor thymus after host T-cell depletion and thymectomy. Immunocompetent mice treated in this way demonstrate recovery of $CD4^+$ T cells in xenogeneic porcine thymic grafts (590). These cells repopulate the periphery, are competent to resist infection (591), and are tolerant of donor antigens, even by the stringent measure of discordant xenogeneic skin grafting (592). Tolerance to both donor and host develops, at least in part, by intrathymic deletional mechanisms in these animals, and this reflects the presence of class II^{high} cells from both species within the thymic graft (592,593). Because MHC restriction is determined by the MHC of the thymus, it is surprising that T cells that differentiated in a xenogeneic thymus are able to respond to peptide antigens presented by host MHC (591). However, the excellent immune function achieved in humans receiving human leukocyte antigen (HLA)-mismatched allogeneic thymic transplantation for the treatment of congenital thymic aplasia (DiGeorge syndrome) suggests that this restriction incompatibility may not be a major obstacle to the achievement of adequate immune function (594). Perhaps this high level of cross-reactivity, even between species, reflects the fact that MHC reactivity is inherent in germline TCR sequences (51).

Transplantation of allogeneic (595) and concordant xenogeneic (596) thymic tissue obtained from fetuses before the time that hematopoietic cells have seeded the organ can also induce a form of tolerance that permits skin graft acceptance. However, the mechanism of tolerance in such animals is unlikely to be deletional because donor-specific MLRs are preserved. Active suppression has been implicated in the allogeneic model (597,598), and studies in the pig to mouse thymic transplantation model described above also suggest a possible role for suppression.

Development of Chimerism and Tolerance Without T Cell–Depleting or Myelosuppressive Treatment Developmentally immunoincompetent recipients. In theory, fetuses might be permissive for engraftment of allogeneic hematopoietic stem cells, not only because of their immunologic immaturity, but because space might be available in their hematopoietic systems, so that engraftment could be achieved without host conditioning. Since prenatal diagnosis of a number of congenital diseases has become possible, there is renewed interest in the possibility of injecting allogeneic or xenogeneic

pleuripotential hematopoietic stem cells (PHSC) into preimmune fetuses. Intrauterine injection of allogeneic hematopoietic stem cells has been used successfully to correct immunodeficiency diseases diagnosed in utero in human fetuses (599,600). However, chimerism was only detected in the T cell compartment afflicted by the congenital deficiency, and not in other hematopoietic lineages. In view of this result and the observation of only low levels of chimerism in preimmune normal mouse fetuses and sheep receiving in utero transplants (601), the concept that hematopoietic space is present in preimmune fetuses is open to question. In a large animal model, successful engraftment of enriched human PHSC populations has been successfully achieved without GVHD (602), raising hopes that this approach could be used for a broader spectrum of disorders in human fetuses. However, the ability of in utero marrow transplantation to induce tolerance is somewhat unpredictable (601,603).

Untreated neonatal rodents can be rendered tolerant of alloantigens by the administration of allogeneic hematopoietic cells shortly after birth. The mechanisms responsible for this phenomenon of neonatal tolerance are slowly being unraveled. Lasting microchimerism has been detected in some neonatally tolerized mice, and evidence to support an intrathymic deletional mechanism has been obtained in some, but not other, strain combinations (604). Furthermore, the presence of microchimerism does not always predict skin graft tolerance in recipients of allogeneic lymphocytes perinatally, and nontolerant animals can still maintain microchimerism after rejection of donor skin grafts (605,606). Thus, it is not surprising that several additional mechanisms have been implicated in rodents in which neonatal tolerance has been induced. First, tolerance cannot be easily broken by the infusion of nontolerant host-type lymphocytes in neonatally tolerized animals (523,604,607), and this has been attributed to the presence of suppressive T-cell populations (523). The ability of neonates to mount host antigraft responses may be essential for the induction of these suppressive cell populations when donor antigen is given. In contrast, when deletional tolerance is induced in animals in which the preexisting peripheral T-cell response has been fully ablated (e.g., mixed chimeras prepared with the lethal or nonlethal regimen described above), the absence of suppressive cell populations makes it easy to abolish tolerance by the infusion of nontolerant host-type lymphocytes (608,609). Second, neonatal mice have a tendency to produce Th2 responses, and these have been implicated in donor-specific skin graft acceptance (537,610). However, neonatal mice are capable of mounting CTL and Th1 responses under certain conditions (611,612). Third, the ability of allogeneic spleen cell infusions to induce tolerance has been suggested to reflect the high ratio of non-costimulatory APCs (T and B cells) in donor inocula to recipient T cells in the neonate, rather than to any unique susceptibility to tolerance induction (613).

Adult recipients. Based on the recent observation that microchimerism can exist for many years in the tissues of human recipients of solid organ allografts who did not receive hematopoietic cell transplants (614), it has been hypothesized that microchimerism, resulting from emigration of passenger leukocytes from the graft to recipient tissues, leads to a state of donor-specific tolerance (615). However, this hypothesis is controversial (616), and it is currently unclear whether chimerism induces tolerance or is even an epiphenomenon that reflects either tolerance or adequate immunosuppressive pharmacotherapy. There are several mechanisms by which microchimerism might in theory induce peripheral T-cell tolerance. These include nonprofessional APC function of donor-derived B or T cells (617–619), which can tolerize responding T cells. In addition, veto activity of T cells, NK cells, and other cell types eliminates CTLs reactive against antigens expressed on the veto cells (620). In addition to these mechanisms by which chimerism might induce peripheral tolerance, donor leukocytes migrating to recipient thymus might induce central tolerance among T cells that develop subsequent to the time of donor engraftment. Recent evidence shows that adult rodent liver grafts contain self-renewing hematopoietic stem cells (621,622), and dendritic cell progenitors have been detected in the marrow of mice that spontaneously accept mouse liver allografts (623). However, lasting microchimerism does not appear to play a role in several animal models of tolerance in which the issue has been carefully examined (624–626). It also has become increasingly clear in humans that microchimerism neither denotes a state of tolerance nor is required to maintain an allograft under all circumstances (616,627–629).

Recently, several groups have evaluated the ability of donor bone marrow cell infusions given without recipient myelosuppression or T-cell depletion to enhance graft survival. Although it is too early to determine whether this approach will be beneficial (630,631), it is clear that such transplants can be associated with significant risks from possible immunosuppressive effects of the transplant and from GVHD (632–634). These studies did not include intentional peripheral T-cell depletion of the hosts. In a primate model that includes recipient pretreatment with antilymphocyte serum for T-cell depletion, and, for optimal results, total lymphoid irradiation, veto cells in donor bone marrow that inactivate recipient CTLp may promote graft acceptance (501). However, only a fraction of recipients show long-term graft acceptance, with the best results obtained when the donor and recipient share a DR class II MHC allele (635).

In the primate BMT model described in the preceding paragraph, no myelosuppressive treatment was included in the host conditioning regimen, and, not surprisingly, only low levels of chimerism were detected. In contrast, macroscopically detectable chimerism has been observed in an otherwise similar primate model that includes a sublethal dose of host irradiation (573). The concept that myelosuppression must be used to create space in the hematopoietic compartment in order to allow donor hematopoietic cells to engraft has long been widely accepted. The mechanism by which myelosuppression promotes marrow engraftment is not fully understood, and could include both the creation of physical niches due to the destruction of host hematopoietic cells, and the upregulation of cytokines that promote hematopoiesis. In syngeneic BMT recipients, a low dose of whole-body irradiation is required to make physiologic space for engraftment of syngeneic marrow cells given in numbers similar to those that could be obtained from marrow of living human allogeneic marrow donors (636). However, this requirement can be overcome by the administration of high doses of syngeneic marrow (637,638). Furthermore, engraftment of high doses of allogeneic marrow can be achieved without myelosuppressive treatment in mice that receive T cell–depleting mAbs (639). However, it is essential to create space in the thymus and to achieve high levels of early donor T-cell repopulation in order to induce permanent skin graft tolerance (639). Apparently, thymic space and peripheral hematopoietic space are regulated independently (638).

Strategies to Achieve Peripheral Tolerance

There are numerous animal models in which peripheral T-cell tolerance has been induced, generally by mechanisms that are not

fully understood. Evidence for anergy as a mechanism of peripheral tolerance has been achieved in several of these models, including transplantation of I-E islet allografts into I-E⁻ recipients after anti-CD4 mAb treatment (451), and in mice receiving allogeneic BMT after treatment with T cell–depleting mAbs (640).

Costimulatory Blockade. Other attempts to induce anergy in transplantation models have included the introduction of alloantigen on non-costimulatory APCs, such as cells whose antigen-presenting activity has been impaired by ultraviolet irradiation (641). It is possible that donor-specific transfusions facilitate tolerance induction (642) because of their B-cell and T cell contents, both of which can present antigen in a manner that induces anergy (618,643). Efforts to induce tolerance by blocking the B7/CD28 costimulatory pathway have enjoyed success in animals receiving vascularized allografts (644–647) or pancreatic islet xenografts (648) under cover of CTLA4Ig, a synthetic soluble molecule that contains the B7-binding portion of CTLA4, one of the T-cell ligands of B7. CTLA4Ig blocks CD28 binding to both B7 molecules, B7-1 and B7-2. This appears to combine with the tolerogenic capacity of primarily vascularized organ allografts in rodents (113,649–652). The ability of differential blocking of B7-1 or B7-2 with specific mAbs to selectively drive Th1-type or Th2-type T-cell responses is controversial (653,654), and the distinct functions of each of these B7 molecules have not been clearly defined. Evidence in a rat renal allograft model suggests that CTLA4Ig may favor the development of Th2 responses, rather than inducing anergy (646).

Recent studies have demonstrated the importance of interactions between CD40 ligand (CD40L) on T cells and CD40, which is expressed not only on activated B cells, but on a variety of APCs. Signaling through the interaction of CD40 on APCs with its T-cell ligand is necessary for the conversion of certain nonprofessional APCs, such as B cells, to functional APCs, in part by upregulating B7 expression. In addition to its important role in providing cognate help for B-cell activation and in activating APCs, this interaction provides important costimulation leading to T cell activation. Blocking CD40L/CD40 interactions can result in graft prolongation that may be associated with a Th2-dominant immune response or with a reduction in the production of nitric oxide, an important mediator produced by activated macrophages (376,655,656). The combination of CTLA4Ig and anti-CD40L antibody seems to provide particularly potent immunosuppression with the ability to markedly prolong the survival of primary skin allografts (459,460). The role of anergy, if any, in these systems, remains to be determined.

T-cell anergy also has been induced in transplantation models by the administration of mAbs that block adhesion molecules (553). Combined treatment with mAbs against LFA-1 and its ligand ICAM-1 has been reported to induce profound tolerance in murine cardiac allograft recipients (657).

Nondepleting Anti–T Cell Antibodies. Th2 cytokines may play a role in the induction of infectious tolerance observed in mice receiving minor antigen-disparate skin allografts under cover of nondepleting anti–T cell mAbs (658–660). Waldmann and colleagues have demonstrated that CD4⁺ T cells, rendered incapable of rejecting the allograft in the original recipients, could render naive T cells unresponsive in secondary recipients, and that these tolerant T cells could, in turn, tolerize naive T cells in tertiary recipients. However, a Th1 to Th2 shift may not fully account for the tolerance in the above model (659).

A Large Animal Model of Peripheral Tolerance Induction

Studies of pig renal transplantation have demonstrated that spontaneous tolerance can be induced by organ grafts in large animals, provided that MHC antigens are matched (40). The ability to achieve such tolerance is dependent on one or possibly two non–MHC-linked genetic loci in the recipient animals (494). The presence of the acceptor phenotype also permits the spontaneous acceptance of single haplotype class I–mismatched kidney grafts (40). Graft acceptance is associated with donor-specific CTL unresponsiveness, apparently due to a deficiency in help for these CTLs, and not due to a deletional mechanism (105). The requirement that class II antigens be matched between donor and recipient in order for this tolerance to be achieved may reflect the influence of a major difference in class II antigen expression that exists between large and small animals. Unlike large animals and humans, in which class II antigens are expressed constitutively on vascular endothelial cells (44), the corresponding endothelial cells of rodent species do not express MHC class II molecules, even in the setting of allograft rejection (37,44). Consistent with this interpretation, the use of a short course of cyclosporine A (CyA) can facilitate the ability of renal allografts to induce tolerance in rodents (661,662) across fully MHC-mismatched barriers, but tolerance induction in swine requires class II matching between donor and recipient for uniform success (663). Thus, in class II–matched, class I–mismatched porcine donor–recipient pairs, a 12-day course of high-dose (10 mg/kg/day) CyA permitted long-term graft acceptance in 100% of cases (663), and animals accepting such allografts became systemically tolerant to the donor's class I and minor antigens, as indicated by the fact that the accepted graft could be removed and replaced by a second donor-matched graft, which was likewise accepted (664). This ability of CyA to facilitate tolerance induction, and the ability of exogenous IL-2 to prevent the induction of tolerance in this model (664), are consistent with the interpretation that induction of tolerance of donor class I–reactive CTLs is due, at least in part, to the absence of adequate T-cell help during the time of initial exposure to antigen. Also consistent was the selective decrease of expression of the Th1-associated cytokine IFN-γ relative to the Th2-associated cytokine IL-10, which has been observed in these accepted grafts (665,666). The thymus appears to play a role in the induction of tolerance among preexisting peripheral T cells in this model because removal of the host thymus before kidney allotransplantation leads to rejection (667). The possible mechanisms responsible for this role of the thymus in inducing peripheral tolerance phenomenon are discussed elsewhere in this chapter.

The Relationship Between Peripheral T-Cell Tolerance and Central Tolerance

The distinction between central and peripheral tolerance may not always be clear. In some systems, passenger leukocytes might emigrate from the graft to the host thymus and tolerize subsequently developing thymocytes. In addition, however, the thymus may be capable of tolerizing T cells that were already in the periphery at the time of organ grafting. In the pig model described above, the thymus appears to play a role in the induction of tolerance among preexisting peripheral T cells (667). It is possible that T cells that are activated in the periphery by the organ allograft recirculate to the thymus as has been described (668) and encounter donor antigen there in ways that inactivate the T cells. This could be a mechanism for ensuring that T cells activated in the periphery of an animal are switched off if the same antigens are present on intrathymic leukocytes. Alternatively, the migration of donor antigen to the thymus may result in the development of T cells that specifically recognize the donor antigen and downregulate the activity of destructive alloreactive T cells when they enter the periphery (522,665).

A second situation in which the boundary between central and peripheral tolerance is blurred arises when donor antigens are injected intrathymically in order to induce tolerance. The initial idea underlying this approach was to use antibody treatment to deplete peripheral T cells and to induce central tolerance among recovering T cells by direct introduction of antigen into the thymus. However, more recent studies have shown that tolerance to soluble alloantigens can be induced by intrathymic injection without peripheral T-cell depletion (669). Because removal of the thymus before or within the first few days of allografting results in rejection of the allograft (255), the thymus must play an active role in tolerizing preexisting peripheral T cells, possibly by one of the mechanisms proposed in the preceding paragraph. Active regulatory cell populations have been reported in rats receiving intrathymic injections of allogeneic bone marrow cells (BMC) (670). These results are consistent with the role of suppressive cell populations in tolerance induced by thymic allografts (597,598) or xenografts.

There is an important role for the allograft in inducing tolerance in animals receiving intrathymic injection, and in other models in which a preexisting peripheral T-cell repertoire must be rendered tolerant. Transferable tolerance is not induced by intrathymic marrow injection alone without an organ allograft in rats (670), suggesting that the graft itself helps to tolerize the preexisting T-cell repertoire. In contrast, pure intrathymic deletional tolerance is not dependent on the continued presence of antigen in the periphery (609). Donor tissue can be grafted at any time, and tolerance is assured. The intrathymic injection approach has not been successful in high responder rat strain combinations and may even induce allosensitization (671,672), and has not successfully allowed xenotolerance induction.

Which Strategy to Achieve Transplantation Tolerance?

Although clinical trials have already begun in which tolerance-inducing strategies are combined with conventional pharmacologic immunosuppression, none of the strategies for achieving transplantation tolerance have been used to replace such chronic therapy in clinical transplantation. In general, short-term results of most organ allograft transplants are excellent, making it essential to have extremely reliable methods of inducing tolerance in order to ethically justify their use in place of conventional chronic immunosuppressive therapies. Although induction of central deletional tolerance with hematopoietic cell grafts is a reliable and durable approach to achieving permanent graft survival, earlier techniques for achieving central tolerance have involved more vigorous ablation of the lymphohematopoietic system than can be safely achieved in larger animals. Thus, the major challenge in bringing this approach to clinical application is to develop highly specific, nontoxic methods of conditioning the host for acceptance of a hematopoietic allograft or xenograft. On the other hand, techniques to achieve peripheral tolerance in larger animals have not generally produced as good results as have been seen in rodent models. Furthermore, peripheral mechanisms alone have not been sufficient to reliably overcome the most stringent transplantation barrier imposed by fully MHC-mismatched primary skin allografts. Conceptually, one major problem with peripheral tolerance strategies is that they cannot prevent the generation of new T cells in the recipient capable of recognizing donor antigens. Although effector cells might be persistently driven toward anergy or deletion by the non-stimulating cells of the graft, the ongoing stimulation of helper cells by professional APCs through the indirect pathway would seem likely to render this a precarious state of tolerance. The only means of completely eliminating the indirect pathway may be through central tolerance induction to the peptides of donor antigens presented in the thymus in association with host MHC antigens. However, thymic APCs appear to be incapable of picking up and re-presenting antigens from lymphoid cells to induce tolerance of T cells that recognize these antigens through the indirect pathway (477). Because superantigens have been shown to be capable of inducing deletional tolerance in the thymus when presented by APCs other than those that produced them (673), further definition of the circumstances under which indirect presentation of hematopoietic cell-derived antigens leads to intrathymic deletion is needed. In addition, the infectious nature of suppressive mechanisms of tolerance makes them potentially attractive as a means of inducing robust and durable tolerance. However, it will be difficult to control the development of such mechanisms until they are better understood. It seems likely that the optimal approach to achieving clinical transplantation tolerance might require combinations of both central and peripheral strategies.

TRANSPLANTATION OF SPECIFIC ORGANS AND TISSUES

Skin Grafting

Although allogeneic skin grafting represents a frequently used experimental model (674), its application in humans is unusual. Most skin transplantation in humans is performed with autologous tissue. Recently, however, artificial skin grafts have been created that consist of stromal elements and cultured cells of allogeneic and even xenogeneic origin. Evidence suggests that these grafts are not rejected, although their components may be replaced by recipient tissues over time.

Skin grafts are frequently used experimentally on small animals to examine rejection because they can be performed rapidly in large numbers. On the one hand, the use of skin grafts has the disadvantage that they are not primarily vascularized and, thus, may not be susceptible to precisely the same mechanisms of rejection as are solid organs. On the other hand, the difficulty in prolonging skin graft survival in rodents more accurately reflects the difficulty in prolonging transplantation of solid organ survival in larger animals than does the transplantation of solid organs in rodents.

Kidney Transplantation

Kidneys have been the most frequently transplanted organs for many years. At present approximately 10,000 kidney transplants are performed annually in the United States. The likelihood that a renal allograft will survive with good function for at least 1 year has slowly been increasing. Patient survival after 1 year is expected to be better than 90%, and the current likelihood of graft function

at 1 year now exceeds 85% in many units, even when organs from totally unrelated donors are used.

Nonetheless, even well-matched recipients of renal transplants must continue to take immunosuppressive medications for the rest of their lives. These patients are susceptible to the complications of their immunosuppressive medications, including increased risks of infection, cancer, hypertension, and metabolic bone disease. Thus, they pay a price for their new organ stemming from our inability to provide specific immunosuppression. The success of clinical transplantation is a double-edged sword. With such good patient and graft survival rates initially, it is difficult to justify risky clinical trials of new approaches to immunosuppression that by achieving antigen-specific tolerance might avoid the long-term need for immunosuppression altogether.

Because of the success of modern nonspecific immunosuppression, the major obstacle to achieving a successful kidney transplant is no longer the rejection of the organ after transplantation. Instead the two major obstacles are now the shortage of organs and the problem of sensitization. Partly because of the increasing success of renal transplantation, the number of candidates for the procedure has continued to grow and now exceeds the supply of available organs. Unlike hearts and livers, where an inadequate supply of organs leads to the death of many candidates, those waiting for renal transplants are instead faced with long periods on dialysis. This waiting time is often 3 or more years even for unsensitized candidates seeking kidneys from cadaver donors. The second major obstacle in obtaining a successful renal transplant stems from the problem of sensitized candidates with broadly reactive antibodies resulting from prior antigen exposure. These highly sensitized individuals may wait many years to obtain a kidney that is cross-match negative, and some never receive a transplant at all.

Liver Transplantation

Transplantation of the liver represents a major technical challenge. For this reason the organ and patient survival rates are not as good as those for renal transplantation. However, successful liver transplantation can now be achieved with survival of about two thirds of the recipients at 1 year (675,676).

From an immunologist's point of view, liver transplantation is of interest first because the organ is apparently quite resistant to immediate antibody-mediated rejection (677). Transplantation across blood group barriers and in the face of a positive cross-match (by retrospective analysis) has generally been successful in the short term (186). There is evidence, however, that long-term organ survival is diminished in blood group–incompatible patients (187). Second, the long-term survival of liver transplants does not appear to be better when better HLA matching between donor and recipient is achieved. In fact, some data have suggested the opposite correlation. The possibility that poorly matched livers may survive better than well-matched ones might be due to an inability of recipient T cells, sensitized to viral pathogens in association with self MHC antigens, to recognize those pathogens in the donor liver presented in association with donor HLA antigens. Thus, poorly matched livers might escape injury caused by immunologic responses to hepatotrophic viruses. Third, transplantation of the liver carries with it large numbers of donor lymphoid cells, thus creating the setting for GVHD. Donor lymphocytes can mediate an antibody-dependent hemolysis of recipient red blood cells in the case of recipient blood group incompatibility with the donor (678).

Thus A or B recipients of O livers have been subject to an immune hemolytic anemia during the early posttransplant period. There also may be other manifestations of GVHD even in blood group–compatible recipients (679).

Heart and Lung Transplantation

Heart transplantation is also a relatively recent component of standard clinical transplantation, with survival rates frequently in excess of 80% at 1 year (680,681). One of the immunologic issues of particular importance in heart transplantation is the high rate of new atherosclerotic disease in the coronary arteries of the donor organ (682). This atherosclerotic disease is probably a manifestation of chronic rejection.

Lung transplantation, either in conjunction with heart transplantation or alone, is a still more recent addition to clinical transplantation (683). Recipients of lung transplants have demonstrated a tendency to develop pathologic changes of bronchiolitis obliterans, which is thought to be a manifestation of chronic rejection.

Pancreas and Islet Transplantation

Transplantation of the whole pancreas met with almost 100% failure until about 1980, largely for technical reasons. More recently, successful pancreas transplantation to treat diabetes mellitus has been achieved using new technical approaches, and with success rates approaching those for kidney transplantation, as long as the two organs are transplanted together (684). The lower survival rates achieved when pancreas transplantation is performed alone probably reflects the difficulty in diagnosing rejection episodes involving this organ. By the time blood sugar levels begin to increase, destruction of the pancreas is generally so far advanced that it cannot be reversed by immunotherapy. Measurement of serum creatinine, reflecting early dysfunction of a simultaneous kidney transplant, allows much earlier detection of rejection activity and, thus, better outcomes (685). On the other hand, simultaneous transplantation of both a kidney and a pancreas from a single donor has demonstrated the interesting phenomenon that rejection activity in one organ is not always associated with rejection activity in the other (686). It is not known whether this occasional dichotomy reflects tissue-specific antigens or localized inflammatory events in one, but not the other organ.

Transplantation of the whole pancreas provides, of course, more tissue than is needed to treat diabetes mellitus. The intriguing aspect of pancreas transplantation, therefore, is the potential that useful results might be accomplished by transplantation of insulin-producing islet cells alone (422). Although islet cell transplants have been successful in animal models, success in humans has been limited (687). Part of the reason that islet transplantation has been so unsuccessful appears to be the autoimmune state of diabetic recipients in addition to their alloreactive response to the transplanted tissue. Thus, patients without previous diabetes, who have undergone islet transplantation at the time of total pancreatectomy, have had much higher success rates than have diabetic patients.

Even if islet transplantation could be performed routinely with current immunosuppressive drugs, it would not dramatically change the course of diabetes for these patients. This is because the primary goal of islet transplantation is to prevent the secondary neurologic, vascular, and retinal complications of diabetes that take many years to develop. However, performance of islet transplantation early in the course of the disease, when it might really affect these processes, would require exchanging insulin therapy for immunosuppressive drugs. Over 20 to 30 years, the latter is at least as damaging to human beings. Thus, even more than for other forms of transplantation, realization of the full potential of islet transplantation will require tolerance induction.

Hematopoietic Cell Transplantation

Bone marrow transplants, and more recently, transplants of hematopoietic stem cells and progenitors mobilized from the marrow into peripheral blood by treatment with cytokines, are used most commonly for the treatment of otherwise incurable leukemias and lymphomas, and for congenital immunodeficiency states. Although autologous stem cell transplants are currently used quite widely in the treatment of malignancies, these will not be considered further here because they do not involve the broaching of any immunologic barriers.

One fundamental difference between hematopoietic cell transplantation and the transplantation of all other organs is that the recipient's treatment for his or her malignancy usually results in ablation of the immune and hematopoietic systems before transplantation. Originally, stem cell allografts were administered only as a means of replacing these ablated host functions. Transplantation for immunodeficiency states does not require such ablation in order to achieve engraftment of allogeneic marrow grafts that reconstitute only the deficient immune system and not other hematopoietic lineages. Another major difference between BMT and solid organ transplantation is that the recovering immune system in BMT recipients is tolerant to the donor alloantigens, so there is no requirement for immunosuppressive therapy to prevent allograft rejection once the initial immune resistance to the allograft has been overcome. A third unique feature of BMT (as well as transplants of other organs that are rich in lymphoid tissue, such as small intestinal grafts and, to a lesser extent, liver grafts) is the ability of T cells in the allograft to mount an immunologic attack on the recipient's tissues, resulting in the condition known as GVHD. Although GVHD rates can be reduced to acceptable levels using prophylaxis with a course of nonspecific immunosuppressive therapy when the donor and recipient are HLA-matched siblings, the frequency and severity of the GVHD that develops when extensive HLA barriers are traversed has essentially precluded the routine performance of such transplants, making BMT unavailable to many for whom no other curative treatment exists. Recently, the establishment of large marrow donor registries has permitted the performance of matched transplants from unrelated donors in a significant fraction of patients, but these transplants are also associated with a high incidence of severe GVHD, due in large part to the existence of HLA mismatches that went undetected by conventional serologic HLA typing techniques.

Bone marrow transplantation for leukemia therapy was originally conceived as a way of providing hematopoietic rescue for patients receiving ablative cytoreductive treatments. However, one of the major benefits of the procedure has proven to be the graft-versus-host immune response, i.e., the recognition by donor T cells of host alloantigens, which are also expressed on leukemic cells. Thus, allogeneic BMT also may be thought of as immunotherapy leading to an attack on the residual leukemic cells that remain in cytoablated hosts. It is not surprising, therefore, that T-cell depletion of the donor has not proved to be an optimal solution to the GVHD problem, primarily because the decreased incidence of GVHD is offset by an increased incidence of leukemic relapse, as well as failure of engraftment (688,689). Rather than depleting donor T cells in this situation, the goal should be to separate the graft-versus-leukemia (GVL) response from the graft-versus-normal host tissue response.

Recently, several new approaches for inhibiting GVHD have been attempted. Some of these make use of similar immunosuppressive regimens to those being evaluated in solid organ transplant recipients, e.g., costimulatory blockade, alone (690,691) or in combination with adhesion molecule blockade (692). Peptides containing the CDR3 portion of the mouse CD4 molecule have been shown to be capable of inhibiting both GVHD (693) and resistance to allogeneic marrow engraftment (694). Treatment with anti-CD40L mAb also has been shown to inhibit GVHD and to promote allogeneic marrow engraftment (655,691). Because these approaches might be expected to block donor antihost responses nonspecifically, including those that eliminate residual leukemia in the host, it seems quite likely that they will also impair GVL responses. Alternative approaches involve immunostimulatory cytokines such as IL-2, IFN-γ, or IL-12, all of which, paradoxically, inhibit GVHD in mouse models (695–697). These cytokines are of interest because they could potentially mediate GVL effects while inhibiting GVHD. Indeed, these cytokines have been shown to preserve or enhance GVL effects while GVHD is inhibited (698–700). The use of nondepleting anti-CD3 F(ab)′2 fragments in vivo has also shown promise in a mouse model for the ability to maintain GVL effects while attenuating GVHD (701). Recently, rodent (702) and humanized (703) anti-CD25 mAbs have been evaluated for the treatment of acute GVHD, with only modest efficacy. In addition, mAbs to proinflammatory cytokines such as TNF-α (704) and an IL-1 receptor antagonist (705) have shown some efficacy in GVHD prophylaxis or treatment in initial clinical trials.

Another approach to separating the GVL potential from the GVHD-inducing capacity of MHC-directed alloreactivity is to separate the hematopoietic cell transplant and the administration of donor T cells in time, so that the T cells are given after some host recovery from the initial conditioning regimen has occurred (706–708). Apparently, host recovery from the injury associated with conditioning or the recovery of regulatory cell populations confers greater resistance to the induction of GVHD at late time points post-BMT compared with that which can be induced by T cells given at the time of conditioning. This resistance may explain the unexpectedly manageable level of GVHD that has been observed in patients who receive delayed donor leukocyte infusions to treat chronic myelogenous leukemia that has relapsed late after allogeneic BMT (709–711).

Several groups have investigated the possibility that CD4+ or CD8+ T-cell subsets could be identified that promote engraftment and GVL effects but not cause GVHD (712–714). Clinical studies involving selective CD8 depletion in HLA-identical sibling transplantation have shown a higher incidence of engraftment failure than is observed for unmanipulated BMT, but the rate was lower than that observed for pan-T cell–depleted transplants, and evidence for an antileukemic effect was obtained (715).

Another approach to separating the beneficial from the harmful effects of allogeneic T cells involves the in vitro expansion and cloning of donor T cells that selectively recognize leukemia-associated antigens but that do not recognize nonmalignant recipient cells. The existence of such CTL clones has been reported in mice

(716) and humans (717–719). Such T cells are probably rare, and in order to separate them from GVHD-producing T cells, prolonged in vitro selection, cloning, and expansion is likely to be required. Such prolonged cultures may be impractical for use in the setting of BMT, in which leukemia-reactive cells must eliminate exponentially expanding leukemic cells. One class of leukemia-specific antigens that has recently stimulated intense research is the idiotypic determinants associated with unique Ig receptors and T-cell receptors on the surface of B- and T-cell malignancies, respectively, which may be particularly effective at immunizing when presented by professional APCs such as dendritic cells (720–722).

Xenogeneic Transplantation

The increasing shortage of cadaver donor organs has evoked a worldwide resurgence of interest in xenotransplantation, i.e., the replacement of human organs or tissues with those from a donor of a different species. Routine clinical application of this therapeutic modality is still in the future. However, recent progress, which will be reviewed briefly here, offers cause for optimism.

Concordant Versus Discordant Xenotransplantation

Xenotransplants have been classified into two groups, concordant and discordant, on the basis of phylogenetic distance between the species combination, speed of the rejection, and levels of detectable preformed antibodies. Animals that are evolutionarily closely related and do not have preformed natural antibodies specific for each other are called concordant, whereas animals that belong to evolutionarily distant species and reject organs in a hyperacute manner are termed discordant. There are, of course, many gradations between these extremes, and there are also a variety of known exceptions to the rule, making this nomenclature less than ideal.

Choice of Donor Species for Clinical Xenotransplantation

From a phylogenetic viewpoint, nonhuman primates would undoubtedly be the most similar to allotransplants immunologically. However, due to considerations of size, availability, and likelihood of transmission of infectious disease, most investigators have decided against the use of primates as a future source of xenogeneic organs. Instead, the discordant species, swine, has been chosen by many as the most suitable xenograft donor. The pig has essentially unlimited availability, as well as favorable breeding characteristics and the similarity of many of its organ systems to those of humans. Partially inbred miniature swine are a particularly attractive choice, because of their size (adult weights of approximately 120 kg), physiology (also similar to humans for many organ systems), and breeding characteristics, which have permitted inbreeding and genetic manipulation (723).

Mechanisms of Xenograft Rejection

Xenografts are subject to all four of the rejection mechanisms described earlier in this chapter and give rise to more powerful immune responses than allografts, probably for each type of rejection. There are two fundamental reasons for this finding. First, xenografts offer more foreign antigens as targets for an immune response. Second, there are frequently molecular incompatibilities between members of different species that prevent the normal function of receptor–ligand interactions. Because in many cases the occurrence of homologous restriction for receptor–ligand pairs has been found to impair the regulatory processes that normally control immune and inflammatory responses, the result is that rejection mechanisms that may be relatively weak in allogeneic combinations become explosive after xenogeneic transplantation.

The well-recognized susceptibility of xenografts toward hyperacute rejection demonstrates both of these fundamental problems. As described earlier, pigs express an endothelial carbohydrate determinant, gal α(1,3) gal, that is not expressed by humans (724). As a result of this additional foreign antigen, pigs, in effect, express a new blood group antigen relative to all human recipients; thus, their organs are subject to hyperacute rejection, initiated by the binding of preformed natural antibodies. However, the hyperacute rejection that occurs with pig-to-primate transplantation is more vigorous than in the case of allogeneic blood group disparities. At least in part, this is because the complement regulatory proteins expressed by pig endothelium are less efficient in controlling human complement activation than are the human regulatory proteins expressed by human organs (180). Thus, these molecular incompatibilities contribute to the increased intensity of the hyperacute rejection mechanism.

Similarly, the factors responsible for accelerated graft rejection are more prominent in xenogeneic than in allogeneic transplantation. The rapid induction of an antibody response against xenografts probably reflects the expression of additional foreign antigens and the existence of preformed antibodies to these antigens, although at levels too low to initiate hyperacute rejection (142–144). In addition, the process of accelerated rejection is magnified considerably in xenografts by the failure of such regulatory molecules as tissue factor protein inhibitor to function effectively with human factor Xa, thus increasing the tendency toward intravascular thrombosis (200). The likely participation of NK cells in this form of xenograft rejection probably also reflects both the presence of additional antigens and the importance of molecular incompatibilities in xenotransplantation because novel carbohydrate determinants on pig endothelium may contribute to NK cell activation, and the molecular incompatibilities between human NK inhibitory receptors and swine class I molecules allows this activation to proceed without inhibition (725).

The available evidence also suggests that cell-mediated immune responses to xenografts are more powerful than to allografts (468). Initially, there was some uncertainty about this point because cell-mediated immune responses to xenogeneic stimulating cells were first studied using mouse T cells, for which molecular incompatibilities between species are actually responsible for a weaker direct recognition of xenogeneic than allogeneic stimulators in vitro (726). In this case, the incompatibilities turned out to involve the accessory molecules that are required for T-cell activation rather than molecules that inhibit a T-cell response. Thus, it seemed that cell-mediated rejection in vivo also might be weak. However, cell-mediated xenograft rejection, even by mice, has consistently been found to be extremely powerful, apparently initiated by CD4+ T cells responding to the many additional antigenic peptides through the indirect pathway (727).

More recently, attention has been directed at investigation of the clinically relevant human–antipig cellular response. In contrast to the murine studies, direct responses by human T cells to pig stim-

ulators can easily be measured in vitro (728,729). In addition, the cell-mediated reaction in vitro has been found to include a significant contribution by NK cells that can lyse pig targets (728,730). Thus, in the human–antipig combination, an important molecular incompatibility is the failure of human NK inhibitory receptors to interact with pig class I molecules. Numerous other molecular interactions that might be important in human–antipig T-cell responses have been examined (Table 6). With the exception of an apparently lower affinity of human CD8 for its binding site on pig class I molecules (which diminishes the direct human CD8+ helper response to pig stimulators, and the failure of human IFN-γ to stimulate pig endothelium), the other molecular interactions appear to be at least partially functional (731).

The results of these studies have suggested that human–antipig T-cell responses are likely to be as great or greater than those in allogeneic combinations. Some investigators have identified a stronger indirect response by human T cells to pig stimulators than to allogeneic stimulators (732). If murine studies are correct in suggesting that the true basis of the strength of cell-mediated xenograft rejection lies in the strength of the indirect sensitization, this stronger indirect proliferation may indicate that human cell-mediated rejection of pig organs, both acutely and chronically, will indeed be more difficult to control than for allografts. Presumably, the source of this stronger indirect response lies partly in the larger number of foreign antigenic peptides generated by the disparate proteins of xenogeneic donors.

Therapeutic Strategies for Xenotransplantation

Three main strategies have been pursued to achieve long-term survival of xenogeneic transplants. The first has been to seek nonspecific immunosuppressive drugs that might prove especially effective for xenotransplantation. This approach was used successfully to achieve the excellent survival of allografts in current clinical practice. However, each new drug that has contributed to better outcomes for allografts has been tested experimentally for xenografts, and none has so far proven to be the magic bullet that might make xenografting possible. Based on our scientific understanding of the immunologic barriers to xenotransplantation, it is unlikely that any such drug exists. Furthermore, the heightened

TABLE 6. *Molecular interactions between human and pig*

Molecular interactions that are at least partially functional	
Human	Pig
TCR	SLA
CD4	SLA class II
CD8	SLA class I (±)
CD2	LFA-3 (±)
LFA-1	ICAM
CD28	B7
VLA-4	VCAM
Fas	FasL

Molecular interactions that are significantly impaired	
Human	Pig
NK KIRs	SLA class I
CD8	SLA class I
IFN-γ	IFN-γ R

immune response to xenografts compared with allografts suggests that larger amounts of exogenous immunosuppression would be required to achieve xenograft survival comparable with that of allografts. Given the narrow therapeutic window that already exists in clinical transplantation, most investigators believe that more than just immunosuppressive drugs will be needed to accomplish widespread clinical application of xenogeneic transplantation.

The second therapeutic approach has been to use genetic engineering of donor animals to lessen the immunologic barriers to xenografts. Because the two features that distinguish xenografts from allografts are the larger number of antigens and the molecular incompatibilities between species, these genetic modifications have been aimed primarily at correcting these two disadvantages of xenografts (Fig. 15). In mice, the technology of homologous recombination has made it possible to eliminate the expression of some of the deleterious genes. For example, knock-out mice have been generated that do not express the galactosyltransferase that is responsible for generating the α (1,3) gal determinant (733,734). However, in larger animals, including pigs, this technology is not currently available, limiting genetic modification of these animals to the insertion of transgenes. The most exciting application of this approach so far has been the creation of so-called hDAF-pigs, which are animals that express the human gene for the DAF complement regulatory protein (735,736). Organs from these animals appear to be significantly less susceptible to hyperacute rejection than are those from wild-type pigs. Numerous other potential transgenes are currently being examined experimentally, including genes for other complement regulatory proteins, genes encoding the human fucosyltransferase that produces the human blood group O determinant from the same substrate used by the pig galactosyltransferase, and genes encoding a glycosidase that might remove the α gal determinant. Almost certainly still other transgenes will be tested that might alter the process of accelerated rejection (perhaps by restoring normal thromboregulation or by promoting accommodation) or that might affect the cell-mediated mechanisms of graft destruction (perhaps by expressing human class I analogs to inhibit NK cells or by expressing downregulating molecules for T cells, such as Fas ligand).

The third strategy to achieve xenotransplantation is to eliminate the immunologic disadvantage of animal donors by inducing tolerance to the donor antigens. Potential applications of this strategy have been described earlier in this chapter. A key feature of this approach is that the techniques to achieve peripheral tolerance induction, which have appeared promising in allogeneic combinations, have generally been less successful even in closely related xenogeneic combinations. Deletional tolerance strategies have been the only ones that have achieved truly long-term xenograft survival using the stringent test of skin graft transplantation (153,154).

There is, of course, no reason to suggest that these three strategies are mutually exclusive, and many investigators believe that some combination of all three will be needed to accomplish xenogeneic organ transplantation on a large scale.

Nonimmunologic Barriers to Xenotransplantation

In addition to the immunologic mechanisms that prevent successful xenografting, there are two other potentially important obstacles to clinical application. First, the same kinds of molecular incompatibilities between species that alter immune responses may cause physiologic dysfunction of xenogeneic organs. For example, it appears that erythropoietin produced by pig kidneys does not function well in primates, causing progressive anemia in recipients with long-surviving pig kidney transplants (737). Presumably, there are many other such examples that will become apparent when long-term survival of metabolically complex organs, such as the liver, can be accomplished using discordant donors. On the other hand, there are also many examples where physiologic function remains intact across species differences, such as the ability of pig insulin to regulate human glucose appropriately. In addition, future examples of physiologic dysfunction are likely to be correctable using transgenic technology. Thus, the physiologic dysfunction of xenogeneic organs is unlikely to be an insurmountable barrier to all forms of xenotransplantation, although it may impair the function of certain types of xenogeneic organs or tissues.

The other nonimmunologic barrier to xenotransplantation is the possibility that successful tissue transplantation may allow the cross-species transfer of infectious agents, potentially creating a public health hazard for society as a whole. This possibility has only recently gained significant attention, and the issue has become confused by enormous uncertainties about the true risks that are involved.

"Zoonosis" is a term that has been used for some time to describe the general process of cross-species infection. More recently, the term "xeno-zoonosis" has been developed to describe

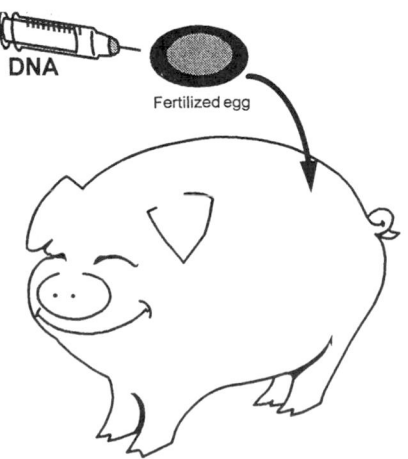

- **Complement inhibition**
  - DAF
  - CD46
  - CD59
- **Antibody binding**
  - Galactosidase
  - Fucosyl transferase
- **Growth factors**
  - pIL-3, pSCF
  - Human GF receptors
- **MHC genes**
  - Class I (NK inhibition)

FIG. 15. Transgenic pigs as xenograft donors. Some of the genes that have been used or have been considered for use in making transgenic pigs for xenograft donor.

infection transmission that might occur as a result of xenotransplantation. It is important to acknowledge that from the point of view of the individual recipient, the risk of transmitting infection by xenotransplantation is likely to be less than by current clinical allotransplantation, both because of the natural resistance to cross-species transmission of infectious diseases and because of the much longer time available to screen prospective donors. It is also important to point out that the risk of infectious transmission is unlikely to come from known pathogens because if the agent is known, it is generally possible to screen for and eliminate its presence.

The major concern, therefore, regarding infections resulting from xenotransplantation is that endogenous retroviral sequences from donor cells might infect the recipient's cells, giving rise themselves, or after recombination with human endogenous retroviral sequences, to previously unrecognized pathogenic viruses. Such new viruses might prove hazardous to other human beings in addition to the xenograft recipient. Although it has seemed to some that cross-species transmission of retroviruses would probably have occurred already in nature if it was likely to happen, others have pointed out that the circumstances of xenotransplantation may create unique conditions favoring this event. In particular, the prolonged coexistence of cells from two different species in patients who are taking immunosuppressive drugs or who have been rendered tolerant to their donors may be especially permissive for cross-species transfer of endogenous retroviruses. This concern has increased as a result of *in vitro* studies showing that pig proviruses can infect human cells when cells from both species are cultured together (738). At this time, however, there is no evidence that such cross-species transfer after a pig-to-human transplant would generate a virus that would be infectious or pathogenic. Because the concern about infections from xenotransplantation involves fear of an event that has never been known to happen, it is impossible to assign an accurate level of risk. Presumably it is low, but on the other hand, the consequences of the unlikely event might prove to be large for the many members of the human species who would receive no direct benefit from xenotransplantation. At this time, therefore, health agencies and members of the transplant community are attempting to design rational approaches for identifying the true risks of xenotransplantation and detecting untoward events rapidly, while at the same time allowing further progress in this potentially enormously important field of transplantation.

Clinical Progress in Xenotransplantation

Given the serious obstacles to successful xenotransplantation described above, it may be surprising that clinical trials using animal donors for humans have been, and are being, conducted. Many of the early efforts took place in the 1960s and involved organ transplants from nonhuman primates (183). One of the patients survived for nine months with normal renal function provided by the kidney of a chimpanzee (739). The most recent clinical trials have involved fetal pig cells transplanted into the brains of patients with Parkinson's or Huntington's diseases. The documented survival of pig tissue 8 months after the transplant in a patient taking only moderate doses of cyclosporine suggests that the blood–brain barrier provides a degree of immunoprotection (740). These studies also suggest that cellular xenotransplantation may be achieved more easily and thus may be performed sooner than solid organ transplants, especially because free cellular transplants lack the

vascular endothelium that is the target for both hyperacute and accelerated rejection.

SOME IMMUNOLOGIC ISSUES IN CLINICAL TRANSPLANTATION

The Effect of Antigen Matching on Graft Survival

Clinical Evidence

Transplantation antigens are defined by their ability to cause graft rejection, and in the absence of transplantation antigen disparities, graft rejection does not occur. Thus, there can be no argument with the statement that antigen matching improves graft survival. Contrary to this simple conclusion, however, the importance of antigen matching is one of the more controversial issues in clinical transplantation. The debate is frequently confused by failure to focus on the relevant quantitative issue of whether improved, but incomplete, antigen matching influences the outcome of organ transplantation sufficiently under current clinical circumstances to warrant its logistic difficulties.

The evidence from transplantation of kidneys using living-related donors provides a clinical demonstration of the importance of antigen matching in subsequent graft survival. Two siblings may share all of their HLA antigens (25% likelihood), half of their HLA antigens (50% likelihood), or none of their HLA antigens (25% likelihood). Identical twins share all of their transplantation antigens, but siblings are generally matched for only about half of the minor antigens, which distinguish their parents, even if they are HLA identical. Table 7 shows one institution's survival rates for kidney grafts after 1 year for HLA-identical and one-haplotype–matched living-related donors. Similar differences have been reported in the UCLA kidney transplant registry (741,742). The data in Table 7 indicate that some graft loss occurs even for HLA-identical siblings (indicating the role of minor histocompatibility antigens even in the face of immunosuppression) and that the outcome of kidney transplantation is better when there is complete HLA matching compared with only partial matching. These data support the basic concept that antigen matching matters, and for related donors, MHC antigen matching is widely agreed to be advantageous.

In the absence of a living-related donor, transplantation is performed with organs from unrelated donors, usually from cadaveric sources. Because of the extensive polymorphism of MHC antigens, unrelated donors selected in a random fashion would not be expected to share many HLA antigens with the recipient. Similarly, there would only be sporadic matching of the minor histocompatibility antigens. Correspondingly, the survival of organs from cadaveric donors has generally been poorer than that of HLA-identical or one-haplotype–matched siblings as shown by the data in

TABLE 7. *One-year kidney graft function*

	1996	1986	1976
HLA identical grafts (living-related)	100%	100%	90%
One-haplotype matched grafts (living-related)	94%	92%	78%
Cadaver–Donor Grafts	86%	83%	58%

Data from the Transplantation Unit, Massachusetts General Hospital, Boston.

Table 7. The clinical issue under these circumstances is whether or not the nonrandom distribution of organs to achieve a larger number of matched antigens would achieve better results.

Figure 16 shows the effect of antigen matching for cadaver donor renal transplantation according to the data in the UCLA kidney transplant registry (741). The results suggest that for cadaver donor transplantation, only near-perfect MHC antigen matching leads to detectable benefit, and that the benefit is probably less than 10% in 1-year allograft survival. Not all studies of the effect of antigen matching in cadaver donor transplantation have shown the same benefit (743–748). Many factors probably affect our ability to measure the influence of antigen matching, including, for example, the finding that the success of transplantation, using poorly matched grafts, has varied considerably in different studies. Centers with poor graft survival might be expected to see greater benefit of antigen matching than centers that achieve high rates of success even under less favorable circumstances. Therefore, although antigen matching matters in the biology of transplantation, it probably matters little in modern clinical medicine.

Over the years the controversy about the impact of antigen matching has focused on several specific issues. Some investigators have suggested that matching for particular alleles of the HLA antigens is especially important, and others have suggested that matching for some loci is more important than for others (749,750). More recently, the issue has been further refined to include the question of whether matching for class II antigens might be more important than matching for class I antigens. There are clinical data suggesting that class II antigen matching is of particular benefit to the outcome of transplantation (751–753). Furthermore, it has recently become possible to perform class II typing with more precise molecular techniques than the serologic methods used in the past. Although the use of this technology could potentially increase the survival benefits associated with class II antigen matching, it would also reduce the likelihood that a matched donor could be found by these more stringent criteria and might increase the time required to perform HLA typing. Thus, it remains unclear that the distribution of organs to achieve such matching is worth the incumbent effort, expense, and increased ischemic time, which also may affect outcome.

Experimental Evidence

A particularly useful large animal model has been developed to test experimentally the importance of antigen matching. Over the past 20 years, three herds of partially inbred miniature swine have been developed for studies of transplantation biology. Each herd has been bred to homozygosity for a different allele at the MHC (termed SLA in swine) (40). Subsequent breeding has been intentionally randomized within herds in order to maintain a variety of segregating minor histocompatibility loci. Transplants among these animals thus resemble the situation within human families, i.e., HLA identical versus nonidentical siblings.

Studies of skin and renal allografts between these animals produced the results shown in Table 8. The difference observed for skin graft survival between SLA matched and mismatched animals was modest. Matching had a much more profound effect on kidney graft survival. One-third of the grafts between SLA-matched animals survived indefinitely without immunosuppression, despite the existence of multiple minor histoincompatibilities. The ability to reject renal allografts across minor differences was found to depend on an Ir gene, inherited in an autosomal-dominant fashion and not linked to the MHC (494).

Intra-MHC recombinants between several NIH minipig haplotypes have been identified, making it possible to examine the relative importance of class I versus class II matching on renal allograft survival in these large animals (40). The survival of renal allografts with class I–only differences and with class II–only differences is shown in Table 8. As in the mouse, both class I and class II differences appeared sufficient to cause prompt skin graft rejection. However, for kidney allografts, class II matching was of particular importance in determining the outcome. In fact, the results for minor plus class I differences were indistinguishable from those for minor histocompatibility antigen differences alone.

These experimental data were obtained without the exogenous immunosuppression always administered in clinical studies. They demonstrate the biologic principle that antigen matching is important to graft survival and further indicate that class II antigen matching is likely to be particularly important. No experimental system is likely to settle the empirical issue in clinical medicine,

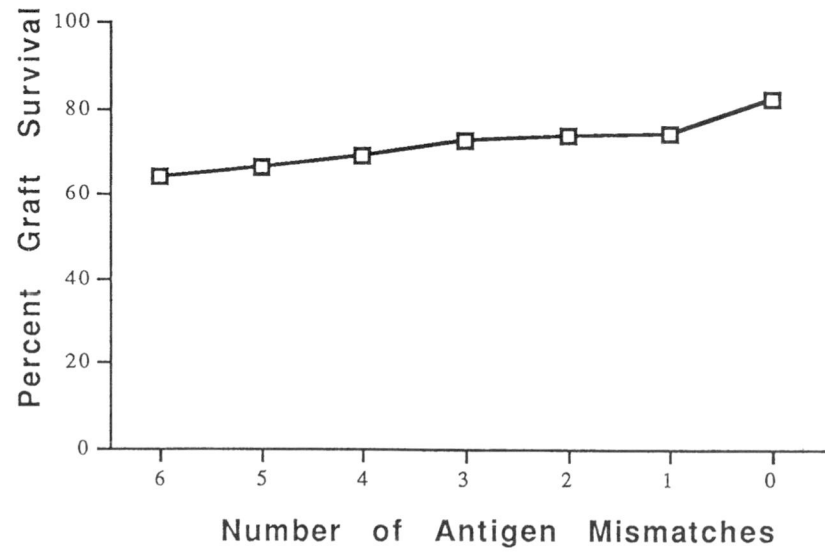

FIG. 16. Effect of antigen matching on graft survival. Three-year graft survival based on number of antigen mismatches.

TABLE 8. *Graft survival and antigen matching in minipigs without immunosuppression*

| Graft | Mismatch | | | |
	Minors only	Major and minors	Class I*	Class II*
Skin	11.8 ± 0.9	7.0 ± 0.4	10.8 ± 2.3	7.8 ± 1.0
Kidney	30.0 ± 15.0 (2/3)	12 ± 1.9	19.5 ± 6.8 (2/3)	21.8 ± 10.4
	>120 (1/3)	12.0	>120 (1/3)	

*a*Single haplotype mismatch
Survival time is shown in days.
Data from reference (40).

however, of how much benefit will be obtained under the conditions of current practice.

The Cross-Match

There are several means of detecting preexisting antibodies in the serum of potential recipients that have specificity for donor antigens. First, it is necessary to determine blood type because clinical transplantation across blood group barriers is never knowingly attempted for those organs susceptible to hyperacute rejection. One exception is the ability to transplant organs from donors of the A2 blood group to recipients of other blood groups (754). Secondly, immediate pretransplant sera from prospective recipients are tested against lymphocytes of potential donors. This test is called a cross-match, and it is not the same as antigen matching discussed above. An individual can have a negative cross-match (meaning that he or she does not have antibodies reactive with donor antigens) but still be completely unmatched with respect to HLA antigens. On the other hand, matching for some HLA antigens may improve the chances of obtaining a negative cross-match for prospective recipients who have developed antibodies reactive with many foreign HLA antigens. The cross-match is generally performed by a two-step antibody-mediated complement-dependent cytotoxicity assay. In many centers, the test is augmented by the intermediate addition of antihuman immunoglobulin to increase the sensitivity for detecting lysis (184,755). More recently, flow cytometry has been used to detect preexisting recipient antibodies with still additional sensitivity, although the data from flow cytometric analysis may be too sensitive to be clinically applicable (756–758).

The Sensitized Candidate for Organ Transplantation

Because kidneys and many other vascularized organs cannot currently be transplanted into recipients with preexisting antibodies, the clinical goal is to avoid the formation of antibodies reactive with donor antigens or to find organs that do not express the particular HLA antigens against which the recipient has been sensitized. Except for blood group antibodies, recipient sensitization to transplantation antigens always occurs by prior exposure to allogeneic tissue. This may occur as a result of blood transfusion, as a result of previous organ transplantation, or, in women, by exposure to paternal antigens during or just after pregnancy. The degree of sensitization of a potential kidney recipient is measured regularly by testing sera on a panel of lymphocytes selected from individuals who collectively express a broad representation of the HLA antigens. Transplantation candidates whose sera react with a high percentage of the cells in this panel (panel reactive antibody) are said to be "highly sensitized." The term may be confusing to immunologists because in the clinical setting it refers only to B-cell sensitization and does not necessarily imply sensitization of cell-mediated effector mechanisms. Highly sensitized candidates may wait years to receive a kidney transplant, and some may never receive one.

If a recipient has detectable antibodies to HLA antigens, they cannot receive an organ bearing these HLA antigens. Prior screening of potential recipients against the panel of HLA antigens can predict some of the determinants against which antibodies already exist. Most highly sensitized individuals actually produce antibodies of relatively limited heterogeneity that are reactive with public epitopes of HLA antigens (759). Thus, the HLA phenotype of unsuitable donors for any given recipient can be predicted with some precision. In this case, HLA tissue typing has value in identifying kidneys that may have a negative cross-match for highly sensitized individuals.

The level of sensitization manifested by transplantation candidates fluctuates over time. As a result, it is possible for recipients to have a negative cross-match with a donor's cells using recently obtained serum, but a positive cross-match using previously collected sera. Transplantation in the face of this historical positive cross-match has been performed successfully (760).

Obtaining cross-match–negative donors by locating well-matched organs or by waiting for a decline in the level of sensitization represent the primary solutions currently available for sensitized patients. Despite numerous trials, no widespread protocol for the active treatment of sensitized individuals to remove antibody has been adopted.

The Diagnosis of Rejection

In clinical organ transplantation, the most obvious manifestation of the rejection process is diminished function of the transplanted organ. Other causes of graft dysfunction exist, however, and it is obviously important to confirm the immunologic origin of the event before increasing immunosuppression. The clinical pattern of dysfunction often helps to suggest the diagnosis of rejection. However, no clinical sign can definitively diagnose rejection. It would be useful, therefore, to determine a means of identifying rejection episodes based on systemic manifestations of the immunologic mechanisms involved. Unfortunately there is not yet a well-established assay to measure rejection activity. Two approaches include the measurement of antidonor antibody production and the sequential measurement of cell-mediated responses to donor antigens. Antibody responses have frequently been documented following graft rejection, but they tend to appear after rejection is complete. *In vitro* cell-mediated responses, both proliferative and cytotoxic, may or may not be present while a graft is in place and are not well correlated with clinical rejection episodes (761,762). Assays of humoral and cellular responses to donor antigens both suffer from the possibility that donor-specific elements of the response may be absorbed by the antigens of the graft, at least until the late stages of rejection. Furthermore, the existence of tissue-specific peptides may allow T-cell responses to occur *in vivo* that cannot be measured *in vitro* when donor lymphocytes are used as stimulators.

The standard procedure in the diagnosis of allograft rejection has always been the biopsy of the transplanted organ itself. Pathologists have been able to identify the abnormal lymphocytic infiltrate within grafts, to grade the intensity of the infiltrate, and, for some organs, to describe histologic findings characterizing the effects of immunologic injury (763–769). Some pathologic changes, including a lymphocytic infiltrate of the vascular wall, seem to be well correlated with rejection activity (769). In addition, pathologic changes suggesting nonimmunologic causes of renal dysfunction may be helpful in patient management.

Despite the widespread reliance on the biopsy to define episodes of rejection, however, differentiation of rejection from its absence is often difficult, particularly when cyclosporine immunosuppression has been used. Because most clinical allograft biopsies are performed when the organ is not functioning well, and only after mechanical causes of dysfunction have been excluded, most organs that are examined via biopsy, by selection, are undergoing rejection. Therefore, inability to detect nonrejection events in a few cases pathologically will still leave an excellent correlation between the diagnosis of rejection and the response to therapy. When routine biopsies of transplanted organs have been done, regardless of organ dysfunction, they have revealed a poor correlation between histologic findings and clinical evidence of rejection (770,771). Experimental studies of skin grafts, as discussed above, have found that the degree of lymphocytic infiltrate in an allograft correlated better with the nature of the antigenic disparity rather than with the intensity of the rejection process (285). Furthermore, several experimental models of tolerance induction have shown intense lymphocytic infiltrates in organs that go on to survive indefinitely in recipients who develop tolerance to the donor antigens (772). These studies suggest that the amount of lymphocytic infiltrate detected pathologically may not be helpful in diagnosing rejection episodes and determining the need for treatment.

How Much Immunosuppression Is Enough?

Although the majority of transplant recipients respond immunologically to their new organ despite immunosuppression, some patients seem never to generate any rejection activity and maintain their transplanted organ with small doses of immunosuppressive drugs. Indeed, a few patients have been known to stop all of their medications but have kept their transplant for years without rejection. On the other hand, some patients seem to require and tolerate high doses of exogenous immunosuppression, whereas others seem to be severely immunocompromised by low doses of these drugs. These observations make it clear that the amount of immunosuppression that is required or that is safe is not the same for every individual or for all grafts. Unfortunately there is no well-established assay to determine the amount of immunosuppression an individual requires and can safely tolerate for their particular transplant.

Recently, a biologic determination of immunocompetence for patients on cyclosporine has been reported. Lymphocytes from transplant recipients were tested for their capacity to generate CD4$^+$ direct helper responses, CD8$^+$ direct helper responses, and CD4$^+$ indirect helper responses to foreign antigens. Those patients whose direct responses were intact appeared to experience more rejection than those who only maintained their indirect responses (36,773). Refinement of assays such as this, especially to incorporate donor-specific responses, would help enable tailoring of immunosuppressive therapy for the individual patient.

CONCLUSION

The great danger in any textbook chapter is that the need to summarize what we think is known will obscure the much greater amount still left to be learned. In recent years enormous progress has been made in the study of the major histocompatibility antigens; yet we still know too little about the products of the numerous other histocompatibility loci that encode the minor antigens. Recently we have gained important insight into the role of APCs in T-cell sensitization; but we still have not explored adequately the role that indirect presentation of alloantigens plays in graft rejection. During the past two decades we have learned much about the generation and function of CTLs and about their likely role in some mechanisms of graft rejection; however, the suspicion is strong that noncytotoxic mechanisms of rejection probably also exist, involving a crucial role for cytokines. Finally, this chapter has outlined several techniques for the generation of immunologic tolerance to alloantigens in experimental systems; yet it is still not possible to accomplish routine organ transplantation in human beings without the use of nonspecific immunosuppression. It is, of course, the great fascination of transplantation immunology that new insights into these and other basic immunologic issues will likely have such important consequences in clinical transplantation.

REFERENCES

1. Russell PS, Monaco AP, eds. *The biology of tissue transplantation.* Boston: Little, Brown, 1965.
2. Morris PS. *Tissue transplantation.* New York: Churchill Livingstone, 1982.
3. Bach FH, Sachs DH. Transplantation immunology. *N Engl J Med* 1987;317:489–492.
4. Rogers BO. Transplantation of skin. In: Peer LA, ed. *Transplantation of tissues.* Baltimore: Williams and Wilkins, 1959:75.
5. Woodruff MFA, ed. *The transplantation of tissues and organs.* Springfield, IL: Charles C. Thomas Publisher, 1960.
6. Gibson T. Zoografting: a curious chapter in the history of plastic surgery. *Br J Plast Surg* 1955;8:234.
7. Billingham RE. Transplantation: past, present and future. *J Invest Dermatol* 1963;41:165.
8. Voronoff S, ed. *Rejuvenation by grafting.* London: George Allen and Unwin, 1925.
9. Carrel A. Transplantation in mass of the kidneys. *J Exp Med* 1908;10:98.
10. Converse JM, Casson PR. The historical background of transplantation. In: Rapaport FT, Dausset J, eds. *Human transplantation.* New York: Grune & Stratton, 1968:7.
11. Medawar PB. The immunology of transplantation. *Harvey Lectures* 1958; 1956–1957:144.
12. Lawler RH, et al. Homotransplantation of the kidney in the human. *JAMA* 1950;147:844.
13. Servelle M. La greffe du rein. *Rev Chir* 1951;70:186.
14. DuBost C. Resultats d'une tentative de greffe renale. *Bull Memoirs Soc Med* 1951;67:1372.
15. Kuss R. Quelques essais de greffe du rein chez l'homme. *Mem Acad Chir* 1951;77:755.
16. Hume DM, Merrill JP, Miller BF. Homologous transplantation of the human kidney. *J Clin Invest* 1952;31:640.
17. Hume DM, Merrill JP, Miller BF, Thorn GW. Experience with renal homotransplantation in the human: report of 9 cases. *J Clin Invest* 1955;34:327–382.

18. Merrill JP, Murray JE, Harrison JH, Guild WR. Successful homotransplantation of human kidney between identical twins. *JAMA* 1956;160:277–282.

19. Groth CG. Landmarks in clinical renal transplantation. *Surg Gynecol Obstet* 1972;134:323.

20. Gibson T, Medawar PB. The fate of skin homografts in man. *J Anat* 1943;77:299.

21. Medawar PB. The behavior and fate of skin autografts and skin homografts in rabbits. *J Anat* 1944;78:176–199.

22. Billingham RE, Brent L, Medawar PB, Sparrow EM. Quantitative studies of transplantation immunity. I. Survival times of skin homografts exchanged between members of different inbred strains of mice. *Proc R Soc Lond [Biol]* 1954;143:43–58.

23. Medawar PB. Second study of behaviour and fate of skin homografts in rabbits. *J Anat* 1945;79:157.

24. Little CC. The genetics of tissue transplantation in mammals. *Cancer Res* 1924;8:75–95.

25. Little CC. A possible mendelian explanation for a type of inheritance apparently non-Mendelian in nature. *Science* 1914;40:904–906.

26. Little CC, Typper EE. Further studies on inheritance of susceptibility to a transplantable tumor of Japanese waltzing mice. *J Med Res* 1916;33:393.

27. Bailey DW. Four approaches to estimating number of histocompatibility loci. *Transplant Proc* 1970;2:32–38.

28. Bailey DW, Mobraaten LE. Estimates of the number of loci contributing to the histoincompatibility between C57BL/6 and BALB/c strains of mice. *Transplantation* 1969;7:394–400.

29. Barnes AD, Krohn PL. Estimation of number of histocompatibility genes controlling successful transplantation of normal skin in mice. *Proc R Soc Lond [Biol]* 1957;146:505–526.

30. Billingham RE, Hodge BA, Silvers WK. Estimate of number of hitocompatibiltiy loci in rat. *Proc Natl Acad Sci U S A* 1962;48:422–433.

31. Little CC. The genetics of tumor transplantation. In: Snell GD, ed. Biology of the laboratory mouse, 1st ed. New York: Dover Publications, 1941:279–309.

32. Stimpfling JH, Reichert AE. Strain C57BL/10ScSn and its congenic resistant sublines. *Transplant Proc* 1970;2:39.

33. Bach FH, Widmer MB, Bach ML, Klein J. Serologically defined and lymphocyte-defined components of the major histocompatibility complex in the mouse. *J Exp Med* 1972;136:1430.

34. Lerner EA, Matis LA, Janeway CA, Jones PP, Schwartz RH, Murphy DB. Monoclonal antibody against an Ir gene product. *J Exp Med* 1980;152:1085.

35. Caughman SW, Sharrow SO, Shimad S, et al. Ia+ murine epidermal Langerhans cells are deficient in surface expression of class I MHC. *Proc Natl Acad Sci U S A* 1986;83:7438–7442.

36. Harris HW, Gill TJ. Expression of class I transplantation antigens. *Transplantation* 1986;42:109.

37. Daar AS, Fuggle SV, Fabre JW, Ting A, Morris PJ. The detailed distribution of MHC class II antigens in normal human organs. *Transplantation* 1984;38:293.

38. Glimcher LH, Kara CJ. Sequences and factors: a guide to MHC class-II transcription. *Ann Rev Immunol* 1992;10:13–49.

39. Pescovitz MD, Sachs DH, Lunney JK, Hsu S-M. Localization of class II MHC antigens on porcine renal vascular endothelium. *Transplantation* 1984;37:627–30.

40. Pescovitz MD, Thistlethwaite JR Jr, Auchincloss H Jr, et al. Effect of class II antigen matching on renal allograft survival in miniature swine. *J Exp Med* 1984;160:1495–1508.

41. Rosenberg A, Mizuochi T, Singer A. Analysis of T-cell subsets in rejection of Kb mutant skin allografts differing at class I MHC. *Nature* 1986;322:829–831.

42. Fischer Lindahl K, Wilson DB. Histocompatibility antigen-activated cytotoxic T lymphocytes II. Estimates of frequency and specificity of precursors. *J Exp Med* 1977;145:508–522.

43. Teh HS, Harley E, Phillips RA, Miller RG. Quantitative studies on the precursors of cytotoxic lymphocytes I. Characterization of a clonal assay and determination of the size of clones derived from single precursors. *J Immunol* 1977;118:1049–1056.

44. Heber-Katz E, Schwartz RH, Matis LA, et al. Contribution of antigen-presenting cell major histocompatibility complex gene products to the specificity of antigen-induced T cell activation. *J Exp Med* 1982;155:1086–1099.

45. Hunig T, Bevan MJ. Specificity of T-cell clones illustrates altered self hypothesis. *Nature* 1981;294:460–62.

46. Ben-Nun A, Lando Z, Dorf MA, Burakoff SJ. Analysis of cross-reactive antigen-specific T cell clones: specific recognition of two major histocompatibility complex (MHC) and two non-MHC antigens by a single clone. *J Exp Med* 1983;157:2147–2153.

47. Zinkernagel RM, Callahan GN, Cooper AS, Klein PA, Klein J. On the thymus in the differentiation of "H-2 self-recognition" by T cells: evidence for dual recognition. *J Exp Med* 1978;147:882.

48. Jerne NK. The somatic generation of immune recognition. *Eur J Immunol* 1971;1:1–9.

49. Blackman M, Yague J, Kubo R, et al. The T cell repertoire may be biased in favor of MHC recognition. *Cell* 1986;47:349–57.

50. Kappler JW, Wade T, White J, et al. A T cell receptor V beta segment that imparts reactivity to a class II major histocompatibility complex product. *Cell* 1987;49:263–271.

51. Zerrahn J, Held W, Raulet DH. The MHC reactivity of the T cell repertoire prior to positive and negative selection. *Cell* 1997;88:627.

52. Surh CD, Lee D-S, Fung-Leung W, Karlsson L, Sprent J. Thymic selection by a single MHC/peptide ligand produces a semidiverse repertoire of CD4+ T cells. *Immunity* 1997;7:209.

53. Bevan MJ. In thymic selection, peptide diversity gives and takes away. *Immunity* 1997;7:175.

54. Tourne S, Miyazaki T, Oxenius A, et al. Selection of a broad repertoire of CD4+ T cells in H-2Ma0/0 mice. *Immunity* 1997;7:187.

55. Grubin CE, Kovats S, deRoos P, Rudensky AY. Deficient positive selection of CD4 T cells in mice displaying altered repertoires of MHC class II-bound self-peptides. *Immunity* 1997;7:197.

56. Sprent J, Lo D, Gao EK, Ron Y. T cell selection in the thymus. *Immunol Rev* 1988;101:173–190.

57. Bevan MJ. High determinant density may explain the phenomenon of alloreactivity. *Immunol Today* 1984;5:128–30.

58. Matzinger P, Bevan MJ. Why do so many lymphocytes respond to major histocompatibility complex antigens? *Cell Immunol* 1977;29:1.

59. Berkowitz N, Braunstein NS. T cell responses specific for subregions of allogenic MHC molecules. *J Immunol* 1992;148:309–317.

60. Muellbacher A, Hill AB, Blanden RV, Cowden WB, King NJC, Tha Hla R. Alloreactive cytotoxic T cells recognize MHC class I antigen without peptide specificity. *J Immunol* 1991;147:1765–1772.

61. Smith PA, Brunmark A, Jackson MR, Potter TA. Peptide-independent recognition by alloreactive cytotoxic T lymphocytes (CTL). *J Exp Med* 1997;185:1023–1033.

62. Demotz S, Sette A, Sakaguchi K, Buchner R, Appella E, Grey HM. Self peptide requirement for class II major histocompatibility complex allorecognition. *Proc Natl Acad Sci U S A* 1991;88:8730–8734.

63. Heath WR, Kane KP, Mescher MF, Sherman LA. Alloreactive T cells discriminate among a diverse set of endogenous peptides. *Proc Natl Acad Sci U S A* 1991;88:5101–5105.

64. Roetzschke O, Falk K, Faath S, Rammensee H-G. On the nature of peptides involved in T cell alloreactivity. *J Exp Med* 1991;174:1059–1071.

65. Weber DA, Terrell NK, Zhang Y, et al. Requirement for peptide in alloreactive CD4+ T cell recognition of class II MHC molecules. *J Immunol* 1995;154:5153–5164.

66. Alexander-Miller MA, Burke K, Koszinowski UH, Hansen TH, Connolly JM. Alloreactive cytotoxic T lymphocytes generated in the presence of viral-derived peptides show exquisite peptide and MHC specificity. *J Immunol* 1993;151:1–10.

67. Smith KD, Huczko E, Engelhard VH, Li Y-Y, Lutz CT. Alloreactive cytotoxic T lymphocytes focus on specific major histocompatibility complex-bound peptides. *Transplantation* 1997;64:351–9.

68. Graff RJ, Bailey DW. The non-H-2 histocompatibility loci and their antigens. *Transplant Rev* 1973;15:26.

69. Loveland B, Simpson E. The non-MHC transplantation antigens: neither weak nor minor. *Immunol Today* 1986;7:223–229.

70. Simpson E. Non-H-2 histocompatibility antigens: can they be retroviral products? *Immunol Today* 1987;8:176–177.

71. Roopenian DC, Widmer MB, Orosz CG, Bach FH. Response against single minor histocompatibility antigens. I. Functional immunogenetic analysis of cloned cytolytic T cells. *J Immunol* 1983;131:2135–2140.

72. Roopenian DC, Orosz CG, Bach FH. Responses against single histocompatibility antigens. II. Analysis of cloned helper T cells. *J Immunol* 1984;132:1080–1084.

73. Tekolf WA, Shaw S. Primary in vitro generation of cytotoxic cells specific for human minor histocompatibility antigens between HLA identical siblings. *J Immunol* 1984;132:1756–1760.

74. Czitrom AA, Gascoigne NR, Edwards S, Waterfield DJ. Induction of minor alloantigen-specific T cell subsets in vivo: recognition of processed antigen by helper but not by cytotoxic T cell precursors. *J Immunol* 1984;133:33–39.

75. Bevan MJ. Cross-priming for a secondary cytotoxic response to minor H antigens with H-2 congenic cells which do not cross-react in the cytotoxic assay. *J Exp Med* 1976;143:1283.

76. Wallny H J, Rammensee H-G. Identification of classical minor histocompatibility antigen as cell-derived peptide. *Nature* 1990;343:275–278.

77. Elliott T, Townsend A, Cerundolo V. Naturally processed peptides. *Nature* 1990;348:195–197.

78. Falk K, Rotzschke O, Rammensee H-G. Cellular peptide composition governed by major histocompatibility complex class I molecules. *Nature* 1990;348:248–251.

79. Lai PK, Waterfield JD, Gascoigne NR, Sharrock CE, Mitchison NA. T-cell responses to minor histocompatibility antigens. *Immunology* 1982;47:371–81.

80. Roopenian DC. What are minor histocompatibility loci? A new look at an old question. *Immunol Today* 1992;13:7–10.

81. Elkins WI. Decreased immunogenicity of a transplantation antigen in hosts sensitized to other isoantigens of its cellular vehicle. *J Immunol* 1964;92:275.

82. Johnson LL, Bailey DW, Mobraaten LE. Antigenic competition between minor (non-H-2) histocompatibility antigens. *Immunogenetics* 1981;13:451–455.

83. Wettstein PJ, Bailey DW. Immunodominance in the immune response to "multiple" histocompatibility antigens. *Immunogenetics* 1982;16:47–58.

84. Wettstein PJ. Immunodominance in the T cell response to multiple non-H-2 histocompatibility antigens III. Single histocompatibility antigens dominate the male antigen. *J Immunol* 1986;137:2073.

85. Lai PK. Antigen competition in cytotoxic T cell response to minor histocompatibility antigens. *Transplantation* 1985;39:638–643.
86. Nevala WK, Wettstein PJ. The preferential cytolytic T lymphocyte response to immunodominant minor histocompatibility antigen peptides. *Transplantation* 1996;62:283–291.
87. Roopenian DC, Widmer MB, Orosz CG, Bach FH. Helper cell-independent cytolytic T lymphocytes specific for a minor histocompatibility antigen. *J Immunol* 1983;130:542–545.
88. Rammensee HG, Klein J. Complexity of the histocompatibility-3 region in the mouse. *J Immunol* 1983;130:2926–2929.
89. Juretic A, Vucak I, Malenica B, Nagy ZA, Klein J. H-41, a new histocompatibility locus. I. Histogenetic analysis. *J Immunol* 1984;133:2950–2954.
90. Ichikawa H, Suzuki H, Hino T, Kubota E, Saito K. In vivo priming of mouse CTL precursors directed to product of a newly defined minor H-42 locus is under a novel control of class II MHC gene. *J Immunol* 1985;135:3681–3685.
91. Gordon RD, Simpson E, Samelson LE. In vitro cell-mediated immune responses to the male specific (H-Y) antigen in mice. *J Exp Med* 1975;142:1108.
92. Simpson E, Gordon RD. Responsiveness to H-Y antigen, Ir gene complementation, and target cell specificity. *Immunol Rev* 1977;35:59.
93. Simpson E. The role of H-Y as a minor transplantation antigen. *Immunol Today* 1982;3:97–106.
94. Roopenian DC, Davis AP, Christianson GJ, Mobraaten LE. The functional basis of minor histocompatibility loci. *J Immunol* 1993;151:4595–4605.
95. Schorle H, Holtschke T, Hunig T, Schimpl A, Horak I. Development and function of T cells in mice rendered interleukin-2 deficient by gene targeting. *Nature* 1991;352:621–624.
96. Arase-Fukushi N, Arase H, Ogasawara K, Good RA, Onoe K. Production of minor lymphocyte stimulatory-1a antigen from activated CD4+ or CD8+ T cells. *J Immunol* 1993;151:4445–4454.
97. Jarvis CD, Germain RN, Hager GL, Damschroder M, Matis LA. Tissue-specific expression of messenger RNAs encoding endogenous viral superantigens. *J Immunol* 1994;152:1032–1038.
98. Moore NC, Anderson G, McLoughlin DEJ, Owen JJT, Jenkinson EJ. Differential expression of Mtv loci in MHC class II-positive thymic stromal cells. *J Immunol* 1994;152:4826–4831.
99. Ardavin C, Waanders G, Ferrero I, Anjurere F, Acha-Orbea H, MacDonald HR. Expression and presentation of endogenous mouse mammary tumor virus superantigens by thymic and splenic dendritic cells and B cells. *J Immunol* 1996;157:2789–2794.
100. Steinmuller D, Wachtel SS. Transplantation biology and immunogenetics of murine skin-specific (Sk) alloantigens. *Transplant Proc* 1980;12:100.
101. Rosengard BR, Kortz EO, Ojikutu CA, et al. The failure of skin grafting to break tolerance to class I–disparate renal allografts in miniature swine despite inducing marked antidonor cellular immunity. *Transplantation* 1991;52:1044–1052.
102. Lorenz R, Allen PM. Processing and presentation of self proteins. *Immunol Rev* 1988;106:115–127.
103. Hadley GA, Rostapshova EA, Bartlett ST. Dominance of tissue-restricted cytotoxic T lymphocytes in the response to allogeneic renal epithelial cell lines. *Transplantation* 1996;62:75–83.
104. Bonomo A, Matzinger P. Thymus epithelium induces tissue-specific tolerance. *J Exp Med* 1993;177:1153–1164.
105. Race RR, Sanger R, eds. Blood groups in man. Oxford, England: Blackwell Scientific, 1958.
106. Oriol R. Tissular expression of ABH and Lewis antigens in humans and animals: expected value of different animal models in the study of ABO-incompatible organ transplants. *Transplant Proc* 1987;19:4416.
107. Szulman AE. The histological distribution of the blood group substances in man as disclosed by immunofluorescence. II. The H antigen and its relation to A and B antigens. *J Exp Med* 1962;115:977–996.
108. Joyce S, Mathew JM, Flye MW, Mohanakumar T. A polymorphic human kidney-specific non-MHC alloantigen. Its possible role in tissue-specific allograft immunity. *Transplantation* 1992;53:1119–1127.
109. Platt JL, Bach FH. The barrier to xenotransplantation. *Transplantation* 1991;52:937–947.
110. Fischel RJ, Bolman RM III, Platt JL, Najarian JS, Bach FH, Matas AJ. Removal of IgM anti-endothelial antibodies results in prolonged cardiac xenograft survival. *Transplant Proc* 1990;22:1077–1078.
111. Kiessling R, Hochman PS, Haller O, Shearer GM, Wigzell H, Cudkowicz G. Evidence for a similar or common mechanism for natural killer activity and resistance to hemopoietic grafts. *Eur J Immunol* 1977;7:655–663.
112. Lafferty KJ, Bootes A, Dart G, Talmage DW. Effect of organ culture on the survival of thyroid allografts in mice. *Transplantation* 1976;22:138–149.
113. Lafferty K, Prowse S, Simeonovic C, Warren HS. Immunobioloby of tissue transplantation: a return to the passenger leucocyte concept. In: Paul WE, Fathman CG, Metzgar H, eds. *Annual review of immunology.* Palo Alto, CA: Annual Reviews, Inc., 1983;143–173.
114. Sollinger HW, Burkholder PM, Rasmus WR, Bach FH. Prolonged survival of xenografts after organ culture. *Surgery* 1977;81:74.
115. Lechler R, Batchelor J. Restoration of immunogeneity to passenger cell depleted kidney allografts by the addition of donor strain dendritic cells. *J Exp Med* 1982;155:31–41.
116. Faustman D, Hauptfeld V, Lacy P, Davie J. Prolongation of murine islet allograft survival by pretreatment of islets with antibody directed to Ia determinants. *Proc Natl Acad Sci U S A* 1981;78:5156–5159.
117. Steinman RM. Dendritic cells. *Transplantation* 1981;31:151.
118. Faustman D, Steinman R, Gebel H, Hauptfeld V, Davie J, Lacy P. Prevention of rejection of murine islet allografts by pre-treatment with anti-dendritic cell antibody. *Proc Natl Acad Sci U S A* 1984;81:3864–3868.
119. Glimcher LH, Kim KJ, Green I, Paul WE. Ia antigen-bearing B cell tumor lines can present protein antigen and alloantigen in a major histocompatibility complex–restricted fashion to antigen-reactive T cells. *J Exp Med* 1982;155:445–59.
120. Janeway CA, Ron J, Katz ME. The B cell is the initiating antigen-presenting cell in peripheral lymph nodes. *J Immunol* 1987;138:1051–1055.
121. Ron Y, Sprent J. T cell priming in vivo: a major role for B cells in presenting antigen to T cells in lymph nodes. *J Immunol* 1987;138:2848–2856.
122. Steinman RM. The dendritic cell system and its role in immunogenicity. *Annu Rev Immunol* 1991;9:271–296.
123. Skoskievicz MJ, Colvin RB, Schneeberger EE, Russell PS. Widespread and selective induction of MHC-determined antigens in vivo by interferon-gamma. *J Exp Med* 1985;162:1645–1664.
124. Benson EM, Colvin RB, Russell PS. Induction of Ia antigens in murine renal transplants. *J Immunol* 1985;134:7.
125. Pober JS, Collins T, Gimbrone MA Jr, Libby P, Reiss CS. Inducible expression of class II major histocompatibility complex antigens and the immunogeneicity of vascular endothelium. *Transplantation* 1986;41:141–146.
126. La Rosa FG, Talmage DW. Synergism between minor and major histocompatibility antigens in the rejection of cultured allografts. *Transplantation* 1985;39:480–485.
127. Parker KE, Dalchau R, Fowler VJ, Priestley CA, Carter CA, Fabre JW. Stimulation of CD4+ T lymphocytes by allogenic MHC peptides presented on autologous antigen-presenting cells. *Transplantation* 1992;53:918–924.
128. Woodward JG, Shegekawa JA, Frelinger JA. Bone marrow–derived cells are responsible for stimulating I region-incompatible skin graft rejection. *Transplantation* 1982;33:254.
129. Katz SI, Tamaki K, Sachs DH. Epidermal Langerhans cells are derived from cells originating in bone marrow. *Nature* 1979;282:324–326.
130. Chen H-D, Raab S, Silvers WK. Influence of major-histocompatibility-complex–compatible and incompatibile Langerhans cells on the survival of H-Y–incompatible skin grafts in rats. *Transplantation* 1985;40:194.
131. Chen H-D, Silvers WK. Influence of Langerhans cells on the survival of H-Y incompatible skin grafts in rats. *J Invest Dermatol* 1983;81:20–23.
132. Gouw AS, Houthoff HJ, Huitema S, Beelen JM, Gips CH, Poppema S. Expression of major histocompatibility complex antigens and replacement of donor cells by recipient ones in human liver grafts. *Transplantation* 1987;43:291–296.
133. Barker CF, Billingham RE. The role of regional lymphatics in the skin homograft response. *Transplantation* 1967;5:962.
134. Tilney NL, Gowans JL. The sensitization of rats by allografts transplanted to alymphatic pedicles of skin. *J Exp Med* 1971;133:951.
135. Hume DM, Egdahl RH. Progressive destruction of renal homografts isolated from the regional lymphatics of the host. *Surgery* 1955;38:194.
136. Pedersen NC, Morris B. The role of the lymphatic system in the rejection of homografts: a study of lymph from renal transplants. *J Exp Med* 1970;131:936–969.
137. Kraal G, Breel M, Janse M, Bruin G. Langerhans cells, veiled cells, and interdigitating cells in the mouse recognized by a monoclonal antibody. *J Exp Med* 1986;163:981–997.
138. Dustin ML, Springer TA. Role of lymphocyte adhesion receptors in transient interactions and cell locomotion. *Ann Rev Immunol* 1991;9:27–66.
139. Springer TA. Adhesion receptors of the immune system. *Nature* 1990;346:425–34.
140. Kirby JA, Cunningham AC. Intragraft antigen presentation: the contribution of bone-marrow derived, epithelial and endothelial presenting cells. *Transplant Rev* 1997;11:127–140.
141. Strober S, Gowans JL. The role of lymphocytes in the sensitization of rats to renal allografts. *J Exp Med* 1965;122:347.
142. van den Bogaerde J, Aspinall R, Wang M-W, et al. Induction of long-term survival of hamster heart xenografts in rats. *Transplantation* 1991;52:15–20.
143. Cramer DV, Chapman FA, Jaffee BD, et al. The prolongation of concordant hamster-to-rat cardiac xenografts by brequinar sodium. *Transplantation* 1992;54:403–408.
144. Xiao F, Chong AS, Foster P, et al. Leflunomide controls rejection in hamster to rat cardiac xenografts. *Transplantation* 1994;58:828–834.
145. Manning DD, Reed ND, Shaffer CF. Maintenance of skin xenografts of widely divergent phylogenetic origin on congenitally athymic (nude) mice. *J Exp Med* 1973;138:488.
146. Rosenberg AS, Mizuochi T, Sharrow SO, Singer A. Phenotype, specificity, and function of T cell subsets and T cell interactions involved in skin allograft rejection. *J Exp Med* 1987;165:1296.
147. Sprent J, Schaefer M, Lo D, Korngold R. Properties of purified T cell subsets. II. In vivo responses to class I vs. class II H-2 differences. *J Exp Med* 1986;163:998–1011.
148. Cosimi AB, Burton RC, Colvin RB, et al. Treatment of acute renal allograft rejection with OKT3 monoclonal antibody. *Transplantation* 1981;32:535–539.
149. Auchincloss H Jr, Ghobrial RRM, Russell PS, Winn HJ. Anti-L3T4 in vivo prevents alloantibody formation after skin grafting without prolonging graft survival. *Transplantation* 1988;45:1118–1123.

150. Keene J-A, Forman J. Helper activity is required for the in vivo generation of cytotoxic T lymphocytes. *J Exp Med* 1982;155:768.

151. Karlhofer FM, Ribaudo RK, Yokoyama WM. MHC class I alloantigen specificity of Ly-49- IL-2- activated natural killer cells. *Nature* 1992;358:66–70.

152. Moretta L, Ciccone E, Moretta A, Hoglund P, Ohlen C, Karre K. Allorecognition by NK cells: nonself or no self? *Immunol Today* 1992;13:300–306.

153. Lee LA, Sergio JJ, Sykes M. Natural killer cells weakly resist engraftment of allogeneic long-term multilineage-repopulating hematopoietic stem cells. *Transplantation* 1996;61:125–132.

154. Sharabi Y, Aksentijevich I, Sundt TM III, Sachs DH, Sykes M. Specific tolerance induction across a xenogeneic barrier: production of mixed rat/mouse lymphohematopoietic chimeras using a nonlethal preparative regimen. *J Exp Med* 1990;172:195–202.

155. Sharabi Y, Sachs DH. Mixed chimerism and permanent specific transplantation tolerance induced by a non-lethal preparative regimen. *J Exp Med* 1989;169:493–502.

156. Bix M, Liao NS, Zijlstra M, Loring J, Jaenisch R, Raulet DH. Rejection of class I MHC-deficient haemopoietic cells by irradiated MHC-matched mice. *Nature* 1991;349:329.

157. Zijlstra M, Auchincloss H Jr, Loring JM, Chase CM, Russell PS, Jaenisch R. Skin graft rejection by beta2-microglobulin–deficient mice. *J Exp Med* 1992;175:885–893.

158. Renard V, Cambiaggi A, Vely F, et al. Transduction of cytotoxic signals in natural killer cells: a general model of fine tuning between activatory and inhibitory pathways in lymphocytes. *Immunol Rev* 1997;155:205–221.

159. Hoglund P, Sundback J, Olsson-Alheim MY, et al. Host MHC class I gene control of NK cell specificity in the mouse. *Immunol Rev* 1997;155:11–28.

160. Goodman DJ, Millan MT, Ferran C, Bach FH. Mechanisms of delayed xenograft rejection. In: Cooper DKC, Kemp E, Platt JL, White DJG, eds. *Xenotransplantation.* Heidelberg: Springer, 1997:77.

161. Inverardi L, PC, Stolzer AL, Bender JR, Sandrin MS, Pardi R. Human natural killer lymphocytes directly recognize evolutionarily conserved oligosaccharide ligands expressed by xenogeneic tissue. *Transplantation* 1997;63:1318–1330.

162. Sykes M, Harty MW, Karlhofer FM, Pearson DA, Yokoyama W. Hematopoietic cells and radioresistant host elements influence natural killer cell differentiation. *J Exp Med* 1993;178:223–229.

163. Johansson MH, Bieberich C, Jay G, Karre K, Hoglund P. Natural killer cell tolerance in mice with mosaic expression of major histocompatibility complex I transgene. *J Exp Med* 1997;186:353–364.

164. Held W, Raulet DH. Ly49A transgenic mice provide evidence for a major histocompatibility complex-dependent education process in natural killer cell development. *J Exp Med* 1997;185:2079–2088.

165. Sykes M. Unusual T cell populations in adult murine bone marrow: prevalence of CD3+CD4-CD8- and αβTCR+NK1.1+ cells. *J Immunol* 1990;145:3209–3215.

166. Kikly K, Dennert G. Evidence for extrathymic development of TNK cells. NK1+CD3+ cells responsible for acute marrow graft rejection are present in thymus-deficient mice. *J Immunol* 1992;149:403–412.

167. Sato K, Ohtsuka K, Hasegawa K, et al. Evidence for extrathymic generation of intermediate T cell receptor cells in the liver revealed in thymectomized, irradiated mice subjected to bone marrow transplantation. *J Exp Med* 1995;182:759–767.

168. Yoshimoto T, Paul WE. CD4pos, NK1.1pos T cells promptly produce interleukin 4 in response to in vivo challenge with anti-CD3. *J Exp Med* 1994;179:1285–1295.

169. Bendelac A, Lantz O, Quimby ME, Yewdell JW, Bennink JR, Brutkiewicz RR. CD1 recognition by mouse NK1+ T lymphocytes. *Science* 1995;268:863–865.

170. Porcelli S, Brenner MB, Greenstein JL, Balk SP, Terhorst C, Bleicher PA. Recognition of cluster of differentiation 1 antigens by human CD4-CD8- cytolytic T lymphocytes. *Nature* 1989;341:447–450.

171. Schmidt-Wolf IGH, Lefterova P, Johnston V, Huhn D, Blume KG, Negrin RS. Propagation of large numbers of T cells with natural killer cell markers. *Br J Hematol* 1994;87:453–458.

172. Lantz O, Bendelac A. An invariant T cell receptor α chain is used by a unique subset of major histocompatibility complex class I-specific CD4+ and CD4-8- T cells in mice and humans. *J Exp Med* 1994;180:1097–1106.

173. Bendelac A. CD1: presenting unusual antigens to unusual T lymphocytes. *Science* 1995;269:185–186.

174. Yankelevich B, Knobloch C, Nowicki M, Dennert G. A novel cell type responsible for marrow graft rejection in mice. T cells with NK phenotype cause acute rejection of marrow grafts. *J Immunol* 1989;142:3423–3430.

175. Blakely ML, Van Der Werf W, Berndt MC, Dalmasso AP, Bach FH, Hancock WW. Activation of intragraft endothelial and mononuclear cells during discordant xenograft rejection. *Transplantation* 1994;58:1059–1066.

176. Myburgh JA, Cohen I, Gecelter L, et al. Hyperacute rejection in human-kidney allografts: Shwartzman or Arthus reaction? *N Engl J Med* 1969;281:131–135.

177. Platt JL, Fischel RJ, Matas AJ, Reif SA, Bolman RM, Bach FH. Immunopathology of hyperacute xenograft rejection in a swine to primate model. *Transplantation* 1991;52:214–220.

178. Platt JL, Bach FH. The barrier to xenotransplantation. *Transplantation* 1991;52:937–947.

179. Pruitt SK, Baldwin WM III, Barth RN, Sanfilippo F. The effect of xenoreactive antibody and B cell depletion on hyperacute rejection of guinea pig-to-rat cardiac xenografts. *Transplantation* 1993;56:1318–1324.

180. Dalmasso AP, Vercellotti GM, Platt JL, Bach FH. Inhibition of complement-mediated endothelial cell cytotoxicity by decay-accelerating factor. *Transplantation* 1991;52:530–533.

181. Borche L, Thibaudeau K, Navenot J-M, Soulillou J-P, Blanchard D. Cytolytic effect of human anti-Gal IgM and complement on porcine endothelial cells: a kinetic analysis. *Xenotransplantation* 1994;1:125–131.

182. Platt JL, Vercellotti GM, Lindman BJ, Oegema TR Jr, Bach FH, Dalmasso AP. Release of heparan sulfate from endothelial cells: implications for pathogenesis of hyperacute rejection. *J Exp Med* 1990;171:1363–1368.

183. Auchincloss H Jr. Xenogeneic transplantation. A review. *Transplantation* 1988;46:1–20.

184. Fuller TC, Cosimi AB, Russell PS. Use of an antiglobulin-ATG reagent for detection of low levels of alloantibody—improvement of allograft survival in presensitized recipients. *Transplant Proc* 1978;10:463.

185. Alexandre GPJ, Squifflet JP, De Bruyere M, et al. Present experiences in a series of 26 ABO-incompatible living donor renal allografts. *Transplant Proc* 1987;19:4538.

186. Gordon RD, Fung JJ, Markus B, et al. The antibody crossmatch in liver transplantation. *Surgery* 1986;100:705–715.

187. Gordon RD, Iwatsuki S, Esquivel CO, Tzakis A, Todo S, Starzl TE. Liver transplantation across blood groups. *Surgery* 1986;100:342–348.

188. Doyle HR, Marino IR, Morelli F, et al. Assessing risk in liver transplantation: special reference to the significance of a positive cytotoxic crossmatch. *Ann Surg* 1996;224:168–177.

189. Jooste SV, Colvin RB, Soper WD, Winn HJ. The vascular bed as the primary target in the destruction of skin grafts by antiserum. I. Resistance of freshly-placed skin grafts to antiserum. *J Exp Med* 1981;154:1319–1331.

190. Baldamus CA, McKenzie IFC, Winn HJ, Russell PS. Acute destruction by humoral antibody of rat skin grafted in mice. *J Immunol* 1973;110:1532–1541.

191. Pierson RN III, Winn HJ, Russell PS, Auchincloss H Jr. Xenogeneic skin graft rejection is especially dependent on CD4+ T cells. *J Exp Med* 1989;170:991–996.

192. Ricordi C, Kneteman NM, Scharp DW, Lacy PE. Transplantation of cryopreserved human pancreatic islets into diabetic nude mice. *World J Surg* 1988;12:861–865.

193. Ricordi C, Scharp DW, Lacy PE. Reversal of diabetes in nude mice after transplantation of fresh and 7-day-cultured (24 degrees C) human pancreatic islets. *Transplantation* 1988;45:994–996.

194. Falqui L, Finke EH, Carel J-C, Scharp DW, Lacy PE. Marked prolongation of human islet xenograft survival (human-to-mouse) by low-temperature culture and temporary immunosuppression with human and mouse anti-lymphocyte sera. *Transplantation* 1991;51:1322–1324.

195. Aksentijevich I, Sachs DH, Sykes M. Natural antibodies against bone marrow cells of a concordant xenogeneic species. *J Immunol* 1991;147:79–85.

196. Trpkov K, Campbell P, Pazderka F, Cockfield S, Solez K, Halloran PF. Pathologic features of acute renal allograft rejection associated with donor-specific antibody. Analysis using the Banff grading schema. *Transplantation* 1996;61:1586–1592.

197. Platt JL. The immunological barriers to xenotransplantation. *Crit Rev Immunol* 1996;16:331–358.

198. Bach FH, Ferran C, Hechenleitner P, et al. Accommodation of vascularized xenografts: expression of "protective genes" by donor endothelial cells in a host Th2 cytokine environment. *Nature Med* 1997;3:196–204.

199. Millan MT, Geczy C, Stuhlmeier KM, Goodman DJ, Ferran C, Bach FH. Human monocytes activate porcine endothelial cells, resulting in increased E-selectin, interleukin-8, monocyte chemotactic protein-1, and plasminogen activator inhibitor-type-1 expression. *Transplantation* 1997;63:421–429.

200. Kopp CW, Siegel JB, Hancock WW, et al. Effect of porcine endothelial tissue factor pathway inhibitor on human coagulation factors. *Transplantation* 1997;63:749–758.

201. Lesnikoski B-A, Candinas D, Otsu I, Metternich R, Bach FH, Robson SC. Thrombin inhibition in discordant xenograft rejection. *Xenotransplantation* 1997;4:140–146.

202. Dorling A, Stocker C, Tsao T, Haskard DO, Lechler RI. In vitro accommodation of immortalized porcine endothelial cells: resistance to complement mediated lysis and down-regulation of VCAM expression induced by low concentrations of polyclonal human IgG antipig antibodies. *Transplantation* 1996;62:1127–1136.

203. The Tricontinental Mycophenolate Mofetil Renal Transplantation Study Group. A blinded, randomized clinical trial of mycophenolate mofetil for the prevention of acute rejection in cadaveric renal transplantation. *Transplantation* 1996;61:1029–1037.

204. Auchincloss H Jr, Mayer T, Ghobrial R, Winn HJ. T cell subsets, bm mutants, and the mechanism of allogeneic skin graft rejection. *Immunol Res* 1989;8:149–164.

205. Mizuochi T, Golding H, Rosenberg AS, Glimcher LH, Malek TR, Singer A. Both L3T4+ and Lyt-2+ helper T cells initiate cytotoxic T lymphocyte responses against allogeneic major histocompatibility antigens but not against trinitrophenyl-modified self. *J Exp Med* 1985;162:427–443.

206. Mizuochi T, Munitz TI, McCarthy S, et al. Differential helper and effector responses of Lyt-2 T cells to H-2Kb mutant (Kbm) determinants and the appearance of thymic influence on anti-Kbm CTL responsiveness. *J Immunol* 1986;137:2740–2747.

207. Mizuochi T, Ono S, Malek TR, Singer A. Characterization of two distinct pri-

mary T cell populations that secrete interleukin 2 upon recognition of class I or class II major histocompatibility antigens. *J Exp Med* 1986;163:603–619.

208. Golding H, Mizuochi T, McCarthy SA, Cleveland CA, Singer A. Relationship among function, phenotype, and specificity in primary allospecific T cell populations: identification of phenotypically identical but functionally distinct primary T cell subsets that differ in their recognition of MHC class I and class II allodeterminants. *J Immunol* 1987;138:10–17.

209. Singer A, Munitz TI, Golding H, Rosenberg AS, Mizuochi T. Recognition requirements for the activation, differentiation, and function of T-helper cells specific for class I MHC alloantigens. *Immunol Rev* 1987;98:143–170.

210. Sprent J, Schaefer M. Properties of purified T cell subsets. I. In vitro responses to class I and class II H-2 alloantigens. *J Exp Med* 1985;162:2068–2088.

211. McCarthy SA, Singer A. Recognition of MHC class I allodeterminants regulates the generation of MHC class II-specific CTL. *J Immunol* 1986;137:3087–3092.

212. Mizuochi T, Hugin AW, Morse HC, Singer A, Buller RML. Role of lymphokine-secreting CD8+ T cells in cytotoxic T lymphocyte responses against vaccinia virus. *J Immunol* 1989;142:270–273.

213. Heath WR, Kjer-Nielsen L, Hoffmann MW. Avidity for antigen can influence the helper dependence of CD8- T lymphocytes. *J Immunol* 1993;151:5993–6001.

214. Wheelahan J, McKenzie IFC. The role of T4+ and Ly-2+ cells in skin graft rejection in the mouse. *Transplantation* 1987;44:273–280.

215. Cobbold SP, Jayasuriya A, Nash A, Prospero TD, Waldmann H. Therapy with monoclonal antibodies by elimination of T cell subsets in vivo. *Nature* 1984;312:548–551.

216. Cobbold S, Waldmann H. Skin allograft rejection by L3T4+ and Lyt-2+ T cell subsets. *Transplantation* 1986;41:634–639.

217. Woodcock J, Wofsy D, Eriksson E, Scott JH, Seaman WE. Rejection of skin grafts and generation of cytotoxic T cells by mice depleted of L3T4+ cells. *Transplantation* 1986;42:636–642.

218. Madsen JC, Peugh WN, Wood KJ, Morris PJ. The effect of anti-L3T4 monoclonal antibody treatment on first-set rejection of murine cardiac allografts. *Transplantation* 1987;44:849–852.

219. Shizuru JA, Gregory AK, Chao CT, Fathman CG. Islet allograft survival after a single course of treatment of recipient with antibody to L3T4. *Science* 1987;237:278–280.

220. Smith DM, Stuart FP, Wemhoff GA, Quintas J, Fitch FW. Cellular pathways for rejection of class-I–MHC-disparate skin and tumor allografts. *Transplantation* 1988;45:168–175.

221. Ichikawa T, Nakayama E, Uenaka A, Monden M, Mori T. Effector cells in allelic H-2 class I–incompatible skin graft rejection. *J Exp Med* 1987;166:982–990.

222. Rosenberg AS, Munitz TI, Maniero TG, Singer A. Cellular basis of skin allograft rejection across a class I major histocompatibility barrier in mice depleted of CD8+ T cells in vivo. *J Exp Med* 1991;173:1463–1471.

223. Rosenberg AS, Singer A. Cellular basis of skin allograft rejection: an in vivo model of immune-mediated tissue destruction. *Annu Rev Immunol* 1992;10:333–358.

224. Wecker H, Grusby MJ, Auchincloss HJr. Effector cells must recognize antigens expressed in the graft to cause efficient skin graft rejection in SCID mice. *Transplantation* 1995;59:1223–1227.

225. Braun YM, McCormack A, Webb G, Batchelor RJ. Mediation of acute but not chronic rejection of MHC-incompatible rat kidney grafts by alloreactive CD4 T cells activated by the direct pathway of sensitization. *Transplantation* 1993;55:117.

226. Krieger NR, Yin DP, Fathman CG. CD4+ but not CD8+ cells are essential for allorejection. *J Exp Med* 1996;184:2013–2018.

227. Lee RS, Grusby MJ, Laufer TM, Colvin R, Glimcher LH, Auchincloss H Jr. CD8+ effector cells responding to residual class I antigens, with help from CD4+ cells stimulated indirectly, cause rejection of "major histocompatibility complex–deficient" skin grafts. *Transplantation* 1997;63:1123–1133.

228. La Rosa FG, Talmage DW. The failure of a major histocompatibility antigen to stimulate a thyroid allograft reaction after culture in oxygen. *J Exp Med.*1983;157:898–906.

229. Bartlett ST, Jennings AS, Yu C, Naji A, Barker CF, Silvers WK. Influence of culturing on the survival of major histocompatibility complex–compatible and –incompatible thyroid grafts in rats. *J Exp Med* 1983;157:348.

230. Gill RG, Rosenberg AS, Lafferty KJ, Singer A. Characterization of primary T cell subsets mediating rejection of pancreatic islet grafts. *J Immunol* 1989;143:2176–2178.

231. Priestley CA, Spencer SC, Sawyer GJ, Fabre JW. Suppression of kidney allograft rejection across full MHC barriers by recipient-specific antibodies to class II MHC antigens. *Transplantation* 1992;53:1024–1032.

232. Fangmann J, Dalchau R, Fabre JW. Rejection of skin allografts by indirect allorecognition of donor class I major histocompatibility complex peptides. *J Exp Med* 1992;175:1521–1529.

233. Auchincloss H Jr, Lee R, Shea S, Markowitz JS, Grusby MJ, Glimcher LH. The role of "indirect" recognition in initiating rejection of skin grafts from major histocompatibility complex class II–deficient mice. *Proc Natl Acad Sci U S A* 1993;90:3373–3377.

234. Bradley JA, Mowat AM, Bolton EM. Processed MHC class I alloantigen as the stimulus for CD4+ T-cell dependent antibody-mediated graft rejection. *Immunol Today* 1992;13:434–438.

235. Kobayashi E, Kawai K, Ikarashi Y, Fujiwara M. Mechanism of the rejection of major histocompatibility complex class I–disparate murine skin grafts: rejection

can be mediated by CD4+ cells activated by allo-class I + II antigen in CD8+ cell-depleted hosts. *J Exp Med* 1992;176:617–621.

236. Kitagawa S, Sato S, Hori S, Hamaoka T, Fujiwara H. Induction of anti–allo-class I H-2 tolerance by inactivation of CD8+ helper T cells, and reversal of tolerance through introduction of third-party helper T cells. *J Exp Med* 1990;172:105–113.

237. Auchincloss H Jr, Winn HJ. Murine CD8+ T cell helper function is particularly sensitive to CsA suppression in vivo. *J Immunol* 1989;143:3940–3943.

238. Fidelus RK, Ferguson RM, Widmer MB, Wee S-L, Bach FH, Orosz CG. Effect of cyclosporin A on murine and human T helper cell clones. *Transplantation* 1982;34:308–311.

239. Orosz CG, Roopenian DC, Widmer MB, Bach FM. Analysis of cloned T cell function. II. Differential blockade of various cloned T cell functions by cyclosporine. *Transplantation* 1983;36:706–711.

240. Rosenberg AS, Mizuochi T, Singer A. Evidence for involvement of dual-function T cells in rejection of MHC class I disparate skin grafts. Assessment of MHC class I alloantigens as in vivo helper determinants. *J Exp Med* 1988;168:33–45.

241. Muluk SC, Clerici M, Via CS, Weir MR, Kimmel PL, Shearer GM. Correlation of in vitro CD4+ T helper cell function with clinical graft status in immunosuppressed kidney transplant recipients. *Transplantation* 1991;52:284–291.

242. Susskind B, Iannotti MR, Shornick MD, Steward NS, Gorka J, Mohanakumar T. Indirect allorecognition of HLA class I peptides by CD4+ cytolytic T lymphocytes. *Hum Immunol* 1996;46:1–9.

243. Benham AM, Sawyer GJ, Fabre JW. Indirect T cell allorecognition of donor antigens contributes to the rejection of vascularized kidney allografts. *Transplantation* 1995;59:1028–1032.

244. Sayegh MH, Watschinger B, Carpenter CB. Mechanisms of T cell recognition of alloantigen: the role of peptides. *Transplantation* 1994;57:1295.

245. Liu Z, Sun Y-K, Xi Y-P, Maffei A, Reed E, Harris P, Suciu-Foca N. Contribution of direct and indirect recognition pathways to T cell alloreactivity. *J Exp Med* 1993;177:1643–1650.

246. Benichou G, Tam RC, Soares LRB, Popov IA, Garovoy MR, Fedoseyeva EV. The influence of two distinct alloresponse pathways on the design of peptide-based strategies for allograft tolerance. *Res Immunol* 1996;147:377–387.

247. Gallon L, Watschinger B, Murphy B, Akalin E, Sayegh MH, Carpenter CB. The indirect pathway of allorecognition: the occurrence of self-restricted T cell recognition of allo-MHC peptides early in acute renal allograft rejection and its inhibition by conventional immunosuppression. *Transplantation* 1995;59:612–616.

248. Shirwan H, Leamer M, Wang HK, Makowka L, Cramer DV. Peptides derived from α-helices of allogeneic class I major histocompatibility complex antigens are potent inducers of CD4+ and CD8+ T cell and B cell responses after cardiac allograft rejection. *Transplantation* 1995;59:401–410.

249. Benichou G, Fedoseyeva E, Lehmann PV, et al. Limited T cell response to donor MHC peptides during allograft rejection: implications for selective immune therapy in transplantation. *J Immunol* 1994;153:938–945.

250. Liu Z, Harris PE, Colovai AI, Reed EF, Maffei A, Suciu-Foca N. Indirect recognition of donor MHC class II antigens in human transplantation. *Clin Immunol Immunopathol* 1996;78:228–235.

251. Molajoni ER, Cinti P, Orlandini A, et al. Mechanisms of liver allograft rejection: the indirect recognition pathway. *Hum Immunol* 1997;53:57–63.

252. Liu Z, Colovai AI, Tugulea S, et al. Indirect recognition of donor HLA-DR peptides in organ allograft rejection. *J Clin Invest* 1996;98:1150–1157.

253. Vella JP, Spadafora-Ferreira M, Murphy B, et al. Indirect allorecognition of major histocompatibility complex allopeptides in human renal transplant recipients with chronic graft dysfunction. *Transplantation* 1997;64:795–800.

254. Tugulea S, Ciubotariu R, Colovai AI, et al. New strategies for early diagnosis of heart allograft rejection. *Transplantation* 1997;64:842–847.

255. Sayegh MH, Perico N, Gallon L, et al. Mechanisms of acquired thymic unresponsiveness to renal allografts. *Transplantation* 1994;58:125–132.

256. Oluwole SF, Chowdhury NC, Jin M, Hardy MA. Induction of transplantation tolerance in rat cardiac allografts by intrathymic inoculation of allogeneic soluble peptides. *Transplantation* 1993;56:1523.

257. Sayegh MH, Perico N, Imberti O, Hancock WW, Carpenter CB, Remuzzi G. Thymic recognition of class II MHC allopeptides induces donor specific unresponsiveness to renal allografts. *Transplantation* 1993;56:461.

258. Sayegh MH, Khoury SK, Hancock WW, Weiner HL, Carpenter CB. Induction of immunity and oral tolerance with polymorphic class II MHC allopeptides in the rat. *Proc Natl Acad Sci U S A* 1992;89:7762–7766.

259. Lechler RI, Batchelor JR. Restoration of immunogenicity to passenger cell-depleted kidney allografts by the addition of donor strain dendritic cells. *J Exp Med* 1982;155:31–41.

260. Monaco JJ. A molecular model of MHC class-I–restricted antigen processing. *Immunol Today* 1992;13:173–178.

261. Neefjes JJ, Ploegh HL. Intracellular transport of MHC class II molecules. *Immunol Today* 1992;13:179–183.

262. Grant EP, Rock KL. MHC class I–restricted presentation of exogenous antigen by thymic antigen-presenting cells in vitro and in vivo. *J Immunol* 1992;148:13–18.

263. Michalek MT, Benacerraf B, Rock KL. The class II MHC-restricted presentation of endogenously synthesized ovalbumin displays clonal variation, requires endosomal/lysosomal processing, and is upregulated by heat shock. *J Immunol* 1992;148:1016–1024.

264. Kurts C, Heath WR, Carbone FR, Allison J, Miller JFAP, Kosaka H. Constitutive

class I–restricted exogenous presentation of self antigens in vivo. *J Exp Med* 1996;184:923–930.

265. Williams NS, Engelhard VH. Perforin-dependent cytotoxic activity and lymphokine secretion by CD4⁺ T cells are regulated by CD8⁺ T cells. *J Immunol* 1997;159:2091–2099.

266. Orosz CG, Bishop DK. Limiting dilution analysis of alloreactive T-cell status and distribution during allograft rejection. *Hum Immunol* 1990;28:72–81.

267. Swain SL. Significance of Lyt phenotypes: Lyt2 antibodies block activities of T cells that recognize class I MHC antigens regardless of their function. *Proc Natl Acad Sci U S A* 1981;78:7101.

268. Swain SL. T cell subsets and the recognition of MHC class. *Immunol Rev* 1983; 74:129–142.

269. Swain SL, Bakke A, English M, Dutton RW. Ly phenotypes and MHC recognition: the alloheper that recognizes K or D is a mature Ly123 cell. *J Immunol* 1979;123:2716–2724.

270. Rosenberg AS, Katz SI, Singer A. Rejection of skin allografts by CD4⁺ T cells is antigen-specific and requires expression of target alloantigen on Ia⁻ epidermal cells. *J Immunol* 1989;143:2452–2456.

271. Rosenberg AS, Finbloom DS, Maniero TG, Van der Meide PH, Singer A. Specific prolongation of MHC class II disparate skin allografts by in vivo administration of anti–IFN-gamma monoclonal antibody. *J Immunol* 1990;144: 4648–4650.

272. Mintz B, Silvers WK. Histocompatiblity antigens on melanoblasts and hair follicle cells: cell-localized homograft rejection in allophenic skin grafts. *Transplantation* 1970;9:497–505.

273. Mintz B, Silvers WK. "Intrinsic" immunological tolerance in allophenic mice. *Science* 1967;158:1484–1486.

274. Rosenberg AS, Singer A. Evidence that the effector mechanism of skin allograft rejection is antigen-specific. *Proc Natl Acad Sci U S A* 1988;85:7739.

275. Doody DP, Stenger KS, Winn HJ. Immunologically nonspecific mechanisms of tissue destruction in the rejection of skin grafts. *J Exp Med* 1994;179: 1645–1652.

276. Roberts PJ, Hayry P. Sponge matrix allografts. A model for analysis of killer cells infiltrating mouse allografts. *Transplantation* 1976;21:437.

277. Strom TB, Tilney NL, Paradyez J, Banceqicz J, Carpenter CB. Cellular components of allograft rejection: Identity, specificity, and cytotoxic function of cells infiltrating acutely rejecting allografts. *J Immunol* 1977;118:2020–2026.

278. Hall B, Dorsch S. Cells mediating allograft rejection. *Immunol Rev* 1984;77:570.

279. Ascher NL, Hoffman R, Hanto D, Simmons R. Cellular basis of allograft rejection. *Immunol Rev* 1984;77:217–232.

280. Hall B, Bishop G, Farnsworth A, et al. Identification of the cellular subpopulations infiltrating rejecting cadaver renal allografts: preponderance of the T4 subset of T cells. *Transplantation* 1984;37:564–570.

281. Hayry P, von Willebrand E, Parthenais E, et al. The inflammatory mechanisms of allograft rejection. *Immunol Rev* 1984;77:85–142.

282. Bradley JA, Bolton EM. The T-cell requirements for allograft rejection. *Transplant Rev* 1992;6:115–129.

283. Prefter FI, Colvin RB, Leary CP, et al. Two color flow cytometry and functional analysis of lymphocytes cultured from human renal allografts: identification of a Leu 2⁺3⁺ subpopulation. *J Immunol* 1986;137:2823–2830.

284. Tilney NL, Strom TB, MacPherson SG, Carpenter CB. Surface properties and functional characteristics of infiltrating cells harvested from acutely rejecting cardiac allografts in inbred rats. *Transplantation* 1975;20:323–330.

285. Mayer TG, Bhan AK, Winn HJ. Immunohistochemical analysis of skin graft rejection in mice: kinetics of lymphocyte infiltration in grafts of limited immunogenetic disparity. *Transplantation* 1988;46:890–899.

286. Mueller C, Gershenfeld HK, Lobe CG, Okada CY, Bleackley RC, Weissman IL. A high proportion of T lymphocytes that infiltrate H-2–incompatible heart allografts in vivo express genes encoding cytotoxic cell–specific serine proteases, but do not express the Mel-14–defined lymph node homing receptor. *J Exp Med* 1988;167:1124–1136.

287. Colvin RB. The renal allograft biopsy. *Kidney Int* 1996;50:1069–1082.

288. Kim B, Rosenstein M, Weiland D, Eberlein TJ, Rosenberg SA. Clonal analysis of the lymphoid cells mediating skin allograft rejection. *Transplantation* 1983;36:525–532.

289. Kilbeck PC, Miceli C, Finn OJ, Bollinger RR, Sanfilippo F. Relationships among renal allograft biopsy infiltrates, growth of T cell lines, and irreversible rejection. *Transplant Proc* 1988;20:303–305.

290. Kilbeck PC, Tatum AH, Sanfilippo F. Relationships among the histologic pattern, intensity, and phenotypes of T cells infiltrating renal allografts. *Transplantation* 1984;38:709–713.

291. Sanfilippo F, Kilbeck PC, Vaughn WK, Bollinger RR. Renal allograft cell infiltrates associated with irreversible rejection. *Transplantation* 1985;40:679–685.

292. Knechtle SJ, Wolfe JA, Burchette J, Sanfilippo F, Bollinger RR. Infiltrating cell phenotypes and patterns associated with hepatic allograft rejection or acceptance. *Transplantation* 1987;43:169–172.

293. Wolfe JA, Knechtle SJ, Burchette J, Bollinger RR, Sanfilippo F. Phenotype and patterns of inflammatory cell infiltration associated with rejection or acceptance of rat liver allografts. *Transplant Proc* 1987;19:364–368

294. Straznickas J, Howell D, Ruiz P, Sanfilippo F. Phenotype and function of T cells propagated from donor-specific blood transfusion enhanced and autologous blood transfused rejecting rat renal allografts. *Transplant Proc* 1988;20: 276–280.

295. Miceli MC, Finn OJ. T cell receptor beta-chain selection in human allograft rejection. *J Immunol* 1989;142:81–86.

296. Moreau JF, Peyrat MA, Vie H, Bonneville M, Soulillou JP. T cell colony-forming frequency of mononucleated cells extracted from rejected human kidney transplants. *Transplantation* 1985;39:649.

297. Bonneville M, Moreau JF, Blokland E, et al. T lymphocyte cloning from rejected human kidney allograft. Recognition repertoire of alloreactive T cell clones. *J Immunol* 1988;141:4187–4195.

298. Miceli MC, Barry TS, Finn OJ. Human renal allograft infiltrating T cells: phenotype-function correlation and clonal heterogeneity. *Transplant Proc* 1988;20: 199.

299. Chen RH, Bushell A, Fuggle SV, Wood KJ, Morris PJ. Expression of granzyme A and perforin in mouse heart transplants immunosuppressed with donor-specific transfusion and anti-CD4 monoclonal antibodies. *Transplantation* 1996; 61:625–629.

300. Kondo T, Novick AC, Toma H, Fairchild RL. Induction of chemokine gene expression during allogeneic skin graft rejection. *Transplantation* 1996;61: 1750–1757.

301. Pavlakis M, Strehlau J, Lipman M, Shapiro M, Maslinski W, Strom TB. Intragraft IL-15 transcripts are increased in human renal allograft rejection. *Transplantation* 1996;62:543–545.

302. Truong LD, Shappell S, Barrios R, Gonzalez J, Suki WN, Solez K. Immunohistochemistry and molecular biology markers of renal transplant rejection: diagnostic applications. *Transplant Rev* 1996;10:187–208.

303. Carlquist JF, Edelman LS, White W, Shelby J, Anderson JL. Cytokines and rejection of mouse cardiac allografts. *Transplantation* 1996;62:1160–1166.

304. O'Connell PJ, Pacheco-Silva A, Nickerson PW, et al. Unmodified pancreatic islet allograft rejection results in the preferential expression of certain T cell activation transcripts. *J Immunol* 1993;150:1093–1104.

305. Strehlau J, Pavlakis M, Lipman M, et al. Quantitative detection of immune activation transcripts as a diagnostic tool in kidney transplantation. *Proc Natl Acad Sci U S A* 1997;94:695–700.

306. Fairchild RL, VanBuskirk AM, Kondo T, Wakely ME, Orosz CG. Expression of chemokine genes during rejection and long-term acceptance of cardiac allografts. *Transplantation* 1997;63:1807–1812.

307. Sharma VK, Bologa RM, Li B, et al. Molecular executors of cell death—differential intrarenal expression of Fas ligand, Fas, granzyme B, and perforin during acute and/or chronic rejection of human renal allografts. *Transplantation* 1996;62:1860–1866.

308. Martinez OM, Krams SM, Sterneck M, et al. Intragraft cytokine profile during human liver allograft rejection. *Transplantation* 1992;53:449–456.

309. Griffiths GM, Mueller C. Expression of perforin and granzymes in vivo: potential diagnostic markers for activated cytotoxic cells. *Immunol Today* 1991;12: 415–418.

310. Griffiths GM, Namikawa R, Mueller C, et al. Granzyme A and perforin as markers for rejection in cardiac transplantation. *Eur J Immunol* 1991;21:687–692.

311. Linsley PS, Brady W, Urnes M, Grosmaire LS, Damle NK, Ledbetter JA. CTLA-4 is a second receptor for the B cell activation antigen B7. *J Exp Med* 1991;174: 561–569.

312. Lipman ML, Stevens CA, Bleackley CR, et al. The strong correlation of cytotoxic T lymphocyte-specific serine protease gene transcripts with renal allograft rejection. *Transplantation* 1992;53:73–79.

313. Thiele DL, Geissler GH, Williams FH, Lipsky PE. The role of leucyl-leucine methyl ester-sensitive cytotoxic cells in skin allograft rejection. *Transplantation* 1992;53:1334–1340.

314. Chen RH, Ivens KW, Alpert S, et al. The use of granzyme A as a marker of heart transplant rejection in cyclosporine or anti-CD4 monoclonal antibody-treated rats. *Transplantation* 1993;55:146–153.

315. Sharma VK, Bologa RM, Li B, et al. Molecular executors of cell death-differential intrarenal expression of Fas ligand, Fas, granzyme B, and perforin during acute and/or chronic rejection of human renal allografts. *Transplantation* 1996; 62:1860–1866.

316. Lipman ML, Stevens AC, Strom TB. Heightened intragraft CTL gene expression in acutely rejecting renal allografts. *J Immunol* 1994;152:5120–5127.

317. Grusby MJ, Auchincloss H Jr, Lee R, et al. Mice lacking major histocompatibility complex class I and class II molecules. *Proc Natl Acad Sci U S A* 1993; 90:3919.

318. Campos L, Naji A, Deli BC, et al. Survival of MHC-deficient mouse heterotopic cardiac allografts. *Transplantation* 1995;59:187–191.

319. Glas R, Franksson L, Ohlen C, et al. Major histocompatibility complex class I–specific and –restricted killing of β2-microglobulin–deficient cells by CD8⁺ cytotoxic T lymphocytes. *Proc Natl Acad Sci U S A* 1993;89:11381.

320. Markmann JF, Bassiri H, Desai NM, et al. Indefinite survival of MHC class I–deficient murine pancreatic islet allografts. *Transplantation* 1992;54: 1085–1089.

321. Markmann JF, Jacobson ID, Choti MA, et al. Modulation of major histocompatibility complex antigens and the immunogenicity of islet allografts. *Transplantation* 1989;48:478–486.

322. Markmann JF, Campos L, Bhandoola A, et al. Genetically engineered grafts to study xenoimmunity: a role for indirect antigen presentation in the destruction of major histocompatibility complex antigen deficient xenografts. *Surgery* 1994; 116:242–249.

323. Osorio RW, Ascher NL, Jaenisch R, Freise CE, Roberts JP, Stock PG. Major his-

tocompatibility complex class I deficiency prolongs islet allograft survival. *Diabetes* 1993;42:1520–1527.

324. Munn SR, Marjoribanks C. Current limitations to use of major histocompatibility complex transgenic donors for islet transplantation. *Transplantation* 1994;57:760–763.

325. Schulz M, Schuurman H-J, Joergensen J, et al. Acute rejection of vascular heart allografts by perforin-deficient mice. *Eur J Immunol* 1995;25:474–480.

326. Selvaggi G, Ricordi C, Podack ER, Inverardi L. The role of the perforin and Fas pathways of cytotoxicity in skin graft rejection. *Transplantation* 1996;62:1912–1915.

327. Steiger J, Nickerson PW, Steurer W, Moscovitch-Lopatin M, Strom TB. IL-2 knockout recipient mice reject islet cell allografts. *J Immunol* 1995;155:489–498.

328. Dalloul AH, Chmouzis E, Ngo K, Fung-Leung W-P. Adoptively transferred CD4+ lymphocytes from CD8−/− mice are sufficient to mediate the rejection of MHC class II or class I disparate skin grafts. *J Immunol* 1996;156:4114–4119.

329. Nickerson P, Zheng XX, Steiger J, et al. Prolonged islet allograft acceptance in the absence of interleukin 4 expression. *Transplant Immunol* 1996;4:81–85.

330. Roy-Chaudhury P, Manfro RC, Steiger J, et al. IL-2 and IL-4 double knock-out mice reject islet allografts: a role for novel T-cell growth factors? *Transplant Proc* 1997;29:1083–1084.

331. Bradley AJ, Bolton EM. The T-cell requirements for allograft rejection. *Transplant Rev* 1992;6:115–129.

332. McCarthy SA, Kaldjian E, Singer A. Induction of anti-CD8 resistant cytotoxic T lymphocytes by anti-CD8 antibodies. Functional evidence for T cell signaling induced by multi-valent cross-linking of CD8 on precursor cells. *J Immunol* 1988;141:3737–3746.

333. Sawada T, Wu Y, Sachs DH, Iacomini J. CD4+ T cells are able to reject class I disparate allografts. *Transplantation* 1997;64:335–340.

334. Hurme M, Hetherington CM, Simpson E. Cytotoxic T-cell responses to H-Y: correlation with the rejection of syngeneic male skin grafts. *J Exp Med* 1978;147:768–775.

335. McKenzie IFC, Henning MM, Michaelides M. Skin graft rejection and delayed-type hypersensitivity responses to H-Y in an I-Ab mutant. *Immunogenetics* 1984;20:475.

336. Gordon RD, Mathieson BJ, Samelson LE, Boyse EA, Simpson E. The effect of allogeneic presensitization on H-Y graft survival and in vitro cell-mediated responses to H-Y antigen. *J Exp Med* 1976;144:810.

337. Bradley JA, Mason DW, Morris PJ. Evidence that rat renal allografts are rejected by cytotoxic T cells and not by nonspecific effectors. *Transplantation* 1985;39:169–175.

338. Hall BM. Cells mediating allograft rejection. *Transplantation* 1991;51:1141–1151.

339. Kitagawa S, Iwata H, Sato S, Shimizu J, Hamaoka T, Fujiwara H. Heterogenous graft rejection pathways in class I major histocompatibility complex–disparate combinations and their differential susceptibility to immunomodulation induced by intravenous presensitization with relevant alloantigens. *J Exp Med* 1991;174:571–581.

340. Mason DW, Dallman MJ, Arthur RP, Morris PJ. Mechanisms of allograft rejection: the roles of cytotoxic T-cells and delayed-type hypersensitivity. *Immunol Rev* 1984;77:177.

341. Mason DW, Morris PJ. Effector mechanisms in allograft rejection. *Ann Rev Immunol* 1986;4:119–145.

342. Peeler JS, Niederkorn JY. Antigen presentation by Langerhans cells in vivo: donor-derived Ia+ Langerhans cells are required for induction of delayed-type hypersenitivity but not for cytotoxic T lymphocyte responses to alloantigens. *J Immunol* 1986;136:4362.

343. Ando K, Moriyama T, Guidotti LG, et al. Mechanisms of class I restricted immunopathology. A transgenic mouse model of fulminant hepatitis. *J Exp Med* 1994;178:1541–1554.

344. Walsh CM, Hayashi F, Saffran DC, Ju S-T, Berke G, Clark WR. Cell-mediated cytotoxicity results from, but may not be critical for, primary allograft rejection. *J Immunol* 1996;156:1436–1441.

345. VanBuskirk AM, Wakely ME, Orosz CG. Acute rejection of cardiac allografts by noncytolytic CD4+ T cell populations. *Transplantation* 1996;62:300–302.

346. Sirak J, Orosz CG, Wakely E, VanBuskirk AM. Alloreactive delayed-type hypersensitivity in graft recipients: complexity of responses and divergence from acute rejection. *Transplantation* 1997;63:1300–1307.

347. Beckerman KP, Rogers HW, Corbett JA, Schreiber RD, McDaniel ML, Unanue ER. Release of nitric oxide during the T cell–independent pathway of macrophage activation. *J Immunol* 1993;150:888.

348. Cecka JM, Terasaki PI, eds. *Clinical transplants 1995*. Los Angeles: UCLA Tissue Typing Laboratory, 1995.

349. Russell PS, Chase CM, Colvin RB. Accelerated atheromatous lesions in mouse hearts transplanted to apolipoprotein-E–deficient recipients. *Am J Pathol* 1996;149:91–99.

350. Schmid C, Heeman U, Tilney NL. Factors contributing to the development of chronic rejection in heterotopic rat heart transplantation. *Transplantation* 1997;64:222–228.

351. Petersen VP, Olsen TS, Kissmeyer-Nielsen F, et al. Late failure of human renal transplants. An analysis of transplant disease and graft failure among 125 recipients surviving for one to eight years. *Medicine* 1975;54:45–71.

352. Reed EF, Hong B, Ho E, Harris PE, Weinberger J, Suciu-Foca N. Monitoring of soluble HLA alloantigens and anti-HLA antibodies identifies heart allograft recipients at risk of transplant-associated coronary artery disease. *Transplantation* 1996;61:566–572.

353. Cosio FG, Pelletier RP, Falkenhain ME, et al. Impact of acute rejection and early allograft function on renal allograft survival. *Transplantation* 1997;63:1611–1615.

354. Russell PS, Chase CM, Winn HJ, Colvin RB. Coronary atherosclerosis in transplanted mouse hearts. I. Time course and immunogenetic and immunopathological considerations. *Am J Pathol* 1994;144:260–274.

355. Russell PS, Chase CM, Colvin RB. Insights regarding the pathogenesis of transplant arteriopathy from experiments with animals. *Transplantation* 1997;64 (*in press*).

356. Geraghty JG, Stoltenberg RL, Sollinger HW, Hullett DA. Vascular smooth muscle cells and neointimal hyperplasia in chronic transplant rejection. *Transplantation* 1996;62:502–509.

357. Utans U, Quist WC, McManus BM, et al. Allograft inflammatory factory-1. A cytokine-responsive macrophage molecule expressed in transplanted human hearts. *Transplantation* 1996;61:1387–1392.

358. Sharma VK, Bologa RM, Xu GP, et al. Intragraft TGF-beta 1 mRNA: a correlate of interstitial fibrosis and chronic allograft nephropathy. *Kidney Int* 1996;49:1297–1303.

359. Molossi S, Clausell N, Sett S, Rabinovitch M. ICAM-1 and VCAM-1 expression in accelerated cardiac allograft arteriopathy and myocardial rejection are influenced differently by cyclosporine A and tumor necrosis factor-α blockade. *J Pathol* 1995;176:175.

360. Russell PS, Chase CM, Colvin RB. Coronary atherosclerosis in transplanted mouse hearts. IV. Effects of treatment with monoclonal antibodies to intercellular adhesion molecule-1 and leukocyte function-associated antigen-1. *Transplantation* 1995;60:724–729.

361. Suthanthiran M. Molecular analyses of human renal allografts: differential intragraft gene expression during rejection. *Kidney Int Suppl* 1997;58:15–21.

362. Russell ME, Wallace AF, Wyner LR, Newell JB, Karnovsky MJ. Upregulation and modulation of inducible nitric oxide synthase in rat cardiac allografts with chronic rejection and transplant atherosclerosis. *Circulation* 1995;92:457–464.

363. Zhao X-M, Blanton RH, Becker YT, et al. Increased expression of acidic fibroblast growth factor (aFGF) and FGF receptor-1 (FGFR-1) in rat cardiac allografts versus isografts and normal hearts. *Circulation* 1994;90(suppl I):361.

364. Motomura N, Lou H, Maurice P, Foegh ML. Acceleration of arteriosclerosis of the rat aorta allograft by insulin growth factor-I. *Transplantation* 1997;63:932–936.

365. Forbes RD, Cernacek P, Zheng S, Gomersall M, Guttmann RD. Increased endothelin expression in a rat cardiac allograft model of chronic vascular rejection. *Transplantation* 1996;61:791–797.

366. Watschinger B, Sayegh MH, Hancock WW, Russell ME. Upregulation of endothelin-1 mRNA and peptide expression in rat cardiac allografts with rejection and arteriosclerosis. *Am J Pathol* 1995;146:1065.

367. Madsen JC, Sachs DH, Fallon JT, Weissman NJ. Cardiac allograft vasculopathy in partially inbred miniature swine. *J Thorac Cardiovasc Surg* 1996;111:1230–1239.

368. Russell PS, Chase CM, Winn HJ, Colvin RB. Coronary atherosclerosis in transplanted mouse hearts. III. Effects of recipient treatment with a monoclonal antibody to interferon-γ. *Transplantation* 1994;57:1367–1371.

369. Russell PS, Chase CM, Winn HJ, Colvin RB. Coronary atherosclerosis in transplanted mouse hearts. II. Importance of humoral immunity. *J Immunol* 1994;152:5135–5141.

370. McLean AG, Hughes M, Welsh KI, et al. Patterns of graft infiltration and cytokine gene expression during the first 10 days of kidney transplantation. *Transplantation* 1997;63:374–379.

371. Matzinger P. Tolerance, danger, and the extended family. *Annu Rev Immunol* 1994;12:991–1045.

372. Harding FA, McArthur JG, Gross JA, Raulet DH, Allison JP. CD28-mediated signalling co-stimulates murine T cells and prevents induction of anergy in T-cell clones. *Nature* 1992;356:607–609.

373. Schwartz RH. Costimulation of T lymphocytes: the role of CD28, CTLA-4, and B7/BB1 in interleukin-2 production and immunotherapy. *Cell* 1992;71:1065–1068.

374. Coulombe M, Yang H, Guerder S, Flavell RA, Lafferty KJ, Gill RG. Tissue immunogenicity: the role of MHC antigen and the lymphocyte costimulator B7-1. *J Immunol* 1996;157:4790–4795.

375. Shuford WW, Klussman K, Tritchler DD, et al. 4-1BB costimulatory signals preferentially induce CD8+ T cell proliferation and lead to the amplification in vivo of cytotoxic T cell responses. *J Exp Med* 1997;186:47–55.

376. Larsen CP, Alexander DZ, Hollenbaugh D, et al. CD40-gp39 interactions play a critical role during allograft rejection. *Transplantation* 1996;61:4–9.

377. Grewel IS, Foellmer HG, Grewel KD, et al. Requirement for CD40 ligand in costimulation induction, T cell activation, and experimental allergic encephalomyelitis. *Science* 1996;273:1864–1867.

378. Yang Y, Wilson JM. CD40 ligand-dependent T cell activation: requirement of B7-CD28 signaling through CD40. *Science* 1996;273:1862–1864.

379. Bluestone JA. New perspectives of CD28-B7–mediated T cell costimulation. *Immunity* 1995;2:555–559.

380. Tivol EA, Borriello F, Schweitzer AN, Lynch WA, Bluestone JA, Sharpe AH. Loss of CTLA-4 leads to massive lymphoproliferation and fatal multiorgan tis-

sue destruction, revealing a critical negative regulatory role of CTLA-4. *Immunity* 1995;3:541–547.

381. Lu L, Qian S, Hershberger PA, Rudert WA, Lynch DH, Thomson AW. Fas ligand (CD95L) and B7 expression on dendritic cells provide counter-regulatory signals for T cell survival and proliferation. *J Immunol* 1997;158:5676–5684.

382. Bellgrau D, Gold D, Selawry H, Moore J, Franzusoff A, Duke RC. A role for CD95 ligand in preventing graft rejection. *Nature* 1995;377:630–632.

383. Kawai K, Shahinian A, Mak TW, Ohashi PS. Skin allograft rejection in CD28-deficient mice. *Transplantation* 1996;61:352.

384. Russell PS, Chase CM, Winn HJ, Colvin RB. Coronary atherosclerosis in transplanted mouse hearts. III. Effects of recipient treatment with a monoclonal antibody to interferon-gamma. *Transplantation* 1994;57:1367–1371.

385. Saleem S, Konieczny BT, Lowry RP, Baddoura FK, Lakkis FG. Acute rejection of vascularized heart allografts in the absence of IFN$\gamma^{1,2}$. *Transplantation* 1996; 62:1908–1911.

386. Goes N, Urmson J, Vincent D, Halloran PF. Acute renal injury in the interferon-gamma gene knockout mouse: effect on cytokine gene expression. *Transplantation* 1995;60:1560–1564.

387. Qin L, Chavin KD, Ding Y, Woodward JF, Favaro JP, Lin J, Bromberg JS. Gene transfer for transplantation: prolongation of allograft survival with transforming growth factor-β1. *Ann Surg* 1994;220:508–519.

388. Qin L, Chavin KD, Ding Y, et al. Retrovirus-mediated transfer of viral IL-10 gene prolongs murine cardiac allograft survival. *J Immunol* 1996;156: 2316–2323.

389. Weimer R, Zipperle S, Daniel V, Carl S, Staehler G, Opelz G. Pretransplant CD4 helper function and Interleukin 10 response predict risk of acute kidney graft rejection. *Transplantation* 1996;62:1606–1614.

390. Zheng XX, Steele AW, Nickerson PW, Steurer W, Steiger J, Strom TB. Administration of noncytolytic IL-10/Fc in murine models of lipopolysaccharide-induced septic shock and allogeneic islet transplantation. *J Immunol* 1995;154: 5590–5600.

391. Sayegh MH, Akalin E, Hancock WW, et al. CD28-B7 blockade after alloantigenic challenge in vivo inhibits Th1 cytokines but spares Th2. *J Exp Med* 1995; 181:1869–1874.

392. Piccotti JR, Chan SY, Goodman RE, Magram J, Eichwald EJ, Bishop DK. IL-12 antagonism induces T helper 2 responses, yet exacerbates cardiac allograft rejection: evidence against a dominant protective role for T helper 2 cytokines in alloimmunity. *J Immunol* 1996;157:1951–1957.

393. Piccotti JR, Chan SY, VanBuskirk AM, Eichwald EJ, Bishop DK. Are Th2 helper T lymphocytes beneficial, deleterious, or irrelevant in promoting allograft survival? *Transplantation* 1997;63:619–624.

394. Strom TB, Roy-Chaudhury P, Manfro R, et al. The Th1/Th2 paradigm and the allograft response. *Curr Opin Immunol* 1996;8:688–693.

395. Nickerson P, Steurer W, Steiger J, Zheng X, Steele AW, Strom TB. Cytokines and the Th1/Th2 paradigm in transplantation. *Curr Opin Immunol* 1994;6:757–764.

396. VanBuskirk AM, Wakely ME, Orosz CG. Transfusion of polarized TH2-like cell populations into SCID mouse cardiac allograft recipients results in acute allograft rejection. *Transplantation* 1996;62:229–238.

397. Mueller R, Davies JD, Krahl T, Sarvetnick N. IL-4 expression by grafts from transgenic mice fails to prevent allograft rejection. *J Immunol* 1997;159: 1599–1603.

398. Russell P, Chase C, Colvin R, Plate J. An analysis of the immune status of mice bearing long-term H-2 incompatible transplants. *J Exp Med* 1979;147: 1449–1468.

399. Russell PS, Chase CM, Colvin RB, Plate JMD. Kidney transplants in mice: an analysis of the immune status of mice bearing long-term H-2 incompatible transplants. *J Exp Med* 1978;147:1449–1468.

400. Qian S, Thai NL, Lu L, Fung JJ, Thomson AW. Liver transplant tolerance: mechanistic insights from animal models, with particular reference to the mouse. *Transplant Rev* 1997;11:151–164.

401. Calne RY, Sells RA, Pena JR, et al. Induction of immunological tolerance by porcine liver allografts. *Nature* 1969;223:472–476.

402. Burdick RC, Russell PS. Antigenic requirement for induced rejection of long-surviving murine heart transplants. *J Immunol* 1982;128:1551–1554.

403. Corry RJ, Winn HJ, Russell PS. Primarily vascularized allografts of hearts in mice. The role of H-2D, H-2K, and non-H-2 antigens in rejection. *Transplantation* 1973;16:343–350.

404. Russell PS, Chase CM, Colvin RB, Plate JMD. Induced immune destruction of long-surviving H-2 incompatible kidney transplants in mice. *J Exp Med* 1978;147:1469–1486.

405. Souillou JP, Peyronnet P, Le Mauff B, et al. Prevention of rejection of kidney transplants by monoclonal antibody directed against interleukin 2. *Lancet* 1987;1:1339–1342.

406. Mitchison NA. An exact comparison between the efficiency of two- and three-cell clusters in mediating helper activity. *Eur J Immunol* 1990;20:699–702.

407. Paul WE. Between two centuries: specificity and regulation in immunology. *J Immunol* 1987;139:1–6.

408. Tucker MJ, Bretscher PA. T cells cooperating in the induction of delayed-type hypersensitivity act via the linked recognition of antigenic determinants. *J Exp Med* 1982;155:1037.

409. Bretscher PA. A cascade of T-T interactions, mediated by the linked recognition of antigen, in the induction of T cells able to help delayed-type hypersensitivity responses. *J Immunol* 1986;137:3726.

410. Mitchison NA, O'Malley C. Three-cell-type clusters of T cells with antigen-presenting cells best explain the epitope linkage and noncognate requirements of the in vivo cytolytic response. *Eur J Immunol* 1987;17:1579–1583.

411. Bennett SRM, Carbone FR, Karamalis F, Miller JFAP, Heath WR. Induction of a CD8$^+$ cytotoxic T lymphocyte response by cross-priming requires cognate CD4$^+$ T cell help. *J Exp Med* 1997;186:65–70.

412. Hori S, Kitagawa S, Iwata H, et al. Cell-cell interaction in graft rejection responses: induction of anti-allo-class I H-2 tolerance is prevented by immune responses against allo-class II H-2 antigens coexpressed on tolerogen. *J Exp Med* 1992;175:99–109.

413. Kelly CM, Benham AM, Sawyer GJ, Dalchau R, Fabre JW. A three-cell cluster hypothesis for noncognate T-B collaboration via direct T cell recognition of allogeneic dendritic cells. *Transplantation* 1996;61:1094–1099.

414. Steele DJR, Laufer TM, Smiley ST, et al. Two levels of help for B cell alloantibody production. *J Exp Med* 1996;183:699–703.

415. Benham AM, Sawyer GJ, Fabre JW. T and B cell responsiveness to donor class I MHC molecules and peptides in long survivors with kidney allografts. *Transplantation* 1996;61:1455–1460.

416. Clement JD, Chan SY, Bishop DK. Allogeneic class I MHC requirement for alloantigen-reactive helper T-lymphocyte responses in vivo: Evidence for indirect presentation of alloantigen. *Transplantation* 1996;62:388–396.

417. MacDonald CM, Bolton EM, Jaques BC, Walker KG, Bradley JA. Reduction of alloantibody response to class I major histocompatibility complex by targeting synthetic allopeptides for presentation by B cells. *Transplantation* 1997;63: 926–932.

418. Lee RS, Grusby MJ, Glimcher LH, Winn HJ, Auchincloss H Jr. Indirect recognition by helper cells can induce donor-specific cytotoxic T lymphocytes in vivo. *J Exp Med* 1994;179:865–872.

419. Lacy PE, Davie JM. Transplantation of pancreatic islets. *Ann Rev Immunol* 1984;2:183.

420. Morrow CE, Sutherland DE, Steffes MW, Najarian JS, Bach FH. Lack of donor-specific tolerance in mice with established anti-Ia treated islet allografts. *Transplantation* 1983;36:691–694.

421. Gores DF, Sutherland DE, Platt JL, Bach FH. Lack of tolerance to donor-strain skin grafts in mice with established islet allografts. *Transplantation* 1987;43:749–750.

422. Bowen KM, Andrus L, Lafferty KJ. Survival of pancreatic islet allografts. *Lancet* 1979;2:585–586.

423. Butcher EC. Leukocyte-endothelial cell recognition: three (or more) steps to specificity and diversity. *Cell* 1991;67:1033–1036.

424. Hutchinson IV. Cellular mechanism of allograft rejection. *Curr Opin Immunol* 1991;3:722–728.

425. Hynes RO. Integrins: versatility, modulation, and signaling in cell adhesion. *Cell* 1992;69:11–25.

426. Shimizu Y, Newman W, Tanaka Y, Shaw S. Lymphocyte interaction with endothelial cells. *Immunol Today* 1992;13:106–111.

427. Tang MLK, Hale LP, Steeber DA, Tedder TF. L-selectin is involved in lymphocyte migration to sites of inflammation in the skin: delayed rejection of allografts in L-selectin deficient mice. *J Immunol* 1997;158:5191–5199.

428. Mobley JL, Dailey MO. Regulation of adhesion molecule expression by CD8 T cells in vivo. *J Immunol* 1992;148:2348–2356.

429. Koster F, McGregor D. The mediators of cellular immunity. II. Migration of immunologically committed lymphocytes into inflammatory exudates. *J Exp Med* 1971;133:400–409.

430. Pelletier RP, Ohye RG, Vanbuskirk A, Sedmak DD, Kincade P, Ferguson RM, Orosz CG. Importance of endothelial VCAM-1 for inflammatory leukocytic infiltration in vivo. *J Exp Med* 1992;149:2473–2481.

431. Wacholtz MC, Patel SS, Lipsky PE. Patterns of costimulation of T cell clones by cross-linking CD3, CD4/CD8, and class I MHC molecules. *J Immunol* 1989; 142:4201–4212.

432. Harding CV, Unanue ER. Modulation of antigen presentation and peptide-MHC-specific, LFA-1–dependent T cell-macrophage adhesion. *J Immunol* 1991;147:767–773.

433. Cosimi AB, Conti D, Delmonico FL, et al. In vivo effects of monoclonal antibody to ICAM-1 (CD54) in nonhuman primates with renal allografts. *J Immunol* 1990;144:4604–4612.

434. Wee SL, Cosimi AB, Preffer FI, et al. Functional consequences of anti-ICAM-1 (CD54) in cynomolgus monkeys. *Transplant Proc* 1991;23:279–280.

435. Suthanthiran M, Morris RE, Strom TB. Immunosuppressants: cellular and molecular mechanisms of action. *Am J Kidney Dis* 1996;28:159–172.

436. European Mycophenolate Mofetil Cooperative Study Group. Placebo-controlled study of mycophenolate mofetil combined with cyclosporin and corticosteroids for prevention of acute rejection. *Lancet* 1995;345:1321–1325.

437. Sollinger HW, for the US Renal Transplant Mycophenolate Mofetil Study Group. Mycophenolate mofetil for the prevention of acute rejection in primary cadaveric renal allograft recipients. *Transplantation* 1995;60:225–232.

438. Shevach EM. The effects of cyclosporin A on the immune system. *Ann Rev Immunol* 1985;3:397.

439. Kahan BD. Cyclosporine. *N Engl J Med* 1989;321:1725–1738.

440. Kahan BD, Van Buren CT, Flechner SM, et al. Clinical and experimental studies with cyclosporine in renal transplantation. *Surgery* 1985;97:125.

441. Goto T, Kino T, Hatanaka H, et al. Discovery of FK-506, a novel immunosuppressant isolated from Streptomyces Tsukubaenisis. *Transplant Proc* 1987; 19(suppl 6):4.

442. Abraham RT, Wiederrecht GJ. Immunopharmacology of rapamycin. *Ann Rev Immunol* 1996;14:483–510.

443. Todo S, Murase N, Kahn D, et al. Effect of 15-deoxyspergualin on experimental organ transplantation. *Transplant Proc* 1988;209(suppl 1):233–236.

444. Yuh D, Gandy KL, Morris RE, et al. Leflunomide prolongs pulmonary allograft and xenograft survival. *J Heart Lung Transplant* 1995;14:1136–1144.

445. Lin Y, Sobis H, Vandeputte M, Waer M. Mechanism of leflunomide-induced prevention of xenoantibody formation and xenograft rejection in the hamster to rat heart transplantation model. *Transplant Proc* 1995;27:305–306.

446. Cosimi AB, Wortis H, Delmonico F, Russell PS. Randomized clinical trial of antitymocyte globulin in cadaver renal allograft recipients. *Surgery* 1976; 80:155–161.

447. Shield CF, Cosimi AB, Tolkoff-Rubin N, Rubin RH, Herrin J, Russell PS. Use of antithymocyte globulin for reversal of acute allograft rejection. *Transplantation* 1979;28:461.

448. Cosimi AB, Colvin RB, Jaffers GJ, et al. Immunologic monitoring of monoclonal antibody therapy: comparison of five antibodies as immunosuppressants of renal allograft rejection. *Transplant Proc* 1984;16:1459–1461.

449. Cosimi AB, Burton RC, Kung PC, et al. Evaluation in primate renal allograft recipients of monoclonal antibody to human T-cell subclasses. *Transplant Proc* 1981;13:499–503.

450. Onodera K, Lehmann M, Akalin E, Volk H-D, Sayegh MH, Kupiec-Weglinski JW. Induction of "infectious" tolerance to MHC-incompatible cardiac allografts in CD4 monoclonal antibody-treated sensitized rat recipients. *J Immunol* 1996; 157:1944–1950.

451. Alters SE, Shizuru JA, Ackerman J, Grossman D, Seydel KB, Fathman CG. Anti-CD4 mediates clonal anergy during transplantation tolerance induction. *J Exp Med* 1991;173: 491

452. Kirkman RL, Barrett LV, Gaulton GN, et al. The effect of anti-interleukin-2 receptor monoclonal antibody on allograft rejection. *Transplantation* 1985;40: 719.

453. Kelley VE, Gaulton GN, Strom TB. Inhibitory effect of anti-interleukin 2 receptor and anti-L3T4 antibodies on delayed type hypersensitivity: the role of complement and epitope. *J Immunol* 1987;138:2771–2775.

454. Reed MH, Shapiro ME, Strom TB, et al. Prolongation of primate renal allografts with anti-Tac monoclonal antibody. *Curr Surg* 1988;45:28–30.

455. Bacha P, Williams DP, Waters C, Williams JM, Murphy JR, Strom TB. Interleukin 2 receptor-targeted cytotoxicity. Interleukin 2 receptor–mediated action of a diphtheria toxin–related interleukin 2 fusion protein. *J Exp Med* 1988;167:612–622.

456. Kirkman RL, Shapiro ME, Carpenter CB, et al. A randomized prospective trial of anti-TAC monoclonal antibody in human renal transplantation. *Transplantation* 1991;51:107–113.

457. Tinubu SA, Hakimi J, Kondas JA, et al. Humanized antibody directed to the IL-2 receptor β-chain prolongs primate cardiac allograft survival. *J Immunol* 1994;153:4330–4338.

458. Turka LA, Linsley PS, Lin H, et al. T-cell activation by the CD28 ligand B7 is required for cardiac allograft rejection in vivo. *Proc Natl Acad Sci U S A* 1992;89:11102

459. Larsen CP, Elwood ET, Alexander DZ, et al. Long-term acceptance of skin and cardiac allografts after blocking CD40 and CD28 pathways. *Nature* 1996;381: 434–438.

460. Kirk AD, Harlan DM, Armstrong NN, et al. CTLA4-Ig and anti-CD40 ligand prevent renal allograft rejection in primates. *Proc Natl Acad Sci U S A* 1997; 94:8789–8794.

461. Cosimi AB, Colvin RB, Burton RC, et al. Use of monoclonal antibodies to T-cell subsets for immunologic monitoring and treatment in recipients of renal allografts. *N Engl J Med* 1981;305:308.

462. Russell PS, Colvin RB, Cosimi AB. Monoclonal antibodies for the diagnosis and treatment of transplant rejection. *Ann Rev Med* 1984;35:63.

463. Hirsch R, Gress RE, Pluznik DH, Eckhaus M, Bluestone JA. Effects of in vivo administration of anti-CD3 monoclonal antibody on T cell function in mice II. In vivo activation of T cells. *J Immunol* 1989;142:737–743.

464. Davis LS, Wacholtz MC, Lipsky PE. The induction of T cell unresponsiveness by rapidly modulating CD3. *J Immunol* 1989;142:1084–1094.

465. Alegre ML, Collins AM, Pulito VL, et al. Effect of a single amino acid mutation on the activating and immunosuppressive properties of a "humanized" OKT3 monoclonal antibody. *J Immunol* 1992;148:3461–3468.

466. Vitetta ES, Uhr JW. The potential use of immunotoxins in transplantation, cancer therapy, and immunoregulation. *Transplantation* 1984;37:535.

467. Knechtle SJ, Vargo D, Fechner J, et al. FN18-CRM9 immunotoxin promotes tolerance in primate renal allografts. *Transplantation* 1997;63:1–6.

468. Auchincloss HA. Why is cell-mediated xenograft rejection so strong? *Xeno* 1995;3:19–22.

469. Goodnow CC. Transgenic mice and analysis of B-cell tolerance. *Ann Rev Immunol* 1992;10:489–518.

470. Hartley SB, Crosbie J, Brink RA, Kantor AB, Basten A, Goodnow CC. Elimination from peripheral lymphoid tissues of self-reactive B lymphocytes recognizing membrane-bound antigens. *Nature* 1991;353:765–769.

471. Murakami M, Tsubata T, Okamoto M, et al. Antigen-induced apoptotic death of Ly-1 B cells is responsible for autoimmune disease in transgenic mice. *Nature* 1992;357:77–80.

472. Allen PM. Peptides in positive and negative selection: a delicate balance. *Cell* 1994;76:593–596.

473. Alam SM, Travers PJ, Wung JL, et al. T-cell-receptor affinity and thymocyte positive selection. *Nature* 1996;381:616–620.

474. Brocker T, Riedinger M, Karjalainen K. Targeted expression of major histocompatibiity complex (MHC) class II molecules demonstrates that dendritic cells can induce negative but not positive selection of thymocytes in vivo. *J Exp Med* 1997;185:541–550.

475. Inaba M, Inaba K, Hosono M, et al. Distinct mechanisms of neonatal tolerance induced by dendritic cells and thymic B cells. *J Exp Med* 1991;173:549–559.

476. Schonrich G, Strauss G, Muller K-P, et al. Distinct requirements of positive and negative selection for selecting cell type and CD8 interaction. *J Immunol* 1993; 151:4098–4105.

477. Schulz R, Mellor AL. Self major histocompatibility complex class I antigens expressed solely in lymphoid cells do not induce tolerance in the CD4+ T cell compartment. *J Exp Med* 1996;184:1573–1578.

478. Oukka M, Colucci-Guyon E, Tran PL, Cohen-Tannoudji M, Kosmatopoulos K. CD4 T cell tolerance to nuclear proteins induced by medullary thymic epithelium. *Immunity* 1996;4:545–553.

479. Matzinger P. Why positive selection? *Immunol Rev* 1993;135:81–117.

480. Ferber I, Schonrich G, Schenkel J, Mellor AL, Hammerling GJ, Arnold B. Levels of peripheral T cell tolerance induced by different doses of tolerogen. *Science* 1994;263:674–676.

481. Webb SR, Hutchinson J, Hayden K, Sprent J. Expansion/deletion of mature T cells exposed to endogenous superantigens in vivo. *J Immunol* 1994;152: 586–597.

482. Rocha B, Von Boehmer H. Peripheral selection of the T cell repertoire. *Science* 1991;251:1225–1228.

483. Ramsdell F, Fowlkes BJ. Clonal deletion versus clonal anergy:the role of the thymus in inducing self tolerance. *Science* 1990;248:1342–1348.

484. Schwartz RH. A cell culture model for T lymphocyte clonal anergy. *Science* 1990;248:1349–1356.

485. Nossal GJV, Pike BL. Clonal anergy: persistence in tolerant mice of antigen-binding B lymphocytes incapable of responding to antigen or mitogen. *Proc Natl Acad Sci U S A* 1980;77:1602–1606.

486. Nossal GJV. Cellular mechanisms of immunologic tolerance. *Ann Rev Immunol* 1983;1:33–62.

487. Zanders ED, Lamb JR, Feldmann M, Green N, Beverley PCL. Tolerance of T-cell clones is associated with membrane antigen changes. *Nature* 1983;303:625–627.

488. Schonrich G, Kalinke U, Momburg F, et al. Down-regulation of T cell receptors on self-reactive T cells as a novel mechanism for extrathymic tolerance induction. *Cell* 1991;65:293–304.

489. Arnold B, Schonrich G, Hammerling GJ. Multiple levels of peripheral tolerance. *Immunol Today* 1993;14:12–14.

490. Rocken M, Urban JF, Shevach EM. Infection breaks T cell tolerance. *Nature* 1992;359:79–82.

491. Rocha B, Tanchot C, Von Boehmer H. Clonal anergy blocks in vivo growth of mature T cells and can be reversed in the absence of antigen. *J Exp Med* 1993; 177:1517–1521.

492. Ramsdell F, Fowlkes BJ. Maintenance of in vivo tolerance by persistence of antigen. *Science* 1992;257:1130–1134.

493. Kohler H. The Immune Network Revisted. In: Kohler H, Urbain J, Cazenave P-A, eds. *Idiotypy in biology and medicine.* Orlando, FL: Academic Press, 1984: 3–14.

494. Pennington LR, Flye MW, Kirkman RL, Thisthlethwaite JR Jr, Williams GM, Sachs DH. Transplantation in miniature swine. X. Evidence for non-SLA linked immune response gene(s) controlling rejection of SLA-matched kidney allografts. *Transplantation* 1981;32:315–320.

495. Bluestone JA, Leo O, Epstein SL, Sachs DH. Idiotypic manipulation of the immune response to transplantation antigens. *Immunol Rev* 1986;90:5–27.

496. Carpenter CB, D'Apice AJF, Abbas AK. The role of antibody in the rejection and enhancement of organ allografts. *Adv Immunol* 1976;22:1.

497. Kaliss N. Immunological enhancement of tumor homografts in mice. A review. *Cancer Res* 1958;18:992.

498. Stuart FP, Fitch FW, Rowley DA. Specific suppression of renal allograft rejection by treatment with antigen and antibody. *Transplant Proc.* 1970;2:483–438.

499. Batchelor JR. The riddle of kidney graft enhancement. *Transplantation* 1978; 26:139–141.

500. French ME, Batchelor JR. Enhancement of renal allografts in rats and man. *Transplant Rev* 1972;13:115–141.

501. Verbanac KM, Carver FM, Haisch CE, Thomas JM. A role for transforming growth factor-beta in the veto mechanism in transplant tolerance. *Transplantation* 1994;57:893–900.

502. Raju GP, Belland SE, Eisen HJ. Prolongation of cardiac allograft survival with transforming growth factor-β1 in rats. *Transplantation* 1994;58:392–396.

503. Langrehr JM, Dull KE, Ochoa JB, et al. Evidence that nitric oxide production by in vivo allosensitized cells inhibits the development of allospecific CTL. *Transplantation* 1992;53:632–640.

504. Langrehr JM, Hoffman RA, Lancaster JR Jr, Simmons RL. Nitric oxide—a new endogenous immunomodulator. *Transplantation* 1993;55:1205–1212.

505. Snijdewint FGM, Kalinski P, Wierenga EA, Bos JD, Kapsenberg ML. Prostaglandin E2 differentially modulates cytokine secretion profiles of human T helper lymphocytes. *J Immunol* 1993;150:5321–5329.

506. Betz M, Fox BS. Prostaglandin E2 inhibits production of Th1 lymphokines but not of Th2 lymphokines. *J Immunol* 1991;146:108–113.

507. Maes LY, York JL, Soderberg LSF. A soluble factor produced by bone marrow natural suppressor cells blocks interleukin 2 production and activity. *Cell Immuol* 1988;116:35–43.

508. Hertel-Wulff B, Strober S. Immunosuppressive lymphokine derived from natural suppressor cells. *J Immunol* 1988;140:2633–2638.

509. Knaan-Shanzer S, Van Bekkum DW. Soluble factors secreted by naturally occurring suppressor cells that iterfere with in vivo graft-vs.-host disease and with T cell responsiveness in vitro. *Eur J Immunol* 1987;17:827–834.

510. Choi KL, Maier T, Holda JH, Claman HN. Suppression of cytotoxic T-cell generation by natural suppressor cells from mice with GVHD is partially reversed by indomethacin. *Cell Immunol* 1988;112:271–278.

511. Weingust RW, McCain GA, Singhal SK. Regulation of autoimmunity in normal and rheumatoid individuals by bone marrow-derived natural suppressor cells and their suppressor factor: BDSF. *Cell Immunol* 1989;122:154–163.

512. Okada S, Strober S. Spleen cells from adult mice given total lymphoid irradiation or from newborn mice have similar regulatory effects in the mixed leukocyte reaction. I. Generation of antigen-specific cells in the mixed leukocyte reaction after the addition of spleen cells from adult mice given total lymphoid irradiation. *J Exp Med* 1982;156:522–538.

513. Okada S, Strober S. Spleen cells from adult mice given total lymphoid irradiation (TLI) or from newborn mice have similar regulatory effects in the mixed leukocyte reaction. II. Generation of antigen-specific suppressor cells in the MLR after the addtion of spleen cells from newborn mice. *J Immunol* 1982;129:1892–1897.

514. Oseroff A, Okada S, Strober S. Natural suppressor (NS) cells found in the spleen of neonatal mice and adult mice given total lymphoid irradiation (TLI) express the null surface phenotype. *J Immunol* 1984;132:101–110.

515. Muraoka S, Miller RG. Cells in bone marrow and in T cell colonies grown from bone marrow can suppress generation of cytotoxic T lymphocytes directed against their self antigens. *J Exp Med* 1980;152:54–71.

516. Miller RG. The veto phenomenon and T-cell regulation. *Immunol Today* 1986;7:112–114.

517. Claesson MH, Miller RG. Functional heterogeneity in allospecific cytotoxic T lymphocyte clones I. CTL clones express strong anti-self suppressive activity. *J Exp Med* 1984;160:1702–1716.

518. Azuma E, Kaplan J. Role of lymphokine-activated killer cells as mediators of veto and natural suppression. *J Immunol* 1988;141:2601–2606.

519. Sambhara SR, Miller RG. Programmed cell death of T cells signaled by the T cell receptor and the alpha-3 domain of class I MHC. *Science* 1991;252:1424–1427.

520. Kaplan DR, Hambor JE, Tykocinski ML. An immunoregulatory function for the CD8 molecule. *Proc Natl Acad Sci U S A* 1989;86:8512

521. Takahashi H, Nakagawa Y, Leggatt GR, et al. Inactivation of human immunodeficiency virus (HIV)-1 envelope-specific CD8⁺ cytotoxic T lymphocytes by free antigenic peptide: a self-veto mechanism? *J Exp Med* 1996;183:879–889.

522. Pearce NW, Spinelli A, Gurley KE, Hall BM. Specific unresponsiveness in rats with prolonged cardiac allograft survival after treatment with cyclosporine. V Dependence of CD4⁺ suppressor cells on the presence of alloantigen and cytokines, including interleukin-2. *Transplantation* 1993;55:374–379.

523. Roser BJ. Cellular mechanisms in neonatal and adult tolerance. *Immunol Rev* 1989;107:179–202.

524. Tomita Y, Mayumi H, Eto M, Nomoto K. Importance of suppressor T cells in cyclophosphamide-induced tolerance to the non–H-2-encoded alloantigens. Is mixed chimerism really required in maintaining a skin allograft tolerance. *J Immunol* 1990;144:463–473

525. Tutschka PJ, Ki PF, Beschorner WE, Hess AD, Santos GW. Suppressor cells in transplantation tolerance. II. Maturation of suppressor cells in the bone marrow chimera. *Transplantation* 1981;32:321

526. Lancaster F, Chui YL, Batchelor JR. Anti-idiotypic T cells suppress rejection of renal allografts in rats. *Nature* 1985;315:336–337.

527. Maki T, Gottshalk R, Wood ML, Monaco AP. Specific unresponsiveness to skin allografts in anti-lymphocyte serum-treated, marrow-injected mice: participation of donor marrow-derived suppressor T cells. *J Immunol* 1981;127:1433–1437.

528. Wood ML, Monaco AP. Suppressor cells in specific unresponsiveness to skin allografts in ALS-treated, marrow-injected mice. *Transplantation* 1980;29:196–200.

529. Wilson DB. Idiotypic regulation of T cells in graft-versus-host disease and autoimmunity. *Immunol Rev* 1989;107:159–176.

530. Koide J, Engleman EG. Differences in surface phenotype and mechanism of action between alloantigen-specific CD8⁺ cytotoxic and suppressor T cell clones. *J Immunol* 1990;144:32–40.

531. Mossman TR, Coffman RL. Th1 and Th2 cells: different patterns of lymphokine secretion to different functional properties. *Ann Rev Immunol* 1989;7:145

532. Kupiec-Weglinski JW, Wasowska B, Papp I, et al. CD4 mAb therapy modulates alloantibody production and intracardiac graft deposition in association with selective inhibition of Th1 lymphokines. *J Immunol* 1993;151:5053–5061

533. Gorczynski RM, Wojcik D. A role for nonspecific (cyclosporin A) or specific (monoclonal antibodies to ICAM-1, LFA-1, and IL-10) immunomodulation in the prolongation of skin allografts after antigen-specific pretransplant immunization or transfusion. *J Immunol* 1994;152:2011–2019.

534. Hancock WW, Sayegh MH, Kwok CA, Weiner HL, Carpenter CB. Oral, but not intravenous, alloantigen prevents accelerated allograft rejection by selective intragraft TH2 activation. *Transplantation* 1993;55:1112–1118.

535. Takeuchi T, Lowry RP, Konieczny B. Heart allografts in murine systems. The differential activation of Th2-like effector cells in peripheral tolerance. *Transplantation* 1992;53:1281–1294.

536. Mottram PL, Han W-R, Purcell LJ, McKenzie IFC, Hancock WW. Increased expression of IL-4 and IL-10 and decreased expression of IL-2 and interferon-gamma in long-surviving mouse heart allografts after brief CD4-monoclonal antibody therapy. *Transplantation* 1995;59:559–565.

537. Chen N, Field EH. Enhanced type 2 and diminished type 1 cytokines in neonatal tolerance. *Transplantation* 1995;59:933–941.

538. Bucy RP, Li J, Huang GQ, Honjo K, Xu XY. Allograft tolerance induced by combined anti–LFA-1 and anti-ICAM-1 mAb is associated with shift from Th1 to Th2 cytokine expression in allograft [Abstract]. *FASEB J* 1995;9:A497.

539. Onodera K, Hancock WW, Graser E, et al. Type 2 helper T cell-type cytokines and the development of "infectious" tolerance in rat cardiac allograft recipients. *J Immunol* 1997;158:1572–1581.

540. Bishop DK, Chan SY, Eichwald EJ. Th1 and Th2 cytokines promote distinct forms of allograft rejection [Abstract]. *FASEB J* 1995;9:497.

541. Martinez OM, Lang T, Villanueva JC, Esquivel CO, So S, Krams SM. Allograft rejection is associated with a Th2-dominant cytokine profile [Abstract]. *FASEB J* 1995;9:497.

542. Alexander DZ, Pearson TC, Ritchie SC, et al. Analysis of the mechanisms of CTLA4-Ig plus bone marrow induced transplantation tolerance [Abstract]. *FASEB J* 1995;9:783.

543. Zheng XX, Steele AW, Nickerson PW, Steurer W, Steiger J, Strom TB. Administration of noncytolytic IL-10/Fc in murine models of lipopolysaccharide-induced septic shock and allogeneic islet transplantation. *J Immunol* 1995;154:5590–5600.

544. Wren SM, Wang SC, Thai NL, et al. Evidence for early Th2 T cell predominance in xenoreactivity *Transplantation* 1993;56:905–911.

545. Groux H, O'Garra A, Bigler M, et al. A CD4⁺ T-cell subset inhibits antigen-specific T-cell responses and prevents colitis. *Nature* 1997;389:737–742.

546. Bohme J, Haskins K, Stecha P, et al. Transgenic mice with I-A on islet cells are normoglycemic but immunologically intolerant. *Science* 1989;244:1179–1183.

547. Ohashi PS, Oehen S, Buerki K, et al. Ablation of "tolerance" and induction of diabetes by virus infection in viral antigen transgenic mice. *Cell* 1991;65:305–317.

548. Hammerling GJ, Schonrich G, Momburg F, et al. Non-deletional mechanisms of peripheral and central tolerance:studies with transgenic mice with tissue-specific expression of a foreign MHC class I antigen. *Immunol Rev* 1991;122:47–66.

549. Picarella DE, Kratz A, Li C, Ruddle NH, Flavell RA. Transgenic tumor necrosis factor (TNF)-α production in pancreatic islets leads to insulinitis, not diabetes: distinct patterns of inflammation in TNF-α and TNF-β transgenic mice. *J Immunol* 1993;150:4136–4150.

550. Heath WR, Allison J, Hoffman MW, et al. Autoimmune diabetes as a consequence of locally produced interleukin-2. *Nature* 1992;359:547–549.

551. von Herrath MG, Guerder S, Lewicki H, Flavell RA, Oldstone MBA. Coexpression of B7-1 and viral ("self") transgenes in pancreatic b cells can break peripheral ignorance and lead to spontaneous autoimmune diabetes. *Immunity* 1995;3:727–738.

552. Lafferty KJ, Babcock SK, Gill RG. Prevention of rejection by treatment of the graft:an overview. *Prog Clin Biol Res* 1986;224:87.

553. Charlton B, Auchincloss H Jr, Fathman CG. Mechanisms of transplantation tolerance. *Annu Rev Immunol* 1994;12:707–734.

554. Orloff MS, Fallon MA, DeMara F, Coppage ML, Leong N, Cerilli J. Induction of specific tolerance to small-bowel allografts. *Surgery* 1994;116:222–228.

555. Auchincloss H Jr, Sachs DH. Mechanisms of tolerance in murine radiation bone marrow chimeras: I. Nonspecific suppression of alloreactivity by spleen cells from early but not late chimeras. *Transplantation* 1983;36:436.

556. Auchincloss H Jr, Sachs DH. Mechanisms of tolerance in murine radiation bone marrow chimeras II. Absence of nonspecific suppression in mature chimeras. *Transplantation* 1983;36:442.

557. Almaraz R, Ballinger W, Sachs DH, Rosenberg SA. The effect of peripheral lymphoid cells on the incidence of lethal graft versus host disease following allogeneic mouse bone marrow transplantation. *J Surg Res* 1983;34:133–144.

558. Sharp TG, Sachs DH, Fauci AS, Messerschmidt GL, Rosenberg SA. T-cell depletion of human bone marrow using monoclonal antibody and complement mediated lysis. *Transplantation* 1983;35:112–120.

559. Martin P. Overview of marrow transplantation immunology. In: Forman SJ, Blume KG, Thomas ED, eds. *Bone marrow transplantation*. Cambridge, England: Blackwell Scientific, 1994:16

560. Singer A, Hathcock KS, Hodes RJ. Self recognition in allogeneic radiation bone marrow chimeras. A radiation-resistant host element dictates the specificity and immune response gene phenotype of T-helper cells. *J Exp Med* 1981;153:1286.

561. Ruedl E, Sykes M, Ildstad ST, et al. Antiviral T cell competence and restriction specificity of mixed allogeneic (P1 + P2 → P1) irradiation chimeras. *Cell Immunol* 1989;121:185–195.

562. Slavin S, Fuks Z, Strober S, Kaplan H, Howard RJ, Sutherland DER. Transplantation tolerance across major histocompatibility barriers after total lymphoid irradiation. *Transplantation* 1979;28:359.

563. Slavin S, Strober S, Fuks Z, Kaplan HS. Induction of specific tissue transplantation tolerance using fractionated total lymphoid irradiation in adult mice:long term survival of allogeneic bone marrow and skin grafts. *J Exp Med* 1977;146:34.

564. Field EH, Rouse TM. Alloantigen priming after total lymphoid irradiation alters alloimmune cytokine responses. *Transplantation* 1995;60:695–702.

565. Zeng D, Ready A, Huie P, et al. Mechanisms of tolerance to rat heart allografts using posttransplant TLI. *Transplantation* 1996;62:510–517.

566. Strober S. Natural suppressor (NS) cells, neonatal tolerance, and total lymphoid irradiation:Exploring obscure relationships. *Ann Rev Immunol* 1984;2:219

567. Najarian JS, Ferguson RM, Sutherland DER, et al. Fractionated total lymphoid irradiation as preparative immunosuppression in high risk renal transplantation: clinical and immunological studies. *Ann Surg* 1982;196:442.

568. Myburgh JA, Meyers AM, Margolius L, et al. Total lymphoid irradiation in clinical renal transplantation—results in 73 patients. *Transplant Proc* 1991;23: 2033–2034.

569. Strober S, Dhillon M, Schubert M, et al. Acquired immune tolerance to cadaveric renal allografts. A study of three patients treated with total lymphoid irradiation. *N Engl J Med* 1989;321:28–33.

570. Thomas J, Alqaisi M, Cunningham P, et al. The development of a posttransplant TLI treatment strategy that promotes organ allograft acceptance without chronic immunosuppression. *Transplantation* 1992;53:247–258.

571. Ildstad ST, Sachs DH. Reconstitution with syngeneic plus allogeneic or xenogeneic bone marrow leads to specific acceptance of allografts or xenografts. *Nature* 1984;307:168–170.

572. Ildstad ST, Wren SM, Bluestone JA, Barbieri SA, Sachs DH. Characterization of mixed allogeneic chimeras: immunocompetence, in vitro reactivity, and genetic specificity of tolerance. *J Exp Med* 1985;162:231–244.

573. Kawai T, Cosimi AB, Colvin RB, et al. Mixed allogeneic chimerism and renal allograft tolerance in cynomologous monkeys. *Transplantation* 1995;59: 256–262.

574. Mayumi H, Good RA. Long-lasting skin allograft tolerance in adult mice induced across fully allogeneic (multimajor H-2 plus multiminor histocompatibility) antigen barriers by a tolerance-inducing method using cyclophosphamide. *J Exp Med* 1989;169:213.

575. De Vries-van der Zwan A, Besseling AC, De Waal LP, Boog CJP. Specific tolerance induction and transplantation: a single-day protocol. *Blood* 1997;89: 2596–2601.

576. Colson YL, Wren SM, Schuchert MJ, et al. A nonlethal conditioning approach to achieve durable multilineage mixed chimerism and tolerance across major, minor, and hematopoietic histocompatibility barriers. *J Immunol* 1995;155: 4179–4188.

577. Nomoto K, Yung-Yun K, Omoto K, Umesue M, Murakami Y, Matsuzaki G. Tolerance induction in a fully allogeneic combination using anti-T cell receptor-αβ monoclonal antibody, low dose irradiation, and donor bone marrow transfusion. *Transplantation* 1995;59:395–401.

578. Vallera DA, Taylor PA, Sprent J, Blazar BR. The role of host T cell subsets in bone marrow rejection directed to isolated major histocompatibility complex class I versus class II differences of bm1 and bm12 mutant mice. *Transplantation* 1994;57:249–256.

579. Sharabi Y, Sachs DH, Sykes M. T cell subsets resisting induction of mixed chimerism across various histocompatibility barriers. In: Gergely J, Benczur M, Falus A, et al., eds. *Progress in immunology VIII. Proceedings of the Eighth International Congress of Immunology, Budapest, 1992.* 1992:801

580. Aguila HL, Weissman IL. Hematopoietic stem cells are not direct cytotoxic targets of natural killer cells. *Blood* 1996;87:1225–1231.

581. Sykes M, Sachs DH, Nienhuis AW, Pearson DA, Moulton AD, Bodine DM. Specific prolongation of skin graft survival following retroviral transduction of bone marrow with an allogeneic MHC gene. *Transplantation* 1993;55:197–202.

582. Emery DW, Sablinski T, Shimada H, et al. Expression of an allogeneic MHC DRB transgene, through retroviral transduction of bone marrow, induces specific reduction of alloreactivity. *Transplantation* 1997 (*in press*).

583. Papayannopoulou T, Craddock C, Nakamoto B, Priestley GV, Wolf NS. The VLA4/VCAM-1 adhesion pathway defines contrasting mechanisms of lodgement of transplanted murine hemopoietic progenitors between bone marrow and spleen. *Proc Natl Acad Sci U S A* 1995;92:9647–9651.

584. Hayashi S-I, Gimble JM, Henley A, Ellingsworth LR, Kincade PW. Differential effects of TGF-β1 on lymphohemopoiesis in long-term bone marrow cultures. *Blood* 1989;74:1711–1717.

585. Lee LA, Sergio JJ, Sykes M. Evidence for non-immune mechanisms in the loss of hematopoietic chimerism in rat-mouse mixed xenogeneic chimeras. *Xenotransplant* 1995;2:57–66.

586. Pallavicini M, Flake AW, Bethel C, et al. Creation of human-mouse xenogeneic chimeras by the in utero transplantation of hemopoietic cells [Abstract]. *First International Congress on Xenotransplantation.* 1991:50.

587. Lapidot T, Pflumia F, Doedens M, Murdoch B, Williams DE, Dick JE. Cytokine stimulation of multilineage hematopoiesis from immature human cells engrafted in SCID mice. *Science* 1992;255:1137–1143.

588. Gritsch HA, Glaser RM, Emery DW, et al. The importance of non-immune factors in reconstitution by discordant xenogeneic hematopoietic cells. *Transplantation* 1994;57:906–917.

589. Yang Y-G, Sergio JJ, Swenson K, Glaser RM, Monroy R, Sykes M. Donor-specific growth factors promote swine hematopoiesis in SCID mice. *Xenotransplant* 1996;3:92–101.

590. Lee LA, Gritsch HA, Sergio JJ, et al. Specific tolerance across a discordant xenogeneic transplantation barrier. *Proc Natl Acad Sci U S A* 1994;91: 10864–10867.

591. Zhao Y, Fishman JA, Sergio JJ, et al. Immune restoration by fetal pig thymus grafts in T cell-depleted, thymectomized mice. *J Immunol* 1997;158:1641–1649.

592. Zhao Y, Swenson K, Sergio JJ, Arn JS, Sachs DH, Sykes M. Skin graft tolerance across a discordant xenogeneic barrier. *Nature Med* 1996;2:1211–1216.

593. Zhao Y, Sergio JJ, Swenson KA, Arn JS, Sachs DH, Sykes M. Positive and negative selection of functional mouse CD4 cells by porcine MHC in pig thymus grafts. *J Immunol* 1997;159:2100–2107.

594. Markert ML, Kostyu DD, Ward FE, et al. Successful formation of a chimeric human thymus allograft following transplantation of cultured postnatal human thymus. *J Immunol* 1997;158:998–1005.

595. Salaun J, Bandeira A, Khazaal I, et al. Thymic epithelium tolerizes for histocompatibility antigens. *Science* 1990;247:1471–1474.

596. Ohki H, Martin C, Corbel C, Coltey M, Le Douarin NM. Tolerance induced by thymic epithelial grafts in birds. *Science* 1987;237:1032–1035.

597. Modigliani Y, Tomas-Vaslin V, Bandeira A, et al. Lymphocytes selected in allogeneic thymic epithelium mediate dominant tolerance toward tissue grafts of the thymic epithelium haplotype. *Proc Natl Acad Sci U S A* 1995;92:7555–7559.

598. Modigliani Y, Pereira P, Thomas-Vaslin V, et al. Regulatory T cells in thymic epithelium-induced tolerance. I. Suppression of mature peripheral non-tolerant T cells. *Eur J Immunol* 1995;25:2563–2571.

599. Touraine JL, Raudrant D, Rebaud A, et al. In utero transplantation of stem cells in humans:immunological aspects and clinical follow-up of patients. *Bone Marrow Transplant* 1992;9(suppl 1):121–126.

600. Flake AW, Roncarolo M-G, Puck JM, et al. Treatment of X-linked severe combined immunodeficiency by in utero transplantation of paternal bone marrow. *N Engl J Med* 1996;335:1806–1810.

601. Carrier E, Lee TH, Busch MP, Cowan MJ. Induction of tolerance in nondefective mice after in utero transplantation of major histocompatibility complex–mismatched fetal hematopoietic stem cells. *Blood* 1995;86:4681–4690.

602. Kawashima I, Zanjani ED, Almaida-Porada G, Flake AW, Zeng H, Ogawa M. CD34+ human marrow cells that express low levels of Kit protein are enriched for long-term marrow-engrafting cells. *Blood* 1996;87:4136–4142.

603. Hedrick MH, Rice HE, MacGillivray TE, Bealer JF, Zanjani ED, Flake AW. Hematopoietic chimerism achieved by in utero hematopietic stem cell injection does not induce donor-specific tolerance for renal allografts in sheep. *Transplantation* 1994;58:110–111.

604. Streilein JW. Neonatal tolerance of H-2 alloantigens. *Transplantation* 1991; 52:1–10.

605. Alard P, Matriano JA, Socarras S, Ortega M-A, Streilein JW. Detection of donor-derived cells by polymerase chain reaction in neonatally tolerant mice. Microchimerism fails to predict tolerance. *Transplantation* 1995;60:1125–1130.

606. Smith JP, Kasten-Jolly J, Field LJ, Thomas JM. Assessment of donor bone marrow cell–derived chimerism in transplantation tolerance using transgenic mice. *Transplantation* 1994;58:324–329.

607. Lubaroff DM, Silvers WK. The importance of chimerism in maintaining tolerance of skin allografts in mice. *J Immunol* 1973;111:65–71.

608. Sykes M, Sheard MA, Sachs DH. Effects of T cell depletion in radiation bone marrow chimeras II. Requirement for allogeneic T cells in the reconstituting bone marrow inoculum for subsequent resistance to breaking of tolerance. *J Exp Med* 1988;168:661–673.

609. Khan A, Tomita Y, Sykes M. Thymic dependence of loss of tolerance in mixed allogeneic bone marrow chimeras after depletion of donor antigen. Peripheral mechanisms do not contribute to maintenance of tolerance. *Transplantation* 1996;62:380–387.

610. Donckier V, Wissing M, Bruyns C, et al. Critical role of interleukin 4 in the induction of neonatal transplantation tolerance. Transplantation 1995;59: 1571–1576.

611. Sarzotti M, Robbins DS, Hoffman PM. Induction of protective CTL responses in newborn mice by a murine retrovirus. *Science* 1996;271:1726–1728.

612. Forsthuber T, Yip HC, Lehmann PV. Induction of Th1 and Th2 immunity in neonatal mice. *Science* 1996;271:1728–1730.

613. Ridge JP, Fuchs EJ, Matzinger P. Neonatal tolerance revisited: turning on newborn T cells with dendritic cells. *Science* 1996;271:1723–1726.

614. Starzl TE, Demetris AJ, Trucco M, et al. Chimerism and donor-specific nonreactivity 27 to 29 years after kidney allotransplantation. *Transplantation* 1993;55: 1272–1277.

615. Anonymous. The lost chord: microchimerism and allograft survival. *Immunol Today* 1996;17:577–584.

616. Wood K, Sachs DH. Chimerism and transplantation tolerance: cause and effect. *Immunol Today* 1996;17:584–588.

617. Eynon EE, Parker DC. Parameters of tolerance induction by antigen targeted to B lymphocytes. *J Immunol* 1993;151:2958–2964.

618. Fuchs EJ, Matzinger P. B cells turn off virgin but not memory T cells. *Science* 1992;258:1156–1159.

619. Lombardi G, Hargreaves R, Sidhu S, et al. Antigen presentation by T cells inhibits IL-2 production and induces IL-4 release due to altered cognate signals. *J Immunol* 1996;156:2769–2775.

620. Burlingham WJ, Grailer AP, Fechner JH Jr, et al. Microchimerism linked to cytotoxic T lymphocyte functional unresponsiveness (clonal anergy) in a tolerant renal transplant recipient. *Transplantation* 1995;59:1147–1155.

621. Murase N, Starzl TE, Ye Q, et al. Multilineage hematopoietic reconstitution of supralethally irradiated rats by syngeneic whole organ transplantation with particular reference to the liver. *Transplantation* 1996;61:1–4.

622. Taniguchi H, Toyoshima T, Fukao K, Nakauchi H. Presence of hematopoietic stem cells in the adult liver. *Nature Med* 1996;2:198–203.

623. Lu L, Rudert WA, Qian SG, et al. Growth of donor-derived dendritic cells from the bone marrow of murine liver allograft recipients in response to granulocyte/macrophage colony-stimulating factor. *J Exp Med* 1995;182:379–387.

624. Bushell A, Pearson TC, Morris PJ, Wood KJ. Donor-recipient microchimerism is not required for tolerance induction following recipient pretreatment with donor-specific transfusion and anti-CD4 antibody. *Transplantation* 1995;59: 1367–1371.

625. Shirwan H, Wang HK, Barwari L, Makowka L, Cramer DV. Pretransplant injection of allograft recipients with donor blood or lymphocytes permits allograft tolerance without the presence of persistent donor microchimerism. *Transplantation* 1996;61:1382–1386.

626. Fisher RA, Cohen DS, Ben-Ezra JM, Sallade RE, Tawes JW, Tarry WC. Induction of long-term graft tolerance and donor/recipient chimerism. *J Surg Res* 1996;60:181–185.

627. Schlitt HJ. Is microchimerism needed for allograft tolerance? *Transplant Proc* 1997;29:82–84.

628. Hisanaga M, Hundrieser J, Boker K, et al. Development, stability, and clinical correlations of allogeneic microchimerism after solid organ transplantation. *Transplantation* 1996;61:40–45.

629. Schlitt HJ, Hundrieser J, Ringe B, Pichlmayr R. Systemic microchimerism of donor-type associated with irreversible acute liver graft rejection eight years after transplantation. *N Engl J Med* 1994;330:646–647.

630. Shapiro R, Rao AS, Fontes P, et al. Combined simultaneous kidney/bone marrow transplantation. *Transplantation* 1995;60:1421–1425.

631. Rolles K, Burroughs AK, Davidson BR, Karatapanis S, Prentice HG, Hamon MD. Donor-specific bone marrow infusion after orthotopic liver transplantation. *Lancet* 1994;343:263–265.

632. Ricordi C, Karatzas T, Nery J, et al. High-dose donor bone marrow infusions to enhance allograft survival. The effect of timing. *Transplantation* 1997;63:7–11.

633. Garcia-Morales R, Carreno M, Mathew JM, et al. The effects of chimeric cells following donor bone marrow infusions as detected by PCR-flow assays in kidney transplant recipients. *J Clin Invest* 1997;99:1118–1129.

634. Mathew JM, Carreno M, Fuller L, Ricordi C, Esquenazi V, Miller J. Modulatory effects of human donor bone marrow cells on allogeneic immune responses. *Transplantation* 1997;63:689–692.

635. Thomas JM, Verbanac KM, Smith JP, et al. The facilitating effect of one-DR antigen sharing in renal allograft tolerance induced by donor bone marrow in rhesus monkeys. *Transplantation* 1995;59:245–255.

636. Tomita Y, Sachs DH, Sykes M. Myelosuppressive conditioning is required to achieve engraftment of pluripotent stem cells contained in moderate doses of syngeneic bone marrow. *Blood* 1994;83:939–948.

637. Ramshaw HS, Crittenden RB, Dooner M, Peters SO, Rao SS, Quesenberry PJ. High levels of engraftment with a single infusion of bone marrow cells into normal unprepared mice. *Biol Blood Marrow Transplant* 1995;1:74–80.

638. Sykes M, Szot GL, Swenson K, Pearson DA. Separate regulation of hematopoietic and thymic engraftment. *Exp Hematol* 1997 (in press).

639. Sykes M, Szot GL, Swenson K, Pearson DA. Induction of high levels of allogeneic hematopoietic reconstitution and donor-specific tolerance without myelosuppressive conditioning. *Nature Med* 1997;3:783–787.

640. Waldmann H, Cobbold S. The use of monoclonal antibodies to achieve immunological tolerance. *Immunol Today* 1993;14:247–251.

641. Kobata T, Ohnishi Y, Urushibara N, Takahashi TA, Sekiguchi S. UV irradiation can induce in vitro clonal anergy in alloreactive cytotoxic T lymphocytes. *Blood* 1993;82:176–181.

642. Wood KJ. Transplantation tolerance with monoclonal antibodies. *Semin Immunol* 1990;2:389–399.

643. Lombardi G, Sidhu S, Batchelor R, Lechler R. Anergic T cells as suppressor cells in vitro. *Science* 1994;264:1587–1589.

644. Pearson TC, Alexander DZ, Winn KJ, Linsley PS, Lowry RP, Larsen CP. Transplantation tolerance induced by CTLA4Ig. *Transplantation* 1994;57:1701–1706.

645. Baliga P, Chavin KD, Qin L, et al. CTLA4Ig prolongs allograft survival while suppressing cell-mediated immunity. *Transplantation* 1994;58:1082–1090.

646. Sayegh MH, Akalin E, Hancock WW, et al. CD28-B7 blockade after alloantigenic challenge in vivo inhibits Th1 cytokines but spares Th2. *J Exp Med* 1995; 181:1869–1874.

647. Yin D, Fathman CG. Induction of tolerance to heart allografts in high responder rats by combining anti-CD4 with CTLA4Ig. *J Immunol* 1995;155:1655–1659.

648. Lenshow DJ, Zeng Y, Thistlethwaite JR, et al. Long-term survival of xenogeneic pancreatic islets induced by CTLA4Ig. *Science* 1992;257:789.

649. Lafferty KJ. A contemporary view of transplantation tolerance: an immunologist's perspective. *Clin Transplant* 1994;8:181–187.

650. Calne R, Davies H. Organ graft tolerance: the liver effect. *Lancet* 1994;343:67–68.

651. Sun J, McCaughan GW, Matsumoto Y, Sheil AGR, Gallagher ND, Bishop GA. Tolerance to rat liver allografts. I. Differences between tolerance and rejection are more marked in the B cell compared with the T cell or cytokine response. *Transplantation* 1994;57:1349–1357.

652. Starzl TE, Murase N, Thomson A, Demetris AJ. Liver transplants contribute to their own success. *Nature Med* 1996;2:163–165.

653. Kuchroo VK, Das MP, Brown JA, et al. B7-1 and B7-2 costimulatory molecules activate differentially the Th1/Th2 developmental pathways: application to autoimmune disease therapy. *Cell* 1995;80:707–718.

654. Schweitzer AN, Borriello F, Wong RCK, Abbas AK, Sharpe AH. Role of costimulators in T cell differentiation. Studies using antigen-presenting cells lacking expression of CD80 or CD86. *J Immunol* 1997;158:2713–2722.

655. Durie FH, Foy TM, Masters SR, Laman JD, Noelle RJ. The role of CD40 in the regulation of humoral and cell-mediated immunity. *Immunol Today* 1994;15: 406–411.

656. Noelle RJ. CD40 and its ligand in host defense. *Immunity* 1996;4:415–419.

657. Isobe M, Yagita H, Okumura K, Ihara A. Specific acceptance of cardiac allograft after treatment with antibodies to ICAM-1 and LFA-1. *Science* 1992;255: 1125–1127.

658. Qin S, Cobbold SP, Pope H, et al. "Infectious" transplantation tolerance. *Science* 1993;259:974–977.

659. Cobbold SP, Adams E, Marshall SE, Davies JD, Waldmann H. Mechanisms of peripheral tolerance and suppression induced by monoclonal antibodies to CD4 and CD8. *Immunol Rev* 1996;149:5–34.

660. Rao SS, Peters SO, Crittenden RB, Stewart FM, Ramshaw HS, Quesenberry PJ. Stem cell transplantation in the normal nonmyeloablated host: relationship between cell dose, schedule, and engraftment. *Exp Hematol* 1997;25:114–121.

661. Homan WP, Fabre JW, Williams KA, Millard PR, Morris PJ. Studies of the immunosuppressive properties of cyclosporin A in rats receiving renal allografts. *Transplantation* 1980;29:360–369.

662. Hall BM, Pearce NW, Gurley K, Dorsch SE. Specific unresponsiveness in rats with prolonged cardiac allograft survival after treatment with cyclosporine. *J Exp Med* 1990;171:141–157.

663. Rosengard BR, Ojikutu CA, Guzetta PC, et al. Induction of specific tolerance to class I-disparate renal allografts in miniature swine with cyclosporine. *Transplantation* 1992,54.490–497.

664. Gianello PR, Blancho G, Fishbein JF, et al. Mechanism of cylosporin-induced tolerance to primarily vascularized allografts in miniature swine. Effect of administratin of exogenous IL-2. *J Immunol* 1994;153:4788–4797.

665. Blancho G, Gianello PR, Germana S, Baetscher M, Sachs DH, LeGuern C. Molecular identification of porcine interleukin-10: regulation of expression in a kidney allograft model. *Proc Natl Acad Sci U S A* 1995;92:2800–2804.

666. Blancho G, Gianello PR, Lorf T, et al. Molecular and cellular events implicated in local tolerance to kidney allografts in miniature swine. *Transplantation* 1997;63:26–33.

667. Yamada K, Gianello PR, Ierino FL, et al. Role of the thymus in transplantation tolerance in miniature swine. I. Requirement of the thymus for rapid and stable induction of tolerance to class I-mismatched renal allografts. *J Exp Med* 1997;186:497–506.

668. Agus DB, Surh CD, Sprent J. Reentry of T cells to the adult thymus is restricted to activated T cells. *J Exp Med* 1991;173:1039–1046.

669. Oluwole SF, Jin M-X, Chowdhury NC, Ohajewkwe OA. Effectiveness of intrathymic inoculation of soluble antigens in the induction of specific unresponsiveness to rat islet allografts without transient recipient immunosuppression. *Transplantation* 1994;58:1077–1081.

670. Odorico JS, O'Connor T, Campos L, Barker CF, Posselt AM, Naji A. Examination of the mechanisms responsible for tolerance induction after intrathymic inoculation of allogeneic bone marrow. *Ann Surg* 1993;218:525–531.

671. Debruin RWF, Vanrossum TJ, Scheringa M, Bonthuis F, Ijzermans JNM, Marquet RL. Intrathymic injection of alloantigen may lead to hyperacute rejection and prolonged graft survival of heart allografts in the rat. *Transplantation* 1996;60:1061–1063.

672. Alfrey EJ, Wang X, Lee L, et al. Tolerance induced by direct inoculation of donor antigen into the thymus in low and high responder rodents. *Transplantation* 1995;59:1171–1176.

673. Speiser DE, Schneider R, Hengartner H, MacDonald HR, Zinkernagel RM. Clonal deletion of self-reactive T cells in irradiation bone marrow chimeras and neonatally tolerant mice. Evidence for intercellular transfer of Mlsa. *J Exp Med* 1989;170:595–600.

674. Billingham RE, Medawar PB. Technique of free skin grafting in mammals. *J Exp Biol* 1951;28:385.

675. Starzl TE, Iwatsuki S, Van Thiel DH, et al. Evolution of liver transplantation. *Hepatology* 1982;2:614.

676. Calne RY. Liver grafting. *Transplantation* 1983;35:109.

677. Russell PS. Some immunological considerations in liver transplantation. *Hepatology* 1984;4(suppl):76–78.

678. Ramsey G, Nusbacher J, Starzl TE, Lindsay GD. Isohemagglutinins of graft origin after ABO-unmatched liver transplantation. *N Engl J Med* 1984;311: 1167–1170.

679. Burdick JF, Vogelsang GB, Smith WJ, et al. Severe graft-versus-host disease in a liver-transplant recipient. *N Engl J Med* 1988;318:689–691.

680. Jamieson SW, Stinson EB, Shumway NE. Cardiac transplantation in 150 patients at Stanford University. *Br Med J* 1979;1:93.

681. Burke CM, Baldwin JC, Morris AJ, et al. Twenty-eight cases of human heart lung transplantation. *Lancet* 1986;1:517.

682. Griepp RB, Stinson EB, Bieber CP, et al. Control of graft arteriosclerosis in human heart transplant recipients. *Surgery* 1977;81:262.

683. Toronto Lung Transplant Group. Unilateral lung transplantation for pulmonary fibrosis. *N Engl J Med* 1986;314:1140.

684. Cosimi AB, Auchincloss H Jr, Delmonico FL, et al. Combined kidney and pancreas transplantation in diabetics. *Arch Surg* 1988;123:621.

685. Pancreas Transplantation in the United States as reported to the United Network

for Organ Sharing (UNOS) and analyzed by the International Pancreas Transplant Registry. In: Cecka and Terasaki, eds. *Clinical transplants 1995.* Los Angeles: UCLA Tissue Typing Laboratory, 1995.

686. Kuhr CS, Davis CL, Barr D, et al. Use of ultrasound and cystoscopically guided pancreatic allograft biopsies and transabdominal renal allograft biopsies: safety and efficacy in kidney-pancreas transplant recipients. *J Urol* 1995;153:316–321.

687. Matas AJ, Sutherland DER, Steffes MW, Najarian JS. Islet transplantation. *Surg Gynecol Obstet* 1977;145:757.

688. Martin PJ, Hansen JA, Torok-Storb B, et al. Graft failure in patients receiving T cell–depleted HLA-identical allogeneic marrow transplants. *Bone Marrow Transplant* 1988;3:445–456.

689. Goldman JM, Gale RP, Horowitz MM, et al. Bone marrow transplantation for chronic myelogenous leukemia in chronic phase: increased risk of relapse associated with T-cell depletion. *Ann Intern Med* 1988;108:806

690. Blazar BR, Taylor PA, Linsley PS, Vallera DA. In vivo blockade of CD28/CTLA4: B7/BB1 interaction with CTLA4-Ig reduces lethal murine graft-versus-host disease across the major histocompatibility complex barrier in mice. *Blood* 1994;83:3815–3825.

691. Blazar BR, Taylor PA, Panoskaltsis-Mortari A, et al. Blockade of CD40 ligand-CD40 interactions impairs CD4⁺ T cell–mediated alloreactivity by inhibiting mature donor T cell expansion and function after bone marrow transplantation. *J Immunol* 1997;158:29–39.

692. Blazar BR, Taylor PA, Panoskaltsis-Mortari A, Gray GS, Vallera DA. Coblockade of the LFA1:ICAM and CD28/CTLA4:B7 pathways is a highly effective means of preventing acute lethal graft-versus-host disease induced by fully major histocompatibility complex–disparate donor grafts. *Blood* 1995;85: 2607–2618.

693. Townsend RM, Briggs C, Marini JC, Murphy GF, Korngold R. Inhibitory effect of a CD4-CDR3 peptide analog on graft-versus-host disease across a major histocompatibility complex–haploidentical barrier. *Blood* 1996;88:3038–3047.

694. Koch U, Korngold R. A synthetic CD4-CDR3 peptide analog enhances bone marrow engraftment across major histocompatibility barriers. *Blood* 1997;89: 2880–2890.

695. Sykes M, Romick ML, Hoyles KA, Sachs DH. In vivo administration of interleukin 2 plus T cell–depleted syngeneic marrow prevents graft-versus-host disease mortality and permits alloengraftment. *J Exp Med* 1990;171:645–658.

696. Brok HPM, Heidt PJ, Van der Meide PH, Zurcher C, Vossen JM. Interferon-gamma prevents graft-versus-host disease after allogeneic bone marrow transplantation in mice. *J Immunol* 1993;151:6451–6459.

697. Sykes M, Szot GL, Nguyen PL, Pearson DA. Interleukin-12 inhibits murine graft-vs-host disease. *Blood* 1995;86:2429–2438.

698. Sykes M, Romick ML, Sachs DH. Interleukin 2 prevents graft-vs-host disease while preserving the graft-vs-leukemia effect of allogeneic T cells. *Proc Natl Acad Sci U S A* 1990;87:5633–5637.

699. Sykes M, Harty MW, Szot GL, Pearson DA. Interleukin-2 inhibits graft-versus-host disease-promoting activity of CD4⁺ cells while preserving CD4- and CD8-mediated graft-versus-leukemia effects. *Blood* 1994;83:2560–2569.

700. Yang Y-G, Sergio JJ, Pearson DA, Szot GL, Sykes M. Interleukin-12 preserves the CD8-mediated graft-vs-leukemia effect of allogeneic T cells while inhibiting graft-vs-host disease. *Blood* 1997 (*in press*)

701. Johnson BD, McCabe C, Hanke CA, Truitt RL. Use of anti-CD3 epsilon F(ab')2 fragments in vivo to modulate graft-versus-host disease without loss of graft-versus-leukemia reactivity after MHC-matched bone marrow transplantation. *J Immunol* 1995;154:5542–5554.

702. Cahn JY, Bordigoni P, Tiberghien P, et al. Treatment of acute graft-versus-host disease with methylprednisolone and cyclosporine with or without an anti–interleukin-2 receptor monoclonal antibody. *Transplantation* 1995;60:939–942.

703. Anasetti C, Hansen JA, Waldmann TA, et al. Treatment of acute graft-versus-host disease with humanized anti-Tac: an antibody that binds to the interleukin-2 receptor. *Blood* 1994;84:1320–1327.

704. Herve P, Flesch M, Tiberghien P, et al. Phase I-II trial of a monoclonal anti-tumor necrosis factor α antibody for the treatment of refractory severe acute graft-versus-host disease. *Blood* 1992;79:3362–3368.

705. Antin JH, Weinstein HJ, Guinan EC, et al. Recombinant human interleukin-1 receptor antagonist in the treatment of steroid-resistant graft-versus-host disease. *Blood* 1994;84:1342–1348.

706. Sykes M, Sheard MA, Sachs DH. Graft-versus-host–related immunosuppression is induced in mixed chimeras by alloresponses against either host or donor lymphohematopoietic cells. *J Exp Med* 1988;168:2391–2396.

707. Sykes M, Chester CH, Sachs DH. Protection from graft-versus-host disease in fully allogeneic chimeras by prior administration of T cell–depleted syngeneic bone marrow. *Transplantation* 1988;46:327–330.

708. Johnson BD, Drobyski WR, Truitt RL. Delayed infusion of normal donor cells after MHC-matched bone marrow transplantation provides and antileukemia reaction without graft-versus-host disease. *Bone Marrow Transplant* 1993;11: 329–336.

709. Kolb HJ, Mittrmuller J, Clemm C, et al. Donor leukocyte transfusions for treatment of recurrent chronic myelogenous leukemia in marrow transplant patients. *Blood* 1990;76:2462–2465.

710. Cullis JO, Jiang YZ, Schwarer AP, Hughes TP, Barrett AJ, Goldman JM. Donor leukocyte infusions for chronic myeloid leukemia in relapse after allogeneic bone marrow transplantation. *Blood* 1992;79:1379–1381.

711. Mackinnon S, Papadopoulos EB, Carabasi MH, et al. Adoptive immunotherapy evaluating escalating doses of donor leukocytes for relapse of chronic myeloid leukemia after bone marrow transplantation: separation of graft-versus-leukemia resonses from graft-versus-host disease. *Blood* 1995;86:1261–1268.

712. Sykes M, Sheard M, Sachs DH. Effects of T cell depletion in radiation bone marrow chimeras. I. Evidence for a donor cell population which increases allogeneic chimerism but which lacks the potential to produce GVHD. *J Immunol* 1988;141:2282–2288.

713. Lapidot T, Faktorowich Y, Lubin I, Reisner Y. Enhancement of T-cell–depleted bone marrow allografts in the absence of graft-versus-host disease is mediated by CD8⁺CD4⁻ and not by CD8⁻CD4⁺ thymocytes. *Blood* 1992;80:2406–2411.

714. Martin PJ. Prevention of allogeneic marrow graft rejection by donor T cells that do not recognize recipient alloantigens: potential role of a veto mechanism. *Blood* 1996;88:962–969.

715. Champlin R, Jansen J, Ho W, et al. Retention of graft-versus-leukemia using selective depletion of CD8-positive T lymphocytes for prevention of graft-versus-host disease following bone marrow transplantation for chronic myelogenous leukemia. *Transplant Proc* 1991;23:1695–1696.

716. Truitt RL, Shih C-Y, LeFever AV, Tempelis LD, Andreani M, Bortin MM. Characterization of alloimmunization-induced T lymphocytes reactive against AKR leukemia in vitro and correlation with graft-versus-leukemia activity in vivo. *J Immunol* 1983;131:2050–2058.

717. van Lochem E, de Gast B, Goulmy E. In vitro separation of host specific graft-versus-host and graft-versus-leukemia cytotoxic T cell activities. *Bone Marrow Transplant* 1992;10:181–183.

718. van der Harst D, Goulmy E, Falkenburg JHF, et al. Recognition of minor histocompatibility antigens on lymphocytic and myeloid leukemic cells by cytotoxic T-cell clones. *Blood* 1994;84:1060–1066.

719. Oettel KR, Wesly OH, Albertini MR, et al. Allogeneic T cell clones able to selectively destroy Philadelphia chromosome (Ph1) bearing human leukemia lines can also recognize Ph1 negative cells from the same patient. *Blood* 1994;83:3390–3402.

720. Kwak LW, Pennington R, Longo DL. Active immunization of murine allogeneic bone marrow transplant donors with B-cell tumor–derived idiotype: a strategy for enhancing the specific antitumor effect of marrow grafts. *Blood* 1996; 87:3053–3060.

721. Hsu FJ, Benike C, Fagnoni F, et al. Vaccination of patients with B-cell lymphoma using autologous antigen-pulsed dendritic cells. *Nature Med* 1996;2:52–58.

722. Hsu FJ, Caspar CB, Czerwinski D, et al. Tumor-specific idiotype vaccines in the treatment of patients with B-cell lymphoma—long-term results of a clinical trial. *Blood* 1997;89:3129–3135.

723. Sachs DH. The pig as a potential xenograft donor. *Vet Immunol Immunopathol* 1994;43:185–191.

724. Oriol R, Ye Y, Koren E, Cooper DKC. Carbohydrate antigens of pig tissues reacting with human natural antibodies as potential targets for hyperacute vascular rejection in pig-to-man organ xenotransplantation. *Transplantation* 1993;56: 1433–1442.

725. Seebach JD, Comrack C, Germana S, LeGuern C, Sachs DH, DerSimonian H. HLA-Cw3 expression on porcine endothelial cells protects against xenogeneic cytotoxicity mediated by a subset of human NK cells. *J Immunol* 1997;159: 3655–3661.

726. Moses RD, Pierson RN III, Winn HJ, Auchincloss H Jr. Xenogeneic proliferation and lymphokine production are dependent on CD4⁺ helper T cells and self antigen-presenting cells in the mouse. *J Exp Med* 1990;172:567–575.

727. Wecker H, Winn HJ, Auchincloss H Jr. CD4⁺ T cells, without CD8⁺ or B lymphocytes, can reject xenogeneic skin grafts. *Xenotransplantation* 1994;1:8–16.

728. Chan DV, Auchincloss H Jr. Human anti-pig cell–mediated cytotoxicity in vitro involves non-T as well as T cell components. *Xenotransplantation* 1996;3:158–165.

729. Yamada K, Seebach JD, DerSimonian H, Sachs DH. Human anti-pig T-cell mediated cytotoxicity. *Xenotransplantation* 1996;3:179–187.

730. Inverardi L, Samaja M, Motterlini R, Mangili F, Bender JR, Pardi R. Early recognition of a discordant xenogeneic organ by human circulating lymphocytes. *J Immunol* 1992;149:1416–1423.

731. Seebach JD, Yamada K, McMorrow IM, Sachs DH, DerSimonian H. Xenogeneic human anti-pig cytotoxicity mediated by activated natural killer cells. *Xenotransplantation* 1996;3:188–197.

732. Dorling A, Binns R, Lechler RI. Cellular xenoresponses: observation of significant primary indirect human T cell anti-pig xenoresponses using co-stimulator–deficient or SLA class II–negative porcine stimulators. *Xenotransplantation* 1996;3:112–119.

733. Dorling A, Binns R, Lechler RI. Significant primary indirect human T-cell anti-pig xenoresponses observed using immature porcine dendritic cells and SLA-class II–negative endothelial cells. *Transplant Proc* 1996;28:654.

734. Tearle RG, Tange MJ, Zannettino ZL, et al. The α-1,3-Galactosyltransferase knockout mouse. *Transplantation* 1996;61:13–19.

735. Platt JL, Logan JS. Use of transgenic animals in xenotransplantation. *Transplant Rev* 1996;10:69–77.

736. Waterworth PD, Cozzi E, Tolan MJ, et al. Pig-to-primate cardiac xenotransplantation and cyclophosphamide therapy. *Transplant Proc* 1997;29:899–900.

737. Storck M, Abendroth D, Prestel R, et al. Morphology of hDAF (CD55) transgenic pig kidneys following ex-vivo hemoperfusion with human blood. *Transplantation* 1997;63:304–310.

738. Patience C, Takeuchi Y, Weiss RA. Infection of human cells by an endogenous retrovirus of pigs. *Nature Med* 1997;3:282–286.

739. Reemtsma K. Renal heterotransplantation from nonhuman primates to man. *Ann N Y Acad Sci* 1969;162:412–418.

740. Deacon T, Schumacher J, Dinsmore J, et al. Histological evidence of fetal pig neural cell survival after transplantation into a patient with Parkinson's disease. *Nature Med* 1997;3:350–353.

741. Terasaki PI, ed. *Clinical transplants, 1987.* Los Angeles: UCLA Tissue Typing Laboratory, 1987.

742. Terasaki PI, ed. *Clinical transplants, 1988.* Los Angeles: UCLA Tissue Typing Laboratory, 1988.

743. Ascher NL, Simmons RL, Fryd D, Noreen H, Najarian JS. Effects of HLA-A and B matching on success of cadaver grafts at a single center. *Transplantation* 1979;28:172.

744. Opelz G. Correlation of HLA matching with kidney graft survival in patients with or without cyclosporine treatment. *Transplantation* 1985;40:240–243.

745. Opelz G, Terasaki PI. International study of histocompatibility in renal transplantation. *Transplantation* 1982;33:87.

746. Persign GG, Cohen B, Lansbergen Q, et al. Effect of HLA-A and HLA-B matching on survival of grafts and recipients after renal transplantation. *N Engl J Med* 1982;307:905.

747. Tiwari JL. HLA matching and kidney graft survival: a review. In: Terasaki PI, ed. *Clinical transplants 1986.* Los Angeles: UCLA Tissue Typing Laboratory, 1986:333–340.

748. Festenstein H, Doyle P, Holmes J. Long-term follow-up in London transplant group recipients of cadaver renal allografts: the influence of HLA matching on transplant outcome. *N Engl J Med* 1986;314:7.

749. Middleton D, Gillespie EL, Doherty CC, Douglas JF, McGeown MG. The influence of HLA A,B, and DR matching on graft survival in primary cadaveric renal transplantation in Belfast. *Transplantation* 1985;39:608–610.

750. Sanfilippo F, Vaughn WK, Spees EK, Heise ER, LeFor WM. The effect of HLA-A,-B matching on cadaver renal allograft rejection comparing public and private specificities. *Transplantation* 1984;38:483–489.

751. Berg B, Moller E. The influence of HLA-DR match on the outcome of cadaver renal transplantation in Stockholm during 1977–1980. *Tissue Antigens* 1981;18:316–328.

752. Morris PJ, Ting A. Studies of HLA DR with relevance to renal transplantation. *Immunol Rev* 1982;66:103.

753. Ayoub G, Terasaki P. HLA-DR matching in multicenter, single-typing laboratory data. *Transplantation* 1982;33:515.

754. Brynger H, Rydberg B, Samuelsson B, Sandberg L. Experience with 14 renal transplants with kidneys from blood group A (subgroup A2) to O recipients. *Transplant Proc* 1984;16:1175–1176.

755. Fuller TC, Phelan D, Gebel HM, Rodey GE. Antigen specificity of antibody reactive in the antiglobulin-augmented lymphocytotoxicity test. *Transplantation* 1982;34:24.

756. Thisthlethwaite JR Jr, Buckingham M, Stuart JK, Gaber AO, Mayes JT, Stuart FP. T cell immunofluorescence flow cytometry cross-match results in renal transplants. *Transplant Proc* 1987,19.722.

757. Cook DJ, Terasaki PI, Iwaki Y, et al. The flow cytometry crossmatch in kidney transplantation. In: Terasaki PI, ed. Clinical Transplants, 1987. Los Angeles: UCLA Tissue Typing Laboratory, 1987.

758. Pelletier RP, Orosz CG, Adams PW, et al. Clinical and economic impact of flow cytometry crossmatching in primary cadaveric kidney and simultaneous pancreas-kidney transplant recipients. *Transplantation* 1997;63:1639–1645.

759. Delmonico FL, Fuller A, Cosimi AB, et al. New approaches to donor crossmatching and successful transplantation of highly sensitized patients. *Transplantation* 1983;36:629.

760. Fuller TC, Forbes JB, Delmonico FL. Renal transplantation with a positive historical donor crossmatch. *Transplant Proc* 1985;17:113–115.

761. Smith WJ. Monitoring the components of the immune system. In: Williams GM, Burdick JF, Solez K, eds. *Kidney transplant rejection:* diagnosis and treatment. New York: Marcel Dekker, 1987:264–282.

762. Stiller C, Sinclair N, McGirr D, Jernikar A, Ullan R. Diagnostic and prognostic value of donor specific posttransplant immune responses: clinical correlates and in vitro variables. *Transplant Proc* 1978;10:525–530.

763. Kincaid-Smith P. Histological diagnosis of rejection of renal homografts in man. *Lancet* 1967;2:849–852.

764. Kiaer H, Hansen HE, Olsen S. The predictive value of percutaneous biopsies from human renal allografts with early impaired function. *Clin Nephrol* 1980; 13:58–63.

765. Banfi G, Imbasciati Etarantino A, Ponticelli C. Prognostic value of renal biopsy in acute rejection of kidney transplantation. *Nephron* 1981;28:222–226.

766. Matas AJ, Sibley R, Mauer M, Sutherland DE, Simmons RL, Najarian JS. The value of needle renal allograft biopsy. I. A retrospective study of biopsies performed during putative rejection episodes. *Ann Surg* 1983;197:226–237.

767. Sibley RK, Rynasiewicz JJ, Ferguson RM, et al. Morphology of cyclosporine nephrotoxicity and acute rejection in patients immunosuppressed with cyclosporine and prednisone. *Surgery* 1983;94:245.

768. Bishop GA, Hall BM, Duggin GG, Horvath JS, Sheil AG, Tiller DJ. Diagnosis of renal allograft rejection by analysis of fine needle aspiration biopsy specimens with immunostains and simple cytology. *Lancet* 1986;2:645–650.

769. Colvin RB Immunopathology of renal allografts. In: Colvin RB, Bhan AK, McCluskey RT, eds. *Diagnostic immunopathology.* New York: Raven Press, 1988:151–197.

770. Burdick JF, Beschorner WE, Smith WJ, McGraw DJ, Bender WL, Williams GM, Solez K. Characteristics of early routine renal allograft biopsies. *Transplantation* 1984;38:679–684.

771. Solez K, McGraw DJ, Beschorner WE, Burdick JF Pathology of "acute tubular necrosis" and acute rejection:Observations on early systematic renal tranplant biopsies. In: Williams GM, Burdick JF, Solez K, eds. *Kidney transplant rejection.* New York: Marcel Dekker, 1986:207 224.

772. Rosengard BR, Kortz EO, Guzzetta PC, et al. Transplantation in miniature swine: analysis of graft-infiltrating lymphocytes provides evidence for local suppression. *Hum Immunol* 1990;28:153–8.

773. Schulick RD, Weir MB, Miller MW, Cohen DJ, Bermas BL, Shearer GM. Longitudinal study of in vitro CD4+ T helper cell function in recently transplanted renal allograft patients undergoing tapering of their immunosuppressive drugs. *Transplantation* 1993;56:590–596.

774. Winn HJ. Laws of transplantation. In: *Human immunogenetics.* New York: Marcel Dekker, 1988.

Fundamental Immunology, Fourth Edition,
edited by William E. Paul
Lippincott–Raven Publishers, Philadelphia © 1999.

CHAPTER 37

Tumor Immunology

Hans Schreiber

The application of the science of immunology to the problems of cancer has fascinated immunologists since the turn of the century. The strongest impetus for the many decades of research in tumor immunology has been the hope that sensitive immunologic techniques might detect tumor-specific material that could be used for prevention, therapy, and/or diagnosis of cancer. Indeed, after the development of inbred mouse strains, tumor transplantation studies in the 1950s and 1960s showed that mice could be immunized against transplants of chemically induced cancers that arose in the same inbred mouse strain. These studies, providing the first evidence for the existence of "tumor-specific" rejection antigens, initiated the modern era of tumor immunology. In the absence of molecular information, it remained, however, unclear whether murine or human tumors indeed expressed truly tumor-specific

antigens (i.e., molecules that are only expressed on the malignant cells and are recognized by the immune system). In recent years, two discoveries have provided a strong foundation for tumor immunology and profoundly altered our perspectives. The first is that T cells can detect intracellular protein antigens that are "processed" and carried as peptides to the cell surface and presented by major histocompatibility complex (MHC) molecules as target structures for clonally selected specific T cells. The second discovery is that truly tumor-specific antigens recognized by T cells and encoded by tumor-specific somatic mutations exist. These two discoveries taken together suggest that clinically useful immunologic differences between malignant and normal cells will be found.

Even though immunologists have not made major breakthroughs in the therapy or diagnosis of cancer, the study of cancer cells and their products with immunologic techniques has led to important discoveries. For example, tumor transplantation studies paved the way for the discovery of the MHC and the development of inbred mouse

H. Schreiber: Department of Pathology, The University of Chicago, Chicago, Illinois 60637.

strains. Immunologic analyses of myeloma proteins (i.e., antibodies produced by malignant plasma cells) led to the chemical and physical characterization of the antibody molecule. There are other examples in which immunologic mechanisms were first observed in a tumor system but were later found to have a much broader application. For example, the phenomenon of antigenic modulation of surface molecules was discovered while studying immune responses to murine leukemias. Analysis of cell surface antigens on malignant hematopoietic cells led to the discovery of markers that permit separation of functionally different lymphocytes. Also, graft enhancement was first demonstrated using tumor transplants. Finally, the search for nonspecific approaches to manipulating tumor immunity led to the discovery of cell types such as natural killer (NK) cells and of cytokines such as tumor necrosis factor (TNF).

At present we are lacking tumor-specific diagnostic markers shared by many or all cancers, so that the only reliable diagnosis of cancer is usually made by the pathologist using histologic or cytologic techniques (1). Although *tumor* simply means "swelling," the term is usually equated with neoplasm, which literally means "new growth." A neoplasm is an abnormal mass of tissue that persists and proliferates after withdrawal of the stimulus that initiated its appearance. There are two types of neoplasms or tumors: benign and malignant. The common term for all malignant tumors is *cancer.* Nearly all benign tumors are encapsulated and never metastasize. In contrast, cancers are almost never encapsulated but invade adjacent tissue by infiltrative destructive growth. Invasive growth may be followed by cancer cells implanted at sites discontinuous with the original tumor, usually by transplantation of cells through lymphatic and/or hematogenous spread. This process, called *metastasis,* unequivocally marks a tumor as malignant, though invasive growth is the most reliable criterion for the diagnosis of cancer because invasive growth usually proceeds metastasis.

Several lines of evidence are consistent with the notion that cancer is not a single disease. However, there are certain important principles that apply to many, if not all, cancers. There is now substantial evidence that cancers in mice and humans are the result of multiple sequential mutations (2,3). Physical and chemical carcinogens are involved in the induction of most human cancers in industrialized countries (4), and many of these carcinogens are mutagens (5). While most of these mutations seem to be acquired (somatic mutations), increasing numbers of germline mutations are being discovered that make individuals prone to develop cancer (2). A cancer may require, in multiple steps, as many as ten or more mutations to develop its full devastating malignant character. This process of cancer development can be divided into three different phases. The first stage is called *tumor initiation,* which is the acquisition of mutations due to carcinogen exposure or germline transmission. Initiated cells do not form tumors unless exposed to promoting agents or conditions during a process called *tumor promotion.* This process represents the second stage, which ends with the appearance of the first neoplastic cells (1). The earlier abnormal cells during the first two stages are referred to as *preneoplastic* or *premalignant. Tumor progression* (1,6–8) refers to the third phase of the multistep process, which begins with development of invasive growth from a premalignant tumorous lesion and usually ends with a highly aggressive, widely metastatic cancer that ultimately kills the host. There is compelling evidence that most cancers are clonal in origin and that in tumor progression, new subpopulations of cells that have acquired additional mutations arise continuously (2,8) due to Darwinian selection of genetic variants that have a growth advantage. During this evolution of a cancer, sequential mutations result in changes in growth morphology, hormone dependence, enzyme and cytokine production, and expression of surface antigens. Some of these changes might be coincidental, but others allow the abnormal cells to escape homeostatic controls or resist destruction by defense mechanisms or treatment.

REJECTION ANTIGENS ON TUMORS

Around the turn of the century, it was discovered that, in some instances, tumors developing spontaneously in experimental animals could be transplanted to other animals of the same species and in this way could be propagated continuously. This finding provided an important experimental tool for cancer research (9). Immediately, scientists began to investigate the possibility of immunizing against such transplantable cancers. Rodents exposed to a small nonlethal challenge of certain tumors became immune to subsequent challenge with large transplants of the same tumor, which regularly killed nonimmunized recipients. Also, complete removal of the tumors after initial growth immunized animals against tumors. (Many experimental tumors do not metastasize readily and can, therefore, be removed completely by ligation of the blood supply or by surgical excision, even though the tumors have grown for considerable time.) These early results seemed to suggest that immunization against cancer was possible. Furthermore, there were certain other spontaneous tumors that were not readily transplantable into other animals of the same species, and this was taken as evidence for *natural resistance* or *natural immunity* against some cancers. Many years later, it became clear that no such conclusions could be drawn from these early studies, because outbred rats or mice had been used. The problem became apparent when it was realized that the immunization with tumor would also immunize the host against normal tissue of the donor and that normal tissues of the donor could also immunize the host against the tumor (10). These experiments, which brought the idea of tumor-specific antigens into disrepute, also started the search for antigens that caused rejection of normal transplanted tissue. This research eventually led to the discovery of the MHC and to the development of inbred mouse strains (10–12). Once inbred mouse strains became available, it was shown that tumors transplanted within an inbred mouse strain usually grew so well that the existence of tumor-specific antigens seemed very unlikely. In fact, transplantability of tumors in syngeneic animals became (and still is) a diagnostic criterion for the malignant phenotype of an experimental tumor. This criterion was especially useful because many rodent tumors are cancers of nonepithelial origin (sarcomas) and also because a clear histologic demonstration of local invasive growth can be especially difficult in such cancers. Furthermore, these tumors are rarely metastatic, a characteristic that is shared by many other experimentally induced tumors in rodents.

Evidence for Tumor-specific Rejection of Transplanted Cancers

The modern era of tumor immunology began with the discovery that inbred mice could be immunized against sarcomas induced by the chemical carcinogen methylcholanthrene (MCA). The first such demonstration of induced immunity to transplanted MCA-induced sarcomas, by Gross, was in 1943 (13); however, it was not until the 1950s that more complete experiments provided unequivocal evidence for "tumor-specific rejection of transplanted cancers (14–19). In particular, the experiments of Prehn and Main (16) in 1957 made it likely that the rejection antigens on the MCA-induced sarcomas were functionally tumor-specific, because transplantation assays could not detect these antigens in normal tissue of the mice used. These investigators showed that the tumor cells did not immunize against normal skin grafts from the mouse of tumor origin, nor did normal tissue of this mouse immunize against the tumor (Fig. 1). These results made it highly unlikely that residual heterozygosity (20), if it existed in these inbred mice, was responsible for the immunogenicity of the transplanted tumors. The notion of tumor

antigenicity was confirmed by further experiments demonstrating that tumor-specific resistance against MCA-induced tumors could be elicited in the autochthonous host (i.e., in the mouse in which the tumor had originated), if the tumors were first removed completely (17). In subsequent years, it was demonstrated that the induction of tumor-specific transplantation resistance was not restricted to tumors induced by MCA because such resistance could also be induced by tumors induced with other chemical or physical [e.g., ultraviolet (UV)] carcinogens or by spontaneous tumors (21–25). While evidence is now robust that animal tumors can express antigens that lead to rejection of tumors, but not rejection of normal tissues, one

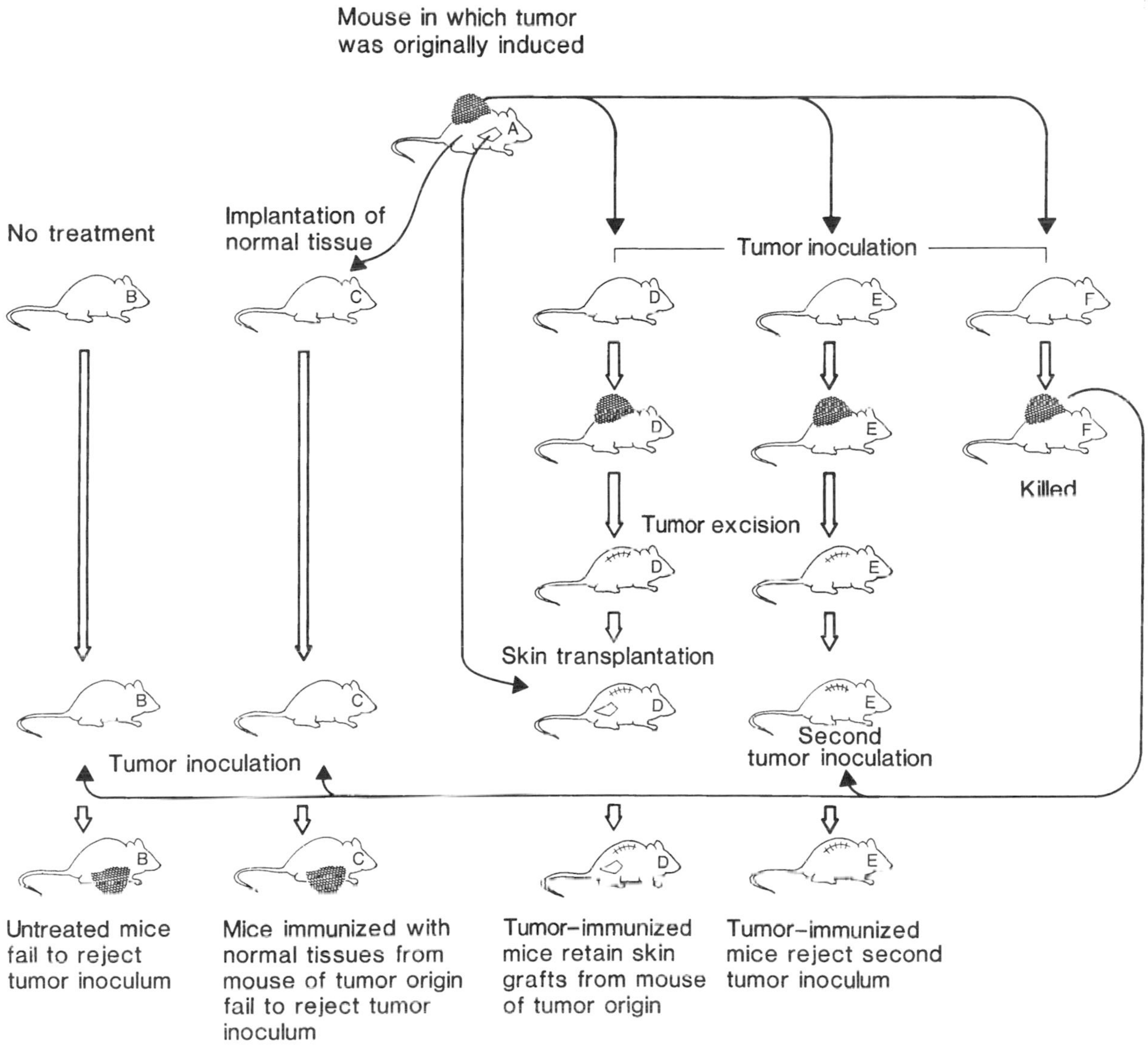

FIG. 1. Transplantation experiments demonstrating the existence of rejection antigens on MCA-induced murine sarcomas (16). Only those mice (E) that had been immunized by previous tumor inoculation and removal rejected the tumor upon second tumor inoculation. Tumor immunized mice (D), however, still accepted normal tissue (skin grafts) of the mouse of tumor origin (A), and normal tissues of this mouse (A) did not protect other mice (C) against tumor challenge. Animal F is used simply to "store" the tumor from mouse A for the period required to immunize other mice (C–F) with normal and malignant tissues. In similar experiments (17) (not shown), the original tumor was removed completely without killing the animal; after an interim period, during which the tumor was stored in a second mouse, the tumor was reimplanted into the original mouse that now rejected the tumor that once originated from that mouse. This suggested that a mouse can be made immune to its autochthonous tumor after it has been removed completely from the animal.

caveat remains: At least some of these antigens may be encoded by normal genes that are only expressed at an undetectable level of normal cells. At present, we are only beginning to identify the genetic origins of the antigens that induce an immune response in the host that results in tumor rejection.

Because protective immunity against the growth of transplanted tumors was used as the criterion for antigenicity, these antigens are also commonly referred to as *transplantation antigens* or *rejection antigens*. Unfortunately, several papers and reviews have been written on the subject of tumor rejection antigens without presenting evidence that the antigens described actually lead to tumor rejection. For example, the term *rejection antigen* is often improperly used for any antigen that is expressed on tumors and supposedly not on normal tissues and is recognized by cytolytic T cells *in vitro*. However, tumors may grow very aggressively, even when tumor antigen-specific T cells can be isolated from such tumors or the peripheral blood of the tumor-bearing hosts (mouse or human), and even when it can be shown that these T cells lyse tumor cells *in vitro;* that is, such findings *in vitro* do not indicate that recognition of these antigen causes tumor rejection.

Antigens Are Unique for an Individual Cancer or Are Shared by Other Cancers

An early objective of the experiments using MCA-induced murine tumors was to search for tumor-specific antigens that were shared by different independently induced tumors. Such shared antigens might be used for either diagnosis or therapy of cancers occurring in different individuals. However, transplantation experiments (15–18, 26,27) revealed that the strongest immunologic protection against challenge with cancer cells was individually tumor-specific. Immunization with one tumor protected effectively only against challenge with the same tumor, but not against challenge with many other tumors tested (Table 1); that is, each cancer was unique, even though the cancers were of the same histologic type and were induced by the same carcinogen in the same organ system in genetically identical individuals. The unique specificity indicated that each tumor had a unique transplantation antigen and/or expressed a unique combination of shared antigens. In fact, careful studies suggested that the antigenic repertoire of these tumors is very large. Because of the impractical prospect of immunizing each patient to the unique antigen of the individual's tumor, studies were undertaken many years

ago to identify shared antigens that could elicit effective and repeatable tumor rejection. The result of those studies was that no wide cross-protection was observed (26). Thus, when searching for antigens shared among ten MCA-induced tumors, no reproducible cross-protection (Fig. 2) was found in 90 tests using mice first immunized with one and then challenged with other syngeneic tumors (26). In addition to MCA, a number of other chemical (19) or physical (21,22) carcinogens, such as 3,4-benzopyrene or UV light, also induce tumors that elicit strong transplantation immunity that is unique (i.e., individually tumor-specific). Unique as well as shared tumor antigens have also been found to be *in vitro* targets of human autologous T cells. However, even when a shared antigen is recognized by cytolytic T cells, transplantation immunity may be individually tumor-specific. For example, the shared antigen P1A (28) is expressed by multiple lineages of tumors as determined by Northern blots and sensitivity to lysis by P1A-specific cytolytic T-cell lines (CTLs), and P1A can induce cross-reactive T cells that are cytolytic for multiple tumor lineages (29). Despite this cross-reactivity, immunologic protection was found to be mediated by unique antigens because there was no cross-protection. This study also cautions us against accepting the recognition of an antigen by CTL as sufficient evidence for calling this antigen a rejection antigen.

Shared antigens might lead to cross-protection between independently induced tumors, and indeed, cross-protection between independently derived tumors is regularly found among murine melanomas induced by UV or chemicals (30). Under selected experimental conditions, cross-protection is also found in the model of MCA or UV-induced murine tumors (16,17,31–33). For example, hyperimmunization with a highly immunogenic regressor tumor led to protective immunity against challenge with several other less immunogenic progressor tumors (31). The finding of cross-protection has been taken as suggesting that the size of the antigenic repertoire may be limited or that common, yet tumor-specific antigens exist. While this is possible, it is also important to note that the resistance induced by immunization with unrelated tumors is usually weak (33), rather short-lived, and sensitive to gamma radiation (33),

TABLE 1. *Characteristics of unique individually distinct rejection antigens on tumors*

1. Specific for each tumor and different from other tumors even when
   (a) of the same histologic type
   (b) induced in the same organ system
   (c) by the same carcinogen
   (d) in the same strain of mice or in the same mouse
2. Not detected on normal syngeneic cells
3. Defined by transplantation assays (not possible in humans)
4. Found predominantly on chemically and physically induced tumors but also on some spontaneous experimental tumors
5. Seemingly endless variety
6. Not known whether caused by
   (a) clonal amplification of preexisting antigens
   (b) activation of previously silent normal genes or
   (c) tumor-specific somatic mutation

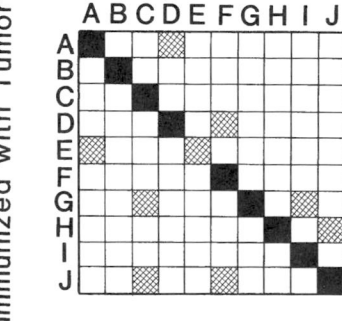

Challenged with Tumor

FIG. 2. Demonstration of the individual (unique) specificity of transplantation antigens on independently derived MCA-induced tumors using transplantation experiments (26). Mice were immunized by injecting nontumorigenic doses of viable cells. One to 3 weeks later, mice were challenged by injection with tumorigenic doses of the same tumor and nine other syngeneic tumors that had been induced independently in syngeneic mice. Protection was specific for the tumor used for immunization, because no repeatable cross-protection was found. *Solid black square,* rejection of the tumor inoculum; *cross-hatched square,* unrepeatable rejections; *white squares,* combinations that showed no rejection. (Adapted from ref. 27.)

or requires hyperimmunization (31); in contrast, resistance induced by immunization with unique antigens is usually long-lived (33) and, like other specific immune responses, becomes relatively radioresistant once immunization has occurred (34). Furthermore, weak resistance against challenge with living tumor cells has sometimes been induced with normal tissue (17). The weak cross-protective effects induced by hyperimmunization with unrelated tumors or normal tissues may, therefore, be due to a nonspecific bolstering of immune responses to specific antigens (17). Alternatively, cross-protection among independently derived tumors could be due to oncofetal, oncospermatogonal, viral, or differentiation antigens (see below) that may be shared by many tumors, but these antigens may not be tumor-specific because they are also found on certain nonmalignant adult tissues or cells. Molecules that are tumor-specific and are shared among independently induced human cancers do exist, however. Examples are the tumor-specific mutant proteins found in certain types of human cancers (see below), but it remains uncertain how effectively shared tumor antigens on human tumors can be used as targets for immunotherapy to achieve rejection (35).

Transplantation Immunity Is Primarily T Cell-mediated

Transplantation immunity elicited by immunization with cancer cells is primarily T cell-mediated (18,36). Cloned CTLs can be generated that represent stable transferable and highly specific probes for rejection antigens. Using such probes, it has been possible sometimes to demonstrate that tumors induced by chemical or physical carcinogens express unique, individually distinct antigenic epitopes (Fig. 3) (37). Using CTL clones *in vitro*, it is also possible to determine whether an antigen recognized by a CTL clone *in vitro* acts as

a rejection antigen *in vivo* (38). This was done in the model of UV-induced regressor tumors that are rejected regularly by normal mice but grow progressively in T cell-deficient mice (39). Antigen loss variants of such tumors were selected *in vitro* for resistance to specific CTLs (Fig. 4). Injection of the variants derived *in vitro* into mice suggested that antigen loss caused a change from a regressor to a progressor phenotype *in vivo* (39). Thus, by isolating tumor variants with selective resistance to a CTL clone, the relative importance of single or several combined antigens or epitopes on the tumor cell in tumor rejection can be indicated.

Multiplicity of Unique Tumor Antigens Expressed on a Single Cancer Cell

CTL clones can also be used to determine whether the antigenicity of a given tumor is due to single or multiple independent components. Such dissection of the antigenic complexity of a tumor can be done by selecting resistant tumor variants and by determining whether these variants have retained any other CTL-recognized antigen or epitopes (41). The results from such studies (37) suggest that CTL-defined tumor antigenicity may be composed of multiple independent, unique epitopes. Thus, the diversity of unique tumor-specific antigens may be even larger than previously anticipated. Whether these multiple CTL-defined epitopes expressed by a single tumor cell reside on one or on different molecules is presently unclear; in any case, these epitopes appear to be functionally independent because CTL clones always selected for variants that had lost only the recognized epitope. This functional independence of epitopes makes this multiplicity important for understanding immune escape and for allowing combination immunotherapy (see section on selection of antigen loss or epitope

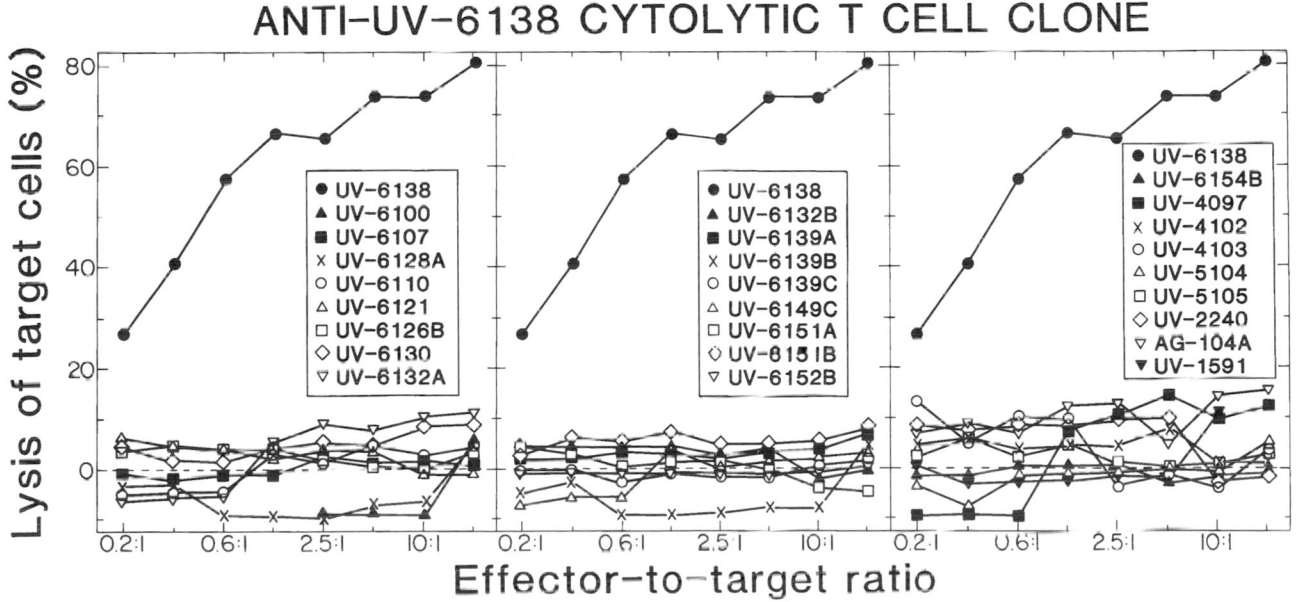

ANTI-UV-6138 CYTOLYTIC T CELL CLONE

FIG. 3. Example of the unique specificity with which cytolytic T-cell clones can lyse cells of a particular UV-induced tumor that had been used for immunization in this case UV-6138. None of the 25 other syngeneic C3H tumor cell lines shown in the three panels lysed which demonstrates the uniqueness of the CTL-defined antigen. Effector cells were incubated with ^{51}Cr-labeled target cells for 4.5 hours, and the amount of the radioisotope released from damaged tumor cells into the supernatant was used to determine the percentage of target cells lysed. (Adapted from ref. 37.)

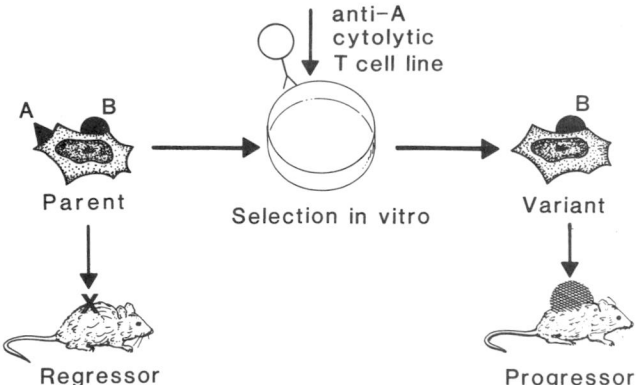

anti-A
cytolytic
T cell line

A B

Parent   Selection in vitro   Variant

Regressor   Progressor

FIG. 4. Scheme of an experiment to test the relevance of a CTL-defined antigen for tumor rejection *in vivo*. Rare antigen loss variants can be selected by exposing the parental tumor cells *in vitro* to a CTL clone. In the example shown here, loss of the A antigen leads to variants showing progressive tumor growth in normal mice, whereas variants selected for loss of the B antigen (not shown) are still rejected by the normal host, like the parental UV-induced regressor tumor (From ref. 40, with permission).

loss variants). Using similar approaches for selecting loss variants with CTL clones, it has been shown that human tumors or murine mast-cell tumor cells can express multiple independent target epitopes (42–44), although cells of the same lineage and MHC class I have not been tested extensively for tumor specificity.

TUMOR ANTIGENS ENCODED BY MUTANT CELLULAR GENES (TUMOR-SPECIFIC ANTIGENS)

Mutations Discovered by Immunologic Analyses

Although unique tumor antigens (see Table 1) were discovered in the 1960s, we have begun to learn about the molecular basis of the diversity of these antigens only since 1995. In principle, there are three possible mechanisms that may lead to the appearance of these antigens: clonal amplification, mutation, or gene activation. Most chemical or physical carcinogens are mutagens (5). Therefore, it is generally assumed that unique tumor antigens on tumors induced by these carcinogens are products of mutated genes, possibly single genes with "hot spots" for mutations. However, Burnet (45) proposed that the uniqueness of carcinogen-induced transplantation antigens on tumors may also be due to clonal amplification of single cells expressing a particular normal antigen. According to this hypothesis, normal precursor cells in the host contain different antigens; these antigens, however, are not sufficient in amount to be recognized by the immune system until amplified by clonal expansion of the cancer cells. [An analogous situation may occur with clonal antigens (see below) when an individual develops a malignancy of B- or T-cell origin; the idiotype, present on relatively few normal cells, may not be sufficient in amount to elicit a response in the normal host, but may serve as target antigen for tumor cells bearing the same idiotype (46).] This possibility has been addressed experimentally (47,48). In one study (48), a nonmalignant fibroblast line was cloned *in vitro,* and then expanded; subclones, all derived from the same precursor cell, were malignantly transformed by MCA in diffusion chambers

implanted into mice. Transplantation experiments showed that the developing tumors all had individually distinct antigens, even though all tumors had been derived from the same precursor cell. These results seemed to indicate the appearance of new antigens (neoantigens) following carcinogen exposure and that the unique antigens were not already expressed on the precursor cell. However, normal cells can generate considerable diversity of surface molecules during clonal expansion from a single precursor (49), and the transformation event caused by the carcinogen may simply fix a particular antigenic phenotype of the cell, giving rise to the malignant clone. Alternatively, normal genes that were previously silent may be activated by the carcinogen. Both mechanisms involving normal genes could produce considerable antigenic diversity of tumors. Therefore, previous experiments have not answered whether the appearance of the individually distinct (unique) antigens was caused by carcinogen-induced somatic mutations of structural DNA sequences, or whether these antigens are encoded by normal genes (50). It was also not clear in what way unique rejection antigens caused by mutagen exposure of cancer cells *in vitro* may serve as a paradigm for individually distinct rejection antigens (51). Furthermore, residual germline heterozygosity and antigenic drift is commonly observed in inbred mouse strains and tumors derived from them (20). Therefore, several unique tumor antigens, claimed to be "tumor-specific" (52–55) and encoded by "mutations," may be encoded by heterozygous germline genes, giving rise to unique, seemingly tumor-specific antigens; in any case, absence of the described mutational changes from autologous normal DNA from the host of tumor origin was not demonstrated. Finally, while one generally assumes that the appearance of unique tumor antigens is a direct result of the exposure to carcinogen, there is no direct evidence for this, except when the antigens are encoded by the transforming genes of oncogenic viruses. Even the fact that unique tumor antigens are often shared by a majority (or all) of the cells in a given tumor only implies that the cells in the tumor arose from a single precursor cell. It is still possible that a precursor expressing the unique tumor antigen arose in a pre- or posttransformational cell population in which the other cells not expressing this antigen were eliminated or overgrown during the continuous evolution of the cancer (8).

Since 1995, the genetic origins of several T cell–recognized unique antigens from murine and human cancers have been identified, and in every case, the antigen was caused by a somatic mutation (i.e., by a genetic change absent from autologous normal DNA) and thus found to be truly tumor-specific (56–61). Table 2 shows that these antigens do not seem to involve a single gene family, but rather involve multiple different unrelated genes. The second fascinating finding is that most of these mutations do not appear to be located in random sites, but rather occur in genes that code for functionally important parts of the expressed protein. For example, the mutation in the cycline-dependent kinase 4 reduces the binding to its inhibitor and tumor-suppressor protein p16INK4a (58), and the same mutation is found in cases of familial melanoma (62). Also, the mutation in the β-catenin appears to prevent the degradation of this oncogene (63); and the mutation in the helicase protein p68 resulted in an amino acid substitution in a functionally important domain of this possible tumor-suppressor gene (61). Finally, for the ribosomal protein L9, loss of heterozygosity (LOH) with loss of the wild-type allele is found (64). At present, it is too early to decide whether a restricted number of genes affected by somatic mutations encodes tumor-specific antigens and how com-

TABLE 2. *Unique tumor antigens recognized by syngeneic or autologous T cells*

Protein from which mutant antigenic peptide originates	Recognizing T-cell subset	Tumor of origin	Somatic mutation/ tumor specificity	Reference
Mouse				
Ribosomal protein L9	CD4+	UV-induced sarcoma	Yes	56
Helicase protein p68	CD8+	UV-induced sarcoma	Yes	61
Human				
MUM-1	CD8+	Melanoma	Yes	57
cdk4	CD8+	Melanoma	Yes	58
β-catenin	CD8+	Melanoma	Yes	59
HLA-A2	CD8+	Renal cell carcinoma	Yes	60

Excluded are unique antigens that lack evidence for somatic mutation and thus tumor specificity because the analyzed genes were from tumors for which nonmalignant control cells were not available to distinguish between germline polymorphism or somatic mutation. These genes include connexin 37, c-akt, activated gag, or the mitogen-activated protein kinase ERK2 (52–55).

monly these tumor-specific alterations play a functional role in malignancy. It would be expected that at some frequency the same mutation may be selected for in another patient, and, indeed, the same somatic mutation in the CDK-4 gene was found in one additional melanoma among 28 analyzed (58). It is also likely that we understand only a fraction of the genetic changes needed to cause the different stages of different types of cancers. Therefore, it is important to note that T cells against unique tumor antigens were used to identify tumor-specific mutations and that these antigens would probably not have been detected by other available technology not relying on immunologic probes. Furthermore, as mentioned earlier, unique antigens can elicit strong tumor-specific rejection of cancers and may therefore be important target antigens for immunotherapy. For both reasons, it will be important to further analyze the genetic origins of unique tumor antigens.

Mutations Discovered by Functional or Genetic Analyses

Most human cancers in industrialized countries are probably not induced by viruses, but rather result from mutations caused by physical or chemical carcinogens (3–5). Some of these mutations may be the immediate result of the initial mutational damage to normal target cells and randomly affect many genes. However, most mutational changes are probably a disadvantage to the cancer cell, so that the mutations that are found when cancers eventually arise are highly selected, probably throughout the long process of carcinogenesis and tumor progression. These selected mutations occur preferentially in certain genes and often in highly selected locations in these genes, many of these mutations are causally related to, and specific for, the malignant process. These mutations were originally discovered because the mutant gene was found (a) to be overexpressed, (b) to cause transformation in transfection assays, or (c) to be involved in a cancer-specific chromosomal translocation. Several of the mutations affect DNA sequences that encode proteins, and therefore result in the appearance of tumor-specific mutant proteins. These novel proteins may be the result of point mutations, internal deletions, or other gene rearrangements, including fusion of genes. The original reason for discovering these mutations was not the antigenicity of the encoded mutant proteins, therefore, these mutant proteins may not necessarily encode tumor-specific antigens. Computerized algorithms have been used [in a process that is also called "reverse immunology" (65)] to predict the likelihood of a particular

mutation resulting in a strong antigen, and several of the mutant proteins and peptides have been used to explore the possibility of inducing tumor-specific immunity. It is interesting that antigens recognized by the host when immunized with tumor cells (direct immunology) have so far always been found to be encoded by different mutations (see previous section). Therefore, an important question is: How commonly are mutant proteins that have been identified initially by nonimmunologic methods recognized by the host as tumor-specific antigens, and can such antigens serve as effective targets for immunologic rejection of cancer cells? Some examples (Table 3) are given below (for review, also see ref. 66).

Mutant RAS Oncogene-encoded Proteins

The tumorigenic potential of the RAS protooncogene can be acquired by *activating mutations,* which occur at selected predictable sites and affect amino acid residue 12 or 61 and, less frequently, residue 13 of the p21 ras protein. Mutant RAS can elicit specific antibody (67,68), but the protein is located at the inner tumor cell membrane, not at the cell surface. However, mutant RAS peptides resulting from proteolytic cleavage can bind to some MHC class molecules and elicit CD4+ or CD8+ T-cell responses (69–73). For example, human CD4+ T cells have been shown to recognize a valine for glycine substitution at position 12 of RAS, which is one of the most common mutations in human cancers (69). The region of the mutant RAS protein from which the peptide was derived is identical for all the three members of the RAS protooncogene family, namely, H-RAS, K-RAS, and N-RAS, which have different prevalence in different cancers. RAS mutations occur in premalignant or malignant cells after thymic deletion of self-reactive clones, and most individuals should therefore have clones that respond to the mutant proteins. In all instances, the T cells have been induced with the purified ras peptide or protein rather than tumor cells. A potential problem is that only in some tumor cells, the peptide–MHC complexes may have sufficient density to be recognized by RAS-specific T cells (74,75). Also, the presentation of ras peptides on MHC molecules has been found to be unconventional (76), and the antigenic specificity of the weak immunity that was found against transplanted tumor cells following immunization with a semipurified mutant ras protein remains unclear (77). Thus, at present, it remains uncertain whether mutant RAS can serve as an effective target for tumor rejection. For example, no immunologic cross-reactivity in protection assays was observed between chemically induced fibrosarcomas that shared the

TABLE 3. *Origin, distribution, and antigenicity of different categories of tumor antigens represented by examples*

Category/Type of antigen	Example	Mechanism of expression in cancer	Contributes to malignant behavior	Normal adult tissue distribution	Occurrence: Cancer specific	Occurrence: Normal precursor lineage	Occurrence: Type of cancer	Shared versus unique	Recognition by: T	Recognition by: B	Rejection antigen
Normal cellular gene products											
Oncospermatogonal antigen											
	MAGE-1	Ectopic expression	?	Testis	—	—	Several	Shared	+	—	
Oncofetal antigen											
	MAGE-3	Ectopic expression	?	Testis/trophoblast	—	—	Several	Shared	+	—	
	P1A	Ectopic expression	?	Testis/trophoblast	—	—	Mastocytoma	Shared	+	—	
	CEA	Amplification of regenerative cell	?	Colon/lactating breast	—	+	Several	Shared	—	+	Weak
Differentiation antigen											
	17-1A	Normal surface glycoprotein	—	Broad	—	+	Several	Shared	—	+	Passive
	PSA	Normal intracellular enzyme	—	Prostate	—	+	Prostate	Shared	—	—	
	Tyrosinase	Normal intracellular enzyme	—	Melanocytes	—	+	Melanoma	Shared	+	+	Passive
	Lewis (carbohydrate)	Aberrant glycosylation	?	Broad	—	+	Several	Shared	—	+	
	HER-2/neu (oncoprotein)	Overexpression	+(?)	Breast/ovary	—	+	Several	Shared	—	+	
	GD2/GD3 ganglioside	Overexpression	?	Broad	—	+	Several	Shared	—	+	Passive
Clonal antigen											
	Immunoglobulin idiotype	Clonal amplification	—	B-cell clone	—	+	B-cell malignancy	Unique	(+)	+	Weak
Mutant cellular gene products											
Primary detection as antigen											
Ribosomal protein	Mut L9	Point mutation	LOH	—	+	—	Fibrosarcoma	Unique	+	+	
Cyclin	Mut cdk4	Point mutation	+	—	+	—	Melanoma	Highly restricted	+	?	
Primary detection as oncogene											
Oncogene product	Mut. p21s	Point mutation	+	—	+[a]	—	Several	Shared	+	+	?
Suppressor gene product	Mut. p53s	Point mutation	+	—	+[b]	—	Several	Unique	?	+	?
Internal fusion protein	Mut. EGFR	Internal deletion	+(?)	—	+	—	Ganglioma	Shared	?	+	?
Chimeric fusion protein	BCR-ABL	Translocation	+	—	+	—	CML	Shared	+	+	?
Viral gene product											
Nuclear protein	E6/E7 of HPV16	Transforming viral gene	+	—	[a]	—	Cervical	Shared	+	+	+

[a] Can also occur in carcinogen-induced benign premalignant lesions (e.g., papillomas).

[b] Also found as germline mutations in the dominantly inherited Li-Fraumeni familiar cancer syndrome.

Mut,, mutant; T, T cells; B, B cells; MCA, methylcholanthrene; CML, chronic myelogenous leukemia; EGFR, epidermal growth factor receptor; HER-2, human epidermal growth factor receptor 2; LOH, loss of heterozygosity; PSA, prostate-specific antigen; HPV, human papilloma virus.

same RAS mutation (78). Nevertheless, clinical trials have been developed (79,80).

Mutant p53 Suppressor Gene–encoded Proteins

Mutations in the p53 suppressor gene are among the most common mutations found in human and experimental cancers. p53 was originally discovered by antibody raised against a mouse sarcoma (81) or against preparations of SV40 T antigen (82,83). The protein was found in a large variety of cancers (including those of no known viral etiology) but was not detected in nonmalignant embryonic or adult cells, thereby implicating a possible central role for p53 in the malignant process (81–83). It is now understood that normal p53 protein, which acts as a suppressor of cell growth, is little expressed in normal cells and therefore generally not detected, whereas the high levels of p53 commonly detected in malignant cells usually represent a mutant p53 protein (84). The mutations in p53 tend to cluster in evolutionarily conserved regions of the gene, but the exact locations of mutations in the p53 gene are highly diverse (85). Different mutations appear to cause common conformational changes (and possibly similar dysfunction), as evidenced by preferential reactivity of different mutant p53 proteins with certain anti-p53 monoclonal antibodies (86). Patients appear to mount an antibody response to mutant p53 proteins, particularly those that associate with heat-shock proteins (87), and the presence of these antibodies correlated with a poor prognosis (88). It is also not known to what extent mutant p53 can be recognized by T cells or serve as a target for tumor rejection. Unlike antibodies, T cells will recognize unique short mutant peptides in which common conformational changes are absent. Exploring mutant p53 proteins as a potential immunologic target for therapy is attractive because T cells with unique specificity appear to mediate the strongest antitumor immunity, and p53-specific T cells have been induced (for review, see ref. 66). However, as with mutant ras, immunization with tumor cells has not induced T cells specific for mutant p53 peptides, suggesting that other unique antigens may usually dominate the response. Nevertheless, tumor immunity in vivo has been induced by vaccination against mutant p53 peptides if given with interleukin-12 (IL-12) (89). Because p53 is commonly overexpressed in cancer cells, T cells directed against normal p53 might preferentially destroy tumor cells. Vaccines designed to immunize against normal p53 would also not require tailoring the vaccines for the individual, highly diverse p53 mutations. However, normal p53 is a self antigen to which individuals are tolerant. Because mouse and human normal p53 sequences are not fully conserved, murine T cells specific for human normal p53 peptides have been induced that lyse human tumor cells (90). Furthermore, p53 knock-out mice generate T cells specific for normal murine p53 that, on adoptive transfer into p53 wild-type mice, can erradicate murine p53-overexpressing tumors without signs of autoimmunity to the host (91).

Fusion Proteins Resulting from Internal Deletions or Chromosomal Translocations

New antigenic determinants can result from the juxtaposition of previously distant amino acid sequences, resulting in a new peptide sequence and possibly a change in conformational structure. Such fusion proteins can result from internal deletions within the coding sequence of a single gene. For example, about 40% of malignant glioblastomas, the most common primary brain malignancy in humans, have an internal deletion of the epidermal growth factor receptor (EGFR) gene, resulting in a fusion protein (92). About half of the patients with this tumor have the same deletion, which generates a new amino acid at the fusion point. The new antigenic determinants on the surface of the cancer cells can be recognized specifically by a monoclonal antibody (93). Such tumor-specific antibody may be therapeutically useful against this cancer, which is untreatable by conventional therapy. Fusion proteins may also result from chromosomal translocations found in a variety of human cancers (94,95). The resulting fusion proteins are chimeric because parts of the same protein are encoded by sequences of two distinct genes. Remarkably, similar translocations and recombinational events may occur in a given type of cancer, which may result in the juxtaposition of exactly the same coding sequences from the two involved chromosomes (95,96). These highly conserved chromosomal breakpoints may therefore result in the same fusion proteins in the same cancers from different individuals. The best examples are the chimeric BCR/ABL fusion proteins found in patients with certain human leukemias (97). In other types of cancers, breakpoints may vary considerably, leading to unique fusion proteins. In some instances, a new codon may be created, resulting in a different or inappropriate amino acid at the fusion point. Fusion proteins can be recognized specifically by antibody (98), and peptides spanning the fusion point may be recognized specifically by human CD4[+] T cells (99). Importantly, many of these fusion proteins are essential for maintaining the malignant state of the cell, and tumor cells may not easily escape therapy by losing expression of fusion proteins. It is uncertain, however, whether these fusion proteins can serve as effective targets for active or passive immunotherapy.

TUMOR ANTIGENS ENCODED BY NORMAL CELLULAR GENES (TUMOR-ASSOCIATED ANTIGENS)

All of the antigens listed in this section are encoded by nonmutant cellular genes that are expressed not only by certain cancer cells, but also by at least one subset of normal adult cells. Therefore, these antigens are not tumor-specific, and they are commonly referred to as tumor-associated antigens. The extent to which these antigens are expressed by normal cells and tissues can vary from widespread expression to extreme restriction to a small population of normal cells (100). Furthermore, the time during development or differentiation when these markers are expressed on normal cells can vary considerably. Some of these antigens have been found only in spermatogonia and spermatocytes and certain cancer cells (oncospermatogonal antigens), but not in normal cells of the tissue of tumor origin, that is, these antigens are expressed in a non lineage-specific fashion. Most tumor-associated antigens, however, are expressed at least at some level on the cell type from which the tumor developed; that is, these antigens are lineage-specific and represent differentiation antigens. Some of these differentiation antigens are only found in a small clone of normal cells from which the malignancy originated (clonal antigens), while other differentiation antigens are also found in embryonic or fetal precursor cells and are, therefore, called carcinoembryonic or oncofetal antigens.

Even though none of the antigens discussed in this section are truly tumor-specific, several mechanisms for an operational relative tumor specificity have been invoked for several tumor-associated antigens: (a) Malignant cells may express a given antigen at much higher levels (e.g., ten- to 100-fold) (101), and some studies suggest that such differences in expression levels between normal and malignant cells can be exploited therapeutically (for review, see ref. 102). (b) Relative tumor specificity may also be attained because of a better access of the antigen-specific effector cells to the malignant cells than to normal cells. (c) For certain antigens, the expression of the epitopes on the normal cells is hidden from the immune system by more complete glycosylation of the target molecule in the normal cells (in the case of epithelial mucins). (d) In the case of oncospermatogonal antigens, lack of expression of MHC molecules by the normal cells may prevent these cells from becoming a direct target for T cells (103). However, indirect presentation of antigens can occur for all antibody as well as T cell–recognized antigen, and a large body of experimental evidence supports the concept that the induction of protective T cell-mediated responses to tumor-specific antigens by active immunization is much more effective than inducing immune responses to target structures that lack tumor specificity (29,35). Nevertheless, passive immunization with a murine monoclonal antibody directed against a human tumor-associated differentiation antigen has been described to be effective (104–106) (see below), and the possibility of achieving therapeutic effects of active immunization against oncospermatogonal antigens is currently being explored.

Oncospermatogonal Antigens

It has been postulated repeatedly that certain normal genes that are completely silent in all nonmalignant cells may be activated exclusively in malignant cells. However, several previous similar claims of selective activation of normal genes in cancer cells leading to tumor-specific antigens have not been substantiated. Usually, at least transient expression of the same antigen by at least one normal cell type was later discovered. For example, the thymic leukemia (TL) antigen is encoded by a normal cellular gene in the MHC locus (107,108). Initially, it was found that the TL gene was not expressed in normal thymocytes of TL-negative mice, but it could be activated specifically in leukemias developing in these strains. However, much later studies demonstrated that the TL antigen was expressed by normal gut epithelium of TL-negative strains (109). As another example, certain CTL-recognized antigens on human melanomas and several other cancers (e.g., MAGE-1, MAGE-2, MAGE-3) were reported to be encoded by normal genes that were found to be expressed only in the malignant cells (110). However, further research revealed that these antigens were also expressed by normal spermatogonia and primary spermatocytes in the testis (111) and possibly other normal cells (112). Similar oncospermatogonal antigens have also been defined using autologous sera of cancer patients as probes (113). Oncospermatogonal antigens may also be found in murine tumor models, and a murine homologue of MAGE is expressed in post-meiotic spermatids (114). Furthermore, a CTL-recognized antigen on mouse mastocytoma P1A was reported to be expressed by a normal gene not expressed by normal cells (28); later work, however, revealed expression of the antigen in normal spermatogonia and trophoblast cells (115). Thus, we lack convincing evidence that normally completely silent genes are specifically activated in cancer cells and can encode truly tumor-specific antigens.

The detection of several of these antigens in spermatogonia and spermatocytes is very interesting, because it may be related to the extensive demethylation of genes (116). Such demethylation takes place rather selectively during spermatogenesis and may lead to expression of a large number of genes. These genes either may be completely silent in other cells, or, more likely, are expressed at some selective stage of cellular development, possibly in a cell type that has escaped observation. Consistent with this explanation is the finding that some tumor-associated antigen, such as P1A, MAGE 3, and MAGE 4, are found not only in spermatogonia, but also in trophoblast cells, and thus represent carcinoembryonic antigens (CEAs) (115,117). In any case, unlike differentiation antigens, oncospermatogonal antigens are observantly expressed in cancer cells in a highly selective non–lineage-specific fashion. Because of their *relative tumor specificity,* the oncospermatogonal antigens may represent important targets for diagnosis of, as well as immunotherapy for, cancer.

Differentiation Antigens

Some antigens expressed on tumor cells are also expressed during at least some stage of differentiation on nonmalignant cells of the cell lineage from which the tumor developed. These *lineage-specific* antigens can, therefore, be considered as differentiation markers. These antigens represent a very diverse group of proteins, glycoproteins (including mucins), and glycolipids (carbohydrate or peptide epitopes); several of these antigens are being explored as potential immunotherapeutic targets (104,105,118–121). Other lines of evidence support the idea that effectors and target structures may not need to have absolute specificity. For example, several chemotherapeutic agents are used successfully against cancer despite potential severe side effects on normal cells. Furthermore, an antibody to a normal surface glycoprotein expressed at similar levels on normal and malignant colonic epithelial cells (122) has been found to be effective in inhibiting the growth of colorectal carcinoma cells in nude mice when given shortly after tumor cell injection (106); the same antibody appears to be effective in reducing the incidence of metastatic disease and in increasing long-term survival in humans when given shortly after surgery to patients with colorectal carcinoma, who have undergone tumor resection with curative intent (104,105). Similarly, passive antibodies against melanocyte-specific differentiation antigens are effective against metastatic spread of melanoma cells in mice when given at the time of seeding of the malignant cells (123), and similar antibodies may have analogous beneficial effects in human melanoma patients (124).

Differentiation markers are found on cancer cells because malignant cells usually express at least some of the genes that are characteristic of normal cell types from which the tumor cell originated. The presence of these normal differentiation antigens can, therefore, help to determine the organ or cell type of origin (lineage) of a cancer (33,125). For example, B-cell tumors express surface immunoglobulin, and T-cell leukemias can be separated into helper and suppressor cell leukemias using T-cell subset-specific monoclonal antibodies (126). Careful diagnostic delineation of different subtypes of cancer is important because different tumor subtypes may have different prognoses and may be susceptible to different therapies. While lineage-specific markers have been particularly useful for subclassifying hematopoietic cancers (126), only very few cell type- or lineage-specific antigens have been found for cells outside the hematopoetic and melanocyte lineage. Instead, some of the other cell types can be characterized by distinct patterns of expression of antigenic markers that have a wider distribution (100). Tumors often acquire less differentiated appearance with progression. In fact, metastatic lesions of tumors of quite different tissue origin are often morphologically so much alike that the retention of a cell type–specific antigen by the metastatic cells may give an important diagnostic clue as to the organ from which the cancer originated (125). However, the use of differentiation markers for histologic or cytologic tumor classification has pitfalls. First, cancer cells occasionally express differentiation antigens normally not expressed in the cell linage from which the tumor originated (aberrant expression). Second, differentiation markers can be lost during tumor progression, leaving no clue as to the cancer's tissue of origin. Some tissue-specific antigens are detected only cyto- or histochemically, whereas other tissue-specific antigens can be used as serum markers; for example, the prostate-specific antigen (PSA), a chymotrypsin-like protease, which is selectively expressed by the normal or malignant epithelial cells of the prostate gland, is elevated in benign hypertrophy of the prostate as well as in prostatic cancer. Therefore, detection of any PSA following complete surgical removal of the prostate indicates residual tumor cells and/or recurrence (for review, see refs. 127, 128). However, there are no immunologic serum markers presently available that are specific for cancer, because levels of presently available serologic markers are also elevated in a variety of nonmalignant diseases and conditions (129).

Several differentiation antigens (such as tyrosinase, the related brown locus protein, gp100, and Melan A/MART-1) appear to be restricted to melanocytes, and all of them are being explored as possible immunotherapeutic targets. Another useful target may be gangliosides GD2 and GD3, which are not only overexpressed in melanoma, but also found in other cells of neurocrest origin and in other tissues (130,131). Pancreatic, breast, and colon cancers express mucins that can be recognized on cancer cells by MHC-unrestricted cytolytic T cells that react specifically with repeated epitopes on the protein core of the mucin molecules exposed because of deficient glycosylation in the malignant cells (132). Finally, overexpression of the human EGFR-2 (HER-2/neu) is observed in some breast and ovarian cancers and other adenocarcinomas, and high levels of expression correlate with a more aggressive clinical course. Antibody as well as helper and cytolytic T-cell responses to the HER-2/neu protein can be induced, and methods are being developed to use this protein as a therapeutic target (66).

Oncofetal and Carcinoembryonic Antigens

Over 50 years ago, human cancer cells were found to express antigens that serologically cross-react with normal embryonic tissue (133). The appearance of these antigens was attributed to *retrodifferentiation,* because the lack of differentiated phenotype of cancer cells was often associated with the appearance of antigens that were expressed at higher levels in embryonic or fetal cells and tissues (134). Some tumors have a highly differentiated appearance, because the tumor stem cells have retained the capability to differentiate like their normal counterparts. However, there is a propensity of tumors to lose their differentiated appearance with tumor progression (134). This loss of differentiation characteristics during tumor progression does not appear to be associated with an orderly acquisition of cell markers characteristic of earlier developmental stages of a cell lineage (135). Therefore, the term *retrodifferentiation* may be confusing. There appear to be two different mechanisms for the appearance of such antigens. In the first mechanism, expression of embryonic or fetal antigens appears to occur as a result of malignant transformation and/or tumor progression. This expression appears to result from an aberrant activation or "depression" of genes that are supposedly completely silent in adult nonmalignant cells of the lineage of tumor cell origin (e.g., due to methylation, see ref. 116) but are normally active in certain fetal and embryonic cells (e.g., trophoblast cells). Examples are *non–lineage-specific* tumor antigens such as MAGE-3 in humans and P1A in mice (115,117). In the second mechanism, the antigens are *lineage-specific* and expressed not only in fetal or embryonic cells, but also already in the normal stem cells of the adult tissue from which the tumor originated. The more mature progeny usually do not express these antigens, at least not at high levels, but these antigens are expressed in nonmalignant adult cells, especially after various types of injury or disease. Tumors seem to represent an amplification and immortalization of such stem cells. An example is one of the best-studied embryonic tumor markers, CEA.

CEA was discovered as a tumor-specific antigen in human colon carcinoma (136) and as a fetal antigen restricted to fetal gut, pancreas, and liver in the first two trimesters of gestation (137). Now it is realized that CEA is also present in low levels in nonmalignant, nonfetal adult tissues such as normal colonic mucosa, lung, and lactating breast tissue (138). Therefore, using the term *embryonic* or *fetal* antigen for these molecules that are also found in adult cells is confusing. CEA was originally described as a 200-kDa membrane-associated glycoprotein that is released into surrounding fluids. Sequence analysis of cDNA clones for CEA revealed three long repeating units that show significant sequence homology with members of the immunoglobulin supergene family (138). At one time, it was hoped that CEA could be used as a marker for early diagnosis of gastrointestinal malignancies; however, elevated serum levels of CEA are found not only in gastrointestinal malignancy, but also in a number of other malignant diseases outside the gastrointestinal tract, such as cancers of the lung and breast. Furthermore, elevated levels of CEA are also found in the absence of malignancy (e.g., in smokers and in inflammatory bowel diseases, such as ulcerative colitis). Though serum levels of CEA are not useful for detecting early cancer, the level of CEA in the blood can be used to monitor the effects of therapy to indicate whether a cancer has been successfully eradicated or has recurred (139). The possibility of using CEA as an immunotherapeutic target is also being explored (140).

Alpha-fetoprotein (AFP) is another example of a fetal or embryonic protein (141), which, though produced by fetal liver and yolk sac cells, is present in small amounts in the serum of normal adults. The amount of this protein is elevated in some patients with cancer of the liver or testis and also in some patients with various nonmalignant liver diseases. Therefore, similar to CEA, using AFP as a marker for the early diagnosis of cancer is difficult (142). Nevertheless, assays of AFP can detect primary liver cancer at a time when the cancer is treatable, and AFP assays are also used for monitoring patients after therapy (142). The fact that fetal and embryonic antigens are often found on nonmalignant adult tissue serum poses particular problems for using these antigens as targets for active or passive immunotherapy (143) and may account for why using such developmental antigens as targets for immunotherapy has so far been unsuccessful or only modestly successful.

Clonal Antigens

Clonal antigens, in contrast to the other differentiation antigens described above, are expressed only on a few normal adult cells, that is, only on the clone of cells from which the tumor originated (46), for example, the idiotype of surface immunoglobulin-positive B-cell malignancies. In this particular case, it is interesting that immunization of mice against the idiotype induces an idiotype-specific transplantation immunity against the growth of the tumors (myeloma, lymphoma) expressing the idiotype (144,145). Human CTLs that express the γδ chains of the T-cell receptor (TCR) and are specific for the idiotype of immunoglobulin on autologous B-cell tumors have been generated (146). Furthermore, idiotype-specific antibodies prevented the growth of idiotype-positive murine myeloma cells *in vivo* (147) or *in vitro* (148). Idiotype-specific antibodies have also been used in the therapy of murine (149) or guinea pig (150) idiotype-positive B-cell leukemias. Finally, idiotype-specific monoclonal antibodies have caused several partial remissions and one complete remission in patients with B-cell lymphoma (151), and active idiotype-specific immunizations are also in clinical trials (152,153). It is necessary to generate different monoclonal antibodies or idiotypic vaccines for each individual cancer to be treated, but the advantage of using such clonal antigens over a less restricted tumor- associated antigen is that only a few normal cells bear the same antigen. For example, normal B-cell clone expressing the idiotype will probably not interfere with the use of the antiidiotypic antibody, nor is it likely that the loss of a normal B-cell clone due to therapy would adversely affect the patient. Except for idiotypes on B-cell and T-cell malignancies, there are presently no candidates for other clonal antigens.

TUMOR ANTIGENS ENCODED BY VIRAL GENES

DNA Tumor Viruses

SV40 and polyoma viruses are cancer-inducing DNA viruses that encode functionally similar, but antigenically distinct, proteins required for the induction and maintenance of malignant transformation. As would be expected, these virally encoded proteins are shared by all tumors induced by the same virus regardless of tissue origin or animal species (154–156). These proteins appear intracellularly as predominantly nuclear antigens, but the same genes that encode these proteins are also required for the expression of the CTL-recognized, virus-specific, MHC-presented peptides acting as transplantation antigens on the tumor cell surface (157,158). The rejection antigens are tumor-specific in the sense that they are not expressed by normal host cells and are not encoded by genes of the host, or presented on the virion particles themselves, which carry viral capsid antigens. In the early 1980s, extensive studies analyzed how the SV40-specific CTL could recognize the nuclear T antigen on the surface of tumor cells (157–160). By transfection of truncated nontransforming portions of the gene encoding the T-antigen epitopes, these studies provided an early hint that MHC class I antigen–restricted CTLs can recognize on the cell surface–processed fragments of proteins that are primarily located intracellularly (157,159).

Similar to the T antigens of SV40 and polyoma virus, adenoviruses and human papilloma virus (HPV) also have so-called early region genes, designated E1A/E1B and E6/E7, respectively, which are transcribed not only during early stages of viral replication, but also in transformed cells, and expression of these antigens is required for maintenance of the transformed phenotype. Thus, DNA viruses, such as SV40, polyoma, papilloma, and adenovirus, show stable but random integration of at least the early-region genes of the virus into the genome of the cells they transform. It is the protein product of the early region rather than the site of integration of the virus into the genome that seems to be important for inducing and maintaining the transformed phenotype. Thus, the early-region proteins are virally encoded, tumor-specific antigens that are clearly related to the transformed phenotype and the establishment of malignant behavior. Several of these antigens induce MHC class I–restricted CTLs. Several types of DNA viruses have been associated with human cancer: certain subtypes of HPVs with cervical cancer and certain other cancers; hepatitis B virus (HBV) with primary liver cancer; and Epstein-Barr virus (EBV) with immunoblastic lymphomas in immunocompromised individuals and with the endemic (African) Burkitt's lymphoma; in addition, SV40 may contribute to the development mesotheliomas, bone tumors, ependymomas, and chorion plexus tumors (for review, see ref. 161). The viral genes involved in the malignant transformation by EBV are largely unknown, but the lymphoma cells usually have integrated viral sequences. EBV can encode a number of CTL-recognized antigens that have been carefully mapped (162). Of particular importance are several EBV-encoded nuclear antigens (EBNAs) and latent membrane proteins (LMPs) that are expressed in latently infected cells. There is strong suggestive evidence that adoptive T-cell immunotherapy in immunosuppressed patients may be effective in eradicating more advanced EBV-associated lymphomas that express the full array of target antigens (163). HPV-associated cervical cancers express the transforming proteins E6 and E7 (for review, see ref. 164), and in mice, active immunization against E6/E7 leads to rejection of transplanted tumor cells expressing these antigens (165).

RNA Tumor Viruses

RNA tumor viruses, which can be of exogenous or endogenous type, integrate into host cell DNA; however, for most of the viral life cycle, exogenous viruses exist and replicate as infectious particles capable of infecting other cells. In contrast, endogenous viruses remain, most of the time, as proviruses integrated into the host's genome and only produce infectious particles when "induced" by ionizing radiation, chemical carcinogens, mutagens, or protein synthesis inhibitors. Genomic DNA of inbred mice contains about 50 copies of normal murine leukemia virus (MULV)-related proviral sequences (166). These proviruses can be categorized into three major groups, which are determined by the range of the host cells that can be infected by the infectious particles derived from these proviruses: ecotropic viruses, which replicate in mouse cells but not in non-mouse cells; xenotropic viruses, which replicate in non-mouse cells but not in mouse cells; and polytropic (amphotropic or dualtropic) viruses, which replicate in both types of cells. The differences in host range of the viruses are determined by differences in their viral envelope (env) genes, which encode a 70-kDa glycoprotein (gp70). Thus, oligonucleotide probes specific for the three types of env genes (167) or antibody probes specific for the three antigenic types of gp70 viral envelope proteins (107,108,168) can be used to group these proviruses into one of the three categories listed above. Apparently, all RNA tumor viruses share a number of antigenic determinants of envelope proteins, even when isolated from different species. This is consistent with the notion that RNA tumor viruses are rather closely related, which is supported by the similar genomic structure of these viruses.

Human T-lymphotropic virus I (HTLV-1) is the only RNA virus presently known to be associated with a human cancer, an endemic adult T-cell leukemia. However, expression of a human endogenous retroviral gene product has been reported in several human cancers, and RNA viruses are associated with several cancers in animals (169). Viral antigens found in these tumors include the virus envelope glycoproteins encoded by the env gene, several viral core proteins encoded by the viral gag gene, and superantigens encoded by an open reading frame (ORF) in the long terminal repeat (LTR) of mouse mammary tumor virus (MMTV) or by the gag gene of MULV. Thus, proteins encoded by RNA tumor viruses are found in the virus particles as well as on the surface of virus-infected or virus-transformed cells. By contrast, proteins encoded by DNA tumor viruses are not expressed on the virus particles, but only by the transformed or infected cells. There is strong evidence that certain proviral genes, such as the env genes encoding gp70 surface glycoproteins of MULV, can be expressed on normal murine cells and on chemically induced or UV-induced tumors without activation of the provirus to produce infectious particles (107,108). Therefore, expression of gp70 is commonly observed on normal cells, where the appearance of these glycoproteins is regulated by the stage of cellular differentiation (170,171).

Injection of MULV or murine sarcoma virus (MSV) into newborn animals induces cancer (172). While antibodies to gp70 can apparently prevent viral infection, rejection of RNA tumor virus–transformed cells depends on MHC-restricted T cells specific for the viral antigens. These T cells detect both viral envelope (e.g., gp70) and viral core proteins (e.g., gag) of the MULV- or MSV-induced tumor cells (173–175). Such proteins can also be recognized by T cells on chemically induced or spontaneously arising murine cancer cells (54,176). These experimental studies have shown that activation of endogenous retroviral sequences can lead to the expression of tumor antigens that are shared (176) or appear to be unique (53,54); but because of the lack of normal control cells from the mouse of tumor origin, it is not clear whether the transcriptional activation was tumor-specific or caused by rearrangements already present in germline genes. Some RNA tumor viruses, such as the MMTV, are vertically transmitted (e.g., during nursing of the neonate), but neonatal exposure to antigens encoded by endogenous MMTV LTR sequences can prevent infection by exogenous MMTV [due to deletion of reactive T cells that act as carriers for the virus (177)] and result in a lower mammary tumor incidence. Transforming genes of DNA tumor viruses are not closely related to normal cellular genes; therefore, the products encoded by these genes elicit a vigorous immune response. In contrast, transforming genes of RNA tumor viruses (also called viral oncogenes) are closely related to, and in

some cases identical to, cellular oncogenes (3); their products, therefore, may also elicit no or only weak responses. Thus, self tolerance may account for why it is more difficult to induce CTLs specific for oncogene products of RNA tumor viruses than for the transforming proteins of SV40, HPV, and adenoviruses.

IMMUNOLOGIC FACTORS INFLUENCING THE INCIDENCE OF CANCER

Immunosurveillance of Tumor Development

Early in this century, it was suggested that cancer would occur at an "incredible frequency" if host defenses did not prevent the outgrowth of cancer cells that arise continuously (9). This hypothesis of immunologic resistance of the host to the outgrowth of primary cancer did not receive major attention until the late 1950s (178) and 1960s, when the problem was restated and redefined. The extended hypothesis (179) suggested that the primary reason for development of T cell–mediated immunity during the evolution of vertebrates was for specific defense against altered self or neoplastic cells. Furthermore, the term *immunosurveillance* was coined to describe the concept of a natural immunologic host resistance against the development of cancer (179). The concept of surveillance was especially attractive in the 1950s and 1960s because it provided evolutionary significance to T cell-mediated cellular immunity, which previously seemed to have no use other than to cause rejection of experimental allografts. We now know that T cell-mediated immunity is necessary for resistance to many viral and, probably, other infections. For example, nude mice, which do not have a thymus and lack functional T-cell immunity, are highly susceptible to viral infections but do not show an increased incidence or a shortened latency of chemically induced cancers (180,181), though the incidence of lymphoreticular tumors is increased in these mice (182). Similarly, patients with certain congenital immunodeficiency diseases may have a markedly (several thousandfold) increased incidence of cancer (183), but mostly of lymphopoietic and reticuloendothelial origin. Most common forms of cancer do not occur earlier or at a significantly higher rate in these individuals than in the general immunocompetent population. It is, therefore, quite possible that the congenital abnormality in these tissues contributed significantly to the high incidence of these particular types of cancers. Most common forms of cancer are also not increased in patients with acquired immune deficiency syndrome (AIDS) or in individuals who have been immunosuppressed by drug treatment because of transplants or other conditions. However, patients with immunodeficiency are usually highly susceptible to viral infections, and Table 4 shows that these individuals have an

TABLE 4. *Malignant neoplasms with an increased incidence in immunodeficiency patients*

Type of immunodeficiency	Cancer	Carcinogen
Primary (Inherited)	B-cell lymphoma	EBV
	Hepatocellular carcinoma	HBV
	Hematological malignancies	Germline
Secondary, drug-induced (patients with or without allograft)	B-cell lymphoma	EBV
	Squamous cell carcinoma (skin)	HPV, UV
	Hepatocellular carcinoma	HBV
	Cervical carcinoma	HPV
AIDS	B-cell lymphoma	EBV
	Cloagenic or oral carcinoma	HPV
	Hepatocellular carcinoma	HBV

EBV, Epstein-Barr virus; HBV, hepatitis B virus; HPV, human papilloma virus; UV, ultraviolet light.

increased incidence of cancers caused by virus or UV light (184). Renal transplant patients show a highly significant increase in skin cancers preferentially on UV-exposed sites of the body, which is independent of the immunosuppressive agent used (185). Even treatment with the immunosuppressive drug cyclosporine (which has not been found to be mutagenic) caused a similar increase. Therefore, the restricted localization of these skin cancers to UV-exposed sites argues against cocarcinogenic effects of the systemic drug treatment; rather, this observation supports the concept that indirect effects of the drug-induced suppression of the host's immune defenses can increase the development of primary skin cancers caused by UV light. In this regard, it is interesting that cyclosporine slightly reduced the latency period of UV-induced skin cancers in mice (186), and it suppressed the rejection of transplanted UV-induced regressor tumors by mice (187).

It appears from the above that T cell-mediated immunity provides a selective advantage for an individual by providing protection against lethal viral diseases and other types of infections. Therefore, immunosurveillance does play an important role in the protection of humans and animals against virally induced or virus-associated malignancies (188). Tumors induced by certain DNA or RNA viruses can be very immunogenic (188). For example, SV40 and polyoma viruses usually do not induce tumors in adult animals because the viruses induce rejection antigens on the transformed cells that are immunogenic enough to elicit rejection without prior immunization. Therefore, the use of immunoincompetent animals, such as very young or newborn animals or nude mice, is required for tumor induction, a finding that led to a breakthrough in studying the tumorigenicity of viruses and of cells transformed by viruses in vitro. Tumors induced by these viruses may, nevertheless, be serially passaged in adult mice, but only when very large numbers of tumor cells are used for transfer. It is important to note that this immunologic resistance of the natural host is directed against virally transformed cells, not against the virus itself. Cells malignantly transformed by oncogenic DNA viruses do not produce (in contrast to oncogenic RNA viruses) viruses, and often tumor formation, not infection by these viruses, is prevented by the immune system. Such resistance to tumor induction by DNA tumor viruses is consistent with the fact that polyoma virus is a common harmless passenger virus in adult mice and is commonly found in wild mice without inducing malignancies (189).

The resistance to tumor induction by oncogenic viruses is genetically determined, as illustrated by the example of the lymphotropic herpes virus saimiri (190). In its natural host, the squirrel monkey, the virus is an innocuous inhabitant. In some other New World monkeys (such as the marmoset or owl monkey) that do not harbor the virus, inoculation of the virus regularly causes malignant lymphomas. It has been found that susceptible monkeys respond to the virally encoded antigens, but too late and only at a time when lymphoma development has already occurred. To some extent, these results suggest that viruses with oncogenic potential select natural hosts that can effectively destroy cells transformed by such viruses, because lethal tumors would eliminate the virus along with the host. A further example of this is the lymphotropic EBV (188), which causes a self-limiting lymphoproliferative disease called mononucleosis in humans, the natural host of EBV. Thereafter, the EBV becomes latent; and while about 90% of adults are latently infected, only immunosuppressed individuals or patients with malaria appear to develop EBV-associated malignant lymphomas. EBV-encoded CTL-recognized antigens must be important for host recognition and tumor rejection because lymphomas expressing

these antigens in immunocompetent individuals have not been found. Instead EBV-associated lymphomas express the full array of CTL-recognized antigens only in immunosuppressed patients, while Burkitt lymphomas, which tend to appear before any obvious impairment of immune function, express only the EBV-encoded target antigen EBNA-1, which is a poor target for CTL. Both types of EBV-associated lymphomas, however, share the same translocation involving the myc and the immunoglobulin loci.

Probably, the term *immunosurveillance* should be reserved for description of effective host resistance to original (i.e., primary) tumors (e.g., certain virus-induced malignancies). Transplantation studies using tumor cells (191) or cells transformed in vitro (192) cannot adequately test the concept of immunosurveillance in the strict sense. Nevertheless, it is important to know that for most tumors a considerable number of tumor cells must be inoculated into a genetically identical animal or into a nude mouse before tumors develop; that is, whatever means of immune suppression is being used, a threshold number of tumor cells is usually needed. Therefore, this barrier to transplantation may well be of a nonimmunologic nature. Certainly, numerous nonimmunologic homeostatic control mechanisms could be responsible for preventing the outgrowth of these transplanted tumor cells.

In conclusion, immunosurveillance is effective against the development of several virally induced cancers, but it does not seem to play a role in preventing the development of most forms of cancers induced by chemical or physical carcinogens, with the possible exception of UV-induced tumors. However, the absence of immunosurveillance of spontaneous cancers or those induced by physical or chemical carcinogens does not imply that these tumors are nonantigenic or insensitive to immunologic destruction. In fact, as will be shown below, there is convincing evidence that cancers carry antigens that are specific (i.e., not present on normal cells) and that some of these antigens may be causally related to the malignant phenotype. In addition, several of these antigens may serve as targets for diagnosis or therapy of cancer. Finally, extensive clinical and experimental evidence suggests that cancers can stimulate immune responses in the tumor-bearing host, even though this response usually fails to prevent cancer from developing.

Stimulation of Tumor Development

In the last century, Virchow (193) suggested a possible functional relationship between inflammatory infiltrates and malignant growth. It is now known that such infiltrates can contribute either to the regression or to the development (and progression) of cancer. However, these differences can not be readily predicted from the histologic appearance of the infiltrates, because inflammatory cellular reactions resulting from tumor destruction may not be easily distinguished histologically from inflammatory infiltrates causing tumor destruction. Futhermore, inflammatory cells, such as macrophages, may look morphologically identical, even though they may secrete different cytokines that have opposite effects on tumor growth. Despite continuous other claims (e.g., ref. 194), measurements of the inflammatory infiltration into tumors appear to remain a histopathologic variable of unproved prognostic significance (195,196). This also applies to the finding of histologically "regressive" areas of progressive primary melanoma lesions, even when such a lesion is associated with an oligoclonal T-cell infiltrate or vitiligo (a depigmentation of normal skin) (196,197). Destruction of parts of a malignant lesion may simply be the result of the infiltrative growth of the cancer cells into the surrounding tissue, which may destroy part of the tumors' blood supply. Thus, tumors have been compared with "wounds that do not heal" (198). Dependent upon the antigens, cell, and cytokine involvement, the result may be either inhibition or stimulation of the growth of the premaligment or malignant cells by acquired and/or innate immunity (Fig. 5). It is likely that cytokines play a central role in the inflammatory reaction. While nonmalignant cells, under physiologic conditions, produce cytokines only transiently for short-term signaling between cells, cancer cells can produce considerable and sustained amounts of various cytokines and chemokines, such as IL-8, transforming growth factor-β (TGF-β) and macrophage chemotactic proteins (MCPs). These cytokines and chemokines may attract nonmalignant host cells and/or induce such cells to produce other cytokines. For example, MCPs released from tumor cells will attract macrophages to the site of tumor growth, and these tumor-associated macrophages can release other cytokines and growth factors, such as platelet-derived growth factor (PDGF) to stimulate tumor growth (199) (for review, see refs. 200, 201) (see Fig. 5). Similarly, latent TGF-β produced continuously by tumor cells can be activated by infiltrating inflammatory cells, such as macro-

phages, and active TGF-β may induce angiogenesis and the production of extracellular matrix and other cytokines by fibroblasts and endothelial cells (for review, see ref. 202). These infiltrating and sessile nonmalignant host cells and the extracellular matrix provide the stroma (literally, "the bed") in which the tumor grows. Therefore, developing approaches to destroy the stroma of tumors may be of central importance for successful therapy of established solid tumors (203).

The mechanisms of the tumor-promoting effects of stromal inflammation have become clearer with experiments using transgenic and knock-out mice. Earlier studies already had shown that the effectiveness of promotion of skin tumor development by chemical (phorbol esters) or physical (wounding) methods correlates directly with the degree of inflammation induced. Thus, strains of mice that have low or poor inflammatory reactions to wounding or phorbol esters are more resistant to tumor development following promotion (204). The induction of prostaglandin H synthase 2 encoded by the gene Cox-2 is of central importance (205). Certain cytokines or chemical promoters induce the transcription of this gene in macrophages and other inflammatory cells, resulting in the local production of prostaglandin E_2 (PGE$_2$)

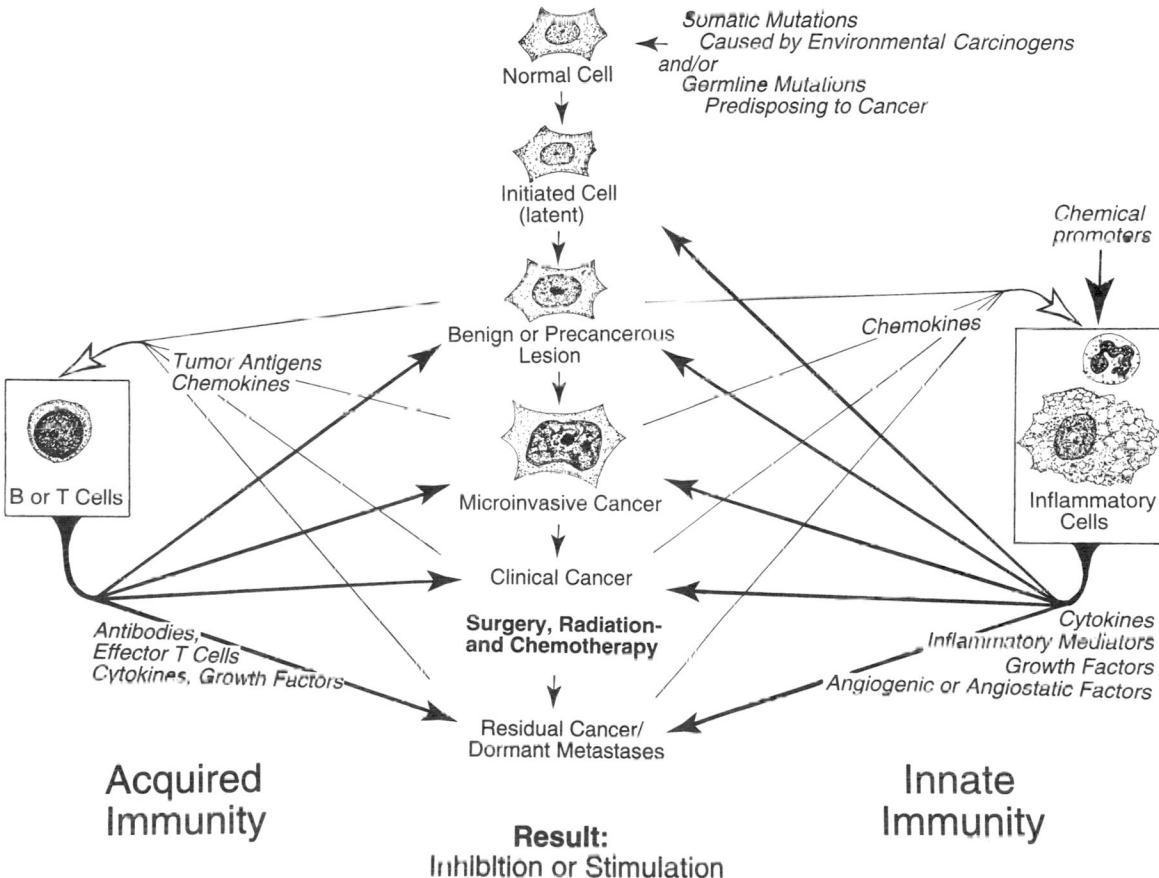

FIG. 5. Both acquired and innate immunity can have significant influence on tumor development and growth. For example, specific T-cell immunity prevents the development of EBV-induced lymphomas in humans, while the presence of particular T-cell subsets helps the development of MMTV-associated mammary tumors in mice. Innate immunity may also either stimulate or inhibit cancer development. For example, BCG-induced inflammation prevents recurrence of bladder cancers in humans, while prostaglandin H synthase 2–dependent inflammation seems to promote the development of certain skin and colon tumors. In principle, the two areas of the immune system can inhibit or stimulate tumor cells in any stage of the multistep process of cancer development and growth.

and other substances, such as reactive oxygen intermediates. PGE_2 can (a) directly stimulate the growth of certain neoplastic cells (including colonic epithelial cells), (b) induce angiogenesis, and (c) block IL-12 and thus interferon-γ (IFN-γ) production. [Both cytokines may reduce the induction of primary cancers by chemical carcinogens (206).] In addition, the reactive oxygen intermediates can cause additional mutations in the initiated cells and thereby help tumors to develop (205). The activity of the prostaglandin synthase-2 is not constitutive but induced in cells such as monocytes and macrophages, which are found as interstitial cells in epithelial tumors (207). Inhibition of the Cox-2–encoded enzyme, by either specific chemicals or genetic knockout, significantly reduces the formation of intestinal tumors in mice prone to develop such neoplasms (207). Similarly, inhibition of prostaglandin production by nonsteroidal antiinflammatory drugs, including aspirin, can inhibit the development of skin papillomas and intestinal neoplasias (207).

Tumor progression may depend on a continued inflammatory reaction, because regression of papillomas is observed when the application of chemical promoters is stopped too soon. Later stages of tumor progression may also be influenced significantly by inflammatory cells. For example, variant cancer cells can acquire much more aggressive growth *in vivo* by acquisition of a paracrine stimulatory loop (208–210) by producing chemokines that attract inflammatory cells; these inflammatory cells in turn may produce cytokines and growth factors that stimulate tumor angiogenesis or the growth of the tumor cells directly. Another example is the discovery that production of viral IL-6 by nonmalignant stromal cells infected with Kaposi's sarcoma-associated herpes virus (KSHV) may play an essential role in the development of multiple myeloma (the second most frequent human malignancy of blood cells). This malignancy of plasma cells develops in about 25% of patients with a premalignant condition called monoclonal gammopathy (211). Other experiments have shown that cancer cells can switch during tumor progression from being inhibited to being stimulated by certain cytokines (e.g., TGF-β or IL-6) (212,213). At later stages of tumor progression, paracrine stimulation may switch to autocrine stimulation when the cancer cells themselves begin to produce the factors (214). This process of variant selection may be hastened by incomplete therapy aimed at destroying the tumor stroma, which provides the paracrine growth factors (215). Certain bacterial substances, such as bacillus Calmette-Guérin (BCG) and certain cytokines, when produced by transfected cancer cells, have antitumor effects that are associated with inflammatory responses, but at present we do not know what determines whether a given inflammatory response suppresses rather than stimulates tumor growth. Once the differences in effector mechanisms and regulatory circuits of inflammatory responses are better understood, we may develop powerful new approaches to prevent as well as treat malignant diseases.

In an interesting example, the presence of a certain T-cell subset has been shown to result in a higher incidence of virally induced mammary tumors in mice. MMTV can be transmitted as milk-borne infection through the nursing mother to the offspring, resulting in mammary carcinoma later in the adult (216,217). A protein, the superantigen ORF, encoded in the ORF of the LTR of the MMTV genome, mediates the Mls response and stimulates or deletes particular T-cell subsets, for example, the Vβ14 subset in the C3H/He mice (218–220). Dividing cells are more readily infected with retrovirus (221,222), and those T cells that are stimulated by ORF are preferentially infected. These T cells appear to be the primary carrier of virus to the mammary gland (223). The importance of this T-cell subset for the development of mammary tumors is demonstrated by the finding that transgenic mice expressing high levels of the ORF superantigen at birth delete the Vβ14 subset and do not become infected with the milk-borne virus. Thus, mice have a lower incidence of mammary tumors, whereas mice expressing lower levels of the same antigen did not delete this T-cell subset and remained susceptible (177). These results are consistent with earlier findings that neonatal thymectomy of mice greatly diminishes the incidence of mammary carcinomas (224). Interestingly, the incidence of breast cancer is reportedly decreased slightly in women who are chronically immunosuppressed after organ transplantation (225).

It has been postulated that, in general, immune responses to tumor antigens, when "weak," stimulate and, when "strong," suppress tumor growth (226,227). However, none of the studies that are used to support this concept have identified the antigens involved. Thus, it remains unclear whether antigen-specific or innate immunity played the significant role. Nevertheless, antigen-specific immune reactions are always accompanied with effector cells of innate immunity, and an acceleration of tumor development by vaccination is a possibility.

FACTORS INFLUENCING TUMOR IMMUNOGENICITY

Differences in Immunogenicity between Spontaneous and Induced Cancers

There is the widely held misconception that human cancers are usually less immunogenic than are murine tumors (228). However, convincing evidence indicates that many human cancers are antigenic, even when growth is progressive. Similarly, even the most antigenic murine "regressor" tumors grow progressively in, and invariably kill, the primary host (Fig. 6). Only transplantation of primary murine tumors into young, syngeneic, immunocompetent recipients reveals the immunogenicity that can be so strong that either the transplanted tumor fragments are rejected at any testable dose without prior immunization (i.e., the tumor is a regressor), or the transplant will grow progressively and the tumor therefore represents a "progressor." Therefore, it is quite possible that some human primary tumors are as immunogenic as murine regressor tumors, because only transplantation (not possible in humans) could reveal such immunogenicity.

The mode of tumor induction greatly influences the immunogenicity of the tumor induced, as measured by transplantation experiments. Spontaneous murine cancers that develop without any known exposure to carcinogens tend to be less immunogenic than cancers induced by DNA tumor viruses or by deliberate exposure to carcinogen (14,15,229–232), even though serially transplanted tumors were used for most of these studies and transplantation may have been selected for less immunogenic variants. If spontaneous murine cancers more closely resembled human cancers, this would suggest that human cancers are poorly immunogenic (232). However, most human cancers are induced by environmental carcinogens and, as already mentioned, the immunogenicity of human tumors cannot be measured in transplantation experiments.

Some UV-induced tumors are among the most immunogenic cancers; transplantation resistance to these so-called regressor tumors appears to be absolute rather than relative. Rejection by normal syn-

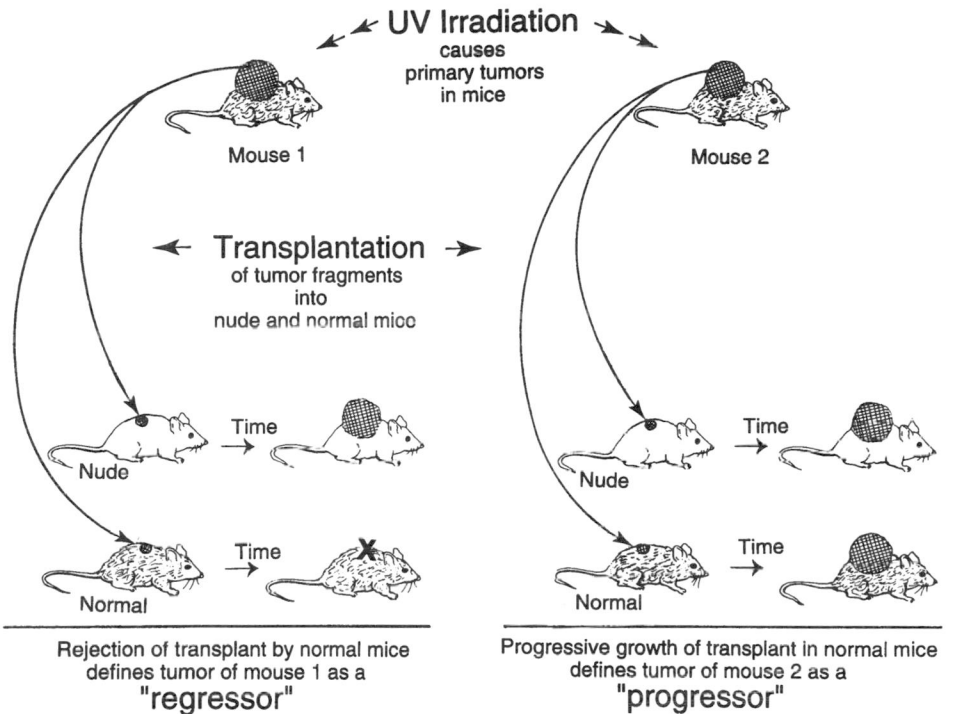

FIG. 6. The growth of primary UV-induced skin cancers is indistinguishable in the primary host, whether or not the tumors are highly immunogenic. Only subsequent transplantations into normal young syngeneic mice define tumors as either regressors or progressors. Growth of the transplanted fragments into nude mice serves as control for the viability of the transplanted tumor fragments and for determining the T-cell dependence of the regressor phenotype.

geneic mice is observed without prior immunization of the mice, even when the largest testable doses of tumor cells or fragments are used (22); these tumor transplants will grow for about a week and then disappear, though small numbers of the same tumor cells will grow and kill athymic nude mice. Most MCA-induced fibrosarcomas display an intermediate degree of immunogenicity (16,17,31). This is shown by the fact that induction of immunologic resistance to most chemically induced tumors requires prior immunization, because the initial graft of the tumor generally produces progressive lethal growth (16). Immunization can be done either by administration of a small nontumorigenic dose of tumor cells or by a complete surgical removal (excision or ligation) of an initial tumor transplant after the tumor has grown for several days or weeks. Immunologic resistance induced by these chemically induced tumors is usually relative rather than absolute and breaks down when the number of tumor cells used for challenge is high.

Effect of Carcinogen Dose, Immunocompetence, and Tumor Latency

Most, if not all, carcinogens are mutagens (4,5), and mutations leading to cancer may also cause the expression of tumor specific antigens. It therefore seems logical to postulate that the immunogenicity of a tumor is proportional to the dose of carcinogen used for induction; this might account for the usually low or absent immunogenicity of "spontaneous" tumors presumably induced by undetectable levels of environmental carcinogens. By analogy, tumors induced with larger doses of physical or chemical carcinogens, as for experimentally induced tumors, would be immuno-

genic. However, it is not clear why tumors induced with the same dose of chemical or physical carcinogen may exhibit quite different degrees of immunogenicity (16,233). One reason might be that the actual local dose of carcinogen that is delivered to a particular target cell or target tissue may vary greatly from animal to animal. Another reason might be that mutations are selected that favor malignant behavior irrespective of the degree of immunogenicity that a resultant mutant protein may have. This might occur because the autochthonous host may not respond to its own tumor unless it is immunized after tumor removal (17). This is consistent with the observation that considerable differences in immunogenicity of primary UV-induced tumors only become apparent after transplantation into secondary hosts (37,233) (see Fig. 6).

Immunocompetence of the host during cancer induction and development may sometimes allow the host to select for variants that have lost antigens (18). Conversely, immunosuppression or immune deficiency of the host during carcinogenesis should allow growth of highly immunogenic tumors (e.g., the appearance of highly antigenic EBV-associated lymphomas in immunosuppressed transplant recipients). So, it may be highly relevant that some carcinogens are immunosuppressive (234). In the mouse, for example, repeated exposures to UV light induce immunosuppression (235–237), which seems to allow the development of highly immunogenic regressor tumors. In contrast, the single injection of MCA required to induce tumors in 100% of mice only induces a short-lived state of immune suppression, thus allowing the host to select for less immunogenic variants during tumor development. This concept, that immunocompetence of a host influences the degree of immunogenicity of the developing tumor, has been tested experimentally by comparing the immunogenicity of MCA-induced tumors occurring in UV-irradiated versus normal mice (238). Indeed, tumors induced with MCA in mice immunosuppressed by UV light were more frequently highly immunogenic regressor tumors than were tumors induced with MCA in mice that were not suppressed by UV radiation.

There is no consistent correlation between the length of the latency period and the degree of immunogenicity when comparing different tumor models. For example, the length of the latency period correlates inversely with the degree of immunogenicity in MCA-induced tumors (18,239), but there is no such correlation in UV-induced tumors (22). The reasons for this inconsistency may be that as the latency period increases, so does the age of the host, and that an age-related decrease in immunocompetence (240–243) may prevent the host from selecting against highly immunogenic tumor cells. Therefore, cancers developing in old individuals after a long latency period may sometimes be very immunogenic.

EFFECTOR MECHANISMS IN CANCER IMMUNITY

Because cancer is not a single disease, it is not surprising that findings using one tumor model may not apply to other tumor models. Considering the antigenic diversity found in tumors, it is also not surprising that the different components of humoral and cell-mediated immunity have been shown to play different roles in the destruction of malignant cells in one or another of the numerous tumor models.

Assays to Study the Importance of Effector Mechanisms *In Vivo*

In principle, four different assays have been used to evaluate the importance of different effector mechanisms *in vivo*. The first type of assay involves transfer of effector cells, cytokines, or antibodies into sublethally irradiated, cyclophosphamide-pretreated, or normal animals challenged with tumor cells. There are certain limitations of this assay. Effector cells may not reach or localize in the tumor unless both the effector cells and cancer cells are injected intravenously and both are trapped in the lungs. Furthermore, if transferred cells or reagents are effective, the assay does not rule out that other effector mechanisms of the host may have been activated by the procedure. In a second procedure, called the *Winn assay* (17,18,244), tumor cells are mixed with effector cells or serum *in vitro*, and then the mixture is injected subcutaneously into an animal to determine whether tumor growth *in vivo* is prevented. Tumor cells are probably killed within minutes before or shortly after the injection, though the read-out takes much longer. Therefore, the Winn assay is, in principle, an *in vitro* cytotoxicity assay, even though the host is used as a receptacle for tumor growth. A third method involves elimination of specific lymphocyte subsets or cytokines *in vivo* by treatment with antibodies specific for different lymphocyte subsets or cytokines (e.g., see refs. 39, 245). Failure of the host to resist a tumor challenge indicates that the particular subsets or cytokines are an essential component of the host resistance. An analysis of tumor variants that have escaped tumor destruction by the host provides a fourth way for determining the importance of immunologic effectors *in vivo* (39,44,191). The phenotypic changes observed in these variants may indicate which effector mechanism was responsible for the selection. Therefore, the type of phenotypic change may give insight into the importance

of a naturally occurring defense mechanism that may function in immunocompetent mice (analogous to deducing the action of an antibiotic from the type of change found in the bacterium that has become drug-resistant). This approach is illustrated using UV light–induced tumors. These cancers have strong tumor-specific antigens and are rejected regularly by syngeneic mice without prior immunization, though these regressor tumors do grow in immunodeficient mice. Rarely, usually in less than 1% of the normal recipients, these tumors escape rejection by undergoing some heritable change. These escape variants, which grow progressively upon reimplantation into normal mice (progressor variants), were tested *in vitro* for changes in sensitivity to T cells, activated macrophages, or NK cells (39,191,246). Some of the progressor variants showed resistance to cytotoxic T cells due to the loss of a unique tumor antigen (39,191) and the increased resistance to activated macrophages (246) and TNF *in vitro*, suggesting that cytolytic T cells and activated macrophages may have tumoricidal activity *in vivo* in this tumor system. However, at least some of the observed changes could be coincidental, and a failure to observe a change in resistance to an effector mechanism does not imply that such effector mechanism was unimportant. For example, the majority of the progressor variants retained the T cell–recognized antigens (39), and other heritable changes, such as establishment of a paracine stimulatory loop, apparently enabled these variants to escape destruction by T cells (208–210).

Antibodies and B Cells

The role of B cells in regulating tumor immunity is poorly understood: In a tumor model in which CD4$^+$ helper T cells are required for tumor rejection, B cells appear to be necessary for efficient T-cell priming and tumor resistance (247). Conversely, in another tumor model, elimination of CD4$^+$ T cells promoted tumor rejection by CD8$^+$ cells, and an absence of B cells improved CTL responses and tumor rejection (248,249).

Human antisera and monoclonal antibodies reactive with autologous tumors have been isolated (108,250). However, a strong humoral response to tumor antigens does not seem to be correlated with demonstrable resistance of the host to the tumors. For example, an experimentally induced humoral immune response to MCA-induced sarcomas does not provide protective immunity against a tumor transplant (251). In another example, TL$^+$ leukemias induce high titers of TL-specific antibodies that are cytotoxic to TL$^+$ leukemia cells *in vitro* in the presence of heterologous complement (108), but TL$^+$ leukemias grow equally well in immunized mice having high titers of TL antigen–specific antibody and in nonimmunized mice (252,253). Obviously, the presence of antibodies for these kinds of tumors has no relevance in predicting whether the host will reject the tumor (251,253). Normal or malignant cells of hematopoietic origin are generally lysed quite effectively by antibody and heterologous complement *in vitro*; however, certain normal or malignant cells derived from solid tissues may be much less affected, even when expressing high levels of antigen. The reasons for this striking difference are still unclear, but differences depending on the source of complement, the antigen distribution, or repair of complement-mediated lesions may be involved. *In vitro*, some solid tumor cells are killed by a process involving coating with antibody, opsonization, and subsequent phagocytosis by macrophages; this process may be enhanced by the presence of complement. Alternatively, antibody-coated tumor cells may be killed in the absence of phagocytosis by antibody-dependent cell-mediated cytotoxicity when cocultured with macrophages, NK cells, or neutrophils. The general relevance of these mechanisms for killing tumor cells *in vivo* is unclear.

T lymphocytes

It has been demonstrated convincingly that T cell–mediated immunity is of critical importance for the rejection of virally (254–256) and chemically induced tumors (17,18,36) by immunized mice, or for the rejection of allogeneic (257) and UV-induced (22,39,236) tumors by normal mice. For example, in the model of murine MCA-induced tumors, it was shown that intravenous injection of immune cells, but not of immune serum, could transfer systemic tumor-specific immunity into sublethally x-irradiated mice (18). In another study, transfer of immunity to a plasma-cell tumor was abolished by pretreatment of the immune cells by anti-T cell antibodies and complement (36). These results are consistent with studies (17) showing that immune cells, but not immune serum, when mixed with tumor cells *in vitro* and then injected subcutaneously, could prevent outgrowth of the tumor; this procedure is a local adoptive transfer assay (the Winn assay) (244). Similarly, T cells are also required for the rejection of UV-induced regressor tumors by nonimmunized (normal) mice (22,39,236,258). The relative importance of various T-cell subsets in tumor rejection has been the subject of repeated, and probably unnecessary, controversies (259). Different tumors are dissimilar enough so that differences would be expected in the T-cell subsets required for rejection. For certain tumors, such as UV-induced tumors, the CD8$^+$ cytolytic T-cell subset appears to be regularly required for rejection (39). Relatively little is known about how the CD4$^+$ T-cell subsets can influence antitumor immunity, but truly tumor-specific CD4$^+$ T cell–recognized tumor antigens exist (56). CD4$^+$ T cells seem to be critical for the development of CD8$^+$ T-cell memory (260) and for the survival of adoptively transferred CD8$^+$ T cells (261). Certain CD4$^+$ subsets may also negatively influence tumor rejection, because elimination of the CD4$^+$ T-cell subset may increase tumor resistance in certain tumor models (248). Murine CTLs that kill tumor targets in a 4- to 5-hour ^{51}Cr release assay can be freshly isolated from mice after repeated intraperitoneal injection of antigenic tumor cells or generated *in vitro* in a 7-day mixed lymphocyte–tumor cell culture. In most experimental tumor models, specific T cells were generated from tumor-free syngeneic mice. Because this approach is not feasible in humans, T lymphocytes from cancer patients have been isolated from peripheral blood (262,263) or from the tumor [tumor-infiltrating lymphocytes (TILs)] (264). Such T cells can react *in vitro* with autologous cancer cells (for review, see ref. 265). When freshly isolated from the patient, these lymphocytes usually require 16 to 48 hours of incubation with the tumor target before a significant level of lysis or growth inhibition of the tumor cells can be observed, whereas lymphocytes that have been grown and restimulated in culture will often lyse the tumor cells in a 4- to 5-hour ^{51}Cr release assay.

Natural Killer Cells and Lymphokine-activated Killer Cells

NK cells (266–271) are a distinct subpopulation of lymphocytes that, without prior sensitization and without the requirement for MHC restriction, can kill some cancer cells (for review, see ref. 272

and Chapter 17). Furthermore, cancer cells that fail to express at least one of the MHC class I alleles of the host are more effectively rejected (273,274) (for review, see ref. 272) by a mechanism involving NK cells (275). Conversely, expression of an MHC allele by cancer cells can protect tumor cells from lysis by NK cells (276). It is now known that ligation of receptors on NK cells recognizing MHC molecules exerts an inhibitory signal to prevent the activation of NK cells for lysis. The cytotoxicity of murine and human NK cells against malignant cells has been most fully characterized *in vitro* using a few highly sensitive cell lines, such as the murine T-cell leukemia line, YAC, and the human erythroleukemia cell line, K562. In addition, studies *in vivo* suggest that NK cells may help reduce metastatic dissemination of intravenously injected cancer cells (277–279). Observations that are consistent with (but do not prove) a role for NK cells *in vivo* include (a) an increased incidence of spontaneous tumors with age in mice at a time when endogenous NK activity is decreasing and (b) the capacity of nude mice, which have NK cells but deficient T-cell immunity, to reject some tumors.

Activation of peripheral blood cells *in vitro* with high doses of IL-2 induce *lymphokine-activated killer* (LAK) cells (280,281). Cancer cells, even when resistant to NK cells, are usually susceptible to killing by LAK cells *in vitro*, whereas most nonmalignant target cells have been reported to be resistant to killing by LAK cells. However, fetal and placental cells and occasionally normal peripheral blood cells (281) have been reported to be susceptible to killing by LAK cells. Intravenous injection of LAK cells early after intravenous seeding of cancer cells into mice reduces the metastatic tumor-cell growth in the lungs, but with this procedure, both LAK and cancer cells are trapped in the lungs (282,283). Antitumor responses have also been reported in humans after adoptive transfer of LAK cells in patients with renal cell carcinoma and melanoma (284). This selectivity is difficult to explain, considering the general susceptibility of cancer cells to LAK cells *in vitro*. The cells that mediate the killing *in vitro* of a broad range of malignant cells are more than 90% activated CD16$^+$/CD3 NK cells (285,286), but which cells have antitumor activity *in vivo* is not fully established. Even though murine LAK cells can be generated from nude mouse spleen cells (287), it has not been demonstrated that LAK cells from nude mice and normal mice have similar therapeutic effects against tumor cells *in vivo*. Other cell types, such as CD3$^+$ lymphocytes, which are regularly present in every preparation of LAK cells (287), may contribute significantly to the killing of tumor cells *in vivo*.

Macrophages and Neutrophils

Macrophages and neutrophils from normal donors are generally not cytotoxic to tumor cells or normal cells *in vitro*; however, macrophages and neutrophil granulocytes can be activated by bacterial products *in vitro* to cause selective cytolysis or cytostasis of malignant cells (288–294). Such tumoricidal activation of macrophages and neutrophils does not seem to occur when using tumor cells that are uncontaminated by bacteria or their products. Apparently, cancer cells lack the "danger signal" (295) necessary for such direct activation of these effector cells of innate immunity (296). Fully activated macrophages require long-term 16- to 72-hour assays to demonstrate *in vitro* tumoricidal activity in isotope-release assays or cytostatic activity in growth-inhibition assays. Some of the cytolytic or cytostatic effects of macrophages on tumor cells involve cell contact and/or the secretion of various cytotoxic substances, but phagocytosis may also play an important role (297).

TNF (298,299) produced by activated macrophages can account for all of the classical tumoricidal effects against some tumors *in vitro* (300). For example, variants that were resistant to TNF were also completely resistant to activated macrophages; in the converse experiment, variants for resistant-to-activated macrophages were completely resistant to TNF (300). Furthermore, macrophage cytotoxicity could be inhibited completely with antibodies to recombinant TNF (300). TNF also seems to be an important effector molecule in the killing of certain tumor cells by human peripheral blood monocytes (301–303). As might be expected because of the plethora of cytotoxic molecules that can be released by macrophages (304), mechanisms not involving TNF are also involved in the killing of some tumor cells. For example, activated macrophages synthesize nitrogen oxides from L-arginine, and these reactive nitrogen intermediates also appear to be mediators of killing of tumor cells by activated macrophages (305,306).

Because of the rather selective cytotoxicity of activated macrophages against malignant cells, numerous studies have considered the potential role of this cell type in immunosurveillance and immunotherapy. It is known that the normal host can select for variant cancer cells resistant to the effects of TNF and activated macrophages *in vitro* (246,300,307–309). However, this selection appears to be dependent on T cells (246), which are known to produce large amounts of TNF on antigenic stimulation. Therefore, there is, at present, no critical evidence to establish or refute the idea that activated macrophages destroy nascent tumors and therefore play a role in immune surveillance (310). The more important question may be whether activated macrophages can be useful in cancer therapy. Experimental evidence indicates that activation of macrophages *in vivo* or adoptive transfer of macrophages activated *in vitro* can eliminate or reduce metastasis in some experimental models (for review, see ref. 311).

Cytokines

The possible stimulatory effects of cytokines produced by the tumor cells or by the nonmalignant host cells in the tumor stroma on tumor growth were discussed earlier in this chapter (see section on stimulation of tumor growth). The effects of locally sustained high levels of various cytokines have been studied by using tumor cells transfected to produce large amounts of certain cytokines. Some cytokines, such as granulocyte colony-stimulating factor (G-CSF) (312), IL-2 (313), IL-4 (314), and TNF (315,316), when secreted in sufficiently large amount by the transfected tumor cells, may lead to significant growth inhibition, even in the absence of T cells. Certain other cytokines, such as IL-1 (317), IL-7 (318), and IFN-γ (319–321), have been shown to inhibit the growth of transfected tumor cells *in vivo*, but this inhibition was dependent on the presence of T cells. However, we are only at the beginning of understanding the mechanisms leading to this growth inhibition. Such mechanisms may be quite different for different cytokines, even though the histologic and ultrastructural appearance of the cellular reactions to the transfected tumor cells may be similar.

TNF provides example of the difficulties in analyzing the mechanism involved the inhibition of tumor growth *in vivo* by a particular cytokine. Variant tumor cells, which are heritably stable and completely macrophage- (246) and TNF-resistant (300) *in vitro*, still form tumors *in vivo* that remain as highly susceptible as the TNF-sensitive parental tumor to hemorrhagic necrosis after injections of TNF. Thus, sensitivity of tumor cells to the direct cytotoxicity of

TNF *in vitro* may not be important *in vivo* for the effects of passive TNF treatment. Tumor products may sensitize the vascular bed of the tumor to become susceptible to hemorrhagic necrosis by TNF. This notion is supported by the finding that tumor cells can produce tissue factors that enhance the procoagulant response to TNF (322), but the precise nature of this signal remains elusive. Tumor cells transfected to produce TNF are also completely resistant to TNF *in vitro* but are arrested by the produced TNF *in vivo*, even in the absence of T-cell immunity. Interestingly, the mechanism of this TNF-mediated growth arrest does not involve hemorrhagic necrosis (316).

Some tumor cells produce a given cytokine constitutively, whereas other tumor cells can be stimulated to produce cytokines by various agents, for example, other cytokines, bacterial products (such as lipopolysaccharide), irradiation, or drugs. Thus, treatments could be aimed at eliciting the release of an inhibitory cytokine from the tumors themselves (323). Such an approach may be advantageous *in vivo*, because targeting every cell with a therapeutic gene seems unrealistic and also because systemic applications of recombinant cytokines may cause major systemic toxicity and/or insufficient local cytokine concentrations at the site of tumor growth. Possibly cytokine gene-transfected T cells that localize in tumors could cause high local levels of a chosen cytokine, but no experimental model exists for this suggestion.

FACTORS LIMITING EFFECTIVE TUMOR IMMUNITY

As might be expected from the diversity of tumors, tumor cells can escape or fail to elicit tumor-specific immune responses by various mechanisms (Table 5). Cancer cells are genetically and phenotypically less stable than normal cells and can rapidly change to escape immune destruction. The following are examples of some of the ways tumors escape or host resistance fails.

Major Histocompatibility Complex Haplotype

Tumor cells may express mutant proteins that are tumor-specific, but these mutant proteins may not serve as an antigen if they lack mutant peptides that can be presented by the MHC molecules or a TCR that recognizes the peptide-MHC complex. For example, depending on the genetic MHC background, only some mouse strains recognize a particular mutant ras protein as an antigen, whereas others do not (70). MHC genes may also regulate immune responses to antigens on cancer cells or to cancer-causing viruses; and since the discovery that the MHC profoundly influences the susceptibility of mice to leukemia (324) (for review, see ref. 325), investigators have searched for a possible association between MHC type and cancer susceptibility in humans and mice. So far, however, no firm association between HLA haplotype and the occurrence of any major human cancer has been established.

Tolerance Versus Ignorance

Even when cancer cells express a potentially antigenic molecule, the host may not respond to the tumor because of tolerance or clonal ignorance. Tolerance to self may explain why oncofetal and carcinoembryonic or oncospermatogonal antigens that are expressed on some normal adult cells induce weaker protection than is usually

TABLE 5. *Mechanisms of tumor escape from immunologic destruction*

I. Tumor-related

1. Failure of the tumor to provide a suitable target (defective immunosensitivity)
   (a) Lack of antigenic epitope
   (b) Lack of MHC class I molecule
   (c) Deficient antigen processing by tumor cell
   (d) Antigenic modulation
   (e) Antigenic masking of the tumor
   (f) Resistance of tumor cell to tumoricidal effector pathway
2. Failure of the tumor to induce an effective immune response (defective immunogenicity)
   (a) Lack of antigenic epitope (see above)
   (b) Decreased MHC or antigen expression by the tumor (see above)
   (c) Lack of costimulatory signal
   (d) Production of inhibitory substances (e.g., cytokines) by the tumor
   (e) Shedding of antigen and tolerance induction
   (f) Induction of apoptosis in T cells by expression of Fas ligand by cancer cells
   (g) Induction of T cell signaling defects by tumor burden
3. Establishment of a paracrine stimulatory loop

II. Host-related

1. Failure of the host to respond to an antigenic tumor
   (a) Immune suppression or deficiency of host including apoptosis and signaling defects of T cells due to carcinogen (physical, chemical), infections, or age
   (b) Deficient presentation of tumor antigens by host antigen-presenting cells
   (c) Failure of host effectors to reach the tumor (e.g., stromal barrier)
2. Failure of host to kill variant tumor cells because of immunodominant antigens on parental tumor cells

found in animals immunized with unique tumor antigens (29,34,35,143). Possibly only those T cells that react with such antigens at low avidity can escape deletion and tolerance (326). It is likely that the T cells in the tumor-bearing host do not simply "ignore" the tumor antigen, because complete removal of a tumor often results in specific immunity to rechallenge with the tumor, even without additional immunization. Thus, these T cells have been exposed to antigen but are anergic either systemically or just locally, and passive treatment of tumor-bearing mice with monoclonal antibodies to the regulatory molecule CTLA-4 or the activation molecule 4-1BB on T cells may overcome this problem (327,328). It is not clear whether, under some conditions, the host may also ignore completely the presence of antigens on tumors. While mutant peptides can be used to elicit T cells with higher affinity (329), a critical problem of low-affinity interaction with the original tumor-derived peptides at the site of tumor growth probably remains.

Tumor Stroma and Other Local Factors

Experiments have shown that stroma is critical for preventing or permitting the immunologic destruction of tumor cells (203), and it is also likely that tumor stroma is an important factor in the rapidly developing resistance of solid tumors to systemic immunity, even at relatively early stages of tumor growth (e.g., see ref.

330). Local factors must explain why tumor-bearing mice fail to reject their primary tumors, even though the animals may be resistant to implants of small numbers of tumor cells at second sites, a phenomenon called *concomitant immunity* (331). Local factors particular to the tumor environment may also explain why mice bearing malignant grafts fail to reject the tumors but reject nonmalignant grafts expressing through gene transfer the same rejection antigen (332). This seems to occur even in TCR transgenic mice in which both the tumor and the nonmalignant graft are recognized by a single type of TCR (333). Thus, T cells in these tumor-bearing mice that fail to reject the tumor are neither clonally exhausted nor systemically anergic (333). The disparity in response to normal and malignant grafts is also not explained by the expression of weaker rejection antigens on the tumor, because tumor and normal grafts express the same antigen. The difference may result from the fact that the stroma of tumors is nonantigenic and interferes as a physical barrier with the rejection of the cancer cells (203); while the presence of an antigenic stroma, as it exists in nonmalignant allografts, can help T cells to destroy also the tumor cells (203). For example, T cell-mediated destruction of allogeneic stroma may not only destroy the vascular support for the tumor and allow T cells to reach the cancer cells by breaking a physical barrier but also generate local help for T cells and other leukocytes needed for tumor rejection. Lack of "help" at the site of tumor growth may be an important reason for the failure of solid tumor to be rejected. The situation might be somewhat analogous to transgenic mice that express allo-MHC class I molecules as self antigen on islet cells and also have autoreactive T cells that infiltrate the islets (334): Even after priming, these autoreactive cells fail to destroy the islet cells unless local help is provided in the form of IL-2 (334). Antigen-specific T cells can infiltrate even tumors growing in immunologically privileged sites, but proper differentiation of the infiltrating T cells is prevented. In fact, it appears that the growing tumor itself can create an immunologically privileged site (335–337). Lack of costimulatory molecules on the malignant cells or expression of Fas ligand by these cells may lead to peripheral anergy (338–340). Indirect presentation by host antigen-presenting cells (APCs) of antigens released from tumor cells can play a significant role (341,342). However, under certain conditions, direct presentation may be more efficient than indirect presentation in inducing a response (343). In addition, transfecting tumor cells to express one of several cytokines or costimulatory molecules (such as B7) can make tumor cells more effective inducers of immune responses (for review, see ref. 118). However, the effectiveness of any induced response is limited by the wild-type (i.e., the untransfected) tumor cells, and the environment surrounding these tumor cells may still counteract tumor destruction for the reasons mentioned above (333). Thus, the critical unresolved problem may be to provide local help and costimulation at the site of tumor growth to accomplish effective tumor destruction (328,333). Finally, as mentioned earlier, the stroma can provide factors essential for the development of certain cancers (211), and the stroma is the site for paracrine stimulatory loops that cause rapid malignant growth and thereby impede immunologic rejection (209).

Changes in Expression of Major Histocompatibility Complex Class I Antigens

In some cancers, changes in MHC class I expression are due to a total or selective loss or downregulation of MHC class I molecules. In other cancers, such changes may be due to mutations in the gene coding for β2-microglobulin (344). These mechanism for escape from host immunity may occur especially in those cancer cells in which the tumor-specific antigen cannot be lost because expression is required for the maintenance of the malignant phenotype (e.g., cancer cells that express E6 and E7 of HPV). Changes in the expression of MHC class I antigens are particularly frequent in metastatic cancers cells (345,346). Thus, studies on MHC class I expression using tissue sections of human metastatic melanoma (347) and metastatic breast (346,348) or colon cancer (349–352) have commonly detected changes in HLA expression; in these studies, loss of a single HLA class I allele was found more commonly than loss of all class I alleles (for review, see ref. 353). Oncogenes such as myc may cause locus-specific suppression of MHC class I antigen expression (354), and results of clinical studies have thus far not supported the concept that downregulation of MHC class I expression is the result of escape from T-cell attack and leads to a poorer clinical prognosis (349). Nevertheless, defective antigen presentation by tumor cells will prevent an effective direct immune attack by effector T cells (355). Even worse, an antigen that no longer serves as a target for destruction, because of loss of the MHC allele presenting it on the tumor cell surface, may prevent an effective immune response to the cancer cells. This may occur because this antigen can still be presented indirectly by host APCs and induce an immunodominant response (see next section) that excludes a response to possible target antigens on the cancer cells (341).

Selection of Antigen Loss or Epitope Loss Variants

During the slow, stepwise development of cancer from the original target cell, host selection should clearly favor the emergence of nonimmunogenic, nonrejectable tumor-cell variants. However, demonstrating such a mechanism by clinical studies is difficult, if not impossible, because the antigenicity cannot be known for the original single cancer cell, and there are no probes for the putative antigens. Nevertheless, a possible example of sequential changes consistent with immune selection in a patient at later stages of malignancy has been reported (356).

Loss of immunogenicity of tumors can be the result of serial transplantation (357,358), and heritable tumor variants showing increased malignant growth can be isolated from mice transplanted with immunogenic tumors. Some of these variants escaped immune destruction by having lost a CTL-recognized target antigen (39,44,191). The finding of such variants is consistent with the notion that selection for antigen loss variants may also occur naturally during tumor progression. However, loss of the antigenicity of the target molecule, rather than loss of its expression, may sometimes be the mechanism of escape. Cytolytic T cells usually recognize only a few discrete epitopes on even a large protein antigen, and point mutations leading to amino acid replacements in the peptide sequence of these epitopes may lead to loss of antigenicity. An example of such a mechanism was demonstrated by SV40 T gene–transformed cancer cells that have escaped destruction by CTLs in vitro (359). Analysis of such variants revealed point mutations in the amino acid sequences representing the CTL-recognized epitopes of the T antigen. This mechanism allowed the cancer cells not only to escape T-cell destruction, but also to continue to express a gene essential for maintaining malignant transformation. At present, it is uncertain whether this mechanism of escape is being used

for other virus-associated cancers. For example, mutational changes in the transforming genes E6 and E7 of HPV have not been observed in cervical cancer cells, while total or allelic loss of HLA class I expression is commonly observed in this cancer (353).

As mentioned earlier, experimental and human tumors have multiple tumor-specific CTL-recognized epitopes that are lost independently by selection with T cells in vitro (37,41,44). However, the host fails to recognize all antigens simultaneously on a tumor cell (360,361); recognition of the second antigen occurred only after the first antigen was lost by most of the tumor cells (360,361). This suggested that an immunodominant antigen by a tumor cell could prevent sensitization to other tumor antigens and in this way prevent immune attack on variants, thereby leading to sequential loss of the antigens from the tumor cells. A hierarchy in the immune response to multiple independent antigens has also been described in the study of immune responses to multiple minor histocompatibility antigens expressed on a single cell (362). The mechanism for this hierarchy is unclear in either system, and understanding how to break the hierarchy could help us to prevent immune selection and tumor escape. For example, studies in vitro using CTL clones suggest that the rate of mutation resulting in the loss of a single antigen from the tumor cells is less than 10^{-6}. Even if the frequency were as high as 10^{-4}, only one tumor cell that had lost four independent antigens would be expected in 10^{16} tumor cells (i.e., in a tumor larger than the human body). Thus, if the immune response of the host could be manipulated so that all four antigens were attacked simultaneously, no escape of tumors should occur. Experimental evidence suggests that immunization with in vitro selected tumor-cell variants expressing selective antigenic components can overcome immunodominance and prevent tumor escape (363).

Partial immune suppression may lead to the rapid selection and outgrowth of antigen loss variants (364). It was found that fully immunocompetent mice regularly rejected highly immunogenic regressor tumors with only very rare exceptions, while mice lacking T cell–mediated immunity (e.g., nude or x-irradiated thymectomized mice) did not select for antigen loss variants. In contrast, the tumors grew in UV-irradiated mice at a very high frequency, but all of the tumors were found to consist of heritably stable variants that had lost the CTL-defined rejection antigen. This was apparently because UV-irradiated mice show a partial immunocompetence, so that the generation of cytolytic T cells was delayed (360,365) until the tumor had reached a size that contained a sufficient number of antigen loss variants so that the tumor could escape. (Incomplete therapy of bacterial infections with antibiotic drugs also favors the outgrowth of variant bacterial strains that show heritable resistance to these drugs, so that, by analogy, partial or incomplete immunotherapy of cancer-bearing individuals may lead to selection of antigen loss variants.)

Antigenic Modulation

The phenomenon of antigenic modulation represents a reversible antibody-induced, complement-independent loss of an antigen from the surface of a cell. This phenomenon was first demonstrated with leukemia cells expressing the TL antigen (252,253,366). Mice expressing the TL antigen at a very low level (81) (TL mice) and immunized with TL+ leukemia cells developed high titers of anti-TL antibodies that lysed TL+ leukemia cells in vitro; nevertheless, the leukemia cells grew in vivo equally well in immunized and nonimmunized mice. Loss of sensitivity to anti-TL antibody and complement occurred because the antibody caused patching, capping, and disappearance of the TL antigen from the cell surface. Surface immunoglobulin is another cell surface protein that modulates upon exposure to specific antibody (367); however, several other cell surface antigens do not modulate, and it is not known why certain surface molecules are more susceptible to antigenic modulation than others.

Immunologic Enhancement and Blocking Factors

In the early days of transplantation immunology, it was found that mice preimmunized with disrupted cells of certain allogeneic tumors failed to reject challenge with the viable tumor, whereas normal mice rejected the same tumor after initial brief growth (368,369). Injecting immune serum into nonimmunized hosts sometimes enhanced tumor allografts also, and this was effective when given at the time of challenge or up to 1 week before or after tumor grafting. Furthermore, alloimmune antisera were found to protect target cells from lysis by allo-sensitized lymphocytes *in vitro* (370), suggesting a possible mechanism for enhancement *in vivo*. While the phenomenon of enhancement has clearly been demonstrated in allogeneic tumor systems, its relevance for immune responses to syngeneic tumors has remained uncertain (371,372). Antibody, complexes of tumor antigen and antibody (372), and shed antigen (373) have all been implicated in this phenomenon of blocking. Complexes of tumor antigen and antibody can induce suppressor T cells (374), which may play a role in the mechanism by which blocking factors function.

Immune Suppression or Immunodeficiency

In the earlier section, on immunosurveillance of tumor development, it was discussed that immune suppression and immune deficiencies [primary (inherited) or secondary (drug-induced) or AIDS] have an increased incidence of virally associated cancers.

Carcinogens

Many chemical and physical carcinogens used in experimental animals are immunosuppressive (234–238); for example, immune suppression by UV irradiation may in part be responsible for the outgrowth of highly immunogenic tumors (236,375). UV irradiation damages DNA, which leads to impaired function of APCs (376). Possibly as a result of this dysfunction, suppressor cells are induced in mice, the action of which can be demonstrated by adoptive transfer assays (375,377). Thus, it was found that lethally x-irradiated mice rejected UV-induced regressor tumors when reconstituted by intravenous injection of spleen and lymph node cells from normal mice; however, transferring a mixture of lymphoid cells from UV-irradiated and normal mice prevented the rejection of the regressor tumors by the recipients. Moreover, adoptive transfer of spleen cells from UV-irradiated mice also appeared to shorten the latency period of development of primary UV-induced tumors in the recipients (378). The UV-induced suppressor cells were not specific for an individual tumor, but instead suppressed immune responses to all syngeneic UV-induced tumors; however, the suppressor cells did not affect the capability of the reconstituted mice to reject allogeneic tumors.

Gamma radiation or certain chemotherapeutic drugs are carcinogenic as well as immunosuppressive in mice and humans. However, it is not clear whether immune suppression induced by chemical or physical carcinogens is important for tumor escape in humans. In most instances, humans are probably exposed to much lower doses of these carcinogens than are commonly given to experimental animals, and this may result in less immune suppression. However, the immunosuppressive effects of carcinogens may differ from species to species. This makes interpretation difficult, because cancer following exposure to these agents could develop as a result of carcinogenic action (379), as a result of suppression of immune responses to transformed cells or as a result of both types of actions.

Oncogenic viruses represent another interesting example of how the immunosuppressive component of a carcinogen can help tumor induction by preventing effective host immunity. For example, the E1A gene of the adenovirus (Ad) strain Ad12 suppresses MHC class I expression, which may permit escape from destruction by CTLs and lead to the formation of a tumor (380). However, reduced levels of MHC class I antigens may not be sufficient to explain the higher oncogenicity of the E1A gene of Ad12. For example, no correlation between the level of MHC class I expression and differences in tumorigenicity of Ad2 and Ad5 in immunocompetent syngeneic adult animals was found when mouse and hamster cells transformed with these viruses were examined (381). Another viral protein, P15E, that is encoded in murine RNA tumor viruses has been studied extensively for its immunosuppressive properties, and a P15E-related immunosuppressive antigen was found in human malignant cells (382).

Tumor Burden

In a number of different experimental tumor models and in humans, it has been well documented that the tumor-bearing host frequently has suppressed immune functions. Sometimes, the tumor cells themselves appear to release substances that are immunosuppressive, for example, prostaglandins, TGF-β, P15E, and probably several other yet-unidentified substances, which may suppress the immune system directly or indirectly. In other cases, tumors can invade the lymphoid tissue and thereby interfere with the immune responses. The mechanisms and magnitude and specificity of tumor-induced suppression probably differ widely for different cancers and at different stages of the cancers (383). The degree of immune suppression caused by a tumor burden can be profound: For example, it was found that mice bearing UV-induced or MCA-induced progressor tumors will fail to reject most immunogenic regressor tumors that are regularly rejected by normal mice (384). The capability of these mice to mount humoral immune responses to conventional antigen or to reject allogeneic tumors or normal skin grafts remained intact. Thus, similar to UV-induced immune suppression, immune responses to a number of independently derived tumors were affected, but other responses in these animals were not.

Tumor-bearing mice and cancer patients can have alterations in the signal-transduction machinery of systemic and/or tumor-associated T cells, beginning with a decrease in the NFkB p65 followed, after continued tumor growth, by loss of TCR ζ chain and p56 lck (385–390), and activated macrophages can secrete substances that induce these structural abnormalities (391). Maintenance of the suppression requires a continuous presence of the cancer, but residual tumor tissues remaining after incomplete tumor removal can be sufficient. However, suppression is short-lived after complete tumor removal and often gives way to specific immunity without further immunization (392). In some animal models, it has been shown convincingly by adoptive transfer experiments that the induction and maintenance of suppression requires T cells (384,393,394). In other tumor models (395), the suppressor cells had the phenotype of B cells or macrophages (396). As might be expected from the diversity of tumors, there also appears to be a large degree of variability in the specificity of the suppression. In some tumor models, immune suppression appeared to be selective for the tumor that induced suppression (394), whereas in other instances, the responses to a broad range of other tumors were suppressed (395). Even responses to conventional antigens can be suppressed, especially in instances in which the tumor originated from or invaded the immune system; for example, in patients with Hodgkin's disease, immune suppression often results in depressed delayed-type hypersensitivity to a wide variety of antigens and increased susceptibility to various types of infections. In certain tumor models, it has been shown that immune suppression by tumor burden may also prevent effective adoptive immunotherapy by immune T cells (397). Therefore, ionizing radiation, cyclophosphamide, or other agents have been used to pretreat animals before adoptive immunotherapy (397).

Radiation or Chemotherapeutic Agents

Treatment of patients with anticancer agents, such as chemotherapeutic radiomimetic drugs or ionizing radiation, can be very immunosuppressive. Lymphocytes are highly sensitive to destruction by many chemotherapeutic drugs and ionizing radiation, and, therefore, these same agents (e.g., cyclophosphamide) are also used to suppress deliberately immune responses for organ transplantation. As expected, the immunosuppression caused by these agents often leads to increased susceptibility to infection. In addition, many anticancer agents, such as cyclophosphamide, are mutagenic and carcinogenic (379). Induction of a second malignancy may therefore follow successful therapy of the first cancer as a late complication of successful chemotherapy or radiation therapy (379). Most second malignancies originate from the hematopoietic, lymphopoietic, and reticuloendothelial systems, which are the most sensitive direct targets of the immunosuppressive anticancer agents; similar types of malignancies are commonly seen in organ transplant patients who are treated with immunosuppressive drugs. The development of these secondary malignancies is related to direct carcinogenic effects of the anticancer agents on the lymphoreticular system or to immune suppression, which permits development of virally associated cancers.

Age

Some immune responses gradually decline with age (398), whereas the incidence of malignancy increases considerably with age. Thus, the increased incidence of cancer in old individuals could result from ineffective immunosurveillance. However, carcinogenesis requires multiple steps, and the length of the latency period of a tumor is usually inversely proportional to the dose of carcinogen. Many cancers may occur late in life simply because they were induced by a very low dose of carcinogens, which is associated with a long latency period, or exposure is cumulative

over many years. Experimentally, there is a decrease in immune responses to transplanted cancer with age. For example, murine UV-induced regressor tumors that are rejected by young syngeneic mice may grow progressively in untreated old mice (241,242). The defective immune responses in old individuals may prevent immune selection and allow tumors developing in old individuals to retain tumor antigens that can serve as targets for therapy. However, the development of effective immunotherapy of cancer in older individuals may also require rescuing the age-dependent immune deficiencies (243).

In summary, the induction, growth, and therapy of cancer are commonly associated with immune suppression and immune deficiencies. However, immune suppression does not lead to an increase in the common types of cancers. Instead, less common lymphoreticular and virally associated malignancies and skin cancer are significantly increased. In addition, the common occurrence of immune suppression and immune defects in cancer patients deserves important consideration when designing protocols for active or passive immunotherapy of cancer.

IMMUNOPREVENTION

As there is convincing evidence that immunosurveillance can prevent or reduce the incidence of cancers associated with certain viruses, active immunization against the viral capsid proteins may prevent infection. For example, DNA-free virus-like particles containing the coat proteins could be used (399). Such an approach is being tested for HPV-associated diseases and for HBV in an attempt to reduce the incidence of cervical and hepatocellular carcinoma. Other cancers, such as Kaposi's sarcoma associated with KSHV and human T-cell leukemia associated with HTLV-1, offer additional opportunities. Once infected, one may still be able to prevent the development of premalignant and malignant cells by immunizing against the viral transforming proteins, if they are expressed by the premalignant and malignant cells. Hamsters, for example, receiving a single inoculation of polyoma or SV40 virus at birth, develop a high incidence of primary tumors several months later (400); however, tumor incidence was reduced if a second dose of the virus, or irradiated tumor cells transformed by this virus, were given during the latency period. The neonatally inoculated hamsters were obviously not tolerant because they generated a protective response when exposed to the same antigen later. With a single inoculation of virus, the neoplastic clones apparently escape unnoticed by the immune system. Additional immunization with a sufficient dose of antigens during the latency period between virus inoculation and tumor development could prevent this problem and reduce the tumor incidence. In HPV-infected humans, cervical cancers may be prevented by inducing immunity to T cell-recognized epitopes on the transforming HPV proteins E6 and E7, expressed by the virus-induced premalignant lesions in patients at early stages of the disease (dysplasia) before carcinoma *in situ* or invasive cancer occurs (for review, see ref. 164). It is important to determine whether cancer may also be prevented by active immunization of cancer-prone individuals carrying a predisposing mutation. An ever-increasing number of such mutations is being identified that encode tumor-specific proteins in cells in these individuals. However, inducing immune responses against them may be problematic because these proteins are self. For example, active immunization against an oncogenic viral protein encoded by a transgene became ineffective in preventing cancer development in the cancer-prone mice when the immunization was begun after the oncogenic protein was expressed in premalignant host tissues, suggesting induction of peripheral tolerance (401).

IMMUNOTHERAPY

Multiple immunotherapeutic strategies involving innate or acquired immunity have been developed to control cancer; they include (a) local application of a live bacterial vaccine, BCG; (b) use of cytokines; (c) active immunization; (d) passive therapy with antibodies; and (e) adoptive transfer of effector cells. Very few immunotherapeutic approaches are clearly effective or the treatment of choice (102). One example is the topical use of BCG for treating patients with residual superficial bladder cancer, which typically recurs following surgery (402). Repeated instillation of the live mycobacteria into the bladder by way of a catheter after surgery has become the treatment of choice for superficial bladder cancer. The local infection with BCG leads to a prolonged inflammatory response in the bladder wall, which reduces significantly the risk of cancer recurrence (402). Interestingly, the first attempts of nonspecific immunotherapy by intratumoral injection of bacteria were more than 100 years ago (403–405). Another approach of nonspecific immunotherapy uses the local or systemic application of cytokines. For example, IL-12 has shown promising antitumor effects in animal experiments (406); some of the effects of this cytokine seem to depend on simultaneous presence of T cells. Cytokines act physiologically at short range between cells, and this may explain the toxicity commonly observed with systemic cytokine applications.

Immunotherapy that uses acquired immunity (i.e., tumor antigens or effector cells and molecules specific for them) can, in principle, be divided into (a) active therapeutic immunization, (b) adoptive transfer of T cells, and (c) passive therapy with antibodies. It is important to know that, by attempting active therapeutic vaccination, tumor immunologists have taken an approach that has been completely abandoned in the clinical management of infectious diseases, except for rabies, which has a particularly long incubation period. Cancer cells have a slower generation time than most infectious organisms, and most of the bulk of the tumor load can often be removed by other therapy (e.g., surgery). At the time when the antigen load is the lowest, the suppressive environment may be removed, and active immunization may lead to an effective therapeutic immune response. The critical question, therefore, is whether residual and dormant cancers can be treated effectively by active immunization.

When considering immunotherapy of cancer, the distinction between immunogenicity and immunosensitivity of cancer cells is important. Certain cancer cells may be fully sensitive to tumor-specific T cells or antibodies but, for various reasons, fail to induce an immune response. Experimental studies suggest that such cancers may still be rejected if specific effector T cells or antibodies can be induced. This requires effective immunization against the relevant target antigen on the tumor cells. The reasons for a poor immunogenicity of the target antigen on the tumor cells may vary; therefore, different methods must be used for different cancers to immunize effectively against it (407). Also, either T cells or antibodies might be most effective therapeutically; therefore, different methods of immunization may have to be used to induce preferentially one or the other. Immunization with viable tumor cells may cause cancer and kill the host, whereas dead and disrupted tumor cells, membrane fractions, or cell extracts are usually poor immunogens and may enhance the growth of the cancer. One way to circumvent this problem is to destroy the proliferative potential of the tumor cells while leaving the cells viable and metabolically active, at least temporarily. For example, this can be done by exposing the cells to gamma radiation or certain cytostatic chemicals, such as mitomycin C. These methods alone are often insufficient to elicit a cytolytic T-cell response to cancer cells. Many strategies have been designed to increase the immunogenicity of the tumor-cell inoculum (Fig. 7). One approach is to increase the antigenicity of the tumor cell by (a) *heterogenization* of the tumor cells by infection with certain viruses (408–410), somatic cell fusion with various nontumorigenic cells (411–413), transfection of self or foreign MHC class I or class II molecules (118,414,415), hapten conjugation (416,417), or exposure to mutagens (418); (b) transfection of tumor cells to express the B7 ligand that can provide a costimulating signal to T cells (415,419,420); (c) coinjection of tumor cells with killed bacteria, such as *Corynebacterium parvum* (421,422); and (d) transfection of tumor cells to produce certain cytokines (423,424), such as IL-2, IFN-γ, IL-4, IL-6, IL-7, G-CSF, granulocyte–macrophage colony-stimulating factor (GM-CSF), or TNF. At present, GM-CSF appears to be particularly attractive, because this cytokine leads to the recruitment and activation of dendritic cells, which are powerful APCs. Finally, tumor cells have been transfected to express antisense RNA of a required growth factor (425). This transfection results in terminal differentiation in the cancer cells and increased immunogenicity for unknown reasons. In fact, irrespective of which particular genetic engineering of the tumor cells is used to decrease their growth potential *in vivo*, rejection of the modified tumor cells is often followed by T cell-mediated immunity against the unmodified tumor cells. It is possible that the growth arrest and ultimate rejection of the altered, but metabolically viable, cancer cells result in a prolonged exposure to the antigen that allows T-cell immunity to develop.

Pure antigens are often ineffective in inducing an acquired (i.e., antigen-specific immune response) unless certain "adjuvants" are used to stimulate innate immunity, which in turn helps the generation of an antigen-specific response. Therefore, numerous approaches are designed to stimulate innate immunity at the site of vaccinations by the use of chemical and/or bacterial agents. Synthetic peptides used in vaccines have to be designed for particular MHC haplotypes and may be ineffective or even "tolerize" the host (426); delivering antigenic peptides after loading to heat-shock protein (or as recombinant virus-like particles) can increase the efficacy of immunization. Effective induction of an immune response requires antigen presentation in an environment that provides appropriate help or secondary signals. Therefore, several experimental designs use dendritic cells pulsed with virus-specific or tumor-associated peptides to induce tumor-reactive T cells and rejection of transplanted tumor cells. Dendritic cells can be loaded with (a) synthetic antigenic peptides or (b) recombinant proteins. Dendritic cells can also be loaded with (a) native peptides stripped from tumor cell surfaces; (b) tumor-derived, peptide-loaded heat-shock proteins; and (c) tumor-derived m-RNA; or (d) by fusion of tumor cells (for review, see ref. 427). One advantage of the latter three strategies is that powerful immunity to (unique) individually distinct tumor antigens, as well as tumor-associated antigen, can be induced without having to identify the antigens. The limitation of these customized approaches that use molecularly unidentified antigens is that the antigen dose cannot be standardized.

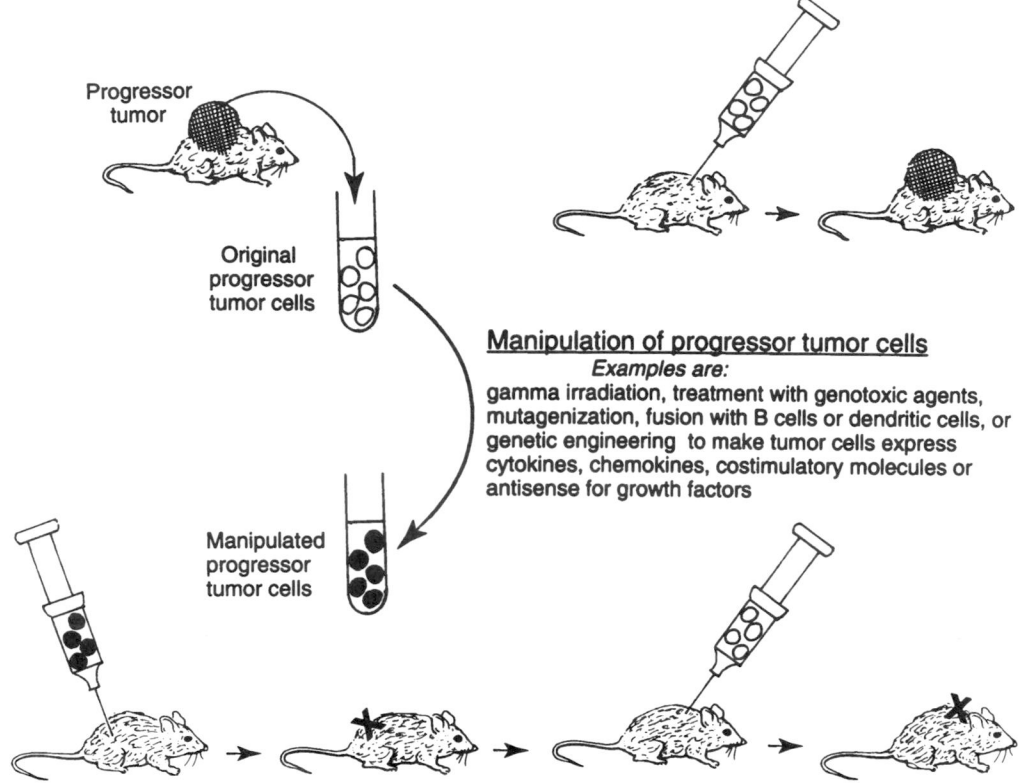

FIG. 7. Many different methods can be used to increase the immunogenicity of spontaneous or experimentally induced tumor cells. Poorly immunogenic tumor cells will kill normal syngeneic hosts when transplanted (progressor tumors). The various manipulations listed in the text and the illustration all result in metabolically active tumor cells that fail to form tumors when injected into normal syngeneic mice [i.e., the inocula are rejected (*x*)]. In addition, these mice are often protected against subsequent challenge with the unmodified tumor cells. Thus, the manipulated tumor cells can serve as a preventive vaccine. However, the use of such manipulated cells for therapeutic vaccination (not shown here) seems to be restricted almost invariably to very early stages of tumor growth, usually a few days to less than 2 weeks to tumor growth. For longer established tumors (which may be more comparable to human cancers when they are clinically detected in the patients), the efficiency of the active therapeutic vaccination using these methods usually is reduced dramatically.

For tumor antigens that are identified molecularly, recombinant vaccines have been developed using vaccinia, *listeria,* or virus-like particles. Other strategies of active immunization include genetic vaccination (428), for example, by injecting naked DNA plasmid constructs, intramuscularly encoding the tumor antigen [whereby the gene for GM-CSF may also be used to improve the presentation of the antigen by dendritic cells at the site of injection 429)], or vaccination with antiidiotypic antibodies, which bear the internal image of a tumor antigen (430). It is hoped that some of these novel ways of active immunization will be effective against cancers, particularly in patients with clinically undetectable (residual or dormant) cancers or premalignant lesions. Whether any of these procedures will be effective against longer established or advanced stages of cancer is questionable because therapeutic effects of active immunization in experimental tumor transplant models are usually limited to early stages of malignant growth.

The major alternative to active immunization is passive antibody therapy or adoptive transfer of tumor-specific T cells. In certain experimental tumor models, passive immunization with antibody can protect against challenge with tumor cells and can be therapeutic when given soon after challenge with the cancer cells (e.g., see ref. 106). Thus, the antibody is usually given simultaneously or

only a few hours or days after tumor-cell challenge. Passive immunization of patients with a murine monoclonal antibody against a tumor-associated antigen on human colon cancer has been found to reduce the incidence of metastatic spread and to increase long-term survival when treatment is begun shortly after surgery in patients with no clinically detectable metastatic spread or residual disease (104,105). Antiidiotypic antibody treatment of an experimental B-cell leukemia appears to be effective in inducing the cancer cells to go into a long-lasting dormant state (431), and antiidiotypic antibodies are being used in the treatment of patients with B-cell lymphoma (151) (also see section on clonal antigens). Some therapeutic effects have also been observed in patients treated with other murine monoclonal antibodies (151,432,433). However, therapeutic effectiveness of monoclonal antibody in treating well-established advanced human cancer is uncertain. It will, therefore, be important to determine the conditions under which antibody therapy can be successful and which of a large number of possible mechanisms are responsible for tumor escape from the therapeutic effects of antibodies. Because antibody-induced tumor regression may occur weeks after treatment (432,433), direct antibody-mediated tumor-cell lysis sometimes may not be the mechanism of the antitumor effect. Other approaches used antibodies to growth factor receptors on cancer cells for inhibiting cancer growth. For example, the oncogene neu-1/HER2 encodes a growth factor receptor that is overexpressed on certain cancers, and monoclonal antibodies to this antigen have been found to inhibit tumor growth (434,435), possibly by inducing differentiation (436). Similarly, antibodies to the IL-2 receptors can cause tumor regression in patients with cutaneous T-cell lymphoma (437). Considerable technologic efforts are being made to enhance the ability of antibodies to kill tumor cells by using them as carriers for cytokines or cytotoxic agents, such as radiochemicals or natural toxins (438,439). The recombinant antibody-cytokine or antibody-toxin fusion proteins may be useful to concentrate these agents in the stroma surrounding the tumor cells, but some of these coupled antibodies may have serious toxicity unless selective delivery of the conjugates to the tumor is achieved. An alternative, possibly fruitful approach is the engineering of bispecific monoclonal antibodies that bind effector cells as well as tumor antigens on the cancer cells. Murine monoclonal antibodies have also been "humanized" to reduce the stimulation of neutralizing antimurine antibodies by the patients. The clinical usefulness of these various engineered antibody molecules will remain unknown until necessary clinical trials in patients have been carried out. Alternative immunotherapeutic approaches that are being developed utilize monoclonal antibodies specific for regulatory and activation molecules expressed on T cells (327,328) to increase their antitumor activity.

With most presently available immunotherapeutic procedures tested in animal experiments, therapeutic efficiency occurs in relatively early stages following tumor transplantation, and experimental studies are lacking that test the therapeutic efficacy in mice with small tumor loads of long established cancer that is dormant and/or remains after surgery or chemotherapy. Adoptive transfer of T cells may be more effective with longer established tumor loads. It is uncertain, however, which antigens will be the most effective target molecules on human cancers and in which way specific T cells should be generated *in vitro* so that they are effective *in vivo* upon adoptive transfer. T cells that have been isolated from the patients can be expanded *in vitro* with IL-2 and then infused into patients who receive IL-2 as well. In a selected group of patients with melanoma, favorable responses were observed in several patients, and an apparent cure was seen in one patient (440). It is not clear whether insufficient specificity of the T cells or failure of these cells to localize specifically is responsible for the difficulty in achieving permanent therapeutic effects. Early evidence suggests that adoptive transfer of T cells may be effective against EBV-associated lymphomas developing in immunocompromized patients (163), but much more work remains before this approach is applicable to other tumors.

CONCLUSIONS

Cancer immunology is at the interphase of two extraordinarily complex fields of research. Cancers generally harbor (and are caused by) multiple cancer-specific mutations, many of which have not been defined but may be detected by T cells. Cancer specific mutations that can be functionally important are the basis for individually distinct (unique) tumor antigens, and it is now certain that truly tumor-specific antigens indeed exist. There are also tumor-nonspecific, nonmutant antigens to which the host can also respond. Some of these normal-self antigens are not found on normal cells of the lineage of tumor origin; instead, the expression of these antigens on normal cells appears to be highly restricted to

spermatogonia and trophoblast cells. These antigens may therefore have a particular diagnostic and therapeutic potential. However, it is uncertain whether immunity to normal-self antigens can be highly effective against cancers without causing deleterious autoimmunity.

Surveillance by adaptive immunity protects us from many infectious agents and prevents, or at least reduces, the incidence of certain cancers caused by viruses such as EBV or HPV. Therefore, researchers are currently trying to prevent infection or the growth of the virally transformed cells by active immunization. However, preventive vaccination, which is extensively used for protecting against infectious diseases, may not be feasible for most cancers. A great diversity of mechanisms has been identified that may contribute to the failure of antigenic cancers to be destroyed by the host's immune system. This understanding of basic regulatory mechanisms and molecules offers hope for finding new ways to counteract tumor escape. Much evidence suggests that the local environment surrounding tumor cells may prevent the effective immunity against established solid tumors, cause dormancy of metastatic cells, or promote recurrence, but the critical mechanisms still need to be defined. In particular, we need a better understanding of the mechanisms whereby inflammation or regulatory T cells can lead to tumor promotion or tumor inhibition. The availability of genetically engineered tumor cells and mouse strains offers many important new models for examining fundamental issues of self-nonself discrimination and inflammation, and elucidates the mechanisms of tumor escape, promotion, and progression, but there still is a lack of models for tumor dormancy and recurrence.

With the rapid advances in biotechnology and in our understanding of cancer and of the immune system, numerous new immunotherapeutic strategies for cancer are being developed and must be examined in preclinical models for their potential usefulness. Even though therapeutic active vaccination has been all but abandoned in the clinical management of infectious disease, numerous novel methods of active immunization are being developed that may prove to be effective in cancer. In addition, passive antibody therapy and adoptive T-cell therapy offer important alternative approaches. Together, there is great promise that tumor immunology can be exploited not only to increase further our understanding of cancer biology and immunology, but also to significantly improve the diagnosis and therapy of cancer, though caution is still very much warranted.

REFERENCES

1. Cotran R, Kumar V, Robbins S. *Neoplasia: pathologic basis of disease.* Philadelphia: WB Saunders, 1994:241–303.
2. Kinzler KW, Vogelstein B. Lessons from hereditary colorectal cancer. *Cell* 1996; 87:159–170.
3. Weinberg RA. How cancer arises. *Sci Am* 1996;275:62–70.
4. Schottenfeld D, Fraumeni JF Jr. *Cancer epidemiology and prevention.* 2nd ed. New York: Oxford University Press, 1996:1–1521.
5. Williams GM, Iatropoulos MJ, Weisburger JH. Chemical carcinogen mechanisms of action and implications for testing methodology. *Exp Toxicol Pathol* 1996;48:101–111.
6. Rous P, Beard J. The progression to carcinoma of virus induced rabbit papillomas (Shope). *J Exp Med* 1935;62:523–528.
7. Foulds L. The experimental study of tumor progression. A review. *Cancer Res* 1954;14:327–339.
8. Nowell PC. Mechanisms of tumor progression. *Cancer Res* 1986;46:2203–2207.
9. Ehrlich P. Über den jetzigen Stand der Karzinomforschung. *Ned Tijdschr Geneeskd* 1909;5:273–290.
10. Woglom WH. Immunity to transplantable tumors. *Cancer Rev* 1929;4:129–214.
11. Gorer PA. Some recent work on tumor immunity. *Adv Cancer Res* 1956;4: 149–186.

12. Andervont HB. The use of pure strain animals in studies on natural resistance to transplantable tumors. *Public Health Rep* 1937;52:1885–1895.

13. Gross L. Intradermal immunization of C3H mice against a sarcoma that originated in an animal of the same line. *Cancer Res* 1943;3:326–333.

14. Foley EJ. Antigenic properties of methylcholanthrene-induced tumors in mice of the strain of origin. *Cancer Res* 1953;13:835–837.

15. Baldwin RW. Immunity to methylcholanthrene-induced tumors-inbred rats following atrophy and regression of implanted tumors. *Br J Cancer* 1955;9: 652–665.

16. Prehn RT, Main JM. Immunity to methylcholanthrene-induced sarcomas. *J Natl Cancer Inst* 1957;18:769–778.

17. Klein G, Sögren HO, Klein E, Hellström KE. Demonstration of resistance against methylcholanthrene-induced sarcomas in the primary autochthonous host. *Cancer Res* 1960;20:1561–1572.

18. Old LJ, Boyse EA, Clarke DA, Carswell EA. Antigenic properties of chemically-induced tumors. *Ann NY Acad Sci* 1962;101:80–106.

19. Globerson A, Feldman M. Antigenic specificity of benzo(a) pyrene-induced sarcomas. *J Natl Cancer Inst* 1964;32:1229–1243.

20. Bailey DW. How pure are inbred strains of mice? *Immunol Today* 1982;3:210–214.

21. Pasternak G, Graffi A, Horn K-H. Der Nachweis individual specifischer Antigenität bei UV-induzierten Sarkomen der Maus. *Acta Biol Med Ger* 1964;13: 276–279.

22. Kripke ML. Antigenicity of murine skin tumors induced by ultraviolet light. *J Natl Cancer Inst* 1974;53:1333–1336.

23. Vaage J. Nonvirus-associated antigens in virus-induced mouse mammary tumors. *Cancer Res* 1968;28:2477–2483.

24. Morton DL, Miller GF, Wood DA. Demonstration of tumor-specific immunity against antigens unrelated to the mammary tumor virus in spontaneous mammary adenocarcinomas. *J Natl Cancer Inst* 1969;42:289–301.

25. Carswell EA, Wanebo HJ, Old U, Boyse EA. Immunogenic properties of reticulum cell sarcomas of SJL/J mice. *J Natl Cancer Inst* 1970;44:1281–1288.

26. Basombrio MA. Search for common antigenicities among twenty-five sarcomas induced by methylcholanthrene. *Cancer Res* 1970;30:2458–2462.

27. Basombrio MA, Prehn RT. Studies on the basis for diversity and time of appearance of antigens in chemically induced tumors. *Natl Cancer Inst Monogr* 1972; 35:117–124.

28. Van den Eynde B, Lethe B, Van Pel A, De Plaen E, Boon T. The gene coding for a major tumor rejection antigen of tumor P815 is identical to the normal gene of syngeneic DBA/2 mice. *J Exp Med* 1991;173:1373–1384.

29. Ramarathinam L, Sarma S, Maric M, et al. Multiple lineages of tumors express a common tumor antigen, P1A, but they are not cross-protected. *J Immunol* 1995;155:5323–5329.

30. Donawho C, Kripke ML. Immunogenicity and cross-reactivity of syngeneic murine melanomas. *Cancer Commun* 1980;2:101–107.

31. Spellman CW, Daynes RA. Ultraviolet light induced murine suppressor lymphocytes dictate specificity of anti-ultraviolet tumor immune responses. *Cell Immunol* 1978;38:25–34.

32. Leffell MS, Coggin JH Jr. Common transplantation antigens on methylcholanthrene-induced murine sarcomas detected by three assays of tumor rejection. *Cancer Res* 1977;37:4112–4119.

33. Van Waes C, Urban JL, Rothstein JL, Ward PL, Schreiber H. Highly malignant tumor variants retain tumor-specific antigens recognized by T helper cells. *J Exp Med* 1986;164:1547–1565.

34. Brent L, Medawar P. Quantitative studies on tissue transplantation immunity. The effects of irradiation. *Proc R Soc Lond B Biol Sci* 1966;165:413–423.

35. Srivastava PK. Do human cancers express shared protective antigens? or the necessity of remembrance of things past. *Semin Immunol* 1996;8:295–302.

36. Rouse BT, Röllinghoff M, Warner NL. Anti-theta serum-induced suppression of the cellular transfer of tumour-specific immunity to a syngeneic plasma cell tumour. *Nat New Biol* 1972;238:116–117.

37. Ward PL, Koeppen H, Hurteau T, Schreiber H. Tumor antigens defined by cloned immunological probes are highly polymorphic and are not detected on autologous normal cells. *J Exp Med* 1989;170:217–232.

38. Wortzel RD, Urban JL, Schreiber H. Malignant growth in the normal host after variant selection in vitro with cytolytic T-cell lines. *Proc Natl Acad Sci USA* 1984;81:2186–2190.

39. Ward PL, Koeppen HK, Hurteau T, Rowley DA, Schreiber H. Major histocompatibility complex class I and unique antigen expression by murine tumors that escaped from CD8+ T-cell-dependent surveillance. *Cancer Res* 1990;50: 3851–2858.

40. Koeppen H, Rowley DA, Schreiber H. Tumor-specific antigens and immunological resistance to cancer. In: Steinman RM, North RJ, eds. *Mechanisms of host resistance for infectious agents, tumors and allografts.* New York: Rockefeller University Press, 1986:359–386.

41. Wortzel RD, Philipps C, Schreiber H. Multiple tumour-specific antigens expressed on a single tumour cell. *Nature* 1983;304:165–167.

42. Knuth A, Wölfel T, Klehmann E, Boon T, Meyer zum Buschenfelde KH. Cytolytic T-cell clones against an autologous human melanoma: specificity study and definition of three antigens by immunoselection. *Proc Natl Acad Sci USA* 1989;86:2804–2808.

43. Van den Eynde B, Hainaut P, Herin M, et al. Presence on a human melanoma of multiple antigens recognized by autologous CTL. *Int J Cancer* 1989;44: 634–640.

44. Uyttenhove C, Maryanski J, Boon T. Escape of mouse mastocytoma P815 after nearly complete rejection is due to antigen-loss variants rather than immunosuppression. *J Exp Med* 1983;157:1040–1052.

45. Burnet FM. A certain symmetry: histocompatibility antigens compared with immunocyte receptors. *Nature* 1970;226:123–126.

46. Lampson LA, Levy R. A role for clonal antigens in cancer diagnosis and therapy. *J Natl Cancer Inst* 1979;62:217–220.

47. Embleton MJ, Heidelberger C. Antigenicity of mouse prostate transformed in vitro. *Int J Cancer* 1972;9:8–18.

48. Basombrio MA, Prehn RT. Antigenic diversity of tumors chemically induced within the progeny of a single cell. *Int J Cancer* 1972;10:1–8.

49. Hood L, Huang HV, Dreyer WJ. The area-code hypothesis: the immune system provides clues to understanding the genetic and molecular basis of cell recognition during development. *J Suprastruct* 1977;7:531–559.

50. Srivastava PK, Old LJ. Individually distinct transplantation antigens of chemically induced mouse tumors. *Immunol Today* 1988;9:78–83.

51. Lurquin C, Van Pel A, Mariame B, et al. Structure of the gene of tum-transplantation antigen P91A: the mutated exon encodes a peptide recognized with Ld by cytolytic T cells. *Cell* 1989;58:293–303.

52. Mandelboim O, Berke G, Fridkin M, Feldman M, Eisenstein M, Eisenbach L. CTL induction by a tumour-associated antigen octapeptide derived from a murine lung carcinoma. *Nature* 1994;369:67–71.

53. Uenaka A, Ono T, Akisawa T, Wada H, Yasuda T, Nakayama E. Identification of a unique antigen peptide pRL1 on BALB/c RL male 1 leukemia recognized by cytotoxic T lymphocytes and its relation to the Akt oncogene. *J Exp Med* 1994;180:1599–1607.

54. de Bergeyck V, De Plaen E, Chomez P, Boon T, Van Pel A. An intracisternal A-particle sequence codes for an antigen recognized by syngeneic cytolytic T lymphocytes on a mouse spontaneous leukemia. *Eur J Immunol* 1994;24: 2203–2212.

55. Ikeda H, Ohta N, Furukawa K, et al. Mutated mitogen-activated protein kinase: a tumor rejection antigen of mouse sarcoma. *Proc Natl Acad Sci USA* 1997;94:6375–6379.

56. Monach PA, Meredith SC, Siegel CT, Schreiber H. A unique tumor antigen produced by a single amino acid substitution. *Immunity* 1995;2:45–59.

57. Coulie PG, Lehmann F, Lethe B, et al. A mutated intron sequence codes for an antigenic peptide recognized by cytolytic T lymphocytes on a human melanoma. *Proc Natl Acad Sci USA* 1995;92:7976–7980.

58. Wölfel T, Hauer M, Schneider J, et al. A p16INK4a-insensitive CDK4 mutant targeted by cytolytic T lymphocytes in a human melanoma. *Science* 1995;269:1281–1284.

59. Robbins PF, El-Gamil M, Li YF, et al. A mutated beta-catenin gene encodes a melanoma-specific antigen recognized by tumor infiltrating lymphocytes. *J Exp Med* 1996;183:1185–1192.

60. Brändle D, Brasseur F, Weynants P, Boon T, Van den Eynde B. A mutated HLA-A2 molecule recognized by autologous cytotoxic T lymphocytes on a human renal cell carcinoma. *J Exp Med* 1996;183:2501–2508.

61. Dubey P, Hendrickson RC, Meredith SC, et al. The immunodominant antigen of an ultraviolet-induced regressor tumor is generated by a somatic point mutation in the DEAD box helicase p68. *J Exp Med* 1997;185:695–705.

62. Zuo L, Weger J, Yang Q, et al. Germline mutations in the p16INK4a binding domain of CDK4 in familial melanoma. *Nat Genet* 1996;12:97–99.

63. Rubinfeld B, Robbins P, El-Gamil M, Albert I, Porfiri E, Polakis P. Stabilization of beta-catenin by genetic defects in melanoma cell lines. *Science* 1997;275:1790–1792.

64. Mumberg D, Wick M, Schreiber H. Unique tumor antigens redefined as mutant tumor-specific antigens. *Semin Immunol* 1996;8:289–293.

65. Boon T, van der Bruggen P. Human tumor antigens recognized by T lymphocytes. *J Exp Med* 1996;183:725–729.

66. Disis ML, Cheever MA. Oncogenic proteins as tumor antigens. *Curr Opin Immunol* 1996;8:637–642.

67. Pullano TG, Sinn E, Carney WP. Characterization of monoclonal antibody R256, specific for activated ras p21 with arginine at 12, and analysis of breast carcinoma of v-Harvey-ras transgenic mouse. *Oncogene* 1989;4:1003–1008.

68. Feramisco JR, Clark R, Wong G, Arnheim N, Milley R, McCormick F. Transient reversion of ras oncogene-induced cell transformation by antibodies specific for amino acid 12 of ras protein. *Nature* 1985;314:639–642.

69. Jung S, Schluesener HJ. Human T lymphocytes recognize a peptide of single point-mutated, oncogenic ras proteins. *J Exp Med* 1991;173:273–276.

70. Peace DJ, Chen W, Nelson H, Cheever MA. T cell recognition of transforming proteins encoded by mutated ras proto-oncogenes. *J Immunol* 1991;146: 2059–2065.

71. Skipper J, Stauss HJ. Identification of two cytotoxic T lymphocyte-recognized epitopes in the Ras protein. *J Exp Med* 1993;177:1493–1498.

72. Peace DJ, Smith JW, Chen W, et al. Lysis of ras oncogene-transformed cells by specific cytotoxic T lymphocytes elicited by primary in vitro immunization with mutated ras peptide. *J Exp Med* 1994;179:473–479.

73. Abrams SI, Stanziale SF, Lunin SD, Zaremba S, Schlom J. Identification of overlapping epitopes in mutant ras oncogene peptides that activate CD4+ and CD8+ T cell responses. *Eur J Immunol* 1996;26:435–443.

74. Van Elsas A, Nijman HW, Van der Minne CE, et al. Induction and characterization of cytotoxic T-lymphocytes recognizing a mutated p21ras peptide presented by HLA-A*0201. *Int J Cancer* 1995;61:389–396.

75. Fossum B, Olsen AC, Thorsby E, Gaudernack G. CD8+ T cells from a patient with colon carcinoma, specific for a mutant p21-Ras-derived peptide (Gly13→Asp), are cytotoxic towards a carcinoma cell line harbouring the same mutation. *Cancer Immunol Immunother* 1995;40:165–172.

76. Yin L, Thomas C, Hsuan JJ, Stauss HJ. Unconventional cytotoxic T lymphocyte recognition of synthetic peptides corresponding to residues 1-23 of Ras protein. *Eur J Immunol* 1994;24:1988–1992.

77. Fenton RG, Keller CJ, Hanna N, Taub DD. Induction of T-cell immunity against Ras oncoproteins by soluble protein or Ras-expressing Escherichia coli. *J Natl Cancer Inst* 1995;87:1853–1861.

78. Carbone G, Borrello MG, Molla A, et al. Activation of ras oncogenes and expression of tumor-specific transplantation antigens in methylcholanthrene-induced murine fibrosarcomas. *Int J Cancer* 1991;47:619–625.

79. Abrams SI, Hand PH, Tsang KY, Schlom J. Mutant ras epitopes as targets for cancer vaccines. *Semin Oncol* 1996;23:118–134.

80. Gjertsen MK, Bakka A, Breivik J, et al. Vaccination with mutant ras peptides and induction of T-cell responsiveness in pancreatic carcinoma patients carrying the corresponding RAS mutation. *Lancet* 1995;346:1399–1400.

81. DeLeo AB, Jay G, Appella E, Dubois GC, Law LW, Old LJ. Detection of a transformation-related antigen in chemically induced sarcomas and other transformed cells of the mouse. *Proc Natl Acad Sci USA* 1979;76:2420–2424.

82. Lane DP, Crawford LV. T antigen is bound to a host protein in SV40-transformed cells. *Nature* 1979;278:261–263.

83. Linzer DI, Maltzman W, Levine AJ. The SV40 A gene product is required for the production of a 54,000 MW cellular tumor antigen. *Virology* 1979;98:308–318.

84. Vogelstein B, Kinzler KW. p53 function and dysfunction. *Cell* 1992;70:523–526.

85. Hollstein M, Sidransky D, Vogelstein B, Harris CC. p53 mutations in human cancers. *Science* 1991;253:49–53.

86. Gannon JV, Greaves R, Iggo R, Lane DP. Activating mutations in p53 produce a common conformational effect. A monoclonal antibody specific for the mutant form. *EMBO J* 1990;9:1595–1602.

87. Davidoff AM, Iglehart JD, Marks JR. Immune response to p53 is dependent upon p53/HSP70 complexes in breast cancers. *Proc Natl Acad Sci USA* 1992;89:3439–3442.

88. Houbiers JG, van der Burg SH, van de Watering LM, et al. Antibodies against p53 are associated with poor prognosis of colorectal cancer. *Br J Cancer* 1995;72:637–641.

89. Noguchi Y, Richards EC, Chen YT, Old LJ. Influence of interleukin 12 on p53 peptide vaccination against established Meth A sarcoma. *Proc Natl Acad Sci USA* 1995;92:2219–2223.

90. Theobald M, Biggs J, Dittmer D, Levine AJ, Sherman LA. Targeting p53 as a general tumor antigen. *Proc Natl Acad Sci USA* 1995;92:11993–11997.

91. Melief CJ, Offringa R, Toes RE, Kast WM. Peptide-based cancer vaccines. *Curr Opin Immunol* 1996;8:651–657.

92. Humphrey PA, Gangarosa LM, Wong AJ, et al. Deletion-mutant epidermal growth factor receptor in human gliomas: effects of type II mutation on receptor function. *Biochem Biophys Res Commun* 1991;178:1413–1420.

93. Humphrey PA, Wong AJ, Vogelstein B, et al. Anti-synthetic peptide antibody reacting at the fusion junction of deletion-mutant epidermal growth factor receptors in human glioblastoma. *Proc Natl Acad Sci USA* 1990;87:4207–4211.

94. Solomon E, Borrow J, Goddard AD. Chromosome aberrations and cancer. *Science* 1991;254:1153–1160.

95. Rowley JD. A new consistent chromosomal abnormality in chronic myelogenous leukaemia identified by quinacrine fluorescence and Giemsa staining. *Nature* 1973;243:290–293.

96. Sato Y, Rowley JD. Chromosome abnormalities in hematologic malignant diseases. In: Nathan DG, Orkin SH, Lantiqua CJ, eds. *Hemotology of infancy and childhood*. Philadelphia: WB Saunders, 1998:1147–1182.

97. Shtivelman E, Lifshitz B, Gale RP, Canaani E. Fused transcript of abl and bcr genes in chronic myelogenous leukaemia. *Nature* 1985;315:550–554.

98. van Denderen J, Hermans A, Meeuwsen T, et al. Antibody recognition of the tumor-specific bcr-abl joining region in chronic myeloid leukemia. *J Exp Med* 1989;169:87–98.

99. Bosch GJ, Joosten AM, Kessler JH, Melief CJ, Leeksma OC. Recognition of BCR-ABL positive leukemic blasts by human CD4+ T cells elicited by primary in vitro immunization with a BCR-ABL breakpoint peptide. *Blood* 1996;88:3522–3527.

100. Rettig WJ, Old LJ. Immunogenetics of human cell surface differentiation. *Annu Rev Immunol* 1989;7:481–511.

101. Brown JP, Woodbury RG, Hart CE, Hellstrom I, Hellstrom KE. Quantitative analysis of melanoma-associated antigen p97 in normal and neoplastic tissues. *Proc Natl Acad Sci USA* 1981;78:539–543.

102. Oettgen HF, Old LJ. The history of cancer immunotherapy. In: DeVita VT, Hellman S, Rosenberg SA, eds. *Biologic therapy of cancer.* Philadelphia: Lippincott, 1991:87–119.

103. Uyttenhove C, Godfraind C, Lethe B, et al. The expression of mouse gene P1A in testis does not prevent safe induction of cytolytic T cells against a P1A-encoded tumor antigen. *Int J Cancer* 1997;70:349–356.

104. Riethmuller G, Holz E, Schlimok G, et al. Monoclonal antibody therapy for resected Dukes' C colorectal cancer: seven-year outcome of a multicenter randomized trial. *J Clin Oncol* 1998;16:1788–1794.

105. Riethmüller G, Schneider-Gadicke E, Schlimok G, et al. Randomised trial of monoclonal antibody for adjuvant therapy of resected Dukes' C colorectal carcinoma. German Cancer Aid 17-1A Study Group. *Lancet* 1994;343:1177–1183.

106. Herlyn DM, Steplewski Z, Herlyn MF, Koprowski H. Inhibition of growth of colorectal carcinoma in nude mice by monoclonal antibody. *Cancer Res* 1980;40:717–721.

107. Chen YT, Obata Y, Stockert E, Takahashi T, Old LJ. Tla-region genes and their products. *Immunol Res* 1987;6:30–45.

108. Old LJ. Cancer immunology: the search for specificity—G. H. A. Clowes Memorial lecture. *Cancer Res* 1981;41:361–375.

109. Wu M, van Kaer L, Itohara S, Tonegawa S. Highly restricted expression of the thymus leukemia antigens on intestinal epithelial cells. *J Exp Med* 1991;174:213–218.

110. van der Bruggen P, Traversari C, Chomez P, et al. A gene encoding an antigen recognized by cytolytic T lymphocytes on a human melanoma. *Science* 1991;254:1643–1647.

111. Takahashi K, Shichijo S, Noguchi M, Hirohata M, Itoh K. Identification of MAGE-1 and MAGE-4 proteins in spermatogonia and primary spermatocytes of testis. *Cancer Res* 1995;55:3478–3482.

112. Becker JC, Gillitzer R, Brocker EB. A member of the melanoma antigen-encoding gene (MAGE) family is expressed in human skin during wound healing. *Int J Cancer* 1994;58:346–348.

113. Chen YT, Scanlan MJ, Sahin U, et al. A testicular antigen aberrantly expressed in human cancers detected by autologous antibody screening. *Proc Natl Acad Sci USA* 1997;94:1914–1918.

114. Chomez P, Williams R, De Backer O, Boon T, Vennstrom B. The SMAGE gene family is expressed in post-meiotic spermatids during mouse germ cell differentiation. *Immunogenetics* 1996;43:97–100.

115. Amar-Costesec A, Godelaine D, Van den Eynde B, Beaufay H. Identification and characterization of the tumor-specific P1A gene product. *Biol Cell* 1994;81:195–203.

116. De Smet C, De Backer O, Faraoni I, Lurquin C, Brasseur F, Boon T. The activation of human gene MAGE-1 in tumor cells is correlated with genome-wide demethylation. *Proc Natl Acad Sci USA* 1996;93:7149–7153.

117. De Plaen E, Arden K, Traversari C, et al. Structure, chromosomal localization, and expression of 12 genes of the MAGE family. *Immunogenetics* 1994;40:360–369.

118. Baskar S. Gene-modified tumor cells as cellular vaccine. *Cancer Immunol Immunother* 1996;43:165–173.

119. Barratt-Boyes SM. Making the most of mucin: a novel target for tumor immunotherapy. *Cancer Immunol Immunother* 1996;43:142–151.

120. Hakomori S, Wang SM, Young WW Jr. Isoantigenic expression of Forssman glycolipid in human gastric and colonic mucosa: its possible identity with "A-like antigen" in human cancer. *Proc Natl Acad Sci USA* 1977;74:3023–3027.

121. Lloyd KO. Philip Levine award lecture. Blood group antigens as markers for normal differentiation and malignant change in human tissues. *Am J Clin Pathol* 1987;87:129–139.

122. Göttlinger HG, Funke I, Johnson JP, Gokel JM, Riethmüller G. The epithelial cell surface antigen 17-1A, a target for antibody-mediated tumor therapy: its biochemical nature, tissue distribution and recognition by different monoclonal antibodies. *Int J Cancer* 1986;38:47–53.

123. Hara I, Takechi Y, Houghton AN. Implicating a role for immune recognition of self in tumor rejection: passive immunization against the brown locus protein. *J Exp Med* 1995;182:1609–1614.

124. Livingston PO. Approaches to augmenting the immunogenicity of melanoma gangliosides: from whole melanoma cells to ganglioside-KLH conjugate vaccines. *Immunol Rev* 1995;145:147–166.

125. DeLellis RA, Dayal Y. The role of immunohistochemistry in the diagnosis of poorly differentiated malignant neoplasms. *Semin Oncol* 1987;14:173–92.

126. Freedman AS, Nadler LM. Cell surface markers in hematologic malignancies. *Semin Oncol* 1987;14:193–212.

127. Garnick MB, Fair WR. Prostate cancer: emerging concepts. *Ann Intern Med* 1996;125:118–125.

128. Kelly WK, Slovin S, Scher HI. Clinical use of posttherapy prostate-specific antigen changes in advanced prostate cancer. *Semin Oncol* 1996;23:8–14.

129. Pandha HS, Waxman J. Tumour markers. *Q J Med* 1995;88:233–241.

130. Garin-Chesa P, Beresford HR, Carrato-Mena A, et al. Cell surface molecules of human melanoma. Immunohistochemical analysis of the gp57, GD3, and mel-CSPG antigenic systems. *Am J Pathol* 1989;134:295–303.

131. Mueller BM, Reisfeld RA. Melanoma antigens and antibodies. *Encycl Hum Biol* 1991;4:957–967.

132. Finn OJ, Jerome KR, Henderson RA, et al. MUC-1 epithelial tumor mucin-based immunity and cancer vaccines. *Immunol Rev* 1995;145:61–89.

133. Hirszfeld L, Halber W, Rosenblat J. Untersuchungen über Verwandtschaftsreaktionen zwischen Embryonal- und Krebsgewebe. II. Menschenembryo und Menschenkrebs. *Z Immunitätsforsch* 1932;75:209–216.

134. Uriel J. Retrodifferentiation and the fetal patterns of gene expression in cancer. *Adv Cancer Res* 1979;29:127–174.

135. Leibson PJ, Loken MR, Panem S, Schreiber H. Clonal evolution of myeloma cells leads to quantitative changes in immunoglobulin secretion and surface antigen expression. *Proc Natl Acad Sci USA* 1979;76:2937–2941.

136. Gold P, Freedman SO. Specific carcinoembryonic antigens of the human digestive system. *J Exp Med* 1965;122:467–481.

137. Gold P, Freedman SO. Specific carcinoembryonic antigens of the human digestive system. *J Exp Med* 1965;122:467–481.

138. Thompson JA. Molecular cloning and expression of carcinoembryonic antigen gene family members. *Tumour Biol* 1995;16:10–16.

139. Northover J. The use of prognostic markers in surgery for colorectal cancer. *Eur J Cancer* 1995;31A:1207–1209.

140. Hodge JW. Carcinoembryonic antigen as a target for cancer vaccines. *Cancer Immunol Immunother* 1996;43:127–134.

141. Abelev GI, Perova SD, Khramkov NI, Postnikova ZA, Irlin IS. Production of embryonal a-globulin by transplantable mouse hepatomas. *Transplantation* 1963;1:174–180.

142. Haydon GH, Hayes PC. Screening for hepatocellular carcinoma. *Eur J Gastroenterol Hepatol* 1996;8:856–860.

143. Medawar PB, Hunt R. Can fetal antigens be used for prophylactic immunization? *Ciba Found Symp* 1983;96:160–181.

144. Lynch RG, Graff RJ, Sirisinha S, Simms ES, Eisen HN. Myeloma proteins as tumor-specific transplantation antigens. *Proc Natl Acad Sci USA* 1972;69:1540–1544.

145. Syrengelas AD, Chen TT, Levy R. DNA immunization induces protective immunity against B-cell lymphoma. *Nat Med* 1996;2:1038–1041.

146. Krensky AM. Cytotoxic T lymphocyte recognition of non-Hodgkin's B cell lymphomas. *Immunol Res* 1996;15:91–97.

147. Beatty PG, Kim BS, Rowley DA, Coppleson LW. Antibody against the antigen receptor of a plasmacytoma prolongs survival of mice bearing the tumor. *J Immunol* 1976;116:1391–1396.

148. Schreiber H, Leibson P. Suppression of myeloma growth in vitro by anti-idiotypic antibodies: inhibition of DNA synthesis and colony formation. *J Natl Cancer Inst* 1978;60:225–233.

149. Krolick KA, Uhr JW, Slavin S, Vitetta ES. In vivo therapy of a murine B cell tumor (BCL1) using antibody-ricin A chain immunotoxins. *J Exp Med* 1982;155:1797–1809.

150. Stevenson FK, Elliott EV, Stevenson GT. Some effects on leukaemic B lymphocytes of antibodies to defined regions of their surface immunoglobulin. *Immunology* 1977;32:549–557.

151. Miller RA, Maloney DG, Warnke R, Levy R. Treatment of B-cell lymphoma with monoclonal anti-idiotype antibody. *N Engl J Med* 1982;306:517–522.

152. Hsu FJ, Benike C, Fagnoni F, et al. Vaccination of patients with B-cell lymphoma using autologous antigen-pulsed dendritic cells. *Nat Med* 1996;2:52–58.

153. Stevenson FK, Zhu D, King CA, Ashworth LJ, Kumar S, Hawkins RE. Idiotypic DNA vaccines against B-cell lymphoma. *Immunol Rev* 1995;145:211–228.

154. Habel K. Resistance of polyoma virus immune animals to transplanted polyoma tumors. *Proc Soc Exp Biol Med* 1961;106:722–725.

155. Sjögren HO, Hellström I, Klein G. Resistance of polyoma virus-immunized mice to transplantation of established mice to transplantation of established polyoma tumors. *Exp Cell Res* 1961;23:204–208.

156. Defendi V. Effects of SV40 virus immunization on growth of transplantable SV40 and polyoma virus tumors in hamsters. *Proc Soc Exp Biol Med* 1963;113:12–16.

157. Tevethia SS, Tevethia MJ, Lewis AJ, Reddy VB, Weissman SM. Biology of simian virus 40 (SV40) transplantation antigen (TrAg). IX. Analysis of TrAg in mouse cells synthesizing truncated SV40 large T antigen. *Virology* 1983;128:319–330.

158. Tevethia SS, Greenfield RS, Flyer DC, Tevethia MJ. SV40 transplantation antigen: relationship to SV40-specific proteins. *Cold Spring Harbor Symp Quant Biol* 1980;44:235–242.

159. O'Connell KA, Gooding LR. Cloned cytotoxic T lymphocytes recognize cells expressing discrete fragments of the SV40 tumor antigen. *J Immunol* 1984;132:953–958.

160. Sharma S, Rodgers L, Brandsma J, Gething MJ, Sambrook J. SV40 T antigen and the exocytotic pathway. *EMBO J* 1985;4:1479–1489.

161. Carbone M, Rizzo P, Grimley PM, et al. Simian virus-40 large- T antigen binds p53 in human mesotheliomas. *Nat Med* 1997;3:908–912.

162. Rickinson AB, Murray RJ, Brooks J, Griffin H, Moss DJ, Masucci MG. T cell recognition of Epstein-Barr virus associated lymphomas. *Cancer Surv* 1992;13:53–80.

163. Smith CA, Ng CY, Loftin SK, et al. Adoptive immunotherapy for Epstein-Barr virus-related lymphoma. *Leuk Lymphoma* 1996;23:213–220.

164. Tindle RW. Human papillomavirus vaccines for cervical cancer. *Curr Opin Immunol* 1996;8:643–650.

165. Mayordomo JI, Zorina T, Storkus WJ, et al. Bone marrow-derived dendritic cells pulsed with synthetic tumour peptides elicit protective and therapeutic antitumour immunity. *Nat Med* 1995;1:1297–1302.

166. Coffin JM. Endogenous retrovirus. In: Weiss R, Teich N, Varmas H, Coffin J, eds. *Molecular biology of tumor viruses, part III. RNA tumor viruses,* 2nd ed. Cold Spring Harbor, NY: Cold Spring Harbor Laboratory, 1984:1109–1203.

167. Stoye JP, Coffin JM. Polymorphism of murine endogenous proviruses revealed by using virus class-specific oligonucleotide probes. *J Virol* 1988;62:168–175.

168. Nowinski RC, Stone MR, Tam MR, Lostrom ME, Burnette WN, O'Donnell PV. Mapping of viral proteins with monoclonal antibodies. In: Kennett RH, McKearn TJ, Bechton KB, eds. *Monoclonal antibodies. Hybridomas: a new dimension in biological analyses.* New York: Plenum Press, 1980:295–316.

169. Löwer R, Löwer J, Kurth R. The viruses in all of us: characteristics and biological significance of human endogenous retrovirus sequences. *Proc Natl Acad Sci USA* 1996;93:5177–5184.

170. Müller R, Slamon DJ, Tremblay JM, Cline MJ, Verma IM. Differential expression of cellular oncogenes during pre- and postnatal development of the mouse. *Nature* 1982;299:640–644.

171. Britt WJ, Chesebro B, Portis JL. Identification of a unique erythroleukemia-associated retroviral gp70 expressed during early stages of normal erythroid differentiation. *J Exp Med* 1984;159:1591–1603.

172. Fefer A, McCoy JL, Glynn JP. Induction and regression of primary moloney sarcoma virus-induced tumors in mice. *Cancer Res* 1967;27:1626–1631.

173. Plata F, Lilly F. Viral specificity of H-2-restricted T killer cells directed against syngeneic tumors induced by Gross, Friend, or Rauscher leukemia virus. *J Exp Med* 1979;150:1174–1186.

174. Plata F, Langlade-Demoyen P, Abastado JP, Berbar T, Kourilsky P. Retrovirus antigens recognized by cytolytic T lymphocytes activate tumor rejection in vivo. *Cell* 1987;48:231–240.

175. Klarnet JP, Kern DE, Okuno K, Holt C, Lilly F, Greenberg PD. FBL-reactive CD8+cytotoxic and CD4+ helper T lymphocytes recognize distinct Friend murine leukemia virus-encoded antigens. *J Exp Med* 1989;169:457–467.

176. Huang AY, Gulden PH, Woods AS, et al. The immunodominant major histocompatibility complex class I-restricted antigen of a murine colon tumor derives from an endogenous retroviral gene product. *Proc Natl Acad Sci USA* 1996;93:9730–9735.

177. Golovkina TV, Chervonsky A, Dudley JP, Ross SR. Transgenic mouse mammary tumor virus superantigen expression prevents viral infection. *Cell* 1992;69:637–645.

178. Thomas L. Discussion of cellular and humoral aspects of the hypersensitive states. In: Lawrence HS, ed. New York: Hoeber-Harper, 1959:529–532.

179. Burnet FM. The concept of immunological surveillance. *Prog Exp Tumor Res* 1970;13:1–27.

180. Outzen HC, Custer RP, Eaton GJ, Prehn RT. Spontaneous and induced tumor incidence in germfree "nude" mice. *J Reticuloendothel Soc* 1975;17:1–9.

181. Stutman O. Tumor development after 3-methylcholanthrene in immunologically deficient athymic nude mice. *Science* 1979;183:534–536.

182. Holland JM, Mitchell TJ, Gipson LC, Whitaker MS. Survival and cause of death in aging germfree athymic nude and normal inbred C3Hf/He mice. *J Natl Cancer Inst* 1978;61:1357–1361.

183. Good R. Relations between immunity and malignancy. *Proc Natl Acad Sci USA* 1972;69:1026–1030.

184. Kinlein LJ. Immunologic factors including AIDS. In: Schottenfield D, Fraumeni JF Jr, eds. *Cancer epidemiology and prevention.* New York: Oxford University Press, 1996:532–545.

185. Bouwes Bavinck JN, Hardie DR, Green A, et al. The risk of skin cancer in renal transplant recipients in Queensland, Australia. A follow-up study. *Transplantation* 1996;61:715–721.

186. Kelly GE, Meikle W, Sheil AG. Effects of immunosuppressive therapy on the induction of skin tumors by ultraviolet irradiation in hairless mice. *Transplantation* 1987;44:429–434.

187. Servilla KS, Burnham DK, Daynes RA. Ability of cyclosporine to promote the growth of transplanted ultraviolet radiation-induced tumors in mice. *Transplantation* 1987;44:291–295.

188. Klein G. Immunological surveillance against neoplasia. *Harvey Lect* 1975;69:71–102.

189. Tooze J. Origins of contemporary tumor virus research. In: *The molecular biology of tumor viruses.* Cold Spring Harbor, NY: Cold Spring Harbor Laboratory, 1973:1–73.

190. Deinhardt FW, Falk LA, Wolfe LG. Simian herpesviruses and neoplasia. *Adv Cancer Res* 1974;19:167–205.

191. Urban JL, Burton RC, Holland JM, Kripke ML, Schreiber H. Mechanisms of syngeneic tumor rejection. Susceptibility of host-selected progressor variants to various immunological effector cells. *J Exp Med* 1982;155:557–573.

192. Collins JL, Patek PQ, Cohn M. In vivo surveillance of tumorigenic cells transformed in vitro. *Nature* 1982;299:169–171.

193. Virchow R. *Aetiologie der neoplastischen Geschwülste/Pathogenie der neoplastischen Geschwülste. Die Krankhaften Geschwülste.* Berlin: Verlag von August Hirschwald, 1863:57–101.

194. Clemente CG, Mihm MC Jr, Bufalino R, Zurrida S, Collini P, Cascinelli N. Prognostic value of tumor infiltrating lymphocytes in the vertical growth phase of primary cutaneous melanoma. *Cancer* 1996;77:1303–1310.

195. Barnhill RL, Mihm MC. Histopathology of malignant melanoma and its precursor lesions. In: Balch CM, Houghton AN, Milton GW, Sober AJ, Soong S, eds. *Cutaneous melanoma.* Philadelphia: Lippincott, 1992:234–263.

196. Berd D, Mastrangelo MJ, Lattime E, Sato T, Maguire HC Jr. Melanoma and vitiligo: immunology's Grecian urn. *Cancer Immunol Immunother* 1996;42:263–267.

197. Mackensen A, Carcelain G, Viel S, et al. Direct evidence to support the immunosurveillance concept in a human regressive melanoma. *J Clin Invest* 1994;93:1397–1402.

198. Dvorak HF. Tumors: wounds that do not heal. Similarities between tumor stroma generation and wound healing. *N Engl J Med* 1986;315:1650–1659.

199. Van Damme J, Proost P, Lenaerts JP, Opdenakker G. Structural and functional identification of two human, tumor-derived monocyte chemotactic proteins (MCP-2 and MCP-3) belonging to the chemokine family. *J Exp Med* 1992;176:59–65.

200. Mantovani A. Tumor-associated macrophages. *Curr Opin Immunol* 1990;2:689–692.

201. Mantovani A, Bottazzi B, Colotta F, Sozzani S, Ruco L. The origin and function of tumor-associated macrophages. *Immunol Today* 1992;13:265–270.

202. Ruoslahti E, Yamaguchi Y. Proteoglycans as modulators of growth factor activities. *Cell* 1991;64:867–869.
203. Singh S, Ross SR, Acena M, Rowley DA, Schreiber H. Stroma is critical for preventing or permitting immunological destruction of antigenic cancer cells. *J Exp Med* 1992;175:139–146.
204. DiGiovanni J, Bhatt TS, Walker SE. C57BL/6 mice are resistant to tumor promotion by full thickness skin wounding. *Carcinogenesis* 1993;14:319–321.
205. Prescott SM, White RL. Self-promotion? Intimate connections between APC and prostaglandin H synthase-2. *Cell* 1996;87:783–786.
206. Noguchi Y, Jungbluth A, Richards EC, Old LJ. Effect of interleukin 12 on tumor induction by 3-methylcholanthrene. *Proc Natl Acad Sci USA* 1996;93: 11798–801.
207. Oshima M, Dinchuk JE, Kargman SL, et al. Suppression of intestinal polyposis in Apc delta716 knockout mice by inhibition of cyclooxygenase 2 (COX-2). *Cell* 1996;87:803–809.
208. Pekarek LA, Starr BA, Toledano AY, Schreiber H. Inhibition of tumor growth by elimination of granulocytes. *J Exp Med* 1995;181:435–440.
209. Seung LP, Rowley DA, Dubey P, Schreiber H. Synergy between T-cell immunity and inhibition of paracrine stimulation causes tumor rejection. *Proc Natl Acad Sci USA* 1995;92:6254–6258.
210. Seung LP, Seung SK, Schreiber H. Antigenic cancer cells that escape immune destruction are stimulated by host cells. *Cancer Res* 1995;55:5094–5100.
211. Rettig MB, Ma HJ, Vescio RA, et al. Kaposi's sarcoma-associated herpesvirus infection of bone marrow dendritic cells from multiple myeloma patients. *Science* 1997;276:1851.
212. Huang F, Hsu S, Yan Z, Winawer S, Friedman E. The capacity for growth stimulation by TGF beta 1 seen only in advanced colon cancers cannot be ascribed to mutations in APC, DCC, p53 or ras. *Oncogene* 1994;9:3701–3706.
213. Okamoto M, Lee C, Oyasu R. Interleukin-6 as a paracrine and autocrine growth factor in human prostatic carcinoma cells in vitro. *Cancer Res* 1997;57:141–146.
214. Lu C, Kerbel RS. Interleukin-6 undergoes transition from paracrine growth inhibitor to autocrine stimulator during human melanoma progression. *J Cell Biol* 1993;120:1281–1288.
215. Mintz B, Silvers WK. Accelerated growth of melanomas after specific immune destruction of tumor stroma in a mouse model. *Cancer Res* 1996;56:463–466.
216. Bittner JJ. Some possible effects of nursing on the mammary gland tumor incidence in mice. *Am J Cancer* 1936;25:162.
217. DeOme KB. The incidence of mammary tumors among low tumor strain C57DLK mice when foster-nursed by high-tumor strain A females. *Am J Cancer* 1940;40:231–234.
218. Choi Y, Kappler JW, Marrack P. A superantigen encoded in the open reading frame of the 3' long terminal repeat of mouse mammary tumour virus. *Nature* 1991;350:203–207.
219. Marrack P, Kushnir E, Kappler J. A maternally inherited superantigen encoded by a mammary tumour virus. *Nature* 1991;349:524–526.
220. Acha-Orbea H, Shakhov AN, Scarpellino L, et al. Clonal deletion of V beta 14-bearing T cells in mice transgenic for mammary tumour virus. *Nature* 1991;350: 207–211.
221. Fritsch EF, Temin HM. Inhibition of viral DNA synthesis in stationary chicken embryo fibroblasts infected with avian retroviruses. *J Virol* 1977;24:461–469.
222. Varmus HE, Padgett T, Heasley S, Simon G, Bishop JM. Cellular functions are required for the synthesis and integration of avian sarcoma virus-specific DNA. *Cell* 1977;11:307–319.
223. Tsubura A, Inaba M, Imai S, et al. Intervention of T-cells in transportation of mouse mammary tumor virus (milk factor) to mammary gland cells in vivo. *Cancer Res* 1988;48.6555–6559.
224. Squartini F, Olivi M, Bolis GB. Mouse strain and breeding stimulation as factors influencing the effect of thymectomy on mammary tumorigenesis. *Cancer Res* 1970;30:2069–2072.
225. Stewart T, Tsai SC, Grayson H, Henderson R, Opelz G. Incidence of de-novo breast cancer in women chronically immunosuppressed after organ transplantation. *Lancet* 1995;346:796–798.
226. Prehn RT. The immune reaction as a stimulator of tumor growth. *Science* 1972; 176:170–171.
227. Prehn RT. Stimulatory effects of immune reactions upon the growths of untransplanted tumors. *Cancer Res* 1994;54:908–914.
228. Rapp HJ. Appropriateness of animal models for the immunology of human cancer. *Cancer Res* 1979;39:4285–4287.
229. Baldwin RW. Tumour specific immunity against spontaneous rat tumours. *Int J Cancer* 1966;1:257 264.
230. Klein G, Klein E. Immune surveillance against virus-induced tumors and nonrejectability of spontaneous tumors: contrasting consequences of host versus tumor evolution. *Proc Natl Acad Sci USA* 1977;74:2121 2125.
231. Hewitt HB, Blake ER, Walder AS. A critique of the evidence for active host defence against cancer, based on personal studies of 27 murine tumours of spontaneous origin. *Br J Cancer* 1976;33:241–259.
232. Hewitt HB. The choice of animal tumors for experimental studies of cancer therapy. *Adv Cancer Res* 1978;27:149–200.
233. Kripke ML. Latency, histology, and antigenicity of tumors induced by ultraviolet light in three inbred mouse strains. *Cancer Res* 1977;37.1395–1400.
234. Malmgren RA, Bennison BE, McKinely TW Jr. Reduced antibody titers in mice treated with carcinogenic and cancer chemotherapeutic agents. *Proc Soc Exp Biol Med* 1952;79:484–488.
235. Kripke ML, Fisher MS. Immunologic parameters of ultraviolet carcinogenesis. *J Natl Cancer Inst* 1976;57:211–215.
236. Spellman CW, Daynes RA. Ultraviolet light, tumors, and suppressor T cells. *Hum Pathol* 1981;12:299–301.
237. Kripke ML. Immunological unresponsiveness induced by ultraviolet radiation. *Immunol Rev* 1984;80:87–102.
238. Roberts LK, Daynes RA. Modification of the immunogenic properties of chemically induced tumors arising in hosts treated concomitantly with ultraviolet light. *J Immunol* 1980;125:438–447.
239. Bartlett GL. Effect of host immunity on the antigenic strength of primary tumors. *J Natl Cancer Inst* 1972;49:493–504.
240. Makinodan T, Kay MM. Age influence on the immune system. *Adv Immunol* 1980;29:287–330.
241. Spellman CW, Daynes RA. Immunoregulation by ultraviolet light-III. Enhancement of suppressor cell activity in older animals. *Exp Gerontol* 1978;13: 141–146.
242. Flood PM, Urban JL, Kripke ML, Schreiber H. Loss of tumor-specific and idiotype-specific immunity with age. *J Exp Med* 1981;154:275–290.
243. Urban JL, Schreiber H. Rescue of the tumor-specific immune response of aged mice in vitro. *J Immunol* 1984;133:527–534.
244. Winn HJ. Immune mechanisms in homotransplantation. II. Quantitative assay of the immunologic activity of lymphoid cells stimulated by tumor homografts. *J Immunol* 1961;86:228–239.
245. North RJ, Havell EA. The antitumor function of tumor necrosis factor (TNF) II. Analysis of the role of endogenous TNF in endotoxin-induced hemorrhagic necrosis and regression of an established sarcoma. *J Exp Med* 1988;167: 1086–1099.
246. Urban JL, Schreiber H. Selection of macrophage-resistant progressor tumor variants by the normal host. Requirement for concomitant T cell-mediated immunity. *J Exp Med* 1983;157:642–656.
247. Schultz KR, Klarnet JP, Gieni RS, HayGlass KT, Greenberg PD. The role of B cells for in vivo T cell responses to a Friend virus-induced leukemia. *Science* 1990;249.921–923.
248. Koeppen HK, Singh S, Stauss HJ, Park BH, Rowley DA, Schreiber H. CD4-positive and B lymphocytes in transplantation immunity. I. Promotion of tumor allograft rejection through elimination of CD4-positive lymphocytes. *Transplantation* 1993;55:1349 1355.
249. Monach PA, Schreiber H, Rowley DA. CD4+ and B lymphocytes in transplantation immunity. II. Augmented rejection of tumor allografts by mice lacking B cells. *Transplantation* 1993;55:1356–1361.
250. Real FX, Mattes MJ, Houghton AN, Oettgen HF, Lloyd KO, Old LJ. Class 1 (unique) tumor antigens of human melanoma. Identification of a 90,000 dalton cell surface glycoprotein by autologous antibody. *J Exp Med* 1984;160: 1219–1233.
251. Brown JP, Klitzman JM, Hellstrom I, Nowinski RC, Hellstrom KE. Antibody response of mice to chemically induced tumors. *Proc Natl Acad Sci USA* 1978; 75:955–958.
252. Old LJ, Boyse EA, Stockert E. Antigenic properties of experimental leukemias. I. Serological studies in vitro with spontaneous and radiation-induced leukemias. *J Natl Cancer Inst* 1963;31:977–986.
253. Boyse FA, Old LJ, Luell S. Antigenic properties of experimental leukemias. II. Immunological studies in vivo with C57Bl/6 radiation-induced leukemias. *J Natl Cancer Inst* 1963;31:987–995.
254. Leclerc JC, Gomard E, Levy JP. Cell-mediated reaction against tumors induced by oncornaviruses. I. Kinetics and specificity of the immune response in murine sarcoma virus (MSV)-induced tumors and transplanted lymphomas. *Int J Cancer* 1972;10:589–601.
255. Tevethia SS, Blasecki JW, Vaneck G, Goldstein AL. Requirement of thymus-derived theta-positive lymphocytes for rejection of DNA virus (SV 40) tumors in mice. *J Immunol* 1974;113:1417–1423.
256. Cheever MA, Thompson DB, Klarnet JP, Greenberg PD. Antigen-driven long term-cultured T cells proliferate in vivo, distribute widely, mediate specific tumor therapy, and persist long-term as functional memory T cells. *J Exp Med* 1986,163:1100–1112.
257. Algire GH, Weaver JM, Prehn RT. Growth of cells in vivo in diffusion chambers. I. Survival of homografts in immunized mice. *J Natl Cancer Inst* 1954;15: 493–507.
258. Kripke ML. Immunologic mechanisms in UV radiation carcinogenesis. *Adv Cancer Res* 1981;34:69–106.
259. Robins RA. T-cell responses at the host-tumour interface. *Biochim Biophys Acta* 1986;865:289–305.
260. Matloubian M, Concepcion RJ, Ahmed R. CD4+ T cells are required to sustain CD8+ cytotoxic T cell responses during chronic viral infection. *J Virol* 1994;68: 8056–8063.
261. Walter EA, Greenberg PD, Gilbert MJ, et al. Reconstitution of cellular immunity against cytomegalovirus in recipients of allogeneic bone marrow by transfer of T-cell clones from the donor. *N Engl J Med* 1995;333:1038–1044.
262. Mukherji B, MacAlister TJ. Clonal analysis of cytotoxic T cell response against human melanoma. *J Exp Med* 1983;158:240–245.
263. Knuth A, Danowski B, Oettgen HF, Old LJ. T-cell-mediated cytotoxicity against autologous malignant melanoma: analysis with interleukin 2-dependent T-cell cultures. *Proc Natl Acad Sci USA* 1984,81:3511–3515.
264. Klein E, Vanky F, Galili U, Vose BM, Fopp M. Separation and characteristics of

tumor-infiltrating lymphocytes in man. *Contemp Top Immunobiol* 1980;10: 79–107.

265. Anichini A, Fossati G, Parmiani G. Clonal analysis of the cytolytic T-cell response to human tumors. *Immunol Today* 1987;8:385–389.

266. Takasugi M, Mickey MR, Terasaki PI. Reactivity of lymphocytes from normal persons on cultured tumor cells. *Cancer Res* 1973;33:2898–2902.

267. Kiessling R, Klein E, Wigzell H. "Natural" killer cells in the mouse. I. Cytotoxic cells with specificity for mouse Moloney leukemia cells. Specificity and distribution according to genotype. *Eur J Immunol* 1975;5:112–117.

268. Herberman RB, Nunn ME, Lavrin DH. Natural cytotoxic reactivity of mouse lymphoid cells against syngeneic acid allogeneic tumors. I. Distribution of reactivity and specificity. *Int J Cancer* 1975;16:216–229.

269. Sendo F, Aoki T, Boyse EA, Buafo CK. Natural occurrence of lymphocytes showing cytotoxic activity to BALB/c radiation-induced leukemia RL male 1 cells. *J Natl Cancer Inst* 1975;55:603–609.

270. Joihdal M, Press H. Surface markers on human B and T lymphocytes VI. Cytotoxicity against cell lines as a functional marker for lymphocyte subpopulations. *Int J Cancer* 1975;15:596.

271. Matthews N, Maclaurin BP, Clarke GN. Characterization of the normal lymphocyte population cytolytic to Burkitt's lymphoma cells of the EB2 cell line. *Aust J Exp Biol Med Sci* 1976;53:389–398.

272. Trinchieri G. Biology of natural killer cells. *Adv Immunol* 1989;47:187–376.

273. Snell GD. Histocompatibility genes of the mouse. II. Production and analysis of isogenic resistant lines. *J Natl Cancer Inst* 1958;21:843–877.

274. Cudkowicz G, Cosgrove GE. Immunologically competent cells in adult mouse liver: studies with parent-to-hybrid radiation chimeras (26113). *Proc Soc Exp Biol Med* 1960;105:336–371.

275. Leibson PJ. Signal transduction during natural killer cell activation: inside the mind of a killer. *Immunity* 1997;6:655–661.

276. Ciccone E, Pende D, Viale O, et al. Involvement of HLA class I alleles in natural killer (NK) cell-specific functions: expression of HLA-Cw3 confers selective protection from lysis by alloreactive NK clones displaying a defined specificity (specificity 2). *J Exp Med* 1992;176:963–971.

277. Hanna N, Fidler IJ. Role of natural killer cells in the destruction of circulating tumor emboli. *J Natl Cancer Inst* 1980;65:801–809.

278. Talmadge JE, Meyers KM, Prieur DJ, Starkey JR. Role of natural killer cells in tumor growth and metastasis: C57BL/6 normal and beige mice. *J Natl Cancer Inst* 1980;65:929–935.

279. Hanna N, Burton RC. Definitive evidence that natural killer (NK) cells inhibit experimental tumor metastases in vivo. *J Immunol* 1981;127:1754–1758.

280. Grimm EA, Mazumder A, Zhang HZ, Rosenberg SA. Lymphokine-activated killer cell phenomenon. Lysis of natural killer-resistant fresh solid tumor cells by interleukin 2-activated autologous human peripheral blood lymphocytes. *J Exp Med* 1982;155:1823–1841.

281. Grimm EA, Rosenberg SA. The human lymphokine-activated killer cell phenomenon. *Lymphokines.* New York: Academic Press, 1984;9:279–311.

282. Eberlein TJ, Rosenstein M, Rosenberg SA. Regression of a disseminated syngeneic solid tumor by systemic transfer of lymphoid cells expanded in interleukin. *J Exp Med* 1982;156:385–397.

283. Mazumder A, Rosenberg SA. Successful immunotherapy of natural killer-resistant established pulmonary melanoma metastases by the intravenous adoptive transfer of syngeneic lymphocytes activated in vitro by interleukin 2. *J Exp Med* 1984;159:495–507.

284. Rosenberg SA, Lotze MT, Muul LM, et al. A progress report on the treatment of 157 patients with advanced cancer using lymphokine-activated killer cells and interleukin-2 or high-dose interleukin-2 alone. *N Engl J Med* 1987;316:889–897.

285. Phillips JH, Lanier LL. Dissection of the lymphokine-activated killer phenomenon. Relative contribution of peripheral blood natural killer cells and T lymphocytes to cytolysis. *J Exp Med* 1986;164:814–825.

286. Ortaldo JR, Mason A, Overton R. Lymphokine-activated killer cells. Analysis of progenitors and effectors. *J Exp Med* 1986;164:1193–1205.

287. Yang JC, Mule JJ, Rosenberg SA. Murine lymphokine-activated killer (LAK) cells: phenotypic characterization of the precursor and effector cells. *J Immunol* 1986;137:715–722.

288. Hibbs JB Jr, Lambert LH Jr, Remington JS. Possible role of macrophage mediated nonspecific cytotoxicity in tumour resistance. *Nat New Biol* 1972;235: 48–50.

289. Hibbs JB Jr, Lambert LH Jr, Remington JS. Control of carcinogenesis: a possible role for the activated macrophage. *Science* 1972;177:998–1000.

290. Evans R, Alexander P. Mechanism of immunologically specific killing of tumour cells by macrophages. *Nature* 1972;236:168–170.

291. Nathan CF, Karnovsky ML, David JR. Alterations of macrophage functions by mediators from lymphocytes. *J Exp Med* 1971;133:1356–1376.

292. Pace JL, Russell SW. Activation of mouse macrophages for tumor cell killing. I. Quantitative analysis of interactions between lymphokine and lipopolysaccharide. *J Immunol* 1981;126:1863–1867.

293. Meltzer MS. Macrophage activation for tumor cytotoxicity: characterization of priming and trigger signals during lymphokine activation. *J Immunol* 1981;127: 179–183.

294. Lichtenstein A. Granulocytes as possible effectors of tumor immunity. *Immunol Allergy Clin North Am* 1990;10:731.

295. Matzinger P. Tolerance, danger, and the extended family. *Annu Rev Immunol* 1994;12:991–1045.

296. Fearon DT, Locksley RM. The instructive role of innate immunity in the acquired immune response. *Science* 1996;272:50–53.

297. Munn DH, Cheung NK. Phagocytosis of tumor cells by human monocytes cultured in recombinant macrophage colony-stimulating factor. *J Exp Med* 1990; 172:231–237.

298. Carswell EA, Old LJ, Kassel RL, Green S, Fiore N, Williamson B. An endotoxin-induced serum factor that causes necrosis of tumors. *Proc Natl Acad Sci USA* 1975;72:3666–3670.

299. Pennica D, Nedwin GE, Hayflick JS, et al. Human tumour necrosis factor: precursor structure, expression and homology to lymphotoxin. *Nature* 1984;312: 724–729.

300. Urban JL, Shepard HM, Rothstein JL, Sugarman BJ, Schreiber H. Tumor necrosis factor: a potent effector molecule for tumor cell killing by activated macrophages. *Proc Natl Acad Sci USA* 1986;83:5233–5237.

301. Philip R, Epstein LB. Tumour necrosis factor as immunomodulator and mediator of monocyte cytotoxicity induced by itself, gamma-interferon and interleukin-1. *Nature* 1986;323:86–89.

302. Ziegler-Heitbrock HWL, Moller A, Linke RP, Haas JG, Rieber EP, Riethmüller G. Tumor necrosis factor as effector molecule in moocyte ediated cytotoxicity. *Cancer Res* 1986;46:5947–5952.

303. Feinman R, Henriksen-DeStefano D, Tsujimoto M, Vilcek J. Tumor necrosis factor is an important mediator of tumor cell killing by human monocytes. *J Immunol* 1987;138:635–640.

304. Nathan CF, Murray HW, Cohn ZA. The macrophage as an effector cell. *N Engl J Med* 1980;303:622–626.

305. Hibbs JB Jr, Taintor RR, Vavrin Z. Macrophage cytotoxicity: role for L-arginine deiminase and imino nitrogen oxidation to nitrite. *Science* 1987;235:473–476.

306. Keller R, Geiges M, Keist R. L-arginine-dependent reactive nitrogen intermediates as mediators of tumor cell killing by activated macrophages. *Cancer Res* 1990;50:1421–1425.

307. Nestel FP, Casson PR, Wiltrout RH, Kerbel RS. Alterations in sensitivity to nonspecific cell-mediated lysis associated with tumor progression: characterization of activated macrophage- and natural killer cell-resistant tumor variants. *J Natl Cancer Inst* 1984;73:483–491.

308. Yamamura Y, Fischer BC, Harnaha JB, Proctor JW. Heterogeneity of murine mammary adenocarcinoma cell subpopulations. In vitro and in vivo resistance to macrophage cytotoxicity and its association with metastatic capacity. *Int J Cancer* 1984;33:67–72.

309. Lattime EC, Stutman O. Tumor growth in vivo selects for resistance to tumor necrosis factor. *J Immunol* 1989;143:4317–4323.

310. Adams DO, Snyderman R. Do macrophages destroy nascent tumors? *J Natl Cancer Inst* 1979;62:1341–1345.

311. Whitworth PW, Pak CC, Esgro J, Kleinerman ES, Fidler IJ. Macrophages and cancer. *Cancer Metastasis Rev* 1990;8:319–351.

312. Colombo MP, Ferrari G, Stoppacciaro A, et al. Granulocyte colony-stimulating factor gene transfer suppresses tumorigenicity of a murine adenocarcinoma in vivo. *J Exp Med* 1991;173:889–897.

313. Bubenik J, Simova J, Jandlova T. Immunotherapy of cancer using local administration of lymphoid cells transformed by IL-2 cDNA and constitutively producing IL-2. *Immunol Lett* 1990;23:287–292.

314. Tepper RI, Pattengale PK, Leder P. Murine interleukin-4 displays potent anti-tumor activity in vivo. *Cell* 1989;57:503–512.

315. Oliff A, Defeo-Jones D, Boyer M, et al. Tumors secreting human TNF/cachectin induce cachexia in mice. *Cell* 1987;50:555–563.

316. Teng MN, Park BH, Koeppen HKW, Tracey KJ, Fendly BM, Schreiber H. Long-term inhibition of tumor growth by tumor necrosis factor in the absence of cachexia or T-cell immunity. *Proc Natl Acad Sci USA* 1991;88:3535–3539.

317. Zöller M, Douvdevani A, Segal S, Apte RN. Interleukin-1 production by transformed fibroblasts. II. Influence on antigen presentation and T-cell-mediated anti-tumor response. *Int J Cancer* 1992;50:450–457.

318. Hock H, Dorsch M, Diamantstein T, Blankenstein T. Interleukin 7 induces CD4+ T cell-dependent tumor rejection. *J Exp Med* 1991;174:1291–1298.

319. Watanabe Y, Kuribayashi K, Miyatake S, et al. Exogenous expression of mouse interferon gamma cDNA in mouse neuroblastoma C1300 cells results in reduced tumorigenicity by augmented anti-tumor immunity. *Proc Natl Acad Sci USA* 1989;86:9456–9460.

320. Gansbacher B, Bannerji R, Daniels B, Zier K, Cronin K, Gilboa E. Retroviral vector-mediated gamma-interferon gene transfer into tumor cells generates potent and long lasting antitumor immunity. *Cancer Res* 1990;50:7820–7825.

321. Restifo NP, Spiess PJ, Karp SE, Mule JJ, Rosenberg SA. A nonimmunogenic sarcoma transduced with the cDNA for interferon gamma elicits CD8+ T cells against the wild-type tumor: correlation with antigen presentation capability. *J Exp Med* 1992;175:1423–1431.

322. Murray JC, Clauss M, Thurston G, Stern D. Tumour-derived factors which induce endothelial tissue factor and enhance the procoagulant response to TNF. *Int J Radiat Biol* 1991;60:273–277.

323. Hallahan DE, Spriggs DR, Beckett MA, Kufe DW, Weichselbaum RR. Increased tumor necrosis factor alpha mRNA after cellular exposure to ionizing radiation. *Proc Natl Acad Sci USA* 1989;86:10104–10107.

324. Lilly F, Boyse EA, Old LJ. Genetic basis of susceptibility to viral leukaemogenesis. *Lancet* 1964;2:1207–1209.

325. Demant P. Histocompatibility and the genetics of tumour resistance. *J Immunogenet* 1986;13:61–67.

326. Gervois N, Guilloux Y, Diez E, Jotereau F. Suboptimal activation of melanoma infiltrating lymphocytes (TIL) due to low avidity of TCR/MHC-tumor peptide interactions. *J Exp Med* 1996;183:2403–2407.

327. Leach DR, Krummel MF, Allison JP. Enhancement of antitumor immunity by CTLA-4 blockade. *Science* 1996;271:1734–1736.

328. Melero I, Shuford WW, Newby SA, et al. Monoclonal antibodies against the 4-1BB T-cell activation molecule eradicate established tumors. *Nat Med* 1997;3:682–685.

329. Topalian SL, Gonzales MI, Parkhurst M, et al. Melanoma-specific CD4+ T cells recognize nonmutated HLA-DR-restricted tyrosinase epitopes. *J Exp Med* 1996;183:1965–1971.

330. Golumbek PT, Lazenby AJ, Levitsky HI, et al. Treatment of established renal cancer by tumor cells engineered to secrete interleukin-4. *Science* 1991;254:713–716.

331. Gorelik E. Concomitant tumor immunity and the resistance to a second tumor challenge. *Adv Cancer Res* 1983;93:71–120.

332. Perdrizet GA, Ross SR, Stauss HJ, Singh S, Koeppen H, Schreiber H. Animals bearing malignant grafts that express through gene transfer the same antigen. *J Exp Med* 1990;171:1205–1220.

333. Wick M, Dubey P, Koeppen H, et al. Antigenic cancer cells can grow progressively in immune hosts without evidence for T cell exhaustion or systemic anergy. *J Exp Med* 1997;186:229–237.

334. Heath WR, Allison J, Hoffmann MW, et al. Autoimmune diabetes as a consequence of locally produced interleukin-2. *Nature* 1992;359:547–549.

335. Ksander BR, Streilein JW. Failure of infiltrating precursor cytotoxic T cells to acquire direct cytotoxic function in immunologically privileged sites. *J Immunol* 1990;145:2057–2063.

336. Ksander BR, Acevedo J, Streilein JW. Local T helper cell signals by lymphocytes infiltrating intraocular tumors. *J Immunol* 1992;148:1955–1963.

337. Streilein JW, Ksander BR, Taylor AW. Immune deviation in relation to ocular immune privilege. *J Immunol* 1997;158:3557–3560.

338. O'Connell J, O'Sullivan GC, Collins JK, Shanahan F. The Fas counterattack: Fas-mediated T cell killing by colon cancer cells expressing Fas ligand. *J Exp Med* 1996;184:1075–1082.

339. Strand S, Hofmann WJ, Hug H, et al. Lymphocyte apoptosis induced by CD95 (APO-1/Fas) ligand-expressing tumor cells—a mechanism of immune evasion? *Nat Med* 1996;2:1361–1366.

340. Hahne M, Rimoldi D, Schroter M, et al. Melanoma cell expression of Fas(Apo-1/CD95) ligand: implications for tumor immune escape. *Science* 1996;274:1363–1366.

341. Seung S, Urban JL, Schreiber H. A tumor escape variant that has lost one major histocompatibility complex class I restriction element induces specific CD8+ T cells to an antigen that no longer serves as a target. *J Exp Med* 1993;178:933–940.

342. Huang AY, Golumbek P, Ahmadzadeh M, Jaffee E, Pardoll D, Levitsky H. Role of bone marrow-derived cells in presenting MHC class I-restricted tumor antigens. *Science* 1994;264:961–965.

343. Kündig TM, Bachmann MF, DiPaolo C, et al. Fibroblasts as efficient antigen-presenting cells in lymphoid organs. *Science* 1995;268:1343–1347.

344. Wang Z, Cao Y, Albino AP, Zeff RA, Houghton A, Ferrone S. Lack of HLA class I antigen expression by melanoma cells SK-MEL-33 caused by a reading frameshift in beta 2-microglobulin messenger RNA. *J Clin Invest* 1993;91:684–692.

345. Trowsdale J, Travers P, Bodmer WF, Patillo RA. Expression of HLA-A, -B, and -C and beta 2-microglobulin antigens in human choriocarcinoma cell lines. *J Exp Med* 1980;152:11s–17s.

346. Travers PJ, Arklie JL, Trowsdale J, Patillo RA, Bodmer WF. Lack of expression of HLA-ABC antigens in choriocarcinoma and other human tumor cell lines. *Natl Cancer Inst Monogr* 1982;60:175–180.

347. Ruiter DJ, Bergman W, Welvaart K, et al. Immunohistochemical analysis of malignant melanomas and nevocellular nevi with monoclonal antibodies to distinct monomorphic determinants of HLA antigens. *Cancer Res* 1984;44:3930–3935.

348. Natali PG, Giacomini P, Bigotti A, et al. Heterogeneity in the expression of HLA and tumor-associated antigens by surgically removed and cultured breast carcinoma cells. *Cancer Res* 1983;43:660–668.

349. Stein B, Momburg F, Schwarz V, Schlag P, Moldenhauer G, Moller P. Reduction or loss of HLA-A,B,C antigens in colorectal carcinoma appears not to influence survival. *Br J Cancer* 1988;57:364–368.

350. Smith ME, Bodmer WF, Bodmer JG. Selective loss of HLA-A,B,C locus products in colorectal adenocarcinoma. *Lancet* 1988;1:823–824.

351. Möller P, Hämmerling GJ. The role of surface HLA-A,B,C molecules in tumour immunity. *Cancer Surv* 1992;13:101–127.

352. Kaklamanis L, Gatter KC, Hill AB, et al. Loss of HLA class I alleles, heavy chains and beta 2-microglobulin in colorectal cancer. *Int J Cancer* 1992;51:379–385.

353. Garrido F, Ruiz-Cabello F, Cabrera T, et al. Implications for immunosurveillance of altered HLA class I phenotypes in human tumours. *Immunol Today* 1997;18:89–95.

354. Versteeg R, Kruse-Wolters KM, Plomp AC, et al. Suppression of class I human histocompatibility leukocyte antigen by c-myc is locus specific. *J Exp Med* 1989;170:621–635.

355. Ferrone S, Marincola FM. Loss of HLA class I antigens by melanoma cells: molecular mechanisms, functional significance and clinical relevance. *Immunol Today* 1995;16:487–494.

356. Lehmann F, Marchand M, Hainaut P, et al. Differences in the antigens recognized by cytolytic T cells on two successive metastases of a melanoma patient are consistent with immune selection. *Eur J Immunol* 1995;25:340–347.

357. Graffi A, Pasternak G, Horn K-H. Die Erzeugung von Resistenz gegen isologe Transplantate UV-induzierter Sarkome der Maus. *Acta Biol Med Ger* 1964;12:726–728.

358. Pasternak G. Immunologische Eigenschaften chemisch und physikalisch induzierter Tumoren. *Arch Geschwulstforsch* 1967;29:113–141.

359. Lill NL, Tevethia MJ, Hendrickson WG, Tevethia SS. Cytotoxic T lymphocytes (CTL) against a transforming gene product select for transformed cells with point mutations within sequences encoding CTL recognition epitopes. *J Exp Med* 1992;176:449–457.

360. Urban JL, Kripke ML, Schreiber H. Stepwise immunologic selection of antigenic variants during tumor growth. *J Immunol* 1986;137:3036–3041.

361. Urban JL, Van Waes C, Schreiber H. Pecking order among tumor-specific antigens. *Eur J Immunol* 1984;14:181–187.

362. Wettstein PJ, Bailey DW. Immunodominance in the immune response to "multiple" histocompatibility antigens. *Immunogenetics* 1982;16:47–58.

363. Van Waes C, Monach PA, Urban JL, Wortzel RD, Schreiber H. Immunodominance deters the response to other tumor antigens thereby favoring escape: prevention by vaccination with tumor variants selected with cloned cytolytic T cells in vitro. *Tissue Antigens* 1996;47:399–407.

364. Urban JL, Holland JM, Kripke ML, Schreiber H. Immunoselection of tumor cell variants by mice suppressed with ultraviolet radiation. *J Exp Med* 1982;156:1025–1041.

365. Daynes RA, Fernandez PA, Woodward JG. Cell-mediated immune response to syngeneic ultraviolet-induced tumors. II. The properties and antigenic specificities of cytotoxic T lymphocytes generated in vitro following removal from syngeneic tumor-immunized mice. *Cell Immunol* 1979;45:398–414.

366. Boyse EA, Old LJ. Some aspects of normal and abnormal cell surface genetics. *Annu Rev Genet* 1969;3:269–290.

367. Takashi T, Old L, McIntire R, Boyse E. Immunoglobulin and other surface antigens of cells of the immune system. *J Exp Med* 1971;134:815–832.

368. Kaliss N. Immunological enhancement of tumor homografts in mice. A review. *Cancer Res* 1957;18:992–1003.

369. Kaliss N. The survival of homografts in mice pretreated with antisera to mouse tissue. *Ann NY Acad Sci* 1957;64:977–993.

370. Möller G. Antagonistic effect of humoral isoantibodies on the in vitro cytotoxicity of immune lymphoid cells. *J Exp Med* 1965;122:11–24.

371. Möller G. Effect on tumour growth in syngeneic recipients of antibodies against tumour-specific antigens in methylcholanthrene-induced mouse sarcomas. *Nature* 1964;204:846–847.

372. Hellström KE, Hellström I. Lymphocyte-mediated cytotoxicity and blocking serum activity to tumor antigens. *Adv Immunol* 1974;18:209–277.

373. Currie G. Immunological aspects of host resistance to the development and growth of cancer. *Biochim Biophys Acta* 1976;458:135–165.

374. Gershon RK, Mokyr MB, Mitchell MS. Activation of suppressor T cells by tumour cells and specific antibody. *Nature* 1974;250:594–596.

375. Fisher MS, Kripke ML. Systemic alteration induced in mice by ultraviolet light irradiation and its relationship to ultraviolet carcinogenesis. *Proc Natl Acad Sci USA* 1977;74:1688–1692.

376. Vink AA, Strickland FM, Bucana C, et al. Localization of DNA damage and its role in altered antigen-presenting cell function in ultraviolet-irradiated mice. *J Exp Med* 1996;183:1491–1500.

377. Daynes RA, Spellman CW. Evidence for the generation of suppressor cells by ultraviolet radiation. *Cell Immunol* 1977;31:182–187.

378. Fisher MS, Kripke ML. Suppressor T lymphocytes control the development of primary skin cancers in ultraviolet-irradiated mice. *Science* 1982;216:1133–1134.

379. Harris CC. A delayed complication of cancer therapy—cancer. *J Natl Cancer Inst* 1979;63:275–277.

380. Schrier PI, Bernards R, Vaessen RT, Houweling A, van der Eb AJ. Expression of class I major histocompatibility antigens switched off by highly oncogenic adenovirus 12 in transformed rat cells. *Nature* 1983;305:771–775.

381. Haddada H, Lewis AM Jr, Sogn JA, et al. Tumorigenicity of hamster and mouse cells transformed by adenovirus types 2 and 5 is not influenced by the level of class I major histocompatibility antigens expressed on the cells. *Proc Natl Acad Sci USA* 1986;83:9684–9688.

382. Snyderman R, Cianciolo GJ. Immunosuppressive activity of the retroviral envelope protein P15E and its possible relationship to neoplasia. *Immunol Today* 1984;5:240–244.

383. Levey DL, Srivastava PK. Alterations in T cells of cancer-bearers: whence specificity? *Immunol Today* 1996;17:365–368.

384. Mullen CA, Urban JL, Van Waes C, Rowley DA, Schreiber H. Multiple cancers. Tumor burden permits the outgrowth of other cancers. *J Exp Med* 1985;162:1665–1682.

385. Mizoguchi H, O'Shea JJ, Longo DL, Loeffler CM, McVicar DW, Ochoa AC. Alterations in signal transduction molecules in T lymphocytes from tumor-bearing mice. *Science* 1992;258:1795–1798.

386. Nakagomi H, Petersson M, Magnusson I, et al. Decreased expression of the signal-transducing zeta chains in tumor-infiltrating T-cells and NK cells of patients with colorectal carcinoma. *Cancer Res* 1993;53:5610–5612.

387. Rabinowich H, Suminami Y, Reichert TE, et al. Expression of cytokine genes or proteins and signaling molecules in lymphocytes associated with human ovarian carcinoma. *Int J Cancer* 1996;68:276–284.

388. Franco JL, Ghosh P, Wiltrout RH, et al. Partial degradation of T-cell signal transduction molecules by contaminating granulocytes during protein extraction of splenic T cells from tumor-bearing mice. *Cancer Res* 1995;55: 3840–3846.

389. Li X, Liu J, Park JK, et al. T cells from renal cell carcinoma patients exhibit an abnormal pattern of kappa B-specific DNA-binding activity: a preliminary report. *Cancer Res* 1994;54:5424–5429.

390. Ghosh P, Sica A, Young HA, et al. Alterations in NF kappa B/Rel family proteins in splenic T-cells from tumor-bearing mice and reversal following therapy. *Cancer Res* 1994;54:2969–2972.

391. Aoe T, Okamoto Y, Saito T. Activated macrophages induce structural abnormalities of the T cell receptor-CD3 complex. *J Exp Med* 1995;181:1881–1886.

392. Mullen CA, Rowley DA, Schreiber H. Highly immunogenic regressor tumor cells can prevent development of postsurgical tumor immunity. *Cell Immunol* 1989;119:101–113.

393. Fujimoto S, Greene MI, Sehon AH. Regulation of the immune response to tumor antigens. I. Immunosuppressor cells in tumor-bearing hosts. *J Immunol* 1976; 116:791–799.

394. Berendt MJ, North RJ. T-cell-mediated suppression of anti-tumor immunity. An explanation for progressive growth of an immunogenic tumor. *J Exp Med* 1980; 151:69–80.

395. Naor D. Suppressor cells: permitters and promoters of malignancy? *Adv Cancer Res* 1979;29:45–125.

396. Ting CC, Rodrigues D. Switching on the macrophage-mediated suppressor mechanism by tumor cells to evade host immune surveillance. *Proc Natl Acad Sci USA* 1980;77:4265–4269.

397. North RJ. Cyclophosphamide-facilitated adoptive immunotherapy of an established tumor depends on elimination of tumor-induced suppressor T cells. *J Exp Med* 1982;155:1063–1074.

398. Miller RA. The aging immune system: primer and prospectus. *Science* 1996;273: 70–74.

399. Suzich JA, Ghim SJ, Palmer-Hill FJ, et al. Systemic immunization with papillomavirus L1 protein completely prevents the development of viral mucosal papillomas. *Proc Natl Acad Sci USA* 1995;92:11553–11557.

400. Deichman GI. Immunological aspects of carcinogenesis by deoxyribonucleic acid tumor viruses. *Adv Cancer Res* 1969;12:101–136.

401. Ye X, McCarrick J, Jewett L, Knowles BB. Timely immunization subverts the development of peripheral nonresponsiveness and suppresses tumor development in simian virus 40 tumor antigen-transgenic mice. *Proc Natl Acad Sci USA* 1994;91:3916–3920.

402. Morales A, Eidinger D, Bruce AW. Intracavitary Bacillus Calmette-Guerin in the treatment of superficial bladder tumors. *J Urol* 1976;116:180–183.

403. Fehleisen F. Über die Züchtung der Erysipel-Kokken auf Künstlichen Nährböden und die Übertragbarkeit auf den Menschen. *Deutsche Med Wochenschr* 1882;8: 553–554.

404. Bruns P. Die Heilwirkung des Erysipels auf Geschwülste. *Beitr Klin Chir* 1887–1888;3:443–466.

405. Coley WB. The treatment of malignant tumors by repeated inoculations of erysipelas: with a report of ten original cases. *Am J Med Sci* 1893;105:487–511.

406. Trinchieri G. Function and clinical use of interleukin-12. *Curr Opin Hematol* 1997;4:59–66.

407. Bartlett GL. In vivo methods for the assessment of cell-mediated tumor immunity. *Natl Cancer Inst Monogr* 1972;35:27–32.

408. Lindenmann J, Klein PA. Viral oncolysis: increased immunogenicity of host cell antigen associated with influenza virus. *J Exp Med* 1967;126:93–108.

409. Austin FC, Boone CW. Virus augmentation of the antigenicity of tumor cell extracts. *Adv Cancer Res* 1979;30:301–345.

410. Haas C, Schirrmacher V. Immunogenicity increase of autologous tumor cell vaccines by virus infection and attachment of bispecific antibodies. *Cancer Immunol Immunother* 1996;43:190–194.

411. Liang W, Cohen EP. Resistance to murine leukemia in mice rejecting syngeneic somatic hybrid-cells. *J Immunol* 1976;116:623–626.

412. Guo Y, Wu M, Chen H, et al. Effective tumor vaccine generated by fusion of hepatoma cells with activated B cells. *Science* 1994;263:518–520.

413. Gong J, Chen D, Kashiwaba M, Kufe D. Induction of antitumor activity by immunization with fusions of dendritic and carcinoma cells. *Nat Med* 1997;3: 558–561.

414. DeBruyne L. Treatment of malignancy by direct gene transfer of a foreign MHC class I molecule. *Cancer Immunol Immunother* 1996;43:180–189.

415. Baskar S, Glimcher L, Nabavi N, Jones RT, Ostrand-Rosenberg S. Major histocompatibility complex class II+ B7-1+ tumor cells are potent vaccines for stimulating tumor rejection in tumor-bearing mice. *J Exp Med* 31995;181:619–629.

416. Mitchison NA. Immunologic approach to cancer. *Transplant Proc* 1970;2: 92–103.

417. Sato T. Active specific immunotherapy with hapten-modified autologous melanoma cell vaccine. *Cancer Immunol Immunother* 1996;43:174–179.

418. Van Pel A, Boon T. Protection against a nonimmunogenic mouse leukemia by an immunogenic variant obtained by mutagenesis. *Proc Natl Acad Sci USA* 1982; 79:4718–4722.

419. Chen L, Ashe S, Brady WA, et al. Costimulation of antitumor immunity by the B7 counter-receptor for the T lymphocyte molecules CD28 and CTLA-4. *Cell* 1992;71:1093–1102.

420. Townsend SE, Allison JP. Tumor rejection after direct costimulation of CD8+ T cells by B7-transfected melanoma cells. *Science* 1993;259:368–370.

421. Woodruff MF, Boak JL. Inhibitory effect of injection of Corynebacterium parvum on the growth of tumour transplants in isogenic hosts. *Br J Cancer* 1966; 20:345–355.

422. Dye ES, North RJ, Mills CD. Mechanisms of anti-tumor action of Corynebacterium parvum. I. Potentiated tumor-specific immunity and its therapeutic limitations. *J Exp Med* 1981;154:609–620.

423. Blankenstein T, Cayeux S, Qin Z. Genetic approaches to cancer immunotherapy. *Rev Physiol Biochem Pharmacol* 1996;129:1–49.

424. Colombo MP, Rodolfo M. Tumor cells engineered to produce cytokines or cofactors as cellular vaccines: do animal studies really support clinical trials? *Cancer Immunol Immunothery* 1995;41:265–270.

425. Trojan J, Johnson TR, Rudin SD, Ilan J, Tykocinski ML, Ilan J. Treatment and prevention of rat glioblastoma by immunogenic C6 cells expressing antisense insulin-like growth factor I RNA. *Science* 1993;259:94–97.

426. Toes RE, Offringa R, Blom RJ, Melief CJ, Kast WM. Peptide vaccination can lead to enhanced tumor growth through specific T-cell tolerance induction. *Proc Natl Acad Sci USA* 1996;93:7855–7860.

427. Shurin MR. Dendritic cells presenting tumor antigen. *Cancer Immunol Immunother* 1996;43:158–164.

428. Donnelly JJ, Ulmer JB, Liu MA. DNA vaccines. *Life Sci* 1997;60:163–172.

429. Syrengelas AD, Chen TT, Levy R. DNA immunization induces protective immunity against B-cell lymphoma. *Nat Med* 1996;2:1038–1041.

430. Mittelman A, Wang X, Matsumoto K, Ferrone S. Antiidiotypic response and clinical course of the disease in patients with malignant melanoma immunized with mouse antiidiotypic monoclonal antibody MK2-23. *Hybridoma* 1995;14:175–181.

431. Uhr JW, Picker LJ, Scheuermann RH, Tucker TF, Vitetta ES, Yefenof E. Cancer dormancy: isolation and characterization of dormant lymphoma cells. 45th Annual Symposium on Fundamental Cancer Research, The University of Texas, MD Anderson Cancer Center. 1992:29–30.

432. Houghton AN, Mintzer D, Cordon-Cardo C, et al. Mouse monoclonal IgG3 antibody detecting GD3 ganglioside: a phase I trial in patients with malignant melanoma. *Proc Natl Acad Sci USA* 1985;82:1242–1246.

433. Goodman GE, Hellström I, Brodzinsky L, et al. Phase I trial of murine monoclonal antibody L6 in breast, colon, ovarian, and lung cancer. *J Clin Oncol* 1990; 8:1083–1092.

434. Drebin JA, Link VC, Weinberg RA, Greene MI. Inhibition of tumor growth by a monoclonal antibody reactive with an oncogene-encoded tumor antigen. *Proc Natl Acad Sci USA* 1986;83:9129–9133.

435. Stancovski I, Hurwitz E, Leitner O, Ullrich A, Yarden Y, Sela M. Mechanistic aspects of the opposing effects of monoclonal antibodies to the ERBB2 receptor on tumor growth. *Proc Natl Acad Sci USA* 1991;88:8691–8695.

436. Bacus SS, Stancovski I, Huberman E, et al. Tumor-inhibitory monoclonal antibodies to the HER-2/Neu receptor induce differentiation of human breast cancer cells. *Cancer Res* 1992;52:2580–2589.

437. Waldmann TA. Multichain interleukin-2 receptor: a target for immunotherapy in lymphoma. *J Natl Cancer Inst* 1989;81:914–923.

438. Ghetie V, Vitetta E. Immunotoxins in the therapy of cancer: from bench to clinic. *Pharmacol Ther* 1994;63:209–234.

439. Reisfeld RA, Gillies SD. Recombinant antibody fusion proteins for cancer immunotherapy. *Curr Top Microbiol Immunol* 1996;213:27–53.

440. Rosenberg SA, Packard BS, Aebersold PM, et al. Use of tumor-infiltrating lymphocytes and interleukin-2 in the immunotherapy of patients with metastatic melanoma. A preliminary report. *N Engl J Med* 1988;319:1676–1680.

Fundamental Immunology, Fourth Edition,
edited by William E. Paul
Published by Lippincott–Raven Publishers, Philadelphia 1999.

CHAPTER 38

Immune Regulation in Parasitic Infection and Disease

Edward J. Pearce, Phillip A. Scott, and Alan Sher

Parasites and the Immune System
Type 1–Type 2 Responses Induced by Natural Infection
Initiation of the Immune Response to Parasites
Influence of Parasitic Infection on Immune Responsiveness and Self-reactivity
Evasion of Effector Responses by Parasites
Vaccination against Parasites
General Conclusions
Acknowledgments
References

PARASITES AND THE IMMUNE SYSTEM

The Nature and Global Health Importance of Parasitic Pathogens

The word *parasite,* although strictly applicable to all infectious agents, is usually understood to refer only to protozoan and metazoan pathogens. Despite the disparate nature of this group, parasites are often (although not always) characterized by their longevity, or chronicity, in the host; their metamorphosis through multiple and usually antigenically distinct life-cycle stages; and their expression of highly evolved immune evasion mechanisms. Cruelly, the most serious parasitic infections tend to occur in developing areas within the tropics, where they continue to be an enormous public health and economic burden. As illustrated by the outbreaks in North America of disease caused by the protozoa

E. J. Pearce: Department of Microbiology and Immunology, Cornell University, College of Veterinary Medicine, Ithaca, New York 14853-4601.

P. A. Scott: Department of Pathobiology, School of Veterinary Medicine, University of Pennsylvania, Philadelphia, Pennsylvania 19104.

A. Sher: Immunobiology Section, Laboratory of Parasitic Diseases, National Institute of Allergy and Infectious Disease, National Institutes of Health, Bethesda, Maryland 20892.

Cryptosporidium (1), *Cyclospora* (2), and *Toxoplasma* (3), parasites also represent a significant emerging threat to populations in more developed regions. The current acquired immunodeficiency syndrome (AIDS) epidemic has also increased the impact of parasitic disease in richer countries, because immunocompromised individuals are uniquely sensitive to some normally tolerated parasites, such as *Toxoplasma gondii.*

Overall, it is clear that, as a group, parasitic diseases remain a major global human health problem and, despite the more rapid deployment of intervention strategies, also continue to exact a heavy toll on livestock worldwide. A list of the most important parasitic infections of humans, along with estimates of their incidence, prevalence, and current control methods, is presented in Table 1. Table 1 emphasizes that after decades of active research there is still no commercially available vaccine for any parasitic infection of humans, a fact that underscores both our deficient understanding of the nature of protective immunity to parasites as well as the sophistication of parasite immune evasion mechanisms. However, it belies the considerable advances in our knowledge of the immune response to parasites which have emerged in recent years, largely from the application of approaches and concepts from fundamental immunology. In turn, studies on parasitic infection models have provided immunology with major insights as well as fre-

TABLE 1. *Primary parasitic infections of humans*

Parasitic disease	New (incidence)	All (prevalence)	Current methods of control
Protozoa			
Malaria	300–500 million	Data not available	Vector control, chemotherapy, bed nets
Chagas disease (*T. cruzi*)	800,000	18 million	Vector control
Leishmaniasis	18 million	12 million	Vector control, chemotherapy
Sleeping sickness	Data not available	300,000	Vector control
(*T. brucei rhodesiense* and *T. gambiense*)			
Helminths	Data not available		
Ascariasis		250 million	Chemotherapy, hygiene
Schistosomiasis		200 million	Chemotherapy, hygiene
Hookworm		151 million	Chemotherapy, hygiene
Filariasis (lymphatic)		120 million	Vector control, chemotherapy
Trichuriasis		46 million	Chemotherapy, hygiene
Onchocerciasis		18 million	Chemotherapy

Data compiled from the 1996 World Health Report.

quent "reality checks" concerning effector and regulatory responses as they occur *in vivo*. This highly productive interface between modern parasitologic and immunologic research is the focus of this chapter.

The Role of T-Cell Subsets in the Response to Parasites

At the time of the preparation of the previous edition of *Fundamental Immunology*, the T cell–subset dichotomy had arisen as the prevailing framework within which to investigate parasite-directed immune responses. This concept, based largely on the seminal work of Mosmann and Coffman (4), divides immunologic effector functions into two major categories based on the pattern of lymphokine expression by CD4 T cells (see Chapter 26). Moreover, the discovery that cytokines produced by the respective T helper 1–T helper 2 (Th1/Th2) lymphocyte subsets cross-inhibit each other's development and function provides a widely applicable, molecularly based rationale for understanding the polarization of immune responses occurring in many infectious diseases. Indeed, the first direct demonstrations of the relevance of the Th1/Th2 paradigm to the regulation of disease *in vivo* were made in studies on the *Leishmania major* mouse model (discussed below). It is now clear that a wide variety of different parasite-induced responses show a dominant Th1 or Th2 cytokine production profile that is frequently associated with either an exacerbative or protective effect on infection. Nevertheless, we now also realize that cells [e.g., CD8, γδ, natural killer (NK cells)] other than CD4 lymphocytes can contribute to the observed *in vivo* cytokine production pattern (5). Accordingly, to be more accurate, immune responses are now often assigned a type 1 or type 2 (as opposed to Th1/Th2) designation, based solely on the cytokine production profile without directly implicating the cellular source (6). While in one sense more appropriate, this type 1–type 2 nomenclature has resulted in considerable confusion, both with the structurally based type 1 and type 2 designations for cytokine families (see Chapter 21) as well as with the type I through IV terminology for hypersensitivity responses, originally established by Coombs and Gel (7). Although in need of revision, we will defer to this now widely accepted categorization and designate parasite-induced responses as type 1 or type 2, based on the dominant cytokine profile.

While a conceptually powerful framework for analyzing effector functions and their regulation, the T cell–cytokine dichotomy often presents an oversimplified view of parasite-induced immune responses and their influence on host resistance or disease. As emphasized below, few of these responses are purely type 1 or type 2 in character, and many are accompanied by cryptic responses of the opposite type, which are downregulated by inhibitory cytokines produced by the dominant subset. As will be discussed, such cross-regulation may have evolved to protect the host against the potential immunopathologic consequences of the suppressed response and/or the unregulated dominant response. Similarly, it is becoming increasingly clear that many host resistance and disease processes, rather than mediated solely by either type 1 or type 2 T cells or their cytokines, actually require an orchestration of both responses. Finally, a number of new mechanisms [e.g., that involving CTLA4-mediated immune response downregulation (8)] have been described in recent years that offer explanations for parasite-triggered immunoregulatory phenomena that invoke neither T-cell subsets nor their cytokines.

TYPE 1–TYPE 2 RESPONSES INDUCED BY NATURAL INFECTION

In describing parasite-directed immune responses, we will first discuss those protective and immunopathologic responses induced by natural infection. A separate section devoted to vaccine-induced immunity is presented later in the chapter. In terms of naturally stimulated host resistance, the most obvious type of protective immune response is that which allows an infected animal to definitively clear its parasites. In reality, most parasites, through their elaborately evolved evasion strategies, produce infections that are chronic or persistent in nature and are seldom completely eliminated by host immunity. The more usual situation and best-case scenario is that the immune response is able to partially protect the host, thereby preventing lethal infection, but in the process, also stimulates immunopathology. The immunologic features of these parasite-induced responses and their role in the induction of both resistance and disease are described below. Conceptual summaries of the inductive and effector phases of parasite-triggered type 1 and type 2 pathways are presented in Figs. 1 and 2.

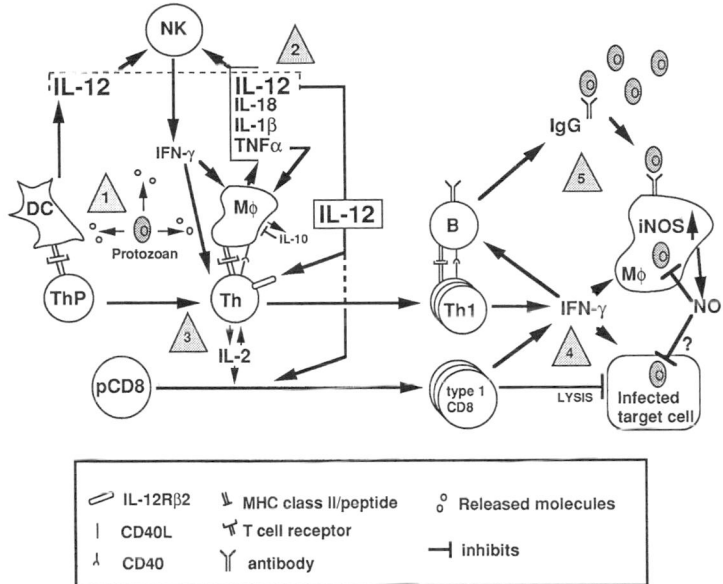

FIG. 1. Type 1 response induction and effector function during protozoan infection. **Step 1:** Early in infection, parasites and/or molecules that they release activate dendritic cells and/or macrophages (or neutrophils) to make IL-12 and other proinflammatory cytokines. **Step 2:** Together, these cytokines activate NK cells to make IFN-γ, which itself functions to promote the production of more IL-12 and, in conjunction with TNF-α, to upregulate iNOS in macrophages (and probably additional cell types). NO plus other reactive nitrogen intermediates act to begin to control parasite growth. IL-10 and possibly other downregulatory cytokine are also synthesized to prevent overproduction of proinflammatory cytokines. **Step 3:** Antigen presentation to ThP cells in an environment rich in IL-12 initiates a STAT4-dependent differentiation step towards a Th1 phenotype (see Chapter 26), and IFN-γ maintains IL-12Rβ2 expression on the differentiating Th cell, allowing it to continue to receive signals from IL-12. IL-2 produced by responding T cells acts as an autocrine growth factor, a growth factor for pCD8 cells, and also promotes NK-cell activation. Activated Th cells express CD40L and through a CD40L-CD40 interaction, can directly activate macrophages to make IL-12, thereby accentuating the type 1 response. IL-12 also promotes the differentiation of precursor CD8 cells into type 1 CD8 cells. **Step 4:** In the later stages of infection following the development of the adaptive response, Th1 and type 1 CD8 cells, by making large amounts of IFN-γ, are able to activate macrophages and other cells to control parasite growth, by the production of mediators such as NO. Type 1 CD8 cells may also be directly cytotoxic towards infected cells. **Step 5:** B cells responding to parasite Ag and receiving help from Th1 cells (or type 1 CD8 cells) produce antibodies that are complement fixing and opsonizing and thus able to target parasites to macrophages for phagocytosis and destruction.

Protective Type 1 Responses

Protozoa

The prototype of a protective type 1 response is that responsible for resistance to *L. major* in the mouse model. In their mammalian hosts, all *Leishmania* species live intracellularly as dividing amastigotes within the phagolysosomal compartments of macrophages. The disease is transmitted by biting sand flies, within which the parasites transform from amastigotes to promastigotes, divide, and differentiate to become once again infectious for mammals.

Experimentally, promastigotes can be grown in tissue culture and, by injection, used to initiate infections. In all strains of mice, *L. major* causes an early lesion of varying magnitude, and, in resistant strains of mice, the lesions resolve. Current evidence suggests that resolution is primarily the result of the activation of

macrophages by interferon-γ (IFN-γ), produced initially by NK cells and then subsequently by Th1 cells (9–12) The central role for CD4 T cells is evident when mice lacking CD4 or CD8 T cells are infected. Thus, major histocompatibility complex (MHC) class II knock-out mice are unable to control *L. major* infections (13), while β2-microglobulin (β2m)$^{-/-}$ mice exhibit a healing infection similar to their wild-type (WT) counterparts (14). Paradoxically, following infection of class II$^{-/-}$ mice with *Leishmania amazonensis,* a species that is less well studied, lesion development is drastically delayed (15). The latter finding suggests that T cells are not only important as effector (Th1) or suppressor (Th2) cells, but with some species of *Leishmania* may be required for maintaining infection by promoting an influx of inflammatory macrophages for the parasites to invade.

The ultimate effector molecules responsible for controlling *Leishmania* growth are reactive nitrogen intermediates generated

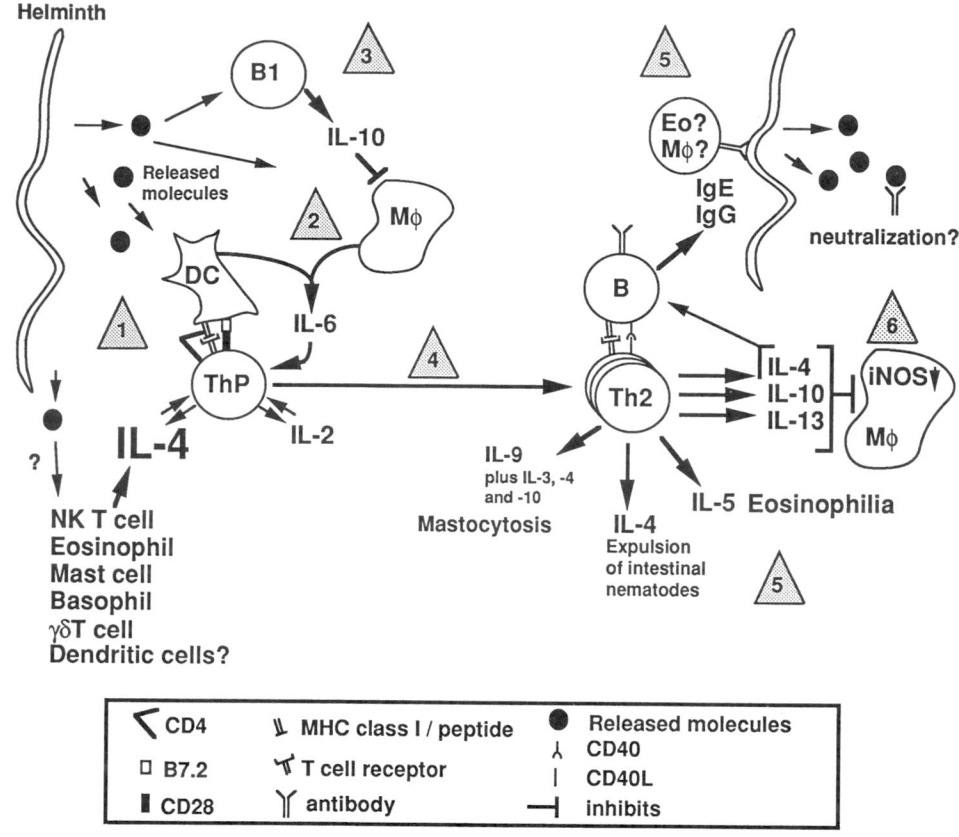

FIG. 2. Type 2 response induction and effector function during helminth infection. **Step 1:** Helminth antigens are presented to specific pTh cells, which either make IL-4 themselves or are triggered by IL-4 from other cell types that have been activated as a consequence of infection. The various cell types implicated in the production of early IL-4 are listed. **Step 2:** IL-4 production by ThP cells may be promoted by macrophage and/or dendritic cell–derived IL-6. **Step 3:** Helminth Ags fail to stimulate substantial IL-12 production by macrophages or dendritic cells, perhaps because they can, in certain instances, induce rapid IL-10 production by B1 or other cells. Additionally, helminths may promote rapid B7-2 upregulation, which can enhance type 2 response development. **Step 4:** IL-4, in a STAT6- (see Chapter 26) and CD4-dependent manner, promotes ThP-cell differentiation towards a Th2 phenotype and simultaneosuly causes IL-12Rβ2 downregulation, thereby extinguishing reponsiveness to IL-12 and consolidating the Th2 response. **Step 5:** Th2 cells orchestrate a panel of responses that, in particular instances, can play protective roles. **Step 6:** In addition to promoting antihelminth effector functions, type 2 responses can also play an important role in limiting the pathogenic effects of type 1 inflammatory responses mediated by macrophages.

by iNOS within infected macrophages activated with IFN-γ (16). IFN-γ is absolutely essential in lesion resolution, as shown by the fact the neither IFN-γ (17) nor IFN-γ receptor (18) knock-out mice are able to control parasite replication. Similarly, disruption of the iNOS⁻/⁻ gene in a normally resistant strain leads to a susceptible phenotype (19). Moreover, prolonged treatment of infected resistant mice with the iNOS inhibitor L-N6-iminoethyl-lysine (L-NIL) also results in susceptibility (20). Interestingly, when inhibitor treatment was started late after resolution of primary infection in resistant animals, lesion reactivation and parasite outgrowth occurred (20), strongly supporting the view that immunity to *Leishmania* is not sterile and is dependent on continued control of parasite replication by iNOS-dependent mechanisms. How parasites are able to persist in the long term in resistant animals remains unclear, but it remains possible that there is a so far undescribed, persistent, metabolically quiescent *Leishmania* stage analogous to the *Toxoplasma* cyst (see below).

The upregulation of iNOS and subsequent production of NO by activated macrophages has, in many systems, been considered

to be tumor necrosis factor-α (TNF-α)–dependent (21,22). However, it is now clear that in *L. major*-infected macrophages, NO can be produced in a TNF-independent manner, because IFN-γ–activated macrophages taken from TNFRI mice can make NO and kill *Leishmania* parasites (23). One interpretation of this finding is that alternative second signals exist for macrophage activation in these animals. Possible substitutes for the TNF signal are CD40, through ligation by CD40L, and/or a parasite immunostimulatory molecule(s) analogous to lipopolysaccharide (LPS) (discussed separately below). Interestingly, studies with the TNFR knock-out animals have revealed an important role independent of parasite killing for TNFRI in lesion resolution (23). Normally, C57BL/6 mice develop a lesion at the site of parasite inoculation that subsequently resolves. Once healed, it is difficult to culture parasites from the lesion [although pretreating the animals with an inhibitor of iNOS facilitates this process (20)]. In C57BL/6 TNFR1⁻/⁻ mice, parasites are eliminated with the same kinetics as in WT mice, but lesion resolution fails to occur. Examination of the cellular composition of the lesion revealed it to be predominantly lymphocytic in nature. One interpretation of these findings is that during normal lesion resolution, TNF-driven apoptosis plays a crucial role in promoting the death of parasite antigen–specific T cells, a function absent in the knock-out animals.

Trypanosoma cruzi, like *Leishmania,* a member of the kinetoplastidae, is also an intracellular parasite that is transmitted by the bite of a hematophagous insect. In the mammalian host, *T. cruzi* is able to invade many different nucleated cell types, and once intracellular, is able to leave the parasitophorous vacuole and enter the cytoplasm. This of course places it in the appropriate subcellular compartment to allow antigen processing through the class I pathway (24), which implies that infection will lead to the induction of a CD8 cell response. That this is the case and that the CD8 cells are likely to play a role in protection were illustrated by the finding that class I–deficient ($\beta2m^{-/-}$ and class I$^{-/-}$) mice are extremely susceptible to infection (25,26). Although antigen-specific cytolytic CD8 cells are generated during infection, it is probable that IFN-γ produced by these cells, rather than classical perforin- and granzyme-mediated cytotoxicity, is playing the dominant role in protection, as the administration to infected mice of IFN-γ, or of a neutralizing mAb anti–IFN-γ, leads to diminished or exacerbated infections, respectively (27). NO is the likely effector molecule induced by IFN-γ (28). Th1 cells and antibody also contribute toward the control of *T. cruzi* infection, the former by producing IFN-γ, and possibly by providing IL-2 for CD8 cells, and the latter by inhibiting the spread of the parasites between host cells (26). During acute *T. cruzi* infection, NK cells also serve as a source of IFN-γ (29). The importance of type 1 responses in resistance to *T. cruzi* is supported by the finding that mouse strains that are highly susceptible to infection can be rendered more resistant by treatment with mAb anti–IL-10 (30).

Apicomplexan parasites, intracellular protozoa characterized by a distinct set of apical organelles, which play a role in invasion, are, like the kinetoplastidae, also susceptible to type 1 mediated immune responses. Malaria, caused by *Plasmodia* species, is undoubtedly the most important parasitic disease of humans. It is transmitted between hosts by infected mosquitoes, which, when they bite, introduce the malaria sporozoite stages, which travel with the blood to the liver, where they rapidly invade hepatocytes and undergo a series of divisions to give rise to merozoites. Merozoites reenter the bloodstream and invade erythrocytes, within which they multiply through several microscopically distinct stages to give rise either to additional merozoites, which, by infecting erythrocytes, continue the infection, or to gametes, which, if taken up by a feeding mosquito, fuse and initiate the sexual stage of the life cycle, which eventually gives rise to sporozoites. This complex life cycle—involving intracellular residence in two distinct host cell types, one of which expresses class I (the hepatocyte) and the other (the erythrocyte) of which does not, and the extracellular existence of several distinct life forms of the parasite—implies that more than one type of immune response may be important for controlling malaria. This has turned out to be the case, with antibodies effective against sporozoite and erythrocytic stages (to be discussed further below) and type 1 cytokine-mediated responses that are functional against the intrahepatic stages. The latter is illustrated perhaps most clearly by the finding that the injection of IL-12 into monkeys or mice 2 days prior to challenge with *P. cynomolgi* or *P. yoelii,* respectively, completely prevents infection (31,32). In the mouse model, this was shown to be due to the production of IFN-γ by NK cells and the upregulation in the liver of iNOS, with NO being the assumed effector mechanism against the intracellular parasite (32). Hepatocytes can express iNOS (33), so presumably the IFN-γ is working directly on these cells to induce the parasite-directed effector response.

While Th2 responses are important for resistance to blood-stage malaria (see below), type 1 responses, under certain circumstances, may also contribute (34). For example, in normally susceptible A/J mice, injection of IL-12 prior to and following exposure to *P. chabaudi*-infected erythrocytes results in decreased parasitemia and, in some cases, increased survival, a mechanism in which Th1 cells, IFN-γ, TNF, and NO are implicated (35). Detailed studies of Th responses from acute to chronic blood-stage infections with *P. chabaudi chabaudi* have revealed that the type 1 response (mediated by NO) is important at earlier time points, but that later in infection, a type 2 response, B cells, and IgG1 antibodies are essential for the complete clearance of the parasite (36).

In humans living in areas endemic for *P. falciparum,* there is evidence of the slow development of immunity. The antibody-based nature of this was demonstrated in experiments in which sera from adults were transferred to children, resulting in a temporary but highly significant reduction in parasitemia (37). The proposed mode of action of this antibody is in so-called antibody-dependent cellular inhibition (ADCI), in which IFN-γ–dependent cytophilic IgG1 and IgG3 in donor serum interact with monocytes or granulocytes via FcR, thereby signaling them to produce TNF-α, which is, in some so far ill-defined way, inhibitory for parasite development. Similar experiments have been performed using the mouse *P. yoelii* or *P. berghei* systems, in which the type 1 response–associated cytophilic IgG2a from the infected animals is able to control an existing infection or prevent new infections (38,39).

T. gondii, an apicomplexan parasite contracted perorally, is, in most individuals, a manageable, although persistent, infection. However, infected individuals who develop AIDS require constant chemotherapy to prevent fatal reactivation (40). It is an unusual parasite inasmuch as it is able to infect a wide variety of different vertebrate hosts (not being restricted to mammals) and is able to live within any nucleated cell type. Unlike *T. cruzi, T. gondii* remains within a membrane-bound compartment [albeit much modified (41)] in the host cell. In immunologically competent intermediate hosts (the cat is the only definitive host for this parasite and will not be discussed here), the infection is chronic and the parasite is found encysted in muscle and central nervous system (CNS) tissue. IFN-γ– and TNF-α–dependent immune pressure, probably manifest as NO production (see below), maintains the organism in this relatively benign state; monoclonal antibody (mAb)-mediated neutralization of either of these cytokines allows the parasites to emerge, invade surrounding tissue, and disseminate (42,43). Animals so treated, like AIDS patients with uncontrolled toxoplasmosis, die of toxoplasmic encephalitis. Careful dissection of the murine immune response to this parasite has shown that both CD4 and CD8 cells are necessary for resistance, because mice made deficient of both these cell types die during the chronic phase of infection (44). Data suggest that CD8 cells are the effectors, while CD4 cells primarily act in a helper capacity (probably providing IL-2 for CD8 cells). While CD8 cells that are cytolytic for *T. gondii*-infected target cells have been identified (45,46), the protective role of this cell type *in vivo* appears to be not due to direct cytotoxicity, as perforin$^{-/-}$ mice are nearly as resistant as WT mice to infection (47). Rather, the CD8 cells appear to be playing a protective role by secreting IFN-γ (48); this is reminiscent of the role of CD8 cells in resistance to malaria and *T. cruzi.*

In vitro studies have pointed toward NO as being a major effector against *T. gondii*, because killing of the parasites by IFN-γ–activated, infected macrophages could be prevented by inhibitors of iNOS (49), and macrophages from iNOS$^{-/-}$ mice are incapable of controlling the parasite (50). However, iNOS$^{-/-}$ mice survived through the acute period of infection and did not succumb until the chronic phase, at which time the parasite has reached and encysted within the brain (50). This finding led to two important conclusions. First, an IFN-γ–dependent iNOS-independent mechanism is responsible for controlling the parasite during the initial stages of infection. Examination of cell types represented in the cellular infiltrate at the site of infection revealed a large granulocyte component, and depletion of these cells, using mAb that targets neutrophils and eosinophils, rendered mice acutely sensitive to infection, strongly implicating these cells in the protective early response (50,51). Further experiments, using IL-5–depleted animals, which were competent to control acute infection, indicated that the antigranulocyte antibody was functioning to abrogate immunity by depleting neutrophils, not eosinophils (50). The second realization from these experiments is that some cell type within the brain, possibly the macrophage-like microglial cell, is utilizing iNOS to control the parasites. As in the *Leishmania* system, this production of iNOS does not require TNFR signaling (52). Interestingly, in humans, IFN-γ is additionally able to mediate killing of parasites infecting nonmacrophage cell types (e.g., fibroblasts) through the intracellular depletion of free tryptophan, an essential amino acid for *T. gondii* (53).

The potency of type 1 immune responses in resistance to *T. gondii* is perhaps exemplified by a vaccine model in which complete protection against the highly virulent RH strain (LD50, one parasite) of the parasite is induced by prior exposure to a temperature-sensitive (avirulent) mutant of the same strain (54). Again, resistance appears to be mediated by CD8 cells through the production of IFN-γ (55). In this system, CD4 cells are essential for the successful induction of the protective immune response by the vaccine, but they play a role as helpers rather than effectors during challenge infection (55). Interestingly, in this model, NK1.1$^+$CD4$^+$ T cells (NK T cells) can substitute for Th cells as a source of help for CD8 cells in class II$^{-/-}$ mice (56), and NK cells can substitute for CD8 cells as a source of IFN-γ in class I–deficient β2m$^{-/-}$ mice (57).

Other apicomplexan parasites that are contracted via the fecal–oral route, but which, unlike *T. gondii*, remain in the intestinal mucosa and normally do not disseminate, are *Cryptosporidium* and *Eimeria* species. Within these genera there are pathogens of considerable veterinary importance, and *C. parvum* is also a pathogen of humans. As for *T. gondii*, type 1 responses play a central role in the control of these parasites, with IL-12 promoting the induction of protective immunity to *Cryptosporidium* (58) and CD4 cells and IFN-γ serving as crucial effector components of the protective response to both pathogens (59–61).

Helminths

The most well-documented example of a host-protective type 1 immune response against helminth infection is provided by the radiation-attenuated vaccine for *Schistosoma mansoni*, discussed in detail below. Further evidence for protective type 1 responses against helminths comes from studies of humans living in areas endemic for *Onchocerca volvulus*, a filarial worm transmitted by hematophagous flies, but who fail to become infected. Peripheral blood mononuclear cells (PBMCs) from these individuals respond to *O. volvulus* Ag by making lower amounts of IL-5 and IL-10 and more IFN-γ than do PBMCs from patients who have patent infections (62).

Exacerbative or Pathologic Type 1 Responses

As we learn more about the relationship of parasites with the immune system, it is becoming increasingly clear that there is an extremely fine balance between an effective, protective immune response and one that causes more damage than it prevents. Indeed, in the case of some parasitic infections, it is not clear whether morbidity is due directly to the parasite itself or is the result of an uncontrolled immune response. It now seems that both type 1 and type 2 responses can, under inappropriate conditions, initiate tissue damage during parasite infections.

Protozoa

There is little doubt that type 1 responses are protective against *T. gondii*, with IL-12 (63–65), IFN-γ, CD4 cells, CD8 cells, NK cells, and iNOS all having been shown to play decisive roles in mediating resistance to infection in several different model systems (see above). However, in studies in which infection in mice has been initiated by peroral administration of cysts, the natural route of infection, it has become apparent that there is great potential for an unregulated type 1 response to cause fatal inflammatory disease in the intestine. This was particularly well demonstrated in a comparison of the outcome of infection with the ME49 strain of *T. gondii* in C57BL/6 and BALB/c mice (66). When challenged perorally with a high dose of cysts, C57BL/6 mice develop a potent type 1 response and severe ileal inflammation that can be averted by a mAb, which neutralizes IFN-γ. In contrast, the type 1 response in the infected BALB/c mice was more subdued, and the animals avoided intestinal damage. IL-4 and/or other antiinflammatory cytokines probably play a role in controlling the magnitude of the type 1 response, because in a mouse strain that is resistant to peroral infection, the absence of a functional IL-4 gene leads to increased mortality (67). Interestingly, in the latter situation, those IL-4$^{-/-}$ mice that survive the acute intestinal disease subsequently exhibit reduced brain pathology and parasite burdens (67). Because iNOS is central to the control of *T. gondii* in the CNS (50), it is likely that in WT mice IL-4 is functioning to inhibit NO production, thereby allowing increased parasite burdens in the brain. The importance of endogenous antiinflammatory cytokine production during infection with pathogens that strongly promote type 1 responses has been demonstrated further using IL-10$^{-/-}$ mice. In these animals, both *T. gondii* (68) (Fig. 3A) and *T. cruzi* (69) induce heightened type 1 cytokine production and enhanced mortality, compared with that seen in WT mice. Tissue damage occurs systemically and, in the case of perorally inoculated *T. gondii*, is accompanied by severe intestinal inflammation, even at low-parasite inocula. In another protozoal infection, that caused by *E. vermiformis*, intestinal inflammation is exaggerated in δ$^{-/-}$ mice, which lack γδT cells, probably due to a type 1 αβT-cell response (which controls parasite numbers) becoming immunopathogenic in the absence of appropriate regulation, raising the interesting possi-

A
Toxoplasma gondii

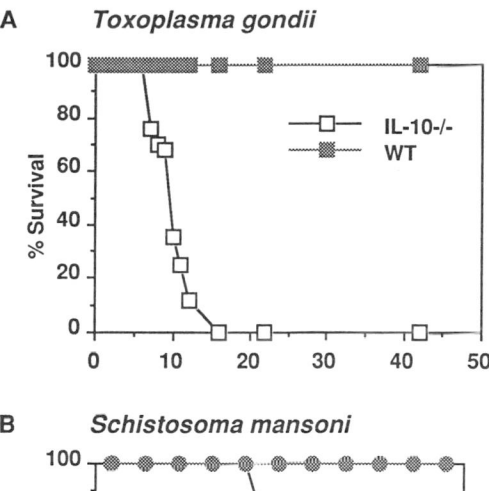

B
Schistosoma mansoni

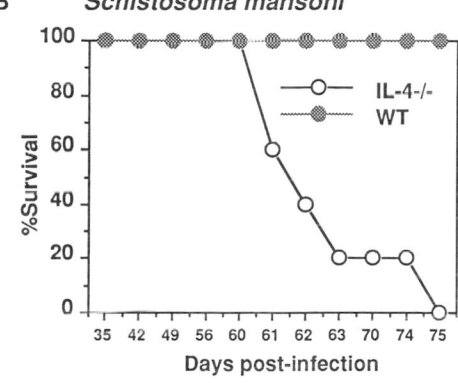

FIG. 3. Experiments illustrating the antiinflammatory roles of type 2 cytokines in protozoan and helminth diseases. **A:** C57BL/10 WT or IL-10$^{-/-}$ mice were each infected with ten to 20 cysts of the *T. gondii* ME-49 strain. While the WT mice survived infection, the IL-10$^{-/-}$ mice succumbed during the acute phase. The animals died with no evidence of enhanced parasite replication, but they did show accentuated tissue pathology. **B:** C57BL/6 WT or IL-4$^{-/-}$ mice were each infected with approximately 30 *S. mansoni* cercariae. At this level of infection, the WT mice all survived, while the IL-4$^{-/-}$ animals became cachectic and succumbed, despite equivalent worm burdens. In both infections, decreased survival is associated with the expression of increased levels of proinflammatory mediators. (Adapted from refs. 68 and 127.)

bility that γδT cells may play a role in producing the cytokines that are known to control intestinal inflammation (70).

While type 1 cytokine production in the absence of regulatory type 2 responses appears to be optimal and nonpathogenic for the control of *Toxoplasma* in the brain, there is, in contrast, a tight correlation between increased TNF-α production and severity of disease during cerebral malaria (CM). In this condition, which is a major cause of death in children infected with *P. falciparum* in sub-Saharan Africa, parasitized erythrocytes adhere to the postcapillary endothelium of blood vessels in the brain, a process that leads to acidosis and reduced local circulation (71,72). In CM patients, high serum TNF levels are prognostic of death (73), and polymorphisms in the TNF-α promoter are associated with susceptibility to CM. It has been postulated that elevated TNF production leads to heightened cerebral NO levels, which may be responsible for the characteristic coma into which severely ill patients lapse (74). In certain strains of mice infected with the ANKA strain of *P. berghei*, which develop a CM-like condition in which brain capillaries and venules become blocked with leukocytes, a neutralizing anti-TNF mAb is able to prevent death (75). These data strongly implicate TNF in CM (for a review of this area, see ref. 76).

In an situation analogous to that seen with *T. gondii* and *T. cruzi*, IL-10$^{-/-}$ mice also exhibit increased susceptibility to *P. chabaudi chabaudi* (77). While type 1 responses play a role early during infection in controlling this parasite, they are normally downregulated and give way to Th2 responses, which then control later blood-stage infection. However, in IL-10$^{-/-}$ mice, the type 1 responses persist and lead to an endotoxin shocklike condition, which can be fatal (77).

Helminths

Studies indicate that type 1 responses have the potential to cause severe disease during helminth infections. Infection with filarial parasites (*Wuchereria bancrofti, Brugia malayi,* and *B. timori*) can lead to a spectrum of conditions, ranging from one in which larval parasites (microfilariae) are present in the blood, but severe pathology associated with adult worms living in the lymphatics is absent, leaving the patient essentially asymptomatic, to one of chronic lymphatic pathology, evident in its most severe form as elephantiasis. Analysis of the cytokines secreted by PBMCs from patients with both types of infection revealed a strong correlation between IFN-γ and severe pathology, and of type 2 cytokines with the microfilaremic condition (78).

The potential for type 1 response–mediated severe disease is also apparent in schistosome infected individuals. *S. mansoni*, which is the most extensively studied of the schistosome species that infect humans, live within the mesenteric veins and migrate to areas adjacent to the intestine to lay their eggs. Through an immune-dependent process, the eggs translocate across the intestinal wall into the lumen of the gut, from there to be excreted to continue the life cycle (79). However, a considerable percentage of the eggs are captured by the blood flow and delivered to the liver, where, due to their size, they become lodged in the sinusoids. The eggs release highly antigenic molecules, which strongly promote the development of Th responses, which then orchestrate the formation of granulomas around the eggs (80,81). The majority (more than 90%) of patients living in areas endemic for schistosomiasis do not suffer from severe disease. However, the minority of infected individuals develop life-threatening hepatosplenomegaly (82). Data indicate that this condition is associated with the ability of PBMCs to make TNF and IFN-γ following *in vitro* stimulation with antigen, whereas PBMCs from low-morbidity patients produce few of these type 1 cytokines, but high levels of IL-5 (83). In this infection, as with lymphatic filariasis, the implication is that a primary role of type 2 responses is to regulate proinflammatory type 1 responses. Analysis of cytokine production by PBMCs from individuals infected with schistosomes or filarial worms, or by spleen cells from schistosome-infected mice, has revealed that cells capable of making IFN-γ in response to antigen are present, but are regulated in their ability to produce this cytokine by other cytokines, such as IL-10 (84–86).

Protective Type 2 Responses

Protozoa

While humoral antibody can play a major role in the immune clearance of protozoa, in most protozoan infections it is difficult to make firm generalizations about the respective roles of Th1- versus Th2-regulated isotypes in protection. One situation in which the Th2 response clearly contributes to host resistance occurs in mice infected with *P. chabaudi chabaudi*. In this model, Th2 and B cells protect against erythrocytic forms of the parasite in the later stages of infection by cooperating in the production of IgG1 antibody (36). The explanation for why antibody of this isotype preferentially mediates resistance is unknown and, as noted above, in a different murine malaria model employing infection with *P. yoelii*, Th1-dependent IgG2a antibodies were found to be protective (38,39).

Helminths

Helminths are unusual in that, in the great majority of cases, they induce strong Th2 responses. This of course is consistent with the long-recognized association between eosinophilia, elevated IgE, and worm infections. For the intestinal helminths in particular, it is clear that elements of the type 2 response are crucial for resistance to infection. Several worms have been studied in detail in this regard: *Trichuris muris,* a natural parasite of the mouse and closely related to human whipworm, *Heligomosoides polygyrus, Trichinella spiralis, Nippostrongylus brasiliensis,* the rat hookworm, and *Strongyloides stercoralis.* Readers are referred to a comprehensive review by Finkelman and colleagues for an in-depth discussion (87).

Both *T. muris* and *H. polygyrus* are transmitted by the oral–fecal route independently of an intermediate host and can cause chronic infections in mice. In the case of the former helminth, different mouse strains are differentially susceptible to infection, with some strains rejecting the parasite shortly after exposure and others (AKR) developing a long-lived infection (88,89). Such genetic control of infection is indicative of the broad range of susceptibilities to whipworm infection evident in human populations, with, in essence, different inbred mouse strains being considered to represent different individuals (90). In this system, resistant mice express type 2 responses, susceptible mice mount Th1 responses (91), and IL-12 causes a switch from a protective type 2 to an infection-permissive type 1 response (92). Most mouse strains are susceptible to a primary *H. polygyrus* infection, but following drug clearance the animals exhibit a strong type 2 response and are highly resistant to a secondary infection. For both *H. polygyrus* and *T. muris,* CD4 cells are required for the induction and/or expression of immunity (93,94). IL-4 can cure primary infections with both *T. muris* and *H. polygyrus* (91,95), anti–IL-4R blocks resistance to both (91,96), and IL-4$^{-/-}$ mice are unable to resist a challenge infection with *H. polygyrus* (87) or a primary infection with *T. muris* (97). It has been found that disruption of the IL-13 gene in a normally resistant strain of mouse leads to susceptibility to *T. muris* in the face of the development of an otherwise "normal" type 2 response, indicating that the earlier finding that mAb anti–IL-4R blocks parasite clearance was probably the result of the inhibition of the binding of IL-13 rather than IL-4 to this receptor (97). Although IL-4 can lead to the expulsion of *N. brasiliensis* from infected severe combined immunodeficiency disease (SCID) or CD4 cell–depleted mice (which normally are unable to expel the usually short-lived adult *N. brasiliensis* parasites) (95), it clearly controls a redundant protective mechanism, as anti–IL-4 mAb–treated mice are as resistant to infection as are WT animals (98). Anti–IL-4R treatment potentiates infection with *T. spiralis*

in the mouse (87), suggesting the possibility that IL-13 also plays a role in the mechanism of host resistance to this infection.

While it is now tempting to extrapolate the findings from these various experimental systems and say that resistance to intestinal nematodes requires Th2-mediated responses, it is far from clear how the type 2 responses are actually functioning to mediate protection. The most simple explanation, and one predicted over many years—that IgE, an isotype of antibodies made by B cells following exposure to IL-4 (99) [and under appropriate situations, other independent signals, possibly CD40L (100)], is protective against intestinal helminths—has, following intensive investigation using mouse models, either been refuted or at least received little direct confirmation. The possibility exists however, that there are host species differences in this regard, because, in rats, "rapid expulsion" (the speedy rejection of a secondary *T. spiralis* infection) can be transferred to naive animals with IgE (101). How IL-4 mediates protection against gastrointestinal nematodes is unclear at present. In uninfected mice, IL-4 has dramatic effects on intestinal physiology, causing decreased peristalsis (102), increased small intestine permeability, and decreased fluid absorption in response to glucose (87). For the most part, these responses appear to be T cell– and mast cell–dependent (87). Their net effect is to increase the intestinal fluid content, a phenomenon whose contribution to parasite rejection remains to be elucidated.

Eosinophils, elevated numbers of which are usually associated with helminth infections, and the production and activation of which are stimulated by the type 2 cytokine IL-5 and inhibited by mAb anti–IL-5 (103,104), have not, at the time of writing, been shown to play any role in protective responses to *T. muris, H. polygyrus* (96), *N. brasiliensis* (103), or *T. spiralis* (105). However, there is evidence from the use of eosinophil-deficient mAb anti–IL-5–treated mice and/or IL-5R α-chain knock-out animals, and from IL-5 transgenic mice that have high levels of ciruclating eosinophils, that eosinophils can be important in protective immune responses directed against tissue-invasive larval forms of *Strongyloides* species (106,107) and *Angiostrongylus cantonensis* (108,109). Moreover, there is a body of literature, primarily from studies in rats and humans, that suggests that eosinophils play a role in protection against (non–gut dwelling) schistosomes (110–112), although mAb anti–IL-5–treated and/or IL-5$^{-/-}$ mice can develop immunity to this parasite (113,114), again suggesting host species differences. Overall, despite the prevailing dogma, the record does not strongly support an indispensable role for eosinophils in immunity to helminths.

Additional prominent components of the type 2 response induced by intestinal helminths are increased IgG1 production and intestinal mastocytosis (87). While IgG1 may play a role in immunity to *T. spiralis* (115) and *H. polygyrus* (116), it plays no obvious protective role in the other intestinal helminthiases. Mast cells, which are implicated in the effects of IL-4 on intestinal physiology (87), appear to play an important role in immunity to *T. spiralis,* as mice treated with mAbs against stem-cell factor (SCF) (a non–T cell–derived cytokine) or c-kit, its receptor (both of which play a central role in mast-cell development), are unable to expulse worms (117). In the latter experiments, there was no effect of the treatment on the CD4 response, and once the mAb treatment was stopped, the parasites were expelled. These data taken together with other findings in this system suggest that a CD4 cell–dependent response cooperates with SCF (a non–T cell–derived cytokine) to promote a mast-cell response that mediates parasite expulsion. Several cytokines made by CD4 cells, including IL-3, IL-4 (118), and IL-9 (119), have been implicated in mastocytosis. Consistent with this, IL-9, when expressed at high levels from a transgene, allows mice to expel *T. spiralis* even more rapidly than is usual (120). Moreover, these mice exhibit an enhanced Th2 response, raising the possibility that IL-4 from mast cells is feeding back to enhance ThP/Th2 differentiation (120) [as has been proposed for IL-4 from basophils in schistosome-infected mice (121)].

In addition to playing a role in immunity to gastrointestinal helminths, there is growing epidemiologic evidence that type 2 responses, particularly in the form of Ag-specific IgE, mediate the resistance to infection with schistosomes that develops with age in endemic areas (122–124). While the exact mechanism by which IgE Abs would mediate protection is unclear, it is possible that they cooperate with eosinophils or macrophages in an ADCC mechanism (125). Consistent with this general hypothesis, data from field studies in Brazil indicate that the ability to resist infection is influenced by a major gene that localizes to a region of chromosome 5 that encodes type 2 cytokines (126).

Studies point to an additional important role for the type 2 response in schistosomiasis in controlling inflammation associated with egg passage across the intestinal wall (127). This process involves the perforation of the mucosal epithelium and, therefore, presumably, an opportunity for bacterial translocation and increased exposure to bacterial toxins. In C57BL/6 IL-4$^{-/-}$ mice, which are Th2 response–defective, infection leads to serious morbidity, characterized by cachexia, leading to death (127) (see Fig. 3B). These animals exhibit more severe intestinal pathology than is normally noted in infected WT mice. Morbidity can be partially ameliorated in these animals with a neutralizing antibody against TNF, and disease severity can be correlated with the level of NO made *in vitro* by their LPS-activated spleen cells. Together, these data indicate that IL-4, and possibly other type 2 antiinflammatory cytokines, such as IL-10 and IL-13, play a crucial role in controlling gut-focused, IFN-γ–exacerbated pathology by inhibiting endotoxin-induced TNF and NO production. Thus, in both mice and humans infected with *S. mansoni*, diminished type 2 and heightened type 1 responses are associated with severe morbidity (83,127).

Exacerbative or Pathologic Type 2 Responses

Protozoa

Following infection of macrophages or dendritic cells by *Leishmania* parasites, the host cell is killed and the parasite progeny infect additional cells within the same lineage. Some species of *Leishmania* are prone, for reasons that may relate to optimal growth temperatures, to metastasizing to visceral organs, where they cause more severe disease, than are others, which remain largely cutaneous (128). As discussed above, *L. major* causes resolving cutaneous leishmaniasis in humans and in the majority of WT mouse strains. In BALB/c mice, however, the infection does not resolve, spreads to the viscera, and is lethal (129). Studies performed during the late 1980s showed that resistance to *L. major* is associated with the development of a marked Th1-like response (10,11), with IFN-γ playing the role of the major effector cytokine, owing to its ability to activate macrophages to kill the intracellular *Leishmania* parasites (9). However, BALB/c mice develop a strong Th2 response following infection and, due in large part to the absence of a macrophage-activating type 1 cytokine (IFN-γ) in combination with the production of the macrophage-deactivating

type 2 cytokines [e.g., IL-4 (130)], develop severe disease. The question of why BALB/c (but not other murine strains) develops Th2 responses following exposure to *L. major* led to the discoveries that naive Th cells from BALB/c mice have an unusual tendency to make IL-4 when stimulated with antigen (131) (Th cells from other strains tend to make less or no IL-4 at this stage of their differentiation) and, moreover, compared to naive Th cells from resistant B10.D2 mice, to become nonreceptive to IL-12 earlier following activation (132).

Although anti–IL-4 treatment can convert a BALB/c mouse into a type 1 responder exhibiting a healing phenotype (133), and similar results have been obtained using IL-4$^{-/-}$ BALB/c animals (134), one paper, showing, unexpectedly, that IL-4$^{-/-}$ BALB/c mice are susceptible to infection (135), has indicated that there are probably multiple factors that contribute to susceptibility. For example, *L. amazonensis* infections do not resolve in mice that can heal following *L. major* infections, and this is not due to the presence of IL-4 (136). Factors that are believed to contribute to the divergent results with the IL-4 knock-out mice include differences in both the *L. major* strain used and the dose of parasites used in the various studies; at very low parasite doses, even BALB/c WT mice can control *L. major* infection (137).

Helminths

Probably the most extensively studied T cell–mediated lesion associated with a parasitic infection is the granuloma that forms around liver-trapped eggs of *S. mansoni*. A considerable body of data indicates that the dominant Th response induced by the eggs is Th2-like, and this is reflected in the composition of the granuloma, which contains a high percentage of eosinophils in addition to macrophages, fibroblasts, and lymphocytes (138). Th cells are essential for granuloma formation (139,140), although all other lymphocyte types examined so far [including B cells (141), CD8 cells (140,142), NK T cells (142), and γδ T cells (143)] are not. Granulomas are pathogenic, primarily not because they cause hepatic failure in the short term, but rather because they precipitate fibrosis, increased portal blood pressure, and the development of portal systemic shunts (144). The role of Th2 cells in these pathologic processes has been shown by experiments in which mice vaccinated with egg antigen plus IL-12 to induce an egg-specific Th1 response upon subsequent infection, developed smaller granulomas and less severe fibrosis than did nonvaccinated infected controls (145). Decreased fibrosis was associated with a diminished Th2-response and accentuated type 1 cytokine production. Additionally, mAb anti–IL-4 treatment of infected mice tends to reduce granuloma size and fibrosis (146), although the same outcome was not observed when different strains of IL-4$^{-/-}$ mice have been studied (127,147). It is important to note that Th1 cytokines (IL-2, IFN-γ) also contribute to granuloma formation, but their role appears to be more prominent in the early stages of the response (80,148–150).

While schistosome egg granulomas are clearly T cell dependent and their expansion is strongly influenced by type 2 cytokines, other elements of the immune response clearly play a role in their development and regulation. Of particular note is an underlying requirement for TNF-α in the pathogenesis of the lesions (151–154). Additionally, as might be expected, chemokines such as MCP-1 (155) and those requiring signaling through the CCR1 receptor family (156) appear to play a role in controlling granuloma formation, although in part perhaps through indirect effects on the Th1/Th2 balance (156,157). Finally, B cell–deficient mice mount exacerbated granulomatous responses and, unlike WT animals, fail to downmodulate pathology late in infection (158). Mice lacking FcγRI have a similar phenotype, suggesting that Ab-mediated signaling events strongly influence the granulomatous response (158).

Although schistosome egg granulomas can clearly lead to pathology (81), they also serve an essential host-protective function (159). This is best illustrated by the observation that a majority of infected SCID mice, which are incapable of mounting granulomatous responses, die of severe hepatocellular necrosis associated with liver-trapped eggs (151). Presumably, the chronic detrimental effects associated with granulomas represent a better alternative (for host and parasite) than that of the host dying soon after parasite egg production begins. Granuloma formation, therefore, seems to be a compromise solution to allow the host to live with the infection.

River blindness, is caused by the migration through the eye of *O. volvulus* microfilarial larvae. While mice are not susceptible to infection with this parasite, they have provided an excellent host for studying the immunopathology of the eye disease, and data suggest an underlying role for type 2 responses in this condition (160,161). In the model employed, mice are immunized subcutaneously with an extract of *O. volvulus* parasites, a process that induces a strong Th2 response, and then challenged intrastromally in the eye with the same antigen. The immunized mice develop severe CD4 cell–dependent corneal opacification and neovascularization, which is averted by treatment with mAb anti–IL-4 and which does not occur in immunized and challenged IL-4$^{-/-}$ animals.

INITIATION OF THE IMMUNE RESPONSE TO PARASITES

Effector Choice Selection

Because of the polarized cytokine profiles induced, there has been a great deal of interest in using parasitic infection models to study how Th1 or Th2 responses are selectively triggered *in vivo*. In the case of Th1 response initiation, most information has come from analysis of experimental infections with the intracellular protozoa *Leishmania* or *T. gondii*. In both models, the early induction of IL-12 has been shown to be crucial to the induction of Th1-dependent host resistance (162–164). As discussed in detail in Chapter 26, this pivotal cytokine provides a link between the innate and adaptive type 1 responses and appears to do so by triggering NK cells to synthesize host-protective IFN-γ while directly promoting the differentiation of naive ThP cells to Th1 cells (165). The IFN-γ stimulated by the IL-12 response is itself immunoregulatory, suppressing Th2 proliferation (166) while providing a positive feedback for greater IL-12 production by macrophages and/or dendritic cells (167).

A major question in this area of research concerns the source of the initial IL-12 triggered by these protozoa to initiate the type 1 response cascade. Activated macrophages are usually considered the major source of the cytokine and *T. gondii* is a stimulator of IL-12 synthesis by these cells *in vitro* (63). Intriguingly, however, the same macrophage populations are not activated to make IL-12 when invaded by *Leishmania* promastigotes (168,169). Instead, the

synthesis of the cytokine is actually inhibited by this parasite (169). On the other hand, evidence from analysis of LN draining sites of *L. major* infection indicate that IL-12 is produced early following infection [although with varying kinetics amongst different resistant mouse strains (163)], raising the possibility that either IL-12 is not coming from macrophages, but rather from some other cell, with the dendritic cell being a likely source (170), or that crucial activating signals are missing in the *in vitro* macrophage culture experiments. The latter possibility is supported by the findings that resistant-strain mice, in which the CD40 or CD40L genes are disrupted, are susceptible to *L. major* infection and fail to mount a Th1 response (171,172). CD40L$^{-/-}$ mice also develop significantly enhanced infections with *L. amazonensis* (173), a species of *Leishmania* to which all mouse strains are susceptible. Mechanistically, decreased resistance to *Leishmania* species in CD40 or CD40L$^{-/-}$ mice appears to be at least partly due to a defect at the level of T cell–dependent IL-12 production by macrophages. In WT mice, activated Th1 cells promote macrophage-mediated IL-12 production through a combination of secreting IFN-γ, a potent macrophage-activating cytokine, and expressing cell surface CD40L, which, by interacting with CD40 on macrophages, plays an important accessory role (171,172). This scenario raises the question of which, in a WT mouse, comes first, the Th1 cell or the IL-12–producing macrophage? A possible sequence of events is that, on interaction with the Ag-presenting macrophage and/or dendritic cell, the naive Th cell upregulates CD40L expression. This, in combination with IFN-γ from another source, probably NK cells (12), provides the necessary signal to promote IL-12 production by the Ag-presenting cells, and thereby initiates the cascade of events that leads to a Th1 response. In contrast, in mice infected with *T. gondii*, CD40/CD40L interactions are not required for the initiation of the IL-12 response *in vivo* (174). In the case of this intracellular protozoan, the initial T cell–independent pulse of IL-12, which starts the type 1 cytokine cascade, appears to derive from unprimed, resting dendritic cells (174).

Parasite infection models have been particularly useful in the study of the events determining Th2 response selection and effector choice. It has been appreciated for some time that IL-4 is the central factor that promotes the differentiation of ThP cells into Th2 cells (133,175–179). By analogy with the Th1 differentiation pathway, where macrophages or dendritic cells make IL-12, it has been hypothesized that a cell of the innate immune system would, upon encounter with antigen, produce early IL-4, which is known to be pivotal in the inductive phase of Th2 responses. At present, it seems unlikely that there will be a universal source of early IL-4 that is important for the development of all Th2 responses (180). Moreover, the developing view is that, in the absence of IL-12, ThP cells themselves make enough IL-4 to allow Th2-lineage commitment (181–183); this appears to be particularly the case in BALB/c mice (131). However, perhaps especially in other mouse strains, other cells, by making IL-4, may play a role in promoting the Th2 response. *In vitro*, IL-6, probably produced by antigen-presenting cells (APCs), promotes IL-4 production by ThP cells, and thus favors Th2 commitment, raising the possibility that this cytokine provides the link between the innate and type 2 adaptive responses (184).

The discovery that NK T cells make IL-4 within 30 minutes of injection of mAb anti-CD3 into naive mice (185) and are crucial for the development of the Th2 response induced by anti-IgD (186) suggested that this cell type might be important in pathogen-induced Th2 responses. However, β2m$^{-/-}$ mice, which, because they fail to express CD1, lack NK T cells, were found to mount normal Th2 responses to *S. mansoni, N. brasiliensis,* and *L. major,* essentially precluding a central role for NK T cells in Th2 induction during parasitic infections (187). Another set of CD4 cells expressing a highly restricted T-cell receptor (TCR) (Vβ4Vα8) does play an important role in producing early IL-4 during the response to *L. major* in BALB/c mice (188). In this model, there is a burst of IL-4 production in the draining LN 16 hours following subcutaneous infection (189). This IL-4 is coming from a population of Vβ4Vα8 CD4 cells, which are responsive to the *Leishmania* antigen LACK (189). The critical importance of this population of cells was inferred by the observation that infected Vβ4-deficient BALB/c mice mount Th1 responses and resolve their lesions (189). The current concept of these LACK-specific cells is that they represent a conventional population of naive CD4 cells (perhaps present in unusually high frequency) and, as is true for BALB/c naive CD4 cells in general, are capable of making physiologically significant levels of IL-4. Thus, the stimulation of lymphoid cells from uninfected BALB/c mice with recombinant LACK leads to the

activation of this cell type, and thus to a substantial early burst of IL-4. The central importance of LACK in the Th2 induction process following infection with *L. major* in BALB/c mice was established when animals of this strain, made tolerant to LACK by the transgenic expression of this protein in their thymus, were found to be resistant to the parasite (Fig. 4A) and to mount diminished type 2 responses (Fig. 4B) (190).

Sources of early IL-4, pivotal in the development of Th2 responses to parasitic helminths, have also been sought. In a model system, in which *S. mansoni* eggs were injected intraperitoneally into naive mice, there was a burst of IL-4 production between 12 and 24 hours (191). This IL-4 was produced by eosinophils, and the data suggested that this cell type was recruited by IL-5 released from mast cells (192). The stimuli for initiating this series of responses is T cell–independent (192), but beyond that, poorly understood. Moreover, the eosinophil-derived IL-4 appears not to be essential for subsequent Th2-cell development, as IL-5$^{-/-}$ mice, which are unable to mount the early eosinophil response, are not Th2 response–defective. In a different model, *N. brasiliensis* larvae, injected intraperitoneally into naive mice, caused a rapid influx of γδ T cells, which stained positively for intracellular IL-4 (193). Because mast cells and basophils also make IL-4, they have been implicated as sources of IL-4 for Th2-cell development (194), but to the best of our knowledge, there is no direct evidence to support their role, and mice deficient in FcεRI, the major signaling receptor for such cells, develop normal Th2 responses after *S. mansoni* infection (195).

Several reports have stressed the importance of appropriate costimulation in priming for Th1 and Th2 responses (196). The most important costimulatory receptor on T cells is CD28, which can bind to either B7.1 (CD80) or B7.2 (CD86) expressed on professional Ag-presenting cells (197,198). Until recently, it was thought that CTLA4 on T cells could also receive a costimulatory signal. Although this may be true in some situations, it now seems clear that the most important role for CTLA4, which is upregulated at the T-cell surface following ligation of CD28 and which binds to both B7 molecules with much higher affinity than does CD28, is to switch off the Th cell and, therefore, to play a role in immune response resolution (8,199). The influence of CTLA4 in dampening immune response development was illustrated when mice treated with a mAb that blocks the interaction of CTLA4 with B7 were shown to be significantly more resistant than control mice to a primary *N. brasiliensis* infection; increased resistance was associated with a more rapid onset and intense Th2 response (200). While initially it was thought that Th2 responses had less of a requirement for costimulation during their development, the findings that CTLA4-Ig, which blocks the interaction of B7 molecules with CD28 and T-cell CTLA4, is able to inhibit the induction of Th2 responses to *H. polygyrus* (201) and *L. major* (202) (with profound effects on the outcome of infection in both cases) firmly established a role for one or both of the B7 molecules in Th2 response induction. Similarly, CD28$^{-/-}$ mice were unable to develop a Th2 response to injected schistosome eggs (203), although IL-4-producing CD4 cells do develop in *L. major*-infected CD28$^{-/-}$ BALB/c mice (204); in the absence of CD28 it is possible that CTLA4 is able to play a costimulatory role (204). The possibility has arisen that B7.1 and B7.2 play preferential roles in Th1 and Th2 priming, respectively (205). This may be true in some settings; for example, blocking B7.2 prevents Th2 responses by *L. major* in BALB/c mice (206) and by schistosome eggs and *B. malayi* microfilariae in C57BL/6 mice (207), although this may

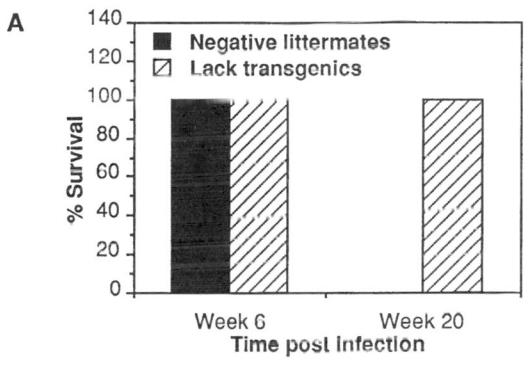

A

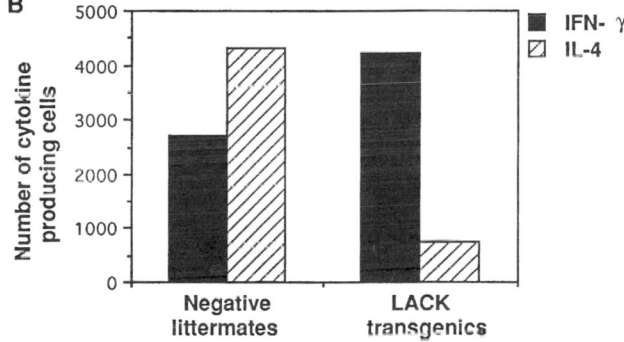

B

FIG. 4. BALB/c mice made tolerant to the *Leishmania* antigen LACK develop a type 1 response and become resistant to infection. Normally, infected BALB/c mice mount a type 2 response and, because of this, succumb. The Th2 response is promoted by the production, early in infection, of a burst of IL-4 by a subpopulation of Vβ4Cα8 CD4 cells that respond to LACK. The importance of this early IL-4 for type 2 response development was demonstrated by an experiment in which BALB/c mice, made tolerant to LACK by transgenic expression of this protein in the thymus, resist infection (**A**). At 8 weeks after infection, the frequency of IL-4-secreting Th cells in the spleens of LACK transgenic mice was greatly reduced, compared with that in LACK-negative littermates (**B**). Concomitantly, there was an increase in IFN-γ-secreting Th cells in the transgenic mice (**B**). The values on the y-axis represent the number of cytokine-secreting cells per 10^6 spleen cells, as determined using ELISPOT. (Adapted from data in ref. 190.)

simply reflect the preferential expression of B7.2 following these Ag challenges. Overall, a central role of B7 molecules in directing the immune response cannot be considered universal, as B7.1 and B7.2 can substitute for each other following exposure to *H. polygyrus* (208) or immunogenic anti-IgD antibodies (196), both of which are strong stimulators of Th2 responses.

In addition to costimulation via CD28, there is a requirement for ligation of the coreceptor CD4 for ThP/Th2 differentiation. In CD4$^{-/-}$ mice, there develops a population of class II–restricted Th cells that are CD4$^-$ and that are defective in their ability to give rise to Th2 cells (209,210). This is true *in vivo*, where BALB/c CD4$^{-/-}$ mice express the opposite phenotype to that of WT mice in being resistant to infection with *L. major* (209,210) and susceptible to *N. brasiliensis* (210). It is also true *in vitro*, where CD4/CD8 double-negative T cells from mice transgenic for a TCR that recognizes the *L. major* antigen LACK$_{156-173}$ peptide in the context of I-Ad fail to differentiate into IL-4–producing cells, even when activated in the presence of IL-4 (209,210). Interestingly, the cytoplasmic region of the CD4 molecule (via which CD4 ligation initiates signaling), is not necessary for Th2-cell differentiation (209). These findings, along with the repeated observation that high-dose antigen is more likely to induce Th2 responses (137,211,212), have led to the still somewhat undefined strength of signal hypothesis (213), wherein it is proposed that differentiation along the Th2 pathway requires more, or qualitatively different, TCR–class II peptide interactions.

Role of Parasite Toxins

It is becoming increasingly clear that many parasites produce molecules that are functionally analogous to endotoxins and super-antigens, that can activate cells such as macrophages and T cells via mechanisms that do not require a recognition event by the antigen-binding site of an antibody or TCR (214). Because these molecules, in essence, act as adjuvants, it may explain why parasites so often induce such strong immune responses. Moreover, if these toxins, as they have been referred to, preferentially activate a cell type that is influential in T-cell subset selection (one that secretes IL-12 or IL-4, for example), they might play a major role in promoting skewing of the immune response. Structurally, these molecules are diverse. Some, such as the malaria (215) and *T. cruzi* (216), *T. brucei* and *Leishmania* (217) toxins, are glycolipids that may stimulate cells such as macrophages, dendritic cells, and neutrophils, via receptors analogous to those involved in LPS triggering (214). The analysis of these factors has been complicated by problems with contamination by mycoplasma which contain lipid-like substances with similar cytokine inducing activities (218). The malaria toxin is implicated in the induction of the inflammatory response that is associated with the development of CM and has been proposed as a target for an antipathology malaria vaccine (219).

In addition to an as yet undefined molecule which triggers IL-12 production (214), *T. gondii* extracts also contain a factor which has superantigen-like activity, being able to stimulate T cells by crosslinking the invariant region of MHC class II to an invariant region of Vβ5 (220). Interestingly, and for yet-unclear reasons, this superantigen preferentially activates CD8 cells. In so doing, it contributes to the induction of large amounts of IFN-γ, which itself may play a role in promoting type 1 bias in the *T. gondii*-induced response. Another parasite-derived immunostimulatory protein is *Leif*, an elongation initiation factor from *Leishmania*, which strongly promotes IL-12 production from human monocytes (221).

This molecule is currently under investigation for development as an adjuvant.

It is clear from studies on *L. major* (12,222,223) and *T. gondii* (224,225) that NK cells, by making IFN-γ, play a crucial role in controlling early parasitemia and promoting type 1 responses. These cells are also involved in the host response to other protozoan parasites, including *Babesia, Cryptosporidium, Eimeria, Plasmodium*, and *Trypanosoma*, and seem likely to play a central role in innate resistance to protozoa and in influencing the adaptive immune system to respond in an appropriate fashion (226). While it is possible that the NK cells are activated directly by parasite-derived molecules or are responding to altered MHC expression on infected or affected cells, the major mechanism for NK-cell activation is likely to be indirect and mediated through IL-12 produced by macrophages and/or dendritic cells (see above), with the potential for further activation by TNF-α (227), IL-β (228), and/or IL-18 (229). Thus, the interactions between parasite toxins and macrophages and/or dendritic cells are the subject of much current research.

While most of the parasite toxins described to date are derived from protozoa, it seems likely that helminths will also produce immunoregulatory molecules that promote Th2 response induction. Schistosome eggs and *Brugia* microfilariae, for example, when injected without adjuvant, induce markedly polarized type 2 responses (230,231). Both of these life forms are characterized by resistant outer structures (the shell and cuticle, respectively), which probably allow the slow release of antigen from within, a process that, when mimicked using minipumps, for unknown reasons, allows normally nondeviating antigen to induce Th2 responses (232). However, soluble extracts of helminths can also be strong type 2 response inducers (160), and the suspicion persists that there are additional reasons why antigens from this type of parasite promote this kind of response. In this context, some schistosome egg proteins have been shown to be modified by a sugar, LNFP-II, which itself is able to promote IL-10 production by B1 cells and to stimulate their proliferation (233). It has been suggested that IL-10 produced by this pathway during infection promotes the immunodeviation towards type 2 responses that occurs following exposure to schistosome eggs (233).

Genetic Influences

It is well established that the host genetic background can have a major influence on the selection of Th1/Th2 responses in parasitic infection. In addition to the well-known paradigm of genetic control of resistance and susceptibility in *L. major* infection, control of other parasites, such as *T. muris*, is also genetically determined and linked to Th selection (see above).

Attempts to understand the susceptibility of BALB/c mice to *L. major* infection have followed two routes. The first, a dedicated genetics approach, has involved the serial back-crossing of disease-resistance genes from resistant B10.D2 mice onto BALB/c over five generations. This has allowed the identification of loci on chromosomes 6, 7, 10, 11, 15, and 16 as being associated with resistance (234). The second approach, more mechanistic, has centered on a functional comparison of BALB/c and B10.D2 Th cells. These studies have revealed two fundamental differences that could account for the observed resistance–susceptibility patterns. First, as alluded to above, under neutral conditions *in vitro* (i.e., with no exogenous cytokines or other immunologic mediators), upon activation, BALB/c ThP cells have the propensity to make more IL-4 than do those from B10.D2 mice (131). This is true even when TCR usage is controlled for through transgenic TCR expression. Second, under these same neutral conditions, following the initial activation signal, ThP cells from B10.D2 mice express the IL-12R β2 chain for prolonged periods, compared with ThP cells from BALB/c mice (235). Thus, the opportunity for responding Th cells to be influenced to differentiate in the Th1 direction persists in B10.D2 at times when responding BALB/c Th cells have become nonresponsive to IL-12 (132,235) and additionally are being exposed to more IL-4 (131). Moreover, because IL-4 inhibits IL-12R β2-chain expression, and IFN-γ maintains responsiveness to IL-12 (236), the tendency for Th responses to become highly skewed by the early production of IL-4 or IFN-γ is clear. A locus on chromosome 11 controls the ability of Th cells from B10.D2 cells to remain responsive to IL-12 for prolonged periods (237), and it is tempting to speculate that this is the same locus as that defined in the serial back-cross study described above (234). The locus on chromosome 11 is syntenic with a locus on human chromosome 5q31.1 (237) that is associated with type 2 responses and that is implicated in regulating resistance to schistosome infection (126) (see above).

While the details of the mechanisms underlying the inability of BALB/c mice to control *L. major* infection are becoming clear, it is perhaps appropriate to point out that this strain of mouse is quite resistant and Th1-competent in the face of other protozoal pathogens, such as *T. gondii* (55). Perhaps this reflects the relative rapidity of the activation of the innate IL-12/IFN-γ axis by *Toxoplasma* compared with *Leishmania* and the subsequent maintenance of IL-12 signaling competence in the emerging Ag-responsive Th population. An additional point to note is that C3H, C57BL/6, and other strains of mice that develop Th1 responses following exposure to *L. major* mount strong Th2 responses when, for example, infected with schistosomes (146,238). A possible explanation to account for this is that prevailing IL-4 levels from non-Th sources are sufficient to inhibit IL-12R β2-chain expression, and thus inhibit Th1 response development.

INFLUENCE OF PARASITIC INFECTION ON IMMUNE RESPONSIVENESS AND SELF-REACTIVITY

Immunosuppression

Immunosuppression, often defined by a failure of T cells from infected animals to proliferate when exposed to specific or polyclonal stimuli, has been described extensively as a characteristic of many parasitic infections, especially those caused by protozoa. Such generalized immunosuppression in human trypanosomiasis, leishmaniasis, and malaria can result in decreased immune responses to unrelated Ag. The historical record of this much-studied area has been reported in considerable detail (239) and will be addressed only in brief here. The clinical significance of the noted immunosuppression is suggested by numerous examples of increased incidence of concurrent infectious diseases in patients with, for example, trypanosomiasis or malaria. While it is tempting to assign many of these phenomena to immune deviation (see below), it appears that, at least in some cases, mechanisms that cannot simply be explained by that paradigm are at work. A common feature of many of the described cases of immunosuppression is that the observed defect is at the level of the APC. In infectious disease models, prostaglandins, NO, IL-10, and/or IL-6 have all been implicated as inhibitors of T-

cell proliferation (240,241), though it seems clear that additional factors can also play a role (242). Due to its profound immunosuppressive effects, it is tempting to speculate that TGF-β will be found to play a significant role in at least some of these states of generalized immunosuppression (see Chapter 22).

Immune Deviation of Concomitant Responses

A logical extension of the early findings that Th1 and Th2 responses counterregulate each other while promoting their own expansion and consolidation, combined with observations that parasites often induce markedly skewed immune responses, is that an infection that leads to, for example, a strong type 2 response might prevent the subsequent induction of a strong type 1 immune response and/or promote the development of a type 2 response to an unrelated microbial agent. The result could be a biasing of effector selection, leading to either enhanced resistance or exacerbated growth of the coinfecting pathogen.

Early studies, showing that helminth-infected animals made IgE responses to antigens that normally did not induce this isotype, were indicative of an influence of existing infection over effector selection against unrelated antigens. Initial studies, aimed at experimentally addressing this phenomenon from the viewpoint of Th1/Th2 selection, showed that immune responses to a model antigen, sperm whale myoglobin in complete Freund's adjuvant (243), to vaccinia virus (244), or to BCG (245), which in normal mice are type 1–like, are inhibited or skewed in the type 2 direction in mice mounting strong type 2 responses to helminth antigen. More recently, the stimulation of a type 2 response in AKR mice, by either infection with schistosomes or the injection of schistosome eggs, was shown to allow these animals to expel a *T. muris* infection (246); normally AKR mice mount a type 1 response to this intestinal nematode and develop a chronic infection (see above).

If preexisting infections can influence effector selection against unrelated Ag, the implications for the effectiveness of vaccination programs, especially in developing countries, may be significant. The relevance of this concern is demonstrated by two studies, one in an area endemic for schistosomiasis (247), and another in an area endemic for onchocerciasis (248), where helminth infection has been shown to inhibit the development of type 1 responses to tetanus toxoid following tetanus vaccination.

Because the type 1 cytokines IL-2 and IFN-γ can cause fetal loss (249), an extension of the ideas discussed above is that biased immune responses induced by parasitic infections might influence the outcome of pregnancy. That this is, in fact, the case was illustrated by studies showing that C57BL/6 mice previously exposed to *L. major,* and mounting a Th1 response, were less able to support pregnancy than were uninfected mice of the same strain, or infected BALB/c animals that mount Th2 responses (250). Failed pregnancy correlated with increased placental IFN-γ and TNF and decreased IL-4 and IL-10 (250). The converse, that pregnancy in C57BL/6 mice makes them more susceptible to infection with *L. major,* has also been reported (251).

Certain autoimmune diseases, especially those for which experimental models exist, have been ascribed to either type 1 or type 2 responses. In particular, organ-specific autoimmunities, such as multiple sclerosis, insulin-dependent diabetes mellitus (IDDM), uveoretinitis, and Hashimoto's thyroiditis, appear to be mediated by type 1 responses, whereas more systemic autoimmunities (e.g., lupus and systemic sclerosis) are associated with type 2 responses (see Chap-

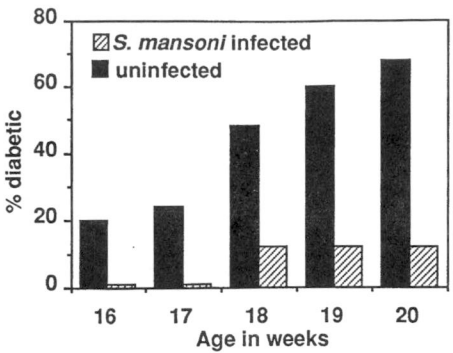

FIG. 5. The spontaneous incidence of insulin-dependent diabetes mellitus (IDDM) in female NOD mice is greatly reduced if the animals are infected with the helminth *S. mansoni*. Six- to 7-week-old female NOD animals were exposed to 50 *S. mansoni* cercariae and, along with uninfected controls, were monitored for diabetes by assaying glucose in the blood and urine. Infection with this helminth significantly inhibits the development of diabetes. It is hypothesized that the schistosome infection, by inducing a strong type 2 response, is modifying the immunologic environment in such a way as to prevent the development of, or inhibit the deleterious expression of, the organ-specific type 1 response, which is associated with this autoimmune disease. (Adapted from ref. 252.)

ter 34). Again, then, the potential exists for parasitic infections, which appear to so strongly skew Th responses, to either ameliorate or exacerbate autoimmune diseases. This has been demonstrated experimentally in the IDDM system, where infection of female NOD mice, which spontaneously develop IDDM, with *S. mansoni* prevents disease onset (252) (Fig. 5), due, it is hypothesized, to the inhibition of type 1 responses directed against the islet cells.

While there are now several published examples of how immune imbalance created by a parasitic infection can affect subsequent responses to disparate immunologic stimuli, it should be noted that, despite provocative reports [e.g., those implicating viral hepatitis in severe malaria (253) and schistosomiasis (254)], there is as yet little substantive evidence supporting a role for immune response bias promoted by one parasitic infection on susceptibility or resistance to other diseases in humans. Nevertheless, given what we know about immune response induction and regulation, it seems naive to expect that immune responses to one pathogen will not influence subsequent immunologic responsiveness. Anecdotally, in tropical developing countries, autoimmunity and allergies seem rare, suggesting that parasitic infections, which in most cases are endemic, may be playing some role in altering the frequency of these disorders that are not uncommon in the developed world. The rapid progression of AIDS in the same global regions offers a pertinent example of a situation in which parasitic infection might be an important cofactor in shaping the course of an unrelated disease (255).

Autoimmunity

It has long been hypothesized that some of the chronic pathologies associated with parasitic infections have an autoimmune etiology. Because so many of the molecules performing basic housekeeping functions are common to different eukaryotes, it is perhaps not surprising that infection with parasites can lead to immune responses to antigens that share homology with host molecules,

with the consequence that the induced response has the potential to target the host as well as the parasite. An example of such a possibility was provided by the discovery that antibody directed towards a γ-glutamyl transpeptidase (initially identified as the Bm2325 allergen) of the filarial worm *B. malayi,* cross-reacts with the human enzyme present in the airway epithelium (256). Because a serious complication of *B. malayi* infection is tropical pulmonary eosinophilia (TPE), a condition in which the lungs become pathologically infiltrated with eosinophils, the implication of this finding is that TPE is an autoimmune manifestation of the immune response to the parasite γ-glutamyl transferase (256,257).

The presence of shared epitopes between heart and neural tissue and *T. cruzi* (258,259) has been taken as an indicator of an autoimmune component in the cardiomyopathy and mega-organ syndromes of chronic Chagas' disease (260). This idea has been supported by the failure of traditional histopathologic examination to detect parasites in diseased tissues (261). However, studies using a parasite strain–mouse strain (Sylvio/C3H) combination, which results in disease that is similar to that seen in *T. cruzi*-infected humans, and taking advantage of a technique in which hearts from healthy mice are transplanted into the subcutaneous tissue of the ear, have produced evidence that argues strongly against the autoimmunity concept (262). In this system, mice chronically infected with *T. cruzi* develop severe heart disease associated with an extensive inflammatory response. Importantly, *in situ* polymerase chain reaction (PCR) for parasite-unique sequences revealed that the damaged heart tissue was significantly infected. Despite the persistence of parasites in the chronically diseased hosts, transplanted hearts failed to become infected, presumably due to the efficacy of the existing immune response in controlling parasite spread, and were not rejected unless directly injected with trypanosomes. PCR has also allowed the detection of *T. cruzi* DNA in the esophageal tissues of patients with chronic digestive Chagas' disease (263). The implications of these findings are significant in that they contraindicate immunosuppressive treatment for chronic Chagas' treatment and suggest that previous concerns about *T. cruzi* vaccines inducing exacerbative autoimmune responses may be unwarranted. The possible induction of autoimmunity is a concern in all vaccines where significant homologies exist between the parasite molecule used for immunization and host molecules, and it can be a significant issue in the decision to develop a given vaccine candidate (see below)

EVASION OF EFFECTOR RESPONSES BY PARASITES

Antigenic Variation

By definition, well-adapted parasites express effective immune evasion mechanisms. Clearly, one of the first protective systems encountered by many parasites is the complement cascade, and there is a large body of literature on how different parasites are able to evade the detrimental consequences of complement activation, from the production of molecules that mimic the activity of decay-accelerating factor (DAF) [*T. cruzi* (264)], the acquisition of DAF itself [*S. mansoni* (265)], the inhibition of complement activation by other mechanisms [the tapeworm *Taenia solium* (266)], or the expression of surface molecules, which physically prevent insertion of the membrane attack complex [*L. major* (267) and *T. brucei* (268)].

Intuitively, the complex life cycles required by many parasites for transmission between mammalian hosts might necessitate the prolonged persistence of the parasite within the host, making the expression of mechanisms that allow evasion of the adaptive immune response a requirement for successful parasitism. The most striking example of such an immune evasion mechanism is perhaps provided by the African trypanosomes (*T. brucei brucei,* the cattle parasite, and the human pathogens *T. brucei rhodesiense* and *T. gambiense*). These parasites, which live extracellularly in the bloodstream, are transmitted between their human or bovine hosts by tsetse flies. The form of the parasite that is parasitic in the mammalian host expresses at its surface in high copy number, so as to form a cohesive coat, the so-called variant surface glycoprotein (VSG). During infection, the host is able to successfully mount a VSG-specific protective antibody response that is able to clear the parasites expressing that antigen. However, within any population, a small percentage of parasites will select from a library of over 100 variants, another VSG-encoding gene for expression, and in so doing will evade the previously established immune response and clonally expand (reviewed in refs. 269, 270). This battle between the immune response and trypanosome can proceed via many VSG variants over several years (in the case of the human trypanosomes), but eventually the untreated host succumbs. Interestingly, in combination with the expression of VSGs, trypanosomes have developed a specialized area of their surface membrane around the flagellar insertion region, called the flagellar pocket, into which necessarily invariant receptor molecules are sequestered. While serum components, including antibodies, can enter this site, the morphology of the pocket precludes access to granulocytes or macrophages, which otherwise could presumably engage in ADCC against the parasite.

Although its discussion is outside the scope of this chapter, the molecular basis for trypanosome surface antigen variation has been investigated and defined in great detail (reviewed in refs. 270, 271). The mechanism of antigen variation in malaria, a phenomenon recognized but underappreciated since 1965 (272,273), was elucidated when the diverse family of VAR genes (50 to 150 variant copies) encoding the *P. falciparum* erythrocyte membrane protein 1 (pfEMP1) was discovered (274–276); pfEMP1 is expressed at the surface of malaria-infected erythrocytes and plays a role in allowing these cells to adhere to the vascular endothelium via molecules such as CD36 and ICAM-1 (277,278). In so doing, the infected cells are prevented from being swept to the spleen, where they would, due to their significantly altered morphology, be recognized as effete and phagocytosed. During the course of infection, the host mounts an antibody response to pfEMP1, which presumably is deleterious for the infected erythrocyte (by either blocking adhesion or promoting ADCC or ADCI reactions). It is to circumvent this possibility that pfEMP1 is variant, undergoing clonal variation at the very high frequency of approximately 2% per generation.

Stealth

Parasites that, unlike malaria, live intracellularly but do not, to the best of our knowledge, extensively modify the host-cell membrane through the insertion of parasite-encoded molecules are thus able to evade antibody responses, but become susceptible to targeting by T cells that recognize parasite-derived peptides in the context of class I or II molecules. A particular problem for *Leishmania* parasites, which infect macrophages, is to invade the cells without activating them. In this context, it has been found that *L. major* metacyclic promastigotes do not induce IL-12 production

(168) but, in fact, actively suppress transcription of the IL-12 (p40) gene (169). Indeed, the parasites are able to inhibit the production of this cytokine by cells exposed to microbial products that are known to be strong inducers of IL-12 (169). This inhibition is not mediated by IL-10, as it can occur in macrophages derived from IL-10$^{-/-}$ mice (169). Moreover, IL-12 suppression is selective, in that macrophages exposed to microbial stimuli plus promastigotes make IL-1α and -β, TNF-α, IL-10, and MCP-1 (169), and, moreover, promastigotes stimulate transient chemokine expression themselves (279). Because IL-12 is a major physiologic promoter of IFN-γ production, and *Leishmania* are highly susceptible to killing by IFN-γ–activated macrophages, this ability to suppress IL-12 production would be expected to provide a clear survival advantage to the parasite.

Camouflage

While once a popular area of research (reviewed in ref. 280), progress in defining helminth immune evasion mechanisms has been limited in recent years. For example, it was clear over 20 years ago that schistosomes acquire a range of host molecules and array them at their surface, and it was proposed that this constituted some form of molecular camouflage that would account for the noted inability of Ab in sera from infected mice to bind to the surface of blood-stage schistosomes. Unfortunately, for the most part, this work has not advanced beyond the descriptive phase. However, the importance for schistosomes of avoiding recognition by antibody was demonstrated in experiments in which praziquantel, the current drug of choice for treating schistosomiasis, was shown to work by altering the parasite surface in such a way that antibodies specific for surface proteins (presumably generated in response to released antigen) could gain access to their previously cryptic epitopes, and in so doing, target the parasite for killing by monocytes and granulocytes (281,282).

Immune Response Deviation

It has been postulated for some time that parasites may either produce or respond to cytokines, and in so doing, influence the immune response. While this area remains largely unstudied, an example of how such a process may work is provided by the *T. muris* system. As discussed above, this parasite can survive for prolonged periods if the host mounts a type 1 response, but it is rapidly expelled by mice that, in response to infection, develop a type 2 response. It is therefore in the parasite's best interest to promote a type 1 response, and the discovery of an IFN-γ–like molecule in *T. muris* suggests that it may be able to influence immune response outcome in its favor (283).

VACCINATION AGAINST PARASITES

The expansion in studies on the immunology of parasitic infections during the seventies and early eighties was driven largely by an expectation that it would be possible to develop effective antiparasite vaccines, and significant advances were made in this area (284). While naturally or artificially attenuated parasites can clearly be used as effective immunizing agents, their deployment as vaccines is limited, for safety reasons, to veterinary applications. Nevertheless, attenuated vaccines continue to be studied, with the expectation that understanding more about the protective immune responses they induce will increase the likelihood of the rational development of successful, defined vaccines.

Of the parasitic diseases of medical importance, it is malaria that is most in need of a successful vaccination method (285). Over the last decade there has been a serious increase in the incidence of drug-resistant malaria, and while new compounds are in development, it seems probable that the days of both effective and affordable mass chemotherapy are limited (285). Thus, development of a vaccine for this parasitic infection has become a matter of urgency. Perhaps because of this urgency, the malaria field has been foremost in adopting and swiftly developing new vaccine technologies, such as multiple antigenic peptides (286) and DNA vaccines (287). The initiative to sequence the *P. falciparum* genome (288) will increase the chances of rapidly identifying new vaccine candidates. Nevertheless, there remain serious hurdles to the development of an anti-malaria vaccine, including the ability of the parasite to evade the immune response through Ag variation (discussed, in part, above) and the lack of good *in vitro* correlates of protection. In addition, there are issues that pertain to malaria but also extend to vaccine development programs for other parasites, including problems associated with the large-scale production of vaccine antigen, the choice of suitable delivery systems and adjuvants, and the difficulty and expense of human trials. Because of its high prevalence and morbidity, schistosomiasis, among human parasitic diseases, ranks second to malaria as a target for vaccine development. While more genetically stable than plasmodia, schistosomes utilize a variety of highly successful immune evasion strategies, which make them equally difficult to attack immunologically (280). For malaria and schistosomiasis, as well as many other parasitic infections, there are four basic vaccine development strategies, based on the part of the life-cycle targeted (Fig. 6): (a) to prevent infection by killing invasive forms, (b) to eliminate or prevent the growth of established stages, (c) to prevent disease in the face of continuing infection (vaccination to prevent pathology), and (d) to block transmission of the parasite. This philosophy, as it pertains to malaria, against which a multicomponent vaccine that unites all four of these strategies is being considered, has been outlined in detail (289,290).

Vaccination to Prevent Infection

Malaria is initiated when the sporozoite stage of the parasite, injected by infected mosquitoes, enters the bloodstream and within 30 to 60 minutes invades an hepatocyte. Studies with an irradiated sporozoite vaccine showed that immunity induced by this stage could protect against infection (reviewed in ref. 291). In part, this protection is due to an antibody response that is directed primarily towards the major surface protein of this stage, the circumsporozite protein (CSP), and that is able to neutralize the parasite before it is able to invade hepatocytes (291). Additionally, this vaccine primes for a specific CD8 response that plays a role in protective immunity by targeting infected hepatocytes (292). As is the case for *T. gondii* and *T. cruzi*, the CD8 cells appear to be working more through secreting IFN-γ than by direct cytotoxicity (293). Indeed, IFN-γ is known to be able to directly activate hepatocytes to make NO (33), which is the likely mediator of resistance (294). In addition to CSP, several other sporozoite proteins, including SSP2/TRAP, STARP, SALSA, LSA-1, Exp-1, and MSP-1, have been implicated as target antigens in the protection induced by the sporozoite immunization, and each of these is under consideration as a vaccine (reviewed in ref. 290). Promisingly, a successful

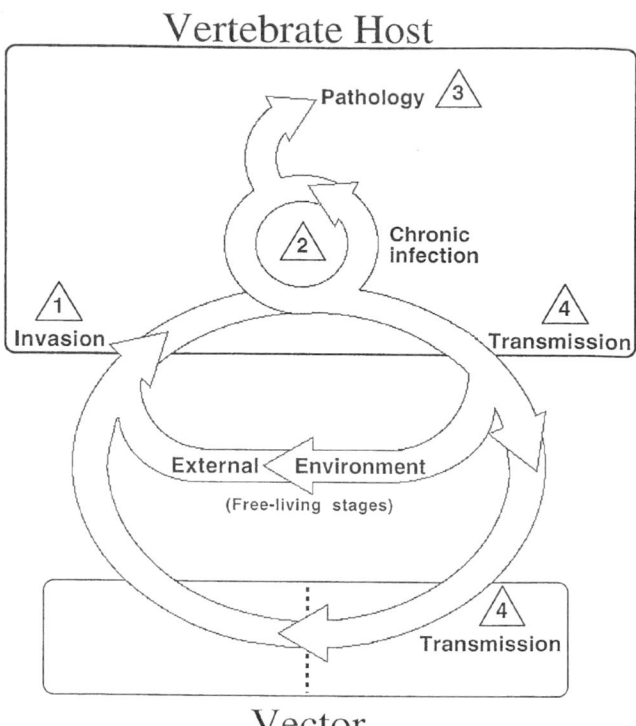

FIG. 6. Stage specificity of vaccine-induced immunity against parasites. Protective responses are directed against (1) invasive stages immediately after host entry, (2) established stages responsible for maintaining chronic infection, (3) pathology-inducing stages, or (4) the life-cycle forms responsible for maintaining transmission. The immunologic effects of the latter can be expressed in the host itself or in the vector by means of antibodies ingested with the blood meal.

human trial of an antisporozoite vaccine, utilizing recombinant CSP fused to hepatitis B surface antigen, was reported (295,296).

Although a debated issue, an antisporozoite vaccine that fails to eradicate all sporozoites can, in principle, allow the escape of fulminant malaria. This concern is not a problem in vaccination against schistosomes, which do not replicate within the mammalian host. Instead, each parasitic worm is acquired as the result of exposure of the host to a single infective larva (cercaria). Thus, a vaccine that is only partly effective at preventing schistosome infection is still useful, and, indeed, given certain assumptions. may be all that is required to eliminate morbidity (297).

Although there have, as yet, been no human trials of defined anti-schistosome vaccines, there is an approach being coordinated by the World Health Organization and USAID, and independently by the Pasteur Institute, to carry forward into human trials the most promising of several antigens that have been demonstrated to confer immunity to rodents in experimental vaccination studies (284). Two of these antigens, IrV-5 (298) and paramyosin (299), were identified either directly or indirectly through studies of an experimental radiation-attenuated vaccine against *S. mansoni*, the most geographically widespread species of schistosome that infects humans. In this system, percutaneous exposure to irradiated cercariae (the infectious stage of the parasite), which migrate to the lungs but die there, results in the development of a CD4 cell–dependent, partially protective immune response, which targets challenge parasites as they migrate through the lungs (300–302). Th cells from vaccinated mice respond to parasite antigens by making IFN-γ and comparatively little IL-4 or IL-5 (238), and mAb-mediated neutralization of IFN-γ in vaccinated mice renders them susceptible to challenge (303,304). Moreover, IFN-γR$^{-/-}$ mice are less protected than are WT animals following immunization with irradiated cercariae (305). Thus, in contrast to expectations from epidemiologic studies, which predict a type 2 response–based immunity (e.g., see ref. 123), vaccine resistance against this helminth appears to involve a Th1 rather than a Th2 response. Consistent with this latter hypothesis, IFN-γ–activated macrophages and endothelial cells have been shown to kill larval schistosomes *in vitro* by an NO-dependent fashion (306) and iNOS inhibitors partially abrogate immunity *in vivo* (301). However, the inability of such compounds to completely abolish resistance and the finding that vaccinated iNOS$^{-/-}$ mice develop significant though reduced immunity indicate that additional factors may be important in the effector arm of this response (302). One candidate factor is TNF-α, as it can directly kill schistosome larvae *in vitro* (307). IL-12, used as an adjuvant, enhances the levels of resistance induced by the irradiated vaccine, presumably by increasing the magnitude and polarization of the Th1 response (308).

While immunity to schistosomes following one vaccination with irradiated cercariae is type 1 in nature, multiple vaccinations, even when given with IL-12 as an adjuvant, lead to a response that has components of both type 1 and type 2 responses (high IFN-γ and IgG1) and is significantly more protective than the response induced by one vaccination alone (309,310). In part, the additional resistance is due to antibody, which is alone effective in passive immunization studies at protecting nonvaccinated mice against infection (311). These vaccination studies may have broad significance in demonstrating that, under the appropriate conditions, IL-12 can act as an adjuvant for both humoral and cell-mediated protective responses against infection (310,312,313).

The use of IL-12 as an adjuvant originated in the *L. major* system, in which vaccination with a crude soluble promastigote extract plus the cytokine was shown to make normally susceptible BALB/c mice highly resistant to challenge infection, most probably by deviating the accompanying response from Th2 to Th1 (314). Similar results have been obtained using IL-12 with the recombinant LACK molecule (315) (see above), and trials of these IL-12–potentiated antileishmanial vaccines in primates are in progress. In related studies, it was also shown that IL-12 may be useful for immunotherapy as well, because treatment of BALB/c mice with established lesions and a Th2 response could be cured by administration of IL-12 with a leishmanicidal drug, while neither of these agents given alone was effective (316). A DNA immunization method, using a plasmid encoding LACK, has been shown to be as effective as the LACK (protein) plus IL-12 vaccine (317).

Vaccination to Control Established Parasites

As inferred above, complete protection may be required for a sporozoite vaccine to prevent malaria infection. Therefore, it has been argued that effective immunity will more likely be achieved by vaccinating against the established, erythrocytic form of the parasite that is directly responsible for the disease (318). Some antigens expressed by this stage undergo extensive variation (see above) and have thus been considered poor targets for vaccination. Nevertheless, naturally acquired immunity to malaria appears to be directed mostly

against blood forms and to be mediated primarily by antibodies (319). The mechanism of action of these protective antibodies is, as yet, not well defined, although they probably function by facilitating the destruction of infected erythrocytes expressing parasite-encoded molecules on their surfaces. Most progress towards a defined vaccine against bloodstream forms of malaria has come from studies on the antigenic targets of the antibodies induced by the protective immunization of monkeys with merozoites in complete Freund's adjuvant and from similar experiments in mice in which protective mAbs have also been raised (reviewed in ref. 318). Based on such investigations, two merozoite proteins, merozoite surface protein 1 (MSP1) and apical membrane antigen 1 (AMA1), have been identified, and they induce partial protection against blood-stage malaria in these hosts (318). An important goal will be to elucidate the mechanism of vaccine resistance and to learn how to enhance its activity by altering the form of antigen-presentation strategies and/or by employing the appropriate adjuvants acceptable for human use.

Transmission-blocking Vaccines

The idea of blocking transmission by immunization has been developed most extensively in the malaria arena, where the approach has been seen as a safety net, capable of preventing the transmission of antigen variant escape mutants emerging in individuals vaccinated against sporozoite or blood-stage targets. Moreover, in geographically isolated areas, where there are no reservoir hosts, a transmission-blocking vaccine might, in itself, be capable of eradicating the parasite. The parasite stages targeted by this approach are the sexual and sporogonic stages within the mosquito, and it is envisaged that Ab consumed with the blood meal acts on the parasite within the gut of the vector to prevent further development (320). Several parasite antigens (Pfs25, Pfs28, Pfs230, and Pfs48/45) that can serve as targets for transmission blocking have been identified, and one of these, Pfs25, the major surface protein of the zygote, is in human clinical trials (320). An interesting and potentially important feature of these antigens is that they tend to be relatively nonvariant, a result, it is postulated, of the absence of prior immune pressure. Transmission-blocking vaccines have also been proposed for filariasis and leishmaniasis but may be less useful in their epidemiologic settings.

Vaccination to Prevent Pathology

Because parasites are so exquisitely adapted to the host immune response, it may be easier and more practical to design immune intervention strategies that prevent parasite-induced immunopathology rather than the infection itself. For example, much of the severe pathology in malaria may be associated with the stimulation of TNF production by parasite toxin(s), and the targeting of these molecules for neutralization by vaccine-induced antibodies has been proposed as a form of disease immunoprophylaxis (321). Although in the theoretical stage, due in large part to the less than fully defined structures of the relevant toxins, this remains an intriguing approach.

Because disease in schistosomiasis is largely due to the granulomatous pathology that develops around parasite eggs trapped in target host tissues, a valid approach towards immunoprophylaxis for schistosomiasis is to vaccinate to minimize granuloma formation or to reduce female schistosome fecundity. In WT mice, granuloma size and intensity are correlated with the intensity of the type 2 response, and immunologic interventions, such as the administration of mAb anti–IL-4, reduces both the size of, and collagen deposition within, granulomas (discussed above). In extensions of these studies, mice preimmunized with parasite eggs plus IL-12 to induce an egg-antigen–specific type 1 response, upon subsequent infection, exhibited far less severe egg-associated liver disease than did infected unimmunized controls (145). In a different line of experiments, the humoral response to glutathione-S-transferase (p28), a major candidate vaccine antigen for preventing schistosome infection (322), has been shown to result in diminished egg production (fecundity) and viability in challenged animals, thus simultaneously reducing both disease and transmission (322,323).

An interesting counterpoint to the experimental antipathology vaccine for schistosomiasis is provided by the attempt to reduce experimental eye disease associated with the type 2 response to *O. volvulus* (see above). In this study, mice were primed with parasite Ag plus IL-12 (to induce a type 1 rather than type 2 response) prior to intraocular injection of antigen (324). In contrast to the findings in the schistosome model, this vaccination protocol failed to confer a beneficial effect, despite the fact that the cytokine did push the induced immune response in a Th1 direction. A likely explanation is that, despite the prevailing type 1 response in these animals, Ag injection into the eyes of vaccinated mice induces a pronounced eosinophil and mononuclear cell infiltrate, similar to that seen in the mice vaccinated with Ag alone. The induction by injected Ag of a series of proinflammatory chemokines, including MIP-1a, MIP-1B, MCP-1, eotaxin, and RANTES, probably accounts for the observed cellular infiltration and associated ocular pathology, and thus vaccine approaches that inhibit the latter responses, rather than simply alter the type 2 cytokine production profile, are needed for immunoprophylaxis in this particular disease setting (324).

GENERAL CONCLUSIONS

It has been traditional in the field of parasite immunology to make sharp distinctions between those effector mechanisms mediating host resistance, on the one hand, and immunopathology on the other. A major theme emerging from the research summarized in this chapter, much, though by no means all of it, from studies using cytokine gene knock-out mice, is that the line between immunity and pathology is often extremely fine, with protective responses often requiring strict regulation if they are not to be pathologic. This is well illustrated by the situation with *T. gondii* infection in mice lacking IL-10. Here, due to an enhanced type 1 response, invading parasites may be eliminated more effectively than in WT mice, but, nevertheless, the animals succumb more rapidly due to the unlimited and extensive inflammation associated with the protective response (68). Thus, in this and other cases (69,77), there is a requirement during the expression of a protective type 1 response for the underlying production of regulatory type 2 cytokines. In some cases, typified by tissue-dwelling helminths, such as filariae and schistosomes, with resilient life-cycle stages that persist for long periods, the importance of avoiding inflammation due to type 1 cytokines is such that the development of dominant type 2 responses appears to be crucial (83,127,325), despite the fact that they cause distinctive pathologies of their own (138,326). Using a battlefield analogy, the issue can be seen as one of how to blow up the enemy without, at the same time, blowing up oneself. Perhaps the generalized immunosuppression seen during many chronic parasitic infections reflects the ultimate last-ditch attempt by the immune system to prevent disease due to inflam-

mation. Important remaining challenges are to understand the parasite and host genetic factors that lead to the induction of the regulatory signals that dictate the balance between the expression of immunity and disease, such that immunomodulatory regimens that mimic or improve on the most well balanced, naturally acquired protective immune responses can be developed.

A second major theme emerging from current studies on the immunology of the host–parasite relationship concerns the redundancy of effector responses. The importance of this concept has been driven home by the numerous studies employing mice with genetically engineered immune deficiencies, in which compensatory mechanisms have been observed to replace those deleted. While hindering the definition of responses required for resistance and pathology, this redundancy has led to the identification of new pathways that would have been difficult to define in functionally intact hosts. For example, IgE production, previously thought to be solely under the control of IL-4, has been shown to occur in IL-4$^{-/-}$ mice infected with *P. chabaudi* (327), and in class II$^{-/-}$ mice vaccinated against *T. gondii*, NK T cells replace conventional Th cells in providing help for CD8 cells (56).

Finally, the ultimate practical goal of the study of immune responses to parasites must be the application of new information to the development of immunotherapeutics or prophylaxis against parasites and extension of these findings to other pathogens. In the conclusion of this chapter in the previous edition of this book, it was suggested that the stage was set for the use of cytokines and/or other immunologic mediators in the development of vaccines or immunotherapeutics. To a certain extent, this has occurred with the use of IL-12, in particular, as an adjuvant and the appreciation that its adjuvant properties extend into the humoral as well as cell-mediated arms of the immune response. With the realization that the recruitment of appropriate costimulatory and cytokine signals at the outset of an immune response can have profound effects on type 1 or type 2 response selection, the time has come for a move away from vaccine selection based solely on antigen identity [an approach that has had limited success; e.g., the SPf66 malaria vaccine (328)] to a more encompassing approach, in which the details of antigen presentation take at least equal precedence.

ACKNOWLEDGMENTS

We wish to express our appreciation to numerous colleagues who contributed their ideas and criticisms during the preparation of this manuscript, and to Drs. Anne Cook, David Dunne, Richard Grencis, and Thomas Nutman for allowing us to refer to their unpublished findings. EJP and PAS are each a recipient of a Burroughs Wellcome New Investigator Award in Molecular Parasitology.

REFERENCES

1. MacKenzie WR, Hoxie NJ, Proctor ME, et al. A massive outbreak in Milwaukee of cryptosporidium infection transmitted through the public water supply. *N Engl J Med* 1994;331:161–167.
2. Herwaldt BL, Ackers ML. An outbreak in 1996 of cyclosporiasis associated with imported raspberries. The Cyclospora Working Group. *N Engl J Med* 1997; 336:1548–1556.
3. Bowie WR, King AS, Werker DH, et al. Outbreak of toxoplasmosis associated with municipal drinking water. The BC toxoplasma investigation team. *Lancet* 1997;350:173–177.
4. Mosmann TR, Coffman RL. TH1 and TH2 cells: different patterns of lymphokine secretion lead to different functional properties. *Annu Rev Immunol* 1989;7:145–173.
5. Mosmann TR, Sad S. The expanding universe of T-cell subsets: Th1, Th2 and more. *Immunol Today* 1996;17:138–146.

6. Clerici M, Shearer G. The Th1-Th2 hypothesis. Immunol Today 1994;15: 575–581.

7. Coombs R, Gell P. Classification of allergic reactions responsible for clinical hypersensitivity and disease. In: Gell P, Coombs R, Lachmann P, eds. *Clinical aspects of immunology.* Oxford: Blackwell Scientific, 1975:761–781.

8. Perez VL, Van Parijs L, Biuckians A, Zheng XX, Strom TB, Abbas AK. Induction of peripheral T cell tolerance in vivo requires CTLA-4 engagement. *Immunity* 1997;6:411–417.

9. Belosevic M, Finbloom DS, Van Der Meide PH, Slayter MV, Nacy CA. Administration of monoclonal anti-IFN-gamma antibodies in vivo abrogates natural resistance of C3H/HeN mice to infection with *Leishmania major. J Immunol* 1989;143:266–274.

10. Heinzel FP, Sadick MD, Holaday BJ, Coffman RL, Locksley RM. Reciprocal expression of interferon-γ or interleukin-4 during the resolution or progression of murine leishmaniasis. *J Exp Med* 1989;169:59–72.

11. Scott P, Natovitz P, Coffman RL, Pearce E, Sher A. Immunoregulation of cutaneous leishmaniasis. *J Exp Med* 1988;168:1675–1684.

12. Scharton TM, Scott P. Natural killer cells are a source of interferon gamma that drives differentiation of CD4+ T cell subsets and induces early resistance to *Leishmania major. J Exp Med* 1993;178:567–577.

13. Erb K, Blank C, Ritter U, Bluethmann H, Moll H. *Leishmania major* infection in major histocompatibility complex class II-deficient mice: CD8+ T cells do not mediate a protective immune response. *Immunobiology* 1996;195:243–260.

14. Wang ZE, Reiner SL, Hatam F, et al. Targeted activation of CD8 cells and infection of beta 2-microglobulin-deficient mice fail to confirm a primary protective role for CD8 cells in experimental leishmaniasis. *J Immunol* 1993;151: 2077–2086.

15. Soong L, Chang CH, Sun J, et al. Role of CD4+ cells in pathogenesis associated with *Leishmania amazonensis* infection. *J Immunol* 1997;158:5374–5383.

16. Green SJ, Meltzer MS, Hibbs JB, Nacy CA. Activated macrophages destroy intracellular *Leishmania major* amastigotes by an L-arginine-dependent killing mechanism. *J Immunol* 1990;144:278–283.

17. Wang ZE, Reiner SL, Zheng S, Dalton DK, Locksley RM. CD4+ effector cells default to the Th2 pathway in interferon gamma deficient mice infected with *Leishmania major. J Exp Med* 1994;179:1367–1371.

18. Swihart K, Fruth U, Meeemer N, et al. Mice from a genetically resistant background lacking the interferon gamma receptor are susceptible to infection with *Leishmania major* but mount a polarized T helper cell 1-type T cell response. *J Exp Med* 1995;181:961–971.

19. Wei XQ, Charles IG, Smith A, et al. Altered immune responses in mice lacking inducible nitric oxide synthase. *Nature* 1995;375:408–411.

20. Stenger S, Donhauser N, Thuring H, Rollinghof M, Bogdan C. Reactivation of latent leishmaniasis by inhibition of inducible nitric oxide synthase. *J Exp Med* 1996;183:1501–1514.

21. Liew FY, Li Y, Millot S. Tumor necrosis factor (TNF-alpha) in leishmaniasis. II. TNF-alpha-induced macrophage leishmanicidal activity is mediated by nitric oxide from L arginine. *Immunology* 1990;71:556–559.

22. Nacy CA, Meierovics AI, Belosevic M, Green SJ. Tumor necrosis factor-alpha: central regulatory cytokine in the induction of macrophage antimicrobial activities. *Pathobiology* 1991;59:182–184.

23. Vieira LQ, Goldschmidt M, Nashleanas M, Pfeffer K, Mak T, Scott P. Mice lacking the TNF receptor p55 fail to resolve lesion caused by infection with *Leishmania major,* but control parasite replication. *J Immunol* 1996;157:827–835.

24. Garg N, Nunes MP, Tarleton RL. Delivery by *Trypanosoma cruzi* of proteins into the MHC class I processing and presentation pathway. *J Immunol* 1997;158:3293–3302.

25. Tarleton RL, Koller BH, Latour A, Postan M. Susceptibility of beta 2-microglobulin-deficient mice to *Trypanosoma cruzi* infection [see comments]. *Nature* 1992;356:338–340.

26. Tarleton RL, Grusby MJ, Postan M, Glimcher LH. *Trypanosoma cruzi* infection in MHC-deficient mice: further evidence for the role of both class I and class II restricted T cells in immune resistance and disease. *Int Immunol* 1996;8:13–22.

27. Silva JS, Morrissey PJ, Grabstein KH, Mohler KM, Anderson D, Reed SG. Interleukin 10 and interferon gamma regulation of experimental *Trypanosoma cruzi* infection. *J Exp Med* 1992;175:169–174.

28. Gazzinelli RT, Oswald IP, Hieny S, James SL, Sher A. The microbicidal activity of interferon-gamma-treated macrophages against *Trypanosoma cruzi* involves an L-arginine-dependent, nitrogen oxide mediated mechanism inhibitable by interleukin-10 and transforming growth factor-B. *Eur J Immunol* 1992;22: 2501–2506.

29. Cardillo F, Voltarelli JC, Reed SG, Silva JS. Regulation of *Trypanosoma cruzi* infection in mice by gamma interferon and interleukin-10: role of NK cells. *Infect Immun* 1996;64:128–135.

30. Reed SG, Brownell CE, Russo DM, Silva JS, Grabstein KH, Morrissey PJ. IL-10 mediates susceptibility to *Trypanosoma cruzi* infection. *J Immunol* 1994;153: 3135–3140.

31. Hoffman SL, Crutcher JM, Puri SK, et al. Sterile protection of monkeys against malaria after administration of interleukin-12. *Nat Med* 1997;3:80–83.

32. Sedegah M, Finkelman F, Hoffman S. Interleukin 12 induction of interferon γ-dependent protection against malaria. *Proc Natl Acad Sci USA* 1994;91: 10700–10702.

33. Nussler AK, Beger H-G, Liu ZZ, Billiar TR. Nitric oxide, hepatocytes and inflammation. *Res Immunol* 1996;146:671–677

34. von der Weid T, Langhorne J. The roles of cytokines produced in immune response to erythrocytic stages of mouse malarias. *Immunobiology* 1993;189: 397–418.

35. Stevenson MM, Tam MF, Wolf FS, Sher A. IL-12 induced protection against blood stage *Plasmodium chabaudi* AS requires IFN-gamma, TNF-alpha and occurs via a nitric oxide-dependent mechanism. *J Immunol* 1995;155:2545–2556.

36. Taylor-Robinson AW, Phillips RS, Severn A, Moncada S, Liew FY. The role of TH1 and TH2 cells in a rodent malaria infection. *Science* 1993;260:1931–1934.

37. Druihle P, Sabcharoen A, Bouharoun-Tayoun H, Oeuvray C, Perignon J-L. In vivo-veritas: lessons from immunoglobulin-transfer experiments in malaria patients. *Ann Trop Med Parasitol* 1997;91[Suppl 1]:S37–S53.

38. White WI, Evans CB, Taylor DW. Antimalarial antibodies of the immunoglobulin G2a isotype modulate parasitemias in mice infected with *Plasmodium yoelii. Infect Immun* 1991;59:5347–5354.

39. Waki S, Uehara S, Kanbe K, Nariuchi H, Suzuki M. Interferon-gamma and the induction of protective IgG2a antibodies in non-lethal *Plasmodium berghei* infections of mice. *Parasite Immunol* 1995;17:503–508.

40. Leport C, Remington J. Toxoplasmosis in AIDS. *Presse Med* 1992;21: 1165–1171.

41. Joiner KA, Bermudes D, Sinai A, Qi H, Polotsky V, Beckers C. Structure and function of the *Toxoplasma gondii* vacuole. *Ann NY Acad Sci* 1996;797:1–7.

42. Suzuki Y, Coneley FS, Remington JS. Importance of endogenous IFN-γ for prevention of toxoplasmic encephalitis in mice. *J Immunol* 1989;143:2045–2052.

43. Gazzinelli RT, Eltoum I, Wynn TA, Sher A. Acute cerebral toxoplasmosis is induced by in vivo neutralization of TNF-alpha and correlates with the down-regulated expression of inducible nitric oxide synthase and other markers of macrophage activation. *J Immunol* 1993;151:3672–3681.

44. Gazzinelli R, Xu Y, Hieny S, Cheever A, Sher A. Simultaneous depletion of CD4+ and CD8+ T lymphocytes is required to reactivate chronic infection with *Toxoplasma gondii. J Immunol* 1992;149:175–180.

45. Hakim FT, Gazzinelli RT, Denkers EY, Hieny S, Shearer FM, Sher A. CD8+ T cells from mice vaccinated against *Toxoplasma gondii* are cytotoxic for parasite infected or antigen-pulsed host cells. *J Immunol* 1991;147:2310–2317.

46. Subauste CS, Koniaris AH, Remington JS. Murine CD8+ cytotoxic T lymphocytes lyse *Toxoplasma gondii* infected cells. *J Immunol* 1991;147:3955–3962.

47. Denkers EY, Yap G, Scharton-Kerston T, et al. Perforin-mediated cytolysis plays a limited role in host resistance to *Toxoplasma gondii. J Immunol* 1997;159: 1903–1908.

48. Suzuki Y, Remington JS. The effect of anti-IFN-γ on the protective effect of lyt-2+ immune T cells against toxoplasmosis in mice. *J Immunol* 1990;144: 1954–1961.

49. Adams LB, Hibbs JB, Taintor RR, Krahenbuhl JS. Microbistatic effect of murine activated macrophages for *Toxoplasma gondii*. Role for synthesis of inorganic nitrogen oxides from L-arginine. *J Immunol* 1990;144:2725–2729.

50. Scharton-Kersten TM, Yap G, Magram J, Sher A. Inducible nitric oxide is essential for host control of persistent but not acute infection with the intracellular pathogen *Toxoplasma gondii. J Exp Med* 1997;185:1261–1273.

51. Sayles PC, Johnson LL. Exacerbation of toxoplasmosis in neutrophil-depleted mice. *Nat Immun* 1997 1998;160:134–1345.

52. Yap GS, Scharton-Kersten T, Charest H, Sher A. Decreased resistance of TNF receptor p55 and p75 deficient mice to chronic toxoplasmosis despite normal activation of iNOS in vivo. *J Immunol* 1998;160:1340–1345.

53. Pfefferkorn R, Eckel M, Rebhun S. Interferon-gamma suppresses the growth of *Toxoplasma gondii* in human fibroblasts by through starvation for tryptophan. *Mol Biochem Parasitol* 1986;20:215–224.

54. Waldeland H, Pfefferkorn ER, Frenkel JK. Temperature-sensitive mutants of *Toxoplasma gondii: pathogenicity and persistence in mice.* J Parasitol 1983;69: 171–175.

55. Gazzinelli RT, Hakim FT, Hieny S, Shearer GM, Sher A. Synergistic role of CD4+ and CD8+ T lymphocytes in IFN-γ production and protective immunity induced by an attenuated *Toxoplasma gondii* vaccine. *J Immunol* 1991;146: 286–292.

56. Denkers EY, Scharton-Kersten T, Barbieri S, Casper P, Sher A. A role for CD4+ NK1.1+ T lymphocytes as major histocompatibility complex class II independent helper cells in the generation of CD8+ effector function against intracellular infection *J Exp Med* 1996;184:131–139.

57. Denkers EY, Gazzinelli RT, Martin D, Sher A. Emergence of NK1.1+ cells as effectors of IFN-γ dependent immunity to *Toxoplasma gondii* in MHC class-I deficient mice. *J Exp Med* 1993;178:1465–1472.

58. Urban JF, Fayer R, Chen S-J, Gause WC, Gately MK, Finkelman FD. IL-12 protects immunocompetent and immunodeficient neonatal mice against infection with *Cryptosporidium parvum. J Immunol* 1996;156:263–268.

59. Ungar BLP, Kao TC, Burris JA, Finkelman FD. *Cryptosporidium* infection in the mouse model: independent roles for IFN-gamma and CD4 T lymphocytes in protective immunity. *J Immunol* 1991;147:1014–1021.

60. Ovington KS, Alleva LM, Kerr EA. Cytokines and immunological control of *Eimeria* spp. *Int J Parasitol* 1995;25:1331–1351.

61. McDonald V, Robinson HA, Kelly A, Bancroft GJ. Immunity to *Cryptosporidium muris* infection in mice is expressed through gut CD4+ intraepithelial lymphocytes. *Infect Immun* 1996;64:2556–2562.

62. Elson LH, Calvopina M, Paredes W, et al. Immunity to onchocerciasis: putative immune persons produce a Th1-like response to *Onchocerca volvulus. J Infect Dis* 1995;171:652–658.

63. Gazzinelli RT, Hieny S, Wynn TA, Wolf S, Sher A. Interleukin 12 is required for the T-lymphocyte-independent induction of interferon gamma by an intracellular parasite and induces resistance in T-cell-deficient hosts. *Proc Natl Acad Sci USA* 1993;90:6115–6119.

64. Hunter C, Candolfi E, Subauste C, Van Cleeve V, Remington JS. The role of IL-12 in acute murine toxoplasmosis. *Immunology* 1995;84:16–20.

65. Khan IA, Matsuura T, Kaspar LH. Interleukin12 enhances murine survival against acute toxoplasmosis. *Infect Immun* 1994;62:1639–1642.

66. Liesenfeld O, Kosek J, Remington JS, Suzuki Y. Association of CD4+ T cell dependent interferon-gamma mediated necrosis of the small intestine with genetic susceptibility of mice to peroral infection with *Toxoplasma gondii*. *J Exp Med* 1996;184:597–607.

67. Roberts CW, Ferguson DJ, Jebbari H, Satoskar A, Bluethman H, Alexander J. Different roles for interleukin-4 during the course of *Toxoplasma gondii*. *Infect Immun* 1996;64:897–904.

68. Gazzinelli RT, Wysocka M, Hieny S, et al. In the absence of endogenous IL-10, mice acutely infected with *Toxoplasma gondii* succumb to a lethal immune response dependent on CD4+ cells and accompanied by overproduction of IL-12, IFN-gamma and TNF-alpha. *J Immunol* 1996;157:798–805.

69. Hunter CA, Ellis-Neyes LA, Slifer T, et al. IL-10 is required to prevent immune hyperactivity during infection with *Trypanosoma cruzi*. *J Immunol* 1997;158:3311–3316.

70. Roberts SJ, Smith AL, West AB, et al. T cell alpha-beta+ and gamma delta+ deficient mice display abnormal but distinct phenotypes towards a natural, widespread infection of the intestinal epithelium. *Proc Natl Acad Sci USA* 1996;93:11774–11779.

71. Kwiatkowski D. Tumour necrosis factor, fever and fatality in falciparum malaria. *Immunol Lett* 1990;25:213–216.

72. Grau GE, Bieler G, Pointaire P, et al. Significance of cytokine production and adhesion molecules in malarial immunopathology. *Immunol Lett* 1990;25:189–194.

73. Kwiatkowski D, Hill AVS, Sambou I, et al. TNF concentration in fatal cerebral, non-fatal cerebral, and uncomplicated *Plasmodium falciparum* malaria. *Lancet* 1990;336:1201–1204.

74. Clark IA, Rockett KA, Cowden WB. Proposed central role of nitric oxide in conditions clinically similar to cerebral malaria. *Lancet* 1992;340:894–895.

75. Grau GE, Kindler V, Piguet PF, Lambert PH, Vassalli P. Prevention of experimental cerebral malaria by anticytokine antibodies. Interleukin 3 and granulocyte macrophage colony-stimulating factor are intermediates in increased tumor necrosis factor production and macrophage accumulation. *J Exp Med* 1988;168:1499–1504.

76. Schlichtherle IM, Treutiger CJ, Fernandez V, Carlson J, Wahlgren M. Molecular aspects of severe malaria. *Parasitol Today* 1996;12:329–332.

77. Linke A, Kuhn R, Muller W, Hornavar N, Li C, Langhorne J. *Plasmodium chabaudi chabaudi*: differential susceptibility of gene-targeted mice deficient in IL-10 to an erythrocytic stage infection. Exp Parasitol 1996;84:253–263.

78. King CL, Mahanty S, Kumaraswami V, et al. Cytokine control of parasite-specific anergy in human lymphatic filariasis. Preferential induction of a regulatory T helper type 2 lymphocyte subset. *J Clin Invest* 1993;92:1667–1673.

79. Doenhoff MJ, Musallam R, Bain J, McGregor A. Studies on the host-parasite relationship in *Schistosoma mansoni*-infected mice: the immunological dependence of parasite egg excretion. *Immunology* 1979;35:771.

80. Boros D. The role of cytokines in formation of the schistosome egg granuloma. *Immunobiology* 1994;191:441–450.

81. Cheever AW. Schistosomiasis: infection versus disease and hypersensitivity versus immunity. *Am J Pathol* 1993;142:699–702.

82. Jordan P, Webbe G, Sturrock RF. *Human schistosomiasis*. Oxon UK: CAB International, 1993.

83. Mwatha JK, Kimani G, Kamau T, et al. High levels of tumor necrosis factor (TNF), soluble TNF receptors, soluble intracellular adhesion molecule-1 and interferon gamma, but low levels of interleukin-5, are associated with hepatosplenic disease in human schistosomiasis mansoni. *J Immunol* 1998;160:1992–1999.

84. Sher A, Fiorentino D, Casper P, Pearce EJ, Mosmann TR. Production of IL-10 by CD4+ T lymphocytes correlates with down regulation of Th1 cytokine synthesis. *J Immunol* 1991;147:2713–2718.

85. King CL, Medhat A, Malhotra I, et al. Cytokine control of parasite-specific anergy in human urinary schistosomiasis. *J Immunol* 1996;156:4715–4721.

86. Mahanty S, Ravichandran M, Raman U, Jayaraman K, Kumaraswami V, Nutman TB. Regulation of parasite antigen-driven immune responses by interleukin-10 (IL-10) and IL-12 in lymphatic filariasis. *Infect Immun* 1997;65:1742–1747.

87. Finkelman FD, Shea-Donohue T, Goldhill J, et al. Cytokine regulation of host defense against parasitic gastrointestinal nematodes: lessons from studies with rodent models. *Annu Rev Immunol* 1997;15:505–533.

88. Wakelin D. Genetic control of immune responses to parasites: immunity to *Trichuris muris* in inbred and random bred strains of mice. *Parasitology* 1975;71:51–60.

89. Else KJ, Hultner L, Grencis RK. Cellular immune responses to the murine nematode parasite *Trichuris muris*. II. Differential induction of T cell subsets in resistant versus susceptible mice. *Immunology* 1992;75:232–237.

90. Kightlinger LK, Seed JR, Kightlinger MB. The epidemiology of *Ascaris lumbricoides, Trichuris trichura,* and hookworm in children in the Ranomafana rainforest, Madagascar. *J Parasitol* 1995;81:159–169.

91. Else KJ, Finkelman FD, Maliszewski CR, Grencis RK. Cytokine-mediated regulation of chronic intestinal helminth infection. *J Exp Med* 1994;179:347–351.

92. Bancroft AJ, Else KJ, Sypek JP, Grencis RK. Interleukin-12 promotes a chronic intestinal heliminth infection. *Eur J Immunol* 1997;27:866–877.

93. Urban JF, Katona IM, FInkelman FD. *Heligmosomoides polygyrus: CD4+ but not CD8+ T cells regulate the IgE response and protective immunity in mice.* Exp Parasitol 1991;73:500–511.

94. Koyama K, Tamauchi H, Ito Y. The role of CD4+ and CD8+ T cells in protective immunity to the murine nematode parasite *Trichuris muris*. *Parasite Immunol* 1995;17:161–165.

95. Urban JF Jr, Maliszewski CR, Madden KB, Katona IM, Finkelman FD. IL-4 treatment can cure established gastrointestinal nematode infections in immunocompetent and immunodeficient mice. *J Immunol* 1995;154:4675–4684.

96. Urban JF Jr, Katona IM, Paul WE, Finkelman FD. Interleukin 4 is important in protective immunity to a gastrointestinal nematode infection in mice. *Proc Natl Acad Sci USA* 1991;88:5513–5517.

97. Bancroft AJ, McKenzie ANJ, Grencis RK. A critical role for IL-13 in resistance to helminth infection. *J Immunol* 1998;160:3453–3461.

98. Finkelman FD, Pearce EJ, Urban JFJ, Sher A. Regulation and biological function of helminth-induced cytokine responses. *Immunol Today* 1991;12:A62–A65.

99. Finkelman FD, Katona IM, Urban JF, Snapper CM, Ohara J, Paul WE. Suppression of in vivo polyclonal IgE responses by monoclonal antibody to the lymphokine B-cell stimulatory factor. *Proc Natl Acad Sci USA* 1986;83:9675–9678.

100. Morawetz RA, Gabriele L, Rizzo LV, et al. Interleukin (IL)-4 independent immunoglobulin class switch to immunoglobulin (Ig)E in the mouse. *J Exp Med* 1996;184:1651–1661.

101. Ahmad A, Wang CH, Bell RG. A role for IgE in intestinal immunity: expression of rapid expulsion of *Trichinella spiralis* from rats transfused with IgE and thoracic duct lymphocytes. *J Immunol* 1984;70:3563–3570.

102. Goldhill J, Morris SC, Maliszewski C, et al. Interleukin-4 modulates cholinergic neural control of mouse small intestinal longitudinal muscle. *Am J Physiol* 1997;272:G1135–G1140.

103. Coffman RL, Seymour BWP, Haduk S, Jackson J, Rennick D. Antibody to interleukin 5 inhibits helminth-induced eosinophilia in mice. *Science* 1989;245:308–310.

104. Weller PF. Eosinophils: structure and function. *Curr Opin Immunol* 1994;6:85–90.

105. Herndon FJ, Kayes SG. Depletion of eosinophils by anti-IL-5 eosinophil antibody treatment of mice infected with *Trichinella spiralis* does not alter parasite burden or immunologic resistance to reinfection. *J Immunol* 1992;149:3642–3647.

106. Rotman HL, Yutanawiboonchai W, Brigandi RA, et al. *Strongyloides stercoralis:* eosinophil-dependent immune-mediated killing of third-stage larvae in BALB/cByJ mice. Exp Parasitol 1996;82:267–278.

107. Korenaga M, Hitoshi Y, Takatsu K, Tada I. Regulatory effect of anti-interleukin 5 monoclonal antibody on intestinal worm burden in a primary infection with *Strongyloides venezuelensis*. *Int J Parasitol* 1994;24:951–957.

108. Sasaki O, Sugaya H, Ishida K, Yoshimura K. Ablation of eosinophils with anti-IL-5 antibody enhances the survival of intracranial worms of *Angiostrongylus cantonensis* in the mouse. *Parasite Immunol* 1993;15:349–354.

109. Sugaya H, Aoki M, Yoshida T, Takatsu K, Yoshimura K. Eosinophilia and intracranial worm reccovery in interleukin-5 transgenic and interleukin-5 receptor alpha-chain knockout mice infected with *Angiostrongylus cantonensis*. *Parasitol Res* 1997;83:583–590.

110. Capron M, Capron A. Effector functions of eosinophils in schistosomiasis. *Mem Inst Oswaldo Cruz* 1992;87[Suppl 4]:167–170.

111. Gounni AS, Lamkhioued B, Ochiai K, et al. High-affinity IgE receptor on eosinophils is involved in defence against parasites. *Nature* 1994;367:183–186.

112. Hagan P. Immunity and morbidity in infection due to *Schistosoma haematobium*. *Am J Trop Med Hyg* 1996;55[5 suppl]:116–120.

113. Sher A, Coffman RL, Hieny S, Scott P, Cheever AW. Interleukin 5 (IL-5) is required for the blood and tissue eosinophilia but not granuloma formation induced by infection with *Schistosoma mansoni*. *Proc Natl Acad Sci USA* 1990;87:61–66.

114. Rosa Brunet L, Kopf M, Pearce EJ. IL-4, but not IL-5 is necessary for resistance to *Schistosoma mansoni* superinfection in mice (*submitted*).

115. Ortega-Pierres G, Mackenzie CD, Parkhouse RM. Protection against *Trichinella spiralis* induced by a monoclonal antibody that promotes killing of newborn larvae by granulocytes. *Parasite Immunol* 1984;6:275–284.

116. Pritchard DI, Williams DJ, Behnke JM, Lee TDG. The role of IgG1 hypergammaglobulinaemia in immunity to the gastrointestinal nematode *Nematospiroides dubius*. The immunochemical purification, antigen specificity and in vivo antiparasite effect of IgG1 from immune serum. *Immunology* 1983;49:353–365.

117. Donaldson LE, Schmitt E, Huntley JF, Newlands GF, Grencis RK. A critical role for stem cell factor and c-kit in host protective immunity to an intestinal helminth. *Int Immunol* 1996;8:559–567.

118. Madden KB, Urban JFJ, Ziltener HJ, Schrader JW, Finkelman FD, Katona IM. Antibodies to IL-3 and IL-4 suppress helminth induced mastocytosis. *J Immunol* 1991;147:1387–1391.

119. Hultner L, Druez C, Moeller J, et al. Mast cell growth-enhancing activity (MEA) is structurally related and functionally identical to the novel mouse T cell growth factor P40/TCGFIII (interleukin 9). *Eur J Immunol* 1990;20:1413–1416.

120. Faulkner HC, Humphreys N, Renauld JC, Van Snick J, Grencis RK. Interleukin-9 is involved in host-protective immunity to intestinal nematode infection. *Eur J Immunol* 1997;27:2536–2540.

121. Kullberg MC, Berzofsky JA, Jankovic DL, et al. T cell-derived IL-3 induces the production of IL-4 by non-B, non-T cells to amplify the Th2-cytokine response to a non-parasite antigen in *Schistosoma mansoni*-infected mice. *J Immunol* 1996;156:1482–1490.

122. Dunne DW, Butterworth AE, Fulford AJC, et al. Immunity after treatment of human schistosomiasis: association between IgE antibodies to adult worm antigens and resistance to reinfection. *Eur J Immunol* 1992;22:1483–1494.

123. Hagan P, Blumenthal UJ, Dunn D, Simpson AJG, Wilkins HA. Human IgE, IgG4 and resistance to reinfection with *Schistosoma haematobium*. *Nature* 1991;349: 243–245.

124. Rihet P, Demeure DE, Bourgois A, Prata A, Dessein AJ. Evidence for an association between human resistance to *Schistosoma mansoni* and high anti-larval IgE levels. *Eur J Immunol* 1991;21:2679–2686.

125. Capron M, Capron A, Joseph M, Verwaerde C. IgE receptors on phagocytic cells and immune response to schistosome infection. *Monogr Allergy* 1983;18:33–44.

126. Marquet S, Abel L, Hillaire D, et al. Genetic localization of a locus controlling the intensity of infection by *Schistosoma mansoni* on chromosome 5q31-q33. *Nat Genet* 1996;14:181–184.

127. Rosa Brunet LR, Finkelman FD, Cheever AW, Kopf MA, Pearce EJ. IL-4 protects against TNF-alpha-mediated cachexia and death during acute schistosomiasis. *J Immunol* 1997;159:777–785.

128. Leiby DA, Kanesa-thasan N, Scott P, Nacy CA. Leishmaniasis. In: Kierszenbaum F, ed. *Parasitic infections and the immune system*. San Diego: Academic Press, 1994.

129. Howard JG, Hale C, Liew FW. Immunological regulation of experimental cutaneous leishmaniasis III. Nature and significance of specific suppression of cell mediated immunity in mice highly susceptible to *Leishmania tropica*. *J Exp Med* 1980;152:594–607.

130. Bogdan C, Vodovotz Y, Paik J, Xie Q, Nathan C. Mechanism of suppression of nitric oxide synthase expression by interleukin-4 in primary mouse macrophages. *J Leukoc Biol* 1994;55:227–233.

131. Hsieh C-S, Macatonia SE, O'Garra A, Murphy KM. T cell genetic background determines default T helper phenotype development in vitro. *J Exp Med* 1995;181:713–721.

132. Guler ML, Gorham JD, Hsieh CS, et al. Genetic susceptibility to *Leishmania*: IL-12 responsiveness in TH1 cell development. *Science* 1996;271:984–987.

133. Sadick MD, Heinzel FP, Holaday BJ, Pu RT, Dawkins RS, Locksley RM. Cure of murine leishmaniasis with anti-interleukin 4 monoclonal antibody. *J Exp Med* 1990;171:115–127.

134. Kopf M, Brombacher F, Kohler G, et al. IL-4-deficient Balb/c mice resist infection with *Leishmania major*. *J Exp Med* 1996;184:1127–1136.

135. Nohen-Trauth N, Kropf P, Muller I. Susceptibility to *Leishmania major* infection in interleukin-4-deficient mice. *Science* 1996;271:987–990.

136. Afonso LC, Scott P. Immune responses associated with susceptibility of C57BL/10 mice to *Leishmania amazonensis*. *Infect Immun* 1993;61:2952–2959.

137. Bretscher PA, Wei G, Menon JN, Bielefeldt-Ohmann H. Establishment of stable, cell-mediated immunity that makes "susceptible" mice resistant to *Leishmania major*. *Science* 1992;257:539–542.

138. Wynn TA, Cheever AW. Cytokine regulation of granuloma formation in schistosomiasis. *Curr Opin Immunol* 1995;7:505–511.

139. Mathew RC, Boros DL. Anti-L3T4 antibody treatment suppresses hepatic granuloma formation and abrogates antigen induced IL-2 production in *Schistosoma mansoni* infection. *Infect Immun* 1986;54:820–824.

140. Hernandez HJ, Wang Y, Tzellas N, Stadecker MJ. Expression of class II, but not class I, major histocompatibility complex molecules is required for granuloma formation in infection with *Schistosoma mansoni*. *Eur J Immunol* 1997;27: 1170–1176.

141. Hernandez HJ, Wang Y, Stadecker MJ. In infection with *Schistosoma mansoni*, B cells are required for T helper type 2 cell responses but not for granuloma formation. *J Immunol* 1997;158:4832–4837.

142. Yap G, Cheever A, Caspar P, Jankovic D, Sher A. Unimpaired down-modulation of the hepatic granulomatous response in CD8 T-cell- and gamma interferon-deficient mice chronically infected with *Schistosoma mansoni*. *Infect Immun* 1997;65:2583–2586.

143. Iacomini J, Ricklan DE, Stadecker MJ. T cells expressing the gamma delta T cell receptor are not required for egg granuloma formation in schistosomiasis. *Eur J Immunol* 1995;25:884–888.

144. Cheever AW, Yap GS. The immunologic basis of disease and disease regulation in schistosomiasis. *Chem Immunol* 1996;66:159–176.

145. Wynn TA, Cheever AW, Jankovic D, et al. An IL-12-based vaccination method for preventing fibrosis induced by schistosome infection. *Nature* 1995;376: 594–596.

146. Cheever AW, Williams ME, Wynn TA, et al. Anti-IL-4 treatment of *Schistosoma mansoni*-infected mice inhibits development of T cells and non-B, non-T cells expressing Th2 cytokines while decreasing egg-induced hepatic fibrosis. *J Immunol* 1994;153:753–759.

147. Pearce EJ, Cheever A, Leonard S, et al. *Schistosoma mansoni* in IL-4 deficient mice. *Int Immunol* 1996;8:435–444.

148. Cheever AW, Finkelman FD, Caspar P, Heiny S, Macedonia JG, Sher A. Treatment with anti-IL-2 antibodies reduces hepatic pathology and eosinophilia in *Schistosoma mansoni*-infected mice while selectively inhibiting T cell IL-5 production. *J Immunol* 1992;148:3244–3248.

149. Wynn TA, Eltoum I, Oswald IP, Cheever AW, Sher A. Endogenous interleukin 12

150. Flores Villanueva PO, Harris TS, Ricklan DE, Stadecker MJ. Macrophages from schistosomal egg granulomas induce unresponsiveness in specific cloned Th-1 lymphocytes in vitro and down-regulate schistosomal granulomatous disease in vivo. *J Immunol* 1994;152:1847–1855.

151. Amiri P, Locksley RM, Parslow TG, et al. Tumour necrosis factor α restores granulomas and induces parasite egg-laying in schistosome-infected SCID mice. *Nature* 1992;356:604–606.

152. Lukacs NW, Chensue SW, Strieter RM, Warmington K, Kunkel SL. Inflammatory granuloma formation is mediated by TNF-α inducible intercellular adhesion molecule-1. *J Immunol* 1994;152:5883–5889.

153. Adewusi OI, Freeman GL, Colley DG, Secor WE. Production of TNF-α by spleen cells of mice with chronic *Schistosoma mansoni* infections. *Am J Trop Med Hyg* 1996;55:A507.

154. Adewusi O, Nix N, Lu X, Colley D, Secor W. *Schistosoma mansoni*: relationship of tumor necrosis factor-alpha to morbidity and collagen deposition in chronic experimental infection. *Exp Parasitol* 1996;84:115–123.

155. Chensue SW, Warmington KS, Lukacs NW, et al. Monocyte chemotactic protein expression during schistosome egg granuloma formation. Sequence of production, localization, contribution, and regulation. *Am J Pathol* 1995;146:130–138.

156. Gao JL, Wynn TA, Chang Y, et al. Impaired host defense, hematopoiesis, granulomatous inflammation and type 1-type 2 cytokine balance in mice lacking CC chemokine receptor 1. *J Exp Med* 1997;185:1959–1968.

157. Lukacs NW, Chensue SW, Karpus WJ, et al. C-C chemokines differentially alter interleukin-4 production from lymphocytes. *Am J Pathol* 1997;150:1861–1868.

158. Jankovic D, Cheever AW, Kullberg M, et al. CD4+ T cell mediated granulomatous pathology in schistosomiasis is down-regulated by a B lymphocyte-dependent mechanism requiring Fc receptor signalling (*submitted*).

159. Dunne DW, Doenhoff MJ. *Schistosoma mansoni* egg antigens and hepatocyte damage in infected T cell-deprived mice. *Contrib Microbiol Immunol* 1983;7: 22–29.

160. Pearlman E, Lass JH, Bardenstein DS, Hazlett FE, Diaconu E, Kazura JW. IL-4 and Th2 cells are required for the development of experimental onchocercal keratitis (river blindness). *J Exp Med* 1995;182:931–940.

161. Pearlman E. Immunopathology of onchocerciasis: a role for eosinophils in onchocercal dermatitis and keratitis. *Chem Immunol* 1997;66:26–40.

162. Heinzel FP, Rerko RM, Ahmed F, Pearlman E. Endogenous IL-12 is required for control of Th2 cytokine responses capable of exacerbating leishmaniasis in normally resistant mice. *J Immunol* 1995;155:730–739.

163. Scharton-Kersten T, Afonso LC, Wysocka M, Trinchieri G, Scott P. IL-12 is required for natural killer cell activation and subsequent T helper 1 cell development in experimental leishmaniasis. *J Immunol* 1995;154:5320–5330.

164. Gazzinelli RT, Wysocka M, Hayashi S, et al. Parasite-induced IL-12 stimulates early IFN gamma synthesis and resistance during acute infection with *Toxoplasma gondii*. *J Immunol* 1994;153:2533–2543.

165. Trinchieri G. Interleukin-12: a proinflammatory cytokine with immunoregulatory functions that bridge innate resistance and antigen-specific adaptive immunity. *Annu Rev Immunol* 1995;13:251–276.

166. Gajewski TF, Joyce J, Fitch FW. Antiproliferative effect of murine IFN γ in immune regulation. III. Differential selection of TH1 and TH2 murine helper T lymphocyte clones using recombinant IL-2 and recombinant IFN-γ. *J Immunol* 1989;143:15–22.

167. Ma X, Chow JM, Gri G, et al. The interleukin 12 p40 gene promoter is primed by interferon gamma in monocytic cells. *J Exp Med* 1996;183:147–157.

168. Reiner SL, Zheng S, Wang Z-E, Stowring L, Locksley RM. Leishmania promastigotes evade interleukin 12 (IL-12) induction by macrophages and stimulate a broad range of cytokines from CD4+ T cells during initiation of infection. *J Exp Med* 1994;179:447–456.

169. Carrera L, Gazzinelli RT, Badolato R, et al. Leishmania promastigotes selectively inhibit interleukin 12 induction in bone marrow-derived macrophages from susceptible and resistant mice. *J Exp Med* 1996;183:515–526.

170. Macatonia SE, Hosken NA, Litton M, et al. Dendritic cells produce IL-12 and direct the development of Th1 cells from naive CD4+ T cells. *J Immunol* 1995;154:5071–5079.

171. Campbell KA, Ovendale PJ, Kennedy MK, Fanslow WC, Reed SG, Maliszewski CR. CD40 ligand is required for protective cell-mediated immunity to *Leishmania major*. *Immunity* 1996;4:283–289.

172. Kamanaka M, Yu P, Yasui T, et al. Protective role of CD40 in *Leishmania major* infection at two distinct phases of cell-mediated immunity. *Immunity* 1996;4: 275–281.

173. Soong L, Xu JC, Grewal IS, et al. Disruption of CD40-CD40 ligand interactions results in an enhanced susceptibility to *Leishmania amazonensis* infection. *Immunity* 1996;4:263–273.

174. Reis e Sousa C, Hieny S, Scharton-Kersten T, et al. In vivo microbial stimulation induced rapid CD40L-independent production of IL-12 by dendritic cells and their re-distribution to T cell areas. *J Exp Med* 1997;186:1819–1829.

175. Le Gros G, Ben-Sasson SZ, Seder R, Finkelman FD, Paul WE. Generation of interleukin 4 (IL-4)-producing cells in vivo and in vitro: IL-2 and IL-4 are required for in vitro generation of IL-4-producing cells. *J Exp Med* 1990;172: 921–929.

176. Hsieh CS, Heimberger AB, Gold JS, O'Garra A, Murphy KM. Differential reg-

ulation of T helper phenotype development by interleukins 4 and 10 in an αβ T-cell-receptor transgenic system. *Proc Natl Acad Sci USA* 1992;89:6065–6069.

177. Seder RA, Paul WE, Davis MM, de St Groth BF. The presence of interleukin 4 during in vitro priming determines the lymphokine-producing potential of CD4+ T cells from T cell receptor transgenic mice. *J Exp Med* 1992;176:1091–1098.

178. Swain SL, Weinberg AD, English M, Huston G. IL-4 directs the development of different subsets of helper T cells. *J Immunol* 1990;145:3796.

179. Kopf M, Le Gros G, Bachmann M, Lamers MC, Bluethmann H, Kohler G. Disruption of the murine IL-4 gene blocks Th2 cytokine responses. *Nature* 1993; 362:245–248.

180. Coffman RL, von der Weid T. Multiple pathways for the initiation of T helper 2 (Th2) responses. *J Exp Med* 1997;185:373–375.

181. Schmitz J, Thiel A, Kuhn R, Rajewsky K, Muller W, Assenmacher M. Induction of interleukin 4 (IL-4) expression in T helper (Th) cells is not dependent on IL-4 from non-Th cells. *J Exp Med* 1994;179:1349–1353.

182. Launois P, Ohteki T, Swihart K, MacDonald HR, Louis JA. In susceptible mice, *Leishmania major* induce very rapid interleukin-4 production by CD4+ T cells which are NK1.1-. *Eur J Immunol* 1995;25:3298–3307.

183. von der Weid T, Beebe AM, Roopenian DC, Coffman RL. Early production of IL-4 and induction of Th responses in the lymph node originate from an MHC class I-independent CD4-NK1.1- T cell population. *J Immunol* 1996;157: 4421–4427.

184. Rincon M, Anguita J, Nakamura T, Fikrig E, Flavell R. Interleukin (IL)-6 directs the differentiation of IL-4 producing CD4+ cells. *J Exp Med* 1997;185:461–469.

185. Yoshimoto TO, Paul WE. CD4+, NK1.1+ T cells promptly produce interleukin 4 in response to in vivo challenge with anti-CD3. *J Exp Med* 1994;179:1285–1295.

186. Yoshimoto T, Bendelac A, Watson C, Hu-Li J, Paul WE. Role of NK1.1+ T cells in a Th2 response and in immunoglobulin E production. *Science* 1995;270: 1845–1847.

187. Brown DR, Fowell DJ, Corry DB, et al. Beta 2-microglobulin-dependent NK1.1+ T cells are not essential for T helper cell 2 immune responses. *J Exp Med* 1996;184:1295–1304.

188. Launois P, Maillard I, Pingel S, et al. IL-4 rapidly produced by V beta 4 V alpha 8 CD4+ T cells instructs Th2 development and susceptibility to *Leishmania major* in BALB/c mice. *Immunity* 1997;6:541–549.

189. Launois P, Swihart KG, Milon G, Louis JA. Early production of IL-4 in susceptible mice infected with *Leishmania major* rapidly induces IL-12 unresponsiveness. *J Immunol* 1997;158:3317–3324.

190. Julia V, Rassoulzadegan M, Glaichenhaus N. Resistance to *Leishmania major* induced by tolerance to a single antigen. *Science* 1996;274:421–423.

191. Sabin EA, Pearce EJ. Early IL-4 production by non-CD4+ cells at the site of antigen deposition predicts the development of a T helper 2 cell response to *Schistosoma mansoni* eggs. *J Immunol* 1995;155:4844–4853.

192. Sabin EA, Kopf MA, Pearce. EJ. *Schistosoma mansoni* egg induced early IL-4 production is dependent upon IL-5 and eosinophils. *J Exp Med* 1996;184: 1871–1878.

193. Ferrick DA, Schrenzel MD, Mulvania T, Hsieh B, Ferlin WG, Lepper H. Differential production of interferon-γ and interleukin-4 in response to Th1- and Th2-stimulating pathogens by γδ T cells in vivo. *Nature* 1995;373:255–257.

194. Paul WE, Seder RA, Plaut M. Lymphokine and cytokine production by FcεRI+ cells. *Adv Immunol* 1993;53:1–29.

195. Jankovic D, Kullberg MC, Dombrowicz D, et al. Fc epsilonRI-deficient mice infected with *Schistosoma mansoni* mount normal Th2-type responses while displaying enhanced liver pathology. *J Immunol* 1997;159:1868–1875.

196. Gause WC, Halvorson MJ, Lu P, et al. The function of costimulatory molecules and the development of IL-4-producing T cells. *Immunol Today* 1997;18: 115–120.

197. Lenschow DL, Walunas TL, Bluestone JA. CD28/B7 system of T cell costimulation. *Annu Rev Immunol* 1996;14:233–258.

198. Chambers CA, Allison JP. Co-stimulation in T cell responses. *Curr Opin Immunol* 1997;9:396–404.

199. Waterhouse P, Marengere LEM, Mittrucker H-W, Mak TW. CTLA-4, a negative regulator of T-lymphocyte activation. *Immunol Rev* 1996;153:183–207.

200. McCoy K, Camberis M, Le Gros G. Protective immunity to nematode infection is induced by CTLA-4 blockade. *J Exp Med* 1997;186:183–188.

201. Lu P, Zhou XD, Chen SJ, et al. Requirement of CTLA-4 counter receptors for IL-4 but not IL-10 elevations during a primary systemic in vivo immune response. *J Immunol* 1995;154:1078–1087.

202. Corry DB, Reiner SL, Linsley PS, Locksley RM. Differential effects of blockade of CD28-B7 on the development of Th1 or Th2 effector cells in experimental leishmaniasis. *J Immunol* 1994;153:4142–4148.

203. King CL, Xianli J, June CH, Abe R, Lee KP. CD28-deficient mice generate an impaired Th2 response to *Schistosoma mansoni* infection. *Eur J Immunol* 1996; 26:2448–2455.

204. Brown DR, Green JM, Moskowitz NH, Davis M, Thompson CB, Reiner SL. Limited role of CD28-mediated signals in T helper subset differentiation. *J Exp Med* 1996;184:803–810.

205. Kuchroo VK, Das MP, Brown JA, et al. B7-1 and B7-2 costimulatory molecules activate differentially the Th1/Th2 developmental pathways: application to autoimmune disease therapy. *Cell* 1995;80:707–718.

206. Brown JA, Titus RG, Nabavi N, Glimcher LH. Blockade of CD86 ameliorates *Leishmania major* infection by down-regulating the Th2 response. *J Infect Dis* 1996;174:1303–1308.

207. Subramanian G, Kazura JW, Pearlman E, Jia X, Malhorta I, King CL. B7-2 requirement for helminth-induced granuloma formation and CD4 type 2 helper cell cytokine expression. *J Immunol* 1997;158:5914–5920.

208. Greenwald RJ, Lu P, Halvorson MJ, et al. Effects of blocking B7-1 and B7-2 interactions during a type 2 in vivo immune response. *J Immunol* 1997;158: 4088–4096.

209. Brown DR, Moskowitz NH, Killeen N, Reiner SL. A role for CD4 in peripheral T cell differentiation. *J Exp Med* 1997;186:101–107.

210. Fowell DJ, Magram J, Turck CW, Killeen N, Locksley RM. Impaired Th2 subset development in the absence of CD4. *Immunity* 1997;6:559–569.

211. Parrish CR. The relationship between humoral and cell-mediated immunity. *Transplant Rev* 1972;13:35–66.

212. Hosken NA, Shibuya K, W. HA, Murphy KM, O'Garra A. The effect of antigen dose on CD4+ T helper cell phenotype development on a T cell receptor-alpha beta-transgenic model. *J Exp Med* 1995;182:1579–1584.

213. Abbas AK, Murphy KM, Sher A. Functional diversity of helper T lymphocytes. *Nature* 1996;383:787–793.

214. Gazzinelli RT, Camargo MM, Almeida IC, et al. Identification and characterization of protozoan products that trigger the synthesis of IL-12 by inflammatory macrophages. *Chem Immunol* 1997;68:136–152

215. Schofield L, Hackett F. Signal transduction in host cells by a glycosylphosphatidylinositol toxin of malaria parasites. *J Exp Med* 1993;177:145–153.

216. Camargo MM, Almeida IC, Pereira ME, Ferguson MA, Travassos LR, Gazzinelli RT. Glycosylphosphatidylinositol-anchored mucin-like glycoproteins isolated from *Trypanosoma cruzi* trypomastigotes initiate the synthesis of proinflammatory cytokines by macrophages. *J Immunol* 1997;158:5890–5901.

217. Tachado SD, Gerold P, Schwarz R, Novakovic S, McConville M, Scofield L. Signal transduction in macrophages by glycosylphosphatidylinositols of *Plasmodium, Trypanosoma* and *Leishmania*: activation of protein tyrosine kinases and protein kinase C by inositolglycan and diacylglycerol moieties. *Proc Natl Acad Sci USA* 1997;94:4022–4027.

218. Turrini F, Giribaldi G, Valente E, Arese P. Mycoplasma contamination of Plasmodium cultures: A case of parasitism. *Parasitology Today*

219. Jakobsen PH, Bate CA, Taverne J, Playfair JH. Malaria: toxins, cytokines and disease. *Parasite Immunol* 1995;17:223–231.

220. Denkers EY, Caspar P, Sher A. *Toxoplasma gondii* possesses a superantigen activity that selectively expands murine T cell receptor Vbeta 5-bearing CD8+ lymphocytes. *J Exp Med* 1994;180:985–994.

221. Skeiky YA, Guderian JA, Benson DR, et al. A recombinant Leishmania antigen that stimulates human peripheral blood mononuclear cells to express a Th1-type cytokine profile and to produce interleukin 12. *J Exp Med* 1995;181:1527–1537.

222. Scharton-Kersten T, Afonso LC, Wysocka M, Trinchieri G, Scott P. IL-12 is required for natural killer cell activation and subsequent T helper 1 cell development in experimental leishmaniasis. *J Immunol* 1995;154:5320–5330.

223. Laskay T, Diefenbach A, Rollinghoff M, Solbach W. Early parasite containment is decisive for resistance to *Leishmania major*. *Eur J Immunol* 1995;25: 2220–2227.

224. Sher A, Denkers EY, Gazzinelli RT. Induction and regulation of host cell-mediated immunity by *Toxoplasma gondii*. In: Mitchison NA, ed. *CIBA Foundation Symposium*. West Sussex: John Wiley and Sons, 1995.

225. Scharton-Kersten T, Denkers EY, Gazzinelli R, Sher A. Role of IL-12 in induction of cell-mediated immunity to *Toxoplasma gondii*. *Res Immunol* 1996;146: 539–545.

226. Scharton-Kersten TM, Sher A. Role of natural killer cells in innate resistance to protozoan infections. *Curr Opin Immunol* 1997;9:44–51.

227. Hunter CA, Subauste CS, Van Cleave VH, Remington JS. Production of gamma interferon by natural killer cells from *Toxoplasma gondii*-infected SCID mice: regulation by interleukin-10, interleukin-12, and tumor necrosis factor alpha. *Infect Immun* 1994;62:2818–2824.

228. Hunter CA, Chizzonite R, Remington JS. IL-1 beta is required for IL-12 to induce production of IFN-gamma by NK cells. A role for IL-1 beta in the T cell-independent mechanism of resistance against intracellular pathogens. *J Immunol* 1995;155:4347–4354.

229. Zhang T, Kawakami K, Qureshi MH, Okamura H, Kurimoto M, Saito A. Interleukin-12 (IL-12) and IL-18 synergistically induce the fungicidal activity of murine peritoneal exudate cells against *Cryptococcus neoformans* through production of gamma interferon by natural killer cells. *Infect Immun* 1997;65: 3594–3599.

230. Vella AT, Pearce EJ. CD4+ Th2 response induced by *Schistosoma mansoni* eggs develops rapidly, through an early, transient, Th0-like stage. *J Immunol* 1992;148:2283–2290.

231. Pearlman E, Hazlett FE Jr, Boom WH, Kazura JW. Induction of murine T-helper-cell responses to the filarial nematode *Brugia malayi*. *Infect Immun* 1993;61: 1105–1112.

232. Guery JC, Galbiati F, Smiroldo S, Adorini L. Selective development of T helper (Th)2 cells induced by continuous administration of low dose soluble proteins to normal or beta(2)-microglobulin-deficient BALB/c mice. *J Exp Med* 1996;183: 485–497.

233. Velupillai P, Harn DA. Oligosaccharide-specific induction of interleukin 10 production by B220+ cells from schistosome-infected mice: a mechanism for regulation of CD4+ T-cell subsets [see comments]. *Proc Natl Acad Sci USA* 1994;91: 18–22.

234. Beebe AM, Mauze S, Schork NJ, Coffman RL. Serial backcross mapping of mul-

tiple loci associated with resistance to *Leishmania major* in mice. *Immunity* 1997;6:551–557.

235. Guler M, Jacobson NG, Gubler U, Murphy KM. T cell genetic background determines maintenance of IL-12 signaling: effects on BALB/c and B10.D2 T helper cell type 1 phenotype development. *J Immunol* 1997;159:1767–1774.

236. Szabo SJ, Dighe AS, Gubler U, Murphy KM. Regulation of the interleukin (IL)-12R beta 2 subunit expression in developing T helper 1 (Th1) and Th2 cells. *J Exp Med* 1997;185:817–824.

237. Gorham JD, Guler ML, Steen RG, et al. Genetic mapping of a murine locus controlling development of T helper 1/T helper 2 type responses. *Proc Natl Acad Sci USA* 1996;93:12467–12472.

238. Pearce EJ, Caspar P, Grzych JM, Lewis FA, Sher A. Downregulation of Th1 cytokine production accompanies induction of Th2 responses by a helminth, *Schistosoma mansoni. J Exp Med* 1991;173:159–165.

239. Kierszenbaum F. *Parasitic infections and the immune system.* San Diego, CA: Academic Press, 1994.

240. Schleifer KW, Mansfield JM. Suppressor macrophages in African trypanosomiasis inhibit T cell proliferative responses by nitric oxide and prostaglandins. *J Immunol* 1993;151:5492–5503.

241. VanHeyningen TK, Collins HL, Russell DG. IL-6 produced by macrophages infected with *Mycobacterium* species suppresses T cell responses. *J Immunol* 1997;158:330–337.

242. Allen JE, Lawrence RA, Maizels RM. APC from mice harbouring the filarial nematode, *Brugia malayi,* prevent cellular proliferation but not cytokine production. *Int Immunol* 1996;8:143–151.

243. Kullberg MC, Pearce EJ, Hieny SA, Sher A, Berzofsky JA. Infection with *Schistosoma mansoni* alters Th1/Th2 cytokine responses to a non-parasite antigen. *J Immunol* 1992;148:3264–3270.

244. Actor JK, Shirai M, Kullberg MC, Buller RM, Sher A, Berzofsky JA. Helminth infection results in decreased virus-specific CD8+ cytotoxic T-cell and Th1 cytokine responses as well as delayed virus clearance. *Proc Natl Acad Sci USA* 1993;90:948–952.

245. Pearlman E, Kazura JW, Hazlett FE Jr, Boom WH. Modulation of murine cytokine responses to mycobacterial antigens by helminth-induced T helper 2 cell responses. *J Immunol* 1993;151:4857–4864.

246. Curry AJ, Else KJ, Jones F, Bancroft A, Grencis RK, Dunne DW. Evidence that cytokine-mediated immune interactions induced by *Schistosoma mansoni* alter disease outcome in mice concurrently infected with *Trichuris muris. J Exp Med* 1995;181:769–774.

247. Sabin EA, Araujo MI, Carvalho EM, Pearce EJ. Impairment of tetanus toxoid-specific Th1-like immune responses in humans infected with *Schistosoma mansoni. J Infect Dis* 1996;173:269–272.

248. Cooper PJ, Espinel I, Paredes W, Guderian RH, Nutman TB. Impaired tetanus specific cellular and humoral responses following tetanus vaccination in human onchocerciasis: a role for IL-10 (*submitted*).

249. Chaouat G, Menu EM, Clark DA, Dy M, Minkowski M, Wegmann TG. Control of fetal survival in CBA X DBA/2 mice by lymphokine therapy. *J Reprod Fertil* 1990;89:447–453.

250. Krishnan L, Guilbert LJ, Wegmann TG, Belosevic M, Mosmann TR. T helper 1 responses against *Leishmania major* in pregnant C57BL/6 mice increases implantation failure and fetal resorptions. Correlation with increased IFN-gamma and TNF and reduced IL-10 production by placental cells. *J Immunol* 1996;156:653–662.

251. Krishnan L, Guilbert LJ, Russell AS, Wegmann TG, Mosmann TR, Belosevic M. Pregnancy impairs resistance of C57BL/6 mice to *Leishmania major* infection and causes decreased antigen-specific IFN-gamma response and increased production of T helper 2 cytokines. *J Immunol* 1996;156:644–652.

252. Cooke A, Tonks P, Jones FM, et al. Infection with *Schistosoma mansoni* prevents insulin dependent diabetes mellitus in NOD mice (*submitted*).

253. Thursz MR, Kwiatkowski D, Torok ME, et al. Association of hepatitis B surface antigen carriage with severe malaria in Gambian children. *Nat Med* 1995;4:374–375.

254. Pereira LM, Melo MC, Saleh MG, et al. Hepatitis C virus infection in schistosomiasis mansoni in Brazil. *J Med Virol* 1995;45:423–428.

255. Bentwich Z, Weisman Z, Moroz C, Bar-Yehuda S, Kalinkovich A. Immune dysregulation in Ethiopian immigrants in Israel: relevance to helminth infections. *Clin Exp Immunol* 1996;103:239–243.

256. Lobos E, Zahn R, Weiss N, Nutman TB. A major allergen of lymphatic filarial nematodes is a parasite homolog of the gamma-glutamyl transpeptidase. *Mol Med* 3 1996;2:712–724.

257. Lobos E, Ondo A, Ottesen EA, Nutman TB. Biochemical and immunologic characterization of a major IgE-inducing filarial antigen of *Brugia malayi* and implications for the pathogenesis of tropical pulmonary eosinophilia. *J Immunol* 1992;149:3029–3034.

258. Cunha-Neto E, Duranti M, Gruber A, et al. Autoimmunity in Chagas disease cardiopathy: biological relevance of a cardiac myosin-specific epitope crossreactive to an immunodominant *Trypanosoma cruzi* antigen. *Proc Natl Acad Sci USA* 1995;92:3541–3545.

259. Van Voorhis WC, Schlekewy L, Trong HL. Molecular mimicry by *Trypanosoma cruzi:* the F1-160 epitope that mimics mammalian nerve can be mapped to a 12-amino acid peptide. *Proc Natl Acad Sci USA* 1991;88:5993–5997.

260. Tanowitz HB, Kirchhoff LV, Simon D, Morris SA, Weiss LM, Wittner M. Chagas' disease. *Clin Microbiol Rev* 1992;5:400–419.

261. Minoprio P, Itohara S, Heusser C, Tonegawa S, Coutinho A. Immunobiology of murine *T. cruzi* infection: the predominance of parasite-nonspecific responses and the activation of TCRI T cells. *Immunol Rev* 1989;112:183–207.

262. Tarleton RL, Zhang L, Downs MO. "Autoimmune rejection" of neonatal heart transplants in experimental Chagas disease is a parasite-specific response to infected host tissue. *Proc Natl Acad Sci USA* 1997;94:3932–3927.

263. Vago AR, Macedo AM, Adad SJ, Reis DD, Correa-Oliveira R. PCR detection of *Trypanosoma cruzi* DNA in oesophageal tissues of patients with chronic digestive Chagas' disease. *Lancet* 1996;348(9031):891–892.

264. Rimoldi MT, Sher A, Heiny S, Lituchy A, Hammer CH, Joiner K. Developmentally regulated expression by *Trypanosoma cruzi* of molecules that accelerate the decay of complement C3 convertases. *Proc Natl Acad Sci USA* 1988;85:193–197.

265. Pearce EJ, Fenton Hall B, Sher A. Host specific evasion of the alternative complement pathway by schistosomes correlates with the presence of a phospholipase C sensitive surface molecule resembling human decay accelerating factor. *J Immunol* 1990;144:2751.

266. Landa A, Laclette JP, Nicholson-Weller A, Shoemaker CB. cDNA cloning and recombinant expression of collagen-binding and complement inhibitor activity of *Taenia solium* paramyosin (AgB). *Mol Biochem Parasitol* 1993;60:343–347.

267. Puentes SM, Sacks DL, da Silva RP, Joiner KA. Complement binding by two developmental stages of Leishmania major promastigotes varying in expression of a surface lipophosphoglycan. *J Exp Med* 1988;167:887–902.

268. Russo DC, Williams DJ, Grab DJ. Mechanisms for the elimination of potentially lytic complement-fixing variable surface glycoprotein antibody-complexes in *Trypanosoma brucei. Parasitol Res* 1994;80:487–492.

269. Pays E, Vanhamme L, Berberof M. Genetic controls for the expression of surface antigens in African trypanosomes. *Annu Rev Microbiol* 1994;48:25–52.

270. Borst P, Rudenko G, Taylor MC, et al. Antigenic variation in trypanosomes. *Arch Med Res* 1996;27:379–388.

271. Barry JD. The relative significance of mechanisms of antigenic variation in African trypanosomes. *Parasitol Today* 1997;13:212–218.

272. Brown KN, Brown IN. Immunity to malaria: antigenic variation in chronic infections of *Plasmodium knowlesi. Nature* 1965;208:1286–1288.

273. Brown KN. Antigenic variation in malaria. *Adv Exp Med Biol* 1977;93:5–25.

274. Su XZ, Heatwole VM, Wertheimer SP, et al. The large diverse gene family var encodes proteins involved in cytoadherence and antigenic variation of *Plasmodium falciparum*-infected erythrocytes. *Cell* 1995;82:89–100.

275. Smith JD, Chitnis CE, Craig AG, et al. Switches in expression of *Plasmodium falciparum* var genes correlate with changes in antigenic and cytoadherent phenotypes of infected erythrocytes. *Cell* 1995;82:101–110.

276. Baruch DI, Pasloske BL, Singh HB, et al. Cloning the *P. falciparum* gene encoding PfEMP1, a malarial variant antigen and adherence receptor on the surface of parasitized human erythrocytes. *Cell* 1995;14:77–87.

277. Gardner JP, Pinches RA, Roberts DJ, Newbold CI. Variant antigens and endothelial receptor adhesion in *Plasmodium falciparum. Proc Natl Acad Sci USA* 1996;93.3503–3508.

278. Baruch DI, Gormely JA, Ma C, Howard RJ, Pasloske BL. *Plasmodium falciparum* erythrocyte membrane protein 1 is a parasitized erythrocyte receptor for adherence to CD36, thrombospondin, and intercellular adhesion molecule 1. *Proc Natl Acad Sci USA* 1996;93:3497–3502.

279. Racoosin EL, Beverley SM. *Leishmania major* promastigotes induce expression of a subset of chemokine genes in murine macrophages. *Exp Parasitol* 1997;85:283–295.

280. Pearce EJ, Sher A. Mechanisms of immune evasion in schistosomiasis. In: Cruse JM, Lewis RE, eds. *Contributions to microbiology and immunology; Antigenic variation: molecular and genetic mechanisms of relapsing disease.* Basel: Karger, 1987, 219–232.

281. Brindley PJ, Sher A. Immunological involvement in the efficacy of praziquantel. *Exp Parasitol* 1990;71:245–248.

282. Fallon PG, Cooper RO, Probert AJ, Doenhoff MJ. Immune-dependent chemotherapy of schistosomiasis. *Parasitology* 1992:S41–S48.

283. Grencis RK, Entwistle GM. Production of an interferon-gamma homologue by an intestinal nematode: functionally significant or interesting artefact? *Parasitology* 1997;115.S101–S106.

284. Engers HD, Bergquist R, Modabber F. Progress on vaccines against parasites. *Dev Biol Stand* 1996;87:73–84.

285. Bruno JM, Feachem R, Godal T, et al. The spirit of Dakar: a call for action on malaria. *Nature* 1997;386:541.

286. Nardin EH, Oliveira GA, Calvo-Calle JM, Nussenzweig RS. The use of multiple antigenic peptides in the analysis and induction of protective immune responses against infectious diseases. *Adv Immunol* 1995;60:105–149.

287. Hoffman SL, Doolan DL, Sedegah M, et al. Strategy for development of a pre erythrocytic *Plasmodium falciparum* DNA vaccine for human use. *Vaccine* 1997;15:842–845.

288. Hoffman SL, Bancroft WH, Gottlieb M, et al. Funding for malaria genome sequencing. *Nature* 1997;387:647.

289. Hoffman SL, Miller LH. Perspective on malaria vaccine development. In: Hoffman SL, ed. *Malaria vaccine development: a multi-immune response approach.* Washington: American Society for Microbiology, 1996, 1–13.

290. Doolan DL, Hoffman SL. Multi-gene vaccination against malaria: a multistage, multi-immune response approach. *Parasite Immunol* 1997;13:171–178.

291. Nussenzweig V, Nussenzweig RS. Rationale for the development of an engineered sporozoite malaria vaccine. *Adv Immunol* 1989;45:283–334.

292. Hoffman SL, Franke ED, Hollingdale MR, Druihle P. Attacking the infected hepatocyte. In: Hoffman SL, ed. *Malaria vaccine development: a multi-immune response approach.* Washington: American Society for Microbiology, 1996, 35–75.

293. Schofield L, Villaquiran J, Ferreira A, Schellekens H, Nussenzweig R, Nussenzweig V. Gamma interferon, CD8+ T cells and antibodies required for immunity to malaria sporozoites. *Nature* 1987;330:664–666.

294. Seguin MC, Klotz FW, Schneider I, et al. Induction of nitric oxide synthase protects against malaria in mice exposed to *Plasmodium berghei* infected mosquitoes: involvement of interferon-gamma and CD8+ cells. *J Exp Med* 1994;180: 353–358.

295. Stoute JA, Slaoui M, Heppner G, et al. A preliminary evaluation of a recombinant circumsporozoite protein vaccine against *Plasmodium falciparum* malaria. *N Engl J Med* 1997;336:86–90.

296. Nussenzweig RS, Zavala F. A malaria vaccine based on a sporozoite antigen. *N Engl J Med* 1997;336:128–130.

297. Chan M-S, Hall BF, Bundy DAP. Modelling of potential schistosomiasis vaccination programmes. *Parasitol Today* 1996;12:457–460.

298. Soisson LM, Masterson CP, Tom TD, McNally MT, Lowell GH, Strand M. Induction of protective immunity in mice using a 62-kDa recombinant fragment of a *Schistosoma mansoni* surface antigen. *J Immunol* 1992;149:3612–3620.

299. Lanar DE, Pearce EJ, James SL, Sher A. Identification of paramyosin as the schistosome antigen recognized by intradermally vaccinated mice. *Science* 1986; 254:593.

300. Wilson RA. Immunity and immunoregulation in helminth infections. *Curr Opin Immunol* 1993;5:538–547.

301. Wynn TA, Oswald IP, Eltoum IA, et al. Elevated expression of Th1 cytokines and nitric oxide synthase in the lungs of vaccinated mice after challenge infection with *Schistosoma mansoni. J Immunol* 1994;153:5200–5209.

302. Coulson PS. The radiation-attenuated vaccine against schistosomes in animal models: paradigm for a human vaccine? *Adv Parasitol* 1997;39:271–336.

303. Sher A, Coffman RL, Hieny S, Cheever AW. Ablation of eosinophil and IgE responses with anti-IL-5 or anti-IL-4 antibodies fails to affect immunity against *Schistosoma mansoni* in the mouse. *J Immunol* 1990;145:3911–3916.

304. Smythies LE, Coulson PS, Wilson RA. Monoclonal antibody to IFN-gamma modifies pulmonary inflammatory responses and abrogates immunity to *Schistosoma mansoni* in mice vaccinated with attenuated cercariae. *J Immunol* 1992;149:3654–3658.

305. Wilson RA, Coulson PS, Betts C, Dowling MA, Smythies LE. Impaired immunity and altered pulmonary responses in mice with a disrupted interferon-gamma receptor gene exposed to the irradiated *Schistosoma mansoni* vaccine. *Immunology* 1996;87:275–282.

306. Oswald IP, Eltoum I, Wynn TA, et al. Endothelial cells are activated by cytokine treatment to kill an intravascular parasite, *Schistosoma mansoni,* through the production of nitric oxide. *Proc Natl Acad Sci USA* 1994;91:999–1003.

307. James SL, Glaven J, Goldenberg S, Meltzer MS, Pearce E. Tumour necrosis factor (TNF) as a mediator of macrophage helminthotoxic activity. *Parasite Immunol* 1990;12:1–13.

308. Wynn TA, Jankovic D, Hieny S, Cheever AW, Sher A. IL-12 enhances vaccine-induced immunity to *Schistosoma mansoni* in mice and decreases T helper 2 cytokine expression, IgE production, and tissue eosinophilia. *J Immunol* 1995;154:4701–4709.

309. Caulada-Benedetti Z, al-Zamel F, Sher A, James S. Comparison of Th1- and Th2-associated immune reactivities stimulated by single versus multiple vaccination of mice with irradiated *Schistosoma mansoni* cercariae. *J Immunol* 1991; 146:1655–1660.

310. Wynn TA, Reynolds A, James S, et al. IL-12 enhances vaccine-induced immunity to schistosomes by augmenting both humoral and cell-mediated immune responses against the parasite. *J Immunol* 1996;157:4068–4078.

311. Mangold BL, Dean DA. Passive transfer with serum and IgG antibodies of irradiated cercariae-induced resistance against *Schistosoma mansoni. J Immunol* 1986;136:2644–2649.

312. Metzger DW, Buchanan JM, Collins JT, et al. Enhancement of humoral immunity by interleukin-12. *Ann NY Acad Sci* 1996;795:100–115.

313. Jankovic D, Caspar P, Zweig M, et al. Adsorption to aluminum hydroxide promotes the activity of IL-12 as an adjuvant for antibody as well as type 1 cytokine responses to HIV-1 gp120. *J Immunol* 1997;159:2409–2417.

314. Afonso LC, Scharton TM, Vieira LQ, Wysocka M, Trinchieri G, Scott P. The adjuvant effect of interleukin-12 in a vaccine against *Leishmania major. Science* 1994;263:235–237.

315. Mougneau E, Altare F, Wakil AE, et al. Expression cloning of a protective Leishmania antigen. *Science* 1995;268:563–566.

316. Nabors GS, Afonso LC, Farrell JP, Scott P. Switch from a type 2 to a type 1 T helper cell response and cure of established *Leishmania major* infection in mice is induced by combined therapy with interleukin 12 and Pentostam. *Proc Natl Acad Sci USA* 1995;92:3142–3146.

317. Guranathan S, Sacks DL, Brown DR, et al. Vaccination with DNA encoding the immunodominant LACK parasite antigen confers protective immunity to mice infected with *Leishmania major. J Exp Med* 1997;186:1137–1147.

318. Good MF, Kaslow DC, Miller LH. Pathways and strategies for developing a malaria blood stage vaccine. *Annu Rev Immunol* 1998;16:57–87.

319. Sabchareon A, Outtara D, Attanah P, et al. Parasitologic and clinical human response to immunoglobulin administration in falciparum malaria. *Am J Trop Med Hyg* 1991;45:297–308.

320. Kaslow DC. Transmission-blocking vaccines: uses and current status of development. *Int J Parasitol* 1997;27:183–189.

321. Jakobsen PH, Bate CAW, Taverne J, Playfair JH. Malaria: toxins, cytokines and disease. *Parasite Immunol* 1995;17:223–231.

322. Capron A, Riveau G, M. GJ, Boulanger D, Capron M, Pierce R. Development of a vaccine strategy against human and bovine schistosomiasis. Background and update. *Trop Geogr Med* 1994;46:242–246.

323. Xu CB, Verwaerde C, Grzych JM, Fontaine J, Capron A. A monoclonal antibody blocking the *Schistosoma mansoni* 28-kDa glutathione S-transferase activity reduces female worm fecundity and egg viability. *Eur J Immunol* 1991;21: 1801–1807.

324. Pearlman E, Lass JH, Bardenstein DS, et al. IL-12 exacerbates helminth-mediated corneal pathology by augmenting inflammatory cell recruitment and chemokine expression. *J Immunol* 1997;158:827–833.

325. Ottesen EA. Immune responsiveness and the pathogenesis of human onchocerciasis. *J Infect Dis* 1995;171:659–671.

326. Ottesen EA, Nutman TB. Tropical pulmonary eosinophilia. *Annu Rev Med* 1992;43:417–424.

327. von der Weid T, Kopf M, Kohler G, Langhorne J. The immune response to *Plasmodium chabaudi* malaria in interleukin-4-deficient mice. *Eur J Immunol* 1994;24:2285.

328. Marshall E. Serious setback for Patarroyo vaccine. *Science* 1996;273:1652.

Fundamental Immunology, Fourth Edition,
edited by William E. Paul
Lippincott–Raven Publishers, Philadelphia © 1999.

CHAPTER 39

Immunity to Viruses

Rafi Ahmed and Christine A. Biron

The science of immunology originated from the study of infectious diseases, and until the early part of the twentieth century, studies on immune responses to viral and microbial infections occupied the center stage of immunology. But as the devastation caused by infectious diseases lessened due to better public health measures and development of antibiotics and vaccines, the interests of immunologists shifted toward the study of well-defined protein and hapten antigens to analyze the immune system. However, there is now once again considerable interest in studying immune responses to viruses. The resurgence in this area is due to several reasons. First, despite the many successes against viruses, most notably the eradication of small pox and the impending one of polio, viral infections continue to be a major cause of human morbidity and mortality (1,2). During the past two decades, several new viral diseases have emerged. This is best exemplified by the global epidemics of human immunodeficiency virus (HIV) and hepatitis B and C viruses (HBV, HCV) and the recent outbreaks of Ebola and hantavirus (1,2). Also, many old viruses continue to take a heavy toll; there are still a large number of respiratory infections due to influenza virus and respiratory syncitial virus (RSV), gastrointestinal diseases due to rotaviruses, and recurrent epidemics of measles, dengue, and hemorrhagic viral infections (1,2). There is a need to characterize immune responses against these viruses, not only for clinical diagnosis and surveillance purposes, but also to understand correlates of protective immunity and to use this information in developing new and improved vaccines against these diseases. In addition to their medical importance, there is now a growing realization among immunologists that viruses are excellent tools for probing the immune system, and that basic studies with well-defined viral models will provide insights into the workings of the immune system. Thus, it is becoming increasingly popular to use viruses to ask fundamental questions about the immune system.

To present the subject of viral immunity, this chapter has been divided into the following sections: The first section provides an overview of the viral life cycle *in vivo* and the patterns of viral infections. This is followed by sections on innate and specific (adaptive) immunity to viruses and effector mechanisms critical to control of viral infections. The following section discusses interplay between innate and specific responses. Next, there is a review of immune memory to viruses and mechanisms of protective immunity. The last two sections are on immunopathology of viral infections and on mechanisms by which viruses evade immune responses and persist *in vivo*.

R. Ahmed: Emory Vaccine Center, Emory University School of Medicine, Atlanta, Georgia 30322.
C. A. Biron: Department of Molecular Microbiology and Immunology, Brown University, Providence, Rhode Island 02912.

VIRAL INFECTIONS: GENERAL CONSIDERATIONS

Entry, Spread, and Transmission of Viruses

Successful propagation of a virus requires the following sequence of events *in vivo:* (a) entry into a susceptible host, (b) replication and spread within the host, (c) shedding to the exterior, and (d) transmission to a new host (Fig. 1). An appreciation of these events is necessary to understand the types of immune responses elicited by different viruses and the mechanisms by which viral infections are controlled. For a detailed description of the viral life cycle *in vivo,* the reader is referred to textbooks in virology (1–4). A general overview of stages of viral infection is given below.

Viral Entry

The first step of infection is entry into the host. This can occur at the following sites: (a) skin, (b) urogenital tract, (c) conjunctiva, (d) respiratory tract, and (e) alimentary tract. The list of viruses that enter at each of these sites is given in Tables 1 through 3. The skin is the largest organ of the body, but it represents a tough barrier for viral entry. It is unlikely that any virus can initiate infection if placed on the intact skin. However, this physical barrier can be bypassed by injection, animal or insect bites, and minor cuts and sores (Table 1). Mucous membranes of the eye and genital tract do not constitute a major physical barrier but are bathed in liquid that can provide some protection because of its viscous nature. However, this is usually not sufficient to prevent infection, and the best protection against viral entry at mucous membranes comes from secretory immunoglobulin. Therefore, there is considerable interest in developing vaccines that will induce potent and long-lasting mucosal immunity.

A large number of viruses initiate infection via the respiratory tract, making this the most common route of infection (Table 2). There are some mechanical barriers in the respiratory tract, such as the mucociliary blanket lining the nasal cavity. Foreign particles (i.e., viruses) can be caught in mucus and carried from the nasal cavity or lungs into the throat and swallowed into the gut (a much more hostile environment for viruses). Also, the nasal turbinates have a narrow and complicated pathway of inspired air and can impede entry of viral particles into the respiratory tract. However, none of these mechanical obstacles in the respiratory tract are particularly effective in preventing viral infection, and the key determining factor is, once again, the presence or absence of the right kind of secretory antibody. The viruses that initiate infection via the respiratory tract can be broken down into two broad groups:

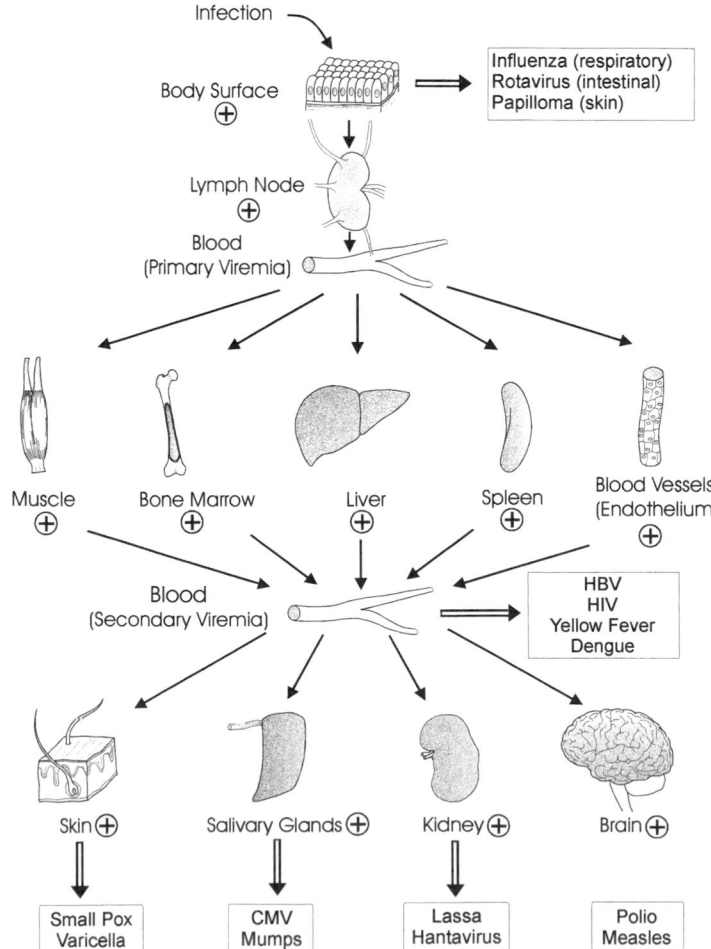

FIG. 1. The virus life cycle *in vivo,* showing entry, spread, and shedding. The symbol (+) indicates possible sites of viral replication, *small arrows* indicate movement of virus, and *large arrows* indicate sites of shedding. Only a few examples of viruses are listed. Transfer from blood is by transfusion in the case of HBV and HIV, and by insect bites for yellow fever and Dengue. This figure does not illustrate neural spread. In addition to hematogenous spread, viruses can also spread to the central nervous system (CNS) via the peripheral nerves. The classic examples of neural spread are HSV, rabies, and VZV. (Adapted from ref. 4.)

TABLE 1. *Viruses that initiate infection via the skin, eye, or genital tract*

Site of infection	Method of infection	Virus family	Examples[a]
Skin	Minor breaks/cuts	Hepadnaviridae	Hepatitis B
		Herpesviridae	Herpes simplex 1
		Papovaviridae	Papillomavirus
		Poxviridae	Vaccinia
	Animal bite	Herpesviridae	Herpes monkey B
		Rhabdoviridae	Rabies
	Vector bite	Bunyaviridae	Rift Valley fever
		Flaviviridae	Yellow fever, Dengue
		Reoviridae	Colorado tick fever
		Togaviridae	Eastern encephalitis
	Injection	Flaviviridae	Hepatitis C
		Hepadnaviridae	Hepatitis B
		Herpesviridae	Cytomegalovirus
		Retroviridae	Human immunodeficiency virus, human T-cell leukemia virus I/II
Conjunctiva	Contact	Adenoviridae	Adenovirus
		Picornaviridae	Enterovirus 70
Genital tract	Contact	Flaviviridae	Hepatitis C
		Hepadnaviridae	Hepatitis B
		Herpesviridae	Herpes simplex 2
		Papovaviridae	Papillomavirus
		Retroviridae	Human immunodeficiency virus

[a]Only selected examples of human viruses are given.
Adapted from Mims CA, White DO. *Viral pathogenesis and immunology.* Oxford: Blackwell Science, 1984.

ones that produce local respiratory symptoms and usually remain confined to the respiratory tract, such as influenza virus, rhinovirus (common cold), and RSV; and ones that do not produce any initial respiratory symptoms but spread to other tissues and produce generalized disease (i.e., measles, mumps, varicella, Lassa, etc).

Viruses that initiate infection via the alimentary tract are listed in Table 3. Some of these viruses produce enteritis (i.e., rotavirus, Norwalk), whereas others produce systemic disease without enteric symptoms (i.e., polio, hepatitis A). The enteric route contains numerous barriers and presents a hostile environment for viruses. To successfully initiate infection by this route, viruses have to resist

the destructive actions of acid, bile, and proteolytic enzymes. Bile destroys lipid and, consequently, enveloped viruses are rapidly inactivated upon contact with bile and acid. In general, only nonenveloped viruses (i.e., those with a protein shell) can survive and initiate infection in the intestinal tract. This is nicely illustrated by hepatitis A and B viruses. Hepatitis A is a nonenveloped virus (like polio virus and rotavirus), whereas hepatitis B is an enveloped virus (like influenza and HIV). Both hepatitis A and B viruses replicate in the liver and are excreted in the bile into the intestinal tract. Hepatitis A survives and is secreted in infectious form in the feces (hence is transmitted enterically), whereas hepatitis B is

TABLE 2. *Viruses that initiate infection via the respiratory tract*

Localization of disease	Virus family	Example[a]
Upper respiratory tract	Adenoviridae	Adenovirus
	Picornaviridae	Rhinoviruses, some enteroviruses
Lower respiratory tract	Bunyaviridae	Sin Nombre
	Coronaviridae	Coronavirus
	Orthomyxoviridae	Influenza
	Paramyxoviridae	Parainfluenza, respiratory syncitial virus
Generalized systemic disease without initial respiratory symptoms	Arenaviridae	Lassa fever
	Bunyaviridae	Hantaan virus
	Herpesviridae	Varicella, cytomegalovirus
	Papovaviridae	BK and JC viruses
	Paramyxoviridae	Mumps, measles
	Poxviridae	Smallpox (extinct)
	Togaviridae	Rubella

[a]Only selected examples of human viruses are given.
Adapted from Mims CA, White DO. *Viral pathogenesis and immunology.* Oxford: Blackwell Science, 1984.

TABLE 3. *Viruses that initiate infection via the alimentary tract*

Site of infection	Virus family	Example[a]
Mouth/oropharynx	Herpesviridae	Herpes simplex, Epstein-Barr virus, cytomegalovirus
Intestinal tract		
Producing enteritis	Adenoviridae	Adenovirus 40, 41
	Astroviridae	Astrovirus
	Caliciviridae	Norwalk agent
	Reoviridae	Rotavirus
Producing generalized disease usually without enteric illness	Picornaviridae	Poliovirus
		Hepatitis A
Usually symptomless	Adenoviridae	Some adenoviruses
	Picornaviridae	Enterovirus
	Reoviridae	Reovirus

[a]Only selected examples of human viruses are given.
Adapted from Mims CA, White DO. *Viral pathogenesis and immunology.* Oxford: Blackwell Science, 1984

rapidly inactivated in the gut. Resistance to proteolytic enzymes is also an important characteristic in determinig whether a virus can initiate infection through the gut. Interestingly, some viruses, such as rotavirus and reovirus, actually take advantage of intestinal proteases to enhance infectivity. Proteolytic cleavage of one of the outer capsid proteins results in virus particles that are more efficient in initiating infection (1,2).

Viral Spread

Following entry into the host, viral infections may remain confined to the site at which the virus entered, or infections may spread through the body. A listing of viruses producing local or systemic disease is given in Table 4. This distinction has an important bear-

TABLE 4. *Relationship between initial site of viral infection and disease production[a]*

Site of infection	Local[b]	Systemic[c]
Oropharynx		Cytomegalovirus
		Epstein-Barr virus
		Herpes simplex 1
Respiratory tract	Influenza virus	Measles
	Respiratory syncitial virus	Mumps
	Rhinovirus	Rubella
		Varicella
		Lassa
Intestinal tract	Norwalk	Hepatitis A
	Rotavirus	Polio
Genital tract	Papillomavirus[d]	Hepatitis B
		Hepatitis C
		HIV

[a]Only selected examples of human viruses are given.
[b]Infections confined to body surfaces. Short incubation period (disease usually in < week).
[c]Infections initiated at body surfaces, followed by spread through the body. Long incubation period (disease in usually > week).
[d]Infection is confined to the initial site of a viral entry, but papilloma development can take several weeks.

ing on the duration of protective immunity. In general, protective immunity is short-lived for viruses causing disease due to local infection and is of much longer duration for viruses producing clinical symptoms after systemic infection. The underlying mechanisms for these differences will be discussed later in the section on immunologic memory.

After initial replication at the point of entry, most viruses spread locally by cell-to-cell transmission (see Fig. 1). Also, free virus or virus particles injested by phagocytic cells are transported by afferent lymphatic drainage from the site of initial infection to regional lymph nodes. This is a critical event in the viral life cycle. Not only is this the first step in dissemination of the infection, but it is also the beginning of the specific immune response. It is very likely that antigen presentation to initiate immune responses first occurs in the regional lymph nodes. An important determinant of viral spread is the ability of the virus to replicate and/or survive in macrophages. Virus particles are taken up by these phagocytic cells in regional lymph nodes, and viruses that replicate well in macrophages tend to spread more efficiently.

The subepithelial invasion and lymphatic spread described above lead to local spread and amplification of the virus, but the most important mechanism for dissemination is the blood, which can transport the virus to any organ in the body. The virus that enters into blood from initial sites of infection and/or via the draining lymph nodes is referred to as *primary viremia.* In most instances, virus levels during primary viremia are very low and not detectable by conventional assays. After entering the blood, viruses may be carried free in plasma or be cell-associated. An advantage of being cell-associated is that it provides a potential means of escape from neutralizing antibody. Different viruses are carried by different cells; for example, Epstein-Barr virus (EBV) is transported by B cells; HIV, by CD4 T cells and monocytes; measles virus, by monocytes and T cells; cytomegalovirus (CMV), by monocytes; and so on (Table 5). In all of these instances, the appropriate receptors and/or coreceptors are present on the target cell, and the virus is able to infect the cell that is carrying it. Substantial amplification of the virus can now occur within these circulating blood cells and in tissues, which subsequently become infected by virus carried through the blood. The target organs seeded by primary viremia include liver, spleen, muscle, bone marrow, and so forth, and different viruses amplify in different tissues. For example, HBV and HCV grow in hepatocytes in the liver, and HIV grows in CD4 T cells and

TABLE 5. *Viruses that infect circulating blood cells*

Cell type	Virus[a]
Monocytes	CMV
	Dengue
	Ebola
	HIV
	Lassa
	Measles
	Rubella
	Yellow fever
B cells	EBV
T cells	HIV
	Human T-cell leukemia virus I/II
	Human herpes 6,7
Erythroblasts	Colorado tick fever[b]

[a]Only selected examples of human viruses are given.
[b]Colorado tick fever virus replicates in erythroblasts in bone marrow and circulates in mature erythrocytes.
Adapted from Nathanson N, ed. *Viral pathogenesis.* Philadelphia: Lippincott–Raven, 1997.

macrophages. Some viruses, especially those causing hemorrhagic fevers (Ebola and Lassa viruses) replicate in endothelial cells of blood vessels. This viral growth in selected target tissues now results in increased virus in the blood (i.e., *secondary viremia*). Virus levels during secondary viremia can be very high and lead to seeding of more distant organs, such as the skin [measles, small pox, varicella-zoster virus (VZV)], salivary glands (mumps, EBV), kidney (measles, CMV, mumps, hantavirus), testes (mumps), brain (polio, HIV, measles), and placenta (rubella, CMV). Invasion of the placenta can lead to infection of the fetus, causing fetal death or congenital abnormalities. It is worth noting that the reticuloendothelial system (RES) is very effective in removing viral particles from blood, and that viremia can only be maintained by continuous virus production within cells that are in contact with blood. These include circulating blood cells, of course, and also organs with extensive sinusoids, such as liver and spleen. Therefore, viruses like HBV, HCV, HIV, measles, Ebola, and yellow fever are found in high levels in blood, whereas influenza virus, whose replication is confined to lung, produces no detectable viremia.

Viral Shedding and Transmission

The last stage of the *in vivo* viral life cycle is shedding and transmission. The biologic imperative for any virus is transmission, because its survival depends on continual infection of susceptible hosts. Some viruses, such as measles, polio, and mumps, survive within a single host, infecting humans only, whereas other viruses, such as influenza, yellow fever, and rabies circulate in more than one species. Shedding occurs via one of the body surfaces involved in entry of viruses, and viral particles can be shed through saliva, coughing, urine, feces, semen, lesions on skin, and so on. The various modes of viral transmission, including zoonoses (i.e., transmission involving animals and insects), are listed in Table 6.

We have covered the salient points of viral entry, spread, and transmission in this chapter on viral immunity because these topics are closely related. It is essential to know how a particular virus enters the host, what kind of cells it infects, and how it is transmitted, in order to fully appreciate what type of immune responses would be most beneficial in controlling the infection.

Patterns of Viral Infection

Viral infections can be divided into three general categories, based on levels of infectious virus detectable in the organism at various times after infection (Fig. 2). The three types of infection are as follows:

1. Acute infection followed by viral clearance due to the host immune response. A large number of viruses fall into this category. They include polio, influenza, rotavirus, mumps, yellow fever, RSV, and so on.

2. Acute infection followed by latent infection, in which virus persists in a noninfectious form, with intermittent periods of viral

TABLE 6. *Viral transmission*

Mode of transmission	Example[a]	Comment
Aerosol/saliva →Respiratory or salivary spread	Influenza virus EBV Measles Mumps	Transmission is difficult to control
Fecal→Oral spread	Polio Rotavirus Hepatitis A	Controllable by public health measures
Venereal spread	HSV HIV HPV	Controllable by appropriate precautions
Zoonoses Insect→Human Animal →Human Animal→Insect→Human	Dengue Rabies Lassa Hantavirus Yellow fever	Human infection can be controlled by controlling vectors (insects) and/or by controlling animal infection. No (or rare) human to human transmission

[a]Only selected examples of human viruses are given

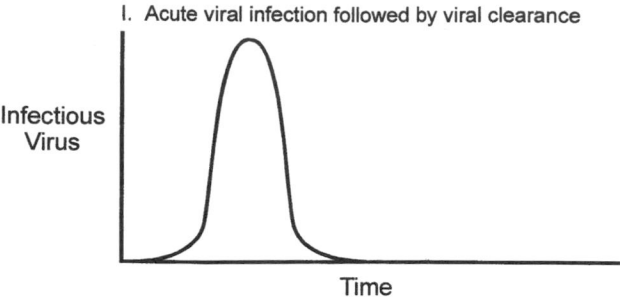

I. Acute viral infection followed by viral clearance

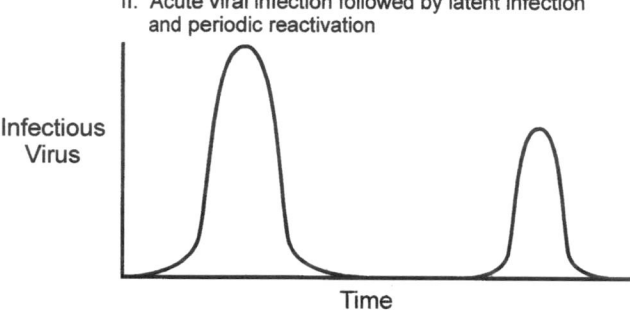

II. Acute viral infection followed by latent infection and periodic reactivation

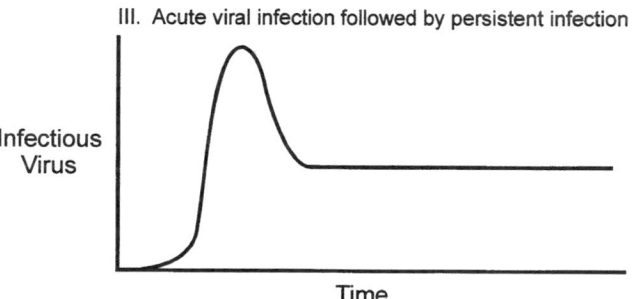

III. Acute viral infection followed by persistent infection

FIG. 2. General patterns of viral infection.

reactivation and shedding. Viruses that establish latent infections with periodic reactivation must be capable of undergoing a productive infection in certain cells or under certain conditions while undergoing a nonpermissive infection in other cells. The classic examples of viruses that establish such infections are the herpesviruses (HSV, VZV, EBV).

3. Acute infection followed by persistent infection, in which infectious virus is continuously shed from or is present in infected tissues. Such infections are established when the host immune response fails to fully eliminate virus produced during the acute stage of infection. Productive infection of host cells during the acute stage may be followed by spread to cells that are less permissive, or by evolution of an immune response that dampens viral replication but cannot completely clear virus from the host. HIV, HBV, and HCV are examples of such infections.

We have defined these idealized patterns of viral infections (see Fig. 2), but sometimes viruses show different patterns of infection in different tissues or cell types, or they combine these general patterns such that their infection of the host does not fit clearly within these definitions. For example, EBV causes a latent infection in B

cells but a productive infection in pharyngeal epithelial cells (1,2). Therefore, the patterns shown in Fig. 1 should be viewed as themes with variations, and not as rigid definitions.

HOST DEFENSE AGAINST VIRUSES

Organization of the Immune System

Other chapters in this book deal extensively with development, structure, and function of the mammalian immune system. However, it is appropriate to make a few general comments about cells of the immune system and the secondary lymphoid tissues (lymph nodes and spleen) in the context of viral immunity.

The cellular mediators of specific immunity are the lymphocytes, which, together with the monocytes, make up the great majority of leukocytes in normal individuals. These cells discriminate self from nonself with a high degree of precision mediated by the specific recognition units on lymphocytes, the T-cell receptors (TCRs) and immunoglobulin (Ig) molecules, the B-cell receptors. The T-cell populations are selected in the thymus to allow the survival of precursors expressing TCRs with low avidity for cells expressing self class I (CD8 subset) or class II (CD4 subset) MHC glycoproteins, and high avidity for somatic cells (encountered later in the extrathymic environment), signaling abnormality or "danger" through surface major histocompatibility (MHC) molecules that have been modified by the binding of peptides processed from nonself (i.e., viral proteins). The viral proteins are degraded from newly synthesized product in cytoplasm (class I, endogenous pathway) or in endosomes–lysosomes, subsequent to phagocytosis (class II mostly, but also class I, exogenous pathway) (5,6). The MHC molecules are among the most polymorphic known, reflecting the need of the species to avoid nonresponsiveness to a novel pathogen after failure to develop an appropriate (i.e., antigenic) peptide–MHC glycoprotein complex.

The antigen-specific TCR on both sets of lymphocytes consists of an αβ heterodimer that cannot be assigned *a priori* to a CD8[+] or CD4[+] T cell simply by looking at sequence variation (7). Both CD4 and CD8 molecules have ancillary binding function for nonvarying regions of the particular MHC molecule, and there are six other TCR-associated chains (the CD3 complex), all of which are thought to have the capacity to transduce signals to the cytoplasm. The alternative TCR, the γδ heterodimer, is expressed on substantial populations of sessile lymphocytes in the skin and various mucosae, and on a low percentage of circulating T cells in mice and humans (8). The γδ T cells are much more prevalent in chickens, pigs, cattle, and sheep (9,10). Although γδ T cells are found in sites of virus-induced inflammatory pathology, it has been difficult to assign a functional role for these cells (11–13). However, one study has shown that γδ T cells may play a role in regulating herpes simplex virus (HSV) infection (14). It is speculated that γδ TCRs may be much more immunoglobulin-like in their binding characteristics with, perhaps, a tendency to recognize heat-shock proteins, which may have bound peptides derived from other proteins. Studies in bacterial systems have shown that γδ T cells can recognize nonpeptide antigens and also peptides with altered (modified) amino acids (15–17). The relevance of such target antigens for viral systems is not known. The B cells are generated in the bone marrow and localize to germinal centers in secondary lymphoid tissue. Their receptor, the immunoglobulin molecule, has the capacity to bind directly to tertiary structures on viral proteins. A central difference between B-cell and T-cell responses is affinity maturation of the immunoglobulin molecule as a consequence of somatic mutation. In contrast, the T-cell repertoire (spectrum of available TCRs) is essentially determined at the time the cells leave the thymus.

Cells of the innate immune system include monocytes and macrophages, natural killer (NK) cells, dendritic cells, and polymorphonuclear leukocytes (PMNs). These populations are dependent on bone marrow for development and maturation. For the most part, NK cells and PMNs preferentially "hang out" in the blood and spleen. However, they can respond to regional and systemic challenges and migrate into tissues. Moreover, although NK cells are not generally found in lymph nodes during systemic viral infections, they have been shown to be called into draining lymph nodes after local challenge with antigen (18) or parasites (19). In contrast, monocytes and macrophages and dendritic cells are generally found at high concentrations in lymph nodes as well as blood and spleen. Localization in lymph nodes and spleen allows these populations to carry out their functions of antigen processing and presentation to stimulate adaptive immune responses. Although PMNs can clearly be identified in histologic sections of virus-infected tissues, study of their effects has been neglected largely because of the broad and likely erroneous generalization that PMN function is of importance during bacterial infections but not viral infections. New reagents have propelled the study of dendritic cells, but information concerning how they function to promote antiviral innate immune responses is still in its infancy. Both populations have the potential to promote innate antiviral immunity because they can be stimulated to make cytokines under certain conditions. In contrast to PMNs and dendritic cells, there is a significant body of knowledge on the activation and function of macrophages and NK cells during viral infections. These cell populations can respond to infections to produce a variety of soluble factors mediating or accessing antiviral mechanisms as well as reciprocally promoting each others responses.

The secondary lymphoid tissue of mammals consists of lymph nodes, spleen, and mucosa-associated lymphoid tissue. All tissues have two forms of drainage: the venous system and the lymph. The former is monitored by the spleen, the latter by the lymph nodes. Extracellular fluid may be collected into the afferent lymphatics and pumped, as a result of normal movement and muscular contraction, to the regional lymph nodes (e.g., cervical, popliteal, axillary). Intradermal injection, for example, can be regarded as essentially intralymphatic. A virus that invades by this route may be taken up by dendritic cells (Langerhans' cells), or by monocytes and macrophages and transported by lymph to the regional node, where primary immune responses then develop. In contrast, virus that gains direct entry into blood is removed from the circulation in the spleen, and, in such instances, initial immune responses occur in spleen and not lymph nodes.

Immunologically naive T and B cells enter lymph nodes through the specialized high endothelial venules, which express specific ligands for the L-selectin (CD62L) molecule on the lymphocyte membrane. Access to the spleen is thought not be controlled by the L-selectin–dependent gating process involving L-selectin. Moreover, memory T cells may express little L-selectin (20–22) and transit to the lymph node in afferent lymph after leaving the blood in the postcapillary venules of solid tissues. T and B cells exit lymph nodes through the efferent lymphatics, which cumulate to larger ducts that drain to the vena cava, and (after passage through the lung) are pumped around the body in the arterial circulation. Antigen-stimulated T and B cells can extravasate into tissue sites supporting virus growth, with B-cell localization being particularly

apparent for viral infections of the central nervous system (CNS) (23). Locally produced immunoglobulin is readily detected in the cerebrospinal fluid and (because neurons do not express MHC glycoproteins) is clearly important for limiting infectious processes in the brain. In general, however, the continuing recirculation from blood to tissue to lymph of the primed lymphocytes that mediate immune surveillance is essentially a function of the T-cell subsets.

Overview of Host Response to Viral Infection

The immune response to viral infections can be broken down into two broad categories: (a) innate or nonspecific responses and (b) adaptive or specific responses. These play critical roles at distinct times in controlling the infection. The innate responses start almost immediately, and within a day after infection, there is induction of type 1 interferons (IFNs) and increased levels of NK-cell activity (Fig. 3). These early nonspecific responses are critical in controlling the overall extent of viral replication and spread. Innate

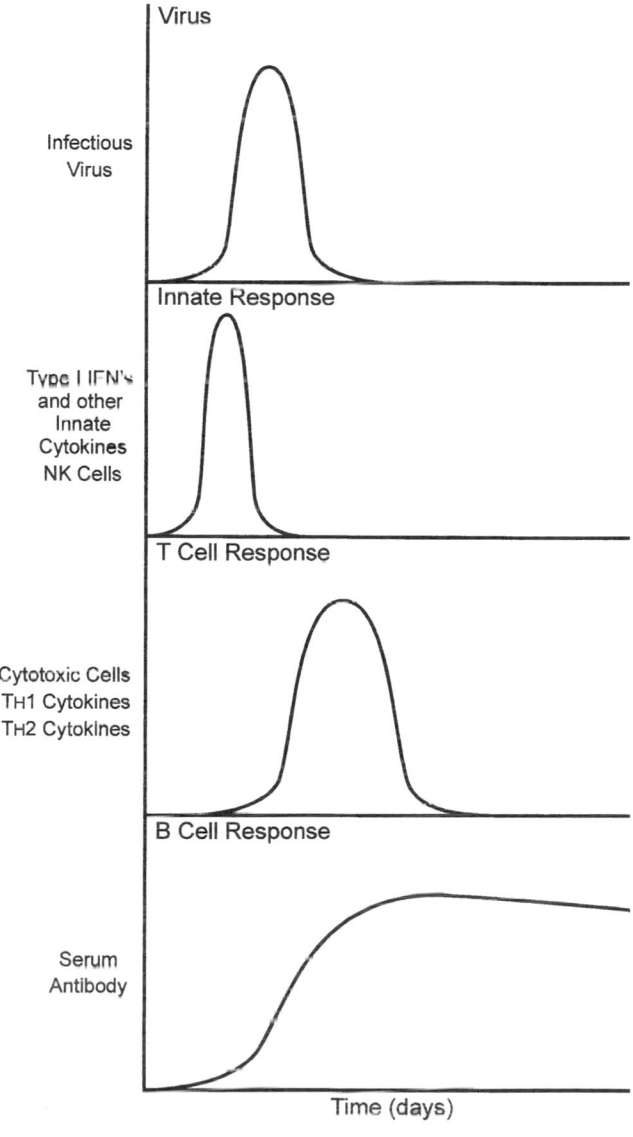

FIG. 3. Kinetics of host responses during a primary acute viral infection.

responses cannot eliminate the virus on their own but provide a crucial first line of defense, especially during infection of naive hosts (i.e., primary infection). Specific responses are essential for clearing the infection and take about a week or so to develop. In general, effector CD4 and CD8 T-cell responses subside as the virus infection is resolved, but antibody production can last for several months to years (20). The following sections cover innate and specific immunity to viruses.

INNATE IMMUNITY

Leukocyte populations, excluding the classical T- and B-lymphocytes of adaptive immune responses, contribute to innate immune responses. However, soluble factors made by both of these immune-cell populations and many different nonimmune tissue cell types are also important players in innate immunity. Because innate immunity can function at times preceding adaptive immunity, it has long been appreciated for its role in defense at early times during primary infections. Components of the innate system can mediate protection by blocking initial virus infection of, inducing conditions inhibiting viral replication within, and/or eliminating virus-infected host cells (Fig. 4). Indeed, adaptive immune responses frequently utilize the components of innate immunity to deliver antiviral effects. During the last few years, however, there has been a growing appreciation for the immunoregulatory roles of innate immune responses both in activating cellular constituents of innate immunity and in setting up conditions to promote and/or shape downstream adaptive immune responses. In addition to immediately activating effector functions of the innate cellular constituents, NK cells and monocytes and macrophages, soluble constituents of innate immune responses can modify cell-trafficking patterns to localize effector cells to sites of infections and to concentrate T and B cells of the adaptive immune system to sites of antigen presentation. Moreover, innate cytokine responses can produce endogenous milieus, preferentially promoting particular T- and B-cell responses (see Fig. 4). Although these cytokine-controlled pathways have been more thoroughly examined in the context of bacterial and parasitic infections directing either T cell helper type 1 (Th1) or helper type 2 (Th2) cytokine responses, comparable or alternative pathways for promoting immune responses during viral infections are being identified. The emerging picture is that different general pathogen characteristics, resulting from unique chemical structures not found in the host, elicit

cytokine responses, which in turn promote the most effective immunity against the agent. As a result, innate immunity functions not only to protect the host from infection while slower adaptive responses are developing, but also to direct the qualitative and quantitative nature of adaptive immunity.

Cytokines

Cytokines are important soluble contributors to defense against viral infections. Effects of individual cytokines are generally pleiotropic, with multiple and distinct consequences. Nevertheless, cytokine responses to infections are frequently observed in cascades with simultaneous or sequential expression of multiple factors. A variety of cell types make cytokines contributing to innate immune responses, and certain cytokines can be produced by infected or activated nonimmune cells such as fibroblasts and endothelial cells. The list of cytokines with the potential to contribute to innate immunity is given in Table 7. A variety of these factors are known to be produced at early times during viral infections and to be important for innate immunity against these agents. Cytokine responses to distinct viral infections can differ in magnitude and composition, and the differences are likely to be important in directing the immune responses most beneficial to the host. The known major cytokine constituents of innate responses to viral infections are reviewed here.

Interferons α and β

The first characterized class of cytokines, and perhaps the best understood in regard to innate defense functions, are the type 1 IFNs. These were identified because of their ability to interfere with virus replication (24). In humans and mice, the multigene members of this cytokine family include those coding for multiple IFN-α and a single IFN-β protein. Many, but not all, viruses are potent inducers of IFN-α/β. Although much remains to be learned about the induction pathways, double-stranded RNA (dsRNA), not detectable in normal cells, can be produced in infected cells as a result of replication of many RNA and DNA viruses, and is a known potent inducer of IFN-α/β. A synthetic analogue of dsRNA, polyinosinic-polycytidylic acid (polyI:C), is a chemical inducer of these IFNs (24,25). However, there appear to be other pathways of induction, including interactions between certain viruses and their

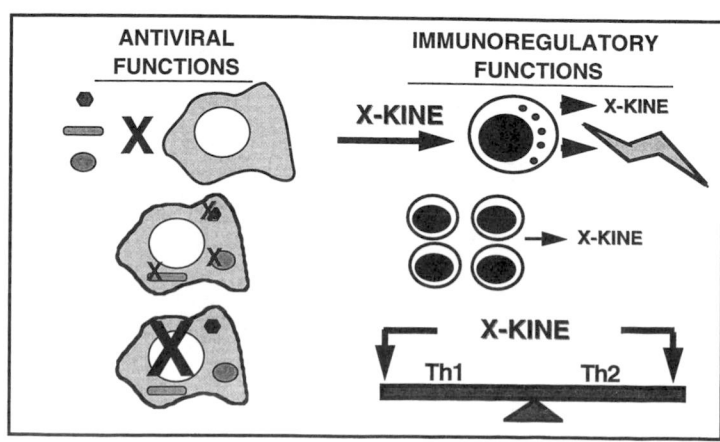

FIG. 4. Functions of innate responses to viral infections. Innate immunity can provide antiviral activity at early times during infections by blocking initial infection of cells, inhibiting virus replication within cells, and/or lysing virus-infected cells. In addition, the cytokine components (*X-KINE*) of the innate immune system can mediate a wide range of immunoregulatory functions. These include activation of the cellular constituents of the innate immune system (i.e., NK cells and monocyte and macrophages) to produce additional cytokines and/or mediate enhanced antiviral activity. In addition, early cytokine responses can modify cell trafficking to help localize immune cells to sites for activation or to sites for delivery of antiviral functions, and set up an endogenous milieu to promote the most beneficial adaptive immune responses, such as preferential Th1- or Th2-type responses.

TABLE 7. *Cytokines with potential to promote innate immunity during viral infections*

Cytokine	Nonadaptive cell sources	Functions	
		Antiviral	Immunoregulatory
IFN-α/β	Monocytes/macrophages	XXX	XXX
	Virus-infected immune and nonimmune cells		
TNF	Monocytes/macrophages	XXX	XXX
	NK Cells		
	Other nonimmune cells		
IFN-γ	NK Cells	XXX	XXX
IL-12	Monocytes, macrophages	XX	XXX
	PMN's, dendritic cells		
IL-1α, IL-1β	Monocytes/macrophages	?	XX
	Other nonimmune cells		
IL-6	Monocytes/macrophages	?	XX
	Other nonimmune cells		
IGIF	Monocytes/macrophages	?	XX
	Other nonimmune cells		
IL-15	Monocytes/macrophages	?	XX
	Other nonimmune cells		
IL-10	Monocytes/macrophages	?	XX
	Other nonimmune cells		
TGF-β	Monocytes/macrophages	X	X
	Other nonimmune cells		

cell surface receptors (26–28). Generally, but not exclusively, leukocytes including macrophages produce more IFN-α than IFN-β, and other cell types, including fibroblast, produce more IFN-β.

The type 1 IFNs are made by infected cells to directly induce antiviral states in neighboring uninfected cells. During the last few years, there has been an explosion of biochemical information concerning the receptor and signal transduction molecules required for induction of IFN-α/β–mediated effects (24,29). The post–ligand-binding intracellular pathways activate specific tyrosine kinases (i.e., Tyk2 and JAK1) and downstream signal transducers and activators of transcription (i.e., STAT1, STAT2, and STAT4). However, the final mediators of defense functions in the cell still are understood incompletely (24). The best-characterized antiviral pathways result from IFN-α/β induction of the (2′-5′)-oligoadenylate synthetase and the dsRNA-dependent protein kinase (PKR). In the presence of dsRNA, these enzymes promote inhibition of host-cell protein synthesis by respectively activating RNase L to degrade mRNA and, by phosphorylating the translation initiation factor elongation factor 2 (eIF2), to block its recycling from an inactive form (Fig. 5). Consequently, they render cells refractory to protein synthesis and inhibit viral replication. Another group of IFN-induced proteins are the Mx molecules, contributing to resistance against certain viral infections. *In vitro* studies also have shown that, at high enough concentrations, the type 1 IFNs inhibit proliferation of cells. A wide range of viruses are sensitive to IFN-α/β–mediated antiviral effects, including the RNA viruses, vesicular stomatitis virus (VSV), influenza virus, picornaviruses, DNA viruses, HSV, and vaccinia virus (VV) (24).

Virus-infected mice neutralized in IFN-α/β functions (30), or rendered either IFN-α/β receptor-deficient (31–33) or deficient in required signal transduction molecules (34) by genetic mutation, have revealed a number of profound resistance effects mediated by IFN-α/β–driven pathways. The most extensive studies have been with lymphocytic choriomeningitis virus (LCMV), VV, and VSV. Lack of IFN-α/β functions dramatically inhibits resistance to these infections. However, in addition to direct antiviral functions in

cells, significant immunoregulatory effects also can be mediated by IFN-α/β. These include dramatic changes in cell distribution (25,35–37), activation of NK cell cytotoxic activity (38), regulation of cytokine and cytokine receptor gene expression (39–41), induction of the class I major histocompatibility molecules (MHC) for promotion of CD8 T-cell responses (42), and *in vivo* induction of modest NK-cell and memory T-cell proliferation (43–45). Thus, multiple mechanisms are likely to be responsible for changes in susceptibility to infection resulting from elimination of the IFN-α/β induction pathway in the host.

Tumor Necrosis Factor-α and Interferon-γ

Additional cytokines produced at early times during certain but not all viral infections with known direct antiviral functions are NK cell–produced IFN-γ and tumor necrosis factor-α (TNF-α) (46–52). The antiviral pathways elicited by these cytokines appear to overlap with those induced by the type 1 IFNs. TNF is much weaker than, but synergizes with, IFN-α/β for these effects. In addition, IFN-γ is a potent activator, and TNF can synergize with IFN-α/β to activate inducible nitric oxide synthase (iNOS) and iNOS-dependent pathways of antiviral defense mediated by macrophage-lineage cells (53). TNF enhances interleukin-12 (IL-12) induction of NK-cell IFN-γ production (54), and both of these cytokines also can mediate a number of other immunoregulatory effects.

Other Cytokines

A variety of other cytokines, with the potential to mediate either antiviral or immunoregulatory functions, can be made by cells of the innate immune system and/or nonimmune cells. These include IL-12, IL-1α, IL-1β, IL-6, IFNγ–inducing factor (IGIF), IL-15, IL-10, and transforming growth factor-β (TGF-β). Most, but not all, of these have been shown to be induced during certain viral infec-

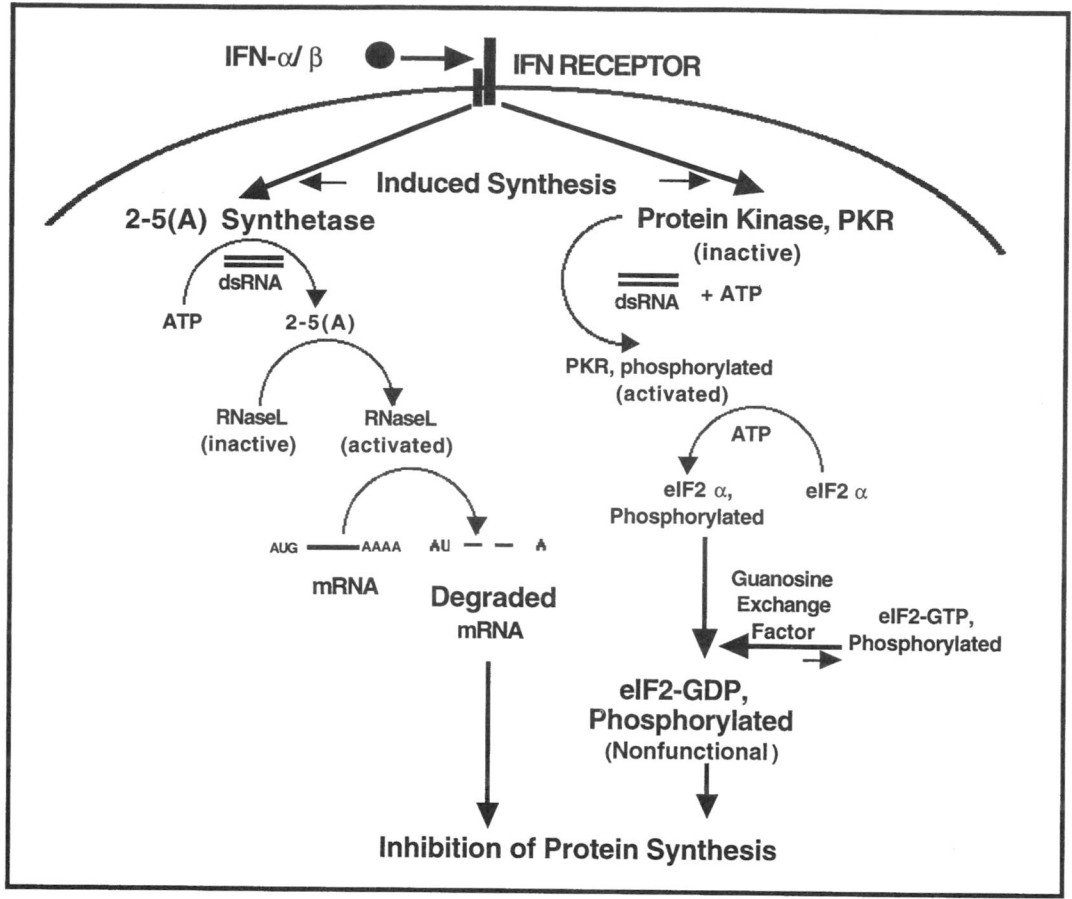

FIG. 5. Pathways of antiviral activity induced by IFN-α/β. These cytokines induce two independent pathways inhibiting translation and, as a consequence, viral replication. Both of these are activated by double stranded RNA (dsRNA). One uses the 2-5(A) synthetase to activate the RNase L to degrade RNA. The other uses the dsRNA-dependent protein kinase (PKR) to phosphorylate the translation initiation factor eIF-2. Phosphorylated eIF-2 cannot recycle, and, as a result, its function is limited in the cell. (Modified from ref. 24.)

tions. IL-12 mRNA is elevated during a range of viral infections. However, biologically active IL-12 protein is detectable in some, but not all, viral infections (39,51,55–58), and its production can be inhibited by IFN-α/β (39). IL-6 protein is induced during many infections, including those with different herpes viruses (51,59–62). TGF-β1 only has been examined in a few viral infections, but it has been shown to be induced at the protein level in these (63,64). Limited numbers of studies suggest that IL-15 expression is induced by human herpesvirus-6 (HSV-6) and human herpesvirus-7 (HSV-7) (65,66), and that IL-10 can be produced in response to viral infections (60). Although certain bacterial products induce high levels of IL-1α and IL-1β, the proteins for these factors appear to induced to more modest levels during CMV infections (51,62). IGIF remains to be tested.

Only a subset of these factors have been shown to mediate antiviral activity. IL-12 is a potent inducer of NK-cell IFN-γ production, and can promote both antiviral and immunoregulatory effects through this pathway (49). However, IL-12 also may mediate IFN-γ–independent effects. Additional pathways for IL-12–mediated defense appear to be in place during VSV (67) and *murine CMV* (MCMV) (50) infections. Because IL-12 can enhance expression of TNF receptors (68), it has the potential of promoting

the antiviral effects mediated by TNF. However, IL-12 may be able to induce different NOSs and plug into NOS-mediated antiviral defense pathways through TNF- and IFN-γ–independent mechanisms (67,69). TGF-β1 inhibits human papillomavirus gene expression (70).

Each of these factors can mediate a variety of immunoregulatory effects to shape adaptive immune responses. In addition, although their relative importance during viral infections has yet to be proven, IL-1α, IL-1β, and IGIF all have been shown to enhance IL-12 induction of NK-cell IFN-γ production (71). Another remarkable function of certain of these cytokines, however, is to alert the neuroendocrine system of high and potentially damaging immune responses to activate the hypothalamic–pituitary–adrenal (HPA) axis and stimulate adrenal gland production of glucocorticoids (GCs) (Fig. 6) (72). The GC hormones themselves mediate a number of immunoregulatory effects. In particular, they can inhibit cytokine expression as a result of activated GC receptor interference with transcriptional regulators (73,74). Interestingly, during MCMV infections, high circulating levels of IL-6 are induced to elicit an endogenous GC response (51). Thus, in addition to downstream immunoregulatory effects on the adaptive immune system, innate cytokine responses to viral infections mediate direct antivi-

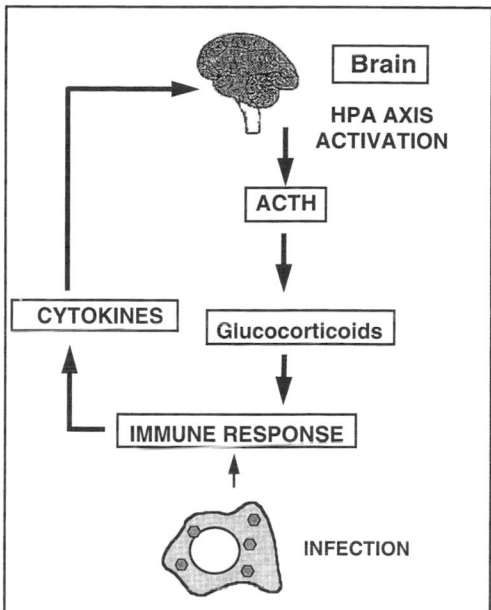

FIG. 6. Communication between the immune and neuroendocrine systems to limit endogenous immune responses during infections. High circulating levels of certain cytokines can induce the hypothalamic–pituitary–adrenal (HPA) axis. An end product of this activation is stimulation of the adrenal glands to produce glucocorticoid hormones. These hormones are known to mediate profound immunoregulatory effects, including inhibition of cytokine gene expression. The pathway can operate in the host to protect against detrimental consequences resulting from high levels of certain cytokines.

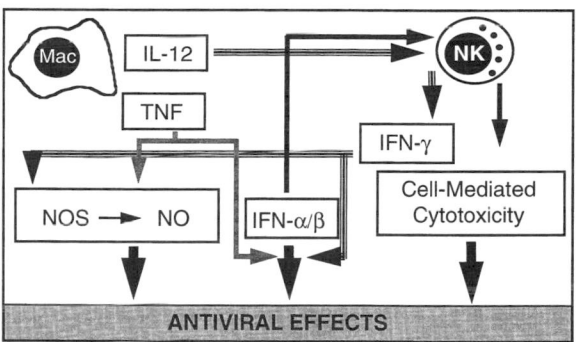

FIG. 7. Roads taken by innate immune responses to fundamental antiviral pathways. There are three known major pathways to antiviral activity (the *dark and broad arrowheads*): IFN-α/β–induced activation of several mechanisms, including those inhibiting protein synthesis; NOS-dependent mechanisms, including those resulting from NO production; and cell-mediated lysis of infected cells by NK cells. Innate immune responses access these pathways through several gates. Although access to IFN-α/β–induced mechanisms is most readily obtained by production of IFN-α/β (*black, narrow arrows*), IFN-γ (*broken-line arrows*) and TNF (*gray arrows*) can access some of the same mechanisms. Because IFN-γ is a good inducer of iNOS, it also is a potent activator of the NOS to NO mechanisms. As IL-12 induces NK-cell IFN-γ production, IL-12 has the potential to plug into both antiviral pathways. TNF can synergize with other factors to activate NOS. Finally, NK cells are induced to mediate elevated cytotoxicity by IFN-α/β. Thus, innate immune responses activate multiple and distinct antiviral activities.

ral effects, activate cells of the innate immune system, and call in hormonal regulators of immune responses.

Cells

Monocytes and macrophages, NK cells, dendritic cells, and PMNs are all cells of the innate immune system. In contrast to the limited information concerning PMN and dendritic cell responses for innate immunity to viral infections, there is a significant body of knowledge on the activation and function of macrophages and NK cells. The responses of these cell populations result in production of a variety of soluble factors. The factors can mediate antiviral mechanisms or access antiviral pathways. Moreover, they also can promote activation of other cell populations (Fig. 7). The known major cellular innate responses to viral infections and their consequences are reviewed here.

Natural Killer Cells

NK cells were discovered because of their ability to spontaneously mediate killing of certain highly sensitive tumor-cell lines (38). The first indication of a possible role for these lymphocytes in defense against viral infections came from the observations that NK cells are activated by virus-induced IFN-α/β to mediate elevated lysis of sensitive target cells and to lyse a broader range of cells, including virus-infected cells (38,75–77), and that their lytic activity is induced endogenously after infections with a number of

different viruses (78–82). Under the conditions generated during primary viral infections, NK cells are activated, in response to endogenously expressed IFN-α/β, at early times preceding adaptive immune responses (30,83). The responding cells do not express the mature components of TCRs for antigen (84,85), and responses occur in the absence of T and B cells. Thus, NK cells are constituents of innate immune responses to viral infections.

The importance of NK cells in early defense against certain viral infections has been established definitively (78,86–91). These cells are significant mediators of protection during herpes group virus infections. Nevertheless, mechanisms for NK cell–mediated effects are not understood completely. NK cells activated *in vivo* by virus-induced IFN-α/β are large granular lymphocytes (LGLs) and use many of the same molecules as cytotoxic T-lymphocytes (CTLs), including perforin (92), to lyse target cells. However, demonstration of this pathway in antiviral defense has been elusive (50,93), and, during certain viral infections, NK cells are induced to mediate elevated cytotoxicity without contributing to viral resistance (88).

The difficulty in documenting antiviral roles for NK cell-mediated cytotoxicity may be, in part, a result of the complex safeguards in place to protect normal cells. Both cell-to-cell contact between NK effector cells and target cells and the presence of positive, as well as the absence of negative, signals to NK cells are required for killing (Fig. 8). Although the molecules responsible for delivery of positive signals during innate responses are poorly characterized, certain viral products may contribute to these (27,94,95). Once adaptive immunity is induced, antibodies specific for viral determinants on infected cells can act to deliver positive signals through Fc receptors class III (FcRIII) (38,96) identified as CD16 (see below). Negative signals are delivered to NK cells by MHC class I

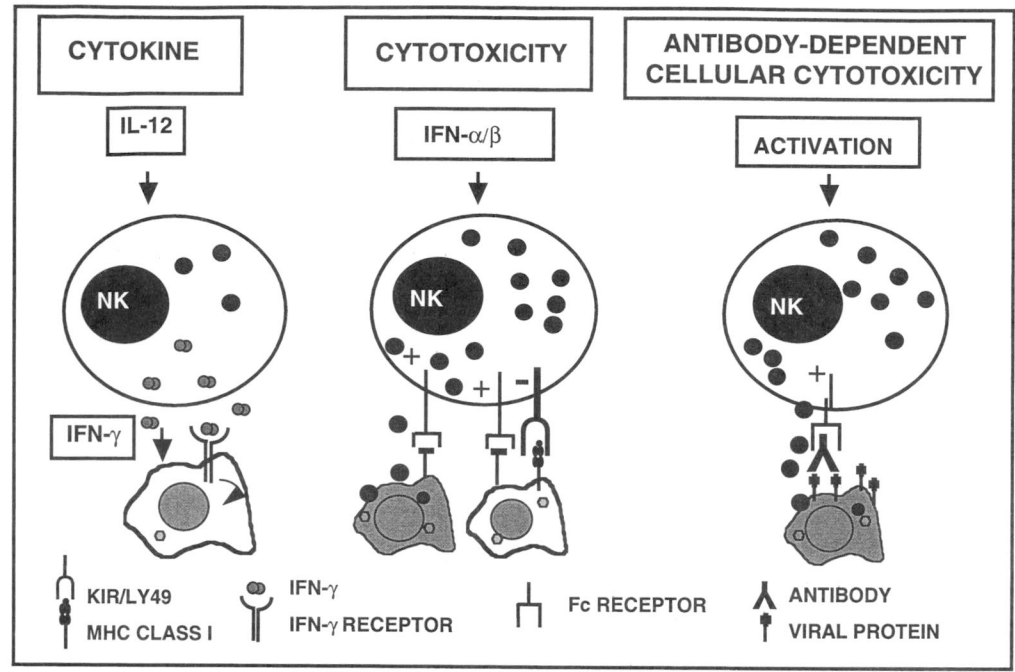

FIG. 8. NK-cell function and regulation during viral infection. NK cells are known to act in three different mechanisms with potentials to contribute to antiviral defense. They can be activated to produce high levels of IFN-γ. The cytokine IL-12 is a particularly good inducer of NK-cell IFN-γ production. NK cells also can be activated by a number of factors to mediate elevated cytotoxicity. In the context of viral infections, IFN-α/β appear to be the major cytokines for inducing cytotoxic activity. Once virus-specific antibodies are induced, NK cells can use their receptors for immunoglobulins to lyse infected target cells through antibody-dependent mechanisms. NK cells are capable of directly lysing cells. MHC class I molecules can deliver negative signals through the KIR/Ly49 molecules on the surfaces of NK cells to inhibit this lysis.

molecules (97–101). Multiple types of NK-cell receptors for the MHC molecules have been identified. In mice, the Ly49 receptors, type II membrane glycoproteins of the C-type lectin superfamily, interact with mouse MHC class I to regulate NK cells. In humans, killing inhibitory receptors (KIRs), type I glycoproteins of the immunoglobulin superfamily, interact with human MHC class I molecules. Both the human and mouse receptors are products of gene clusters with several homologous genes. Individual receptors have ligand specificity for different groups of MHC class I alleles. They are able to deliver negative signals to NK cells through intracellular tyrosine-based inhibitory motifs (ITIMs), which recruit tyrosine phosphatases to cut off proximal positive-signaling pathways (102–104). Although these inhibitory receptors were identified first on NK cells, other cell populations, including certain T-cell subsets, can express the regulatory molecules. In addition, the receptors have the potential to inhibit a number of cellular responses in addition to cytotoxicity, including induction of cytokine production, provided that the negative signals are delivered in the vicinity of the positive signals (105,106). A related human molecule with ITIM sequences and the ability to bind class I, named the *leukocyte immunoglobulin-like receptor* (LIR-1), has been cloned and shown to be expressed primarily on monocytic and B-cell lineage populations (107). Moreover, an additional negative receptor complex, CD94/NKG2A, has been identified on human NK cells and shown to recognize MHC leader sequence peptide presented by the nonclassical MHC molecule, HLA-E (108). Thus, there is a growing list of receptors, which, as a result of interacting with class I MHC molecules, transduce negative signals to regulate immune cell responses, and the best studied of these inhibit NK cell–mediated cytotoxicity.

Many viruses, most notably the herpes group viruses, have evolved strategies to decrease class I expression and avoid recognition by T cells (103,109–113). It is believed that such reduced levels of class I on virus-infected cell surfaces may allow NK cell–mediated lysis, and thus, use of NK cells for defense under conditions of suboptimal T-cell effectiveness. Correlation of the ability to sabotage class I expression and the role for NK cells in defense suggests but does not prove cause and effect during herpes infections. Interestingly, CMVs of the herpes group have genes coding for class I homologues, for example, UL18 in *human CMV* (HCMV) and m144 in MCMV, which may serve as decoys to deliver negative signals and protect virus-infected cells, with blocked class I expression, from immune cell functions, including NK cell-mediated lysis (107,114,115). Although work is needed to definitively prove this mechanism for immune avoidance, it is interesting to note that NK cell surface receptors for class I molecules are organized in known genetic clusters, and certain viral resistance genes have been mapped to one such region in the mouse (116,117). Thus, even though much remains to be learned about the significance of NK cell-positive and -negative receptor signaling for antiviral defense, evidence is accumulating to indicate that these signaling pathways are involved in regulating NK cell-mediated effects in the host.

In addition to lysing target cells, NK cells can produce a variety of cytokines, including IFN-γ, TNF, and granulocyte–macrophage colony stimulating factor (GM-CSF). A potent inducer of NK-cell

IFN-γ production is IL-12 (118–120), and IL-12 is elicited at early times during some, but not all, viral infections (50,51,55–58). In contrast to the NK cell–mediated cytotoxicity driven by IFN-α/β, NK-cell IFN-γ production during infection is IL-12–dependent (57). The role for NK cell–produced IFN-γ in antiviral defense has been established definitively during CMV infections (49). Protection may result from both direct and indirect mechanisms, as the virus is sensitive to either IFN-γ-mediated inhibition of replication (47) or iNOS-dependent pathways (93) thought to be delivered by IFN-γ-activated macrophages (53,121). The antiviral role for NK cell–produced IFN-γ could be more important or more easy to define than the role for NK cell-mediated lysis, because IL-12 can override localized negative signaling at sites of infected cell contact by globally stimulating NK cell surfaces (see Fig. 8), and/or because the IFN-γ pathway can avoid negative signals from infected cells by acting away from the immediate site of production. Consistent with these possibilities are the observations that certain viral infections induce high circulating levels of IL-12 and NK cell–produced IFN-γ (51,57). However, even under these conditions, peak antiviral functions in tissues appear to require proximity of NK cells to infected cells (122). NK cell–produced IFN-γ also has potential to promote important immunoregulatory functions through effects on the expression of cytokines and cytokine receptors (123–125) (see below).

NK cells can use their Fc receptors for antibodies to mediate antibody-dependent cell-mediated cytotoxicity (ADCC) (38). As this defense pathway for antiviral functions requires virus-specific antibody attachment to infected target cells, NK cell-mediated ADCC could only come into play after antibody production at late times after primary, or during secondary, infections. To date, ADCC has been poorly characterized for effectiveness as an *in vivo* antiviral defense mechanism (126,127). Interesting new studies, however, indicate that NK cell-mediated ADCC contributes to the rate of CD4+ T-cell decline during HIV disease (128). Although this observation suggests a pathway by which NK cells mediate or promote pathology, it also provides evidence supporting the delivery of NK cell-mediated ADCC *in vivo*.

Macrophages

Macrophages can play a role in antiviral defense, but a conflicting contribution of these cells to viral spread, as a result of serving as initial hosts for infections, has been appreciated for some time (129–134). In addition, because of the ability of these cells to traffic to a variety of host compartments, including the brain, virus-infected macrophages have been proposed to facilitate viral spread throughout the host (64,135). Interestingly, development of increased resistance to infection with age frequently correlates with increasing resistance of macrophages to viral infections. As examples, macrophages from young mice are more susceptible than those from older mice to infections with a number of viruses, including herpes viruses (136–140), and human neonatal macrophages derived from cord blood are more sensitive than those from adults to infections with different viruses, including HIV (141–143). Thus, under certain conditions, macrophages may promote viral replication and spread.

The role for macrophages in defense against viral infection has been suggested in a number of different systems (144–146). However, it has been difficult to conclusively define their contributions as direct or indirect and to characterize the mechanisms for such

contributions. Macrophages can make the antiviral cytokine TNF-α. However, evidence indicates that macrophages also can mediate resistance against viral infections through the iNOS-dependent pathways that are so effective in destruction of intracellular bacteria. Interestingly, IFN-γ and TNF-α promote macrophage activation during herpes group virus infections, and this can occur through T cell-independent pathways (121). Moreover, iNOS, alternatively identified as NOS2, can be expressed in activated macrophages. Although many of the studies characterizing iNOS induction have been done in the mouse, inflammatory macrophages from humans are known to express iNOS (53,147). NOS enzymes catalyze production of NO, with L-citruline as a second product, through biochemical pathways with NADPH to oxidize and consume L-arginine (53). NO is a lipid- and water-soluble gas, which can react with oxygen and its intermediates to yield a number of other reactive molecules. The iNOS-dependent pathways have been shown to contribute to defense during a range of infections, including those with the DNA viruses, VV, EBV, HSV, and MCMV (53,93,148), and the RNA virus, VSV (53,69). Because of the variety of reactive intermediates and products, NO has the potential to modify a number of downstream target molecules to mediate antiviral activity. Although there still is much to be learned about iNOS-dependent effects, NO has been shown to interrupt VV replication and late protein synthesis by blocking required enzymes and intermediates (149,150) and to promote maintenance of EBV latency by downregulating an intermediate-early transactivator protein (151).

In addition to apparently direct antiviral functions, macrophages can mediate a number of important immunoregulatory effects. These cells are a source of a variety of immunoregulatory cytokines, including IL-12, TNF-α, and IL-1α. Furthermore, they can be important in the processing and presentation of antigen to cells of the adaptive immune system. Thus, macrophages have the ability to promote antiviral immunity, and they are likely to do so through a range of direct and indirect mechanisms.

Chemokines

A growing number of small molecular chemotactic factors, called chemokines, are being characterized (152–154). These factors can be made by a variety of immune and nonimmune cell types, have important proinflammatory functions, and have been shown to be induced during infections with VV, LCMV, mouse hepatitis virus (MHV), and MCMV (122,155–157). The chemokine identified as macrophage inflammatory protein 1α (MIP-1α) contributes to tissue inflammation at times associated with adaptive immunity after infections of mice with influenza or Coxsackie viruses (158). Studies have shown that this chemokine also is important for innate defense. During infections of mice with MCMV, inflammatory foci are at sites of viral replication in livers (Fig. 9A), and NK cells preferentially accumulate at (Fig. 9B), and traffic to (Fig. 9C), these locations. Absence or inhibition of MIP-1α functions blocks these NK-cell inflammatory responses (Fig. 9D) and results in decreased protection at this tissue site (122). Thus, chemokines have immunoregulatory functions and contribute to innate immunity during viral infections by promoting cell trafficking of leukocytes to appropriate sites. However, under specific circumstances, chemokines also may mediate direct antiviral effects by blocking infection (154,159). HIV uses chemokine receptors as coreceptors with CD4 molecules for virus infection

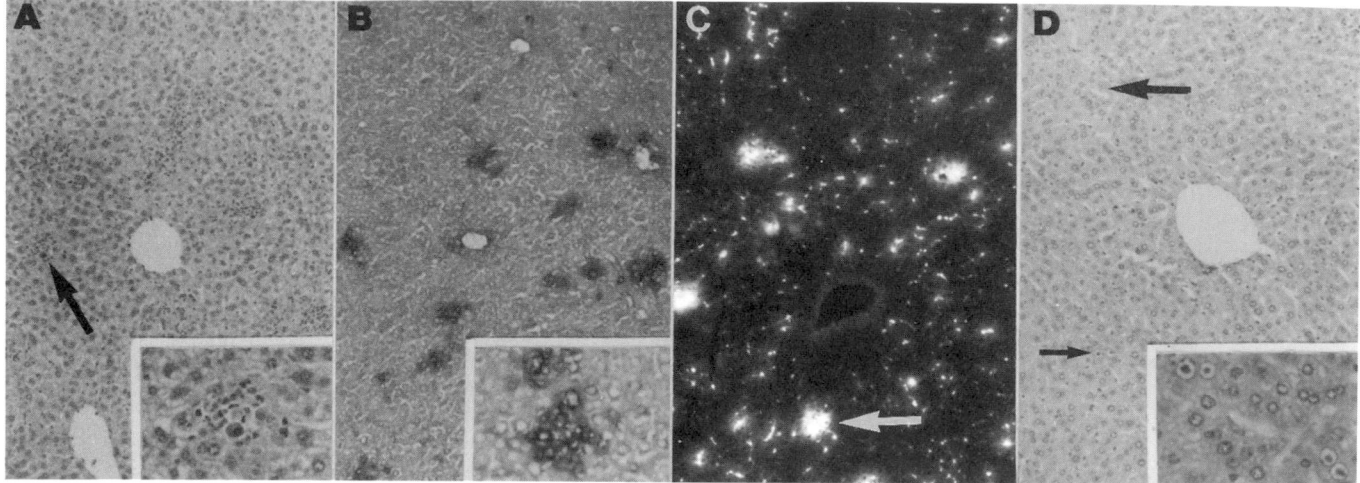

FIG. 9. MIP-1α–dependent NK-cell focal inflammation in livers of MCMV-infected mice. Early focal inflammation is induced by MCMV infection in immunocompetent mice and mice lacking T and B, but not NK, cells. The morphology of H&E-stained liver sections prepared from day-2 MCMV-infected C57BL/6 SCID mice is shown in (**A**). Inflammatory foci are comprised primarily of NK cells. An immunohistochemically stained frozen section, from day-2 MCMV-infected C57BL/6-SCID mice, localizing viral antigen expression relative to NK cells is shown in (**B**). MCMV antigen expression is detected using virus-specific antibody and appears as diffuse light staining, and NK cells are identified by staining for AGM1 marker and appear as dark focal staining. NK cells are induced to traffic to the inflammatory foci during viral infections. Bone marrow leukocytes, harvested from uninfected mice and labeled with the fluorescent dyes, accumulate in livers after intravenous transfer. The focal trafficking and accumulation pattern, induced by MCMV infection and dependent on NK cells in a donor-cell population, is shown in (**C**). This NK-cell inflammation in liver is dependent on MIP-1α. The morphology of H&E-stained liver sections prepared from day-2 MCMV-infected C57BL/6-MIP-1α–deficient mice is shown in (**D**). *Large arrow* in **Panel A** denotes inflammatory foci shown in insert. *Large arrow* in **Panel B** identifies a focal accumulation of trafficking cells. **Panel D:** *Large arrow* denotes cluster of cells shown in insert, having the morphologic characteristics of MCMV-infected cells (i.e., cytomegalic inclusion bodies). (Results are taken from ref. 122. Copyright 1998, by the Rockefeller University Press, 0022-1007/98/01/1/14.)

(154,160,161). The natural chemokine ligands for these specific receptors can block HIV infection (154,159). Although T cells were first shown to be capable of delivering this chemokine-mediated mechanism of protection (159), other cell types, including those contributing to innate immunity, can make chemokines. Thus, innate responses have the potential to deliver these virus receptor blockade–protective effects during HIV infections.

SPECIFIC IMMUNITY

Antibodies and T cells are the two main antigen-specific effector systems for resolving viral infections (20,23,162,163). It is useful to review how these cells control viral infections and to define the critical molecules involved in recognition of viral materials by T cells and antibodies (Table 8). Antibodies can recognize free

TABLE 8. *Antiviral T-cell and B-cell immunity*

Effector system	Recognition molecule	Mechanism of viral control
Antibody	Surface glycoproteins or outer capsid proteins of virus particle	Neutralization of virus
		Opsonization of virus particles
	Viral glycoproteins expressed on membrane of infected cells	Antibody complement-mediated and antibody-dependent cell-mediated cytotoxicity of virus infected cells.
		Downregulation of intracellular viral gene expression
CD4 T cells	Viral peptides (10–20 mers) presented by MHC class II molecules. This could be any viral protein (surface, internal, or nonstructural). Peptides presented by MHC class II molecules usually are derived from exogenous proteins.	Release of antiviral cytokines (IFN-γ, TNF)
		Activation/recruitment of macrophages
		Help for antiviral antibody production
		Help for CD8 CTL responses
		Killing of virus-infected cells?
CD8 T cells	Viral peptides (8–10 mers) presented by MHC class I molecules. This could be any viral protein. Peptides presented by MHC class I are usually derived from endogenous proteins, but evidence suggests that the exogenous pathway is also quite efficient in loading MHC class I molecules.	Killing of virus-infected cells
		Release of antiviral cytokines (IFN-γ, TNF)
		Activation/recruitment of macrophages

virus or virus-infected cells. They control virus infections by neutralizing virus particles and by killing infected cells through complement-mediated cytotoxicity or ADCC. The critical viral proteins recognized in these processes are surface glycoproteins or outer capsid proteins, and although antibodies against internal and nonstructural viral proteins also are made, these do not participate in viral neutralization or antibody-mediated killing of infected cells. Antibody binding to viral glycoproteins at the cell surface also can downregulate the expression of viral genes inside infected cells, but the mechanism by which this effect occurs is not well understood. This interesting phenomenon, first described for measles virus-infected cells in culture (164), also may operate *in vivo* in controlling Sindbis virus infection in neurons (165). Similar observations have been made using antibodies to the surface glycoproteins of rabies virus and Sendai virus (166,167). These studies have also suggested that antibodies can neutralize virus inside the cell (165–167). Thus, antibodies can control viral infections by several different mechanisms, and the critical recognition molecules appear to be viral surface glycoproteins or outer capsid proteins. Changes in the structure or expression of these viral outer capsid or surface glycoproteins could be important mechanisms by which viruses avoid elimination by antibodies. Alterations in other viral proteins (internal and nonstructural) probably are not critical in escape from humoral immunity. However, there are a few reports of antibodies to internal or core proteins playing a role in protection (168).

In contrast to antibodies, which recognize viral proteins by themselves, T cells only see viral antigen in association with host MHC molecules. The antigen-specific TCR recognizes short viral peptides bound to cellular MHC molecules. An important consequence of this mode of recognition is that T cells cannot recognize free virus, and their antiviral activities are confined to infected cells. The T-cell arm of the immune system has evolved for surveillance of infected cells, whereas antibody serves as the primary defense against free virus. T cells are subdivided further into two subsets, CD4 and CD8 T cells. CD4 T cells recognize viral peptides in association with MHC class II antigens, whereas CD8 T cells recognize viral peptides bound to MHC class I antigens. These peptide fragments can be derived from any viral protein, structural (surface or internal) or nonstructural. Thus, all viral proteins are potential targets for T-cell recognition. The limiting factors are intracellular processing of the protein and capability of the peptides to bind to MHC molecules (i.e., their affinity for various MHC molecules). The interaction of virus-specific T cells with virus-infected cells depends on binding of the antigen-specific TCR with the MHC-peptide complex and on several other accessory molecules that increase adherence between T cells and their infected target cells (169). How do T cells control virus infections (Fig. 10)? The primary mechanism used by CD8 T cells is killing of virus-infected cells (92,170–172). CD8 T cells also control virus growth by producing antiviral cytokines such as IFN-γ and TNF, which interfere intracellularly with virus replication (173). CD4 T cells play a central role in antiviral immunity and contribute to viral control in many different ways: They produce antiviral cytokines, are involved in the activation and recruitment of macrophages, and provide cytokine-mediated help for both antibody production and CD8 CTL responses (20,23,174). Virus-specific CD4 CTLs also have been described in several systems, but the contribution of killing per *se* by CD4 T cells in eliminating virus infections *in vivo* is not clear (163,175,176)

Historically, there has been great interest in determining the relative importance of T- versus B-cell immunity in controlling viral infections. This has resulted in much debate and considerable experimentation to assess the role of T- and B-cell responses in viral elimination and in protection from reinfection (20,23,162). When examining this issue, one must remember that antibodies and T cells have evolved to perform entirely different functions. The business of antibodies is to deal with virus particles and that of T cells is to deal with infected cells. In some ways, the argument of which is more important is not a particularly useful one, because

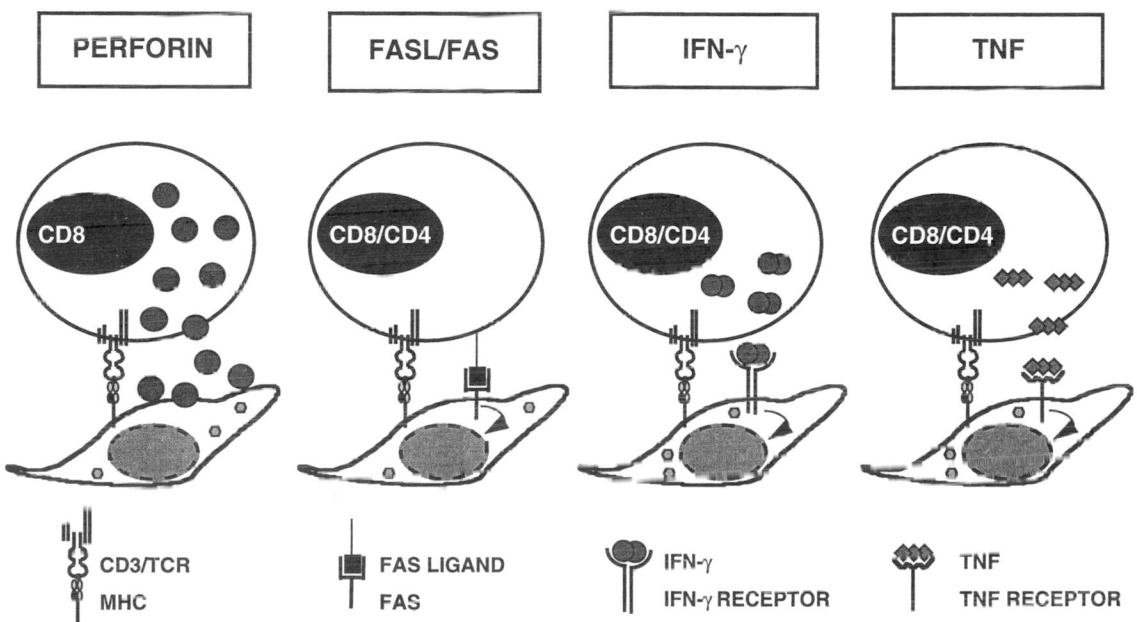

FIG. 10. Effector mechanisms used by T cells to control viral infections.

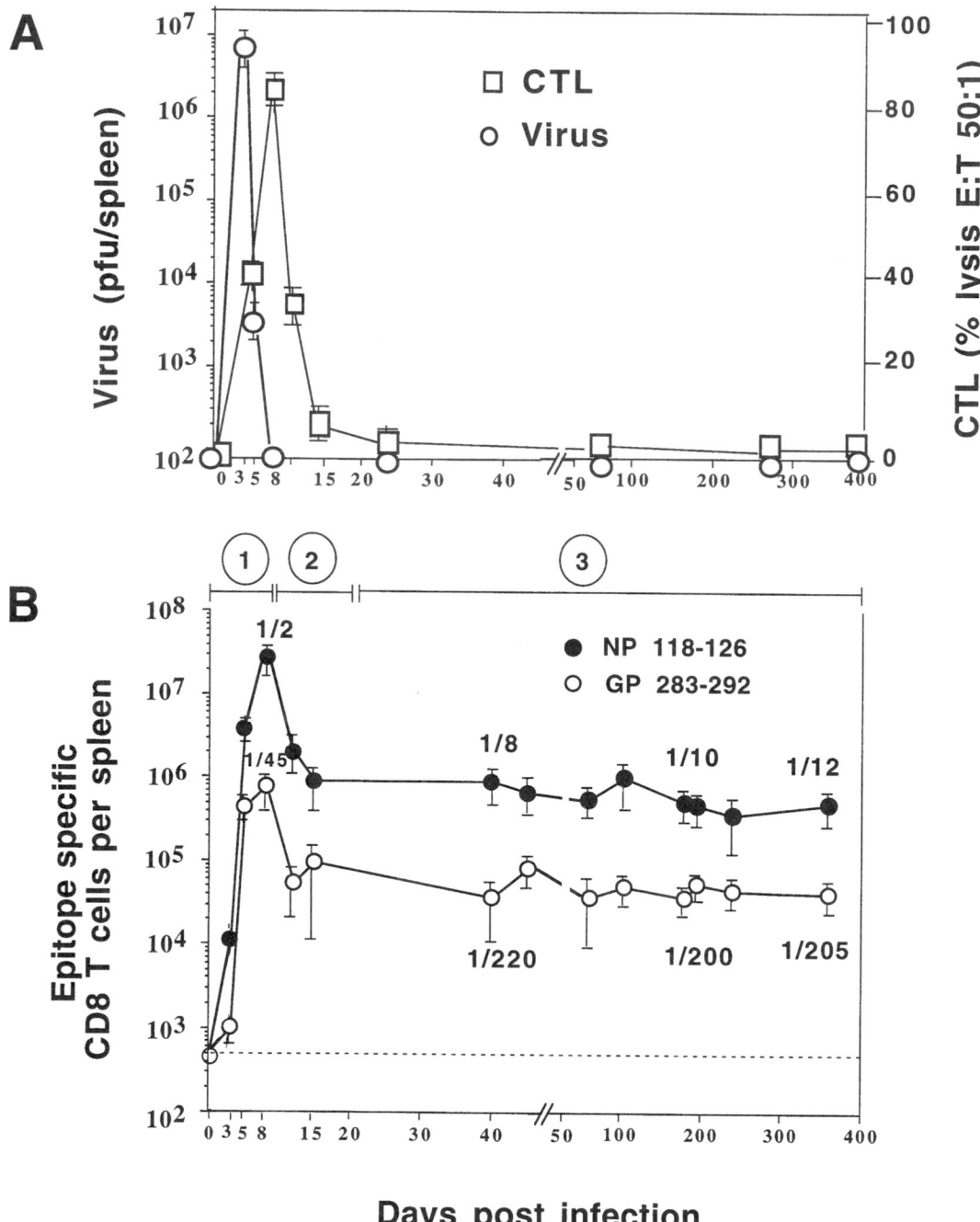

FIG. 11. Kinetics of CTL response, viral clearance, and *in vivo* dynamics of antigen-specific CD8 T cells at different stages after acute viral infection. **A:** BALB/c mice were infected with LCMV, and the virus level and direct *ex vivo* CTL activity in the spleen were analyzed at the indicated time points. **B:** Antigen-specific CD8 T cells against a dominant viral epitope (NP 118-126) and a subdominant epitope (GP 283-292) were quantitated at indicated time points by MHC class I tetramer binding and by assays measuring IFN-γ production at the single-cell level (see Figs. 12 and 13). The frequencies of peptide-specific cells–total CD8 T cells are indicated for each of the epitopes at selected time points. The expansion, death, and memory phases of the CD8 T-cell responses are marked as *1, 2, 3 in circles.* Note that the expansion, death, and formation of memory pool for both dominant and subdominant epitope-specific cells follow similar kinetics. This shows that the size of the memory T cell pool (*phase 3*) is determined by the original burst size (*phase 1*) and emphasizes the importance of initial priming in inducing long-term immunity. (Adapted from ref. 183.)

the two antiviral defense mechanisms perform such distinct functions. Antibodies are our only specific defense against free virus, and T cells are by far the most efficient means of eliminating virus-infected cells.

CD8 T-Cell Responses

Primary CD8 T-cell responses to acute viral infections consist of three distinct phases: (a) activation and expansion, (b) death, and (c) stability or memory (20) (Fig. 11). During the initial phase, which typically lasts about a week, there is antigen-driven expansion of the specific T cells and their differentiation into effector CTLs (i.e., direct *ex vivo* killers). In several viral systems examined, there is between 100-fold and 10,000-fold expansion of virus-specific CD8 T cells (20,23,162). A period of death then ensues (between weeks 1 and 2), when most of the activated T cells undergo apoptosis and effector activity subsides as antigen level declines (20). This contraction of the T-cell response is as dramatic as the expansion, and in most instances, 95% or more of the antigen-specific T cells disappear. This phenomenon, termed *activation-induced cell death* (AICD), serves as a mechanism for regulating cell numbers and maintaining homeostasis. Apoptosis resulting from Fas (CD95)/Fas ligand (FasL) interactions has been implicated in AICD, and a role for TNF in the apoptosis of activated CD8 T cells has also been documented (177–179). The third phase of the T-cell response is characterized by a stable pool of memory cells that can persist for many years (20,180–182). On rechallenge, the same three phases (expansion, death, and stability) are seen once again, but with accelerated kinetics (180,183). In some instances, recall responses, as measured by cytokine production, direct killer activity, and cell proliferation, can be detected as early as 1 to 2 days after reinfection (180,183). This rapid anamnestic response results in faster elimination of virus upon reinfection.

Size of the Virus-specific CD8 T-Cell Response

Viral infections can induce extensive proliferation of CD8 T cells *in vivo* ( ). This is seen in humans during the acute phase of infection with viruses that replicate systemically, such as HIV, EBV, measles, and CMV (184–191). Expansions of CD8 T cells are also seen in experimental models, such as infection of mice with VV, VSV, murine γ herpesvirus, and LCMV (180,183,192–199). There has been considerable interest in determining how much of this expansion represents virus-specific CD8 T cells and how much of it is due to activation of T cells not specific to the immunizing antigen (45,196,200–203). Limiting dilution analysis (LDA) to quantitate virus-specific CTLs has shown that only a small fraction (1% to 5% at most) of the activated CD8 T cells are antigen-specific at the peak of the primary response (20,23,162). This has led to the hypothesis that most of the CD8 T-cell expansion is not antigen specific and represents bystander activation and/or cross-reactive stimulation of non-specific cells (45). However, studies using more sensitive techniques to quantitate antigen-specific CD8 T cells have shown that the size of the antiviral response is considerably larger than the estimates obtained by LDA, and that much of the CD8 T-cell expansion seen during viral infection represents antigen-specific cells (183,205). The most powerful of these new techniques is one using fluorescent labeled tetramers of MHC class I molecules containing the nominal antigenic peptide to stain specific CD8 T cells (Figs. 12 and 13) (183,204). This approach allows direct visualization of antigen-spe-

cific CD8 T cells, and the analysis can be done on freshly explanted cells without any *in vitro* manipulations. Other sensitive new techniques involve measuring cytokine production at the single-cell level by intracellular staining or by ELISPOT assay (183) (see Fig. 13). Studies using these techniques to analyze CD8 T-cell responses during acute LCMV infection of mice have shown that 50% to 70% of the activated CD8 T cells are virus-specific (183,205). This represents a greater than 10,000 fold increase in 8 days, with the peak expansion occurring between days 3 and 5, during which period virus-specific CD8 T cells have an estimated division time of approximately 8 hours. These results document the enormous capacity of CD8 T cells to expand during virus infection.

Why have previous studies underestimated the size of the virus-specific T-cell response? In almost all viral systems examined to date, the LDA has been used to quantitate virus-specific CTL$_p$ (20,23,162). This technique involves plating graded numbers of cells in 96-well plates and stimulating them for 1 to 2 weeks in the presence of antigen plus IL-2. At the end of the culture period, the contents of each well are tested for the presence of antigen-specific killer cells. An important caveat of this widely used assay is that only cells that are capable of dividing and surviving during the 1- to 2-week *in vitro* culture period will score as positive. Several studies have shown that activated T cells are prone to apoptosis upon restimulation with antigen (177). Thus, it is likely that many antigen-specific T cells either die or do not divide to a sufficient extent to score as positive in the LDA assay. In contrast, techniques using MHC class I tetramers and the cytokine assays do not have this limitation. This is especially true of staining with MHC class I tetramers, a method that involves no *in vitro* manipulations and allows direct visualization of the antigen-specific T cells. Also, the cytokine functional assays require only a short period of *in vitro* stimulation (5 hours for intracellular stain and 24 to 36 hours for ELISPOT), and neither technique is dependent on long-term cell survival or proliferation.

It will be interesting to see if findings from the LCMV model can be generalized to other viral infections, including those by

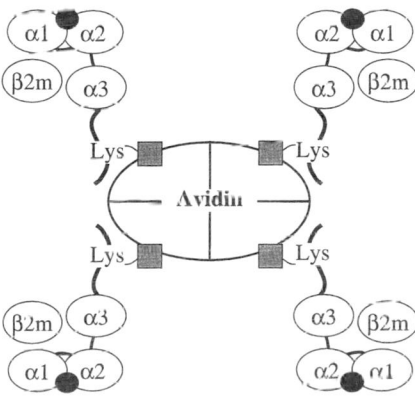

FIG. 12. Tetrameric MHC molecules have high avidity for antigen-specific T cells. The soluble domains of a class I MHC molecule are enzymatically biotinylated on a BirA substrate peptide fused to the carboxy-terminal end of the α3 domain. Singly biotinylated MHC molecules containing the nominal antigenic peptide are mixed with fluorescently labeled streptavidin at a 4:1 molar ratio to form MHC tetramers, which are used for identification of antigen-specific T cells by flow cytometry (183,204).

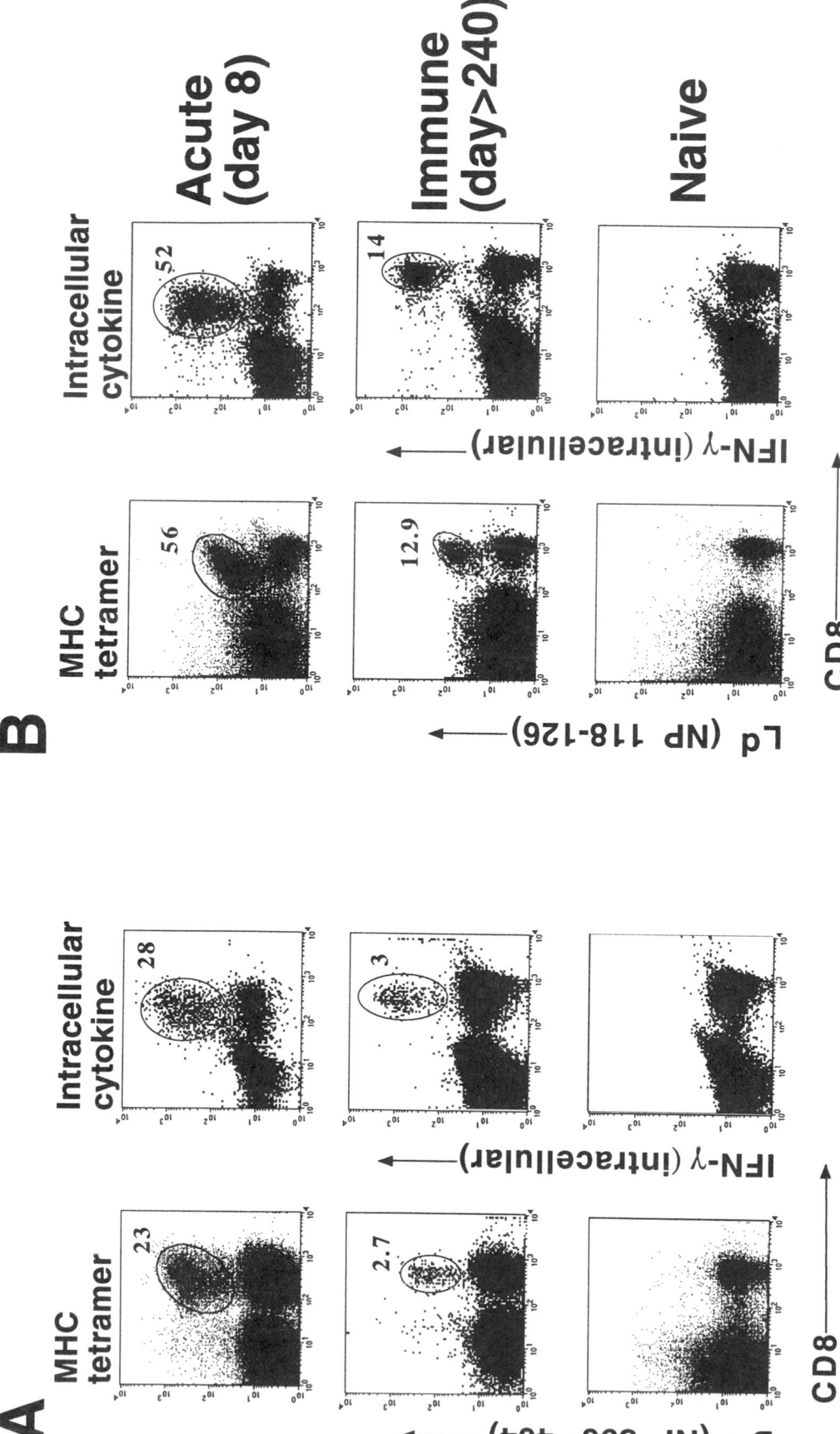

FIG. 13. Quantitation and visualization of antigen-specific CD8 T cells during primary and memory phases after acute virus infection. C57BL/6 (**A**) and BALB/c (**B**) mice were infected with LCMV, and spleen cells were checked for antigen-specific CD8 T cells at acute (day 8) and memory (after day 240) phases after infection. As a control, cells from naive mice were used. Antigen-specific CD8 T cells were visualized either by staining freshly explanted spleen cells with tetramers of MHC class I molecules containing the nominal antigenic peptide (D^b-restricted LCMV NP 396-404 peptide in the case of C57BL/6 and L^d-restricted NP 118-126 in the case of BALB/c) or by intracellular IFN-γ stain. Intracellular IFN-γ stain was done after culturing the spleen cells *in vitro* for 5 hours with NP 396-404 (**A**) or NP 118-126 (**B**). Numbers represent the percentage of CD8 T cells that are antigen-specific. Note that both techniques (tetramer binding and intracellular IFN-γ stain) give similar frequencies of antigen-specific CD8 T cells. (Adapted from ref. 183.)

human pathogens. In this context, it is worth noting that it has been known for many years that acute EBV infection (infectious mononucleosis) is characterized by a massive increase in the number of CD8 T cells (187), and more recently it has also been shown that substantial CD8 T-cell expansion occurs during primary HIV infection (184,185). Increased numbers of activated CD8 T cells in the blood and cerebrospinal fluid of patients infected with human T-cell leukemia virus-1 (HTLV-1) have also been reported (206). It is possible that the majority of the expanded CD8 T cells are EBV-, HTLV-1, and HIV-specific. In fact, studies analyzing TCR usage by CD8 T cells during acute EBV and HIV infections have shown expansions of a few dominant clones (185,187). Such oligoclonal populations are most consistent with antigen-driven expansion of T cells. It will be of interest to see what frequencies are obtained in these human viral infections employing the sensitive techniques used in the LCMV study. Even with viral infections that provide a much weaker stimulus to CD8 T cells, such as HSV, it is possible that most of the responding cells are virus-specific. A study (207) analyzing CD8 T-cell responses in lymph nodes draining the site of HSV infection has documented expansion of CD8 T cells expressing a restricted TCR, suggesting that a large proportion of the blasting cells may be HSV-specific. Thus, it is likely that findings from the LCMV system, showing that most of the proliferating CD8 T cells are virus-specific, will be a paradigm for viral infections in general.

CD8 T-Cell Epitopes

A large number of epitopes have been identified in several different viral systems (208–212). The search for these epitopes has been greatly facilitated by identification of allele-specific sequence motifs for MHC-binding peptides for several murine and human class I molecules (213–216). The class I motifs usually consist of two or three conserved anchor residues and comprise between eight and 11 amino acids. Using these allele-specific sequence motifs, it is possible to predict which peptides of a viral protein have the capacity to bind to an MHC class I molecule. However, it should be noted that only a minority of motif-fitting peptides is immunogenic. Although a protein may contain multiple motif-fitting peptides, CTL responses are usually directed against a limited number of epitopes (211,217,223). There are several factors that determine whether a T-cell response is actually made against a potential epitope. First, not all motif-containing peptides bind MHC class I, and those that do bind do so with a wide range of binding affinities. This is presumably due to the existence of

secondary anchor residues and other secondary effects. Second, intracellular processing of peptides determines whether a particular peptide will be presented at the cell surface and at what level (210,218–222). Finally, holes in the T-cell repertoire may restrict CTL responses. As a result of these limitations, only about 10% of motif-containing peptides end up being CTL epitopes during a viral infection (211,223). An example of this is illustrated in Table 9. The LCMV nucleoprotein and glycoprotein contain a total of 88 motif-fitting peptides for the murine MHC class I molecules D^b, K^b, D^d, and K^d. Out of these 88 peptides, 29 (32%) bind the respective MHC molecule and only eight (9%) are actually recognized as epitopes during LCMV infection. It is interesting to examine the relationship between binding affinity and the likelihood of being a CD8 T-cell epitope. None (0/14) of the low-affinity binders are epitopes, whereas six of ten of the intermediate binders and two of five of the high-affinity binders are epitopes. Thus, among the peptides that have good affinity for MHC molecules, approximately 50% end up being actual CTL epitopes.

CD8 T-Cell Effector Mechanisms

A major function of virus-specific CD8 T cells is to kill infected cells. CTLs can kill their targets by two distinct mechanisms: (a) a secretory and membranolytic pathway involving perforin and granzymes and (b) a nonsecretory receptor-mediated pathway involving Fas (CD95) (170,224,225). Alternative mechanisms of killing, such as cytotoxicity mediated by TNF and secreted adenosinel triphosphate, have also been postulated, but there is now a general consensus that perforin- and Fas-mediated pathways are the two major killing mechanisms used by CTL (226–229). Perforin, a 65-kDa protein with sequence homology to complement components C6–C9, is stored in cytoplasmic granules of CTL and plays a major role in the secretory pathway. Upon binding of CTL to the target cell and appropriate engagement of the TCR, the cytoplasmic granules containing perforin and granzymes (serine proteases) are released vectorially onto the target cell. Perforin monomers assemble into polymeric pore structures that insert into target-cell plasma membranes, making the membrane permeable to water and small ions. This "hole punching", along with the effects of granzymes, eventually leads to apoptotic death of the target cell (170,225,226,230,231). Studies with perforin-deficient mice have shown that perforin-mediated cytotoxicity is essential for controlling LCMV infection in vivo (92,172). These studies have clearly established that, at least in this system, killing per se is critical in controlling the infection and that perforin-mediated cytotoxicity is

TABLE 9. *Predictive value of MHC class I allele specific motifs and binding affinity in identifying CD8 T-cell epitopes during viral infection*

MHC class I allele	Total number of motif-fitting peptides in LCMV glycoprotein and nucleoprotein	Number of MHC class I binders[a]			Number of CTL epitopes during LCMV infection (% of total motif-fitting peptides)
		High $IC_{50} < 50$ nM	Intermediate IC_{50} 50–500	Low IC_{50} 500–5,000	
D^b	26	2 (2)[b]	3 (2)	3 (0)	4 (15)
K^b	28	2 (0)	4 (2)	6 (0)	2 (7)
D^d	18	0	0	3 (0)	0 (0)
K^d	16	1 (0)	4 (2)	2 (0)	2 (12)
Total	88	5 (2)	11 (6)	14 (0)	8 (9)

[a]Peptides are distributed among high-, intermediate-, and low-affinity binders for MHC class I molecules.
[b]Numbers in parentheses indicate CTL epitopes during LCMV infection.
Adapted from refs. 211, 223.

the dominant killing pathway *in vivo*. A role for perforin has also been suggested in regulating *Listeria monocytogenes* infection and in eliminating certain tumors (92,225).

Similar to the perforin pathway, the Fas-dependent pathway is initiated by engagement of the TCR by appropriate antigen (177,179,232,233). This interaction results in upregulation of FasL expression on the T cell. Binding and cross-linking of FasL with Fas molecules expressed on the target cells leads to apoptosis of Fas-positive cells. A death-inducing cytoplasmic domain of the Fas protein triggers an intracellular apoptotic program in the target cells involving IL-1β–converting enzyme (ICE) and/or other ICE-related proteases (234,235). One study has implicated Fas-mediated killing in controlling HBV infection in a transgenic mouse model (236,237). However, it is worth noting that mice deficient in Fas (lpr mice) or FasL (gld mice) do not exhibit enhanced susceptibility to viruses. Moreover, Fas is only expressed on certain cell types (hepatocytes, activated T cells, etc.), and it is therefore unlikely that Fas-mediated killing can be a major effector mechanism *in vivo* when a large number of cells and tissues do not express this molecule and cannot be killed by this mechanism. Such a limitation does not apply to the perforin pathway. It is likely that the primary function of Fas-mediated killing is in immune regulation and maintaining homeostasis and not as an effector mechanism (172,177,179,225,232,233).

In addition to killing infected cells, CD8 T cells also secrete several antiviral cytokines (173,188,238,239). The best characterized of these cytokines are IFN-γ and TNF (173). (See the section on innate immunity for a discussion of how cytokines regulate virus growth). Several studies have documented the importance of IFN-γ in controlling virus infections, and the most extensive and mechanistic analysis has been done in the HBV transgenic mouse model (238). What are the relative contributions of killing versus cytokine-mediated effects in controlling virus infection? Killing is likely to be of importance in eliminating noncytolytic viruses. Such viruses, best exemplified by LCMV and HBV, can replicate and produce infectious progeny without killing the cell. Thus, killing *per se* is the most efficient mechanism of getting rid of infected cells. Cytokines, acting by themselves, can inhibit viral growth but are unlikely to clear infections by noncytolytic viruses. In contrast, cytolytic viruses (i.e., vaccinia, polio, VSV, etc.) kill the cell they grow in and in this way eliminate their own factories. Continued virus propagation then becomes dependent on infecting new cells. In such a setting, cytokines can be of critical importance. IFN-γ can induce an antiviral state and make cells resistant to virus infection. Thus, with cytolytic viruses, cytokines acting alone can eliminate the infection. However, these generalizations should be taken with caution, and the most likely scenario is that both T cell-mediated killing and cytokine effects are important in virus infections. Even with cytolytic viruses, killing of an infected cell by CTL during the initial stages of the virus life cycle will reduce the viral burst size and help in controlling the infection. Similarly, with noncytolytic viruses, cytokines do play a role in the overall regulation of virus infection (173,188,238,239). Thus, in summary, both mechanisms are important, but, for cytolytic viruses, the dominant T-cell effector mechanism is cytokines, whereas, for noncytolytic viruses, the dominant mechanism is killing.

CD4 T-Cell Responses

CD4 T cells are of central importance in viral immunity. They are necessary for optimal antibody and CD8 T-cell responses and can act as effectors themselves by producing antiviral cytokines such as IFN-γ and TNF (163,173,239,241,242). CD4 deficiency has profound consequences on the ability to control viral infections. This has been shown in several experimental systems using CD4 or MHC class II–deficient mice (163,242–245) and is most dramatically illustrated in humans with AIDS, in which CD4 dysfunction is associated with increased susceptibility to viral infections (185,246,247).

An important role of CD4 T cells in virus infections is to provide help for clonal expansion and differentiation of virus-specific B cells. Although some virus-specific antibody responses are T-independent (20), in general, antibody responses are severely compromised in the absence of CD4 T cells (174,248,249). This can result in enhanced susceptibility to viruses such as influenza, Sendai, and VSV (163,250). The CD4 response in viral infections is often dominated by a Th1-type profile, characterized by IFN-γ and IL-2 production, which leads to a prominent IgG2a response (163). However, it should be noted that Th2-type responses, characterized by IL-4, and IL-5 secretion are also seen during virus infections (251,252). Thus, unlike some parasitic infections that show highly polarized Th1 or Th2 responses, viral infections appear to have a "mixed" response (236,253–255).

The requirement of CD4 T-cell help in the induction of CD8 T-cell responses has been found to vary depending on the viral system. CTL responses to viruses such as LCMV and ectromelia, which provide a strong stimulus to CD8 T cells, are relatively CD4-independent (174,248,256). CD4-deficient mice infected with LCMV generate a CTL response that is about twofold lower in precursor frequency than the response of normal mice, but it is still potent enough to resolve the acute LCMV infection (174,248). In contrast, CTL responses to VSV, influenza virus, and HSV are much more CD4-dependent. The precise reasons why some virus-specific CD8 responses are CD4-dependent and others less so are not known. One possibility is that viruses such as LCMV and ectromelia activate such a large number of CD8 T cells that some of these CD8 T cells can provide the necessary cytokines for expansion and differentiation of CTLs. On the other hand, influenza virus and HSV are known to activate fewer CD8 T cells and may therefore be more dependent on CD4 help. It has also been suggested that antigen density per cell can determine whether CD8 activation requires CD4 help (259,260). An LCMV- or ectromelia virus–infected antigen-presenting cell (APC) contains a large number of viral peptide–MHC complexes and will engage many TCRs of the CD8 T cell, rendering the activation of these cells less dependent on CD4 T cells and also on costimulatory signals. However, viruses that do not replicate efficiently in APCs will engage fewer TCRs on the CD8 T cell, making the responses more dependent on CD4 T cells and/or costimulation.

Although CD4 help is dispensible for induction of CTL responses during some acute viral infections, there is now a general consensus that CD4 T cells are essential for sustaining CD8 T-cell responses during chronic viral infections (174,249,257,258). This critical observation, initially made with studies on LCMV and Moloney murine leukemia virus, has been extended to other viral systems, including HIV infection of humans (257,258). It has been shown that even in the presence of an overwhelming infection of the immune system, CD8 T cells can remain active for long periods and eventually resolve and/or keep the virus infection in check. In contrast, CD8 T-cell responses are rapidly lost under conditions of CD4 deficiency, and there is no control of virus infection (Fig. 14) (174,197,257). How do CD4 T cells sustain CD8 T-cell

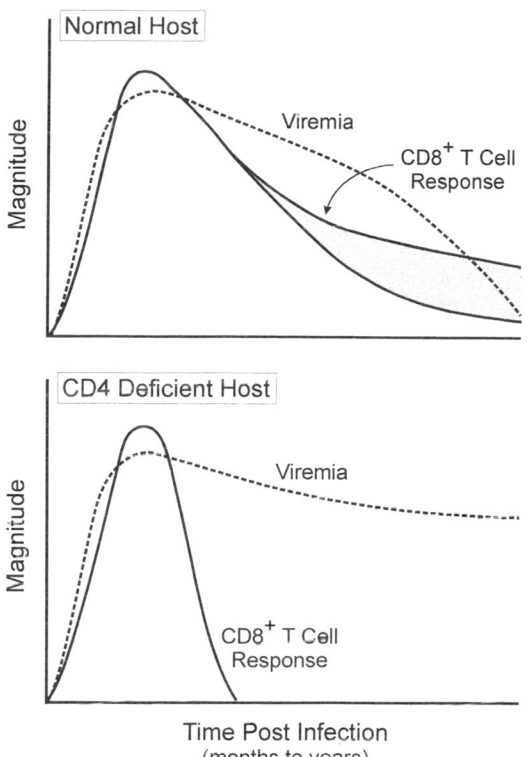

Normal Host

Magnitude

Viremia

CD8⁺ T Cell Response

CD4 Deficient Host

Magnitude

Viremia

CD8⁺ T Cell Response

Time Post Infection
(months to years)

FIG. 14. CD4 T cells are necessary to maintain CD8 T-cell responses during chronic viral infection. (Adapted from ref. 174.)

responses under conditions of a chronic stimulus? One possibility is that CD4 T cells make cytokines, such as IL-2, that are necessary for survival of CD8 T cells. It is known that cytokine deprivation can result in apoptosis of activated T cells (261). Alternatively, through direct cell-to-cell interaction with APCs, CD4 T cells may increase expression of costimulatory molecules, such as B7-1 and B7-2, on APCs. Because CD8 T cells also interact directly with APCs, upregulation of these critical costimulatory molecules by CD4 T cells may be essential in prevention of CTL "exhaustion" under conditions of chronic stimulation (174,262,263).

Despite the enormous importance of CD4 T cells in viral infections, very few quantitative studies have been done to analyze the kinetics and longevity of virus-specific CD4 T-cell responses (264). Some quantitation of CD4 T-cell precursors has been performed following acute infection of mice with Sendai virus and influenza virus (265,266). These studies suggest that the burst size of the antiviral CD4 response is not as large as the CD8 response, but the overall pattern of the two responses is similar (265). The CD4 response exhibits the same three phases as the CD8 response: (a) the activation and expansion phase during the first week of infection, (b) a death phase during the second week following viral clearance, and (c) a memory phase that lasts for an extended period.

B-Cell Responses

Virus-specific antibody plays a major role in preventing reinfection and in controlling the extent of viral spread. If neutralizing antibody is present at sufficiently high concentration at the site of viral entry (i.e., IgA antibody at mucosal surfaces), then the virus infection can be stopped cold in its tracks. However, even if this is not possible, IgG antibody in the serum can limit viral spread within the body and prevent disease. An example of this is illustrated by the inactivated polio virus (Salk) vaccine (1). The inactivated vaccine induces high levels of polio virus–specific IgG in the serum, but little or no IgA in the gut (the site of entry for polio virus). In this instance, polio virus infects the gut, but its hematogenic spread to the CNS and poliomyelitis are prevented by serum antibody. In addition to their importance in preventing infection and/or disease upon reinfection, antibody responses can also be crucial in recovery from primary infection (250,265–269).

During a virus infection, antibodies are generated against many viral proteins. The most critical of these are those directed against the viral surface proteins. However, not all antibodies that bind to viral surface glycoproteins can neutralize virus infectivity. In fact, in some instances, most of the antibody produced is nonneutralizing; this is seen in antibody responses to HIV gp120 (270,271). Only antibodies that prevent binding of the virus to the cellular receptor and/or prevent penetration and uncoating of the virus are able to block infection. It is worth noting that virus neutralization *in vitro,* as measured by inhibition of plaque formation or cytopathic effect on cell lines, does not always correlate well with protection *in vivo* (239,268,272). Complement can act in concert with antibody to enhance virus neutralization. Binding of complement to virus–antibody complexes can result in enhanced uptake and subsequent degradation of virus particles by phagocytic cells. Also, antibody plus complement can directly lyse enveloped viruses. Paradoxically, in some instances, antibodies can actually enhance virus infectivity. This phenomenon has been documented with several viruses, including Dengue, RSV, and HIV (273–276). The precise mechanism of this antibody-mediated enhancement is not known, but the working model is that antibody–virus complexes can now infect macrophages and other cell types via Fc or complement receptors, thereby broadening their host range.

Some virus-specific antibody responses are T-independent, but most responses that switch from IgM to IgG are T-dependent (277,278). The IgG subclass is determined by the cytokines produced, and virus infections tend to induce IgG2a antibody responses, reflecting the influence of IFN-γ (279–281). The majority of serum antibody is produced by terminally differentiated plasma cells. These nondividing cells differ from memory B cells in many respects. For instance, plasma cells downregulate surface expression of many typical B-cell markers, including major MHC class II and surface immunoglobulin (282,283). These changes indicate that, unlike memory B cells, mature plasma cells are unlikely to participate in antigen processing and presentation. Instead, the main function of a plasma cell is to continuously secrete large quantities of specific antibody. Plasma-cell secretion rates have been estimated to be as high as 5,000 molecules per second (284,285). In contrast, memory B cells do not spontaneously secrete antibody; rather, following appropriate stimulation, these cells proliferate and differentiate into antibody-secreting cells (ASCs). Because protection against viral infection often relies on the level of preexisting antibody in the serum or mucosal surfaces, the number and specificity of preexisting plasma cells are critical components of protective immunity.

The kinetics and anatomic location of antibody production after an acute viral infection are shown in Fig. 15. The IgM response is transient, but the serum IgG response is long-lived and can persist for many years (Table 10). Antibody is initially produced by ASCs

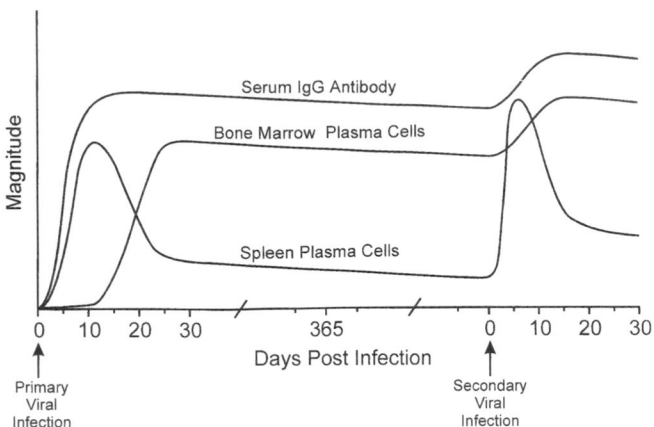

FIG. 15. Kinetics and anatomic site of antibody production after acute viral infection. Initial antibody production is by plasma cells within germinal centers in the spleen and lymph nodes, but after resolving the viral infection, the bone marrow becomes the site of long-term antibody production. After secondary viral infection, the spleen mounts a rapid but transient antibody response, and after returning to homeostasis, the bone marrow is again the predominant source of virus-specific plasma cells. (Adapted from ref. 287)

occur in the spleen and lymph nodes, because most of the memory B cells reside in these organs. After secondary viral infection, the memory B cells in spleen and lymph nodes proliferate and/or differentiate into plasma cells, resulting in a transient increase in the number of ASCs in the spleen. However, once the secondary infection is cleared, this response subsides, and, once again, the bone marrow becomes the predominant site of antibody production. It is worth noting the anatomic segregation between virus-specific plasma cells (reside mostly in the bone marrow) and virus-specific memory B cells that are found predominantly in spleen and lymph nodes after viral infection has been resolved and homeostasis is reestablished. One way of looking at this is to consider the spleen and lymph nodes as "factories" where B-cell differentiation into plasma cells occurs, and the bone marrow as the storehouse where the products (i.e., plasma cells) are kept. It makes sense that the B cells should reside in the vicinity of the factories so they can be quickly mobilized into action as the need arises, and that the plasma cells are shipped out to the bone marrow to make room in the factory. Plasma cells residing in the bone marrow go on with their business of making antibodies, which end up in the blood and can protect against reinfection.

in germinal centers in the spleen and draining lymph nodes. The antibody response in these organs peaks during the first 2 weeks and then declines within 2 to 4 weeks after infection. The decline in plasma cells appears to be due to selection for higher affinity plasma cells and apoptotic loss of low-affinity cells. As splenic plasma-cell populations decline, antigen-specific plasma cells begin to migrate and/or accumulate in the bone marrow compartment. After the germinal center reaction subsides, the bone marrow becomes the predominant site of antibody production, with 80% to 90% of the host's plasma cells located in this anatomic compartment (198,286). Plasma-cell longevity studies have indicated that the initial antibody response is due to short-lived plasma cells, whereas long-term antibody is maintained by long-lived plasma cells (287,288). Upon reinfection, antibody responses once again

REGULATION OF IMMUNE RESPONSES

Immune responses to infections are activated, shaped, and regulated by complex cytokine and cellular interactions. In the context of primary infections, innate responses act on cell populations, with limited diversity and requirements for proliferation, to mediate or promote effector functions. In contrast, the adaptive responses of T- and B-cell populations require engagement of antigen-specific receptors and conditions supporting extensive expansion of low-frequency cells, as well as development of different effector functions. Both innate and adaptive responses must be tightly regulated to achieve the balance required to promote particular protective effector mechanisms and to protect the host from detrimental consequences resulting from "too much of a good thing." Much progress has been made toward understanding regulation of immune responses in the context of nonviral infections

TABLE 10. *Humoral response to acute viral infection in humans*

Example	Serum antibody (yr)	Mucosal antibody[a] (mo)	Ref.
Systemic infections			
Dengue	32		439
Yellow fever	75		440
Measles	65		441
Mumps	12		442
Polio	40		443
Hepatitis A	25		444
Smallpox	40		445
Vaccinia	15		446
Rubella	14		447
Mucosal infections			
Coronavirus		12	448
Influenza virus		30	449
Respiratory syncytial virus		3	450
Rotavirus		12	451, 452

[a]The duration of the secretory antibody response of the respiratory or gastrointestinal tract is shown. The duration of the serum antibody response after a single infection is difficult to determine because of the high frequency of reinfection by this group of viruses.

with intracellular bacteria, such as *Listeria monocytogenes,* or protozoan parasites, such as *Leishmania major* and *Toxoplasma gondii,* as well as with extracellular parasites, such as nematodes (118,120). In general, defense against the nonviral intracellular pathogens is mediated by cytokines activating macrophages. Antigens from such organisms are primarily presented by MHC class II molecules, and protective responses depend on development of Th1 CD4 T cells producing IFN-γ. Failure to elicit these responses and/or substitution with development of Th2 CD4 T cells producing IL-4 and IL-5 renders the host more susceptible to infection and/or to infection-induced disease. If the intracellular organisms have protein products accessing MHC class I presentation pathways, a CD8 T-cell contribution to protection can sometimes be demonstrated. With extracellular parasites, development of Th2 CD4 T cells producing IL-4 and IL-5 can promote defense. The IL-5 response can elicit production and recruitment of eosinophils. Shaping of endogenous T-cell responses to these agents appears to be controlled by certain innate cytokine responses. In particular, early IL-12 expression and IL-12–induced NK-cell IFN-γ production are known to promote CD4 Th1-type responses (289,290).

Interesting studies indicate that this, at least in part, can be the result of IFN-γ–mediated facilitation of IL-12 receptor expression on Th1 cells to allow their preferential expansion in the presence of IL-12 (125).

Although immune responses to viruses include an assortment of those also observed during infections with other organisms, they often have components unique to, and/or uniquely dominant during, viral infections. As described above, these include high circulating levels of IFN-α/β and IFN-α/β-mediated effects. Moreover, because many viral protein products are readily available for processing and presentation by MHC class I molecules, CD8 T cells can have dramatic responses and play prominent roles during viral infections. This section reviews the known major innate and adaptive immunoregulatory pathways in place during viral infections. Emphasis is placed on regulation of acute primary responses to infections and the cytokine effects not discussed earlier in the chapter. A schematic representation of the players and their effects is given in Fig. 16. It is important to recall, however, that just as different viruses do not fit clearly into idealized patterns of infections, host responses adapt to the different conditions in attempts to acti-

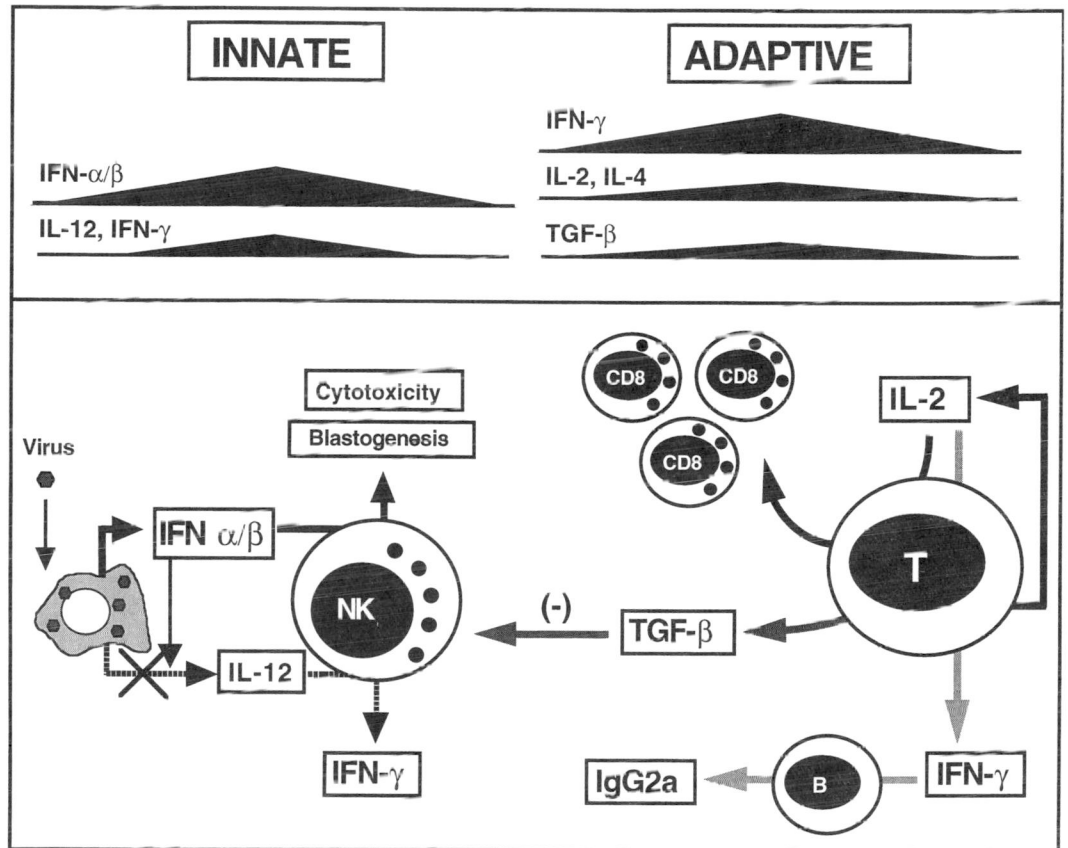

FIG. 16. Regulation of immune responses to viral infections. Early, after many viral infections, IFN-α/β is induced to activate NK cell–mediated cytotoxicity and blastogenesis. Some, but not all, viral infections also elicit detectable IL-12 and NK-cell IFN-γ production. IFN-α/β inhibits IL-12 expression. These are major constituents of innate responses to viral infections. Adaptive responses to viral infections include CD4 T-, CD8 T-, and B-cell activation, with induction of T-cell CTL function and B-cell antibody production. Major T-cell cytokine responses associated with virus-elicited adaptive immunity are IFN-γ, IL-2, and IL-4 expression. The IFN-γ response is the most easily detectable and plays a role in skewing virus-specific antibody responses to the IgG2a isotype. Both the IL-2 and IL-4 responses have demonstrable immunoregulatory functions. IL-2 is particularly important for supporting CD8 T-cell proliferation. The activation of T-cell responses also can facilitate the production of biologically active TGF-β, and this response appears to contribute to the negative regulation of NK-cell responses.

vate better or more appropriate defense mechanisms. Thus, many different variations can arise.

Innate Responses

Innate responses are both mediators and recipients of immunoregulatory pathways. They (a) active and mediate early defense, (b) have the potential to promote particular protective adaptive immune responses, and (c) receive negative regulation.

Interferons a and b and Interleukin-12

The IFN-α/β cytokines have the potential to mediate a broad range of immunoregulatory functions, affecting both innate and adaptive responses. In contrast, although the importance for innate expression of early IL-12 and IL-12–induced NK-cell IFN-γ in shaping protective Th1 responses to intracellular bacteria and protozoan parasites has been established, the pathway's contribution to promoting protective T-cell responses to viral infections is less clear. In the context of viral infections, IFN-α/β can become dominant for induction of NK cell–mediated cytotoxicity (38,50,57,75,83). Some, but not all, viruses induce IL-12 protein, and NK-cell IFN-γ production during viral infection is dependent on this response (57). However, the downstream effects on T-cell responses mediated by early IL-12 and IFN-γ have yet to be defined. Interestingly, LCMV infections induce dramatic CD8 T-cell responses but fail to elicit detectable IL-12 protein expression (39,57). Moreover, the T-cell responses during this infection, including IFN-γ production, are not inhibited by IL-12 neutralization (57). Thus, there must be other pathways in place to promote a variety of T-cell responses during viral infections.

In addition to the inability to demonstrate expression and function, there are other indications that IL-12 can be detrimental to antiviral T-cell responses, and that components of innate immune responses to viral infection can act to negatively regulate IL-12 expression. IL-12 administration during LCMV infection interferes with, and is toxic for, CD8 T-cell expansion and induction of CTL function (291,292). This results, in part, from synergism for enhanced induction of multiple cytokines, including TNF, between IL-12 and virus-induced IL-2, and a sensitivity of responding CD8 T cells to TNF-mediated effects (292). Interestingly, a virus inducing more modest T-cell responses, MCMV, does induce high early IL-12 expression (57). These observations suggest that it may be particularly important to regulate IL-12 expression during viral infections eliciting CD8 T-cell responses. Indeed, although IFN-α can facilitate IL-12 receptor expression and act to enhance Th1-type responses (40,41,293), IFN-α and IFN-β concentrations equivalent to those observed in serum during viral infections inhibit IL-12 expression (39). Thus, innate immune responses to viral infections include induction of cytokines with the potential to negatively regulate IL-12 and IL-12–dependent effects.

The mechanisms by which adaptive responses to viral infections are regulated are not completely understood, and it is not clear how innate immune responses set up conditions to selectively expand and develop protective CD8 T-cell responses. Effects could be mediated at a number of different levels, including induction of relevant enhancing cytokine expression, protection of cells against inhibitory mechanisms, activation of appropriate T-cell subsets for responsiveness to particular enhancing cytokines, and/or inhibition of inappropriate T-cell responses. As IFN-α/β can enhance antigen processing and presentation through the class I pathway (42), these cytokines presumably promote CD8 T-cell responses by facilitating stimulation through their T-cell receptors for antigen. However, endogenous expression of these cytokines also has been shown to result in conditions promoting limited blastogenesis and expansion of specific lymphocyte subsets, including NK cells (43,44,294) and memory T cells (45). As IFN-α/β are not growth factors in and of themselves, intermediaries in the *in vivo* proliferative responses induced by these cytokines need to be identified.

Negative Regulation of Natural Killer-Cell Responses

In contrast to the known role for T-cell IFN-γ production in activation of macrophages, adaptive immune responses to viral infections appear to preferentially induce and/or result in a number of immunoregulatory pathways turning off NK-cell responses. Certain of these pathways induce cells consuming cytokines with potential to enhance NK-cell responses. For example, although IL-2 can activate and support proliferation of NK cells during acute viral infections, the cytokine is expressed at times subsequent to peak NK-cell responses (295). Moreover, most NK cells express the low-affinity IL-2 receptor, whereas activated T cells express the high-affinity receptor containing the IL-2 α chain (294–297). As a result, T cells have a competitive advantage for IL-2 consumption, and virus-induced IL-2–dependent NK-cell responses can only be identified in the absence of proliferating CD8 T-cell responses (298). Other pathways promote production of cytokines with potential to negatively regulate NK cells. For example, NK cells are sensitive to TGF-β–mediated inhibition of proliferation, cytotoxic activity, and cytokine production (299–305), and T-cell responses to viral infection can promote production of the biologically active form of this molecule (63). A variety of other T-cell cytokines reported to be produced during viral infections, such as IL-4, are known to mediate NK immunoregulatory effects, but they remain to be evaluated in regard to their *in vivo* significance for NK-cell control.

T-Cell Responses

It is not yet clear whether the same or overlapping populations of T cells are capable of mediating the multiple effector functions carried out by these populations (see Fig. 10). The best-studied examples of effector T-cell induction during viral infections are CD8 T-cell responses associated with profound CD8 T-cell expansion (see above). Characterized CD4 T-cell responses appear to be more limited in magnitudes. They are, however, clearly associated with cytokine expression, in particular IFN-γ, IL-2, and IL-4. These cytokines are known to contribute to immunoregulatory pathways for T-cell activation and proliferation. Negative regulation of these responses is likely, in large part, to be mediated by antigen clearance and a resulting lack of continued T-cell antigen receptor stimulation. Other active pathways, discussed above, for induction of cell death also appear to be in place to decrease peak numbers of responding T cells.

Interferon-γ, Interleukin-2, and Interleukin-4

Although a clear dichotomy of Th1- and Th2-type responses has been identified in several nonviral infections, the picture has not been so clear in regard to T-cell responses to viral infections. Despite a general perception of classification as Th1 type, a number of different viral infections in mouse and human have been reported to express both the Th1 cytokines IL-2 and IFN-γ and the Th2 cytokine IL-4 at some level, including HIV (306), HSV (307), influenza (308), LCMV (297,309), RSV (310), Sendai (60), and Sindbis (311). Indeed, based on results with cloned T cells from HIV-seropositive, as compared with those from HIV-seronegative, individuals, it has been suggested that T-cell responses to HIV infection are of a Th0 phenotype, with concurrent expression of both the Th1 and Th2 cytokines (312,313). Some of the discrepancy in classification of cytokine responses may result from level of production and/or sensitivity of quantitation assays. Generally, IFN-γ is expressed at high levels and readily detected as either mRNA or protein, whereas IL-2 and IL-4 are more difficult to measure. Moreover, the latter cytokines appear to be easily consumed by the T-cell populations producing them. For example, although IL-4 is difficult to detect, it can be revealed if consumption is blocked by addition of antibody to the receptor (309) and/or in ELISPOT assays with antibody capture of factor (60). Alternatively or additionally, there may be regional differences with local environments mediating selective effects on cytokine expression (307). Nevertheless, if taken together, the results indicate that T-cell IFN-γ responses are frequent and major responses to viral infections, whereas IL-2 and IL-4 are more difficult to measure but are often present.

T-cell production of IFN-γ is an effector mechanism for antiviral defense, and this is likely to be the most important function for the response. The cytokine does not appear to be necessary for CTL induction (33,314,315). Although both CD8 and CD4 T cells can make IFN-γ during viral infections (60,308,309,316,317), at least in response to LCMV infections preferentially inducing CD8 T-cell expansion, CD8 T cells are the primary producers of IFN-γ, accounting for 60% to 90% of the T cells expressing the factor (309). Almost all of the other cells expressing IFN-γ are CD4 T cells. Depending on proportions of individual subsets responding to particular viruses, the relative contributions of CD8 and CD4 T cells to IFN-γ responses are likely to vary during different infections. Nevertheless, the responses to LCMV infections demonstrate that CD8 T cells can be significant contributors to virus-induced IFN-γ responses.

IL-2 is a potent T-cell growth factor and primarily an immunoregulatory cytokine. Although both T-cell populations have been shown to be induced to express IL-2 mRNA during certain viral infections (297,316,318), CD4 T cells appear to be the major producers, whereas CD8 T cells appear to be the major consumers of the factor (309,318). The role for IL-2 in promoting endogenous T-cell responses has been extensively studied during LCMV infections. In this system, neither CD4 T cells (248,309,318,319) nor B cells (320) are required for acute virus-induced CD8 T-cell expansion or CTL activation, but CD4 T cells do support conditions promoting peak IFN-γ expression (309). IL-2 contributed by other cell types, presumably CD8 T cells, is biologically important because, in contrast to CD4 T cell–deficient conditions, absence of the factor profoundly inhibits CD8 T-cell expansion and net CTL induction as well as CD8 T cell IFN-γ production (194,309). Effects of IL-2 on CTLs appear to be secondary to its role in supporting T-cell expansion, as CTL functions can be induced at lower levels in the absence of the factor (194,321). Effects of IL-2 on CD8 T-cell IFN-γ responses are at the levels of both supporting T-cell expansion and facilitating continued cytokine production by activated cells (309). The critical requirements for CTL induction during viral infections have yet to be identified. IL-4 deficiency has no

detectable effect on CTL responses during LCMV or VV infections (322). Comparison of CTL responses during infections with these viruses in the absence of both IL-4 and IL-2 indicate that different cytokines are likely to be more or less important under different conditions. Although CTL activity is almost completely blocked during VV under these conditions, it can still be detected, albeit to lower levels, during LCMV infections (322). In defining particular roles for endogenous IL-2 and IL-4, these studies also demonstrate that the factors must be expressed and exerting biologic functions during viral infections.

Interleukin-5

Less is known about expression and function of the Th2 cytokine IL-5 during viral infections. The major activities associated with this factor are induction and activation of eosinophils. However, these cells have not been observed frequently or reported to mediate defense during viral infections. They have been detected during certain respiratory infections, in particular those with RSV (323). It is now known that immunization with the heavily glycosylated G protein from this virus can predispose mice to respond with Th2 cytokines, including IL-5, under certain conditions of secondary cell stimulation (324) and upon infection (325–327). These immunizations also can result in pulmonary eosinophilia during challenge infections (326,328). The clinical relevance of such immunization-induced immune modulation first came to light during the 1960s because of the appearance of detrimental immune responses during natural infections of infants previously vaccinated with formalin-inactivated RSV (329). In the experimental models, predisposition to Th2 responses with IL-5 production may depend on unique characteristics of the RSV G protein, as vaccination with other RSV proteins under similar responses do not elicit similar responses (324–326,328). The protein is unusual in its extensive glycosylation, and it is reported to be a poor inducer of CD8 T-cell responses (330). Nevertheless, it is somewhat surprising that the conditions resulting from RSV infection do not overcome the predisposition to Th2 responses induced by vaccination with G protein. Interesting studies indicate that inclusion of RSV epitopes for presentation to CD8 T cells during vaccination with G protein results in priming for CD8 T-cell responses, and that the presence of the primed CD8 T-cell responses during challenge infection inhibits development of the presumably primed Th2 responses and associated eosinophilia (330). Thus, in this system, there appears to be a requirement for concurrent priming and recall activation of CD8 T-cell responses to negatively regulate Th2 type responses.

B-Cell Responses

Cytokines can modulate B-cell antibody responses to viruses. Systemic virus-specific antibody responses, during infections of immunocompetent mice, are comprised of mixed isotypes, but are skewed through IFN-γ–dependent mechanisms to IgG2a (33,314,315). In the absence of IFN-γ, more IgG1 is produced (33). Although T cell–independent IgG2a antibody responses have been reported (277), peak induction of B cell responses for antibody production to viral infections requires the presence of CD4 T cells (163,197,248,319). There is general consensus concerning the importance of functional interactions between CD40L on activated T cells and its receptor CD40 on B cells for antibody responses (331–334). A remarkable CTL-mediated pathway regulating early induction of antibodies neutralizing virus has been demonstrated. This pathway is thought to be in place as a result of B-cell infection, facilitated by neutralizing antibody receptors, with subsequent presentation of antigen on class I MHC to CTLs (335).

IMMUNOLOGIC MEMORY

Acute viral infections induce both T- and B-cell memory (20,23,162). However, the nature of T- and B-cell memory is different (Fig. 17). Antiviral B-cell memory is usually manifested by continuous antibody production, even after resolution of the disease. Prolonged antibody production (lasting for decades) after infection or vaccination has been observed with many human (see Table 10) and animal viruses (20,23,162). In contrast, the effector phase of the T-cell response is short-lived (a few weeks), and "memory" in the T-cell compartment results from the presence of memory T cells, which are found at higher frequencies and can respond faster and develop into effector cells (i.e., CTL or cytokine producers) more efficiently than can naive T cells (20,23,162,183,336–338). This

dichotomy in the humoral and cellular responses is a feature of most acute viral infections (also of immunization, in general) and makes teleologic sense. Sustained secretion or overproduction of cytokines can have deleterious effects on the immune system, and the presence of fully active killers could result in immunopathologic damage if some of these CTLs were cross-reactive with self antigens. Thus, maintaining T-cell immunity by sustaining the effector phase carries a high price tag. Because memory T cells can rapidly develop into effectors and quickly gain access to sites of infection, it is not essential, in most instances, to have preexisting effector T cells to provide protection. An exception to this might be certain mucosal infections (see section on protective immunity).

T-Cell Memory

Accelerated T-cell responses seen on reexposure to virus are due to increases in the frequencies of antigen-specific T cells and to qualitative changes in memory T cells (20,23,162,183,269,339,340). Because memory cells express increased levels of adhesion mole-

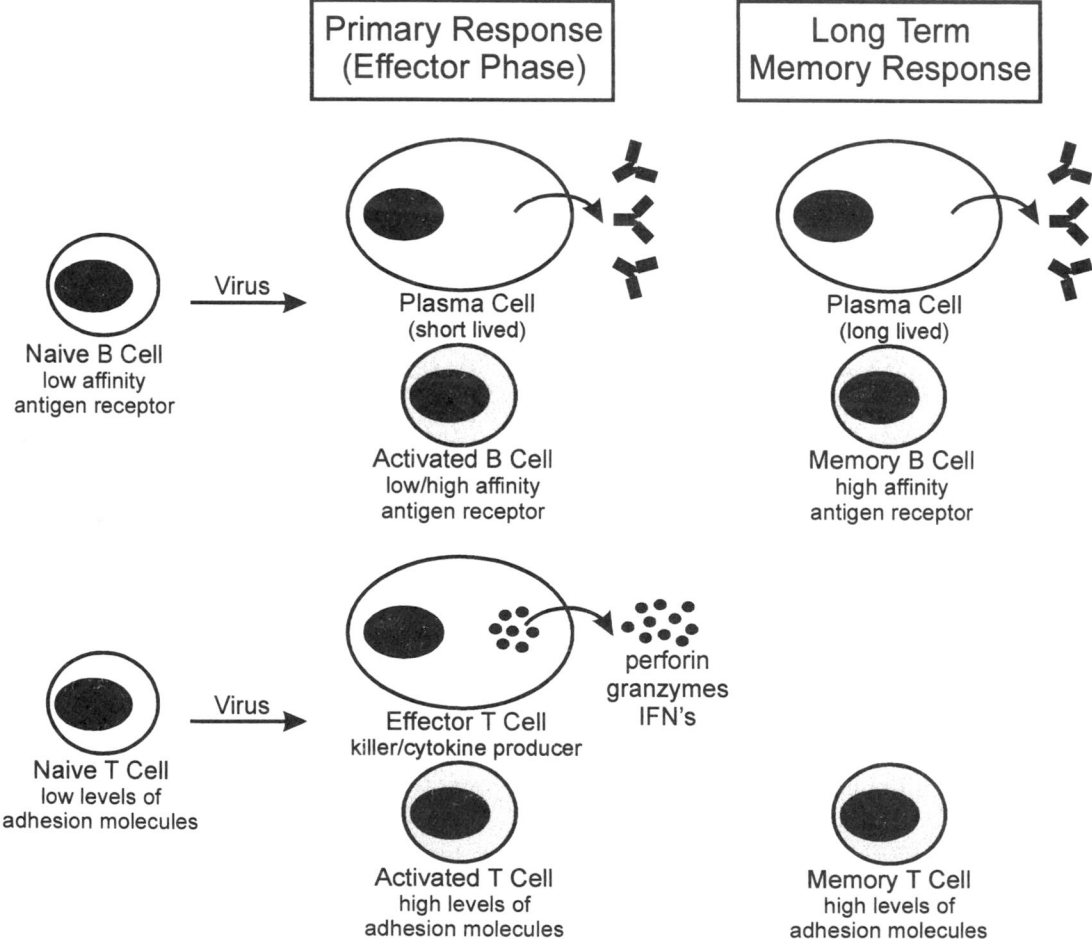

FIG. 17. Antiviral immunity after resolution of acute viral infection. The nature of T-cell and B-cell memory is different. B-cell memory is manifested by the presence of memory B cells and by continuous antibody production. This preexisting antibody provides the first line of defense against reinfection and is a key aspect of protective immunity against viral infections. In contrast, the effector phase of the T-cell response is short-lived, and long-term T-cell memory is due to the persistence of antigen-specific memory T cells that are present at higher frequencies and express increased levels of cell surface adhesion molecules. This increased frequency of virus-specific memory T cells and the ability of these cells to rapidly proliferate and develop into effector T cells provide a highly effective second line of defense against viruses. The memory T-cell response does not prevent infection per *se*, but it is crucial in limiting the severity of infection and eliminating virally infected cells.

cules, they are likely to adhere to APCs more efficiently. This may explain why memory cells are activated more readily than are naive cells and are able to respond to lower doses of antigen, as compared with naive cells (180,183,265,341–344). This increased responsiveness might also be due to higher affinity IL-2 receptors. The altered expression of adhesion molecules on memory T cells will also affect the circulation and/or homing of these cells. In this context, it is worth noting that CD44 and CD62L, two markers whose expression is changed on memory T cells, are both homing receptors (265,343,344). These changes influencing the circulation of memory T cells may result in better surveillance against viruses.

There has been considerable debate regarding the role of specific antigen in maintaining T-cell memory (20,162,345–349). At the outset, it should be stated that the presence of antigen is essential to maintain effector T cells. It should also be said that periodic reexposure to antigen enhances the level of T-cell memory; experiments showing increases in the number of memory T cells (or level of protective immunity) after reintroduction of viral antigen should not be taken as evidence that memory is strictly antigen-dependent. The real question is whether the pool of memory T cells formed after infection or immunization can remain relatively stable in the absence of an endogenous depot of specific antigen or is strictly dependent on stimulation by specific antigen. This chronic stimulus could come from a low-grade viral infection and/or from antigen persisting on follicular dendritic cells (FDCs) (20,350). Resolution of this issue is important for practical reasons (vaccines) and also because it addresses a fundamental issue of immune memory.

The experimental approach commonly used to examine the antigen dependence of T-cell memory is to adoptively transfer primed T cells into naive recipients and follow their survival in the apparent absence of antigen (20,23,162,180,344). The availability of B cell-deficient mice has provided an additional approach to this question since antigen-antibody complexes on FDCs have been implicated in sustaining T-cell memory (20,350). FDCs can trap antigen in the form of antigen–antibody complexes and retain it on their cell surfaces for long periods. It has been postulated that B cells or other APCs pick up this trapped antigen and present it to T cells (350). This mode of antigen loading favors MHC class II presentation, but there is now increasing evidence that macrophages and dendritic cells can process and present exogenous antigen on MHC class I molecules (351–356). Thus, antigen depots on FDCs could potentially play a role in sustaining both CD4 and CD8 T-cell memory. Both experimental approaches (i.e., adoptive transfers and infection of B cell-deficient mice) have been used to examine the antigen dependence of CD8 and CD4 T-cell memory. More extensive studies have been done on CD8 memory, and the consensus is that CD8 memory cells can persist in the absence of specific viral antigen (20,23,180–182,320,357–361). Convincing evidence for persistence of CD8 memory in the absence of specific antigen was provided by Lau et al. (180). In these experiments, LCMV-specific memory CD8 cells, which were free of any viral genetic material (polymerase chain reaction–negative), were adoptively transferred into uninfected mice and shown to persist and provide protective immunity for more than 2 years. Mullbacher (181) and Hou et al. (182), studying CTL responses to influenza virus and Sendai virus, have come to similar conclusions. Several groups have analyzed CD8 responses in B cell-deficient mice and found that CTL memory does not wane in these mice (20,320,362). Thus, it appears that neither B cells nor antigen–antibody complexes are essential for maintaining CD8 T-cell memory. In addi-

tion to these experimental systems, there is evidence for long-term CTL persistence in humans in the apparent absence of specific antigen. A study (357) has shown that VV-specific memory CTLs can be detected in individuals vaccinated more than 30 years earlier. It is unlikely that this long-term CTL memory is due to antigen persistence, because VV does not cause a chronic or latent infection in humans and there is no possibility of reexposure to VV, because vaccination against smallpox virus was stopped in 1977. Long-lasting (30 years or more) CD8 T-cell memory is also seen after acute HBV infection (363,364). However, in this instance, a role for antigen cannot be ruled out, because some of the subjects contained trace levels of HBV DNA. Very few studies have investigated whether antigen is required for the maintenance of CD4 T-cell memory. In one study, it was shown that CD4 T-cell memory to influenza virus was intact in the absence of B cells (269). However, additional studies are clearly needed, and it will be of interest to determine if the rules for maintaining CD4 and CD8 T-cell memory are the same or different (20).

B-Cell Memory

Viral infections not only induce memory B cells that persist for many years, but also are characterized by chronic antibody production that can last for decades (see Table 10). Although antibody levels in the serum do decline over time, it is remarkable that circulating antibody can still be detected 25 to 50 years after infection and/or vaccination (20,23,162,239). Since the half-life of free immunoglobulin is less than 3 weeks (365,366), continuous antibody production is necessary to sustain antigen-specific immunoglobulin levels in the serum. How is this long-term antibody production maintained? Conventional models suggest that long-term antibody responses are the result of continuous memory B-cell differentiation into antibody-secreting plasma cells. This is based on the notion that plasma cells are short-lived and need to be continually replenished by memory B cells. The antigenic stimulus for this continuous differentiation of virus-specific memory B cells into plasma cells could come from a variety of sources. These include reexposure to viruses, a low-grade chronic infection, antigen–antibody complexes on FDCs, and cross-reactivity to self or environmental antigens (Table 11). It is possible that one or more of these mechanisms is responsible for the long-term antibody responses seen after viral infections. However, a study has documented the existence of long-lived plasma cells and provided a new mechanism for maintaining humoral immunity (287).

Protection: Systemic Versus Mucosal Immunity

As mentioned above, antiviral antibody in the serum can persist for decades after viral infection. In contrast, mucosal antibody responses are relatively short-lived (usually a few months to a year or so) (see Table 10). This has profound consequences for protective immunity against mucosal infections. It is not coincidental that short-lived immunity is often associated with localized mucosal infections (e.g., rotavirus, RSV, rhinoviruses, and so on), whereas long-term protective immunity is a feature of many systemic infections (such as measles, yellow fever, polio, mumps, and smallpox) (72). The reasons for the marked differences in the durations of mucosal versus systemic antibody responses are not known. Most of the antibody present in serum comes from plasma cells residing in the bone marrow (1,20), whereas mucosal antibody levels

TABLE 11. *Models of long-term antibody production*

Mechanism	Comment

Reexposure to virus
  Persistent viral infection
  Immune complexes on follicular dendritic cells
  Cross-reactivity to self or environmental antigens
  Idiotypic networks
	Conventional models for maintaining humoral immunity in which short-lived plasma cells are continuously replenished by memory B cells proliferating and differentiating into plasma cells

Long-lived plasma cells	Long-lived plasma cells provide an additional mechanism for maintaining persistent antibody production

mostly reflect the number of plasma cells present at mucosal sites. It is possible that plasma cells have very different life spans at these two anatomic locations. The bone marrow microenvironment may provide the signals and cytokines to sustain plasma cells for long periods, perhaps for several years (287,288). On the other hand, plasma cells at mucosal surfaces may be short-lived. By identifying the factors that prolong plasma cell survival, it may be possible to increase the potency of suboptimal vaccines and thereby decrease the number of booster vaccinations required to sustain protective immunity against mucosal infections.

Memory B and T cells do not prevent infection *per se,* but they quickly proliferate and differentiate into effectors on reexposure to pathogens; this rapid recall response is critical in controlling the extent of infection and preventing disease (20,198). However, memory responses, in general, are more effective in preventing disease due to systemic infection than to mucosal infection. With viruses such as measles and polio, virus replication at the site of entry (the respiratory tract for measles and the intestinal tract for polio) does not produce any clinical symptoms; disease results from viral spread to other tissues (1,2). In such systemic infections, there is enough time for memory T and B cells to expand, differentiate into effectors, control the infection, and prevent clinical disease. The window of opportunity is much shorter for pathogens that produce disease by replicating and causing tissue damage at the site of entry (e.g., rotavirus in the gut and RSV in the respiratory tract) (1,2). In such mucosal infections, clinical symptoms appear so quickly (within 1 or 2 days) that there is not sufficient time for memory T cells to come into play. By the time memory T cells expand, differentiate into effectors, and get to the site of infection, part or most of the damage is already done. In such situations, effector T cells at mucosal sites may be required to prevent disease. This may be the case in experimental models of RSV and rotavirus infections, in which it was reported that protective CTL immunity is short-lived (367,368). Because effector CTLs are strictly dependent on antigen, it is not surprising that this response waned rapidly as amounts of antigen declined. Thus, in mucosal infections, immunologic memory can remain intact, but protective immunity starts waning with the decline of effector cells at mucosal sites.

IMMUNOPATHOLOGY OF VIRAL INFECTIONS

The immune response is a two-edged sword, and a certain amount of tissue damage is nearly always associated with control of viral infections. In most instances, this is well tolerated and does not produce any overt disease. However, there are situations in which a substantial amount of tissue damage and disease is due to the immune response directed against the virus (242,369–371). In this section, we briefly review some examples of virus-induced immunopathology. For a detailed description of immunopathologic mechanisms, see the chapters on inflammation and autoimmunity in this book (Chapters 31, 32, 33, and 34).

Immune Complex Disease

Continuous antibody production during a chronic viral infection results in the formation of soluble viral antigen–antibody complexes that are deposited in kidneys and arterioles. This continuous trapping of immune complexes in renal glomeruli, arteries, and choroid plexus can lead to glomerulonephritis, arteritis, and choroiditis (372,373). Various manifestations of immune complex disease have been described in chronic infections of animals (LCMV in mice, aleutian disease virus in minks, equine infectious anemia virus in horses) and humans (HBV, HIV, HCV).

T Cell- and Cytokine-mediated Damage

The classic example of T cell–mediated damage is LCMV infection of mice (225,374,375). Because LCMV is a noncytolytic virus, most diseases seen in this model (meningitis, hepatitis, diabetes, etc.) are the result of the T-cell response against LCMV and can be prevented by suppressing the immune response. The major mediators of this tissue damage are virus-specific CD8 T cells and both perforin-mediated killing and IFN-γ production have been implicated in causing the immunopathology (225,369). It has been shown that CD4 T cells can cause a chronic wasting syndrome during persistent LCMV infection (256). The best-documented example of T cell–mediated injury in humans is during chronic HBV infection (376,377). Periodic flare-ups of "chronic active hepatitis" in HBV carriers are the result of liver damage by HBV-specific T cells (376,377). The mechanism of this liver injury has been studied extensively in the HBV transgenic model. It has been proposed that the profound loss of CD4 T cells seen during AIDS is mediated by killing of infected CD4 T cells by HIV-specific CD8 T cells (378). Experiments examining *in vivo* dynamics of T-cell turnover and virus load during HIV infection do not support this simple model of AIDS (247,379,380). Nevertheless, the issue of immune-mediated damage during HIV infection merits attention. HIV persists in CD4 T cells, macrophages and monocytes, and dendritic cells—all crucial components of the immune system. At the same time, there are large numbers of HIV-specific CD8 T cells setting up a scenario of chronic infection and chronic immune activation (247). Such conditions of chronic immune activation may result in altered T-cell homeostasis, eventually leading to loss of T cells and immune dysfunction. In this context, it is worth noting that activated T cells and certain cytokines can suppress bone marrow function.

Cytokines made during innate immune response can also cause immunopathology. This is well appreciated for bacterial infections. For example, there are detrimental consequences due to cytokines made during gram-negative bacterial sepsis and after exposure to lipopolysaccharide (LPS) (381), as well as in response to gram-positive bacterial toxins, as represented by the staphylococcal enterotoxins (382) [i.e., staphylococcal enterotoxin A (SEA) and staphylococcal enterotoxin B (SEB)]. In general, high-level exposure to the first class of agents induces proinflammatory cytokines by innate immune response mechanisms, whereas exposure to the second activates large proportions of T-cell subsets to produce cytokines amplifying the proinflammatory innate cytokine cascades. If uncontrolled, the conditions can result in coagulation, vascular collapse, and multiorgan failure. Although these responses are clearly of major significance to health outcomes, little attention has been paid to their activation during viral infections. MCMV infections have been shown to induce systemic proinflammatory cytokines overlapping with, but not exactly identical to, those known to be induced under conditions of LPS exposure, that is, IL-12, IFN-γ, TNF, and IL-6 levels are significant, but IL-1 responses are low to undetectable during MCMV infection (49–51). Under these conditions, an adaptive immune response–independent but TNF-dependent liver necrosis is induced and results in significant organ damage (383). Such a pathway may contribute to liver disease during other viral infections. In particular, infection with mouse hepatitis virus type 3 (MHV-3) induces liver necrosis and disease associated with macrophage activation and coagulation (384–386). Treatments with IL-12 suggest that there

may be conditions under which T-cell responses to viral infections also might promote cytokine-mediated or cytokine-dependent disease during viral infections (292). Although such pathways are likely to contribute to pathology during Dengue virus infection (387, 388), they remain to be thoroughly investigated.

EVASION OF HOST IMMUNITY

Viruses have developed various strategies to evade host immune responses and persist *in vivo* (Tables 12 and 13). As can be seen from Table 12, the ability to persist is not confined to a particular virus group, and a variety of DNA- and RNA-containing viruses can establish long-term infections. Persistent viruses now cause an increasing proportion of the viral disease burden borne by humans—AIDS caused by HIV, chronic hepatitis and hepatocellular carcinoma due to HBV and HCV, anogenital cancer associated with human papillomaviruses (HPVs), disseminated HSV type 2 infection in the newborn, and so on (1,2).

Viral Evasion Strategies

Immune evasion is the essence of viral persistence. The many strategies used by viruses to avoid detection and elimination by the immune system are described below and summarized in Table 13.

TABLE 12. *Viruses that persist in humans*

Virus group	Site of persistence	Consequences
DNA viruses		
Adenovirus	Adenoids, tonsils, lymphocytes	None known
CMV	Kidneys, salivary glands, lymphocytes?, macrophages, stromal cells	Pneumonia, retinitis
EBV	Pharyngeal epithelial cells, B cells	Infectious mononucleosis, Burkitt's lymphoma, nonpharyngeal carcinoma, non-Hodgkin's lymphoma, oral hairy leukoplakia
Herpes simplex virus 1 and 2	Sensory ganglia neurons	Cold sores, genital herpes, encephalitis, keratosis
Human herpesvirus 6	Lymphocytes	Exantem subiturn
Human herpesvirus 8	PBMC? Endothelial spindle cells?	Kaposi sarcoma
Varicella zoster virus	Sensory ganglia neurons and/or satellite cells	Varicella zoster
Hepatitis B virus	Hepatocytes	Hepatitis, hepatocellular carcinoma
Hepatitis D virus	Hepatocytes	Exacerbation of chronic HBV infection
Papillomavirus	Epithelial skin cells	Papilloma, carcinomas
Parvovirus B19	Erythroid progenitor cells in bone marrow	Aplastic crisis in hemolytic anemia, chronic bone marrow deficiency
Polyomavirus BK	Kidney	Hemorrhagic cystitis
Polyomavirus JC	Kidney, oligodendrocytes in CNS	Progressive multifocal leukoencephalopathy
RNA viruses		
Hepatitis C virus	Hepatocytes	Hepatitis, hepatocellular carcinomas
Measles virus[a]	Neurons and supporting cells in CNS	Subacute sclerosing panencephalitis, measles-inclusion body encephalitis
Rubella virus[a]	CNS	Progressive rubella panencephalitis, insulin-dependent diabetes? juvenile arthritis?
HIV	CD4 T cells, monocytes/macrophages, microglia	AIDS
Human T-cell leukemia virus I	T cells	T-cell leukemia, tropical spastic paraparesis, polymyositis
Human T cell leukemia virus II	T cells	None known

[a]Measles and rubella viruses typically cause acute infections. However, in rare instances, these viruses have been shown to persist in the CNS.

TABLE 13. *Viral strategies for evading the immune system*

Escape mechanism	Example[a]
Restricted gene expression; virus remains latent in the cell with minimal to no expression of viral proteins	HSV and VZV in latently infected neurons, EBV in B cells, HIV in resting T cells
Infection of sites not readily accessible to the immune system	HSV, VZV, measles, and rubella persistence in neurons/CNS
	CMV, polyomaviruses BK and JC in the kidney
	EBV and CMV in the salivary gland
	Papillomaviruses in the epidermis
Inhibition of NK function	CMV protein UL18 is a MHC class I homologue that inhibits NK activity.
Antigenic variation; virus rapidly evolves and mutates antigenic sites that are critical for recognition by antibody and T cells	Antibody escape variants in lentiviruses
	CTL escape variants in HIV, EBV, and HBV
	T-cell receptor antagonism by HIV and HBV variants
Suppression of cell surface molecules required for T-cell recognition	Suppression of MHC class I molecules by adenoviruses, CMV, HSV, and HIV
	Decreased expression of cell adhesion molecules LFA-3 and ICAM-1 by EBV
	Suppression of MHC class II molecules by CMV, HIV, and measles
Interference with antigen processing and presentation	HSV ICP47 protein and CMV U6 protein interfere with TAP to inhibit MHC class I antigen presentation.
	EBV protein EBNA-1 contains gly-ala repeats that confer resistance to proteasome mediated degradation and subsequent MHC class I presentation.
	CMV protein pp65 phosphorylates the CMV immediate–early (IE) protein and inhibits its processing and/or presentation.
Viral "defense" molecules that interfere with the function of antiviral cytokines and chemokines	Adenovirus proteins E3 and E1B protect infected cells from lysis by TNF.
	Adenovirus VA RNA, EBV EBER RNA, and HIV TAR RNA inhibit function of interferon.
	EBV protein BCRF1 (a homologue of IL-10) blocks synthesis of cytokines such as IL-2 and interferon gamma.
Immunologic tolerance	Clonal deletion–anergy of virus-specific CTLs in HBV carriers, HIV(?)
Cell-to-cell spread by snycytia	SSPE caused by measles

[a]Only examples of viruses known to persist in humans are cited.

Restricted Expression of Viral Genes

Restricted viral gene expression provides a simple and highly effective mechanism by which infected cells escape detection by the host's immune response. This strategy is used to varying degrees by nearly all of the viruses that persist *in vivo*. However, it is exemplified best by the herpesviruses and retroviruses. The most extensively analyzed system is latent infection of neurons by HSV, in which viral gene expression is turned off completely, except for transcription from one region of the genome, and there appear to be no viral proteins expressed in the infected neurons (389,390). Under such conditions, the virus essentially becomes invisible to the immune system, and absolute latency is an ideal way of evading host immunity. However, this is not always feasible because, often, certain viral proteins are essential for replicating viral DNA during latency. For example, during latent infection of B cells by EBV, expression of one of the EBV proteins, called EBNA-1, is necessary for propagating the episomal EBV genome through cycles of cell division. Further, a permanent state of latency is not in the best interest of the virus in terms of transmission. Without the production of infectious virus, there can be no horizontal spread—an important mode of viral transmission. As a result, even viruses that are highly efficient in establishing latent infections go through intermittent phases of productive infection.

Infection of Immunologically Privileged Sites

Another strategy used by viruses is infection of tissues and cell types that are not readily accessible to the immune system (391).

A site of persistence favored by many viruses is the CNS. At least two factors favor viral persistence in the CNS: the presence of the blood–brain barrier, which limits lymphocyte trafficking through the CNS, and the presence of specialized cells, such as neurons, which express little or no MHC class I and no class II molecules, and therefore cannot be recognized efficiently by T cells (392–395). The kidney is another organ in which viruses tend to persist (392,396,397). The human polyomaviruses BK and JC replicate in the kidney, with almost lifelong shedding into the urine. CMV is also found in the kidney and is shed for long periods. It is not fully understood why the immune system is less effective in eliminating microbes from the kidney, because no blood–kidney barrier exists and there is extensive trafficking of lymphocytes through the kidney. However, a study has shown that, although T cells infiltrate the kidney, they have limited access to infected epithelial cells (398). These cells are protected by an intact basement membrane and microvascular endothelium, and this barrier has to be broken before T cells can have direct contact with their target cells. This limitation of T-cell access would also apply to the epithelial surfaces of other secretory or excretory glands, and it is notable that the salivary gland, a secretory tissue, is a favored site of persistence for viruses such as CMV and EBV. Replication of papillomaviruses in the epidermis provides another example of persistence at an immunologically privileged site. The productive cycle only occurs in differentiating keratinocytes, and, as a result, the infected cell and the viral particles are physically separated from the host's immune response by a basement membrane.

Viral Escape from Antibody Recognition

There are many examples of antibody-resistant variants, and mutation of viral proteins at sites critical for antibody recognition is a highly effective means of escape from neutralizing antibody. The classic example of this is the antigenic "shift" and "drift" seen among influenza viruses (399,400). These antigenic changes are the result of alterations in the two surface glycoproteins of influenza virus, the hemagglutinin and the neuraminidase. Influenza virus does not establish a persistent infection in individuals, but the emergence of antigenic variants contributes to the survival of influenza virus at the population level. The best examples of antigenic variation during a persistent infection come from the lentiviruses. Antigenic variants have been shown to emerge during persistence of equine infectious anemia virus in horses, visna virus in sheep, caprine arthritis encephalitis virus in goats, simian immunodeficiency virus in monkeys, and HIV in humans (401–404). However, the biologic importance of antigenic variation in these viruses is not fully understood. With the possible exception of equine infectious anemia virus, in which the recurrent episodes of disease (clinical symptoms associated with bursts of viremia) correlate with the emergence of antibody escape variants, the phenomenon of antigenic variation among lentiviruses does not seem to be essential for the persistence or induction of disease. In many cases, the "parental" virus continues to persist along with the variants in the infected host, in spite of the presence of neutralizing antibodies. Although neutralizing antibodies select antigenic variants, they are unable to eliminate completely the parental wild-type virus, and variant and wild-type viruses often coexist in the persistently infected host.

Viral Escape from T-Cell Recognition

Antigenic variation in viral peptides at residues involved in the processing and binding of the peptides to MHC molecules or alterations in viral peptides at sequences that directly contact the TCR can result in loss of recognition by the appropriate T cell. Theoretically, such alterations can occur in viral peptides presented by MHC class I or class II molecules, resulting in escape from CD8 and CD4 T cells, respectively. Few studies have systematically analyzed antigenic variation within viral epitopes recognized by CD4 T cells. In large part, this is because of the paucity of information on viral peptides seen by CD4 T cells. In contrast, there is more information on CD8 T-cell epitopes, and there are several well-documented examples of antigenic variation resulting in viral escape from CTL recognition (405). CTL escape variants were first demonstrated using the LCMV system (406). In this study, it was shown that a single amino acid change can abrogate CTL recognition, leading to persistence of the mutant virus in vivo. However, this profound biologic effect of the CTL escape variant was seen in transgenic mice that expressed a single LCMV-specific TCR and could only make a monoclonal CTL response. It remains to be seen whether CTL escape variants will have a similar advantage under more physiologic conditions, when antiviral CTL responses are likely to be polyclonal and multispecific.

CTL escape variants have been shown to occur in several viruses infecting humans, including HIV, EBV, and HBV (405–409). There is substantial evidence that CTLs play a role in controlling, at least to some degree, infections by all three of these viruses. It is tempting to propose that, in these cases, generation of CTL escape variants is critical for maintenance of the persistent infection. However,

in most of the studies in which CTL escape variants were identified, these variants did not go on to become the predominant viral species (405). In addition, in a longitudinal study of HIV-infected individuals, no escape variants were detected over a 14-month period, demonstrating that the presence of such variants may not be essential for HIV persistence (410). Similar observations have been made with simian immunodeficiency virus (411). Although these studies question the role of CTL escape variants in viral persistence, escape from CTLs also can occur by several other mechanisms (see later). CTL lysis also may be avoided if the density of viral peptides present on the cell surface is too low to trigger efficient lysis of the target cells. A study has provided evidence for this by showing that the low density of certain HIV peptides on naturally infected cells limits the effectiveness of HIV-specific CTLs (412).

Two studies on HIV and HBV have provided evidence for a novel strategy for foiling the CTL response (413,414). These studies have identified mutants of HIV and HBV that can interfere with CTL function in vitro. These variants have alterations in epitopes recognized by CTLs. However, unlike CTL escape variants that are not recognized by CTLs (i.e., are invisible to the TCR), these mutant epitopes can still interact with the TCR, but, instead of giving a stimulatory signal, they act as antagonists and render the CTLs nonfunctional. This phenomenon has been termed *TCR antagonism,* and although the mechanism is not fully undertood, it provides a highly effective means of evading the CTL response (415,416). An important aspect of this strategy is that the "antagonistic" variants can block CTL-mediated lysis of cells that are coinfected with viruses containing wild-type sequences. This would provide a possible explanation for the survival of wild-type virus in the face of an ongoing CTL response. The one caveat to these exciting observations is that it is not known whether TCR antagonism is effective *in vivo.*

Suppression of Cell Surface Molecules Required for T-Cell Recognition

Viruses can escape T-cell recognition by downregulating expression of cell surface molecules necessary for efficient T-cell recognition of virus-infected cells. These include host MHC class I (for CD8 cells) or class II (for CD4 cells) molecules and several adhesion molecules, such as ICAM-1 and LFA-3. Viruses have developed strategies for disrupting this multimeric interaction by selectively inhibiting the expression of these critical host-cell molecules.

The reduction of MHC class I antigen expression on host cells as a consequence of viral infection has been reported for several viruses (417–419). The best-documented examples of virus-mediated suppression of MHC class I antigens are by adenoviruses and CMV (418,420). Human adenoviruses can downregulate MHC expression by two distinct mechanisms. One of the early proteins of adenovirus type 2, the E3 protein, can bind to and form a complex with MHC antigens. The formation of this E3–MHC class I complex prevents the MHC antigens from being processed correctly by inhibiting their terminal glycosylation. This results in reduced cell surface expression of the class I antigen. Another early protein, the E1 protein of adenovirus type 12, prevents MHC class I expression by a different mechanism, which involves a transcriptional block or lack of export of messenger RNA (mRNA) from the nucleus. Both HCMV and MCMV contain several genes that interfere with MHC class I expression (109,110,112,113,418). The MCMV gpm152 proteins cause retention of MHC class I molecules in a pre-Golgi compartment, and MCMV gpm04 associates with MHC class I in the endoplasmic reticulum, travels with it to the surface, and, by a mechanism currently not well understood, inhibits MHC class I function. HCMV encodes two genes, US2 and US11, that mediate rapid degradation of newly synthesized MHC class I. This occurs because these viral proteins cause extrusion of newly made MHC class I molecules into the cytoplasm, where they get deglycosylated by the enzyme N-glycan. This deglycosylation makes the MHC class I molecules more sensitive to proteolytic degradation. HCMV encodes another protein, gpUS3, that binds class I and retains it in the endoplasmic reticulum.

Numerous reports have documented virus-mediated suppression of MHC class II antigens (417,418). Among the viruses infecting humans, CMV, HIV, and measles virus have been shown to interfere with MHC class II expression. The mechanism of viral interference is not understood, but, in all the cases examined, viral infection does not affect basal level expression of MHC class II molecules. Instead, the viral effect is directed toward inhibiting the interferon-γ-mediated upregulation of MHC class II mRNA transcription. Increased expression of MHC class II may play a role in antigen presentation, and interference with this step may prevent the generation of an effective immune response against the virus.

EBV can downregulate the expression of cell surface adhesion molecules LFA-3 and ICAM-1 (421). As a result of this inhibition, certain Burkitt's lymphoma cell lines are not efficiently killed by CTL. The mechanism involved in selective suppression of these adhesion molecules is not known, but these studies illustrate yet another viral strategy of circumventing the immune response.

Interference with Antigen Presentation

Studies have described a novel mechanism by which HSV inhibits antigen presentation by MHC class I molecules (418). ICP47, one of the early proteins of HSV, binds to the transporter associated with antigen processing (TAP), and prevents peptide translocation into the endoplasmic reticulum. As a result, peptide loading onto MHC class I molecules does not take place and the empty class I molecules remain stuck in the endoplasmic reticulum and are not displayed on the cell surface. It will be of interest to determine the role of ICP47 in HSV persistence and pathogenesis *in vivo*. Studies with ICP47 mutants in appropriate animal models should shed light on this issue. In this context, it is notable that the site of HSV latency is the neuron—a cell that expresses little or no MHC class I molecules. Residence of HSV in neurons during latency or during primary infection, when there is productive infection, may not be influenced by the ability of ICP47 to inhibit antigen presentation by MHC class I molecules. It is more likely that this novel function of ICP47 is of importance when HSV replicates in cells (epithelial cells, fibroblasts) that do express MHC class I molecules and otherwise would be recognized and killed by HSV-specifc CD8 CTLs. The ability of ICP47 to interfere with TAP function and inhibit antigen presentation in these cells would result in increased HSV shedding and more efficient transmission to new hosts. CMV also encodes a protein, U6, that can inhibit TAP function (418,422). Although the precise mechanism is not known, it has been shown that U6 glycoprotein interacts with TAP at the lumenal surface. This is different from the HSV ICP47 that binds to the cytoplasmic surface of TAP. Thus, it appears that these two viral proteins acheive the same end (i.e., inhibition of TAP function), but by different mechanisms.

There are also examples of viral proteins being inherently resistant to antigen processing. The EBNA-1 protein of EBV contains repeats of the gly-ala sequence that confers resistance to degradation in the proteasome (418,423,424). As a result of this, peptides from EBNA-1 are not endogenously presented to CD8 T cells. It should be pointed out that expression of EBNA-1 is essential for replicating the EBV genome in latently infected B cells. Thus, inhibiting the presentation of EBNA-1 may be crucial for EBV persistence *in vivo*. A study has shown that some CD8 T-cell responses are made against the EBNA-1 protein, and this is due to exogenous processing of the EBNA-1 protein (423). However, in this instance, even though CTLs are induced (by cross-priming), these EBNA-1 specific CD8 T cells cannot recognize latently infected cells because EBNA-1 is not endogenously processed within the infected B cell. The pp65 protein of CMV uses a different strategy. Unlike EBNA-1, pp65 is efficiently presented to CD8 T cells, but pp65 phosphorylates the major immediate-early protein of CMV and prevents the presentation of this intermediate-early protein (418,425).

Interference with Cytokine and Chemokine Function

Viral proteins that can interfere with cytokine function have been identified in several different viruses (420,426–429). Some of the adenovirus early proteins (E3, E1B) can protect virus-infected cells from lysis by TNF. The poxviruses also encode a protein, T2, that inhibits the action of TNF. The poxvirus T2 protein is a homologue of the cellular receptor for TNF and is released from infected cells, serving as a decoy. T2 binds TNF and could potentially prevent TNF from binding its true cellular receptor and exerting its antiviral effects. Other examples of viral defense molecules include the EBV protein BCRF1, which is a homologue of IL-10 and can block the synthesis of IL-2 and interferon-γ, and a secretory protein encoded by myxoma virus, which binds interferon-γ (430,431). In some instances, viral RNA itself can function as a defense molecule. The adenovirus VA RNA, the HIV TAR RNA, and the EBV EBER RNA can inhibit the antiviral effects of IFN-α/β. IFNs induce the synthesis of a phosphoprotein called DAI, which, in the presence of dsRNA, phosphorylates initiation factor eIF-2 and prevents the initiation of translation (see Fig. 5). The extensive secondary structure of these viral RNAs allows them to bind to DAI, inhibiting dsRNA binding and interfering with the action of IFN.

Certain viruses have genes with homology to chemokines and/or chemokine receptors and other gene products with chemokine-binding activities (429,432–435). It is not yet clear whether all of these function to help virus escape from immune defense. In soluble forms, they could act as chemokine receptor antagonists or blockers. However, chemokine homologues also might promote virus spread by recruiting sensitive mobile cells to sites of initial infections. If expressed on cell surfaces, homologues for chemokine receptors might act as dominant negatives in binding host chemokines and blocking signaling through the natural receptor and/or act to receive host chemokine signals enhancing virus infection in the cell. In the case of myxovirus infection, however, it has been demonstrated that certain viral products with chemokine-binding activity are virulence factor for infections and interfere with recruitment of leukocytes into virus-infected tissues.

Immunologic Tolerance

Perhaps the most efficient means of establishing and maintaining a persistent infection is to selectively silence the effector system responsible for clearing the virus. The classic example of this is the suppression of LCMV-specific CTL responses in congenitally infected carrier mice (20,239). Adult mice infected with LCMV mount a vigorous cellular and humoral response against the virus and clear the infection within 2 weeks. This clearance is mediated primarily by LCMV-specific CD8 CTLs (20,239). In contrast to the acute infection seen in adults, mice infected with LCMV at birth or *in utero* become chronically infected, showing life-long viremia with high levels of infectious virus and viral antigen in most of their major organs. The persistence of LCMV in these carrier mice is accompanied by the lack of a T-cell response to the virus. This is a highly specific defect. Such persistently infected mice exhibit no generalized immune supresion and respond normally to other antigens, but they show no detectable T-cell respones against LCMV because the virus-specific T cells have been clonally deleted within the thymus on seeing viral antigen (396,436). The inability of the carrier mice to eliminate virus results primarily from this T-cell defect because adoptive transfer of LCMV-specific T cells results in viral clearance (20,239).

Immuologic tolerance also plays a role in the establishment of chronic HBV infections. Most children (more than 90%) born to HBV-infected mothers go on to become HBV carriers. It is probable that, in these neontally infected carriers, at least some of the HBV-specific T cells undergo clonal deletion within the thymus or in the periphery. Even during adult onset of HBV infection, it is possible that some of the virus-specific T cells may be deleted in the periphery as a result of overstimulation by high doses of viral antigen, as has been documented during infection of adult mice with macrophage-tropic and invasive strains of LCMV that rapidly produce a high antigen load in many tissues (130,263,437). Under these conditions, virus-specific CD8 CTLs are overstimulated and driven to clonal exhaustion (deletion) in the periphery. Studies have shown that CD4 T cells play a critical role in sustaining CD8 CTL responses during chronic infection; under conditions of CD4 T-cell deficiency, there is rapid exhaustion of LCMV-specific CTLs in the periphery (174,438) (see Fig. 14). These findings have implications for chronic viral infections in general and may provide a possible explanation for the loss of HIV-specific CTL activity that is seen during the late stages of AIDS, when CD4 T cells become limiting and their numbers fall below a critical threshold necessary for maintaining CTL function.

The various viral evasion mechanisms that have been discussed are summarized in Table 13. Although specific examples have been cited to illustrate the different strategies, it is unlikely that a single mechanism can account for the persistence of a given virus. It is more probable that a combination of these strategies, plus other, unknown mechanisms, contribute to the persistence of virus in an otherwise immunocompetent host.

ACKNOWLEDGMENTS

We thank Kaja Murali-Krishna, Khuong B Nguyen, and Joe Blattman for their help with this article, and John Altman for providing Fig. 12, and Ganes Sen, Barney Graham, and Mark Hogarth for helpful comments.

REFERENCES

1. Fields BN. *Fields' virology.* Philadelphia: Lippincott–Raven Publishers, 1996.
2. Nathenson N, ed. *Viral pathogenesis.* Philadelphia: Lippincott–Raven Publishers, 1996.
3. Mims CA, ed. *The pathogenesis of infectious disease.* 3rd ed. London: Academic Press, 1987.
4. Mims CA, White DO, eds. *Viral pathogenesis and immunology.* Oxford: Blackwell Science, 1984.
5. Watts C. Capture and processing of exogenous antigens for presentation on MHC molecules. *Annu Rev Immunol* 1997;15:821–850.
6. York IA, Rock KL. Antigen processing and presentation by the class I major histocompatibility complex. *Annu Rev Immunol* 1996;14:369–396.
7. Bentley GA. The structure of the T cell antigen receptor. *Annu Rev Immunol* 1996;14:563–590.
8. Haas W, Pereira P, Tonegawa S. Gamma/delta cells. *Annu Rev Immunol* 1993;11:637–685.
9. Bucy RP, Chen CH, Cooper MD. Ontogeny of T cell receptors in the chicken thymus. *J Immunol* 1990;144:1161–1168.
10. Hein WR, Mackay CR. Prominence of gamma delta T cells in the ruminant immune system. *Immunol Today* 1991;12:30–34.
11. Eichelberger M, Allan W, Carding SR, Bottomly K, Doherty PC. Activation status of the CD4⁻8⁻ cells recovered from mice with influenza pneumonia. *J Immunol* 1991;147:2069–2074.
12. Hou S, Katz JM, Doherty PC, Carding SR. Extent of gamma delta T cell involvement in the pneumonia caused by Sendai virus. *Cell Immunol* 1992;143:183–193.
13. Welsh RM, Lin MY, Lohman BL, Varga SM, Zarozinski CC, Selin LK. Alpha beta and gamma delta T-cell networks and their roles in natural resistance to viral infections. *Immunol Rev* 1997;159:79–93.
14. Sciammas R, Kodukula P, Tang Q, Hendricks RL, Bluestone JA. T cell receptor-gamma/delta cells protect mice from herpes simplex virus type 1-induced lethal encephalitis. *J Exp Med* 1997;185:1969–1975.
15. Tanaka Y, Sano S, Nieves E, et al. Nonpeptide ligands for human gamma delta T cells. *Proc Natl Acad Sci USA* 1994;91:8175–8179.
16. Lenz LL, Dere B, Bevan MJ. Identification of an H2-M3-restricted Listeria epitope: implications for antigen presentation by M3. *Immunity* 1996;5:63–72.
17. Gulden PH, Fischer P III, Sherman NE, et al. A Listeria monocytogenes pentapeptide is presented to cytolytic T lymphocytes by the H2-M3 MHC class Ib molecule. *Immunity* 1996;5:73–79.
18. Bogen SA, Fogelman I, Abbas AK. Analysis of IL-2, IL-4, and IFN-gamma-producing cells in situ during immune responses to protein antigens. *J Immunol* 1993;150:4197–4205.
19. Scharton TM, Scott P. Natural killer cells are a source of interferon gamma that drives differentiation of CD4+ T cell subsets and induces early resistance to Leishmania major in mice. *J Exp Med* 1993;178:567–577.
20. Ahmed R, Gray D. Immunological memory and protective immunity: understanding their relation. *Science* 1996;272:54–60.
21. Bradley LM, Watson SR, Swain SL. Entry of naive CD4 T cells into peripheral lymph nodes requires L-selectin. *J Exp Med* 1994;180:2401–2406.
22. Hou S, Doherty PC. Partitioning of responder CD8+ T cells in lymph node and lung of mice with Sendai virus pneumonia by LECAM-1 and CD45RB phenotype. *J Immunol* 1993;150:5494–5500.
23. Doherty PC, Allan W, Eichelberger M, Carding SR. Roles of alpha beta and gamma delta T cell subsets in viral immunity. *Annu Rev Immunol* 1992;10:123–151.
24. Vilcek J, Sen GC. Interferons and other cytokines. In: Fields BN, Knipe DM, Howley PM, eds. *Fundamental Virology.* 3rd ed. Philadelphia: Lippincott–Raven Publishers, 1996:341–365.
25. Ishikawa R, Biron CA. IFN induction and associated changes in splenic leukocyte distribution. *J Immunol* 1993;150:3713–3727.
26. Feldman SB, Ferraro M, Zheng H-M, Patel N, Gould-Fogerite, Fitzgerald-Bocarsly P. Viral induction of low frequency interferon-α producing cells. *Virology* 1994;201:1–7.
27. Fitzgerald-Bocarsly P, Howell DM, Pettera L, Tehrani S, Lopez-C. Immediate-early gene expression is sufficient for induction of natural killer cell-mediated lysis of herpes simplex virus type 1-infected fibroblasts. *J Virol* 1991;65:3151–3160.
28. Lebon P. Inhibition of herpes simplex virus type-1 induced interferon synthesis by monoclonal antibodies against viral glycoprotein D and by lysosomotropic drugs. *J Gen Virol* 1985;66:2781–2786.
29. Darnell, JE. STATS and gene regulation. *Science* 1997;277:1630–1635.
30. Rivière Y, Gresser I, Guillon JC, Tovey MG. Inhibition by anti-interferon serum of lymphocytic choriomeningitis virus disease in suckling mice. *Proc Natl Acad Sci USA* 1977;74:2135–2139.
31. Fiette L, Aubert C, Muller U, et al. Theiler's virus infection of 129Sv mice that lack the interferon alpha/beta or interferon gamma receptors. *J Exp Med* 1995;181:2069–2076.
32. Müller U, Steinhoff U, Reis LFL, et al. Functional role of type I and type II interferons in antiviral defense. *Science* 1994;264:1918–1921.
33. van den Broek MF, Müller U, Huang S, Aguet M, Zinkernagel RM. Antiviral defense in mice lacking both alpha/beta, and gamma interferon receptors. *J Virol* 1995;69:4792–4796.

34. Meraz MA, White JM, Sheehan KC, et al. Targeted disruption of the Stat1 gene in mice reveals unexpected physiologic specificity in the JAK-STAT signaling pathway. *Cell* 1996;84:431–442.

35. Gresser I, Guy-Grand D, Maury C, Maunoury MT. Interferon induces peripheral lymphademopathy in mice. *J Immunol* 1981;127:1569–1575.

36. Korngold R, Blank KJ, Murasko DM. Effect of interferon on thoracic duct lymphocyte output: induction with either polyI:polyC or vaccinia virus. *J Immunol* 1983;130:2236–2240.

37. Woodruff JF, Woodruff JJ. Virus-induced alterations of lymphocyte tissues. I. Modification of the recirculating pool of small lymphocytes by Newcastle Disease Virus. *Cell Immunol* 1970;1:333–354.

38. Trinchieri G. Biology of natural killer cells. *Adv Immunol* 1989;47:187–376.

39. Cousens LP, Orange JS, Su HC, Biron CA. Interferon-α/β inhibition of interleukin 12 and interferon-γ production *in vitro* and endogenously during viral infection. *Proc Natl Acad Sci USA* 1997;94:634–639.

40. Manetti R, Annuziato F, Tomasevic L, et al. Polyinosinic acid: polycytidylic acid promotes T helper type 1-specific immune responses by stimulating macrophage production of interferon-alpha and interleukin-12. *Eur J Immunol* 1995;25:2656–2660.

41. Rogge L, Barberis-Maino L, Biffi M, et al. Selective expression of an interleukin-12 receptor component by human T helper 1 cells. *J Exp Med* 1997;185:825–831.

42. Lindahl P, Gresser I, Leary P, Tovey M. Interferon treatment of mice. Enhanced expression of histocompatibility antigens on lymphoid cells. *Proc Natl Acad Sci USA* 1976;73:1284–1287.

43. Biron CA, Welsh RM. Blastogenesis of natural killer cells during viral infection in vivo. *J Immunol* 1982;129:2788–2795.

44. Biron CA, Sonnenfeld G, Welsh RM. Interferon induces natural killer cell blastogenesis in vivo. *J Leukoc Biol* 1984;35:31–37.

45. Tough DF, Borrow P, Sprent J. Induction of bystander T cell proliferation by viruses and type I interferon in vivo. *Science* 1996;272:1947–1950.

46. Gilles PN, Fey G, Chisari FV. Tumor necrosis factor alpha negatively regulates hepatitis B virus gene expression in transgenic mice. *J Virol* 1992;66:3955–3960.

47. Lucin P, Jonjic S, Messerle M, Polic B, Hengel H, Koszinowski UH. Late phase inhibition of murine cytomegalovirus replication by synergistic action of interferon-gamma and tumour necrosis factor. *J Gen Virol* 1994;75:101–110.

48. Neuzil KM, Tang YW, Graham BS. Protective Role of TNF-alpha in respiratory syncytial virus infection in vitro and in vivo. *Am J Med Sci* 1996;311:201–204.

49. Orange JS, Wang B, Terhorst C, Biron CA. Requirement for natural killer (NK) cell-produced interferon γ in defense against murine cytomegalovirus infection and enhancement of this defense pathway by interelukin 12 administration. *J Exp Med* 1995;182:1045–1056.

50. Orange JS, Biron CA. Characterization of early IL-12, IFN-α/β, and TNF effects on antiviral state and NK cell responses during murine cytomegalovirus infection. *J Immunol* 1996;156:4746–4756.

51. Ruzek MC, Miller AH, Opal SM, Pearce BD, Biron CA. Characterization of early cytokine responses and an interleukin (IL)-6-dependent pathway of endogenous glucocorticoid induction during murine cytomegalovirus infection. *J Exp Med* 1997;185:1185–1192.

52. Wong GHW, Goeddel DV. Tumor necrosis factors alpha and beta inhibit virus replication and synergize with interferons. *Nature* 1986;323:819–822.

53. MacMicking J, Xie QW, Nathan C. Nitric oxide and macrophage function. *Annu Rev Immunol* 1997;15:323–350.

54. Chan SH, Perussia B, Gupta JW, et al. Induction of interferon gamma production by natural killer cell stimulatory factor: characterization of the responder cells and synergy with other inducers. *J Exp Med* 1991;173:869–879.

55. Coutelier JP, Van Broeck J, Wolf SF. Interleukin-12 gene expression after viral infection in the mouse. *J Virol* 1995;69:1955–1958.

56. Kanangat S, Thomas J, Gangappa S, Babu JS, Rouse BT. Herpes simplex virus type 1-mediated up-regulation of IL-12 (p40) mRNA expression. Implications in immunopathogenesis and protection. *J Immunol* 1996;156:1110–1116.

57. Orange JS, Biron CA. An absolute and restricted requirement for IL-12 in natural killer cell IFN-γ production and antiviral defense. Studies of natural killer and T cell responses in contrasting situations of viral infections. *J Immunol* 1996;156:1138–1142.

58. Schijns VECJ, Wierda CMH, van Hoeij M, Horzinek MC. Exacerbated viral hepatitis in IFN-γ receptor-deficient mice is not suppressed by IL-12. *J Immunol* 1996;157:815–821.

59. Kanangat S, Babu JS, Knipe DM, Rouse BT. HSV-1-mediated modulation of cytokine gene expression in a permissive cell line: selective upregulation of IL-6 gene expression. *Virology* 1996;219:295–300.

60. Mo XY, Sarawar SR, Doherty PC. Induction of cytokines in mice with parainfluenza pneumonia. *J Virol* 1995;69:1288–1291.

61. Moskophidis D, Frei K, Lohler J, Fontana A, Zinkernagel RM. Production of random classes of immunoglobulins in brain tissue during persistent viral infection paralleled by secretion of interleukin-6 (IL-6) but not IL-4, IL-5, and gamma interferon. *J Virol* 1991;65:1364–1369.

62. Pulliam L, Moore D, West DC. Human cytomegalovirus induces IL-6 and TNF alpha from macrophages and microglial cells: possible role in neurotoxicity. *J Neurovirol* 1995;1:219–227.

63. Su HC, Ishikawa R, Biron CA. Transforming growth factor-β expression and natural killer cell responses during virus infection of normal, nude, and SCID mice. *J Immunol* 1993;151:4874–4890.

64. Wahl SM, Allen JB, McCartney-Francis N, et al. Macrophage- and astrocyte-derived transforming growth factor beta as a mediator of central nervous system dysfunction in acquired immune deficiency syndrome. *J Exp Med* 1991;173:981–991.

65. Atedzoe BN, Ahmad A, Menezes J. Enhancement of natural killer cell cytotoxicity by the human herpesvirus-7 via IL-15 induction. *J Immunol* 1997;159:4966–4972.

66. Flamand L, Stefanescu I, Menezes J. Human herpesvirus-6 enhances natural killer cell cytotoxicity via IL-15. *J Clin Invest* 1996;97:1373–1378.

67. Komatsu T, Reiss CS. IFN-γ is not required in the IL-12 response to vesicular stomatitis virus infeciton of the olfactory bulb. *J Immunol* 1997;159:3444–3452.

68. Naume B, Johnsen AC, Espevik T, Sundan A. Gene expression and secretion of cytokines and cytokine receptors from highly purified CD56+ natural killer cells stimulated with interleukin-2, interleukin-7 and interleukin-12. *Eur J Immunol* 1993;23:1831–1838.

69. Bi Z, Reiss CS. Inhibition of vesicular stomatits virus infection by nitric oxide. *J Virol* 1995;69:2208–2213.

70. Braun L, Durst M, Mikumo R, Crowley A, Robinson M. Regulation of growth and gene expression in human papillomavirus-transformed keratinocytes by transforming growth factor-beta: implications for the control of papillomavirus infection. *Mol Carcinog* 1992;6:100–111.

71. Hunter CA, Timans J, Pisacane P, et al. Comparison of the effects of interleukin-1 alpha, interleukin-1 beta and interferon-gamma-inducing factor on the production of interferon-gamma by natural killer. *Eur J Immunol* 1997;27:2787–2792.

72. McEwen BS, Biron CA, Brunson KW, et al. The role of adrenocorticoids as modulators of immune function in health and disease: neural, endocrine and immune interactions. *Brain Res Brain Res Rev* 1997;23:79–133.

73. Vacca A, Felli MP, Farina AR, et al. Glucocorticoid receptor-mediated suppression of the interleukin 2 gene expression through impairment of the cooperativity between nuclear factor of activated T cells and AP-1 enhancer elements. *J Exp Med* 1992;175:637–646.

74. Scheinman RI, Cogswell PC, Lofquist AK, Baldwin AS Jr. Role of transcriptional activation of I kappa B alpha in mediation of immunosuppression by glucocorticoids. *Science* 1995;270:283–286.

75. Biron CA. Activation and function of natural killer cell responses during viral infections. *Curr Opin Immunol* 1997;9:24–34.

76. Gidlund M, Örn A, Wigzell H, Senik A, Gresser I. Enhanced NK cell activity in mice injected with interferon and interferon inducers. *Nature* 1978;273:759–761.

77. Santoli D, Trinchieri G, Koprowski H. Cell-mediated cytotoxicity against virus-infected target cells in humans. II. Interferon induction and activation of natural killer cells. *J Immunol* 1978;121:532–538.

78. Bancroft GJ, Shellam GR, Chalmer JE. Genetic influences on the augmentation of natural killer (NK) cells during murine cytomegalovirus infection: correlation with patterns of resistance. *J Immunol* 1981;126:988–994.

79. Macfarlan RI, Burns WH, White DO. Two cytotoxic cells in peritoneal cavity of virus-infected mice: antibody-dependent macrophages and non-specific killer cells. *J Immunol* 1977;119:1569–1574.

80. Pfizenmaier K, Trostmann H, Rollinghoff M, Wagner H. Temporary presence of self-reactive cytotoxic T-lymphocytes during murine lymphocytic choriomeningitis virus infection. *Nature* 1975;258:238–240.

81. Shellam GR, Allan JE, Papadimitriou JM, Bancroft GJ. Increased susceptibility to cytomegalovirus infection in beige mutant mice. *Proc Natl Acad Sci USA* 1981;78:5104–5108.

82. Welsh RM. Cytotoxic cells induced during lymphocytic choriomeningitis virus infection of mice. I. Characterization of natural killer cell induction. *J Exp Med* 1978;148:163–181.

83. Grundy (Chalmer) JE, Trapman J, Allan JE, Shellam GR, Melief CJM. Evidence for a protective role of interferon in resistance to murine cytomegalovirus and its control by non-H-2-linked genes. *Infect Immun* 1982;37:143–150.

84. Biron CA, van den Elsen P, Tutt MM, Medveczky P, Kumar V, Terhorst C. Murine natural killer cells stimulated *in vivo* do not express the T cell receptor α, β, T3δ, or T3ε genes. *J Immunol* 1987;139:1704–1710.

85. Wang B, Biron C, She J, et al. A block in both early T lymphocyte and natural killer cell development in transgenic mice with high-copy numbers of the human CD3ε gene. *Proc Natl Acad Sci USA* 1994;91:9402–9406.

86. Biron CA, Byron KS, Sullivan JL. Severe herpesvirus infections in an adolescent without natural killer cells. *N Engl J Med* 1989;320:1731–1735.

87. Bonavida B, Katz J, Gottlieb M. Mechanism of defective NK cell activity in patients with acquired immunodeficiency syndrome (AIDS) and AIDS-related complex. *J Immunol* 1986;137:1157–1163.

88. Bukowski JF, Woda BA, Habu S, Okumura K, Welsh RM. Natural killer cell depletion enhances virus synthesis and virus-induced hepatitis in vivo. *J Immunol* 1983;131:1531–1538.

89. Habu S, Akamatsu K, Tamaoki N, Okumura K. *In vivo* significance of NK cells on resistance against virus (HSV-1) infections in mice. *J Immunol* 1984;133:2743–2747.

90. Rager-Zisman B, Quan P-C, Rosner M, Moller JR, Bloom BR. Role of NK cells in protection of mice against herpes simplex virus-1 infection. *J Immunol* 1987;138:884–888.

91. Sullivan JL, Byron KS, Brewster FE, Purtillo DT. Deficient natural killer cell activity in the X-linked lymphoproliferative syndrome. *Science* 1980;210:543–545.

92. Kägi D, Ledermann B, Burki K, et al. Cytotoxicity mediated by T cells and natural killer cells is greatly impaired in perforin-deficient mice. *Nature* 1994;369: 31–37.

93. Tay CH, Welsh RM. Distinct organ-dependent mechanisms for the control of murine cytomegalovirus infection by natural killer cells. *J Virol* 1997;71:267–275.

94. Borysiewicz LK, Rodgers B, Morris S, Graham S, Sissons JG. Lysis of human cytomegalovirus infected fibroblasts by natural killer cells: demonstration of an interferon-independent component requiring expression of early viral proteins and characterization of effector cells. *J Immunol* 1985;134:2695–2701.

95. Welsh RM, Hallenbeck LA. Effect of virus infections on target cell susceptibility to natural killer cell-mediated lysis. *J Immunol* 1980;124:2491–2497.

96. Perussia B, Tutt MM, Qiu WQ, et al. Murine natural killer cells express functional Fc gamma receptor II encoded by the Fc gamma R alpha gene. *J Exp Med* 1989;170:73–86.

97. Yokoyama WM. Right-side-up and up-side-down NK cell-receptors. *Curr Biol* 1995;5:982–985.

98. Colonna M. Natural killer cell receptors specific for MHC class I molecules. *Curr Opin Immunol* 1996;8:101–107.

99. Lanier, LL. Natural killer cell receptors and MHC class I interactions. *Curr Opin Immunol* 1997,9.126–131.

100. Moretta A, Moretta L. HLA class I specific inhibitory receptors. *Curr Opin Immunol* 1997;9:694–701.

101. Parham P, ed. NK cells, MHC class I antigens and missing self. *Immunol Rev* 1997;155:1–221.

102. Burshtyn DN, Scharenberg AM, Wagtmann N, et al. Recruitment of tyrosine phosphatase HCP by the killer cell inhibitor receptor. *Immunity* 1996; 4:77–85.

103. Campbell AE, Slater JS. Down-regulation of major histocompatibility complex class I synthesis by murine cytomegalovirus early gene expression. *J Virol* 1994;68:1805–1811.

104. Olcese L, Lang P, Vély F, et al. Human and mouse killer-cell inhibitory receptors recruit PTP1C and PTP1D protein tyrosine phosphatases. *J Immunol* 1996;156: 4531–4534.

105. D'Andrea A, Chang C, Phillips JH, Lanier LL. Regulation of T cell lymphokine production by killer cell inhibitory receptor recognition of self HLA class I alleles. *J Exp Med* 1996;184:789–794.

106. Ortaldo JR, Mason LH, Gregorio TA, Stoll J, Winkler-Pickett RT. The Ly-49 family: regulation of cytokine production in murine NK cells. *J Leukoc Biol* 1997,62.381–388.

107. Cosman D, Fanger N, Borges L, et al. A novel immunoglobulin superfamily receptor for cellular and viral MHC class I molecules. *Immunity* 1997;7: 273–282.

108. Braud VM, Allan SJ, O'Callaghan CA, et al. HLA-E binds to natural killer cell receptors CD94/NKG2A, B, and C. *Nature* 1998;391:795–799.

109. Del Val M, Hengel H, Häcker H, et al. Cytomegalovirus prevents antigen presentation by blocking the transport of peptide-loaded major histocompatibility complex class I molecules into the medial-golgi compartment. *J Exp Med* 1992;176:729–738.

110. Hengel H, Koszinowski UH. Interference with antigen processing by viruses. *Curr Opin Immunol* 1997;9:470–476.

111. Hill A, Jugovic P, York I, et al. Herpes simplex virus turns off the TAP to evade host immunity. *Nature* 1995;375:411–515.

112. Jones TR, Hanson LK, Sun L, Slater JS, Stenberg RM, Campbell AE. Multiple independent loci within the human cytomegalovirus unique short region down-regulate expression of major histocompatibility complex class I heavy chains. *J Virol* 1995;69:4830–4841.

113. Wiertz EJHJ, Jones TR, Sun L, Bogyo M, Geuze HJ, Ploegh HL. The human cytomegalovirus US11 gene product dislocates MHC class I heavy chains from the endoplasmic reticulum to the cytosol. *Cell* 1996;84:769–779.

114. Farrell HE, Hally H, Lynch DM, et al. Inhibition of natural killer cells by a cytomegalovirus MHC class I homologue in vivo. *Nature* 1997;386:510–514.

115. Reyburn HT, Mandelboim O, Valès-Gomez M, Davis DM, Pazmani L, Strominger JL. The class I MHC homologue of human cytomegalovirus inhibits attack by natural killer cells. *Nature* 1997;386:514–517.

116. Scalzo AA, Lyons PA, Fitzgerald NA, Forbes CA, Yokoyama WM, Shellam GR. Genetic mapping of Cmv1 in the region of mouse chromosome 6 encoding the NK gene complex-associated loci Ly49 and musNKR-P1. *Genomics* 1995;27: 435–441.

117. Delano ML, Brownstein DG. Innate resistance to lethal mousepox is genetically linked to the NK gene complex on chromosome 6 and correlates with early restriction of virus replication by cells with an NK phenotype. *J Virol* 1995;69: 5875–5877.

118. Biron CA, Gazzinelli RT. Effects of IL-12 on immune responses to microbial infections: a key mediator in regulating disease outcome. *Curr Opin Immunol* 1995;7:485–496.

119. Kobayashi M, Fitz L, Ryan M, et al. Identification and purification of natural killer cell stimulatory factor (NKSF), a cytokine with multiple biologic effects on human lymphocytes. *J Exp Med* 1989;170:827–845.

120. Romani L, Puccetti P, Distoni F. Interleukin-12 in infectious diseases. *Clin Microbiol Rev* 1997;10:611–636.

121. Heise MT, Virgin IV HW. The T cell independent role of gamma interferon and tumor necrosis factor alpha in macrophage activation during murine cytomegalovirus and herpes simplex virus infections. *J Virol* 1995;69:904–909.

122. Salazar-Mather TP, Orange JS, Diron CA. Early murine cytomegalovirus

123. Gollob JA, Kawasaki H, Ritz J. Interferon-gamma and interleukin-4 regulate T cell interleukin-12 responsiveness through the differential modulation of high-affinity interleukin-12 receptor expression. *Eur J Immunol* 1997;27:647–652.

124. Ma X, Chow JM, Gri G, et al. The interleukin 12 p40 gene promoter is primed by interferon gamma in monocytic cells. *J Exp Med* 1996;183:147–157.

125. Szabo SJ, Dighe AS, Gubler U, Murphy KM. Regulation of the interleukin (IL)-12R beta 2 subunit expression in developing T helper 1 (Th1) and Th2 cells. *J Exp Med* 1997;185:817–824.

126. Allison AC. Interactions of antibodies, complement components and various cell types in immunity against viruses and pyogenic bacteria. *Transplant Rev* 1974; 19:3–55.

127. Ching C, Lopez C. Natural killing of herpes simplex virus type-1 infected target cells: normal human responses and influence of antiviral antibody. *Infect Immun* 1979;26:49–56.

128. Skowron G, Cole BF, Zheng D, Accetta G, Yen-Lieberman B. gp120-directed antibody-dependent cellular cytotoxicity as a major determinant of the rate of decline in CD4 percentage in HIV-1 disease. *AIDS* 1997;11:1807–1814.

129. Brautigam AR, Dutko FJ, Olding LB, Oldstone MBA. Pathogenesis of murine cytomegalovirus infection: the macrophage as a permissive cell for cytomegalovirus infection, replication and latency. *J Gen Virol* 1979;44:349–359.

130. Matloubian M, Kolhekar SR, Somasundaram T, Ahmed R. Molecular determinants of macrophage-tropism and viral persistence: importance of single amino acid changes in the polymcrase and glycoprotein of lymphocytic choriomeningitis virus. *J Virol* 1993;67:7340–7349.

131. Mims CA, Gould J. The role of macrophages in mice infected with murine cytomegalovirus. *J Gen Virol* 1978;41:143–153.

132. Mims CA, Murphy FA. Parainfluenza virus Sendai infection in macrophages, ependyma, choroid plexus, vascular endothelium, and respiratory tract of mice. *Am J Pathol* 1973;70:315–328.

133. Narayan O, Kennedy-Stoskopf S, Sheffer D, Griffin DE, Clements JE. Activation of caprine arthritis-encephalitis virus expression during maturation of monocytes to macrophages. *Infect Immun* 1983;41:67–73.

134. Roberts JA. Growth of virulent and attenuated ectromelia virus in cultured macrophages from normal and ectromelia-immune mice. *J Immunol* 1964;92: 837–842.

135. Cafruny WA, Bradley SE. Trojan Horse macrophages: studies with the murine lactate dehydrogenase-elevating virus and implications for sexually transmitted infection. *J Gen Virol* 1996;77:3005–3012.

136. Bang FB. Genetics of resistance of animal to viruses: I. Introduction and studies in mice. *Adv Virus Res* 1978;23:269–348.

137. Bang FB, Warwick A. Mouse macrophages as host cells for the mouse hepatitis virus and genetic basis of their susceptibility. *Proc Natl Acad Sci USA* 1960;46. 1065–1075.

138. Ben-Hur T, Hadar J, Shtram Y, Gilden DH, Becker Y. Neurovirulence of herpes simplex virus type 1 depends on age in mice and thymidine kinase expression. *Arch Virol* 1983;78:303–308.

139. Goodman GT, Koprowski H. Macrophages as a cellular expression of inherited natural resistance. *Proc Natl Acad Sci USA* 1961;48:160–165.

140. Mogensen SC. Role of marophages in natural resistance to virus infections. *Microbiol Rev* 1979;43:1–26.

141. Ho WZ, Lioy J, Song L, Cutilli JR, Polin RA, Douglas SD. Infection of cord blood monocyte-derived macrophages with human immunodeficiency virus type 1. *J Virol* 1992;66:573–579.

142. Sperduto AR, Bryson YJ, Chen IS. Increased susceptibility of neonatal monocyte/macrophages to HIV-1 infection. *AIDS Res Hum Retroviruses* 1993;9: 1277–1285.

143. Sullivan JL, Barry DW, Lucas SJ, Albrecht P. Measles infection of human mononuclear cells. I. Acute infection of peripheral blood lymphocytes and monocytes. *J Exp Med* 1975;142:773–784.

144. Selgrade MK, Osborn JE. Role of macrophages in resistance to murine cytomegalovirus. *Infect Immun* 1974;10:1383–1390.

145. Zisman B, Hirsch MS, Allison AC. Selective effects of anti-macrophage serum, silica and anti-lymphocyte serum on pathogenesis of herpes virus infection of young adult mice. *J Immunol* 1970;104:1155–1159.

146. Zisman D, Wheelock EF, Allison AC. Role of macrophages and antibody in resistance of mice against yellow fever virus. *J Immunol* 1971;107:236–243.

147. Nicholson S, Bonecini-Almeida M-da-G, Lapa-e-Silva JR, et al. Inducible nitric oxide synthase in pulmonary alveolar macrophages from patients with tuberculosis. *J Exp Med* 1996;183:2293–2302.

148. Karupiah G, Xie QW, Buller RM, Nathan C, Duarte C, MacMicking JD. Inhibition of viral replication by interferon-gamma-induced nitric oxide synthase. *Science* 1993;261:1445–1448.

149. Melkova Z, Esteban M. Inhibition of vaccinia virus DNA replication by inducible expression of nitric oxide synthase. *J Immunol* 1995;155:5711–5718.

150. Karupiah G, Harris N. Inhibition of viral replication by nitric oxide and its reversal by ferrous sulfate and tricarboxylic acid cycle metabolites. *J Exp Med* 1995; 181:2171–2179.

151. Mannick JB, Asano K, Izumi K, Kieff E, Stamler JS. Nitric oxide produced by human B lymphocytes inhibits apoptosis and Epstein-Barr virus reactivation. *Cell* 1994;79:1137–1146.

152. Oppenheim JJ, Zachariae COC, Mukaida N, Matsushima K. Properties of the novel proinflammatory supergene "intercrine" cytokine family. *Annu Rev Immunol* 1991;9:617–648.

153. Schall TJ, Bacon KB. Chemokines, leukocyte trafficking, and inflammation. *Curr Opin Immunol* 1994:6:865–873.

154. Berger EA. HIV entry and tropism: the chemokine receptor connection. *AIDS* 1997;11:S3–S16.

155. Asensio VC, Campbell IL. Chemokine gene expression in the brains of mice with lymphocytic choriomeningitis. *Virology* 1997;71:7832–7840.

156. Lane TE, Asensio VC, Yu N, Paoletti AD, Campbell IL, Buchmeir MJ. Dynamic regulation of alpha- and beta-chemokine expression in the central nervous system during mouse hepatitis virus-induced demyelinating disease. *J Immunol* 1998;160:970–978.

157. Amichay D, Gazzinelli RT, Karupiah G, Moench TR, Sher A, Farber JM. Genes for chemokines mumig and crg-2 are induced in protozoan and viral infections in response to IFN-gamma with patterns of tissue expression that suggest nonredundant roles in vivo. *J Immunol* 1996;157:4511–4520.

158. Cook DN, Beck MA, Coffman TM, et al. Requirement of MIP-1α for an inflammatory response to viral infection. *Science* 1995;268:1583–1585.

159. Cocchi F, DeVico AL, Garzino-Demo A, Arya SK, Gallo RC, Lusso P. Identification of RANTES, MIP-1 alpha, and MIP-1 beta as the major HIV-suppressive factors produced by CD8+ T cells. *Science* 1995;270:1811–1815.

160. Alkhatib G, Combadiere C, Broder CC, et al. CC CKR5: a RANTES, MIP-1alpha, MIP-1beta receptor as a fusion cofactor for macrophage-tropic HIV-1. *Science* 1996;272:1955–1958.

161. Endres MJ, Clapham PR, Marsh M, et al. CD4-independent infection by HIV-2 is mediated by fusin/CXCR4. *Cell* 1996;87:745–756.

162. Zinkernagel RM, Bachmann MF, Kundig TM, Oehen S, Pircher H, Hengartner H. On immunological memory. *Annu Rev Immunol* 1996;14:333–367.

163. Doherty PC, Topham DJ, Tripp RA, Cardin RD, Brooks JW, Stevenson PG. Effector CD4+ and CD8+ T-cell mechanisms in the control of respiratory virus infections. *Immunol Rev* 1997;159:105–117.

164. Fujinami RS, Oldstone MBA. Antibody initiates virus persistence:immune modulation and measles virus infection. In: Nokins AL, Oldstone MBA, eds. *Concepts in viral pathogenesis*. New York: Springer-Verlag, 1984:187–193.

165. Levine B, Hadwick JM, Trapp BD, Crawford TO, Bollinger RC, Griffin DE. Antibody-mediated clearance of alphavirus infection from neurons. *Science* 1991;254:856–860.

166. Dietzschold B, Kao M, Zheng YM, et al. Delineation of putative mechanisms involved in antibody-mediated clearance of rabies virus from the central nervous system. *Proc Natl Acad Sci USA* 1992;89:7252–7256.

167. Mazanec MB, Kaetzel CS, Lamm ME, Fletcher D, Nedrud JG. Intracellular neutralisation of virus by immunoglobulin A antibodies. *Proc Natl Acad Sci USA* 1992;89:6901–6905.

168. Lodmell DL, Esposito JJ, Ewalt LC. Rabies virus antinucleoprotein antibody protects against rabies virus challenge in vivo and inhibits rabies virus replication in vitro. *J Virol* 1993;67:6080–6086.

169. Springer TA. Adhesion receptors of the immune system. *Nature* 1990; 346:425–433.

170. Berke G. The binding and lysis of target cells by cytotoxic lymphocytes: molecular and cellular targets. *Annu Rev Immunol* 1994;12:735–773.

171. Kagi D, Vignaux F, Ledermann B, et al. Fas and perforin pathways as major mechanisms of T-cell mediated cytotoxicity. *Science* 1994;265:528–530.

172. Walsh CM, Matloubian M, Liu C-C, et al. Immune function in mice lacking the perforin gene. *Proc Natl Acad Sci USA* 1994;91:10854–10858.

173. Biron CA. Cytokines in the generation of immune responses to and resolution of virus infection. *Curr Opin Immunol* 1994;6:530–538.

174. Matloubian M, Concepcion RJ, Ahmed R. CD4+ T cells are required to sustain CD8+ cytotoxic T-cell responses during chronic viral infection. *J Virol* 1994; 68:8056–8063.

175. LehmanGrube F, Lohler J, Utermohlen O, Gegin C. Antiviral immune responses of lymphocytic choriomeningitis virus-infected mice lacking CD8+ T lymphocytes because of disruption of the b2-microglobulin gene. *J Virol* 1993;67: 332–339.

176. Muller D, Koller BH, Whitton JL, LaPan KE, Brigman KK, Frelinger JA. LCMV-specific, class II restricted cytotoxic T cells in b2-microglobulin-deficient mice. *Science* 1992;255:1576–1578.

177. Nagata S, Golstein P. The Fas death factor. *Science* 1995;267:1449–1456.

178. Zheng L, Fisher G, Miller RE, Peschon J, Lynch DH, Lenardo MJ. Induction of apoptosis in mature T cells by tumour necrosis factor. *Nature* 1995;377: 348–351.

179. Singer GG, Abbas AK. The fas antigen is involved in peripheral but not thymic deletion of T lymphocytes in T cell receptor transgenic mice. *Immunity* 1994;1: 365–371.

180. Lau LL, Jamieson BD, Somasundaram T, Ahmed R. Cytotoxic T-cell memory without antigen. *Nature* 1994;369:648–652.

181. Mullbacher A. The long-term maintenance of cytotoxic T cell memory does not require persistence of antigen. *J Exp Med* 1994;179:317–321.

182. Hou S, Hyland L, Ryan KW, Portner A, Doherty PC. Virus-specific CD8+ T-cell memory determined by clonal burst size. *Nature* 1994;369:652–654.

183. Murali-Krishna K, Altman JD, Suresh M, et al. Counting antigen-specific CD8 T cells: a reevaluation of bystander activation during viral infection. *Immunity* 1998;8:177–187.

184. Koup RA, Safrit JT, Cao Y, et al. Temporal association of cellular immune responses with the initial control of viremia in primary human immunodeficiency virus type 1 syndrome. *J Virol* 1994;68:4650–4655.

185. Pantaleo G, Graziosi C, Fauci AS. Virologic and immunologic events in primary HIV infection. *Springer Semin Immunopathol* 1997;18:257–266.

186. Griffin DE. Immune responses during measles virus infection. *Curr Top Microbiol Immunol* 1995;191:117–134.

187. Callan MF, Steven N, Krausa P, et al. Large clonal expansions of CD8+ T cells in acute infectious mononucleosis. *Nat Med* 1996;2:906–911.

188. Oldstone MB. Virus-lymphoid cell interactions. *Proc Natl Acad Sci USA* 1996;93:12756–12758.

189. Wills MR, Carmichael AJ, Mynard K, Jin X, et al. The human cytotoxic T-lymphocyte (CTL) response to cytomegalovirus is dominated by structural protein pp65: frequency, specificity, and T-cell receptor usage of pp65-specific CTL. *J Virol* 1996;70:7569–7579.

190. Borrow P, Lewicki H, Wei X, et al. Antiviral pressure exerted by HIV-1-specific cytotoxic T lymphocytes (CTLs) during primary infection demonstrated by rapid selection of CTL escape virus. *Nat Med* 1997;3:205–211.

191. Steven NM, Annels NE, Kumar A, Leese AM, Kurilla MG, Rickinson AB. Immediate early and early lytic cycle proteins are frequent targets of the Epstein-Barr virus-induced cytotoxic T cell response. *J Exp Med* 1997;185:1605–1617.

192. Sunil-Chandra NP, Arno J, Fazakerley J, Nash AA. Lymphoproliferative disease in mice infected with murine gammaherpesvirus 68. *Am J Pathol* 1994;145: 818–826.

193. Bi Z, Barna M, Komatsu T, Reiss CS. Vesicular stomatitis virus infection of the central nervous system activates both innate and acquired immunity. *J Virol* 1995;69:6466–6472.

194. Cousens LP, Orange JS, Biron CA. Endogenous IL-2 contributes to T cell expansion and IFN-γ production during lymphocytic choriomeningitis virus infection. *J Immunol* 1995;155:5690–5699.

195. Murata K, Garcia-Sastre A, Tsuji M, et al. Characterization of in vivo primary and secondary CD8+ T cell responses induced by recombinant influenza and vaccinia viruses. *Cell Immunol* 1996;173:96–107.

196. Selin LK, Vergilis K, Welsh RM, Nahill SR. Reduction of otherwise remarkably stable virus-specific cytotoxic T lymphocyte memory by heterologous viral infections. *J Exp Med* 1996;183:2489–2499.

197. Doherty PC, Tripp RA, Hamilton-Easton AM, Cardin RD, Woodland DL, Blackman MA. Tuning into immunological dissonance: an experimental model for infectious mononucleosis. *Curr Opin Immunol* 1997;9:477–483.

198. Slifka MK, Whitmire JK, Ahmed R. Bone marrow contains virus-specific cytotoxic T lymphocytes. *Blood* 1997;90:2103–2108.

199. Biron CA, Pederson KF, Welsh RM. Aberrant T cells in beige mutant mice. *J Immunol* 1987;138:2050–2056.

200. Nahill SR, Welsh RM. High frequency of cross-reactive cytotoxic T lymphocytes elicited during the virus-induced polyclonal cytotoxic T lymphocyte response. *J Exp Med* 1993;177:317–327.

201. Razvi ES, Welsh RM, McFarland HI. In vivo state of antiviral CTL precursors. Characterization of a cycling cell population containing CTL precursors in immune mice. *J Immunol* 1995;154:620–632.

202. Ehl S, Hombach J, Aichele P, Hengartner H, Zinkernagel RM. Bystander activation of cytotoxic T cells: studies on the mechanism and evaluation of in vivo significance in a transgenic mouse model. *J Exp Med* 1997;185:1241–1251.

203. Zarozinski CC, Welsh RM. Minimal bystander activation of CD8 T cells during the virus-induced polyclonal T cell response. *J Exp Med* 1997;185:1629–1639.

204. Altman JD, Moss PAH, Goulder PJR, et al. Phenotypic analysis of antigen-specific T lymphocytes. *Science* 1996;274:94–96.

205. Butz EA, Bevan MJ. Massive expansion of antigen-specific CD8+ cells during an acute virus infection. *Immunity* 1998;8:167–175.

206. Utz U, Banks D, Jacobson S, Biddison WE. Analysis of the T-cell receptor repertoire of human T-cell leukemia virus type 1 (HTLV-1) Tax-specific CD8+ cytotoxic T lymphocytes from patients with HTLV-1-associated disease: evidence for oligoclonal expansion. *J Virol* 1996;70:843–851.

207. Cose SC, Jones CM, Wallace ME, Heath WR, Carbone FR. Antigen-specific CD8+ T cell subset distribution in lymph nodes draining the site of herpes simplex virus infection. *Eur J Immunol* 1997;27:2310–2316.

208. Feltkamp MC, Vreugdenhil GR, Vierboom MP, et al. Cytotoxic T lymphocytes raised against a subdominant epitope offered as a synthetic peptide eradicate human papillomavirus type 16-induced tumors. *Eur J Immunol* 1995;25: 2638–2642.

209. Jameson SC, Bevan MJ. Dissection of major histocompatibility complex (MHC) and T cell receptor contact residues in a Kb-restricted ovalbumin peptide and an assessment of the predictive power of MHC-binding motifs. *Eur J Immunol* 1992;22:2663–2667.

210. Oukka M, Riche N, Kosmatopoulos K. A nonimmunodominant nucleoprotein-derived peptide is presented by influenza A virus-infected H-2b cells. *J Immunol* 1994;152:4843–4851.

211. van der Most RG, Murali-Krishna K, Whitton JL, et al. Identification of Db- and Kb-restricted subdominant cytotoxic T-cell responses in lymphocytic choriomeningitis virus-infected mice. *Virology* 1998;240:158–167.

212. Vitiello A, Yuan L, Chesnut RW, et al. Immunodominance analysis of CTL responses to influenza PR8 virus reveals two new dominant and subdominant Kb-restricted epitopes. *J Immunol* 1996;157:5555–5562.

213. Falk K, Rotzschke O, Stevanovic S, Jung G, Rammensee HG. Allele-specific

motifs revealed by sequencing of self-peptides eluted from MHC molecules. *Nature* 1991;351:290–296.

214. Rotzschke O, Falk K, Deres K, et al. Isolation and analysis of naturally processed viral peptides as recognized by cytotoxic T cells. *Nature* 1990;348:252–254.

215. Corr M, Boyd LF, Padlan EA, Margulies DH. H-2Dd exploits a four residue peptide binding motif. *J Exp Med* 1993;178:1877–1892.

216. Rammensee HG, Friede T, Stevanoviic S. MHC ligands and peptide motifs: first listing. *Immunogenetics* 1995;41:178–228.

217. Barber LD, Parham P. The essence of epitopes. *J Exp Med* 1994;180:1191–1194.

218. Sette A, Vitiello A, Reherman B, et al. The relationship between class I binding affinity and immunogenicity of potential cytotoxic T cell epitopes. *J Immunol* 1994;153:5586–5592.

219. Feltkamp MC, Vierboom MP, Kast WM, Melief CJ. Efficient MHC class I-peptide binding is required but does not ensure MHC class I-restricted immunogenicity. *Mol Immunol* 1994;31:1391–1401.

220. Chen W, Khilko S, Fecondo J, Margulies DH, McCluskey J. Determinant selection of major histocompatibility complex class I-restricted antigenic peptides is explained by class I-peptide affinity and is strongly influenced by nondominant anchor residues. *J Exp Med* 1994;180:1471–1483.

221. Ruppert J, Sidney J, Celis E, Kubo RT, Grey HM, Sette A. Prominent role of secondary anchor residues in peptide binding to HLA-A2.1 molecules. *Cell* 1993; 74:929–937.

222. Sadovnikova E, Zhu X, Collins SM, et al. Limitations of predictive motifs revealed by cytotoxic T lymphocyte epitope mapping of the human papilloma virus E7 protein. *Int Immunol* 1994;6:289–296.

223. van der Most RG, Sette A, Oseroff C, et al. Analysis of cytotoxic T cell responses to dominant and subdominant epitopes during acute and chronic lymphocytic choriomeningitis virus infection. *J Immunol* 1996;157:5543–5554.

224. Clark WR, Walsh CM, Glass AA, Hayashi F, Matloubian M, Ahmed R. Molecular pathways of CTL-mediated cytotoxicity. *Immunol Rev* 1995;146:33–44.

225. Kägi D, Ledermann B, Burki K, Zinkernagel RM, Hengartner H. Molecular mechanisms of lymphocyte-mediated cytotoxicity and their role in immunological protection and pathogenesis in vivo. *Annu Rev Immunol* 1996;14:207–232.

226. Liu C, Walsh CM, Young JD. Perforin: structure and function. *Immunol Today* 1995;16:194–201.

227. Di Virgilio F, Pizzo P, Zanovello P, Bronte V, Collavo D. Extracellular ATP as a possible mediator of cell-mediated cytotoxicity. *Immunol Today* 1990;11: 274–276.

228. Filipini A, Traffs RA, Sitovsky MV. Extracellular ATP in T-lymphocyte activation: possible role in effector functions. *Proc Natl Acad Sci USA* 1990;87: 8267–8271.

229. Tian Q, Streuli M, Saito H, Schlossman SF, Anderson P. A polyadenylate binding protein localized to the granules of cytolytic lymphocytes induces DNA fragmentation in target cells. *Cell* 1991;67:629–639.

230. Heusel JW, Wesselschmidt RL, Shresta S, Russell JH, Ley TJ. Cytotoxic lymphocytes require granzyme B for the rapid induction of DNA fragmentation and apoptosis in allogeneic target cells. *Cell* 1994;76:977–987.

231. Shresta S, Heusel JW, Macivor DM, Wesselschmidt RL, Russell JH, Ley TJ. Granzyme B plays a critical role in cytotoxic lymphocyte induced apoptosis. *Immunol Rev* 1995;146:211–221.

232. Lenardo MJ. Fas and the art of lymphocyte maintenance. *J Exp Med* 1996;183: 721–724.

233. Lynch DH, Ramsdell F, Alderson MR. Fas and FasL in the homeostatic regulation of immune responses. *Immunol Today* 1995;16:569–574.

234. Henkart PA. ICE family proteases: mediators of all apoptotic death? *Immunity* 1996;4:195–201.

235. Hyland L, Sangster M, Sealy R, Coleclough C. Respiratory virus infection of mice provokes a permanent humoral immune response. *J Virol* 1994;68: 6083–6086.

236. Chisari FV. Hepatitis B virus transgenic mice: models of viral immunobiology and pathogenesis. *Curr Top Microbiol Immunol* 1996;206:149–173.

237. Guidotti LG, Ishikawa T, Hobbs MV, Matzke B, Schreiber R, Chisari FV. Intracellular inactivation of the hepatitis B virus by cytotoxic T lymphocytes. *Immunity* 1996;4:25–36.

238. Chisari FV, Klopchin K, Moriyama T, et al. Molecular pathogenesis of hepatocellular carcinoma in hepatitis B virus transgenic mice. *Cell* 1989;59:1145–1156.

239. Zinkernagel RM. Immunology taught by viruses. *Science* 1996;271:173–178

240. Belyakov IM, Derby MA, Ahlers JD, et al. Mucosal immunization with HIV-1 peptide vaccine induces mucosal and systemic cytotoxic T lymphocytes and protective immunity in mice against intrarectal recombinant HIV-vaccinia challenge. *Proc Natl Acad Sci USA* 1998;95:1709–1714.

241. Koszinowski UH, Reddehase MJ, Jonjic S. The role of CD4 and CD8 T cells in viral infections. *Curr Opin Immunol* 1991;3:471–475.

242. von Herrath MG, Oldstone MB. Interferon-gamma is essential for destruction of beta cells and development of insulin-dependent diabetes mellitus. *J Exp Med* 1997;185:531–539.

243. Ghiasi H, Cai S, Nesburn AB, Wechsler SL. MIIC-II but not MHC-I responses are required for vaccine induced protection against ocular challenge with HSV-1. *Curr Eye Res* 1997;16:1152–1158.

244. Thomsen AR, Johansen J, Marker O, Christensen JP. Exhaustion of CTL memory and recrudescence of viremia in lymphocytic choriomeningitis virus-infected MHC class II-deficient mice and B cell-deficient mice. *J Immunol* 1996;157:3074–3080.

245. Christensen JP, Marker O, Thomsen AR. The role of CD4+ T cells in cell-mediated immunity to LCMV: studies in MHC class I and class II deficient mice. *Scand J Immunol* 1994;40:373–382.

246. McMichael AJ, Phillips RE. Escape of human immunodeficiency virus from immune control. *Annu Rev Immunol* 1997;15:271–296.

247. Perelson AS, Essunger P, Ho DD. Dynamics of HIV-1 and CD4+ lymphocytes in vivo. *AIDS* 1997;11:S17–S24.

248. Ahmed R, Butler LD, Bhatti L. T4+ T helper cell function in vivo: differential requirement for induction of antiviral cytotoxic T-cell and antibody responses. *J Virol* 1988;62:2102–2106.

249. Cardin RD, Brooks JW, Sarawar SR, Doherty PC. Progressive loss of CD8+ T cell-mediated control of a gamma-herpesvirus in the absence of CD4+ T cells. *J Exp Med* 1996;184:863–871.

250. Graham MB, Braciale TJ. Resistance to and recovery from lethal influenza virus infection in B lymphocyte-deficient mice. *J Exp Med* 1997;186:2063–2068.

251. Cohen J. T cell shift: key to AIDS therapy? *Science* 1993;262:175–176.

252. Fujimura T, Yamanashi R, Masuzawa M, et al. Conversion of the CD4+ T cell profile from T(H2)-dominant type to T(H1)-dominant type after varicella-zoster virus infection in atopic dermatitis. *J Allergy Clin Immunol* 1997;100:274–282.

253. Wasik TJ, Jagodzinski PP, Hyjek EM, et al. Diminished HIV-specific CTL activity is associated with lower type 1 and enhanced type 2 responses to HIV-specific peptides during perinatal HIV infection. *J Immunol* 1997;158:6029–6036.

254. Alonso K, Pontiggia P, Medenica R, Rizzo S. Cytokine patterns in adults with AIDS. *Immunol Invest* 1997;26:341–350.

255. Peterson JD, Waltenbaugh C, Miller SD. IgG subclass responses to Theiler's murine encephalomyelitis virus infection and immunization suggest a dominant role for Th1 cells in susceptible mouse strains. *Immunology* 1992;75:652–658.

256. Doherty PC. Virus infections in mice with targeted gene disruptions. *Curr Opin Immunol* 1993;5:479–483.

257. Rosenberg ES, Billingsley JM, Caliendo AM, et al. Vigorous HIV-1-specific CD4+ T cell responses associated with control of viremia. *Science* 1997;278:1447–1450.

258. Saha K, Wong PK. Protective role of cytotoxic lymphocytes against murine leukemia virus-induced neurologic disease and immunodeficiency is enhanced by the presence of helper T cells. *Virology* 1992;188:921–925.

259. Viola A, Lanzavecchia A. T cell activation determined by T cell receptor number and tunable thresholds. *Science* 1996;273:104–106.

260. Sebzda E, Choi M, Fung-Leung WP, Mak TW, Ohashi PS. Peptide-induced positive selection of TCR transgenic thymocytes in a coreceptor-independent manner. *Immunity* 1997;6:643–653.

261. Akbar AN, Salmon M. Cellular environments and apoptosis: tissue microenvironments control activated T cell death. *Immunol Today* 1997;18:72–76.

262. Wodarz D, Klenerman P, Nowak MA. Dynamics of cytotoxic T-lymphocyte exhaustion. *Proc R Soc Lond B Biol Sci* 1998;265:191–203.

263. Moskophidis D, Lechner F, Pircher H, Zinkernagel RM. Virus persistence in acutely infected immunocompetent mice by exhaustion of antiviral cytotoxic effector T cells. *Nature* 1993;362:758–761.

264. Doherty PC, Topham DJ, Tripp RA. Establishment and persistence of virus-specific CD4+ and CD8+ T cell memory. *Immunol Rev* 1996;150:23–44.

265. Topham DJ, Tripp RA, Hamilton-Easton AM, Sarawar SR, Doherty PC. Quantitative analysis of the influenza virus-specific CD4+ T cell memory in the absence of B cells and Ig. *J Immunol* 1996;157:2947–2952.

266. Ewing C, Topham DJ, Doherty PC. Prevalence and activation phenotype of Sendai virus-specific CD4+ T cells. *Virology* 1995;210:179–185.

267. Mozdzanowska K, Furchner M, Maiese K, Gerhard W. CD4+ T cells are ineffective in clearing a pulmonary infection with influenza type A virus in the absence of B cells. *Virology* 1997;239:217–225.

268. Bachmann MF, Kalinke U, Althage A, et al. The role of antibody concentration and avidity in antiviral protection. *Science* 1997;276:2024–2027.

269. Topham DJ, Doherty PC. Clearance of an influenza A virus by CD4+ T cells is inefficient in the absence of B cells. *J Virol* 1998;72:882–885.

270. Farzadegan H. HIV-1 antibodies and serology. *Clin Lab Med* 1994;14:257–269.

271. Kent KA. Neutralising epitopes of simian immunodeficiency virus envelope glycoprotein. *J Med Primatol* 1995;24:145–149.

272. Buchmeier MJ, Welsh RM, Dutko FJ, Oldstone MBA. The virology and immunobiology of lymphocytic choriomeningitis virus infection. *Adv Immunol* 1980;30:275–331.

273. Bielefeldt-Ohmann H. Pathogenesis of dengue virus diseases: missing pieces in the jigsaw. *Trends Microbiol* 1997;5:409–413.

274. Morens DM. Antibody-dependent enhancement of infection and the pathogenesis of viral disease. *Clin Infect Dis* 1994;19:500–512.

275. Osiowy C, Horne D, Anderson R. Antibody-dependent enhancement of respiratory syncytial virus infection by sera from young infants. *Clin Diagn Lab Immunol* 1994;1:670–677.

276. Gimenez HB, Chisholm S, Dornan J, Cash P. Neutralizing and enhancing activities of human respiratory syncytial virus-specific antibodies. *Clin Diagn Lab Immunol* 1996;3:280–286.

277. Szomolanyi-Tsuda E, Welsh RM. T cell-independent antibody-mediated clearance of polyoma virus in T cell-deficient mice. *J Exp Med* 1996;183:403–411.

278. Mond JJ, Lees A, Snapper CM. T cell-independent antigens type 2. *Annu Rev Immunol* 1995;13:655–692.

279. Coutelier JP, Coulie PG, Wauters P, Heremans H, van der Logt JT. In vivo polyclonal B-lymphocyte activation elicited by murine viruses. *J Virol* 1990; 64:5383–5388.

280. Maloy KJ, Odermatt B, Hengartner H, Zinkernagel RM. Interferon gamma-producing gammadelta T cell-dependent antibody isotype switching in the absence of germinal center formation during virus infection. *Proc Natl Acad Sci USA* 1998;95:1160–1165.

281. Sarawar SR, Sangster M, Coffman RL, Doherty PC. Administration of anti-IFN-gamma antibody to beta 2-microglobulin-deficient mice delays influenza virus clearance but does not switch the response to a T helper cell 2 phenotype. *J Immunol* 1994;153:1246–1253.

282. Abney ER, Cooper MD, Kearney JF, Lawton AR, Parkhouse RM. Sequential expression of immunoglobulin on developing mouse B lymphocytes: a systematic survey that suggests a model for the generation of immunoglobulin isotype diversity. *J Immunol* 1978;120:2041–2049.

283. Halper J, Fu SM, Wang CY, Winchester R, Kunkel HG. Patterns of expression of human "Ia-like" antigens during the terminal stages of B cell development. *J Immunol* 1978;120:1480–1484.

284. Helmreich E, Kern M, Eisen HN, The secretion of antibody by isolated lymph node cells. *J Biol Chem* 1961;236:464–473.

285. Hibi T, Dosch HM. Limiting dilution analysis of the B cell compartment in human bone marrow. *Eur J Immunol* 1986;16:139–145.

286. Hyland L, Sangster M, Sealy R, Coleclough C. Respiratory virus infection of mice provokes a permanent humoral immune response. *J Virol* 1994;68: 6083–6086.

287. Slifka MK, Antia R, Whitmire JK, Ahmed R. Humoral immunity due to long lived plasma cells. *Immunity* 1998;8:177–187.

288. Manz RA, Thiel A, Radbruch A. Lifetime of plasma cells in the bone marrow. *Nature* 1997;388:133–134.

289. Manetti R, Parronchi P, Giudizi MG, et al. Natural killer cell stimulatory factor (interleukin 12 [IL-12]) induces T helper type 1 (Th1)-specific immune responses and inhibits the development of IL-4 producing Th cells. *J Exp Med* 1993;177:1199–1204.

290. Seder RA, Gazzinelli R, Sher A, Paul WE. IL-12 acts directly on CD4+ T cells to enhance priming for IFN-γ production and diminishes IL-4 inhibition of such priming. *Proc Natl Acad Sci USA* 1993;90:10188–10192.

291. Orange JS, Wolf SF, Biron CA. Effects of IL-12 on the response and susceptibility to experimental viral infections. *J Immunol* 1994;152:1253–1264.

292. Orange JS, Salazar-Mather TP, Opal SM, et al. Mechanism of interleukin 12-mediated toxicities during experimental viral infections: role of tumor necrosis factor and glucocorticoids. *J Exp Med* 1995;181:901–914.

293. Brinkmann V, Geiger T, Alkan S, Heusser CH. Interferon alpha increases the frequency of interferon gamma-producing human CD4+ T cells. *J Exp Med* 1993; 178:1655–1663.

294. Biron CA, Young HA, Kasaian MT. Interleukin 2-induced proliferation of murine natural killer cells in vivo. *J Exp Med* 1990;171:173–188.

295. Kasaian MT, Biron CA. Effects of cyclosporin A on IL-2 production and lymphocyte proliferation during infection of mice with lymphocytic choriomeningitis virus. *J Immunol* 1990;144:299–306.

296. Caligiuri MA, Zmuidzinas A, Manley TJ, Levine H, Smith KA, Ritz J. Functional consequences of interleukin 2 receptor expression on resting human lymphocytes. Identification of a novel natural killer cell subset with high affinity receptors. *J Exp Med* 1990;171:1509–1526.

297. Kasaian MT, Biron CA. The activation of IL-2 transcription in L3T4+ and Lyt-2+ lymphocytes during virus infection *in vivo. J Immunol* 1989;142:1287–1292.

298. Su HC, Orange JS, Fast LD, et al. IL-2-dependent NK cell responses discovered in virus-infected beta 2-microglobulin-deficient mice. *J Immunol* 1994;153: 5674–5681.

299. Bellone G, Aste-Amezaga M, Trinchieri G, Rodeck U. Regulation of NK cell functions by TGF-β1. *J Immunol* 1995;155:1066–1073.

300. Hunter CA, Bermudez L, Beernink H, Waegell W, Remington JS. Transforming growth factor-beta inhibits interleukin-12-induced production of interferon-gamma by natural killer cells: a role for transforming growth factor-beta in the regulation of T cell-independent resistance to Toxoplasma gondii. *Eur J Immunol* 1995;25:994–1000.

301. Rook AH, Kehrl JH, Wakefield LM, et al. Effects of transforming growth factor beta on the functions of natural killer cells: depressed cytolytic activity and blunting of interferon responsiveness. *J Immunol* 1986;136:3916–3920.

302. Migliorati G, Cannarile L, Herberman RB, Riccardi C. Effect of various cytokines and growth factors on the interleukin-2-dependent in vitro differentiation of natural killer cells from bone marrow. *Nat Immun Cell Growth Regul* 1989;8:48–55.

303. Ortaldo JR, Mason AT, O'Shea JJ, et al. Mechanistic studies of transforming growth factor-beta inhibition of IL-2-dependent activation of CD3– large granular lymphocyte functions. Regulation of IL-2R beta (p75) signal transduction. *J Immunol* 1991;146:3791–3798.

304. Scharton-Kersten T, Afonso LC, Wysocka M, Trinchieri G, Scott P. IL-12 is required for natural killer cell activation and subsequent T helper 1 cell development in experimental leishmaniasis. *J Immunol* 1995;154:5320–5330.

305. Su HC, Leite-Morris KA, Braun L, Biron CA. A role for transforming growth factor-β1 in regulating natural killer cell and T lymphocyte proliferative responses during acute infection with lymphocytic choriomeningitis virus. *J Immunol* 1991;147:2717–2727.

306. Graziosi C, Pantaleo G, Gantt KR, et al. Lack of evidence for the dichotomy of TH1 and TH2 predominance in HIV-infected individuals. *Science* 1994;265: 248–252.

307. Niemialtowski MG, Rouse BT. Predominance of Th1 cells in ocular tissues during herpetic stromal keratitis. *J Immunol* 1992;149:3035–3039.

308. Sarawar SR, Doherty PC. Concurrent production of interleukin-2, interleukin-10, and gamma interferon in the regional lymph nodes of mice with influenza pneumonia. *J Virol* 1994;68:3112–3119.

309. Su HC, Cousens LP, Fast LD, et al. CD4+ and CD8+ T cell interactions in IFN-γ and IL-4 responses to viral infections: requirements for IL-2. *J Immunol* 1998; 160:5007–5017.

310. Hussell T, Spender LC, Georgiou A, O'Garra A, Openshaw PJ. Th1 and Th2 cytokine induction in pulmonary T cells during infection with respiratory syncytial virus. *J Gen Virol* 1996;77:2447–2455.

311. Wesselingh SL, Levine B, Fox RJ, Choi S, Griffin DE. Intracerebral cytokine mRNA expression during fatal and nonfatal alphavirus encephalitis suggests a predominant type 2 T cell response. *J Immunol* 1994;152:1289–1297.

312. Maggi E, Manetti R, Annunziato F, et al. Functional characterization and modulation of cytokine production by CD8+ T cells from human immunodeficiency virus-infected individuals. *Blood* 1997;89:3672–3681.

313. Romagnani S, Del-Prete G, Manetti R, et al. Role of TH1/TH2 cytokines in HIV infection. *Immunol Rev* 1994;140:73–92.

314. Graham MB, Dalton DK, Giltinan D, Braciale VL, Stewart TA, Braciale TJ. Response to influenza infection in mice with a targeted disruption in the interferon gamma gene. *J Exp Med* 1993;178:1725–1732.

315. Huang S, Hendriks W, Althage A, et al. Immune response in mice that lack the interferon-γ receptor. *Science* 1993;259:1742–1745.

316. Carding SR, Allan W, McMickle A, Doherty PC. Activation of cytokine genes in T cells during primary and secondary murine influenza pneumonia. *J Exp Med* 1993;177:475–482.

317. Gessner A, Moskophidis D, Lehmann-Grube F. Enumeration of single IFN-γ producing cells in mice during viral and bacterial infection. *J Immunol* 1989;142:1293–1298.

318. Kasaian MT, Leite-Morris KA, Biron CA. The role of CD4+ cells in sustaining lymphocyte proliferation during lymphocytic choriomenigitis virus infection. *J Immunol* 1991;146:1955–1963.

319. Rahemtulla A, Fung-Leung WP, Schilham MW, et al. Normal development and function of CD8+ cells but markedly decreased helper cell activity in mice lacking CD4. *Nature* 1991;353:180–184.

320. Asano MS, Ahmed R. CD8 T cell memory in B cell-deficient mice. *J Exp Med* 1996;183:2165–2174.

321. Kündig TM, Schorle H, Bachmann MF, Hengartner H, Zinkernagel RM, Horak I. Immune responses in interleukin-2-deficient mice. *Science* 1993;262: 1059–1061.

322. Bachmann MF, Schorle H, Kuhn R, et al. Antiviral immune responses in mice deficient for both interleukin-2 and interleukin-4. *J Virol* 1995;69:4842–4846.

323. Garofalo R, Kimpen JL, Welliver RC, Ogra PL. Eosinophil degranulation in the respiratory tract during naturally acquired respiratory syncytial virus infection. *J Pediatr* 1992;120:28–32.

324. Alwan WH, Kozlowska WJ, Openshaw PJ. Distinct types of lung disease caused by functional subsets of antiviral T cells. *J Exp Med* 1994;179:81–89.

325. Hancock GE, Speelman DJ, Heers K, Bortell E, Smith J, Cosco C. Generation of atypical pulmonary inflammatory responses in BALB/c mice after immunization with the native attachment (G) glycoprotein of respiratory syncytial virus. *J Virol* 1996;70:7783–7791.

326. Srikiatkhachorn A, Braciale TJ. Virus-specific CD8+ T lymphocytes downregulate T helper cell type 2 cytokine secretion and pulmonary eosinophilia during experimental murine respiratory syncytial virus infection. *J Exp Med* 1997; 186:421–432.

327. Waris ME, Tsou C, Erdman DD, Zaki SR, Anderson LJ. Respiratory synctial virus infection in BALB/c mice previously immunized with formalin-inactivated virus induces enhanced pulmonary inflammatory response with a predominant Th2-like cytokine pattern. *J Virol* 1996;70:2852–2860.

328. Openshaw PJ, Clarke SL, Record FM. Pulmonary eosinophilic response to respiratory syncytial virus infection in mice sensitized to the major surface glycoprotein G. *Int Immunol* 1992;4:493–500.

329. Graham BS. Pathogenesis of respiratory syncytial virus vaccine-augmented pathology. *Am J Respir Crit Care Med* 1995;152:S63–S66.

330. Srikiatkhachorn A, Braciale TJ. Virus-specific CD8+ T lymphocytes downregulate T helper cell type 2 cytokine secretion and pulmonary eosinophilia during experimental murine respiratory syncytial virus infection. *J Exp Med* 1997a; 186:421–432.

331. Borrow P, Tishon A, Lee S, et al. CD40L-deficient mice show deficits in antiviral immunity and have an impaired memory CD8+ CTL response. *J Exp Med* 1996;183:2129–2142.

332. Oxenius A, Campbell KA, Maliszewski CR, et al. CD40-CD40 ligand interactions are critical in T-B cooperation but not for other anti-viral CD4+ T cell functions. *J Exp Med* 1996;183:2209–2218.

333. Yang Y, Su Q, Grewal IS, Schilz R, Flavell RA, Wilson JM. Transient subversion of CD40 ligand function diminishes immune responses to adenovirus vectors in mouse liver and lung tissues. *J Virol* 1996;70:6370.

334. Whitmire JK, Slifka MK, Grewal IS, Flavell RA, Ahmed R. CD40 ligand-deficient mice generate a normal primary cytotoxic T-lymphocyte response but a defective humoral response to a viral infection. *J Virol* 1996;70:8375–8381.

335. Planz O, Seiler P, Hengartner H, Zinkernagel RM. Specific cytotoxic T cells eliminate cells producing neutralizing antibodies. *Nature* 1996;382:726–729.

336. Lalvani A, Brookes R, Hambleton S, Britton WJ, Hill AV, McMichael AJ. Rapid effector function in CD8+ memory T cells. *J Exp Med* 1997;186:859–865.

337. Pihlgren M, Dubois PM, Tomkowiak M, Sjogren T, Marvel J. Resting memory CD8+ T cells are hyperreactive to antigenic challenge in vitro. *J Exp Med* 1996;184:2141–2151.

338. McHeyzer-Williams MG, Davis MM. Antigen-specific development of primary and memory T cells in vivo. *Science* 1995;268:106–111.

339. Morimoto C, Schlossman SF. P. Rambotti lecture. Human naive and memory T cells revisited: new markers (CD31 and CD27) that help define CD4+ T cell subsets. *Clin Exp Rheumatol* 1993;11:241–247.

340. Mitchison A, Sieper J. Immunological basis of oral tolerance. *Z Rheumatol* 1995;54:141–144.

341. Pape KA, Kearney ER, Khoruts A, et al. Use of adoptive transfer of T-cell-antigen-receptor-transgenic T cell for the study of T-cell activation in vivo. *Immunol Rev* 1997;156:67–78.

342. Ingulli E, Mondino A, Khoruts A, Jenkins MK. In vivo detection of dendritic cell antigen presentation to CD4(+) T cells. *J Exp Med* 1997;185:2133–214.

343. Wang L, Robb CW, Cloyd MW. HIV induces homing of resting T lymphocytes to lymph nodes. *Virology* 1997;228:141–152.

344. Zimmerman C, Brduscha-Riem K, Blaser C, Zinkernagel RM, Pircher H. Visualization, characterization, and turnover of CD8+ memory T cells in virus-infected hosts. *J Exp Med* 1996;183:1367–1375.

345. Mackay CR. Immunological memory. *Adv Immunol* 1993;53:217–265.

346. Sprent J, Webb SR. Function and specificity of T cell subsets in the mouse. *Adv Immunol* 1987;41:39–133.

347. Beverley PC. Human T-cell memory. *Curr Top Microbiol Immunol* 1990;159:111–122.

348. Vitetta ES, Berton MT, Burger C, Kepron M, Lee WT, Yin XM. Memory B and T cells. *Annu Rev Immunol* 1991;9:193–217.

349. Swain SL, Bradley LM, Croft M, et al. Helper T-cell subsets: phenotype, function and the role of lymphokines in regulating their development. *Immunol Rev* 1991;123:115–144.

350. MacLennan IC. Germinal centers. *Annu Rev Immunol* 1994;12:117–139.

351. Albert ML, Sauter B, Bhardwaj N. Dendritic cells acquire antigen from apoptotic cells and induce class I-restricted CTLs. *Nature* 1998;5:392:86–89.

352. Germain RN. MHC-dependent antigen processing and peptide presentation: providing ligands for T lymphocyte activation. *Cell* 1994;76:287–299.

353. Bevan MJ. Antigen presentation to cytotoxic T lymphocytes in vivo. *J Exp Med* 1995;182:639–641.

354. Rock KL. A new foreign policy: MHC class I molecules monitor the outside world. *Immunol Today* 1996;17:131–137.

355. Shen H, Miller JF, Fan X, Kolwyck D, Ahmed R, Harty JT. Compartmentalization of bacterial antigens: differential effects on priming of CD8 T cells and protective immunity. *Cell* 1998;92:535–545.

356. Albert M, Sauter B, Bharadwaj N. Dendritic cells acquire antigen from apoptotic cells and induce class I restricted CTLs. *Nature* 1998;392:82–89.

357. Demkowicz WE Jr, Littaua RA, Wang J, Ennis FA. Human cytotoxic T-cell memory: long-lived responses to vaccinia virus. *J Virol* 1996;70:2627–2631.

358. Oehen S, Waldner H, Kundig TM, Hengartner H, Zinkernagel RM. Antivirally protective cytotoxic T cell memory to lymphocytic choriomeningitis virus is governed by persisting antigen. *J Exp Med* 1992;176:1273–1281.

359. Di Rosa F, Matzinger P. Long-lasting CD8 T cell memory in the absence of CD4 T cells or B cells. *J Exp Med* 1996;183:2153–2163.

360. Bruno L, Kirberg J, von Boehmer H. On the cellular basis of immunological T cell memory. *Immunity* 1995;2:37–43.

361. Gray D, Matzinger P. T cell memory is short-lived in the absence of antigen. *J Exp Med* 1991;174:969–974.

362. Brundler MA, Aichele P, Bachmann M, Kitamura D, Rajewsky K, Zinkernagel RM. Immunity to viruses in B cell-deficient mice: influence of antibodies on virus persistence and on T cell memory. *Eur J Immunol* 1996;26:2257–2262.

363. Rehermann B, Ferrari C, Pasquinelli C, Chisari FV. The hepatitis B virus persists for decades after patients' recovery from acute viral hepatitis despite active maintenance of a cytotoxic T-lymphocyte response. *Nat Med* 1996;2:1104–1108.

364. Penna A, Artini M, Cavalli A, et al. Long-lasting memory T cell responses following self-limited acute hepatitis B. *J Clin Invest* 1996;98:1185–1194.

365. Talbot PJ, Buchmeier MJ. Catabolism of homologous murine monoclonal hybridoma IgG antibodies in mice. *Immunology* 1987;60:485–489.

366. Vieira P, Rajewsky K. The half lives of serum immunoglobulins in adult mice. *Eur J Immunol* 1988;18:313–316.

367. Kulkarni AB, Connors M, Firestone CY, Morse HC III, Murphy BR. The cytolytic activity of pulmonary CD8+ lymphocytes, induced by infection with a vaccinia virus recombinant expressing the M2 protein of respiratory syncytial virus (RSV), correlates with resistance to RSV infection in mice. *J Virol* 1993;67:1044–1049.

368. Franco MA, Greenberg H. Immunity to rotavirus in T cell deficient mice. *Virology* 1997;238:169–179.

369. von Herrath MG, Homann D, Gairin JE, Oldstone MB. Pathogenesis and treatment of virus-induced autoimmune diabetes: novel insights gained from the RIP-LCMV transgenic mouse model. *Biochem Soc Trans* 1997;25:630–635.

370. Aichele P, Bachmann MF, Hengartner H, Zinkernagel RM. Immunopathology or organ-specific autoimmunity as a consequence of virus infection. *Immunol Rev* 1996;152:21–45.

371. Zinkernagel RM. Immune protection vs. immunopathology vs. autoimmunity: a question of balance and of knowledge. *Brain Pathol* 1993;3:115–121.

372. Oldstone MB. Virus neutralization and virus-induced immune complex disease. Virus-antibody union resulting in immunoprotection or immunologic injury—two sides of the same coin. *Prog Med Virol* 1975;19:84–119.

373. Oldstone MB, Tishon A, Buchmeier MJ. Virus-induced immune complex disease: genetic control of C1q binding complexes in the circulation of mice persistently infected with lymphocytic choriomeningitis virus. *J Immunol* 1983;130:912–918.

374. Rall GF, Mucke L, Oldstone MB. Consequences of cytotoxic T lymphocyte interaction with major histocompatibility complex class I-expressing neurons in vivo. *J Exp Med* 1995;182:1201–1212.

375. Asano MS, Ahmed R. Immune conflicts in lymphocytic choriomeningitis virus. *Springer Semin Immunopathol* 1995;17:247–259.

376. Ferrari C, Penna A, Bertoletti A, et al. Immune pathogenesis of hepatitis B. *Arch Virol* 1992;4:11–18.

377. Eddleston AL. Virus- and immune-mediated liver damage in hepatitis. *Intervirology* 1993;35:122–132.

378. Zinkernagel RM. Are HIV-specific CTL responses salutary or pathogenic? *Curr Opin Immunol* 1995;7:462–470.

379. Miedema F. Immunological abnormalities in the natural history of HIV infection: mechanisms and clinical relevance. *Immunodefic Rev* 1992;3:173–193.

380. Ho DD. Viral counts count in HIV infection. *Science* 1996;272:1124–1125.

381. Gutierrez-Ramos JC, Bluethmann H. Molecules and mechanisms operating in septic shock: lessons from knockout mice. *Immunol Today* 1997;18:329–334.

382. Marrack P, Kappler J. The staphylococcal enterotoxins and their relatives. *Science* 1990;248:705–711.

383. Orange JS, Salazar-Mather TP, Opal SM, Biron CA. Mechanisms for virus-induced liver disease: tumor necrosis factor-mediated pathology independent of natural killer and T cells during murine cytomegalovirus infection. *J Virol* 1997;71:9248–9258.

384. Ding JW, Ning Q, Liu MF, et al. Fulminant hepatic failure in murine hepatitis virus strain 3 infection: tissue-specific expression of a novel fgl2 prothrombinase. *J Virol* 1997;71:9223–9230.

385. Levy GA, Leibowitz JL, Edgington TS. Induction of monocyte procoagulant activity by murine hepatitis virus type 3 parallels disease susceptibility in mice. *J Exp Med* 1981;154:1150–1163.

386. Li C, Fung LS, Chung S, et al. Monoclonal antiprothrombinase (3D4.3) prevents mortality from murine hepatitis virus (MHV-3) infection. *J Exp Med* 1992;176:689–697.

387. Kurane I, Innis BL, Nimmannitya S, et al. Activation of T lymphocytes in dengue virus infections. High levels of soluble interleukin 2 receptor, soluble CD4, soluble CD8, interleukin 2, and interferon-γ in sera of children with dengue. *J Clin Invest* 1991;88:1473–1480.

388. Kurane I, Rothman AL, Livingston PG, et al. Immunopathologic mechanisms of dengue hemorrhagic fever and dengue shock syndrome. *Arch Virol Suppl* 1994;9:59–64.

389. Stevens JG. Human herpesviruses: a consideration of the latent state. *Microbiol Rev* 1989;53:318–332.

390. Stevens JG. Overview of herpesvirus latency. *Semin Virol* 1994;5:191–196.

391. Barker CF, Billingham RE. Immunologically privileged sites. *Adv Immunol* 1977;25:1–54.

392. Ahmed R, Jamieson BD, Porter DD. Immune therapy of a persistent and disseminated viral infection. *J Virol* 1987;61:3920.

393. Joly E, Mucke L, Oldstone MB. Viral persistence in neuron explained by lack of major histocompatibility class I expression. *Science* 1991;253:1283–1285.

394. Jamieson BD, Butler LD, Ahmed R. Effective clearance of a persistent viral infection requires cooperation between virus-specific Lyt2+ T cells and nonspecific bone marrow-derived cells. *J Virol* 1987;61:3930–3937.

395. Oldstone MBA, Blount P, Southern P. Cytoimmunotherapy for persistent virus infection reveals a unique clearance pattern from the central nervous system. *Nature* 1986;321:239–243.

396. Jamieson BD, Somasundaram T, Ahmed R. Abrogation of tolerance to a chronic viral infection. *J Immunol* 1991;147:3521–3529.

397. Butler JC, Peters CJ. Hantaviruses and hantavirus pulmonary syndrome. *Clin Infect Dis* 1994;19:387–394.

398. Ando K, Guidotti LG, Cerny A, et al. CTL access to tissue antigen is restricted in vivo. *J Immunol* 1994;153:482–488.

399. Palese P, Young JF. Variation of influenza A, B, and C viruses. *Science* 1982;215:1468–1474.

400. Webster RG, Laver WG, Air GM, Schild GC. Molecular mechanisms of variation in influenza viruses. *Nature* 1982;296:115–121.

401. Burns DP, Collignon C, Desrosiers RC. Simian immunodeficiency virus mutants resistent to serum neutralization arise during persistent infection of rhesus monkeys. *J Virol* 1993;67:4104–4113.

402. Fauci A. Immunopathogenesis of HIV infection. *AIDS* 1993;6:655–662.

403. Narayan O, Zink MC, Huso D, et al. Lentiviruses of animals are biological models of the human immunodeficiency viruses. *Microb Pathog* 1988;5:149–157.

404. Montelaro CR, Parekh B, Orrego A, Issel CJ. Antigenic variation during persistent infection by equine infectious anemia virus, a retrovirus. *J Biol Chem* 1984;259:10539–10544.

405. Koup RA. Virus escape from CTL recognition. *J Exp Med* 1994;180:779.

406. Pircher H, Moskophidis D, Rohrer U, Burki K, Hengartner H, Zinkernagel RM.

Viral escape by selection of cytotoxic T cell-resistant virus variants *in vivo*. *Nature* 1990;346:629.

407. de Campos-Lima P-O, Levitsky V, Brooks J, et al. T cell responses and virus evolution: loss of HLA A11-restricted CTL epitopes in Epstein-Barr virus isolates from highly A11-positive populations by selective mutation at anchor residues. *J Exp Med* 1994;179:1297.

408. Eisenlohr LC, Yewdell JW, Bennink JR. Flanking sequences influence the presentation of an endogenously synthesized peptide to cytotoxic T lymphocytes. *J Exp Med* 1992;175:481.

409. Lill NL, Tevethia MJ, Hendrickson WG, Tevethia SS. Cytotoxic T lymphocytes (CTL) against a transforming gene product select for transformed cells with point mutations within sequences encoding CTL recognition epitopes. *J Exp Med* 1992;176:449.

410. Meyerhans A, Dadaglio G, Vartanian J-P, et al. *In vivo* persistence of a HIV-1-encoded HLA-B27-restricted cytotoxic T lymphocyte epitope despite specific *in vitro* reactivity. *Eur J Immunol* 1991;21:2637–2640.

411. Chen AX, Shen L, Miller MD, Ghim SH, Hughes AL, Letvin NL. Cytotoxic T lymphocytes do not appear to select for mutations in an immunodominant epitope of simian immunodeficiency virus gag. *J Immunol* 1992;149:4060.

412. Tsomides TH, Aldovini A, Johnson RP, Walker BD, Young RA, Eisen HN. Naturally processed viral peptides recognized by cytotoxic T lymphocytes on cells chronically infected by human immunodeficiency virus type 1. *J Exp Med* 1994;180:1283–1293.

413. Bertoletti A, Sette A, Chisari FV, et al. Natural variants of cytotoxic epitopes are T cell receptor antagonists for antiviral cytotoxic T cells. *Nature* 1994;369:407.

414. Klenerman P, Rowland-Jones S, McAdams S, et al. Cytotoxic T cell activity antagonized by naturally occurring HIV-1 gag variants. *Nature* 1994;369:403.

415. Jameson SC, Carbone FR, Bevan MJ. Clone-specific T cell receptor antagonists of major histocompatibility complex class-I-restricted cytotoxic T cells. *J Exp Med* 1993;177:1541.

416. Sloan-Lancaster J, Evavold BD, Allen PM. Induction of T-cell anergy by altered T-cell-receptor ligands on live antigen presenting cells. *Nature* 1993;363:156.

417. Rinaldo CR Jr. Modulation of major histocompatibility complex antigen expression by viral infection. *Am J Pathol* 1994;144:637–650.

418. Johnson DC, Hill AB. Herpesviruses and immune evasion. *Curr Top Microbiol Immunol* 1998 (*in press*).

419. Collins KL, Chen BK, Kalams SA, Walker BD, Baltimore D. HIV-1 Nef protein protects infected primary cells against killing by cytotoxic T lymphocytes. *Nature* 1998;391:397–401.

420. Wold WSM, Gooding LR. Region E3 of adenovirus: a cassette of genes involved in host immunosurveillance and virus-cell interactions. *Virology* 1991;184:1–8.

421. Gregory CD, Murray RJ, Edwards CF, Rickinson AB. Down regulation of cell adhesion molecules LFA-3 and ICAM-1 in Epstein-Barr virus-positive Burkitt's lymphoma underlies tumor cell escape from virus-specific T cell surveillance. *J Exp Med* 1988;167:1811–1824.

422. Ahn K, Gruhler A, Galocha B, et al. The ER-luminal domain of the HCMV glycoprotein US6 inhibits peptide translocation by TAP. *Immunity* 1997;6:613–621.

423. Blake N, Lee S, Redchenko I, et al. Human CD8+ T cell responses to EBV EBNA1: HLA class I presentation of the (Gly-Ala)-containing protein requires exogenous processing. *Immunity* 1997;7:791–802

424. Levitskaya J, Coram M, Levitsky V, et al. Inhibition of antigen processing by the internal repeat region of the Epstein-Barr virus nuclear antigen-1. *Nature* 1995;375:685–688.

425. Gilbert MJ, Riddell SR, Plachter B, Greenberg PD. Cytomegalovirus selectively blocks antigen processing and presentation of its immediate-early gene product. *Nature* 1996;383:720–722.

426. Marrack P, Kappler J. Subversion of the immune system by pathogens. *Cell* 1994;76:323–332.

427. Spriggs MK. Cytokine and cytokine receptor genes captured by viruses. *Curr Opin Immunol* 1994;6:526–529.

428. Gooding LR. Virus proteins that counteract host immune defenses. *Cell* 1992; 71:5–7.

429. Smith GL. Virus proteins that bind cytokines, chemokines or interferons. *Curr Opin Immunol* 1996;8:467–471.

430. Upton C, Mossman K, McFadden G. Encoding of a homolog of the IFN-receptor by myxoma virus. *Science* 1992;258:1369–1372.

431. Moore KW, O'Garra A, de Waal Malefyt R, Vieira P, Mosmann TR. Interleukin-10. *Annu Rev Immunol* 1993;11:165–190.

432. Lalani AS, Graham K, Mossman K, et al. The purified myxoma virus gamma interferon receptor homolog M-T7 interacts with the heparin-binding domains of chemokines. *J Virol* 1997;71:4356–4363.

433. McDonald MR, Li XY, Virgin HW. Late expression of a beta chemokine homolog by murine cytomegalovirus. *J Virol* 1997;71:1671–1678.

434. Gao JL, Murphy PM. Human cytomegalovirus open reading frame US28 encodes a functional B chemokine receptor. *J Biol Chem* 1994;268: 28539–28542.

435. Graham KA, Lalani AS, Macen JL, et al. The T1/35KDa family of poxvirus-secreted proteins bind chemokines and modulate leukocyte influx into virus-infected tissues. *Virology* 1997;229:12–24.

436. Pircher H, Burki K, Lang R, Hengartner H, Zinkernagel RM. Tolerance induction in double specific T-cell receptor transgenic mice varies with antigen. *Nature* 1989;342:559–561.

437. Ahmed R, Salmi A, Butler LD, Chiller JM, Oldstone MBA. Selection of genetic variants of lymphocytic choriomeningitis virus in spleens of persistently infected mice: role in suppression of cytotoxic T lymphocyte response and viral persistence. *J Exp Med* 1984;60:521–540.

438. Battegay M, Moskophidis D, Rahemtulla A, Hengartner H, Mak TW, Zinkernagel RM. Enhanced establishment of a virus carrier state in adult CD4+ T-cell-deficient mice. *J Virol* 1994;68:4700–4704.

439. Fujita N, Yoshida K. Follow-up studies on Dengue endemic in Nagasaki, Japan: detection of specific antibodies in serum taken more than 30 years after a single attack of dengue. *Kobe J Med Sci* 1979;25:217–224.

440. Sawyer WA. Persistence of yellow fever immunity. *J Prev Med* 1930;5:413–428.

441. Panum PL. Beobachtungen uber das Maserncontagium. *Virchows Arch* 1847; 1:492–503.

442. Weibel RE, Buynak EB, Mclean AA, Hilleman MR. Follow-up surveillance for antibody in human subjects following live attenuated measles, mumps, and rubella virus vaccines (40675). *Proc Soc Exp Biol Med* 1979;162:328–332.

443. Paul JR, Riiordan JT, Melnick JL. Antibodies to three different antigenic types of poliomyelitis virus in sera from North Alaskan Eskimos. *Am J Hyg* 1951;54:275–285.

444. Jia XY, Summers DF, Ehrenfeld E. Host antibody response to viral stuctural and nonstructural proteins after hepatitis A virus infection. *J Infect Dis* 1992;165: 273–280.

445. Burnet FM, Fenner F. *The production of antibodies.* Melbourne: Macmillan, 1949.

446. Cooney EL, Collier AC, Greenberg PD, et al. Safety of and immunological response to a recombinant vaccinia virus vaccine expressing HIV envelope glycoprotein. *Lancet* 1991;337:567–572.

447. Plotkin SA, Buser F. History of RA27/3 rubella vaccine. *Rev Infect Dis* 1985; 7:S77–S78.

448. Callow KA, Parry HF, Sergeant M, Tyrrell DAJ. The time course of the immune response to experimental coronavirus infection of man. *Epidemiol Infect* 1990;105:435–446.

449. Johnson PRJ, Feldman S, Thompson M, Mahoney JD, Wright PF. Comparison of long-term systemic and secretory antibody responses in children given live, attenuated, or inactivated influenza A vaccine. *J Med Virol* 1985;17:325–335.

450. Hornsleth A, Friis B, Grauballe C, Krasilnikof A. Detection by ELISA of IgA and IgM antibodies in secretion and IgM antibodies in serum in primary lower respiratory syncytial virus infection. *J Med Virol* 1984;13:149–161.

451. Coulson BS, Grimwood K, Masendycz PJ, et al. Comparison of rotavirus immunoglobin A coproconversion with other indices of rotavirus infection in a longitudinal study in childhood. *J Clin Microbiol* 1990;28:1367–1374.

452. Davidson GP, Hogg RJ, Kirubakaran CP. Serum and intestinal immune response to rotavirus enteritis in children. *Infect Immun* 1983;40:447–452.

Fundamental Immunology, Fourth Edition,
edited by William E. Paul
Lippincott–Raven Publishers, Philadelphia © 1999.

CHAPTER **40**

Immunity to Intracellular Bacteria

Stefan H.E. Kaufmann

This chapter focuses on infections with intracellular bacteria, emphasizing, in particular, the general immune mechanisms underlying protection and pathogenicity Intracellular bacteria comprise numerous pathogens, some of which are of utmost medical importance, whereas others play only an inferior role. Ancient (but still existent) as well as newly emerging diseases are caused by intracellular bacteria. Of paramount significance for humans are *Mycobacterium tuberculosis, M. leprae, Salmonella enterica* serovar typhi, and *Chlamydia trachomatis,* the etiologic agents of tuberculosis, leprosy, typhoid, and trachoma, respectively, which, together, afflict more than 600 million individuals. Some opportunistic pathogens, such as *M. avium* and *M. intracellulare,* are gaining increasing significance with the growing number of immunodeficient patients, such as acquired immune deficiency syndrome (AIDS) sufferers.

As can be deduced from their name, intracellular bacteria live inside host cells for most of their lives (1,2). *Intracellular living* implies coexistence with the abused host cells; accordingly, many

S.H.E. Kaufmann: Department of Immunology, Max-Planck-Institute for Infection Biology, 10117 Berlin, Germany.

intracellular bacteria are of low toxicity by themselves. These characteristic features have direct consequences for the immune response evoked. Because of their intracellular location, these pathogens are relatively well shielded from humoral immunity. However, during intracellular living, microbial proteins are processed and peptides presented in the context of major histocompatibility complex (MHC) molecules, thus promoting activation of T-lymphocytes. Accordingly, acquired resistance against and pathogenesis of intracellular bacterial infections crucially depend on T-lymphocytes (1). Although CD4 T-lymphocytes are central to acquired resistance, evidence suggests contribution by CD8 T cells as well as additional unconventional T cells. Moreover, while macrophage activation by interferon γ (IFN-γ) is crucial for antibacterial protection, further mechanisms are often required for clearance of infection.

GENERAL PRINCIPLES OF PATHOGENICITY AND VIRULENCE OF INTRACELLULAR BACTERIA

Characteristic Features of Intracellular Bacteria

Bacterial pathogens are microorganisms that cause disease in a given host species. The term *pathogenicity* embodies the quality of a whole microbial species comprising several strains of varying virulence—that is, of varying disease-causing strength. Only rarely is infectious disease the direct and invariable consequence of an encounter between host and pathogen. Rather, it is the eventual outcome of complex interactions between them. Because this is particularly relevant to our understanding of infections with intracellular bacteria, the principal steps will be discussed briefly.

Some intracellular bacteria, in particular *Rickettsia* species, are introduced directly into the bloodstream by insect bites, from where they have ready access to internal tissues. Most intracellular bacteria, however, enter the host through the mucosa, and bacterial entry is frequently initiated by adhesion to cells of the epithelial mucosa (3–6). Major ports of entry are the lung for airborne pathogens, such as *M. tuberculosis* and *Legionella pneumophila,* and the intestine for food-borne pathogens, such as *S. enterica* and *L. monocytogenes.* Subsequently, intracellular bacteria pass through the epithelial layers. Either they actively induce transcytosis (i.e., endo- and exocytosis) through the epithelial cells, or they are passively translocated within macrophages. Bacteria may be removed by nonspecific defense mechanisms such as mucociliary movements and gut peristalsis, or they may be destroyed by professional phagocytes without necessitating the specific attention of the immune system. Cells that survive these nonspecific defense reactions colonize deeper tissue sites and stably infect a suitable niche. At this stage, the host generally pays sufficient attention to the infectious agent, as indicated by the development of a specific immune response.

Infection is abortive when the immune system succeeds in eliminating the pathogen before overt clinical disease develops. Alternatively, tissue damage increases to a significant level before the immune system succeeds in controlling the pathogen effectively, and clinical disease develops. This is the case with many extracellular bacteria that cause diseases of acute type, but is less common in the case of intracellular bacteria. Finally, it is possible that the immune response restrains the infectious agent but fails to completely eradicate it. Under these conditions, a long-lasting equilib-

rium between microbial persistence and the immune response unfolds. This balance, however, remains labile and can be tipped in favor of the pathogen at a later time point, converting infection into disease.

The time lapse between host entry and expression of clinical disease is often termed *incubation time,* and from what has been said above, it follows that in many intracellular bacterial infections the incubation times are long-lasting to lifelong. By improving the immune response or by impairing bacterial growth (typically accomplished by chemotherapy), or both, disease can be overcome. Ideally, sterile bacterial eradication is achieved; alternatively, some dormant bacteria continue to persist in niches that are poorly accessible to the immune response.

To reemphasize, the relevant steps leading to diseases caused by intracellular bacteria are the following: (a) Commonly, infection is clearly separated from disease, and the immune response is already induced at the stage of infection. (b) Infection persists in the face of dynamic interactions between pathogen and immune mechanisms. (c) The host–pathogen relationship represents a highly sophisticated form of parasitism, which need not necessarily lead to disease but, rather, allows for long-lasting coexistence. (d) Infection, however, includes the potential to harm the host severely at a later stage, and pathogenesis is strongly influenced by the immune response.

Hallmarks of an "Idealized" Intracellular Bacterium

Although this chapter focuses on general mechanisms underlying immunity to intracellular bacteria, it is important to emphasize that this group is extremely heterogeneous, despite several commonalities. Therefore, the major hallmarks of intracellular bacterial infections will first be described for a nonexistent "idealized" intracellular bacterium and compared with an "idealized" extracellular bacterium (Table 1). Subsequently, characteristics of selected intracellular bacteria will be specified.

- Hallmark 1: As implied by the name, the intracellular lifestyle represents the distinguishing feature of intracellular bacteria. Yet, invasion of host cells is not restricted to these pathogens, and transient trespassing through epithelial cells is a common invasion mechanism of both intracellular and extracellular pathogens.
- Hallmark 2: T cells are the central mediators of protection against intracellular bacterial infections. These T cells do not interact with microbes directly, but, instead, interact with the infected host cell. In contrast, antibodies that recognize microbial antigens directly are of exquisite importance for defense against extracellular bacteria.

TABLE 1. *Hallmarks of the intracellular bacterial infections*

Essential
Intracellular habitat
T cell-mediated protection
Delayed type hypersensitivity
Granulomatous tissue reaction
Conditional
Low intrinsic toxicity / Immune pathology
Labile balance between infection and protective immunity
Protracted incubation time/chronic disease
Dissociation of infection from disease

- Hallmark 3: Infections with intracellular bacteria are accompanied by delayed-type hypersensitivity (DTH), which expresses itself after local administration of soluble antigens as a delayed tissue reaction mediated by T cells and effected by macrophages.
- Hallmark 4: Tissue reactions against intracellular bacteria are granulomatous, and protection against, as well as pathology caused by, intracellular bacteria are centered on these lesions. Rupture of a granuloma promotes bacterial dissemination and formation of additional lesions at distinct tissue sites. In contrast, tissue reactions against extracellular bacteria are purulent and lead to abscess formation or systemic reactions.
- Hallmark 5: Intracellular bacteria express little or no toxicity for host cells by themselves, and the pathology is primarily a result of immune reactions, particularly those mediated by T-lymphocytes. In contrast, extracellular bacteria produce various toxins, which are directly responsible for tissue damage.
- Hallmark 6: Intracellular bacteria coexist with their cellular habitat for long periods. A labile balance develops between persistent infection and protective immunity, resulting in long incubation time and in chronic disease. Accordingly, infection is clearly dissociated from disease. In contrast, extracellular bacteria typically cause acute diseases, which develop soon after their entry into the host and are terminated once the immune response has developed. Thus, the transition of infection into clinical disease occurs rapidly.

Hallmarks 1 to 4 should be considered essential, and hallmarks 5 and 6 conditional, criteria for defining intracellular bacteria. Of course, the ideal intracellular bacterium, as characterized above, does not exist. *M. tuberculosis* probably resembles it most. Yet, at the height of active tuberculosis, tubercle bacilli replicate extracellularly in the detritus of dissolved host cells in an unrestricted way (7). Experimental listeriosis of mice fulfills many criteria (though not all) but takes an acute course of disease (8). In typhoid, antibodies probably participate in the protective immune response, and in leprosy they contribute to pathogenesis.

Two Types of Intracellular Bacteria: Facultative and Obligate Intracellular

With respect to their preferred habitat, intracellular bacteria can be divided into two groups: Those pathogens that do not essentially depend on the intracellular habitat include *M. tuberculosis, M. bovis, M. leprae, S. enterica, Brucella* species, *L. pneumophila, L. monocytogenes,* and *Francisella tularensis* (Table 2) (1,7,9–15). Although these pathogens favor mononuclear phagocytes (MPs) as

their biotope, other types of host cells are misused as well. *M. leprae,* for example, lives in numerous host-cell types, notably in Schwann cells, and hepatocytes serve as an important reservoir for *L. monocytogenes.* Although *M. tuberculosis* can infect a variety of mammalian cells *in vitro, in vivo* it seems to restrict itself to macrophages.

So-called obligate intracellular bacteria fail to survive outside host cells (2). These bacteria prefer nonprofessional phagocytes as biotope—for example, endothelial and epithelial cells. Nevertheless, they are sometimes found in MPs, as well. Rickettsiae and Chlamydiae are representatives of this group. They include *R. prowazekii, R. rickettsii, R. typhi, R. tsutsugamushi,* and *Coxiella burnetii,* the etiologic agents of louse-borne typhus, Rocky Mountain spotted fever, typhus, scrub typhus, and Q-fever, respectively (16). Different biovars of *C. trachomatis* that are responsible for trachoma, conjunctivitis, urogenital infections, and lymphogranuloma venerum, as well as *C. psittaci* and *C. pneumoniae,* causative agents of psittacosis or rare types of pneumonia, respectively, also belong to this group (Table 3) (17–19). Although evidence, at present, is still scarce, *C. pneumoniae* infection has been suggested as cofactor in the development of atherosclerotic cardiovascular disease (20).

Preferential living in macrophages does not depend on specific invasion mechanisms but, rather, on highly sophisticated intracellular survival strategies. Yet, most facultative intracellular bacteria express specific invasion factors, if only to cross epithelial layers. In contrast, selection of nonprofessional phagocytes as habitat essentially depends on invasion molecules, whereas survival inside these cells is generally less hazardous.

Because this chapter focuses on general mechanisms underlying the immune response to intracellular bacteria, some selectivity is required, and major emphasis will be given to

1. Experimental listeriosis of mice, because this model has proven most productive in the exploration of the immune mechanisms responsible for acquired resistance against intracellular bacteria
2. Human tuberculosis, which not only represents the paradigm of intracellular bacterial infections, but also is of paramount medical importance
3. Human leprosy, which is characterized by different disease forms
4. *S. enterica* infection, which is increasingly used for elucidating the intracellular lifestyle of bacteria

Where appropriate, other infections will be included in the discussion.

TABLE 2. *Major infections of humans caused by facultative intracellular bacteria*

Pathogen	Disease	Preferred target cell	Preferred location in host cell	Preferred port of entry
Mycobacterium tuberculosis/M. bovis	Tuberculosis	Macrophages	Phagosome	Lung
Myocabacterium leprae	Leprosy	Macrophages, Schwann cells, numerous other host cells	Phagolysosome (?)	Nasopharyngeal mucosa
Salmonella enterica serovar Typhi	Typhoid fever	Macrophages	Phagosome	Gut
Brucella sp.	Brucellosis	Macrophages	Phagolysosome	Mucosa
Legionella pneumophila	Legionnaire's disease	Macrophages	Phagosome	Lung
Listeria monocytogenes	Listeriosis	Macrophages, hepatocytes	Cytosol	Gut
Francisella tularensis	Tularaemia	Macrophages	Phagosome	Skin, mucosa, lung

TABLE 3. *Major infections of humans caused by obligate intracellular bacteria*

Pathogen	Disease	Preferred target cell	Preferred location in host cell	Preferred port of entry
Rickettsia rickettsii	Rocky Mountain spotted fever	Endothelial cells, smooth muscle cell	Cytosol	Blood vessel (tick bite)
Rickettsia prowazekii	Endemic typhus	Endothelial cells	Cytosol	Broken skin, mucosa
Rickettsia typhi	Typhus	Endothelial cells	Cytosol	Blood vessel (flea bite)
Rickettsia tsutsugamushi	Scrub typhus	Endothelial cells	Cytosol	Blood vessel (mite bite)
Coxiella burnetii	Q-fever	Macrophages, lung parenchyma cells	Late phagosome	Lung
Chlamydia trachomatis	Urogenital infection, conjunctivitis, trachoma, lymphogranuloma venerum (different serovars)	Epithelial cells	Phagosome	Eye, urogenital mucosa
Chlamydia psittaci	Psittacosis	Macrophages, lung parenchyma cells	Phagosome	Lung
Chlamydia pneumoniae	Pneumonia, coronary heart disease (?)	Lung parenchyma cells	Phagosome	Lung

SPECIFIC FEATURES AND EXAMPLES

Mycobacterium tuberculosis and Tuberculosis

This paradigm intracellular bacterium is an acid-fast bacillus with a replication time of approximately 12 hours. Tubercle bacilli are obligate aerobes and hence prefer tissue sites with high pO values, such as the lung. *M. tuberculosis,* as well as other mycobacteria, contain abundant lipids, glycolipids, and waxes, which are responsible not only for the hydrophobic character of the mycobacteria, but also for their acid-fastness, strong adjuvanticity (mycobacteria are the crucial components of Freund's complete adjuvant), resistance against complement lysis, and resistance against acids, alkalines, and simple disinfectants. Most importantly, these lipoids are central to intracellular survival inside activated MPs. More recent findings have revealed that certain mycobacterial lipids and lipoglycans serve as antigenic targets for a small population of unconventional T cells in humans. *M. tuberculosis* and, to a lesser extent, *M. bovis* cause tuberculosis, which is of paramount medical importance globally (7,21–23). The disease is characterized by long incubation time, dormant infection, and protracted course of disease. It is estimated that, globally, 60 million people suffer from tuberculosis and that every year 8 million new cases arise. Annually, 3 million people die of this disease, making *M. tuberculosis* the major killer among all infectious agents. On the other hand, it has been estimated that one-third of the entire world population (2 billion people) are infected with *M. tuberculosis.* Infected individuals harbor *M. tuberculosis* inside small granulomas at sequestered tissue sites. Persistence of *M. tuberculosis* in these seclusions does not remain unrecognized by the immune system; rather, it is controlled by T cells (24). Hence, the vast majority (more than 90%) of infected people remain healthy, and only a minority develop disease following weakening of the immune response. Primary infection generally proceeds via the aerosol route, and the lung remains the principal site of infection as well as disease. Nevertheless, any other tissue site can be infected following reactivation of dormant foci and hematogenic–lymphogenic dissemination. Tuberculosis of adults primarily develops through reactivation of dormant foci; only rarely does reinfection of individuals already harboring dormant *M. tuberculosis* cause disease. In 1927, Calmette and Guérin developed an attenuated strain of *M. bovis,* termed *bacille Calmette-Guérin* (BCG). At present, this strain is the most widely used viable vaccine globally (25). However, its protective efficacy in adults is insufficient (26).

Mycobacterium leprae and Leprosy

This pathogen can still not be grown in artificial media. It has an extremely slow growth rate of 11 to 30 days in the mouse footpad; probably in patients, the doubling time is even slower (11). *M. leprae* grows best at relatively low temperatures (27°C to 30°C). This feature may be responsible for its predilection for peripheral nerves. *M. leprae* is also rich in the lipoids described above, with phenolic glycolipid I being the most abundant one. It is estimated that approximately 12 million people suffer from leprosy (11,27). Leprosy is a chronic infectious disease characterized by long incubation time and protracted course of illness. It is a spectral disease, ranging from a tuberculoid pole characterized by strong T cell–mediated immunity and paucibacillary lesions to a lepromatous pole with deficient cell-mediated immunity and multibacillary lesions (11,27,28). The immune mechanisms effective in tuberculoid leprosy resemble those active in tuberculosis. Toward the lepromatous pole, however, suppressive immune mechanisms develop that are characteristic for this disease. Because leprosy generally affects the skin, lesions are easily accessible, and immune histologic analyses of leprosy skin lesions have provided deep insight into the mechanisms operative in a granulomatous lesion.

Listeria monocytogenes and Listeriosis

This bacterium is a gram-positive, non–spore-forming, facultatively anaerobic rod. Molecular biology analyses have revealed several virulence factors of *L. monocytogenes* that are instrumental for cell invasion, intracellular replication, and cell-to-cell spread (29,30). Listeriolysin is a sulfhydril-activated, pore-forming cytolysin, which is active at the low pH existing in the phagosome and promotes evasion from the phagosomal into the cytoplasmic compartment (31,32). Two different phospholipase C molecules and a lecithinase contribute to the escape of *L. mono-*

cytogenes into the cytoplasm and to cell-to-cell spread (33–35). Transition from the phagosome into the cytosol not only is essential for virulence, but also markedly influences the type of T-cell response evoked, because it promotes loading of MHC class I molecules with antigenic peptides. The actA gene product is involved in intracellular movements and promotes cell-to-cell spreading, while intracellular survival may be further facilitated by a metalloprotease (36–38). Internalin and a secreted 60-kDa protein encoded by the iap gene are involved in invasion of non-phagocytic host cells (39,40). The prfA gene encodes a protein that positively regulates expression of several virulence factors such as listeriolysin, lecithinase, and phospholipase C (41). Listeriosis is primarily a disease of sheep and cattle and only rarely occurs in humans (14,42). *L. monocytogenes* infection of experimental mice has provided an extremely helpful tool for elucidating the mechanisms central to our understanding of immunity to intracellular bacteria (1,8). Despite the capacity of *L. monocytogenes* organisms to survive in resting macrophages, they are readily killed once macrophages are activated. Therefore, murine listeriosis is an acute infection that is easily terminated following T-cell activation. Even in the absence of T cells, listeriosis is quite efficiently, if incompletely, controlled (43). These features must be kept in mind in interpreting data from murine listeriosis experiments.

Salmonella enterica *and Salmonellosis*

According to the latest nomenclature, all salmonellae belong to a single species termed *S. enterica* (15,44–46). This species encompasses more than 2,000 serovars, including *S. enterica* serovar *typhi,* the causative agent of human typhoid, and *S. enterica typhimurium,* which is responsible for a similar disease in mice. The salmonellae are widespread in nature and infect a vast variety of animals, including mammals, reptiles, and birds. Some salmonellae, such as *S. enterica typhimurium,* have a broad host range; others are highly restricted, such as *S. enterica typhi,* which is almost exclusively restricted to humans. Typically, salmonellosis is food-borne, and, in the susceptible host, the pathogens cause diseases ranging from mild enterocolitis to severe diarrhea. Some salmonellae, having passed through the gut epithelium, can cause bacteremia, which sometimes results in enteric fever or typhoid. Although human typhoid causes severe health problems globally, it is now much better controlled than it was in the past. The diarrheal diseases caused by various *S. enterica* serovars are a major threat to humankind. The findings, described in the remaining part of this chapter, are almost exclusively derived from experiments with *S. enterica typhimurium.* Although the species designation *S. enterica* is being used throughout the text, it must be kept in mind that some of these findings cannot be extrapolated to other serovars of *S. enterica,* including typhi.

ENTRY INTO, KILLING BY, AND SURVIVAL IN HOST CELLS

For intracellular bacteria, entry into host cells represents the central requirement for survival in, as well as elimination by, the host (1,2). Host cell-directed uptake is called *phagocytosis: It is a feature of the so-called professional phagocytes, which comprise polymorphonuclear granulocytes (PNGs) and MPs. Entry induced by*

the pathogen is termed invasion: It allows entry into nonphagocytic cells (nonprofessional phagocytes). Contact between host cells and pathogens proceeds either directly via receptor-ligand interactions or indirectly via deposition on the surface of the pathogen of host molecules for which physiologic receptors exist on the target cell.

Depending on the cellular target, the final outcome of host-cell entry varies markedly:

1. PNGs are short-lived. Because they are highly phagocytic and express potent antibacterial activities constitutively, uptake by PNGs is generally fatal for the pathogen.

2. Nonprofessional phagocytes are nonphagocytic, and hence entry depends on expression of surface receptors, which can be misused for invasion. Because of their low antibacterial activities, they primarily serve as a habitat.

3. MPs are phagocytic and express medium-to-high antibacterial activities, depending on their activation status. Accordingly, they serve as both habitat and effector cell.

In the following, the major steps from uptake to bacterial elimination by, or survival in, host cells will be described, with emphasis on the major target of intracellular bacteria, the MPs (Fig. 1; see also Table 4).

Adhesion and Invasion

Adhesion to mammalian cells is a common feature of bacterial pathogens (47–49). It is a prerequisite for extracellular colonization and for host-cell invasion. Bacterial adhesins, which solely expedite adhesion to host cells, are expressed by numerous extracellular bacteria. In contrast, invasion-inducing molecules are a feature of bacteria that permanently or transiently enter host cells. The intracellular bacteria covered here live in host cells permanently, whereas other pathogens, such as *Shigella* species and *Yersinia* species intrude host cells transiently (15,47,49–53).

Although induced by the bacterium, invasion is ultimately a function of the host cell. Following adhesion, invasion can be induced in either of the following two ways: First, cell signaling by host-cell receptors misused for adhesion induces uptake; second, uptake is induced independently of the molecules that mediate adhesion (49,50,54). The term *zipper mechanism* has been suggested for the highly selective receptor-mediated bacterial entry, whereas the term *trigger mechanism* has been proposed for indiscriminate, apparently adhesion-independent uptake (54).

Entry by Zipper Mechanisms

Host-cell invasion by *Yersinia* species and *L. monocytogenes* is an example of invasion via the zipper mechanism (49,55). Invasion of *Yersinia* species is specific for an integrin receptor. Its binding induces phagocytic mechanisms in nonprofessional phagocytes similar to those that are constitutively operative in MPs. Host entry of *L. monocytogenes* through the intestinal epithelia is mediated by internalin on the surface of this pathogen and E cadherin on epithelial cells (49,56). Schwann cells, a major target of *M. leprae,* are shielded by a basal lamina composed of laminin, collagen, and proteoglycans. Evidence suggests that the unique tropism of *M. leprae* for peripheral nerves is due to bacterial binding to laminin. This molecule, which serves as natural ligand for integrins, thus provides a link between pathogen and Schwann cell (57).

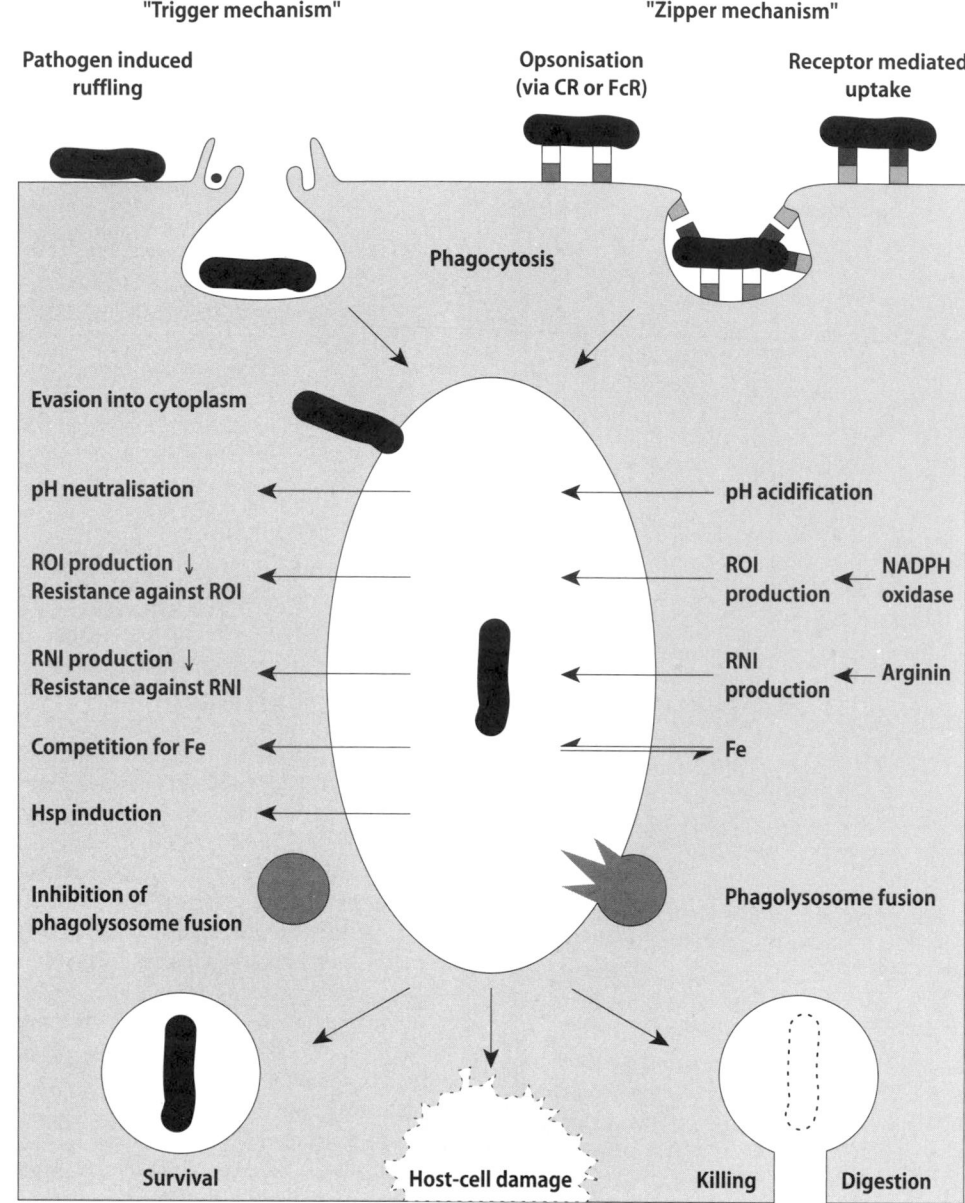

FIG. 1. The multiple encounters between mononuclear phagocytes (MPs) and intracellular bacteria.

Entry by Trigger Mechanisms

Different molecules and mechanisms participate in host-cell entry by *S. enterica*. Interactions between *S. enterica* and host cells cause "membrane ruffling" at the site of attachment, followed by bacterial entry (49,51,52). Ruffling induces indiscriminate uptake, even of other particles in the vicinity of *S. enterica*. This process has been termed *macropinocytosis*. *S. enterica* triggers its uptake by exploiting the "signaling machinery" of the host cell, thus inducing cytoskeletal rearrangements. However, the exact nature of the receptor(s) for *S. enterica* is still unclear. In certain mouse cells, *S. enterica* induces phosphorylation of the receptor for the epidermal growth factor (EGF) (58). Yet, *S. enterica* can also enter cells that do not express the EGF receptor (15,52). This pathogen possesses a type III secretion apparatus, which allows it to directly manipulate the intracellular signaling cascade in host cells (15,49). Interaction with the small guanosine triphosphate (GTP)-binding

protein CDC42 of the Ras superfamily has been implied in bacterial invasion through membrane ruffling (59).

Phagocytosis by Professional Phagocytes

Professional phagocytes express receptors that recognize molecular structures on microbial pathogens that are normally absent from the mammalian host. Binding to these receptors induces phagocytosis in professional phagocytes. By means of these so-called pattern-recognition receptors, professional phagocytes are endowed with the capacity to promptly identify bacterial invaders (60). These pattern-recognition receptors include

- Lectin-like glycoproteins with specificity for sugars commonly expressed on the bacterial cell surface (61)
- Surface molecules, notably CD14, with specificity for glycolipids, such as lipopolysaccharide (LPS) of gram-negative bacte-

TABLE 4. *Major antibacterial capacities of activated macrophages and microbial evasion mechanisms*

Macrophage effector capacity	Microbial evasion mechanism
Defensins	Unknown
Phagosome acidification	Phagosome neutralization
Phagosome–lysosome fusion	Inhibition of phagosome–lysosome fusion
Lysosomal enzymes	Resistance against enzymes
Intraphagolysosomal killing	Evasion into cytosol Robust cell wall
ROI	CR-mediated uptake, ROI detoxifiers, ROI scavengers
RNI	Unknown (ROI detoxifiers probably interfere with RNI)
Iron starvation	Microbial iron scavengers (e.g., siderophores)
Tryptophan starvation	Unknown

ROI, reactive oxygen intermediates; RNI, reactive nitrogen intermediates.

ria and certain lipoarabinomannans (LAMs) of mycobacteria (62–64).

Three types of lectin-like receptors can be distinguished (61,65): The mannose-type receptor recognizes *N*-acetylglucosamine, mannose, glucose, and L-fucose; the galactose-type receptor is specific for *N*-acetylgalactosamine and galactose; and the fucose-type receptor is specific for L-fucose. Broad distribution of these sugars on various microbes guarantees the broad target spectrum of professional phagocytes. LAM with terminal mannan (ManLAM) is primarily recognized by the mannose-type receptor (66). In contrast, LAM lacking these mannose caps and having terminal arabinose cannot be recognized through these receptors. Evidence has been presented that CD14 is involved in recognition of these AraLAM moieties (66).

A group of receptors that are collectively termed *scavenger receptors* react with host serum lipoproteins (67,68). Some of these receptors also bind microbial surface molecules, and circumstantial evidence suggests that they may participate in host defense against bacterial infection (67,69,69a).

Indirect binding of bacteria to professional phagocytes involves immunoglobulin G (IgG), breakdown products of the complement component C3, or fibronectin as ligands, the Fc receptor (FcR) and the complement receptors, CR1, CR3, and CR4 or the fibronectin receptor (FnR), respectively, on the part of the host cell (70–73). Binding of specific IgG antibodies to bacteria promotes phagocytosis via FcR and—after complement activation—by CR1, CR3, or CR4, in addition. FcR binding generally activates the respiratory burst, resulting in the activation of reactive oxygen intermediates (ROIs; see below) (74,75). Many intracellular bacteria, such as *M tuberculosis, M. leprae*, and *L. pneumophila*, induce breakdown of C3 and—as a corollary—their own uptake (76–79). The phenolic glycolipid of *M. leprae* and the major outer membrane protein of *L. pneumophila*, for example, promote uptake via CR through C3 fixation (76,78). C3 fixation and activation by *M. leprae* surface glycolipid either proceed through the antibody-independent alternative pathway or are promoted by low concentrations of cross-reactive serum antibodies through the classical pathway of complement activation. C3b deposition on the cell wall of the pathogenic mycobacteria *M. tuberculosis, M. leprae*, and *M. avium* was found to be pro-

moted by the natural complement component C2a. Apparently, these microbes first cleave serum C2 to become the C3 convertase, C2a, which then causes formation from C3 of C3b and its fixation (79a). Some intracellular bacteria directly bind to CR3 independent of C3 activation (80,80a). Direct binding to CR3 involves either the RGD sequence or a lectin-like binding site for β-glucan. Thus, CR3 serves as both—as pattern-recognition receptor and as a receptor for host molecules. CR-promoted uptake may interfere with the generation of ROIs in MPs, and hence may represent a bacterial evasion mechanism (see below) (76–78).

Some intracellular bacteria, such as *L. pneumophila* and *C. psittaci*, enter MPs by an unusual engulfment process, called "coiling phagocytosis" (76,81). Coiling is promoted by C3 breakdown products and does not stimulate ROI secretion. In contrast, FcR-facilitated uptake of *L. pneumophila* is normal and induces neither coiling nor interference with the ROI burst. CR-mediated uptake of particles does not trigger the oxidative burst, suggesting that it represents a general evasion mechanism, which facilitates intracellular survival.

Fibronectin also binds to FnR through an RGD-containing sequence, so that intracellular bacteria expressing fibronectin-binding molecules may be taken up via this pathway. For example, *M. tuberculosis* secretes a family of 32-kDa molecules with fibronectin-binding activity (82,83). Fibronectin, however, appears to be a weak and inefficient inducer of phagocytosis that requires additional internalization mechanisms (71,84,85). In fact, more recent studies have provided compelling evidence that members of the 32-kDa molecular complex act as mycolyl transferase, and thus are involved in cell wall biosynthesis rather than in host-cell adhesion of mycobacteria (85a). Probably, intracellular bacteria misuse a variety of other proteins present in serum or secretion. Thus, *M. tuberculosis* was found to bind to heparin or to surfactant protein, which may promote adhesion and perhaps uptake by host cells in the lung (85b,85c).

Invasion of Nonprofessional Phagocytes

Intracellular bacteria generally do not attempt to avoid phagocytosis; rather, they often promote their own engulfment. Microbe-directed uptake allows for misuse of nonphagocytic cells, and hence can be seen as an evasion mechanism from phagocytosis by professional phagocytes. The target spectrum of intracellular bacteria ranges from very broad to highly specific. *M. leprae* is found in a large variety of host cells, and hence shows a broad target-cell spectrum (27,86). *L. monocytogenes* enters the host through the gut epithelium, and its major target, besides MPs, is the hepatocyte (87,88); *M. tuberculosis* is almost, if not exclusively, restricted to MPs. For the obligate intracellular bacteria, nonprofessional phagocytes, rather than MPs, represent the preferred biotope (2). They are primarily found in endothelial and epithelial cells (17).

Phagosome Maturation, Acidification, and Phagosome–Lysosome Fusion

Phagocytosis of inert particles initiates a series of events that ultimately lead to the formation of a phagolysosome (49,89,90). Three major stages can be distinguished.

- The early phagosome, characterized by a slightly acidic pH 6 and membrane markers such as mannose receptor, transferrin, and transferrin receptor.

- The late phagosome, characterized by pH less than 5.5 and the acquisition of the vacuolar adenosine triphosphatase (ATPase) proton pump
- The phagolysosome, as the result of fusion between phagosomes and lysosomes, characterized by pH less than 5.5, high density of lysosome-associated membrane proteins (LAMPs), and typical lysosomal enzymes.

It should be kept in mind that the three stages are not distinctly separated, but form a continuum involving sorting of membrane proteins, as well as budding of and fusion with other vesicles. During this dynamic process, the phagosomes successively interact with the corresponding endosomes and subsequently with lysosomes (91).

The intraphagosomal pH is controlled by a vacuolar ATPase proton pump, which is responsible for acidification (92). Immediately after phagocytosis, the phagosome becomes alkaline for a short time before acidification is initiated. The basic milieu is optimal for the activity of defensins and basic proteins, whereas the acidic pH is optimal for lysosomal enzymes (93). Defensins are small (3.5 to 4.0 kDa) peptides rich in arginine and cysteine (94,95). They are abundant in PNGs and present in some, though not all, MPs (depending on species and tissue location). Purified defensins are microbicidal for certain intracellular bacteria, such as *S. enterica* and *L. monocytogenes*. A virulence factor of *S. enterica* for mice, phoP, has been implicated in resistance against defensins (95,96). Contribution of lysosomal enzymes to bacterial killing is small. Their major task is the degradation of already-killed bacteria. These enzymes reside in the lysosome and are delivered into the phagosome during maturation through several independent waves, and they reach their optimum activity during later stages (i.e., in the phagolysosome).

Most intracellular bacteria interfere with phagosome maturation (89,90,97,98). These include *L. pneumophila, M. tuberculosis, S. enterica,* and *C. psittaci*. Although mechanistically incompletely understood, mycobacterial sulfatides and some mycobacterial glycolipids impede phagolysosome fusion (99–102). Antibody-coated *M. tuberculosis* organisms lose their capacity to block discharge of lysosomal enzymes, suggesting an auxiliary function of antibodies in cell-mediated protection against tuberculosis (103). Finally, the robust, lipid-rich cell wall of mycobacteria renders them highly resistant against enzymatic attack. *M. tuberculosis* as well as *M. avium* restrict phagosome acidification via the exclusion of the proton pump from the phagosome (92,104). Additional mechanisms may contribute to this event, such as $NH4^+$ production by *M. tuberculosis* (105). Consistent with intraphagosomal $NH4^+$ production, the urease of *M. tuberculosis* is active at low pH. It has long been known that $NH4^+$ also interfers with phagosome lysosome fusion. Exogenous ATP has been shown to promote phagolysosome fusion, resulting in concomitant death of macrophages and killing of *M. bovis* BCG (105a,105b).

Phagosome maturation is somewhere arrested between the early and the late stages by *M. tuberculosis, M. bovis* BCG, *L. pneumophila, S. enterica,* and *C. trachomatis,* which all replicate in nonacidified vacuoles. Phagosomes containing *S. enterica, M. bovis* BCG, or *C. trachomatis* appear uncoupled from the maturation process through which phagosomes containing inert particles proceed (81,106–109). *S. enterica* remains in the spacious membrane-bound phagosome that is formed after uptake by the trigger mechanism. The vacuole containing *C. trachomatis,* which lacks any specific phagosome markers, is loaded with ATP by an unknown mechanism, which is required by *C. trachomatis* (109).

The *L. pneumophila*–containing phagosome is surrounded by mitochondria, and later by ribosomes connected with the endoplasmic reticulum (110). Evidence has been presented that *L. pneumophila* exploits an intracellular compartment with some features of autophagosomes (110,111).

Intracellular Iron

Intracellular bacteria require iron, and production of ROIs and reactive nitrogen intermediates (RNIs) also depends on iron. Thus, competition for the intracellular iron pool between the intracellular pathogen and the host cell markedly influences the outcome of their relationship (112–116). To improve their iron supply, mammalian cells utilize specific molecules. In the intracellular milieu, iron is bound to ferritin, heme, and iron sulfur proteins (117). In the extracellular host milieu, iron is tightly bound to transferrin and lactoferrin and taken up by host cells via transferrin receptors. As mentioned above, transferrin and transferrin receptors have been identified in the early phagosome. The transferrin receptor takes up iron-loaded transferrin, which releases its iron under the reducing conditions of the early phagosome. It has been suggested that the NRAMP system is involved in iron transport into the phagosome. Accordingly, iron availability is controlled in multiple ways, including transferrin receptor expression on the cell surface and in the phagosome, lactoferrin release, and intracytosolic ferritin concentrations. To successfully compete for iron, many bacteria possess iron-binding proteins. They first secrete low-molecular-weight iron scavengers, termed *siderophores*. IFN-γ–activated MPs downmodulate transferrin receptor expression and intracellular ferritin, resulting in reduced iron availability within the phagosome. Studies with *L. pneumophila* revealed that sufficient iron is available in the phagosome of the resting MPs. However, the available iron is markedly reduced in IFN-γ–activated MPs, and, as a consequence, *L. pneumophila,* which lacks efficient iron uptake mechanisms, starves from iron deprivation. In contrast, *M. tuberculosis* possesses a potent iron acquisition system comprising exochelins and mycobactins. The exochelins successfully compete for iron under limiting conditions and transfer it to mycobactins in the cell wall (118,119).

Tryptophan Degradation

Increased degradation of the amino acid tryptophan has been associated with killing of *C. psittaci* and the intracellular protozoan pathogen, *Toxoplasma gondii* (120,121). Although it is possible that limiting the intracellular availability of essential amino acids provides a potent antimicrobial mechanism, little is known about its general role in resistance against intracellular bacteria.

Toxic Effector Molecules

Killing of intracellular bacteria by MPs and/or PNGs is primarily accomplished by highly reactive toxic molecules, particularly ROIs and RNIs (74,75,122–126). Many bacteria are susceptible to ROIs *in vitro*. Yet, the contribution of ROIs to killing of intracellular bacteria by MPs remains unclear; in murine macrophages, RNIs appear more important (122,126–131). Consistent with a central role of RNI in antibacterial defense, gene knock-out (KO) mice with a deficient inducible NO synthase (iNOS) (which is responsible for RNI production; see below) suffer from exacerbated listeriosis and tuberculosis (126,130,132). On the other hand, production of RNIs by human MPs at levels sufficiently high for bacterial killing remains controversial (126,133–138). However, evidence is now accumulating that human MPs from the site of intracellular bacterial infection possess the potential to produce RNIs (126,138). Using antibodies with exquisite specificity for human iNOS, for example, this enzyme could be detected in a large proportion of alveolar macrophages from tuberculosis patients (138). Because RNI production represents the major effector mechanism in tuberculostasis by murine macrophages, it may be speculated that relatively low RNI production in human macrophages is, at least partially, related to the higher susceptibility of humans for tuberculosis.

ROI production is initiated by a membrane-bound NADPH oxidase, which is activated by IFN-γ and by IgG/FcR binding:

$$O_2 + NADPH \xrightarrow{NADPH\ oxidase} NADP + O_2^- + H^+$$

O_2^- is further metabolized by superoxide dismutase (SOD):

$$O_2^- + H^+ \xrightarrow{SOD} O_2 + H_2O_2$$

In the presence of appropriate iron catalysts, the Haber-Weiss reaction takes place:

$$O_2^- + Fe^{3+} \rightarrow O_2 + Fe^{2+}$$

$$H_2O_2 + Fe^{2+} \rightarrow {}^{\cdot}OH + OH^- + Fe^{3+}$$

$$O_2^- + H_2O_2 \rightarrow {}^{\cdot}OH + OH^- + O_2$$

In addition, O_2^- is transformed into ${}^1O_2$. The ${}^1O_2$ and ${}^{\cdot}OH$ radicals are short-lived, powerful oxidants with high antibactericidal activity, causing damage to DNA, membrane lipids, and proteins (O_2^-, hyperoxide anion; ${}^{\cdot}OH$, hydroxyl radical containing a free electron; ${}^1O_2$, singlet oxygen, a highly reactive form of O_2).

Granulocytes and blood monocytes, but not tissue macrophages, possess myeloperoxidase (MPO), thus allowing halogenation of microbial proteins (74):

$$H_2O_2 + Cl^- \xrightarrow{MPO} OCl^- + H_2O$$

In addition to hypochlorous acid, chloramines are formed, and both agents further increase the bactericidal power of the ROI system by destroying biologically important proteins through chlorination.

Nitric oxide (NO) is exclusively derived from the terminal guanidino-nitrogen atom of L-arginine (Fig. 2) (123,124). This reaction is catalyzed by iNOS, which leads to the formation of L-citrulline and NO·.

NO· can act as oxidizing agent alone, or it interacts with O_2^- to form the unstable peroxynitrite (ONOO⁻). This then may be transformed to the more stable anions, NO_2^- and NO_3^-, or decomposed to NO·:

$$O_2^- + NO^{\cdot} \rightarrow ONOO^-$$

$$ONOO^- + H^+ \rightarrow NO_2^- + {}^{\cdot}OH$$

$$NO_2^- + {}^{\cdot}OH \rightarrow NO_3^- + H^+$$

$$ONOO^- + H^+ \rightarrow {}^{\cdot}OH + NO^{\cdot}$$

NO· and ONOO⁻ are highly reactive antimicrobial agents. NO· may be transformed to nitrosothiols expressing the most potent antimicrobial activity. In contrast, NO_2^- and NO_3^- are without notable effects on microorganisms.

Production of NO· is NADPH-dependent and requires tetrahydrobiopterin as cofactor. Three distinct NOS isoenzymes are known. The two constitutive NOSs (cNOSs) exist in various host cells and account for basal NO synthesis, whereas iNOS is primarily found in professional phagocytes and is responsible for microbial killing (126). Its induction is controlled by exogenous stimuli such as IFN-γ. This iNOS stimulation results in a burst of high RNI concentrations required for microbial killing, whereas the low NO levels produced by cNOS perform physiologic functions. The RNIs exert their bactericidal activities by directly inactivating iron-sulfur–containing enzymes, by S-nitrosylating proteins, by damaging DNA, or by synergizing with ROIs.

Evasion from Killing by Reactive Oxygen Intermediates and Reactive Nitrogen Intermediates

Binding to CR1/CR3 does not induce the respiratory burst and ROI production (76,78,79,114). The CR therefore provide a less dangerous way of entry for intracellular bacteria. Low-molecular-weight fractions, particularly of mycobacteria, such as phenolic glycolipid 1 of M. leprae, scavenge ROIs (139,140). Some intracellular bacteria may block the respiratory burst by interfering with protein kinase C activity. Such a mechanism also affects iNOS activity. Finally, many intracellular bacteria produce superoxide dismutase and catalase, which detoxify O_2^- and H_2O_2, respectively (141). Production of ROI detoxifying molecules by intracellular bacteria is not constitutive; rather, expression of these enzymes is controlled by regulators such as soxR or oxyR, which sense for concentrations of O_2^- or H_2O_2, respectively. Accordingly, several transposon mutants of S. enterica, which fail to survive inside murine MPs, are highly sensitive to ROIs in vitro (142). Although less is known about specific mechanisms by which intracellular bacteria may interfere with killing by RNIs, catalase and other antioxidative enzymes may indirectly inhibit RNI functions (143, 144). Because both ROIs and RNIs also affect host molecules,

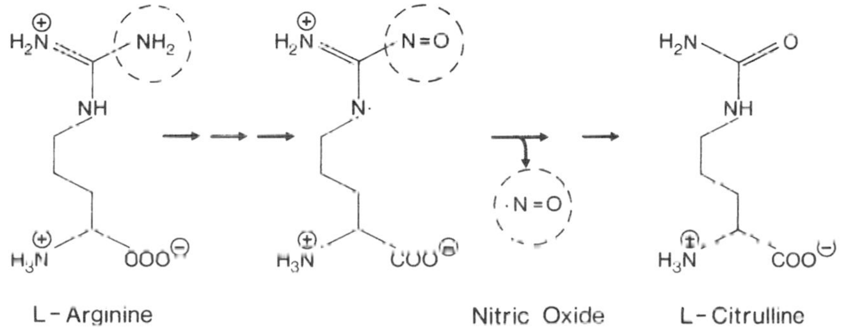

FIG. 2. Generation of nitric oxide from L-arginine.

L - Arginine   Nitric Oxide   L-Citrulline

excess generation of these effector molecules is dangerous for the host as well.

Evasion into the Cytoplasm

Evasion from the phagosomal into the cytoplasmic compartment represents a highly successful microbial survival strategy, because bacterial killing is focused on the phagolysosome in order to limit self-damage of MPs. This egression has been extensively studied in

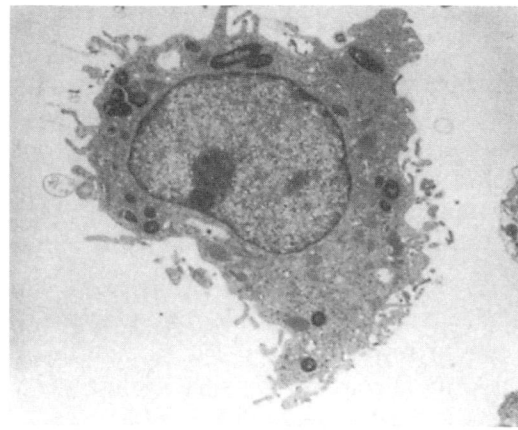

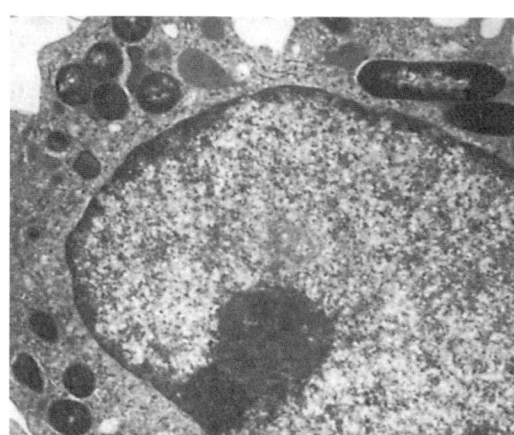

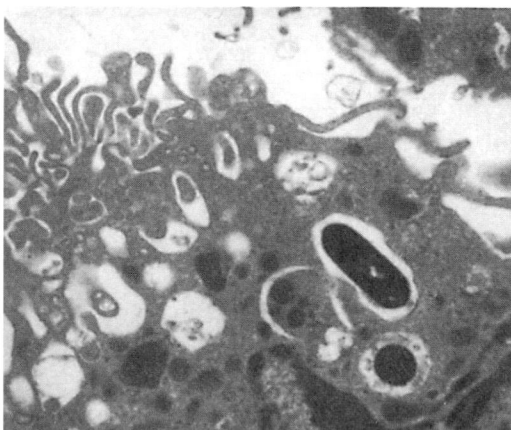

FIG. 3. Localization of *L. monocytogenes* inside mononuclear phagocytes (MPs). **Top:** Electron photomicrograph of an *L. monocytogenes*-infected macrophage. **Middle:** *L. monocytogenes* in the cytoplasm. **Bottom:** *L. monocytogenes* in the phagosome. (Provided by G. Szalay, S.H.E. Kaufmann, and J. Golecki.)

L. monocytogenes, but it may also be utilized by other intracellular pathogens (Fig. 3) (29–32,145–149). Cytoplasmic invasion by *L. monocytogenes* depends on listeriolysin, an SH-activated cytolysin. Deletion of the responsible gene renders *L. monocytogenes* avirulent. Probably, other cytolysins, such as phospholipases, lecithinase, and metalloprotease, are involved in membrane transition but are insufficient on their own. Evasion of *L. monocytogenes* into the cytoplasmic compartment is, however, markedly reduced in IFN-γ–activated macrophages, in which the microbe entrapped in the phagosome rapidly succumbs to attack by ROIs, RNIs, and/or defensins (150).

Cell-to-Cell Spreading

L. monocytogenes is cleared from the blood by Kupffer cells, and from here it spreads to adjacent hepatocytes without reentering the extracellular milieu (87,151,152). This mechanism of cell-to-cell spreading has been carefully studied *in vitro* (152–154). Having entered the cytoplasm, *L. monocytogenes* is surrounded by fibrillar material, which subsequently forms a tail composed of actin filaments. In this way, *L. monocytogenes* is pushed forward to the outer regions of the cell, where it induces pseudopod formation. Intracellular movement is achieved by coordinated actin polymerization at, and polarized release from, the bacterial surface. The actA gene encodes a 90-kDa protein located on the bacterial surface, which is responsible for these actin-based movements (36,38). A host cytosolic complex composed of eight polypeptides has been identified, which, on binding ActA, induces actin polymerization (155). The pseudopod-containing *L. monocytogenes* is engulfed by the adjacent cell, and the microbe reaches the phagosome of the recipient cell still enclosed by the cytoskeletal material from the donor cell. The bacterium then traverses the double membrane and enters the cytoplasm of the recipient cell. Thus, *L. monocytogenes* can infect numerous cells without contacting extracellular defense mechanisms. Although less well understood, a similar spreading mechanism seems to be employed by *R. rickettsii,* but not by *R. prowazekii* and *R. typhi* (16).

Apoptosis

Death of mammalian cells occurs by two different forms: accidental or programmed cell death, which results in necrosis and apoptosis, respectively (156). Necrosis is the result of cell destruction caused by various exogenous effector mechanisms, including those mediated by complement and cytolytic T-lymphocytes (CTLs). Apoptosis, in contrast, is initiated by intrinsic mechanisms within the dying cell itself. This programmed cell death involves a series of enzymatic events, notably intracellular proteases of the caspase family. Studies have revealed that several bacterial pathogens, including *M. tuberculosis, S. enterica,* and *L. monocytogenes,* can activate the apoptotic machinery in cells after their uptake (157–163). *S. enterica* has been found to induce apoptosis in macrophages, whereas *L. monocytogenes* causes apoptosis in hepatocytes and dendritic cells, but not in macrophages (159–161,164). The responsible molecules and mechanisms are incompletely understood in these cases. Perhaps the formation of small pores by listeriolysin from *L. monocytogenes* and by SipB of *S. enterica* initiate apoptosis (165). However, apoptosis induced by *Shigella flexneri* has been studied in more detail, and it was found that its virulence factor, IpaB, not only participates in pore formation, but also interacts with the apoptotic machinery by binding to and activating members of the caspase family (166,167). It remains to be established whether it is the host or the pathogen that primarily benefits from apoptosis. Exogenous ATP causes death of host cells harboring *M. bovis* BCG, which, in turn, results in mycobacterial killing (105a,105b). Although this macrophage death has some resemblance with apoptosis, it is also distinct from conventional apoptosis induced through CD95 and mediated by caspases.

Controlled Expression of Genes Involved in Intracellular Survival

Increasing evidence suggests that rather than expressing their virulence genes constitutively, bacterial pathogens do so only when required (168–170). *S. enterica, M. tuberculosis* and *M. bovis, L. monocytogenes,* and *L. pneumophila* are not restricted to the mammalian host and survive in the environment for a considerable part of their life span. In the environment, many virulence factors are not required, making their constitutive expression unnecessary. Similarly, living conditions for rickettsiae markedly differ from insects to humans. Expression of virulence factors is controlled by specific sensors, which enable intracellular bacteria to express the appropriate factors in a coordinated way (168–170). Although the external stimuli responsible for virulence gene expression are not fully understood, it is probable that they include changes in pH, pO_2, osmolarity, temperature, N_2, or phosphate. Such sensors include the PhoP/PhoQ system of *S. enterica* and the regulatory gene prfA of *L. monocytogenes,* which positively regulates the expression of a variety of factors involved in intracellular survival, including listeriolysin (168–171). Also, HSP70 has been proposed to serve as a sensor for stress situations (172).

Heat-Shock Proteins as Broad Survival Factors of Intracellular Bacteria

Heat-shock proteins (HSPs) are produced at increased levels when a cell is insulted by various stress stimuli, such as altered pO_2, pH, or temperature and various starvation phenomena (173–175). Inside MPs, intracellular bacteria face several of these stress stimuli, and one of their responses is to increase HSP synthesis (176). Accordingly, *S. enterica* mutants deficient in HSP expression are more susceptible to killing by MPs *in vitro* and *in vivo* (142,177,178). HSPs are involved in protein folding and assembly of protein complexes. Conversely, they prevent or retard protein unfolding. As a result of the attack by toxic effector molecules, protein unfolding and/or disassembly of protein complexes occur, which are at least partially impeded by HSPs. Thus, HSPs promote intracellular survival in a general manner.

PROFESSIONAL PHAGOCYTES

Mononuclear Phagocytes

Metchnikoff (179) was the first to realize the importance of professional phagocytes in acquired resistance against bacterial infections. He observed that leukocytes accumulated at the site of inflammation and bacterial growth, where they were heavily engaged in microbial engulfment and destruction. Metchnikoff distinguished two types of phagocytes: (a) the early-appearing and short-lived microphages, which are now called PNGs; and (b) the later-appearing, long-lived macrophages, still known under this name. The preferential localization of tubercle bacilli inside macrophages, as already discovered by Koch (180) and Metch-

nikoff (179), pointed to the central role of these phagocytes in defense against intracellular bacteria. Metchnikoff also observed that, during infection, macrophages are nonspecifically activated (179). Macrophage activation as an important factor of acquired resistance against bacterial infections was further substantiated by Lurie (181) and shown to be under the control of lymphocytes by Mackaness and Blanden (182). Later, cytokines were identified as the mediators of macrophage activation (183–186).

It is now clear that many of the antibacterial activities described above and summarized in Table 4 are not constitutively expressed in MPs. Rather, expression of full antibacterial activities by MPs depends on appropriate stimulation by cytokines, with IFN-γ being of paramount importance (93,184,186). Furthermore, significant differences exist among MPs of different maturation status or from different species. For example, human blood monocytes, but not tissue macrophages, possess myeloperoxidase activity. High RNI levels are produced by murine MPs and probably by human MPs under certain conditions. Activation of MPs coincides with increased phagocytosis, elevated CR, reduced FcR expression, and a higher overall metabolic rate, to name but a few inducible activities. Most importantly, during macrophage activation, iNOS and NADPH oxidase, which initiate RNI or ROI production, respectively, are stimulated. In other words, activation by cytokines results in transition of MPs from a habitat supporting microbial replication into an effector cell capable of terminating, or at least restricting, microbial survival (187).

Polymorphonuclear Granulocytes

Although the role of PNGs in intracellular bacterial infections has often been neglected, their high antibacterial potential allows them to kill many intracellular bacteria (188,189). However, PNGs are short-lived, and intracellular bacteria are sequestered in intracellular niches; hence the overall contribution of PNGs to defense against chronic infections remains small. Yet, during the early acute inflammatory response, they help to reduce the initial bacterial load (190). This is particularly evident in experimental listeriosis, which is an acute disease: The first day of infection is characterized by extensive PNG infiltration at sites of listerial growth (87,191), and elimination of PNG by mAb treatment remarkably exacerbates listeriosis (192,193). While the listerial burden in the liver of mAb-treated mice was dramatically increased, that in the spleen remained virtually unchanged. This finding shows an organ-specific role of PNG in early antilisterial resistance.

PNGs are also potent secretors of ROIs and hypochlorous acid, as well as of proteolytic enzymes such as elastase (a serine proteinase), collagenase, and gelatinase (74,189). These secretion products act as mediators of tissue destruction. In the extracellular milieu, protease inhibitors are normally present, preventing tissue damage by these proteases. However, the concomitant secretion of hypochlorous acid inactivates these proteinase inhibitors, thus promoting cell lysis. Accordingly, PNGs have been shown to cause inflammatory liver damage by destroying infected hepatocytes during early listeriosis (191). MPs are less potent secretors of proteinases and fail to produce the major inactivator of proteinase inhibitors, hypochlorous acid. Thus, established granulomas, such as productive granulomas in chronic tuberculosis, are dominated by MPs and are characterized by necrosis and fibrosis and lack signs of tissue liquefaction. During reactivation, however, PNGs may eventually be recruited to tuberculous granulomas and then contribute to granuloma caseation and liquefaction.

THE CENTRAL ROLE OF T CELLS

Acquisition of resistance against intracellular bacteria crucially depends on T-lymphocytes, which, ideally, accomplish sterile bacterial eradication. When a "normal" immune status is provided, bacterial clearance is rapidly achieved in the case of susceptible bacteria, such as *L. monocytogenes*. In the case of resistant pathogens, such as *M. tuberculosis,* clearance frequently remains incomplete and is arrested at the stage of bacterial containment to, and growth control at, distinct foci. Bacterial containment and eradication occur in granulomatous lesions. The longer the struggle between host and microbial pathogen continues, the more essential the granuloma becomes. Granuloma formation and perpetuation are orchestrated by T-lymphocytes. The cross-talk in the granuloma between T-lymphocytes, MPs, and the other cells is promoted by cytokines.

The T-cell requisite is probably best exemplified by the high incidence of tuberculosis and other intracellular bacterial infections in patients suffering from T-cell deficiencies, particularly AIDS. It is not contradicted by experiments showing transient resistance of nu/nu and severe combined immunodeficient (SCID) mice against experimental listeriosis (43,194). Although these T cell-deficient mice are capable of controlling experimental listeriosis for relatively long periods, they ultimately fail to eradicate their pathogens. In the long run, therefore, these animals succumb to disseminated listeriosis.

At the same time, T-lymphocytes are an unavoidable element of the pathogenesis of intracellular bacterial infections. First, expanding granulomas impair tissue functions by occupying space and affecting surrounding cells. Second, the physiologic functioning of infected host cells may be affected by specific T-lymphocytes.

Historical Perspective

The role of antibodies in antibacterial protection has become increasingly clear since the demonstration by Behring and Kitasato, before the turn of the century, that passive transfer of serum from immune animals protects against diseases caused by toxin-producing bacteria (195). Although subsequent claims had been published that antituberculous immunity can be transferred with sera from immune animals, most investigations provided evidence to the contrary (1). It was not until the 1960s that scientists, most notably G.B. Mackaness, revealed that acquired resistance against intracellular bacteria can be transferred with viable lymphocytes from immune donor animals (8,182). Mackaness and his coworkers established the model of experimental listeriosis in mice, which proved extremely helpful.

Mice are infected intravenously with a sublethal dose of *L. monocytogenes*. At various time points thereafter, they are killed, and their spleens and livers are removed. Numbers of bacteria are determined in organ homogenates after serial dilution and plating on agar plates. Fifteen minutes after injection, more than 95% of all bacteria are removed from the circulation and are found in these organs. After a prompt but transient drop in bacterial numbers, listeriae grow continuously until days 4 to 6. Afterward, bacterial numbers rapidly decline and become undetectable by days 8 to 10. The turnaround on days 5 to 6 correlates with the emergence of specific T-lymphocytes capable of transferring protection upon naive recipients. Infection with *L. monocytogenes* induces protective immunity. Mice that overcome primary sublethal infection are able to defeat a second, much higher and normally lethal, dose of *L. monocytogenes* (see Fig. 4). Although tuberculosis can be studied similarly in mice, it is far more laborious, and significant differences between immune and naive mice are less dramatic and often seen only after several weeks to months.

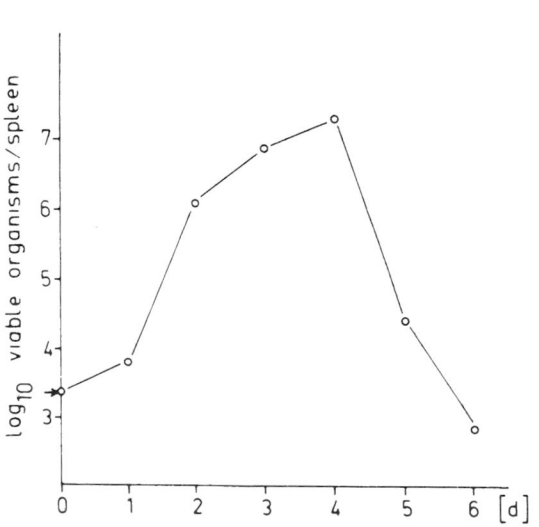

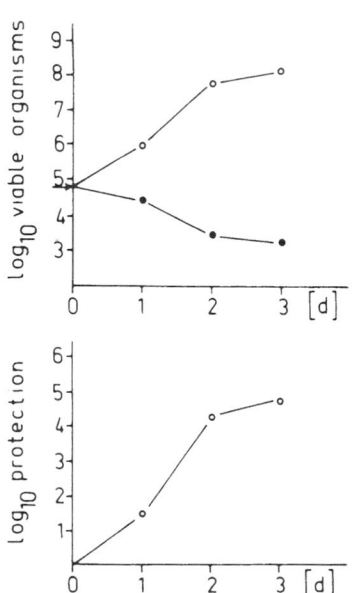

FIG. 4. Course of experimental listeriosis in mice. **Left-hand panel:** Primary listeriosis following infection with a sublethal dose (5 × 10³ i.v.) of *L. monocytogenes*. Infection is monitored by counting colony-forming units (*CFUs*) of *L. monocytogenes* in spleens and livers. Only spleen CFUs are shown. **Upper right-hand panel:** Comparison of primary listeriosis in naive mice (*open circles*) and secondary listeriosis in already immune (vaccinated) mice (*closed circles*) following a lethal dose of *L. monocytogenes*. **Lower right-hand panel:** The difference in CFUs between naive and vaccinated mice is termed *protection*.

TABLE 5. *Conventional and unconventional T cells in antibacterial immunity*

| T-cell population | Antigen-presenting molecule | | | Ligand | Site of ligand loading |
	Type	Tissue distribution	Polymorphism		
CD4 αβ T cell	MHC class II	Restricted (APC)	High	12–20mer peptide	Endosome
CD8 αβ T cell	MHC class Ia (+ β2m)	Broad	High	Nonapeptide	Cytosol
CD8 αβ T cell	MHC class Ib (+ β2m)	Broad	Low	N-f-met-pentapeptide	Endosome, cytosol (?)
DN (CD8) αβ T cell	Group 1 CD1 (+ β2m)	Restricted (APC)	Low	Lipid, lipoglycan	Endosome
CD4 (DN) αβ T cell	Group 2 CD1 (+ β2m)	Intermediate	Low	?	?
DN γδ T cell	No presentation molecule known	Not applicable	Not applicable	Phospholigands and others	?

T-Cell Subpopulations

The peripheral T-cell system comprises several phenotypically distinct and stable populations (196,197) (Tables 5 and 6). T-lymphocytes expressing the αβ T-cell receptor (TCR) make up more than 90% of all T cells in secondary lymphoid organs and peripheral blood of humans and experimental mice. They are further subdivided into (a) CD4 αβ T cells, which recognize antigenic peptides presented by gene products of the MHC class II; and (b) CD8 αβ T cells, which interact with antigenic peptides in the context of MHC class I molecules.

Undoubtedly, these conventional αβ T cells are of primary importance for antibacterial resistance, although good evidence exists that unconventional T cells additionally participate in control of intracellular bacteria (197,198). These unconventional T-cell populations encompass

1. CD8 αβ T cells, which recognize bacterial peptides presented by nonclassical MHC class Ib molecules
2. Double-negative (DN) or CD8 αβ T cells, which recognize bacterial lipids or glycolipids presented by group 1 CD1 molecules
3. CD4 or DN αβ T cells, which coexpress the natural killer (NK) marker and are specific for group 2 CD1 molecules
4. γδ T-lymphocytes with specificity for antigenic ligands presented in very different ways.

Conventional CD4 and CD8 αβ T Cells

Both MHC class II–restricted CD4 αβ T cells and MHC class I–restricted CD8 αβ T cells participate in acquired resistance against intracellular bacteria. This has been most extensively studied in *L. monocytogenes*-infected mice:

1. Adoptive transfer of antilisterial immunity depends on compatibility between transferred T cells and recipient mice in MHC class II and in MHC class I gene loci (199,200).
2. *In vitro* depletion of CD4 and of CD8 T cells from *Listeria*-immune lymphocyte populations markedly impairs adoptive transfer of protection against *L. monocytogenes* (201–204).
3. Both CD4 and CD8 T-cell clones with specificity for *L. monocytogenes* and capable of adoptively transferring protection have been isolated from infected mice (205–207).
4. Both MHC class II– and MHC class I–deficient gene-deletion mutant mice (so-called KO mice) lacking conventional CD4 or CD8 T cells, respectively, suffer from exacerbated listeriosis (208).

Most intracellular bacteria primarily reside in the phagosomal compartment of MPs, and hence pathogen-derived peptides have ready access to the MHC class II presentation pathway (Fig. 5). However, some microbes are capable of egressing into the cytosol (see above). Accordingly, intracellular bacteria can be grouped as phagosomal pathogens or cytosolic pathogens (209,210). The phagosomal pathogens encompass most intracellular bacteria, with the exception of *Rickettsia* species and *L. monocytogenes,* which are clearly cytosolic pathogens (32,149,211). Controversy exists whether *M. leprae* and *M. tuberculosis* can leave the phagosome under rare circumstances (145–148,212,213). Obviously, antigens from cytosolic pathogens can be readily introduced into the MHC class I–processing pathway, thus promoting activation of CD8 T cells (209,211, 214–216). Yet, CD8 T cells have also been isolated from mice infected with phagosomal pathogens, such as *M. bovis* and *S. enterica* (217–219). The following speculative and not mutually exclusive pathways for antigen translocation from the phagosome into the cytosol, independent of bacterial egression into the cytosol, are possible:

TABLE 6. *Conventional and unconventional T cells in antibacterial immunity*

T-cell population	Species	Major *in vitro* function	Role in antibacterial protection	Comment
CD4 αβ T cell	Human, murine	IFN-γ, CTL	Proven	Control of "endosomal pathogens"
CD8 αβ T cell (MHC 1a)	Human, murine	CTL, IFN-γ	Proven	Control of "cytosolic pathogens"
CD8 αβ T cell (MHC 1b)	Human	CTL, IFN-γ	Proven	Well characterized in murine listeriosis
DN (CD8) αβ T cell	Human	CTL, IFN-γ	Likely	Specificity for mycobacteria (and related species?); known ligands: mycolic acid, LAM
CD4 (DN) αβ T cell	Human, murine	IL-4, IFN-γ	Unknown (regulatory ?)	No microbial ligand known; recognition of CD1 proper possible; surface expression of CD1 may be influenced by infection
DN γδ T cell	Human	IFN-γ, CTL	Proven (compensatory, regulatory)	Known ligand in human system: isopentenyl-pyrophosphate and alkyl derivatives (present in pro- and eukaryotes); murine γδ T cell with reactivity for phospholigands unknown

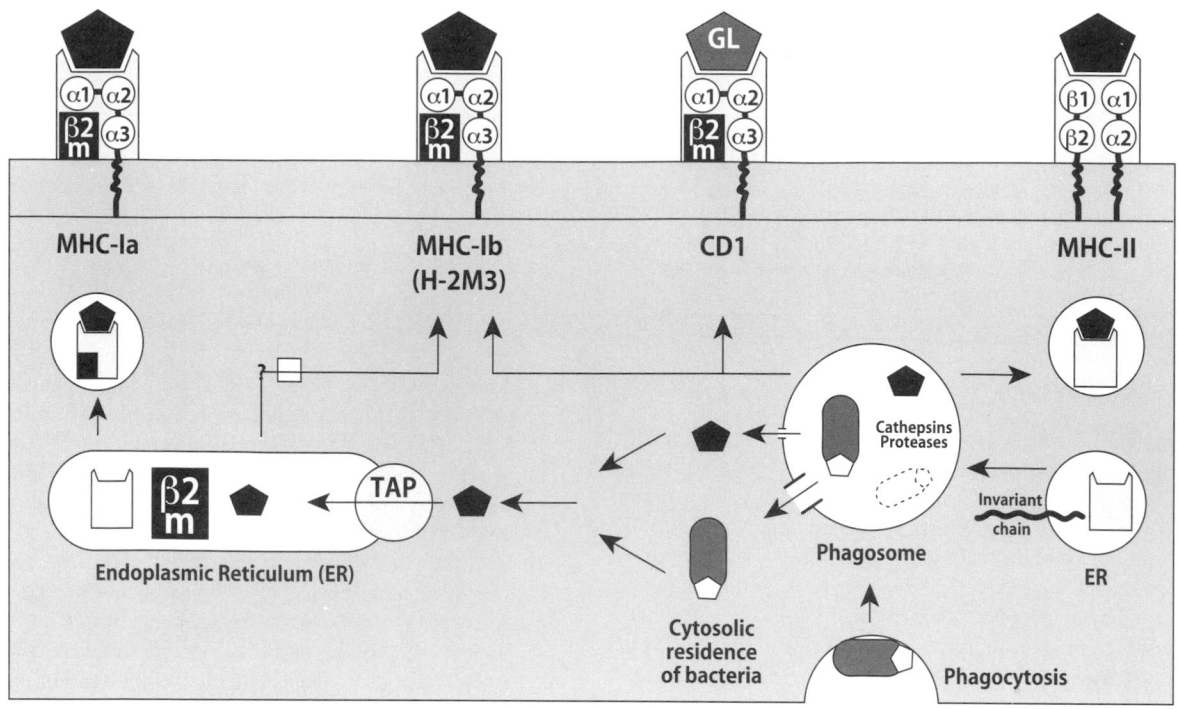

FIG. 5. Multiple antigen-processing pathways for stimulation of T cells during bacterial infections. Note that at least three different presentation molecules (MHC II, MHC Ib, CD1) are loaded in the phagosome. GL, glycolipid.

1. Some intracellular bacteria possess cytolysins, which would permit translocation into the cytosol of secreted proteins or peptides without requiring bacterial egression from the phagosome. Such a mechanism, for example, has been claimed for *M. tuberculosis* (220).

2. The early phagosome harboring *M. tuberculosis* retains MHC class I molecules, which may allow direct loading of *M. tuberculosis*-derived peptides (213).

3. Some phagosomal bacteria, such as *S. enterica,* possess a specific secretion apparatus, which may promote protein translocation into the cytosol of host cells (15).

4. Bacteria containing phagosomes have thorough exchange with corresponding endosomes, which may allow peptide loading of vacuolar MHC class I molecules (221).

5. Antigens from bacteria that persist in the phagosome may leak into the cytosolic compartment (222).

6. Antigenic peptides from phagosomal bacteria are loaded to surface-expressed MHC class I molecules by regurgitation (221,223). This pathway may involve sensitization of bystander cells (224).

It is now beyond doubt that alternative pathways of MHC class I antigen presentation exist (209,224–226). Even killed bacteria, denatured proteins, and proteins coupled to inert particles, such as latex beads, can be processed and loaded to the MHC class I pathway (224). Yet, the different antigen-processing pathways for MHC class I remarkably differ in their efficacy. The most efficacious means for antigen introduction into the MHC class I–processing machinery is bacterial egression into the cytosol. Accordingly, cytosolic pathogens are the most potent stimulators of CD8 T cells, whereas CD4 T-lymphocytes are primarily stimulated by phagosomal pathogens. Reciprocally, phagosomal or cytosolic pathogens are primarily controlled by CD4 or CD8 T cells, respectively.

Intracellular bacteria also invade nonprofessional phagocytes, some of which do not express MHC class II molecules constitu-

tively. Consequently, such cells remain unrecognized by CD4 T-lymphocytes and provide a hiding place for intracellular bacteria—a situation that has consequences for the course of disease. Because MHC class I molecules are expressed by almost every cell, CD8 T-lymphocytes have the potential of surveying the whole body. This is particularly important for those intracellular bacteria that hide in MHC class II⁻ host cells. Obviously, recognition of these cells depends on CD8 T-lymphocytes (and perhaps unconventional T cells; see below). *L. monocytogenes,* on the one hand, resides in nonprofessional phagocytes with low antibacterial potential and, on the other hand, promotes MHC class I presentation of its antigens. This may explain the predominance of MHC class I–restricted CD8 T-lymphocytes in defense against experimental listeriosis, both by number and by biologic relevance (208,211). In contrast, *M. bovis* is primarily restricted to MPs and remains in the phagosome. This is compatible with its preferential control by MHC class II–restricted CD4 T-lymphocytes (227). Although *M. tuberculosis* resides primarily in MPs, its high resistance to antibacterial effector mechanisms may require the concerted action of both CD4 and CD8 T cells (228,229). *M. leprae* also seems to be a weak stimulator of MHC class I–restricted CD8 T cells; yet, it lives in a variety of host cells. In these situations, a discrepancy may arise between strong dependence on CD8 T cells and insufficient activation of these cells. Principally, CD4 T cells and CD8 T cells with specificity for bacterial antigens express similar biologic functions, and differences in the spectrum of the target cells may be of greater importance.

Unconventional T Cells

During recent years, several populations of unconventional T-lymphocytes have been identified, some of them showing unique specificity for bacterial ligands. Some of these T cells do not follow the rule of MHC–peptide recognition by the TCR and recognize unusual ligands, either directly or in the context of nonclassical MHC class Ib or CD1 molecules. In some cases, unconventional T cells recognize ligands unique to bacteria, suggesting an important role for these T cells in antibacterial resistance. This also provides strong evidence that these unconventional T cells are the result of a long-lasting coevolution between bacterial pathogens and their mammalian host. It is conceivable that specificity for ligands that are unique to bacteria provides a powerful means of distinguishing foreign invaders from self antigens.

Major Histocompatibility Complex Class Ib–restricted CD8 T Cells

In murine listeriosis, CD8 T cells with protective activity have been identified that are not restricted by the classical MHC class Ia molecules (230,231). These CD8 T cells recognize N-formylmethionine (N-f-met)–containing peptides presented by nonclassical MHC class Ib gene products (232,233). In mammalian cells, only few N-formylated proteins exist, these being of mitochondrial origin. In contrast, many bacterial proteins contain the N-f-met sequence. (Furthermore, N-f-met–containing peptides have proinflammatory activity for MPs and PNGs; see below.) Thus, it appears that MHC class Ib gene products are specialized for presentation of bacterial antigens (234). The peptide-binding groove of the responsible mouse MHC class Ib molecule, H2-M3, has room for small peptides only (235). Consistent with this, the recently identified N-f-met peptides from $L.$ $monocytogenes$ are penta- or hexapeptides, as compared with the nonapeptides typically presented by classical MHC class Ia molecules (236,237). While the nonclassical MHC class Ib molecules are covalently bound to $\beta 2$-microglobulin ($\beta 2m$) on the cell surface, as are classical MHC class Ia molecules, N-f-met peptide presentation seems to originate in the phagosome (see Fig. 5) (237,238). Consistent with this notion, killed listeriae are a source of N-f-met peptides for H2-M3 presentation (238). Stimulation of unconventional CD8 T-lymphocytes through this pathway probably contributes to protection, which is induced by vaccination with heat-killed $L.$ $monocytogenes$ (239). Yet, it appears likely that N-f-met peptides can also be loaded to H2-M3 from listeriae residing in the cytosol (238). MHC class Ia–independent CD8 T cells have also been isolated from mice infected with $M.$ $bovis$ or immunized with killed $M.$ $tuberculosis$ (217). Thus, activation of MHC class Ib–restricted, N-f-met peptide–specific CD8 T cells may be a general phenomenon of intracellular bacterial infections in mice. It remains to be established, however, whether a similar type of unconventional CD8 T cells also exists in humans.

CD1 Molecules and Antigen Presentation

Although the CD1 polypeptides share several features with MHC class Ia/Ib molecules, they are encoded outside of the MHC (240). On the one hand, CD1 and MHC class Ia or Ib heavy chains have some homologies, and both CD1 and MHC class I molecules are generally surface-expressed in association with $\beta 2m$. On the other hand, their unique functional features and their genomic location outside the MHC define CD1 polypeptides as a distinct family of nonpolymorphic antigen-presenting molecules. In humans, four major types of CD1 molecules can be distinguished (CD1a to

CD1d), and they fall into two groups: Group 1 encompasses CD1a/b/c, and group 2 comprises CD1d. The group 1 CD1 molecules, which are primarily expressed on conventional antigen-presenting cells (APCs), are capable of presenting mycobacterial lipids and glycolipids to T cells (241–243). The distribution and functional role of group 2 CD1 molecules is less well understood (240). However, group 2 CD1 molecules have been identified on numerous host cells. Only group 2 CD1 molecules exist in the mouse (termed $CD1.1$ and $CD1.2$). These group 2 CD1 molecules are recognized by murine NK T cells, described below (244). More recent evidence suggests that all CD1 molecules form a hydrophobic cleft in which hydrophobic peptides or lipid–lipoglycans could be accommodated (245).

Group 1 CD1-restricted Double-negative or CD8 T Cells

In humans, an unconventional $\alpha\beta$ T cell of DN or CD8 phenotype has been described that has the unique capacity to recognize mycobacterial lipids or glycolipids presented by CD1 (241–243). Antigen presentation by group 1 CD1 molecules commences in the late endosomal compartment (see Fig. 5) (241,242,246). Two mycobacterial ligands have thus far been identified, these being mycolic acids from $M.$ $tuberculosis$ and LAM from $M.$ $leprae$ (241,242). Both molecular entities are important components of the cell wall of mycobacteria and some related genera, such as nocardiae and corynebacteriae (247). Lipoids from different species show structural differences, which are apparently distinguished by the distinct TCRs (242). These unconventional glycolipid-specific $\alpha\beta$ T cells produce IFN-γ and lyse target cells, strongly suggesting that they participate in antiinfective immunity. Similar T-lymphocytes have not been identified in the mouse—probably due to the lack of group 1 CD1 molecules in this species. In the absence of an appropriate mouse model, a clear role for group 1 CD1–restricted T cells in antibacterial immunity has not yet been shown. Nevertheless, the data obtained with the human T cells demonstrate the paramount impact of bacterial pathogens on the evolution of the T-lymphocyte system, which apparently resulted in a highly specialized T-cell population with exquisite specificity for bacterial components.

Natural Killer T Cells with Specificity for Group 2 CD1 Molecules

In mice, lymphocytes have been identified that coexpress the $\alpha\beta$ TCR and the NK-cell marker, NK1 (244). Thus, these cells share characteristic phenotypic features with NK cells and $\alpha\beta$ T cells. The NK T cells are specific for group 2 CD1 (the only CD1 molecules that exist in mice) (248–251). Although binding of highly hydrophobic peptides to CD1d and apparent T-cell recognition of this MHC–peptide complex has been described (245), it remains an open question whether NK T cells recognize group 2 CD1 molecules directly or a self or nonself ligand presented by these molecules (244). Accordingly, it is unclear whether antigens from intracellular bacteria can be presented by group 2 CD1 gene products. Use of a restricted TCR repertoire and of an invariant $V\alpha 14/J\alpha 281$ chain would be consistent with direct recognition of CD1 proper or of highly conserved antigenic ligands (244). It is possible that infectious agents regulate group 2 CD1 surface expression, thus influencing NK T-cell stimulation indirectly (252). Glycosylceramides encompassing long-chain fatty acid and sphingosine base have been identified as ligands for murine NK T cells (252a). Because these compounds are rare in mammals and bacteria, the natural ligands for these NK T cells in host, invading pathogens, or both remain to be identified. Thus far, the evidence suggesting a role of these NK T cells in antiinfective immunity stems from their potent and rapid cytokine production upon stimulation through their TCR with a bias towards IL-4 (253). As will be discussed in more detail below, these cells may, therefore, participate in the regulation of antiinfective immunity. Although characterization of NK T cells was mostly done in the mouse system, T-lymphocytes expressing a homologous invariant Vα chain have been described in humans (244). Thus, similar cells may exist in humans.

γδ T cells

A minor T-cell population in the peripheral blood and lymphoid organs of humans expresses an alternative TCR made up of a γ and a δ chain. Although the role of these γδ T cells in antibacterial immunity has not been fully revealed, recent years have witnessed compelling evidence that γδ T cells play a prominent role in antibacterial immunity (254).

γδ T cells from the peripheral blood of healthy individuals are strongly reactive to mycobacterial components *in vitro* (255–257). The responsible entities have been identified as small-molecular-weight, nonproteinaceous molecules comprising phosphate as essential component (258–262). Isopentenyl pyrophosphate and alkyl derivatives thereof have been defined as natural ligands, but other components, including phosphosugars, phosphoesters, and nucleotides, probably serve as antigenic ligands as well. These phospholigands stimulate the major subset of γδ T cells in humans, expressing the Vγ2Vδ2 TCR combination with high junctional diversity. Despite this oligoclonal activation, a conserved TCR-binding site is required for stimulation. The isopentenyl pyrophosphate represents a ubiquitous precursor of various metabolites, both in prokaryotes and eukaroytes. Apparently, it is presented to γδ T cells on the host-cell membrane independently of known antigen-presenting molecules encoded by MHC or CD1 genes (263). The most likely explanation for these findings is direct recognition of phospholigands by the TCRγδ. In contrast to the human system, murine γδ T cells are not stimulated by these phospholigands (254,264).

Studies with γδ T cell–deficient TCRδ gene-deletion mutant mice or with mice treated with anti-γδ TCR mAb suggest an auxiliary role of γδ T cells in antilisterial protection (265–268). More profound effects of γδ T-cell deficiency were observed in γδ T cell–deficient KO mice, which die of a high inoculum of *M. tuberculosis* (269,270). At present, it is safe to state that γδ T cells participate in antibacterial immunity. However, in most cases, they seem to perform auxiliary rather than essential functions.

Increased numbers of γδ T cells have been frequently identified at sites of inflammation. In particular, an increased proportion of γδ T cells has been noted in lesions of leprosy patients during reactional stages and at the sites of DTH reaction to lepromin (271). In TCRδ KO mice infected with the intracellular bacteria, *L. monocytogenes* or *M. tuberculosis,* the characteristic granulomas do not develop (267,269,270). Instead, inflammatory abscess-like lesions emerge, reminiscent of the characteristic tissue response to purulent extracellular pathogens. Taken together, these findings indicate a regulatory role of γδ T cells in inflammation, and particularly in granuloma formation.

Because γδ T cells are activated prior to αβ T cells, they could potentially fill a gap between early, nonspecific resistance mediated by the innate immune system and the later highly specific acquired immune responses mediated by αβ T cells. The major role of γδ T cells, however, seems to be of a regulatory nature. In particular, γδ T cells seem to regulate inflammatory responses at the site of microbial implantation (e.g., granuloma formation). Recognition of ubiquitous phospholigands by human Vγ2Vδ2 T cells is consistent with a regulatory role of these cells in inflammation and maintenance of homeostasis during infection. Although γδ T cells represent a minor population of all T cells in peripheral blood and lymphoid organs, bacterial pathogens can stimulate high numbers of γδ T cells. Oligoclonal stimulation of approximately 80% of all γδ T cells by phospholigands, as compared with clonal stimulation of antigen-specific αβ T cells, accounts for this phenomenon. Finally, in the complete absence of αβ T cells, γδ T cells can assume biologic effector functions, which are performed by αβ T cells under normal conditions. Thus, γδ T cells possess a high compensatory plasticity.

The γδ T cells make up a large proportion of all T cells in mucosal epithelia, both in human and mouse (272). Because mucosal epithelia represent the major port of entry for many intracellular bacteria, a role in first-line defense of intraepithelial γδ T cells in gut and lung may be assumed. Although this is an intriguing assumption, convincing evidence to support this hypothesis is still missing.

T-CELL FUNCTIONS DURING THE COURSE OF INFECTION

T-Cell Functions

Generally speaking, T-lymphocytes perform three major functions: cytolytic functions and helper functions of T helper (Th) 1 or Th2 type. Th cells produce various cytokines, with Th1 cells being characterized by potent IL-2 and IFN-γ secretion, and Th2 cells by potent IL-4 and IL-5 production (273). The CTLs lyse infected target cells by direct cell contact (274). Although each of the T-cell populations, as described above, can, in principle, perform numerous biologic functions, some preference can be observed. CD8 T cells (either MHC class Ia– or MHC class Ib–restricted) are preferentially cytolytic (275). A role for CTLs in immunity against *L. monocytogenes* has been demonstrated by the use of KO mice with deficient CTL functions (276). CD4 T cells as well as γδ T cells are typically cytokine-producing Th cells. Similarly, the human group 1 CD1–restricted αβ T cells and the murine group 2 CD1–specific NK T cells are potent cytokine producers. IFN-γ–producing Th1 cells are of paramount importance for acquired immunity against intracellular bacteria. In contrast to Th1 cells, Th2 cells do not contribute to acquired resistance against intracellular bacteria measurably, and if default Th2-cell activation occurs, disease is exacerbated.

Contribution of Conventional and Unconventional T Cells to Protection: Implications for Vaccine Design

The findings described above emphasize that a number of distinct T-lymphocyte populations participate in the antibacterial host response. Without doubt, a hierarchy exists regarding the contribution of T-cell sets, with the conventional CD4 and CD8 αβ T cells being of highest importance. Yet, unconventional T cells, which make up only a minor population, are probably required for efficient control to occur. This may be particularly important for combat of highly resistant bacteria, such as *M. tuberculosis*. Thus, although our knowledge about unconventional T cells is still limited, their participiation in the antibacterial immune response can no longer be ignored. Specificity of DN αβ T cells to unique components of certain bacteria, on the one hand, and oligoclonal reactivity of γδ T cells to components that are ubiquitous in the biosphere, on the other hand, illustrate the flexibility of the antiinfective immune response. In principle, each of the different T-cell populations is capable of expressing all the biologic functions relevant to antibacterial immunity. Thus, other differences must exist if one considers high functional redundancy an insufficient explanation. These differences include

- Differential tissue expression of the restricting elements (MHC class I being broadly distributed, MHC class II and group 1 CD1 having a restricted tissue expression with preference for APCs)
- Differential origin of the antigen-processing pathway (MHC class Ia starting in the cytosol; MHC class II, MHC class Ib, and group 1 CD1 originating in the endosome)
- Differential kinetics of activation (γδ T cells frequently preceding conventional αβ T cells)
- Differential physicochemical nature of the ligands (peptides being presented by MHC class I and MHC class II; glycolipids being presented by CD1; phospholigands being recognized by γδ T cells directly)

Identification of the spectrum of T-cell sets involved in antibacterial immunity, as well as characterization of the stimulatory antigenic ligands, form the basis for rational design of effective vaccines directed against intracellular bacteria. With regard to activation of conventional CD4 and CD8 T cells, two major issues deserve particular consideration (Fig. 6). First, localization of the bacterial pathogen within the host cell influences the relative contribution of CD4 or CD8 T cells to antibacterial protection. Consequently, the use of vaccines, which are preferentially localized in the endosome and, thus, predominantly activate CD4 T cells, may be insufficient for control of microbial pathogens that are primarily defeated by CD8 T cells (277). Such discrepancy may explain the low efficacy of BCG against tuberculosis. Yet, as discussed before, alternative pathways exist that allow introduction of antigens from endosomal vaccines into the MHC class I-processing machinery. Second, a profound impact of antigen display in secreted or somatic form on vaccine efficacy has been described (278). *S. enterica* vaccine carriers secreting or retaining, within their soma, the same listerial antigens conferred protection against *L. monocytogenes* infection only when the vaccine displayed the antigens in secreted form. Because intracellular bacteria only survive within resting macrophages, secreted proteins are already available for antigen processing in the initial phase of infection. Accordingly, only T cells directed against such secreted antigens can be activated. Once MPs have been activated by T cells, they can kill and degrade the intracellular pathogens, and, thus, somatic proteins become available for antigen processing. Accordingly, at later times of infection, T-cell responses against somatic antigens arise. Because efficacious vaccines must activate the T-cell response promptly after infection, secreted proteins are superior vaccine antigen candidates over somatic ones. Antigenic ligands presented by MHC class Ib or group 1 CD1 molecules have two potential advantages: First, the nonpolymorphic nature of the encoding genes circumvents problems associated with genetic variations among vaccinees, as is the case for peptides presented by the highly polymorphic classical MHC molecules. Second, absence of the antigenic ligands from host cells significantly reduces the risk of autoimmune responses. Obviously, uncovering the rules underlying antigen processing and activation of distinct T-cell subsets will promote rational design of vaccines against intracellular bacteria.

Kinetics of Infection

The course of infection with intracellular bacteria can be conveniently separated into three stages (Fig. 7). At each stage, cytokines are produced that perform two functions: First, they execute effector functions directed at reducing the microbial burden, and, second, they express regulatory functions that influence the subsequent course of infection (279,280). The early stage is initiated within minutes after microbial entry and dominated by cells of the innate immune system, in particular, PNG and MPs, which are attracted to the site of bacterial replication by chemokines and proinflammatory cytokines. Phagocytosis and intracellular killing of bacterial pathogens by these PNGs and MPs probably represent the predominant effector function at this early stage. Cytokines produced during this early stage (in particular, IL-12 from MPs) influence the subsequent stages by promoting induction of the protective acquired immune response. The intermediate stage is characterized by NK cells and γδ T cells, both of which produce IFN-γ. It links the early (innate) with the late (acquired) immune response. At the late stage, αβ T cells are operative that mobilize and sustain host defense mechanisms primarily in granulomatous lesions that result in effective control and, ideally, sterile eradication of the pathogen.

The length and importance of each stage are markedly influenced by the type of intracellular pathogen. In experimental listeriosis of mice, the complete sequence of host response lasts for less

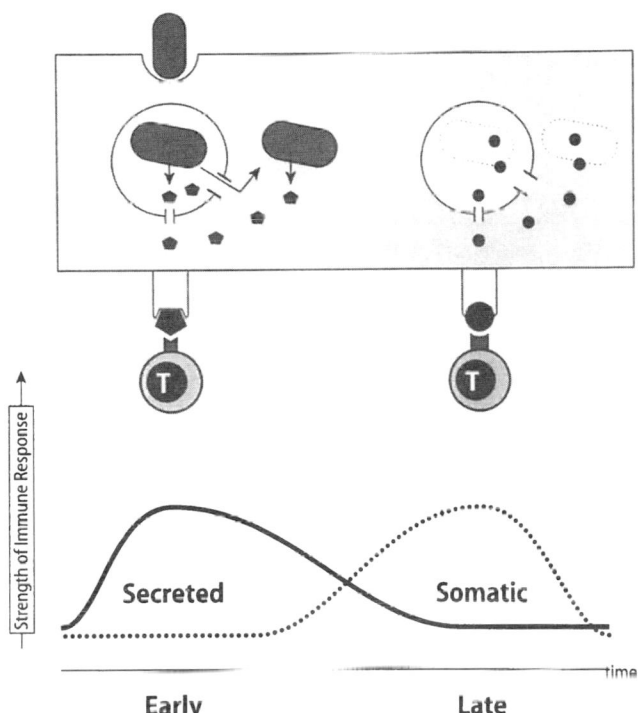

FIG. 6. Influence of intracellular localization and antigen display on the protective T cell response.

Strength of Immune Response

Secreted   Somatic

Early   Late

time

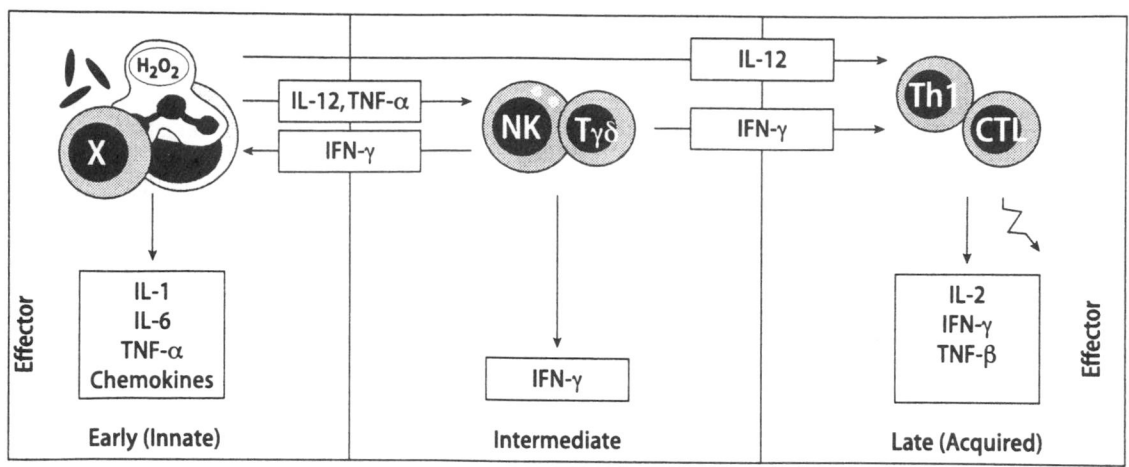

FIG. 7. The three stages of the immune response against intracellular bacteria.

than 10 days, whereas, in tuberculosis of humans, it may endure for several years. The early stage is particulary important for control of *L. monocytogenes* organisms, which divide rapidly and, at the same time, are highly susceptible to intracellular killing. The more robust and slowly dividing *M. tuberculosis* organisms are less vulnerable to this early stage of response. The relevance of the intermediate stage to microbial control is significantly influenced by the strength of the innate and the acquired immune responses. The broader the window between these two stages, the more important the intermediate stage becomes. In T cell–deficient mice (e.g., nu/nu mice, SCID mice, or RAG KO mice), the late stage fails to develop, and, accordingly, the intermediate stage has to compensate for this lack (43,281). Such mice, therefore, provide a useful model for analyzing the role of NK cells in antibacterial immunity.

CYTOKINES IN ANTIBACTERIAL DEFENSE

Cytokines are central to resistance against intracellular bacteria (Table 7). At all stages, cytokines are produced that perform regulator and/or effector functions. Although cytokines are essential for control of infection, they can also cause harm to the host. To avoid such harmful consequences, downregulation of the immune response is required at later stages of infection. Neutralization of

cytokines with specific antibodies and application of KO mice lacking defined cytokine or cytokine receptor genes have provided deep insights into the role of single cytokines. Identification of cytokines in lesions, in particular those from leprosy patients, has provided further information about the role of cytokines in antibacterial immunity. Cytokines control the following highly intertwined steps of the antiinfectious host response:

- Leukocyte recruitment to the site of bacterial deposition
- Formation of granulomatous lesions
- Activation of antibacterial functions in MPs at the site of bacterial replication
- Induction of a protective T-cell response
- Downregulation of the antibacterial host response to avoid harmful sequelae of an exaggerated immune response

Leukocyte Recruitment

Influx of inflammatory phagocytes occurs prior to the appearance of specific T-lymphocytes, and, accordingly, the relevant cytokines are primarily produced by MPs, as well as by epithelial and endothelial cells, in response to microbial invasion. Early produced cytokines with effector functions include the proinflammatory cytokines, tumor necrosis factor (TNF), IL-1, and IL-6, and

TABLE 7. *Cytokines in antibacterial immunity*

Cytokine	Contribution to antibacterial protection	Major cellular source in bacterial infection	Major function in bacterial infection
Chemokines	Likely	Epithelial cell, endothelial cell, macrophage, PNG	Leukocyte recruitment and activation
IL-1	Important role proven	Macrophage	Leukocyte recruitment and stimulation
IL-6	Essential role proven	Macrophage, T cell	Leukocyte recruitment, T-cell differentiation
TNF-α	Essential role proven	Macrophage, mast cell	Leukocyte recruitment, NK-cell activation, granuloma formation, IFN-γ costimulation
IFN-γ	Essential role proven	Th 1 cell, NK cell	Macrophage activation, granuloma formation
IL-12	Important role proven	Macrophage	Th 1-cell, NK-cell stimulation
IL-18	Likely, not proven	Macrophage	Th 1-cell stimulation
IL-4	Exacerbation	NK T cell, Th2 cell, basophil (?), Eosinophil (?)	Th 1-cell inhibition
IL-10	Exacerbation	Macrophage	Macrophage inhibition
TGF-β	Exacerbation likely, not proven	Macrophage	Macrophage inhibition

the still-expanding family of chemokines (282–288). The chemokine superfamily encompasses more than 50 related small-molecular-weight polypeptides (288–290). Three subgroups can be distinguished on the basis of a conserved cysteine motif: the CC chemokines, with two unseparated terminal cysteine residues; the CXC chemokines, with a nonconserved amino acid separating the two terminal cysteine residues; and the C chemokine, with only one terminal cysteine (C chemokine), which comprises only one member thus far (lymphotactin). Grouping of the large chemokine family can be further extended on the basis of different chemokine receptors (291). The CC chemokines (also termed β *chemokines*) preferentially act on MPs, whereas PNGs are primarily activated by CXC chemokines (also termed α *chemokines*). Other leukocytes, including lymphocytes, eosinophils, and basophils, may also be stimulated by these chemokines. The C chemokine (γ *chemokine*), lymphotactin, primarily recruits lymphocytes.

Although definite proof for the important role of chemokines in defense against intracellular bacteria is still scarce, one can assume that chemokines as a group play an important role in early mobilization of host defense (292,293). Generation of KO mice lacking the receptor for the CC chemokine MCP-1 revealed elevated susceptibility of these mice to listeriosis (291a). Experiments in other systems have revealed a central role of chemokines in early inflammation, in particular, PNG and monocyte extravasation (see also Fig. 10). In addition, some chemokines activate professional phagocytes and in this way probably promote early reduction of the bacterial load. The proinflammatory cytokines, IL-1, IL-6, and TNF, are also involved in the early accumulation of inflammatory phagocytes at the site of bacterial growth (282–285,287). The essential role of IL-6 and TNF in antibacterial immunity is dramatically demonstrated by the extreme susceptibility to listeriosis and tuberculosis of KO mice with a deficient IL-6 or TNF type 1 receptor (TNF-R1) gene (294–299). The proinflammatory cytokines, when produced in high amounts, cause acute-phase responses by inducing release of various plasma proteins from hepatocytes. However, they serve as endogenous pyrogens that stimulate fever, and TNF is also responsible for cachexia, the characteristic feature of wasting in infections with many intracellular bacteria, notably tuberculosis. Clinical trials showing that detrimental effects of excessive TNF production in tuberculosis and leprosy patients can be ameliorated by treatment with thalidomide emphasize the double-sided role of TNF in chronic infections (300–302).

Granuloma Formation

Experiments utilizing KO mice with a deficient IFN-γ or TNF-R1 gene emphasize a role of IFN-γ and TNF in granuloma formation during tuberculosis (299,303,304). Although in both types of mouse mutants necrotic lesions develop, they apparently fail to contain tubercle bacilli, resulting in disseminated tuberculosis. Hereditary IFN-γR deficiency has been described in humans, and these immunodeficient patients severely suffer and ultimately die of infections with intracellular bacteria (305,306). This high susceptibility was accompanied by impaired granuloma formation. Conversely, evidence has been presented that transforming growth factor-β (TGF-β) and IL-10 counteract granuloma development (307–311). Probably, these cytokines minimize immunopathology by preventing formation of extensive lesions. Premature inhibition of granuloma formation, however, may interfere with optimum protection. The relatively easy access to clinical leprosy lesions has provided often complementary insights into the function of cytokines in granulomatous

lesions. Analysis of cytokine mRNA patterns in tuberculoid leprosy lesions has revealed abundant IL-1, TNF, granulocyte–macrophage colony-stimulating factor (GM-CSF), TGF-β, IL-6, IL-2, IL-12, and IFN-γ mRNA, indicating an involvement of these cytokines in the control of granuloma perpetuation (311–313). In contrast, IL-4, IL-5, and IL-10 mRNA levels are low to undetectable in these granulomas, but they are relatively high in lepromatous lesions, suggesting a role of these cytokines in granuloma downregulation.

Macrophage Activation

The activation of antibacterial macrophage properties by cytokines represents a central step in acquired resistance against intracellular bacteria. This step has been extensively studied *in vitro* using murine macrophages, and IFN-γ has been identified as the major cytokine of MP activation (314–316). IFN-γ-activated macrophages rapidly kill susceptible intracellular bacteria, such as *L. monocytogenes* (317). Although the question as to whether IFN-γ-stimulated MPs actually kill *M. tuberculosis* remains a matter of controversy, they markedly inhibit growth of these pathogens (314,318). RNIs are the major effectors of bacteriostatic–bactericidal MP activities against most intracellular bacteria (126,132), although some bacterial pathogens may be more susceptible to ROIs. IFN-γ-stimulated MPs often produce TNF, which synergizes with IFN-γ in the activation of antibacterial macrophage functions (319). Consistent with such a central role of IFN-γ in antibacterial immunity, IFN-γ- or IFN-γR-deficient KO mice rapidly succumb to infections with *L. monocytogenes, M. tuberculosis, S. enterica,* and other intracellular pathogens (303,304,320–322). The activation by cytokines of antibacterial functions in human MPs is less well understood. First, the production of high levels of RNIs by human MPs remains a matter of debate, although more recent data consolidate profound RNI synthesis by MP from patients with infectious disease (126,132,138). Second, IFN-γ fails to consistently induce tuberculostasis in human macrophages (323–326). Some tuberculostasis has been achieved in human MPs by costimulation with IFN-γ and TNF (323), and maximum tuberculostasis can apparently be achieved by further addition of 1,25-dihydroxyvitamin D3, the biologically active metabolite of vitamin D3 (323–326). This latter steroid is either taken up in the diet or produced in the skin after exposure to ultraviolet (UV) light (327). By 1α-hydroxylation, vitamin D3 is converted to its circulating metabolite, 1α-hydroxyvitamin D3. Further hydroxylation at C25 yields 1,25-dihydroxyvitamin D3, the biologically active component. Macrophages possess 1α-hydroxylase activity, which is controlled by IFN-γ. It is therefore likely that *in situ* IFN-γ can induce the autocrine 1,25-dihydroxyvitamin D3 production, which may be missing in certain *in vitro* systems. Further support for the central role of IFN-γ in control of intracellular bacterial infections in humans stems from the identification of hereditary IFN-γR deficiency in young children who succumbed to infections with various intracellular bacteria, or even to *M. bovis* BCG vaccination (305,306). Conversely, IFN-γ treatment in adjunct to chemotherapy has been used successfully in the treatment of leprosy, tuberculosis, and atypical mycobacteriosis (328–331). Hence, also in humans, IFN-γ plays a central role in host defense against intracellular bacteria. This cytokine is produced by different cells, which infiltrate the lesion in a sequential order. These are NK cells, γδ T cells, and αβ T cells of CD4, CD8, or DN phenotype (43,206,266, 332,333). In experimental listeriosis of mice, NK cells produce IFN-γ 1 day after infection; IFN-γ-producing γδ T cells appear by day 2, and IFN-γ–secreting CD4 and CD8 αβ T cells are demonstrable by day 5 (see Fig. 6).

Induction of a Protective T-Cell Response

The type of immune response, and hence the course and ultimate fate of infection, is determined soon after bacterial entry into the host (280). IL-12 is the crucial promoter of the protective immune response (334,335). It is rapidly produced by macrophages infected with intracellular bacteria, activates NK cells and stimulates maturation of Th1 cells (334–337). In either case, IFN-γ production is the result. TNF-α produced by infected macrophages synergizes with IL-12 for NK-cell activation, and IFN-γ from activated NK cells further promotes IL-12 secretion via a positive-feedback mechanism (338). In infections with microbes of weak stimulatory potential, IFN-γ may be required for appreciable IL-12 secretion (339–341). In murine listeriosis, IL-12 is apparently essential for generation of a protective primary immune response, whereas secondary challenge with *L. monocytogenes* of previously vaccinated mice shows partial IL-12 independence (342). Similarly, IL-12 seems to be an important, but not absolute, requirement for immunity against tuberculosis (343,344,344a). These findings argue against exclusive IL-12 dependency of IFN-γ induction. Perhaps the more recently identified cytokine, IL-18 [IFN-γ-inducing factor (IGIF)], is responsible for this partial IL-12 independence (345). Consistent with studies in the mouse system, patients with an intrinsic IL-12 defect suffer from lowered IFN-γ titers, accompanied by disseminated *M. avium* complex infections (346).

Downregulation of the Antibacterial Host Response to Avoid Its Harmful Sequelae

Generally, IL-4–producing Th2 cells are not significantly activated in intracellular bacterial infections. Nevertheless, counterregulatory cytokines are produced during infection. IL-10 is secreted rapidly after infection and probably serves to control Th1-cell development (338,347). Both murine and human macrophages produce IL-10 comcomitantly with IL-12 in response to bacterial infections, and, in both systems, IL-10 was found to decrease IL-12 secretion and, as a corollary, IFN-γ production (334,335). Consistent with a downregulatory role of IL-10 in antibacterial immunity, IL-10–deficient KO mice control listeriosis more efficiently, this being correlated with elevated production of numerous cytokines of relevance to protection, including IL-12 and IFN-γ (348). Precedent exists in murine toxoplasmosis for the importance of IL-10 in the control of antimicrobial immunity by preventing immunopathology caused by exaggerated IL-12 and IFN-γ responses. Once the bacterial pathogen is successfully defeated, the ongoing immune response must be confined to avoid severe harm to the host. In certain systems, IL-4–producing Th2 cells have been detected at later stages of chronic infections with bacterial pathogens, probably to counteract IFN-γ–producing Th1 cells (349,350). Macrophage deactivation and Th1-cell inhibition by TGF-β and IL-10 may further contribute to this event (308,309,319,338,351,352). Although downregulation of the antiinfective immune response has been largely ignored, it is probably essential for bringing back the activated immune response to normal levels. On the other hand, premature mobilization of downregulatory immune mechanisms prior to successful pathogen defeat may cause disease exacerbation. As will be discussed later, such an aberrant situation may lead to the lepromatous form of leprosy.

PREDOMINANCE OF T HELPER 1 OVER T HELPER 2 CELL ACTIVITIES IN INTRACELLULAR BACTERIAL INFECTIONS: THE INFLUENCE OF THE INNATE IMMUNE SYSTEM

The kind of infectious agent has a decisive influence on the type of cytokine-producing Th cells that develop as the most appropriate defense mechanisms (Fig. 8) (273,280,353). The two Th populations that arise, Th1 cells characterized by IFN-γ and IL-2 secretion and Th2 cells typically producing IL-4 and IL-5, are derived from a common precursor cell, designated *Th0 cell* (354,355). Th1 cells combat intracellular pathogens, including bacteria, protozoa, and fungi, while Th2 cells are responsible for control of helminths (273,356,357). Microbes and virions present in the extracellular milieu are also largely controlled by Th2 cells, although Th1 cells are involved, in addition. Conversely, uncontrolled Th1 or Th2 responses have been made responsible for autoimmune or allergic diseases, respectively. The distinction between Th1 and Th2 cells is made operationally on the basis of the type of cytokines produced, and it is, by no means, absolute. Stable surface markers that distinguish Th1 and Th2 cells have not been identified unequivocally (355). Although CD30 has been claimed to be a characteristic marker of human Th2 cells, IFN-γ–producing Th cells with reactivity for intracellular bacteria have been found to coexpress CD30, arguing that this molecule cannot be used as a specific Th2 marker, at least in intracellular bacterial infections (358,359). More recent evidence suggests that the β2 chain of the IL-12 receptor (IL-12Rβ2) is distinctive for Th1 cells in the human and murine systems (360,361).

Th1- and Th2-cell differentiation progresses through several stages, which are initiated promptly after microbial entry into the host (see Fig. 7). Under the counterregulatory influence of Th1 and Th2 cytokines, gradually polarization becomes more stable (273). It is now clear that the innate immune system, by promptly reacting to microbial components, determines the generation of the appropriate immune response (280). Default recognition of the infectious agent by the innate immune system, therefore, results in development of an inappropriate immune response, thus causing exacerbation of, rather than protection from, pathology. This has been best studied in the model of experimental infection of mice with the intracellular protozoal pathogen, *Leishmania major* (362). C57BL/6 mice, when challenged with *L. major,* build up a potent Th1 response and are protected. In contrast, BALB/c mice develop a Th2 response accompanied by increased susceptibility to leishmaniasis.

As was said above, in infections with almost all intracellular bacteria, potent Th1 responses develop, and Th2 responses are virtually absent. The prominent Th1 response caused by these infections has even been claimed to antagonize development of allergic diseases (363). Only in the case of leprosy does polarization towards a resistant tuberculoid or susceptible lepromatous pole occur, and some evidence suggests that a Th1/Th2 dichotomy underlies this polarization—at least in part.

How is the predominant Th1 response achieved at the different stages of antiinfective immunity? At the early stage of infection, IL-12 is produced rapidly by macrophages after microbial entry into the host, which serves as the central signal for Th1-cell development (334,335). In contrast, prompt IL-4 secretion, presumably by basophils, mast cells, eosinophils, and NK T cells, is low and short-lived (253,273,354,364). The microbial entities responsible for rapid IL-12 secretion are being identified. Carbohydrates, lipids, and gly-

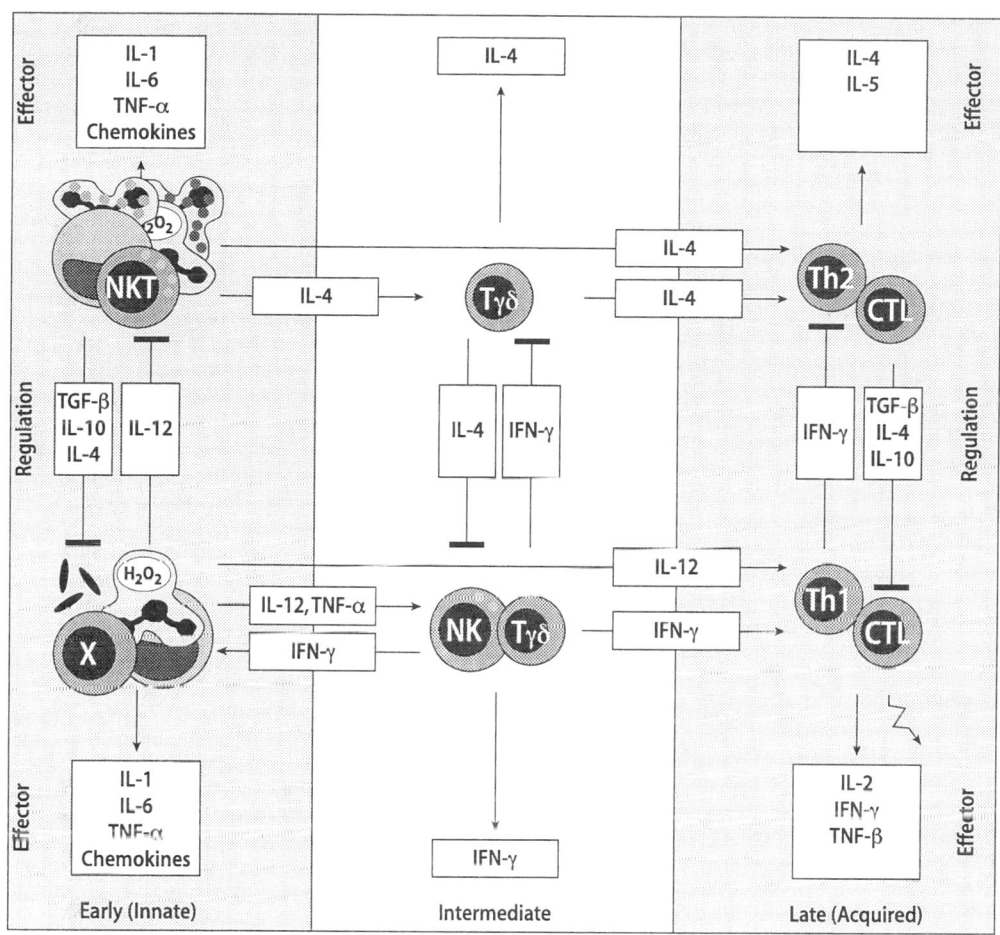

FIG. 8. Predominance of Th1- over Th2-cell activities at the three stages of the immune response against intracellular bacteria.

colipids, which are regular components of the bacterial cell wall, can induce IL-12 secretion. Thus, LPSs of gram-negative bacteria, lipoteichoic acids of gram-positive bacteria, as well as trehalose dimycolate, and LAM from mycobacteria have been shown to induce IL-12 secretion (365–367). Because MPs express pattern-recognition receptors for these lipoglycans, such as CD14, they can promptly react to bacterial invaders. Although direct recognition of bacteria-specific patterns appears to be the central mechanism that instructs the innate immune system, additional mechanisms may contribute (60). First, bacterial carbohydrates, lipids, and glycolipids also activate complement via the alternative pathway (280). Binding of the resulting C3b to its CR may further promote macrophage activation. (Note, however, that this mechanism may facilitate microbial entry into macrophages, avoiding the respiratory burst that results in ROI production.) Second, it is likely that pathogen-induced host-cell killing can result in proinflammatory cytokine release, and thus further support Th1-cell development. Third, oligonucleotides containing unmethylated CpG motifs, which are abundant in bacterial DNA, are potent IL-12 inducers (367a).

IL-12 acts not only on Th1 cells, but also on NK cells and γδ T cells, the central players at the intermediate stage of infection. Activation of both cell types profits from costimulation with TNF-α, which is secreted by activated macrophages concomitantly with IL-12. The IFN-γ from NK cells further increases IL-12 production by macrophages via a positive-feedback loop, thus greatly enhancing

IL-12 production. Under the concerted action of IFN-γ and IL-12, stable Th1-cell development is achieved. Conventional CD4 and CD8 T cells, as well as MHC class Ib-restricted CD8 T cells, group 1 CD1 controlled T cells, and γδ T cells, all acquire a Th1 phenotype during intracellular bacterial infections.

In vitro studies have revealed a dominance of IL-4 over IL-12, suggesting that Th2 cells develop in the presence of both cytokines (368). Moreover, NK T cells have been found to produce IL-4 promptly after their stimulation (253). Why, then, does one generally see unconstrained Th1-cell development in intracellular bacterial infections? This is probably promoted by downmodulation of the IL-4–producing NK T cells and of IL-4–producing Th2 cells (279). In support of this notion, infections with intracellular bacteria downregulate IL-4 production by NK T cells via IL-12 (369). NK T cells, upon long-lasting stimulation, apparently shift their cytokine pattern from IL-4 to IFN-γ production (279,369a; Emoto et al., in preparation). Thus, NK T cells may promote rather than interfere with Th1-cell polarization during infection with intracellular bacteria. Moreover, IL-4–producing Th2 cells develop profoundly in *L. monocytogenes*-infected IFN-γR-deficient mice, and the IL-4 produced further aggravates the already high susceptibility of IFN-γR−/− KO mice to listeriosis (370). The IL-12Rβ2 may be involved in Th1 polarization (360,361): While the IL-12Rβ2-chain expression remains high on Th1 cells, Th2 cells lose this chain successively during maturation, thus losing the capacity to respond to IL-12. This is consistent with convertibility of Th2 and Th1 cells in the early phase of polarization and increasing unresponsiveness to IL-12 of Th2 cells at later stages.

Although cytokines are the prime signal transmitters in Th polarization, cognate receptor interactions participate in this process. The most important ones are the CD40/CD40 ligand (CD40L) system and the B7/CD28/CTLA-4 system (371–375). The CD40/CD40L system was originally identified as an important regulator of B-cell activation and immunoglobulin class switching (376). Later it was found that interactions between CD40 on macrophages and CD40L (now termed *CD154*) on T cells provide a bidirectional cross-talk, which participates in activation of either partner cell. Thus, during the whole course of the antiinfective Th1 response—from its initiation to the execution of effector functions—CD40/CD40L interactions may participate. In KO mice with deficient CD40 or CD40L genes, IL-12 and IFN-γ secretion are impaired, resulting in increased susceptibility to the intracellular protozoan parasite, *L. major* (377–379). Yet, such a disease exacerbation has not been observed in experimental listeriosis of a CD40L-deficient mouse mutant (380). The B7 system comprises the B7-1 (now CD80) and the B7-2 (now CD86) molecules on macrophages and other APCs and the CD28 and CTLA-4 (now CD152) receptors on T cells (371,372,374,375). The cross-talk between these receptors–coreceptors supports, but is not essential for, induction of primary T-cell responses. Microbial carbohydrates, lipids, and glycolipids regulate surface expression of B7 molecules, and the relative density of B7-1 and B7-2 molecules on the surface of APCs may provide costimulatory signals for Th0 cells, directing them toward either the Th1 or the Th2 pole (252).

Employing both cytokines and cognate interactions provides the means for balanced amplification and tight control of the antiinfective immune response. Cytokines promote the broad-spectrum signaling that is required for accumulation and activation of leukocytes at the site of microbial replication. Cognate interactions between cell surface receptors are more restricted, and hence avoid activation of bystander cells, which may cause undesirable tissue reactions or even activation of autoimmune responses.

DEATH OF INFECTED CELLS

Several lines of evidence suggest that the death of infected cells plays an important role in protection against, and pathogenesis caused by, intracellular bacteria (Fig. 9) (157,158,187,191,211). First, several intracellular bacteria, including *S. enterica, Mycobacterium* species, and *L. monocytogenes,* have exploited ways to induce apoptosis in infected host cells (see above). *L. monocytogenes*-infected hepatocytes and dendritic cells rapidly undergo apoptosis, causing an inflammatory milieu that attracts PNGs to the site of bacterial replication (160,161). In contrast, macrophages apparently do not become apoptotic after *L. monocytogenes* infection (164). Subsequently, different host cells with killer potential enter the stage in succession. These are in the order of their appearance: PNGs, NK cells, γδ T cells, and αβ T cells (see Fig. 6). PNGs rapidly infiltrate the *L. monocytogenes*-infected liver, where they contribute not only to listerial killing, but also to hepatocyte damage (190,191). Elimination of these PNGs markedly exacerbates listeriosis (192,193). Hepatocytes are highly permissive to listerial growth, and both *L. monocytogenes*-induced apoptosis and PNG-mediated lysis of these host cells appear to play an important role in the early antilisterial defense (281). NK cells are activated during intracellular bacterial infections (281,381). *In vitro*, activated NK

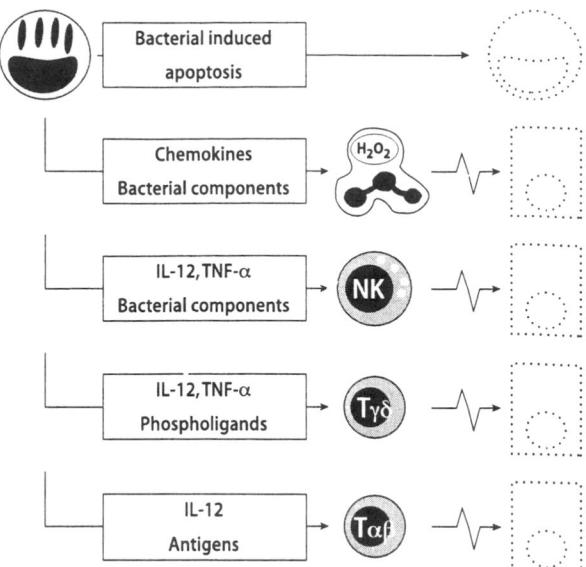

FIG. 9. Cell death in bacterial infections.

cells lyse MPs infected with a variety of intracellular bacteria, leaving uninfected target cells unaffected (382–385). Activated γδ T cells and group 1 CD1–restricted αβ T cells are also capable of lysing bacteria-infected target cells (386,387). MHC Ia– and MHC Ib–restricted CD8 T cells, as well as MHC class II–restricted CD4 T cells from mice infected with intracellular bacteria, rapidly express cytolytic activities after restimulation *in vitro* (211,238). Similarly, CD8 and CD4 T cells expressing specific cytolytic activity have been isolated from patients suffering from bacterial infections (388–391). A role of CTLs in antilisterial resistance has been corroborated by the finding that perforin-deficient KO mice with impaired CTL activity suffer from exacerbated listeriosis (276). At the same time, evidence has been presented that CD8 T cells cause liver damage in experimental listeriosis, resulting in elevated transaminase serum levels (392). CD4 and CD8 T cells in lesions of tuberculoid leprosy patients express phenotypic markers indicative of cytolytic activities (330,393,394). CTLs generally employ two forms of killer mechanism: apoptosis through Fas/Fas ligand (FasL) interactions and lysis via perforin-dependent mechanisms (274). In the mouse model, killing of infected macrophages by CTLs is accompanied by mycobacteriostasis (217). Using human CTL clones expressing either form of cytolytic mechanism, evidence was presented that perforin-dependent, but not apoptotic, macrophage death participated in growth inhibition of *M. tuberculosis* (387). Using mouse mutants, no major role for conventional CTL activity mediated by perforin or Fas/FasL interactions in the control of tuberculosis has been found thus far (395,396). Yet, macrophage death caused by ATP has been shown to result in mycobacteriostasis (105a,105b). CTLs can induce cell death via secretion of ATP, and, through this way, they may participate in mycobacteriostasis (396a). Binding of exogenous ATP to the P2Z receptor apparently causes fusion of phagosomes harboring mycobacteria within lysosomes, and this fusion results in both cell death and mycobacteriostasis, independent of RNI and ROI. Although analysis of this novel mycobacteriostatic pathway has thus far been restricted to *M. bovis* BCG and not analyzed using *M. tuberculosis,* it may represent an important control mechanism in tuberculosis.

Taken together, these findings suggest the participation of cell-destructive mechanisms in intracellular bacterial infections. On the one hand, phagocyte killing may directly impair growth of intracellular pathogens; on the other hand, death of nonprofessional phagocytes may contribute to pathogenesis by affecting physiologic organ functions. In addition, lysis of MPs is potentially harmful, because it could facilitate microbial dissemination. Many tissue MPs, such as alveolar macrophages and Kupffer cells, are insufficiently equipped to eliminate intracellular pathogens. Moreover, MPs may be further deactivated by microbial components, which interfere with macrophage functions. Destruction of MPs could breach this containment, thus promoting bacterial dissemination. On the other hand, lysis could contribute to sterile bacterial elimination. By facilitating release from incapacitated host cells (be they nonprofessional phagocytes or deactivated MPs), lysis promotes bacterial killing by more potent effector mechanisms. Thus, bacteria taken up by blood monocytes immediately after their release from incapacitated cells could be killed more efficiently (211).

THE GRANULOMATOUS LESION

"Idealized Granuloma"

The encounter between intracellular bacteria and host defense is a local event centered on the granulomatous lesion, which forms the focus of antibacterial protection (397,398). Failure to develop a granuloma or breakdown of an organized granuloma generally leads to disease exacerbation, often with fatal consequences. At the same time, expanding granulomas impair physiologic tissue function and therefore are central to pathogenesis. The "idealized" granuloma is a well-structured and organized lesion composed of T-lymphocytes of diverse phenotype and MPs at differing maturation and differentiation stages (Fig. 10). These include multinucle-

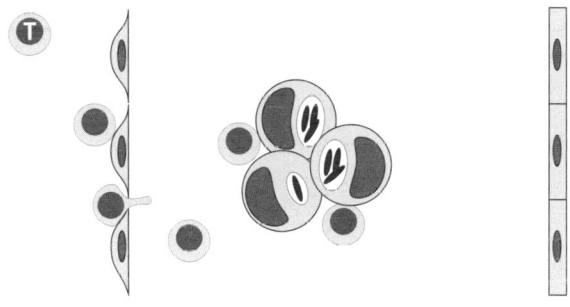

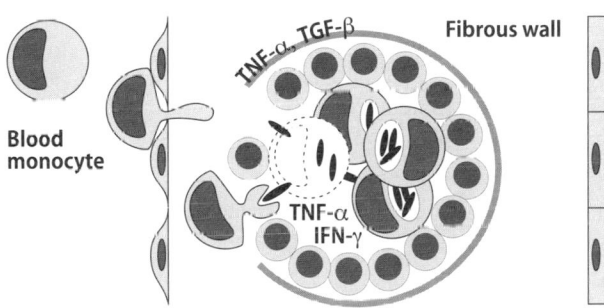

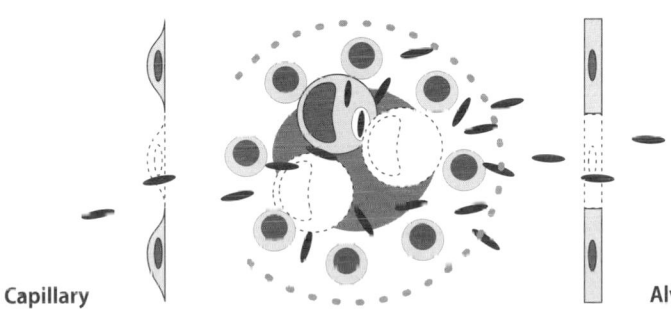

FIG. 10. Cellular interactions in an "idealized" granuloma.

ated giant cells, epithelioid cells, freshly immigrant monocytes, and mature MPs (398), among which, numerous CD4 T cells are interspersed. The whole is surrounded by an outer mantle primarily composed of CD8 T-lymphocytes (330,394,399). Microorganisms are located inside the granuloma MPs. As a result of necrotic death of the inner cells, a caseous, but still solid, center develops. Eventually, the lesion is encapsulated by fibrosis and calcification. In the following, the development of an idealized granuloma will first be described; subsequently, different forms of granulomatous lesions will be discussed.

Leukocyte Extravasation

In the early phase of granuloma formation, extravasation of (and invasion by) PNGs and, subsequently, blood monocytes is induced by proinflammatory signals mediated by bacterial components (N-f-met–containing peptides, such as f-Met-Leu-Phe, or oligonucleotides containing unmethylated CpG motifs), complement components (C5a), and cytokines (Fig. 11). Infected MPs produce numerous proinflammatory cytokines, such as IL-1, IL-6, and TNF-α, as well as various chemokines, which stimulate local endothelial cells and blood phagocytes (286,400–403). In the lung, substance P, a neuropeptide produced by sensory neuronal cells, and macrophage migration inhibitory factor (MIF) may further promote the inflammatory process (404,404a). The inflamed endothelium around the primary lesion expresses elevated levels of adhesion molecules, thus promoting extravasation of inflammatory phagocytes (see Fig. 11) (400,405–408). Extravasation is mediated by interactions between leukocytes and endothelial cells by means of adhesion molecules (400,408). These include selectins, integrins, and members of the immunoglobulin superfamily (see Fig. 11).

The L-selectins are found on leukocytes, whereas the P- and E-selectins are expressed by endothelial cells. Selectins are lectins that bind to carbohydrate ligands on the corresponding cell type. The integrins are heterodimers expressed on many cell types, including leukocytes and endothelial cells. At least six different integrins on leukocytes mediate binding to endothelial cells, notably LFA-1, Mac-1, and VLA-4. The ICAMs are members of the immunoglobulin superfamily, which includes ICAM-1, ICAM-2, ICAM-3, VCAM-1, and PECAM-1. ICAM-1 is strongly induced on leukocytes and endothelial cells. Endothelial cells constitutively express ICAM-2, VCAM-1, and PECAM-1, whereas resting leukocytes bear ICAM-3 and PECAM-1 on their surfaces. ICAM-1 interacts with the integrins LFA-1 and Mac-1; ICAM-2 and ICAM-3, with LFA-1; VCAM-1 with VLA-4; and PECAM-1 is engaged in homophilic interactions.

Contact between leukocytes and endothelial cells is initiated when the blood vessel is suddenly broadened in diameter at sites of inflammation (400). Activated endothelial cells and leukocytes upregulate surface expression of adhesion molecules, and thus promote leukocyte binding to the endothelium. This sets into motion the cascade of adhesion events. Selectin-mediated interactions result in leukocyte tethering and rolling. Subsequently, integrin interactions with immunoglobulin superfamily molecules cause tight leukocyte adhesion to endothelial cells. Once leukocytes firmly adhere to the endothelium, transmigration to the inflammatory focus occurs. Upregulation of P- and E-selectin expression primarily promotes PNG extravasation. In contrast, the L-selectins are constitutively expressed on virtually all leukocytes. Activated and memory T cells, as well as inflammatory phagocytes, however, express higher levels of integrins, such as LFA-1 and VLA-4, and activated endothelial cells show elevated expression of immunoglobulin superfamily molecules. ICAM-1 and VCAM-1 upregulation is primarily important for monocyte and T-cell transmigration to inflammatory foci. In summary, selectin-induced tethering and rolling, which is then succeeded by tight adhesion and subsequent extravasation of leukocytes, results in leukocyte accumulation at the site of microbial colonization, which forms the basis for granuloma formation.

Granuloma Formation

Although inflammatory PNGs and monocytes restrict bacterial replication, they frequently fail to eradicate their pathogens. At the same time, these phagocytes release proteolytic enzymes, which cause tissue damage (87,189,191). The early lesion, therefore, is often exudative. Eventually, specific T-lymphocytes are activated in the draining lymph nodes. Recirculating T-lymphocytes passing by the inflammatory lesion are recruited by proinflammatory cytokines and chemokines through mechanisms described above (286,400,405–408).

Gradually, infiltrating cells become organized and form a granuloma predominantly consisting of MPs. TNF and IFN-γ appear to be of crucial importance for this event. Although αβ T cells are the dominant T-lymphocyte population throughout all stages of granuloma formation, a significant proportion of γδ T cells has been observed in the initial phase (271). These γδ T cells apparently play an important role in the organization of a tight and well-structured granulomatous lesion, because, in their absence, more loosely structured or even abscess-like lesions develop that represent the characteristic tissue reactions against purulent bacteria (265,267, 270). Moreover, group 1 CD1–restricted DN αβ T cells have been isolated from skin lesions of leprosy patients, indicating their participation in this tissue reaction (242). Upon antigen-specific interactions with infected MPs, T-lymphocytes produce IFN-γ, thus activating antimicrobial macrophage functions.

Granulomas are at the forefront of protection by restricting bacterial replication at, as well as confining pathogens to, discrete foci. This is achieved by the following:

1. Activated MPs capable of inhibiting bacterial growth
2. Encapsulation promoted by fibrosis and calcification
3. Necrosis leading to a reduced nutrient and oxygen supply

Yet, frequently, microbial pathogens are not fully eradicated, and some organisms survive in a dormant form. A labile balance between microbial persistence and antibacterial defense develops that lasts for long periods.

Macrophage activation strongly relies on IFN-γ, which is sufficient in the mouse but requires support by TNF and 1,25-dihydroxyvitamin D3 in the human system. Fibrosis and necrosis are primarily promoted by TNF (285). MPs are deactivated by various microbial components. Under the influence of these factors, immigrant blood monocytes mature into epithelioid cells and multinucleated giant cells. Eradication of bacteria sequestered in granuloma MPs may be facilitated by controlled uptake by immigrant monocytes following their release from destroyed macrophages. Furthermore, release into the nutrient- and oxygen-deficient necrotic center may restrict bacterial survival. Although the granulomatous lesion may impair tissue functions, detriment to the host usually remains limited and infection does not necessarily cause clinical disease.

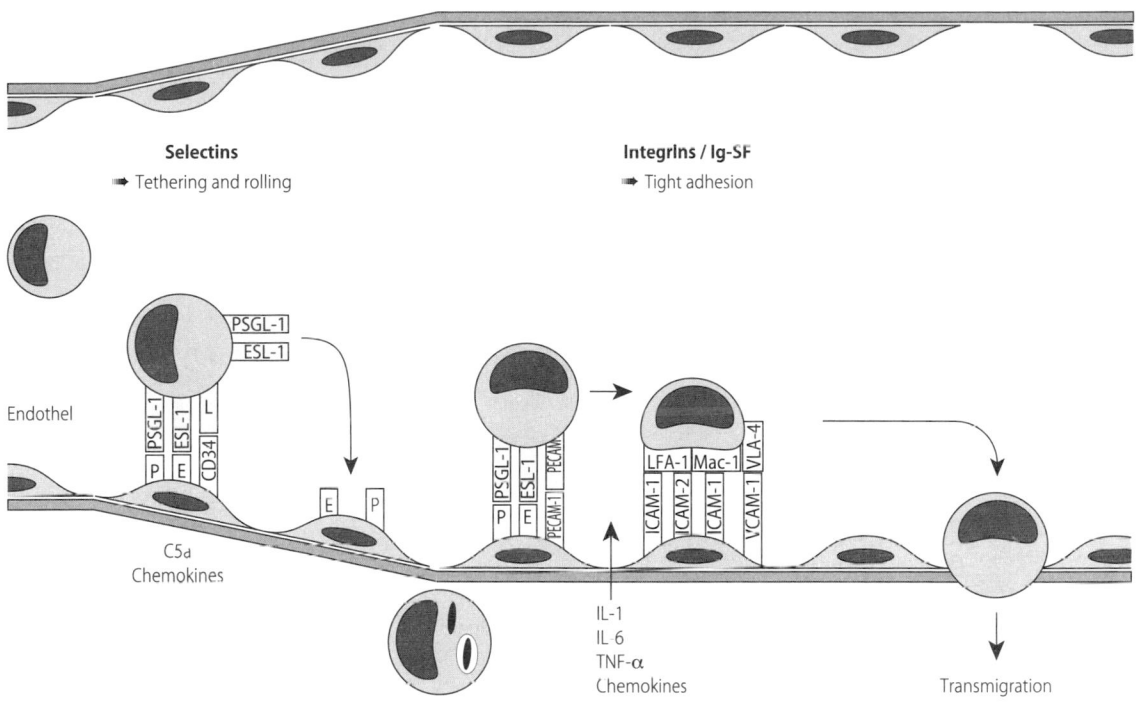

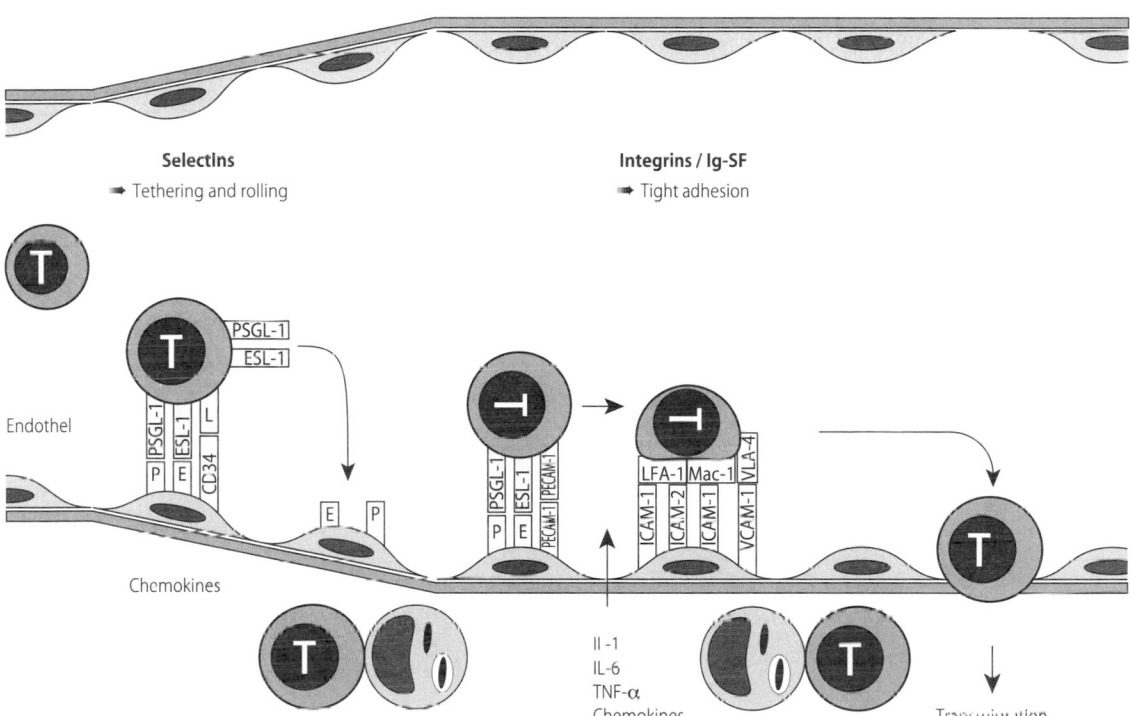

FIG. 11. Influx of phagocytes and T-lymphocytes from the blood to the site of bacterial growth. Selectins and their receptors: E, E-selectin; P, P-selectin; L, L-selectin; ESL-1, E-selectin ligand; PSGL-1, P-selectin ligand. Integrins: LFA-1, Mac-1, VLA-4. Immunoglobulin superfamily molecules: ICAM-1, ICAM-2, VCAM-1, PECAM-1.

Tuberculosis

The productive and proliferative granuloma, which effectively controls *M. tuberculosis,* best resembles the idealized granuloma described above. This lesion can then progress in five directions (7, 187,397):

1. The labile balance between microbial persistence and local protection remains equilibrated and succeeds in perpetuating stable immunity in the absence of disease. In more than 90% of *M. tuberculosis*-infected individuals, infection is arrested at this stage.

2. In rare cases, the proliferative granuloma succeeds in fully eradicating the microbial pathogens and disappears.

3. In the face of a strong immune response, necrotic reactions prevail, thereby extending tissue injury. Extensive secretion of fibrogenic cytokines, including TNF and TGF, may then lead to lung fibrosis (285). Yet, bacteria frequently remain restricted within the necrotic lesion. The clinical disease is thus confined to the affected organ (typically the lung), takes a more benign form, and is usually noncontagious.

4. Provided that cell-destructive mechanisms endure, the granuloma becomes exudative and subsequently liquefies. In the liquefied cellular detritus, *M. tuberculosis* grows in an uncontrolled manner, and extensive tissue damage markedly impairs the affected organ. It is in this cell detritus, in which huge numbers (up to 10^9) of *M. tuberculosis* organisms emerge, that multi–drug-resistant tubercle bacilli develop under incomplete chemotherapy. Microbial dissemination through the blood circulation promotes infection of secondary organs, and rupture into the bronchoalveolar system facilitates spreading into the environment. Excessive TNF may be released into the circulation and cause cachexia (283). The disease takes a malignant form and is highly contagious.

5. In cases of insufficient or deficient T-cell immunity, the granuloma soon breaks down, and bacteria are disseminated. In cases of severe immunodeficiency, as seen in AIDS patients or in newborns, productive granulomas do not develop at all, and infection directly progresses to disseminated, generally fatal, miliary tuberculosis.

Experimental Listeriosis

In experimental listeriosis, development of lesions is arrested at the stage of infiltration by inflammatory phagocytes and specific T-lymphocytes. Because *L. monocytogenes* is rapidly eradicated, a highly structured granuloma does not develop (409–411). In fact, formation of lesions is not essentially required for elimination of *L. monocytogenes*. On the other hand, infiltration of PNGs, MPs, and T cells causes hepatocyte damage, which impairs liver function. Hence, in experimental listeriosis, lesions have a strong pathologic component (392).

Leprosy

The lesions in tuberculoid leprosy have much resemblance to those in tuberculosis (28,86,330,394,412). Towards the lepromatous pole, suppressive mechanisms dictate the fate of the granuloma (see below). Lepromatous leprosy lesions are characterized by the presence of abundant *M. leprae* organisms and deactivated MPs, such as foamy macrophages, as well as a few T-lymphocytes expressing phenotypic markers characteristic for T cells with suppressor functions (CD8$^+$, CD28$^-$) (28). Evidence for involvement of TH2-like activities in lepromatous leprosy lesions has been presented (see below).

DELAYED-TYPE HYPERSENSITIVITY

An individual immune to an intracellular bacterium will develop a skin reaction at the site of local administration of soluble antigens from this agent. The reaction is characterized by monocyte infiltration and develops after 24 to 72 hours; that is, it is delayed. The first description of a DTH reaction against bacterial antigens was given in 1890 by R. Koch (180), who showed that guinea pigs infected with *M. tuberculosis* develop a specific inflammatory response against locally applied soluble culture filtrate, which he called *tuberculin.* In the 1930s, F. Seibert [cited in ref. (22)] produced a purified protein derivative (PPD) by removing the bulk of carbohydrates and enriching for proteins and peptides; PPD is still widely used.

It is now clear that DTH to antigens of intracellular bacteria is mediated by T cells primarily of the CD4 phenotype. Because soluble protein antigens generally fail to enter the MHC class Ia pathway, the contribution of conventional CD8 T cells to the DTH reaction must be considered low to absent. An auxiliary role of γδ T cells, however, appears likely (271). It is not yet clear whether these γδ T cells respond to specific antigens or whether they are nonspecifically activated by inflammatory stimuli. Although the DTH reaction, like the granulomatous lesion, primarily consists of MPs and is dependent on T-lymphocytes, it is a short-lived response, lasting for the few days it takes for the proteins to have been degraded. Accordingly, pathology of a DTH reaction is generally minimal. Application of high antigen doses into the skin of individuals with active tuberculosis, however, can cause marked necrotic reactions, leading to significant tissue damage.

SPECIFIC AND NONSPECIFIC UNRESPONSIVENESS IN INTRACELLULAR BACTERIAL INFECTIONS

Impaired immune responses are occasionally observed during chronic bacterial infections. They are most prominent in leprosy, which, towards its lepromatous pole, is characterized by immunologic unresponsiveness. Because unresponsiveness is central to the course of disease in leprosy, emphasis is laid on this disease (28,412). Although not as prominent, unresponsiveness may occur in other bacterial infections, particularly in severe active tuberculosis. While the phenomenon of immunologic unresponsiveness in leprosy is undoubted, the underlying mechanisms remain just as elusive as they are in other types of suppression.

Absent Delayed-type Hypersensitivity

Absence of DTH reactions in patients suffering from tuberculosis and leprosy is a well-established phenomenon (413–418). Proliferative responses, as well as IL-2 and IFN-γ production *in vitro,* are frequently reduced in such patients (414–419). DTH can be absent in up to 50% of tuberculosis patients before chemotherapy (420). In addition, in a certain percentage of BCG vaccinees, conversion to PPD$^+$ does not occur. These observations of specific unresponsiveness are thought to reflect insufficient protection and are taken as a negative prognostic indicator. In some individuals and in certain experimental animal models, efficient protection against intracellular bacteria has been observed, despite missing DTH responses, arguing that it is not a useful predictor. DTH responses are often reduced or absent during the height of protection. At least three explanations can account for segregation between DTH and acquired resistance:

1. DTH reactions elicited by soluble antigens are a function of CD4 T cells, whereas acquired resistance against most intracellular bacteria additionally involves CD8 T-lymphocytes and, perhaps, unconventional T-cell subsets. Therefore, impaired CD4 T-cell responses will have a greater effect on DTH than on resistance.
2. PPD does not contain all the antigens derived from *M. tuberculosis,* and hence does not fully reflect immunity against the pathogen.
3. T-lymphocytes may be trapped in granulomas during reactivation. This could be beneficial rather than detrimental, because it reflects T-cell accumulation at the site of antibacterial defense at the cost of irrelevant sites in the periphery.

Specific Unresponsiveness

M. leprae–specific unresponsiveness is frequently associated with less extreme forms of lepromatous leprosy (28,421,422). Lesions of these patients still contain significant numbers of T-lymphocytes (primarily of the CD8 phenotype), but they also contain abundant *M. leprae* organisms and macrophages lacking signs of activation (330,394,399). DTH reactions, as well as T-cell proliferation and IL-2 and IFN-γ secretion *in vitro,* are only negative in response to *M. leprae* antigens, but they can be induced by other antigens, even by the closely related PPD. Following biochemical separation of *M. leprae* antigens, T-cell responses against certain proteins in lepromatous leprosy patients are revealed. These findings indicate association of unique and specific antigens in *M. leprae* with suppression.

Direct administration of PPD into lepromatous leprosy lesions, as well as therapeutic vaccination with BCG and certain other mycobacteria, can cause remission towards the tuberculoid pole (423–425). Such a beneficial effect has also been reported after local administration of IL-2 and IFN-γ into lesions (394,423,426). Despite extensive efforts by several groups, the mechanisms underlying specific unresponsiveness have still not been elucidated completely. However, because specific unresponsiveness could be reversed by immune intervention, it cannot be due to deletion of *M. leprae*–specific T cells, but must be caused by active mechanisms.

Nonspecific Unresponsiveness

Nonspecific unresponsiveness, comprising T cells and/or macrophages, is observed *in vitro* and *in vivo* in severe cases of miliary tuberculosis and at the extreme pole of lepromatous leprosy (414,416,418,427). Patients suffering from nonspecific unresponsiveness fail to express DTH reactions, not only toward the relevant test antigen (lepromin in the case of lepromatous leprosy), but also toward unrelated antigens, such as PPD, histoplasmin, or contact sensitizers (e.g., picryl chloride). Similarly, T cells from such patients fail to proliferate and produce the cytokines IL-2 and IFN-γ in response to a variety of bacterial antigens (419,428–430). Although, in some cases, exogenous IL-2 has been shown to reconstitute IFN-γ production, often, nonspecific unresponsiveness could not be reversed (428).

Nonspecific unresponsiveness at the T-cell and macrophage levels is primarily caused by direct inhibitory effects of microbial components. Several constituents of *M. leprae* have been implicated in nonspecific unresponsiveness, including phenolic glycolipid, LAM, and sulfatides (101,430–433). Phenolic glycolipid has been shown to scavenge ROIs, thus hampering the antimicrobial functions of MPs (134,136). Furthermore, these and other mycobacterial components cause MPs to secrete factors that inhibit T-cell activation, including IFN-γ, RNIs, and prostaglandins. Nonspecific unresponsiveness affecting MPs and T cells towards various antigens is a rare event, which only occurs towards the extreme pole of lepromatous leprosy and in severe forms of miliary tuberculosis. It is virtually irreversible and, prognostically, extremely ominous. Lesions in polar lepromatous leprosy patients are characterized by a large burden of acid-fast bacilli, markedly reduced T-cell numbers, and few macrophages lacking signs of activation.

Mechanisms Involved in Specific Unresponsiveness

The mechanisms underlying specific unresponsiveness, though incompletely understood, may be best explained within the framework of current concepts of T-cell anergy. Such mechanisms, which are highly intertwined, include

- A shift from Th1 to Th2 polarization
- Default costimulatory cytokine signals
- Default signaling through costimulatory molecules

Comparative analysis, by polymerase chain reaction (PCR), of tuberculoid and lepromatous leprosy lesions has provided evidence for abundant mRNA of Th1 cytokines in tuberculoid lesions and higher mRNA levels of Th2 cytokines in lepromatous lesions (311–313,412) (see above). In particular, lepromatous lesions are characterized by high IL-10 and low IL-12 expression, whereas tuberculoid lesions show the opposite pattern. These findings are suggestive of a role of Th2-like cytokines in the development and/or perpetuation of lepromatous leprosy. CD8 T cells seem to be the primary source of IL-4 in human leprosy, and suppression of CD4 Th1 cells by CD8 T cells could be reversed by neutralizing anti–IL-4 antibodies *in vitro* (28,312,412,434). The potential role of the B7/CD28/CTLA-4 and the CD40/CD40L systems in Th1/Th2 polarization has already been discussed (371–374,380). Although direct evidence for their role in unresponsiveness in infections with intracellular bacteria is still missing, differential surface expression of CD40 and B7 molecules on cells infected with intracellular bacteria is a likely possibility (252). CD8 T cells isolated from lepromatous leprosy lesions lack the CD28 molecule, suggesting that the B7/CD28 costimulation is impaired in these cells. Such CD8+ CD28− T cells have been found to suppress Th-cell responses *in vitro* after *M. leprae*–specific activation (28,394,399,412,422).

It should be reemphasized here that—aside from lepromatous leprosy—unresponsiveness is a rare event in infections with intracellular bacteria, which are potent stimulators of Th1-type cytokines. Therefore, the question as to how *M. leprae* outwits the immune system in some patients, causing it to develop towards the lepromatous pole, remains central to our understanding of this disease. Although *M. leprae* contains abundant lipoglycans, which *per se* are potent IL-12 stimulators, monocyte infection with *M. leprae* seems to favor IL-10 secretion (311). It remains to be established how far an early imbalance between IL-10 and IL-12 contributes to polarization towards lepromatous leprosy. Most likely, unresponsiveness is not a defined entity determined by a single cell. Rather, it is multifactorial and variable and ranges from antigen-specific to antigen-nonspecific unresponsiveness. The former form is transient and can be reversed by appropriate immune intervention, whereas the latter is associated with decreased T-cell numbers and total macrophage failure.

GENETIC CONTROL OF RESISTANCE AGAINST INTRACELLULAR BACTERIA

Resistance against intracellular bacteria is genetically controlled, and inherited factors are of particular importance in chronic infections with a broad clinical spectrum, such as tuberculosis and leprosy. The significance of genetic factors was perhaps most dramatically illustrated by the terrible Luebeck disaster, which occurred in 1927, when 251 babies had been vaccinated accidentally with viable *M. tuberculosis* instead of BCG. At the end of the 6-year observation period, six children (2%) still suffered from tuberculosis, 129 (51%) had become ill but recovered, and 77 (31%) had died, and in 39 children (16%), clinical signs of tuberculosis had never developed (435).

In the 1940s, Lurie studied native resistance to tuberculosis in rabbits, and, by selective inbreeding, he succeeded in establishing strains of rabbits that differed remarkably in their susceptibility to infection with *M. tuberculosis* (181). Similarly, congenic mouse strains that differ in their susceptibility to experimental infection with several intracellular bacteria have been developed (436).

At least three levels of the host–pathogen relationship serve as potential targets for genetic control:

1. Genetic factors decide whether infection becomes abortive or establishes itself in a stable form. Convincing evidence for genetic control at this level does not exist.

2. Genetic factors control transition from infection to disease. This control step segregates "susceptible" from "resistant" individuals. Such inherited influences are well proven in the mouse and are most likely in the human population.

3. Severity and/or form of disease are controlled by genetic factors. It is generally accepted that MHC class II–encoded factors influence the development of leprosy towards the tuberculoid or the lepromatous pole. An association with a disturbed Th1/Th2 balance has been proposed (see above).

Control of Innate Antibacterial Resistance by the Nramp1 Gene

Studies in the mouse system have revealed a single dominant autosomal gene on chromosome 1 that is responsible for resistance against *M. bovis* BCG, *M. lepraemurium,* and *M. avium* and *M. intracellulare* (436–440). This gene, which has been termed Bcg, is identical with the Ity and the Lsh genes, which encode murine resistance against *S. enterica* and against the protozoan pathogen *L. donovani* (438,441). In contrast, murine resistance against other intracellular bacteria, most remarkably *M. tuberculosis,* is apparently not controlled by the Bcg/Ity gene (442–444). Positional cloning led to the identification of a full-length cDNA sequence. The responsible gene has been renamed Nramp1 (for natural resistance–associated macrophage protein) (445,446). The gene belongs to a family of genes that also encompasses Nramp2 on mouse chromosome 15. The human syntenic genes NRAMP1 and NRAMP2 have been identified on chromosomes 2q and 12q,

respectively (447). The Nramp1 gene product shows 85% identity and 92% similarity with its murine cognate. Regarding the role of Nramp1 in controlling infectious disease in humans, almost nothing is known thus far, and controversy exists whether Nramp1 serves as a susceptibility locus for leprosy (448–451). Most recent data, however, suggest an association between Nramp1 and susceptibility to tuberculosis (451a).

The functional importance of Nramp1 could be proven using transfected macrophage cell lines and by the generation of gene-disruption mutant mice (452,453). Differential susceptibility of Bcgs and Bcgr mouse strains can be traced to a single, nonconservative glycine to aspartic acid substitution at position 169 of the Nramp1 gene product. Importantly, transfer of the glycine 169 allele of Nramp1 into animals of susceptible background reestablishes resistance to *M. bovis* BCG infection.

Studies with congenic mouse strains and Nramp1 gene-deletion mutant mice have provided deeper insights into the mechanisms encoded by the Nramp1 gene. Differences between Bcgr and Bcgs strains are most obvious during the first weeks of infection; once T-lymphocytes have entered the picture, differences are less marked. Bcgr macrophages produce higher levels of ROI and RNI, as well as proinflammatory cytokines and some chemokines, after IFN-γ stimulation and/or infection. Furthermore, they express higher levels of MHC class II molecules, indicating that they are more potent antigen presenters for CD4 T cells. Indeed, CD4 T-cell responses seem to be elevated in Bcgr mice. In contrast, B-cell responses are higher in Bcgs mice.

Expression of the Nramp1 gene product is restricted to professional phagocytes, whereas the Nramp2 product is found in various cell types. The Nramp1 polypeptide is an integral membrane protein that contains several phosphorylation sites. It is found in the late endosome rather than on the outer surface of macrophages (453,454). Because the Nramp1 polypeptide has characteristic features of transporter molecules, it may be assumed that it participates in the transport of molecule(s) involved in intraphagosomal growth inhibition of microorganisms. It has been suggested that the Nramp1 polypeptide participates in ion (in particular, iron) transport into the pathogen-containing phagosome (454a,454b).

Major Histocompatibility Complex Control of the Severity and Form of Disease

Human malaria caused by the protozoan parasite *Plasmodium* species represents the best example of the impact of MHC molecules on the severity of disease. Moreover, these studies emphasize the profound influence of natural selection against infection on MHC polymorphism (455–457). Segregation analyses in various human populations also indicate linkage of human leukocyte antigen (HLA) types with severity of tuberculosis and leprosy (451,458–463). Strong evidence exists to suggest an influence of the HLA on the development towards the tuberculoid or the lepromatous pole of leprosy (464,465). Although some linkage with MHC class I molecules has been observed in certain populations, MHC class II control appears to be more important. Originally, it was found that HLA-DR2 and HLA-DQ1 are linked with increased incidences of lepromatous leprosy and that HLA-DR3 represents a linkage marker for tuberculoid leprosy. Population-based association studies, however, have provided evidence for an association between HLA-DR2 and susceptibility to tuberculoid leprosy (466). With more data from different population groups being available, it is becoming increasingly clear that HLA-DR associations with distinct disease forms differ in different population groups, thus making it impossible to generalize from one to another population group. More refined molecular typing suggests preferential association of susceptibility to tuberculoid leprosy with the presence of arginine at position 13 or 70-71 of HLA-DR2 (451,466). These residues may participate in peptide binding. Hence, selection of unique *M. leprae* peptides may influence susceptibility to leprosy. In tuberculosis, evidence for positive association of HLA-DR2 and HLA-DQ1 with pulmonary tuberculosis has been found (462,467).

Genetic Control of Listeriosis and Legionellosis in the Mouse

Resistance of mice to some intracellular bacteria, such as *L. monocytogenes* and *L. pneumophila* infection, is not influenced by the Nramp1 gene. Susceptibility to listeriosis, as seen most markedly in A/J mice, was found to associate with a deficiency in the complement component C5 (468–470). C5 breakdown gives rise to the anaphylatoxin C5a, which plays a major role in the attraction of inflammatory phagocytes to sites of inflammation. As described above, early influx of professional phagocytes to the site of listerial growth is a decisive factor for resistance. In the C5-sufficient congenic A/J mouse strain, antilisterial resistance is fully reestablished, although the inflammatory response still remains imperfect. This finding suggests that a slight inflammatory reaction suffices for correcting susceptibility against *L. monocytogenes* and that local MP activation is less important. Gene-deletion mutant mice with a deficient C5a receptor suffer from exacerbated *Pseudomonas aeruginosa* pneumonia (471). The availability of these mouse mutants will allow definite characterization of the role of C5a in listeriosis.

Macrophages from A/J mice are also more susceptible to *L. pneumophila* infection, as compared with MPs from most other inbred mouse strains, although distinct gene products are apparently responsible for resistance to *L. monocytogenes* and *L. pneumophila* (472). The gene responsible for permissiveness to *L. pneumophila* has been identified on chromosome 13 and termed *Lgn1* (473–475).

Differential genetic control of natural resistance against *M. bovis* BCG, *M. tuberculosis*, *L. monocytogenes,* and *L. pneumophila* further serves to underline the different types of disease forms caused by intracellular bacteria. In addition to the inherited factors described, several other genes are involved in control of resistance against intracellular bacteria (476).

CONCLUSIONS AND OUTLOOK

It is hoped that the reader of this chapter not only has become familiar with the principal mechanisms underlying immunity against intracellular bacteria, but also realizes the great complexity of this system. Understanding intracellular bacterial infections requires knowledge not only of immunology, but also of the molecular biology of the infectious agent and the biology of the target cell. *In vitro* analyses can only provide incomplete answers to the questions relevant to antibacterial immunity and must be complemented by *in vivo* experiments.

Despite the high degree of complexity, such interdisciplinary research efforts almost certainly will provide rewards. First, understanding the performance of the immune system in bacterial infections can provide clues to the answers of questions pertinent to basic immunology. Knowledge of the rules underlying the extraordinary plasticity and adaptability of the immune system, required for coping with transmutable "viable antigens," which developed during millenia of coexistence, will provide deeper insights into the immunoregulation and the evolution of the immune system. Second, applied questions will benefit equally well from these approaches. With the increasing inadequacy of chemotherapy in the control of bacterial infections, the need for adjunctive immune measures is gaining further importance. Rational strategies towards vaccination and immunotherapy will benefit from the deeper understanding of the immune mechanisms operative in intracellular bacterial infections. The reader may find it ironic that this brings us back to the roots of immunology, which started as an approach to the intervention of bacterial infections.

ACKNOWLEDGMENTS

The author acknowledges financial support from the German Science Foundation (SFB 322 and Project Ka 573/3-1/2), the BMBF Joint Project "Mycobacterial Infections," the Interdisciplinary Center for Clinical Research, and the German Leprosy Relief Association. The author is grateful to his colleagues at the Max-Planck-Institute for Infection Biology for critical comments, and he thanks Mrs. R. Mahmoudi for excellent secretarial assistance and Dr. K. Miksits (Institute for Infection Medicine, Berlin) for computer graphics.

REFERENCES

1. Hahn H, Kaufmann SHE. The role of cell mediated immunity in bacterial infections. *Rev Infect Dis* 1981;3:1221–1250.
2. Moulder JW. Comparative biology of intracellular parasitism. *Microbiol Rev* 1985;49:298–337.
3. Reynolds HY. Immunologic system in the respiratory tract. *Physiol Rev* 1991;71:1117–1133.
4. Brandtzaeg P, Sollid LM, Thrane PS, et al. Lymphoepithelial interactions in the mucosal immune system. *Gut* 1988;29:1116–1130.
5. Neutra MR, Pringault E, Kraehenbuhl J-P. Antigen sampling across epithelial barriers and induction of mucosal immune responses. *Annu Rev Immunol* 1996;14:275–300.
6. Lipscomb MF, Bice DE, Lyons CR, Schuyler MR, Wilkes D. The regulation of pulmonary immunity. *Adv Immunol* 1995;59:369–455.
7. Schlossberg D. *Tuberculosis.* 3rd ed. New York: Springer-Verlag, 1988.
8. Mackaness GD. Cellular resistance to infection. *J Exp Med* 1962;116:381–406.
9. Eisenstein BI, Engleberg NC. Genetics and molecular pathogenesis of *Legionella pneumophila*, an intracellular parasite of macrophages. *Mol Biol Med* 1989;6:409–424.
10. Finlay BB, Falkow S. Salmonella as an intracellular parasite. *Mol Microbiol* 1989;3:1833–1841.
11. Hastings RC. *Leprosy.* 2nd ed. Edinburgh: Churchill Livingstone, 1994.
12. Smith LD, Ficht TA. Pathogenesis of Brucella. *Crit Rev Microbiol* 1990;17:209–230.
13. Sandström G. The tularaemia vaccine. *J Chem Tech Biotechnol* 1994;59:315–320.
14. Southwick FS, Purich DL. Intracellular pathogenesis of listeriosis. *N Engl J Med* 1996;334:770–776.
15. Jones BD, Falkow S. Salmonellosis: host immune responses and bacterial virulence. *Annu Rev Immunol* 1996;14:533–562.
16. Hackstadt T. The biology of rickettsiae. *Infect Agents Dis* 1996;5:127–143.
17. Moulder JW. Interaction of Chlamydiae and host cells in vitro. *Microbiol Rev* 1991;55:143–190.
18. Ward ME. The immunobiology and immunopathology of chlamydial infections. *APMIS* 1995;103:769–796.
19. Beatty WL, Morrison RP, Byrne GI. Persistent chlamydiae: from cell culture to a paradigm for chlamydial pathogenesis. *Microbiol Rev* 1994;58:686–699.
20. Jackson LA, Grayston JT. Chlamydia pneumoniae and Mycoplasma pneumoniae infections. *Curr Opin Infect Dis* 1996;9:89–93.
21. Bloom BR, Murray CJL. Tuberculosis: commentary on reemergent killer. *Science* 1992;257:1055–1064.
22. Kaufmann SHE, Young DB. Vaccination against tuberculosis and leprosy. *Immunobiology* 1992;184:208–229.

23. Bloom BR. *Tuberculosis: pathogenesis, protection, and control.* Washington DC: American Society for Microbiology, 1994.

24. Kaufmann SHE, Andersen P. Immunity to mycobacteria with emphasis on tuberculosis: implications for rational design of an effective tuberculosis vaccine. *Chem Immunol* 1998;70:21–59.

25. Fine PE. Variation in protection by BCG: implications of and for heterologous immunity. *Lancet* 1995;346:1339–1345 [erratum in *Lancet* 1996;347:340].

26. Colditz GA, Brewer TF, Berkey CS, et al. Efficacy of BCG vaccine in the prevention of tuberculosis. Meta-analysis of the published literature. *JAMA* 1994; 271:698–702.

27. Kaufmann SHE. Immunology of leprosy: new facts, future perspectives. *Microb Pathog* 1986;1:107–114.

28. Bloom BR, Modlin RL, Salgame P. Stigma variations: observations on suppressor T cells and leprosy. *Annu Rev Immunol* 1992;10:453–488.

29. Cossart P, Mengaud J. *Listeria monocytogenes.* A model system for the molecular study of intracellular parasitism. *Mol Biol Med* 1989;6:463–474.

30. Portnoy DA, Chakraborty T, Goebel W, Cossart P. Molecular determinants of *Listeria monocytogenes* pathogenesis. *Infect Immun* 1992;60:1263–1267.

31. Mengaud J, Chenevert J, Geoffroy C, Gaillard J-L, Cossart P. Identification of the structural gene encoding the SH-activated hemolysin of *Listeria monocytogenes: listeriolysin O* is homologous to streptolysin O and pneumolysin. *Infect Immun* 1987;55:3225–3227.

32. Portnoy DA, Jacks PS, Hinrichs DJ. Role of hemolysin for the intracellular growth of *Listeria monocytogenes. J Exp Med* 1988;167:1459–1471.

33. Camilli A, Goldfine H, Portnoy DA. *Listeria monocytogenes* mutants lacking phosphatidylinositol-specific phospholipase C are avirulent. *J Exp Med* 1991; 173:751–754.

34. Geoffroy C, Raveneau J, Beretti J-L, et al. Purification and characterization of an extracellular 29-kilodalton phospholipase C from *Listeria monocytogenes. Infect Immun* 1991;59:2382–2388.

35. Leimeister-Wächter M, Domann E, Chakraborty T. Detection of a gene encoding a phosphatidylinositol-specific phospholipase C that is co-ordinately expressed with listeriolysin in *Listeria monocytogenes. Mol Microbiol* 1991;5: 361–366.

36. Domann E, Wehland J, Rohde M, et al. A novel bacterial virulence gene in *Listeria monocytogenes* required for host cell microfilament interaction with homology to the proline-rich region of vinculin. *EMBO J* 1992;11:1981–1990.

37. Domann E, Leimeister-Wachter M, Goebel W, Chakraborty T. Molecular cloning, sequencing, and identification of a metalloprotease gene from *Listeria monocytogenes* that is species specific and physically linked to the listeriolysin gene. *Infect Immun* 1991;59:65–72.

38. Kocks C, Gouin E, Tabouret M, Berche P, Ohayon H, Cossart P. *L.monocytogenes*-induced actin assembly requires the actA gene product, a surface protein. *Cell* 1992;68:521–531.

39. Gaillard J-L, Berche P, Frehel C, Gouin E, Cossart P. Entry of *L. monocytogenes* into cells is mediated by internalin, a repeat protein reminiscent of surface antigens from gram-positive cocci. *Cell* 1991;65:1127–1141.

40. Kuhn M, Goebel W. Identification of an extracellular protein of *Listeria monocytogenes* possibly involved in intracellular uptake by mammalian cells. *Infect Immun* 1989;57:55–61.

41. Leimeister-Wächter M, Haffner C, Domann E, Goebel W, Chakraborty T. Identification of a gene that positively regulates expression of listeriolysin, the major virulence factor of *Listeria monocytogenes. Proc Natl Acad Sci USA* 1990;87:8336–8340.

42. Kaufmann SHE. Listeriosis: new findings—current concern. *Microb Pathog* 1988;5:225–231.

43. Bancroft GJ, Schreiber RD, Unanue ER. Natural immunity: a T-cell-independent pathway of macrophage activation, defined in the *scid* mouse. *Immunol Rev* 1991;124:5–24.

44. Le Minor L. Typing of Salmonella species. *Eur J Clin Microbiol Infect Dis* 1988;7:214–218.

45. Richter-Dahlfors AA, Finlay BB. *Salmonella* interactions with host cells. In: Kaufmann SHE, ed. *Host response to intracellular pathogens.* Austin, TX: R.G. Landes Company, 1997;251–270.

46. Mäkelä PH, Hormaeche CE. Immunity to *Salmonella.* In: Kaufmann SHE, ed. *Host response to intracellular pathogens.* Austin, TX: R.G. Landes Company, 1997;143–166.

47. Isberg RR. Discrimination between intracellular uptake and surface adhesion of bacterial pathogens. *Science* 1991;252:934–938.

48. Hoepelman AIM, Tuomanen EI. Consequences of microbial attachment: directing host cell functions with adhesins. *Infect Immun* 1992;60:1729–1733.

49. Finlay BB, Cossart P. Exploitation of mammalian host cell functions by bacterial pathogens. *Science* 1997;276:718–725.

50. Bliska JB, Galán JE, Falkow S. Signal transduction in the mammalian cell curing bacterial attachment and entry. *Cell* 1993;73:903–920.

51. Galán JE, Bliska JB. Cross-talk between bacterial pathogens and their host cells. *Annu Rev Cell Biol* 1996;12.221–256.

52. Finlay BB. Interactions between *Salmonella typhimurium,* enteropathogenic *Escherichia coli* (EPEC), and host epithelial cells. *Adv Dent Res* 1995;9:31–36.

53. Sansonetti P, Phalipon A. Shigellosis: from molecular pathogenesis of infection to protective immunity and vaccine development. *Res Immunol* 1996;147:595–612.

54. Swanson JA, Baer SC. Phagocytosis by zippers and triggers. *Trends Cell Biol* 1995;5:89–92.

55. Isberg RR, Van Nhieu GT. The mechanism of phagocytic uptake promoted by invasin-integrin interaction. *Trends Cell Biol* 1995;5:120–124.

56. Mengaud J, Ohayon H, Gounon P, Mege R, Cossart P. E-cadherin is the receptor for internalin, a surface protein required for entry of *L. monocytogenes* into epithelial cells. *Cell* 1996;84:923–932.

57. Rambukkana A, Salzer JL, Yurchenco PD, Tuomanen EI. Neural targeting of *Mycobacterium leprae* mediated by the G domain of the laminin-α2 chain. *Cell* 1997;88:811–821.

58. Galán JE, Pace J, Hayman MJ. Involvement of the epidermal growth factor receptor in the invasion of cultured mammalian cells by *Salmonella typhimurium. Nature* 1992;357:588–589.

59. Chen L-M, Hobbie S, Galán JE. Requirement of CDC42 for Salmonella-induced cytoskeletal and nuclear responses. *Science* 1996;274:2115–2118.

60. Janeway CA. The immune system evolved to discriminate infectious nonself from noninfectious self. *Immunol Today* 1992;13:11–16.

61. Stahl PD. The mannose receptor and other macrophage lectins. *Curr Opin Immunol* 1992;4:49–52.

62. Ulevitch RJ, Tobias PS. Receptor-dependent mechanisms of cell stimulation by bacterial endotoxin. *Annu Rev Immunol* 1995;13:437–457.

63. Lynn WA, Golenbock DT. Lipopolysaccharide antagonists. *Immunol Today* 1992;13:271–276.

64. Wright SD. CD14 and innate recognition of bacteria. *J Immunol* 1995;155:6–8.

65. Ofek I, Sharon N. Lectinophagocytosis: a molecular mechanism of recognition between cell surface sugars and lectins in the phagocytosis of bacteria. *Infect Immun* 1988;56:539–547.

66. Schlesinger LS. Role of mononuclear phagocytes in *M tuberculosis* pathogenesis. *J Invest Med* 1996;44:312–323.

67. Pearson AM. Scavenger receptors in innate immunity. *Curr Opin Immunol* 1996;8:20–28.

68. Krieger M, Herz J. Structures and functions of multiligand lipoprotein receptors: macrophage scavenger receptors and LDL receptor-related protein (LRP). *Annu Rev Biochem* 1994;63:601–637.

69. Suzuki H, Kurihara Y, Takeya M, et al. A role for macrophage scavenger receptors in atherosclerosis and susceptibility to infection. *Nature* 1997;386:292–296.

69a. Haworth R, Platt N, Keshav S, et al. The macrophage scavenger receptor type A is expressed by activated macrophages and protects the host against lethal endotoxic shock. *J Exp Med* 1997;186:1431–1439.

70. Brown EJ. Complement receptors and phagocytosis. *Curr Opin Immunol* 1991; 3:76–83.

71. Ruoslahti E. Fibronectin and its receptors. *Annu Rev Biochem* 1988;57: 375–413.

72. Unkeless JC, Scigliano E, Freedman VH. Structure and function of human and murine receptors for IgG. *Annu Rev Immunol* 1988;6:251–281.

73. Daëron M. Fc receptor biology. *Annu Rev Immunol* 1997;15:203–234.

74. Elsbach P, Weiss J. A reevaluation of the roles of the O_2-dependent and O_2-independent microbicidal systems of phagocytes. *Rev Infect Dis* 1983;5:843–853.

75. Nathan CF. Macrophage microbicidal mechanisms. *Trans R Soc Trop Med Hyg* 1983;77:620–630.

76. Horwitz MA. Phagocytosis of the Legionnaires' disease bacterium (*Legionella pneumophila*) occurs by a novel mechanism: engulfment within a pseudopod coil. *Cell* 1984;36:27–33.

77. Payne NR, Horwitz MA. Phagocytosis of *L. pneumophila* is mediated by human monocyte complement receptors. *J Exp Med* 1987;166:1377–1389.

78. Schlesinger LS, Horwitz MA. Phenolic glycolipid-1 of *Mycobacterium leprae* binds complement component C3 in serum and mediates phagocytosis by human monocytes. *J Exp Med* 1991;174:1031–1038.

79. Schlesinger LS, Bellinger-Kawahara CG, Payne NR, Horwitz MA. Phagocytosis of *Mycobacterium tuberculosis* is mediated by human monocyte complement receptors and complement component C3′. *J Immunol* 1990;144:2771–2780.

79a. Schorey JS, Carroll MC, Brown EJ. A macrophage invasion mechanism of pathogenic mycobacteria. *Science* 1997;277:1091–1093.

80. Kaufmann SHE, Reddehase MJ. Infection of phagocytic cells. *Curr Opin Immunol* 1989;2:43–49.

80a. Cywes C, Godenir NL, Hoppe HC, et al. Nonopsonic binding of *Mycobacterium tuberculosis* to human complement receptor type 3 expressed in Chinese hamster ovary cells. *Infect Immun* 1996;64:5373–5383.

81. Wyrick PB, Brownridge EA. Growth of *Chlamydia psittaci* in macrophages. *Infect Immun* 1978;19:1054–1060.

82. Abou-Zeid C, Ratliff TL, Wiker HG, Harboe M, Bennedsen J, Rook GAW. Characterization of fibronectin-binding antigens released by *Mycobacterium tuberculosis* and *Mycobacterium bovis* BCG. *Infect Immun* 1988;56:3046–3051.

83. Borremans M, de Wit L, Volckaert G, et al. Cloning, sequence determination and expression of a 32-kilodalton protein gene of *Mycobacterium tuberculosis. Infect Immun* 1989;57:3123–3130.

84. Hynes RO. *Fibronectins.* New York: Springer-Verlag, 1990.

85. Yamada KM. Adhesive recognition sequences. *J Biol Chem* 1991;266: 12809–12912.

85a. Belisle JT, Vissa VD, Sievert T, Takayama K, Brennan PJ, Besra GS. Role of the major antigen of *Mycobacterium tuberculosis* in cell wall biogenesis. *Science* 1997;276:1420–1422.

85b. Menozzi FD, Rouse JH, Alavi M, et al. Identification of a heparin-binding hemagglutinin present in mycobacteria. *J Exp Med* 1996;184:993–1001.

85c. Downing JF, Pasula R, Wright JR, Twigg HL, Martin WJ. Surfactant protein a promotes attachment of *Mycobacterium tuberculosis* to alveolar macrophages during infection with human immunodeficiency virus. *Proc Natl Acad Sci USA* 1995;92:4848–4852.

86. Kaplan G, Cohn ZA. Leprosy and cell-mediated immunity. *Curr Opin Immunol* 1991;3:91–96.

87. North RJ. The relative importance of blood monocytes and fixed macrophages to the expression of cell-mediated immunity to infection. *J Exp Med* 1970;132:521–524.

88. Racz P, Tenner K, Mero E. Experimental Listeria enteritis. I. An electron microscopic study of the epithelial phase in experimental listeria infection. *Lab Invest* 1972;26:694–700.

89. Russell DG. Mycobacterium and leishmania: stowaways in the endosomal network. *Trends Cell Biol* 1995;5:125–128.

90. Clemens DL. Characterization of the *Mycobacterium tuberculosis* phagosome. *Trends Microbiol* 1996;4:113–118.

91. Mellman I. Endocytosis and molecular sorting. *Ann Rev Cell Dev Biol* 1996;12:575–625.

92. Sturgill-Koszycki S, Schlesinger PH, Chakraborty P, et al. Lack of acidification in *Mycobacterium* phagosomes produced by exclusion of the vesicular proton-ATPase. *Science* 1994;263:678–681.

93. Adams DO, Hamilton TA. The cell biology of macrophage activation. *Annu Rev Immunol* 1984;2:283–318.

94. Lehrer RI, Ganz T, Selsted ME. Defensins: endogenous antibiotic peptides of animal cells. *Cell* 1991;64:229–230.

95. Selsted ME, Ouellette AJ. Defensins in granules of phagocytic and non-phagocytic cells. *Trends Cell Biol* 1995;5:114–119.

96. Fields PI, Groisman EA, Heffron F. A Salmonella locus that controls resistance to microbicidal proteins from phagocytic cells. *Science* 1989;243:1059–1062.

97. Small PL, Ramakrishnan L, Falkow S. Remodeling schemes of intracellular pathogens. *Science* 1994;263:637–639.

98. Berón W, Alvarez-Dominguez C, Mayorga L, Stahl PD. Membrane trafficking along the phagocytic pathway. *Trends Cell Biol* 1995;5:100–104.

99. Goren MB, D'Arcy Hart P, Young MR, Armstrong JA. Prevention of phagosome-lysosome fusion in cultured macrophages by sulfatides of *Mycobacterium tuberculosis*. *Proc Natl Acad Sci USA* 1976;73:2510–2514.

100. Pabst MJ, Gross JM, Brozna JP, Goren MB. Inhibition of macrophage priming by sulfatide from *Mycobacterium tuberculosis*. *J Immunol* 1988;140:634–640.

101. Sibley LD, Hunter SW, Brennan PJ, Krahenbuhl JL. Mycobacterial lipoarabinomannan inhibits gamma interferon-mediated activation of macrophages. *Infect Immun* 1988;56:1232–1236.

102. Zhang L, Goren MB, Holzer TJ, Andersen BR. Effect of *Mycobacterium tuberculosis*-derived sulfolipid I on human phagocytic cells. *Infect Immun* 1988;56:2876–83.

103. Armstrong JA, D'Arcy Hart P. Response of cultured macrophages to *Mycobacterium tuberculosis*, with observations on fusion of lysosomes with phagosomes. *J Exp Med* 1971;134:713–740.

104. Russell DG, Dant J, Sturgill-Koszycki S. *Mycobacterium avium*- and *Mycobacterium tuberculosis*-containing vacuoles are dynamic, fusion-competent vesicles that are accessible to glycosphingolipids from the host cell plasmalemma. *J Immunol* 1996;156:4764–4773.

105. Gordon AH, D'Arcy Hart P, Young MR. Ammonia inhibits phagosome-lysosome fusion in macrophages. *Nature* 1980;286:79–80.

105a. Lammas DA, Stober C, Harvey CJ, Kendrick N, Panchalingam S, Kumararatne DS. ATP-induced killing of mycobacteria by human macrophages is mediated by purinergic P2Z(P2X7) receptors. *Immunity* 1997;7:433–444

105b. Molloy A, Laochumroonvorapong P, Kaplan G. Apoptosis, but not necrosis, of infected monocytes is coupled with killing of intracellular Bacillus Calmette-Guérin. *J Exp Med* 1994;180:1499–1509.

106. Hasan Z, Schlax C, Kuhn L, et al. Isolation and characterization of the mycobacterial phagosome: segregation from the endosomal/lysosomal pathway. *Mol Microbiol* 1997;24:545–553.

107. Heinzen RA, Scidmore MA, Rockey DD, Hackstadt T. Differential interaction with endocytic and exocytic pathways distinguish parasitophorous vacuoles of *Coxiella burnetii* and *Chlamydia trachomatis*. *Infect Immun* 1996;64:796–809.

108. Garcia-del Portillo F, Finlay BB. Targeting of *Salmonella typhimurium* to vesicles containing lysosomal membrane glycoproteins bypasses compartments with mannose 6-phosphate receptors. *J Cell Biol* 1995;129:81–97.

109. Hackstadt T, Scidmore MA, Rockey DD. Lipid metabolism in *Chlamydia trachomatis*-infected cells: directed trafficking of Golgi-derived sphingolipids to the chlamydial inclusion. *Proc Natl Acad Sci USA* 1995;92:4877–4881.

110. Swanson MS, Isberg RR. Association of *Legionella pneumophila* with the macrophage endoplasmic reticulum. *Infect Immun* 1995;63:3609–3620.

111. Berger KH, Merriam JJ, Isberg RR. Altered intracellular targeting properties associated with mutations in the *Legionella pneumophila* dotA gene. *Mol Microbiol* 1994;14:809–822.

112. Alford CE, King TEJ, Campbell PA. Role of transferrin, transferrin receptors, and iron in macrophage listericidal activity. *J Exp Med* 1991;174:459–466.

113. Byrd TF, Horwitz MA. Interferon gamma-activated human monocytes downregulate transferrin receptors and inhibit the intracellular multiplication of *Legionella pneumophila* by limiting the availability of iron. *J Clin Invest* 1989;83:1457–1465.

114. Payne SM, Lawlor KM. Molecular studies on iron acquisition by non-

Escherichia coli species. In: Iglewski BH, Clark VL, eds. *Molecular basis of bacterial pathogenesis*. San Diego: Academic Press, 1990;225–248.

115. Payne SM. Iron acquisition in microbial pathogenesis. *Trends Microbiol* 1993;1:66–69.

116. Cornelissen CN, Sparling PF. Iron piracy: acquisition of transferrin-bound iron by bacterial pathogens. *Mol Microbiol* 1994;14:843–850.

117. Harrison PM, Arosio P. The ferritins: molecular properties, iron storage function and cellular regulation. *Biochim Biophys Acta* 1996;1275:161–203.

118. Gobin J, Moore CH, Reeve JR Jr, Wong DK, Gibson BW, Horwitz MA. Iron acquisition by *Mycobacterium tuberculosis*: isolation and characterization of a family of iron-binding exochelins. *Proc Natl Acad Sci USA* 1995;92:5189–5193.

119. Gobin J, Horwitz MA. Exochelins of *Mycobacterium tuberculosis* remove iron from human iron-binding proteins and donate iron to mycobactins in the *M. tuberculosis* cell wall. *J Exp Med* 1996;183:1527–1532.

120. Byrne GL, Lehmann LK, Landry GJ. Induction of tryptophan catabolism is the mechanism for gamma-interferon-mediated inhibition of intracellular *Chlamydia psittaci* replication in T24 cells. *Infect Immun* 1986;53:347–351.

121. Pfefferkorn ER. Interferon blocks the growth of *Toxoplasma gondii* in cultured fibroblasts by inducing the host cells to degrade tryptophan. *Proc Natl Acad Sci USA* 1984;81:908–912.

122. Flesch IEA, Kaufmann SHE. Attempts to characterize the mechanisms involved in mycobacterial growth inhibition by interferon-γ activated bone marrow macrophages. *Infect Immun* 1988;56:1464–1469.

123. Marletta MA. Nitric oxide: biosynthesis and biological significance. *TIBS* 1989;14:488–492.

124. Nathan CF, Hibbs JB Jr. Role of nitric oxide synthesis in macrophage antimicrobial activity. *Curr Opin Immunol* 1991;3:65–70.

125. Miller RA, Britigan BE. Role of oxidants in microbial pathophysiology. *Clin Microbiol Rev* 1997;10:1–18.

126. MacMicking J, Xie Q, Nathan C. Nitric oxide and macrophage function. *Annu Rev Immunol* 1997;15:323–350.

127. Chan J, Xing Y, Magliozzo RS, Bloom BR. Killing of virulent *Mycobacterium tuberculosis* by reactive nitrogen intermediates produced by activated murine macrophages. *J Exp Med* 1992;175:1111–1122.

128. Denis M. Interferon-gamma-treated murine macrophages inhibit growth of tubercle bacilli via the generation of reactive nitrogen intermediates. *Cell Immunol* 1991;132:150–157.

129. Flesch IEA, Kaufmann SHE. Mechanisms involved in mycobacterial growth inhibition by gamma-interferon activated bone marrow macrophages: role of reactive nitrogen intermediates. *Infect Immun* 1991;59:3213–3218.

130. MacMicking JD, Nathan C, Hom G, et al. Altered responses to bacterial infection and endotoxic shock in mice lacking inducible nitric oxide synthase. *Cell* 1995;81:641–650.

131. Chan J, Tanaka K, Carroll D, Flynn J, Bloom BR. Effects of nitric oxide synthase inhibitors on murine infection with *Mycobacterium tuberculosis*. *Infect Immun* 1995;63:736–740.

132. MacMicking JD, North RJ, LaCourse R, Mudgett JS, Shah SK, Nathan CF. Identification of nitric oxide synthase as a protective locus against tuberculosis. *Proc Natl Acad Sci USA* 1997;94:5243–5248.

133. Denis M. Tumor necrosis factor and granulocyte macrophage colony stimulating factor stimulate human macrophages to restrict growth of virulent *Mycobacterium avium* and to kill avirulent *M. avium*: killing effector mechanism depends on the generation of reactive nitrogen intermediates. *J Leukoc Biol* 1991;49:380–387.

134. Munoz-Fernández MA, Fernández MA, Fresno M. Activation of human macrophages for the killing of intracellular *Trypanosoma cruzi* by TNF-α and IFN-γ through a nitric oxide-dependent mechanism. *Immunol Lett* 1992;33:35–40.

135. Padgett EL, Bruett SB. Evaluation of nitrite production by human monocyte-derived macrophages. *Biochem Biophys Res Comm* 1992;186:775–781.

136. Sherman MP, Loro ML, Wong VZ, Tashkin DP. Cytokine- and *Pneumocystis carinii*-induced L-arginine oxidation by murine and human pulmonary alveolar macrophages. *J Protozool* 1991;38:234S–236S.

137. Vouldoukis I, Riveros-Moreno V, Dugas B, et al. The killing of *Leishmania major* by human macrophages is mediated by nitric oxide induced after ligation of the Fc RII/CD23 surface antigen. *Proc Natl Acad Sci USA* 1995;92:7804–7808.

138. Nicholson S, Bonecini-Almeida M da G, Lapa e Silva JR, et al. Inducible nitric oxide synthase in pulmonary alveolar macrophages from patients with tuberculosis. *J Exp Med* 1996;183:2293–2302.

139. Chan J, Fujiwara T, Brennan P, et al. Microbial glycolipids: possible virulence factors that scavenge oxygen radicals. *Proc Natl Acad Sci USA* 1989;86:2453–2457.

140. Neill MA, Klebanoff SJ. The effect of phenolic glycolipid-1 from *Mycobacterium leprae* on the antimicrobial activity of human macrophages. *J Exp Med* 1988;167:30–42.

141. Storz G, Tartaglia LA, Farr SB, Ames BN. Bacterial defenses against oxidative stress. *Trends Genet* 1990;6:363–368.

142. Fields PI, Swanson RV, Haidaris CG, Heffron F. Mutants of *Salmonella typhimurium* that cannot survive within the macrophage are avirulent. *Proc Natl Acad Sci USA* 1986;83:5189–5193.

143. De Groote MA, Granger D, Xu Y, Campbell G, Prince R, Fang FC. Genetic and redox determinants of nitric oxide cytotoxicity in a *Salmonella typhimurium* model. *Proc Natl Acad Sci USA* 1995;92:6399–6403.

144. De Groote MA, Testerman T, Xu Y, Stauffer G, Fang FC. Homocysteine antagonism of nitric oxide-related cytostasis in *Salmonella typhimurium*. *Science* 1996;272:414–417.

145. Myrvik QN, Leake ES, Wright MJ. Disruption of phagosomal membranes of normal alveolar macrophages by the H37Rv strain of *Mycobacterium tuberculosis*. A correlate of virulence. *Am Rev Respir Dis* 1984;129:322–328.

146. McDonough KA, Kress Y, Bloom BR. Pathogenesis of tuberculosis: interaction of *Mycobacterium tuberculosis* with macrophages. *Infect Immun* 1993;61: 2763–2773.

147. Leake ES, Myrvik QN, Wright MJ. Phagosomal membranes of *Mycobacterium bovis* BCG-immune alveolar macrophages are resistant to disruption by *Mycobacterium tuberculosis*. *Infect Immun* 1984;45:443–446.

148. Mor N. Intracellular location of *Mycobacterium leprae* in macrophages of normal and immune-deficient mice and effect of rifampin. *Infect Immun* 1983;42: 802–811.

149. Winkler HH. *Rickettsia prowazekii,* ribosomes and slow growth. *Trends Microbiol* 1995;3:196–198.

150. Portnoy DA, Schreiber RD, Connelly P, Tilney LG. Gamma interferon limits access of *Listeria monocytogenes* to the macrophage cytoplasm. *J Exp Med* 1989;170:2141–2146.

151. Lepay DA, Nathan CF, Steinman RM, Murray HW, Cohn ZA. Murine Kupffer cells. Mononuclear phagocytes deficient in the generation of reactive oxygen intermediates. *J Exp Med* 1985;161:1079–1096.

152. Tilney LG, Connelly PS, Portnoy DA. Actin filament nucleation by the bacterial pathogen, *Listeria monocytogenes*. *J Cell Biol* 1990;111:2979–2988.

153. Sanders MC, Theriot JA. Tails from the hall of infection: actin-based motility of pathogens. *Trends Microbiol* 1996;4:211–213.

154. Lasa I, Cossart P. Actin-based bacterial motility: towards a definition of the minimal requirements. *Trends Cell Biol* 1996;6:109–114.

155. Welch MD, Iwamatsu A, Mitchison TJ. Actin polymerization is induced by Arp2/3 protein complex at the surface of *Listeria monocytogenes*. *Nature* 1997; 385:265–269.

156. Majno G, Joris I. Apoptosis, oncosis, and necrosis. An overview of cell death. *Am J Pathol* 1995;146:3–15.

157. Zychlinsky A. Programmed cell death in infectious diseases. *Trends Microbiol* 1993;1:114–117.

158. Chen Y, Zychlinsky A. Apoptosis induced by bacterial pathogens. *Microb Pathog* 1994;17:203–212.

159. Monack DM, Raupach B, Hromockyj AE, Falkow S. *Salmonella typhimurium* invasion induces apoptosis in infected macrophages. *Proc Natl Acad Sci USA* 1996;93:9833–9838.

160. Rogers HW, Callery MP, Deck B, Unanue ER. *Listeria monocytogenes* induces apoptosis of infected hepatocytes. *J Immunol* 1996;156:679–684.

161. Guzman CA, Domann E, Rohde M, et al. Apoptosis of mouse dendritic cells is triggered by listeriolysin, the major virulence determinant of *Listeria monocytogenes*. *Mol Microbiol* 1996;20:119–126.

162. Keane J, Balcewicz-Sablinska MK, Remold HG, et al. Infection by *Mycobacterium tuberculosis* promotes human alveolar macrophage apoptosis. *Infect Immun* 1997;65:298–304.

163. Zychlinsky A, Sansonetti PJ. Apoptosis as a proinflammatory event: what can we learn from bacteria-induced cell death? *Trends Microbiol* 1997;5:201–204.

164. Barsig J, Kaufmann SHE. The mechanism of cell death in *Listeria monocytogenes*-infected murine macrophages is distinct from apoptosis. *Infect Immun* 1997;65:4075–4081.

165. Hermant D, Menard R, Arricau N, Parsot C, Popoff MY. Functional conservation of the Salmonella and Shigella effectors of entry into epithelial cells. *Mol Microbiol* 1995;17:781–789.

166. Zychlinsky A, Prevost MC, Sansonetti PJ. *Shigella flexneri* induces apoptosis in infected macrophages. *Nature* 1992;358:167–169.

167. Chen Y, Smith MR, Thirumalai K, Zychlinsky A. A bacterial invasin induces macrophage apoptosis by binding directly to ICE. *EMBO J* 1996;15:3853–3860.

168. Finlay BB, Falkow S. Common themes in microbial pathogenicity. *Microbiol Rev* 1989;53:210–230.

169. Gross R, Aricò B, Rappuoli R. Families of bacterial signal-transducing proteins. *Mol Microbiol* 1989;3:1661–1667.

170. Finlay BB, Falkow S. Common themes in microbial pathogenicity revisited. *Microbiol Mol Biol Rev* 1997;61:136–169.

171. Leimeister-Wächter M, Domann E, Chakraborty T. The expression of virulence genes in *Listeria monocytogenes* is thermoregulated. *J Bacteriol* 1992;174: 947–952.

172. Craig EA, Gross CA. Is hsp70 the cellular thermometer? *Trends Biochem Sci* 1991;16:135–140.

173. Kaufmann SHE. Heat shock proteins and pathogenesis of bacterial infections. *Springer Semin Immunopathol* 1991;13:25–36.

174. Kaufmann SHE. Heat shock proteins and the immune response. *Immunol Today* 1990;11:129–136.

175. Schoel B, Kaufmann SHE. The unique role of hsp in infections. In: van Eden W, Young D, eds. *Stress proteins in medicine*. New York: Marcel Dekker Inc, 1996:27–51.

176. Buchmeier NA, Heffron F. Induction of *Salmonella* stress proteins upon infection of macrophages. *Science* 1990;248:730–732.

177. Johnson K, Charles I, Dougan G, et al. The role of a stress-response protein in *Salmonella typhimurium* virulence. *Mol Microbiol* 1991;5:401–407.

178. Morgan RW, Christman MF, Jacobson FS, Storz G, Ames BN. Hydrogen peroxide-inducible proteins in *Salmonella typhimurium* overlap with heat shock and other stress proteins. *Proc Natl Acad Sci USA* 1986;83:8059–8063.

179. Metchnikoff E. *Immunity to infectious diseases*. London: Cambridge University Press, 1905.

180. Koch R. Weitere Mitteilungen über ein Heilmittel gegen Tuberkulose. *Dtsch Med Wochenschr* 1890;16:1029–1032.

181. Lurie MB. *Resistance to tuberculosis*. Cambridge, MA: Harvard University Press, 1964.

182. Mackaness GB, Blanden RV. Cellular immunity. *Prog Allergy* 1967;11:89–140.

183. Bloom BR, Bennett B. Mechanism of a reaction in vitro associated with delayed-type hypersensitivity. *Science* 1966;153:80–82.

184. Cohn ZA. The activation of mononuclear phagocytes: fact, fancy, and future. *J Immunol* 1978;121:813–816.

185. David JR. Delayed hypersensitivity in vitro: its mediation by cell-free substances formed by lymphoid cell-antigen interaction. *Proc Natl Acad Sci USA* 1966;56:72–77.

186. Nathan CF, Murray HW, Wiebe ME, Rubin BY. Identification of interferon-γ as the lymphokine that activates human macrophage oxidative metabolism and antimicrobial activity. *J Exp Med* 1983;158:670–689.

187. Kaufmann SHE. Immunity to intracellular bacteria. *Annu Rev Immunol* 1993;11:129–163.

188. Haslett C, Savill JS, Meagher L. The neutrophil. *Curr Opin Immunol* 1989;2: 10–18.

189. Weiss SJ. Tissue destruction by neutrophils. *N Engl J Med* 1989;320:365–376.

190. Conlan JW. Critical roles of neutrophils in host defense against experimental systemic infections of mice by *Listeria monocytogenes, Salmonella typhimurium,* and *Yersinia enterocolitica*. *Infect Immun* 1997;65:630–635.

191. Conlan JW, North RJ. Neutrophil-mediated dissolution of infected host cells as a defense strategy against a facultative intracellular bacterium. *J Exp Med* 1991; 174:741–744.

192. Rogers HW, Unanue ER. Neutrophils are involved in acute, nonspecific resistance to *Listeria monocytogenes* in mice. *Infect Immun* 1993;61:5090–5096.

193. Conlan JW, North RJ. Neutrophils are essential for early anti-*Listeria* defense in the liver, but not in the spleen or peritoneal cavity, as revealed by a granulocyte-depleting monoclonal antibody. *J Exp Med* 1994;179:259–268.

194. Emmerling P, Finger H, Bockemühl J. *Listeria monocytogenes* infection in nude mice. *Infect Immun* 1974;12:437–439.

195. von Behring E. E. v. *Behring's gesammelte Abhandlungen*. Bonn: A. Marcus & E. Webers Verlag, 1915.

196. Janeway CA. The T cell receptor as a multicomponent signalling machine: CD4/CD8 coreceptors and CD45 in T cell activation. *Annu Rev Immunol* 1992; 10:645–674.

197. Kaufmann SHE. The roles of conventional and unconventional T cells in antibacterial immunity. *ASM News* 1997;63:251–255.

198. Kaufmann SHE. Immunity to intracellular bacteria and protozoa. *Immunologist* 1995;3:221–225.

199. Cheers C, Sandrin MS. Restriction in adoptive transfer of resistance to *Listeria monocytogenes*. *Cell Immunol* 1983;7:199–205.

200. Zinkernagel RM. Restriction by H-2 gene complex of transfer of cell-mediated immunity to *Listeria monocytogenes*. *Nature* 1974;251:230–233.

201. Kaufmann SHE, Hug E, Väth U, Müller I. Effective protection against *Listeria monocytogenes* and delayed-type hypersensitivity to listerial antigens depend on cooperation between specific L3T4+ and Lyt2+ T cells. *Infect Immun* 1985; 48:263–266.

202. Kaufmann SHE, Simon MM, Hahn H. Specific Lyt 123 T cells are involved in protection against *Listeria monocytogenes* and in delayed-type hypersensitivity to listerial antigens. *J Exp Med* 1979;150:1033–1038.

203. Lukacs K, Kurlander R. Lyt-2+ T cell-mediated protection against listeriosis. Protection correlates with phagocyte depletion but not with IFN-γ production. *J Immunol* 1989;142:2879–2886.

204. Lukacs K, Kurlander RJ. MHC-unrestricted transfer of antilisterial immunity by freshly isolated immune CD8 spleen cells. *J Immunol* 1989;143:3731–3736.

205. Kaufmann SHE, Hug E, DeLibero G. *Listeria monocytogenes*-reactive T lymphocyte clones with cytolytic activity against infected target cells. *J Exp Med* 1986;164:363–368.

206. Kaufmann SHE. Effective antibacterial protection induced by *Listeria monocytogenes*-specific T cell clone and its lymphokines. *Infect Immun* 1983;39: 1265–1270.

207. Kaufmann SHE, Hahn H. Biological functions of T cell lines with specificity for the intracellular bacterium *Listeria monocytogenes* in vitro und in vivo. *J Exp Med* 1982;155:1754–1765.

208. Ladel CH, Flesch IEA, Arnoldi J, Kaufmann SHE. Studies with MHC deficient knock-out mice reveal impact of both MHC I and MHC II dependent T cell responses in *Listeria monocytogenes* infection. *J Immunol* 1994;153:3116–3122.

209. Reimann J, Kaufmann SHE. Alternative antigen processing pathways in anti-infective immunity. *Curr Opin Immunol* 1997;9:462–469.

210. Harding CV. Alternate pathways of MHC-I antigen processing. In: Kaufmann SHE, ed. *Host response to intracellular pathogens*. Austin, TX: Landes Company, 1997:37–46.

211. Kaufmann SHE. CD8+ T lymphocytes in intracellular microbial infections. *Immunol Today* 1988;9:168–174.

212. Xu S, Cooper A, Sturgill-Koszycki S, et al. Intracellular trafficking in

Mycobacterium tuberculosis and *Mycobacterium avium*-infected macrophages. *J Immunol* 1994;153:2568–2576.

213. Clemens DL, Horwitz MA. Characterization of the *Mycobacterium tuberculosis* phagosome and evidence that phagosomal maturation is inhibited. *J Exp Med* 1995;181:257–270.

214. Bouwer HGA, Nelson CS, Gibbins BL, Portnoy DA, Hinrichs DJ. Listeriolysin O is a target of the immune response to *Listeria monocytogenes*. *J Exp Med* 1992;175:1467–1471.

215. Brunt LM, Portnoy DA, Unanue ER. Presentation of *Listeria monocytogenes* to CD8+ T cells requires secretion of hemolysin and intracellular bacterial growth. *J Immunol* 1990;145:3540–3546.

216. Harty JT, Bevan MJ. CD8+ T cells specific for a single nonamer epitope of *Listeria monocytogenes* are protective in vivo. *J Exp Med* 1992;175:1531–1538.

217. DeLibero G, Flesch I, Kaufmann SHE. Mycobacteria reactive Lyt2+ T cell lines. *Eur J Immunol* 1988;18:59–66.

218. Pope M, Kotlarski I. Detection of *Salmonella*-specific L3T4+ and Lyt-2+ T cells which can proliferate *in vitro* and mediate delayed-type hypersensitivity reactivity. *Immunology* 1994;81:183–191.

219. Pope M, Kotlarski I, Doherty K. Induction of Lyt-2+ cytotoxic T lymphocytes following primary and secondary *Salmonella* infection. *Immunology* 1994;81:177–182.

220. Mazzaccaro RJ, Gedde M, Jensen ER, et al. Major histocompatibility class I presentation of soluble antigen facilitated by *Mycobacterium tuberculosis* infection. *Proc Natl Acad Sci USA* 1996;93:11786–11791.

221. Pfeifer JD, Wick MJ, Roberts RL, Findlay K, Normark SJ, Harding CV. Phagocytic processing of bacterial antigens for class I MHC presentation to T cells. *Nature* 1993;361:359–362.

222. Kovacsovics-Bankowski M, Rock KL. A phagosome-to-cytosol pathway for exogenous antigens presented on MHC class I molecules. *Science* 1995;267:243–246.

223. Harding CV, Song R. Phagocytic processing of exogenous particulate antigens by macrophages for presentation by class I MHC molecules. *J Immunol* 1994;153:4925–4933.

224. Jondal M, Schirmbeck R, Reimann J. MHC class I-restricted CTL responses to exogenous antigens. *Immunity* 1996;5:295–302.

225. Watts C. Capture and processing of exogenous antigens for presentation on MHC molecules. *Annu Rev Immunol* 1997;15:821–850.

226. York IA, Rock KL. Antigen processing and presentation by the class I major histocompatibility complex. *Annu Rev Immunol* 1996;14:369–396.

227. Ladel CH, Daugelat S, Kaufmann SHE. Immune response to *Mycobacterium bovis* bacille Calmette Guerin infection in major histocompatibility complex class I- and II-deficient knock-out mice: contribution of CD4 and CD8 T cells to acquired resistance. *Eur J Immunol* 1995;25:377–384.

228. Flynn JL, Goldstein MM, Triebold KJ, Koller B, Bloom BR. Major histocompatibility complex class I-restricted T cells are required for resistance to *Mycobacterium tuberculosis* infection. *Proc Natl Acad Sci USA* 1992;89:12013–12017.

229. Müller I, Cobbold SP, Waldmann H, Kaufmann SHE. Impaired resistance against *Mycobacterium tuberculosis* infection after selective in-vivo depletion of L3T4+ and Lyt2+ T cells. *Infect Immun* 1987;55:2037–2041.

230. Kaufmann SHE, Rodewald HR, Hug E, De Libero G. Cloned *Listeria monocytogenes* specific non-MHC-restricted Lyt2+ T cells with cytolytic and protective activity. *J Immunol* 1988;140:3173–3179.

231. DeLibero G, Kaufmann SHE. Antigen-specific Lyt2+ cytolytic T lymphocytes from mice infected with the intracellular bacterium *Listeria monocytogenes*. *J Immunol* 1986;137:2688–2694.

232. Pamer EG, Wang C-R, Flaherty L, Fischer Lindahl K, Bevan MJ. H-2M3 presents a *Listeria monocytogenes* peptide to cytotoxic T lymphocytes. *Cell* 1992;70:215–223.

233. Kurlander RJ, Shawar SM, Brown ML, Rich RR. Specialized role for a murine class I-b MHC molecule in prokaryotic host defenses. *Science* 1992;257:678–679.

234. Lindahl KF, Byers DE, Dabhi VM, et al. H2-M3, a full-service class Ib histocompatibility antigen. *Annu Rev Immunol* 1997;15:851–879.

235. Wang C-R, Castano AR, Peterson PA, Slaughter C, Fischer Lindahl K, Deisenhofer J. Nonclassical binding of formylated peptide in crystal structure of the MHC class Ib molecule H2-M3. *Cell* 1995;82:655–664.

236. Gulden PH, Fischer P III, Sherman NE, et al. A *Listeria monocytogenes* pentapeptide is presented to cytolytic T lymphocytes by the H2-M3 MHC class Ib molecule. *Immunity* 1996;5:73–79.

237. Lenz LL, Dere B, Bevan MJ. Identification of an H2-M3-restricted listeria epitope: implications for antigen presentation by M3. *Immunity* 1996;5:63–72.

238. Lenz LL, Bevan MJ. H2-M3 restricted presentation of *Listeria monocytogenes* antigens. *Immunol Rev* 1996;151:107–121.

239. Szalay G, Ladel CH, Kaufmann SHE. Stimulation of protective CD8+ T lymphocytes by vaccination with nonliving bacteria. *Proc Natl Acad Sci USA* 1995;92:12389–12392.

240. Porcelli SA. The CD1 family: a third lineage of antigen-presenting molecules. *Adv Immunol* 1995;59:1–98.

241. Beckman EM, Porcelli SA, Morita CT, Behar SM, Furlong ST, Brenner MB. Recognition of a lipid antigen by CD1-restricted αβ+ T cells. *Nature* 1994;372:691–694.

242. Sieling PA, Chatterjee D, Porcelli SA, et al. CD1-restricted T cell recognition of microbial lipoglycan antigens. *Science* 1995;269:227–230.

243. Beckman EM, Melian AM, Behar SM, et al. CD1c restricts responses of mycobacteria-specific T cells: evidence for antigen presentation by a second member of the human CD1 family. *J Immunol* 1996;157:2803.

244. Bendelac A, Rivera MN, Park SH, Roark JH. Mouse CD1-specific NK1 T cells: development, specificity, and function. *Annu Rev Immunol* 1997;15:535–562.

245. Castano AR, Tangri S, Miller JEW, et al. Peptide binding and presentation by mouse CD1. *Science* 1995;269:223–226.

246. Prigozy TI, Sieling PA, Clemens D, et al. The mannose receptor delivers lipoglycan antigens to endosomes for presentation to T cells by CD1b molecules. *Immunity* 1997;6:187–197.

247. Brennan PJ, Nikaido H. The envelope of mycobacteria. *Annu Rev Biochem* 1995;64:29–63.

248. Smiley ST, Kaplan MH, Grusby MJ. Immunoglobulin E production in the absence of interleukin-4-secreting CD1-dependent cells. *Science* 1997;275:977–979.

249. Mendiratta SK, Martin WD, Hong S, Boesteanu A, Joyce S, Van Kaer L. CD1d1 mutant mice are deficient in natural T cells that promptly produce IL-4. *Immunity* 1997;6:469–477.

250. Chen YH, Chiu NM, Mandal M, Wang N, Wang CR. Impaired NK1+ T cell development and early IL-4 production in CD1- deficient mice. *Immunity* 1997;6:459–467.

251. Bendelac A, Lantz O, Quimby ME, Yewdell JW, Bennink JR, Brutkiewicz RR. CD1 recognition by mouse NK1+ T lymphocytes. *Science* 1995;268:863–865.

252. Medzhitov R, Janeway CA Jr. Innate immunity: impact on the adaptive immune response. *Curr Opin Immunol* 1997;9.4–9.

252a. Kawano T, Cui J, Koezuka Y, et al. CD1d-restricted and TCR-mediated activation of VαNK1 cells by glycosylceramides. *Science* 1997;278:1626–1629.

253. Yoshimoto T, Paul WE. CD4pos, NK1.1pos T cells promptly produce interleukin 4 in response to in vivo challenge with anti-CD3. *J Exp Med* 1994;179:1285–1295.

254. Kaufmann SHE. γ/δ and other unconventional T lymphocytes: what do they see and what do they do? *Proc Natl Acad Sci USA* 1996;93:2272–2279.

255. DeLibero G, Casorati G, Giachino C, et al. Selection by two powerful antigens may account for the presence of the major population of human peripheral γ/δ T cells. *J Exp Med* 1991;173:1311–1322.

256. Kabelitz D, Bender A, Prospero T, Wesselborg S, Janssen O, Pechhold K. The primary response of human γ/δ+ T cells to *Mycobacterium tuberculosis* is restricted to Vγ9-bearing cells. *J Exp Med* 1991;173:1331–1338.

257. Kabelitz D, Bender A, Schondelmaier S, Schoel B, Kaufmann SHE. A large fraction of human peripheral blood γ/δ+ T cells is activated by *Mycobacterium tuberculosis* but not by its 65-kD heat shock protein. *J Exp Med* 1990;171:667–679.

258. Pfeffer K, Schoel B, Gulle H, Kaufmann SHE, Wagner H. Primary responses of human T cells to mycobacteria: a frequent set of γ/δ T cells are stimulated by protease-resistant ligands. *Eur J Immunol* 1990;20:1175–1179.

259. Schoel B, Zügel U, Ruppert T, Kaufmann SHE. Elongated peptides, not the predicted nonapeptide stimulate a major histocompatibility complex class I-restricted cytotoxic T lymphocyte clone with specificity for a bacterial heat shock protein. *Eur J Immunol* 1994;24:3161–3169.

260. Constant P, Davodeau F, Peyrat M-A, et al. Stimulation of human γδ T cells by nonpeptidic mycobacterial ligands. *Science* 1994;264:267–270.

261. Tanaka Y, Sano S, Nieves E, et al. Nonpeptide ligands for human γδ T cells. *Proc Natl Acad Sci USA* 1994;91:8175–8179.

262. Tanaka Y, Morita CT, Nieves E, Brenner MB, Bloom BR. Natural and synthetic non-peptide antigens recognized by human γδ T cells. *Nature* 1995;375:155–158.

263. Morita CT, Beckman EM, Bukowski JF, et al. Direct presentation of nonpeptide prenyl pyrophosphate antigens to human γδ T cells. *Immunity* 1995;3:495–508.

264. Chien Y-H, Jores R, Crowley MP. Recognition by γ/δ T cells. *Annu Rev Immunol* 1996;14:511–532.

265. Mombaerts P, Arnoldi J, Russ F, Tonegawa S, Kaufmann SHE. Different roles of αβ and γ/δ T cells in immunity against an intracellular bacterial pathogen. *Nature* 1993;365:53–56.

266. Hiromatsu K, Yoshikai Y, Matsuzaki G, et al. A protective role of γ/δ T cells in primary infection with *Listeria monocytogenes* in mice. *J Exp Med* 1992;175:49–56.

267. Fu Y-X, Roark CE, Kelly K, et al. Immune protection and control of inflammatory tissue necrosis by γδ T cells. *J Immunol* 1994;153:3101–3115.

268. Skeen MJ, Ziegler HK. Induction of murine peritoneal γ/δ T cells and their role in resistance to bacterial infection. *J Exp Med* 1993;178:971–984.

269. Ladel CH, Blum C, Dreher A, Reifenberg K, Kaufmann SHE. Protective role of γ/δ T cells and α/β T cells in tuberculosis. *Eur J Immunol* 1995;25:2877.

270. D'Souza CD, Cooper AM, Frank AA, Mazzaccaro RJ, Bloom BR, Orme IM. An anti-inflammatory role for γδ T lymphocytes in acquired immunity to *Mycobacterium tuberculosis*. *J Immunol* 1997;158:1217–1221.

271. Modlin RL, Pirmez C, Hofmann FM, et al. Lymphocytes bearing antigen-specific γ/δ T-cell receptors accumulate in human infectious disease lesions. *Nature* 1989;339:544–548.

272. Sim G-K. Intraepithelial lymphocytes and the immune system. *Adv Immunol* 1995;58:297–343.

273. Abbas AK, Murphy KM, Sher A. Functional diversity of helper T lymphocytes. *Nature* 1996;383:787–793.

274. Liu C-C, Young LHY, Young JDE. Mechanisms of disease. Lymphocyte-mediated cytolysis and disease. *N Engl J Med* 1996;335:1651–1659.

275. Kägi D, Ledermann B, Bürki K, Zinkernagel RM, Hengartner H. Molecular mechanisms of lymphocyte-mediated cytotoxicity and their role in immunological protection and pathogenesis in vivo. *Annu Rev Immunol* 1996;14:207–232.

276. Kägi D, Ledermann B, Bürki K, Hengartner H, Zinkernagel RM. CD8⁺ T cell-mediated protection against an intracellular bacterium by perforin-dependent cytotoxicity. *Eur J Immunol* 1994;24:3068–3072.

277. Kaufmann SHE. Antibacterial vaccines: impact of antigen handling and immune response. *J Mol Med* 1997;75:360–363.

278. Hess J, Gentschev I, Miko D, et al. Superior efficacy of secreted over somatic antigen display in recombinant Salmonella vaccine induced protection against listeriosis. *Proc Natl Acad Sci USA* 1996;93:1458–1463.

279. Kaufmann SHE, Emoto M, Szalay G, Barsig J, Flesch IEA. Interleukin 4 and listeriosis. *Immunol Rev* 1997;158:95–105.

280. Fearon DT, Locksley RM. The instructive role of innate immunity in the acquired immune response. *Science* 1996;272:50–54.

281. Unanue ER. Macrophages, NK cells and neutrophils in the cytokine loop of Listeria resistance. *Res Immunol* 1996;147:499–504.

282. Dinarello CA. Role of interleukin-1 in infectious diseases. *Immunol Rev* 1992;127:119–146.

283. Tracey KJ, Cerami A. Cachectin/tumor necrosis factor and other cytokines in infectious disease. *Curr Opin Immunol* 1989;1:454–461.

284. Van Snick J. Interleukin-6: An overview. *Annu Rev Immunol* 1990;8:253–278.

285. Vassalli P. The pathophysiology of tumor necrosis factors. *Annu Rev Immunol* 1992;10:411–452.

286. Ward PA, Marks RM. The acute inflammatory reaction. *Curr Opin Immunol* 1989;2:5–9.

287. Taga T, Kishimoto T. GP130 and the interleukin-6 family of cytokines. *Annu Rev Immunol* 1997;15:797–819.

288. Baggiolini M, Dewald B, Moser B. Human chemokines: an update. *Annu Rev Immunol* 1997;15:675–705.

289. Vaddi K, Keller M, Newton RC. *The chemokine factsbook*. San Diego: Academic Press, 1997.

290. Schluger NW, Rom WN. Early responses in infection: chemokines as mediators of inflammation. *Curr Opin Immunol* 1997;9:504–508.

291. Premack BA, Schall TJ. Chemokine receptors: gateways to inflammation and infection. *Nat Med* 1996;2:1174–1178.

291a. Kurihara T, Warr G, Loy J, Bravo R. Defects in M macrophage recruitment and host defense in mice lacking the CCR2 chemokine receptor. *J Exp Med* 1997;186:1757–1762.

292. Rollins BJ. Monocyte chemoattractant protein 1: a potential regulator of monocyte recruitment in inflammatory disease. *Mol Med Today* 1996;2:198–204.

293. Rutledge BJ, Rayburn H, Rosenberg R, et al. High level monocyte chemoattractant protein-1 expression in transgenic mice increases their susceptibility to intracellular pathogens. *J Immunol* 1995;155:4838–4843.

294. Kopf M, Baumann H, Freer G, et al. Impaired immune and acute phase responses in interleukin-6 deficient mice. *Nature* 1994;368:339–341.

295. Dalrymple SA, Lucian LA, Slattery R, et al. Interleukin-6-deficient mice are highly susceptible to *Listeria monocytogenes* infection: correlation with inefficient neutrophilia. *Infect Immun* 1995;63:2262–2268.

296. Ladel CH, Blum C, Dreher A, Reifenberg K, Kopf M, Kaufmann SHE. Lethal tuberculosis in interleukin-6 deficient mutant mice. *Infect Immun* 1997;65:4843–4849.

297. Pfeffer K, Matsuyama T, Kündig TM, et al. Mice deficient for the 55 kd tumor necrosis factor receptor are resistant to endotoxic shock, yet succumb to *L. monocytogenes* infection. *Cell* 1993;73:457–467.

298. Rothe J, Lesslauer W, Lötscher H, et al. Mice lacking the tumour necrosis factor receptor 1 are resistant to TNF-mediated toxicity but highly susceptible to infection by *Listeria monocytogenes*. *Nature* 1993;364:798–802.

299. Flynn JL, Goldstein MM, Chan J, et al. Tumor necrosis factor-α is required in the protective immune response against *Mycobacterium tuberculosis* in mice. *Immunity* 1995;2:561–572.

300. Kaplan G, Freedman VH. The role of cytokines in the immune response to tuberculosis. *Res Immunol* 1997;147:565–571.

301. Tramontana JM, Utaipat U, Molloy A, et al. Thalidomide treatment reduces tumor necrosis factor alpha production and enhances weight gain in patients with pulmonary tuberculosis. *Mol Med* 1995;1:384–397.

302. Sampaio EP, Kaplan G, Miranda A, et al. The influence of thalidomide on the clinical and immunologic manifestation of erythema nodosum leprosum. *J Infect Dis* 1993;168:408–414.

303. Flynn JL, Chan J, Triebold KJ, Dalton DK, Stewart TA, Bloom BR. An essential role for interferon-γ in resistance to *Mycobacterium tuberculosis* infection. *J Exp Med* 1993;178:2249–2254.

304. Cooper AM, Dalton DK, Stewart TA, Griffin JP, Russell DG, Orme IM. Disseminated tuberculosis in interferon-γ gene-disrupted mice. *J Exp Med* 1993;178:2243–2247.

305. Jouanguy E, Altare F, Lamhamedi S, et al. Interferon-γ-receptor deficiency in an infant with fatal bacille Calmette-Guérin infection. *N Engl J Med* 1996;335:1956–1961.

306. Newport MJ, Huxley CM, Huston S, et al. A mutation in the interferon-γ-receptor gene and susceptibility to mycobacterial infection. *N Engl J Med* 1996;335:1941–1949.

307. Maeda J, Ueki N, Ohkawa T, et al. Local production and localization of trans-forming growth factor-beta in tuberculous pleurisy. *Clin Exp Immunol* 1993;92:32–38.

308. Hirsch CS, Hussain R, Toossi Z, Dawood G, Shahid F, Ellner JJ. Cross-modulation by transforming growth factor beta in human tuberculosis: suppression of antigen-driven blastogenesis and interferon gamma production. *Proc Natl Acad Sci USA* 1996;93:3193–3198.

309. Lin Y, Zhang M, Hofman FM, Gong J, Barnes PF. Absence of a prominent Th2 cytokine response in human tuberculosis. *Infect Immun* 1996;64:1351–1356.

310. Toossi Z, Gogate P, Shiratsuchi H, Young T, Ellner JJ. Enhanced production of TGF-β by blood monocytes from patients with active tuberculosis and presence of TGF-β in tuberculous granulomatous lung lesions. *J Immunol* 1995;154:465–473.

311. Libraty DH, Airan LE, Uyemura K, et al. Interferon-γ differentially regulates interleukin-12 and interleukin-10 production in leprosy. *J Clin Invest* 1997;99:336–341.

312. Yamamura M, Uyemura K, Deans RJ, et al. Defining protective responses to pathogens: cytokine profiles in leprosy lesions. *Science* 1991;254:277–279.

313. Sieling PA, Wang X-H, Gately MK, et al. IL-12 regulates T helper type 1 cytokine responses in human infectious disease. *J Immunol* 1994;153:3639–3647.

314. Kaufmann SHE, Flesch I. The role of T cell-macrophage interactions in tuberculosis. *Springer Semin Immunopathol* 1988;10:337–358.

315. Boehm U, Klamp T, Groot M, Howard JC. Cellular responses to interferon-gamma. *Annu Rev Immunol* 1997;15:749–795.

316. Murray HW. Interferon-gamma and host antimicrobial defense: current and future clinical applications. *Am J Med* 1994;97:459–467.

317. Denis M, Gregg EO. Studies on cytokine activation of listericidal activity in murine macrophages. *Can J Microbiol* 1990;36:671–675.

318. Flesch I, Kaufmann SHE. Mycobacterial growth inhibition by interferon-γ-activated bone marrow macrophages and differential susceptibility among strains of *Mycobacterium tuberculosis*. *J Immunol* 1987;138:4408–4413.

319. Flesch IEA, Hess JH, Kaufmann SHE. Growth inhibition of *Mycobacterium bovis* by IFN-γ stimulated macrophages: regulation by endogenous tumor necrosis factor-α and interleukin 10. *Int Immunol* 1994;6:693–700.

320. Hess J, Ladel C, Miko D, Kaufmann SH. *Salmonella typhimurium* aroA⁻ infection in gene-targeted immunodeficient mice. Major role of CD4⁺ TCR-αβ cells and IFN-γ in bacterial clearance independent of intracellular location. *J Immunol* 1996;156:3321–3326.

321. Dalton DK, Pitts-Meek S, Keshav S, Figari IS, Bradley A, Stewart TA. Multiple defects of immune cell function in mice with disrupted interferon-γ genes. *Science* 1993;259:1739–1742.

322. Kamijo R, Shapiro D, Le J, Huang S, Aguet M, Vilcek J. Generation of nitric oxide and induction of major histocompatibility complex class II antigen in macrophages from mice lacking the interferon-γ receptor. *Proc Natl Acad Sci USA* 1993;90:6626–6630.

323. Crowle AJ, Ross EJ, May MH. Inhibition by 1,25(OH)₂-vitamin D3 of the multiplication of virulent tubercle bacilli in cultured human macrophages. *Infect Immun* 1987;55:2945–2950.

324. Denis M. Killing of *Mycobacterium tuberculosis* within human monocytes: activation by cytokines and calcitriol. *Clin Exp Immunol* 1991;84:200–206.

325. Douvas GS, Looker DL, Vatter AE, Crowle AJ. Gamma interferon activates human macrophages to become tumoricidal and leishmanicidal but enhances replication of macrophage-associated mycobacteria. *Infect Immun* 1985;50:1–8.

326. Rook GAW, Taverne J, Leveton C, Steele J. The role of gamma-interferon, vitamin D3 metabolites and tumor necrosis factor in the pathogenesis of tuberculosis. *Immunology* 1987;62:229–234.

327. Rigby WFC. The immunobiology of vitamin D. *Immunol Today* 1988;9:33–63.

328. Holland SM, Eisenstein EM, Kuhns DB, et al. Treatment of refractory disseminated nontuberculous mycobacterial infection with interferon gamma. A preliminary report. *N Engl J Med* 1994;330:1348–1355.

329. Raad I, Hachem R, Leeds N, Sawaya R, Salem Z, Atweh S. Use of adjunctive treatment with interferon-gamma in an immunocompromised patient who had refractory multidrug-resistant tuberculosis of the brain. *Clin Infect Dis* 1996;22:572–574.

330. Nathan CF, Kaplan G, Levis WR, et al. Local and systemic effects of intradermal recombinant interferon-γ in patients with lepromatous leprosy. *N Engl J Med* 1986;316:6–15.

331. Holland SM. Therapy of mycobacterial infections. *Res Immunol* 1996;147:572–581.

332. Kaufmann SHE, Hahn H, Berger R, Kirchner H. Interferon-γ production by *Listeria monocytogenes*-specific T cells active in antibacterial immunity. *Eur J Immunol* 1983;13:265–268.

333. Nakane A, Numata A, Asano M, Kohanawa M, Chen Y, Minagawa T. Evidence that endogenous gamma interferon is produced early in *Listeria monocytogenes* infection. *Infect Immun* 1990;58:2386–2388.

334. Trinchieri G. Interleukin-12: a proinflammatory cytokine with immunoregulatory functions that bridge innate resistance and antigen-specific adaptive immunity. *Annu Rev Immunol* 1995;13:251–276.

335. Trinchieri G, Gerosa F. Immunoregulation by interleukin-12. *J Leukoc Biol* 1996;59:505–511.

336. Magram J, Connaughton SE, Warrier RR, et al. IL-12-deficient mice are defective in IFN-γ production and type 1 cytokine responses. *Immunity* 1996;4:471–481.

337. Zhang M, Gately MK, Wang E, et al. Interleukin 12 at the site of disease in tuberculosis. *J Clin Invest* 1994;93:1733–1739.

338. Tripp CS, Wolf SF, Unanue ER. Interleukin 12 and tumor necrosis factor α are costimulators of interferon-γ production by natural killer cells in severe combined immunodeficiency mice with listeriosis, and interleukin 10 is a physiologic antagonist. *Proc Natl Acad Sci USA* 1993;90:3725–3729.

339. Flesch IEA, Hess JH, Huang S, et al. Early interleukin-12 production by macrophages in response to mycobacterial infection depends on interferon-γ and tumor necrosis factor-α. *J Exp Med* 1995;181:1615–1622.

340. Hayes MP, Wang J, Norcross MA. Regulation of interleukin-12 expression in human monocytes: selective priming by interferon-gamma of lipopolysaccharide-inducible p35 and p40 genes. *Blood* 1995;86:646–650.

341. Ma X, Chow JM, Gri G, et al. The interleukin 12 p40 gene promoter is primed by interferon gamma in monocytic cells. *J Exp Med* 1996;183:147–157.

342. Tripp CS, Gately MK, Hakimi J, Ling P, Unanue ER. Neutralization of IL-12 decreases resistance to *Listeria* in SCID and C.B-17 mice. *J Immunol* 1994;152:1883–1887.

343. Cooper AM, Roberts AD, Rhoades ER, Callahan JE, Getzy DM, Orme IM. The role of interleukin-12 in acquired immunity to *Mycobacterium tuberculosis* infection. *Immunology* 1995;85:423–432.

344. Flynn JL, Goldstein MM, Triebold KJ, Sypek J, Wolf S, Bloom BR. IL-12 increases resistance of BALB/c mice to *Mycobacterium tuberculosis* infection. *J Immunol* 1995;155:2515–2524.

344a. Cooper AM, Magram J, Ferrante J, Orme IM. Interleukin 12 (IL-12) is crucial to the development of protective immunity in mice intravenously infected with *Mycobacterium tuberculosis*. *J Exp Med* 1997;186:39 45.

345. Okamura H, Tsutsi H, Komatsu T, et al. Cloning of a new cytokine that induces IFN-gamma production by T cells. *Nature* 1995;378:88–91.

346. Frucht DM, Holland SM. Defective monocyte costimulation for IFN-gamma production in familial disseminated *Mycobacterium avium* complex infection: abnormal IL-12 regulation. *J Immunol* 1996;157:411–416.

347. Flesch IEA, Kaufmann SHE. Role of macrophages and α/β T lymphocytes in early interleukin-10 production during *Listeria monocytogenes* infection. *Int Immunol* 1994;6:463–468.

348. Dai WJ, Kohler G, Brombacher F. Both innate and acquired immunity to *Listeria monocytogenes* infection are increased in IL-10-deficient mice. *J Immunol* 1997;158:2259–2267.

349. Orme IM, Roberts AD, Griffin JP, Abrams JS. Cytokine secretion by CD4 T lymphocytes acquired in response to *Mycobacterium tuberculosis* infection. *J Immunol* 1993;151:518–325.

350. Surcel H-M, Troye-Blomberg M, Paulie S, Andersson G, Moreno C, Pasvol G. Th1/Th2 profiles in tuberculosis, based on the proliferation and cytokine response of blood lymphocytes to mycobacterial antigens. *Immunology* 1994;81:171–176.

351. Hirsch CS, Ellner JJ, Blinkhorn R, Toossi Z. In vitro restoration of T cell responses in tuberculosis and augmentation of monocyte effector function against *Mycobacterium tuberculosis* by natural inhibitors of transforming growth factor β. *Proc Natl Acad Sci USA* 1997;94:3926–3931.

352. Toossi Z, Ellner JJ. Mechanisms of anergy in tuberculosis. *Curr Top Microbiol Immunol* 1996;215:221–238.

353. Kaufmann SHE. Immunity to intracellular microbial pathogens. *Immunol Today* 1995;16:338–342.

354. Seder RA, Paul WE. Acquisition of lymphokine-producing phenotype by CD4+ T cells. *Annu Rev Immunol* 1994;12:635–673.

355. Romagnani S. Lymphokine production by human T cells in disease states. *Annu Rev Immunol* 1994;12:227–257.

356. Daugelat S, Kaufmann SHE. Role of Th1 and Th2 cells in bacterial infections. In: Romagnani S, ed. *Th1 and Th2 Cells in health and disease.* Basel: Karger, 1996:66–97.

357. Finkelman FD, Shea-Donohue T, Goldhill J, et al. Cytokine regulation of host defense against parasitic gastrointestinal nematodes. *Annu Rev Immunol* 1997;15:505–534.

358. Del Prete G, De Carli M, Almerigogna F, et al. Preferential expression of CD30 by human CD4+ T cells producing Th2-type cytokines. *FASEB J* 1995;9:81–86.

359. Munk ME, Kern P, Kaufmann SHE. Human CD30+ cells are induced by *Mycobacterium tuberculosis* and present in tuberculosis lesions. *Int Immunol* 1997;9:713–720.

360. Rogge L, Barberis-Maino L, Biffi M, et al. Selective expression of an interleukin-12 receptor component by human T helper 1 cells. *J Exp Med* 1997;185:825–831.

361. Szabo SJ, Dighe AS, Gubler U, Murphy KM. Regulation of the interleukin (IL)-12Rβ2 subunit expression in developing T helper 1 (Th1) and Th2 cells. *J Exp Med* 1997;185:817–824.

362. Reiner SL, Locksley RM. The regulation of immunity to *Leishmania major*. *Annu Rev Immunol* 1995;13:151–177.

363. Shirakawa T, Enomoto T, Shimazu S, Hopkin JM. The inverse association between tuberculin responses and atopic disorder. *Science* 1997;275:77–79.

364. Aoki I, Kinzer C, Shirai A, Paul WE, Klinman DM. IgE receptor-positive non-B/non-T cells dominate the production of interleukin 4 and interleukin 6 in immunized mice. *Proc Natl Acad Sci USA* 1995;92:2534–2538.

365. Cleveland MG, Gorham JD, Murphy TL, Tuomanen E, Murphy KM. Lipoteichoic acid preparations of gram-positive bacteria induce interleukin-12 through a CD14-dependent pathway. *Infect Immun* 1996;64:1906–1912.

366. Yoshida A, Koide Y. Arabinofuranosyl-terminated and mannosylated lipoarabinomannans from *Mycobacterium tuberculosis* induce different levels of interleukin-12 expression in murine macrophages. *Infect Immun* 1997;65:1953–1955.

367. Oswald IP, Dozois CM, Petit J-F, Lemaire G. Interleukin-12 synthesis is a required step in trehalose dimycolate-induced activation of mouse peritoneal macrophages. *Infect Immun* 1997;65:1364–1369.

368. Hsieh C-S, Macatonia SE, Tripp CS, Wolf SF, O'Garra A, Murphy KM. Development of TH1 CD4+ T cells through IL-12 produced by Listeria-induced macrophages. *Science* 1993;260:547–549.

369. Emoto M, Emoto Y, Kaufmann SHE. Bacille Calmette Guérin and interleukin-12 (IL-12) down-modulate IL-4-producing CD4+ NK1+ T lymphocytes. *Eur J Immunol* 1997;27:183–188.

369a. Chen H, Paul WE. Cultured NK1.1+ CD4+ T cells produce large amounts of IL-4 and IFN-γ upon activation by anti-CD3 or CD1. *J Immunol* 1997;159:2240–2249.

370. Szalay G, Ladel C, Blum C, Kaufmann SHE. IL-4 neutralization or TNF-α treatment ameliorates disease by a bacterial Th1 pathogen in IFN-γ receptor deficient mice. *J Immunol* 1996;157:4746–4750.

371. Grewal IS, Flavell RA. A central role of CD40 ligand in the regulation of CD4+ T-cell responses. *Immunol Today* 1996;17:410–414.

372. Bluestone JA. New perspectives of CD28-B7-mediated T cell costimulation. *Immunity* 1995;2:555–559.

373. Noelle RJ. CD40 and its ligand in host defense. *Immunity* 1996;4:415–419.

374. Constant SL, Bottomly K. Induction of Th1 and Th2 CD4+ T cell responses. the alternative approaches. *Annu Rev Immunol* 1997;15.297–322.

375. Lenschow DJ, Walunas TL, Bluestone JA. CD28/B7 system of T cell costimulation. *Annu Rev Immunol* 1996;14:233–258.

376. Banchereau J, Bazan F, Blanchard D, et al. The CD40 antigen and its ligand. *Annu Rev Immunol* 1994;12:881 922.

377. Soong L, Xu JC, Grewal IS, et al. Disruption of CD40-CD40 ligand interactions results in an enhanced susceptibility to *Leishmania amazonensis* infection. *Immunity* 1996;4:263–273.

378. Campbell KA, Ovendale PJ, Kennedy MK, Fanslow WC, Reed SG, Maliszewski CR. CD40 ligand is required for protective cell-mediated immunity to *Leishmania major*. *Immunity* 1996;4:283–289.

379. Kamanaka M, Yu P, Yasui T, et al. Protective role of CD40 in *Leishmania major* infection at two distinct phases of cell-mediated immunity. *Immunity* 1996;4:275–281.

380. Grewal IS, Borrow P, Pamer EG, Oldstone MBA, Flavell RA. The CD40/CD154 system in anti-infective host defense. *Curr Opin Immunol* 1997;9:491 497.

381. Holmberg LA, Ault KA. Characterization of *Listeria monocytogenes*-induced murine natural killer cells. *Immunol Res* 1986;5:50–60.

382. Blanchard DK, Michelini-Norris MB, Friedman H, Djeu JY. Lysis of mycobacteria-infected monocytes by IL-2-activated killer cells: role of LFA-1. *Cell Immunol* 1989;119:402–411.

383. Blanchard DK, Stewart WEII, Klein TW, Friedman H, Djeu JY. Cytolytic activity of human peripheral blood leukocytes against *Legionella pneumophila*-infected monocytes: characterization of the effector cell and augmentation by interleukin 2. *J Immunol* 1987;139:551–556.

384. Carl M, Dasch GA. Characterization of human cytotoxic lymphocytes against cells infected with typhus group Rickettsiae: evidence for lymphokine activation of effectors. *J Immunol* 1986;136:2654–2661.

385. Rollwagen FM, Dasch GA, Jerrells TR. Mechanisms of immunity to Rickettsial infection: characterization of a cytotoxic effector cell. *J Immunol* 1986;136:1418–1421.

386. Munk ME, Gatrill A, Kaufmann SHE. Antigen-specific target cell lysis and interleukin-2 secretion by *Mycobacterium tuberculosis*-activated γ/δ T cells. *J Immunol* 1990;145:2434–2439.

387. Stenger S, Uyemura K, Cho S, et al. Differential effects of cytolytic T cell subsets on intracellular infection. *Science* 1997;276:1684–1687.

388. Kumararatne DS, Pithie AS, Drysdale P, et al. Specific lysis of mycobacterial antigen-bearing macrophages by class II MHC-restricted polyclonal T cell lines in healthy donors or patients with tuberculosis. *Clin Exp Immunol* 1990;80:314–323.

389. Mustafa AS, Godal T. BCG induced CD4+ cytotoxic T cells from BCG vaccinated healthy subjects: relation between cytotoxicity and suppression in vitro. *Clin Exp Immunol* 1987;69:255–262.

390. Rees ADM, Scoging A, Mehlert A, Young DB, Ivanyi J. Specificity of proliferative response of human CD8 clones to mycobacterial antigens. *Eur J Immunol* 1988;18:1881–1887.

391. Turner J, Dockrell HM. Stimulation of human peripheral blood mononuclear cells with live *Mycobacterium bovis* BCG activates cytolytic CD8+ T cells in vitro. *Immunology* 1996;87:339–342.

392. Sasaki T, Mieno M, Udono H, et al. Roles of CD4+ and CD8+ cells, and the effect of administration of recombinant murine interferon-γ in listerial infection. *J Exp Med* 1990;171.1141.

393. Cooper CL, Mueller C, Sinchaisri TA, et al. Analysis of naturally occurring delayed type hypersensitivity reactions in leprosy by in situ hybridization. *J Exp Med* 1989;169.1565–1581.

394. Mehra V, Modlin RL. T lymphocytes in leprosy lesions. *Curr Top Microbiol Immunol* 1989;155:97 109.

395. Laochumroonvorapong P, Wang J, Liu C-C, et al. Perforin, a cytotoxic molecule which mediates cell necrosis, is not required for the early control of mycobacterial infection in mice. *Infect Immun* 1997;65:127–132.

396. Cooper AM, D'Souza C, Frank AA, Orme IM. The course of *Mycobacterium tuberculosis* infection in the lungs of mice lacking expression of either perforin- or granzyme-mediated cytolytic mechanisms. *Infect Immun* 1997;65:1317–1320.

396a. Blanchard DK, Wei S, Duan C, Pericle F, Diaz JI, Djeu JY. Role of extracellular adenosine triphosphate in the cytotoxic T-lymphocyte-mediated lysis of antigen presenting cells. *Blood* 1995;85:3173–3182.

397. Dannenberg AM Jr. Delayed-type hypersensitivity and cell-mediated immunity in the pathogenesis of tuberculosis. *Immunol Today* 1991;12:228–233.

398. Warren KS. A functional classification of granulomatous inflammation. *Ann NY Acad Sci* 1976;278:7–18.

399. Modlin RL, Melancon-Kaplan J, Young SMM, et al. Learning from lesions: patterns of tissue inflammation in leprosy. *Proc Natl Acad Sci USA* 1988;85:1213–1217.

400. Salmi M, Jalkanen S. How do lymphocytes know where to go: current concepts and enigmas of lymphocyte homing. *Adv Immunol* 1997;64:139–218.

401. Barnes PF, Fong S-J, Brennan PJ, Twomey PE, Mazumder A, Modlin RL. Local production of tumor necrosis factor and IFN-γ in tuberculous pleuritis. *J Immunol* 1990;145:149–154.

402. Friedland JS, Remick DG, Shattock R, Griffin GE. Secretion of interleukin-8 following phagocytosis of *Mycobacterium tuberculosis* by human monocyte cell lines. *Eur J Immunol* 1992;22:1373–1378.

403. Ogawa T, Uchida H, Kusumoto Y, Mori Y, Yamamura Y, Hamada S. Increase in tumor necrosis factor alpha- and interleukin-6-secreting cells in peripheral blood mononuclear cells from subjects infected with *Mycobacterium tuberculosis*. *Infect Immun* 1991;59:3021–3025.

404. Colten HR, Krause JE. Pulmonary inflammation—a balancing act. *N Engl J Med* 1997;336:1094–1096.

404a. Donnelly SC, Bucala R. Macrophage migration inhibitory factor: a regulator of glucocorticoid activity with a critial role in inflammatory disease. *Mol Med Today* 1997;3:502–507.

405. Dustin ML, Springer TA. Role of lymphocyte adhesion receptors in transient interactions and cell locomotion. *Annu Rev Immunol* 1991;9:27–66.

406. Lasky LA. Selectins: interpreters of cell-specific carbohydrate information during inflammation. *Science* 1992;258:964–969.

407. McEver RP. Leukocyte-endothelial cell interactions. *Curr Opin Cell* Biol 1992;4:840–849.

408. Imhof BA, Dunon D. Leukocyte migration and adhesion. *Adv Immunol* 1995;58:345–416.

409. Mielke MEA, Rosen H, Brocke S, Peters C, Hahn H. Protective immunity and granuloma formation are mediated by two distinct tumor necrosis factor alpha- and gamma-interferon-dependent T cell-phagocyte interactions in murine listeriosis: dissociation on the basis of phagocyte adhesion mechanisms. *Infect Immun* 1992;60:1875–1882.

410. Mielke MEA, Niedobitek G, Stein H, Hahn H. Acquired resistance to *Listeria monocytogenes* is mediated by Lyt-2+ T cells independently of the influx of monocytes into granulomatous lesions. *J Exp Med* 1989;170:589–594.

411. Mielke MEA, Ehlers S, Hahn H. T-cell subsets in delayed-type hypersensitivity, protectin, and granuloma formation in primary and secondary Listeria infection in mice: superior role of Lyt-2+ cells in acquired immunity. *Infect Immun* 1988;56:1920–1925.

412. Modlin RL. Th1-Th2 paradigm: insights from leprosy. *J Invest Dermatol* 1994;102:828–832.

413. Gaylord H, Brennan PJ. Leprosy and the leprosy bacillus: recent developments in characterization of antigens in immunology of the disease. *Annu Rev Microbiol* 1987;41:645–675.

414. Godal T, Myrvang B, Fröland SS, Shao J, Melaku G. Evidence that the mechanism of immunological tolerance ("central failure") is operative in the lack of host resistance in lepromatous leprosy. *Scand J Immunol* 1972;1:311–321.

415. Myrvang B, Godal T, Ridley DS, Froland SS, Song YK. Immune responsiveness of *Mycobacterium leprae* and other mycobacterial antigens throughout the clinical and histopathological spectrum of leprosy. *Clin Exp Immunol* 1973;14:541–553.

416. Rees RJW. The significance of the lepromin reaction in man. *Prog Allergy* 1964;8:224–258.

417. Turk JL, Waters MFR. Cell-mediated immunity in patients with leprosy. *Lancet* 1969;ii:243–246.

418. Waldorf DS, Sheagren JN, Trautman JR, Block JB. Impaired delayed hypersensitivity in patients with lepromatous leprosy. *Lancet* 1966;ii:733–776.

419. Horwitz MA, Levis WR, Cohn ZA. Defective production of monocyte activating lymphokines in lepromatous leprosy. *J Exp Med* 1984;159:666–678.

420. Maes HH, Causse JE, Maes RF. Mycobacterial infections: are the observed enigmas and paradoxes explained by immunosuppression and immunodeficiency? *Med Hypotheses* 1996;46:163–171.

421. Bloom BR, Mehra V. Immunological unresponsiveness in leprosy. *Immunol Rev* 1984;80:5–28.

422. Modlin RL, Brenner MB, Krangel MS, Duby AD, Bloom BR. T-cell receptors of human suppressor cells. *Nature* 1987;329:541–545.

423. Kaplan G, Sampaio EP, Walsh GP, et al. Influence of *Mycobacterium leprae* and its soluble products on the cutaneous responsiveness of leprosy patients to antigen and recombinant interleukin 2. *Proc Natl Acad Sci USA* 1989;86:6269–6273.

424. Kaplan G, Sheftel G, Job CK, Mathur NK, Nath I, Cohn ZA. Efficacy of a cell-mediated reaction to the purified protein derivative of tuberculin in the disposal of *Mycobacterium leprae* from human skin. *Proc Natl Acad Sci USA* 1988;85:5210–5214.

425. Kaplan G, Laal S, Sheftel G, et al. The nature and kinetics of a delayed immune response to purified protein derivative of tuberculin in the skin of lepromatous leprosy patients. *J Exp Med* 1988;168:1811–1824.

426. Kaplan G, Kiessling R, Teklemariam S, et al. The reconstitution of cell-mediated immunity in the cutaneous lesions of lepromatous leprosy by recombinant interleukin 2. *J Exp Med* 1989;169:893–907.

427. Bullock WJ. Studies of immune mechanisms in leprosy. I. Depression of delayed allergic response to skin test antigens. *N Engl J Med* 1968;278:298.

428. Haregewoin A, Mustafa AS, Helle I, Waters MFR, Leiker DL, Godal T. Reversal by interleukin-2 of the T cell unresponsiveness of lepromatous leprosy to *Mycobacterium leprae*. *Immunol Rev* 1984;80:77–86.

429. Kaplan G, Weinstein DE, Steinman RM, et al. An analysis of in vitro T cell responsiveness in lepromatous leprosy. *J Exp Med* 1985;162:917–929.

430. Nogueira N, Kaplan G, Levy E, Sarno E, Kushner P. Defective γ-interferon production in leprosy. Reversal with antigen and interleukin 2. *J Exp Med* 1983;158:2165–2170.

431. Ellner JJ, Daniel TM. Immunosuppression by mycobacterial arabinomannan. *Clin Exp Immunol* 1979;35:250–257.

432. Hunter SW, Gaylord H, Brennan PJ. Structure and antigenicity of the phosphorylated lipopolysaccharides of the tubercle and leprosy bacilli. *J Biol Chem* 1986;261:12345–12351.

433. Prasad HK, Mishra RS, Nath I. Phenolic glycolipid-1 of *Mycobacterium leprae* induces general suppression of *in vitro* concanavalin A responses unrelated to leprosy type. *J Exp Med* 1987;165:239–244.

434. Salgame PR, Abrams JS, Clayberger C, et al. Differing lymphokine profiles of functional subsets of human CD4 and CD8 T cell clones. *Science* 1991;254:279–282.

435. Reiter H, Ed. Die Säuglingstuberkulose in Lübeck. Berlin: Julius Springer, 1935.

436. Schurr E, Malo D, Radzioch D, et al. Genetic control of innate resistance to mycobacterial infections. *Immunol Today* 1991;12:A42–A45.

437. Schurr E, Buschman E, Malo D, Gros P, Skamene E. Immunogenetics of mycobacterial infections: mouse-human homologies. *J Infect Dis* 1990;161:634–639.

438. Skamene E, Pietrangeli CE. Genetics of the immune response to infectious pathogens. *Curr Opin Immunol* 1991;3:511–517.

439. Malo D, Skamene E. Genetic control of host resistance to infection. *Trends Genet* 1994;10:365–371.

440. Buschman E, Schurr E, Skamene E. Constitutional resistance to mycobacterial infection: role of genetic factors in resistance to infection. In: Verduin CM, Watson DA, van Dijk H, Verhoef J, eds. *Constitutional resistance to infection*. Austin, TX: R.G. Landes Company, 1995:55–81.

441. Plant J, Glynn AA. Genetics of resistance to infection with *Salmonella typhimurium* in mice. *J Infect Dis* 1976;133:72–78.

442. Nikonenko BV, Apt AS, Mezhlumova MB, Avdienko VG, Yeremeev VV, Moroz AM. Influence of the mouse Bcg, Tbc-1 and xid genes on resistance and immune responses to tuberculosis infection and efficacy of bacille Calmette-Guerin (BCG) vaccination. *Clin Exp Immunol* 1996;104:37–43.

443. Medina E, North RJ. Evidence inconsistent with a role for the Bcg gene (Nramp1) in resistance of mice to infection with virulent *Mycobacterium tuberculosis*. *J Exp Med* 1996;183:1045–1051.

444. Medina E, Rogerson BJ, North RJ. The *Nramp1* antimicrobial resistance gene segregates independently of resistance to virulent *Mycobacterium tuberculosis*. *Immunology* 1996;88:479–481.

445. Vidal SM, Malo D, Vogan K, Skamene E, Gros P. Natural resistance to infection with intracellular parasites: isolation of a candidate for BCG. *Cell* 1993;73:469–485.

446. Cellier M, Govoni G, Vidal S, et al. Human natural resistance-associated macrophage protein: cDNA cloning, chromosomal mapping, genomic organization, and tissue-specific expression. *J Exp Med* 1994;180:1741–1752.

447. Blackwell JM, Barton CH, White JK, et al. Genomic organization and sequence of the human NRAMP gene: identification and mapping of a promoter region polymorphism. *Mol Med* 1995;1:194–205.

448. Abel L, Vu DL, Oberti J, et al. Complex segregation analysis of leprosy in southern Vietnam. *Genet Epidemiol* 1995;12:63–82.

449. Shaw MA, Atkinson S, Dockrell H, et al. An RFLP map for 2q33-q37 from multicase mycobacterial and leishmanial disease families: no evidence for an Lsh/Ity/Bcg gene homologue influencing susceptibility to leprosy. *Ann Hum Genet* 1993;57:251–271.

450. Levee G, Liu J, Gicquel B, Chanteau S, Schurr E. Genetic control of susceptibility to leprosy in French Polynesia; no evidence for linkage with markers on telomeric human chromosome 2. *Int J Lepr Other Mycobact Dis* 1994;62:499–511.

451. Abel L, Dessein AJ. The impact of host genetics on susceptibility to human infectious diseases. *Curr Opin Immunol* 1997;9:509–516.

451a. Bellamy R, Ruwende C, Corrah T, McAdam KPWJ, Whittle HC, Hill AVS. Variations in the *NRAMP1* gene and susceptibility to tuberculosis in West Africans. *N Eng J Med* 1998;338:640–644.

452. Vidal S, Tremblay ML, Govoni G, et al. The *Ity/Lsh/Bcg* locus: natural resistance to infection with intracellular parasites is abrogated by disruption of the *Nramp1* gene. *J Exp Med* 1995;182:655–666.

453. Govoni G, Vidal S, Gauthier S, Skamene E, Malo D, Gros P. The *Bcg/Ity/Lsh* locus: genetic transfer of resistance to infections in C57BL/6J mice transgenic for the *Nramp1*[Gly169] allele. *Infect Immun* 1996;64:2923–2929.

454. Gruenheid S, Pinner E, Desjardins M, Gros P. Natural resistance to infection with intracellular pathogens: the *Nramp1* protein is recruited to the membrane of the phagosome. *J Exp Med* 1997;185:717–730.

454a. Atkinson GP, Blackwell JM, Barton HC. Nramp1 locus encodes a 65 kDa interferon-γ-inducible protein in murine macrophages. *Biochem J* 1997;325:779–786.

454b. Gunshin H, Mackenzie B, v Berger U, et al. Cloning and characterization of a mammalian proton-coupled metal-ion transporter. *Nature* 1997;388:482–488.

455. Hill AV, Allsopp CE, Kwiatkowski D, et al. Common west African HLA antigens are associated with protection from severe malaria. *Nature* 1991;352:595–600.

456. Hill AV, Elvin J, Willis AC, et al. Molecular analysis of the association of HLA-B53 and resistance to severe malaria. *Nature* 1992;360:434–439.

457. Hill AVS. MHC polymorphism and susceptibility to intracellular infections in humans. In: Kaufmann SHE, ed. *Host response to intracellular pathogens.* Austin, TX: R.G. Landes Company, 1997:47–60.

458. Mehra NK. Role of HLA-linked factors in governing susceptibility to leprosy and tuberculosis. *Trop Med Parasitol* 1990;41:352–354.

459. Pitchappan RM. Genetics of tuberculosis susceptibility. *Trop Med Parasitol* 1990;41:355–356.

460. van Eden W, DeVries RRP. HLA and leprosy: re-evaluation. *Lepr Rev* 1984;55:89–104.

461. Kaslow RA, Shaw S. The role of histocompatibility antigens (IILA) in infection. *Epidemiol Rev* 1981,3.90–114.

462. Bothamley GH, Beck JS, Schreuder GM, et al. Association of tuberculosis and *M. tuberculosis*-specific antibody levels with HLA. *J Infect Dis* 1989;159:549–555.

463. Todd JR, West BC, McDonald JC. Human leukocyte antigen and leprosy: study in northern Louisiana and review. *Rev Infect Dis* 1990;12:63–74.

464. van Eden W, Gonzalez NM, de Vries RR, Convit J, van Rood JJ. HLA-linked control of predisposition to lepromatous leprosy. *J Infect Dis* 1985;151:9–14.

465. Ottenhoff TH, de Vries RR. HLA class II immune response and suppression genes in leprosy. *Int J Lepr Other Mycobact Dis* 1987;55:521–534.

466. Zerva L, Cizman B, Mehra NK, et al. Arginine at positions 13 or 70-71 in pocket 4 of HLA-DRB1 alleles is associated with susceptibility to tuberculoid leprosy. *J Exp Med* 1996;183:829–836.

467. Rajalingam R, Mehra NK, Jain RC, Myneedu VP, Pande JN. Polymerase chain reaction—based sequence-specific oligonucleotide hybridization analysis of HLA class II antigens in pulmonary tuberculosis: relevance to chemotherapy and disease severity. *J Infect Dis* 1996;173:669–676.

468. Cheers C, McKenzie IFC, Pavlov H, Waid C, York J. Resistance and susceptibility of mice in bacterial infection: course of listeriosis in resistant or susceptible mice. *Infect Immun* 1978;19:763–777.

469. Stevenson MM, Kongshavn PAL, Skamene E. Genetic linkage of resistance to *Listeria monocytogenes* with macrophage inflammatory responses. *J Immunol* 1981;127:402–407.

470. Gervais F, Desforges C, Skamene E. The C5-sufficient A/J congenic mouse strain. Inflammatory response and resistance to *Listeria monocytogenes*. *J Immunol* 1989;142:2057–2060.

471. Höpken UE, Lu B, Gerard NP, Gerard C. The C5a chemoattractant receptor mediates mucosal defence to infection. *Nature* 1996;383:86–89.

472. Yoshida S, Goto Y, Mizuguchi Y, Nomoto K, Skamene E. Genetic control of natural resistance in mouse macrophages regulating intracellular Legionella pneumophila multiplication in vitro. *Infect Immun* 1991;59:428–432.

473. Dietrich WF, Damron DM, Isberg RR, Lander ES, Swanson MS. *Lgn1,* a gene that determines susceptibility to *Legionella pneumophila,* maps to mouse chromosome 13. *Genomics* 1995;26:443–450.

474. Beckers M-C, Ernst E, Diez E, et al. High-resolution linkage map of mouse chromosome 13 in the vicinity of the host resistance locus *Lgn1*. *Genomics* 1997;39:254–263.

475. Scharf JM, Damron D, Frisella A, et al. The mouse region syntenic for human spinal muscular atrophy lies within the *Lgn1* critical interval and contains multiple copies of *Naip* exon 5. *Genomics* 1996;38:405–417.

476. Biozzi G, Mouton D, Stiffel C, Bouthillier Y. Macrophage in regulation of immunoresponsiveness. *Adv Immunol* 1984;36:189–234.

Fundamental Immunology, Fourth Edition,
edited by William E. Paul
Lippincott–Raven Publishers, Philadelphia © 1999.

CHAPTER 41

Immunity to Extracellular Bacteria

Moon H. Nahm, Michael A. Apicella, and David E. Briles

Human bacterial pathogens are extremely diverse. Based on the pathogenesis of infection and the resulting immune response, these bacteria can be categorized into two general types: those causing intracellular infections and those causing extracellular infections. Most bacteria causing intracellular infections avoid being killed after phagocytosis by either interfering with phagosome–lysosome fusion or by escaping from the phagosome and into the cytoplasm. Against intracellular bacteria, cellular immunity is critical (see Chapter 40). In contrast, the bacteria causing extracellular infections survive in the host by avoiding phagocytosis. They do this by presenting a surface that minimizes the opsonic and lytic effects of antibody and complement. Although extracellular bacteria do have the ability to enter and pass through cells as a means of moving from one *in vivo* environment to another, they are readily killed once captured by phagocytes. Accordingly, the host defense against extracellular bacteria is critically dependent on complement and the production of specific antibody. Table 1 lists many of the important bacteria that can cause extracellular infections in humans along with the disease they cause and some of their major virulence factors. In this chapter we describe the surface structures of many of these bacteria and provide some examples of how they are able to infect their hosts and cause disease. We also describe the salient aspects of the innate immunity and antigen-induced immunity important in the host's defense against these bacteria.

M. H. Nahm: Departments of Pediatrics, Pathology, and Internal Medicine, University of Rochester, Rochester, New York 14642-8777.
M. A. Apicella: Department of Microbiology, University of Iowa, Iowa City, Iowa 52242.
D. E. Briles: Department of Microbiology, University of Alabama, Birmingham, Alabama 35294.

BACTERIAL SURFACE STRUCTURE OF GRAM-POSITIVE AND GRAM-NEGATIVE BACTERIA

Extracellular, as well as intracellular, pathogenic bacteria can be divided into two major tribes (Gram negative and Gram positive) based on the characteristics of Gram staining. To illustrate the surface of bacteria in the two tribes, the surface structure of *Streptococcus pneumoniae* and *Neisseria meningitidis* are shown in Fig. 1A and B, respectively. Three layers are commonly recognized: cytoplasmic membrane, cell wall, and outer layer. Although these layers are described below in detail, it is important to note that these definitions are operational and that in reality the layers are not entirely distinct. Molecules anchored in the cytoplasmic membrane or cell wall may extend into or through other layers. Thus, there are molecules other than peptidoglycan and capsular polysaccharide (PS) in the cell wall and the outer layer, respectively. It is also important to note that the capsule, O-antigens, and cell wall are not contiguous shields but are open enough to be permeable to secreted products and nutrients, as well as some immunologic factors (e.g., antibodies and complement) (Fig. 1).

A cell wall is found in all pathogenic bacteria of both tribes, with the exception of mollicutes (which include mycoplasma). The cell wall surrounds the cytoplasmic membrane and is made of peptidoglycan, which is a highly cross-linked polymer of amino sugars (N-acetyl glucosamine and muramic acid) and amino acids. The peptidoglycan polymerization is performed by the enzymes, many of which are also referred to as penicillin-binding proteins. Compared with Gram-negative bacteria, Gram-positive organisms have a thicker cell wall (20 to 30 nm compared with 2 to 4 nm) layer than do Gram-negative organisms and can thus retain the Gram stain dye better. The cell walls help protect the bacteria from the

TABLE 1. *Bacteria commonly associated with extracellular disease*

Species	Diseases	Important virulence structures/molecules	Special adaptations critical to host infection
Neisseria gonorrhoeae	Urethritis, cervicitis, salpingitis, endometritis, prostatitis, arthritis, proctitis, pharyngitis	Lipopolysaccharide, fimbria, peptidoglycan, Opa protein, unidentified adhesins and invasins	Phase and antigenic variation, molecular mimicry of human antigens
Neisseria meningitidis	Meningitis, meningococcemia, arthritis, pneumonia, asymptomatic carriage	Capsular polysaccharide, lipopolysaccharide, fimbria, membrane proteins, unidentified adhesins and invasins	Phase and antigenic variation, molecular mimicry of human antigens
Haemophilus influenzae type b	Meningitis, sepsis, arthritis, epiglottitis, asymptomatic carriage	Capsular polysaccharide, lipopolysaccharide, fimbria, peptidoglycan	Asymptomatic colonization, phase and antigenic variation, molecular mimicry of human antigens
Nontypeable *Haemophilus influenzae*	Otitis media, bronchitis, pneumonia, neonatal sepsis, endometritis, asymptomatic carriage	Lipopolysaccharide, fimbria, adhesive fibrils, peptidoglycan	Phase and antigenic variation, molecular mimicry of human antigens
Haemophilus ducreyi	Genital ulcer disease	Lipopolysaccharide (?), adhesive fibrils, hemolysin	Molecular mimicry of human antigens
Bordetella pertussis	Whooping cough in children, chronic cough syndrome in adults	Pertussis toxin, pertactin, filamentous hemagglutinin, fimbria, ciliary toxin	Coordinate regulation of toxin expression
Pseudomonas aeruginosa	Infections in compromised hosts, pneumonia, sepsis	Lipopolysaccharide, proteases, lipases, lecithinases, exotoxin A, elastase	Relatively large genomic size (~6 megabases) allows considerable adaptibility to changes in environmental conditions
Escherichia coli	Urinary tract infection, sepsis, traveler's diarrhea, dysentery, meningitis, hemolytic-uremic syndrome	Capsular polysaccharide, lipopolysaccharide, fimbria, toxins	Antigenic heterogeneity of capsule and lipopolysaccharide
Vibrio cholera	Diarrhea	Cholera toxin, fimbria	Bacterial dispersal via cholera toxin, which induces copious watery diarrhea
Helicobacter pylori	Peptic ulcer disease	Urease, flagella	Ability to survive at low pH provides a niche lacking bacterial competition or efficient immune surveillance
Treponema pallidum	Local genital ulcer disease, disseminated infection, tertiary disease	Endoflagella, rare outer membrane proteins	Limited exposed antigenic sites
Streptococcus pneumoniae	Pneumonia, otitis media, meningitis, sinusitis	Capsular polysaccharide, PspA, pneumolysin, neuraminidase, PsaA, hyaluronidase, teichoic acids	Symptomatic colonization, genetic transformation permitting continual generation of new genotypes
Staphylococcus aureus	Impetigo, folliculitis, boils, cellulitis, wound infections, toxic shock, osteomyelitis, endocarditis, bacteremia, pneumonia, food poisoning	Tissue-degrading enzymes, alpha toxin and other membrane damaging toxins, epidermolytic toxins, enterotoxins, capsule	Resistant to dehydration, asymptomatic colonization, regulation of virulence factor expression
Streptococcus pyogenes	Acute pharyngitis, scarlet fever, necrotizing fasciitis, streptococcal toxic shock syndrome, rheumatic fever, and glomerulonephritis	Hyaluronic acid capsule, M protein, streptococcal pyrogenic exotoxins, streptolysin O, streptolysin S,	Molecular mimicry of human antigens, high diversity of M proteins, phage-associated virulence properties
Streptococcus agalactiae	Bacteremia, pneumonia, otitis media, and other focal infections	Capsule, beta hemolysin, hyaluronidase	Asymptomatic colonization, acquisition by infants during parturition
Corynebacterium diphtheria	Diphtheria (pharyngitis/tonsillitis)	Diphtheria toxin	Toxin gene contained in temperate phage and expression regulated by iron concentration
Clostridium tetani	Tetanus (lock jaw)	Tetanus toxin (affects central nervous system)	Opportunities infection by a spore-forming soil anaerobe
Closridium perfringens	Gas gangrene, anaerobic cellulitis, endometritis, food poisoning	More than 10 exotoxins	Opportunistic infection of wounds

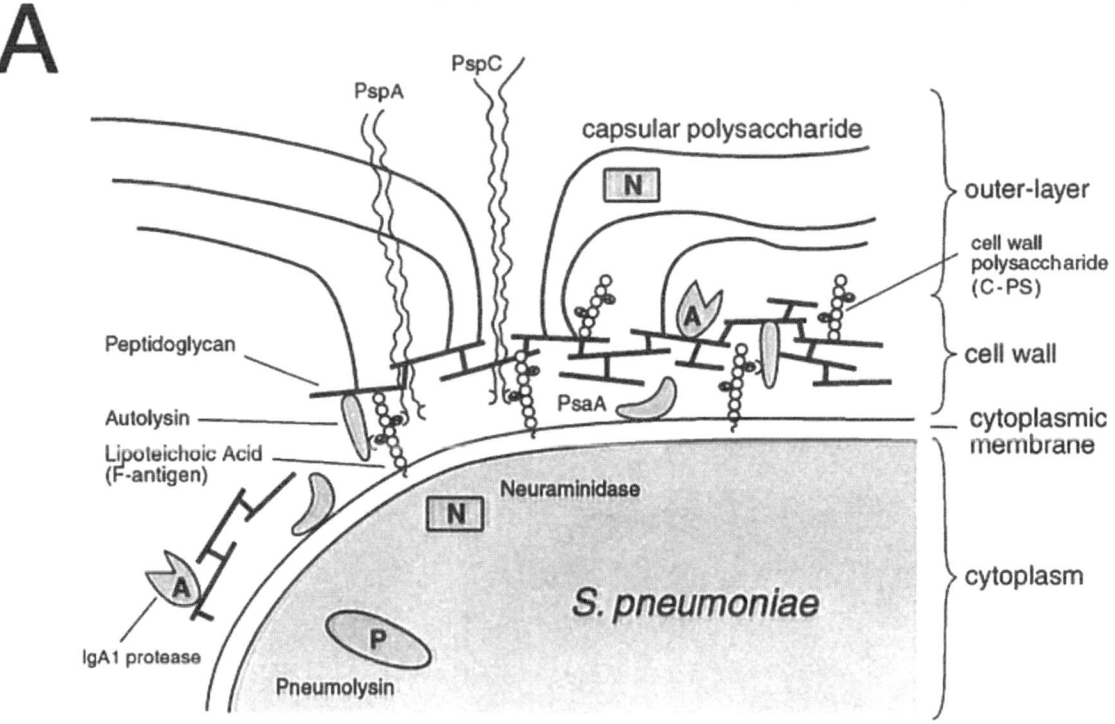

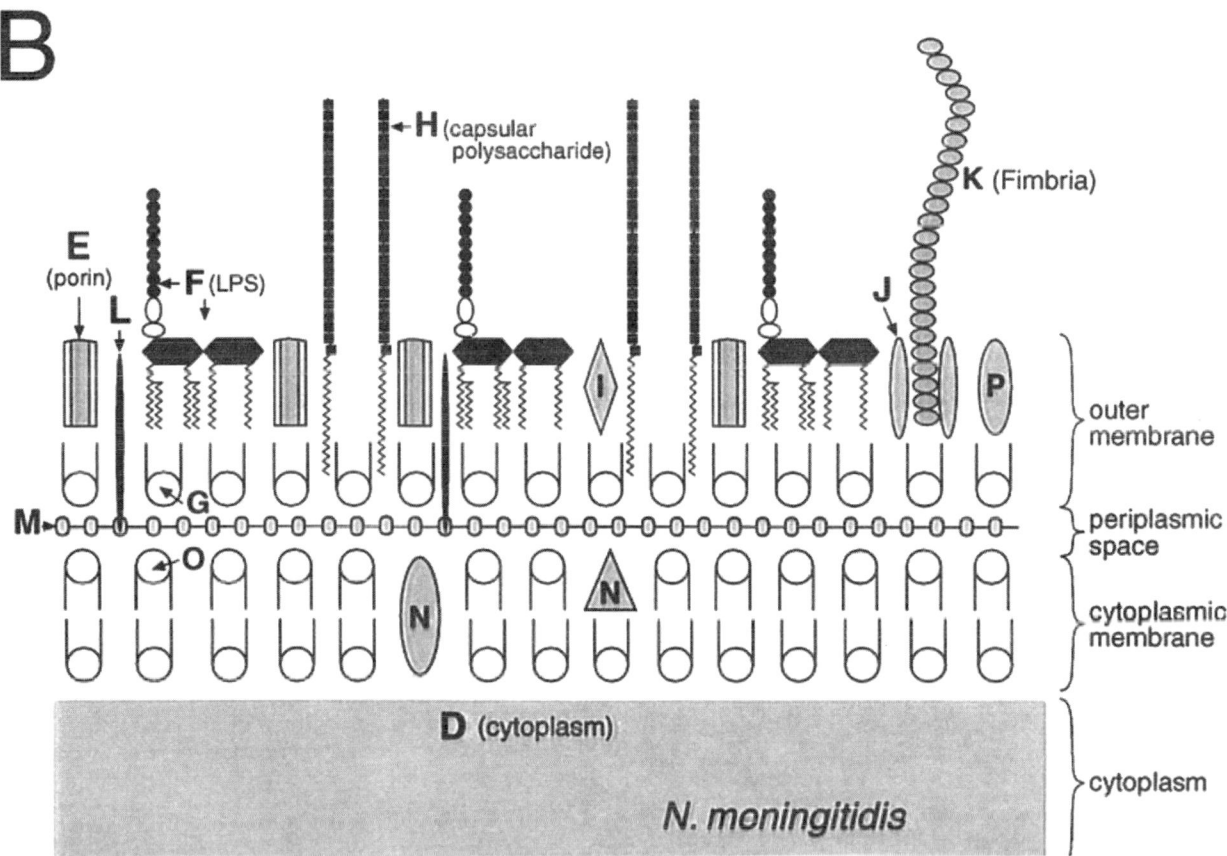

FIG. 1. Schematic representation of a Gram-positive (A) and Gram-negative (B) bacteria. D, cytoplasm; E, porin proteins; F, LPS; G, membrane phospholipids; H, capsular polysaccharide; I and P, outer membrane proteins; J, fimbrial channel; K, fimbria; L, peptidoglycan associated proteins, M, peptidoglycan; N, cytoplasmic membrane proteins; O, membrane phospholipids. Cell wall polysaccharide of *S. pneumoniae* is often called C-PS.

extremes of the environment (especially differences in osmolarity). In the case of Gram-positive bacteria, the cell wall provides protection from complement-mediated lysis.

In addition to peptidoglycan, many bacteria have polysaccharides associated with their cell walls, and these cell wall polysaccharides often extend into the capsular area. The cell wall polysaccharides of Gram-positive bacteria vary among different bacteria, and the structure of the cell wall polysaccharide has been used to distinguish many different species of streptococci (i.e., group A, B, C, etc.) (1,2). In the pneumococcus, cell wall polysaccharides are teichoic acid (labeled as C-polysaccharide in Fig. 1A). C-polysaccharide is invariant among pneumococcal strains (3,4). In Gram-positive bacteria, lipoteichoic acid is also often found attached to the cytoplasmic membrane and extending out through the cell wall (5). In pneumococci, the overall polysaccharide structure of lipoteichoic acid (also called F-antigen) and cell wall teichoic acid are very similar. They are thought to differ only in their mode of attachment to the bacterial surface (6).

The cell wall and outer layer of Gram-positive bacteria are also the location of a number of cell surface proteins involved in a variety of functions, including, but not limited to, adherence, enzyme activity against host substrates, nutrient transport, and interference with complement deposition. For instance, *Streptococcus pneumoniae* has PspA (7,8), PspC (7), PsaA (9), autolysin (10), and IgA1 protease (11,12), as well as less well-characterized proteins such as C3 protease (13) and HSP72 (14). C3 protease is able to inactivate native C3 in serum. PspA also may interfere with complement fixation (7), and may also play a role in colonization (15). PspA, autolysin, HSP72, and PsaA have all been shown to elicit protective immune responses in mice (9,14,16–18). In addition to pneumococci, many other extracellular bacteria, including *Neisseria* and *Haemophilus,* produce a protease of IgA1 (the most common form of human secretory IgA) (11,12). *Streptococcus pyogenes* has highly variable and strain-specific M proteins, which interfere with complement activation.

In the pneumococcus, many of the proteins presently identified in the cell wall and outer layer have choline binding sites through which they attach to phosphocholine residues in the teichoic and lipoteichoic acids (7,19). In other Gram-positive bacteria such as group A streptococci and staphylococci, most surface proteins have a peptide motif of LPXTGX, which precedes a hydrophobic stretch referred to as a stop-transfer sequence. In staphylococci, the LPXTGX sequence is cleaved carboxyl to the threonine and covalently linked to the free amino group of a pentaglycine cross-bridge in the bacterial cell wall (20,21), thus covalently attaching the protein to the cell wall. Some of these surface proteins have become candidates for the development of new protein-based vaccines (22).

Gram-negative bacteria have typically thinner cell walls than those of Gram-positive bacteria. Another major difference between Gram-negative and Gram-positive bacteria is the presence of an outer membrane on Gram-negative bacteria. The outer membrane is an asymmetrical bilayer: the inner leaflet is primarily phospholipid and the outer leaflet contains the lipid A component of lipopolysaccharide (LPS). In addition to enclosing the cell, the outer membrane contains proteins, enzymes, invasins, adhesins, and toxins, which are important in pathogenesis as well as recognition targets for the host cells, bacteriophage, and bacterial conjugation. Although the membrane is a selective barrier to various molecules, it is more permeable to ions than a cytoplasmic membrane and is relatively resistant to osmotic rupture. The space between the cell wall and the outer membrane is called periplasmic gel and contains a variety of hydrolytic enzymes and proteins that act to bind and transport substrates against a gradient. This space also contains cytoplasmic membrane-derived oligosaccharides, which help to regulate cellular osmolarity.

Gram-negative bacteria have LPS (also called endotoxin) in the outer membrane. LPS is an amphipathic molecule with four distinct regions: lipid A, the inner core, the outer core, and the O-antigen. Lipid A is composed of a dihexosamine backbone to which are attached through amide and ester linkages between five and seven saturated (12 to 16 carbon) fatty acids. Lipid A is the principle toxin associated with most Gram-negative bacteria. Lipid A is the major lipid component of the outer leaflet, and the acyl portion of lipid A is embedded in the phospholipid inner leaflet. The carbohydrate portion of the LPS is attached to the lipid A through a molecule unique to Gram-negative bacteria called keto-deoxyoctanoate. This sugar, along with three heptose moieties, forms the inner core of the LPS. The outer core is composed of seven to 10 monosaccharide units whose arrangement is relatively conserved among Gram-negative species (23).

In most Gram-negative bacteria, the outer core of LPS is connected to a repeating series of tetramer to hexamer of carbohydrates called the O-antigen. The O-antigen forms a hydrophilic shield around the bacterium and forms a barrier to complement deposition on the bacterial cell surface. The O-antigen is variable in length and antigenically diverse and confers serotypic specificity. The O antigens of *Escherichia coli, Klebsiella,* and *Salmonella* have as many as 30 repeating units composed of four to six sugars each (23). In the case of pathogenic *Neisseria, Haemophilus influenzae,* and *Haemophilus ducreyi,* the LPS lacks O-antigens and the size of the carbohydrate region does not exceed 7,000 daltons. The LPS of these organisms have been called *lipo-oligosaccharides* (LOS) to distinguish them from their long-chain forming relatives (24).

In addition to LPS, a number of proteins are found in the outer membrane. *E. coli* or *Neisseria* may have 20 to 30 distinct proteins in the outer membrane, whereas *Treponema pallidum* has very few proteins. A major group of outer membrane proteins are porins, which facilitate the diffusion of small hydrophilic molecules through the outer membrane. The basic porin structure is a homotrimer arranged to form a channel with a discrete pore size through the outer-leaflet. Although most porins are nonselective, some porins are components in transport systems for specific metabolites [e.g., the LamB porin of *E. coli,* which mediates maltose transport (23)]. The expression of selective porins is generally regulated by the presence or absence of substrate in the environment. Some proteins in the outer leaflet form components of the pumping systems for removal of hydrophobic compounds (e.g., tetracycline) or form a specialized pore through which pili exit the membrane (23,25).

For both Gram-positive and Gram-negative bacteria, polysaccharide dominates the outer layer. *S. pneumoniae* has capsular PS that is covalently attached to the cell wall. In Gram-negative bacteria, this layer is composed mainly of LPS and capsular PS. The capsule polysaccharide is anchored to the outer leaflet by acyl chains in *Neisseria meningitidis.* The outer layer is well developed in bacteria causing extracellular infections and has many features that help the bacteria circumvent the host immune system. First, the outer layer has properties that reduce the attachment of extracellular bacteria to eukaryotic surfaces, including those of phagocytes. Generally, the polysaccharide capsules render the bacteria hydrophilic and negatively charged like eukaryote cell surfaces that are rich in sialic acid. The negatively charged polysaccharide surfaces provided by most capsular PS also present surfaces that are at least partly resistant to alternative pathway complement fixation, because of their ability to enhance the degradation of C3b (26). Second, the elicitation of antibody is minimized in some cases because the polysaccharide capsule or LPS mimics host antigens, as is more fully described later in this chapter. This mimicry also may reduce interactions of the bacteria with host surfaces. Third, the outer layer can physically mask most of the other bacterial surface components and thus provide a minimal number of exposed epitopes that can be recognized by the antibody and complement. Although the capsule is porous to antibodies and complement, the binding of antibodies and fixation of complement beneath the capsule surface generally is relatively ineffective at promoting opsonophagocytosis and blood clearance (27). Lastly, the shielding function of the outer layer is further augmented by the presence of proteins that can interfere with complement deposition.

The polysaccharide and protein molecules at the surface of bacteria are often genetically diverse, even within a single bacterial species. If antibodies made to antigens produced by one allele cross-reacts poorly or not at all with antigens made by most other alleles, this polymorphism provides a way for the bacteria to escape antigen specific immunity elicited by prior infection. For instance, pneumococci have 90 serologically distinct capsular PS (28), and over 20 non–cross-reactive groups of pneumococci are common in human disease (29). This situation allows many of the invading pneumococci to escape recognition by anticapsular antibodies produced in response to previous pneumococcal infections with other serotypes. Similarly, there are at least 100 different serologic types of M proteins of *S. pyogenes* (30). Antibodies to one serotype of M protein do not provide protection against strains expressing other serotypes (31). Other serologically variable proteins include immunoglobulin (Ig)A1 protease and PspA of pneumococci. Unlike antibodies to M proteins, antibodies to one PspA type usually cross-react at least weakly with most other types of PspA (18,32).

The polymorphism of surface antigens is achieved by various genetic mechanisms. Variation in M proteins is the result of sequence differences in the N-terminal (but not the C-terminal) half of M-proteins (33). *S. pneumoniae* has the genes for synthesizing capsular PS as a genetic cassette, which can be exchanged among different strains (34,34a). In *Neisseria* genetic machinery exist for rapid genetic rearrangement of genes encoding surface pili (35). Lipooligosaccharides of *N. gonorrhoeae* can be modified by host enzymes and host substances, presumably resulting in enhancement of bacterial survival in the host (36). In addition, the bacteria have the genetic machinery to adapt to different host environments. Extracellular bacteria (including *Neisseria, H. influenzae,* group B streptococci, and *S. pneumoniae*) can undergo spontaneous reversible phase changes that permit them to modify their cell surfaces to adapt to different host environments (37–41). Bacteria also can regulate the expression of different virulence components in response to environmental stimuli (42), thus permitting them to readily adapt to transitions from free living versus *in vivo* environments as well as transitions from mucosal versus invasive host environments. This genetic flexibility to express different surface properties, transport systems, and metabolic pathways permits a single organism to be able to successfully evade host immune system and survive in many niches outside as well as inside the host.

BACTERIAL INVASION OF THE HOST

Both the keratinized skin and mucosal surfaces have inherent nonimmune defense mechanisms that modulate bacterial growth and minimize the risk of invasion. Healthy human skin is an effective physical barrier to infection by most human extracellular and intracellular pathogens. The keratinization of fully differentiated skin epithelium results in a relatively impermeable surface. In addition, the combination of lysozyme, toxic lipids, and hydrogen ions secreted by cutaneous glands offers bacteriostatic protection for cutaneous pores and hair follicles (43). Occasionally, these defenses can be breached by extracellular bacteria such as *S. pyogenes* or *S. aureus*, causing cellulitis and abscess. More commonly, bacterial invasion through intact skin requires physical damage such as abrasions, burns, or other trauma. For instance, *Staphylococcus epidermidis,* a member of the commensal skin flora, can infect indwelling catheters by spreading through the puncture site of the skin and then occasionally lead to a bacteremia or colonization of prosthetic devices, including artificial heart valves and shunts. A major factor allowing these bacteria to cause disease is their ability to elaborate a slime, which facilitates its adhesion, is antiphagocytic, and acts as a barrier to antibiotic penetration (44).

Unlike the skin, the mucosal epithelium is not keratinized. Instead, it is moist and nutritionally rich. Thus, it is not surprising that many mucosal areas such as the gastrointestinal tract, the nasopharynx, upper airway, and vagina can be colonized by bacteria. Most of the bacteria found at these sites are either harmless normal flora or pathogens that are asymptotically colonizing the mucosal tissue. Colonization refers to the asymptotic presence of the organism on the mucosal surface for extended periods of time, ranging from days to months. Infection refers to bacterial presence that is associated with symptomatic and or deleterious disease conditions. However, many potentially pathogenic bacteria found in mucosal areas of healthy individuals do not usually cause symptoms. *S. pneumoniae, N. meningitidis, H. influenzae,* and *S. aureus* are examples of extracellular bacteria that are frequently carried in the nasopharynx of healthy individuals. For instance, during nonepidemic periods, approximately 5% to 10% of the population are carriers of *N. meningitidis* organisms, which are mostly nonencapsulated (45). During epidemics, 30% to 60% of the population may carry the meningococci, which are mostly encapsulated and the majority of which are the same capsular type as the case strain causing the epidemic (46). Group B streptococci on the other hand are Gram-positive bacteria that are carried asymptotically in the lower intestine and the female genital tract, but can be acquired by infants during parturition and cause life-threatening bacteremia and sepsis (47). The presence of *N. gonorrhoeae* in the female genital tract is frequently asymptomatic, whereas in other individuals symptomatic and often deleterious disease is observed (48,49). Simultaneous presence of many bacterial species limits the overexpansion of one bacterial species. For instance, the destruction of the normal gastrointestinal bacterial flora with a number of antibiotics can be associated with a selective expansion of *Clostridium difficile* and development of pseudomembranous colitis (50).

To survive and colonize in the mucosal environment and in the blood, extracellular bacteria elaborate many molecules to facilitate their survival and proliferation. These molecules are often called virulence factors or toxins. One group of virulence factors helps bacteria to acquire essential nutrients. Mucosal fluid and blood is low in free iron due to the presence of iron-binding proteins such as lactoferrin and transferrin. To successfully compete with the host for this vital metabolite, *N. meningitidis, N. gonorrhoeae,* and *H. influenzae* have complex surface transport systems that can transport iron-binding human transferrin, lactoferrin, and hemoglobin into the cell (51–54). *E. coli* and *Salmonella* use a different mechanism to acquire iron. They secrete a low molecular weight iron chelator, called a siderophore, which removes iron from human proteins in the environment surrounding the bacteria. The iron–siderophore complex is then taken up by the bacterium, and the siderophore is degraded so that the iron can be freed for utilization (55,56).

In some cases, the bacterial virulence factors neutralize host defenses. Pneumolysin from *S. pneumoniae* is a cytoplasmic protein that is released during pneumococcal growth, presumably by autolysis of some of the bacteria. It exhibits its biologic effects by consuming complement at a distance from the pneumococci and by interfering with the function of phagocytes (57). Its presence also appears to impair the development of protective host responses against pneumococci (58). Immunization with pneumolysin increases the resistance of mice to pneumococcal infection (57). *S. pyogenes* and group B streptococci produce C5a peptidase that inhibits chemotaxis of host phagocytes to the sites of infections (59,60). Some bacteria also produce C3 protease (61) or IgA1 protease (11,12,62).

Another important class of the virulence factors is involved in the adherence of bacteria to the host cells. The adherence mechanisms are potential targets for vaccine developments, and many different adhesions have been described. Carriage of pneumococci is mediated largely by adherence to the host molecules N-acetyl-D-glucosamine 1-3 galactose, N-acetyl-D-glucosamine 1-4 galactose, and the receptor for the platelet activation factor (PAF receptor) (63,64). Moreover, adherence of pneumococci is enhanced by the phase shift from opaque to transparent colony morphology as well as the activation of host lung and vascular endothelial cells (64). Pili are important in adhesion for many bacteria. They express specific adhesion molecules that selectively bind host antigens. Pap pilus of *E. coli* binds the Galα4Gal unit of cell surface globoside of urethral epithelial cells (65). The *Vibrio cholerae* pilus allows attachment of the bacterium to the enterocyte for efficient toxin delivery (66,67). *Bordetella pertussis* has three adherence factors: a filamentous hemagglutinin, pertactin, and a pilus (fimbriae), which allows it to attach to ciliated respiratory epithelial cells in the trachea and bronchi, and thus resists the cleansing action of mucus flow (68,69).

N. gonorrhoeae exhibits novel mechanisms of adhesion and invasion into urethral epithelial cells (70). Initial attachment of *N. gonorrhoeae* is accomplished through pili (71). Through a unique genetic recombination system, gonococcal pili can undergo antigenic variation at a very high rate, and an individual organism can express pili with different antigenic characteristics simultaneously. The number of potential pilus antigen variants within a single organism is estimated to be greater than 100,000 (72). In addition, *N. gonorrhoeae* expresses outer membrane surface proteins designated Opa proteins, which can bind human cell surface proteoglycans on the surface of the epithelial cell (41). This binding leads to the fusion of the bacterial and epithelial cells' membranes and the internalization of the bacterium into vacuoles in the epithelial cell.

The gene for each Opa protein has a series of CTCTT within the Opa open reading frame. Recombination between CTCTT sequences varies the number of repeats (73). The number of repeats determines the transitional frame of the gene and the ultimate expression of the complete protein. Due to slip-strand mispairing, the Opa proteins can phase vary at a rapid rate. A single bacteria can express many variant Opa proteins on their surface. Upon contact with the epithelial surface, the meningococcus facilitates its entry into the epithelial cells by shutting down the synthesis of capsular PS (74), which is hydrophilic, is negatively charged, and prevents the entry into mucosal epithelial cells. Upon emergence from the epithelial cell in the submucosa, capsular synthesis is resumed.

Expression of virulence factors is often closely regulated by bacteria to accommodate the changes in the environmental stimuli. In staphylococci it has been shown that the amount of capsule is regulated in response to environmental stimuli (75,76). One of the best studied such regulatory systems is the BvgAS two-component regulatory system in *Bordetella pertussis* (77). This system regulates the expression of adhesins, toxins, and other virulence factors. The system is controlled by external signals, including Mg^{2+}, temperature, and nicotinic acid. Two proteins are involved in this regulatory system, BvgS and BvgA. BvgS, the sensor, is a kinase and is able to autophosphorylate itself in response to the environmental signal. BvgA is in turn phosphorylated by BvgS. Phosphorylated BvgA is able to activate transcription of virulence genes through a change in its interaction with a 70-bp consensus sequence repeated in *bvg*-regulated promoters (77). Two-component regulatory systems are one of the mechanisms frequently used to regulate the expression of genes associated with virulence (78).

The pathogenic extracellular bacteria are generally able to colonize the mucosal tracts without causing any harm to the host but occasionally cause focal infections at less well defended sites. For instance, *S. pneumoniae* and *H. influenzae* type b (Hib) are often carried in the nasopharyngeal space, but they can infect fluid-filled cavities (e.g., lungs and middle ear). Aspiration of bacteria from the nasopharynx into the lung undoubtedly occurs frequently with no ill effects. However, the chance of an infection increases as the result of a pulmonary blockage (such as aspirated food), damage to the epithelial surface (one cause is smoking), or viral infection (RSV or influenzae) (2,79). Viral infections are important because they can lead to the expression by the host of molecules adhesive to pneumococci in addition to the loss of host ciliary action (2,80). Some bacteria produce molecules that modify the host cell surfaces and reduce mucosal flow through the upper airways. Some Gram-positive bacteria produce hyaluronidase and neuraminidase (81–83), which modify the host cell surfaces, release host sugars to the bacteria, and destroy host tissues important for drainage. Staphylococci and *S. pyogenes* are effectively cleared from the blood but can be present as transient bacteremia due to breaks in the mucosal surface or in the skin. These circulating bacteria under rare conditions can cause focal infections, including cellulitis in damaged (or bruised) tissue when the blood flow is interrupted (84).

In some cases, the virulence factors are highly toxic to the host and can account almost completely for the detrimental symptoms of their respective infections. For example, diphtheria toxin is carried throughout the body from the site of the local infection (the throat) and blocks protein synthesis in multiple cell types (85). Cholera toxins block the uptake of sodium in the intestine and are responsible for a severe diarrhea that, if not treated, can be fatal owing to dehydration. Tetanus toxin causes central nervous system paralysis (86). Staphylococcal enterotoxin A, which is one of five membrane-damaging toxins produced by staphylococci, is the primary cause of staphylococcal food poisoning and plays a major role in invasive infections (87). Some strains of *E. coli* produce verotoxin, which may damage the microvasculature of kidney and cause hemolytic uremic syndrome (88,89). In many cases, if the host can be protected from the toxins by neutralizing antibodies, which allow the host to survive, then the host can easily eradicate the infecting bacteria. For example, vaccines eliciting antibody to tetanus toxin and diphtheria toxin are highly efficacious even though they do not elicit antibody to the organism's surface.

ANTIGEN-NONSPECIFIC HOST DEFENSE RESPONSE

To protect the host from infections caused by highly adaptable bacteria, the host employs a multilayered defense. They include the mechanical barriers described above as well as phagocytes, complement fixation, lysozyme, and (cytokine-mediated) local inflammation. In addition, the host is protected with antigen-specific antibody (see section below on Antigen-Specific Host Defense Response) and T cell–mediated cellular immunity. Antigen-specific immunity, although powerfully protective, takes at least several days to weeks to develop after exposure to a pathogen. Consequently, the primary defense against bacteria during the early phase of infection still remains the antigen-nonspecific host immunity. The importance and significance of nonspecific immunity is readily demonstrated by the relative ease with which one can maintain SCID mice that lack antigen-specific immunity (90), even in the presence of normally nonpathogenic bacteria. This section describes several antigen-nonspecific host defense mechanisms.

Mucosal Defense

Although mucosal areas are rich with nutrients for bacteria, the uncontrolled proliferation of bacteria in the mucosal areas is largely checked by mechanical cleansing actions. In the gastrointestinal tract, normal peristaltic motility, the secretion of mucus, and the detergent action of bile limit the number of bacteria. The movements of cilia along the bronchial tree continually remove aspirated bacteria along with the mucus from the lower respiratory tracts. Normal epithelial and tissue architecture is essential for draining and expulsion of bacteria, and the disruption of this mechanism by smoking, viral infections (e.g., influenza), or bacterial infection (e.g., pertussis) makes the host markedly susceptible to infection by bacteria that normally just colonizes the upper airway. The increased frequency of lower respiratory tract infections in the elderly is due in large part to loss of function of the mucociliary elevator and increased aspiration of secretions containing bacteria from the upper respiratory tract (91,92).

In addition to the removal of bacteria by mucus flow, mucosal fluid contains many antibacterial products such as lysozyme, lactoferrin, lactoperoxidase, and mucin (see Chapter 27) (93). Body fluids such as milk, saliva, and tears have lactoferrin, which binds iron and lowers the level of available iron (especially in areas with low pH) (94). Lysozyme reduces bacterial load by cleaving 1-4 linkage of N-acetyl muramic acid in the bacterial peptidoglycan. Mucin traps the microbes and facilitates their removal. IgA antibodies in mucosal fluid may inhibit colonization by blocking microbial adherence sites and by inactivating toxins. Paneth cells in the crypts of small intestines can participate in the mucosal defense by producing lysozyme and cryptdins (95).

Local Response to Bacterial Invasion (Acute Inflammation)

Upon entry, many bacterial products initiate local inflammatory processes (see Chapter 32). The list of the bacterial products initiating these processes includes peptidoglycan, LPS, formyl-methionyl peptides (e.g. f-met-leu-phe), lipoteichoic acid, exotoxins, lipoproteins, and glycolipids (96). LPS binds CD14 and triggers macrophages and monocytes (see Chapter 32). Some exotoxins, such as S. aureus enterotoxin B, activate a large subset of T cells to release cytokines. The peptide f-met-leu-phe is a chemotactic factor of neutrophils. Bacterial DNA is rich with a sequence motif that can stimulate lymphocytes (97) and macrophages (98). Many components of bacteria (e.g., peptidoglycan) nonspecifically trigger the complement by the alternative pathway (99) and enhance the activation of the inflammatory process.

During the initial phase of inflammation after a bacterial invasion, many cell types residing in the mucosa or skin (e.g., keratinocytes) may produce molecules important in controlling infections. Several recent studies showed that mast cells are one of the important resident host cells. Mast cells are abundant along the bronchial tree and epidermis of the skin and are classically known as stores of histamine and serotonin (100). They are now known to contain preformed tumor necrosis factor (TNF)-α as well as to be a major source of various cytokines. They account for 90% of IL-4– and IL-6–producing cells in the nasal cavity (101). Upon exposure to various bacterial products (e.g., LPS), they release these cytokines, which are essential for the recruitment of neutrophils to the site of inflammation. The absence of mast cells can increase the susceptibility of animals to bacterial infections in the peritoneum or the lung, and their absence can be partially compensated by administration of TNF-α (102,103).

Inflammatory processes trigger various types of cells to release many cytokines. The released cytokines trigger other cells and initiate the cascade of cytokine release. The cytokines produced during the acute inflammation can be divided into two groups: proinflammatory cytokines (e.g., IL-1 and TNF-α) and antiinflammatory cytokines (e.g., IL-4) (see Chapter 32). The molecules produced during inflammation can induce the expression of CD62E, intracellular adhesion molecule (ICAM), and vascular cell adhesion molecule (VCAM) on endothelial cells and selectins and integrins in leukocytes (see Chapter 32). These molecular changes increase the migration of neutrophils to the sites of inflammation (104,105). In prolonged cases of inflammation, macrophages also become attracted to the focus of infection (see Chapter 39). Upon arrival at the site of infection, neutrophils and macrophages become activated by the bacterial products (e.g., LPS) and cytokines. Neutrophils and macrophages can rapidly phagocytize and kill the bacteria (see Chapter 30 for a detailed description of phagocytosis). Phagocytosis can occur by recognizing certain native molecular structures of the bacteria such as lectins, polysaccharides, and peptides (RGD sequence) (106). Alternatively, the phagocytosis can occur by recognizing the host opsonins on the bacterial surface with CR3 and Fc receptors.

Systemic Response to Bacterial Invasion

Once the bacteria enter the systemic circulation, they are removed by the lymph nodes, spleen, or liver. Persons lacking splenic function (sickle cell disease and splenectomy) are at greatly increased risk of pneumococcal sepsis (107,108). Clearance of bacteria from the blood is facilitated by preexisting, cross-reactive antibodies (109) and nonspecific, alternative pathway, complement fixation. The bacteria release many inflammatory bacterial products to the systemic circulation and trigger many systemic changes such as fever and accumulation of leukocytes at sites of infection.

Cytokines (e.g., IL-6, IL-1) and glucocorticoids trigger the acute phase response by stimulating hepatocytes to produce and secrete a variety of molecules that are termed acute-phase reactants, such as coagulation factors, serum amyloid A protein, C reactive protein, and collectins (110). Collectin molecules have a C-type lectin motif and a collagenlike motif, and they can bind to the surface of bacteria, activate the complement along the classical pathway, and opsonize bacteria. For instance, mannose-binding protein, a collectin, binds glycoproteins with mannose and N-acetyl glucosamine on the surface of bacteria. Individuals with one specific allele of mannose-binding protein have been associated with increased incidence of infections (111,112).

One systemic response to infection is to lower the serum concentration of iron (94). This is achieved by an increase in the transferrin concentration in serum and by an increase in iron storage of tissues. Iron at the site of inflammation may be reduced by neutrophil-secreted lactoferrin. The reduction in iron available to bacteria can be a significant defensive measure. Moreover, a moderate reduction of iron intake (113) or the use of iron chelator (114) have proven beneficial against infections with extracellular bacteria.

ANTIGEN-SPECIFIC HOST DEFENSE RESPONSE

Patients with Bruton's agammaglobulinemia lack serum antibody but have relatively normal numbers of T cells. These patients suffer mostly from infections with extracellular bacteria and are successfully treated with passive administration of pooled gammaglobulin (115). This clinical observation emphasizes the importance of antibodies in the defense against this class of bacteria. The importance of antibodies in protection is further demonstrated by the efficacy of passive antibodies to the pneumococcal polysaccharide capsule as a therapy against pneumococcal infections. Reactivity of antibody with various surface components and/or virulence factors can result in protection against specific bacteria. A well-known group of the target antigens are toxins, including tetanus toxin and diphtheria toxin. Antibodies neutralize the toxins by preventing its binding to the host cell receptors or by increasing the removal rate of the toxin. Antibodies to LPS can protect against Gram-negative infection and LPS-induced shock (116). Although antibodies to lipid A can apparently provide some protection, they appear to be much less protective than antibodies to the O-antigens (117). Another group of the target antigens are the capsular PS of many of the extracellular bacteria. Antibodies to the capsule polysaccharide neutralize the shielding effect of capsule from host immunity. Other protective antibodies react with a host of different virulence factors. For instance, antibodies to an *E. coli* adhesin can prevent experimental infections of *E. coli* (118), and antibody to M protein neutralizes its ability to interfere with complement and provides protection against infections by *S. pyogenes*.

Among these target antigens, the polysaccharide capsule is often an elusive target for the host immune system because polysaccharide antigens are less immunogenic than protein antigens (119). This property contributes to the ability of surface polysaccharides to shield bacteria from the host immune system. Young children do not produce antibodies to many polysaccharide antigens until they are over two years old (29), and they are particularly susceptible to infections by the encapsulated bacteria (120). Polysaccharide antigens generally stimulate a subset of B cells (121) with minimal T-cell help (122), do not usually cause the formation of germinal centers (123,124), elicit poor immune memory (125), and easily tolerize B cells (125,126). Polysaccharide antigens commonly elicit oligoclonal antibodies that use a restricted number of V region genes (127–130), even among genetically unrelated humans (131,132). In addition, the antibodies to polysaccharide exhibit few somatic mutations (132,133) and generally have low affinity (134,135). Because the capsular PS presents repeating epitopes, even low-affinity antibody can bind with enough avidity to fix complement and cause opsonization and bacteriolysis.

Antibodies to a given polysaccharide often cross-react with structurally similar polysaccharide (136–138). Such cross-reactions may sometimes play an important role in protecting the host against their first exposure to a bacterial species. Human adults carry detectable amounts of antibodies to the *H. influenzae* type b polysaccharide (Hib-PS), even in the absence of vaccination, and are relatively resistant to *H. influenzae* infections (120). Although some of the antibodies may be the result of immunization by subclinical infections, the majority of human preimmune (but not postimmune) anti–Hib-PS antibody cross-reacts with *E. coli* K100, whose polysaccharide capsule is an isopolymer of Hib-PS (139). Experimental colonization of rats with *E. coli* K100 can protect them against Hib (140). About 1% of human IgG binds a carbohydrate epitope (galα1→3gal) (141), and this antibody can kill *Trypanosoma* and *Leishmania in vitro* (142). Cross-reactive antibodies binding the LPS core components are thought to be responsible for the protection from bacteremic dissemination of gonococci in nonimmune patients (109), although they cannot prevent infection of the genital tract (109). Antibodies in the normal serum react with a phosphocholine epitope found on pneumococci, *H. influenzae* and *Wuchereria bancrofti* (a tissue nematode) (143–145). These antibodies may reduce the susceptibility of mice to pneumococcal infection (146,147). The normal gut flora may be the antigenic stimulus for many of the cross-reactive antipolysaccharide antibodies. *E. coli* K100 is carried by about 1% of the population in the gut at any moment (148). Antibodies to (galα1→3gal) are found to bind many species of bacteria isolated from normal stool specimens (141). Interestingly, in animals such as chickens and rabbits, microbial colonization of the gut appears to be necessary for the normal development of antibody V region repertoires (149).

Complement-fixing antibodies can protect the host by causing bacteriolysis and opsonization. Bacteriolysis pathway can be significant *in vivo* in the protection against Gram-negative bacteria, as is illustrated by the fact that persons with deficiencies of C5-9 components are susceptible to infection by *N. meningitidis* (150). Gram-positive bacteria do not undergo bacteriolysis *in vitro* (99). Even though Gram-positive bacteria bearing surface antibody and complement are not lysed, the antibody and complement fragments on the bacteria are recognized with CD16b and CR3 (CD11b/CD18) and induce the phagocytosis and intracellular killing of bacteria. Protection mediated by this antibody/complement-mediated opsonization is probably very important *in vivo* because both complement deficiency and agammaglobulinemia predispose individuals to the infections of many different extracellular bacteria (115,150). To be effective for opsonization, the epitope of the surface antigens must be exposed on the surface of the bacteria. Effective antibodies to the porins of *N. meningitidis* recognize the surface loop of the molecule (151). In most pneumococci, C-PS is mostly buried underneath the polysaccharide capsule. Although antibodies to C-PS can fix complement (27), anti–C-PS is not so effective against *S. pneumoniae* (152). Antibodies to C-PS are much more protective, however, against capsular type 27 pneumococci, where the capsule itself contains C-PS epitopes (153).

Because antibody-mediated opsonization and bacterolysis are dependent on the complement-fixing properties of the Fc region, the relative efficacy of antibodies of different immunoglobulin isotypes have been compared. IgM antibodies, which are produced early in the course of infections and should be important in the early phase of infections because they fix complement very efficiently and can opsonize the bacteria. Studies found that specific IgM antibodies agglutinate erythrocytes, fix complement, and lyse erythrocytes more readily than IgG antibodies (154), and IgM antibodies are more effective in complement-mediated bacteriolysis (155). However, IgG antibodies are more effective than IgM antibodies at preventing infection of mice with pneumococci (156,157) or in opsonizing *H. influenzae* type b *in vitro* (158). Moreover some IgG subclasses have been reported to be more protective against specific viral (159) and fungal (160) infections than antibodies to other subclasses. These results suggest that optimal opsonization requires not only complement receptors but also Fc receptors for IgG. In the absence of inflammation, IgM antibodies are confined to the intravascular space, whereas IgG antibodies can enter the extracellular space. However, inflammation can make the vessels at the infection site permeable, and antibodies of all isotypes may enter the site of infection. IgG antibodies may be especially efficient at neutralizing toxins because compared with IgM antibodies they have longer half-lives and generally have a higher affinity and are already present in extravascular spaces before infection (161).

IgG subclasses differ in their ability to fix complement and to bind Fc receptors (162,163). Studes have shown that antibodies of one of the four subclasses has been found to provide the best protection against a viral (159) and a fungal infection (160). Consequently, the fact that antibodies to bacterial polysaccharide are found to be restricted largely to a single IgG subclass (IgG2 in human and IgG3 in mice) has led to many studies of differences in the protective properties of antipolysaccharide antibodies of different isotypes. Mouse IgG3 (but not other IgG subclasses) antibodies can associate with each other through their Fc regions (164), and this feature may make the IgG3 antibodies to polysaccharide with low affinity more effective in binding the antigen than antibodies of other isotypes of the same affinity. Although the above observations provide a theoretical advantage for mouse IgG3, this same aggregation phenomenon has not been observed for human IgG2 antibodies. The full significance of IgG3 aggregation is not clear, however, because antipolysaccharide antibodies of the IgG3 isotype have not been observed to be any more efficacious against pneumococcal infections than antibodies of other isotypes (165). Also in contrast to expectation, many studies found that human IgG1 antibodies are slightly more effective than human IgG2 antibodies for opsonization and bacteriolysis (163,166–168). However, neither of these isotypes appears to be essential because individuals lacking IgG1 and IgG2 subclass genes are healthy (169). Furthermore, human IgG2 antibodies bind less strongly to CD16, CD32, and CD64 than do IgG1 or IgG3 (170) and may not be effective for opsonization by neutrophils from the individuals homozygous for a specific CD32 allele (168). These observations, taken together, strongly suggest that human IgG2 (or mouse IgG3) subclass does not provide any unique advantage in defense against bacteria.

Although it has been reported that IgA can opsonize (171,171a), fix complement (172), and facilitate the lysis of *N. meningitidis* (173), other studies have found that IgA does not fix complement *in vitro* (174) and may even inhibit IgG-mediated complement-dependent killing (175,176). Nevertheless, bacteria that commonly colonize or infect mucosal areas often produce IgA1 protease, and IgA antibody has been found to be able to provide protection in at least some cases (177). These findings suggest that IgA may play an important role as a part of the complex mucosal immune defense (see Chapter 27). It may function by aggregating the bacteria and facilitating their expulsion from mucosal areas. IgA also may block the invasion of bacteria through the mucosal epithelial cells because endocytosed IgA was found to block the transport of virus through the epithelial cells (178). However, IgA-deficient persons or mice with defective IgA genes are relatively healthy, and IgA-deficient mice could elicit normal protective immunity to experimental infections with influenzae virus. It has been suggested that IgM antibodies may function as secretory antibodies in IgA-deficient individuals (179).

IgG (but not IgM and IgA) antibodies are transported across the placenta to the fetus during the late phase of gestation. The maternal antibodies provide significant amounts of protection to the neonates from many extracellular bacterial infections. Neonates with Bruton's agammaglobulinemia are generally healthy for about 6 to 9 months, until their maternal antibodies are catabolized. Among IgG subclasses, IgG1 concentration in the cord blood is higher (1.8-fold) than that in mother's blood, whereas IgG2 concentrations are comparable in both sites (180). Recent studies suggest that IgG antibodies are actively transported across the placenta by FcRn, which is structurally similar to the class I MHC molecules (181). This molecule may also be responsible for the rescue of the antibody molecules from intracellular catabolism (182).

Vaccine Development

Efforts to develop vaccines against extracellular bacteria often focus on eliciting immunity to capsular PS, which is well known for its ability to increase bacterial virulence. Recently, capsular PS has been made more immunogenic by conjugating it to protein molecules, and the conjugate vaccines inducing antibodies to Hib PS in young children have virtually eliminated Hib meningitis (183) as well as oropharyngeal colonization by Hib (184). Similar conjugate vaccine approaches are being used to improve the currently available pneumococcal vaccine, which contains polysaccharide of the 23 most common capsular types. Although the approach is likely to succeed, the new pneumococcal conjugate vaccine will need to contain a large subset of the 23 polysaccharides coupled to carrier protein molecules. This will make the pneumococcal conjugate vaccine highly complex and relatively expensive.

Recent studies of bacterial virulence factors are providing target antigens other than the capsular PS. Fatal pneumococcal sepsis in animal models can be prevented with antibodies induced with PspA, pneumolysin, or PsaA. These antigens are being investigated as a potential replacement for the expensive pneumococcal conjugate vaccines. Additional target antigens that are being investigated for the vaccines include bacterial adhesion molecules, (118,185), complement-cleaving enzymes, IgA1 protease, and iron-transport systems (52–54).

Although the identification of these antigens greatly increases the potential candidates for vaccines, the successful development of a vaccine is complex. The target antigen must be exposed on the cell surface or be a virulence factor that can be inhibited by antibody *in vivo*. Ideally the target antigens should be both protection eliciting and of limited polymorphism. They should also not induce antibodies to the host antigen. For instance, even though the protective epitopes of the M protein of *S. pyogenes* have been identified (22), there are over 100 M protein serotypes, and immunity to at least some M proteins has been shown to elicit host cross-reactive antibodies.

DELETERIOUS HOST RESPONSE

Inflammatory response by the host inevitably causes some tissue damage, and in some bacterial infections such as pneumonia and meningitis this damage plays a significant role in disease pathology and symptoms. For instance, it has been shown with animal models of meningitis that inflammation associated with bacterial products (primarily cell walls) is the primary cause of neurologic damage. Treatment of animals with antibiotics alone can eradicate the bacteria but does not prevent neurologic damage. In contrast, when the inflammation was controlled by coadministered steroids along with the antibiotic, the amount of neurologic damage was considerably reduced (186).

Antigen-Nonspecific Deleterious Response

Uncontrolled inflammation at the systemic level can produce a septic shock. The septic shock can be triggered by several factors, including exotoxins (e.g., staphylococcal enterotoxin B) of Gram-positive bacteria or LPS. Staphylococcal enterotoxin B binds MHC-particular class II molecules of the host and are able to stimulate large numbers of helper T cells to release cytokines. Such toxins are termed superantigens because they often are able to stimulate all T cells expressing one particular VβTCR family (see Chapter 10). Septic shock also can be initiated when LPS from Gram-negative bacteria binds CD14 and stimulates macrophages or monocytes to secrete inflammatory cytokines (see Chapter 32). In addition to cytokines, the stimulation of host cells by bacterial products leads to the release of other mediators of inflammation such as arachidonic acid metabolites, activate complement, and coagulation cascades. Excess release of the mediators leads to the collapse of the vascular system and finally the failure of multiple organ systems. Studies using transgenic mice with defective genes identified several molecules critical in developing the septic shock, such as TNF-α, one of its receptors (TNFRI), IL-1–converting enzyme, and ICAM-1 (187). This approach also showed that CD14 is critical for LPS-induced septic shock and that CD28, a T-cell costimulation molecule, is necessary for superantigen-induced septic shock (187).

Although inflammation is frequently a cause of significant morbidity and mortality, it also must be regarded as a primary savior of the host from bacterial infections. Evidence from this hypothesis comes from studies with Lps^d mice which although nonreactive to LPS and completely resistant to LPS shock, are more susceptible to infection with Gram-negative bacteria than mice that are fully responsive to LPS (188,189). Perhaps LPS is toxic because the host has evolved to use this common bacterial component as a trigger for host responses.

Antigen-Specific Deleterious Response

Many bacterial antigens express the epitopes cross-reactive with host antigens and thus have the potential to elicit antibodies during infections that cross-react with host tissue. For instance, the PS capsule of *N. meningitidis* group B mimics epitopes expressed in the central nervous system (190), such as N-acetylneuramic acid, an epitope in the embryonic neuronal cell adhesion molecule (N-CAM) (191). The LPS of *N. meningitidis, N. gonorrhoeae, H. influenzae, H. ducreyi, Campylobacter jejuni,* and *Helicobacter pylori* express epitopes with immunochemical identity to a number of human blood group antigens such as paragloboside, antigen, pk, and Lewis X, respectively (192). Epidemiologic studies associated infections with *C. jejuni* with the development of an autoimmune

disease (193). Studies with experimental animals found that immunizations with *S. pneumoniae* can elicit antibodies to C-PS that can react with mouse kidney glomerulus and cause proteinuria (194). Further studies of this observation suggest that the B cells producing antibodies cross-reacting with autoantigens may be normally eliminated by apoptosis (195).

Although the association between the above noted examples of cross-reacting bacterial antigens and autoimmunity is unclear, *S. pyogenes* infection is associated with rheumatic fever and acute glomerulonephritis. Studies found that *S. pyogenes* can be divided into two classes with a monoclonal antibody to M protein (196) and that rheumatic fever develops only after an infection of *S. pyogenes* with class I strains (196). Class I and class II strains of *S. pyogenes* can also be readily distinguished by the linkage relationship of the M protein genes with genes encoding related surface proteins (196,197). M proteins from class I *S. pyogenes* express the epitopes highly cross-reactive with epitopes of cardiac myosin, tropomyosin, vimentin, laminin, and keratin (198–200). An antibody molecule may bind to all of these protein molecules because a major portion of these proteins is coiled-coil α-helix (200). The polyreactive antibodies to M protein may directly damage myocardial and endothelial cells (201). In addition to antibodies, CD4+ and CD8+ T cells are found at the rheumatic heart valves (202), and the T cells proliferate to M protein peptides and heart proteins (203). These observations suggest that the T cells with cross-reactivity between M protein and myosin may be involved in the pathogenesis of rheumatic fever as well.

In addition to M protein, group A polysaccharide of *S. pyogenes* has now been shown to express epitopes cross-reactive with myosin. This antibody to group A polysaccharide also binds M protein and other α-helical molecules (200,204,205). This antibody to group A polysaccharide also may be cytotoxic to cardiac myocardium and endothelium. Interestingly, the V region of antibodies to group A polysaccharide with myosin cross-reactivity is encoded by the same germline V genes used for the antibodies binding only group A polysaccharide (206).

FUTURE OUTLOOK

Although humoral immunity is the main immune defense against the extracellular bacteria, some roles of T-cell immunity may emerge in the future. For instance, T-cell immunity to pertussis is being investigated because the immune protection elicited by pertussis vaccines so far does not correlate well with the antibody levels. It has been shown that some bacteria (e.g., *H. influenzae*) can produce capsular PS associated with lipid (207), which T cells can directly recognize (208). Lastly, recent studies suggest that several of the bacteria we classify as extracellular may in fact spend an extended period of time within human cells (see A *Neisseria* story on the next page).

Two recent technologic developments should greatly facilitate the future studies of the immune response to extracellular bacteria. One is that the whole bacterial genome of many bacteria has been sequenced and the sequence information has begun to yield information about pathogenetic factors. The other is the availability of transgenic mice lacking specific genes. Studies using these mice should permit critical tests of the role of select features of immune system in host responses to infection. Examples include mice lacking cytokine genes or specific cell populations. These technologic innovations would help determine how our multi-layered immune system protects our body, a walking incubator, against ubiquitous extracellular bacteria.

A *NEISSERIA* STORY

Although *Neisseria* species of bacteria are classical extracellular bacteria, increasing evidence supports the notion that they can reside within the host cells. Stephens and co-workers demonstrated that *N. meningitidis* entered human mucosal epithelial cells in experimental infections in human adenoidal explants (209). Using a fallopian tube model, Melly showed that gonococci can also enter nonciliated mucosal cells in a fashion similar to that described above for meningococci (210). During the invasion, meningococci produce low levels of C-PS (74), and gonococci initiate cortical actin polymerization in addition to focal actin polymerization around the bacterium. Once within the cell, both species of *Neisseria* appear to enter vacuoles, where the organisms survive and proliferate. Magdalene So and co-workers have shown that IgA1 protease may play a role in protecting the meningococcus during its intravacuolar existence by cleaving LAMP1 (74). LAMP1 is a membrane glycoprotein of the late endosomes and lysosomes that is thought to play a role in maintaining the stability of these compartments (211). The vacuoles are transported to the basolateral surface of the mucosal epithelial cell. Organisms have been seen to exit the vacuole and the epithelial cell from the basolateral surface (212). Because studies of exudates from males with urethritis have demonstrated that the urethral epithelial cell is invaded by the gonococcus (70), the intracellular existence of the gonococcus may not be limited to fallopian tube cells.

Bactericidal anticapsular antibody is a key factor in protection from systemic infections with *Neisseria* (213–215). Artenstein, Goldschlich, and Goldschneider were studying the military trainees at the U.S. Army basic training center at Fort Dix, New Jersey, when an epidemic of meningococcal disease occurred. To obtain the baseline bacterial studies, these investigators obtained blood samples from over 15,000 recruits when they arrived at the base. Nasopharyngeal cultures were obtained from all recruits at regular intervals during their training. Eventually, five cases of *N. meningitidis* serogroup C infection were identified among members of the same training battalion. Nasopharyngeal cultures obtained before the outbreak indicated that 53 were colonized with *N. meningitidis* serogroup C, considered to be the case strain. Thirteen of these colonized recruits lacked bactericidal antibody to the case strain. The five cases of systemic meningococcal infection were among the 13 who lacked bactericidal antibody and had nasopharyngeal colonization with the case strain. Thus, in a meningococcal epidemic situation, if a person acquires the case strain in the nasopharynx and lacks bactericidal antibody, the risk of serious infection is approximately 30% to 40%. These studies indicated the importance of bactericidal antibody in protection against serious meningococcal disease. These findings also led to the development and use of a tetravalent meningococcal capsular vaccine in military recruits that has prevented epidemics in basic training centers since 1973.

REFERENCES

1. M. The streptococcal cell wall. *Harvey Lect* 1971;65:73.
2. Gray BM. Streptococcal infection. In: Brachman PE, ed. Bacterial infection, 3rd ed. New York: Plenum Publishing, 1997.
3. Tomasz A. Choline in the cell wall of a bacterium: novel type of polymer-linked choline in *Pneumococcus*. *Science* 1967;57:694–697.
4. Brundish DE, Baddiley J. Pneumococcal C-substance, a ribitol teichoic acid containing choline phosphate. *Biochem J* 1968;110:573–582.
5. Fischer W. Teichoic acid and lipoglycans. *New Compr Biochem* 1994;27:199–215.
6. Fisher W, Behr T, Hartmann R, Peter-Katalinic J, Egge H. Teichoic acid and lipoteichoic acid of *Streptococcus pneumoniae* have identical chain structures. A reinvestigation of teichoic acid (C-polysaccharide). *Eur J Biochem* 1993;215:851–857.
7. Briles DE, Hollingshead SK, Swiatlo E, al. PspA and PspC: their potential for use as pneumococcal vaccines. *Microb Drug Resist* 1997;3:401–408.
8. Briles DE, Tart RC, Wu HY, Ralph BA, Russell MW, McDaniel LS. Systemic and mucosal protective immunity to pneumococcal surface protein A. *N Y Acad Sci* 1996;797:118–126.
9. Talkington DF, Brown BG, Tharpe JA, Koening A, Russell H. Protection of mice against fatal pneumococcal challenge by immunization with pneumococcal surface adhesion A (PsaA). *Microb Pathog* 1996;21:17–22.
10. Canvin JR, Marvin AP, Sivakumaran M, et al. The role of pneumolysin and autolysin in the pathology of pneumoniae and septicemia in mice infected with a type 2 pneumococcus. *J Infect Dis* 1995;172:119–123.
11. Wani JH, Gilbert JV, Plaut AG, Weiser JN. Identification, cloning, and sequencing of the immunoglobulin A1 protease gene of *Streptococcus pneumoniae*. *Infect Immun* 1996;64:3967–3974.
12. Poulsen K, Reinholdt J, Kilian M. Characterization of the *Streptococcus pneumoniae* immunoglobulin A1 protease gene and its translation product. *Infect Immun* 1996;64:3957–3966.
13. Nandiwada LS, Hostetter MK, Dunny GM. Genetic analysis of a C3 degrading proteinase in *Streptococcus pneumoniae* [Abstract B-134]. ASM meeting, New Orleans, 1996:177.
14. Hamel J, Martin D, Brodeur BB. Heat shock response of Streptococcus pneumoniae: identification of immunoreactive stress proteins. *Microb Pathog* 1997;23:11–21.
15. Wu HY, Nahm MH, Guo Y, Russell M, Briles DE. Intranasal immunization of mice with PspA (pneumococcal surface protein A) can prevent intranasal carriage and infection with *Streptococcus pneumoniae*. *J Infect Dis* 1997;175:893–846.
16. Hamel J, Rioux CR, Martin D, Brodeur BR. Protection from experimental *Streptococcus pneumoniae* infection by vaccination with recombinant HSP70 antigens [Abstract]. ASM meeting, Miami FL. 1997;43.
17. Lock RA, Hansman D, Paton JC. Comparative efficacy of autolysin and pneumolysin as immunogens protecting mice against infection by *Streptococcus pneumoniae*. *Microb Pathog* 1992;12:137–143.
18. Tart RC, McDaniel LS, Ralph BA, Briles DE. Truncated Streptococcus pneumoniae PspA molecules elicit cross-protective immunity against pneumococcal challenge in mice. *J Infect Dis* 1996;173:380–386.
19. Briese T, Hakenbeck R. Interaction of the pneumococcal amidase with lipoteichoic acid and choline. *Eur J Biochem* 1985;146:417–427.
20. Schneewind O, Fowler A, Faull KF. Structure of cell wall anchor of cell surface proteins in *Staphylococcus aureus*. *Science* 1995;268:103–106.
21. Fischetti VA, Pancholi V, Schneewind O. Conservation of a hexapeptide sequence in the anchor region of surface proteins from Gram-positive cocci. *Mol Microbiol* 1990;4:1603–1605.
22. Dale JB, Chiang EY, Lederer JW. Recombinant tetravalent group A streptococcal M protein vaccine. *J Immunol* 1993;151:2188–2194.
23. Nikaido H. Outer membrane. In: Neidhardt FC, ed. Escherichia coli and Salmonella: cellular and molecular biology. Washington, DC: ASM Press, 1996:29–47.
24. Preston A, Mandrell RE, Gibson BW, Apicella MA. The lipooligosaccharides of pathogenic Gram-negative bacteria. *Crit Rev Microbiol* 1996;22:139–180.
25. Jap BK, Walian PJ. Structure and function of porins. *Physiol Rev* 1996;76:1073–1088.
26. Kazatchkine MD, Fearon DT, Austen KF. Human alternative complement pathway: membrane-associated sialic acid regulates the competition between B and beta 1H for cell-bound C3b. *J Immunol* 1979;122:75–81.
27. Brown EJ, Hosea SW, Hammer CH, Burch CG. A quantitative analysis of the interactions of antipneumococcal antibody and complement in experimental pneumococcal bacteremia. *J Clin Invest* 1982;69:85–98.
28. Henrichsen J. Six newly recognized types of *Streptococcus pneumoniae*. *J Clin Microbiol* 1995;33:2759–2762.
29. Robbins JB, Austrian R, Lee CJ, et al. Considerations for formulating the second-generation pneumococcal capsular polysaccharide vaccine with emphasis on the cross-reactive types within groups. *J Infect Dis* 1983;148:1136–1159.
30. Fischetti VA. Streptococcal M protein: molecular design and biological behavior. *Clin Microbiol Rev* 1989;2:286–314.
31. Lancefield RC. Current knowledge of the type specific M antigens of group A streptococci. *J Immunol* 1962;89:307–313.
32. Crain MI, Waltman WD II, Turner JS, et al. Pneumococcal surface protein A (PspA) is serologically highly variable and is expressed by all clinically important capsular serotypes of *Streptococcus pneumoniae*. *Infect Immun* 1990;58:3293–3299.
33. Fischetti VA, Bessen DE, Schneewind O, Hruby DE. Protection against streptococcal pharyngeal colonization with vaccines composed of M protein conserved regions. *Adv Exp Med Biol* 1991;303:159–167.
34. Dillard JP, Vandersea MW, Yother J. Characterization of the cassette containing genes for type 3 capsular polysaccharide biosynthesis in *Streptococcus pneumoniae*. *J Exp Med* 1995;181:973–983.
34a. Coffey TJ, Enright MC, Daniels M, et al. Recombinatorial exchanges at the capsular polysaccharide biosynthetic locus lead to frequent serotype changes among natural isolates of *Streptococcus pneumoniae*. *Molecular Microbiol* 1998;27:73–83.
35. Zhang QY, DeRyckere D, Lauer P, Koomey M. Gene conversion in *Neisseria gonorrhoeae*: evidence for its role in pilus antigenic variation. *Proc Natl Acad Sci U S A* 1992;89:5366–5370.
36. Mandrell RE, Apicella MA. Lipo-oligosaccharides (LOS) of mucosal pathogens:

molecular mimicry and host-modifications of LOS. *Immunobiology* 1993;187: 382–402.

37. Gray BM, Pritchard DG. Phase variation in the pathogenesis of group B streptococcal infections. *Zentralbl Bakt* 1992;22(suppl):452–454.

38. Jonsson AB, Nyberg G, Normark S. Phase variation of gonococcal pili by frameshift mutation in pili C, a novel gene for pilus assembly. *EMBO J* 1991;10: 477–488.

39. Weiser JN, Markiewicz A, Tuomanen EI, Wani JH. Relationship between phase variation in colony morphology, intrastrain variation in cell wall physiology, and nasopharyngeal colonization by *Streptococcus pneumoniae*. *Infect Immun* 1996; 64:2240–2245.

40. Weiser JN. Relationship between colony morphology and the life cycle of Haemophilus influenzae: the contribution of lipopolysaccharide phase variation to pathogenesis. *J Infect Dis* 1993;168:672–680.

41. Bos MP, Grunert F, Belland RJ. Differential recognition of members of the carcinoembryonic antigen family by Opa variants of *Neisseria gonorrhoeae*. *Infect Immun* 1997;65:2353–2361.

42. Mekalanos JJ. Environmental signals controlling expression of virulence gene determinants in bacteria. *J Bacteriol* 1992;174:1–7.

43. Salyers AA, Whitt DD. *Bacterial pathogenesis, a molecular approach.* Washington, DC: ASM Press, 1994.

44. Rupp ME, Archer GL. Coagulase-negative staphylococci. *Clin Infect Dis* 1994; 19:231–245.

45. Caugant DA, Hoiby EA, Magnus P, et al. Asymptomatic carriage of *Neisseria meningitidis* in a randomly sampled population. *J Clin Microbiol* 1994;32: 323–330.

46. Kuhns DM, Nelson CT, Feldman HA, et al. The prophylactic value of sulfadiazine in the control of meningococcic meningitis. *Am J Hygiene* 1948;47177–47186.

47. Zangwill KM, Schuchat A, Wenger JD. Group B streptococcal disease in the United States, 1990: report from a multistate active surveillance system. *MMWR* 1992;41:25–32.

48. Rein MF. Epidemiology of gonococcal infections. In: Roberts RB, ed. *The gonococcus.* New York: John Wiley and Sons, 1977:1–31.

49. Handsfield HH, Lipman TO, Harnisch JP, Tronca E, Holmes KK. Asymptomatic gonorrhea in men: diagnosis, natural course, prelavence, and significance. *N Engl J Med* 1974;290:117–123.

50. Bartlett JG, Chang TW, Taylor NS, Onderdonk AB. Colitis induced by *Clostridium difficile*. *Rev Infect Dis* 1979;1:370–378.

51. Stojiljkovic I, Srinivasan N. *Neisseria meningitidis* tonB, exbB and exbD genes: ton-dependent utilization of protein-bound iron in *Neisseriae*. *J Bacteriol* 1997; 179:805–812.

52. Lewis LA, Gray E, Wang YP, Roe BA, Dyer DW. Molecular characterization of hpuAB, the haemoglobin-haptoglobin-utilization operon of *Neisseria meningitidis*. *Mol Microbiol* 1997;23:737–749.

53. Pettersson A, Poolman JT, van der Ley P, Tommassen J. Response of *Neisseria meningitidis* to iron limitation. *Antonie Van Leeuwenhoek* 1997;71:129–136.

54. Thomas CE, Sparling PF. Isolation and analysis of a fur mutant of *Neisseria gonorrhoeae*. *J Bacteriol* 1996;178:4224–4232.

55. Earhart CF. Uptake and metabolism of iron and molybdenum. In: Neidhardt FC, ed. Escherichia coli *and* Salmonella: *cellular and molecular biology.* Washington, DC: ASM Press, 1996:1075–1090.

56. Neilands JB. Siderophores: structure and function of microbial iron transport compounds. *J Biol Chem* 1995;270:26723–26726.

57. Paton JS. The contribution of pneumolysin to the pathogenecity of *Streptococcus pneumoniae*. *Trends Microbiol* 1996;4:103–106.

58. Benton KA, Everson MP, Briles DE. A pneumolysin-negative mutant of *Streptococcus pneumoniae* causes chronic bacteremia rather than acute sepsis in mice. *Infect Immun* 1995;63:448–455.

59. Ji Y, Carlson B, Kondugunta A, Cleary PP. Intranasal immunization with C5a peptidase prevents nasopharyngeal colonization of mice by the group A *Streptococcus*. *Infect Immun* 1997;65:2080–2087.

60. Bohnsack JF, Widjaja K, Ghazizadeh S, et al. A role for C5 and C5a-ase in the acute neutrophile response to group B streptococcal infections. *J Infect Dis* 1997;175:847–855.

61. Angel CS, Ruzek M, Hostetter MK. Degradation of C3 by *Streptococcus pneumoniae*. *J Infect Dis* 1994;170:600–608.

62. Kilian M, Mestecky J, Kulhavy R, Tomana M, Butler WT. IgA1 proteases from *Haemophilus influenzae, Streptococcus pneumoniae, Neisseria meningitidis,* and *Streptococcus sanguis:* comparative immunochemical studies. *J Immunol* 1980;124:2596–2596.

63. Andersson B, Dahmen J, Frejd T, Leffler H, Magnusson G, Norri G, et al. Identification of an active disaccharide unit of a glycoconjugate receptor for pneumococci attaching to human pharyngeal epithelial cells. *J Exp Med* 1983;158: 559–570.

64. Cundell DR, Weiser JN, Shen J, Young A, Tuomanen EI. Relationship between colonial morphology and adherence of *Streptococcus pneumoniae*. *Infect Immun* 1995;63:757–761.

65. Striker R, Nilsson U, Stonecipher A, Magnusson G, Hultgren SJ. Structural requirements for the glycolipid receptor of human uropathogenic *Escherichia coli*. *Mol Microbiol* 1995;16:1021–1029.

66. Sengupta TK, Sengupta DK, Ghose AC. A 20-kDa pilus protein with haemagglutination and intestinal adherence properties expressed by a clinical isolate of a non-01 *Vibrio cholerae*. *FEMS Microbiol Lett* 1993;112:237–242.

67. Chiang SL, Taylor RK, Koomey M, Mekalanos JJ. Single amino acid substitu-

68. Brennan MJ, Shahin RD. Pertussis antigens that abrogate bacterial adherence and elicit immunity. *Am J Respir Crit Care Med* 1996;154:S145–S149

69. Geuijen CA, Willems RJ, Bongaerts M, Top J, Gielen H, Mooi FR. Role of the *Bordetella pertussis*; minor fimbrial subunit, FimD, in colonization of the mouse respiratory tract. *Infect Immun* 1997;65:4222–4228.

70. Apicella MA, Ketterer M, Lee FKN, Zhou D, Rice PA, Blake MS. The pathogenesis of gonococcal urethritis in men: confocal and immunoelectron microscopic analysis of urethral exudates from men infected with *Neisseria gonorrhoeae*. *J Infect Dis* 1996;173:636–646.

71. Swanson J, Kraus SJ, Gotschlich EC. Studies on gonococcus infection. I. Pili and zone of adhesion: their relation to gonococcal growth patterns. *J Exp Med* 1997; 134:886–906.

72. Seifert HS. Questions about gonococcal pilus phase- and antigenic variation. *Mol Microbiol* 1997;2:433–440.

73. Stern A, Meyer TF. Common mechanisms controlling phase and antigenic variation in pathogenic *Neisseria*. *Mol Microbiol* 1987;1:5–12.

74. Hammerschmidt SMA, Sillmann H, Muhlenhoff M, Borrow R, Fox A, van Putten J, et al. Capsule phase variation in *Neisseria meningitidis* serogroup B by slipped-strand mispairing in the polysialyltransferase gene (siaD): correlation with bacterial invasion and the outbreak of meningococcal disease. *Mol Microbiol* 1996;20:1211–1220.

75. Dassy B, Hogan T, Foster TJ, Fournier JM. Involvement of the accessory gene regulator (agr) in expression of type-5 capsular polysaccharide by *Staphylococcus aureus*. *J Gen Microbiol* 1993;139:1301–1306.

76. Lee JC, Takeda S, Livolsi PJ, Paoletti LC. Effects of in vitro and in vivo growth conditions on expression of type-8 capsular polysaccharide by *Staphylococcus aureus*. *Infect Immun* 1993;61:1853–1858.

77. Uhl MA, Miller JF. Autophosphorylation and phosphotransfer in the *Bordetella pertussis* BvgAS siganl transduction cascade. *Proc Natl Acad Sci U S A* 1994;91: 1163–1167.

78. Hoch JA, Silhavy TJ. *Two-component signal transduction.* Washington, DC: ASM Press, 1995.

79. Musher DM. Infections caused by *Streptococcus pneumoniae*: clinical spectrum, pathogenesis, immunity, and treatment. *Clin Infect Dis* 1992;14:801–809.

80. Tuomanen EI. The biology of pneumococcal infection. *Pediatr Res* 1997;42: 253–258.

81. Berry AM, Lock RA, Paton JC. Cloning and characterization of nanB, a second *Streptococcus pnuemoniae* neuraminidase gene, and purification of the NanB enzyme from recombinant *Escherichia coli*. *J Bacteriol* 1996;178: 4854–4860.

82. Berry AM, Lock RA, Thomas SM, Rajan DP, Hansman D, Paton J. Cloning and nucleotide sequence of the *Streptococcus pneumoniae* hyaluronidase gene and purification of the enzyme from recombinant *Escherichia coli*. *Infect Immun* 1994;62:1101–1108.

83. Lin B, Hollingshead SK, Coligan JE, Egan ML, Baker JR, Pritchard DG. Cloning and expression of the gene for group B streptococcal hyaluronate lyase. *J Biol Chem* 1994;269:30113–30116.

84. Swartz MN. Skin and soft tissue infections. In: Mandell GL, Bennett JE, Dolin R, eds. *Principles and practice of infectious diseases,* 4th ed. New York: Churchill Livingstone, 1995:909–929.

85. MacGregor RR. *Corynebacterium diphtheriae*. In: Mandell GL, Bennet JE, Dolin R, eds. *Principles and practice of infectious diseases,* 4th ed. New York: Churchill Livingstone, 1995:1865–1872.

86. Salyers AA, Whitt DD. *Bacterial pathogenesis.* Washington, DC: ASM Press, 1994.

87. Barg NL, Harris T. Toxin-mediated syndromes. In: Crossely KB, ed. *The staphylococci.* New York: Churchill Livingstone, 1997:527–543.

88. Noel JM, Boedeker EC. Enterohemorrhagic *Escherichia coli*: a family of emerging pathogens. *Dig Dis* 1997;15:67–91.

89. Lingwood CA. Verotoxin-binding in human renal sections. *Nephron* 1994;66: 21–28.

90. Bancroft GJ, Kelly JP. Macrophage activation and innate resistance to infection in SCID mice. *Immunobiology* 1994;191:424–431.

91. Musher DM. *Streptococcus pneumoniae*. In: Mandell GL, Bennett JE, Dolin R, eds. *Principles and practice of infectious diseases,* 4th ed. New York: Churchill Livingstone, 1995:1811–1826.

92. Donowitz GR, Mandell GL. Acute pneumonia. In: Mandell GL, Bennett JE, Dolin R, eds. *Principles and practices of infectious diseases,* 4th ed. New York: Churchill Livingstone, 1995:619–637.

93. Pruitt KM, Rahemtulla F, Mansson-Rahemtulla B. Innate humoral factors. In: Ogra PL, ed. *Handbook of mucosal immunology.* New York: Academic Press, 1994:53–70.

94. Weinberg ED. Iron withholding: a defense against infection and neoplasia. *Physiol Rev* 1984;64:65–101.

95. Eisenhauer PB, Harwig SS, Lehrer RI. Cryptdins: antimicrobial defensins of the murine small intestine. *Infect Immun* 1992;60:3556–3565.

96. Henderson B, Poole S, Wilson M. Bacterial modulins: a novel class of virulence factors which cause host tissue pathology by inducing cytokine synthesis. *Microbiol Rev* 1996;60:316–341.

97. Klinman DM, Yi A-K, Beaucage SL, Conover J, Krieg AM. CpG motifs present in bacterial DNA rapidly induce lymphocytes to secrete interleukin 6, interleukin 12, and interferon gamma. *Proc Natl Acad Sci U S A* 1996;93:2879–2883.

98. Sparwasser T, Miethke T, Lipford G, et al. Bacterial DNA causes septic shock. *Nature* 1997;386:336–337.

99. Frank MM, Fries LF. The role of complement in defense against bacterial disease. *Baillieres Clin Immunol Allergy* 1988;2:335–361.

100. Galli SJ. New concepts about the mast cell. *N Engl J Med* 1993;328:257–265.

101. Bradding P, Feather IH, Wilson S, et al. Immunolocalization of cytokines in the nasal mucosa of normal and perennial rhinitic subjects. The mast cell as a source of IL-4, IL-5, and IL-6 in human allergic mucosal inflammation. *J Immunol* 1993;151:3853–3865.

102. Malaviya R, Ross EA, MacGregor JI, et al. Mast cell phagocytosis of fimH-expressing enterobacteria. *J Immunol* 1994;152:1907–1914.

103. Malaviya R, Ikeda T, Ross E, Abraham SN. Mast cell modulation of neutrophil influx and bacterial clearance at sites of infection through TNF-alpha. *Nature* 1996;381:21–22.

104. Ming WJ, Bersani L, Mantovani A. Tumor necrosis factor is chemotactic for monocytes and polymorphonuclear leukocytes. *J Immunol* 1987;138:1469–1474.

105. Sayers TJ, Wiltrout TA, Bull CA, Denn AC, Pilaro AM, Lokesh B. Effect of cytokines on polymorphonuclear neutrophil infiltration in the mouse. Prostaglandin- and leukotriene-independent induction of infiltration by IL-1 and tumor necrosis factor. *J Immunol* 1988;141:1670–1677.

106. Ofek I, Goldhar J, Keisari Y, Sharon N. Nonopsonic phagocytosis of microorganisms. *Ann Rev Microbiol* 1995;49:239–276.

107. Styrt B. Infection associated with asplenia: risks, mechanisms, and prevention. *Am J Med* 1990;88:33N–42N.

108. Van Wyck DB, Witte MH, Witte CL. Synergism between the spleen and serum complement in experimental pneumococcemia. *J Infect Dis* 1982;145:514–519.

109. Apicella MA, Westerink MAJ, Morse SA, Schneider H, Rice PA, Griffiss JM. Bactericidal antibody response of normal human serum to the lipooligosaccharide of *Neisseria gonorrhoeae*. *J Infect Dis* 1997;153:520–526.

110. Steel DM, Whitehead AS. The major acute phase reactants: C-reactive protein, serum amyloid P component and serum amyloid A protein. *Immunol Today* 1994;15:81–88.

111. Turner MW. Mannose-binding lectin: the pluripotent molecule of the innate immune system. *Immunol Today* 1996;17:532–540.

112. Lau YL, Chan SY, Turner MW, Fong J, Karlberg J. Mannose-binding protein in preterm infants: developmental profile and clinical significance. *Clin Exp Immunol* 1995;102:649–654.

113. Weinberg ED, Weinberg GA. The role of iron in infection. *Curr Opin Infect Dis* 1997;8:164–169.

114. Jones RL, Peterson CM, Grady RW, Kumbaraci T, Cerami A, Graziano JH. Effects of iron chelators and iron overload on *Salmonella* infection. *Nature* 1977;267:63–65.

115. Lederman HM, Winkelstein JA. X-linked agammaglobulinemia: an analysis of 96 patients. *Medicine* 1985;64:145–156.

116. Singh SP, Williams YU, Benjamin WH, Klebba PE, Boyd D. Immunoprotection by monoclonal antibodies to the porins and lipopolysaccharide of *Salmonella typhimurium*. *Microb Pathog* 1996;21:249–263.

117. Hoffman WD, Pollack M, Banks SM, et al. Distinct functional activities in canine septic shock of monoclonal antibodies specific for the O-polysaccharide and core regions of *Escherichia coli* lipopolysaccharide. *J Infect Dis* 1994;169:553–561.

118. Langermann S, Palaszynski S, Barnhart M, et al. Prevention of mucosal *Escherichia coli* infection by FimH-adhesin-based systemic vaccination. *Science* 1997;276:533–534.

119. Mond JJ, Lees A, Snapper CM. T cell-independent antigens type 2. *Ann Rev Immunol* 1995,13.655–692.

120. Fothergill LD, Wright J. Influenzal meningitis: the regulation of age incidence to the bactericidal power of blood against the causal organism. *J Immunol* 1933;24:273–284.

121. Herzenberg LA, Stall AM, Lalor PA, Sidman C, Moore WA, Parks DR. The LY-1 B cell lineage. *Immunol Rev* 1986;93:81–102.

122. Humphrey JH, Parrott DMV, East J. Studies of globulin and antibody production in mice thymectomized at birth. *Immunology* 1964;7:419–439.

123. Weissman IL, Gutman GA, Friedberg SH, Jerabek L. Lymphoid tissue architecture. III. Germinal centers, T cells, and thymus-dependent vs thymus-independent antigens. *Adv Exp Med Biol* 1976;66:229–237.

124. Davies AJS, Carter RL, Leuchars E, Wallis V, Dietrich FM. The morphology of immune reactions in normal, thymectomized and reconstituted mice. III. Response to bacterial antigens: salmonellal flagellar antigen and pneumococcal polysaccharide. *Immunology* 1970;19:945–957.

125. Baker PJ, Stashak PW, Amsbaugh DF, Prescott B. Characterization of the antibody response to type III pneumococcal polysaccharide at the cellular level. I. Dose-response studies and the effect of prior immunization on the magnitude of the antibody response. *Immunology* 1971;20:469–480.

126. Klaus GGB, Humphrey JH. The immunological properties of haptens coupled to thymus-independent carrier molecules. I. The characteristics of the immune response to dinitrophenol-lysine-substituted pneumococcal polysaccharide (SIII) and levan. *Eur J Immunol* 1974;4:370–377.

127. Crews S, Griffin J, Huang H, Calame K, Hood L. A single V_H gene segment encodes the immune response to phosphorylcholine: somatic mutation is correlated with the class of the antibody. *Cell* 1981;25:59–66.

128. Carroll WL, Adderson EE, Lucas AH, et al. Molecular basis of antibody diversity. In: Ellis RW, Granoff DM, eds. *Development and clinical uses of Haemophilus b conjugate vaccines*, 1st ed. New York: Marcel Dekker, 1994:207–229.

129. Claflin JL, Hudak S, Maddalena A. Anti-phosphocholine hybridoma antibodies. I. Direct evidence for three distinct families of antibodies in the murine response. *J Exp Med* 1981;153:352–364.

130. Briles DE, Davie JM. Clonal dominance. I. Restricted nature of the IgM antibody response to group A streptococcal carbohydrate in mice. *J Exp Med* 1975;141:1291–1307.

131. Insel RA, Kittelberger A, Anderson P. Isoelectric focusing of human antibody to the *Haemophilus influenzae* b capsular polysaccharide: restricted and identical spectrotypes in adults. *J Immunol* 1985;135:2810–2816.

132. Scott MG, Crimmins DL, McCourt DW, et al. Clonal characterization of the human IgG antibody repertoire to *Haemophilus influenzae* type b polysaccharide. III. A single VKII gene and one of several JK genes are joined by an invariant arginine to form the most common L chain V region. *J Immunol* 1989;143:4110–4116.

133. Gearhart PJ, Johnson ND, Douglas R, Hood L. IgG antibodies to phosphorylcholine exhibit more diversity than their IgM counterparts. *Nature* 1981;291:29–34.

134. Sharon J, Kabat EA, Morrison S. Association constants of hybridoma antibodies specific for alpha (1-6) linked dextran determined by affinity electrophoresis. *Mol Immunol* 1982;19:389–397.

135. Hetherington SV. The intrinsic affinity constant (K) of anticapsular antibody to oligosaccharides of *Haemophilus influenzae* type b. *J Immunol* 1988;140:3966–3970.

136. Heidelberger M, Rebers PA. Immunochemistry of the pneumococcal types II, V, and VI. The relation of type II to type II and other correlations between chemical constitution and precipitation in antisera to type VI. *J Bacteriol* 1960;80:145–153.

137. MacPherson CFC, Heidelberger M, Alexander HE, Leidy G. The specific polysaccharides of types A,B,C,D, and F *Haemophilus influenzae*. *J Immunol* 1946;52:207–219.

138. Heidelberger M, Bernheimer AW. Cross-reactions of polysaccharides of fungi, molds, and yeasts in anti-pneumococcal and other antisera. *Proc Natl Acad Sci U S A* 1984;81:5247–5249.

139. Lucas AH, Langley RJ, Granoff DM, Nahm MH, Kitamura MY, Scott MG. An idiotypic marker associated with a germ-line encoded kappa light chain variable region that predominates the vaccine-induced human antibody response to the *Haemophilus influenzae* b polysaccharide. *J Clin Invest* 1991;88:1811–1818.

140. Moxon ER, Anderson P. Meningitis caused by *Haemophilus influenzae* in infant rats: protective immunity and antibody priming by gastrointestinal colonization with *Escherichia coli*. *J Infect Dis* 1979;140:471–478.

141. Galili U, Mandrell RE, Hamadeh RM, Shohet SB, Griffiss JM. Interaction between human natural anti–alpha-galactosyl immunoglobulin G and bacteria of the human flora. *Infect Immun* 1988;56:1730–1737.

142. Avila JL, Rojas M, Galili U. Immunogenic Gal-alpha-1-3Gal carbohydrate epitopes are present on pathogenic American *Trypanosoma* and *Leishmania*. *J Immunol* 1989;142:2828–2834.

143. Lal RB, Paranjape RS, Briles DE, Nutman TB, Ottesen EA. Circulating parasite antigen(s) in lymphatic filariasis: use of monoclonal antibodies to phosphocholine for immunodiagnosis. *J Immunol* 1987;138:3454–3460.

144. Briles DE, Nahm M, Schroer K, et al. Antiphosphocholine antibodies found in normal mouse serum are protective against intravenous infection with type 3 *Streptococcus pneumoniae*. *J Exp Med* 1981;153:694–705.

145. Weiser JN, Shchepetov M, Chong ST. Decoration of lipopolysaccharide with phosphorylcholine: a phase-variable characteristic of *Haemophilus influenzae*. *Infect Immun* 1997;65:943–950.

146. Tsukada M, Spicer SS. Heterogeneity of macrophages evidenced by variability in their glycoconjugates. *J Leukoc Biol* 1988;43:455–467.

147. Hashimoto S, Ogata T. Blood vascular organization of the human appendix: a scanning electron microscopic study of corrosion casts. *Tohoku J Exp Med* 1988;154:271–283.

148. Ginsburg CM, McCracken Jr. GH, Schneerson R, Robbins JB, Parke JC Jr. Association between cross-reacting *Escherichia coli* K100 and disease caused by *Haemophilus influenzae* type b. *Infect Immun* 1978;22:339–342.

149. Knight KL, Crane MA. Generating the antibody repertoire in rabbit. *Adv Immunol* 1994;56:179–218.

150. Winkelstein JA. The complement system. In: Gorbach SL, Bartlett JG, Blacklow NR, eds. *Infectious diseases*, 1st ed. Philadelphia: WB Saunders, 1992:37–43.

151. Van der Ley P, Heckels JE, Virji M, Hoogerhout P, Poolman JT. Topology of outer membrane porins in pathogenic *Neisseria* spp. *Infect Immun* 1991;59:2963–2971.

152. Nielsen SV, Sorensen UBS, Henrichsen J. Antibodies against pneumococcal C-polysaccharide are not protective. *Microb Pathog* 1993;14:299–305.

153. Briles DE, Forman C, Horowitz JC, et al. Antipneumococcal effects of C-reactive protein and monoclonal antibodies to pneumococcal cell wall and capsular antigens. *Infect Immun* 1989;57:1457–1464.

154. Cooper NR. The classical complement pathway: activation and regulation of the first complement component. *Adv Immunol* 1985;37:151–216.

155. Mostov KE. Transepithelial transport of immunoglobulins. *Ann Rev Immunol* 1997;12:63–84.

156. McDaniel LS, Benjamin WH, Forman C, Briles DE. Blood clearance by anti phosphocholine antibodies as a mechanism of protection in experimental pneumococcal bacteremia. *J Immunol* 1984;133:3308–3312.

157. Briles DE, Claflin JL, Schroer K, Forman C. Mouse IgG3 antibodies are highly protective against infection with *Streptococcus pneumoniae*. *Nature* 1981;294:88–90.

158. Schreiber JR, Barrus V, Cates KL, Siber GR. Functional characterization of human IgG, IgM, and IgA antibody directed to the capsule of *Haemophilus influenzae* type b. *J Infect Dis* 1986;153:8–16.

159. Schlesinger JJ, Foltzer M, Chapman S. The Fc portion of antibody to yellow fever virus NS1 is a determinant of protection against YF encephalitis in mice. *Virology* 1993;192:132–141.

160. Yuan R, Casadevall A, Spira G, Scharff MD. Isotype switching from IgG3 to IgG1 converts a nonprotective murine antibody to Cryptococcus neoformans into a protective antibody. *J Immunol* 1995;154:1810–1816.

161. Possee RD, Schild GC, Dimmock NJ. Studies on the mechanism of neutralization of influenza virus by antibody: evidence that neutralizing antibody inactivates influenza virus by inhibiting virion transcriptase activity. *J Gen Virol* 1997;58:373–386.

162. Jefferis R, Pound J, Lund J, Goodall M. Effector mechanisms activated by human IgG subclass antibodies: clinical and molecular aspects. *Ann Biol Clin* 1994;52:57–65.

163. Burton DR, Woof JM. Human antibody effector function. *Adv Immunol* 1992;51:1–84.

164. Cooper LJ, Shikhman AR, Glass DD, Kangisser D, Cunningham MW, Greenspan NS. Role of heavy chain constant domains in antibody–antigen interaction. Apparent specificity differences among streptococcal IgG antibodies expressing identical variable domains. *J Immunol* 1993;150:2231–2242.

165. Briles DE, Forman C, Hudak S, Claflin JL. The effects of subclass on the ability of anti-phosphocholine antibodies to protect mice from fatal infection with *Streptococcus pneumoniae*. *J Mol Cell Immunol* 1984;1:305–309.

166. Amir J, Scott MG, Nahm MH, Granoff DM. Bactericidal and opsonic activity of IgG1 and IgG2 anticapsular antibodies to *Haemophilus influenzae* type b. *J Infect Dis* 1990;162:163–171.

167. Weinberg GA, Granoff DM, Nahm MH, Shackelford PG. Functional activity of different IgG subclass antibodies against type b capsular polysaccharide of *Haemophilus influenzae*. *J Immunol* 1986;136:4232–4236.

168. Bredius RGM, de Vries CEE, Troelstra A, et al. Phagocytosis of *Staphylococcus aureus* and *Haemophilus influenzae* type b opsonized with polyclonal human IgG1 and IgG2 antibodies. *J Immunol* 1993;151:1463–1472.

169. Lefranc M, Lefranc G, Rabbitts TH. Inherited deletion of immunoglobulin heavy chain constant region genes in normal human individuals. *Nature* 1982;300:760–762.

170. Ravetch JV, Kinet J. Fc Receptors. *Ann Rev Immunol* 1991;9:457–492.

171. Gorter A, Hiemstra PS, Leijh PCJ, et al. IgA- and secretory IgA-opsonized *S. aureus* induce a respiratory burst and phagocytosis by polymorphonuclear leucocytes. *Immunology* 1987;61:303–309.

172. Hiemstra PS, Gorter A, Stuurman ME, van Es LA, Daha MR. Activation of alternative pathway of complement by human serum IgA. *Eur J Immunol* 1987;17:321–326.

173. Jarvis GA, Griffiss JM. Human IgA1 initiates complement-mediated killing of *Neisseria meningitidis*. *J Immunol* 1989;143:1703–1709.

174. Imai H, Chen RJ, Wyatt RJ, Rifai A. Lack of complement activation by human IgA immune complexes. *Clin Exp Immunol* 1988;73:479–483.

175. Jarvis GA, Griffiss JM. Human IgA1 blockade of IgG-initiated lysis of Neisseria meningitidis is a function of antigen-binding fragment binding to the polysaccharide capsule. *J Immunol* 1991;147:1962–1967.

176. Griffiss JM, Bertram MA. Immunoepidemiology of menigococcal disease in military recruits. II. Blocking of serum bactericidal activity by circulating IgA early in the course of invasive disease. *J Infect Dis* 1977;136:733–739.

177. Michetti P, Mahan MJ, Slauch JM, Mekalanos JJ, Neutra MR. Monoclonal secretory immunoglobulin A protects mice against oral challenge with the invasive pathogen *Salmonella typhimurium*. *Infect Immun* 1992;60:1786–1792.

178. Lamm ME. Interaction of antigens and antibodies at mucosal surfaces. *Ann Rev Microbiol* 1997;51:311–340.

179. Brandtzaeg P, Fjellanger I, Gjeruldsen ST. Immunoglobulin M: local synthesis and selective secretion in patients with immunoglobulin A deficiency. *Science* 1968;160:789–791.

180. Einhorn MS, Granoff DM, Nahm MH, Quinn A, Shackelford PG. Concentrations of antibodies in paired maternal and infant sera: relationship to IgG subclass. *J Pediatr* 1987;111:783–788.

181. Leach JL, Sedmak DD, Osborne JM, Rahill B, Lairmore MD, Anderson CL. Isolation from human placenta of the IgG transporter, FcRn, and localization to the syncytiotrophoblast: implications for maternal–fetal antibody transport. *J Immunol* 1996;157:3317–3322.

182. Ravetch JV, Margulies DH. New tricks for old molecules. *Nature* 1997;372:323–324.

183. Adams WG, Deaver KA, Cochi SL, et al. Decline of childhood *Haemophilus influenzae* Type b (Hib) disease in the Hib vaccine era. *JAMA* 1993;269:221–226.

184. Takala AK, Eskola J, Leinonen M, et al. Reduction of oropharyngeal carriage of *Haemophilus influenzae* type b (Hib) in children immunized with an Hib conjugate vaccine. *J Infect Dis* 1991;164:982–986.

185. Briles DE, Swiatlo E, Edwards K. Vaccine strategies for *Streptococcus pneumoniae*. In: Stevens DL, ed. *Streptococci*. New York: Oxford University Press, 1999.

186. Bhatt SM, Cabellos C, Nadol JB Jr, et al. The impact of dexamethasone on hearing loss in experimental pneumococcal meningitis. *Pediatr Infect Dis J* 1995;14:93–96.

187. Gutierrez-Ramos JC, Bluethmann H. Molecules and mechanisms operating in septic shock: lessons from knockout mice. *Immunol Today* 1997;18:329–334.

188. O'Brien AD, Rosenstreich DL, Scher I, Campbell GH, MacDermott RP, Formal SB. Genetic control of susceptibility to *Salmonella typhimurium* in mice: role of the Lps gene. *J Immunol* 1980;124:20–24.

189. Hagberg L, Briles DE, Eden CS. Evidence for separate genetic defects in C3H/HeJ and C3HeB/FeJ mice, that affect susceptibility to Gram-negative infections. *J Immunol* 1985;134:4118–4122.

190. Finne J, Leinonen M, Makela PH. Antigenic similarities between brain components and bacteria causing meningitis. Implications for vaccine development and pathogenesis. *Lancet* 1983;2:355–357.

191. Rougon G, Dubois C, Buckley N, Magnani JL, Zollinger W. A monoclonal antibody against meningococcus group B polysaccharides distinguishes embryonic from adult N-CAM. *J Cell Biol* 1986;103:2429–2437.

192. Moran AP, Prendergast MM, Appelmelk BJ. Molecular mimicry of host structures by bacterial lipopolysaccharides and its contribution to disease. *FEMS Immunol Med Microbiol* 1997;16:105–115.

193. Rees JH, Soudain SE, Gregson NA, Hughes RA. *Campylobacter jejuni* infection and Guillain-Barré syndrome. *N Engl J Med* 1995;333:1374–1379.

194. Limpanasithikul W, Ray S, Diamond B. Cross-reactive antibodies have both protective and pathogenic potential. *J Immunol* 1995;155:967–973.

195. Ray SK, Putterman C, Diamond B. Pathogenic autoantibodies are routinely generated during the response to foreign antigen: a paradigm for autoimmune disease. *Proc Natl Acad Sci U S A* 1996;93:2019–2024.

196. Bessen D, Jones KF, Fischetti VA. Evidence for two distinct classes of streptococcal M protein and their relationship to rheumatic fever. *J Exp Med* 1989;169:269–283.

197. Hollingshead SK, Bessen DE. Evolution of the emm gene family: virulence gene clusters in group A streptococci. *Dev Biol Stand* 1995;85:163–169.

198. Cunningham MW, McCormack JM, Fenderson PG, Ho M-K, Beachey EH, Dale JB. Human and murine antibodies cross-reactive with streptococcal M protein and myosin recognize the sequence gln-lys-ser-lys-gln in M protein. *J Immunol* 1989;143:2677–2683.

199. Cunningham MW, Antone SM, Gulizia JM, McManus BA, Gauntt CJ. Alpha-helical coiled-coil molecules: a role in autoimmunity against the heart. *Clin Immunol Immunopathol* 1993;68:118–123.

200. Cunningham MW. Streptococci and rheumatic fever. In: Friedman H, Rose NR, Bendinelli M, eds. *Microorganisms and autoimmune disease*. New York: Plenum, 1996:13–66.

201. Cunningham MW, Antone SM, Gulizia JM, McManus BM, Fischetti VA, Gauntt CJ. Cytotoxic and viral neutralizing antibodies crossreact with streptococcal M protein, enteroviruses and human cardiac myosin. *Proc Natl Acad Sci U S A* 1992;89:1320–1324.

202. Chow LH, Yuling Y, Linder J, McManus BM. Phenotype analysis of infiltrating cells in human myocarditis. *Arch Pathol Lab Med* 1989;113:1357–1362.

203. Guilherme L, Chuna-Neto E, Coelho V, et al. Human heart-infiltrating T cell clones from rheumatic heart disease patients recognize both streptococcal and cardiac proteins. *Circulation* 1995;92:415–446.

204. Shikhman AR, Greenspan NS, Cunningham MW. A subset of mouse monoclonal antibodies cross-reactive with cytoskeletal proteins and group A streptococcal M proteins recognizes N-acetyl-β-D-glucosamine. *J Immunol* 1993;151:3902–3913.

205. Shikhman AR, Cunningham MW. Immunological mimicry between N-acetyl-β-d-glucosamine and cytokeratin peptides. *J Immunol* 1994;152:4375–4387.

206. Quinn A, Adderson EE, Shackelford PG, Carroll WL, Cunningham MW. Autoantibody germline gene segment encodes VH and VL regions of a human anti-streptococcal Mab recognizing streptococcal M protein and human cardiac myosin epitopes. *J Immunol* 1994;154:4203–4212.

207. Kuo JS-C, Doelling VW, Graveline JF, McCoy DW. Evidence for covalent attachment of phospholipid to the capsular polysaccharide of *Haemophilus influenzae* type b. *J Bacteriol* 1985;163:769–773.

208. Sieling PA, Chatterjee D, Porcelli SA, et al. CD1-restricted T cell recognition of microbial lipoglycan antigens. *Science* 1995;269:227–230.

209. Stephens DS, Hoffman LH, McGee ZA. Interaction of *Neisseria meningitidis* with human nasopharyngeal mucosa: attachment and entry into columnar epithelial cells. *J Infect Dis* 1983;148:369–376.

210. Melly MA, McGee ZA, Rosenthal RS. Ability of monomeric peptidoglycan fragments from *Neisseria gonorrhoeae* to damage human fallopian-tube mucosa. *J Infect Dis* 1984;149:378–386.

211. Lin L, Ayala F, Larson J, et al. The *Neisseria* type 2 IgA1 protease cleaves LAMP1 and promotes survival of bacteria within epithelial cells. *Mol Microbiol* 1997;24:1083–1094.

212. Stephens DS, Whitney AM, Melly MA, Hoffman LH, Farley MM, Frasch CE. Analysis of damage to human ciliated nasopharyngeal epithelium by *Neisseria meningitidis*. *Infect Immun* 1986;51:579–585.

213. Gotschlich EC, Goldschneider I, Artenstein MS. Human immunity to the meningococcus. V. The effect of immunization with meningococcal group C polysaccharide on the carrier state. *J Exp Med* 1969;129:1385–1395.

214. Gotschlich EC, Goldschneider I, Artenstein MS. Human immunity to the meningococcus. IV. Immunogenicity of group A and group C meningococcal polysaccharides in human volunteers. *J Exp Med* 1969;129:1367–1384.

215. Gotschlich EC, Liu TY, Artenstein MS. Human immunity to the meningococcus. 3. Preparation and immunochemical properties of the group A, group B, and group C meningococcal polysaccharides. *J Exp Med* 1969;129:1349–1365.

Fundamental Immunology, Fourth Edition,
edited by William E. Paul
Lippincott–Raven Publishers, Philadelphia © 1999.

CHAPTER 42

Vaccines

G.J.V. Nossal

Historical Perspectives
Classification of Vaccines
Adjuvants and Principles of Mucosal Immunity
Bacterial Vaccines
Viral Vaccines
Vaccines against Parasitic Diseases
Vaccines against Cancer
Birth-control Vaccines
Negative Vaccines in Autoimmunity and Allergy
Adverse Effects of Vaccines
The Future
Acknowledgments
References

Vaccines are history's most cost-effective public health tool. In fact, some vaccines have so reduced disease prevalence as to make community complacency a significant problem. It is curious to reflect on how little academic immunology has contributed to vaccine development over the last 40 years. In the period following Pasteur's introduction of rabies vaccination, immunology was clearly seen as part of medical microbiology, but it began to take on a life of its own when it was realized that, as well as microbes, foreign cells and small organic molecules could also function as antigens. The rapid development from the 1950s of transplantation immunology and autoimmunity research, and the simultaneous

growth in interest in the puzzle of antibody diversity, served to take academic immunology far from its traditional roots. Thus, great triumphs, such as poliomyelitis and hepatitis vaccines, came from other disciplines; the ever-expanding peer group that attended the International Congresses of Immunology, or that contributed to the three previous editions of this textbook, displayed relatively little interest in immunization. Over the last decade, this has begun to change. It is hard to point to a single cause. The devastating impact of the human immunodeficiency virus (HIV) and acquired immunodeficiency syndrome (AIDS) has certainly been a major factor, as has the active role of the World Health Organization (WHO) in pushing for an expanded vaccine research and development effort. Perhaps most importantly, as the focus of academic interest in immunology shifts more and more to the rules governing regula-

G. J. V. Nossal: Department of Pathology, The University of Melbourne, Parkville, Victoria 3052, Australia.

tion and guidance of the immune response, scientists have come to recognize the enormity of the contribution they can make to rational design of vaccines and immune adjuvants. Partly as a result of this reawakening of interest among many of our top immunologists, and partly because of a renewed research commitment by half a dozen or so major international vaccine manufacturers, we have seen new and improved vaccines emerging, with many more in the pipeline. This poses two huge challenges: how to administer the new vaccines without burdening populations with an unacceptable number of injections; and how to achieve an equitable distribution of the benefits, including to citizens of the developing countries.

This chapter attempts to summarize the basic principles of vaccination, including a consideration of the elaborate mechanisms that some pathogens have evolved to foil the immune response. Its primary focus is on communicable diseases. However, in the long term, vaccine approaches may be important to widely differing problems, such as cancer and birth control. Furthermore, as antigen can cause tolerance as well as immunity, the possibility exists that suitably administered antigenic preparations can control autoimmunity, allergy, and transplant rejection. The mechanisms that could underpin such "negative vaccines" are addressed, though more cursorily.

Like much of clinical medicine, vaccinology is an amalgam of scientific design and accumulated empirical experience. Some aspects, such as the search for suitable adjuvants, are tilted towards the latter. As we now know much more about what kind of immune response is required to control a particular kind of infection, vaccines and adjuvants should increasingly be designed to guide lymphocytes down the most appropriate pathway. At the experimental level, cytokines have powerfully helped in the guidance process; it remains to be seen whether the use of these agents, or of genes coding for them, will find a role in practice. Cytokines are but one example of new, rational approaches to immunogenicity.

This chapter is not meant as a compendium of current or likely future vaccines. There are excellent works that fulfil this purpose (1–3). Rather, the examples of vaccines described are meant to be illustrative of the diverse processes capable of leading to protection, and of the immense public benefits obtainable. The fact that it has been necessary to cite quite a few diseases reflects the protean nature and rich promise of the field.

HISTORICAL PERSPECTIVES

Early civilizations that left written records, such as those of Egypt, India, Greece, and China, made references to infectious diseases, but the accuracy of diagnosis is frequently questionable. Thus, it is now believed that the "leprosy" referred to in the Bible may well have represented a dermatologic condition such as psoriasis. In their monumental work on smallpox and its eradication (4), Fenner et al. conclude that "unmistakable descriptions of smallpox did not appear until the fourth century A.D. in China." Nevertheless, the specificity of immunity and its frequent lifelong duration were known, for example, to the ancient Greeks. The word *immunity* was first used in the fourteenth century with reference to plague. In the absence of knowledge of the microbial origin of infections, including epidemics, little could be done to make use of the concept.

One exception was the practice of variolation as a procedure to prevent smallpox. This most feared of diseases causes a case fatality of 20% to 30% and leaves its other victims scarred for life. As early as the tenth century A.D., the pustular fluid from smallpox

lesions, or the dried scabs from healing sores, were given to susceptible individuals to make them immune. In India, inoculation was into the skin, but in China, into the nose. For reasons that are not entirely clear, variolation resulted in less severe disease than did natural infection. There was usually a nasty lesion at the inoculation site, some satellite blisters, frequently a mild rash, and constitutional symptoms. However, the mortality rate at 1% to 2% was relatively low, and there was much less scarring than following a regular attack. There were other serious constraints. For example, contacts of variolated people not infrequently developed the full, natural infection. Despite this, no less august a body than the Royal Society of London debated the subject in the early eighteenth century. There is no doubt that variolation worked, in the sense of conferring immunity. Still the medical profession as a whole remained sceptical.

Lady Mary Montagu is usually credited for introducing variolation into Great Britain, although the importance of her promotional work has been called into question (5). As the wife of the British Ambassador in Constantinople, she had been sufficiently impressed with the common local practice to have her own 6-year-old son variolated in 1718. Returning to London, she interested several prominent members of the Royal College of Physicians in the practice as they struggled with the terrible smallpox epidemic of 1721. The President of the College, Sir Hans Sloane, became a convert following some experiments on convicted felons, and arranged the variolation of two royal princesses. Despite several successes, variolation never became a truly widespread practice in Great Britain or Europe. However, certain failures of variolation to "take" ushered in the vaccine era.

The Jennerian Era

In the 1760s and 1770s, several physicians drew attention to the fact that milkmaids were rarely pockmarked. Frequently, they had developed sores on their hands because they had caught an infection from the teat of a cow. The relevant cow disease bore some similarity to human smallpox. It was found that these milkmaids could not be successfully variolated. Several people, subsequent to Jenner's triumph, claimed to have inoculated cowpox material into their children because of this series of observations. Be that as it may, it was Edward Jenner (6) who not only published first but also actually tested immunity by challenge with smallpox. Sarah Nelmes donated a little fluid from her cowpox-infected hands, and Jenner, on May 14, 1796, inoculated James Phipps with this material, which took at the inoculation site. As Jenner noted:

> Notwithstanding the resemblance which the pustule, thus excited on the boy's arm, bore to variolous inoculation, yet as the indisposition attending it was barely perceptible, I could scarcely persuade myself the patient was secure from the smallpox. However, on his being inoculated some months afterwards, it proved that he was secure (7).

A further challenge with smallpox material 5 years later confirmed maintenance of immunity. Jenner failed to get his work into the *Transactions of The Royal Society* (5) and published his "Inquiry" (6) privately. Soon after, vaccination, as the practice came to be called, took off. It spread to Europe, to the United States, and thence throughout the world. Vaccination became compulsory in several European countries in the early years of the nineteenth century, and as a result, the number of smallpox deaths fell dramatically. For example, in Sweden, there were 5,126 deaths per million population in 1800 but 100-fold fewer by 1821 (4). In

Great Britain, vaccination became compulsory in 1853. The source of vaccine material changed from human to calf-derived in the second half of the nineteenth century, and revaccination also became popular. In 1896, Great Britain extensively celebrated the centenary of the James Phipps experiment, secure in the knowledge that vaccination had proven brilliantly successful. The final chapter in the smallpox drama is so compelling that it will require a section of it own. Let us simply record here that the Gloucestershire general practitioner has been recognized by statues and memorials in many parts of the world. He sits in state in Kensington Gardens, London, the statue there representing a focal point for the extensive 1996 bicentenary celebrations. The plaque under the statue refers to "the country doctor who benefited mankind." Who could have guessed that more than 80 years had to elapse before the next big advance in immunization?

The Pasteurian Era: Action and Reaction

Jenner had no overarching theory for how vaccination provided immunity to smallpox. Two great giants established the true etiologic cause of infectious diseases—Louis Pasteur (1822–1895) and Robert Koch (1843–1910)—and thus set the scene for a better understanding of the specificity of immunity. Pasteur (8) destroyed the spontaneous generation theory of bacteria, and Koch, his arch-rival and debating opponent, enunciated his famous postulates, which, if fulfilled, established an agent as the cause of a disease. Pasteur made the critically important observation that bacteria grown for substantial periods in artificial media lost their virulence. For example, *Pasteurella septica,* the cause of fowl cholera, when attenuated *in vitro,* no longer caused disease. Rather, injection of such attenuated bacteria protected chickens from the effects of fresh, virulent cultures (9). With surprising speed, the idea was tested in a real-life setting. In 1881, the first tests of an attenuated anthrax vaccine were run, and in 1882, 85,000 sheep were immunized (10). Pasteur coined the word *vaccine* as a general one for immunizing preparations in homage to Edward Jenner and his use of vaccinia virus. Even though Pasteur did not know that rabies was caused by a virus rather than a bacterium, and had to attenuate it in rabbit spinal cord rather than through culture, his introduction of rabies immunization on little Jacob Meister had a galvanic effect and was soon widely practiced. Crowned heads from all over the world came to pay honor to Pasteur, and he was able to build the Pasteur Institute in Paris entirely from benefactions. Founded in 1888, this Institute is of huge historic significance, as it was the first human institution entirely devoted to biomedical research.

Other live, attenuated bacterial vaccines to come on stream were several failed cholera vaccines: for example, those of Ferran and Halfkine (11) and an interesting variant of Koch's tubercle bacillus. Calmette and Guerin (12) started with an isolate of tuberculosis from a cow. After an amazing series of 213 subcultures over a period of 13 years, they intrepidly tried the culture orally in a newborn infant. Thus, bacille Calmette Guerin (BCG) was born. It was soon given intradermally rather than orally, and was clearly effective in infants for the prevention of miliary tuberculosis (TB) and tuberculous meningitis, though its capacity to prevent adult pulmonary TB, the real killer in TB, is much more controversial.

Pasteur originally believed that microbes had to be alive to cause immunity. Nevertheless, killed whole-cell bacterial vaccines against cholera, typhoid, and plague were introduced as early as 1896, and essentially similar vaccines were shown to be effective, at least partially, in a variety of trials in the first half of the twentieth century. Another major step forward came with the recognition that certain diseases, such as diphtheria and tetanus, resulted from the secretion of powerful exotoxins by the relevant bacteria. Von Behring and Kitasato (13) discovered antibodies in 1890, and had some success in the passive immunotherapy of diphtheria, with antidiphtheria toxin antibodies from horses. This resulted in the first-ever Nobel Prize in Medicine. Antitoxin could be mixed with the relatively crude toxin preparations available from culture supernatants, and the first active immunization against diphtheria or tetanus involved toxin–antitoxin mixtures. Much more satisfactory and consistent results were obtained when it was realized that toxins could be neutralized through denaturation with formaldehyde, yet could still be protectively immunogenic. These so-called toxoids were good vaccines (14) and their progressive introduction into the industrialized countries from 1930 on lowered the impact of these infections to a marked degree.

It could be argued that the first golden age of immunology (say 1880–1910) was accompanied by a certain degree of hubris. There was a time when it almost appeared that all that was needed to conquer communicable diseases was to isolate the causative agent, establish Koch's postulates, attenuate or kill the agent, and immunize. Yet, from the earliest trials (e.g., those of Pasteur on rabies), there was controversy. Levine (11) notes a number of historic disasters arising from vaccines, and it is clear that several of the early preparations were neither as safe nor as protective as their protagonists claimed. It must be remembered that neither production facilities nor regulatory agencies were well developed at this time, and the design of many of the clinical trials left much to be desired. In the broad, particular triumphs notwithstanding, the early promise of vaccines was not fully realized in the first golden age. There were significant professional reservations about vaccines and, in certain quarters, a distinctly antagonistic community reaction. The author was born in 1931, and it is quite clear that at that time, educated parents were by no means convinced about the advantages of immunization as a whole.

The Virus Revolution: Salk and Sabin

Growth of viruses on the chorioallantoic membrane of chick embryos resulted in the production of two useful vaccines in the 1930s, namely those against yellow fever (a live, attenuated, and very effective vaccine) and influenza (a killed vaccine with a lower success rate). However, the revolution in antiviral vaccines really began with the development of tissue culture, resulting in the successful growth of the poliomyelitis virus by Enders and his colleagues (15), followed shortly by the development of the Salk vaccine.

It is difficult now to reconstruct the fear that surrounded poliomyelitis before 1955. While the disease was epidemic in nature, waxing and waning with the summer seasons of maximum spread, it never went away. During a high incidence year, mothers feared to send their children to the cinema or the swimming pool. Polio was a dreaded enemy. In the United States, for example, there were typically 20,000 or more cases of paralytic poliomyelitis per year. The Salk inactivated poliomyelitis vaccine was introduced in 1955, and between 1955 and 1961, 300 million doses of the vaccine were administered, and the incidence of the disease fell tenfold. There was the infamous Cutter Incident, in which faulty production techniques allowed two lots of vaccine to slip through with inadequate formalin inactivation, resulting in 149 cases of polio, a disaster that lent impetus to the development of the live, attenuated oral poliomyelitis vaccine of Sabin, first introduced in 1961. By 1965, this latter vaccine had essentially replaced the Salk vaccine in the United States, and soon after, in most countries, though not in The Netherlands, Iceland, and Sweden. Being orally active, it was more convenient to use, and containing far fewer virions, it was also much cheaper. It is somewhat ironic that the very rare reversions to neurovirulence, particularly in poliomyelitis virus type 3 (estimated at one case of acute flaccid paralysis per 2.7 million doses of oral poliomyelitis vaccine administered), have now prompted U.S. health authorities to recommend initial immunization with injectable poliomyelitis vaccine to minimize risk. The late Jonas Salk campaigned tirelessly for this reversion, the rivalry between him and Albert Sabin being legendary.

The great adventure of polio eradication will be discussed later, but there is no doubt that the dramatic success of polio immunization paved the way for a number of other live, attenuated virus vaccines, again dependent on the principle of attenuation in tissue culture. Enders' original Edmondston strain of measles vaccine, first introduced in 1963, was a little bit "hot." When the author's younger son was born in 1964, the recommendation was to use this vaccine, but to coadminister gamma globulin containing antimeasles antibodies! The problem was solved through the introduction of the more attenuated Moraten and Schwartz derivatives of the original Enders strain. This excellent measles vaccine was followed by a mumps vaccine, first introduced in 1967, and a live, attenuated rubella vaccine in 1968. Hilleman (16) recorded that a combined measles–mumps–rubella vaccine was the realization of a long-term dream, achieved in 1969 and licenced in 1971. Now we are on the threshold of a measles–mumps–rubella–varicella quadrivalent vaccine having the potential to eradicate all four diseases from the industrialized countries. In several European countries, measles, mumps, and rubella transmission appears to have ceased.

Smallpox Eradication

By the mid-1960s, the societal scepticism about vaccines had largely evaporated; the polio success was in the vanguard in reshaping public opinion. But, no matter how successful any vaccine had been, there was no example of a disease having actually been eradicated from the globe. Interestingly, Edward Jenner had speculated about this with respect to smallpox. But, despite the good efforts of many countries, global eradication was not a subject of much discussion before the formation of the WHO. Because Europe had essentially managed to beat this scourge by 1953, and similarly North and Central America by 1951, global eradication seemed feasible. Progress in many of the countries of Asia was also good, but by 1960 smallpox was still a serious matter in Africa and most of the Indian subcontinent.

A heady decision was taken by the Twelfth World Health Assembly in May 1959. Global eradication of smallpox was set as a new goal for the WHO. At that time, 977 million people lived in smallpox endemic areas. The preamble to the 1959 resolution mentioned a wildly optimistic timetable of 4 to 5 years. In the event, little happened between 1959 and 1966, when at last a significant budgetary allocation was made for a major WHO effort to be begin on January 1, 1967. The plan of that time called for 220 million people to be vaccinated in 1967 at a total cost of some $US 180 million (including indigenous country costs). Dr D.A. Henderson was appointed Head of the Smallpox Eradication Unit at WHO in 1966, with Dr. Isao Arita as his Medical Officer. Setting themselves a target of a decade for eradication, and with an external budget averaging $US 7 million per year (in addition to the countries' own efforts), the team attacked their ambitious goal, realizing the vital challenge in vaccine requirements and quality control, disease surveillance, data collection, training programs needed for mass vaccination campaigns, the requirements for WHO's own reference laboratories, and a host of similar practical problems. Sufficient progress towards global eradication had been made by 1971 for both the United States and the United Kingdom to cease their routine vaccination programs. Still, Africa and the Indian subcontinent remained problematic. This led to a greatly intensified effort in these regions in 1973, and, by 1975, the virus was eliminated from Asia, with Ethiopia now the only real problem area. War broke out between Ethiopia and Somalia, and smallpox reestablished itself in the latter. A large-scale emergency effort got on top of the problem, and the last case of naturally occuring smallpox was recorded in Merca, Somalia, on October 26, 1977.

The certification of smallpox eradication was no easy task. A Global Commission had to tread warily amid the sensitivities of several countries. On December 9, 1979, the Global Commission certified that eradication had been achieved (Fig. 1). Unfortunately, in the Birmingham outbreak of 1978, a medical photographer died of the disease, apparently through catching it somehow from the smallpox laboratory one floor below her in the medical school. This highlighted the danger of variola virus stocks in laboratories. The 49-year-old head of the smallpox laboratory, Prof. H.S. Bedson, died soon after, apparently of suicide. At the time of writing, the last stocks of smallpox virus remaining in the United States and Russia have still not been destroyed. Nevertheless, the eradication

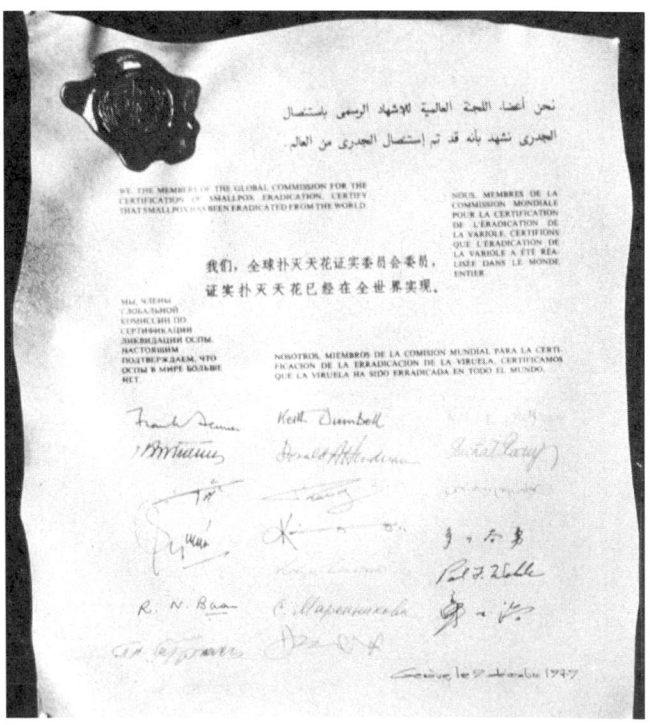

FIG. 1. Frontispiece picture of the official parchment certifying the global eradication of smallpox. (Reprinted with permission of the World Health Organization.)

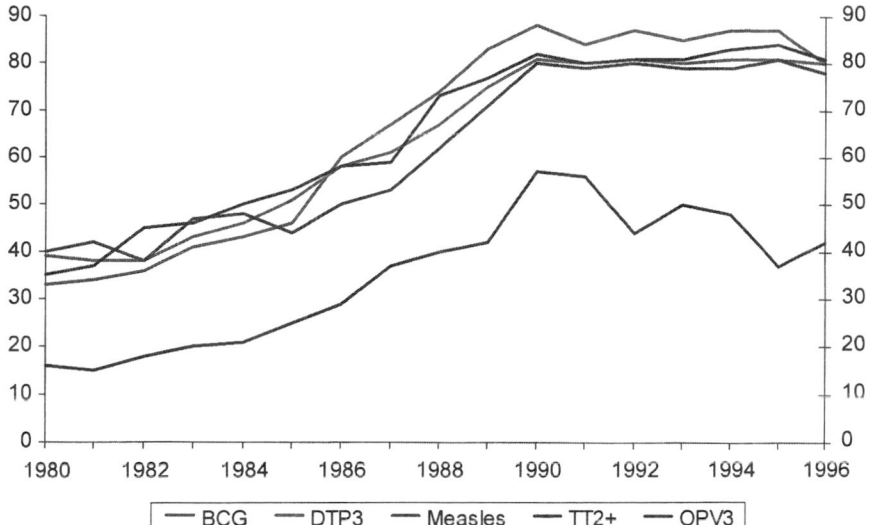

FIG. 2. World Health Organization Expanded Program on Immunization: Reported coverage from 1980 to 1996 for bacillus Calmette-Guérin (BCG), three doses of diphtheria, measles, three doses of oral poliomyelitis vaccine, and two doses of tetanus toxoid (TT) to pregnant women. The slight downturn for 1996 represents some areas that have not reported full data. Note the tendency for a plateauing around 80% coverage. Tetanus toxoid coverage is still much lower than is desirable. (Reprinted with permission from the World Health Organization.)

of the natural disease, more than 4,000 years after its first appearance, and 181 years after the first use of an effective vaccine, must count as one of humanity's noblest achievements. The total costs of smallpox eradication to industrialized and developing countries together have been estimated as $US 300 million over an 11-year period. This compares with an annual cost of smallpox to the world of $US 1,350 million per annum in 1967 dollars.

Dawn of the Molecular Era: Hepatitis B

Hepatitis B vaccine represented a watershed from several points of view. While the toxoids and polysaccharide meningococcal vaccines are molecular or subunit vaccines from one point of view, use of the surface antigen of the hepatitis B virus (HBsAg) represented a new degree of purity of a single protein as a vaccine. It was also the first vaccine manufactured through recombinant DNA technology. It was the first example of a protein, the tendency of which, for self-assembly into 22-nM virion-like particles, greatly aided immunogenicity. Less obviously, it was the first time that a vaccine was introduced to the market as an expensive "boutique" vaccine for special risk groups, such as doctors, nurses, and blood bank workers, later to become a much cheaper public health tool of immense significance for developing countries. Given that there are 250 million carriers of hepatitis B worldwide and that 20% to 25% of carriers develop chronic liver disease, and a substantial proportion of these go on to primary hepatocellular carcinoma, the hepatitis B vaccine is the first anticancer vaccine in history (see also the section on vaccines against cancer). It is also unique in that the relevant antigen was originally thought to represent a protein polymorphism (Australia antigen) (17) and only later was recognized as a viral component (18).

The great success of the hepatitis B vaccine has stilled many of society's fears about the use of recombinant DNA products and has certainly helped usher in the new era, where genetic engineering approaches have become the norm in vaccine research and development. It is to be hoped that the 18-year gap between Blumberg's discovery of Australia antigen and the development of the first-generation blood-derived vaccine (19) will not be repeated. Indeed, the time gap between cloning HBsAg and the yeast-derived vaccine was much shorter (20), and expression systems have improved enormously since that time.

Expanded Program on Immunization

It is appropriate to end this historical overview with a relatively recent development. What was the WHO to do as an encore to smallpox eradication? As the end was nearing, it was decided in 1974 to apply the experience gained with smallpox to launch a stronger attack against other vaccine-preventable diseases. Dr Ralph H. Henderson (no relation to D.A. Henderson of smallpox eradication fame) was appointed Head of an Expanded Program on Immunization (EPI) with the objective of providing, for all of the 120 million children born annually into the world, protection against six diseases: diphtheria, pertussis, tetanus, measles, poliomyelitis, and TB. Though the program only swung into top gear 3 years later, when the smallpox task was over, it has achieved some remarkable successes. Figures 2 through 4 tell the story. As vaccine coverage has risen, so reported cases of diseases have fallen. In 1988, the World Health Assembly gave EPI a further challenge: Eradicate polio by the year 2000. In 1991, hepatitis B was added to the list of diseases to be attacked, with a hoped-for

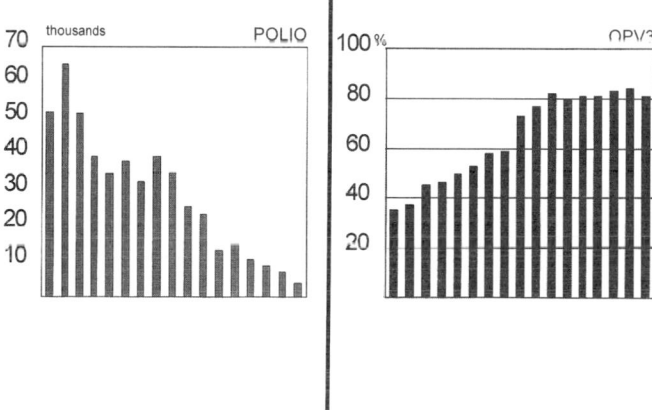

FIG. 3. Fall in reported poliomyelitis cases as a result of global immunization. The dramatic fall over the last 10 years is due not only to the programs of infant immunization, which have stabilized at just over 80% of infants worldwide, but also to the introduction of National Immunization Days (NIDs) in many countries. (Reprinted with permission from the World Health Organization.)

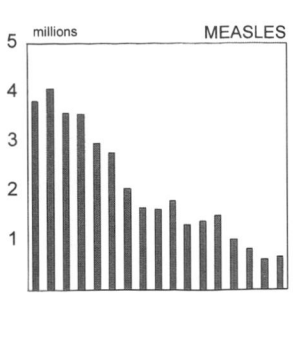
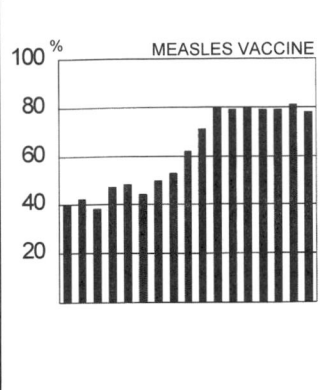

FIG. 4. Fall in reported measles cases as a result of global immunization. The declines over the last 3 or 4 years indicate a major effort in some countries where transmission has been interrupted through national catch-up campaigns. (Reprinted with permission from the World Health Organization.)

introduction of immunization programs in all countries with a carrier rate of 8% by 1995, and in all countries by 1997. Yellow fever was also made a target in certain countries. For reasons that will be covered in the section on vaccines against parasitic diseases, these deadlines have not been fully met, but substantial progress has nevertheless been made. The section on parasitic diseases will also cover further exciting organizational changes in world vaccinology.

Two hundred years after Jenner's breakthrough and 100 years after Pasteur's death, the world is at last taking their legacy seriously. But, as the next sections will show, much more remains to be done.

CLASSIFICATION OF VACCINES

The purpose of a vaccine is to stimulate the immune response without subjecting a person to the risk of actual infection. An ideal vaccine would confer the same degree of immunity as natural infection for those diseases for which immunity is solid, or to do better than nature for those diseases for which it is not. Because most vaccines fall short of this ideal, it is frequently necessary to give vaccines more than once, making use of the phenomenon of immunologic memory, namely the capacity to respond more strongly to an antigen on reexposure to it. Vaccines can elicit every kind of immune response, including antibody formation, T helper 1 (Th1)- and Th2-type CD4$^+$ T-cell responses, and CD8$^+$ T-cell responses, but most practical vaccine development programs have relied on the vaccine's capacity to evoke antibody formation. This may change as more ambitious targets are set, and as capacity to guide immune responses down particular pathways improves.

Vaccines are primarily designed to prevent infection, although one of the first vaccines, that against rabies, was given after infection had been initiated. There is now increasing research on therapeutic vaccines, that is, vaccines administered after infection has been established. Such vaccines are designed to strengthen an immune response that is inadequate, particularly in cases of chronic or recurrent disease.

Obviously, microorganisms possess thousands of molecules that are foreign to a host animal or person, and that are thus antigenic. Immune responses against the majority of these are entirely irrele-

vant to the prevention of infection. Therefore, increasing attention is being given to the identification, purification, and, frequently, molecular cloning of those antigens that evoke host-protective responses. With more complex pathogens, such as parasites, it is not immediately apparent which antigens these are, and detective work needs to be done to establish correlates of immunity. When the correct antigen has been identified, this is not the end of the story, because many pure, soluble proteins are poorly immunogenic. In fact, there is the need to balance the greater immunogenicity of whole microorganisms against the lower reactogenicity and greater conceptual elegance of molecular vaccines. This needs to be dissected on a case-by-case basis, although with more recent vaccines, such as *Haemophilus influenzae B* (Hib) and acellular pertussis, the balance appears to be swinging in the latter direction.

Vaccines have potential usefulness beyond communicable diseases. In later sections, anticancer vaccines, birth control vaccines, and vaccines aimed at lowering immune responses (e.g., in autoimmunity or allergy) will be discussed. A classification of vaccines and some examples of licensed or experimental vaccines is presented in Table 1.

Live, Attenuated Vaccines

Ever since Jenner's smallpox vaccine, live, attenuated vaccines have occupied a special place in the pantheon of vaccinology. Many viral vaccines of this type have an efficacy of greater than 90%, and protection frequently lasts for many years. This is perhaps not surprising, because the multiplication of the pathogen in the host creates an antigenic stimulus not unlike that of a natural infection in terms of antigen amount, character, and location. This key advantage is also the source of potential disadvantage, as the "miniversion" of the relevant disease can assume dangerous proportions (e.g., generalized vaccinia or BCG spread in immunodeficient or immunosuppressed children). In some vaccines, the mutations causing loss of virulence are not known. Further, mutations can restore virulence, as we have noted in the case of poliomyelitis. Much recent research has centered on more rationally planned attenuation based on an understanding of the molecular determinants of virulence. Relevant genetic engineering can result in improved vaccines whereby reversion to virulence is impossible.

It must be recognized that the success of live, attenuated vaccines poses some problems as to correct maintenance of immune status. For example, in many countries, measles vaccine is given once only, and nowhere is it mandated more than twice. Will this confer the same life-long immunity as an attack of measles? We cannot be sure, and until disease eradication is achieved, we must maintain a level of alertness about booster doses in adult life. This has not been a priority area for live, attenuated or any other kind of vaccine, but it is currently the subject of much debate.

Vaccines Consisting of Killed Microorganisms

As these are nonreplicating antigens, booster doses are essential. Some are excellent vaccines with high efficacy and safety, such as the Salk injectable poliomyelitis vaccine (IPV) or the hepatitis A vaccine. Others are of poor efficacy and short duration, such as the whole cell killed injectable cholera vaccine, which has all but been abandoned. Others are partially effective, but require improvement in terms of percent protection and/or duration of immunity. These include the conventional killed influenza and typhoid vaccines. Many of these vaccines will eventually be over-

TABLE 1. *Classification of vaccines*

Types of vaccine	Some Examples of Disease		
	Viral	Bacterial	Parasitic (all x)
Live, attenuated organism	Polio, measles, mumps, rubella, varicella, yellow fever, rotavirus (x),dengue (x), hepatitis A (x)	Tuberculosis, typhoid, cholera (x), shigellosis (x), leprosy (x)	
Killed organism	Polio, influenza, rabies, Japanese B encephalitis, hepatitis A	Pertussis, typhoid, cholera, leprosy (x), Helicobacter disease (x)	Malaria (x)
Antitoxins		Diphtheria, tetanus, shigellosis (x), enterotoxic *E. coli* (x)	
Subunit vaccines, including peptide vaccines	Hepatitis B, herpes simplex type 2 (x), influenza (x), human papilloma virus (x), HIV (x), rabies (x)	*Hemophilus influenzae* B, pertussis, *H. pylori* (x), meningococci, pneumococci, typhoid	Malaria (x), schistosomiasis (x), leishmaniasis (x)
Vectored vaccines (all x)	HIV (x), measles (x), rabies (x)	Typhoid (x), cholera (x), tuberculosis (x), shigellosis (x)	Malaria (x),
Nucleic acid vaccine (all x)	HIV (x), influenza (x), herpes simplex type 2 (x), rabies (x), hepatitis B (x), hepatitis C (x), hepatitis D (x), papilloma virus (x), HTLV1 (x), cytomegalovirus (x), St. Louis encephalitis (x)	Tyhpoid (x), tuberculosis (x)	Malaria (x), schistosomiasis (x), leishmaniasis (x)

x, experimental.

taken by new and improved versions, chiefly vectored vaccines and subunit vaccines.

Antitoxins

Where disease pathology is predominantly due to a powerful exotoxin or enterotoxin, antitoxin vaccines make good sense. In some cases, an exotoxin is a bacterium's device to create sufficient tissue destruction to permit a rich growth medium to develop. That is the case in tetanus, diphtheria, and gas gangrene. Here the relevant toxoids make good vaccines. Toxoids from enterotoxins have, in general, been less successful. Now, however, a genetically detoxified derivative of the heat-labile enterotoxin (LT) of enterotoxigenic *E. coli* is showing great promise as a possible traveller's diarrhea vaccine (21). This has been achieved through site-directed mutagenesis to inactivate the adenosine diphosphate (ADP)-ribosyltransferase activity of the A subunit of LT. Equivalent mutants of cholera toxin (CT) may eventually prove even more important.

As Rappuoli has pointed out (22), our current conventional diphtheria and tetanus vaccines contain many impurities, and, furthermore, the formaldehyde treatment needed to turn the toxins into toxoids also causes cross-linkage of beef peptides present in the culture medium, resulting in unnecessary antigens being present in the final preparation. Scientifically, one could mount an argument for a mutant, nontoxic pure molecule, such as CRM197, as a new vaccine. CRM197 is a cross-reacting material to diphtheria toxin, containing a single glycine to glutamic acid substitution at position 52, rendering the toxin inactive. Despite scientific attractiveness, there is not much commercial pressure for changing vaccines that are working well. Doubtless, if the acellular pertussis component of DPT continues to impress with its lack of reactogenicity, more pressure may build up for the D and T components to be free of side effects, so ongoing research should be encouraged.

Subunit Vaccines, Including Peptide Vaccines

The recombinant DNA era has brought forward a plethora of antigenic molecules that are pure and that have been chosen in animal models through their capacity to provoke an immune response that is host-protective. Some subunit vaccines, such as Hib and acellular pertussis, result from extremely elegant research, which warrants description in its own right (see the sections on viral and bacterial vaccines) Whereas some subunit vaccines, such as HBsAg, are highly immunogenic at low dose, others have been of disappointing strength, and require adjuvants more powerful than the aluminium salts currently used to adsorb pure proteins onto small particles. As a group, subunit vaccines have been more expensive than older vaccines. This is a major barrier to use in developing countries, but it need not be a permanent situation. The new-generation vaccines have been the result of extensive and expensive research, costs that must be recouped. Furthermore, they have not yet enjoyed the huge volume of sales of, say, the six traditional EPI vaccines. Doubtless, mass production technology will drive costs down, as will increased competition on expiration of patent protection.

Peptide vaccines, usually synthesized rather than genetically engineered, have not really taken off, though they retain their ardent proponents. The most interesting relevant research is in HIV and malaria. A further future use may be in cancer vaccines, where quite a few tumor-associated T-cell epitopes have been identified. Relevant aspects will be taken up in later sections.

Vectored Vaccines

Bernard Moss and Enzo Paoletti independently opened up a major chapter in vaccinology when they demonstrated that genes for important antigens could be introduced into the vaccinia virus without perturbing its replication, and could be expressed in host cells where the virus was dividing (23–25). This "Trojan horse" concept, in which harmless microorganisms act as vectors for antigen genes, has now been extended in innumerable directions. Among other important vectors in use experimentally are vaccinia variants, avipoxviruses, adenoviruses, polio viruses, herpes viruses, *Salmonella, Shigella,* and BCG bacterial species, and doubtless many more. The power of the concept is that it combines the best of two worlds: the force of a live, attenuated vaccine and the scientific precision of the rational subunit vaccine approach. Furthermore, given the large size of the vaccinia genome, or, for that matter, the genomes of some of the other vectors, it is feasible to consider the insertion of quite a few antigen genes, thus covering several diseases at once. It is also straightforward to incorporate one or more cytokine genes in the construct, should this be desirable for either the strength of the immune response or the direction it should take.

It is now 15 years since the concept was first introduced, but no relevant vaccine is yet on the market. Clinical investigation has been somewhat limited so far. There are understandable reservations about the use of unmodified vaccinia, particularly in an age in which HIV is rife, because it can be dangerous in people with an ineffective T-cell system, a reservation that could be countered by the inclusion of the interleukin-2 (IL-2) gene in the construct, which prevents athymic nude mice from succumbing to vaccinia (26). A number of vaccinia strains lacking genes that contribute to virulence have been prepared and are in clinical trial. Also, non-replicating viral vectors, such as canary-pox in humans, can be considered (27). The field has doubtless been slowed up somewhat by poor responses in early clinical trials of experimental HIV and malaria vaccines. Still, the overwhelming weight of preclinical data, with disease protection against at least 20 pathogens in at least 15 species, suggests that further research must eventually be crowned with success. It should be noted that the approach induces excellent T-cell, including cytotoxic T-cell, immunity.

Experimentation with bacterial vectors is not yet as far advanced, but examples will be taken up when we consider enteric and intracellular pathogens.

Nucleic Acid Vaccines

Few areas of experimental vaccinology have emerged as surprisingly and developed as explosively as that of nucleic acid vaccines, also known as DNA vaccines or naked DNA vaccines. Two preludes to the actual discovery warrant mention. Wolff et al. (28), using plasmid DNA coding for a reporter gene, found that DNA injected as a saline solution and without the adjunct agents normally used for transfection, could cause synthesis of the reporter protein in the recipient animal. This surprising finding came from a control group where the real hope for the experimental group was uptake of liposomes containing DNA. Of various injection sites tested, intramuscular injection worked best. The total number of myotubes transfected within the injection region is 1% to 5%. The second prelude relates to a DNA delivery system, originally developed by an agricultural firm, Agrecetus, first used as a means of transfecting plant cells. This Accell gene delivery system, also termed the *gene gun,* consists of a helium gas pressure-driven device capable of delivering into very superficial layers of tissue tiny gold particles coated with plasmid DNA. These DNA-coated microprojectiles could, for example, be delivered to the skin of mice, resulting in the synthesis of the relevant protein (29). It was not long before each of these two approaches was used to

elicit immune responses in the mouse. The gene gun approach induced antibody formation against human growth hormone and human α1 antitrypsin in the first demonstration that DNA immunization could work (30). Furthermore, the prolonged persistence of encoded protein in the serum signaled the probability of continued antigenic stimulation. The first demonstration of a host-protective immune response came from the intramuscular injection approach (31). Mice were injected with plasmids encoding the nucleoprotein of influenza A virus. They developed both antibodies and major histocompatibility complex (MHC) class I–restricted cytotoxic T-lymphocytes (CTLs). Upon challenge with a virulent influenza A strain, PR/8, 100% of treated mice survived, whereas 100% of controls were dead by day 9 (32). Almost simultaneously, Fynan et al. (33) also protected mice against PR/8, using the gene gun and DNA encoding the relevant hemagglutinin as the antigen. Following these two striking results, the field really took off. A scant 4 years later, Donnelly et al. (34) were able to review an extraordinary range of preclinical studies showing humoral and T-cell responses protective against a wide range of viruses, bacteria, and parasites, as well as various tumor models. Furthermore, the approach worked in a range of species including subhuman primates.

What are the essential features of nucleic acid vaccines? The key difference from the live vector approach is that the DNA encoding the antigen of interest cannot replicate in the human or animal body. The plasmids concerned are usually grown in *E. coli.* Their origin of replication is not suitable for mammalian cells. It is important to include a strong promoter element suitable for high-level gene expression in mammalian cells, for example, the immediate–early promoter of the human cytomegalovirus (CMV) (35) works well. The construct should also have an appropriate mRNA transcript termination–polyadenylation sequence. After intramuscular injection, the DNA enters the cytoplasm and then the nucleus of the myocyte, but it is not integrated into the genome. Neither muscle cells nor the dendritic cells (DCs), which are the target of the gene gun approach, have a high rate of division, nor do they show extensive homology with the plasmid, so homologous recombination is highly unlikely. Random integration remains a formal possibility, but, so far, no adverse effects have been noted. Gene expression is probably not at a high level. There are virtually no quantative data on this question, but it seems likely that antigen would leak out of myocytes for long periods, whereas, in the case of the gene gun, the gold particles deposited in the epidermis would soon find their way into Langerhans' cells, which would then make their way to local lymph nodes. In the case of intramuscular injection, it is clear that it is not the myocyte itself that is the inducer of immune responses. This was approached by Fu et al. (36) in an ingenious experiment. Parental into F1 bone marrow chimeric mice were prepared such that the myocytes carried both parental MHC haplocytes, but the professional antigen-presenting cells (APCs), such as DCs, being (after an appropriate period) bone marrow–derived, carried only the bone marrow donor parental haplotype. Following reconstitution, the chimeric mice were given plasmid DNA coding for influenza virus nucleoprotein to generate CTLs. According to the rules of MHC restriction, as the mice possessed the thymic epithelial framework of the F1, their peripheral T cells, though of parental genotype, should be capable of recognizing antigen in the context of *both* parental haplotypes. Yet, when the CTLs were tested *in vitro,* they were clearly restricted only by the MHC alleles of the bone marrow donor. Had myocytes been the APCs creating the CTLs *in vivo,* this would not have been the case.

Furthermore, in further chimeras, transplantation studies were done with an NP gene-transfected myoblast cell line. With appropriate choice of strains, it could be shown that H-2 incompatible myoblasts could induce CTL responses, but these, when analyzed, were restricted to the MHC haplocyte, not of the myoblast donor, but of the bone marrow donor. This clearly showed that the myoblasts acted as a source of antigen that was somehow transferred to APCs in a way that allowed processing for the MHC class I pathway. This apparent exception to the dual pathway rules is an example of cross-priming, which has been noted in other systems (37). The efficacy of DNA vaccines in generating CTLs has been a common feature of most examples so far studied.

The potential advantages of nucleic acid vaccines are numerous. The subunit approach to pure molecular vaccines can be seriously hampered by incorrect folding and/or glycosylation of antigens, which can present formidable problems and add to the cost of such vaccines. This should be largely obviated in DNA vaccines. Once an appropriate DNA vaccine has been engineered, it should be stable and batch variation should be minimal, facilitating quality control procedures. In terms of actual manufacturing procedure, nucleic acid vaccines should be relatively cheap. Multivalency could be achieved either by coinjection of a mixture of plasmids (38) or by constructing complex plasmids, though this appears not to have been attempted. Theoretically, the persistence of antigen synthesis should lessen the need for booster injections, though, in practice, nearly all of the preclinical work has involved a number of DNA doses. It does appear, however, that excellent CTL priming can be achieved with remarkably small amounts of DNA, sometimes in the nanogram range.

Close scrutiny of published results shows, not unexpectedly, a variation in efficacy of DNA vaccines from antigen to antigen and from species to species. The initial combination of mice and influenzal antigens appears to have been a particularly felicitous one, inducing high and persistent antibody levels and strong CTL responses. Some of the early studies with the genes for HIV envelope protein were quantitatively inferior. For example, Robinson's group found that antibody titers to the envelope protein were moderate and declined after boosting (39). This has prompted investigation into the combined effects of DNA and protein immunization. It is generally believed that an effective AIDS vaccine will need to elicit both strong neutralizing antibody and a strong CTL response to destroy HIV-infected cells. A study by Letvin et al. (40) has shown that rhesus monkeys can develop powerful and persistent HIV-1 envelope-specific CTL responses following DNA immunization, but with disappointing levels of neutralizing antibody. However, the addition of HIV-1 envelope protein itself, combined with the DNA preparation, constitutes a most effective booster, resulting in high levels of neutralizing antibody. In a small number of monkeys, a DNA prime/DNA + protein boost protected monkeys from infection with an HIV-1–simian immunodeficiency virus (SIV) chimeric virus. Obviously, the need for a protein as well as DNA complicates the protocol and would add greatly to expense.

It is clear that something as novel as nucleic vaccines will present substantial problems for the regulatory agencies. As well as the carcinogenicity–insertional mutagenesis possibility, the conjectural hazards include autoimmunity to DNA or as a result of immune-mediated destruction of antigen-expressing cells. The latter could lead to damage directly and/or could occasion the release of intracellular antigens, which would then provoke autoimmunity. In practice, however, induction of autoimmunity to autologous constituents is quite difficult and proceeds only with the use of strong adjuvants like Freund's complete adjuvant. Another objection that has been raised is the possibility that a constant leak of small quantities of antigen over a prolonged period could lead to immunologic tolerance, thus making the recipient incapable of responding to the antigen in question. This has not been encountered in any situation so far.

In the event, clinical experimentation has been allowed to begin, though with due caution. At the time of writing, the author is aware of three clinical trials that have begun—two with HIV vaccines and one with an influenza vaccine—and there are almost certainly more studies underway. None of these have yet been reported, although they may well be in the public domain by the time this volume is printed. Considering the youth of the field, progress has been remarkable. Very little attention has yet been given to augmenting DNA uptake, optimizing in vivo gene expression, or modulating resultant responses. One particularly encouraging exception was the combined use of IL-12 and HIV antigen in a single plasmid, which markedly increased the antigen-specific CTL response and shifted immunity towards Th1 in a mouse model (41). It is difficult to avoid real excitement about the promise of this field. At the same time, informal information is leaking out that, quantitatively, the responses in humans are much weaker than in mice. This could well be primarily a dosage effect. Clearly, a great deal more research is required to turn dream into reality.

Edible Vaccines

The idea of edible vaccines, resulting from the expression of antigenic proteins in transgenic plants, comes from Arntzen and colleagues (42). In the first instance, the gene for HBsAg was inserted into cells of tobacco plants, and these produced antigen that was immunogenic on injection. The heat-labile enterotoxin of E. coli has been engineered into potatoes, which accumulate 1 mg per raw potato. The virus capsid antigen of Norwalk virus has been similarly engineered, and 5-g samples were fed to mice, which produced serum and secretory antibodies. Currently, effort is being directed at the genetic engineering of bananas. The long-term hope is the possibility of a multisubunit vaccine, including an oral adjuvant, which could be eaten, and could be cheap and acceptable in a Third World setting.

ADJUVANTS AND PRINCIPLES OF MUCOSAL IMMUNITY

There is a surprising degree of variability in the immunogenicity of pure proteins. Something like a foreign serum protein is very poorly immunogenic in pure, soluble form. Yet, highly purified bacterial flagellins, injected without adjuvants of any kind, are immunogenic in picogram amounts (43). There has been relatively little systematic study of this paradox. Factors such as capacity to activate the alternative complement pathway or the preexistence of natural antibodies, thus permitting uptake via C3 or Fc receptors, certainly play a role. A variety of scavenger receptors also exist on APCs, facilitating uptake of molecules or particles capable of recognizing these. The "degree of foreignness" (i.e., multiplicity of epitopes not subject to self-tolerance) also comes into play. Whatever the details may be, antigens have to be associated with APCs in order to be immunogenic. Even as simple a matter as route of administration can be determining, with intravenous injection of soluble, deaggregated antigen favoring tolerance induction, but subcutaneous injection permitting sufficient association with APCs to result in immunity. As early as 1926, Glenny et al. (44) noted that alum precipitation of diphtheria toxoid (DT), creating a mico-particulate antigen, considerably increased immunogenicity.

The immune system evolved (at least chiefly) to deal with microbes, and it was realized quite early that microbes had several advantages as immunogens. Their particulate nature and degree of foreignness helped, but, beyond that, they possessed molecules that nonspecifically raised immune responsiveness. Killed tubercle bacilli were rich in this property, and, when combined with the absorption-delaying effects of mineral oil, create the strong but too toxic Freund's complete adjuvant (45). Ever since Freund, the search has been on for bacteria-derived immune response–strengthening molecules that are safe and lacking in side effects. Even in Freund's day, it was realized that the exact formulation of an adjuvant could guide the immune response. Freund's complete adjuvant promotes both antibody formation and delayed-type hypersensitivity (DTH) reactions to the antigen with which it is mixed, but Freund's incomplete adjuvant, lacking the mycobacteria, promotes antibody formation only.

Adjuvants, then, are substances and formulations that have the capacity to increase the immune response to an antigen. While a number of adjuvants are licensed for veterinary use, aluminium salts are currently the only adjuvants allowed to be used in humans, and alum is not registered as such but only as a part of each specific vaccine formulation. In asking why this may be so, two chief reasons come to mind. First, it has clearly proven extremely difficult to preserve immunogenicity while losing toxicity. Second, the field of research has been somewhat chaotic, not commanding the same academic respect as, for example, molecular or cellular immunology, thus lacking the quality of discovery building on discovery. On the whole, each commercial firm interested in the field has simply gone its own way, with little collaboration between the groups. One has the impression that both of these reasons are losing their force as vaccinology moves forward.

A classification of adjuvants is difficult because, in practice, most adjuvants make use of several different principles. Table 2 presents several different principles by which adjuvants act. It is immediately apparent that the headings overlap.

Rendering Antigens Particulate

Alum precipitation, as already mentioned, was introduced early into vaccinology and underlies diphtheria, tetanus, hepatitis B, and other vaccines. With the use of aluminium hydroxide or aluminium phosphate, the antigen in question becomes incorporated into an insoluble, gel-like precipitate or else is bound to preformed gel by electrostatic interactions. The particles that form are 0.1 to 1 µM in diameter. Alum-precipitated antigens cause good antibody formation, including IgE, but little DTH or CD8$^+$ T cell–mediated cyto-

TABLE 2. *Some factors promoting the immunogenicity of antigens*

Rendering antigens particulate
Polymers and polymerization of antigens
Emulsions and adjuvant formulations
Microencapsulation of antigens
Bacteria and bacterial products
Other chemical adjuvants
Cytokines
Agents targeting antigens to APC

toxicity. Equally early, it was noted that poorly immunogenic proteins could be made more immunogenic by simple mild heat aggregation. But modern particles are much more sophisticated.

One very useful property is that of self-assembly. For example, flagellin readily self-assembles into polymerized flagellin, which possesses many of the physical characteristics of flagella. HBsAg self-assembles into a virus-like particle. This helps not only its own immunogenicity, but also that of other antigens associated with it.

Liposomes, virosomes, and immunostaining complexes (ISCOMs) are other examples of particulate entities that have been used as adjuvants. We shall begin with a description of ISCOMs, because there is currently a major effort going into making them a commercially viable concept.

ISCOMs consist of submicron particles, which form when virus preparations are treated with saponin. Such an ISCOM consists essentially of cholesterol, saponin, phospholipid, and viral envelope proteins. Morein's group (46) noted that these cagelike structures could be used as a general adjuvant to which other proteins could become associated. ISCOMs formed in the absence of viral proteins are hollow, spherical, negatively charged particles with a mean particle size of 40 nM. Such preformed ISCOMs or ISCOM matrix particles can be used as a carrier, even for peptide vaccines (47). Critical to the success of the ISCOM is the saponin, which forms 60% to 70% of the composition by weight. Saponins are plant derivatives, and it was found that saponins derived from the South American tree *Quillaia saponaria* were particularly effective at nonspecifically stimulating immune responses (48). A semipurified fraction, Quil A, has been chiefly used in ISCOMs to date. However, Quil A can be further purified into a least 22 fractions, of which one, QS21, appears to be the best (49). Cholesterol is equally important in ISCOMs, as it is the only lipid that, reacting with saponin, produces the cagelike structure. A small amount of phospholipid, such as phosphatidyl choline or phosphatidylethanolamine, is also essential to create the ISCOM matrix. The antigens that have been most prominently incorporated into ISCOMs are proteins possessing a hydrophobic transmembrane domain. These amphipathic molecules are integrated into the lipid–saponin structure when the detergent is removed. Incorporation of nonamphipathic molecules (ovalbumin, peptides) can be achieved after acid treatment, but this may well be simply an association rather than a true insertion into the structure. A great deal of research on how to achieve true incorporation is being conducted (48). No totally satisfactory method to predictably insert high levels of hydrophilic proteins has yet been designed.

ISCOMS promote not only antibody formation, but also good DTH and CTL formation. Like liposomes, some ISCOMs appear to enter the APCs without going through the endocytic pathway. Thus, they achieve the necessary class I–restricted antigen presentation. Because of this efficacy in multiple limbs of immunity, ISCOMs have proven valuable in many experimental animal models, including vaccines against viruses, bacteria, and parasites. There is a registered veterinary ISCOM-based vaccine for equine influenza, and CSL in Australia has commenced phase I clinical trial work in humans with an ISCOM-influenza vaccine.

Liposomes have some but not all of the features of ISCOMs. Alving's group has obtained a good adjuvant effect using liposomes with cholera and malaria antigens. They have also obtained quite promising results using envelope protein peptides in a macaque monkey SIV trial (50). The liposomes contain dimyristoyl phosphatidyl choline, dimyristoyl phosphatidyl glycerol, cholesterol, and monophosphoryl lipid A. In some experiments, liposomes were alum-adsorbed. Liposomes have also acted as adjuvants for DT (51), tetanus toxoid (TT) (52), and a variety of hepatitis antigens (52). There is a great capacity to vary the particle size of liposomes, from about 20 nM up to more than 10 μM in diameter. In general, liposomes are best used in combination with some other adjuvant.

Virosomes are multimeric aggregates of virus-derived transmembrane proteins (e.g., influenza hemagglutinin), and proteosomes are similar multimers of bacterial transmembrane proteins. They consist of 60- to 100-nM vesicles or membrane vesicle fragments. Amphipathic immunogens can be incorporated into these structures. These agents do not induce cell-mediated immunity unless an appropriate further adjuvant is added. Microencapsulation represents a special kind of particle that will be discussed further below.

Polymers and Polymerization of Antigens

There are other ways of effecting a polymerization of antigens, such as association with polymers. Nonionic block copolymers, usually used as additives to adjuvants employing an emulsion, are polymers of polyoxypropylene and polyoxyethylene, with which antigen can be associated. They have been used as components of complex adjuvant formulations by both Syntex (SAF-1, Syntex Adjuvant Formulation-1) and Ribi Chemical Co. These formulations induce a good Th1 response.

Carbohydrate polymers of mannose (e.g., mannan) or of β1-3 glucose (e.g., glucan) have been used in similar fashion (53,54). It is possible to conjugate peptides to mannan via an aminocaproic spacer, and thereby to produce a good antibody response (55). Mannan can also enhance the adjuvant properties of lipopolysaccharides (LPSs) (56). Part of the action may be due to the stimulation of macrophages, which have a mannan-binding receptor. An interesting series of studies from McKenzie's group has demonstrated that the way an antigen is conjugated to mannan can be very important. It had previously been shown (57) that proteins coupled to mannan can stimulate good cell-mediated immune responses. Apostoulopoulos et al. (58), working with mice, claim that if the conjugation of antigen to mannan is done under oxidizing conditions, the resultant conjugated polymer selectively stimulates Th1 responses, with good DTH, marked CTL generation, but low antibody titers, and T cells secreting predominantly interferon-γ (IFN-γ). When reducing conditions are used, the reverse is true: This polymer selects for a Th2 response, with IL-4 production, good IgG1 antibody production, but poor CTL generation. Obviously, the former preparation should prove far superior as a cancer vaccine, and the group is currently testing this, using Muc-1 as a tumor-associated antigen.

Jackson's group (59) has reported a generic method for the assembly of multipeptide polymers, which results in highly antigenic preparations. The basic principle is that peptides are synthesized in the solid phase, the N-terminal residue is acryloylated, and after cleavage, the derivitized peptides are polymerized by free radical-induced polymerization. The peptides used can be the same or different. Multiple B- and T-cell epitopes can be incorporated into the final construct. The approach has been validated with peptides from influenza virus, malaria parasites, tetanus toxin, and various model proteins.

Tripalmitoyl-S-glycerine cysteine (Pam₃Cys), derived from a lipoprotein of *E. coli,* has strong adjuvant properties. This can be covalently coupled to peptides, creating a "built-in" adjuvant (60).

Pam₃Cys has also been used by Tam's group (61), who introduced the concept of multiple antigen peptide (MAP), using an oligomeric branching lysine as the core. There are many variations on this theme of peptide polymerization. This lively field will be of particular relevance as more disease-protective T-cell epitopes are defined.

Promoting Slow Antigen Release

An antigen depot was one of the major ideas behind Freund's adjuvants. Thus, emulsions and emulsifying agents have been central to adjuvant research. Extensive clinical trials were done early on with Freund's incomplete adjuvant in influenza vaccine trials, but regulatory approval was not forthcoming (62). These water-in-oil emulsions consist of tiny droplets of water stabilized by a surfactant such as mannide monooleate in a continuous phase of mineral oil or other oils, such as squalene or squalane. Obviously, water-soluble immunostimulants can be incorporated into the watery droplets. An alternative approach is to use oil-in-water emulsions. Extensive work has been done with a preparation of Chiron's, known as MF59 (63). In this adjuvant, the oil droplets consist of the metabolizable oil squalene and are 150 nM in diameter. The emulsifying agents are a carefully chosen mixture of Tween 80 and Span 85, and chemical immunomodulators such as the derivative of muramyl dipeptide, muramyl tripeptide–phosphatidyl ethanolamine (MTP-PE), can be added or not, as desired (64). Small amounts of polysorbate 80 and sorbitan trioleate are also present. The antigen does not associate firmly with the oil droplets, yet somehow the adjuvant markedly helps lymph node localization of antigen. MF59 is a good promoter of antibody formation and stimulates Th1 cells. It induces CTLs in some but not all situations. MF59 has now been administered to some 8,000 people in trials of HIV, herpes simplex virus (HSV), CMV, and hepatitis B virus (HBV) vaccines sponsored by Chiron. It is impressively safe and minimally reactogenic without MTP-PE. The addition of MTP-PE does increase reactogenicity, but this seems not to have been a problem in the context of HIV-seropositive persons included in a therapeutic HIV vaccine trial.

SAF-1 (65) is Syntex's oil-in-water adjuvant, consisting of Pluronic L121, squalene, and Tween 80, to which appropriate concentrations of immunomodulators are added. SAF emulsion and the antigen solution are then gently mixed for 2 to 3 minutes. This adjuvant has been successful in inducing antibody formation in at least 11 species, using at least ten antigens.

Microencapsulation of Antigens

This idea combines several desirable principles for adjuvants. Biodegradable microcapsules are particulate. They can enclose immunostimulatory molecules as well as antigen. They delay absorption of antigen and act as long-term depots. Best of all, they offer the hope that different chemical compositions will create particles that release their antigen as a pulse at various defined times after injection. Variables that affect the timing of release include particle size and the composition of the polymer. An ideal preparation would be a mixture of particles dissolving at intervals to mimic a primary dose and two different booster doses.

Several laboratories share the credit for the development of controlled-release vaccine through encapsulation. The idea of biodegradable microcapsules containing antigens was promoted by Chang (66) and put into practice by Langer (67). The currently most popular material, the polymer poly (lactide-co-glycolide)

(PLG), was first used by O'Hagan et al. (68) and Eldridge et al. (69). This material was a happy choice, as PLG has been used for many years as a biodegradable suture material. In that context, it has shown itself to be safe and nonreactogenic. PLG degrades by hydrolysis. How long this takes is determined both by chain length and by the ratio of lactide to glycolide in the polymer (70). The WHO has sponsored a considerable amount of work on PLG, in the hope of coming up with a "one-shot" formulation, which, in the first instance, could be applied to the problem of neonatal tetanus in developing countries. As infant immunization rates were low for women of child-bearing age, WHO programs aim to immunize pregnant women with TT so that the newborn infant would be protected by antibodies crossing the placenta. However, it is difficult to persuade women to make three trips to their local health center, which may require hours of walking. Once the controlled-release strategy has been perfected for this purpose, it could be adapted to other vaccines, such as hepatitis B or Hib.

Many frustrating problems were encountered in this endeavor that are gradually being overcome one by one (71–73). The most important one relates to stability of antigens in microparticles, during both the manufacturing process and *in vivo*. Furthermore, while the lactide-to-glycolide ratio in PLG affects degradation rate, it was found in practice that a mixture of two different sets of microcapsules did not result in sharp peaks of antigen release, but continuous release over a period. This seems to produce satisfactory antibody responses (74,75). It is now clear that, in preclinical studies, one injection of antigen in microcapsules can lead to higher and more sustained antibody formation than two injections of antigen adsorbed onto alum.

Cox's group at CSL in Australia have come up with an experimental one-shot method in their formulation of a single-dose but two-component experimental influenza vaccine (76). There is an immediate-release component, which is produced by spray-drying the antigen, with or without adjuvant, in the presence of a stabilizer (e.g., trehalose). The delayed-release component consists of antigen that is encapsulated in a PLG matrix. An aqueous solution of influenza A/PR8 virus, ISCOMs, and trehalose is emulsified into a solution of PLG in methylene chloride. The resultant water-in-oil emulsion is also spray-dried. Shortly before use, the two components are mixed and suspended in buffer with 0.1% Tween 80. Such a formulation significantly outperformed a single injection of a liquid preparation and, in fact, resembled two spaced doses in efficacy.

Cyanoacrylates are another form of biodegradable polymer. For example, poly (butyl-2-cyanoacrylate) has been used as an adjuvant for oral immunization (77).

The use of PLG and other microparticles is under extensive investigation for the mucosal administration of vaccines. Particles of very small size (nanoparticles) may be even more suitable. Digestion in the stomach needs to be combated, perhaps by enteric coated polymers, and coating with substances that increase intestinal absorption may be necessary. Delivery via the respiratory tract (e.g., via intranasal immunization or aerosol administration) is a good possibility for respiratory pathogens. Rectal and vaginal delivery is also possible. As there is a great deal of "cross-talk" between the various components of the mucosal immune system, and as oral delivery is, by far, the most practical, this deserves full experimental exploration in the first instance.

Biodegradable microparticles can induce T-cell immunity, including CD8+ CTLs, as well as just antibody formation. For example, HIV envelope proteins contained in PLG particles induced HIV-specific CD4+ and CD8+ T-cell responses in mice

(78). Similarly, microparticles out-performed incomplete Freund's adjuvant in promoting Th1 CD4+ T-cell responses using a subunit antigen from *M. tuberculosis* (79). The addition of cytokines or chemical adjuvants to further enhance these T-cell effects remains to be explored.

Bacteria and Bacterial Products

In experimental immunology, various bacteria other than killed *M. tuberculosis* are used as adjuvants. It appears that if a killed bacterial preparation is itself highly antigenic, the adjuvant power spills over to the response to an antigen coadministered with it. Some guidance may also be given to the response. Killed *Bordetella pertussis* organisms are a strong Th2–antibody formation adjuvant for pure protein antigens. *Corynebacterium parvum* is more of a Th1 adjuvant. Turning to a parasite, *Nippostrongylus brasiliensis* has long been used if one wishes to elicit powerful IgE responses.

Review of the large older literature on the results of extracting bacteria and seeking the immunopotentiating agent is beyond the scope of this chapter. Both peptide and lipid components are important. Since the early work of Lederer's group (80), *N*-acetyl-muramyl-*L*-analyl-*D*-isoglutamine, or muramyl dipeptide (MDP), has been used as a cell-mediated immunity (CMI) and antibody-inducing adjuvant. Chedid et al. (81) have proposed a less pyrogenic, less toxic synthetic MDP (murabutide), whereas Allison and Byars favor threonyl MDP (82) and, as already described, MTP-PE has been used by the Chiron group. The lipid adjuvants are portions of the LPS endotoxins of gram-negative bacteria, such as *Escherichia, Salmonella,* and *Pseudomonas.* These LPS molecules are powerful adjuvants but much too toxic. The lipid A structure has been chemically modified to lower toxicity but retain adjuvanticity. Monophosphoryl lipid A (MPL) is the best product remaining from this line of research (83). The enterotoxins as adjuvants will be taken up below.

Other Chemical Adjuvants

Many chemicals have been used as immunopotentiators from time to time (84). These include the polynucleotide poly-I:C and poly-A:U; vitamin D3, dextran sulphate, inulin, dimethyl dioctadecyl ammonium bromide (DDA), avridine, carbohydrate polymers similar to mannan (already discussed), and trehalose dimycolate, to name just a few. Which, if any, of these progress towards the marketplace will largely depend on the pharmaceutical companies. Two very interesting new chemical adjuvants are being promoted by two biotechnology companies. These are polyphosphazines (initially introduced as slow release–promoting agents) and a *Leishmania* protein, LeIF.

Cytokines

The effect of cytokines on immune responses needs to be considered at three levels. First, cytokines can stimulate APCs, activating them and/or causing their division. Second, cytokines can help in the activation and multiplication of lymphocytes. Third, cytokines can guide the immune response, for example, influencing the question of whether antigen causes more a "Th1" or a "Th2"type of CD4+ T-cell response, or influencing the antibody isotype formed. Despite the great interest in this field, there has not yet been much clinical exploration of the issue. Of course, cytokines as such are expensive and can be quite toxic. The use of cytokine genes in vectored vaccines is an alternative approach.

IL-2 was the first cytokine investigated for adjuvant potential. In a vaccinia model, it turns out that IL-2 can potentiate the immune response in monkeys (85) and in congenitally athymic nude mice, but not in euthymic mice (26). Some limited clinical experimentation suggests that IL-2 can enhance the human antibody response to influenza virus. IL-2 can also be helpful if injected into lesions of lepromatous leprosy, reverting the status to one more akin to tuberculoid leprosy. IL-2 is very toxic in high dose.

IL-4 is a very interesting cytokine with multiple effects on the immune system. If IL-4 is present early during a T-cell response, it veers the response in a Th2 direction, causing the production of more IL-4, constituting a positive-feedback loop (86,87). At the same time, there is a suppression of Th1 T-cell development (e.g., a marked inhibition of IFN-γ production). The sources of the early surge of IL-4 are controversial, with conventional CD4$^+$ T cells, NKI-1$^+$, T cells, basophils, and eosinophils being the main contenders. IL-10 has a somewhat similar effect. In contrast, IL-12 has a completely opposite effect (88). Monocytes and macrophages are the chief producers of IL-12, but DCs also make it (89). Bacteria can directly infect macrophages, leading to IL-12 production, and bacterial products can stimulate macrophages to produce IL-12. Particularly if IL-4 is not present, or is neutralized by anti–IL-4 antibodies, IL-12 drives Th1 T-cell development, leading to high levels of IFN-γ and to cell-mediated immunity. Thus, the relative levels of IL-4 later produced by Th2 cells themselves and IL-12 (produced by macrophages and DCs) determine the Th2/Th1 balance of immunity.

IL-4 is also a key influence on B cells, being involved in their early activation from the resting state and in the isotope switch from predominant IgM production to the synthesis of IgG1 and IgE (90). A variety of other cytokines can drive the B-cell response in different directions. Thus transforming growth factor-β (TGF-β) is implicated in the switch to IgA (91), and IFN-γ in the switch to IgG2a.

IL-6 is a potent stimulator of terminal differentiation of plasma cells, and thus of antibody formation. It has also been suggested that IL-6 can stimulate IL-4 production and might be an influence in the early IL-4 surge that leads to a Th2 response. IL-6 is itself too toxic to be seriously considered as an adjuvant.

IL-10 is a cytokine with possible therapeutic potential in that it can damp down Th1-type inflammatory responses. It also down-regulates tumor necrosis factor-α (TNF-α) and IL-1 production. Currently, the focus is chiefly on IL-10 as a possible therapy in autoimmunity, and it is not under consideration as an adjuvant.

The cytokine granulocyte–macrophage colony-stimulating factor (GM-CSF) and the cell-associated FLT-3 ligand are stimulators of DCs. Their adjuvant potential will be considered in the section on cancer vaccines. Suffice it to say here that soluble FLT-3 ligand given with protein antigens markedly enhances T-cell and serum antibody responses (B. Pulendran, personal communication).

One example of the effects of cytokines exogenously administered together with a vaccine is the work of Schijns et al. (92). They investigated the effects of TNF-α, IL-1α, IL-2, and IFN-γ on the response of mice to an inactivated rabies virus vaccine. While all the cytokines increased virus-specific IgG responses, TNF-α and IL-1α did not enhance virus-neutralizing antibody and only marginally raised resistance to challenge infection. In contrast, IL-2 and IFN-γ did raise neutralizing antibody levels and allowed lower levels of antigen to protect mice. A combination of IFN-γ and IL-2

acted synergistically. These particular investigators were optimistic about the role of cytokines in vaccination.

Clearly, the field of cytokines as adjuvants is in a very early exploratory stage. It seems more likely that existing adjuvants stimulating the formation of particular cytokines or cytokine combinations will constitute a more practical focus of interest than cytokines as such. In the longer term, however, cytokine genes might well find a place in the more sophisticated vectored or DNA vaccines.

Molecular Targeting of Antigens

Many of the strategies considered above depend on efficient ways of bringing antigens to the APCs. The role of C3 and Fc receptors on APCs is critical. An experiment of Fearon's group documents the point (93). Mice were immunized either with hen egg lysozyme (HEL) prepared through recombinant DNA technology, or, alternatively, with HEL fused to one, two, or three copies of C3d. It is known that C3d binds to CR2 receptors. HEL itself and the three model antigens were injected into mice at various doses and without any adjuvant. HEL-C3d$_1$ was found to suppress the T-dependent IgG1 antibody response, but not consistently, so this construct was dropped from the study. No dose of HEL under 500 pmol caused antibody formation, but 5 fmol of HEL-C3d$_3$ and 500 fmol of HEL-C3d$_2$ elicited a primary response. In terms of ELISA titer, HEL-C3d$_2$ was about 1,000-fold and HEL-C3d$_3$ about 10,000-fold a stronger immunogen than was HEL. In that respect, attachment of C3d was about 100-fold more effective than Freund's complete adjuvant. When mice were given a booster dose of 50 pmol of HEL in incomplete Freund's adjuvant, these relative differences were approximately maintained. Thus, the targeting of antigen to APCs including follicular DCs is equally effective in augmenting primary antibody responses and immunologic memory. The feasibility of such targeting in a "real life" vaccination setting certainly warrants early preclinical exploration.

This general approach of covalent association of a targeting molecule with an antigen is validated in a mucosal model to be explored further below. Sun et al. (94) coupled minute amounts of antigens covalently to the B subunit of CT (CTB), a known powerful mucosal adjuvant. A single dose of the conjugate given orally markedly suppressed the systemic immune response capacity of unimmunized mice, as measured both by DTH induction and antibody formation. The preparation was up to 500-fold more effective than unconjugated antigen. Even mice that had been preimmunized could be rendered tolerant by feeding CTB antigen. The technique works not just for pure proteins but also for autoantigens (95), alloantigens, and haptens. It may thus have relevance to autoimmune diseases, transplant rejection, and allergy.

Adjuvants for Mucosal Surfaces

It has been estimated that the combined surface area of the mucosas of the gastrointestinal, respiratory, and urogenital tracts is 400 M^2 (96). The total lymphocyte complement of the mucosal immune system is greater than that of the lymph nodes and spleen. The mucosal immune system includes organized collections of lymphoid tissue, such as the tonsils, adenoids, Peyer's patches, and appendix, and also single lymphoid follicles. These collections contain macrophages and DCs, sample antigens, and generate both T- and B-cell responses, including germinal center formation. There is a high proportion of IgA in the antibody formed. There is also extensive infiltration of epithelia and the lamina propria with lymphocytes and plasma cells. It is believed that these represent effector cells and that there is no immune induction within these latter sites.

Two types of antigen-capturing cells are of importance in mucosal immunity. These are the intraepithelial DCs and M cells. In stratified or pseudostratified epithelia, there are DCs that serve much the same function as skin Langerhans' cells, and that extend right to the surface. In tracheal epithelium, for example, there are up to 700 such cells per mm², forming an almost contiguous network (97). As in the case of Langerhans' cells, these DCs take antigen to draining lymph nodes for immune induction (98). The M cells are unique features of the mucosal immune system. They exist in the epithelium overlying organized collections such as Peyer's patches. Their job is to take up antigens from the mucosa and to deliver them to the mucosal lymphoid tissue (99) via a specialized pocket in the epithelium. M cells are active in taking up both macromolecular antigens and particulate antigens such as bacteria (100) and essentially serve to channel them to professional APCs in the lymphoid collections beneath. M-cell membranes contain the glycolipid GM1, to which CT can bind, and a variety of other carbohydrate structures with selective binding activity. Bacteria and viruses can also exploit this capacity of M cells to take them up efficiently to infect mucosae (101). This probably includes sexual transmission of HIV.

The lymphocyte traffic pattern differs for the mucosal immune system and the conventional immune system (102). There is a distinct tendency for mucosa-associated cells to home back to mucosal tissue, but not necessarily to the same mucosa. The possibility therefore exists that one could immunize via one mucosal surface but protect an unrelated one. Nevertheless, there is some compartmentalization within the system (103).

Stimulation of immune responses via mucosal surfaces, leading to local IgA production and a variety of systemic B- and T-cell effects, suffers from the difficulty that most nonreplicating antigens lead to immune responses only after large and multiple antigen doses, and these responses are of short duration. Even natural infection may lead to shorter-lived immunity than in the case of a systemic infection. This makes the field of mucosal adjuvants particularly important.

Mucosal adjuvants include any substance or process that enhances uptake of antigen by mucosal lymphoid tissue. For example, bacteria are capable of recruiting large numbers of DCs into tracheal epithelium, and these DCs are critical to the induction of an immune response (104). Similarly, viruses can bring DCs into epithelia and can stimulate subsequent migration to draining lymph nodes (105). It has been argued that the increased susceptibility of neonates to respiratory infections is due to the hyporesponsiveness of their immature DCs to such signals (106). In more mature individuals, the inherent immunogenicity of microorganisms suggests that the use of live vectors, be they bacterial or viral, engineered to express the antigen of interest, may in itself provide sufficient adjuvanticity, albeit perhaps with a limited duration of immunity.

We have already briefly encountered the second main strategy, namely the use of particulate antigens such as liposomes and biodegradable PLG microspheres. Variations on this theme include polyphosphazenes, polyalginates, or other excipients with incorporated or adsorbed antigens.

The third main strategy is the use of lectin-like molecules endowed with immunostimulatory properties. CT is the most powerful mucosal adjuvant yet developed (107,108). *E. coli* LT is also powerful (109). Fragment C of tetanus toxin may have a somewhat

similar effect (110). These work whether the antigen in question is conjugated to them, or whether the two agents are simply coadministered (111). Chemical coupling, as already noted, can enhance effectiveness, and so can a fusion through genetic engineering.

The CTB has been strongly promoted as a mucosal adjuvant, but there is a possibility that this property might, in some instances, have been due to small amounts of contaminating CT (94). Further, it appears that CTB can act as a powerful toleragen. Is there a paradox here? Not really, because given orally, CTB plus antigen induces a powerful mucosal immunity but a systemic tolerance. Within the gut there are many "Th0" cells making IFN-γ and IL-4. Whatever the mechanism, the protective efficacy of oral inactivated whole cell cholera vaccine, administered together with a recombinant CTB (112), is thoroughly established. One possibility is that of a genuine synergy in immunogenesis between CTB and CT (113).

Obviously, the toxicity of CT and LT limits their usefulness as adjuvants. A clever strategy has been developed by Rappuoli's group, involving genetic modification of CT and LT, resulting in derivatives that are still able to assemble into a holotoxin but that have greatly diminished toxicity (21). These mutants act not only as mucosal immunogens, but also as adjuvants for coadministered bystander antigens. Two equivalent derivatives of CT and LT, known as CTK63 and LTK63, have been prepared by substitution of a single, identical amino acid. The substitution is near the NAD-binding cleft. Interestingly, LTK63 worked much better than CTK63, both for the facilitation of serum antibody and as a coinducer of IgA in nasal or lung lavages of mice, being only slightly inferior to CT itself (114). The reasons for this difference are currently entirely obscure. Indeed, the mechanisms whereby the toxins mediate immunity are poorly understood. The nature of the coadministered antigen is clearly important; there is a hierarchy of immunogenicity, as for injected antigens (114). Capacity of the adjuvant to bind to M cells is obviously essential.

The reader will by now have gathered that the field of adjuvants is not too rich in simplifying or overarching paradigms. It seems likely that empirical research will continue to dominate for some time. It may be well to end on a positive note. Combinations of the principles we have been discussing seem to be the way of the future. There have been any number of disappointing clinical trials of a malaria vaccine based on the *P. falciparum* circumsporozoite protein (CSP). Only when three separate principles of adjuvanticity were combined did a vaccine capable of protecting six of seven volunteers against mosquito-bite challenge result (115). The antigen in question is amino acids 207 to 395 of CSP, fused to the HBsAg. A corresponding DNA was prepared and yeast cells were simultaneously transfected with this construct and one coding for HBsAg itself, resulting in the production of virion-like, self-assembled particles containing CSP-specific immunogenicity. The second principle was to incorporate this in an oil-in-water emulsion. The third was to add two strong immune stimulants, MPL and QS21. All the included components were essential for protective immunity. This breakthrough, after more than a decade of frustration, has infused new hope into an extremely important field.

BACTERIAL VACCINES

The particular vaccines discussed in the next three sections are not meant as a comprehensive list of important vaccines. Rather, they are chosen to reveal recent major research achievements and to highlight future challenges.

Diphtheria and Acellular Pertussis

Historically, the diphtheria–pertussis–tetanus (DPT) combination has come to be well accepted, with perhaps 2% of the population harboring serious reservations. In view of its importance in a Third World setting and the fact that health systems are geared to it, DPT has been regarded as a "platform" on which further vaccines, such as hepatitis B, Hib, and perhaps injectable poliomyelitis vaccine, could be placed. Different countries follow different schedules for a primary course of DPT—for example, at 2, 3, or 4 months of age; 2, 4, and 6 months; or, in a developing-country setting, 6, 10, and 14 weeks. It is generally agreed that there should be three doses administered by 6 months of age. There is also variability between countries on the timing of a booster dose (e.g., 18 months or DT only at 3 to 5 years). TT plus a low dose of DT is advised again at school-leaving age, and, ideally, a further booster should be given if a person suffers a penetrating wound (for tetanus), or travels to an epidemic or endemic area (for diphtheria). As regards tetanus, five doses are regarded as conferring life-long immunity, but, as we shall see in the section on the future, this may not be correct. For diphtheria, a major recent epidemic in the countries of the former Soviet Union, including many cases among adults, has shown that initial immunization had been inadequate and/or that immunity does wane with time. In the United Kingdom, 25% of blood donors aged 20 to 29, but 53% of those aged 50 to 59, were found to have inadequate antibodies to diphtheria toxin. There has been relatively little attention given to adult reimmunization, but a movement for more aggressive immunization of older persons has begun.

We have already mentioned that genetic detoxification of diphtheria and tetanus toxins is possible, but that there has been little pressure to modify the traditional toxoid vaccines. Such is not the case for pertussis, however, which has a reputation for being reactogenic and perhaps of causing rare, more serious side effects, as will be discussed in the section on the adverse effects of vaccines. Whole, killed *B. pertussis* organisms are irritating and do cause local reactions and pyrexia in a significant proportion of infants.

For these reasons, there has been pressure for a subunit vaccine containing, not killed bacteria, but pure antigens derived from the bacteria. In fact, acellular pertussis vaccines have been in routine use in Japan since 1981 (116). Renewed interest in the United States and in Europe has resulted in the testing of no fewer than 13 acellular pertussis vaccines (117). The key antigen is pertussis toxoid (PT) (118), and other important antigens for protection are filamentous hemagglutinin (119) and pertactin. Typical of the extensive clinical research that has been done on acellular pertussis vaccines is a trial in Italy, where immunization rates are low (around 40%) and in which 2 acellular vaccines from Smith, Kline Beecham and Chiron Biocine were compared with a whole cell vaccine from Connaught Laboratories. The double-blind, randomized controlled trial involved 14,751 infants enrolled over a 1-year period between 1992 and 1993 (120). It involved 62 public health clinics and follow-up for an average of 17 months. Pertussis infection was confirmed by culture and quantitative serology. Unfortunately, the Connaught vaccine behaved quite atypically, giving only 36% protection. The two acellular vaccines behaved equivalently, giving 84% protection. Local and systemic adverse events were significantly less frequent with the two acellular vaccines, and were similar to those of a DT vaccine without the pertussis component.

The chief difference between these two vaccines was that in the Smith, Kline Beecham vaccine, the PT was detoxified by chemical treatment, whereas the Chiron Biocine vaccine contained a mutated, nontoxic form of PT that had been genetically detoxified. Site-directed mutagenesis introduced two point mutations (Arg9 → Lys and Glu129 → Gly) in the enzymic site of the PT. This vaccine caused a higher anti-PT response than that containing chemically inactivated PT, and continued blinded observation for a further year showed significantly fewer pertussis cases in the Chiron Biocine group (121). A brief review by Rappuoli (122) gives a sobering insight into what is involved in bringing a new vaccine to the market. The project started in 1984. The cloning and sequencing of the PT gene was achieved in 1985; the identification of amino acids needing to be changed to remove toxicity happened in 1987; the filamentous hemagglutinin was cloned in 1988; and the *B. pertussis* strain producing the nontoxic PT was constructed in 1989. Phased clinical trials were started as follows: phase I, 1989; phase II, 1990; phase III, 1992; end of phase III, 1995; and filing of worldwide product license application worldwide, 1996. Introduction of new and improved vaccines is not for the fainthearted!

An analysis of six different acellular pertussis vaccines from nine different trials has been presented by Klein (123). In all of these, the acellular vaccine was either statistically no different from nor more protective than the whole cell vaccine. In three of the trials, the acellular vaccine was about 10% less protective (84% versus 93%, 89% versus 98%, 85% versus 96%), but the differences did not reach statistical significance. The author is not aware of any metaanalysis of these data. It is anticipated that several of these vaccines will soon be licensed for broad use in the United States. Some are already available in Europe and elsewhere.

At the moment, different firms are going forward with vaccines containing anything from two to five (124) acellular components, the ones not yet mentioned being fimbrial antigens 2 and 3. It is too early to say whether including more antigens than two improves protective efficacy. Among other questions, it remains to be determined how long protection lasts with these newer vaccines. At the moment, there is no compelling reason to switch over to these more expensive vaccines in developing countries.

Diarrheal Disease Vaccines: Typhoid, Cholera, and *Shigella*

The search for better, orally active diarrheal disease vaccines has also been a long one, but here major success is fast approaching. The challenge will be to make these vaccines available to those who most need them, at a price that is not too formidable.

Typhoid Vaccines

Typhoid fever causes 600,000 deaths annually. A truly effective typhoid vaccine would thus be a potent public health tool. Attenuated *S. typhi* can be used as a live, oral vaccine. At the moment, the strain Ty21a, derived from wild *S. typhi* by mutagenesis, is registered in most countries. It requires three or four spaced doses, and in many markets competes with a vaccine based on a single dose of a parenteral vaccine containing the Vi polysaccharide antigen from the capsule of the organism. An analysis of the protective efficacy and immunogenicity of the Vi antigen in a South African trial was presented 3 years after its administration (125). Vaccine efficacy was estimated at 55% (95% confidence limits 30% to 71%), with persisting, significantly raised antibody levels. Given that this result is not overwhelming, the search has been on for considerably more immunogenic, but still well-tolerated, vaccines. As early as

1981, Hoiseth and Stocker (126) demonstrated that aromatic-dependent *Salmonella* bacteria, such as *S. typhimurium,* are non-virulent but nevertheless efficient immunogens. Precise deletion mutations can be engineered, for example, in the genes *aroC* and *aroD*, which render the bacteria nutritionally dependent on substrates paraaminobenzoic acid and 2,3-dihydroxy-benzoate, which are not present in high concentrations in human tissues. Such mutants and others like them have been the subject of extensive research, not only for the creation of vaccines against the organism, but also as potential vectors for other antigen genes.

One attenuated *S. typhi* strain of this type is CVD908, which has been the subject of early clinical trials (127). A dose of 5×10^7 bacteria gives impressive rises in anti-O antibody titers in serum, as well as inducing intestinal IgA formation (128). However, it does induce silent, asymptomatic, and time-limited vaccinemias, a characteristic shared by the early strains of Stocker. A modified strain, CVD908 *htr*A, a deletion mutant lacking a particular serine protease, has been developed by Chatfield et al. (129) on the basis of experimentation in an *S. typhimurium* mouse model. This attenuated variant does not cause vaccinemia but is equally immunogenic, and thus appears particularly promising as a typhoid vaccine candidate.

Both CVD908 and CVD908 *htr*A can be used as live vectors for other antigens. For example, important antigens of enterotoxigenic *E. coli* have been successfully inserted (110), and other successes have involved the carriage of tetanus, diphtheria, *Schistosoma*, and malaria antigens. Furthermore, oral feeding of CVD908 can induce cellular immunity, including CD8+ CTLs (130). It seems that this strain could prove to be a highly versatile vector with oral activity.

Cholera Vaccines

There is no satisfactory cholera vaccine on the market. Experimentally, however, there has been much progress, and, again, it may be that reasonably satisfactory answers will emerge without great expense. For example, Trach et al. (131) reported on an oral, killed, whole cell *Vibrio cholerae* vaccine, being two doses of a mixture of Inaba and Ogawa strains, which was trialled in 134,453 people in Vietnam. This vaccine was locally produced in Hanoi and was quite inexpensive (about U.S. 10 cents per dose). During an epidemic some 8 months after immunization, it proved 66% protective. Despite some admitted limitations in the trial protocol, the results are promising.

Extensive work has been done on a Swedish vaccine consisting of a mixture of the CTB and killed whole cells. In a large clinical trial in Bangladesh, conducted among 62,285 children and female adults, involving three doses, a 5-year follow-up showed a 49% efficacy of the vaccine, but, interestingly, the whole cell vaccine without CTB performed just as well (132). This result was different from what was noted in the first 6 months, when the combined vaccine worked much better. Protection was evident only during the first 3 of the 5 years, with protection better in the first 2 years than in the third. In fact, protection against *V. cholerae* 01 was 85% for 6 months and 60% for 3 years with the combined vaccine. Since this trial was initiated, a further variant of cholera emerged in Madras, India. This *V. cholerae* serogroup 0139 has spread rapidly in India, Bangladesh, and adjacent countries, and has reached as far as Malaysia, Thailand, and China. Accordingly, formalin-killed 0139 vibrios were added to the existing 01 vaccine, and intestinal and systemic immune response against both strains were elicited in a majority of human volunteers (133). This suggests that the devel-

opment of a bivalent vaccine will be relatively straightforward.

There are also live, attenuated, orally active cholera vaccines undergoing clinical trial. CVD103-HgR is a live oral cholera vaccine strain constructed by recombinant DNA methods from a classical Inaba strain in which the A subunit of CT has been deleted. This was safe and immunogenic in North American volunteers (134), provided significant protection against experimental challenge (135), and in 1993, a large scale, randomized, placebo-controlled field trial was initiated in North Jakarta involving a single oral dose of vaccine. Some 67,000 subjects aged 2 to 42 are involved. As surveillance is planned for at least 3 years, results are not available but are eagerly awaited. An attenuated 0139 live oral vaccine, known as CD112, has also been prepared and confers good protection against challenge with wild-type 0139 (136).

Pearson and colleagues (137) have constructed a new series of live, attenuated, oral cholera vaccines based on the deletion of a whole "virulence cassette" (137). Instead of deleting just the CT gene, additional associated virulence factors are deleted. These include the genes for Zot (zona occludence toxin), Ace (auxiliary cholera enterotoxin), and Cep (core-encoded pilus). Certain sequences encouraging recombination were also deleted to prevent the strain regaining CT genes. Furthermore, mobility-deficient variants were found to be less reactogenic. Volunteer studies with two of these, Peru-15 for *V. cholerae* 01 (138) and Bengal-15 for *V. cholerae* 0139, look promising for a one-dose oral vaccine.

Shigella Vaccines

Shigellosis, or bacillary dysentery, is one of the most serious causes of diarrheal disease in the world. There are many millions of cases per year, and 600,000 to 800,000 deaths are ascribable annually to this cause. The most important pathogens are *Shigella flexneri, Shigella sonnei,* and *Shigella dysenteriae*. Each exists in diverse serotypes, but in each case, certain serotypes are of prime importance (e.g., serotype 2a for *S. flexneri*). This is a more crucial public health problem than cholera, with a case mortality of the order of 10%. *Shigella* is, in fact, a facultative intracellular parasite that invades the colonic and rectal mucosa. Invasion of M cells and other APCs occurs, and lymphoid collections can be rapidly destroyed. Systemic and mucosal humoral immune responses are elicited by an infection, and the LPS of the organism is of great importance, as antibodies to it can protect against bacterial challenge (139). Thus, much of the search for an effective vaccine has centered on the LPS O antigen, and more recently on the development of orally administered, live, attenuated vaccines. There are at least five major efforts ongoing, involving academic and industrial partners. A conjugate vaccine of *S. sonnei* works well in soldiers. An attenuated *S. flexneri* strain, carrying both an auxotrophic mutation and one diminishing virulence, is particularly promising on the basis of human volunteer trials (140). An attractive feature is that oral administration of as little as 10^3 to 10^4 organisms elicits a good local immune response against LPS. Another interesting strain is SC599, derived from *S. dysenteriae* 1, in which three deletions have been introduced to reduce virulence (141).

Another live, attenuated strain of promise is CVD1203, which is derived from wild-type *S. flexneri* 2a and contains deletions of both an auxotrophic type (*aro*A deletions) and a virulence-loss type (*virG* deletion). This strain can invade intestinal epithelial cells but replicates poorly and cannot spread to adjacent cells. In a guinea pig model, it is immunogenic and protective (142). This strain can also be used as a vector to deliver antigens of enterotoxigenic *E. coli* (143). It is, however, rather reactogenic in humans (144). A further variant, CVD105, has been prepared. This involved introducing a further mutation affecting the guanine nucleotide synthesis pathway. This has reduced reactogenicity, with good immunogenicity in mice and guinea pigs (145), but it has not yet been in clinical trial. A challenge will be to perfect an at least trivalent vaccine.

Helicobacter pylori Vaccines

Helicobacter pylori has been identified as a causative factor in chronic gastritis, peptic ulcer, and gastric carcinoma and lymphoma (146,147). This is a widespread microorganism, but 10% of the infected population develop peptic ulcer disease. It is not clear why the infection is silent in most people; strain variation may be a factor. Antibiotic intervention can eradicate the infection, particularly if triple therapy with omeprazole (a protein pump inhibitor), metronidazole, and amoxycillin is used. This is an arduous and expensive therapeutic regimen; a vaccine would represent an attractive alternative, particularly as antibiotic resistance is on the increase. One could consider either population-wide prophylactic vaccination or a therapeutic vaccine designed to eradicate the organism from already infected people.

Clearly, an animal model of *H. pylori* would be required to advance knowledge of the potential of the vaccine approach. Lee et al. (148) isolated a gastric spiral bacterium from cats, and this organism, *H. felis,* can colonize mouse stomach and cause gastritis (149), and even lymphoma. With this model in place, it was soon shown that a sonicate of *H. felis* was a protective vaccine in mice giving 96% protection against oral challenge (150). A further important development was that of adapting fresh clinical isolates of *H. pylori* to grow in the mouse stomach by 2-weekly serial passage through specific pathogen-free mice (151). This resulted in the development of a strain, derived from a type I clinical isolate, which caused gastric pathology mimicking that of the human, and development of another strain, derived from a type II clinical isolate, which caused only a mild inflammatory infiltrate without erosive lesions. The difference between type I and type II isolates is that the former express a vacuolating cytotoxin, VacA, which damages epithelial cells, and also a cytotoxin-associated antigen, CagA, of unknown function. Type II strains lack this expression.

These considerations naturally led to the possibility of subunit vaccines. *H. pylori* urease was the first antigen in clinical trial, as it confers protection in animal models. The results of the first studies were not too impressive, though there was some reduction in the bacterial load. Antigens expressed only in type I strains are obviously of great interest. Both CagA and VacA are being assessed as possible oral immunogens in the *H. pylori* mouse model, with the addition of the genetically detoxified *E. coli* heat-labile enterotoxin, LTK63, as a mucosal adjuvant. Early results with VacA appear encouraging, as do those with CagA and urease as single agents with this adjuvant (151). A combination of VacA and urease with LTK63 appears even better.

What about therapeutic intervention? Doidge et al. (152) achieved eradication of *H. felis* in infected mice with an oral administration of *H. felis* sonicate and CT as a mucosal adjuvant. Similarly, Corthesy-Theulaz et al. (153) successfully used the *H. pylori* urease B subunit as an oral treatment in mice. This gives encouragement for the early commencement of clinical therapeutic vaccine trials. It is probable that Th1 T cells are responsible for much of the inflammatory damage in the stomach, and a change in the balance towards a greater proportion of Th2 cells may be helpful. This accentuates the importance of a safe and effective adjuvant suitable for human use. The Sydney strain of *H. pylori* is being used for impending clinical trials (154).

Vaccines against Encapsulated Organisms

Haemophilus influenzae *B, Meningococci, and Pneumococci*

Vaccines traditionally available for encapsulated organisms such as the above have been prepared from purified capsular polysaccharide antigen. These vaccines suffer from two major disadvantages (3). Being polysaccharide in nature, they do not engage the T-cell limb of the immune response. This means that the antibodies are chiefly IgM, affinity maturation does not occur, and, most importantly, young infants do not respond well. As the peak incidence of Hib meningitis is at around 10 to 11 months of age, a vaccine that is not really effective below the age of 18 to 24 months is far from ideal.

The first generation Hib vaccine, based on the polyribosylribitol phosphate (PRP) capsule, was developed almost simultaneously by Anderson et al. (155) and Rodrigues et al. (156). An extensive clinical trial involving 130,178 Finnish children was performed by Peltala et al. (157). No protection was noted in children under 18 months of age, even in those given a booster dose, but even a single dose in children 18 months to 5 years of age gave good protection against invasive Hib disease.

The second problem for these vaccines is that, in each case, there are multiple serotypes. With Hib, six capsular serotypes, a through f, are capable of causing disease in humans, but fortunately, 99% of typeable strains causing invasive disease are type b. With pneumococci, on the other hand, there are 84 capsular types. Though eight to ten cause 70% of the serious infections, the present carbohydrate vaccine is a cocktail of no fewer than 23 serotypes! This covers more than 90% of serious infections. With *Neisseria meningitidis* there are five main antigenically distinct groups, of which, groups A, B, and C are the most important. Group B strains account for about two-thirds of cases of meningococcal meningitis in industrialized countries. Group A strains cause epidemic disease, particular in the "meningitis belt" of Sub-Sahara Africa. Polysaccharide outer capsule vaccines are available for group A and C organisms.

The same groups that pioneered the carbohydrate vaccine were involved in the breakthrough that gave us the extremely effective Hib conjugate vaccine (158,159). This made use of the principle of conjugating antigenic Hib PRP saccharides to protein carriers in order to induce a T-dependent response, which matures much earlier in the human than the T-independent response to saccharides alone. Different-length saccharides and different carriers were used by different companies, with small, medium, and large polysaccharides attached, with or without linkers, to DT, the diphtheria toxin variant CRM$_{197}$, TT, or the group B meningococcal outer membrane complex. Once again Mäkelä led the way with a clinical trial in Finland (1986 to 1987) (160), in which the vaccine was 83% effective and also eliminated oropharyngeal carriage. A further trial (1988 to 1990) with an improved vaccine showed higher, more persistent antibody levels and better efficacy. From about 1990 on, there has been an increasing number of countries with national vaccination programs, and the result has been a dramatic decline in invasive Hib disease due to immunity, herd immunity, and lowered pathogen carriage rates (161). By 1991, meningitis incidence had decreased by 82% in the United States (162). In many countries, Hib meningitis is simply no longer seen. It may not be too early to contemplate the eventual eradication of this pathogen. Particularly encouraging is the fact that the conjugate vaccine works well in a developing-country setting. Mullholland et al. (163) performed a double-blind randomized trial in The Gambia, involving 42,848 infants who were given either DPT alone at 2, 3, and 4 months or DPT mixed with Hib polysaccharide–tetanus protein (PRP-T). Hib meningitis, Hib pneumonia, and five other forms of invasive Hib disease were encountered over a 3-year period. For those children (83%) who received all three doses, the efficacy of the vaccine for the prevention of all invasive Hib disease was 95%; for the prevention of Hib pneumonia, 100%; and for meningitis, 92%. Furthermore, there was a 21.1% reduction of *all* cases of radiologically defined pneumonia. Given the importance of acute respiratory disease as a killer of infants in developing countries, this is an important finding. It is probable that the conjugate Hib vaccine will become the ninth vaccine recommended for all children. Some developing Latin American countries have already begun to deploy it.

There still remains the problem of untypeable and non–type B serotypes of *H. influenzae*. A promising vaccine candidate outer membrane protein known as D15 has been cloned by Thomas' group (164). It is present in sarcosyl-insoluble outer membrane protein preparations in every one of 36 *H. influenzae* isolates tested. Affinity-purified antibodies against cloned D15 were protective in a rat pup model. There is a 98% conservation between all serotypes in this 778-amino acid, 85-kDa molecule (W.R. Thomas, personal communication). No homologous protein has been found in data banks (165). This protein could represent a "universal" recurrent otitis media vaccine candidate.

Obviously, the same principles that apply to Hib are being applied to create conjugate vaccines for *Streptococcus pneumoniae* and *Neisseria meningitidis*. A pneumococcal polysaccharide–CRM$_{197}$ vaccine induces a good T-dependent immune response in children (166), and the vaccine was well tolerated in HIV-infected children, although their antibody response was lower (167). A seven-valent vaccine would cover 70% of cases and an 11-valent one, 82%. Several companies are moving towards nine-valent or 11-valent conjugates. Progress towards group A and C conjugate meningococcal vaccines is also good. A Cuban-produced serogroup B meningococcal vaccine based on outer membrane proteins was 74% effective in children over 4 years and in adults, but it was less effective in very young infants (168).

Intracellular Pathogens, Especially Tuberculosis and Leprosy

Bacteria that exploit the scavenger cell system and successfully learn to live inside cells present special challenges to the vaccine developer. Organisms of this sort include *M. tuberculosis, M. leprae,* and *L. monocytogenes.* Robust T-cell responses are the key to immune protection here, involving Th1-type CD4$^+$ cells and CD8$^+$ CTLs as well as γ/δ T cells and natural killer (NK) cells, each of which has been shown to be of importance in animal models (169). Because of its great public health importance, we shall consider mainly TB.

TB may be the single greatest communicable disease killer in the world. About 2 billion people harbor the bacterium somewhere

in their system, of whom fewer than 10% will develop active disease. However, there are about 8 million new active cases each year and about 3 million annual deaths. Two huge threats are combined infection with HIV and TB, from which death can occur within weeks of infection, and the increased prevalence of strains of *M. tuberculosis* that are resistant to one or more antimicrobial agents. For example, in the United States, 13% of new cases of TB are resistant to at least one first-line drug, and 3% are resistant to both isoniazid and rifampycin, the two most important drugs (170).

BCG was introduced in 1921 and reaches nearly 90% of the world's children, being the most widely used EPI vaccine. Its protective efficacy in childhood TB (e.g., TB meningitis and miliary TB) ranges from 50% to 80% in various trials. Its capacity to prevent adult pulmonary TB is more controversial, reasonably good early European results contrasting with poor developing country results, including an entirely negative large trial in India. One possible reason relates to the presence of cross-reacting mycobacteria in a developing-country setting, which may already have caused some immunity without BCG.

There is no shortage of good ideas in this field. Three broad areas of research are commanding most attention: DNA vaccines, subunit vaccines, and genetically engineered Mycobacteria, including BCG and *M. tuberculosis*. These areas are being underpinned by a massive effort to sequence the whole of the *M. tuberculosis* genome which, *inter alia,* will result in a compendium of possible candidate antigens (1).

There is a substantial number of credible candidates for a subunit vaccine. Information from several laboratories has highlighted the potential of antigens secreted into the culture medium by *M. tuberculosis*. A mixture of secreted antigens can lead to protective immunity in animal models, and high-resolution separation techniques have identified a number of effective single secreted antigens, of which, the most effective is ESAT-6 (171,172). This antigen is expressed only in virulent mycobacterial strains and has been deleted during the attenuation of *M. bovis* to BCG. This antigen is a dominant T-cell target when T cells are extracted from TB lesions or local lymph nodes. ESAT-6 has proven to be an effective vaccine in both mouse and guinea pig models.

Another important antigen is antigen 85, which is actually a complex of three related proteins, Ag85A, B, and C. These 30- to 32-kDa molecules are secreted by all mycobacterial species (173). Patients with active pulmonary TB do not have strong anti-Ag85 T-cell responses, but healthy tuberculin-positive individuals do, and purified Ag85 with adjuvant is protective in the guinea pig model. A further candidate antigen is HSP60 (174). This is homologous to the chaperone HSP65 of other species. It is recognized by T cells both after infection and after immunization, but its usefulness as a vaccine candidate may be compromised by its (at least theoretical) capacity to cause autoimmunity through cross-reactivity with human HSP65. A number of other secreted proteins are also of interest, including HSP70, PRA, 35-kDa proline-rich antigen, and MPT83 (175,176).

A DNA vaccine encoding Ag85A has been used in mice and protects against intravenous administration of live *M. bovis* (BCG) or aerosol administration of *M. tuberculosis* (177). In both cases, protection was similar to that achieved with BCG. The vaccine induced both humoral (chiefly IgG1 and IgG2a) and cell-mediated (chiefly Th1 and CTL) responses against Ag85A. Apart from this encouraging result, the DNA vaccine approach should help to define other protective antigens. Plasmid DNA expressing HSP65 gives long-lasting protection, believed to be due to CD8$^+$ CD44-high memory CTL clones.

The live genetically engineered vaccines include a variant BCG into which *M. tuberculosis* genes for candidate antigens have been introduced. Another variant includes constructs encoding immunostimulatory cytokines. Another approach is starting with live, virulent *M. tuberculosis* but carefully targeting and deleting genes believed to be associated with virulence. These approaches are still at an early stage. It is possible that environmentally acquired immunity to cross-reacting mycobacteria might limit the replication of such vaccines, and thus limit their efficacy.

M. leprae has many similarities to *M. tuberculosis*. There is some evidence that BCG is partially effective as a leprosy vaccine. Convit has pioneered research on a vaccine consisting of heat-killed, armadillo-derived *M. leprae* and live BCG. It has not been excluded that the partial protective effects of this vaccine are due to the BCG component. An atypical *Mycobacterium,* known as *Mycobacterium w.* is another vaccine candidate. *M. w.* is a readily cultivatable, rapidly growing *Mycobacterium* resembling but not identical to bacteria in Runyon's group IV.

Autoclaved whole bacteria were well tolerated in a phase I trial, and large scale field trials on 414,000 inhabitants of the Uttar Pradesh state in India are under way. It will be some time until this immunoprophylactic trial can be interpreted, but, in the meantime, the first results of an immunotherapy trial have been reported (178). Ninety-three multibacillary leprosy patients received 10^9 killed bacteria intradermally initially, followed by seven doses of 5 × 10^8 bacteria at 3-monthly intervals. One hundred seven patients served as controls. All 200 sufferers received standard multidrug therapy. The trial was double-blinded and randomized, the placebo injections consisting of autoclaved micronized starch. The vaccinated patients showed significantly more rapid and more complete bacteriologic clearance, accelerated clinical regression of lesions, and higher lepromin conversion rates. Clinical improvement, as measured by Ramu's scores, was significantly greater. There were some significant side effects but no increase in neuritis or deformity. The authors recommend the treatment as an adjunct to chemotherapy.

Vaccines against Group A Streptococci

Somewhat amazingly, nearly 60 years after the development of penicillin, rheumatic fever and rheumatic heart disease remain common in many developing countries, the prevalence being up to 20 per 1,000. *Streptococcus pyogenes* infections can also be followed by acute and chronic glomerulonephritis and otitis media. A good vaccine candidate would be the M protein, which varies greatly between strains. A conserved 20-amino acid peptide has been identified near the carboxy-terminal end of the protein, which may be less exposed on the streptococcal surface and thus less immunogenic. Antibodies specific for this peptide were effective in opsonization assays and bacteriocidal assays, suggesting the possibility that the peptide could form the basis of a streptococcal vaccine (179), particularly early in childhood. There is a gradual, age-related development of antibodies to group A streptococci in areas of high incidence of infection. This appears to parallel the acquisition of antibodies to the specific peptide of the M protein. Further research has defined a still smaller epitope, of only 12 amino acids, that is specific for opsonic activity. Use of a minimal peptide should minimize the risk of using as a vaccine epitopes shared between streptococci and heart muscle, which of course would risk causing rather than preventing autoimmune

complications (180). In fact, T cells isolated from mice immunized with this peptide do not proliferate in the presence of heart extract, myosin, tropomyosin, or keratin, suggesting it is not likely to cause deleterious effects.

VIRAL VACCINES

Viral vaccines have proven particularly effective and underlie current disease eradication strategies, hopefully soon for poliomyelitis and then for measles (and mumps, rubella, and varicella in due course). Some aspects of this subject have already been touched on, and others will be covered in the sections on vaccines against cancer and the future. It is neither feasible nor necessary to deal at length with the many improved viral vaccines that are working their way through the research-and-development pipeline. Rather, we wish to highlight some of the complexities, challenges, and frustrations that have emerged during this research and to draw some lessons from these experiences.

Hepatitis A, B, and C

These three viruses show an interesting spectrum of solved and unsolved problems that confront the vaccinologist. Hilleman (181) cites literature suggesting that contagious jaundice has been known to occur since the fifth century B.C. It became clear in the 1950s that "infectious hepatitis" and "homologous serum jaundice" had differing features, and this was cemented in the 1960s (182). Since the isolation of hepatitis A and B viruses and good serologic tests for their recent presence, other forms of fecal-orally and of blood-transmitted hepatitis have been discovered, of which, the most important enterically transmitted agent is hepatitis E, and the most important parenterally transmitted is hepatitis C (183,184).

Hepatitis A is one of a group of diseases, which also includes infectious mononucleosis, that is mild or entirely asymptomatic in young children but more severe in adolescent or adult life. It can rarely cause fulminant hepatitis, but is usually less severe, though causing illness for up to several months. As it is now only moderately common in industrialized countries, but very common in many developing countries, immunization is a good idea for travelers, and active immunization has largely replaced passive administration of gamma-globulin for this purpose.

The virus initially proved very difficult to grow, and early studies depended on its identification in fecal extracts by electron microscopy (185). It was eventually grown in marmoset liver cells and a human hepatoma cell line (186), following which, a range of cells were successfully infected. Growth of the virus in LLC-MK2 cells and availability of a marmoset model for vaccine testing led to a formalin-inactivated, killed whole virus vaccine (187), which, however, was not acceptable at that time because malignant cells were involved in growing the virus. Two groups eventually succeeded in obtaining growth in human diploid lung fibroblasts, and the resultant vaccines from Smith, Kline Beecham and Merck Sharp and Dohme work well. However, as virus yields are not enormous, hepatitis A is an expensive vaccine, and a live, attenuated vaccine would be most beneficial in a Third World setting. Several candidate vaccines exist, one has been extensively tested in China and found to be highly effective (188), but none has yet made it through to full registration.

Hepatitis B carrier rates vary from less than 0.1% to 15% of the population in different countries. The acute attack is mild or insignificant, but 20% to 25% of carriers develop chronic liver disease, and some go on to cancer. Hepatitis B vaccine has already been briefly described. The virus does not grow in tissue culture, and there are two sources of vaccine, HBsAg isolated from chronic carriers of the virus and the same material molecularly cloned in yeast (20) or Chinese hamster ovary cells (189). The carrier-derived vaccine was, for a long time, by far cheaper, and, as it is an excellent and perfectly safe product, it has been widely used in developing countries. Now the recombinant vaccine is becoming much cheaper, and estimates are that it could be made for $0.50 (U.S.) per dose if the demand were sufficient, in which case, it would probably replace the human-derived material. Both vaccines are about equally effective; response rates to protective levels of antibody vary from 85% to 95% in different studies. Protection may be achieved with lower levels of antibody than those generally believed to be protective, perhaps because of CD8$^+$ T-cell effects. One worry is that some vaccinated people become carriers of what have been called "escape mutants," which persist despite the presence of good antibody levels to the native virus (190). The most common change is an arginine-for-glycine substitution in the *a* loop, against which antibodies are usually directed. While it is not yet certain that the mutation changes the virus to one of lower infectivity, M.H. Kane points out (personal communication) that there is no evidence, yet, of escape mutants having spread from one person to another. There is therefore no need to worry about the univalency of the current vaccine. Presumably, if escape mutants become a problem, but if the number of different serotypes is limited, the variants could be included in a recombinant vaccine.

The hepatitis C virus (HCV) was the first of the non-A–non-B viruses identified, yet it has not been grown in tissue culture nor visualized in the electron microscope. Hepatitis C is transmitted like hepatitis B, but it is an even nastier disease, as about 80% of people who contract the infection become chronic carriers, and the majority of these go on to develop chronic liver disease. Furthermore, a significant proportion develop hepatocellular carcinoma—in Japan, where about 2% of people are carriers, hepatitis C is a more common cause of liver cancer than is hepatitis B.

Because of the frustrations surrounding the difficulty of isolating this virus, the cloning of the virus by Choo et al. (191) was considered a major triumph, particularly because it soon led to the development of an assay for antibodies useful in screening blood donations (192). However, development of a vaccine against hepatitis C faces difficulties. The virus is a rapidly mutating RNA virus with a single open reading frame encoding a polyprotein of about 3000 amino acids. There are two putative envelope proteins, E1 and E2, identified by analogy with other flaviviruses, which presumably are produced by proteolytic cleavage. Study of these by genomic analysis of hepatitis C cloned from patients in different parts of the world shows a great degree of structural (and, therefore, presumably antigenic) diversity (193). Furthermore, experimentation on vaccine candidates is rendered difficult by the fact that the only animal model is in the chimpanzee. This makes it hard to characterize and quantitate neutralizing antibodies, although it is known that plasma from a chronic carrier can protect chimpanzees from infection (194). An assay has been developed that shows great promise as a surrogate neutralization assay (195). It is the neutralization of binding (NOB) assay. HCV recombinant envelope antigen E2 was expressed in HeLa or CHO cells, and it bound with high affinity to MOLT-4 cells, a human cell line that may allow low-level replication of HCV. The degree of binding can be readily assessed through the use of a sandwich fluorescent antibody technique to detect E2 antigen. Unknown serum can then be assayed for its ability to neutralize this binding. Chimpanzees immunized with E1 and E2 show varying degrees of protection to challenge. It was found that the degree of protection correlated with the NOB titer. Also, the assay showed cross-neutralization of binding between greatly disparate isolates, leading to the hope that binding (and hence presumably neutralization) is at least partly independent of E2 antigenic variation. It has also been found that high titers of NOB antibodies correlate with resolution of HCV infection in patients. Of 34 patients with acute hepatitis C, 29 developed chronic hepatitis, but seven of these gradually resolved. In six of these seven, the emergence and persistence of high serum titers of NOB antibodies coincided with virus clearance and clinical resolution, while continuing chronic patients not showing resolution had low or undetectable NOB antibody levels (196). This was quite different than ELISA tests against HCV structural proteins, which showed no such correlation. T-lymphocyte responses, particularly to the core antigen, may also be critical for a benign course of an HCV infection (197). These correlations should be helpful to the design of further experiments seeking a vaccine against this important pathogen.

Rotavirus Vaccines

Rotavirus is an important cause of diarrheal disease in infants and young children. In the industrialized world, it is a leading cause of hospitalization for diarrhea, but intravenous fluid and electrolyte replacement usually allow the child to turn the corner. In the developing countries, rotavirus is devastating, causing an estimated 870,000 deaths per year (1). Virtually all children have been infected by the age of 5 years, so vaccination would obviously have to be at a very young age. It appears that the long search for an effective rotavirus vaccine is at last coming to an end.

There are seven serogroups of rotaviruses, but only three (A, B, and C) have been associated with diarrhea in the human. Group A is by far the most important in young children. The two vaccines that are at the most advanced stage of development (one is about to be licensed), are both "reassortant" vaccines. They are live, attenuated vaccines, administered orally, and are based on an animal strain of rotavirus—rhesus monkey in one case and bovine in the other. These have been modified by the insertion of genes from the human viruses, coding for outer capsid proteins. In two multicenter trials of tetravalent vaccines in the United States, each involving over 1,000 infants aged 1 to 6 months, the vaccine produced 57% protection against diarrhea but 87% protection against severe disease. The present, suggested three-dose schedule could be given at the same time as oral polio vaccine. The tests of a large trial in Venezuela are eagerly awaited to see if the vaccine is effective in a less developed country. But there is little doubt that the "Jennerian" vaccine will find a real place (198).

Other approaches are also being pursued. These include baculovirus-expressed subunit antigens, which self-assemble into virus-like particles. These are highly immunogenic in rabbits; preparations containing capsid proteins VP2, VP4, VP6, and VP7, or just VP2, VP6, and VP7, were protective against homotypic challenge (199). This vaccine could follow or precede the live, attenuated vaccine. Further research is in train on an attenuated human rotavirus vaccine, RV3, isolated from a human infant with asymptomatic infection in a hospital nursery. This vaccine strain, grown in the AGMK cell line, has been shown to be safe at 10^5 virions per dose in neonates, children, and adults, and further clinical trials are planned. Microencapsulated vaccines, consisting of live or killed virus, or DNA vaccines are also the subjects of research. Rotavirus genes for VP4 and VP7 have also been inserted into recombinant Sabin polio virus 3 (200) or vaccinia. As no studies have shown the Jennerian vaccine to be 100% effective, these efforts should be continued. Further priority activities include a better definition of the burden of rotavirus disease and the prevalence of the various strains.

Respiratory Syncytial Virus Vaccines

Respiratory syncytial virus (RSV) is a highly contagious virus of infants and young children. It is the largest single cause of lower respiratory tract infections in this age group in the industrialized countries, and it kills about 900,000 children annually in the Third World (1). There it is often complicated by Hib or pneumococcal infection.

RSV also presents a threat to immunosuppressed patients (e.g., those undergoing transplantation) and to elderly and chronically ill subjects (201). Furthermore, children with bronchopulmonary dysplasia, congenital heart disease, or prematurity may benefit from immunoprophylaxis mediated by immunoglobulin with a high anti-RSV titer or with humanized murine monoclonal antibodies.

RSV is an enveloped RNA paramyxovirus. Two major groups of strains, A and B, exist, which are probably too far apart for cross-protection by a vaccine. A formalin-inactivated RSV vaccine was tested nearly 30 years ago, and, for reasons that are still not clear, vaccinated children exposed to natural infection actually developed a higher incidence and a greater severity of RSV disease (202). This could have been due to immune complex deposition. This naturally slowed progress of vaccine research, but renewed efforts are being mounted. Two cold-adapted, temperature-sensitive strains of A and B serotypes have been isolated as potential live, attenuated vaccine candidates (203). Given intranasally, the putative vaccine stimulates fusion (F) protein–specific IgA and IgG antibody formation and a Th1-type T-cell response. CTLs were also present in the lungs. The vaccine was protective against wild-type RSV challenge, as measured by virus growth in the lungs. The analysis of mutant strains suggests that loss of virulence may be associated with mutations in the virus' polymerase gene and/or F gene (204). Early clinical trials are under way.

A subunit vaccine based on the purified F protein has undergone a double-blinded, placebo-controlled study in children with cystic fibrosis (205). Vaccine-enhanced disease was not observed. Protection against infection, as such, was not achieved, but there was a significant reduction in mean number of lower respiratory tract illnesses and in their severity. Paradiso et al. (206) also report safety and immunogenicity of an F protein subunit vaccine in children aged 24 to 48 months. Live vector vaccines incorporating F or the other envelope glycoprotein, G, into adenovirus or vaccinia are also in preclinical research.

Vaccines against Human Immunodeficiency Virus and Acquired Immunodeficiency Syndrome

The human immunodeficiency virus-1 (HIV-1) has developed some devilishly clever strategies to foil the human immune response. It exhibits an astonishing rate of mutation, particularly in that portion of its envelope protein involved in infectivity, allowing the virus to escape the antibody response. It finds several levels of "safe haven" refuges that are unreachable by antibodies (e.g., persistence within macrophages and DCs or penetration into the brain). Further to that, integration of provirus DNA into the host-cell genome, with no external evidence of the virus' presence, represents an escape resistant to CTL attack. It targets the first lymphocyte in the immune cascade, the CD4$^+$ T cell, a factor that may delay an effective immune response and will certainly facilitate the disastrous upsurge in viral load late in the disease, as T-cell levels fall so low that resistance essentially disappears. It has an extraordinarily high rate of replication. We now know that the immune system is a pitched battleground from the first entry of the virus. Large numbers of CD4$^+$ lymphocytes are infected, die, and are replaced. CD8$^+$ CTLs help to control the early infection and bring the viral load down to one-thousandth of the peak level, but the repeated cycles of infection and death of CD4$^+$ cells and CD8$^+$ cell activation to control infected cell numbers continue (207). In fact, the degree to which the viral load can be driven down is an important prognostic factor (208). At the same time, high rates of HIV replication continue in lymphatic tissues (209).

The early history of attempts to develop an AIDS vaccine has been depressing, but an interesting "experiment of nature" suggests we should not despair. There is a small subset of Gambian prostitutes who are repeatedly exposed to the virus but who, unlike the majority of their sisters, do not seroconvert and do not develop HIV/AIDS (210). These women show a robust HIV-specific CTL response. Similarly, some spouses of HIV-positive partners do not seroconvert but display CD4$^+$ immunity of the Th1 type (211). Presumably, these rare individuals have managed so to activate their immune systems early after first exposure (and before seroconversion) as to eliminate the virus altogether. An effective vaccine would be one that could consistently cause such a state of immunity in the majority of recipients.

The early clinical trials of vaccines all involved HIV-1 envelope protein preparations, either the full molecule (gp160) or the portion lacking the transmembrane domain (gp120). There were two big disappointments in these trials, namely a small number of "breakthrough" infections despite vaccination and a failure of the antibodies arising from immunization to neutralize fresh isolates of HIV, as opposed to laboratory passage strains. As a result, a series of more elaborate trials that had been planned did not go forward. In retrospect, these results are not too surprising. First, any natural source of virus would have mutant virions, which might not have been neutralized by antibodies predominantly directed at a particular clade. As a matter of fact, in a feline immunodeficiency virus model, immunization with an envelope glycoprotein subunit vaccine actually *enhanced* infectivity of the virus after challenge (212). Furthermore, vaccine-induced virus-neutralizing antibodies failed to protect macaque monkeys from SIV (213). Second, there can be no assurance that parenteral vaccination would have achieved enough mucosal antibodies in the rectum (or vagina) to neutralize every last virus. Even one HIV particle slipping through could have entered a CD4$^+$ lymphocyte or APC and have initiated the replicative cycle mentioned above. It is a pity that it has not been possible to ascertain whether this type of vaccine actually lowered (though not eliminating) the risk of infection, or lowered the initial virus load, thus perhaps prompting a longer disease-free interval. Of many possible explanations for the poor neutralization capacity of vaccinees' sera, problems of assay sensitivity is one. A study of volunteers given gp120, using a new neutralization assay, showed a capacity to neutralize a primary clade B isolate closely related to the immunizing strain (214). For this reason, it is pleasing to note a large, WHO-sponsored trial of recombinant gp120 vaccine in Thailand, using the correct clade E for that part of the world. Such a trial can proceed only if (a) the government of the country is in favor of it and (b) certain ethical norms are met. The trial would have to be acceptable to the population under study; the vaccine would have to be appropriate to the particular population; and the product, if effective, would have to be made available to the population. Of course, it is essential that all participants in any prevention trial be counselled vigorously on the use of established prevention methods. There are also a number of phase I trials of peptides from the V3 loop of gp160 or of whole inactivated HIV virions in progress at the time of writing.

There are good reasons to believe that CD8+ CTLs play a role in limiting HIV spread (209,210). This conclusion is supported by the finding that HIV-1–specific CTL appearance coincides with a fall in virus levels in HIV-1–infected macrophages (215). If so, it would be important to include in a vaccine virally encoded proteins produced in the cytosol of the infected cell, so that peptide fragments of such proteins could be presented at the surface of the infected cell in association with class I MHC molecules. Furthermore, it would be advantageous to use adjuvants or other techniques known to favor CD8+ T-cell production. Third, use of a multiplicity of antigens might counteract mutations occurring in any single component within the virus-infected cells that should be eliminated. Finally, a procedure evoking mucosal as well as lymph node and splenic CTLs would be ideal. In fact, in a resurgent AIDS vaccine effort, a large number of antigens or genes for antigens have been the subject of basic research and/or of protective trials in animal models. The antigens, used in various combinations, include (as well as *env*) *gag, pol, nef, rev,* and protease (2). The vector systems used include vaccinia, canary pox, adenovirus, poliovirus, mengovirus, Venezuelan equine encephalitis virus, *Salmonella, Listeria,* BCG, and *Shigella.* Some of these trials have yielded disappointment in phase I in terms of the strength and type of immunity. Only a combined avipox/gp120 ("prime-boost") vaccine has yet progressed to phase II.

Obviously, the DNA vaccine approach has attractions, given its capacity to induce Th1 and CTL immunity. There are already two phase I trials under way, an amazing fact, given that this approach is so new, and these should have been reported by the time this volume is in print. In one preclinical study in mice and African green monkeys and rhesus monkeys, promising results have been reported (216). A plasmid DNA was prepared encoding gp120 and the HIV regulatory protein *rev.* This induced Th1 responses for both proteins and a good CTL response against gp120. Significant levels of gp120-specific antibody were also achieved in all species. With lower doses of DNA, some animals failed to make antibody but still had a Th1 response. However, antisera from African green monkeys showed only low to moderate levels of virus-neutralizing antibodies. Of course, finding that antibodies can neutralize primary HIV isolates *in vitro* is no guarantee that such antibodies will be protective in a real-life setting. Schutten et al. (217) have demonstrated (in a human to irradiated mouse model) that quite high levels of passively administered antibodies fail to achieve this goal. This casts some doubt on the use of neutralizing antibody titers in the assessment of vaccine candidates.

There has been much discussion of an immunization strategy based on vectored or DNA vaccine priming followed by a subunit vaccine booster to raise antibody levels. This has received support from a chimpanzee protection experiment involving HIV-1 (218). This goal had previously been achieved only with prolonged courses of gp120 immunization. Chimpanzees were primed intranasally with adenovirus recombinant vectors carrying the HIV-1 gp160 gene. Subsequently, they were boosted parenterally

by gp120. The animals developed high-titered neutralizing antibodies and strong CTL responses, and they showed protection to HIV-1 challenge for periods of 1 year or longer. In further work, other antigens, such as *gag* and *nef,* will be included. Whether adenovirus vectors or nucleic acid vaccines will emerge as more effective remains to be seen.

The concept of a live, attenuated vaccine, difficult though it may prove to implement in practice, has received renewed interest. It has been known for some years (219) that monkeys can be protected from a large dose of SIV by a live, attenuated strain of SIV containing an engineered deletion of the regulatory *nef* gene. This is not as hopeful as it seems, because the defective virus can cause AIDS in newborn monkeys, and, moreover, continues to proliferate within the simian host. Montagnier (220) has discussed the possible value of Nef vaccination against HIV. A curious finding in humans has many similarities (221). In 1989, a review of the registry of the Red Cross Blood Transfusion Service in Sydney led to the identification of a male homosexual blood donor who had contracted HIV in late 1980 or early 1981 and who had donated blood between February 1981 and July 1984. Neither the donor nor seven blood recipients who converted to seropositive status have developed any AIDS-related illness and have stable, normal CD4+ lymphocyte counts 13 to 16 years after seroconversion. An eighth infectee, a woman with systemic lupus erythematosus on high-dose steroid treatment, died. It is not clear whether her death was attributable to HIV infection, lupus, or a combination of the two. When a genomic analysis was performed from either virus isolates or peripheral blood cells of the healthy individuals, similar deletions in the *nef* gene and the nef-LTR overlap region were found. The mutant virus replicates poorly *in vitro,* and the HIV-1 DNA copy number per 10^5 CD4+ cells from the infected individuals is low, varying from less than 10 to 400. Although the continuing presence of replicating HIV (however attenuated) is hard to contemplate, it should be remembered that yellow fever strain 17D, a brilliant vaccine virus, can be recovered from vaccinees 30 years after immunization. Apart from the possibility of a live, attenuated vaccine, the Sydney cohort focuses attention on the importance of *nef* and LTR in virulence, prompting a search for drugs specific for these regions.

New hope has entered the HIV/AIDS arena since the demonstration that a combination of three drugs, two reverse-transcriptase inhibitors and one HIV protease inhibitor, can markedly lower viral load, frequently to undetectable levels and for a prolonged period. This raises the very real possibility that a therapeutic vaccine approach following chemotherapy and targeted towards CTL activation may eliminate the last few virus-infected cells or keep them under control indefinitely.

Perhaps the greatest single problem in HIV vaccine research, apart from rapid mutation, is the question of how vaccine efficacy can be tested. Strong though the evidence implicating CD8+ T cells in protection may be, the correlates of protection remain uncertain. Following encouraging phase I studies, where to then? Given the partial control of the pandemic in industrialized countries, the answer may have to be within high-incidence developing countries, after the strictest possible ethical scrutiny of protocols. Maternal-to-infant transmission remains a big problem, particularly as AZT, which is effective in this regard, may be too expensive for general use in poorer countries. In the section on the future, we shall review a possible way of inducing Th1 and CTL activity in newborns.

Obviously, the complex issue of HIV immunization requires more analysis than is possible in this chapter. The article by Heeney et al. (222) provides a useful summary of the key issues.

VACCINES AGAINST PARASITIC DISEASES

If viruses and bacteria have evolved elaborate strategies to defeat the vertebrate immune system, parasites, with their much larger complement of DNA, possess an even wider and more diverse range (223). Although no vaccine against any human parasitic disease has been licensed, the feasibility of such vaccines has been demonstrated in the veterinary field, where a range of successful vaccines is in use to deal with both protozoan and metazoan infestations. The difficulty of overcoming all of the necessary hurdles for human vaccines is evidenced by the fact that over the last 20 years some of the best minds in vaccinology have applied themselves to the problem, but only in malaria has one vaccine moved to the stage of phase III trials, and that, with dubious success. Nevertheless, parasitism is so important from a public health viewpoint, and the recent progress in understanding of parasite molecular biology and genetics so significant, that the research effort must continue. Moveover, the progressive resistance of some parasites to chemotherapy and of vectors to insecticides highlights the importance of vaccines for disease control.

Malaria Vaccines

Malaria is the most prevalent vector-borne disease in the world. It is caused by protozoa of four different species of *Plasmodium*. It threatens 2 billion people in 90 countries and causes of the order of 500 million clinical cases and 2 million deaths per year. Overwhelmingly, the worst continent for malaria is Africa, where 90% of the deaths occur, chiefly in children under 5 years. *P. falciparum* is, by far, the most dangerous of the four species that affect humans, and cerebral malaria, in which parasitozed erythrocytes develop cytoadherence antigens and block up cerebral arterioles, is the most prominent cause of death. It is known that antibodies can be therapeutic, and the hope that a vaccine will eventually be developed is sustained by the observation that inhabitants of endemic areas eventually become relatively immune to attacks.

There are four stages in the life cycle of the parasite wherein intervention by the immune system could have a big impact. The mosquito injects a lifeform known as a *sporozoite*. This exhibits a prominent circumsporozoite protein (CSP) on its surface as a dominant antigen. A feature of this antigen is that it exhibits multiple tandem repeats of the sequence NANP, which is the target of a large proportion of the antibody content of both the serum of patients or of CSP (or irradiated sporozoite)-immunized persons. Yet, early attempts to protect against infection by CSP immunization failed, perhaps because the antibody content of anti-CSP sera was too low.

Sporozoites move quickly to the liver, and the antigens presented on the surface of the infected liver cell present good targets for CTL attack. These are essentially peptides from the sporozoites and, more particularly, the merozoites, which develop in the liver cells. These are being progressively defined. Once the liver cells rupture and release merozoites, the asexual cycle of red blood cell replication begins. Vaccines against the erythrocyte stage of the cycle are particularly important, as this is the stage that causes disease. It could be argued that a vaccine capable of lowering sporozoite entry into the liver by 70% would not achieve very much, but one that lowered intensity of erythrocyte production of merozoites by 70% would significantly lower parasitic burden and thus morbidity and mortality. The erythrocytic cycle produces predominantly merozoites, but it is also responsible for the production of gametocytes, which are taken up by the mosquito in a blood meal

and mature into gametes in the mosquito. A vaccine capable of producing antigametocyte antibodies could destroy gametocytes in the blood and/or prevent the gametocytes maturing within the mosquito. Thus, if widely deployed in a population, it could lower transmission rates without actually benefiting the person who received the vaccine. It has generally been argued that a successful malaria vaccine would include antigens from at least three, if not all four, of these stages.

One feature of malarial antigens is the prominence of multiple tandem repeats of short stretches of peptide in the majority of the proteins that have been isolated. This has prompted the view that these are the epitopes that the parasite "wants" the immune system to see. Moreover, the strong T-independent stimulus represented by these multivalent epitopes may "lock" the response into relatively low-affinity IgM antibody formation, which does not undergo adequate affinity maturation, particularly as there are many such antigens that cross-react to greater or lesser degrees (224). Mutant antibody molecules *not* possessing raised affinity might be preserved through restimulation by a cross-reacting protein.

A second feature of many malarial antigens is considerable variability between different isolates, presumably as the parasite mutates away from the initial antibody attack. This has led to a search for conserved portions of the antigens concerned.

As far as CSP is concerned, there were about 20 disappointing clinical trials before the encouraging breakthrough described in the section on adjuvants and principles of mucosal immunity. Some other approaches are still being pursued, including CSP expressed in several different vectors and a synthetic MAP vaccine.

An interesting candidate vaccine was SPf66, developed by Patarroyo and colleagues (225). This includes peptides from both CSP and blood-stage antigens and has been tested in a large number of volunteers in Colombia and Africa. In areas of relatively low endemicity, protection of the order of 30% has been obtained, but in a hyperendemic area, such as The Gambia, the vaccine has not been significantly effective statistically.

A further ambitious vaccine candidate consisted of seven different antigens from three stages of the parasite life cycle, made by a genetically recombined attenuated vaccinia virus. Phase I and II trials of this vaccine have been disappointing.

Moving to asexual blood-stage vaccines, there are at least half a dozen candidate molecules being trialed preclinically or clinically for efficacy. The first of these was merozoite surface antigen 1 (MSA-1), which has been found to be an effective immunogen that is protective in a number of animal species (226,227). A 19-kDa fragment from the C-terminal portion provokes antibodies that inhibit *in vitro* invasion of erythrocytes by *P. falciparum* merozoites (228). Antibodies to an analogous region of murine malaria were protective in a passive transfer model in mice (229). This fragment, prepared from *P. yoelii* expressed in yeast, can induce complete protection in mice, and careful analysis has shown that this is completely dependent on a high antibody titer and not on T cells (230). Another important antigen is MSA-2, also expressed on the merozoite surface (231). An extremely promising vaccine candidate on the basis of preclinical trials is apical membrane antigen 1 (AMA-1) (232), which is expressed at the apical surface of the merozoite just before it is ready to invade. This protein seems to be derived from the rhoptries, organelles believed to be involved in merozoite invasion of erythrocytes, during late schizogeny. AMA-1 consists of three disulphide-bonded domains, and the most C-terminal of these, which is relatively conserved, is undergoing preclinical testing. The ring erythrocytes surface antigen (RESA) is a micronemederived protein that is also involved in invasion, and it, too, has shown promise in *in vitro* and preclinical work (224,233). Several other products of the rhoptries are at less advanced stages of research. Various combinations of the above molecules are in early clinical trial as subunit vaccines.

Once again, and not surprisingly, given the importance of the problem, a variety of vectors, adjuvants, and DNA approaches are being deployed for erythrocytic-stage antigens.

The best developed of the sexual stage antigens is Pfs25, a protein of about 25 kDa, derived from gametocytes, which turns out to be surprisingly immunogenic, compared with many other malarial proteins. This prevents the further development of gametocytes, which the mosquito ingests. Pfs25 has come to be known as the "unselfish" vaccine and would really only be practical as part of a cocktail.

In some ways, the pace of malaria vaccine research has been disappointing, but the field is full of activity at the moment, and the DNA vaccine approach, in particular, has infused it with new energy. The breakthrough of the Walter Reed–Smith, Kline Beecham group, described in an earlier section, will galvanize it further.

Leishmaniasis Vaccines

Leishmania parasites, especially *L. tropica, L. major,* and *L. donovani,* are vector-borne protozoa that cause a variety of serious diseases. Immunologic interest in leishmaniasis was first aroused by the realization that cutaneous leishmaniasis (tropical sore) caused solid immunity to reinfection when it eventually healed. On the other hand, visceral leishmaniasis causing kala azar is frequently progressive and fatal. A second fascinating observation in leishmaniasis arises from the murine model, in which some of the first evidence was gathered that Th1-type immunity helps cure, but Th2-type immunity leads to increasing lesions and death (234).

In a procedure reminiscent of variolation (see the earlier section covering historical perspectives), there was an ancient practice known as leishmanization, in which material from an active lesion was used to produce a self-limited sore on normal people. Prophylactic immunization with killed *Leishmania* was used in the 1940s. Animal experimentation showed the feasibility of live, attenuated vaccines (235), and work is continuing on an attenuated *L. major* lacking the dihydrofolate reductase–thymidilate synthetase gene (236). But subunit vaccines are receiving the most attention, not only in a variety of adjuvants, but also via the vectored and DNA delivery approaches.

Gp63 is a surface protease of *L. major,* the gene for which has been engineered into auxotrophic mutants of *S. typhimurium.* This produced an orally active vectored vaccine, which protected the genetically susceptible BALB/c mouse strain (237). This has also been used successfully in a DNA vaccine (238). The promastigote surface antigen known as PSA-2 can also be protective if delivered so as to induce a Th1 response (239). Other proteins and peptides are also under investigation.

An unusual antigen of considerable interest is not a protein but a glycolipid, the abundant lipophosphoglycan (LPG) of promastigotes, which possesses one or more determinants involved in the penetration of the promastigote into the macrophage (240). Immunization with *L. major* LPG is protective in mouse models.

As with other vaccines for which Th1 immunity is required, the IL-12 gene could well form a part of an eventual gene construct.

An unanswered question is whether sufficient support can be mustered for an applied research and development effort after the basic research on leishmania vaccines has been concluded. This could be an area for which the oil-rich nations of the Middle East could be asked for a major contribution, as the vaccine is not of enormous interest to commercial companies.

Schistosomiasis

Schistosomiasis, or bilharzia, also called snail fever, is the worst human disease caused by a metazoan parasite. It is due to five different species of *Schistosoma,* of which the three most important are *S. mansoni, S. hematobium,* and *S. japonicum.* Freshwater snails are the intermediate host for the parasite, and they release free-swimming cercariae, which penetrate human skin. There are also plentiful animal hosts; schistosomiasis is a zoonosis, which makes control of transmission much harder. In quite a complex migratory process, adult worms eventually develop and lodge in the veins, the predominant organs depending on the species. The male and female conjugate, and the female lays up to thousands of eggs per day. These ova are the real inducers of immunopathology. They penetrate the tissues and reach the gastrointestinal tract or the urinary tract, thus being excreted into feces or urine. The life cycle is completed if water sources are contaminated and snails become infested. At the same time, ova lodge in organs such as the liver or the bladder and cause granuloma formation and fibrosis. Induction of cirrhosis of the liver caused by *S. japonicum* is the most fatal manifestation of schistosomiasis. As the adult worms consume blood, anemia is a complication. Bladder cancer in young men, associated with schistosomiasis, is common in Egypt. It has been estimated that 200 million people are infested with schistosomes. Twenty million are seriously ill, and 200,000 die each year. Controlling the snail intermediate host has been a major effort in China, but the highly effective drug praziquantel represents a more effective control measure (1). A vaccine to prevent reinfection after drug therapy would represent a major new tool.

Two isoforms of the schistosome enzyme glutathione-*S*-transferase have been extensively investigated as vaccine candidates, especially by Capron's group (241). They are highly effective in a rat model, for reasons that are not entirely clear. Other molecules of interest include two surface antigens from the migratory larval stage of *S. mansoni* parasites, which look promising in animal models, and two different parasite muscle proteins. While none of these antigens has yet reached clinical trial, the WHO is actively promoting consensus choice of the most promising antigen and linkage with a commercial partner to spearhead eventual vaccine testing and production.

In conclusion, parasitism is so grave a problem that it must be tackled on many fronts simultaneously. Protection from vectors is obviously important, as is chemical and biologic control of vectors. Drug therapy is highly effective in many cases, but always fraught with the danger of development of resistance. Vaccines are still, in many respects, a distant dream, but one that must be sustained.

VACCINES AGAINST CANCER

Few fields have been as controversial as tumor immunology, and, moreover, the field tends to oscillate between optimism and pessimism, dependent both on the time frame and on the perspectives of individual investigators. Tumor immunology became an independent discipline in the mid to late 1950s when it was shown that carcinogen or virally induced experimental tumors were highly immunogenic in syngeneic mice and rats. This observation prompted a veritable spate of experiments in which such tumors were rendered nonviable and were used as quite effective cancer prophylactic vaccines. Enthusiasm for this approach gave way to disappointment when it was realized that spontaneously emerging tumors of rodents were either poorly or not at all immunogenic. This was particularly true for cancers of great importance to the human host (e.g., breast or lung cancer). Nevertheless, a host of empirical immunotherapy approaches were tried in humans, frequently involving the use of nonspecific immunostimulatory agents such as BCG, together with irradiated malignant cells or chemical extracts from them. There was also a wave of enthusiasm for the use of BCG or other adjuvants, theoretically designed to enhance the body's own, but inadequate, anticancer responses. This did indeed result in some spectacular remissions, but it was soon realized that these were mainly confined to a few types of tumor (e.g., malignant melanoma, renal carcinoma, acute myelogenous leukemia, retinoblastoma, and chorionic carcinoma). Interestingly, these are cancers in which spontaneous remissions and long disease-free intervals can occur. It was realized that the good results from immunotherapy were quite unpredictable.

Following this empirical research, modern molecular biology is identifying authentic tumor antigens and is increasingly able to measure the cytotoxic T-cell response to them. Furthermore, rather than relying on the cancer cell itself as the vaccine substance, tumor cells are being genetically manipulated to render them more immunogenic. As a result, a new, cautious optimism has entered the field.

There is certainly no shortage of immunologic mechanisms for killing tumor cells. Antibody alone can lead to complement fixation and tumor-cell lysis. Alternatively, antibody can promote opsonization of cancer cells and can engender antibody-dependent cellular cytotoxicity. Antibody can also be used to bring a drug, a toxin, or an isotope onto, or even into, a tumor cell through appropriate conjugation. CTLs can be powerful killing agents, and a greater degree of specificity can be ensured by manipulation of tumor-infiltrating lymphocytes. Other cells with anticancer potential include NK cells, natural cytotoxic cells, and lymphocyte-activated killer cells. Macrophages have long been known to be able to kill tumors, particularly via their products, such as TNF-α and oxygen free radicals.

However, it should be noted that there are also numerous mechanisms by which tumor cells can escape from immunologic attack, particularly the attack of CTLs. Many of these have been noted in experimental situations. For example, the tumor-associated antigen in question can be downregulated or completely lost from the tumor cell. Similarly, a downregulation of MHC class I molecules can occur, such that the cytotoxic T cell has many fewer MHC-peptide targets to attack. As rapidly growing cancer cells are subject to many mutations, the tumor-associated antigen itself could mutate, thus affecting its immunogenicity. Finally, it should be noted that the human subject receiving immunotherapy might be immunologically impaired, for example, by drugs, radiotherapy, the growth of the tumor itself, or by the ageing process, many cancer victims being advanced in years. All of the above act as potential and actual barriers to immunotherapy being universally effective.

Vaccines against Cancer-related Viruses

The causation of cancer is complex and multifactorial, but the association between certain cancers and prior virus infections is so strong as to leave little doubt that infection with the virus is a condition precedent to the later development of the specific cancer. Thus, chronic carriers of hepatitis B or C frequently develop chronic liver disease, multiple nodular hyperplasia, hepatic cirrhosis, and, eventually, primary hepatocellular carcinoma. Viral genes can readily be detected in the cancer cells. In some countries (e.g., China for hepatitis B, Japan for hepatitis C), liver cancer is sufficiently common to be acknowledged as a major public health concern. Moreover, antiviral treatments such as acyclovir or IFN-α are not effective in eliminating the virus in a sufficient percentage of patients to constitute a satisfactory cancer prophylactic strategy. Thus, vaccination to prevent virus infection in the first place would be the preferred alternative.

For hepatitis B, this is now a relatively straightforward matter. In some countries, the infection that leads to carrier status is acquired during passage through the birth canal or, conceivably, via breast milk in the very nearly neonatal period. Here, the ideal treatment is "passive–active," or an injection of hepatitis B–specific gamma-globulin as well as an injection of hepatitis B vaccine, both given at birth or, at the latest, within 48 hours of birth. This is feasible in an industrialized country such as Japan, where the carrier rate is around 2%, where all pregnant women can be tested for carrier status, and where the above protocol has been deemed preferable to immunization of all infants. In many countries, this is not yet practical, so only active immunization is given, with three injections of hepatitis B vaccine (e.g., at 0, 1, and 6 months). This works well to prevent the carrier state. In certain countries, acquisition of the infection appears to be community-based in the majority of instances, and here it is feasible to delay active immunization until the first administration of DTP vaccine, at 6 to 8 weeks of age. Using DTP as a "platform" for the addition of further vaccines affords a simplification of vaccine schedules. A pentavalent DTP–hepatitis B–H. influenzae B vaccine is currently in clinical trial. For hepatitis C, no vaccine currently exists, but one is badly required. It appears as though 80% of patients infected with hepatitis C become chronic carriers (a percentage that begins to approach that in HIV), and the majority of these will eventually go on to develop chronic liver disease.

Epstein-Barr virus (EBV) represents another interesting case. This virus, which is virtually ubiquitous, is involved in nasopharyngeal carcinoma, Burkitt's lymphoma, and probably some other forms of lymphoma and leukemia. It is not known why the great majority of people recover from EBV infection either with no obvious illness (particularly if the virus is encountered in early childhood) or with a self-limited case of glandular fever, while a few go on to these vicious cancers. In some countries (e.g., Southern China), a prophylactic EBV vaccine should be a worthwhile public health intervention.

A great deal of work has been done on human papilloma viruses (HPVs), particularly types HPV-16 and HPV-18, as causative agents of carcinoma of the cervix. Two different kinds of vaccines are under active investigation, one that would prevent infection with the virus in the first place, and that could thus be targeted at teenagers who are not yet sexually active; and a therapeutic vaccine, where the HPV gene products E6 and E7 make attractive targets. These genes are clearly involved in the transforming ability of the viruses and continue to be expressed in cervical cancer cells, including metastases. Active research is exploring the possibility that recombinant DNA-derived forms of these antigens could strengthen the T-cell attack in this disease.

Capsid proteins are the most logical candidates for vaccines designed to protect against infection with HPV. The major capsid protein L1, as a virus-like particle, is particularly attractive. The range of candidates for a therapeutic vaccine is wider. Keratinocytes infected with papilloma viruses express six to eight virally encoded proteins that, however, do not form part of the mature virus. Of these so-called early antigens, two, namely E6 and E7, are consistently expressed in cervical cancer cells. Their abundance is higher than that of E1 and E2, and E4 is only abundant in terminal keratinocytes. Class I–restricted T-cell epitopes have been identified for E6 and E7. The induction of CTL responses against them by peptide, protein, or vectored vaccines has been shown to be effective in tumor elimination in animal models (242). Studies of mice transgenic for these antigens from HPV-16 spontaneously develop squamous cell carcinomas and lenticular tumors, supporting the view that these gene products are directly involved in malignant transformation (243).

In view of the above success, two phase I trials of immunotherapy of cervical cancer have been reported. A vaccinia virus construct encoding E6 and E7 of HPV-16 and 18 induced specific antibodies in three of eight subjects and circulating CTL precursors in one (244). The injection of HPV-16 E7 protein, using "Algammulin" as adjuvant, into five subjects led to antibodies to E7 in all five, and measurable T cell–proliferative response in two, but no specific CTLs were demonstrated in any patient (245). The immunogenicity of E7 in humans should encourage further clinical experimentation with other adjuvants, vectors, or DNA vaccine constructs. For example, three human CTL epitopes from E7 of HPV-16 have been expressed conjointly with hepatitis B core antigen in aroA⁻ aroD⁻ S. typhimurium as a preclinical orally active vaccine. This imaginative approach is well worth following up.

The International Agency for Research on Cancer has attempted to estimate what proportion of cancer is attributable to virus infection. This adds up to 15% globally and 20% in developing countries. Fifty-five percent of stomach cancers could be attributable to H. pylori (500,000 cases per annum); 84% of liver cancers, to hepatits B and C (400,000 cases per annum); and 89% of cervical cancers, to HPV (400,000 cases per annum). Control via community-wide immunization represents an attractive approach.

Vaccines against Tumor-specific and Tumor-associated Antigens

The hypothesis underlying all anticancer vaccines is that the cancer cell, being biochemically different from normal tissue, may display one or more antigens not expressed in normal cells. If that antigen could be injected into the host in a form suitable for eliciting an appropriate immune response, an attack more powerful than that mounted against the tumor cells as such could ensue. While most recent attention has focused on manipulations that evoke CD8⁺ T-lymphocytes, antibodies, CD4⁺ T cells, and macrophages can all be involved in antitumor immunity.

Not so many years ago, it was thought that an antigen had to be an integral membrane protein or some other key constituent of the plasma membrane if it were to serve as a useful target for antitumor surveillance. Now we know that self proteins are processed into peptides and can be presented at the cell surface in association with self class I MHC. Thus, intracellular proteins become potentially important. Given the power of CTLs to lyse target cells, then to move away and to strike again, CTLs could be effective against a wide range of possible tumor antigens. Basically, the antigens against which an antitumor immune attack can be mounted fall into four categories.

Mutant Antigens

First there are truly tumor-specific antigens; these are cases in which a somatic point mutation has taken place in a protein of the cancer cell, and in which peptides derived from that protein can be presented on a class I MHC molecule of the cell, thus constituting a T-cell epitope unique to the tumor and not possessed by any other cell. In a pivotal series of studies, Boon's group (246) showed that mutated housekeeping genes could lead to the appearance of antigenic T-cell epitopes on the tumor cell surface, which served as the target of a CTL attack. Similar mutations occur in human tumors (247) (e.g., CDK4 and MuM1). As mutations will occur in different proteins and various parts of the same protein in different individuals, such mutant peptides would have to be identified and formulated into vaccines separately for each patient. This serious practical disadvantage could only be overcome by major advances in technology. However, two advantages of such vaccines would be the absolute lack of effect against normal cells and the absence of prior immunologic tolerance against what is essentially a new antigen.

Shared Antigens Not Expressed in Normal Tissues, Frequently Oncofetal Antigens

These are proteins that are not normally expressed in adult tissues, but are present in tumors, frequently of a variety of origins. They are products of unmutated genes, some of which have been shown to be normally expressed in fetal life. This category of oncofetal antigen has been the subject of study in murine systems for more than three decades, but it has assumed a new importance since the identification of a number of examples in human tumors. The greatest body of knowledge has built up around malignant melanoma. Here, CTLs from the patient were used as detectives to identify components of a tumor-derived cosmid library made from the DNA of the antigenic melanoma. Transfected cells, which themselves had lost the antigen in question, were tested for capacity to stimulate CTLs. Once the right gene has been isolated, further cycles of transfection, using fragments of the gene, can lead to the identification of the relevant class I–restricted CTL epitope. The antigen MAGE-1 was the first thus identified (248). This HLA-A1 restricted epitope was a nonamer with the sequence EADPTGHSY. It was soon realized that MAGE-1 belonged to a multigene family with at least 12 members (249). Using basically the same approach, other genes coding for tumor-rejection antigens, such as the BAGE and GAGE genes, have been identified. These are both members of multigene families and have no sequence homology to any other known gene or to one another. To date, seven different antigenic peptides have been established as capable of stimulating CTLs from these three types of genes, and, in each case, the peptide sequence and the HLA restriction element are known (250). Some antigens possess more than one T-cell epitope. For example, MAGE-3 encodes antigenic peptides, restricted by HLA-A1, -A2 and -B44, respectively. More than 60% of melanomas from Caucasians are positive for at least one of the above antigens. Reverse-transcriptase polymerase chain reaction (RT-PCR) shows that they can also be expressed, though at lower frequency, in cells from non–small cell lung cancers, bladder cancers, breast cancers, squamous cell carcinomas, and prostatic carcinomas. They are rarely expressed in colorectal cancers and virtually never in leukemia and/or lymphoma.

Would immunization with one of these peptides damage normal tissues? MAGE, BAGE, and GAGE can be expressed in testis or placenta (249) but apparently only in cells lacking HLA class I, such as spermatogonia, spermatocytes, or labyrinthine trophoblast cells. Thus side effects appear to be unlikely. Moreover, no problems were encountered in a small phase I trial with a MAGE-3 peptide (251), which gave some promising preliminary results in metastatic melanoma. A murine gene, *PIA,* shares some features with the present group of human tumor antigens, in that it is expressed in murine mastocytoma cells and some other cancers, but not in normal adult tissues, except for testis and placenta. Immunization of mice with this antigen did not result in autoimmune orchitis, nor was normal gestation interfered with (252). Obviously PIA is only a model. The matter will have to be followed carefully in clinical trials on a case-by-case basis.

This group of antigens presents some favorable features for further clinical experimentation. First, knowing the patient's HLA genotype and the expression pattern of the particular tumor, rational peptide choices can be made. Second, quantitative evaluation of specific CTL responses (or, for that matter, antibody and CD4+ T-cell responses) will progressively allow information on the immunologic correlates of tumor progression or latency to build-up. Third, knowing the peptide of interest, comparisons can be made between vaccines using live vectors, different forms of adjuvants, protein carriers, or other types of immunomanipulation. Finally, because many tumors carry more than one antigen, combinations of antigenic peptides may delay or eliminate the problem of antigen-loss mutants, as two antigens would rarely be lost simultaneously.

The search for CTL-identifiable autologous antigens is far from over. Boon's group has discovered some exciting variations on the theme. About 50% of melanomas abnormally activate the *N*-acetyl-glucosaminyltransferase gene, such that an HLA-A2–restricted peptide encoded by an intronic sequence is produced (253). Furthermore, RAGE is a new gene coding for an antigen of human renal carcinoma, again identified by autologous CTL (254). In all, 12 important potential vaccine peptides of this type have been described (249).

What event prompts the activation of MAGE or other genes in a melanoma cell? This may be due to demethylation of the relevant promoter, which may be a random consequence of a genome-wide demethylation that is frequently seen in tumor cells (255).

Differentiation Antigens

Another type of antigen that could conceivably be used as a cancer vaccine is an antigen expressed by the malignant cell and by the normal counterpart of that cell. A very particular kind of differentiation antigen is the idiotype of a B-cell lymphoma, the unique immunoglobulin receptor clonally expressed on all of the cancer cells, and this molecule has been the target of both passive and active immunotherapy, with some limited success (256). Similarly, molecules such as CD19 and CD20, present on only certain differentiation stages of lymphocytes, belong in this general category. Of broader and more recent interest are antigens recognized on melanoma cells by autologous T cells, but also present on normal melanocytes. The first of these was tyrosinase (257), in which five class I–restricted and two class II–restricted peptides have been identified (250). Tyrosinase peptides have been the targets for some tumor-infiltrating lymphocytes (258). Three other genes of this type are Melan-A/Mast1, gp100/8P and 17, and gp75/TPR-1. Obviously, immunotherapy targeted against such antigens endangers normal melanocytes. Indeed, vitiligo has been noticed in some patients who appear to respond well to melanoma immunotherapy. Of greater concern is the presence of melanocytes in the choroid layers of the retina. To date, no retinal problems have been encountered in the many subjects who have had immunotherapy of one type or another for melanoma. In all, 15 peptides using five different restriction elements constitute this group of potential vaccine molecules (250).

Tumor-associated Mucins

Epithelial cell mucins assumed a new importance when it was noted that human T-lymphocytes could recognize and kill pancreatic tumor cells (259). An extensive series of experiments from Finn's group (260) has resulted in a working hypothesis, which has been reviewed. The antigen epithelial cell mucin is encoded by the gene Muc-1, and is a heavily glycosylated, high-molecular-weight glycoprotein produced by normal epithelial cells to lubricate mucosal surfaces. Typically, Muc-1 protein is confined to the luminal side of the epithelial cell. O-linked carbohydrate chains, many ending in sialic acid residues, project from the serine and threonine residues of Muc-1. One could image that this dense carbohydrate coat could sterically hinder the access of T-cell receptors (TCRs) to the protein core of Muc-1. When malignant transformation of an epithelial cell takes place, as in epithelial adenocarcinomas such as those of breast, pancreas, or colon, important changes in the mucins are noted. Expression is not polarized, but uniform, over the cell surface. The amount of mucin is up to ten times higher than normal. Furthermore, the mucin is poorly glycosylated, and thus the protein core of the integral membrane protein becomes more exposed. A number of groups cloned Muc-1 almost simultaneously (e.g., see refs. 261, 262), whereupon it became clear that the molecule contained a large number of tandem repeats with the sequence PDTRPAPGSTAPPAHGVTSA. There is a polymorphism resulting in different individuals possessing anywhere from 20 to 125 such repeats. The repeats display a stable polyproline β-turn helix (263). Remarkably, CTLs isolated from patients with various carcinomas (e.g., breast, ovary, or pancreas) are capable of recognizing multiple tandem repeats of the 20-mer in an HLA-unrestricted fashion. The T cells isolated from patients are typical αβ TCR T cells, and antibodies against the TCR inhibit T-cell recognition of the mucin core. The postulate is that the multiple TCRs on a T cell engaging the multiple sets of 20-mer on a tumor cell involves such a high degree of multivalency that the relatively low affinity of the TCRs for a single repeat does not matter.

Following extensive preclinical investigation, a number of early clinical trials of Muc-1 as a cancer vaccine have been reported. Goydos et al. (264) tested a synthetic 105-aminoacid peptide consisting of five repeated immunodominant epitopes plus a linker, administered mixed with BCG. Patients received 100 mg initially and then two further vaccinations at 3-week intervals. Patients had advanced adenocarcinomas of the pancreas, breast, or colon. As expected, there was local ulceration at the injection site, but patients tolerated the therapy reasonably well. About a third of patients tested had a two- to fourfold increase in Muc-1 CTL pre-cursor cells; two-thirds had flulike symptoms, possibly associated with secretion of IL-6; and many patients had profound DTH reactions to mucin-specific peptides. Three of 63 patients showed stabilization of disease. Future work will concentrate on less toxic adjuvants. Under consideration is the use of autologous APCs, such as DCs (265) or EBV-treated B cells (266) engineered to express high levels of Muc-1, as a cellular vaccine.

Other approaches, which have been briefly summarized (267), include 1.5 tandem repeats covalently linked to keyhole limpet hemocyanin (KLH) together with the adjuvant molecule QS21, in which nine breast cancer patients showed impressive antibody production but no CTL generation, a situation perhaps capable of dealing with micrometastases; and live vaccinia virus vector/Muc-1/IL-2 constructs, in which a phase I trial involving nine stage 3/4 breast cancer patients is in train.

McKenzie's group (268) has used an oxidized mannan–Muc-1 F protein that elicits strong CTL responses in the mouse. In a clinical trial involving 25 patients, cellular responses were less common than hoped, but humoral responses were observed in more than 70%. Interestingly, when this group immunized mice with human Muc-1, the CTLs that were obtained were quite clearly MHC-restricted. The reasons for the difference are not clear, but it will be of interest to see whether *evoked* CTLs in the human (as opposed to spontaneously occurring ones) show MHC restriction (268).

Clearly the above represents examples only. The field of tumor antigens is very active, and there are many other candidates on the list. It is good to see the previous clinical empiricism (for which there will always be a place) now being buttressed by a good deal of hard cellular and molecular science.

Cellular Vaccines

Defined molecular vaccines are attractive because of their precision, but an argument could be mounted that a vaccine should make use not just of one antigen, but of every possible antigen that the cancer may possess, in case selection of antigen-loss mutants frustrates the purpose of the more precise vaccine. There is an extensive literature concerning vaccines dependent on the use of whole irradiated tumor cells, tumor cell lines, extracts therefrom, or proteins shed from tumor cells in culture. The most popular tumor under investigation was melanoma, and there is no doubt that, in a small minority of patients, substantial tumor regression was achieved. The most frequently used adjuvant was BCG or bacterial products derived from BCG. Some of these trials achieved sufficiently good results in terms of documented induction of antitumor T-cell reactivity and prolongation of survival to warrant follow-up work (269–271). While injection of vaccinia or BCG directly into cutaneous metastases of melanoma occasionally led to dramatic short-term resolution of lesions, injected and noninjected, there is no evidence that long-term cures resulted. The history of this whole field is long and turbulent, and it is hard to believe that the crude approaches will survive without significant modification.

An extensive study of the transfection of tumor cells by cytokine genes has been undertaken to see whether the delivery of a cytokine concomitantly and in an identical site to putative tumor antigens could increase the antitumor T-cell response (272). Of 30 cytokines or related molecules, GM-CSF was found to be the only truly impressive agent. GM-CSF causes division and activation of DCs, thus strengthening the afferent limb of the immune response.

In the human situation, it might be necessary to use the melanoma cells of the particular patient involved—to obtain metastatic tissue, place it into culture, transduce the GM-CSF gene, and irradiate tumor-cell populations prior to a series of autologous vaccine injections. The first patient thus treated (273) did indeed produce extra CTL precursors, though briefly, and some clinical and radiologic features suggested infiltration of metastatic lesions, but, unfortunately, the patient died without real clinical improvement. Another DC stimulant is the flt-3 ligand, which is well worthy of close examination (274). This is a strong *in vitro* and *in vivo* DC stimulant and is a potent T-cell adjuvant. In the long run, it may not be practical to individualize treatment to the extent demanded by autologous tumor-cell vaccines. Another patient-specific technique is growth and cytokine transduction of tumor-infiltrating lymphocytes, followed by their return to the patient, or growth of DCs and pulsing these *in vitro* with either crude tumor sonicates or more specific peptide antigens. As DCs can be grown in large numbers from peripheral blood in the presence of GM-CSF and IL-4, this may not be too formidable logistically. Alternatively and more generically, a number of model systems are now exploring the value of GM-CSF or soluble flt-3 ligand, using the patient's own *in situ* tumor as the antigen source.

There has not yet been much research on the approaches covered in this section as methods to deal with minimal residual disease. The author repeats his belief that this will be the most appropriate target for tumor immunotherapy, which he further believes holds rich promise as an adjuvant therapy.

Immunotoxins and Antibodies as Antitumor Agents

Whereas this chapter is primarily about active immunization, a few remarks about passive immunotherapy of cancer may be in order. The conjugation of a drug, toxin, or isotope to an antibody molecule directed against some antigen on a tumor cell has been extensively studied in experimental systems as a tumor-ablative therapy, and a modest amount of clinical experimentation utilizing this principle has also been performed. A good example of the approach is the work of Vitetta's group (275). In what she terms *second-generation* immunotoxins, many of the problems of the approach, such as hepatotoxicity, rapid catabolism, and poor efficacy of the antibody, have been overcome by various experimental manipulations. For example, an antibody directed at either CD19 or CD22, present on most B-cell lymphomas, can be conjugated to a deglycosylated ricin A chain to create an immunotoxin that is reasonably well tolerated and that is effective in limited clinical studies in reducing the tumor burden in a significant proportion of patients, particularly those for which the tumor mass present at the initiation of therapy is not too large. While the results with these bulky tumors may appear moderate, the trials have delineated acceptable dosage levels and have established a certain credibility. Viewed in this light, the results look quite promising for an attack on minimal residual disease.

Micrometastases were indeed the target of an interesting study by Riethmueller's group (summarized in 276). They chose to use antibody alone, not conjugated to any toxin, because they believed that complement or ADCC can do a good job if small nests of cells constituting micrometastases were the target of therapy. Using the unconjugated murine monoclonal antibody 17-1A, an IgG2A antibody against a widely expressed epithelial glycoprotein, patients with colon cancer were treated. In a randomized trial of 189 cases of Duke's stage C colon cancer, with a median follow-up period of 5 years, 500 mg of antibody given postsurgery and then 100 mg given monthly for a further four doses decreased the death rate by 30% and the recurrence rates by 27%. Furthermore, the decrease in recurrences was confined to distant, but not local, return of tumor. This substantiated the viewpoint that micrometastases, rather than substantial local residual collections of tumor cells, were the target of therapy. This trial was very encouraging, because the antibody was an early one, no attempts at humanization having taken place. The effect on mortality was approximately equivalent to that achieved with adjuvant chemotherapy, which has become more or less mandatory in recent years for this kind of tumor. It is difficult to escape the conclusion that results would improve still further if antibody treatment were combined with adjuvant chemotherapy. Such trials are now ongoing.

From these examples, it is evident that passive immunotherapy with antibodies is sufficiently promising to warrant a great deal of further exploration.

Conclusions

It is appropriate that students of tumor immunotherapy have learned a certain degree of modesty. The swashbuckling, exaggerated claims are a thing of yesteryear. A more cautious and scientific approach is being taken, with a realization that successes will be slow in coming and probably confined to particular stages of particular cancers in the first instance. At least the tools are now at hand for an intelligent series of assays. These involve identification of tumor antigens, measurement of T-cell responses, assessment of susceptibility to antibody, and careful logging of antitumor responses. Within such constraints, the field is ripe for much more preclinical and clinical research. Given the volume of work that is progressing, it is also quite probable that variations on the above themes will come forward, and as we learn more about immunoregulation, so the approaches should become more powerful.

BIRTH-CONTROL VACCINES

It is not the author's intent to launch into an extensive review of this important subject. Rather, it is introduced to illustrate the point that the induction of an immune response can be employed in a realm far removed from communicable diseases or oncology, and to alert the reader that there may be other surprises in store in the future.

What is required is a vaccine, the effects of which last for a reasonable period, say, up to 3 years, but which is reversible. If designed for women, it should not perturb the regular menstrual cycle nor cause excessive bleeding. It should most certainly not cause any autoimmune pathology. One prominent candidate for women has been human chorionic gonadotrophin (hCG). This hormone is made by the ovary very soon after fertilization of the ovum and is essential for implantation into the uterine wall a few days later. Interference with hCG has no effects on ovulation or on steroid hormones. There is one disadvantage, however, in that hCG is a heterodimer consisting of an α and a β chain. The β chain is unique, but the α chain is shared with several other hormones. Some limited clinical research has been done with the β chain conjugated to protein, but the most hopeful results have been obtained with an artificial hormone consisting of the β chain of hCG non covalently associated with the α chain of ovine luteinizing hormone. This heterospecies dimer (HSD) was, in turn, conjugated

covalently to DT or TT. This vaccine has been trialled in 148 women over 1,224 menstrual cycles (277). The women chosen all had at least two children, were sexually active, and had presented at family planning clinics. Immunization consisted of three injections of HSD adsorbed onto alum. For the first injection, 1 mg of the sodium phthalyl derivative of LPS was included as an adjuvant. The DT and TT preparations were used alternatively. Women were regularly monitored for the level of anti-hCG antibodies, as it had been determined that the bioneutralizing levels of anti-hCG was about 50 ng per ml of antibody. For the 80% of women who produced levels above this threshold, only one pregnancy resulted. Most women had to receive booster injections to maintain this level for prolonged periods. In the absence of boosters, most women lost protection from pregnancy after a year or less.

The proof of principle was certainly there in this phase II study. However, a stronger adjuvant is needed, one that promotes better serum antibody formation. As the vaccine seems entirely safe, and reversible, it is to be hoped that clinical research can continue.

Another interesting vaccine candidate is the decapeptide luteinizing hormone-releasing hormone (LH-RH), also known as gonadotrophin-releasing hormone (GnRH). This hormone is common to males and females and controls the production of gametes and sex steroids in both sexes. A synthetic vaccine, in which a glycine is replaced at position 6 by *D*-lysine, and in which the peptides are conjugated to DT, could be an effective, reversible fertility control agent for domestic pets. In humans, this vaccine has been in phase I and II trials for advanced prostate cancer as an alternative to orchidectomy. Prostate-specific antigen and acid phosphatase levels fell in five of six and four of six patients, respectively, receiving the vaccine at 400-μg doses three times. Clinical and radiologic improvement was noted in some but not all patients (278). Delivery in PLG microspheres is under investigation.

A different approach is to immunize against critical molecules of spermatozoa (279). Antibodies that agglutinate, immobilize, or coat the sperm surface would inhibit sperm function. In principle, immunization with sperm antigens could target the male or the female. The number of sperms that enter the oviduct after intercourse is only in the 10s or 100s, and it should be straightforward to neutralize these few by immunizing women. On the other hand, women have for too long carried the major responsibility for birth control, so immunization of men should also be considered. Virtually all vasectomized males make antisperm antibodies, which clearly do them no harm. Six or seven key candidate sperm antigens have already been identified, and about 200 proteins on the surface of sperm are accessible to sperm surface radioiodination or biotinylation. A promising candidate antigen is sperm-agglutinating antigen-1 (SAGA-1), which appears to cover the entire sperm surface (280). Naturally, it will be important to determine that candidate antigens are truly sperm-specific. A clinical trial on SAGA-1 is in the late planning stage.

NEGATIVE VACCINES IN AUTOIMMUNITY AND ALLERGY

A vaccine is a preparation that induces a desirable immune response. There are, of course, some situations in which therapy demands switching off an immune response rather than switching one on. The three most common of these are autoimmune disease, allergy, and transplantation. To the extent that immunologic tolerance involves the deletion or negative selection of immunocytes, or the induction of a state of clonal anergy within them (281), using the word *vaccine* in relation to the toleragen may stretch the definition. But, in addition to these classical ways of tolerance induction (282), we now recognize that there are other ways of modulating or abrogating an immune response. The phrase *suppressor T cells* is now used with caution, though there are many undoubted examples of infectious tolerance, actively mediated by T-cell populations, in the litertaure. More recently, it has become clear that guiding an immune response away from the proinflammatory Th1 T-cell pathway can strongly modulate the propensity to develop autoimmunity and can even reverse established autoimmune aggression. Perhaps no field illustrates the point better than that of oral tolerance (as an example of mucosal tolerance). Given that this is clearly due to the induction of a regulatory T-cell population, it seems legitimate to refer to such treatment as a negative vaccine. This topic is somewhat peripheral to the main thrust of this chapter, so it will be dealt with only briefly.

Treatment of Autoimmunity

We owe a considerable debt to Hafler and Weiner for reawakening interest in the old topic (283) of oral tolerance (284); and also to Holt et al. (285) for similar observations on the respiratory tract. It has been shown that the oral administration of the appropriate antigen can suppress experimental autoimmune encephalomyelitis, collagen-induced arthritis, autoimmune uveitis, and autoimmune diabetes in nonobese diabetic mice. While more than one mechanism is at work, the induction of a regulatory population of T cells may be the most important. These cells have two key characteristics. While generated in the mesenteric lymph nodes and other gut-associated lymphoid tissue, they migrate to the target organs and tissues where the oral toleragen is expressed. Further, on meeting "their" antigen, they secrete TGF-β1, and they may or may not secrete IL-4 and IL-10 as well. Such T cells have come to be referred to as Th3 cells (286). TGF–β1 is an interesting regulatory molecule, as, on the one hand, it is a powerful inhibitor of division among both T and B cells, while, on the other, it increases IgA synthesis. Any accompanying IL-4 production would also favor a reduction of Th1 T-cell development, and thus a reduction in T cell–mediated inflammation. Moreover, while a Th3 cell may be specific for antigen A, and may be attracted to a tissue in which antigen A is expressed, on arrival there, its antiinflammatory action is nonspecific, so cells with specificity for an antigen B that happens to be coexpressed in the same tissue will also be inhibited. This bystander suppression is important in autoimmune situations in which more than one antigen is the target.

These principles, worked out in mice, have led to the initiation of phase I trials of oral toleragens as negative vaccines in multiple sclerosis, uveitis, and rheumatoid arthritis. This work has been sufficiently encouraging to lead to a phase III multicenter trial with myelin antigens in multiple sclerosis. The results of this, announced to the press but not yet published, were curious, in that the placebo group registered a 58% beneficial response, statistically not different from that of the control group. Two different phase II trials of type II collagen in rheumatoid arthritis were also disappointing.

Aerosol administration of autoantigens represents another way of inducing immunologic tolerance. Harrison's group (287) have administered insulin as an aerosol to NOD mice during the preclinical, insulitis phase of their disease and have found a substantial reduction both in the incidence of clinical diabetes and in the severity of insulitis lesions in the pancreas. Interestingly, while proliferation among splenic T cells to the most important peptide was essentially abrogated, that to a separate β cell autoantigen, glutamic acid decarboxylase, was also significantly reduced. While this suggests a final effector mechanism of a nonspecific nature, as in the above studies, a vital difference was noted. The regulatory cells in Harrison's work appear to have been CD8+ γδ T cells, not CD4+ Th3 cells. These were powerfully effective in preventing diabetes in an adoptive cotransfer model.

Some clinical trial work on oral insulin in high-risk islet-cell antibody-positive first-degree relatives of known diabetics has begun, but the code has not yet been broken.

A further indication that tolerance to a single protein may prevent an autoimmune disease associated with multiple autoantibodies comes from the work of French et al. (288). NOD mice transgenic for the mouse proinsulin II gene were constructed, the promoter being an MHC class II promoter, so that (*inter alia*) DCs in the thymus might express the antigen. Insulitis and diabetes were almost completely prevented. This finding suggests that particular antigens may be central in the development of an autoimmune disease, with other antigens coming into the picture via cascade effects.

We have already mentioned the work of Sun et al. (94), which has shown that CTB can powerfully augment the capacity of proteins to induce oral tolerance when covalently coupled to the protein. This treatment strongly inhibits the early, initiation phases of the DTH reaction as well as the later effector stages, and inhibition can be adoptively transferred. The treatment works in immunotherapeutic models of autoimmunity, such as myelin basic protein-induced EAE, NOD mouse diabetes with insulin conjugated to CTB (289), and collagen type II arthritis, in which an *aerosol* of as little as 25 μg of collagen coupled to CTB effectively prevented arthritis, even when given a week *after* the lesion-inducing injection (290). Finally, allogenic thymocytes coupled to CTB significantly prolonged the survival of heart allografts. As a result of these encouraging findings, early clinical work with CTB has begun, showing that doses up to 100 μg are well tolerated intranasally.

Treatment of Allergy

While desensitization with allergens is a procedure that has been used for many decades, the molecular definition of the major allergenic molecules (with a few exceptions) had to await the gene-cloning era. Most of the important molecules have been cloned, and allelic polymorphisms are being addressed (291). IgE formation is intimately dependent on T-cell help and IL-4 production, so much emphasis has been placed on defining T-cell epitopes and inducing tolerance with them. In line with the observations in the previous section, it might be anticipated that oral tolerance to a peptide might shut off the immune response to the whole allergen. For example, a major allergen from the house dust mite is a 222-amino acid protein Der p 1. When mice are immunized with this protein, T cells can be produced with specificity for at least four T-cell epitopes, and further cryptic epitopes can be identified. Feeding peptides can markedly inhibit the ability of the whole antigen to immunize mice, including preventing the emergence of T-cell immunity to epitopes that are not included in the fed peptides (292). Subcutaneous injection of allergens, the traditional form of desensitization, is now thought to act, at least in part, by modulation of the IL-4–secreting CD4+ T cells, which act as helpers in IgE induction (293). In a murine model of allergy to the major birch pollen antigen Bet v 1, it was shown that the subcutaneous injection of large amounts of an immunodominant T-cell epitope, BV139, could diminish T-cell reactivity to the whole protein (294). Interestingly, a DNA immunization approach to allergy may hold some promise (295). Rats were injected intramuscularly with a plasmid coding for the house dust mite allergen Der p 5, resulting in IgG2a and IgG1 but no IgE antibodies. The DNA vaccine prevented the induction of IgE synthesis and airway hyperresponsiveness, which normally follows aerosol challenge. While this type of result is consistent with shifting T-cell responses from Th2 to Th1 (296), the possible involvement of CD8$^+$ $\gamma\delta$ cells in inhibition of allergic phenomena must be borne in mind.

Data on the use of peptides for human desensitization have so far only been reported at meetings (W.R. Thomas, personal communication), but promising results with injections are coming forward in bee venom and cat dander allergies. The injections of peptides are certainly very well tolerated.

While the above negative vaccines for allergy have been designed for the treatment of established disease, an even more ambitious goal would be to prevent the initial sensitization to environmental allergens. This, in essence, would mean the prevention of Th2 T-cell induction to common allergens.

Holt (297) argues that, in view of the increasing incidence of asthma in many industrialized countries and the economic impact of atopy taken as a whole, large scale preventative strategies should be taken seriously. Most children initiate IgG antibody production to common food and inhaled allergens very early in life, before 3 months of age. This response wanes with time, presumably because of some form of antigen-mediated downregulation. Low-level IgE production to food allergens is also noted early and wanes in nonatopic individuals. The rise and fall of IgE to aeroallergens is much slower. Atopy may be due to the gradual dominance of Th2 over Th1 clones in some individuals. This is much rarer for food allergens than for inhaled allergens, probably because of dosage differences. Holt describes the protective mechanisms of immune deviation to Th1 and of T-cell anergy as "highly efficient" for inhaled antigens but "approaching perfection" in the gastrointestinal tract. So the putative strategy for preventing respiratory allergy, and thus much of asthma, would be to administer an oral negative vaccine of natural or recombinant major antigens (chosen for each region). A limited number of antigens is responsible for the bulk of disease, and the bystander effects already discussed might do the rest. A cocktail of synthetic peptides could also be considered, as could the arguably more efficient intranasal route. The progressive identification of the genes responsible for human atopy might make it possible to confine the approach to susceptible individuals. As exposure to high levels of inhaled allergens during the first 3 months of life predisposes to sensitization and to locking the response into a Th2 direction, measures to minimize levels of inhalant allergens in the nursery may also be important (298). Interestingly, frequent respiratory infections may facilitate an environment favorable to Th1 induction, and thus militate against the establishment of the allergic state. Of course, this is not a circumstance to be encouraged!

ADVERSE EFFECTS OF VACCINES

Three considerations dictate that adverse effects of vaccines must be taken very seriously. First, vaccines are normally given to healthy individuals in opposition to most other biopharmaceuticals, which are given to the sick. Second, most vaccines are given to infants and young children, deemed to be both very precious and very vulnerable. Third, in the industrialized countries, the very success of immunization programs, combined with good personal hygiene, environmental sanitation, and improved living conditions, has made epidemic disease seem like something unfamiliar, and perhaps something that antibiotics and other medical treatments can cope with. In other words, opponents of immunization can be excused for not understanding the risk–benefit equation of vaccines because of a lack of personal experience. This has to be countered by good education.

Fortunately, serious adverse events are rare with currently used vaccines. This creates what, at first sight, seems to be a curious problem. Given that nearly all children get quite a few vaccine injections in the first year of life, a reasonable proportion of all infants coming down with some rare complaint (say, encephalitis) will have had an immunization within, for example, a week of this illness. The assumption of a causative rather than coincidental relationship is quite human and can only be contested by statistical arguments, which are unfamiliar to most people. We shall consider first the more serious claimed side effects.

The most controversial vaccine from the viewpoint of side effects has been DPT containing whole killed pertussis bacteria. Reactions such as fever, irritability, local redness, swelling and pain, anorexia, and drowsiness are quite common, though of short duration and easily ameliorated by a drug such as paracetamol. Febrile convulsions occur in about one case in 2,000 to 3,000, and they cause no long-term harm. Follow-up has shown no evidence of neurologic damage or intellectual impairment. The question of serious acute neurologic illness (e.g., encephalopathy) has caused the most concern. It was put at one case per 330,000 vaccine doses in the United Kingdom in 1981, but reanalysis of the data, coupled with a large study in United States by the Institute of Medicine, challenged this conclusion. The American Academy of Pediatrics (299) found that although "the data accumulated to date may not prove that pertussis vaccine can never cause brain damage, they indicate that if it does so, such occurrences must be exceedingly rare." The U.S. Institute of Medicine concluded that the risk of serious neurologic complications was somewhere between zero and one in 200,000. As the number of cases of whooping cough has fallen by a factor of 50 in the United States since the introduction of the vaccine, and as the disease is accompanied by permanent brain damage in about 1% of cases and by death in 0.1% to 4.0% of cases, depending on the study, the risk–benefit equation is still enormously on the side of vaccination, even on the worst assumptions about brain damage from vaccination.

The acellular pertussis vaccine has certainly caused less acute reactogenicity, as measured by the superficial parameters of local pain, swelling, redness, and so forth. It will, however, take a great deal of experience in the actual deployment phase of this vaccine to determine whether the alleged serious side reactions are less frequent with this purer vaccine.

The Institute of Medicine study determined that the following alleged adverse events of the DTP (whole cell pertussis) were *not* supported by the evidence: infantile spasms, hypsarrhythmia, Reye's syndrome, and sudden infant death syndrome. However, an association with "protracted, inconsolable crying" as a rare complication seems established.

The next important area of concern is poliomyelitis. Adverse reactions to this vaccine are of particular importance, as there have been no cases of wild poliomyelitis in the industrialized countries for many years. In fact, poliomyelitis transmission ceased in the Western Hemisphere in 1991. This makes even a single case of vaccine-associated poliomyelitis a tragedy. Unfortunately, a reversion to neurovirulence of the Sabin polio virus, though excessively rare, is not absolutely unknown. It would appear that once for approximately 2.7 million doses of the oral polio virus vaccine, there is a case of paralytic polio, most commonly of Sabin type 3. On average, there have been about five such cases in the United States per year. Some have been in vaccinees, and some in their contacts.

A major survey of paralytic poliomyelitis in England and Wales between 1985 and 1991 was reported by Joce et al. (300). A total of 21 confirmed cases were found. Thirteen were vaccine-associated, with nine being vaccinees and four being contacts. Five were imported cases, and three were cases with the source of infection unknown. The estimated risk of vaccine-associated paralysis was 1.46 per million for the first dose, but 0.49 per 10^6 for the second and zero for the third and fourth. In all, nine cases of paralysis arose over 18.4 million doses of vaccine administered over 7 years, with a risk of paralysis of 0.49% per 10^6 immunizations, remarkably similar to the U.S. figure of one per 2.7 million. Two vaccine-associated cases were immunodeficient children for whom inactivated poliomyelitis vaccine (IPV) should have been offered.

Whereas the risks of oral polio vaccine (OPV) are truly minuscule, the United States has now suggested either 2 IPV, followed by 2 OPV, or else 4 IPV, as the prophylactic of choice for this affluent population. It is important to bear in mind that the mortality of paralytic poliomyelitis was 5% to 10%, chiefly through bulbar polio. Again the equation works out remarkably in favor of the vaccine.

One can draw up a panoply of other "accusations" against vaccines. Certainly, live, attenuated virus vaccines can cause damage in immunodeficient or immunosuppressed children—generalized vaccinia was probably the worst example. Now that smallpox has been eradicated, this risk has disappeared. If a vaccinia variant is rescued as a vaccine vector, it will be one of lessened virulence.

One can go through the existing vaccines one by one and identify claims for side reactions. Mild measles rash can follow the measles vaccine. Certainly, measles is a nasty disease for the unimmunized, with a case fatality rate in the Third World of about 2% to 3% in unimmunized infants. In the industrialized world, measles deaths are vastly lower, at 0.01% to 0.02%. However, nonfatal complications are common, including otitis media, pneumonia, and subacute sclerosing pan-encephalitis (SSPE). As far as the live, attenuated vaccine is concerned, encephalitis and similar problems are very occasionally reported but have been hard to pin down, and the feasibility of reducing these rare, conjectural complications as well as the acknowledged more common ones (e.g., febrile convulsions) remains problematic at this stage.

Both the measles vaccine and its companions (mumps, rubella, and soon, perhaps, varicella) have good track records in *not* causing serious complications. Suffice it to say that these are live, attenuated vaccines, which can cause problems in particular patients. Reactions are mild and include malaise, fever, mild rash, and (rarely) febrile convulsions. A report (301) has surveyed the incidence of thrombocytopenic purpura after measles, mumps, and rubella vaccination. This was one per 500,000 for measles or rubella alone, one per 120,000 for measles and rubella, and one per 105,000 for the combined measles, mumps, and rubella vaccine. The syndrome resembled the purpura, which can occur after natural measles or rubella infections. Complete recovery occurred in

89.5% of cases; normalization followed by relapse was noted in 7%. No deaths have been reported. This French study accords with conclusions reached in several other countries. While a plausible causal relationship can be argued, the usually favorable outcome ensures that this rare complication does not modify the risk–benefit equation significantly. The mumps vaccine may occasionally cause aseptic meningitis (302).

Vaccinia, while used, was a reasonably reactogenic vaccine and quite dangerous in immunodeficient–immunosuppressed children. Fortunately, this is no longer a problem since smallpox eradication. In general terms, severe reactions against BCG, varicella, measles, or other live vaccines can occur in such individuals.

Excipients in the vaccine or adjuvant substances can occasion side reactions varying from inflammation to abscess formation. More seriously, vaccines can occasionally cause anaphylaxis, thrombocytopenia (as already mentioned), or acute arthritis. These serious complications occur in less than one case in 100,000.

In summary, vaccines that have been through the current stringent regulatory process are incredibly safe. This fact deserves to be widely promulgated, and particularly the media need to be educated via a consistent and nonconfrontational effort.

THE FUTURE

As this chapter has shown, there is a considerable renaissance in vaccinology. The present, surprisingly extensive preclinical research effort will lead to new and improved products. Future developments in the field will center on three areas of uncertainty. How many of the current preclinical research projects will actually lead to marketable products? To what extent will combination vaccines and new vaccination approaches simplify immunization schedules (in the absence of which infant programs could become too arduous)? At what rate will it be possible to make the benefits of new vaccines available to all of the world's children and adults, and not just to the citizens of richer countries? This last question is the most important of all, not just because of its obvious humanitarian aspect, but also because eradication of diseases, possible in theory for many major pathogens, demands global coverage. It is clear that the future of vaccinology is not just in the hands of research scientists or public health officials, but rather depends on societal attitudes and political considerations. That being so, it is incumbent on the immunology community, including the readers of this volume, to be firm and articulate advocates of global immunization.

Global Program for Vaccines and Immunization

In 1993, conscious of the great progress that the EPI was making, WHO decided to place nearly all of its efforts in the vaccine field under one roof, the Global Programme for Vaccines and Immunization (GPV). This united two existing programs, EPI and a research promotion and coordination program formerly known as PVD, as well as a new program designed to promote a consistent adequate supply of vaccines of acceptable quality. Furthermore, the World Summit for Children, held in New York in 1990, had led to the formation of an umbrella body known as the Children's Vaccine Initiative, which represented a coalition of all of the major players in the vaccine field, not only WHO. In 1993, it was decided that the same person, Dr. J.W. Lee, should act as the director of GPV and administrative head of CVI, to provide the best cooperation between the interacting bodies. It was also decided to have a single Scientific Advisory Group of Experts (SAGE) to provide scientific guidance to both GPV and CVI. The director-general of WHO did the present author the great honor of asking him to act as chairman of SAGE. It remained to ensure that those efforts not under GPV, namely AIDS vaccines and antiparasite vaccines, proceeded in full knowledge of what GPV was doing and *vice versa*. This has been done by formal and informal links with the two relevant organizations: UNAIDS, under Dr. Peter Piot; and the Tropical Diseases Research Programme, under Dr. Tore Godal. To the greatest extent possible, GPV and SAGE create a series of lively interfaces with the larger national and regional research efforts and with industry, which is seen as an essential partner. In an imperfect world, the global effort to produce new and improved vaccines and to deliver them appropriately is now reasonably well coordinated. Resource constraints remain the factor limiting more rapid progress. The relatively slow take-up of the only two new vaccines recommended for EPI over its 23-year history, for hepatitis B and yellow fever, is a sobering reminder of how far there is to go.

The Challenge of Disease Eradication

The smallpox triumph showed that the total eradication of a disease from the globe was possible. Provided that there is an effective vaccine, no animal or other reservoir in the biosphere, and a genuine worldwide commitment, eradication of quite a number of diseases should prove possible. Perhaps the first century of the third millennium will be the time when humanity takes this issue seriously.

In 1985, 11 years after the EPI was launched, the Pan-American Health Organization adopted the goal of polio eradication. There were three overarching elements to the strategy (303): first, achieving and maintaining high OPV immunization levels; second, effective surveillance and accurate diagnosis; third, area-wide vaccination around all new cases. Cuba was the first country to mount a major national campaign. By 1989, an 86% decline from the 1986 figure had been achieved in all of the Americas, and by 1990, only 18 cases were reported. "Operation Mop-up" started in 1989, involving special house-to-house campaigns in areas deemed still at risk. In the event, the last case of polio occurred in Peru in August 1991, and in 1994 an International Commission certified that polio had been eradicated from the Western Hemisphere (304).

WHO has set its cap at the global eradication of poliomyelitis by the year 2000. Immunization of about 82% of infants in their first 6 months of life is being achieved, but this alone will not do the job. An extremely valuable tool has been the establishment of National Immunization Days (NIDs). These are particular days, usually in winter, when natural transmission of polio is at its seasonal low, when a whole country mobilizes a massive effort to immunize all children of a particular age (usually less than 5 years of age), regardless of previous immunization history, the aim being to catch the normally hard-to-reach and thus not-yet-immunized. These NIDs have been spectacularly successful and are a great credit to the health officials and political leaders in the relevant countries; to Rotary International, which, through its Polio Plus campaign, has raised hundreds of millions of private dollars and has played a big role in mobilizing local voluntary support, and to the literally millions of volunteers involved in the effort.

China has also been a remarkable success story. NIDs were held in December 1993 and January 1994 and again over the next 2

years. In 1996, there were only three confirmed cases of polio in China, all imported. In Laos and Cambodia, there were four. One of the most remarkable stories is India. The subcontinent began its effort in December 1995. In January 1997, the author was in New Delhi on the second of two NIDs for that season. Unbelievably, a total of 167 million children under 5 years of age received the vaccine, not only in India, but also in all of the other countries of the subcontinent. This involved 3.5 million volunteers and 650,000 immunization stations. An 18-nation grouping from the Middle East, the Caucasus, and the Central Asian Republics, known as MECACAR, also achieved a success rate of over 95% in most of the countries during their NIDs. In Africa, the winter of 1996 to 1997 saw Nelson Mandela assume the presidency of the "Kick Polio Out of Africa" campaign, with 42 countries running NIDs under the auspices of the Organization for African Unity and the strong backing of the African Regional Office of WHO. These efforts suggest that eradication by the year 2000 or somewhat later is still possible.

One aspect of great importance in achieving eradication is disease surveillance. This involves a reporting system for all cases of acute flaccid paralysis, as well as a network of laboratories to provide confirmation of the diagnosis by examination of stool samples. Good surveillance is necessary for the intensive "mopping up" immunizations necessary when chains of transmission are confined to a few geographic pockets. Follow-up surveillance for several years is required when transmission has ceased, to be sure that the disease is really gone, before eradication can be certified.

Despite the great infectiousness of measles, many of the lessons learned from polio eradication can be applied to this disease. The WHO Regional Office for the Americas has made measles eradication a goal by the year 2000. In many countries, a 95% coverage rate has been achieved in infants. Already, transmission has ceased in Cuba, the countries of the English-speaking Carribean, and Chile. The Carribean countries have been measles-free for 6 years. Measles, mumps, and rubella transmission has ceased in some of the Scandinavian countries. An experience in the United Kingdom is worth recording (3). In 1993, small outbreaks of measles in secondary school children and epidemiologic study of the probable pool of susceptible subjects, using reasonable assumptions about vaccine efficacy rates, suggested the possibility of a brisk epidemic among schoolchildren. Accordingly, in November 1994, a national immunization campaign was mounted, targeted at children aged 5 to 16 years, who received a measles–rubella vaccine. This achieved greater than 90% coverage, 8 million children being immunized by a mobilized workforce of nurses. Reports of serious adverse reactions were rare, at seven per 100,000. As a result, measles has very nearly disappeared from the United Kingdom, the rare cases that have been confirmed since arising from imported cases.

WHO has not set a target date for global measles eradication, but may well do so when polio is gone. Surveillance will again be of great importance, as many rashes can resemble the exanthem of measles. Given that the present vaccine is not effective before 9 months of age, some experts feel that a population of susceptibles aged between 4 to 6 months (when maternally derived passive immunity wanes) and 9 months may frustrate eradication efforts. For this reason, research is being directed at vaccine formulations that are effective even in the presence of maternal antibodies.

Eradication efforts and NIDs have been criticized as representing vertical programs with the possibility of drawing resources away from more broadly based health initiatives. In many instances, however, NIDs have also given opportunities for extended activities, such as provision of vitamin A supplements or administration of vaccines other than that for the target disease. Moreover, the social mobilization required for NIDs tends to raise a community's health consciousness, which is of benefit to regular health programs. In the last analysis, the permanence of eradication makes it a supremely cost-effective endeavor.

Vaccination of the Very Young and the Old

Both extremes of age offer special challenges for the designer of new and improved vaccines. Some vaccines should be delivered very early in life (e.g., at birth) to be maximally useful. These include vaccines for diseases carried by the mother, such as hepatitis B, hepatitis C, HIV, or CMV. Traditionally, BCG has also been given, in developing countries, within a few days of birth. Other vaccines are recommended for the elderly, including (in many countries) influenza and pneumococcal vaccines. There has been an upsurge of interest in protecting the elderly.

As regards the newborn, a significant degree of immaturity of the immune system exists in both mice and humans (305). Furthermore, there is a bias towards Th2-type responses in the mouse, which persists if boosters are given later. Induction of CTLs is also difficult in the very young. The observed Th2/Th1 imbalance can be partly corrected by selected adjuvants, such as water-in-oil emulsions containing block copolymer, though accompanied by significant local toxicity (306). A more exciting finding is that a single DNA immunization at 1 week of age in the mouse can lead to both a Th1-biased, IgG2a-dominated antibody response and to Th1-type cytokine secretion on restimulation of T cells *in vitro* (307). Furthermore, a specific CTL response also resulted. Each of three DNA vaccines behaved similarly, namely constructs coding for measles virus hemagglutinin, fragment C of tetanus toxin, or Sendai virus nucleoprotein. However, this adult-like pattern of response to DNA immunization could not be achieved when mice had been primed in the newborn period with a Th2-biased immunization. This represents another example of how responses can get locked into a pattern. The capacity of DNA vaccines to yield Th1 immunity might be particularly favorable for the development of a human AIDS or TB vaccine based on the DNA approach. On the other hand, trials in human newborns have not begun.

At the other end of life, several factors militate against robust immune responses. The thymic cortex is largely replaced by fat, and few or no new T cells are exported from there. Thus T-cell immunity to new antigens must depend on cross-reactions with previously encountered ones. Similarly, the number of progenitors of B cells in the bone marrow is also reduced, though not as markedly. Interestingly, DCs from the peripheral blood of individuals over 65 years of age are present in somewhat *increased* numbers, are normal in appearance and surface markers, and are unimpaired in antigen-presenting function (308). This may partly militate against the reduced proliferative capacity of aged T cells (309). Overall, the capacity to mount a serum antibody response may be reduced by up to tenfold in old age.

It is well known that the elderly are relatively more susceptible to infections such as tuberculosis, influenza, and pneumonia. An interesting, though infrequent, problem relates to tetanus. It has been estimated that only 25% (310) to 40% (311) of the healthy elderly have protective levels of antitetanus antibodies in their serum, as opposed to 92% in subjects under 30 years of age. This is mainly due to a failure to receive the recommended booster injections every 10 years. It is possible, however, that the frequency of boosters may have to be greater after 70 years of age. The fact that immunization against influenza and pneumococci significantly reduces the burden of these infections in the elderly should prompt an examination of what other vaccines might be useful in this age group, given the emergence of many antibiotic-resistant strains of bacteria and the ever-present threat of many viruses. For example, the effects of boosting with the varicella vaccine on the later incidence of herpes zoster require urgent investigation.

New Vaccination Approaches

Of the new vaccination approaches discussed in this chapter, DNA vaccines, superior adjuvant formulations, microencapsulation, and mucosal immunity are among the more promising. Despite his great enthusiasm for them, the author is also aware of the fact that changes to national immunization programs can be made only after very extensive clinical research, particularly in cases in which an effective vaccine already exists. The future will therefore represent a judicious balance between conservatism in a measure already regarded skeptically by a minority and cautious activism, as thorough research documents the value of each new and improved vaccine. Nor should a healthy pluralism be opposed. Some countries will move faster on some vaccines because of their particular perspectives and problems. All of this will mean that the widespread introduction of the rich panoply of vaccines coming from the research sector will probably be slower than the scientific community would like. But, in the long run, the approach to many communicable diseases will be revolutionized by the new vaccinology. The legacy of Jenner and Pasteur is in good hands.

ACKNOWLEDGMENTS

The author would like to thank many kind colleagues for providing reprints, preprints, and permission to cite unpublished results. He would also like to thank the World Health Organization for providing the figures and permission to use them. Dr. P.-H. Lambert deserves special thanks for being the author's chief tutor in vaccinology.

REFERENCES

1. *State of the world's vaccines and immunization, 1996.* Geneva: World Health Organization and United Nations Children's Fund, Publication WHO/GPV/96.04, 1996:161 pp.
2. Baker PJ, ed. *The Jordan Report. Accelerated development of vaccines.* Bethesda, MD: Division of Microbiology and Infectious Diseases, NIAID, NIH, 1996:79 pp.
3. Salisbury DM, Begg NT, eds. *Immunization against infectious disease, Edward Jenner Bicentenary Edition.* London: Department of Health, 1996.
4. Fenner F, Henderson DA, Arita I, Jezek Z, Ladnyi ID. *Smallpox and its eradication.* Geneva: World Health Organization, 1988:1460 pp.
5. Silverstein AM. The royal experiment on immunity, 1721–1722. *In: A history of immunology.* San Diego: Academic Press, 1989:24–37.
6. Jenner E. *An inquiry into the causes and effects of the variolae vaccinae, a disease discovered in some of the western counties of England, particularly Gloucestershire, and known by the name of cow pox.* London: Published privately, 1778.
7. Jenner E. *The origin of the vaccine inoculation.* London: DN Shury, 1801.
8. Pasteur L, Joubert J, Chamberland C. The germ theory of disease. *C R Hebd Seances Acad Sci* 1878;86:1037–1052.
9. Pasteur L. De l'attenuation du virus du cholera des poules. *C R Acad Sci Paris* 1880;91:673–680.
10. Pasteur L, Chamberland CE, Roux E. Sur la vaccination charbonneuse. *C R Acad Sci Paris* 1881;92:1378–1383.
11. Levine MR. Vaccines and vaccination in the historical perspective. In: Woodrow

GC, Levine MM, eds. *New generation vaccines*. New York: Marcel Dekker Inc, 1990:3–17.

12. Calmette LCA, Guérin C, Weill-Hallé B. Essai d'immunisation contre l'infection tuberculeuse. *Bull Acad Med (Paris)* 1924;91:787–796.

13. von Behring EA, Kitasato S. Ueber das Zustandekommen der Diphtherie-Immunität und der Tetanus-Immunität bei Thieren. *Dtsch Med Wochenschr* 1890;16:1113–1114.

14. Glenny AT, Hopkins BE. Diphtheria toxoid as an immunising agent. *Br J Exp Pathol* 1923–1924;4:283–288.

15. Enders JF, Weller TH, Robbins RC. Cultivation of the Lansing strain of poliomyelitis virus in cultures of various human embryonic tissues. *Science* 1949;109:85–87.

16. Hilleman MR. The development of live attenuated mumps virus vaccine in historic perspective and its role in the evolution of combined measles-mumps-rubella in vaccinia, vaccination and vaccinology. In: Plotkin S, Fantini B, eds. *Jenner, Pasteur and their successors*. Paris: Elsevier Science, 1996:283–291.

17. Blumberg BS, Alter HJ, Visnich S. A "new" antigen in leukemia sera. *JAMA* 1965;191:541–546.

18. Blumberg BS. Australia antigen, hepatitis, and leukemia. *Tokyo J Med Sci* 1968; 76:1.

19. Hilleman MR, McAleer WJ, Buynak EB McLean AA. The preparation and safety of hepatitis B vaccine. *J Infect* 1983;7:3–8.

20. Valenzuela P, Medina A, Rutter WJ, Ammerer G, Hall BD. Synthesis and assembly of hepatitis B virus surface antigen particles in yeast. *Nature* 1982; 298: 347–350.

21. Pizza M, Fontana MR, Giuliani MM, et al. A genetically detoxified derivative of heat-labile *Escherichia coli* enterotoxin induces neutralizing antibodies against the A subunit. *J Exp Med* 1994;180:2147–2153.

22. Rappuoli R. New and improved vaccines against diphtheria and tetanus. In: Woodrow GC, Levine MM, eds. *New generation vaccines*. New York: Marcel Dekker Inc, 1990:251–268.

23. Mackett M, Smith GL, Moss B. Vaccinia virus: a selectable eukaryotic cloning and expression vector. *Proc Natl Acad Sci USA* 1982;79:7415–7419.

24. Panicali D, Paoletti E. Construction of pox viruses as cloning vectors: insertion of the thymidine kinase gene from herpes simplex virus into the DNA of infectious vaccinia virus. *Proc Natl Acad Sci USA* 1982;79:4927–4931.

25. Moss B, Flexner C. Vaccinia virus expression vectors. *Annu Rev Immunol* 1987; 5:305–324.

26. Ramshaw IA, Andrew ME, Phillips SM, Boyle DB, Coupar BEH. Recovery of immunodeficient mice from a vaccinia/IL-2 recombinant infection. *Nature* 1987;329:545–546.

27. Taylor J, Weinberg R, Tartaglia J, et al. Nonreplicating viral vectors as potential vaccines: recombinant canary pox virus expressing measles virus fusion (F) and hemagglutinin (HA) glycoproteins. *Virology* 1992;187:321–328.

28. Wolff JA, Malone RW, Williams P, et al. Direct gene transfer into mouse muscle *in vivo*. *Science* 1990;247:1465–1468.

29. Williams RS, Johnstone SA, Reidy M, Devit MJ, McElligott SG, Sanford JC. Introduction of foreign genes into tissues of living mice by DNA-coated microprojectiles. *Proc Natl Acad Sci USA* 1991;88.2726–2730.

30. Tang DC, Devit M, Johnston SA. Genetic immunization is a simple method for eliciting an immune response. *Nature* 1992;356:152–154.

31. Ulmer JB, Donnelly JJ, Parker SE, et al. Heterologous protection against influenza by injection of DNA encoding a viral protein. *Science* 1993;259:1745–1749.

32. Montgomery DL, Shiver JW, Leander KR, et al. Heterologous and homologous protection against influenza-A by DNA vaccination-optimization of DNA vectors. *DNA Cell Biol* 1993;12:777–783.

33. Fynan EF, Webster RG, Fuller DH, Haynes JR, Santoro JC, Robinson HL. DNA vaccines—protective immunizations by parenteral, mucosal and gene-gun inoculations. *Proc Natl Acad Sci USA* 1993;90:11478–11482.

34. Donnelly JJ, Ulmer JB, Shiver JW, Liu MA. DNA vaccines. *Annu Rev Immunol* 1997;15:617–648.

35. Boshart M, Weber F, John G, Dorsch-Hasler K, Fleckenstein B, Schaffner W. A very strong enhancer is located upstream of an immediate early gene of human cytomegalovirus. *Cell* 1985;41:521–530.

36. Fu T-M, Ulmer JB, Caulfield MJ, et al. Priming of CTL by DNA vaccines: requirement for professional APCs and evidence for antigen transfer from myocytes. *Mol Med* 1997;3:362–371.

37. Bevan MJ. Antigen presentation to cytotoxic T lymphocytes *in vivo*. *J Exp Med* 1995;182:639–641.

38. Donnelly JJ, Friedman A, Martinez D, et al. Preclinical efficacy of a prototype DNA vaccine-enhanced protection against antigenic drift in influenza virus. *Nat Med* 1995;1:583–587.

39. Lu S, Santoro JC, Fuller DH, Haynes JR, Robinson HL. Use of DNAs expressing HIV-1 env and non-infectious HIV-1 particles to raise antibody responses in mice. *Virology* 1995;209:147–154.

40. Letvin NL, Montefiori DC, Yasutomi Y, et al. Potent, protective anti-HIV immune responses generated by bimodal HIV DNA protein vaccination. *Proc Natl Acad Sci USA* 1997;94:9378–9383.

41. Kim JJ, Ayyavoo V, Bagarazzi ML, et al. *In vivo* engineering of a cellular immune response by coadministration of IL-12 expression vector with a DNA immunogen. *J Immunol* 1997;158:816–826.

42. Arntzen CJ. Edible vaccines produced in transgenic plants. In: Baker PJ, ed. *The*

Jordan Report. Accelerated development of vaccines. Bethesda, MD: Division of Microbiology and Infectious Diseases, NIAID, NIH, 1996:43–48.

43. Nossal GJV, Ada GL, Austin CM. Antigens in immunity. II. Immunogenic properties of flagella, polymerized flagellin and flagellin in the primary response. *Aust J Exp Biol* 1964;42:283–294.

44. Glenny AT, Pope CG, Waddington H, Wallace V. The antigenic value of toxoid precipitated by potassium alum. *J Pathol Bacteriol* 1926;29:38–45.

45. Freund J, McDermott K. Sensitization to horse serum by means of adjuvants. *Proc Soc Exp Biol Med* 1942;49:548–553.

46. Morein B, Sundquist B, Höglund S, Dalsgaard K, Osterhaus A. Iscom, a novel structure for antigenic presentation of membrane proteins from enveloped viruses. *Nature* 1984;308:457–460.

47. Lövgren K, Lindmark J, Pipkorn R, Morein B. Antigenic presentation of small molecules and synthetic peptides conjugated to a preformed iscom as carrier. *J Immunol Methods* 1987;98:137–143.

48. Barr IG, Mitchell GF. ISCOMs (immune stimulating complexes): the first decade. *Immunol Cell Biol* 1996;74:8–25.

49. Weiss HP, Stitz L, Becht H. Immunogenic properties of ISCOMs prepared with influenza virus glycoprotein. *Arch Virol* 1990;114:109–120.

50. Alving CR, Detrick B, Richards RL, Lewis MG, Shafferman A, Eddy GA. Novel adjuvant strategies for experimental malaria and AIDS vaccines. *Ann NY Acad Sci* 1993;690:265–275.

51. Allison AC, Gregoriades G. Liposomes as immunologic adjuvants. *Nature* 1974; 252:252.

52. Sanchez Y, Ionescu-Matiu I, Dressman GR, et al. Humoral and cellular immunity to hepatitis B virus-derived antigens: comparative activity of Freund's complete adjuvant, alum and liposomes. *Infect Immun* 1980;30:728–733.

53. Chinnap AD, Baig MA, Tizard IR, Kemp MC. Antigen-dependent adjuvant activity of a polydispersed β-(1-4)-linked acetylated mannan (acemannan). *Vaccine* 1992;10:551–557.

54. Hamuro J, Chihara G. Lentinan, a T cell-oriented immunopotentiator. In: Fenichel RL, Chirigos MA, eds. *Immune modulation agents and their mechanisms*. New York: Marcel Dekker Inc, 1984:409–436.

55. Okawa Y, Howard CR, Steward MW. Production of anti-peptide antibody in mice following immunization of mice with peptides conjugated to mannan. *J Immunol Methods* 1992;142:127–131.

56. Ohta M, Kido N, Hasegawa T, et al. Contribution of the mannan side chains to the adjuvant action of lipopolysaccharides. *Immunology* 1987;60:503–507.

57. Lett E, Gangloff S, Zimmermann M, Wachsmann D, Klein JP. Immunogenicity of polysaccharides conjugated to peptides containing T- and B-cell epitopes. *Infect Immun* 1994;62:785–792.

58. Apostoulopoulos V, Pietersz G, Loveland BE, Sandro MS, McKenzie IFC. Oxidative/reductive conjugation of mannan to antigen selects for T_1 or T_2 immune responses. *Proc Natl Acad Sci USA* 1995;92:10128–10132.

59. O'Brien-Simpson NM, Ede NJ, Brown LE, Swan J, Jackson DC. Polymerization of unprotected synthetic peptides: a view towards synthetic peptide vaccines. *J Am Chem Soc* 1997;119:1183–1188.

60. Zeng W, Jackson DC, Rose K. Synthesis of a new template with a built-in adjuvant and its use in constructing peptide vaccine candidates through polyoxime chemistry. *J Peptide Sci* 1996;2:66–72.

61. Tam JP. Synthetic peptide vaccine design: synthesis and properties of a high-density multiple antigenic peptide system. *Proc Natl Acad Sci USA* 1988;85:5409–5413.

62. Davenport RM. Seventeen years experience with mineral oil adjuvant influenza virus vaccines. *Ann Allergy* 1968;26:288–292.

63. Ott G, Barchfeld GL, Chernoff D, Radhakrishnan R, van Hoogevest P, Van Nest G. MF59: design and evaluation of a safe and potent adjuvant for human vaccines. In: Powell MF, Newman MJ, eds. *Vaccine design: the subunit and adjuvant approach*. New York: Plenum Press, 1995:277–296.

64. Valensi J-PM, Carlson JR, Van Nest GA. Systemic cytokine profiles in Balb/c mice immunized with trivalent influenza vaccine containing MF59 oil emulsion and other advanced adjuvants. *J Immunol* 1994;153:4029–4039.

65. Byars NE, Allison AC. Adjuvant formulation for use in vaccines to elicit both cell-mediated and humoral immunity. *Vaccine* 1987;5:223–228.

66. Chang TMS. Biodegradable, semi-permeable microcapsules containing enzymes hormones, vaccines and other biologicals. *J Bioeng* 1976;1:25–32.

67. Langer R. Polymers for the sustained release of macromolecules: their use in a single-step method of immunization. *Methods Enzymol* 1981;73:57–75.

68. O'Hagan DT, Rakman D, McGee JP, et al. Biodegradable microparticles as controlled release antigen delivery systems. *Immunology* 1991;73:239–242.

69. Eldridge JH, Staas JK, Meulbrock JA, et al. Biodegradable and biocompatible poly (DL-lactide-co-glycolide) microspheres as an adjuvant for staphylococcal enterotoxin B toxoid which enhances the level of toxin-neutralizing antibodies. *Infect Immun* 1991;59:2978–2986.

70. Aguado MT, Lambert PH. Controlled-release vaccines—biodegradable polylactide/polyglycolide (PL/PG) microspheres as antigen vehicles. *Immunobiology* 1992;184:113–125.

71. Schwendeman SP, Gupta RK, Constantino HR. Stabilization of tetanus and diphtheria toxoids against moisture-induced aggregation. *Proc Natl Acad Sci USA* 1995;92:11234–11238.

72. Chang A-C, Gupta RK. Stabilization of tetanus toxoid in poly (DL-lactide-co-glycolic acid) microspheres for the controlled release of antigen. *J Pharm Sci* 1996;85:129–132.

73. Sanchez A, Gupta RK, Alonso MJ, et al. Pulsed controlled-release system for potential use in vaccine delivery. *J Pharm Sci* 1996;85:547–552.

74. McGee JP, Davis SS, O'Hagan DT. The immunogenicity of a model protein entrapped in poly (lactide-co-glycolide) microparticles prepared by a novel phase-separation technique. *J Cont Rel* 1994;31:55–60.

75. Sah H, Toddywalla R, Chien YW. Continuous release of proteins from biodegradable microcapsules and *in vivo* evaluation of their potential as a vaccine adjuvant. *J Cont Rel* 1995;35:137–144.

76. Macdonald L, Kleinig M, Cox J. A single dose (two component) experimental influenza vaccine. *Proc Intern Symp Control Rel Bioact Mater* 1997;24:1–2.

77. O'Hagan DT, Palin KJ, Davis SS. Poly (butyl-2-cyanoacrylate) particles as adjuvants for oral immunization. *Vaccine* 1989;7:213–216.

78. Moore A, McGuirk P, Adams S, et al. Immunization with a soluble recombinant HIV protein entrapped in biodegradable microparticles induces HIV-specific CD8[+] cytotoxic T lymphocytes and CD4[+] Th1 cells. *Vaccine* 1995;13:1741–1749.

79. Vordermeier HM, Coombes AGA, Jenkins P, et al. Synthetic delivery system for tuberculosis vaccines: immunological evaluation of the *M. tuberculosis* 38 kDa protein entrapped in biodegradable PLG microparticles. *Vaccine* 1995;13:1576–1582.

80. Ellouz F, Adam A, Ciorbaru R, Lederer E. Minimal structural requirements for adjuvant activity of bacterial peptidoglycans. *Biochem Biophys Res Commun* 1974;59:1317–1325.

81. Chedid L, Parant MA, Audibert FM, et al. Biological activity of a new synthetic muramyl dipeptide devoid of pyrogenicity. *Infect Immun* 1982;35:417–424.

82. Allison AC, Byars NE. An adjuvant formulation that selectively elicits the formation of antibodies of protective isotypes and cell-mediated immunity. *J Immunol Methods* 1986;95:157–168.

83. Johnson AG, Tomai M, Solem L, Beck L, Ribi E. Characterization of non-toxic monophosphoryl lipid. *Rev Infect Dis* 1987;9:S512.

84. Morein B, Lövgren-Bengtsson K, Cox J. Modern adjuvants: functional aspects. In: Kaufmann SHE, ed. *Concepts in vaccine development.* Berlin: Walter de Gruyter, 1996:243–263.

85. Ruby J, Brinkman C, Jones S, Ramshaw IA. Response of monkeys to vaccination with recombinant vaccinia virus which co-express HIV gp160 and human interleukin-2. *Immunol Cell Biol* 1990;68:113–117.

86. Swain SL, Weinberg AD, English M, Huston G. IL-4 directs the development of Th-2-like helper effectors. *J Immunol* 1990;145:3796–3806.

87. Seder RA, Paul WE, Davis MM, Fazekas-de St Groth B. The presence of interleukin 4 during *in vitro* priming determines the lymphokine-producing potential of CD4[+] T cells from T cell receptor transgenic mice. *J Exp Med* 1992;176:1091–1098.

88. Hsieh C-S, Macatonia SE, Tripp CS, Wolff SF, O'Garra A, Murphy KM. Development of TH-1 CD4[+] T cells through IL-12 produced by *Listeria*-induced macrophages. *Science* 1993;260:547–549.

89. Macatonia SE, Hoskin NA, Litton M, et al. Dendritic cells produce IL-12 and direct the development of Th1 cells from naive CD4[+] T cells. *J Immunol* 1995;154:5071–5079.

90. Snapper CM, Paul WE. Interferon-γ and B cell stimulatory factor-1 reciprocally regulate Ig isotype production. *Science* 1987;236:944–947.

91. Defrance T, Vanbervliet B, Briere F, Durand I, Bousset F, Banchereau J. Interleukin 10 and transforming growth factor β cooperate to induce anti-CD40-activated naive human B cells to secrete immunoglobulin A. *J Exp Med* 1992;175:671–682.

92. Schijns VE, Claassen IJ, Vermeulen AA, Horzinek MC, Osterhaus AD. Modulation of anti-viral immune responses by exogenous cytokines. *J Gen Virol* 1994;75:55–63.

93. Dempsey PW, Allison MED, Akkaraju S, Goodnow CC, Fearon DT. C3d of complement as a molecular adjuvant: bridging innate and acquired immunity. *Science* 1996;271:348–350.

94. Sun J-B, Holmgren J, Czerkinsky C. Cholera toxin B subunit: an efficient transmucosal carrier-delivery system for induction of peripheral immunological tolerance. *Proc Natl Acad Sci USA* 1994;91:10795–10799.

95. Sun J-B, Rask C, Olsson T, Holmgren J, Czerkinsky C. Treatment of experimental autoimmune encephalomyelitis by feeding myelin basic protein conjugated to cholera toxin B subunit. *Proc Natl Acad Sci USA* 1996;93:7196–7201.

96. Neutra MR, Pringault E, Krahenbuhl J-P. Antigen sampling across epithelial barriers and induction of mucosal immune responses. *Annu Rev Immunol* 1996;14:275–300.

97. Holt PG, Schon-Hegrad MA, McMenamin PG. Dendritic cells in the respiratory tract. *Int Rev Immunol* 1990;6:139–149.

98. Holt PG, Haining S, Nelson DJ, Sedgwick JD. Origin and steady state turnover of class II MHC-bearing dendritic cells in the epithelium of the conducting airways. *J Immunol* 1994;153:256–261.

99. Neutra MN, Krahenbuhl J-P. Transepithelial transport and mucosal defence. I. The role of M cells. *Trends Cell Biol* 1992;2:134–138.

100. Ermak TH, Dougherty EP, Bhagat HR, Kabok Z, Pappo J. Uptake and transport of copolymer biodegradable microspheres by rabbit Peyer's patch M cells. *Cell Tissue Res* 1995;279:433–436.

101. Neutra MR, Giannasca PJ, Giannasca KT, Krahenbuhl J-P. M cells and microbial pathogens. In: Blaser M, Smith P, Ravdin J, Greenberg HG, Guerrat R, eds. *Infections of the G-I tract.* New York: Raven Press, 1994:163–178.

102. Picker LJ, Butcher EC. Physiological and molecular mechanisms of lymphocyte homing. *Annu Rev Immunol* 1994;62:561–569.

103. Czerkinsky C, Holmgren J. The mucosal immune system and prospects for anti-infectious and anti-inflammatory vaccines. *Immunologist* 1995;3:97–103.

104. McWilliam AS, Nelson D, Thomas JA, Holt PG. Rapid dendritic cell recruitment is a hallmark of the acute inflammatory response at mucosal surfaces. *J Exp Med* 1994;179:1331–1336.

105. McWilliams AS, Marsh AM, Holt PG. Inflammatory infiltration of the upper airway epithelium during Sendai virus infection: involvement of epithelial dendritic cells. *J Virol* 1997;71:226–236.

106. Nelson DJ, Holt PG. Defective regional immunity in the respiratory tract of neonates is attributable to hyporesponsiveness of local dendritic cells to activation signals. *J Immunol* 1995;155:3517–3524.

107. Elson CJ, Ealding W. Generalized systemic and mucosal immunity in mice after mucosal stimulation with cholera toxin. *J Immunol* 1984;132:2736–2743.

108. Holmgren J, Lycke N, Czerkinsky C. Cholera toxin and cholera B subunit as oral-mucosal adjuvant and antigen vector systems. *Vaccine* 1993;11:1179–1184.

109. Clements JD, Hartzog NM, Lyon FL. Adjuvant activity of *Escherichia coli* heat-labile enterotoxin and effect on the induction of oral tolerance in mice to unrelated protein antigens. *Vaccine* 1988;6:269–277.

110. Gomez-Duarte OG, Galen J, Chatfield SN, Rappuoli R, Eidels L, Levine MM. Expression of fragment C of tetanus toxin fused to a carboxyl-terminal fragment of diphtheria toxin in *Salmonella typhi* CVD 908 vaccine strain. *Vaccine* 1995;13:1596–1602.

111. Holmgren J, Czerkinsky C, Lycke N, Svennerholm A-M. Strategies for the induction of immune responses at mucosal surfaces making use of cholera toxin B subunit as immunogen, carrier and adjuvant. *Am J Trop Med Hyg* 1994;50:42–54.

112. Sanchez JL, Vasquez B, Begue RE, et al. Protective efficacy of oral whole cell/recombinant B subunit cholera vaccine in Peruvian military recruits. *Lancet* 1994;344:1273–1276.

113. Tamura S, Yamanaka A, Shimohara M, et al. Synergistic action of cholera toxin B subunit (and *Escherichia coli* heat-labile toxin B subunit) and a trace amount of cholera whole toxin as an adjuvant for nasal influenza vaccine. *Vaccine* 1994;12:419–426.

114. Douce G, Fontana M, Pizza M, Rappuoli R, Dougan G. Mucosal immunogenicity and adjuvanticity of site-directed mutant derivatives of cholera toxin. *Infect Immun* 1997;65:2821–2828.

115. Stoute JA, Slaoui M, Heppner DG, et al. A preliminary evaluation of a recombinant circumsporozoite protein vaccine against *Plasmodium falciparum* malaria. *N Engl J Med* 1997;336:86–91.

116. Mortimer EA, Kimura M, Cherry JD, et al. Protective efficacy of the Takeda acellular pertussis vaccine combined with diphtheria and tetanus toxoids following household exposure of Japanese children. *Am J Dis Child* 1990;144:899–904.

117. Edwards KM, Meade BD, Decker MD, et al. Comparison of 13 acellular pertussis vaccines: overview and serologic response. *Pediatrics* 1995;96:548–557.

118. Trollfors B, Taranger J, Lagergard T, et al. A placebo-controlled trial of a pertussis toxoid vaccine. *N Engl J Med* 1995;333:1045–1050.

119. Simondon F, Yam A, Gagnepain JY, Wassilak S, Danve B, Cadoz M. Comparative safety and immunogenicity of an acellular versus whole-cell pertussis component of diphtheria-tetanus-pertussis vaccines in Senegalese infants. *Eur J Clin Microbiol Infect Dis* 1996;15:927–932.

120. Greco D, Salmaso S, Mastrantonio P, et al. A controlled trial of two acellular vaccines and one whole cell vaccine against pertussis. *N Engl J Med* 1996;334:341–348.

121. Greco D, Salmaso S, Mastrantonia P, et al. A difference in relative efficacy of two DTaP vaccines in continued blinded observation of children following a clinical trial. *Pediatr Res* 1996;39:173A.

122. Rappuoli R. Rational design of vaccines. *Nat Med* 1997;3:1–3.

123. Klein D. Pertussis vaccines: a continuing saga. In: Baker PJ, ed. *The Jordan Report. Accelerated development of vaccines.* Bethesda, MD: Division of Microbiology and Infectious Diseases, NIAID, NIH, 1996:29–32.

124. Gustafsson L, Hallander HO, Olin P, Reizenstein E, Storsaeter J. A controlled trial of a two-component acellular, a five-component acellular, and a whole-cell pertussis vaccine. *N Engl J Med* 1996;334:349–355.

125. Klugman KP, Koornhof HJ, Robbins JB, Le Cam NN. Immunogenicity, efficacy and serological correlate of protection of *Salmonella typhi* Vi capsular polysaccharide vaccine three years after immunization. *Vaccine* 1996;14:435–438.

126. Hoiseth SK, Stocker BAD. Aromatic-dependent *Salmonella typhimurium* are non-virulent and effective as a vaccine. *Nature* 1981;291:238–241.

127. Tacket CO, Hone DM, Losonsky G, Guers L, Edelman R, Levine MM. Clinical acceptability and immunogenicity of CVD908 *Salmonella typhi* vaccine strain. *Vaccine* 1992;10:443–446.

128. Levine MM, Galeu J, Barry E, et al. Attenuated *Salmonella* as live oral vaccines against typhoid fever and as live vectors. *J Biotechnol* 1996;44:193–196.

129. Chatfield S, Strahan K, Pickard D, Charles IG, Hormaeche CE, Dougan G. Evaluation of *Salmonella typhimurium* strains harboring defined mutations in htrA and aroA in the murine salmonellosis model. *Microb Pathog* 1992;12:145–151.

130. Sztein MB, Tanner MK, Polotsky Y, Orenstein JM, Levine MM. Cytotoxic T lymphocytes after oral immunization with attenuated vaccine strains of *Salmonella typhi* in humans. *J Immunol* 1995;155:3987–3993.

131. Trach DD, Clements JD, Ke NT, et al. Field trial of a locally produced, killed oral cholera vaccine in Vietnam. *Lancet* 1997;349:231–235.

132. van Leon FPL, Clemens JD, Chakraborty J, et al. Field trial of inactivated oral cholera vaccines in Bangladesh: results from 5 years of follow-up. *Vaccine* 1996;14:162–166.

133. Jertborn M, Svennerholm A-M, Holmgren J. Intestinal and systemic immune responses in humans after oral immunization with a bivalent B subunit—01/0139 whole cell cholera vaccine. *Vaccine* 1996;14:1459–1465.

134. Kotloff KL, Wasserman SS, O'Donnell S, Losonsky GA, Cryz SJ, Levine MM. Safety and immunogenicity in North Americans of a single dose of live oral cholera vaccine CVD 103-HgR: results of a randomized, placebo-controlled, double-blind crossover trial. *Infect Immun* 1992;60:4430–4432.

135. Tacket CO, Losonsky G, Nataro JP, et al. Onset and duration of protective immunity in challenged volunteers after vaccination with live oral cholera vaccine CVD103 HgR. *J Infect Dis* 1992;166:837–841.

136. Tacket CO, Losonsky G, Nataro JP, et al. Initial clinical studies of CVD112 *Vibrio cholerae* O139 live oral vaccine: safety and efficacy against experimental challenge. *J Infect Dis* 1995;172:883–886.

137. Pearson GDN, Woods A, Chiang SL, Mekalanos JJ. CTX genetic element encodes a site-specific recombination system and an intestinal colonization factor. *Proc Natl Acad Sci USA* 1993;90:3750–3754.

138. Kenner JR, Coster TS, Taylor DN, et al. Peru 15, an improved live attenuated oral vaccine candidate for *Vibrio cholerae* O1. *J Infect Dis* 1995;172:1126–1129.

139. Phalipon A, Kaufmann M, Michett P, et al. Monoclonal immunoglobulin A antibody directed against serotype-specific epitope of *Shigella flexneri* lipopolysaccharide protects against murine experimental shigellosis. *J Exp Med* 1995;182:769–778.

140. Barzu S, Fontaine A, Sansonetti PJ, Phalipon A. Induction of local anti-IpaC antibody response in mice by the use of a *Shigella flexneri* 2a vaccine candidate: implications for use of IpaC as a protein carrier. *Infect Immun* 1996;64:1990–1196.

141. Fontaine A, Arondel J, Sansonetti PJ. Construction and evaluation of live attenuated vaccine strains of *Shigella flexneri* and *Shigella dysenteriae* 1. *Res Microbiol* 1990;141:907–912.

142. Noriega FR, Wang JY, Losonsky G, Maneval DR, Hone DM, Levine MM. Construction and characterization of attenuated *CaroA CvirG Shigella flexneri* 2a strain CVD 1203, a prototype live oral vaccine. *Infect Immun* 1994;62:5168–5172.

143. Noriega FR, Losonsky G, Wang JY, Formal SB, Levine MM. Further characterization of *CaroA CvirG Shigella flexneri* 2a strain CVD 1203 as a mucosal *Shigella* vaccine and as a live vector vaccine for delivering antigens of enterotoxigenic *Escherichia coli*. *Infect Immun* 1996;64:23–27.

144. Kotloff KL, Noriega F, Losonsky GA, et al. Safety, immunogenicity, and transmissibility in humans of CVD 1203, a live oral *Shigella flexneri* 2a vaccine candidate attenuated by deletions in aroA and virG. *Infect Immun* 1996;64:4542–4548.

145. Noriega FR, Losonsky G, Lauderbaugh C, Liao FM, Wang JY, Levine MM. Engineered *CguaB-A, CvirG Shigella flexneri* 2a strain CVD 1205: construction, safety, immunogenicity, and potential efficacy as a mucosal vaccine. *Infect Immun* 1996;64:3055–3061.

146. Marshall BJ, Warren JR. Unidentified curved bacilli in the stomach of patients with gastritis and peptic ulceration. *Lancet* 1983;1:1311–1315.

147. Parsonnet J, Hansen S, Rodriguez L, et al. *Helicobacter pylori* infection and gastric lymphoma. *N Engl J Med* 1994;330:1267–1271.

148. Lee A, Hazell SL, O'Rourke J, Kouprach S. Isolation of a spiral-shaped bacterium from the cat stomach. *Infect Immun* 1988;56:2843–2850.

149. Lee A, Fox JG, Otto G, Murphy J. A small animal model of human *Helicobacter pylori* active chronic gastritis. *Gastroenterology* 1990;99:1315–1323.

150. Chen M, Lee A, Hazell S. Immunization against gastric *Helicobacter* infection in a mouse/*Helicobacter felis* model. *Lancet* 1992;339:1120–1121.

151. Marchetti M, Arico B, Burroni D, Figura N, Rappuoli R, Ghiara P. Development of a mouse model of *Helicobacter pylori* infection that mimics the human disease. *Science* 1995;267:1655–1658.

152. Doidge C, Gust I, Lee A, Buck F, Hazell S, Manne U. Therapeutic immunization against *Helicobacter* infection—the first evidence. *Lancet* 1994;343:914–915.

153. Corthesy Theulaz I, Porta N, Glauser M, et al. Oral immunization with *Helicobacter pylori* urease B subunit as a treatment against *Helicobacter* infection in mice. *Gastroenterology* 1995;109:115–1121.

154. Lee A, Orourke J, Deungria MC, Robertson B, Daskalopoulos G, Dixon MF. A standardized mouse model of *Helicobacter pylori* infection—introducing the Sydney strain. *Gastroenterology* 1997;112:1386–1397.

155. Anderson P, Peter G, Johnston RB, Wetterlow LH, Smith DH. Immunization of humans with polyribophosphate, the capsular antigen of *Hemophilus influenzae*, type b. *J Clin Invest* 1972;51:39–44.

156. Rodrigues LP, Schneerson R, Robbins JB. Immunity to *Haemophilus influenzae* type b. I. The isolation and some physico-chemical, serologic, and biologic properties of the capsular polysaccharide of *Haemophilus influenzae* type b. *J Immunol* 1971;107:1071–1080.

157. Peltala H, Käyhty H, Sivonen A, Mäkelä PH. *Haemophilus influenzae* type b capsular polysaccharide vaccine in children: a double-blind field study of 100,000 vaccinees 3 months to 5 years of age in Finland. *Pediatrics* 1977;60:730–737.

158. Anderson P. Antibody responses to *Haemophilus influenzae* type b and diphtheria toxin induced by conjugates of oligosaccharides of the type b capsule with the non-toxic protein CRM197. *Infect Immun* 1983;39:233–238.

159. Schneerson R, Robbins JB, Chu C, Sutton A, Schiffman G, Vann WF. Semisynthetic vaccines composed of capsular polysaccharides of pathogenic bacteria covalently bound to proteins for the prevention of invasive diseases. *Prog Allergy* 1983;33:144–158.

160. Eskola J, Käyhty H, Takala AK, et al. A randomized prospective field trial of a conjugate vaccine in the protection of infants and young children against invasive *Haemophilus influenzae* type b disease. *N Engl J Med* 1990;323:1381–1387.

161. Madore DV. Impact of immunization on *Haemophilus influenzae* type b disease. *Infect Agents Dis* 1996;5:8–20.

162. Adams WG, Deaver KA, Cochi SL, et al. Decline of childhood *Haemophilus influenzae* type b (Hib) disease in the Hib vaccine era. *JAMA* 1993;169:221–226.

163. Mulholland K, Hilton S, Adegbola R, et al. Randomised trial of *Haemophilus influenza* type-b tetanus protein conjugate for prevention of pneumonia and meningitis in Gambian infants. *Lancet* 1997;349:1191–1197.

164. Thomas WR, Callow MG, Dilworth RJ, Audesho AA. Expression in *Escherichia coli* of a high molecular weight protective surface antigen found in nontypeable and type b *Haemophilus influenza*. *Infect Immun* 1990;58:1909–1913.

165. Flack FS, Loosmore S, Chang P, Thomas WR. The sequencing of the 80-kDa D15 protective surface antigen of *Haemophilus influenzae*. *Gene* 1995;156:97–99.

166. O'Brien KL, Steinhoff MC, Edwards K, Keyserling H, Thoms ML, Madore D. Immunologic priming of young children by pneumococcal glycoprotein conjugate, but not polysaccharide, vaccines. *Pediatr Infect Dis J* 1996;15:425–430.

167. King JC, Vink PE, Farley JJ, et al. Comparison of the safety and immunogenicity of a pneumococcal conjugate with a licensed polysaccharide vaccine in human immunodeficiency virus and non-human immunodeficiency virus-infected children. *Pediatr Infect Dis J* 1996;15:192–196.

168. de Moracs JC, Perkins BA, Camargo MC, et al. Protective efficacy of a serogroup B meningococcal vaccine in Sao Paulo, Brazil. *Lancet* 1992;340:1074–1078.

169. Kaufmann SHE. Immunity to intracellular bacteria. *Annu Rev Immunol* 1993;11:129–163.

170. Musser JM. Antimicrobial agent resistance in mycobacteria: molecular genetic insights. *Clin Microbiol Rev* 1995;8:496–514.

171. Andersen P, Askgaard D, Ljungqvist L, Bennedsen J, Heron I. Proteins released from *Mycobacterium tuberculosis* during growth. *Infect Immun* 1991;59:1905–1910.

172. Andersen P, Andersen AB, Sorensen AL, Nagai S. Recall of long-lived immunity to *Mycobacterium tuberculosis* infection in mice. *J Immunol* 1995;154:3359–3372.

173. Wiker HG, Harboe M. The antigen 85 complex: a major secretion product of *Mycobacterium tuberculosis*. *Microbiol Rev* 1992;56:648–661.

174. Kaufmann SHE, Schoel B, van Embden JD, et al. Heat-shock protein 60: implications for pathogenesis of and protection against bacterial infections. *Immunol Rev* 1991;121:67–90.

175. Andersen P. Effective vaccination of mice against *Mycobacterium tuberculosis* infection with a soluble mixture of secreted mycobacterial proteins. *Infect Immun* 1994;62:2536–2544.

176. Tascon RE, Colston MJ, Ragno S, Stavropoulos E, Gregory D, Lowrie DB. Vaccination against tuberculosis by DNA injection. *Nat Med* 1996;2:888–892.

177. Huygen K, Content J, Denis O, et al. Immunogenicity and protective efficacy of a tuberculosis DNA vaccine. *Nat Med* 1996;2:893–898.

178. Zaheer SA, Beena KR, Kar HK. Addition of immunotherapy with *Mycobacterium w* vaccine to multi-drug therapy benefits multibacillary leprosy patients. *Vaccine* 1995;13:1102–1110.

179. Brandt ER, Hayman WA, Currie B, et al. Opsonic human antibodies from an endemic population specific for a conserved epitope on the M protein of group A streptococci. *Immunology* 1996;89:331–337.

180. Brandt ER, Hayman WA, Currie B, Pruksakorn S, Good MF. Human antibodies to the conserved region of the M protein: opsonization of heterologous strains of group A streptococci. *Vaccine* 1997;15:1805–1812.

181. Hilleman MR. Hepatitis and hepatitis A vaccine: a glimpse of history. *J Hepatol* 1993;18:S5–S10.

182. Krugman S, Giles JP, Hammond J. Infectious hepatitis. Evidence for two distinctive clinical, epidemiological, and immunological types of infection. *JAMA* 1967;200:365–373.

183. Bradley DW, Krawczynski K, Beach MJ, Purdy MA. Non-A, non-B hepatitis. Toward the discovery of hepatitis C and E viruses. *Semin Liver Dis* 1991;11:128–146.

184. Houghton M, Wiener A, Han J, Kuo G, Chao Q-L. Molecular biology of the hepatitis C viruses: implications for diagnosis, development and control of viral disease. *Hepatology* 1991;14:381–388.

185. Gust ID, Coulepsis AG, Feinstone SM, et al. Taxonomic classification of hepatitis A virus. *Intervirology* 1983;20:1–7.

186. Frösner GG, Deinhardt F, Scheid R, et al. Propagation of human hepatitis A virus in hepatoma cell line. *Infection* 1979;7:303–304.

187. Provost PJ, Hughes JV, Miller WJ, et al. An inactivated hepatitis A viral vaccine of cell culture origin. *J Med Virol* 1986;19:23–31.

188. Mao J-S, Dong D-Y, Zhang II-Y, Chai N-C. Primary study of attenuated live hepatitis A vaccine (H2 strain) in humans. *J Infect Dis* 1989;159:621–624.

189. Adamowicz Ph, Tron F, Vinas R, et al. Hepatitis B vaccine containing the S and PreS-2 antigens produced in Chinese hamster ovary cells. In: Zuckerman AJ, ed. *Viral hepatitis and liver disease*. New York: Alan R Liss, 1988:982–988.

190. Corman W, Thomas H, Domingo E. Viral genetic variation: hepatitis B virus as a clinical example. *Lancet* 1993;341:349–353.

191. Choo Q-L, Richman KH, Han JH, et al. Genetic organization and diversity of the hepatitis C virus. *Proc Natl Acad Sci USA* 1991;88:2451–2455.

192. Kuo G, Choo QL, Alter HJ, et al. An assay for circulating antibodies to a major etiologic virus of human non-A, non-B hepatitis. *Science* 1989;244:362–364.

193. Weiner AJ, Brauer MJ, Rosenblatt J, et al. Variable and hypervariable domains are found in the regions of HCV corresponding to the flavivirus envelope and NS1 proteins and the pestivirus envelope glycoproteins. *Virology* 1991;180:842–848.

194. Farci P, Alter HJ, Wong D, et al. Prevention of hepatitis C virus infection in chimpanzees after antibody-mediated *in vitro* neutralization. *Proc Natl Acad Sci USA* 1994;91:7792–7796.

195. Rosa D, Campagnoli S, Moretto C, et al. A quantitative test to estimate neutralizing antibodies to the hepatitis C virus: cytofluorometric assessment of envelope glycoprotein 2 binding to target cells. *Proc Natl Acad Sci USA* 1996;93: 1759–1763.

196. Ishii K, Rosa D, Watanabe Y, et al. High titres of envelope neutralizing antibodies correlate with natural resolution of chronic hepatitis C. *Hepatology* 1998; (in press).

197. Botarelli P, Brunetto MR, Minutello MA, et al. T-lymphocyte response to hepatitis C virus in different clinical courses of infection. *Gastroenterology* 1993;104: 580–587.

198. Kapikian AZ, Hoshino Y, Channock RM, Perez-Schael I. Jennerian and modified Jennerian approach to vaccination against rotavirus diarrhea using a quadrivalent rhesus rotavirus (RRV) and human-RRV reassortant vaccine. *Arch Virol* 1996;12: 163–175.

199. Conner ME, Zarley CD, Hu B, et al. Virus-like particles as a rotavirus subunit vaccine. *J Infect Dis* 1996;174:S88–S92.

200. Mattion NM, Reilly PA, Composano E, et al. Characterization of recombinant polioviruses expressing regions of rotavirus VP4, hepatitis B surface antigen, and herpes simplex virus type 2 glycoprotein D. *J Virol* 1995;69:5132–5137.

201. Mills J. Immunotherapy and immunoprophylaxis of respiratory syncytial virus infections. *Curr Opin Infect Dis* 1995;8:473–478.

202. Kapikian AZ, Mitchell RH, Channock RM, Shreddof RA, Stewart CE. An epidemiologic study of altered clinical reactivity to respiratory syncytial (RS) virus infection in children previously vaccinated with an inactivated RS virus vaccine. *Am J Epidemiol* 1969;89:405–421.

203. Palladino G, York LJ, Adams SM, Giorgio DP, Randolph V, Mishkin EM. The immunogenicity of two cold-adapted, temperature-sensitive strains of respiratory syncytial virus in mice. *Vaccine Res* 1996;5:57–67.

204. Tolley KP, Marriott AC, Simpson A, et al. Identification of mutations contributing to the reduced virulence of a modified strain of respiratory syncytial virus. *Vaccine* 1996;14:1637–1646.

205. Piedra PA, Grace S, Jewell A, et al. Purified fusion protein vaccine protects against lower respiratory tract illness during respiratory syncytial virus season in children with cystic fibrosis. *Pediatr Infect Dis J* 1996;15:23–31.

206. Paradiso PR, Hildreth SW, Hogerman DA, et al. Safety and immunogenicity of a subunit respiratory syncytial virus vaccine in children 24-48 months old. *Pediatr Infect Dis J* 1994;13:792–798.

207. Ho DD, Neumann AU, Perelson AS, Chen W, Leonard JM, Markowitz M. Rapid turnover of plasma virions and CD4 lymphocytes in HIV-1 infection. *Nature* 1995;373:123–126.

208. Mellors JW, Rinaldo CJ, Gupta P, White RM, Todd JA, Kingsley LA. Prognosis in HIV-1 infection predicted by the quantity of virus in plasma. *Science* 1996; 272:1167–1170.

209. Pantaleo G, Grziosi C, Demarest JF, et al. HIV infection is active and progressive in lymphoid tissue during the clinically latent stage of disease. *Nature* 1993; 362:355–358.

210. Rowland-Jones S, Sutton J, Ariyoshi K, et al. HIV-specific cytotoxic T cells in HIV-exposed but uninfected Gambian women. *Nat Med.* 1995;1:59–64.

211. Clerici M, Shearer GM. The Th1-Th2 hypothesis of HIV infection: new insights. *Immunol Today* 1994;15:575–581.

212. Siebelink KHJ, Tijhaar E, Huisman RC, et al. Enhancement of feline immunodeficiency virus infection after immunization with envelope glycoprotein subunit vaccines. *J Virol* 1995;69:3704–3711.

213. Hulskotte EG, Geretti AM, Siebelink KHJ, et al. Vaccine-induced virus neutralizing antibodies and cytotoxic T cells do not protect macaques from experimental infection with simian immunodeficiency virus SIVmac32H (J5). *J Virol* 1995;69:6289–6296.

214. Zolla-Pazner S, Alving C, Belshe R, et al. Neutralization of a clade B primary isolate by sera from human immunodeficiency virus-uninfected recipients of candidate AIDS vaccines. *J Infect Dis* 1997;175:764–774.

215. Kent SJ, Woodward A, Zhao A. HIV-specific T cell responses correlate with control of acute HIV-1 infection in macaques. *J Infect Dis* 1997;176:1188–1197.

216. Shiver JW, Davies M-E, Perry HC, Freed DC Liu M. Humoral and cellular immunities elicited by HIV-1 DNA vaccination. *J Pharmaceut Sci* 1996;85: 1317–1324.

217. Schutten M, Tenner-Racz K, Racz P, van Bekkum DW, Osterhaus ADME. Human antibodies that neutralize primary human immunodeficiency virus type 1 *in vitro* do not provide protection in an *in vivo* model. *J Gen Virol* 1996;77: 1667–1675.

218. Lubeck MD, Natuk RN, Myagkikh M, et al. Long-term protection of chimpanzees against high-dose HIV-1 challenge induced by immunization. *Nat Med* 1997;3:651–658.

219. Daniel MD, Kirchoff F, Czajak SC, Schgal PK, Desrosiers RC. Protective effects of a live attenuated SIV-1 vaccine with a deletion in the *nef* gene. *Science* 1992; 258:1938–1940.

220. Montagnier L. Nef vaccination against HIV disease. *Lancet* 1995;346:1170.

221. Deacon NJ, Tsykin A, Solomon A, et al. Genomic structure of an attenuated quasi species of HIV-1 from a blood transfusion donor and recipients. *Science* 1995;270:988–991.

222. Heeney JL, Bruck C, Goudsmit J, et al. Immune correlates of protection from HIV infection and AIDS. *Immunol Today* 1997;18:4–8.

223. Mitchell GF. Problems specific to parasite vaccines. *Parasitology* 1989;98: S49–S60.

224. Anders RF, Saul AJ. Candidate antigens for an asexual blood stage vaccine against falciparum malaria. In: Good MJ, Saul AJ, eds. *Molecular immunological considerations in malaria vaccine development.* Boca Raton, FL: CRC Press, 1994:169.

225. Patarroyo ME, Amado R, Clavijo P, et al. A synthetic vaccine protects humans against challenge with asexual blood stages of *Plasmodium falciparum* malaria. *Nature* 1988;332:158–161.

226. Holder AA, Freeman RR. Immunization against blood-stage rodent malaria using purified parasite antigens. *Nature* 1981;294:361–364.

227. Siddiqui WA, Tam LQ, Kramer KJ, et al. Merozoite surface coat precursor completely protects Aotus monkeys against *Plasmodium falciparum* malaria. *Proc Natl Acad Sci USA* 1987;84:3014–3018.

228. Daly TM, Long CA. A recombinant 15-kilodalton carboxyl-terminal fragment of *Plasmodium yoelii yoelii* 17XL merozoite surface protein 1 induces a protective immune response in mice. *Infect Immun* 1993;61:2462–2467.

229. Daly TM, Long CA. Humoral response to a carboxyl-terminal region of the merozoite surface protein-1 plays a predominant role in controlling blood-stage infection in rodent malaria. *J Immunol* 1995;155:236–243.

230. Hirunpetcharat C, Tian J-H, Kaslow DC, et al. Complete protective immunity induced in mice by immunization with 19 kDa carboxylterminal fragment of the merozoite surface protein-1 (MSP$_{19}$) of *Plasmodium yoelii* expressed in *Saccharomyces cerevisiae*: correlation of protection with antigen-specific antibody titer, but not effector CD4$^+$ T cells. *J Immunol* 1997;159:3400–3411.

231. Smythe JA, Coppel RL, Brown GV, Ramasamy R, Kemp DJ, Anders RF. Identification of two integral membrane proteins of *Plasmodium falciparum*. *Proc Natl Acad Sci USA* 1988;85:5195–5199.

232. Peterson MG, Marshall VM, Smythe JA, et al. Integral membrane protein located in the apical complex of *Plasmodium falciparum*. *Mol Cell Biol* 1989;9: 3151–3154

233. Perlmann H, Berzins K, Wahlgren M, et al. Antibodies in malarial sera to parasite antigens in the membrane of erythrocytes infected with early asexual stages of *Plasmodium falciparum*. *J Exp Med* 1984;159:1686–1704.

234. Locksley RM, Louis JA. Immunology of leishmaniasis. *Curr Opin Immunol* 1992;4:413–418.

235. Handman E, McConville MJ. Vaccines against leishmania. In: Woodrow GC, Levine MM, eds. *New generation vaccines*. New York: Marcel Dekker Inc, 1990: 545–564.

236. Titus RG, Gueiros-Filho FJ, de Freitas LA. Development of a safe live Leishmania vaccine line by gene replacement. *Proc Natl Acad Sci USA* 1995;92: 10267–10271.

237. Xu D, McSorley SJ, Chatfield SN, et al. Protection against *Leishmania major* infection in genetically susceptible BALB/c mice by gp63 delivered orally in attenuated *Salmonella typhimurium* (AroA- AroD−). *Immunology* 1995;85:1–7.

238. Xu D, Liew FY. Protection against leishmaniasis by injection of DNA encoding a major surface glycoprotein, gp63 of *L. major*. *Immunology* 1995;84:173–176.

239. Handman E, Symons FM, Baldwin TM, et al. Protective vaccination with promastigote surface antigen 2 from *Leishmania major* is mediated by a TH1 type of immune response. *Infect Immun* 1995;63:4261–4267.

240. Kelleher M, Bacic A, Handman E. Identification of a macrophage-binding determinant on lipophosphoglycan from *Leishmania major* promastigotes. *Proc Natl Acad Sci USA* 1992;89:6–10.

241. Capron A, Riveau G, Grzych J-M, Boulanger D, Capron M, Pierce R. Development of a vaccine strategy against human and bovine schistosomiasis. *Trop Geogr Med* 1994;46:242–246.

242. Frazer IH. Immunology of papillomavirus infection. *Curr Opin Immunol* 1996; 8:484–491.

243. Frazer IH, Leippe DM, Dunn LA, et al. Immunological responses in human papillomavirus 16 E6/E7-transgenic mice to E7 protein correlate with the presence of skin disease. *Cancer Res* 1995;55:2635–2639.

244. Borysiewicz LK, Fiander A, Nimako M, et al. A recombinant vaccinia virus encoding human papillomavirus types 16 and 18, E6 and E7 proteins as immunotherapy for cervical cancer. *Lancet* 1996;347:1523–1527.

245. Frazer IH. Strategies for immunoprophylaxis and immunotherapy of papillomaviruses. *Clin Dermatol* 1997;15:285–297.

246. Boon T. Toward a genetic analysis of tumor rejection antigens. *Adv Cancer Res* 1992;58:177–210.

247. Wölfel T, Hauer M, Schneider J, et al. A p16INK4a-insensitive CDK4 mutant targeted by cytolytic T lymphocytes in a human melanoma. *Science* 1995;269: 1281–1284.

248. van der Bruggen P, Traversari C, Chomez P, et al. A gene encoding an antigen recognized by cytolytic T lymphocytes on a human melanoma. *Science* 1991; 254:1643–1647.

249. Wölfel T, Van Pel A, Brichard V, et al. Two tyrosinase nonapeptides recognized on HLA-A2 melanomas by autologous cytolytic T lymphocytes. *Eur J Immunol* 1994;24:759–764.

250. Van den Eynde BJ, Boon T. Tumor antigens recognized by T lymphocytes. *Int J Clin Lab Res* 1997;27:81–86.

251. Marchand M, Weynants P, Rankin E, et al. Tumor regression responses in melanoma patients treated with a peptide encoded by gene MAGE-3. *Int J Cancer* 1995;63:883–885.

252. Uyttenhove C, Godfraind C, Lethé B, et al. The expression of mouse gene P1A in testis does not prevent safe induction of cytolytic T cells against a P1A-encoded tumor antigen. *Int J Cancer* 1997;70:349–356.

253. Guilloux Y, Lucas S, Brichard VG, et al. A peptide recognized by human cytolytic T lymphocytes on HLA-A2 melanomas is encoded by an intron sequence of the N-acetylglucosaminyltransferase V gene. *J Exp Med* 1996;183:1173–1183.

254. Gaugler B, Brouwenstijn N, Vantomme V, et al. A new gene coding for an antigen recognized by autologous cytolytic T lymphocytes on a human renal carcinoma. *Immunogenetics* 1996;44:323–330.

255. de Smet C, de Backer O, Faraoni I, Lurquin C, Brasseur F, Boon T. The activation of human gene MAGE-1 in tumor cells is correlated with genome-wide demethylation. *Proc Natl Acad Sci USA* 1996;93:7149–7153.

256. Levy R, Miller R. Therapy of lymphoma directed at idiotypes. *J Natl Cancer Inst* 1990;10:61–68.

257. Brichard V, Ban Pel A, Wölfel T, et al. The tyrosine gene codes for an antigen recognized by autologous cytolytic T lymphocytes on HLA-A2 melanomas. *J Exp Med* 1993;178:489–495.

258. Kang X, Kawakami Y, El-Gamil M, et al. Identification of a tyrosinase epitope recognized by HLA-A2-restricted, tumor-infiltrating lymphocytes. *J Immunol* 1995;155:1343–1348.

259. Barnd DL, Lan M, Metzgar RS, Finn OJ. Specific, MHC-unrestricted recognition of tumor-associated mucins by human cytotoxic T cells. *Proc Natl Acad Sci USA* 1989;86:7159–7163.

260. Finn OJ, Jerome KR, Henderson RA, et al. MUC-1 epithelial tumor mucin-based immunity and cancer vaccines. *Immunol Rev* 1995;145:61–89.

261. Gendler S, Lancaster C, Taylor-Papadimitriou J, et al. Molecular cloning and expression of human tumor-associated polymorphic epithelial mucin. *J Biol Chem* 1990;265:15286–15293.

262. Wreschner DH, Hareuveni M, Tsarfaty I, et al. Human epithelial cell tumor antigen cDNA sequences. *Eur J Biochem* 1990;189:463–473.

263. Fontenot JD, Finn OJ, Dales N, Andrews PC, Montelaro RC. Synthesis of large multideterminant peptide immunogens using a poly-proline beta-turn helix motif. *Pept Res* 1993;6:330–336.

264. Goydos JS, Elder E, Whiteside TL, Finn OJ, Lotze MT. A phase 1 trial of a synthetic mucin peptide vaccine. *J Surg Res* 1996;63:298–304.

265. Henderson RA, Nimgaonkar MT, Watkins SC, Robbins PD, Ball ED, Finn OJ. Human dendritic cells genetically engineered to express high levels of the human epithelial tumor antigen mucin (MUC-1). *Cancer Res* 1996;56:3763–3770.

266. Pecher G, Finn OJ. Induction of cellular immunity in chimpanzees to human tumor-associated mucin by vaccination with MUC-1 cDNA-transfected Epstein-Barr virus-immortalized autologous B cells. *Proc Natl Acad Sci USA* 1996;93:1699–1704.

267. Fricker J. Mucin-based vaccines and cancer. *Mol Med Today* 1997;3:47.

268. Apostolopoulos V, Loveland BE, Pietersz GA, McKenzie IFC. CTL in mice immunized with human mucin 1 are MHC-restricted. *J Immunol* 1995;155:5089–5094.

269. Morton DL, Foshag LJ, Hoon DSB, et al. Prolongation of survival in metastatic melanoma after active specific immunotherapy with a new polyvalent melanoma vaccine. *Ann Surg* 1992;216:463–482.

270. Barth A, Hoon DSB, Leland J, et al. Polyvalent melanoma cell vaccine induces delayed-type hypersensitivity and *in vitro* cellular immune responses. *Cancer Res* 1994;54:3342–3345.

271. Bystryn JC. Clinical activity of a polyvalent melanoma antigen vaccine. *Recent Results Cancer Res* 1995;239:333–345.

272. Dranoff G, Jaffee E, Lazenby A, et al. Vaccination with irradiated tumor cells engineered to secrete murine granulocyte-macrophage colony-stimulating factor stimulates potent, specific, and long-lasting anti-tumor immunity. *Proc Natl Acad Sci USA* 1993;93:3539–3543.

273. Herr W, Wölfel T, Heike M, Méyer zum Buschenfelde K-H, Knuth A. Frequency analysis of tumor reactive cytotoxic T lymphocytes in peripheral blood of a melanoma patient vaccinated with autologous tumor cells. *Cancer Immunol Immunother* 1994;39:93–99.

274. Maraskovsky E, Brasel K, Teepe M, et al. Dramatic increase in the numbers of functionally mature dendritic cells in Flt3 ligand-treated mice: multiple dendritic cell subpopulations identified. *J Exp Med* 1996;184:1953–1962.

275. Thrush GR, Lark LR, Clinchy BC, Vitetta ES. Immunotoxins: an update. *Annu Rev Immunol* 1996;14:49–71.

276. Nossal GJV. Minimal residual disease as the target for immunotherapy of cancer. *Lancet* 1994;343:1172–1173.

277. Talwar GP, Singh O, Pal R, et al. A vaccine that prevents pregnancy in women. *Proc Natl Acad Sci USA* 1994;91:8532–8536.

278. Talwar GP, Diwan M, Davar H, Frick J, Sharma SK, Wadha SN. Counter GnRH vaccine. In: Rajalakshmi M, Griffin PD, eds. *Male contraception—present and future.* New Delhi: New Age International, 1998;309–318.

279. Primakoff P, Lathrop W, Woolman L, Cowan A, Myles D. Fully effective contraception in male and female guinea pigs immunized with the sperm protein PH-20. *Nature* 1988;335:543–546.

280. Diekman AB, Herr JC. Sperm antigens and their use in the development of an immunocontraceptive. *Am J Reprod Immun* 1997;37:111–117.

281. Nossal GJV, Pike BL. Clonal anergy: persistence in tolerant mice of antigen-binding B lymphocytes incapable of responding to antigen or mitogen. *Proc Natl Acad Sci USA* 1980;77:1602–1606.

282. Nossal GJV. Cellular mechanisms of immunological tolerance. *Annu Rev Immunol* 1983;1:33–62.

283. Chase MW. Inhibition of experimental drug allergy by prior feeding of the sensitizing agent. *Proc Soc Exp Biol Med* 1946;61:257–259.

284. Hafler DA, Weiner HL. Immunological mechanisms and therapy in multiple sclerosis. *Immunol Rev* 1995;144:75–107.

285. Holt PG, Batty JE, Turner KJ. Inhibition of specific IgE responses in mice by pre-exposure to inhaled antigen. *Immunology* 1981;42:409–417.

286. Chen Y, Kuchroo VK, Inobe J-I, Hafler DA, Weiner HL. Regulatory T cell clones induced by oral tolerance: suppression of autoimmune encephalomyelitis. *Science* 1994;265:1237–1240.

287. Harrison LC, Dempsey-Collier M, Kramer DR, Takahashi K. Aerosol insulin induces regulatory CD8 γδ T cells that prevent murine insulin-dependent diabetes. *J Exp Med* 1996;184:2167–2174.

288. French MB, Allison J, Cram DS, et al. Transgenic expression of mouse proinsulin II prevents diabetes in nonobese diabetic mice. *Diabetes* 1997;46:34–39.

289. Bergerot I, Ploix C, Petersen J, et al. A cholera toxoid-insulin conjugate as an oral vaccine against spontaneous autoimmune diabetes. *Proc Natl Acad Sci USA* 1997;94:4610–4614.

290. Holmgren J, Czerkinsky C, Sun JB, Svennerholm A-M. Oral vaccination, mucosal immunity and oral tolerance with special reference to cholera toxin. In: Kaufmann SHE, ed. *Concept in vaccine development.* New York: Walter de Gruyter, 1996:437–458.

291. Thomas WR, Smith W, Hales BJ, Carter MD. Functional effects of polymorphisms of house dust mite allergens. *Int Arch Allergy Immunol* 1997;908:113:96–98.

292. Hoyne GF, Callow MG, Kuo M-C, Thomas WR. Inhibition of T-cell responses by feeding peptides containing major and cryptic epitopes: studies with Der p 1 allergen. *Immunology* 1994;83:190–195.

293. O'Brien RM, Byron KA, Varigos GA, Thomas WR. House dust mite immunotherapy results in a decrease in Der p 2-specific IFN-γ and IL-4 expression by circulating T lymphocytes. *Clin Exp Allergy* 1997;27:46–51.

294. Bauer L, Bohle B, Jahn-Schmid B, et al. Modulation of the allergic immune response in Balb/c mice by subcutaneous injection of the dominant T cell epitope from the major birch pollen allergen Bet v 1. *Clin Exp Immunol* 1997;107:536–541.

295. Hsu C-H, Chua K-Y, Tao M-H, et al. Immunoprophylaxis of allergen-induced IgE synthesis and airway hyperresponsiveness *in vivo* by genetic immunization. *Nat Med* 1996;2:540–544.

296. O'Hehir RE, Hoyne GF, Thomas WR, Lamb JR. House dust mite allergy: from T cell epitopes to immunotherapy. *Eur J Clin Invest* 1993;23:763–772.

297. Holt PG. Immunoprophylaxis of atopy: light at the end of the tunnel? *Immunol Today* 1994;15:484–489.

298. Holt PG, Sly PD. Allergic respiratory disease: strategic targets for primary prevention during childhood. *Thorax* 1997;52:1–4.

299. American Academy of Pediatrics Committee on Infectious Diseases. The relationship between pertussis vaccine and brain damage: reassessment. *Pediatrics* 1991;88:397–400.

300. Joce R, Wood D, Brown D, Begg M. Paralytic poliomyelitis in England and Wales 1985–1991. *BMJ* 1992;305:79–82.

301. Jonville-Béra AP, Autret E, Galy-Eyraud C, Hessel L. Thrombocytopenic purpura after measles, mumps and rubella vaccination: a retrospective survey by the French Regional Pharmacovigilance Centres and Pasteur-Mérieux Sérums et Vaccins. *Pediatr Infect Dis J* 1996;15:44–48.

302. Jonville-Béra AP, Autret E, Galy-Eyraud C, Hessel L. Aseptic meningitis following mumps vaccine. *Pharmacoepidemiol Drug Safety* 1996;5:33–37.

303. de Quadros CA, Andrus JK, Olivé J-M, de Macedo CG. Polio eradication from the Western Hemisphere. *Annu Rev Public Health* 1992;13:239–252.

304. Robbins FC, deQuadros CA. Certification of the eradication of indigenous transmission of wild poliovirus in the Americas. *J Infect Dis* 1997;175:S281–S285.

305. Barrios C, Brawand P, Berney M, Brandt C, Lambert P-H, Siegrist C-A. Neonatal and early life immune responses to various forms of vaccine antigens qualitatively differ from adult responses: predominance of a Th2-biased pattern which persists after adult boosting. *Eur J Immunol* 1996;26:1489–1496.

306. Barrios C, Brandt C, Berney M, Lambert P-H, Siegrist C-A. Partial correction of the TH2/TH1 imbalance in neonatal murine responses to vaccine antigens through selective adjuvant effects. *Eur J Immunol* 1996;26:2666–2670.

307. Martinez X, Brandt C, Saddallah F, et al. DNA immunization circumvents deficient induction of TH1 and CTL responses in neonates and during early life. *Proc Natl Acad Sci USA* 1997;94:8726–8731.

308. Steger MM, Maczek C, Grubeck-Loebenstein B. Morphologically and functionally intact dendritic cells can be derived from the peripheral blood of aged individuals. *Clin Exp Immunol* 1996;105:544–550.

309. Steger MM, Maczek C, Grubeck-Loubenstein B. Peripheral blood dendritic cells reinduce proliferation in *in vitro* aged T cell populations. *Mech Ageing Dev* 1997;93:125–130.

310. Albright JW. The challenge of vaccinating the elderly. In: Baker PJ, ed. *The Jordan Report. Accelerated development of vaccines.* Bethesda, MD: Division of Microbiology and Infectious Diseases, NIAID, NIH, 1996:37–42.

311. Steger MM, Maczek C, Berger P, Grubeck-Loebenstein B. Vaccination against tetanus in the elderly: do recommended vaccination strategies give sufficient protection? *Lancet* 1996;348:762.

Fundamental Immunology, Fourth Edition,
edited by William E. Paul
Lippincott–Raven Publishers, Philadelphia © 1999.

CHAPTER 43

Primary Immunodeficiency Diseases

Rebecca H. Buckley

Recognition of the first human primary immunodeficiency disease four and a half decades ago (1) set the stage for an exponential increase in information about the functions of the various components of the immune system. This discovery was soon complemented by results of experimental deletions of the thymus and bursa of Fabricious in animals, leading to the concept of cellular and humoral compartmentalization of the immune system. Since then, more than 70 primary immunodeficiency disorders have been recognized in humans (2), and a number of naturally occurring immune defects have been described in various experimental animals, each providing unique insights into the intricate workings of the immune system. Recently, molecular manipulations of the immune system, creating knock-out mice by inserting mutant genes for selected immune components, have seemingly opened the door to the ultimate dissection of the immune system (3).

Primary (or genetically determined) immunodeficiency disorders may affect one or more components of the immune system, including T-, B-, and natural killer (NK)-lymphocytes, as well as phagocytic cells and complement proteins. This chapter will focus on the currently understood genetic bases of and faulty immunologic mechanisms underlying some of the most important human immunodeficiency diseases involving lymphocytes (Table 1). This

will be supplemented by information derived from naturally occurring animal models and from mutant mice.

Immunodeficiency diseases are characterized by undue susceptibility to infection. Paradoxically, many immunodeficiency syndromes are also characterized by autoimmune diseases and excessive production of IgE antibodies. Due to the ability of modern antibiotics to control many types of infections, autoimmune diseases now account for significant morbidity among immunodeficiency patients. Finally, there is an increased incidence of malignancy in patients with immunodeficiency diseases (4,5). Whether the latter is due to increased susceptibility to infection with agents predisposing to malignancy or to defective tumor immunosurveillance is unknown.

With the exception of selective immunoglobulin (Ig)A deficiency, genetically determined immunodeficiency is rare (2). B-cell defects far outnumber those affecting T cells, phagocytic cells, or complement proteins. Although general population statistics are not available in the United States, it has been estimated that agammaglobulinemia occurs with a frequency of 1:50,000 and *severe combined immunodeficiency* (SCID) with a frequency of 1:100,000 to 1:500,000 live births. Selective absence of serum and secretory IgA is the most common defect, with reported incidences ranging from 1:333 to 1:700 (6,7). Primary immunodeficiency is seen more often in infants and children than in adults. During childhood, there is a 5:1 male:female sex predominance for these

R.H. Buckley: Departments of Pediatrics and Immunology, Duke University School of Medicine, Durham, North Carolina 27710-0001.

TABLE 1. *Abnormal genes known to cause human primary immunodeficiency*

Chromosome	Disease
1q	MHC Class II antigen deficiency due to RFX5 mutation[a]
1q25	Chronic granulomatous disease (CGD) due to gp67[phox] deficiency[a]
1q42-43	Chediak-Higashi syndrome[a]
2p11	Kappa chain deficiency[a]
2q12	CD8 lymphocytopenia due to ZAP70 deficiency[a]
6p21.3	MHC class I antigen defect due to mutations in *TAP2*[a]
6p21.3	(?)Common variable immunodeficiency and selective IgA deficiency
6q22-q23	Interferon γR1 mutations[a]
7q11.23	CGD due to gp47[phox] deficiency[a]
8q21	Nijmegen breakage syndrome
9p21-p13	Cartilage hair hypoplasia
10p13	DiGeorge/velocardiofacial syndrome
10p14-15	IL-2 receptor alpha chain deficiency[a]
11	CD3 gamma or epsilon chain deficiency[a]
11p13	Severe combined immunodeficiency (SCID) due to RAG1 or RAG2 deficiencies[a]
11q22.3	Ataxia-telangiectasia (AT), due to AT mutation, causing deficiency of DNA-dependent kinase[a]
14q13.1	Purine nucleoside phosphorylase (PNP) deficiency[a]
14q32.3	Immunoglobulin heavy chain deletions[a]
16p13	MHC class II antigen deficiency due to CIITA mutation[a]
16q24	CGD, due to gp22[phox] deficiency[a]
19p13.1	SCID due to Janus kinase 3 (Jak 3) deficiency[a]
20q13.11	SCID due to adenosine deaminase (ADA) deficiency[a]
21q22.3	Leukocyte adhesion deficiency, type 1 (LAD1) due to CD18 deficiency[a]
22q11.2	DiGeorge syndrome
Xp21.1	CGD due to gp91[phox] deficiency[a]
Xp11.23	Wiskott-Aldrich syndrome (WAS) due to WAS protein (WASP) deficiency[a]
Xp11.3-p21.1	Properdin deficiency[a]
Xq13.1	X-linked SCID due to common cytokine receptor gamma-chain (τ_c) deficiency[a]
Xq22	X-linked agammaglobulinemia due to Bruton tyrosine kinase (Btk) deficiency[a]
Xq24-26	X-linked lymphoproliferative syndrome
Xq26	Immunodeficiency with hyper-IgM due to CD154 (CD40 ligand) deficiency[a]

[a]Gene cloned and sequenced, gene product known.

disorders. This later reverses so that there is a slight predominance (1:1.4) in women in adulthood.

MOLECULAR GENETICS OF PRIMARY IMMUNODEFICIENCY

Human Immunodeficiency Diseases

Until the past few years, there was little insight into the fundamental problems underlying a majority of these conditions. Many have now been mapped to specific chromosomal locations, and the fundamental biologic errors have been identified in an impressive number since the last edition of this book was published (Table 1) (8–12). These remarkable advances have been made possible through a combination of new knowledge in molecular and cellular immunology and of greatly improved approaches to disease loci mapping and detection within the human genome.

Within the past 5 years the molecular bases of four X-linked immunodeficiency disorders have been discovered: X-linked agammaglobulinemia, X-linked immunodeficiency with hyper-IgM, the Wiskott-Aldrich syndrome (WAS), and X-linked SCID (Fig. 1 and Table 1) (8–11). The abnormal gene in X-linked chronic granulomatous disease (CGD) had been identified several years earlier (13), and the gene encoding properdin (mutated in prop-

erdin deficiency) has also been cloned (14). The faulty gene in X-linked lymphoproliferative disease has been localized to a specific site on the X chromosome but has not yet been identified (Fig. 1) (15,16).

Autosomal-recessive immunodeficiencies for which the molecular bases have been discovered include leukocyte adhesion deficiency type 1 (LAD 1) (17,18); adenosine deaminase (ADA) deficiency (19); purine nucleoside phosphorylase (PNP) deficiency (20); ataxia-telangiectasia (21); DiGeorge's syndrome (22–24); major histocompatibility complex (MHC) antigen deficiency (25,26); ZAP-70 deficiency (27); interleukin-2 receptor alpha (IL-2Rα) chain deficiency (28); Jak3 deficiency (29); and interferon receptor deficiency (Table 1) (30,31). The discovery and cloning of the genes for these diseases have obvious implications for the potential of gene therapy. The rapidity of these advances suggests that there will soon be many more to come.

A Committee of the World Health Organization (WHO) has published several versions of a classification of primary immunodeficiency diseases over the past three decades, with the most recent having been reported in 1997 (2). Table 1 lists a number of conditions for which the molecular bases are already known. Table 2 classifies these diseases according to the type of molecular defect present. As the fundamental causes of more of these disorders are identified, it is likely that future classifications will be mutation based.

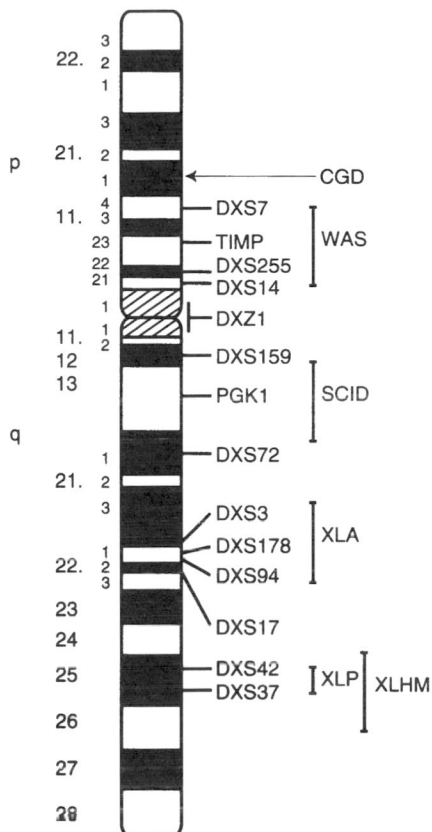

FIG. 1. Locations of the X-linked immunodeficiency disease loci. Correspondence with the cytogenetic map of the X chromosome is indicated on the left. Modified with permission from deSaint-Basile and Fischer.

TABLE 2. *Classification of known molecular defects causing human primary immunodeficiency*

I. Deficiencies of signaling molecules:
  A. Tyrosine kinases
    1. Bruton tyrosine kinase (btk). Disease: X-linked agammaglobulinemia.
    2. Zeta-associated protein (ZAP)-70. Disease: CD8 lymphocytopenia.
    3. Janus kinase (Jak) 3. Disease: Autosomal-recessive severe combined immunodeficiency (SCID)
  B. Other intracellular molecules
    1. Vesicle membrane component. Disease: Chediak-Higashi syndrome
    2. Proline-rich protein. Disease: Wiskott-Aldrich syndrome protein
    3. DNA-dependent protein kinase: Disease: Ataxia telangiectasia
    4. Recombinase activating gene (RAG1, RAG2) products. Disease: T-B-SCID
    5. Transporter protein (*TAP*) 1. Disease: MHC class I deficiency
II. Transcription factor deficiencies
  A. X-box binding protein (RFX5). Disease: MHC class II deficiency
  B. Class II transactivator (CIITA). Disease: MHC class II deficiency
  C. Nuclear factor of activated T cells (NF-AT). Disease: Cytokine deficiencies.
III. Deficiencies of cytokine receptor chains
  A. Common cytokine receptor γ chain. Disease: X-linked SCID
  B. IL-2 receptor α chain (CD25). Disease: Lymphoproliferative T-cell deficiency
  C. IFN-γ receptor chain 1 (IFN-γ R1). Disease: Disseminated mycobacterial disease
IV. Deficiencies of adhesion molecules or member of ligand pairs
  A. CD18 deficiency. Disease: Leukocyte adhesion deficiency type I (LAD1)
  B. CD154 deficiency. Disease: X-linked hyper-IgM (hyper-IgM)
V. Structural gene deficiencies
  A. CD3 γ or ε chain deficiency. Disease: CD3 deficiency
  B. Kappa-chain deficiency. Disease: All immunoglobulins bear lambda chains
  C. Immunoglobulin heavy-chain gene deficiency. Disease: B cell–negative agammaglobulinemia due to μ chain mutations; other chain deficiencies lead to absence of the isotype
VI. Metabolic defects
  A. Adenosine deaminase (ADA) deficiency. Disease: SCID
  B. Purine; nucleoside phosphorylase deficiency. Disease: Combined immunodeficiency (CID)

Animal Models of Immunodeficiency

For many years, a limited number of animal models of some human primary immunodeficiency diseases have been recognized. The application of techniques of gene targeting by homologous recombination to the study of genes involved in immune system development has resulted in the creation of a much larger number of animal models, each revealing the biologic consequences of the specific mutation (3). Many of these mutant mice have no known counterpart among the currently recognized human immunodeficiency diseases. A compendium of the T-, B-, and NK-cell abnormalities in mice mutated for one of each of 129 genes involved in the development and function of the immune system has recently been published (Table 3) (3). This data base should be of great value to all investigating humans with potential genetically determined immunodeficiencies for which the molecular basis has not yet been determined. Several of these knock-out mice bear mutations in genes known to be responsible for human primary immunodeficiency diseases. From these, it has been learned that, for some mutations, the phenotypes are similar in mice and humans. Examples of the gene defects for which there is phenotypic concordance between the immunologic abnormalities in the mouse mutant and the human disease include

CD18, RAG1, RAG2, and *class II transactivator* (CIITA). However, there are many others, including Btk, CD154, γc, Jak3, ZAP-70, and ADA mutant mice, in which the phenotype is either less or more severe and sometimes quite different from the immunodeficiency in the human disease counterpart (3). Thus, there are limitations to the use of these animals to elucidate diseases of unknown cause. Because of space limitations, immunologic abnormalities in only a few of the mutant mice (Table 3) and in only some of the naturally occurring animal models will be described in this chapter.

TABLE 3. *Human chromosome locations of genes with immunological phenotypes in mouse mutants*

Human chromosome	Genes
1	CD2, CD3 η, CD3 ζ, CD30, CD45, CR2, E-selectin, FasL, FcγRII, FcγRIII, FcRγ, IL-10, L-selectin, Lyst, p56 lck
2	CD8 α, CD8 β, CD28, CTLA-4, IL-1 β, IL-8R, kappa chain, Ku80, substance P receptor, ZAP-70
3	B7-1, IL-5R α
4	IL-2, IRF-2, NF-κB (p50 subunit)
5	CD14, GM-CSF, granzyme A, IL-4, IL-5, IL-7R, IL-12 p40, IRF-1, itk, 1i (invariant chain), Tcf-1
6	c-myb, C4, IFN-γ receptor α, LMP-2, LMP-7, MHC class II, p 59 fyn, Pim-1, SOX-4, TAP1, TNF-β
7	Ikaros, IL-6, TCR β chain
8	DNA-dependent kinase (p350), DNA polymerase β, IL-7, Lyn
9	abl, Pax5/BSAP, Syk
10	Fas/CD95, IL-2R α, PBSF/SDF-1, Perforin, TDT
11	ATM, CD3 ε, CD5, ETS-1, NF-κB (p65/Rel-A subunit), RAG-1, RAG-2
12	β7 integrin, CD4, GATA-2, IFN-γ, Lag3, P-selectin, p27 kip1, TNFR p55 (α), STAT-6
13	flk-2
14	c-fos, IgD, IgE, IgM, Ig Gm-2b, JH, switch γ1, TCR α chain, TCR δ chain
15	β2 microglobulin, p50 csk
16	CD19, CD43, PKC β
18	Bcl-2
19	Bax, C/EBP β, C3, C5aR, CD23, E2A, ICAM-1, Jak-3, OCT-2, TGF-β 1, Vav
20	ADA, CD40, NFAT1
21	CD18
22	IL-2R β, IL-3/GMCSF/IL-5 R β, lambda 5
X	btk, CD40L/CD154, IL-2Rγ

Reprinted with permission from Kokron CM, Bonilla FA, Oettgen HC, Ramesh N, Geha RS, Pandolfi F. Searching for genes involved in the pathogenesis of primary immunodeficiency diseases: Lessons from mouse knockouts. *J Clin Immunol* 1997;17: 109–126.

DEFECTS CHARACTERIZED BY ANTIBODY DEFICIENCY

X-linked Agammaglobulinemia

Most boys afflicted with X-linked agammaglobulinemia (XLA), also known as Bruton's agammaglobulinemia (1), remain well during the first 6 to 9 months of life by virtue of maternally transmitted IgG antibodies (32). Thereafter, they repeatedly acquire infections with extracellular pyogenic organisms such as pneumococci, streptococci, and haemophilus unless given prophylactic antibiotics or gammaglobulin therapy. Chronic fungal infections are not usually present, and *Pneumocystis carinii* pneumonia rarely occurs unless there is an associated neutropenia (33). Viral infections are also usually handled normally, with the notable exceptions of the hepatitis viruses and the enteroviruses (34,35). In addition to septic arthritis, patients with this condition may have joint inflammation similar to that seen in rheumatoid arthritis (36). Infections with *Ureaplasma urealyticum* (37,38) and viral agents such as echoviruses, coxsackie viruses, and adenovirus have been identified from joint fluid cultures of patients even on IVIG replacement therapy (36). These observations suggest a primary role for antibody, particularly secretory IgA, in host defense against this group of viruses because normal T-cell numbers and function have been present in all individuals with XLA with persistent enterovirus infections reported thus far. Concentrations of immunoglobulins of all isotypes are very low, and circulating B cells are usually absent. Pre-B cells are present in reduced numbers in the bone marrow. Tonsils are usually very small and lymph nodes are rarely palpable due to absence of germinal centers from these lymphoid tissues. Thymus architecture, including Hassall's corpuscles, is normal, as are the thymus-dependent areas of spleen and lymph nodes. In 1993, two

groups of investigators independently and almost simultaneously discovered the mutated gene in XLA. Because XLA had been precisely mapped to position Xq22 (Fig. 1), one group successfully used the technique of positional cloning to identify an abnormal gene in patients with this defect (Table 1) (39). For other reasons, the second group had sought and found a B cell–specific tyrosine kinase important in murine B-lymphocyte signaling (40); the kinase was found to be encoded by a gene on the mouse X chromosome. When the human gene counterpart was cloned, it was found to reside at Xq22 and the gene product was identical to that found by the first group. This intracellular signaling tyrosine kinase has been named *Bruton tyrosine kinase* (Btk) in honor of Dr. Bruton. Btk is a member of the Tec family of cytoplasmic protein tyrosine kinases (41). It is expressed at high levels in all B-lineage cells, including pre-B cells. This kinase appears to be necessary for pre-B cell expansion and maturation into surface Ig–expressing B cells, but probably has a role at all stages of B-cell development (42). It has not been detected in any cells of T lineage, but it has been found in cells of the myeloid series (40). Thus far, all males with known XLA (by family history) have had low or undetectable Btk messenger RNA (mRNA) and kinase activity. To date, more than 250 different mutations in the human Btk gene have been recognized (41,43–46). These have encompassed most parts of the coding portions of the gene, and there has been no clear correlation between the location of the mutation and the clinical phenotype (45,47–50).

Female carriers of XLA can be identified by the finding of nonrandom X chromosome inactivation in their B cells or by the detection of the mutated gene (if known in the family) (8,47). Prenatal diagnosis of affected or nonaffected male fetuses also has been accomplished by detection of the mutated gene in chorionic villous or amniocentesis samples. Studies of Btk protein, enzymatic activity, or mRNA also have permitted identification of X-linked inheritance in some agammaglobulinemic boys with no family history (8). The fact that Btk is also expressed in cells of myeloid lineage is of interest in light of the well-known occurrence of intermittent neutropenia in boys with XLA, particularly at the onset of an acute infection (51,52). It is conceivable that Btk is only one of several signaling molecules participating in myeloid maturation and that neutropenia would be observed in XLA only when rapid production of such cells is needed. XLA also has been reported in association with growth hormone deficiency in nine cases (53–56).

A condition that resembles XLA phenotypically (i.e., there is an absence of circulating B cells) occurs in some agammaglobulinemic females (57–59). The molecular basis for this autosomal-recessive defect has recently been shown to be mutations in the μ heavy chain gene on chromosome 14 (59). The latter indicates the fundamental necessity for expression of intact membrane-bound μ chains for B-cell maturation.

X-linked Immunodeficiency in Mice

The animal model for human XLA is the X-linked immunodeficiency (Xid) mutation in CBA/N mice (60). Xid mice have normal numbers of pre-B cells in their bone marrow but abnormally low numbers of B cells in their lymphoid tissues (60). These animals have low serum IgG and IgM concentrations and fail to produce antipolysaccharide antibodies to thymus-independent (TI) antigens type 2 (TI-2). Unlike most humans with XLA, Xid mice have some B cells of mature phenotype, and they produce some antibodies to TI-1 antigens. However, B cells from Xid mice do not proliferate after ligation of CD40, even in the presence of IL-4 or anti-Ig reagents (61). A mutation at position 28 of the murine btk gene has been shown to be the basis for the B-cell defect in CBA/N mice (62,63). Because such mice have a much milder antibody deficiency than boys with XLA, speculation had been that humans with mutations in the non–kinase-encoding part of the Btk gene might have a less severe immunodeficiency. However, humans with classic X-linked agammaglobulinemia have been identified with mutations affecting the same residue as in CBA/N mice (64). Again, as in female carriers of human XLA, female mice heterozygous for Xid display nonrandom X-chromosome inactivation in their B cells.

Immunodeficiency with Elevated IgM (Hyper-IgM)

Like boys with XLA, patients with hyper-IgM may become symptomatic during the first or second year of life with recurrent pyogenic infections, including otitis media, sinusitis, pneumonia, and tonsillitis (2,65). In contrast to patients with XLA, however, the frequent presence of lymphoid hyperplasia in patients with hyper-IgM is often misleading. Until the fundamental cause of this condition was discovered, coexistent neutropenia had been considered a possible explanation for the occurrence of *Pneumocystis carinii* pneumonia (PCP) and extensive verruca vulgaris lesions in some such patients (2,65).

Hyper-IgM is characterized by very low serum IgG, IgA, and IgE but either a normal or, more frequently, a markedly elevated concentration of polyclonal IgM. Some of these patients have low molecular weight IgM molecules that give falsely high IgM values in radial immunodiffusion assays. Even more than with some of the other antibody deficiency syndromes, there is an increased frequency of autoimmune disorders in the hyper-IgM syndrome

(2,65). Lymph node histology is abnormal, showing only abortive germinal center formation and a severe depletion and phenotypic abnormalities of follicular dendritic cells (66). However, thymic-dependent lymphoid tissues and T-cell functions, as assessed by standard testing, had formerly been considered to be normal.

Normal or only slightly reduced numbers of IgM or IgD B-lymphocytes have been found in the blood of these patients. Until recently, this condition was classified as a B-cell defect because only IgM is produced. However, normal numbers of B-lymphocytes are usually present in the circulation of these patients, and B cells from some such patients were shown over a decade ago to have the capacity to synthesize IgM, IgA, and IgG normally when cocultured with a switch T-cell line, suggesting that in those patients the defect lay in T-lineage cells (67).

The abnormal gene in X-linked hyper-IgM was localized to Xq26 (68) (Fig. 1) and identified by six groups almost simultaneously in 1993 (69–72). The gene product is a surface molecule now known as CD154 (or CD40 ligand) on the surfaces of activated helper T cells (73), which interacts with CD40 molecules on B cells (Table 1) (69). CD40 is a type I integral membrane glycoprotein belonging to the tumor necrosis factor (TNF)/nerve growth factor receptor family; it is expressed on B cells, monocytes, some carcinomas, and a few other types of cells. Cross-linking of CD40 on either normal or X-linked hyper-IgM B cells with a monoclonal antibody to CD40 or with soluble CD154 in the presence of cytokines (IL-2, IL-4, or IL-10), causes the B cells to undergo proliferation and isotype switching and to secrete various types of immunoglobulins. CD154 is a type II integral membrane glycoprotein with significant sequence homology to TNF; it is found only on activated T cells, primarily of the CD4 phenotype (73). Mutations in the gene encoding CD154 in X-linked hyper-IgM patients result in a lack of signaling of their B cells by their activated T cells. Therefore, hyper-IgM B cells fail to undergo isotype switching and produce only IgM.

Of further relevance to the defective immune responses of these patients, the lack of stimulation of CD40 also results in these patients' B cells not upregulating CD80 and CD86. The latter are important costimulatory molecules that interact with CD28/CTLA4 on T cells (74). The failure of interaction of the molecules of those pathways results in a propensity for tolerogenic T-cell signaling. Many distinct point mutations or deletions in the gene encoding CD154 have been identified, giving rise to frame shifts, premature stop codons, and single amino acid substitutions, most of which were clustered in the TNF homology domain located in the carboxy-terminal region (75,76). There is an increased incidence of both autoimmunity and malignancy in this condition. Mutations in the gene encoding CD154 are thought to account for both defective negative selection of autoreactive thymocytes and defective recognition of tumor cells due to tolerogenic signaling of peripheral T cells. A highly polymorphic microsatellite dinucleotide (CA) repeat region in the 3' untranslated end of the gene for CD154 is useful for detecting carriers of X-linked hyper-IgM and for making a prenatal diagnosis of this condition (77).

CD154 mutant mice are similar to humans with X-linked hyper-IgM in many respects, including their susceptibility to PCP (78). Unlike the inability to isotype-switch in the human defect, however, such mice can produce IgG3 when immunized with polysaccharide antigens.

Not all males with hyper-IgM have a mutation in the gene encoding CD154 (79), and there are several examples in females (80), indicating that this condition has more than one genetic cause. In such patients, the B cells are not able to switch from IgM-secreting to IgG-, IgA-, or IgE-secreting cells, even when cocultured with monoclonal antibodies to CD40 and a variety of cytokines (79). Thus, in those patients, the condition truly is a B-cell defect. CD40 has been present on the surfaces of the B cells in such patients, ruling out deficiency of that protein as the defect. However, there is currently an intense search in several laboratories for one or more B cell-specific, CD40-associated signaling molecule defects in those patients.

Common Variable Immunodeficiency

Common variable immunodeficiency (CVID), also known as acquired hypogammaglobulinemia, may appear similar clinically in many respects to XLA (2,81). The kinds of infections experienced and bacterial etiologic agents involved are generally the same for the two defects. Fortunately, however, for unknown reasons echovirus meningoencephalitis does not occur as frequently in patients with CVID (35). In comparing the two defects further, it is noted that in CVID there is an almost equal sex distribution, generally a later age of onset of infections, which are somewhat less severe, a tendency to autoantibody formation, normal-sized or enlarged tonsils and lymph nodes, and splenomegaly in approximately 25% of affected individuals. Lymphoid interstitial pneumonia, pseudolymphoma, amyloidosis, and noncaseating granulomata of the lungs, spleen, skin, and liver also have been seen. There is a 438-fold increase in lymphomas in affected women in the fifth and sixth decades of life (82).

The serum immunoglobulin and antibody deficiencies in CVID may be as profound as in XLA. Despite normal numbers of circulating immunoglobulin-bearing B-lymphocytes and the presence of lymphoid cortical follicles, blood B-lymphocytes from CVID patients do not differentiate into immunoglobulin-producing cells when stimulated with pokeweed mitogen (PWM) *in vitro,* even when cocultured with normal T cells (81), and they are L-selectin negative, possibly due to aberrant lymphocyte activation (83). From these observations, it was thought that the defect(s) in this syndrome are intrinsic to the B cell (81). In keeping with this are recent studies showing a lack of protein kinase C activation and translocation to the plasma membrane when CVID B cells are stimulated with phorbol ester or anti-μ (84). However, CVID B cells can be stimulated to both isotype-switch and to synthesize and secrete immunoglobulin when stimulated with anti-CD40 plus IL-4 or IL-10 (85,86).

T cells and T-cell subsets are usually present in normal percentages, but a dominance of γδ T cells has been observed in some patients (87), and depressed T-cell function has been reported in others (88–92). Mitogen-activated T cells from some CVID patients also were found to be deficient in expression of genes for several lymphokines, while retaining a normal capacity to proliferate (93). In addition, a decreased number and function of antigen-specific T cells was noted in CVID patients immunized with KLH (94). One group of CVID patients was reported to have significantly depressed (but not absent) expression of CD40 ligand (CD154) mRNA and surface protein in their activated T-lymphocytes, suggesting that inefficient signaling by poorly expressed CD154 on their T cells could account for failure of their B cells to differentiate (95). Tonsils and lymph nodes are either normal-sized or enlarged, and splenomegaly occurs in approximately 25% of patients with CVID. In addition, there is a tendency toward autoantibody formation, and several cases of lupus erythematosus converting to CVID have been reported (96). Rarely, CVID has been reported to resolve transiently or permanently when some such patients acquired HIV infection (97).

Because this disorder occurs in first-degree relatives of patients with selective IgA deficiency (A Def) and some patients with A Def later became panhypogammaglobulinemic (98), it has long been suspected that these diseases have a common genetic basis (99,100). The high incidences of abnormal immunoglobulin concentrations, autoantibodies, autoimmune disease, and malignancy in families of both types of patients also suggested a shared hereditary influence (101). This concept is supported by the finding of a high incidence of C4-A gene deletions and C2 rare gene alleles in the class III MHC region in individuals with either A Def (101,102) or CVID (103,104), suggesting that there is a susceptibility gene in this region on chromosome 6. However, the abnormal gene has not yet been identified. These studies also have shown that a small number of human leukocyte antigen (HLA) haplotypes are shared by individuals affected with CVID and A Def, with at least one of two particular haplotypes being present in 77% of those affected (104). In one large family with 13 members, two had A Def and three had CVID (99). All of the immunodeficient patients in the family had at least one copy of an MHC haplotype shown to be abnormally frequent in A Def and CVID: HLA-DQB1 *0201, HLA-DR3, C4B-Sf, C4A-deleted, G11-15, Bf-0.4, C2a, HSP70-7.5, TNFα-5, HLA-B8 and HLA-A1 (105). However, four immunologically normal members of the pedigree also possessed this haplotype, indicating that its presence alone is not sufficient for expression of the defects (99). Environmental factors, particularly drugs such as phenytoin, have been suspected as providing the triggers for disease expression in individuals with the permissive genetic background. The prognosis for patients with CVID is reasonably good unless severe autoimmune disease or malignancy develop (82).

Selective IgA Deficiency

An isolated absence or near-absence (i.e., less than 10 mg/dl) of serum and secretory IgA is thought to be the most common well-defined immunodeficiency disorder, a frequency of 1:333 being reported among some blood donors (6,7,102). Although this disorder has been observed in apparently healthy individuals (6), it is commonly associated with ill health. As would be expected when there is a deficiency of the major immunoglobulin of external secretions, infections occur predominantly in the respiratory, gastrointestinal and urogenital tracts (7). Bacterial agents responsible are essentially the same as in other types of antibody deficiency syndromes. There is no clear evidence that patients with this disorder have an undue susceptibility to viral agents. Similar to CVID, there is a frequent association of A Def with collagen-vascular and autoimmune diseases (101). In further similarity to patients with CVID, there is an increased incidence of malignancy.

Serum concentrations of other immunoglobulins are usually normal in patients with A Def, although IgG2 subclass deficiency has been reported (101,106,107) and IgM (usually elevated) may be monomeric. Children with A Def vaccinated with killed poliovirus intranasally produced local IgM and IgG antibodies. Of possible etiologic and great clinical significance is the presence of antibodies to IgA in the sera of as high as 44% of patients with A Def (6). IgG anti-IgA antibodies can fix complement and remove IgA from the circulation four to 20 times faster than the normal catabolic rate for IgA. A number of A Def patients have had severe or fatal anaphylactic reactions after intravenous administration of blood products containing IgA, and anti-IgA antibodies [particularly IgE anti-IgA antibodies (108)] have been implicated. For this reason, only five times washed (in 200 ml volumes) normal donor erythrocytes or blood products from other IgA absent individuals should be administered to these patients. Patients with A Def also frequently have IgG antibodies against cow milk and ruminant serum proteins (109). These antiruminant antibodies often falsely detect "IgA" in immunoassays that use goat (but not rabbit) antisera (7). A high incidence of autoantibodies also has been noted (110).

The basic defect leading to A Def is unknown. *In vitro* cultures of B cells from some IgA-deficient patients could be stimulated to produce IgA by the combination of anti-CD40 and IL-10; those whose B cells did not produce IgA with these treatments appeared to be more infection prone (111,112). Treatment with dilantin, sulfasalazine (113), d-penicillamine, or gold has been suspected as being the cause of A Def; the condition also has been known to remit after discontinuation of dilantin therapy or spontaneously (114,115). Usually when this happens the remission is permanent. The occurrence of A Def in both males and females and in families is consistent with autosomal inheritance; in most families this appears to be dominant with variable expressivity (99). As already noted, this defect occurs in pedigrees with CVID patients, some patients with IgA deficiency have gone on to develop CVID (98), and recent studies suggest that the susceptibility genes for these two defects may reside in the MHC class III region as an allelic condition on chromosome 6 (Table 1) (99,100,104,105).

Immunodeficiency with Thymoma

Patients with immunodeficiency with thymoma are adults who almost simultaneously develop recurrent infections, panhypogammaglobulinemia, deficits in cell-mediated immunity, and benign thymoma (2). They may also have eosinophilia or eosinopenia, aregenerative or hemolytic anemia, agranulocytosis, thrombocytopenia, or pancytopenia. Antibody formation is poor, and progressive lymphopenia develops, although percentages of Ig-bearing B-lymphocytes are usually normal. The thymomas are predominantly of the spindle cell variety, although other types of benign and malignant thymic tumors also have been seen.

IgG Subclass Deficiencies

A number of patients have been reported to have deficiencies of one or more subclasses of IgG, despite normal or elevated total IgG serum concentrations (107,116,117). IgG_2 deficiency would be suspected if patients had repeated problems with encapsulated bacterial pathogens, because a majority of the antipolysaccharide antibody molecules are of the IgG_2 isotype. Most of those with absent or very low concentrations of IgG_2 have been patients with A Def (106,107). However, not all A Def patients who have recurrent infections have IgG_2 deficiency, and some A Def patients have defective antipolysaccharide antibody responses despite normal levels of IgG_2. Similarly, patients with WAS, who have a profound antipolysaccharide antibody deficiency, have normal levels of IgG_2. Marked deficiencies of antipolysaccharide antibodies also have been noted in other non-WAS children and adults with recurrent infections who had normal concentrations of IgG_2, as well as normal concentrations of all of the other immunoglobulin isotypes (118). Conversely, a number of healthy children have been described who had low levels of IgG_2 but normal responses to polysaccharide antigens when immunized

(119). In other patients with IgG_2 deficiency, continued follow-up showed an evolving pattern of immunodeficiency (such as into CVID), suggesting that the presence of IgG subclass deficiency may be a marker for more general immune dysfunction (120). Thus, the more relevant question to ask is, "What is the capacity of the patient to make specific antibodies to protein and polysaccharide antigens?" It is therefore difficult to know the biologic significance of the multiple moderate deficiencies of IgG subclasses that have been reported, particularly when completely asymptomatic individuals have been described who totally lacked IgG_1, IgG_2, IgG_4, and IgG_1 due to gene deletion (Table 1) (121).

X-linked Lymphoproliferative Disease

X-linked lymphoproliferative disease (XLP), also referred to as Duncan's disease (after the original kindred in which it was described), is a recessive trait characterized by an inadequate immune response to infection with *Epstein-Barr virus* (EBV) (15,122). Affected individuals are apparently healthy until they experience infectious mononucleosis (15). Through the use of RFLP probes in linkage with XLP, it has recently become possible to identify affected males before they develop primary EBV infection (122). Immunologic studies demonstrated elevated IgA or IgM and/or variable deficiency of IgG, IgG_1, and IgG_3 in 13 of 13 RFLP-positive but in none of 14 RFLP-negative, EBV-negative males (122). Thus, the immunodeficiency in affected boys may not all be due to EBV infection, and the preexisting abnormalities found may be related to their inadequate response to EBV. The mean age of presentation is less than 5 years. The most common form of presentation (75%) is severe mononucleosis, of which 80% of cases are fatal, primarily due to extensive liver necrosis caused by polyclonally activated alloreactive cytotoxic T cells that recognize EBV-infected autologous B cells (15). Most patients surviving the primary infection developed global cellular immune defects involving T, B, and NK cells, lymphomas, or hypogammaglobulinemia. There is a marked impairment in production of antibodies to the *EBV nuclear antigen* (EBNA), whereas titers of antibodies to the viral capsid antigen have ranged from zero to markedly elevated. *Antibody-dependent cell-mediated cytotoxicity* (ADCC) against EBV-infected cells has been low in many, and NK function is also depressed. There is also a deficiency in long-lived T-cell immunity to EBV. Studies of T-lymphocyte subpopulations with monoclonal antibodies have frequently shown elevated percentages of CD8-positive cells. Immunoglobulin synthesis in response to PWM stimulation *in vitro* is markedly depressed (15). Thus, both EBV-specific and -nonspecific immunologic abnormalities occur in these patients. The defective gene in XLP has been localized to the Xq26-q27 region but as of this writing has not yet been identified (Fig. 1, Table 1) (15,16). Approximately half of the limited number of patients with XLP given HLA-identical related or unrelated unfractionated bone marrow transplants are currently surviving without sign of the disease (123).

T-CELL DEFECTS

In general, patients with partial or absolute defects in T-cell function have infections or other clinical problems for which there is no effective treatment or which are of a more severe nature than those with antibody deficiency disorders. It is also rare that such individuals survive beyond infancy or childhood.

DiGeorge's Syndrome

Thymic hypoplasia results from dysmorphogenesis of the third and fourth pharyngeal pouches during early embryogenesis, leading to hypoplasia or aplasia of the thymus and parathyroid glands (2,124). Other structures forming at the same age are also frequently affected, resulting in anomalies of the great vessels (right-sided aortic arch), esophageal atresia, bifid uvula, upper limb malformations (125), congenital heart disease (atrial and ventricular septal defects), a short philtrum of the upper lip, hypertelorism, an antimongoloid slant to the eyes, mandibular hypoplasia, and low-set, often notched ears. There are clinical similarities between DiGeorge's syndrome and fetal alcohol syndrome (124). The diagnosis of DiGeorge's syndrome is usually first suggested by the presence of hypocalcemic seizures during the neonatal period. Since the original description of the syndrome, it has become apparent that a variable degree of hypoplasia is more frequent than total aplasia of the thymus and parathyroid glands. Some children have little trouble with life-threatening infections and grow normally; such patients are often referred to as having partial DiGeorge's syndrome (126,127). Those with complete DiGeorge's syndrome may resemble patients with SCID in their susceptibility to infections with opportunistic pathogens (i.e., fungi, viruses, and *Pneumocystis carinii*) and to graft-versus-host disease (GVHD) from nonirradiated blood transfusions.

DiGeorge's patients are usually only mildly lymphopenic (126, 127). However, the percentage of T cells is variably decreased; as a result, there is a relative increase in the percentage of B cells. B-cell function is impaired only to the extent of needing helper T cells. Immunoglobulin concentrations are usually normal, although sometimes IgE is elevated and IgA may be low (126,127). Monoclonal antibody analyses of blood lymphocytes have demonstrated that, despite a decreased number of CD3+ T cells, there are usually normal proportions of CD4 and CD8+ cells. Responses of blood lymphocytes after mitogen stimulation have been absent, reduced, or normal, depending on the degree of thymic deficiency, suggesting that the T-lymphocytes that are present are intrinsically normal (126,127). Thymic tissue, when found, does contain Hassall's corpuscles and a normal density of thymocytes; corticomedullary distinction is present. Lymphoid follicles are usually present, but lymph node paracortical areas and thymus-dependent regions of the spleen show variable degrees of depletion.

DiGeorge's syndrome has occurred in both males and females. It is rarely familial, but three cases of apparent autosomal-dominant inheritance have been reported. Microdeletions of specific DNA sequences from chromosome 22q11.2 (the DiGeorge's chromosomal region or DGCR) have been shown in a majority of patients (24,128,129) (Table 1), and PCR-based genotyping using microsatellite DNA markers located within the commonly deleted region permits rapid detection of such microdeletions (130). Several candidate genes have been identified in this region (22,24,131,132). There appears to be an excess of 22q11.2 deletions of maternal origin (133). There are similarities between DiGeorge's syndrome, the velocardiofacial syndrome (VCFS) (134), and the conotruncal anomaly face syndrome (CTAFS) (135) because all three have conotruncal heart defects and 22q deletions. The so-called CATCH 22 syndrome (cardiac, abnormal facies, thymic hypoplasia, cleft palate, and hypocalcemia) includes the broad clinical spectrum of conditions with 22q11.2 deletions (136). Another deletion associated with DiGeorge's and velocardiofacial syndromes has been identified on chromosome 10p13 (Table 1) (23,137,138).

No immunologic treatment is needed for the partial form. If they do not have a severe cardiac lesion, they have few clinical problems except that some experience seizures and developmental delay. Because of variability in the severity of the immunodeficiency, it is difficult to evaluate claimed benefits of fetal thymus transplantation (139). Transplantation of HLA-DR–matched cultured mature thymic epithelial explants has successfully reconstituted the immune function of some such infants (140). Three patients have experienced immunologic reconstitution after unfractionated HLA-identical bone marrow transplantation (141).

Nude Mice and Rats

The animals with functional immune defects most closely resembling that of infants with DiGeorge's syndrome are nude mice (142) and rats (143). However, in contrast to the DiGeorge's anomaly, the defect in nude mice is in their epithelial cells, resulting in hairlessness (144) and a lack of thymic development (145). It has been found that the nude phenotype is caused by mutations in a gene on murine chromosome 11 that encodes a novel winged helix or fork head domain transcription factor, whn (146). Of much greater relevance to patients with the DiGeorge's or velocardiofacial syndromes is a 150-kb region on mouse chromosome 16 that was recently found to be syntenic to the most commonly deleted portion of 22qll.2 in those syndromes (147). Seven genes have been identified in that region, most interesting of which are two serine/threonine kinase genes and a novel goosecoidlike homeobox gene (Gscl). These genes will be the objects of future targeted mutations in order to determine whether haploinsufficiencies in the mutated mice will cause field defects characteristic of this syndrome.

COMBINED IMMUNODEFICIENCY DISORDERS

X-linked Recessive Severe Combined Immunodeficiency Disease

Severe combined immunodeficiency is a rare, fatal syndrome characterized by profound deficiencies of T- and B-cell function (2,148). In the 48 years since the initial description of SCID in 1950 (149), it has become evident that the genetic origins of this condition are quite diverse (Table 1). X-linked SCID (XSCID) is the most common form, accounting for approximately 42% of cases in the United States (150). Figure 2 shows the frequency of the various genetic forms of SCID evaluated by the author over the past three decades. Affected infants present within the first few months of life with frequent episodes of diarrhea, pneumonia, otitis, sepsis, and cutaneous infections. Growth may appear normal initially, but extreme wasting usually develops after infections and diarrhea begin. Persistent infections with opportunistic organisms such as *Candida albicans, Pneumocystis carinii*, varicella, measles, parainfluenzae 3, cytomegalovirus, EBV, and bacillus Calmette-Guerin (BCG) lead to death. These infants also lack the ability to reject foreign tissue and are therefore at risk for GVHD. GVHD can result from maternal T cells that cross into the fetal circulation while the SCID infant is *in utero* or from T-lymphocytes in nonirradiated blood products or allogeneic bone marrow (123).

Infants with SCID are lymphopenic (Fig. 3) (150,151). They have an absence of lymphocyte proliferative responses to mitogens, antigens, and allogeneic cells *in vitro*, even on samples collected *in*

108 SCID INFANTS

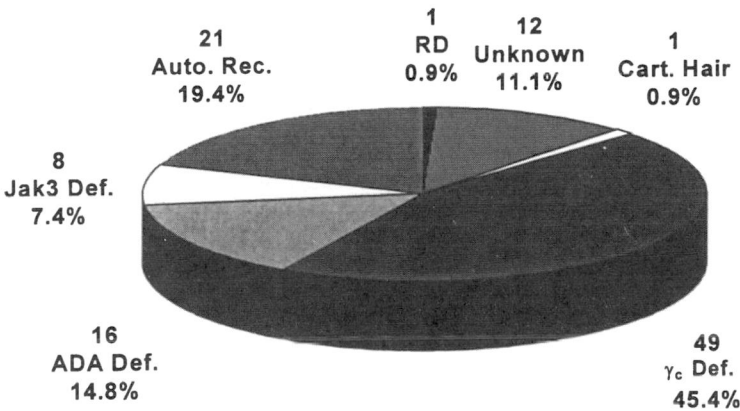

88 SCID FAMILIES

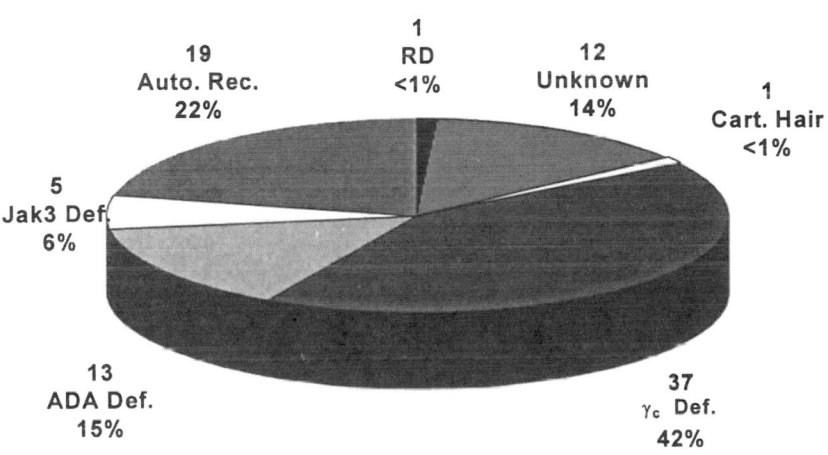

FIG. 2. Relative frequencies of the different genetic types of SCID among 108 patients seen consecutively by the author over three decades and the 88 families of origin. Reprinted with permission from Buckley RH, Schiff RI, Schiff SE, et al. *J Pediatr* 1997;l130:380.

utero or from the cord blood. Therefore, physicians caring for newborns need to be aware of what the normal range for the cord blood absolute lymphocyte count is (2,000 to 11,000/mm³) and thus arrange for functional studies to be performed on blood from neonates with values below this range (150,152,153). The normal absolute lymphocyte count is much higher at the age when most patients with SCID are diagnosed (6 to 7 months), however, so that any count below 4,000/mm³ is lymphopenic (Fig. 3) (154). Serum immunoglobulin concentrations are diminished to absent, and no antibody formation occurs after immunization.

Despite the uniformly profound lack of T- or B-cell function, patients with XSCID usually have elevated percentages of B cells (Fig. 4) (150,152,153,155). However, these B cells do not produce immunoglobulin normally, even after T-cell reconstitution by bone marrow transplantation. By contrast, all but those with transpla-

centally acquired maternal T cells have few or no T cells, and NK cells and function are usually very low or totally lacking in patients with XSCID (Fig. 4) (150,156). Typically, all SCID patients have very small thymuses (usually less than 1 g), which fail to descend from the neck, contain few thymocytes, and lack corticomedullary distinction and Hassall's corpuscles. However, the thymic epithelium is normal, and it is apparent from the outcomes of bone marrow stem cell transplantation that these tiny thymuses are capable of supporting normal T-cell development. Thymus-dependent areas of the spleen are depleted of lymphocytes in SCID patients, and lymph nodes, tonsils, adenoids, and Peyer's patches are absent or extremely underdeveloped.

The abnormal gene in XSCID was mapped by RFLP analysis to the Xq13 region (157) (Fig. 1) and later identified as the gene encoding a common gamma chain (γc) shared by several cytokine

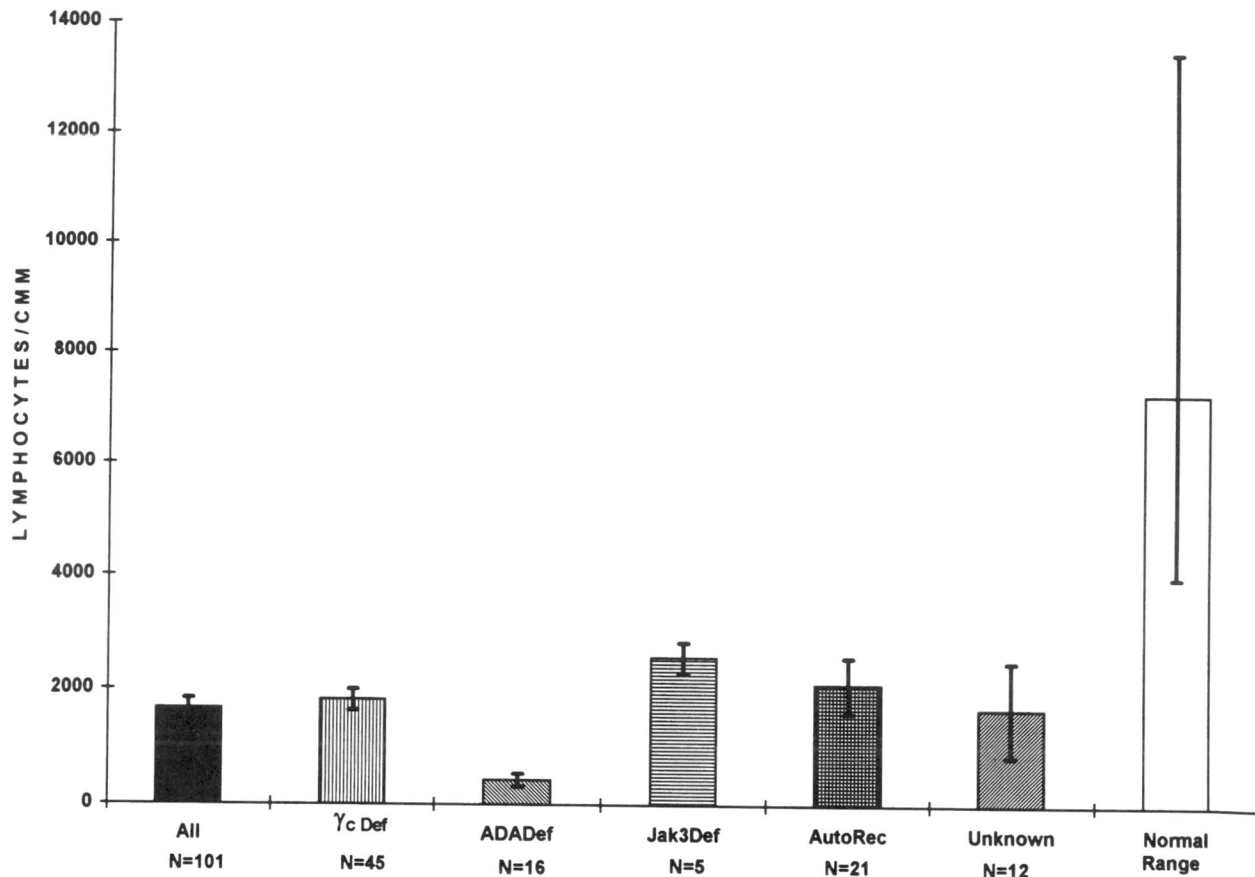

FIG. 3. Mean ± SEM absolute blood lymphocyte counts at initial evaluation for the different types of SCID. The normal mean blood lymphocyte count at age 6 months is 7,300/mm³, and the normal range is 4,000 to 13,500/mm³. Infants with ADA deficiency had significantly lower lymphocyte counts than those in the other groups. Reprinted with permission from Buckley RH, Schiff RI, Schiff SE, et al. *J Pediatr* 1997;130:382.

receptors (Table 1, Fig. 5), including those for IL-2, IL-4, IL-7, IL-9, and IL-15 (Fig. 6) (158–161). This is the most common form of SCID in the United States (Fig. 2). Of the first 136 patients studied, 95 distinct mutations spanning all eight IL-2RG exons were identified, most of them consisting of small changes at the level of one to a few nucleotides (Fig. 5) (162–164). These mutations resulted in abnormal γc chains in two thirds of the cases and absent γc protein in the remainder. Despite the fact that infants with XSCID do not produce immunoglobulins normally even after successful marrow stem cell transplantation, the author (165) and others (166) have found that XSCID B cells are capable of isotype-switching and producing IgE when they are cultured with anti-CD40 and IL-4 or IL-13 *in vitro*. Carriers of XSCID can be detected by the demonstration of nonrandom X-chromosome inactivation in T-lymphocytes (8). Results of X-chromosome inactivation studies had suggested earlier that the genetic defect affects XSCID B lineage cells as well as those of NK and T lineage (167,168). The finding that the mutated gene results in faulty signaling through several cytokine receptors explains how multiple cell types can be affected by a single mutation (169–172). Mutations in γc causing XSCID can be screened via *single-strand conformation polymorphism analysis* (SSCP) (163,173). As more patients are studied, it is likely that atypical cases will be found, such as one recently reported who had an apparent reversion of a documented mutation in the gene encoding γc (174).

SCID is a pediatric emergency (150). Replacement therapy with IVIG fails to halt the progressively downhill course (175). Unless bone marrow transplantation from HLA-identical or -haploidentical donors can be performed, death usually occurs before the patient's first birthday and almost invariably before the second. On the other hand, transplantation in the first 3 months of life offers a greater than 95% chance of survival (176). Therefore, early diagnosis is essential. Affected infants exhibit lymphopenia in the cord blood (150,177). This should alert the physician to perform studies of T-cell function and to examine cord blood mononuclear cells for expression of γc (178). Currently, there are more than 375 SCID patients surviving worldwide as a result of successful bone marrow transplantation (123).

XSCID also exists in dogs (179). Like human SCID infants, affected pups all die or are euthanized by 5 months of age with bacterial or viral infections, including canine distemper, infectious hepatitis, severe pyoderma, and bacterial pneumonia. In further similarity to human XSCIDs, these dogs have elevated numbers of circulating B-lymphocytes. Serum IgM concentrations are normal, but there are low or absent concentrations of serum IgG and IgA. Like human XSCID patients, dogs with XSCID are nearly devoid of T cells in the first 3 weeks of life, but unlike their human counterparts, approximately half go on to develop approximately one third the normal number of T cells (180). Nevertheless, the T cells have severely depressed proliferative responses to T-cell mitogens

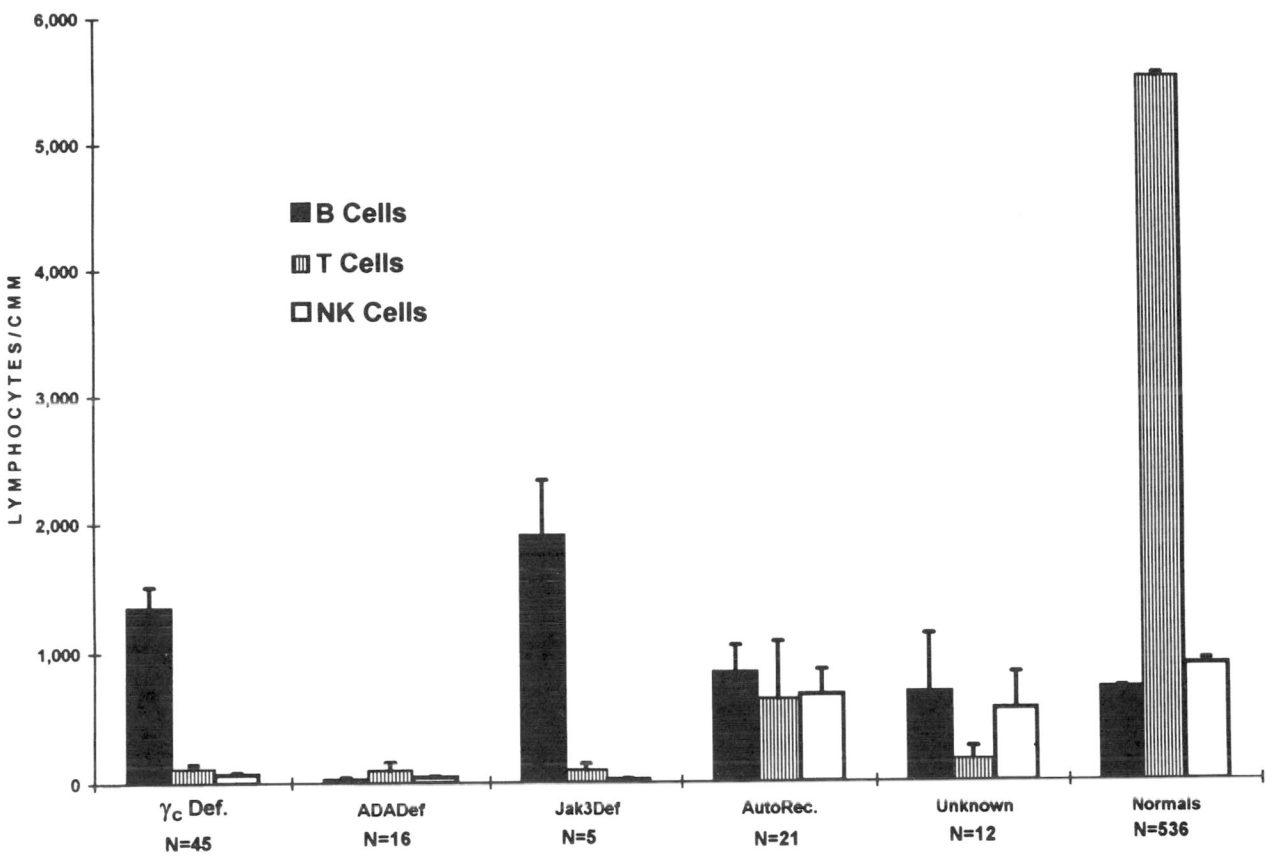

FIG. 4. Means ± SEM of CD20⁺ B cells, CD3⁺ T cells, and CD16⁺ NK cells at initial evaluation for the different types of SCID, as compared with means ± SEM for normal controls. Reprinted with permission from Buckley RH, Schiff RI, Schiff SE, et al. *J Pediatr* 1997;130:383.

despite undergoing a rapid switch from CD45RA to CD45RO (180), and the thymuses and lymphoid tissues are hypoplastic at postmortem examination (179). Unlike human XSCIDs, however, Hassall's corpuscles were present in the thymus, and occasionally normal corticomedullary junctions could be seen. Two different mutations in the canine IL-2RG gene have been identified (181, 182).

Mutant mice with disrupted IL-2RG genes also have hypoplastic thymuses and are devoid of NK cells (183,184). However, they differ from both human and dog XSCIDs in that they have greatly reduced numbers of B cells. Like the dogs, they have some CD4⁺ T cells that respond to γc-independent but not γc-dependent mitogens.

Autosomal-Recessive Severe Combined Immunodeficiency Diseases

This was the first pattern of inheritance noted in SCID, reported initially by Swiss workers in 1958 (149). This type of inheritance is less common in the United States than in European (Fig. 2) (150,153). Mutated genes on autosomal chromosomes have been identified in three forms of SCID: adenosine deaminase (ADA) deficiency, Janus kinase 3 (Jak3) deficiency, and RAG1 or 2 deficiency, and there are likely other causes yet to be discovered (Table 1, Fig. 2) (164,185).

Autosomal-Recessive Severe Combined Immunodeficiency Disease Due to Adenosine Deaminase Deficiency

An absence of the enzyme ADA has been observed in approximately 15% of patients with SCID (Fig. 2) (19,150). Patients with ADA deficiency have the same clinical problems of susceptibility to opportunistic bacterial, viral, and parasitic diseases as described above for XSCID and the same susceptibility to GVHD from allogeneic T cells in blood products or bone marrow. However, there are certain distinguishing features of ADA deficiency, including the presence of rib cage abnormalities similar to a rachitic rosary and multiple skeletal abnormalities of chondro-osseous dysplasia on radiographic examination; these occur predominantly at the costochondral junctions, at the apophyses of the iliac bones, and in the vertebral bodies.

ADA-deficient patients usually have a much more profound lymphopenia than do infants with other types of SCID, with mean absolute lymphocyte counts of less than 500/mm³ (Fig. 3); they rarely have elevated percentages of B or NK cells (Fig. 4) (150). They do have normal NK function (150,152), and after T cell function is conferred by bone marrow transplantation without pretransplant chemotherapy, they generally have excellent B-cell function. This is due to the fact that ADA deficiency affects primarily T-cell function, which is absent just as in all of the other forms of SCID.

IL2RG MUTATIONS IN 87 FAMILIES WITH X-LINKED SCID

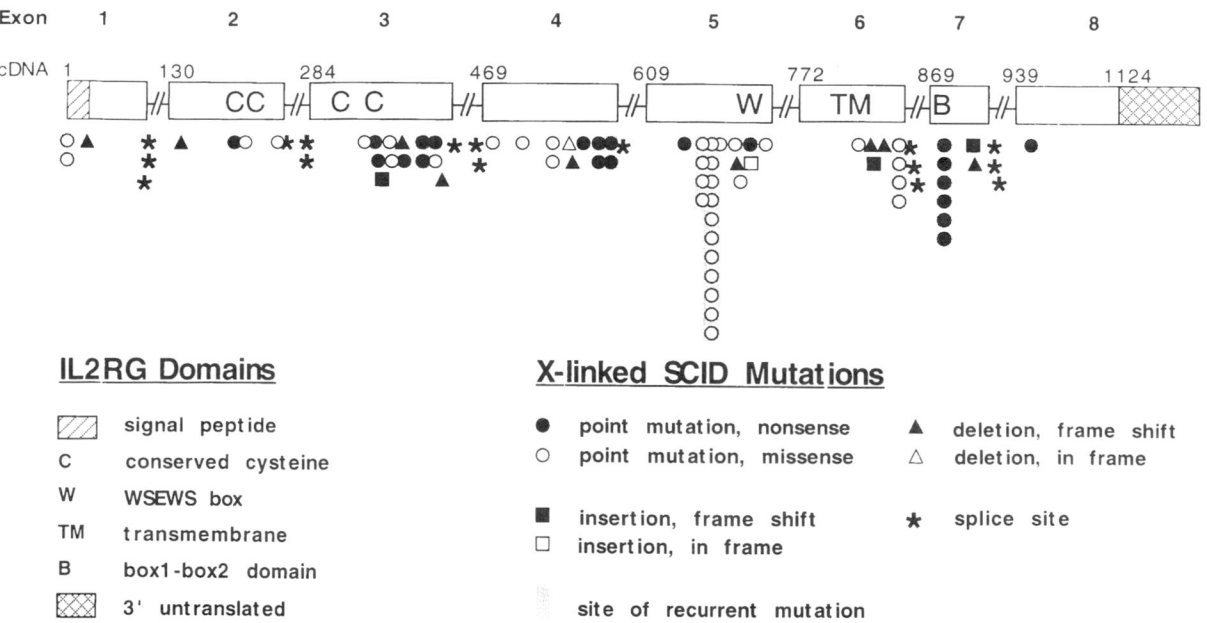

IL2RG Domains

▨	signal peptide
C	conserved cysteine
W	WSEWS box
TM	transmembrane
B	box1-box2 domain
▨	3' untranslated

X-linked SCID Mutations

●	point mutation, nonsense	▲	deletion, frame shift
○	point mutation, missense	△	deletion, in frame
■	insertion, frame shift	★	splice site
□	insertion, in frame		
	site of recurrent mutation		

FIG. 5. IL-2RG cDNA map showing exons, cDNA numbers corresponding to the first coding nucleotide of each exon, protein domains, and sites of mutations found in 87 unrelated families with XSCID. Identical mutations found in unrelated patients are surrounded by shaded boxes. Reprinted with permission from Puck JM, Pepper AE, Henthorn PS, et al. *Blood* 1997;89:1970.

In further contrast to infants with other types of SCID, however, a few ADA-deficient patients have been found to have rare Hassall's corpuscles in their thymuses and changes suggestive of early thymic differentiation (19). Moreover, milder forms of this condition have been reported, leading to delayed diagnosis of immunodeficiency even to adulthood (186).

The gene encoding ADA was mapped to chromosome 20q13-ter and it was cloned and sequenced over a decade ago (Table 1) (19). The ADA deficiency caused by mutations in this gene results in marked accumulations of adenosine, 2'-deoxyadenosine, and 2'-O-methyladenosine (187). The latter directly or indirectly lead to lymphocyte toxicity, which causes the immunodeficiency. Adenosine and deoxyadenosine are apparent suicide inactivators of the enzyme S-adenosylhomocysteine (SAH) hydrolase, resulting in the accumulation of SAH. SAH is a potent inhibitor of virtually all cellular methylation reactions.

As with other types of SCID, ADA-deficiency can be cured by HLA-identical or -haploidentical T cell–depleted bone marrow transplantation without the need for pre- or posttransplant chemotherapy; this remains the treatment of choice (123,152,188). Enzyme replacement therapy with polyethylene glycol-modified bovine ADA (PEG-ADA) administered subcutaneously once weekly has resulted in both clinical and immunologic improvement in more than 40 ADA-deficient patients (189–191). However, the immunocompetence achieved is not nearly as effective as with bone marrow transplantation (123). In view of this, PEG-ADA therapy should not be initiated if bone marrow transplantation is contemplated, because it will confer graft-rejection capability upon the infant. ADA deficiency is the first genetic defect in which gene therapy was attempted; however, those particular efforts have not been very suc-

cessful thus far (192–196). Recently there was a report of a spontaneous *in vivo* reversion to normal of a mutation in the ADA gene (197,198).

Unlike their human counterparts, mice with disrupted ADA genes do not survive beyond the immediate perinatal period; they die of hepatocellular and small bowel necrosis and of atelectasis (199).

Autosomal Recessive Severe Combined Immunodeficiency Disease Due to Janus Kinase 3 Deficiency

SCID patients with this very recently discovered defect resemble all other types in their susceptibility to infection and to GVHD from allogeneic T cells. However, they have lymphocyte characteristics most closely resembling those of patients with XSCID, including an elevated percentage of B cells and very low percentages of T and NK cells (Fig. 4) (150). Because Jak3 is the only signaling molecule known to be associated with γc, it was a candidate gene for mutations leading to autosomal-recessive SCID not due to ADA deficiency (Table 1, Fig. 6) (200–205). Thus far, 15 patients have been identified who lack Jak3 (29,150,206). Like XSCID patients, they have very low or no NK activity. Even after successful T-cell reconstitution by transplantation of haploidentical stem cells, they fail to develop NK cells (123). Moreover, as with XSCID patients, they fail to develop normal B-cell function posttransplantation despite their high numbers of B cells. The reason for their failure to develop NK cells or B-cell function is unknown but is thought to be related to the defective function of the multiple types of cytokine receptors that share γc (Fig. 6) (207).

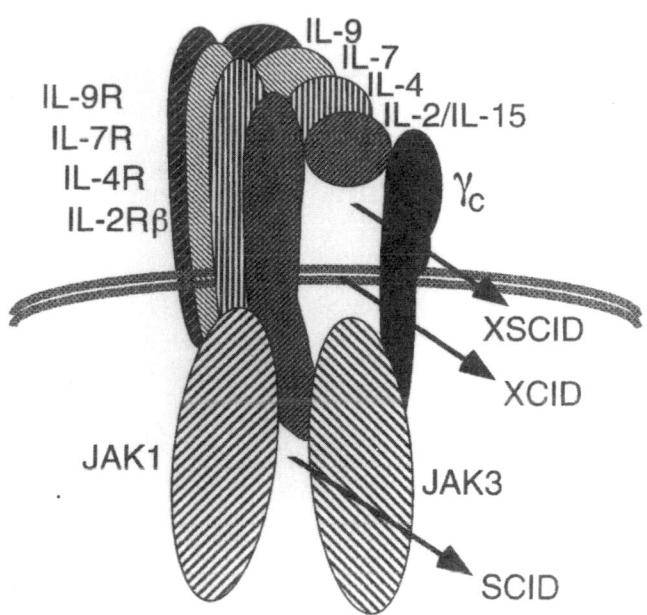

FIG. 6. Cartoon showing that Jak3 is the major signal transducer for the common gamma chain (γ_c) shared by multiple cytokine receptors. Mutations in the gene encoding Jak3 result in a form of autosomal-recessive SCID that mimics XSCID phenotypically. Figure courtesy of Drs. Sarah Russell and Warren Leonard.

Unlike humans with Jak3 deficiency (but similar to the situation in IL-2RG mutant mice), Jak3 knock-out mice have very few B cells (208). Similar to the human Jak3-deficient infant, they have few or no T or NK cells.

Autosomal-Recessive Severe Combined Immunodeficiency Due to RAG1 or RAG2 Deficiencies

Infants with this most recently discovered cause of SCID resemble all others in their infection susceptibility and complete absence of T- or B-cell function. However, their lymphocyte phenotype differs from those of patients with SCID due to γ_c, Jak3, or ADA deficiencies in that they lack both B- and T-lymphocytes (so-called T-B- SCID) and have primarily NK cells in their circulation (Fig. 4). This suggested a problem with their antigen receptor genes, and, indeed, some patients with this phenotype were found to have mutations in the genes that encode the recombinase activating genes RAG1 or RAG2 (Table 1) (209). Such mutations result in a functional inability to form antigen receptors through genetic recombination, as had been noted in the comparable RAG1 or RAG2 mutant mice (210,211). The latter have very small lymphoid organs containing immature lymphoid cells that all fail to rearrange their immunoglobulin or *T-cell receptor* (TCR) loci.

Until recently the Bosma SCID mouse had been considered to be a likely animal model for human T-B- SCID (212). As in human SCIDs with RAG1 or RAG2 mutations (209), these mice have a small epithelial thymus containing sparse lymphoid elements, but there is a virtual absence of T and B cells in the blood and in all peripheral lymphoid tissues due to defective rearrangement of antigen receptor genes in both lineages (213). "Leaky" SCID mice have an incomplete block in antigen receptor rearrangement, resulting in the presence of B cells, immunoglobulins, and some

functional T cells (214). However, like RAG1 or RAG2 mutants, bone marrow–derived myeloid cells and natural killer cells are present in normal number (215). The Bosma SCID mouse defect is now known to be due to a nonsense mutation in the gene on murine chromosome 16 encoding the catalytic subunit of a DNA-dependent protein kinase, p350, or the Ku protein (216,217). A human gene encoding a similar protein has been assigned to human chromosome 8p12→q22, but thus far no human SCID has been identified with this type of mutation (218).

Arabian horses have been known for over 20 years to carry a recessive gene for SCID, and recently the mode of inheritance has been confirmed as autosomal recessive (219). The heterozygous state occurs in thoroughbred horses at a frequency of one in four (219,220). In contrast to humans with autosomal-recessive SCID, however, the basic thymic architecture of Arabian horses afflicted with SCID is normal except for a small number of lymphoid elements. However, the foals are profoundly lymphopenic and hypogammaglobulinemic, they lack all cell-mediated and humoral immunity, and they usually die from infection before the fifth month of life (219,221). Recent studies suggest that the same gene may be mutated in the Arabian horse as is mutated in the Bosma SCID mouse (222).

Reticular dysgenesis was first described in 1959 in identical twin male infants who exhibited a total lack of both lymphocytes and granulocytes in their peripheral blood and bone marrow. Seven of the eight infants thus far reported with this defect died between 3 and 119 days of age from overwhelming infections; the eighth underwent complete immunologic reconstitution from a bone marrow transplant (2). Mature, normal-appearing granulocytes (although markedly reduced in number) were noted in three patients, and a normal percentage of E rosetting T cells in the cord blood of a fourth patient, arguing against a total failure of stem cell differentiation in this defect. However, despite the normal percentage of T cells in the latter patient's cord blood, the cells failed to give an *in vitro* proliferative response to mitogens. The thymus glands have all weighed less than 1 g, no Hassall's corpuscles have been present, and few or no thymocytes have been seen. The molecular basis of this autosomal-recessive disorder is unknown.

Combined Immunodeficiency

Combined immunodeficiency (CID) is a syndrome characterized by low but not absent T-cell function. Patients with CID present during infancy with recurrent or chronic pulmonary infections, failure to thrive, oral or cutaneous candidiasis, chronic diarrhea, recurrent skin infections, Gram-negative sepsis, urinary tract infections, or severe varicella (2).

Serum immunoglobulins may be normal or elevated for all classes, but selective IgA deficiency, marked elevation of IgE, and elevated IgD levels have been found in some cases. Although antibody-forming capacity has been impaired in a majority, it has not been absent and has been apparently normal in roughly one third of the reported cases. Moreover, plasma cells are usually abundant in the lamina propria and lymph nodes of many of these patients. Other findings include neutropenia and eosinophilia.

Studies of cellular immune function have shown delayed cutaneous anergy to ubiquitous antigens in all such patients, lymphopenia, and extremely low but not absent lymphocyte proliferative responses to mitogens and allogeneic cells *in vitro*. CID patients have profound deficiencies of CD3+ T cells, but usually normal proportions of CD4 and CD8+ cells, in contrast to patients with AIDS, who characteristically have a selective deficiency of CD4+ cells. Peripheral lymphoid tissues demonstrate paracortical lymphocyte depletion. The thymuses are very small and have a paucity of thymocytes and usually no Hassall's corpuscles; however, thymic epithelium is intact. An autosomal-recessive pattern of inheritance is often seen.

Patients with CID usually survive longer than do infants with SCID, but they fail to thrive and die early in life. Some have been successfully reconstituted by unfractionated matched sibling or unrelated adult donor bone marrow transplants or cord blood transplants, but T cell–depleted haploidentical marrow stem cell transplants have not been very successful because they require chemoablation before transplantation to achieve graft acceptance and there is resistance to engraftment.

Purine Nucleoside Phosphorylase Deficiency

More than 40 patients with CID have been found to have purine nucleoside phosphorylase (PNP) deficiency (Table 1) (20). Although ADA and PNP are both purine salvage pathway enzymes, PNP deficiency does not lead to as severe an immunodeficiency as in ADA deficiency. In further contrast to ADA deficiency, no characteristic physical or skeletal abnormalities have been noted in PNP deficiency. Deaths have occurred from generalized vaccinia, varicella, lymphosarcoma, and GVHD mediated by T cells from nonirradiated allogeneic blood or bone marrow. Two thirds of patients have had neurologic abnormalities ranging from spasticity to mental retardation. One third of patients developed autoimmune diseases, the most common of which is autoimmune hemolytic anemia. Idiopathic thrombocytopenic purpura and systemic lupus erythematosus also have been reported.

Most patients have normal or elevated concentrations of all serum immunoglobulins, although there are exceptions. PNP-deficient patients are as profoundly lymphopenic as those with ADA deficiency, with absolute lymphocyte counts usually less than 500/mm³. Analyses of lymphocyte subpopulations with monoclonal antibodies have demonstrated a marked deficiency of T cells and of T-cell subsets but increased numbers of cells with NK phenotype and function. T-cell function is low but not absent and is variable with time.

The gene encoding PNP is on chromosome 14q13.1, and it has been cloned and sequenced. A variety of mutations have been found in the PNP gene in patients with PNP deficiency (223). Unlike ADA deficiency, serum and urinary uric acid are markedly deficient because PNP is needed to form the urate precursors hypoxanthine and xanthine. Unlike most patients with CID, the thymuses of PNP-deficient patients have had occasional Hassall's corpuscles at postmortem examination, reminiscent of some patients with ADA deficiency. Prenatal diagnosis is possible.

Attempts to correct the immunologic and enzymatic deficiencies of PNP-deficient patients by enzyme replacement or deoxycytidine therapy have not been successful. This condition is invariably fatal in childhood unless immunologic reconstitution can be achieved. Bone marrow transplantation is the treatment of choice but has thus far been successful in only three such patients (224). Gene therapy may be an option in the future (196).

Cartilage-Hair Hypoplasia

In 1965, an unusual form of short-limbed dwarfism with frequent and severe infections was reported among the Pennsylvania Amish; non-Amish cases have since been described (2,225). These patients have short and pudgy hands with redundant skin; metaphyseal chondrodysplasia; hyperextensible joints of hands and feet but an inability to extend the elbows completely; and fine, sparse light hair and eyebrows. These features led to the name cartilage-hair hypoplasia (CHH). Radiographically, the bones show scalloping and sclerotic or cystic changes in the metaphyses. In contrast to ADA deficiency, in which the predominant changes are in the apophyses of the iliac bones, the ribs, and vertebral bodies, the chondrodysplasia in CHH principally affects the limbs. Severe and often fatal varicella infections, progressive vaccinia, and vaccine-associated poliomyelitis have been observed. Associated conditions include deficient erythrogenesis, Hirschsprung's disease, and an increased risk of malignancies.

Three patterns of immune dysfunction have emerged: defective antibody-mediated immunity, defective cellular immunity (most common form), and SCID. NK cells, however, are increased in number and function.

CHH is an autosomal-recessive condition, and the defective gene has recently been mapped to chromosome 9p21-p13 in Amish and Finnish families (Table 1) (226). The gene has not been identified as yet, however, so the fundamental molecular abnormality is unknown. In vitro studies have shown decreased numbers of T cells and defective T-cell proliferation, owing to an intrinsic defect related to the G1 phase, resulting in a longer cell cycle for individual cells (225,227). This abnormality also occurs in fibroblasts from these patients and in in vitro colony formation in erythroid, myeloid, and megakaryocytic lineages, suggesting a common cell proliferation defect in CHH (228). Bone marrow transplantation has resulted in immunologic reconstitution in some CHH patients with the SCID phenotype. Those with milder types of immune deficiency have lived to adulthood, some even to old age.

Immunodeficiency with Thrombocytopenia and Eczema (Wiskott-Aldrich Syndrome)

Wiskott-Aldrich syndrome is an X-linked recessive syndrome characterized by eczema, thrombocytopenic purpura with normal-appearing megakaryocytes but small defective platelets, and undue susceptibility to infection (2,229). Patients usually present during infancy with either prolonged bleeding from the circumcision site, bloody diarrhea, or excessive bruising. The thrombocytopenia is caused by an intrinsic platelet abnormality, leading to decreased survival of autologous but not homologous ⁵¹Cr-labeled platelets.

Atopic dermatitis and recurrent infections usually also develop during the first year of life. Asthma and other diseases may be seen. In younger patients, infections are usually those produced by pneumococci and other encapsulated bacteria, resulting in otitis media, pneumonia, meningitis, or sepsis. Later, infections with opportunistic agents such as Pneumocystis carinii and the herpes viruses become more problematic. Autoimmune cytopenias and vasculitis are common in those who live beyond infancy. There may be considerable variability in the degree of infection susceptibility or in the extent to which atopic manifestations are expressed. However, survival beyond the teens is rare; infections and bleeding are major causes of death, but there is also a 12% incidence of fatal malignancy in this condition.

Patients with WAS have an impaired humoral immune response to polysaccharide antigens, as evidenced by absent or markedly diminished isohemagglutinins and poor or absent antibody responses to polysaccharide antigens (2). In addition, antibody titers to protein antigens decrease with time, and anamnestic responses are often poor or absent. There is an accelerated rate of synthesis as well as hypercatabolism of albumin, IgG, IgA, and IgM, resulting in highly variable immunoglobulin concentrations (230). Most often there is a low serum IgM, elevated IgA, and IgE, and a normal or slightly low IgG concentration. Flow cytometry of blood lymphocytes has shown moderately reduced percentages of CD3-, CD4-, and CD8-bearing T cells, and lymphocyte responses to mitogens are moderately depressed. The CD8 molecules of peripheral blood T cells of WAS patients have decreased expression of the α/β heterodimer and an increase in those expressing the α/α homodimer, possibly explaining part of the defective lymphocyte function (231).

The mutated gene responsible for this defect was mapped to Xp11.22-11.23 (232) (Fig. 1) and isolated in 1994 by Derry and coworkers (Table 1) (9). It was found to be limited in expression to lymphocytic and megakaryocyte lineages (9). The gene product, a 501–amino acid proline-rich protein that lacks a hydrophobic transmembrane domain, was designated WASP (WAS protein). It has been shown to bind CDC42H2 and rac, members of the Rho family of GTPases important in actin polymerization (233,234). In addition, it was found to physically associate with Nck through Src homology 3 domains (235) and with tyrosine-phosphorylated Shc (236). WASP appears to control the assembly of actin filaments required for microvesicle formation downstream from protein kinase C and tyrosine kinase signaling (236). A large and varied number of mutations in the WASP gene have been identified in WAS patients (237,238), with some correlation of the site of the mutation with severity of infection susceptibility or other problems in one series (Ochs, personal communication), but not in the other (239). Isolated X-linked thrombocytopenia is also caused by mutations in the WASP gene (240). Carriers can be detected by the finding of nonrandom X chromosome inactivation in several hematopoietic cell lineages or by detection of the mutated gene (if known in the family) (241–243). Prenatal diagnosis of WAS also can be made by chorionic villous sampling or amniocentesis if the mutation is known in that family. Recently two families with apparent autosomal inheritance of a clinical phenotype similar to WAS have been reported (244,245).

A number of patients with WAS have had complete corrections of both the platelet and the immunologic abnormalities by HLA-identical sibling bone marrow transplants after being conditioned with irradiation or busulfan and cyclophosphamide (123). Success has been minimal with T cell–depleted haploidentical stem cell transplants in WAS, primarily because of the requirement for pretransplant immunosuppression to permit engraftment, the long time course to immunoreconstitution when T cells are depleted, resistance to engraftment, and a high mortality rate from preexisting opportunistic infections in that setting (123). Recently, some success has been achieved in the treatment of WAS with matched unrelated donor transplants when performed in patients under the age of 5 years (246). It is likely that matched cord blood transplants will be similarly successful because in both cases T cells can be left in the donor cell suspension. Unless immunologic reconstitution can be achieved, patients with the clinically more severe forms of WAS usually die in childhood. Vasculitis is a major problem in many older children with WAS. Several patients who required splenectomy for uncontrollable bleeding had impressive increases in their platelet counts and have done well clinically while on prophylactic antibiotics and IVIG (247,248). The higher platelet counts also permitted the use of high-dose aspirin or other nonsteroidal antiinflammatory agents in the control of vasculitis. Unless

the patient is under the age of 5 years and an appropriate unrelated matched donor exists, splenectomy is likely to remain the treatment of choice for WAS patients lacking an HLA-identical donor until gene therapy can be perfected (196). The most common cause of death in WAS patients currently is EBV-induced lymphoreticular malignancy.

The X-chromosome linked scurfy (Sf) mouse mutant resembles humans with WAS somewhat by having scaly skin, low platelet and erythrocyte counts, and gastrointestinal bleeding (249). They also exhibit a fatal lymphoreticular disease mediated by CD4+ T cells that overexpress cytokine genes for IL-4, IL-6, IL-7, and TNF-α (250,251). It is not known whether such mice have an immunodeficiency. However, the loci of the Sf mutant mouse gene and human WAS lie in homologous segments of the X-chromosome (252).

Ataxia Telangiectasia

Ataxia telangiectasia (AT) is a complex combined immunodeficiency syndrome with associated neurologic, endocrinologic, hepatic, and cutaneous abnormalities (2,253). The most prominent features are progressive cerebellar ataxia, oculocutaneous telangiectasias, chronic sinopulmonary disease, a high incidence of malignancy (254), and variable humoral and cellular immunodeficiency. The ataxia typically becomes evident shortly after the child begins to walk and progresses until he or she is confined to a wheelchair, usually by the age of 10 to 12 years. The telangiectasias develop at 3 to 6 years of age. Recurrent, usually bacterial, sinopulmonary infections occur in roughly 80% of these patients. Fatal varicella occurred in one of the author's patients, and transfusion-associated GVHD also has been reported (255).

Selective IgA deficiency is found in 50% to 80% of affected individuals; in some patients this may be due in part to hypercatabolism of IgA (253). IgE concentrations are usually low, and the IgM may be of the low molecular weight variety. IgG_2 or total IgG may be decreased. Specific antibody titers may be decreased or normal. Cell-mediated immunity is impaired, as evidenced by delayed skin test anergy and prolonged allograft survival. In vitro tests of lymphocyte function have generally shown moderately depressed proliferative responses to T- and B-cell mitogens. The percentages of CD3+ and CD4+ T cells are only modestly low, and there are usually normal or increased percentages of CD8+ T cells and (sometimes) elevated numbers of gamma/delta TCR-positive cells. Studies of immunoglobulin synthesis have shown both helper T cell and intrinsic B-cell defects. The thymus is hypoplastic, exhibits poor organization, and is lacking in Hassall's corpuscles.

Cells from patients as well as those of heterozygous carriers have increased sensitivity to ionizing radiation, defective DNA repair, and frequent chromosomal abnormalities (253,256,257). The sites of chromosomal breakage in more than 50% of cases involve the genes that encode the TCR on chromosome 7 and the immunoglobulin heavy chains on chromosome 14, most likely accounting for the combined T- and B-cell abnormalities seen. These rearrangements may be clonal and may either be stable or undergo malignant transformation. The malignancies reported in this condition have usually been of the lymphoreticular type, but adenocarcinoma and other forms also have been seen; there is also an increased incidence of malignancy in unaffected relatives.

Inheritance of AT follows an autosomal recessive pattern. The mutated gene (ATM) responsible for this defect was mapped by RFLP analysis to the long arm of chromosome 11 (11q22-23) and was recently cloned (Table 1) (21,253,256,258). The gene product is a DNA-dependent protein kinase localized predominantly to the nucleus and thought to be involved in mitogenic signal transduction, meiotic recombination, and cell cycle control (259–261). Of the mutations identified to date, a majority were expected to completely inactivate the ATM protein by truncating it, by abolishing correct initiation or termination of translation, or by deleting large segments (262,263). An ATM knock-out mouse has been generated (264).

No satisfactory definitive treatment has been found (253). The prognosis is exceedingly poor for patients with this condition, although a number have reached adulthood. The most common causes of death are lymphoreticular malignancy and progressive neurologic disease (264).

Nijmegen Breakage Syndrome

This is a rare autosomal-recessive condition in which the immunologic, cytogenetic, and radiation sensitivity findings are almost identical to those in AT (265–267). However, the patients are quite distinct from AT clinically in that they have short stature, a bird-like facies and microcephaly from birth. They lack the classic clinical features of AT, including ataxia and telangiectasia, and they have normal serum alpha fetoprotein levels. Intelligence can vary from normal to moderate mental retardation. The immunodeficiency appears to be more severe than in AT. Most of the patients have had recurrent respiratory infections, and the tendency to express rearrangements of chromosomes 7 and 14 and to develop a malignancy is much higher than in AT. More than 40 patients from approximately 30 families have been reported, and most are of Eastern European origin (265,267). Complementation studies have indicated that patients with this syndrome are genetically distinct from those with AT. The abnormal gene in this condition has been mapped to chromosome 8q21 (Table 1) (268).

Defective Expression of Major Histocompatibility Complex Antigens

There are two main forms: (a) class I MHC antigen deficiency (bare lymphocyte syndrome) and (b) class II MHC antigen deficiency (269).

MHC Class I Antigen Deficiency

An isolated deficiency of MHC class I antigens is rare, and the resulting immunodeficiency is much milder than in SCID, contributing to a later age of presentation. Sera from affected children contain normal quantities of class I MHC antigens and β2 microglobulin, but class I MHC antigens are not detected on any cells in the body. There is a deficiency of CD8+ but not of CD4+ T cells. Recently, two siblings from a Moroccan family presented with relatively late onset recurrent, severe bacterial pulmonary infections and were found to have a nonsense mutation in one of two genes within the MHC locus on chromosome 6 that encode the antigenic peptide transporter protein known as TAP (25,270). The genes are designated TAP1 and TAP2; the affected siblings had a nonsense mutation in TAP2 (Table 1). Both siblings had a deficiency of CD8+ cells and lacked MHC class I antigens on their lymphocytes. TAP functions to transport antigenic peptides from the cytoplasm across the Golgi apparatus membrane to join the α chain of MHC class 1 antigens and β2 microglobulin. These are then all assembled into an MHC class I complex that can then move to the cell surface. If the assembly of the complex cannot be completed because there is no antigenic peptide, the MHC class I complex is destroyed in the cytoplasm (271).

MHC Class II Antigen Deficiency

Many affected with this autosomal-recessive syndrome are of North African descent (269,272). Patients with the different genetic forms of this condition present with persistent diarrhea in early infancy. The latter is often associated with cryptosporidiosis, infections with enteroviruses (polio, coxsackie), herpes or other viral agents, and oral candidiasis. They also experience bacterial pneumonia, pneumocystis, and septicemia. Nevertheless, their immunodeficiency is not as severe as in SCID, as evidenced by their failure to develop BCG-osis or GVHD from nonirradiated blood transfusions (269).

MHC class II–deficient patients have a very low number of CD4+ T cells but normal or elevated numbers of CD8+ T cells. Lymphopenia is only moderate. The MHC class II antigens HLA-DP, -DQ, and -DR are undectable on blood B cells and monocytes, even though B cells are present in normal number. The patients are nevertheless hypogammaglobulinemic due to impaired antigen-specific responses caused by the absence of these antigen-presenting molecules. In addition, MHC antigen-deficient B cells fail to stimulate allogeneic cells in mixed leukocyte culture. Lymphocyte proliferation studies show normal responses to mitogens but no response to antigens. The thymus and other lymphoid organs are severely hypoplastic, and the lack of class II molecules results in abnormal thymic selection. The latter results in circulating CD4+ T cells that have altered CDR3 profiles (272,273). The associated defects of both B- and T-cell immunity and of HLA expression emphasize the important biologic role for HLA determinants in effective immune cell cooperation.

MHC class II antigen deficiency is genetically heterogeneous, with at least four different complementation groups having been reported (26,272,274–276). The molecular defects thus far described affect the regulation of expression of class II genes rather than causing abnormalities of the coding regions for HLA-DP, -DQ, or -DR, and they do not segregate with the MHC genes on chromosome 6. Two different molecular defects were identified by complementation cloning (276); both cause impairment in the coordinate expression of MHC class II molecules on the surface of B cells and macrophages (274,277). In one there is a mutation in the gene on chromosome 1q that encodes a protein called RFX5, a promoter protein that binds to the MHC class II gene promoter region X-box (Table 1) (278). In the other, there is a mutation in the gene on chromosome 16p13 that encodes a novel MHC CIITA, which coordinates the binding of proteins to the MHC Class II gene promoter region (276,277,279,280). A mouse with a targeted deletion of CIITA shows phenotypic concordance with humans who have this defect (281).

Leukocyte Adhesion Deficiencies

Leukocyte Adhesion Deficiency 1

This condition is due to mutations in the gene on chromosome 21 at position q22.3 encoding CD18, a 95-kDa beta subunit shared by three adhesive heterodimers: LFA-1 on B-, T-, and NK-lymphocytes; complement receptor type 3 (CR3) on neutrophils, monocytes, macrophages, eosinophils, and NK cells; and p150,95 (another complement receptor) (17,18,282). The alpha chains of these three molecules (encoded by genes on chromosome 16) are not expressed because of the abnormal beta chain. Those so affected have histories of delayed separation of the umbilical cord, omphalitis, gingivitis, recurrent skin infections, repeated otitis media, pneumonia, septicemia, ileocolitis (283,284), peritonitis, perianal abscesses, and impaired wound healing. Life-threatening bacterial and fungal infections account for the high mortality. Affected people do not have increased susceptibility to viral infections or malignancy. Blood neutrophil counts are usually significantly elevated even when no infection is present, owing to an inability of the cells to adhere to vascular endothelium and migrate out of the intravascular compartment. All cytotoxic lymphocyte functions are markedly impaired because of a lack of the adhesion protein LFA-1; deficiency of LFA-1 also interferes with immune cell interaction and immune recognition. CR3 binds fixed iC3b fragments of C3 and β-glucans; its absence causes abnormal phagocytic cell adherence and chemotaxis and a reduced respiratory burst with phagocytosis. Deficiencies of these glycoproteins can be screened via cytofluorography of blood leukocytes with monoclonal antibodies to CD18 or to CD11a, b, or c. Because the CD18 gene has been cloned and sequenced (Table 1), this disorder is another potential candidate for gene therapy (196,282). A gene-targeted mouse deficient in CD18 shows many similarities to patients with this defect (285).

Leukocyte Adhesion Deficiency 2

Leukocyte adhesion deficiency 2 (LAD2) is due to the absence of neutrophil Sialyl-Lewis X, a ligand of E-selectin on vascular endothelium (18,286). This disorder was discovered in two unrelated Israeli boys, aged three and five years, each the offspring of consanguinous parents. Both have severe mental retardation, short stature, a distinctive facial appearance, and the Bombay (hh) blood phenotype, and both are secretor and Lewis negative. They both have had recurrent severe bacterial infections similar to those seen in patients with LAD1, including pneumonia, peridontitis, otitis media, and localized cellulitis. Similar to patients with LAD1, their infections have been accompanied by marked leukocytosis (30,000 to 150,000/mm³) but an absence of pus formation at sites of recurrent cellulitis. *In vitro* studies revealed a marked defect in neutrophil motility. Because the genes for the red cell H antigen and for the secretor status encode for distinct α1,2-fucosyltransferases and the synthesis of Sialyl-Lewis X requires an α1,3-fucosyltransferase, the authors have postulated a general defect in fucose metabolism as the basis for this disorder (286). The abnormal gene in this condition has not yet been identified.

Interleukin 2 Receptor α Chain (CD25) Mutation

A male infant born of a consanguinous union presented at 6 months of age with cytomegalovirus pneumonia, persistent oral and esophageal candidiasis, adenoviral gastroenteritis, and failure to thrive. He developed lymphadenopathy, hepatosplenomegaly, and chronic inflammation of his lungs and mandible. Biopsies showed extensive lymphocytic infiltration of his lung, liver, gut, and bone. Serum IgG and IgM were elevated, but IgA was low. He had a T-cell lymphocytopenia, with an even CD4:CD8 ratio. The T cells responded poorly to anti-CD3, phytohemagglutinin and other mitogens, and to IL-2. He was found to have a truncated mutation of the IL-2R α chain (CD25) (Table 1) (28). He could not reject an

allogeneic skin graft. He was given a successful allogeneic bone marrow transplant after cytoreduction.

Young mutant mice lacking the IL-2R α chain have phenotypically normal T- and B-cell development (287). However, as adults they develop massive lymphoid organ enlargement and polyclonal T- and B-cell expansion attributed to defective apoptosis. They also develop autoimmune disorders, including hemolytic anemia and inflammatory bowel disease. Similarly, gene targeted mice lacking the IL-2R β chain develop exhaustive differentiation of B cells into plasma cells, elevated IgG₁ and IgE, and autoantibodies that cause hemolytic anemia (288). T cells did not respond to polyclonal or antigen-specific activators. It is known that IL-2 programs murine αβ T-lymphocytes for apoptosis (289). From these observations, it is deduced that both IL-2R α and β chains play an important role in influencing the activation programs of T cells, the balance between clonal expansion and cell death after lymphocyte activation, and the prevention of autoimmunity.

Interferon Gamma Receptor 1 Mutations

Disseminated BCG infections occur in infants with SCID or with other severe T-cell defects. However, in approximately half the cases no specific host defect has been found. Recently, one possible explanation for this predilection was found in a 2.5-month-old Tunisian female infant who had fatal idiopathic disseminated BCG infection (30) and in four children from Malta who had disseminated atypical mycobacterial infection in the absence of a recognized immunodeficiency (31). In the case of all five children, there was consanguinity in their pedigrees. All affected were found to have a functional defect in the upregulation of TNF-α production by their blood macrophages in response to stimulation with interferon-γ (IFN-γ). Furthermore, they all lacked expression of IFN-γ receptors on their blood monocytes or lymphocytes, and each was found to have a mutation in the gene on chromosome 6q22-q23 that encodes IFN-γR1 (Table 1). Interestingly, these children did not appear to be susceptible to infection with agents other than mycobacteria. Th1 responses appeared to be normal in these patients. The susceptibility of these children to mycobacterial infections thus apparently results from an intrinsic impairment of the IFN-γ pathway response to these particular intracellular pathogens, showing that IFN-γ is obligatory for efficient macrophage antimycobacterial activity (30,31).

Mutant mice with disrupted IFN-γR had no overt abnormalities and their immune system appeared to develop normally (290). However, they had increased susceptibility to infections with *Listeria monocytogenes* or vaccinia virus despite normal cytotoxic and helper T-cell responses to these agents. They also failed to make a normal antigen-specific IgG₂a antibody response. Similarly, mice with a targeted disruption of the gene encoding IFN-γ died from a sublethal dose of *Mycobacterium bovis*. Splenocytes from these animals exhibited uncontrolled proliferation in response to mitogen and alloantigen stimulation *in vitro*, and increased cytotoxic T-cell responses after mixed lymphocyte culture, whereas resting NK cell activity was reduced (291). Thus, IFN-γ and its receptor appear to be essential for the function of or the negative regulation of several types of immune system cells.

Chediak-Higashi Syndrome

This rare disease is characterized by oculocutaneous albinism and susceptibility to recurrent respiratory tract and other types of infections (292). The hallmark of the disease is giant lysosomal granules, not only in neutrophils, but also in most of the other cells of the body, including melanocytes (293), neural Schwann cells, renal tubular cells, gastric mucosa, pneumatocytes, hepatocytes, Langerhans' cells of the skin, and adrenal cells (294). The granules in neutrophils are positive for peroxidase, acid phosphatase, and esterase. The abnormal lysosomes are unable to fuse with phagosomes, so that ingested bacteria cannot be lysed normally. In addition, there is nearly complete absence of cytotoxic T-lymphocyte and NK cell activity as a result of abnormal lysosomal granule function (295,296). Abnormal chemotaxis also has been reported, and there is evidence of a profound alteration of the cytoskeleton of the neutrophils. There are reports of a decreased number of centriole-associated microtubules and abnormalities in tubulin tyrosinolation.

The fundamental defect in this autosomal-recessive disorder was recently found to be caused by mutations in a gene on human chromosome 1 at position q42-43 (Table 1) (297,298). This gene is similar to the one mutated in the murine beige defect (299–301). The gene is postulated to function with other genes as components of a vesicle membrane-associated signal transduction complex that regulates intracellular protein trafficking (297). Approximately 85% of the patients develop an accelerated phase of the disease, with fever, jaundice, hepatosplenomegaly, lymphadenopathy, pancytopenia, bleeding diathesis, and neurologic changes (302). Once the accelerated phase occurs, the disease is usually fatal within 30

months unless successful treatment with an unfractionated HLA-identical bone marrow transplant after cytoreductive conditioning can be accomplished (123,303).

T-CELL ACTIVATION DEFECTS

These conditions are characterized by the presence of normal or elevated numbers of blood T cells that appear phenotypically normal but that fail to proliferate or produce cytokines in response to stimulation with mitogens, antigens, or other signals delivered to the T-cell antigen receptor (TCR) due to defective signal transduction from the TCR to intracellular metabolic pathways (Fig. 7) (304). These patients have problems similar to those of other T cell–deficient individuals, and some with severe T-cell activation defects may resemble SCID patients clinically (Figs. 8 and 9).

CD8 Lymphocytopenia Due to ZAP-70 Deficiency

Patients with this condition present during infancy with severe, recurrent, often fatal infections similar to those of SCID patients. Eight cases have been reported, and a majority were diagnosed in Mennonites (27,305,306). They have normal or elevated numbers of circulating CD3$^+$CD4$^+$ T-lymphocytes, but essentially no CD8$^+$ T cells. These T cells fail to respond to mitogens or to allogeneic cells *in vitro* or to generate cytotoxic T-lymphocytes. By contrast, NK

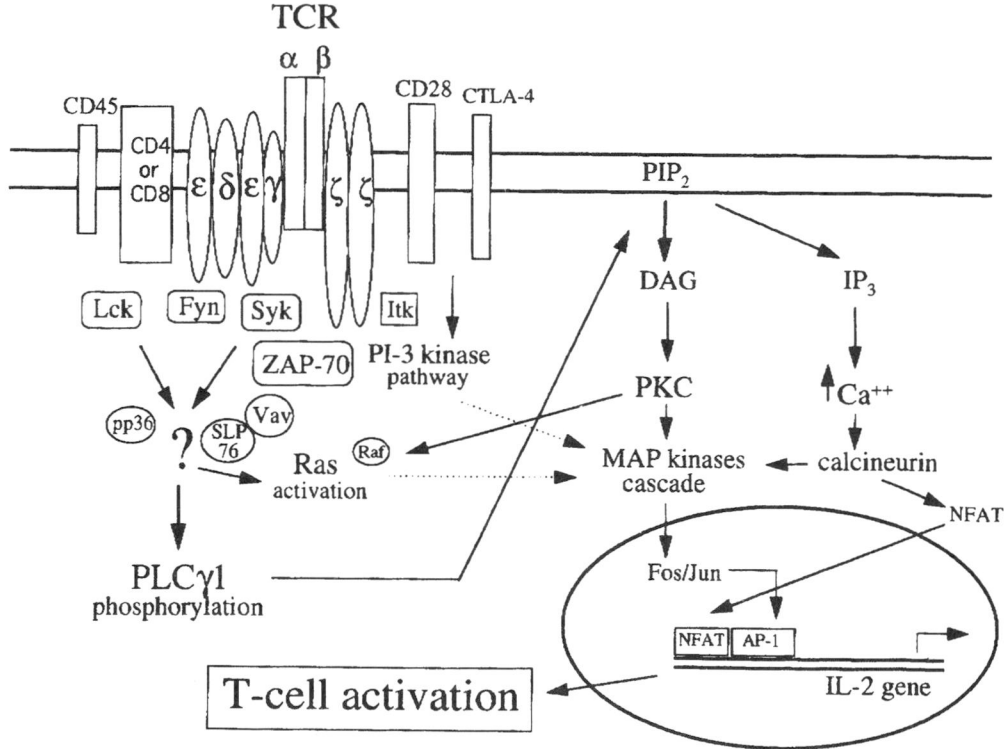

FIG. 7. T-cell signal transduction pathway. The TCR spans the plasma membrane in association with CD3 and ζ, CD4 or CD8, CD28 and CD45. Cytoplasmic protein tyrosine kinases (PTK) associated with the TCR are activated upon antigen binding to the TCR. These PTK include Lck, Fyn, ZAP-70, and Syk. PTK activation results in the phosphorylation of phospholipase Cγ1 and the activation of other signaling molecules. Distal signaling events, including PKC activation and Ca^{2+} mobilization, result in the transcription of genes encoding IL-2 and other proteins, culminating in T-cell activation, differentiation, and proliferation. Ionomycin and phorbol myristate acetate (PMA) can be used to mimic distal signaling events. Mutations in the gene encoding ZAP-70 result in markedly impaired T-cell activation, in addition to abnormal thymic selection resulting in CD8 deficiency. Modified with permission from Elder ME. *Pediatr Res* 1996;39:744, courtesy of Dr. Melissa Elder.

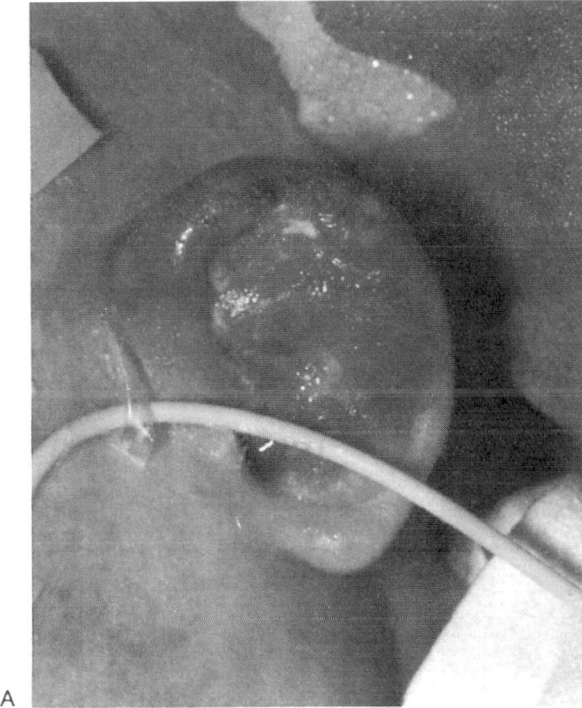
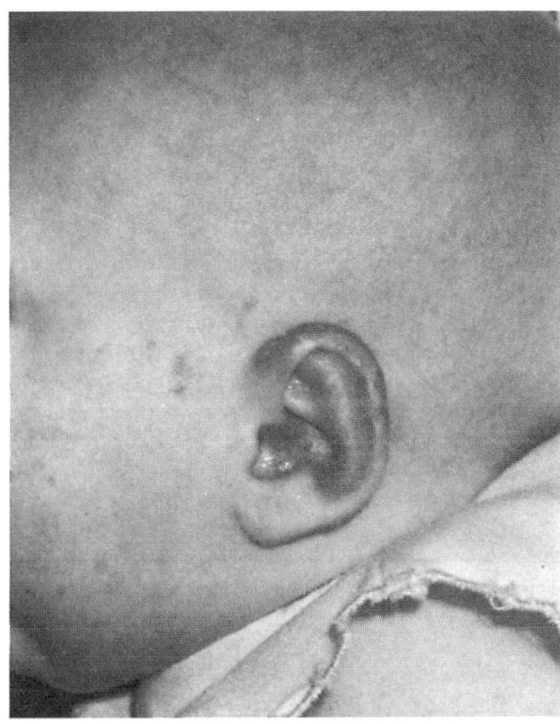

FIG. 8. **A:** Pyoderma gangrenosum in an infant with a T-cell activation defect of as yet unknown molecular cause resulting in failure to produce IL-2. **B:** After 2 weeks of therapy with recombinant IL-2.

activity is normal, and they have normal or elevated numbers of B cells and low to elevated serum immunoglobulin concentrations. The thymus of one patient exhibited normal architecture; there were normal numbers of double-positive (CD4+CD8+) thymocytes, but an absence of CD8 single-positive thymocytes. This condition has been shown to be due to mutations in the gene encoding ZAP-70, a non-src family protein tyrosine kinase important in T-cell signaling (Fig. 7) (27,305). The gene is on chromosome 2 at position q12 (Table 1). ZAP-70 has been shown to have an essential role in both positive and negative selection in the thymus (Fig. 7) (307). The hypothesis as to why there are normal numbers of CD4+ T cells is that thymocytes can use the other member of the same tyrosine kinase family, i.e., Syk, to facilitate positive selection of CD4+ cells. In addition, there is a stronger association of Lck with CD4+ than with CD8+ cells. Syk is present at fourfold higher levels in thymocytes than in peripheral T cells, possibly accounting for the lack of normal responses by the CD4+ blood T cells.

ZAP-70 knock-out mice differ from humans with ZAP-70 deficiency in that they have reduced numbers of both CD4+ and CD8+ T cells. This suggests that ZAP-70 plays an essential role in the development of CD4+ as well as CD8+ T cells in the mouse (307). Mutant mice that do not express the thymic isoform of p59fyn, another protein tyrosine kinase important in lymphocyte signaling, also have been generated by homologous recombination (308,309). The fyn− thymocytes showed limited clonal deletion to the Mls-1a self-superantigen but not to staphylococcal enterotoxin A, suggesting that some thymic selection does take place in these mice (308). Thymocytes of these mice are refractile to stimulation through the TCR by mitogen or antigen, whereas peripheral T and B cells reacquire some antigen-receptor signaling capabilities. These mice confirm the importance of p59fyn in TCR signal transduction. p59fyn does not appear to be involved in sIgM-coupled signaling events;

however, signaling of B cells through the IL-5 receptor, which ordinarily provides a comitogenic stimulus with antiimmunoglobulin, is completely blocked (310). Mutant mice lacking p56lck have pronounced thymic atrophy, a dramatic reduction in double positive (CD4+CD8+) thymocytes, no detectable single-positive thymocytes, and only a few peripheral T cells. Thus far, no human defects involving p59fyn or p56lck have been described (Fig. 7).

Defective Expression of the T-Cell Receptor–CD3 Complex

The first type of this disorder was found in two male siblings in a Spanish family (311). The proband presented with severe infections and died at 31 months of age with autoimmune hemolytic anemia and viral pneumonia. His lymphocytes had responded poorly to mitogens and to anti-CD3 in vitro and could not be stimulated to develop cytotoxic T cells. However, his antibody responses to protein antigens had been normal, indicating normal T-helper cell function. His 12-year-old brother is healthy but he has almost no CD3-bearing T cells and has IgG2 deficiency similar to his sibling. The defect in this family was shown to be due to mutations in the CD3 chain (Table 1) (311). The second phenotype of CD3 deficiency was found in a 4-year-old French boy who had recurrent Hemophilus influenzae pneumonia and otitis media in early life but is now healthy. He has a partial defect in expression of the TCR–CD3 (Ti–CD3) complex, resulting in an about half normal percentage of CD3+ cells, all with very low CD3 staining on flow cytometry. His T cells do not proliferate in response to anti-CD3 or anti-CD2, nor do they express the IL-2 receptor or have normal calcium influx after these treatments. However, they do respond normally to costimulation with anti-CD28 or antigens, such as tetanus toxoid (312). The defect

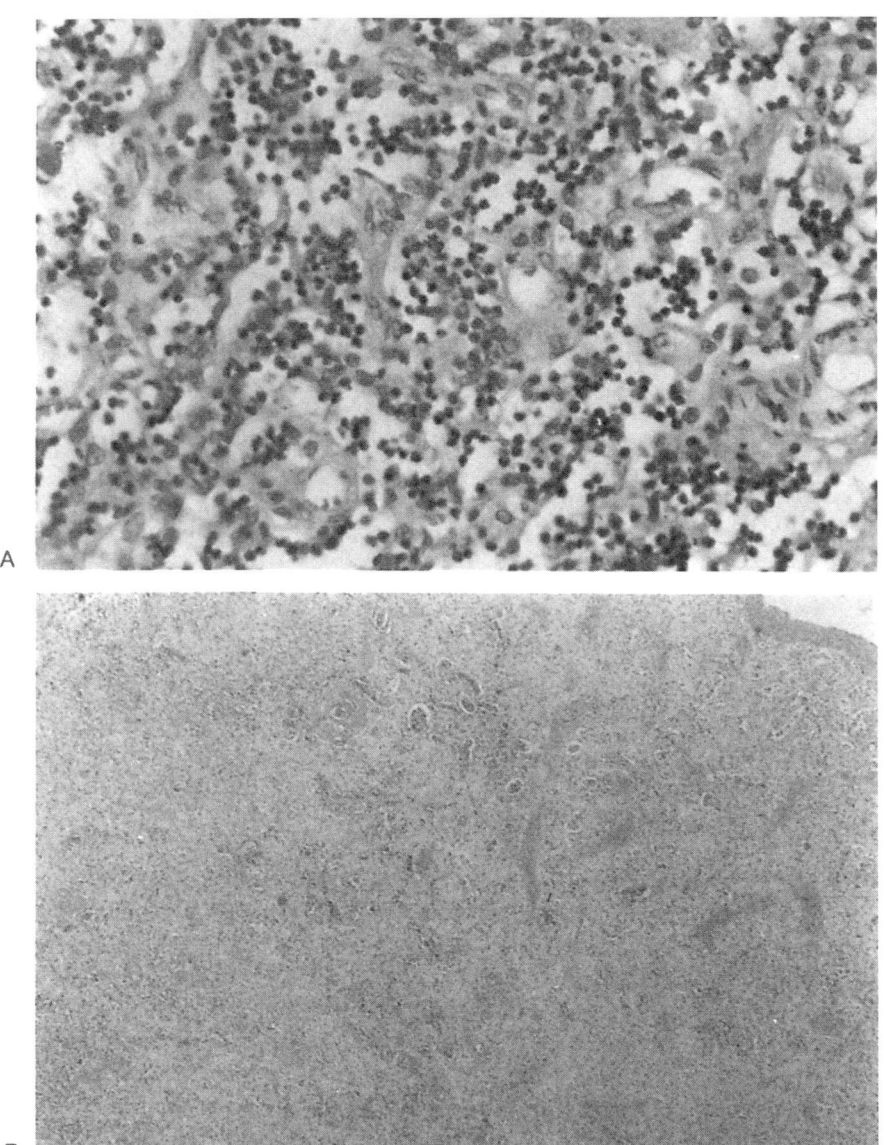

FIG. 9. Photomicrograph of thymus (**A**) and spleen (**B**) from the infant in Fig. 8 with persistent leukocytosis and lymphocytosis and recurrent bacterial infections. Thymocytes are abundant in thymus but lacking in spleen.

was shown to be due to two independent CD3ε gene mutations, leading to defective CD3ε chain synthesis and preventing normal association and membrane expression of the TCR–CD3 complex (Table 1) (313).

Thymocytes of mice with a targeted mutation of the CD3ε gene do not progress beyond the CD44$^-$/lowCD25$^+$ triple-negative stage and appear to be arrested at the same stage as RAG-deficient thymocytes (314). However, it is possible that these mice may have been deficient in other elements of the Ti–CD3 receptor complex. They do rearrange their TCR gene segments and produce low levels of full-length TCR transcripts but have few productive TCR gene rearrangements. The absence of intact CD3ε polypeptides had no effect on the completion of TCR γ or δ gene rearrangements (314). Gene-targeted mice deficient in the CD3ζ chain had few CD4$^+$CD8$^+$ thymocytes and impaired but not absent generation of CD4$^+$ and CD8$^+$ single-positive T cells. Peripheral T cells expressed small amounts of CD5 and few TCRs. From these mice, it was concluded that expression of the CD3 chain influences thymocyte differentiation but is not absolutely required for the generation of single-positive T cells (315).

Gene-targeted mice deficient in the pre-TCR α gene (316) or in the TCR α or β chain genes (317) demonstrate blockages of thymocyte development at different stages. TCR β gene–deficient mice were unable to differentiate CD4$^-$CD8$^-$ thymocytes into CD4$^+$CD8$^+$ thymocytes or expand the latter population normally. Similarly, mice deficient in the pre-TCR α gene evinced a severe inability to differentiate CD4$^-$CD8$^-$ thymocytes into CD4$^+$CD8$^+$ thymocytes and to develop αβ T cells (316). Mice homozygous for a disrupted TCR α gene could develop CD4$^-$CD8$^-$ thymocytes into CD4$^+$CD8$^+$ thymocytes but had a loss of the thymic medulla and failed to develop αβ$^+$ T cells (318). Nevertheless, whether the mice were deficient in the pre-TCR α gene or in the TCR α or β chain genes, they all developed γδ T cells normally.

Defective Cytokine Production

Two main types of defects in cytokine production are known. The first is a selective inability to produce IL-2. In the two reported cases, patients had severe recurrent infections in infancy (319,320). The IL-2 gene was present in both, but no IL-2 message or protein were produced. Other T-cell cytokines were produced normally. The second type was seen in a single patient who also presented during infancy with severe recurrent infections and failure to thrive (321). She had defective transcription of several lymphokine genes, including IL-2, IL-3, IL-4, and IL-5, possibly due to abnormal binding of *nuclear factor of activated T cells* (NF-AT) to response elements in IL-2 and IL-4 enhancer (321). She was treated with recombinant IL-2 with some clinical improvement. The molecular defects have not been identified in either type of cytokine deficiency. Recently, two male infants born to consanguinous parents had SCID-like infection susceptibility despite phenotypically normal blood lymphocytes. However, their T cells were unable to produce IL-2, IFN-γ, IL-4 and TNF-α. Electrophoretic mobility shift assays were used to examine the DNA binding of AP-1, Oct, CREB, SP1, NF-κB, and NF-AT, and the binding of all but NF-AT was normal. In the case of NF-AT, the binding of it to its IL-2 promoter response element was barely detectable before and after T-cell stimulation (322). The finding suggests that the NF-AT/DNA binding defect is responsible for the multiple cytokine deficiency in these two boys.

A number of mutant mice lacking genes encoding cytokines have been generated by homologous recombination (3). IL-2 knock-out mice have been generated (323). Such mice were reported to undergo normal thymic development and to have a normal distribution of lymphocyte subsets in spleen and lymph nodes until 3 to 4 weeks of age. Immunization of these mice with TNP-KLH resulted in the production of a high titer of IgG antibody to KLH and in the generation of T cells that proliferated when stimulated with TNP-KLH. However, there was a marked increase in the production of IgG1 and IgE, and T cells were predominantly of the Th2 type. T-cell proliferation was reduced but not completely abrogated; however, there was a selective deficiency of cytotoxic T-lymphocytes. Later the animals developed lymphadenopathy, splenomegaly, and alterations of splenic T-cell subsets, as well as immature B cells in the spleen. They also developed severe autoimmune disease, including hemolytic anemia and ulcerative colitis, caused by uncontrolled activation and proliferation of CD4+ T cells (324,325). From these observations, it was suggested that an essential role of IL-2 *in vivo* is the maintenance of self tolerance.

OMENN'S SYNDROME

This severe immunodeficiency is characterized by the development soon after birth of a generalized erythroderma and desquamation, failure to thrive, protracted diarrhea, hepatosplenomegaly, hypereosinophilia, and markedly elevated serum IgE levels (326). The condition has been seen in association with neonatal minimal change nephrotic syndrome (327). Paradoxically, there are increased circulating and tissue-infiltrating activated T-lymphocytes that do not respond normally to mitogens or antigens *in vitro;* these T cells are both oligoclonal and polyclonal (328–330). Circulating B cells are not found, and there is hypogammaglobulinemia except for IgE. Superficial lymph node architecture is highly abnormal due to a proliferation of interdigitating S-100 protein–positive nonphagocytic reticulum cells and a depletion of B-lymphocytes (331,332). Evidence has been presented to suggest that this is a Th2-mediated condition, but the fundamental problem has not yet been discovered (333–335). The condition is fatal in the first 5 months of life unless corrected by bone marrow transplantation after chemoablation (123).

HYPERIMMUNOGLOBULINEMIA E SYNDROME

The hyperimmunoglobulinemia E (hyper-IgE) syndrome is a relatively rare primary immunodeficiency syndrome characterized by recurrent severe staphylococcal abscesses of the skin, lungs, and viscera and markedly elevated levels of serum IgE (Fig. 8) (336,337). The disorder was first reported by the author and her co-workers in two young boys in 1972 (336); since then she has evaluated over 30 patients with the condition, and many other examples have been reported (337). These patients all have histories of staphylococcal abscesses involving the skin, lungs, joints, and other sites from infancy; persistent pneumatoceles develop as a result of their recurrent pneumonias (Fig. 9). The pruritic dermatitis that occurs is not typical atopic eczema, and it does not always persist; respiratory allergic symptoms are usually absent.

Laboratory features include exceptionally high serum IgE; elevated serum IgD; usually normal concentrations of IgG, IgA, and IgM; pronounced blood and sputum eosinophilia; abnormally low anamnestic antibody responses to booster immunizations; and poor antibody-mediated and cell-mediated responses to neoantigens. *In vitro* studies have shown normal percentages of CD2+, CD3+, CD4+, and CD8+ lymphocytes, and there is no increase in the percentage of IgE-bearing B-lymphocytes. Most have normal lymphocyte proliferative responses to mitogens but very low or absent responses to antigens or allogeneic cells from family members. Blood, sputum, and histologic sections of lymph nodes, spleen, and lung cysts show striking eosinophilia. Hassall's corpuscles and normal thymic architecture were observed at postmortem examination of one patient.

Phagocytic cell ingestion, metabolism, killing, and total hemolytic complement activity have been normal in all patients. Variable defects of mononuclear or polymorphonuclear chemotaxis have been present in some but not all patients and hence are not the basic problem in these patients (337).

The fundamental problem in this condition is unknown despite intense study. Possibly related to these patients' impaired anamnestic antibody responses, impaired antigen-specific T-cell responses and abnormal mixed leukocyte response is the observation by the author of a decreased percentage of T cells with the memory (CD45RO) phenotype in the blood of these patients. Paradoxically, B cells from these patients do not produce as much IgE as do normal or atopic B cells when they are cultured with IL-4 and anti-CD40 *in vitro* (338). The latter suggests that the B cells had already been exposed to IL-4 *in vivo* and were no longer sensitive to it because they had already isotype-switched *in vivo*. Due to the very short half-life of IL-4, serum levels cannot be detected; therefore, it has been difficult to prove that the condition is caused by excessive IL-4 production. The presence of increased numbers of eosinophils in blood, sputum, and tissues suggests that some of the pathology seen may be eosinophil mediated. The fact that both men and women have been affected, as have members of succeeding generations, suggests an autosomal-dominant form of inheritance with incomplete penetrance.

The most effective management for this condition consists of long-term therapy with a penicillinase-resistant penicillin or cephalosporin, with the addition of other antibiotics or antifungal agents as required for specific infections, and appropriate thoracic surgery for superinfected pneumatoceles or those persisting beyond 6 months. IFN-γ therapy has been tried but had no clinical benefit (339). If the diagnosis is made early and antistaphylococcal antibiotic therapy is rendered in treatment doses continuously, the prognosis is good. The prognosis is poor, primarily because of progressive lung disease, in those who are not so treated. Three patients are known to have died of lymphoreticular malignancy, and three have experienced cryptococcal meningitis.

Stat4 Knock-Out Mice

Of potential relevance to the fundamental problem in patients with the hyper-IgE syndrome are mice that were made deficient in the signal-transducer and activator of transcription protein number 4 (Stat4) by gene targeting. This protein is tyrosine phosphorylated only after stimulation of T cells with IL-12. Stat4-deficient mice were found to have a disruption of all IL-12 funtions, including the induction of IFN-γ, mitogenesis, enhancement of NK cytolytic function, and Th1 differentiation. As a consequence, they have a Th2 dominance due to their failure to produce in response to IL-12 (340,341). Stat4 deficiency could thus be one potential fundamental cause for human diseases characterized by a Th2 dominance, such as the hyper-IgE syndrome. Alternately, some other component of the signaling pathway for IL-12 could be at fault.

CONCLUSIONS

Since the discovery of X-linked agammaglobulinemia four and a half decades ago, a panoply of genetically determined immunodeficiencies has been identified, and the list is rapidly growing. Recent research has led to major breakthroughs in the definition of the molecular bases of a large number of these disorders and, undoubtedly, this will soon be the case for many others. This information will obviously be of great value in clarifying variant forms of these diseases, in carrier detection, in prenatal diagnosis, and, hopefully, eventually in permitting gene therapy for many of these conditions (196).

In addition to the knowledge gained about the immune system from studying the clinical and immunologic features of these rare patients, even greater information about the functioning of the immune system should come from the integrated and comparative study of immune abnormalities in patients and those in gene-targeted mutant mice. In addition, these studies should lead to the design of more specific and effective therapies, even if gene therapy does not become possible.

Although treatment of these rare defects has not advanced as rapidly as the discovery of new primary immunodeficiency diseases and the fundamental causes of a large number of them, major therapeutic advances have been made over the past 16 years. These include (a) the development of safe intravenous forms of human immunoglobulin that make it possible to deliver high quantities of missing antibodies to antibody-deficient patients and (b) the development of T-cell depletion techniques that permit the use of half-matched parents as donors of corrective stem cells for human infants with SCID. Moreover, the chimeras created by the latter technique are making possible the study of early human T- and B-cell ontogeny, tolerance induction, and MHC restriction mechanisms (i.e., thymic education) in a manner heretofore not possible. In the next few years these enormously informative patients, as well as the artificially created immunodeficient animals, will undoubtedly provide many more insights into the normal workings of the immune system.

REFERENCES

1. Bruton OC. Agammaglobulinemia. *Pediatrics* 1952;9:722–728.
2. WHO Scientific Group. Primary immunodeficiency diseases: report of a WHO scientific group. *Clin Exp Immunol* 1997;99:1–124.
3. Kokron CM, Bonilla FA, Oettgen HC, Ramesh N, Geha RS, Pandolfi F. Searching for genes involved in the pathogenesis of primary immunodeficiency diseases: lessons from mouse knockouts. *J Clin Immunol* 1997;17:109–126.
4. Filipovich AH, Mathur A, Kamat D, Shapiro RS. Primary immunodeficiencies: genetic risk factors for lymphoma. *Cancer Res* 1992;52:5465s–5467s.
5. Elenitoba-Johnson KSJ, Jaffe ES. Lymphoproliferative disorders associated with congenital immunodeficiencies. *Semin Diagn Pathol* 1997;14:35–47.
6. Clark JA, Callicoat PA, Brenner NA. Selective IgA deficiency in blood donors. *Am J Clin Pathol* 1983;80:210–213.
7. Buckley RH. Clinical and immunologic features of selective IgA deficiency. In: Bergsma D, Good RA, Finstad J, Paul NW, eds. *Immunodeficiency in man and animals.* Stamford, CT: Sinauer Associates, 1975:134–142.
8. Puck JM. Molecular and genetic basis of X-linked immunodeficiency disorders. *J Clin Immunol* 1994;14:81–89.
9. Derry JMJ, Ochs HD, Francke U. Isolation of a novel gene mutated in Wiskott-Aldrich syndrome. *Cell* 1994;78:635–644.
10. Rosen FS, Cooper MD, Wedgwood RJ. The primary immunodeficiencies. *N Engl J Med* 1995;333:431–440.
11. Buckley RH. Breakthroughs in the understanding and therapy of primary immunodeficiency. *Pediatr Clin North Am* 1994;41:665–690.
12. Fischer A, Arnaiz-Villena A. Immunodeficiencies of genetic origin. *Immunol Today* 1995;16:510–514.
13. Dinauer MC, Orkin SH, Brown R. The glycoprotein encoded by the X-linked chronic granulomatous disease locus is a component of the neutrophil cytochrome b complex. *Nature* 1987;327:717
14. Westberg J, Fredrikson GN, Truedsson L, Sjoholm AG, Uhlen M. Sequence-based analysis of properdin deficiency: identification of point mutations in two phenotypic forms of an X-linked immunodeficiency. *Genomics* 1995;29:1–8.
15. Sullivan JL, Woda BA. X-linked lymphoproliferative syndrome. *Immunodef Rev* 1989;1:325–347.
16. Schuster V, Seidenspinner S, Grimm T, et al. Molecular genetic haplotype segregation studies in three families with X-linked lymphoproliferative disease. *Eur J Pediatr* 1994;153:432–437.
17. Fischer A, Lisowska-Grospierre B, Anderson DC, Springer TA. Leukocyte adhesion deficiency: molecular basis and functional consequences. *Immunodef Rev* 1988;1:39–54.
18. Etzioni A. Adhesion molecule deficiencies and their clinical significance. *Cell Adhesion Commun* 1994;2:257–260.
19. Hirschhorn R. Adenosine deaminase deficiency. *Immunol Rev* 1991;3:45–81.
20. Markert ML. Purine nucleoside phosphorylase deficiency. *Immunodef Rev* 1991; 3:45–81.
21. Savitsky K, Bar-Shira A, Gilad S, et al. A single ataxia telangiectasia gene with a product similar to PI-3 kinase. *Science* 1995;268:1749–1753.
22. Budarf ML, Collins J, Gong W, et al. Cloning a balanced translocation associated with DiGeorge syndrome and identification of a disrupted candidate gene. *Nature Genet* 1995;10:269–278.
23. Daw SC, Taylor C, Kraman M, et al. A common region of 10p deleted in DiGeorge and velocardiofacial syndromes. *Nature Genet* 1996;13:458–460.
24. Gong W, Emanuel BS, Collins J, Kim DH, Wang Z. A transcription map of the DiGeorge and velo-cardio-facial syndrome minimal critical region on 22q11. *Hum Mol Genet* 1996;5:789–800.
25. de la Salle H, Hanau D, Fricker D. Homozygous human TAP peptide transporter mutation in HLA class I deficiency. *Science* 1994;265:237–241.
26. Steimle V, Reith W, Mach B. Major histocompatibility complex class II deficiency: a disease of gene regulation. *Adv Immunol* 1996;61:327–340.
27. Elder ME, Lin D, Clever J, et al. Human severe combined immunodeficiency due to a defect in ZAP-70, a T cell tyrosine kinase. *Science* 1994;264:1596–1599.
28. Sharfe N, Dadi HK, Shahar M, Roifman CM. Human immune disorder arising from mutation of the alpha chain of the interleukin-2 receptor. *Proc Natl Acad Sci U S A* 1997;94:3168–3171.
29. Russell SM, Tayebi N, Nakajima H, et al. Mutation of Jak3 in a patient with SCID: essential role of Jak3 in lymphoid development. *Science* 1995;270: 797–799.
30. Jouanguy E, Altare F, Lamhamedi S, et al. Interferon-gamma-receptor deficiency in an infant with fatal bacille Calmette-Guerin infection. *N Engl J Med* 1996;335:1956–1961.
31. Newport MJ, Huxley CM, Huston S, et al. A mutation in the interferon-gamma-receptor gene and susceptibility to mycobacterial infection. *N Engl J Med* 1996; 335:1941–1949.
32. Timmers E, DeWeers M, Alt FW, Kendriks RW, Schuurman RKB. X-linked agammaglobulinemia. *Clin Immunol Immunopathol* 1991;61(suppl):83–93.
33. Kozlowski C, Evans DIK. Neutropenia associated with X-linked agammaglobulinaemia. *J Clin Pathol* 1991;44:388–390.
34. Wilfert CM, Buckley RH, Mohanakumar T, et al. Persistent and fatal central nervous system Echovirus infections in patients with agammaglobulinemia. *N Engl J Med* 1977;296:1485–1489.
35. McKinney RE, Katz SL, Wilfert CM. Chronic enteroviral meningoencephalitis in agammaglobulinemic patients. *Rev Infect Dis* 1987;9:334–356.

36. Lederman HM, Winkelstein JA. X-linked agammaglobulinemia: an analysis of 96 patients. *Medicine* 1985;64:145–156.

37. Roberts D, Murray AE, Pratt BC, Meigh RE. Mycoplasma hominis as a respiratory pathogen in X-linked hypogammaglobulinemia. *J Infect* 1989;18:175–177.

38. Mohiuddin AA, Corren J, Harbeck RJ, Teague JL, Volz M, Gelfand EW. Ureaplasma urealyticum chronic osteomyelitis in a patient with hypogammaglobulinemia. *J Allergy Clin Immunol* 1991;87:104–107.

39. Vetrie D, Vorechovsky I, Sideras P, et al. The gene involved in X-linked agammaglobulinaemia is a member of the src family of protein-tyrosine kinases. *Nature* 1993;361:226–233.

40. Tsukada S, Saffran DC, Rawlings DJ, et al. Deficient expression of a B cell cytoplasmic tyrosine kinase in human X-linked agammaglobulinemia. *Cell* 1993;72:279–290.

41. Haire RN, Ohta Y, Strong SJ, et al. Unusual patterns of exon skipping in Bruton tyrosine kinase are associated with mutations involving the intron 17 3′ splice site. *Am J Hum Genet* 1997;60:798–807.

42. de Weers M, Verschuren MCM, Kraakman MEM, et al. The Bruton's tyrosine kinase gene is expressed throughout B cell differentiation, from early precursor B cell stages preceding immunoglobulin gene rearrangement up to mature B cell stages. *Eur J Immunol* 1993;23:3109–3114.

43. Hashimoto S, Tsukada S, Matsushita M, et al. Identification of Bruton's tyrosine kinase (Btk) gene mutations and characterization of the derived proteins in 35 X-linked agammaglobulinemia families: a nationwide study of Btk deficiency in Japan. *Blood* 1996;88:561–573.

44. Vihinen M, Iwata T, Kinnon C, et al. BTKbase, mutation database for X-linked agammaglobulinemia (XLA). *Nucleic Acids Res* 1996;24:160–165.

45. Vihinen M. BTKbase: XLA mutation registry. *Immunol Today* 1996;17:502–506.

46. Vorechovsky I, Vihinen M, de Saint Basile G, et al. DNA-based mutation analysis of Bruton's tyrosine kinase gene in patients with X-linked agammaglobulinaemia. *Hum Mol Genet* 1995;4:51–58.

47. Sideras P, Smith CIE. Molecular and cellular aspects of X-linked agammaglobulinemia. *Adv Immunol* 1995;59:135–223.

48. Bykowsky MJ, Haire RN, Ohta Y, et al. Discordant phenotype in siblings with X-linked agammaglobulinemia. *Am J Hum Genet* 1996;58:477–483.

49. Jones A, Bradley L, Alterman L, et al. X linked agammaglobulinaemia with a "leaky" phenotype. *Arch Dis Child* 1996;74:548–549.

50. Satterthwaite AB, Witte ON. Lessons from human genetic variants in the study of B cell differentiation. *Curr Opin Immunol* 1996;8:454–458.

51. Buckley RH, Rowlands DR. Allergy rounds: agammaglobulinemia, neutropenia, fever and abdominal pain. *J Allergy Clin Immunol* 1973;51:308–318.

52. Farrar JE, Rohrer J, Conley ME. Neutropenia in X-linked agammaglobulinemia. *Clin Immunol Immunopathol* 1996;81:271–276.

53. Conley ME, Burks AW, Herrod HG, Puck JM. Molecular analysis of X-linked agammaglobulinemia with growth hormone deficiency. *J Pediatr* 1991;119:392–397.

54. Fleisher TA, White RM, Broder S, et al. X-linked hypogammaglobulinemia and isolated growth hormone deficiency. *N Engl J Med* 1980;302:1429–1434.

55. Sitz KV, Burks AW, Williams LW, Kemp SF, Steele RW. Confirmation of X-linked hypogammaglobulinemia with isolated growth hormone deficiency as a disease entity. *J Pediatr* 1990;116:292–294.

56. Monafo V, Maghnie M, Terracciano L, Valtorta A, Massa M, Severi F. X-linked agammaglobulinemia and isolated growth hormone deficiency. *Acta Paediatr Scand* 1991;80:563–566.

57. Conley ME, Sweinberg SK. Females with a disorder phenotypically identical to X-linked agammaglobulinemia. *J Clin Immunol* 1992;12:139–143.

58. Meffre E, LeDeist F, de Saint Basile G, et al. A human non-XLA immunodeficiency disease characterized by blockage of B cell development at an early proB cell stage. *J Clin Invest* 1996;98:1519–1526.

59. Yel L, Minegishi Y, Coustan-Smith E, et al. Mutations in the mu heavy chain gene in patients with agammaglobulinemia. *N Engl J Med* 1996;335:1486–1493.

60. Scher I. The CBA/N mouse strain: an experimental model illustrating the influence of X-chromosome on immunity. *Adv Immunol* 1982;33:1

61. Hasbold J, Klaus GG. B cells from CBA/N mice do not proliferate following ligation of CD40. *Eur J Immunol* 1997;24:152–157.

62. Thomas JD, Sideras P, Smith CIE, Vorechovsky I, Chapman V, Paul WE. Colocalization of X-linked agammaglobulinemia and X-linked immunodeficiency genes. *Science* 1993;261:355–361.

63. Rawlings DJ, Saffran DC, Tsudaka S, et al. Mutation of unique region of Bruton's tyrosine kinase in immunodeficient XID mice. *Science* 1993;261:358

64. de Weers M, Mensink RGJ, Kraakman MEM, Schuurman RKB, Hendriks RW. Mutation analysis of the Bruton's tyrosine kinase gene in X-linked agammaglobulinemia: identification of a mutation which affects the same codon as is altered in immunodeficient xid mice. *Hum Mol Genet* 1994;3:161–166.

65. Notarangelo LD, Duse M, Ugazio AG. Immunodeficiency with hyper-IgM (HIM). *Immunodef Rev* 1992;3:101–121.

66. Facchetti F, Appiani C, Salvi L, Levy J, Notarangelo LD. Immunohistologic analysis of ineffective CD40-CD40 ligand interaction in lymphoid tissues from patients with X-linked immunodeficiency with hyper IgM. *J Immunol* 1995;154:6624–6633.

67. Mayer L, Swan SP, Thompson C. Evidence for a defect in "switch" T cells in patients with immunodeficiency and hyperimmunoglobulinemia M. *N Engl J Med* 1986;314:409–413.

68. Padayachee M, Feighery C, Finn A, et al. Mapping of the X-linked form of hyper IgM syndrome (HIGM1) to Xq26 by close linkage to HPRT. *Genomics* 1992;14:551–553.

69. Allen RC, Armitage RJ, Conley ME, et al. CD40 ligand gene defects responsible for X-linked hyper IgM syndrome. *Science* 1993;259:990–993.

70. Di Santo JP, Bonnefoy JY, Gauchat JF, Fischer A, de Saint Basile G. CD40 ligand mutations in X-linked immunodeficiency with hyper IgM. *Nature* 1993;361:541–543.

71. Aruffo A, Farrington M, Hollenbaugh D. The CD40 ligand, gp39, is defective in activated T cells from patients with X-linked hyper IgM syndrome. *Cell* 1993;72:291–300.

72. Korthauer U, Graf D, Mages HW. Defective expression of T cell CD40 ligand causes X-linked immunodeficiency with hyper IgM. *Nature* 1993;361:539–541.

73. Noelle RJ, Roy M, Shepherd DM, Stamenkovic I, Ledbetter JA, Aruffo A. A 39-kDa protein on activated helper T cells binds CD40 and transduces the signal for cognate activation of B cells. *Proc Natl Acad Sci U S A* 1992;89:6550–6554.

74. Yang Y, Wilson JM. CD40 ligand-dependent T cell activation: requirement of B7-CD28 signaling through CD40. *Science* 1996;273:1862–1864.

75. Notarangelo LD, Peitsch MC. CD40Lbase: a database of CD40L gene mutations causing X-linked hyper-IgM syndrome. *Immunol Today* 1996;17:511–517.

76. Katz F, Hinshelwood S, Rutland P, Jones A, Kinnon C, Morgan G. Mutation analysis in CD40 ligand deficiency leading to X-linked hypogammaglobulinemia with hyper IgM syndrome. *Hum Mutation* 1996;8:223–228.

77. Disanto JP, Markiewicz S, Gauchat J, Bonnefoy J, Fischer A, de Saint Basile G. Brief report: prenatal diagnosis of X-linked hyper IgM syndrome. *N Engl J Med* 1994;330:969–973.

78. Grewal IS, Xu J, Flavell RA. Impairment of antigen-specific T-cell priming in mice lacking CD40 ligand. *Nature* 1995;378:617–620.

79. Conley ME, Larche M, Bonagura VR, et al. Hyper IgM syndrome associated with defective CD40-mediated B cell activation. *J Clin Invest* 1994;94:1404–1409.

80. Oliva A, Quinti I, Scala E, et al. Immunodeficiency with hyperimmunoglobulinemia M in two female patients is not associated with abnormalities of CD40 or CD40 ligand expression. *J Allergy Clin Immunol* 1995;96:403–410.

81. Cunningham-Rundles C. Clinical and immunologic analyses of 103 patients with common variable immunodeficiency. *J Clin Immunol* 1989;9:22–33.

82. Cunningham-Rundles C, Siegal FP, Cunningham-Rundles S, Lieberman P. Incidence of cancer in 98 patients with common varied immunodeficiency. *J Clin Immunol* 1987;7:294–298.

83. Zhang JG, Morgan L, Spickett GP. L-selectin in patients with common variable immunodeficiency (CVID): a comparative study with normal individuals. *Clin Exp Immunol* 1996;104:275–279.

84. Kaneko H, Katagiri-Kawade M, Motoyoshi F, Tashita H, Teramoto T, Kondo N. Abnormal B cell response of protein kinase C in some common variable immunodeficiency. *Exp Clin Immunogenet* 1996;13:36–42.

85. Nonoyama S, Farrington M, Ochs HM. Activated B cells from patients with common variable immunodeficiency proliferate and synthesize immunoglobulin. *J Clin Invest* 1993;92:1281–1287.

86. Punnonen J, Kainulainen L, Ruuskanen O, Nikoskelainen J, Arvilommi H. IL-4 synergizes with IL-10 and anti-CD40 MoAbs to induce B cell differentiation in patients with common variable immunodeficiency. *Scand J Immunol* 1997;45:203–212.

87. Katial RK, Lieberman MM, Muehlbauer SL, Lust JA, Hamilos DL. δ T lymphocytosis associated with common variable immunodeficiency. *J Clin Immunol* 1997;17:34–42.

88. Spickett GP, Webster ADB, Farrant J. Cellular abnormalities in common variable immunodeficiency. *Immunodef Rev* 1990;2:199–219.

89. Pandolfi F, Trentin L, San Martin JE, Wong JT, Kurnick JT, Moscicki RA. T cell heterogeneity in patients with common variable immunodeficiency as assessed by abnormal T cell subpopulations and T cell receptor gene analysis. *Clin Exp Immunol* 1989;89:198–203.

90. Jaffe JS, Strober W, Sneller MC. Functional abnormalities of CD8⁻ T cells define a unique subset of patients with common variable immunodeficiency. *Blood* 1993;82:192–201.

91. Funauchi M, Farrant J, Moreno C, Webster ADB. Defects in antigen-driven lymphocyte responses in common variable immunodeficiency (CVID) are due to a reduction in the number of antigen-specific CD4⁺ T cells. *Clin Exp Immunol* 1995;101:82–88.

92. Fischer MB, Wolf HM, Hauber I, et al. Activation via the antigen receptor is impaired in T cells, but not in B cells from patients with common variable immunodeficiency. *Eur J Immunol* 1996;26:231–237.

93. Eisenstein EM, Jaffe JS, Strober W. Reduced interleukin-2 (IL-2) production in common variable immunodeficiency is due to a primary abnormality of CD4⁺ T cell differentiation. *J Clin Immunol* 1993,13.247–258.

94. Kondratenko I, Amlot PL, Webster ADB, Farrant J. Lack of specific antibody response in common variable immunodeficiency (CVID) associated with failure in production of antigen-specific memory T cells. *Clin Exp Immunol* 1997;108:9–13.

95. Farrington M, Grosmaire LS, Nonoyama S, et al. CD40 ligand expression is defective in a subset of patients with common variable immunodeficiency. *Proc Natl Acad Sci U S A* 1994;91:1099–1103.

96. Baum CG, Chiorazzi N, Frankel S, Shepherd GM. Conversion of systemic lupus erythematosus to common variable hypogammaglobulinemia. *Am J Med* 1989;87:449–456.

97. Wright JJ, Birx DL, Wagner DK, Waldmann TA, Blaese RM, Fleisher TA. Normalization of antibody responsiveness in a patient with common variable hypogammaglobulinemia and HIV infection. *N Engl J Med* 1987;317:1516–1519.

98. Slyper AH, Pietryga D. Conversion of selective IgA deficiency to common variable immunodeficiency in an adolescent female with 18q deletion syndrome. *Eur J Pediatr* 1997;155:155–159.

99. Ashman RF, Schaffer FM, Kemp JD, et al. Genetic and immunologic analysis of a family containing five patients with common variable immune deficiency or selective IgA deficiency. *J Clin Immunol* 1992;12:406–414.

100. Truedsson L, Baskin B, Pan Q, et al. Genetics of IgA deficiency. *APMIS* 1995;103:833–842.

101. French MA, Dawkins RL. Central MHC genes, IgA deficiency and autoimmune diseases. *Immunol Today* 1990;11:271–274.

102. Schaffer FM, Monteiro RC, Volanakis JE, Cooper MD. IgA deficiency. *Immunodef Rev* 1991;3:15–44.

103. Howe HS, So AKL, Farrant J, Webster ADB. Common variable immunodeficiency is associated with polymorphic markers in the human major histocompatibility complex. *Clin Exp Immunol* 1991;84:387–390.

104. Volanakis JE, Zhu Z, Schaffer FM, et al. Major histocompatibility complex class III genes and susceptibility to immunoglobulin A deficiency and common variable immunodeficiency. *J Clin Invest* 1992;89:1914–1922.

105. Fiore M, Pera C, Delfino L, Scotese I, Ferrara GB, Pignata C. DNA typing of DQ and DR alleles in IgA deficient subjects. *Eur J Immunogenet* 1995;22:403–411.

106. Oxelius VA, Laurell AB, Lindquist B. IgG subclasses in selective IgA deficiency. *N Engl J Med* 1981;304:1476–1477.

107. Cunningham-Rundles C, Fotino M, Rosina O, Peter JB. Selective IgA deficiency, IgG subclass deficiency, and the major histocompatibility complex. *Clin Immunol Immunopathol* 1991;61(suppl):61–69.

108. Burks AW, Sampson HA, Buckley RH. Anaphylactic reactions after gamma globulin administration in patients with hypogammaglobulinemia. *N Engl J Med* 1986;314:560–564.

109. Buckley RH, Dees SC. The correlation of milk precipitins with IgA deficiency. *N Engl J Med* 1969;281:465–469.

110. Goshen E, Livne A, Krupp M, et al. Antinuclear and related autoantibodies in sera of healthy subjects with IgA deficiency. *J Autoimmun* 1989;2:51–60.

111. Briere F, Bridon JM, Chevet D, et al. Interleukin 10 induces B lymphocytes from IgA-deficient patients to secrete IgA. *J Clin Invest* 1994;94:97–104.

112. Friman V, Hanson LA, Bridon JM, Tarkowski A, Banchereau J, Briere F. IL-10–driven immunoglobulin production by B lymphocytes from IgA-deficient individuals correlates to infection proneness. *Clin Exp Immunol* 1996;104:432–438.

113. Leickly FE, Buckley RH. Development of IgA and IgG2 subclass deficiency after sulfasalazine therapy. *J Pediatr* 1986;108:481–482.

114. Plebani A, Monafo V, Ugazio AG, Burgio GR. Clinical heterogeneity and reversibility of selective immunoglobulin A deficiency in 80 children. *Lancet* 1986;1:829–831.

115. DeLaat PCJ, Weemaes CMR, Bakkeren JAJM. Immunoglobulin levels during follow-up of children with selective IgA deficiency. *Scand J Immunol* 1992;35:719–725.

116. Preud'Homme JL, Hanson LA. IgG subclass deficiency. *Immunodef Rev* 1990;2:129–149.

117. Shield JPH, Strobel S, Levinsky RJ, Morgan G. Immunodeficiency presenting as hypergammaglobulinaemia with IgG2 subclass deficiency. *Lancet* 1992;340:448–450.

118. Ambrosino DM, Umetsu DT, Siber GR, et al. Selective defect in the antibody response to *Haemophilus influenzae* type b in children with recurrent infections and normal IgG subclass levels. *J Allergy Clin Immunol* 1988;81:1175–1179.

119. Shackelford PG. IgG subclasses: importance in pediatric practice. *Pediatr Rev* 1993;14:291–296.

120. Shackelford PG, Granoff DM, Polmar SH, et al. Subnormal serum concentrations of IgG2 in children with frequent infections associated with varied patters of immunologic dysfunction. *J Pediatr* 1990;116:529–538.

121. Lefranc MP, Hammarstrom L, Smith CIE, Lefranc G. Gene deletions in the human immunoglobulin heavy chain constant region locus: molecular and immunological analysis. *Immunol Rev* 1991;2:265–281.

122. Grierson HL, Skare J, Hawk J, Pauza M, Purtilo DT. Immunoglobulin class and subclass deficiencies prior to Epstein-Barr virus infection in males with X-linked lymphoproliferative disease. *Am J Med Genet* 1991;40:294–297.

123. Buckley RH. Bone marrow transplantation in primary immunodeficiency. In: Rich RR, ed. *Clinical immunology: principles and practice.* St. Louis: CV Mosby, 1995:1813–1830.

124. Hong R. The DiGeorge anomaly. *Immunodef Rev* 1991;3:1–14.

125. Prasad C, Quackenbush EJ, Whiteman D, Korf B. Limb anomalies in DiGeorge and CHARGE syndromes. *Am J Med Genet* 1997;68:179–181.

126. Junker AK, Driscoll DA. Humoral immunity in DiGeorge syndrome. *J Pediatr* 1995;127:231–237.

127. Muller W, Peter HH, Kallfelz HC, Franz A, Rieger CH. The DiGeorge sequence. II. Immunologic findings in partial and complete forms of the disorder. *Eur J Pediatr* 1989;149:96–103.

128. Driscoll DA, Budarf ML, Emanuel BS. A genetic etiology for DiGeorge syndrome: consistent deletions and microdeletions of 22q11. *Am J Hum Genet* 1992;50:924–933.

129. Webber SA, Hatchwell E, Barber JCK, et al. Importance of microdeletions of

130. Bonnet D, Cormier-Daire V, Kachaner J, et al. Microsatellite DNA markers detects 95% of chromosome 22q11 deletions. *Am J Med Genet* 1997;68:182–184.

131. Kkurahashi H, Akagi K, Inazawa J, et al. Isolation and characterization of a novel gene deleted in DiGeorge syndrome. *Hum Mol Genet* 1995;4:541–549.

132. Llevadot R, Scambler P, Estivill X, Pritchard M. Genomic organization of TUPLE1/HIRA: a gene implicated in DiGeorge syndrome. *Mammalian Genome* 1996;7:911–914.

133. Demczuk S, Levy A, Aubry M, Croquette M, et al. Excess of deletions of maternal origin in the DiGeorge/velo-cardio-facial syndromes. A study of 22 new patients and review of the literature. *Hum Genet* 1995;96:9–13.

134. Goldmuntz E, Emanuel BS. Genetic disorders of cardiac morphogenesis—the DiGeorge and velocardiofacial syndromes. *Circ Res* 1997;80:437–443.

135. Pierpont JW, Erickson RP, Thompson FH, Yang JM. Size of 22q deletions in four previously reported patients with conotruncal anomaly face syndrome. *Clin Genet* 1996;50:545–547.

136. Wilson DI, Burn J, Scambler P, Goodship J. Syndrome of the month. DiGeorge syndrome: part of CATCH 22. *J Med Genet* 1993;30:852–856.

137. Schuffenhauer S, Seidel H, Oechsler H, et al. DiGeorge syndrome and partial monosomy 10p: case report and review. *Ann Genet* 1995;38:162–167.

138. Lipson A, Fagan K, Colley A, Colley P, Sholler G, Issacs D. Velo-cardio-facial and partial DiGeorge phenotype in a child with interstitial deletion at 10p13—implications for cytogenetics and molecular biology. *Am J Med Genet* 1996;65:304–306.

139. Cleveland WW, Fogel BJ, Brown WR, Kay HEM. Fetal thymus transplant in a case of DiGeorge's syndrome. *Lancet* 1968;2:1211–1214.

140. Davis CM, McLaughlin TM, Watson TJ, et al. Normalization of the peripheral blood T cell receptor V repertoire after cultured postnatal human thymic transplantation in DiGeorge syndrome. *J Clin Immunol* 1997;17:167–175.

141. Goldsobel AB, Haas A, Stiehm ER. Bone marrow transplantation in DiGeorge syndrome. *J Pediatr* 1987;111:40–44.

142. Wortis HH. Immunological responses of "nude" mice. *Clin Exp Immunol* 1971;8:305.

143. Festing MFW, May D, Connors TA, Lovell D, Sparrow S. An athymic nude mutation in the rat. *Nature* 1978;274:365.

144. Flanagan SP. "Nude," a new hairless gene with pleiotropic effects in the mouse. *Genet Res* 1966;8:295.

145. Pantelouris EM. Absence of thymus in a mouse mutant. *Nature* 1968;217:370

146. Segre JA, Nemhauser JL, Taylor BA, Nadeau JH, Lander ES. Positional cloning of the nude locus: genetic, physical, and transcription maps of the region and mutations in the mouse and rat. *Genomics* 1995;28:549–559.

147. Galili N, Baldwin HS, Lund J, et al. A region of mouse chromosome 16 is syntenic to the DiGeorge, velocardiofacial syndrome minimal critical region. *Genome Res* 1997;7:17–26.

148. Bortin MM, Rimm AA. Severe combined immunodeficiency disease. Characterization of the disease and results of transplantation. *JAMA* 1977;238:591–600.

149. Glanzmann E, Riniker P. Essentielle lymphocytophtose. Ein neues krankeitsbild aus der Sauglingspathologie. *Ann Paediat* 1950;174:1–5.

150. Buckley RH, Schiff RI, Schiff SE, et al. Human severe combined immunodeficiency (SCID): genetic, phenotypic and functional diversity in 108 infants. *J Pediatr* 1997;130:378–387.

151. Gossage DL, Buckley RH. Prevalence of lymphocytopenia in severe combined immunodeficiency. *N Engl J Med* 1990;323:1422–1423.

152. Buckley RH, Schiff SE, Sampson HA, et al. Development of immunity in human severe primary T cell deficiency following haploidentical bone marrow stem cell transplantation. *J Immunol* 1986;136:2398–2407.

153. Stephan JL, Vlekova V, Le Deist F, et al. Severe combined immunodeficiency: a retrospective single-center study of clinical presentation and outcome in 117 cases. *J Pediatr* 1993;123:564–572.

154. Altman PL. Blood leukocyte values: man. In: Dittmer DS, ed. *Blood and other body fluids.* Washington DC: Federation of American Societies for Experimental Biology, 1961:125–126.

155. Conley ME, Buckley RH, Hong R, et al. X-linked severe combined immunodeficiency. Diagnosis in males with sporadic severe combined immunodeficiency and clarification of clinical findings. *J Clin Invest* 1990;85:1548–1554.

156. Schiff SE, Buckley RH. Variation in natural killer (NK) lymphocyte function among the different molecular forms of severe combined immunodeficiency (SCID). *J Allergy Clin Immunol* 1994;93:273

157. Puck JM, Conley ME, Bailey LC. Refinement of linkage of human severe combined immunodeficiency (SCIDXI) to polymorphic markers in Xq13. *Am J Hum Genet* 1993;53:176–184.

158. Puck JM, Deschenes SM, Porter JC, et al. The interleukin-2 receptor gamma chain maps to Xq13.1 and is mutated in X-linked severe combined immunodeficiency, SCIDX1. *Hum Mol Genet* 1993;2:1099–1104.

159. Noguchi M, Yi H, Rosenblatt HM, et al. Interleukin-2 receptor gamma chain mutation results in X-linked severe combined immunodeficiency in humans. *Cell* 1993;73:147–157.

160. Sugamura K, Asao H, Kondo M, et al. The interleukin-2 receptor gamma chain: its role in the multiple cytokine receptor complexes and T cell development in XSCID. *Ann Rev Immunol* 1996;14:179–205.

161. Leonard WJ. Dysfunctional cytokine receptor signaling in severe combined immunodeficiency. *J Invest Med* 1996;44:304–311.

chromosomal region 22q11 as a cause of selected malformations of the ventricular outflow tracts and aortic arch: a three year prospective study. *J Pediatr* 1996;129:26–32.

162. Puck JM. IL2RGbase: a database of gamma c-chain defects causing human X-SCID. *Immunol Today* 1996;17:506–511.

163. Puck JM, Pepper AE, Henthorn PS, et al. Mutation analysis of IL2RG in human X-linked severe combined immunodeficiency. *Blood* 1997;89:1968–1977.

164. O'Marcaigh AS, Puck JM, Pepper AE, de Santes K, Cowan MJ. Maternal mosaicism for a novel interleukin-2 receptor gamma chain mutation causing X-linked severe combined immunodeficiency in a Navajo kindred. *J Clin Immunol* 1997;17:29–33.

165. Nash DR, Levine AD, Buckley RH. B cells from most patients with either X-linked (XL) or autosomal recessive (AR) forms of severe combined immunodeficiency (SCID) produce IgE and other isotypes normally when stimulated with anti-CD40 mAb and IL-4. *J Allergy Clin Immunol* 1994;93:273

166. Matthews DJ, Clark PA, Herbert J, et al. Function of the interleukin-2 (IL-2) receptor gamma chain in biologic responses of X-linked severe combined immunodeficient B cells to IL-2, IL-4, IL-13 and IL-15. *Blood* 1995;85:38–42.

167. Conley ME, Lavoie A, Briggs C, Brown P, Guerra C, Puck JM. Nonrandom X chromosome inactivation in B cells from carriers of X chromosome-linked severe combined immunodeficiency. *Proc Natl Acad Sci U S A* 1988;85:3090–3094.

168. Wengler SG, Allen RC, Parolini O, Smith H, Conley ME. Nonrandom X chromosome inactivation in natural killer cells from obligate carriers of X-linked severe combined immunodeficiency. *J Immunol* 1993;150:700–704.

169. Disanto JP, Dautry-Varsat A, Certain S, Fischer A, de Saint Basile G. Interleukin-2 (IL-2) receptor chain mutations in X-linked severe combined immunodeficiency disease result in the loss of high-affinity IL-2 receptor binding. *Eur J Immunol* 1994;24.475–479.

170. Russell SM, Keegan AD, Harada N, et al. Interleukin-2 receptor gamma chain: a functional component of the interleukin-4 receptor. *Science* 1993;262:1880–1883.

171. Noguchi M, Nakamura Y, Russell SM, et al. Interleukin-2 receptor gamma chain: a functional component of the interleukin-7 receptor. *Science* 1993;262: 1977–1980.

172. Voss SD, Hong R, Sondel PM. Severe combined immunodeficiency, interleukin-2 (IL-2), and the IL-2 receptor: experiments of nature continue to point the way. *Blood* 1994;83:626–635.

173. Clark PA, Lester T, Genet S, et al. Screening for mutations causing X-linked severe combined immunodeficiency in the IL-2R gamma chain gene by single strand conformation polymorphism analysis. *Hum Genet* 1995;96:427–432.

174. Stephan V, Wahn V, LeDeist F, et al. Atypical X-linked severe combined immunodeficiency due to possible spontaneous reversion of the genetic defect in T cells. *N Engl J Med* 1996;335:1563–1567.

175. Buckley RH, Schiff RI. The use of intravenous immunoglobulin in immunodeficiency diseases. *N Engl J Med* 1991;325:110–117.

176. Myers LA, Riester DE, Schiff RI, et al. Bone marrow transplantation for SCID in the neonatal period. *J Allergy Clin Immunol* 1997;99(suppl):101

177. Hague RA, Rassam S, Morgan G, Cant AJ. Early diagnosis of severe combined immunodeficiency syndrome. *Arch Dis Child* 1994;70:260–263.

178. Saito S, Morii T, Umekage H, et al. Expression of the interleukin-2 receptor gamma chain on cord blood mononuclear cells. *Blood* 1996;87:3344–3350.

179. Jefyk PF, Felsburg PJ, Haskins ME, Patterson DF. X-linked severe combined immunodeficiency in the dog. *Clin Immunol Immunopathol* 1989;52:173–189.

180. Somberg RL, Tipold A, Hartnett BJ, Moore PF, Henthorn PS, Felsburg PJ. Postnatal development of T cells in dogs with X-linked severe combined immunodeficiency. *J Immunol* 1996;156:1431–1435.

181. Henthorn PS, Somberg RL, Fimiani VM, Puck JM, Patterson DF, Felsburg PJ. IL-2R gene microdeletion demonstrates that canine X-linked severe combined immunodeficiency is a homologue of the human disease. *Genomics* 1994;23: 69–74

182. Somberg RL, Pullen RP, Casal ML, Patterson DF, Felsburg PJ, Henthorn PS. A single nucleotide insertion in the canine interleukin-2 receptor gamma chain results in X-linked severe combined immunodeficiency disease. *Vet Immunol Immunopathol* 1995;47:203–213.

183. Disanto JP, Muller W, Guy GD, Fischer A, Rajewsky K. Lymphoid development in mice with a targeted deletion of the interleukin 2 receptor gamma chain. *Proc Natl Acad Sci U S A* 1995;92:377–381.

184. Cao X, Shores EW, Hu-Li J, et al. Defective lymphoid development in mice lacking expression of the common cytokine receptor gamma chain. *Immunity* 1995; 2:223–238.

185. Taccioli GE, Alt FW. Potential targets for autosomal SCID mutations. *Curr Opin Immunol* 1995;7:436–440.

186. Shovlin CL, Simmonds HA, Fairbanks LD, et al. Adult onset immunodeficiency caused by inherited adenosine deaminase deficiency. *J Immunol* 1994;153: 2331–2339.

187. Hirschhorn R. Adenosine deaminase deficiency: molecular basis and recent developments. *Clin Immunol Immunopathol* 1995;76(suppl).219–227.

188. Buckley RH, Schiff SE, Schiff RI, et al. Haploidentical bone marrow stem cell transplantation in human severe combined immunodeficiency. *Semin Hematol* 1993;30:92–104.

189. Hershfield MS, Buckley RH, Greenberg ML, et al. Treatment of adenosine deaminase deficiency with polyethylene glycol modified adenosine deaminase (PEG-ADA). *N Engl J Med* 1987;316:589–596.

190. Hershfield MS, Chaffee S, Sorensen RU. Enzyme replacement therapy with polyethylene glycol-adenosine deaminase in adenosine deaminase deficiency: overview and case reports of three patients, including two now receiving gene therapy. *Pediatr Res* 1993;33(suppl):42–48.

191. Hershfield MS. PEG-ADA replacement therapy for adenosine deaminase deficiency: an update after 8.5 years. *Clin Immunol Immunopathol* 1995;76(suppl): 228–232.

192. Bordignon C, Notarangelo LD, Nobili N, et al. Gene therapy in peripheral blood lymphocytes and bone marrow for ADA- immunodeficient patients. *Science* 1995;270:470–475.

193. Hoogerbrugge PM, van Beusechem VW, Fischer A, et al. Bone marrow gene transfer in three patients with adenosine deaminase deficiency. *Gene Ther* 1996; 3:179–183.

194. Mullen CA, Snitzer K, Culver KW, Morgan R, Anderson WF, Blaese RM. Molecular analysis of T lymphocyte-directed gene therapy for adenosine deaminase deficiency: long-term expression *in vivo* of genes introduced with a retroviral vector. *Hum Gene Ther* 1996;7:1123–1129.

195. Kohn DB, Weinberg KI, Nolta JA, et al. Engraftment of gene-modified umbilical cord blood cells in neonates with adenosine deaminase deficiency. *Nat Med* 1995;1:1017–1023.

196. Fischer A, de Saint Basile G, Disanto JP, Hacein-Bey S, Sharara L, Cavazzana-Calvo M. Gene therapy of primary immunodeficiencies. *Adv Nephrol* 1997;26: 107–120.

197. Hirschhorn R, Yang DR, Israni A, Huie ML, Ownby DR. Somatic mosaicism for a newly identified splice-site mutation in a patient with adenosine deaminase immunodeficiency and spontaneous clinical recovery. *Am J Hum Genet* 1994;55:59–68.

198. Hirschhorn R, Yang DR, Puck JM, Huie ML, Jiang CK, Kurlandsky LE. Spontaneous in vivo reversion to normal of an inherited mutation in a patient with adenosine deaminase deficiency. *Nature Genetics* 1996;13:290–295.

199. Migchielsen AA, Breuer ML, van Roon RM, et al. Adenosine-deaminase-deficient mice die perinatally and exhibit liver-cell degeneration, atelectasis and small intestinal cell death. *Nature Genet* 1995;10:279–287.

200. Kawamura M, McVicar DW, Johnston JA, et al. Molecular cloning of L-Jak, a Janus family protein tyrosine kinase expressed in natural killer cells and activated leukocytes. *Proc Natl Acad Sci U S A* 1994;91:6374–6378.

201. Johnston JA, Kawamura M, Kirken RA, et al. Phosphorylation and activation of the Jak-3 Janus kinase in response to interleukin-2. *Nature* 1994;370:151–153.

202. Miyazaki T, Kawahara A, Jujii H, et al. Functional activation of Jak1 and Jak3 by selective association with IL-2 receptor subunits. *Science* 1994;266:1045–1047.

203. Russell SM, Johnston JA, Noguchi M, et al. Interaction of IL-2R and gamma c chains with Jak1 and Jak3: implications for XSCID and XCID. *Science* 1994; 266;1042–1045.

204. Ihle JN, Kerr IM. JAKs and STATs in signaling by the cytokine receptor superfamily. *Trends Genet* 1995;11:69–72.

205. Johnston JA, Bacon CM, Riedy MC, O'Shea JJ. Signaling by IL-2 and related cytokines: JAKs, STATs, and relationship to immunodeficiency. *J Leukoc Biol* 1996;60:441–452.

206. Macchi P, Villa A, Gillani S, et al. Mutations of Jak-3 gene in patients with autosomal severe combined immune deficiency (SCID). *Nature* 1995;377:65–68.

207. Sharfe N, Dadi HK, Roifman CM. Jak3 protein tyrosine kinase mediates interleukin-7-induced activation of phosphatidylinositol-3' kinase. *Blood* 1995;86: 2077–2085.

208. Nosaka T, van Deursen DJ, Tripp RA, et al. Defective lymphoid development in mice lacking Jak3. *Science* 1995;270:800–802.

209. Schwarz K, Gauss GH, Ludwig L, et al. RAG mutations in human B cell–negative SCID. *Science* 1996;274:97–99.

210. Mombaerts P, Iacomini J, Johnson RS, Herrup K, Tonegawa S, Papaioannou VE. RAG-1–deficient mice have no mature B and T lymphocytes. *Cell* 1992;68: 869–877.

211. Shinkai Y, Rathbun G, Lam K, et al. RAG-2 deficient mice lack mature lymphocytes owing to inability to initiate V(D)J rearrangement. *Cell* 1992;68: 855–867.

212. Bosma GC, Custer RP, Bosma MJ. A severe combined immunodeficiency mutation in the mouse. *Nature* 1983;301:527–530.

213. Schuler W, Weiler IJ, Schuler A, et al. Rearrangement of antigen receptor genes is defective in mice with severe combined immune deficiency. *Cell* 1986;46: 963–972.

214. Bosma MJ. B and T cell leakiness in the SCID mouse mutant. *Immunodef Rev* 1992;3:261–276.

215. Dorshkind K, Pollack SB, Bosma MJ, Phillips RA. Natural killer cells are present in mice with severe combined immunodeficiency (SCID). *J Immunol* 1985; 134.3798

216. Miller RD, Hogg J, Ozaki JH, Gell D, Jackson SP, Riblet R. Gene for catalytic subunit of mouse DNA-dependent protein kinase maps to the scid locus. *Proc Natl Acad Sci U S A* 1995;92:10792–10795.

217. Araki R, Fujimori A, Hamatani K, et al. Nonsense mutation at Tyr-4046 in the DNA-dependent protein kinase catalytic subunit of severe combined immune deficiency mice. *Proc Natl Acad Sci U S A* 1997;94:2438–2443.

218. Itoh M, Hamatani K, Komatsu K, Araki R, Takayama K, Abe M. Human chromosome 8(p12- q22) complements radiosensitivity in the severe combined immune deficiency (SCID) mouse. *Radiat Res* 1993;134:364–368.

219. Felsburg PJ, Somberg RL, Perryman LE. Domestic animal models of severe combined immunodeficiency: canine X-linked severe combined immunodeficiency and severe combined immunodeficiency in horses. *Immunodef Rev* 1992; 3:277–303.

220. Poppie MJ, McGuire TC. Combined immunodeficiency in foals of Arabian breeding: evaluation of mode of inheritance and estimation of prevalence of affected foals and carrier mares and stallions. *J Am Vet Med Assoc* 1977;170:31

221. McGuire TC, Banks KL, Poppie MJ. Combined immunodeficiency in horses: characterization of the lymphocyte defect. *Clin Immunol Immunopatholh* 1975; 3:555

222. Wiler R, Leber R, Moore BB, VanDyk LF, Perryman LE, Meek K. Equine severe combined immunodeficiency: A defect in V(D)J recombination and DNA-dependent protein kinase activity. *Proc Natl Acad Sci U S A* 1995;92:11485–11489.

223. Pannicke U, Tuchschmid P, Friedrich W, Bartram CR, Schwarz K. Two novel missense and frameshift mutations in exons 5 and 6 of the purine nucleoside phosphorylase (PNP) gene in a severe combined immunodeficiency (SCID) patient. *Hum Genet* 1996;98:706–709.

224. Broome CB, Graham ML, Saulsbury FT, Hershfield MS, Buckley RH. Correction of purine nucleoside phosphorylase deficiency by transplantation of allogeneic bone marrow from a sibling. *J Pediatr* 1996;128:373–376.

225. Polmar SH, Pierce GF. Cartilage hair hypoplasia: immunological aspects and their clinical implications. *Clin Immunol Immunopathol* 1986;40:87–93.

226. Sulisalo T, van der Burgt I, Rimoin DL, Bonaventure J. Genetic homogeneity of cartilage-hair hypoplasia. *Hum Genet* 1995;95:157–160.

227. Pierce GF, Polmar SH. Lymphocyte dysfunction in cartilage hair hypoplasia. II. Evidence for a cell cycle specific defect in T cell growth. *Clin Exp Immunol* 1982;50:621

228. Juvonen E, Makitie O, Makipernaa A, Ruutu T. Defective in-vitro colony formation of haematopoietic progenitors in patients with cartilage-hair hypoplasia and history of anaemia. *Eur J Pediatr* 1995;154:30–34.

229. Remold-O'Donnell E, Rosen FS. Sialophorin (CD43) and the Wiskott-Aldrich syndrome. *Immunodef Rev* 1990;2:151–174.

230. Inoue R, Kondo N, Kuwabara N, Orii T. Aberrant patterns of immunoglobulin levels in Wiskott-Aldrich syndrome. *Scand J Immunol* 1995;41:188–193.

231. Kawabata K, Nagasawa M, Morio T, Okawa H, Yata J. Decreased α/β heterodimer among CD8 molecules of peripheral blood T cells in Wiskott-Aldrich syndrome. *Clin Immunol Immunopathol* 1996;81:129–135.

232. de Saint Basile G, Fraser NJ, Craig IW, et al. Close linkage of hypervariable marker DXS255 to disease locus of Wiskott-Aldrich syndrome. *Lancet* 1989;2: 1319–1320.

233. Symons M, Derry JMJ, Karlak B, et al. Wiskott-Aldrich syndrome protein, a novel effector for the GTPase CDC42H2, is implicated in actin polymerization. *Cell* 1996;84:723–734.

234. Aspenstrom P, Lindberg U, Hall A. Two GTPases, cdc42 and rac, bind directly to a protein implicated in the immunodeficiency disorder Wiskott-Aldrich syndrome. *Curr Biol* 1996;6:70

235. Finan PM, Soames CJ, Wilson L, et al. Identification of regions of the Wiskott-Aldrich syndrome protein responsible for association with selected Src homology 3 domains. *J Biol Chem* 1996;271:25646–25656.

236. Miki H, Nonoyama S, Zhu Q, Aruffo A, Ochs HD, Takenawa T. Tyrosine kinase signaling regulates Wiskott-Aldrich syndrome protein function, which is essential for megakaryocyte differentiation. *Cell Growth Differentiation* 1997;8:195–202.

237. Schwarz K. WASPbase: a database of WAS- and XLT-causing mutations. *Immunol Today* 1996;17:496–502.

238. Schwartz M, Bekassy A, Donner M, et al. Mutation spectrum in patients with Wiskott-Aldrich syndrome and X-linked thrombocytopenia: identification of twelve different mutations in the WASP gene. *Thromb Haemost* 1996;75:546–550.

239. Greer WL, Shehabeldin A, Schulman J, Junker A, Siminovitch KA. Identification of WASP mutations, mutation hotspots and genotype-phenotype disparities in 24 patients with Wiskott-Aldrich syndrome. *Hum Genet* 1996;98:685–690.

240. de Saint Basile G, Lagelouse RD, Lambert N, et al. Isolated X-linked thrombocytopenia in two unrelated families is associated with point mutations in the Wiskott-Aldrich syndrome gene. *J Pediatr* 1996;129:56–62.

241. Wengler G, Gorlin JB, Williamson JM, Rosen FS, Bing DH. Non-random inactivation of the X chromosome in early lineage hematopoietic cells in carriers of Wiskott-Aldrich syndrome. *Blood* 1995;85:2471–2477.

242. Kwan SP, Hagemann TL, Radtke BE, Blaese RM, Rosen FS. Identification of mutations in the Wiskott-Aldrich syndrome gene and characterization of a polymorphic dinucleotide repeat at the DXS6940, adjacent to the disease gene. *Proc Natl Acad Sci U S A* 1995;92:4706–4710.

243. Ariga T, Yamada M, Sakiyama Y. Mutation analysis of five Japanese families with Wiskott-Aldrich syndrome and determination of the family members' carrier status using three different methods. *Pediatr Res* 1997;41:535–540.

244. Kondoh T, Hayashi K, Matsumoto T, et al. Two sisters with clinical diagnosis of Wiskott-Aldrich syndrome: Is the condition in the family autosomal recessive? *Am J Med Genet* 1995;60:364–369.

245. Rocca B, Bellacosa A, de Cristofaro R, et al. Wiskott-Aldrich syndrome: report of an autosomal dominant variant. *Blood* 1996;87:4538–4543.

246. Filipovich AH, Pelz C, Sobocinski K, Ireland M, Kollman C, Horowitz MM. Allogeneic bone marrow transplantation (BMT) for Wiskott Aldrich syndrome (WAS): comparison of outcomes by donor type. *J Allergy Clin Immunol* 1997; 99S:102

247. Mullen CA, Anderson KD, Blaese RM. Splenectomy and/or bone marrow transplantation in the management of the Wiskott-Aldrich syndrome: long-term follow-up of 62 cases. *Blood* 1993;82:2961–2966.

248. Litzman J, Jones A, Hann I, Chapel H, Strobel S, Morgan G. Intravenous immunoglobulin, splenectomy, and antibiotic prophylaxis in Wiskott-Aldrich syndrome. *Arch Dis Child* 1996;75:436–439.

249. Lyon MF, Peters J, Glenister PH, Ball S, Wright E. The scurfy mouse mutant has previously unrecognized hematological abnormalities and resembles Wiskott-Aldrich syndrome. *Proc Natl Acad Sci U S A* 1990;87:2433–2437.

250. Blair PJ, Bultman SJ, Haas JC, Rouse BT, Wilkinson JE, Godfrey VL. CD4⁺CD8⁻ T cells are the effector cells in disease pathogenesis in the scurfy (sf) mouse. *J Immunol* 1994;153:3764–3774.

251. Kanangat S, Blair P, Reddy R, et al. Disease in the scurfy (sf) mouse is associated with overexpression of cytokine genes. *Eur J Immunol* 1996;26:161–165.

252. Derry JMJ, Wiedemann P, Blair P, et al. The mouse homolog of the Wiskott-Aldrich syndrome protein (WASP) gene is highly conserved and maps near the scurfy (sf) mutation on the X chromosome. *Genomics* 1995;29:471–477.

253. Gatti RA, Boder E, Vinters HV, Sparkes RS, Norman A, Lange K. Ataxia-telangiectasia: an interdisciplinary approach to pathogenesis. *Medicine* 1991;70:99–117.

254. Taylor AMR, Metcalfe JA, Thick J, Mak Y. Leukemia and lymphoma in ataxia telangiectasia. *Blood* 1996;87:423–438.

255. Watson HG, McLaren KM, Todd A, Wallace WH. Transfusion associated graft-versus-host disease in ataxia telangiectasia. *Lancet* 1997;349:179

256. Swift M. Genetic aspects of ataxia telangiectasia. *Immunodef Rev* 1990;2:67–81.

257. Beamish H, Williams R, Chen P, Lavin MF. Defect in multiple cell cycle checkpoints in ataxia telangiectasis postirradiation. *J Biol Chem* 1996;271: 20486–20493.

258. Lavin MF, Shiloh Y. Ataxia telangiectasia: a multifaceted genetic disorder associated with defective signal transduction. *Curr Opin Immunol* 1996;8:459–464.

259. Hartley KO, Gell D, Smith GC, et al. DNA-dependent protein kinase catalytic subunit: a relative of phosphatidylinositol 3-kinase and the ataxia telangiectasia gene product. *Cell* 1995;82:849–856.

260. Xu Y, Baltimore D. Dual roles of ATM in the cellular response to radiation and in cell growth control. *Genes Dev* 1996;10:2401–2410.

261. Heintz N. Ataxia telangiectasia: cell signaling, cell death and the cell cycle. *Curr Opin Neurol* 1996;9:137–140.

262. Gilad S, Khosravi R, Shkedy D, et al. Predominance of null mutations in ataxia telangiectasia. *Hum Mol Genet* 1996;5:433–439.

263. Wright J, Teraoka S, Onengut S, et al. A high frequency of distinct ATM gene mutations in ataxia telangiectasia. *Am J Hum Genet* 1996;59:839–846.

264. Barlow C, Hirotsune S, Paylor R, et al. Atm-deficient mice: a paradigm of ataxia telangiectasia. *Cell* 1996;86:159–171.

265. Weemaes CMR, Smeets DFCM, van der Burgt CJAM. Nijmegen breakage syndrome: a progress report. *Int J Radiat Biol* 1994;66(suppl):185–188.

266. Kleijer WJ, van der Kraan M, Los FJ, Jaspers NGJ. Prenatal diagnosis of ataxia telangiectasia and Nijmegen breakage syndrome by the assay of radioresistant DNA synthesis. *Int J Radiat Biol* 1994;66(suppl):167–174.

267. Chrzanowska KH, Kleijer WJ, Krajewska-Walasek M, et al. Eleven Polish patients with microcephaly, immunodeficiency, and chromosomal instability: the Nijmegen breakage syndrome. *Am J Med Genet* 1995;57:462–471.

268. Saar K, Chrzanowska KH, Stumm M, et al. The gene for the ataxia-telangiectasia variant, Nijmegen breakage syndrome, maps to a 1-cM interval on chromosome 8q21. *Am J Hum Genet* 1997;60:605–610.

269. Klein C, Lisowska-Grospierre B, LeDeist F, Fischer A, Griscelli C. Major histocompatibility complex class II deficiency: clinical manifestations, immunologic features, and outcome. *J Pediatr* 1993;123:921–928.

270. Donato L, de la Salle H, Hanau D, et al. Association of HLA class I antigen deficiency related to a TAP2 gene mutation with familial bronchiectasis. *J Pediatr* 1995;127:895–900.

271. Grandea AG, Androlewicz MJ, Athwal RS, Geraghty DE, Spies T. Dependence of peptide binding by MHC class I molecules on their interaction with TAP. *Science* 1995;270:105–108.

272. Elhasid R, Etzioni A. Major histocompatibility complex class II deficiency: a clinical review. *Blood Rev* 1996;10:242–248.

273. Henwood J, van Eggermond MC, van Boxel-Dezaire AN, et al. Human T cell repertoire generation in the absence of MHC class II expression results in a circulating CD4⁺CD8⁻ population with altered physicochemical properties of complementarity-determining region 3. *J Immunol* 1996;156:895–906.

274. Reith W, Steimle V, Mach B. Molecular defects in the bare lymphocyte syndrome and regulation of MHC class II genes. *Immunol Today* 1995;16:539–546.

275. Peijnenburg A, Godthelp B, van Boxel-Dezaire A, van den Elsen P. Definition of a novel complementation group in MHC class II deficiency. *Immunogenetics* 1995;41:287–294.

276. Mach B, Steimle V, Martinez-Soria E, Reith W. Regulation of MHC class II genes: lessons from a disease. *Annu Rev Immunol* 1996;14:301–331.

277. Steimle V, Otten LA, Zufferey M, Mach B. Complementation cloning of an MHC class II transactivator mutated in hereditary MHC class II deficiency (or bare lymphocyte syndrome). *Cell* 1993;75:135–146.

278. Reith W, Barras E, Satola S. Cloning of the major histocompatibility complex class II promoter binding protein affected in a hereditary defect in class II gene regulation. *Proc Natl Acad Sci U S A* 1989;86:4200

279. Steimle V, Siegrist CA, Mottet A, Lisowska-Grospierre B, Mach B. Regulation of MHC class II expression by interferon-γ mediated by the transactivator gene CIITA. *Science* 1994;265:106–109.

280. Zhou H, Glimcher LH. Human MHC class II gene transcription directed by the carboxyl terminus of CIITA, one of the defective genes in type II MHC combined immune deficiency. *Immunity* 1995;2:545–553.

281. Chang C-H, Guerder S, Hong S-C, van Ewijk W, Flavell RA. Mice lacking the MHC class II transactivator (CIITA) show tissue-specific impairment of MHC class II expression. *Immunity* 1996;4:167–178.

282. Kishimoto TK, Springer TA. Human leukocyte adhesion deficiency: molecular basis for a defective immune response to infections of the skin. *Curr Prob Dermatol* 1989;18:106.

283. D'Agata ID, Paradis K, Chad Z, Bonny Y, Seidman E. Leucocyte adhesion deficiency presenting as a chronic ileocolitis. *Gut* 1996;39:605–608.

284. Rivera-Matos IR, Rakita RM, Mariscalco MM, Elder FFB, Dreyer SA, Cleary TG. Leukocyte adhesion deficiency mimicking Hirschsprung disease. *J Pediatr* 1995;127:755–757.

285. Wilson RW, Ballantyne CM, Smith CW, et al. Gene targeting yields a CD18-mutant mouse for study of inflammation. *J Immunol* 1993;151:1571–1578.

286. Etzioni A, Frydman M, Pollack S, et al. Brief report: recurrent severe infections caused by a novel leukocyte adhesion deficiency. *N Engl J Med* 1992;327: 1789–1792.

287. Willerford DM, Chem J, Ferry JA, Davidson L, Ma A, Alt FW. Interleukin-2 receptor α chain regulates the size and content of the peripheral lymphoid compartment. *Immunity* 1995;3:521–530.

288. Suzuki H, Kundig TM, Furlonger C, et al. Deregulated T cell activation and autoimmunity in mice lacking interleukin-2 receptor. *Science* 1995;268:1472–1476.

289. Lenardo MJ. Interleukin-2 programs mouse α T lymphocytes for apoptosis. *Nature* 1991;353:858–861.

290. Huang S, Hendriks W, Althage A, et al. Immune response in mice that lack the interferon-γ receptor. *Science* 1993;259:1742–1745.

291. Dalton DK, Pitts-Meek S, Keshav S, Figari IS, Bradley A, Stewart TA. Multiple defects of immune cell function in mice with disrupted interferon-γ genes. *Science* 1993;259:1739–1742.

292. Stolz W, Graubner U, Gerstmeier J, Burg G, Belohradsky BH. Chediak syndrome: approaches to diagnosis and treatment. *Curr Prob Dermatol* 1989;18:93

293. Zhao H, Boissy YL, Abdel-Malek Z, King RA, Nordlund JJ, Boissy RE. On the analysis of the pathophysiology of Chediak-Higashi syndrome—defects expressed by cultured melanocytes. *Lab Invest* 1994;71:25–34.

294. Holcombe RF, Jones KL, Stewart RM. Lysosomal enzyme activities in Chediak-Higashi syndrome: evaluation of lymphoblastoid cell lines and review of the literature. *Immunodeficiency* 1994;5:131–140.

295. Merino F, Esparza B, Sabino E. Chediak-Higashi syndrome natural killer cells: a protein kinase C defective activation/regulation defect? *Eur J Pediatr* 1996; 155:254–258.

296. Baetz K, Isaaz S, Griffiths GM. Loss of cytotoxic T lymphocyte function in Chediak-Higashi syndrome arises from a secretory defect that prevents lytic granule exocytosis. *J Immunol* 1995;154:6122–6131.

297. Nagle DL, Karim MA, Woolf EA, et al. Identification and mutation analysis of the complete gene for Chediak-Higashi syndrome. *Nature Genet* 1996,14. 307–311.

298. Barrat FJ, Auloge L, Pastural E, et al. Genetic and physical mapping of the Chediak-Higashi syndrome on chromosome 1q42-43. *Am J Hum Genet* 1996;59: 625–632.

299. Perou CM, Moore KJ, Nagle DL, et al. Identification of the murine beige gene by YAC complementation and positional cloning. *Nature Genet* 1996;13: 303–308.

300. Barbosa MDFS, Nguyen QA, Tchernev VT, et al. Identification of the homologous beige and Chediak-Higashi syndrome genes. *Nature* 1996;382:262–265.

301. Fukai K, Oh J, Karim MA, et al. Homozygosity mapping of the gene for Chediak-Higashi syndrome to chromosome 1q42-q44 in a segment of conserved synteny that includes the mouse beige locus (bg). *Am J Hum Genet* 1996;59:620–624.

302. Aslan Y, Erduran E, Gedik Y, Mocan H, Yildiran A. The role of high dose methylprednisolone and splenectomy in the accelerated phase of Chediak-Higashi syndrome. *Acta Haematol* 1996;96:105–107.

303. Haddad E, Le Deist F, Blanche S, et al. Treatment of Chediak-Higashi syndrome by allogenic bone marrow transplantation: report of 10 cases. *Blood* 1995;85: 3328–3333.

304. Chatila T, Wong R, Young M, Miller R, Terhorst C, Geha RS. An immunodeficiency characterized by defective signal transduction in T lymphocytes. *N Engl J Med* 1989;320:696–702.

305. Arpaia E, Shahar M, Dadi H, Cohen A, Roifman CM. Defective T cell receptor signaling and CD8+ thymic selection in humans lacking zap-70 kinase. *Cell* 1994;76:947–958.

306. Elder ME. Severe combined immunodeficiency due to a defect in the tyrosine kinase ZAP-70. *Pediatr Res* 1996;39:743–748.

307. Negishi I, Motoyama N, Nakayama K, et al. Essential role for ZAP-70 in both positive and negative selection of thymocytes. *Nature* 1995;376:435–438.

308. Stein PL, Lee H, Rich S, Soriano P. p59fyn mutant mice display differential signaling in thymocytes and peripheral T cells. *Cell* 1992;70:741–750.

309. Appleby MW, Gross JA, Cooke MP, Levin SD, Qian X, Perlmutter RM. Defective T cell receptor signaling in mice lacking the thymic isoform of p59fyn. *Cell* 1992;70:751–761.

310. Appleby MW, Kerner JD, Chien S, Maliszewski CR, Bondada S, Perlmutter RM. Involvement of p59fynT in interleukin-5 receptor signaling. *J Exp Med* 1995; 182:811–820.

311. Arnaiz-Villena A, Timon M, Corell A, Perez-Aciego P, Martin-Villa JM, Regueiro JR. Brief report: primary immunodeficiency caused by mutations in the gene encoding the CD3-γ subunit of the T lymphocyte receptor. *N Engl J Med* 1992;327:529–533.

312. Thoenes G, Soudais C, Le Deist F, Griscelli C, Fischer A, Lisowska-Grospierre B. Structural analysis of low TCR-CD3 complex expression in T cells of an immunodeficient patient. *J Biol Chem* 1992;267:487–493.

313. Soudais C, de Villartay J, Le Deist F, Fischer A, Lisowska-Grospierre B. Independent mutations of the human CD3-ε gene resulting in a T cell receptor/CD3 complex immunodeficiency. *Nature Genet* 1993;3:77–81.

314. Malissen M, Gillet A, Ardouin L, et al. Altered T cell development in mice with a targeted mutation of the CD3-ε gene. *EMBO J* 1995;14:4641–4653.

315. Love PE, Shores EW, Johnson MD, et al. T cell development in mice that lack the chain of the T cell antigen receptor complex. *Science* 1993;261:918–921.

316. Fehling HJ, Krotkova A, Saint-Ruf C, Von Boehmer H. Crucial role of the pre-T-cell receptor α gene in development of α but not δ T cells. *Nature* 1995;375: 795–798.

317. Mombaerts P, Clarke AR, Rudnicki MA, et al. Mutations in T cell antigen receptor genes α and thymocyte development at different stages. *Nature* 1992;360: 225–231.

318. Philpott KL, Viney JL, Kay G, et al. Lymphoid development in mice congenitally lacking T cell receptor αβ-expressing cells. *Science* 1992;256:1448–1452.

319. Weinberg K, Parkman R. Severe combined immunodeficiency due to a specific defect in the production of interleukin-2. *N Engl J Med* 1990;322:1718–1723.

320. Disanto JP, Keever CA, Small TN, Nichols GL, O'Reilly RJ, Flomenberg N. Absence of interleukin 2 production in a severe combined immunodeficiency disease syndrome with T cells. *J Exp Med* 1990;171:1697–1704.

321. Castigli E, Pahwa R, Good RA, Geha RS, Chatila TA. Molecular basis of a multiple lymphokine deficiency in a patient with severe combined immunodeficiency. *Proc Natl Acad Sci U S A* 1993;90:4728–4732.

322. Feske S, Muller JM, Graf D, et al. Severe combined immunodeficiency due to defective binding of the nuclear factor of activated T cells in T lymphocytes of two male siblings. *Eur J Immunol* 1996;26:2119–2126.

323. Schorle H, Holtschke T, Hunig T, Schimpl A, Horak I. Development and function of T cells in mice rendered interleukin-2 deficient by gene targeting. *Nature* 1991;352:621–624.

324. Sadlack B, Lohler J, Schorle H, et al. Generalized autoimmune disease in interleukin-2-deficient mice is triggered by an uncontrolled activation and proliferation of CD4+ T cells. *Eur J Immunol* 1995;25:3053–3059.

325. Sadlack B, Merz H, Schorle H, Schimpl A, Feller AC, Horak I. Ulcerative colitis-like disease in mice with a disrupted interleukin-2 gene. *Cell* 1993;75: 253–261.

326. Businco L, Di Frazio A, Ziruolo MG, et al. Clinical and immunologic findings in four infants with Omenn's syndrome: a form of severe combined immunodeficiency with phenotypically normal T cells, elevated IgE, and eosinophilia. *Clin Immunol Immunopathol* 1987;44:123–133.

327. Rybojad M, Cambiaghi S, Moraillon I, et al. Omenn's reticulosis associated with the nephrotic syndrome. *Br J Dermatol* 1996;135:124–127.

328. Karol RA, Eng J, Cooper JB, et al. Imbalances in subsets of T lymphocytes in an inbred pedigree with Omenn's syndrome. *Clin Immunol Immunopathol* 1983;27: 412–427.

329. de Saint-Basile G, Le Deist F, de Vallartay J, et al. Restricted heterogeneity of T lymphocytes in combined immunodeficiency with hypereosinophilia (Omenn's syndrome). *J Clin Invest* 1991;87:1352–1359.

330. Mathioudakis G, Good RA, Chernajovsky Y, Day NK, Platsoucas CD. Selective gamma-chain T cell receptor gene rearrangements in a patient with Omenn's syndrome: absence of V-II subgroup (V 9) transcripts. *Clin Diagn Lab Immunol* 1996;3:616–619.

331. Ruco LP, Stoppacciaro A, Pezzella F, et al. The Omenn's syndrome: histological, immunohistochemical and ultrastructural evidence for a partial T cell deficiency evolving in an abnormal proliferation of T lymphocytes and S-100+/T-6+ Langerhans like cells. *Virchows Arch* 1985;407:69–82.

332. Martin JV, Willoughby PB, Giusti V, Price G, Cerezo L. The lymph node pathology of Omenn's syndrome. *Am J Surg Pathol* 1995;19:1082–1087.

333. Melamed I, Cohen A, Roifman CM. Expansion of CD3+ CD4- CD8- T cell population expression high levels of IL5 in Omenn's syndrome. *Clin Exp Immunol* 1994;95:14–21.

334. Schandene L, Ferster A, Mascart-Lemone F, et al. T helper type 2-like cells and therapeutic effects of interferon gamma in combined immunodeficiency with hypereosinophilia (Omenn's syndrome). *Eur J Immunol* 1993;23:56–60.

335. Chilosi M, Facchetti F, Notarangelo LD, et al. CD30 cell expression and abnormal soluble CD30 serum accumulation in Omenn's syndrome: evidence for a T helper 2-mediated condition. *Eur J Immunol* 1996;26:329–334.

336. Buckley RH, Wray BB, Belmaker EZ. Extreme hyperimmunoglobulinemia E and undue susceptibility to infection. *Pediatrics* 1972;49:59–70.

337. Buckley RH, Sampson HA. The hyperimmunoglobulinemia E syndrome. In: Franklin EC, ed. *Clinical immunology update.* New York: Elsevier North-Holland, 1981:147–167.

338. Claassen JL, Levine AD, Schiff SE, Buckley RH. Mononuclear cells from patients with the hyper IgE syndrome produce little IgE when stimulated with recombinant interleukin 4 in vitro. *J Allergy Clin Immunol* 1991;88:713–721.

339. King CL, Gallin JI, Malech HL, Abramson SL, Nutman TB. Regulation of immunoglobulin production in hyperimmunoglobulin E recurrent infection syndrome by interferon. *Proc Natl Acad Sci U S A* 1989;86:10085–10089.

340. Kaplan MH, Sun YL, Hoey T, Grusby MJ. Impaired IL-12 responses and enhanced development of Th2 cells in stat4–deficient mice. *Nature* 1996;382: 174–177.

341. Thierfelder WE, van Deursen JM, Yamamoto K, et al. Requirement for stat4 in interleukin-12–mediated responses of natural killer and T cells. *Nature* 1996, 382:171–173.

Fundamental Immunology, Fourth Edition,
edited by William E. Paul
Published by Lippincott–Raven Publishers, Philadelphia 1999.

CHAPTER 44

The Immunopathogenesis of HIV Infection

Oren Cohen, Drew Weissman, and Anthony S. Fauci

The human immunodeficiency virus (HIV) was first identified in 1983, and in 1984 it was shown to be the cause of the acquired immunodeficiency syndrome (AIDS) (1–3). HIV infection is characterized by the depletion of the CD4+ helper/inducer subset of T-lymphocytes, leading to severe immunosuppression, constitutional symptoms, neurologic disease, and opportunistic infections and neoplasms (4). Twenty-nine million individuals are

O. Cohen and A. S. Fauci: Laboratory of Immunoregulation, National Institute of Allergy and Infectious Diseases, National Institutes of Health, Bethesda, Maryland 20892.
D. Weissman: Division of Infectious Diseases, University of Pennsylvania Medical Center, Philadelphia, Pennsylvania 19104.

thought to have been infected with HIV throughout the world, and approximately 650,000 to 900,000 of these individuals are currently living in the United States (5,6). It is estimated that by the year 2000, between 40 and 100 million people will have been infected with HIV worldwide. Between 1981, when the first AIDS patients were described, and June 1997, more than 600,000 cases of AIDS have been diagnosed in the United States and more than 60% of these patients have died (7). HIV is transmitted by sexual contact, parenteral (and rarely mucosal) exposure to blood or blood products, during pregnancy or the perinatal period, and by breast feeding (8). Rectal trauma and the presence of ulcerative genital lesions increase the risk of HIV transmission during sexual contact (8–14).

This chapter describes the biology of HIV and the interaction of the virus with its target cells, the spectrum of clinical entities that results from infection with HIV, the immunologic defects observed during the course of HIV infection, the mechanisms of immunopathogenesis, the host immune responses to infection, and newly described genetic modifiers of HIV disease. As discussed in detail below, HIV infection is predominantly an infection of the human immune system; its mechanisms of pathogenesis are intricately intertwined with normal immune processes.

THE CLINICAL SPECTRUM OF HIV INFECTION

Approximately 3 to 6 weeks after exposure and primary infection with HIV, at least 50% of individuals experience an acute, self-limited syndrome that typically persists from 1 to several weeks and usually resolves spontaneously (15). This acute HIV syndrome is associated with a burst of viremia; concomitantly, the level of CD4+ T cells in peripheral blood declines, sometimes precipitously, but then usually returns to near-normal or lower-than-normal levels (16) (Fig. 1). In some cases the initial transient decline in CD4+ T cell levels is so profound, and the levels of plasma viremia so high, that opportunistic infections have occurred during the acute HIV syndrome (17). The levels of CD8+ T cells and B cells also decline during the acute HIV syndrome; however, the levels of CD8+ T cells usually increase to normal or higher-than-normal levels within 3 to 4 weeks after the onset of illness (16). Because the CD8+ T cell count rebounds faster than the CD4+ T cell level, an inversion of the normal CD4:CD8 ratio occurs during the later phases of the acute syndrome and is maintained after resolution of the acute syndrome, even in the unusual setting of a normal CD4+ T cell count (4). It is likely that these changes occur to a greater or lesser degree in most patients after primary HIV infection, even in the absence of clinical symptoms.

HIV disease comprises a spectrum from the asymptomatic state to advanced immunodeficiency and clinical disease. The median time between primary HIV infection and the development of AIDS is approximately 10 years (18). During this period, CD4+ T cell counts usually decrease gradually until they reach a level at which the risk of opportunistic diseases is high (19) (Fig. 1). Before the onset of opportunistic diseases, HIV-infected individuals may experience various constitutional signs and symptoms (4). Neurologic disease in the form of AIDS encephalopathy may occur in HIV-infected individuals in the absence of opportunistic diseases (20). Conditions indicative of advanced immunodeficiency include a variety of opportunistic infections and neoplasms (4). The incidence of opportunistic infections has declined with the advent of earlier diagnosis of HIV infection, more potent antiretroviral therapy, and improved prophylaxis against opportunistic infections. However, an increased incidence of late lymphoid malignancies has been observed, likely as a result of the increased survival times experienced by patients with advanced immunodeficiency.

Epidemiology

The current estimate of the number of individuals worldwide who have become infected with HIV exceeds 29 million (5). The epidemic has occurred in multiple waves depending on the timing of introduction of the virus into a population and the demographics of the population in question. In parts of the world the incidence of infection has recently plateaued, whereas in other regions incidence rates continue to increase (Fig. 2). In certain regions of sub-Saharan Africa, the prevalence of HIV infection may be as high as 10% of the entire population; similar rates may be seen in the near future in regions of Asia where the epidemic is accelerating. In the United States, male-to-male sexual contact is the most common mechanism of HIV transmission; however, injection drug use accounts for an increasing proportion of cases of HIV transmis-

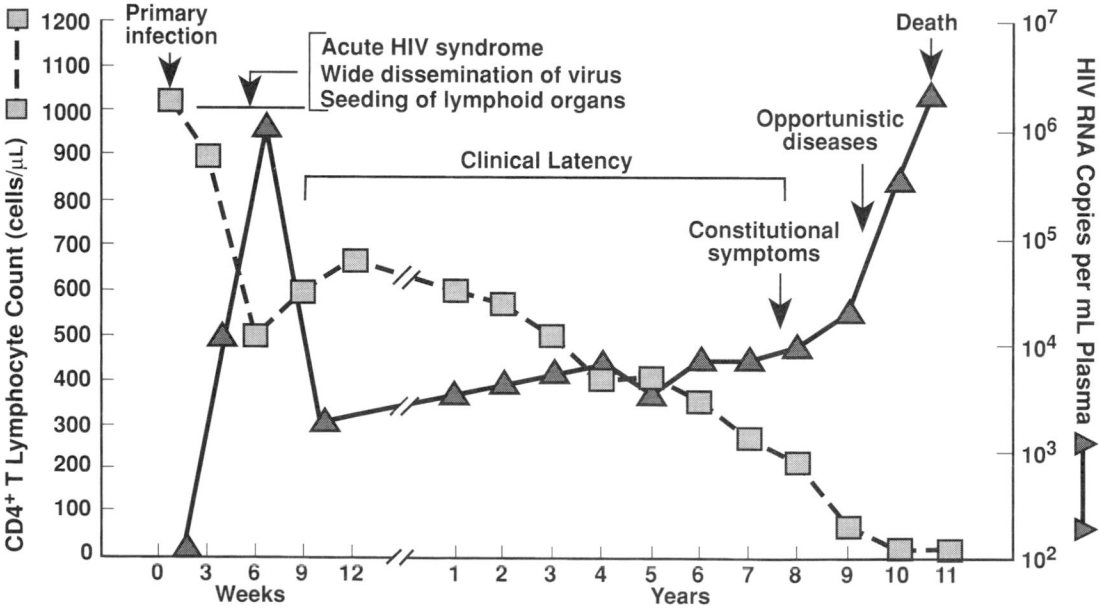

FIG. 1. The typical clinical course of an HIV-infected individual. After primary HIV infection, a burst of plasma viremia occurs in concert with a transient decline in the CD4+ T-cell count. Partial immune control over viral replication ensues, resulting in a variable period of clinical latency. As the CD4+ T-cell count declines, the risk of developing constitutional symptoms and opportunistic diseases increases. Adapted with permission from Fauci AS, et al. *Ann Intern Med* 1996;124:654.

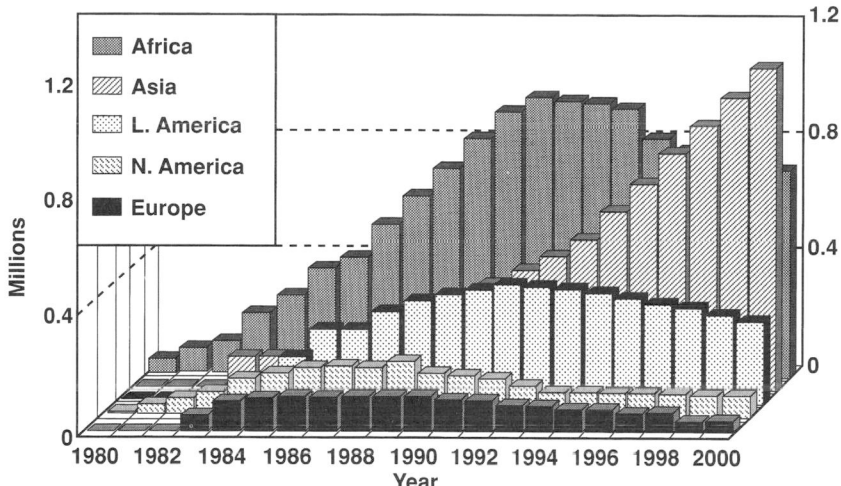

FIG. 2. Projected incidence of adult HIV infections by geographic region (data obtained from the World Health Organization).

sion, as does heterosexual transmission, particularly to women who are the sexual partners of injection drug users (7).

Globally, different subtypes, or clades, of HIV have been identified (Fig. 3). Phylogenetic analysis of HIV proviral sequences reveals two major genetic groups of HIVs: the M (major) and O (outlier) groups. The relatively rare O group viruses are concentrated in west Africa and may elude detection by standard antibody tests for HIV-1. Within the M group, related HIV variants are classified into clades (currently designated A through J) according to their degree of genetic similarity (21). The biochemical basis of the generation of viral diversity is the relative infidelity of the viral reverse transcriptase (RT) enzyme. At the nucleotide level, viral subtypes differ from each other by about 14% in their *gag* (viral core) coding sequences, and by about 30% in their envelope coding sequences (21). Subtype A viruses are the most common worldwide; they are prevalent in central Africa and are also found in Europe, Russia, east Asia, and South America. Subtype B viruses comprise the overwhelming majority of viruses isolated in the United States, likely as a result of a dominant founder effect. Subtype B viruses also are prevalent in Europe, Australia, and South America; variant subtype B viruses have been isolated in Thailand, China, Malaysia, and Japan. Eastern and southern Africa and India are the major foci of infections with subtype C viruses, although such viruses also have been isolated in Europe, Russia, China, and Brazil. Subtype D viruses circulate primarily in central Africa, whereas subtype E viruses are isolated predominantly in the rapidly expanding epidemic in southeast Asia. HIV viral subtypes G, H, and J have been isolated in central Africa; however, all three of these subtypes are uncommon. Finally, subtype I viruses have been isolated from patients in Cyprus, although these viruses may actually be recombinants of other viral subtypes (22).

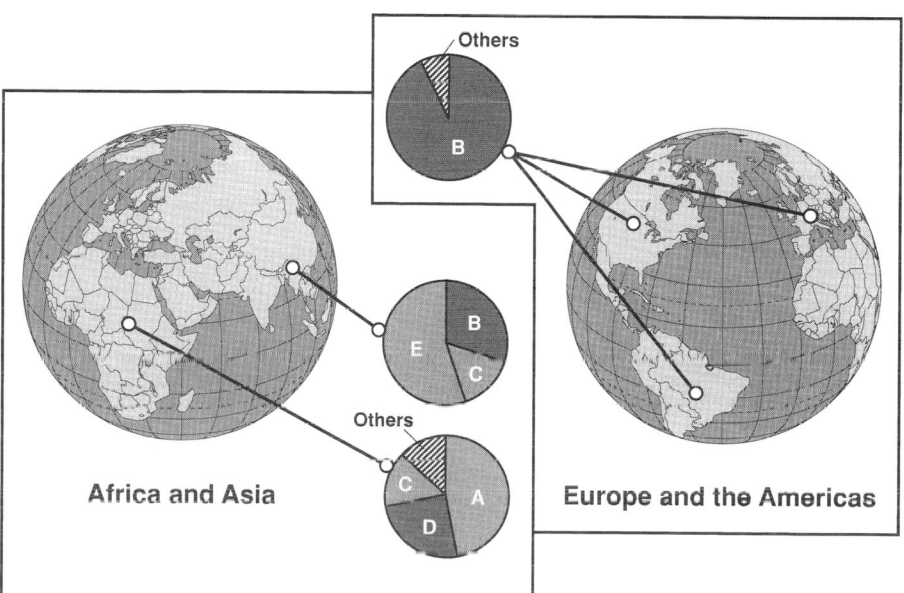

FIG. 3. Distribution of HIV-1 clades (subtypes) by geographic region. Although clade B viruses predominate in the Americas and in Europe, they are responsible for a minority of infections in Asia and Africa. Courtesy of Drs. Francine E. McCutchan and Mika O. Salminen of The Henry Jackson Foundation for the Advancement of Military Medicine and Col. Donald S. Burke of the Walter Reed Army Institute of Research.

TABLE 1. *Human immunodeficiency virus proteins*

Name	Size	Function	Localization
Gag MA	p17	Membrane anchoring, envelope interaction, nuclear transport of viral core (myristylated protein)	Virion
Gag CA	p24	Core capsid	Virion
Gag NC	p7	Nucleocapsid, binds RNA	Virion
	p6	Binds Vpr	Virion
Env	gp 120/gp41	External viral glycoproteins, binds to CD4 and coreceptor	Plasma membrane, virion envelope
Protease	p15	Gag-Pol cleavage and maturation	Virion
Reverse transcriptase	p66/p51 (heterodimer)	Reverse transcription, RNase H activity	Virion
Integrase		DNA provirus integration	Virion
Tat	p16/p14	Viral transcriptional transactivator	Primarily in nucleolus–nucleus
Rev	p19	RNA transport	Primarily in nucleolus–nucleus, shuttles between nucleolus and cytoplasm
Vif	p23	Promotes virion maturation and infectivity	Cytoplasm (cytosol, membranes), virion
Vpr	p10–15	Promotes nuclear localization of preintegration complex, inhibits cell division, arrests infected cells at G2/M	Virion, nucleus
Vpu	p16	Promotes extracellular release of viral particles, degrades CD4 in the endoplasmic reticulum	Integral membrane protein
Nef	p27/25	CD4 downregulation (myristylated protein)	Plasma membrane, cytoplasm, virion

Viral Life Cycle

HIV is a member of the Retroviridae family, which is characterized by a unique enzyme, RT, that allows the virus to copy its RNA into double-stranded DNA in order to replicate (23,24). Within the Retroviridae family, HIV is classified as a lentivirus. The three major coding regions for HIV and all lentiviruses encode core (*gag*), polymerase (*pol*), and envelope (*env*) gene products (Table 1 and Fig. 4). The HIV genome additionally encodes several other proteins, initially termed accessory proteins, that may play key roles in the pathogenesis of HIV infection. The viral life cycle (Fig. 5) begins with the binding of the glycoprotein (gp)120 component of the viral envelope to target cells via CD4 (25–28) and a seven-transmembrane core-ceptor (29). Fusion of the viral lipid envelope to the cellular membrane occurs through the fusion domain of gp41, another component of the envelope gp160 protein (30,31). The viral core enters the cell and the viral RNA is reverse transcribed into double-stranded DNA in the cytoplasm by virally encoded RT. Double-stranded HIV DNA, complexed with the viral enzyme integrase, a product of the *pol* gene, travels to the nucleus and is inserted into chromosomal DNA (32). In the setting of cellular activation, viral messenger RNA (mRNA) production ensues, and new virions are produced. The outer surface of the virion contains the envelope glycoprotein encoded by HIV (Table 1). In addition, as the HIV virion buds through the plasma membrane, it incorporates portions of the membrane, including cellular proteins derived from the infected cell (33).

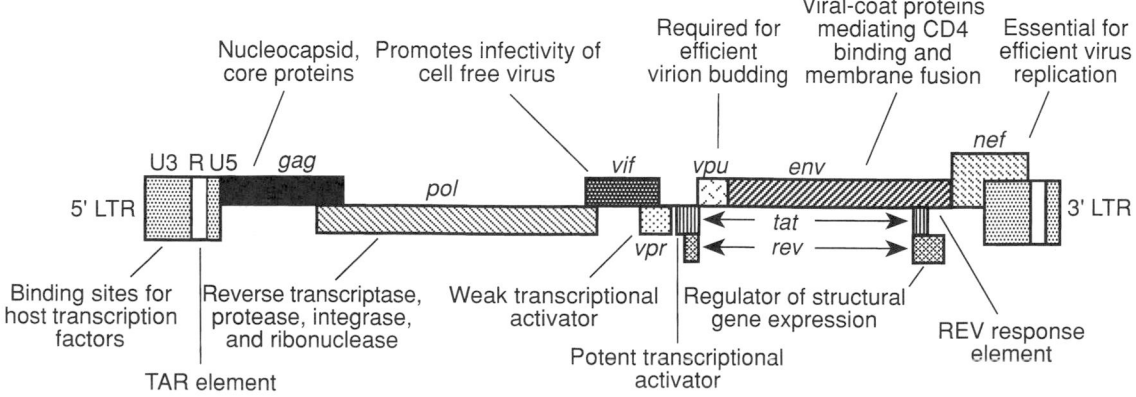

FIG. 4. The genomic organization of HIV. Typical elements of retroviral genomes include the LTRs and genes for core proteins (*gag*), reverse transciptase (*pol*), and the viral envelope (*env*). Genes encoding accessory proteins are also depicted with descriptions of some of their known functions. Adapted with permission from Greene WC. *N Engl J Med* 1991;324:308.

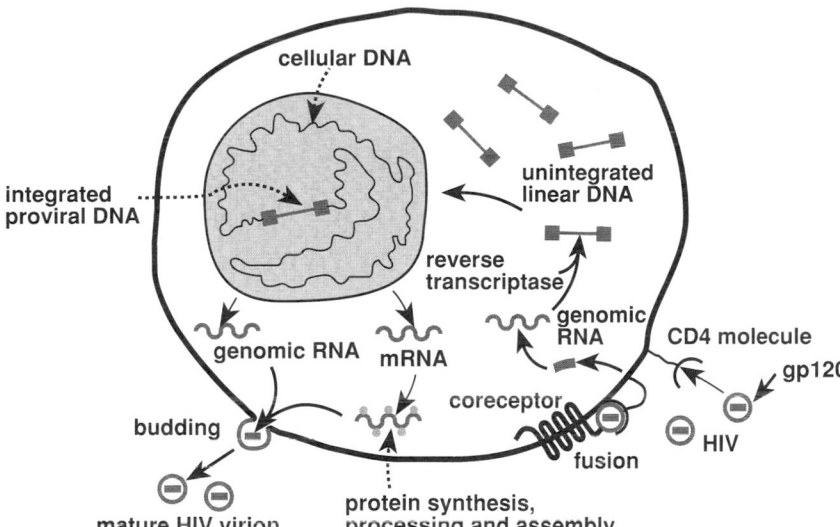

FIG. 5. The life cycle of HIV. Viral attachment to CD4 and an appropriate coreceptor molecule leads to a conformational change that allows fusion to occur. Viral genomic RNA is reverse transcribed, and the resulting DNA is transported to the nucleus, where integration into host DNA occurs. Transcription of viral genes ensues, followed by assembly of viral components and budding through the cell membrane.

HIV Entry

The observation that monoclonal antibodies directed against CD4 inhibited HIV infection of cells *in vitro* led to the discovery that CD4 was the major receptor involved in the binding and entry of HIV into target cells (25–28,34). However, studies involving transfection of human CD4 into nonhuman cells suggested that other coreceptors also were required for efficient entry of the HIV virion (34). The recent discovery of the chemokine receptors as HIV coreceptors has clarified the events required for entry of HIV.

Currently, it is thought that the fusion of HIV with a target cell begins with the interaction between the envelope glycoprotein of the virus and CD4. This interaction induces a conformational change in the viral envelope, allowing binding to a coreceptor molecule (35,36) and exposure of portions of gp41 consisting of a bundle of six helices with three interior regions and three highly conserved hydrophobic grooves. This model is similar to the low-pH–induced conformational change of influenza hemagglutinin that fuses with the plasma membrane (37). After fusion, the HIV nucleoprotein core is released into the cytoplasm, where reverse transcription occurs.

Reverse Transcription

Retroviruses are defined by their unique life cycle, in which the viral RNA genome is reverse transcribed by RT to proviral DNA. Before release of virions from the host cell, viral RT and a host transfer RNA (tRNA) become associated with viral RNA. The host tRNA has a sequence complementary to HIV and is used by RT as a primer, starting at the 5′ R-U5 region of the viral long terminal repeat (LTR), to produce a negative DNA strand. The RNase H activity of RT degrades the 5′ R region and induces the newly synthesized negative strand to rehybridize with the same or another genomic RNA. Reverse transcription continues through the *env*, *pol*, and *gag* genes. Positive strand synthesis begins by replicating the 3′ LTR; another intramolecular jump allows the completion of reverse transcription and the generation of flanking LTRs. The reverse transcription process is inefficient and generates mutations and intermolecular strand switches in the progeny viruses. *In vitro*

assays demonstrate an error rate of one per 6,000 nucleotides and an *in vivo* mutation rate of approximately 1 base per genome per round of replication (38,39). The extent of reverse transcription depends on the state of activation of the target cell; in quiescent CD4+ T cells, reverse transcription is incomplete. Activation of a quiescent cell soon after infection results in the completion of reverse transcription; otherwise, the partially reverse-transcribed HIV genome is degraded (40,41).

Integration

After the completion of reverse transcription, a complex of double-stranded HIV DNA, matrix protein, integrase, and RT from the original infecting virion is present in the cytoplasm (32,42). The p17 matrix protein has at least two nuclear localization sequences, and the Vpr protein also may be involved in the subsequent translocation of the preintegration complex to the nucleus (43).

In the nucleus, HIV integrase removes the last two 3′ nucleotides from both ends of the linear double-stranded DNA provirus (44) and also nonspecifically cuts the host chromosomal DNA to generate a 5′ five-nucleotide overhang. Cellular DNA repair enzymes complete the integration process and fill in the missing nucleotides.

Transcription of Proviral DNA

After integration, and possibly in certain cell types in extrachromosomal circular unintegrated HIV DNA as well, transcription of viral RNA begins. The initiation of transcription occurs in the 5′ LTR

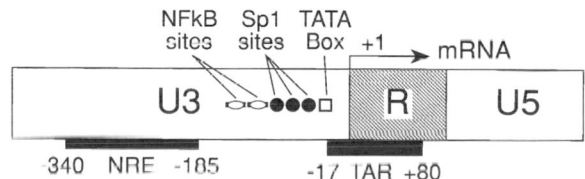

FIG. 6. Transcriptional regulatory elements of the HIV LTR. Adapted with permission from Poli G, Fauci AS. *AIDS Res Hum Retrovir* 1992;8:191.

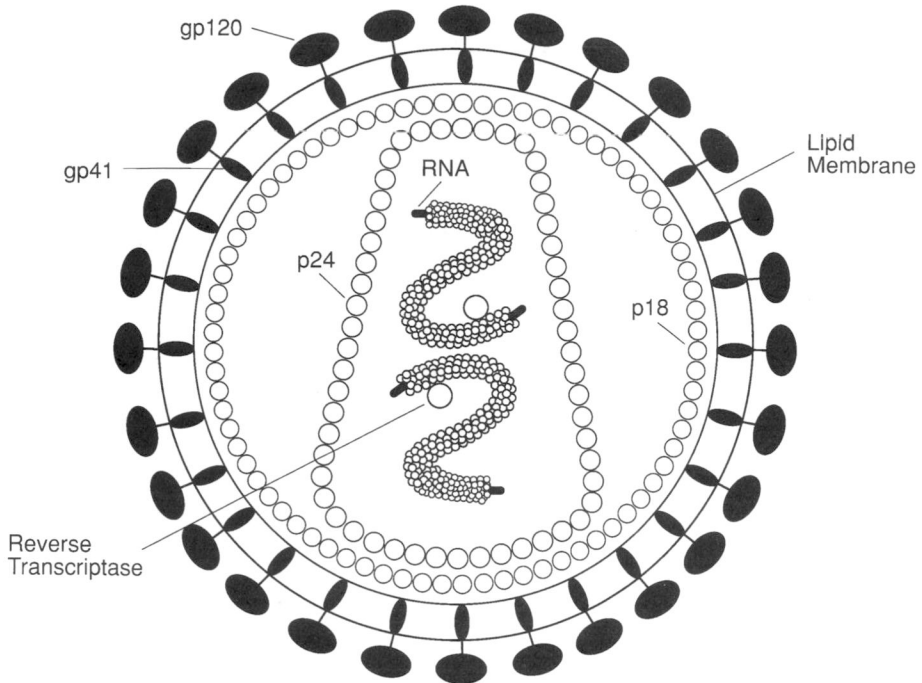

FIG. 7. Organization of the HIV-1 virion.

at the beginning of the R region and terminates in the 3' LTR at the end of the R region. Transcription is controlled by multiple cis- and trans-acting factors derived from both the virus and the host.

The viral regulatory sequences in the LTR (Fig. 6) include a TATA box, which facilitates assembly of transcription initiation complexes (45,46), three Sp-1 sites, and two NF-κB sites. Other sites that bind cellular factors include NF-AT, AP-2, AP-1, HIP-1, and cortisol responsive elements. The NFκB sites bind members of the *rel* oncogene family (47,48) and are important in cellular activation and cytokine modulation of HIV expression (49–51).

The Tat protein binds to the trans-activating response region (TAR) of the LTR (Fig. 6), which leads to a dramatic increase in viral transcription. Viral transcription products can be divided into two classes that comprise over 30 different members. The first class includes unspliced and singly spliced RNAs that contain the Rev-responsive element (RRE) and are dependent on the viral protein Rev to transport these RNAs into the cytoplasm. This class of RNAs encode Gag, Pol, Env, and the regulatory proteins Vif, Vpr, Vpu, and Tat-1. The second class of RNAs encode the multiply spliced species that lack the RRE and include Tat, Rev, and Nef.

Virion Assembly

HIV begins its assembly at the plasma membrane or within intracytoplasmic vacuoles. The Gag p55 protein oligomerizes (52) and is transported to the plasma membrane by the p17 matrix protein. The nucleocapsid domain of p55 causes two copies of HIV genomic RNA to assemble (53). The Gag-Pol polyprotein and a host tRNA^{lys} associate with the matrix RNA and form the mature, cone-shaped viral core (54) (Fig. 7). The viral protease processes multiple viral proteins, and gp160 envelope protein is transported to the surface as noncovalently linked gp120 and gp41. The virion assimilates the gp160 protein as part of the lipid outer layer during budding from the cell.

CELLULAR TARGETS OF HIV INFECTION

CD4+ T-lymphocytes and cells of the monocyte lineage are the principal targets of HIV infection. However, virtually any cell that expresses the CD4 molecule together with an appropriate coreceptor molecule (see section below on HIV Coreceptors) can potentially be infected with HIV. In addition, HIV has been reported to infect *in vitro* a wide range of primary cells and cell lines that may or may not express CD4 or HIV coreceptors (55). These include follicular dendritic cells (FDCs), microglial cells, megakaryocytes, eosinophils, CD8+ T cells, B cells, natural killer (NK) cells, thymus and bone marrow stromal cells, astrocytes, oligodendrocytes, renal epithelial cells, cervical cells, trophoblastic cells, rectal and bowel mucosal cells, and parenchymal cells from a variety of organs such as heart, muscle, liver, lung, salivary gland, eye, testis, prostate, and adrenal gland. However, *in vivo* the only cells unequivocally shown to be infected with HIV are CD4+ T-lymphocytes and cells of the monocyte/macrophage lineage, suggesting that the clinical relevance of *in vitro* infection of other cell types may be marginal.

HIV cellular tropism is described in terms of the ability of certain viral isolates to grow in macrophages or transformed T-cell lines *in vitro*. Isolates that can grow in macrophages and peripheral blood mononuclear cells (PBMCs) but not in T-cell lines are classified as *macrophage (M) tropic*, whereas isolates that can grow in PBMC and T-cell lines but not in macrophages are called *T tropic* (56–58); isolates that can grow in both macrophages and T-cell lines are referred to as *dual tropic*. In addition, certain HIV isolates are termed *syncytium inducing* (SI) because of their ability to induce giant cell, or syncytium, formation in certain T-cell lines *in vitro*, whereas others that lack this ability are referred to as *nonsyncytium inducing (NSI)*. Considerable but incomplete overlap exists between T tropism and the SI phenotype and between M tropism and the NSI phenotype. The viral determinant of cellular tropism maps to the gp120 envelope protein of HIV-1, mostly to the third variable region (V3 loop) (59–68), which is also the major determinant for coreceptor usage (69) (see section below on HIV Coreceptors).

Changes in viral phenotype have been observed at different stages of HIV infection. M-tropic/NSI viruses are found at the time of initial infection and at most stages of infection (70,71). In approximately 50% of HIV-infected individuals, the appearance of T-tropic/SI HIV isolates late in the course of disease heralds accelerated CD4+ T-cell decline and clinical disease progression (72–76). The transition from an NSI to SI virus may occur by mutation of only a few amino acid residues predominantly in the envelope V3 loop (59–65,68); given the high error rate of RT and the rapid kinetics of HIV replication, the surprising failure of such mutants to emerge until late in the disease process indicates a change in the selective advantage of such a mutation during the course of disease progression. The nature of such a selective advantage is currently unknown; however, it may relate to the ability of SI viruses to use an expanded repertoire of coreceptor molecules for cellular entry (see sections below on HIV Coreceptors and Viral Sequence Diversity).

HIV CORECEPTORS

CD4 was identified as the major receptor for HIV fusion and entry in 1984 (25–28). Transfection of CD4 into CD4- human cells rendered them infectable with HIV (34); however, transfection of human CD4 into murine cell lines did not render these cells susceptible to HIV infection despite gp120 binding to CD4, suggesting that other factor(s) were necessary for HIV fusion and entry (77,78). These additional factors remained elusive for many years.

In late 1995 and early 1996, a series of papers were published that altered our understanding of how HIV enters a target cell. The first report by Cocchi and co-workers (79) identified the β-chemokines, macrophage inflammatory protein (MIP)-1α, MIP-1β, and RANTES (regulated on activation, normal T cell expressed and secreted), as major components of CD8+ T cell–derived HIV suppressor factors (see section below on Immune Responses). They observed that these chemokines in combination could inhibit the infection of activated CD4+ T cells by certain strains of HIV-1, HIV-2, and simian immunodeficiency virus (SIV). Of note, these β-chemokines did not block infection with HIV-IIIB, the prototypic T-cell line–adapted strain of HIV. Subsequently, the isolation of a gene from a HeLa cell mRNA library was described whose expression allowed gp160-mediated cell fusion in the presence of CD4 (80,81). The protein, called fusin (later renamed CXCR4), is a seven-transmembrane chemokine receptor. This receptor, together with CD4, was required for T-tropic envelope fusion, but was not used by M-tropic strains. The natural ligand for CXCR4 was later determined to be stromal cell–derived factor (SDF)-1 (82,83) (Fig. 8).

In a separate line of research, Paxton and co-workers were studying a population of individuals who had been multiply exposed to HIV-infected partners but remained uninfected (84). They identified two subjects whose CD4+ T cells were refractory to infection with M-tropic strains of HIV but were easily infectable with T-tropic cell-line adapted strains. In addition, cells from these individuals produced high levels of MIP-1α, MIP-1β, and RANTES, the same chemokines previously identified as suppressors of HIV infection. Subsequently, a new β-chemokine receptor, CC chemokine receptor (CCR)-5, was identified: the natural ligands that bind to this receptor were shown to be MIP-1α, MIP-1β, and RANTES (85–87). In light of the previous work showing that the CCR5 ligands inhibit cellular entry of M-tropic strains of HIV, the obvious question that arose was whether CCR5 might function as a coreceptor for such strains. A series of five papers simultaneously showed this to be the case (88–92) (Fig. 8). Other chemokine receptors, including CCR1, CCR2b, and CCR3, also were identified in these reports as potential coreceptors for certain HIV strains. Recently, other orphan receptors of the chemokine receptor class have been shown to be potential HIV coreceptors (93–95).

With very few exceptions, and even across HIV clades, primary M-tropic HIV isolates use CCR5 for entry. Primary T-tropic HIV isolates use both CCR5 and CXCR4, and T-cell line–adapted strains such as IIIB use CXCR4 exclusively (96,97). An analysis of HIV tropism during disease progression showed that virus isolation from individuals with early-stage HIV disease yielded almost exclusively M-tropic viruses that use CCR5. With disease progression, the spec-

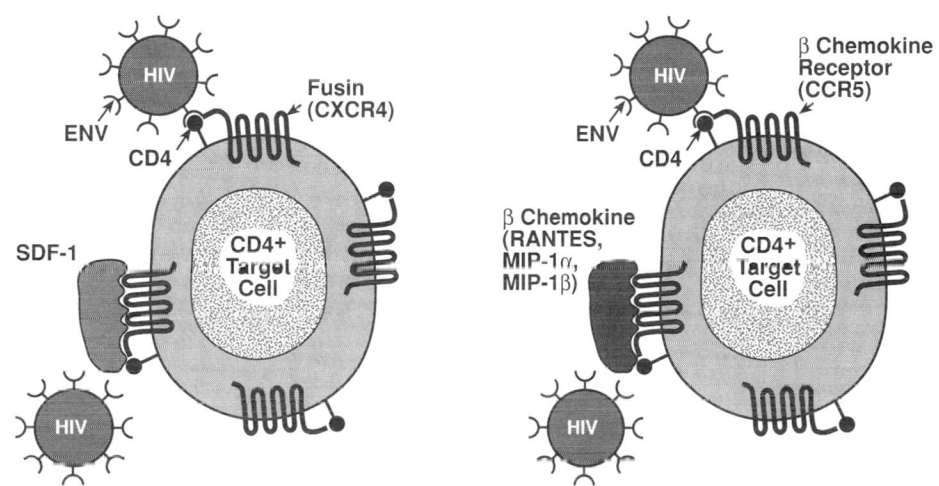

T Cell Line-Tropic Strain of HIV-1   **Macrophage-Tropic Strain of HIV-1**

FIG. 8. Model of coreceptor (CCR5 and CXCR4) usage and inhibition of HIV binding by coreceptor ligands. Entry of M-tropic strains of HIV is blocked by the CCR5 ligands MIP-1α, MIP-1β, and RANTES. Entry of T-tropic strains is blocked by the CXCR4 ligand SDF-1. Adapted with permission from Fauci AS. *Nature* 1996;384:529.

trum of coreceptor usage by HIV expands to include CCR2b and CCR3, and finally, CXCR4 (98). Of note is the fact that it is rare for a primary viral isolate to lose the ability to use CCR5 (98).

The identification of CCR5 as the predominant coreceptor for M-tropic strains of HIV and the observation that M-tropic strains but not T-tropic strains were responsible for most new infections with HIV set the stage for the identification of the genetic defect in a subset of exposed, uninfected subjects whose cells were uninfectable with M-tropic virus *in vitro*. Two exposed, uninfected individuals were shown to be homozygous for identical 32–base pair (bp) deletions in the *CCR5* gene (*CCR5-Δ32*), resulting in a truncated version of the receptor that was not expressed at the cell surface (99). Large-scale screenings for this deletion in HIV-uninfected populations found that approximately 20% of white individuals of northern and western European background were heterozygous for the mutation and 1% were homozygous (100–103). Among HIV-infected whites, no subjects homozygous for the 32-bp deletion were initially identified, suggesting complete protection from infection (100–103); however, rare cases of infection of homozygous individuals subsequently have been reported (104–106). Although *CCR5-Δ32* heterozygotes are not protected against HIV infection, they are afforded a modest degree of protection against disease progression and are overrepresented among cohorts of long-term nonprogressors (see section below on Long-Term Nonprogressors). The mechanism of delayed disease progression in *CCR5-Δ32* heterozygotes may involve a lower viral load "set point" after acute HIV infection, and a slower rate of CD4+ T-cell depletion (102). These effects may be due to a decrease in expression of CCR5 on CD4+ cells from *CCR5-Δ32* heterozygotes (107,108) or an inhibitory transdominant activity of the 32-bp deleted CCR5 protein (G. Scala et al., unpublished data). The *CCR5-Δ32* allele has not been found in African, Asian, or Indian populations, and no immunologic abnormalities have been identified in subjects who carry two copies of the defective *CCR5* gene.

Studies recently have begun to delineate the interactions between the HIV envelope, CD4, and the chemokine receptors (35,36). In this regard, MIP-1α, MIP-1β, and RANTES appear to block infection with M-tropic strains of HIV by a competitive physical mechanism (Fig. 8) (89). Signaling through CCR5 by the chemokines is not necessary for inhibition of viral entry (109–111), although it may influence postentry events in the viral life cycle (A. Kinter and A.S. Fauci, unpublished data).

The interaction between T-tropic HIV envelope and its coreceptors is similar in many respects to the interaction between M-tropic HIV envelope and its coreceptors; however, differences exist that may be important in the evolution of these viruses with disease progression. T-tropic gp120 has been demonstrated by immunoprecipitation to physically interact with CD4 and CXCR4 (112). The natural ligand for CXCR4, SDF-1, inhibits T-tropic viral infection via CXCR4 with no effect on M-tropic viruses (Fig. 8) (82,83). In addition, a monoclonal antibody against CXCR4 has been demonstrated to inhibit infection with T-tropic viral strains, and gp120 from T-tropic HIV blocks the binding of this antibody to CXCR4 (113,114). Of note, certain HIV-2 and T-cell line–adapted HIV-1 viruses can directly use CXCR4 for entry in the absence of CD4 (114).

Viral envelope gp120 binding to CD4 and a coreceptor molecule likely occurs by one of two different mechanisms. In the case of CCR5, either the binding of gp120 to CD4 increases the avidity of binding to neighboring CCR5 molecules [an avidity that in the absence of CD4 would be very low (36)], or the binding to CD4

induces a conformational change in gp120 that increases its affinity for CCR5 (35). T-tropic HIV isolates derived from patients are relatively inefficient at infecting cells with low levels of CD4, suggesting a strong dependence on CD4 for infection. Adaptation of T-tropic strains of HIV for growth in T-cell lines is associated with an increase in the affinity of the viral envelope for CD4 (115). M-tropic viruses derived from patients' efficiently infected cells with low levels of CD4, suggesting a lesser dependence on CD4 for infection (115). These observations suggest that the physical interaction between gp160 and CD4 and CCR5 or CXCR4 may be similar, although differences are seen in the affinities of interaction between the various components.

The regions of CCR5, CXCR4, and gp120 that are important for binding have been only partially identified. Multiple strains of HIV-1, HIV-2, and SIV can bind to CCR5 (36,91,97,116,117), but no sequence has been identified that defines a common binding motif. In fact, different strains of virus use different CCR5 domains for binding. The V3 loop of gp120 is an important determinant of binding to CXCR4 and CCR5 and at least partially determines M versus T tropism (69,84,91). Various deletions within gp120 have highlighted the important regions involved in binding to the coreceptors. Deletion of the first and second variable regions of gp120 does not interfere with binding to CCR5 (35); however, deletion of the V3 loop eliminates binding to CCR5 (35,36). Antibodies directed against the V3 loop abolish the binding of gp120 to CCR5; however, two antibodies that neutralize HIV infectivity but do not bind to the V3 region of gp120 also inhibit viral binding (35,36). Together, these data suggest that multiple sites may exist within gp120 that are important for binding to CCR5; additionally, the binding of one region may influence interactions in other domains.

In order to further define the domains of CCR5 used in gp120 binding, chimeras between human CCR5 and murine CCR5 or human CCR2 have been developed. The results of these studies have not identified a specific region or domain necessary for fusion and entry, but have demonstrated that these sites are complex and discontinuous (109,118–120), as has been observed previously for IL-8 binding to CXCR1 (121,122).

T-tropic strains of SIV also use CCR5 for entry (97,117,120). Before the identification of the chemokine coreceptors, it was known that both M- and T-tropic SIV entered macrophages with equal efficiency, yet only M-tropic strains replicated efficiently (123). M-tropic strains of SIV preferentially use the N-terminus of CCR5, whereas T-tropic strains depend on the second extracellular loop (120).

HIV coreceptor usage in macrophages appears to be more complex than that in CD4+ T cells. Studies of macrophages from individuals homozygous for *CCR5-Δ32* demonstrated that these cells were not infectable with M-tropic strains of HIV (124,125), suggesting that CCR5 is essential for M-tropic viral entry into macrophages as well as CD4+ T cells. However, HIV infection of macrophages cannot be blocked with the β-chemokine ligands of CCR5 (89,126), suggesting an alternate usage of CCR5 or the usage of other coreceptors. The inability of T-tropic strains of HIV to establish infection in macrophages has been demonstrated to be both a pre- and postfusion phenomenon (123,127). The relative inability of T-tropic viruses to enter blood monocytes and cultured mature macrophages is curious, given that both express mRNA for CXCR4 and have surface expression of the CXCR4 protein (83,128). Finally, microglia (brain macrophages) have been demonstrated to express both CCR5 and CCR3, and infection by certain strains of HIV is potently inhibited by eotaxin, a CCR3 ligand (129).

Dendritic cells (DCs) are likely responsible for initiating HIV infection by carrying virus from the site of exposure to draining lymphoid organs, where CD4+ T cells become infected and virus disseminates (see section below on HIV Infection and the Development of HIV Disease) (130). Tissue DCs and certain preparations of blood DCs express CD4 and multiple chemokine receptors, including CCR5, CCR3, CCR2b, and CCR1 (131) (A. Rubbert et al., unpublished data). Most, but not all, preparations of DCs are infectable with M- and T-tropic strains of HIV, although there is disagreement regarding the productivity of infection. Initial studies using mature DCs demonstrated that infection with T-tropic strains was blocked by SDF-1 and infection with M-tropic strains was blocked by MIP-1α, MIP-1β, and RANTES. DCs from individuals homozygous for the 32-bp deletion in CCR5 were infectable with T-tropic but not M-tropic strains of HIV (131). Follow-up studies using immature DCs, which resemble Langerhans' cells (LCs; DCs that reside in the epidermis), demonstrated that CCR3 also could be used by certain strains of HIV for entry. In addition, an alternative non-CXCR4, SDF-1–sensitive receptor could be used by both T- and M-tropic strains of HIV. Immature DCs from individuals homozygous for the 32-bp CCR5 deletion can be infected not only with T-tropic strains of HIV, but also with strains of HIV that appear to be CCR5 dependent in other cells (A. Rubbert et al., unpublished data). Thus, the expression of multiple chemokine receptors by these cells may provide a variety of pathways that HIV can exploit in order to gain entry.

VIRAL DYNAMICS

The development of sensitive, quantitative assays for plasma viremia has enabled investigators to better understand the dynamics of viral replication during the course of HIV infection. Measures of viral load, including plasma viremia, remain relatively constant in a given patient over a period of weeks (132–135). This steady state is due to an equilibrium between production and clearance of virus. The use of new antiretroviral agents that target the HIV-1 protease enzyme and can inhibit viral replication by an average of 99% allows for perturbation of the viral load steady state and estimation of the in vivo dynamics of HIV infection. Because antiretroviral agents block de novo infection of cells, frequent measurement of plasma viremia after administration of these agents yields a decay curve that reflects the clearance rate of virions from plasma as well as the elimination rate of HIV-producing cells. Using different drugs, studies from two groups found the half-life of plasma virus to be approximately 2 days (136,137). In a follow-up study that included more frequent measurements of plasma viremia after drug administration, Perelson and co-workers estimated the half-life of plasma virus to be 5.8 hours (138), although further analyses suggest that the half-life may be even shorter. Because virus production is proportional to the number of productively infected cells and the number of virions produced per cell, these data imply that the steady-state level of plasma viremia is fueled by rapid and continuous infection of target cells. In fact, the average production of HIV virions was estimated to be nearly 10^{10} virions per day, the average generation time of HIV in vivo (i.e., the time from virion release from an infected cell to the time of virus production from a cell infected by the first virion) was approximately 2.6 days, and the half-life of productively infected cells was about 1.6 days (138). Although a substantial number of assumptions are built into the mathematical formulae used to derive these estimates, the clear conclusion of these data is that the steady-state level of plasma viremia is dependent on viral replication from a pool of newly infected cells that is rapidly turning over.

The decay curve of plasma viremia during potent antiretroviral therapy is actually biphasic. The estimates of half-life discussed above were derived from the rapid first phase of decay that occurs over the first week of therapy. Subsequently, the decay curve of plasma viremia becomes significantly less steep, indicating the existence of secondary sources of plasma viremia with a longer half-life. Based on the observed exponential decay during therapy of 99% of plasma viremia derived from newly infected lymphocytes, secondary sources of viremia must contribute only about 1% to steady-state pretreatment levels of plasma viremia. The half-life of the secondary sources of plasma viremia has been estimated to be approximately 14 days; these sources may include long-lived HIV-infected cells (i.e., macrophages or dendritic cells), latently infected cells that become activated, or the release of trapped virions from the surface of the FDC network in lymphoid tissue (139). Although these secondary sources of viremia may account for only a small fraction of the steady-state level of plasma viremia, they nonetheless may be major contributors to disease pathogenesis. In this regard, it is likely that virions trapped on the surface of FDCs are infectious (140) and may facilitate the infection of activated CD4+ T cells trafficking through germinal centers (see section below on Lymphoid Tissue in the Pathogenesis of HIV Disease). Without such facilitation, the primary source of plasma viremia (newly infected T cells in a rapid state of turnover) might be quantitatively far smaller.

Estimation of the half-life of the secondary source of viremia allows for a minimum estimate of the time necessary for elimination of HIV with a therapeutic regimen able to completely inhibit HIV replication; one such estimate is 2.3 to 3.1 years (139), although other estimates are considerably longer (T-W. Chun and A.S. Fauci, unpublished data). Mathematical modeling of viral dynamics during treatment with therapeutic regimens that do not completely suppress viral replication leads to the prediction that suppression of plasma viremia should be quite transient due to de novo infections of an increased population of uninfected target cells. The prolonged suppression of viremia that occurs during highly active antiretroviral therapy (HAART) may be explained by the immune response against HIV, depletion of uninfected target cells by mechanisms other than direct infection or differential effects of the drugs used on different cell types such that viral replication is eliminated in some tissue compartments but not in others (141). The existence of a latently infected and inducible population of resting CD4+ T cells as well as evidence of persistent virus replication in individuals receiving HAART with levels of plasma viremia that are below the limits of detectability indicate that estimates of durations of therapy required for HIV eradication are somewhat premature (T-W. Chun and A.S. Fauci, unpublished data).

The increases in CD4+ T-cell counts that occur during potent antiretroviral therapy can be modeled in order to obtain an estimate of CD4+ T-cell turnover at steady state. Estimates that approximately 2×10^9 CD4+ T cells are destroyed and replenished each day (136,137) are likely flawed for a number of reasons. The assumption that the increases in CD4+ T-cell counts during therapy reflect production of new cells from progenitor cells or proliferation of mature cells ignores the possibility that cells may be trafficking from lymphoid organs into the periphery. The large extrapolation between sampling the peripheral blood CD4+ T-cell count and the total body CD4+ T-cell count further weakens assumptions regarding the origin of the increased number of circulating CD4+

T cells (142). Failure to repair damage to the T-cell repertoire during therapy with interleukin (IL)-2 plus antiretroviral agents argues against repopulation via differentiation of stem cells (143). Instead, proliferation of mature cells or trafficking of cells into peripheral blood are more likely explanations.

Another assay of CD4+ T-cell turnover measures telomeric terminal restriction fragment (TRF) length, a marker of cellular replicative history. After each round of cell division, telomeric sequence is lost, eventually leading to replicative senescence. Increased turnover within the CD4+ T-cell pool would be expected to result in shortening of the TRF length over time; however, measurement of TRF length in CD4+ T cells from HIV-infected patients and uninfected controls revealed no change over time in TRF length in either group (144). In another study, TRF lengths were compared in CD4+ T cells from monozygotic twins discordant for HIV infection. In that study, TRF lengths were actually greater in the HIV-infected twins compared with their uninfected siblings; this finding could not be explained by differences in telomerase activity (an enzyme that adds hexanucleotide telomeric repeats to chromosomes) or differences in numbers of CD4+ naive cells (which have shorter replicative histories and therefore longer telomeres compared with memory cells) between the groups (145). Overall, current data do not suggest increased turnover of CD4+ T cells during HIV infection. The relative contributions of lymphocyte redistribution and peripheral expansion of lymphocytes to the observed increases in CD4+ T-cell counts during antiretroviral therapy remain to be determined.

VIRAL SEQUENCE DIVERSITY

Examination of the genetic diversity of HIV in patients yields important information about the epidemiology of the HIV epidemic, the dynamics of viral replication, the pressure exerted by the host immune response or by antiretroviral therapy, and the compartmentalization of viral replication within the host. Furthermore, studies of HIV genetic diversity have implications for the development of vaccines as well as strategies to prevent and overcome drug resistance.

A high degree of HIV sequence diversity within an infected host (intrahost variation) and within populations of infected individuals (interhost variation) has been reported by many groups (146–153). Analysis of interhost sequence variation is particularly useful in epidemiologic studies of viral transmission within and between populations, and analysis of intrahost sequence variation can yield valuable insight into the complex interactions between host and virus over time. The biochemical mechanism responsible for the observed sequence diversity is the error-prone viral RT (38,39). The rapid dynamics of HIV replication also contribute directly to HIV sequence diversity due to the enormous number of generations of viral replication in an infected individual. Host factors also may exert selective pressure on the evolution of viral diversity by means of cell-mediated and humoral immune responses. Host factors involved in viral cell tropism (i.e., cell- and tissue-specific regulation of coreceptor usage) also help to shape viral diversity. Some investigators discount the potential role of selective pressure in determining viral diversity and invoke mechanisms such as mutation-driven evolution (154), neutral evolution (155), and chance stimulation of cells harboring variant proviruses (156,157). However, early studies showing that the greatest degree of sequence diversity is concentrated within the HIV envelope gene (148,152,158) suggested that the generation of sequence diversity was not a neutral or chance event.

The degree to which selective pressures drive the evolution of HIV sequence diversity can be assessed by analysis of synonymous (amino acid–preserving) and nonsynonymous (amino acid–changing) mutations. Were sequence variation a purely random process driven entirely by an error-prone polymerase and a large number of replication cycles, then a similar number of synonymous (ds) and nonsynonymous (dn) mutations would result. However, many authors have observed high ratios of nonsynonymous to synonymous mutations, strongly suggesting the existence of dominant host selection pressures that result in viral escape mutants (159). These results are consistent with the hypothesis that selective pressure for viral diversification due to viral-specific immune responses is proportional to the intactness of the immune system; however, the data also may be a reflection of a plateau in adaptation by the virus for various cell tropisms during disease progression. This latter possibility is tenable in light of the observed "bottleneck" in viral transmission in which homogeneous V3 sequences encoding NSI viruses are selected (70,71), followed by diversification toward multiple coreceptor usage and hence, multiple cell tropisms (96,98,116).

Whether viral diversification is driven by attempts to escape from host immune responses or antiviral drug pressure (160–162), or by a change in coreceptor usage (61,98,163), any selective advantage gained by a virus with a particular mutation will have a strong impact on the subsequent generation of viral genomes (164). The observed patterns of HIV sequence diversity argue against a purely neutral mechanism (165). Models of disease pathogenesis that invoke the appearance of a specific viral mutation (e.g., appearance of SI variants) are also difficult to support. As previously discussed (see section above on Cellular Targets of HIV Infection), the transition from an NSI to an SI virus may occur by mutation of only a few amino acid residues in the V3 loop of the viral envelope. Given the error rate of viral RT and the rapid dynamics of viral replication, the failure of such mutants to emerge until late in the disease process indicates a change in the selective advantage of such a mutation during the course of disease progression. Because SI variants are able to use a broader range of entry coreceptors (e.g., CXCR4) compared with NSI viruses, it is possible that SI variants emerge in response to high levels of β-chemokines, which block cellular entry of viruses that use CCR5 (i.e., predominantly NSI viruses) (96,98,163). Emergence of SI variants also may represent an escape from neutralizing antibodies, which may interfere with the interaction between the HIV envelope and CCR5 (35,36). The situation is no doubt more complex, and multiple host factors as well as regulatory aspects of coreceptor expression in different tissue compartments likely determine the environment in which selection for NSI or SI variants is made (107,166,167).

A number of studies suggest that effective host immune responses result in a higher degree of sequence diversity, and slower rates of disease progression. Analysis of genetic diversity of proviral quasispecies (genetically distinct HIV sequences within an individual) by heteroduplex mobility assay suggested that a higher degree of viral sequence diversity was associated with a slower rate of CD4+ T-cell decline, whereas a lower degree of viral sequence diversity, perhaps reflective of the relative inability to exert immune pressure on the virus, was associated with a more rapid rate of CD4+ T-cell depletion (168). Lukashov and co-workers studied sequence diversity of viral RNA in the sera of patients obtained at seroconversion and 5 years later. Nonsynonymous mutations in the envelope V3 region were more common among nonprogressors compared with progressors (0.011 ± 0.001 versus 0.007 ± 0.001 nonsynonymous mutations per site per year), whereas the number of synonymous mutations per site per year was no different between progressors and nonprogressors. Thus, the ratio of nonsynonymous to synonymous mutations, a reflection of the selective pressure exerted by the host immune response, was significantly higher in nonprogressors (2.86 versus 1.61) (169). Similar results were obtained by others who found that increasing diversity in proviral V3-V5 and C1-C3 envelope sequences correlated with slower disease progression (170,171). In one of these studies, high frequencies of cytolytic T-cell (CTL) precursors were associated with slower progression, and viral mutations within relevant HLA class I restricted epitopes occurred frequently in these slow progressors (170). The lesser degree of sequence diversity generated in rapid progressors appeared to be a consequence of the low frequency of CTL precursors and, therefore, a relative inability to exert immune pressure on the virus.

An alternative view of the relationship between viral sequence heterogeneity and disease progression derives from the antigenic diversity threshold theory. This view holds that over time, increasing viral sequence diversity weakens immune control over virus replication, leading to high viral load and disease progression (172–174). According to this theory, rapid progressors have a low sequence diversity threshold. The inability of the immune responses of rapid progressors to exert selective pressure on viral replication allows for rapid increases in viral load without the need for immune escape mutations. The higher diversity threshold presumed to exist in slow progressors is related to a higher degree of plasticity of immune responses in these individuals. Immune responses lower viral load and select for escape mutants; however, the host is able to generate waves of secondary immune responses that are able to partially control the emergent viral quasispecies. If the virus can "lead" the host immune response farther and farther away from immunodominant epitopes while retaining a reasonable degree of fitness, a certain diversity threshold is surpassed, and the virus overcomes the ability of the host to recruit any further effective immune response (173). HIV disease is thus viewed as a Darwinian struggle between the host's ability to generate effective immune responses against a continuously mutating target and the virus' ability to escape immune responses without suffering a lethal blow to its replicative fitness. This theory is difficult to test experimentally, although some support can be found in data suggesting that CTL responses of limited clonotypic scope are associated with rapid progression after primary HIV infection (175).

A major caveat associated with studies of viral sequence diversity relates to compartmentalization of viral replication and immune responses. Measurement of viral sequence diversity in proviruses from PBMC yields a different result compared with sequence diversity in viral RNA from plasma or PBMCs (176–178); even within a microenvironment, for example, from one splenic white pulp to another, diversity can be striking (156,157). Analysis of viral sequence diversity in HIV RNA from plasma and in HIV DNA from PBMCs of the same patients over time showed that sequences that initially appeared in plasma eventually became the predominant PBMC proviral sequences (176). This finding suggested that PBMC proviral sequences were archival, reflecting quasispecies that had previously been actively replicated and sampled in plasma (176,177). Analysis of viral sequence diversity in various tissues obtained at autopsy as well as in PBMCs and plasma demonstrated that quasispecies from lymph node, bone marrow, and plasma, but not PBMCs, were related

(179). These data support the concept that lymphoid tissue and bone marrow are important sites of active viral replication that are reflected in plasma viremia.

Perhaps the clearest evidence for compartmentalization of viral quasispecies evolution is provided by analysis of sequences derived from central nervous system (CNS) tissue. Comparison of HIV LTR, *pol*, and *env* sequences from the same individuals shows distinct clustering of sequences derived from the CNS compared with sequences derived from other anatomic compartments (179–184). Thus, selective pressures appear to be quite different in the CNS compared with lymphoid tissue or bone marrow. Similar evidence of compartmentalization of viral replication has been found in lungs (185) and genital secretions (186) as well. These findings highlight the likelihood that sequence diversity in each microenvironment evolves in the context of selective pressures. In the CNS, selective pressure may exist predominantly for expanded coreceptor usage (129), whereas selective pressure in the lungs may involve a combination of selection for strains capable of infecting alveolar macrophages as well as evading systemic and local immune responses.

HIV INFECTION AND THE DEVELOPMENT OF HIV DISEASE

Primary Infection

Primary infection with HIV is followed by a series of events including rapid dissemination of virus throughout the body and the subsequent induction of immune responses that partially control viral replication (187). The events that occur during primary HIV infection involve both viral and host factors and are important in determining the course of HIV disease. Depending on the route of exposure, the mechanisms of initial infection may vary, although there are no obvious differences in disease manifestations in individuals infected by blood-borne versus mucosal routes. This suggests that even if the initial target cells of HIV infection are different, the subsequent rounds of viral spread occur in similar cells with a similar outcome. HIV introduced directly into the bloodstream (i.e., by transfusion, maternal-to-fetal transmission, or injection drug use with contaminated needles) is probably cleared from the circulation by the reticuloendothelial system of the spleen, liver, and lungs. However, lymphoid tissues in these regions become infected, leading to continued HIV replication, a burst of viremia, and spread of the virus to other lymphoid organs.

It remains unclear which cell type in the blood, lymphoid tissue, spleen, or mucosa is the first to actually become infected with HIV; however, studies during chronic HIV infection indicate that the major reservoir of HIV is contained within the CD4+ T-cell population (188). In studies of macaques exposed to SIV intravaginally, bone marrow–derived DCs in the vaginal mucosa are the first cells to contain SIV DNA, which is detectable 2 days after exposure. In subsequent examinations of lymphoid organs, the pattern of appearance and spread of SIV mirrored the course that DCs take upon migrating from peripheral tissues to lymphoid organs (189). DCs function by binding antigens in the peripheral tissues, processing them into peptides that are associated with major histocompatibility complex (MHC) antigens, migrating to lymphoid organs via afferent lymphatics into the paracortical regions, and activating T cells (see Chapter 16). DCs can retain infectious virus on their surface for extended periods of time (190). Thus, their role in the initiation of HIV infection likely includes capturing virions at sites of entry, carrying HIV to the paracortical regions of lymphoid organs, and delivering virus to CD4+ T cells that become activated through their interaction with DCs (Fig. 9).

The precise nature of the early events during primary HIV and SIV infection that lead to viral replication in lymphoid tissue have not been elucidated. DCs express low levels of CD4, and it is generally agreed that these cells can be infected by HIV only at a low level (see section below on Immune Dysfunction Caused by HIV Infection). *In vitro* studies have demonstrated that DCs and CD4+ T cells form conjugates and that active viral replication takes place in these conjugates (191). Similar conjugates of DCs and CD4+ T cells containing HIV antigen have been identified *in vivo* in tonsil biopsy specimens from individuals infected with HIV (192), in the peripheral blood at low quantities (190), and in the submucosal tissue after vaginal exposure of SIV (189). It is likely that DCs carry HIV from tissues in which the initial rounds of viral replication occur to the regional lymph nodes, where CD4+ T cells become infected after contact with DCs. This leads to subsequent rounds of virus replication and spread in the absence of HIV-specific immune responses.

Immune Response and Downregulation of HIV Replication

Vigorous anti-HIV responses can be detected soon after primary infection and are very likely involved in the downregulation and substantial but incomplete clearance of circulating virus (193–197). These responses can be categorized as HIV-specific antibody responses, HIV-specific cell-mediated cytotoxicity, and cytokine responses (Fig. 10). The relative role of humoral versus cellular immunity in the downregulation of viral replication is a subject of considerable debate; however, both appear to be important.

The primary immune response to HIV is characterized by the appearance of high titers of HIV-specific antibodies, which are first observed at the time of the peak of plasma viremia or soon thereafter (195,198). Interestingly, this initial antibody response does not include measurable amounts of neutralizing antibody (196,197). However, this lack of neutralizing activity should not be construed to indicate that the primary antibody response is not important in downregulating viral replication. The initial antibodies produced after HIV infection may downregulate HIV replication and plasma viremia through complement-mediated lysis, antibody-dependent cellular cytotoxicity (ADCC), clearance of the virus by complement receptor–dependent trapping in the FDC network of lymphoid tissue germinal centers (199), or in the reticuloendothelial system (196,197,200,201) (Fig. 11A). Such a scenario has been observed in the macaque model of SIV infection, in which the decline in SIV antigenemia correlates with the appearance of complement-fixing antibodies and viral trapping in FDC networks in lymphoid tissue (200,202,203). Neutralizing antibodies typically appear during the transition from the acute phase to the chronic, clinically latent phase of HIV disease (197,204,205). Interestingly, the neutralizing antibodies detected in HIV-infected individuals react strongly with laboratory adapted or T-tropic isolates but less efficiently if at all with autologous virus or M-tropic primary isolates (see section below on Immune Responses).

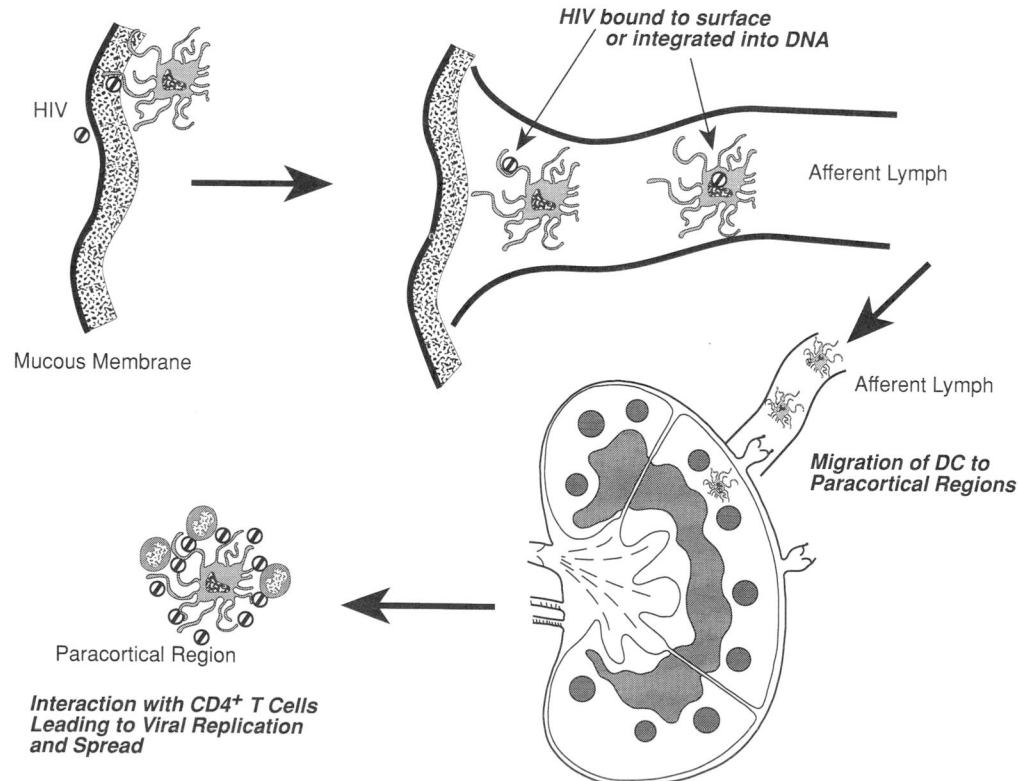

FIG. 9. The role of DCs in the initiation of HIV replication. DCs at the site of exposure transport HIV to the paracortical regions of draining lymphoid tissues, leading to infection of CD4+ T cells. Reprinted with permission from Weissman D, Fauci AS. *Clin Microbiol Rev* 1997;10:358.

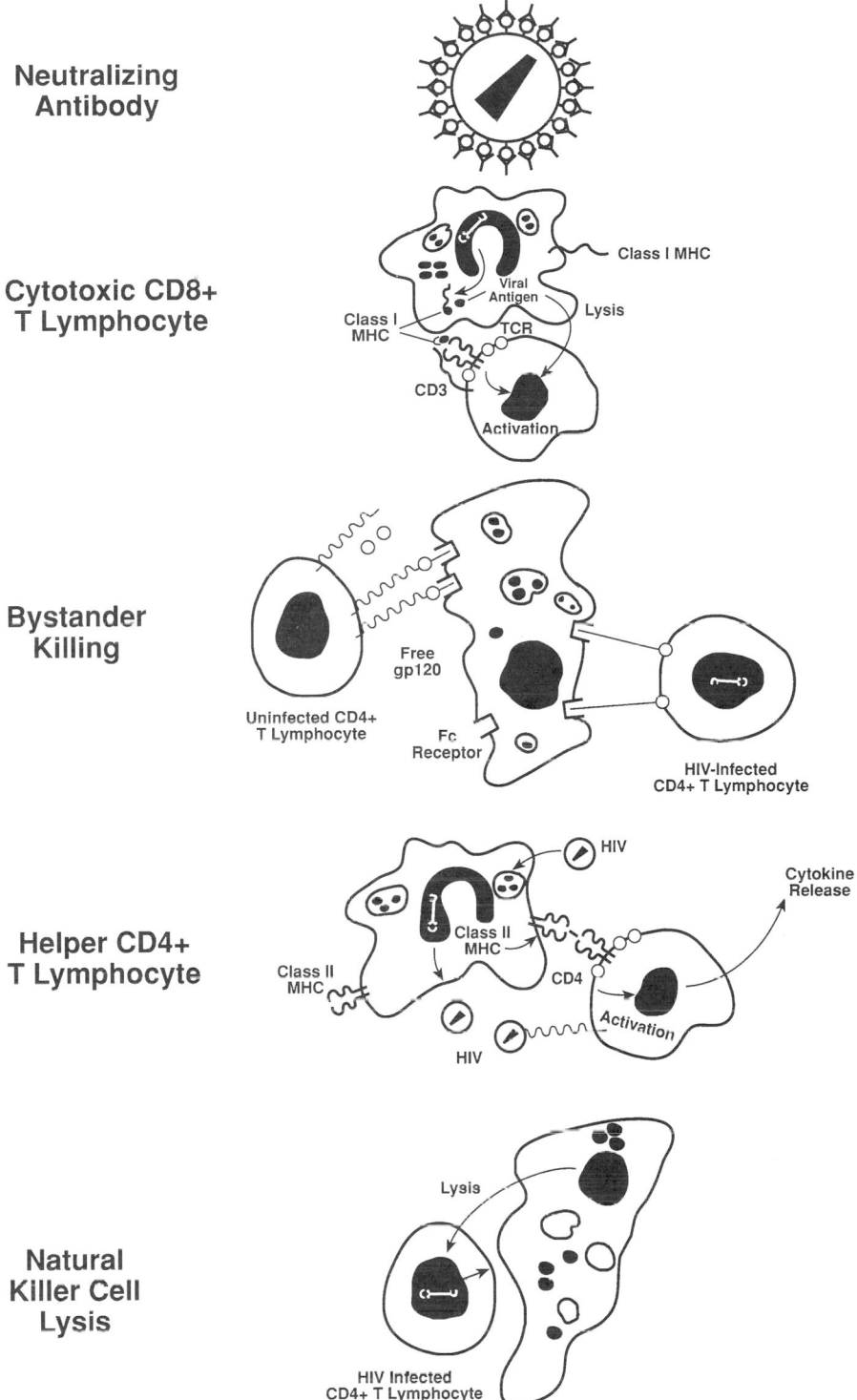

Neutralizing Antibody

Cytotoxic CD8+ T Lymphocyte

Bystander Killing

Helper CD4+ T Lymphocyte

Natural Killer Cell Lysis

FIG. 10. Possible mechanisms of down-regulation of HIV replication by immune responses. Neutralizing antibodies bind to virion components and prevent attachment to target cells. Classical CD8+ cytotoxic T-lymphocytes recognize viral determinants on infected cells in the context of MHC class I presentation and are able to directly lyse these cells. ADCC results not only in Fc receptor–mediated elimination of infected cells, but also in elimination of uninfected cells that are coated by HIV gp120 and antibody. Recognition by CD4+ T cells of viral determinants on the surface of infected cells occurs in the context of MHC class II presentation. The release of cytokines may in part control viral replication. NK cells also may directly lyse HIV-infected cells. Reprinted with permission from Fauci AS, Lane HC. Human immunodeficiency virus (HIV) disease: AIDS and related disorders. In: Fauci AS, et al., eds. *Harrison's Principles of Internal Medicine*, 14th ed. 1998. Chapter 308, pp.1791–1856.

HIV-specific cell-mediated immune responses can be detected at the time of the acute viral syndrome and correlate with the down-regulation of plasma viremia (193,194,197) (Fig. 11B). During primary infection the precursor frequency of HIV-specific CTLs may be as high as one per 100 cells (197); the CTLs mainly recognize structural HIV proteins. Noncytolytic, CD8+ T cell-mediated, MHC-unrestricted HIV suppressive activity also has been identified (see section below on Immune Responses) (206).

Molecular analysis has demonstrated that clones of HIV-specific CD8+ CTLs initially expand during primary HIV infection, then decrease after their initial expansion. CD8+ T-cell subsets can be categorized according to the expression of different variable (V) regions of the T cell receptor Vβ chain. There are 24 Vβ families in the T-cell receptor repertoire (see Chapter 10). Three patterns of CD8+ CTL expansions may occur during the acute stages of HIV infection, and these patterns correlate with rates of disease pro-

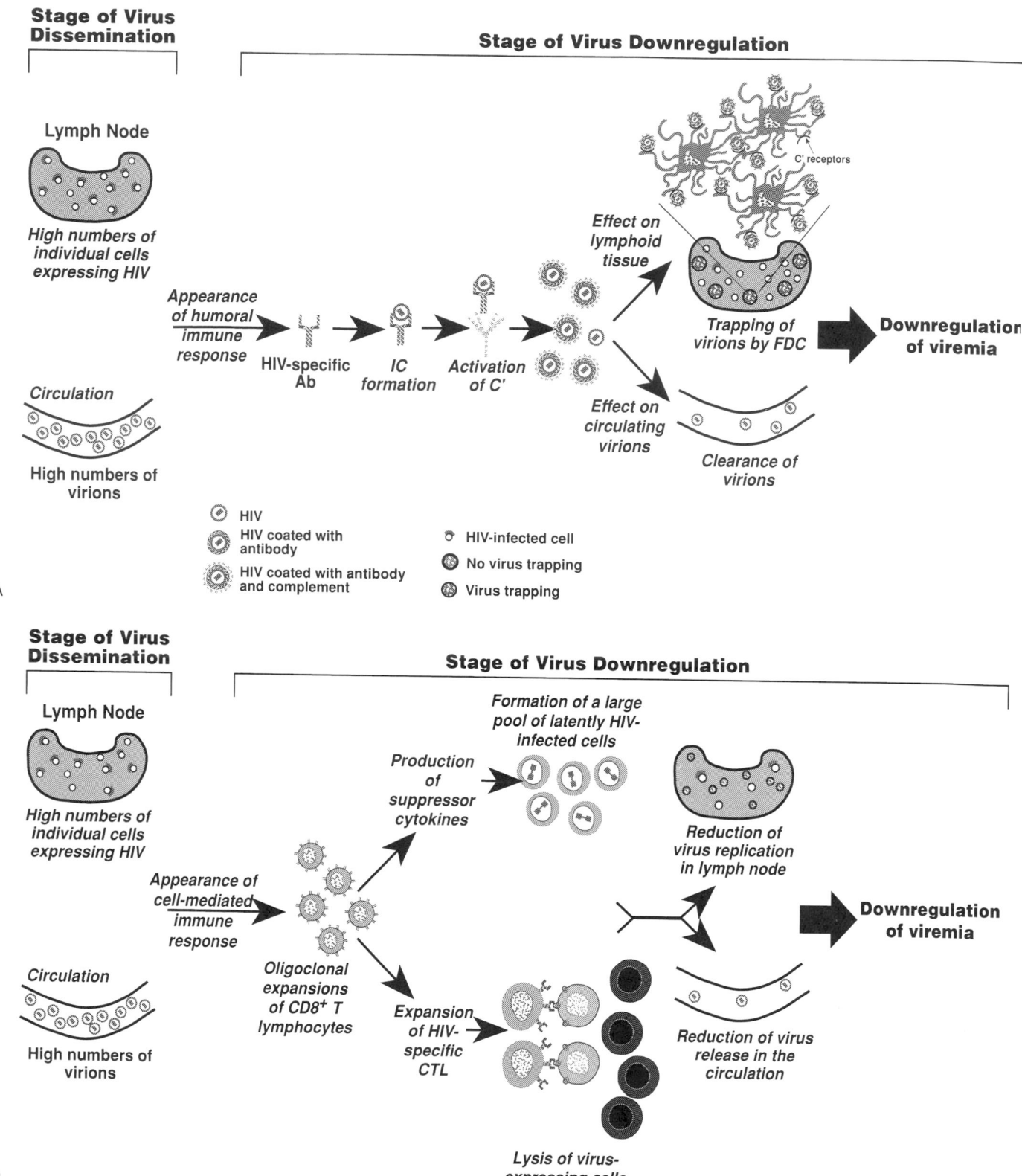

FIG. 11. A: Downregulation of plasma viremia and fixation of viral immune complexes to follicular dendritic cells in lymph node germinal centers. HIV-specific antibodies (Ab) combine with virions to form immune complexes (IC). Complement (C') binds to the immune complexes, which are then trapped in the FDC network by the C3b and C3d complement receptors. Adapted with permission from Pantaleo G, et al. *Immunol Rev* 1994;140:105. **B:** Downregulation of plasma viremia and establishment of a chronic viral reservoir in lymph nodes after primary HIV infection. Emergence of cell-mediated immune responses against HIV leads to elimination of a large number of productively infected cells within the lymph node. This in turn is partly responsible for the reduction in plasma viremia. Adapted with permission from Pantaleo G, et al. *Immunol Rev* 1994;140:105.

gression. In the first pattern of CTL expansion, a major expansion of 1 or 2 Vβ families occurs. This pattern of expansion is associated with rapid disease progression, with subjects often developing AIDS within 1 to 2 years. The second pattern of CTL expansion includes smaller expansions of three or four Vβ families and is associated with a more moderate rate of disease progression. The third pattern, with minor, diffuse, or no significant expansions of Vβ families, is associated with the most favorable prognosis (175). Expansions of particular Vβ families usually disappear over time; interestingly, the disappearance of expanded CTL clones occurs in the absence of viral mutations that affect the relevant CTL epitope (207). The cause of the loss of the expanded clones is unknown but may be due to clonal exhaustion or deletion (207). These data suggest that the ability to recruit a broad-spectrum CTL response against HIV during primary infection is associated with better control of viral replication and an improved prognosis compared with mobilization of a large wave of CTLs with a very narrow spectrum of epitope specificity.

The cytokine responses to HIV infection during the initial phases of infection have been determined in both peripheral blood and lymphoid cells. The earliest response consists of high levels of interferon (IFN)-γ, tumor necrosis factor (TNF)-α, and IL-10; IL-2, IL-4, and IL-6 are generally not increased in the PBMCs or lymph node mononuclear cells (208). In the macaque model, acute SIV infection leads to consistent increases in IL-6, TNF-α, IL-10, and IFN-γ in most animals (209–211).

Chronic Persistent Infection

HIV is a lentivirus, a family of viruses characterized by chronic persistent infection with development of pathologic consequences in the later stages of disease. Similar to other lentiviruses, and despite potent cellular and humoral immune responses that develop after primary infection, HIV is not completely cleared from the body. Instead, chronic infection develops that persists for approximately 10 years before the patient becomes clinically symptomatic (18). Ongoing virus replication can be detected in the plasma and in lymphoid tissue during the course of chronic infection (see section below on Laboratory Markers of HIV Infection).

In other chronic viral infections, such as hepatitis B, a defective immune response to a particular portion of the virion has been associated with the development of chronic infection. In HIV disease, chronic infection is the norm and no immune response has been identified that is completely protective. Important factors in the ability of the virus to avoid immune clearance are the extraordinary replication kinetics of HIV replication (136–139), and the high error rate of RT (38,39), which allow for the constant generation of viral genomes with new mutations.

HIV-infected individuals have HIV-specific CTL activity in their peripheral blood that is detectable upon direct *ex vivo* isolation of CD8+ T cells (212,213); this situation is not observed in other disease states or viral infections. During acute infection with HIV, activated HIV-specific CTLs and CTL precursors are segregated in the peripheral blood (207), where very little active virus replication takes place, but not in the lymphoid tissue, the predominant site of virus replication and spread. This segregation of CTL responses in anatomic compartments distinct from sites of viral replication is an additional mechanism by which HIV may evade the host immune response.

HIV infection can cause cell lysis *in vitro* and can establish a population of cells (i.e., CD4+ T cells and monocytes/macrophages) that become latently infected. A similar situation occurs *in vivo*. In certain tissues of the body (e.g., CNS microglia), high numbers of HIV-infected cells can be found. These cells are not killed by acute HIV infection and may become viral reservoirs. Such reservoirs are involved in the pathogenesis of complications of HIV disease such as AIDS dementia and other neurologic syndromes (see section below on Cytokines and HIV) (214–217). Similarly, a population of CD4+ T cells that are not killed by HIV infection is generated. Studies of these latently infected cells, which harbor chromosomally integrated HIV DNA, demonstrate that their number is low (one in 50,000 at later stages of disease); however, upon restimulation of the cells, production of virions may ensue (218). Other reservoirs of HIV include antibody and complement-bound virions, which may remain infectious even after attachment to FDCs (140). Thus, despite the generation of potent immune responses leading to downregulation of virus replication after primary infection, HIV in most instances establishes a state of chronic infection characterized by variable degrees of active virus replication and persistence of reservoirs of latently infected cells.

Advanced HIV Disease (AIDS)

Clinical Aspects

Progression of HIV disease is associated with depletion of CD4+ T cells and consequent increased risk for the development of opportunistic AIDS-defining diseases (19). The loss of integrity of cell-mediated immune responses allows ubiquitous environmental organisms with limited virulence (e.g., *Pneumocystis carinii* and *Mycobacterium avium*) to become life-threatening pathogens. Syndromes indicative of depressed cell-mediated immunity in HIV infection that are not AIDS defining include oropharyngeal and recurrent vulvovaginal candidiasis, bacillary angiomatosis (usually due to infection with *Bartonella henselae*), recurrent or multidermatomal herpes zoster, listeriosis, infections due to *Rhodococccus equi*, pelvic inflammatory disease, oral hairy leukoplakia associated with Epstein-Barr virus (EBV), cervical dysplasia (usually associated with human papillomavirus infection), constitutional symptoms such as unexplained fever or diarrhea lasting more than 1 month, idiopathic thrombocytopenic purpura, and peripheral neuropathy (219). More severe conditions indicative of depressed cell-mediated immunity due to HIV infection constitute the Centers for Disease Control and Prevention (CDC) surveillance case definition of AIDS. These conditions include fungal infections (e.g., esophageal or pulmonary candidiasis; extrapulmonary cryptococcosis, histoplasmosis, or coccidioidomycosis; and pulmonary or extrapulmonary *Pneumocystis carinii* infection), viral infections (e.g., cytomegalovirus retinitis, esophagitis, pneumonia, myelitis, pancreatitis, or adrenalitis; and herpes simplex virus bronchitis, pneumonia, esophagitis, or chronic skin ulcers), bacterial and mycobacterial infections (e.g., pulmonary tuberculosis; extrapulmonary infection due to any mycobacterium; recurrent bacterial pneumonia; and recurrent *Salmonella septicemia*), protozoal infections (e.g., gastrointestinal syndromes due to infection with *Cryptosporidium* or *Isospora*, and toxoplasmic encephalitis), neoplasia (e.g., invasive cervical cancer; Burkitt's, immunoblastic, or primary CNS lymphoma; and Kaposi's sarcoma), as well as HIV-related encephalopathy, progressive multifocal leukoencephalopathy (due to reactivation of JC virus), and wasting syndrome (219).

HIV-associated diseases indicative of severe impairment of cell-mediated immunity but not included in the current case definition of AIDS include chronic microsporidiosis, gastrointestinal infection with *Cyclospora cayetanensis,* disseminated *Penicillium marneffei* infection (endemic to southeast Asia), cerebral or disseminated *Trypanosoma cruzi* infection (endemic to Latin America), relapsing or chronic visceral leishmaniasis, anal carcinoma, and EBV-positive cases of leiosarcoma, leiomyosarcoma, and Hodgkin's disease (220). Nearly all of these HIV-associated illnesses, including the malignancies, are now known to be caused by infection with or reactivation of opportunistic organisms. In this regard, human papillomaviruses, EBV, and human herpes virus-8 appear to play causative roles in the AIDS-defining malignancies, cervical cancer, lymphomas, and Kaposi's sarcoma, respectively (221–225).

The degree to which an infection or reactivation syndrome can be considered opportunistic can be inferred by the CD4+ T-cell counts at which it occurs (19,226,227). Oral candidiasis and tuberculosis tend to occur as the CD4+ T-cell count falls into the 250 to 500 cells/μl range. Cryptosporidiosis generally does not occur until the CD4+ T-cell count is less than 200 cells/μl. *Pneumocystis carinii* pneumonia, disseminated *Mycobacterium avium* complex infection, cryptococcosis, and toxoplasmosis are indicative of more severe immunodeficiency. At the more extreme end of the opportunistic disease spectrum, cytomegalovirus (CMV) retinitis is usually diagnosed after the CD4+ T-cell count has fallen below 50 cells/μl. The steep increase in the risk of developing AIDS-defining illnesses associated with a CD4+ T-cell count of less than 200 cells/μl led to the 1993 revision of the CDC definition of AIDS, which now includes a low CD4+ T-cell count (less than 200 cells/μl) as an AIDS-defining criterion (219).

The clinical management of HIV-infected patients with advanced-stage disease requires intense vigilance because complications directly related to HIV or opportunistic diseases may affect virtually any organ system. The combination of antiretroviral therapy, prophylaxis against opportunistic infections, and aggressive treatment of opportunistic diseases as they occur has led to a significant increase in survival and quality of life after diagnosis of AIDS (228–230).

Immunologic Aspects

A wide array of immune system deficits are associated with the advanced stages of HIV infection. Abnormalities in the function of all limbs of the immune system, including T- and B-lymphocytes, antigen-presenting cells, NK cells, and neutrophils, have been described (see section below on Immune Dysfunction Caused by HIV Infection). Immunodeficiency may become sufficiently profound in the late stages of disease that the HIV-specific antibody and cytolytic T-lymphocyte responses diminish in the face of high levels of ongoing viral replication. The loss of immune competence during the course of HIV disease progression can be gauged by the sequential loss of *in vitro* proliferative responses of peripheral blood lymphocytes to recall antigens, alloantigens, and finally, to mitogens (231).

A variety of mechanisms, both directly and indirectly related to HIV infection of CD4+ T cells, are likely responsible for the observed defects in T-cell colony formation, autologous mixed lymphocyte reactions, expression of IL-2 receptors, and IL-2 production (232). Interference with CD4 expression by HIV gp120 (233), Nef (234), and Vpu (235,236), may impair the ability of the infected CD4+ T cell to interact with appropriate MHC class II molecules. Preferential infection by HIV of CD4+CD45RO+ memory cells or the preferential susceptibility of these cells to the cytopathic effects of HIV infection may in part explain the loss of memory responses to soluble antigens and consequent increase in the risk of infection with opportunistic organisms (237,238). Circulating gp120 molecules may deliver aberrant immunologic signals and dysregulate expression of costimulatory molecules in uninfected CD4+ cells, rendering these cells anergic (239–248).

A more incisive view of the qualitative nature of the immunodeficiency that occurs in the late stages of HIV infection is provided by study of the CD4+ T-cell receptor Vβ repertoire. Polymerase chain reaction (PCR) amplification across the CDR3 region with primers specific for the T-cell receptor Vβ families yields products of different lengths depending on the recombination of variable, diversity, and junctional gene segments. Failure to detect some of these products within a Vβ family indicates disruption of the Vβ repertoire. Such disruptions are seen with increased frequency in CD4+ T cells from patients in advanced stage HIV disease, particularly with CD4+ T-cell counts of less than 200 cells/μl (143). Interestingly, increases in CD4+ T-cell counts associated with antiretroviral or IL-2 therapy do not result in restoration of Vβ subfamily disruptions (143). These data imply that HIV-induced holes in the T-cell receptor repertoire may be permanent or may take a substantial amount of time to regenerate and suggest that prophylaxis against opportunistic infections may need to be continued in patients with AIDS who experience significant increases in CD4+ T-cell counts associated with therapy.

Ultimately, the immunodeficiency induced by HIV must be considered in the context of the microenvironment in which immune responses are generated. The advanced stages of HIV infection are marked by striking disruption of lymphoid tissue architecture (249–256). Follicular involution, hypervascularity, and fibrosis are some of the pathologic changes evident in lymph nodes from patients with advanced HIV disease. The loss of FDCs, resulting in follicular involution, has important implications with regard to the pathogenesis of HIV-related immunodeficiency. The ability to mount immune responses against new antigens and the ability to maintain memory responses are severely impaired in the absence of an intact FDC network (257). This loss of functional substrate for the generation and maintenance of immune responses results in loss of containment of HIV replication and enhanced susceptibility to opportunistic infections.

Virologic Aspects

The increase in plasma viremia that occurs during the progression of HIV disease likely results from the loss of HIV trapping capacity in lymph nodes (due to involution of the FDC network) as well as the deterioration of HIV-specific immune responses (200). However, qualitative differences in the virus also appear to play an important role in the pathogenesis of late-stage HIV infection. As previously discussed, viruses isolated from patients with advanced HIV infection often display increased cytopathicity and the ability to replicate in a wider range of target cell types (see section above on Cellular Targets of HIV Infection and HIV Coreceptors) (72–76). Emergence of SI strains of HIV occurs in nearly 50% of individuals at a mean CD4+ T-cell count of 50 cells/μl and heralds accelerated loss of CD4+ T cells (75). The transition from NSI to SI viruses has recently been correlated with a change in HIV core-

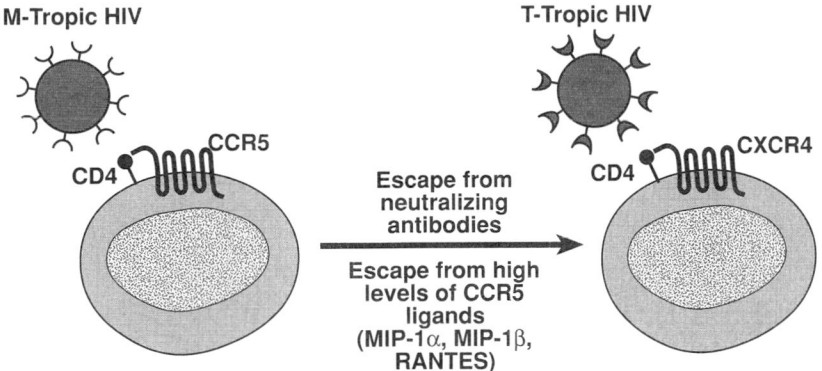

FIG. 12. Potential mechanisms of expanded tropism with HIV disease progression.

ceptor usage of these viruses (see section above on HIV Coreceptors) (98). NSI viruses predominantly use CCR5 to gain entry into cells, whereas SI viruses can use CXCR4 (96,98,116). The transitions in viral phenotype from NSI to SI and in viral coreceptor usage from CCR5 to CXCR4 correspond to mutations in the V3 loop of the HIV envelope, wherein uncharged amino acid residues are exchanged for positively charged residues (see section above on Cellular Targets of HIV Infection). These mutations do not appear to be simply a consequence of increasing diversity of envelope sequences over time because slow progressors with a high degree of sequence diversity in the envelope gene maintain NSI viruses that use CCR5. As previously discussed, changes in host factors that select for viruses with tropism for coreceptors other than CCR5 may be responsible for this transition in viral phenotype (Fig. 12).

LABORATORY MARKERS OF HIV INFECTION

Appreciation of the natural history and the pathogenesis of HIV infection has led to a search for laboratory parameters that serve as indicators of disease activity before the development of overt clinical disease (Table 2). The ideal laboratory marker should be easily and reproducibly measurable in all individuals with the disease (258). Furthermore, it should worsen with progression of disease and improve with positive responses to therapy. Although no ideal marker currently exists, several have been of critical importance in the clinical management of patients, especially with regard to establishing standards of care for initiation of antiretroviral therapy and prophylaxis against opportunistic infections.

TABLE 2. *Laboratory markers of HIV disease*

Markers of immune depletion and dysregulation	Markers of viral load
CD4+ T cell count	Viral burden (i.e., HIV DNA PCR+ cells)
β2-microglobulin levels	
Neopterin levels	Cell-associated virus (detected by culture or by molecular quantitation)
TNF-α receptor levels	
Anti-CD3 proliferative responses of T cells *in vitro*	HIV RNA splicing pattern
Delayed type hypersensitivity responses to antigen *in vivo*	Plasma viremia (detected by culture or by molecular quantitation)
CD38 expression on CD8+ T cells	
	p24 antigenemia

Markers of Immune Depletion and Immune Dysregulation

Because CD4+ T cells are the primary targets of HIV infection and because depletion of CD4+ T cells is the immunologic hallmark of HIV disease progression, measurement of CD4+ T cells should be an excellent marker of HIV infection. Indeed, studies of the natural history of HIV infection demonstrate that nearly 90% of individuals with a CD4+ T-cell count of less than 200 cells/μl experience an AIDS-defining illness within 4 years, whereas one half to two thirds with CD4+ T-cell counts of 200 to 400 cells/μl and only 15% to 20% of those with CD4 counts of greater than 400 cells/μl progress to clinical AIDS over the same period of time (259–261). Similar trends are evident across all HIV risk groups, including individuals with hemophilia (262,263) and injecting drug users (264). In addition to the absolute CD4+ T-cell count, the peripheral blood CD4+ T-cell percentage and the slope of the CD4+ T-cell count over time also function as valid laboratory markers of disease progression (265–267).

CD4+ T-cell counts frequently increase in response to antiretroviral therapy, and this salutary response has been used as a criterion in the licensing of new anti-HIV drugs (268–271). However, caution is warranted in concluding that increases in CD4+ T-cell counts during antiretroviral therapy necessarily lead to improvements in prognosis (258,272–274).

Markers of generalized immune activation such as serum levels of β2 microglobulin and neopterin are also valid markers of HIV disease progression. β2 microglobulin is an 11-kDa protein that associates with MHC class I molecules on the surface of most nucleated cells in the body. Serum levels of free β2 microglobulin derive mainly from lymphocytes and are elevated in conditions associated with lymphocyte activation or destruction such as lymphoproliferative syndromes, autoimmune diseases, and viral infections. A direct correlation exists between serum levels of β2 microglobulin and the risk of progression to AIDS (275). The β2 microglobulin level is a risk factor for the development of AIDS independent of the CD4+ T-cell count. In one large study, only 1% of participants with CD4+ T-cell counts of more than 300 cells/μl and β2 microglobulin levels of less than 4 mg/L developed AIDS after 1 year, compared with 18% of those with similar CD4+ T-cell counts but β2 microglobulin levels of more than 4 mg/L. Among participants with CD4+ T cell counts of less than 300 cells/μl, the corresponding rates of progression to AIDS for the low and high β2 microglobulin groups were 18% and 33%, respectively (276).

Neopterin is a metabolite of guanosine triphosphate that is produced largely by cells of the monocyte/macrophage lineage and lymphocytes during tetrahydrobiopterin synthesis. Elevated levels of serum neopterin are seen in patients with autoimmune diseases and viral infections. Like β2 microglobulin, an elevated serum neopterin level is a predictor of progression to AIDS independent of the CD4+ T cell count (277,278). The combination of a CD4+ T-cell count plus either a β2 microglobulin or neopterin level has more predictive value for disease progression than any of the three measurements taken individually (261).

The extracellular domains of the receptors for TNF-α are released from the cell membrane by proteolytic cleavage and are detectable in soluble form in serum. Levels of these soluble TNF receptors may reflect levels of TNF activity. Insofar as TNF has a critical role in upregulating HIV replication (see section below on Cytokines and HIV) (279,280), it is not surprising that levels of soluble TNF receptors serve as a valid surrogate marker of HIV disease progression. In separate studies, levels of soluble TNF receptor type II were found to correlate strongly with plasma viremia and with progression to AIDS (281,282); however, levels of soluble TNF receptors do not appear to serve as reliable markers of therapeutic efficacy during antiretroviral therapy (283).

A number of other indicators of immune dysregulation correlate with HIV disease progression. The diminished proliferative response of T cells to anti-CD3 antibodies *in vitro* serves as an indicator of immunodeficiency (284,285) as does diminished delayed-type hypersensitivity response to recall antigens *in vivo* (286–288). The percentage of peripheral blood CD8+ T cells bearing the activation marker CD38 is positively correlated with disease progression (289,290). CD8+CD38+ cells mediate cytolytic activity, and increased numbers of these cells in the chronic phase of HIV infection likely reflect a high viral load. Additional markers of HIV disease activity include hematocrit, serum levels of immunoglobulin (Ig)A, and serum levels of 1,25-vitamin D (291,292).

Markers of Viral Load

Before the development of currently available sensitive molecular techniques for the quantitation of HIV RNA molecules, direct culture of HIV from plasma or mononuclear cells was found to correlate with stage of disease (293–295). Changes in levels of culturable plasma viremia further serve as reliable indicators of activity of antiretroviral agents (296); however, these assays are extremely labor intensive and less sensitive than currently available molecular diagnostic tests.

During viral replication, the viral core protein p24 is shed into plasma and can be measured by immunoassay. Measurement of p24 antigenemia is relatively insensitive; however, positivity of a p24 antigen test does herald accelerated decline in CD4+ T-cell counts and the likelihood of progression to AIDS. In the Multicenter AIDS Cohort Study, 61% of HIV+ individuals who progressed to AIDS over 4 years had detectable p24 antigenemia, compared with 17% of those who did not develop AIDS (260). In the subset of patients who developed AIDS, p24 antigenemia was first detected an average of 16.8 months before an AIDS diagnosis. Detection of p24 antigenemia was associated with accelerated decline in CD4+ T-cell counts, from an average loss of 119 cells/μl/year in those who remained negative for p24 antigenemia to 157 cells/μl/year in those with p24 antigenemia. Although a positive test for p24 antigenemia has prognostic value with regard to progression of disease, changes in levels of p24 antigenemia during antiretroviral therapy do not serve as an accurate surrogate for therapeutic efficacy (297).

The frequency of HIV-infected cells can be quantified using PCR for detection of HIV-1 DNA, and this measurement has some predictive value with regard to HIV disease progression. Several investigators found increases of approximately one to two orders of magnitude in the frequency of HIV-infected cells in peripheral blood among patients who progressed to AIDS (298–301). Only modest decreases or no change in the frequency of infected cells have been detected during antiretroviral therapy (135,302–308). Changes in the frequency of infected cells during antiretroviral therapy, however, are difficult to interpret for a number of reasons. Cells harboring defective proviruses may be detected by DNA PCR; however, their contribution to the pathogenesis of HIV disease remains unclear, and a decrease in their number would not necessarily be expected during antiretroviral therapy. In addition, the decay in frequency of infected cells during antiretroviral therapy may be an insensitive indicator of therapeutic efficacy because cells harboring integrated proviruses may be long lived. In this regard, measurement of unintegrated viral DNA may be a more dynamic marker for following the effects of RT inhibitor antiretroviral therapy (309). Unintegrated viral DNA is the immediate product of reverse transcription of viral RNA and has a relatively short half-life during which either integration into host DNA or degradation occurs (40,41).

Measurement of cell-associated HIV mRNA in peripheral blood, although technically demanding, has been shown by several groups to serve as an independent predictor of disease progression. Particularly impressive is the ability of this marker to predict disease progression in patients with early stage HIV disease and relatively high CD4+ T-cell counts. In a study of patients with more than 600 CD4+ T cells/μl, those with no detectable HIV mRNA in PBMCs all remained AIDS free for 8 years, whereas approximately 50% of those with 101 to 4,500 HIV mRNA copies per μg total RNA and 80% of those with more than 4,500 HIV mRNA copies per μg total RNA progressed to AIDS during the same period (310). Determination of the splicing pattern of HIV mRNA in PBMCs can add further predictive value with regard to disease progression. Thus, although levels of multiply-spliced and unspliced HIV mRNAs increase with disease progression, a disproportionate increase in unspliced HIV mRNA is most predictive of accelerated loss of CD4+ T cells and clinical disease progression (311–315). Studies of the effect of antiretroviral therapy on the frequency of infected cells in lymphoid tissue, a major *in vivo* reservoir and site of HIV replication, demonstrated that decreases in levels of unspliced HIV mRNA correlated well with decreases in plasma viremia during therapy (134,316). This finding, combined with the fact that HIV mRNAs are orders of magnitude more abundant in lymph node mononuclear cells compared with peripheral blood mononuclear cells, supports the concept that changes in plasma viremia during antiretroviral therapy are reflective of changes in cell-associated viral mRNA production in lymphoid tissue (134,316,317).

The ability to assess the level of viral replication with quantitative assays of HIV RNA in plasma (i.e., plasma viremia) has revolutionized the use of laboratory markers for HIV disease. Measurement of the CD4+ T-cell count yields information regarding the degree of immunodeficiency and short-term risk of opportunistic disease (i.e., a reflection of the damage already sustained by the immune system). In contrast, quantitation of HIV RNA in plasma yields information that predicts what is likely to happen subsequently to the immune system. Technology currently available for reproducible measurement of plasma viremia in clinical specimens includes PCR (132,318), nucleic acid sequence-based amplification (NASBA) (319), and branched DNA (b-DNA) assays (320). PCR and NASBA are both cycle-based target amplification systems, whereas b-DNA is a single-step signal amplification system that uses multiple HIV-specific nucleic acid target probes, each of which can be bound to an amplifier molecule containing multiple oligonucleotides. Each oligonucleotide in this array can in turn hybridize to an enzyme-labeled complementary probe, and detection is accomplished by addition of substrate. Each of these assays (PCR, NASBA, and b-DNA) can detect as few as approximately 20 to 50 molecules of HIV RNA per ml of plasma, and each has a dynamic range of several orders of magnitude.

The recognition that high levels of HIV replication are sustained throughout the course of infection occurred with a convergence of several lines of data. The enhanced sensitivity of PCR compared with conventional viral detection techniques enabled Bagnarelli and co-workers in 1992 to report that the mean levels of plasma viremia in patients with early, intermediate, and late-stage disease were approximately 21,000 HIV RNA copies/ml, 43,000 HIV RNA copies/ml, and 270,000 HIV RNA copies/ml, respectively (299). Piatak and co-workers found that plasma viremia levels determined by PCR correlated with those determined by endpoint dilution culture in the same patient; however, levels of plasma viremia determined by PCR were found to exceed those determined by culture by an average of 60,000-fold (132). Further evidence that high levels of HIV replication occur even during the clinically latent period of disease came from the demonstration of massive levels of viral burden and viral replication in lymphoid tissue compared with peripheral blood (256,321).

The predictive value of plasma viremia as a marker for disease progression was demonstrated in the Multicenter AIDS Cohort Study, where individuals were stratified by quartiles according to baseline plasma viremia levels. The proportion of patients who progressed to AIDS within 5 years after entry into the study with plasma viremia levels in the lowest through highest quartiles was 8%, 26%, 49%, and 62% respectively (322) (Fig. 13). Plasma viremia was also shown to predict progression of disease independently from CD4+ T-cell counts; this measurement was in fact superior to the predictive value of CD4+ T-cell counts. In this regard, patients with a mean CD4+ T-cell count of approximately 780 cells/µl and plasma viremia

levels of greater than 10,190 HIV RNA copies/ml had a median survival time of 6.8 years compared with greater than 10 years in individuals with the same mean CD4+ T-cell count but plasma viremia levels of less than 10,190 HIV RNA copies/ml (322). Further validation of the use of plasma viremia measurement as a predictor of disease progression was provided by the AIDS Clinical Trials Group, which found that baseline measurements of plasma viremia as well as changes in viremia over time were predictive of disease progression (323,324).

The impressive decreases in plasma viremia during combination antiretroviral therapy reported by many groups suggested that this measurement might serve as a valid marker not only for predicting progression but also for monitoring therapy in HIV-infected individuals. The link between decreased plasma viremia in individuals receiving therapy and improved clinical outcome was established by the Veteran's Affairs Cooperative Study Group on AIDS (325), which found that a 75% reduction in plasma viremia over the first 6 months of antiretroviral therapy accounted for 59% of the clinical benefit of treatment (i.e., the lack of progression to AIDS). Finally, data indicating that decreases in plasma viremia during therapy are reflective of decreases in viral replication in lymphoid tissue further validates the use of plasma viremia as a laboratory marker of a critical aspect of HIV pathogenesis (134,316).

Levels of plasma viremia become predictive of disease progression after stabilization of viremia (i.e. achievement of a viral load set point) in the months after primary HIV infection. Mellors and co-workers found that the level of plasma viremia within 6 months of seroconversion was significantly higher in patients who developed AIDS within approximately 5 years of follow-up (74,000 HIV RNA copies/ml) compared with levels in those who did not develop AIDS during the same period (19,000 HIV RNA copies/ml) (326). A plasma viremia level of more than 100,000 HIV RNA copies/ml within 6 months of seroconversion was associated with an odds ratio of 10.8 for the development of AIDS. Schacker and co-workers found that levels of plasma viremia stabilize at a later time point than that reported by Mellors. Plasma viremia levels obtained 0 to 6 months after seroconversion did not correlate with subsequent clinical outcome; however, the level of plasma viremia at 7 to 12 months after seroconversion was a strong predictor of CD4+ T-cell depletion during follow-up (327). These results are in agreement with a previous study in which levels of plasma viremia obtained around the time of seroconversion were also not predictive of the subsequent clinical course (328). Stabilization of plasma viremia to the so-called set point after primary infection likely reflects the ability of the early anti-HIV immune response to contain viral replication, although it has been argued that the viral load set point occurs independently of the host immune response (329).

The development of sensitive, quantitative assays for plasma viremia, and the ability of this marker to predict progression of disease and to serve as an indicator of therapeutic efficacy, has added an important dimension to decisions regarding initiation and maintenance of antiretroviral therapy in HIV-infected individuals. The variation in plasma viremia by several orders of magnitude in patients with early stage HIV disease with similar CD4+ T-cell counts allows for the initiation of early therapeutic intervention in those who are most likely to progress. In patients with low CD4+ T-cell counts who are being treated, a low level of plasma viremia militates against a change in the therapeutic regimen. Current recommendations regarding the initiation and maintenance of antiretroviral therapy rely heavily on the two best laboratory markers

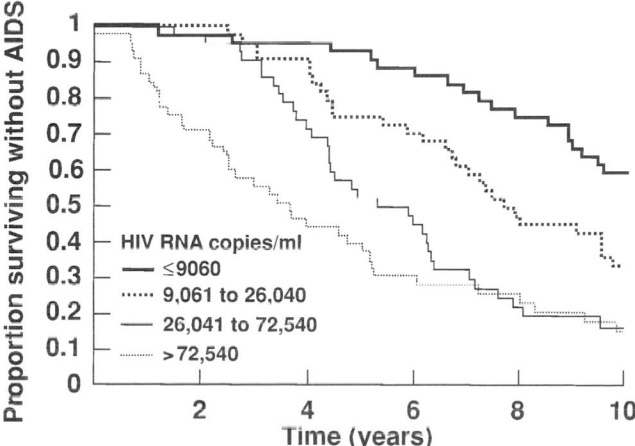

FIG. 13. Relationship between levels of plasma viral load and disease progression. Adapted with permission from Mellors J, et al. *Science* 1996;272:1167.

for HIV disease progression: the CD4+ T-cell count and the level of plasma viremia (330–332).

ANTIRETROVIRAL THERAPY

Recent progress in understanding the pathogenesis of HIV disease combined with the development of potent antiretroviral agents have resulted in an abundance of treatment options for HIV-infected individuals. The recognition that virus continuously replicates in lymphoid tissue throughout the course of HIV infection even during the clinically latent stage strengthened the rationale for early intervention (256,321). Quantitative estimates of the extraordinary rate of viral replication *in vivo* have further strengthened the rationale for early therapy with combination antiretroviral regimens (136–139). The rapid rate of viral replication together with the high rate of mutation leads to a high probability of the evolution of drug-resistant mutants if replication is not completely suppressed by antiretroviral drug regimens (164). Thus, the failure of antiretroviral monotherapy to significantly impact viral load in lymphoid tissue is not surprising in light of these viral dynamics (135). More recently, however, trials have shown rapid and significant reductions in viral load in peripheral blood and lymphoid tissue of individuals treated with combination therapy including inhibitors of the HIV-1 protease (139,333–337). The availability of clinical laboratory tests to monitor plasma viremia also has allowed for timely modification of antiretroviral regimens because an effective regimen should rapidly decrease viral load (136–139).

Viral Life Cycle and Antiretroviral Agents

A number of steps of the viral life cycle can be targeted by agents that are either currently available or under investigation (Fig. 14). Previous disappointment with the use of soluble CD4 as a means of inhibiting viral attachment and entry (338,339) has yielded to optimism that interference with viral coreceptors may represent an effective therapeutic modality targeted to the earliest stage of the viral life cycle (111,340,341).

Inhibitors of viral RT were the first agents to be developed for the treatment of HIV infection; they remain important components of the anti-HIV therapeutic armamentarium. Most RT inhibitors are nucleoside analogs; these agents act as DNA chain terminators by virtue of their structures that lack the 3′ hydroxyl moiety necessary for chain elongation. Nonnucleoside RT inhibitors are also used clinically. RT inhibitors as a group suffer from several disadvantages, including their association with multiple neurologic and hematologic side effects, the rapidity with which they select for resistant viral variants when used alone, and their lack of effect on cells already infected with HIV, which no longer require RT in order to complete the viral life cycle.

HIV-1 protease cleaves the Gag precursor polyprotein into the p24 and p17 virion components necessary for viral infectivity (342). Development of HIV-1 protease inhibitors based on the crystal structure of the protease was a triumph for rational drug design (343,344). The combination of agents that can inhibit *de novo* infection of cells (i.e., RT inhibitors) with agents that lead to the release of defective, noninfectious virions from cells already infected by HIV (i.e., protease inhibitors) results in potent antiviral activity. Protease inhibitors have rapidly become drugs of choice for the treatment of HIV infection in combination with RT inhibitors.

Integration of reverse-transcribed viral DNA (provirus) into the host DNA is facilitated by the viral enzyme integrase. The recent determination of the crystal structure of integrase (345) has stimulated a search for inhibitors of this enzyme, which should lead to the availability of clinically useful agents in the near future (346).

Targeting the accessory proteins of HIV has been hampered by the difficulty in delineating the precise biochemical activities of these proteins. A clinical trial of the Tat antagonist Ro24-7429 failed to demonstrate antiviral activity for this agent (347); however, agents targeting the HIV-1 Rev and Nef proteins are being developed.

Treatment of Primary HIV Infection

Treatment of HIV infection before its wide dissemination to lymphoid tissue and hence before establishment of the viral load set point is an approach supported by our current understanding of the pathogenesis of early events in HIV infection (200). The window of opportunity for treatment of primary HIV infection may actually extend to 12 to 18 months after acute infection; this possibility is based on the persistence of high numbers of productively infected cells in lymphoid tissue during this period, despite attainment of the apparent set point of plasma viremia (G. Pantaleo et al., unpublished data).

A trial of zidovudine therapy versus placebo given for 6 months after primary HIV infection showed that those patients assigned to active treatment maintained higher CD4+ T-cell counts, lower levels of plasma viremia, and slower progression to minor clinical endpoints (e.g., oral candidiasis, herpes zoster, and oral hairy leukoplakia) over a mean follow-up period of 15 months (348). Treatment of patients with recent (i.e., within 90 days) HIV infection with a combination of zidovudine, lamivudine, and a protease inhibitor is currently under study. Preliminary results suggest that plasma viremia can be suppressed to less than 20 HIV RNA copies/ml for a prolonged (more than 1 year at present) period by this drug combination (334).

Mathematical models suggest that treatment of acute as well as established HIV infection with a potent combination drug regimen that completely suppresses viral replication for approximately 3 years may eradicate infection (see section above on Viral Dynamics) (139). These models indicate that the slow second-phase decay of plasma viremia during therapy derives from long-lived infected cells rather than from activation of latently infected cells. However, experimental data suggest that activation of latently infected cells may be a viable mechanism for viral persistence even during potent combination therapy (T-W. Chun and A.S. Fauci, unpublished data). Another assumption inherent in models of virus eradication is that the therapeutic regimen is completely effective in inhibiting viral replication. The fact that traces of viral replication can be detected in lymphoid tissue from individuals who are receiving therapy and in whom plasma viremia is undetectable indicates that suppression of viral replication is not complete (335). Despite highly encouraging results from clinical trials, many questions remain to be answered regarding the treatment of acute HIV infection with potent combination antiretroviral regimens, including what constitutes the optimal antiretroviral regimen and the duration of therapy. In addition, long-term follow-up will be necessary to determine whether eradication of HIV is possible, and what the clinical outcome will be in patients in whom viral suppression is incomplete.

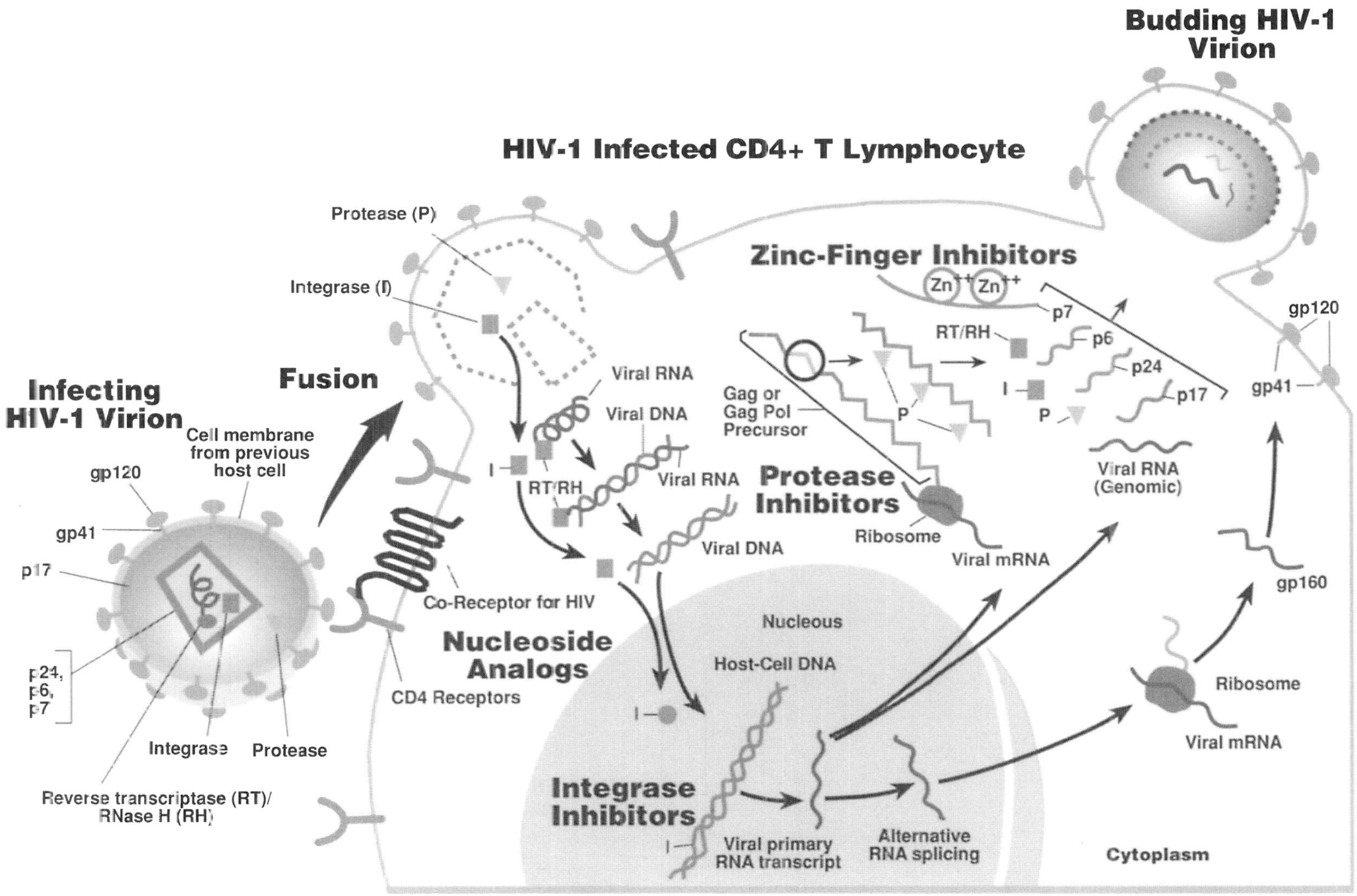

FIG. 14. Viral and cellular targets of anti-HIV therapy. Strategies that interfere with HIV fusion and entry into the CD4+ T cell are being developed, following the identification of chemokine receptors that function as HIV entry coreceptors. Agents that interfere with the viral enzymes RT, protease, and integrase are either in use or in development.

Treatment of Chronic HIV Infection

Early studies of zidovudine monotherapy demonstrated improvements in laboratory markers of HIV disease activity, and delayed progression of disease in individuals with symptomatic HIV disease as well as in asymptomatic individuals with relatively low CD4+ T-cell counts (268–271,349). Subsequent studies demonstrated that switching from zidovudine to didanosine therapy further delayed progression of disease (350–354) and that combination therapy with two nucleoside analogs is generally superior compared with monotherapy (354–358).

More potent combination antiretroviral drug regimens capable of prolonged suppression of viral replication have recently become available. For example, treatment of patients with advanced HIV disease with the combination of zidovudine and lamivudine results in a 0.5- to 1-log decrease in plasma viremia that is sustained over a period of at least 6 months to a year (359–362). Of note, the potency of this regimen appears to derive from the preferential selection for a viral mutation that simultaneously confers resistance to lamivudine and restores sensitivity to zidovudine (363).

The addition of protease inhibitors to the antiretroviral armamentarium has resulted in cautious optimism that significant improvements in the prognosis for HIV-infected individuals are at hand. The protease inhibitors saquinavir, ritonavir, indinavir, and nelfinavir are all potent antiretrovirals, particularly when used in combination with nucleoside analog RT inhibitors (139,333, 364–368). Such combination therapy is now considered the treatment of choice for HIV infection (331,332). Addition of ritonavir to the existing antiretroviral regimen in patients with CD4+ T-cell counts of less than 100 cells/μl resulted in a 50% reduction in the rate of progression to AIDS or death compared with addition of placebo (369). Treatment of patients in the advanced stage of HIV disease (i.e., CD4+ T-cell counts of less than 400 cells/μl and plasma viremia of more than 20,000 HIV RNA copies/ml of plasma) with indinavir, zidovudine, and lamivudine resulted in sustained suppression of viremia to less than 500 HIV RNA copies/ml of plasma through 24 weeks in 90% of those treated (336). Among those treated with indinavir alone, 43% had suppression of plasma viremia to less than 500 HIV RNA copies/ml through 24 weeks, whereas no patients treated with zidovudine and lamivudine had this degree of suppression of viremia (336). In another study of HIV-infected patients with CD4+ T-cell counts of less than 200 cells/μl, treatment with a combination of indinavir, zidovudine, and lamivudine significantly delayed the progression to AIDS or death compared with the regimen of zidovudine and lamivudine without a protease inhibitor (337). The rapid and profound reductions in plasma viremia observed during treatment with protease inhibitor/RT inhibitor combinations are likely due to the rapid elimination of productively infected cells from lymphoid tissue and of virions bound to FDCs in germinal centers (335). In addition, the number of cells that are truly latently infected with HIV appears to be quite low (218). These data are encouraging regarding the prospect of long-term control over viral replication; however, the rapidity with which massive viral replication can reappear when suppression of viremia is incomplete is troublesome (370).

Ultimately, the success of long-term antiretroviral therapy depends not only on suppression of viral replication, but also on at least partial restoration of immune function. Immune competence prevents the onset of HIV-related opportunistic diseases and may synergize with antiviral agents to control viral replication. Cau-

tious optimism appears to be warranted in this regard in light of a recent study showing improved CD4+ T-cell function during HAART (371); however, the failure to reconstitute the T-cell receptor Vβ repertoire during therapy with IL-2 and antiretroviral agents leaves open the question of whether a threshold level of damage to the immune system may exist beyond which immune reconstitution may not be possible (143).

Although potent combination antiretroviral regimens will likely lead to significant improvements in the prognosis for HIV-infected patients treated soon after acute infection as well as in the intermediate-to-late stages of disease, uncertainty remains regarding treatment strategies for early asymptomatic HIV infection. In this regard, it is unclear whether the difficulties associated with long-term adherence to a therapeutic regimen that disrupts life-style, causes toxic side effects, and may promote the emergence of drug resistant mutants will outweigh the potential clinical benefits (332).

LYMPHOID TISSUE IN THE PATHOGENESIS OF HIV DISEASE

Acute HIV Infection

In animal models of SIV infection, the lymphoid organs have been implicated in the initial establishment of infection. Virus can be detected in peripheral lymph nodes within 1 week of infection (202,203). *In situ* hybridization studies show that nearly all of the SIV RNA at this time is cell associated, originating from productively infected cells in lymph nodes. This production of virus by individually infected cells in lymphoid tissue precedes and likely is responsible for the peak of SIV p26 antigenemia. A decrease in the frequency of productively infected cells is seen during the second week after infection coincident with the appearance of SIV-specific immune responses. By 4 weeks after infection, antigenemia begins to decrease as a result of further elimination of productively infected cells by SIV-specific cell-mediated immune responses and clearance of circulating virions by the formation of immune complexes consisting of virus, antibody, and complement that are trapped within lymphoid germinal centers (202,203).

Cross-sectional studies in patients evaluated soon after acute HIV infection corroborate the findings in the SIV model (Fig. 15). The kinetics of HIV viremia and HIV-specific immune responses in peripheral blood parallel those in the SIV model (194,195,197,198, 208). Preliminary data from a limited number of lymph node biopsies obtained from acutely infected individuals suggest that the SIV model is valid in depicting the early events associated with HIV infection in lymphoid tissue as well (G. Pantaleo et al., unpublished data). In the weeks to months after acute HIV infection, a sharp decline in the frequency of productively infected cells is evident in lymphoid tissue. Germinal center formation within lymphoid follicles becomes pronounced and viral RNA corresponding to extracellular virions complexed with antibody and complement is detected in the network of FDC processes (200,256,372–374). As noted above, the immune system is capable of efficient elimination of productively infected cells in lymphoid tissue and potent downregulation of viremia. However, the massive numbers of virions trapped within the germinal center FDC network as well as the latently infected cells that harbor proviral DNA but do not express viral proteins, and thus elude the immune response, represent potential continuous sources of virus for *de novo* infection of CD4+ T-lymphocytes that are resident in or migrating through lymphoid tissue (140,218,375).

Stage of Disease:

Acute	Early	Intermediate	Late

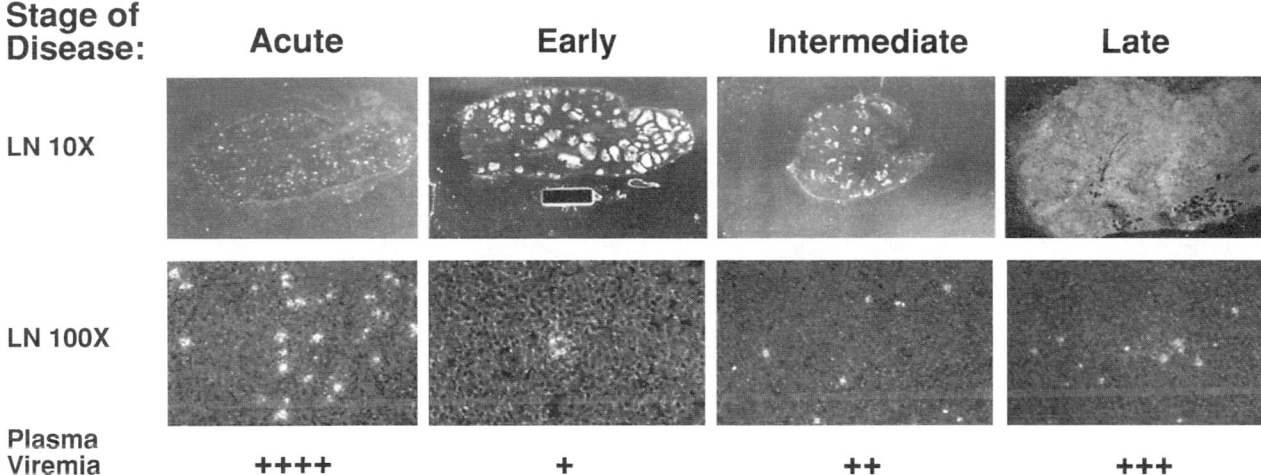

LN 10X

LN 100X

Plasma Viremia

++++	+	++	+++

FIG. 15. Patterns of HIV RNA expression in lymph nodes obtained at various stages of HIV disease. *In situ* hybridization was performed to detect HIV RNA, which appears as white grains in these dark field micrographs. In the acute phase of HIV infection, HIV RNA is detected mostly in association with productively infected paracortical T cells. The level of plasma viremia is high before the development of HIV-specific immune responses. In the early chronic phase of disease, emergence of HIV-specific immune responses leads to the elimination of most productively infected cells in the lymph node, downregulation of plasma viremia, and trapping of HIV-containing immune complexes in germinal centers. In the intermediate and late stages of disease, progressive follicular involution and loss of control over viral replication lead to loss of the viral trapping capacity in germinal centers, an increase in the frequency of productively infected paracortical T cells, and an increase in plasma viremia.

Chronic Infection: The Clinically Latent Period

The early chronic stage of HIV disease is characterized by a dichotomy in viral load between peripheral blood and lymphoid tissue. In this regard, the frequency of infected cells in lymph nodes exceeds that in peripheral blood by five- to 10-fold; differences in levels of viral replication are generally 10- to 100-fold (135,201, 256). Embretson and co-workers used *in situ* PCR to demonstrate that up to 25% of CD4+ T lymphocytes present in lymph node germinal centers harbor HIV DNA, further emphasizing the role of lymphoid tissue as a critical reservoir for HIV *in vivo* (321). The continuous state of rapid high-level turnover of plasma viremia discussed previously (more than 10^9 virions produced daily; see section above on Viral Dynamics) derives in large measure from viral replication in lymphoid tissue (134,316,317,335).

The dichotomy in viral burden and replication between lymph node and peripheral blood is created in part by the normal process of follicular hyperplasia within lymphoid germinal centers after antigenic challenge (252–255,372). The expansion of the FDC network within hyperplastic lymphoid follicles is an efficient mechanism for viral trapping via interactions between antibody and complement-coated virions with the complement receptor molecules C3b and C3d on the surface of FDCs. In addition to this mechanical phenomenon, immunologic mechanisms may play a major role in maintaining the dichotomy between lymph node and peripheral blood. The microenvironment of the lymph node is ideally suited to maintain a high degree of immune activation. Close contact between immune effector cells and the resultant high levels of proinflammatory cytokines produced in lymph nodes that harbor efficiently trapped virions favors viral replication in several ways. Activated CD4+ T-lymphocytes migrating through lymphoid tissue in response to antigens serve as ideal targets for *de novo* infection with HIV (375–380). Activation signals such as those delivered by proinflammatory cytokines, found in abundance within activated lymph nodes, are potent inducers of HIV replication in latently infected cells (40,41,218,381–383) and can increase the pool of activated HIV-susceptible cells (see section below on Cytokines and HIV) (379,381,382). Another example of the ability of HIV to subvert the immune system for its own replicative advantage is the immune hyperactivation induced by the virus itself (380). Sequestration of HIV-infected cells within lymphoid tissue also may contribute to the dichotomy between lymph node and peripheral blood. This sequestration may result from defective egress of cells due to histopathologic abnormalities and cytokine imbalances (384).

During the stage of viral burden dichotomy between lymph node and peripheral blood, there is a progressive shift in the lymphoid histopathologic pattern from follicular hyperplasia to follicular involution. This shift in histopathology is associated with important changes in viral distribution. Disruption of the FDC network is characteristic during the transition from follicular hyperplasia to involution, leading to a decrease in the efficiency of viral trapping in germinal centers and a resultant increase in plasma viremia (200,256). Sequestration of infected cells within lymphoid tissue also becomes less efficient during follicular involution. Thus, changes in the levels of viral burden and replication in lymph node and peripheral blood may be dependent, at least in part, on redistribution of viral load between these two compartments.

Advanced Stage Disease

All measures of viral load increase as HIV disease progresses. As the CD4+ T-lymphocyte count falls below 200 cells/µl, there is a tendency for viral load to increase more rapidly in the peripheral blood compartment, leading to equilibration between lymph node and peripheral blood. As noted above, disruption of the FDC network and the consequent loss of the ability to trap virions may contribute significantly to the process of equilibration of viral load between these compartments. Destruction of lymphoid tissue certainly is a major mechanism responsible for the severe immune dysfunction and loss of the ability to inhibit viral replication observed in advanced-stage HIV disease. The ability to maintain an effective immune response to HIV is severely impaired in the absence of intact lymphoid tissue architecture. As a consequence, increased cell-associated viral RNA is evident in the paracortical regions of lymph nodes, reflecting increased viral replication. Thus, during progression of HIV disease there is a reversal in the predominant forms of virus in lymph nodes, with progressive diminution of the extracellular form (i.e., trapped virus) and an increase in cell-associated virus (i.e., cells expressing HIV) (200,256). In the advanced stage of disease there is almost total dissolution of lymphoid architecture. Follicular involution, fibrosis, frank lymphocyte depletion, and fatty infiltration herald complete loss of functional lymphoid tissue, contributing to the state of immunodeficiency and the dramatically enhanced susceptibility to opportunistic infections.

Disruption of the lymphoid microenvironment during the course of HIV infection remains an enigmatic process with considerable implications for future therapeutic interventions. Productive infection of FDCs by HIV may occur, particularly in the late stages of HIV infection (385); however, the majority of data suggest that productive infection of FDCs is rare during the period of intermediate stage disease when dissolution of the FDC network begins (386). Direct toxicity of viral gene products may contribute to loss of FDC network integrity. Tat and gp120 have been shown to be capable of disrupting normal intracellular signaling (245,246) as well as inducing apoptosis (387–389), although these effects have been studied largely in CD4+ T cells and little is known regarding the normal physiology of FDCs and their interactions with HIV proteins. Tat, Nef, and Vpu have been found to downregulate MHC class I expression (386,390,391), which may interfere with normal cell–cell interactions in the lymphoid microenvironment. Depletion of CD4+ T cells during the course of HIV disease also could lead to withdrawal of a trophic factor necessary for FDC survival. Induction of tissue-damaging gene products by HIV may contribute to disruption of the FDC network over time: candidate mediators include nitric oxide (392–394) and matrix metalloproteinases (MMP) such as MMP-9 (395,396). An innocent bystander phenomenon is also a possibility, wherein cells such as CD8+ T cells or macrophages infiltrating into hyperplastic lymph nodes elaborate substances such as TNF-α that may be toxic at high sustained concentrations.

IMMUNE DYSFUNCTION CAUSED BY HIV INFECTION

Dysfunction of virtually every component of the immune system can be demonstrated during the course of HIV infection. Dysfunction of CD4+ T cells may be the result of direct infection with HIV, but it also may be caused indirectly by exposure of uninfected cells to various viral proteins. Because CD4+ T cells play a critical role in the orchestration of normal immune responses, it is not surprising that many of the immune defects that are observed during HIV disease are secondary to the progressive decline in the number and function of CD4+ T cells.

CD4+ T Cells

CD4+ T-cell dysfunction is the hallmark of HIV disease. The opportunistic infections observed with advancing disease are primarily due to defects in T-cell number and function that result directly or indirectly from HIV infection. Direct effects of HIV on CD4+ T-cell function include infection and resultant cytotoxicity with loss of absolute cell numbers. Indirect effects of HIV infection result in decreased CD4+ T-cell proliferation and differentiation, dysregulation and decreased production of IL-2 and other cytokines, decreased IL-2 receptor expression, and defective colony formation and other precursor defects.

HIV disease is characterized by an inversion of the ratio of CD4+ to CD8+ T cells, due primarily to depletion of CD4+ T cells. Until the very late stages of disease, the total number of CD3+ T cells remains relatively constant with an increase in CD8+ T cells counterbalancing the loss of CD4+ T cells (397). This phenomenon has been called T-cell homeostasis (398) and has been observed in other diseases. In this model, when T cells are lost, irrespective of whether they are CD4+ or CD8+, the body produces more CD3+ T cells at a constant ratio of CD4+ T cells to CD8+ T cells. If a selective loss of CD4+ T cells occurs, as in HIV disease, replacement of both CD4+ and CD8+ T cells leads to a net loss of CD4+ T cells and increase in CD8+ T cells (397–400). In the later stages of disease, overriding defects in lymphopoiesis result in an inability to maintain T-cell homeostasis with a subsequent loss of both CD4+ and CD8+ T cells.

A relentless loss of CD4+ T-cell function is observed with progression of HIV disease. Among the first abnormalities noted are a loss of response to common recall antigens such as tetanus toxoid, and decreased IL-2 production, followed by defects in T-cell proliferative responses to alloantigens. Subsequently, with the continued decline in CD4+ T cells, defects in response to mitogenic stimulation occur (231).

The mechanisms responsible for the CD4+ T-cell defects are only partially understood. Viral proteins have been demonstrated to directly alter T-cell function. gp41 has been observed to inhibit antigen- and mitogen-induced proliferation of PBMCs (401). The interaction between gp120 and CD4 leads to a state of altered cellular activation whereby a second activation signal leads to apoptosis of the cell. Apoptosis can be induced *in vitro* using CD4 cross-linking antibodies or trimeric HIV envelope protein (387,402,403; J. Arthros and A.S. Fauci, unpublished data). This CD4-induced effect can be overridden by CD28 or CD2 cross-linking (402,404). In addition, cells from HIV-infected individuals may be anergic and undergo apoptosis in response to CD4 cross-linking more readily than do cells from normal individuals (387,388,403,405–408).

T cells from HIV-infected individuals manifest a variety of phenotypic abnormalities. The percentage of CD4+ T cells expressing CD28, the ligand for B-7 and a major coactivation signal necessary for activation of T cells, is reduced compared with uninfected individuals (68% in cells from patients with AIDS versus 96% in cells from healthy, uninfected subjects) (409). CD28- cells do not respond to activation signals, including anti-CD3 monoclonal antibodies or mitogens, and express markers of terminal activation, including HLA-DR, CD38, and CD45RO (410). HIV-infected individuals develop an increase in CD45RO expressing memory cells and a loss of naive, CD45RA-expressing cells. Of note, the CD45RO cells appear to be the main source of HIV replication *in vivo* and produce much more HIV *in vitro* compared with CD45RA cells (237,411).

Defects in T-cell colony formation have been observed in HIV-infected individuals, and infection of CD34+ bone marrow progenitor cells and thymocytes has been demonstrated; in addition, myelodysplasticlike changes have been noted in the bone marrow. These defects may contribute to the lack of reconstitution of T cells in later stages of disease.

Mechanisms of CD4+ T-Cell Depletion

Direct Infection

Dysfunction and depletion of CD4+ T cells are the hallmarks of HIV infection and the predominant causes of immunodeficiency. The observations that CD4+ T cells are the principal targets of HIV infection *in vivo* (188,412) and that HIV infection of CD4+ T cells *in vitro* causes cytopathicity (1,2,146,413–417) led to a reasonable assumption that direct infection of CD4+ T cells *in vivo* results in their depletion. However, quantitative studies of the frequency of HIV-infected cells *in vivo* suggest that single cell killing by direct infection with HIV may not be the predominant mechanism of CD4+ T-cell depletion. In this regard, the proportion of HIV-infected peripheral blood CD4+ T cells in individuals in the early asymptomatic stage of HIV infection is typically in the range of one in 1,000 to one in 10,000 (201,298,412,418, 419). Although this frequency increases with disease progression, the proportion of HIV-infected peripheral blood CD4+ T cells rarely exceeds one in 100 even in patients with AIDS (298–300,311,418). In the early stages of disease, the frequency of HIV-infected cells in lymphoid tissue exceeds that in peripheral blood by 0.5 to 1 log. In the advanced stage of disease, equilibration in viral burden between these compartments is seen (201,256). In lymphoid tissue, the percentage of cells harboring HIV DNA and actively expressing viral mRNA is generally less than 1% (321). Although viral burden and expression are clearly far greater than earlier estimates based on standard *in situ* hybridization methods (420), the data illustrate the difficulty in accounting for CD4+ T-cell depletion solely by direct mechanisms; however, it should be pointed out that considerable CD4+ T-cell depletion could result from the death of a small but rapidly turning over population of cells that are recently infected, produce virus that infects other cells, and die (136–139). This population of cells might not be readily detected by currently available techniques and represents an area of intense investigation.

Multiple mechanisms of cell death appear to be operative after infection of a CD4+ T cell with HIV (Table 3). Early events in the viral life cycle, such as accumulation of reverse-transcribed viral DNA in the cytoplasm, have been associated with cell death in other retroviral systems (421,422) and also may contribute to cell killing in HIV infection (146); however, accumulation of unintegrated DNA is clearly not the sole mechanism responsible for single-cell killing by HIV (423). High levels of viral RNA and aberrant RNA molecules also are present in the cytoplasm of infected cells and possibly interfere with normal cellular RNA processing (424,425).

The intracellular concentration of envelope gp120 molecules is high during the process of virion assembly in an HIV-infected cell. Several studies have suggested that intracellular gp120 may interact with intracellular CD4 molecules and that this interaction may induce cell death (415,426). The mechanism of cell death as a consequence of this intracellular gp120–CD4 interaction may be autofusion events that disrupt the integrity of the cell membrane (427). Cell membrane integrity also may be compromised by the budding of virions from an infected cell (428,429) and by HIV-induced increases in the concentration of intracellular monovalent cations (430).

TABLE 3. *Mechanisms of CD4+ T-cell depletion–dysfunction*

Direct infection	Indirect mechanisms
Accumulation of unintegrated viral DNA	Syncytium formation
Interference with cellular RNA processing	Autoimmunity (i.e., molecular mimicry of host proteins by viral components)
Intracellular gp120–CD4 autofusion events	Superantigenic stimulation
Loss of plasma membrane integrity due to viral budding	Elimination of HIV gp120-coated cells by HIV-specific immune effectors (i.e., "innocent bystander" killing)
Elimination of infected cells by HIV-specific immune effectors	Apoptosis
	Infection of stem cells and interference with lymphopoiesis

HIV-infected cells also may die as a consequence of viral-specific immune responses that occur before the cell succumbs directly to viral infection. Multiple effector mechanisms may be involved in the killing of HIV-infected cells, including cytotoxic T-lymphocyte responses, ADCC, and NK cell responses (see Fig. 10 and section below on Immune Responses).

Indirect Mechanisms

Syncytium Formation

By virtue of its ability to interact with molecules essential to normal immune function, the envelope glycoprotein of HIV-1 is an important mediator of pathogenic events. HIV envelope glycoprotein molecules are inserted into the host cell membrane during virion assembly and are shed by infected cells into the surrounding milieu. Interaction of these HIV envelope glycoprotein molecules with uninfected cells may be responsible for a significant amount of cell death.

The molecular events associated with viral entry that lead to fusion between the viral coat and cell membrane involve the interaction of the HIV envelope glycoprotein, CD4, and a coreceptor molecule (see section above on HIV Coreceptors). Similar events may occur when an infected cell bearing HIV envelope glycoprotein molecules on its surface encounters an uninfected CD4+ cell with an appropriate coreceptor. Fusion between infected and uninfected cells, resulting in multinucleated giant cells or syncytia has long been observed *in vitro* (414,416,417,431–433). Other molecules implicated in syncytium formation include leukocyte function-associated antigen (LFA)-1 (434,435), CD7 (436), and HLA class I molecules (437). Syncytia have been observed only rarely in tissues obtained from HIV-infected individuals (192,253,438–442); thus, it is unlikely that syncytium formation is a major pathogenic mechanism of CD4+ T-cell depletion.

Autoimmunity

Autoimmune phenomena occur in HIV-infected individuals and may contribute to CD4+ T-cell depletion. Autoimmunity may occur as a result of molecular mimicry by viral components and by abnormal release of nuclear antigens from cells dying by apoptosis. Highly homologous regions exist in the carboxy terminus of the HIV-1 envelope glycoprotein and the amino-terminal domains of different HLA-DR and -DQ alleles (443). Monoclonal antibodies generated using the HIV envelope peptide as immunogen can recognize native gp160 and MHC class II molecules (444). Sera from one third of HIV-infected individuals were found to react with the gp41 and MIIC class II determinants. These sera were capable of inhibiting normal antigen-specific proliferative responses and also eliminated class II–bearing cells by ADCC (444). Similar instances of molecular mimicry between HIV-1 envelope constituents and host proteins that may result in pathogenic autoimmune responses include the collagenlike region of complement component C1q-A (445), MHC class I heavy chains (446), HLA-DR4 and -DR2 alleles (447), variable regions of the T-cell receptor alpha, beta, and gamma chains (447), Fas (447), functional domains of IgG and IgA (447), denatured collagen (448), and a number of nuclear antigens (449,450).

Superantigens

Superantigens can bind to the T-cell receptor Vβ chain and an MHC class II molecule and are therefore able to stimulate virtually any T cell from a particular Vβ family. The consequences of superantigenic stimulation involve perturbations (expansions, deletions, and functional impairment) of cells from particular T-cell receptor Vβ families. Superantigens specific for a number of different T-cell receptor Vβ families are mediators of disease pathogenesis for a number of pathogens, including staphylococcus (451), mycoplasma (452), toxoplasma (453), and mouse mammary tumor virus (454).

The discovery that the pathogenesis of murine leukemia virus–induced immunodeficiency syndrome in mice was linked to the presence of a virally encoded superantigen (455) led to the investigation of a similar scenario in HIV infection. Depletion of various sets of T-cell receptor Vβ families in peripheral blood from HIV-infected patients further suggested that HIV may encode superantigens (456). Anergy of Vβ8+ T cells in HIV-infected individuals and preferential infectability of CD4+ Vβ12+ T cells with HIV also supported a possible role for a superantigen (457–460). However, these latter observations were shown to be due to a putative CMV-encoded superantigen rather than one encoded by HIV itself (461). The superantigen-mediated pathogenesis hypothesis in HIV infection is tenuous given the number of studies that have found no evidence of superantigenlike effects in HIV-infected patients. Several studies have found no selective loss of particular Vβ families of T cells during HIV infection (462,463). Other studies have found variable perturbations of the T-cell receptor Vβ repertoire that are inconsistent with superantigen-mediated effects (143,175,193,464).

Innocent Bystander Phenomena

Immune responses that target HIV determinants on infected cells also may contribute to elimination of uninfected cells bearing HIV proteins (e.g., gp120) on their surface. Targeting of such "innocent bystander" cells by antibody and cellular immune responses has been described (465–467).

Apoptosis

Apoptosis is the morphologic description of a form of programmed cell death critical to physiologic homeostasis in virtually every organ system (405,468). Apoptotic cell death is characterized by plasma membrane blebbing, nuclear condensation, DNA fragmentation, and release of cellular contents in the form of small,

dense apoptotic bodies. Ingestion of apoptotic bodies by phagocytes completes the apoptotic death process without the inflammation associated with spillage of cellular contents that occurs in nonphysiologic necrotic cell death. A wide array of physiologic stimuli serve as positive and negative regulators of apoptosis. Important inhibitors of apoptosis include growth factors, extracellular matrix, and CD40 ligand, whereas important activators of apoptosis include CD95 (Fas) ligand, TNF, transforming growth factor (TGF)-β, neurotransmitters, and withdrawal of growth factor. The discoveries that the bcl-2 gene plays an important pathogenic role in lymphomagenesis through its ability to prevent cells from undergoing apoptosis (469–471), and that the p53 gene is necessary for initiation of apoptosis (472–474), established the paradigm that diseases associated with increased cell survival or increased cell death may result from dysregulation in normal pathways of apoptosis.

Ascher and Sheppard suggested in 1990 that HIV pathogenesis was largely caused by the inappropriate signals delivered to T cells by HIV envelope molecules (475). Subsequently, Ameisen and Capron proposed in 1991 that apoptosis may be a pathogenic mechanism of CD4+ T-cell depletion during HIV infection (476). Acute infection of T cells with HIV in vitro was shown to induce apoptosis (408,477), and T cells from HIV-infected patients were demonstrated to undergo enhanced rates of apoptosis in vitro compared with normal T cells, particularly after activation (407,478). Cross-linking of CD4 followed by ligation of the T-cell receptor is sufficient to induce apoptosis, suggesting that uninfected CD4+ T cells could be depleted inappropriately upon encountering antigen if CD4 had been cross-linked by gp120 (387,479). The viral Tat protein also can lead to apoptotic cell death, possibly by upregulation of CD95 ligand or by enhancing activation of cyclin-dependent kinases (388,389).

It remains uncertain whether HIV-induced apoptosis plays an important role in vivo in CD4+ T-cell depletion. The frequency of apoptotic CD4+ and CD8+ T cells as well as B cells is significantly higher in lymphoid tissue from HIV-infected individuals compared with uninfected controls (480). The intensity of apoptosis is related to the degree of immune activation and is observed predominantly in uninfected bystander cells (480,481). Although some data support a positive correlation between the stage of HIV disease and susceptibility of peripheral blood T cells to apoptosis (482), another study found no such correlation (483); Muro-Cacho and co-workers found that the intensity of apoptosis in lymphoid tissue was independent of the peripheral CD4+ T-cell count and level of plasma viremia (480). Perhaps the most compelling evidence that apoptosis may play a role in HIV pathogenesis is that an increased frequency of apoptosis in CD4+ T cells is seen in HIV-infected humans and in primates infected with pathogenic strains of SIV, but not in primates infected with nonpathogenic strains of SIV (406).

Infection of Progenitor Cells and Inhibition of Hematopoiesis

Failure of normal hematopoiesis is an obvious candidate mechanism to account for depletion of CD4+ T cells during HIV infection. A subset of CD34+ progenitor cells express CD4 and are infectable in vitro with HIV-1 (484–486). Whether or not CD34+ progenitor cells represent a substantial in vivo reservoir for HIV is controversial. A number of studies have failed to detect HIV-infected CD34+ progenitor cells in most HIV-infected individuals (487–490); however, a large study by Stanley and co-workers showed that a substantial minority of HIV-infected patients with severe CD4+ T-cell depletion have a reservoir of HIV-infected CD34+ progenitor cells (491). Recent reports demonstrating expression of CXCR4 on CD34+ progenitor cells (492) suggest that the CD4+ subset of these cells may be infectable with T-tropic strains of HIV (i.e., strains that predominate in the later stages of HIV disease), further substantiating the earlier findings of Stanley and co-workers.

Although the role of direct infection of CD34+ progenitor cells in HIV pathogenesis remains controversial, a large body of evidence suggests that viral proteins and HIV-induced cytokines can impair the survival and clonogenic potential of these cells. CD34+ cells cultured in the presence of HIV exhibit defective clonogenic potential (493); uninfected CD34+ cells purified from bone marrow of HIV-infected patients are also defective in clonogenic potential (490,494,495) and are committed to apoptotic death in culture (496). The HIV envelope gp120 and Tat proteins have been implicated in these effects on CD34+ progenitor cells (497,498), possibly due to gp120 and Tat-mediated upregulation of TGF-β (498,499), or gp120-mediated upregulation of TNF-α (500).

Disruption of the thymic microenvironment (501) and HIV-induced thymocyte depletion also may contribute to the failure of CD4+ T cell replenishment. Thymic epithelial cells normally secrete IL-6, which can in turn increase HIV replication in infected cells (502). Subpopulations of thymic CD3⁻CD4⁻CD8⁻ cells are susceptible to infection with HIV in vitro (503), and thymic CD3⁻CD4+CD8⁻ progenitor cells from HIV-infected patients are infected in vivo. Finally, uninfected thymocytes from HIV-infected individuals are primed for apoptotic death, suggesting that indirect mechanisms of defective thymopoiesis are operative as well (504).

CD8+ T Cells

Levels of CD8+ T cells vary throughout the course of HIV disease. After acute primary infection, CD8+ T-cell counts usually rebound to supernormal levels and may remain elevated for prolonged periods. Increases in CD8+ T cells during all but the late stages of disease may, in part, reflect the expansion of HIV-specific CD8+ CTLs.

HIV-specific CD8+ CTLs have been identified in HIV-infected individuals early in the course of disease, and their activity can be measured in peripheral blood lymphocytes without prior in vitro stimulation (212,213). During HIV disease progression, CD8+ T cells assume an abnormal phenotype characterized by the expression of certain activation markers and the absence of expression of the CD25 IL-2 receptor. Alterations in the phenotype of CD8+ T cells in HIV-infected individuals may have prognostic significance. In particular, individuals whose CD8+ T cells express HLA-DR but not CD38 after seroconversion experience a stabilization of their CD4+ T-cell counts and a less fulminant disease course, whereas individuals whose CD8+ T cells express both HLA-DR and CD38+ experience a more aggressive course with rapid CD4+ T-cell depletion and a poorer prognosis (290,505,506). CD8+ T cells lacking CD28 expression are also increased in HIV disease (507), possibly reflecting the expansion of the CD8+CD28⁻CD57+ T-cell subset containing in vivo activated CTLs (508). The loss of CTL activity with disease progression is not restricted to HIV-specific CTLs: a loss of cytotoxic activity to other common antigens including EBV and Mycobacterium tuberculosis also has been observed (509,510).

In addition to CTL activity, other CD8+ T-cell functions are impaired during HIV disease progression, including loss of noncytolytic non-MHC restricted CD8+ T cell–derived HIV suppression.

Analyses of factors released by CD8+ T cells demonstrate that in certain in vitro systems the CD8+ T cell-associated suppressor activity termed CD8 antiviral factor (CAF) decreases with disease progression (see section below on Immune Responses) (206). In contrast, levels of MIP-1α, MIP-1β, and RANTES, factors produced by CD8+ T cells that also suppress HIV replication (79), are not reduced with progression of HIV disease (511–518).

Dendritic Cells

DCs are the first cells infected by SIV after vaginal mucosal exposure and, as previously discussed (see section above on HIV Infection and the Development of HIV Disease), likely are responsible for transporting the virus to lymphoid organs, resulting in infection of CD4+ T cells and viral dissemination. The role of DCs in HIV infection is somewhat controversial, mainly due to the multiple lineages of DCs and the differences in in vitro assay systems used in different studies.

In Vitro *Infectability and* In Vivo *Infection of DCs with HIV*

DCs derived from the peripheral blood of normal volunteers were initially found to be highly infectable with HIV in vitro, and DCs from HIV-infected individuals were found to be HIV-infected in vivo; however, these early studies used relatively impure populations of cells (519–522). Follow-up studies of DCs from uninfected normal volunteers were discordant in their results: some groups found that DCs obtained by negative selection from peripheral blood were easily and productively infected in vitro with multiple strains of HIV (523–527), whereas other groups found that peripheral blood DCs isolated by similar methods were not infectable (190,528,529). Identification of multiple populations of cells with dendritic morphology in peripheral blood is a likely reason for these differing results (190,530,531). When three different populations of peripheral blood DCs were analyzed for infectability with HIV, only one was easily and productively infected in vitro with HIV (190). Studies of DCs from HIV-infected individuals have yielded similarly conflicting results: some authors found high levels of infection in DCs isolated ex vivo from peripheral blood (520), whereas others did not (532,533).

A number of studies have demonstrated that productive infection of tissue DCs with HIV is rare. There is general agreement that LCs (DCs resident in the epidermis) from the skin of HIV-infected individuals are occasionally infected; however, such infection occurs at a very low frequency, rarely approaching the level of infection found in peripheral blood CD4+ T cells and often 10 to 100 times less (534–543). Study of DC infection in lymphoid organs has been more limited. In one study, the frequency of HIV-infected splenic DCs was approximately two orders of magnitude less than that observed in CD4+ T cells from the same individuals (543). In an analysis of lymph node biopsies, tissue sections from HIV-infected individuals at various stages of disease were stained for DC markers by immunohistochemistry and for HIV RNA by in situ hybridization (130). No cells that stained for both DC markers and HIV were observed, suggesting that DCs in these organs were rarely, if ever, infected with HIV at any stage of disease. These data suggest that in the tissues where DCs reside for the purposes of obtaining antigen, and in the lymphoid organs where they activate T cells, DCs are rarely productively infected.

LCs from normal skin appear to be infectable with HIV, although viral production is very low (535,536,544,545). Interestingly, infectability of LCs may be dependent on viral subtype. Clade B viruses, which are predominant in the United States and Europe, replicate poorly in LCs *in vitro,* whereas clade E viruses, which are predominant in Southeast Asia, replicate well in these cells (546). This finding may in part explain the differences in the epidemiology of HIV infection in the United States and Europe versus sub-Saharan Africa, Asia, and India. In the United States and Europe, the majority of HIV infections occur in homosexuals and injection drug users, whereas in sub-Saharan Africa, Asia, and India, more than 90% of infections are spread via heterosexual contact (547–556). Thus, an HIV subtype that can replicate well in LCs, likely a major cell type involved in the initiation of viral infection through mucosal contact (189), may be more efficiently transmitted heterosexually. These findings are controversial, and further studies are required to establish whether preferential cellular tropism of different clades of HIV plays a role in the global epidemiology of HIV spread.

Depletion and Dysfunction of DCs in HIV Infection

The question of depletion and dysfunction of DCs in HIV disease follows the same controversy as discussed above for infectability. Studies of the number of DCs present in peripheral blood of HIV-infected individuals compared with uninfected individuals have demonstrated a decrease (520), increase (557), or no change (558). Most studies have found no decrease in the percentage of LCs in skin cell preparations when comparing infected to uninfected individuals or when comparing HIV-infected individuals at various stages of disease (542). In a study of lymphoid organs, sections of lymph node tissue from HIV-infected individuals at various stages of disease were stained for DC markers and examined by light microscopy. Visual analysis did not suggest a selective loss in the number of DCs populating the paracortical regions of the lymph node; rather, loss of DCs from the lymph node occurred in parallel with the loss of lymphoid architecture and the development of fibrosis (130).

With regard to DC function, studies of the effect of HIV infection on the ability of DCs to activate T cells also have yielded conflicting results. Several studies found that peripheral blood DCs from HIV-infected individuals were much less efficient in activating T cells than DCs from uninfected individuals (520,525,559, 560), whereas another report found no difference in the ability of peripheral blood DCs from HIV-infected versus uninfected individuals to activate allogeneic CD4+ T cells (558). All of these studies used peripheral blood DCs that have the confounding variables of a requirement for *in vitro* maturation, long purification processes, and the existence of multiple subpopulations in blood. In a study using identical twins discordant for HIV infection, DCs were obtained from each sibling and cocultured with their own CD4+ T cells, the CD4+ T cells of their sibling, or allogeneic CD4+ T cells. No defects were found in the ability of the DCs from the HIV-infected sibling to present antigen to the uninfected T cells as compared with the DCs from the uninfected sibling. The only defect observed in DCs from the HIV-infected sibling was a decreased ability to activate allogeneic T cells (542). Further studies are needed to clarify the possible role of DC depletion and dysfunction in the pathogenesis of HIV disease.

B Lymphocytes

The number of circulating B cells may be decreased in primary HIV infection (561); however, this is usually a transient phenome-non and likely reflects, at least in part, a redistribution of cells into lymphoid tissues. Soon after the resolution of acute HIV infection, hypergammaglobulinemia and B-lymphocyte hyperactivation are noted. The increase in immunoglobulins occurs for all classes of antibody. A large component of the immunoglobulin specificity, at least in early-stage disease, is directed against HIV antigens. It has been suggested that a majority of activated B cells produce antibodies directed against HIV during this stage of infection (562). The ability of B cells to respond in a primary or secondary fashion to both protein and polysaccharide antigens is reduced, likely due in part to the loss of CD4+ T-cell help. Dysregulation of B-cell activation and the decreased ability of these cells to respond to antigen are likely responsible in part for the increase in certain bacterial infections seen in advanced HIV disease in adults, as well as for the morbidity and mortality associated with bacterial infections in HIV-infected children who cannot mount an adequate humoral response to common bacterial pathogens.

B cells from HIV-infected individuals secrete increased amounts of TNF-α and IL-6, cytokines known to enhance HIV replication (563–565), and express surface-bound TNF-α that can induce the production of HIV from infected CD4+ T cells (566). The secretion of proinflammatory cytokines and the expression of surface-bound TNF-α by B cells in the lymphoid microenvironment may contribute to T-cell activation and HIV replication in these tissues.

HIV gp120 has been observed to directly bind to an immunoglobulin variable chain (VH3) and activate these B cells in much the same manner as a superantigen (567,568). This antigen-independent polyclonal activation leads in part to the hypergammaglobulinemia and B-lymphocyte hyperactivation of HIV infection. Other portions of HIV, including gp41, directly activate B cells in a non–superantigen-mediated manner (569). Correlates of B-cell dysfunction observed in HIV-infected individuals include an increase in spontaneous EBV transformation *in vitro* and may contribute to the observed increased frequency of EBV-induced lymphomas (570–572).

Several studies have found an overall increase in IgE levels among HIV-infected individuals, likely reflecting a spectrum of IgE regulatory dysfunction. The mechanisms of this increase are unclear but may include B-cell hyperactivation and cytokine dysregulation. Levels of IgE continue to increase with disease progression (573,574). An increase in aeroallergen specific IgE has not been associated with the increase in total IgE; in one study, allergen-specific IgE decreased with HIV disease progression in all but the subgroup with the highest total IgE level (573). An overall increase in IgE levels was noted in pediatric HIV infection without an increase in allergen-specific IgE, suggesting polyclonal activation. An association between elevated levels of IgE and emergence of SI viruses was also noted (575). In HIV-infected children, an expanded minor population of B-lymphocytes has been identified that does not express CD23 (IgE receptor) and CD62L (L-selectin) and may be involved in the pathogenesis of IgE dysregulation (576).

Polymorphonuclear Leukocytes

Defects in neutrophil function have been observed at all stages of HIV disease. Neutrophils isolated from asymptomatic HIV-infected individuals have an increase in nitroblue tetrazolium (NBT) reduction, suggesting a state of increased cellular activation (577). Plasma from these individuals activates neutrophils from healthy, uninfected individuals, suggesting the presence of a plasma neutrophil-activating factor. In addition, plasma from the same individuals was found to be low in N-acetyl cysteine, indicating that depletion of antioxidants may occur due to increased oxygen radical production (578). The oxidative capacity of neutrophils after priming with granulocyte/macrophage (GM) colony-stimulating factor (CSF) also was increased in HIV-infected individuals with CD4+ T-cell counts greater than 200/μl (579). There is some controversy regarding neutrophil defects in HIV infection; this may be due to differences in in vitro preparation and analysis of cells. In a flow cytometric analysis of neutrophils in whole blood, which obviates the need for purification, neutrophils from HIV-infected subjects demonstrated increased expression of adhesion molecules, decreased expression of CD62L, and increased actin polymerization and H_2O_2 production (577), indicating activation of neutrophils. Opsonizing activity of neutrophils was significantly impaired, and this correlated with disease progression (580). Neutrophils from AIDS patients also undergo apoptosis at an increased rate compared with those from normal controls. Unlike the neutrophil activating factor described above, serum from HIV-infected individuals could not transfer the increased apoptosis activity to neutrophils from healthy, uninfected individuals (581). The addition of GM-CSF to the assay system significantly decreased apoptosis in neutrophils from patients with AIDS (581). Neutrophils from HIV-infected individuals also produce more TNF-α and IL-6 in response to lipopolysaccharide (LPS) or Candida antigen compared with neutrophils from normal donors (582).

Dysfunction of neutrophils in HIV-infected individuals has several clinical implications. HIV infection, especially in women, is characterized by an increase in the incidence and severity of Candida infections. In a study comparing the ability of neutrophils from HIV-infected patients and normal controls to phagocytize and kill Candida albicans, neutrophils from patients with AIDS showed an increased ability to phagocytize the organism, a similar ability to generate reactive oxygen, but a decreased ability to kill Candida, suggesting a defect in nonoxidative killing (583). A potential mechanism for the decreased ability of neutrophils to kill Candida organisms has been suggested by the finding that IL-10, shown in some studies to be increased in HIV disease, inhibits neutrophil killing of Candida (584).

Abnormalities in eosinophils also have been observed in HIV infection. Eosinophil counts in HIV-infected individuals are preserved in the setting of decreases in other blood cells; however, they may be increased in a subgroup of patients (585). Eosinophils express low levels of CD4 and are infectable with HIV in vitro, leading to productive infection and apoptosis (586). The significance of eosinophil infection in vivo, if it in fact occurs, is unclear at present.

Monocytes and Macrophages

Monocytes are important in HIV infection as reservoirs of infection, mediators of certain pathologic processes in tissues, and immune modulators in the destruction of intracellular pathogens and activation of other cell types. Peripheral blood monocytes are generally normal in number in HIV-infected individuals. Because monocytes express CD4 and numerous HIV coreceptors, including CCR5, CXCR4, and CCR3 on their surface (129), they are potential targets of HIV infection. Unlike infection of CD4+ T cells, which generally results in cell lysis, HIV cytopathicity for cells of the monocyte lineage is low and HIV can replicate extensively in these cells (587,588). Circulating monocytes are rarely

found to be infected in vivo and are difficult to infect in vitro (188,588,589); however, infection can readily be demonstrated in tissue macrophages, including resident microglial cells in the brain, pulmonary alveolar macrophages, and mature macrophages derived from blood monocytes in vitro (213,590–592). In addition, infection of monocytic precursors in bone marrow may be directly or indirectly responsible for certain of the hematologic abnormalities observed in HIV-infected individuals.

Treatment of normal monocytes in vitro with HIV gp120 or Tat leads to abnormal activation of these cells (593). In vitro infection of monocytes from healthy individuals leads to a decrease in ADCC and killing of intracellular Candida pseudotropicalis (594) as well as to decreased Fc- and C3-mediated phagocytosis (595). Monocytes isolated from HIV-infected subjects exhibit a number of functional abnormalities as well. A decrease in the oxidative burst has been observed in individuals with both early- and advanced-stage disease (596,597). In addition, impairment of chemotaxis and migration has been observed in monocytes from patients with AIDS (44,598,599).

Natural Killer Cells

The presumed role of NK cells is to provide immunosurveillance against allogeneic cells, virus-infected cells, and certain tumor cells (see Chapter 17). Abnormalities of NK cells are observed throughout the course of HIV disease, and these abnormalities increase with disease progression. Most studies report that NK cells are normal in numbers and phenotype in HIV-infected individuals; however, decreases in numbers of the CD16+/CD56+ subpopulation of NK cells with an associated increase in activation markers have been reported (600,601). NK cells from HIV-infected individuals are defective in their ability to kill typical NK target cells as well as gp160-expressing cells. The abnormality in NK cell lysis is thought to occur after binding of the NK cell to its target (602). Otherwise, the NK lytic machinery appears to be capable of functioning normally because NK cells from HIV-infected individuals are able to mediate ADCC (603). A possible mechanism for defective NK activity includes a lack of cytokines necessary for optimal function. Addition of either IL-2, IL-12, or IFN-α to cultures enhances the defective in vitro NK cell function of HIV-infected individuals (604).

ROLE OF CELLULAR ACTIVATION IN HIV PATHOGENESIS

The primary function of the immune system is to recognize foreign antigens, mobilize a response to pathogenic substances, clear them, and then return to a resting state in order to respond efficiently to other antigens or to a second challenge of the same antigen with increased efficiency (anamnestic response). In HIV infection the immune system is chronically activated in response to persistent HIV replication. HIV subverts the immune system by inducing immune activation and utilizing this milieu toward its own replicative advantage (166,376,381,475). Manifestations of an activated immune system include hyperactivation of B cells leading to hypergammaglobulinemia; spontaneous lymphocyte proliferation; activation of monocytes; an increase in the expression of activation markers on CD4+ and CD8+ T cells; lymphoid hyperplasia, particularly early in the course of disease; increased secretion of proinflammatory cytokines; elevated levels of neopterin, β2 microglobulin, acid-labile interferon, and soluble IL-2 receptors; as well as autoimmune phenomena.

A number of experiments suggest that HIV replication *in vivo* is dependent on antigen-driven activation of CD4+ T cells. HIV-infected individuals who had intercurrent infections, or who were immunized with various vaccines, experienced transient increases in plasma viremia that correlated with the degree of immune activation that was induced; similar observations have been made in SIV-infected macaques (605–610). The amount of viral replication observed after vaccination with influenza vaccine or tetanus toxoid, or during active infection with *Mycobacterium tuberculosis,* correlated inversely with the stage of HIV disease (607,609,610). Individuals with late-stage HIV disease had a moderate increase in viral replication, whereas individuals with early stage disease had a much greater increase in plasma viremia over baseline, suggesting a correlation between the ability of the immune system to respond to antigen and the magnitude of viral induction (609,610). Furthermore, when PBMCs from tetanus toxoid–immunized, HIV-infected individuals were stimulated *in vitro* with tetanus antigen, or when PBMCs from purified protein derivative (PPD)-positive, HIV-infected individuals were stimulated *in vitro* with PPD or live *Mycobacterium tuberculosis,* subjects with early-stage disease manifested a much stronger proliferative response to the respective antigens with a larger increase in viral replication *in vitro* than did individuals with advanced-stage disease (607,609,611). These studies suggest that the level of viral replication correlates with the level of immune system activation in response to an antigen. Other experiments have analyzed lymphoid tissue from HIV-infected individuals. Within individual splenic white pulps, a restricted number of individual antigen-specific immune responses occurred (defined by the analysis of T-cell receptor Vβ gene usage), and each of the immune responses contained a single or limited number of HIV quasispecies (157). These data support the theory that within the context of individual antigen-specific immune responses, a single quasispecies of HIV, which was present at the initiation of the reaction, spread among the newly activated T cells. Thus, it is likely that the continuous daily production of HIV occurs in newly activated CD4+ T cells that are being driven by antigen-specific activation.

The potential deleterious consequences of chronic immune activation are numerous. From an immunologic standpoint, activation of the immune system in response to antigenic stimuli is critical for normal immune function. However, chronic, persistent exposure of the immune system to a particular antigen over an extended period of time may lead to a decreased ability to maintain an adequate immune response to the antigen in question. Additionally, the functional capability of the immune system to respond to a broad spectrum of antigens may be compromised. From a virologic standpoint, although quiescent CD4+ T cells can be infected with HIV, reverse transcription, integration, and virus spread are much more efficient in activated cells (40,41). In addition, it has been demonstrated that cellular activation induces expression of virus in latently infected CD4+ T cells (218). These observations highlight the extraordinary capacity of HIV to exploit immune activation for its own replicative advantage.

CYTOKINES AND HIV

Cytokines (see Chapters 21 and 22) are the soluble mediators of inflammation, activation, differentiation, and chemotaxis. They have complex effects on the replication of HIV (166,612,613) (Fig. 16); certain cytokines (e.g., TNF-α) can directly induce HIV expression through the activation of NF-κB, whereas others act by altering the state of activation or differentiation of target cells. HIV infection induces the production of TNF-α and IL-6, as well as other cytokines, which act in an autocrine and paracrine manner to upregulate HIV replication. HIV envelope proteins also can directly induce the release of many cytokines, suggesting that HIV infection of a cell is not required to induce the release of certain cytokines. *In vitro* studies in a variety of model systems have assigned general HIV-regulatory activities to individual cytokines; certain of these cytokines can either induce or suppress HIV, depending on the *in vitro* system that is used. The *in vivo* effects of a cytokine on HIV replication are difficult to predict because most *in vitro* systems reflect a small fraction of the possible interactions in an entire immune system. However, it is likely that cytokines are important modulators of HIV replication *in vivo* and that the balance between HIV-inductive and HIV-suppressive cytokines is important in determining the steady-state level of viral replication that occurs in an HIV-infected individual (166,612,613) (Fig. 17). Alterations in cellular activation and the resultant change in the cytokine milieu, as well as the administration of antiinflammatory cytokines, have been shown to have substantial effects on HIV replication.

Effect of Cytokines on HIV Replication

Multiple cytokines, including IL-1β, IL-2, IL-3, IL-6, IL-12, TNF-α and -β, macrophage (M)-CSF, and GM-CSF, induce HIV replication in *in vitro* systems. Other cytokines, including IL-4, TGF-β, IL-10, and IFN-γ, have dual effects depending on the system used in their study, and some cytokines, including IFN-α and -β and IL-13, have only been observed to suppress HIV replication (614) (Table 4). The α- and β-chemokines also have profound effects on virus replication. Most of these effects are suppressive; however, under certain circumstances these cytokines can upregulate virus replication (166). Cell culture systems used to study cytokine regulation can be broadly divided into transformed cell lines and primary cells. These can be further divided into acute infection systems, where HIV is added to uninfected cell lines or to cells from healthy, uninfected individuals, and endogenous infection systems, where chronically infected cell lines or cells from HIV-infected subjects are used and the virus that replicates is produced by the infected cells. A number of *in vitro* model systems of chronically infected monocytic or T-cell lines, primary cultures of peripheral blood or lymph node mononuclear cells from HIV-infected individuals, and acutely infected primary cell cultures have been used to demonstrate the role of cytokines in the regulation of HIV expression. In addition, modulation of HIV expression has been demonstrated either by manipulating endogenous cytokines or by adding exogenous cytokines to culture.

The best studied activators of HIV replication are the proinflammatory cytokines, TNF-α, IL-1β, and IL-6. HIV infection directly upregulates TNF-α production *in vitro,* and TNF-α increases HIV replication in multiple *in vitro* systems (614). Initial studies of the effect of TNF-α on HIV were conducted in cell lines chronically infected with HIV with low level or no baseline level of virus production. The addition of TNF-α to these cell lines resulted in an increase in virion RNA, protein, and particle production (279,615). This enhancement of HIV replication was found to be due to TNF activation of NF-κB proteins, which bind to tandem NF-κB sites

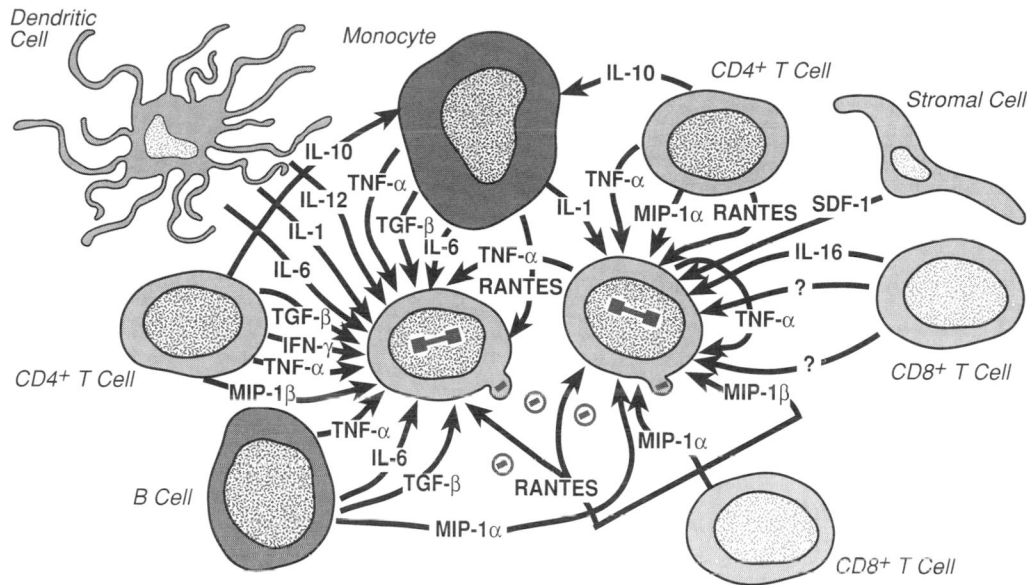

FIG. 16. Cytokine regulatory networks that affect HIV. Endogenous cytokines regulate viral replication in CD4+ T cells. Numerous cytokines, particularly the proinflammatory cytokines TNF-α, IL-1β, and IL-6, strongly upregulate viral replication. TGF-β and IL-10 downregulate viral replication; in the case of IL-10, this effect is at least in part due to downregulation of proinflammatory cytokines. The β-chemokines, which are secreted by a variety of cell types, including CD8+ and CD8- mononuclear cells, strongly inhibit infection by M-tropic strains of HIV-1, whereas SDF-1 inhibits infection with T-tropic strains. Adapted with permission from Fauci AS. *Nature* 1996;384:529.

on the viral LTR and increase transcription (49,616,617). Addition of exogenous TNF-α to monocyte-derived macrophages (MDMs) or activated PBMCs also resulted in enhancement of HIV replication; inhibition of the endogenously produced TNF-α by the addition of neutralizing antibodies or soluble receptors resulted in inhibition of HIV replication (618,619). Another member of the TNF receptor family, CD30, can stimulate HIV replication in a chronically infected T-cell line in an NF-κB–dependent, TNF-independent manner (620,621).

IL-1β directly activates HIV replication in monocytic cell lines by transcriptional and posttranscriptional mechanisms independent of NF-κB. It synergizes with multiple cytokines, including IL-4 and IL-6, to induce HIV expression in the chronically HIV-infected promonocytic U1 cell line; this effect can be inhibited with IL-1 receptor antagonist (ra) (587,622,623). Inhibition of endogenously

produced IL-1β in activated PBMCs by the addition of neutralizing antibodies or IL-1ra to the culture leads to inhibition of viral replication (619). IL-6 induces HIV replication in chronically infected monocytic cell lines and synergizes with other cytokines, including TNF-α. In the U1 promonocytic cell line, the mechanism of IL-6 action on HIV appears to be mainly posttranscriptional; however, when IL-6 was added to TNF-α–stimulated cells, enhancement of transcription was also observed (622). Inhibition of endogenously produced IL-6 in cultures of stimulated PBMCs results in a decrease in viral replication (619).

IL-2 is the most potent stimulator of HIV replication in activated CD4+ T cells, due to the dependence of HIV replication on T-cell proliferation (1,3). IL-2 does not appear to have an enhancing effect on HIV in the absence of T-cell proliferation (624). The addition of IL-2 to acutely infected PBMCs or CD8+ T cell–depleted

HIV-specific immune response

CD8+ T cell-derived suppressor factors (? identity)

RANTES, MIP-1α, MIP-1β (macrophage-tropic HIV strains)

SDF-1 (T cell tropic HIV strains)

Inhibitory cytokines (IL-10, TGF-β)

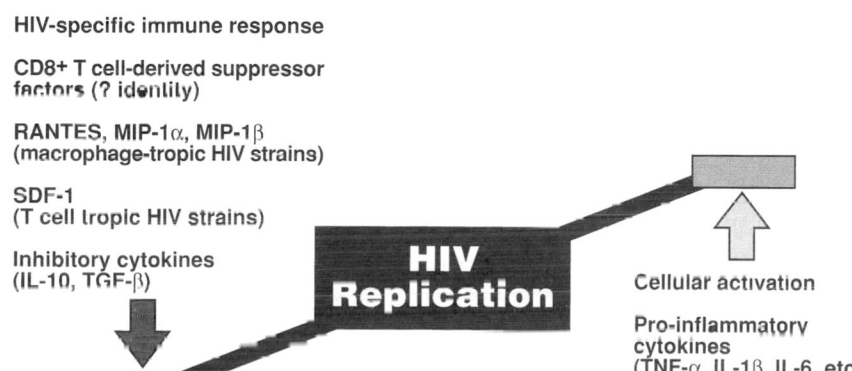

Cellular activation

Pro-inflammatory cytokines (TNF-α, IL-1β, IL-6, etc.)

FIG. 17. A delicate balance of host factors determines the net rate of HIV replication. Some of the HIV-inductive and HIV-suppressive factors are depicted. Adapted with permission from Fauci AS. *Nature* 1996;384:529.

TABLE 4. *Cytokine and cytokine-related molecules with regulatory effects on HIV replication*

Cytokine	Effects on	
	T cells	Macrophages
IL-1β	↑	↑
IL-2	↑	nd
IL-3	nd	↑
IL-4	↑	↑↓
IL-6	nd	↑
IL-10	↓	↑↓
IL-12	↑	nd
IL-13	nd	↓
IL-15	↑	nd
IFN-α	↓	↓
IFN-γ	↑↓	↑↓
TGF-β	↑↓	↑↓
GM-CSF	nd	↑
M-CSF	nd	↑
TNF-α/β	↑	↑
CD30 (ligand)	↑	↑

↑, enhancement of HIV replication; ↓, suppression of HIV replication; nd, not tested or no substantial effects have been reported.

PBMCs from HIV-infected individuals results in the production of multiple cytokines, including IL-1β, IL-6, TNF-α, and IFN-γ. Neutralization of these endogenous cytokines blocks viral replication, suggesting that IL-2 can induce an autocrine and paracrine loop of HIV-inductive cytokines (618,619,625). However, IL-2 also can increase HIV replication in systems that are relatively independent of proinflammatory cytokines, suggesting multiple mechanisms of IL-2–induced HIV replication (626). Although IL-2 can increase the expression of the M-tropic HIV coreceptor CCR5 on CD4⁺ T cells (107), it does not result in a net increase in plasma viremia when administered to HIV-infected subjects, as discussed below.

IL-15 is produced by antigen-presenting cells, including monocytes/macrophages and DCs, and uses portions of the IL-2 receptor (the β chain) for signaling. In both HIV+ and HIV- individuals, IL-15 induces many of the same LAK-activating and IFN-γ–enhancing activities as IL-2. Similarly, both cytokines induce HIV replication in PBMCs, although some reports suggest that IL-15 induces less p24 production compared with that induced by IL-2 (627,628). It also has been suggested that IL-15 plays a role in the hypergamma-globulinemia observed in HIV-infected subjects (629).

IL-4, IL-10, IL-13, TGF-β, and IL-1ra all have antiinflammatory activities in that they inhibit the production or action of the inflammatory mediators IL-1β, IL-6, and TNF-α. In addition to their antiinflammatory effect, each has different and partially overlapping immune activities (see Chapter 21) and each can modulate expression of HIV. IL-4 has both enhancing and suppressing activities on HIV infection of MDMs, depending on the culture conditions (587,630–632). IL-4, either alone or in combination with IL-2, is a very potent stimulator of HIV replication in CD4+ T cells, likely by increasing the growth rate of these cells through its T-cell growth factor activities (626). IL-10 potently inhibits HIV replication in acute and endogenous infection systems of CD4+ T cells. One of its mechanisms of action is an inhibition of activation and proliferation of T cells (626). IL-10 also inhibits HIV replication in MDMs (633–639). At high concentrations, IL-10 inhibits the release of HIV-induced TNF-α and IL-6; exogenous supplementa-

tion of these cytokines restores viral replication (639). At lower concentrations of IL-10, inhibition of TNF-α and IL-6 is incomplete, no inhibition of HIV replication is observed, and modest enhancement may be seen (639). In the chronically HIV-infected U1 cell line, IL-10 alone has no effect on HIV replication; however, it can synergize with multiple cytokines, including IL-1β, IL-4, IL-6, TNF-α, and GM-CSF to increase viral production (640–642). IL-13 has been found to inhibit HIV infection of MDMs by unknown mechanisms (630,643); this effect may be dependent on the stage of maturation of the infected cells (644). TGF-β has dichotomous effects on HIV replication in acutely infected MDMs, depending on when the cytokine is added to the culture relative to infection (645,646). In chronically infected monocytic cell lines, TGF-β blocks phorbol 12-myristate 13-acetate (PMA)- or IL-6–induced production of HIV (645). IL-1ra inhibits HIV replication in IL-2–stimulated PBMCs through its blockade of IL-1β (619). In addition, IL-4, IL-13, and TGF-β inhibit HIV expression in LPS- and GM-CSF–stimulated chronically infected monocytic cell lines by increasing the ratio of expression of endogenous IL-1ra to IL-1β (647). Thus, although each of these antiinflammatory cytokines has multiple effects on HIV replication in different systems, they share the ability to inhibit at least a portion of the proinflammatory cytokine response, thereby inhibiting HIV production.

The colony-stimulating factors GM-CSF and M-CSF are both potent stimulators of HIV replication in MDMs. Initial studies of MDM infection with HIV used M-CSF and GM-CSF to promote the *in vitro* maturation of the macrophages and allow for efficient infection (648–652). GM-CSF has been used in clinical trials for leukopenia in advanced HIV disease; it resulted in a greater than twofold increase in total leukocytes, monocytes, and neutrophils, which was maintained throughout therapy, and no adverse events or significant increases in plasma viremia were detected (653,654). Likewise, a study of GM-CSF therapy in HIV-infected children found similar increases in leukocyte and neutrophil counts (655). Thus, although GM-CSF has been demonstrated to be a potent inducer of HIV replication in MDMs *in vitro*, no increases in viral replication were noted in adults or children receiving this cytokine. This status may have been observed because most patients were concomitantly receiving antiretroviral therapy.

The interferons have potent effects on HIV replication in various *in vitro* systems. IFN-α and -β suppress HIV replication at multiple steps in the viral life cycle in both activated CD4+ T cells and MDMs. In acute infection systems of activated T cells and monocytes, the major level of blockade occurs before formation and integration of the provirus (656). In chronically infected cell lines, at least two mechanisms of inhibition have been identified. One is a block in viral assembly and release (657), and the second is the inhibition of viral transcription (658). IFN-γ enhances HIV replication in CD4+ T cells in an autocrine manner (619). In MDMs and chronically infected monocytic cell lines, it enhances viral replication when added before infection and inhibits replication when added after infection (659). Inhibition of viral replication occurs by a mechanism similar to that observed for the alpha-interferons (657). Clinical trials with IFN-α, generally used to treat Kaposi's sarcoma, have not generally shown a favorable impact on progression of HIV disease (660).

MIP-1α, MIP-1β, and RANTES inhibit M-tropic HIV infection of CD4+ T cells by blocking the interaction of gp160 with CCR5 and subsequent fusion of the virus with the cell membrane (79). However, these chemokines also can enhance viral replication of T-tropic viruses that use CXCR4 for entry into cells (A. Kinter and

A.S. Fauci, unpublished data). They also enhance the replication of M-tropic virus in MDMs (661). Levels of MIP-1α, MIP-1β, and RANTES have varied from individual to individual in most studies; however, no significant differences in plasma levels or in levels from mitogen-stimulated PBMCs were noted among HIV-infected individuals at various stages of disease (511–518). SDF-1, a ligand for CXCR4, the major coreceptor for T-tropic strains of HIV, has been shown to block infection of T-tropic viruses by blocking fusion and entry of the virus (82,83).

Effect of HIV on Cytokine Production and Networks

HIV has multiple effects on cytokine production *in vivo* and *in vitro*. These include direct effects due to infection of cells or binding of the virus to the cell surface, and indirect effects mediated by responses to the viral infection. Soluble viral proteins also can directly induce certain cytokines. The role of HIV-induced dysregulation of cytokine networks in disease pathogenesis is likely multifactorial; many of the alterations in cytokine production, such as the increases in proinflammatory cytokines, favor HIV replication, whereas others, such as the decrease in IL-2 production, have effects that are less clear (613).

As noted above, HIV infection of cells *in vitro* induces the secretion of TNF-α, IL-1β, and IL-6. These proinflammatory cytokines then act on the cell to increase HIV replication, forming an autocrine/paracrine loop (618,619,625). Production of these cytokines is not dependent on infection because the addition of HIV envelope protein alone induces these cytokines through ligation of cell surface CD4 on monocytes and MDMs (639,662). During acute infection with HIV in humans and SIV in macaques, elevated levels of both TNF-α and IL-6 have been observed. During the clinically latent stages of disease, levels of TNF-α, IL-1β, IFN-γ, and IL-6 have been observed to be elevated in some but not all studies (564,618,662–664). PBMCs, CD4+ T cells, monocytes/macrophages, and alveolar macrophages from HIV-infected subjects produce more TNF-α *in vitro* compared with cells from healthy, uninfected control subjects (665–667). Certain studies have demonstrated that, with disease progression, levels of TNF-α increase, suggesting a pathogenic role for this cytokine.

Dysregulation of IL-2 production has long been recognized as a characteristic of HIV infection (668). HIV infection of CD4+ T cells *in vitro* results in a decreased ability to produce IL-2; indeed, CD4+ T cells isolated from HIV-infected individuals produce abnormally low levels of IL-2 in response to mitogenic or antigenic stimulation (383). A decrease in IL-2 production and loss of antigen-specific T cells are hallmarks of the immune deficiency of HIV infection. IL-2 protein and mRNA levels are reduced in both PBMCs and lymph node cells from HIV-infected individuals compared with levels found in healthy, uninfected control subjects (383,665). Loss of IL-2 secretion in response to mitogens, alloantigens, and recall antigens correlates with the loss of CD4+ T cells and disease progression (669–671).

T helper (Th)-1 cells are characterized by the secretion of IL-2 and IFN-γ and favor cell-mediated immune responses, whereas Th2 cells secrete IL-4, IL-5, and IL-6 and preferentially support humoral immune responses, although clones of each type can support either activity. Although it is clear that the Th1 limb of cellular immune responses is impaired during the course of HIV infection (669,672–674), controversy surrounds the proposed dominance of Th2-like responses (i.e., secretion of IL-4, IL-5, and IL-10) during progression of HIV disease. Clerici and co-workers showed that stimulated PBMCs from HIV-infected patients exhibit a preferential Th2 pattern of cytokine secretion with disease progression (669,672,675,676); however, other investigators have found a skewing of the cytokine secretion pattern of T cells from HIV-infected patients toward a Th0 state (i.e., secretion of cytokines characteristic of both Th1 and Th2 patterns) rather than toward a Th2 state (383,673,674). In either case, the finding that HIV replication is more efficient in Th0 compared with Th1 clones (673,677) highlights the potential importance of impaired Th1 responses in the pathogenesis of HIV disease (678).

In vitro studies of the effect of various cytokines on HIV replication provide models to understand possible pathogenic mechanisms; however, the complexity of the *in vivo* cytokine network renders the interpretation of the role of individual cytokines in HIV pathogenesis quite difficult. In this regard, a number of cytokines have been used therapeutically in HIV-infected individuals; these include IL-2, IL-4, IL-10, IFN-α, and GM-CSF.

IL-2 is currently being studied in clinical trials using a regimen of continuous intravenous or daily subcutaneous dosing for 3 to 5 days followed by a rest period of approximately 8 weeks. In phase I and II studies, many subjects had a significant increase in their CD4+ T-cell counts, often to ranges of 800 to 1,000/ml (679,680) (Fig. 18). Administration of IL-2 was associated with multiple, transient adverse effects that correlated in part with IL-2–induced secretion of TNF-α. A transient increase in plasma viremia that returned to baseline was also noted in the acute setting of IL-2 administration. All patients who received IL-2 were also receiving some form of antiretroviral therapy, and levels of baseline viremia were no different from those in comparable patients who were receiving antiretroviral therapy without IL-2. In subjects with low CD4+ T-cell counts (i.e., less than 200 cells/ml) who received IL-2, CD4+ T-cell counts failed to increase and levels of plasma viremia increased (679,680). This latter finding likely relates to the fact that patients with lower CD4+ T cell counts were more likely to harbor a virus that was resistant to the antiretroviral drugs that they were receiving. In addition, patients with advanced stage HIV disease have substantial depletion of multiple CD4+ T-cell clones, a situation apparently not reversed by IL-2 therapy (see section above on HIV Infection and the Development of HIV Disease) (143). In cells isolated from patients with moderate immunodeficiency, IL-2 *in vitro* selectively and preferentially induces the noncytolytic CD8 suppressor effect discussed previously, rather than increasing virus replication (681). The addition of combination antiviral drugs, including protease inhibitors, to IL-2 therapy resulted in a more sustained increase in CD4+ T-cell counts, a blunted transient burst in plasma viremia, and increases in CD4+ T-cell counts in patients with initial counts below 200 cells/μl. Increases in CD4+ T cells during IL-2 therapy appear to result from extrathymic expansion of the existing CD4+ T-cell repertoire because PCR analysis of the T-cell receptor repertoire indicated that deleted clones are not regenerated and that the repertoire remains skewed as it expands (143).

IL-10 has been used in phase 1 clinical trials in HIV-infected subjects. In subjects receiving 1 μg/kg as a single intravenous dose, a transient decrease in plasma viremia was noted (average decrease 70%) that returned to baseline in 24 to 48 hours (D. Weissman and A.S. Fauci, unpublished data). In addition, inhibition of *in vitro* LPS-induced secretion of proinflammatory cytokines (e.g., TNF-α, IL-1β, IL-6) was observed. Potential mechanisms responsible for the IL-10–induced decrease in plasma viremia include suppression of HIV-inducing proinflam-

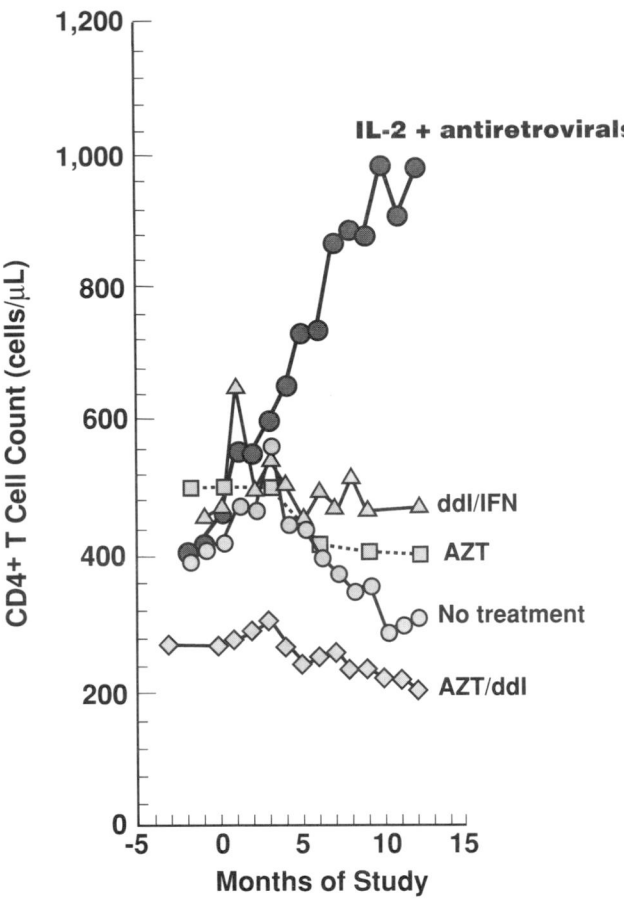

FIG. 18. IL-2 administration in combination with antiretroviral agents induces sustained increases in CD4+ T-cell counts compared with antiretroviral therapy alone or no treatment.

matory cytokines, a decrease in cellular activation, and increased clearance of virions from plasma.

IL-4 has been used in the treatment of Kaposi's sarcoma. No increases in plasma viral load were observed during treatment, again demonstrating the differences between *in vitro* systems and *in vivo* action.

HIV Infection and Cytokine Networks in the Central Nervous System

HIV-induced CNS disease likely is a result of the complex interaction of cytokine networks and activation of the targets of HIV infection, including microglial cells. HIV infection of brain microglial cells, derived from the monocytic lineage, may lead to certain of the manifestations of HIV nervous system disease. HIV infection of microglial cells, like that of CD4+ T cells, results in a higher level of cytopathicity than that seen in macrophages (682). The manifestations of HIV infection of microglial cells include encephalopathy and neuropathy (214), astrocytosis (215), and cerebral vasculitis (216,217). IL-1β and TNF-α, both induced by HIV, have neurotoxic activities (683–686). TGF-β, an antiinflammatory cytokine, has been demonstrated to have both a neuroprotective (687) and a neurotoxic effect (688). IL-10 has a macrophage-deactivating and antiproinflammatory effect on CNS microglia, resulting in a decrease in neurotoxin release (689).

New insights into the pathogenesis of AIDS-associated CMV encephalitis highlight the complex interactions between cytokines, HIV coreceptors, and HIV. Bernasconi and co-workers reported that levels of the chemokine monocyte chemotactic protein (MCP)-1, were markedly elevated in the cerebrospinal fluid of patients with AIDS who had CMV encephalitis (690). Subsequently, it was shown that CMV encodes a chemokine receptor, US28, that is homologous to CCR2 (691). This receptor is triggered by MCP-1 and also can be used by HIV as a co-receptor for cell entry. Thus, the high levels of MCP-1 that are found in cerebrospinal fluid during CMV encephalitis may be responsible for recruitment and activation of monocytes; these cells can elaborate proinflammatory cytokines and thereby enhance HIV replication and induce neuropathologic disease. Furthermore, expression of US28 on CMV-infected cells may provide HIV with an expanded range of target cells for infection.

IMMUNE RESPONSES

The absence of known correlates of protective immunity to HIV infection presents a major obstacle to the development of effective immunotherapies and vaccines. Some evidence suggests that particular immune responses to HIV may actually be harmful to the host. Certain antienvelope gp41 antibodies present in the sera of HIV-infected individuals enhance rather than inhibit HIV replication *in vitro* (692,693); the presence of these HIV-enhancing antibodies correlates with progression to AIDS (694). In addition, antibody responses to a specific epitope (residues 503 to 528) within the carboxy terminus of gp120 are associated with disease progression (695). Anti-HIV CTL responses may be pathogenic in HIV-related inflammatory syndromes such as lymphocytic alveolitis (696,697). It also has been suggested that HIV-specific CTLs may play a central role in HIV pathogenesis by killing HIV-infected antigen-presenting cells in lymph nodes, bone marrow, and thymus, thus impairing the generation of immune responses (698).

A larger body of evidence supports a salutary role for most HIV-specific immune responses. The profound decrease in plasma viremia after acute HIV infection is associated with the appearance of HIV-specific cellular (194,197) and humoral (198,699–701) immune responses. The correlation of slow progression with vigorous HIV-specific immune responses also argues strongly in favor of a salutary role for these responses (see section below on Long-Term Nonprogressors).

Humoral Immune Responses

Anti-p24 Antibodies

Antibodies against the viral core protein p24 develop within weeks of acute HIV infection and may play a role in the decline of plasma viremia associated with primary infection (198,700,702, 703). Loss of anti-p24 antibodies is associated with progression of HIV disease (198,700,702–705).

Neutralizing Antibodies

Antibodies that neutralize HIV infectivity *in vitro* are likely an important host mechanism responsible for at least partial control of viral replication *in vivo* (700,705–709). Neutralizing antibodies may be type specific (i.e., specific for one viral isolate) or group specific (i.e., specific for a broad range of viral isolates). Most type-specific neutralizing antibodies recognize the V3 region of the

HIV envelope gp120 protein (710–715). These neutralizing anti-V3 loop antibodies may prevent cleavage and conformational changes within gp120 necessary for HIV entry or for cell–cell fusion (713,716–719). Group-specific neutralizing antibodies recognize epitopes within the HIV envelope gp41 protein (720–722), discontinuous conformational epitopes around the CD4 binding site of gp120 (723–726) or carbohydrate determinants (727). Both type- and group-specific neutralizing antibodies are more efficient in neutralizing laboratory strains of HIV grown in T-cell lines as opposed to primary isolates grown in PBMCs; this is likely due to differential exposure of the V3 loop and CD4 binding domain epitopes (728–731). Some neutralizing antibodies interfere with the interaction between the HIV envelope and CCR5, thereby inhibiting cellular entry of M-tropic strains of HIV (35,36).

The type of neutralizing antibody most relevant to the course of HIV infection is that which neutralizes autologous viral isolates (732–734). The regularity with which viral variants emerge that resist neutralization suggests that such autologous neutralizing antibodies are potent impediments to viral replication (732, 735–737). This cycle of neutralization followed by escape may be continuous over the course of infection because serum from a given time point may neutralize contemporaneously isolated virus, but not virus isolated at a later time point (735,736,738).

There is disagreement surrounding the potential correlation between the presence of HIV-neutralizing antibodies and course of disease. This is not surprising given the many different types of neutralizing antibodies that can be detected and the wide variety of assays for neutralization. Several studies do, however, suggest that the presence of neutralizing antibodies with broad specificity is correlated with a more favorable prognosis (199,204,699,709,739, 740).

Antibodies that Mediate ADCC

Some anti-HIV antibodies bind to IgG Fc receptor–positive cells and sensitize them to mediate ADCC against HIV-infected or HIV-coated cells (741–744). Most of these antibodies are directed against HIV envelope gp120 or gp41 proteins (741,743–747). CD16+ NK cells are important mediators of ADCC (744,748), although monocytes also may mediate this activity (749). Anti-HIV ADCC antibodies develop soon after primary infection and are detectable throughout the course of HIV disease, with some decrease in titers with the onset of AIDS (750–752).

Cellular Immune Responses

Cytotoxic T-Lymphocytes

In HIV-infected individuals, classical MHC class I–restricted, HIV-specific, CD8+ CTL responses have been demonstrated (212, 213,753) against a variety of HIV target proteins (754), including core proteins (755,756), RT (757–759), envelope proteins (759–762), and regulatory proteins (763). An extraordinarily high frequency of HIV-specific CTLs and CTL precursors (up to 1% of peripheral blood T cells) has been observed in asymptomatic HIV-infected patients (764,765).

A critical role for CTLs in the suppression of viral replication in HIV-infected individuals is suggested by the close correlation between emergence of an HIV-specific CTL response and downregulation of viremia after acute infection (194,197), the decline in HIV-specific CTL activity with disease progression (212,764), and

the association of vigorous HIV-specific CTL responses with slow progression of HIV disease (199,766–769). A beneficial role for HIV-specific CTLs is also suggested by their presence in the peripheral blood of individuals who are frequently exposed to HIV yet remain uninfected (770), and the depletion of HIV-specific CTLs from lymph nodes of patients with advanced HIV disease (771). These data argue against an immunopathogenic role for CTLs in HIV disease (698), although, as previously noted, CTL responses may be involved in the pathogenesis of some of the HIV-related inflammatory syndromes (696,697).

Qualitative aspects of the HIV-specific CTL response are also important determinants of the efficacy of these responses in controlling viral replication. Maintenance of CTL responses specific for viral core proteins is associated with a decreased risk of disease progression (769,772); however, similar associations have not been observed for CTL responses against other viral proteins. CTL recognition of immunodominant HIV epitopes presented by certain MHC class I alleles may result in potent anti-HIV activity (773) and may in part explain the association of certain MHC class I alleles with slower progression of HIV disease (774–776). Furthermore, examination of the skewing of the CD8+ T-cell receptor Vβ repertoire in HIV-infected individuals suggests that the ability to recruit an HIV-specific CTL response composed of a diverse group of Vβ families during primary infection is associated with better control of viral replication and an improved prognosis compared with a restricted CTL expansion from only one or two Vβ families (see section above on HIV Infection and the Development of HIV Disease) (175).

The loss of HIV-specific CTL activity in patients with progressive disease is likely a result of several factors. The viral accessory proteins Tat, Nef, and Vpu can downregulate cellular expression of MHC class I molecules that are necessary for CTL recognition of infected cells (386,390,391). Another mechanism responsible for the loss of CTL activity is the selective accumulation of CD8+DR+ HIV-specific CTLs that lack the IL-2 receptor and are defective in clonogenic potential (756,777,778). Finally, the ability of HIV to escape CTL responses by viral mutation or by exhaustion of CTL clones due to high concentration of antigen help explain the loss of CTL-mediated control over viral replication (207).

The host CTL response against HIV is constrained by the ability of the MHC class I alleles to bind to various viral epitopes, whereas the virus is constrained by the degree to which an escape mutation impairs viral fitness. These host–virus dynamics are extraordinarily complex given the large number of permutations of viral epitopes and MHC class I alleles. Viral mutations within CTL recognition epitopes (i.e., escape mutants) are associated with increased levels of viral replication and progression of HIV disease (779–782). Viral escape mutants may thrive due to the release of CTL control over their replication and may inhibit CTL responses against the preescape viral epitope (783,784). Itescu and co-workers suggested that some viral escape mutations are costly to viral fitness. These investigators found that diffuse infiltrative CD8 lymphocytosis in HIV infection was associated with certain HLA types that apparently constrain evolution of viral sequence diversity in the envelope V3 loop (785). Other studies have highlighted the constraints on the host CTL response imposed by MHC class I alleles. Kalams and co-workers demonstrated in an HIV-infected individual that CTL clones specific for an HLA-B14–restricted epitope of gp41 displayed limited diversity of T-cell receptor utilization (786). These investigators further demonstrated the limited plasticity of certain CTL responses in individuals with viral escape mutants in whom the dominant CTL response may remain largely directed at the preescape viral epitope (787,788). Other studies demonstrated that increased plasticity of the CTL response (i.e., generation of vigorous escape mutant–specific CTLs) may allow the host to maintain more continuous and effective control over viral replication (170,789). A mathematical model of CTL-virus dynamics was provided by Nowak and co-workers who described disease progression as a result of viral sequence variation that escapes an immunodominant CTL response and shifts the host response toward a weaker epitope (173). In this scenario, disease progression may be the result of fitness of viral escape mutants outpacing the plasticity of the host CTL response, with slow progression resulting from CTL plasticity overpowering viral escape mutants with limited fitness.

A further mechanism for loss of CTL control over viral replication may be clonal exhaustion. This appears to be a strategy for viral persistence used by other viruses, such as certain strains of lymphocytic choriomeningitis virus that rapidly and completely mobilize the host CTL response resulting in CTL exhaustion (i.e., high zone tolerance) (790). CTL exhaustion also may occur to some degree in HIV infection: the disappearance of some CTL clonotypes can be demonstrated in the absence of viral escape mutations, which might otherwise explain the phenomenon (207).

CD8 Soluble Suppressor Factors

A variety of soluble antiviral factors are elaborated by CD8+ T cells. CD8 antiviral factor (CAF) (791–793) is noncytolytic, acts in a non–MHC-restricted manner, inhibits viral replication at the level of HIV LTR transcription (794–796), and lacks identity to known cytokines (797). CAF activity decreases with disease progression but remains potent in long-term nonprogressors (517,739,798). The combination of RANTES, MIP-1α, and MIP-1β (the natural ligands for CCR5, a major coreceptor for M-tropic strains of HIV) are also important soluble antiviral factors and are secreted by CD8+ T cells and other cell types (79,681). These β-chemokines inhibit viral replication primarily at the level of cell entry. Conflicting data have been obtained regarding a relationship between levels of these chemokines and progression of HIV disease (511–518). A recent report, however, does support a possible role for the β-chemokines in the protection of some exposed-uninfected individuals against HIV infection. Upon stimulation with HIV antigens, CD4+ T cells from these individuals secreted high levels of β-chemokines that were capable of inhibiting the replication of M-tropic strains of HIV in vitro (799). Finally, IL-16 has been reported to be a soluble antiviral factor (800); however, a relationship between IL-16 production and disease progression remains to be established (515,517).

CD4+ T-Cell Responses

HIV proteins contain helper T cell epitopes that may be presented by MHC class II alleles (801–803). Recognition of these epitopes by CD4+ T cells results in IL-2 secretion and cellular proliferation. These responses decrease with HIV disease progression (804); however, it is uncertain whether CD4+ T-cell proliferative responses to HIV of themselves play any definitive protective or deleterious role in HIV-specific immunity. In this regard, it is likely that IL-2 produced during these responses augments HIV-specific CTL responses; however, IL-2 also may indirectly enhance HIV replication by inducing secretion of proinflammatory cytokines (619,625).

GENETIC FACTORS IN HIV PATHOGENESIS

Host genetic factors influence the rate of disease progression in HIV infection. Multiple reports have described MHC alleles, including class I, II, and III, and other host factors that may influence the pathogenesis and course of HIV disease. Associations with certain HIV-related manifestations such as Kaposi's sarcoma and diffuse lymphadenopathy, and with the rate of clinical disease progression, have been reported for particular alleles (774–776, 805). Certain MHC haplotypes (i.e., DQ2, DR3, B8, Cw7, A1) show an association with more rapid progression to AIDS in pediatric HIV infection (806). Additionally, in pediatric HIV infection the DR3 haplotypes DRB1*0301, DQA1*0501, and DQB1*0201 correlate with an increased risk of encephalopathy, greater CD4+ T cell loss, and death before age 2 (807). Among HIV-infected adults, HLA-B27, B57, and B51 are most strongly associated with a slower rate of disease progression, whereas HLA-A23, B37, and B49 are associated with rapid progression (776). In a study of hemophilic twins, the presence of certain class II haplotypes also was significantly associated with the rate of disease progression (808). Transporter-associated with antigen-presenting (TAP) genes, which are members of the MHC class III family of alleles, also have been observed to play a role in determining the rate of disease progression in HIV infection. In this regard, HLA profiles that reflect certain combinations of MHC-encoded TAP genes and class I and class II genes are strongly associated with different rates of HIV disease progression. TAP genes such as TAP1.4 and the combination of TAP1.4 and 2.3 have been found to be significantly increased in individuals who have been exposed to HIV-1 but do not become infected (809).

A number of different mechanisms may be responsible for the observed associations between certain HLA haplotypes and different rates of HIV disease progression (774–776,805). Some HLA molecules may be associated with slow disease progression due to their ability to efficiently present immunodominant epitopes for antiviral cell-mediated immune responses. Other HLA molecules may promote immunopathogenic responses associated with more rapid disease progression.

Alloantigen-specific immune responses may protect some individuals with rare MHC haplotypes from HIV infection. Alloantigen-stimulated lymphocytes have been shown to inhibit HIV replication in vitro (810); certain rare MHC class I and class II alleles therefore might allow for the rapid recognition of HIV-infected cells from the HIV-infected partner and promote rejection of these cells by alloreactive responses before HIV infection can occur. Similarly, common shared MHC alleles may lead to less effective removal of HIV-infected allogeneic cells, contributing to an increased efficiency of infection.

As previously discussed, CCR5 is a major coreceptor for M-tropic strains of HIV-1 (see section above on HIV Coreceptors) (88–92). A mutant allele of the CCR5 gene, which contains an internal 32–base pair deletion resulting in a truncated nonfunctional coreceptor for HIV fusion (100,103,811), is associated with slower rates of HIV disease progression. Homozygosity for the CCR5 mutation results in near-total protection from HIV-1 infection (100–106). Heterozygosity for the CCR5 mutation results in decreased expression of CCR5 on the cell surface and reduced infectability of T cells with M-tropic strains of HIV-1 compared with cells from CCR5 wild-type individuals (108). Although heterozygosity for CCR5 does not appear to afford protection against HIV-1 infection, it may result in partial protection against disease progression in HIV-infected individuals (101–103,167,812,813). Protection against disease progression in *CCR5* heterozygotes is due in part to the lower viral load set point after HIV seroconversion, and a slower rate of CD4+ T-cell depletion compared with CCR5 wild-type individuals (102). In addition, heterozygosity for the *CCR5* mutation is significantly more common in cohorts of HIV-infected long-term nonprogressors compared with HIV-infected control populations (103,167,812,813).

Other genetic polymorphisms may influence susceptibility to HIV infection and rates of disease progression. Polymorphisms in cytokine genes may influence the response to HIV, as has been demonstrated with other pathogens. In this regard, certain strains of mice have a Th2 response to pathogens while other strains respond in a Th1 fashion. Depending on the pathogen, a Th1 or Th2 response may be protective or lethal (see Chapter 38). Other genetic factors reported to affect rates of HIV disease progression include allelic forms of the vitamin D binding factor Gc (814), variant alleles of mannose-binding lectin (815), and the TNF c2 microsatellite allele (816).

LONG-TERM NONPROGRESSORS

The mean time between infection with HIV and development of AIDS is approximately 10 years; however, rates of disease progression vary widely among individuals. In recent years, it has become clear that in a small percentage of HIV-infected individuals no evidence of disease progression can be detected over a long period of time (199,516,739,817–823). Studies of such long-term nonprogressors have contributed to our understanding of the pathogenesis of disease progression and have increased optimism that some forms of protective immunity may indeed exist in HIV infection.

Definitions of long-term nonprogressors have varied; however, a reasonable consensus may include documented HIV infection for more than 7 years; CD4+ T-cell count greater than 600 cells/µl without significant decline over time; no symptoms of HIV disease; and no history of antiretroviral therapy (824). Because definitions of long-term nonprogressors were created empirically, it is not surprising that such individuals constitute a heterogeneous group. Long-term nonprogressors have been identified in all HIV risk groups, and no demographic features reliably distinguish them from typical progressors. Mechanisms that may determine a nonprogressive course during HIV infection include host genetic factors, effective immunologic control of virus replication, or infection with an attenuated strain of HIV (Table 5). Certain HLA haplotypes as well as heterozygosity for a defective *CCR5* gene are associated with slow progression; however, these factors do not appear to be dominant. Compared with individuals with progressive HIV disease, nonprogressors tend to have lower viral loads, higher numbers of circulating CD8+ T cells, and more vigorous antiviral humoral and cell-mediated immune responses. However, measurement of any of these parameters in nonprogressors reveals a great deal of heterogeneity as well as some degree of overlap with measurements in progressors. In this regard, it is likely that determinants of nonprogression are multifactorial. It is currently uncertain whether nonprogressors represent the extreme tail of the normal distribution of the rate of disease progression (slow progressors), or whether some may actually never experience disease progression (true nonprogressors).

TABLE 5. *Possible mechanisms of long-term nonprogression with HIV infection*

Host genetic factors
  Slow progressor HLA profile
  Heterozygosity for 32–bp deletion in CC chemokine receptor 5
  Mannose binding lectin alleles
  Tumor necrosis factor c2 microsatellite alleles
  Gc vitamin D–binding factor alleles
Host immune response factors
  Effective CTL responses
  Secretion of CD8 antiviral factor
  Secretion of chemokines that block HIV entry coreceptors CCR5 (e.g., MIP-1α, MIP-1β, and RANTES) and CXCR4 (e.g. SDF-1)
  Secretion of IL-16
  Effective humoral immune response
  Maintenance of functional lymphoid tissue architecture
Virologic factors
  Infection with attenuated strains of HIV

Host Genetic Factors

As previously discussed, an HIV-infected individual's MHC haplotype plays an important role in determining his or her rate of disease progression (see section above on Genetic Factors in HIV Pathogenesis). In addition, *CCR5* genotype has an impact on rates of progression of HIV-induced disease; individuals who harbor one copy of the mutant *CCR5-Δ32* allele have an increased chance of experiencing a slow rate of disease progression compared with individuals who inherit only the wild-type alleles (see section above on Genetic Factors in HIV Pathogenesis) (101–103,167,812, 813). Despite the association between *CCR5* genotype and nonprogressive HIV infection, this factor does not appear to be a dominant influence in the determination of the state of long-term nonprogression. In this regard, although the frequency of *CCR5* heterozygotes is increased twofold among nonprogressors compared with HIV-infected controls, fewer than 50% of nonprogressors are *CCR5* heterozygotes (103). The possibility that *CCR5* heterozygotes might constitute a subgroup among nonprogressors with the lowest viral loads and most preserved CD4+ T-cell counts was investigated; however, the immunologic and virologic profile of *CCR5* wild-type and *CCR5* heterozygous nonprogressors was indistinguishable (812). These data indicate that although *CCR5* heterozygotes have an increased chance of becoming nonprogressors, HIV-infected *CCR5* wild-type individuals may arrive at the same phenotype by other means.

Host Immune Response Factors

Precursor frequencies of HIV-specific CTLs with broad specificity have been consistently detected at higher levels in long-term nonprogressors compared with progressors (199,766–769). This observation has a number of important implications regarding the pathogenesis of HIV disease progression. The maintenance of high precursor frequencies of HIV-specific CTLs in the face of low or undetectable levels of plasma viremia indicates that HIV replication is active (i.e., in lymphoid tissue) in long-term nonprogressors (199). The presence of CTLs in nonprogressors also argues against a proposed immunopathogenic role for CTLs in HIV disease (698). It is likely that HIV-specific CTLs play at least some role in the maintenance of low viral load and the state of nonprogression. This inference follows from the demonstrated role of CTLs in reducing levels of plasma viremia during primary HIV infection (194,197), and the association of progression to AIDS with late viral escape from a long-lived (9 to 12 years) immunodominant CTL response (782). Further support for the salutary role of CTLs comes from a longitudinal study in which maintenance of HIV Gag-specific CTL precursors was associated with nonprogression, whereas loss of these CTLs was associated with increasing viral load and CD4+ T-cell depletion (769).

Soluble antiviral factors elaborated by CD8+ T cells also may play a role in nonprogression of HIV infection, as previously discussed (see section above on Immune Responses). In this regard, CAF activity correlates with stage of disease (798), and studies of long-term nonprogressors have demonstrated more potent CD8+ T cell–derived soluble antiviral responses compared with progressors (517,739).

RANTES, MIP-1α, and MIP-1β are also important antiviral soluble factors secreted by CD8+ T cells as well as other cell types (79,681). These chemokines are natural ligands for CCR5, a coreceptor for M-tropic strains of HIV-1, and inhibit viral replication primarily at the level of cell entry. Conflicting data have been obtained regarding a relationship between levels of these chemokines and progression of HIV disease (511–518). Finally, IL-16 has been reported to be a soluble antiviral factor (800); a relationship between IL-16 production and disease progression remains to be established (515,517).

The relationship between humoral immune responses to HIV and disease progression remains uncertain (825). Nonprogressive HIV infection has been associated with lack of an antibody response to an epitope (residues 503 to 528) within the carboxy terminus of gp120 (695), with maintenance of high levels of p24-specific antibodies (704), and with maintenance of neutralizing antibodies (199,204,739). Sei and co-workers showed that the presence of HIV IIIB–neutralizing antibodies correlated with a more favorable prognosis (699). Subsequent studies demonstrated that the presence of neutralizing antibodies to primary HIV isolates and to autologous virus was associated with nonprogression (205,737). Furthermore, viral escape from neutralizing antibody responses is associated with emergence of the SI phenotype of HIV and with disease progression (735,737). Although HIV-infected long-term nonprogressors tend to maintain antibody responses that can neutralize a broad panel of primary isolates and autologous virus isolates, they are a heterogeneous group with regard to these neutralizing antibody responses (204,205). Whether the maintenance of neutralizing antibodies in nonprogressors is simply a marker for a relatively intact immune system or whether these antibodies play an active role in determining the state of nonprogression remains unclear.

The morphologic abnormalities of lymphoid tissue associated with HIV disease progression are important determinants of immunodeficiency (249–256). Despite the long period of HIV infection in long-term nonprogressors, histopathologic examination of lymph node biopsy samples from these individuals shows only mild HIV-related abnormalities such as follicular hyperplasia (199,826). The follicular involution, fibrosis, and lymphocyte depletion associated with progressive HIV disease are lacking in lymph nodes from nonprogressors. The degree of follicular hyperplasia seen in nonprogressors is significantly less than that seen in progressors and is qualitatively distinct as well, without evidence of large geographic germinal centers extending into the nodal medulla (199,826). It is likely that preservation of lymphoid architecture in nonprogressors is a reflection of the lower levels of viral replication over time. Regardless of the mechanisms responsible

for lower levels of viral replication in nonprogressors, preservation of lymphoid tissue architecture is a critical component of their immunocompetence. This further highlights the need to understand the mechanisms responsible for the destruction of lymphoid architecture during progression of HIV disease. If immunorestorative strategies in advanced HIV infection are to be successful, substrate for the generation of immune responses (i.e., intact lymphoid tissue) must be present, necessitating the prevention or reversal of the histopathologic abnormalities of lymphoid tissue associated with HIV disease progression.

Virologic Factors

Infection with attenuated strains of HIV may result in nonprogression in a small subset of individuals. The strongest evidence for an association of attenuated viral strains and nonprogression comes from an Australian cohort of nonprogressors who were infected by transfusion from a common donor, himself a nonprogressor (827,828). Viruses from these individuals frequently contained deletions in the *nef* gene and in the *nef*/U3 LTR overlap region, as well as duplications and rearrangements of NF-κB/SP-1 sites in the viral LTR (828). Another isolated nonprogressor with viruses containing deletions within the *nef* gene was reported by Kirchhoff et al. (829). Although these cases argue strongly that nonprogression may be due to infection with viral strains containing attenuated *nef* genes, this scenario appears to be uncommon even among long-term nonprogressors (830–832). Other anecdotes implicate defective *rev, vif, vpr, vpu,* and *tat* genes in the pathogenesis of nonprogression (833,834); however, such instances appear to be the exception rather than the rule (835,836). Recent studies of the HIV *env* genes from long-term nonprogressors suggest the presence of functional defects in the ability to mediate viral entry in some individuals, as well as some unique mutations in the V3 region (837) (S. Menzo and O. Cohen, unpublished data).

VACCINES

Given the current magnitude of the global HIV pandemic (i.e., 22.6 million people living with HIV infection) and the projected increase to more than 40 million cumulative infections by the year 2000, the development of safe and effective prophylactic vaccines is essential. There are a number of formidable challenges to the development of an HIV vaccine. One of the most important is the lack of clear-cut correlates of protective immunity (838). The virus has a high degree of antigenic variability due to the high error rate of RT; in addition, infection can be transmitted by cell-free or cell-associated virus.

Despite gaps in our understanding of the correlates of protective immunity in HIV infection, a number of observations suggest that such protective immune responses may exist. As noted above, individuals who remain uninfected and seronegative despite multiple exposures to HIV have been identified, suggesting that immunologic elements of protection exist but may not be readily detectable by standard measures of immune response. This group is likely heterogeneous with regard to the mechanisms of resistance to HIV infection (839).

A prophylactic HIV vaccine ideally would prevent infection; however, a vaccine that significantly altered the course of HIV disease and decreased infectiousness of a vaccinated individual who subsequently became infected could have an impact both on that individual and on the spread of the infection in the community

(840). At present, multiple types of immune responses have been generated with prophylactic vaccines. It has been proposed that vaccines that induce (a) a strong CTL response, (b) specific neutralizing antibodies, and (c) mucosal immunity may afford some level of protection (838).

A useful animal model for vaccine development is SIV infection of macaques. SIV is closely related to HIV-2 and causes an acute infection that leads to CD4+ T-cell depletion, immunodeficiency, opportunistic infections, and death in susceptible animals. A number of studies using different preparations of SIV vaccines have demonstrated protection from infection, although the mechanisms of protection are not always understood and are not necessarily directed against viral components. Macaques infected with an SIV lacking the *nef* gene develop a nonpathogenic infection and are protected from a subsequent challenge with a pathogenic SIV containing an active *nef* gene (841). The mechanism of protection of the attenuated *nef*-deleted SIV is unknown. Of note, when the attenuated *nef*-deleted virus was given to neonatal macaques, a pathogenic infection ensued (842), suggesting that the attenuated virus is pathogenic under certain circumstances. However, disagreement exists regarding this question because others have safely given attenuated SIV to neonatal animals (843).

Vaccines using inactivated SIV or viral proteins in various delivery vectors have afforded protection from subsequent challenge with a pathogenic virus. In studies using antigens that did not result in complete protection from infection, progression of the disease that developed after infection appeared to be slowed (844,845). Again, the mechanisms responsible for protection from infection in immunized animals are not clear. In certain studies using inactivated virus vaccines, the protective elements of the immune response were not directed toward the virus itself but toward components of the cells used in growing the viral stocks (i.e., cellular proteins that were incorporated into the viral envelope as the virions budded from the cells) (846–848). These data suggest that antibodies or immune responses to certain cell surface proteins that participate in SIV binding may provide excellent protection against infection (847,848). In addition, allogeneic responses to the cells used to produce the pathogenic challenge viral stock may play a role in the protection from infection (810). Vaccine studies using envelope-expressing recombinant vaccinia virus as a primary immunization and recombinant envelope as a booster immunization suggest that an immune response to the envelope is potentially protective (841,849–851).

The most suitable animal model for HIV infection is the chimpanzee; however, chimpanzees are an endangered species, they are expensive, and when infected with HIV they rarely develop any manifestations of HIV-induced disease. Unless a candidate vaccine prevents infection in this model, its overall impact on disease progression cannot be readily assessed. Recently, immunization of chimpanzees with either whole inactivated virus followed by protein or peptide boosting or with recombinant envelope proteins conferred protection against subsequent infection with HIV-1 (852,853). A DNA vaccine containing the HIV-1 *env, rev,* and *gag/pol* genes protected vaccinated chimpanzees from infection with a heterologous HIV-1 challenge (854). These data suggest the feasibility of inducing at least partial protection against HIV infection in humans by vaccination.

Clinical trials of potential HIV vaccines in both uninfected and HIV infected individuals have been undertaken (855–857). Recombinant envelope proteins and recombinant non-HIV viruses expressing HIV envelope proteins have proven safe and immunogenic in healthy uninfected volunteers. Some of these approaches

also have been assessed as active immunotherapy in patients who are already infected. The type of immune response that develops from a particular vaccine depends on multiple properties, including the composition, route of delivery, dose, and adjuvant. Live virus vaccines (canarypox or vaccinia genetically modified to express HIV proteins) or DNA vaccines, in which the viral antigens are synthesized within the host cell, usually result in the generation of cytotoxic T-cell responses. Killed virus vaccines and recombinant proteins tend to promote antibody responses, although this appears to be dose-dependent.

The first generation of candidate HIV vaccines were composed of recombinant envelope proteins derived from HIV-LAV, the prototypic T-cell line–tropic strain of HIV. The predominant immune response to these immunizations in uninfected individuals was humoral (858), and antibodies induced by these immunogens varied in the level of their neutralizing activity. A major drawback of these initial vaccine candidates was that the antibodies induced could only neutralize T-tropic viruses. As discussed above, a significant difference between M-tropic primary isolates and T-cell line–adapted laboratory isolates, in addition to the coreceptor they use for cellular entry, is that T-tropic viruses are easily neutralized by antibodies, whereas M-tropic viruses are poorly neutralized (857). A further confounding issue is that different clades or subtypes of HIV are present throughout the world. Clade B is predominant in North America and western Europe but not in Africa, India, or Asia, where most of the HIV-infected individuals reside and where the epidemic is spreading most rapidly. Vaccines based on clade B viruses may not necessarily induce immunity that will be effective against other clades. In an experiment in which chimpanzees were immunized with a clade B–based vaccine that had previously been shown to be protective against clade B virus challenge, subsequent challenge with a clade E virus led to the development of infection, demonstrating a lack of cross-clade protection (859).

Studies of long-term nonprogressors suggest that a vigorous CTL response may contribute to the protection against disease progression (199,766–769). Given the failure of protein antigens to induce a potent CTL response, a number of alternate approaches have been used to favor the generation of HIV-specific CTLs. Foremost among these approaches are DNA vaccines, in which HIV genes are injected directly into the recipient. Another approach is the use of viral vectors, such as canarypox. These vectors carry a portion of the HIV genome into host cells, where HIV antigens are produced. HIV gp160 expressed in a poxvirus vector with or without other components of HIV, given as multiple administrations with or without subsequent boosting with purified gp160, has induced CTL activity in several human trials. The CTLs that developed were able to lyse HIV-infected autologous cells (850,860–862), suggesting the possibility of inducing protective responses. Of note, a canarypox vector vaccine using a clade B gp160 induced CTLs that lysed target cells infected with multiple non-B clade viruses (861).

These vaccine approaches rely on the production and expression of HIV proteins by host cells that leads to a predominant CTL response as well as a humoral response. The CTL response is dependent on the HLA haplotype of the individual in that different peptides of the administered protein will be recognized depending on the context of HLA class I presentation (861,863).

Naked DNA is readily taken up by cells and transcribed, and the expressed proteins are processed and presented on MHC class I antigens, resulting in the induction of CD8+ CTL responses. Initial studies in animals indicate that these vaccines produce a potent cell-mediated as well as a neutralizing antibody response (864–865). As previously discussed, trials in chimpanzees have demonstrated protection from challenge with HIV after DNA immunization (854).

CONCLUSIONS

Great strides have been made in the clinical management of HIV disease; although these advances have greatly improved the quality of life for many HIV-infected individuals, it is likely that further advances will be dependent on a fuller understanding of the immunopathogenesis of HIV infection. In this regard, the discovery that certain chemokine receptors function as coreceptors for cellular entry by HIV has greatly expanded the range of host factors that can be targeted for therapeutic intervention. As more is learned about the expression and regulation of these chemokine receptors in tissues and about the complex effects that these receptors and their ligands have on the trafficking of cells that may play central roles in the pathogenesis of HIV disease, no doubt more opportunities for therapeutic intervention will arise. Many other questions linger regarding the pathogenesis of HIV disease. The dynamics of CD4+ T-cell production, trafficking, and death during the course of HIV infection and after initiation of antiretroviral therapy remain enigmatic. Many mechanisms of HIV-induced CD4+ T-cell death appear to be operative *in vitro*; however, debate continues regarding the precise mechanisms of CD4+ T-cell depletion *in vivo*. Studies of individuals who are frequently exposed to HIV infection yet remain uninfected, and HIV-infected long-term nonprogressors should yield important insights into the nature of protective immunity in HIV infection. Answers to these central questions in HIV pathogenesis will facilitate the rational development of vaccines, antiretroviral agents, and immunorestorative strategies.

ACKNOWLEDGMENTS

We gratefully acknowledge helpful discussions with Dr. Shari-lyn Stanley and Greg Folkers, and the expert editorial assistance of Mary Rust and Patricia Walsh.

REFERENCES

1. Gallo R, Salahuddin S, Popovic M, et al. Frequent detection and isolation of cytopathic retroviruses (HTLV-III) from patients with AIDS and at risk for AIDS. *Science* 1984;224:500–503.
2. Levy J, Hoffman A, Kramer S, Landis J, Shimabukuro J, Oshiro L. Isolation of lymphocytopathic retroviruses from San Francisco patients with AIDS. *Science* 1984;225:840–842.
3. Barre-Sinoussi F, Chermann JC, Rey F, et al. Isolation of a T-lymphotropic retrovirus from a patient at risk for acquired immune deficiency syndrome (AIDS). *Science* 1983;220:868–871.
4. Fauci AS, Lane HC. Human immunodeficiency virus (HIV) disease: AIDS and related disorders. In: Fauci AS, Isselbacher KJ, Wilson JD, et al., eds. *Harrison's principles of internal medicine,* 14th ed. New York: McGraw-Hill, 1998: 1791–1856.
5. World Health Organization. *Wkly Epidemiol Rec* 1997;72:17–24.
6. Karon J, Rosenberg P, McQuillan G, Khare M, Gwinn M, Petersen L. Prevalence of HIV infection in the United States, 1984 to 1992. *JAMA* 1996;276:126–131.
7. Centers for Disease Control amd Prevention. *HIV/AIDS Surveillance Rep* 1997; 9:1–37.
8. Curran JW, Jaffe HW, Hardy AM, Morgan WM, Selik RM, Dondero TJ. Epidemiology of HIV infection and AIDS in the United States. *Science* 1988;239: 610–616.
9. George S, Jacob M, John TJ, et al. A case-control analysis of risk factors in HIV transmission in South India. *J AIDS Hum Retrovir* 1997;14:290–293.
10. Dickerson MC, Johnston J, Delea TE, White A, Andrews E. The causal role for genital ulcer disease as a risk factor for transmission of human immunodeficiency virus. An application of the Bradford Hill criteria. *Sex Transm Dis* 1996; 23:429–440.
11. Tyndall MW, Ronald AR, Agoki E, et al. Increased risk of infection with human immunodeficiency virus type 1 among uncircumcised men presenting with genital ulcer disease in Kenya. *Clin Infect Dis* 1996;23:449–453.
12. Bassett MT, McFarland WC, Ray S, et al. Risk factors for HIV infection at enrollment in an urban male factory cohort in Harare, Zimbabwe. *J AIDS Hum Retrovir* 1996;13:287–293.
13. Rodrigues JJ, Mehendale SM, Shepherd ME, et al. Risk factors for HIV infection in people attending clinics for sexually transmitted diseases in India. *Br Med J* 1995;311:283–286.
14. Hayes RJ, Schulz KF, Plummer FA, et al. The cofactor effect of genital ulcers on the per-exposure risk of HIV transmission in sub-Saharan Africa HIV-1 seroconversion in patients with and without genital ulcer disease. A prospective study. *J Trop Med Hyg* 1995;98:1–8.
15. Tindall B, Cooper DA. Primary HIV infection: host responses and intervention strategies. *AIDS* 1991;5:1–14.
16. Gaines H, von Sydow MA, von Stedingk LV, et al. Immunological changes in primary HIV-1 infection. *AIDS* 1990;4:995–999.
17. Tindall B, Hing M, Edwards P, Barnes T, Mackie A, Cooper DA. Severe clinical manifestations of primary HIV infection. *AIDS* 1989;3:747–749.
18. Lemp GF, Payne SF, Rutherford GW, et al. Projections of AIDS morbidity and mortality in San Francisco. *JAMA* 1990;263:1497–1501.
19. Masur H, Ognibene F, Yarchoan R, et al. CD4 counts as predictors of opportunistic pneumonias in human immunodeficiency virus (HIV) infection. *Ann Intern Med* 1989;111:223–231.
20. Price RW, Brew B, Sidtis J, Rosenblum M, Scheck AC, Cleary P. The brain in AIDS: central nervous system HIV-1 infection and AIDS dementia complex. *Science* 1988;239:586–592.
21. Leitner T. Genetic subtypes of HIV-1. In: Myers G, Foley B, Mellors J, Korber B, Jeang K, Wain-Hobson S, eds. *Human retroviruses and AIDS 1996.* Los Alamos, NM: Los Alamos National Laboratory, 1996:28–40.
22. Kostrikis LG, Bagdades E, Cao Y, Zhang L, Dimitriou D, Ho DD. Genetic analysis of human immunodeficiency virus type 1 strains from patients in Cyprus: identification of a new subtype designated subtype I. *J Virol* 1995;69: 6122–6130.
23. Baltimore D. RNA-dependent DNA polymerase in virions of RNA tumour viruses. *Nature* 1970;226:1209–1211.
24. Temin H, Mizutani S. RNA-dependent DNA polymerase in virions of Rous sarcoma virus. *Nature* 1970;226:1211–1213.
25. McDougal J, Kennedy M, Sligh J, Cort S, Mawle A, Nicholson J. Binding of HTLV-III/LAV to T4+ T cells by a complex of the 110K viral protein and the T4 molecule. *Science* 1986;231:382–385.
26. Dalgleish AG, Beverly PC, Clapham PR, Crawford DH, Greaves MF, Weiss RA. The CD4(T4) antigen is an essential component of the receptor for the AIDS retrovirus. *Nature* 1984;312:763–767.
27. Klatzmann D, Barre-Sinoussi F, Nugeyre MT, et al. Selective tropism of lymphadenopathy-associated virus (LAV) for helper-inducer T-lymphocytes. *Science* 1984;225:59–63.
28. Klatzmann D, Champagne E, Chamaret S, et al. T-lymphocyte T4 molecule behaves as receptor for human retrovirus LAV. *Nature* 1984;312:767–768.
29. Moore J. Coreceptors: implications for HIV pathogenesis and therapy. *Science* 1997;276:51–52.
30. Hunter E, Swanstrom R. Retrovirus envelope glycoproteins. In: Swanstrom RVP, ed. *Retroviruses: strategies of replication.* Berlin: Springer-Verlag, 1990:187.
31. Maddon PJ, McDougal JS, Clapham PR, et al. HIV infection does not require endocytosis of its receptor, CD4. *Cell* 1988;54:865–874.
32. Bukrinsky MI, Sharova N, Dempsey MP, et al. Active nuclear import of human immunodeficiency virus type 1 preintegration complexes. *Proc Natl Acad Sci U S A* 1992;89:6580–6584.
33. Arthur L, Bess JJ, Sowder RN, et al. Cellular proteins bound to immunodeficiency viruses: implications for pathogenesis and vaccines. *Science* 1992;258: 1935–1938.
34. Maddon PJ, Dalgleish AG, McDougal JS, Clapham PR, Weiss RA, Axel RA. The T4 gene encodes the AIDS virus receptor and is expressed in the immune system and the brain. *Cell* 1986;47:333–348.
35. Wu L, Gerard N, Wyatt R, et al. CD4-induced interaction of primary HIV-1 gp120 glycoproteins with the chemokine receptor CCR-5. *Nature* 1996;384: 179–183.
36. Trkola A, Dragic T, Arthos J, et al. CD4-dependent, antibody-sensitive interactions between HIV-1 and its co-receptor CCR-5. *Nature* 1996;384:184–187.
37. Chan DC, Fass D, Berger JM, Kim PS. Core structure of gp41 from the HIV envelope glycoprotein. *Cell* 1997;89:263–273.
38. Roberts JD, Benbenek K, Kunkel TA. The accuracy of reverse transcriptase from HIV-1. *Science* 1988;242:1171–1173.
39. Takeuchi Y, Nagumo T, Hoshino H. Low fidelity of cell-free DNA synthesis by reverse transcriptase of human immunodeficiency virus. *J Virol* 1989;62: 3900–3902.
40. Zack JA, Arrigo SJ, Weitsman SR, Go AS, Haislip A, Chen IS. HIV-1 entry into quiescent primary lymphocytes: molecular analysis reveals a labile, latent viral structure. *Cell* 1990;61:213–222.
41. Bukrinsky M, Stanwick T, Dempsey M, Stevenson M. Quiescent T lymphocytes as an inducible virus reservoir in HIV-1 infection. *Science* 1991;254:423–427.

42. Stevenson M. Identification of factors that govern HIV-1 replication in nondividing host cells. *AIDS Res Hum Retrovir* 1994;10(suppl 1):11–15.

43. Myers G, Foley B, Mellors J, Korber B, Jeang K, Wain-Hobson S. *Human retroviruses and AIDS 1996*. Los Alamos, NM: Los Alamos National Laboratory, 1996.

44. Pauza CD, Galindo J. Persistent human immunodeficiency virus type 1 infection of monoblastoid cells lead to accumulation of self-integrated viral DNA and to production of defective virions. *J Virol* 1989;63:3700–3707.

45. Peterson MG, Tanese N, Pugh BF, Tijan R. Functional domains and upstream activation properties of cloned human TATA binding protein. *Science* 1990;248:1625–1630.

46. Maldonado E, Ha I, Cortes P, Weis L, Reinberg D. Factors involved in specific transcription by mammalian RNA polymerase II: role of transcription factors IIA, IID, IIB during formation of a transcription-competent complex. *Mol Cell Biol* 1990;10:6335–6347.

47. Kieran M, Blank V, Logeat F, et al. The DNA binding subunit of NFkB is identical to factor KBF1 and homologous to the rel oncogene product. *Cell* 1990;62:1007–1018.

48. Bours V, Villalobos J, Burd PR, Kelly K, Siebenlist U. Cloning of mitogen-inducible gene encoding a kB DNA-binding protein with homology to the rel oncogene and to cell-cycle motifs. *Nature* 1990;348:76–80.

49. Nabel G, Baltimore D. An inducible transcription factor activates expression of human immunodeficiency virus in T cells. *Nature* 1987;326:711–713.

50. Franza BR, Josephs SF, Gilman MZ, Ryan W, Clarkson B. Characterization of cellular proteins recognizing the HIV enhancer using a microscale DNA-affinity precipitation assay. *Nature* 1987;330:391–395.

51. Kawakami K, Scheidereit C, Roeder RG. Identification and purification of a human immunoglobulin-enhancer–binding protein (NFkB) that activates transcription from a human immunodeficiency virus type I promotor in vivo. *Proc Natl Acad Sci U S A* 1988;85:4700–4704.

52. Trono D, Feinberg MG, Baltimore D. HIV-1 Gag mutants can dominantly interfere with the replication of the wild-type virus. *Cell* 1989;59:113–120.

53. South TL, Blake PR, Sowder RC, Arthur LO, Henderson LE, Summers MF. The nucleocapsid protein isolated from HIV-1 particles binds zinc and forms retroviral-type zinc fingers. *Biochemistry* 1990;29:7786–7789.

54. Dorfman T, Burkovsky A, Ohagen A, Hoglund S, Gottlinger HG. Functional domains of the capsid protein of human immunodeficiency virus type 1. *J Virol* 1994;68:8180–8187.

55. Levy J, Shimabukuro J, McHugh T, Casavant C, Stites D, Oshiro L. AIDS-associated retroviruses (ARV) can productively infect other cells besides human T helper cells. *Virology* 1985;147:441–448.

56. Sakai K, Dewhurst S, Ma XY, Volsky DJ. Differences in cytopathogenicity and host cell range among infectious molecular clones of human immunodeficiency virus type 1 simultaneously isolated from an individual. *J Virol* 1988;62:4078–4085.

57. Cheng-Mayer C, Levy JA. Distinct biological and serological properties of human immunodeficiency viruses from the brain. *Ann Neurol* 1988;23(suppl):58–61.

58. Fenyo EM, Albert J, Asjo B. Replicative capacity, cytopathic effect and cell tropism of HIV. *AIDS* 1989;3(suppl 1):5–12.

59. York-Higgins D, Cheng-Mayer C, Bauer D, Levy JA, Dina D. Human immunodeficiency virus type 1 cellular host range, replication, cytopathicity are linked to the envelope region of the viral genome. *J Virol* 1990;64:4016–4020.

60. deJong JJ, Goudsmit J, Keulen W, et al. Human immunodeficiency virus type 1 clones chimeric for the envelope V3 domain differ in syncytium formation and replication capacity. *J Virol* 1992;66:757–765.

61. Kuiken CL, deJong JJ, Baan E, Keulen W, Tersmette M, Goudsmit J. Evolution of the V3 envelope domain in proviral sequences and isolates of human immunodeficiency virus type 1 during transition of the viral biological phenotype. *J Virol* 1992;66:4622–4627.

62. Hwang SS, Boyle TJ, Lyerly HK, Cullen BR. Identification of the envelope V3 loop as the primary determinant of cell tropism in HIV-1. *Science* 1991;253:71–74.

63. Takeuchi Y, Akutsu M, Murayama K, Shimuzu N, Hoshino H. Host range mutant of human immunodeficiency virus type 1: modification of cell tropism by a single point mutation at the neutralization epitope in the env gene. *J Virol* 1991;65:1710–1718.

64. Cheng-Mayer C, Shioda T, Levy JA. Host range, replicative, and cytopathic properties of human immunodeficiency virus type 1 are determined by a very few amino acid changes in tat and gp120. *J Virol* 1991;65:6931–6941.

65. Fouchier RA, Groenink M, Koostra NA, et al. Phenotype-associated sequence variation in the third variable domain of the human immunodeficiency virus type 1 gp120 molecule. *J Virol* 1992;66:3183–3187.

66. Gu R, Westervelt P, Ratner L. Role of HIV-1 envelope V3 loop cleavage in cell tropism. *AIDS Res Hum Retrovir* 1993;9:1007–1015.

67. Ebenbichler C, Westervelt P, Carrillo A, Henkel T, Johnson D, Ratner L. Structure-function relationships of the HIV-1 envelope V3 loop tropism determinant: evidence for two distinct conformations. *AIDS* 1993;7:639–646.

68. Bhattacharyya D, Brooks BR, Callahan L. Positioning of positively charged residues in the V3 loop correlates with HIV type 1 syncytium-inducing phenotype. *AIDS Res Hum Retrovir* 1996;12:83–90.

69. Cocchi F, DeVico AL, Garzino-Demo A, Cara A, Gallo RC, Lusso P. The V3 domain of the HIV-1 gp120 envelope glycoprotein is critical for chemokine-mediated blockade of infection. *Nat Med* 1996;2:1244–1247.

70. Zhang LQ, Mackenzie P, Cleland A, Holmes EC, Leigh-Brown AJ, Simmonds P. Selection for specific sequences in the external envelope protein of human immunodeficiency virus type 1 upon primary infection. *J Virol* 1993;67:3345–3356.

71. Zhu T, Mo H, Wang N, et al. Genotypic and phenotypic characterization of HIV-1 in patients with primary infection. *Science* 1993;261:1179–1181.

72. Tersmette M, Lange JMA, DeGoede REY, et al. Association between biological properties of human immunodeficiency virus variants and risk for AIDS and AIDS mortality. *Lancet* 1989;1:983–985.

73. Tersmette M, Gruters RA, DeWolf F, et al. Evidence for a role of virulent human immunodeficiency virus (HIV) variants in the pathogenesis of acquired immunodeficiency syndrome: studies on sequential HIV isolates. *J Virol* 1989;63:2118–2125.

74. Cheng-Mayer C, Seto D, Tateno M, Levy JA. Biologic features of HIV-1 that correlate with virulence in the host. *Science* 1988;240:80–82.

75. Koot M, Keet IPM, Vos AHV, et al. Prognostic value of HIV-1 syncytium-inducing phenotype for rate of CD4+ cell depletion and progression to AIDS. *Ann Intern Med* 1993;118:681–688.

76. Richman DD, Bozzette SA. The impact of the syncytium-inducing phenotype of human immunodeficiency virus on disease progression. *J Infect Dis* 1994;169:968–974.

77. Alkhatib G, Broder CC, Berger EA. Cell type-specific fusion cofactors determine human immunodeficiency virus type 1 tropism for T-cell lines versus primary macrophages. *J Virol* 1996;70:5487–5494.

78. Broder CC, Berger EA. Fusogenic selectivity of the envelope glycoprotein is a major determinant of human immunodeficiency virus type 1 tropism for CD4-T-cell lines vs. primary macrophages. *Proc Natl Acad Sci U S A* 1995;92:9004–9008.

79. Cocchi F, DeVico A, Garzino-Demo A, Arya S, Gallo R, Lusso P. Identification of RANTES, MIP-1α, and MIP-1β as the major HIV suppressive factors produced by CD8+ T cells. *Science* 1995;270:1811–1815.

80. Feng Y, Broder C, Kennedy P, Berger E. HIV-1 entry cofactor: functional cDNA cloning of a seven-transmembrane domain, G-protein coupled receptor. *Science* 1996;272:872–877.

81. Berson J, Long D, Doranz B, Rucker J, Jirik F, Doms R. A seven-transmembrane domain receptor involved in fusion and entry of T-cell-tropic human immunodeficiency virus type 1 strains. *J Virol* 1996;70:6288–6295.

82. Bleul CC, Farzan M, Choe H, et al. The lymphocyte chemoattractant SDF-1 is a ligand for LESTR/fusin and blocks HIV-1 entry. *Nature* 1996;382:829–833.

83. Oberlin E, Amara A, Bachelerie F, et al. The CXC chemokine SDF-1 is the ligand for LESTR/fusin and prevents infection by T-cell-line–adapted HIV-1. *Nature* 1996;382:833–835.

84. Paxton WA, Martin SR, Tse D, et al. Relative resistance to HIV-1 infection of CD4 lymphocytes from persons who remain uninfected despite multiple high-risk sexual exposures. *Nat Med* 1996;2:412–417.

85. Samson M, Labbe O, Mollereau C, Vassart G, Parmentier M. Molecular cloning and functional expression of a new human CC-chemokine receptor gene. *Biochemistry* 1996;35:3362–3367.

86. Combadiere C, Ahuja SK, Tiffany HL, Murphy PM. Cloning and functional expression of CC CKR5, a human monocyte CC chemokine receptor selective for MIP-1(alpha), MIP-1(beta), and RANTES. *J Leukoc Biol* 1996;60:147–152.

87. Raport C, Gosling J, Schweickart V, Gray P, Charo I. Molecular cloning and functional characterization of a novel human CC chemokine receptor (CCR5) for RANTES, MIP-1beta, and MIP-1alpha. *J Biol Chem* 1996;271:17161–17166.

88. Deng H, Liu R, Ellmeier W, et al. Identification of a major co-receptor for primary isolates of HIV-1. *Nature* 1996;381:661–666.

89. Dragic T, Litwin V, Allaway G, et al. HIV-1 entry into CD4+ cells is mediated by the chemokine receptor CC-CKR-5. *Nature* 1996;381:667–673.

90. Alkhatib G, Combadiere C, Broder C, et al. CC CKR5: A RANTES, MIP-1α, MIP-1β receptor as a fusion cofactor for macrophage-tropic HIV-1. *Science* 1996;272:1955–1958.

91. Choe H, Farzan M, Sun Y, et al. The β-chemokine receptors CCR3 and CCR5 facilitate infection by primary HIV-1 isolates. *Cell* 1996;85:1135–1138.

92. Doranz B, Rucker J, Yi Y, et al. A dual-tropic primary HIV-1 isolate that uses fusin and the β-chemokine receptors CKR-5, CKR-3, and CKR-2β as fusion cofactors. *Cell* 1996;85:1149-1158.

93. Alkhatib G, Liao F, Berger EA, Farber JM, Peden KW. A new SIV co-receptor, STRL33. *Nature* 1997;388:238.

94. Liao F, Alkhatib G, Peden KW, Sharma G, Berger EA, Farber JM. STRL33, a novel chemokine receptor–like protein, functions as a fusion cofactor for both macrophage-tropic and T cell line–tropic HIV-1. *J Exp Med* 1997;185:2015–2023.

95. Deng HK, Unutmaz D, KewalRamani VN, Littman DR. Expression cloning of new receptors used by simian and human immunodeficiency viruses. *Nature* 1997;388:296–300.

96. Simmons G, Wilkinson D, Reeves J, et al. Primary, syncytium-inducing human immunodeficiency virus type 1 isolates are dual-tropic and most can use either Lestr or CCR5 as coreceptors for virus entry. *J Virol* 1996;70:8355–8360.

97. Chen Z, Zhou P, Ho DD, Landau NR, Marx PA. Genetically divergent strains of simian immunodeficiency virus use CCR5 as a coreceptor for entry. *J Virol* 1997;71:2705–2714.

98. Connor RI, Sheridan KE, Ceradini D, Choe S, Landau NR. Change in coreceptor use correlates with disease progression in HIV-1–infected individuals. *J Exp Med* 1997;185:621–628.

99. Liu R, Paxton WA, Choe S, et al. Homozygous defect in HIV-1 coreceptor accounts for resistance of some multiply-exposed individuals to HIV-1 infection. *Cell* 1996;86:367–378.

100. Samson M, Libert F, Doranz B, et al. Resistance to HIV-1 infection in caucasian individuals bearing mutant alleles of the CCR-5 chemokine receptor gene. *Nature* 1996;382:722–725.

101. Dean M, Carrington M, Winkler C, et al. Genetic restriction of HIV 1 infection and progression to AIDS by a deletion allele of the CKR5 structural gene. *Science* 1996;273:1856–1862.

102. Huang Y, Paxton W, Wolinsky S, et al. The role of a mutant CCR5 allele in HIV-1 transmission and disease progression. *Nat Med* 1996;2:1240–1243.

103. Zimmerman P, Buckler-White A, Alkhatib G, et al. Inherited resistance to HIV-1 conferred by an inactivating mutation in CC chemokine receptor 5: studies in populations with contrasting clinical phenotypes, defined racial backgrounds and quantified risks. *Mol Med* 1997;3:23–36.

104. Biti R, French R, Young J, Bennetts B, Stewart G, Liang T. HIV-1 infection in an individual homozygous for the CCR5 deletion allele. *Nat Med* 1997;3:252–253.

105. Theodorou I, Meyer L, Magierowska M, Katlama C, Rouzioux C. HIV-1 infection in an individual homozygous for CCR5∆32. *Lancet* 1997;349:1219–1220.

106. O'Brien T, Winkler C, Dean M, et al. HIV-1 infection in a man homozygous for CCR5∆32. *Lancet* 1997;349:1219.

107. Bleul C, Wu L, Hoxie J, Springer T, MacKay C. The HIV coreceptors CXCR4 and CCR5 are differentially expressed and regulated on human T lymphocytes. *Proc Natl Acad Sci U S A* 1997;94:1925–1930.

108. Wu L, Paxton WA, Kassam N, et al. CCR5 levels and expression pattern correlate with infectability by macrophage-tropic HIV-1, in vitro. *J Exp Med* 1997;185:1681–1692.

109. Atchison RE, Gosling J, Monteclaro FS, et al. Multiple extracellular elements of CCR5 and HIV-1 entry: dissociation from response to chemokines. *Science* 1996;274:1924–1926.

110. Oravecz T, Pall M, Norcross MA. B-chemokine inhibition of monocytotropic HIV-1 infection. Interference with a postbinding fusion step. *J Immunol* 1996;157:1329–1332.

111. Simmons G, Clapham PR, Picard L, et al. Potent inhibition of HIV-1 infectivity in macrophages and lymphocytes by a novel CCR5 antagonist. *Science* 1997;276:276–279.

112. Lapham C, Ouyang J, Chadrasekhar B, Nguyen N, Dimitrov D, Golding H. Evidence for cell-surface association between fusin and CD4–gp120 complex in human cell lines. *Science* 1996;274:602–605.

113. Ugolini S, Moulard M, Mondor I, et al. HIV-1 gp120 from T cell line tropic viruses induces and association between CD4 and the chemokine receptor CXCR4. *J Immunol* 1997;159:3000–3008.

114. Endres MJ, Clapham PR, Marsh M, et al. CD4-independent infection by HIV-2 is mediated by fusin/CXCR4. *Cell* 1996;87:745–756.

115. Kozak SL, Platt EJ, Madani N, Ferro FE Jr, Peden K, Kabat D. CD4, CXCR-4, and CCR-5 dependencies for infections by primary patient and laboratory-adapted isolates of human immunodeficiency virus type 1. *J Virol* 1997;71:873–882.

116. Zhang L, Huang Y, He T, Cao Y, Ho D. HIV-1 subtype and second receptor use. *Nature* 1996;383:768.

117. Marcon L, Choe H, Martin KA, et al. Utilization of C-C chemokine receptor 5 by the envelope glycoproteins of a pathogenic simian immunodeficiency virus, SIVmac239. *J Virol* 1997;71:2522–2527.

118. Rucker J, Samson M, Doranz BJ, et al. Regions in β-chemokine receptors CCR5 and CCR2b that determine HIV-1 cofactor specificity. *Cell* 1996;87:437–446.

119. Bieniasz PD, Fridell RA, Aramori I, Ferguson SSG, Caron MG, Cullen BR. HIV-1 induced cell fusion is mediated by multiple regions within both the viral envelope and the CCR-5 co-receptor. *EMBO J* 1997;16:2599–2609.

120. Edinger AL, Amedee A, Miller K, et al. Differential utilization of CCR5 by macrophage and T cell tropic simian immunodeficiency virus strains. *Proc Natl Acad Sci U S A* 1997;94:4005–4010.

121. Wu L, Ruffing N, Shi X, et al. Discrete steps in binding and signaling of interleukin-8 with its receptor. *J Biol Chem* 1996;271:31202–31209.

122. Ahuja SK, Lee JC, Murphy PM. CXC chemokines bind to unique sets of selectivity determinants that can function independently and are broadly distributed on multiple domains of human interleukin-8 receptor B. Determinants of high affinity binding and receptor activation are distinct. *J Biol Chem* 1996;271:225–232.

123. Mori K, Ringler DJ, Desrosiers RC. Restricted replication of simian immunodeficiency virus strain 239 in macrophages is determined by env but is not due to restricted entry. *J Virol* 1993;67:2807–2814.

124. Connor RI, Paxton WA, Sheridan KE, Koup RA. Macrophages and CD4+ T-lymphocytes from multiply exposed, uninfected individuals resist infection with primary non–syncytium-inducing isolates of human immunodeficiency virus type 1. *J Virol* 1996;70:8758–8764.

125. Rana S, Besson G, Cook DG, et al. Role of CCR5 in infection of primary macrophages and lymphocytes by macrophage-tropic strains of HIV: resistance to patient-derived and prototype isolates resulting from the delta CCR5 mutation. *J Virol* 1997;71:3219–3227.

126. Moriuchi M, Moriuchi H, Combadiere C, Murphy PM, Fauci AS. CD8+ T-cell–derived factor(s), but not β-chemokines RANTES, MIP-1 alpha and MIP-1 beta, suppress HIV-1 replication in monocyte/macrophages. *Proc Natl Acad Sci U S A* 1996;93:15341–15345.

127. Hirsch I, de Mareuil J, Salaun D, Chermann JC. Genetic control of infection of primary macrophages with T-cell–tropic strains of HIV-1. *Virology* 1996;219:257–261.

128. McKnight A, Wilkinson D, Simmons G, et al. Inhibition of human immunodeficiency virus fusion by a monoclonal antibody to a coreceptor (CXCR4) is both cell type and virus strain dependent. *J Virol* 1997;71:1692–1696.

129. He J, Chen Y, Farzan M, et al. CCR3 and CCR5 are co-receptors for HIV-1 infection of microglia. *Nature* 1997;385:645–649.

130. Weissman D, Fauci AS. Role of dendritic cells in immunopathogenesis of human immunodeficiency virus infection. *Clin Microbiol Rev* 1997;10:358–367.

131. Granelli-Piperno A, Moser B, Pope M, et al. Efficient interaction of HIV-1 with purified dendritic cells via multiple chemokine coreceptors. *J Exp Med* 1996;184:2433–2438.

132. Piatak M, Saag MS, Yang LC, et al. High levels of HIV-1 in plasma during all stages of infection determined by competitive PCR. *Science* 1993;259:1749–1754.

133. Winters MA, Tan LB, Katzenstein DA, Merigan TC. Biological variation and quality control of plasma human immunodeficiency virus type 1 RNA quantitation by reverse transcriptase polymerase chain reaction. *J Clin Microbiol* 1993;31:2960–2966.

134. Cohen OJ, Pantaleo G, Holodniy M, et al. Decreased HIV-1 plasma viremia during antiretroviral therapy reflects downregulation of viral replication in lymphoid tissue. *Proc Natl Acad Sci U S A* 1995;92:6017–6021.

135. Cohen O, Pantaleo G, Holodniy M, et al. Antiretroviral monotherapy in early stage human immunodeficiency virus disease has no detectable effect on virus load in peripheral blood and lymph nodes. *J Infect Dis* 1996;173:849–856.

136. Ho DD, Neumann AU, Perelson AS, Chen W, Leonard JM, Markowitz M. Rapid turnover of plasma virions and CD4 lymphocytes in HIV-1 infection. *Nature* 1995;373:123–126.

137. Wei X, Ghosh SK, Taylor ME, et al. Viral dynamics in human immunodeficiency virus type 1 infection. *Nature* 1995;373:117–122.

138. Perelson AS, Neumann AU, Markowitz M, Leonard JM, Ho DD. HIV-1 dynamics in vivo: virion clearance rate, infected cell life-span, and viral generation time. *Science* 1996;271:1582–1586.

139. Perelson AS, Essunger P, Cao Y, et al. Decay characteristics of HIV-1 infected compartments during combination therapy. *Nature* 1997;387:188–191.

140. Heath SL, Tew JG, Tew JG, Szakal AK, Burton GF. Follicular dendritic cells and human immunodeficiency virus infectivity. *Nature* 1995;377:740–744.

141. Bonhoeffer S, Coffin JM, Nowak MA. Human immunodeficiency virus drug therapy and virus load. *J Virol* 1997;71:3275–3278.

142. Westermann J, Pabst R. Lymphocyte subsets in the blood: a diagnostic window on the lymphoid system? *Immunol Today* 1990;11:406–410.

143. Connors M, Kovacs JA, Krevat S, et al. HIV infection induces changes in CD4+ T-cell phenotype and depletions within the CD4+ T-cell repertoire that are not immediately restored by antiviral or immune-based therapies. *Nat Med* 1997;3:533–540.

144. Wolthers KC, Wisman GBA, Otto SA, et al. T cell telomere length in HIV-1 infection: no evidence for increased CD4+ T cell turnover. *Science* 1996;274:1543–1547.

145. Palmer LD, Weng N, Levine BL, June CH, Lane HC, Hodes RJ. Telomere length, telomerase activity, and replicative potential in HIV infection: analysis of CD4+ and CD8+ T cells from HIV-discordant monozygotic twins. *J Exp Med* 1997;185:1381–1386.

146. Shaw GM, Hahn BH, Arya SK, Groopman JE, Gallo RC, Wong-Staal F. Molecular characterization of human T-cell leukemia (lymphotropic) virus type III in the acquired immune deficiency syndrome. *Science* 1984;226:1165–1171.

147. Wong-Staal F, Shaw GM, Hahn BH, et al. Genomic diversity of human T-lymphotropic virus type III. *Science* 1985;229:759–762.

148. Hahn BH, Gonda MA, Shaw GM, et al. Genomic diversity of the acquired immune deficiency syndrome virus HTLV-III: different viruses exhibit greatest divergence in their envelope genes. *Proc Natl Acad Sci U S A* 1985;82:4813–4817.

149. Benn S, Rutledge R, Folks T, et al. Genomic heterogeneity of AIDS retroviral isolates from North America and Zaire. *Science* 1985;230:949–951.

150. Ratner L, Haseltine W, Patarca R, et al. Complete nucleotide sequence of the AIDS virus, HTLV-III. *Nature* 1985;313:277–284.

151. Rabson AB, Martin MA. Molecular organization of the AIDS retrovirus. *Cell* 1985;40:477–480.

152. Starcich BR, Hahn BH, Shaw GM, et al. Identification and characterization of conserved and variable regions in the envelope gene of HTLV-III/LAV, the retrovirus of AIDS. *Cell* 1986;45:637–648.

153. Hahn BH, Shaw GM, Taylor ME, et al. Genetic variation in HTLV-III/LAV over time in patients with AIDS or at risk for AIDS. *Science* 1986;232:1548–1553.

154. Temin HW. Is HIV unique or merely different? *J AIDS* 1989;2:1–9.

155. Gojobori T, Moriyama EN, Kimura M. Molecular clock of viral evolution, and the neutral theory. *Proc Natl Acad Sci U S A* 1990;87:10015–10018.

156. Delassus S, Cheynier R, Wain-Hobson S. Nonhomogeneous distribution of human immunodeficiency virus type 1 proviruses in the spleen. *J Virol* 1992;66:5642–5645.

157. Cheynier R, Henrichwark S, Hadida F, et al. HIV and T cell expansion in splenic white pulps is accompanied by infiltration of HIV-specific cytotoxic T lymphocytes. *Cell* 1994;78:373–387.

158. Fisher AG, Ensoli B, Looney D, et al. Biologically diverse molecular variants within a single HIV-1 isolate. *Nature* 1988;334:444–447.

159. Bonhoeffer S, Holmes EC, Nowak MA. Causes of HIV diversity. *Nature* 1995;376:125.

160. Larder B, Kemp S. Multiple mutations in HIV-1 reverse transcriptase confer high-level resistance to zidovudine (AZT). *Science* 1989;246:1155–1158.

161. Simmonds P, Balfe P, Ludlam CA, Bishop JO, Brown AJ. Analysis of sequence diversity in hypervariable regions of the external glycoprotein of human immunodeficiency virus type 1. *J Virol* 1990;64:5840–5850.

162. Kliks SC, Shioda T, Haigwood NL, Levy JA. V3 variability can influence the ability of an antibody to neutralize or enhance infection by diverse strains of human immunodeficiency virus type 1. *Proc Natl Acad Sci U S A* 1993;90:11518–11522.

163. Jansson M, Popovic M, Karlsson A, et al. Sensitivity to inhibition by β-chemokines correlates with biological phenotypes of primary HIV-1 isolates. *Proc Natl Acad Sci U S A* 1996;93:15382–15387.

164. Coffin JM. HIV population dynamics in vivo: implications for genetic variation, pathogenesis, and therapy. *Science* 1995;267:483–489.

165. Zhang L, Diaz RS, Ho DD, Mosley JW, Busch MP, Mayer A. Host-specific driving force in human immunodeficiency virus type 1 evolution in vivo. *J Virol* 1997;71:2555–2561.

166. Fauci A. Host factors and the pathogenesis of HIV-induced disease. *Nature* 1996;384:529–534.

167. Michael N, Chang G, Louie L, et al. The role of viral phenotype and CCR-5 gene defects in HIV-1 transmission and disease progression. *Nat Med* 1997;3:338–340.

168. Delwart EL, Sheppard HW, Walker BD, Goudsmit J, Mullins JI. Human immunodeficiency virus type 1 evolution in vivo tracked by DNA heteroduplex mobility assays. *J Virol* 1994;68:6672–6683.

169. Lukashov VV, Kuiken CL, Goudsmit J. Intrahost human immunodeficiency virus type 1 evolution is related to length of the immunocompetent period. *J Virol* 1995;69:6911–6916.

170. Wolinsky SM, Korber BTM, Neumann AU, et al. Adaptive evolution of human immunodeficiency virus-type 1 during the natural course of infection. *Science* 1996;272:537–542.

171. McDonald RA, Mayers DL, Chung RC-Y, et al. Evolution of human immunodeficiency virus type 1 env sequence variation in patients with diverse rates of disease progression and T-cell function. *J Virol* 1997;71:1871–1879.

172. Nowak MA, Anderson RM, McLean AR, Wolfs TF, Goudsmit J, May RM. Antigenic diversity thresholds and the development of AIDS. *Science* 1991;254:963 941.

173. Nowak MA, May RM, Phillips RE, et al. Antigenic oscillations and shifting immunodominance in HIV-1 infections. *Nature* 1995;375:606–611.

174. Nowak MA, Bangham CRM. Population dynamics of immune responses to persistent viruses. *Science* 1996;272:74–79.

175. Pantaleo G, Demarest JF, Schacker T, et al. The qualitative nature of the primary immune response to HIV infection is a prognosticator of disease progression independent of the initial level of plasma viremia. *Proc Natl Acad Sci U S A* 1997;94:254–258.

176. Simmonds P, Zhang LQ, McOmish F, Balfe P, Ludlam CA, Brown AJL. Discontinuous sequence change of human immunodeficiency virus (HIV) type 1 env sequences in plasma viral and lymphocyte-associated proviral populations in vivo: implications for models of HIV pathogenesis. *J Virol* 1991;65:6266–6276.

177. Zhang Y-M, Dawson SC, Landsman D, Lane HC, Salzman NP. Persistence of four related human immunodeficiency virus subtypes during the course of zidovudine therapy: relationship between virion RNA and proviral DNA. *J Virol* 1994;68:425–432.

178. Michael NL, Chang G, Ehrenberg PK, Vahey MT, Redfield RR. HIV-1 proviral genotypes from the peripheral blood mononuclear cells of an infected patient are differentially represented in expressed sequences. *J AIDS* 1993;6:1073–1085.

179. Ball JK, Holmes EC, Whitwell H, Desselberger U. Genomic variation of human immunodeficiency virus type 1 (HIV-1): molecular analyses of HIV-1 in sequential blood samples and various organs obtained at autopsy. *J Gen Virol* 1994;75:867–879.

180. Cheng-Mayer C, Weiss C, Seto D, Levy JA. Isolates of human immunodeficiency virus type 1 from the brain may constitute a special group of the AIDS virus. *Proc Natl Acad Sci U S A* 1989;80:8575–8579.

181. Epstein LG, Kuiken C, Blumberg BM, et al. HIV-1 V3 domain variation in brain and spleen of children with AIDS: tissue-specific evolution within host-determined quasispecies. *Virology* 1991;180:583–590.

182. Pang S, Vinters HV, Akashi T, O'Brien WA, Chen ISY. HIV-1 Env sequence variation in brain tissue of patients with AIDS-related neurologic disease. *J AIDS* 1991;4:1082–1092.

183. Ait-Khaled M, McLaughlin JE, Johnson MA, Emery VC. Distinct HIV-1 long terminal repeat quasispecies present in nervous tissues compared to that in lung, blood and lymphoid tissues of an AIDS patients. *AIDS* 1994;91:

184. Wong JK, Ignacio CC, Torriani F, Havlir D, Fitch NJS, Richman DD. In vivo compartmentalization of human immunodeficiency virus: evidence from the examination of pol sequences from autopsy tissues. *J Virol* 1997;71:2059–2071.

185. Itescu S, Simonelli PF, Winchester RJ, Ginsberg HS. Human immunodeficiency virus type 1 strains in the lungs of infected individuals evolve independently from those in peripheral blood and are highly conserved in the C-terminal region of the envelope V3 loop. *Proc Natl Acad Sci U S A* 1994;91:11378–11382.

186. Zhu T, Wang N, Carr A, et al. Genetic characterization of human immunodeficiency virus type 1 in blood and genital secretions: evidence for viral compartmentalization and selection during sexual transmission. *J Virol* 1996;70:3098–3107.

187. Pantaleo G, Graziosi C, Fauci A. Virologic and immunologic events in primary HIV infection. *Springer Semin Immunopathol* 1997;18:257–266.

188. Schnittman SM, Psallidopoulos MC, Lane HC, et al. The reservoir for HIV-1 in human peripheral blood is a T cell that maintains expression of CD4. *Science* 1989;245:305–308.

189. Spira AI, Marx PA, Patterson BK, et al. Cellular targets of infection and route of viral dissemination after an intravaginal inoculation of simian immunodeficiency virus into rhesus macaques. *J Exp Med* 1996;183:215–225.

190. Weissman D, Li Y, Ananworanich J, et al. Three populations of cells with dendritic morphology exist in peripheral blood, only one of which is infectable with human immunodeficiency virus type 1. *Proc Natl Acad Sci U S A* 1995;92:826–830.

191. Pope M, Betjes MG, Romani N, et al. Conjugates of dendritic cells and memory T lymphocytes from skin facilitate productive infection with HIV-1. *Cell* 1994;78:389–398.

192. Frankel SS, Wenig BM, Burke AP, et al. Replication of HIV-1 in dendritic cell–derived syncytia at the mucosal surface of the adenoid. *Science* 1996;272:115–117.

193. Pantaleo G, Demarest JF, Soudeyns H, et al. Major expansion of CD8+ T cells with a predominant V beta usage during the primary immune response to HIV. *Nature* 1994;370:463–467.

194. Borrow P, Lewicki H, Hahn BH, Shaw GM, Oldstone MBA. Virus-specific CD8+ cytotoxic T-lymphocyte activity associated with control of viremia in primary human immunodeficiency virus type 1 infection. *J Virol* 1994;68:6103–6110.

195. Daar ES, Moudgil T, Meyer RD, Ho DD. Transient high levels of viremia in patients with primary human immunodeficiency virus type 1 infection. *N Engl J Med* 1991;324:961–964.

196. Moore JP, Cao Y, Ho DD, Koup RA. Development of the anti-gp120 antibody response during seroconversion to human immunodeficiency virus type 1. *J Virol* 1994;68:5142–5155.

197. Koup RA, Safrit JT, Cao Y, et al. Temporal association of cellular immune responses with the initial control of viremia in primary human immunodeficiency virus type 1 syndrome. *J Virol* 1994;68:4650–4655.

198. Clark SJ, Saag MS, Decker WD, et al. High titers of cytopathic virus in plasma of patients with symptomatic primary HIV-1 infection. *N Engl J Med* 1991;324:954–960.

199. Pantaleo G, Menzo S, Vaccarezza M, et al. Studies in subject with long-term nonprogressive human immunodeficiency virus infection. *N Engl J Med* 1995;332:209–216.

200. Pantaleo G, Graziosi C, Demarest J, et al. Role of lymphoid organs in the pathogenesis of human immunodeficiency virus (HIV) infection. *Immunol Rev* 1994;140:105–130.

201. Pantaleo G, Graziosi C, Butini L, et al. Lymphoid organs function as major reservoirs for human immunodeficiency virus. *Proc Natl Acad Sci* 1991;88:9838–9842.

202. Chakrabarti L, Isola P, Cumont M, Claessens-Maire M, Hurtrel M, Montagnier L. Early stages of simian immunodeficiency virus infection in lymph nodes. Evidence for high viral load and successive populations of target cells. *Am J Pathol* 1994;144:1226–1237.

203. Reimann KA, Tenner-Racz K, Racz P. Immunopathogenic events in acute infection of Rhesus monkeys with simian immunodeficiency virus of macaques. *J Virol* 1994;68:2362–2370.

204. Montefiori DC, Pantaleo G, Fink LM, et al. Neutralizing and infection-enhancing antibody responses to human immunodeficiency virus type 1 in long-term nonprogressors. *J Infect Dis* 1996;173:60–67.

205. Pilgrim A, Pantaleo G, Cohen O, et al. Neutralizing antibody responses at various stages of infection with human immunodeficiency virus type 1. *J Infect Dis* 1997;176:924–932.

206. Mackewicz CE, Yang LC, Lifson JD, Levy JA. Non-cytolytic CD8 T-cell anti-HIV responses in primary HIV-1 infection. *Lancet* 1994;344:1671–1673.

207. Pantaleo G, Soudeyns H, Demarest J, et al. Evidence for rapid disappearance of initially expanded HIV-specific CD8+ T cell clones during primary HIV infection. *Proc Natl Acad Sci U S A* 1997;94:9848–9853.

208. Graziosi C, Pantaleo G, Butini L, et al. Kinetics of human immunodeficiency virus type 1 (HIV-1) DNA and RNA synthesis during primary HIV-1 infection. *Proc Natl Acad Sci U S A* 1993;90:6405–6409.

209. Clayette P, Le Grand R, Noack O, et al. Tumor necrosis factor-alpha in serum of macaques during SIVmac251 acute infection. *J Med Primatol* 1995;24:94–100.

210. Cheret A, Le Grand R, Caufour P, et al. Cytokine mRNA expression in mononuclear cells from different tissues during acute SIVmac251 infection of macaques. *AIDS Res Hum Retrovir* 1996;12:1263–1272.

211. Benveniste O, Vaslin B, Le Grand R, et al. Interleukin 1 beta, interleukin 6, tumor necrosis factor alpha, and interleukin 10 responses in peripheral blood mononuclear cells of cynomolgus macaques during acute infection with SIVmac251. *AIDS Res Hum Retrovir* 1996;12:241–250.

212. Walker BD, Chakrabarti S, Moss B, et al. HIV-specific cytotoxic T lymphocytes in seropositive individuals. *Nature* 1987;328:345–348.

213. Plata F, Autran B, Martins LP, et al. AIDS virus–specific cytotoxic T lymphocytes in lung disorders. *Nature* 1987;328:348–351.

214. Britton CB, Miller JR. Neurological complications in acquired immunodeficiency syndrome (AIDS). *Neurol Clin* 1984;2:315–339.

215. Nielson SL, Petito CK, Urmacher CD, Posner JB. Subacute encephalitis in acquired immune deficiency syndrome: a postmortem study. *Am J Clin Pathol* 1984;82:678–682.

216. Faulstich M. Acquired immune deficiency syndrome: an overview of central nervous system complications and neuropsychological sequelae. *Int J Neurosci* 1986;30:249–254.

217. Gabuza DH, Ho DD, de la Monte SM, Hirsch MS, Rota TR, Sobel RA. Immunohistochemical identification of HTLV-III antigen in brains of patients with AIDS. *Ann Neurol* 1986;20:289–295.

218. Chun T-W, Carruth L, Finzi D, et al. Quantification of latent tissue reservoirs and total body viral load in HIV infection. *Nature* 1997;387:183–187.

219. Centers for Disease Control and Prevention. 1993 revised classification system for HIV infection and expanded surveillance case definition for AIDS among adolescents and adults. *MMWR* 1992;41:1–19.

220. Albrecht H. Redefining AIDS: towards a modification of the current AIDS case definition. *Clin Infect Dis* 1997;24:64–74.

221. Cinque P, Brytting M, Vago L, et al. Epstein-Barr virus DNA in cerebrospinal fluid from patients with AIDS-related primary lymphoma of the central nervous system. *Lancet* 1993;342:398–401.

222. Laga M, Icenogle J, Marsella R, et al. Genital papillomavirus infection and cervical dysplasia—opportunistic complications of HIV infection. *Int J Cancer* 1992;50:45–48.

223. Schrager L, Friedland G, Maude D, et al. Cervical and vaginal squamous cell abnormalities in women infected with human immunodeficiency virus. *J AIDS* 1989;2:570–575.

224. Moore PS, Chang Y. Detection of herpesvirus-like DNA sequences in Kaposi's sarcoma in patients with and without HIV infection. *N Engl J Med* 1995;332:1181–1185.

225. Schalling M, Ekman M, Kaaya EE, Linde A, Biberfeld P. A role for a new herpes virus (KSHV) in different forms of Kaposi's sarcoma. *Nat Med* 1995;1:707–708.

226. Crowe S, Carlin J, Stewart K, Lucas C, Hoy J. Predicitve value of CD4 lymphocyte numbers for the development of opportunistic infections and malignancies in HIV-infected persons. *J AIDS* 1991;4:770–776.

227. Moore R, Chaisson R. Natural history of opportunistic disease in an HIV-infected urban clinical cohort. *Ann Intern Med* 1996;124:633–642.

228. Enger C, Graham N, Peng Y, et al. Survival from early, intermediate, and late stages of HIV infection. *JAMA* 1996;275:1329–1334.

229. Chiasson M, Berenson L, Li W, Stewart S, Mojica B, Hamburg M. Declining AIDS mortality in New York City [Abstract 376]. Fourth Conference on Retroviruses and Opportunistic Infections, Washington, DC, 1997.

230. Graham N, Zeger S, Park L, et al. The effects on survival of early treatment of human immunodeficiency virus infection. *N Engl J Med* 1992;326:1037–1042.

231. Clerici M, Stocks NI, Zajac RA, et al. Detection of three distinct patterns of T helper cell dysfunction in asymptomatic, human immunodeficiency virus–seropositive patients independent of CD4⁺ cell numbers and clinical settings. *J Clin Invest* 1989;84:1892–1899.

232. Pantaleo G, Fauci AS. Immunopathogenesis of HIV infection. *Annu Rev Microbiol* 1996;50:825–854.

233. Stevenson M, Meier C, Mann AM, Chapman N, Wasiak A. Envelope glycoprotein of HIV induces interference and cytolysis resistance in CD4⁺ cells: mechanisms for persistence in AIDS. *Cell* 1988;53:483–496.

234. Garcia JV, Miller AD. Serine phosphorylation-independent downregulation of cell-surface CD4 by nef. *Nature* 1991;350:508–511.

235. Willey RL, Maldarelli F, Martin MA, Strebel K. Human immunodeficiency virus type 1 Vpu protein induces rapid degradation of CD4. *J Virol* 1992;66:7193–7200.

236. Yao XJ, Friborg J, Checroune F, et al. Degradation of CD4 induced by human immunodeficiency virus type 1 Vpu protein: a predicted alpha-helix structure in the proximal cytoplasmic regin of CD4 contributes to Vpu sensitivity. *Virology* 1995;209:615–623.

237. Schnittman SM, Lane HC, Greenhouse J, Justement JS, Baseler M, Fauci AS. Preferential infection of CD4⁺ memory T cells by human immunodeficiency virus type 1: evidence for a role in the selective T-cell functional defects observed in infected individuals. *Proc Natl Acad Sci U S A* 1990;87:6058–6062.

238. Chun T-W, Chadwick K, Margolick J, Siliciano R. Differential susceptibility of naive and memory CD4⁺ T cells to the cytopathic effects of infection with human immunodeficiency virus type 1 strain LAI. *J Virol* 1997;71:4436–4444.

239. Gupta S, Vayuvegula B. Human immunodeficiency virus–associated changes in signal transduction. *J Clin Immunol* 1987;7:486–489.

240. Linette GP, Hartzman RJ, Ledbetter JA, June CH. HIV-1–infected T cells show a selective signaling defect after perturbation of CD3/antigen receptor. *Science* 1988;241:573–576.

241. Cefai D, Debre P, Kaczorek M, Idziorek T, Autran B, Bismuth G. Human immunodeficiency virus-1 glycoproteins gp120 and gp160 specifically inhibit the CD3/T cell-antigen receptor phosphoinositide transduction pathway. *J Clin Invest* 1990;86:2117–2124.

242. Gaulton GN, Brass LF, Kozbor D, Pletcher CH, Hoxie JA. Inhibition of T cell antigen receptor–dependent phosphorylation of CD4 in human immunodeficiency virus type 1 infected cells. *J Biol Chem* 1992;267:4102–4109.

243. Cohen DI, Tani Y, Tian H, Boone E, Samelson LE, Lane HC. Participation of tyrosine phosphorylation in the cytopathic effect of human immunodeficiency virus-1. *Science* 1992;256:542–545.

244. Cefai D, Ferrer M, Serpente N, et al. Internalization of HIV glycoprotein gp120 is associated with down-modulation of membrane CD4 and p56lck together with impairment of T cell activation. *J Immunol* 1992;149:285–294.

245. Hivroz C, Mazerolles F, Soula M, et al. Human immunodeficiency virus gp120 and derived peptides activate protein tyrosine kinase p56lck in human CD4 T lymphocytes. *Eur J Immunol* 1993;23:600–607.

246. Goldman F, Jensen W, Johnson G, Heasley L, Cambier J. gp120 ligation of CD4 induces p56lck activation and TCR desensitization independent of TCR tyrosine phosphorylation. *J Immunol* 1994;153:2905–2917.

247. Chirmule N, McCloskey TW, Hu R, Kalyanaraman VS, Pahwa S. HIV gp120 inhibits T cell activation by interfering with expression of costimulatory molecules CD40 ligand and CD80 (B7-1). *J Immunol* 1995;155:917–924.

248. Guntermann C, Dye J, Nye KE. Human immunodeficiency virus infection abolishes CD4-dependent activation of ZAP-70 by inhibition of p56lck. *J AIDS Hum Retrovir* 1997;14:204–212.

249. Ioachim HL, Lerner CW, Tapper ML. The lymphoid lesions associated with the acquired immunodeficiency syndrome. *Am J Surg Pathol* 1983;7:543–553.

250. Fernandez R, Mouradian J, Metroka C, Davies J. The prognostic value of histopathology in persistent generalized lymphadenopathy in homosexual men. *N Engl J Med* 1983;309:185–186.

251. Janossy G, Pinching AJ, Bofill M, et al. An immunohistological approach to persistent lymphadenopathy and its relevance to AIDS. *Clin Exp Immunol* 1985;59:257–266.

252. Biberfeld P, Chayt K, Marselle L, Biberfeld G, Gallo R, Harper M. HTLV-III expression in infected lymph nodes and relevance to pathogenesis of lymphadenopathy. *Am J Pathol* 1986;125:436–442.

253. Racz P, Tenner-Racz K, Kahl C, Feller AC, Kern P, Dietrich M. Spectrum of morphologic changes of lymph nodes from patients with AIDS or AIDS-related complexes. *Prog Allergy* 1986;37:81–181.

254. Pallesen G, Gerstoft J, Mathiesen L. Stages in LAV/HTLV-III lymphadenitis: I. Histological and immunohistological classification. *Scand J Immunol* 1987;25:83–91.

255. Turner R, Levine A, Gill P, Parker J, Meyer P. Progressive histopathologic abnormalities in the persistent generalized lymphadenopathy syndrome. *Am J Surg Pathol* 1987;11:625–632.

256. Pantaleo G, Graziosi C, Demarest JF, et al. HIV infection is active and progressive in lymphoid tissue during the clinically latent stage of disease. *Nature* 1993;362:355–358.

257. Tew JG, Burton GF, Kupp LI, Szakal A. Follicular dendritic cells in germinal center reactions. *Adv Exp Med Biol* 1993;329:461–465.

258. Fleming TR, DeMets DL. Surrogate endpoints in clinical trials: are we being misled? *Ann Intern Med* 1996;125:605–613.

259. Moss A, Bacchetti P, Osmond D, et al. Seropositivity for HIV and the development of AIDS or AIDS related condition: three year follow up of the San Francisco General Hospital cohort. *Br Med J* 1988;296:745–750.

260. MacDonnell K, Chmiel J, Poggensee L, Wu S, Phair J. Predicting progression to AIDS: combined usefulness of CD4 lymphocyte counts and p24 antigenemia. *Am J Med* 1990;89:706–712.

261. Fahey J, Taylor J, Detels R, et al. The prognostic value of cellular and serologic markers in infection with human immunodeficiency virus type 1. *N Engl J Med* 1990;322:166–172.

262. Eyster M, Gail M, Ballard J, Al-Mondhiry H, Goedert J. Natural history of human immunodeficiency virus infections in hemophiliacs: effects of T-cell subsets, platelet counts, and age. *Ann Intern Med* 1987;107:1–6.

263. Goedert J, Kessler C, Aledort L, et al. A prospective study of human immunodeficiency virus type 1 infection and the development of AIDS in subjects with hemophilia. *N Engl J Med* 1989;321:1141–1148.

264. Munoz A, Vlahov D, Solomon L, et al. Prognostic indicators for development of AIDS among intravenous drug users. *J AIDS* 1992;5:694–700.

265. Taylor J, Fahey J, Detels R, Giorgi J. CD4 percentage, CD4 number, and CD4:CD8 ratio in HIV infection: which to choose and how to use. *J AIDS* 1989;2:114–124.

266. Stein D, Korvick J, Vermund S. CD4⁺ lymphocyte cell enumeration for prediction of clinical course of human immunodeficiency virus disease: a review. *J Infect Dis* 1992;165:352–363.

267. Phillips A, Lee C, Elford J, et al. Serial CD4 lymphocyte counts and the development of AIDS. *Lancet* 1991;337:389–392.

268. Yarchoan R, Weinhold K, Lyerly H, et al. Administration of 3′-azido-3′-deoxythymidine, an inhibitor of HTLV-III/LAV replication, to patients with AIDS or AIDS-related complex. *Lancet* 1986;1:575–580.

269. Fischl M, Richman D, Grieco M, et al. The efficacy of azidothymidine (AZT) in the treatment of patients with AIDS and AIDS-related complex. A double-blind, placebo-controlled trial. *N Engl J Med* 1987;317:185–191.

270. Fischl M, Richman D, Hansen N, et al. The safety and efficacy of zidovudine (AZT) in the treatment of subjects with mildly symptomatic human immunodeficiency virus type 1 (HIV) infection. A double-blind, placebo-controlled trial. *Ann Intern Med* 1990;112:727–737.

271. Volberding P, Lagakos S, Koch M, et al. Zidovudine in asymptomatic human immunodeficiency virus infection. A controlled trial in persons with fewer than 500 CD4-positive cells per cubic millimeter. *N Engl J Med* 1990;322:941–949.

272. Choi S, Lagakos S, Schooley R, Volberding P. CD4⁺ lymphocytes are an incomplete surrogate marker for clinical progression in persons with asymptomatic HIV infection taking zidovudine. *Ann Intern Med* 1993;118:674–680.

273. Concorde Coordinating Commitee. Concorde: MRC/ANRS randomised double-blind controlled trial of immediate and deferred zidovudine in symptom-free HIV infection. *Lancet* 1994;343:871–881.

274. Volberding P, Lagakos S, Grimes J, et al. A comparison of immediate with deferred zidovudine therapy for asymptomatic HIV-infected adults with CD4 cell counts of 500 or more per cubic millimeter. *N Engl J Med* 1995;333:401–407.

275. Anderson R, Lang W, Shiboski S, Royce R, Jewell N, Winkelstein W. Use of β₂-microglobulin level and CD4 lymphocyte count to predict development of acquired immunodeficiency syndrome in persons with human immunodeficiency virus infection. *Arch Intern Med* 1990;150:73–77.

276. Lifson A, Hessol N, Buchbinder S, et al. Serum β₂-microglobulin and prediction of progression to AIDS in HIV infection. *Lancet* 1992;339:1436–1440.

277. Kramer A, Wiktor S, Fuchs D, et al. Neopterin: a predictive marker of acquired immune deficiency syndrome in human immunodeficiency virus infection. *J AIDS* 1989;2:291–296.

278. Melmed R, Taylor J, Detels R, Bozorgmehri M, Fahey J. Serum neopterin changes in HIV-infected subjects: indicator of significant pathology, CD4 T cell changes, and the development of AIDS. *J AIDS* 1989;2:70–76.

279. Folks TM, Clouse KA, Justement J, et al. Tumor necrosis factor alpha induces expression of human immunodeficiency virus in a chronically infected T-cell clone. *Proc Natl Acad Sci U S A* 1989;86:2365–2368.

280. Poli G, Kinter A, Justement JS, et al. Tumor necrosis factor alpha functions in an autocrine manner in the induction of human immunodeficiency virus expression. *Proc Natl Acad Sci U S A* 1990;87:782–785.

281. Godfried MH, vanderPoll T, Weverling GJ, et al. Soluble receptors for tumor necrosis factor as predictors of progression to AIDS in asymptomatic human immunodeficiency virus type 1 infection. *J Infect Dis* 1994;169:739–745.

282. Bilello JA, Stellrecht K, Drusano GL, Stein DS. Soluble tumor necrosis factor-alpha receptor type II (sTNF alpha RII) correlates with human immunodeficiency virus (HIV) RNA copy number in HIV-infected patients. *J Infect Dis* 1996;173:464–467.

283. Frissen PH, Weverling GJ, Endert E, Jansen J, Sauerwein HP, Lange JM. Predictive value for survival of soluble tumor necrosis factor receptors p55 and p75 during zidovudine-containing treatment in symptomatic human immunodeficiency virus type 1 infection. *J AIDS Hum Retrovir* 1996;15:482–488.

284. Miedema F, Petit AJ, Terpstra FG, et al. Immunological abnormalities in human immunodeficiency virus (HIV)-infected asymptomatic homosexual men. HIV affects the immune system before CD4⁺ T helper cell depletion occurs. *J Clin Invest* 1988;82:1908–1914.

285. Gruters RA, Terpstra FG, DeJong R, Noesel CJV, Lier RAV, Miedema F. Selective loss of T cell functions in different stages of HIV infection. Early loss of anti-CD3-induced T cell proliferation followed by decreased anti-CD3-induced cytotoxic T lymphocyte generation in AIDS-related complex and AIDS. *Eur J Immunol* 1990;20:1039–1044.

286. Blatt SP, Hendrix CW, Butzin CA, et al. Delayed-type hypersensitivity skin testing predicts progression to AIDS in HIV-infected patients. *Ann Intern Med* 1993;119:177–184.

287. Dolan MJ, Clerici M, Blatt SP, et al. In vitro T cell function, delayed-type hypersensitivity skin testing, and CD4⁺ T cell subset phenotyping independently predict survival time in patients infected with human immunodeficiency virus. *J Infect Dis* 1995;172:79–87.

288. Gordin FM, Hartigan PM, Klimas NG, Zolla-Pazner SB, Simberkoff MS, Hamilton JD. Delayed-type hypersensitivity skin tests are an independent predictor of human immunodeficiency virus disease progression. *J Infect Dis* 1994;169:893–897.

289. Giorgi JV, Liu Z, Hultin LE, Cumberland WG, Hennessey K, Detels R. Elevated levels of CD38⁺CD8⁺ T cells in HIV infection add to the prognostic value of low CD4⁺ T cell levels: results of 6 years of follow-up. *J AIDS* 1993;6:904–912.

290. Giorgi JV, Ho H-N, Hirji K, et al. CD8⁺ lymphocyte activation at human immunodeficiency virus type 1 seroconversion: development of HLA-DR⁺ CD38⁻ CD8⁺ cells is associated with subsequent stable CD4⁺ cell levels. *J Infect Dis* 1994;170:775–781.

291. Haug C, Muller F, Aukrust P, Froland SS. Subnormal serum concentration of 1,25-vitamin D in human immunodeficiency virus infection: correlation with degree of immune deficiency and survival. *J Infect Dis* 1994;169:889–893.

292. Polis MA, Masur H. Predicting the progression to AIDS. *Am J Med* 1990;89:701–705.

293. Ho D, Moudgil T, Alam M. Quantitation of human immunodeficiency virus type 1 in the blood of infected persons. *N Engl J Med* 1989;321:1621–1625.

294. Coombs R, Collier A, Allain J, et al. Plasma viremia in human immunodeficiency virus infection. *N Engl J Med* 1989;321:1626–1631.

295. Saag M, Crain M, Decker W, et al. High-level viremia in adults and children infected with human immunodeficiency virus: relation to disease stage and CD4⁺ lymphocyte levels. *J Infect Dis* 1991;164:72–80.

296. Davey RT, Dewar RL, Reed GF, et al. Plasma viremia as a sensitive indicator of the antiretroviral activity of L-697,661. *Proc Natl Acad Sci U S A* 1993;90:5608–5612.

297. DeGruttola V, Beckett L, Coombs R, et al. Serum p24 antigen level as an intermediate end point in clinical trials of zidovudine in people infected with human immunodeficiency virus type 1. *J Infect Dis* 1994;169:713–721.

298. Schnittman SM, Greenhouse JJ, Psallidopoulos MC, et al. Increasing viral burden in CD4⁺ T cells from patients with human immunodeficiency virus (HIV) infection reflects rapidly progressive immunosuppression and clinical disease. *Ann Intern Med* 1990;113:438–443.

299. Bagnarelli P, Menzo S, Valenza A, et al. Molecular profile of human immunodeficiency virus type 1 infection in symptomless patients and in patients with AIDS. *J Virol* 1992;66:7328–7335.

300. Connor RI, Mohri H, Cao Y, Ho DD. Increased viral burden and cytopathicity correlate temporally with CD4⁺ T-lymphocyte decline and clinical progression in human immunodeficiency virus type 1–infected individuals. *J Virol* 1993;67:1772–1777.

301. Chevret S, Kirsteter M, Mariotti M, Lefrere F, Frottier J, Lefrere J-J. Provirus copy number to predict disease progression in asymptomatic human immunodeficiency virus type 1 infection. *J Infect Dis* 1994;169:882–885.

302. Aoki S, Yarchoan R, Thomas RV, et al. Quantitative analysis of HIV-1 proviral DNA in peripheral blood mononuclear cells from patients with AIDS or ARC: decrease of proviral DNA content following treatment with 2′,3′-dideoxyinosine (ddI). *AIDS Res Hum Retrovir* 1990;6:1331–1339.

303. Clark AGB, Holodniy M, Schwartz DH, Katzenstein DA, Merigan TC. Decrease in HIV provirus in peripheral blood mononuclear cells during zidovudine and human rIL-2 administration. *J AIDS* 1992;5:52–59.

304. Edlin BR, Weinstein RA, Whaling SM, et al. Zidovudine–interferon-alpha combination therapy in patients with advanced human immunodeficiency virus type 1 infection: biphasic response of p24 antigen and quantitative polymerase chain reaction. *J Infect Dis* 1992;165:793–798.

305. Donovan RM, Dickover RE, Goldstein E, Huth RG, Carlson JR. HIV-1 proviral copy number in blood mononuclear cells from AIDS patients on zidovudine therapy. *J AIDS* 1991;4:766–769.

306. Furtado MR, Murphy R, Wolinsky SM. Quantification of human immunodeficiency virus type 1 tat mRNA as a marker for assessing the efficacy of antiretroviral therapy. *J Infect Dis* 1993;167:213–216.

307. Katzenstein DA, Winters M, Bubp J, Israelski D, Winger E, Merigan TC. Quantitation of human immunodeficiency virus by culture and polymerase chain reaction in response to didanosine after long-term therapy with zidovudine. *J Infect Dis* 1994;169:416–419.

308. Bagnarelli P, Menzo S, Valenza A, et al. Quantitative molecular monitoring of human immunodeficiency virus type 1 activity during therapy with specific antiretroviral compounds. *J Clin Microbiol* 1995;33:16–23.

309. Donovan RM, Bush CE, Smereck SM, Baxa DM, Markowitz NP, Saravolatz LD. Rapid decrease in unintegrated human immunodeficiency virus DNA after the initiation of nucleoside therapy. *J Infect Dis* 1994;170:202–205.

310. Saksela K, Stevens CE, Rubinstein P, Taylor PE, Baltimore D. HIV-1 messenger RNA in peripheral blood mononuclear cells as an early marker of risk for progression to AIDS. *Ann Intern Med* 1995;123:726–727.

311. Michael NL, Vahey M, Burke RS, Redfield RR. Viral DNA and mRNA expression correlate with the stage of human immunodeficiency virus (HIV) type 1 infection in humans: evidence for viral replication in all stages of HIV disease. *J Virol* 1992;66:310–316.

312. Seshamma T, Bagasra O, Trono D, Baltimore D, Pomerantz RJ. Blocked early-stage latency in the peripheral blood cells of certain individuals infected with human immunodeficiency virus type 1. *Proc Natl Acad Sci U S A* 1992;89:10663–10667.

313. Gupta P, Kingsley L, Armstrong J, Ding M, Cottrill M, Rinaldo C. Enhanced expression of human immunodeficiency virus type 1 correlates with development of AIDS. *Virology* 1993;196:586–595.

314. Michael NL, Mo T, Merzouki A, et al. Human immunodeficiency virus type 1 cellular RNA load and splicing patterns predict disease progression in a longitudinally studied cohort. *J Virol* 1995;69:1868–1877.

315. Furtado MR, Kingsley LA, Wolinsky SM. Changes in the viral mRNA expression pattern correlate with a rapid rate of CD4⁻ T-cell number decline in human immunodeficiency virus type 1 infected individuals. *J Virol* 1995;69:2092–2100.

316. Lafeuillade A, Poggi C, Profizi N, Tamalet C, Costes O. Human immunodeficiency virus type 1 kinetics in lymph nodes compared with plasma. *J Infect Dis* 1996;174:404–407.

317. Haase AT, Henry K, Zupancic M, et al. Quantitative image analysis of HIV-1 infection in lymphoid tissue. *Science* 1996;274:985–989.

318. Hewlett I, Gregg R, Ou C, et al. Detection in plasma of HIV-1 specific DNA and RNA by polymerase chain reaction before and after seroconversion. *J Clin Immunoassay* 1988;11:161–164.

319. Kievits T, vanGemen B, vanStrijp D, et al. NASBA isothermal enzymatic in vitro nucleic acid amplification optimized for the diagnosis of HIV-1 infection. *J Virol Methods* 1991;35:273–286.

320. Urdea MS, Wilber JC, Yeghiazarian T, et al. Direct and quantitative detection of HIV-1 RNA in human plasma with a branched DNA signal amplification assay. *AIDS* 1993;7(suppl 2):11–14.

321. Embretson J, Zupancic M, Ribas J, et al. Massive covert infection of helper T lymphocytes and macrophages by HIV during the incubation period of AIDS. *Nature* 1993;362:359–362.

322. Mellors JW, Rinaldo CR, Gupta P, White RM, Todd JA, Kingsley LA. Prognosis in HIV-1 infection predicted by the quantity of virus in plasma. *Science* 1996;272:1167–1170.

323. Coombs RW, Welles SL, Hooper C, et al. Association of plasma human immunodeficiency virus type 1 RNA level with risk of clinical progression in patients with advanced infection. *J Infect Dis* 1996;174:704–712.

324. Welles SL, Jackson JB, Yen-Lieberman B, et al. Prognostic value of plasma human immunodeficiency virus type 1 (HIV-1) RNA levels in patients with advanced HIV-1 disease and with little or no prior zidovudine therapy. *J Infect Dis* 1996;174:696–703.

325. O'Brien WA, Hartigan PM, Martin D, et al. Changes in plasma HIV-1 RNA and CD4$^+$ lymphocyte counts and the risk of progression to AIDS. *N Engl J Med* 1996;334:426–431.

326. Mellors JW, Kingsley LA, Rinaldo CR, et al. Quantitation of HIV-1 RNA in plasma predicts outcome after seroconversion. *Ann Intern Med* 1995;122:573–579.

327. Schacker TW, Hughes J, Shea T, Corey L. Virologic course of primary HIV Infection [Abstract 480]. 3rd Conference on Retroviruses and Opportunistic Infections, 1996.

328. Jurriaans S, vanGemen B, Weverling GJ, et al. The natural history of HIV-1 infection: virus load and virus phenotype independent determinants of clinical course? *Virology* 1994;204:223–233.

329. Phillips AN. Reduction of HIV concentration during acute infection: independence from a specific immune response. *Science* 1996;271:497–499.

330. Carpenter CCJ, Fischl MA, Hammer SM, et al. Antiretroviral therapy for HIV infection in 1996. *JAMA* 1996;276:146–154.

331. Carpenter C, Fischl M, Hammer S, et al. Antiretroviral therapy for HIV infection in 1997—updated recommendations of the International AIDS Society USA panel. *JAMA* 1997;277:1962–1969.

332. Department of Health and Human Services/Henry J. Kaiser Family Foundation Panel on Clinical Practices for Treatment of HIV Infection. Guidelines for the use of antiretroviral agents in HIV-infected adults and adolescents. *MMWR* 1998;47(RR-5):43–82.

333. Collier AC, Coombs RW, Schoenfeld DA, et al. Treatment of human immunodeficiency virus infection with saquinavir, zidovudine, and zalcitabine. *N Engl J Med* 1996;334:1011–1017.

334. Markowitz M, Cao Y, Hurley A, et al. Triple therapy with AZT, 3TC, and ritonavir in 12 subjects newly infected with HIV-1 [Abstract Th.B.933]. Eleventh International Conference on AIDS, 1996.

335. Cavert W, Notermans DW, Staskus K, et al. Kinetics of response in lymphoid tissues to antiretroviral therapy of HIV-1 infection. *Science* 1997;276:960–963.

336. Gulick R, Mellors J, Havlir D, et al. Treatment with indinavir, zidovudine, and lamivudine in adults with human immunodeficiency virus infection and prior antiretroviral therapy. *N Engl J Med* 1997;337:734–739.

337. Hammer S, Squires K, Hughes M, et al. A controlled trial of two nucleoside analogues plus indinavir in persons with human immunodeficiency virus infection and CD4 cell counts of 200 per cubic millimeter or less. *N Engl J Med* 1997;337:725–733.

338. Kahn J, Allan J, Hodges T, et al. The safety and pharmacokinetics of recombinant soluble CD4 (rCD4) in subjects with the acquired immunodeficiency syndrome (AIDS) and AIDS-related complex. A phase 1 study. *Ann Intern Med* 1990;112:254–261.

339. Schooley R, Merigan T, Gaut P, et al. Recombinant soluble CD4 therapy in patients with acquired immunodeficiency syndrome (AIDS) and AIDS-related complex. A phase I–II escalating dosage trial. *Ann Intern Med* 1990;112:247–253.

340. Arenzana-Seisdedos F, Virelizier J-L, Rousset D, et al. HIV blocked by chemokine antagonist. *Nature* 1996;383:400.

341. Schols D, Cabrera C, Henson G, Clotet B, DeClerq E. Inhibition of HIV-1 replication by the bicyclam AMD3100, a CXCR4 antagonist. Interscience Conference on Antimicrobial Agents and Chemotherapy, 1997 (Abstract I-66.)

342. Kohl NE, Emini EA, Schleif WA, et al. Active human immunodeficiency virus protease is required for viral infectivity. *Proc Natl Acad Sci U S A* 1988;85:4686–4690.

343. Navia MA, Fitzgerald PM, McKeever BM, et al. Three-dimensional structure of aspartyl protease from human immunodeficiency virus HIV-1. *Nature* 1989;337:615–620.

344. Wlodawer A, Miller M, Jaskolski M, et al. Conserved folding in retroviral proteases: crystal structure of a synthetic HIV-1 protease. *Science* 1989;245:616–621.

345. Dyda F, Hickman AB, Jenkins TM, Engelman A, Craigie R, Davies DR. Crystal structure of the catalytic domain of HIV-1 integrase: similarity to other polynucleotidyl transferases. *Science* 1994;266:1981–1986.

346. Farnet CM, Bushman FD. HIV cDNA integration: molecular biology and inhibitor development. *AIDS* 1996;10(suppl A):3–11.

347. Haubrich RH, Flexner C, Lederman MM, et al. A randomized trial of the acitivity and safety of Ro 24-7429 (Tat antagonist) versus nucleoside for human immunodeficiency virus infection. The AIDS Clinical Trials Group 213 Team. *J Infect Dis* 1995;172:1246–1252.

348. Kinloch-DeLoes S, Hirschel BJ, Hoen B, et al. A controlled trial of zidovudine in primary human immunodeficiency virus infection. *N Engl J Med* 1995;333:408–413.

349. Volberding P, Lagakos S, Grimes J, et al. The duration of zidovudine benefit in persons with asymptomatic HIV infection. *JAMA* 1994;272:437–442.

350. Kahn J, Lagakos S, Richman D, et al. A controlled trial comparing continued zidovudine with didanosine in human immunodeficiency virus infection. *N Engl J Med* 1992;327:581–587.

351. Spruance SL, Pavia AT, Peterson D, et al. Didanosine compared with continuation of zidovudine in HIV-infected patients with signs of clinical deterioration while receiving zidovudine. *Ann Intern Med* 1994;120:360–368.

352. Abrams DI, Goldman AI, Launer C, et al. A comparative trial of didanosine or zalcitabine after treatment with zidovudine in patients with human immunodeficiency virus infection. *N Engl J Med* 1994;330:657–662.

353. Montaner JSG, Schechter MT, Rachlis A, et al. Didanosine compared with continued zidovudine therapy for HIV-infected patients with 200 to 500 CD4 cells/mm^3. *Ann Intern Med* 1995;123:561–571.

354. Hammer SM, Katzenstein DA, Hughes MD, et al. A trial comparing nucleoside monotherapy with combination therapy in HIV-infected adults with CD4 cell counts from 200 to 500 per cubic millimeter. AIDS Clinical Trials Group Study 175 Study Team. *N Engl J Med* 1996;335:1081–1090.

355. Collier AC, Coombs RW, Fischl MA, et al. Combination therapy with zidovudine and didanosine compared with zidovudine alone in HIV-1 infection. *Ann Intern Med* 1993;119:786–793.

356. Graham NMH, Hoover DR, Park LP, et al. Survival in HIV-infected patients who have received zidovudine: comparison of combination therapy with sequential monotherapy and continued zidovudine monotherapy. *Ann Intern Med* 1996;124:1031–1038.

357. D'Aquila RT, Hughes MD, Johnson VA, et al. Nevirapine, zidovudine, and didanosine compared with zidovudine and didanosine in patients with HIV-1 infection. *Ann Intern Med* 1996;124:1019–1030.

358. Delta Coordinating Committee. Delta: a randomised double-blind controlled trial comparing combinations of zidovudine plus didanosine or zalcitabine with zidovudine alone in HIV-infected individuals. *Lancet* 1996;348:283–291.

359. Eron JJ, Benoit SL, Jemsek J, et al. Treatment with lamivudine, zidovudine, or both in HIV-positive patients with 200 to 500 CD4$^+$ cells per cubic millimeter. North American HIV working party. *N Engl J Med* 1995;333:1662–1669.

360. Staszewski S, Loveday C, Picazo JJ, et al. Safety and efficacy of lamivudine–zidovudine combination therapy in zidovudine-experienced patients. A randomized controlled comparison with zidovudine monotherapy. Lamivudine European HIV Working Group. *JAMA* 1996;276:111–117.

361. Katlama C, Ingrand D, Loveday C, et al. Safety and efficacy of lamivudine–zidovudine combination therapy in antiretroviral-naive patients. A randomized controlled comparison with zidovudine monotherapy. Lamivudine European HIV Working Group. *JAMA* 1996;276:118–125.

362. Bartlett JA, Benoit SL, Johnson VA, et al. Lamivudine plus zidovudine compared with zalcitabine plus zidovudine in patients with HIV infection. *Ann Intern Med* 1996;125:161–172.

363. Larder B, Kemp S, Harrigan R. Potential mechanism for sustained antiretroviral efficacy of AZT–3TC combination therapy. *Science* 1995;269:696–699.

364. Markowitz M, Saag M, Powderly WG, et al. A preliminary study of ritonavir, an inhibitor of HIV-1 protease, to treat HIV-1 infection. *N Engl J Med* 1995;333:1534–1539.

365. Danner SA, Carr A, Leonard JM, et al. A short-term of the safety, pharmacokinetics, and efficacy of ritonavir, an inhibitor of HIV-1 protease. European–Australian Collaborative Ritonavir Study Group. *N Engl J Med* 1995;333:1528–1533.

366. Schapiro JA, Winters MA, Stewart F, et al. The effect of high-dose saquinavir on viral load and CD4$^+$ T-cell counts in HIV-infected patients. *Ann Intern Med* 1996;124:1039–1050.

367. Stein DS, Fish DG, Bilello JA, Preston SL, Martineau GL, Drusano GL. A 24-week open-label phase I/II evaluation of the HIV protease inhibitor MK-639 (indinavir). *AIDS* 1996;10:485–492.

368. Deeks SG, Smith M, Holodniy M, Kahn JO. HIV-1 protease inhibitors. A review for clinicians. *JAMA* 1997;277:145–153.

369. Cameron D, Heath-Chiozzi M, Kravick S, Mills R, Potthoff A, Henry D. Prolongation of life and prevention of AIDS complications in advanced HIV immunodeficiency with Ritonavir [Abstract MoB411]. Eleventh International Conference on AIDS, 1996.

370. Stellbrink HJ, Zoller B, Fenner T, et al. Rapid plasma virus and CD4$^+$ T-cell turnover in HIV-1 infection: evidence for an only transient interruption by treatment. *AIDS* 1996;10:849–857.

371. Autran B, Carcelain G, Li T, et al. Positive effects of combined antiretroviral therapy on CD4$^+$ T cell homeostasis and function in advanced HIV disease. *Science* 1997;277:112–116.

372. Fox C, Tenner-Rácz K, Rácz P, Firpo A, Pizzo P, Fauci A. Lymphoid germinal centers are reservoirs of human immunodeficiency virus type 1 RNA. *J Infect Dis* 1991;164:1051–1057.

373. Spiegel H, Herbst H, Niedobitek G, Foss H, Stein H. Follicular dendritic cells are a major reservoir for human immunodeficiency virus type 1 in lymphoid tissues facilitating infection of CD4$^+$ T-helper cells. *Am J Pathol* 1992;140:15–22.

374. Joling P, Bakker L, Van Strijp J, et al. Binding of human immunodeficiency virus type-1 to follicular dendritic cells in vitro is complement dependent. *J Immunol* 1993;150:1065–1073.

375. Hufert FT, vanLunzen J, Janossy G, et al. Germinal center CD4$^+$ T cells are an important site of HIV replication in vivo. *AIDS* 1997;11:849–857.

376. Ascher M, Sheppard H. AIDS as immune system activation: a model for pathogenesis. *Clin Exp Immunol* 1988;73:165–167.

377. Sheppard HW, Ascher MS, McRae B, Anderson RE, Lang W, Allain JP. The initial immune response to HIV and immune system activation determine the outcome of HIV disease. *J AIDS* 1991;4:704–712.

378. Bass H, Nishanian P, Hardy W, et al. Immune changes in HIV infection: significant correlations and differences in serum markers and lymphoid phenotypic antigens. *Clin Immunol Immunopathol* 1992;64:63–70.

379. Weissman D, Barker TD, Fauci AS. The efficiency of acute infection of CD4$^+$ T cells is markedly enhanced in the setting of antigen-specific immune activation. *J Exp Med* 1996;183:687–692.

380. Ott M, Emiliani S, VanLint C, et al. Immune hyperactivation of HIV-1–infected T cells mediated by tat and the CD28 pathway. *Science* 1997;275:1481–1485.

381. Fauci A. The human immunodeficiency virus: infectivity and mechanisms of pathogenesis. *Science* 1988;239:617–622.

382. Fauci A. Multifactorial nature of human immunodeficiency virus diseases: implications for therapy. *Science* 1993;262:1011–1018.

383. Graziosi C, Pantaleo G, Gantt KR, et al. Lack of evidence for the dichotomy of TH1 and TH2 predominance in HIV-infected individuals. *Science* 1994;265:248–252.

384. Westermann J, Persin S, Matyas J, van der Meide P, Pabst R. Migration of so-called naive and memory T lymphocytes from blood to lymph in the rat. The influence of IFN-gamma on the circulation pattern. *J Immunol* 1994;152:1744–1750.

385. Sprenger R, Toellner KM, Schmetz C, et al. Follicular dendritic cells productively infected with immunodeficiency viruses transmit infection to T cells. *Med Microbiol Immunol* 1995;184:129–134.

386. Schmitz J, van Lunzen J, Tenner-Racz K, et al. Follicular dendritic cells retain HIV-1 particles on their plasma membrane, but are not productively infected in asymptomatic patients with follicular hyperplasia. *J Immunol* 1994;153:1352–1359.

387. Banda NK, Bernier J, Kurahara DK, et al. Crosslinking CD4 by human immunodeficiency virus gp120 primes T cells for activation-induced apoptosis. *J Exp Med* 1992;176:1099–1106.

388. Li CJ, Friedman DJ, Wang C, Metelev V, Pardee AB. Induction of apoptosis in uninfected lymphocytes by HIV-1 tat protein. *Science* 1995;268:429–431.

389. Westendorp MO, Frank R, Ochsenbauer C, et al. Sensitization of T cells to CD95-mediated apoptosis by HIV-1 tat and gp120. *Nature* 1995;375:497–500.

390. Howcroft T, Strebel K, Martin M, Singer D. Repression of MHC class I gene promoter activity by two-exon tat of HIV. *Science* 1993;260:1320–1322.

391. Kerkau T, Bacik I, Bennink JR, et al. The human immunodeficiency virus type 1 (HIV-1) vpu protein interferes with an early step in the biosynthesis of major histocompatibility complex (MHC) class I molecules. *J Exp Med* 1997;185:1295–1305.

392. Dawson V, Dawson T, Uhl G, Snyder S. Human immunodeficiency virus type 1 coat protein neurotoxicity mediated by nitric oxide in primary cortical cultures. *Proc Natl Acad Sci U S A* 1993;90:3256–3259.

393. Pietraforte D, Tritarelli E, Testa U, Minetti M. gp120 HIV envelope glycoprotein increases the production of nitric oxide in human monocyte-derived macrophages. *J Leukoc Biol* 1994;55:175–182.

394. Bukrinsky M, Nottet H, Schmidtmayerova H, et al. Regulation of nitric oxide synthase activity in human immunodeficiency virus type 1 (HIV-1)–infected monocytes: Implications for HIV associated neurological disease. *J Exp Med* 1995;181:735–745.

395. Weeks B, Klotman M, Holloway E, Stetler-Stevenson W, Kleinman H, Klotman P. HIV-1 infection stimulates T cell invasiveness and synthesis of the 92-kDa type IV collagenase. *AIDS Res Hum Retrovir* 1993;9:513–518.

396. Lafrenie R, Wahl L, Epstein J, Hewlett I, Yamada K, Dhawan S. HIV-1 tat modulates the function of monocytes and alters their interactions with microvessel endothelial cells. *J Immunol* 1996;156:1638–1645.

397. Margolick JB, Munoz A, Donnenberg AD, et al. Failure of T-cell homeostasis preceding AIDS in HIV-1 infection. The Multicenter AIDS Cohort Study. *Nat Med* 1995;1:674–680.

398. Stanley SK, Fauci AS. T-cell homeostasis in HIV infection: part of the solution, or part of the problem? *J AIDS* 1993;6.142–143.

399. Grossman Z, Herberman RB, Adleman LM, Wofsy D. T-cell homeostasis in HIV infection is neither failing nor blind: modified cell counts reflect an adaptive response of the host. *Nat Med* 1997;3:486–490.

400. Adleman LM, Wofsy D. T-cell homeostasis: implications in HIV infection. *J AIDS* 1993;6:144–152.

401. Chen YH, Christiansen A, Dierich MP. HIV-1 gp41 selectively inhibits spontaneous cell proliferation of human cell lines and mitogen- and recall antigen-induced lymphocyte proliferation. *Immunol Lett* 1995;48:39–44.

402. Tuosto L, Piazza C, Moretti S, et al. Ligation of either CD2 or CD28 rescues CD4+ T cells from HIV-gp120–induced apoptosis. *Eur J Immunol* 1995;25:2917–2922.

403. Tian H, Lempicki R, King L, Donoghue E, Samelson LE, Cohen DI. HIV envelope directed signaling aberrancies and cell death of CD4+ T cells in the absence of TCR co-stimulation. *Int Immunol* 1996;8:65–74.

404. Faith A, Yssel H, O'Hehir RE, Lamb JR. Reversal of the inhibitory effects of HIV-gp120 on CD4+ T cells by stimulation through the CD28 pathway. *Clin Exp Immunol* 1996;105:225–230.

405. Cohen JJ. Apoptosis. *Immunol Today* 1993;14:126 130.

406. Estaquier J, Idziorek T, DeBels F, et al. Programmed cell death and AIDS: significance of T-cell apoptosis in pathogenic and nonpathogenic primate lentiviral infections. *Proc Natl Acad Sci U S A* 1994;91:9431–9435.

407. Groux H, Torpier G, Monte D, Mouton Y, Capron A, Ameisen JC. Activation-induced death by apoptosis in CD4+ T cells from human immunodeficiency virus–infected asymptomatic individuals. *J Exp Med* 1992;175:331–340.

408. Laurent-Crawford AG, Krust B, Muller S, et al. The cytopathic effect of HIV is associated with apoptosis. *Virology* 1991;185:829–839.

409. Choremi-Papadopoulou H, Viglis V, Gargalianos P, Kordossis T, Iniotaki-Theodoraki A, Kosmidis J. Downregulation of CD28 surface antigen on CD4+ and CD8+ T lymphocytes during HIV-1 infection. *J AIDS* 1994;7:245–253.

410. Borthwick NJ, Bofill M, Gombert WM, et al. Lymphocyte activation in HIV-1 infection. II. Functional defects of CD28- T cells. *AIDS* 1994;8:431–441.

411. Spina CA, Prince HE, Richman DD. Preferential replication of HIV-1 in the CD45RO memory cell subset of primary CD4 lymphocytes in vitro. *J Clin Invest* 1997;99:1774–1785.

412. Psallidopoulos MC, Schnittman SM, Thompson LM, et al. Integrated proviral human immunodeficiency virus type is present in CD4- peripheral blood lymphocytes in healthy seropositive individuals. *J Virol* 1989;63:4626–4631.

413. Popovic M, Sarngadharan M, Read E, Gallo R. Detection, isolation, and continuous production of cytopathic retroviruses (HTLV-III) from patients with AIDS and pre-AIDS. *Science* 1984;224:497–500.

414. Sodroski J, Goh WC, Rosen K, Campbell K, Haseltine WA. Role of the HTLV-III/LAV envelope in syncytium formation and cytopathicity. *Nature* 1986;322:470–474.

415. DeRossi A, Franchini G, Aldovini A, et al. Differential response to the cytopathic effects of human T-cell lymphotropic virus type III (HTLV-III) superinfection in T4+ (helper) and T8+ (suppressor) T-cell clones transformed by HTLV-1. *Proc Natl Acad Sci U S A* 1986;83:4297–4301.

416. Lifson JD, Reyes GR, McGrath MS, Stein BS, Engleman EG. AIDS retrovirus induced cytopathology: giant cell formation and involvement of CD4 antigen. *Science* 1986;232:1123–1127.

417. Lifson JD, Feinberg MB, Reyes GR, et al. Induction of CD4-dependent cell fusion by the HTLV-III/LAV envelope glycoprotein. *Nature* 1986;323:725–728.

418. Poznansky MC, Walker B, Haseltine WA, Sodroski J, Langhoff E. A rapid method for quantitating the frequency of peripheral blood cells containing HIV-1 DNA. *J AIDS* 1991;4:368–373.

419. Brinchmann JE, Albert J, Vartdal F. Few infected CD4+ T cells but a high proportion of replication-competent provirus copies in asymptomatic human immunodeficiency virus type 1 infection. *J Virol* 1991;65:2019–2023.

420. Harper ME, Marselle LM, Gallo RC, Wong-Staal F. Detection of lymphocytes expressing human T-lymphotropic virus type III in lymph nodes and peripheral blood from infected individuals by in situ hybridization. *Proc Natl Acad Sci U S A* 1986;83:772–776.

421. Weller SK, Joy AE, Temin HM. Correlation between cell killing and massive second round superinfecton by members of some subgroups of avian leukosis virus. *J Virol* 1980;33:494–506.

422. Keshet E, Temin HM. Cell killing by spleen necrosis virus is correlated with a transient accumulation of spleen necrosis virus DNA. *J Virol* 1979;31:376–388.

423. Bergeron L, Sodroski J. Dissociation of unintegrated viral DNA accumulation from single-cell lysis induced by human immunodeficiency virus type 1. *J Virol* 1992;66:5777–5787.

424. Somasundaran M, Robinson HL. Unexpectedly high levels of HIV-1 RNA and protein synthesis in a cytocidal infection. *Science* 1988;242:1554–1557.

425. Koga Y, Lindstrom E, Fenyo EM, Wigzell H, Mak TW. High levels of heterodisperse RNAs accumulate in T cells infected with human immunodeficiency virus and in normal thymocytes. *Proc Natl Acad Sci U S A* 1988;85:4521–4525.

426. Koga Y, Sasaki M, Yoshida H, Wigzell H, Kimura G, Nomoto K. Cytopathic effect determined by the amount of CD4 molecules in human cell lines expressing envelope glycoprotein of HIV. *J Immunol* 1990;144:94–102.

427. Cao J, Park IW, Cooper A, Sodroski J. Molecular determinants of acute single-cell lysis by human immunodeficiency virus type 1. *J Virol* 1996;70:1340–1354.

428. Leonard R, Zagury D, Desportes I, Bernard J, Zagury JF, Gallo RC. Cytopathic effect of human immunodeficiency virus in T4 cells is linked to the last stage of virus infection. *Proc Natl Acad Sci U S A* 1988;85:3357–3574.

429. Lynn WS, Tweedale A, Cloyd MW. Human immunodeficiency virus (HIV-1) cytotoxicity: perturbation of the cell membrane and depression of phospholipid synthesis. *Virol* 1988;163:43–51.

430. Voss TG, Fermin CD, Levy JA, Vigh S, Choi B, Garry RF. Alteration of intracellular potassium and sodium concentrations correlates with induction of cytopathic effects by human immunodeficiency virus. *J Virol* 1996;70:5447–5454.

431. Yoffe B, Lewis DE, Petrie BL, Noonan CA, Melnick JL, Hollinger FB. Fusion as a mediator of cytolysis in mixtures of uninfected CD4+ lymphocytes and cells infected by human immunodeficiency virus. *Proc Natl Acad Sci U S A* 1987;84:1429–1433.

432. Crowe S, Mills J, Elbeik T, et al. Human immunodeficiency virus–infected monocyte-derived macrophages express surface gp120 and fuse with CD4 lymphoid cells in vitro: a possible mechanism of T lymphocyte depletion in vivo. *Clin Immunol Immunopathol* 1992;65:143–151.

433. Hart TK, Truneh A, Bugelski PJ. Characterization of CD4-gp120 activation intermediates during human immunodeficiency virus type 1 syncytium formation. *AIDS Res Hum Retrovir* 1996;12:1305–1313.

434. Hildreth JE, Orentas RJ. Involvement of a leukocyte adhesion receptor (LFA-1) in HIV-induced syncytium formation. *Science* 1989;244:1075–1078.

435. Pantaleo G, Butini L, Graziosi C, et al. Human immunodeficiency virus (HIV) infection in CD4+ T lymphocytes genetically deficient in LFA-1: LFA-1 is required form HIV-mediated cell fusion but not for viral transmission. *J Exp Med* 1991;173:511–514.

436. Sato AI, Balamuth FB, Ugen KE, Williams WV, Weiner DB. Identification of CD7 glycoprotein as an accessory molecule in HIV-1–mediated syncytium formation and cell-free infection. *J Immunol* 1994;152:5142–5152.

437. deSantis C, Robbioni P, Longhi R, Carrow E, Siccardi AG, Beretta A. Role of HLA class I in HIV type 1–induced syncytium formation. *AIDS Res Hum Retrovir* 1996;12:1031–1040.

438. Burke AP, Benson W, Ribas JL, et al. Postmortem localization of HIV-1 RNA by in situ hybridization in lymphoid tissues of intravenous drug addicts who died unexpectedly. *Am J Pathol* 1993;142:1701–1713.

439. Burke AP, Anderson D, Mannan P, et al. Systemic lymphadenopathic histology in human immunodeficiency virus-1–seropositive drug addicts without apparent acquired immunodeficiency syndrome. *Hum Pathol* 1994;25:248–256.

440. Sharer LR, Cho ES, Epstein LG. Multinucleated giant cells and HTLV-III in AIDS encephalopathy. *Hum Pathol* 1985;16:760.

441. Maier H, Budka H, Lassmann H, Pohl P. Vacuolar myelopathy with multinucleated giant cells in the acquired immune deficiency syndrome (AIDS). Light and electron microscopic distribution of human immunodeficiency virus (HIV) antigens. *Acta Neuropathol* 1989;78:497–503.

442. Teo I, Veryard C, Barnes H, et al. Circular forms of unintegrated human immunodeficiency virus type 1 DNA and high levels of viral protein expression: association with dementia and multinucleated giant cells in the brains of patients with AIDS. *J Virol* 1997;71:2928–2933.

443. Golding H, Robey FA, Gates FT, et al. Identification of homologous regions in human immunodeficiency virus I gp41 and human MHC class II beta 1 domain. I. Monoclonal antibodies against the gp41-derived peptide and patient's sera react with native HLA class II antigens, suggesting a role for autoimmunity in the pathogenesis of acquired immune deficiency syndrome. *J Exp Med* 1988; 167:914–923.

444. Golding H, Shearer G, Hillman K, et al. Common epitope in human immunodeficiency virus (HIV)1 gp41 and HLA class II elicits immunosuppressive autoantibodies capable of contributing to immune dysfunction in HIV 1–infected individuals. *J Clin Invest* 1989;83:1430–1435.

445. Metlas R, Skerl V, Veljkovic V, Colombatti A, Pongor S. Immunoglobulin-like domain of HIV-1 envelope glycoprotein gp120 encodes putative internal image of some common human proteins. *Viral Immunol* 1994;7:215–219.

446. Grassi F, Meneveri R, Gullberg M, et al. Human immunodeficiency virus type 1 gp120 mimics a hidden monomorphic epitope borne by class I major histocompatibility complex heavy chains. *J Exp Med* 1991;174:53–62.

447. Silvestris F, Williams RC, Dammacco F. Autoreactivity in HIV-1 infections: the role of molecular mimicry. *Clin Immunol Immunopathol* 1995;75:197–205.

448. Grant MD, Weaver MS, Tsoukas C, Hoffmann GW. Distribution of antibodies against denatured collagen in AIDS risk groups and homosexual AIDS patients suggests a link between autoimmunity and the immunopathogenesis of AIDS. *J Immunol* 1990;144:1241–1250.

449. Muller S, Richalet P, Laurent-Crawford A, et al. Autoantibodies typical of non–organ-specific autoimmune diseases in HIV-seropositive patients. *AIDS* 1992;6:933–942.

450. Cassani F, Baffoni L, Raise E, et al. Serum non-organ specific autoantibodies in human immunodeficiency virus 1 infection. *J Clin Pathol* 1991;44:64–68.

451. Kappler J, Kotzin B, Gelfand LHW, et al. V beta-specific stimulation of human T cells by staphylococcal toxins. *Science* 1989;244:811–813.

452. Cole BC, Kartchner DR, Wells DJ. Stimulation of mouse lymphocytes by a mitogen derived from *Mycoplasma arthritidis* (MAM). VII. Selective activation of T cells expressing distinct V beta T cell receptors from various strains of mice by the "superantigen" MAM. *J Immunol* 1990;144:425–431.

453. Denkers EY, Caspar P, Sher A. *Toxoplasma gondii* possesses a superantigen activity that selectively expands murine T cell receptor V beta 5–bearing CD8+ lymphocytes. *J Exp Med* 1994;180:985–994.

454. Choi Y, Kappler JW, Marrack P. A superantigen encoded in the open reading frame of the 3′ long terminal repeat of mouse mammary tumour virus. *Nature* 1991;350:203–207.

455. Hugin AW, Vacchio MS, Morse HC. A virus-encoded "superantigen" in a retrovirus-induced immunodeficiency syndrome of mice. *Science* 1991;252:424–427.

456. Imberti L, Sottini A, Bettinardi A, Puoti M, Primi D. Selective depletion in HIV infection of T cells that bear specific T cell receptor V beta sequences. *Science* 1991;254:860–862.

457. Garcia S, Dadaglio G, Cilote V, Chenal H, Bondurand A, Gougeon ML. Evidence for an in vivo superantigenic activity in human immunodeficiency virus–infected individuals. *Blood* 1996;88:2151–2161.

458. Laurence J, Hodtsev AS, Posnett DN. Superantigen implicated in dependence of HIV-1 replication in T cells on TCR V beta expression. *Nature* 1992;358:255–259.

459. Posnett DN, Kabak S, Dobrescu D, Hodtsev AS. The HIV-1 reservoir in distinct V beta subsets of CD4 T cells: evidence for a putative superantigen. *J Clin Immunol* 1995;15(suppl):18–21.

460. Dobrescu D, Kabak S, Mehta K, et al. Human immunodeficiency virus 1 reservoir in CD4+ T cells is restricted to certian V beta subsets. *Proc Natl Acad Sci U S A* 1995;92:5563–5567.

461. Dobrescu D, Ursea B, Pope M, Asch AS, Posnett DN. Enhanced HIV-1 replication in V beta 12 T cells due to human cytomegalovirus in monocytes: evidence for a putative herpesvirus superantigen. *Cell* 1995;82:753–763.

462. Boyer V, Smith LR, Ferre F, et al. T cell receptor V beta repertoire in HIV-infected individuals: lack of evidence for selective V beta deletion. *Clin Exp Immunol* 1993;92:437–441.

463. Posnett DN, Kabak S, Hodtsev A, Goldberg EA, Asch A. T-cell antigen receptor V beta subsets are not preferentially deleted in AIDS. *AIDS* 1993;7:625–631.

464. Boldt-Houle DM, Rinaldo CR, Ehrlich GD. Random depletion of T cells that bear specific T cell receptor V beta sequences in AIDS patients. *J Leukoc Biol* 1993;54:486–491.

465. Weinhold KJ, Lyerly HK, Stanley SD, Austin AA, Matthews TJ, Bolognesi DP. HIV-1 GP120-mediated immune suppression and lymphocyte destruction in the absence of viral infection. *J Immunol* 1989;142:3091–3097.

466. Zarling JM, Ledbetter JA, Sias J, et al. HIV-infected humans, but not chimpanzees, have circulating cytotoxic T lymphocytes that lyse uninfected CD4+ cells. *J Immunol* 1990;144:2992–2998.

467. Manca F, Habeshaw JA, Dalgleish AG. HIV envelope glycoprotein, antigen specific T-cell responses, and soluble CD4. *Lancet* 1990;335:811–815.

468. Thompson CB. Apoptosis in the pathogenesis and treatment of disease. *Science* 1995;267:1456–1462.

469. Vaux DL, Cory S, Adams JM. Bcl-2 gene promotes haemopoietic cell survival and cooperates with c-myc to immortalize pre-B cells. *Nature* 1988;335:440–442.

470. Nunez G, London L, Hockenbery D, Alexander M, McKearn JP, Korsmeyer SJ. Deregulated Bcl-2 gene expression selectively prolongs survival of growth factor–deprived hemopoietic cell lines. *J Immunol* 1990;144:3602–3610.

471. Hockenbery D, Nunez G, Milliman C, Schrieber RD, Korsmeyer SJ. Bcl-2 is an inner mitochondrial membrane protein that blocks programmed cell death. *Nature* 1990;348:334–336.

472. Lowe SW, Schmitt EM, Smith SW, Osborne BA, Jacks T. p53 is required for radiation-induced apoptosis in mouse thymocytes. *Nature* 1993;362:847–849.

473. Clarke AR, Purdie CA, Harrison DJ, et al. Thymocyte apoptosis induced by p53-dependent and independent pathways. *Nature* 1993;362:849–852.

474. Lee JM, Bernstein A. p53 mutatons increase resistance to ionizing radiation. *Proc Natl Acad Sci U S A* 1993;90:5742–5746.

475. Ascher MS, Sheppard HW. AIDS as immune system activation. II. The panergic imnesia hypothesis. *J AIDS* 1990;3:177–191.

476. Ameisen JC, Capron A. Cell dysfunction and depletion in AIDS: the programmed cell death hypothesis. *Immunol Today* 1991;12:102–105.

477. Terai C, Kornbluth RS, Pauza CD, Richman DD, Carson DA. Apoptosis as a mechanism of cell death in cultured T lymphoblasts acutely infected with HIV-1. *J Clin Invest* 1991;87:1700–1705.

478. Meyaard L, Otto SA, Jonker RR, Mijnster MJ, Keet RPM, Miedema F. Programmed death of T cells in HIV-1 infection. *Science* 1992;257:217–219.

479. Oyaizu N, McCloskey TW, Coronesi M, Chirmule N, Kalyanaraman VS, Pahwa S. Accelerated apoptosis in peripheral blood mononuclear cells (PBMCs) from human immunodeficiency virus type-1 infected patients and in CD4 cross-linked PBMCs from normal individuals. *Blood* 1993;82:3392–3400.

480. Muro-Cacho CA, Pantaleo G, Fauci AS. Analysis of apoptosis in lymph nodes of HIV-infected persons. *J Immunol* 1995;154:5555–5566.

481. Finkel TH, Tudor-Williams G, Banda NK, et al. Apoptosis occurs predominantly in bystander cells and not in productively infected cells of HIV- and SIV-infected lymph nodes. *Nat Med* 1995;1:129–134.

482. Gougeon M-L, Lecoeur H, Dulioust A, et al. Programmed cell death in peripheral lymphocytes from HIV-infected persons. *J Immunol* 1996;156:3509–3520.

483. Meyaard L, Otto SA, Keet IP, Roos MT, Miedema F. Programmed death of T cells in human immunodeficiency virus infection. No correlation with progression to disease. *J Clin Invest* 1994;93:982–988.

484. Folks TM, Kessler SW, Orenstein JM, Justement JS, Jaffe ES, Fauci AS. Infection and replication of HIV-1 in purified progenitor cells of normal human bone marrow. *Science* 1988;242:919–922.

485. Steinberg HN, Crumpacker CS, Chatis PA. In vitro suppression of normal human bone marrow progenitor cells by human immunodeficiency virus. *J Virol* 1991; 65:1765–1769.

486. Chelucci C, Hassan JH, Locardi C, et al. In vitro human immunodeficiency virus-1 infection of purified hematopoietic progenitors in single-cell culture. *Blood* 1995;85:1181–1187.

487. vonLaer D, Hufert FT, Fenner TE, et al. CD34+ hematopoietic progenitor cells are not a major reservoir of the human immunodeficiency virus. *Blood* 1990;76: 1281–1286.

488. Davis BR, Schwartz DH, Marx JC, et al. Absent or rare human immunodeficiency virus infection of bone marrow stem/progenitor cells in vivo. *J Virol* 1991;65:1985–1990.

489. Neal TF, Holland HK, Baum CM, et al. CD34+ progenitor cells from asymptomatic patients are not a major reservoir for human immunodeficiency virus-1. *Blood* 1995;86:1749–1756.

490. Marandin A, Katz A, Oksenhendler E, et al. Loss of primitive hematopoietic progenitors in patients with human immunodeficiency virus infection. *Blood* 1996;88:4568–4578.

491. Stanley SK, Kessler SW, Justement JS, et al. CD34+ bone marrow cells are infected with HIV in a subset of seropositive individuals. *J Immunol* 1992;149:689–697.

492. Deichmann M, Kronenwett R, Haas R. Expression of the human immunodeficiency virus type-1 coreceptors CXCR-4 (fusin, LESTR) and CKR-5 in CD34+ hematopoietic progenitor cells. *Blood* 1997;89:3522–3528.

493. Zauli G, Re MC, Furlini G, Giovannini M, LaPlaca M. Evidence for an HIV-1 mediated suppression of in vitro growth of enriched (CD34+) hematopoietic progenitors. *J AIDS* 1991;4:1251–1253.

494. Louache F, Henri A, Bettaieb A, et al. Role of human immunodeficiency virus replication in defective in vitro growth of hematopoietic progenitors. *Blood* 1992;80:2991–2999.

495. DeLuca A, Teofili L, Antinori A, et al. Haemopoietic CD34+ progenitor cells are not infected by HIV-1 in vivo but show impaired clonogenesis. *Br J Haematol* 1993;85:20–24.

496. Re MC, Zauli G, Gibellini D, et al. Uninfected haematopoietic progenitor (CD34+) cells purified from the bone marrow of AIDS patients are committed to apoptotic cell death in culture. *AIDS* 1993;7:1049–1055.

497. Zauli G, Re MC, Furlini G, Giovannini M, LaPlaca M. Human immunodefi-

ciency virus type 1 envelope glycoprotein gp120-mediated killing of human haematopoietic progenitors (CD34+ cells). *J Gen Virol* 1992;73:417–421.

498. Zauli G, Davis BR, Re MC, Visani G, Furlini G, LaPlaca M. Tat protein stimulates production of transforming growth factor-β1 by marrow macrophages: a potential mechanism for human immunodeficiency virus-1–induced hematopoietic suppression. *Blood* 1992;80:3036–3043.

499. Zauli G, Vitale M, Gibellini D, Capitani S. Inhibition of purified CD34+ hematopoietic progenitor cells by human immunodeficiency virus 1 or gp120 mediated by endogenous transforming growth factor beta 1. *J Exp Med* 1996; 183:99–108.

500. Maciejewski JP, Weichold FF, Young NS. HIV-1 suppression of hematopoiesis in vitro mediated by envelope glycoprotein and TNF-α. *J Immunol* 1994;153: 4303–4310.

501. Stanley S, McCune J, Kaneshima H, et al. Human immunodeficiency virus infection of the human thymus and disruption of the thymic microenvironment in the SCID-hu mouse. *J Exp Med* 1993;178:1151–1163.

502. Schnittman SM, Singer KH, Greenhouse JJ, et al. Thymic microenvironment induces HIV expression. Physiologic secretion of IL-6 by thymic epithelial cells up-regulates virus expression in chronically infected cells. *J Immunol* 1991; 147: 2553–2558.

503. Valentin H, Nugeyre MT, Vuillier F, et al. Two subpopulations of human triple-negative thymic cells are susceptible to infection by human immunodeficiency virus type 1 in vitro. *J Virol* 1994;68:3041–3050.

504. Su L, Kaneshima H, Bonyhadi M, et al. HIV-1–induced thymocyte depletion is associated with indirect cytopathogenicity and infection of progenitor cells in vivo. *Immunity* 1995;2:25–36.

505. Mocroft A, Bofill M, Lipman M, et al. CD8+,CD38+ lymphocyte percent: a useful immunological marker for monitoring HIV-1–infected patients. *J AIDS Hum Retrovir* 1997;14:158–162.

506. Liu Z, Hultin LE, Cumberland WG, et al. Elevated relative fluorescence intensity of CD38 antigen expression on CD8+ T cells is a marker of poor prognosis in HIV infection: results of 6 years of follow-up. *Cytometry* 1996;26:1–7.

507. Kammerer R, Iten A, Frei PC, Burgisser P. Expansion of T cells negative for CD28 expression in HIV infection. Relation to activation markers and cell adhesion molecules, and correlation with prognostic markers. *Med Microbiol Immunol (Berl)* 1996;185:19–25.

508. Vingerhoets JH, Vanham GL, Kestens LL, et al. Increased cytolytic T lymphocyte activity and decreased B7 responsiveness are associated with CD28 down-regulation on CD8+ T cells from HIV-infected subjects. *Clin Exp Immunol* 1995; 100:425–433.

509. Carmichael A, Jin X, Sissons P, Borysiewicz L. Quantitative analysis of the human immunodeficiency virus type 1 (HIV-1)–specific cytotoxic T lymphocyte (CTL) response at different stages of HIV-1 infection: differential CTL responses to HIV-1 and Epstein-Barr virus in late disease. *J Exp Med* 1993;177:249–256.

510. Forte M, Maartens G, Rahelu M, et al. Cytolytic T-cell activity against mycobacterial antigens in HIV. *AIDS* 1992;6:407–411.

511. McKenzie S, Dallalio G, North M, Frame P, Means R. Serum chemokine levels in patients with non-progressing HIV infection. *AIDS* 1996;10:29–33.

512. Zanussi S, D'Andrea M, Simonelli C, Tirelli U, DePaoli P. Serum levels of RANTES and MIP-1a in HIV-positive long-term survivors and progressor patients. *AIDS* 1996;10:1431–1432.

513. Clerici M, Balotta C, Trabattoni D, et al. Chemokine production in HIV-seropositive long-term asymptomatic individuals. *AIDS* 1996;10:1432–1433.

514. Chen Y, Gupta P. CD8+ T-cell–mediated suppression of HIV-1 infection may not be due to chemokines RANTES, MIP-1α, and MIP-1β. *AIDS* 1996;10:1434–1435.

515. Blazevic V, Heino M, Ranki A, Jussila T, Krohn K. RANTES, MIP, and interleukin-16 in HIV infection. *AIDS* 1996;10:1435–1436.

516. Vicenzi E, Bagnarelli P, Santagostino E, et al. Hemophilia and nonprogressing human immunodeficiency virus type 1 infection. *Blood* 1997;89:191–200.

517. Scala E, D'Offizi G, Rosso R, et al. C-C chemokines, IL-16, and soluble antiviral factor activity are increased in cloned T cells from subjects with long-term nonprogressive HIV infection. *J Immunol* 1997;158:4485–4492.

518. Rubbert A, Weissman D, Combadiere C, et al. Multifactorial nature of noncytolytic CD8+ T cell–mediated suppression of HIV replication: beta-chemokine–dependent and –independent effects. *AIDS Res Hum Retrovir* 1997;13:63–69.

519. Knight SC, Macatonia SE. Dendritic cells and viruses. *Immunol Lett* 1988;19: 177–181.

520. Macatonia SE, Lau R, Patterson S, Pinching AJ, Knight SC. Dendritic cell infection, depletion and dysfunction in HIV-infected individuals. *Immunology* 1990; 71:38–45.

521. Knight SC, Macatonia SE, Patterson S. HIV-1 infection of dendritic cells. *Int Rev Immunol* 1990;6:163–175.

522. Patterson S, Knight SC. Susceptibility of human peripheral blood dendritic cells to infection by human immunodeficiency virus. *J Gen Virol* 1987;68:1177–1181.

523. Langhoff E, Terwilliger EF, Bos HJ, et al. Replication of human immunodeficiency virus type 1 in primary dendritic cell cultures. *Proc Natl Acad Sci U S A* 1991;88:7998–8002.

524. Langhoff E, Haseltine WA. Infection of accessory dendritic cells by human immunodeficiency virus type 1. *J Invest Dermatol* 1992;99:89S–94S.

525. Chehimi J, Prakash K, Shanmugam V, Jackson SJ, Bandyopadhyay S, Starr SE. In-vitro infection of peripheral blood dendritic cells with human immunodeficiency virus-1 causes impairment of accessory functions. *Adv Exp Med Biol* 1993;329:521–526.

526. Chehimi J, Prakash K, Shanmugam V, et al. CD4-independent infection of human peripheral blood dendritic cells with isolates of human immunodeficiency virus type 1. *J Gen Virol* 1993;74:1277–1285.

527. Knight SC. Infection of dendritic cells with HIV type 1. *AIDS Res Hum Retrovir* 1994;10:1591–1592.

528. Cameron PU, Freudenthal PS, Barker JM, Gezelter S, Inaba K, Steinman RM. Dendritic cells exposed to human immunodeficiency virus type-1 transmit a vigorous cytopathic infection to CD4+ T cells. *Science* 1992;257:383–387.

529. Pinchuk LM, Polacino PS, Agy MB, Klaus SJ, Clark EA. The Role Of CD40 and CD80 accessory cell molecules in dendritic cell–dependent HIV-1 infection. *Immunity* 1994;1:317–325.

530. O'Doherty U, Steinman RM, Peng M, et al. Dendritic cells freshly isolated from human blood express CD4 and mature into typical immunostimulatory dendritic cells after culture in monocyte-conditioned medium. *J Exp Med* 1993;178: 1067–1076.

531. Thomas R, Lipsky PE. Human peripheral blood dendritic cell subsets—isolation and characterization of precursor and mature antigen-presenting cells. *J Immunol* 1994;153:4016–4028.

532. Karhumaki E, Viljanen ME, Cottler-Fox M, Ranki A, Fox CH, Krohn KJ. An improved enrichment method for functionally competent, highly purified peripheral blood dendritic cells and its application to HIV-infected blood samples. *Clin Exp Immunol* 1993;91:482–488.

533. Hsia K, Tsai V, Zvaifler NJ, Spector SA. Low prevalence of HIV-1 proviral DNA in peripheral blood monocytes and dendritic cells from HIV-1–infected individuals. *AIDS* 1995;9:398–399.

534. Dezutter-Dambuyant C, Schmitt D. Epidermal Langerhans cells and HIV-1 infection. *Immunol Lett* 1993;39:33–37.

535. Dezutter-Dambuyant C, Charbonnier AS, Schmitt D. In vivo and in vitro HIV-1 infection of epithelial dendritic cells. *Pathol Biol* 1995;43:882–888.

536. Zambruno G, Giannetti A, Bertazzoni U, Girolomoni G. Langerhans cells and HIV infection. *Immunol Today* 1995;16:520–524.

537. Charbonnier AS, Mallet F, Fiers MM, Desgranges C, Dezutterdambuyant C, Schmitt D. Detection of HIV-specific DNA sequences in epidermal Langerhans cells infected in vitro by means of a cell-free system. *Arch Dermatol Res* 1994; 287:36–41.

538. Schmitt D, Dezutterdambuyant C. Epidermal and mucosal dendritic cells and HIV1 infection. *Pathol Res Pract* 1994;190:955–959.

539. Giannetti A, Zambruno G, Cimarelli A, et al. Direct detection of HIV-1 RNA in epidermal Langerhans cells of HIV-infected patients. *J AIDS* 1993;6:329–333.

540. Muller H, Weier S, Kojouharoff G, et al. Distribution and infection of Langerhans cells in the skin of HIV-infected healthy subjects and AIDS patients. *Res Virol* 1993;144:59–67.

541. Sala M, Zambruno G, Vartanian J-P, et al. Discontinuous distribution of HIV-1 quasispecies in epidermal Langerhans cells of an AIDS patient and evidence for double infection. In: Banchereau J, Schmitt D, eds. *Dendritic cells in fundamental and clinical immunology*. Vol. 2. New York: Plenum Publishing, 1995.

542. Blauvelt A, Katz SI. The skin as target, vector, and effector organ in human immunodeficiency virus disease. *J Invest Dermatol* 1995;105:122S–126S.

543. McIlroy D, Autran B, Cheynier R, et al. Infection frequency of dendritic cells and CD4(+) T lymphocytes in spleens of human immunodeficiency virus–positive patients. *J Virol* 1995;69:4737–4745.

544. Ayehunie S, Groves RW, Bruzzese AM, Ruprecht RM, Kupper TS, Langhoff E. Acutely infected Langerhans cells are more efficient than T cells in disseminating HIV type 1 to activated T cells following a short cell–cell contact. *AIDS Res Hum Retrovir* 1995;11:877–884.

545. Ramazzotti E, Marconi A, Re MC, et al. In vitro infection of human epidermal Langerhans' cells with HIV-1. *Immunology* 1995;85:94–98.

546. Soto-Ramirez LE, Renjifo B, McLane MF, et al. HIV-1 Langerhans' cell tropism associated with heterosexual transmission of HIV. *Science* 1996;271:1291–1293.

547. Bollinger RC, Tripathy SP, Quinn TC. The human immunodeficiency virus epidemic in India. Current magnitude and future projections. *Medicine (Baltimore)* 1995;74:97–106.

548. Cassol S, Weniger BG, Babu PG, et al. Detection of HIV type 1 env subtypes A, B, C, and E in Asia using dried blood spots: a new surveillance tool for molecular epidemiology. *AIDS Res Hum Retrovir* 1996;12:1435–1441.

549. Hu DJ, Dondero TJ, Rayfield MA, et al. The emerging genetic diversity of HIV. The importance of global surveillance for diagnostics, research, and prevention. *JAMA* 1996;275:210–216.

550. Janssens W, Heyndrickx L, Fransen K, et al. Genetic variability of HIV type 1 in Kenya. *AIDS Res Hum Retrovir* 1994;10:1577–1579.

551. Nkengasong JN, Janssens W, Heyndrickx L, et al. Genotypic subtypes of HIV-1 in Cameroon. *AIDS* 1994;8:1405–1412.

552. Quinn TC. Population migration and the spread of types 1 and 2 human immunodeficiency viruses. *Proc Natl Acad Sci U S A* 1994;91:2407–2414.

553. Quinn TC. The epidemiology of the acquired immunodeficiency syndrome in the 1990s. *Emerg Med Clin North Am* 1995;13:1–25.

554. Quinn TC. Global burden of the HIV pandemic. The epidemiology of the acquired immunodeficiency syndrome in the 1990s. *Lancet* 1996;348:99–106.

555. Schechter MT, Laga M. AIDS 1995. Epidemiology: overview. *AIDS* 1995; 9(suppl A):55–57.

556. Weniger BG, Takebe Y, Ou CY, Yamazaki S. The molecular epidemiology of HIV in Asia. *AIDS* 1994;8(suppl 2):13–28.

557. Ree HJ, Liau S, Yancovitz SR, Qureshi MN, Khan AA, Teplitz C. The number of

CD1a+ large low-density cells with dendritic cell features is increased in the peripheral blood of HIV+ patients. *Clin Immunol Immunopathol* 1994;70: 190–197.

558. Cameron PU, Forsum U, Teppler H, Granelli-Piperno A, Steinman RM. During HIV-1 infection most blood dendritic cells are not productively infected and can induce allogeneic CD4+ T cells clonal expansion. *Clin Exp Immunol* 1992;88: 226–236.

559. Roberts M, Gompels M, Pinching AJ, Knight SC. Dendritic cells from HIV-1 infected individuals show reduced capacity to stimulate autologous T-cell proliferation. *Immunol Lett* 1994;43:39–43.

560. Macatonia SE, Gompels M, Pinching AJ, Patterson S, Knight SC. Antigen-presentation by macrophages but not by dendritic cells in human immunodeficiency virus (HIV) infection. *Immunology* 1992;75:576–581.

561. Reddy M, Goetz R, Gorman J, Grieco M, Chess L, Lederman S. Human immunodeficiency virus type-1 infection of homosexual men is accompanied by a decrease in circulating B cells. *J AIDS* 1991;4:428–434.

562. Amadori A, Chieco-Bianchi L. B-cell activation and HIV-1 infection: deeds and misdeeds. *Immunol Today* 1990;11:374–379.

563. Kehrl JH, Rieckmann P, Kozlow E, Fauci AS. Lymphokine production by B cells from normal and HIV-infected individuals. *Ann N Y Acad Sci* 1992;651:220–227.

564. Rieckmann P, Poli G, Fox CH, Kehrl JH, Fauci AS. Recombinant gp120 specifically enhances tumor necrosis factor-alpha production and Ig secretion in B lymphocytes from HIV-infected individuals but not from seronegative donors. *J Immunol* 1991;147:2922–2927.

565. Rieckmann P, Poli G, Kehrl JH, Fauci AS. Activated B lymphocytes from human immunodeficiency virus–infected individuals induce virus expression in infected T cells and a promonocytic cell line, U1. *J Exp Med* 1991;173:1–5.

566. Macchia D, Almerigogna F, Parronchi P, Ravina A, Maggi E, Romagnani S. Membrane tumour necrosis factor-alpha is involved in the polyclonal B-cell activation induced by HIV-infected human T cells. *Nature* 1993;363:464–466.

567. Goodglick L, Zevit N, Neshat MS, Braun J. Mapping the Ig superantigen-binding site of HIV-1 gp120. *J Immunol* 1995;155:5151–5159.

568. Berberian L, Goodglick L, Kipps TJ, Braun J. Immunoglobulin VH3 gene products: natural ligands for HIV gp120. *Science* 1993;261:1588–1591.

569. Chirmule N, Kalyanaraman VS, Saxinger C, Wong-Staal F, Ghrayeb J, Pahwa S. Localization of B-cell stimulatory activity of HIV-1 to the carboxyl terminus of gp41. *AIDS Res Hum Retrovir* 1990;6:299–305.

570. Dolcetti R, Gloghini A, De Vita S, et al. Characteristics of EBV-infected cells in HIV-related lymphadenopathy: implications for the pathogenesis of EBV-associated and EBV-unrelated lymphomas of HIV-seropositive individuals. *Int J Cancer* 1995;63:652–659.

571. Monroe JG, Silberstein LE. HIV-mediated B-lymphocyte activation and lymphomagenesis. *J Clin Immunol* 1995;15:61–68.

572. Yao QY, Tierney RJ, Croom-Carter D, et al. Frequency of multiple Epstein-Barr virus infections in T-cell–immunocompromised individuals. *J Virol* 1996;70: 4884–4894.

573. Goetz DW, Webb EL Jr, Whisman BA, Freeman TM. Aeroallergen-specific IgE changes in individuals with rapid human immunodeficiency virus disease progression. *Ann Allergy Asthma Immunol* 1997;78:301–306.

574. Mazza DS, Grieco MH, Reddy MM, Meriney D. Serum IgE in patients with human immunodeficiency virus infection. *Ann Allergy Asthma Immunol* 1995; 74:411–414.

575. Vigano A, Balotta C, Trabattoni D, et al. Virologic and immunologic markers of disease progression in pediatric HIV infection. *AIDS Res Hum Retrovir* 1996;12: 1255–1262.

576. Rodriguez C, Thomas JK, O'Rourke S, Stiehm ER, Plaeger S. HIV disease in children is associated with a selective decrease in CD23+ and CD62L+ B cells. *Clin Immunol Immunopathol* 1996;81:191–199.

577. Elbim C, Prevot MH, Bouscarat F, et al. Impairment of polymorphonuclear neutrophil function in HIV-infected patients. *J Cardiovasc Pharmacol* 1995; 25(suppl 2):66–70.

578. Jarstrand C, Akerlund B. Oxygen radical release by neutrophils of HIV-infected patients. *Chem Biol Interact* 1994;91:141–146.

579. Meyer CN, Nielsen H. Priming of neutrophil and monocyte activation in human immunodeficiency virus infection. Comparison of granulocyte colony-stimulating factor, granulocyte-macrophage colony-stimulating factor and interferon-gamma. *APMIS* 1996;104:640–646.

580. Tachavanich K, Pattanapanyasat K, Sarasombath S, Suwannagool S, Suvattee V. Opsonophagocytosis and intracellular killing activity of neutrophils in patients with human immunodeficiency virus infection. *Asian Pac J Allergy Immunol* 1996;14:49–56.

581. Pitrak DL, Tsai HC, Mullane KM, Sutton SH, Stevens P. Accelerated neutrophil apoptosis in the acquired immunodeficiency syndrome. *J Clin Invest* 1996;98: 2714–2719.

582. Torosantucci A, Chiani P, Quinti I, Ausiello CM, Mezzaroma I, Cassone A. Responsiveness of human polymorphonuclear cells (PMNL) to stimulation by a mannoprotein fraction (MP-F2) of *Candida albicans*: enhanced production of IL-6 and tumour necrosis factor-alpha (TNF-alpha) by MP-F2–stimulated PMNL from HIV-infected subjects. *Clin Exp Immunol* 1997;107:451–457.

583. Wenisch C, Parschalk B, Zedwitz-Liebenstein K, Graninger W, Rieger A. Dysregulation of the polymorphonuclear leukocyte—*Candida* spp. interaction in HIV-positive patients. *AIDS* 1996;10:983–987.

584. Tascini C, Baldelli F, Monari C, et al. Inhibition of fungicidal activity of poly-

585. Cohen AJ, Steigbigel RT. Eosinophilia in patients infected with human immunodeficiency virus. *J Infect Dis* 1996;174:615–618.

586. Weller PF, Marshall WL, Lucey DR, Rand TH, Dvorak AM, Finberg RW. Infection, apoptosis, and killing of mature human eosinophils by human immunodeficiency virus-1. *Am J Respir Cell Mol Biol* 1995;13:610–620.

587. Schuitemaker H, Kootstra NA, Koppelman MHGM, et al. Proliferation-dependent HIV-1 infection of monocytes occurs during differentiation into macrophages. *J Clin Invest* 1992;89:1154–1160.

588. Weinberg JB, Matthews TJ, Cullen BR, Malim MH. Productive human immunodeficiency virus type1 (HIV-1) infection of nonproliferating human monocytes. *J Exp Med* 1991;174:1477–1482.

589. Valentin A, Gegerfelt AV, Matsuda S, Nilsson K, Asjo B. In vitro maturation of mononuclear phagocytes and susceptibility to HIV-1 infection. *J AIDS Syndr Hum Retrovir* 1991;4:751–759.

590. Collman R, Hassan NF, Walker R, et al. Infection of monocyte-derived macrophages with human immunodeficiency virus type 1 (HIV-1). *J Exp Med* 1989;170.

591. Koenig S, Gendelman HE, Orenstein JM, et al. Detection of AIDS virus in macrophages in brain tissue from AIDS patients with encephalopathy. *Science* 1986;233:1089–1093.

592. Armstrong J, Horne R. Follicular dendritic cells and virus-like particles in AIDS-related lymphadenopathy. *Lancet* 1984;2:370–372.

593. Lafrenie RM, Wahl LM, Epstein JS, Hewlett IK, Yamada KM, Dhawan S. HIV-1-Tat protein promotes chemotaxis and invasive behavior by monocytes. *J Immunol* 1996;157:974–977.

594. Baldwin GC, Fleischmann J, Chung Y, Koyanagi Y, Chen IS, Golde DW. Human immunodeficiency virus causes mononuclear phagocyte dysfunction. *Proc Natl Acad Sci U S A* 1990;87:3933–3937.

595. Bender BS, Augor FA, Quinn TC, Redfield R, Gold J, Folks TM. Impaired antibody-dependent cell-mediated cytotoxic activity in patients with the acquired immunodeficiency syndrome. *Clin Exp Immunol* 1986;64:166–172.

596. Muller F, Rollag H, Froland SS. Reduced oxidative burst responses in monocytes and monocyte-derived macrophages from HIV-infected individuals. *Clin Immunol Immunopathol* 1990;82:10–15.

597. Spear GT, Kessler HA, Rothberg L, Phair J, Landay AL. Decreased oxidative burst activity of monocytes from asymptomatic HIV-infected individuals. *Clin Immunol Immunopathol* 1990;54:184–191.

598. Poli G, Botazzi B, Acero R, et al. Monocyte function in intravenous drug abusers with lymphadenopathy syndrome and in patients with acquired immunodeficiency syndrome: selective impairment of chemotaxis. *Clin Exp Immunol* 1985; 62:136–142.

599. Gendelman HE, Freidman RM, Joe S, et al. A selective defect of IFN-α production in HIV-infected monocytes. *J Exp Med* 1990;172:1433–1442.

600. Hu PF, Hultin LE, Hultin P, et al. Natural killer cell immunodeficiency in HIV disease is manifest by profoundly decreased numbers of CD16+CD56+ cells and expansion of a population of CD16dimCD56- cells with low lytic activity. *J AIDS Hum Retrovir* 1995;10:331–340.

601. Lucia B, Jennings C, Cauda R, Ortona L, Landay AL. Evidence of a selective depletion of a CD16+ CD56+ CD8+ natural killer cell subset during HIV infection. *Cytometry* 1995;22:10–15.

602. Ahmad A, Menezes J. Defective killing activity against gp120/41-expressing human erythroleukaemic K562 cell line by monocytes and natural killer cells from HIV-infected individuals. *AIDS* 1996;10:143–149.

603. Ahmad A, Menezes J. Antibody-dependent cellular cytotoxicity in HIV infections. *FASEB J* 1996;10:258–266.

604. Ullum H, Gotzsche PC, Victor J, Dickmeiss E, Skinhoj P, Pedersen BK. Defective natural immunity: an early manifestation of human immunodeficiency virus infection. *J Exp Med* 1995;182:789–799.

605. Claydon EJ, Bennett J, Gor D, Forster SM. Transient elevation of serum HIV antigen levels associated with intercurrent infection. *AIDS* 1991;5:11311–11314.

606. Fultz PN, Gluckman JC, Muchmore E, Girard M. Transient increases in numbers of infectious cells in an HIV-infected chimpanzee following immune stimulation. *AIDS Res Hum Retrovir* 1992;8:313–317.

607. Goletti D, Weissman D, Jackson RW, et al. Effect of Mycobacterium tuberculosis on HIV replication. Role of immune activation. *J Immunol* 1996;157: 1271–1278.

608. Ho DD. HIV-1 viremia and influenza. *Lancet* 1992;339:1549.

609. Stanley S, Ostrowski MA, Justement JS, et al. Effect of immunization with a common recall antigen on viral expression in patients infected with human immunodeficiency virus type 1. *N Engl J Med* 1996;334:1222–1230.

610. O'Brien WA, Grovit-Ferbas K, Namazi A, et al. Human immunodeficiency virus-type 1 replication can be increased in peripheral blood of seropositive patients after influenza vaccination. *Blood* 1995;86:1082–1089.

611. Ostrowski MA, Stanley SK, Justement JS, Gantt K, Goletti D, Fauci AS. Increased in vitro tetanus-induced production of HIV type 1 following in vivo immunization of HIV type 1–infected individuals with tetanus toxoid. *AIDS Res Hum Retrovir* 1997;13:473–480.

612. Poli G, Fauci A. Role of cytokines in the pathogenesis of human immunodeficiency virus infection. In: Aggarwal B, Puri R, eds. *Human cytokines: their role in disease and therapy.* Cambridge, MA: Blackwell Science, 1995:421–449.

613. Cohen O, Kinter A, Fauci A. Host factors in the pathogenesis of HIV infection. *Immunol Rev* 1997;159:31–48.

614. Poli G, Kinter AL, Vicenzi E, Fauci AS. Cytokine regulation of acute and chronic HIV infection in vitro: from cell lines to primary mononuclear cells. *Res Immunol* 1994;145:578–582.

615. Clouse KA, Powell D, Washington I, et al. Monokine regulation of human immunodeficiency virus-1 expression in a chronically infected human T cell clone. *J Immunol* 1989;142:431–438.

616. Duh EJ, Maury WJ, Folks TM, Fauci AS, Rabson AB. Tumor necrosis factor alpha activates human immunodeficiency virus type 1 through induction of nuclear factor binding to the NF-kappa B sites in the long terminal repeat. *Proc Natl Acad Sci U S A* 1989;86:5974–5978.

617. Israel N, Hazan U, Alcami J, et al. Tumor necrosis factor stimulates transcription of HIV-1 in human T lymphocytes, independently and synergistically with mitogens. *J Immunol* 1989;143:3956–3960.

618. Vyakarnam A, McKeating J, Meager A, Beverley PC. Tumour necrosis factors (alpha, beta) induced by HIV-1 in peripheral blood mononuclear cells potentiate virus replication. *AIDS* 1990;4:21–27.

619. Kinter AL, Poli G, Fox L, Hardy E, Fauci AS. HIV replication in IL-2–stimulated peripheral blood mononuclear cells is driven in an autocrine/paracrine manner by endogenous cytokines. *J Immunol* 1995;154:2448–2459.

620. Biswas P, Smith CA, Goletti D, Hardy EC, Jackson RW, Fauci AS. Cross-linking of CD30 induces HIV expression in chronically infected T cells. *Immunity* 1995; 2:587–596.

621. Maggi E, Annunziato F, Manetti R, et al. Activation of HIV expression by CD30 triggering in CD4+ T cells from HIV-infected individuals. *Immunity* 1995;3: 251–255.

622. Poli G, Bressler P, Kinter A, et al. Interleukin 6 induces human immunodeficiency virus expression in infected monocytic cells alone and in synergy with tumor necrosis factor alpha by transcriptional and posttranscriptional mechanisms. *J Exp Med* 1990;172:151–158.

623. Poli G, Kinter AL, Vicenzi E, Fauci AS. Cytokine regulation of acute and chronic HIV infection in vitro: from cell lines to primary mononuclear cells. 60th Forum in Immunology. 1994:578–582.

624. Hazan U, Thomas D, Alcami J, et al. Stimulation of a human T-cell clone with anti-CD3 or tumor necrosis factor induces NF-kappa B translocation but not human immunodeficiency virus 1 enhancer–dependent transcription. *Proc Natl Acad Sci U S A* 1990;87:7861–7865.

625. Ramilo O, Bell KD, Uhr JW, Vitetta ES. Role of CD25+ and CD25- T cells in acute HIV infection in vitro. *J Immunol* 1993;150:5202–5208.

626. Weissman D, Daugher J, Barker T, Adelsberger J, Baseler M, Fauci AS. Cytokine regulation of HIV replication induced by dendritic cell–CD4-positive T cell interactions. *AIDS Res Hum Retrovir* 1996;12:759–767.

627. Lucey DR, Pinto LA, Bethke FR, et al. In vitro immunologic and virologic effects of interleukin 15 on peripheral blood mononuclear cells from normal donors and human immunodeficiency virus type 1–infected patients. *Clin Diagn Lab Immunol* 1997;4:43–48.

628. Bayard-McNeeley M, Doo H, He S, Hafner A, Johnson WD Jr, Ho JL. Differential effects of interleukin-12, interleukin-15, and interleukin-2 on human immunodeficiency virus type 1 replication in vitro. *Clin Diagn Lab Immunol* 1996;3:547–553.

629. Kacani L, Stoiber H, Dierich MP. Role of IL-15 in HIV-1–associated hypergammaglobulinaemia. *Clin Exp Immunol* 1997;108:14–18.

630. Mikovits JA, Meyers AM, Ortaldo JR, et al. IL-4 and IL-13 have overlapping but distinct effects on HIV production in monocytes. *J Leukoc Biol* 1994;56: 340–346.

631. Kazazi F, Mathijs JM, Chang J, et al. Recombinant interleukin 4 stimulates human immunodeficiency virus production by infected monocytes and macrophages. *J Gen Virol* 1992;73:941–949.

632. Novak RM, Holzer TJ, Kennedy MM, Heynen CA, Dawson G. The effect of interleukin 4 (BSF-1) on infection of peripheral blood monocyte–derived macrophages with HIV-1. *AIDS Res Hum Retrovir* 1990;6:973–976.

633. Akridge RE, Oyafuso LK, Reed SG. IL-10 is induced during HIV-1 infection and is capable of decreasing viral replication in human macrophages. *J Immunol* 1994;153:5782–5789.

634. Kollmann TR, Pettoello-Mantovani M, Katopodis NF, et al. Inhibition of acute in vivo human immunodeficiency virus infection by human interleukin 10 treatment of SCID mice implanted with human fetal thymus and liver. *Proc Natl Acad Sci U S A* 1996;93:3126–3131.

635. Kootstra NA, van't Wout A, Huisman HG, Miedema F, Schuitemaker H. Interference of interleukin 10 with human immunodeficiency virus type 1 replication in primary monocyte-derived macrophages. *J Virol* 1994;68:6967–6975.

636. Masood R, Lunardi-Iskandar Y, Moudgil T, et al. IL-10 inhibits HIV-1 replication and is induced by tat. *Biochem Biophys Res Commun* 1994;202:374–383.

637. Montaner LJ, Griffin P, Gordon S. Interleukin-10 inhibits initial reverse transcription of human immunodeficiency virus type 1 and mediates a virostatic latent state in primary blood-derived human macrophages in vitro. *J Gen Virol* 1994;75:3393–3400.

638. Saville MW, Taga K, Foli A, Broder S, Tosato G, Yarchoan R. Interleukin-10 suppresses human immunodeficiency virus-1 replication in vitro in cells of the monocyte/macrophage lineage. *Blood* 1994;83:3591–3599.

639. Weissman D, Poli G, Fauci AS. Interleukin 10 blocks HIV replication in macrophages by inhibiting the autocrine loop of tumor necrosis factor alpha and interleukin 6 induction of virus. *AIDS Res Hum Retrovir* 1994;10:1199–1206.

640. Weissman D, Poli G, Fauci AS. IL-10 synergizes with multiple cytokines in enhancing HIV production in cells of monocytic lineage. *J AIDS Hum Retrovir* 1995;9:442–449.

641. Finnegan A, Roebuck KA, Nakai BE, et al. IL-10 cooperates with TNF-alpha to activate HIV-1 from latently and acutely infected cells of monocyte/macrophage lineage. *J Immunol* 1996;156:841–851.

642. Angel JB, Saget BM, Wang MZ, Wang A, Dinarello CA, Skolnik PR. Interleukin-10 enhances human immunodeficiency virus type 1 expression in a chronically infected promonocytic cell line (U1) by a tumor necrosis factor alpha-independent mechanism. *J Interferon Cytokine Res* 1995;15:575–584.

643. Montaner LJ, Gordon S. Th2-mediated HIV1 virostatic state: macrophage-specific regulation in vitro. *Res Immunol* 1994;145:583–587.

644. Naif HM, Li S, Ho-Shon M, Mathijs JM, Williamson P, Cunningham AL. The state of maturation of monocytes into macrophages determines the effects of IL-4 and IL-13 on HIV replication. *J Immunol* 1997;158:501–511.

645. Poli G, Kinter AL, Justement JS, Bressler P, Kehrl JH, Fauci AS. Transforming growth factor beta suppresses human immunodeficiency virus expression and replication in infected cells of the monocyte/macrophage lineage. *J Exp Med* 1991;173:589–597.

646. Lazdins JK, Klimkait T, Alteri E, et al. TGF-beta: upregulator of HIV replication in macrophages. *Res Virol* 1991;142:239–242.

647. Goletti D, Kinter AL, Hardy EC, Poli G, Fauci AS. Modulation of endogenous IL-1 beta and IL-1 receptor antagonist results in opposing effects on HIV expression in chronically infected monocytic cells. *J Immunol* 1996;156:3501–3508.

648. Perno CF, Yarchoan R, Cooney DA, et al. Replication of human immunodeficiency virus in monocytes. Granulocyte/macrophage colony-stimulating factor (GM-CSF) potentiates viral production yet enhances the antiviral effect mediated by 3'-azido-2'3'-dideoxythymidine (AZT) and other dideoxynucleoside congeners of thymidine. *J Exp Med* 1989;169:933–951.

649. Koyanagi Y, O'Brien WA, Zhao JQ, Golde DW, Gasson JC, Chen IS. Cytokines alter production of HIV-1 from primary mononuclear phagocytes. *Science* 1988; 241:1673–1675.

650. Meltzer MS, Gendelman HE. Effects of colony stimulating factors on the interaction of monocytes and the human immunodeficiency virus. *Immunol Lett* 1988,19.193–198.

651. Gendelman HE, Orenstein JM, Martin MA, et al. Efficient isolation and propagation of human immunodeficiency virus on recombinant colony-stimulating factor 1–treated monocytes. *J Exp Med* 1988;167:1428–1441.

652. Gruber MF, Weih KA, Boone EJ, Smith PD, Clouse KA. Endogenous macrophage CSF production is associated with viral replication in HIV-1-infected human monocyte-derived macrophages. *J Immunol* 1995;154: 5528–5535.

653. Manfredi R, Mastroianni A, Coronado O, Chiodo F. Recombinant human granulocyte-macrophage colony-stimulating factor (rHuGM-CSF) in leukopenic patients with advanced HIV disease. *J Chemother* 1996,8.214–220.

654. Manfredi R, Cariani T, Latini F, Chiodo F. Recombinant granulocyte-macrophage colony-stimulating factor in the treatment of HIV-related leucopenia. *Acta Paediatr* 1995;84:943–944.

655. Zuccotti GV, Plebani A, Biasucci G, et al. Granulocyte-colony stimulating factor and erythropoietin therapy in children with human immunodeficiency virus infection. *J Int Med Res* 1996,24.113–121.

656. Shirazi Y, Pitha PM. Alpha interferon inhibits early stages of the human immunodeficiency virus type 1 replication cycle. *J Virol* 1992;66:1321–1328.

657. Poli G, Orenstein JM, Kinter A, Folks TM, Fauci AS. Interferon-alpha but not AZT suppresses HIV expression in chronically infected cell lines. *Science* 1989; 244:575–577.

658. Shirazi Y, Pitha PM. Interferon alpha–mediated inhibition of human immunodeficiency virus type 1 provirus synthesis in T-cells. *Virology* 1993;193:303–312.

659. Poli G, Biswas P, Fauci AS. Interferons in the pathogenesis and treatment of human immunodeficiency virus infection. *Antiviral Res* 1994;24:221–233.

660. Kovacs J, Bechtel C, Davey RJ, et al. Combination therapy with didanosine and interferon-alpha in human immunodeficiency virus–infected patients: results of a phase I/II trial. *J Infect Dis* 1996;173:840–848.

661. Schmidtmayerova H, Sherry B, Bukrinsky M. Chemokines and HIV replication. *Nature* 1996;382:767.

662. Merrill JE, Koyanagi Y, Chen ISY. Interleukin-1 and tumor necrosis factor-alpha can be induced from mononuclear phagocytes by human immunodeficiency virus type 1 binding to the CD4 receptor. *J Virol* 1989;63:4404–4408.

663. von Sydow M, Sonnerborg A, Gaines H, Strannegard O. Interferon-alpha and tumor necrosis factor-alpha in serum of patients in various stages of HIV-1 infection. *AIDS Res Hum Retrovir* 1991;7:375–380.

664. Rautonen J, Rautonen N, Martin NL, Philip R, Wara DW. Serum interleukin-6 concentrations are elevated and associated with elevated tumor necrosis factor-alpha and immunoglobulin G and A concentrations in children with HIV infection. *AIDS* 1991;5:1319–1325.

665. Graziosi C, Pantaleo G, Fauci AS. Comparative analysis of constitutive cytokine expression in peripheral blood and lymph nodes of HIV-infected individuals. *Res Immunol* 1994;145:602–605.

666. Israel-Biet D, Cadranel J, Beldjord K, Andrieu JM, Jeffrey A, Even P. Tumor necrosis factor production in HIV-seropositive subjects. Relationship with lung opportunistic infections and HIV expression in alveolar macrophages. *J Immunol* 1991;147:490–494.

667. Millar AB, Miller RF, Foley NM, Meager A, Semple SJ, Rook GA. Production of tumor necrosis factor-alpha by blood and lung mononuclear phagocytes from

patients with human immunodeficiency virus–related lung disease. *Am J Respir Cell Mol Biol* 1991;5:144–148.

668. Lane HC, Depper JM, Greene WC, Whalen G, Waldmann TA, Fauci AS. Qualitative analysis of immune function in patients with the acquired immunodeficiency syndrome. Evidence for a selective defect in soluble antigen recognition. *N Engl J Med* 1985;313:79–84.

669. Clerici M, Hakim FT, Venzon DJ, et al. Changes in interleukin-2 and interleukin-4 production in asymptomatic, human immunodeficiency virus–seropositive individuals. *J Clin Invest* 1993;91:759–765.

670. Clerici M, Sarin A, Coffman RL, et al. Type 1/type 2 cytokine modulation of T-cell programmed cell death as a model for human immunodeficiency virus pathogenesis. *Proc Natl Acad Sci U S A* 1994;91:11811–11815.

671. Clerici M, Shearer GM. The Th1-Th2 hypothesis of HIV infection: new insights. *Immunol Today* 1994;15:575–581.

672. Clerici M, Shearer G. A TH1-TH2 switch is a critical step in the etiology of HIV infection. *Immunol Today* 1993;14:107–111.

673. Maggi E, Mazzetti M, Ravina A, et al. Ability of HIV to promote a TH1 to TH0 shift and to replicate preferentially in TH2 and TH0 cells. *Science* 1994;265:244–248.

674. Meyaard L, Otto S, Keet I, vanLier R, Miedema F. Changes in cytokine secretion patterns of CD4+ T-cell clones in human immunodeficiency virus infection. *Blood* 1994;84:4262–4268.

675. Clerici M, Lucey D, Berzofsky J, et al. Restoration of HIV-specific cell–mediated immune responses by interleukin-12 in vitro. *Science* 1993;262:1721–1724.

676. Clerici M, Wynn T, Berzofsky J, et al. Role of interleukin-10 in T helper cell dysfunction in asymptomatic individuals infected with the human immunodeficiency virus. *J Clin Invest* 1994;93:768–775.

677. Vyakarnam A, Matear P, Martin S, Wagstaff M. Th1 cells specific for HIV-1 gag p24 are less efficient than Th0 cells in supporting HIV replication, and inhibit virus replication in Th0 cells. *Immunology* 1995;86:85–96.

678. Clerici M, Balotta C, Meroni L, et al. Type 1 cytokine production and low prevalence of viral isolation correlate with long-term non-progression in HIV infection. *AIDS Res Hum Retrovir* 1996;12:1053–1061.

679. Kovacs JA, Baseler M, Dewar RJ, et al. Increases in CD4 T lymphocytes with intermittent courses of interleukin-2 in patients with human immunodeficiency virus infection. A preliminary study. *N Engl J Med* 1995;332:567–575.

680. Kovacs JA, Vogel S, Albert JM, et al. Controlled trial of interleukin-2 infusions in patients infected with the human immunodeficiency virus. *N Engl J Med* 1996;335:1350–1356.

681. Kinter AL, Ostrowski M, Goletti D, et al. HIV replication in CD4+ T cells of HIV-infected individuals is regulated by a balance between the viral suppressive effects of endogenous beta-chemokines and the viral inductive effects of other endogenous cytokines. *Proc Natl Acad Sci U S A* 1996;93:14076–14081.

682. Watkins BA, Dorn HH, Kelly W, et al. Specific tropism of HIV-1 for microglial cells in primary human brain cultures. *Science* 1990;249:549–553.

683. Selmaj KW, Raine CS. Tumor necrosis factor mediates myelin and oligodendrocyte damage in vitro. *Ann Neurol* 1988;23:339–346.

684. Rutka JT, Giblin JRT, Berens ME, et al. The effects of human recombinant tumor necrosis factor on glioma-derived cell lines: cellular proliferation, cytotoxicity, morphological and radioreceptor studies. *Int J Cancer* 1988;41:573–582.

685. Mastroianni CM, Paoletti F, Valenti C, Vullo V, Jirillo E, Delia S. Tumour necrosis factor (TNF-α) and neurological disorder in HIV infection. *J Neurol Neurosurg Psychiatry* 1992;55:219–221.

686. Giulian D, Vaca K, Noonan CA. Secretion of neurotoxins by mononuclear phagocytes infected with HIV-1. *Science* 1990;250:1593–1596.

687. Meucci O, Miller RJ. gp120-induced neurotoxicity in hippocampal pyramidal neuron cultures: protective action of TGF-beta1. *J Neurosci* 1996;16:4080–4088.

688. da Cunha A, Jackson RW, Vitkovic L. HIV-1 non-specifically stimulates production of transforming growth factor-beta 1 transfer in primary astrocytes. *J Neuroimmunol* 1995;60:125–133.

689. Benveniste EN. Cytokine circuits in brain. Implications for AIDS dementia complex. *Res Publ Assoc Res Nerv Ment Dis* 1994;72:71–88.

690. Bernasconi S, Cinque P, Peri G, et al. Selective elevation of monocyte chemotactic protein-1 in the cerebrospinal fluid of AIDS patients with cytomegalovirus encephalitis. *J Infect Dis* 1996;174:1098–1101.

691. Pleskoff O, Treboute C, Brelot A, Heveker N, Seman M, Alizon M. Identification of a chemokine receptor encoded by human cytomegalovirus as a cofactor for HIV-1 entry. *Science* 1997;276:1874–1878.

692. Robinson WE, Montefiori DC, Mitchell WM. Antibody-dependent enhancement of human immunodeficiency virus type 1 infection. *Lancet* 1988;1:790–794.

693. Robinson WE, Kawamura T, Gorny MK, et al. Human monoclonal antibodies to the human immunodeficiency virus type 1 (HIV-1) transmembrane glycoprotein gp41 enhance HIV-1 infection in vitro. *Proc Natl Acad Sci USA* 1990;87:3185–3189.

694. Homsy J, Meyer M, Levy JA. Serum enhancement of human immunodeficiency virus (HIV) infection correlates with disease in HIV-infected individuals. *J Virol* 1990;64:1437–1440.

695. Wong MT, Warren RQ, Anderson SA, et al. Longitudinal analysis of the humoral immune response to human immunodeficiency virus type 1 (HIV-1) gp160 epitopes in rapidly progressing and nonprogressing HIV-1–uninfected subjects. *J Infect Dis* 1993;168:1523–1527.

696. Autran B, Mayaud CM, Raphael M, et al. Evidence for a cytotoxic T-lymphocyte

697. Guillon JM, Autran B, Denis M, et al. Human immunodeficiency virus–related lymphocytic alveolitis. *Chest* 1988;94:1264–1270.

698. Zinkernagel RM, Hengartner H. T-cell–mediated immunopathology versus direct cytolysis by virus: implications for HIV and AIDS. *Immunol Today* 1994;15:262–268.

699. Sei Y, Tsang PH, Roboz JP, Sarin PS, Wallace JI, Bekesi JG. Neutralizing antibodies as a prognostic indicator in the progression of acquired immune deficiency syndrome (AIDS)-related disorders: a double-blind study. *J Clin Immunol* 1988;8:464–472.

700. Sei Y, Tsang PH, Chu FN, et al. Inverse relationship between HIV-1 p24 antigenemia, anti-p24 antibody and neutralizing antibody response in all stages of HIV-1 infection. *Immunol Lett* 1989;20:223–230.

701. Lathey JL, Pratt RD, Spector SA. Appearance of autologous neutralizing antibody correlates with reduction in virus load and phenotype switch during primary infection with human immunodeficiency virus type I. *J Infect Dis* 1997;175:231–232.

702. Allain JP, Laurian Y, Paul DA, Senn D. Serological markers in early stages of human immunodeficiency virus infection in haemophiliacs. *Lancet* 1986;2:1233–1236.

703. Paul DA, Falk LA, Kessler HA, et al. Correlation of serum HIV antigen and antibody with clinical status in HIV-infected patients. *J Med Virol* 1987;22:357–363.

704. Hogervorst E, Jurriaans S, deWolf F, et al. Predictors for non- and slow progression in human immunodeficiency virus (HIV) type 1 infection: low viral RNA copy numbers in serum and maintenance of high HIV-1 p24-specific but not V3-specific antibody levels. *J Infect Dis* 1995;171:811–821.

705. Weber JN, Clapham PR, Weiss RA, et al. Human immunodeficiency virus infection in two cohorts of homosexual men: neutralizing sera and association of anti-gag antibody with prognosis. *Lancet* 1987;1:119–122.

706. Weiss RA, Clapham PR, Cheingsong-Popov R, et al. Neutralization of human T-lymphotropic virus type III by sera of AIDS and AIDS-risk patients. *Nature* 1985;316:69–72.

707. Robert-Guroff M, Brown M, Gallo RC. HTLV-III–neutralizing antibodies in patients with AIDS and AIDS-related complex. *Nature* 1985;316:72–74.

708. Alesi DR, Ajello F, Lupo G, et al. Neutralizing antibody and clinical status of human immunodeficiency virus (HIV)–infected individuals. *J Med Virol* 1989;27:7–12.

709. Fenyo EM, Putkonen P. Broad cross-neutralizing activity in serum is associated with slow progression and low risk of transmission in primate lentivirus infections. *Immunol Lett* 1996;51:95–99.

710. Matthews TJ, Langlois AJ, Robey WG, et al. Restricted neutralization of divergent human T-lymphotropic virus type III isolates by antibodies to the major envelope glycoprotein. *Proc Natl Acad Sci U S A* 1986;83:9709–9713.

711. Putney SD, Matthews TJ, Robey WG, et al. HTLV-III/LAV–neutralizing antibodies to an *E. coli*–produced fragment of the virus envelope. *Science* 1986;234:1392–1395.

712. Palker TJ, Clark ME, Langlois AJ, et al. Type-specific neutralization of the human immunodeficiency virus with antibodies to env-encoded synthetic peptides. *Proc Natl Acad Sci U S A* 1988;85:1932–1936.

713. Rusche JR, Javaherian K, McDanal C, et al. Antibodies that inhibit fusion of human immunodeficiency virus–infected cells bind a 24–amino acid sequence of the viral envelope, gp120. *Proc Natl Acad Sci U S A* 1988;85:3198–3202.

714. Goudsmit J, Debouck C, Meloen RH, et al. Human immunodeficiency virus type 1 neutralization epitope with conserved architecture elicits early type-specific antibodies in experimentally infected chimpanzees. *Proc Natl Acad Sci U S A* 1988;85:4478–4482.

715. Javaherian K, Langlois AJ, McDanal C, et al. Principal neutralizing domain of the human immunodeficiency virus type 1 envelope protein. *Proc Natl Acad Sci U S A* 1989;86:6768–6772.

716. Kido H, Fukutomi A, Katunuma N. A novel membrane-bound serine esterase in human T4+ lymphocytes immunologically reactive with antibody inhibiting syncytia induced by HIV-1. Purification and characterization. *J Biol Chem* 1990;265:21979–21985.

717. Clements GJ, Price-Jones MJ, Stephens PE, et al. The V3 loops of the HIV-1 and HIV-2 surface glycoproteins contain proteolytic cleavage sites: a possible function in viral fusion? *AIDS Res Hum Retrovir* 1991;7:3–16.

718. Freed EO, Myers DJ, Risser R. Identification of the principal neutralizing determinant of human immunodeficiency virus type 1 as a fusion domain. *J Virol* 1991;65:190–194.

719. Niwa Y, Yano M, Futaki S, Okumura Y, Kido H. T-cell membrane–associated serine protease, tryptase TL2, binds human immunodeficiency virus type 1 gp120 and cleaves the third-variable-domain loop of gp120. Neutralizing antibodies of human immunodeficiency virus type 1 inhibit cleavage of gp120. *Eur J Biochem* 1996;237:64–70.

720. Muster T, Steindl F, Purtscher M, et al. A conserved neutralizing epitipe on gp41 of human immunodeficiency virus type 1. *J Virol* 1993;67:6642–6647.

721. Conley AJ, Kessler JA, Boots LJ, et al. Neutralization of divergent human immunodeficiency virus type 1 variants and primary isolates by IAM-41-2F5, an anti-gp41 human monoclonal antibody. *Proc Natl Acad Sci U S A* 1994;91:3348–3352.

722. Reitz MS, Wilson C, Naugle C, Gallo RC, Robert-Guroff M. Generation of a

neutralization-resistant variant of HIV-1 is due to selection for a point mutation in the envelope gene. *Cell* 1988;54:57–63.

723. Back NK, Thiriart C, Delers A, Ramautarsing C, Bruck C, Goudsmit J. Association of antibodies blocking HIV1 gp160-sCD4 attachment with virus neutralizing activity in human sera. *J Med Virol* 1990;31:200–208.

724. Steimer KS, Scandella C, Skiles PV, Haigwood NL. Neutralization of divergent HIV-1 isolates by conformation-dependent human antibodies to Gp120. *Science* 1991;254:105–108.

725. Ho DD, Fung MS, Cao YZ, et al. Another discontinuous epitope on glycoprotein gp120 that is important in human immunodeficiency virus type 1 neutralization is identified by a monoclonal antibody. *Proc Natl Acad Sci U S A* 1991;88:8949–8952.

726. Thali M, Olshevsky U, Furman C, Gabuzda D, Posner M, Sodroski J. Characterization of a discontinuous human immunodeficiency virus type 1 gp120 epitope recognized by a broadly reactive neutralizing human monoclonal antibody. *J Virol* 1991;65:6188–6193.

727. Hansen JE, Clausen H, Nielsen C, et al. Inhibition of human immunodeficiency virus (HIV) infection in vitro by anticarbohydrate monoclonal antibodies: peripheral glycosylation of HIV envelope glycoprotein gp120 may be a target for virus neutralization. *J Virol* 1990;64:2833–2340.

728. Mascola JR, Snyder SW, Weislow OS, et al. Immunization with envelope subunit vaccine products elicits neutralizing antibodies against laboratory-adapted but not primary isolates of human immunodeficiency virus type 1. The National Institute of Allergy and Infectious Diseases AIDS Vaccine Evaluation Group. *J Infect Dis* 1996;173:340–348.

729. Arendrup M, Akerblom L, Heegaard PM, Nielsen JO, Hansen JE. The HIV-1 V3 domain on field isolates: participation in generation of escape virus in vivo and accessibility to neutralizing antibodies. *Arch Virol* 1995;140:655–670.

730. Sullivan N, Sun Y, Li J, Hofmann W, Sodroski J. Replicative function and neutralization sensitivity of envelope glycoproteins from primary and T-cell line–passaged human immunodeficiency virus type 1 isolates. *J Virol* 1995;69:4413–4422.

731. Bou-Habib DC, Roderiquez G, Oravecz T, Berman PW, Lusso P, Norcross MA. Cryptic nature of envelope V3 region epitopes protects primary monocytotropic human immunodeficiency virus type 1 from antibody neutralization. *J Virol* 1994;68:6006–6013.

732. Albert J, Abrahamsson B, Nagy K, et al. Rapid development of isolate-specific neutralizing antibodies after primary HIV-1 infection and consequent emergence of virus variants which resist neutralization by autologous sera. *AIDS* 1990;4:107–112.

733. VonGegerfelt A, Albert J, Morfeldt-Manson L, Broliden K, Fenyo EM. Isolate-specific neutralizing antibodies in patients with progressive HIV-1–related disease. *Virology* 1991;185:162–168.

734. Lu W, Shih JW, Tourani JM, Eme D, Alter HJ, Andrieu JM. Lack of isolate-specific neutralizing activity is correlated with an increased viral burden in rapidly progressing HIV-1–infected patients. *AIDS* 1993;7(suppl 2):91–99

735. Arendrup M, Nielsen C, Hansen J-ES, Pedersen C, Mathiesen L, Nielsen JO. Autologous HIV-1 neutralizing antibodies: emergence of neutralization-resistant escape virus and subsequent development of escape virus neutralizing antibodies. *AIDS* 1992;5:303–307.

736. Tremblay M, Wainberg MA. Neutralization of multiple HIV-1 isolates from a single subject by autologous sequential sera. *J Infect Dis* 1990;162:735–737.

737. Tsang ML, Evans LA, McQueen P, et al. Neutralizing antibodies against sequential autologous human immunodeficiency virus type 1 isolates after seroconversion. *J Infect Dis* 1994;170:1141–1147.

738. Wrin T, Crawford L, Sawyer L, Weber P, Sheppard HW, Hanson CV. Neutralizing antibody responses to autologous and heterologous isolates of human immunodeficiency virus. *J AIDS* 1994;7:211–219.

739. Cao Y, Qin L, Zhang L, Safrit J, Ho DD. Virologic and immunologic characterization of long-term survivors of human immunodeficiency virus type 1 infection. *N Engl J Med* 1995;332:201–208.

740. Scarlatti G, Leitner T, Hodara V, et al. Interplay of HIV-1 phenotype and neutralizing antibody response in pathogenesis of AIDS. *Immunol Lett* 1996;51:23–28.

741. Lyerly HK, Matthews TJ, Langlois AJ, Bolognesi DP, Weinhold KJ. Human T-cell lymphotropic virus IIIB glycoprotein (gp120) bound to CD4 determinants on normal lymphocytes and expressed by infected cells serves as target for immune attack. *Proc Natl Acad Sci U S A* 1987;84:4601–4605.

742. Ojo-Amaize EA, Nishanian P, Keith DE, et al. Antibodies to human immunodeficiency virus in human sera induce cell-mediated lysis of human immunodeficiency virus–infected cells. *J Immunol* 1987;139:2458–2463.

743. Weinhold KJ, Lyerly HK, Matthews TJ, et al. Cellular anti-GP120 cytolytic reactivites in HIV-1 seropositive individuals. *Lancet* 1988;1:902–905

744. Tyler DS, Nastala CL, Stanley SD, et al. GP120 specific cellular cytotoxicity in HIV-1 seropositive individuals. Evidence for circulating CD16+ effector cells armed in vivo and cytophilic antibody. *J Immunol* 1989;142:1177–1182.

745. Tyler DS, Stanley SD, Zolla-Pazner S, et al. Identification of sites within gp41 that serve as targets for antibody-dependent cellular cytotoxicity by using human monoclonal antibodies. *J Immunol* 1990;145:3276–3282.

746. Koup RA, Sullivan JL, Levine PH, et al. Antigenic specificity of antibody dependent cell-mediated cytotoxicity directed against human immunodeficiency virus in antibody-positive sera. *J Virol* 1989;63:584–590.

747. Tanneau F, McChesney M, Lopez O, Sansonetti P, Montagnier L, Riviere Y. Primary cytotoxicity against the envelope glycoprotein of human immunodeficiency virus-1: evidence for antibody-dependent cellular cytotoxicity in vivo. *J Infect Dis* 1990;162:837–843.

748. Murayama T, Cai Q, Rinaldo CR. Antibody-dependent cellular cytotoxicity mediated by CD16+ lymphocytes from HIV-seropositive homosexual men. *Clin Immunol Immunopathol* 1990;55:297–304.

749. Jewett A, Giorgi JV, Bonavida B. Antibody-dependent cellular cytoxicity against HIV-coated target cells by peripheral blood monocytes from HIV seropositive asymptomatic patients. *J Immunol* 1990;145:4065–4071.

750. Tyler DS, Stanley SD, Nastala CA, et al. Alterations in antibody-dependent cellular cytotoxicity during the course of HIV-1 infection. Humoral and cellular defects. *J Immunol* 1990;144:3375–3384.

751. Ljunggren K, Karlson A, Fenyo EM, Jondal J. Natural and antibody-dependent cytotoxicity in different clinical stage of human immunodeficiency virus type 1 infection. *Clin Exp Immunol* 1989;75:184–189.

752. Ojo-Amaize E, Nishanian PG, Heitjan DF, et al. Serum and effector-cell antibody-dependent cellular cytotoxicity (ADCC) activity remains high during human immunodeficiency virus (HIV) disease progression. *J Clin Immunol* 1989;9:454–461.

753. Koup RA, Sullivan JL, Levine PH, et al. Detection of major histocompatibility complex I–restricted, HIV-specific cytotoxic T lymphocytes in the blood of infected hemophiliacs. *Blood* 1989;73:1909–1914.

754. Riviere Y, Tanneau-Salvadori F, Regnault A, et al. Human immunodeficiency virus–specific cytotoxic responses of seropositive individuals: distinct types of effector cells mediate killing of targets expressing gag and env proteins. *J Virol* 1989;63:2270–2277.

755. Nixon DF, Townsend AR, Elvin JG, Rizza CR, Gallwey J, McMichael AJ. HIV-1 gag-specific cytotoxic T lymphocytes defined with recombinant vaccinia virus and synthetic peptides. *Nature* 1988;336:484–487.

756. Gotch FM, Nixon DF, Alp N, McMichael AJ, Borysiewicz LK. High frequency of memory and effector gag specific cytotoxic T lymphocytes in HIV seropositive individuals. *Int Immunol* 1990;2:707–712.

757. Walker BD, Flexner C, Paradis TJ, et al. HIV-1 reverse transcriptase is a target for cytotoxic T lymphocytes in infected individuals. *Science* 1988;240:64–66.

758. Hosmalin A, Clerici M, Houghten R, et al. An epitope in human immunodeficiency virus 1 reverse transcriptase recognized by both mouse and human cytotoxic T lymphocytes. *Proc Natl Acad Sci U S A* 1990;87:2344–2348.

759. Lieberman J, Fabry JA, Kuo MC, Earl P, Moss B, Skolnik PR. Cytotoxic T lymphocytes from HIV-1 seropositive individuals recognize immunodominant epitopes in Gp160 and reverse transcriptase. *J Immunol* 1992;148:2738–2747.

760. Koenig S, Earl P, Powell D, et al. Group-specific, major histocompatibility complex class I–restricted cytotoxic responses to human immunodeficiency virus 1 (HIV-1) envelope proteins by cloned peripheral blood T cells from an HIV-1–infected individual. *Proc Natl Acad Sci U S A* 1988;85:8638–8642.

761. Hammond SA, Obah E, Stanhope P, et al. Characterization of a conserved T cell epitope in HIV-1 gp41 recognized by vaccine-induced human cytolytic T cells. *J Immunol* 1991;146:1470–1477.

762. Clerici M, Lucey DR, Zajac RA, et al. Detection of cytotoxic T lymphocytes specific for synthetic peptides of gp160 in HIV-seropositive individuals. *J Immunol* 1991;146:2214–2219.

763. Koenig S, Fuerst TR, Wood LV, et al. Mapping the fine specificity of a cytolytic T cell response to HIV-1 nef protein. *J Immunol* 1990;145:127–135.

764. Hoffenbach A, Langlade Demoyen P, Dadaglio G, et al. Unusually high frequencies of HIV-specific cytotoxic T lymphocytes in humans. *J Immunol* 1989;142:452–462.

765. Moss PA, Rowland-Jones SL, Frodsham PM, et al. Persistent high frequency of human immunodeficiency virus–specific cytotoxic T cells in peripheral blood of infected donors. *Proc Natl Acad Sci U S A* 1995;92:5773–5777.

766. Harrer T, Harrer E, Kalams SA, et al. Cytotoxic T lymphocytes in asymptomatic long-term nonprogressing HIV-1 infection. Breadth and specificity of the response and relation to in vivo viral quasispecies in a person with prolonged infection and low viral load. *J Immunol* 1996;156:2616–2623.

767. Harrer T, Harrer E, Kalams SA, et al. Strong cytotoxic T cell and weak neutralizing antibody responses in a subset of persons with stable nonprogressing HIV type 1 infection. *AIDS Res Hum Retrovir* 1996;12:585–592.

768. Rinaldo C, Huang X-L, Fan Z, et al. High levels of anti–human immunodeficiency virus type 1 (HIV-1) memory cytotoxic T-lymphocyte activity and low viral load are associated with lack of disease in HIV-1–infected long-term nonprogressors. *J Virol* 1995;69:5838–5842.

769. Klein MR, vanBaalen CA, Holwerda AM, et al. Kinetics of gag-specific cytotoxic T lymphocyte responses during the clinical course of HIV-1 infection: a longitudinal analysis of rapid progressors and long-term asymptomatics. *J Exp Med* 1995;181:1365–1372.

770. Rowland-Jones S, Sutton J, Ariyoshi K, et al. HIV-specific cytotoxic T-cells in HIV-exposed but uninfected Gambian women. *Nat Med* 1995;1:59–64.

771. Tenner-Racz K, Racz P, Thome C, et al. Cytotoxic effector cell granules recognized by the monoclonal antibody TIA-1 are present in CD8+ lymphocytes in lymph nodes of human immunodeficiency virus-1–infected patients. *Am J Pathol* 1993;142:1750–1758.

772. Riviere Y, McChesney MB, Porrot F, et al. Gag-specific cytotoxic responses to HIV type 1 are associated with a decreased risk of progression to AIDS-related complex or AIDS. *AIDS Res Hum Retrovir* 1995;11:903–907.

773. Goulder PJ, Bunce M, Krausa P, et al. Novel, cross-restricted, conserved, and

immunodominant cytotoxic T lymphocyte epitopes in slow progressors in HIV type 1 infection. *AIDS Res Hum Retrovir* 1996;12:1691–1698.

774. Klein MR, Keet IPM, D'Amaro J, et al. Associations between HLA frequencies and pathogenic features of human immunodeficiency virus type 1 infection in seroconverters from the Amsterdam Cohort of Homosexual Men. *J Infect Dis* 1994;169:1244–1249.

775. Keet IP, Klein MR, Just JJ, Kaslow RA. The role of host genetics in the natural history of HIV-1 infection: the needles in the haystack. *AIDS* 1996;10(suppl A): 59–67.

776. Kaslow RA, Carrington M, Apple R, et al. Influence of combinations of human major histocompatibility complex genes on the course of HIV-1 infection. *Nat Med* 1996;2:405–411.

777. Pantaleo G, DeMaria A, Koenig S, et al. CD8+ T lymphocytes of patients with AIDS maintain normal broad cytolytic function despite the loss of human immunodeficiency virus–specific cytotoxicity. *Proc Natl Acad Sci U S A* 1990; 87:4818–4822.

778. Pantaleo G, Koenig S, Baseler M, Lane HC, Fauci AS. Defective clonogenic potential of CD8+ T lymphocytes in patients with AIDS. *J Immunol* 1990;144: 1696–1704.

779. Phillips RE, Rowland-Jones S, Nixon DF, et al. Human immunodeficiency virus genetic variation that can escape cytotoxic T cell recognition. *Nature* 1991;354: 433–434.

780. Koenig S, Conley AJ, Brewah YA, et al. Transfer of HIV-1–specific cytotoxic T lymphocytes to an AIDS patient leads to selection for mutant HIV variants and subsequent disease progression. *Nat Med* 1995;1:330–336.

781. Borrow P, Lewicki H, Wei X, et al. Antiviral pressure exerted by HIV-1–specific cytotoxic T lymphocytes (CTLs) during primary infection demonstrated by rapid selection of CTL escape virus. *Nat Med* 1997;3:205–211.

782. Goulder PJR, Phillips RE, Colbert RA, et al. Late escape from an immunodominant cytotoxic T-lymphocyte response associated with progression to AIDS. *Nat Med* 1997;3:212–217.

783. Klenerman P, Rowland-Jones S, McAdam S, et al. Cytotoxic T-cell activity antagonized by naturally occurring HIV-1 Gag variants. *Nature* 1994;369:403–407.

784. Meier U-C, Klenerman P, Griffin P, et al. Cytotoxic T lymphocyte lysis inhibited by viable HIV mutants. *Science* 1995;270:1360–1362.

785. Itescu S, Rose S, Dwyer E, Winchester R. Certain HLA-DR5 and-DR6 major histocompatibility complex class II alleles are associated with a CD8 lymphocytic host response to human immunodeficiency virus type 1 characterized by low viral strain heterogeneity and slow disease progression. *Proc Natl Acad Sci U S A* 1994;91:11472–11476.

786. Kalams SA, Johnson RP, Trocha AK, et al. Longitudinal analysis of T cell receptor (TCR) gene usage by human immunodeficiency virus 1 envelope-specific cytotoxic T lymphocyte clone reveals a limited TCR repertoire. *J Exp Med* 1994; 179:1261–1271.

787. Kalams SA, Johnson RP, Dynan MJ, et al. T cell receptor usage and fine specificity of human immunodeficiency virus 1–specific cytotoxic T lymphocyte clones: analysis of quasispecies recognition reveals a dominant response directed against a minor in vivo variant. *J Exp Med* 1996;183:1669–1679.

788. Wilson CC, Kalams SA, Wilkes BM, et al. Overlapping epitopes in human immunodeficiency virus type 1 gp120 presented by HLA A, B, and C molecules: effects of viral variation on cytotoxic T-lymphocyte recognition. *J Virol* 1997;71: 1256–1264.

789. Haas G, Plikat U, Debre P, et al. Dynamics of viral variants in HIV-1 Nef and specific cytotoxic T lymphocytes in vivo. *J Immunol* 1996;157:4212–4221.

790. Moskophidis D, Lechner F, Pircher H, Zinkernagel RM. Virus persistence in acutely infected immunocompetent mice by exhaustion of antiviral cytotoxic effector T cells. *Nature* 1993;362:758–761.

791. Walker CM, Moody DJ, Stites DP, Levy JA. CD8+ lymphocytes can control HIV infection in vitro by suppressing virus replication. *Science* 1986;234:1563–1566.

792. Walker CM, Levy JA. A diffusible lymphokine produced by CD8+ T lymphocytes suppresses HIV replication. *Immunology* 1989;66:628–630.

793. Walker CM, Erickson AL, Hsueh FC, Levy JA. Inhibition of human immunodeficiency virus replication in acutely infected CD4+ cells by CD8+ cells involves a noncytotoxic mechanism. *J Virol* 1991;65:5921–5927.

794. Chen CH, Weinhold KJ, Bartlett JA, Bolognesi DP, Greenberg ML. CD8+ T lymphocyte-mediated inhibition of HIV-1 long terminal repeat transcription: a novel antiviral mechanism. *AIDS Res Hum Retrovir* 1993;9:1079–1086.

795. Copeland KF, McKay PJ, Rosenthal KL. Suppression of activation of the human immunodeficiency virus long terminal repeat by CD8+ T cells is not lentivirus specific. *AIDS Res Hum Retrovir* 1995;11:1321–1326.

796. Mackewicz C, Balckbourn DJ, Levy JA. CD8+ T cells suppress human immunodeficiency virus replicaton by inhibiting viral transcription. *Proc Natl Acad Sci U S A* 1995;92:2308–2312.

797. Mackewicz CE, Oretega H, Levy JA. Effect of cytokines on HIV replication in CD4+ lymphocytes: lack of identity with the CD8+ cell antiviral factor. *Cell Immunol* 1994;153:329–343.

798. Mackewicz CE, Ortega HW, Levy JA. CD8+ cell anti-HIV activity correlates with the clinical state of the infected individual. *J Clin Invest* 1991;87:1462–1466.

799. Furci L, Scarlatti G, Burastero S, et al. Antigen-driven C-C chemokine-mediated HIV-1 suppression by CD4(+) T cells from exposed uninfected individuals expressing the wild-type CCR-5 allele. *J Exp Med* 1997;186:455–460.

800. Baier M, Werner A, Bannert N, Metzner K, Kurth R. HIV suppression by interleukin-16. *Nature* 1995;378:563.

801. Clerici M, Stocks NI, Zajac RA, et al. Interleukin-2 production used to detect antigenic peptide recognition by T-helper lymphocytes from asymptomatic HIV-seropositive individuals. *Nature* 1989;339:383–385.

802. Schrier RD, Gnann JW, Landes R, et al. T cell recognition of HIV synthetic peptides in a natural infection. *J Immunol* 1989;142:1166–1176.

803. Cease KB, Margalit H, Cornette JL, et al. Helper T-cell antigenic site identification in the acquired immunodeficiency syndrome virus gp120 envelope protein and induction of immunity in mice to the native protein using a 16-residue synthetic peptide. *Proc Natl Acad Sci U S A* 1987;84:4249–4253.

804. Torseth JW, Berman PW, Merigan TC. Recombinant HIV structural proteins detect specific cellular immunity in vitro in infected individuals. *AIDS Res Hum Retrovir* 1988;4:23–30.

805. Kaslow RA, Duquesnoy R, VanRaden M, et al. A1, Cw7, B8, DR3 HLA antigen combination associated with rapid decline of T-helper lymphocytes in HIV-1 infection. *Lancet* 1990;335:927–930.

806. Just JJ, Abrams E, Louie LG, et al. Influence of host genotype on progression to acquired immunodeficiency syndrome among children infected with human immunodeficiency virus type 1. *J Pediatr* 1995;127:544–549.

807. Just JJ, Casabona J, Bertran J, et al. MHC class II alleles associated with clinical and immunological manifestations of HIV-1 infection among children in Catalonia, Spain. *Tissue Antigens* 1996;47:313–318.

808. Kroner BL, Rosenberg PS, Aledort LM, Alvord WG, Goedert JJ. HIV-1 infection incidence among persons with hemophilia in the United States and western Europe, 1978–1990. Multicenter Hemophilia Cohort Study. *J AIDS* 1994;7: 279–286.

809. Detels R, Mann D, Carrington M, et al. Resistance to HIV infection may be genetically mediated. *AIDS* 1996;10:102–104.

810. Bruhl P, Kerschbaum A, Zimmermann K, Eibl MM, Mannhalter JW. Allostimulated lymphocytes inhibit replication of HIV type 1. *AIDS Res Hum Retrovir* 1996;12:31–37.

811. Liu R, Paxton W, Choe S, et al. Homozygous defect in HIV-1 coreceptor accounts for resistance of some multiply-exposed individuals to HIV-1 infection. *Cell* 1996;86:367–377.

812. Cohen O, Vaccarezza M, Lam G, et al. Heterozygosity for a defective gene for CC chemokine receptor 5 is not the sole determinant for the immunologic and virologic phenotype of HIV-infected long term non-progressors. *J Clin Invest* 1997;100:1581–1589.

813. Eugen-Olsen J, Iversen AKN, Garred P, et al. Heterozygosity for a deletion in the CKR-5 gene leads to prolonged AIDS free survival and slower CD4 T cell fall in a cohort of HIV seropositive individuals. *AIDS* 1997;11:305–310.

814. Eales L-J, Nye KE, Parkin JM, et al. Association of different allelic forms of group specific component with susceptibility to and clinical manifestation of human immunodeficiency virus infection. *Lancet* 1987;1:999–1002.

815. Garred P, Madsen HO, Balslev U, et al. Susceptibility to HIV infection and progression of AIDS in relation to variant allels of mannose-binding lectin. *Lancet* 1997;349:236–240.

816. Khoo SH, Pepper L, Snowdon N, et al. The TNF c2 microsatellite allele is associated with the rate of HIV disease progression. *AIDS* 1997;11:423–428.

817. Lifson AR, Buchbinder SP, Sheppard HW, et al. Long-term human immunodeficiency virus infection in asymptomatic homosexual and bisexual men with normal CD4+ lymphocyte counts: immunologic and virologic characteristics. *J Infect Dis* 1991;163:959–965.

818. Sheppard HW, Lang W, Ascher MS, Vittinghoff E, Winkelstein W. The characterization of non-progressors: long-term HIV-1 infection with stable CD4+ T-cell levels. *AIDS* 1993;7:1159–1166.

819. Levy JA. HIV pathogenesis and long-term survival. *AIDS* 1993;7:1401–1410.

820. Buchbinder SP, Katz MH, Hessol NA, O'Malley PM, Holmberg SD. Long-term HIV-1 infection without immunologic progression. *AIDS* 1994;8:1123–1128.

821. Keet IP, Krol A, Klein MR, et al. Characteristics of long-term asymptomatic infection with human immunodeficiency virus type 1 in men with normal and low CD4+ cell counts. *J Infect Dis* 1994;169:1236–1243.

822. Munoz A, Kirby AJ, He YD, et al. Long-term survivors with HIV-1 infection: incubation period and longitudinal patterns of CD4+ lymphocytes. *J AIDS Hum Retrovir* 1995;8:496–505.

823. Balotta C, Bagnarelli P, Riva C, et al. Comparable biological and molecular determinants in HIV type 1–infected long-term nonprogressors and recently infected individuals. *AIDS Res Hum Retrovir* 1997;13:337–341.

824. Schrager L, Young J, Fowler M, Mathieson B, Vermund S. Long-term survivors of HIV-1 infection: definitions and research challenges. *AIDS* 1994;8(suppl 1): 95–108.

825. Zwart G, VanderHoek L, Valk M, et al. Antibody responses to HIV-1 envelope and gag epitopes in HIV-1 seroconverters with rapid versus slow disease progression. *Virology* 1994;201:285–293.

826. Pantaleo G, Vaccarezza M, Graziosi C, Cohen OJ, Fauci AS. Antiviral immunity in HIV-1 infected long-term non-progressors (LTNPs). *Semin Virol* 1996;7:131–138.

827. Learmont J, Tindall B, Evans L, et al. Long-term symptomless HIV-1 infection in recipients of blood products from a single donor. *Lancet* 1992;340:863–867.

828. Deacon NJ, Tsykin A, Solomon A, et al. Genomic structure of an attenuated quasi species of HIV-1 from a blood transfusion donor and recipients. *Science* 1995;270:988–991.

829. Kirchhoff F, Greenough TC, Brettler DB, Sullivan JL, Desrosiers RC. Brief report: absence of intact nef sequences in a long-term survivor with nonprogressive HIV-1 infection. *N Engl J Med* 1995;332:228–232.

830. Michael NL, Chang G, D'arcy LA, Tseng CJ, Birx DL, Sheppard HW. Functional characterization of human immunodeficiency virus type 1 nef genes in patients with divergent rates of disease progression. *J Virol* 1995;69:6758–6769.

831. Huang Y, Zhang L, Ho DD. Characterization of nef sequences in long-term survivors of human immunodeficiency virus type 1 infection. *J Virol* 1995;69:93–100.

832. Huang Y, Zhang L, Ho D. Biological characterization of nef in long term survivors of human immunodeficiency virus type 1 infection. *J Virol* 1995;69:8142–8146.

833. Iversen AKN, Shpaer EG, Rodrigo AG, et al. Persistence of attenuated rev genes in a human immunodeficiency virus type 1–infected asymptomatic individual. *J Virol* 1995;69:5743–5753.

834. Michael NL, Chang G, D'arcy LA, et al. Defective accessory genes in a human immunodeficiency virus type 1–infected long-term survivor lacking recoverable virus. *J Virol* 1995;69:4228–4236.

835. Cornelissen M, Kuiken C, Zorgdrager F, Hartman S, Goudsmit J. Gross defects in the vpr and vpu genes of HIV type 1 cannot explain the differences in RNA copy number between long-term asymptomatics and progressors. *AIDS Res Hum Retrovir* 1997;13:247–252.

836. Zhang LQ, Huang YX, Yuan HN, Tuttleton S, Ho DD. Genetic characterization of vif, vpr, and vpu sequences from long-term survivors of human immunodeficiency virus type 1 infection. *Virology* 1997;228:340–349.

837. Connor RI, Sheridan KE, Lai C, Zhang L, Ho DD. Characterization of the functional properties of env genes from long-term survivors of human immunodeficiency virus type 1 infection. *J Virol* 1996;70:5306–5311.

838. Haynes B, Pantaleo G, Fauci A. Toward an understanding of the correlates of protective immunity to HIV infection. *Science* 1996;271:324–328.

839. Shearer GM, Clerici M, Clerici M, et al. Protective immunity against HIV infection: has nature done the experiment for us? HIV-specific T-helper activity in seronegative health care workers exposed to contaminated blood. *Immunol Today* 1996;17:21–24.

840. Rida WN. Assessing the effect of HIV vaccination on infectiousness. *Stat Med* 1996;15:2393–2404.

841. Daniel MD, Kirchhoff F, Czajak SC, Sehgal PK, Desrosiers RC. Protective effects of a live attenuated SIV vaccine with a deletion in the nef gene. *Science* 1992;258:1938–1941.

842. Ruprecht RM, Baba TW, Liska V. Attenuated HIV vaccine: caveats. *Science* 1996;271:1790–1792.

843. Wyand MS, Manson KH, Lackner AA, Desrosiers RC. Resistance of neonatal monkeys to live attenuated vaccine strains of simian immunodeficiency virus. *Nat Med* 1997;3:32–36.

844. Shafferman A, Lewis MG, McCutchan FE, et al. Prevention of transmission of simian immunodeficiency virus from vaccinated macaques that developed transient virus infection following challenge. *Vaccine* 1993;11:848–852.

845. Lewis MG, Bellah S, McKinnon K, et al. Titration and characterization of two rhesus-derived SIVmac challenge stocks. *AIDS Res Hum Retrovir* 1994;10:213–220.

846. Stott E, Chan W, Mills K, et al. Preliminary report: protection of cynomolgus macaques against simian immunodeficiency virus by fixed infected-cell vaccine. *Lancet* 1990;336:1538–1541.

847. Stott E. Anti-cell antibodies in macaques. *Nature* 1991;353:393.

848. Chan WL, Rodgers A, Grief C, et al. Immunization with class I human histocompatibility leukocyte antigen can protect macaques against challenge infection with SIVmac-32H. *AIDS* 1995;9:223–228.

849. Abimiku AG, Franchini G, Tartaglia J, et al. HIV-1 recombinant poxvirus vaccine induces cross-protection against HIV-2 challenge in rhesus macaques. *Nat Med* 1995;1:321–329.

850. Egan MA, Pavlat WA, Tartaglia J, et al. Induction of human immunodeficiency virus type 1 (HIV-1)–specific cytolytic T lymphocyte responses in seronegative adults by a nonreplicating, host-range–restricted canarypox vector (ALVAC) carrying the HIV-1MN env gene. *J Infect Dis* 1995;171:1623–1627.

851. Cole K, Rowles J, Jagerski B, et al. Evolution of envelope-specific antibody responses in monkeys experimentally infected or immunized with simian immunodeficiency virus and its association with the development of protective immunity. *J Virol* 1997;71:5069–5079.

852. Girard M, Meignier B, Barre-Sinoussi F, et al. Vaccine-induced protection of chimpanzees against infection by a heterologous human immunodeficiency virus type 1. *J Virol* 1995;69:6239–6248.

853. el-Amad Z, Murthy KK, Higgins K, et al. Resistance of chimpanzees immunized with recombinant gp120SF2 to challenge by HIV-1SF2. *AIDS* 1995;9:1313–1322.

854. Boyer JD, Ugen KE, Wang B, et al. Protection of chimpanzees from high-dose heterologous HIV-1 challenge by DNA vaccination. *Nat Med* 1997;3:526–532.

855. Bolognesi D. Overview of HIV vaccine development. *Antibiot Chemother* 1996;48:63–67.

856. Esparza J, Heyward W, Osmanov S. HIV vaccine development: from basic research to human trials. *AIDS* 1996;10(suppl A):123–132.

857. Haynes BF. HIV vaccines: where we are and where we are going. *Lancet* 1996;348:933–937.

858. Pincus SH, Messer KG, Cole R, et al. Vaccine-specific antibody responses induced by HIV-1 envelope subunit vaccines. *J Immunol* 1997;158:3511–3520.

859. Girard M, Yue L, Barre-Sinoussi F, et al. Failure of a human immunodeficiency virus type 1 (HIV-1) subtype B–derived vaccine to prevent infection of chimpanzees by an HIV-1 subtype E strain. *J Virol* 1996;70:8229–8233.

860. Fleury B, Janvier G, Pialoux G, et al. Memory cytotoxic T lymphocyte responses in human immunodeficiency virus type 1 (HIV-1)–negative volunteers immunized with a recombinant canarypox expressing gp 160 of HIV-1 and boosted with a recombinant gp160. *J Infect Dis* 1996;174:734–738.

861. Ferrari G, Humphrey W, McElrath MJ, et al. Clade B–based HIV-1 vaccines elicit cross-clade cytotoxic T lymphocyte reactivities in uninfected volunteers. *Proc Natl Acad Sci U S A* 1997;94:1396–1401.

862. Perales MA, Schwartz DH, Fabry JA, Lieberman J. A vaccinia-gp160–based vaccine but not a gp160 protein vaccine elicits anti-gp160 cytotoxic T lymphocytes in some HIV-1 seronegative vaccinees. *J AIDS Hum Retrovir* 1995;10:27–35.

863. Gorse GJ, Patel GB, Newman FK, Mandava M, Belshe RB. Recombinant gp160 vaccination schedule and MHC HLA type as factors influencing cellular responses to HIV-1 envelope glycoprotein. NIAID AIDS Vaccine Clinical Trials Network. *Vaccine* 1995;13:1170–1179.

864. Tsuji T, Fukushima J, Hamajima K, et al. HIV-1–specific cell-mediated immunity is enhanced by co-inoculation of TCA3 expression plasmid with DNA vaccine. *Immunology* 1997;90:1–6.

865. Okuda K, Bukawa H, Hamajima K, et al. Induction of potent humoral and cell-mediated immune responses following direct injection of DNA encoding the HIV type 1 env and rev gene products. *AIDS Res Hum Retrovir* 1995;11:933–943.

Fundamental Immunology, Fourth Edition,
edited by William E. Paul
Lippincott–Raven Publishers, Philadelphia © 1999.

CHAPTER 45

Immunotherapy

Herman Waldmann, Lisa K. Gilliland, Stephen P. Cobbold, and Geoffrey Hale

---

INTRODUCTION

The immune system has evolved a most sophisticated set of responses designed to protect against infectious microbes. Detailed knowledge of the cellular and molecular components of these reactions has opened up opportunities for new forms of therapeutics, often involving *biologic agents* derived from the immune system itself. Obvious targets for the newly emerging immunotherapy are the numerous disease conditions which conventional small-drug therapy cannot cure or control long-term. These embrace transplantation, autoimmunity, cancer, cardiovascular diseases, and inflammatory bowel diseases, among others.

The biologic agents can be divided into three categories: (a) cellular products [exemplified by transplantation of allogeneic bone marrow (BMT) and tumor-infiltrating lymphocytes (TILs)], (b) proteins (e.g., antibodies and cytokines), and (c) gene therapeutics (e.g., for enhancing tumor immunogenicity). As gene therapy is

H. Waldmann, L.K. Gilliland, S.P. Cobbold, and G. Hale: Sir William Dunn School of Pathology, University of Oxford, OX1 3RE Oxford, United Kingdom.

still largely at the experimental stage, it will only receive limited coverage here.

These biologic therapeutics have been useful in four ways: First, for so-called acute events:

1. Cellular deficiencies arising from chemo- or radiotherapy, whereby survival is enabled by reconstitution of stem cells, or by administration of growth factors to escalate the rate of natural reconstitution of desired hemopoietic cell lineages
2. Acute inflammatory episodes, such as injury from ischemia–reperfusion (which can been seen in myocardial infarction, in strokes, and in vessel damage that inevitably occurs in organ transplantation), or in the control of septic shock arising from gram-negative bacterial infections, or for reversing an acute rejection episode in transplantation

Second, these agents have been used to debulk tumor masses or as adjuvant therapy to eliminate residual cancer cells left after surgical extirpation, chemotherapy, or radiotherapy. In as far as it is unlikely that every single tumor cell can be eliminated by such procedures, there is an unspoken assumption that long-term remissions might arise wherein any residual tumor cells become dormant, or come under some sort of growth control by natural host processes.

Third, these agents have been used to bring various manifestations of a range of chronic inflammatory diseases under some control. For example, in rheumatoid arthritis, many signs and symptoms of the disease can be controlled by biologics that neutralize tumor necrosis factor-α (TNF-α), although without evidence yet that the underlying cartilage destructive processes are altered. In multiple sclerosis, agents such as interferon-β (IFN-β) may impact by diminishing the incidence of new acute inflammatory lesions, and in a proportion of patients, delay the disease process without necessarily being able to cure.

Fourth, and perhaps the most exciting prospect for immunotherapy, is the possibility of inducing immunologic tolerance through a short-term therapeutic maneuver. This has been demonstrated in numerous rodent models of transplantation and autoimmunity, and with a more complete understanding of underlying mechanisms, should be applicable to humans.

Why Immunotherapy?

The initial interest in harnessing products of the immune system undoubtedly relates to the goal of achieving a substantial specificity and, consequently, therapeutic index for a defined target structure. In addition, cells of the hemopoietic and lymphoid systems are easily isolated as single-cell suspensions and are therefore amenable to well-controlled and reproducible cell manipulations *in vitro* (including cell expansion) prior to their use as *in vivo* therapeutics.

Why the Emphasis on Antibodies?

Every new antibody for every cell surface molecule represents a potential therapeutic drug. This is a far greater "hit rate" than can be achieved for drug discovery in any other way. Additionally, the application of monoclonal antibodies and related protein products to human disease processes has dual benefits resulting from their use both as probes and as therapeutics. As probes, they provide evidence, through demonstration of therapeutic efficacy, as to which cells or cell surface molecules are involved in particular pathologic processes, so defining these as targets for future therapeutic agents.

Antibodies Can Give Long-term Benefit from Short-term Therapy

Although the magic bullet concept may have provided the driving force to harness lytic antibodies as therapeutic tools, it has become clear, in the context of therapeutic immunosuppression, that non-lytic antibodies can also be used to guide or polarize the immune response to antigen into various modes of nonaggression. The latter strategy we have termed *reprogramming* (1) The short-term use of nonlytic antibodies to block T-cell responses to defined antigens may result in the T-cell population as a whole becoming long-term unresponsive to just those same antigens. Furthermore, it appears that among the various mechanisms that determine therapeutic tolerance is that of dominant tolerance, whereby regulatory T cells prevent aggressive responses to the target antigen. It is becoming quite clear that there are indeed many ways to engage the immune system to obtain reprogramming. For example, the mucosal administration

of antigens, and peptides derived from them, to ameliorate experimental autoimmunity has opened up opportunites for antigen- and tissue-specific therapy that could truly achieve a high therapeutic index with little risk of adverse reactions.

The realization that tumor cells and lymphocytes are never exempt from apoptosis offers further opportunities to use biologic approaches to eliminate particular cell types, by ensuring that the signals of assisted suicide dominate over the signals of survival (2–4).

Finally, one study suggests that tissues surviving aggressive encounters with the immune system may themselves change so as to be more resistant to immune attack (5). These principles, learned from studying mechanisms in xenotransplantation and infectious tolerance, may have far broader application in control of immune-mediated tissue damage in general.

Paving the Way with Monoclonal Antibodies

Much of the renewed interest in biologics as therapeutics has come from the application of monoclonal antibodies. It is inevitable, at this time, that a chapter in this fourth edition of *Fundamental Immunology* should have a major emphasis on therapeutic antibodies. The explosion of technologies for engineering antibodies, to design them for the desired effect *in vivo,* as well as reducing their immunogenicity, has been crucial to the rapid progress of this field. Yet, the number of good ideas for biologic products and therapeutic strategies far outweighs the number that can eventually come to the clinic. In these next sections, we hope to provide the reader with a sense of what those ideas and strategies are. In the last part of the chapter, we will discuss why so few of the ideas and innovations make it into clinical practice.

A MAJOR GOAL FOR IMMUNOTHERAPY: SHORT-TERM THERAPY FOR A LONG-TERM EFFECT

Short-term Antigen Administration Can Protect against Autoimmune Disease

Without doubt, the ideal strategy for achieving therapeutic tolerance in autoimmune disease or transplantation would be to identify the key target antigens and to administer them in tolerogenic form. Concerns have always centered on the following:

1. It may not be possible to identify all of the target antigens in any particular disease process (especially in the case of transplantation).
2. It may not be practicable to isolate the quantities of tolerogenic fragments or synthetic peptides required for each individual antigen.
3. The tolerogens may need to persist to maintain their effects, and this may be hard to achieve with molecules whose half-lives are short.

These concerns have been partially allayed through the demonstrations in so-called mucosal tolerance that low-dose tolerance induced to single antigens or peptides from a tissue can result in bystander tolerance to other antigens in that same tissue (6–8). This form of tolerance depends on active regulation by T cells. The fact that one need use only one of the many antigens of a tissue as a tolerogenic vaccine to ensure tolerance to all of the tissue antigens makes this very attractive. As the dose of antigen seems to influence whether tolerance is regulatory or deletional in type, so must the therapeutic application take account of these issues.

Other systemic routes of vaccination can also achieve the same. For example, the identification of heat-shock proteins (HSPs) as potential targets for attack in murine models of diabetes has led to the successful use of tolerogenic HSP-derived peptides to prevent the development of diabetes in NOD mice (9).

An alternative to giving antigen from *without* is to take advantage of the antigen *within,* by treating the host so as to alter the way in which the immune system perceives that antigen. Short-term therapy with antibodies has been able to achieve just that. In the next section, we will discuss the mechanisms that underlie *antibody reprogramming.*

Short-term Antibody Treatment Can Produce Long-term Tolerance

Depleting Antibodies

From the time that Medawar, Brent, and Billingham demonstrated that tolerance could be imposed upon the newborn mouse by infusion of allogeneic marrow, many investigators have tried to develop low-impact procedures that might permit comparable tolerance in the adult. In 1986, it was shown that it was possible to do this in adult rodents, where donor marrow was transplanted into recipients conditioned with a nonlethal dose of irradiation (600 rads) (10), together with a combination of lytic CD4 and CD8 antibodies to prevent graft-versus-host disease (GVHD) and graft rejection. Tolerance involved substantive donor chimerism. The need for irradiation was, in part, related to a requirement for host myeloablation to create hemopoietic space, as relatively nonimmunosuppressive doses of the alkylating agent dimethylmyeleran (DMM) could fully substitute for irradiation (11). "Hemopoietic space" might be required to ensure that more donor stem cells can engraft and generate sufficient donor cells to overwhelm residual host resistance mechanisms before these are able to reject the graft.

The dose of conditioning irradiation could be reduced to as little as 300 rads, if supplemented with 700 rads applied to the thymus

(12,13), or by increasing the level of antibody immunosuppression, either by addition of supplementary anti-LFA-1 antibodies to the CD4 and CD8 antibody cocktail (14), or by extending the period of antibody therapy (15).

Although tolerance with depleting protocols of antibody therapy looks feasible, a major concern for application to humans is the fact that CD4 T cells do not reconstitute efficiently in adult life, probably because of thymic involution. For that reason, there is a growing interest in achieving tolerance without T-cell depletion.

Nondepleting Antibodies

The demonstration in rodents in the mid-1980s that a short course of treatment with nonlytic CD4 antibodies resulted in long-term T-cell tolerance to foreign immunoglobulins (16–22) raised the more general possibility that short-term antibody blockade of T-cell function might lead to long-term tolerance. Tolerance with nonlytic CD4 antibodies could be extended to models involving transplants of bone marrow, heart, and skin (21–24). Not only could tolerance be induced in naive individuals, but also in previously sensitized recipients (25,26) (Fig. 1). In the context of autoimmunity, CD4 antibody therapy could also prevent the development of diabetes in NOD mice if given sufficiently early in the disease process (27–29).

Since those initial findings, many other antibodies and immunoglobulin-based blockading agents have been shown capable of producing transplantation tolerance, or of modulating the long-term outcome of autoimmunity. These include CTLA4-immunoglobulin, antibodies to CD11a, CD2, CD25, CD3, CD40 ligand (CD40L), and others (30–42). Remarkably, among these, CD3 antibodies have even proved potent in reversing the disease in overt murine diabetes when given in the short window before complete islet-cell destruction (36).

What Mechanisms Determine Tolerance through Antibody Blockade?

Most of the models of tolerance induced with nonlytic CD4 antibodies involve peripheral mechanisms, as they can be elicited in adult thymectomized (ATx) mice. A common feature of most model

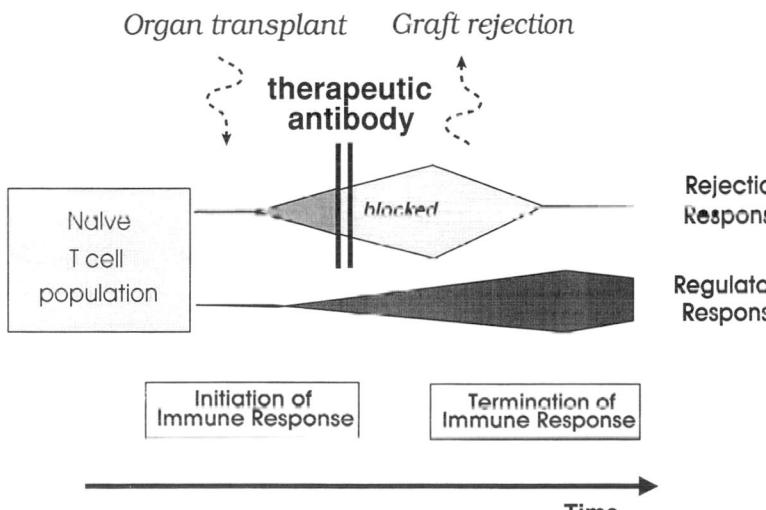

FIG. 1. Two stages in the evolution of "reprogramming." CD4 antibodies stop the induction of immune reactivity to the antigen while permitting regulatory T-cells to develop. Once CD4 antibody is withdrawn, the dominance of regulatory T-cells maintains that tolerant state through infectious tolerance. Persistence of antigen is needed to sustain these tolerance processes.

systems is that tolerance, once induced, cannot be broken by infusion of naive lymphocytes, although sufficient primed cells can do so (43,44). Antibody ablation of host CD4$^+$ T cells removes this *resistance* (26,43), while CD4$^+$ T cells from tolerant animals are able to prevent naive cells from rejecting grafts on adoptive transfer (26,45–50). This is the evidence of a role for *dominant tolerance.*

Animals tolerized to one set of transplantation antigens often show evidence of *linked suppression* (49,51). In other words, they exhibit an impaired response to subsequent third-party grafts when the third-party antigens are *presented* together on the same cells as the tolerated antigens. Linked suppression predicts that regulation must operate in a local microenvironment where antigen focuses naive antigen-specific T cells into the proximity and influence of regulatory T cells.

Infectious Tolerance

For dominant tolerance to operate throughout the life of the individual, either the first cohort of regulators must survive indefinitely, or their regulatory behavior must be endowed on new cohorts of T cells that develop later. Evidence for the latter scenario came with the demonstration that naive T cells became tolerant following cohabitation with (gentically marked) tolerant T cells in the presence of the graft antigens (45,49,50). Not only did naive T cells become tolerant, they also gained the ability to regulate the responses of further cohorts of naive T cells (Fig. 2). In studies involving vascularized heart grafts, infectious tolerance could be demonstrated over at least ten generations of recipient animals, showing it to be a robust and sustainable process.

Deletional Tolerance Can Also Be Induced with Nonlytic Antibodies

Studies with marrow transplants in rodents have suggested that the dose of marrow can determine whether deletion or regulation operates as the major mechanism of tolerance. High doses of marrow produced *deletional* tolerance, while low doses promoted *dominant* and *infectious* tolerance (50).

Is There an Overall Hypothesis for How Short-term Blockade by Antibodies Leads to Tolerance?

The accumulating evidence suggests that the different antibodies work by creating a sort of ceasefire (52), in which further aggres-

sion is prevented. Within this ceasefire, antigen-specific T cells remain able to recognize antigen and are signaled to become anergic or regulatory or to die, depending on the context and dose of antigen they experience (Fig. 3). If the outcome is to promote regulatory T cells, then the eventual numerical dominance of these cells, and their continuous interaction with antigen, ensure that the individual's response remains polarized towards that (nonaggressive) status. In some cases, the outcome could be polarization towards a T helper 2 (Th2) phenotype. In other situations, the outcome may be to some other form of regulatory T-cell activity hitherto unrecognized by immunologists. It is indeed becoming clear that other forms of regulatory CD4 T cells (e.g., Th3) can be isolated in different biologic contexts (7). We anticipate that identification of the various regulatory modes of CD4 T cells will become an important scientific growth area for understanding peripheral tolerance, and for clarification of the diverse phenomena that have been carried under the label of *T-cell suppression.*

Two-stage Tolerance Protocols

The above studies have been concerned with the development of tolerance to tissues transplanted under the umbrella of therapeutic antibodies. In those situations, the tissues were at risk of damage while simultaneously providing a source of tolerogen. To confer a greater level of protection for the transplanted tissue, there has been growing interest in the use of a two-stage process, whereby tolerance is initiated by infusion of nonvital cells and reinforced by subsequent transplantation of the donor organ. The use of CD4 antibodies to enhance the tolerogenic potential of blood transfusions in two stage prophylactic therapy for transplantation has been promoted by Wood and coworkers (53,54). This group has also shown that transfectants expressing single major histocompatibility complex (MHC) class I or MHC class II molecules can also be used in conjunction with CD4 monoclonal antibodies to induce tolerance and linked suppression, to enable acceptance of fully MHC-mismatched vascularized heart grafts.

The attraction of using nonlytic antibodies to induce tolerance is that one need not know the complete identity of all antigens to which the immune system is exposed. Therapy with blockading antibodies can be seen as simply altering some aspect of the way the immune system perceives the antigens to which it is reacting, so as to become reprogrammed. Tolerance is induced only to antigens given under the antibody umbrella. The period of global immunosuppression lasts only as long as there is antibody remaining in the

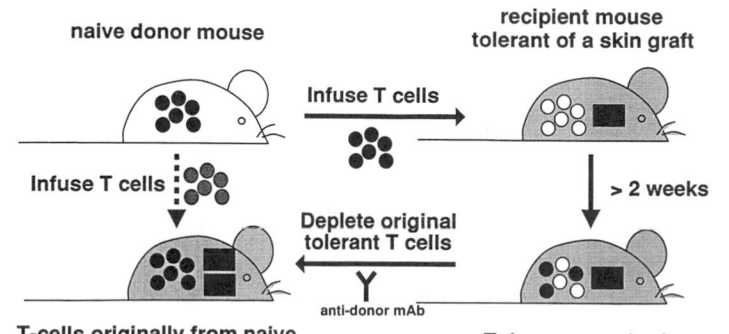

FIG. 2. Experimental demonstration of infectious tolerance in which a tolerant T cells guide naive T cells towards tolerance. As a result of this, the second cohort of T cells becomes able to stop other naive T cells from rejecting the grafts.

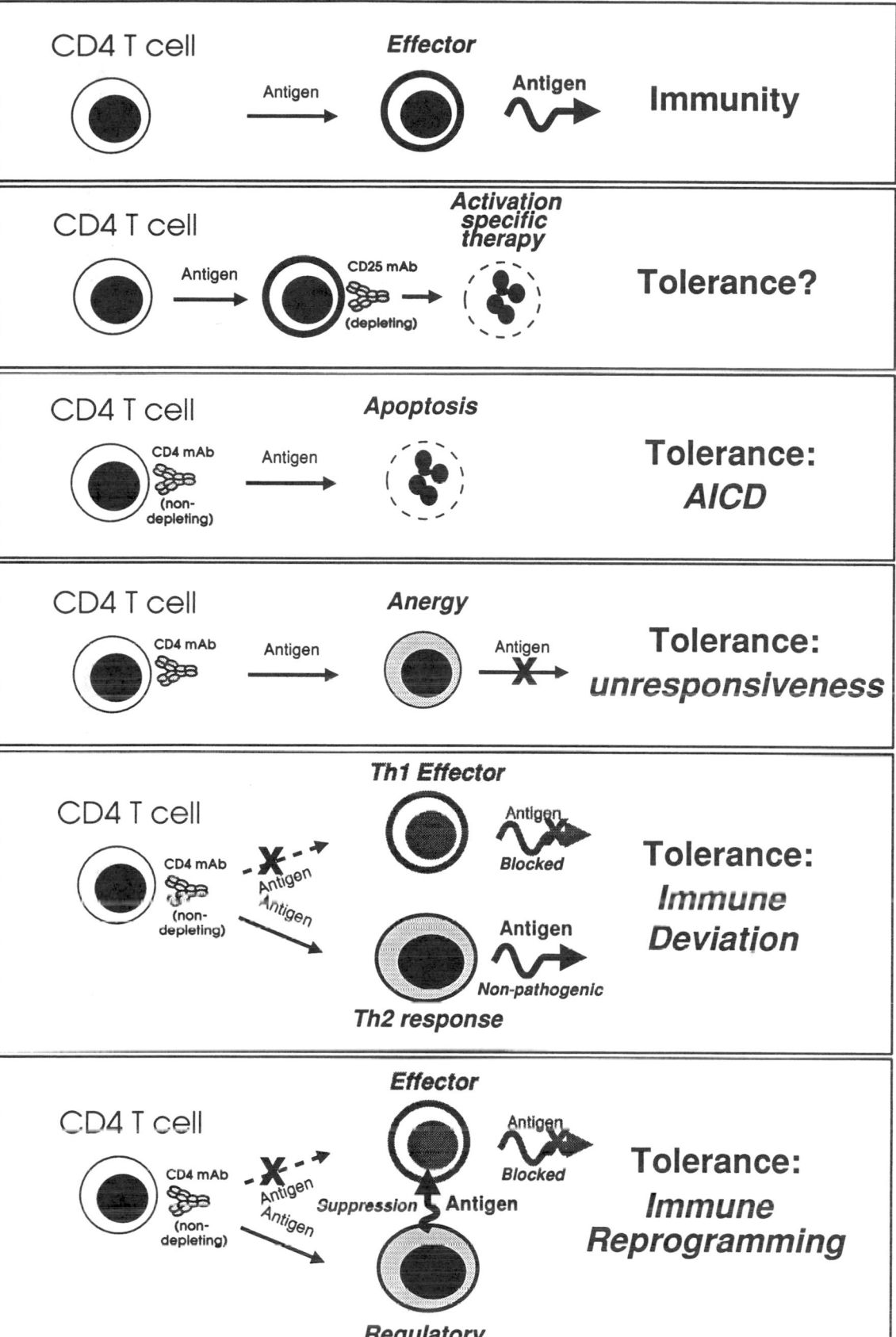

FIG. 3. Proposed mechanisms of specific tolerance induced by antibodies. Some antibodies may selectively eliminate clones of T cells that have been activated by antigen. Nondepleting CD4 antibodies may prevent T-cells from getting full signals that drive them to aggression. As a result, T-cells may become tolerant through any of the mechanisms of deletion, anergy, activation-induced cell death (AICD), immune deviation, or infectious tolerance (reprogramming).

Tolerance Induction

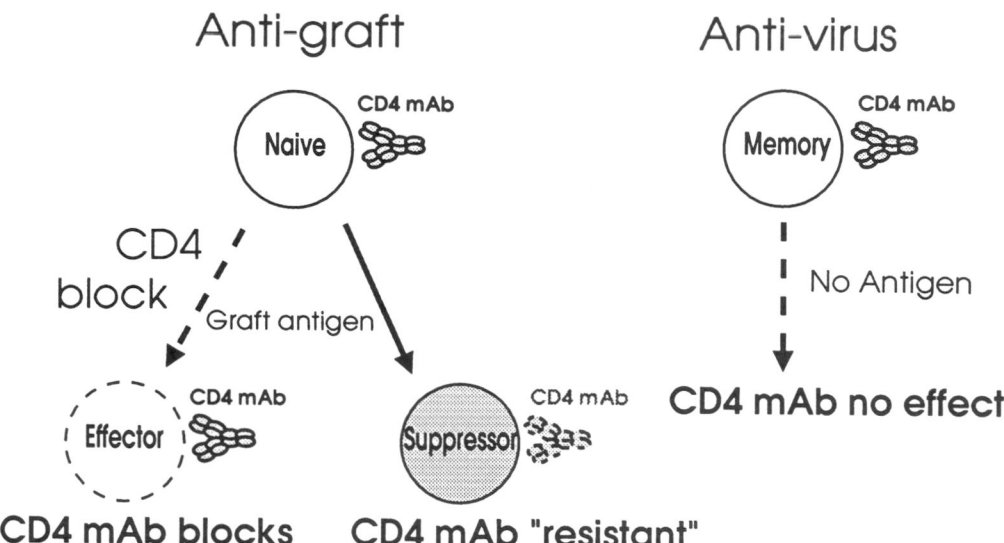

Tolerance maintenance

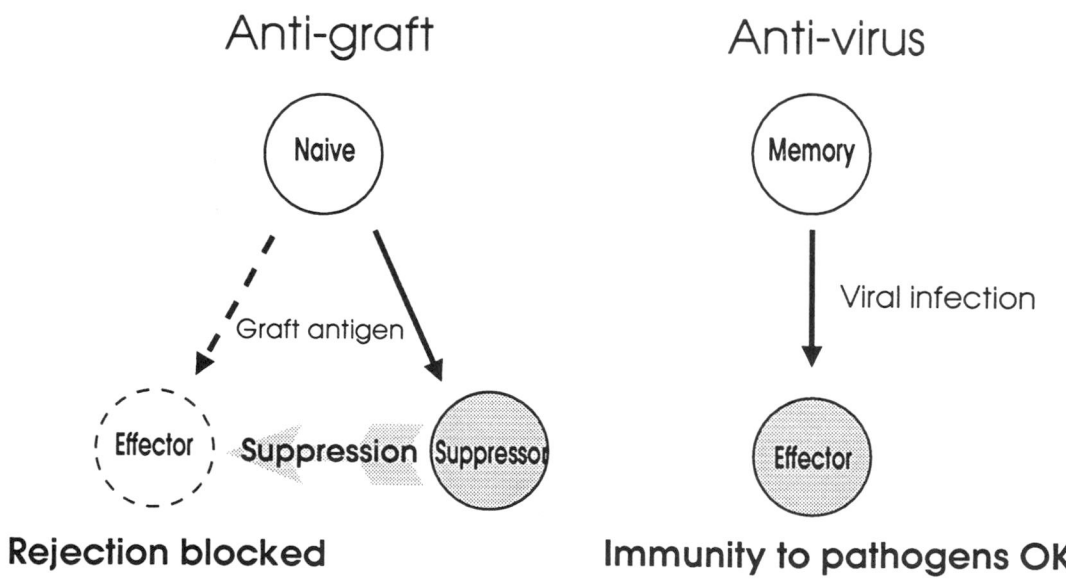

FIG. 4. How selectivity for antigen is maintained in tolerance through "reprogramming." In the induction phase, when the short course of antibody is given, the whole immune system is suppressed. However, tolerance is induced only to antigens given under the antibody umbrella. Once antibody is withdrawn and dominant tolerance is in place, there is no reason why regulatory T cells should, in any way, interfere with memory responses to any pathogen.

host. As antibody clears, then so should immune competence return to all antigens other than those to which tolerance has been induced (Fig. 4). The attraction of dominant and infectious tolerance for clinical application is that one may not need, at the outset, to establish tolerance to all antigenic peptides in the target tissue. Rather, if one could establish a dominant regulatory mechanism early on, then a limited set of antigens within the target tissue could serve to promote linked suppression and infectious tolerance, and disseminate tolerance to other antigens in that same tissue.

Ultimately, the clinician will be looking for diagnostic markers of tolerance before attempting to withdraw immunosuppressive drugs. If there were markers of regulatory cells, or unique products that could be monitored in the blood, then these might be very helpful prognostically as well as diagnostically. Tolerance without regulation would not be amenable to such analysis, and could only be confirmed following judicious withdrawal of immunosuppression. For this reason, and because the induction of this form of tolerance need not involve high-impact therapy, we anticipate that the harnessing of regulatory mechanisms will prove to be the most attractive target for immunosuppression in the next millenium.

CELLULAR THERAPEUTICS

There are numerous ideas and animal models of immunotherapy involving cell transplants to control leukemia and solid tumor growth. Rather than list all, we will discuss allogeneic BMT to exemplify many of the issues and complexity of cellular therapies.

Allogeneic Marrow Transplantation

Transplantation of bone marrow is the best established form of cellular immunotherapy but still remains a complex and crude procedure, fraught with numerous potential complications. Many of the experimental developments over the last 20 years have been aimed at reducing these complications, using cytokines or monoclonal antibodies to manipulate the composition of the bone marrow graft or the immunologic environment in the recipient, in order to overcome the problems that currently limit its clinical applications (Fig. 5).

Much of the original impetus for research on grafting allogeneic bone marrow came from work to treat the victims of radiation poisoning, because hemopoietic stem cells are among the tissues most vulnerable to radiation damage. Today, BMT is regularly used to treat patients suffering from severe inborn or acquired deficits in the blood system (immunodeficiencies or anemias) and to rescue leukemia and other cancer patients from the otherwise lethal effects of high-dose chemotherapy and radiotherapy. However, there are three principal complications, which have already been described in Chapter 36, namely (a) GVHD, caused by the immune attack of donor T cells on recipient tissues; (b) rejection, caused by residual recipient T cells; and (c) slow or abnormal immune reconstitution, mainly as a result of the limited capacity of the adult thymus to process new T cells. All of these complications are interrelated and dependent on the degree of tissue matching between donor and recipient. Apart from an identical twin, the best donor is a human leukocyte antigen (HLA)-matched sibling, but this option is restricted to only a minority of patients, and still many of them will suffer significant morbidity and mortality from GVHD, even if they are given long-term immunosuppressive drugs. If these complications could be prevented, marrow transplantation might be used to treat a much wider range of patients suffering from severe, but not necessarily life-threatening, diseases, for example, thalassaemia, sickle cell anemia, and, possibly, a large spectrum of autoimmune diseases.

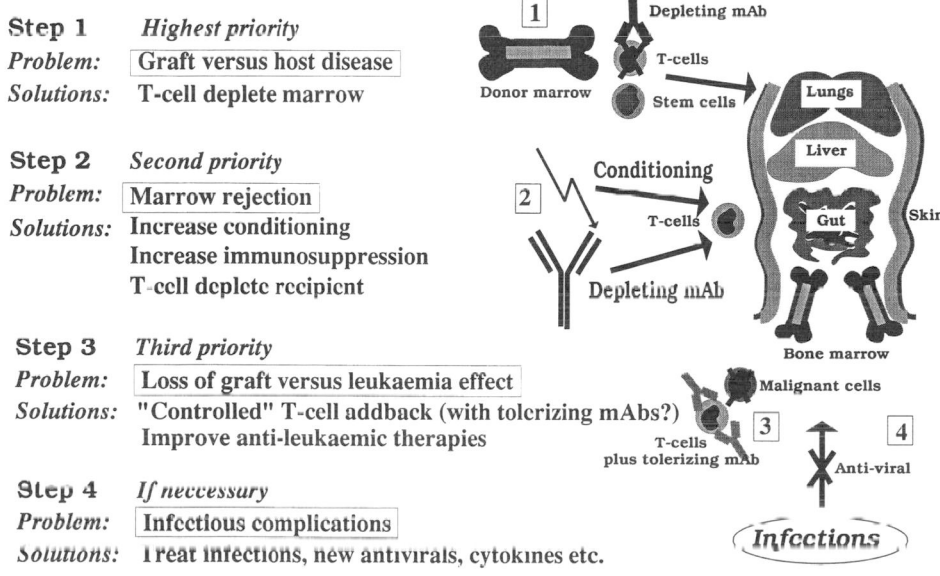

Bone Marrow Transplantation
The logical approach - solving one problem at a time

Step 1   *Highest priority*
Problem: Graft versus host disease
Solutions: T-cell deplete marrow

Step 2   *Second priority*
Problem: Marrow rejection
Solutions: Increase conditioning
Increase immunosuppression
T-cell deplete recipient

Step 3   *Third priority*
Problem: Loss of graft versus leukaemia effect
Solutions: "Controlled" T-cell addback (with tolerizing mAbs?)
Improve anti-leukaemic therapies

Step 4   *If neccessary*
Problem: Infectious complications
Solutions: Treat infections, new antivirals, cytokines etc.

FIG. 5. Allogeneic bone marrow transplantation: The problems and possible solutions.

Depletion of T Cells to Prevent Graft-Versus-Host Disease

The realization that GVHD is caused by mature donor T cells led to many efforts to eliminate them from the bone marrow graft, and this was one of the first therapeutic applications for monoclonal antibodies in the early 1980s. Antibodies to T-cell antigens, such as CD2, CD3, CD5, and CD7, as well as antibodies that recognize T and B cells, such as CD52, have been used in a variety of ways to deplete donor T cells, while sparing the hemopoietic stem. Some techniques did not give an adequate level of depletion, and it was found that fewer than 1% of the donor T cells could still cause significant GVHD. One of the most widely used techniques, because of its simplicity and effectiveness, has used the monoclonal antibody CAMPATH-1M, a rat IgM against the CD52 antigen (55,56). Unlike most other monoclonal antibodies to human cells, it is exceptionally able to lyse cells using human complement, and so no other manipulation is required to deplete the T cells, other than to add some donor serum. Human cells normally evade lysis by homologous complement via several different membrane-bound inhibitors (see Chapter 29). CD52 antibodies may be able to overcome this restriction, because the antigen is exceptionally abundant and because the antigenic epitope lies close to the cell membrane.

Without posttransplant immunosuppression, the risk of severe GVHD is probably more than 80%, and even with the best drugs, it is still about 40%. By effective depletion of T cells, it can be reduced to less than 10%. However, at the time of writing, no method of T-cell depletion has been approved for use, for reasons that will be explained below.

Overcoming Marrow Graft Rejection by Additional Immunosuppression

Graft rejection is normally very infrequent following allogeneic marrow transplantation, because the recipient's immune system is generally ablated by the high-dose chemotherapy and radiotherapy used to eradicate the primary disease. However, there is a reciprocal interaction between GVHD and rejection (10) (see Chapter 36), so that when donor T cells are removed, there is a significantly higher risk of rejection.

Experimental studies have shown that this rejection is caused by residual recipient T cells. To some extent, this can be overcome by increasing the stem-cell dose (57). Alternatively, rejection can be avoided by depletion of host T cells, using the same type of monoclonal antibodies that have been used to treat the donor marrow (10). Complement lysis alone is not an effective way to eliminate cells *in vivo*, partly because of the high concentrations of complement-regulatory factors. However, other effector functions can come into play, such as antibody-dependent cellular cytotoxicity (ADCC), which rely on antibody binding to Fc receptors (FcRs) on effector cells such as natural killer (NK) cells or macrophages. A rat IgG2b CD52 antibody, CAMPATH-1G, which can interact with human FcRs, is particularly efficient at lysing residual lymphocytes *in vivo*, comparable in activity to polyclonal antilymphocyte globulin (ALG) from horses or rabbits, but without the side effects of those reagents. Studies with CAMPATH-1G have shown that it is possible to obtain a low risk of GVHD and rejection, resulting in a significant reduction in the morbidity and mortality of the transplant procedure.

The Antileukemic Effect of Allogeneic T Cells

Elimination of transplant complications is likely to deliver a better long-term outcome for patients transplanted for nonmalignant disorders, such as the inborn errors of metabolism or hemopoiesis. Unfortunately, this is not guaranteed for patients with malignant diseases, because there is evidence that the donor T cells are sometimes responsible for the curative effect of the transplant, possibly by eliminating residual tumor cells that escaped the conditioning regime (58,59). This would be the true immunotherapeutic role of marrow transplantation, mediated not by the stem cells, but by the same T-cell population that will cause GVHD. This antitumor effect of T-cells has only been conclusively demonstrated in two diseases—chronic myeloid leukemia (CML) and Epstein-Barr virus (EBV)–induced B-cell lymphoproliferative disease (BLPD)—though many authors infer that it may be a contributory factor in other leukemias.

CML is a malignancy of hemopoietic stem cells themselves and can be cured only by allogeneic marrow transplantation. Removal of donor T cells results in a great increase in the risk of relapse (59). However, the disease can be closely monitored by molecular detection of the unique clonally rearranged gene bcr-abl, and, if donor lymphocytes are infused at the first sign of relapse, the malignant clone can be eliminated. The price, of course, is a high risk of reinducing GVHD. Much effort has been spent in trying to delineate T cells causing GVHD from those responsible for the graft-versus-leukemia (GVL) effect, but there are still few theoretical guidelines for clinical application (60).

BLPD is a different case, because this is almost exclusively an iatrogenic disease, induced by extensive and selective depletion of T-lymphocytes. EBV is latent in the B cells of most adults, and, in the absence of T cells, it can give rise to rapid oligoclonal proliferation, leading to malignant transformation to a lethal lymphoma. The disease can readily be brought under complete control if donor T cells are infused in time.

Immune Reconstitution after Allogeneic Marrow Transplantation

For 2 to 4 weeks following ablative chemo- and/or radiotherapy, the whole blood system is severely depressed until new elements are formed from the donor stem cells. Red cells and platelets can be maintained by transfusions, but the most severe risk is from bacterial infection due to the lack of granulocytes. Transfusions are of little use, as the cells are so short-lived, but a significant acceleration in the production of new granulocytes may be achieved by administration of the recombinant growth factor, granulocyte colony-stimulating factor (G-CSF), which stimulates proliferation and differentiation of the granulocyte precursor cells.

The long-term consequences of marrow transplantation for the immune system are still not fully understood, but it is evident that restoration of "normal" levels of blood lymphocytes is slow, particularly when the donor lymphocytes are depleted. It seems that the thymus of adults is not very effective in processing of new T cells; in any case, immunologic memory will likely derive from the residual donor T cells. If the initial numbers of T cells are small, there may then be only a restricted repertoire, resulting in increased risk of infections or even autoimmune disease. While there is no doubt that marrow transplant recipients are at increased risk of these long-term complications, compared with normal individuals, it is perhaps remarkable that the reported incidence is not substantial and the great majority of long-term survivors remain healthy. The most vulnerable period for infections is probably during the first 6 months posttransplant, when reactivation of viruses such as EBV (see above) and cytomegalovirus (CMV) is a frequent occurrence. Current research aims to provide donor T cells stimulated *in vitro* against viral antigens (e.g., CMV) as specific immunotherapy for such complications, without inducing a major risk of GVHD.

Autologous Bone Marrow Transplantation

One way to avoid all of the immunologic problems of allogeneic marrow transplantation is to use the patient's own bone marrow, previously cryopreserved, to rescue from the otherwise lethal effects of the treatment regime. Clearly, this is inappropriate for diseases that affect the stem cell, severe aplastic anemia or CML. However, for other malignancies, or for autoimmune diseases, it is an attractive proposition, and even for inborn errors it is possible to conceive of correcting the defect by gene therapy. The problem now is one of eliminating the undesirable cells from the bone marrow infusion, whether they are tumor cells or lymphocytes responsible for autoimmune disease. The same ingenuity that was applied to T-cell depletion has been used to exploit the specificity of monoclonal antibodies in various ways for tumor-cell depletion. However, seemingly more attractive technologies have emerged, relying on positive selection of stem cells using CD34 antibodies (61). The CD34 antigen is selectively expressed on about 1% of bone marrow cells, including multipotential and committed stem cells, but it is not found on the majority of tumor-cell types, nor on mature blood cells. At the time of writing, there are three commercial systems, licensed or close to being approved, that use CD34 variously coupled to different types of support for the enrichment of bone marrow stem cells. Nevertheless, although it can be demonstrated that some logs of tumor-cell depletion can be achieved, it is not known whether infusion of this depleted bone marrow will improve patient survival, compared with undepleted bone marrow. The major difficulty is that we generally cannot differentiate between relapse occurring from reinfused tumor cells or from cells that survived the conditioning treatment.

Application of this type of approach to the treatment of autoimmune diseases is still highly experimental, and we doubt whether marrow ablative therapy is really necessary, given that it might be possible to selectively eliminate or modulate the function of lymphocytes *in vitro* by using monoclonal antibodies or other biologic agents.

New Developments in Bone Marrow Transplantation

Hemopoietic stem cells are normally found in the bone marrow and have traditionally been obtained for transplantation by aspiration from pelvic bones. This is a painful procedure, which must be carried out under general anesthetic. In recent years it has been discovered that large numbers of stem cells become mobilized into the peripheral blood following treatment with cytotoxic drugs or hemopoietic growth factors such as G-CSF. They can be harvested by cytopheresis, and this will probably supplant marrow aspiration within the next few years (62,63). Greater numbers of stem cells are obtained, which results in more rapid and reliable engraftment. The procedure is now routine for autologous transplants, but for allogeneic transplants, there is a potential problem due to the higher number of T cells. However, the risks of GVHD do not

appear to be increased, and it is still possible to deplete the T cells. The one remaining concern is whether there is any long-term hazard associated with administration of growth factors to the donor, but this does not currently seem to be a serious problem, especially when considering the known risks of anesthesia.

Gene Therapy

Because of the ready accessibility of bone marrow stem cells, they have been studied as one of the first targets for gene therapy. The adenosine deaminase (ADA) gene, which is defective in one type of severe immunodeficiency (see Chapter 43), was an obvious candidate for replacement. However, the field is still limited by the relative inefficiency of current methods for gene transduction and the great rarity of many of the diseases that are straightforward candidates for treatment.

Conclusions

Stem-cell transplantation is very fertile ground for the development of new therapeutic strategies involving monoclonal antibodies and cytokines. Many of the initial targets have been iatrogenic complications of the transplant procedure, rather than the underlying disease. This is perhaps not unreasonable, because the complications were predictable and often due to a single cause that was quite well understood. By solving one problem at a time, the complex interrelationships of GVHD, rejection, relapse, and infection are being broken down to yield an improvement in the overall results (60). This will, in turn, mean that curative transplant procedures can be offered to more patients, including those with less well matched donors and those with chronic but not immediately life-threatening diseases. Furthermore, the lessons learned about the application of these biologic therapies can be applied to direct treatment of leukemias, cancers, and immunologic diseases, as exemplified in the other sections of this chapter.

ANTIBODY THERAPEUTICS

As discussed in the previous sections, the fine specificity of monoclonal antibodies has attracted a great deal of research into development of antibody-based therapies for cancer and for modulation of the immune response. Antibodies are capable of highly specific interactions with a wide variety of ligands, both in their variable and constant domains, thus providing vast potential to engineer suitable therapeutics to treat a diverse range of diseases. Areas in which recombinant DNA technology are being applied to the design of therapeutic antibodies include (a) reducing immunogenicity so that antibody therapy can be used over extended periods (e.g., the treatment of autoimmune diseases); (b) adding extrinsic effector functions to a therapeutic or removing or modifying the intrinsic effector functions; (c) increasing antibody affinity, and the generation of novel specificities, using phage antibody technology; and (d) efficient production of stable recombinant antibodies at high levels in a cost-effective manner.

Potential for "Tailor-made" Therapeutics

Antibodies are composed of structurally distinct domains that provide different functions. Antibody engineering allows the creation of "designer" therapeutics, tailor-made to best fit the application at hand. Individual immunoglobulin domains retain their native structures when isolated from the whole antibody, and the functions associated with each domain can be recovered. Moreover, each antibody domain is encoded by a different exon, and recombinant antobodies can be built by genetically fusing the desired exons together. The modular arrangement of antibody domains (VH and VL bind antigen, while the Fc domains mediate effector functions) has allowed for a "mix and match" approach to designing antibody-based therapeutics (Fig. 6). Thus, functional domains providing specific antigen-binding or effector functions can be exchanged between antibodies, expressed as separate units with biologic activity or used as building blocks to construct novel fusion proteins. The exons encoding the antibody specificity of interest can be obtained by polymerase chain reaction (PCR) by a number of different methods. Expressed VL and VH domains pair appropriately, driven by their hydrophobic surface charges.

Variable Regions: Antigen Binding

The specificity and affinity of an antibody are dictated by the three hypervariable loops of the VL and the three hypervariable loops of the VH located on each arm of that antibody. Variations in the lengths and sequences of these loops define the antibody-combining site (ACS). Antibodies that bind small haptens typically have binding sites shaped as grooves or pockets, while antibodies that bind proteins typically have large, planar surfaces forming the ACS. In contrast to the variability found in the loop structures, the framework supporting the loops is a relatively invariant β-sheet structure.

Constant Regions: Antibody Effector Function and Catabolism

The constant domains include the Fc region that mediates the effector functions of the antibody. Effector functions can be divided into (a) those that operate after binding of antibody to antigen and are responsible for recruiting other cells or molecules to remove the antigen, and (b) those that are independent of antigen binding, including antibody catabolism and transcytosis (64). Together with the antigen-binding affinity and specificity conferred by the variable regions, the antigen-dependent Fc effector functions are responsible for the protective effect of antibody in host defense by recruiting FcR-positive cells and complement components following antigen binding. These in turn remove and/or destroy the antigen through opsonization, ADCC, or complement-mediated cytotoxicity (CMC). The antigen-independent property of binding to the FcRn salvage receptor is involved in regulating the half-life of the antibody in serum (65–68). In addition to exploiting their functions in whole antibody, Fc domains have also been genetically linked to ligands to create immunoglobulin fusion proteins. For example, a portion of human CD4 was fused with the hinge CH2/CH3 regions of human IgG1, and the expressed dimeric CD4 immunoglobulin protein had a serum half-life (48 hours) in rabbits that was significantly better than CD4 alone (25 minutes) (69).

Potential for Therapeutic Application

Passive antibody therapy has been used successfully for many years to protect patients who are susceptible to infectious agents. Gamma-globulins, from naive or immunized human volunteers, have been used to transfer immunity to patients with primary and secondary immunodeficiencies. Monoclonal antibodies are beginning to replace some of the requirements for pooled gamma-globulin, offering advantages in terms of potency, reproducibility, and minimal contaminants. In the foreseeable future, monoclonal antibodies will likely replace polyclonal sera for prophylaxis of Rhesus disease of the newborn.

This need, together with the potential of antibody therapy in the fields of cancer and immunosuppression, has catalyzed the application of protein engineering technologies to make antibodies more adaptable to the tasks required of them.

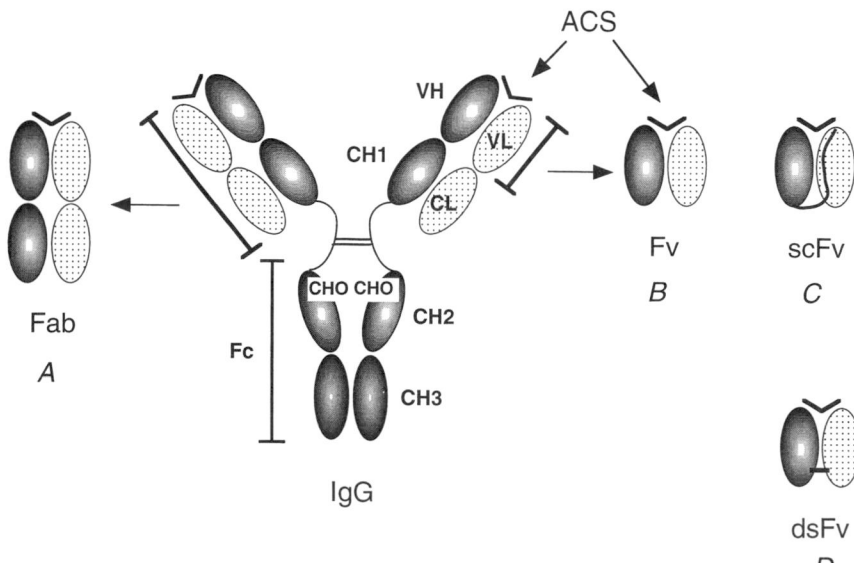

FIG. 6. An antibody IgG molecule and commonly used antigen-binding derivatives. Each immunoglobulin heavy and light chain is structurally divided into domains of variable (VL and VH) or constant (CL, CH1, CH2, CH3) regions. The CH2 domain contains the N-linked glycosylation site at Asn297. The Fab region (**A**) comprises VL/CL and VH/CH1. The Fv region (**B**) consists of the VL + CL only. The Fv can be expressed in recombinant form as a single-chain Fv (scFv) with a flexible peptide linker (**C**) or as a disulfide-stabilized Fv (dsFv) (**D**). ACS, antibody-combining site.

Lytic and Blocking Antibodies

Therapeutic antibodies act in one of two ways. Depleting antibodies kill lymphocytes *in vivo* by targeting them for destruction. Such antibodies should possess high specificity and affinity–avidity for target antigen, efficient effector functions for recruiting FcR-positive cells and complement, as well as a long serum half-life. Nonlytic antibodies act by blocking the function of the target antigen without killing the cell that bears it. These antibodies can be engineered for loss of antigen-dependent effector functions while retaining the capacity for long serum half-life, as the catabolic sites are located at the CH2 and CH3 domain interface (64), while the residues involved in complement binding (70) or interaction with FcγR (71–74) lie elsewhere in the Fc region. Alternatively, an antibody isotype with poor effector function can be used to achieve binding without depletion. For example human IgG4 is very poor in initiating CMC (75,76). IgG4 has been shown to bind weakly to FcγRI and does not mediate ADCC in many people (77,78). However, in some individuals, IgG4 has been shown to be as effective as IgG1 for ADCC (79). Therefore, a more reliable strategy for generating nondepleting antibodies may be mutation of the residues involved in mediating CMC and binding to FcRs. For example, removing the glycosylation site in CH2 has a profoundly detrimental effect on constant region–associated effector functions (80–82).

The Role of Antibody Isotype

Antibody isotype has a clear impact on the capacity of the antibodies to harness natural effector mechanisms. This has been well demonstrated with rat, mouse, and human antibodies, both *in vitro* and *in vivo,* through the use of class-switch variants of hybridomas or through construction of chimeric antibodies with the same V region. The first *in vivo* demonstration of the importance of antibody isotype on tumor-cell lysis is shown in Fig. 7. A patient with a prolymphocytic leukemia did not respond to treatment with either rat IgM or IgG2a antibody to the CD52 antigen. In contrast, a class-switch variant from rat IgG2a to rat IgG2b was potently lymphocytic and produced a complete therapeutic response (83). The human IgG1 isotype was shown to be the most effective in both CMC and ADCC in experiments using a matched set of antibodies with identical specificity but varying in antibody heavy-chain isotype (77). For CMC, human IgG1 bound less C1q than human IgG3, but deposition of C4b on the cell surface was more efficient for IgG1, which accounted for its effective target-cell lysis (75). Table 1 displays the known interactions of the human IgG subclasses with C1q and different FcRs.

Although murine IgG2a, rat IgG2b, and human IgG1 and IgG3 are considered the most potent isotypes, lysis *in vivo* cannot be guaranteed and is very much dependent on the target antigen. The relative roles of complement and FcR-dependent mechanisms may vary, depending on the antigenic target, but an analysis of various mutant and isotype variant Fc regions suggested that FcR-mediated destruction was probably a more universal mechanism for destruction of nucleated cells (84).

The Nature of the Target Antigen

Not all cell surface antigens are equal in their capacity to harness natural effector mechanisms. Antigen density and capacity to modulate may be important. However, some antigens are good targets for lysis by natural effector mechanisms, without any definitive explanation as yet (e.g., CD52 and CD20 on lymphocytes).

Specificity

For specificity in cancer therapy, the ideal target antigen would be expressed on the surface of tumor cells but not on normal cells. In reality, there are very few tumor-specific antigens, perhaps the closest being idiotype on B-cell lymphomas (85,86). What matters is whether the expression of tumor-associated antigens would render the tumor more susceptible to damage than normal tissue, and whether loss of normal tissue would itself be problematic. For example, elimination of normal B cells as a price for eradicating a B-cell lymphoma might be acceptable, especially as new B cells could eventually develop from stem cells.

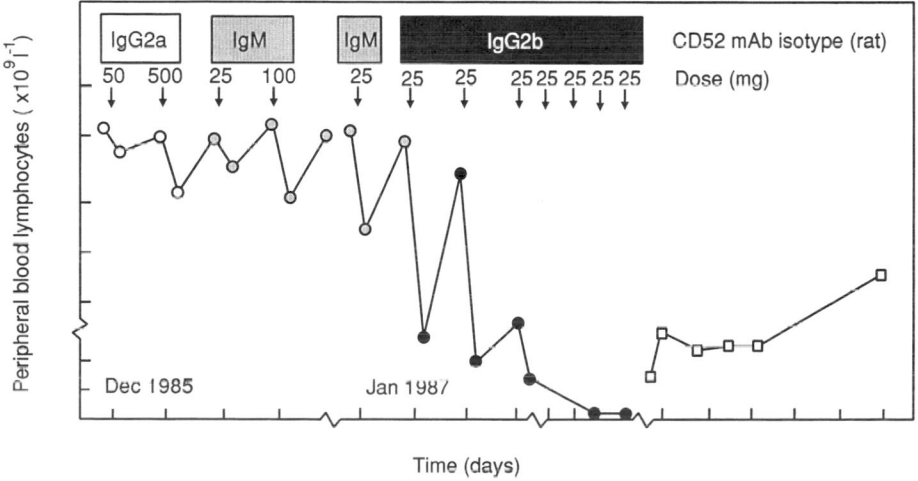

FIG. 7. The effect of rat antibody isotype on the clearance of peripheral lymphocyte cells in a patient with chronic B-cell leukemia. The antibody specificity was directed to the CD52 antigen (83).

TABLE 1. *The interaction of human IgG isotypes with human C1q and FcγR*

Isotype	C1q	FcγRI	FcγRII	FcγRIII
IgG1	+	+	+	+
IgG2	Weak	–	–	–
IgG3	+	+	+	+
IgG4	–	Weak	–	–

It is also desirable that any antigen loss mutants be disadvantageous for growth of the targeted cell. This requirement may be hard to meet for many tumors. It may, however, be relevant to the success of targeting idiotypic determinants on B-cell lymphomas. The latter has proven to be one of the more rewarding arenas of tumor targeting, and one that has provided great insight into tumor immunotherapy in general (85,86).

Tumor-associated antigens usually emerge as one of the following:

1. Oncofoetal antigens: antigens that otherwise are found in the developing foetus
2. Differentiation antigens: reflecting cells frozen at a particular stage of development
3. Overexpressed surface molecules, such as receptors for growth factors
4. Cryptic antigens, which are exposed as a consequence of altered glycosylation

Antigen Internalization and Shedding

Some cell surface antigens are internalized rapidly following binding by bivalent antibodies (e.g., CD3), while others are relatively immobile (e.g., CD52) (87). For clinical applications requiring lysis by the naked antibody, a nonmodulating antigen might be preferred. Some investigators have used chemically engineered univalent antibodies to enhance lysis towards antigens that have demonstrated that univalent antibodies derived by somatic cell fusion (88) or by genetic engineering (89) are better able to activate complement than is the wild-type modulating form. In contrast, optimal delivery of a toxin or chemotherapeutic might benefit from internalization. Antigens that shed from the cell surface (e.g., carcinoembryonic antigen or idiotype) can be problematic, because free antigen could compete for binding of the therapeutic reagent to cancer cells.

Converting Poor Antigens to Good Ones: Synergistic Lysis

Some antigens, even very abundant ones, prove poor targets for exploiting the natural effector mechanisms of antibodies. Synergistic pairs of lytic antibodies of a permissive isotype, directed to two distinct epitopes on the same target molecule, proved capable of activating homologous complement where each individual antibody had failed (90,91). Synergistic pairs of antibodies can also achieve better depletion *in vivo* through FcR-mediated effector mechanisms than can each antibody alone. There are, as yet, no published clinical studies of the utility of synergistic pairs.

Signaling Dormancy and Cell Death

Certain cell surface molecules, targeted by bivalent antibody, are capable of delivering signals to cells that can lead to tumor dormancy (92,93), and others may provide death signals that can lead to apoptosis (2,4). There is a need to define the molecular basis of dormancy-signaling and to understand fully the "survival signals" that enable many cells to resist "death signals." Pharmacologic intervention to disrupt survival signals might help tumor cells to commit suicide.

ENGINEERED ANTIBODIES FOR THERAPY

Modifying Variable Regions

X-ray crystallography has revealed the important aspects of the antibody–antigen interaction (94,95). The six complementarity-determining regions (CDRs) (96) provide most of the contacts necessary to bind antigen, but they do not contribute equally. Generally, four or more CDRs are used to bind antigen, and VH contributes more buried surface area to Ag binding than does VL (97). The H3 loop contained within CDR3 of VH often makes essential contacts with antigen and has been shown to undergo a major change in position upon binding (98). The importance of this loop in the diversity of the antibody repertoire is underscored by the sequence variation found in H3, which ranges from two to 26 residues (99). Each CDR is a loop connecting two framework β strands of fixed orientation, and these loops cluster at the end of the Fv. Due to their close proximity, structural changes due to mutations within a CDR may be propagated to adjacent CDRs or to the framework itself (100). Additionally, CDR/CDR interactions in the VL/VH interface may prevent correct domain assembly (101), and thus may disrupt expression of the antibody and limit its commercial production. Because the orientation of the CDR loops is critically involved in antibody specificity and affinity, a model (or preferably a structure) is important to guide rational design for desired goals with respect to antigen binding and production.

Although thousands of V-region gene fragments have been cloned, few structures have been solved, the majority of these being in the uncomplexed form. Molecular modeling of antibody structure has grown into a discipline in its own right, as considerable improvements in homology-based methods and conformational searches have allowed increasingly accurate structural predictions (100,102).

Two routes have been taken to optimize antibody for a therapeutic application:

1. Improvement on those available rodent antibodies that have shown some success in the clinic, often relying heavily on computer-assisted three-dimensional models to predict the effects of point mutations introduced in the ACS, or to assess perturbations to CDR loop positions during humanization
2. Generation of a new human antibody with high specificity and affinity for the target antigen, likely then to be less immunogenic in humans

It is worth noting that novel ACS shapes and chemical constitutions that have not yet been formed through natural evolution can be generated by replacement of residues or whole CDRs by rational design (100) or by using the combinatorial library approaches.

Improving Rodent Antibodies

Most of the currently available antibody therapeutics are reengineered versions of rodent antibody derived by conventional hybridoma technology. Any genetic manipulation of the rodent antibody requires that its V-region genes are isolated from the parent hybridoma. Antibody engineering has progressed rapidly following the development of PCR-based techniques for isolation and amplification of V-region sequences from hybridomas (103–105). Of particular interest (106) is a method for cloning antibody cDNA from single lymphocytes producing antibody against rare, defined, target antigens.

New Specificities and Increased Affinities through Phage Display

There may be times when a desired specificity is difficult to produce through the hybridoma technology, or when the affinity of a particular antibody is too low to be of use *in vivo*. Phage display technology (107,108) represents a powerful tool for overcoming these problems. Phage libraries enable screening or selection of the best antibody derivative with regards to binding affinity, epitope recognition, and VL/VH pairing. Very large libraries not only increase the likelihood of recovering the original pairs of heavy and light chains expressed in individual B cells, but also increase the probability of isolating high-affinity antibody. For example, it is difficult to produce antibody specific for estradiol by conventional hybridoma technology, yet an antiestradiol antibody isolated by phage display from a very large library binds to estradiol in the nanomolar range, but only weakly to a number of related steroids. Whereas generation of antibody by conventional hybridoma technology is subject to constraints of the immune system, some (109) have used phage display to isolate antibody against compounds that are normally toxic or immunosuppressive, including a high-affinity antibody against doxorubicin.

Phage display can be used to mimic *in vitro* many of the *in vivo* processes that the immune system uses to generate high-affinity antibody. Consequently, high-affinity antibody can be produced without prior immunization or use of conventional hybridoma technology. For example, artificial affinity maturation of phage antibody repertoires has generated affinities suitable for therapeutic use, in the nanomolar to picomolar range (110–113). This has been achieved by shuffling the heavy or light chains (114) by random or directed mutagenesis of CDR (115–117), by error-prone PCR (118,119), or by repeated cycling of repertoires through bacterial mutator strains (120). These techniques can be time consuming but may not be neccesary if the repertoire is very large. Vaughan et al. (109) described the construction of a library of 1.4×10^{10} clones of human sFv fragments displayed on the surface of phage. The tightest binders had dissociation constants (K_d) in the subnanomolar range, higher than previously reported for a nonimmunzed library and comparable to high-affiinity antibody derived from hybridomas.

Engineering Constant Regions

Identification of Functional Sites

Studies with domain-shuffled variants (121) have emphasized that the CH2 domain has a crucial role in determining functions of the Fc region. Mutagenesis within the CH2 domain has identified critical sites involved in the binding of C1q and FcR. Consequently, mutant isotypes can be adapted for particular clinical uses, for which there is a need to avoid one or other of the natural effector mechanisms, to avoid cell destruction or to minimize toxicity (e.g., avoidance of the cytokine release syndrome with CD3 antibodies).

Introduction of Multiple Effector Domains in the One-antibody Molecule

Introduction of cysteine residues into the CH3 domain of antibodies has allowed the creation of dimers through reduction and oxidation of the heavy chains *in vitro* (122,123). Such dimers are more efficient in mediating complement lysis. No *in vivo* efficacy studies are published for such dimeric antibodies. The introduction of extra CH2 domains in tandem within the same heavy chain did not, however, improve effector function (123).

A Single Mutation to Produce an Aglycosyl Antibody Serves to Prevent C1q and FcR Binding

Carbohydrate is found at conserved positions in the constant regions of antibody heavy chains, with each isotype displaying a distinct array of N-linked carbohydrate structures that affect protein assembly, secretion, and/or function (124). The heavy chain of human IgG has a single, large N-linked biantennary carbohydrate structure at Asn297 that is buried between the two CH2 domains and forms extensive contacts with residues in that domain (125).

Removal of carbohydrate by site-directed mutagenesis of Asn297 to Gln (126) or Ala (82) does not affect interaction of the Fc region with *Staphylococcus* protein A; however, C1q binding is greatly reduced or undetectable, and FcR binding is substantially reduced. The *in vivo* half-life of Gln297 IgG1 was not affected by lack of carbohydrate (126), and *in vivo* clearance of Ala297 IgG2a was indistinguishable from that of wild-type (127). These studies suggest that while removal of carbohydrate at Asn297 diminishes IgG binding to FcR and greatly reduces its ability to fix complement, it does not significantly alter the antibody structure nor its stability. An aglycosylated humanized therapeutic antibody against CD3 is in early clinical trials for treatment of renal allograft rejection (82). It remains fully competent to reverse graft rejection, but, compared with the wild-type antibody, it exhibits greatly reduced toxicity from cytokine release (where the toxicity is known to be dependent on FcR binding).

Engineering Serum Half-life

The persistence of antibody in the blood is governed by two overlapping processes. Initially, there is rapid decay in the serum concentration of antibodies, reaching equilibrium during the first day after administration. This is followed by natural catabolism of antibody, which results in its disappearance from serum. Persistence of IgG in the serum for extended periods of time relative to proteins of similar size led to the proposal of the existence of a specific salvage receptor (128) that could capture IgG inside endosomes and recycle it back into the plasma. The neonatal FcR (FcRn) has been identified as that salvage receptor (68). Tight binding of FcRn to IgG in the acidic endosomes protects IgG molecules from catabolic degradation, and recycles them by dissociation into the neutral extracellular fluid. The implication for therapeutics is that (a) serum persistence of whole antibody may be extended by mutagenesis of residues to ensure good binding to human FcRn, and (b) the half-life of smaller antibody fragments (e.g., sFv) could be enhanced by including a tag that contains the FcRn interaction site. For mouse IgG1, this site has been mapped to amino acids Ile253, His310, His435, and His436, located at the CH2/CH3 domain interface (129–131). To this end, Ghetie et al. (67) have designed a recombinant murine immunoglobulin fragment with a significantly increased serum half-life in mice by increasing the binding affinity of the antibody for FcRn.

Novel Antibodies and Antibody Derivatives for Human Therapy

The genes encoding VL and VH can be expressed linked together by an intervening flexible peptide linker to form a single-chain Fv (scFv) molecule (132,133). ScFv proteins can be expressed in either VH linker–VL or VL linker–VH orientations, have a molecular weight of 27 kDa, and are the smallest molecules to retain full antibody-binding function (although the binding is monovalent). Expressing antibody as scFv has become a popular and versatile approach: The sFv gene cassette can then be used alone, to express a monovalent antigen-binding molecule, or in combination with other genes to create artificial adhesion receptors (134), immunotoxins (135,136), bispecific antibody (137–144), intracellular targeting molecules (145–148), or gene fusions with cytokines (149).

Bispecific Antibodies

Bispecific antibodies (BsAbs) (150) were developed for redirecting or enhancing immune effector response towards tumors and to induce killing of target cells in a non–MHC-restricted manner (151,152). One arm of the BsAb recognizes a cell surface antigen on a cytotoxic effector cell (ususaly CD3, CD16, or CD64), while the other arm is specific for a tumor antigen. The first BsAbs were prepared by chemical cross-linking of antibody containing effector specificity with antibody having antitumor specificity, or by cell fusion of the corresponding hybridomas. Recruited effector cells include CTLs, lymphokine-activated killer (LAK) cells, TILs, NK cells, and monocytes and macrophages. Cytokine release triggered by BsAb binding to such effector cells potentiates the cytotoxic effects (153,154).

Preclinical *in vivo* studies have shown that BsAb directed against B-cell idiotype can sometimes be effective in prolonging the survival of tumor-bearing mice. Modest but encouraging effects have been observed in several small-scale clinical trials (reviewed in ref. 155).

There have been also been some encouraging claims for BsAb that target monocytes and macrophages through CD64 (FcγRI) to tumor cells overexpressing the Her2/neu oncogene product on breast, ovarian, and prostate cancers. The monocytes and macrophages armed with the CD64 × Her2 BsAbs penetrate tumors and induce transient inflammation, as measured by release of cytokines such as TNF-α, interleukin-6 (IL-6), IL-8, and granulocyte–macrophage colony-stimulating factor (GM-CSF).

The application of DNA recombinant technology to the construction of BsAb fragments will facilitate more extensive clinical evaluation of these types of molecules (reviewed in ref. 156). Recombinant BsAbs have been generated in the form of bispecific scFv, minibodies, diabodies, and multivalent BsAb (157–160) (Figs. 8, 9). Single-chain BsAbs are composed of linked variable domains fused to human Fc domains (104,138,140). Miniantibodies comprise an scFv joined by a linker to a dimerization domain (160), while diabodies exploit the intrinsic nature of VH and VL domains within an Fv to pair. VH/VL dimer association is spontaneous and has a binding constant of about 10^{-10} M (100). This high affinity is due to the close complementarity of conserved residues at the domain interface. The use of short linkers or no (zero) linkers in an scFv forces the intramolecular pairing of VH and VL within the same chain (158). Zero-linker diabody libraries have been constructed in phagemids (159) to generate and analyze thousands of different bispecific molecules. In addition to the intrinsic pairing of diabodies, multimerization domains also can be used to generate antibody with multiple specificities. These domains or tags include amphipathic helices (160), CH3 (161,162) or Fc (dimers), TNF (trimers), or helix–turn–helix motifs (163). Overall, though, the clinical utility of these agents remains to be shown.

Antibody Expression for the Manufacturing Process

None of the benefits of antibody engineering are meaningful if antibody cannot be produced on a large scale and purified free of contaminants. This necessitates high-level expression. The

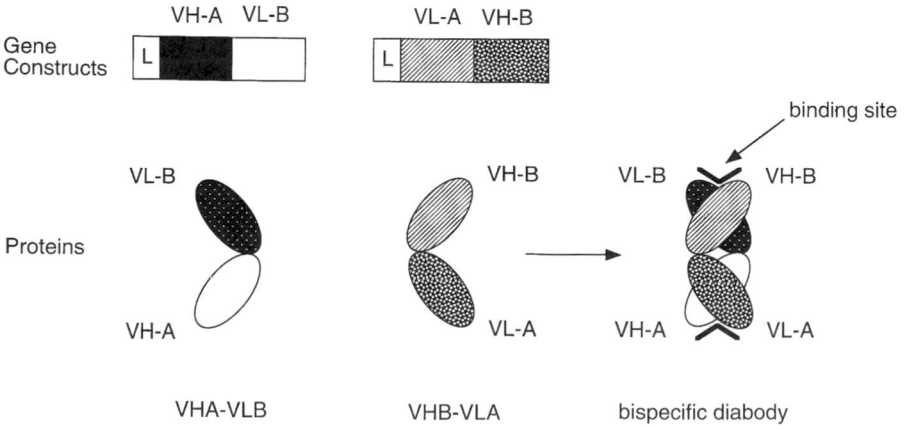

FIG. 8. Bispecific diabodies.

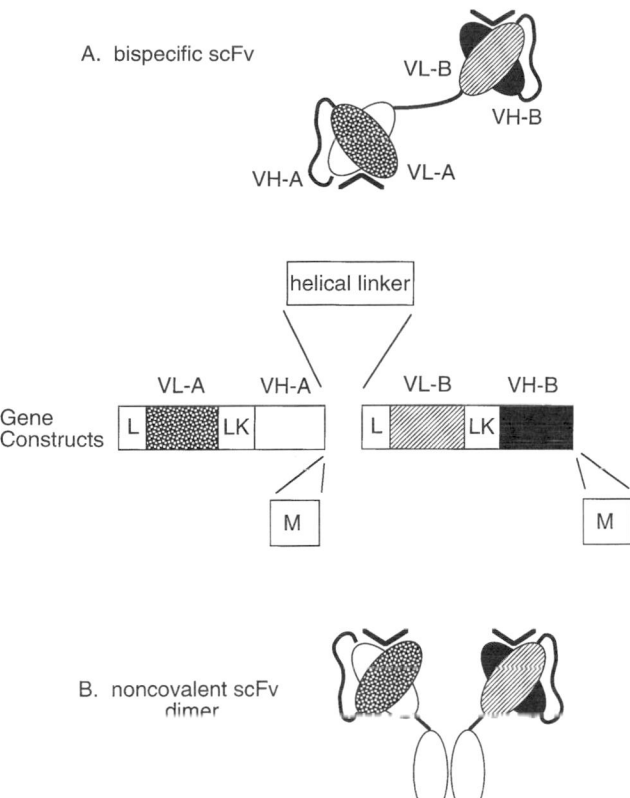

A. bispecific scFv

VL-B

VH-B

VH-A   VL-A

helical linker

VL-A   VH-A   VL-B   VH-B

Gene
Constructs   L   LK   L   LK

M   M

B. noncovalent scFv
dimer

FIG. 9. **A:** Single-chain bispecific scFv. The gene construct consists of two scFv gene cassettes separated by sequence encoding a "helical" linker (220). Expression of this construct generates a single-chain protein in which the two scFvs are tethered. **B:** Noncovalently linked scFv dimer. Each scFv gene cassette is fused to a multimerization domain (M) and expressed separately. Bispecificity is achieved by noncovalent association of the multimerization domains.

sequence of antibody chains may have a major effect on folding, transport, and aggregation of antibodies intracellularly. Therefore, good engineering must proceed with the end in mind to provide "high producers."

Initial attempts to express antibody intracellularly in *E. coli* produced very low yields of functional antibody (164,165). These proteins were retained in inclusion bodies, and it was presumed that the highly reducing intracellular environment of *E. coli* was not conducive to disulphide bond formation. *In vitro* denaturation and refolding is required to obtain functional native antibody from the material in inclusion bodies (166,167). An alternative approach is to use the signal sequences (ompA and pho) to direct expressed domains into the periplasmic space, where the oxidizing environment permits authentic disulphide bond formation (166,168). The scFv format has been adopted for the expression of Fv domains to overcome the tendency of the noncovalently associated VH and VL domains to dissociate (132,133).

THE PROBLEM OF IMMUNOGENICITY

Because the first cohort of therapeutic monoclonal antibodies was of mouse or rat origin, a major drawback of early antibody-based therapy was that the monoclonal antibodies were recognized

as foreign by the patient's immune system, leading to a humoral immune response against the therapeutic. That antiglobulin comprises an antiidiotypic component (anti-id) directed against the variable regions of the antibody and/or an antiisotype component (anti-iso) directed against the constant region.

The antiglobulin response is a major obstacle in the routine use of antibody in the clinic, both by neutralizing the therapeutic and by removing it in the form of complexes from circulation, so rendering the treatment ineffective (reviewed in ref. 169). Additionally, some patients can experience life-threatening anaphylaxis if treatment is continued (170). However, therapy may still be possible in some patients with preexisting antiglobulin antibodies, if plasmapheresis is to reduce antilevels.

This, however, is far from being the ideal solution. The problem of immunogenicity could be avoided if we could design antibody that could evade "recognition" by the human immune system. Substantial effort has been directed towards achieving this goal. It is easier to prevent the primary antiimmunoglobulin response than to arrest it once it has started, and it is in *prevention* that most progress has been made.

Administration of the therapeutic antibody, together with immunosuppressive drugs (171), can reduce the antiimmunoglobulin response. However, such nonspecific suppression of the patient's immune system somewhat negates the selective nature of antibody therapy unless it forms part of a synergistic drug combination for a particular disease process.

Antibody Engineering to Reduce Immunogenicity

Chimerization and Humanization

Chimerization and CDR grafting were developed in attempts to "humanize" rodent antibody. The amount of "foreign" sequence is reduced by swapping the rodent antibody constant regions (chimerization) and the variable-domain framework regions (humanization) for sequences found in human antibody.

The first therapeutic antibody to be humanized was the rat anti-human CD52 antibody, CAMPATH-1H (172). In this case, the rat CDRs were grafted onto the human frameworks NEWM for VH and REI for VL because the structures of these V regions had been solved. Although the first version of the humanized antibody had a much lower affinity than the original rat antibody, this could be restored when two framework residues in the VH were back-mutated to the rodent sequence (172). The appropriate human framework to serve as "acceptor" sequence can be chosen to increase the chance of obtaining a humanized antibody with antigen-binding affinity as close to the rodent antibody as is possible (173,174). The rodent V-region family subgroup is assigned on the basis of amino acid homology, and it is then compared with the consensus sequence for that subgroup to identify unusual residues that may have been introduced during *in vivo* affinity maturation. These residues, which may be required for correct orientation of the CDRs, are introduced into the human framework. The framework is also compared with its subgroup consensus sequence to identify and remove unusual amino acids. The human and rodent sequences are then compared so as to eliminate species differences that would change charge, size, or hydrophobicity.

Other approaches to humanization include *hyperchimerization* and *resurfacing*. Hyperchimerization is a process by which the human sequence that is most homologous to the rodent sequence is identified by homology searches and is used as the acceptor sequence. The human sequence is scanned for idiosyncratic residues, which are replaced by consensus residues to generate a more generic framework. Structural modeling is used to identify framework residues that may need to be substituted to preserve the CDR loop conformations (175). Resurfacing involves changing only the surface-exposed foreign residues to the equivalent human residues from the sequence of highest homology. Only a limited number of surface residues differ between human and mouse variable domains, and the strategy preserves the packing residues between the VL and VH domains (176,177).

Human Antibody from the Outset

The generation of human antibody by traditional hybridoma technology has proven extremely difficult (178). In the few instances in which immunization of humans has occurred, it has been difficult to obtain stable human hybridomas expressing high levels of antibody. Phage display technology and transgenic approaches have provided useful ways of overriding this problem.

Phage Display

In phage display, antibody fragment gene repertoires (rearranged variable, diversity, and joining genes) are expressed on the surface of filamentous phage, and the clones with desired antigen specificity are selected by a *wholly in vitro* procedure. The system mimics the key features of the humoral immune response. As a result, high-affinity antibody can be produced without immunization or the use of conventional hybridoma technology. By using natural (179) or synthetic (111) human repertoires, it is possible to create and affinity mature human antibody to many different antigens. Ideally, a large antibody repertoire would generate enough diversity to select high-affinity antibody to antigens of interest. Human antibody to a diverse range of antigens, including TT, hepatitis B, gp120, and RSV, have been isolated by phage display, many from asymptomatic individuals.

Transgenic Mice

Transgenic mice have also been used to produce human antibodies (180–182). Human germline V-gene segments can be rearranged and expressed in mice. By crossing these mice with heavy-chain knock-out mice, in which the endogenous mouse immunoglobulin loci have been silenced by gene targeting, strains are created that produce human antibody. The human IgH translocus "rescues" the development of mouse B cells (arrested due to lack of mIg), and, therefore, essentially all of the B cells in these animals express human immunoglobulin chains.

Xenochimeric Mice to Rescue Human Antibodies

Another ingenious approach to rescue human antibodies from immunized donors has been to transfer human lymphocytes to irradiated mice, which can then be boosted with defined antigens, and primed lymphoid tissues used to provide cells for fusion with myeloma cells lines (183)

Are Humanized Antibodies Nonimmunogenic?

It is already clear that humanized antibodies are immunogenic in some patients over repeated courses of treatment (184,185). The immunogenicty of therapeutic antibodies, even humanized ones, is due in part to their cell-binding ability (17). Non–cell-binding antibodies are far less immunogenic. To be confident that no antiidiotypic responses can ever arise, it will be essential to engineer antibodies further. One approach, involving a novel two-stage strategy to induce immunologic tolerance to the therapeutic antibody, is described below.

Prophylactic Induction of Tolerance to Therapeutic Antibodies

This novel strategy is based on (a) historical studies showing that deaggregated immunoglobulin can induce *in vivo* tolerance to an aggregated (immunogenic) form, if administered prior to the aggregate; (b) the antiimmunoglobulin response being a typical CD4+ T cell–dependent B-cell response (186); and (c) the relative ease of tolerance induction to a *non–cell-binding* antibody. Previous studies have shown that mice could be easily tolerized to xenogeneic IgG if this did not bind to cells. Tolerance could not be induced to *cell-binding* antibodies (17).

Consequently, it might be possible to induce T-cell tolerance to a therapeutic antibody by presenting all of the potential light-chain and heavy-chain helper epitopes in a nonimmunogenic way in the form of *non–cell-binding* mutants, prior to administration of the wild-type *cell-binding* form (186).

PCR mutagenesis was used to change one or two residues of CAMPATH-1H to create a nonbinding form. Such a minimal mutation destroys antigen binding but can still preserve the B-cell epitopes that are dependent on correct heavy–light pairing and retain most of the T-cell epitopes of the wild-type antibody.

The deaggregated mutant non–cell-binding form of CAMPATH-1H, injected into transgenic mice expressing CDw52, tolerized these mice for any response to wild-type cell-binding antibody. This finding may have important implications in the long-term administration of therapeutic proteins to humans.

ENGINEERING ANTIBODIES FOR CANCER THERAPY

Overview

Progress in the treatment of cancer with antibody-based therapies has been slower than for their application in immunosuppression. One reason is that immune reactivity against tumor cells requires more than blocking of receptor function, as the primary goal is cell death. The antibody may induce cytotoxicity in a number of ways, for example, through induction of host effector functions via the Fc region or by delivery of a toxic moiety (e.g., radionuclide or toxin) to the tumor site. Although these killing mechanisms can be very powerful *in vitro,* the effectivity *in vivo* is often limited by tumor accessibility. In general, antibody-based cancer therapy has been more successful against leukemias and lymphomas than against poorly vascularized solid tumors.

Diversity of Experimental Strategies

For a review of the diversity of experimental strategies, see the work by Wawrzynczak (187). Antibody can be engineered to kill tumor cells in several ways: (a) They can be modified so as to best recruit the natural effector mechanisms, or to invoke apoptosis or dormancy through intracellular signaling, or to block the binding of necessary growth factors. (b) Modified antibody can be designed to carry radionuclides, toxins, or cytotoxic drugs to tumor cells. Additionally, bispecific antibody can be used to recruit effector cells to tumor sites. (c) In the future, it may even be possible to use the gene therapy approach to express intracellular antibody that bind to key targets that inhibit tumor growth. These "intrabodies" can be expressed intracellularly in precise locations within mammalian cells by modifying the intrabody genes (in scFv or Fab format) with sequence-encoding classical intracellular trafficking signals (e.g., KDEL) (145,188,189). Some well-characterized tumors are known to be dependent on certain growth factors or hormones, and genes encoding neutralizing antibody to those factors could be delivered to cells at the tumor site. ErbB2 is overexpressed in a variety of human tumors, including breast and ovarian carcinomas, and its expression correlates with unfavorable prognosis (190). Endoplasmic reticulum–targeted scFv intrabodies have been reported to inhibit expression of the ErbB2 transmembrane protein (146,190) and, ultimately, to trigger apoptosis in target cells (146,147). ScFvs have also been targeted to the cell surface via fusion to cytoplasmic and transmembrane domains and can function as artificial ligands. Cell surface–expressed CD28-specific scFv, expressed on several different cell types, can induce costimulation of CD28+ T cells (104,134).

All of these approaches are intellectually satisfying, but, in the end, they need to make their mark in the clinic. Perhaps only few will survive to that stage.

The Trade-off between Antibody Size and Function

Although certain therapeutic antibodies have demonstrable benefit in the treatment of leukemia and some lymphomas, antibodies have had limited utility in the treatment of solid tumors. The main reason is that poor tumor penetration and poor target specificity result in only a small fraction of the antibody reaching the tumor (191). Decreasing the size of the antibody would allow better penetration, although this may never be equivalent to that possible with the diffusion of small drugs. sFvs have been shown to permeate more rapidly and deeper into tumors than does whole IgG (192). However, loss of the effector functions naturally associated with the Fc means that any desired effector-function cytotoxic agent or domain will have to be added, so removing the benefit of size reduction. The challenge for antibody-based cancer therapeutics is, therefore, to create small molecules that demonstrate good tumor penetration, but that bind strongly to the antigen through improved avidity.

If the size issue is compromised, then stability conferred by bivalent binding can increase the functional affinity for antigen up to 1,000-fold higher for IgG compared with Fab'. One approach is to make multivalent sFvs through the use of amphipathic helix tags that covalently associate to force dimerization of the sFv (160). These proteins, however, still lack Fc-associated functions. An approach has been described (162) in which an sFv is fused to either a whole antibody or a F(ab')2-like molecule to produce tetravalent, bispecific molecules with opportunities for improved effector functions.

Antibody Targeting of Cytotoxic Agents

Many cytotoxic agents have a low therapeutic index (benefit versus damage), which means that the dose needed to give maximal kill of tumor will damage normal tissue. Antibody targeting of cytotoxic agents could, in principle, localize the cytotoxic activity to the disease site, so enhancing that therapeutic index. Such agents include conjugates of radioisotopes, chemotherapeutic drugs, enzymes, toxins, and/or a second antibody arm to localize the effector molecule in a two-stage process.

Radionuclides. The most effective radionuclides are those that have long half-lives and deliver high doses of irradiation; these include α and β emitters such as astatine 211 and yttrium 90, respectively, and Auger electron emitters such as iodine 125.

Chemotherapeutics. Effective conjugates of antibodies with chemotherapeutics require that the drug get access to its intracellular target. For this to happen, covalent conjugates need to be internalized by endocytosis and then released by cleavage, usually within the lysosomal compartment. The limitations on dose of chemotherapeutic agent that can be provided this way remain an obstacle.

Immunotoxins. Conjugates of antibodies with protein toxins based on ricin, gelonin, saporin, diphtheria, and *Pseudomonas* toxins use the antibody to locate the toxin chain to a cell surface target, and then require that the toxin become internalized. Translocation of the toxic moiety into the cytosol will result in interference with the protein synthetic process, leading to death. A great deal of toxin modification and molecular engineering has attempted to improve these toxins for therapeutic purposes, often eliminating the "natural" cell-binding component so as to ensure that any cell binding occurs through the ACS and that linkage to antibody remains stable.

Progress in this field can be be exemplified with the *Pseudomonas* exotoxin. The initial immunotoxins (ITs) were composed of tumor-specific antibody coupled to the full (holo) toxin. These ITs were shown to be highly cytotoxic, as only a few molecules reaching the cytoplasm of a cell could kill it. However, their efficacy was limited by poor tumor penetration, due to their large size, and by nonspecific toxicity towards normal cells. Tumor penetration was improved by developing scFv forms of the tumor-specific antibody (193). As the mechanisms of toxin killing became elucidated, it was possible to alter these toxin moieties to increase specificity. *Pseudomonas* exotoxin is composed of three domains: The N-terminal domain I binds to surface proteins on cells, domain II is involved in translocation across the membrane of the endosome, and domain III inhibits protein synthesis (194). Truncated forms of *Pseudomonas* exotoxin, such as PE40, that lack domain I cannot bind to normal cells (194). Recombinant ITs are therefore constructed using scFv, dsFv (disulfide bond–stabilized scFv), or Fab fragments fused to genes encoding a truncated toxin. In addition to the advantage of smaller size for increased tumor penetration (in comparison to early ITs), these antibody derivatives avoid "innocent bystander" killing of FcR+ cells such as macrophages and B-cells because they lack Fc regions. Recombinant ITs are showing some promise in the clinic.

One of the major limitations of recombinant ITs is their immunogenicity. Although humanized V-region components can be used to construct the antibody portion of the ITs, the toxin component is itself immunogenic, and the effectiveness of the IT is often neutralized by the host immune response about 10 days following administration (195). As an alternative to the bacterial or plant toxins, human enzymes, such as nucleases, are being explored as potentially less immunogenic domains (196,197).

All of the signs with these sorts of molecule look encouraging, but the challenge, at least in the case of tumor therapy, is to aim for very high therapeutic ratios to ensure substantial tumor kill with minimal toxicity before immunogenicity renders the drug ineffective. The right context for many of these agents may come to be in synergy with other drugs or as adjuvant therapy.

Two-stage Strategies

A number of other approaches have been taken to add cytotoxic "payloads" to antibody to obtain killing of target cells. In antibody-directed enzyme prodrug therapy (ADEPT), an antibody is used to target an enzyme to the tumor, and unbound reagent is allowed to clear. A nontoxic prodrug is then given, and this is activated by the enzyme to generate a cytotoxic drug at the tumor site (198,199). Target-site conversion of prodrugs to active drugs has been shown to be an effective means of killing target cells while minimizing systemic toxic side effects. An important aspect of ADEPT is the generation of bystander killing. Because the drugs are activated extracellularly by the antibody–enzyme complex, neighboring cells can also be killed by a mechanism that does not require translocation across intracellular membranes. In contrast, immunotoxins kill only the cell to which they bind, and killing is limited by the efficiency of endocytosis and translocation.

THE CLINICAL APPLICATION OF ANTIBODIES

Why Are There So Few Antibodies in Clinical Practice?

Although monoclonal antibodies were discovered in 1975, it has been a relatively slow process for them to achieve respectability as therapeutics. There are probably many reasons for this.

1. Antibodies are often species-specific, and so preclinical toxicology and efficacy studies cannot always be done in the same way as has been possible for small molecule therapeutics.

2. The early trials with antibodies showed them to be quite immunogenic, raising concerns as to long-term utility. In the past 9 years, numerous strategies have evolved to overcome this, and they have restored confidence.

3. There was initially a certain naiveté in expectation of potential efficacy, often before good animal models had indicated the best therapeutic strategies. We now know how important it is to engage in an iterative process of drug improvement before deciding that an agent is worthless.

4. Many antibodies with therapeutic potential may not make it to clinical development because the disease targets are not sufficiently attractive to pharmaceutical companies to cover the development costs and potential liabilities.

5. In part, the community is suffering from the partial success of "small drugs," such that it is becoming increasingly difficult to demonstrate efficacy of therapeutic antibody without major clinical trials over extended periods.

6. The need to administer antibodies parenterally has perceived disadvantages over orally administered drugs.

7. Patent issues in various aspects of antibody manufacture impact profit margins, and, therefore, pharmaceutical companies feel obliged to target potential "blockbuster" areas.

8. Few have grappled with the issue of what if short-term therapy could give long-term tolerance. How could one put a price on

such therapy to recoup development costs and so forth? We recall one head of a major pharmaceutical company, light-headed with dinner wine, confiding that his company could "never take on any such curative therapy because it would be hard to put a profitable price on it."

9. Initial failures with antibodies in the biotechnology sector limited investor confidence in the field at large. With the registration of an increasing number of new therapeutic antibodies, this will now surely change.

Regulatory Issues for Antibodies

All pharmaceutical products are subject to regulations that ensure safety, efficacy, consistency, and stability of a drug. This guides both the manufacturing process that is performed under conditions of good manufacturing practice (GMP) and the nature of the clinical studies that are required to enable the drug to be licensed for use. Compliance with these regulations requires a substantial financial commitment, and this does impose constraints on the number of therapeutic antibodies that can emerge into routine clinical practice.

The clinical studies required for a drug to be granted a product license involve three phases. Phase I studies are required to provide an initial assessment of safety and to ascertain some of the pharmacologic features of the drug. Phase II studies are designed to provide further safety data and to obtain some information on efficacy based on established endpoints and indices of disease activity. Ideally, comparison with placebo in double-blinded, randomized control studies provides the most convincing data. Phase III studies are designed to demonstrate clear-cut benefit of a drug in appropriately selected patient groups. Attention is paid to appropriate comparisons with patient groups receiving either placebo or established drugs. Long-term efficacy and safety can also be evaluated during these trials.

Features of Biologics and Antibodies That Make Them Likely to Become Drugs

All of the above factors lead to the obvious conclusion that, for any new biologic product to be developed into the clinical arena, one requires the following:

1. Clear-cut demonstration of therapeutic (safety and efficacy) superiority over conventional agents, either alone or in synergy with other agents.
2. Evidence that the effects can be controlled and therapy suspended when desirable (with implications, say, for gene therapy).
3. Simplicity and economy in production and use will have an advantage.
4. Cost effectiveness of the therapy (which is increasingly becoming a major issue to be considered by health providers).
5. Elimination of any immunogenicity problem, to enable repeated usage, if required.
6. Evidence that short-term therapy can give long-term benefit (if pharmaceutical companies find a way to put a price on such treatments!).
7. Opportunism, single-mindedness, good sense, and good luck in championing a product through to final registration.

Some Clinical Highlights

It was not the intention of the authors to review the numerous clinical studies that have been performed with antibodies. We will give examples that emphasize certain themes only.

Immunosuppression

Autoimmune Disease

Vasculitis. Certain autoimmune diseases, such as Wegener's granulomatosis, have a relentless course and become increasingly difficult to manage with current antiinflammatory and immunosuppressive regimens, eventually requiring therapy with cytotoxic agents if other agents fail. This category of diseases offers an unfortunate but ideal opportunity for assessment of immunosuppressive antibodies. The studies of Lockwood and coworkers (200) with the CD52 antibody CAMPATH-1H suggest that, for this disease, short-term therapy can give very long-term effects. Relapses can be treated by further courses of antibodies and remissions reinduced. Many patients are reported as off of virtually all drug therapy other than adrenal-maintenance doses of steroids.

Whether this can be considered therapeutic tolerance is debatable. As is the case for many lympholytic regimens, CD4 T-cell reconstitution into the peripheral blood is very slow, and so the overall level of immunocompetence of the immune system may possibly be diminished. This is not, however, reflected in the rate of significant infections in such patients.

Rheumatoid Arthritis. Rheumatoid arthritis has long been a major target for the pharmaceutical industry. Very few biologic agents, including antibodies, have demonstrated the efficacy of some of the more conventional small drugs, although many such studies were possible only in patients who had failed on other disease-modifying drugs. The demonstration that TNF-α is a major proinflammatory cyokine in this disease has led to studies designed to neutralize TNF-α activity with either antibody or fusion proteins of immunoglobulin with TNF-α receptors (201,202). Indices of disease activity show clear-cut medium-term benefit. Recurrence of disease could also be managed by repeat treatment.

The outstanding question is whether anti-TNF therapy can actually control the erosive aspect of the disease process. There are opportunities for new synergistic combinations between this agent and other biologics that may target different aspects of disease pathophysiology to ensure control of cartilage erosion.

It may well be that other biologic agents could be more effective if tested at an earlier stage of the disease process, but ethical constraints limit their evaluation. There is a need to define a poor-prognosis subgroup of patients, who might benefit from experimental intervention at an earlier stage, even at disease presentation.

Multiple Sclerosis. Multiple sclerosis is another disease offering a challenge to the development of new therapeutics. Here, the important question has been how one can demonstrate benefit without having to complete large clinical trials over long periods. The development of modern imaging techniques has provided surrogate endpoints that can score the number of acute inflammatory lesions as evidence of therapeutic benefit (203). The measures of clinical improvement may not necessarily reflect the efficacy of an immunosuppressive drug—especially in progressive stages of the disease—either because old damage may be irreversible and hard to repair, or because there may be aspects of the disease progression that do not depend solely on immunology.

Thus far, the applications of antibodies or other biologic strategies to this disease have not been impressive enough to represent breakthroughs.

Organ Transplantation

Antibodies have been widely investigated in organ transplantation, both as prophylactics and as therapeutics to reverse rejection. The justification for searching for new agents is that, although current drug immunosuppression is effective in the short term, the survival of grafts in the long term is poor. Chronic rejection still poses the major challenge to immunosuppressive therapy.

Prophylaxis. The philosophy behind improved prophylactic therapy is that the early events in the life of a graft influence its long-term fate. These early events probably begin from the very time the graft is put in place, with ischemia–reperfusion injury and direct vascular damage as starting a process that may smolder but eventually become uncontrollable. In addition, antibodies and strategies aimed at preventing such very early damage may have great impact in both allogeneic and xeno-transplantation.

Any reduction of acute rejection episodes is also considered beneficial, both in reducing the risk of chronic rejection and of sparing the use of steroids, with all of their attendant side effects.

Because renal transplant patients currently require life-long immunosuppressive therapy, cost issues are becoming very important. The addition of new biologics (such as anti–IL-2R antibodies) to current immunosuppressive regimens may reduce the incidence of acute rejection episodes beyond that achieved by the conventional agents, but any biologic that obviated the need for other drugs would have a significant advantage.

It is of great interest that a short course of treatment with an antibody to CD40L was able to permit long-term engraftment of mismatched kidney grafts in primates without recourse to other drug therapy (204). This finding provides some optimism for the future, as it fulfils some of the predictions from the many rodent studies showing that short term therapy can give long-term tolerance.

Rejection Reversal. OKT3, the first licensed murine antibody, has proven very effective at reversing episodes of acute rejection, even those refractory to steroids. The major disadvantage of its use has been the cytokine-release syndrome, which results from triggering through the T-cell receptor complex, following the interaction of the antibody Fc region with FcRs on a variety of cell types. Elimination of the cytokine release syndrome would greatly enhance the utility of anti-CD3 antibodies, and even expand their use within the area of autoimmune diseases.

As previously mentioned, a number of anti-CD3 antibodies have now been humanized and mutated to abolish FcR binding and, consequently, their propensity for cyokine release. Such agents have been shown to be less immunogenic and less toxic and should now replace the murine form in the clinic (82,205).

Cardiovascular Disease

Undoubtedly, one of the major success stories of antibody therapeutics has been the demonstration that acute administration of a chimeric antibody to the gpIIb/IIIa receptor on platelets is of benefit in reducing the complications of ischemia–reperfusion injury in angioplasty and of myocardial infarction (206,207). The immunogenicity of the antibody in some patients suggests that improvements are needed if repeated retreatment is to be optimal.

Cancer Therapy

The relative accessibility of leukemias and lymphomas to antibodies has encouraged numerous trials with native as well as conjugated antibodies. With unconjugated antibodies, notable responses to therapy have been obtained with the humanized CD52 antibody CAMPATH-1H in chronic B-cell leukemia and prolymphocytic T-cell leukemia (208–210), and with a CD20 antibody in non-Hodgkin's lymphoma and postlymphoproliferative disease (211,212). Why these individual antibodies should be somewhat selective for the B-cell leukemias they kill is unclear, as the target antigens exist on all B cells. The possibility exists that, in addition to natural effector mechanisms, these antibodies recruit distinct apoptotic processes that are only available in subsets of B-cell leukemias. In one subset of leukemia, the adult T-cell leukemia, a CD25 antibody (anti-Tac) was able to induce responses in a third of the treated patients (213).

In solid tumors, a major intellectual breakthrough seemed to emerge in the use of the murine antibody 17-1A, which is a tumor-associated antigen in colorectal cancer. By conducting a phase II study in patients with minimal residual disease, Riethmuller and colleagues (214) were able to show clinical benefit and objective evidence of reduced incidence of micrometastases. This study highlights the importance of exploiting antibodies when tumor cells are most accessible and as adjuvant therapy after, say, surgical removal of, or radiotherapy to, the main tumor mass.

Studies with toxin conjugates have also shown efficacy, although the toxicity from endothelial damage resulting in a vascular leak syndrome remains an obstacle requiring resolution (215,216). For the present, this may limit the utility of immunotoxins to localized tumor masses in closed spaces, until such a time as toxicity is engineered out or prevented.

The dose-limiting factor for radioimmunoconjugates has been toxicity for the hemopoietic system, and, again, responses to some forms of leukemia and/or lymphoma have been encouraging (217,218). For some solid tumors, there have also been notable responses in which radioconjugates have been given as locoregional administration or into closed cavities (219).

CONCLUDING REMARKS

There can be little doubt that monoclonal antibodies will find their place in therapeutics. The affinities of interaction of antibodies with their target antigens, and their long half-lives may be hard to match with small drugs derived from synthetic chemistry approaches.

Perhaps most important of all is the fact that monoclonal antibodies have been crucial in helping to define the pathophysiology of a number of disease processes. With this knowledge, it has become much easier to define the most appropriate targets for rational intervention.

The use of short-term therapy with antibodies to obtain modulatory long-term effects on the immune system must remain one of the most exciting and challenging prospects for the future of antibody therapy. There can be little doubt that this will have an impact on management of autoimmune diseases and on acceptance of transplants.

In the area of cancer therapeutics, one has to be impressed with the ingenious and dedicated approaches that are being taken. There are major challenges in persuading tumor cells to die or to stop growing, but we can be confident that antibodies will surely have an increasing part to play in the armamentarium of the oncologist.

REFERENCES

1. Cobbold SP, Qin S, Leong LYW, Martin G, Waldmann H. Reprogramming the immune system for peripheral tolerance with CD4 and CD8 monoclonal antibodies. *Immunol Rev* 1992;129:165–201.
2. Coney LR, Daniel PT, Sanborn D, et al. Apoptotic cell death induced by a mouse-human anti-APO-1 chimeric antibody leads to tumor regression. *Int J Cancer* 1994;58;562–567.
3. Thome M, Schneider P, Hofmann K, et al. Viral FLICE-inhibitory proteins (FLIPs) prevent apoptosis induced by death receptors. *Nature* 1997;386:517–521.
4. Matiba B, Mariani SM, Krammer PH. The CD95 system and the death of a lymphocyte. *Semin Immunol* 1997;9:59–68.
5. Bach FH, Ferran C, Hechenleitner P, et al. Accommodation of vascularized xenografts: expression of "protective genes" by donor endothelial cells in a host Th2 cytokine environment. *Nat Med* 1997;3:196–204.
6. Weiner HL, Friedman A, Miller A, et al. Oral tolerance: immunologic mechanisms and treatment of animal and human organ-specific autoimmune diseases by oral administration of autoantigens. *Annu Rev Immunol* 1994;12:809–837.
7. Weiner HL. Oral tolerance: immune mechanisms and treatment of autoimmune diseases. *Immunol Today* 1997;18:335–343.
8. Metzler B, Wraith DC. Mucosal tolerance in a murine model of experimental autoimmune encephalomyelitis. *Ann NY Acad Sci* 1996;778:228–242.
9. Elias D, Meilin OS, Carmi S, Konen-Waisman ?, Cohen IR. Hsp60 peptide therapy of NOD mouse diabetes induces a Th2 cytokine burst and downregulates autoimmunity to various β-cell antigens. *Diabetes* 1997;46:758–764.
10. Cobbold, SP, Martin G, Qin S, Waldmann H. Monoclonal antibodies to promote marrow engraftment and tissue graft tolerance. *Nature* 1986;323;164–166.
11. Leong LYW, Qin S, Cobbold SP, Waldmann H. Classical transplantation tolerance in the adult. The interaction between myeloablation and immunosuppression. *Eur J Immunol* 1992;22:2825–2830.
12. Sharabi Y, Sachs, DH. Mixed chimerism and permanent specific transplantation tolerance induced by a nonlethal preparative regimen. *J Exp Med* 1989;169:493.
13. Sharabi Y, Abraham VS, Sykes M, Sachs DH. Mixed allogeneic chimeras prepared by a non-myeloablative regimen: requirement for chimerism to maintain tolerance. *Bone Marrow Transplant* 1996;3:191–196.
14. Waldmann H, Hale G, Cobbold S, et al. Monoclonal antibody therapy for the prevention of graft-vs.-host disease. *Hematology* 1990;22:277–293.
15. Tomita Y, Sachs DH, Khan A, Sykes M. Additional monoclonal antibody (mAB) injections can replace thymic irradiation to allow induction of mixed chimerism and tolerance in mice receiving bone marrow transplantation after conditioning with anti-T cell mABs and 3-Gy whole body irradiation. *Transplantation* 1996; 61:469–475.
16. Benjamin RJ, Waldmann H. Induction of tolerance by monoclonal antibody therapy. *Nature* 1986;320:449–451.
17. Benjamin RJ, Cobbold SP, Clark MR, Waldmann H. Tolerance of rat monoclonal antibodies: implications for serotherapy. *J Exp Med* 1986;163:1539–1552.
18. Gutstein NL, Seaman WE, Scott JH, Wofsy D. Induction of immune tolerance by administration of monoclonal antibody to L3T4. *J Immunol* 1986;137:1127–1132.
19. Carteron NL, Wofsy D, Seaman WE. Induction of immune tolerance during administration of monoclonal antibody to L3T4 does not depend on depletion of L3T4+ cells. *J Immunol* 1988;140:713–716.
20. Carteron NL, Schimenti CL, Wofsy D. Treatment of murine lupus with F(ab′)2 fragments of monoclonal antibody to L3T4. Suppression of autoimmunity does not depend on T helper cell depletion. *J Immunol* 1989;142:1470–1476.
21. Qin S, Wise MP, Cobbold SP, et al. Induction of tolerance in peripheral T cells with monoclonal antibodies. *Eur J Immunol* 1990;20:2737–2745.
22. Qin S, Cobbold SP, Tighe H, Benjamin R, Waldmann H. CD4 monoclonal antibody pairs for immunosuppression and tolerance induction. *Eur J Immunol* 1987;17:1159–1165.
23. Qin S, Cobbold S, Benjamin R, Waldmann H. Induction of classical transplantation tolerance in the adult. *J Exp Med* 1989;169:779–794.
24. Chen Z, Cobbold SP, Metcalfe S, Waldmann H. Tolerance in the mouse to MHC mismatched heart allografts, and to rat heart xenografts, using monoclonal antibodies to CD4 and CD8. *Eur J Immunol* 1992;22:805–810.
25. Cobbold SP, Martin G, Waldmann H. The induction of skin graft tolerance in MHC-mismatched or primed recipients: primed T-cells can be tolerized in the periphery with CD4 and CD8 antibodies. *Eur J Immunol* 1990;20:2747–2755.
26. Marshall SE, Cobbold SP, Davies JD, Martin GM, Phillips JM, Waldmann H. Tolerance and suppression in a primed immune system. *Transplantation* 1996;62:1614–1621.
27. Hayward AR, Shriber M, Cooke A, Waldmann H. Prevention of diabetes but not insulitis in NOD mice injected with antibody to CD4. *J Autoimmun* 1993;6:301–310.
28. Hutchings P, O'Reilly L, Parish NM, Waldmann H, Cooke A. The use of a non-depleting anti-CD4 monoclonal antibody to re-establish tolerance to b cells in NOD mice. *Eur J Immunol* 1992;22:1913–1918.
29. Parish NM, Hutchings PR, Waldmann H, Cooke A. Tolerance to IDDM induced by CD4 antibodies in nonobese diabetic mice is reversed by cyclophosphamide. *Diabetes* 1993;42:1601–1605.
30. Benjamin RJ, Quin S, Wise MP, Cobbold SP, Waldmann H. Mechanisms of monoclonal antibody-facilitated tolerance induction: a possible role for the CD4 (L3T4) and CD11a (LFA-1) molecules in self-non-self discrimination. *Eur J Immunol* 1988;8:1079–1088.

31. Isobe M, Yagita H, Okumura K, Ihara A. Specific acceptance of cardiac allograft after treatment with antibodies to ICAM-1 and LFA-1. *Science* 1992;255: 1125–1127.

32. Isobe M, Suzuki J, Yamazaki S, Sekiguchi M. Acceptance of primary skin graft after treatment with anti-intercellular adhesion molecule-1 and anti-leukocyte function-associated antigen-1 monoclonal antibodies in mice. *Transplantation* 1996;62:411–413.

33. Tran HM, Nickerson PW, Restif AC, et al. Distinct mechanisms for the induction and maintenance of allograft tolerance with CTLA-4 Fc treatment. *J. Immunol.* 1997;159:2232–2239.

34. Chavin KD, Qin L, Lin J, Yagita H, Bromberg JS. Combined anti-CD2 and anti-CD3 receptor monoclonal antibodies induce donor-specific tolerance in a cardiac transplant model. *J Immunol* 1993;151:7249–7259.

35. Krieger NR, Most D, Bromberg JS, et al. Coexistence of Th1- and Th2-type cytokine profiles in anti-CD2 monoclonal antibody-induced tolerance. *Transplantation* 1996;62:1285–1292.

36. Chatenoud L, Thervett E, Primo J, Bach JF. Anti-CD3 antibody induces long-term remission of overt autoimmunity in non-obese diabetic mice. *Proc Natl Acad Sci USA* 1994;91:123–127.

37. Lenschow DJ, Zeng Y, Thistlethwaite JR, et al. Long-term survival of xenogeneic pancreatic islet grafts induced by CTLA4Ig. *Science* 1992;57:789–792.

38. Pearson TC, Alexander DZ, Winn KJ, Linsley PS, Lowry RP, Larsen CP. Transplantation tolerance induced by CTLA4-Ig. *Transplantation* 1994;57:1701–1706.

39. Steurer W, Nickerson PW, Steele AW, Steiger J, Zheng XX, Strom TB. Ex vivo coating of islet cell allografts with murine CTLA4/Fc promotes graft tolerance. *J Immunol* 1995;155:1165–1174.

40. Bolling SF, Lin H, Wei RQ, Turka LA. Preventing allograft rejection with CTLA4IG: effect of donor-specific transfusion route or timing. *J Heart Lung Transplant* 1996;15:928–935.

41. Judge TA, Tang A, Spain LM, Deans Gratiot J, Sayegh MH, Turka LA. The in vivo mechanism of action of CTLA4Ig. *J Immunol* 1996;156:2294–2299.

42. Pearson TC, Alexander DZ, Hendrix R, et al. CTLA4-Ig plus bone marrow induces long-term allograft survival and donor specific unresponsiveness in the murine model. Evidence for hematopoietic chimerism. *Transplantation* 1996;61:997–1002.

43. Wise MP, Benjamin R, Qin S, Cobbold S, Waldmann H. Tolerance induction in the peripheral immune system. In: Vogel H, Alt F, eds. *Molecular mechanisms of immunological self-recognition.* New York: Academic Press, 1997:149–155.

44. Scully R, Qin S, Cobbold SP, Waldmann H. Mechanisms in CD4 antibody-mediated transplantation tolerance: kinetics of induction, antigen dependency and role of regulatory T cells. *Eur J Immunol* 1994;27:2383–2392.

45. Qin S, Cobbold SP, Pope H, Elliott J, Kioussis D, Waldmann H. Infectious transplantation tolerance. *Science* 1993;259:974–977.

46. Davies JD, Martin G, Phillips J, Marshall SE, Cobbold SP, Waldmann H. T cell regulation in adult transplantation tolerance. *J Immunol* 1996;157:529–533.

47. Yin D, Fathman GD. CD4+ suppressor cells block allotransplant rejection. *J Immunol* 1995;154:6339–6345.

48. Cobbold SP, Adams E, Marshall SE, Davies JD, Waldmann H. Mechanisms of peripheral tolerance and suppression induced by monoclonal antibodies to CD4 and CD8. *Immunol Rev* 1996;149.5–33.

49. Chen ZK, Cobbold SP, Waldmann H, Metcalfe S. Amplification of natural regulatory immune mechanisms for transplantation tolerance. *Transplantation* 1996; 62:1200–1206.

50. Bemelman F, Honey K, Adams E, Cobbold SP, Waldmann H. Bone marrow transplantation induces either clonal deletion or infectious disease tolerance depending on the dose. *J Immunol* 1998;160:2645–2648.

51. Davies JD, Leong LYW, Mellor A, Cobbold SP, Waldmann H. T-cell suppression in transplantation tolerance through linked recognition. *J Immunol* 1996;156: 3602–3607.

52. Waldmann H, Cobbold S. How may immunosuppression lead to tolerance? The war analogy. In: Banchereau J, Dodet B, Schwartz R, Trannoy E, eds. *Immune tolerance.* Paris: Elsevier Science, 1996:221–227.

53. Wood KJ. The induction of tolerance to alloantigens using MHC class I molecules. *Curr Opin Immunol* 1993;5:759–762.

54. Saitovitch D, Morris PJ, Wood KJ. Recipient cells expressing single donor MHC locus products can substitute for donor-specific transfusion in the induction of transplantation tolerance when retreatment is combined with anti-CD4 monoclonal antibody. Evidence for a vital role of CD4+ T cells in the induction of tolerance to class I molecules. *Transplantation* 1996;61:1532–1536.

55. Waldmann H, Or R, Hale G, et al. Elimination of graft versus host disease by in vitro depletion of alloreactive lymphocytes using a monoclonal rat anti-human lymphocyte antibody (CAMPATH-1). *Lancet* 1984;2:483–486.

56. Hale G, Waldmann H. For CAMPATH users CAMPATH 1 monoclonal antibodies in bone marrow transplantation. *Hematotherapy* 1994;3:15–31.

57. Reisner Y, Martelli MF. Bone marrow transplantation across HLA barriers by increasing the number of transplanted cell. *Immunol Today* 1995;16:437–440.

58. O'Reilly RJ, Lacerda JF, Lucas KG, Rosenfield NS, Small TN, Papadopoulos EB. Adoptive cell therapy with donor lymphocytes for EBV-associated lymphomas developing after allogeneic marrow transplants. *Important Adv Oncol* 1996;149–161.

59. MacKinnon S, Papadopoulos EP, Carabasi MH, et al. Adoptive immunotherapy evaluating escalating dose of donor leukocytes for relapse of chronic myeloid leukaemia following bone marrow transplantation: separation of graft-versus-leukaemia responses from graft-versus-host disease. *Blood* 1995;86:1261–1268.

60. Waldmann H, Cobbold S, Hale G. What can be done to prevent graft-versus-host disease? *Curr Opin Immunol* 1994;6:777–783.

61. Holyoake TL, Alcorn MJ. CD34+ positive haemopoietic cells: biology and clinical applications. *Blood Rev* 1994;8:113–124.

62. Korbling M. Autologous and allogeneic blood stem cell transplantation: potential advantage of blood-over marrow-derived stem cell grafts. *Cancer Invest* 15: 127–137.

63. Mielcarek M, Torok Storb B. Phenotype and engraftment potential of cytokine-mobilized peripheral blood mononuclear cells. *Curr Opin Hematol* 1997;16P: 437–440.

64. Ward ES, Ghetie V. The effector functions of immunoglobulins: implications for therapy. *Ther Immunol* 1995;2:77–94.

65. Clark MC. One IgG receptor, two different functions. *Lancet* 1996;347:1104.

66. Ghetie V, Hubbard JG, Kim JK, et al. Abnormally short serum half-lives of IgG in b2-microglobulin deficient mice. *Eur J Immunol* 1996;26:690–696.

67. Ghetie V, Popov S, Borvak J, et al. Increasing the serum persistence of an IgG fragment by random mutagenesis. *Nat Biotech* 1997;15:637–640.

68. Junghans RP, Anderson CL. The protection receptor for IgG catabolism is the b2-microglobulin containing neonatal intestinal transport receptor. *Proc Natl Acad Sci USA* 1996;93:5512–5516.

69. Capon DJ, Chamow SM, Mordenti J, Marsters SA. Designing CD4 immunoadhesins for AIDS therapy. *Nature* 1989;337:525–530.

70. Duncan AR, Winter G. The binding site for C1q on IgG. *Nature* 1988;332:738–740.

71. Duncan AR, Woof JM, Partridge LJ, et al. Localization of the binding site for the high affinity Fc receptor on IgG. *Nature* 1988;332:563–564.

72. Jefferis R, Lund J, Pound J. Molecular definition of interaction sites on human IgG for Fc receptors. *Mol Immunol* 1990;27:1237–1240.

73. Lund J, Winter G, Jones PT, et al. Human FcgRI and FcgRII interact with distinct but overlapping sites in human IgG. *J Immunol* 1991;147:2657–2662.

74. Sarmay G, Lund J, Rozsnyay Z, et al. Mapping and comparison of the interaction sites on the Fc region of IgG responsible for triggering antibody dependent cellular cytotoxicity (ADCC) through different types of human Fcg receptor. *Mol Immunol* 1992;29:633–639.

75. Bindon CI, Hale G, Bruggemann M, et al. Human monoclonal IgG isotypes differ in complement activating function at the level of C4 as well as C1q. *J Exp Med* 1988;168:127–142.

76. Michaelsen TE, Garred P, Aase A. Human IgG subclass pattern of inducing complement mediated cytolysis depends on antigen concentration and to a lesser extent on epitope patchiness, antibody affinity and complement concentration. *Eur J Immunol* 1991;21:11–16.

77. Bruggemann M, Willilams GT, Bindon CI, et al. Comparison of the effector functions of human immunoglobulins using a matched set of chimeric antibodies. *J Exp Med* 1987;166:1351–1361.

78. Adair JR. Engineering antibodies for therapy. *Immunol Rev* 1992;130:5–40.

79. Greenwood J, Clark M, Waldmann H. Structural motifs involved in human IgG antibody effector functions. *Eur J Immunol* 1993;5:1098–1104.

80. Tao MH, Morrison SL. Studies of aglycosylated chimeric mouse human IgG: role of carbohydrate in the structure and effector functions mediated by the human IgG constant region. *J Immunol* 1989;143:2595–2601.

81. Lund J, Tanaka T, Takahashi N, et al. A protein structural change in aglycosylated IgG3 relates with loss of huFcgRI and huFcgRIII binding and/or activation. *Mol Immunol* 1990;27:1145–1153.

82. Bolt S, Routledge E, Lloyd I, et al. The generation of a humanized, non-mitogenic CD3 monoclonal antibody which retains in vitro immunosuppressive properties. *Eur J Immunol* 1993;23:403–411.

83. Dyer MJS, Hale G, Hayhoe FGJ, Waldmann H. Effects of CAMPATH-1 Antibodies in vivo in patients with lymphoid malignancies: influence of antibody isotype. *Blood* 1989;73:1431–1439.

84. Isaacs JD, Clark MR, Greenwood J, Waldmann H. Therapy with monoclonal antibodies. An in vivo model for the assessment of therapeutic potential. *J Immunol* 1992;148:3062–3071.

85. Maloney DG, Brown S, Czerwinski DK, et al. Monoclonal anti-idiotype antibody therapy of B-cell lymphoma: the addition of a short course of chemotherapy does not interfere with the antitumor effect nor prevent the emergence of idiotype-negative variant cells. *Blood* 1992;80:1502–1510.

86. Stevenson GT, Glennie MJ, Kank S. Chemically engineered chimeric and multi-Fab antibodies. In: Clark M, ed. *Protein engineering of antibody molecules for prophylactic and therapeutic applications in man.* Nottingham, UK: Academic Titles, 1992:127–141.

87. Xia MQ, Tone M, Packman L, et al. Characterization of the CAMPATH-1 (CDw52) antigen: biochemical analysis and cDNA cloning reveal an unusually small peptide backbone. *Eur J Immunol* 1991;21:1677–1684.

88. Clark M, Bindon C, Dyer M, et al. The improved lytic function and in vivo efficacy of monovalent monoclonal CD3 antibodies. *Eur J Immunol* 1989; 19:381–388.

89. Routledge EG, Lloyd I, Gorman S, Clark M, Waldmann H. A humanized monovalent CD3 antibody which can activate homologous complement. *Eur J Immunol* 1991;21:2717–2725.

90. Hughes-Jones NC, Gorrick BD, Howard JC. The mechanism of synergistic complement lysis of rat red cells by monoclonal IgG antibodies. *Eur J Immunol* 1983;13:635–641.

91. Bindon CI, Hale G, Hughes-Jones N, Gorick B, Waldmann H. Synergistic complement lysis by monoclonal antibodies to the human leukocyte common antigen

requires both the classical and alternative pathways. *Mol Immunol* 1987;24: 587–594.

92. Ghetie MA, Podar EM, Ilgen A, Gordon BE, Uhr JW, Vitetta ES. Homodimerization of tumor-reactive monoclonal antibodies markedly increases their ability to induce growth arrest or apoptosis of tumor cells. *Proc Natl Acad Sci USA* 1997;94:7509–7514.

93. Racila E, Hsueh R, Marches R, et al. Tumor dormancy and cell signaling: antimu-induced apoptosis in human B-lymphoma cells is not caused by an APO-1-APO-1 ligand interaction. *Proc Natl Acad Sci USA* 1996;3:2165–2168.

94. Davies DR, Padlan EA, Sheriff S. Antibody-antigen complexes. *Annu Rev Biochem* 1990;59:439–448.

95. Wilson IA, Stanfield RL, Rini JM, et al. Structural aspects of antibodies and antibody-antigen complexes. *Ciba Found Symp* 1991;159:13–39.

96. Wu TT, Kabat EA. An analysis of the sequences of the variable regions of Bence Jones and myeloma light chains and their implications for antibody complementarity. *J Exp Med* 1970;132:211–250.

97. Wilson IA, Stanfield RL. Antibody-antigen interactions: new structures and new conformational changes. *Curr Opin Struct Biol* 1994;3:857–867.

98. Rini JM, Schulze-Gahmen U, Wilson IA. Structural evidence for induced fit as a mechanism for antibody-antigen recognition. *Science* 1992;255:959–965.

99. Wu TT, Johnson G, Kabat EA. Length distribution of CDRH3 in antibodies. *Proteins* 1993;16:1–7.

100. Searle SJ, Pedersen JT, Henry AH, et al. Antibody structure and function. In: Borrebaeck CAK, ed. *Antibody engineering.* 2nd ed. Oxford: Oxford University Press, 1995:3–51.

101. Steipe B, Pluckthun A, Huber R. Refined crystal structure of a recombinant immunoglobulin domain and a complementarity-determining region 1-grafted mutant. *J Mol Biol* 1992;225:739–753.

102. Bajorath J, Novotny J. Model building of antibody combining sites. *Ther Immunol* 1995;2:95–103.

103. Gilliland LK, Norris NA, Marquardt H, et al. Rapid and reliable cloning of antibody V regions and generation of recombinant single chain antibody fragments. *Tissue Antigens* 1996;47:1–20.

104. Hayden MS, Gilliland LK, Ledbetter JA. Antibody engineering. *Curr Opin Immunol* 1997;9:201–212.

105. Orlandi R, Gussow DH, Jones PT, Winter G. Cloning of immunoglobin variable domains for expression by the polymerase chain reaction. *Proc Natl Acad Sci USA* 1989;86:3833–3837.

106. Babcook JS, Leslie KB, Olsen OA, et al. A novel strategy for generating monoclonal antibodies from single, isolated lymphocytes producing antibodies of defined specificities. *Proc Natl Acad Sci USA* 1996;93:7843–7848.

107. McCafferty J, Griffiths AD, Winter G, Chiswell DJ. Phage antibodies: filamentous phage displaying antibody variable domains. *Nature* 1990;348:552–554.

108. Clackson T, Hoogenboom HR, Griffiths AD, Winter G. Making antibody fragments using phage display libraries. *Nature* 1991;352:624–628.

109. Vaughan TJ, Williams AJ, Pritchard K, et al. Human antibodies with subnanomolar affinities isolated from a large non-immunized phage display library. *Nat Biotech* 1996;14:309–314.

110. Foote J, Eisen HN. Kinetic and affinity limits on antibodies produced during immune responses. *Proc Natl Acad Sci USA* 1995;92:1254–1256.

111. Griffiths AD, Williams SC, Hartley O, et al. Isolation of high-affinity human antibodies directly from large synthetic repertoires. *EMBO J* 1994;13:3245–3260.

112. Barbas CF III, Burton DR. Selection and evolution of high-affinity human antiviral antibodies. *Trends Biotechnol* 1996;14:230–234.

113. Barbas CF III. Synthetic human antibodies. *Nat Med* 1995;1:837–839.

114. Marks JD, Griffiths AD, Malmquist M, et al. By-passing immunization: building high-affinity human antibodies by chain shuffling. *Biotechnology* 1992;10: 779–783.

115. Yelton DE, Rosok MJ, Cruz G, et al. Affinity maturation of the BR96 anti-carcinoma antibody by codon-based mutagenesis. *J Immunol* 1995;155:1994–2004.

116. Barbas CF III, Hu D, Dunlop N, et al. In vitro evolution of a neutralizing human antibody to human immunodeficiency virus type 1 to enhance affinity and broaden strain cross-reactivity. *Proc Natl Acad Sci USA* 1994;91:3809–3813.

117. Yang WP, Green K, Pinz-Sweeney S, et al. CDR walking mutagenesis for the affinity maturation of a potent human anti-HIV-1 antibody into the picomolar range. *J Mol Biol* 1995;254:392–403.

118. Hawkins RE, Russell SJ, Winter G. Selection of phage antibodies by binding affinity: mimicking affinity maturation. *J Mol Biol* 1992;226:889–896.

119. Gram H, Marconi LA, Barbas CF III, et al. In vitro selection and affinity maturation of antibodies from a naive combinatorial immunoglobulin library. *Proc Natl Acad Sci USA* 1992;89:3576–3580.

120. Low NM, Holliger PH, Winter G. Mimicking somatic hypermutation: affinity maturation of antibodies displayed on bacteriophage using a bacterial mutator strain. *J Mol Biol* 1996;260:359–368.

121. Greenwood J, Clark M, Waldmann H. Structural motifs involved in human IgG antibody effector functions. *Eur J Immunol* 1993;5:1098–1104.

122. Shopes B. A genetically engineered human IgG mutant with enhanced cytolytic activity. *J Immunol* 1992;148:2918–2922.

123. Greenwood J, Gorman SD, Routledge EG, Lloyd IS, Waldmann H. Engineering multiple domain forms of the therapeutic antibody CAMPATH-1H; effects on complement lysis. *Ther Immunol* 1994;1:247–265.

124. Carayannopoulos L, Capra JD. Immunoglobulins: structure and function. In: Paul WE, ed. *Fundamental immunology.* 3rd ed. New York: Raven Press, 1993: 283–314.

125. Jefferis R, Lund J, Goodall M. Recognition sites on human IgG for Fc γ receptors: the role of glycosylation. *Immunol Lett* 1995;44:111–117.

126. Tao MH, Morrison SL. Studies of aglycosylated chimeric mouse human IgG: role of carbohydrate in the structure and effector functions mediated by the human IgG constant region. *J Immunol* 1989;143:2595–2601.

127. Hobbs SM, Jackson LE, Hoadley J. Interaction of aglycosyl immunoglobulins with the IgG Fc transport receptor from neonatal gut: comparison of deglycosylation by tunicamycin treatment and genetic engineering. *Mol Immunol* 1992;29:949–956.

128. Brambell FWR, Hemmings WA, Morris IG. A theoretical model of gamma-globulin catabolism. *Nature* 1964;203:1352–1355.

129. Kim JK, Tsen MF, Ghetie V, Ward ES. Localization of the site of the murine IgG1 molecule that is involved in binding to the murine intestinal Fc receptor. *Eur J Immunol* 1994;24:2429–2434.

130. Medesan C, Radu C, Kim JK, et al. Localization of the site of the IgG molecule that regulates maternofetal transmission in mice. *Eur J Immunol* 1996;26: 2533–2536.

131. Medesan C, Matesoi D, Radu C, et al. Delineation of the amino acid residues involved in transcytosis and catabolism of mouse IgG1. *J Immunol* 1997;158: 2211–2217.

132. Bird RE, Hardman KD, Jacobson JW, et al. Single-chain antigen-binding proteins. *Science* 1998;242:423–426.

133. Huston JS, Levinson D, Mudgett-Hunter M, et al. Protein engineering of antibody binding sites: recovery of specific activity in an anti-digoxin single-chain Fv analogue produced in Escherichia coli. *Proc Natl Acad Sci USA* 1988;85: 5879–5883.

134. Winberg G, Grosmaire LS, Klussman K, et al. Surface expression of CD28 single chain Fv for costimulation by tumour cells. *Immunol Rev* 1996;153:6–14.

135. Francisco JA, Gilliland LK, Stebbins MR, et al. Activity of a single-chain immunotoxin that selectively kills lymphoma and other B-lineage cells expressing the CD40 antigen. *Cancer Res* 1995;55:3099–3104.

136. Siegall CB. Targeted therapy of carcinomas using BR96 sFv-PE40, a single chain immunotoxin that binds to the Le^y antigen. *Semin Cancer Biol* 1995; 6:289–295.

137. Demanet C, Brissinck J, De Jonge J, Thielemans K. Bispecific antibody-mediated immunotherapy of the BCL$_1$ lymphoma: increased efficacy with multiple injections and CD28-induced costimulation. *Blood* 1996;87:4390–4398.

138. Hayden MS, Linsley PS, Gayle MG, et al. Single chain mono- and bispecific antibody derivatives with novel biological properties and anti-tumor activity from a COS cell transient expression system. *Ther Immunol* 1994;1:3–15.

139. Hayden MS, Grosmaire LS, Norris NA, et al. Costimulation by CD28 sFv expressed on the tumor cell surface or as a soluble bispecific molecule targeted to the L6 carcinoma antigen. *Tissue Antigens* 1996;48:242–254.

140. Jost CR, Titus JA, Kurucz I, Segal DM. A single-chain bispecific Fv$_2$ molecule produced in mammalian cells redirects lysis by activated CTL. *Mol Immunol* 1996;33:211–219.

141. Kurucz I, Titus JA, Jost CR, et al. Retargeting of CTL by an efficiently refolded bispecific single-chain Fv dimer produced in bacteria. *J Immunol* 1995;154: 4576–4582.

142. Mack M, Riethmuller G, Kufer P. A small bispecific antibody construct expressed as a functional single-chain molecule with high tumor cell cytotoxicity. *Proc Natl Acad Sci USA* 1995;92:7021–7025.

143. Weiner LM, Clark JI, Davey M, et al. Phase I trial of 2B1, a bispecific monoclonal antibody targeting c-erbB-2 and FcgRIII. *Cancer Res* 1995;55: 4586–4593.

144. Zhu Z, Lewis GD, Carter P. Engineering high-affinity humanized anti-p185^{HER2}/anti-CD3 bispecific F(ab′)$_2$ for efficient lysis of p185^{HER2} overexpressing tumor cells. *Int J Cancer* 1995;62:319–324.

145. Duan L, Bagasra O, Laughlin MA, et al. Potent inhibition of human immunodeficiency virus type 1 replication by an intracellular anti-Rev single chain antibody. *Proc Natl Acad Sci USA* 1994;91:5075–5079.

146. Deshane J, Cabrera G, Grim JE, et al. Targeted eradication of ovarian cancer mediated by intracelluar expression of anti-erb-2 single-chain antibody. *Gynecol Oncol* 1995;59:8–14.

147. Deshane J, Siegal GP, Alvarez RD, et al. Targeted tumor killing via an intracellular antibody against erbB-2. *J Clin Invest* 1995;96:2980–2989.

148. Biocca S, Cattaneo A. Intracellular immunization: antibody targeting to subcellular compartments. *Trends Cell Biol* 1995;5:248–252.

149. Sabzevari H, Gillies SD, Mueller BM, et al. A recombinant antibody-interleukin 2 fusion protein suppresses growth of hepatic human neuroblastoma metastases in severe combined immunodeficiency mice. *Proc Natl Acad Sci USA* 1994;91: 9626–9630.

150. Staerz UD, Kanagawa O, Bevan MJ. Hybrid antibodies can target sites for attack by T cells. *Nature* 1985;314:628–631.

151. Clark MR, Waldmann H. T cell killing of target cells induced by hybrid ntibodies: a comparison of two bispecific monoclonal antibodies. *J Natl Cancer Inst* 1987;79:1393–1401.

152. Gilliland LK, Clark MR, Waldmann H. Universal bispecific antibody for targeting tumour cells for destruction by cytotoxic T cells. *Proc Natl Acad Sci USA* 1988;85:7719–7723.

153. Perez P, Hoffman RW, Shaw S, et al. Specific targeting of cytotoxic T cells by anti-T3 linked to anti-target cell antibody. *Nature* 1985:316:354–356.

154. Waldmann TA. Monoclonal antibodies in diagnosis and therapy. *Science* 1991;252:1657–1662.

155. Carter P, Ridgway J, Zhu Z. Toward the production of bispecific antibody fragments for clinical applications. *J Hematother* 1995;4:463–470.

156. Holliger P, Winter G. Engineering bispecific antibodies. *Curr Opin Biotechnol* 1993;4:446–449.

157. Hoogenboom HR. Mix and match: building manifold binding sites. *Nat Biotechnol* 1997;15:125–126.

158. Holliger P, Prospero T, Winter G. "Diabodies": small bivalent and bispecific antibody fragments. *Proc Natl Acad Sci USA* 1993;90:6444–6448.

159. McGuinness BT, Walter G, FitzGerald K, et al. Phage diabody repertoires for selection of large numbers of bispecific antibody fragments. *Nat Biotechnol* 1996;14:1149–1154.

160. Pack P, Pluckthun A. Miniantibodies: use of amphipathic helices to produce functional, flexibly linked dimeric Fv fragments with high avidity in Escherischia coli. *Biochemistry* 1992;31:1579–1584.

161. Ridgway JBB, Presta LG, Carter P. "Knobs-into-holes" engineering of antibody CH3 domains for heavy chain heterodimerization. *Protein Eng* 1996;9:617–621.

162. Coloma MJ, Morrison SL. Design and production of novel tetravalent bispecific antibodies. *Nat Biotechnol* 1997;15:159–163.

163. Pack P, Muller K, Zahn R, Plunkthun A. Tetravalent miniantibodies with high avidity assembling in Escherichia coli. *J Mol Biol* 1995;246:28–34.

164. Cabilly S, Riggs AD, Pande H, et al. Generation of antibody activity from immunoglobulin polypeptide chains produced in Escherichia coli. *Proc Natl Acad Sci USA* 1984;81:3273–3277.

165. Boss MA, Kenton JH, Wood CR, Emtage JS. Assembly of functional antibodies from immunoglobulin heavy and light chains synthesized in E. coli. *Nucleic Acids Res* 1984;12:3791–3806.

166. Guise AD, West SM, Chaudhuri JB. Protein folding in vivo and renaturation of recombinant proteins from inclusion bodies. *Mol Biotechnol* 1996;6:53–64.

167. Huston JS, George AJT, Tai M-S, et al. Single-chain Fv design and production by preparative folding. In: Borrebaeck CAK, ed. *Antibody engineering.* 2nd ed. Oxford: Oxford University Press, 1995:185–209.

168. Ge L, Knappick, Pack P, et al. Expressing antibodies in E. coli. In: Borrebaeck CAK, ed. *Antibody engineering.* 2nd ed. Oxford: Oxford University Press, 1995:229–243.

169. Isaacs, JD. The antiglobulin response to therapeutic antibodies. *Semin Immunol* 1990;2:449–456.

170. Bertram JH, Gill PS, Levine AM, et al. Monoclonal antibody T101 in T cell malignancies: a clinical, pharmacokinetic and immunologic correlation. *Blood* 1986;68:752–761.

171. Hricik PR, Zarconi J, Schulak JA. Influence of low-dose cyclosporine on the outcome of treatment with OKT3 for acute renal allograft rejection. *Transplantation* 1989;47:272–277.

172. Riechmann L, Clark M, Waldmann H, Winter G. Reshaping human antibodies for therapy. *Nature* 1988;332:323–327.

173. Verhoeyen M, Milstein C, Winter G. Reshaping human antibodies: grafting an anti-lysozyme activity. *Science* 1988;239:1534–1536.

174. Gussow D, Seemann G. Humanization of monoclonal antibodies. *Methods Enzymol* 1991;203:99–121.

175. Queen C, Schneider WP, Selick HE, et al. A humanized antibody that binds to the interleukin-2 receptor. *Proc Natl Acad Sci USA* 1989;86:10029–10033.

176. Roguska MA, Pedersen JT, Henry AH, et al. A comparison of two murine monoclonal antibodies humanized by CDR-grafting and variable domain resurfacing. *Protein Eng* 1996;9:895–904.

177. Roguska MA, Pedersen JT, Keddy CA, et al. Humanization of murine monoclonal antibodies through variable domain resurfacing. *Proc Natl Acad Sci USA* 1994;91:969–973.

178. James K, Bell GI. Human monoclonal antibody production: current status and future prospects. *J Immunol Methods* 1987;100:5–40.

179. Marks JD, Hoogenboom HR, Bonnert TP, et al. By passing immunization. Human antibodies from V gene libraries displayed on phage. *J Mol Biol* 1991;222:581–597.

180. Bruggemann M, Caskey HM, Teale C, et al. A repertoire of monoclonal antibodies with human heavy-chains from transgenic mice. *Proc Natl Acad Sci USA* 1989;86:6709–6713.

181. Jakobovits A. Production of fully human antibodies by transgenic mice. *Curr Opin Biotechnol* 1995;6:561–566.

182. Bruggemann MS, Neuberger MS. Strategies for expressing human antibody repertoires in transgenic mice. *Immunol Today* 1996;17:391–397.

183. Lubin I, Segall H, Marcus H, et al. Engraftment of human peripheral blood lymphocytes in normal strains of mice. *Blood* 1994;83:2368–2381.

184. Isaacs JD, Watts RA, Hazleman BL, et al. Humanized monoclonal antibody therapy for rheumatoid arthritis. *Lancet* 1992;340:748–752.

185. Lockwood CM, Thiru S, Isaacs JD, et al. Long-term remission of intractable systemic vasculitis with monoclonal antibody therapy. *Lancet* 1993;341:1620–1622.

186. Isaacs JD, Waldmann H. Helplessness as a strategy for avoiding antiglobulin responses to therapeutic monoclonal antibodies. *Ther Immunol* 1994;1:303–312.

187. Wawrzynczak EJ. *Antibody therapy.* Oxford, UK: Bios Scientific Publishers, 1995.

188. Marasco WA. Intrabodies: turning the humoral immune system outside in for intracellular immunization. *Gene Ther* 1997;4:11–15.

189. Richardson JH, Marasco WA. Intracellular antibodies: development and therapeutic potential. *Trends Biotechnol* 1995;13:306–310.

190. Graus-Porta D, Beerli RR, Hynes NE. Single-chain antibody-mediated intracellular retention of ErbB-2 impairs Neu differentiation factor and epidermal growth factor signalling. *Mol Cell Biol* 1995;15:1182–1191.

191. Chester KA, Hawkins RE. Clinical issues in antibody design. *Trends Biotechnol* 1995;13:294–300.

192. Yokata T, Milenic DE, Whitlow M, Schlom J. Rapid tumour penetration of a single chain Fv and comparison with other immunoglobulin forms. *Cancer Res* 1992;52:3402–3408.

193. Brinkmann U, Pastan I. Immunotoxins against cancer. *Biochim Biophys Acta* 1994;1198:27–45.

194. Hwang J, FitzGerald DJ, Adhya S, Pastan I. Functional domains of Pseudomonas exotoxin identified by deletion analysis of the gene expressed in E. coli. *Cell* 1987;48:129–136.

195. Pastan I, FitzGerald D. Recombinant toxins for cancer treatment. *Science* 1991;254:1173–1177.

196. Rybak SM, Hoogenboom HR, Meade HM, et al. Humanization of immunotoxins. *Proc Natl Acad Sci USA* 1992;89:3165–3169.

197. Newton DL, Xue Y, Olson KA, et al. Angiogenin single-chain immunofusions: influence of peptide linkers and spacers between fusion protein domains. *Biochemistry* 1996;35:545–553.

198. Bagshawe KD. The first Bagshawe lecture: towards generating cytotoxic agents at cancer sites. *Br J Cancer* 1989;60:275–281.

199. Bagshawe KD, Sharma SK, Springer CJ, Antoniw P. *Tumour Targeting* 1995;1:17–29.

200. Lockwood CM, Thiru S, Steard S, et al. Treatment of refractory Wegener's granulomatosis with humanized monoclonal antibodies. *Q J Med* 1996;89:903–912.

201. Elliott MJ, Maini RN, Feldmann M, et al. Randomised double-blind comparison of chimeric monoclonal antibody to tumour necrosis factor alpha (cA2) versus placebo in rheumatoid arthritis. *Lancet* 1994;344:1105–1110.

202. Elliott MJ, Maini RN, Feldmann M, et al. Repeated therapy with monoclonal antibody to tumour necrosis factor alpha (cA2) inpatients with rheumatoid arthritis. *Lancet* 1994;344:1125–1127.

203. Moreau T, Thorpe J, Miller D, et al. Preliminary evidence from magnetic resonance imaging for reduction in disease activity after lymphocyte depletion in multiple sclerosis. *Lancet* 1994;344:298–301.

204. Kirk AD, Harlan DM, Armstrong NN, et al. CTLA4-Ig and anti-CD40 ligand prevent renal allograft rejection in primates. *Proc Natl Acad Sci USA* 1997;94:8789–8794.

205. Routledge E, Waldmann H. The effect of aglycosylation on the immunogenicity of a humanised therapeutic CD3 antibody. *Transplantation* 1995;60:847.

206. Schultz RD, Heuser RR, Hatler C, Frey D. Use of c7E3 Fab in conjunction with primary coronary stenting for acute myocardial infarctions complicated by cardiogenic shock. *Cathet Cardiovasc Diagn* 1996;39:143–148.

207. Simoons ML, de Boer MJ, van den-Brand MJ, et al. European Cooperative Study Group. Randomized trial of a GPIIb/IIIa platelet receptor blocker in refractory unstable angina. *Circulation* 1994;89:596–603.

208. Pawson R, Dyer MJ, Barge R, et al. Treatment of T-cell prolymphocytic leukemia with human CD52 antibody. *J Clin Oncol* 1997;15:2667–2672.

209. Dyer MJ, Kelsey SM, Mackay HJ, et al. In vivo 'purging' of residual disease in CLL with Campath-1H. *Br J Haematol* 1997;91:669–672.

210. Osterborg A, Dyer MJ, Bunjes D, et al. Phase II multicenter study of human CD52 antibody in previously treated chronic lymphocytic leukemia. European Study Group of CAMPATH-1H treatment in chronic lymphocytic leukemia. *J Clin Oncol* 1997;15:1567–1574.

211. Antoine C, Garnier JL, Dubhoust A, Bariety J, Stevenson G, Glotz D. Successful treatment of posttransplant lymphoproliferative disorder with renal graft preservation by monoclonal antibody therapy. *Transplant Proc* 1996;28:2825–2826.

212. Maloney DG, Grillo Lopez AJ, White CA, et al. C2B8 (Rituximab) anti-CD20 monoclonal antibody therapy in patients with relapsed low-grade non-Hodgkin's lymphoma. *Blood* 1997;90:2188–2195.

213. Waldmann TA, White JD, Goldman CK, et al. The interleukin-2 receptor: a target for monoclonal antibody treatment of human T-cell lymphotrophic virus I-induced adult T-cell leukemia. *Blood* 1993;82:1701–1712.

214. Riethmuller G, Schneider Gadicke E, Schlimok G, et al. Randomised trial of monoclonal antibody for adjuvant therapy of resected Dukes' colorectal carcinoma. German Cancer Aid 17-1A Study Group. *Lancet* 1994;343:1177–1183.

215. Engert A, Diehl V, Schnell R, et al. A phase-I study of an anti-CD25 ricin A-chain immunotoxin (RFT5 SMPT-dgA) in patients with refractory Hodgkin's lymphoma. *Blood* 1997;89:403–410.

216. Stone MJ, Sausville EA, Fay JW, et al. A phase I study of bolus versus continuous infusion of the anti-CD19 immunotoxin, IgG-HD37-dgA, in patients with B-cell lymphoma. *Blood* 1996;88:1188–1197.

217. Press OW, Eary JF, Appelbaum FR, et al. Radiolabeled-antibody therapy of B-cell lymphoma with autologous bone marrow support. *N Engl J Med* 1993;329:1219–1224.

218. Kaminski MS, Zasadny KR, Francis IR, et al. Radioimmunotherapy of B-cell lymphoma with [131I]anti-B1 (anti-CD20) antibody. *N Engl J Med* 1993;329:459–465.

219. Hird V, Maraveyas A, Snook D, et al. Juvant therapy of ovarian cancer with radioactive monoclonal antibody. *Br J Cancer* 1993;68:403–406.

220. Hayden MS, Linsley PS, Gayle MA, et al. Single-chain mono and bispecific antibody derivatives with novel biological properties and anti-tumour activity form a COS cell transient expression system. *Ther Immunol* 1994;1:3–15.

Subject Index

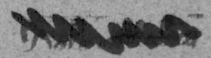